MARTINDALE

The Extra Pharmacopoeia

MARTINDALE

The Extra Pharmacopoeia

Twenty-eighth Edition

Edited by James E. F. Reynolds

Assistant Editor Anne B. Prasad

Published by direction of the Council of
The Pharmaceutical Society of Great Britain and prepared
in the Society's Department of Pharmaceutical Sciences

London
THE PHARMACEUTICAL PRESS
1982

 Published by The Pharmaceutical Press, 1 Lambeth High Street, London SE1 7JN, England.

The first edition of the Extra Pharmacopoeia was published in July 1883. The twenty-seventh edition was published in June 1977. This current (twenty-eighth) edition was published in December 1982.

International Standard Book Number (ISBN): 0 85369 160 6. International Standard Serial Number (ISSN): 0263-5364.

Keystroke capture by Page Bros (Norwich) Ltd., Norwich, Norfolk; database system design and operation, and computer composition by Peter Peregrinus Ltd., Hitchin, Hertfordshire; phototypesetting output by Unwin Brothers Ltd., Old Woking, Surrey. Printed and bound in the USA by R. R. Donnelley & Sons Company.

THE COUNCIL OF THE PHARMACEUTICAL SOCIETY OF GREAT BRITAIN 1982–1983

DEPARTMENT OF PHARMACEUTICAL SCIENCES

Martindale Editorial Staff

Contents

Preface

Ninety-nine years have passed since William Martindale produced the first edition of the Extra Pharmacopoeia—now better known as 'Martindale'. It was his aim and it is still our aim to provide a concise summary of the properties, actions, and uses of drugs and medicines for the practising pharmacist and medical practitioner. However, over these years his 'little book' has so grown that now it covers most of the drugs in clinical use throughout the world.

The quantity of information about drugs continues to increase and there seems to have been no reduction in the number of new drugs released during the preparation of the 28th edition. Martindale has increased in content by about 25%, but by rearranging the typographical layout and careful selection of paper we have managed to produce this edition within a single volume.

All the material in this edition has been revised and much of it rewritten. While we have always been very careful to ensure that our dosage information is accurate, increased effort has been made during this revision to provide guidance on the administration of drugs to infants, children, pregnant women, the elderly, and patients with hepatic or renal impairment. There are often differing views on the actions and uses of drugs and as a further development we have tried to provide comprehensive details of those controversies that are still not resolved. We have also attempted to include more detailed information on the mode of action of each drug. Since Martindale is widely used throughout the world, we have included very many more proprietary names from most parts of the world.

The last 5 years has seen a more cautious approach in the management of diseases both in terms of total patient care and in controlling or monitoring drug therapy. Advances have been made in the treatment of Gram-negative, anaerobic, and viral infections. Better responses and more prolonged remissions are being achieved in cancer therapy. Organ transplants carry less risk of rejection while hypertension and cardiovascular disorders should be more easily managed as should parenteral nutrition and diabetes mellitus. Genetic engineering which is already yielding insulin and interferons holds great promise for the development and production of biological materials.

We have rearranged some of the monographs in this edition. This has led to new chapters entitled Anthelmintics and Schistosomicides; Electrolytes; Metoclopramide and some other Anti-emetics; Metronidazole and some other Antiprotozoal Agents; and Sodium Cromoglycate and related Anti-allergic Agents. A few chapters have been renamed, and new titles include Antidepressants; Antihypertensives; and Idoxuridine and some other Antiviral Agents. We have added more than 900 monographs to this edition. Many of these are for drugs still under investigation. We have deleted 97 monographs.

Martindale is based on published information and has no official status; it is not a book of standards. Inclusion of a substance or a preparation is not to be considered as a recommendation for use, indeed some monographs are included by virtue of the substances' toxicity. While every effort has been made to check all the material in Martindale, the publisher cannot accept any responsibility for errors or omissions.

A major development in this edition has been the use made of computer techniques to organise the contents for printing and for retrieval from computerised information systems where our information will be held in a databank known as Martindale Online. The only indication of this development to the reader of the book is the inclusion of a Martindale Identity Number in each monograph. However, readers with access to these systems, through their own terminals or through various information services, will be able to pluck from Martindale Online sections of monographs that answer their specific questions in much the same way as some imaginary reader could answer questions if he had memorised comprehensively the whole of this edition. Martindale Online will be updated regularly with newly revised chapters while the book will continue with its current cycle of publication.

Arrangement

PART 1 (pages 1–1671) contains monographs on some 3990 substances arranged in 105 chapters. These chapters generally bring together drugs that have similar uses or actions. Cross-references are used to guide the reader to drugs that may be of interest in related chapters. Most chapters now have an introduction which provides background information on that group of drugs. Some drugs such as the corticosteroids can be considered readily as a group with its members having many common actions; in such cases the introduction provides much of the information for that chapter.

Monographs follow the introduction in alphabetical order, unless a chapter has the name of a substance in the title when the monograph for that substance appears first.

PART 2 (pages 1673–1771) consists of a series of short monographs on some 1120 drugs and ancillary substances arranged in the alphabetical order of their main titles. It includes monographs on new drugs, on drugs under investigation, on drugs not easily classified, and on obsolescent drugs still of interest. There are also some monographs on toxic substances, the effects of which may require drug therapy.

PART 3 (pages 1773–89) gives the composition of some 900 proprietary medicines that are advertised to the public in Great Britain and that are usually supplied on demand. The formulas are generally as described by the manufacturers. Herbal medicines have been omitted. As in earlier editions of Martindale, the claims made for these products and their recommended doses are not included.

The number of 'counter' proprietary medicines has declined considerably over the last 5 years. Nevertheless, there is still a large number of preparations with 'product licences of right' and it is expected that further preparations will be discontinued as review of these licences progresses.

Indexes

DIRECTORY OF MANUFACTURERS. Throughout the text the names of manufacturers and distributors are abbreviated. Their full names are given in this directory together with the full address if it is available. Because of our continued expansion of the number of proprietary names, the directory has considerably increased from about 1400 entries to over 3000.

INDEX TO CLINICAL USES. This index is a guide to the uses described in the text; it should not be used otherwise and is not a comprehensive therapeutic index. It refers the reader to the chapters and monographs where the listed diseases are mentioned. The drugs under each disease heading are listed in order of page number and not of preference.

INDEX TO MARTINDALE IDENTITY NUMBERS. Each monograph in Martindale now has an identity number which is used in our computer manipulation. These identity numbers will be referred to in the databank (Martindale Online) and will mainly be of value to the user of the online service; however, they may also be of some value to the user of the book. The numbers have no structure and are not significant in themselves. The index lists the identity number followed by the relevant monograph title and the page on which it appears. Identity numbers for chapter introductions have also been included.

GENERAL INDEX. To make fullest use of the contents of Martindale the general index should always be consulted. The exhaustive index to the drugs, preparations, compounds, and pharmacological and therapeutic groups in the book has been compiled to exacting standards and this has resulted in an index of about 50 000 entries. As in previous editions, the index is arranged alphabetically 'word-by-word' rather than 'letter-by-letter'.

In order to save space we have omitted the inverted entries for pharmaceutical forms which in earlier editions resulted in long lists of tablets, capsules, etc.

Nomenclature

MARTINDALE IDENTITY NUMBERS. Each monograph begins with an identity number which consists of a maximum of 6 figures followed by a check character. These numbers are used in our computer manipulation and their sole purpose is to identify monographs in Martindale. They are referred to in the databank and will mainly be of value to the user of the online service; however, they may also be of value to the reader of the book.

TITLES. The title of each monograph is in English, with preference being given to British Approved Names, United States Adopted Names, International Nonproprietary Names, and names used in the *European Pharmacopoeia*. Other names given as synonyms include commonly-used abbreviated names; English, American, and Latin synonyms; French, German, Scandinavian, Spanish, Portuguese, Italian, and other names from the relevant pharmacopoeias when these may not be readily identifiable; manufacturers' code numbers; and trivial chemical names. In some approved names it is now general policy to use 'f' for 'ph' in sulpha, 't' for 'th', and 'i' for 'y'; for this reason entries in alphabetical lists and indexes should be sought in alternative spellings if the expected spellings are not found. A table of abbreviated names for radicals and groups used in approved names and titles is given on page xx.

BOTANICAL NAMES. The nomenclature follows the International Rules of Botanical Nomenclature.

CHEMICAL NAMES. The nomenclature generally follows the definitive rules issued by the International Union of Pure and Applied Chemistry, 1979.

NAMES OF MICRO-ORGANISMS. The nomenclature used is principally that of the *Catalogue of the National Collection of Type Cultures—1972* (Public Health Laboratory Service Board, London, HM Stationery Office, 1972); *Nomenclature of Fungi Pathogenic to Man and Animals* (Medical Research Council Memorandum No. 23, 4th Edn, HM Stationery Office, 1977); *Index Bergeyana* (London, E. & S. Livingstone, 1966); and *Approved Lists of Bacterial Names* (V.B.D. Skerman *et al.* (Ed.), *Int. J. syst. Bacteriol.*, 1980, *30*, 225).

CAS REGISTRY NUMBERS. Chemical Abstracts Service (CAS) registry numbers are provided, where available, for each monograph substance to help readers refer to other information systems. Numbers for various forms of the monograph substance are listed with the variation in form given in parenthesis.

Pharmacopoeias

The titles of substances included in the *British Pharmacopoeia* or the *British Pharmacopoeia (Veterinary)* are followed in parentheses by the initials *B.P.* or *B.P. Vet.* respectively; those not included in these pharmacopoeias but included in the *British Pharmaceutical Codex* or the *British Veterinary Codex* are followed by *B.P.C. 1973* (or earlier) or *B. Vet. C. 1965* respectively. Substances which are the subject of monographs in the *European Pharmacopoeia*, the *United States Pharma-*

copeia, or the *United States National Formulary* are similarly indicated by the abbreviations *Eur. P.*, *U.S.P.*, or *U.S.N.F.* after the main title or synonyms.

The pharmacopoeias in which each substance appears are listed and differences of chemical, pharmaceutical, or therapeutic significance are usually indicated. Current and amended copies of the pharmacopoeias should be consulted for confirmation and for details of standards.

The pharmacopoeias covered include: Argentine, *Austrian* (*Supplement II*), *Belgian* (*Supplements I* and *II*), *Brazilian*, *British* (including *Addendum 1981*), *British Veterinary* (including *amendments 1977*), *Chinese*, *Czechoslovakian* (*Addendum 1976*), *European* (*Supplement 1977*), *French* (*Amendments 1976*), *German*, Hungarian, *Indian* (*Supplement 1975*), International, *Italian* (*Supplement 1978*), *Japanese*, Jugoslavian, Mexican, *Netherlands*, *Nordic* (*Addenda* to *1976*), Polish, Portuguese, *Roumanian*, Russian, Spanish, *Swiss* (*Supplements 1973, 1976*, and *1977*), *Turkish*, and *United States* (including the *Formulary* and *Supplements 1, 1a, 2*, and *2a*). Those *italicised* in the above list either appeared as new editions or were revised by supplements (as shown in brackets) since the last edition of Martindale, and have been examined for this 28th edition.

Atomic and Molecular Weights

Atomic weights are based on the table of Atomic Weights as revised in 1977 by the Commission on Atomic Weights, XXIX International Union of Pure and Applied Chemistry General Assembly and based on the ^{12}C scale (see page xxx). Molecular weights are given corrected to one place of decimals or to four significant figures for relative weights of less than 100.

Pharmaceutical Information

Chemical and physical properties likely to be of use or interest are given for each drug. This information is culled from a variety of sources and is not definitive in the pharmacopoeial sense. Special attention has been paid to the collection of data on the stability of drugs and on incompatibilities with drugs and preparations of drugs, particularly those likely to occur in solutions for intravenous administration.

ISO-OSMOTIC SOLUTIONS. The term iso-osmotic is used for solutions which exert the same osmotic pressure as serum and does not necessarily indicate that such solutions would be in osmotic equilibrium with red blood cells. It is used in preference to the more generally employed term 'isotonic' which in pharmaceutical practice has not always been correctly used to indicate osmotic equilibrium with red blood cells. Care is necessary if solutions not in osmotic equilibrium with red blood cells are administered by rapid intravenous infusion. The osmotic activity of the blood or its components is sometimes expressed in milliosmoles (mosmol). An osmole has the molal concentration in moles per 1000 g of solvent [molar concentration is in moles per 1000 g of solution] of an ideal solution of a non-dissociating substance which exerts the same osmotic pressure as the solution under consideration; it is calculated as the weight of any solute that depresses the freezing point of water by 1.86°. For real solutions correction factors have to be applied.

PERCENTAGE STRENGTHS. Unless otherwise stated, solutions of solids in liquids are expressed as percentage w/v, of liquids in liquids as percentage v/v, and of gases in liquids as percentage w/w.

SOLUBILITY. The figures given for solubility in each monograph have generally been obtained from the major pharmacopoeias in which the drug is described or from the manufacturers. These sources have not always used comparable materials or methods of determination and the figures should not be considered absolute. Unless otherwise indicated in the text, the figures are for solubility at 'ordinary room temperature'. At one time this was considered to be in the range 15° to 20° but 20° to 25° is the probable range in most laboratories today. In this edition, the solubility terms used by most of the world's pharmacopoeias have been adopted:

solubility	
very soluble	1 in less than 1
freely soluble	1 in 1 to 1 in 10
soluble	1 in 10 to 1 in 30
sparingly soluble	1 in 30 to 1 in 100
slightly soluble	1 in 100 to 1 in 1000
very slightly soluble	1 in 1000 to 1 in 10 000
practically insoluble	1 in more than 10 000

STORAGE. Substances and preparations should be stored under conditions which prevent contamination and diminish deterioration, and the conditions of storage given in the text indicate the precautions which should be taken in specific cases. The term 'a cool place' is generally used to describe a place in which the temperature does not exceed 15°. Unless otherwise specified, all injections should be stored in alkali-free containers.

TEMPERATURE. Temperatures are expressed in degrees Celsius (centigrade) unless otherwise indicated.

Pharmacological and Therapeutic Information

Information on the adverse effects, treatment of adverse effects, precautions, absorption and fate, and uses of each substance is provided by concise statements under these headings and these are elaborated and expanded by abstracts from published papers and reviews. In compiling these statements the intention has been to present unbiased summaries and, where views are conflicting, to represent these as fairly as possible by a suitable selection of abstracts and in some instances by providing a review of the conflict.

The abstracts of medical and pharmaceutical literature have been a characteristic and valuable feature of Martindale since the book was first published. During revision for this edition a wider selection of journals was used than for any previous edition and out of the large store of abstracts created from these journals about 57000 were selected for inclusion as abstracts or references. Some abstract journals were used to lead the editorial staff to the original publication. When it was not possible to obtain the original, an abstract was prepared from the abstract journal and a reference supplied both to that journal and to the original journal.

Much information has been found in sources such as World Health Organization publications, government reports and legislation, and other official and standard publications. Manufacturers' literature has been considered in the light of other available information.

The risks of administering drugs in pregnancy are well known and the general principle is to give a drug only when the benefit to the individual mother outweighs the risk to the foetus. Where there is a clear risk it is noted under the Precautions or Adverse Effects heading but safety should not be inferred from the absence of a statement for any drug.

Interactions are described under the Precautions heading with detailed information being provided in the monograph for the drug that is being affected.

Doses

Doses are described under the Uses heading with as much detail as is necessary and available. The abbreviated 'Dose' section near the beginning of each monograph of previous editions has been deleted. Unless otherwise stated the doses represent the average range of quantities which are generally regarded as suitable for adults when administered by mouth and may usually be repeated three or four times in twenty-four hours. If it is usual to administer a drug by a method other than by mouth, the dose suitable for that method of administration is stated. More information on doses and drug administration may be given in the abstracts and under the Preparations section. Unless otherwise specified, dextrose injection is 5% w/v, sodium chloride injection is 0.9% w/v, and water is purified water.

When doses for children are expressed as a range of quantities within specified age limits, the lower dose applies at the lower age and the higher dose at the higher age.

Formulas

Formulas are given for preparations in current editions of the *British Pharmacopoeia*, and the *United States Pharmacopeia* and *National Formulary*. Formulas from the *British Pharmaceutical Codex 1973* are included if not yet covered by the *British Pharmacopoeia* and formulas from other pharmacopoeias and national formularies are also included if they are considered to be of special interest. Selected formulas from hospital formularies and from the medical and pharmaceutical literature are included for their special interest to those pharmacists required to formulate comparable preparations.

Ingredients of preparations are named according to the title under which they are described in Martindale. The term 'freshly prepared' is used to indicate that a preparation must be made not more than twenty-four hours before issue for use, and the term 'recently prepared' indicates that deterioration is likely if the preparation is stored for more than a few weeks at temperate room conditions.

Proprietary Preparations

In Parts 1 and 2, the information on proprietary preparations available in Great Britain is presented in the same manner as in the last edition, each product being described at the end of the monograph on its principal ingredient. The proprietary names of single-ingredient preparations have been included for Argentina, Australia, Belgium, Canada, Denmark, France, Germany, Italy, the Netherlands, Norway, South Africa, Spain, Sweden, Switzerland, the United States of America, and for some other countries. It is hoped that the inclusion of this increased number of proprietary names will assist pharmacists and physicians in identifying the active ingredients used; the route of administration and dose may not be comparable.

The proprietary preparations described in Parts 1 and 2 are mostly those intended for supply on prescription. Most proprietary medicines which are advertised in Great Britain to the public and supplied on demand are described in Part 3.

The information on composition, dosage, and uses of proprietary preparations is mainly taken from the literature issued by the manufacturers or their distributing agents and has been confirmed by them, but no responsibility can be accepted for the accuracy of this information.

Information on diluents suggested for liquid proprietary preparations for oral administration has been provided by the manufacturers or taken from the *Diluent Directory* issued by the National Pharmaceutical Association (formerly National Pharmaceutical Union).

Acknowledgements

The Editor gratefully acknowledges the advice and assistance of the many experts who have suggested amendments to the text, particularly Professor H.A.F. Dudley, Heather M. Elliston, and Margaret J. Gilmour. Thanks are due to many hospital pharmacists for advice and information, to community pharmacists for information on counter proprietaries, to manufacturers for providing information on their products and checking entries relating to them, to the British Pharmacopoeia Commission, and to the Medicines Division of the Department of Health and Social Security.

Martindale staff have been able to call freely on the expertise of other members of the Pharmaceutical Society's staff. In particular the Editor is grateful to Ainley Wade for encouragement and advice, Pamela M. North and the staff of the library and information department for helping to collect our sources of information, Janet

M. Batson for help with chemical names and CAS registry numbers, Sheenagh M. Langtry for checking preparation statements, W. Lund of the Pharmaceutical Society's Pharmaceutics Laboratory, G.E. Appelbe and the staff of the Law Department, and B. J. Yates, Publications Manager of the Pharmaceutical Society.

The organisation of this edition into a computerised databank is a significant development and the assistance of B. Tarry of Peter Peregrinus Ltd in this project is gratefully acknowledged.

The Editor welcomes this opportunity to record his warmest appreciation of the dedicated services rendered by the editorial staff P. Blake, Rosalind Dixon, Chloe Loewe, Theresa Ormiston, Anne V. Parsons, Marion Savva, D. Shenton, S. Sweetman, and especially of the senior staff Anne B. Prasad, G.E. Diaper and Kathleen Parfitt. Revision of Martindale normally calls for many talents and a wide range of knowledge from the staff; computerisation of this edition made considerable additional demands.

Thanks are due to the following who provided extra assistance with proofreading and some editorial tasks: Candida A. Chaplin, Clare Cronin, Jane Dickson, Pamela Francis, Jennifer M. Hallson, Linda Hanrahan, A. Holme, Louise Kiff, Patricia Purdy, Christine Simpson, Susan E. Reynolds, and Susan Young. Thanks are also due to Wiesia Smiechowska and Linda Bailey for typing and clerical assistance and especially to Cathleen Hussein who for the second successive edition has efficiently typed most of the manuscript.

London SE1
August 1982

Abbreviations

The titles of journals are abbreviated according to the general style of *World List of Scientific Periodicals* (London, Butterworths, 1963–80).

For abbreviations of the names of manufacturers or their distributors, see Directory of Manufacturers, p.1791.

≈—approximately equals.
α—alpha. Also used in radiation data for alpha particles.
A—ampere(s).
Å—ångström(s).
aa—*ana*, 'of each'.
Aberdeen Roy. Infirm.—Aberdeen Royal Infirmary, Scotland.
ABPI—Association of the British Pharmaceutical Industry.
Addenbrooke's Hosp.—Addenbrooke's Hospital, Cambridge, England.
Adelaide Child. Hosp.—The Adelaide Children's Hospital Inc., Australia.
ADI—acceptable daily intake.
A.D.T.—Accepted Dental Therapeutics, published by the American Dental Association.
Afghan.—Afghanistan.
agg.—aggregate (in botanical names), including 2 or more species which resemble each other closely.
Ala—alanine.
Alg.—Algeria.
a.m.—*ante meridiem*, 'before noon'.
AMA—American Medical Association.
A.P.F.—Australian Pharmaceutical Formulary and Handbook, 1978.
Arg—arginine.
Arg.—Argentina, Argentine, *or* Argentinian.
Arg. P.—Argentinian Pharmacopoeia 1966 (Farmacopea Nacional Argentina, Quinta Edicion).
Asn—asparagine.
Asp—aspartic acid.
Aust.—Austria *or* Austrian.
Aust. P.—Austrian Pharmacopoeia 1960 (Österreichisches Ärzneibuch, 9 Ausgabe) and Supplements I (1966) and II (1975).
Austral.—Australia.
β^+—beta particles: positrons.
β^-—beta particles: electrons.
B.—*Bacillus, Bacteroides*, or *Bordetella.*
BAN—British Approved Name.
Barb.—Barbados.
Belg.—Belgium *or* Belgian.
Belg. P.—Belgian Pharmacopoeia 1962 (Pharmacopée Belge, Cinquième Édition) and Supplements I (1966) and II (1969).
B.N.F.—British National Formulary.
Bol.—Bolivia.
Born.—Borneo.
B.P.—British Pharmacopoeia. Unless otherwise specified in the text, *B.P.* references are to the 1980 Edn, including the addendum 1981.
b.p.—boiling point.
B.P. Vet.—British Pharmacopoeia (Veterinary) 1977 and amendments 1977.
B.P.C.—British Pharmaceutical Codex.
Bq—becquerel(s).
Br.—British *or Brucella.*
Braz.—Brazil *or* Brazilian.
Braz. P.—Brazilian Pharmacopoeia 1977 (Farmacopéia Brasileira, 3ª Edição).
Bristol Roy. Infirm.—Bristol Royal Infirmary, England.
Brompton Hosp.—Brompton Hospital, London, England.
BS—British Standard (specification).
BSI—British Standards Institution.
BUN—Blood-urea-nitrogen.
B. Vet. C.—British Veterinary Codex.
°C—degrees Celsius (centigrade). Unless otherwise indicated in the text, temperatures are expressed in this thermometric scale.
C.—*Campylobacter, Candida*, or *Corynebacterium.*
Canad.—Canada.
CAS—Chemical Abstracts Service.
CCID50—cell-culture-infective dose 50 (the dose of the micro-organism which infects 50% of cell cultures inoculated).
Charing Cross Hosp.—Charing Cross Hospital (Fulham), London, England.
Chin.—Chinese.
Chin. P.—Chinese Pharmacopoeia.
CI—Colour Index (Colour Index, 3rd Edn 1971 and supplements.)
Ci—curie(s).
CIA—Chemical Industries Association (UK).
Cl.—*Clostridium.*
CM—Chick-Martin (coefficient).
cm—centimetre(s).
cm^2—square centimetre(s).
cm^3—cubic centimetre(s).
CNS—central nervous system.
Col.—Colombia.
cP—centipoise(s).
CRM—Committee on the Review of Medicines (UK).
CSF—cerebrospinal fluid.
CSM—Committee on Safety of Medicines (UK).
cSt—centistokes.
Curac.—Curaçao.
Cys—cysteine.
Cz.—Czechoslovakia *or* Czechoslovak.
Cz. P.—Czechoslovak Pharmacopoeia 1970 (Československý Lékopis, Vydání třetí; Pharmacopoea Bohemoslovenica, Editio tertia) and Addendum 1976.
D & C—designation applied in USA to dyes permitted for use in drugs and cosmetics.
Dan.—Danish.
Dan. Disp.—Danish Dispensatory 1963 (Dispensatorium Danicum) including all amendments to 1973.
d.c.—direct current.
Denm.—Denmark.
DHSS—Department of Health and Social Security (UK).
DNA—deoxyribonucleic acid.
Dom. Rep.—Dominican Republic.
D.P.F.—Dental Practitioners' Formulary.
D.T.F.—Drug Tariff Formulary: Drug Tariff, 1981 (National Health Service, Department of Health and Social Security, UK).
E.—*Escherichia.*
EC—electron capture.
ECG—electrocardiogram.
ECT—electroconvulsive therapy.
Ecuad.—Ecuador.
Ed.—editor(s) *or* edited by.
Edn—edition.
EEC—European Economic Community.
EEG—electro-encephalogram.
e.g.—*exempli gratia*, 'for example'.
EID50—egg-infective dose 50 (the dose of the micro-organism which infects 50% of the eggs inoculated).
El Salv.—El Salvador.

ENL—erythema nodosum leprosum.
ENT—ear, nose and throat.
ESR—erythrocyte sedimentation-rate.
et al.—*et alii*, 'and others': for three or more co-authors or co-workers.
Eur.—European.
Eur. P.—European Pharmacopoeia vol. I 1969, vol. II 1971, vol. III 1975, and Supplements 1973 and 1977.
eV—electronvolt(s).
Ext. D & C—designation applied in USA to dyes permitted for use in external drug and cosmetic preparations.
°F—degrees Fahrenheit.
FAC—Food Additives and Contaminants Committee of the Ministry of Agriculture, Fisheries and Food (UK).
FAO—Food and Agriculture Organization of the United Nations.
FAO/WHO—Food and Agriculture Organization of the United Nations *and the* World Health Organization.
FDA—Food and Drug Administration of USA.
F D & C—designation applied in USA to dyes permitted for use in foods, drugs, and cosmetics.
FDD—Food and Drug Directorate of Canada.
FEV_1—forced expiratory volume in 1 second.
Fin.—Finland.
fl—femtolitre(s).
fl oz—fluid ounce(s).
F. N. Belg.—The Belgian National Formulary 1977 (Formularium Nationale, Editio Quinta).
F. N. Fr.—The National Formulary of France 1974 (Formulaire National, Ire Édition) and Supplement 1976.
f.p.—freezing point.
FPA—Family Planning Association (UK).
Fr.—France *or* French.
Fr. P.—French Pharmacopoeia 1972 (Pharmacopée Française, IXe Edition) and amendments 1974 and 1976.
FSC—Food Standards Committee of the Ministry of Agriculture, Fisheries and Food (UK).
ft—foot (feet).
ft^2—square foot (feet).
γ—gamma. Also used in radiation data for gamma-radiation.
g—gram(s).
gal—gallon(s).
Ger.—W. Germany *or* W. German.
Ger. P.—West German Pharmacopoeia 1978 (Deutsches Arzneibuch, 8 Ausgabe).
GFR—glomerular filtration-rate.
Gib.—Gibraltar.
Gln—glutamine.
Glu—glutamic acid.
Gly—glycine.
GRAS—generally recognised as safe. A designation applied to food additives.
Groote Schuur Hosp.—Groote Schuur Hospital, S. Africa.
Gt Ormond St Child. Hosp.—The Hospitals for Sick Children, Great Ormond Street, London, England.
Guat.—Guatemala.
Guy's Hosp.—Guy's Hospital, London, England.
Gy—Gray.
H.—*Haemophilus.*
Hadassah Univ. Hosp.—Hadassah University Hospital, Jerusalem, Israel.
Hb—haemoglobin.
HDL—high-density lipoproteins.
His—histidine.
HLB—hydrophilic-lipophilic balance.
Hond.—Honduras.
Hung.—Hungary *or* Hungarian.
Hung. P.—VIth Hungarian Pharmacopoeia 1967 (Magyar Gyógyszerkönyv).
Hz—hertz.
IAEA—International Atomic Energy Agency.
ibid.—*ibidem*, 'in the same place (journal or book)'.
ICRP—International Commission on Radiological Protection.
ICRU—International Commission on Radiation Units and Measurements.
idem—'the same': used for the same authors and titles.
i.e.—*id est*, 'that is'.
Ig—immunoglobulin.
Ile—isoleucine.
in—inch(es).
in^2—square inch(es).
Ind.—India *or* Indian.
Ind. P.—Pharmacopoeia of India, 2nd Edn, 1966 and Supplement 1975.
Int.—International.
Int. P.—International Pharmacopoeia 1967 (Specifications for the Quality Control of Pharmaceutical Preparations, 2nd Edn) and Supplement 1971.
IQ—intelligence quotient.
i.r.—infra-red.
ISO—International Organization for Standardization.
IT—isomeric transition.
It.—Italian.
It. P.—Italian Pharmacopoeia 1972 (Farmacopea Ufficiale della Repubblica Italiana, Ottava Edizione) and Supplement 1978.
Ital.—Italy.
iu—international unit(s).
IUB—International Union of Biochemistry.
IUD—intra-uterine device.
IUPAC—International Union of Pure and Applied Chemistry.
J—joule(s).
Jam.—Jamaica.
Jap.—Japan *or* Japanese.
Jap. P.—The Pharmacopoeia of Japan, 9th Edn, 1976.
Jug.—Jugoslav.
Jug. P.—Jugoslav Pharmacopoeia 1972 (Farmakopeja SFRJ; Pharmacopoea Jugoslavica, Editio Tertia).
K—kelvin.
kcal—kilocalorie(s).
keV—kiloelectronvolt(s).
kg—kilogram(s).
King's Coll. Hosp.—King's College Hospital, London, England.
kJ—kilojoule(s).
Kleb.—*Klebsiella.*
Kor.—Korea.
kPa—kilopascal(s).
L.—*Listeria.*
lb—pound(s) avoirdupois.
LD50—a dose lethal to 50% of the specified animals or micro-organisms.
LDL—low-density lipoproteins.
Leeds Gen. Infirm.—The General Infirmary, Leeds, England.
Leu—leucine.
Lf—limit flocculation.
loc. cit.—*loco citato*, 'in the place cited'.
Lux.—Luxembourg.
Lys—lysine.
m—metre(s).
m^2—square metre(s).
m^3—cubic metre(s).
M—molar.
M.—*Mycobacterium* or *Mycoplasma.*
mA—milliampere(s).
Malay.—Malaysia.
MAOI—monoamine oxidase inhibitor.
max.—maximum.
MB 1959: Sweden—MB Formulary 1959 (Apotekarsocietetens Förlag, Stockholm).
MBC—minimum bactericidal concentration.
mCi—millicurie(s).
mEq—milliequivalent(s).

Met—methionine.
MeV—megaelectronvolt(s).
Mex.—Mexico *or* Mexican.
Mex. P.—Mexican Pharmacopoeia 1952 (Farmacopea Nacional de los Estados Unidos Mexicanos, Segunda Edicion).
mg—milligram(s).
MIC—minimum inhibitory concentration.
Middlesex Hosp.—The Middlesex Hospital, London, England.
min—minute.
min.—minimum.
MJ—megajoule(s).
ml—millilitre(s).
mm—millimetre(s).
mm^2—square millimetre(s).
mm^3—cubic millimetre(s).
mmHg—millimetre(s) of mercury.
mmol—millimole.
mol—mole.
mol. wt—molecular weight.
Moorfields Eye Hosp.—Moorfields Eye Hospital, London, England.
Mor.—Morocco.
mosmol—milliosmole.
m.p.—melting point.
Mrad—megarad.
MRC—Medical Research Council (UK).
mrem—millíröntgen-equivalent-man.
μCi—microcurie(s).
μg—microgram(s).
μl—microlitre(s).
μm—micrometre(s).
N.—*Neisseria.*
nCi—nanocurie(s).
NCTC—National Collection of Type Cultures (Central Public Health Laboratory, London, England).
Neth.—The Netherlands.
Neth. P.—Netherlands Pharmacopoeia 1978 (Nederlandse Farmacopee, Achtste Uitgave).
ng—nanogram(s).
NIH—National Institutes of Health (USA).
nm—nanometre(s).
Nord.—Nordic.
Nord. P.—Nordic Pharmacopoeia 1963 (Pharmacopoea Nordica) including all addenda published up to 1976.
Norw.—Norway.
NPU—National Pharmaceutical Union, now the National Pharmaceutical Association (NPA).
NRPB—National Radiological Protection Board, Harwell, Oxfordshire, England.
NZ—New Zealand.
OECD—Organisation for Economic Co-operation and Development.
OP—over proof.
Orsett Hosp.—Orsett Hospital, Grays, Essex, England.
o/w—oil-in-water.
oz—ounce(s).
P—probability.
Pa—pascal(s).
Parag.—Paraguay.
PBI—protein-bound iodine.
pCO_2—plasma partial pressure (concentration) of carbon dioxide.
p_aCO_2—arterial plasma partial pressure (concentration) of carbon dioxide.
per—'through'.
pg—picogram(s).
pH—the negative logarithm of the hydrogen ion concentration.
Phe—phenylalanine.
Pharm. Soc. Lab. Rep.—Pharmaceutical Society's Laboratory Report.
Phillipp.—Phillippines.
pK_a—the negative logarithm of the dissociation constant.
p.m.—*post meridiem*, 'afternoon'.
pO_2—plasma partial pressure (concentration) of oxygen.
P_aO_2—arterial plasma partial pressure (concentration) of oxygen.
Pol.—Poland *or* Polish.
Pol. P.—Polish Pharmacopoeia 1965 (Farmakopea Polska IV).
Port.—Portugal *or* Portuguese.
Port. P.—Portuguese Pharmacopoeia 1946 (Farmacopeia Portuguesa IV) and Supplements 1961 and 1967.
ppm—parts per million.
Pr.—*Proteus.*
P.R.—Puerto Rico.
Pro—proline.
Ps.—*Pseudomonas.*
PSGB—The Pharmaceutical Society of Great Britain.
q.s.—*quantum sufficit*, 'as much as suffices'.
Queen Eliz. Hosp., S. Australia—The Queen Elizabeth Hospital, South Australia.
q.v.—*quod vide*, 'which see'.
R—röntgen.
rad—radiation absorbed dose.
RCGP—Royal College of General Practitioners (UK).
REM sleep—rapid-eye-movement sleep.
rem—röntgen-equivalent-man.
RNA—ribonucleic acid.
Rochester Methodist Hosp.—Rochester Methodist Hospital, Minnesota, USA.
Roum.—Roumanian.
Roum. P.—Roumanian Pharmacopoeia 1976 (Farmacopeea Românǎ. Editia A. IX-A).
Roy. Free Hosp.—The Royal Free Hospital, London, England.
Roy. Hallamshire Hosp.—Royal Hallamshire Hospital, Sheffield, England.
Roy. Marsden Hosp.—The Royal Marsden Hospital, London, England.
Roy. Melb. Hosp.—The Royal Melbourne Hospital, Australia.
Roy. Nat. Orthopaedic Hosp.—Royal National Orthopaedic Hospital, Stanmore, Middx, England.
Roy. Nat. T. N. and E. Hosp.—The Royal National Throat, Nose and Ear Hospital, London, England.
Roy. Victoria Hosp.—Royal Victoria Hospital, Belfast, Northern Ireland.
Roy. Victoria Infirm.—The Royal Victoria Infirmary, Newcastle-upon-Tyne, England.
Rus.—Russian.
Rus. P.—Russian Pharmacopoeia (State Pharmacopoeia of the USSR, Tenth Edition).
RW—Rideal-Walker (coefficient).
S.—*Salmonella* or *Serratia.*
S. Afr.—South Africa.
St. Bart.'s Hosp.—St. Bartholomew's Hospital, London, England.
St. John's Hosp.—St. John's Hospital for Diseases of the Skin, London, England.
St. Mark's Hosp.—St. Mark's Hospital, London, England.
St. Mary's Hosp.—St. Mary's Hospital, London, England.
St. Thomas' Hosp.—St. Thomas' Hospital, London, England.
Scand.—Scandinavian.
SCI—Society of Chemical Industry (UK).
Ser—serine.
SGOT—serum glutamic oxaloacetic transaminase (serum aspartate aminotransferase *now preferred*).
SGPT—serum glutamic pyruvic transaminase (serum alanine aminotransferase *now preferred*).
Sh.—*Shigella.*
SI—Statutory Instrument *or* Système International d'Unités (International System of Units).
SLE—systemic lupus erythematosus.
sp.—species (plural spp.).

sp. gr.—specific gravity.
Span.—Spanish.
Span. P.—Spanish Pharmacopoeia 1954 (Farmacopea Oficial Española, Novena Edicion).
St—stokes.
Staph.—*Staphylococcus.*
Stoke Mandeville Hosp.—Stoke Mandeville Hospital, Aylesbury, Bucks, England.
Str.—*Streptococcus.*
Suppl.—supplement(s).
Sv—sievert.
Swed.—Sweden.
Swiss P.—Swiss Pharmacopoeia 1971 (Pharmacopoea Helvetica, Editio Sexta, Édition Française) and Supplements 1973, 1976, and 1977.
Switz.—Switzerland.
Tanz.—Tanzania.
TCID—tissue-culture-infective dose.
TCID50—tissue-culture-infective dose 50 (the dose of the micro-organism which infects 50% of tissue cultures inoculated).
Thai.—Thailand.
Thr—threonine.
Trp—tryptophan.
Tun.—Tunisia.
Turk.—Turkey *or* Turkish.
Turk. P.—Turkish Pharmacopoeia 1974 (Türk Farmakopesi).
Tyr—tyrosine.
UK—United Kingdom.
UKAEA—United Kingdom Atomic Energy Authority.
Univ. Coll. Hosp.—University College Hospital, London, England.
UP—under proof.
Urug.—Uruguay.
US and *USA*—United States of America.
USAID—United States Agency for International Development.
USAN—United States Adopted Name.
U.S.N.F.—The United States 'National Formulary XV', 1980, and Supplements 1 (1980), 1a (1980), 2 (1981), and 2a (1981).
U.S.P.—The United States Pharmacopeia XX, 1980, and Supplements 1 (1980), 1a (1980), 2 (1981), and 2a (1981).
U.S.P. units—units defined in the United States Pharmacopeia.
USSR—Union of Soviet Socialist Republics.
u.v.—ultraviolet.
V—volt(s).
V.—*Vibrio.*
Val—valine.
var.—variety.
Venez.—Venezuela.
Viet.—Vietnam.
VLDL—very low-density lipoproteins.
vol.—volume(s).
v/v—volume in volume.
v/w—volume in weight.
WHO—World Health Organization.
w/o—water-in-oil.
wt—weight.
wt per ml—weight per millilitre.
w/v—weight in volume.
w/w—weight in weight.
Wycombe Gen. Hosp.—Wycombe General Hospital, High Wycombe, Bucks, England.
Y.—*Yersinia.*

Abbreviated Names for Radicals and Groups

The following abbreviated names for radicals and groups are used in approved names and titles:

Abbreviated Name	*Chemical Name*
acetonide	isopropylidene ether of a dihydric alcohol
acetophenide	methylphenylmethylene ether of a dihydric alcohol
aceturate	*N*-acetylglycinate
amsonate	4,4′-diaminostilbene-2,2′-disulphonate
benetonide	acetonide 3-benzamido-2-methylpropionate (as in triamcinolone benetonide)
besylate	benzenesulphonate
bunapsylate	3,7-di-*tert*-butylnapthalene-1,5-disulphonate
camsylate	camphor-10-sulphonate
caproate	hexanoate
carbesilate	4-carboxybenzenesulphonate
closylate	4-chlorobenzenesulphonate
cromacate	[(6-hydroxy-4-methyl-2-oxo-2*H*-chromen-7-yl)oxy]-acetate
cromesilate	6,7-dihydroxycoumarin-4-methanesulphonate
cyclotate	4-methylbicyclo[2.2.2]oct-2-ene-1-carboxylate
cypionate	3-cyclopentylpropionate
dibudinate	2,6-di-*tert*-butylnapthalene-1,5-disulphonate
diolamine	diethanolamine
edetate	ethylenediamine-*NNN′N′*-tetra-acetate
edisylate	ethane-1,2-disulphonate
eglumine	*N*-ethylglucamine
embonate	4,4′-methylenebis(3-hydroxy-2-naphthoate) (= pamoate)
enanthate	heptanoate
estolate	propionate dodecyl sulphate
esylate	ethanesulphonate
fendizoate	2-[(2′-hydroxy-4-biphenylyl)-carbonyl]benzoate
gluceptate	glucoheptonate
hybenzate	2-(4-hydroxybenzoyl)benzoate
hyclate	monohydrochloride hemi-ethanolate hemihydrate
isethionate	2-hydroxyethanesulphonate
lauryl sulphate	dodecyl sulphate
megallate	3,4,5-trimethoxybenzoate
meglumine	*N*-methylglucamine
mesylate	methanesulphonate
napadisylate	naphthalene-1,5-disulphonate
napsylate	naphthalene-2-sulphonate
olamine	ethanolamine
oxoglurate	2-oxoglutarate
pamoate	4,4′-methylenebis(3-hydroxy-2-naphthoate) (=embonate)
phenpropionate	3-phenylpropionate
pivalate	trimethylacetate
steaglate	stearoyloxyacetate
tebutate	*tert*-butylacetate
teprosilate	3-(theophyllin-7-yl)propane-sulphonate
theoclate	8-chlorotheophyllinate
tofesilate	2-(theophyllin-7-yl)ethane-sulphonate
tosylate	toluene-4-sulphonate
triclofenate	2,4,5-trichlorophenolate
trolamine	triethanolamine
troxundate	3,6,9-trioxaundecanoate

Weights and Measures

The International System of Units

The International System of Units (Système International d'Unités; SI) was established by resolutions of the Eleventh General Conference on Weights and Measures, 1960; some additions and changes have been made by later resolutions. The SI units are of 3 types: *base*; *supplementary*; and *derived*. The base units for the seven physical quantities which are regarded as dimensionally independent, are:

metre (m) (length)
kilogram (kg) (mass)
second (s) (time)
ampere (A) (electric current)
kelvin (K) (thermodynamic temperature)
mole (mol) (amount of substance)
candela (cd) (luminous intensity)

There are supplementary units for plane angle (radian = rad) and solid angle (steradian = sr).

The derived unit for any other physical quantity is that obtained by the dimensionally appropriate multiplication and division of the base units. Many of the derived units have special names and symbols. They include:

hertz	$Hz=s^{-1}$	frequency
newton	$N=m\ kg\ s^{-2}$	force
pascal	$Pa=m^{-1}\ kg\ s^{-2}$	pressure
joule	$J=m^{2}\ kg\ s^{-2}$	energy
watt	$W=m^{2}\ kg\ s^{-3}$	power
coulomb	$C=s\ A$	quantity of electricity, electric charge
volt	$V=m^{2}\ kg\ s^{-3}\ A^{-1}$	electric potential
ohm	$\Omega=m^{2}\ kg\ s^{-3}\ A^{-2}$	electric resistance
siemens	$S=m^{-2}\ kg^{-1}\ s^{3}\ A^{2}$	electric conductance
farad	$F=m^{-2}\ kg^{-1}\ s^{4}\ A^{2}$	electric capacitance
degrees Celsius	°C=K	Celsius temperature
becquerel	$Bq=s^{-1}$	activity of a radioactive source
gray	$Gy=J\ kg^{-1}$	absorbed dose of ionising radiation
sievert	$Sv=J\ kg^{-1}$	dose equivalent

In addition there are units which although not part of SI will continue to be used in appropriate contexts, such as the minute (min), hour (h), day (d) (time); and electronvolt (energy) and units which although not part of SI will continue in use for a limited time. They include:

ångström	Å	length
curie	Ci	activity of a radioactive source
rad	rad	absorbed dose of ionising radiation
röntgen	R	exposure to ionising radiation

It is recommended that some units be not generally used with SI units. They include:

dyne	dyn	force
erg	erg	energy
poise	P	dynamic viscosity
stokes	St	kinematic viscosity

The use of other units not part of SI is generally deprecated; the values of some that may be encountered are defined in the equivalent tables below.

In the European Communities a directive (80/181/EEC, as amended) requires, with various exceptions, that SI units be used as legal units of measurements and specifies dates after which some non-SI units may not be used.

The following prefixes may be used to construct decimal submultiples and multiples of units.

Factor	Prefix	Symbol
10^{-18}	atto	a
10^{-15}	femto	f
10^{-12}	pico	p
10^{-9}	nano	n
10^{-6}	micro	μ
10^{-3}	milli	m
10^{-2}	centi	c
10^{-1}	deci	d
10	deca	da
10^{2}	hecto	h
10^{3}	kilo	k
10^{6}	mega	M
10^{9}	giga	G
10^{12}	tera	T
10^{15}	peta	P
10^{18}	exa	E

Thousandfold multiples are to be preferred, e.g. gram, milligram, microgram, nanogram; μg per ml, mg per litre; joule, kilojoule, megajoule.

Millimoles and Milliequivalents

The mole (mol) is the amount of substance of a system which contains as many elementary entities (atoms, molecules, ions, electrons, or other particles or specified groups of such particles) as there are atoms in 0.012 kilogram of carbon-12. A millimole is one thousandth this amount and for ions is the ionic mass (the sum of the relative atomic masses of the elements of an ion) expressed in milligrams. A milliequivalent is this quantity divided by the valency of the ion.

1 Millimole (mmol) = 10^{-3} mole

For ions, 1 millimole (mmol) = 1 milliequivalent (mEq) × valency of the ion.

The following terms, though not strictly correct, are still in common use:

ionic weight, for ionic mass
atomic weight, for relative atomic mass
molecular weight, for relative molecular mass.

Concentration

In the SI units, concentration may be expressed either as mass concentration (e.g. g per dm^3, conventionally expressed as g per litre) or as 'amount of substance' concentration (e.g. mol per litre). The term 'molar' or the symbol M, to describe a solution containing one mole per dm^3, should not be used.

Mass concentration is used for the measurement of the concentration of mixtures or of substances with an indefinite or unknown molecular weight. It is recommended that mass concentration should not be expressed using 100 ml (1 dl) as the unit of volume. Common exceptions are measurements of blood alcohol and haemoglobin which are usually expressed as mg per 100 ml (mg per dl) and g per 100 ml (g per dl), respectively.

The amount of substance concentration should be used for the measurement of the concentration of substances with defined molecular weights. Equivalent concentration (mEq per litre) should no longer be used.

In medical and pharmaceutical practice amount of substance concentration is only in current use for expressing the strength of parenteral electrolyte infusions and dialysis solutions and for laboratory results. Prescribing and dispensing continue to be carried out in terms of mass concentration. In this edition of Martindale values of mmol and mEq per gram are stated in monographs for electrolytes.

SI Unit Equivalents of Imperial and other Units

LENGTH

1 ångström (Å)	= 10^{-10} metre = 10^{-1} nanometre
1 micron	= 10^{-6} metre
1 inch (in)	= 2.54×10^{-2} metre
1 foot (ft)	= 3.048×10^{-1} metre
1 yard (yd)	= 9.144×10^{-1} metre
1 mile	= 1.60934×10^{3} metres

MASS

1 grain (gr)	= 6.47989×10^{-2} gram
1 ounce (avoirdupois) (oz) (= 437.5 grains)	= 2.83495×10 grams
1 ounce (apothecaries') (= 480 grains)	= 3.11035×10 grams
1 pound (avoirdupois)	= 4.53592×10^{2} grams
1 ton	= 1.01605×10^{3} kg
1 tonne	= 10^{3} kg

AREA

1 are (a)	= 100 square metres
1 square inch (in^2)	= 6.4516×10^{-4} square metre
1 square foot (ft^2)	= 9.29030×10^{-2} square metre
1 square yard (yd^2)	= 8.36127×10^{-1} square metre
1 square mile	= 2.58999×10^{6} square metres

VOLUME

1 millilitre (ml)	= 1 cubic centimetre
1 litre*	= 1 cubic decimetre
1 cubic inch (in^3)	= 1.63871×10^{-5} cubic metre
1 cubic foot (ft^3)	= 2.83168×10^{-2} cubic metre
1 cubic yard (yd^3)	= 7.64555×10^{-1} cubic metre
1 minim (UK)	= 5.91939×10^{-8} cubic metre
1 fluid ounce (UK) (fl oz)	= 2.8413×10^{-5} cubic metre
1 pint	= 5.68261×10^{-4} cubic metre
1 gallon (UK)	= 4.54609×10^{-3} cubic metre
1 fluid ounce (US)	= 2.95735×10^{-5} cubic metre
1 liquid pint (US)	= 4.73176×10^{-4} cubic metre
1 gallon (US)	= 3.78541×10^{-3} cubic metre

* The litre has been redefined as 1 cubic decimetre, which represents a decrease from its former value of 1.000028 cubic decimetres. The litre should not be used for measurements of high precision.

ENERGY

1 kilocalorie, thermochemical (kcal)	= 4.1840×10^{3} joules
1 erg (erg)	= 10^{-7} joule
1 electronvolt (eV)	= 1.60219×10^{-19} joule
1 thousand (kilo) electronvolt (keV)	= 1.60219×10^{-16} joule
1 million (mega) electronvolt (MeV)	= 1.60219×10^{-13} joule
1 British thermal unit (Btu)	= 1.05506×10^{3} joules

PRESSURE

1 millimetre of mercury (mmHg)	= 1.33322×10^{2} pascals
1 bar (bar)	= 10^{5} pascals
1 pound-force per square inch	= 6.89476×10^{3} pascals
1 atmosphere (atm)	= 1.01325×10^{5} pascals

VISCOSITY, DYNAMIC

1 poise (P)	= 10^{-1} pascal second 10^{-1} newton second per square metre

VISCOSITY, KINEMATIC

1 centistokes (cSt)	= 10^{-6} square metre per second
1 stokes (St)	= 10^{-4} square metre per second

TEMPERATURE

1 degree Fahrenheit (°F)	= $\frac{5}{9}$ kelvin.

Imperial and other Equivalents of SI Units

LENGTH

1 metre (m)	= 10^{10} ångströms 10^{6} microns 39.3701 inches 3.28084 feet 1.09361 yards
1 kilometre (km)	= 0.621372 mile

MASS

1 gram (g)	= 15.4324 grains 0.032151 ounce (apothecaries') 0.035274 ounce (avoirdupois)
1 kilogram (kg)	= 35.274 ounces (avoirdupois) 2.20462 pounds

AREA

1 square metre (m^2)	= 1550 square inches 10.7639 square feet 1.196 square yards 3.86102×10^{-7} square mile

VOLUME

1 cubic metre (m^3)	= 6.10236×10^4 cubic inches 35.3147 cubic feet 1.30795 cubic yards
1 cubic centimetre* (cm^3)	= 1 millilitre 16.8934 minims (UK)
1 cubic decimetre (dm^3)	= 1 litre 35.1952 fluid ounces 1.75976 pints 0.21997 gallon (UK)

*The abbreviations 'cc', 'ccm', and 'cu cm' should not be used.

FORCE

1 newton (N)	= 10^5 dynes 1.01972×10^2 gram-force 1.01972×10^{-1} kilogram-force 7.23301 poundals

ENERGY

1 joule (J)	= 2.39006×10^{-4} kilocalorie 10^7 ergs 6.2415×10^{18} electronvolts 9.47813×10^{-4} British thermal unit

PRESSURE

1 pascal (Pa)	= 7.50064×10^{-3} millimetre of mercury 1.45038×10^{-4} pound-force per square inch 9.86923×10^{-6} atmosphere
1 kilopascal (kPa)	= 7.50064 millimetres of mercury

VISCOSITY, DYNAMIC

1 pascal second (Pa s)	= 10.0 poises

VISCOSITY, KINEMATIC

1 square metre per second ($m^2 s^{-1}$)	= 10^4 stokes

TEMPERATURE

1 kelvin (K)	= $^9/_5$ degrees Fahrenheit

SI Unit Equivalents of Radiation Units

ACTIVITY OF A RADIOACTIVE SOURCE

1 nanocurie (nCi)	= 3.7×10 becquerels
1 microcurie (μCi)	= 3.7×10^4 becquerels
1 millicurie (mCi)	= 3.7×10^7 becquerels
1 curie (Ci)	= 3.7×10^{10} becquerels

ABSORBED DOSE OF IONISING RADIATION

1 rad (rad)	= 10^{-2} gray
1 megarad (Mrad)	= 10^4 grays

ABSORBED DOSE RATE

1 rad per second (rad s^{-1})	= 10^{-2} gray per second

EXPOSURE TO IONISING RADIATIONS

1 röntgen (R)	= 2.58×10^{-4} coulomb per kilogram

DOSE EQUIVALENT

1 millirem (mrem)	= 10^{-5} sievert
1 rem (rem)	= 10^{-2} sievert

Radiation Unit Equivalents of SI Units

ACTIVITY OF A RADIOACTIVE SOURCE

1 becquerel (Bq)	= 2.7027×10^{-2} nanocurie 2.7027×10^{-5} microcurie 2.7027×10^{-8} millicurie 2.7027×10^{-11} curie

ABSORBED DOSE OF IONISING RADIATION

1 gray (Gy)	= 100 rads

EXPOSURE TO IONISING RADIATIONS

1 coulomb per kilogram (C kg^{-1})	= 3.876×10^3 röntgens

DOSE EQUIVALENT

1 sievert (Sv)	= 100 rems

References: D.A. Lowe, *A Guide to International Recommendations on Names and Symbols for Quantities and on Units of Measurement*, World Health Organization, Geneva, 1975; Report by the Symbols Committee of the Royal Society, *Quantities, Units, and Symbols*, 2nd Edn, London, The Royal Society, 1975; *The International System of Units (SI)* 1970 (BS 3763: 1976); *SI Units and Recommendations for the Use of their Multiples and of certain other Units* (BS 5555: 1976); *SI: The International System of Units*, (C.H. Page and P. Vigoureux, Ed.), National Physical Laboratory, London, HM Stationery Office, 1977; *The Use of SI Units*, British Standards Institution, PD 5686: 1978.

The use of SI units in medicine.—D.N. Baron, *Br. med. J.*, 1974, *4*, 509.

The use of SI units in hospital laboratories.—D.N. Baron *et al.*, *J. clin. Path.*, 1974, *27*, 590.

Dissociation Constants

The pK_a values given are for some of the drugs and ancillary substances included in Parts 1 and 2. They are derived from official publications and published papers, but as they are largely unconfirmed they should be taken as approximate values only. The temperature is specified where it is known.

Acebutolol	9.4
Acetanilide (25°)	0.6
Acetarsol	3.7
	7.9
	9.3
Acetazolamide (25°)	7.2
	9.0
Acetic Acid, Glacial (25°)	4.8
Aconitine (25°)	8.1
Acriflavine (25°)	9.1
Adrenaline (20°)	8.7
	10.2
	12.0
Ajmaline	8.2
Alclofenac	4.6
Allobarbitone (25°)	7.8
Allopurinol	9.4
Alphaprodine (20°)	8.7
Alprenolol (20°)	9.5
Amantadine	10.4
Ametazole (20°)	2.2
	9.6
Amethocaine (20°)	8.5
Amidephrine	9.1
Amidopyrine (20°)	5.1
Amiloride	8.7
Aminacrine (25°)	9.5
Aminobenzoic Acid (25°)	2.4
	4.9
Aminocaproic Acid (25°)	4.4
	10.8
Aminocephalosporanic Acid (35°)	2.0
	4.4
Aminodeacetoxycephalosporanic Acid (35°)	3.0
	4.9
Aminohippuric Acid	3.6
Aminophylline	5.0
Aminopterin	5.5
Aminosalicylic Acid (20°)	
($-NH_2$)	1.8
(−COOH)	3.6
Amiodarone	5.6
Amitriptyline (25°)	9.4
Amoxycillin	2.4
	7.4
	9.6
Amphetamine (20°)	9.9
Amphotericin	5.5
	10.0
Ampicillin (25°) (−COOH)	2.5
($-NH_2$)	7.3
Amylobarbitone (25°)	7.9
Amylocaine (25°)	8.4
Anileridine	3.7
	7.5
Aniline (25°)	4.6
Antazoline (25°)	2.5
	10.1
Apomorphine (15°)	7.2
	8.9
Aprobarbitone (25°)	8.0
Arecoline (20°)	7.4
Arsthinol	9.5
Ascorbic Acid (25°)	4.2
	11.6
Aspirin (25°)	3.5
Atenolol (24°)	9.6
Atropine (20°)	9.9
Baclofen	3.9
	9.6
Bamethan (25°)	9.0
	10.2
Barbitone (25°)	8.0
Bemegride	11.6
Benactyzine	6.6
Bendrofluazide (25°)	8.5
Benoxaprofen	3.5
Benzocaine (20°)	2.5
Benzoic Acid (25°)	4.2
Benzphetamine	6.6
Benzquinamide	5.9
Benztropine (20°)	10.0
Benzylmorphine (20°)	8.1
Benzylpenicillin (25°)	2.8
Betahistine	3.5
	9.7
Betaine (25°)	1.8
Bethanidine	10.6
(20°)	12.0
Boric Acid (25°)	9.2
Brilliant Green (25°)	7.9
Bromazepam	2.9
	11.0
Bromocriptine	4.9
Bromodiphenhydramine (25°)	8.6
Brompheniramine	3.9
Bromvaletone	10.8
Brucine (25°)	2.3
	8.0
Bupivacaine	8.1
Buprenorphine	8.5
	10.0
Burimamide	7.5
Butacaine	9.0
Butalbital (20°)	7.6
Butobarbitone (25°)	8.0
Cacodylic Acid (25°)	1.6
	6.2
Caffeine (40°)	0.6
(25°)	14.0
Capreomycin	6.2
	8.2
	10.1
	13.3
Carbachol	4.8
Carbenicillin	2.6
	2.7
	3.3
Carbenoxolone	6.7
	7.1
Carbinoxamine (25°)	8.1
Carbonic Acid (25°)	6.4
	10.3
Carbutamide (20°)	6.0
Cefapirin	2.2
Cefoxitin (25°)	3.5
Cefuroxime	2.5
Cephacetrile	2.0
Cephalexin	2.5
	5.2
	7.3
Cephaloglycin	1.9
	4.6
	7.1
Cephaloridine (35°)	1.7
	3.4
Cephalothin (35°)	2.2
Cephazolin (35°)	2.5
Cephradine (35°)	2.5
	7.3
Chloral Hydrate	10.0
Chlorambucil	5.8
	8.0
Chloramphenicol	5.5
Chlorcyclizine (25°)	2.4
	7.8
Chlordiazepoxide (20°)	4.6
Chlormethiazole	3.2
Chlorocresol (20°)	9.2
Chloroprocaine	8.7
Chloropyrilene (25°)	8.4
Chloroquine (20°)	8.4
	10.8
Chlorothiazide (20°)	6.7
	9.5
Chlorpheniramine	4.0
	9.2
Chlorphentermine	9.6
Chlorpromazine (20°)	9.3
Chlorpropamide (20°)	5.0
Chlorprothixene	8.8
Chlortetracycline (25°)	3.3
	7.4
	9.3
Chlorthalidone	9.4
Chlorzoxazone (20°)	8.0
Choline	8.9
Ciclacillin (25°)	2.7
Cimetidine	6.8
	7.1
Cinchocaine (20°)	7.5
	8.3
Citric Acid (25°)	3.1
	4.7
	6.4
Clindamycin (25°)	7.7
Clofibrate	3.0
Clonazepam	1.5
	10.5
Clonidine	8.2
Clorazepate	3.5
	12.5

Cloxacillin (25°)	2.7
Cocaine (20°)	8.6
Codeine (20°)	8.2
Colchicine	1.7
	12.4
m-Cresol (25°)	10.1
o-Cresol (25°)	10.3
p-Cresol (25°)	10.3
Crystal Violet (25°)	9.4
Cyacetazide (20°)	2.3
	11.2
Cyclizine	2.4
	7.8
Cyclobarbitone (20°)	7.6
Cyclopentamine	10.5
	11.5
Cyclopentolate	7.9
Cycloserine	4.5
	7.4
Cyclothiazide	9.1
	10.5
Cytarabine	4.3
Dacarbazine	4.4
Dantrolene	7.5
Dapsone	1.3
	2.5
Daunorubicin	8.2
Debrisoquine	11.9
Dehydrocholic Acid	5.1
Demeclocycline (25°)	3.3
	7.2
	9.2
Demoxepam	4.5
	10.6
Deserpidine	6.7
Desipramine (24°)	10.2
Desmethylchlordiazepoxide	4.4
Dexamphetamine	9.9
Dexchlorpheniramine (20°)	9.0
Dextromethorphan	8.3
Dextromoramide (25°)	7.1
Dextropropoxyphene	6.3
Diamorphine (23°)	7.6
Diatrizoic Acid (20°)	3.4
Diazepam (20°)	3.3
Diazoxide	8.5
Dichlorphenamide	7.4
	8.6
Dicloxacillin (25°)	2.7
Dicoumarol	4.4
	8.0
Diethazine (20°)	9.1
Diethylcarbamazine (20°)	7.7
Dihydrocodeine (25°)	8.8
Dihydroergocornine (24°)	6.9
Dihydroergocristine (24°)	6.9
Dihydroergocryptine (24°)	6.9
Dihydroergotamine (24°)	6.8
Dihydrostreptomycin	7.8
Dinoprost	4.9
Diodone (20°)	2.8
Diphenhydramine (25°)	9.0
Diphenoxylate	7.1
Dipipanone (25°)	8.5
Dipyridamole	6.4
Disopyramide	8.4
	9.6
Dixyrazine (25°)	7.8
Dopamine (20°)	8.8
	10.6
Doxepin	8.0
	9.0
Doxorubicin	8.2
	10.2
Doxycycline (20°)	3.5
	7.7
	9.5
Doxylamine	4.4
	9.2
Droperidol	7.6
Emetine (25°)	7.4
	8.3
Ephedrine (25°)	9.6
Ergometrine (20°)	6.8
(25°)	7.2
Ergotamine (24°)	6.3
Erythromycin	8.9
Ethacrynic Acid (20°)	3.5
Ethambutol (20°)	6.3
	9.5
Ethanolamine (25°)	9.4
Ethebenecid (25°)	3.3
Ethoheptazine	8.5
Ethopropazine (20°)	9.6
Ethosuximide (20°)	9.5
Ethyl Biscoumacetate	3.1
Ethylenediamine (20°)	7.2
	10.0
Ethylmorphine (20°)	8.2
Ethylnoradrenaline (25°)	8.4
Etidocaine	7.7
Etilefrine (25°)	9.0
	10.2
Etomidate	4.2
Eugenol (20°)	9.8
Fencamfamin (25°)	8.7
Fenclofenac	5.5
Fenfluramine (25°)	9.1
Fenoprofen (25°)	4.5
Fentanyl	7.8
	8.4
Floxuridine	7.7
Flucloxacillin	2.7
Flucytosine	2.9
	10.7
Flufenamic Acid	3.9
Flumizole	10.7
Flunitrazepam	1.8
Fluopromazine (24°)	9.2
Fluorouracil	8.0
	13.0
Fluphenazine	3.9
	8.1
Flurazepam	1.9
	8.2
Fomocaine	7.1
Formic Acid (25°)	3.8
Frusemide (20°)	3.9
Fumaric Acid (25°)	3.0
	4.5
Fusidic Acid	5.4
Gentamicin	8.2
Glibenclamide	5.3
Gliclazide	5.8
Glutethimide	4.5
	9.2
Glycerophosphoric Acid (25°)	1.5
	6.2
Glycine (25°)	2.3
	9.8
Guanethidine (20°)	8.3
	11.4
Guanoxan	12.3
Haloperidol	8.3
Harmine (20°)	7.6
Heptabarbitone (20°)	7.4
Hexetidine	8.3
Hexobarbitone (20°)	8.2
Hippuric Acid (25°)	3.8
Histamine (25°)	5.9
	9.7
Homatropine (20°)	9.9
Hydralazine	0.5
	7.1
Hydrastine (25°)	6.2
Hydrochlorothiazide	7.0
	9.2
Hydrocodone (20°)	8.3
Hydrocortisone Sodium Succinate	5.1
Hydroflumethiazide (20°)	8.5
	10.0
Hydromorphone (20°)	8.2
Hydroxyamphetamine (25°)	9.3
p-Hydroxybenzoic Acid	4.5
Hydroxyquinoline (20°)	5.0
	9.9
Hydroxyzine	2.1
	7.1
Hyoscine (23°)	7.6
Hyoscyamine (21°)	9.7
Hypochlorous Acid (17°)	7.4
Ibomal (20°)	7.7
Ibuprofen	4.4
	5.2
Idoxuridine	8.3
Imipramine (24°)	9.5
Imipramine Oxide (20°)	4.7
Indomethacin	4.5
Indoramin	7.7
Iodipamide	3.5
Iprindole	8.2
Isocarboxazid	10.4
Isoniazid (20°)	1.8
	3.5
	10.8
Isoprenaline (20°)	8.6
	10.1
	12.0
Isoxsuprine	8.0
	9.8
Kanamycin	7.2
Ketamine	7.5
Ketobemidone (20°)	8.7
Labetalol	7.4
Lactic Acid (25°)	3.9
Levallorphan	4.5
	6.9
Levamisole	8.0
Levodopa (25°)	2.3
	8.7
	9.7
	13.4
Levorphanol (20°)	8.2
Lignocaine (25°)	7.9
Lincomycin	7.5
Liothyronine	8.5
Lithium Carbonate (20°)	6.5
	10.3
Lorazepam (20°)	1.3
	11.5

Loxapine	6.6
Lysergide	7.5
Mandelic Acid (25°)	3.4
Mazindol	8.6
Mebhydrolin	6.7
Mecamylamine	11.3
Mecillinam	3.4
	8.9
Meclozine (25°)	3.1
	6.2
Medazepam (20°)	4.4
(37°)	6.2
Mefenamic Acid	4.2
Meglumine (20°)	9.5
Mepacrine (20°)	7.7
	10.3
Mephentermine	10.4
Mepivacaine (20°)	7.7
Mepyramine (25°)	4.0
	8.9
Mercaptomerin	3.7
	5.1
Mercaptopurine (20°)	7.7
	11.0
Metaraminol	8.6
Metformin (32°)	2.8
	11.5
Methacycline (20°)	3.1
	7.6
	9.5
Methadone (20°)	8.3
Methapyrilene (25°)	3.7
	8.9
Methaqualone	2.5
Metharbitone (20°)	8.3
Methazolamide	7.3
Methdilazine	7.5
Methetoin	8.1
Methicillin (25°)	2.8
L-Methionine	2.3
	9.2
Methohexitone	8.3
Methotrexate	3.8
	4.8
	5.6
Methotrimeprazine	9.2
Methoxamine (25°)	9.2
Methoxyphenamine	10.1
Methyclothiazide	9.4
Methyl Hydroxybenzoate (22°)	8.4
Methyl Nicotinate (22°)	3.1
Methylamphetamine	10.1
Methyldopa (25°) (−COOH)	2.2
(−OH)	9.2
($-NH_2$)	10.6
(−OH)	12.0
Methylene Blue	3.8
Methylephedrine (25°)	9.3
Methylergometrine (24°)	6.7
Methylphenidate	8.8
Methylphenobarbitone (20°)	7.8
Methylthiouracil (20°)	8.2
Methyprylone	12.0
Methysergide (24°)	6.6
Metoclopramide	7.3
	9.0
Metolazone	9.7
Metoprolol	9.7
Metronidazole	2.5
Mexiletine	9.1
Miconazole	6.7
Minocycline	2.8
	5.0
	7.8
	9.5
Molindone (25°)	6.9
Morphine (20°)	8.0
	9.9
Mustine (25°)	6.4
Nafcillin (25°)	2.7
Naftidrofuryl (30°)	8.2
Nalidixic Acid	6.0
Nalorphine (20°)	7.8
Naloxone	7.9
Naphazoline (20°)	10.9
Naphthol (20°)	8.8
Naproxen (25°)	4.2
Narceine (20°)	3.8
Narcotine	6.2
Nealbarbitone (20°)	7.2
Nefopam	9.2
Neostigmine	12.0
Nicotinamide (20°)	3.3
Nicotine (25°)	3.1
	7.9
Nicotinic Acid (25°) (−N=)	2.0
(−COOH)	4.8
Nicoumalone	4.7
Nifenalol	8.8
Nikethamide (20°)	3.5
Nitrazepam (20°)	3.2
	10.8
Nitrofurantoin (25°)	7.2
Noradrenaline (20°)	8.6
	9.8
	12.0
Norcodeine	5.7
Nordazepam	3.5
	12.0
Nordefrin (20°)	8.8
	9.8
Normethadone	9.2
Norpseudoephedrine (25°)	9.4
Nortriptyline	9.7
Noscapine (20°)	6.2
Novobiocin (25°)	4.2
	9.1
Obidoxime (25°)	7.6
	8.3
Opipramol	3.8
Orciprenaline (25°) (−OH)	9.0
(−NH−)	10.1
(−OH)	11.4
Orphenadrine	8.4
Oxacillin	2.8
Oxalic Acid (25°)	1.2
	4.2
Oxazepam (20°)	1.7
	11.6
Oxazolam	5.3
	11.9
Oxedrine (25°) (−OH)	9.3
(−NH−)	10.2
Oxprenolol	9.5
Oxycodone (20°)	8.9
Oxyfedrine (20°)	7.5
Oxymorphone	4.8
	8.5
	9.3
Oxyphenbutazone (22°)	4.7
Oxypurinol	7.7
Oxytetracycline (25°)	3.3
	7.3
	9.1
Pamaquin	8.7
Papaverine (25°)	6.4
Paracetamol (25°)	9.5
Parachlorophenol (20°)	9.2
Pargyline	6.9
Pecazine (24°)	9.7
Pemoline	10.5
Pempidine	2.8
	11.0
Penicillamine	1.8
	7.9
	10.5
Pentazocine (20°)	8.5
	10.0
Pentobarbitone (20°)	8.0
Perphenazine (24°)	3.7
	7.8
Pethidine (20°)	8.7
Phenadoxone (20°)	6.9
Phenazocine	8.5
Phenazone (25°)	1.5
Phencyclidine	8.5
Phendimetrazine	7.6
Phenethicillin (25°)	2.7
Phenformin (32°)	2.7
	11.8
Phenindamine (25°)	8.3
Pheniramine (25°)	4.2
	9.3
Phenmetrazine (25°)	8.4
Phenobarbitone (25°)	7.4
Phenol (25°)	10.0
Phenolphthalein (25°)	9.7
Phenolsulphonphthalein	7.9
Phenoxymethylpenicillin (25°)	2.7
Phentermine	10.1
Phentolamine	7.7
Phenylbutazone (20°)	4.4
Phenylephrine (20°) (−OH)	8.9
(−NH−)	10.1
Phenylmercuric Nitrate (20°)	3.3
Phenylmethylbarbituric Acid (25°)	7.7
Phenylpropanolamine (20°)	9.4
Phenyltoloxamine	9.1
Phenyramidol	5.9
Phenytoin (25°) (−OH)	8.3
Pholcodine (37°)	8.0
	9.3
Pholedrine (25°)	9.4
Phosphoric Acid (25°)	2.1
	7.2
	12.7
Physostigmine (25°)	1.8
	7.9
Pilocarpine (15°)	1.6
	7.1
Pimozide	7.3
	8.6
Pindolol	8.8
(24°)	9.7
Pipamazine	8.6
Piperazine (25°)	5.6
	9.8
Pirbuterol	3.0
	7.0
	10.3

Pivampicillin	7.0
Pivmecillinam	8.9
Pizotifen	7.0
Polymyxin B	8.9
Practolol (20°)	9.5
Pralidoxime (25°)	8.0
Prazepam	2.7
Prazosin	6.5
Prilocaine (25°)	7.9
Probenecid (20°)	3.4
Procainamide (20°)	9.2
Procaine (25°)	9.0
Procarbazine	6.8
Prochlorperazine	3.7
	8.1
Proguanil (22.5°)	2.3
	10.4
Promazine (25°)	9.4
Promethazine (25°)	9.1
Propicillin (25°)	2.7
Propiomazine	6.6
Propionic Acid	4.9
Propoxycaine	8.6
Propranolol	9.5
Propyl Hydroxybenzoate (22°)	8.4
Propylhexedrine (25°)	10.7
Propylthiouracil (20°)	8.3
Prothipendyl (25°)	2.3
Pseudoephedrine	9.8
Pyrantel (20°)	11.0
Pyrathiazine	8.9
	9.4
Pyrazinamide	0.5
Pyridoxine (25°) (−N=)	5.0
(−OH)	9.0
Pyrimethamine (20°)	7.0
Pyrrobutamine (25°)	8.8
Quinalbarbitone (20°)	7.9
Quinethazone	9.3
	10.7
Quinidine (20°)	4.2
	8.8
Quinine (20°)	4.1
	8.5
Reserpine (25°)	6.6
Resorcinol (20°)	9.5
	10.1
Riboflavine (20°)	1.9
	10.2
Riboflavine Phosphate (Sodium Salt) (20°)	2.5
	6.5
	10.3
Rifampicin	1.7
	7.9
Rolitetracycline	7.4
Saccharin (25°)	1.6
Salbutamol	9.3
	10.3
Salicylamide (37°)	8.2
Salicylic Acid (25°)	3.0
	13.4
Secbutobarbitone (20°)	8.0
Serotonin	9.1
	9.8
Sodium Calciumedetate (20°)	2.0
	2.7
	6.2
	10.3
Sodium Cromoglycate (20°)	2.5
Sodium Monofluorophosphate (20°)	2.5
	4.5
Sotalol	8.3
	9.8
Spectinomycin	7.0
	8.7
Spiramycin	8.0
Strychnine (25°)	2.3
	8.0
Sulfamerazine (25°)	7.1
Sulfametopyrazine	7.0
Sulfaquinoxaline (20°)	5.5
Sulphacetamide	1.8
	5.4
Sulphadiazine (25°)	6.5
Sulphadimethoxine (25°)	5.9
Sulphadimidine (25°)	7.4
Sulphaethidole	5.6
Sulphafurazole (25°)	4.9
Sulphaguanidine	11.3
	12.1
Sulphamethizole (25°)	5.3
Sulphamethoxazole (25°)	5.6
Sulphamethoxydiazine	7.0
Sulphamethoxypyridazine (25°)	7.2
Sulphamoxole	7.4
Sulphanilamide (20°)	10.4
Sulphaphenazole	6.5
Sulphapyridine (25°)	8.4
Sulphasalazine	0.6
	2.4
	9.7
	11.8
Sulphasomidine (27°)	7.5
Sulphathiazole (25°)	7.1
Sulphinpyrazone (22°)	2.8
Sulthiame	10.0
Talbutal (20°)	7.9
Tartaric Acid (25°)	3.0
	4.4
Taurine (25°)	1.5
Temazepam	1.6
Terbutaline (20°)	8.7
	10.0
	11.0
Tetracycline (25°) (acidic)	3.3
(acidic)	7.7
(basic)	9.7
Tetrahydrocannabinol	10.6
Tetramisole (20°)	7.8
Thebaine (20°)	8.2
Thenyldiamine (25°)	3.9
	8.9
Theobromine (25°)	<1
	10.0
Theophylline (25°)	<1
	8.6
Thiamine	4.8
	9.0
Thiamphenicol	7.2
Thiamylal	7.5
Thiopentone (20°)	7.6
Thiopropazate (24°)	7.3
Thioridazine (24°)	9.5
Thiouracil (25°)	7.5
Thonzylamine (25°)	2.1
	8.9
Ticarcillin	2.5
	3.4
Tobramycin	6.7
	8.3
	9.9
Tolamolol	9.2
Tolazamide	3.5
	5.7
Tolazoline (20°)	10.6
Tolbutamide (25°)	5.3
Tolmetin	3.5
Tranexamic Acid (20°)	4.5
	10.5
Tranylcypromine	8.2
Triamterene	6.2
Trichlormethiazide	8.6
Trichloroacetic Acid (25°)	<1
Triethanolamine (25°)	7.8
Trifluoperazine (24°)	8.1
Trimethobenzamide	8.3
Trimethoprim	7.2
Trimustine (25°)	4.4
Tripelennamine (25°)	3.9
	9.0
Triprolidine	6.5
Trometamol (20°)	8.2
Tropacocaine (15°)	9.7
Tropicamide	5.2
Tuaminoheptane	10.5
Tubocurarine (22°)	8.0
	9.2
Urea (25°)	0.2
Valproic Acid	5.0
Vanillin (20°)	7.4
Viloxazine	8.1
Vinbarbitone (20°)	7.5
Vinblastine	5.4
	7.4
Vincristine	5.0
	7.4
Viomycin	8.2
	10.3
Warfarin (20°)	5.0
Zimelidine	3.8

Determination of Body Surface Area from Height and Weight

Because of the variable relationship between the size and weight of patients it is sometimes more satisfactory to adjust dosage of medicaments to body surface area rather than to weight. The average normal body surface area for an adult man is 1.8 square metres. The following tables set out the relationship between the three functions, height (in feet or in centimetres), weight (in pounds or in kilograms), and body surface area (in square metres).

The values given are calculated from the formula of Dubois and Dubois (*Archs intern. Med.*, 1916, *17*, 863),

$$S = W^{0.425} \times H^{0.725} \times 71.84 \text{ (a constant)},$$

where S = surface area in square centimetres (expressed in the tables as square metres), W = weight in kilograms, and H = height in centimetres.

Height ft in / Weight lb	3′0″	3′2″	3′4″	3′6″	3′8″	3′10″	4′0″	4′2″	4′4″	4′6″	4′8″	4′10″	5′0″	5′2″	5′4″	5′6″	5′8″	5′10″	6′0″	6′2″	6′4″	6′6″
14	0.42																					
21	0.50	0.51																				
28	0.56	0.58	0.60	0.63																		
35	0.62	0.64	0.66	0.69	0.71	0.73																
42	0.66	0.69	0.72	0.74	0.77	0.79	0.82	0.84														
49		0.74	0.77	0.79	0.82	0.85	0.87	0.90	0.93													
56		0.78	0.81	0.84	0.87	0.90	0.92	0.95	0.98	1.01												
63				0.88	0.91	0.94	0.97	1.00	1.03	1.06	1.09											
70					0.95	0.98	1.02	1.05	1.08	1.11	1.14											
77					0.99	1.03	1.06	1.09	1.12	1.15	1.18	1.21	1.25	1.28								
84						1.06	1.10	1.13	1.16	1.20	1.23	1.26	1.29	1.32	1.35							
91							1.14	1.17	1.20	1.24	1.27	1.30	1.34	1.37	1.40	1.43	1.46					
98								1.21	1.24	1.28	1.31	1.35	1.38	1.41	1.45	1.48	1.51	1.54				
105									1.28	1.32	1.35	1.39	1.42	1.45	1.49	1.52	1.55	1.59	1.62			
112											1.39	1.42	1.46	1.50	1.53	1.56	1.60	1.63	1.67	1.70		
119											1.42	1.46	1.50	1.53	1.57	1.60	1.64	1.67	1.71	1.74	1.78	
126											1.46	1.50	1.53	1.57	1.61	1.64	1.68	1.72	1.75	1.79	1.82	1.86
133												1.53	1.57	1.61	1.65	1.68	1.72	1.76	1.79	1.83	1.86	1.90
140												1.57	1.60	1.64	1.68	1.72	1.76	1.79	1.83	1.87	1.90	1.94
147													1.64	1.68	1.72	1.76	1.79	1.83	1.87	1.91	1.94	1.98
154														1.71	1.75	1.79	1.83	1.87	1.91	1.95	1.98	2.02
161														1.74	1.78	1.82	1.86	1.90	1.94	1.98	2.02	2.06
168															1.82	1.86	1.90	1.94	1.98	2.02	2.06	2.10
175															1.85	1.89	1.93	1.97	2.01	2.05	2.09	2.13
182																1.92	1.96	2.01	2.05	2.09	2.13	2.17
189																1.95	2.00	2.04	2.08	2.12	2.16	2.21
196																	2.03	2.07	2.11	2.16	2.20	2.24
203																	2.06	2.10	2.14	2.19	2.23	2.27
210																		2.13	2.18	2.22	2.26	2.31
217																		2.16	2.21	2.25	2.29	2.34
224																			2.24	2.28	2.33	2.37
231																				2.31	2.36	2.40
238																					2.39	2.43

Height cm / Weight kg	90	95	100	105	110	115	120	125	130	135	140	145	150	155	160	165	170	175	180	185	190	195
10	0.50	0.52	0.54	0.56																		
12·5	0.55	0.57	0.59	0.61	0.64																	
15	0.59	0.62	0.64	0.66	0.69	0.71	0.73															
17.5	0.63	0.66	0.68	0.71	0.73	0.76	0.78	0.80														
20	0.67	0.70	0.72	0.75	0.78	0.80	0.83	0.85	0.88	0.90												
22.5			0.76	0.79	0.82	0.84	0.87	0.89	0.92	0.95	0.97	1.00										
25				0.82	0.85	0.88	0.91	0.94	0.96	0.99	1.02	1.04	1.07									
27.5				0.86	0.89	0.92	0.95	0.97	1.00	1.03	1.06	1.08	1.11	1.14	1.16							
30					0.92	0.95	0.98	1.01	1.04	1.07	1.10	1.13	1.15	1.18	1.21	1.24						
32.5					0.95	0.98	1.02	1.05	1.08	1.11	1.14	1.16	1.19	1.22	1.25	1.28	1.31					
35						1.02	1.05	1.08	1.11	1.14	1.17	1.20	1.23	1.26	1.29	1.32	1.35					
37.5							1.08	1.11	1.14	1.17	1.21	1.24	1.27	1.30	1.33	1.36	1.39	1.42				
40								1.14	1.17	1.21	1.24	1.27	1.30	1.33	1.37	1.40	1.43	1.46				
42.5								1.17	1.21	1.24	1.27	1.30	1.34	1.37	1.40	1.43	1.46	1.50	1.53			
45									1.24	1.27	1.30	1.34	1.37	1.40	1.44	1.47	1.50	1.53	1.56			
47.5									1.26	1.30	1.33	1.37	1.40	1.44	1.47	1.50	1.53	1.57	1.60	1.63		
50									1.29	1.33	1.36	1.40	1.43	1.47	1.50	1.54	1.57	1.60	1.64	1.67	1.70	
52.5										1.36	1.39	1.43	1.46	1.50	1.53	1.57	1.60	1.64	1.67	1.70	1.74	1.77
55										1.38	1.42	1.46	1.49	1.53	1.56	1.60	1.63	1.67	1.70	1.74	1.77	1.80
57.5											1.45	1.48	1.52	1.56	1.59	1.63	1.66	1.70	1.74	1.77	1.80	1.84
60											1.47	1.51	1.55	1.59	1.62	1.66	1.70	1.73	1.77	1.80	1.84	1.87
62.5												1.54	1.58	1.61	1.65	1.69	1.72	1.76	1.80	1.83	1.87	1.91
65												1.56	1.60	1.64	1.68	1.72	1.75	1.79	1.83	1.86	1.90	1.94
67.5													1.63	1.67	1.71	1.74	1.78	1.82	1.86	1.90	1.93	1.97
70													1.65	1.69	1.73	1.77	1.81	1.85	1.89	1.92	1.96	2.00
72.5														1.72	1.76	1.80	1.84	1.88	1.91	1.95	1.99	2.03
75														1.74	1.78	1.82	1.86	1.90	1.94	1.98	2.02	2.06
77.5															1.81	1.85	1.89	1.93	1.97	2.01	2.05	2.09
80															1.83	1.87	1.92	1.96	2.00	2.04	2.08	2.12
82.5																1.90	1.94	1.98	2.02	2.06	2.10	2.14
85																	1.96	2.01	2.05	2.09	2.13	2.17
87.5																	1.99	2.03	2.07	2.12	2.16	2.20
90																		2.06	2.10	2.14	2.18	2.22
92.5																		2.08	2.12	2.17	2.21	2.25
95																			2.15	2.19	2.23	2.28
97.5																			2.17	2.22	2.26	2.30
100																				2.24	2.28	2.33
102.5																				2.26	2.31	2.35
105																					2.33	2.38
107.5																						2.40

Atomic Weights of the Elements— $^{12}C=12$

Atomic Number	Name	Symbol	Atomic Weight
89	*Actinium	Ac	227.0278
13	Aluminium	Al	26.98154
95	Americium	Am	(243)
51	Antimony	Sb	121.75
18	Argon	Ar	39.948
33	Arsenic	As	74.9216
85	Astatine	At	(210)
56	Barium	Ba	137.34
97	Berkelium	Bk	(247)
4	Beryllium	Be	9.01218
83	Bismuth	Bi	208.9804
5	Boron	B	10.81
35	Bromine	Br	79.904
48	Cadmium	Cd	112.41
55	Caesium	Cs	132.9054
20	Calcium	Ca	40.08
98	Californium	Cf	(251)
6	Carbon	C	12.011
58	Cerium	Ce	140.12
17	Chlorine	Cl	35.453
24	Chromium	Cr	51.996
27	Cobalt	Co	58.9332
29	Copper	Cu	63.546
96	Curium	Cm	(247)
66	Dysprosium	Dy	162.50
99	Einsteinium	Es	(252)
68	Erbium	Er	167.26
63	Europium	Eu	151.96
100	Fermium	Fm	(257)
9	Fluorine	F	18.998403
87	Francium	Fr	(223)
64	Gadolinium	Gd	157.25
31	Gallium	Ga	69.72
32	Germanium	Ge	72.59
79	Gold	Au	196.9665
72	Hafnium	Hf	178.49
2	Helium	He	4.00260
67	Holmium	Ho	164.9304
1	Hydrogen	H	1.0079
49	Indium	In	114.82
53	Iodine	I	126.9045
77	Iridium	Ir	192.22
26	Iron	Fe	55.847
36	Krypton	Kr	83.80
57	Lanthanum	La	138.9055
103	Lawrencium	Lr	(260)
82	Lead	Pb	207.2
3	Lithium	Li	6.941
71	Lutetium	Lu	174.967
12	Magnesium	Mg	24.305
25	Manganese	Mn	54.9380
101	Mendelevium	Md	(258)
80	Mercury	Hg	200.59
42	Molybdenum	Mo	95.94
60	Neodymium	Nd	144.24
10	Neon	Ne	20.179
93	*Neptunium	Np	237.0482

Atomic Number	Name	Symbol	Atomic Weight
28	Nickel	Ni	58.70
41	Niobium	Nb	92.9064
7	Nitrogen	N	14.0067
102	Nobelium	No	(259)
76	Osmium	Os	190.2
8	Oxygen	O	15.9994
46	Palladium	Pd	106.4
15	Phosphorus	P	30.97376
78	Platinum	Pt	195.09
94	Plutonium	Pu	(244)
84	Polonium	Po	(209)
19	Potassium	K	39.0983
59	Praesodymium	Pr	140.9077
61	Promethium	Pm	(145)
91	*Protactinium	Pa	231.0359
88	*Radium	Ra	226.0254
86	Radon	Rn	(222)
75	Rhenium	Re	186.207
45	Rhodium	Rh	102.9055
37	Rubidium	Rb	85.4678
44	Ruthenium	Ru	101.07
62	Samarium	Sm	150.4
21	Scandium	Sc	44.9559
34	Selenium	Se	78.96
14	Silicon	Si	28.0855
47	Silver	Ag	107.868
11	Sodium	Na	22.98977
38	Strontium	Sr	87.62
16	Sulphur	S	32.06
73	Tantalum	Ta	180.9479
43	Technetium	Tc	(98)
52	Tellurium	Te	127.60
65	Terbium	Tb	158.9254
81	Thallium	Tl	204.37
90	*Thorium	Th	232.0381
69	Thulium	Tm	168.9342
50	Tin	Sn	118.69
22	Titanium	Ti	47.90
74	Tungsten	W	183.85
106	Unnilhexium	Unh	(263)
105	Unnilpentium	Unp	(262)
104	Unnilquadium	Unq	(261)
92	Uranium	U	238.029
23	Vanadium	V	50.9415
54	Xenon	Xe	131.30
70	Ytterbium	Yb	173.04
39	Yttrium	Y	88.9059
30	Zinc	Zn	65.38
40	Zirconium	Zr	91.22

Values in parentheses are used for certain radioactive elements whose atomic weights cannot be quoted precisely without knowledge of origin; the value given is the atomic mass number of the isotope of that element of longest known half-life. The atomic weight of elements marked (*) is that of the radioisotope of longest half-life.

Part 1

Monographs on Drugs and Ancillary Substances

Adrenaline and some other Sympathomimetics

2040-z

Sympathomimetic agents have actions similar to those which follow stimulation of postganglionic sympathetic or adrenergic nerves. They are sometimes termed sympathicomimetic agents.

The main effects of sympathomimetic agents include:

1. cardiac stimulation, resulting in an increase in the rate and force of contraction of the heart;
2. central nervous system stimulation, resulting in increased wakefulness, increased rate and volume of respiration, and reduced appetite;
3. metabolic stimulation, resulting in increased oxygen consumption, increased liver and muscle glycogenolysis, and increased blood concentrations of glucose and free fatty acids;
4. smooth muscle stimulation, increasing smooth muscle tone in peripheral blood vessels supplying the skin and mucous membranes;
5. smooth muscle inhibition, decreasing smooth muscle tone in blood vessels supplying skeletal muscle and decreasing the tone of some smooth muscle of the respiratory system and intestinal tract.

The 3 naturally occurring sympathomimetic agents are adrenaline, dopamine, and noradrenaline. All 3 are catecholamines, i.e. their aromatic portion is catechol (which is characterised by hydroxy groups at adjacent positions of a benzene ring), and the aliphatic portion is an amine. Despite the widespread use of the term 'adrenergic' for sympathetic, it is noradrenaline which is the endogenous neurotransmitter at postganglionic sympathetic nerves and within the central nervous system. The physiological properties of adrenaline itself are predominantly metabolic, although it can act directly as a neurotransmitter. Dopamine is predominantly a neurotransmitter within the central nervous system, although it also has peripheral effects. In the biosynthesis of the endogenous catecholamines L-tyrosine is converted into L-dopa (levodopa) by tyrosine hydroxylase, L-dopa is converted into dopamine by L-dopa decarboxylase, dopamine is converted into noradrenaline by dopamine β-hydroxylase, and noradrenaline is converted into adrenaline by phenylethanolamine *N*-methyltransferase. Hence, dopamine is a precursor of noradrenaline, and noradrenaline is a precursor of adrenaline.

Sympathomimetic agents differ in the intensity and duration of their actions and qualitatively according to the predominance of a particular effect. For those with predominantly stimulating effects on the central nervous system and which may be used to depress appetite, see Anorectics, p.65.

The type of effect a sympathomimetic agent exerts at peripheral sympathetic sites is largely determined by the receptor through which it acts. It was postulated (Ahlquist, *Am. J. Physiol.*, 1948, *153*, 586) that there are alpha and beta adrenergic receptors (or adrenoceptors). Stimulation of the alpha receptors, which is the predominant effect of the catecholamine, noradrenaline, results in vasoconstriction of arterioles of the skin and splanchnic area, producing an increase in blood pressure, dilatation of the pupils, and relaxation of the gut. Predominant alpha-adrenergic effects are also shown by metaraminol, methoxamine, and phenylephrine. The existence of alpha-adrenoceptor subtypes has been postulated.

Stimulation of the beta receptors, which is the predominant effect of isoprenaline, results in increased cardiac output, excitability, and rate, dilation of arterioles supplying skeletal muscles, and relaxation of the uterus, intestine, and bronchial muscle. When sympathomimetics combine with beta-adrenoceptors they activate the enzyme, adenylate cyclase leading to increased synthesis of cyclic adenosine monophosphate (cyclic AMP); this brings about the final beta-adrenergic response. In turn, cyclic AMP is broken down by phosphodiesterases. Caffeine and similar xanthines inhibit phosphodiesterases, and elicit responses, such as bronchodilatation and cardiac stimulation, similar to those of beta-adrenoceptor stimulants.

The relative potencies of beta-adrenoceptor stimulating agents has led to the hypothesis that beta-adrenoceptor subtypes exist. Thus, the effects on the heart appear to be mediated by a receptor termed $beta_1$ while a receptor termed $beta_2$ is involved in bronchodilatation. Dobutamine, which has prominent effects on the heart, is an example of a $beta_1$-adrenoceptor stimulant. Salbutamol and terbutaline, which have prominent effects on the lungs at doses which have little effect on the heart, are examples of $beta_2$-adrenoceptor stimulants.

Although their mode of action differs, adrenaline and ephedrine both show marked alpha- and beta-adrenergic activity. Other sympathomimetic agents differ quantitatively in their action on alpha and beta receptors. Thus sympathomimetic agents may be arranged in order of decreasing alpha-adrenergic activity and increasing beta-adrenergic activity from predominantly alpha-adrenergic activity to predominantly beta-adrenergic activity.

Dopamine possesses, in addition to alpha- and beta-adrenergic effects, the ability to dilate renal and mesenteric vessels by mechanisms not believed to require alpha- or beta-adrenergic receptors.

Alpha-receptor effects are selectively blocked by alpha-adrenoceptor blocking agents such as phentolamine, phenoxybenzamine, and tolazoline. Beta-receptor effects are selectively blocked by beta-adrenoceptor blocking agents such as acebutolol, oxprenolol, and propranolol.

Adrenergic receptors at other than peripheral sites, such as in the central nervous system or in tissues producing the metabolic effects of sympathetic stimulation, are not so readily classifiable into types.

Sympathomimetic agents are classed as direct acting when they act directly on adrenergic receptors, e.g. isoprenaline and noradrenaline. Some sympathomimetic agents, such as amphetamine, methylamphetamine, and mephentermine, act mainly indirectly by releasing noradrenaline from storage sites in adrenergic nerve endings; hence their actions are largely those of noradrenaline. Many sympathomimetic agents, such as ephedrine and metaraminol are dependent partly on direct action and partly on indirect action for their effects.

Therapeutically, sympathomimetic agents may be broadly classified into the following groups:

Sympathomimetic agents with prominent bronchodilatory effects used in the treatment of asthma and similar conditions including: adrenaline, p.1, ephedrine, p.10, isoetharine, p.14, isoprenaline, p.15, methoxyphenamine, p.19, methylephedrine, p.20, orciprenaline, p.22, phenylephrine, p.23, phenylpropanolamine, p.25, pseudoephedrine, p.27, rimiterol, p.28, salbutamol, p.29, terbutaline, p.31.

CAUTION. *Excessive usage of aerosols containing sympathomimetic agents has been associated with sudden death in asthmatics*—see p.15.

Sympathomimetic agents that have been used in the treatment of heart block and similar conditions including: adrenaline, p.1, ephedrine, p.10, isoprenaline, p.15.

Sympathomimetic agents used in the treatment of nasal congestion including: ephedrine, p.10, hydroxyamphetamine, p.14, mephentermine, p.18, methoxamine, p.19, naphazoline, p.20, oxymetazoline, p.23, phenylephrine, p.23, phenylpropanolamine, p.25, pseudoephedrine, p.27, tetrahydrozoline, p.33, tuaminoheptane, p.33, xylometazoline, p.33.

Sympathomimetic agents used in the treatment of hypotension including: angiotensin amide, p.6, dopamine, p.9, ephedrine, p.10, mephentermine, p.18, metaraminol, p.18, methoxamine, p.19, noradrenaline, p.20, oxedrine, p.23, phenylephrine, p.23, phenylpropanolamine, p.25.

Sympathomimetic agents used in the prevention of premature labour including: fenoterol, p.13, ritodrine, p.28, salbutamol, p.29, terbutaline, p.31.

A discussion on the pharmacology of the catecholamines and their role in disease.— R. Laverty, *Drugs*, 1978, *16*, 418.

Further reviews of the physiology and pharmacology of adrenaline (epinephrine) and other sympathomimetic agents: J. H. Burn, *J. Pharm. Pharmac.*, 1976, *28*, 342; *idem*, 1977, *29*, 325; L. Landsberg and J. B. Young, *New Engl. J. Med.*, 1978, *298*, 1295; R. J. Lefkowitz, *Ann. intern. Med.*, 1979, *91*, 450; B. B. Hoffman and R. J. Lefkowitz, *New Engl. J. Med.*, 1980, *302*, 1390; P. E. Cryer, *ibid.*, *303*, 436; *Br. med. J.*, 1981, *283*, 173.

CAUTION. *Care is necessary if a sympathomimetic agent is given to a patient being treated with a monoamine oxidase inhibitor (or within 14 days of stopping such treatment) or a tricyclic antidepressant (or within several days of stopping such treatment). Care is also necessary if a sympathomimetic agent is given to a patient receiving antihypertensive therapy.*

2041-c

Adrenaline *(B.P.)*. Adren.; Epinefrina; Epinephrinum; Epinephrine *(U.S.P.)*; Epirenamine; Levorenin; Suprarenin; Adrenalin. (*R*)-1-(3,4-Dihydroxyphenyl)-2-methylaminoethanol. $C_9H_{13}NO_3$=183.2.

CAS — 51-43-4.

NOTE. Racepinephrine is racemic adrenaline.

Pharmacopoeias. In *Arg.*, *Belg.*, *Br.*, *Braz.*, *Chin.*,

Hung., Ind., Int., It., Jap., Mex., Neth., Nord., Pol., Port., Roum., Span., Turk., and *U.S.*

Adrenaline is an active principle of the medulla of the suprarenal gland. It may be obtained from the glands of certain mammals or it may be prepared synthetically.

A white or creamy-white, odourless, crystalline powder or granules with a slightly bitter, numbing taste. It darkens in colour on exposure to air and light. M.p. about 212° with decomposition.

Sparingly **soluble** in water; freely soluble in solutions of mineral acids and boric acid solution, and in solutions of sodium or potassium hydroxide. Practically insoluble in alcohol, chloroform, ether, light petroleum, liquid paraffin, many other organic solvents, solutions of ammonia or alkali carbonates, and fixed and volatile oils. Oleic acid is a poor solvent. A solution in M hydrochloric acid is laevorotatory. Solutions in water are alkaline to litmus. It is not precipitated by ordinary alkaloidal reagents.

Incompatible with alkalis, copper, iron, silver, zinc, and other metals, gums, oxidising agents, and tannin. It is unstable in neutral or alkaline solution which rapidly becomes red on exposure to air. **Store** in airtight containers, preferably in which the air has been replaced by nitrogen. Protect from light.

2042-k

Adrenaline Acid Tartrate *(B.P., B.P. Vet., Eur. P.).*

Adren. Tart.; Adrenaline Tartrate; Epinephrini Bitartras; Adrenaline Bitartrate; Epinephrine Bitartrate *(U.S.P.)*; Epirenamine Bitartrate; Adrenalini Bitartras; Adrenalinii Tartras; Adrenalinium Hydrogentartaricum.

$C_9H_{13}NO_3,C_4H_6O_6$=333.3.

CAS — 51-42-3.

Pharmacopoeias. In *Aust., Belg., Br., Braz., Cz., Eur., Fr., Ger., Ind., Int., It., Jug., Neth., Nord., Rus., Swiss, Turk.,* and *U.S.*

A white to greyish-white or light brownish-grey, odourless, crystalline powder. It slowly darkens on exposure to air and light. M.p. 147° to 152° with decomposition. Adrenaline acid tartrate 1.8 mg is approximately equivalent to 1 mg of adrenaline.

Soluble 1 in 3 of water and 1 in 520 of alcohol; practically insoluble in chloroform and ether. A 5% solution in water has a pH of 3 to 4. A 5.7% solution is iso-osmotic with serum. Solutions are **sterilised** by autoclaving or by filtration; they should contain 0.1% of sodium metabisulphite.

Incompatible with alkalis, copper, iron, silver, zinc, and other metals, gums, oxidising agents, and tannin. Aqueous solutions have their optimum stability at about pH 3.6. **Store** in airtight containers, preferably in a vacuum-sealed tube or in an atmosphere of inert gas. Protect from light.

An aqueous solution of adrenaline acid tartrate iso-osmotic with serum (5.7%) caused 100% haemolysis of erythrocytes cultured in it for 45 minutes. The solution turned dark brown.— E. R. Hammarlund and K. Pedersen-Bjergaard, *J. pharm. Sci.*, 1961, *50*, 24.

Incompatibility. Adrenaline hydrochloride was incompatible with mephentermine sulphate.— R. C. Bogash, *Bull. Am. Soc. Hosp. Pharmsts*, 1955, *12*, 445.

There was loss of clarity when intravenous solutions of adrenaline were mixed with hyaluronidase, novobiocin sodium, or (in dextrose injection) warfarin sodium.— J. A. Patel and G. L. Phillips, *Am. J. Hosp. Pharm.*, 1966, *23*, 409.

Preservatives. Benzalkonium chloride 0.01% was a suitable preservative for adrenaline eye-drops sterilised by heating at 98° to 100° for 30 minutes, or chlorhexidine gluconate 0.02% when sterilised by filtration.— M. Van Ooteghem, *Pharm. Tijdschr. Belg.*, 1968, *45*, 69.

Stability. A solution of adrenaline 0.1% (as acid tartrate) and sodium metabisulphite 0.1% with a pH of 3.6 in full 2-ml ampoules was sterilised by autoclaving. Bio-assay showed little loss of potency after storage for 6 years at room temperature in the dark. Over the same period slightly greater losses occurred at pH 3 and 4.2.— G. B. West, *J. Pharm. Pharmac.*, 1950, *2*, 864.

Degradation of adrenaline solutions stored in an oxygen-free atmosphere proceeded at a faster rate in the presence of sodium metabisulphite than in its absence probably due to the formation of an addition compound.— L. C. Schroeter *et al.*, *J. Am. pharm. Ass., scient. Edn*, 1958, *47*, 723. See also T. Higuchi and L. C. Schroeter, *ibid.*, 1959, *48*, 535. It was postulated that boric acid stabilised adrenaline against degradation by sodium metabisulphite in an oxygen-free atmosphere, and that this was due to chelation of the adrenaline by the boric acid; the degree of chelation and the consequent stability of the adrenaline increased with rise of pH. If, however, a solution of adrenaline with sodium metabisulphite was exposed to atmospheric oxygen, oxidation was not prevented by the addition of boric acid. At a pH above 4.5 the metabisulphite was oxidised even in the dark; after this oxidation was complete the adrenaline was stable for several days, if kept in the dark, but quickly started to oxidise with the development of a red colour on exposure to light.— S. Riegelman and E. Z. Fischer, *J. pharm. Sci.*, 1962, *51*, 206 and 210.

The stability during storage of adrenaline injection 1 in 10 000 was investigated. Solutions were prepared to the following formulas: (1) adrenaline acid tartrate 18 mg, sodium metabisulphite 100 mg, sodium chloride 800 mg, Water for Injections to 100 ml (pH 4.15); (2) as formula 1, but with the addition of 50 mg of tartaric acid. Both solutions were autoclaved at 115° for 30 minutes. The percentage losses after autoclaving, after 2 weeks' and after 5 weeks' storage at 37° were respectively 1.3, 3.9, and 6% for formula 1, and 0.4, 2.8, and 5.6% for formula 2.— Pharm. Soc. Lab. Rep. No. 21, 1964.

Adrenaline injection 0.1% (pH 3.6), containing adrenaline acid tartrate 0.182%, sodium chloride 0.8%, sodium metabisulphite 0.05%, and Water for Injections to 100 ml (K. Backe-Hansen *et al.*, *J. Pharm. Pharmac.*, 1963, *15*, 804), and sterilised by autoclaving at 120° for 20 minutes showed no decrease in biological activity after storage for 5 years in the dark at 4°. Non-stabilised injections (pH 3) had lost about 10% activity.— K. Backe-Hansen *et al.*, *Acta pharm. suec.*, 1966, *3*, 269.

The shelf-life of 1 and 2% lignocaine hydrochloride injections containing adrenaline 0.001%, sodium metabisulphite 0.05%, methyl hydroxybenzoate 0.1%, 0.03M acetate buffer to pH 4.0 or 4.4, and sodium chloride sufficient to produce an iso-osmotic solution was studied by accelerated storage tests. It was estimated that adrenaline would lose 15% of its potency anaerobically at pH 4.4 in 15 months at 30°, 11 years at 15°, and 31 years at 8°. As *U.S.P.* injections could have a pH of up to 5.5, injections should be stored in a cold place and the upper limit of pH should be 4.4.— B. R. Hajratwala, *Drug Dev. ind. Pharm.*, 1977, *3*, 65. See also *idem, J. pharm. Sci.*, 1975, *64*, 45. Earlier reference: P. C. M. Hoevanaars, *Pharm. Weekbl. Ned.*, 1965, *100*, 1151.

Adverse Effects and Precautions. Side-effects such as anxiety, dyspnoea, hyperglycaemia, restlessness, palpitations, tachycardia, tremors, weakness, dizziness, headache, and coldness of the extremities may occur even with small doses of adrenaline. Overdosage may cause cardiac arrhythmias, cerebral haemorrhage, and pulmonary oedema; these effects have also been reported with normal doses in susceptible or hypersensitive individuals. Hypersusceptibility occurs especially in psychoneurotic patients, in patients of nervous temperament, and most markedly in those with hyperthyroidism.

In patients with hypertension or arteriosclerosis, adrenaline may cause cerebral haemorrhage. In patients with angina pectoris it may precipitate an attack and ventricular fibrillations may be induced if there is organic heart disease. Ventricular fibrillations may also occur if adrenaline is given with excessive doses of cardiac glycosides, mercurial diuretics, or other drugs that sensitise the heart to arrhythmias.

Gangrene may follow the infiltration of local anaesthetic solutions containing adrenaline into digits. In the presence of microbial contamination, the favourable environment of lowered oxygen tension induced by intramuscular injection of long-acting adrenaline preparations has led to gas gangrene.

Adrenaline is contra-indicated in narrow-angle glaucoma since the resulting dilatation of the pupil could increase the intra-ocular pressure. Melanin-like deposits in the cornea and conjunctiva may follow the use of eye-drops of adrenaline and have also caused obstruction of the naso-lachrymal ducts. Repeated ocular administration of adrenaline may cause oedema, hyperaemia, and inflammation of the eyes.

It has been suggested that the hyperglycaemic effect of adrenaline may call for increased insulin or oral hypoglycaemic therapy.

Inhalation of adrenaline may cause epigastric pain and the mouth and throat should be rinsed with water after inhaling.

Ventricular fibrillations may occur if adrenaline is used during anaesthesia with chloroform, cyclopropane, ethyl chloride, fluroxene, halothane, methoxyflurane or trichloroethylene, and it is contra-indicated with these agents except possibly in very dilute solution for the control of local haemorrhage (see below).

Adrenaline has been reported to have an enhanced action in patients receiving reserpine (whereas the reverse is the case for the indirectly acting sympathomimetic agents), and it should be used with extreme caution in patients receiving guanethidine or related antihypertensive agents since it may have a markedly enhanced action. Interactions between adrenaline and beta-adrenoceptor blocking agents are complex: whereas propranolol reverses the bronchodilating properties of adrenaline, and adrenaline reverses the antihypertensive properties of propranolol, adrenaline also markedly enhances propranolol-induced bradycardia and peripheral vasoconstriction. Similarly complex interactions occur with alpha-adrenoceptor blocking agents: thus adrenaline enhances both the cardiac-accelerating and the antihypertensive effects of phenoxybenzamine, whereas use has been made of phenoxybenzamine to reverse hypertension in adrenaline overdosage. Cocaine and adrenaline enhance one another's stimulatory effects; such an association should be avoided, preferably even on topical administration. Similarly, the association of adrenaline and thyroid should be avoided. The potentially catastrophic interaction, however, that may occur between the indirectly acting sympathomimetics, such as tyramine (p.526) and monoamine oxidase inhibitors (see Phenelzine Sulphate, p.128) is less of a problem with adrenaline, which is not solely dependent upon monoamine oxidase for its inactivation; nevertheless, subjects receiving monoamine oxidase inhibitors may be sensitive to the general sympathomimetic properties of adrenaline, so there remains a need for caution. Where possible, adrenaline should be avoided in patients receiving tricyclic antidepressants (or within several days of their discontinuation) since concurrent administration may induce hazardous cardiac arrhythmias. For further details see under the precautions for each drug.

CAUTION. *Excessive usage of aerosols of sympathomimetic agents has been associated with sudden death in asthmatics*—see p.15.

An account of rare individuals whose sensitivity to adrenaline was so great that they developed acute fulminating pulmonary oedema upon injection of even small amounts of adrenaline 1 in 200 000 while under general anaesthesia.— N. M. Woldorf and P. N. Pastore, *Archs Otolar.*, 1972, *96*, 272.

Of 229 patients who received intra-osseous injections of procaine 2%, trimecaine 2%, or lignocaine 1% with a vasoconstrictor, usually adrenaline, for dental anaesthesia, 24 had reactions which included fainting, anxiety, and tremor of hands or knees and were attributed to the sympathomimetic. These reactions occurred more frequently with adrenaline 1 in 50 000 than with lower concentrations of 1 in 100 000 and 1 in 200 000.— A. Z. Petrikas (letter), *Br. dent. J.*, 1973, *135*, 146. An account of adverse reactions to local anaesthetics and vasoconstrictor drugs.— P. J. Verrill, *Practitioner*, 1975, *214*, 380.

Further references: R. K. Lansche, *Am. J. Ophthal.*, 1966, *61*, 95 (serious systemic toxicity following the instillation of 2 drops of 2% adrenaline eye-drops in 2 patients); D. A. Dantes and J. W. Winkelman (letter), *Lancet*, 1972, *1*, 450 (systemic effects associated with long-term use of eye-drops); B. Lilienthal and A. K.

Reynolds, *Oral Surg.*, 1975, *40*, 574 (cardiovascular effects associated with intra-osseous injection in dentistry).

Bronchospasm. For a comment on bronchospasm associated with the inhalation of solutions of adrenaline that were not fresh, see under Preparations (below).

Effects on the eyes. Black localised punctate conjunctival pigmentation in patients treated for at least a year with adrenaline eye-drops for open-angle glaucoma was found to be due to the deposition of melanin. It appeared that adrenaline was oxidised to adrenochrome and then to melanin in pre-existing conjunctival pockets or cysts.— M. E. Corwin and W. H. Spencer, *Archs Ophthal., N.Y.*, 1963, *69*, 317. Black corneal lesions were found in 2 patients who had been treated with adrenaline eye-drops for glaucoma. In 1 of the patients, pigmentation was noticed after about 8 weeks' treatment.— A. P. Ferry and L. E. Zimmerman, *Am. J. Ophthal.*, 1964, *58*, 205. See also J. Sugar, *Archs Ophthal., N.Y.*, 1974, *91*, 11.

During 4 years, 15 patients showed reactions to adrenaline eye-drops, usually 2% of the hydrochloride or acid tartrate, while some used 1% epinephryl borate. Blurring and distortion of vision were followed by decreased visual acuity, and by the appearance of oedema and sometimes haemorrhage in the macular region. A few patients developed cysts near the fovea. These effects appeared within a few weeks of, or several months after, commencement of therapy and were usually reversible. All except 1 of the patients were aphakic (devoid of lens). In a study of 200 consecutive patients receiving adrenaline therapy, 23 were aphakic, and 7 experienced these reactions to adrenaline.— A. E. Kolker and B. Becker, *Archs Ophthal., N.Y.*, 1968, *79*, 552. Further references to macular oedema associated with the use of adrenaline eye-drops in aphakic eyes: R. J. Mackool *et al.*, *Archs Ophthal., N.Y.*, 1977, *95*, 791; J. V. Thomas *et al.*, *ibid.*, 1978, *96*, 625.

Corneal endothelial changes associated with long-term use of adrenaline eye-drops.— S. R. Waltman *et al.*, *Archs Ophthal., N.Y.*, 1977, *95*, 1357.

Effects of the heart. An account of the adverse effects of various drugs, including sympathomimetics, on the heart.— S. M. Deglin *et al.*, *Drugs*, 1977, *14*, 29. See also I. M. Lightbody, *Practitioner*, 1980, *224*, 275.

Effects on the salivary glands. Non-inflammatory enlargement of salivary glands (termed sialosis) is sometimes encountered in asthmatic patients having sustained treatment with sympathomimetic drugs.— D. K. Mason and M. M. Ferguson, *Practitioner*, 1978, *221*, 571.

Gas gangrene associated with intramuscular injection. A fatal occurrence of gas gangrene after the intramuscular injection of adrenaline in oil in the left buttock.— R. Van Hook and A. G. Vandevelde (letter), *Ann. intern. Med.*, 1975, *83*, 669. Further references: W. B. Maguire and N. F. Langley, *Med. J. Aust.*, 1967, *1*, 973; P. W. Harvey and G. V. Purnell, *Br. med. J.*, 1968, *1*, 744; H. Gaylis (letter), *ibid.*, 1968, *3*, 59.

Interactions. A review of the factors and interactions affecting the use of vasoconstrictors in local anaesthetics. There is no special risk in patients on *monoamine oxidase inhibitors*, since inactivation depends chiefly on uptake into nerves and tissues and not upon metabolism; patients taking these drugs have a normal response to intravenous doses of adrenaline and noradrenaline, though they are at risk from a pressor crisis if noradrenaline-releasing agents, such as tyramine are used. Drugs that blockade adrenergic neurones increase sensitivity to circulating catecholamines several-fold, as do the *tricyclic antidepressants* such as imipramine, which block the uptake of adrenaline and noradrenaline into nerves; in each case enhancement of the effect of the catecholamines is likely to be important only if a dose is injected intravenously.— *Br. med. J.*, 1970, *4*, 633.

See also Phenelzine Sulphate, p.130.

Anaesthetic agents. Sensitisation of the myocardium to β-adrenergic stimulation caused by some anaesthetics was of clinical importance when adrenaline was injected into an operation area to reduce bleeding. It had been considered that adrenaline could not be given when the patient had been anaesthetised with cyclopropane, halothane, or similar anaesthetics. However, it was now evident that adrenaline could safely be used so long as the dose was small and other factors likely to increase the irritability of the myocardium, such as carbon-dioxide retention, hypoxia, or the simultaneous use of cocaine were avoided. The conclusions of R.L. Katz and G.J. Katz (*Br. J. Anaesth.*, 1966, *38*, 712) were that provided the solution of adrenaline was not stronger than 1 in 100 000 and that the rate of injection did not exceed 10 ml per 10 minutes or 30 ml an hour no serious results should ensue under halothane or trichloroethylene anaesthesia. The technique should not be used with cyclopropane. Where a high risk of intravascular injection occurred, such as in the sub-occipital area, the neck, the broad ligaments of the uterus, and in the erectile tissue of the external genitalia in both sexes, a vasoconstrictor drug which would not produce arrhythmias, such as felypressin, might be valuable.— *Lancet*, 1967, *1*, 484. Cyclopropane could also be used although the risk of arrhythmias was higher than with halothane or trichloroethylene.— R. L. Katz and R. A. Epstein, *Anesthesiology*, 1968, *29*, 763.

In 19 patients undergoing cataract removal under halothane anaesthesia, with lignocaine used to provide topical anaesthesia of the larynx, adrenaline 0.4 to 68 µg per kg body-weight by intra-ocular injection did not increase the incidence of cardiac arrhythmias compared with a control group.— R. B. Smith *et al.*, *Br. J. Anaesth.*, 1972, *44*, 1314. See also A. P. Melgrave, *Can. Anaesth. Soc. J.*, 1970, *17*, 256.

Further references: L. S. Reisner and M. Lippmann, *Anesth. Analg. curr. Res.*, 1975, *54*, 468 (ventricular arrhythmias associated with subcutaneous adrenaline during halothane and enflurane anaesthesia); W. Mattig and G. Radam, *Dte GesundhWes.*, 1977, *32*, 953 (cardiac arrest associated with topical adrenaline during halothane anaesthesia).

Antihypertensives. For the effect of adrenaline on debrisoquine, see Debrisoquine, p.142.

Tricyclic antidepressants. An exaggerated cardiac response to adrenaline in a local anaesthetic may have been due to an interaction with amitriptyline.— *Med. J. Aust.*, 1979, *2*, 553.

See also under Phenylephrine (p.24).

Overdosage. An account of the response to a 5-mg overdose of adrenaline injected subcutaneously during an operative procedure. The initial hypertensive episode lasted for 10 minutes and was followed by severe hypotension 20 minutes after the injection, which is a characteristic response to larger doses of adrenaline. An unexpected finding was high urinary excretion of noradrenaline during the first 30 minutes, which may have been a response to the hypotensive episode or may have represented noradrenaline displaced from the tissues by the injected adrenaline. One hour after the overdose the patient was alert and responsive. Treatment included rapid digitalisation with digoxin 1 mg intravenously in divided doses.— B. T. Carter *et al.*, *Anesth. Analg. curr. Res.*, 1971, *50*, 175.

For further reports of adrenaline overdosage and its treatment see under Treatment of Adverse Effects (below).

Pregnancy and the neonate. *Postpartum haemorrhage.* An unrecognised cause of postpartum haemorrhage is the excessive use of local anaesthetics containing adrenaline. If large amounts are used as much as 250 µg of adrenaline may be administered. With this amount there is, in some cases, inhibiton of uterine contractions with postpartum blood loss. Similarly, a patient who is extremely apprehensive may release enough adrenaline to produce uterine atony and haemorrhage.— N. W. Fugo, *W. Virginia med. J.*, 1969, *65*, 374.

Transplacental diffusion. Controlled studies in 11 women given adrenaline before and during delivery indicated that adrenaline diffused across the placenta.— F. P. Zuspan *et al.*, *Am. J. Obstet. Gynec.*, 1966, *95*, 284.

Treatment of Adverse Effects. Because of the rapid onset and short duration of adrenaline action, severe toxic reactions due to the accidental administration of an overdose or to hypersensitivity should be treated with an immediate intravenous injection of a quick-acting alpha-adrenoceptor blocking agent, such as 5 to 10 mg of phentolamine mesylate, followed by a beta-adrenoceptor blocking agent such as 2.5 to 5 mg of propranolol. Amyl nitrite, glyceryl trinitrate, phenoxybenzamine, or chlorpromazine have also been used as alternatives in an emergency.

Glyceryl trinitrate was used to treat a severe pressor response to adrenaline (2 ml of 0.1% solution given intramuscularly) in a 45-year-old man. His blood pressure had risen rapidly to 250/140 mmHg and frequent, premature, ventricular beats developed which were controlled within 15 seconds of the sublingual administration of glyceryl trinitrate. His blood pressure fell progressively during the next half-hour.— Y. -C. Lee and N. V. Brazauskas (letter), *J. Am. med. Ass.*, 1967, *202*, 367. Glyceryl trinitrate sublingually produced rapid vasodilatation and could be used to counteract the pressor effects produced by adrenaline or noradrenaline and would also have a beneficial effect on ventricular arrhythmias. It was more convenient for use in dentistry than adrenergic blocking agents.— P. J. Verrill, *Practitioner*, 1975, *214*, 380.

A 23-year-old woman, who was inadvertently given during anaesthesia a subcutaneous injection of 16 ml of a 1 in 1000 solution of adrenaline (16 mg), developed hypertension, tachycardia, and vasoconstriction. Treatment with trimetaphan camsylate, 500 mg by intravenous injection, was aimed at rapidly reducing the systolic blood pressure. Phentolamine was given concurrently. Hypotension which lasted for about 2 days then followed despite administration of hydrocortisone and methylamphetamine. The heart-rate took about 4 days to settle.— M. A. Lewis, *Br. med. J.*, 1967, *4*, 38. Accidental overdosage of adrenaline should be treated by intravenous injection of phenoxybenzamine 20 mg followed by intravenous injection of propranolol 5 mg. Subsequent dosage should be given according to diastolic pressure and heart-rate.— W. E. Glover and R. G. Shanks (letter), *ibid.*, 293.

A 38-year-old man was accidentally given 30 mg of adrenaline, intravenously, as 1 in 1000 solution, over 1 minute. He experienced abdominal pain, haematemesis, hypertension followed by hypotension, pulmonary oedema, and severe impairment of renal function. He recovered after treatment with oxygen, aminophylline intravenously, lanatoside C, noradrenaline, and dialysis.— H. S. Novey and L. N. Meleyco, *J. Am. med. Ass.*, 1969, *207*, 2435.

A report of the successful use of chlorpromazine intravenously to reverse adrenaline-induced pulmonary oedema due to acute overdosage during anaesthesia.— N. Ersoz and S. C. Finestone, *Br. J. Anaesth.*, 1971, *43*, 709.

Further references: K. Kolendorf and B. B. Moller, *Acta med. scand.*, 1974, *196*, 465 (lactic acidosis in adrenaline poisoning).

Absorption and Fate. As a result of enzymatic degradation in the gut and first-pass metabolism in the liver, adrenaline is almost totally inactive when given by mouth. It acts rapidly following subcutaneous or intramuscular injection, although absorption is slowed by local vasoconstriction (it can be hastened by massaging the injection site). Most adrenaline that is either injected into the body or released into the circulation from the adrenal medulla, is very rapidly inactivated by processes which include uptake into adrenergic neurones, diffusion, adsorption onto plasma proteins, and enzymatic degradation in the liver and body tissues. One of the enzymes responsible for the chemical inactivation of this exogenous or hormonal adrenaline is catechol-*O*-methyltransferase (COMT), the other is monoamine oxidase (MAO). In general, adrenaline is methylated to metanephrine by COMT followed by oxidative deamination by MAO to 4-hydroxy-3-methoxymandelic acid (formerly termed vanillylmandelic acid; VMA), or oxidatively deaminated by MAO to 3,4-dihydroxymandelic acid which, in turn, is methylated by COMT, once again to 4-hydroxy-3-methoxymandelic acid; the metabolites are excreted in the urine mainly as their glucuronide and ethereal sulphate conjugates.

The ability of catechol-*O*-methyltransferase to effect introduction of a methyl group is an important step in the chemical inactivation of adrenaline and similar catecholamines (in particular, noradrenaline). It means that the termination of the pharmacological response of catecholamines is not simply dependent upon monoamine oxidase.In its role of neurotransmitter intraneuronal catecholamine (mainly noradrenaline) is, however, enzymatically regulated by monoamine oxidase.

An account of the catabolism of catecholamines and a review of studies.— D. F. Sharman, *Br. med. Bull.*, 1973, *29*, 110. Biochemical aspects of monoamine oxidase.— K. F. Tipton, *ibid.*, 116. Catecholamine uptake processes.— L. L. Iversen, *ibid.*, 130. Uptake of noradrenaline by smooth muscle.— J. S. Gillespie, *ibid.*, 136.

Pregnancy and the neonate. For a reference to transplacental diffusion see under Adverse Effects and Precautions, above.

Protein binding. A brief review of studies on the binding of catecholamines to plasma proteins.— J. J. Vallner, *J. pharm. Sci.*, 1977, *66*, 447.

Uses. Adrenaline is a direct-acting sympathomimetic agent with pronounced effects on alpha- and beta-adrenergic receptors. Its effects are similar to most of those of sympathetic nerve stimulation (with the notable exception of sweating). In fact, however, its action should be likened to the hormonal role of endogenous adrenaline, released from the adrenal medulla in response to severe physiological stress, rather than to the immediate sympathetic stress response mediated by increased sympathetic nerve discharge (mainly noradrenaline released in its role of neurotransmitter in adrenergic nerves). Moreover, adrenaline has a more marked effect on beta-adrenoceptors than on alpha-adrenoceptors, and this property explains many aspects of its pharmacology; in addition, its actions vary considerably according to the dose given, and the consequent reflex compensating responses of the body.

In practice, major effects of adrenaline include increased speed and force of cardiac contraction (with lower doses this causes increased systolic pressure yet reduced diastolic pressure since overall peripheral resistance is lowered, but with higher doses both systolic and diastolic pressure are increased as stimulation of peripheral alpha-receptors increases peripheral resistance); blood flow to skeletal muscle is increased (reduced with higher doses); hepatic blood flow is increased, and metabolic effects include increased glucose output as well as markedly increased oxygen consumption; blood flow in the kidneys, mucosa, and skin is reduced; there is little direct effect on cerebral blood flow.

Aqueous solutions of adrenaline are usually prepared using the acid tartrate or the hydrochloride but the dosage is generally stated in terms of the equivalent content of adrenaline. In general, aqueous injections have an adrenaline content equivalent to 1 in 1000 (1 mg per ml). The recommended *B.P.* dose of an aqueous injection containing the equivalent of adrenaline 1 in 1000 is 0.2 to 0.5 ml (200 to 500 μg) by subcutaneous injection as a single dose.

Adrenaline relaxes the bronchial musculature and may be injected subcutaneously to relieve bronchial spasm in acute attacks of bronchial asthma. The adult dose is 0.2 to 0.5 ml of a 1 in 1000 aqueous solution (200 to 500 μg); children should receive 0.01 ml (10 μg) per kg body-weight to a maximum total dose of 0.5 ml (500 μg). Benefit usually occurs within 3 to 5 minutes but if the dose fails to control the attack, it may be repeated at 15- to 20-minute intervals for 2 doses, then subsequently every 4 hours if needed. The attack is more effectively treated with small doses of adrenaline at first than with larger doses at the peak. Tolerance or refractoriness may develop; for detailed recommendations relating to the emergency management of severe asthma, including a recommendation to use $beta_2$-selective sympathomimetic agents rather than adrenaline, see Corticosteroids, p.453.

For prolonged control of asthmatic attacks adrenaline has been given by intramuscular injection of a 1 in 500 oily suspension or by subcutaneous injection of a 1 in 200 aqueous suspension. Such injections have been associated with tissue necrosis owing to their prolonged vasoconstrictor properties and, in particular, the oily injections have been associated with gas gangrene (see under Adverse Effects and Precautions). The use of sympathomimetics with an intrinsically prolonged duration of action is accordingly preferable to such retard-action preparations of adrenaline.

Aqueous solutions with an adrenaline content equivalent to 1 in 100 have been used by inhalation as a spray to alleviate asthmatic spasms; these solutions must never be confused with the weaker strength used for injection. Pressurised aerosols delivering metered doses of 280 μg of adrenaline acid tartrate (equivalent to approximately 160 μg of adrenaline) are more convenient; the recommended adult dosage is 1 to 3 metered doses repeated, if necessary, after 30 minutes up to a maximum of 8 metered doses in 24 hours. If more than 1 metered dose is inhaled at a time, at least 1 or 2 minutes should elapse between any 2 inhalations. In the 1960s overuse of pressurised aerosol inhalers was an associated factor in an increase in sudden deaths among asthmatic patients (for further details see under Adverse Effects of Isoprenaline, p.15). It is therefore essential to instruct the patients in the correct use of such preparations; if relief is not obtained the dose should not be increased and alternate therapy should be given. Swallowing adrenaline may cause some epigastric pain and it is advisable to rinse the mouth and throat with water after using the inhalation.

Subcutaneous or intramuscular injection of 0.2 to 0.5 ml (200 to 500 μg) of adrenaline (1 in 1000) gives symptomatic relief in acute allergy and may be life-saving in anaphylactic shock. Up to 1 ml (1 mg) may be given, and more than one dose may be required (for further details see under Allergy and Anaphylaxis, below).

Subcutaneous or intramuscular adrenaline is also indicated for cardiovascular resuscitation procedures. Although very hazardous, in extreme emergencies a dilute solution of adrenaline may be given by very slow intravenous injection; in some circumstances intracardiac injection may be required (for further details see under Cardiac Resuscitation, below). The use of adrenaline by very slow intravenous infusion (in dextrose injection), usually in a concentration of 1 in 500 000 and not exceeding 1 in 100 000, has been recorded.

In general, the use of adrenaline in asthma has been superseded by $beta_2$-selective sympathomimetic agents, such as salbutamol (p.30) which can alleviate bronchospasm with fewer effects on the heart.

Adrenaline was formerly given intramuscularly in the emergency treatment of hypoglycaemia, but treatment with dextrose or glucagon is generally preferred.

Adrenaline is frequently added to local anaesthetics, such as lignocaine hydrochloride (p.904), and procaine hydrochloride (p.921), to retard diffusion and limit absorption, to prolong the duration of effect, and to lessen the danger of toxicity. A concentration of 1 in 200 000 (5 μg per ml) is usually effective for infiltration injections; as little as 1 in 500 000 may be adequate though in some preparations 1 in 50 000 continues to be available. Even the 1 in 200 000 concentration should not be used for digits, ears, nose, penis, or scrotum owing to the risk of tissue necrosis. Adrenaline has also been added to injections for spinal anaesthesia to delay absorption and prolong the effect but its use is not recommended because of the danger of reducing the blood supply to the cord. For further details of the appropriate concentrations and doses of adrenaline in local anaesthetic preparations see under Lignocaine and other Local Anaesthetics, p.899.

Adrenaline constricts arterioles and capillaries and causes blanching when applied locally to mucous membranes and exposed tissues. It is used as an aqueous solution in a 1 in 100 000 to 1 in 1000 dilution to check capillary bleeding, epistaxis, and bleeding from superficial wounds and abrasions, and after tooth extraction, but it does not stop internal haemorrhage. It is usually applied as a spray or on pledgets of cotton wool or gauze. The vasoconstriction lasts about ½ to 2 hours. It is also used as a 1 in 200 000 to 1 in 80 000 solution during surgical operations, especially on the eye, ear, nose, throat, or larynx to produce ischaemia of the operative field but this may make tying off of bleeding points difficult.

An aqueous solution of adrenaline (1 in 10 000 to 1 in 5000) has been applied to the nasal mucous membrane in the form of a spray in acute coryza, allergic rhinitis, hay fever, and sinusitis. Adrenaline, however, causes rebound congestion and may lead to a drug-induced rhinitis.

In ophthalmology, adrenaline 1 in 20 000 to 1 in 1000 is used to reduce conjunctival congestion, and 1 in 100 is used to reduce intra-ocular pressure in simple glaucoma. It is a poor mydriatic.

Adrenaline cream (1 in 5000) has been used by massage in the treatment of fibrositis but claims for its superior value over other creams or massage have not been substantiated.

Adrenaline, in suppositories or ointment, has been used as a vasoconstrictor in haemorrhoids and inflammatory conditions of the anus and rectum.

Allergy and anaphylaxis. General symptoms of hypersensitivity to an insect sting should be treated with adrenaline, which can be inhaled as a pressurised aerosol of adrenaline acid tartrate or injected subcutaneously in a dose of 0.5 to 1 ml of 1 in 1000 solution (Adrenaline Injection *B.P.*). Whichever preparation is favoured it should be given at the first sign of untoward symptoms. In life-threatening anaphylaxis 1 ml of adrenaline injection (1 in 1000) should be given intramuscularly without delay, followed by methylprednisolone sodium succinate 125 mg intravenously; if there is no sign of improvement in 3 minutes the adrenaline injection should be repeated.— H. R. C. Riches, *Practitioner*, 1978, *220*, 511. Emphasis that adrenaline injection should always be given subcutaneously except in life-threatening anaphylaxis when the intramuscular route may be used. Intravenous adrenaline is *extremely hazardous* because it provokes a pressor reaction with alarming hypertension, bradycardia or tachycardia, and cardiac arrhythmia; cerebral vascular catastrophes have been precipitated. Antihistamines are of little value in the treatment of anaphylaxis, but they do help to control the irritation of urticaria which sometimes follows the immediate reaction; chlorpheniramine maleate 8 mg by mouth or 10 mg intramuscularly can be given to an adult. Adrenaline, antihistamines, and corticosteroids can be expected to control general hypersensitivity symptoms but do not usually produce any immediate resolution of the local swelling around the sting which may take from 24 to 72 hours to disappear.— *idem*, 1977, *218*, 337.

Allergic reactions to insect stings can include urticaria, bronchospasm, laryngeal oedema, hypotension, and death. The insects whose stings most often cause anaphylactic reactions are the *Hymenoptera* spp., including bees (honey-bees), wasps, hornets, fire ants, and yellow-jackets. Adrenaline is the most effective drug for treatment of a systemic reaction and is usually given in a subcutaneous injection of 0.3 ml of a 1 in 1000 solution (0.1 to 0.2 ml for children). Adrenaline does not always relieve shock, however, and it may be necessary for some patients to be treated in hospital with intravenous fluids and electrolytes, pressor agents, or other measures. A minority of patients with systemic reactions who respond to initial treatment with adrenaline subsequently develop recurrent pruritus or urticaria; they should be treated with antihistamines or, if symptoms are severe or persistent, with corticosteroids.— *Med. Lett.*, 1978, *20*, 54.

Patients who are at risk from severe sting reactions should have available a disposable syringe and needles and a 1-ml ampoule of adrenaline 1 in 1000. Half of this ampoule should be given as a deep subcutaneous injection near to the sting site if possible; they should be fully instructed in self-administration. Tourniquets are usually not practical and are not advised. Since 80% of deaths are due to high airways obstruction, patients should carry with them a salbutamol bronchodilator spray such as asthmatic patients use.— *Br. med. J.*, 1979, *1*, 726. Patients acutely sensitive to wasp and bee stings are recommended to inhale 3 metered doses of adrenaline (Medihaler-Epi) immediately after a sting; this can be repeated if necessary after 20 to 25 minutes.— M. A. Ganderton (letter), *Br. med. J.*, 1979, *1*, 1216. Inhalation of adrenaline from a Medihaler-Epi does not provide a therapeutically useful amount of adrenaline for the relief of anaphylactic shock. Syringes precharged with adrenaline are available from American pharmaceutical firms.— J. F. Ackroyd (letter), *Lancet*, 1980, *2*, 1190. Comment on the availability of pre-filled adrenaline syringes in the UK.— R. Wright (letter), *ibid.*, 1981, *1*, 155.

Comment on leukotrienes, slow-reacting substances of anaphylaxis.— *Lancet*, 1980, *1*, 1226. See also M. C. Holroyde *et al.*, *Lancet*, 1981, *2*, 17.

Comment on the causes, symptoms, and management of anaphylactic shock and the key role of adrenaline. As soon as the reaction is recognised 0.5 to 1 mg (0.5 to

1 ml of so-called 1:1000) should be injected intramuscularly (not subcutaneously because absorption is too slow, especially in the presence of shock). A slow intravenous injection of a histamine H_1-receptor antagonist, such as chlorpheniramine 10 to 20 mg, should be given immediately after the intramuscular adrenaline and repeated over the subsequent 24 to 48 hours to prevent relapse. Although histamine H_1-receptor antagonists are particularly effective in the management of angio-oedema, pruritus, and urticaria, they remain second-line treatment. Local injection of adrenaline into the site of antigen administration is beneficial only in the early stages of the reaction. Intravenous corticosteroids have little place in the immediate management of anaphylaxis, since their beneficial effects are delayed for several hours but in severely ill patients early administration may help prevent deterioration after the primary treatment has been given. Continuing deterioration with circulatory collapse, bronchospasm, or laryngeal oedema requires further treatment including intravenous fluids, intravenous aminophylline, a nebulised β_2-agonist (such as salbutamol or terbutaline), oxygen, assisted respiration (if necessary), and possibly, emergency tracheostomy. If electrolyte solutions are used for volume replacement large amounts may be necessary because it has been reported that the plasma loss in severe anaphylactic shock may constitute 20 to 40% of the plasma volume. Colloid solutions, such as plasma protein fraction or dextran are theoretically preferable, but they may themselves release histamine, although in severe anaphylaxis intracellular stores of histamine are likely to have been depleted.— *Br. med. J.*, 1981, *282,* 1011.

Further references: D. A. Warrell, *Prescribers' J.*, 1979, *19,* 190; *Lancet,* 1980, *2,* 956; H. M. Brown (letter), *ibid.*, 1082; C. A. Frazier (letter), *ibid.*, 1981, *1,* 53.

For information on desensitisation procedures for allergic subjects, see Allergens and Specific Desensitisation, p.1322.

Urticaria. Although subcutaneous or intramuscular injections of 0.5 to 1 ml of adrenaline 1 in 1000 were the initial treatment of choice for violent attacks of urticaria or angioneurotic oedema they were less valuable in the treatment of chronic urticaria. A few patients found that isoprenaline sulphate sublingually could abort recurrent acute attacks of urticaria, and ephedrine 15 to 30 mg once or twice daily sometimes helped to control resistant chronic urticaria.— R. H. Champion, *Br. med. J.*, 1973, *4,* 730.

See also under Corticosteroids, p.459.

Angioneurotic oedema. A report of beneficial results with high doses of adrenaline in an 18-year-old girl and her 23-year-old brother with hereditary angioneurotic oedema. Adrenaline 1 in 1000 given subcutaneously in a dose of 1 ml every hour for episodes threatening the upper airway, resulted in both subjective and objective improvement of signs and symptoms. On one occasion the girl was admitted to hospital for a 20-hour period and received a total of 11 ml of 1 in 1000 adrenaline subcutaneously on an hourly basis over this period; she also had 3 units of fresh frozen plasma during her second hour of treatment; her symptoms abated about 11 hours after admission.— M. Roth *et al.*, *Ann. Allergy,* 1975, *35,* 175.

Asthma. A discussion on the avoidance of asthma fatalities with emphasis on the importance of the prompt treatment of severe acute asthma. Concerning the choice of a bronchodilator drug, there seems to be no place for subcutaneous adrenaline.— *Br. med. J.*, 1978, *1,* 873. A defence of the use of subcutaneous adrenaline in asthma, and the view that it still remains an effective first-line drug for the hospital management of the young acute asthmatic.— T. Waterston (letter), *ibid.*, 1350. Comment on the value of subcutaneous terbutaline.— I. M. Slessor and H. Davies, *Astra* (letter), *ibid.*, *2,* 505.

Further references: M. S. Karetzky, *Am. J. med. Sci.*, 1978, *275,* 319.

Bleeding. In 11 patients with bleeding of the gastro-intestinal tract, bleeding was arrested in 10 by the infusion, into the artery supplying the haemorrhagic site, of adrenaline, usually preceded by propranolol. A suitable dose of adrenaline was 6 to 12 μg per minute for 5 to 10 minutes, repeated if necessary at 10-minute intervals.— J. Rösch *et al.*, *Gastroenterology,* 1970, *59,* 341.

Cardiac resuscitation. Standards developed and recommended at the National Conference on Standards for Cardiopulmonary Resuscitation and Emergency Cardiac Care held in May 1973. For purposes of the Conference recommendations, drugs considered essential were: sodium bicarbonate, adrenaline, atropine sulphate, lignocaine, morphine sulphate, calcium chloride, and oxygen; drugs considered useful were: noradrenaline, metaraminol, isoprenaline, propranolol, and corticosteroids. Drugs are usually administered intravenously during the cardiopulmonary resuscitation emergency to ensure their delivery into the cardiovascular system as artificial circulation is provided. Intracardiac injections are sometimes used, but this route is usually limited to adrenaline (epinephrine) early in the cardiac arrest and before an intravenous infusion has become available. Although adrenaline can be shown experimentally to produce ventricular fibrillation, its actions in restoring electrical activity in asystole and in enhancing defibrillation in ventricular fibrillation are also well documented. Adrenaline increases myocardial contractility, elevates perfusion pressure, lowers defibrillation threshold and, in some instances, restores myocardial contractility in electromechanical dissociation. A dose of 0.5 ml of a 1 in 1000 solution diluted to 10 ml, or 5 ml of a 1 in 10 000 solution, should be administered intravenously every 5 minutes during a resuscitation effort. Intracardiac administration may be utilised by personnel well trained in the technique if there has not been sufficient time to establish an intravenous route. When prompt establishment of an intravenous lifeline is not possible, adrenaline 1 to 2 mg per 10 ml sterile distilled water (1 in 10 000 to 1 in 5000) can be effective when instilled directly into the tracheobronchial tree through an endotracheal tube.— American Heart Association and the National Academy of Sciences–National Research Council, *J. Am. med. Ass.*, 1974, *227, Suppl.*, 833–868. A brief discussion on the risk of coronary artery lacerations associated with intracardiac injection of adrenaline, and an explanation of the perilous nature of the obsolete technique of transthoracic injection.— D. C. Schechter, *ibid.*, 1975, *234,* 1184.

Further references to the hazards of intracardiac adrenaline: M. Eliastam (letter), *New Engl. J. Med.*, 1978, *298,* 1313; J. C. Baldwin (letter), *ibid.*, 1314.

Diagnostic use. *Angiography.* The injection of a few μg of adrenaline into the renal artery shortly before introducing a contrast medium would often differentiate normal from tumour arteries, which were thin-walled, deficient in muscle, and failed to constrict in response to adrenaline. Adrenaline was not useful in conjunction with nephrotomography.— J. J. Pollard and R. A. Nebesar, *New Engl. J. Med.*, 1968, *279,* 1035. See also P. C. Kahn, *Radiology,* 1967, *88,* 686; M. A. Bosniak *et al.*, *Am. J. Roentg.*, 1977, *129,* 647; H. P. Jander and I. L. Tonkin, *Radiology,* 1979, *132,* 61.

Breast cancer. Comment on infiltration of the breast tissues with 1 in 200 000 adrenaline solution as a useful aid in a selective biopsy technique when screening for breast cancer.— *Br. med. J.*, 1978, *2,* 153. References: A. W. M. C. Owen *et al.*, *Br. J. Surg.*, 1977, *64,* 725.

Epiglottitis, laryngitis, and croup. Intermittent positive-pressure breathing with racemic adrenaline 2.25% (Vaponefrin) diluted 1 to 8 with water and administered from the nebuliser of a Mark VII Bird Respirator, reduced the need for tracheostomy for 359 children with acute laryngotracheitis admitted during 1973 and 1974; improvement occurred within 10 to 15 minutes of commencing treatment, and no ill effects were reported.— O. P. Singer and W. J. Wilson, *Can. med. Ass. J.*, 1976, *115,* 132. See also C. R. Westley *et al.*, *Am. J. Dis. Child.*, 1978, *132,* 484.

Ocular disorders. Neutral adrenaline eye-drops 1% are commonly used in chronic simple glaucoma as they lower the intra-ocular pressure by reducing the production of aqueous humour by the ciliary body. They produce a mild pupillary dilatation which is advantageous in elderly patients with central lens opacities who would otherwise be visually handicapped by the pupillary constriction of miotics. Adrenaline eye-drops are contra-indicated in narrow-angle glaucoma.— S. I. Davidson, *Prescribers' J.*, 1978, *18,* 139.

Reports and studies on adrenaline eye-drops: D. Vaughan *et al.*, *Archs Ophthal., N.Y.*, 1961, *66,* 232 (neutral adrenaline); B. Becker and W. R. Morton, *Am. J. Ophthal.*, 1966, *62,* 272 (neutral adrenaline); B. Becker and D. H. Shin, *Archs Ophthal., N.Y.*, 1976, *94,* 2057 (long-term study of response to adrenaline); M. B. Koback *et al.*, *Am. J. Ophthal.*, 1976, *81,* 768 (dipivefrin—dipivalyl adrenaline); D. H. Shin *et al.*, *Archs Ophthal., N.Y.*, 1976, *94,* 2059 (long-term therapy); B. Becker *et al.*, *Archs Ophthal., N.Y.*, 1977, *95,* 789 (increased ocular and cardiac responsiveness to adrenaline in primary open-angle glaucoma); M. E. Yablonski *et al.*, *Archs Ophthal., N.Y.*, 1977, *95,* 2157 (tolerance of dipivefrin—dipivalyl adrenaline, by adrenaline-intolerant eyes); P. F. J. Hoyng and C. L. Dake, *Br. J. Ophthal.*, 1979, *63,* 56 (with guanethidine); D. E. P. Jones *et al.*, *Br. J. Ophthal.*, 1979, *63,* 813 (with guanethidine); J. Romano and G. Patterson, *Br. J. Ophthal.*, 1979, *63,* 52 (with guanethidine); A. J. Flach and S. G. Kramer, *Archs Ophthal., N.Y.*, 1980, *98,* 482 (increased sensitivity after long-term therapy).

Pregnancy and the neonate. A report of the use of adrenaline or isoprenaline by intravenous infusion at the rate of up to 1 μg per kg body-weight per minute, for their immediate effect on muscle contractility, during the treatment of postoperative heart failure in infants and neonates.— J. Stark, *Postgrad. med. J.*, 1972, *48,* 478.

A long-acting aqueous suspension of adrenaline given by intramuscular injection to hypoglycaemic infants born of diabetic mothers had no advantage over administration of dextrose solution 25%. It had the adverse effect of raising the lactate concentration in the blood, and lactic acidosis was observed in 2 of 11 infants.— J. C. Haworth *et al.*, *J. Pediat.*, 1973, *82,* 94.

Shock. See under Allergy and Anaphylaxis (above).

Preparations

Creams

Adrenaline Cream 1 in 5000 *(D.T.F.).* Crem. Adrenal. Adrenaline solution 20 ml, dilute hydrochloric acid 0.04 ml, sodium metabisulphite 40 mg, chlorocresol 100 mg, emulsifying ointment 30 g, water to 100 g.

From the results of therapeutic trials arranged by the Research Subcommittee of the Empire Rheumatism Council it was concluded that there was no demonstrable difference between the effects of adrenaline cream and a similar cream without adrenaline.— E. G. L. Bywaters, *Pharm. J.*, 1951, *2,* 35.

Eye-drops

Adrenaline Eye Drops Strong *(A.P.F.).* Adrenaline 1 g, boric acid 500 mg, sodium metabisulphite 100 mg, disodium edetate 100 mg, phenylmercuric nitrate 2 mg, Water for Injections to 100 ml. Sterilise by filtration. Protect from light. These eye-drops should be recently prepared.

Adrenaline Neutral 1% Eye-drops *(Moorfields Eye Hosp.).* Adrenaline 1.2, boric acid 1, borax 0.6, sodium metabisulphite 0.3, disodium edetate 0.1, ascorbic acid 0.2, hypromellose '4000' 0.25, chlorhexidine acetate 0.01, Water for Injections to 100. Sterilise by maintaining at 98° to 100° for 30 minutes.

Epinephrine Bitartrate for Ophthalmic Solution *(U.S.P.).* A sterile dry mixture of adrenaline acid tartrate and suitable antioxidants, prepared by freeze-drying. The solution is prepared by the addition of diluent before use. Potency is expressed in terms of the equivalent amount of adrenaline.

Epinephrine Bitartrate Ophthalmic Solution *(U.S.P.).* A sterile, buffered, aqueous solution of adrenaline acid tartrate, with a suitable antibacterial agent. It may contain suitable preservatives. Potency is expressed in terms of the equivalent amount of adrenaline. pH 3 to 3.8. Store in small well-filled airtight containers. Protect from light. It should not be used if it is brown or contains a precipitate.

Epinephrine Ophthalmic Solution *(U.S.P.).* A sterile aqueous solution of adrenaline prepared with the aid of hydrochloric acid; it contains a suitable antibacterial agent and may contain an antioxidant, suitable buffers, chelating agents, and agents to adjust the osmotic pressure. pH 2.2 to 4.5. Store in airtight containers. Protect from light. It should not be used if it is brown or contains a precipitate.

Epinephryl Borate Ophthalmic Solution *(U.S.P.).* A sterile aqueous solution containing adrenaline as a borate complex (known as epinephryl borate, $C_9H_{12}BNO_4$ = 209.0), a suitable antibacterial agent, and one or more suitable preservatives and buffers. pH 5.5 to 7.6. Potency is expressed in terms of the equivalent amount of adrenaline. Store in small well-filled airtight containers. Protect from light. It should not be used if it is brown or contains a precipitate.

Neutral Adrenaline Eye-drops *(B.P.C. 1973).* A sterile solution containing adrenaline 1%, with sodium metabisulphite, 8-hydroxyquinoline sulphate, and other pharmaceutical adjuvants in a borate buffer solution adjusted to pH 7.4 (limits: 7.2 to 7.6) with sodium hydroxide in containers in which the air has been replaced with nitrogen or other inert gas. Store in a cool place. Protect from light.

Zinc and Adrenaline Eye Drops *(A.P.F.).* BZA Eye Drops. Adrenaline solution 10 ml, zinc sulphate 250 mg, boric acid 1.5 g, sodium metabisulphite 50 mg, chlorbutol 500 mg, glycerol 1 ml, Water for Injections to 100 ml. Sterilise by autoclaving. Protect from light.

Zinc and Adrenaline Eye-drops *(Moorfields Eye Hosp.).* Gutt. Zinc. et Adren. Adrenaline solution 50, zinc sulphate 0.25, boric acid 2, phenylmercuric nitrate (0.002%) solution to 100.

Zinc Sulphate and Adrenaline Eye Drops *(B.P.).* A sterile solution of adrenaline acid tartrate 90 mg, zinc sulphate 250 mg, sodium metabisulphite 50 mg, phenylmercuric acetate or nitrate 2 mg, in water to 100 ml.

Store at a temperature not exceeding 25°. Protect from light. If intended for use on more than one occasion they should not be used more than one month after first opening the container.

Studies of the stability and compatibility of benzalkonium chloride and phenethyl alcohol as preservatives of Zinc Sulphate Eye-drops and Zinc Sulphate and Adrenaline Eye-drops.— Pharm. Soc. Lab. Rep. P/74/9, P/74/10, P/74/11, 1974.

Inhalations

Epinephrine Bitartrate Inhalation Aerosol *(U.S.P.)*. An aerosol spray in a pressurised container containing a fine suspension of adrenaline acid tartrate in propellents. Store in containers with metered-dose valves and oral inhalation actuators. Protect from light.

Epinephrine Inhalation *(U.S.P.)*. A solution of adrenaline 0.9 to 1.15% in water, prepared with the aid of hydrochloric acid. Store in small well-filled airtight containers. Protect from light. It should not be used if it is brown or contains a precipitate.

Injections

Adrenaline Injection *(B.P.)*. Adren. Inj.; Adrenaline Tartrate Injection. Adrenaline acid tartrate 180 mg, sodium metabisulphite 100 mg, sodium chloride 800 mg, Water for Injections to 100 ml; sterilised by autoclaving; potency is expressed as adrenaline 1 in 1000. pH 2.8 to 3.6. Protect from light.

Adrenaline injection in 0.5-ml ampoules could be autoclaved at 134° for 3.75 minutes up to 6 times without loss of potency.— T. R. Lowther and J. King, *J. Hosp. Pharm.*, 1973, *31*, 218.

Epinephrine Injection *(U.S.P.)*. A sterile solution of adrenaline in Water for Injections prepared with the aid of hydrochloric acid. pH 2.5 to 5. Protect from light. It should not be used if it is brown or contains a precipitate.

Sterile Epinephrine Oil Suspension *(U.S.P.)*. A sterile suspension of adrenaline, 1.8 to 2.4 mg per ml, in a suitable vegetable oil. Protect from light.

Solutions

Adrenaline Solution *(B.P.)*. Adren. Soln.; Adrenaline Tartrate Solution. Adrenaline acid tartrate 180 mg, chlorbutol 400 mg, chlorocresol 100 mg, sodium metabisulphite 100 mg, sodium chloride 800 mg in water to 100 ml; it contains the equivalent of adrenaline 1 in 1000. pH 2.7 to 3.6. Store in well-filled, well-closed containers. Protect from light.

NOTE. The *B.P.* states that when Solution of Adrenaline Hydrochloride is prescribed or demanded, Adrenaline Solution may be dispensed or supplied.

Epinephrine Nasal Solution *(U.S.P.)*. A solution of adrenaline 0.09 to 0.115% in water, prepared with the aid of hydrochloric acid. Store in small well-filled airtight containers. Protect from light. It should not be used if it is brown or contains a precipitate.

Sprays

Compound Adrenaline and Atropine Spray *(B.P.)*. Adrenaline and Atropine Compound Spray; Nebula Adrenalinae et Atropinae Composita. Adrenaline acid tartrate 800 mg, atropine methonitrate 100 mg, papaverine hydrochloride 800 mg, chlorbutol 500 mg, sodium metabisulphite 100 mg, propylene glycol 5 ml, freshly boiled and cooled water to 100 ml. Store in well-filled containers. Protect from light.

Bronchoconstriction accompanied by wheezing and slight breathlessness lasting 2 to 3 minutes had been observed in patients given inhalations of adrenaline. The effect appeared to be due to a colourless oxidation product of adrenaline which appeared to produce the effect only in a small proportion of asthmatics. It was suggested that only fresh solutions of adrenaline should be used for inhalation and mixing other preparations with adrenaline solutions should be avoided.— R. S. Jones (letter), *Lancet*, 1966, *2*, 593.

Proprietary Preparations of Adrenaline and its Salts

Asma-Vydrin *(Lewis, UK)*. A solution for inhalation containing adrenaline 0.55%, atropine methonitrate 0.14%, papaverine hydrochloride 0.88%, and chlorbutol 0.5%. For bronchospasm.

Brovon Inhalant Solution *(Napp, UK)*. Contains adrenaline 0.5%, atropine methonitrate 0.14%, papaverine hydrochloride 0.88%, and chlorbutol 0.5%. **Brovon Pressurised Inhalant.** Contains adrenaline 0.5% and atropine methonitrate 0.1% with propellents. Each metered dose provides adrenaline 250 µg and atropine methonitrate 50 µg. For bronchospasm.

Epifrin *(Allergan, UK)*. Eye-drops containing adrenaline hydrochloride equivalent to adrenaline 1 or 2%. (Also available as Epifrin in *Austral., Belg., Canad., S.Afr., Switz., USA*).

Eppy *(Smith & Nephew Pharmaceuticals, UK)*. Eye-drops of pH 7.4 containing adrenaline 1% in a buffered solution of boric acid, iso-osmotic with serum. For reducing intra-ocular pressure in simple (open-angle) and secondary glaucoma primarily by reducing the rate of aqueous humour production. (Also available as Eppy in *Fr., Ital., S.Afr., Swed.*, and as Eppy/N in *Austral., Canad., Switz.*).

Isopto Epinal *(Alcon, UK: Farillon, UK)*. Eye-drops containing adrenaline 0.5 or 1%, with hypromellose 0.5%. (Also available as Isopto Epinal in *Neth., Switz.* and as Isopto-Epinal in *Norw., Swed.*).

Medihaler Epi *(Riker, UK)*. A pressurised spray for inhalation containing in each ml adrenaline acid tartrate 14 mg and delivering 280 µg in each metered dose. For bronchial asthma and similar conditions. (Also available as Medihaler Epi in *Austral.* and as Medihaler-Epi in *Canad., S.Afr., USA*).

Min-I-Jet Adrenaline 1:1000 Injection *(IMS, UK)*. A cartridge assembly containing a sterile solution of adrenaline hydrochloride 1 mg per ml (1 in 1000), in disposable syringes of 0.5 and 1 ml. The 0.5-ml size is suitable for self-administration.

For comment on the importance of 1 in 1000 adrenaline in the emergency treatment of anaphylactic shock, see under Allergy and Anaphylaxis (above).

Min-I-Jet Adrenaline 1:10 000 Injection *(IMS, UK)*. A cartridge assembly containing a sterile solution of adrenaline hydrochloride 100 µg per ml (1 in 10 000), in vials of 10 ml and paediatric vials of 3 ml.

For comment on the role of 1 in 10 000 adrenaline in cardiac resuscitation, see under Cardiac Resuscitation (above).

Riddobron Inhalant *(Seaford, UK)*. Contains adrenaline hydrochloride 0.5%, atropine methonitrate 0.14%, papaverine hydrochloride 0.88%, aqueous pituitary extract (1:20) 0.4%, chlorbutol 0.5%, sodium nitrate 0.08%, and glycerol 15%. For asthma and hay fever.

Riddofan *(Seaford, UK)*. An inhalant containing adrenaline hydrochloride 1%, racephedrine 0.5%, papaverine hydrochloride 0.25%, atropine 0.14%, amethocaine hydrochloride 1%, and glycerol 15%. For bronchospasm.

Riddovydrin Inhalant *(Seaford, UK)*. Contains adrenaline 1%, papaverine 0.88%, atropine 0.075%, ascorbic acid 1%, pituitary extract (1:8) 0.5%, chlorbutol 0.5%, and glycerol 20%. For bronchospasm.

Rybarvin *(Rybar, UK)*. An inhalant containing adrenaline 0.4%, atropine methonitrate 0.1%, papaverine hydrochloride 0.08%, and benzocaine 0.08%, in a saline basis. For bronchospasm.

Silbe Inhalant *(Berk Pharmaceuticals, UK)*. A solution containing adrenaline acid tartrate 1%, papaverine hydrochloride 0.95%, atropine methonitrate 0.125%, hyoscine hydrobromide 0.05%, chlorbutol 1%, glycerol 35%, and water to 100%. For bronchospasm.

Simplene *(Smith & Nephew Pharmaceuticals, UK)*. Eye-drops containing adrenaline 0.5 or 1% in a buffered iso-osmotic solution. (Also available as Simplene in *S.Afr.*).

Welder's Flash Drops *(Industrial Pharmaceutical, UK)*. Eye-drops containing zinc sulphate 0.25% and adrenaline acid tartrate 0.09%.

Other Proprietary Names

Arg.—Epifrina; *Austral.*—Epinal (borate complex) (see also under Alclofenac), Glaucon, Micronefrin (racemic); *Canad.*—Bronkaid Mistometer, Epinal (borate complex) (see also under Alclofenac), Epitrate, Glaucon, Sus-Phrine, Vaponefrin (racemic); *Denm.*—Adrenaline-Isopto (borate complex), Adrenalin-Medihaler, Adrenalintråd, Hektalin; *Fr.*—Glauposine P.O.S.; *Ger.*—Epiglaufrin, Glyirenan, Suprarenin; *Ital.*—Dyspne-Inhal, Liadren; *Neth.*—Epirest; *Norw.*—Adrenalin Medihaler, Adrenalintråd, Levocon; *S.Afr.*—Epinal (borate complex) (see also under Alclofenac), Epitrate, Micronefrin (racemic); *Swed.*—Adrenalintråd; *Switz.*—Dyspné-Inhal, Glaucon, Glauposine; *USA*—E1, E2, Epitrate, Glaucon, Micronefrin (racemic), Sus-Phrine, Vaponefrin (racemic).

Adrenaline and its salts were also formerly marketed in Great Britain under the proprietary names Adrenapax Cream (*Sinclair*), Lloyd's Cream with Adrenaline (*Howard Lloyd*, now *Lloyds Pharmaceuticals*), and Lyophrin (*Alcon*). Preparations containing adrenaline or its salts were also formerly marketed in Great Britain under the proprietary names Asthmasan (*Riddell*, now *Seaford*), Asthmosana (*Riddell*, now *Seaford*), Cremor Urical Co. (*Sinclair*), Drenalgin (*Lloyds Pharmaceuticals*), and Rybarex (*Riddell*, now *Seaford*).

2043-a

Amidephrine Mesylate. Amidefrine Mesilate. 3-(1-Hydroxy-2-methylaminoethyl)methanesulphonanilide methanesulphonate.

$C_{10}H_{16}N_2O_3S,CH_4O_3S = 340.4$.

CAS — 3354-67-4 (amidephrine); 1421-68-7 (mesylate).

A white crystalline solid. **Soluble** 1 in about 5 of water.

Uses. Amidephrine mesylate is a vasoconstrictor and nasal decongestant.

Proprietary Names

Fentrinol *(Mead Johnson, Arg.)*.

Amidephrine mesylate was formerly marketed in Great Britain under the proprietary name Dricol (*Bristol*).

2044-t

Angiotensin Amide. Angiotensinamide. Asn-Arg-Val-Tyr-Val-His-Pro-Phe; [1-Asparagine, 5-valine]-angiotensin II.

$C_{49}H_{70}N_{14}O_{11} = 1031.2$.

CAS — 11128-99-7 (angiotensin II); 53-73-6 (amide).

A white or almost white odourless powder. **Soluble** in water, alcohol, and propylene glycol; practically insoluble in chloroform and ether. **Incompatible** with blood and plasma. **Store** in airtight containers. Protect from light.

Adverse Effects. Rapid infusion of angiotensin amide may readily cause very severe hypertension and bradycardia but ventricular arrhythmias are uncommon unless high doses are used. Coronary insufficiency and chest pain have been reported. Dizziness, headache, and mild urticarial reactions may occur.

A fatality arising from acute hypertension has been reported in a healthy volunteer given a prolonged intravenous infusion of angiotensin.— C. T. Dollery, *Prescribers' J.*, 1977, *17*, 126.

Precautions. Angiotensin amide should not be given to patients being treated with a monoamine oxidase inhibitor or within 14 days of stopping such treatment (see Precautions for Phenelzine Sulphate p.128). It should not be given to patients receiving oxytocic agents and should be given with caution to patients with cardiovascular disease or cardiac insufficiency.

Interactions. *Anaesthetic agents.* Lack of hazardous interaction with halothane.— J. M. Wallace, *Am. Heart J.*, 1967, *73*, 326, per *J. Am. med. Ass.*, 1967, *200* (May 22), A187.

Absorption and Fate. Angiotensin amide is rapidly inactivated in the tissues and circulation by peptidases. When given by intravenous injection it has a duration of action of about 4 minutes.

Uses. Angiotensin amide is a pressor agent related to the naturally occurring peptide angiotensin II. It increases the peripheral resistance mainly in cutaneous, splanchnic, and renal blood vessels. The increased blood pressure is accompanied by a reflex reduction in heart-rate, and cardiac output may also be reduced. These effects on heart-rate and cardiac output are reversed by atropine.

Angiotensin amide has been used in the treatment of hypotensive states, such as may follow surgical operations or trauma and occur in toxic shock, but it has not achieved general acceptance as a satisfactory alternative to sympathomimetic agents. Its value in hypotension following cardiac infarction has not been established.

Angiotensin amide has been used (with due caution) to restore blood pressure in hypotensive crises during anaesthesia with chloroform, cyclopropane, halothane, and other halogenated anaesthetics.

It is given by continuous intravenous infusion usually in a concentration of 1 mg per litre of sodium chloride injection or dextrose injection at a usual rate varying between 1 and 10 µg per minute according to the blood pressure response. Until a continuous drip infusion can be set up, an intravenous injection, administered slowly, may be given and repeated if necessary; the single adult dose is 5 to 20 µg.

Reviews of the physiology and pharmacology of angiotensin: A. P. Somlyo and A. V. Somlyo, *Pharmac. Rev.*, 1970, *22*, 249; W. B. Severs and A. E. D. Severs, *ibid.*, 1973, *25*, 415; D. Regoli *et al.*, *ibid.*, 1974, *26*, 69; M. J. Peach, *Physiol. Rev.*, 1977, *57*, 313; R. L. Malvin, *Fedn Proc.*, 1979, *38*, 2253.

Diagnostic use. *Angiography.* The use of angiotensin for angiographic enhancement of bone and soft-tissue tumours.— L. Ekelund *et al.*, *Radiology*, 1977, *122*, 95.

Cardiac disorders. In 66 patients with confirmed diagnosis and 16 healthy subjects, angiotensin amide, 75 ng per kg body-weight injected intravenously over a period of 30 seconds as a 1-µg per ml solution in sodium chloride injection, was found to be superior to methoxamine for differential phonocardiography of left-heart murmurs. Side-effects were minimal, and the brief duration of action of angiotensin amide (5 minutes) was an additional advantage.— H. Yamamoto *et al., Am. Heart J.,* 1971, *81,* 29. See also L. J. Krovetz *et al., Circulation,* 1968, *37,* 729.

Hypertension. The possibility that in renovascular disease increases in the circulatory levels of angiotensin would occur and lead to an increase in the patient's tolerance of angiotensin was used as the basis of a test to distinguish hypertension of renovascular origin from that due to other causes. Intravenous infusions of dextrose injection were given for 30 minutes to establish basal blood-pressure levels, and were followed by the slow infusion of a solution of angiotensin amide 200 µg per litre of dextrose injection. The rate of infusion was increased at 10-minute intervals from 0.2 to 0.4 ml per minute until a sustained rise of diastolic blood pressure of 20 mmHg was obtained or until an infusion rate of 16 ng per kg body-weight per minute was reached. The test was then repeated using an angiotensin amide infusion of double strength. Renovascular hypertension was considered to be strongly suggested whenever more than 10 ng per kg per minute of angiotensin was necessary to produce the desired increase in blood pressure.— A. G. Hocken *et al., Lancet,* 1966, *1,* 5. See also J. A. Nicotero *et al., New Engl. J. Med.,* 1966, *274,* 1464; J. G. Silar *et al., Can. med. Ass. J.,* 1967, *96,* 1397.

In patients with hypertension the response to an intravenous infusion of angiotensin amide was not sufficiently precise to differentiate between renovascular hypertension and essential hypertension.— B. Weeke and A. R. Krogsgaard, *Acta med. scand.,* 1966, *180,* 349.

The mean dose of angiotensin amide required to increase diastolic blood pressure by 20 mmHg was 9 to 11 ng per kg body-weight per minute in 29 pregnant women with chronic essential hypertension and studied from week 21 of gestation. In 34 similar women who later developed pregnancy-induced hypertension the mean dose of angiotensin amide was 9.8 ng per kg per minute at 23 to 24 weeks; it fell by the 27th week and was significantly reduced by the 30th week. Further study was necessary to determine whether this increased sensitivity to angiotensin amide could be used as a screening test to detect those who would later develop pregnancy-induced hypertension.— N. F. Gant *et al., Am. J. Obstet. Gynec.,* 1977, *127,* 369. Experience with 26 pregnant women did not confirm that the pressor response to infused angiotensin was predictive of patients at risk of developing pregnancy-induced hypertension.— J. A. Morris *et al., Am. J. Obstet. Gynec.,* 1978, *130,* 379. Further references: R. B. Everett *et al., Am. J. Obstet. Gynec.,* 1978, *132,* 359.

Hyperkalaemia. The use of angiotensin amide in a patient with hyperkalaemia due to aldosterone deficiency.— J. J. Brown *et al., Br. med. J.,* 1973, *1,* 650.

Shock. In 12 patients in shock the effect of angiotensin was compared with noradrenaline and metaraminol. It was found that there was significantly lower cardiac output and urine flow and a disproportionate increase of peripheral vascular resistance when angiotensin was employed and the rationale for its use in the treatment of shock was questioned.— V. N. Udhoji and M. H. Weil, *New Engl. J. Med.,* 1964, *270,* 501. See also P. Lichtlen *et al., Schweiz. med. Wschr.,* 1962, *92,* 639; J. P. Nolan *et al., Clin. Pharmac. Ther.,* 1967, *8,* 235.

Proprietary Names

Hypertensin *(Ciba, Austral.; Ciba, Ger.).*

Angiotensin amide was formerly marketed in Great Britain under the proprietary name Hypertensin-Ciba (*Ciba*).

2045-x

Butethamate Citrate. Butetamate Citrate. 2-Diethylaminoethyl 2-phenylbutyrate citrate.
$C_{16}H_{25}NO_2,C_6H_8O_7=455.5.$

CAS — 14007-64-8 (butethamate); 13900-12-4 (citrate).

A crystalline solid. Freely **soluble** in water and alcohol.

Uses. Butethamate citrate is reported to be an antispasmodic and bronchodilator and has been used in mixtures and tablets for the symptomatic treatment of asthma and bronchitis. It has been given in doses of 6 to 30 mg thrice daily.

It is an ingredient of CAM, see under Proprietary Preparations of Ephedrine and its Salts, p.12.

2046-r

Carbuterol Hydrochloride. SKF 40383-A.

[5-(2-*tert*-Butylamino-1-hydroxyethyl)-2-hydroxyphenyl]urea hydrochloride.
$C_{13}H_{21}N_3O_3,HCl=303.8.$

CAS — 34866-47-2 (carbuterol); 34866-46-1 (hydrochloride).

Carbuterol hydrochloride is a direct-acting sympathomimetic agent with general properties similar to those of salbutamol (p.29). It has been used as a bronchodilator in doses of 1 to 3 mg three or four times daily by mouth, or by inhalation in doses of 100 to 200 µg at intervals of not less than 3 hours.

Animal pharmacology of carbuterol: J. R. Wardell *et al., J. Pharmac. exp. Ther.,* 1974, *189,* 167; D. F. Colella *et al., Eur. J. Pharmac.,* 1977, *46,* 229.

Asthma. Clinical studies on the bronchodilator effects of carbuterol: P. R. Saleeby and M. M. Ziskind, *Curr. ther. Res.,* 1975, *17,* 225; D. W. Cockcroft *et al., ibid.,* 1976, *19,* 170; M. A. Sackner *et al., Chest,* 1976, *69,* 593; D. H. Drachler *et al., J. clin. Pharmac.,* 1977, *17,* 734; J. Miller *et al., Ann. Allergy,* 1977, *39,* 12; J. P. Sanders *et al., J. Allergy clin. Immunol.,* 1977, *60,* 174; H. M. Beumer *et al., Respiration,* 1978, *35,* 220; G. B. Irsigler and J. Ker, *S.Afr. med. J.,* 1978, *53,* 571; A. Van As *et al., ibid.,* 1011; T. D. James and H. A. Lyons, *J. Am. med. Ass.,* 1979, *241,* 704; J. S. Guleria *et al., Ann. Allergy,* 1979, *43,* 123.

Proprietary Names

Bronsecur *(Warner, S.Afr.).*

2047-f

Clenbuterol Hydrochloride. NAB 365.

1-(4-Amino-3,5-dichlorophenyl)-2-*tert*-butylaminoethanol hydrochloride.
$C_{12}H_{18}Cl_2N_2O,HCl=313.7.$

CAS — 37148-27-9 (clenbuterol); 21898-19-1 (hydrochloride).

A colourless crystalline powder. Readily **soluble** in water, alcohol, and methyl alcohol; slightly soluble in chloroform. M.p. about 184° with decomposition.

Adverse Effects. As for Salbutamol, p.29.

Some conflicting reports on the incidence of side-effects, such as anxiety, agitation, and muscle tremor in patients receiving clenbuterol: P. L. Kamburoff *et al., Br. J. clin. Pharmac.,* 1977, *4,* 67; C. Mazzola and C. Vibelli, *Curr. ther. Res.,* 1978, *23,* 231; T. L. Whitsett *et al., Clin. Pharmac. Ther.,* 1980, *27,* 294.

Treatment of Adverse Effects. As for Isoprenaline, p.15.

Precautions. As for Salbutamol, p.29.

CAUTION. *Excessive usage of aerosols of sympathomimetic agents has been associated with sudden death in asthmatics,* see p.15.

Absorption and Fate. Clenbuterol is reported to be readily absorbed from the gastro-intestinal tract and to be excreted largely unchanged in the urine.

Uses. Clenbuterol hydrochloride is a direct-acting sympathomimetic agent with general properties similar to those of salbutamol (p.30). It has been used as a bronchodilator in doses of 20 to 30 µg twice daily.

Animal pharmacology of clenbuterol: J. Aravani and G. N. Melville, *Arzneimittel-Forsch.,* 1974, *24,* 849; V. Adhami, *ibid.,* 860; G. Engelhardt, *ibid.,* 1976, *26,* 1404; S. R. O'Donnell, *Archs int. Pharmacodyn. Ther.,* 1976, *224,* 190; K. Bohmer *et al., Clin. exp. Pharmac. Physiol.,* 1977, *4,* 224; *idem,* 383.

Asthma. Clinical studies on the bronchodilator effects of clenbuterol: O. Uhl, *Arzneimittel-Forsch.,* 1974, *24,* 855; D. Nolte *et al., ibid.,* 858; Y. Salorinne *et al., Eur. J. clin. Pharmac.,* 1975, *8,* 189; G. Anderson and E. Wilkins, *Thorax,* 1977, *32,* 717; N. Del Bono *et al., Curr. ther. Res.,* 1977, *22,* 376; P. Dorow, *Arzneimittel-Forsch.,* 1977, *27,* 2020; A. Baronti *et al., Eur. J. clin. Pharmac.,* 1978, *13,* 171; V. Brusasco *et al., Int. J. clin. Pharmac. Biopharm.,* 1978, *16,* 589; J. Cummiskey *et al., J. Irish med. Ass.,* 1978, *71,* 123; N. Del Bono *et al., Curr. med. Res. Opinion,* 1979, *6,* 237; P. C. Curti and C. Vibelli, *Curr. ther. Res.,* 1979, *25,* 465; C. Pasotti and C. Vibelli, *ibid.,* 473; C. Pasotti *et al., Int. J. clin. Pharmac. Biopharm.,* 1979, *17,* 176; A. Baronti *et al., Int. J. clin. Pharmac. Biopharm.,* 1980, *18,* 21; V. Brusasco *et al., Curr. med. Res. Opinion,* 1980, *6,* 449.

Proprietary Names

Spiropent *(Thomae, Ger.).*

2048-d

Clorprenaline Hydrochloride. Chlorprenaline Hydrochloride; Isoprophenamine Hydrochloride. 1-(2-Chlorophenyl)-2-isopropylaminoethanol hydrochloride monohydrate.
$C_{11}H_{16}ClNO,HCl,H_2O=268.2.$

CAS — 3811-25-4 (clorprenaline); 6933-90-0 (hydrochloride, anhydrous); 5588-22-7 (hydrochloride, monohydrate).

Uses. Clorprenaline hydrochloride is a sympathomimetic agent with general properties similar to those of isoprenaline (p.15). It has been given in doses of 10 or 20 mg three or four times daily for the prophylaxis of asthma, increased to up to 30 mg every 3 or 4 hours for acute attacks.

Reference to the metabolism of clorprenaline.— K. Tatsumi *et al., Chem. pharm. Bull., Tokyo,* 1970, *18,* 1254.

Proprietary Names

Asthone, Bazarl, Broncon, Cosmoline, Kalutein, Pentadoll, Restanolon *(all Jap.).*

A preparation containing clorprenaline hydrochloride was formerly marketed in Great Britain under the proprietary name Vortel (*Lilly*).

2049-n

Coumazoline Hydrochloride. L 5818. 2-(2-Ethylbenzofuran-3-ylmethyl)-2-imidazoline hydrochloride.
$C_{14}H_{16}N_2O,HCl=264.8.$

CAS — 37681-00-8 (coumazoline).

Uses. Coumazoline hydrochloride is a sympathomimetic agent used topically as a nasal vasoconstrictor.

Proprietary Names

Galenyl *(Labaz, Belg.);* Gayenil *(Labaz, Spain).*

2050-k

Cyclopentamine Hydrochloride *(U.S.P.).* Cyclopentadrin Hydrochloride; Cyclopentaminium Chloride. 2-Cyclopentyl-1,*N*-dimethylethylamine hydrochloride.
$C_9H_{19}N,HCl=177.7.$

CAS — 102-45-4 (cyclopentamine); 538-02-3 (hydrochloride).

A white crystalline powder with a slight characteristic odour and a bitter taste. M.p. 111° to 117° with a range of not more than 2°. **Soluble** 1 in 1 of water, 1 in 2 of alcohol, and 1 in 1 of chloroform; slightly soluble in ether. A 1% solution in water has a pH of about 6. A 2.68% solution in water is iso-osmotic with serum. **Store** in airtight containers.

A solution of cyclopentamine hydrochloride iso-osmotic with serum (2.68%) caused 100% haemolysis of erythrocytes cultured in it for 45 minutes.— E. R. Hammarlund and K. Pedersen-Bjergaard, *J. pharm. Sci.,* 1961, *50,* 24.

Cyclopentamine hydrochloride is a sympathomimetic agent with an action similar to that of ephedrine (p.10), but claimed to produce only slight stimulating effects on the central nervous system.

It has been used as a nasal decongestant in the form of a 0.5 or 1% solution and, in doses of 25 mg intramuscularly or 5 to 10 mg by slow intravenous injection, as a pressor agent.

Preparations

Cyclopentamine Hydrochloride Nasal Solution *(U.S.P.)*. Cyclopentamine Hydrochloride Solution. A solution of cyclopentamine hydrochloride in a suitable iso-osmotic vehicle. Store in airtight containers.

Cyclopentamine hydrochloride is an ingredient of Co-Pyronil: see under Pyrrobutamine Phosphate, p.1318.

2051-a

Dimetofrine Hydrochloride. Dimethophrine Hydrochloride. 1-(4-Hydroxy-3,5-dimethoxyphenyl)-2-methylaminoethanol hydrochloride.
$C_{11}H_{17}NO_4,HCl = 263.7$.

CAS — 22950-29-4 (dimetofrine); 22775-12-8 (hydrochloride).

Dimetofrine hydrochloride is a sympathomimetic agent which has been used for the treatment of hypotension.

The pharmacokinetics of dimetofrine following oral administration.— M. Benedetti *et al.*, *Arzneimittel-Forsch.*, 1977, *27*, 158.

Proprietary Names of Dimetofrine or Dimetofrine Hydrochloride
Dovida *(Zambeletti, Spain)*; Pressamina *(Zambeletti, Ital.)*; Superten *(Beta, Arg.)*.

2052-t

Dobutamine Hydrochloride *(U.S.P.)*. 46236; Compound 81929 (dobutamine). (±)-4-{2-[3-(4-Hydroxyphenyl)-1-methylpropylamino]ethyl}-pyrocatechol hydrochloride; (±)-4-{2-[3-(4-Hydroxyphenyl)-1-methylpropylamino]ethyl}-benzene-1,2-diol hydrochloride.
$C_{18}H_{23}NO_3,HCl = 337.8$.

CAS — 34368-04-2 (dobutamine); 52663-81-7 (hydrochloride).

Pharmacopoeias. In *U.S.* which also includes Dobutamine Hydrochloride for Injection.

A white powder. **Soluble** in water. **Incompatible** with alkalis, oxidising agents, and sodium metabisulphite. **Store** at 15° to 30° in airtight containers.

Adverse Effects. Side-effects associated with dobutamine include raised blood pressure, tachycardia, and increased premature ventricular beats. Other side-effects reported are nausea, headache, anginal and non-specific chest pain, palpitations, and dyspnoea. High doses have been associated with nervousness and tachycardia.

The most serious adverse effect of all the sympathomimetic amines is the precipitation of arrhythmias; it is claimed that dobutamine causes a lower incidence of arrhythmias compared with isoprenaline and dopamine. If rapid ventricular rates occur in the presence of obstructive coronary artery disease, ischaemia can be induced or worsened. Dobutamine may cause a marked increase in heart-rate or systolic blood pressure. Approximately 10% of patients in clinical studies have had rate increases of 30 beats per minute or more, and about 7.5% have had an increase of systolic blood pressure of 50 mmHg or higher. Reduction of dosage usually reverses these effects promptly. Because dobutamine facilitates atrioventricular conduction, patients with atrial fibrillation may be at risk of developing a rapid ventricular response. Other side-effects reported in 1 to 3% of patients include nausea, headache, anginal pain, palpitation, and shortness of breath. No abnormal laboratory values have been attributable to dobutamine, and infusions of up to 72 hours have revealed no adverse effects other than those seen with shorter infusions.— E. H. Sonnenblick *et al.*, *New Engl. J. Med.*, 1979, *300*, 17.

Diabetogenic effect. Dobutamine and increased insulin requirement.— S. M. Wood *et al.*, *Br. med. J.*, 1981, *282*, 946.

Ischaemia. None of 4 patients showed local signs of ischaemia on extravasation of dobutamine 30 to 60 mg, but one complained of an aching pain over the site.— C. V. Leier *et al.*, *Circulation*, 1977, *56*, 468.

Extravasation and dermal necrosis were associated with the intravenous infusion of dobutamine in a 68-year-old diabetic woman. The extravasation was further complicated by cellulitis, which responded to warm soaks. Infiltration with phentolamine mesylate might help to prevent necrosis if extravasation is noticed in time.— J. V. Hoff *et al.* (letter), *New Engl. J. Med.*, 1979, *300*, 1280.

Treatment of Adverse Effects. Since the half-life of dobutamine is only about 2 minutes most adverse effects can be corrected by discontinuing or reducing the rate of infusion.

Precautions. Dobutamine hydrochloride should be avoided or only used with great caution in patients with idiopathic hypertrophic subaortic stenosis. It is contra-indicated in patients with uncorrected tachycardia or ventricular fibrillation; hypovolaemia should be corrected before treatment. Dobutamine hydrochloride should be used with special caution in hypersusceptible patients or those with acute myocardial infarction, arteriosclerosis, or hypertension; hyperthyroid patients may be particularly sensitive.

Although it is less likely than adrenaline to produce ventricular arrhythmias, dobutamine should be avoided or only used with extreme caution during anaesthesia with cyclopropane, halothane, and other halogenated anaesthetics (see p.3). The inotropic effects of dobutamine on the heart are reversed by concomitant administration of beta-adrenoceptor blocking agents. Dobutamine may be ineffective in patients who have recently received beta-adrenoceptor blocking agents and may have a slight vasoconstricting effect.

Interactions. Reversal of the effects of dobutamine by metoprolol and the effects of metoprolol by dobutamine.— F. Waagstein *et al.*, *Br. J. clin. Pharmac.*, 1978, *5*, 515.

Absorption and Fate. For a brief outline of the absorption and fate of a catecholamine, see Adrenaline, p.3.

Like adrenaline, dobutamine is inactive when given by mouth, and it is rapidly inactivated in the body by similar processes.

A study of the pharmacokinetics of dobutamine in 7 patients with severe heart failure. The elimination half-life after intravenous infusion was less than 3 minutes. From the limited data available the volume of distribution of dobutamine appeared to be related to the extent of oedema.— R. E. Kates and C. V. Leier, *Clin. Pharmac. Ther.*, 1978, *24*, 537.

Further references: D. W. McKennon and R. E. Kates, *J. pharm. Sci.*, 1978, *67*, 1756 (plasma concentrations).

Uses. Dobutamine is a sympathomimetic agent with direct effects on beta$_1$-adrenergic receptors, which confer upon it a prominent inotropic action on the heart. Dobutamine differs from dopamine in not having the specific dopaminergic properties of dopamine which induce renal mesenteric vasodilatation; it is reported not to have indirect effects on alpha-adrenergic receptors. Like dopamine, the inotropic action of dobutamine on the heart is associated with less cardiac-accelerating effect than that of isoprenaline.

Dobutamine is used as the hydrochloride in the management of heart failure associated with organic heart disease, myocardial infarction, and cardiac surgery. It is administered as a dilute solution, in dextrose injection, sodium chloride injection, or sodium lactate injection, by intravenous infusion. The usual rate is 2.5 to 10 µg per kg body-weight per minute, according to the patient's heart-rate, blood pressure, cardiac output, and urine output. Up to 40 µg per kg per minute may occasionally be required. It has been recommended that treatment with dobutamine should be discontinued gradually.

Regret for the similarity between the names of dopamine and dobutamine since, although both have an inotropic action, there are important differences between them.— A. Yates (letter), *Br. med. J.*, 1978, *1*, 1622. Criticism of the differences cited.— L. I. Goldberg (letter), *ibid.*, *2*, 1163. Reply.— A. Yates (letter), *ibid.*

General reviews and publications on the clinical role of dobutamine: *Am. J. Med.*, 1978, *65*, 101–216 (symposium); *Med. Lett.*, 1979, *21*, 15 (actions and uses); E. H. Sonnenblick *et al.*, *New Engl. J. Med.*, 1979, *300*, 17 (actions and uses); L. H. Opie, *Lancet*, 1980, *1*, 912 (drugs acting on the heart, including dobutamine).

Cardiac disorders. In a study of 22 patients undergoing open-heart surgery dobutamine increased cardiac output with little effect on heart-rate or peripheral blood vessels.— *J. Am. med. Ass.*, 1973, *226*, 1406.

The cardiovascular effects of dobutamine in doses of 2.5, 5, and 10 µg per kg body-weight infused each minute for 10 minutes were compared with those of isoprenaline 20, 40, and 80 ng per kg per minute for 10 minutes in a study of 17 patients. Both agents produced comparable increases in left ventricular ejection but dobutamine did not significantly increase the heart-rate. Dobutamine at 10 µg per kg also increased the systolic arterial pressure without significantly affecting diastolic arterial pressure and significantly increased cardiac output and stroke volume. There was a significant reduction in peripheral resistance with the 5- and 10-µg doses. Dobutamine was considered to have more powerful inotropic than chronotropic actions.— D. Jewitt *et al.*, *Lancet*, 1974, *2*, 363. See also *idem*, *Am. J. Med.*, 1978, *65*, 197.

The haemodynamic effects of dobutamine and sodium nitroprusside were compared in 19 patients with low cardiac output. At doses producing similar increases in the cardiac index, dobutamine caused only slight changes in blood pressure but it fell significantly with sodium nitroprusside. Dobutamine might therefore be advantageous in patients where hypotension could limit coronary or other blood flow. Sodium nitroprusside significantly lowered arterial systolic and wedge pressures and did not increase heart-rate, and might be preferable when reduction in myocardial oxygen consumption or pulmonary congestion was desired.— C. Berkowitz *et al.*, *Circulation*, 1977, *56*, 918.

In 25 patients with severe left ventricular failure dobutamine, 2.5 µg per kg body-weight per minute increased progressively to 10 to 15 µg per kg and maintained for 72 hours, improved left ventricular contractile performance, increased cardiac output (9 patients evaluated), and reduced pulmonary capillary wedge pressure (9 patients). BUN and creatinine concentrations fell and the urine flow was increased. Twenty of the patients were subjectively improved; improvement persisted for a week in 17. In one patient inadvertently given 30 µg per kg per minute for 2 hours there was mild nervousness and heart-rate increased from 96 to 106 beats per minute. In a second patient given 80 µg per kg per minute for 5 minutes heart-rate rose from 88 to 132 beats per minute and the patient experienced marked nervousness, with fatigue and headache; symptoms abated rapidly.— C. V. Leier *et al.*, *Circulation*, 1977, *56*, 468. See also *idem*, *Am. J. Med.*, 1979, *66*, 238.

A comparison of the haemodynamic effects of dobutamine and digoxin, administered intravenously to 6 normotensive patients with heart failure associated with acute myocardial infarction. Dobutamine increased cardiac output by 33% while preload and afterload were decreased; heart-rate and blood pressure were not significantly affected. In contrast, digoxin increased cardiac output by only 9% and did not affect preload or afterload, thus doing little to relieve the symptoms of pulmonary congestion.— R. A. Goldstein *et al.*, *New Engl. J. Med.*, 1980, *303*, 846.

Further reports and studies on the role of dobutamine in cardiac disorders: W. Delius *et al.*, *Dt. med. Wschr.*, 1976, *101*, 1747 (haemodynamics); S. L. Meyer *et al.*, *Am. J. Cardiol.*, 1976, *38* 103 (haemodynamics); J. H. Tinker *et al.*, *Anesthesiology*, 1976, *44*, 281 (cardiac surgery); J. J. Andy *et al.*, *Am. Heart J.*, 1977, *94*, 175 (haemodynamics); T. A. Gillespie *et al.*, *Am. J. Cardiol.*, 1977, *39*, 588 (myocardial infarction); H. S. Loeb *et al.*, *Circulation*, 1977, *55*, 375 (comparison with dopamine); B. Magnani *et al.*, *J. int. med. Res.*, 1977, *5*, 10 (haemodynamics); T. Sakamoto and T. Yamada, *Circulation*, 1977, *55*, 525 (cardiac surgery); J. D. Stoner *et al.*, *Br. Heart J.*, 1977, *39*, 536 (comparison with dopamine); G. R. J. Lewis *et al.*, *Am. Heart J.*, 1978, *95*, 301 (cardiac surgery); A. Wirtzfeld *et al.*, *Dt. med. Wschr.*, 1978, *103*, 1915 (comparison with dopamine); D. J. Driscoll *et al.*, *Am. J. Cardiol.*, 1979, *43*, 581 (paediatric use); J. Stephens *et al.*, *Br. Heart J.*, 1979, *42*, 43 (comparison with dopamine and isoprenaline); G. Clark *et al.*, *Chest*, 1980, *77*, 220 (myocardial infarction); E. C. H. Keung *et al.*, *J. Am. med. Ass.*, 1981, *245*, 144 (myocardial infarction).

Preparations

Dobutamine Hydrochloride for Injection *(U.S.P.)*. A sterile mixture of dobutamine hydrochloride with suitable diluents. Potency is expressed in terms of the equivalent amount of dobutamine. Store at 15° to 30°.

Dobutrex *(Lilly, UK)*. Dobutamine hydrochloride, available as powder for preparing infusions, in vials each containing the equivalent of 250 mg of dobutamine. (Also available as Dobutrex in *Austral., Canad., Ger., Neth., S.Afr., Switz., USA*).

2053-x

Dopamine Hydrochloride.

ASL 279; 3-Hydroxytyramine Hydrochloride. 4-(2-Aminoethyl)pyrocatechol hydrochloride; 4-(2-Aminoethyl)benzene-1,2-diol hydrochloride.
$C_8H_{11}NO_2,HCl=189.6$.

CAS — 51-61-6 (dopamine); 62-31-7 (hydrochloride).

Pharmacopoeias. In *Chin.*

A white odourless crystalline powder. M.p. about 241° with decomposition. **Soluble** in water and alcohol.

Incompatible with alkalis, iron salts, and oxidising agents. **Store** in airtight containers. Protect from light.

Dopamine hydrochloride was stable for 48 hours at 25° in 8 intravenous fluids of pH 5.4 to 6.85. It was incompatible with sodium bicarbonate and the solution became pink in colour.— L. A. Gardella *et al.* , *Arnar-Stone, Am. J. Hosp. Pharm.*, 1975, *32*, 575. Dopamine hydrochloride in dextrose injection was physically incompatible (precipitate) with amphotericin; with ampicillin sodium a pink colour appeared 3 hours after admixture; dopamine potency was maintained for 24 hours in the presence of benzylpenicillin potassium, cephalothin sodium, and gentamicin sulphate but the antibiotic potencies were not maintained beyond 6 hours.— *idem*, 1976, *33*, 537. Evidence (that has been confirmed) of a much lower loss of gentamicin.— S. S. Chrai *et al.* (letter), *ibid.*, 1977, *34*, 348. Dopamine hydrochloride in dextrose injection was physically compatible for 24 hours, unprotected from light, with heparin sodium, lignocaine hydrochloride, neutral cephalothin sodium, oxacillin sodium, gentamicin sulphate, methylprednisolone sodium succinate, hydrocortisone sodium succinate, potassium chloride, calcium chloride, or calcium gluceptate.— L. A. Gardella *et al.*, *Am. J. Hosp. Pharm.*, 1978, *35*, 581.

Adverse Effects. Extravasation of dopamine during infusion may cause ischaemic necrosis and sloughing; gangrene has occurred.

Systemic side-effects associated with dopamine include nausea and vomiting, ectopic beats, palpitations, tachycardia, anginal pain, dyspnoea, and headache. Low doses may cause hypotension due to the predominance of the vasodilator effect of dopamine, whereas high doses may cause excessive vasoconstriction and hypertension due to the predominance of the vasoconstrictor effect. Other side-effects that have been very occasionally associated with dopamine infusion, include bradycardia and aberrant conduction, and piloerection; raised BUN has also been reported.

Ischaemia and gangrene. Cyanosis, progressing to gangrene, developed in the feet and toes of a 51-year-old man during a 2-day infusion of dopamine 10 µg per kg body-weight per minute after a mitral valve replacement operation. He had previously suffered 3 episodes of frost-bite in his feet. It was suggested that dopamine should be used with caution in elderly patients with pre-existing vascular damage.— C. S. Alexander *et al.*, *New Engl. J. Med.*, 1975, *293*, 591. Massive local arterial and venous vasoconstriction followed infiltration of dopamine from an infusion into the dorsum of the left hand using a 21-gauge scalp-vein needle. There was no response to local injection of phentolamine or systemic injection of papaverine and the patient required partial amputation of the index finger and debridement followed by skin grafting of the entire dorsum of the left hand. Administration of dopamine had since been allowed only through indwelling venous catheters.— R. S. Boltax *et al.* (letter), *ibid.*, 1977, *296*, 823.

A 58-year-old woman with mild diabetes was treated for cardiogenic shock with dopamine hydrochloride. Gangrenous changes followed initial dopamine therapy and administration of very high doses of dopamine led to rapid progression of these changes.— N. K. Julka and J. R. Nora (letter), *J. Am. med. Ass.*, 1976, *235*, 2812.

Further reports and comments on ischaemia and gangrene associated with dopamine therapy: S. I. Greene and J. W. Smith (letter), *New Engl. J. Med.*, 1976, *294*, 114; Tj. Ebels and J. N. Homan van der Heide (letter), *Lancet*, 1977, *2*, 762; J. B. Stetson and G. P. Reading, *Can. Anaesth. Soc. J.*, 1977, *24*, 727; F. L. Golbranson *et al.*, *J. Am. med. Ass.*, 1980, *243*, 1145; *idem*, *244*, 1095.

Polyuria. Two patients with Gram-negative infections developed polyuria during treatment of hypotension with infusions of dopamine.— R. S. Flis *et al.*, *Archs intern. Med.*, 1977, *137*, 1547.

Treatment of Adverse Effects. Since the half-life of dopamine is only about 2 minutes most adverse effects can be corrected by discontinuing or reducing the rate of infusion. If these measures fail excessive vasoconstriction and hypertension may be treated with an alpha-adrenoceptor blocking agent such as 5 to 10 mg of phentolamine mesylate intravenously, repeated as necessary.

Relief from tissue necrosis and pain may be given by immediate infiltration with phentolamine and local anaesthetics, and by the application of hot packs.

Digital ischaemia during infusion of dopamine was controlled within minutes by intravenous administration of chlorpromazine 10 mg followed by infusion of 600 µg per minute (7.3 µg per kg body-weight per minute) for a total of 5½ hours. High doses of dopamine were required for a further 25 hours but the digital ischaemia did not recur suggesting that intermittent bolus administration might also be effective.— M. E. Valdes (letter), *New Engl. J. Med.*, 1976, *295*, 1081. See also D. Stevens and B. Stegall (letter), *Am. J. Hosp. Pharm.*, 1978, *35*, 521.

Precautions. Dopamine hydrochloride is contra-indicated in patients with phaeochromocytoma or uncorrected tachycardia or ventricular fibrillation; hypovolaemia should be corrected before treatment. Dopamine hydrochloride should be used with special caution in hypersusceptible patients or those with acute myocardial infarction, arteriosclerosis and hypertension, and occlusive vascular disorders, such as Raynaud's disease; hyperthyroid patients may be particularly sensitive, and it should be used with caution in diabetes.

Although it is less likely than adrenaline to produce ventricular arrhythmias, dopamine should be avoided or only used with extreme caution during anaesthesia with cyclopropane, halothane, and other halogenated anaesthetics (see p.3). If given to patients taking monoamine oxidase inhibitors the initial dose should be reduced to at least one-tenth of the usual dose; special caution is also necessary in patients receiving tricyclic antidepressants. Reversal of the action of many antihypertensive agents occurs in patients given sympathomimetics, therefore special care is advisable in patients receiving antihypertensive therapy.

Interactions. Animal studies demonstrating that *haloperidol* selectively attenuates the renal and mesenteric vasodilating actions of dopamine.— B. K. Yeh *et al.*, *J. Pharmac. exp. Ther.*, 1969, *168*, 303. See also J. L. McNay and L. I. Goldberg, *ibid.*, 1966, *151*, 23.

Following a report in 1976 to the FDA by R.P. Rapp of hypotension in patients given phenytoin in addition to dopamine infusion R.D. Smith and T.E. Lomas (*Toxic. appl. Pharmac.*, 1978, *45*, 665) studied the potential interaction, and found that dopamine given by intravenous infusion concomitantly with phenytoin infusion to *dogs*, did not alter the CNS effects of phenytoin nor result in hypotension and cardiovascular collapse. Large doses of phenytoin alone, had a reproducible hypotensive effect which was reduced by dopamine, suggesting a possible supportive role in phenytoin-induced hypotension. Further references: B. A. Bivins *et al.*, *Archs Surg., Chicago*, 1978, *113*, 245.

Fatal paradoxical hypotension in a man given *tolazoline* in addition to dopamine.— G. C. Carlon, *Chest*, 1979, *76*, 336.

Absorption and Fate. For a brief outline of the absorption and fate of a catecholamine, see Adrenaline, p.3.

The vasoconstrictor properties of dopamine preclude its administration by subcutaneous or intramuscular administration. Like adrenaline it is inactive when given by mouth, and it is rapidly inactivated in the body by similar processes. Dopamine is a metabolic precursor of noradrenaline and a proportion is excreted as the metabolic products of noradrenaline. Nevertheless, the majority appears to be directly metabolised into dopamine-related metabolic products.

A study of the metabolism of dopamine infused into 6 healthy subjects. Approximately 75% of the infused dopamine was directly metabolised into dopamine-related metabolic products. The remainder was synthesised into noradrenaline and appeared in the urine as noradrenaline or its metabolic products, principally the latter.— M. Goodall and H. Alton, *Biochem. Pharmac.*, 1968, *17*, 905. An account of the catabolism of catecholamines and a review of studies.— D. F. Sharman, *Br. med. Bull.*, 1973, *29*, 110. Biochemical aspects of monoamine oxidase.— K. F. Tipton, *ibid.*, 116. Catecholamine uptake processes.— L. L. Iverson, *ibid.*, 130.

Uses. The catecholamine, dopamine, is a sympathomimetic agent with direct effects on beta-adrenergic receptors and indirect effects on alpha-adrenergic receptors. It is formed in the body by the decarboxylation of levodopa, and is both a neurotransmitter in its own right (notably in the brain) and a precursor of noradrenaline. Dopamine differs from adrenaline and noradrenaline in dilating renal and mesenteric blood vessels and increasing urine output, apparently by a specific dopaminergic mechanism. Moreover, the inotropic action of dopamine on the heart is associated with less cardiac-accelerating effect than that of isoprenaline. In the treatment of shock this dual action of dopamine has the advantage that it can correct haemodynamic imbalance by exerting an inotropic effect on the heart, without undue tachycardia, and at the same time improve renal perfusion. It also confers upon dopamine an increased complexity of action compared with other sympathomimetics, since at low doses the inotropic and renal effects predominate, whereas with higher doses the alpha-adrenergic properties of dopamine may predominate leading to increased peripheral resistance which may ultimately dominate over the renal vasodilatation.

Concentrations of dopamine are reduced in the brains of patients with Parkinson's disease; increased brain-dopamine concentrations are accordingly beneficial in this condition. In practice, as dopamine is not active by mouth and does not readily cross the blood-brain barrier, its precursor, levodopa (p.886) is given for treatment.

Dopamine also inhibits release of prolactin from the anterior pituary and has been identified with the prolactin-inhibiting factor (PIF or PRIF), see Prolactin, p.1275.

Dopamine is used as the hydrochloride in the treatment of shock unresponsive to replacement of fluid loss. It is used to correct haemodynamic imbalances associated with myocardial infarction, trauma, septic shock, and cardiac surgery; it is also used in the management of congestive heart failure. It is administered as a dilute solution, in dextrose injection, sodium chloride injection, or sodium lactate injection, by intravenous infusion. The initial rate is 2 to 5 µg per kg body-weight per minute, gradually increased by 5 to 10 µg per kg per minute according to the patient's blood pressure, cardiac output, and urine output. Up to 20 to 50 µg per kg per minute may be required in seriously ill patients; higher doses have been given. A reduction in urine flow, without hypotension, may indicate a need to reduce the dose. To avoid tissue necrosis dopamine is best administered through a fine catheter into a large vein high up in a limb, preferably the arm. It has been recommended that on gradual discontinuation of dopamine care should be taken to avoid undue hypotension associated with very low dosage levels where vasodilatation could predominate.

Reports, studies, and comments on the endogenous role of dopamine: I. J. Kopin *et al.*, *Ann. intern. Med.*, 1976, *85*, 211 (studies on dopamine-β-hydroxylase the enzyme responsible for converting dopamine to noradrenaline); J. E. Valenzuela *et al.*, *Gastroenterology*, 1976, *76*, 323 (inhibition of gastric acid secretion); G. Delitala (letter), *Lancet*, 1977, *2*, 760 (inhibition of thyrotrophin secretion); S. G. Ball and M. R. Lee, *Br. J. clin. Pharmac.*, 1977, *4*, 115 (natriuretic properties); S. M. Antelman and A. R. Caggiula, *Science*, 1977, *195*, 646 (role in stress); R. Caldara *et al.*, *Gut*, 1978, *19*, 724 (regulation of gastric acid secretion); F. Owen *et al.*, *Lancet*, 1978, *2*, 223; A. V. P. Mackay *et al.* (letter), *ibid.*, 1980, *2*, 915; G. P. Reynolds *et al.* (letter), *ibid.*, 1251 (dopamine receptors and schizophrenia); S. Szabo, *Lancet*, 1979, *2*, 880; M. G. Bramble (letter), *ibid.*, 1190; R. Caldara *et al.* (letter), *ibid.*, 1980, *1*, 95 (inhibition of gastric acid secretion).

General reviews and publications on the clinical role of dopamine: L. I. Goldberg, *Pharmac. Rev.*, 1972, *24*, 1 (pharmacology); L. I. Goldberg, *New Engl. J. Med.*, 1974, *291*, 707 (clinical applications); *Br. med. J.*, 1977, *2*, 1563 (cardiac failure and shock); *Lancet*, 1977, *2*, 231 (cardiac failure); *Proc. R. Soc. Med.*, 1977, *70*, *Suppl.* 2 (symposium); *Drug & Ther. Bull.*, 1978, *16*, 79 (cardiac failure and shock); *Br. med. J.*, 1979, *2*, 160 (cardiac failure).

Administration. A recommendation to calculate an individual concentration of dopamine so that 1 µg per kg body-weight per minute is equivalent to 1 drop per minute. Thus, with a drip set delivering 60 drops per ml, the amount of dopamine in mg in 100 ml of infusion must be 6 times the patient's weight in kg. The method may be adapted for other drip sets by ensuring that the dopamine content of each drop in µg is the same numerically as the patient's weight in kg, when the same drop-to-dose relationship will apply. Children or infants may require double or fourfold concentration to reduce fluid input, but the essential simplicity remains.— J. M. Chapman and J. R. Davies (letter), *Br. med. J.*, 1978, *2*, 437. A similar recommendation.— J. M. Nappi (letter), *Am. J. Hosp. Pharm.*, 1979, *36*, 881.

Asthma. Dopamine at doses that had been reported to increase cardiac contractility, cardiac output and renal blood flow, had no acute effect on airways resistance in 9 healthy subjects and 12 patients with bronchial asthma. There was also no effect when dopamine was given with thymoxamine to 3 of the asthmatics compared with thymoxamine alone.— N. C. Thomson and K. R. Patel, *Br. J. clin. Pharmac.*, 1978, *5*, 421.

Bleeding. A report of the successful use of a regional intra-arterial infusion of dopamine in 4 patients for the management of traumatic haemorrhage. In one patient with a fracture of the right pubic bone, noradrenaline controlled the haemorrhage, but caused anuria. The noradrenaline was stopped and dopamine 7.5 µg per kg body-weight per minute was infused into the right hypogastric artery. Haemostasis was maintained and renal function returned. The infusion was tapered over 14 hours and the patient made an uneventful recovery.— H. J. Mud and H. A. Bruining (letter), *New Engl. J. Med.*, 1980, *303*, 754. See also *idem*, *Ned. Tijdschr. Geneesk.*, 1980, *124*, 333.

Cardiac disorders. Reports and studies on the role of dopamine in cardiac disorders: R. Rosenblum *et al.*, *J. Pharmac. exp. Ther.*, 1972, *183*, 256 (haemodynamics); C. Crexells *et al.*, *Cardiovasc. Res.*, 1973, *7*, 438 (haemodynamics); E. L. Holloway *et al.*, *Br. Heart J.*, 1975, *37*, 482 (haemodynamics); H. S. Loeb *et al.*, *Circulation*, 1977, *55*, 375 (haemodynamics; comparison with dobutamine); R. R. Miller *et al.*, *Circulation*, 1977, *55*, 881 (use with sodium nitroprusside); J. S. Wright *et al.*, *Med. J. Aust.*, 1977, *1*, 651 (cardiac surgery); D. J. Driscoll *et al.*, *J. Pediat.*, 1978, *92*, 309 (paediatric use); S. K. Durairaj and L. J. Haywood, *Clin. Pharmac. Ther.*, 1978, *24*, 175 (haemodynamics); D. R. Stemple *et al.*, *Am. J. Cardiol.*, 1978, *42*, 267 (use with sodium nitroprusside); D. J. Driscoll *et al.*, *J. thorac. cardiovasc. Surg.*, 1979, *78*, 765 (paediatric use); W. Hess *et al.*, *Br. J. Anaesth.*, 1979, *51*, 1063 (use with glyceryl trinitrate in cardiac surgery); P. Lang *et al.*, *J. Pediat.*, 1980, *96*, 630 (haemodynamics in children).

Diagnostic use. Huntington's chorea. Increased dopamine uptake by the platelets of patients with Huntington's chorea. If confirmed by others, these observations could be of value for a predictive test.— M. J. Aminoff *et al.*, *Lancet*, 1974, *2*, 1115. The findings could not be confirmed. It is unlikely that this method could be used as a predictive test for Huntington's chorea.— E. Bonilla *et al.* (letter), *Lancet*, 1978, *2*, 161.

Hepatic disorders. Dopamine hydrochloride increased urine output and urinary-sodium concentration in a 50-year-old woman with a history of alcohol abuse who was being treated for hepatorenal syndrome.— J. R. Wilson, *J. Am. med. Ass.*, 1977, *238*, 2719. See also D. E. Bernado *et al.*, *Gastroenterology*, 1970, *58*, 524.

Renal disorders. Infusion of low doses of dopamine hydrochloride (1 µg per kg body-weight per minute) significantly increased urine output in early oliguric acute tubular necrosis in 11 patients. It was concluded that infusion of low doses of dopamine is worthy of further trial in oliguric states.— I. S. Henderson *et al.*, *Lancet*, 1980, *2*, 827. Comments on the role of the frusemide which was also given.— G. Graziani *et al.* (letter), *ibid.*, 1301; C. Brun-Buisson and J. R. Le Gall (letter), *ibid.* Similar findings using a dose of 2 µg per kg per minute. Irrespective of the primary pathology, continuous infusion of dopamine has been found to promote a diuresis, reducing dialysis requirements and simplifying management. The use of dopamine has been extended to prophylaxis in high-risk patients. Thus, a low-dose infusion of dopamine is started in all patients with acute pancreatitis, bacterial toxaemia, haemorrhagic shock, and severe trauma requiring admission to the intensive care unit. As yet there is insufficient data for statistical analysis, but acute renal failure seems to have been averted in some patients.— A. R. Luksza and S. T. Atherton (letter), *ibid.*, 1036.

Further references: C. M. Perkins *et al.* (letter), *Lancet*, 1980, *2*, 1370.

Shock. In a haemodynamic study of 22 patients suffering from shock of differing aetiology, infusion of dopamine hydrochloride, 1 to 18 µg per kg body-weight per minute in dextrose injection, was superior to isoprenaline in 7 with normal or low peripheral resistance in whom isoprenaline was associated with unacceptably low blood pressure. Infusion of isoprenaline hydrochloride, 10 to 160 ng per kg per minute in dextrose injection was superior in 3 in whom dopamine did not increase cardiac output.— R. C. Talley *et al.*, *Circulation*, 1969, *39*, 361. Only 1 patient of 6 with endotoxic shock reported by R.C. Talley *et al.* survived after treatment with dopamine. Although dopamine has been approved for use in endotoxic shock, further investigation is necessary to determine if it is the drug of choice; in particular, dopamine would not treat the usually fatal pulmonary complications of endotoxic shock.— R. H. Schwarz and D. M. Aviado, *J. clin. Pharmac.*, 1976, *16*, 88. For a long-term study involving the use of sympathomimetic agents in septic shock, see Isoprenaline, p.17.

The most successful application of dopamine was in cardiogenic shock where it could be effective either alone or with other pressor or diuretic agents. A sterile solution in dextrose injection containing 800 µg of dopamine hydrochloride per ml should be infused initially at the rate of 1 to 2 µg per kg body-weight per minute. The dose should be increased by 1 to 4 µg per kg per minute every 15 to 30 minutes, until an optimal effect was obtained as judged by urine output and systemic arterial pressure. Although infusion rates as high as 50 µg per kg per minute might be reached, survival was unusual when such large doses were required. Maintenance doses in surviving patients averaged approximately 9 µg per kg per minute.— J. S. Karliner, *J. Am. med. Ass.*, 1973, *226*, 1217.

The use of dopamine to treat circulatory shock in 34 patients. Shock was attributed to a cardiogenic cause in 19 patients, bacterial infection in 9, and massive blood or fluid loss in 5. In those who ultimately survived, concentrations of arterial blood lactate were normal or only mildy raised. In those with established shock and substantial increases in concentrations of arterial blood lactate, dopamine infusion did not increase peripheral perfusion, reverse lacticacidaemia, or improve survival.— C. E. Ruiz *et al.*, *J. Am. med. Ass.*, 1979, *242*, 165.

Further references to the use of dopamine in shock: J. Holzer *et al.*, *Am. J. Cardiol.*, 1973, *32*, 79 (cardiogenic shock); E. J. Winslow *et al.*, *Am. J. Med.*, 1973, *54*, 421 (septic shock); P. Théroux *et al.*, *Can. med. Ass. J.*, 1977, *116*, 645 (cardiogenic shock); P. G. Lankisch and H. Koop, *Dt. med. Wschr.*, 1978, *103*, 391 (potential role in shock of acute pancreatitis); A. T. Raftery and R. W. G. Johnson, *Br. med. J.*, 1979, *1*, 522 (unstable kidney donors); M. Hemmer and P. M. Suter, *Anesthesiology*, 1979, *50*, 399 (shock of acute pulmonary failure); A. D. Timmis *et al.*, *Br. med. J.*, 1981, *282*, 7 (cardiogenic shock).

Subarachnoid haemorrhage. A report of an arousal phenomenon which occurred in 9 of 14 patients with subarachnoid haemorrhage immediately intracranial infusion of dopamine was begun.— D. J. Boullin *et al.* (letter), *Br. J. clin. Pharmac.*, 1978, *6*, 369. See also *idem*, *Proc. R. Soc. Med.*, 1977, *70*, *Suppl.* 2, 55.

Proprietary Preparations

Intropin *(American Hospital Supply, UK)*. Dopamine hydrochloride, available as sterile solutions containing 40 mg per ml with sodium metabisulphite 1%, in ampoules or syringes of 5 ml; and 160 mg per ml with sodium metabisulphite 1%, in ampoules of 5 ml. For preparing infusion solutions. (Also available as Intropin in *Austral.*, *Canad.*, *Neth.*, *S.Afr.*, *USA*).

Select-A-Jet Dopamine Hydrochloride Injection *(IMS, UK)*. A cartridge assembly containing a solution of dopamine hydrochloride 40 mg per ml, in vials of 5 and 10 ml. For preparing intravenous infusions.

Other Proprietary Names

Aprical-Dopamina *(Spain)*; Dynatra *(Belg.)*; Hettytropin *(Arg.)*; Inotropin *(Arg.)*; Inovan *(Jap.)*; Revimine *(Canad.)*; Revivan *(Ital.)*.

2054-r

Ephedra *(B.P.C. 1954)*. Ma-huang.

Pharmacopoeias. In *Chin.*, *Ind.*, and *Jap.*

Ephedra consists of the dried young branches of *Ephedra sinica*, *E. equisetina*, and *E. gerardiana* (including *E. nebrodensis*) (Ephedraceae), containing not less than 1.25% of alkaloids, calculated as ephedrine. (*Jap. P.* specifies not less than 0.6%). **Store** in airtight containers. Protect from light.

The action of ephedra is due to the presence of ephedrine and pseudoephedrine. It is mainly used as a source of the alkaloids.

Comment on the abuse of 'Ma-Huang Incense').— R. K. Siegel (letter), *New Engl. J. Med.*, 1980, *302*, 817.

2055-f

Ephedrine *(B.P., Eur. P.)*. Ephedrinum; Hydrated Ephedrine; Ephedrinum Hydratum; Ephedrina; Efedrina. (1*R*,2*S*)-2-Methylamino-1-phenylpropan-1-ol hemihydrate. $C_{10}H_{15}NO,\frac{1}{2}H_2O = 174.2$.

CAS — 50906-05-3 (hemihydrate).

Pharmacopoeias. In *Belg.*, *Br.*, *Eur.*, *Fr.*, *Ger.*, *Ind.*, *It.*, *Neth.*, and *Swiss. Braz.*, *Mex.*, and *U.S.* specify anhydrous or hemihydrate. *Arg.* and *Span.* specify anhydrous only.

An alkaloid obtained from species of *Ephedra*, or prepared synthetically. Colourless crystals or white crystalline powder or granules with a bitter taste and either odourless or with a slight aromatic odour. M.p. 40° to 43° without previous drying; in warm weather it slowly volatilises. **Soluble** 1 in 20 of water and 1 in less than 1 of alcohol; soluble in chloroform with turbidity due to separation of water; soluble in ether; soluble in 1 in 20 of glycerol, 1 in 25 of olive oil, and 1 in 100 of liquid paraffin, slowly, with separation of water; the anhydrous alkaloid forms clear solutions in liquid paraffin. A solution in diluted hydrochloric acid is laevorotatory. Solutions in water are strongly alkaline to litmus. **Incompatible** with chlorbutol, iodine, silver salts, and tannic acid. Ephedrine decomposes on exposure to light; solutions in oil may develop an alliaceous odour. **Store** at a temperature not exceeding 8° in airtight containers. Protect from light.

The rate of release of ephedrine and its hydrochloride from theobroma oil suppositories containing 5% of various nonionic surfactants was determined by a dialysis method. Surfactants with an HLB above 9 generally increased the release-rates compared with theobroma oil basis. Ephedrine was released and dialysed at a much lower rate than its hydrochloride.— J. M. Plaxco *et al.*, *J. pharm. Sci.*, 1967, *56*, 809. Surfactants did not impair the release of ephedrine from an oil-surfactant-ephedrine dispersion but did inhibit the release of ephedrine from an ephedrine-surfactant-water system.— W. G. Waggoner and J. H. Fincher, *ibid.*, 1971, *60*, 1830.

Solubility in light liquid paraffin. A clear solution of ephedrine (hemihydrate) 1% in light liquid paraffin could be produced by the addition of sorbitan trioleate 2% v/v.— I. J. Bellafiore, *J. Am. pharm. Ass.*, 1965, *5*, 557.

2056-d

Anhydrous Ephedrine *(B.P., Eur. P.)*.

Ephed. Anhydros.; Ephedrinum Anhydricum; Ephedrine; Efedrina. The anhydrous alkaloid prepared by vacuum distillation of the hydrate.

CAS — 299-42-3.

Pharmacopoeias. In *Arg., Br., Eur., Fr., Ger., It., Neth.,* and *Span.*

NOTE. Ephedrine *U.S.P.* is anhydrous or the hemihydrate

Unctous deliquescent colourless crystals or white crystalline powder, odourless or with a slight aromatic odour. It rapidly absorbs carbon dioxide. M.p. about 38°.

Soluble 1 in 20 of water; very soluble in alcohol; freely soluble in ether; soluble in chloroform, glycerol, olive oil, and liquid paraffin. Solutions in water are strongly alkaline to litmus. Solutions in oil are free from turbidity. Ephedrine decomposes on exposure to light. **Store** at a temperature not exceeding 8° in airtight containers. Protect from light.

2057-n

Ephedrine Hydrochloride *(B.P., Eur. P., U.S.P.)*.

Ephed. Hydrochlor.; Ephedrini Hydrochloridum; Ephedrinae Hydrochloridum; Ephedrinium Chloratum; *l*-Ephedrinum Hydrochloricum.

$C_{10}H_{15}NO,HCl=201.7$.

CAS — 50-98-6.

Pharmacopoeias. In all pharmacopoeias examined. *Hung. P.* includes only the racemic form (racephedrine hydrochloride).

Odourless colourless crystals or white crystalline powder with a bitter taste. M.p. 217° to 220°.

Soluble 1 in 3 or 4 of water, 1 in 14 or 17 of alcohol, and 1 in 60 of glycerol; very slightly soluble in chloroform; practically insoluble in ether; insoluble in olive oil and liquid paraffin. A solution in water is laevorotatory. A 3.2% solution in water is iso-osmotic with serum. Solutions are **sterilised** by autoclaving or by filtration. **Store** in airtight containers. Protect from light.

2058-h

Ephedrine Sulphate.

Ephedrine Sulfate *(U.S.P.)*.

$(C_{10}H_{15}NO)_2,H_2SO_4=428.5$.

CAS — 134-72-5.

Pharmacopoeias. In *Arg., Braz.,* and *U.S.*

Fine white odourless crystals or powder. It darkens on exposure to light. **Soluble** 1 in 1.3 of water, 1 in 90 of alcohol, and 1 in 60 of glycerol; insoluble in oils. A 5% solution in water is laevorotatory. A 4.54% solution in water is iso-osmotic with serum. Solutions are **sterilised** by autoclaving or by filtration. **Store** in airtight containers. Protect from light.

Incompatibility. There was loss of clarity when intravenous solutions of ephedrine sulphate were mixed with those of hydrocortisone sodium succinate, pentobarbitone sodium, phenobarbitone sodium, quinalbarbitone sodium, or thiopentone sodium.— J. A. Patel and G. L. Phillips, *Am. J. Hosp. Pharm.*, 1966, *23,* 409.

Adverse Effects. In large doses ephedrine may give rise to side-effects such as giddiness, headache, nausea, vomiting, sweating, thirst, tachycardia, precordial pain, palpitations, difficulty in micturition, muscular weakness and tremors, anxiety, restlessness, and insomnia; some patients may exhibit these symptoms with the usual therapeutic doses.

Hypertension and ventricular arrhythmias occur more rarely but can follow intravenous injection of ephedrine. Injection of ephedrine during labour can cause foetal tachycardia.

Paranoid psychosis, delusions, and hallucinations may also follow ephedrine overdosage. Prolonged administration has no cumulative effect, but tolerance with dependence has been reported.

In hypersensitive patients local application of the drug may cause a contact dermatitis.

Abuse. Two patients with toxic psychosis and delusions associated with excessive self-medication with ephedrine. A 65-year-old man had taken up to 200 ephedrine tablets (60 mg) a week for several years and a 54-year-old woman had taken increasing quantities of ephedrine over 20 years, latterly up to 15 tablets (30 mg) 5 times a day during asthma attacks.— C. F. Herridge and M. F. a'Brook, *Br. med. J.*, 1968, *2,* 160.

Further references to ephedrine abuse: F. J. Kane and R. Florenzano (letter), *J. Am. med. Ass.*, 1971, *215,* 2116; K. A. Karlsson *et al., Läkartidningen,* 1971, *68,* 713 (intravenous abuse); M. G. Roxanas and J. Spalding, *Med. J. Aust.*, 1977, *2,* 639.

Epileptiform effect. The Boston Collaborative Drug Surveillance Program monitored consecutively 32 812 medical inpatients. Drug-induced convulsions occurred in 1 of 79 patients given ephedrine.— J. Porter and H. Jick, *Lancet,* 1977, *1,* 587.

Overdosage. A 15-year-old girl took about 30 tablets of Franol. Four hours later she was found to be flushed, sweating, and vomiting profusely. Her heart-rate was 140 per minute. The main effect was apparently due to the ephedrine content of the tablets and bore some similarity to the symptoms and signs of diabetic precoma. The effects persisted for about 18 hours and then gradually subsided.— P. E. M. Jarrett (letter), *Lancet,* 1966, *2,* 1190.

Symptoms of cardiomyopathy, with clinical, haemodynamic, and ECG features resembling those of phaeochromocytoma, occurred in a 34-year-old man after chronic excessive intake of ephedrine. Symptoms slowly regressed after prolonged bed rest.— W. Van Mieghem *et al., Br. med. J.*, 1978, *1,* 816.

Urinary retention. Urinary retention associated with ephedrine.— R. S. Glidden and F. J. DiBona, *J. Pediat.*, 1977, *90,* 1013.

Treatment of Adverse Effects. In general the management of overdosage with ephedrine involves supportive and symptomatic therapy.

In severe overdosage the stomach should be emptied by aspiration and lavage. Diazepam may be given to control central nervous system stimulation and convulsions. For marked excitement or hallucinations chlorpromazine may be necessary and, in addition, its alpha-adrenoceptor blocking properties may be useful for the management of hypertension. Severe hypertension may call for the administration of an alpha-adrenoceptor blocking agent, such as phentolamine. A beta-adrenoceptor blocking agent, such as propranolol, may be required to control cardiac arrhythmias; in asthmatic patients a more cardioselective beta-adrenoceptor blocking agent may be more suitable.

It has been found that acidification of the urine enhances the elimination of ephedrine, but for comments on the hazards of procedures such as forced acid diuresis, see Dexamphetamine, p.362.

Precautions. Ephedrine should be avoided in patients with most types of cardiovascular disease, hypertension, hyperthyroidism, hyperexcitability, phaeochromocytoma, and closed-angle glaucoma. In patients with prostatic enlargement, it may increase difficulty with micturition.

Due to its stimulant effects on the central nervous system ephedrine should not usually be given after about 4 pm. Children, however, are less susceptible to this stimulant effect.

Ephedrine should not be given to patients being treated with a monoamine oxidase inhibitor or within 14 days of stopping such treatment (see Precautions for Phenelzine Sulphate, p.128), although the 2 drugs have been given together in narcolepsy.

Although ephedrine is less likely to provoke ventricular arrhythmias than adrenaline (see p.3) it should be used with caution in patients receiving chloroform, cyclopropane, halothane, or other halogenated anaesthetics.

The effects of epehdrine are diminshed by guanethidine, reserpine, and probably methyldopa and may be diminished or enhanced by tricyclic antidepressants. Ephedrine may also diminish the effects of guanethidine and may increase the possibility of arrhythmias in digitalised patients.

Interactions. *Corticosteroids.* For the effect of ephedrine on corticosteroids, see Corticosteroids, p.450.

Tachyphylaxis. A report of tolerance to ephedrine developing in a 12-year-old boy on 3 occasions within only a few days of starting therapy for bronchospasm.— P. Rangsithienchai and R. W. Newcomb (letter), *J. Am. med. Ass.*, 1978, *240,* 20.

Absorption and Fate. Ephedrine is readily and completely absorbed from the gastro-intestinal tract, peak plasma concentrations being achieved about an hour after oral administration. It is resistant to metabolism by monoamine oxidase and is largely excreted unchanged in the urine, with some deaminated metabolites and some as the *N*-demethylated metabolite. Ephedrine has been variously reported to have a plasma half-life ranging from 3 to 6 hours; elimination is enhanced and half-life accordingly shorter in acid urine.

The absorption, metabolism, and excretion of ephedrine, norephedrine, and methylephedrine under constant acidic urine control.— G. R. Wilkinson and A. H. Beckett, *J. pharm. Sci.*, 1968, *57,* 1933. See also *idem, J. Pharmac. exp. Ther.*, 1968, *162,* 139. Urinary excretion of ephedrine in healthy subjects without pH control of urine.— P. G. Welling *et al., J. pharm. Sci.*, 1971, *60,* 1629. Metabolism of ephedrine in healthy subjects.— P. S. Sever *et al., Eur. J. clin. Pharmac.*, 1975, *9,* 193. Pharmacokinetics of ephedrine in asthmatic subjects.— M. E. Pickup *et al., Br. J. clin. Pharmac.*, 1976, *3,* 123. Absorption and excretion of ephedrine in one healthy subject.— K. K. Midha *et al., J. pharm. Sci.*, 1979, *68,* 557.

Uses. Ephedrine is a sympathomimetic agent with direct and indirect effects on adrenergic receptors. It has alpha- and beta-adrenergic activity and has pronounced stimulating effects on the central nervous system. It has a more prolonged though less potent action than adrenaline. In therapeutic doses it raises the blood pressure by increasing cardiac output and also by inducing peripheral vasoconstriction; this effect is slower and more sustained than after adrenaline. Tachycardia may occur but is less frequent than with adrenaline. Ephedrine also causes bronchodilatation, reduces intestinal tone and motility, relaxes the bladder wall while contracting the sphincter muscle but relaxes the detrusor muscle of the bladder and usually reduces the activity of the uterus. It has a stimulant action on the respiratory centre. It dilates the pupil but does not affect the light reflexes. After ephedrine has been used for a short while, tachyphylaxis may develop.

Ephedrine hydrochloride or sulphate, in doses of 15 to 60 mg by mouth 3 or 4 times a day, is of value in preventing bronchial spasm in asthma, but the more $beta_2$-selective sympathomimetic bronchodilating agents, such as salbutamol (p.30) are now preferred. Similar doses have been given by subcutaneous or intramuscular injection. A suggested dose for children is 500 µg per kg body-weight three or four times daily.

Ephedrine salts, in doses of up to 60 mg thrice daily are occasionally used in the treatment of narcolepsy, and doses of 25 or 30 mg thrice daily (usually as an adjunct to neostigmine) were formerly used in the management of myasthenia gravis; doses of 15 to 60 mg have been given at night for enuresis.

Ephedrine hydrochloride or sulphate has been given by subcutaneous or intramuscular injection to combat a fall in blood pressure during spinal anaesthesia. Ephedrine is of little value in hypotensive crises due to shock, circulatory collapse, or haemorrhage. It is no longer generally advocated for orthostatic hypotension.

For allergic disorders, such as hay fever or urticaria, ephedrine salts have been given by mouth or by inhalation as a spray or an aerosol; eye-drops containing 0.1% have been used to relieve the conjunctival congestion of hay fever. Nasal drops or, preferably, sprays usually containing 0.5% are used to relieve rhinitis and sinusitis, but their continued use is liable to aggravate the condition and may lead to rebound congestion and drug-induced rhinitis. A 0.25% or 0.5% strength is used for infants and young children.

For preparing solutions in oil, anhydrous ephedrine was formerly preferred but oily sprays and nasal drops should no longer be used since they reduce ciliary activity and may cause lipoid pneumonia.

Ephedrine has been used as a mydriatic; solutions containing 4 or 5% dilate the pupil fully within 15 to 30 minutes but accommodation is not significantly affected and ephedrine does not cause increased intra-ocular pressure. The effect lasts several hours. Ephedrine is often ineffective in the presence of iritis or iridocyclitis and also in highly pigmented eyes.

Ephedrine has also been given as the camsylate.

Allergy. For the use of ephedrine in chronic resistant urticaria, see Adrenaline (Allergy and Anaphylaxis), p.5.

Anaesthesia. Results of a double-blind study in 17 women undergoing spinal anaesthesia for caesarean section indicated that prophylactic deep intramuscular administration of ephedrine 50 mg reduced the incidence of maternal hypotension, as well as nausea and vomiting.— B. B. Gutsche, *Anesthesiology*, 1976, *45*, 462.

Asthma. A recommendation that non-selective oral bronchodilator drugs such as ephedrine should not be used for bronchodilatation.— A. B. X. Breslin, *Drugs*, 1979, *18*, 103.

Reports and studies of ephedrine in asthma and bronchitis: B. Badiei *et al.*, *Ann. Allergy*, 1975, *35*, 32; S. Chodosh and S. Doraiswami, *Curr. ther. Res.*, 1975, *18*, 773; C. J. Falliers and C. F. Katsampes, *Ann. Allergy*, 1976, *36*, 99; D. G. Tinkelman and S. E. Avner, *J. Am. med. Ass.*, 1977, *237*, 553; M. Weinberger (letter), *ibid.*, *238*, 1148.

Cardiac disorders. Haemodynamic effects of ephedrine in cardiac disorders.— J. A. Franciosa and J. N. Cohn, *Am. J. Cardiol.*, 1979, *43*, 79.

ENT disorders. Comment on the use of nasal drops, sprays, and inhalations. Since all vasoconstrictor drugs will, by virtue of the very action for which they are employed, rapidly produce some degree of 'rebound' vasodilatation their use should be restricted to not longer than one week. Ephedrine is usually prescribed as 0.5% and 1% drops in physiological saline; shrinking of the mucous membrane occurs within 15 minutes but the effect lasts only 3 hours. There is slow vasodilatation and little irritation, but continued use can still cause 'rhinitis medicamentosa'.— D. F. N. Harrison, *Prescribers' J.*, 1976, *16*, 69.

Further references: J. G. Fraser *et al.*, *J. Lar. Otol.*, 1977, *91*, 757 (otitis media).

Hypoglycaemia. Ephedrine in hypoglycaemia.— A. L. Rosenbloom and C. M. Tiwary, *Archs Dis. Childh.*, 1972, *47*, 924. See also J. M. Court *et al.*, *ibid.*, 1974, *49*, 63.

Further references: A. L. Rosenbloom (letter), *New Engl. J. Med.*, 1967, *276*, 638; T. R. Mereu *et al.* (letter), *ibid.*, 1156.

Hypotension. Ephedrine in doses of 30 mg abolished the postural symptoms in 4 patients with orthostatic hypotension but also produced recumbent hypertension. The long-term use of ephedrine for this condition was considered hazardous.— B. Davies *et al.*, *Lancet*, 1978, *1*, 172. Administration of ephedrine in association with propranolol had no beneficial effect in 4 patients with idiopathic orthostatic hypotension (Shy-Drager syndrome) and 1 with orthostatic hypotension believed to be of different origin.— M. S. Kochar and H. D. Itskovitz, *ibid.*, 1011.

Myasthenia gravis. The beneficial effect of ephedrine in myasthenia gravis has long been recognised, though the response is rarely striking. A dose of 30 mg thrice daily should be tried if the response to anticholinesterase agents is inadequate.— C. W. H. Havard, *Br. med. J.*, 1977, *2*, 1008.

Narcolepsy. Ephedrine, up to 150 mg daily, and nialamide, up to 100 mg daily, given to 3 patients with narcolepsy increased their drive and alertness, produced greater emotional stability, and fewer cataleptic attacks. No serious side-effects occurred though sympathetic function was enhanced.— H. G. Baumgarten and W. Bushart, *Eur. Neurol.*, 1970, *3*, 97.

Preparations of Ephedrine and its Salts

Capsules

Ephedrine Sulfate and Phenobarbital Capsules *(U.S.P.)*. Capsules containing ephedrine sulphate and phenobarbitone.

Ephedrine Sulfate Capsules *(U.S.P.)*. Capsules containing ephedrine sulphate. The *U.S.P.* requires 80% dissolution in 30 minutes. Store in airtight containers. Protect from light.

Elixirs

Ephedrine and Phenobarbitone Elixir *(A.P.F.)*. Ephedrine hydrochloride 20 mg, phenobarbitone sodium 15 mg, red syrup 2 ml, concentrated chloroform water 0.1 ml, water to 5 ml. *Dose.* 5 to 10 ml; children, 1 to 4 years, 2.5 ml.

Ephedrine Elixir *(A.P.F.)*. Ephedrine hydrochloride 20 mg, aromatic syrup 2 ml, concentrated chloroform water 0.1 ml, water to 5 ml. *Dose.* 5 to 10 ml; children, 1 to 4 years, 2.5 ml.

Ephedrine Hydrochloride Elixir *(B.P.)*. Ephedrine Elixir. Ephedrine hydrochloride 15 mg, water 0.3 ml, glycerol 1 ml, alcohol (90%) 0.5 ml, chloroform spirit 0.2 ml, compound tartrazine solution 0.05 ml, lemon spirit 0.001 ml, invert syrup 1 ml, syrup to 5 ml. When a dose less than or not a multiple of 5 ml is prescribed the elixir should be diluted to 5 ml, or a multiple, with syrup. Such dilutions must be freshly prepared and not used more than 2 weeks after issue.

Injections

Ephedrine Sulfate Injection *(U.S.P.)*. A sterile solution of ephedrine sulphate in Water for Injections. pH 4.5 to 7. Protect from light.

Mixtures

Ephedrine and Codeine Mixture *(A.P.F.)*. Ephedrine hydrochloride 10 mg, codeine phosphate 10 mg, squill oxymel 1 ml, tolu syrup 1 ml, concentrated anise water 0.25 ml, concentrated chloroform water 0.25 ml, water to 10 ml. *Dose.* 10 ml.

Nasal Drops

Ephedrine Instillation *(A.P.F.)*. Ephedrine Nasal Drops; Ephedrine Nasal Spray. Ephedrine hydrochloride 1 g, sodium chloride 500 mg, chlorbutol 500 mg, propylene glycol 5 ml, freshly boiled and cooled water to 100 ml.

Ephedrine Nasal Drops *(B.P.C. 1973)*. Ephedrine Aqueous Spray; Nebula Ephedrinae; Neb. Ephed. Aquos. Ephedrine hydrochloride 500 mg, sodium chloride 500 mg, chlorbutol 500 mg, freshly boiled and cooled water to 100 ml.

Solutions

Ephedrine Sulfate Nasal Solution *(U.S.P.)*. A solution containing ephedrine sulphate. Store in airtight containers.

Syrups

Ephedrine Sulfate Syrup *(U.S.P.)*. A syrup containing ephedrine sulphate 18 to 22 mg in each 5 ml, with alcohol 2 to 4%. Store at a temperature not exceeding 40° in airtight containers. Protect from light.

Tablets

Ephedrine Hydrochloride Tablets *(B.P.)*. Ephed. Hydrochlor. Tab.; Ephedrine Tablets; Compressi Ephedrini Hydrochloridi. Tablets containing ephedrine hydrochloride.

Ephedrine Sulfate Tablets *(U.S.P.)*. Tablets containing ephedrine sulphate.

Proprietary Preparations of Ephedrine and its Salts

Amesec *(Lilly, UK)*. Capsules each containing ephedrine hydrochloride 25 mg and aminophylline 130 mg. For asthma. *Dose.* 1 capsule once to thrice daily.

Asmapax *(Nicholas, UK)*. Scored sustained-release tablets each containing ephedrine resinate equivalent to ephedrine hydrochloride 50 mg and theophylline hydrate 65 mg. For chronic bronchitis and bronchial asthma. *Dose.* 1 to 2 tablets twice or thrice daily; children, half a tablet.

Asthma Dellipsoids D17 *(Pilsworth, UK)*. Tablets each containing ephedrine hydrochloride 20 mg, theobromine and calcium salicylate 100 mg, calcium iodide 20 mg, phenazone 125 mg, and prepared digitalis 12.5 mg.

Bronchial Dellipsoids D15 *(Pilsworth, UK)*. Tablets each containing ephedrine hydrochloride 20 mg, caffeine 30 mg, sodium benzoate 60 mg, prepared ipecacuanha 30 mg, and grindelia extract 125 mg. For bronchial asthma, bronchitis and colds.

Bronchotone *(Rorer, UK)*. A mixture containing in each 5 ml ephedrine hydrochloride 22.89 mg, caffeine 86.5 mg, sodium salicylate 91.85 mg, sodium iodide 57.04 mg, and belladonna tincture 0.52 ml. For asthma and bronchitis. *Dose.* Asthma, up to 15 ml every 4 hours; bronchitis, 5 to 10 ml.

CAM (Children's Antispasmodic Mixture) *(Rybar, UK)*. An aqueous liquid containing in each 5 ml ephedrine hydrochloride 4 mg and butethamate citrate 4 mg (suggested diluent water). For asthma and bronchitis. *Dose.* Children, up to 2 years, 2.5 ml thrice daily; 2 to 4 years, 5 ml; over 4 years, 10 ml.

Expansyl Spansule *(Smith Kline & French, UK)*. Sustained-release capsules each containing ephedrine sulphate 50 mg, trifluoperazine hydrochloride equivalent to trifluoperazine 2 mg, and diphenylpyraline hydrochloride 5 mg. For bronchospasm. *Dose.* 1 capsule night and morning; not more than 3 capsules in 24 hours.

Franol (known in some countries as Franyl) *(Winthrop, UK)*. Tablets each containing ephedrine hydrochloride 11 mg, phenobarbitone 8 mg, and theophylline 120 mg. For asthma and chronic bronchitis. *Dose.* 1 tablet thrice daily; children, one-third to one-half the adult dose.

Franol Expect *(Winthrop, UK)*. A linctus containing in each 10 ml ephedrine 9.5 mg, theophylline monohydrate 130 mg, guaiphenesin 50 mg, and phenobarbitone 8 mg (suggested diluent, syrup). For chronic bronchitis, bronchial asthma, and coughs. *Dose.* 10 ml thrice daily and at bedtime if required; children, one-third to one-half the adult dose.

Franol Plus *(Winthrop, UK)*. Tablets each containing ephedrine sulphate 15 mg, theophylline 120 mg, phenobarbitone 8 mg, and thenyldiamine hydrochloride 10 mg. For chronic bronchitis, asthma, and hay fever. *Dose.* 1 tablet thrice daily and 1 at bedtime where there are nocturnal asthma attacks; children, one-third to one-half the adult dose.

Iodo-Ephedrine *(Philip Harris, UK)*. A mixture containing ephedrine hydrochloride 8 mg, caffeine 90 mg, sodium iodide 90 mg, glycerol 0.9 ml, and decoction of coffee to 5 ml. For asthma. *Dose.* 5 to 10 ml thrice daily.

Norgotin Ear Drops *(Norgine, UK)*. Contain ephedrine hydrochloride 1%, chlorhexidine acetate 0.1%, and amethocaine hydrochloride 1%, in propylene glycol. For otitis media dnd otitis externa.

Phyldrox Tablets *(Carlton Laboratories, UK)*. Each contains ephedrine hydrochloride 12 mg, theophylline 128 mg, and phenobarbitone 8 mg; supplied **Plain** for prompt action and **Enteric-coated** for delayed action. For chronic bronchitis and bronchial asthma. *Dose.* 1 plain tablet thrice daily; 1 plain tablet and 1 coated tablet on retiring.

Tedral *(General Diagnostics, UK)*. **Tablets** each containing ephedrine hydrochloride 24 mg and theophylline 120 mg and **Suspension** containing the equivalent of half a tablet in each 5 ml (suggested diluent, syrup). For asthma, bronchitis, and hay fever. *Dose.* 1 tablet or 10 ml of suspension every 4 hours after food.

Tedral Expect. Linctus containing in each 10 ml ephedrine hydrochloride 20 mg, diprophylline 200 mg, and guaiphenesin 100 mg (suggested diluent, syrup). For chronic bronchitis and cough. *Dose.* 10 ml every 4 hours, after food; children, 6 to 12 years, 5 ml.

Tedral SA. Sustained-release tablets each containing ephedrine hydrochloride 48 mg and theophylline 180 mg. For asthma, chronic bronchitis, and hay fever. *Dose.* 1 tablet every 12 hours.

Other Proprietary Names

Ectasule Minus *(sulphate) (USA)*; Ephedral *(hydrochloride) (Belg.)*; Roter *(hydrochloride) (*see also under Bismuth Subnitrate*) (Neth.)*.

Ephedrine hydrochloride was also formerly marketed in Great Britain under the proprietary name Minims Ephedrine Hydrochloride (*Smith & Nephew Pharmaceuticals*).

Ephedrine sulphate was also formerly marketed in Great Britain under the proprietary name Spaneph (*Smith Kline & French*).

Preparations containing ephedrine hydrochloride were also formerly marketed in Great Britain under the proprietary names Asmal (*Norton*), Nomaze (*Fisons*), and Taumasthman (*Wallace Mfg Chem.*).

2059-m

Etafedrine Hydrochloride. Ethylephedrine Hydrochloride. (−)-2-(Ethylmethylamino)-1-phenylpropan-1-ol hydrochloride.
$C_{12}H_{19}NO,HCl=229.7$.

CAS — 48141-64-6 (etafedrine); 5591-29-7 (hydrochloride).

Soluble 1 in 1.5 of water and 1 in 8 of alcohol.

Etafedrine hydrochloride is a sympathomimetic agent with an action similar to that of ephedrine (p.10). It has been used for asthma in doses of 80 to 200 mg daily.

Proprietary Preparations

Nethaprin Dospan *(Merrell, UK).* Scored sustained-release tablets each containing etafedrine hydrochloride 50 mg, bufylline 180 mg, doxylamine succinate 25 mg, and phenylephrine hydrochloride 25 mg. For bronchospasm in bronchial asthma and chronic bronchitis. *Dose.* 1 tablet every 12 hours; children, 6 to 12 years, half a tablet.

Nethaprin Expectorant *(Merrell, UK).* Contains in each 5 ml etafedrine hydrochloride 20 mg, bufylline 60 mg, doxylamine succinate 6 mg, and guaiphenesin 100 mg. For unproductive cough and wheezing. *Dose.* 5 to 10 ml every 3 or 4 hours; children, 6 to 12 years, 5 ml.

2060-t

Ethylnoradrenaline Hydrochloride. Ethylnorepinephrine Hydrochloride *(U.S.P.).* 2-Amino-1-(3,4-dihydroxyphenyl)butan-1-ol hydrochloride.
$C_{10}H_{15}NO_3,HCl=233.7$.

CAS — 536-24-3 (ethylnoradrenaline); 3198-07-0 (hydrochloride).

Pharmacopoeias. In *U.S.*

A crystalline solid. M.p. 189° to 194°. **Soluble** in water. A 3.32% solution in water is iso-osmotic with serum. **Protect** from light.

Uses. Ethylnoradrenaline is a sympathomimetic agent with predominantly beta-adrenergic activity. Its actions are similar to those of isoprenaline (p.15) but it is reported to have only about one-tenth the bronchodilator activity of isoprenaline. Ethylnoradrenaline hydrochloride is usually given by subcutaneous or intramuscular injection in doses of 1 to 2 mg for its bronchodilator action in bronchial asthma.

Preparations

Ethylnorepinephrine Hydrochloride Injection *(U.S.P.).* A sterile solution of ethylnoradrenaline hydrochloride in Water for Injections. pH 2.5 to 5. Protect from light. It should not be used if it is brown or contains a deposit.

Proprietary Names

Bronkephrine *(Winthrop, Austral.; Breon, USA).*

2061-x

Etilefrine Hydrochloride. Ethyladrianol Hydrochloride; Ethylnorphenylephrine Hydrochloride; M-I-36. 2-Ethylamino-1-(3-hydroxyphenyl)ethanol hydrochloride.
$C_{10}H_{15}NO_2,HCl=217.7$.

CAS — 709-55-7 (etilefrine); 943-17-9 (hydrochloride).

Pharmacopoeias. In *Jap.*

Etilefrine hydrochloride is a sympathomimetic agent which has been used for the treatment of hypotension.

A comparative study in 6 healthy subjects of absorption time and rate, blood concentration, and biological half-life of etilefrine hydrochloride from a standard and a sustained-release preparation.— M. Donike *et al., Arzneimittel-Forsch.,* 1978, *28,* 856.

Hypotension. A double-blind controlled trial in 9 patients, aged 13 to 25 years, with orthostatic hypotension showed that a single daily dose of etilefrine hydrochloride 50 mg, as a prolonged-action preparation, was significantly more effective than a placebo in controlling blood pressure. No side-effects were observed. Etilefrine had an effect on α- and β-adrenergic receptors.— J. Ankerhus and E. Hansen, *Curr. ther. Res.,* 1969, *11,* 338. Of 15 patients with postural hypotension during treatment with levodopa 14 responded to treatment with etilefrine 15 mg daily. The mean reduction in systolic blood pressure on assuming an upright position was reduced from 26.3 to 4.3% and diastolic pressure from 14.2 to 1.2%.— E. Miller *et al., Archs Neurol., Chicago,* 1973, *29,* 99.

Further references: V. Lund *et al., Curr. ther. Res.,* 1972, *14,* 252 (in geriatrics); A. J. Coleman *et al., Eur. J. clin. Pharmac.,* 1975, *8,* 41 (cardiovascular effects).

Proprietary Names

Circupon RR *(Tropon, Ger.; Medichemie, Switz.)*; Effoless *(Jap.)*; Effortil *(Boehringer Sohn, Arg.; Boehringer Ingelheim, Belg.; Boehringer Ingelheim, Denm.; Boehringer Ingelheim, Fr.; Boehringer Ingelheim, Ger.; Boehringer Ingelheim, Ital.; Boehringer Ingelheim, Neth.; Boehringer Ingelheim, Norw.; Boehringer Ingelheim, S.Afr.; Boehringer Ingelheim, Swed.; Boehringer Sohn, Switz.)*; Efortil *(Boehringer Sohn, Spain)*; Presotona *(Erco, Denm.)*; Pressoton *(Erco, Swed.)*; Sanlephrin *(Jap.)*; Tensio Retard *(Trenker, Belg.)*; Tensofar *(Alet, Arg.)*; Tonus-forte-Tablinen *(Sanorania, Ger.)*; Tri-Effortil *(Boehringer Ingelheim, Ital.).*

2062-r

Etilefrine Pivalate Hydrochloride. K-30052. The hydrochloride of the 3-pivalate ester of etilefrine.
$C_{15}H_{23}NO_3,HCl=301.8$.

CAS — 42145-91-5.

Etilefrine pivalate hydrochloride is a sympathomimetic agent; it may be better absorbed than etilefrine hydrochloride.

Manufacturers

Klinge, Ger.

2063-f

Fenoterol Hydrobromide. TH 1165a. 1-(3,5-Dihydroxyphenyl)-2-(4-hydroxy-α-methylphenethylamino)ethanol hydrobromide.
$C_{17}H_{21}NO_4,HBr=384.3$.

CAS — 13392-18-2 (fenoterol); 1944-12-3 (hydrobromide).

A white odourless crystalline powder with a bitter taste. M.p. about 232°. Slightly **soluble** in alcohol.

Adverse Effects. As for Salbutamol, p.29.

Effects on the heart. Angina pectoris associated with the use of a fenoterol inhaler.— *Med. J. Aust.,* 1979, *2,* 92.

Treatment of Adverse Effects. As for Isoprenaline, p.15.

Precautions. As for Salbutamol, p.29.

CAUTION. *Excessive usage of aerosols of sympathomimetic agents has been associated with sudden death in asthmatics,* see p.15.

Absorption and Fate. Fenoterol is incompletely absorbed from the gastro-intestinal tract and is also subject to extensive first-pass metabolism by sulphate conjugation. It is excreted in the urine and bile almost entirely as the inactive sulphate conjugate.

A study of the pharmacokinetics of fenoterol after administration to *animals* and man. Fenoterol was readily absorbed from the gastro-intestinal tract; the half-life in man was estimated as 6 to 7 hours.— K. L. Rominger and W. Pollmann, *Arzneimittel-Forsch.,* 1972, *22,* 1190. Pharmacokinetics of fenoterol following inhalation.— C. D. Laros *et al., Respiration,* 1977, *34,* 131.

Uses. Fenoterol hydrobromide is a direct-acting sympathomimetic agent with actions and uses similar to those of salbutamol (p.30).

In the treatment of bronchial asthma fenoterol hydrobromide is used by inhalation in a dose of 1 or 2 inhalations of 200 µg, delivering at the mouthpiece 180 µg, thrice daily; up to 2 inhalations (400 µg, delivering at the mouthpiece 360 µg) may be used every 4 hours if necessary. A suggested dose for children is 1 inhalation of 180 µg thrice daily, increased to a maximum of every 4 hours if necessary. It has been given to adults by mouth in doses of 5 mg three or four times daily.

Fenoterol is also used similarly to salbutamol in the management of premature labour.

An extensive review of fenoterol, including details of its pharmacology, its pharmacokinetics, and its therapeutic potential in asthma.— R. C. Heel *et al., Drugs,* 1978, *15,* 3.

Allergy. Studies on the use of fenoterol intranasally in hay fever: P. Borum and N. Mygind, *J. Allergy & clin. Immunol.,* 1980, *66,* 25; M. J. Schumacher, *ibid.,* 33.

Asthma. Fenoterol and terbutaline in doses of 5 mg two to four times daily produced similar responses in a study of 30 patients with chronic bronchial asthma.— P. Chervinsky, *Ann. Allergy,* 1978, *40,* 189.

Further reviews, comments, and studies on the role of fenoterol in the management of asthma: S. C. Shore and E. G. Weinberg (letter), *Br. med. J.,* 1973, *3,* 350; M. I. Blackhall *et al., Med. J. Aust.,* 1976, *2,* 439; T. Morony (letter), *ibid.,* 1977, *2,* 688; S. N. Steen *et al., IRCS Med. Sci.,* 1977, *5,* 491; M. L. Brandon, *Ann. Allergy,* 1978, *40,* 86; E. Huhti and A. Poukkula, *Chest,* 1978, *73,* 348; G. E. Marlin *et al.* (letter), *Br. J. clin. Pharmac.,* 1978, *6,* 547; R. E. Ruffin *et al., Clin. Pharmac. Ther.,* 1978, *23,* 338; E. W. Watson, *Med. J. Aust.,* 1978, *2,* 230; M. Deloughery and D. Gilmore (letter), *ibid.,* 1979, *1,* 341; G. J. Addis *et al., Eur. J. clin. Pharmac.,* 1979, *16,* 97; S. P. Hanley and A. J. Nunn, *Clin. Trials J.,* 1979, *16,* 34; B. W. Madsen *et al., Br. J. clin. Pharmac.,* 1979, *8,* 75; P. Ravez *et al., Clin. Trials J.,* 1979, *16,* 147; R. E. Ruffin *et al., Clin. Pharmac. Ther.,* 1979, *25,* 821; S. L. Spector, *J. Allergy & clin. Immunol.,* 1979, *64,* 23; P. W. Trembath *et al., ibid.,* *63,* 395; S. Chambers *et al., Archs Dis. Childh.,* 1980, *55,* 73; S. S. Chatterjee and A. E. Ross, *Clin. Trials J.,* 1980, *17,* 7; W. C. Miller and D. L. Rice, *Ann. Allergy,* 1980, *44,* 15; T. Sasaki *et al., J. int. med. Res.,* 1980, *8,* 205; M. K. Tandon, *Chest,* 1980, *77,* 429; R. Yeung *et al., Pediatrics,* 1980, *66,* 109.

Pregnancy and the neonate. For comments on the efficacy of beta$_2$-selective adrenoceptor stimulants in the prevention of premature labour, see Salbutamol, p.31.

Studies of fenoterol in premature labour: J. Lipshitz and P. Baillie, *Br. J. Obstet. Gynaec.,* 1976, *83,* 864; J. Lipshitz, *ibid.,* 1977, *84,* 737; M. Marivate *et al., Am. J. Obstet. Gynec.,* 1977, *128,* 707; R. Richter, *ibid.,* *127,* 482; H. J. Seewald and V. Kuhnert, *Dte. GesundhWes.,* 1977, *32,* 107; G. G. M. Essed *et al., Eur. J. Obstet. Gynec. reprod. Biol.,* 1978, *8,* 341; K. D. Gunston and D. A. Davey, *S. Afr. med. J.,* 1978, *54,* 1141; M. F. Epstein *et al., J. Pediat.,* 1979, *94,* 449; R. Richter and M. J. Hinselmann, *Obstet. Gynec.,* 1979, *53,* 81.

Proprietary Preparations

Berotec *(WB Pharmaceuticals, UK: Boehringer Ingelheim, UK).* A pressurised spray for inhalation containing fenoterol hydrobromide and delivering 200 µg in each metered dose, of which 180 µg is available to the patient. (Also available as Berotec in *Arg., Austral., Belg., Canad., Denm., Ger., Neth., Norw., S.Afr., Spain, Swed., Switz.*).

Other Proprietary Names

Partusisten *(Arg., Belg., Ger., Neth., NZ, S.Afr., Switz.).*

2064-d

Fenoxazoline Hydrochloride. 2-(2-Isopropylphenoxymethyl)-2-imidazoline hydrochloride.
$C_{13}H_{18}N_2O,HCl=254.8$.

CAS — 4846-91-7 (fenoxazoline); 21370-21-8 (hydrochloride).

Uses. A 0.05 or 0.1% solution of fenoxazoline hydrochloride has been applied to the nasal mucosa as a nasal decongestant.

Proprietary Names

Aturgyl *(Dausse, Fr.)*; Nebulicina *(Castejon, Spain)*; Snup *(Karlspharma, Ger.).*

2065-n

Hexoprenaline Hydrochloride. ST 1512. *NN'*-Hexamethylenebis[4-(2-amino-1-hydroxyethyl)pyrocatechol] dihydrochloride; *NN'*-Hexamethylenebis[2-amino-1-(3,4-dihydroxyphenyl)ethanol] dihydrochloride.
$C_{22}H_{32}N_2O_6,2HCl=493.4$.

CAS — 3215-70-1 (hexoprenaline); 4323-43-7 (hydrochloride).

2066-h

Hexoprenaline Sulphate.
$C_{22}H_{32}N_2O_6,H_2SO_4=518.6$.

CAS — 32266-10-7.

Hexoprenaline is a direct-acting sympathomimetic agent with general properties similar to those of salbutamol (p.29). The sulphate has been used as a bronchodilator in doses of 250 to 500 µg thrice daily by mouth.

An evaluation of hexoprenaline including details of its absorption and fate.— R. M. Pinder *et al.*, *Drugs*, 1977, *14*, 1.

Asthma. Studies of hexoprenaline in asthma: C. Benjamin and A. Van As, *S. Afr. med. J.*, 1972, *46*, 599; A. Olinsky and J. Wolfsdorf, *ibid.*, 609; J. C. Vermaak *et al.*, *ibid.*, 1999; W. T. Ulmer, *Arzneimittel-Forsch.*, 1974, *24*, 840; S. D. Anderson *et al.*, *Med. J. Aust.*, 1977, *2*, 825; M. Schonell *et al.*, *ibid.*, 828; G. B. Irsigler and J. Ker, *S. Afr. med. J.*, 1978, *53*, 571; M. R. Harris *et al.* (letter), *Med. J. Aust.*, 1979, *2*, 545.

Pregnancy and the neonate. A favourable report of the use of bolus injections of hexoprenaline 10 µg to improve the foetal heart-rate in labour in 6 patients.— J. Lipshitz, *Am. J. Obstet. Gynec.*, 1977, *129*, 31. Studies suggesting that the metabolic effects produced by an infusion of hexoprenaline 10 µg in women in the third trimester of pregnancy would be beneficial to the foetus, especially in cases of acute foetal distress.— J. Lipshitz *et al.*, *ibid.*, 1978, *130*, 761. For criticisms of recommendations that a similar beta-adrenoceptor stimulant, ritodrine, should be used for the treatment of foetal distress, see *Drug & Ther. Bull.*, 1975, *13*, 26. See also *ibid.*, 1978, *16*, 83.

Proprietary Names of Hexoprenaline Salts

Bronalin (sulphate) *(Byk Liprandi, Arg.)*; Etoscol (sulphate) *(Byk Gulden, Ger.; Jap.)*; Ipradol (base, hydrochloride, or sulphate) *(Chemie-Linz, Aust.; Rosco, Denm.; Petersen, S.Afr.; Lacer, Spain)*; Leanol (sulphate) *(Jap.)*.

2067-m

Hydroxyamphetamine Hydrobromide *(U.S.P.)*. Oxamphetamine Hydrobromide; Bromhidrato de Hidroxianfetamina. (±)-4-(2-Aminopropyl)phenol hydrobromide.
$C_9H_{13}NO,HBr=232.1$.

CAS — 103-86-6 (hydroxyamphetamine); 1518-86-1 (hydroxyamphetamine, ±); 306-21-8 (hydrobromide); 140-36-3 (hydrobromide, ±).

Pharmacopoeias. In *Arg.* and *U.S.*

A white crystalline powder. M.p. 189° to 192°. **Soluble** about 1 in 1 of water and 1 in 2.5 of alcohol; slightly soluble in chloroform; practically insoluble in ether. Solutions in water have a pH of about 5. A 3.71% solution is iso-osmotic with serum. **Store** in airtight containers. Protect from light.

An aqueous solution of hydroxyamphetamine hydrobromide iso-osmotic with serum (3.71%) caused 92% haemolysis of erythrocytes cultured in it for 45 minutes.— E. R. Hammarlund and K. Pedersen-Bjergaard, *J. pharm. Sci.*, 1961, *50*, 24.

Adverse Effects, Treatment, and Precautions. As for Ephedrine, p.11. Hydroxyamphetamine has less central nervous system stimulant activity than ephedrine.

Absorption and Fate. Hydroxyamphetamine is readily absorbed from the gastro-intestinal tract. About one-third is excreted in a conjugated form and about one-third is excreted unchanged.

In 2 men given radioactive hydroxyamphetamine 92% of the radioactivity was excreted in the urine in 24 hours and 97% in 3 days. Excretion in the first 24 hours was almost entirely free and conjugated drug (88%) and free and conjugated 4'-hydroxynorephedrine (4%). In 1 subject given hydroxyamphetamine intravenously 75% of the dose was excreted in the urine in the first 5 days.— P. S. Sever *et al.*, *Trans. biochem. Soc.*, 1973, *1*, 1158.

Uses. Hydroxyamphetamine hydrobromide is a sympathomimetic agent with an action similar to that of ephedrine (p.11), but it has little or no stimulant effect on the central nervous system. It has been used topically as a vasoconstrictor, but does not produce vasoconstriction on injection and has not been employed to prolong the absorption of local anaesthetics. It has been used as a pressor agent and in the management of some cardiac disorders. The dosage has ranged from 20 to 60 mg three or four times daily for orthostatic hypotension and heart block.

In ophthalmology, hydroxyamphetamine hydrobromide is used in a 1% solution as a mydriatic.

Ocular disorders. For a comparison of the mydriatic effects of hydroxyamphetamine hydrobromide with those of 3 other commonly used mydriatics, see Homatropine Hydrobromide, p.301.

Preparations

Hydroxyamphetamine Hydrobromide Ophthalmic Solution *(U.S.P.)*. A sterile buffered aqueous solution of hydroxyamphetamine hydrobromide; it contains a suitable antimicrobial agent. pH 4.2 to 6. Store in airtight containers. Protect from light.

Proprietary Names

Paredrine *(Smith Kline & French, USA)*.

A preparation containing hydroxyamphetamine hydrobromide was formerly marketed in Great Britain under the proprietary name Vasocort *(Smith Kline & French)*.

2068-b

Hydroxyephedrine. *p*-Hydroxyephedrine; Methylsynephrine; Oxyephedrine. 1-(4-Hydroxyphenyl)-2-methylaminopropan-1-ol.
$C_{10}H_{15}NO_2=181.2$.

CAS — 365-26-4.

A crystalline powder. M.p. 152° to 154°. Sparingly **soluble** in water, alcohol, and ether; readily soluble in dilute acids and sodium hydroxide solution.

Hydroxyephedrine is a sympathomimetic agent with an action similar to that of ephedrine (p.10). The hydrochloride and the salicylate have been used in antitussive preparations.

2069-v

Ibuterol Hydrochloride. KWD 2058. 2-*tert*-Butylamino-1-(3,5-di-isobutyryloxyphenyl)ethanol hydrochloride; 5-(2-*tert*-Butylamino-1-hydroxyethyl)-*m*-phenylene di-isobutyrate hydrochloride.
$C_{20}H_{31}NO_5,HCl=401.9$.

CAS — 53034-85-8 (ibuterol); 61435-51-6 (hydrochloride).

Ibuterol is an inactive ester of terbutaline (p.31). After absorption into the body it is hydrolysed into terbutaline. It has been given as a bronchodilator by mouth as the hydrochloride in doses of 2 and 4 mg.

Studies on ibuterol in healthy subjects. It was found to be qualitatively identical to terbutaline but slightly less active after subcutaneous injection; by mouth it had a more rapid onset of action and was 2 to 3 times more active. Its greater efficiency by oral route might be related to different physicochemical properties, ibuterol being lipophilic whereas terbutaline is hydrophilic. It could be regarded as a pro-drug to terbutaline and might give more rapid and predictable therapeutic effects by mouth.— E. Höglund *et al.*, *Br. J. Pharmac.*, 1976, *58*, 43. The short duration of action following ibuterol administration appears to demand 5 times daily dosage in order to maintain an adequate serum concentration of active terbutaline during the 24-hour period.— Y. Hörnblad *et al.*, *Eur. J. clin. Pharmac.*, 1976, *10*, 9.

Asthma. Studies of ibuterol in asthma.— N. M. Johnson and S. W. Clarke, *Br. med. J.*, 1977, *1*, 1006; S. Larsson and N. Svedmyr, *Eur. J. clin. Pharmac.*, 1977, *11*, 429.

2070-r

Isoetharine Hydrochloride *(U.S.P.)*. Etyprenalinum Hydrochloridum; *N*-Isopropylethylnoradrenaline Hydrochloride. 1-(3,4-Dihydroxyphenyl)-2-isopropylaminobutan-1-ol hydrochloride.
$C_{13}H_{21}NO_3,HCl=275.8$.

CAS — 530-08-5 (isoetharine); 50-96-4 (hydrochloride).

Pharmacopoeias. In *U.S.*

A white to off-white odourless crystalline solid. M.p. 196° to 208° with decomposition. **Soluble** in water; sparingly soluble in alcohol; practically insoluble in ether. A 1% solution in water has a pH of 4 to 5.6. **Store** in airtight containers.

2071-f

Isoetharine Mesylate *(U.S.P.)*. Isoetarine Mesilate; Isoetharine Methanesulphonate; *N*-Isopropylethylnoradrenaline Mesylate.
$C_{13}H_{21}NO_3,CH_4O_3S=335.4$.

CAS — 7279-75-6.

Pharmacopoeias. In *U.S.*

White or almost white odourless crystals with a bitter salty taste. M.p. 162° to 168°. Freely **soluble** in water; soluble in alcohol; practically insoluble in acetone and ether. A 1% solution in water has a pH of 4.5 to 5.5. **Store** in airtight containers.

Adverse Effects, Treatment, and Precautions. As for Isoprenaline Sulphate, pp.15-6.

Interactions. *Anaesthetic agents.* The cardiovascular effects of isoetharine during cyclopropane anaesthesia were studied in 14 patients. Isoetharine, 1 to 15 µg per kg body-weight intravenously, caused a decrease in systolic and diastolic arterial pressures and an increase in heart-rate. Premature ventricular contractions did not occur. It was suggested that the drug could be used for treating bronchospasm developing during anaesthesia.— M. Shulman *et al.*, *Br. J. Anaesth.*, 1970, *42*, 439.

Uses. Isoetharine hydrochloride is a sympathomimetic agent with predominantly beta-adrenergic activity. It is used similarly to isoprenaline (see p.16) as a bronchodilator. The usual dose is 10 or 20 mg three or four times daily in a sustained-release tablet. Isoetharine mesylate is used in aerosol inhalations.

Asthma. Studies of isoetharine in asthma.— J. Kiviloog and N. Svedmyr, *J. int. Med. Res.*, 1976, *4*, 69; S. L. Spector *et al.*, *J. Allergy & clin. Immunol.*, 1977, *59*, 371; R. Imbruce and S. Nair, *J. clin. Pharmac.*, 1979, *19*, 662; J. Kaimal *et al.*, *Ann. Allergy*, 1979, *43*, 151.

Preparations of Isoetharine Salts

Isoetharine Hydrochloride Inhalation *(U.S.P.)*. A solution of isoetharine hydrochloride in water, rendered iso-osmotic by the addition of sodium chloride. pH 2.5 to 5.5. Store in small well-filled airtight containers. Protect from light.

Isoetharine Mesylate Inhalation Aerosol *(U.S.P.)*. An aerosol spray in a pressurised container containing a solution of isoetharine mesylate in alcohol, in an inert propellent basis. Store in small containers with metered-dose valves and oral inhalation actuators. Protect from light.

Proprietary Preparations of Isoetharine Salts

Bronchilator *(Sterling Research, UK)*. An aerosol inhalant containing isoetharine mesylate 0.6%, phenylephrine hydrochloride 0.125%, and thenyldiamine hydrochloride 0.05%, with saccharin, menthol, ascorbic acid, alcohol, and propellents, in an oral nebuliser delivering measured doses containing isoetharine mesylate 350 µg, phenylephrine hydrochloride 70 µg, and thenyldiamine hydrochloride 28 µg. For bronchospasm. *Dose.* 1 or 2 inhalations, repeated up to 8 times in 24 hours.

Numotac *(Riker, UK)*. Isoetharine hydrochloride, available as tablets of 10 mg, in a porous plastic basis. (Also available as Numotac in *Belg., Neth., Norw.*).

Other Proprietary Names

Asthmalitan Depot (hydrochloride) *(Ger.)*; Bronkometer (mesylate) *(USA)*; Bronkosol (hydrochloride) *(USA)*.

2072-d

Isometheptene Hydrochloride. 1,5,*N*-Trimethylhex-4-enylamine hydrochloride.
$C_9H_{19}N,HCl=177.7$.

CAS — 503-01-5 (isometheptene); 6168-86-1

(hydrochloride).

An almost white very hygroscopic crystalline powder. M.p. about 68°. **Soluble** in water and alcohol. **Store** in airtight containers.

2073-n

Isometheptene Mucate.

Isometheptene galactarate.

$(C_9H_{19}N)_2,C_6H_{10}O_8$=492.7.

CAS — 7492-31-1.

A white crystalline powder with a bitter taste. Freely **soluble** in water; soluble in alcohol; practically insoluble in chloroform and ether. A 4.95% solution in water is iso-osmotic with serum.

Adverse Effects, Treatment, and Precautions. As for Adrenaline, pp.2-3.

Uses. Isometheptene is a sympathomimetic agent which has been advocated for the relaxation of spasms. It has been given as the hydrochloride and as the mucate. It is given for a vasoconstrictor effect in migraine.

Migraine. Comment on the value of a preparation containing isometheptene mucate in the management of migraine.— *Drug & Ther. Bull.*, 1972, *10*, 64. Further references.— P. O. Behan, *Practitioner*, 1978, *221*, 937.

Proprietary Preparations

Midrid Capsules *(Carnrick, UK).* Each contains isometheptene mucate 65 mg, dichloralphenazone 100 mg, and paracetamol 325 mg. *Dose.* For migraine headaches, 2 capsules initially, followed by 1 capsule every hour up to a maximum of 5 capsules in 12 hours; for tension headaches, 2 capsules initially, followed by 1 or 2 capsules every 4 hours up to a maximum of 8 capsules per day.

Other Proprietary Names

Octinum *(hydrochloride and mucate) (Ital., Switz.).*

2074-h

Isoprenaline Hydrochloride *(B.P.).*

Isoprenalini Hydrochloridum; Isoproterenol Hydrochloride *(U.S.P.)*; Isopropylarterenol Hydrochloride; Isopropylnoradrenaline Hydrochloride. 1-(3,4-Dihydroxyphenyl)-2-isopropylaminoethanol hydrochloride.

$C_{11}H_{17}NO_3,HCl$=247.7.

CAS — 7683-59-2 (isoprenaline); 51-30-9 (hydrochloride).

Pharmacopoeias. In *Arg., Br., Braz., Chin., Hung., Int., Roum., Turk.*, and *U.S.*

A white or almost white, odourless or almost odourless, crystalline powder with a slightly bitter taste. It gradually darkens on exposure to air and light. M.p. 165° to 170° with decomposition. **Soluble** 1 in less than 1 of water and 1 in 50 to 55 of alcohol; less soluble in dehydrated alcohol; practically insoluble in chloroform and ether. A 1% solution in water has a pH of about 5. Solutions are **sterilised** by filtration and stored in ampoules, the air in which is replaced by nitrogen or other suitable gas. Solutions become pink to brownish-pink on standing exposed to air and almost immediately so when made alkaline. **Store** in airtight containers. Protect from light.

2075-m

Isoprenaline Sulphate *(B.P.).*

Isoprenalini Sulfas; Isopropylarterenol Sulphate; Isopropylnoradrenaline Sulphate; Isoproterenol Sulfate *(U.S.P.).*

$(C_{11}H_{17}NO_3)_2,H_2SO_4,2H_2O$=556.6.

CAS — 299-95-6 (anhydrous); 6700-39-6 (dihydrate).

Pharmacopoeias. In *Br., Cz., Fr., Ger., Ind., Int., It., Neth., Nord., Pol., Swiss, Turk.*, and *U.S.*

A white or almost white, odourless or almost odourless, crystalline powder with an astringent and somewhat bitter taste. It gradually darkens on exposure to light and air. M.p. about 128° with decomposition. **Soluble** 1 in 4 of water; slightly soluble in alcohol; practically insoluble in chloroform and ether. A 1% solution in water has a pH of 4 to 5.5. A 6.65% solution in water is iso-osmotic with serum.

Solutions are **sterilised** by autoclaving or by filtration. Solutions become pink to brownish-pink on standing exposed to air, and almost immediately so when made alkaline. Solutions should contain sodium metabisulphite as an antoxidant and should not be allowed to come into contact with metal, which causes discoloration and loss of activity; solutions for inhalation should be used in all-glass atomisers. **Store** in airtight containers. Protect from light.

Stability. The addition of sodium metabisulphite 0.1% reduced the discoloration and deposition of particles in an injection containing isoprenaline sulphate 0.02% in water, water adjusted to pH 3 with hydrochloric acid, or in McIlvaine's citrate-phosphate buffer solution pH 3. Solutions made using the buffer were more stable than those adjusted with acid. Autoclaving a solution adjusted with hydrochloric acid to pH 3 led to a 30% loss of potency. If sodium metabisulphite or McIlvaine's buffer solution was used the loss was about 7%. During storage, solutions sterilised by filtration lost no potency at 0° to 4°, about 2 to 10% at 25° over 24 weeks, and 5 to 23% at 37° over 8 weeks. A 0.02% injection of isoprenaline sulphate containing sodium metabisulphite 0.1%, buffered to pH 3 and sterilised by filtration, could be expected to maintain its appearance and potency for up to 6 months when stored in a refrigerator.— Pharm. Soc. Lab. Rep. P/77/2, 1977.

Adverse Effects. Side-effects associated with isoprenaline include nervousness, tachycardia, palpitations, and precordial pain. Other side-effects are hypotension with dizziness and fainting, headache, flushing of the skin, cardiac arrhythmias, tremor, weakness, and nausea and vomiting. Sweating may occasionally occur.

In the late 1960s, reports from many parts of the world indicated that the mortality-rate in patients suffering from asthma was increasing, particularly in asthmatics below 20 years of age. Sudden and unexpected death in asthmatics was also becoming more frequent and in many cases had followed excessive use of aerosols of bronchodilator drugs. Following warnings, use of the aerosols and deaths from asthma declined again. Because of the risk of tolerance and severe bronchoconstriction and the possibility of sudden death following the excessive use of sympathomimetic agents in aerosol form, the instructions for dosage should be followed carefully (see Uses, p.16).

Prolonged use of isoprenaline may lead to resistance, and eventual deterioration, with hypoxia in asthmatic patients.

Prolonged use of isoprenaline tablets sublingually has been reported to cause severe damage to the teeth.

Bronchospasm. Twelve of 41 patients with intractable asthma who were known not to be isoprenaline abusers developed paradoxical bronchospasm after inhalation of isoprenaline. They had not used isoprenaline aerosol for a year prior to evaluation. Furthermore, they consistently showed the expected bronchodilatory response when repeatedly challenged with terbutaline aerosol.— J. Trantlein *et al.*, *Chest*, 1976, *70*, 711. Discussion on the possible reason for such a paradoxical response (including a possible reaction to the aerosol propellent), and comments on the need for further information.— J. W. Jenne and T. W. Chick, *ibid.*, 691.

Effects on the heart. Investigations in 10 healthy subjects indicated that induced respiratory acidosis could alter the usual cardiovascular effects of isoprenaline given intravenously.— C. Xanalatos *et al.*, *Clin. Pharmac. Ther.*, 1973, *14*, 21.

The cardiac effect of repeated inhaled doses of isoprenaline was studied in 18 patients with moderate to severe asthma. Only 1 patient experienced a significant increase in heart-rate immediately after a therapeutic dose of isoprenaline. Arrhythmias did not develop even after repeated inhalations every 5 to 20 minutes.— C. Shim and M. H. Williams, *Ann. intern. Med.*, 1975, *83*, 208. See also J. W. Paterson *et al.*, *Lancet*, 1968, *2*, 426.

A review of patient records revealed 8 cases of documented isoprenaline cardiotoxicity at therapeutic dosages. Two patients developed acute myocardial infarction; a 3-year-old child developed reversible subendocardial ischaemia on receiving an isoprenaline infusion following cardiac surgery; and 5 patients with bronchial asthma demonstrated periods of transient myocardial ischaemia.— T. Winsor *et al.*, *Am. Heart J.*, 1975, *89*, 814.

Individual reports of adverse effects of isoprenaline on the heart: J. R. Matson *et al.*, *J. Pediat.*, 1978, *92*, 776 (myocardial ischaemia in a child); G. Kurland *et al.*, *J. Allergy & clin. Immunol.*, 1979, *63*, 407 (myocardial necrosis).

Animal studies on the adverse effects of isoprenaline on the heart, including induction of cardiac necrosis: M. F. Lockett, *Lancet*, 1965, *2*, 104; G. P. Leszkovszky and G. Gál, *J. Pharm. Pharmac.*, 1967, *19*, 226; T. Balazs *et al.*, *Toxic. appl. Pharmac.*, 1973, *26*, 407; D. G. McDevitt *et al.*, *Br. J. Pharmac.*, 1974, *50*, 335.

Effects on the teeth. A 12-year-old girl, who had been taking isoprenaline sulphate tablets sublingually for 6 years, developed discoloration and destruction of her permanent incisor and canine teeth. They were discoloured a chalky-white with a loss of the natural enamel translucency. Similar results were obtained with experimental teeth when they were immersed for 2 weeks in a solution of isoprenaline sulphate.— J. S. Ball (letter), *Br. med. J.*, 1965, *1*, 1189.

Overdosage. A 64-year-old patient who had been taking up to 260 mg of isoprenaline daily as sublingual tablets for bronchitis developed tremors, incoordination, a disturbing sleep pattern, and deep ulceration of the tongue. When isoprenaline was withdrawn the patient improved and after 4 weeks the ulcer had healed.— R. D. Brown and G. Bolas, *Br. dent. J.*, 1973, *134*, 336.

For controversy surrounding the role of overuse of isoprenaline aerosols and sudden death in asthmatics, see under Sudden Death (below).

Pulmonary oedema. For reference to pulmonary oedema associated with regimens incorporating beta-sympathomimetic drugs for the prevention of premature labour, see Ritodrine Hydrochloride, p.28 and Terbutaline Sulphate, p.32.

Sudden death. Between 1961 and 1966, rapid growth in the sales of pressurised aerosols of sympathomimetics in England and Wales corresponded with an increase in mortality due to asthma. The increase was greatest in children aged 10 to 14 years. Since March 1967, there had been a sharp fall in deaths due to asthma, together with a reduction in the use of pressurised aerosols.— W. H. W. Inman and A. M. Adelstein, *Lancet*, 1969, *2*, 279. See also H. E. Lewis, *Riker* (letter), *ibid.*, 799; *ibid.*, 800. For a similar report for Eire, see W. D. Linehan (letter), *Br. med. J.*, 1969, *4*, 172.

Comment on the surge in asthma fatalities that occurred in the 1960s and the growing realisation that pressurised aerosols were probably not the main culprit.— *Lancet*, 1979, *2*, 337. Strong disagreement with the view that the evidence is declining that pressurised aerosols were reponsible for the epidemic of asthma deaths in the 1960s.— P. D. Stolley and R. Schinnar (letter), *ibid.*, 897. Overuse of isoprenaline aerosols results in tolerance, not toxicity and the conclusion from this and other data can only be that the rise and fall of asthma mortality has a multifactorial aetiology which is only partly known.— H. Herxheimer (letter), *ibid.*, 1084. Following a general alert and warning on aerosol canisters, asthma mortality quickly declined to its former level.— A. M. Adelstein (letter), *Lancet*, 1979, *2*, 1247.

Early information from the British Thoracic Association's confidential enquiry into asthma deaths has indicated that, in general, patients die from asthma rather than from its treatment. When excessive use of bronchodilators does occasionally coincide with asthma death, it is likely that this indicates the need for further treatment by other drugs such as corticosteroids and is not itself the cause of death.— C. J. Stewart *et al.* (letter), *Lancet*, 1981, *2*, 747.

For earlier references to asthma fatalities in patients using isoprenaline aerosols, see Martindale 27th Edn, p. 16.

For a discussion on the avoidance of asthma fatalities with emphasis on the importance of the prompt treatment of severe acute asthma, see Corticosteroids, p.453.

Treatment of Adverse Effects. Most toxic effects of isoprenaline subside rapidly when treatment is stopped. Tachycardia and cardiac arrhythmias induced by isoprenaline may be diminished by propranolol but it must not be given to asthmatics because of the risk of increasing bronchoconstriction. Cautious use of a cardioselective beta-adrenoceptor blocking agent may be indicated in asthmatic patients.

Precautions. Isoprenaline should be avoided or only used with great caution in hypersusceptible patients or those with hyperthyroidism, and in serious cardiovascular disorders such as acute coronary disease or cardiac asthma. It should be used with caution in patients with diabetes mellitus or hypertension. It should never be given at the same time as adrenaline but may be used alternately. Isoprenaline may be used simultaneously with phenylephrine or dopamine.

Some asthmatics become tolerant to the actions of isoprenaline administered as an aerosol leading to their eventual deterioration from loss of sympathetic drive to the bronchi; in such cases the dosage should not be increased but alternative therapy including corticosteroids (see p.453) should be instituted promptly.

Isoprenaline is contra-indicated in digitalis intoxication and during anaesthesia with chloroform, cyclopropane, halothane, and other halogenated anaesthetics since it may provoke or worsen ventricular arrhythmias (see under Adrenaline, p.3). Isoprenaline exacerbates the adverse cardiovascular effects of tricyclic antidepressants, such as imipramine, and whenever possible concurrent administration should be avoided. Propranolol and other beta-adrenoceptor blocking agents antagonise the effects of isoprenaline. The effects of isoprenaline may be enhanced by concomitant administration of aminophylline.

The saliva or sputum of patients using isoprenaline inhalations may be coloured pink or red.

Interactions. Concomitant administration with isoprenaline of drugs, such as salicylamide, which are themselves extensively conjugated with sulphate, could increase the pharmacological effects of isoprenaline. Conjugation of isoprenaline in the gut wall could be decreased by salicylamide, thus increasing the amount of pharmacologically active isoprenaline absorbed.— M. E. Conolly *et al., Br. J. Pharmac.*, 1972, *46*, 458. See also C. F. George *et al., J. Pharm. Pharmac.*, 1974, *26*, 265.

Monoamine oxidase inhibitors. In 4 volunteers pretreated with phenelzine or tranylcypromine for 7 days, the pressor effects of isoprenaline were not enhanced and isoprenaline-induced tachycardia was significantly reduced. Imipramine increased isoprenaline-induced tachycardia two-fold in one of the subjects.— A. J. Boakes *et al., Br. med. J.*, 1973, *1*, 311.

Tricyclic antidepressants. The bronchodilator responses of isoprenaline in asthmatic patients had been reported to be enhanced and prolonged by imipramine. The anticholinergic effects of imipramine might be one of the factors accounting for the subjective feelings of improvement described by the patients.— M. J. Mattila and A. Muittara, *Annls Med. intern. Fenn.*, 1968, *57*, 185, per *Pharm. J.*, 1972, *1*, 559.

Absorption and Fate. As a result of sulphate conjugation in the gut, isoprenaline is very considerably less active following administration by mouth than following parenteral administration. It is absorbed through the oral mucosa and is accordingly given sublingually, but absorption by this route remains very erratic. This explains the wide difference between oral and parenteral doses of isoprenaline.

Pharmacologically active free isoprenaline in the body is resistant to metabolism by monoamine oxidase, but is metabolised by catechol-*O*-methyltransferase, this metabolite being subsequently conjugated before excretion in the urine. Whereas the sulphate conjugate of isoprenaline is inactive the methylated metabolite exhibits weak activity. Isoprenaline is also rapidly inactivated by processes involving uptake into tissues; it has been shown to be metabolised by catechol-*O*-methyltransferase in the lung.

Following intravenous injection isoprenaline has a plasma half-life of about one to several minutes according to whether the rate of injection is rapid or slow; it then has a terminal half-life lasting some hours, and is almost entirely excreted in the urine unchanged and in the form of its metabolites within 24 hours. A much slower onset of action and a more extended initial half-life has been demonstrated following oral administration. Isoprenaline is reported to have a duration of action of about 2 hours after inhalation; it has been demonstrated that a large proportion of an inhaled dose is swallowed.

References to studies on the absorption and fate of isoprenaline: E. W. Blackwell *et al., Br. J. Pharmac.*, 1970, *39*, 194P (metabolism following inhalation); C. T. Dollery *et al., Ann. N.Y. Acad. Sci.*, 1971, *179*, 108 (metabolism following inhalation); M. E. Conolly *et al., Br. J. Pharmac.*, 1972, *46*, 458 (metabolism in dogs and man); E. W. Blackwell *et al., Br. J. Pharmac.*, 1974, *50*, 587 (metabolism in the lungs); C. F. George *et al., J. Pharm. Pharmac.*, 1974, *26*, 265 (metabolism in the intestine); D. Kadar *et al., Clin. Pharmac. Ther.*, 1974, *16*, 789 (metabolic studies in brain-damaged children); J. G. Kelly and D. G. McDevitt, *Br. J. clin. Pharmac.*, 1977, *4*, 628P; *idem*, 1978, *6*, 123 (plasma-protein binding studies).

Uses. Isoprenaline is a sympathomimetic agent which acts almost exclusively on beta-adrenergic receptors. It stimulates the central nervous system. It has a powerful stimulating action on the heart and increases cardiac output, excitability, and rate; it also causes peripheral vasodilatation and produces a fall in diastolic blood pressure and usually maintains or slightly increases systolic blood pressure. It is used for the symptomatic relief of bronchial asthma although the $beta_2$-selective sympathomimetic agents, such as salbutamol are now generally preferred. Resistance to isoprenaline may develop and it is dangerous in the presence of hypoxia; for detailed recommendations relating to the emergency management of severe asthma, including a recommendation to use $beta_2$selective sympathomimetic agents, see Corticosteroids, p.453.

It is used in the treatment of bradycardia in patients with heart block, as a stimulant following cardiac arrest, and to control attacks of Stokes-Adams syndrome. In cardiogenic and endotoxic shock, isoprenaline has been used to treat patients who have failed to respond to replacement of electrolyte and water deficiencies.

Isoprenaline is usually administered sublingually or by inhalation, as the hydrochloride or sulphate, for its bronchodilator effects.

Pressurised aerosols containing isoprenaline and delivering metered doses of 80 micrograms of the sulphate are a commonly used form of inhaler. The hydrochloride is also used. The recommended adult dosage is 1 to 3 inhalations of 80 µg repeated, if necessary, after not less than 30 minutes up to a maximum of 8 inhalations in 24 hours. If more than 1 inhalation is taken at a time, at least 1 minute should elapse between any 2 inhalations.A stronger aerosol inhaler which delivers metered doses of 400 µg is also available in Great Britain. In the 1960s overuse of pressurised aerosol inhalers was an associated factor in an increase in sudden deaths among asthmatic patients (see under Adverse Effects, p.15). It is therefore essential to instruct the patients in the correct use of such preparations. If relief is not obtained the dose should not be increased and alternative therapy should be given.

Solutions containing 0.5 and 1% or more of isoprenaline sulphate have been inhaled in the form of a fine mist using an all-glass nebuliser, and the very finely powdered solid has also been inhaled.

Isoprenaline has been given by sublingual administration in the management of bronchospasm as the hydrochloride or the sulphate in usual doses of 10 to 20 mg thrice daily. The tablets were allowed to dissolve under the tongue without being sucked and as little saliva as possible was swallowed. Relief was usually felt within 2 to 4 minutes. It was recommended that isoprenaline should not be given more than four times daily by this route, and an interval of not less than 3 hours should be allowed between doses. A suggested dose for children was 5 to 10 mg sublingually thrice daily.

Doses of 10 to 30 mg have been administered sublingually 4 to 6 times daily to prevent cardiac stand-still in patients with a hyperactive carotid sinus reflex or in the treatment of heart block.

Sustained-release tablets of isoprenaline hydrochloride have been administered by mouth (*not* sublingually) in a dose of 30 mg thrice daily increased until the heart is sufficiently accelerated to a daily dose which may range from 90 to 840 mg daily, divided into a dosage frequency which may vary from every 2 to every 8 hours.

Isoprenaline, usually as 5 or 10 mg of the sulphate has also been given in suppositories for cardiac disorders.

Isoprenaline has also been given cautiously under ECG control, usually as a solution of the hydrochloride containing 1 mg in 500 ml of dextrose injection by slow intravenous infusion in the treatment of heart block, cardiogenic and endotoxic shock, and as a test of cardiac function. Concentrations of up to 10 mg in 500 ml have been used where limitation of volume is essential. The infusion-rate should provide 0.5 to 10 µg per minute, according to the patient's need; up to 40 µg per minute may be required for monitoring patients with heart block. It has been given subcutaneously or intramuscularly in doses of 200 µg as a 0.02% solution (1 ml) and in emergencies may be given by slow intravenous injection of 10 to 60 µg as a 0.002% solution (0.5 to 3 ml). Intracardiac injections of 20 µg as a 0.02% solution (0.1 ml) or 100 µg as a 0.001% solution (10 ml) have been used.

Allergy. Isoprenaline sulphate sublingually could sometimes abort recurrent acute attacks of urticaria.— R. H. Champion, *Br. med. J.*, 1973, *4*, 730. Comment on the treatment of reactions to bee and wasp stings. For portability, ease of administration, and speed of action in the relief of bronchospasm it would be difficult to improve on sublingually administered isoprenaline.— B. J. Freedman (letter), *ibid.*, 1979, *2*, 798.

See also under Adrenaline, p.4.

Asthma and bronchitis. Reports and studies of isoprenaline in asthma and bronchitis.— R. J. Knudson and H. P. Constantine, *J. appl. Physiol.*, 1967, *22*, 402 (inhalation); E. Tai and J. Read, *Thorax*, 1967, *22*, 543 (inhalation); K. N. V. Palmer and M. L. Diament (letter), *Lancet*, 1968, *1*, 1372 (inhalation); E. H. Chester *et al., Chest*, 1972, *62*, 394 (inhalation); H. Keltz *et al., Archs intern. Med.*, 1972, *130*, 44 (inhalation); D. W. Wood *et al., J. Allergy & clin. Immunol.*, 1972, *50*, 75 (intravenous infusion); D. W. Wood and J. J. Downes, *Ann. Allergy*, 1973, *31*, 607 (intravenous infusion); B. Dübi *et al., Schweiz. med. Wschr.*, 1974, *104*, 1244 (sublingual and inhalation); A. -H. E. Rubin *et al., Chest*, 1974, *66*, 133 (inhalation); M. S. Segal and S. Ishikawa, *Ann. Allergy*, 1975, *34*, 205 (inhalation); W. B. Klaustermeyer *et al., J. Allergy & clin. Immunol.*, 1975, *55*, 325 (intravenous infusion); W. H. Parry *et al., Am. J. Dis. Child.*, 1976, *130*, 39 (intravenous infusion); D. P. Tashkin *et al., Ann. Allergy*, 1977, *39*, 311 (inhalation); W. C. Posey and D. G. Tinkelman, *J. Allergy & clin. Immunol.*, 1979, *63*, 258 (inhalation); T. H. Rossing *et al., Am. Rev. resp. Dis.*, 1980, *122*, 365 (inhalation).

Cardiac disorders. *Heart block and Stokes-Adams syndrome.* A.J. Linenthal and P.M. Zoll (*Circulation*, 1963, *27*, 5) reported that attacks of Stokes-Adams syndrome could be successfully treated with intravenous infusions of isoprenaline or adrenaline at rates of 4 to 8 µg per minute although occasionally higher rates might be necessary. S. Dack (*Am. Heart J.*, 1963, *66*, 579) recommended injection of isoprenaline 200 µg or Adrenaline Injection 0.5 ml for immediate resuscitative measures, followed by intracardiac injection of isoprenaline or adrenaline 100 µg in 10 ml of Water for Injections if this was unsuccessful; an infusion of isoprenaline or adrenaline, 2 mg in a litre of dextrose injection, should then be given at a rate of 4 µg per minute or more according to the ventricle-rate; after stabilisation of the cardiac rhythm the infusion could be gradually reduced and replaced by intermittent intramuscular injections of isoprenaline 200 µg or adrenaline 500 µg, supplemented by isoprenaline orally. Similar therapy using weaker solutions and slower infusion-rates was recommended for Stokes-Adams syndrome precipitated by ventricular tachycardia or fibrillation. Isoprenaline as sustained-action tablets was recommended for long-term maintenance therapy in chronic atrioventricular block, side-effects being less evident than with sublingual treatment. Because of the risk of prolonged periods of arrhythmias precipitated by sustained-action isoprenaline an initial course of isoprenaline sublingually or intravenously was advocated by R. Bluestone and A. Harris (*Lancet*, 1965, *1*, 1299), and D. Redwood (*Br. med. J.*, 1968, *1*, 419) stated that the development of cardiac arrhythmias following a brief intravenous infusion of isoprenaline, 10 to 20 µg per minute, indicated when treatment with isoprenaline by mouth could be dangerous. Isoprenaline by intravenous route was more reliable than oral or sublingual administration for stimulating the higher pacemaker centres but constant ECG monitoring was needed to detect isoprenaline-induced ectopic tachycardia (R.M. Stanzler, *New Engl. J. Med.*, 1966, *274*, 1307). Despite well-documented reports of the value of long-acting isoprenaline hydrochloride tablets in carefully selected patients with chronic heart-block (D. Redwood, *Br. med. J.*, 1969, *1*, 26) it has been suggested that the mortality-rate remained lower in patients with endocardial pacing (M.E. Scott *et al.*, *Lancet*, 1967, *2*, 1382). Further references.— H. A. Fleming and S. M. Bailey, *Br. Heart J.*, 1972, *34*, 309.

Myocardial infarction. A review of the role of inotropic agents and infarct size. Isoprenaline is traditionally used to treat 2 specific complications of acute myocardial infarction: cardiogenic shock and bradycardia. In fact, its use in pump failure syndromes in acute myocardial infarction appears to be contra-indicated. Nor is it the treatment of choice to accelerate cardiac-rate when asymptomatic bradycardia complicates acute myocardial infarction. However, if atropine is ineffective and pacemaker therapy either unavailable or must be delayed, isoprenaline should not be withheld if it reverses bradycardia-induced hypotension, since the unequivocal risks of sustained hypotension far outweigh those of any potential extension of infarct size.— M. Lesch, *Am. J. Cardiol.*, 1976, *37*, 508.

Ocular disorders. The effect of isoprenaline eye-drops on raised intra-ocular pressure.— R. A. Ross and S. M. Drance, *Archs Ophthal., N.Y.*, 1970, *83*, 39.

A report of permanent visual impairment in 2 patients, associated with severe attacks of migraine. In a further 4 patients transient visual loss associated with attacks of migraine was alleviated by prompt inhalation of isoprenaline. Prophylactic inhalation of isoprenaline by migraine patients with visual symptoms may prevent transient visual loss, and possibly avoid permanent visual impairment.— M. J. Kupersmith *et al.*, *Stroke*, 1979, *10*, 299.

Diagnostic use. *Cardiac disorders.* Infusion of isoprenaline 1 to 2 µg per minute as a solution containing 2 µg per ml in dextrose solution was comparable to a treadmill exercise test in causing S-T depression of the ischaemic type, predictive of the presence of coronary artery disease. In 35 patients about to undergo coronary arteriography correct predictions were made in 71 and 68% respectively of the patients.— D. T. Combs and C. M. Martin, *Am. Heart J.*, 1974, *87*, 711. See also S. Mazzoni *et al.*, *Schweiz. med. Wschr.*, 1973, *103*, 1809. Exercise studies remain the method of choice for the complete evaluation of patients with aortic or pulmonary stenosis. The infusion of isoprenaline constitutes a practical alternative in those children in whom exercise studies are not practicable.— N. J. Truccone *et al.*, *Circulation*, 1977, *56*, 79.

Hypertension. The isoprenaline sensitivity test in patients with borderline hypertension.— G. M. London *et al.*, *J. clin. Pharmac.*, 1976, *16*, 174. See also C. R. Cleaveland *et al.*, *Archs intern. Med.*, 1972, *130*, 47; C. F. George *et al.*, *ibid.*, 361.

Pulmonary hypertension. A patient with primary pulmonary hypertension obtained a sustained beneficial response to administration of isoprenaline 20 mg sublingually every 2 hours with supplementary doses as needed; there were no unpleasant side-effects.— U. R. Shettigar *et al.*, *New Engl. J. Med.*, 1976, *295*, 1414. Marked symptomatic improvement was achieved in a 32-year-old woman with primary pulmonary hypertension by the administration of isoprenaline sublingually, taken to the limit of tolerance. Sudden death occurred after her condition had remained stable for about 2 years on isoprenaline 5 to 7.5 mg every 2 hours.— J. A. Pantano (letter), *New Engl. J. Med.*, 1980, *302*, 919. Isoprenaline caused exacerbation in a 46-year-old man; amelioration by isoprenaline is the exception not the rule, and monitoring of the pulmonary vascular pressures is mandatory to avoid aggravating the condition.— M. J. Belman *et al.* (letter), *ibid.*, 1978, *298*, 51. Reply.— H. N. Hultgren and U. R. Shettigar (letter), *ibid.*, 52.

Shock. In a 3-year prospective study involving 113 patients with septic shock considerable reduction in the death-rate was attributed to earlier positive-pressure ventilation and aggressive surgery in association with conventional therapy with fluids, oxygen, and antibiotics. Digoxin was given with increasing frequency and towards the end of the 3-year period digitalisation became almost routine; gentamicin and lincomycin became the initial antibiotics with others, usually carbenicillin, being added subsequently where appropriate. Isoprenaline was given to 20% of the patients during each of the 3 years and thymoxamine was given to 34% of the third-year group. Although corticosteroids (other than initial small physiological doses) and aprotinin were not given and heparin was only given to selected patients of the third-year group in the acute phase, only 2 deaths were attributed to continuing shock; this finding did not support suggestions that heparin, aprotinin, and glucocorticoids might reduce the incidence of deaths from shock, and the precise role of these agents remained to be established.— I. M. Ledingham and C. S. McArdle, *Lancet*, 1978, *1*, 1194.

Further references to the use of regimens incorporating isoprenaline in the management of septic shock.— G. G. Kardos, *New Engl. J. Med.*, 1966, *274*, 868; L. Weinstein and A. S. Klainer, *ibid.*, 950; H. J. du Toit *et al.*, *Lancet*, 1966, *2*, 143; E. J. Winslow *et al.*, *Am. J. Med.*, 1973, *54*, 421.

For a comment on the disappointing role of isoprenaline in cardiogenic shock, see under Cardiac Disorders (above).

Skin disorders. Reactivity to skin tests was reduced by iontophoresis with isoprenaline. This was consistent with a modification of the local synthesis of cyclic AMP.— R. H. Shereff *et al.*, *J. Allergy & clin. Immunol.*, 1973, *52*, 328.

Psoriasis. The daily application for 10 days of isoprenaline sulphate 0.1% in white soft paraffin to skin lesions of 12 patients with psoriasis caused a fall in the mean content of skin-glycogen, and a decrease in scaling. Remissions continued in 9 patients for up to 6 months and 3 other patients relapsed within 2 months. No changes in skin-glycogen content occurred in a further 3 patients treated with white soft paraffin alone.— N. S. Das *et al.*, *Br. J. Derm.*, 1978, *99*, 197.

Urticaria. For a comment on sublingual isoprenaline for recurrent urticaria, see under Allergy (above).

Preparations of Isoprenaline Salts

Inhalations

Isoprenaline Aerosol Inhalation *(B.P.C. 1973).* An aerosol spray in a pressurised container containing a fine suspension of isoprenaline sulphate in a suitable mixture of aerosol propellents. It may contain a surfactant, stabilising agents, and other adjuvants. Each metered dose delivers 80 µg of isoprenaline sulphate to the patient. Store in a cool place. *Dose.* 1 to 3 inhalations, repeated, if necessary, after 30 minutes, to a max. of 8 in 24 hours.

Isoproterenol Hydrochloride and Phenylephrine Bitartrate Inhalation Aerosol *(U.S.P.).* An aerosol spray in a pressurised container containing a fine suspension of isoprenaline hydrochloride and phenylephrine acid tartrate ($C_9H_{13}NO_2,C_4H_6O_6$ = 317.3) in suitable propellents. Store in small containers with metered-dose valves and oral inhalation actuators. Protect from light.

Isoproterenol Hydrochloride Inhalation *(U.S.P.).* A solution of isoprenaline hydrochloride in water, made iso-osmotic with sodium chloride. It should not be used if it is brown in colour or contains a precipitate. Store in small well-filled airtight containers. Protect from light.

Isoproterenol Hydrochloride Inhalation Aerosol *(U.S.P.).* An aerosol spray in a pressurised container containing a solution of isoprenaline hydrochloride in alcohol in an inert propellent vehicle. Store in small containers with metered-dose valves and oral inhalation actuators. Protect from light.

Isoproterenol Sulfate Inhalation Aerosol *(U.S.P.).* Isoproterenol Sulfate Aerosol. A suspension of microfine isoprenaline sulphate in fluorochlorohydrocarbon propellents in a pressurised container. Potency is expressed in terms of anhydrous isoprenaline sulphate. Store in small containers with metered-dose valves and oral inhalation actuators. Protect from light.

Isoproterenol Sulfate Inhalation Solution *(U.S.P.).* A solution of isoprenaline sulphate in water, rendered iso-osmotic by the addition of sodium chloride. Potency is expressed in terms of anhydrous isoprenaline sulphate. It should not be used if is brown in colour or contains a precipitate. Store in small well-filled airtight containers. Protect from light.

Strong Isoprenaline Aerosol Inhalation *(B.P.C. 1973).* An aerosol spray in a pressurised container containing a fine suspension of isoprenaline sulphate in a suitable mixture of aerosol propellents. It may contain a surfactant, stabilising agents, and other adjuvants. Each metered dose delivers 400 µg of isoprenaline sulphate to the patient. Store in a cool place. *Dose.* 1 to 3 inhalations, repeated, if necessary, after 30 minutes to a max. of 8 in 24 hours.

CAUTION. This preparation is approximately 5 times as strong as Isoprenaline Aerosol Inhalation (*B.P.C. 1973*).

Injections

Isoprenaline Hydrochloride Injection *(B.P.).* Isoprenaline Hydrochlor. Inj.; Isoprenaline Injection. A sterile solution of isoprenaline hydrochloride in Water for Injections containing suitable stabilisers. pH 2.5 to 3. Sterilise by filtration and distribute in ampoules in which the air is replaced by nitrogen or other suitable gas. Store in a cool place. Protect from light.

Isoproterenol Hydrochloride Injection *(U.S.P.).* Isoprenaline Hydrochloride Injection. A sterile solution of isoprenaline hydrochloride 180 to 230 µg per ml in Water for Injections. pH 3.5 to 4.5. It should not be used if it is brown in colour or contains a precipitate. Protect from light.

Tablets

Isoprenaline Tablets *(B.P. 1973).* Isoprenaline Sulphate Tablets. They contain isoprenaline sulphate together with citric acid monohydrate 1% and sodium metabisulphite 1%. They should be allowed to dissolve under the tongue. Store in airtight containers. Protect from light.

Isoproterenol Hydrochloride Tablets *(U.S.P.).* Tablets containing isoprenaline hydrochloride. Protect from light.

Proprietary Preparations of Isoprenaline Salts

Aleudrin *(Lewis, UK).* Isoprenaline sulphate, available as **Solution** containing 1% for inhalation, and as **Sublingual Tablets** of 20 mg. (Also available as Aleudrin in *Neth.*, *Switz.*).

Brontisol *(Brocades, UK).* A pressurised inhalant containing isoprenaline hydrochloride 0.3%, and deptropine citrate 0.2% in an inert propellent and providing in each metered dose isoprenaline hydrochloride 150 µg and deptropine citrate 100 µg. For bronchospasm. *Dose.* 1 to 3 inhalations.

Duo-Autohaler *(Riker, UK).* A breath-operated inhaler containing in each ml isoprenaline hydrochloride 8 mg and phenylephrine bitartrate 12 mg, delivering isoprenaline hydrochloride 160 µg and phenylephrine bitartrate 240 µg in each metered dose. For bronchospasm. *Dose.* 1 to 3 inhalations.

Iso-Autohaler *(Riker, UK).* A breath-operated inhaler containing isoprenaline sulphate 4 mg per ml, delivering 80 µg in each metered dose. (Also available as Iso-Autohaler in *Austral.*).

Medihaler Iso *(Riker, UK).* A pressurised spray for inhalation containing isoprenaline sulphate 4 mg per ml, providing 80 µg in each metered dose. (Also available as Medihaler Iso in *Austral.*, as Medihaler ISO in *Switz.*, and as Medihaler-Iso in *Belg.*, *Canad.*, *Neth.*, *S.Afr.*, *USA*).

Medihaler Iso Forte *(Riker, UK).* A pressurised spray for inhalation containing isoprenaline sulphate 20 mg per ml, providing 400 µg in each metered dose.

Medihaler-duo *(Riker, UK).* A pressurised spray for inhalation containing in each ml isoprenaline hydrochloride 8 mg and phenylephrine acid tartrate 12 mg, providing in each metered dose 160 and 240 µg respectively. For bronchospasm. *Dose.* 1 to 3 inhalations.

Min-I-Jet Isoprenaline Hydrochloride Injection *(IMS, UK).* A cartridge assembly containing a solution of isoprenaline hydrochloride 20 µg per ml, in vials of 10 ml.

PIB (Pressurised Iso-Brovon) *(Napp, UK).* Contains isoprenaline hydrochloride 0.35% and atropine methonitrate 0.1%, with propellents. Each metered dose provides isoprenaline hydrochloride 180 µg and atropine methonitrate 50 µg. **PIB Plus** contains isoprenaline hydrochloride 1% and atropine methonitrate 0.1% and provides in each metered dose isoprenaline hydrochloride 500 µg and atropine methonitrate 50 µg. For bronchospasm. *Dose.* 1 or 2 inhalations.

Saventrine *(Pharmax, UK).* Isoprenaline hydrochloride, available as sustained-action tablets of 30 mg. *Dose.* 1 tablet every 8 hours increased according to the needs of the patient; the tablets must be swallowed whole. (Also available as Saventrine in *Austral.*, *Norw.*, *S.Afr.*, *Switz.*).

Saventrine IV *(Pharmax, UK).* Isoprenaline hydrochloride, available as an injection containing 1 mg per ml, in ampoules of 2 ml. For the preparation of solutions for infusion. Saventrine IV was formerly known as Suscardia.

Select-A-Jet Isoprenaline Hydrochloride Injection *(IMS, UK).* A cartridge assembly containing a solution of isoprenaline hydrochloride 200 µg per ml, in vials of 5 and 10 ml. For preparing intravenous infusions.

Other Proprietary Names of Isoprenaline Salts

Arg.—Proterenal *(hydrochloride); Austral.*—Isuprel *(hydrochloride); Belg.*—Aleudrine *(sulphate)*, Isuprel *(hydrochloride)*, Proternol *(hydrochloride); Canad.*—Isuprel *(hydrochloride); Fr.*—Aleudrine *(sulphate)*, Isuprel *(hydrochloride); Ger.*—Aludrin *(sulphate)*, Bellasthman Medihaler *(sulphate)*, Ingelan *(sulphate); Jap.*—Isomenyl *(hydrochloride); S.Afr.*—Isuprel, Norisodrine *(hydrochloride); Spain*—Aleudrina *(sulphate); Swed.*—Isopropydrin *(sulphate)*, Mistaprel *(hydrochloride); Switz.*—Isuprel *(hydrochloride)*, Proternol *(hydrochloride)*, Suscardia *(hydrochloride); USA*—Aerolone *(hydrochloride)*, Isuprel *(hydrochloride)*, Norisodrine *(hydrochloride and sulphate)*, Proternol *(hydrochloride).*

Isoprenaline sulphate was also formerly marketed in Great Britain under the proprietary names Lomupren (*Fisons*) and Prenomiser (*Fisons*).
Preparations containing isoprenaline sulphate were also formerly marketed in Great Britain under the proprietary names Iso-Bronchisan (*Berk Pharmaceuticals*), Prenomiser Plus (*Fisons*), and Riddobron (*Riddell*, now *Seaford*).

2076-b

Levonordefrin *(U.S.P.).* *l*-3,4-Dihydroxynorephedrine. The laevo- form of nordefrin. (−)-2-Amino-1-(3,4-dihydroxyphenyl)propan-1-ol.
$C_9H_{13}NO_3$=183.2.

CAS — 829-74-3.

Pharmacopoeias. In *U.S.*

It is a white to buff-coloured, odourless, crystalline powder. M.p. about 210°. Practically **insoluble** in water; slightly soluble in alcohol, acetone, chloroform, and ether; freely soluble in aqueous solutions of mineral acids. A solution in diluted hydrochloric acid is laevorotatory.

Levonordefrin has general properties similar to those of adrenaline (p.1). It has been used as a vasoconstrictor in dentistry in a concentration of 1 in 20 000 in solutions of local anaesthetics.

2077-v

Mephentermine. *Nαα*-Trimethylphenethylamine.
$C_{11}H_{17}N$=163.3.

CAS — 100-92-5.

A clear colourless to pale yellow liquid with a fishy odour. Practically **insoluble** in water; very soluble in alcohol.

2078-g

Mephentermine Sulphate *(B.P. 1973).* Mephentermini Sulfas; Mephetedrine Sulphate; Sulfato de Mefentermina. *Nαα*-Trimethylphenethylamine sulphate dihydrate.
$(C_{11}H_{17}N)_2,H_2SO_4,2H_20$=460.6.

CAS — 1212-72-2 (anhydrous); 6190-60-9 (dihydrate).

Pharmacopoeias. In *Arg., Chin., Int., Ind.,* and *Turk. U.S.* has anhydrous or $2H_2O$.

Odourless colourless crystals or white crystalline powder. Mephentermine base 15 mg is approximately equivalent to 21 mg of mephentermine sulphate. **Soluble** 1 in 18 to 20 of water and 1 in 150 of alcohol; practically insoluble in chloroform and ether. A 2% solution in water has a pH of 4 to 6.5. A 4.74% solution is iso-osmotic with serum. Solutions are **sterilised** by autoclaving or by filtration. **Store** in airtight containers. Protect from light.

Incompatibility. Adrenaline hydrochloride is incompatible with mephentermine sulphate. Mephentermine sulphate is discoloured in the presence of oxidants.— R. C. Bogash, *Bull. Am. Soc. Hosp. Pharmsts,* 1955, *12,* 445.
A yellow colour was produced when mephentermine sulphate 120 mg per litre was mixed with hydralazine hydrochloride 80 mg per litre in dextrose injection.— B. B. Riley, *J. Hosp. Pharm.,* 1970, *28,* 228.

Adverse Effects and Treatment. Mephentermine may occasionally cause transient anxiety. Hypertension with headache, vomiting, and palpitations, is associated with overdosage.
The hypertensive effects of mephentermine may be treated with an alpha-adrenergic blocking agent such as 5 to 10 mg of phentolamine mesylate intravenously, repeated as necessary.

Abuse. Paranoid hallucinations, which seemed to be identical to amphetamine psychosis or acute paranoid schizophrenia, occurred in 3 patients after abuse of mephentermine aerosols.— B. M. Angrist *et al., Am. J. Psychiat.,* 1970, *126,* 1315.

Precautions. Mephentermine sulphate should be used with caution in patients with hypertension, hyperthyroidism, or severe cardiovascular disease. Its use is contra-indicated in peripheral vascular collapse following severe haemorrhage until fluid loss has been replaced, and in the treatment of hypotension caused by chlorpromazine, as it may further lower the blood pressure.
It should not be given to patients being treated with a monoamine oxidase inhibitor or within 14 days of stopping such treatment (see Precautions for Phenelzine Sulphate p.128); caution is also necessary in patients receiving tricyclic antidepressants. Although the central nervous stimulant effects of mephentermine are much less than those of methylamphetamine its use may lead to dependence of the amphetamine type.
Mutual antagonism may exist between the effects of mephentermine and antihypertensives such as guanethidine, reserpine, and methyldopa.

Absorption and Fate. Mephentermine is readily absorbed from the gastro-intestinal tract. It acts in about 10 minutes following intramuscular injection and has a duration of action of about 2 hours or more, and almost immediately following intravenous injection with a duration of action of about 30 minutes. It is rapidly metabolised in the body by demethylation; hydroxylation may follow.

Uses. Mephentermine sulphate is a sympathomimetic agent with mainly indirect effects on adrenergic receptors. It has alpha- and beta-adrenergic activity, and a slight stimulating effect on the central nervous system.
Mephentermine sulphate has been used to maintain blood pressure in hypotensive states, for example following surgical operations or spinal anaesthesia. For this purpose the equivalent of 15 to 60 mg of mephentermine base was injected slowly over 1 or 2 minutes into a vein followed, if necessary, by an intravenous infusion of 600 mg in 500 ml of dextrose injection at a rate sufficient to maintain the pressure, or by 15 to 30 mg intramuscularly.
Mephentermine sulphate was also formerly given by mouth for its mood-elevating effects. A 0.5% solution of mephentermine sulphate was applied locally as a nasal decongestant.

Mephentermine sulphate, 750 µg per kg body-weight, given by intravenous injection over 20 seconds to 5 healthy volunteers caused an increase in arterial pressure during the first minute, followed by a gradual fall. No change in heart-rate, cardiac output or stroke-volume occurred, but the systemic vascular resistance doubled and there was gradual increase in left ventricular minute work, accompanied by a feeling of relaxation in all and some analgesia in 2 of the recipients, for 1 hour. Given 10 to 15 minutes after atropine 1 to 2 mg, mephentermine maintained the cardiac output above the initial value in 4 of the 5 volunteers, but this dose of atropine produced too great an increase in heart-rate and a fall in stroke-volume.— N. T. Smith, *Br. J. Anaesth.,* 1972, *44,* 452.

Further references to the use of mephentermine sulphate.— J. S. Gravenstein, *Clin. Anaesth.,* 1963, *3,* 13 (test for sympathetic reactivity); V. N. Udhoji and M. H. Weil, *Am. J. Cardiol.,* 1965, *16,* 841 (endotoxic shock); R. F. Cucchiara *et al., Anesthiology,* 1973, *39,* 109 (hypertensive in spinal anaesthesia).

Preparations

Mephentermine Injection *(B.P. 1973).* Mephentermine Inj. A sterile solution of mephentermine sulphate in Water for Injections containing suitable buffering agents. pH 4 to 6.5.

Mephentermine Sulfate Injection *(U.S.P.).* A sterile solution of mephentermine sulphate in Water for Injections. Potency is expressed in terms of the equivalent amount of mephentermine. pH 4 to 6.5.

Proprietary Names

Wyamine *(sulphate) (Wyeth, Belg.; Wyeth, Neth.);* Wyamine Sulfate *(sulphate) (Wyeth, USA).*

Mephentermine sulphate was formerly marketed in Great Britain under the proprietary name Mephine (*Wyeth*).

2079-q

Metaraminol Tartrate *(B.P.).* Metaraminol Acid Tartrate; Metaraminol Bitartrate *(U.S.P.);* Metaradrini Bitartras; Hydroxynorephedrine Bitartrate. (−)-2-Amino-1-(3-hydroxyphenyl)propan-1-ol hydrogen tartrate.
$C_9H_{13}NO_2,C_4H_6O_6$=317.3.

CAS — 54-49-9 (metaraminol); 33402-03-8 (tartrate).

Pharmacopoeias. In *Br., Braz., Chin., Nord., Turk.,* and *U.S.*

An almost odourless, white, crystalline powder with a bitter taste. M.p. 171° to 178°. Metaraminol tartrate 9.5 mg is approximately equivalent to 5 mg of metaraminol. **Soluble** 1 in 3 of water and 1 in 100 of alcohol; practically insoluble in chloroform and ether. A solution in water is laevorotatory. A 5% solution in water has a pH of 3.2 to 3.5. A 5.17% solution is iso-osmotic with serum. Solutions are **sterilised** by filtration. **Store** in airtight containers.

Incompatibility. Metaraminol 20 mg was 'physically incompatible' with fibrinogen 200 mg, thiopentone sodium 250 mg, or warfarin sodium 10 mg in 100 ml of dextrose injection.— R. D. Dunworth and F. R. Kenna, *Am. J. Hosp. Pharm.,* 1965, *22,* 190. There was loss of clarity when intravenous solutions of metaraminol tartrate were mixed with those of benzylpenicillin, hydrocortisone sodium succinate, methicillin sodium, or phenytoin sodium, or (in dextrose injection) thiopentone sodium or warfarin sodium.— J. A. Patel and G. L. Phillips, *ibid.,* 1966, *23,* 409. See also R. Misgen, *ibid.,* 1965, *22,* 92. Nitrofurantoin sodium in dextrose injection was incompatible with metaraminol tartrate; the pH fell to 7.2 and a brown precipitate was formed.— M. Edward, *ibid.,* 1967, *24,* 440. A report of compatibility for 24 hours.— E. A. Parker, *ibid.,* 1970, *27,* 672. A haze developed over 3 hours when metaraminol tartrate 200 mg per litre was mixed with amphotericin 200 mg per litre in dextrose injection; a crystalline precipitate occurred with sulphadiazine sodium 4 g per litre in dextrose injection or sodium chloride injection.— B. B. Riley, *J. Hosp. Pharm.,* 1970, *28,* 228. Metaraminol tartrate was physically incompatible with methylprednisolone sodium succinate, hydrocortisone sodium succinate, prednisolone sodium phosphate, and dexamethasone sodium phosphate in sodium chloride injection and dextrose injection. However, metaraminol appeared to be compatible with hydrocortisone and hydrocortisone 21-phosphate.— F. E. Turner and J. C. King, *Am. J. Hosp. Pharm.,* 1973, *30,* 128.

Stability. Metaraminol tartrate 100 mg per litre had good chemical and biological stability in intravenous fluids at pH 3.75 to 6.25 for up to 48 hours at room temperature.— E. A. Parker, *Am. J. Hosp. Pharm.,* 1967, *24,* 425. Metaraminol tartrate was stable under the following conditions for at least 48 hours at concentrations commonly used in intravenous fluids at pH values from 2.1 to 9.9; in conjunction with hydrocortisone sodium succinate; in conjunction with dextrose 5% in sodium chloride injection; and in conjunction with both hydrocortisone sodium succinate and dextrose 5% in sodium chloride injection.— R. W. Anderson and C. J. Latiolais, *ibid.,* 1970, *27,* 540.

Adverse Effects and Treatment. Side-effects include headache, dizziness, tremor, nausea and vomiting, palpitations, tachycardia and other cardiac arrhythmias. They are usually due to induced hypertension and subside as the blood pressure reaches more normal levels.
Tissue necrosis can occur as a result of accidental extravasation during intravenous injection.
The hypertensive effects of metaraminol may be treated with an alpha-adrenoceptor blocking agent such as 5 to 10 mg of phentolamine mesylate intravenously repeated as necessary.

Precautions. Care is required when using metaraminol tartrate in patients with severe coronary disease, diabetes mellitus, hypertension, or hyperthyroidism. Where necessary volume expanders should be given before injection. It should not be given to patients being treated with a monoamine oxidase inhibitor or within 14 days of stopping such treatment (see Precautions for Phenelzine Sulphate, p.128).

Although metaraminol is less likely than adrenaline to provoke cardiac arrhythmias in patients receiving cyclopropane and halothane or other halogenated anaesthetics, concurrent use should be avoided when possible (see p.3). Metaraminol may increase the possibility of arrhythmias in digitalised patients.

After metaraminol has been infused for some time, withdrawal may lead to recurrent hypotension; it has been suggested that an infusion of noradrenaline may restore responsiveness.

Mutual antagonism may exist between the effects of metaraminol and antihypertensives, but patients receiving guanethidine or reserpine may be particularly susceptible to the hypertensive properties of metaraminol.

Absorption and Fate. Metaraminol is absorbed when taken by mouth but considerably greater amounts are necessary to equal the effects of intramuscular or intravenous injections. It acts 5 to 15 minutes after subcutaneous or intramuscular injection and has a duration of action of about 1 hour and 1 to 2 minutes after intravenous injection with a duration of action of about 20 minutes. It is not acted on by monoamine oxidase.

Uses. Metaraminol tartrate is a sympathomimetic agent with direct and indirect effects on adrenergic receptors. It has alpha- and beta-adrenergic activity, the former being predominant. Metaraminol increases cardiac output, peripheral resistance, and blood pressure. Coronary blood flow is increased and the heart-rate slowed. Its pressor action varies from 20 to 60 minutes according to the route of administration. In doses equivalent to metaraminol 2 to 10 mg by subcutaneous or intramuscular injection, metaraminol tartrate is used for its pressor action in hypotensive states, e.g. following surgical operation or spinal anaesthesia. As the maximum effects are not immediately apparent, at least 10 minutes should elapse before repeating a dose and the possibility of a cumulative effect should be borne in mind. An intravenous infusion of 15 to 100 mg per 500 ml of dextrose injection or sodium chloride injection may also be used for maintaining the blood pressure. In an emergency a dose of 0.5 to 5 mg may be given by direct intravenous injection.

Suggested doses for children are the equivalent of 100 µg per kg body-weight by subcutaneous or intramuscular injection, the equivalent of 400 µg per kg by intravenous infusion at a rate determined by the blood pressure, or the equivalent of 10 µg per kg by intravenous injection.

Cardiac disorders. Patients with paroxysmal supraventricular tachycardia but without organic heart disease had been treated for some years with carotid sinus pressure, or, if necessary, 5 mg of metaraminol given subcutaneously. If the paroxysms continued for more than 20 minutes, 2 mg made up to 2 ml with the patient's venous blood was slowly injected intravenously while monitoring the heart beat for conversion to sinus rhythm. In cases where this failed, sedation and digitalis were given.— D. Bowers (letter), *Can. med. Ass. J.*, 1968, *99*, 868.

Shock. In the treatment of septic shock, pressor agents had been used only in those patients whose blood pressure was unrecordable. Small doses of metaraminol had been given until the arterial pressure had risen to 35 to 40 mmHg in order to establish the peripheral circulation for other medicaments. For the most part, the administration of noradrenaline had been abandoned.— L. Weinstein and A. S. Klainer, *New Engl. J. Med.*, 1966, *274*, 950. For a long-term study involving the use of sympathomimetic agents in septic shock, see Isoprenaline, p.17.

Preparations

Metaraminol Bitartrate Injection *(U.S.P.)*. A sterile solution of metaraminol tartrate in Water for Injections. It contains the equivalent of 9 to 11 mg of metaraminol per ml. pH 3.2 to 4.5. Protect from light.

Metaraminol Injection *(B.P.)*. Metaraminol Acid Tartrate Injection. A sterile solution of metaraminol tartrate in Water for Injections containing a suitable stabilising agent. Sterilised by filtration. pH 3.2 to 4.5. Potency is expressed in terms of the equivalent amount of metaraminol. Protect from light.

Aramine *(Merck Sharp & Dohme, UK)*. Metaraminol tartrate, available as an injection containing the equivalent of 10 mg of metaraminol per ml, in ampoules of 1 ml and vials of 10 ml. (Also available as Aramine in *Austral., Belg., Canad., Denm., Fr., Norw., Swed., USA*).

Other Proprietary Names

Araminum *(Ger.)*; Levicor *(Ital.)*.

2080-d

Methoxamine Hydrochloride *(B.P., U.S.P.)*.

Methoxamini Hydrochloridum; Methoxamini Chloridum; Methoxamedrine Hydrochloride. 2-Amino-1-(2,5-dimethoxyphenyl)propan-1-ol hydrochloride.

$C_{11}H_{17}NO_3,HCl = 247.7$.

CAS — 390-28-3 (methoxamine); 61-16-5 (hydrochloride).

Pharmacopoeias. In *Br., Chin., Int., Nord.*, and *U.S.*

Colourless or white plate-like crystals or white crystalline powder; odourless or with a slight odour, and a bitter taste. M.p. 214° to 219°. **Soluble** 1 in 2.5 of water and 1 in 12 of alcohol; very slightly soluble in chloroform and ether. A 2% solution in water has a pH of 4 to 6. A 3.82% solution is iso-osmotic with serum. Solutions are **sterilised** by autoclaving or by filtration; before autoclaving or after filtration, the solution is distributed into ampoules, the air in which is replaced by nitrogen or other suitable gas. **Incompatible** with alkalis. **Store** in airtight containers. Protect from light.

An aqueous solution of methoxamine hydrochloride iso-osmotic with serum (3.82%) caused 88% haemolysis of erythrocytes cultured in it for 45 minutes.— E. R. Hammarlund and K. Pedersen-Bjergaard, *J. pharm. Sci.*, 1961, *50*, 24.

Adverse Effects and Treatment. Fluid losses should be replaced where necessary before injection. Methoxamine hydrochloride may produce an undesirably high blood pressure which causes headache and vomiting. Reflex bradycardia may occasionally occur which may be prevented or abolished with atropine although there may still be some residual slowing possibly due to a beta-adrenoceptor blocking effect of methoxamine. Methoxamine may also induce a desire to micturate and a pilomotor reaction (goose flesh). The hypertensive effects of methoxamine may be treated with an alpha-adrenoceptor blocking agent such as 5 to 10 mg of phentolamine mesylate intravenously, repeated as necessary.

Precautions. Methoxamine hydrochloride is contra-indicated in severe coronary disease, and should be avoided or only used with extreme caution in hypertension, cardiovascular disease, or hyperthyroidism.

It should not be given to patients being treated with a monoamine oxidase inhibitor, or within 14 days of stopping such treatment (see Precautions for Phenelzine Sulphate, p.128); caution is also necessary in patients receiving tricyclic antidepressants.

Mutual antagonism may exist between the effects of methoxamine and antihypertensives, but patients receiving guanethidine or reserpine may be particularly susceptible to the hypertensive properties of methoxamine.

Absorption and Fate. Methoxamine acts about 1 to 2 minutes after intravenous injection and within about 15 to 20 minutes of intramuscular injection and lasts for about 1 hour and about 1½ hours respectively. It is not acted on by monoamine oxidase.

Uses. Methoxamine hydrochloride is a sympathomimetic agent with mainly direct effects on adrenergic receptors. It has alpha-adrenergic activity entirely; beta-adrenergic activity is not demonstrable and beta-adrenoceptor blockade effect has been reported.

Methoxamine hydrochloride causes prolonged peripheral vasoconstriction and consequently a rise in arterial blood pressure. It has little effect on the heart, though reflex bradycardia may occur. It has a marked pilomotor effect but does not stimulate the central nervous system or cause bronchodilatation. It markedly reduces blood flow to the kidney.

In usual doses of 10 to 15 mg intramuscularly (range 5 to 20 mg), methoxamine hydrochloride is used for its pressor action in hypotensive states, e.g. following surgical operation or spinal anaesthesia; it may be used in patients who have received cyclopropane or halothane anaesthesia. As the maximum effects are not immediately apparent, about 15 minutes should elapse before repeating a dose. In an emergency 3 to 5 mg may be given by slow intravenous injection. It may be given for paroxysmal supraventricular tachycardia in doses of 10 mg intravenously.

Methoxamine hydrochloride has been used for nasal vasoconstriction and decongestion as a solution containing 0.25%.

Preparations

Methoxamine Hydrochloride Injection *(U.S.P.)*. A sterile solution in Water for Injections. pH 3 to 5. Protect from light.

Methoxamine Injection *(B.P.)*. Methoxamine Hydrochloride Injection. Methoxamine hydrochloride 2 g, sodium chloride 430 mg, Water for Injections to 100 ml. Distribute into ampoules, replace the air by nitrogen or other suitable gas, seal, and sterilise by autoclaving.

Vasoxine *(Calmic, UK)*. Methoxamine hydrochloride, available as an injection containing 20 mg per ml, in ampoules of 1 ml. (Also available as Vasoxine in *Ital.*).

Other Proprietary Names

Idasal *(Spain)*; Vasoxyl *(Canad., USA)*; Vasylox Junior *(Austral.)*.

Methoxamine hydrochloride was also formerly marketed in Great Britain under the proprietary name Vasylox (*Wellcome Consumer Division*).

2081-n

Methoxyphenamine Hydrochloride *(U.S.P.)*. Methoxiphenadrin Hydrochloride; Mexyphamine Hydrochloride. 2-Methoxy-*N*α-dimethylphenethylamine hydrochloride.

$C_{11}H_{17}NO,HCl = 215.7$.

CAS — 93-30-1 (methoxyphenamine); 5588-10-3 (hydrochloride).

Pharmacopoeias. In *U.S.*

White or off-white crystals or powder with a faint characteristic odour and a bitter taste. M.p. about 130°. Freely **soluble** in water, alcohol, and chloroform; slightly soluble in ether. A 5% solution in water has a pH of about 5.5. A 3.47% solution is iso-osmotic with serum. **Store** in airtight containers. Protect from light.

Adverse Effects, Treatment, and Precautions. As for Isoprenaline, pp.15-6. It may occasionally cause drowsiness.

Uses. Methoxyphenamine hydrochloride is a sympathomimetic agent with predominantly beta-adrenergic activity. It also has weak antihistamine properties. It has been given as a bronchodilator in doses of 50 to 100 mg every 4 hours.

Identification of metabolites of methoxyphenamine in man.— I. J. McGilveray *et al.*, *J. Pharm. Pharmac.*, 1976, *28, Suppl.*, 55P.

Proprietary Preparations

Orthoxine *(Upjohn, UK)*. Methoxyphenamine hydrochloride, available as scored tablets of 100 mg. (Also available as Orthoxine in *Austral., Belg., S.Afr.*). **Orthoxicol**. A syrup containing in each 5 ml methoxyphenamine hydrochloride 16.9 mg, codeine phosphate 10.95 mg, and sodium citrate 325 mg (suggested diluent, syrup). For coughs. *Dose.* 5 to 10 ml every 3 or 4 hours.

Other Proprietary Names
Denm.—Asmi; *Ital.*—Euspirol, Metasma, Mimexina, Proasma; *Jap.*—Oxynarin.

2082-h

Methylaminoheptane Hydrochloride. 1,*N*-Dimethylhexylamine hydrochloride.
$C_8H_{19}N,HCl=165.7$.

CAS — 540-43-2 (methylaminoheptane).

A white crystalline powder, freely **soluble** in water.

Methylaminoheptane hydrochloride is a sympathomimetic agent with an action similar to that of ephedrine (p.10). It has been used as a pressor agent. The sulphate has been applied topically as a nasal decongestant.

2083-m

Methylephedrine Hydrochloride. *l*-Methylephedrine Hydrochloride; *l*-*N*-Methylephedrine Hydrochloride. (−)-2-Dimethylamino-1-phenylpropan-1-ol hydrochloride.
$C_{11}H_{17}NO,HCl=215.7$.

CAS — 552-79-4 (methylephedrine, −); 1201-56-5 (methylephedrine, ±); 38455-90-2 (hydrochloride, −); 942-46-1; 18760-80-0 (both hydrochloride, ±).

Pharmacopoeias. In *Jap.*, which also includes the (±)-form, *dl*-Methylephedrine Hydrochloride.

A white odourless crystalline powder with a bitter taste. M.p. 190° to 195°. Freely **soluble** in water; soluble in alcohol; practically insoluble in ether. **Protect** from light.

Methylephedrine hydrochloride is a sympathomimetic agent with an action similar to that of ephedrine (p.10). It has been used in bronchial asthma, the usual dose being 40 mg thrice daily and 40 to 80 mg at bedtime. Enuresis in children was formerly treated with a dose of 40 to 80 mg at bedtime.
Methylephedrine has also been given as the camsylate.

Proprietary Names
Tybraïne (camsylate) *(Cooper, Switz.).*

Methylephedrine hydrochloride was formerly marketed in Great Britain under the proprietary name Metheph (*Napp*).

2084-b

Methylhexaneamine. Methylhexamine. 1,3-Dimethylpentylamine.
$C_7H_{17}N=115.2$.

CAS — 105-41-9.

A colourless to pale yellow liquid with an ammoniacal odour. Very slightly **soluble** in water; freely soluble in alcohol, chloroform, ether, and dilute mineral acids.

Uses. Methylhexaneamine is a volatile sympathomimetic agent with a vasoconstrictor action. As the carbonate, it has been used in inhalers for the symptomatic relief of nasal congestion.

2085-v

Naphazoline Hydrochloride *(U.S.P., B.P. 1968).*

Cloridrato de Nafazolina; Naphtazolini Hydrochloridum. 2-(1-Naphthylmethyl)-2-imidazoline hydrochloride.
$C_{14}H_{14}N_2,HCl=246.7$.

CAS — 835-31-4 (naphazoline); 550-99-2 (hydrochloride).

Pharmacopoeias. In *Arg., Aust., Belg., Braz., Jap., Nord., Port., Roum.*, and *U.S.*

A white or almost white, odourless, crystalline powder with a bitter taste. M.p. about 255° with decomposition. **Soluble** 1 in 6 of water and 1 in 15 of alcohol; very slightly soluble in chloroform; practically insoluble in ether. A 1% solution in water has a pH of 5 to 6.6. A 3.99% solution is iso-osmotic with serum. Solutions are **sterilised** by maintaining at 98° to 100° for 30 minutes with a bactericide or by filtration. **Incompatible** with aluminium metal, alkalis, and heavy metal ions. **Store** in airtight containers. Protect from light.

An aqueous solution of naphazoline hydrochloride iso-osmotic with serum (3.99%) caused 100% haemolysis of erythrocytes cultured in it for 45 minutes.— E. R. Hammarlund and K. Pedersen-Bjergaard, *J. pharm. Sci.*, 1961, *50*, 24.

Benzalkonium chloride 0.01% or chlorhexidine gluconate 0.02% were suitable preservatives for naphazoline hydrochloride eye-drops sterilised by filtration.— M. Van Ooteghem, *Pharm. Tijdschr. Belg.*, 1968, *45*, 69.

2086-g

Naphazoline Nitrate *(B.P.).*

Naphazolini Nitras; Naphazolinium Nitricum; Nafazolina Nitrato; Naphthizinum *(Rus.P.)*. 2-(1-Naphthylmethyl)-2-imidazoline nitrate.
$C_{14}H_{14}N_2,HNO_3=273.3$.

CAS — 5144-52-5.

Pharmacopoeias. In *Aust., Br., Cz., Fr., It., Jap., Jug., Neth., Rus.*, and *Swiss.*

A white or almost white, odourless or almost odourless, crystalline powder with a bitter taste. M.p. about 168°. **Soluble** 1 in 36 of water and 1 in 16 of alcohol; very slightly soluble in chloroform; practically insoluble in ether. A 1% solution in water has a pH of 5 to 6.5. Solutions may be **sterilised** by maintaining at 98° to 100° for 30 minutes with a bactericide or by filtration. **Incompatible** with alkalis and heavy metal ions. **Store** in airtight containers. Protect from light.

Adverse Effects and Treatment. After local use of naphazoline transient irritation may occur. Nausea and headache have been reported. Overdosage or accidental administration by mouth may cause depression of the central nervous system with marked reduction of body temperature and symptoms of bradycardia, sweating, drowsiness, and coma, particularly in children; hypertension may be followed by rebound hypotension. Treatment of side-effects is symptomatic.

Overdosage. Symptoms including bradypnoea, cold damp skin, somnolence, and tachycardia occurred in a boy after taking an emulsion containing about 8 mg of naphazoline nitrate. Most symptoms had disappeared 10 hours later but tachycardia persisted for 4 days.— J. Kliment, *Čslká Pediat.*, 1965, *20*, 900, per *Int. pharm. Abstr.*, 1966, *3*, 1152. A 3-month-old boy was given about 7 ml of 0.1% naphazoline nasal drops. He had bradycardia, hypothermia, and irregular respiration but recovered after treatment.— L. Krajci, *Čslká Pediat.*, 1966, *21*, 277, per *Pharm. J.*, 1967, *2*, 533.

Precautions. Naphazoline should be used with caution in patients with cardiac disorders, hypertension, and hyperthyroidism. It should be used with special caution in children. Use of naphazoline on the nasal mucous membranes for more than a few days is associated with severe rebound congestion and rhinorrhoea.
The eye-drops must not be used in narrow-angle glaucoma.

Absorption and Fate. Systemic absorption has been reported following topical application of solutions of naphazoline. It is not used systemically, but it is readily absorbed from the gastro-intestinal tract.

Uses. Naphazoline is a sympathomimetic agent with marked alpha-adrenergic activity. It is a vasoconstrictor with a rapid and prolonged action in reducing swelling and congestion when applied to mucous membranes. Rebound congestion and rhinorrhoea may occur after frequent or prolonged use. It is used for the symptomatic relief of rhinitis and sinusitis. Nasal drops are used as a 0.05% aqueous solution of the hydrochloride or nitrate, 2 drops being instilled in each nostril not more often than every 3 hours.
A 0.1% solution has been instilled into the eye as a conjunctival decongestant.

Preparations of Naphazoline Salts

Naphazoline Hydrochloride Nasal Solution *(U.S.P.)*. A solution of naphazoline hydrochloride in water, adjusted to a suitable pH and osmolarity. Store in airtight containers. Protect from light.

Naphazoline Hydrochloride Ophthalmic Solution *(U.S.P.)*. A sterile buffered solution of naphazoline hydrochloride in water, adjusted to a suitable osmolarity. It contains a suitable preservative. pH 5.5 to 7. Store in airtight containers.

Proprietary Names of Naphazoline Salts
Albalon (hydrochloride) *(Allergan, Austral.; Allergan, Canad.; Bournonville, Neth.)*; Clear Eyes (hydrochloride) *(Abbott, USA)*; Clera (hydrochloride) *(Person & Covey, USA)*; Colirio Alfa (nitrate) *(Rovi, Spain)*; Dazolin (hydrochloride) *(Roux-Ocefa, Arg.)*; Degest 2 (hydrochloride) *(Barnes-Hind, Canad.)*; Imidazyl (nitrate) *(Tubi Lux, Ital.)*; Imizol (nitrate) *(Farmigea, Ital.)*; Naftazolina (hydrochloride) *(Bruschettini, Ital.)*; Naphcon Forte (hydrochloride) *(Alcon, Canad.; Alcon, USA)*; Nasal Yer (hydrochloride) *(Yer, Spain)*; Otrivin (see also under Xylometazoline Hydrochloride) (hydrochloride) *(Ciba, Spain)*; Privin (nitrate) *(Ciba, Denm.; Ciba, Switz.)*; Privina (either as base or nitrate) *(Ciba, Arg.; Ciba, Ital.; Ciba, Spain)*; Privine (either as hydrochloride or nitrate) *(Ciba, Austral.; Ciba, Belg.; Ciba, Canad.; Ciba, Neth.; Ciba, USA)*; Ran (hydrochloride) *(Corvi, Ital.)*; Rhino-Mex-N (hydrochloride) *(Charton, Canad.)*; Rhinospray (hydrochloride) *(Boehringer Sohn, Spain)*; Rimidol (hydrochloride) *(Leo, Swed.)*; Rinazina (nitrate) *(Maggioni, Ital.; Maggioni, Switz.)*; Vasocon (hydrochloride) *(Cooper, Canad.; Cooper, Ger.; Cooper-vision, USA)*; Vasoconstrictor (hydrochloride) *(Pensa, Spain)*.

Naphazoline nitrate was formerly marketed in Great Britain under the proprietary name Privine (*Ciba*).

2087-q

Noradrenaline Acid Tartrate *(B.P.).*

Noradren. Tart.; Noradrenaline Tartrate *(Eur. P.)*; Levarterenol Acid Tartrate; Norepinephrine Bitartrate *(U.S.P.)*; *l*-Arterenol Bitartrate; Levarterenol Bitartrate; Levarterenoli Bitartras; Noradrenalini Tartras; Noradrenaline Bitartrate; *l*-Norepinephrine Bitartrate. (*R*)-2-Amino-1-(3,4-dihydroxyphenyl)ethanol hydrogen tartrate monohydrate.
$C_8H_{11}NO_3,C_4H_6O_6,H_2O=337.3$.

CAS — 51-41-2 (noradrenaline); 51-40-1 (acid tartrate, anhydrous); 69815-49-2 (acid tartrate, monohydrate).

Pharmacopoeias. In *Arg., Aust., Br., Braz., Chin., Eur., Fr., Ger., Hung., Ind., Int., It., Jug., Neth., Nord., Pol., Roum., Rus., Swiss., Turk.*, and *U.S. Ger.* also includes the hydrochloride. *Cz.* and *Fr.* include the base (Noradrenalinum). *Jap.* includes the base in the racemic form (Norepinephrinum; Norepirenamine).

A white or faintly grey, odourless, crystalline powder with a bitter taste. M.p. 98° to 104° with decomposition. It darkens on exposure to air and light. Noradrenaline acid tartrate 2 micrograms is approximately equivalent to 1 microgram of noradrenaline. **Soluble** 1 in 2.5 of water and 1 in 300 of alcohol; practically insoluble in chloroform and ether. A solution in water is laevorotatory. A 1% solution in water has a pH of 3 to 5. Solutions are **sterilised** by autoclaving or by filtration and should contain 0.1% sodium metabisulphite. **Incompatible** with alkalis and oxidising agents. **Store** in airtight containers. Protect from light.

Incompatibility. There was loss of clarity when intravenous solutions of noradrenaline acid tartrate were mixed with those of amylobarbitone sodium, chlorpheniramine maleate, chlorothiazide sodium, nitrofurantoin sodium, novobiocin sodium, pentobarbitone sodium, phenobarbitone sodium, phenytoin sodium, quinalbarbitone sodium, sodium bicarbonate, sodium iodide, streptomycin sulphate, sulphadiazine sodium, sulphafurazole diethanolamine, or thiopentone sodium.— J. A. Patel and G. L. Phillips, *Am. J. Hosp. Pharm.*, 1966, *23*, 409. Noradrenaline acid tartrate is incompatible with cephalothin.— B. Flouvat and P. Lechat, *Thérapie*, 1974, *29*, 337. Solutions of noradrenaline acid tartrate lost 15% of their potency in 4 hours when mixed with solutions of cefapirin sodium.— V. K. Prasad *et al.*, *Curr. ther. Res.*, 1974, *16*, 540.

Stability of solutions. Solutions of noradrenaline acid tartrate (pH 3.6) with sodium metabisulphite 0.1%, enclosed in well-filled ampoules, could be sterilised by autoclaving at 115° for 30 minutes with negligible loss of activity. Dilutions of these solutions in 5% dextrose solutions, distilled water, or plasma, might be stored at room temperature for up to 24 hours with little loss of activity; these dilutions were more stable than those in saline solution or blood.— G. B. West, *J. Pharm. Pharmac.*, 1952, *4*, 560. Less oxidation and racemisation of noradrenaline occurred in injection solutions when air was replaced by carbon dioxide. Autoclaving did not cause significant degradation immediately or on storage if air was excluded.— P. Buri *et al.*, *Pharm. Acta Helv.*, 1969, *44*, 764. See also U. Kesselring and L. Kapétanidis, *ibid.*, 1966, *41*, 428.

Intravenous solutions of noradrenaline should be diluted with dextrose injection or 5% dextrose in sodium chloride injection to minimise oxidation.— J. M. Meisler and M. W. Skolaut, *Am. J. Hosp. Pharm.*, 1966, *23*, 557. At a room temperature of 29° to 30.5°, noradrenaline acid tartrate, 4 mg per 540 ml, was found to be stable for 4 hours in solutions of dextrose 5% in water or dextrose 5% in normal saline but there was significant loss of activity of noradrenaline in solutions of normal saline.— C. W. Ogle (letter), *Br. med. J.*, 1968, *2*, 490. Noradrenaline acid tartrate was stable for about 24 hours in dextrose injection at pH 3.6 to 6.— E. A. Parker, *Am. J. Hosp. Pharm.*, 1975, *32*, 214. The stability of noradrenaline in physiological saline solutions.— I. E. Hughes and J. A. Smith, *J. Pharm. Pharmac.*, 1978, *30*, 124.

Adverse Effects. Noradrenaline acid tartrate is a severe tissue irritant and only very dilute solutions may be injected. The needle must be inserted well into the vein and extravasation must be avoided, otherwise severe phlebitis and sloughing may occur. Necrosis of the skin overlying the tip of the cannula has been reported. The blood pressure must be monitored constantly as cerebral haemorrhage may be caused by the sudden rise in pressure.

Noradrenaline may occasionally cause anxiety, transient headache, palpitations, and respiratory difficulty; it may produce reflex bradycardia which is abolished by atropine. Overdosage or normal dosage in a hypersensitive patient has also resulted in severe hypertension, photophobia, retrosternal and pharyngeal pain, sweating, and vomiting.

The Committee on the Safety of Medicines had received 11 reports of severe occipital headache, with fatal cerebral haemorrhage in 1 patient, in dental patients who had injections of lignocaine 2% with noradrenaline 1 in 25 000 (Xylestesin). Similar symptoms occurred in a patient given butanilicaine and procaine with noradrenaline 1 in 25 000 (Hostacain NOR). The effects of these preparations were compared in 35 dental patients with lignocaine with adrenaline or noradrenaline 1 in 80 000 and prilocaine with felypressin 0.03 units per ml. Noradrenaline 1 in 25 000 produced increases of 21 to 92% in the blood pressure and its use at this strength could not be justified. Of the patients in the 11 original case reports, 1 was taking desipramine, 1 nortriptyline, and 1 might have been taking desipramine or protriptyline; these antidepressants could have enhanced the pressor effects. Felypressin was the vasoconstrictor of choice in such patients.— A. J. Boakes *et al.*, *Br. dent. J.*, 1972, *133*, 137. A discussion of the hazards and precautions to be taken when vasoconstrictors are used in conjunction with local anaesthetics.— *Lancet*, 1972, *2*, 584. Comment.— F. Reynolds (letter), *ibid.*, 764 and 834. See also P. J. Verrill, *Practitioner*, 1975, *214*, 380.

Treatment of Adverse Effects. The hypertensive effects of noradrenaline may be treated with an alpha-adrenoceptor blocking agent such as 5 to 10 mg of phentolamine mesylate intravenously, repeated as necessary; usually somewhat larger doses are required to reduce the blood pressure than are needed for similar states caused by adrenaline. Relief from tissue necrosis and pain may be given by immediate infiltration with phentolamine and local anaesthetics, and by the application of hot packs.

Any ischaemic areas should be infiltrated subcutaneously with 5 to 10 ml of saline solution containing 2.5 mg of phentolamine hydrochloride and 300 units of hyaluronidase. For areas larger than 30 cm^2 half the area should be infiltrated and the other half infiltrated 30 minutes later. The phentolamine infiltration was used 26 times in 20 patients and in no case was there any systemic manifestation due to the phentolamine and in none of the patients did a slough occur.— A. S. Close, *J. Am. med. Ass.*, 1959, *170*, 1916. Extravasation of noradrenaline into the dorsum of the hand in 2 patients produced uncontrollable oedema with venous occlusion of the hands and ischaemic necrosis of the fingers. Both patients later died. Phentolamine injected locally within 12 hours after extravasation of noradrenaline prevented tissue necrosis. Between 12 and 18 hours after extravasation its effect was less predictable, and after 18 hours it was of no value.— P. M. Weeks, *J. Am. med. Ass.*, 1966, *196*, 288. See also R. R. de Alvarez *et al.*, *Am. Surg.*, 1957, *23*, 619.

Precautions. Noradrenaline should be avoided or only used with extreme caution in hypersusceptible patients or those with aneurysms, hypertension, arteriosclerosis, and cardiovascular disorders. Hyperthyroid patients may be particularly sensitive and it should be used with caution in diabetes.

In late pregnancy noradrenaline provokes uterine contractions which can result in foetal asphyxia.

Although it is less likely than adrenaline to produce ventricular arrhythmias, noradrenaline should not be used during anaesthesia with cyclopropane or halothane and other halogenated anaesthetics (see p.3). Arrhythmias may also occur if it is given to patients receiving excessive doses of digitalis, mercurial diuretics, or other drugs that sensitise the heart to arrhythmias. Patients receiving guanethidine and similar adrenergic neurone blocking agents are extremely sensitive to the hypertensive effects of noradrenaline; noradrenaline also markedly reverses the hypotensive effects of reserpine and methyldopa. For details of the differing effects of monoamine oxidase inhibitors and tricyclic antidepressants on noradrenaline, see Adrenaline, p.3.

Interactions. A small increase in the pressor action of noradrenaline in some patients given *methyldopa*. This effect was inconstant and less striking than the prolongation of action seen in every case.— C. T. Dollery *et al.*, *Br. Heart J.*, 1963, *25*, 670.

When given 1 hour before noradrenaline acid tartrate in *rats*, *chlorpheniramine hydrochloride*, *tripelennamine hydrochloride*, and *desipramine*, but not mepyramine, significantly increased the toxicity of noradrenaline. Some antihistamines blocked the uptake of catecholamines by peripheral tissues and enhanced the toxicity of exogenous noradrenaline.— A. Jori (letter), *J. Pharm. Pharmac.*, 1966, *18*, 824. Studies *in vitro* of the nerve uptake of noradrenaline demonstrated an inhibition by *imipramine*, *desipramine*, *amitriptyline*, *nortriptyline*, and *chlorpromazine*. Studies *in vivo* showed that the pressor effects of tyramine were blocked by chlorpromazine, desipramine, and nortriptyline.— D. Tuck *et al.* (letter), *Lancet*, 1972, *2*, 492.

Administration of noradrenaline concurrently with *guanethidine* or *bethanidine* was not advisable since both depleted the adrenergic nerves of noradrenaline, thus enhancing the effect of exogenous noradrenaline.— A. Herxheimer, *Prescribers' J.*, 1969, *9*, 62.

Studies of the effect of noradrenaline on *beta-blockade* alone and in the presence of *atropine*.— D. A. Richards *et al.*, *Br. J. clin. Pharmac.*, 1979, *7*, 429P.

For the effect of *monoamine oxidase inhibitors* and *tricyclic antidepressants* on noradrenaline in local anaesthetics, see Adrenaline, p.3.

Absorption and Fate. For a brief outline of the absorption and fate of a catecholamine, see Adrenaline, p.3.

Noradrenaline cannot be given by subcutaneous or intramuscular injection owing to its powerful vasoconstrictor properties. Like adrenaline it is inactive when given by mouth, and it is rapidly inactivated in the body by similar processes. Only small amounts of noradrenaline are excreted unchanged in the urine of healthy subjects. The proportion of unchanged noradrenaline in the urine increases considerably in subjects with phaeochromocytoma.

An account of the catabolism of catecholamines and a review of studies.— D. F. Sharman, *Br. med. Bull.*, 1973, *29*, 110. Biochemical aspects of monoamine oxidase.— K. F. Tipton, *ibid.*, 116. Mechanisms involved in the release of noradrenaline from sympathetic nerves.— A. D. Smith, *ibid.*, 123. Catecholamine uptake processes.— L. L. Iversen, *ibid.*, 130. Uptake of noradrenaline by smooth muscle.— J. S. Gillespie, *ibid.*, 136. Factors affecting plasma-noradrenaline concentrations, including various neurological disorders, such as the Shy-Drager syndrome.— I. J. Kopin *et al.*, *Ann. intern. Med.*, 1978, *88*, 671. Kinetics of infused noradrenaline in healthy subjects.— G. A. FitzGerald *et al.*, *Clin. Pharmac. Ther.*, 1979, *26*, 669.

Uses. The catecholamine, noradrenaline, is a direct-acting sympathomimetic agent with pronounced effects on alpha-adrenergic receptors and less marked effects on beta-adrenergic receptors. It is a neurotransmitter, stored in granules in nerve axons, which is released at the terminations of post-ganglionic adrenergic nerve fibres when they are stimulated; some is also present in the adrenal medulla from which it is liberated together with adrenaline. A major effect of noradrenaline is to raise systolic and diastolic blood pressure (which is accompanied by reflex slowing of the heart-rate). This is a result of its alpha-stimulant effects which cause vasoconstriction, with reduced blood flow in the kidneys, liver, skin, and usually skeletal muscle. Other effects include contraction of the spleen, and decreased motility of the stomach and intestine, with contraction of the sphincters including those of the bladder; the pregnant uterus also contracts; high doses liberate glucose from the liver and have other hormonal effects similar to those of adrenaline; there is little stimulation of the central nervous system; noradrenaline is a mydriatic. Beta-stimulant effects of noradrenaline have a positive inotropic action on the heart, but there is little bronchodilator effect.

Noradrenaline may be used in concentrations of 1 in 100 000 to 1 in 50 000 to diminish the absorption and localise the effects of local anaesthetics, and to reduce haemorrhage during the subsequent operation. For the control of capillary bleeding, the local application of a 1 in 10 000 solution has been used.

Noradrenaline has been used in the treatment of hypotensive states in which the blood volume is adequate, such as after the removal of a phaeochromocytoma, and in myocardial infarction. To avoid tissue necrosis it is best administered through a fine catheter into a large vein high up in a limb, preferably the arm; some sources have suggested that addition of phentolamine 5 to 10 mg to the infusion may prevent sloughing without affecting the vasopressor action.

Noradrenaline acid tartrate is usually administered by intravenous infusion as a solution containing 8 µg, equivalent to 4 µg of the base, per ml of dextrose injection or sodium chloride and dextrose injection; it is less stable in plasma, blood, or sodium chloride injection. This solution is usually given initially at a rate of 2 to 3 ml per minute and adjusted according to the response so as to maintain the desired blood pressure, the blood pressure being initially recorded every 2 minutes, and the rate of infusion being continuously monitored. The average maintenance dose is 0.5 to 1 ml per minute, but there is a wide variation. According to the patient's fluid requirements the concentration of the infusion may need increasing or decreasing. On some occasions the infusion may be continued for days; it must not be stopped suddenly but should be gradually withdrawn to guard against disastrous falls in blood pressure. A rapid intravenous or intracardiac injection of 0.5 to 0.75 ml of a solution containing noradrenaline acid tartrate 200 µg per ml, equivalent to 100 µg of noradrenaline base per ml has been suggested as an adjunct in the treatment of cardiac arrest (50 to 75 µg of noradrenaline base). For comments on drugs recommended for cardiopulmonary arrest, see Adrenaline (Cardiac Resuscitation), p.5.

Administration. Addition of phentolamine 5 or 10 mg per litre of noradrenaline infusion in order to protect from noradrenaline-induced ischaemic necrosis.— G. Zucker *et al.*, *Circulation*, 1960, *22*, 935.

Cardiac disorders. Infusion of noradrenaline to control paroxysmal tachycardia.— B. R. Rubanovskij, *Sov. Med.*, 1967, *30*, 117.

Myocardial infarction. A review of the role of inotropic agents and infarct size in the management of myocardial infarction. Since *animal* studies suggest that noradrenaline may extend infarct size in normotensive subjects, the unequivocal diagnosis of hypotension and shock is an absolute prerequisite for the clinical use of this drug.— M. Lesch, *Am. J. Cardiol.*, 1976, *37*, 508.

Studies of the role of noradrenaline in cardiogenic shock.— H. Mueller *et al.*, *Circulation*, 1972, *45*, 335 (improved myocardial perfusion and oxygenation but unchanged mortality).

Gastro-intestinal disorders. Massive upper gastro-intestinal haemorrhage occurring in 12 patients with advanced malignant disease was controlled by noradrenaline acid tartrate in 11. In 11 patients noradrenaline was administered by naso-gastric tube as a 0.008% solution in iso-osmotic saline and in 1 patient by intraperitoneal infusion of a 0.0016% solution in iso-osmotic saline. Intraperitoneal administration of noradrenaline led to transient rise in blood pressure.— H. O. Douglass, *J. Am. med. Ass.*, 1974, *230*, 1653. See also H. H. LeVeen *et al.*, *Ann. Surg.*, 1972, *175*, 459; M. C. Kiselow and M. Wagner, *Archs Surg., Chicago*, 1973, *107*, 387.

A 59-year-old man with a history of chronic alcohol and analgesic abuse developed severe gastric bleeding from a 1-cm longitudinal Mallory-Weiss mucosal laceration just below the cardio-oesophaegeal junction. He required 7 units of whole blood, and gastric lavage with 500 ml of cold normal saline containing noradrenaline 1 mg failed to arrest the bleeding. Noradrenaline 1 mg in 10 ml of physiological saline was then applied directly on the lesion, the mucosa around the lesion blanched and oozing ceased immediately. No further haematemesis or passage of fresh blood per rectum occurred and repeat endoscopy before discharge demonstrated complete healing of the lesion.— D. Curran *et al.* (letter), *Lancet*, 1980, *1*, 538.

Ocular disorders. The use of noradrenaline 4% to reduce intra-ocular pressure. Effects lasted for up to 20 weeks; many patients experienced conjunctival hyperaemia.— I. P. Pollock and H. Rossi, *Archs Ophthal., N.Y.*, 1975, *93*, 173. Comment on the role of topical noradrenaline in glaucoma. It reduces the formation of aqueous humour by the ciliary body but it also has a mild dilating effect on the pupil so that patients do not suffer the visual defects of miosis. The eye-drops need to be instilled only twice daily (night and morning) and in elderly glaucoma patients with lenticular opacities their vision may be considerably improved by the resultant mild pupillary dilatation. Noradrenaline must not, of course, be used in patients with closed-angle glaucoma.— S. I. Davidson, *Practitioner*, 1976, *217*, 596.

Shock. The use of intravenous noradrenaline was considered to provide little or no benefit in treating the cold hypotensive symptoms of shock.— G. K. McGowan and G. Walters, *Lancet*, 1966, *1*, 611.

For comments on the role of noradrenaline in cardiogenic shock see under Cardiac Disorders (above).

Preparations

Noradrenaline Injection *(B.P.)*. Noradrenaline Acid Tartrate Injection. A sterile solution of noradrenaline acid tartrate, prepared immediately before use by diluting Strong Sterile Noradrenaline Solution to 250 times its volume with Sodium Chloride and Dextrose Intravenous Infusion or Dextrose Intravenous Infusion. It contains 8 µg of noradrenaline acid tartrate, equivalent to approximately 4 µg of noradrenaline, in 1 ml.

Norepinephrine Bitartrate Injection *(U.S.P.)*. Levarterenol Bitartrate Injection. A sterile solution of noradrenaline acid tartrate in Water for Injections. pH 3 to 4.5. Potency is expressed in terms of the equivalent amount of noradrenaline. It should not be used if the solution is brown or contains a precipitate. Protect from light.

Strong Sterile Noradrenaline Solution *(B.P.)*. A sterile solution of noradrenaline acid tartrate 200 mg, sodium metabisulphite 100 mg, and sodium chloride 800 mg in Water for Injections to 100 ml. Sterilised by autoclaving. pH3 to 4.6. It contains the equivalent of approximately 0.1% of noradrenaline. It must be diluted before administration. It should not be used if it is brown in colour. Protect from light.

Proprietary Preparations

Levophed *(Winthrop, UK)*. Noradrenaline acid tartrate, available as **Solution** containing the equivalent of 0.1% of noradrenaline, in ampoules of 2 and 4 ml, and as **Special Solution** containing the equivalent of 0.01% of noradrenaline, in ampoules of 2 ml. (Also available as Levophed in *Austral., Belg., Canad., Denm., Fr., USA*).

Other Proprietary Names

Adrenor *(Spain)*; Arterenol *(hydrochloride) (Ger.)*; Noradrec *(Ital.)*; Reargon *(base) (Spain)*.

2088-p

Nordefrin Hydrochloride. Corbadrine Hydrochloride; *dl*-3,4-Dihydroxynorephedrine Hydrochloride; Dihydroxyphenylaminopropanol Hydrochloride; Nordephrinium Chloratum. (±)-2-Amino-1-(3,4-dihydroxyphenyl)propan-1-ol hydrochloride.
$C_9H_{13}NO_3,HCl=219.7$.

CAS — 6539-57-7 (nordefrin); 138-61-4 (hydrochloride); 61-96-1 (hydrochloride, ±).

Pharmacopoeias. In *Aust.*, *Cz.*, and *Pol.*

A white odourless crystalline powder which slowly darkens on exposure to air and light. M.p. about 177°. **soluble** 1 in 2 of water and 1 in 12 of alcohol; practically insoluble in chloroform and ether. **Incompatible** with alkalis and oxygen. **Store** in airtight containers. Protect from light.

Nordefrin hydrochloride has been used as a vasoconstrictor in dentistry. Nearly all the vasoconstrictor activity is possessed by the laevo-isomer, levonordefrin (see p.18).

2089-s

Norfenefrine Hydrochloride. Norphenylephrine Hydrochloride; *m*-Norsynephrine Hydrochloride. 2-Amino-1-(3-hydroxyphenyl)ethanol hydrochloride.
$C_8H_{11}NO_2,HCl=189.6$.

CAS — 536-21-0 (norfenefrine); 15308-34-6 (hydrochloride).

NOTE. *m*-Octopamine has been used as a synonym for norfenefrine. Care should be taken to avoid confusion between the 2 compounds.

Crystals. M.p. 159° to 160°. Freely **soluble** in water.

Uses. Norfenefrine is a sympathomimetic agent with predominantly alpha-adrenergic activity, and general properties similar to those of phenylephrine (p.23).
It has been used in the treatment of hypotension, in doses of 12 to 27 mg daily in divided doses, by mouth; it has been given in doses of 10 mg by injection.

The bioavailability of norfenefrine in man, related to its metabolism.— J. H. Hengstmann *et al.*, *Eur. J. clin. Pharmac.*, 1975, *8*, 33.

Proprietary Names

Coritat *(Jap.)*; Depot-Novadral *(Gödecke, Ger.; Gödecke, Switz.)*; Euro-cir *(Virgiliano, Ital.)*; Molycor-R *(Mepha, Switz.)*; Nevadral *(Pharmacia, Swed.)*; Norenol *(sulphate) (UCB-Pevya, Spain)*; Normetolo *(Selvi, Ital.)*; Novadral *(Warner, Arg.; Pharmacia, Denm.; Gödecke, Ger.; Gödecke, Switz.)*; Stagural *(Stada-Chemie, Ger.)*; Tonolift *(Jap.)*; Zondel *(Jap.)*.

2090-h

Octopamine. WV 569; *p*-Norsynephrine; Noroxedrine; *p*-Hydroxymandelamine; β,4-Dihydroxyphenethylamine. 2-Amino-1-(4-hydroxyphenyl)ethanol.
$C_8H_{11}NO_2=153.2$.

CAS — 104-14-3.

Adverse Effects, Treatment, and Precautions. As for Phenylephrine Hydrochloride, p.24.

Absorption and Fate. Octopamine has reduced bioavailability from the gastro-intestinal tract owing to first-pass metabolism by monoamine oxidase in the gut wall. In addition to deamination it is also conjugated.

The physiological disposition of octopamine in man.— J. H. Hengstmann *et al.*, *Archs Pharmac.*, 1974, *283*, 93.

Uses. Octopamine is a sympathomimetic agent with predominantly alpha-adrenergic activity. It has been used as the hydrochloride or the tartrate in the treatment of hypotension.

Evidence of small amounts of octopamine in mammals.— P. Molinoff and J. Axelrod, *Science*, 1969, *164*, 428. The presence of octopamine in the lobster nervous system.— D. L. Barker *et al.*, *Nature New Biol.*, 1972, *236*, 61.

Further references.— K. C. Lam *et al.*, *Scand. J. Gastroenterol.*, 1973, *8*, 465; D. L. Murphy *et al.*, *Clin. Pharmac. Ther.*, 1975, *18*, 587.

Proprietary Names

Norden *(hydrochloride) (Byk Gulden, Ital.)*; Norfen *(hydrochloride) (Jap.)*; Norphen *(hydrochloride and tartrate) (Byk Gulden, Ger.; Byk Gulden, Switz.)*.

2091-m

Orciprenaline Sulphate *(B.P.)*.

Metaproterenol Sulphate; Th 152. (±)-1-(3,5-Dihydroxyphenyl)-2-isopropylaminoethanol sulphate.
$(C_{11}H_{17}NO_3)_2,H_2SO_4=520.6$.

CAS — 586-06-1 (orciprenaline); 5874-97-5 (sulphate).

Pharmacopoeias. In *Br.* and *Cz.*

A white odourless crystalline powder with a bitter taste. It contains up to 6% of water and methyl alcohol of crystallisation of which not more than 2% is water. M.p. about 205°.
Soluble 1 in 2 of water, 1 in 1 of alcohol; practically insoluble in chloroform and ether. A 10% solution in water has a pH of 4 to 5.5. Solutions are **sterilised** by autoclaving or by filtration and kept in ampoules. **Incompatible** with alkalis, heavy metal ions, and oxidising agents. **Store** in airtight containers. Protect from light.

Adverse Effects. As for Salbutamol, p.29. Orciprenaline is less beta$_2$-selective than salbutamol.

Adverse effects were not severe after inhalations or oral doses of up to 100 mg daily of orciprenaline sulphate. Above this dose adverse effects were frequent, continuous, and severe; trembling and palpitations were common. Three patients receiving 120 mg daily had a rise of systolic blood pressure; in 2 of these patients the rise occurred once only and in the third a rise of 30 mmHg systolic persisted for 48 hours and then settled spontaneously while treatment was continued.— G. Edwards, *Br. med. J.*, 1964, *1*, 1015. Muscular cramps that had occurred in about 8% of patients receiving orciprenaline disappeared when potassium was given concomitantly. Extrasystoles or tachycardia and severe headaches which occurred as side-effects of treatment with orciprenaline were also found to decrease or disappear in patients who were given potassium supplements.— L. Lotzof (letter), *Med. J. Aust.*, 1968, *1*, 1105.

Precautions. As for Salbutamol, p.29.
Orciprenaline is more liable to induce tachycardia.

CAUTION. *Excessive usage of aerosols of sympathomimetic agents has been associated with sudden death in asthmatics, see p.15.*

Absorption and Fate. Orciprenaline is incompletely absorbed from the gastro-intestinal tract and is excreted in the urine primarily as the glucuronide conjugate.

Pharmacokinetics of orciprenaline after administration in sustained-release form.— H. J. Gilfrich *et al.*, *Arzneimittel-Forsch.*, 1979, *29*, 967.

Uses. Orciprenaline sulphate is a direct-acting sympathomimetic agent with actions and uses similar to those of salbutamol (p.30).
In the treatment of bronchial asthma it is given by mouth in a dose of 20 mg four times daily. A suggested dose for children is: up to 1 year, 5 to 10 mg thrice daily; 1 to 3 years, 5 to 10 mg four times daily; 3 to 12 years, 10 mg four times daily to 20 mg thrice daily.
Orciprenaline sulphate may be inhaled in 5% solution from a hand nebuliser, the adult dose being 5 to 10 inhalations; if the solution is used with any other nebulising device the maximum single adult dose is the equivalent of a 1-minute

administration of nebulised 5% solution diluted with sterile water or physiological saline. Adequate oxygenation is necessary to avoid hypoxaemia. Pressurised aerosols providing 750 µg in each metered dose, delivering at the mouthpiece 670 µg, are the usual method of inhalation. The usual adult dosage is 1 or 2 inhalations, repeated, if required, after not less than 30 minutes, to a maximum of 12 inhalations in 24 hours.

In the treatment of severe forms of bronchospasm orciprenaline sulphate 500 µg may be given by intramuscular injection; the injection may be repeated if necessary after 30 minutes. Adequate oxygenation is necessary to avoid hypoxaemia. A suggested dose by intramuscular injection for children aged less than 6 years is 250 µg.

Orciprenaline has also been used similarly to salbutamol in the management of premature labour. The initial dose is 2.5 µg of orciprenaline sulphate per minute for 5 minutes, administered by intravenous infusion of a solution containing 5 mg in 500 ml of dextrose injection. If this has little effect on the maternal heart-rate the dose may be increased until uterine contractions are suppressed. The maternal heart-rate should not exceed 130 per minute and the dose should not exceed 60 µg per minute. Up to 3 infusions of about 20 minutes may be given to a maximum dose of 2.5 mg daily. The foetal heart-rate should also be monitored regularly.

In a comparison of the cardiovascular effects of various intravenous doses of orciprenaline and isoprenaline in 3 healthy men, isoprenaline was found to be between 10 and 40 times as potent as orciprenaline. Both drugs increased the heart-rate and forearm blood flow and acted by stimulating β-adrenergic receptors.— R. G. Shanks *et al.*, *Br. med. J.*, 1967, *1*, 610.

Asthma. Results of a double-blind study completed by 17 asthma patients confirmed the impression that orciprenaline is far better tolerated following inhalation of the aerosol than following administration of the tablets.— C. Shim and M. H. Williams, *Ann. intern. Med.*, 1980, *93*, 428.

Further reviews, comments, and studies on the role of orciprenaline in the management of asthma.— G. Edwards, *Br. med. J.*, 1964, *1*, 1015; A. S. Rebuck and J. Read, *Med. J. Aust.*, 1969, *1*, 445; A. Hurst, *Ann. Allergy*, 1973, *31*, 460; J. S. Hyde *et al.*, *Clin. Pharmac. Ther.*, 1976, *20*, 207; B. Garra *et al.*, *J. Allergy & clin. Immunol.*, 1977, *60*, 63; S. P. Galant *et al.*, *ibid.*, 1978, *61*, 73; B. W. Madsen *et al.*, *Br. J. clin. Pharmac.*, 1979, *8*, 75; D. Heimer *et al.*, *J. Allergy & clin. Immunol.*, 1980, *66*, 75; J. M. Rodgers *et al.*, *Curr. ther. Res.*, 1980, *28*, 147.

Musculoskeletal disorders. Orciprenaline increased the speed of relaxation of electrically stimulated muscle contraction and caused a decrease in the resting muscle tone when given to 6 spastic patients.— E. Zaimis, *Lancet*, 1973, *1*, 403.

Pregnancy and the neonate. For comments on the efficacy of beta$_2$-selective adrenoceptor stimulants in the prevention of premature labour, see Salbutamol, p.31.

Studies of orciprenaline in premature labour.— P. Baillie *et al.*, *Br. med. J.*, 1970, *4*, 154.

Preparations

Orciprenaline Aerosol Inhalation *(B.P.C. 1973)*. An aerosol spray in a pressurised canister containing a fine suspension of orciprenaline sulphate in a suitable mixture of aerosol propellents. It may contain a surfactant, stabilising agents, and other adjuvants. Store in a cool place. *Dose.* 1 or 2 inhalations, each of 670 µg, repeated, if necessary, after 30 minutes to a max. of 12 in 24 hours.

Orciprenaline Elixir *(B.P.C. 1973)*. Orciprenaline Sulphate Elixir; Orciprenaline Syrup. A solution of orciprenaline sulphate in a suitable flavoured vehicle. Store in a cool place. Protect from light. When a dose less than 5 ml is prescribed the elixir should be diluted to 5 ml with syrup. Such dilutions must be freshly prepared and not used more than 2 weeks after issue. *Dose.* Orciprenaline sulphate, children up to 1 year, 5 to 10 mg thrice daily; 1 to 5 years, 5 to 10 mg four times daily.

Orciprenaline Injection *(B.P.)*. A sterile solution of orciprenaline sulphate in Water for Injections, containing suitable stabilising agents. pH 3 to 4. Sterilised by autoclaving. Protect from light.

Orciprenaline Tablets *(B.P.)*. Orciprenaline Sulphate Tablets. Tablets containing orciprenaline sulphate. Protect from light.

Proprietary Preparations

Alupent *(Boehringer Ingelheim, UK)*. Orciprenaline sulphate, available in 1-ml **Ampoules** of an injection containing 500 µg per ml; as **Inhalant** solution containing 5%, in bottles of 7.5 ml; as **Syrup** containing 10 mg in each 5 ml (suggested diluent, syrup or Sorbitol Solution); and as scored **Tablets** of 20 mg. (Also available as Alupent in *Arg., Austral., Belg., Canad., Denm., Fr., Ger., Ital., Neth., Norw., S. Afr., Spain, Swed., Switz., USA*).

Alupent Expectorant *(Boehringer Ingelheim, UK)*. **Mixture** containing in each 5 ml orciprenaline sulphate 10 mg and bromhexine hydrochloride 4 mg (suggested diluent, syrup or Sorbitol Solution) and scored **Tablets** each containing orciprenaline sulphate 20 mg and bromhexine hydrochloride 8 mg. For asthma and chronic bronchitis. *Dose.* 10 ml of mixture or 1 tablet 4 times daily; children, under 5 years, 5 ml of mixture twice daily; 5 to 10 years, 5 ml of mixture or half a tablet 3 or 4 times daily.

Alupent Metered Aerosol *(Boehringer Ingelheim, UK)*. A pressurised spray containing orciprenaline sulphate 225 mg suspended in a propellent, providing 750 µg of orciprenaline sulphate in each metered dose, of which 670 µg is available to the patient.

Alupent Obstetric *(Boehringer Ingelheim, UK)*. Orciprenaline sulphate, available as an iso-osmotic solution containing 5 mg in each 10 ml, with disodium edetate 0.05% and sodium metabisulphite 0.01%, in ampoules of 10 ml, for dilution with 500 ml of dextrose injection for intravenous infusion.

Other Proprietary Names

Dosalupent *(Ital.)*; Metaprel *(USA)*; Novasmasol *(Ital.)*.

2092-b

Oxedrine Tartrate *(B.P., Eur. P.)*.

Oxedrini Tartras; Aetaphen. Tartrat.; Synephrine Tartrate; Aethaphenum Tartaricum; Oxyphenylmethylaminoethanol Tartrate; Sinefrina Tartrato. (±)-1-(4-Hydroxyphenyl)-2-methylaminoethanol tartrate.

$(C_9H_{13}NO_2)_2,C_4H_6O_6=484.5$.

CAS — 94-07-5 (oxedrine); 16589-24-5 (tartrate); 67-04-9 (tartrate, ±).

NOTE. *m*-Synephrine has been used as a synonym for phenylephrine. Care should be taken to avoid confusion between the 2 compounds.

Pharmacopoeias. In *Aust., Br., Eur., Fr., Ger., It., Jug., Neth., Nord.*, and *Swiss.*

Sympaethaminum (*Hung.*) is the base.

Odourless colourless crystals or white crystalline powder with a somewhat salty bitter taste. M.p. about 185° with decomposition. **Soluble** 1 in 2 of water and 1 in 400 of alcohol; practically insoluble in chloroform and ether. A 5% solution in water is dextrorotatory and has a pH of 5.6 to 6.5. **Incompatible** with alkalis, ferric salts, and oxidising agents. **Store** in airtight containers. Protect from light.

Oxedrine has general properties similar to those of phenylephrine (p.23). It has been given in hypotensive states in doses of about 100 mg thrice daily by mouth; it has also been given by subcutaneous, intramuscular, or intravenous injection in doses of 60 to 120 mg. The tartrate has been used as an ocular decongestant.

Pharmacokinetics and metabolism of oxedrine tartrate.— J. H. Hengstmann and H. Aulepp, *Arzneimittel-Forsch.*, 1978, *28*, 2326.

Proprietary Preparations

Sympatol *(Lewis, UK)*. Oxedrine tartrate, available as **Liquid** containing 10% and as 1-ml **Ampoules** of an injection containing 60 mg. (Also available as Sympatol in *Belg., Ger., Ital., Switz.*).

Other Proprietary Names

Cardiodinamin *(Ital.)*; Dulcidrine *(Fr.)*; Simpadren *(Arg.)*; Sympacor *(Switz.)*; Sympalept *(Switz.)*.

A preparation containing oxedrine tartrate was also formerly marketed in Great Britain under the proprietary name Chibro-Boraline Collyrium (*Chibret, Fr.*).

2093-v

Oxymetazoline Hydrochloride *(U.S.P.)*.

H990. 2-(4-*tert*-Butyl-3-hydroxy-2,6-dimethylbenzyl)-2-imidazoline hydrochloride; 6-*tert*-Butyl-3-(2-imidazolin-2-ylmethyl)2,4-xylenol hydrochloride.

$C_{16}H_{24}N_2O,HCl=296.8$.

CAS — 1491-59-4 (oxymetazoline); 2315-02-8 (hydrochloride).

Pharmacopoeias. In *Braz.* and *U.S.*

A white or almost white, odourless, hygroscopic, crystalline powder with a bitter taste. M.p. about 300° with decomposition. **Soluble** 1 in 6.7 of water and 1 in 3.6 of alcohol; practically insoluble in chloroform and ether. A 5% solution in water has a pH of 4 to 6.5. **Store** in airtight containers.

Adverse Effects and Precautions. It may occasionally cause local stinging or burning, sneezing, and dryness of the mouth and throat. Prolonged use may cause rebound congestion and drug-induced rhinitis.

Uses. Oxymetazoline hydrochloride is used in 0.05% solution as a vasoconstrictor to relieve nasal congestion. It acts within a few minutes and the effect lasts for several hours.

Preparations

Oxymetazoline Hydrochloride Nasal Solution *(U.S.P.)*. An aqueous solution of oxymetazoline hydrochloride adjusted to a suitable osmolarity. pH 4 to 6.5. Store in airtight containers.

Afrazine *(Kirby-Warrick, UK)*. Oxymetazoline hydrochloride, available as **Nasal Drops** and as **Nasal Spray** each containing 0.05%, and as **Paediatric Nasal Drops** containing 0.025%.

Iliadin-Mini *(E. Merck, UK)*. Nasal drops containing oxymetazoline hydrochloride 0.05% in single-dose disposable applicators (half for each nostril). **Iliadin-Mini Paediatric.** Contains oxymetazoline hydrochloride 0.025% in single-dose disposable applicators.

Other Proprietary Names

Arg.—Lidil; *Austral.*—Drixine, Durazol, Hazol, Iliadin; *Belg.*—Nesivine; *Canad.*—Nafrine; *Fr.*—Iliadine; *Ger.*—Nasivin, Rhinolitan; *Ital.*—Nasivin; *Neth.*—Nasivin; *Norw.*—Iliadin; *S.Afr.*— Drixine, Iliadin; *Swed.*—Nezeril; *Spain*—Nasofarma, Respibien, Respir, Utabon; *USA*—Afrin.

2094-g

Phenylephrine Hydrochloride *(B.P., U.S.P.)*.

m-Synephrine Hydrochloride; Mesatonum; Metaoxedrini Chloridum; Phenylephrinium Chloratum; Néosynéphrine Chlorhydrate; Fenilefrina Cloridrato. (*S*)-1-(3-Hydroxyphenyl)-2-methylaminoethanol hydrochloride.

$C_9H_{13}NO_2,HCl=203.7$.

CAS — 59-42-7 (phenylephrine); 61-76-7 (hydrochloride).

NOTE. Synephrine has been used as a synonym for oxedrine. Care should be taken to avoid confusion between the 2 compounds.

Pharmacopoeias. In *Br., Braz., Chin., Jap., Neth., Nord., Port., Rus., Swiss, Turk.*, and *U.S.*

White or almost white, odourless, crystalline powder with a bitter taste. M.p. 140° to 145°. **Soluble** 1 in 2 of water, 1 in 4 of alcohol, and 1 in 2 of glycerol; practically insoluble in arachis oil. A solution in water is laevorotatory. A 1% solution in water has a pH of about 5. A 3% solution is iso-osmotic with serum.

Solutions are **sterilised** by filtration and distributed into ampoules in which the air has been replaced by nitrogen or other suitable gas. **Incompatible** with butacaine, alkalis, ferric salts, and oxidising agents. **Store** in airtight containers. Protect from light.

Incompatibility. Particulate matter was observed within 2 hours when 1 ml of commercial phenylephrine hydrochloride injection was mixed with 5 ml of sterile water and 1 ml of commercial phenytoin sodium injection.— R. Misgen, *Am. J. Hosp. Pharm.*, 1965, *22*, 92. See also J. A. Patel and G. L. Phillips, *Am. J. Hosp. Pharm.*, 1966, *23*, 409.

Stability of solutions. No detectable loss occurred in a solution at pH 2 kept at 97° for longer than 10 days, but a rise in pH, particularly above pH 9, accelerated decomposition.— H. A. M. El-Shibini *et al.*, *Arzneimittel-Forsch.*, 1969, *19*, 676. See also *idem*, 1613. Yellow discoloration of phenylephrine solutions was an indication of appreciable degradation. Metals, especially copper, when present in 10 ppm concentration, accelerated degradation, though calcium had no influence and magnesium increased stability. Heavy metals might combine with phenylephrine to yield auto-oxidisable complexes. This could be prevented by adding edetic acid 500 μg per ml.— *idem*, 828.

Phenylephrine hydrochloride 250 mg was stable for 84 days at up to 60° in Water for Injections 100 ml; in sodium chloride injection 100 ml; with chloramphenicol succinate 50 mg in sodium chloride injection 100 ml; with chloramphenicol succinate 50 mg in dextrose injection 100 ml (pH 6); and with potassium chloride 4 mmol (4 mEq) in dextrose injection 100 ml. With chloramphenicol succinate 50 mg and sodium bicarbonate 750 mg in dextrose injection 100 ml (pH 8.2), phenylephrine hydrochloride was stable for 84 days only when stored at 22° and unstable at higher temperatures.— C. R. Weber and V. D. Gupta, *J. Hosp. Pharm.*, 1970, *28*, 200.

Nasal drops containing 0.5% phenylephrine hydrochloride with 0.1% sodium metabisulphite and 0.03% hydroxybenzoates, in 0.05M phosphate buffers were stable for up to 18 months when stored at room temperature at pH 5 to 6. Discoloration and loss of preservative occurred at higher pH.— V. D. Gupta and R. L. Mosier, *Am. J. Hosp. Pharm.*, 1972, *29*, 870.

Use in eye-drops. When eye-drops containing 1% phenylephrine hydrochloride and 0.1% cyclopentolate hydrochloride buffered to pH 9.2 with a 2.6% solution of borax were used the mydriatic response was similar to that obtained when eye-drops containing 10% phenylephrine hydrochloride and 1% cyclopentolate hydrochloride without borax were used. No irritation of the eye occurred, but there was some loss of potency on standing for 3 days.— E. S. N. Wang and E. R. Hammarlund, *J. pharm. Sci.*, 1970, *59*, 1559.

Adverse Effects. Phenylephrine hydrochloride may produce an undesirably high blood pressure with headache, vomiting, and, rarely, palpitations. Reflex bradycardia may occur which can be prevented or abolished with atropine.

Overdosage of phenylephrine injection in patients with paroxysmal tachycardia may induce ventricular dysrrhythmias, a sensation of fullness in the head, and tingling and coolness of the skin. Phenylephrine hydrochloride is irritant and may cause local discomfort at the site of application; extravasation of the injection may even cause local tissue necrosis.

When 1 drop of a 10% solution of phenylephrine eye-drops was instilled into the eyes of low birth-weight infants, their systolic and diastolic pressures were increased considerably. This effect lasted for 70 minutes or more and could be hazardous if a left-to-right shunt existed. It was suggested that the 10% solution should be replaced by a 2.5% solution, not only in neonates but in all other patients.— V. Borromeo-McGrail *et al.*, *Pediatrics*, 1973, *51*, 1032. See also *Br. med. J.*, 1974, *1*, 2. One drop of phenylephrine 10% eye-drops instilled into each eye of an infant produced acute pulmonary oedema with associated hypertension.— T. G. Matthews *et al.* (letter), *Lancet*, 1977, *2*, 827.

An 8-year-old boy who received 14 to 18 mg of phenylephrine as eye-drops to stop excessive bleeding developed severe hypertension, and ventricular arrhythmias which were eventually controlled with lignocaine administered intravenously. Absorption from mucosal surfaces was almost as rapid as with intravenous administration and thus the amount of phenylephrine administered was an overdose.— R. W. Vaughan, *Anesth. Analg. curr. Res.*, 1973, *52*, 161.

Persistent hypertension in a 7.5-week-old infant with a respiratory infection was associated with the use during the previous 7 days of phenylephrine in nasal drops together with a preparation containing pseudoephedrine given 4 times daily by mouth.— R. Saken *et al.*, *J. Pediat.*, 1979, *95*, 1077.

Data on 32 patients who suffered systemic reactions possibly associated with phenylephrine given by topical application of 10% eye-drops, on a cotton pledget, by subconjunctival injection, or by irrigation of the lachrymal sac. Of 15 patients with myocardial infarct (9 of whom had a previous history of cardiovascular disease), 11 died; 7 additional patients required cardiopulmonary resuscitation for cardiac arrhythmia or cardia arrests; the remainder of the adverse reactions were severe increase of systemic blood pressure, tachycardia, and reflex bradycardia. The following guidelines are suggested for the clinical use of phenylephrine: use 10% phenylephrine with caution in patients with known cardiac disease, hypertension, aneurysms, and advanced arteriosclerosis; only use the 2.5% solutions in infants and the elderly; the use of 10% phenylephrine to irrigate, with a conjunctival pledget, or injected subconjunctivally should be discouraged; only one application is allowable per hour to each eye; contra-indicated in patients taking monoamine oxidase inhibitors and tricyclic antidepressants; be aware that pressor effects and tachycardia can be induced in the atropinised patient.— F. T. Fraunfelder and A. F. Scafidi, *Am. J. Ophthal.*, 1978, *85*, 447. Results of a prospective double-blind study indicated that the incidence of severe hypertensive response to topically administered ocular 10% phenylephrine is very low.— M. M. Brown *et al.*, *Archs Ophthal.*, 1980, *98*, 487. See also R. B. Smith *et al.*, *Eye Ear Nose Throat Month.*, 1976, *55*, 133.

Treatment of Adverse Effects. The hypertensive effects of phenylephrine may be treated with an alpha-adrenoceptor blocking agent such as phentolamine mesylate, 5 to 10 mg intravenously, repeated as necessary.

Precautions. Phenylephrine should be avoided or only used with great caution in hypersusceptible patients or those with hyperthyroidism, aneurysm, hypertension, arteriosclerosis, and cardiovascular disorders, such as ventricular tachycardia, myocardial disease, or bradycardia. In late pregnancy noradrenaline (p.21) provokes uterine changes which can result in foetal asphyxia; any alpha-adrenoceptor stimulant might have a similar contractile action.

Phenylephrine eye-drops are contra-indicated in narrow-angle glaucoma; they should be avoided or only used with extreme caution in infants since they can have powerful systemic effects.

Excessive use of phenylephrine nasal drops can lead to rebound congestion.

Phenylephrine should not be given to patients being treated with a monoamine oxidase inhibitor or within 14 days of stopping such treatment (see Precautions for Phenelzine Sulphate, p.128; it should also be avoided in patients receiving tricyclic antidepressants. Patients receiving guanethidine and similar adrenergic neurone blocking agents are extremely sensitive to the hypertensive (and mydriatic) effects of phenylephrine; phenylephrine may also markedly reverse the hypotensive effects of reserpine and methyldopa.

Although phenylephrine is less liable than adrenaline and noradrenaline to induce fibrillation if used as a pressor agent during anaesthesia with chloroform, cyclopropane, halothane, and trichloroethylene, nevertheless, caution is necessary.

Interactions. A 46-year-old man taking *debrisoquine* 20 mg thrice daily for hypertension with satisfactory control was given phenylephrine 50 mg by mouth. Marked hypertension occurred which was reduced by phentolamine.— J. Aminu *et al.* (letter), *Lancet*, 1970, *2*, 935. Investigations in 4 healthy subjects indicated that the hypertensive effect of phenylephrine could be markedly enhanced by administration of *debrisoquine*.— W. Allum *et al.*, *Br. J. clin. Pharmac.*, 1974, *1*, 51.

In 4 volunteers pretreated with *imipramine*, 25 mg thrice daily for 5 days, the pressor effect of phenylephrine was enhanced by a factor of 2 to 3, that of adrenaline by a factor of 2 to 4, and that of noradrenaline by a factor of 4 to 8, with no significant difference in the response to isoprenaline. All 4 subjects experienced cardiac arrhythmias when given adrenaline. Felypressin might be a more suitable vasoconstrictor for use in patients taking tricyclic antidepressants. When they were pretreated with monoamine oxidase inhibitors (phenelzine 15 mg thrice daily or tranylcypromine 10 mg thrice daily) for 7 days the pressor effect of *phenylephrine* was significantly enhanced but there was no significant change in the response to *adrenaline*, *noradrenaline*, or *isoprenaline*. Isoprenaline-induced tachycardia was significantly reduced. It was unlikely that patients taking monoamine oxidase inhibitors would be seriously at risk if given noradrenaline in local anaesthetic solutions.— A. J. Boakes *et al.*, *Br. med. J.*, 1973, *1*, 311. The finding that imipramine enhanced the pressor effects of sympathomimetic agents to a greater degree than did monoamine oxidase inhibitors was at variance with clinical experience.— G. G. Wallis (letter), *ibid.*, 549.

Pressor effects and tachycardia can be induced in the *atropinised* patient given phenylephrine eye-drops.— F. T. Fraunfelder and A. F. Scafidi, *Am. J. Ophthal.*, 1978, *85*, 447.

A study indicating that pre-operative phenylephrine eye-drops can be hazardous in patients with sympathetic denervation such as those with long-standing insulin-dependent diabetes or hypertensive patients receiving *reserpine* or *guanethidine*.— J. M. Kim *et al.*, *Am. J. Ophthal.*, 1978, *85*, 862.

A report of a fatality occurring in a 49-year-old woman with asymptomatic hypertension on a regimen of hydrochlorothiazide 50 mg twice daily and propranolol hydrochloride 40 mg four times daily following the instillation of one drop of 10% phenylephrine hydrochloride solution in each eye during an ophthalmological examination.— E. Cass *et al.*, *Can. med. Ass. J.*, 1979, *120*, 1261.

Absorption and Fate. Phenylephrine has reduced bioavailability from the gastro-intestinal tract owing to first-pass metabolism by monoamine oxidase in the gut and liver. When injected intramuscularly it takes 10 to 15 minutes to act and subcutaneous and intramuscular injections are effective for about an hour. Intravenous injections are effective for about 20 minutes.

Pregnancy and the neonate. A study in pregnant *dogs* indicated that phenylephrine produces different effects in the foetus than those in the mother, and that it is not likely that any sizeable amount crosses the placenta.— D. M. Linkie *et al.*, *Am. J. med. Sci.*, 1966, *252*, 277.

Uses. Phenylephrine hydrochloride is a sympathomimetic agent with mainly direct effects on adrenergic receptors. It has predominantly alpha-adrenergic activity and is without stimulating effects on the central nervous system. Its pressor activity is weaker than that of noradrenaline (see p.21) but of longer duration. After injection it produces peripheral vasoconstriction and increased arterial pressure; it also causes reflex bradycardia. It reduces blood flow to the skin and to the kidneys.

Phenylephrine has been used in the treatment of hypotensive states, e.g. circulatory failure, spinal anaesthesia, or hypotension following the use of chlorpromazine and other phenothiazines. It has been administered in a dose of 2 to 5 mg subcutaneously or intramuscularly with further doses of 1 to 10 mg if necessary, or in a dose of 100 to 500 μg by slow intravenous injection as a 0.1% solution, repeated as necessary after at least 15 minutes. Alternatively, 5 to 20 mg in 500 ml of dextrose injection or sodium chloride injection has been infused intravenously, initially at a rate of up to 180 μg per minute, reduced, according to the response, to 30 to 60 μg per minute. A suggested dose for children is 100 μg per kg body-weight, subcutaneously or intramuscularly.

Phenylephrine has been given by intravenous injection to stop paroxysmal supraventricular tachycardia. The initial dose is usually not greater than 500 μg given as a 0.1% solution with subsequent doses gradually increased up to 1 mg if necessary.

Phenylephrine was formerly given by mouth in initial doses of 150 mg daily subsequently reduced to 60 mg daily for the management of orthostatic hypotension, but this use is no longer recommended.

Phenylephrine hydrochloride may be given in preparations for the relief of nasal congestion in doses of 10 mg three or four times daily by mouth. It was formerly tried as an inhalation in bronchial asthma; a 1% solution was employed in a nebuliser for this purpose. The acid tartrate has also been used. Phenylephrine hydrochloride has been used in a concentration of 1 in 20 000 as a vasoconstrictor with local anaesthetics.

Locally, phenylephrine hydrochloride is used as a

nasal decongestant in rhinitis and sinusitis. For this purpose 2 to 3 drops of a 0.25 to 0.5% solution may be instilled into each nostril every 3 to 4 hours. It may cause local irritation; overuse causes rebound congestion.

In ophthalmology, phenylephrine hydrochloride is employed as a mydriatic and conjunctival decongestant as a 0.1% to 10% solution. The effect lasts several hours. Solutions stronger than 2% may cause intense irritation and a local anaesthetic other than butacaine should be added to these. In open-angle glaucoma it is sometimes used to lower intra-ocular pressure temporarily. Owing to the risk of systemic effects the 10% strength is contra-indicated in infants and in patients with aneurysms or other risk factors such as hypertension or coronary heart disease.

Anaesthesia. The injection of vasoconstrictor drugs together with amethocaine into the subarachnoid space of 8852 patients receiving spinal block was found to prolong the anaesthesia safely and consistently. The addition of adrenaline, 0.2 ml of a 1 in 1000 solution, prolonged the block by 50%; phenylephrine, 0.5 ml of a 1% solution, prolonged it by 100%. No systemic effects were noted with either drug, though with phenylephrine occasional hypoaesthesias of the legs and feet lasting 8 to 12 hours occurred. There was no damage to the spinal cord.— D. C. Moore and L. D. Bridenbaugh, *J. Am. med. Ass.*, 1966, *195*, 907.

Cardiac disorders. Phenylephrine terminated ventricular tachycardia in 12 of 13 patients. In 4 patients extensively studied doses of 0.4 to 1 mg were required. The required dose was reduced by a factor of at least 2 when edrophonium hydrochloride 10 to 20 mg was first given; the required dose was increased by a similar factor when atropine 2.4 mg was first given. Carotid sinus massage alone did not break ventricular tachycardia but was effective after edrophonium in doses of 15 or 20 mg. A vagal mechanism was considered to be involved.— M. B. Waxman and R. W. Wald, *Circulation*, 1977, *56*, 385.

ENT disorders. Nebulised phenylephrine produced a short-lasting reduction in respiratory resistance in 7 of 8 infants with symptoms of acute viral croup; the remaining infant was later shown to have acute epiglottitis. Longer-acting alpha-adrenergic stimulants should be investigated.— W. Lenney and A. D. Milner, *Archs Dis. Childh.*, 1978, *53*, 704.

Hypotension. Phenylephrine in doses of 30 mg abolished the postural symptoms in 4 patients with orthostatic hypotension but also produced recumbent hypertension. The long-term use of phenylephrine for this condition is considered hazardous.— B. Davies *et al.*, *Lancet*, 1978, *1*, 172. See also D. Robertson *et al.*, *Am. J. Ophthal.*, 1979, *87*, 819.

Ocular disorders. Phenylephrine 10% dilates the pupils adequately for ophthalmoscopy; pupillary dilatation is produced without loss of accommodation. After the instillation of phenylephrine miosis can be achieved with 1% pilocarpine. As phenylephrine will partially overcome the miosis produced by even the strongest miotics and does not jeopardise control of intra-ocular pressure in chronic open-angle glaucoma, it is useful for ophthalmoscopy in patients with chronic open-angle glaucoma on miotic therapy.— S. I. Davidson, *Prescribers' J.*, 1978, *18*, 139.

Studies of the ocular effects of phenylephrine.— H. D. Gambill *et al.*, *Archs Ophthal., N.Y.*, 1967, *77*, 740; M. J. Mattila *et al.*, *Farmaceutiskt Notisbl.*, 1968, *77*, 205; N. J. Haddad *et al.*, *Am. J. Ophthal.*, 1970, *70*, 729; R. B. Smith *et al.*, *Eye Ear Nose Throat Month.*, 1976, *55*, 133.

For a report of phenylephrine being used in conjunction with eucatropine to induce mydriasis, see Eucatropine Hydrochloride, p.300.

Retrograde ejaculation. A satisfactory result was achieved in 1 of 6 young men with retrograde ejaculation treated with intravenous phenylephrine. Findings in the other 5, who had a predominant disorder of emission and therefore diminished sperm counts in the postcoital urine, indicated that restitution of vas deferens function cannot be achieved pharmacologically.— K. Stockamp *et al.*, *Fert. Steril.*, 1974, *25*, 817.

Preparations

Eye Preparations

Phenylephrine Eye-drops *(B.P.C. 1973)*. PHNL. Phenylephrine hydrochloride 10 g, sodium metabisulphite 500 mg, sodium citrate 300 mg, benzalkonium chloride solution 0.02 ml, water to 100 ml. Sterilised by filtration. Protect from light.

Phenylephrine Eye-drops Strong *(A.P.F.)*. Gutt. Phenylephrin. Fort. Phenylephrine hydrochloride 10 g, sodium metabisulphite 100 mg, disodium edetate 50 mg, benzalkonium chloride solution 0.02 ml, Water for Injections to 100 ml. Sterilised by autoclaving. Protect from light.

Phenylephrine Eye-drops Weak *(A.P.F.)*. Gutt. Phenylephrin. Phenylephrine hydrochloride 125 mg, sodium metabisulphite 100 mg, disodium edetate 50 mg, sodium chloride 700 mg, benzalkonium chloride solution 0.02 ml, Water for Injections to 100 ml. Sterilised by autoclaving. Protect from light.

Phenylephrine Hydrochloride Ophthalmic Solution *(U.S.P.)*. A sterile aqueous solution of phenylephrine hydrochloride. It may contain a suitable antimicrobial agent, buffer, and suitable antioxidants. pH 4 to 7.5 (buffered); 3 to 4.5 (unbuffered). Store in airtight containers. Protect from light.

Injections

Phenylephrine Hydrochloride Injection *(U.S.P.)*. A sterile solution of phenylephrine hydrochloride in Water for Injections. pH 3 to 6.5. Protect from light.

Phenylephrine Injection *(B.P.)*. A sterile solution of phenylephrine hydrochloride in Water for Injections. Sterilise by filtration and store in ampoules in which the air has been replaced by nitrogen or other suitable gas. pH 4.5 to 6.5. Protect from light.

Nasal Preparations

Phenylephrine Hydrochloride Nasal Solution *(U.S.P.)*. A solution of phenylephrine hydrochloride. Store in airtight containers. Protect from light.

Phenylephrine Instillation *(A.P.F.)*. Phenylephrine Nasal Drops; Phenylephrine Nasal Spray. Phenylephrine hydrochloride 250 mg, sodium metabisulphite 100 mg, sodium chloride 600 mg, chlorbutol 500 mg, propylene glycol 5 ml, freshly boiled and cooled water to 100 ml. Store in small, well-filled, airtight containers. Protect from light.

Phenylephrine Instillation Strong *(A.P.F.)*. Strong Phenylephrine Nasal Drops; Strong Phenylephrine Nasal Spray. Phenylephrine hydrochloride 1 g, sodium metabisulphite 100 mg, sodium chloride 400 mg, chlorbutol 500 mg, propylene glycol 5 ml, freshly boiled and cooled water to 100 ml. Store in small, well-filled, airtight containers. Protect from light.

Proprietary Preparations

Biomydrin *(Warner, UK)*. A nasal spray containing phenylephrine hydrochloride 0.25%, thonzylamine hydrochloride 1%, neomycin sulphate 0.1%, and gramicidin 0.005%. For nasal congestion.

Hayphryn *(Winthrop, UK)*. A nasal spray containing phenylephrine hydrochloride 0.5% and thenyldiamine hydrochloride 0.1%. For nasal congestion especially of allergic origin.

Isopto Frin *(Alcon, UK: Farillon, UK)*. Eye-drops containing phenylephrine hydrochloride 0.12% and hypromellose 0.5%. For minor irritation of the eye in the absence of infection. (Also available as Isopto Frin in *Austral.*, *Canad.* and as Isopto-Frin in *S.Afr.*, *Switz.*).

Minims Phenylephrine Hydrochloride *(Smith & Nephew Pharmaceuticals, UK)*. Sterile eye-drops containing phenylephrine hydrochloride 10%, in single-use disposable applicators. (Also available as Minims Phenylephrine Hydrochloride in *Austral.*).

Neophryn *(Winthrop, UK)*. Phenylephrine hydrochloride, available as **Nasal Drops** containing 0.25% and as **Nasal Spray** containing 0.5%. Neophryn is known in some countries as Neosynephrine.

Prefrin Liquifilm *(Allergan, UK)*. Eye-drops containing phenylephrine hydrochloride 0.12%.

Uniflu *(Unigreg, UK: Vestric, UK)*. Tablets each containing phenylephrine hydrochloride 10 mg, caffeine 30 mg, codeine phosphate 10 mg, diphenhydramine hydrochloride 15 mg, and paracetamol 500 mg, supplied with an equal number of **Gregovite C** tablets each containing ascorbic acid 300 mg. For colds and influenza. *Dose.* 1 of each every 4 hours; children, over 12 years, 1 of each thrice daily.

Vibrocil *(Zyma, UK)*. Contains phenylephrine base 0.25%, dimethindene maleate 0.025%, and neomycin sulphate 0.35%, available as **Nasal Drops, Nasal Gel,** and **Nasal Spray.** For the common cold, rhinitis, sinusitis, and hay fever.

Other Proprietary Names

Arg.— Poen-Efrina; *Austral.*— I-Care, Isopto Phenylephrine, Mistol Mist, Phenephrin, Visopt; *Belg.*— Rinex, Visadron; *Canad.*— Mydfrin, Optocrymal, Soothe; *Ital.*— Fenilfar, Isonefrine, Isotropina, Visadron; *Neth.*— Boraline, Visadron; *Norw.*— Metaoxedrinklorid Minims; *S.Afr.*— Nasalmed; *Spain*— Neosinefrina; *Swed.*— Neosyn; *USA*— Isophrin, Mydfrin.

Phenylephrine hydrochloride was also formerly marketed in Great Britain under the proprietary name Narex (*Norton: Vestric*).

A preparation containing phenylephrine hydrochloride was also formerly marketed in Great Britain under the proprietary name Nez (*Rybar*).

2095-q

Phenylpropanolamine Hydrochloride *(B.P., U.S.P.)*.

Cloridrato de Fenilpropanolamine; Mydriatin; *dl*-Norephedrine Hydrochloride.

(±)-2-Amino-1-phenylpropan-1-ol hydrochloride.

$C_9H_{13}NO,HCl = 187.7$.

CAS — 14838-15-4 (phenylpropanolamine); 154-41-6 (hydrochloride).

Pharmacopoeias. In *Br.*, *Braz.*, and *U.S.*

A white to creamy-white crystalline powder, odourless or with a slight aromatic odour and with a bitter taste. M.p. 191° to 196°.

Soluble 1 in 2.5 of water, 1 in 9 of alcohol; practically insoluble in chloroform and ether. A 3% solution in water has a pH of 4.2 to 6. A 2.6% solution is iso-osmotic with serum. Solutions are **sterilised** by autoclaving or by filtration. **Store** in airtight containers. Protect from light.

An aqueous solution of phenylpropanolamine iso-osmotic with serum (2.6%) caused 95% haemolysis of erythrocytes cultured in it for 45 minutes.— E. R. Hammarlund and K. Pedersen-Bjergaard, *J. pharm. Sci.*, 1961, *50*, 24.

Adverse Effects, Treatment, and Precautions. As for Ephedrine, p.11.

Severe hypertensive episodes have followed phenylpropanolamine ingestion.

Abuse. See under Effects on Mental State (below).

Effects on the kidneys. A report of acute interstitial nephritis in a young woman who had taken an appetite suppressant containing phenylpropanolamine (Fullstop) over the previous 3 weeks. She had also taken 2 or 3 tablets containing aspirin 325 mg, and paracetamol 650 mg.— W. M. Bennett (letter), *Lancet*, 1979, *2*, 42.

Effects on mental state. During 1979 the Swedish Adverse Drug Reaction Committee received several reports of psychic disturbances during treatment with phenylpropanolamine. Of 61 cases reported, 48 were in children aged 0 to 15 years. The dominant symptoms were restlessness, irritability, aggression (especially in younger children), and sleep disturbances. Five cases of psychotic episodes have also been reported. These included 2 boys aged 3 and 8 years who were confused and unable to recognise their parents a few hours after taking phenylpropanolamine (Rinexin, *Leo*); a 4-year-old girl who had episodes of visual hallucinosis and a grand-mal seizure after phenylpropanolamine in association with the antihistamine, brompheniramine (Lunerin, *Draco*); a 25-year-old woman who became increasingly excited and lacking in concentration with sleep/wakefulness disturbances during treatment with phenylpropanolamine (Monydrin, *Draco*), after 9 days experiencing vivid paranoid misconceptions and episodic muscular twitchings in the legs, her symptoms disappearing within 24 hours of stopping the drug; and a 17-year-old who was admitted to mental hospital on 3 occasions with signs and symptoms of acute mania-like psychosis with excessive motor excitement, aggressive behaviour, and elevated mood with uncontrollable thought and speech, and hallucinosis and confusion on the third admission, who on recovery was found to have taken large quantities of phenylpropanolamine (Rinexin) and brompheniramine (Rinomar, *Leo*) before each episode.— G. Norvenius *et al.* (letter), *Lancet*, 1979, *2*, 1367.

Further references.— F. J. Kane and B. Q. Green, *Am. J. Psychiat.*, 1966, *123*, 484; B. K. Wharton, *Br. J. Psychiat.*, 1970, *117*, 439.

Hypertension. All of 37 healthy normotensive young adults had a rise in blood pressure within an hour of taking a capsule of an anorectic preparation containing phenylpropanolamine 85 mg (Trimolets); in 12 of the 37, peak supine diastolic blood pressures of 100 mmHg or more were recorded compared with 1 of 35 similar subjects who took matching placebo. Three of the 12 subjects required antihypertensive therapy. Symptoms reported by the subjects receiving phenylpropanolamine were: tingling feelings in head (6); dizziness which was not postural (5); postural dizziness (4); palpitations (5); headache (6); chest tightness (3); rash (3); tremor (2); nausea (2); lassitude (1); tinnitus (1); 'hot feeling' (1); 17 of those receiving active drug did not report symptoms. One subject in the placebo group reported nausea. Because of these blood pressure effects, study of Trimolets was discontinued and a preparation containing less phenylpropanolamine was investigated instead (capsules of Contac 500, which contain phenylpropanolamine 50 mg and belladonna alkaloids 250 µg). In 34 subjects who took one Contac 500 capsule there was a small mean rise in blood pressure, and 4 developed supine diastolic blood pressures of 100 mmHg or more, compared with none of 35 who took matching placebo. No subjects in either group reported symptoms. These results indicate that the availability of high-dose phenylpropanolamine-containing preparations without medical advice is potentially hazardous. Although the second preparation produced far less dramatic effects, it would also be likely to induce dangerous degrees of hypertension if more than one capsule were taken.— J. D. Horowitz *et al.*, *Lancet*, 1980, *1*, 60. Hypertensive episodes appear to be more likely with preparations containing phenylpropanolamine in the free form rather than in the slow-release form.— M. F. Cuthbert (letter), *Lancet*, 1980, *1*, 367.

Individual reports of hypertension, sometimes in association with cardiac arrhythmias, in patients taking preparations containing phenylpropanolamine.— P. H. Livingston (letter), *J. Am. med. Ass.*, 1966, *196*, 1159; W. F. C. Duvernoy, *New Engl. J. Med.*, 1969, *280*, 877; S. R. Shapiro (letter), *ibid.*, 1363; R. B. Peterson and L. A. Vasquez (letter), *J. Am. med. Ass.*, 1973, *223*, 324; D. B. Frewin *et al.*, *Med. J. Aust.*, 1978, *2*, 497.

Interactions. Phenylpropanolamine 50 mg by mouth in 3 healthy men produced a rise of 18 to 26 mmHg in systolic blood pressure, but this dose in a slow-release form with an atropine-like compound had no significant effect. After tranylcypromine 30 mg daily had been taken for 20 to 30 days, phenylpropanolamine 50 mg caused a rapid and potentially dangerous rise of blood pressure with an associated bradycardia and intense throbbing headache. Phentolamine was used to lower the blood pressure. When a capsule containing phenylpropanolamine 50 mg and isopropamide 2.5 mg in a slow-release form was taken after tranylcypromine, a gradual rise of blood pressure to 150 to 160 mmHg systolic and 95 to 100 mmHg diastolic occurred over 90 minutes and fell after 2 hours. Severe hypertensive episodes were more likely to occur when preparations containing phenylpropanolamine in a free form rather than slow-release form were taken by patients receiving monoamine oxidase inhibitors.— M. F. Cuthbert *et al.*, *Br. med. J.*, 1969, *1*, 404.

Severe headache, visions of coloured lights, tightness of the chest, and heart pounding were reported by a patient who had taken phenylpropanolamine 64 mg after eating a meal which included cheese. His blood pressure was 180/110 mmHg after 20 minutes but fell rapidly towards normal.— G. J. Gibson and D. A. Warrell (letter), *Lancet*, 1972, *2*, 492.

A 27-year-old woman with schizophrenia and T-wave abnormality of the heart, who had responded to thioridazine 100 mg daily with procyclidine 2.5 mg twice daily, died from ventricular fibrillation within 2 hours of taking a single dose of a preparation reported to contain chlorpheniramine maleate 4 mg with phenylpropanolamine hydrochloride 50 mg (Contac C), concurrently with thioridazine.— G. Chouinard *et al.*, *Can. med. Ass. J.*, 1978, *119*, 729.

A 27-year-old woman who had been taking D-phenylpropanolamine [sic.] 85 mg daily for some months, experienced severe hypertension when she also took indomethacin 25 mg. In a placebo-controlled challenge neither drug alone caused any significant rise in blood pressure, but administration of phenylpropanolamine followed 40 minutes later by indomethacin, caused very severe hypertension within half an hour. Administration of diazepam caused sedation without affecting the blood pressure, whereas phentolamine rapidly reduced it. It was considered that the inhibition of prostaglandin by indomethacin might have caused enhancement of the sympathomimetic effect of phenylpropanolamine.— K. Y. Lee *et al.*, *Lancet*, 1979, *1*, 1110. See also *idem* (letter), *Med. J. Aust.*, 1979, *1*, 525.

For the effect of phenylpropanolamine on antihypertensive therapy, see Methyldopa, p.153.

Overdosage. A report of hypertension associated with severe postural hypotension occurring in a 17-year-old girl who had ingested 6 capsules of an anorectic preparation containing 85 mg phenylpropanolamine with 15 mg ferrous gluconate and various vitamin additives. During a double-blind crossover study in 6 healthy subjects clinically significant hypertension occurred in all subjects after each had ingested one similar capsule although major degrees of postural hypotension did not occur.— J. D. Horowitz *et al.*, *Med. J. Aust.*. 1979, *1*, 175.

Absorption and Fate. Phenylpropanolamine is readily and completely absorbed from the gastro-intestinal tract, peak plasma concentrations being achieved about an hour or two after oral administration. It is excreted almost entirely unchanged in the urine.

About 94% of a 25-mg dose of radioactive phenylpropanolamine was excreted in the urine in 24 hours; nearly 90% of the dose was excreted unchanged. Of 1 to 7% of the dose which was metabolised at least one-third was metabolised to hippuric acid.— J. E. Sinsheimer *et al.*, *Trans. biochem. Soc.*, 1973, *1*, 1160.

Plasma-phenylpropanolamine concentrations in 2 subjects after oral ingestion.— L. Neelakantan and H. B. Kostenbauder, *J. pharm. Sci.*, 1976, *65*, 740.

Uses. Phenylpropanolamine hydrochloride is a sympathomimetic agent with an action similar to that of ephedrine (p.11) but less active as a central nervous stimulant. It is given in usual doses of 25 or 30 mg three or four times daily for the symptomatic relief of nasal congestion; sustained-release preparations are given in doses of 50 to 100 mg every 12 hours in conjunction with an antihistamine. It has also been given to control urinary incontinence, and was formerly advocated for appetite reduction.

A 1 to 3% solution or nasal jelly has been used for nasal decongestion.

Headache. Cluster headaches in 3 patients were successfully treated with decongestant tablets containing paracetamol, phenyltoloxamine citrate, and phenylpropanolamine hydrochloride (Sinutabs) after numerous other medications including ergot, propranolol, methysergide, and codeine had failed. Phenylpropanolamine was considered to be the active ingredient.— K. L. Cohen (letter), *New Engl. J. Med.*, 1980, *303*, 107.

Obesity. There is no good evidence to indicate that phenylpropanolamine can help obese patients achieve long-term weight reduction.— *Med. Lett.*, 1979, *21*, 65.

Retrograde ejaculation. Reports of the use of preparations containing phenylpropanolamine to correct retrograde ejaculation: B. H. Stewart and J. A. Bergant, *Fert. Steril.*, 1974, *25*, 1073; S. Thiagarajah *et al.*, *ibid.*, 1978, *30*, 96.

Urinary incontinence. Preparations containing phenylpropanolamine may be of benefit in male incontinence.— P. H. L. Worth, *Practitioner*, 1979, *223*, 325. See also S. A. Awad *et al.*, *Br. J. Urol.*, 1978, *50*, 332 (phenylpropanolamine alone).

Proprietary Preparations

Eskornade Spansule *(Smith Kline & French, UK)*. Sustained-release capsules each containing phenylpropanolamine hydrochloride 50 mg, isopropamide iodide equivalent to isopropamide 2.5 mg, and diphenylpyraline hydrochloride 5 mg. For nasal congestion. **Eskornade Syrup**. Contains in each 5 ml phenylpropanolamine hydrochloride 15 mg, isopropamide iodide equivalent to isopropamide 750 µg, and diphenylpyraline hydrochloride 1.5 mg (suggested diluent, syrup). *Dose*. Eskornade Spansules: 1 every 12 hours. Eskornade Syrup: 10 ml thrice daily.

Pholcolix *(Warner, UK)*. Syrup containing in each 5 ml phenylpropanolamine hydrochloride 12.5 mg, paracetamol 150 mg, and pholcodine 5 mg (suggested diluent, syrup). For colds complicated by cough. *Dose*. 10 ml four times daily; children, 2 to 5 years, 2.5 ml; 6 to 12 years, 5 ml.

Rinurel Linctus *(Warner, UK)*. Contains in each 5 ml phenylpropanolamine hydrochloride 12.5 mg, paracetamol 150 mg, phenyltoloxamine citrate 11 mg, and pholcodine 5 mg (suggested diluent, syrup). For the common cold accompanied by cough. **Rinurel Tablets**. Scored tablets each containing phenylpropanolamine hydrochloride 25 mg, paracetamol 300 mg, and phenyltoloxamine citrate 22 mg. For sinus headache, the common cold, hay fever, and rhinitis. **Rinurel SA**. Sustained-action tablets each containing phenylpropanolamine hydrochloride 100 mg, paracetamol 600 mg, and phenyltoloxamine citrate 66 mg. *Dose*. Rinurel linctus: 10 ml 4 times daily; children, 2 to 5 years, 2.5 ml; 5 to 12 years, 5 ml. Rinurel tablets: 2 initially, then 1 every 4 hours; children, 5 to 12 years, half the adult dose. Rinurel SA tablets: 1 every 12 hours.

Totolin *(Galen, UK)*. Syrup containing in each 5 ml phenylpropanolamine hydrochloride 7.5 mg and guaiphenesin 30 mg. Bronchodilator and expectorant. *Dose*. Children, 1 to 5 years, 5 ml every 4 to 6 hours; 6 to 12 years, 10 ml.

Triogesic Elixir *(Wander, UK)*. Contains in each 5 ml phenylpropanolamine hydrochloride 3 mg, paracetamol 125 mg, and alcohol (95%) 0.5 ml (suggested diluent, water or syrup). For sinusitis, otitis media, and coryza. **Triogesic Tablets**. Scored tablets each containing phenylpropanolamine hydrochloride 12.5 mg and paracetamol 500 mg. *Dose*. Elixir: 20 ml every 3 or 4 hours; children, 5 to 10 ml thrice daily. Tablets: 1 or 2 every 3 or 4 hours.

Triominic *(Wander, UK)*. Sustained-release **Tablets** each containing phenylpropanolamine hydrochloride 50 mg, mepyramine maleate 25 mg, and pheniramine maleate 25 mg. For symptomatic relief of hay fever or other forms of rhinitis. **Triominic Syrup**. Contains in each 5 ml the equivalent of one-quarter tablet (suggested diluent, water or syrup). *Dose*. Tablets: 1 every 6 to 8 hours; not more than 3 in 24 hours. Syrup: 10 ml every 4 hours up to 4 times in 24 hours; children, over 6 years, 5 ml.

Triotussic Suspension *(Wander, UK)*. Contains in each 5 ml phenylpropanolamine hydrochloride 12.5 mg, mepyramine maleate 6.25 mg, pheniramine maleate 6.25 mg, noscapine hydrochloride 20 mg, terpin hydrate 90 mg, and paracetamol 160 mg (suggested diluent, syrup). For colds complicated by cough. *Dose*. 5 to 10 ml every 3 to 4 hours up to 4 times in 24 hours; children, over 6 years, 2.5 to 5 ml 4 times daily.

Other Proprietary Names

Coldecon *(Canad.)*; Control *(USA)*; Monydrin *(Norw., Swed.)*; Propadrine, Rhindecon *(both USA)*; Rinexin *(Norw., Swed.)*; Tepanil *(see also under Diethylpropion Hydrochloride, p.66) (Austral.)*.

2096-p

Pholedrine Sulphate *(B.P.C. 1949)*. Isodrine Sulphate; Sympropaminum *(pholedrine)*. 4-(2-Methylaminopropyl)phenol sulphate.
$(C_{10}H_{15}NO)_2,H_2SO_4$=428.5.

CAS — 370-14-9 (pholedrine); 6114-26-7 (sulphate).

Pharmacopoeias. Hung. includes pholedrine.

A white odourless crystalline powder. M.p. about 321° with decomposition. **Soluble** 1 in 20 of water (pH about 6); practically insoluble in alcohol, chloroform, and ether. Solutions are **sterilised** by autoclaving or by filtration.

Pholedrine sulphate is a sympathomimetic agent with an action similar to that of ephedrine (p.10), but it is reported to have little or no stimulant effect on the central nervous system. It has been given by injection as a vasopressor in doses of 10 to 20 mg intramuscularly or subcutaneously, and 5 to 20 mg intravenously. It has also been used topically as a mydriatic.

Proprietary Names

Veritol *(Knoll, Arg.; Knoll, Ger.; Knoll, Ital.; Knoll, Switz.)*.

2097-s

Protokylol Hydrochloride. JB 251; Protochylol Hydrochloride. 1-(3,4-Dihydroxyphenyl)-2-(α-methyl-3,4-methylenedioxyphenethylamino)ethanol hydrochloride.
$C_{18}H_{21}NO_5,HCl$=367.8.

CAS — 136-70-9 (protokylol); 136-69-6 (hydrochloride).

A white crystalline powder. M.p. about 126°. **Soluble** in water.

Adverse Effects, Treatment, and Precautions. As for Isoprenaline, pp.15-6.
Dermatitis has also been reported.

Uses. Protokylol hydrochloride is a sympathomimetic agent with predominantly beta-adrenergic activity and actions and uses similar to those of isoprenaline (p.16). It has been given by mouth as a bronchodilator in doses of 2 to 4 mg four times daily. It has also been given parenterally and by inhalation.

Proprietary Names
Asmetil *(Benvegna, Ital.)*; Beres *(Simes, Ital.)*; Palison *(Farmasimes, Spain)*.

2098-w

Pseudoephedrine Hydrochloride *(B.P., U.S.P.)*.

d-Ψ-Ephedrine Hydrochloride; *d*-Isoephedrine Hydrochloride. (1*S*,2*S*)-2-Methylamino-1-phenylpropan-1-ol hydrochloride. $C_{10}H_{15}NO,HCl=201.7$.

CAS — 90-82-4 (pseudoephedrine); 345-78-8 (hydrochloride).

Pharmacopoeias. In *Br.* and *U.S.*

The hydrochloride of an alkaloid obtained from *Ephedra* spp. White or off-white crystals or powder, with a faint characteristic odour and with a bitter taste. M.p. 182° to 186° with a range of not more than 2°.

Soluble 1 in 1.6 of water, 1 in 4 of alcohol, and 1 in 60 of chloroform; very slightly soluble in ether. A solution in water is dextrorotatory. A 0.5% solution in water has a pH of 4.6 to 6. **Store** in airtight containers. Protect from light.

2099-e

Pseudoephedrine Sulphate.

Pseudoephedrine Sulfate *(U.S.P.)*; Sch 4855. $(C_{10}H_{15}NO)_2,H_2SO_4=428.5$.

CAS — 7460-12-0.

Pharmacopoeias. In *U.S.*

A white crystalline powder. M.p. 174° to 179° with a range of not more than 2°. **Soluble** in water. A 5% solution in water is dextrorotatory and has a pH of 5 to 6.5. **Store** in airtight containers. Protect from light.

Adverse Effects, Treatment, and Precautions. As for Ephedrine, p.11.

A 17-year-old youth became unconscious and developed transient hypertension after taking one 60-mg tablet of pseudoephedrine hydrochloride.— H. R. Rutstein, *Archs Otolar.*, 1963, *77*, 145. A report of a 10-month-old infant with phenylketonuria who appeared to be unduly sensitive to pseudoephedrine. He was noted to be excited and crying for no apparent reason, within an hour of taking a 15-mg dose. A second dose 6 hours later was followed by increased screaming, extreme agitation, and confusion. A third dose the following morning resulted in a return of the abnormal behaviour.—S. P. Spielberg and J. D. Schulman, *J. Pediat.*, 1977, *90*, 1026.

In 34 healthy males given pseudoephedrine 120 or 150 mg, as a sustained-release preparation, twice daily for 7 days mean plasma concentrations were about 450 and 510 ng per ml respectively. Side-effects (dry mouth, anorexia, insomnia, anxiety, tension, restlessness, tachycardia, palpitations) were common; there was some evidence of tachyphylaxis.— J. Dickerson *et al.*, *Eur. J. clin. Pharmac.*, 1978, *14*, 253.

Allergy. Within 2 hours of swallowing one 60-mg tablet of pseudoephedrine hydrochloride a woman developed a severe generalised allergic rash, rigors, joint swelling, faintness, and tachycardia.— *Practitioner*, 1973, *211*, 828.

Effects on the heart. Asymptomatic multifocal ventricular premature contractions in a pilot were attributed to the pseudoephedrine in Actifed, of which he had taken 2 tablets every 4 hours day and night for several days.— C. E. Billings *et al.*, *Aerospace Med.*, 1974, *45*, 551.

Interactions. The absorption rate of pseudoephedrine hydrochloride was increased by the concomitant administration of aluminium hydroxide mixture.— R. L. Lucarotti *et al.*, *J. pharm. Sci.*, 1972, *61*, 903.

Absorption and Fate. Pseudoephedrine is readily and completely absorbed from the gastro-intestinal tract. It is resistant to metabolism by mono-amine oxidase and is largely excreted unchanged in the urine. It has a half-life of several hours; elimination is enhanced and half-life accordingly shorter in acid urine.

The plasma half-lives in 3 subjects given pseudoephedrine 180 mg by mouth were 5.2, 7.6, and 8 hours when their urinary pH was between 5.6 and 6. When the pH was increased to 8 the plasma half-lives lengthened to 9.2, 16, and 15 hours and when the pH was reduced the half-lives shortened.— R. G. Kuntzman *et al.*, *Clin. Pharmac. Ther.*, 1971, *12*, 62. Pseudoephedrine has been shown to accumulate to toxic concentrations in children with renal tubular acidosis, in whom a persistently alkaline urine favoured passive reabsorption of the drug.— D. C. Brater, *Drugs*, 1980, *19*, 31. See also D. C. Brater *et al.*, *Clin. Pharmac. Ther.*, 1980, *28*, 690.

Under steady-state conditions in 5 healthy subjects given pseudoephedrine hydrochloride 120 mg with chlorpheniramine maleate 8 mg as a sustained-release preparation twice daily for 8 days 91% of a pseudoephedrine dose administered was excreted unchanged in the urine between successive doses.— C. M. Lai *et al.*, *J. pharm. Sci.*, 1979, *68*, 1243. See also D. M. Baaske *et al.*, *J. pharm. Sci.*, 1979, *68*, 1472; A. Yacobi *et al.*, *ibid.*, 1980, *69*, 1077.

Uses. Pseudoephedrine is a stereoisomer of ephedrine (p.10) and has a similar action, but has been stated to have less pressor activity and central nervous system effects. The hydrochloride is used as a nasal and bronchial decongestant, usually in doses of 60 mg three or four times daily. Sustained-release preparations are given in a usual dose of 120 mg every 12 hours. Pseudoephedrine sulphate is also used. A suggested dose of pseudoephedrine hydrochloride or sulphate for children is 1 mg per kg body-weight 4 times daily.

Asthma. The bronchodilator effect of pseudoephedrine was less than half that of ephedrine in 9 patients with reversible airways obstruction.— C. D. M. Drew *et al.*, *Br. J. clin. Pharmac.*, 1978, *6*, 221.

ENT disorders. A double-blind study involving 466 adults indicating that pseudoephedrine alone or in combination with triprolidine relieved symptoms of the common cold.— C. E. Bye *et al.*, *Br. med. J.*, 1980, *281*, 189.

Preparations

Pseudoephedrine Hydrochloride Syrup *(U.S.P.)*. A syrup containing pseudoephedrine hydrochloride. It is acid to litmus. Store in airtight containers. Protect from light.

Pseudoephedrine Hydrochloride Tablets *(U.S.P.)*. Tablets containing pseudoephedrine hydrochloride. Store in airtight containers.

Proprietary Preparations

Actifed *(Wellcome, UK)*. **Syrup** containing in each 5 ml pseudoephedrine hydrochloride 30 mg and triprolidine hydrochloride 1.25 mg (suggested diluent, syrup), and **Tablets** each containing pseudoephedrine hydrochloride 60 mg and triprolidine hydrochloride 2.5 mg. For nasal and respiratory congestion. *Dose.* 1 tablet or 10 ml of syrup thrice daily; children, 3 months to 1 year, 2.5 ml; 1 to 6 years, 5 ml; 6 to 12 years, 7.5 ml.

Actifed Compound Linctus *(Wellcome, UK)*. Contains in each 5 ml pseudoephedrine hydrochloride 30 mg, triprolidine hydrochloride 1.25 mg, and codeine phosphate 10 mg (suggested diluent, syrup). For cough associated with congestion. *Dose.* 10 ml thrice daily; children, 1 to 6 years, 5 ml; 6 to 12 years, 7.5 ml.

A 3-month-old infant who had been born prematurely developed near-fatal apnoea after two 5-ml doses of Actifed Compound Linctus. Even if the recommended dose of 2.5 ml thrice daily for a 3-month-old infant had been given, the codeine intake would have been dangerously high; there is clearly an urgent need to revise the dose recommendations for this product as they apply to young infants. Moreover, when prescribing for infants, prematurity should be taken into account.— T. C. R. Wilkes *et al.* (letter), *Lancet*, 1981, *1*, 1166.

Actifed Expectorant *(Wellcome, UK)*. Elixir containing in each 5 ml pseudoephedrine hydrochloride 30 mg, guaiphenesin 100 mg, and triprolidine hydrochloride 1.25 mg (suggested diluent, syrup). Expectorant and decongestant. *Dose.* 10 ml thrice daily; children, 1 to 6 years, 2.5 ml; 6 to 12 years, 5 ml.

Extil Compound Linctus *(Duncan, Flockhart, UK)*. Contains in each 5 ml pseudoephedrine 24.6 mg (equivalent to pseudophedrine hydrochloride 30 mg), carbinoxamine maleate 3 mg, and noscapine 12.5 mg (dilution not recommended). For cough accompanied by bronchospasm or congestion of the upper respiratory tract. *Dose.* 10 ml 3 or 4 times daily; children, 2 to 12 years, 2.5 to 5 ml.

Linctifed Expectorant *(Wellcome, UK)*. Contains in each 5 ml pseudoephedrine hydrochloride 20 mg, triprolidine hydrochloride 1.25 mg, codeine phosphate 7.5 mg, and guaiphenesin 100 mg. For cough and congestion of the respiratory tract. **Linctifed Expectorant Paediatric.** Contains in each 5 ml pseudoephedrine hydrochloride 12 mg, triprolidine hydrochloride 600 µg, codeine phosphate 3 mg, and guaiphenesin 50 mg (suggested diluent, syrup). *Dose.* Linctifed expectorant: adults and children over 12 years, 10 ml thrice daily. Linctifed paediatric expectorant: children 1 to 6 years, 5 ml thrice daily; 6 to 12 years, 10 ml.

Paragesic *(Sandoz, UK)*. Effervescent tablets each containing pseudoephedrine hydrochloride 20 mg, paracetamol 500 mg, and caffeine 10 mg. For the common cold. *Dose.* 1 or 2 tablets, dissolved in water, every 4 hours; not more than 8 tablets in 24 hours.

Sudafed *(Calmic, UK)*. Pseudoephedrine hydrochloride, available as **Elixir** containing 30 mg in each 5 ml (suggested diluent, syrup) and as **Tablets** of 60 mg. (Also available as Sudafed in *Austral.*, *Canad.*, *S.Afr.*, *USA*).

Sudafed Expectorant *(Calmic, UK)*. Syrup containing in each 5 ml pseudoephedrine hydrochloride 30 mg and guaiphenesin 100 mg (suggested diluent, syrup). For cough and congestion of the respiratory tract. *Dose.* 10 ml 3 times daily; children, 1 to 6 years, 2.5 ml; 6 to 12 years, 5 ml.

Sudafed-Co *(Calmic, UK)*. Scored tablets each containing pseudoephedrine hydrochloride 60 mg and paracetamol 500 mg. For upper respiratory congestion with pain or pyrexia. *Dose.* 1 tablet thrice daily; children, 6 to 12 years, half a tablet.

Other Proprietary Names

Austral.—Drixora Repetabs *(sulphate)*, Sudelix *(hydrochloride)*; *Braz.*—Isofedrin *(hydrochloride)*; *Canad.*—Eltor *(hydrochloride)*, Robidrine *(hydrochloride)*; *USA*—Afrinol *(sulphate)*, D-Feda *(hydrochloride)*, Novafed *(hydrochloride)*, Sinufed *(hydrochloride)*.

A preparation containing pseudoephedrine hydrochloride was also formerly marketed in Great Britain under the proprietary name Emprazil (*Calmic*).

2100-e

Racephedrine Hydrochloride.

dl-Ephedrine Hydrochloride; *dl*-Ephedrinium Chloride; Racemic Ephedrine Hydrochloride; Ephedrinum Hydrochloricum *(Hung. P.)*. (±)-2-Methylamino-1-phenylpropan-1-ol hydrochloride. $C_{10}H_{15}NO,HCl=201.7$.

CAS — 90-81-3 (racephedrine); 134-71-4 (hydrochloride).

Pharmacopoeias. In *Hung.* and *Pol.*

Fine white odourless crystals or powder. Solutions in water are optically inactive.

Soluble 1 in about 4 of water and 1 in about 25 of alcohol; practically insoluble in ether. A 5% solution in water has a pH of 4.5 to 7. A 3.07% solution is iso-osmotic with serum. **Store** in airtight containers. Protect from light.

An aqueous solution of racephedrine hydrochloride iso-osmotic with serum (3.07%) caused 94% haemolysis of erythrocytes cultured in it for 45 minutes.— E. R. Hammarlund and K. Pedersen-Bjergaard, *J. pharm. Sci.*, 1961, *50*, 24.

Racephedrine hydrochloride has the actions and uses of ephedrine, p.10, and is given in the same dosage as ephedrine hydrochloride.

Proprietary Names
Efetonina *(Bracco, Ital.)*; Ephetonin *(E. Merck, Ger.)*.

2101-l

Reproterol Hydrochloride.

7-{3-[(3,5,β-Trihydroxyphenethyl)amino]propyl}theophylline hydrochloride. $C_{18}H_{23}N_5O_5,HCl=425.9$.

CAS — 54063-54-6 (reproterol); 13055-82-8 (hydrochloride).

Reproterol hydrochloride is a direct-acting sympathomimetic agent with general properties similar to those of salbutamol (p.29). It is given as a bronchodilator, by mouth, in doses of 10 to 20 mg thrice daily , or by inhalation, in doses of 0.5 to 1 mg, at intervals of 3 to 6 hours if required. It has also been given by injection.

References to reproterol.— *Arzneimittel-Forsch.*, 1977, *27*, 1–76; G. Niebch *et al.*, *ibid.*, 1978, *28*, 765; J. R.

M. Bateman *et al., Clin. Trials J.*, 1979, *16*, 37; F. J. Prime *et al., Curr. med. Res. Opinion*, 1979, *6*, 364; H. Voss and R. Aurich, *Dt. med. Wschr.*, 1979, *104*, 1041.

Proprietary Preparations

Bronchodil *(Keymer, UK)*. Reproterol hydrochloride, available as a pressurised **Aerosol** delivering 500 µg in each metered dose and as scored **Tablets** of 20 mg.

Other Proprietary Names

Bronchospasmin *(Ger.)*.

2102-y

Rimiterol Hydrobromide.

erythro-3,4-Dihydroxy-α-(2-piperidyl)benzyl alcohol hydrobromide; *erythro*-(3,4-Dihydroxyphenyl) (2-piperidyl)methanol hydrobromide.

$C_{12}H_{17}NO_3,HBr = 304.2$.

CAS — 32953-89-2 (rimiterol); 31842-61-2 (hydrobromide).

A white or pale grey odourless crystalline powder. **Soluble** 1 in 10 of water and 1 in 20 of methyl alcohol.

Adverse Effects. As for Salbutamol, p.29.

A study of the metabolic and cardiovascular side-effects of salbutamol and rimiterol in healthy subjects.— P. J. Phillips *et al., Br. J. clin. Pharmac.*, 1980, *9*, 483.

Treatment of Adverse Effects. As for Isoprenaline, p.15.

Precautions. As for Salbutamol, p.29.

CAUTION. *Excessive usage of aerosols of sympathomimetic agents has been associated with sudden death in asthmatics, see p.15.*

Absorption and Fate. Rimiterol is readily absorbed from the gastro-intestinal tract. It is subject not only to extensive first-pass metabolism by sulphate and glucuronide conjugation, but also to metabolism by catechol-*O*-methyltransferase and therefore has a very short plasma half-life. Rimiterol also appears to be metabolised by catechol-*O*-methyltransferase in the lungs. It is excreted in both the urine and the bile.

In studies in 4 subjects rimiterol had 18 to 80 times less chronotropic action on the heart than isoprenaline. Its half-life after intravenous injection was similar to that of isoprenaline. Urinary excretion included unchanged drug, glucuronide, and 3-*O*-methyl derivatives. Mean faecal excretion over 72 hours was about 45%.— J. P. Griffin *et al., Clin. Trials J.*, 1973, *10* (1), 13.

Difference in the pattern of 3-*O*-methylation and conjugation of rimiterol following administration by mouth and by inhalation.— M. E. Evans *et al., Br. J. Pharmac.*, 1973, *49*, 153P. Evidence that rimiterol might be partially metabolised in the lung.— G. M. Shenfield *et al., Br. J. clin. Pharmac.*, 1976, *3*, 583.

Uses. Rimiterol hydrobromide is a direct-acting sympathomimetic agent with general properties similar to those of salbutamol (p.30).

In the treatment of bronchial asthma it is given as an aerosol in a dose of 1 to 3 inhalations of 200 µg; if more than 1 inhalation is taken at a time, at least 1 minute should elapse between any 2 inhalations. This treatment dose should not be repeated in less than 30 minutes. No more than 8 treatments should be taken in any 24-hour period.

Asthma. In 15 patients with asthma the inhalation of an aerosol of salbutamol 0.5% in 40% oxygen by intermittent positive-pressure ventilation led to a marked increase in forced expiratory volume in 1 second (FEV_1), the effect being sustained for 3 or 4 hours. Rimiterol 0.5 or 1% aerosol similarly inhaled produced a similar increase in FEV_1, but the effect declined rapidly. The heart-rate was significantly increased by salbutamol; the increase after rimiterol was less and of shorter duration.— N. J. Cooke *et al., Br. med. J.*, 1974, *2*, 250. Inhalation of an aerosol of rimiterol 0.5% in the same manner produced similar increases in mean peak FEV_1, and in heart-rate to those produced by inhalation of salbutamol 0.25% in a study of 16 patients with chronic asthma. Both effects were of significantly shorter duration after rimiterol than after salbutamol. Inhalation of rimiterol 0.5% in two doses, the second 2 hours after the first, did not produce the same sustained degree of bronchodilation as salbutamol 0.25%.— I. C. Paterson *et al., Br. J. clin. Pharmac.*, 1977, *4*, 605.

Further references.— F. J. Prime and P. L. Kamburoff (letter), *Lancet*, 1972, *1*, 753; G. E. Marlin and P. Turner, *Br. med. J.*, 1975, *2*, 715; *idem, Br. J. clin. Pharmac.*, 1975, *2*, 41; A. D. Mackay and A. T. Axford, *Clin. Trials J.*, 1977, *14*, 73; G. E. Marlin *et al.* (letter), *Br. J. clin. Pharmac.*, 1977, *4*, 77; I. C. Paterson *et al., ibid.*, 605; M. I. Blackhall *et al., Br. J. clin. Pharmac.*, 1978, *6*, 59; B. J. Freedman, *Practitioner*, 1978, *220*, 476; G. E. Marlin *et al., Br. J. clin. Pharmac.*, 1978, *5*, 45; A. Muittari, *Respiration*, 1978, *35*, 165.

Cardiac disorders. The cardiovascular effects of infusions of rimiterol and isoprenaline were compared in patients with suspected coronary artery disease. Rimiterol 100 to 200 ng per kg body-weight per minute for 10 minutes was given by intravenous infusion to 10 patients. Isoprenaline 5 to 50 ng per kg per minute was infused into 5 similar patients to produce changes in cardiac output similar to those seen with rimiterol. Both drugs produced significant dose-related increases in cardiac output accompanied by similar increases in heart-rate and myocardial oxygen consumption. Isoprenaline produced greater increases in coronary sinus flow. Unlike isoprenaline, rimiterol did not cause direct coronary vasodilatation and might be preferable to isoprenaline in the treatment of patients with left ventricular failure when there was regional myocardial ischaemia.— J. D. Stephens *et al., Br. J. clin. Pharmac.*, 1978, *6*, 163.

Proprietary Preparations

Pulmadil Auto *(Riker, UK)*. A breath-operated inhaler containing rimiterol hydrobromide 10 mg per ml, delivering 200 µg in each metered dose.

Pulmadil Inhaler *(Riker, UK)*. A pressurised spray for inhalation containing rimiterol hydrobromide 10 mg per ml, delivering 200 µg in each metered dose. (Also available as Pulmadil in *Austral., Belg., Denm., Neth., Norw., NZ, S.Afr., Switz.*).

Other Proprietary Names

Asmaten *(Arg.)*.

2103-j

Ritodrine Hydrochloride.

DU 21220.

erythro-2-(4-Hydroxyphenethylamino)-1-(4-hydroxyphenyl)propan-1-ol hydrochloride.

$C_{17}H_{21}NO_3,HCl = 323.8$.

CAS — 26652-09-5 (ritodrine); 23239-51-2 (hydrochloride).

Adverse Effects. As for Salbutamol, p.29.

Metabolic effects. Adverse metabolic effects of ritodrine.— W. N. Spellacy *et al., Am. J. Obstet. Gynec.*, 1978, *131*, 637. Comments on the successful use of ritodrine in pregnant diabetic patients.— T. C. G. Smith, *Duphar* (letter), *Br. med. J.*, 1977, *2*, 124 and 770. See also J. M. Steel and J. Parboosingh, *ibid.*, 1977, *1*, 880; C. J. Chandler (letter), *ibid.*, 1159.

Pregnancy and the neonate. Eleven hours after delivery, a 24-year-old woman who had received ritodrine, indomethacin, and betamethasone for premature labour, developed acute pulmonary oedema. Patients receiving such therapy should be monitored not only during treatment but for at least 24 hours after it stops.— D. J. Tinga and J. G. Aarnoudse (letter), *Lancet*, 1979, *1*, 1026. A diabetic woman given intravenous ritodrine in an attempt to prevent premature labour developed metabolic acidosis. The infusion of ritodrine was stopped and measures taken to correct the mother's condition; she was delivered of a still-born foetus. When prevention of preterm delivery is essential the mother's blood glucose and acid base balance must be carfully balanced and insulin administration by continuous infusion should be considered.— M. S. Schilthuis and J. G. Aarnoudse (letter), *Lancet*, 1980, *1*, 1145.

Further references.— H. Freysz *et al., J. perinat. Med.*, 1977, *5*, 94 (absence of harm to offspring); D. Desir *et al., Br. med. J.*, 1978, *2*, 1194 (severe acidosis and elevated lactate concentrations); H. R. Elliott *et al., Br. med. J.*, 1978, *2*, 799 (pulmonary oedema).

Treatment of Adverse Effects. As for Isoprenaline, p.15.

Precautions. As for Salbutamol, p.29.

Absorption and Fate. Ritodrine is readily absorbed from the gastro-intestinal tract but is subject to fairly extensive first-pass metabolism.

A study of the pharmacokinetics of ritodrine in healthy subjects following administration by intravenous infusion, intramuscularly, and by mouth; and a comparison of the pharmacokinetics of ritodrine with those of fenoterol, salbutamol, and terbutaline. Following oral administration the bioavailability of ritodrine was 30% indicating a first-pass effect. The dominant half-life after intramuscular injection was 2 hours while in the oral study half-lives of 1.3 hours and 20 hours were discernible. The half-life of salbutamol is about the same as that of ritodrine and the half-life of terbutaline seems to be slightly longer. Studies in women given ritodrine to arrest preterm labour indicated that ritodrine crosses the placental barrier and enters the foetal circulation.— R. Gandar *et al., Eur. J. clin. Pharmac.*, 1980, *17*, 117.

Further references.— C. Romanini *et al., Pharmatherapeutica*, 1977, *1*, 546 (transplacental diffusion).

Uses. Ritodrine hydrochloride is a direct-acting sympathomimetic agent with general properties similar to those of salbutamol (p.30). It is given by intravenous infusion to arrest premature labour; infusion rates are usually 150 to 350 µg per minute, according to the patient's response. The recommended initial rate of infusion is 50 µg per minute increased at intervals of 10 minutes by 50-µg increments until there is evidence of patient response. The infusion should be continued for 12 to 48 hours after the contractions have stopped; where intravenous infusion is inappropriate 10 mg may be given intramuscularly every 3 to 8 hours and continued for 12 to 48 hours after the contractions have stopped. The maternal pulse should be monitored throughout the infusion and the rate adjusted to avoid a maternal heart-rate of more than 140 beats per minute. Ritodrine hydrochloride may subsequently be given by mouth in an initial dose of 10 mg every 2 hours followed by 10 to 20 mg every 4 to 6 hours according to the patient's response; the first dose may be given 30 minutes before the end of the infusion. The total daily dose by mouth should not exceed 120 mg.

Ritodrine hydrochloride has also been given intravenously to the mother as an emergency means of alleviating foetal asphyxia while other procedures are being arranged.

Pregnancy and the neonate. For comments on the efficacy of $beta_2$-selective adrenoceptor stimulants in the prevention of premature labour, see Salbutamol, p.31.

Reviews of ritodrine in the management of premature labour.— *Drug & Ther. Bull.*, 1980, *18*, 34; *Med. Lett.*, 1980, *22*, 89.

Studies of ritodrine in the management of premature labour.— A. Wesselius-de Casparis *et al., Br. med. J.*, 1971, *3*, 144; T. P. Barden, *Am. J. Obstet. Gynec.*, 1972, *112*, 645; J. Bieniarz *et al., Obstet. Gynec.*, 1972, *40*, 65; F. M. Miller *et al., Obstet. Gynec.*, 1976, *47*, 50; N. H. Lauresen *et al., Am. J. Obstet. Gynec.*, 1977, *127*, 837; R. Richter, *ibid.*, 482; W. A. Walters and C. Wood, *Br. J. Obstet. Gynaec.*, 1977, *84*, 26; G. G. M. Essed *et al., Eur. J. Obstet. Gynec. reprod. Biol.*, 1978, *8*, 341; G. Hastwell and B. E. Lambert, *Curr. med. Res. Opinion*, 1979, *5*, 785; N. Ragni *et al., Br. J. Obstet. Gynaec.*, 1979, *86*, 866; R. Richter and M. J. Hinselmann, *Obstet. Gynec.*, 1979, *53*, 81; I. R. Merkatz *et al., ibid.*, 1980, *56*, 7.

Foetal distress. A report of the use of ritodrine by infusion in a case of severe foetal distress occurring during labour. Propranolol was given to the mother after delivery to slow her increased heart-rate.— A. Schoenfeld *et al., Br. J. Anaesth.*, 1978, *50*, 969. Criticism of recommendations that ritodrine should be used for the treatment of foetal distress.— *Drug & Ther. Bull.*, 1975, *13*, 26. See also *ibid.*, 1978, *16*, 83.

Further references.— G. Boog *et al., Br. J. Obstet. Gynaec.*, 1975, *82*, 285 (respiratory distress syndrome); J. Campbell *et al., Aust. N.Z. J. Obstet. Gynaec.*, 1978, *18*, 110 (foetal respiratory acidosis); S. Suonio *et al., Am. J. Obstet. Gynec.*, 1978, *130*, 745 (placental insufficiency); T. H. Lippert *et al., Int. J. clin. Pharmac. Biopharm.*, 1980, *18*, 15 (hyperactive ischaemic uterus).

Proprietary Preparations

Yutopar *(Duphar, UK)*. Ritodrine hydrochloride, available as **Injection** containing 10 mg per ml, in ampoules of 1 and 5 ml, and as scored **Tablets** of 10 mg. (Also available as Yutopar in *Austral.*).

Other Proprietary Names

Pre-Par *(Aust., Belg., Fr., Ger., Ind., Ital., Jug., Neth., Spain)*; Utopar *(Denm., Iceland, Norw., Swed.)*.

2104-z

Salbutamol *(B.P.)*. AH 3365; Albuterol. 2-*tert*-Butylamino-1-(4-hydroxy-3-hydroxymethylphenyl)ethanol.

$C_{13}H_{21}NO_3$=239.3.

CAS — 18559-94-9.

Pharmacopoeias. In *Br.*

A white or almost white, odourless, almost tasteless, crystalline powder. M.p. about 156°. **Soluble** 1 in 70 of water and 1 in 25 of alcohol; slightly soluble in ether. **Protect** from light.

2105-c

Salbutamol Sulphate *(B.P.)*. Albuterol Sulphate.

$C_{13}H_{21}NO_3,\frac{1}{2}H_2SO_4$=288.4.

CAS — 51022-70-9.

Pharmacopoeias. In *Br.*

A white or almost white odourless powder with a slightly bitter taste. Salbutamol sulphate 1.2 mg is approximately equivalent to 1 mg of salbutamol. **Soluble** 1 in 4 of water; slightly soluble in alcohol, chloroform, and ether. **Protect** from light.

Stability. The stability of salbutamol sulphate in aqueous phosphate buffers decreased with increase in pH above 6.9. In dextrose solution 5%, salbutamol was more stable and lost 10% potency in about 19.9 weeks at 50°.— B. P. Wall and V. B. Sunderland, *Aust. J. Hosp. Pharm.*, 1976, *6*, 156.

Adverse Effects. Salbutamol may cause fine tremor of skeletal muscle (particularly the hands), palpitations, and muscle cramps. Slight tachycardia, tenseness, headaches, and peripheral vasodilatation have been reported after large doses.

The high doses of salbutamol used intravenously to delay premature labour have been associated with nausea and vomiting, and with adverse cardiac and metabolic effects.

A report on the nature and incidence of side-effects of salbutamol in 50 patients with chronic airflow obstruction who had been taking 4 mg thrice daily for a year. The incidence of side-effects was: finger tremor 42%, palpitation 20%, muscle cramp 46%, and other symptoms 6%. Although finger tremor and palpitation are well recognised, muscle cramp is not; patients should be warned of this possibility. In view of this rather high incidence of side-effects when salbutamol is taken by mouth, it should be used by inhalation whenever possible.— K. N. V. Palmer (letter), *Br. med. J.*, 1978, *2*, 833.

Abuse. Acute atypical psychosis in a 51-year-old woman was attributed to the excessive use of salbutamol; she had been taking 30 to 40 mg daily and using at least 12 inhalations daily for 10 days before admission to hospital. The patient claimed that salbutamol made her bright, alert, and forgetful of her anxieties.— L. Gluckman, *N.Z. med. J.*, 1974, *80*, 411, per *Practitioner*, 1975, *214*, 600.

Further references: M. Gaultier *et al.*, *Thérapie*, 1976, *31*, 465 (inhaler); J. G. Edwards and S. T. Holgate, *Br. J. Psychiat.*, 1979, *134*, 624 (inhaler).

Carcinogenicity. A statement attempting to put into perspective findings that long-term administration of very high doses of salbutamol has been associated with the development of benign mesovarian leiomyomas in some species of *rats*, who are known to respond aberrantly to beta-stimulants. There is no evidence that salbutamol is carcinogenic in any species, and much evidence that it is unlikely to be so.— D. Poynter *et al.* , *Allen & Hanburys* (letter), *Br. med. J.*, 1978, *1*, 46. Reply.— M. J. Finkel, *US Food and Drug Administration* (letter), *ibid.*, 649.

Effects on the heart. Following intravenous infusion of salbutamol 10 µg per minute in a placebo-controlled study of 7 healthy subjects the ventilatory response to carbon dioxide was increased in both hypoxia and hyperoxia; a pronounced increase in heart-rate occurred which was more marked when hypoxia was associated with hypercapnia; a pronounced fall in plasma-potassium concentration occurred with a concomitant rise in plasma-glucose and serum-insulin concentrations. It was suggested that if salbutamol was infused intravenously in the management of severe asthma both the plasma potassium and the ECG should be carefully monitored as there might be a predisposition to cardiac arrhythmias.— A. G. Leitch *et al.*, *Br. med. J.*, 1976, *1*, 365. Comment on tachycardia associated with the intravenous administration of salbutamol and the view that it should be administered intravenously slowly over at least 5 minutes.— A. J. Johnson *et al.* (letter), *ibid.*, 1977, *1*, 772. Evidence that salbutamol aerosol causes a tachycardia due to the inhaled rather than the swallowed fraction.— J. G. Collier *et al.* (letter), *Br. J. clin. Pharmac.*, 1980, *9*, 273.

Further references: M. Santo *et al.* (letter), *S. Afr. med. J.*, 1980, *58*, 394.

Metabolic effects. Salbutamol sulphate given as a bolus intravenous injection of 50 to 150 µg in 9 volunteers increased heart-rate, stimulated the release of free fatty acids and insulin, produced a moderate rise in plasma-lactate concentrations, and a small increase in plasma-glucose concentrations. Growth-hormone concentrations were not affected. Pretreatment with the β_1-adrenergic blocker practolol reduced or abolished these changes except for release of free fatty acids.— R. Goldberg *et al.*, *Postgrad. med. J.*, 1975, *51*, 53. Salbutamol 150 ng per kg body-weight per minute given as an intravenous infusion for 60 minutes increased the heart-rate, release of insulin, and reduced the serum concentration of potassium in 4 healthy subjects. Serum-potassium concentrations should be monitored when salbutamol is administered since the hypokalaemic effect produced could provoke cardiac dysrhythmias particularly in patients receiving digoxin.— N. Berend and G. E. Marlin, *Br. J. clin. Pharmac.*, 1978, *5*, 207. Further references: S. G. Nogrady *et al.*, *Thorax*, 1977, *32*, 559 (infusion).

Since hypokalaemia had been reported following the inhalation or intravenous administration of salbutamol plasma-potassium concentrations were studied in 6 healthy subjects and 16 patients given salbutamol by mouth. The healthy subjects received single doses of 4 mg and the patients 5-day courses of 6 to 16 mg daily. There was no significant hypokalaemic effect and digitalised patients were not considered to be at special risk from salbutamol by mouth.— S. P. Deacon (letter), *Lancet*, 1976, *1*, 1302. Increased insulin and glucose concentrations following oral administration of salbutamol to healthy subjects.— M. W. Taylor *et al.*, *Br. med. J.*, 1976, *1*, 22.

There were no significant changes in the plasma concentrations of non-esterified fatty acids, triglyceride, glucose, insulin, or hydrocortisone in 7 of 8 patients with asthma or chronic bronchitis, up to 4 hours after they inhaled salbutamol 5 mg by intermittent positive-pressure ventilation. Plasma concentrations of insulin were elevated up to 4 hours after inhalation in the eighth patient.— S. M. Bateman *et al.*, *Br. J. clin. Pharmac.*, 1978, *5*, 127.

Individual reports of adverse metabolic effects associated with salbutamol: D. Leopold and A. McEvoy (letter), *Br. med. J.*, 1977, *2*, 1152 (hyperglycaemia and ketosis associated with infusion for asthma).

See also under Pregnancy and the Neonate (below).

Overdosage. A 44-year-old asthmatic woman with depressive symptoms swallowed 100 salbutamol tablets 2 mg. When admitted to hospital 2 hours 45 minutes later there was peripheral vasodilatation, increased pulse-rate, sinus tachycardia, and agitation with increased irritability of skeletal muscle. An insignificant amount of salbutamol was recovered following gastric lavage. The patient was managed successfully with practolol, propranolol, and diazepam.— G. W. Morrison and M. J. B. Farebrother (letter), *Lancet*, 1973, *2*, 681.

Hypokalaemia associated with salbutamol overdosage.— I. A. D. O'Brien *et al.*, *Br. med. J.*, 1981, *282*, 1515.

Pregnancy and the neonate. Profuse uterine bleeding has been reported by P.S. Vinall and D.M. Jenkins (*Lancet*, 1977, *2*, 1355) following uterine evacuation in an asthmatic woman who inhaled salbutamol prior to the termination of her 13-week pregnancy. Most adverse effects associated with salbutamol in pregnancy relate, however, to the cardiovascular and metabolic effects of the very high doses given by intravenous infusion in attempts to delay premature labour. Thus, M.I. Whitehead *et al.* (*Lancet*, 1979, *2*, 904) have reported myocardial ischaemia on stopping an infusion, and W.C. Chew and L.C. Lew (*Lancet*, 1979, *2*, 1383) have reported unifocal ventricular ectopics associated with the hypokalaemic response to intravenous salbutamol. A further report by M.I. Whitehead *et al.* (*Br. med. J.*, 1980, *280*, 1221) concerning congestive heart failure in a hypertensive woman aroused controversy surrounding the management of such patients, including comment on the possible enhancement of the adverse effects of salbutamol by ergometrine (see P.A. Poole-Wilson, *Br. med. J.*, 1980, *281*, 226; A.J. Fogarty, *ibid.*; P.D.O. Davies, *ibid.*; M. Robertson and A.E. Davies, *ibid.*, 227; P. Crowley, *ibid.*; M.I. Whitehead *et al.*, *ibid.*). Metabolic acidosis following salbutamol infusions in diabetic women has been reported by M.G. Chapman (*Br. med. J.*, 1977, *1*, 639) and D.J.B. Thomas *et al.* (*Br. med. J.*, 1977, *2*, 438). That this problem is a particular hazard in diabetic women, particularly those given corticosteroids to promote foetal surfactant production, has subsequently been emphasised by a study by A.S. Gündoğdu *et al.* (*Lancet*, 1979, *2*, 1317). Further references: D. Leslie and P. M. Coats (letter), *Br. med. j.*, 1977, *2*, 768 (ketoacidosis); N. O. Lunell *et al.*, *Acta obstet. gynec. scand.*, 1977, *56*, 475 (metabolic effects); D. J. B. Thomas *et al.*, *Br. J. Obstet. Gynaec.*, 1977, *84*, 497 (metabolic effects); S. K. Smith, *Br. J. Obstet. Gynaec.*, 1977, *84*, 344 (hypokalaemia); C. Borberg *et al.*, *Br. J. Obstet. Gynaec.*, 1978, *85*, 184 (metabolic effects); B. B. Fredholm *et al.*, *Diabetologia*, 1978, *14*, 235 (metabolic effects); N. O. Lunell *et al.*, *Eur. J. clin. Pharmac.*, 1978, *14*, 95 (metabolic effects); A. E. Davies and M. J. S. Robertson, *Br. J. Obstet. Gynaec.*, 1980, *87*, 539 (pulmonary oedema).

Urinary retention. Beta-receptor stimulants such as salbutamol and terbutaline are unlikely to produce urinary retention when administered by inhalation, but may do so when given by mouth or intravenously.— P. Turner, *Prescribers' J.*, 1978, *18*, 94.

Treatment of Adverse Effects. As for Isoprenaline, p.15.

In 40 patients who had taken overdoses of salbutamol (5 to 100 mg in those under 10 years; 14 to 240 mg in older patients) symptoms included muscle tremor, flushing, agitation, palpitations, sinus tachycardia, and hypokalaemia. No patient developed convulsions or ventricular arrhythmias. Treatment included gastric lavage or emesis in 20, and the use of beta-adrenoceptor blocking agents, usually propranolol, in 10, though propranolol was probably not necessary.— J. G. Prior *et al.*, *Br. med. J.*, 1981, *282*, 1932.

Precautions. Salbutamol should be used with caution in hypersusceptible patients or those with hyperthyroidism, and in patients with diabetes mellitus, serious cardiovascular disorders, or hypertension.

In asthmatic patients whose condition deteriorates despite salbutamol therapy the dosage should not merely be increased, but alternative or additional therapy, including corticosteroids (p.453) should be instituted promptly.

Salbutamol is not indicated for the prevention of premature labour associated with toxaemia of pregnancy or antepartum haemorrhage, nor should it be used for threatened abortion during the first and second trimesters of pregnancy.

Adverse metabolic effects of high doses of salbutamol may be exacerbated by concomitant administration of high doses of corticosteroids; patients should therefore be monitored carefully when the 2 forms of therapy are used together. Propranolol and other beta-adrenoceptor blocking agents antagonise the effects of salbutamol. Hypokalaemia associated with high doses of salbutamol may result in increased susceptibility to digitalis-induced cardiac arrhythmias. The effects of salbutamol may be enhanced by concomitant administration of aminophylline.

CAUTION. *Excessive usage of aerosols of sympathomimetic agents has been associated with sudden death in asthmatics,* see p.15.

Tolerance. In healthy subjects specific airway conductance was progressively reduced when salbutamol up to 400 µg four times daily was inhaled over 4 to 5 weeks. Hydrocortisone 200 mg intravenously or aminophylline restored the response.— A. E. Tattersfield and S. T. Holgate (letter), *Lancet*, 1976, *1*, 422. See also S. T. Holgate *et al.*, *Lancet*, 1977, *2*, 375; *idem*, *Clin. Sci.*, 1980, *59*, 155.

Absorption and Fate. Salbutamol is readily absorbed from the gastro-intestinal tract and, unlike isoprenaline, is not subject to sulphate conjugation in the gut. It is subject to first-pass metabolism in the liver; about a half is excreted in the urine as an inactive sulphate conjugate, following oral administration (the rest being unchanged salbutamol), whereas less than a third is excreted as the conjugate following intravenous administration. Salbutamol does not appear to be metabolised in the lung, therefore its behaviour following inhalation depends upon the delivery method used, which determines the proportion of inhaled salbutamol relative to the proportion inadvertently swallowed.

The plasma half-life of salbutamol has been estimated to range from about 2 to as much as 7 hours. In general the shorter values have followed intravenous administration, the intermediate values oral administration, and the longer values aerosol inhalation. It has been suggested that the slightly extended half-life following inhalation may reflect slow removal of active drug from the lungs.

Tritiated salbutamol given by mouth in a dose of 4 or 8 mg to 6 patients with asthma was well absorbed giving peak plasma concentrations within 3 hours and up to 78% being excreted in the urine within 24 hours. Measurements in 4 patients showed that 1.2 to 7% was excreted in the faeces. When given by aerosol to another 6 asthmatic patients in doses estimated at 40 to 100 µg, peak plasma concentrations were obtained at 3 to 5 hours; up to 89.6% was excreted in the urine within 24 hours, and in 2 patients 10.2 and 12% of the dose was recovered from the faeces. In both groups just under half the dose was excreted in the urine as a metabolite at the same rate as salbutamol. There was an increase in the 1-second forced expiratory volume (FEV_1) in both groups but this correlated with the dose only in those given salbutamol by mouth. In 5 of the 6 given salbutamol by inhalation, the maximum increase in FEV_1 occurred within 15 minutes, indicating a local effect.— S. W. Walker *et al.*, *Clin. Pharmac. Ther.*, 1972, *13*, 861. See also M. E. Evans *et al.*, *Xenobiotica*, 1973, *3*, 113.

Further references to the absorption and fate of salbutamol: G. L. Snider and R. Laguarda, *J. Am. med. Ass.*, 1972, *221*, 682 (duration of action of the aerosol); G. M. Shenfield *et al.*, *Br. J. clin. Pharmac.*, 1974, *1*, 295 (influence of delivery method on the absorption and metabolism of salbutamol); M. R. Hetzel and T. J. H. Clark, *Br. med. J.*, 1976, *2*, 919 (comparison of intravenous and aerosol routes); S. P. Deacon (letter), *Br. med. J.*, 1976, *2*, 1134; *idem*, 1977, *1*, 639 (comments on the metabolism following oral, intravenous, and aerosol administration); G. M. Shenfield *et al.*, *Br. J. clin. Pharmac.*, 1976, *3*, 583 (salbutamol and absorption in the lung); C. Lin *et al.*, *Drug Metab. & Disposit.*, 1977, *5*, 234 (isolation and identification of the major metabolite).

Uses. Salbutamol is a direct-acting sympathomimetic agent with predominantly beta-adrenergic activity and a selective action on $beta_2$ receptors. It is used similarly to isoprenaline sulphate (see p.16) as a bronchodilator. It has more prolonged actions than isoprenaline and also, as a predominantly $beta_2$-receptor stimulant, has a more selective action, its bronchodilating action being relatively more prominent than its effect on the heart. Such $beta_2$-adrenoceptor stimulants are preferred to isoprenaline for the management of asthma.

Salbutamol is used as the base in aerosol inhalers and as the sulphate in other preparations and its dosage is expressed in terms of salbutamol base. In the treatment of bronchial asthma it is given by mouth in a dose of 2 to 4 mg three or four times daily; some patients may require doses of up to 8 mg. Elderly patients should be given the lower doses initially. A dose of 1 to 2 mg three or four times daily is suggested for children aged 2 to 6 years or 2 mg for older children.

Salbutamol is given as an aerosol for the chronic management or prophylactic therapy of bronchial asthma, in a dose of 2 inhalations of 100 µg of salbutamol 3 or 4 times daily; for the relief of acute bronchospasm or for managing intermittent episodes of asthma 1 or 2 inhalations of 100 µg may be administered as a single dose when required (the bronchodilator effects last at least 4 hours). Exercise-induced bronchospasm may be prevented by 2 inhalations of 100µg before exertion. Children should be given 1 inhalation of 100 µg of salbutamol 3 or 4 times daily for routine maintenance or prophylactic therapy, increased to 2 inhalations if necessary. Worsening asthma should not be treated by increased doses of salbutamol (see Precautions).

Although salbutamol is generally inhaled in aerosol form, inhalation capsules of salbutamol sulphate are available for patients who experience difficulty in using the aerosol. Owing to differences in the relative bioavailability to the lungs of the 2 preparations a 200 µg dose (expressed in terms of salbutamol) from an inhalation capsule is approximately equivalent in activity to a 100-µg dose from an aerosol. The recommended dose for the chronic management or prophylactic therapy of bronchial asthma is therefore 400 µg three or four times daily by inhalation; for the relief of acute bronchospasm or for managing intermittent episodes of asthma, 200 or 400 µg may be inhaled as a single dose when required (the bronchodilator effects last at least 4 hours). Exercise-induced bronchospasm may be prevented by inhalation of 400 µg before exertion. Children should inhale a 200-µg inhalation capsule dose 3 to 4 times daily for routine maintenance or prophylactic therapy; they may similarly inhale a 200-µg inhalation capsule dose when required for the relief of acute bronchospasm or for managing intermittent episodes of asthma, or to prevent exercise-induced asthma.

Together with other forms of therapy (see Corticosteroids, p.453), in the treatment of status asthmaticus or other forms of severe bronchospasm, 2 ml of salbutamol sulphate solution containing the equivalent of salbutamol 0.5% (10 mg) may be inhaled up to 4 times daily as a mist in oxygen-enriched air through an intermittent positive-pressure ventilator over a period of about 3 minutes; similarly a 0.005 to 0.01% solution in sterile water may be administered as a mist by means of an intermittent positive-pressure ventilator at the rate of 1 to 2 mg of salbutamol per hour. Adequate oxygenation is essential to avoid hypoxaemia. Alternatively, salbutamol may be given in a dose of 500 µg by subcutaneous or intramuscular injection repeated every 4 hours as required, or by slow intravenous injection of 250 µg as a solution containing 50 µg per ml. It may also be given as a solution containing 5 mg in 500 ml (10 µg per ml) in infusions such as sodium chloride and dextrose intravenous infusion. The infusion rate should provide 3 to 20 µg per minute according to the patient's need; higher dosages have been used in patients with respiratory failure.

Infusions containing 5 mg in 500 ml (10 µg per ml) are also given to arrest premature labour (but see Precautions); infusion rates are usually 10 to 45 µg per minute, according to the patient's response. The recommended initial rate of infusion is 10 µg per minute increased at intervals of 10 minutes until there is evidence of patient response as shown by reduction in strength, frequency, or duration of contractions; the rate is then increased slowly until contractions cease. The infusion should be maintained at the rate at which contractions cease for one hour, then reduced by decrements of 50% at intervals of 6 hours. The maternal pulse should be monitored throughout the infusion and the rate adjusted to avoid a maternal heart-rate of more than 140 beats per minute. Salbutamol may subsequently be given by mouth in a dose of 4 mg three or four times daily.

As an alternative procedure, or to counteract inadvertent overdosage with oxytocic drugs, salbutamol may be given as a single injection by slow intravenous or intramuscular injection of 100 to 250 µg, repeated according to the patient's response.

In *dogs* and *guinea-pigs* (−)-salbutamol was much more potent than (+)-salbutamol on beta-adrenergic receptors. Both (−)- and (+)-salbutamol showed high selectivity for beta-adrenergic receptors in bronchial muscle compared to cardiac muscle, in this way resembling racemic salbutamol.— R. T. Brittain *et al.*, *Br. J. Pharmac.*, 1973, *48*, 144.

Further pharmacological studies: R. Wiggins *et al.*, *Br. J. clin. Pharmac.*, 1978, *5*, 213 (partial antagonist properties).

Asthma. In the management of asthma, salbutamol and similar $beta_2$-selective sympathomimetic agents have the great advantage over isoprenaline, of a pronounced effect on bronchospasm at doses which have little effect on the heart. Furthermore, inhalation of salbutamol appears to provide an even more specific effect on bronchospasm than administration by mouth. The route of choice for the prophylactic and therapeutic management of bronchial spasms has therefore become inhalation of the aerosol preparation. A large number of children and some adults, however, are unable to use aerosol inhalations in the manner necessary to provide an adequate dose to the lungs and, although tachycardia is not a significant feature of standard oral doses of salbutamol, the incidence of other side-effects, such as muscle tremor and palpitations, may be higher. For such patients, an inhalation-activated device which provides salbutamol in the form of a power mixed with lactose, has been developed; alternatively they will require administration of salbutamol by mouth.

The hospital patient with severe asthma requiring emergency supportive respiratory care until corticosteroid therapy has taken effect may also be unable to respond to inhaled salbutamol, probably owing to factors such as mucous plugs in the lungs. Since adverse cardiovascular effects, notably tachycardia, can occur following parenteral administration of salbutamol, several delivery methods have been studied which supply moist inhalations of salbutamol to enhance penetration in the lungs. In general, the parenteral route may be necessary for the acute emergency, but once the patient can cough and produce sputum moist inhalation methods are preferred. References: M. R. Hetzel and T. J. H. Clark, *Br. med. J.*, 1976, *2*, 919; A. Neville *et al.*, *ibid.*, 1977, *1*, 413; I. C. Paterson *et al.*, *Br. J. clin. Pharmac.*, 1977, *4*, 605; S. Williams and A. Seaton, *Thorax*, 1977, *32*, 555; C. J. Bacon (letter), *Lancet*, 1978, *1*, 158; W. Lenney (letter), *ibid.*, 440; S. J. Connellan and R. S. E. Wilson (letter), *ibid.*, 662; I. A. Campbell *et al.*, *Br. med. J.*, 1978, *1*, 1186; *Drug & Ther. Bull.*, 1978, *16*, 59; *Lancet*, 1978, *1*, 80; P. Lawford and J. S. Milledge (letter), *ibid.*, 269; P. Lawford *et al.*, *Br. med. J.*, 1978, *1*, 84; P. Bloomfield *et al.*, *Br. med. J.*, 1979, *1*, 848; J. F. Costello and D. Honeybourne (letter), *ibid.*, 1284; P. B. Anderson (letter), *ibid.*, 1284; I. D. Starke and R. A. Parker (letter), *Lancet*, 1980, *1*, 266.

Further reviews, comments, and studies on the role of salbutamol in the management of asthma: D. Duncan *et al.*, *Br. J. clin. Pharmac.*, 1977, *4*, 669; J. P. R. Hartley *et al.*, *ibid.*, 673 (comparisons between inhalation of dry powder and aerosol); D. Femi-Pearse *et al.*, *Br. med. J.*, 1977, *1*, 491 (comparison of intravenous salbutamol and intravenous aminophylline); P. Thompson and M. Friedman, *Archs Dis. Childh.*, 1977, *52*, 551 (intramuscular administration in children); R. M. Cayton *et al.*, *Br. J. Dis. Chest*, 1978, *72*, 222 (comparison of aerosol and nebuliser); R. A. Clark and P. B. Anderson, *Lancet*, 1978, *2*, 70; P. D. J. Handslip and J. P. R. Hartley (letter), *ibid.*, 481; P. B. Anderson and R. A. Clark (letter), *ibid.*, 577 (adjunct use before corticosteroid inhalation); A. J. Johnson *et al.*, *Br. med. J.*, 1978, *1*, 1013; I. W. B. Grant (letter), *ibid.*, 1620; H. R. Anderson (letter), *ibid.*; S. G. Spiro and S. W. Clarke (letter), *ibid* (comparison of intravenous salbutamol and intravenous aminophylline); W. Lenney and A. D. Milner, *Archs Dis. Childh.*, 1978, *53*, 532; P. König (letter), *ibid.*, 1979, *54*, 649; A. D. Milner (letter), *ibid.*, 650 (nebulised salbutamol in children); W. Lenney *et al.*, *Archs Dis. Childh.*, 1978, *53*, 958 (salbutamol powder in children); S. J. Connellan and R. S. E. Wilson, *Br. J. clin. Pract.*, 1979, *33*, 135 (emphysema); D. Duncan *et al.*, *Practitioner*, 1979, *223*, 843 (comparison of dry powder, aerosol, and nebulised solution); G. Hambleton and M. J. Stone, *Archs Dis. Childh.*, 1979, *54*, 391; I. Blumenthal and W. P. Tormey (letter), *ibid.*, 983; G. Hambleton and M. J. Stone (letter), *ibid* (comparison of intravenous salbutamol and intravenous aminophylline in children); J. P. R. Hartley *et al.*, *Br. J. Dis. Chest*, 1979, *73*, 271 (comparison of dry powder and aerosol); R. Monie and W. V. Evans (letter), *Br. med. J.*, 1979, *2*, 334 (comment on intravenous aminophylline or intravenous salbutamol); G. E. Marlin (letter), *Br. J.*

clin. Pharmac., 1979, *8*, 595 (inhaled salbutamol or oral theophylline); S. A. McKenzie *et al.*, *Archs Dis. Childh.*, 1979, *54*, 581 (nebulised salbutamol); G. J. Addis *et al.*, *Br. J. clin. Pharmac.*, 1980, *9*, 289P (effect of salbutamol following maximal response to theophylline); P. W. J. Francis *et al.*, *Pediatrics*, 1980, *66*, 103 (comparison of aerosol and tablets in children); P. J. Phillips *et al.*, *Br. J. clin. Pharmac.*, 1980, *9*, 483 (comparison of salbutamol and rimiterol infusions in healthy subjects); C. R. Pullan and A. J. Martin, *Br. med. J.*, 1980, *280*, 364 (dosage of salbutamol inhalation powder in children); M. K. Tandon, *Chest*, 1980, *77*, 429 (comparison with fenoterol); K. Grimwood *et al.*, *Br. med. J.*, 1981, *282*, 105 (comparison of tablets, inhalation powder, and nebulised salbutamol in children); *Lancet*, 1981, *1*, 23 (correct use of aerosol bronchodilators); *Lancet*, 1981, *1*, 313 (problem of severe acute asthma).

For earlier reports of the actions and uses of salbutamol in asthmatic patients, see Martindale 27th Edn, p. 33.

Cardiac disorders. In 11 patients with acute myocardial infarction complicated by left ventricular failure the infusion of salbutamol 10, 20, or 40 µg per minute increased cardiac output while the mean systemic arterial pressure fell slightly; heart-rate increased by only 10 beats per minute. While salbutamol increases cardiac output in patients in whom poor perfusion is the most important haemodynamic disturbance, it fails to reduce left ventricular filling pressure and cannot be recommended for patients with pulmonary oedema after acute infarction.— A. D. Timmis *et al.*, *Br. med. J.*, 1979, *2*, 1101. See also M. B. Fowler *et al.*, *Br. med. J.*, 1980, *280*, 435 (comparison with sodium nitroprusside); A. D. Timmis *et al.*, *Br. med. J.*, 1981, *282*, 7 (comparison with dopamine).

Further references: S. D. Wyse *et al.*, *Br. med. J.*, 1974, *3*, 502 (after cardiovascular surgery); P. A. Poole-Wilson *et al.*, *Br. Heart J.*, 1977, *39*, 721 (comparison with nitroprusside after cardiac surgery); P. D. V. Bourdillon *et al.*, *Br. Heart J.*, 1980, *43*, 206 (haemodynamic effects in chronic heart failure).

Depression. Salbutamol had an antidepressant effect in 9 of 10 patients with endogenous depression, a response being achieved as early as 48 hours after starting treatment.— D. Widlöcher *et al.* (letter), *Lancet*, 1977, *2*, 767. See also Y. Lecrubier *et al.*, *Br. J. Psychiat.*, 1980, *136*, 354.

For reports of psychic dependence on the mental effects of salbutamol, see Abuse, under Adverse Effects (above).

Epiglottitis, laryngitis, and croup. There was a higher rate of recovery from pertussis in children given erythromycin plus salbutamol than in those given erythromycin and a placebo.— D. Pavesio and A. Ponzone (letter), *Lancet*, 1977, *1*, 150.

Hyperkalaemia. Salbutamol in 2 inhalations of 200 µg every 15 minutes for up to 1 hour successfully controlled hyperkalaemic paralysis in 13 patients. It had insufficient effect in another patient.— P. Wang and T. Clausen, *Lancet*, 1976, *1*, 221.

Musculoskeletal disorders. In a study in 15 spastic patients, a combination of salbutamol 2 mg thrice daily with baclofen, up to 20 mg thrice daily, was no more effective than baclofen alone in alleviating spasticity.— U. Tolonen *et al.*, *Curr. ther. Res.*, 1979, *25*, 251.

Ocular disorders. One instillation of a solution of salbutamol sulphate 4.8% (equivalent to salbutamol 4%) lowered intra-ocular pressure in 15 glaucomatous patients. In a further study with 4 patients the fall in pressure was equivalent to that produced by adrenaline 1%. However, with a twice daily instillation intolerable hyperaemia with irritation developed in about half the patients.— G. D. Paterson and G. Paterson, *Br. J. Ophthal.*, 1972, *56*, 288.

Pregnancy and the neonate. A very large number of studies have been carried out into the efficacy of salbutamol and similar beta$_2$-selective adrenoceptor stimulants, particularly fenoterol and ritodrine, for the prevention of premature labour. In a review of 18 of these E. Hemminki and B. Starfield (*Br. J. Obstet. Gynec.*, 1978, *85*, 411) found few that did not contain any methodological drawbacks: only 5 were therapeutic rather than prophylactic studies, and in only 2 of these was the active drug more effective than placebo, moreover, a favourable effect in terms of foetal outcome was found in only one. Nevertheless, in what Hemminki and Starfield considered to be one of the more satisfactory studies, A. Wesselius-de Casparis *et al.* (*Br. med. J.*, 1971, *3*, 144) did find a postponement of preterm labour in 80% of patients receiving ritodrine compared with 48% in the placebo group.

Further reviews of the role of salbutamol and similar beta$_2$-selective adrenoceptor stimulants in the management of premature labour: *Br. med. J.*, 1977, *1*, 1118; *ibid.*, 1618; A. H. A. Wynn (letter), *ibid.*, *2*, 579; *Br. med. J.*, 1979, *1*, 71; *Drug & Ther. Bull.*, 1980, *18*, 34; *Br. med. J.*, 1981, *283*, 395.

Studies of salbutamol in premature labour: A. R. Korda *et al.*, *Med. J. Aust.*, 1974, *1*, 744; K. H. Ng and D. K. Sen (letter), *Br. med. J.*, 1974, *3*, 257; D. G. McDevitt *et al.*, *Br. J. Obstet. Gynaec.*, 1975, *82*, 442; A. M. Dawson, *ibid.*, 1977, *84*, 348; G. Hastwell (letter), *Lancet*, 1977, *2*, 354; G. Ryden, *Acta obstet. gynec. scand.*, 1977, *56*, 293; J. G. Bibby *et al.*, *Br. J. Obstet. Gynaec.*, 1978, *85*, 425; I. E. Boyd *et al.*, *Br. J. clin. Pharmac.*, 1978, *5*, 360P; G. B. Hastwell *et al.*, *Med. J. Aust.*, 1978, *1*, 465; T. F. Coyle (letter), *ibid.*, 1978, *2*, 71; J. W Reynolds, *Aust. N.Z. J. Obstet. Gynaec.*, 1978, *18*, 107; C. D. Sims *et al.*, *Br. J. Obstet. Gynaec.*, 1978, *85*, 761; T. R. Eggers *et al.*, *Med. J. Aust.*, 1979, *1*, 213; G. Spearing, *Obstet. Gynec.*, 1979, *53*, 171; T. Lind *et al.*, *Lancet*, 1980, *2*, 1165; P. Boylan and K. O'Driscoll (letter), *ibid.*, 1374; G. J. Addis (letter), *ibid.*, 1981, *1*, 42 (report of prolonged continuous salbutamol infusion and severe criticisms).

For adverse effects associated with the use of salbutamol in premature labour, see under Adverse Effects (above).

Urinary incontinence. Ineffectiveness of salbutamol in urinary incontinence.— C. M. Castleden and B. Morgan, *Br. J. clin. Pharmac.*, 1980, *10*, 619.

Preparations

Salbutamol Aerosol Inhalation *(B.P.C. 1973)*. An aerosol spray in a pressurised canister containing a fine suspension of salbutamol in a suitable mixture of aerosol propellents. It may contain a surfactant, stabilising agents, and other adjuvants. Store in a cool place. *Dose.* 1 or 2 inhalations, each of 100 µg, every 3 or 4 hours to a max. of 8 in 24 hours.

Salbutamol Sulphate Injection *(B.P.)*. Salbutamol Sulph. Inj. A sterile solution of salbutamol sulphate in Water for Injections containing suitable stabilising agents. The solution is distributed in containers, the air in which is replaced by nitrogen or other suitable gas, and sterilised by autoclaving. Potency is expressed in terms of the equivalent amount of salbutamol. pH 3.4 to 5.

Salbutamol Tablets *(B.P.)*. Tablets containing salbutamol sulphate. Potency is expressed in terms of the equivalent amount of salbutamol.

Proprietary Preparations

Ventolin *(Allen & Hanburys, UK)*. Salbutamol sulphate, available as **Spandets** (sustained-release tablets) each containing the equivalent of 8 mg of salbutamol; as **Syrup** (suggested diluent, syrup free from preservatives) containing the equivalent of 2 mg of salbutamol in each 5 ml; and as **Tablets** each containing the equivalent of 2 or 4 mg of salbutamol. (Also available as Ventolin in *Arg., Austral., Belg., Canad., Ital., Neth., Norw., S.Afr., Spain, Switz., USA*).

Ventolin Inhaler *(Allen & Hanburys, UK)*. A pressurised aerosol providing salbutamol 100 µg in each metered dose.

Ventolin Injection *(Allen & Hanburys, UK)*. Contains salbutamol sulphate equivalent to salbutamol 50 µg per ml in ampoules of 5 ml, and 500 µg per ml in ampoules of 1 ml. **Ventolin Solution for Intravenous Infusion** contains salbutamol sulphate equivalent to salbutamol 1 mg per ml, in ampoules of 5 ml.

Ventolin Respirator Solution *(Allen & Hanburys, UK)*. Contains salbutamol sulphate equivalent to salbutamol 0.5% (suggested diluent, sodium chloride injection or Water for Injections).

Ventolin Rotacaps *(Allen & Hanburys, UK)*. Cartridges each containing salbutamol sulphate equivalent to 200 or 400 µg of salbutamol, in a lactose basis, for administration by inhalation by means of a specially designed inhaler (Rotahaler).

NOTE. The availability of salbutamol to the lungs depends upon the formulation used; Ventolin Inhaler and Ventolin Rotacaps differ in this respect. For further details see under Uses (above).

Other Proprietary Names

Asmatol *(Arg.)*; Asmidon *(Jap.)*; Broncovaleas *(Ital.)*; Buto-Asma *(Spain)*; Salbutan *(Ital.)*; Salbuvent *(Norw.)*; Sultanol *(Ger., Jap.)*; Venetlin *(Jap.)*; Ventoline *(Denm., Fr.)*.

2106-k

Salmefamol. AH 3923. 1-(4-Hydroxy-3-hydroxymethylphenyl)-2-(4-methoxy-α-methylphenethylamino)ethanol.
$C_{19}H_{25}NO_4$=331.4.

CAS — 18910-65-1.

White crystals. M.p. about 82°.

Salmefamol is a direct-acting sympathomimetic agent with general properties similar to those of salbutamol (p.29). It has been given for the relief of bronchospasm in doses of 100 to 200 µg by inhalation and 1 to 2 mg by mouth.

Salmefamol 1 or 2 mg was well absorbed orally, peak plasma concentrations occurring 30 to 120 minutes after administration. A rapid rise in FEV$_1$ was noted after aerosol administration of salmefamol 220 to 340 µg, the plasma and urinary metabolites following this route were similar to those seen after administration by mouth, suggesting that most of the dose had been swallowed. Nearly all the dose of salmefamol was present in plasma or urine in the form of metabolites one of which may have been active.— M. E. Evans *et al.*, *Br. J. clin. Pharmac.*, 1974, *1*, 391. Evidence that salmefamol may be partly metabolised in the lung.— G. M. Shenfield *et al.*, *ibid.*, 1976, *3*, 583.

Asthma. In a double-blind trial in 24 patients salmefamol 100 µg by inhalation had a bronchodilator effect which lasted for at least 4 hours.— D. Bainbridge *et al.*, *Postgrad. med. J.*, 1975, *51*, 627. In a double-blind crossover study in 12 patients with chronic asthma salmefamol 1 mg and 2 mg taken by mouth produced a 40 to 50% increase in peak expiratory flow-rate and FEV$_1$; significant improvement lasted for 3 to 4 hours and 20% improvement for 4 to 6 hours. After the larger dose diastolic blood pressure fell 1 to 1½ hours after the dose.— R. W. Sillett *et al.*, *Eur. J. clin. Pharmac.*, 1976, *9*, 281.

Further references: I. A. Campbell *et al.*, *Br. J. clin. Pharmac.*, 1976, *3*, 151; E. Hills *et al.*, *Br. J. Dis. Chest*, 1976, *70*, 78; A. J. Dyson and I. A. Campbell, *Br. J. clin. Pharmac.*, 1977, *4*, 677.

Manufacturers
Glaxo, UK.

2107-a

Terbutaline Sulphate *(B.P.)*.
Terbutaline Sulfate *(U.S.P)*; KWD 2019; Terbutalini Sulphas.
2-*tert*-Butylamino-1-(3,5-dihydroxyphenyl)ethanol sulphate.
$C_{12}H_{19}NO_3,½H_2SO_4$=274.3.

CAS — 23031-25-6 (terbutaline); 23031-32-5 (sulphate).

Pharmacopoeias. In *Br.*,*Nord.*, and *U.S.*

A white to greyish-white odourless or almost odourless crystalline powder with a bitter taste. M.p. about 255°.

Soluble 1 in 4 of water; slightly soluble in alcohol; practically insoluble in chloroform and ether. **Store** at 15° to 30°. Protect from light.

Terbutaline sulphate was very stable to oxidative degradation in solution at pH 5.— L. -Å. Svensson, *Acta pharm. suec.*, 1972, *9*, 141.

Adverse Effects. As for Salbutamol, p.29.

Ten asthmatic patients received terbutaline 250 µg subcutaneously, 5 mg by mouth, and 10 mg by mouth, on separate days. In a dose of 10 mg, terbutaline caused a disproportionate increase in heart-rate compared with the small ventilatory advantage over a 5-mg dose. Side-effects were slight and included tremor and, in 3 patients, prolonged sleep.— B. J. Freedman, *Br. med. J.*, 1971, *1*, 633. In 16 patients with reversible airway disease, administration of terbutaline sulphate 500 µg thrice daily by inhalation was associated with a high incidence of side-effects—headache (9), nervousness (9), dizziness (8), pounding in chest (5), nausea (5), somnolence (5), diarrhoea (4), flushing (4), insomnia (3), tremors (3), sweating (3), and constipation (1).— J. Trautlein *et al.*, *J. clin. Pharmac.*, 1977, *17*, 76. A report in 1 patient of muscle twitching and cramp associated with the use of terbutaline sulphate 5 mg thrice daily.— S. Zelman (letter), *J. Am. med. Ass.*, 1978, *239*, 930.

Effects on the heart. A report of ventricular arrhythmias in a man with coronary heart disease, following oral administration of terbutaline sulphate 5 mg by mouth.— E. L. Kinney (letter), *J. Am. med. Ass.*, 1978, *240*, 2247. See also A. S. Banner *et al.*, *Archs intern. Med.*, 1979, *139*, 434.

Effects on muscles. Terbutaline 5 and 10 mg produced a significant increase in tremor which paralleled its bronchodilator action.— A. Richens and J. M. Watson, *Br. J. Pharmac.*, 1973, *49*, 187P. See also H. -K. Giesen and H. Illig, *Medsche Klin.*, 1972, *67*, 1045.

Overdosage. Tremor and tachycardia persisted for 24 hours after a 77-year-old man had taken an overdose of 20 tablets of terbutaline 2.5 mg and 9 tablets of flurazepam 15 mg.— I. Gomolin and J. A. Ingelfinger (letter), *New Engl. J. Med.*, 1979, *300*, 143.

Lactic acidosis, high plasma-glucose concentrations, and hypokalaemia occurred in a 28-year-old woman who took an overdose of terbutaline 225 mg, together with clomipramine, oxazepam, chloral hydrate, and wine.— M. Fahlén and L. Lapidus (letter), *Br. med. J.*, 1980, *281*, 390.

In an attempt to arrest premature labour a 35-year-old insulin-dependent diabetic woman was given an intravenous infusion of terbutaline 250 µg hourly for 12 hours, during which time her heart-rate varied between 90 to 114 beats per minute. Her terbutaline was then changed to the subcutaneous route and an hour later she was inadvertently given 2.5 mg, instead of 250 µg, subcutaneously. Ten minutes later non-radiating substernal chest pressure developed with a tachycardia of 150 beats per minute. ECG changes were noted and she was admitted to coronary care to rule out a myocardial infarction. She was given no medication except insulin and her cardiac course remained essentially benign. The tachycardia resolved after 10 hours and the cardiac enzymes over 2 days were essentially normal; the ECG reverted to normal over these 2 days. The terbutaline was not successful in preventing an abortion.— R. D. Brandstetter and V. Gotz (letter), *Lancet*, 1980, *1*, 485. The potentially dangerous cardiac effects could have been treated with a beta-adrenoceptor antagonist, such as propranolol.— R. J. Walden (letter), *ibid.*, 709. A further report of the inadvertent administration of terbutaline sulphate 2.5 mg subcutaneously instead of 250 µg.— C. Lawyer and A. Pond (letter), *New Engl. J. Med.*, 1977, *296*, 821.

Pregnancy and the neonate. A report of pulmonary oedema in 3 women given terbutaline, dexamethasone, and antibiotics to prevent premature delivery. Pulmonary oedema developed on discontinuation of terbutaline. Six other cases were known to have occurred in other hospitals in Northern California. About one in six of patients given this regimen have complained of substernal pain which may be a prodromal symptom.— P. Rogge *et al.* (letter), *Lancet*, 1979, *1*, 1026. See also P. G. Stubblefield, *Am. J. Obstet. Gynec.*, 1978, *132*, 341.

Angina pectoris in an 18-year-old woman given terbutaline intravenously and by mouth for premature labour.— K. -H. Tye *et al.*, *J. Am. med. Ass.*, 1980, *244*, 692.

Treatment of Adverse Effects. As for Isoprenaline, p.15.

Precautions. As for Salbutamol, p.29.

CAUTION. *Excessive usage of aerosols of sympathomimetic agents has been associated with sudden death in asthmatics, see* p.15.

Interference with diagnostic tests. Evidence that terbutaline does not interfere with allergy skin tests.— S. A. Imbeau *et al.*, *J. Allergy & clin. Immunol.*, 1978, *62*, 193.

Tolerance. There was no evidence of tolerance in 5 asthmatic patients treated with terbutaline aerosol for 2 years.— P. L. Kamburoff and F. J. Prime, *Postgrad. med. J.*, 1976, *52*, 205. See also S. Larsson *et al.*, *J. Allergy & clin. Immunol.*, 1977, *59*, 93.

Absorption and Fate. Terbutaline is incompletely absorbed from the gastro-intestinal tract and is also subject to fairly extensive first-pass metabolism by sulphate (and some glucuronide) conjugation in the liver and possibly the gut wall. It is accordingly excreted in the urine partly as the inactive conjugates and partly as unchanged terbutaline, the ratio depending upon whether it was given by mouth or intravenously.

In 7 hypertensive subjects the metabolism of radioactive terbutaline was dependent on the route of administration. After intravenous dosing unchanged drug accounted for most of the radioactivity in plasma. More than 80% of the dose was excreted in urine, mainly (68%) as terbutaline with only 14% as the sulphate conjugate; only 2 to 3% of the dose was excreted in faeces. After dosing by mouth an average of 47% of the radioactivity was recovered in faeces as unchanged drug indicating that terbutaline was incompletely absorbed; less than 15% of the plasma radioactivity was unchanged terbutaline and 70% of the radioactivity excreted in urine was a conjugate of terbutaline.— D. S. Davies *et al.*, *Br. J. clin. Pharmac.*, 1974, *1*, 129. See also H. T. Nilsson *et al.*, *Xenobiotica*, 1972, *2*, 363; K. Persson and K. Persson, *ibid.*, 375.

Further references: H. T. Nilsson *et al.*, *Eur. J. clin. Pharmac.*, 1976, *10*, 1 (aerosol inhalation); Y. Hörnblad *et al.*, *Eur. J. clin. Pharmac.*, 1976, *10*, 9 (comparison with fate of its pro-drug, ibuterol); D. S. Sitar *et al.*, *Curr. ther. Res.*, 1976, *19*, 266 (bioavailability of tablet and elixir preparations).

Uses. Terbutaline sulphate is a direct-acting sympathomimetic agent with actions and uses similar to those of salbutamol (p.30).

In the treatment of bronchial asthma terbutaline sulphate is given by mouth in a dose of 5 mg twice or thrice daily; for children aged 3 to 7 years a dose of 0.75 to 1.5 mg thrice daily is suggested, or 1.5 to 3 mg for older children.

Terbutaline sulphate may also be used as an aerosol in a dose of 1 or 2 inhalations of 250 µg about every 4 hours as required, to a maximum of 8 inhalations in 24 hours; a short interval is recommended between inhalations.

In the treatment of severe forms of bronchospasm terbutaline sulphate 250 µg may be given by subcutaneous, intramuscular, or slow intravenous injection up to 4 times daily; if required the dose may be doubled. Adequate oxygenation is necessary to avoid hypoxaemia. A suggested dose by injection for children aged 2 to 15 years is 10 µg per kg body-weight to a maximum total dose of 300 µg.

Recommended doses of terbutaline sulphate by inhalation as a mist depend on the ventilator machine used, and include 2 to 5 mg, or in severe cases up to 10 mg, in a volume of about 3 to 5 ml; alternatively dilution to a 0.01% solution in sterile physiological saline is recommended for chronic administration at a rate of 1 to 2 mg per hour.

Administration in renal failure. Terbutaline could be given in usual doses by mouth to patients with renal failure. It could be given in usual doses intravenously in patients with a glomerular filtration-rate of more than 50 ml per minute, but doses should be reduced to half in those with a glomerular filtration-rate of 10 to 50 ml per minute, and it should be avoided intravenously in those with a glomerular filtration-rate of less than 10 ml per minute.— W. M. Bennett *et al.*, *Ann. intern. Med.*, 1980, *93*, 286.

Allergy. Beneficial results in patients with chronic urticaria following administration of terbutaline 1.25 mg thrice daily.— B. Kennes *et al.*, *Clin. Allergy*, 1977, *7*, 35. Benefit in conjunction with ketotifen.— E. M. Saihan, *Br. J. Derm.*, 1981, *104*, 205.

Asthma. In a placebo-controlled double-blind crossover study involving 17 patients with moderate to severe asthma, terbutaline 5 mg was comparable in action and side-effects to aminophylline 400 mg; concurrent administration of terbutaline 5 mg with aminophylline 400 mg had at least a partially additive bronchodilator effect. The effect of aminophylline 200 mg with terbutaline 2.5 mg was equivalent to that of the higher doses of either drug used alone and it was hoped might have been associated with a lower incidence of side-effects although in practice this was not demonstrated.— J. D. Wolfe *et al.*, *New Engl. J. Med.*, 1978, *298*, 363. See also R. Levi (letter), *ibid.*, 1314; J. E. Jacobson (letter), *ibid.*; D. J. Salberg (letter), *ibid.*; M. Weinberger (letter), *ibid.*, 1315. Replies.— G. L. Snider (letter), *ibid.*; J. D. Wolfe and D. P. Tashkin (letter), *ibid.*, 1316.

Further reviews, comments, and studies on the role of terbutaline in the management of asthma: J. Allegra *et al.*, *J. clin. Pharmac.*, 1976, *16*, 367 and 444; R. M. Sly (letter), *ibid.*, 1977, *17*, 266; J. J. Trautlein (letter), *ibid.*, 267 (exercise-induced bronchospasm); J. L. C. Morse *et al.*, *Am. Rev. resp. Dis.*, 1976, *113*, 89 (exercise-induced bronchospasm); H. J. Schwartz *et al.*, *J. Allergy & clin. Immunol.*, 1976, *58*, 516 (comparison of subcutaneous terbutaline with subcutaneous adrenaline); B. F. Bachus and G. L. Snider, *J. Am. med. Ass.*, 1977, *238*, 2277; J. J. Trautlein (letter), *ibid.*, 1978, *239*, 1744 (terbutaline inhalation); M. Z. Blumberg *et al.*, *Pediatrics*, 1977, *60*, 14 (comparison of oral doses, with oral ephedrine, in children); W. J. Davis *et al.*, *Chest*, 1977, *72*, 614 (comparison of subcutaneous terbutaline with subcutaneous adrenaline, in children); B. J. S. Hartnett and G. E. Marlin, *Aust. N.Z. J. Med.*, 1977, *7*, 13 (comparison of terbutaline and salbutamol aerosol inhalers); S. Ishikawa *et al.*, *Ann. Allergy*, 1977, *39*, 303 (inhalation in older patients); L. M. Pang *et al.*, *Chest*, 1977, *72*, 469 (subcutaneous terbutaline in children with status asthmaticus); M. A. Sackner *et al.*, *Chest*, 1978, *73*, 802 (terbutaline aerosol); D. J. Birrell *et al.*, *Med. J. Aust.*, 1978, *2*, 231 (wet aerosol inhalation); V. Capecchi *et al.*, *Int. J. clin. Pharmac.*, 1978, *16*, 310 (comparison of terbutaline and salbutamol aerosols); S. Husby *et al.*, *Scand. J. resp. Dis.*, 1978, *59*, 277 (oral terbutaline in chronic bronchitis); E. D. Michaelson *et al.*, *J. Allergy & clin. Immunol.*, 1978, *61*, 365 (oral terbutaline in children); B. Ardal *et al.*, *J. Pediat.*, 1978, *93*, 305 (oral dosage in children); B. W. Madsen *et al.*, *Br. J. clin. Pharmac.*, 1979, *8*, 75 (crossover comparison of fenoterol, orciprenaline, salbutamol, and terbutaline aerosols); F. E. R. Simons *et al.*, *Ann. Allergy*, 1979, *43*, 275 (oral dosage in children); P. W. Trembath *et al.*, *J. Allergy & clin. Immunol.*, 1979, *63*, 395 (comparison with fenoterol aerosol); R. W. Weber *et al.*, *J. Allergy & clin. Immunol.*, 1979, *63*, 116 (comparison of different inhalation methods); E. H. Chester *et al.*, *Clin. Pharmac. Ther.*, 1978, *23*, 630 (comparison of isoprenaline, orciprenaline, and terbutaline aerosols); W. C. Miller and D. L. Rice, *Ann. Allergy*, 1980, *44*, 15 (comparison of oral fenoterol and terbutaline); J. E. Spicer *et al.* (letter), *Lancet*, 1980, *2*, 1248 (comparison of different inhalation methods); D. P. Tashkin *et al.*, *Am. J. Med.*, 1980, *68*, 14 (comparison of subcutaneous and inhaled terbutaline).

For earlier reports of the actions and uses of terbutaline in asthmatic patients, see Martindale 27th Edn, p. 35.

Dysmenorrhoea. Relief of menstrual pain followed intravenous administration of terbutaline 250 to 500 µg. The pain gradually returned after 1 to 2 hours. The mean heart-rate increased from 81 beats per minute before administration to 109 beats per minute after administration and a few patients reported slight palpitations on enquiry. The clinical usefulness of terbutaline in dysmenorrhoea seems limited, because in a pilot study using terbutaline 2.5 mg thrice daily by mouth several patients benefited but stopped taking the drug because of side-effects, primarily tremor.— M. Åkerlund *et al.*, *Br. J. Obstet. Gynaec.*, 1976, *83*, 673.

Pregnancy and the neonate. For comments on the efficacy of beta$_2$-selective adrenoceptor stimulants in the prevention of premature labour, see Salbutamol, p.31.

Studies of terbutaline in premature labour: K. E. Andersson *et al.*, *Br. J. Obstet. Gynaec.*, 1975, *82*, 745; I. Ingermarsson, *Am. J. Obstet. Gynec.*, 1976, *125*, 520; G. Ryden, *Acta obstet. gynec. scand.*, 1977, *56*, 293; F. Arias, *Am. J. Obstet. Gynec.*, 1978, *131*, 39; M. F. Epstein *et al.*, *J. Pediat.*, 1979, *94*, 449.

Preparations

Terbutaline Sulfate Injection *(U.S.P.)*. A sterile solution of terbutaline sulphate in Water for Injections. pH 3 to 5. It should not be used if it is discolored. Store at 15° to 30°. Protect from light.

Terbutaline Sulfate Tablets *(U.S.P.)*. Tablets containing terbutaline sulphate. Store at 15° to 30° in airtight containers.

Proprietary Preparations

Bricanyl *(Astra, UK)*. Terbutaline sulphate, available as 1-ml **Ampoules** of an injection containing 500 µg per ml; as **Syrup** containing 1.5 mg in each 5 ml in a sugar-free basis (suggested diluent, water); and as scored **Tablets** of 5 mg. **Bricanyl Inhaler.** A pressurised spray providing terbutaline sulphate 250 µg in each metered dose; also available with extended mouthpiece as Bricanyl Spacer inhaler. **Bricanyl Respirator Solution.** Contains terbutaline sulphate 10 mg per ml (suggested diluent, sodium chloride injection or Water for Injections). (Terbutaline sulphate is also available as Bricanyl in *Arg.*, *Austral.*, *Belg.*, *Canad.*, *Denm.*, *Fr.*, *Ger.*, *Neth.*, *Norw.*, *S.Afr.*, *Swed.*, *Switz.*, *USA*).

NOTE. In some countries ampoules have been marketed which contain terbutaline sulphate 1 mg in 1 ml. This practice has been criticised as being both wasteful and hazardous and a plea has been made for the introduction of ampoules containing 250 µg only, in order to lessen the risk of overdosage. References: C. Lawyer and A. Pond (letter), *New Engl. J. Med.*, 1977, *296*, 821; R.B. Burtch (letter), *ibid.*, 1237; R.D. Brandstetter and V. Gotz (letter), *Lancet*, 1980, *1*, 485.

Bricanyl Compound Tablets *(Astra, UK)*. Tablets each containing terbutaline sulphate 2.5 mg and guaiphenesin 100 mg. **Bricanyl Expectorant** (suggested diluent water) contains in each 5 ml terbutaline sulphate 1.5 mg and guaiphenesin 66.5 mg. For bronchial asthma and bronchitis. *Dose.* Bricanyl Expectorant: 10 to 15 ml thrice daily; Bricanyl Compound Tablets: 2 thrice daily.

Bricanyl SA *(Astra, UK).* Sustained-release tablets each containing terbutaline sulphate 7.5 mg. *Dose.* 1 every 12 hours.

Other Proprietary Names

Brethine *(USA)*; Bristurin *(Jap.)*; Feevone *(Austral.)*; Terbasmin *(Ital., Spain).*

Terbutaline sulphate was also formerly marketed in Great Britain under the proprietary name Filair (*Riker*).

2108-t

Tetrahydrozoline Hydrochloride *(U.S.P.).*

Cloridrato de Tetrizolina; Tetryzoline Hydrochloride. 2-(1,2,3,4-Tetrahydro-1-naphthyl)-2-imidazoline hydrochloride.

$C_{13}H_{16}N_2,HCl=236.7.$

CAS — 84-22-0 (tetrahydrozoline); 522-48-5 (hydrochloride).

Pharmacopoeias. In *Braz.* and *U.S.*

A white odourless crystalline powder. M.p. about 256° with decomposition. **Soluble** 1 in 3.5 of water and 1 in 7.5 of alcohol; very slightly soluble in chloroform; practically insoluble in ether. A 1% solution in water has a pH of about 6. **Store** in airtight containers.

Adverse Effects, Treatment, and Precautions. As for Naphazoline, p.20.

A 1-year-old girl became drowsy and had cold extremities with slowed respiration and heart-rate after swallowing about 2 to 4 ml of tetrahydrozoline hydrochloride 0.05% eye-drops. She was kept warm, and recovered after 24 hours.— R. L. Mindlin (letter), *New Engl. J. Med.*, 1966, *275,* 112. A further 3 cases of poisoning had been associated with tetrahydrozoline eye-drops, none involving death or serious illness. Children had taken up to 30 ml of the solution by accident.— G. W. Rogers, *Pfizer* (letter), *ibid.*, 447.

Absorption and Fate. Systemic absorption may follow topical administration of solutions of tetrahydrozoline. It is not used systemically, but it is readily absorbed from the gastro-intestinal tract.

Uses. Tetrahydrozoline hydrochloride is a sympathomimetic agent with marked alpha-adrenergic activity. It has actions and uses similar to those of naphazoline (p.20). Nasal drops are used as a 0.1% solution, 2 to 4 drops being instilled in each nostril not more often than every 3 hours for the symptomatic relief of rhinitis and sinusitis. Children aged 2 to 6 years of age may be given 2 to 3 drops of a 0.05% solution instilled in each nostril not more often than every 3 hours.

Solutions containing 0.05% are used as a conjunctival decongestant.

Ocular disorders. Instillation of a solution containing tetrahydrozoline hydrochloride (Visine, *USA*) alleviated droopy eyelid in a 52-year-old man with Horner's syndrome.— W. W. Campbell and T. A. Hill (letter), *New Engl. J. Med.*, 1978, *299,* 835.

Preparations

Tetrahydrozoline Hydrochloride Nasal Solution *(U.S.P.).* A solution of tetrahydrozoline hydrochloride in water, adjusted to a suitable osmolarity. pH 5.3 to 6.5. Store in airtight containers.

Tetrahydrozoline Hydrochloride Ophthalmic Solution *(U.S.P.).* A sterile iso-osmotic solution of tetrahydrozoline hydrochloride in water. pH 5.8 to 6.5. Store in airtight containers.

Proprietary Names

Ischemol *(Farmila, Ital.)*; Murine Plus *(Abbott, USA)*; Rhinopront *(Mack, Illert., Ger.)*; Tyzanol *(Pfizer, Norw.)*; Tyzine *(Pfizer, Austral.*; *Roerig, Belg.*; *Pfizer, Denm.*; *Pfizer, Ger.*; *Pfizer, S.Afr.*; *Pfizer, Spain*; *Pfizer, Switz.*; *Key, USA)*; Visina *(Pfizer, Spain)*; Visine *(Pfizer, Austral.*; *Pfizer, Ital.*; *Pfizer, Switz.*; *Lederle, USA)*; Visumetilen (tetrahydrozoline phosphate) *(LOA, Arg.)*; Yxin *(Pfizer, Ger.).* Also Visine *(Unicliffe, UK).*

NOTE. The name Rhinopront is also used for a preparation containing carbinoxamine maleate and either phenylephrine hydrochloride or phenylpropanolamine.

2109-x

Tramazoline Hydrochloride. 2-(5,6,7,8-Tetrahydro-1-naphthylamino)-2-imidazoline hydrochloride.

$C_{13}H_{17}N_3,HCl=251.8.$

CAS — 1082-57-1 (tramazoline); 3715-90-0 (hydrochloride).

Soluble 1 in 6 of water.

Tramazoline hydrochloride is a nasal decongestant similar to naphazoline (p.20).

ENT disorders. In 88 of 93 patients undergoing nasal surgery the use of a nasal spray containing tramazoline, dexamethasone isonicotinate, and neomycin sulphate (Tobispray) was a very good alternative to nasal packing.— L. W. Wing, *Med. J. Aust.*, 1977, *1,* 752.

Proprietary Preparations

Dexa-Rhinaspray *(Boehringer Ingelheim, UK).* An aerosol nasal spray providing in each metered dose tramazoline hydrochloride 120 µg, dexamethasone isonicotinate 20 µg, and neomycin sulphate 100 µg. For allergic rhinitis. *Dose.* 1 metered dose in each nostril up to 6 times daily.

Other Proprietary Names

Biciron *(Ger.)*; Rhinogutt *(Ger., Neth.)*; Rhinospray *(Belg., Ger., Neth.)*; Spray-Tish *(Austral.).*

2110-y

Tretoquinol Hydrochloride. Ro 07-5965; Trimethoquinol Hydrochloride; Trimetoquinol Hydrochloride. (−)-1,2,3,4-Tetrahydro-1-(3,4,5-trimethoxybenzyl)isoquinoline-6,7-diol hydrochloride monohydrate.

$C_{19}H_{23}NO_5,HCl,H_2O=399.9.$

CAS — 30418-38-3 (tretoquinol); 18559-59-6 (hydrochloride, anhydrous).

White or almost white odourless crystals or crystalline powder with a bitter taste. M.p. about 151° with decomposition. Sparingly **soluble** in water; slightly soluble in methyl alcohol; practically insoluble in acetone, chloroform, and ether.

Tretoquinol is reported to be a direct-acting sympathomimetic agent with general properties similar to those of salbutamol (p.29). It has been given by mouth in doses of 2 to 4 mg twice or thrice daily. It has also been given by inhalation and by injection.

References: Y. Yamamura and S. Kishimoto, *Ann. Allergy*, 1968, *26,* 504; M. Scherrer and H. Bachofen, *Schweiz. med. Wschr.*, 1972, *102,* 909; D. E. MacIntyre and A. L. Willis, *Br. J. Pharmac.*, 1978, *63,* 361P.

Proprietary Names

Inolin *(Tanabe, Jap.*; *Tanabe-Seiyaku, Neth.*; *Tanabe, Switz.)*; Vems *(ISF, Ital.).*

2111-j

Tuaminoheptane *(U.S.P.).* 1-Methylhexylamine.

$C_7H_{17}N=115.2.$

CAS — 123-82-0.

Pharmacopoeias. In *U.S.*

A colourless or pale yellow volatile liquid with an amine-like odour. It absorbs carbon dioxide on exposure to air, forming a white precipitate of tuaminoheptane carbonate. Specific gravity 0.760 to 0.763. **Soluble** 1 in 100 of water, 1 in 25 of alcohol, and 1 in 20 of chloroform; freely soluble in ether. A 1% solution in water has a pH of about 11.5. **Store** in a cool place in airtight containers.

2112-z

Tuaminoheptane Sulfate *(U.S.P.).* 1-Methylhexylamine sulphate.

$(C_7H_{17}N)_2,H_2SO_4=328.5.$

CAS — 6411-75-2.

Pharmacopoeias. In *U.S.*

A white odourless powder. **Soluble** 1 in 105 of water, 1 in 53 of alcohol, 1 in 10 of methyl alcohol, 1 in 3.5 of chloroform, and 1 in 30 of ether. A 1% solution in water has a pH of about 5.4. A 3.4% solution is iso-osmotic with serum. Phenylmercuric nitrate, 0.002%, is a suitable preservative for aqueous solutions. **Store** in airtight containers.

Adverse Effects and Precautions. Excessive use of tuaminoheptane may cause tachycardia and hypertension; care is needed in the presence of cardiovascular disease. Rebound congestion and rhinorrhoea may occur after frequent or prolonged use.

Uses. Tuaminoheptane is a volatile sympathomimetic agent with marked alpha-adrenergic activity and is claimed to be virtually free of central stimulating action. It has been used in inhalers for the symptomatic relief of nasal congestion. The sulphate has been used as a 1% solution for nasal drops or spray in the symptomatic treatment of rhinitis and sinusitis. A 2% solution, applied on pledgets of cotton wool, has been employed for diagnostic procedures and to clear the operative field in nasopharyngeal surgery. For displacement therapy or direct instillation into the sinuses a 0.2% solution was considered suitable.

Preparations

Tuaminoheptane Inhalant *(U.S.P.).* Cylindrical rolls of suitable fibrous material impregnated with tuaminoheptane (as the carbonate), usually with aromatics, and contained in a suitable inhaler. Store at a temperature not exceeding 40° in airtight containers.

Tuaminoheptane Sulfate Nasal Solution *(U.S.P.).* Tuaminoheptane Sulfate Solution. Tuaminoheptane sulphate 1 g, sodium hydroxide 22.7 mg, phenylmercuric nitrate 2 mg, potassium acid phosphate 680 mg, sodium chloride 90 mg, water to 100 ml, adjusted if necessary to pH 5.8 to 6.2. Store in airtight containers.

Proprietary Names

Heptedrine (sulphate) *(Bellon, Belg.)*; Tuamine Sulfate (sulphate) *(Lilly, NZ).*

2113-c

Tymazoline Hydrochloride. 2-Thymyloxymethyl-2-imidazoline Hydrochloride. 2-(2-Isopropyl-5-methylphenoxymethyl)-2-imidazoline hydrochloride.

$C_{14}H_{20}N_2O,HCl=268.8.$

CAS — 24243-97-8 (tymazoline); 28120-03-8 (hydrochloride).

A crystalline solid. M.p. about 216°.

Tymazoline hydrochloride is a sympathomimetic agent with marked alpha-adrenergic activity. A solution containing 0.05% is used as a nasal decongestant. It is not considered suitable for young children.

Proprietary Names

Pernazène *(Robert et Carrière, Fr.).*

2114-k

Xylometazoline Hydrochloride *(B.P., U.S.P.).*

2-(4-*tert*-Butyl-2,6-dimethylbenzyl)-2-imidazoline hydrochloride.

$C_{16}H_{24}N_2,HCl=280.8.$

CAS — 526-36-3 (xylometazoline); 1218-35-5 (hydrochloride).

Pharmacopoeias. In *Br.* and *U.S.*

A white to off-white odourless crystalline powder. M.p. above 300° with decomposition. **Soluble** 1 in 12 of water, 1 in 4 of alcohol, and 1 in 25 of chloroform; practically insoluble in ether. A 5% solution in water has a pH of 5 to 6.6. A 4.68% solution is iso-osmotic with serum. **Store** in airtight containers. Protect from light.

Adverse Effects, Treatment, and Precautions. As for Naphazoline, p.20.

A 1-month-old child was sedated and had hypertension and impaired respiration after the use of xylometazoline nose-drops. The dose administered was 3 times the adult dose.— R. E. Thompson (letter), *J. Am. med. Ass.*, 1970, *211,* 123.

Uses. Xylometazoline hydrochloride is a sympathomimetic agent with marked alpha-adrenergic activity. It is a vasoconstrictor with a rapid and prolonged action and is used in 0.1% solution twice or thrice daily for the relief of nasal congestion caused by rhinitis and sinusitis; 2 or 3 drops of the solution or 1 or 2 applications of spray are used in each nostril. A 0.05% solution is used once or twice daily for infants and children less than 12 years of age; 1 or 2 drops of the solution are used in each nostril.

A 0.05% solution has been instilled into the eye as a conjunctival decongestant.

Preparations

Xylometazoline Hydrochloride Nasal Drops *(B.P.)*. A solution of xylometazoline hydrochloride in water containing suitable antimicrobial preservatives and adjusted to pH 5 to 6.6.

Xylometazoline Hydrochloride Nasal Solution *(U.S.P.)*. Xylometazoline Hydrochloride Solution. An iso-osmotic solution of xylometazoline hydrochloride in water. pH 5 to 7.5. Store in airtight containers. Protect from light.

Proprietary Preparations

Otrivine *(Ciba, UK)*. Xylometazoline hydrochloride, available as **Nasal Drops** and as **Nasal Spray** each containing 0.1% and as **Paediatric Nasal Drops** containing 0.05%. (Also available as Otrivine in *Belg.*).

Otrivine-Antistin *(Ciba, UK)*. An aqueous solution containing xylometazoline hydrochloride 0.05% and antazoline sulphate 0.05%, available as **Nasal Drops** and **Nasal Spray**. Vasoconstrictor and antihistaminic.

Otrivine-Antistin Eye Drops *(Zyma, UK)*. Contain xylometazoline hydrochloride 0.05% and antazoline sulphate 0.05%. Vasoconstrictor and antihistaminic.

Other Proprietary Names

4-Way *(USA)*; Long Acting Neo-Synephrine *(USA)*; Otriven *(Ger.)*; Otrivin (see also under Naphazoline Hydrochloride) *(Austral., Denm., Ital., Neth., Norw., S.Afr., Switz., USA)*; Otrivina *(Arg.)*; Otrix *(Austral.)*; Sinex Long-Acting *(USA)*; Sinutab *(Canad.)*.

Alcohols

550-r

Most of the alcohols described in this section are used as solvents; for other solvents see the section on Solvents, p.1450.

The strength of individual alcoholic beverages varies considerably; the approximate alcoholic (C_2H_6O) content of some typical beverages is: beer 500 ml, 18 g; champagne and red and white wines 180 ml, 18 g; port 50 ml, 8 g; sherry 80 ml, 12.5 g; brandy, gin, and whisky 25 ml, 8 g.

551-f

Alcohol *(U.S.P.).* Ethanol (96 per cent) *(B.P.)*; Alcohol (96 per cent); Ethanolum; Ethyl Alcohol; Alcool; Aethanolum; Spiritus; Spiritus Aethylicus; Spiritus Alcoholisatus; Spiritus Concentratissimus; Spiritus Fortis; Spiritus Vini Rectificatus; Weingeist; Alcohol Etílico.

$C_2H_5OH = 46.07$.

Pharmacopoeias. Alcohol is included in all the pharmacopoeias examined except *Braz., Eur.,* and *Fr.,* the specified strengths ranging from about 89% to 97% v/v.

The *B.P.* specifies under Ethanol (96 per cent) not less than 96% and not more than 96.6% v/v; 93.8 to 94.7% w/w of C_2H_6O. The *B.P. 1973* specified under Alcohol (95 per cent) not less than 94.7% and not more than 95.2% v/v; 92 to 92.7% w/w of C_2H_6O. The *U.S.P.* specifies under Alcohol not less than 94.9% and not more than 96.0% v/v; 92.3 to 93.8% w/w of C_2H_6O.

In *Martindale* the term alcohol is used for alcohol 95 or 96% v/v.

A mixture of ethyl alcohol and water. A clear, colourless, mobile, volatile, readily inflammable liquid with a characteristic spirituous odour and burning taste. B.p. about 78°. The *B.P.* specifies sp. gr. (20°/20°) 0.8062 to 0.8087; the *U.S.P.* specifies 0.812 to 0.816 at 15.56°. Flash-point 14° (closed-cup test).

Miscible with water (with rise of temperature and contraction of volume), acetone, chloroform, ether, glycerol, and almost all other organic solvents. A 1.39% solution of alcohol (95%) in water is iso-osmotic with serum. It is **sterilised** by autoclaving in sealed ampoules or by filtration. **Store** in a cool place in airtight containers.

The **dilute alcohols** of the *B.P.* are of the following strengths and they may be prepared by diluting the specified quantity of alcohol (96%) to 1 litre with water. Before the final adjustment of volume is made, the mixture should be cooled to the same temperature, about 20°, as that at which the alcohol (96%) was measured.

Alcohol (90%)[Ethanol (90%); Rectified Spirit; Spiritus Rectificatus; SVR; Spiritus Vini Rectificatus], 934 ml;
Alcohol (80%) [Ethanol (80%)], 831 ml;
Alcohol (70%) [Ethanol (70%)], 727 ml;
Alcohol (60%) [Ethanol (60%)], 623 ml;
Alcohol (50%)[Ethanol (50%)], 519 ml;
Alcohol (45%) [Ethanol (45%)], 468 ml;
Alcohol (25%) [Ethanol (25%)], 259 ml;
Alcohol (20%) [Ethanol (20%)], 207 ml.

Diluted Alcohol *U.S.N.F.* contains 48.4 to 49.5% v/v or 41 to 42% w/w and is prepared by mixing equal volumes of alcohol and water.

Dilute alcohols of varying strengths are included in most foreign pharmacopoeias.

A directive of the Council of the European Communities requires that, with effect from not later than 1 January 1980, alcoholic strength be expressed only as alcoholic strength by volume (% vol) or alcoholic strength by mass (% mas).

A directive provides a specification for alcoholometers and alcohol hydrometers for the determination of alcoholic strength. The Alcoholometers and Alcohol Hydrometers (EEC Requirements) Regulations 1977 (SI 1977: No. 1753) provides for the verification of such instruments in the UK. British Standard Specifications for alcohol hydrometers and thermometers for use therewith (BS 5470: 1977 and BS 5471: 1977 respectively) are published by the British Standards Institution.

Alcoholic strength was previously often expressed in terms of *proof spirit* (spiritus tenuior). Proof spirit contained about 57.1% v/v or 49.2% w/w of C_2H_6O, and was defined legally as 'that which at the temperature of 51°, F weighs exactly twelve-thirteenth parts of an equal measure of distilled water'. Sp. gr. (60°/60°F) 0.9198.

Spirit of such a strength that 100 volumes contained as much ethyl alcohol as 160 volumes of proof spirit was described as '60 OP' (over proof). Spirit of which 100 volumes contained as much alcohol as 40 volumes of proof spirit was described as '60 UP' (under proof). An alternative method of indicating spirit strength was used on the labels of alcoholic beverages; the strength was given as a number of degrees, proof spirit being taken as 100°.

For the purposes of Customs and Excise the quantity of spirit was formerly expressed in proof gallons. For 100 gallons this figure was obtained by adding 100 to the number of degrees over proof. Hence the figure for the number of proof gallons was no direct indication of the volume of the spirit.

In USA proof spirit contains 50% v/v of C_2H_6O.

The sale of intoxicating liquor is limited in Great Britain to persons holding an appropriate excise licence and, where applicable, a retailer's licence. A licence is not normally required for the sale by pharmacists of spirits or wine for medical or scientific purposes; not more than 142 ml may be sold at any one time.

Spirits and goods containing spirits are liable to excise duty; a reduced rate of duty is payable, subject to the observance of the prescribed conditions, in respect of articles used for medical or scientific purposes.

CAUTION. *In Great Britain it is recommended that scalp lotions or shampoos containing 50% or more of alcohol or containing a more inflammable solvent should carry the following warning:* CAUTION. This preparation is highly flammable. Do not use it, or dry the hair, near a fire or naked flame. *Other inflammable preparations which are sold or dispensed should also carry the label:* Highly flammable.

Complete haemolysis or denaturation of human erythrocytes occurred in all aqueous alcohol solutions after 45 minutes at 37°. Addition of sodium chloride 0.9% prevented haemolysis in solutions containing less than 11% of ethanol.— S. H. Ku and D. E. Cadwallader, *J. pharm. Sci.*, 1974, *63*, 60. The maximum concentration of alcohol in sodium chloride 0.9% which was not associated with haemolysis was 10.1% v/v.— D. E. Cadwallader (letter), *Br. J. Anaesth.*, 1978, *50*, 81. See also E. R. Hammarlund and K. Pedersen-Bjergaard, *J. pharm. Sci.*, 1961, *50*, 24.

Dependence. Dependence of the barbiturate-alcohol type (see p.792) is liable to occur in susceptible persons.

Adverse clinical and behavioural manifestations, including dependence and cirrhosis of the liver, tended to become apparent in persons with an average daily consumption of more than 150 ml of absolute alcohol for prolonged periods. Studies of selected groups of heavy drinkers (total about 12 500) showed that the death-rate from all causes was 2 to 4 times higher than in the general population. Alcohol was a significant causal factor in traffic and other accidents.— Twentieth Report of the WHO Expert Committee on Drug Dependence, *Tech. Rep. Ser. Wld Hlth Org. No. 551*, 1974.

Seven patients undergoing long-term haemodialysis became addicted to vapours of denatured alcohol. Withdrawal symptoms occurred in 2 patients who tried unsuccessfully to stop the practice.— N. G. de Santo *et al.*, *J. Am. med. Ass.*, 1975, *234*, 841.

For a discussion of the alcohol dependence syndrome and a lexicon of terms related to alcohol consumption, see *Alcohol-related Disabilities, WHO Offset Publication No. 32*, G. Edwards *et al.* (Ed.), Geneva, World Health Organization, 1977.

References and reviews.— J. H. Mendelson, *New Engl. J. Med.*, 1970, *283*, 24 and 71; H. Kalant *et al.*, *Pharmac. Rev.*, 1971, *23*, 135; *Lancet*, 1972, *2*, 24; *Alcoholism*, The Standing Medical Advisory Committee, London, Department of Health and Social Security, 1973; M. Evans, *Practitioner*, 1974, *212*, 801; E. M. Sellers and H. Kalant, *New Engl. J. Med.*, 1976, *294*, 757 and 1464; G. Edwards and M. M. Gross, *Br. med. J.*, 1976, *1*, 1058; R. M. Murray, *ibid.*, *2*, 1537; D. B. Goldstein, *Life Sci.*, 1976, *18*, 553; A. D. Wright, *Br. dent. J.*, 1977, *143*, 339; *Br. med. J.*, 1977, *2*, 914; *ibid.*, 1371; J. M. S. Pearce, *Br. J. Hosp. Med.*, 1977, *18*, 132; *Alcoholism, New Knowledge and New Responses*, G. Edwards and M. Grant (Ed.), London, Croom Helm, 1977; Report on a WHO Conference, *Public Health Aspects of Alcohol and Drug Dependence*, Copenhagen, WHO, 1979; Report of a Special Committee of the Royal College of Psychiatrists, *Alcohol and Alcoholism*, London, Tavistock, 1979.

Adverse Effects. In mild alcoholic intoxication symptoms include euphoria, loss of judgement, emotional lability, slurred speech, aggression, diuresis, and ataxia.

The well-known 'morning-after' or hangover effects following such a bout constitute mild withdrawal symptoms and may include nausea, thirst, gastric pain, headache, dizziness, fatigue, tremor, pallor, and sweating.

In acute alcoholic intoxication the patient is stuporous or comatose. The skin is cold and clammy, the body temperature low, respiration is slow and noisy, the pupils are usually dilated, and the heart-rate quickened. Hypoglycaemia may occur, and there may be raised intracranial pressure and circulatory collapse. Death is rare but deep coma persisting for over 12 hours is dangerous. Acute alcoholic intoxication may be followed by acute gastritis and pancreatitis.

Alcohol in small doses depresses the activity of the central nervous system and impairs the higher faculties, including judgement and coordination. For this reason it has become an offence in many countries for motorists to drive when the blood-alcohol concentration is above a stated value; in the United Kingdom this value is 80 mg per 100 ml and in most states of the USA it is 100 mg per 100 ml. The alcohol concentration in expired air and urine can be used to estimate the blood-alcohol concentration.

Chronic intoxication with alcohol, or alcoholism, may lead to gastritis and gastric haemorrhage, acute pancreatitis, hepatic cirrhosis, cardiomyopathy, and muscle wasting; hypertension and hyperuricaemia may also occur. Some of these effects may be enhanced by an inadequate diet.

Alcohol may cause brain damage leading to Korsakoff's syndrome and Wernicke's encephalopathy. Fat deposits may occur in the liver and there may be a reduction in various blood-cell counts. A foetal alcohol syndrome has been described.

Maximum permissible atmospheric concentration 1000 ppm.

A review of the metabolic and hepatic effects of alcohol.— K. J. Isselbacher, *New Engl. J. Med.*, 1977, *296*, 612. See also K. G. M. M. Alberti and M. Nattrass, *Lancet*, 1977, *2*, 25.

Alcoholism had been reported to be associated with avascular necrosis of the hip.— D. S. Owen (letter), *J. Am. med. Ass.*, 1977, *238*, 29.

A discussion of the chronic effects of alcohol.— *Br. med. J.*, 1978, *2*, 381.

Alcohol in the blood. The handling of motor vehicles was impaired by 100 mg per 100 ml of alcohol in the blood, stupor might result from 300 mg per 100 ml, and respiratory failure and sometimes death from 400 mg or more per 100 ml. The fatal dose was about 1 litre of 50% v/v spirit ingested over a short period. In conjunction with other drugs, low concentrations of alcohol might provoke significant toxic effects.— A. J. McBay, *New Engl. J. Med.*, 1966, *274*, 1257.

The results of a survey indicated that when blood-alcohol concentrations were 40 to 50 mg per 100 ml there was a significant increase in the accident-rate in car drivers, and the rate increased rapidly at concentrations up to 80 mg per 100 ml. At blood concentrations of 100 mg per 100 ml the probability of causing an accident was 6 or 7 times greater than that of drivers with less than 10 mg per 100 ml and at 150 mg per 100 ml the probability was 25 times greater.— *Research on the Effects of Alcohol and Drugs on Driver Behaviour*, Report by the Organisation for Economic Cooperation and Development, Paris, 1968.

The influence of alcohol on road and other accidents.— D. Hossack and G. Brown, *Med. J. Aust.*, 1974, *2*, 473; *Br. med. J.*, 1977, *1*, 665; *ibid.*, 1977, *2*, 1295; J. D. J. Havard, *ibid.*, 1978, *1*, 1595; *ibid.*, 1980, *280*, 135.

Amenorrhoea. Amenorrhoea associated with chronic alcohol consumption in 2 women.— R. S. Ryback (letter), *J. Am. med. Ass.*, 1977, *238*, 2143.

Choreoathetosis. Choreoathetotic movements, more usually affecting the upper half of the body, developed in 12 patients with alcoholism. The condition lasted from a few hours to a year, and might have been related to alcohol withdrawal.— P. J. Mullin *et al.*, *Br. med. J.*, 1970, *4*, 278. See also J. M. Kellett (letter), *ibid.*, 434.

Depression. A brief discussion of the role of alcohol in causing depression.— F. A. Whitlock and L. E. J. Evans, *Drugs*, 1978, *15*, 53.

Effect on blood. A discussion of the effects of alcohol on blood.— *Br. med. J.*, 1978, *1*, 1504.

Reports of thrombocytopenia.— J. Lindenbaum and C. S. Lieber, *New Engl. J. Med.*, 1969, *281*, 333; E. C. MacLeod and I. Michaels (letter), *Lancet*, 1969, *2*, 1198; M. A. Sahud, *New Engl. J. Med.*, 1972, *286*, 355. Rebound thrombocytosis.— T. L. Moffatt and A. Schwartz (letter), *New Engl. J. Med.*, 1976, *295*, 1322; E. M. Haselager and J. Vreeken, *Lancet*, 1977, *1*, 774.

Nine leucopenic episodes in 6 alcoholics.— Y. K. Liu, *Am. J. Med.*, 1973, *54*, 605, per *J. Am. med. Ass.*, 1973, *225*, 651.

Macrocytosis in 56 alcoholics.— A. Wu *et al.*, *Lancet*, 1974, *1*, 829.

Reduction in the production of red blood cells, granulocytes, and platelets had been reported in chronic alcoholics, and could produce diagnostic difficulties.— *Lancet*, 1977, *2*, 806 and 988. See also S. Wallerstedt (letter), *ibid.*, 1178.

Results of a study in 7710 apparently healthy men indicated that a relationship existed between alcohol consumption, smoking, and certain blood parameters. For smokers, red blood cell counts were significantly decreased and mean corpuscular volume increased with alcohol consumption; for non-smokers white blood cell counts were significantly increased with alcohol consumption but there was no increase in red blood cell counts; mean corpuscular volume was also significantly increased with alcoholic consumption but to a smaller degree than in smokers.— E. Eschwege *et al.*, *J. clin. Path.*, 1978, *31*, 654.

Stroke. Analysis of 76 patients under 40 years of age with ischaemic infarction, indicated that alcohol intoxication increases the risk of brain infarction 2 to 3 times for men and 3 to 4 times for women.— M. Hillbom and M. Kaste, *Lancet*, 1978, *2*, 1181.

Effect on brain. Alcohol caused brain damage which might be common. Visual-motor and visual-spatial functions were affected and were important particularly in relation to the driving of motor vehicles.— *Br. med. J.*, 1976, *1*, 1168.

A study of the incidence of alcohol-induced brain damage in 37 men under the age of 35 who had drunk at least 50 g of ethanol daily over the preceeding year. Twenty-two (59%) showed signs of intellectual deterioration; 18 had cerebral atrophy, 4 of whom also had central atrophy. Cirrhosis was found in only 19% of the 37 patients. Intellectual impairment may be the earliest sign of alcohol abuse.— K. Lee *et al.*, *Lancet*, 1979, *2*, 759.

Comment on alcoholic brain damage.— *Lancet*, 1981, *1*, 477.

Other references: R. H. Ehrensing *et al.*, *Q. J. Stud. Alcohol*, 1970, *31*, 851, per *Abstr. Wld Med.*, 1971, *45*, 614; J. E. Manno *et al.*, *Clin. Pharmac. Ther.*, 1971, *12*, 202; C. Brewer and L. Perrett, *Br. J. Addict. Alcohol*, 1971, *66*, 170, per *Abstr. Hyg.*, 1972, *47*, 657; R. M. Hoy, *Br. J. Addict. Alcohol*, 1973, *68*, 201, per *Abstr. Hyg.*, 1974, *49*, 169; S. A. Lisman, *Archs gen. Psychiat.*, 1974, *30*, 46, per *J. Am. med. Ass.*, 1974, *227*, 458; E. S. Parker *et al.*, *Archs gen. Psychiat.*, 1974, *31*, 824, per *J. Am. med. Ass.*, 1974, *230*, 1743.

See also Stroke under Effect on Blood, above.

Effect on heart. Reviews of alcoholic cardiomyopathy: *Br. med. J.*, 1979, *2*, 1457; E. Rubin, *New Engl. J. Med.*, 1979, *301*, 28; *Lancet*, 1980, *1*, 961.

See also under Hypomagnesaemia and under Uses.

Effect on sexual function. A discussion of feminisation in alcoholic men.— D. H. Van Thiel and R. Lester, *New Engl. J. Med.*, 1976, *295*, 835. Decreased testosterone concentrations in healthy men given about 3 g of alcohol per kg body-weight daily for up to 4 weeks.— G. G. Gordon *et al.*, *ibid.*, 793. Increased reductase activity might enhance the removal of testosterone.— E. Rubin *et al.*, *Science*, 1976, *191*, 563.

Hyperglycaemia. A significant rise in blood-glucose concentrations and a significant delay in insulin secretion were observed in 12 healthy subjects 1 hour after drinking 50 ml of alcohol.— S. Wapnick and J. J. Jones (letter), *Lancet*, 1972, *2*, 180. Higher blood-glucose concentrations were also observed in 20 patients given alcohol 0.8 to 1 g per kg body-weight intravenously.— J. W. Dundee (letter), *ibid.*, 433.

No deterioration of diabetic control was observed in 20 diabetic patients given alcohol 35 ml.— C. H. Walsh and D. J. O'Sullivan, *Diabetes*, 1974, *23*, 440, per *J. Am. med. Ass.*, 1974, *229*, 723.

Hyperlipidaemia. In 909 men without diabetes, plasma-triglyceride concentrations were higher in those with an alcohol consumption of more than 180 ml per week, but the incidence of coronary-artery occlusion was lower. Plasma concentrations of cholesterol were not consistently affected.— J. J. Barboriak *et al.*, *Br. Heart J.*, 1977, *39*, 289, per *J. Am. med. Ass.*, 1977, *238*, 439.

In a study of about 3800 subjects without known heart disease there was a moderate correlation between alcohol consumption and elevation of plasma-triglyceride concentrations, a stronger correlation with depression of low-density lipoprotein cholesterol, and a strong association with elevation of high-density lipoprotein cholesterol; there was no appreciable correlation with very low-density lipoprotein cholesterol.— W. P. Castelli *et al.*, *Lancet*, 1977, *2*, 153. See also H. Ginsberg *et al.*, *Ann. intern. Med.*, 1974, *80*, 143; L. D. Ostrander *et al.*, *Archs intern. Med.*, 1974, *134*, 451, per *J. Am. med. Ass.*, 1974, *229*, 1823.

See also under Uses (Effect on Cardiovascular System), p.38.

Hypertension. Data from 83 947 men and women of various races indicated that regular intake of 3 or more alcoholic drinks daily was associated with raised blood pressure. This association was independent of age, sex, race, smoking habits, ingestion of coffee, previous heavy drinking, educational attainment, or obesity.— A. L. Klatsky *et al.*, *New Engl. J. Med.*, 1977, *296*, 1194. Criticisms and comments.— T. A. Rustin (letter), *ibid.*, *297*, 450; S. Fisch (letter), *ibid.*; J. Dahlgren (letter), *ibid.*; L. D. Peterson (letter), *ibid.*, 451; H. K. Thompson (letter), *ibid.*

Hypomagnesaemia. Nine of 10 chronic alcoholics had magnesium deficiency.— P. Lim and E. Jacob, *Metabolism*, 1972, *21*, 1045, per *J. Am. med. Ass.*, 1973, *223*, 457.

Life-threatening ventricular tachyarrhythmias in an alcholic associated with hypokalaemia and hypomagnesaemia.— J. Fischer and J. Abrams, *Archs intern. Med.*, 1977, *137*, 1238.

Hypophosphataemia. A report of hypophosphataemia in 11 patients with chronic alcoholism.— M. C. Territo and K. R. Tanaka, *Archs intern. Med.*, 1974, *134*, 445, per *J. Am. med. Ass.*, 1974, *229*, 1823.

Immunosuppression. The adverse effects of alcohol on host defences in 6 non-cirrhotic alcoholic subjects.— S. J. Gluckman *et al.*, *Archs intern. Med.*, 1977, *137*, 1539.

Ketoacidosis and lactic acidosis. A report of 7 episodes of alcoholic ketoacidosis in 6 women.— M. T. Cooperman *et al.*, *Diabetes*, 1974, *23*, 433, per *J. Am. med. Ass.*, 1974, *229*, 722.

A brief discussion of lactic acidosis occurring with alcohol. Diabetic patients appear to be a special risk.— R. A. Kreisberg, *Ann. intern. Med.*, 1980, *92*, 227. See also R. D. Cohen, *Adverse Drug React. Bull.*, 1978, June, 248.

Liver damage. A review by an international group, of the morphological manifestations of alcoholic liver disease.— *Lancet*, 1981, *1*, 707.

There was a 50% chance that cirrhosis would develop in a person who consumed 170 g of alcohol daily for 25 years. Protein malnutrition was not considered a significant factor. Factors involved in liver damage were a rise in intracellular protein; enhanced microsomal enzyme activity probably increasing the hepatotoxicity of environmental compounds; decreased conversion of acetaldehyde to acetate possibly permitting acetaldehyde to exert toxic effects on brain, heart, and other tissues; alterations in the redox state causing hypoglycaemia, hyperlactacidaemia, acidosis, hyperuricaemia, and decreased lipid oxidation; and immunological factors. The activity of serum glutamic dehydrogenase correlated with the degree of liver necrosis and inflammation.— C. S. Lieber, *New Engl. J. Med.*, 1978, *298*, 888.

Neoplasms. Cancers of the mouth, pharynx, larynx, and oesophagus, and primary cancer of the liver appeared to be definitely related to heavy consumption of alcohol in the USA—Report from the National Institute on Alcohol Abuse and Alcoholism, *J. Am. med. Ass.*, 1974, *229*, 1023.

Of 58 patients with cancer of the tonsil, tongue, base of the tongue, pharynx, neck node, and floor of the mouth, 51 were alcoholics and the other 7 were heavy drinkers. Of 14 with supraglottic tumours, 8 were alcoholics and some of the others were believed to be heavy drinkers. Of 28 patients with cancer of the vocal cord, nasopharynx, or buccal mucosa, however, only 1 was an alcoholic. Alcoholism either alone or enhanced by smoking was the most important cause of cancer in certain sites of the head and neck.— W. S. Lowry, *Laryngoscope, St Louis*, 1975, *85*, 1275, per *Practitioner*, 1976, *216*, 5. See also *J. Am. med. Ass.*, 1976, *236*, 435.

There was no correlation between WHO figures on alcohol consumption in 14 countries and on the incidence of malignant neoplasm of the breast.— E. E. Pochin (letter), *Lancet*, 1976, *1*, 1137.

Increases in laryngeal cancer in Britain and Australia were related to increased alcohol consumption.— A. J. McMichael, *Lancet*, 1978, *1*, 1244.

Neurotoxicity. In a study of 145 patients treated for 'alcoholic polyneuropathy', the lack of uniformity of histological and clinical symptoms suggested different pathogenic factors; the toxic effects of alcohol and its metabolites on axons and nutritional deficiency were possible causative factors.— A. Bischoff, *Dt. med. Wschr.*, 1971, *96*, 317.

Evidence of vagal neuropathy in chronic alcoholics.— G. Duncan *et al.*, *Lancet*, 1980, *2*, 1053. See also D. M. Turnbull *et al.* (letter), *ibid.*, 1381.

Pain. The incidence of pain on infusion and venous sequelae (phlebitis, thrombosis, or both) was studied in 400 patients who received alcohol by rapid intravenous injection for the induction of anaesthesia. For concentrations of 5 and 10% w/v the incidence of mild pain was 12 and 32%, of severe pain 0 and 23%, and of venous sequelae 8 and 30%.— M. Isaac and J. W. Dundee, *Br. J. Anaesth.*, 1969, *41*, 1070.

Pregnancy and the neonate. *Pregnancy.* Discussions on the foetal alcohol syndrome.— *Lancet*, 1976, *1*, 1335; *Br. med. J.*, 1976, *2*, 1404; J. J. Mulvihill and A. M. Yeager, *Teratology*, 1976, *13*, 345, per *Int. pharm. Abstr.*, 1976, *13*, 1179; *FDA Drug Bull.*, 1977, *7*, 18; G. Turner, *Med. J. Aust.*, 1978, *1*, 18; N. Gordon, *Postgrad. med. J.*, 1978, *54*, 796; *Br. med. J.*, 1978, *2*, 76; S. K. Clarren and D. W. Smith, *New Engl. J. Med.*, 1978, *298*, 1063.

A characteristic pattern of abnormalities (the foetal alcohol syndrome) was recognised in infants born to alcoholic women; the pattern included characteristic facial features including narrow palpebral fissures, prenatal and postnatal growth deficiency, postnatal brain-growth deficiency, shown by reduced head circumference, developmental delay or mental deficiency, jitteriness or irritability in the neonatal period occasionally leading to permanent impairment of fine motor function. Structural anomalies might occur in 30 to 40% of infants born to heavy drinkers and might include cardiac defects, cleft palate, ocular abnormalities, and limb deformities. A prospective study of 1500 pregnant women had shown that recognisable alterations in growth and morphogenesis might occur in 10% of infants born to mothers taking the equivalent of 30 to 60 ml of absolute alcohol daily in the earliest part of pregnancy.— J. W. Hanson, *Br. J. Hosp. Med.*, 1977, *18*, 126.

In 322 infants congenital abnormalities were noted in 32% of those born to heavy drinkers, 14% born to moderate drinkers, and 9% of the abstinent. Only 2 of 27 women who drank heavily throughout pregnancy had infants who were considered normal at birth.— E. M. Ouellette *et al.*, *New Engl. J. med.*, 1977, *297*, 528.

Two of 163 infants examined had definite signs of the foetal alcohol syndrome; another 9 had some signs and of these 7 were born to women who reported drinking 30 ml or more of alcohol daily in the month before pregnancy was diagnosed. Moderate as well as heavy alcohol intake may harm the early conceptus.— J. W.

Hanson *et al.*, *J. Pediat.*, 1978, *92*, 457.

Experience with over a hundred instances of the foetal alcohol syndrome includes none in which the mother had not been drinking heavily for at least the first trimester of pregnancy.— D. W. Smith and J. M. Graham (letter), *Lancet*, 1979, *2*, 527.

Responsibility for the foetal alcohol syndrome is ascribed to acetaldehyde at maternal concentrations exceeding 35 μmol per litre and this is probably due to an inherited or acquired defect of a specific aldehyde dehydrogenase.— P. V. Véghelyi *et al.* (letter), *Br. med. J.*, 1978, *2*, 1365. If the foetal alcohol syndrome is caused by acetaldehyde rather than by alcohol itself then infants of women with an inherited or acquired defect of mitochondrial aldehyde dehydrogenase, who ingest even moderate amounts of alcohol, may be at risk. Moreover, all drugs that inhibit alcohol dehydrogenase should be avoided during pregnancy. In addition to disulfiram, these include metronidazole, procarbazine, nifuratel, and possibly also tolazoline, mepacrine, and chloramphenicol.— P. M. Dunn *et al.* (letter), *Lancet*, 1979, *2*, 144.

Evidence from a prospective study involving 32 019 pregnant women, that regular drinking of one or more alcoholic beverages daily, is associated with an increased risk of abortion S. Harlap and P. H. Shiono, *Lancet*, 1980, *2*, 173. A similar conclusion from a study of 616 women who aborted spontaneously and 632 who delivered after at least 28 weeks' gestation.— J. Kline *et al.*, *ibid.*, 176. Although there is an increased risk with heavy drinking, one must seriously question the interpretation that this association also applies to moderate or occasional drinking.— R. J. Sokol (letter), *ibid.*, 1079.

A view that features of the foetal alcohol syndrome are not unique. A study of the children of women with phenylketonuria has shown that they have similar features.— A. H. Lipson *et al.* (letter), *Lancet*, 1981, *1*, 717.

Further references to the foetal alcohol syndrome: K. L. Jones *et al.*, *Lancet*, 1973, *1*, 1267; K. L. Jones and D. W. Smith, *ibid.*, 1973, *2*, 999; R. H. Palmer, *Pediatrics*, 1974, *53*, 490, per *J. Am. med. Ass.*, 1974, *229*, 596; J. J. Mulvihill *et al.*, *Am. J. Obstet. Gynec.*, 1976, *125*, 937, per *J. Am. med. Ass.*, 1976, *236*, 2687; F. Majewski *et al.*, *Münch. med. Wschr.*, 1976, *118*, 1635, per *Abstr. Hyg.*, 1977, *52*, 143; M. M. DeBeukelaer *et al.*, *J. Pediat.*, 1977, *91*, 759, per *Abstr. Hyg.*, 1978, *53*, 449; A. P. Streissguth *et al.*, *J. Pediat.*, 1978, *92*, 363, per *Abstr. Hyg.*, 1978, *53*, 622; E. Collins and G. Turner, *Med. J. Aust.*, 1978, *2*, 606; P. J. Lewis and P. Boylan (letter), *Lancet*, 1979, *1*, 388; B. F. Habbick *et al.*, *ibid.*, 580; J. Møller *et al.* (letter), *ibid.*, 605.

Lactation. Cushingoid signs in a suckling infant. The mother's milk contained 1 mg of alcohol per ml. Growth improved when the mother stopped taking alcohol.— A. Binkiewicz *et al.*, *J. Pediat.*, 1978, *93*, 965.

Warnings against alcohol ingestion by nursing mothers appear to be based on one case, reported in 1936, of infant intoxication following ingestion by the nursing mother of 750 ml of port wine in 24 hours.— *Med. Lett.*, 1979, *21*, 21.

Respiratory depression. From studies in patients with chronic alcoholism, it was shown that blood concentrations of alcohol in the range of 350 to 450 mg per 100 ml could cause respiratory depression.— R. E. Johnstone and R. L. Witt (letter), *J. Am. med. Ass.*, 1972, *222*, 486.

Treatment of Adverse Effects. In acute poisoning the stomach should be emptied by aspiration and lavage, care being taken to prevent pulmonary aspiration of the return flow. If respiration is depressed, assisted respiration may be necessary. It is important to provide good supportive treatment and to keep the patient warm. Fluid balance should be maintained by the use of suitable electrolyte solutions, and dextrose may be needed for the treatment of hypoglycaemia. The value of intravenous infusions of laevulose is controversial (see also under Absorption and Fate). Haemodialysis or peritoneal dialysis is of value in severe alcoholic intoxication.

In chronic alcoholics withdrawal syndromes occurring in the presence of declining plasma concentrations of alcohol vary from mild to the possibly fatal delirium tremens. Sedatives should be given to prevent or suppress withdrawal symptoms; agents commonly used include diazepam (p.1523), chlordiazepoxide (p.1508), or chlormethiazole (p.798); phenothiazines are generally considered to be less effective in controlling convulsions. Thiamine (p.1639) and other B-group vitamins are often given in conjunction with sedatives.

For the long-term treatment of alcoholics, see disulfiram (p.579) and citrated calcium carbimide (p.580).

Recovery of a 23-year-old woman with a blood-alcohol concentration of 780 mg per 100 ml after treatment with gastric lavage, instillation of charcoal, and diuresis.— K. G. Hammond *et al.*, *J. Am. med. Ass.*, 1973, *226*, 63.

Haemodialysis reduced the blood-alcohol concentration from 440 to 255 mg per 100 ml in 3 hours in a 23-year-old man; dialysis was continued for 8½ hours.— R. W. Elliott and P. R. Hunter, *Postgrad. med. J.*, 1974, *50*, 515.

The popular belief that coffee relieved the depressant effects of alcohol appeared to be unfounded.— *Med. Lett.*, 1977, *19*, 47.

A study confirming that naloxone in doses of up to 1.2 mg can reverse alcohol-induced coma in some patients. The advice of the National Poisons Information Service recommending cautious intravenous administration of naloxone 0.4 to 1.2 mg to patients with suspected opiate poisoning, has now been extended to cover patients with suspected alcohol poisoning.— D. B. Jefferys *et al.* (letter), *Lancet*, 1980, *1*, 308. See also S. C. Sørensen and K. Mattisson (letter), *ibid.*, 1978, *2*, 688; A. I. Mackenzie (letter), *ibid.*, 1979, *1*, 733.

Evidence that naloxone is not an effective antagonist of alcohol.— M. J. Mattila *et al.* (letter), *Lancet*, 1981, *1*, 775. Comment, and the view that naloxone can be an effective antagonist of alcohol, and that in some circumstances this may even be clinically important.— W. J. Jeffcoate *et al.* (letter), *ibid.*, 1052. Failure of naloxone to reverse alcohol intoxication.— D. M. Catley *et al.* (letter), *ibid.*, 1263.

Precautions. Peripheral vasodilatation produced by alcohol leads to heat loss, and in elderly persons severe hypothermia may occur. Alcohol may aggravate peptic ulcer, impaired liver function, and diabetes mellitus.

Reports of the interactions between alcohol and other drugs are not consistent, possibly because acute alcohol intake may inhibit drug metabolism while chronic alcohol intake may enhance the induction of drug-metabolising enzymes in the liver. Alcoholic beverages containing tyramine, such as Chianti, may cause reactions when taken by patients receiving monoamine oxidase inhibitors. Alcohol may enhance the acute effects of drugs which depress the central nervous system, such as hypnotics, antihistamines, muscle relaxants, antidepressants, and tranquillisers. In turn the effects of alcohol may be enhanced by these drugs. Unpleasant reactions, similar to those occurring with disulfiram (see p.579), may occur when alcohol is taken concomitantly with chlorpropamide or metronidazole and some antibiotics, such as cephamandole.

Alcohol may cause hypoglycaemic reactions in patients receiving sulphonylurea antidiabetic agents, phenformin, or insulin, and may cause orthostatic hypotension in patients taking antihypertensives such as guanethidine.

The regular ingestion of large amounts of alcohol should certainly be avoided by pregnant women; it is still debatable whether the ingestion of regular or sporadic small amounts should be avoided.

In chronic alcoholics or those receiving regular high doses of alcohol, there is tolerance to the effects of alcohol and other central nervous system depressants including general anaesthetics. All processes requiring judgement and coordination are affected by alcohol and these include the driving of any form of transport and the operating of machinery.

Two of 11 premature infants given alcohol intravenously as a nutrient had toxic blood-alcohol concentrations, apparently due to inability to utilise alcohol.— V. H. Peden *et al.*, *J. Pediat.*, 1973, *83*, 490, per *Int. pharm. Abstr.*, 1974, *11*, 251.

At least 3 months' abstention from alcohol was considered reasonable in patients with acute infectious hepatitis. Thereafter a gradual and moderate intake might be allowed as long as the patient felt well and had no continuing clinical or biochemical signs of liver disease. Alcohol should not be taken by patients with cirrhotic liver failure or chronic active hepatitis.— *Drug & Ther. Bull.*, 1975, *13*, 87. See also *Br. med. J.*, 1974, *1*, 156.

Parenteral nutrition with infusions containing alcohol was not advisable in patients with heart disease. Alcohol was claimed to provoke changes in cardiac ultrastructure with possible impairment of cardiac function.— H. Klein and D. Harmjanz, *Postgrad. med. J.*, 1975, *51*, 325.

Patients with severe myocardial damage or chronic congestive heart failure should not drink alcohol. Other cardiac patients should be limited to about 1 drink a day. Those with coronary-artery disease should refrain from strenuous activity for about 2 hours after drinking lest angina be induced.— L. D. Horwitz, *J. Am. med. Ass.*, 1975, *232*, 959. In a double-blind study of 12 men with stable exertional angina pectoris and evidence of severe coronary artery disease, about 60 or 150 ml of alcohol significantly decreased exercise-time to angina. Alcohol was associated with significant ischaemic ST-segment depression following exercise-induced angina and might mask the early recognition of angina pain.— J. Orlando *et al.*, *Ann. intern. Med.*, 1976, *84*, 652.

Alcohol had been reported to precipitate attacks of porphyria.— *Drug & Ther. Bull.*, 1976, *14*, 55.

The effect of drinking patterns on enzyme screening tests for alcoholism.— S. M. Wiseman and J. Spencer-Peet, *Practitioner*, 1977, *219*, 243.

Corticosteroid hypersecretion associated with excessive alcohol ingestion in 4 patients led initially to a false diagnosis of Cushing's syndrome.— L. H. Rees *et al.*, *Lancet*, 1977, *1*, 726. Similar reports.— A. G. Smals *et al.*, *Br. med. J.*, 1976, *2*, 1298; A. Paton (letter), *ibid.*, 1504; R. Frajria and A. Angeli (letter), *Lancet*, 1977, *1*, 1050; A. Smals and P. Kloppenborg (letter), *ibid.*, 1369.

Interactions. Reviews of interactions between alcohol and drugs: M. Linnoila *et al.*, *Drugs*, 1979, *18*, 299; *Br. med. J.*, 1980, *280*, 507.

Interactions between monoamine oxidase inhibitors and alcohol seemed to be mainly due to the tyramine content of certain alcoholic beverages.— I. H. Stockley, *Pharm. J.*, 1973, *2*, 95. For further details, see Phenelzine Sulphate, p.129.

Vomiting, headache, prostration, tachycardia, bradycardia, reddening of the conjunctivae, skin pallor, sweating, behavioural impairment, and psychological distress after the concomitant use of cannabis and alcohol.— A. Sulkowski, *Am. J. Psychiat.*, 1977, *134*, 691, per *Int. pharm. Abstr.*, 1977, *14*, 1191.

A report of isoniazid reducing tolerance to alcohol.— C. -P. Siegers, *Dt. med. Wschr.*, 1977, *102*, 629.

For the effect of alcohol and diazepam on driving skills, see under Diazepam, p.1522.

For a report of a disulfiram-like effect with alcohol and cephamandole, see Cephamandole, p.1131.

Vasoconstriction. Alcohol injected into the brachial artery of normal subjects caused vasoconstriction of the skin and muscle vessels. Administration by mouth caused reduced blood flow through the forearm muscles. Intra-arterial administration was contra-indicated in peripheral vascular disease and administration by mouth could be a disadvantage in the presence of muscle ischaemia.— J. D. Fewings *et al.*, *Br. J. Pharmac. Chemother.*, 1966, *27*, 93.

Absorption and Fate. Alcohol is absorbed from the stomach and small intestine and is rapidly distributed throughout the body fluids. It readily crosses the placenta. Alcohol vapour may be absorbed through the lungs.

Alcohol is mainly metabolised in the liver; it is converted by alcohol dehydrogenase to acetaldehyde and is then further oxidised to acetate. A hepatic microsomal oxidising system is also involved. Over 90% is oxidised and the remainder is excreted by the lungs and in the urine, saliva, sweat, and other secretions. The body can metabolise about 10 to 15 ml of alcohol per hour and the effects of alcohol may be prolonged until an accumulation of alcohol has been metabolised. Admixture of the alcohol with food may delay absorption for some hours. Small volumes of alcohol are rapidly absorbed from an empty stomach.

The rate of metabolism may be accelerated following repeated excessive use.

A study of factors affecting the absorption, blood concentration, and effect of alcohol in 505 volunteers.— J. Lereboullet *et al.*, *Bull. Acad. natn. Méd.*, 1971, *155*, 423, per *Abstr. Hyg.*, 1971, *46*, 1130.

Peak concentrations of alcohol were reduced by 25 to 50% after the prior consumption of 570 ml of milk, by 65% after 570 ml of yogurt, and by 65 to 70% by a 2-course meal.— A. H. Beckett *et al.*, *Autocar*, 1971, *135*, 34, per *Br. med. J.*, 1972, *4*, 744. The absorption of alcohol was not more delayed by the consumption of 285 ml of milk than by 285 ml of water.— E. D. Janus and J. R. Sharman, *N.Z. med. J.*, 1972, *75*, 339, per *Br. med. J.*, 1972, *4*, 744. In 6 healthy subjects absorption of alcohol was reduced by about 96% after a carbohydrate meal, by 90% by fat, and 75% by protein, compared with absorption in the fasting state.— P. G. Welling *et al.*, *J. clin. Pharmac.*, 1977, *17*, 199.

Blood-alcohol concentrations rose higher in patients who had undergone partial gastrectomy or vagotomy with pyloroplasty than in controls. Absorption was slower in the coeliac syndrome.— P. B. Cotton and G. Walker, *Postgrad. med. J.*, 1973, *49*, 27.

There was a significant correlation between hepatic alcohol-dehydrogenase activity and white blood-cell concentrations of ascorbic acid in 12 patients with non-alcoholic liver disease. The elimination of alcohol was also hastened in healthy subjects who had raised white blood-cell concentrations of ascorbic acid following ingestion of ascorbic acid 1 g daily for 2 weeks.— N. Krasner *et al.*, *Lancet*, 1974, *2*, 693.

A detailed study in 7 subjects of blood-alcohol concentrations during and following constant-rate intravenous infusion of alcohol.— P. K. Wilkinson *et al.*, *Clin. Pharmac. Ther.*, 1976, *19*, 213.

Dose-dependent elimination kinetics.— R. E. Rangno and D. S. Sitar, *Clin. Pharmac. Ther.*, 1977, *21*, 115.

Effect of age. In 50 healthy subjects the rates of alcohol elimination were not affected by age but higher peak alcohol concentrations occurred in the older patients probably due to their smaller volume of body-water and decreased lean body-mass.— R. E. Vestal *et al.*, *Clin. Pharmac. Ther.*, 1977, *21*, 343.

Effect of laevulose. Early work by F. Lundquist and H. Wolthers (*Acta pharmac. tox.*, 1958, *14*, 290) and G.L.S. Pawan (*Nature*, 1968, *220*, 374) demonstrated that laevulose increased the rate of metabolism of alcohol, and blood-alcohol concentrations were found to be reduced by about 25% by L.M. Lowenstein *et al.* (*J. Am. med. Ass.*, 1970, *213*, 1899) and S.S. Brown *et al.* (*Lancet*, 1972, *2*, 898) following infusions of 10% and 40% solutions respectively. An alternative mechanism was put forward by E.R. Clark *et al.* (*J. Pharm. Pharmac.*, 1973, *25*, 319) who considered that laevulose might exert its effect by altering alcohol absorption. J.W. Dundee *et al.* (*Medicine Sci. Law*, 1971, *11*, 146) published less favourable results, an infusion of a 20% solution having increased the rate of elimination of alcohol by only 14% while producing chest pain and tightness. Both R.D. Cohen (*Lancet*, 1972, *2*, 1086) and I. Hessov (*ibid.*, 1204) have indicated the risk of lactic acidosis from laevulose and alcohol, and increases in serum concentrations of uric acid and lactate were reported by R. Levy *et al.* (*Archs intern. Med.*, 1977, *137*, 1175) who also found that infusions of laevulose 10% had no effect on the clinical status or rate of alcohol metabolism in 10 alcoholic patients.

Metabolism. In 7 sets of identical twins there was no difference in the rate of metabolism of a single dose of alcohol 1 ml per kg body-weight, but there were significant differences in fraternal twins.— E. S. Vesell *et al.*, *Ann. N.Y. Acad. Sci.*, 1971, *179*, 752. See also *idem*, *Clin. Pharmac. Ther.*, 1971, *12*, 192.

Further references: J. H. Mendelson, *New Engl. J. Med.*, 1970, *283*, 24 and 71; *idem*, 1971, *284*, 104; R. D. Hawkins and H. Kalant, *Pharmac. Rev.*, 1972, *24*, 67; M. N. Shah *et al.*, *Am. J. clin. Nutr.*, 1972, *25*, 135, per *J. Am. med. Ass.*, 1972, *220*, 434; *Metabolic Aspects of Alcoholism*, C.S. Lieber (Ed.), Lancaster, MTP Press, 1977.

Screening tests for alcoholism.— *Lancet*, 1980, *2*, 1117.

Pregnancy and the neonate. A review of excretion in breast milk.— J. T. Wilson *et al.*, *Clin. Pharmacokinet.*, 1980, *5*, 1.

The pharmacokinetics of alcohol given to mothers during childbirth.— R. L. Nation, *Clin. Pharmacokinet.*, 1980, *5*, 340.

Uses. Alcohol has a depressant action on the central nervous system, particularly on the cerebral cortex and on its inhibitory functions. By masking hesitancy, circumspection, and self criticism, alcohol in small doses may appear initially to stimulate, especially in surroundings conducive to excitement; without such an environment its action is usually hypnotic. The ingestion of small amounts of alcohol may postpone the onset of fatigue and increase the work done, as long as the task involved is simple. If the task involves discrimination or selection, accuracy is diminished and the amount of work done may be reduced even though the subject considers efficiency to be undiminished. Such loss of efficiency is important when the control of vehicles or hazardous machinery is concerned.

The slow rate of oxidation and the action of alcohol on the central nervous system limit its food value, but it is useful in illness and convalescence when appetite is deficient and assimilation of ordinary food is impaired. Preparations containing high concentrations of alcohol irritate the stomach and produce gastritis if taken habitually but small amounts, adequately diluted, help digestion by inhibiting emotions such as anxiety and anger. Alcohol also produces peripheral vasodilatation which increases heat loss.

A limited tolerance to the action of alcohol on the brain may develop and dependence usually involves tolerance to other sedatives and anaesthetics.

Alcohol is also given as an energy source in mixed preparations for parenteral nutrition, see Some Proprietary Amino-acid Preparations for Intravenous Administration, p.62. Each g of alcohol represents approximately 29 kJ (7 kcal).

Alcohol has also been given intravenously for surgical anaesthesia, but more effective agents are now available.

Alcohol is sometimes injected into the pituitary, ganglia, or around nerve trunks to relieve severe and chronic pain including that of trigeminal neuralgia and terminal cancer. It has also been injected to relieve spasticity.

Alcohol has been claimed to be of use by inhalation as an anti-foaming agent in the treatment of attacks of acute pulmonary oedema, the alcohol being administered as a vapour in oxygen by means of a face mask, nasal catheter, or respirator.

For external use, alcohol is usually employed as industrial methylated spirit, diluted in evaporating lotions, or as Surgical Spirit, for the treatment of various lesions of the skin, for the prevention of bedsores, for hardening the skin, and to diminish sweating.

It has a bactericidal action against most vegetative organisms at concentrations between 60 and 95%, but it is not effective against bacterial spores. A concentration usually of 70% w/w is employed, either alone or containing chlorhexidine or iodine, for the disinfection of the skin in preparation for injection, venepuncture, or surgical procedures.

Alcohol is widely used as a solvent and preservative in pharmaceutical preparations and as a menstruum in the manufacture of tinctures and other galenicals.

The Food Additives and Contaminants Committee recommended that alcohol should continue to be a permitted solvent in food.— *Report on the Review of Solvents in Food*, FAC/REP/25, Ministry of Agriculture, Fisheries and Food, London, HM Stationery Office, 1978.

Anaesthesia. A report of the use of alcohol for the induction of anaesthesia.— J. W. Dundee *et al.*, *Br. J. Anaesth.*, 1970, *42*, 300.

Use with diazepam.— M. Isaac *et al.*, *Br. J. Anaesth.*, 1970, *42*, 521.

Use with morphine in open-heart surgery.— W. H. Mannaeimer, *Sth. med. J.*, 1971, *64*, 1125, per *Int. pharm. Abstr.*, 1972, *9*, 280.

Disinfection of equipment. The disinfection of syringes by alcohol was *not* recommended. The only circumstances in which it might still be considered permissible were those of the diabetic patient who administered his own insulin. For all other purposes the method should be condemned.— The Sterilisation, Use and Care of Syringes, *MRC Mem.*, *No. 41*, 1962. For a report of abscesses associated with the use of surgical spirit instead of industrial methylated spirit for the storage of insulin syringes, see under Surgical Spirit, p.41. However, with the ready availability of sterilised disposable syringes sterilisation by alcohol is no longer justified.

A high degree of disinfection was achieved in mechanical respirators by flushing the circuit with nitrogen for 10 minutes to reduce the oxygen concentration and then pumping through an aerosol, of particle size less than 1 µm diameter, of either ethyl or isopropyl alcohol for 2 hours. After disinfection, residual alcohol was flushed from the circuit with nitrogen, since mixtures of alcohol with air were explosive.— G. Spencer *et al.*, *Lancet*, 1968, *2*, 667.

Effect on cardiovascular system. In a study of factors associated with cardiac mortality in 18 developed countries, a strong and specific negative correlation was found between deaths from heart disease and alcohol consumption. The consumption of wine appears to account for the entire alcohol effect.— A. S. St Leger *et al.*, *Lancet*, 1979, *1*, 1017. Correspondence: J. McMichael (letter), *ibid.*, 1186; A. S. St Leger *et al.* (letter), *ibid.*, 1294; J. J. Segall (letter), *ibid.;* N. G. P. Slater (letter), *ibid.;* H. Tyrrell (letter), *ibid.;* G. Ricci and F. Angelico (letter), *ibid.*, 1404; M. S. Manku *et al.* (letter), *ibid.*

Details of increased mortality associated with increased consumption of alcohol in Canada in the years 1965–77.— R. P. Gallagher and J. M. Elwood (letter), *Lancet*, 1980, *1*, 775.

Over 10 years of follow-up of civil servants the mortality rate was lower in men reporting moderate alcohol intake than in non-drinkers or in heavier drinkers.— M. G. Marmot *et al.*, *Lancet*, 1981, *1*, 580. Correspondence: J. C. Bignall (letter), *ibid.*, 719; W. J. Wigfield and W. J. Hill (letter), *ibid.*, 1052; M. G. Marmot *et al.* (letter), *ibid.*, 1159.

Further references: C. H. Hennekens *et al.*, *Am. J. Epidem.*, 1978, *107*, 196; D. Kozararevic *et al.*, *Lancet*, 1980, *1*, 613; R. M. Parr (letter), *ibid.*, 1087; M. E. Jennings and J. M. H. Howard (letter), *ibid.*, *2*, 90; J. Werth (letter), *ibid.*, 1141; R. E. LaPorte and J. A. Cauley (letter), *ibid.*, 1981, *1*, 105; W. Willett *et al.*, *New Engl. J. Med.*, 1980, *303*, 1159; K. Kreiss and M. M. Zack (letter), *ibid.*, 1981, *304*, 539.

Effect on intra-ocular pressure. The equivalent of 50 ml of alcohol reduced intra-ocular pressure in glaucomatous patients by up to 30 mmHg. In healthy subjects the reduction was only 1 to 6 mmHg. This effect had been used prior to surgery in 2 patients unable to tolerate other agents.— *J. Am. med. Ass.*, 1967, *199* (Mar. 20), A45.

Fat embolism. Contradictory evidence on the value of alcohol in the management of fat embolism. Some reports indicate a beneficial prophylactic effect, another report fails to show any benefit in treating experimental fat embolism. Further assessment is required.— *Br. med. J.*, 1978, *1*, 1232.

Hyperbilirubinaemia. For reference to alcohol in hyperbilirubinaemia see under Pregnancy and the Neonate, below.

Induction of abortion. Abortion was induced in 11 of 12 women in mid-trimester by the intra-amniotic infusion, after amniocentesis, of 100 to 170 ml of alcohol 47.5%. There were no significant complications.— V. Gomel and C. W. Carpenter, *Obstet. Gynec.*, 1973, *41*, 455, per *Int. pharm. Abstr.*, 1974, *11*, 292.

Pain. The subarachnoid injection of alcohol in 322 patients with intractable pain from malignant disease gave long-lasting marked relief in 187 and partial relief in 84.— E. Y. Kuzucu *et al.*, *J. Am. med. Ass.*, 1966, *195*, 541.

Coeliac-plexus block with alcohol 50%.— G. E. Thompson *et al.*, *Anesth. Analg. curr. Res.*, 1977, *56*, 1, per *J. Am. med. Ass.*, 1977, *237*, 2760.

Chemical hypophysectomy with dehydrated alcohol.— J. Katz and A. B. Levin, *Anesthesiology*, 1977, *46*, 115. Another report.— G. Corssen *et al.*, *Anesth. Analg. curr. Res.*, 1977, *56*, 414.

In 7 healthy subjects alcohol 0.75 ml per kg body-weight as 10% solution in sodium chloride injection intravenously increased the pain threshold to an extent and for a time similar to that after morphine 200 µg per kg.— M. F. M. James *et al.*, *Br. J. Anaesth.*, 1978, *50*, 139.

Further references to the use of alcohol for the relief of pain.— W. W. Mushin *et al.*, *Practitioner*, 1977, *218*, 439; *Br. med. J.*, 1977, *2*, 718; J. W. Lloyd, *ibid.*, 1980, *281*, 432.

Parenteral nutrition. A study of the metabolic effects of alcohol; its use in parenteral nutrition might have serious consequences in hypoglycaemia, lactic acidosis, or hypokalaemia.— N. M. Wilson *et al.*, *Br. med. J.*, 1981, *282*, 849. Criticism.— M. J. Spurr (letter), *ibid.*, 2058. Reply.— P. M. Brown *et al.* (letter), *ibid.*

Peripheral vascular disease. There is no evidence that alcohol increases blood flow in most patients with obstructive arterial disease. Although alcohol may relieve vasospasm, large amounts must often be used.— J. D. Coffman, *New Engl. J. Med.*, 1979, *300*, 713.

See also under Precautions (Vasoconstriction).

Pregnancy and the neonate. Intravenous administration of alcohol might effectively arrest premature labour in some patients. The infusion caused severe inebriation with frequent nausea and vomiting; aspiration was a serious danger; constant nursing care was required.— *Med. Lett.*, 1976, *18*, 42.

A study favouring ritodrine over alcohol in the management of premature labour. Patients receiving alcohol had a higher incidence of nausea, vomiting, and urinary incontinence.— N. H. Lauersen *et al.*, *Am. J. Obstet. Gynec.*, 1977, *127*, 837. For comments on the efficacy of cardioselective beta-adrenoceptor stimulants in the prevention of premature labour, see Salbutamol, p.31.

Hyperbilirubinaemia. Alcohol, 100 to 115 g as a 14.25% solution in sodium chloride injection, administered intravenously at 2 to 4 ml per minute to pregnant women from 3 to 96 hours before delivery, resulted in significantly lower concentrations of bilirubin in the serum of term, or near term, infants.— R. Waltman *et al.*, *Lancet*, 1969, *2*, 1265; *idem* (letter), 108. Comments.— M. Isaac and J. W. Dundee (letter), *ibid.*, 1970, *1*, 37. Alcohol had no consistently beneficial effect on hyperbilirubinaemia in 14 patients.— L. Okolicsanyi *et al.* (letter), *ibid.*, 1972, *1*, 450.

Pruritus ani. Alcohol 40% might rarely be used in treating the most persistent cases of pruritus ani. It was injected under a general anaesthetic at 4 sites spaced equidistantly about 10 cm apart around the anus, 5 to 10 ml being given at each site. Sloughing of the skin or sepsis might occur in about one-third of the patients; sloughing was likely to occur if the injection was made too superficially.— W. W. Slac, *Practitioner*, 1969, *202*, 178.

Pruritus vulvae. Local injection of alcohol was used with success in the treatment of pruritus vulvae.— J. D. Woodruff and B. Thompson, *Obstet. Gynec.*, 1972, *40*, 18, per *Int. pharm. Abstr.*, 1973, *10*, 148; G. D. Ward and J. R. Sutherst (letter), *Br. med. J.*, 1973, *2*, 243.

Multiple intradermal injections of dehydrated alcohol 0.1 to 0.2 ml in the ano-genital area completely relieved 6 of 25 patients with pruritus vulvae followed for a period of 1 year after the injections and gave marked symptomatic relief in 13, and some relief in 3. There was superficial blistering in 2 patients and mild cellulitis in 1.— G. D. Ward and J. R. Sutherst, *Br. J. Derm.*, 1975, *93*, 201.

Spasticity. Injection of alcohol 45% into spastic muscles reduced the frequency of sudden spasms, background spasticity with associated pain, and functional disability in 10 patients.— J. Cockin *et al.*, *Br. J. clin. Pract.*, 1971, *25*, 73.

Fifteen patients with hemifacial spasm had been successfully treated with the injection of alcohol 90% into the distal branches of the facial nerve.— C. J. Blumenthal (letter), *Br. med. J.*, 1973, *2*, 548.

It is doubtful whether alcohol or phenol have any place in peripheral nerve blocks as the analgesia is commonly patchy and there is a definite incidence of neuritis, but one exception is the injection of alcohol 40% into the muscle sheath of patients with painful muscular spasms in multiple sclerosis.— J. W. Lloyd, *Br. med. J.*, 1980, *281*, 432.

Tremor. Severe familial tremor affecting some old people was sometimes alleviated by the administration of alcohol when other drugs such as barbiturates or diazepam had been of no value.— G. Bousfield (letter), *Br. med. J.*, 1970, *4*, 560.

Relief of essential tremor in 19 of 25 patients.— E. Critchley, *J. Neurol. Neurosurg. Psychiat.*, 1972, *35*, 365.

A comment that beta-adrenoceptor blocking agents and alcohol are the only effective agents for essential tremor.— *Lancet*, 1979, *2*, 1280.

Preparations

Alcohol and Dextrose Injection *(U.S.P.)*. A sterile solution of alcohol and dextrose in Water for Injections. Potency is expressed in terms of C_2H_5OH and dextrose monohydrate. pH, of a solution containing not more than 5% of dextrose, 3.5 to 6.5.

Ethanol for Disinfection *(Jap. P.)*. Ethanol. pro Desinfect. Contains 76.9 to 81.4% v/v.

Evaporating Lotion *(B.P.C. 1954)*. Lot. Evap. Alcohol (90%) (or industrial methylated spirit) 12.5 ml, ammonium chloride 3.43 g, water to 100 ml.

High-alcoholic Elixir *(U.S.N.F.)*. Compound orange spirit 0.4 ml, saccharin 300 mg, glycerol 20 ml, alcohol to 100 ml. It contains 73 to 78% v/v of C_2H_6O. Store in airtight containers.

Iso-alcoholic Elixir *(U.S.N.F.)*. This elixir is intended to serve as a general vehicle for various medicaments that require solvents of different alcoholic strengths. It is prepared by mixing together suitable volumes of low-alcoholic elixir and high-alcoholic elixir to produce an elixir of the required alcoholic strength.

Low-alcoholic Elixir *(U.S.N.F.)*. Compound orange spirit 1 ml, alcohol 10 ml, glycerol 20 ml, sucrose 32 g, water to 100 ml. It contains 8 to 10% v/v of C_2H_6O. Store in airtight containers.

Spirit Ear-drops *(B.P.C. 1973)*. Auristillae Spiritus. Alcohol 50 ml, water to 100 ml. *A.P.F.* (Spirit Ear Drops) has alcohol (90%) 50 ml, freshly boiled and cooled water to 100 ml.

For proprietary preparations for parenteral nutrition containing alcohol, see Some Proprietary Amino-acid Preparations for Intravenous Administration, p.62..

Alcoholic Beverages

Brandy. Spiritus e Vino *(Swiss P.)*; Spiritus Vini Saporus *(Span. P.)*; Eau de Vie de Vin; Weinbrand. The liquid obtained by distillation of the wine of grapes and matured by age. It contains 40 to 50% v/v, or more, of alcohol.

Rum. Rhum; Spiritus e Saccharo *(Swiss P.)*. Prepared by fermentation and distillation from the juice of the sugar cane or from sugar syrups or molasses. Rum sold in Great Britain usually contains about 40% v/v of alcohol.

Whisky. Whiskey; Spiritus Frumenti. Prepared by distillation of fermented grain—barley, wheat, rye, or maize. Whisky sold in Great Britain usually contains about 40% v/v of alcohol.

The minimum alcohol content for brandy, rum, and whisky, under the Food and Drugs Act 1955, Section 3 (4), is 37% v/v.

552-d

Dehydrated Alcohol *(U.S.P.)*. Ethanol *(B.P.)*; Absolute Alcohol; Dehydrated Ethanol; Ethanol; Ethanolum Absolutum; Spiritus Absolutus.

CAS — 64-17-5.

Pharmacopoeias. In *Arg., Aust., Br., Ind., Int., Jap., Mex., Nord., Port., Swiss, Turk.*, and *U.S.*

A clear, colourless, mobile, volatile, very hygroscopic, readily inflammable liquid with a characteristic spirituous odour and a burning taste. The *B.P.* specifies 99.4 to 100% v/v or 99 to 100% w/w of C_2H_6O; the *U.S.P.* specifies not less than 99.5% v/v or 99.2% w/w. The *B.P.* specifies sp. gr. (20°/20°) 0.7904 to 0.7935; the *U.S.P.* specifies not more than 0.7964 at 15.56°. B.p. about 78°. Flash-point 12° (closed-cup test). A 1.28% solution in water is iso-osmotic with serum. **Store** in a cool place in airtight containers.

Preparations

Dehydrated Alcohol Injection *(U.S.P.)*. Dehydrated alcohol suitable for parenteral use.

553-n

Amyl Alcohol *(B.P.C. 1934)*. Amylic Alcohol.

$C_5H_{12}O$=88.15.

CAS — 123-51-3 (3-methylbutan-1-ol); 137-32-6 (2-methylbutan-1-ol).

Obtained by purifying fusel oil, and consists of a mixture of mainly 3-methylbutan-1-ol (primary isoamyl alcohol), $(CH_3)_2CH.CH_2.CH_2OH$, with some 2-methylbutan-1-ol (primary active amyl alcohol), $CH_3.CH_2.CH(CH_3)CH_2OH$. A colourless liquid with a characteristic odour. B.p. 128° to 132°. Wt per ml about 0.81 g. Slightly **soluble** in water; miscible with fixed and volatile oils and with alcohol, chloroform, ether, and most organic solvents.

Amyl alcohol has an action similar to that of ethyl alcohol but is a more pronounced local irritant, its vapours rapidly producing intense irritation of nose, eyes, and throat; exposure to excessive concentrations causes headache and nausea. Taken by mouth it is fairly toxic, the symptoms being similar to those produced by isopropyl alcohol. It is used chiefly as a solvent.

Maximum permissible atmospheric concentration of isoamyl alcohol 100 ppm.

Estimated acceptable daily intake of isoamyl alcohol: up to 3.7 mg per kg body-weight.— Twenty-third Report of Joint FAO/WHO Expert Committee on Food Additives, *Tech. Rep. Ser. Wld Hlth Org. No. 648*, 1980.

554-h

Benzyl Alcohol *(B.P., U.S.N.F.)*. Alcohol Benzylicum; Phenylcarbinol; Phenylmethanol; Alcool Benzylique.

$C_6H_5.CH_2OH$=108.1.

CAS — 100-51-6.

Pharmacopoeias. In *Arg., Aust., Belg., Br., Cz., Fr., Hung., Ind., Jap., Neth., Nord., Port.*, and *Swiss*. Also in *U.S.N.F.*

A colourless liquid with a faint aromatic odour and a sharp burning taste. B.p. 203° to 208°. Wt per ml 1.043 to 1.046 g.

Soluble 1 in 25 of water; miscible with alcohol, chloroform, ether, and fixed and volatile oils. A solution in water is neutral to litmus. Solutions are **sterilised** by autoclaving. It is slowly oxidised to benzaldehyde and benzoic acid on exposure to air; **incompatible** with oxidising agents. **Store** at a temperature not exceeding 40° in airtight containers. Protect from light.

Total haemolysis occurred when erythrocytes were cultured for 45 minutes in a 1.2% solution of benzyl alcohol in sodium chloride injection. Only slight haemolysis occurred when the strength was reduced to 1.05%.— H. C. Ansel and D. E. Cadwallader, *J. pharm. Sci.*, 1964, *53*, 169.

Incompatibility. There was loss of clarity when intravenous solutions of benzyl alcohol and chloramphenicol sodium succinate were mixed.— J. A. Patel and G. L. Phillips, *Am. J. Hosp. Pharm.*, 1966, *23*, 409.

Stability. Benzaldehyde was present in many samples after autoclaving parenteral solutions containing benzyl alcohol. Oxidation was reduced by saturating preparations with nitrogen before and during the solution of benzyl alcohol and by replacing air with nitrogen.— R. G. Challen (letter), *Australas. J. Pharm.*, 1971, *52*, S47.

Uses. Benzyl alcohol is a weak local anaesthetic with disinfectant properties. It may be used either by injection or by application to mucous membranes; strong solutions may cause oedema and pain when injected. It is converted in the body to hippuric acid. For topical anaesthesia it is used in concentrations of up to 10%. A lotion of equal parts of benzyl alcohol, alcohol, and water has also been used. It has been used for toothache, a few drops being applied to the cavity or exposed nerve. Benzyl alcohol is included in solutions for subcutaneous or intramuscular injection for its disinfectant and anaesthetic actions, usually at a concentration of 1%. Benzyl alcohol is also included as a preservative in some small-volume preparations for intravenous administration.

After heating at 100° for 30 minutes at pH 5 to 6, benzyl alcohol 1% was about as effective as phenylmercuric nitrate 0.002% in killing the spores of *Bacillus stearothermophilus*. At higher pH values it had less effect and at pH 8.6 it had a negligible effect.— R. A. Anderson, *J. Hosp. Pharm.*, 1969, *26*, 48.

In leukaemic patients indwelling cardiac catheters with a non-return slit valve inserted into a tributary of the subclavian vein had been kept free of infection for up to 3 months by filling with benzyl alcohol 0.9% in Water for Injections when not in use.— A. S. D. Spiers, *Br.*

med. J., 1973, *3*, 528.

An inoculation of *Pseudomonas aeruginosa* could not be detected after 1 hour in simple eye ointment containing benzyl alcohol 2%. The preservative effect was slightly reduced after 6 months.— J. Dankert *et al.*, *Pharm. Weekbl. Ned.*, 1975, *110*, 189.

Benzyl alcohol 0.9% in normal saline injected intradermally provided brief anaesthesia suitable for many procedures and caused less discomfort than lignocaine.— M. A. Wightman and R. Vaughan, *Anesthesiology*, 1976, *45*, 687.

The Food Additives and Contaminants Committee recommended that benzyl alcohol be temporarily permitted for use as a solvent in food and recommended a maximum concentration of use in food as consumed of 500 ppm. Further toxicity studies were required.— *Report on the Review of Solvents in Food*, FAC/REP/25, Ministry of Agriculture, Fisheries and Food, London, HM Stationery Office, 1978.

Estimated acceptable daily intake of the benzyl/benzoic moiety: up to 5 mg per kg body-weight.— Twenty-third Report of Joint FAO/WHO Expert Committee on Food Additives, *Tech. Rep. Ser. Wld Hlth Org. No. 648*, 1980.

555-m

Isopropyl Alcohol *(B.P., U.S.P.)*.

Isopropanol; 2-Propanol; Alcohol Isopropylicus; Dimethyl Carbinol; Secondary Propyl Alcohol. Propan-2-ol. $(CH_3)_2CHOH=60.10$.

CAS — 67-63-0.

Pharmacopoeias. In *Aust., Belg., Br., Jap., Swiss,*and *U.S.*

A clear, colourless, mobile, volatile, inflammable liquid with a characteristic spirituous odour and a burning slightly bitter taste. B.p. 81° to 83°. Wt per ml 0.784 to 0.786 g. Flash-point 12° (closed-cup test).

Miscible with water, alcohol, chloroform, ether, and glycerol. It may be salted out from aqueous mixtures by the addition of salts or sodium hydroxide. **Store** in a cool place in airtight containers.

Complete haemolysis or denaturation of human erythrocytes occurred in all aqueous isopropyl alcohol solutions after 45 minutes at 37°. Addition of sodium chloride 0.9% prevented haemolysis in solutions containing less than 8% of isopropyl alcohol.— S. H. Ku and D. E. Cadwallader, *J. pharm. Sci.*, 1974, *63*, 60.

Adverse Effects. The toxicity of isopropyl alcohol is about twice that of ethyl alcohol and the symptoms of intoxication appear to be similar, except that isopropyl alcohol has no initial euphoric action and gastritis and vomiting are more prominent. A dose of 16 ml has been ingested daily for 3 days without discomfort but acute symptoms have been observed following a dose of 25 ml. Skin reactions have occasionally been attributed to the application of isopropyl alcohol. Maximum permissible atmospheric concentration 400 ppm.

Transient acute renal failure, haemolysis, and myopathy occurred in a 35-year-old alcoholic, and were attributed to the ingestion of isopropyl alcohol. The presence of acetone in body fluids, in the absence of glycosuria and hyperglycaemia, could furnish a clue for differential diagnosis.— L. Juncos and J. T. Taguchi, *J. Am. med. Ass.*, 1968, *204*, 732.

A 20-year-old man attempted suicide by the rectal administration of about 500 ml of isopropyl alcohol. Stupor was followed, 16 hours after admission to hospital, by periods of generalised tremors and agitation, progressing to a schizophrenic syndrome.— J. Corbett and G. Meier, *J. Am. med. Ass.*, 1968, *206*, 2320.

Coma. An infant developed coma following topical applications of isopropyl alcohol for the relief of fever. The alcohol was presumably absorbed mainly by inhalation.— S. W. McFadden and J. E. Haddow, *Pediatrics*, 1969, *43*, 622.

Skin reaction. A patient developed an eczematous reaction to isopropyl alcohol.— A. McInnes (letter), *Br. med. J.*, 1973, *1*, 357.

Reaction to swabs impregnated with isopropyl alcohol; propylene oxide used to sterilise the swabs might be responsible.— P. R. Bateman (letter), *Med. J. Aust.*, 1977, *2*, 841.

Treatment of Adverse Effects. As for Alcohol, p.37.

A 28-year-old man who ingested about 1 litre of a 70% solution of isopropyl alcohol (rubbing alcohol) was successfully treated by haemodialysis. The initial blood concentration of isopropyl alcohol was 440 mg per 100 ml and this was reduced to 100 mg per 100 ml after 5 hours of dialysis. Further recovery was uncomplicated.— L. H. King *et al.* (letter), *J. Am. med. Ass.*, 1970, *211*, 1855. For other similar reports, see A. W. Freireich *et al.*, *New Engl. J. Med.*, 1967, *277*, 699; S. L. Dua (letter), *J. Am. med. Ass.*, 1974, *230*, 35.

Absorption and Fate. Isopropyl alcohol is readily absorbed from the gastro-intestinal tract and persists in the circulation rather longer than ethyl alcohol. There appears to be little absorption through intact skin. Some isopropyl alcohol is converted in the body to acetone, which is slowly excreted in the breath and urine; acetone may be further oxidised to acetate, formate, and carbon dioxide. Unchanged isopropyl alcohol and its glucuronide may be excreted in the urine, especially after large doses.

Uses. Because of its unpleasant taste and its toxicity, isopropyl alcohol is not used internally. Externally it is used for pre-operative skin cleansing and as an ingredient of lotions but its marked degreasing properties may limit its usefulness in preparations used repeatedly. Its disinfectant properties at concentrations of 70% are similar to those of alcohol. It is largely used as a solvent, especially in cosmetics and perfumes, and as a vehicle for culinary essences. It is a satisfactory non-aqueous agent for tablet granulation.

Isopropyl alcohol may be used in place of ethyl alcohol for preserving pathological specimens and for dehydrating tissues. When a 10% solution of the alcohol is frozen in a rubber container the contents may be easily broken into small pieces by mild pressure on the container; this permits the preparation of pliable ice-packs.

Two applications of isopropyl alcohol (70%) appeared to be as effective for skin disinfection as an application of iodine tincture followed by an application of alcohol.— S. Lee *et al.*, *Am. J. clin. Path.*, 1967, *47*, 646, per *J. Am. med. Ass.*, 1967, *200* (May 29), A157.

The Food Additives and Contaminants Committee recommended that isopropyl alcohol should continue to be a permitted solvent in food.— *Report on the Review of Solvents in Food*, FAC/REP/25, Ministry of Agriculture, Fisheries and Food, London, HM Stationery Office, 1978.

Disinfection of equipment. For the use of isopropyl alcohol to disinfect equipment, see p.38.

Preparations

Isopropyl Rubbing Alcohol *(U.S.P.)*. Isopropanol Rubbing Compound. Contains 68 to 72% v/v of isopropyl alcohol, the remainder consisting of water with or without suitable colouring agents, stabilisers, and perfume oils. Store in a cool place in airtight containers. Rubefacient.

Proprietary Preparations

Avantine *(Laporte, UK)*. A brand of isopropyl alcohol, food grade.

IPS.1 *(Shell Chemicals)*. A brand of isopropyl alcohol.

IPS/C *(Shell Chemicals)*. A brand of isopropyl alcohol.

Sterets *(Schering-Prebbles, UK)*. Swabs saturated with 70% isopropyl alcohol. For skin cleansing prior to injection.

Sterile Pack Fluid *(Ethicon, UK)*. A fluid for sterilising the outside of foil suture packs, containing isopropyl alcohol 97%, formaldehyde 1%, sodium nitrite 0.05%, 2-(diethylamino)ethanol 0.05%, and water to 100%.

Other Proprietary Names

Alcojel *(Canad.)*.

556-b

Methyl Alcohol *(U.S.N.F., B.P.C. 1949)*.

Methyl Alcohol (Acetone-free); Methanol. $CH_3OH=32.04$.

CAS — 67-56-1.

Pharmacopoeias. In *U.S.N.F.*

A clear colourless highly inflammable liquid with a characteristic spirituous odour and a burning taste. B.p. 63.5° to 65.7° with a range of not more than 1°. Sp. gr. (15.5°/15.5°) not higher than 0.799. Flash-point 10° (closed-cup test). **Miscible** with water, alcohol, ether, and most other organic solvents. **Store** in a cool place in airtight containers. If dehydrated and 'acetone-free', methyl alcohol has sp. gr. not more than 0.790. The commercial substance known as 'wood naphtha', 'pyroxylic spirit', or 'wood spirit', contains 60 to 90% of methyl alcohol, together with acetone and other empyreumatic impurities. The variety used for denaturing alcohol contains not less than 72% v/v of methyl alcohol.

Complete haemolysis or denaturation of human erythrocytes occurred in all aqueous methyl alcohol solutions after 45 minutes at 37°. Addition of sodium chloride 0.9% prevented haemolysis in solutions containing less than 18% methyl alcohol.— S. H. Ku and D. E. Cadwallader, *J. pharm. Sci.*, 1974, *63*, 60.

Adverse Effects. The symptoms of acute poisoning resemble those of alcohol intoxication, the main differences being delayed onset (possibly up to 36 hours), wide variation in response to a particular dose, presence of severe upper abdominal pain, visual disturbance often proceeding to irreversible blindness, severe metabolic acidosis due to formic acid, and prolonged coma which may terminate in death from respiratory failure. The fatal dose is probably 100 to 200 ml; permanent blindness had been caused by as little as 10 ml. Maximum permissible atmospheric concentration 200 ppm.

A study of the ocular manifestations and complications of acute methyl alcohol intoxication.— R. Dethlefs and S. Naraqi, *Med. J. Aust.*, 1978, *2*, 483.

A report of fatal poisoning with methyl alcohol in an 8-month-old boy. As part of a cold remedy the child had been treated twice daily for 2 days with pads soaked in methyl alcohol; the pads had been set on fire, rapidly extinguished and then applied to the chest. The child developed respiratory difficulties and was later admitted to hospital in a coma and with severe metabolic acidosis. Subsequent analysis indicated the presence of 400 µg per ml of methyl alcohol in the blood. Due to the late start, treatment with alcohol and peritoneal dialysis was unsuccessful. Poisoning was presumably due to percutaneous absorption although inhalation could not be excluded.— A. Kahn and D. Blum, *J. Pediat.*, 1979, *94*, 841.

Treatment of Adverse Effects. Recent ingestion should be treated by aspiration and lavage; sodium bicarbonate solution 5% should be left in the stomach. The outstanding feature of methyl alcohol poisoning is acidosis, which should be corrected with sodium bicarbonate, in severe cases administered intravenously. Alcohol, 25 ml of a 50% solution, should be given by mouth every 3 hours to delay the oxidation of methyl alcohol, and should be continued at least until the acidosis has been corrected. The patient should be kept warm and the eyes protected from strong light. If the response is unsatisfactory, peritoneal dialysis or haemodialysis may be effective. Laevulose should not be used (see p.54).

A man who had ingested 400 to 500 ml of methyl alcohol recovered after prolonged intensive treatment including peritoneal and hemodialysis.— T. J. Humphery, *Med. J. Aust.*, 1974, *1*, 833.

Of 3 patients treated for methyl alcohol poisoning by peritoneal dialysis and intravenous administration of sodium bicarbonate and ethyl alcohol, 1 died and another was permanently blinded. Another 3 treated with haemodialysis recovered rapidly and had no residual effects.— H. Keyvan-Larijarni and A. M. Tannenberg, *Archs intern. Med.*, 1974, *134*, 293, per *Pharm. J.*, 1975, *1*, 158. These observations support the experimental evidence that peritoneal dialysis should be used only when haemodialysis is not available. In a review of the efficacy of haemodialysis in methyl alcohol poisoning A. Gonda *et al.* (*Am. J. Med.*, 1978, *64*, 749) concluded that haemodialysis should be started if the concentration of methyl alcohol in the blood exceeds 500 µg per ml, if there is a metabolic acidosis, or mental, visual, or fundoscopic anomalies attributable to methyl alcohol are present, or if more than 30 ml has been ingested. Treatment should be continued until the concentration of methyl alcohol is less than 250 µg per ml.— *Lancet*, 1978, *2*, 510.

Comment on the potential role of 4-methylpyrazole, a potent inhibitor of alcohol dehydrogenase, in the treatment of poisoning with methyl alcohol.— R. N. Zahlten (letter), *New Engl. J. Med.*, 1981, *304*, 977.

Absorption and Fate. Methyl alcohol is readily absorbed from the gastro-intestinal tract and distributed throughout the body fluids before oxidation to formaldehyde, formic acid, and possibly other products, mainly in the liver and kidney. It may also be absorbed by inhalation. Metabolism is much slower than for ethyl alcohol. Oxidation to formaldehyde is probably accomplished by alcohol dehydrogenase; ethyl alcohol competitively inhibits the metabolism of methyl alcohol. Maximum concentrations of formic acid in the blood and urine occur 2 to 3 days after ingestion.

Uses. Methyl alcohol is used as wood naphtha to denature alcohol in the preparation of industrial methylated spirit, and as a solvent.

The Food Additives and Contaminants Committee recommended that methyl alcohol should be used as a solvent in food solely for extraction purposes, and recommended a maximum concentration in food, after such use, of 2 ppm.— *Report on the Review of Solvents in Food*, FAC/REP/25, Ministry of Agriculture, Fisheries and Food, London, HM Stationery Office, 1978.

557-v

Methylated Spirits

Five varieties of methylated spirits are recognised under the Methylated Spirits Regulations, 1952 (SI 1952: No. 2230). They are: mineralised methylated spirits, industrial methylated spirits, industrial methylated spirits (pyridinised), industrial methylated spirits (Q grade), and power methylated spirits.

Mineralised methylated spirits is alcohol mixed with wood naphtha 9.5% and crude pyridine 0.5% and to every 100 gallons of this mixture is added ⅜ gallon of mineral naphtha (petroleum oil) and not less than one-fortieth of an ounce of methyl violet. Industrial methylated spirits is alcohol mixed with wood naphtha 5%. Industrial methylated spirits (pyridinised) is alcohol mixed with wood naphtha 5% and to every 100 parts of this mixture is added ½ a part of crude pyridine. Industrial methylated spirits (Q grade), which is used in the manufacture of perfumes, is alcohol mixed with pure methyl alcohol 5% and to every gallon of this mixture is added 175 minims of standardised quassin solution. Power methylated spirits is a mixture of alcohol 100 parts with wood naphtha 2½ parts, crude pyridine ½ part, and petrol or benzol not less than 5 parts, all by volume, and to this mixture is added ¼ oz of 'Spirit Red III' dye to every 1000 gallons.

Mineralised methylated spirits is the only variety that may be sold by retail in Great Britain for general use. It is not suitable for local use, e.g. for bed-sores, as it may cause dermatitis. It forms an opaque mixture with water.

Inflammable: keep away from an open flame.

558-g

Industrial Methylated Spirit *(B.P.)*.

Spiritus Methylatus Industrialis; Industrial Methylated Spirits; IMS; Specially Denatured Spirit.

A mixture of alcohol of an appropriate strength 19 volumes with approved wood naphtha 1 volume. It is of the quality known as '66 OP Industrial Methylated Spirit' or '74 OP Industrial Methylated Spirit'; 'Absolute Industrial Methylated Spirit'.

CAS — 8013-52-3 (ethanol-methanol mixture).

Pharmacopoeias. In *Br.* and *Ind.*

It is a clear, colourless, mobile, volatile, highly inflammable liquid with a characteristic odour of alcohol and wood naphtha and with a burning taste. B.p. about 78°. Sp. gr. (20°/20°), for '66 OP', not greater than 0.814; for '74 OP', not greater than 0.795. **Incompatible** with iodine if acetone is present.

559-q

Industrial Methylated Spirit (Ketone-free) *(B.P.)*.

Industrial Methylated Spirit (Acetone-free); Sp. Meth. Indust. s. Aceton.

Pharmacopoeias. In *Br.*

It is of the same strength as Industrial Methylated Spirit *B.P.*, but contains not more than 500 ppm of acetone. **Compatible** with iodine.

560-d

Surgical Spirit *(B.P.)*.

Surgical Spirit No. 1; Spiritus Chirurgicalis; Sp. Chir. Castor oil 2.5 ml, diethyl phthalate 2 ml, methyl salicylate 0.5 ml, industrial methylated spirit to 100 ml.

Pharmacopoeias. In *Br.*

A colourless inflammable liquid. **Store** in a cool place in airtight containers.

The above formula is the only one approved by the Board of Customs and Excise. Surgical spirit made to any other formula may be supplied on prescription only; it cannot be purchased from the wholesaler but must be made by the pharmacist as required and is subject to the statutory regulations relating to dispensing prescriptions for preparations containing Industrial Methylated Spirit.

The possible use of isopropyl alcohol in place of industrial methylated spirit in formulas for surgical spirit was investigated. Its main disadvantage was its somewhat unpleasant odour, which resembled a mixture of acetone and ethyl alcohol.—Pharm. Soc. Lab. Rep., *Pharm. J.*, 1961, *2*, 187.

Adverse Effects and Treatment. As for Methyl Alcohol, p.40.

Bilateral abscesses of the thigh in a diabetic patient appeared to be associated with the use of surgical spirit instead of industrial methylated spirit for the storage of insulin syringes. It was considered that the additives such as castor oil, methyl salicylate, and diethyl phthalate in surgical spirit could produce oily residues on the inner surface of the syringe and that these residues would be sufficiently miscible with certain types of insulin to be deposited with the latter at the site of injection.— D. A. Leigh and G. W. Hough, *Br. med. J.*, 1980, *281*, 541.

Uses. Industrial methylated spirit and surgical spirit are applied externally for their astringent action, but mucous membranes and excoriated skin surfaces must be protected from such applications. Industrial methylated spirit and surgical spirit must *not* be administered internally because of the toxic effects caused by the methyl alcohol they contain.

In Great Britain, the Board of Customs and Excise permit, subject to the observance of the conditions laid down in their regulations, the use of industrial duty-free spirit in the preparation of a range of specified preparations intended for external use only. Industrial methylated spirit may also be used in the preparation of certain extracts, resins, and surgical dressings, provided that in each case no alcohol remains in the finished product.

Industrial methylated spirit may contain small amounts of acetone and should not then be used for the preparation of iodine solutions, since an irritating compound is formed by reaction between iodine and acetone; for such preparations industrial methylated spirit (ketone-free) should be used.

Preparations

Rubbing Alcohol *(U.S.P.)*. Alcohol Rubbing Compound. Prepared from specially denatured alcohol and containing 68.5 to 71.5% v/v of dehydrated alcohol, the remainder consisting of water, acetone, methyl isobutyl ketone, and either sucrose octa-acetate (not less than 0.355% w/v) or denatonium benzoate (not less than 0.0014%), with or without suitable colouring agents and perfume oils; it may contain a suitable stabiliser. Store in a cool place in airtight containers. It is applied to the skin as a rubefacient.

The denatured alcohol, Formula 23-H, consists of acetone 8 parts v/v, methyl isobutyl ketone 1.5 parts v/v, and alcohol 100 parts.

561-n

Propyl Alcohol.

Propanolum; Propanol; Normal *(or* Primary*)* Propyl Alcohol. Propan-1-ol.
$CH_3.CH_2.CH_2OH=60.10$.

CAS — 71-23-8.

Pharmacopoeias. In *Nord.*

A clear, colourless, inflammable liquid with a characteristic spirituous odour and a burning taste. Wt per ml about 0.804 g. B.p. 96° to 100°. Flash-point 15° (closed-cup test). **Miscible** with water, alcohol, chloroform, and ether.

Complete haemolysis or denaturation of human erythrocytes occurred in all aqueous propyl alcohol solutions after 45 minutes at 37°. Addition of sodium chloride 0.9% prevented haemolysis in solutions containing less than 4% of propyl alcohol.— S. H. Ku and D. E. Cadwallader, *J. pharm. Sci.*, 1974, *63*, 60.

Propyl alcohol is slightly more toxic than isopropyl alcohol and is unsuitable for employment in any preparation intended for internal use. Maximum permissible atmospheric concentration 200 ppm. It is applied locally as a disinfectant and is used as a solvent.

The Food Additives and Contaminants Committee recommended that propyl alcohol be temporarily permitted for use as a solvent in food and recommended a maximum concentration of use in food as consumed of 5 ppm. Further toxicity studies were required.— *Report on the Review of Solvents in Food*, FAC/REP/25, Ministry of Agriculture, Fisheries and Food, London, HM Stationery Office, 1978.

Proprietary Names

Satinazid *(Mack, Illert., Ger.)*.

Alkalis and Organic Bases

200-f

The inorganic alkalis have been used to remove warts and, in dilute solutions, in the treatment of certain scaly skin conditions. They are employed as water softeners and as absorbents of carbon dioxide in anaesthetic practice. The organic bases are used as sclerosants, emulsifiers, and solubilisers.

201-d

Strong Ammonia Solution *(B.P.)*. Liquor Ammoniae Fortis; Liq. Ammon. Fort.; Stronger Ammonia Water; Stronger Ammonium Hydroxide Solution; Ammoniacum; Ammoniaca; Solutio Ammoniaci Concentrata; Ammoniaque Officinale.

CAS — 7664-41-7 (NH_3).

Pharmacopoeias. In *Arg.* (31 to 33.5%), *Aust.* (24 to 26%), *Belg.* (16 to 17%), *Br.*, *Fr.* (not less than 20%), *Hung.* (22 to 30%), *Ind.*, *It.*, and *Mex.* (all with 27 to 30%), *Nord.* (23 to 26%), *Port.* (20 to 22%), and *Span.* (20.18%). Also in *U.S.N.F.* which has 27 to 31%.

A clear colourless liquid with a very pungent characteristic odour, containing 27 to 30% w/w of NH_3. Wt per ml 0.892 to 0.901 g. '0.880 ammonia' contains about 35% w/w.

Miscible with water and alcohol. **Incompatible** with iodine, hypochlorites, salts of heavy metals, notably mercuric chloride and silver salts, alkaloidal salts, and tannins. **Store** at a temperature not exceeding 20° in airtight containers.

CAUTION. *Strong preparations of ammonia should be handled with great care as exposure to the concentrated vapour may cause injury to the eyes and inflammation of the respiratory tract or spasm of the glottis with resulting asphyxia. It is advisable to cool bottles before opening.*

Stability. At tropical temperatures (about 30°) a solution containing 27.5% w/w of NH_3 was safe, but should preferably be diluted to 10% before storage and use.— A. B. Elliott and P. L. K. Siong, *Malay. pharm. J.*, 1955, *4*, 269.

202-n

Dilute Ammonia Solution *(B.P.)*. Liquor Ammoniae Dilutus; Liq. Ammon. Dil.; Ammonia Solution; Ammonia Water; Diluted Ammonium Hydroxide Solution; Ammonium Hydricum Solutum; Liquor Ammoniae; Liquor Ammonii Caustici; Ammoniaque Officinale Diluée.

Pharmacopoeias. In *Arg.*, *Br.*, *Cz.*, *Hung.*, *Ind.*, *Jap.*, *Pol.*, *Roum.*, and *Swiss* (all about 10%); in *Aust.* (10.2 to 11%), in *Mex.* (9 to 10%), and in *Port.* (10 to 11%).

Strong Ammonia Solution 37.5 ml, freshly boiled and cooled water to 100 ml. It contains 9.5 to 10.5% w/w of NH_3. Wt per ml 0.955 to 0.959 g. **Store** at a temperature not exceeding 20° in airtight containers.

NOTE. The *B.P.* directs that when Ammonia Solution is prescribed or demanded, Dilute Ammonia Solution shall be dispensed or supplied.

Adverse Effects. Ingestion of strong solutions of ammonia causes severe pain in the mouth, throat, and gastro-intestinal tract, with cough, vomiting, and shock. Convulsions may follow. There may be oesophageal and gastro-intestinal strictures or there may be perforation. Ingestion may also cause oedema of the respiratory tract and pneumonitis, though this may not develop for a few hours.

Inhalation of ammonia vapour causes sneezing and coughing and in high concentration causes pulmonary oedema. Asphyxia has been reported following oedema or spasm of the glottis. Ammonia vapour is irritant to the eyes and causes weeping; there may be conjunctival swelling and temporary blindness. Strong solutions on the conjunctiva may cause a severe reaction with conjunctival oedema, corneal damage, and possibly delayed atrophy of the retina and iris. Severe local reactions have resulted from treating insect bites and stings with the strong solution, and even with the dilute solution, especially if a dressing is subsequently applied.

Maximum permissible atmospheric concentration (of NH_3) 25 ppm.

Of 7 patients who suffered acute ammonia poisoning, 1 died with congestion and oedema of the respiratory mucosa, with complete stripping of the bronchial epithelium. Persisting but not debilitating respiratory impairment was found 5 years later in 5 of the 6 survivors, some of whom were tobacco smokers.— M. Walton, *Br. J. ind. Med.*, 1973, *30*, 78.

Ammonia toxicity and pH. In most biological fluids ammonia existed in 2 forms, the relative proportions of which were determined primarily by the pH of the solution. Toxicity depended on the non-ionised ammonia which entered the organism and thence the cell. In a medium of low pH ammonia was toxic only in high volumes whereas in a medium of high pH far smaller amounts might be lethal.— K. S. Warren, *Nature*, 1962, *195*, 47.

Treatment of Adverse Effects. Ingestion should not be treated by lavage or emesis. Give copious drinks of water and follow this with demulcents. Pain may be relieved by morphine 10 mg intramuscularly. Appropriate measures should be taken to alleviate shock and pulmonary oedema, and maintain an airway; tracheotomy may be necessary. It has been recommended that corticosteroid therapy may prevent the development of oesophageal strictures.

Contaminated skin and eyes should be flooded with water for at least 15 minutes. Any affected clothing should be removed while flooding is being carried out. Eye-drops of liquid paraffin have been instilled after the thorough washing of affected eyes.

Severe eye damage followed ammonia attack in 2 patients. There was recurring raised intra-ocular pressure requiring regular treatment with acetazolamide.— V. N. Highman, *Br. med. J.*, 1969, *1*, 359.

Immediate irrigation of the eyes with any bland fluid might prevent any permanent visual defect after ammonia had been thrown in the eyes during assaults.— A. G. Cross (letter), *Br. med. J.*, 1969, *1*, 638; *idem* (letter), *Lancet*, 1969, *1*, 534. See also A. H. Osmond and C. J. Tallents (letter), *Br. med. J.*, 1968, *3*, 740.

Uses. Dilute solutions of ammonia have been used as reflex stimulants either as smelling salts or solutions for oral administration. They have also been used as rubefacients and counter-irritants and to neutralise insect stings. Users should always be aware of the irritant properties of ammonia.

The use of ammonia in cosmetics and toiletries is restricted under the Cosmetic Product Regulations 1978 (SI 1978: No. 1354).

For a report of the cardiovascular effects of inhalations of ammonia pertaining to its remedial value in the treatment of the simple faint, see R. S. Zitnik *et al.*, *Am. J. Cardiol.*, 1969, *24*, 187, per *Abstr. Wld Med.*, 1970, *44*, 92.

Under normal circumstances the use of smelling salts or ammonia inhalants in adrenaline-sensitive individuals was a safe and effective treatment for fainting.— *J. Am. med. Ass.*, 1974, *228*, 1170.

Stings. Bathers who were stung after intercepting an armada of Portuguese men-of-war (*Physalia physalis*) were rapidly and effectively relieved of discomfort, paresis, irritation, and other symptoms by the application of aromatic ammonia spirit compresses. Such applications had been found to be quickly effective in cases where other agents had given no relief after 5 days' treatment.— I. G. Frohman (letter), *J. Am. med. Ass.*, 1966, *197*, 733.

Preparations

Liniments

Linimentum Ammoniae *(B.P.C. 1949)*. Lin. Ammon.; Ammonia Liniment. Dilute Ammonia Solution 25 ml, oleic acid 2.5 ml, liquid paraffin to 100 ml. Ammonia liniment is usually supplied for 'hartshorn and oil'.

Similar liniments, with a vegetable oil (olive, sesame, or sunflower oil) in place of liquid paraffin, are included in some pharmacopoeias.

Solutions

Aromatic Ammonia Solution *(B.P.)*. Sal Volatile Solution. Ammonium bicarbonate, strong ammonia solution, oils of lemon and nutmeg, alcohol (90%), and water. Store at a temperature not exceeding 25° in airtight containers.

It is of the same ammoniacal strength as aromatic ammonia spirit, but it gives a clear mixture with distilled water, as distinct from the spirit, and it is not so pungent to the taste. *Dose.* 1 to 5 ml diluted with water.

'Cloudy' Ammonia is made with tap water—for this the gravity of the preparation must not be too low, otherwise the lime salts constituting the 'cloud' will settle down. The following is a suitable formula: dissolve hard soap 1.3 in water 60, and add strong ammonia solution 27, lime water 0.6, and tap water to 100. Used as a cleansing agent for general domestic purposes.

Household Ammonia. Liquor Ammoniae Domesticus. Oleic acid 1, alcohol 1; mix and add strong ammonia solution 7, water 7, shake well. For general domestic purposes.

Liq. Ammon. Anisat *(B.P.C. 1934)*. Anisated Solution of Ammonia; Anisated Spirit of Ammonia. Dilute ammonia solution 5, anise oil 1, alcohol (90%) to 30, by vol. *Dose.* 1 to 4 ml.

Similar formulas are given in *Arg. P.*, *Belg. P.*, *Pol. P.*, *Port. P.*, *Rus. P.*, *Span. P.*, and *Swiss P.*

Spirits

Aromatic Ammonia Spirit *(B.P.)*. Sp. Ammon. Aromat.; Sal Volatile Spirit; Spirit of Sal Volatile. Ammonium bicarbonate dissolved in a mixture of strong ammonia solution with a distillate of lemon oil, nutmeg oil, alcohol, and water. It contains 1.12 to 1.3% w/v of free ammonia and 2.76 to 3.24% w/v of ammonium carbonate, $(NH_4)_2CO_3$. Store at a temperature not exceeding 25° in airtight containers.

Storage in the tropics. Aromatic Ammonia Spirit should be stored in small, well-filled well-closed bottles, in a cool place. Glass stoppers could be used but rubber stoppers were unsuitable because they absorbed ammonia.— A. B. Dutta, *Pharm. J.*, 1956, *1*, 214.

Aromatic Ammonia Spirit *(U.S.P.)*. Prepared by dissolving oils of lemon, lavender, and nutmeg in alcohol, adding a solution of ammonium carbonate and diluted ammonia solution, and filtering after 24 hours. It contains 1.7 to 2.1% w/v of total NH_3, and 3.5 to 4.5% w/v of $(NH_4)_2CO_3$. Store at a temperature not exceeding 30° in airtight containers. Protect from light.

203-h

Barium Hydroxide Lime *(U.S.P.)*. A mixture of barium hydroxide octahydrate [$Ba(OH)_2,8H_2O$=315.5] and calcium hydroxide; it may also contain potassium hydroxide.

CAS — 17194-00-2 (barium hydroxide, anhydrous); 12230-71-6 (barium hydroxide, octahydrate).

Pharmacopoeias. In *U.S.*

White or greyish-white granules, or coloured with an indicator to show when absorptive power is exhausted. It absorbs not less than 19% of its weight of carbon dioxide. It loses 11 to 16% of its weight when dried. **Store** in airtight containers.

It is used similarly to soda lime to absorb carbon dioxide in closed-circuit anaesthetic apparatus. Barium hydroxide lime is toxic if swallowed.

204-m

Calcium Hydroxide *(B.P., U.S.P.)*. Calc. Hydrox.; Calcium Hydrate; Slaked Lime. $Ca(OH)_2$=74.09.

CAS — 1305-62-0.

Pharmacopoeias. In *Aust.*, *Br.*, *Ind.*, *It.*, *Jap.*, *Mex.*,

Nord., and *U.S.*

A soft white powder with a slightly bitter alkaline taste. The *B.P.* specifies not less than 90% of $Ca(OH)_2$; the *U.S.P.* specifies 95 to 100.5%.

Almost entirely **soluble** 1 in 600 of water; less soluble in hot water; soluble in aqueous solutions of glycerol and sugars; practically insoluble in alcohol. A solution in water is alkaline to phenolphthalein and readily absorbs carbon dioxide. **Sterilise** by maintaining the whole of the powder at a temperature of at least 160° for 1 hour. **Store** in airtight containers.

Uses. Calcium hydroxide is a weak alkali. It is used in the form of Calcium Hydroxide Solution (lime water) in some skin lotions and oily preparations to form calcium soaps of fatty acids which produce water-in-oil emulsions. The solution was formerly used as an antacid and astringent.

Calcium Hydroxide Solution has been given in doses of 30 to 120 ml.

Maximum permissible atmospheric concentration 5 mg per m^3.

Calcium hydroxide eliminated poliomyelitis virus from experimentally infected human sewage.— S. A. Sattar *et al.*, *Can. J. publ. Hlth*, 1976, *67*, 221, per *Abstr. Hyg.*, 1976, *51*, 930.

A review of the use of calcium hydroxide in root canal therapy.— D. M. Martin and H. S. M. Crabb, *Br. dent. J.*, 1977, *142*, 277. See also G. G. Stewart, *J. Am. dent. Ass.*, 1975, *90*, 793, per *Int. pharm. Abstr.*, 1976, *13*, 538.

A study of the differing antibacterial action of 2 calcium hydroxide base materials used beneath silver amalgam fillings.— F. J. Fisher and J. F. McCabe, *Br. dent. J.*, 1978, *144*, 341.

Preparations

Calcium Hydroxide Solution *(B.P.)*. Liquor Calcii Hydroxidi; Lime Water; Liquor Calcis; Aqua Calcariae; Eau de Chaux; Kalkwasser. A clear colourless liquid with an alkaline taste, containing not less than 0.15% of $Ca(OH)_2$. It may be prepared by thoroughly and repeatedly shaking together calcium hydroxide 10 g and freshly boiled and cooled water 1000 ml and then allowing the excess calcium hydroxide to settle. Only the clear supernatant liquid should be dispensed; it may be drawn off with a siphon as required. It absorbs carbon dioxide from the air, a film of calcium carbonate forming on the surface. Store in well-filled airtight containers.

The solubility of calcium hydroxide varies with the temperature at which the solution is stored, being about 170 mg per 100 ml at 15°, and less at higher temperatures. The undissolved portion of the calcium hydroxide is not suitable for preparing additional quantities of the solution.

Similar solutions are included in many other pharmacopoeias.

Calcium Hydroxide Topical Solution *(U.S.P.)*. Calcium Hydroxide Solution. A solution containing, in each 100 ml, not less than 140 mg of $Ca(OH)_2$, prepared by vigorously and repeatedly shaking together calcium hydroxide 3 g and water 1000 ml, and allowing the excess calcium hydroxide to settle. Store at a temperature not exceeding 25° in well-filled airtight containers.

205-b

Diethanolamine. Diaethanolamin; Diolamine. Bis(2-hydroxyethyl)amine; 2,2′-Iminobisethanol.
$C_4H_{11}NO_2$=105.1.

CAS — 111-42-2.

Pharmacopoeias. In *Swiss.* Also in *U.S.N.F.* which describes a mixture of ethanolamines, consisting largely of diethanolamine.

A clear, colourless to slightly yellowish, viscous liquid with a faint ammoniacal odour. It solidifies below 20° to a white or almost white crystalline mass. **Miscible** with water, alcohol, acetone, and chloroform; soluble 1 in 200 of ether. A 5% solution in water has a pH of 10.2 to 11.4. Solutions are **sterilised** by autoclaving. **Store** in airtight containers. Protect from light.

Diethanolamine is used as an emulsifying and dispersing agent.

It is used to solubilise, by the formation of the diethanolamine salt, fusidic acid. It has been used for the preparation of salts of iodinated organic acids used as contrast media. It may be irritating to the skin and mucous membranes.

206-v

Diisopropanolamine *(U.S.N.F.)*.

CAS — 110-97-4 (diisopropanolamine).

Pharmacopoeias. In U.S.N.F.

A mixture of isopropanolamines, consisting largely of diisopropanolamine [1,1′-iminobis(propan-2-ol), $C_6H_{15}NO_2$=133.2]. **Store** in airtight containers. Protect from light.

Diisopropanolamine is used as a neutralising agent in cosmetics and toiletries.

207-g

Ethanolamine *(B.P.)*. Olamine; Aethanolaminum; Monoethanolamine *(U.S.N.F.)*. 2-Hydroxyethylamine; 2-Aminoethanol.

C_2H_7NO=61.08.

CAS — 141-43-5.

Pharmacopoeias. In *Aust.*, *Br.*, and *Ind.* Also in *U.S.N.F.*

A clear colourless or pale yellow viscous liquid with a slight ammoniacal odour. It is alkaline to litmus and combines with fatty acids to form soaps. Wt per ml 1.014 to 1.023 g. B.p. about 170°.

Miscible with water, alcohol, acetone, chloroform, and glycerol; slightly soluble in ether; it is immiscible with light petroleum and fixed oils but it will dissolve many essential oils. A 1.76% solution in water is iso-osmotic with serum. Solutions are **sterilised** by autoclaving; a bactericide need not be added to multidose containers. **Store** in airtight containers. Protect from light.

An aqueous solution of ethanolamine iso-osmotic with serum (1.76%) caused 100% haemolysis of erythrocytes cultured in it for 45 minutes.— E. R. Hammarlund and K. Pedersen-Bjergaard, *J. pharm. Sci.*, 1961, *50*, 24.

Adverse Effects. It is claimed that the use of ethanolamine oleate causes less sloughing than some sclerosants in the event of an accidental leakage into the perivenous tissues. Allergic reactions have been reported.

Maximum permissible atmospheric concentration 3 ppm.

At an inquest on a 56-year-old woman who had received an injection of ethanolamine oleate for varicose veins, it was stated that death had been due to hypersensitivity to the drug.— *Pharm. J.*, 1965, *1*, 603. A nonfatal allergic reaction.— C. C. M. Watson (letter), *Br. med. J.*, 1958, *1*, 1481.

Nephrotoxicity. Acute renal failure, which cleared spontaneously within 3 weeks, occurred in 2 obese women given sclerosing injections of 15 to 20 ml of a solution containing ethanolamine oleate 5% and benzyl alcohol 2%.— T. J. B. Maling and M. J. Cretney, *N.Z. med. J.*, 1975, *82*, 269.

Precautions. Use of ethanolamine is contra-indicated where there is thrombosis of the deep veins of the leg, acute phlebitis, or other affection in the region of the varices.

Uses. Ethanolamine, combined with oleic acid, is used as a sclerosing agent in the injection treatment of varicose veins. It is administered intravenously as Ethanolamine Oleate Injection in a dose of 2 to 5 ml, this dose being divided into 3 or 4 portions which are injected at different sites. The treatment is repeated at weekly intervals until the varices have been completely occluded.

Thirty-six patients with cirrhosis and recent variceal haemorrhage received ethanolamine oleate injection sclerotherapy by means of a flexible oesophageal sheath, while 28 similar patients acted as controls. In 24 (67%) of the patients in the sclerotherapy group, there was no further bleeding over a mean follow-up period of 9.5 months and, in 3 of the 12 patients with further episodes of bleeding, the bleeding was from gastric varices, follow-up endoscopy having shown complete eradication of oesophageal varices. Haemorrhage from oesophageal varices in the other 9 patients occurred before there had been a significant reduction in size of the vessels, and in 3 this was because of delays in sclerotherapy due to slow healing of oesophageal ulcers. The frequency of rebleeding in the control group was much higher, occurring in 19 (68%) patients over a mean follow-up period of 8.8 months. Analysis of the frequency of rebleeding in the control group indicated that the risk factor per patient month was more than 3 times that of the sclerotherapy group. There was a significant improvement in the one-year survival without rebleeding in the sclerotherapy group (46%) compared with the control group (6%) although the difference in overall survival assessed by cumulative life-table analysis was not statistically significant. In 10 patients who received sclerotherapy oesophageal ulcers developed; in 4 of these oesophageal strictures, which required dilatation, formed 2 to 8 weeks after healing of the ulcer. Minor complications from the procedure included retrosternal chest pain, pyrexia, and basal lung changes on the chest X-ray during the first 48 hours after sclerotherapy, which required only simple analgesia and physiotherapy.— A. W. Clark *et al.*, *Lancet*, 1980, *2*, 552. Results in 21 patients using paravasal injection. General anaesthesia was not required and no gastric rebleeding occurred.— E. -H. Egberts and H. Schomerus (letter), *ibid.*, 797.

Preparations

Ethanolamine Oleate Injection *(B.P.)*. A sterile aqueous solution prepared from ethanolamine 910 mg, oleic acid 4.23 g, benzyl alcohol 2 ml, and Water for Injections to 100 ml. Sterilised by autoclaving. pH 8 to 9. It contains about 5% of ethanolamine oleate. Protect from light.

Manufacturers

Evans Medical, UK; Macarthys, UK.

Proprietary Names

Ethamolin *(oleate)* *(Austral.)*; Etolein *(oleate)* *(Swed.)*.

208-q

Ethylenediamine Hydrate *(B.P.)*. Ethylenediam. Hydr.; Ethylenediamini Hydras; Aethylendiamini Hydras.

$C_2H_4(NH_2)_2,H_2O$=78.11.

CAS — 107-15-3 (anhydrous); 6780-13-8 (monohydrate).

Pharmacopoeias. In *Aust.*, *Br.*, *Hung.*, *Ind.*, *Int.*, *Nord.*, *Swiss*, and *Turk. Jap.* and *U.S.* include anhydrous ethylenediamine.

A clear, colourless or slightly yellow, strongly alkaline liquid with an ammoniacal odour. It solidifies on cooling to a crystalline mass (m.p. 10°). B.p. about 120°. Wt per ml about 0.96 g. It is hygroscopic and absorbs carbon dioxide from the air. **Miscible** with water and alcohol; soluble 1 in 130 of chloroform; slightly soluble in ether. Solutions are **sterilised** by autoclaving or by filtration. **Store** in airtight containers. Protect from light.

Adverse Effects. It is irritant to the skin and to mucous membranes, and contact dermatitis has been reported from the use of preparations containing ethylenediamine. Concentrated solutions cause skin burns. Headache, dizziness, shortness of breath, nausea, and vomiting have also been reported following exposure to fumes. Maximum permissible atmospheric concentration 10 ppm.

Of 600 persons with dermatitis or eczema submitted to patch testing with 1% aqueous solution of ethylenediamine, 3.3% gave a positive reaction.— E. Rudzki and D. Kleniewska, *Br. J. Derm.*, 1970, *83*, 543. See also A. A. Fisher *et al.*, *Archs Derm.*, 1971, *104*, 286.

A 36-year-old man, one-third of whose skin was contaminated with ethylenediamine, developed erythema covering the whole body, hyperkalaemia, tachycardia, cough, abdominal cramps, pyrexia, hypotension, and anuria, and died 55 hours after exposure.— J. Niveau and J. Painchaux, *Archs Mal. prof. Méd. trav.*, 1973, *34*, 523, per *Abstr. Hyg.*, 1974, *49*, 469.

Treatment of Adverse Effects. Ethylenediamine splashed on to the skin or eyes should be removed by rinsing with large volumes of water.

Precautions. Skin reactions may occur in patients given aminophylline after they have become sensitised to ethylenediamine. Cross-sensitivity with edetic acid and with antihistamines has been reported.

Thirteen patients with contact dermatitis had positive reactions to skin tests with 1% ethylenediamine; 12 had used a corticosteroid-antibiotic preparation containing ethylenediamine and 2 had an exacerbation of their eruption when given aminophylline.— T. T. Provost and O. F. Jillson, *Archs Derm.*, 1967, *96*, 231, per *J. Am. med. Ass.*, 1967, *201* (Sept. 18), A176. For a similar effect in 1 patient see J. W. Petrozzi and R. N. Shore, *Archs Derm.*, 1976, *112*, 525.

Ethylenediamine and edetic acid were sensitisers which cross-reacted with each other and with antihistamines.— K. E. Eriksen (letter), *Archs Derm.*, 1975, *111*, 791.

Of 159 patients with contact dermatitis, 20 were sensitive to ethylenediamine; all had used Tri-Adcortyl cream which contained ethylenediamine.— M. I. White *et al.*, *Br. med. J.*, 1978, *1*, 415.

Uses. Ethylenediamine hydrate is used in the manufacture of aminophylline and in the preparation of aminophylline injections. Ethylenediamine hydrochloride is used as an acidifying agent in veterinary practice.

209-p

Meglumine *(B.P., U.S.P.)*. *N*-Methylglucamine; 1-Methylamino-1-deoxy-D-glucitol.

$C_7H_{17}NO_5$=195.2.

CAS — 6284-40-8.

Pharmacopoeias. In *Br., Braz., Chin., Cz., Jap., Nord.,* and *U.S.*

A white or faintly yellowish micro-crystalline powder or crystals, odourless or with a slight odour and a slightly bitter taste. M.p. 128° to 132°. **Soluble** 1 in 1 of water and 1 in 100 of alcohol; slightly soluble in methyl alcohol; practically insoluble in chloroform and ether. A solution in water is laevorotatory. A 10% solution in water has a pH of between 11 and 12. A 5.02% solution in water is iso-osmotic with serum. **Store** in airtight containers.

Uses. Meglumine is an organic base which is used for the preparation of salts of iodinated organic acids used as contrast media; for example, it is used in the preparation of Iodipamide Meglumine Injection, Meglumine Diatrizoate Injection, and Meglumine Iothalamate Injection.

210-n

Potassium Carbonate *(B.P.C. 1949)*. Pot. Carb.; Salt of Tartar; Kalii Carbonas; Kalium Carbonicum.

$K_2CO_3,1\frac{1}{2}H_2O$=165.2.

CAS — 584-08-7 (anhydrous); 6381-79-9 (sesquihydrate).

'Pearl-ash' and 'American potash' are forms of crude potassium carbonate.

Pharmacopoeias. In *Arg., Mex.,* and *Port.* (all with $1\frac{1}{2}H_2O$); and in *Aust., Belg., Fr., Hung., Jap., Jug., Nord., Pol., Roum., Span.,* and *Swiss* (all anhydrous).

A very deliquescent, white, odourless, crystalline powder with a strongly alkaline taste. **Soluble** 1 in 1 of water; practically insoluble in alcohol.

The properties of potassium carbonate resemble those of potassium bicarbonate but it is more caustic and irritating and is rarely given internally. It has been applied externally as a lotion (0.35%) in the treatment of eczema and urticaria.

211-h

Potassium Hydroxide *(B.P., U.S.N.F.)*. Pot. Hydrox.; Kalii Hydroxydum; Potassii Hydroxidum; Caustic Potash; Kalium Hydroxydatum; Ätzkali.

KOH=56.11.

CAS — 1310-58-3.

Pharmacopoeias. In *Aust., Br., Hung., Ind., Int., Jap., Jug., Mex., Nord., Port., Span., Swiss,* and *Turk.* Also in *U.S.N.F.*

Dry, white or almost white sticks, pellets, flakes, or fused masses. It is strongly alkaline and corrosive, and rapidly destroys organic tissues. It contains not less than 85% of total alkali calculated as KOH and not more than 4% of K_2CO_3 (*U.S.N.F.* 3.5%). It rapidly absorbs moisture and carbon dioxide from the air with the formation of potassium carbonate. It may be freed from carbonate by solution in alcohol, filtration, and evaporation of the solution.

Soluble or almost completely soluble 1 in 1 of water, 1 in 3 of alcohol, and 1 in 2.5 of glycerol; very soluble in boiling dehydrated alcohol; very slightly soluble in ether. **Store** in airtight containers; if they are made of glass they should be closed by waxed corks or plastic-lined screw caps.

Adverse Effects. Swallowing caustic alkalis causes immediate burning pain in the mouth, throat, and stomach, and the lining membranes become swollen and detached. Vomiting and purging may occur, the vomitus having a brown colour from altered blood. There is intense pain and shock. Stricture of the oesophagus can develop. In severe cases, circulatory failure, oesophageal perforation and peritonitis, or pneumonia may occur.

Maximum permissible atmospheric concentration 2 mg per m³.

Treatment of Adverse Effects. Ingestion should not be treated by lavage or emesis. Give copious drinks of water and follow this with demulcents. Pain may be relieved by morphine 10 mg intramuscularly. Maintain an airway and alleviate shock. It has been recommended that corticosteroid therapy may prevent the development of oesophageal strictures; periodic checks should be made for the late development of oesophageal damage.

Contaminated skin and eyes should be immediately flooded with copious amounts of water and for skin burns this may be followed by dilute acetic acid. Any affected clothing should be removed while flooding is being carried out.

Oesophageal examination of 209 patients who had swallowed corrosive substances revealed that 35% had lesions which had often been insufficiently indicated during ordinary clinical examination. Immediate admission to hospital was recommended in all cases of corrosive poisoning and oral or intravenous corticosteroid treatment with the equivalent of 5 to 10 mg per kg body-weight of cortisone daily. If oesophageal examination 24 hours after admission failed to reveal any lesions, corticosteroid therapy should be stopped.— A. Genot *et al.*, *Un. méd. Can.*, 1968, *97*, 279, per *Pharm. J.*, 1968, *2*, 193.

Brief discussions on the management of alkali burns of the oesophagus: *Med. Lett.*, 1972, *14*, 18; D. W. Gilmore *et al.*, *Med. J. Aust.*, 1976, *2*, 212.

Uses. Potassium hydroxide is a powerful caustic which has been used to remove warts. A 2.5% solution in glycerol may be used as a cuticle solvent.

The use of potassium hydroxide in cosmetics and toiletries is restricted under the Cosmetic Product Regulations 1978 (SI 1978: No. 1354).

Preparations

Potassium Hydroxide Solution *(B.P.)*. Pot. Hydrox. Soln; Liquor Potassii Hydroxidi; Solutio Kalii Hydroxydi; Potash Solution. An aqueous solution containing 4.9 to 5.1% w/v of total alkali. Store in airtight containers of lead-free glass or of a suitable plastic.

A solution of potassium hydroxide is included in *Aust. P.* (10% w/w), *Ind. P.* (5% w/v), and *Swiss P.* (40% w/w).

Vienna Paste. Pasta Potassae et Calcis. Potassium hydroxide 5 and calcium hydroxide 6, reduced to a fine powder and kept in a well-stoppered bottle. To be made into a paste with alcohol (90%) when required. An escharotic. Similar to London Paste (q.v.).

Proprietary Names

Cerumenol *(Jorba, Spain)*.

NOTE. A preparation containing turpentine oil, paradichlorobenzene, and chlorbutol, in arachis oil was formerly marketed in Great Britain under the name of Cerumenol (see under Cerumol, p.695).

212-m

Soda Lime *(B.P.)*. Calx Sodica; Cal Sodada; Calcaria Compositio; Chaux Sodée. A mixture of calcium hydroxide with sodium hydroxide or sodium hydroxide and potassium hydroxide; it may be prepared by fusion and subsequent granulation of the fused mass.

CAS — 8006-28-8.

Pharmacopoeias. In *Arg., Br., Fr., Ind., Mex.,* and *Pol.* Also in *U.S.N.F.* which specifies a mixture of calcium hydroxide with sodium or potassium hydroxide or both (loss on drying 12 to 19%).

White or greyish-white granules, or coloured with an indicator to show when absorptive power is exhausted. Suitable indicators include phenolphthalein, potassium permanganate, and methyl violet. Soda lime absorbs about 20% of its weight of carbon dioxide. It loses 14 to 21% of its weight when dried. Partly **soluble** in water; almost completely soluble in acetic acid (6 per cent). A suspension in water is strongly alkaline to litmus. **Incompatible** with trichloroethylene. **Store** in airtight containers.

Uses. Soda lime is used to absorb carbon dioxide in closed-circuit anaesthetic apparatus. Limits are specified for particle size to eliminate small granules, which cause excessive resistance to respiration, and large granules, which give inefficient absorption. The granules should also be free from dust which otherwise would be inhaled and cause irritation.

The containers for soda lime attached to the machines usually hold about 0.5 or 2 kg; if used continuously, 500 g of soda lime will absorb carbon dioxide for 2 to 3 hours, in which time the granules will become coated with carbonate and further absorption prevented. After an interval of an hour, the soda lime will partially recover its absorptive capacity and may be used again. By using it intermittently in this way 500 g of soda lime will provide efficient absorption for a total period of about 7 to 8 hours. The condition of the soda lime may be judged from the colour of the indicator which is usually incorporated, but this may not be entirely reliable and close observation of the anaesthetised patient is necessary.

Absorption of carbon dioxide by soda lime is accompanied by the evolution of heat, the temperature of the container usually reaching about 40°; if it becomes much hotter than this the soda lime should be rejected.

It is preferable to change the 500-g container after each operation; this allows the soda lime to cool and to regenerate. Large containers may be used continuously for many hours; their larger cross-section allows dissipation of heat and regeneration is not necessary. It is also advisable to moisten the soda lime with a few millilitres of water when filling the containers, since this increases the rate of absorption. Further moisture will be supplied by the water vapour exhaled by the patient.

Soda lime is similarly used to absorb carbon dioxide during determination of the basal metabolic-rate.

Soda lime must not be used with trichloroethylene, since this is decomposed by warm alkali into dichloroacetylene which is very toxic and gives rise to lesions of the nervous system. Soda lime is used in gas respirators to absorb acid gases.

For reviews of the use of soda lime, see D. E. Hale, *Anesth. Analg. curr. Res.*, 1967, *46*, 648; A. Bracken and L. A. Cox, *Br. J. Anaesth.*, 1968, *40*, 660.

Proprietary Preparations

Durasorb *(Medical & Industrial, UK)*. A brand of soda lime, for use in anaesthetic equipment.

Medisorb *(BOC Medishield, UK)*. A brand of soda lime, for use in anaesthetic equipment.

213-b

Anhydrous Sodium Carbonate *(B.P.C. 1968)*.

Anhyd. Sod. Carb.; Exsiccated Sodium Carbonate; Natrium Carbonicum Calcinatum; Natrium Carbonicum Siccatum; Cenizas de Soda.

Na_2CO_3=106.0.

CAS — 497-19-8.

Pharmacopoeias. In *Arg., Hung., Jap., Pol.*, and *Port.*
NOTE. Sodium Carbonate (*U.S.N.F.*) is anhydrous or the monohydrate.

An odourless white hygroscopic powder with a strongly alkaline taste. When exposed to air it slowly absorbs moisture, forming the monohydrate. **Soluble** 1 in 5 of water and 1 in 10 of glycerol; practically insoluble in alcohol. A 1.32% solution in water is iso-osmotic with serum. **Store** in airtight containers.

Uses. Anhydrous sodium carbonate is used in Thiopentone Injection and was used in the preparation of capsules, pills, and tablets of ferrous carbonate. It is used as a water softener.

214-v

Sodium Carbonate Decahydrate *(B.P., Eur. P.)*.

Sodium Carbonate; Sod. Carb.; Natrii Carbonas; Natrii Carbonas Decahydricus; Natrium Carbonicum Crystallisatum; Cristales de Sosa.

$Na_2CO_3,10H_2O$=286.1.

CAS — 6132-02-1.

NOTE. Soda and washing soda are synonyms for technical grades of sodium carbonate.

Pharmacopoeias. In *Arg., Aust., Belg., Br., Eur., Fr., Ger., Hung., Ind., It., Jap., Jug., Neth., Nord., Pol., Span.*, and *Swiss.*
NOTE. Sodium Carbonate (*U.S.N.F.*) is anhydrous or the monohydrate.

Odourless, colourless, efflorescent crystals or white crystalline powder with a strongly alkaline taste. **Soluble** 1 in 2 of water, 1 in less than 1 of boiling water, and 1 in about 1 of glycerol; practically insoluble in alcohol. A 10% solution in water has a pH greater than 10. Solutions are **sterilised** by autoclaving. **Incompatible** with acids, ammonium salts, calcium hydroxide solution, salts of heavy metals, many alkaloidal salts, and chloral hydrate. **Store** in airtight containers.

Uses. Sodium carbonate decahydrate has been used in the preparation of alkaline baths (about 250 g in 150 litres) for scaly skin diseases. It is also used in the preparation of Surgical Chlorinated Soda Solution and as a water softener. A lotion (0.5%), applied with a compress, has been used for softening incrustations and relieving irritation in eczema.

Use of disinfectants on farms. In Great Britain, sodium carbonate decahydrate, complying with BS 3674 of 1963, 1 in 24 in water is an approved disinfectant for foot-and-mouth disease under The Diseases of Animals (Approved Disinfectants) Order 1978 (SI 1978: No. 32), as amended (SI 1978: No. 934).

215-g

Sodium Carbonate Monohydrate *(B.P., Eur. P.)*.

Natrii Carbonas Monohydricus.

Na_2CO_3,H_2O=124.0.

CAS — 5968-11-6.

Pharmacopoeias. In *Aust., Belg., Br., Braz., Eur., Fr., Ger., It., Neth.*, and *Swiss.*
NOTE. Sodium Carbonate (*U.S.N.F.*) is the anhydrous or the monohydrate.

Odourless, colourless crystals or white crystalline powder with an alkaline salty taste. It is stable in air under ordinary conditions but effloresces when exposed to dry air above 50°. **Soluble** 1 in 3 of water and 1 in 2 of boiling water; practically insoluble in alcohol. A 10% solution in water has a pH greater than 10. A 1.56% solution in water is iso-osmotic with serum. **Store** in airtight containers.

Sodium carbonate monohydrate is used for the same purpose as anhydrous sodium carbonate.

216-q

Sodium Hydroxide *(B.P., U.S.N.F.)*.

Sod. Hydrox.; Natrium Hydroxydatum; Natrium Hydricum; Ätznatron; Caustic Soda.

NaOH=40.00.

CAS — 1310-73-2.

Pharmacopoeias. In *Aust., Br., Chin., Hung., Ind., Jap., Jug., Mex., Nord., Port., Span., Swiss*, and *Turk.* Also in *U.S.N.F.*

Dry, white or almost white sticks, pellets, fused masses, or scales. It is strongly alkaline and corrosive, and rapidly destroys organic tissues. It contains not less than 97.5% of total alkali calculated as NaOH and not more than 2.5% of Na_2CO_3 (*U.S.N.F.* 3%). When exposed to air it rapidly absorbs moisture and liquefies, but subsequently becomes solid again due to absorption of carbon dioxide and formation of sodium carbonate, and effloresces.
Completely or almost completely **soluble** 1 in 1 of water, with the evolution of much heat; very soluble in alcohol; soluble in glycerol. **Store** in airtight containers; if they are of glass they should be closed by waxed corks or plastic-lined screw caps.

Storage. Tenth molar sodium hydroxide solution stored in soda-glass bottles and polyethylene bottles over a period of 15 months increased in strength by 1.4% in the glass bottles, but there was no apparent change in the strength of solution in polyethylene containers.— W. C. Easterbrook and A. B. Cameron (letter), *Chemy Ind.*, 1957, *76*, 1155.

Adverse Effects and Treatment. As for Potassium Hydroxide, p.44. Maximum permissible atmospheric concentration 2 mg per m^3.

Uses. Sodium hydroxide is a powerful caustic which is used for the same purposes as potassium hydroxide. It is also used for adjusting the pH of solutions and as a disinfectant in veterinary practice. The use of sodium hydroxide in cosmetics and toiletries is restricted under the Cosmetic Product Regulations 1978 (SI 1978: No. 1354).

Pseudomonal overgrowth occurred in artificial lenses disinfected with sodium hydroxide.— H. Bauer *et al.*, *Morb. Mortal.*, 1976, *25*, 369, per *Int. pharm. Abstr.*, 1977, *14*, 247.

Use of disinfectants on farms. In Great Britain, sodium hydroxide 1 in 100 of water is an approved disinfectant for swine vesicular disease under the Diseases of Animals (Approved Disinfectants) Order 1978 (SI 1978: No. 32), as amended (SI 1978: No. 934).

Preparations

Sodium Hydroxide Solution *(B.P.C. 1954)*. Liq. Sod. Hydrox. It contains 3.56% w/v of total alkali calculated as NaOH. Store in well-closed bottles of lead-free glass.
A solution of sodium hydroxide is included in *Swiss P.* (30% w/w) and 2 solutions are included in *Aust. P.* (29.5 to 30.5% w/w and 7.3 to 7.5% w/w).

217-p

Sodium Sesquicarbonate.

$Na_2CO_3,NaHCO_3,2H_2O$=226.0.

CAS — 6106-20-3.

Silky crystals or white powder. **Soluble** 1 in about 7 of water and 1 in 2.5 of boiling water.

Sodium sesquicarbonate is used as a water softener.

218-s

Triethanolamine *(B.P.)*.

Trolamine.

CAS — 102-71-6 (triethanolamine)

Pharmacopoeias. In *Aust., Br., Braz., Cz., Fr., Hung., Ind., It., Jap., Mex., Neth., Pol.*, and *Swiss.*
Also in *U.S.N.F.* as Trolamine, a mixture of alkanolamines consisting largely of triethanolamine, with some diethanolamine and ethanolamine, and containing 99 to 107.4% of alkanolamines calculated on the anhydrous basis as triethanolamine.

A variable mixture of bases containing not less than 80% of triethanolamine [tris(2-hydroxyethyl)amine, $(CH_2OH.CH_2)_3N$] with diethanolamine and smaller amounts of ethanolamine; it contains not less than 99% and not more than the equivalent of 110% of total bases calculated as triethanolamine.
It is a clear, colourless or pale yellow, odourless or almost odourless, viscous, hygroscopic liquid; it volatilises slowly at 100°. Wt per ml 1.12 to 1.13 g.
Triethanolamine forms crystalline salts with mineral acids, the hydrochloride and the hydriodide being sparingly soluble in alcohol. With the higher fatty or olefinic acids it forms salts which are soluble in water and have the general characteristics of soaps.
Miscible with water, alcohol, and glycerol; soluble in chloroform; slightly soluble in ether. A 10% solution in water is strongly alkaline to litmus; 1 g of triethanolamine has an alkalinity equivalent to about 7 ml of 1M hydrochloric acid. **Store** in airtight containers. Protect from light.

Adverse Effects. It may be irritating to the skin and mucous membranes.

Of 100 patients with allergic contact dermatitis, 2 gave positive reactions to patch testing with triethanolamine 5% in soft paraffin.— A. A. Fisher *et al.*, *Archs Derm.*, 1971, *104*, 286. See also under Xerumenex, below.

Uses. Triethanolamine is used mainly combined with fatty acids such as stearic and oleic acids; equimolecular proportions of base and fatty acid form a soap which can be used as an emulsifying agent to produce stable, fine-grained, oil-in-water emulsions with a pH of about 8.
Preparations made with triethanolamine soaps tend to darken on keeping; discoloration can be reduced by storage in the dark and by avoiding contact with metals.

Use of ear-drops containing triethanolamine polypeptide oleate-condensate (Xerumenex) and water syringing was more effective than syringing alone in the removal of cerumen in a controlled trial with 45 patients.— P. G. Harris (letter), *Br. med. J.*, 1968, *4*, 775.

A double-blind trial on 67 ears showed that single applications of triethanolamine polypeptide oleate-condensate (Xerumenex) or olive oil were equally effective in facilitating the removal of impacted wax.— D. M. C. de Saintonge and C. I. Johnstone, *Br. J. clin. Pract.*, 1973, *27*, 454.

Further references: F. De S. Donnan, *Practitioner*, 1968, *200*, 574; J. Proudfoot, *Br. J. clin. Pract.*, 1968, *22*, 69.

Preparations

Triethanolamine Stearate Cream *(F.N. Belg.)*. Cremor Triaethanolamini Stearatis. Triethanolamine 1.2 g, stearic acid 24 g, glycerol 13.5 g, and water 61.3 g.

Proprietary Preparations of Triethanolamine Compounds

Xerumenex *(Napp, UK)*. Ear-drops containing triethanolamine polypeptide oleate-condensate 10% and chlorbutol 0.5% in propylene glycol. For the removal of wax from the ear. *Directions.* Fill the ear canal with the drops and allow to remain for not more than 30 minutes before gentle syringing. (Also available in some countries as Cerumenex).

A 43-year-old man developed bilateral acute otitis externa with swelling of the eyelids and dermatitis of the face, neck, and upper chest. He had previously instilled Xerumenex once into each ear and had probably left it in the ear overnight. A patch test showed sensitivity to Xerumenex. Of 8 other patients tested 3 showed slight reactions and 1 a moderate reaction.— K. Grice and C. I. Johnstone (letter), *Br. med. J.*, 1972, *1*, 508.

Amino Acids and Nutritional Agents

570-h

The total daily energy requirements are dependent upon the energy expended on physical activity and growth and the amount of energy required to maintain body temperature and essential physiological functions (basal metabolism). For persons of average weight the total daily energy requirements, depending upon the type of work performed, are 11 000 to 17 000 kJ (2700 to 4000 kcal) for men and 8400 to 13 000 kJ (2000 to 3000 kcal) for women. The daily energy requirements for maintenance of normal body temperature and physiological functions are about 6700 kJ (1600 kcal) for men and about 5400 kJ (1300 kcal) for women. Energy requirements are relatively higher during pregnancy and lactation, for growth during childhood, and in patients with malnutrition, trauma, sepsis, or burns. Most of the energy requirements are derived from *carbohydrates* and *fats*. Each g of carbohydrate (as monosaccharide) provides about 16 kJ (3.75 kcal) and each g of fat 38 kJ (9 kcal). When calculated from polysaccharide content, each g of carbohydrate provides 18 kJ (4.2 kcal). Protein can be used as an energy source and provides 17 kJ (4 kcal) per g. Alcohol, which provides about 30 kJ (7.1 kcal) per g, can also be used as a source of energy but the body can only metabolise about 10 to 15 ml per hour.

Proteins or their constituent amino acids are required for the maintenance of body tissues and for the growth of infants and children. A Joint FAO/WHO Expert Group on Protein Requirements (*Tech. Rep. Ser. Wld Hlth Org. No. 301*, 1965) stated that 0.71 g per kg body-weight daily would cover the requirements of all but a very small proportion of the population, with larger requirements, up to 1.06 g per kg, for children and infants. These values assumed 100% net protein utilisation; for 70% utilisation they would be increased to 1.01 g per kg and 1.5 g per kg respectively. The recommended protein intake for the United Kingdom given in the Report by the Committee on Medical Aspects of Food Policy (*Report on Health and Social Subjects No. 15*, London, HM Stationery Office, 1979) ranged from 54 to 84 g daily for men and 42 to 69 g daily for women according to age, occupational category, and whether they were pregnant or lactating.

A report by a Joint FAO/WHO *ad hoc* Expert Committee on Energy and Protein Requirements (*Tech. Rep. Ser. Wld Hlth Org. No. 522*, 1973) related requirements to measurements of the lowest protein intake at which nitrogen equilibrium could be achieved in adults or satisfactory growth and nitrogen retention in children. The 'safe level of protein intake', assuming 100% net protein utilisation was considered to be 520 mg per kg body-weight daily for an adult woman, increasing to 570 mg per kg for a man and 1.53 g per kg for an infant. These average intakes would need to be increased to correct nitrogen imbalance in patients with extensive burns or those recovering following major surgery.

The amino acids with which the body must be supplied, and which are therefore described as essential, are isoleucine, leucine, lysine, methionine, phenylalanine, threonine, tryptophan, and valine; arginine, cysteine, and histidine are required in addition for infant growth.

For a review of the pharmacology and toxicity of amino acids, see M. D. Milne, *Clin. Pharmac. Ther.*, 1968, *9*, 484.

For a review of factors limiting the use of sugars in paediatric formulations, see R. H. Leach, *Pharm. J.*, 1970, *2*, 227.

For information on energy requirements and nutrition, see *Tech. Rep. Ser. Wld Hlth Org. No. 522*, 1973; *Manual of Nutrition*, London, HM Stationery Office, 1976.

Proteins were metabolised chiefly by pancreatic enzymes—by endopeptidases, such as trypsin and chymotrypsin, breaking amino-acid chains into smaller fragments, and by exopeptidases, such as carboxypeptidases A and B, splitting off amino acids from the ends of chains. Free amino acids were absorbed after hydrolysis of the protein within the intestine. Contrary to the view long held it was now established that dipeptides and tripeptides were also absorbed with subsequent hydrolysis by peptidases probably within the mucosal cells. Impairment of amino-acid absorption did not necessarily involve impairment of dipeptide absorption. The use of diets containing only amino acids could be dangerous in patients with impairment of amino-acid absorption.— D. M. Matthews, *J. clin. Path.*, 1971, *24, Suppl.* 5, 29.

Discussion of problems encountered in the implementation of WHO recommendations.—Recommendations by a joint FAO/WHO informal gathering of experts, *Food Nutr.*, 1975, *1* (2), 11.

A joint FAO/WHO memorandum on protein and energy requirements.— *Bull. Wld Hlth Org.*, 1979, *57*, 65.

General references on nutrition: *Lancet*, 1975, *2*, 263; F. F. Thompson, *Practitioner*, 1975, *215*, 632; *Med. J. Aust.*, 1975, *1*, 49; G. L. Blackburn *et al.*, *Anesthesiology*, 1977, *47*, 181; R. C. Serfass, *J. Am. pharm. Ass.*, 1977, *NS17*, 516; M. Winick, *J. Am. pharm. Ass.*, 1977, *NS17*, 585; M. H. Sleisenger and Y. S. Kim, *New Engl. J. Med.*, 1979, *300*, 659; *Med. Lett.*, 1979, *21*, 62; R. K. Chandra, *Bull. Wld Hlth Org.*, 1979, *57*, 167.

A discussion of enteral feeding.— *Drug & Ther. Bull.*, 1980, *18*, 77.

Trace Elements. Fourteen trace elements are believed to be essential for animal life.

Chromium is considered to be involved in the activation of insulin; deficiency states have been described; trivalent chromium is generally well tolerated; no accurate estimate of daily requirement can be made.

Cobalt is active in man as vitamin B_{12}; there may be a link with iodine and thyroid hormonogenesis; cobalt causes polycythaemia and thyroid hyperplasia; the dietary intake is generally well below that required to cause toxic effects.

Copper is a component of several amine oxidases and is probably essential for haemopoiesis; copper deficiency has been reported in infants; tolerance to copper is generally good. A daily intake of 80 µg per kg body-weight has been suggested for infants and young children with 40 and 30 µg per kg respectively for older children and adults.

Manganese is considered essential for animal life, but deficiency in man has not been demonstrated. Industrial toxicity has been reported; otherwise manganese is well tolerated. A daily intake of 2 to 3 mg maintains a positive manganese balance.

Molybdenum is a component of several enzymes; there is some evidence to suggest an association between gout and a high intake of molybdenum; molybdenum equilibrium appears to be maintained with a daily intake of 2 µg per kg body-weight.

Nickel deficiency has been reported in *animals* and *birds*; deficiency is unlikely in humans taking a conventional diet; the margin between required and toxic concentrations is wide.

Selenium deficiency or excess causes disease in *animals* and *birds*; selenium deficiency has also been reported in man, a safe and adequate intake is considered to be 50 to 200 µg daily for adults. It may be involved in the functioning of membranes and the synthesis of amino acids. Dietary intake varies widely.

Tin deficiency has not been recognised in man; the daily intake (adults) is estimated to be at least 3.5 mg; ingestion of 5 to 7 mg per kg body-weight has caused mild toxicity; canned food might contribute to the intake.

Vanadium deficiency has been reported in *animals* and *birds*; the metabolic role is not clear; dietary exposure in man appears to be well below toxic concentrations.

Zinc is a component of some enzymes; others are zinc-dependent; zinc deficiency causes a number of pathological states in man; the range between dietary intake and toxic concentrations is wide; provisional estimates of daily requirements of available zinc are 1.1 to 1.25 mg for infants, up to 2.65 to 2.8 mg for children, 2.2 mg for adult males and females, with higher amounts in pregnancy and lactation. Additional zinc is necessary in some diets.

Fluorine, *iodine*, *iron*, and *silicon* are also considered essential.

References: *Trace Elements in Human Nutrition*, Report of a WHO Expert Committee, *Tech. Rep. Ser. Wld Hlth Org. No. 532*, 1973; W. Mertz, *Clin. Chem.*, 1975, *21*, 468; J. G. Reinhold, *ibid.*, 476; R. E. Burch *et al.*, *ibid.*, 501; D. D. Ulmer, *New Engl. J. Med.*, 1977, *297*, 318; A. S. Prasad, *Trace Elements and Iron in Human Metabolism*, Chichester, John Wiley, 1978; W. Gooddy, *Practitioner*, 1979, *222*, 637.

Infant Feeding. There is a variety of preparations used as alternatives to breast milk in the feeding of infants and the composition and use of these preparations has caused much controversy. Special care is needed to avoid hypernatraemia, hyperosmolality, and cerebral dehydration.

Reviews and discussions of infant feeding.— *Br. med. J.*, 1973, *2*, 727. See also J. C. L. Shaw *et al.*, *ibid.*, 12; P. W. Wilkinson *et al.*, *ibid.*, 15; R. K. Oates, *ibid.*, 762; R. W. Logan *et al.*, *Archs Dis. Childh.*, 1974, *49*, 200; *Postgrad. med. J.*, 1975, *51, Suppl.* 3, 1–78; D. P. Addy, *Br. med. J.*, 1976, *1*, 1268; B. A. Wharton and H. M. Berger, *ibid.*, 1326; A. E. Mettler, *Postgrad. med. J.*, 1976, *52, Suppl.* 8;; J. Barley and O. G. Brooke (letter), *Lancet*, 1976, *2*, 799; G. T. Lealman *et al.*, *Archs Dis. Childh.*, 1976, *51*, 377; J. D. Mitchell *et al.*, *Lancet*, 1977, *1*, 500; D. J. Naismith *et al.*, *Archs Dis. Childh.*, 1978, *53*, 845; E. M. Widdowson, *Postgrad. med. J.*, 1978, *54*, 176; O. G. Brooke, *Practitioner*, 1978, *221*, 314; *Lancet*, 1978, *1*, 1250; *ibid.*, 1240; D. B. Jelliffe and E. F. P. Jelliffe (letter), *ibid.*, 1978, *2*, 263; *Br. med. J.*, 1978, *2*, 781; G. McEnery and B. Chattopadhyay, *ibid.*, 794; C. W. Woodruff, *J. Am. med. Ass.*, 1978, *240*, 657; J. H. Tripp *et al.*, *Br. med. J.*, 1979, *2*, 707; E. W. Saunders (letter), *Lancet*, 1980, *2*, 42; S. Sjölin (letter), *ibid.*, 1981, *1*, 612.

Possible reduced incidence of coeliac disease in childhood related to changes in infant feeding practices.— J. M. Littlewood *et al.*, *Lancet*, 1980, *2*, 1359.

Modified Diets. Diet may need to be modified in some disorders including diabetes mellitus, obesity, porphyria, and renal disease.

The treatment of acute hepatic porphyria and the role of a high carbohydrate intake.— *Lancet*, 1978, *1*, 1024.

Diet in the management of chronic renal failure.— *Drug & Ther. Bull.*, 1978, *16*, 61.

The nutritional management of enterocutaneous fistulas.— *Lancet*, 1979, *2*, 507.

A review of the use of elemental diets.— R. I. Russell and M. J. Hall, *Practitioner*, 1979, *222*, 631.

The use of elemental diets and whole-protein diets in 40 unconscious patients with head injury.— D. C. Jones *et al.*, *Br. med. J.*, 1980, *280*, 1493.

Hyperkinesis. An 'elimination diet' (Kaiser-Permanente diet, KP diet, Feingold diet), free from artificial colours and flavours and claimed to reduce hyperkinesis, was being evaluated scientifically. Meanwhile the American Academy of Pediatrics urged parents not to use the diet on a long-term basis.— T. Larkin, *FDA Consumer*, 1977, (Mar.), 19.

Criticism of the Feingold diet.— T. H. Jukes, *New Engl. J. Med.*, 1977, *297*, 427.

There was no good evidence to indicate that the use of a Feingold diet, which excluded artificial colours, artificial flavours, and sometimes salicylates, was effective in the treatment of hyperactivity in children.— *Med. Lett.*, 1978, *20*, 55. A similar conclusion from a small double-blind study.— F. Levy *et al.*, *Med. J. Aust.*, 1978, *1*, 61.

The limited value of elimination diets in childhood.— *Br. med. J.*, 1980, *280*, 138.

Obesity. A weight-reducing regimen of supplemented fasting with a protein-sugar diet and added potassium and multivitamins was successfully used in a large-scale outpatient programme involving 519 massively obese patients. When the programme was enlarged to 1300 patients 4 sudden deaths occurred, 3 of which were of patients who had showed evidence of coronary disease. It was suggested that patients who had ECG evidence of ischaemia or of ventricular irritability should be thoroughly evaluated before being accepted for a supplemented fasting programme.— V. Vertes *et al.*, *J. Am. med. Ass.*, 1977, *238*, 2142 and 2151.

A discussion of the clinical use of a protein-sparing modified fast.— B. R. Bistrian, *J. Am. med. Ass.*, 1978, *240*, 2299.

Low-energy protein diets. Low-energy protein diets (also termed low-calorie protein diets were marketed under various trade names. Descriptions included 'last chance diet', 'predigested liquid protein', 'PDLP', 'protein-sparing fast', 'protein supplement', 'amino acids', 'collagen', and 'gelatin with tryptophan'. Most consisted of modified proteins or hydrolysates of low nutritional quality, sometimes fortified with amino acids, vitamins, and minerals. Common complaints included nausea, vomiting, diarrhoea, constipation, faintness, muscle cramps, fatigue, irritability, cold intolerance, decreased libido, amenorrhoea, hair loss, and dry skin. More serious were cardiac arrhythmias, recurrence of gout, dehydration, and hypokalaemia; 40 deaths had occurred; for 15 no underlying cause was found; 11 occurred while on the diet and 4 within 2 weeks of returning to a normal diet. Careful medical supervision was essential and these diets should not generally be used in patients taking specified potent drugs, in those with significant renal, hepatic, cardiovascular, or cerebrovascular disease, in pregnancy or lactation, in psychiatric disease, or in children. The efficacy of such diets over diets of equivalent protein content was not established; older patients were at risk, particularly from orthostatic hypotension; supplementation with vitamins, minerals, and potassium was essential; return to normal diet should be gradual over 1 to 3 weeks. A mandatory warning label was proposed.— *FDA Drug Bull.*, 1978, *8*, 2. Deaths reported now totalled 58.— *ibid.*, 18.

Further references: *Med. Lett.*, 1977, *19*, 69; P. Felig, *New Engl. J. Med.*, 1978, *298*, 1025; *Lancet*, 1978, *2*, 976; T. B. Van Itallie, *J. Am. med. Ass.*, 1978, *240*, 144.

A report of 6 women aged 21 to 67 years who developed thrombophlebitis within 1 to 3 weeks of starting a liquid-protein diet.— H. J. Roberts (letter), *New Engl. J. Med.*, 1978, *298*, 165.

A report on a liquid dietary regimen believed to be safe if used with caution and for restricted periods.— I. M. Baird *et al.* (letter), *Lancet*, 1979, *1*, 618.

Adverse Effects. Adverse reactions have occurred to a large number of components of food and to food additives; symptoms vary widely. Reactions may be caused by immunological processes or by a deficiency of specific enzymes. Deficiency of enzymes may be congenital. Components of food have been suggested as being involved in the aetiology of various diseases.

References.— M. Harrison *et al.*, *Br. med. J.*, 1976, *1*, 1501; J. A. Walker-Smith, *Practitioner*, 1978, *220*, 562; *Lancet*, 1978, *2*, 715; C. J. Glueck *et al.*, *New Engl. J. Med.*, 1978, *298*, 1471; L. J. Bennion and S. M. Grundy, *ibid.*, 1978, *299*, 1221; *Lancet*, 1979, *1*, 249; *Lancet*, 1980, *2*, 1344.

The neurotoxic effects of some amino acids and their analogues.— J. S. Kizer *et al.*, *Pharmac. Rev.*, 1977, *29*, 301.

Parenteral Nutrition. Parenteral nutrition (parenteral alimentation; intravenous hyperalimentation) is used when adequate nutrition is impossible or undesirable by mouth, by gastric or duodenal tube, or by ostomy. The object is (a) to maintain a positive nitrogen balance (particularly for those at risk from increased catabolism caused by stress, sepsis, trauma, and burns), and (b) to provide an adequate source of energy (the requirements for which are also increased), vitamins, trace elements, and other essential factors, particularly in long-term treatment.

The indications are many and varied and include pre-operative supplemental feeding, postoperative feeding in patients unable to take food by mouth 72 to 96 hours after surgery, gastro-intestinal fistulas, postoperative renal failure, neoplastic disease, burns, severe inflammatory bowel disease, and in those who no longer have a functioning small bowel.

For short-term treatment for up to about one week access may be by a cannula placed in a peripheral vein though because of the hyperosmolality of the solution a catheter placed in a central vein may be preferred. For longer-term treatment access is by catheter. Arteriovenous shunts can be used. The use of an infusion pump is desirable.

Protein may be supplied as protein hydrolysates (solutions of amino acids and peptides, see p.58) or as solutions of amino acids, usually the latter.

Energy is supplied as dextrose, laevulose, alcohol, or fat. Dextrose is the preferred carbohydrate. Because of the high energy value of fat and the low osmolality of fat emulsions it is usual to supply up to 50% of the energy requirement as a fat emulsion.

Vitamins and trace elements may need to be added to the solutions; requirements of trace elements may be met for short periods by infusions of blood or plasma; essential fatty acid requirements are usually met by the fat emulsion.

Treatment should be related to the needs of the individual patient; factors to be considered include the total volume to be infused, the electrolyte balance, the acid-base balance, and the ability of the plasma to clear fat. Technique must be meticulous to avoid damage to veins or inadvertent intra-arterial injection, and to reduce the risk of bacterial or fungous infection.

Thrombophlebitis is nearly always a problem in peripheral veins. Folate deficiency may lead to pancytopenia and megaloblastic anaemia. Hypophosphataemia, disturbance of liver function, and fatty acid deficiency may occur. The use of large amounts of dextrose may lead to hyperglycaemia and necessitate the use of insulin.

Raised intracranial pressure occurred in 3 of 12 children given hyperalimentation intravenously.— L. A. O'Tuama *et al.* (letter), *Lancet*, 1973, *2*, 1101.

Hyperammonaemia was a hazard of parenteral alimentation.— V. D. Larkin (letter), *Pediatrics*, 1973, *51*, 584.

The properties of some amino-acid solutions for intravenous use.— D. Tweedle, *Br. J. Hosp. Med.*, 1975, *13*, 81.

A rational approach to parenteral nutrition.— B. W. Ellis *et al.*, *Br. med. J.*, 1976, *1*, 1388.

A discussion of intravenous feeding in infancy.— *Br. med. J.*, 1977, *1*, 1490. See also V. Y. H. Yu *et al.*, *Archs Dis. Childh.*, 1979, *54*, 653.

The umbilical artery or vein was an acceptable route of administration for total parenteral nutrition in infants.— R. T. Hall and P. G. Rhodes, *Archs Dis. Childh.*, 1977, *51*, 929.

Parenteral nutrition in the newborn.— F. Cockburn, *Br. J. Hosp. Med.*, 1977, *18*, 191.

Metabolic aspects of intensive care.— S. P. Allison, *Br. J. Anaesth.*, 1977, *49*, 689.

Deficiencies in parenteral nutrition, with special reference to vitamins and trace metals.— *Br. med. J.*, 1978, *2*, 913.

A report of long-term total parenteral nutrition in the home in 19 patients.— K. Ladefoged and S. Jarnum, *Br. med. J.*, 1978, *2*, 262.

Further references to parenteral nutrition in the home: D. G. Miller *et al.*, *Ann. intern. Med.*, 1979, *91*, 858; *Br. med. J.*, 1980, *281*, 1407; S. Grundfest and E. Steiger, *J. Am. med. Ass.*, 1980, *244*, 1701.

Use in patients with malignant disease.— S. J. Dudrick *et al.*, *Cancer Res.*, 1977, *37*, 2440; B. Eriksson and H. O. Douglass, *J. Am. med. Ass.*, 1980, *243*, 2049.

Use in patients with leucopenia.— A. Dindogru *et al.*, *J. Am. med. Ass.*, 1980, *244*, 680.

A discussion of parenteral nutrition before surgery.— *Br. med. J.*, 1979, *2*, 1529.

Beneficial effect in patients with alcoholic hepatitis.— S. M. Nasrallah and J. T. Galambos, *Lancet*, 1980, *2*, 1276.

A review of the possible hazards associated with intravenous feeding.— *Adverse Drug React. Bull.*, 1979, Aug., 276. See also M. Shike *et al.*, *Ann. intern. Med.*, 1980, *92*, 343 (osteomalacia).

Other references and reviews.— J. T. Harries, *Archs Dis. Childh.*, 1971, *46*, 855; S. J. Dudrick and R. L. Ruberg, *Gastroenterology*, 1971, *61*, 901; H. L. Flack *et al.*, *Am. J. Hosp. Pharm.*, 1971, *28*, 326; *Parenteral Nutrition*, An International Symposium, London, 1971, A.W. Wilkinson (Ed.), London, Churchill Livingstone, 1972; F. D. Moore and M. F. Brennan, *New Engl. J. Med.*, 1972, *287*, 862; *Med. Lett.*, 1972, *14*, 73; *Drug & Ther. Bull.*, 1972, *10*, 49; M. E. Shils, *J. Am. med. Ass.*, 1972, *220*, 1721 (AMA Council on Foods and Nutrition); C. F. Anderson *et al.*, *ibid.*, 1973, *223*, 68; *Lancet*, 1973, *2*, 1179; P. J. Benjamin, *Med. J. Aust.*, 1974, *2*, 295; M. J. T. Peaston, *Practitioner*, 1974, *212*, 552; P. Puri *et al.*, *Archs Dis. Childh.*, 1975, *50*, 133; H. A. Lee and T. F. Hartley, *Postgrad. med. J.*, 1975, *51*, 441; O. Juhl, *Nutr. Metab.*, 1976, *20*, *Suppl.* 1, 6; D. V. Feliciano and R. L. Telander, *Mayo Clin. Proc.*, 1976, *51*, 647; J. J. Skillman *et al.*, *New Engl. J. Med.*, 1976, *295*, 1037; R. P. Craig *et al.*, *Lancet*, 1977, *2*, 8; D. H. Law, *New Engl. J. Med.*, 1977, *297*, 1104; M. Deitel *et al.*, *Can. J. Hosp. Pharm.*, 1977, *30*, 175; *Current Concepts in Parenteral Nutrition*, J.M. Greep *et al.* (Ed.), The Hague, Martinus Nijhoff, 1977; *Advances in Parenteral Nutrition*, I.D.A. Johnston (Ed.), Lancaster, MTP Press, 1978; J. Powell-Tuck *et al.*, *Lancet*, 1978, *2*, 825; H. Fromm *et al.*, *Dt. med. Wschr.*, 1978, *103*, 377; R. Sorkness, *J. parent. Drug Ass.*, 1980, *34*, 80; *Drug & Ther. Bull.*, 1980, *18*, 85.

Trace elements in parenteral nutrition. Following routine administration of a dextrose solution containing in each 500 ml, zinc 40 µmol, calcium 7.5 mmol, and magnesium 9.0 mmol, zinc supplementation had been necessary in only 1 of 76 surgical patients. A similar solution containing phosphate 30 mmol and potassium 30 mmol per 500 ml was also available.— B. W. Ellis *et al.* (letter), *Lancet*, 1978, *2*, 380.

Guidelines for essential trace element preparations for parenteral use.— *J. Am. med. Ass.*, 1979, *241*, 2051.

Other references.— B. E. James and R. A. MacMahon, *Aust. paediat. J.*, 1976, *12*, 154; C. A. Shearer and R. C. Bozian, *Drug Intell. & clin. Pharm.*, 1977, *11*, 465; R. L. Hull and D. Cassidy, *ibid.*, 536; M. A. L. Odne *et al.*, *Am. J. Hosp. Pharm.*, 1978, *35*, 1057.

571-m

Acetylmethionine. Methionamine. DL-2-Acetamido-4-(methylthio)butyric acid.
$C_7H_{13}NO_3S$=191.2.

CAS — 1115-47-5.

Pharmacopoeias. In *Aust.* and *Braz.*

A white crystalline powder with a characteristic odour and a slightly bitter disagreeable taste. M.p. about 114° **Soluble** 1 in 6 of water and 1 in 2 of alcohol; soluble in acetone. **Protect** from light.

Uses. Acetylmethionine has been used as an adjuvant in the treatment of liver disease.

572-b

Alanine *(U.S.P.).* L-Alanine. L-2-Aminopropionic acid.
$C_3H_7NO_2$=89.09.

CAS — 56-41-7.

Pharmacopoeias. In *U.S.*

A white odourless crystalline powder with a sweetish taste. **Soluble** 1 in about 6 of water; sparingly soluble in alcohol; practically insoluble in ether. A solution in hydrochloric acid is dextrorotatory. A 5% solution in water has a pH of 5.5 to 7. **Protect** from light.

Uses. Alanine is an amino acid present in many foods and has been used as a dietary supplement. DL-Alanine is similarly used.

Alanine 50 g daily by mouth in divided doses reversed hypoglycaemia and ketosis and reduced muscle catabolism in obese subjects starved for 2 weeks.— S. M. Genuth, *Metabolism*, 1973, *22*, 927.

Alanine, a potent stimulant of glucagon secretion, was used in a study of glucagon secretion in patients with acute and chronic pancreatitis. Plasma-pancreatic glucagon concentrations were measured in the basal state and after intravenous infusion of alanine 150 mg per kg body-weight over 2 to 4 minutes.— M. Donowitz *et al.*, *Ann. intern. Med.*, 1975, *83*, 778.

573-v

Arginine *(U.S.P.).* L-Arginine. L-2-Amino-5-guanidinovaleric acid.
$C_6H_{14}N_4O_2$=173.2.

CAS — 74-79-3.

Pharmacopoeias. In *Cz.* and *U.S.*

White, almost odourless crystals. Freely **soluble** in water; sparingly soluble in alcohol; practically insoluble in ether. A solution in hydrochloric acid is dextrorotatory.

Uses. Arginine is an amino acid used in solutions of amino acids for intravenous use.

574-g

Arginine Glutamate.

The L-arginine salt of L-glutamic acid.
$C_6H_{14}N_4O_2,C_5H_9NO_4$=321.3.

CAS — 4320-30-3.

A white crystalline powder. **Soluble** in water. A 5.37% solution in water is iso-osmotic with serum.

Incompatibility. Arginine glutamate 2.5 g was 'physically incompatible' with thiopentone sodium 250 mg in 100 ml of dextrose injection.— R. D. Dunworth and F. R. Kenna, *Am. J. Hosp. Pharm.*, 1965, *22*, 190.

Uses. Arginine glutamate has been used in conjunction with other therapeutic measures in the treatment of hyperammonaemia. It is administered by intravenous infusion in a dose of 25 g in 500 or 1000 ml of Dextrose Intravenous Infusion 5 or 10% infused over 1 to 4 hours; more rapid infusions may cause vomiting. The dose may be repeated after 8 to 12 hours if needed.

Homocystinuria. A 20-fold increase in homocystine excretion and a 7-fold increase in cystine excretion following an intravenous infusion of arginine glutamate suggested that renal tubular reabsorption of homocystine and cystine was reduced during the infusion, probably by the arginine.— D. C. Cusworth and A. Gattereau (letter), *Lancet*, 1968, *2*, 916.

575-q

Arginine Hydrochloride

(U.S.P.). L-Arginine Hydrochloride.
$C_6H_{14}N_4O_2,HCl$=210.7.

CAS — 1119-34-2.

Pharmacopoeias. In *U.S.*

A white or almost white odourless crystalline powder. M.p. about 235° with decomposition. Each g represents approximately 4.7 mmol (4.7 mEq) of chloride. Freely **soluble** in water; slightly soluble in hot alcohol; practically insoluble in ether. A solution in hydrochloric acid is dextrorotatory. **Protect** from light.

Adverse Effects. Vomiting may occur if solutions are administered too rapidly. The chloride content may cause hyperchloraemic acidosis. Concentrations of urea, creatine, and creatinine may be elevated.

A 10-year-old boy experienced an anaphylactic reaction 5 minutes after the start of an infusion of a 5% arginine hydrochloride solution in a test for growth-hormone output.— C. M. Tiwary *et al.* (letter), *New Engl. J. Med.*, 1973, *288*, 218.

Precautions. Arginine hydrochloride should not be given to patients with anuria.

Two alcoholic patients with severe liver disease and moderate renal insufficiency developed severe hyperkalaemia following administration of arginine hydrochloride and one died. Both patients had received a total dose of 300 mg of spironolactone some time before arginine hydrochloride administration, but the contribution of spironolactone to the hyperkalaemia was not known. Caution in the administration of arginine hydrochloride to patients with hepatic or renal insufficiency was advised.— D. A. Bushinsky and F. J. Gennari, *Ann. intern. Med.*, 1978, *89*, 632.

Uses. Arginine hydrochloride is used similarly to sodium glutamate (see p.59) in the treatment of hyperammonaemia, and may be better tolerated, but the presence of a chloride ion may be detrimental in some conditions. The usual dose of arginine hydrochloride is 20 g by intravenous infusion in 500 to 1000 ml of Dextrose Intravenous Infusion 5 or 10% over 1 to 4 hours. The dose may be repeated after 8 to 12 hours if needed.

Arginine is an amino acid which may be essential to the growth of infants.

The intravenous infusion of arginine hydrochloride in doses of 25 g, or 500 mg per kg body-weight, in 500 ml of Water for Injections usually stimulates the release of growth hormone by the pituitary gland and is used as a test of pituitary function.

The aspartate has also been used.

It is also used as a food supplement.

Studies in healthy subjects showed that arginine produced a marked increase in the urinary excretion of proteins, possibly due to an inhibition of tubular reabsorption.— C. E. Mogensen *et al.*, *Lancet*, 1975, *2*, 581.

Cystic fibrosis. Arginine hydrochloride aerosol was used as a mucolytic in the treatment of 24 children with cystic fibrosis. They had previously been using acetylcysteine. Five children had to withdraw owing to severe deterioration of their condition and appearance of a severe cough. Bronchoscopy 4 to 10 weeks later showed a deterioration in the endoscopic picture in most of the other children and hypersecretion had increased in 15. It was considered that arginine was not an effective mucolytic agent.— H. -J. Dietzsch *et al.*, *Pediatrics*, 1975, *55*, 96. For earlier reports see C. C. Solomons *et al.*, *ibid.*, 1971, *47*, 384; J. Kattwinkel *et al.*, *ibid.*, 1972, *50*, 133.

Hepatic encephalopathy. In a group of 32 patients, 29 of whom had cirrhosis of the liver, the effect of intravenous infusion of 30 g of arginine hydrochloride in 500 ml of water was compared with that of 500 ml of Dextrose Intravenous Infusion. There was no significant difference between the effects of the 2 solutions on the clinical status or blood-ammonia concentrations.— T. B. Reynolds *et al.*, *Am. J. Med.*, 1958, *25*, 359.

Hepatitis. Vigorous medical management of acute fulminant hepatitis included the intravenous administration of arginine hydrochloride (Argivene) for rapid correction of alkalosis.— M. O. Auslander and G. L. Gitnick, *Archs intern. Med.*, 1977, *137*, 599.

Hyperammonaemia. Apparent recovery of an infant with hyperammonaemia, due to argininosuccinase deficiency, after treatment with arginine.— S. W. Brusilow and M. L. Batshaw, *Lancet*, 1979, *1*, 124. See also C. Bachmann *et al.* (letter), *New Engl. J. Med.*, 1981, *304*, 543.

Infertility. A study in 18 men with infertility, of whom 15 were followed up, did not confirm early reports of the value of arginine. The sperm count rose in only one patient after treatment for 1 to 2 months with arginine 4 g daily.— M. L. Jungling and R. G. Bunge, *Fert. Steril.*, 1976, *27*, 282. See also J. P. Pryor *et al.*, *Br. J. Urol.*, 1978, *50*, 47.

Test in diabetes mellitus. Intravenous infusion of 30 g of arginine hydrochloride over 30 minutes increased the blood-glucose concentration markedly in patients with prematurity-onset diabetes, moderately in patients with maturity-onset diabetes, and only slightly in healthy persons. Compared with healthy persons, the response of immunoreactive serum insulin in maturity-onset diabetics was poor following the infusion. Arginine appeared to be useful in the study of diabetes; it enabled abnormalities to be detected even in mild forms of the disease.— L. L. Sparks *et al.*, *Diabetes*, 1967, *16*, 268. See also T. J. Merimee *et al.* (preliminary communication), *Lancet*, 1966, *1*, 1300; G. Tchobroutsky *et al.* (letter), *Lancet*, 1966, *2*, 498.

Preparations

Arginine Hydrochloride Injection *(U.S.P.).* A sterile solution of arginine hydrochloride 9.5 to 10.5% in Water for Injections; it contains no antimicrobial agents. pH 5 to 6.5.

Proprietary Names

Argamin *(Rio, S.Afr.)*; R-Gene *(Cutter, USA)*; Spermargin (arginine) *(Farber-Ref, Ital.)*.

A preparation containing arginine hydrochloride and dihydrate was formerly marketed in Great Britain under the proprietary name Arginine-Sorbitol (EGIC) *(Servier)*.

576-p

Aspartic Acid. L-Aspartic acid. L-Aminosuccinic acid.
$C_4H_7NO_4$=133.1.

CAS — 56-84-8.

White odourless crystals with an acidic taste. M.p. about 271°. **Soluble** 1 in about 200 of water; practically insoluble in alcohol and ether; soluble in acids and alkalis. **Protect** from light.

Uses. Aspartic acid is an amino acid present in many foods. DL-Aspartic acid is used as a dietary supplement.

A 12-year study of the effects of aspartic acid in chronic hepatitis.— O. Fodor *et al.*, *Acta hepato-splenol.*, 1971, *18*, 383.

The development of physical dependence and tolerance to morphine in *rats* was prevented by aspartic acid.— H. Koyuncuoglu *et al.*, *Arzneimittel-Forsch.*, 1977, *27*, 1676.

577-s

Carbocisteine.

Carbocysteine; AHR-3053; LJ 206. *S*-Carboxymethyl-L-cysteine.
$C_5H_9NO_4S$=179.2.

CAS — 2387-59-9; 638-23-3 (L).

Carbocisteine is **incompatible** with Pholcodine Linctus.

Adverse Effects. Nausea, headache, gastric discomfort, diarrhoea, gastro-intestinal bleeding, and skin rash have occasionally occurred.

Precautions. It is recommended that carbocisteine be used with caution in patients with a history of peptic ulcer and be avoided in patients with active ulceration.

Uses. Carbocisteine is used similarly to methyl cysteine hydrochloride (see p.57) in the treatment of disorders of the respiratory tract associated with excessive mucus. The usual dose in 750 mg thrice daily, reduced by one-third when a response is obtained. A suggested dose for children aged 2 to 5 years is 62.5 to 125 mg four times daily and for those aged 5 to 12 years 250 mg thrice daily.

In 11 healthy subjects given carbocisteine 1 g mean plasma concentrations were about 13 and 2 µg per ml 2 and 10 hours respectively after administration.— W. R. Maynard *et al.*, *J. pharm. Sci.*, 1978, *67*, 1753.

Evidence that sulphoxidation of carbocisteine (Mucodyne) is regulated by the same gene that controls the oxidation of debrisoquine and other drugs.— R. H. Waring *et al.* (letter), *Lancet*, 1981, *1*, 778.

Bronchitis. In a double-blind study in 28 patients with chronic bronchitis carbocisteine 750 mg thrice daily or bromhexine 16 mg thrice daily both increased sputum volume and 'pourability' of sputum, without improving ventilatory capacity or peak expiratory flow-rates. Clinical benefit was considered to be greater after carbocisteine and the effect of carbocisteine appeared to be more rapid.— M. Aylward, *Curr. med. Res. Opinion*, 1973, *1*, 219.

A critical evaluation. — *Drug & Ther. Bull.*, 1975, *13*, 11.

Carbocisteine or bromhexine were no more effective than a placebo in improving ventilatory function in 30 patients with chronic obstructive lung disease, though carbocisteine reduced sputum viscosity.— A. Muittari and M. Linnoila, *Curr. ther. Res.*, 1977, *22*, 246.

In a double-blind study in 20 patients with stable chronic bronchitis there was a significant mean clinical improvement in those given carbocisteine 1 g thrice daily for 2 weeks compared with those given a placebo. Sputum viscosity was increased. Carbocisteine should be considered a mucoregulator, not a mucolytic.— E. Puchelle *et al.*, *Eur. J. clin. Pharmac.*, 1978, *14*, 177.

Further references: M. Aylward, *Curr. med. Res. Opinion*, 1974, *2*, 387; R. Glosauer *et al.*, *Therapiewoche*, 1976, *26*, 6533.

Otitis media. A favourable report of the use of carbocisteine in secretory otitis media (glue ear).— P. H. Taylor and N. Dareshani, *Br. J. clin. Pract.*, 1975, *29*, 177. See also R. J. McGuiness, *ibid.*, 1977, *31*, 105.

In a double-blind study in 52 children with seromucinous otitis media (glue ear) there was no statistical evidence of benefit from carbocisteine over placebo in 44 children treated for 1 month or in 37 treated for 3 months. Doses used were: aged 3 to 4 years, 250 mg twice daily; 5 to 10 years, 250 mg thrice daily.— R. T. Ramsden *et al.*, *J. Lar. Otol.*, 1977, *91*, 847.

Proprietary Preparations

Mucodyne *(Berk Pharmaceuticals, UK)*. Carbocisteine, available as **Capsules** of 375 mg; as **Paediatric Syrup** containing 125 mg in each 5 ml; and as **Syrup** containing 250 mg in each 5 ml.

Mucolex *(Warner, UK)*. Carbocisteine, available as **Syrup** containing 250 mg in each 5 ml and as **Tablets** of 375 mg.

Other Proprietary Names

Actithiol, Broncodeterge Simple, Pectox *(all Spain)*; Bronchipect *(Neth.)*; Fluifort, Lisomucil, Mucojet *(all Ital.)*; Mucocaps, Mucosirop *(both S.Afr.)*; Mucolitic *(Arg.)*; Mucopront, Transbronchin *(both Ger.)*; Rhinathiol *(Fr., Neth., Switz.)*.

A preparation containing carbocisteine was formerly marketed in Great Britain under the proprietary name Visclair S (*Sinclair*).

578-w

Casein. An amphoteric phosphoprotein which may be prepared by the action of acid or rennet on caseinogen, the principal protein occurring in milk, which is the main commercial source.

CAS — 9000-71-9.

Pharmacopoeias. In *Hung.*

Casein contains about 15% of nitrogen, about 0.7% of phosphorus, and about 0.8% of sulphur. It occurs as an odourless, tasteless, white or yellowish-white powder or granules. Practically **insoluble** in water, alcohol, and ether; soluble, with turbidity, in solutions of alkali hydroxides. **Store** in airtight containers.

Uses. Casein may be used in the preparation of protein hydrolysates and, usually in the form of its calcium, potassium, or sodium salts, it is used in various nutritive preparations and proprietary foods, see p.63.

579-e

Cysteine Hydrochloride *(U.S.P.)*. L-Cysteine Hydrochloride. L-2-Amino-3-mercaptopropionic acid hydrochloride monohydrate.
$C_3H_7NO_2S,HCl,H_2O$=175.6.

CAS — 52-90-4 (cysteine); 52-89-1 (hydrochloride, anhydrous); 7048-04-6 (hydrochloride, monohydrate).

Pharmacopoeias. In *Cz.* and *U.S. Fr.* permits anhydrous or monohydrate. *Cz.* also includes DL-Cysteine Hydrochloride.

White crystals or crystalline powder with a slight characteristic odour and acid taste. M.p. about 175° with decomposition. **Soluble** in water, alcohol, and acetone; practically insoluble in ether. It is unstable in solution forming cystine on exposure to air. A solution in hydrochloric acid is dextrorotatory. **Store** in a cool place in airtight containers. Protect from light.

Uses. Cysteine is an amino acid occurring naturally in glutathione (see p.53). It is used topically in ophthalmology. Cysteine has also been used in some proprietary antibiotic preparations applied topically in the treatment of damaged skin. It is also used as a dietary supplement.

Perforations of the cornea occurred in only 1 of 33 eyes severely burnt with alkali which were treated with 0.2M cysteine solution applied as 2 drops 6 times daily after 7 days' routine treatment with antibiotics and cycloplegics; perforations occurred in 5 of 7 eyes not treated with cysteine. Progress of corneal ulcers in 3 badly burnt eyes was arrested immediately after the use of cysteine eye-drops.— S. I. Brown *et al.*, *Am. J. Ophthal.*, 1972, *74*, 316.

Preparations

Cysteine Eye-drops *(Moorfields Eye Hosp.)*. Cysteine hydrochloride 1.576 g and benzalkonium chloride 10 mg in iso-osmotic solution to 100 ml. Contain 100 mmol per litre. Eye-drops containing 200 and 300 mmol per litre are also used. For inactivation of collagenase and for stromal corneal melting.

580-b

Cystine. L-Cystine; Di(α-aminopropionic)-β-disulphide; β,β'-Dithiodialanine. L-3,3'-Dithiobis(2-aminopropionic acid).
$C_6H_{12}N_2O_4S_2$=240.3.

CAS — 56-89-3.

Colourless practically odourless crystals. Very slightly **soluble** in water and alcohol; soluble in dilute mineral acids and alkaline solutions.

Uses. Cystine is an amino acid present in many foods; it has been used in the treatment of congenital homocystinuria and as a dietary supplement.

The biological half-life of cystine was reported to be 43 days.— W. A. Ritschel, *Drug Intell. & clin. Pharm.*, 1970, *4*, 332.

The preparation of cystine eye-drops.— J. R. B. J. Brouwers, *Pharm. Weekbl. Ned.*, 1977, *112*, 155.

Homocystinuria. A diet providing only 10 mg of methionine daily per kg body-weight in conjunction with treatment with cystine 1.5 g daily and choline dihydrogen citrate 10 g daily in divided doses, decreased plasma concentrations of methionine and homocystine in 3 children with homocystinuria. In addition, a 3-year-old child treated with a low-methionine diet and cystine since early infancy had remained mentally and physically normal. Choline might facilitate enzymic remethylation of homocystine to methionine.— T. L. Perry *et al.*, *Lancet*, 1968, *2*, 474.

Three children with homocystinuria responded to treatment with a low-methionine diet and supplements of cystine over an 8-month period.— I. B. Sardharwalla *et al.*, *Can. med. Ass. J.*, 1968, *99*, 731.

Proprietary Names

Gélucystine *(Sarep-Pharmeurop, Fr.)*.

581-v

Dextrin. British Gum; Starch Gum.

CAS — 9004-53-9.

Pharmacopoeias. In *Aust.*, *Chin.*, *Cz.*, *Ger.*, *Jap.*, *Jug.*, *Pol.*, *Port.*, and *Span.*

An intermediate product in the ultimate hydrolysis of starch, made by heating starch, which has been moistened with a small quantity of dilute nitric acid, at 110° to 115°.

A white or yellowish amorphous powder or granules with a slight characteristic odour and a sweet taste. It does not reduce Fehling's solution. Slowly **soluble** in cold water and readily soluble in boiling water forming a mucilaginous solution; practically insoluble in alcohol, chloroform, and ether. **Store** in airtight containers.

Uses. Dextrin is an ingredient of some infant foods and is used as an adhesive and stiffening agent for surgical dressings. It has many industrial uses as a binding and thickening agent.

Proprietary Preparations

Caloreen *(Roussel, UK)*. A water-soluble mixture of dextrins consisting predominantly of polysaccharides containing an average of 5 glucose molecules, with sodium less than 1.8 mmol per 100 g and potassium less than 0.3 mmol per 100 g. For use as a source of carbohydrate. (Also available as Caloreen in *Austral.*, *Denm.*).

Caloreen had a mean molecular weight of about 840 which did not change after heating. No increase in the reducing sugar content occurred after 4 hours at 115° to 116°. A 22% solution was iso-osmotic with serum.— D. E. Bott *et al.*, *Pharm. J.*, 1970, *1*, 583.

The use of Caloreen and Albumaid by nasogastric tube.— A. M. J. Woolfson *et al.*, *Postgrad. med. J.*, 1976, *52*, 678.

Crystal Gum S *(Laing-National, UK)*. A brand of dextrin containing carbohydrate not less than 98% of dry weight.

Maxijul *(Scientific Hospital Supplies, UK)*. A water-soluble mixture of dextrins consisting predominantly of polysaccharides containing an average of 5 glucose molecules, providing in each 100 g sodium 2 mmol and potassium 0.1 mmol. For use in certain malabsorption syndromes. **Maxijul LE** is a similar preparation, providing sodium and potassium 0.01 mmol per 100 g. For use as a source of carbohydrate when electrolyte restriction is necessary.

582-g

Anhydrous Dextrose *(B.P., B.P. Vet.)*.

Anhydrous Dextrose for Parenteral Use *(Eur. P.)*; D-Glucose; Anhydrous Glucose; Anhydrous Grape Sugar; Dextrosum Anhydricum ad Usum Parenterale; Glucosum; Glycosum; Saccharum Amylaceum. D-(+)-Glucopyranose.
$C_6H_{12}O_6$=180.2.

CAS — 50-99-7.

Pharmacopoeias. In *Aust.*, *Belg.*, *Br.*, *Cz.*, *Eur.*, *Fr.*, *Ger.*, *Hung.*, *Jap.*, *Neth.*, *Pol.*, *Port.*, *Roum.*, *Span.*, and *Swiss*. *Arg.*, *Braz.*, *Ind.*, *It.*, *Jug.*, and *U.S.* specify anhydrous or monohydrate.

Colourless crystals or a white odourless crystalline or granular powder with a sweet taste. At relative humidities between about 35 and 85% at 25° it absorbs significant amounts of moisture and the monohydrate is formed at the higher humidities; at relative humidities below 35% and above 85%, insignificant and substantial amounts of moisture are absorbed respectively.

Soluble 1 in 1 of water and 1 in 200 of alcohol; soluble in glycerol; practically insoluble in ether. A solution in water is dextrorotatory. A 5.05% solution in water is iso-osmotic with serum. Solutions are **sterilised,** immediately after preparation, by autoclaving or by filtration. **Store** in airtight containers.

NOTE. The *B.P.* directs that when Anhydrous Dextrose is prescribed or demanded, Anhydrous Dextrose or an equivalent amount of Dextrose Monohydrate for Parenteral Use may be dispensed or supplied.

583-q

Dextrose Monohydrate *(B.P., B.P. Vet.)*.

Dextrose; Glucose; Glucosum; Medicinal Glucose; Purified Glucose; Grape Sugar; Glycosum Hydratum; Traubenzucker. D-(+)-Glucopyranose monohydrate.
$C_6H_{12}O_6,H_2O$=198.2.

CAS — 14431-43-7.

Pharmacopoeias. In *Aust.*, *Br.*, *Chin.*, *Hung.*, *Int.*, *Mex.*, *Nord.*, and *Rus.* Dextrose (*U.S.P.*) is the monohydrate or the anhydrous material. *Arg.*, *Braz.*, *Ind.*, *It.*, and *Jug.* also specify anhydrous or monohydrate.
U.S. also includes Dextrose Excipient—dextrose monohydrate for non-parenteral use.

Odourless colourless cyrstals or a white or cream-coloured crystalline or granular powder with a sweet taste. **Soluble** 1 in 1 of water and 1 in 200 of alcohol; soluble in glycerol; practically insoluble in ether. A solution in water is dextrorotatory. A 5.51% solution in water is iso-osmotic with serum.

NOTE. The *B.P.* directs that when Medicinal Glucose or Purified Glucose is prescribed or demanded, Dextrose Monohydrate be dispensed or supplied.

Solutions for injection are prepared from Anhydrous Dextrose or Dextrose Monohydrate for Parenteral Use.

584-p

Dextrose Monohydrate for Parenteral Use *(B.P., Eur. P.)*.

Glucose for Parenteral Use; Dextrosum Monohydricum ad Usum Parenterale.
$C_6H_{12}O_6,H_2O$=198.2.

Pharmacopoeias. In *Br.*, *Eur.*, *Fr.*, *Ger.*, *Neth.*, *Swiss*, and *Turk*.

A white odourless crystalline powder with a sweet taste. Dextrose monohydrate 1.1 g is approximately equivalent to anhydrous dextrose 1 g. **Solubility, Sterilisation,** and **Storage** as for Anhydrous Dextrose (above).

NOTE. The *B.P.* directs that when Anhydrous

Dextrose is prescribed or demanded, Anhydrous Dextrose or an equivalent amount of Dextrose Monohydrate for Parenteral Use may be dispensed or supplied.

Decomposition on sterilisation. The fall in pH observed during the autoclaving of dextrose solutions was due to the degradation of dextrose to a product which had not yet been isolated. This product was subsequently degraded to 5-hydroxymethylfurfural and finally, it was believed, to formic and laevulinic acids.— R. B. Taylor *et al.*, *J. Pharm. Pharmac.*, 1972, *24*, 121. See also R. B. Taylor and V. C. Sood, *ibid.*, 1978, *30*, 510.

The reduced content of dextrose in autoclaved dextrose-lactate solutions was probably due mainly to decomposition of the dextrose. This decomposition could be reduced to negligible levels by adjusting the pH to about 4 before autoclaving.— Pharm. Soc. Lab. Rep. P/74/12, 1975.

Furfural had been identified as a decomposition product of dextrose solution after prolonged heating.— H. Ogata *et al.* (letter), *J. Pharm. Pharmac.*, 1978, *30*, 668.

Effect of gamma-irradiation. Gamma-irradiation at 20 000 Gy changed the colour of dextrose from white to cream; the specific rotation of a solution showed no significant change.— *The Use of Gamma Radiation Sources for the Sterilisation of Pharmaceutical Products*, London, ABPI, 1960.

Incompatibility. There was loss of clarity when intravenous solutions of dextrose were mixed with those of cyanocobalamin, kanamycin sulphate, novobiocin sodium, or warfarin sodium.— J. A. Patel and G. L. Phillips, *Am. J. Hosp. Pharm.*, 1966, *23*, 409.

The wide range of pH allowed (3.5 to 6.5) for Dextrose Injection *U.S.P.* could be a disadvantage since an additive could be stable in one bottle of injection but not in another. Erythromycin gluceptate was stable only between pH 6 and 7.5, and lost 70 to 80% of its potency at pH 4.5 in 15 minutes without any visible sign of degradation. Only if the pH of the dextrose injection were greater than 5.05 could stability be assured.— M. Edward, *Am. J. Hosp. Pharm.*, 1967, *24*, 440.

Stability with alcohol. An intravenous solution of dextrose (5%) containing 7.5% of alcohol, sterilised by autoclaving at 115° for 45 minutes, was stable at room temperature for 14 months.—Pharm. Soc. Lab. Rep., *Pharm. J.*, 1959, *1*, 9.

Tablet excipient. The use of a commercial food grade of dextrose monohydrate compared with spray-dried lactose as an excipient in the preparation of tablets by direct compression.— R. N. Duvall *et al.*, *J. pharm. Sci*, 1965, *54*, 1196.

Dextrose 95 to 96% in conjunction with 4 to 5% of higher saccharides (dextrates: Celutab, *Penick & Ford, USA*) was a suitable agent for direct compression tablet making.— N. L. Henderson and A. J. Bruno, *J. pharm. Sci.*, 1970, *59*, 1336. See also E. J. Mendell, *Mfg Chem.*, 1972, *43* (May), 43.

Adverse Effects. Concentrated dextrose solutions given by mouth may cause nausea and vomiting.

Intravenous infusions of concentrated dextrose injections are liable to cause local vein irritation. Thrombophlebitis has followed the intravenous infusion of iso-osmotic dextrose injections with low pH due to overheating during sterilisation. Hypophosphataemia may occur after prolonged use.

Intravascular haemolysis occurred in an 18-year-old black male with hereditary spherocytosis given dextrose 5% in sodium chloride 0.225%, and dextrose 5% intravenously, after splenectomy.— S. K. Minn *et al.* (letter), *Blood*, 1972, *40*, 297, per *Int. pharm. Abstr.*, 1973, *10*, 758.

In a 55-year-old man with hypopituitarism, syncope and hypotension occurred on 2 occasions within 30 minutes of ingestion of glucose during a standard glucose-tolerance test. This reaction was attributed to inadequate adrenocortical response to hypovolaemia in a patient already hypovolaemic and hypotensive.— J. Sagel and J. A. Colwell, *J. Am. med Ass.*, 1973, *226*, 667.

A 6-year-old girl, accidentally given 380 ml of 50% dextrose intravenously in an hour, developed headache, seizures and respiratory arrest and was successfully resuscitated. The blood-glucose concentration was 18.5 mg per ml and serum osmolality was 372 milliosmoles. She suffered irreversible brain damage.— C. A. Stanley and L. Baker, *J. Pediat.*, 1974, *84*, 270.

Toxicity of autoclaved solutions. The use of dextrose injection sterilised by autoclaving, as opposed to the use of an injection sterilised by filtration, had been suggested as a cause of thrombophlebitis following intravenous infusion. Though an attempt had been made to divorce the method of sterilisation from the production of this condition (T.J. McNair and H.A.F. Dudley, *Lancet*, 1959, *2*, 365), D.W. Vere and others (*ibid.*, 1960, *2*, 627) showed that thrombophlebitis was more than twice as common with an autoclaved solution (pH about 3.5) as with a solution sterilised by filtration (pH about 6). Neutralisation of 5% dextrose solution to pH 6.8 with phosphate buffer resulted in the incidence of thrombophlebitis being reduced from about 20 to 1% when solutions were given intravenously in 220 controlled infusions.— G. Elfving *et al.* (letter), *Lancet*, 1966, *2*, 226.

The incidence of phlebitis after infusion of dextrose solutions had been reduced to 7 to 10% in adults and virtually eliminated in infants by adding sufficient sodium bicarbonate to raise the pH of the infusion above 7. Each litre of 5% dextrose in water required about 8 ml of 7.5% sodium bicarbonate injection.— E. W. Fonkalsrud (letter), *New Engl. J. Med.*, 1969, *280*, 1480.

Precautions. Dextrose is contra-indicated in patients with the glucose-galactose malabsorption syndrome. Dextrose tolerance may be impaired in patients with renal failure and in the early post-traumatic state or in those with severe sepsis.

Dextrose infusions, even if iso-osmotic, should not be mixed with whole blood; haemolysis and clumping has occurred.

Intravenous feeding with solutions containing insulin and dextrose was followed by deterioration in chronically malnourished patients. Severe hypophosphataemia and cellular overhydration often leading to cerebral oedema were observed.— P. D. Wright (letter), *Lancet*, 1973, *2*, 1335.

In a controlled study of 50 women in the first stage of labour with ketonuria and ketonaemia, it was confirmed that not only treatment with infusion of hyperosmotic laevulose solution, but also treatment with infusion of hyperosmotic sorbitol and dextrose solutions carried a risk of exacerbating pre-existing lactic acidosis and precipitating foetal distress.— A. C. Ames *et al.*, *Br. med. J.*, 1975, *4*, 611. Dextrose with added insulin would fulfil the requirement for the treatment of ketonaemia without raising the blood-lactic acid concentration.— S. J. Tovey (letter), *ibid.*, 1976, *1*, 222.

Effect on ECG. Electrocardiograms of some women given dextrose showed significant changes in rate, rhythm, ST-segment level, or T-wave amplitude. Routine ECG tracings should not be recorded for several hours after ingestion of dextrose.— L. D. Ostrander, *Am. J. med. Sci.*, 1966, *251*, 399.

Effect on gastric acid. Dextrose injection 5% significantly suppressed gastric acid secretion in 15 volunteers compared with saline infusion. Tests of gastric acid function could be affected by dextrose infusion.— J. G. Moore, *Gastroenterology*, 1973, *64*, 1106.

Gastrectomy. The glucose-tolerance test, when carried out in gastrectomised patients, might precipitate a 'dumping' syndrome resulting in profound shock and minor symptoms including nausea and weakness. In such patients glucose should be given intravenously.— H. N. Naumann (letter), *J. Am. med. Ass.*, 1966, *195*, 700.

Hyperkalaemia. Administration of dextrose 50 g by mouth to 8 insulin-dependent subjects who had not received insulin for about 12 to 26 hours provoked a paradoxical rise in plasma-potassium concentrations compared with the expected fall in control subjects. Intravenous administration of dextrose as a therapeutic test in comatose diabetic patients might aggravate hyperkalaemia in insulin-deprived subjects and should perhaps be abandoned.— G. C. Viberti, *Lancet*, 1978, *1*, 690. See also S. Goldfarb *et al.*, *Ann. intern. Med.*, 1976, *84*, 426.

Intolerance. Glucose intolerance was noted in patients undergoing repeated dialysis for uraemia.— R. H. Hutchings *et al.*, *Ann. intern. Med.*, 1966, *65*, 275.

In patients being treated with peritoneal dialysis or haemodialysis there was an inverse relationship between blood-sugar and plasma-potassium concentrations; 4 patients who developed hyperglycaemia when large concentrations of dextrose were added to the dialysate fluid also had low plasma-potassium concentrations. Correction of potassium deficiency was necessary if large amounts of dextrose were used in dialysate fluids.— Y. K. Seedat, *Lancet*, 1968, *2*, 1166. Secreted insulin could have lowered plasma-potassium concentrations without affecting the hyperglycaemia.— B. J. Boucher and L. Strunin (letter), *ibid.*, 1969, *1*, 55. A reply.— Y. K. Seedat (letter), *ibid.*, 104.

Glucose intolerance, hyperglycaemia, failure of insulin secretion, and high concentrations of free fatty acids were found in 12 patients undergoing glucose-tolerance tests within 15 hours of cardiac infarction.— S. P. Allison *et al.*, *Br. med. J.*, 1969, *4*, 776.

Pregnancy and the neonate. The likelihood of early neonatal hypoglycaemia was diminished when the rate of administration of dextrose to diabetic mothers in labour was decreased.— I. J. Light *et al.*, *Am. J. Obstet. Gynec.*, 1972, *113*, 345.

A study indicating that prolonged intravenous infusions of more than 10 g of dextrose per hour to mothers in labour, can cause considerable stimulation of foetal insulin secretion.— A. Lucas *et al.* (letter), *Lancet*, 1980, *1*, 144. In women undergoing caesarean section the rate should not exceed 5 g per hour.— N. B. Kenepp *et al.* (letter), *ibid.*, 645.

Absorption and Fate. Dextrose is absorbed from the gastro-intestinal tract. Three pathways of metabolism are established: glycolysis leading to the formation of pyruvate (aerobic) or lactate (anaerobic), followed by the Krebs tricarboxylic acid cycle (citric acid cycle), leading to metabolism to carbon dioxide and water; a pentose phosphate pathway leads also to carbon dixoide and water. Energy is released in these processes. Dextrose is also stored as glycogen in the liver and muscle. Blood-glucose concentrations are maintained, in healthy persons, within normal limits by insulin, which facilitates the passage of glucose through cell membranes, and other homoeostatic mechanisms. The body can metabolise about 800 mg per kg body-weight hourly.

Uses. Dextrose is given by mouth as a readily absorbed carbohydrate in conditions associated with insufficiency of carbohydrates; it provides a rapidly available source of energy. It also reduces the need for the metabolism of fats and thus prevents ketonaemia. In the absence of sufficient dextrose the amount of fat oxidised is greatly increased and intermediate products such as hydroxybutyric acid and acetoacetic acid accumulate in the blood giving rise to ketosis.

In fevers and other conditions where the nitrogen excretion is raised, the administration of dextrose can diminish nitrogen loss, but this is limited.

Dextrose, with electrolytes, is given orally or parenterally to treat diarrhoea and vomiting in infancy.

A 5% solution of dextrose is given intravenously to replete or maintain body water; when it is desired to replace excessive salt loss, sodium chloride must be added to the solution. A suitable solution contains 4% of anydrous dextrose and 0.18% of sodium chloride.

Hyperosmotic dextrose solutions (10 to 50%) for parenteral nutrition are given by central venous catheter to minimise reactions. Similar solutions are given by intravenous injection to provide temporary relief from the symptoms of cerebral oedema, and for hypoglycaemic coma, but such solutions are liable to cause venous thrombosis at the site of injection. Hyperosmotic dextrose with or without insulin may correct hyperkalaemia in renal failure and also some forms of hyponatraemia.

Concentrated (50% or more) solutions have been used for the injection treatment of varicose veins, but recanalisation and pulmonary embolism are likely to occur.

Dextrose is given by mouth or intravenously in glucose-tolerance tests to aid in the diagnosis of diabetes mellitus (for further details see under Insulin and other Antidiabetic Agents, p.843).

Dextrose may be administered by mouth in solution or, when necessary, a 5% solution may be given rectally as a retention enema. When dextrose is required in infant feeding to supplement the carbohydrate content of cows' milk, dextrose monohydrate is usually employed.

Dextrose may be used to adjust the osmotic pressure of dialysis fluids and injections.

Dextrose 150 g daily reduced the ileostomy fluid losses by 1 litre daily in a patient who had undergone jejunostomy and colectomy.— M. J. Kendall and C. F. Hawkins, *Lancet*, 1971, *2*, 411. See also C. D. Gerson, *ibid.*, 1972, *2*, 353; D. R. Nalin (letter), *ibid.*, 596; C. D. Gerson (letter), *ibid.*, 762.

For the use of 200 ml of 50% dextrose solution by mouth as a dumping provocation test, see J. P. S. Thomson *et al.*, *Gut*, 1974, *15*, 200.

In 89 patients with multiple injuries serum concentrations of cholesterol, free fatty acids, and total lipids fell after the intravenous administration of hyperosmotic dextrose solution; no case of fat embolism occurred.— R. H. Horne and J. H. Horne, *Archs intern. Med.*, 1974, *132*, 288, per *J. Am. med. Ass.*, 1974, *227*, 816.

Cholera. A discussion of dextrose and electrolyte solutions given by mouth for cholera and acute diarrhoea.— *Lancet*, 1975, *1*, 79.

See also under Sodium Chloride, p.637.

Diagnosis of growth-hormone deficiency. A prolonged glucose-tolerance test detected growth-hormone deficiency.— L. Stimmler *et al.*, *Can. med. Ass. J.*, 1967, *97*, 1159. See also G. Boden *et al.*, *Metabolism*, 1968, *17*, 1.

Dialysis. Despite reports that carbohydrate intolerance, common in uraemia, was improved by regular haemodialysis, studies in 10 patients showed that the ability to dispose of an acute glucose load was no better 6 hours after dialysis than 77 hours after dialysis. The acute effects of haemodialysis on glucose tolerance were probably weak, transitory, and unpredictable.— E. Ferrannini *et al.*, *Br. med. J.*, 1977, *2*, 803.

In a double-blind study, infusion of 50 ml (or less) of Strong Dextrose Injection over 5 minutes relieved 17 of 26 episodes of dialysis-induced muscle cramps in 15 chronically uraemic patients, although infusion of sodium chloride injection 50 ml relieved only 5 of 18 similar episodes of muscle cramps.— J. Milutinovich *et al.*, *Ann. intern. Med.*, 1979, *90*, 926.

Glucose-tolerance test. Tests in 133 persons showed that the intravenous injection of 50 g of dextrose per 1.73 m^2 body-surface in a 25% solution over 4 to 6 minutes provided a more sensitive test of glucose tolerance than the use of dextrose by mouth.— D. R. Dyck and J. A. Moorhouse, *J. clin. Endocr. Metab.*, 1966, *26*, 1032, per *Abstr. Wld Med.*, 1967, *41*, 469.

In a study of 33 healthy men and women subjected to 3 oral glucose-tolerance tests (50 g) over a period of 2 weeks, glucose tolerance was better after a 12-hour fast than after an 8-hour or 4-hour fast in those aged over 40 years but not in younger persons. The fasting period before tests should be standardised and in the case of potential diabetics should be 12 hours as recommended by the British Diabetic Association.— C. H. Walsh *et al.*, *Br. med. J.*, 1973, *2*, 691. Oral glucose tests in 17 healthy men aged 22 to 24 years showed that late mild reactive hypoglycaemia occurred after a 12-hour but not after a 4-hour pre-test fast.— P. M. Trenchard, *Br. J. clin. Pract.*, 1975, *29*, 173.

The intravenous glucose-tolerance test was reproducible during the second and third trimesters of pregnancy, but not during the puerperium. In neonates an intravenous glucose-tolerance test was performed by using 500 mg of dextrose per kg body-weight given as a 20% solution through a catheter in the umbilical vein.— H. W. Sutherland *et al.*, *Br. med. J.*, 1973, *3*, 9.

Abnormal glucose-tolerance tests in patients with obstructive jaundice.— N. G. Soler *et al.*, *Br. med. J.*, 1974, *4*, 447.

A discussion on the interpretation of results of glucose-tolerance tests.— C. Reynolds and D. B. Orchard, *Can. med. Ass. J.*, 1977, *116*, 1223.

For details of the WHO recommendations for glucose-tolerance tests see under Insulin and other Antidiabetic Agents, p.843.

Hypoglycaemia. A review of the treatment of spontaneous hypoglycaemia.— V. Marks, *Br. med. J.*, 1972, *1*, 430.

A discussion on the treatment of hyperglycaemic and hypoglycaemic crises.— S. R. Newmark *et al.*, *J. Am. med. Ass.*, 1975, *231*, 185.

Myocardial infarction. For the use of dextrose in conjunction with potassium chloride and insulin in the treatment of myocardial infarction, see under Potassium Chloride, p.630.

Pneumothorax. An episode of pneumothorax in a patient with cystic fibrosis was successfully treated with closed thoracotomy and the intrapleural instillation of 25% dextrose solution, but the pneumothorax recurred 11 days later. The patient experienced transient chest pain.— T. F. Boat *et al.*, *J. Am. med. Ass.*, 1969, *209*, 1498.

Pregnancy and the neonate. In 148 and 111 pregnant patients with low urinary oestriol excretion the infusion of dextrose 25% raised the concentration to normal values in 65 and 59% respectively. The incidence of foetal growth retardation and malformation was independent of the response to dextrose.— N. A. Beischer *et al.*, *Med. J. Aust.*, 1977, *2*, 641. See also A. Chang *et al.*, *Am. J. Obstet. Gynec.*, 1977, *127*, 793.

For reference to the risks of foetal insulin secretion following maternal administration of dextrose see under Precautions (Pregnancy and the Neonate).

Test of insulin productive capacity. As a test of pancreatic beta-cell reserve in patients with chronic pancreatitis, a dose of 75 g of dextrose was followed 30 minutes later by a rapid intravenous injection of 500 mg of tolbutamide and 1 mg of glucagon. In healthy persons, peak serum-immunoreactive-insulin concentrations exceeded 750 micro-units per ml; in patients with chronic pancreatitis the response was significantly less.— B. I. Joffe *et al.*, *Lancet*, 1968, *2*, 890.

Preparations of Anhydrous Dextrose and Dextrose Monohydrate

Dextrose and Glycerol Instillation *(A.P.F.)*. Glucose and Glycerin Nasal Drops. Dextrose [monohydrate] 20 g, glycerol to 100 ml. Store in well-filled airtight containers.

Dextrose Intravenous Infusion *(B.P.)*. Dextrose Injection. A sterile solution of anhydrous dextrose or dextrose monohydrate for parenteral use in Water for Injections. Sterilised, immediately after preparation, by autoclaving. Potency is expressed in terms of anhydrous dextrose. pH 3.5 to 5.5. Store at a temperature not exceeding 25°. Similar injections of various strengths are included in many other pharmacopoeias. In *Martindale*, dextrose injection is 5% unless otherwise specified.

NOTE. The *B.P.* directs that when dextrose injection is required as a diluent for official injections, Dextrose Intravenous Infusion 5% shall be used.

Dextrose Injection *(U.S.P.)*. A sterile solution of anhydrous dextrose or dextrose monohydrate for parenteral use in Water for Injections; it contains no antimicrobial agents. Potency is expressed in terms of dextrose monohydrate. pH of a solution containing not more than 5% of dextrose, 3.5 to 6.5.

Glucose 25% in Glycerol Nasal Drops *(Roy. Nat. T. N. and E. Hosp.)*. Dextrose monohydrate 25 g, glycerol to 100 ml. Heat together over a water-bath, with shaking, to dissolve (solution is slow). Sterilise by maintaining at 150° for 1 hour; fill aseptically into sterile containers.

Strong Dextrose Injection *(B.P.C. 1973)*. A sterile 50% solution of anhydrous dextrose (or an equivalent quantity of dextrose monohydrate for parenteral use) in Water for Injections. pH 3.5 to 5.5. Store in a cool place.

For irreversible brain damage associated with 50% dextrose infusion, see p.51.

Proprietary Preparations

Emdex *(Mendell, USA: K & K-Greeff, UK)*. Contains dextrose monohydrate 90 to 93% and maltose 2 to 5%, with higher glucose saccharides. For use as a tablet excipient.

Glucodin *(Farley, UK)*. A powder containing dextrose monohydrate, with ascorbic acid 50 mg in each 100 g.

GluCoplex 1000 *(Geistlich, UK)*. A solution containing anhydrous dextrose 240 g per litre and electrolytes, providing 4200 kJ and the following ions: sodium 50 mmol, potassium 30 mmol, magnesium 2.5 mmol, chloride 67 mmol, dihydrogen phosphate 18 mmol, and a trace amount of zinc. For use as an energy source in intravenous nutrition. **GluCoplex 1600.** A similar solution containing anhydrous dextrose 400 g per litre, providing 6700 kJ and the same ions.

Other Proprietary Names

Dextromon *(Ger.)*; Dextropur *(Denm.)*; Glutose *(USA)*; Nutrosa *(hydrochloride) (Arg.)*.

A preparation containing dextrose monohydrate for glucose-tolerance testing was formerly marketed in Great Britain under the proprietary name Pal-A-Dex *(Diamed)*.

585-s

Liquid Glucose *(U.S.N.F., B.P.C. 1963)*. Liq. Glucos.; Corn Syrup.

CAS — 8027-56-3.

Pharmacopoeias. In *Chin.*, *Fr.*, and *Hung.* Also in *U.S.N.F.*

A colourless or yellowish, odourless or almost odourless, very viscous syrup with a sweet taste obtained by the incomplete hydrolysis of starch. It consists chiefly of a mixture of dextrose, maltose, dextrins, and water. The dextrose content is only 10 to 20%. **Miscible** with water; sparingly soluble in alcohol. **Store** in airtight containers.

Isoglucose is the name used to describe a glucose syrup with a high fructose content; obtained from starch processed to glucose; a substitute for liquid sugar obtained from sugar-beet or cane. Defined as 'the syrup obtained from glucose syrups with a content by weight in the dry state of at least 10% of fructose and at least 1% in total of oligosaccharides and polysaccharides'.

The preparation of liquid glucose.— J. D. Commerford, in *Symposium: Sweeteners*, G.E. Inglett (Ed.), Westport, AVI, 1974, p. 78. For details of a form of liquid glucose containing a high concentration of laevulose see J. M. Newton and E. K. Wardrip, *ibid.*, p. 87; G. A. Brooks *et al.*, *ibid.*, p. 97.

Adverse Effects and Precautions. As for Dextrose, p.51.

Uses. Liquid glucose is sometimes used instead of dextrose for oral administration. It has also been used as a pill excipient, either alone or as liquid glucose syrup. It is not suitable for injection.

Preparations

Liquid Glucose Syrup *(B.P.C. 1963)*. Syr. Glucos. Liq.; Glucose Syrup. Liquid glucose 33.3% w/w in syrup.

NOTE. Glucose Syrup as defined by the Specified Sugar Products Regulations 1976 (SI 1976: No. 509) consists of a purified concentrated aqueous solution of nutritive saccharides obtained from starch and contains not less than 70% of dry matter of which not less than 20% consists of dextrose.

Hycal *(Beecham Foods, UK)*. A protein-free, low-electrolyte, liquid carbohydrate preparation based on demineralised liquid glucose syrup, containing 49.5% of carbohydrates and providing 1000 kJ (244 kcal) per 100 ml; available in 4 flavours. For the management of patients with acute or chronic renal failure, and for other conditions requiring a high-energy, low-fluid, and low-electrolyte diet.

586-w

Glutamic Acid. Glutaminic Acid. L-(+)-2-Aminoglutaric acid.

$C_5H_9NO_4$=147.1.

CAS — 56-86-0.

Pharmacopoeias. In *Aust.*, *Belg.*, *Chin.*, *Cz.*, *It.*, *Jug.*, *Pol.*, *Port.*, *Roum.*, *Rus.*, and *Swiss.*

A white crystalline powder with an acid taste. M.p. 185° to 205° with decomposition. **Soluble** 1 in 140 of water and 1 in 7 of boiling water; practically insoluble in alcohol, acetone, chloroform, ether, and glacial acetic acid. A saturated solution in water has a pH of about 3.2. **Protect** from light.

Adverse Effects.

For background toxicological information, see *Fd Add. Ser. Wld Hlth Org. No. 5*, 1974.

Uses. Glutamic acid has been given by mouth in the treatment of hyperammonaemia in conditions such as hepatic encephalopathy, usually following a short course of therapy with sodium glutamate intravenously (see p.59).

Glutamic acid was also formerly employed to reduce attacks of petit mal and to increase mental and physical alertness in mentally retarded patients, but its value in these conditions has not been established.

It has been given in doses of 5 to 12 g daily in divided doses.

It has been used as a salt substitute and as a dietary supplement.

For a review of the effects of glutamic acid on cognitive behaviour, see W. Vogel *et al.*, *Psychol. Bull.*, 1966, *65*, 367.

Estimated acceptable daily intake for adults, and children over 12 weeks: up to 120 mg, additional to that from all natural sources, per kg body-weight.— Seventeenth Report of the FAO/WHO Expert Committee on Food Additives, *Tech. Rep. Ser. Wld Hlth Org. No. 539*, 1974.

Mental retardation. There was no acceptable evidence that glutamic acid supplements were of any value in brain-damaged children.— *Br. med. J.*, 1975, *1*, 202.

Proprietary Names

Glutacid (see also under Glutamic Acid Hydrochloride) *(Treupha, Switz.)*; Glutamin *(Verla, Ger.)*; Glutaminol *(Laroche Navarron, Fr.)*.

587-e

Glutamic Acid Hydrochloride. Aciglumin. L-(+)-2-Aminoglutaric acid hydrochloride.
$C_5H_9NO_4,HCl=183.6$.

CAS — 138-15-8.

Pharmacopoeias. In *Nord.* and *Roum.*

A white crystalline powder with a characteristic odour and a sour taste. **Soluble** 1 in 3 of water; practically insoluble in alcohol, chloroform, and ether. Solutions in water are acid to litmus. **Incompatible** with alkalis and magnesium. **Protect** from light.

Uses. Glutamic acid hydrochloride, in aqueous solution, releases hydrochloric acid. It was formerly employed similarly to Dilute Hydrochloric Acid in the treatment of achlorhydria and hypochlorhydria but is no longer considered to be effective. It was usually administered in capsules or tablets, in a dose of 0.6 to 1.8 g, with or immediately after meals.
It is also used as a salt substitute and flavouring agent.

Preparations

Aciglumin Tablets *(Nord. P.)*. Tablettae Aciglumini. Each contains glutamic acid hydrochloride 300 mg.

Muripsin *(Norgine, UK)*. Tablets each containing glutamic acid hydrochloride 500 mg and pepsin 35 mg. For achlorhydria and hypochlorhydria. *Dose.* 1 or 2 tablets with each meal.

Other Proprietary Names

Acidogene *(Spain)*; Acidulin *(Austral., Canad., S.Afr., USA)*; Glutacid (see also under Glutamic Acid) *(Norw.)*; Hypochylin *(Swed.)*.

Glutamic acid hydrochloride was also formerly marketed in Great Britain under the proprietary name Muripsin Plain (*Norgine*).

588-l

Glutathione. Glutathione SH; GSH. *N*-(*N*-L-γ-Glutamyl-L-cysteinyl)glycine.
$C_{10}H_{17}N_3O_6S=307.3$.

CAS — 70-18-8.

A naturally occurring tripeptide, which takes part in detoxication mechanisms in the body. Glutathione is freely **soluble** in water and in dilute alcohol. M.p. about 195° with decomposition.

Uses. Glutathione has been given to patients with hepatic cirrhosis with the object of aiding liver function but results have been disappointing (G.C. Cook and S. Sherlock, *Gut*, 1965, *6*, 472). It has also been used in the treatment of alcoholism, and has been suggested for use in the treatment of infectious hepatitis, of certain skin diseases, and of poisoning by exogenous substances that block the action of enzymes containing thiol (–SH) groups.

Proprietary Names

Glutathiol *(Joullié, Fr.)*; Agifutol S, Atomolan, Beamthion, Detoxan, Estathion, Hydrathion, Ledac, Mohathion, Panaron, Tathiclon, Tathion, Torichion (all *Jap.)*; Reglution (reduced glutathione) *(LEFA, Spain)*; Tition (reduced glutathione) *(Jorba, Spain)*.

589-y

Glycine *(B.P.)*. Aminoacetic Acid *(U.S.P.)*; Acidum Aminoaceticum; Glycocol; Sucre de Gélatine.

$NH_2.CH_2.CO_2H=75.07$.

CAS — 56-40-6.

Pharmacopoeias. In *Arg., Br., Braz., Cz., Jap., Mex., Turk.,* and *U.S.*

A white odourless crystalline powder with a sweet taste. M.p. about 234° with decomposition. **Soluble** 1 in 4 of water; very slightly soluble in alcohol and ether; practically insoluble in dehydrated alcohol. A 5% solution in water has a pH of 5.9 to 6.3. A 2.19% solution in water is iso-osmotic with serum. Solutions may be **sterilised** by autoclaving.

Uses. Glycine is the simplest of the amino acids. It is sometimes used in conjunction with calcium carbonate and other antacids in the treatment of gastric hyperacidity. It is also used as an ingredient of some aspirin tablets with the object of reducing gastric irritation. Sterile solutions of glycine 1.5% in water are used for bladder irrigation during genito-urinary surgery.
Doses of up to 30 g daily, in divided doses, have been given.

The biological half-life of glycine was reported to be 240 hours.— W. A. Ritschel, *Drug Intell. & clin. Pharm.*, 1970, *4*, 332.

Glycine, 10 g thrice daily with food, has been used in the treatment of a child with hyperprolinaemia, the daily proline content of the diet being maintained at about 10 mg per kg body-weight.— J. R. Cooke and D. N. Raine, in *Treatment of Inborn Errors of Metabolism*, J.W.T. Seakins *et al.* (Ed.), London, Churchill Livingstone, 1973.

Isovaleric acidaemia, an inborn error of leucine metabolism, was successfully treated with glycine 250 mg per kg body-weight daily by mouth in 2 infants who became seriously ill during the first 2 weeks of life. Serum concentrations of isovaleric acid declined sharply within 3 days of starting treatment but clinical improvement was slower. Neurological function was not restored to normal for about 2 weeks and pancytopenia persisted until the third week. Treatment was continued for about 6 and 12 months respectively after leaving hospital and glycine 800 mg daily, as a 10% solution in water, in 4 divided doses, was well tolerated. The development of each infant was normal.— R. M. Cohn *et al.*, *New Engl. J. Med.*, 1978, *299*, 996. See also A. Velazquez and E. C. Prieto (letter), *Lancet*, 1980, *1*, 313.

Glycine might be useful in the treatment of poisoning by the unripe fruits of the Jamaican akee.— H. S. A. Sherratt and S. S. Al-Bassam (letter), *Lancet*, 1976, *2*, 1243.

Cholera. In a study in 136 patients with severe dehydration due to cholera, a solution containing glycine 110 mmol, dextrose 110 mmol, bicarbonate 48 mmol, chloride 72 mmol, citrate 8.3 mmol, potassium 25 mmol, and sodium 120 mmol per litre was given by mouth or nasogastric tube to 68, after rehydration with intravenous fluids, until the blood pressure was normal. The solution was absorbed sufficiently well to provide maintenance fluid and electrolytes, and reduced the duration and volume of diarrhoea compared with a similar solution containing no glycine given to the other 68 patients.— D. R. Nalin *et al.*, *Gut*, 1970, *11*, 768. See also D. R. Nalin and R. A. Cash, *Trans. R. Soc. trop. Med. Hyg.*, 1970, *64*, 769.

Glycine-tolerance test. A detailed account of a modified glycine-tolerance test. A dose of 10 g of free glycine per 70 kg body-weight or the equivalent of the peptides, glycylglycine and glycylglycylglycine, was followed by serial estimations of glycine and alpha-amino nitrogen in peripheral plasma. Patients after gastrectomy or with a non-functional pylorus absorbed glycine and glycylglycine more rapidly than normal, while 3 of 7 patients with idiopathic steatorrhoea had extremely depressed curves suggesting severe retardation of absorption.— I. L. Craft *et al.*, *Gut*, 1968, *9*, 425.

Preparations

Aminoacetic Acid Irrigation *(U.S.P.)*. A sterile solution of glycine in Water for Injections. pH 4.5 to 6.5.

Glycine Urological Irrigating Solution *(Travenol, UK)*. Contains 1.5%.

Other Proprietary Names

Glicoamin *(Ital.)*; Glykokoll *(Swed.)*.

590-g

Histidine *(U.S.P.)*. L-Histidine. L-2-Amino-3-(1*H*-imidazol-4-yl)propionic acid.
$C_6H_9N_3O_2=155.2$.

CAS — 71-00-1.

Pharmacopoeias. In *U.S.P.*

White odourless crystals with a bitter taste. **Soluble** in water; very slightly soluble in alcohol; practically insoluble in ether. A solution in hydrochloric acid is dextrorotatory. A 10% solution in water has a pH of 3.5 to 4.5.

591-q

Histidine Hydrochloride. Histidine Monohydrochloride; Histidinium Chloride. L-Histidine hydrochloride monohydrate.
$C_6H_9N_3O_2,HCl,H_2O=209.6$.

CAS — 645-35-2 (anhydrous).

Pharmacopoeias. In *Aust., Span.,* and *Swiss.*

Colourless almost odourless crystals with a slightly acid bitter taste. M.p., after drying, about 250° with decomposition. **Soluble** 1 in 8 of water; practically insoluble in alcohol, chloroform, and ether. A solution in water is acid to litmus.

Uses. Histidine is an essential amino acid for infants and growing children but is not considered essential for adults. In infants with histidinaemia, a rare disease caused by faulty histidine metabolism, a diet low in histidine may be given up to the age of 2 years and then reviewed.
It is given by mouth, usually in a single dose of 15 g, in the investigation of folate deficiency, and is used as a dietary supplement.

Histidine loading test. For the investigation of folate deficiency, histidine hydrochloride 15 g was given as a single dose by mouth, or in a dose of 120 mg per lb body-weight. Urine was collected for the next 8 hours in a bottle containing hydrochloric acid to prevent the hydrolysis of formimino-glutamic acid (FIGLU), the amount of this substance and urocanic acid in the urine being assessed quantitatively. Active folate was required for the catabolism of histidine to FIGLU to glutamic acid, and in folate deficiency there was a block to the further metabolism of FIGLU which accumulated and was excreted in the urine. Other factors might also affect the excretion of FIGLU and urocanic acid after a loading dose of histidine, and a positive result required careful interpretation.— *Br. med. J.*, 1969, *2*, 100.

Proprietary Names

Laristine (hydrochloride) *(Roche, Fr.)*; Larostidine (hydrochloride) *(Roche, Belg.)*; Plexamine (hydrochloride) *(Biodica, Fr.)*; Ulcusemol (ascorbate) *(Saet, Spain)*.

Histidine hydrochloride was formerly marketed in Great Britain under the proprietary name Histicaps (*Geistlich*).

592-p

Purified Honey *(B.P.)*. Mel Depuratum; Clarified Honey; Strained Honey; Mel Despumatum; Miel Blanc; Gereinigter Honig.

CAS — 8028-66-8 (honey).

Pharmacopoeias. In *Arg., Br., Chin., Ind., Jap., Port.,* and *Span.*

Purified honey is obtained from the honey from the comb of the hive bee, *Apis mellifera* and other species of *Apis* (Apidae). It is prepared by melting the honey at a temperature not exceeding 80°, allowing to stand, skimming off the scum rising to the surface, and adjusting the wt per ml to 1.35 to 1.36 g by adding water.
It is a thick syrupy translucent pale yellow or yellowish-brown liquid with a sweet characteristic taste and a pleasant characteristic odour. It contains 70 to 80% of dextrose and laevulose, together with water, sucrose, dextrin, wax, proteins, volatile oil, and formic acid. Pollen and flocculent matter are usually present in suspension and tend to induce fermentation.

Honey had an acid reaction, pH about 3.7. When the pH was raised, honey became darker and its aroma somewhat unpleasant. These effects were especially pronounced above pH 7 and were ascribed to degradation of the sugars in honey. To prevent microbial deterioration in aqueous preparations of honey, 0.05% of sorbic acid (or potassium sorbate) was found effective and superior to sodium benzoate 0.1% and to a mixture of methyl hydroxybenzoate 0.2% and propyl hydroxybenzoate 0.05%. If the concentration of sorbic acid was increased to 0.1%, precipitation of some of the sorbic acid occurred in solutions containing a high proportion of honey.— N. Rubin *et al.*, *Am. J. Pharm.*, 1959, *131*, 246.

It is used as a demulcent and sweetening agent, especially in linctuses and cough mixtures.

The use of a mixture of equal parts of povidone-iodine ointment 10% and honey for the treatment of abrasions and varicose ulcers.— N. Lawrence (letter), *J.R. Coll. gen. Pract.*, 1976, *26*, 843.

Of 43 cases of infant botulinism in California since 1976 thirteen had a history of ingestion of honey. *Clostridium botulinum* (but not preformed toxin) was found in some of the ingested honey and in 13% of 60 samples examined. Other risk factors were involved, but it was recommended that honey should not be given to infants under 1 year of age; its safety for older children and adults was not questioned.— *Morb. Mortal.*, 1978, *27*, 249.

The use of honey to soothe dermal lesions and necrotic malignant breast ulcers was deprecated.— D. A. A. Mossel (letter), *Lancet*, 1980, *2*, 1091.

Preparations

Oxymel *(B.P.C. 1973)*. Acetic acid 15 ml, freshly boiled and cooled water 15 ml, purified honey to 100 ml. *Dose*. 2.5 to 10 ml.

Proprietary Names

M2 Woelm *(Woelm, Ger.)*.

593-s

Isoleucine *(U.S.P.)*. L-Isoleucine. L-2-Amino-3-methylvaleric acid.
$C_6H_{13}NO_2$=131.2.

CAS — 73-32-5.

Pharmacopoeias. In *Jap.* and *U.S.*

An almost odourless white crystalline powder with a slightly bitter taste. It sublimes at about 169°. M.p. about 284° with decomposition. **Soluble** 1 in 25 of water; slightly soluble in hot alcohol; practically insoluble in ether. A solution in hydrochloric acid is dextrorotatory. A 1% solution in water has a pH of 5.5 to 7.

Uses. Isoleucine is an amino acid which is an essential constituent of the diet. It is used as a dietary supplement.

Pellagra considered to be due to the high leucine content of a diet of maize or sorghum improved in 16 patients who were given DL-isoleucine 5 g daily for 10 days followed, if necessary, by 3 g daily for 5 to 7 days. EEG patterns were abnormal in 11 of 14 and after isoleucine some showed improvement.— K. Krishnaswamy and C. Gopalan, *Lancet*, 1971, *2*, 1167.

594-w

Lactose *(B.P., Eur. P.)*. Lactosum; Milk Sugar; Saccharum Lactis; Lattosio. 4-*O*-β-D-Galactopyranosyl-α-D-glucopyranose monohydrate.

$C_{12}H_{22}O_{11},H_2O$=360.3.

CAS — 63-42-3 (anhydrous); 5989-81-1 (monohydrate).

Pharmacopoeias. In all pharmacopoeias examined, except *Int. Braz.* and *U.S.* specify anhydrous or monohydrate.

A disaccharide obtained from the whey of milk. White or creamy-white odourless crystalline masses or powder with a slightly sweet taste. It readily absorbs odours. Lactose exists in 2 modifications corresponding to the α- and β-isomerides. Lactose used in pharmacy is chiefly α-lactose. β-Lactose is also obtainable; it is anhydrous, more soluble than α-lactose, and passes into the α-form in solution.

Soluble 1 in 6 of water and more soluble in hot water; practically insoluble in alcohol, chloroform, and ether. A solution in water is dextrorotatory. A 10% solution in water has a pH of 4 to 6.5. A 9.75% solution in water is iso-osmotic with serum. It may be **sterilised** by drying at 105° and then maintaining at 150° for 1 hour. It absorbs insignificant amounts of moisture at 25° at relative humidities up to about 90%.

Studies *in vitro* indicated that solubility of a drug was the major factor controlling its release from hard gelatin capsules; for soluble drugs, lactose, rather than starch or Primojel, would be the better diluent if required for use in large quantities.— J. M. Newton and F. M. Razzo, *J. Pharm. Pharmac.*, 1977, *29*, 205.

Effect of gamma-irradiation. Gamma-irradiation at 25 000 Gy changed the colour of lactose from white to pale creamy-yellow; at 250 000 Gy colour changed to deep cream and a caramel odour developed. Irradiation caused a significant increase in the acidity of a 10% solution and the specific rotation decreased.— *The Use of Gamma Radiation Sources for the Sterilisation of Pharmaceutical Products*, London, ABPI 1960.

Spray-dried lactose. Tablets could be prepared with spray-dried lactose without moist granulation or slugging; they were harder, less friable, and disintegrated slightly more rapidly than tablets made with conventionally processed lactose. Spray-dried lactose darkened more readily than conventionally processed lactose and the discoloration was increased at elevated temperatures.— W. C. Gunsel and L. Lachman, *J. pharm. Sci.*, 1963, *52*, 178. See also R. A. Castello and A. M. Mattocks, *ibid.*, 1962, *51*, 106; C. A. Brownley and L. Lachman, *ibid.*, 1964, *53*, 452.

For the use of lactose in tablet manufacture by direct compression, see E. J. Mendell, *Mfg Chem.*, 1972, *43* (May), 43.

Adverse Effects and Precautions. Lactose intolerance which occurs in patients with a deficiency of intestinal lactase is considered to exist if a clinical syndrome of abdominal pain, diarrhoea, distension, and flatulence occurs after the ingestion of lactose, 2 g per kg body-weight or 50 g per m^2 body-surface to a maximum of 50 g, as a 20% solution. Failure of the blood-glucose concentration to rise by 260 μg per ml represents lactose malabsorption.

Lactose is contra-indicated in patients with galactosaemia, the glucose-galactose malabsorption syndrome, or congenital lactase deficiency. Some patients with primary or secondary lactose intolerance may tolerate milk in quantities that are nutritiously useful.

Lactose intolerance. The practical significance of lactose intolerance in children from the Committee on Nutrition of the American Academy of Pediatrics.— *Pediatrics*, 1978, *62*, 240.

A discussion on lactose malabsorption and lactose intolerance.— *Lancet*, 1979, *2*, 831.

A study of healthy Japanese subjects indicated that infants and children under 2 years could absorb lactose completely. Lactase deficiency appeared to develop at 3 years and gradually increased with age, at least 85% of the children over 6 years and adults showing lactose malabsorption.— O. Nose *et al.*, *Archs Dis. Childh.*, 1979, *54*, 436.

Breath-hydrogen tests for the detection of lactose intolerance.— R. G. Barr *et al.*, *New Engl. J. Med.*, 1979, *300*, 1449. Lactose intolerance (assessed by the lactose-hydrogen breath test) in 3 of 26 children with recurrent abdominal pain. In only 1 were symptoms induced by lactose and relieved by its removal from the diet.— I. Blumenthal *et al.*, *Br. med. J.*, 1981, *282*, 2013.

Further references: S. -S. Huang and T. N. Bayless, *New Engl. J. Med.*, 1967, *276*, 1283; A. D. Newcomer, *Mayo Clin. Proc.*, 1973, *48*, 648; *Br. med. J.*, 1975, *2*, 351; *Postgrad. med. J.*, 1977, *53*, *Suppl.* 2, 57; J. Lieb and D. J. Kazienko (letter), *New Engl. J. Med.*, 1978, *299*, 314; T. Sahi, *Gut*, 1978, *19*, 1074.

Absorption and Fate. Lactose is hydrolysed by lactase in the small intestine to dextrose and galactose, which are then absorbed. Defective absorption is very common in adults. Lactose is excreted unchanged when given intravenously.

Lactose absorption was diminished in 9 of 19 osteoporotic patients. The calcium deficiency resulting from prolonged avoidance of milk, which provoked the symptoms of lactose intolerance, was believed to be responsible, at least in part, for the development of the osteoporosis.— S. J. Birge *et al.*, *New Engl. J. Med.*, 1967, *276*, 445.

Uses. Lactose is less sweet than sucrose. It is used in infant feeding to adjust the carbohydrate content of diluted cows' milk to that of human milk, but it should not be used excessively since it is a laxative and makes the stools too acid. Cows' milk contains about 50 g of lactose per litre.

Lactose is widely used as a diluent to give bulk to powders and as a diluent in compressed tablets. Sterilised lactose is used as a diluent for antibiotic powders.

Hepatic encephalopathy. Lactose in doses of from 80 to 150 g daily improved the condition of 3 of 4 lactose-deficient patients with hepatic encephalopathy by lowering the pH of the intestine.— J. D. Welsh and D. L. Langdon (letter), *New Engl. J. Med.*, 1972, *286*, 436.

595-e

Laevulose *(B.P., Eur. P.)*. Laevulosum; Diabetin; D-Fructose; Fructose *(U.S.P.)*; Fruit Sugar. D-(−)-Fructopyranose.

$C_6H_{12}O_6$=180.2.

CAS — 57-48-7.

Pharmacopoeias. In *Aust.*, *Br.*, *Eur.*, *Fr.*, *Ger.*, *It.*, *Jap.*, *Jug.*, *Neth.*, *Port.*, *Swiss*, and *U.S.*
NOTE. *Nord.* includes Laevulose for Infusion (Fructosum ad Infundibilia).

Odourless colourless crystals or a white crystalline or granular powder with a very sweet taste. **Soluble** 1 in 0.3 of water, 1 in 15 of alcohol, and 1 in 14 of methyl alcohol; practically insoluble in chloroform and ether. A solution in water is laevorotatory. An aqueous solution is almost neutral. A 5.05% solution in water is iso-osmotic with serum. Solutions are **sterilised** immediately after preparation by autoclaving or by filtration. **Store** at a temperature not exceeding 25° in airtight containers.

Incompatibility. Chlortetracycline was incompatible with solutions of laevulose (10%) in saline.— R. C. Bogash, *Bull. Am. Soc. Hosp. Pharm.*, 1955, *12*, 445.

Adverse Effects. Large doses of laevulose given by mouth may cause abdominal pain and diarrhoea. The intravenous infusion of large doses may cause facial flushing, epigastric pain, and sweating. The rapid injection of concentrated solutions may cause thrombophlebitis. Lactic acidosis and hyperuricaemia with gout may follow intravenous infusions; fatalities have occurred.

Intolerance in some persons may lead to a hypoglycaemic syndrome and may be followed by liver and kidney damage.

Reports of hyperuricaemia.— J. Perheentupa and K. Raivio, *Lancet*, 1967, *2*, 528; H. Mehnert and H. Förster (letter), *ibid.*, 1205; F. Stirpe *et al.* (letter), *ibid.*, 1970, *2*, 1310; M. J. T. Peaston (letter), *Lancet*, 1973, *1*, 266.

Intolerance. Reports of intolerance: J. D. Swales and A. D. M. Smith, *Q.J. Med.*, 1966, *35*, 455; J. A. Black and K. Simpson, *Br. med. J.*, 1967, *4*, 138; R. C. Morris and I. Ueki, *J. clin. Invest.*, 1968, *47*, 1648; B. Levin *et al.*, *Am. J. Med.*, 1968, *45*, 826.

Lactic acidosis. Infusions of laevulose could cause raised blood concentrations of lactate. The Australian Drug Evaluation Committee had recommended that simple solutions of laevulose be banned from the Australian market and that combination solutions be permitted only if the concentration of laevulose, or laevulose plus sorbitol if both were present, did not exceed 5%.— *Med. J. Aust.*, 1976, *1*, 582.

Reports and reviews of lactic acidosis associated with laevulose: G. M. Craig and C. W. Crane, *Br. med. J.*, 1971, *4*, 211; H. F. Woods and K. G. M. M. Alberti, *Lancet*, 1972, *2*, 1354; *Med. J. Aust.*, 1972, *2*, 1220; *Can. med. Ass. J.*, 1973, *108*, 1208; J. W. S. Rickett and D. G. Bowen (letter), *Lancet*, 1973, *1*, 489.

Precautions. Laevulose should not be given to patients with laevulose intolerance. It should not be administered to patients with methyl alcohol poisoning since it enhances the oxidation of methyl alcohol to formaldehyde.

It should be given with caution to patients with impaired kidney function or severe liver damage.

Absorption and Fate. Laevulose is absorbed from the gastro-intestinal tract but more slowly than dextrose. It is metabolised more rapidly than dextrose, mainly in the liver where it is phosphorylated and a part is converted to dextrose. Insulin is considered not to be necessary for its metabolism. Laevulose produces little effect upon the blood-sugar concentration, except in diabetic patients, who may metabolise it to dextrose to a greater extent than do non-diabetic subjects; the quantitative advantages are not great.

For a detailed review of the metabolism of laevulose, see F. Leuthardt and H. P. Wolf, *Proceedings of an International Symposium on the Clinical and Metabolic Aspects of Laevulose*, The Royal Society of Medicine, Apr. 1963, p. 4. See also E. R. Froesch and U. Keller, in *Parenteral Nutrition*, A.W. Wilkinson (Ed.), London, Churchill Livingstone, 1972, p. 105.

Laevulose was converted into glycerol phosphate at a more rapid rate than was dextrose and the enzymes required were present in human liver. The conversion avoided the slow catalysis by hexokinase and phosphofructokinase which occurred with dextrose. This indicated why laevulose rather than dextrose favoured the formation of glycerides.— *Lancet*, 1968, *2*, 1178.

Uses. Laevulose is sweeter than sucrose. It is utilised or converted into glycogen in the absence of insulin. It has been employed similarly to dextrose by intravenous infusion in conditions associated with carbohydrate insufficiency. The dosage is determined in accordance with the condition and needs of the patient. A suggested dose by intravenous infusion as a calorie source for parenteral feeding is 50 to 400 g daily. Laevulose should be administered slowly.

Laevulose has been claimed to accelerate the rate of metabolism of ethyl alcohol and has been given by intravenous injection in the treatment of acute alcohol poisoning (see Alcohol, p.37). It is also given intravenously as a source of energy in patients with renal failure, since tolerance to dextrose, but not laevulose, may be impaired, and it has been infused as a 40% solution for the prevention or treatment of cerebral oedema.

In neonatal hypoglycaemia, which may occur in newborn infants of diabetic mothers receiving large doses of insulin, injection of laevulose into the umbilical vein produces a more prolonged rise in blood sugar than does dextrose. Laevulose was formerly used in conditions such as debility, muscular dystrophy, and vomiting of pregnancy.

Because of its slow absorption and rapid metabolism laevulose has been used in limited quantities as a source of carbohydrate for the diabetic.

The effects of high-dose (1 g per kg body-weight per hour) infusions of dextrose, laevulose, and xylitol.— H. Förster and D. Zagel, *Dt. med. Wschr.*, 1974, *99*, 1300.

The effects of infusions of dextrose, laevulose, and xylitol—250 mg per kg body-weight over 48 hours.— H. Förster *et al.*, *Dt. med. Wschr.*, 1974, *99*, 1723.

The limited usefulness of laevulose in diabetes.— *Drug & Ther. Bull.*, 1980, *18*, 67.

Dialysis. Peritoneal dialysis with a solution containing laevulose 7% was compared in 14 patients with a similar solution containing dextrose 7%. Hyperosmolality and hyperglycaemia were less marked with laevulose. The use of dialysis solutions containing laevulose might be of value in diabetic patients.— R. M. Raja *et al.*, *Ann. intern. Med.*, 1973, *79*, 511.

Laevulose-tolerance test. In the laevulose-tolerance test, 1 g per kg body-weight of laevulose in 240 ml of water was given by mouth to the fasting patient and venous blood samples were taken before and at 15-minute intervals for 1 hour after the dose for determination of the serum-laevulose concentration. From studies in 23 patients with cirrhosis this test was considered a safe and practical alternative to the ammonia-tolerance test in the evaluation of portal-systemic collateral circulation and of portal hypertension.— N. D. Grace *et al.*, *Archs intern. Med.*, 1969, *124*, 330.

Preparations

Fructose and Sodium Chloride Injection *(U.S.P.)*. Laevulose and Sodium Chloride Injection. A sterile solution of laevulose and sodium chloride in Water for Injections. It contains no antimicrobial agents. pH 3 to 6.

Fructose Injection *(U.S.P.)*. Laevulose Injection. A sterile solution of laevulose in Water for Injections. It contains no antimicrobial agents. pH 3 to 6.

Laevulose Intravenous Infusion *(B.P.)*. Laevulose Injection. A sterile solution of laevulose in Water for Injections. Sterilised, immediately after preparation, by autoclaving. pH 3 to 5.5. Store at a temperature not exceeding 25°.

Proprietary Preparations

Laevuflex *(Geistlich, UK)*. Laevulose, available as solution for intravenous use containing 20%.

Levugen *(Travenol, UK)*. Laevulose, available as solutions for intravenous use containing 5, 10, and 20%.

Other Proprietary Names

Fructal, Fructopiran, Levo-Husci 20%, Levupan, Venosio *(all Ital.)*; Inulon *(Spain)*; Laevoral *(Ger., Ital., Switz.)*; Laevosan *(Austral., Belg., Ger., Ital., Switz.)*.

A preparation containing laevulose was also formerly marketed in Great Britain under the proprietary name Ethulose (*Geistlich*).

596-1

Lecithins.
A group of phosphatides also known as phospholipids.

CAS — 8002-43-5.

Pharmacopoeias. Aust. and *Swiss* include Vegetable Lecithin or Soya Lecithin. *Port.* and *Span.* include Egg Lecithin or Ovolecithin.

Lecithins consist chiefly of phosphatidyl esters, with varying amounts of other substances such as triglycerides, fatty acids, and carbohydrates. The phosphatidyl esters are formed from phosphatidic acids esterified with choline, ethanolamine, serine, or inositol. The phosphatidic acids are derived from glycerophosphoric acid by esterification of 2 hydroxyl groups with fatty acids, chiefly stearic, palmitic, oleic, linoleic, and arachidonic acids. Lecithins occur in all animal and vegetable cells and vary in composition according to the source from which they are obtained and the method of fractionation used. The main commercial varieties are *egg Lecithin*, and *vegetable lecithin*, derived from various vegetable sources, particularly leguminous seeds such as soya bean and groundnuts.

Lecithins have no clear therapeutic role.

In the light of biochemical and nutritional experience, the acceptable daily intake of lecithin was not limited.— Seventeenth Report of the Joint FAO/WHO Expert Committee on Food Additives, *Tech. Rep. Ser. Wld Hlth Org. No. 539*, 1974.

For reference to the suitability of lecithins as components of liposomal preparations for drug carriers, see G. Gregoriadis, *New Engl. J. Med.*, 1976, *295*, 704.

The addition of lecithin 0.5 or 1% to aqueous suspensions of fluspirilene 2 mg per ml for intramuscular injection solubilised a high proportion of the fluspirilene over 12 to 20 months. Where the ratio of drug to lecithin was low a suspension could change in physical properties, thus affecting absorption.— C. A. Janicki and W. D. Walkling, *Drug Dev. ind. Pharm.*, 1977, *3*, 339.

Lecithin produced higher and more prolonged serum concentrations of free choline than choline itself in a study of 10 healthy subjects and might be more effective in clinical situations where choline might be used.— R. J. Wurtman *et al.* (preliminary commmunication), *Lancet*, 1977, *2*, 68.

Anaemia. Eight patients with spur-cell anaemia associated with liver disease were given infusions of polyunsaturated phosphatidyl choline 2 g daily for 5 days. The percentage of spur cells was reduced and the cholesterol:phospholipids ratio of red blood cells fell significantly. Low doses of infused lecithin might change the composition and shape of spur cells, and thus ameliorate haemolytic anaemia.— G. Salvioli *et al.*, *Gut*, 1978, *19*, 844.

Gall-stones. Soya-bean lecithin 750 mg and cholic acid 250 mg were given thrice daily by mouth for 6 months to 11 patients with radiolucent gall-stones; the stones disappeared in 2 patients.— J. Toouli *et al.* (preliminary communication), *Lancet*, 1975, *2*, 1124.

Gilles de la Tourette syndrome. In a controlled study of 6 patients with Gilles de la Tourette's syndrome, treatment with lecithin up to 45 g daily for up to 4 weeks induced a variety of individual responses but there was no discernable benefit for the group as a whole.— R. J. Polinsky *et al.* (letter), *New Engl. J. Med.*, 1980, *302*, 1310. Considerable improvement was achieved in 3 young men with Gilles de la Tourette's syndrome when they were given lecithin (20% phosphatidyl choline) 40 to 50 g daily for at least 18 months in addition to haloperidol. Treatment with haloperidol was gradually reduced and could be stopped completely in one patient.— A. Barbeau (letter), *ibid.* Similar findings in 2 patients given choline chloride 20 g daily and in 6 given physostigmine.— S. M. Stahl and P. A. Berger (letter), *ibid.*, 1311.

Hyperlipidaemia. There was no acceptable evidence that lecithin lowered serum-cholesterol concentrations.— D. C. Fletcher, *J. Am. med. Ass.*, 1977, *238*, 64.

Reduction of serum-cholesterol concentrations by 10 to 18% in 3 of 10 persons given lecithin 20 to 30 g daily. The effect might be due to the content of linoleic acid.— L. A. Simons *et al.*, *Aust. N.Z. J. Med.*, 1977, *7*, 262.

Polyenyl phosphatidyl choline 1.8 g daily given in conjunction with clofibrate 1.2 g daily to 67 patients, in a double-blind crossover trial, prevented the elevation of low-density-lipoprotein induced by clofibrate treatment.— J. Schneider *et al.*, *Eur. J. clin. Pharmac.*, 1979, *15*, 15.

Mania. Possible value in mania.— B. M. Cohen *et al.*, *Am. J. Psychiat.*, 1980, *137*, 242.

Neurological disorders. Administration of choline, in the form of lecithin powder containing 3.7 g of choline per 100 g of lecithin (Centrolex-F), appeared to have some beneficial effect in 3 of 7 patients with Alzheimer's disease.— P. Etienne *et al.* (letter), *Lancet*, 1978, *2*, 1206.

Lecithin (60 to 80 g daily, or 40 g of partially purified lecithin) reduced tardive dyskinesia in 3 patients. Choline was the precursor of acetylcholine and serum-choline concentrations rose significantly.— J. H. Growdon *et al.* (letter), *New Engl. J. Med.*, 1978, *298*, 1029. Criticism.— S. Fahn (letter), *ibid.*, *299*, 202.

Lecithin, in daily doses of 3.6 to 49 g, reduced abnormal movements in 2 patients with tardive dyskinesia, produced only mild improvement in 3 patients with Huntington's chorea, no improvement in 6 patients with spastic spinocerebellar degeneration, and significant improvement in 10 patients with Friedreich's ataxia.— A. Barbeau (letter), *New Engl. J. Med.*, 1978, *299*, 200. A 12-week double-blind crossover study in 12 patients with Friedreich's ataxia failed to show any benefit from treatment with lecithin 25 g daily.— B. Pentland *et al.*, *Br. med. J.*, 1981, *282*, 1197.

Further references: A. J. Gelenberg *et al.*, *Am. J. Psychiat.*, 1979, *136*, 772; *Lancet*, 1980, *1*, 293.

Respiratory distress syndrome. Endotracheal administration of an artificial surfactant consisting of a mixture of naturally occurring surfactant lipids and synthetic lipids containing dipalmitoyl lecithin and phosphatidyl glycerol in the phosphorus molar ratios of 1 to 0.65 to 0.12, appeared to have a beneficial effect on hyaline membrane disease, in a study of 10 affected premature infants.— T. Fujiwara *et al.*, *Lancet*, 1980, *1*, 55. Criticism.— C. J. Morley and J. A. Davis (letter), *ibid.*, 252.

A single dose of an artificial lung surfactant consisting of pure dipalmitoyl phosphatidyl choline and phosphatidyl glycerol in a ratio of 7:3 as a dry powder, was blown down an endotracheal tube into the lungs of 22 very premature babies at birth. Compared with 33 control infants fewer needed ventilation and those who did required lower pressures in the first 6 hours of life. None of the treated infants died, but 8 of the control infants did. None of the treated infants had problems which could be attributed to the artificial surfactant.— C. J. Morley *et al.*, *Lancet*, 1981, *1*, 64. Correspondence: M. Ikegami (letter), *ibid.*, 379; D. James and A. Harkes (letter), *ibid.*, 555; D. L. Phelps (letter), *ibid.*; C. J. Morley (letter), *ibid.*

Manufacturers

Vis, Ital.

597-y

Leucine *(U.S.P.)*. L-Leucine; α-Aminoisocaproic acid. L-2-Amino-4-methylvaleric acid.
$C_6H_{13}NO_2$=131.2.

CAS — 61-90-5.

Pharmacopoeias. In *Jap.* and *U.S.*

A white odourless or almost odourless crystalline powder with a slightly bitter taste. It sublimes at about 150°. Sparingly **soluble** in water and glacial acetic acid; practically insoluble in alcohol, chloroform, and ether. A solution in hydrochloric acid is dextrorotatory. A 1% solution in water has a pH of 5.5 to 7.

Uses. Leucine is an amino acid which is an essential constituent of the diet. It is used in the diagnosis and treatment of idiopathic hyperglycaemia of infancy. Defects in the metabolism of keto acids formed from leucine, isoleucine, and valine give rise to maple-syrup-urine disease (leucinosis), a genetic disorder.
Leucine is used as a dietary supplement; DL-leucine is similarly used.

Leucinosis. The normal initial plasma concentration of leucine in infants was less than 0.18 mmol per litre, while in infants aged 7 to 17 days showing leucinosis it was 3 to 6 mmol per litre. The normal range of tolerance of infants to leucine was between 400 and 1400 mg daily while among infants with classic leucinosis it was 200 to 600 mg daily. Individual requirements of isoleucine and valine were also reduced.— *Can. med. Ass. J.*, 1976, *115*, 1005.

Pellagra. Excess of dietary leucine appeared to be involved in the pathogenesis of pellagra. Leucine interfered with the metabolism of tryptophan and nicotinic acid, and pellagra could therefore be considered as a nutritional deficiency disease mediated by leucine imbalance.— C. Gopalan, *Lancet*, 1969, *1*, 197. See also J. P. DesGioseilliers and N. J. Shiffman, *Can. med. Ass. J.*, 1976, *115*, 768.

See also under Isoleucine, p.54.

598-j

Levoglutamide. Levoglutamine; L-Glutamine. L-Glutamic acid 5-amide; L-(+)-2-Aminoglutaramic acid.
$C_5H_{10}N_2O_3$=146.1.

CAS — 56-85-9.

A white crystalline powder. M.p. about 184°. **Soluble** in water; practically insoluble in alcohol, acetone, chloroform, and ether. Levoglutamide slowly decomposes in aqueous solution with the formation of ammonia.

Uses. Levoglutamide has been used similarly to glutamic acid (see p.52) in the treatment of mental disorders and alcoholism in doses of 120 to 720 mg daily.

Cystinuria. Benefit in one patient with cystinuria.— K. Miyagi *et al.*, *New Engl. J. Med.*, 1979, *301*, 196. No benefit in 5 adult patients with typical cystinuria.— F. Skovby *et al.* (letter), *ibid.*, 1980, *302*, 236.

Levoglutamide 30 to 60 g daily had been well tolerated when taken for several months to over 3 years; the main side-effects were transient elevations of blood urea nitrogen and creatinine.— J. Korein (letter), *New Engl. J. Med.*, 1979, *301*, 1066.

Proprietary Names
Energlut *(Ital Suisse, Ital.)*; Glutacerebro *(AFOM, Ital.)*; Glutaven *(Falorni, Ital.)*; Iperphos *(Kalopharma, Ital.)*; Memoril *(Brocchieri, Ital.)*; Multidin *(Radiumfarma, Ital.)*; Sintoglutam *(Von Boch, Ital.)*.

669-y

Lysine Acetate *(U.S.P.)*. L-Lysine Monoacetate. L-2,6-Diaminohexanoic acid acetate.
$C_6H_{14}N_2O_2,C_2H_4O_2$=206.2.

CAS — 57282-49-2.

Pharmacopoeias. In *U.S.*

White odourless crystals or crystalline powder, with an acid taste. Freely **soluble** in water. A solution in water is dextrorotatory.

599-z

Lysine Hydrochloride *(U.S.P.)*. L-Lysine Monohydrochloride. L-2,6-Diaminohexanoic acid hydrochloride.
$C_6H_{14}N_2O_2,HCl$=182.6.

CAS — 56-87-1 (lysine); 657-27-2 (hydrochloride).

Pharmacopoeias. In *U.S.* Also in *Jap.* which does not state the configuration.

A white almost odourless crystalline powder. M.p. about 260° with decomposition. Each g represents approximately 5.5 mmol (5.5 mEq) of chloride. Freely **soluble** in water; practically insoluble in alcohol and ether. A solution in hydrochloric acid is dextrorotatory.

Precautions. The danger of severe metabolic acidosis is reported to be considerably greater with lysine hydrochloride than with ammonium chloride.
Lysine hydrochloride should be administered with caution to patients with hyperchloraemic acidosis or impaired renal function.

Uses. Lysine is an amino acid which is an essential constituent of the diet. The hydrochloride has been used in the treatment of hypochloraemic alkalosis.
Lysine is also used as a dietary supplement.

Six volunteers took 1 capsule containing lysine hydrochloride 205 mg and tryptophan 69 mg thrice daily after meals for up to 60 days. In each subject there was a reduction, significant in 3, in plasma-triglyceride concentration and a reduction in plasma-cholesterol concentration in 5 of the 6.— P. K. Raja and C. I. Jarowski, *J. pharm. Sci.*, 1975, *64*, 691.

Alkalosis. In patients for whom potassium chloride could not be used, ammonium chloride and lysine hydrochloride were convenient sources of chloride ion. They could be given safely, provided their potential for causing acidosis was borne in mind.— W. B. Schwartz *et al.*, *New Engl. J. Med.*, 1968, *279*, 630.

Herpes simplex. Lysine 390 mg given by mouth as soon as oral or vulval lesions were apparent produced rapid resolution of herpes lesions.— C. Kagan (letter), *Lancet*, 1974, *1*, 137.

In 45 patients with recurrent herpes simplex infection the condition was suppressed in 41 and decreased in 2 by treatment with lysine hydrochloride 0.312 to 1.248 g daily; maintenance doses were usually 312 to 500 mg daily. The rationale appeared to depend on increase of the lysine : arginine ratio.— R. S. Griffith *et al.*, *Dermatologica*, 1978, *156*, 257.

In a double-blind study involving 119 patients with recurrent prolabial or perioral herpes simplex, administration of lysine hydrochloride 1 g at the first symptom of an attack, then 500 mg twice daily for a further 9 doses, had no beneficial effect compared with placebo. An investigation of lysine prophylaxis had been started.— N. Milman *et al.* (letter), *Lancet*, 1978, *2*, 942.

Further references: N. Milman *et al.*, *Acta derm.-vener., Stockh.*, 1980, *60*, 85.

Proprietary Names
Enisyl *(Person & Covey, USA)*.

600-z

Magnesium Aspartate. Magnesium aminosuccinate tetrahydrate.
$C_8H_{12}MgN_2O_8,4H_2O$=360.6.

CAS — 7018-07-7 (tetrahydrate).

A mixture of magnesium and potassium aspartates has been claimed to be of value in the management of fatigue. See under Potassium Aspartate, p.58.

Proprietary Names
Magnesiocard (magnesium aspartate hydrochloride) *(Verla, Ger.)*.

601-c

Malt Extract *(B.P.C. 1973)*. Extractum Bynes.

CAS — 8002-48-0.

Pharmacopoeias. In *Arg.* and *Ind.* Both incorporate 10% w/w of glycerol.

An amber or yellowish-brown viscous liquid with an agreeable characteristic odour and sweet taste, containing nitrogen equivalent to not less than 4% w/w of protein. It contains 50% or more of maltose, together with dextrin, dextrose, and small amounts of other carbohydrates. It is prepared from malted grain of barley (*Hordeum distichon* or *H. vulgare*) or a mixture of this with not more than 33% of malted grain of wheat (*Triticum aestivum*). Wt per ml about 1.4 g. **Miscible** with water forming a translucent solution.

Uses. Malt extract has nutritive properties. It is chiefly used as a vehicle in preparations containing cod-liver oil and halibut-liver oil. It is a useful flavouring agent for masking bitter tastes.

Preparations

Malt Extract with Cod-liver Oil *(B.P.C. 1973)*. Extractum Malti cum Oleo Morrhuae. Cod-liver oil 10% w/w (about 4.5 ml in 30 ml) in malt extract. Store in a cool place in well-filled airtight containers. Protect from light. *Dose.* 10 to 30 ml daily.

Malt Extract with Halibut-liver Oil *(B.P.C. 1973)*. Extractum Malti cum Oleo Hippoglossi. Malt extract with 2.5% v/w of a mixture of arachis oil and sufficient halibut-liver oil to give not less than 60 units of vitamin-A activity per g (not less than 2500 units in 30 ml). Store in a cool place in well-filled airtight containers. Protect from light. *Dose.* 5 to 30 ml daily.

Malt Liquid Extract *(B.P.C. 1954)*. Ext. Malt. Liq. It contains about 67.5% v/v of malt extract in a mixture of alcohol and water. Wt per ml about 1.23 g. It was considered a useful vehicle for the administration of iron salts and cascara liquid extract. *Dose.* 4 to 16 ml.

Shark Liver Oil with Malt Extract *(Ind. P.)*. Shark-liver oil 5% w/w in malt extract. It contains not less than 300 units of vitamin-A activity per g. *Dose.* 4 to 16 ml.

Proprietary Preparations

Virol *(Optrex, UK)*. A preparation of malt extract with vegetable oil, maltose, sugar, maltodextrins, glucose syrup, egg, orange juice, phosphoric acid, calcium phosphate, iron phosphate, sodium iodide, vitamins, and flavouring; it contains in each 100 g, vitamin A 5200 units, thiamine hydrochloride 2.4 mg, riboflavine 3.8 mg, vitamin D 1400 units, nicotinic acid 24 mg, iron 28 mg, and iodine 260 µg.

Vitanorm *(Wallace Mfg Chem., UK: Farillon, UK)*. Malt extract preparation containing in 5 ml vitamin A 400 units, ascorbic acid 4 mg, ergocalciferol 40 units, cyanocobalamin 0.4 µg, panthenol 160 µg, ferric ammonium citrate 190 mg, halibut-liver oil 20 mg, nicotinamide 1 mg, pyridoxine hydrochloride 80 µg, riboflavine 80 µg, and thiamine hydrochloride 160 µg. *Dose.* 20 ml twice daily; children 10 ml daily.

Other Proprietary Names
Maltsupex *(USA)*.

602-k

Maltodextrin *(B.P.C. 1949)*. A mixture of dextrins and maltose prepared by the limited hydrolysis of starch.

CAS — 9050-36-6.

A slightly hygroscopic white powder with a slight odour and sweet taste. **Soluble** 2 in 1 of water; partly soluble in alcohol. **Store** in airtight containers.

Uses. Maltodextrin is more readily digested than starch and it has been used in infant feeding in place of lactose for adjusting the carbohydrate content of diluted cows' milk to that of human milk. Similar preparations are used in a number of proprietary foods.

603-a

Maltose *(B.P.C. 1949).* 4-*O*-α-D-Glucopyranosyl-β-D-glucopyranose monohydrate.
$C_{12}H_{22}O_{11},H_2O=360.3$.

CAS — 69-79-4 (anhydrous); 6363-53-7 (monohydrate).

A white crystalline powder with a slight odour and sweet taste. It is obtained from starch by hydrolysis with diastase. Very **soluble** in water; soluble in alcohol; practically insoluble in ether. **Store** in airtight containers.

Uses. Maltose is used in bacteriological culture media.

The mean blood concentrations of glucose in 9 healthy adults at 20 minutes and 2 hours after the ingestion of maltose 90 g per 70 kg body-weight in 500 ml of water were only slightly greater than concentrations found after similar doses of dextrose.— D. M. Matthews *et al.* (letter), *Lancet*, 1968, *2*, 49.

604-t

Manna *(B.P.C. 1934).* Manne en Larmes.

Pharmacopoeias. In *Aust., Fr., It., Port.,* and *Span. It.* and *Port.* permit other *Fraxinus* species.

The dried saccharine juice exuded from the stems of the European flowering ash, *Fraxinus ornus* (Oleaceae), usually containing from 40 to 75% of mannitol.
It occurs as yellowish-white, brittle, stalactitic masses with a slight agreeable odour and a sweet taste. Freely **soluble** in water; slightly soluble in alcohol.

Uses. Manna has mild laxative properties but it may cause flatulence and griping.

605-x

Methionine *(U.S.P.).* L-Methionine. L-2-Amino-4-(methylthio)butyric acid.

$C_5H_{11}NO_2S=149.2$.

CAS — 63-68-3.

Pharmacopoeias. In *Cz., Jap.,* and *U.S.*

White crystals with a characteristic odour and taste.
Soluble in water, in warm dilute alcohol, and in dilute mineral acids; very slightly soluble in alcohol; practically insoluble in acetone, dehydrated alcohol, and ether. A solution in hydrochloric acid is dextrorotatory. A 1% solution in water has a pH of 5.6 to 6.1.

606-r

Racemethionine *(U.S.P.).* DL-Methionine. DL-2-Amino-4-(methylthio)butyric acid.

$C_5H_{11}NO_2S=149.2$.

CAS — 59-51-8.

NOTE. The name methionine (see above) has often been applied to racemethionine.

Pharmacopoeias. In *Aust., Belg., Braz., Cz., Ger., It., Pol., Port., Roum., Rus., Span.,* and *U.S.*

White crystalline platelets or powder with a characteristic odour. M.p. about 270° with decomposition.
Soluble 1 in 30 of water; soluble in dilute acids and solutions of alkali hydroxides; very slightly soluble in alcohol; practically insoluble in ether. A 1% solution in water has a pH of 5.6 to 6.1. **Protect** from light.

Adverse Effects and Precautions. Methionine, given intravenously, may cause nausea, vomiting, drowsiness, and irritability. Large doses by mouth may cause nausea and vomiting. Methionine may precipitate hepatic encephalopathy in patients with established liver disease; it should not be used in paracetamol poisoning if more than 10 hours have elapsed since ingestion of the overdose.

For the effect of methionine(L) in reversing the effectiveness of levodopa in parkinsonism, see Levodopa.

Effect with a monoamine oxidase inhibitor. When schizophrenic patients being treated with a monoamine oxidase inhibitor were given methionine(L) in a dose of 300 mg per kg body-weight daily they experienced the superimposed symptoms of intoxication, such as delirium, visual hallucinations, ataxia, speech disturbance, increased salivation, and hyperhidrosis.— Y. Kikimoto *et al.* (letter), *Nature*, 1967, *216*, 1110.

Absorption and Fate. About 80% of methionine(L) ingested is converted to inorganic sulphate which is excreted in the urine. In the biosynthesis of cystine, methionine is converted by demethylation to homocysteine which by enzymic condensation with serine forms cystathionine. In patients with homocystinuria the condensation process cannot proceed and homocysteine is converted to homocystine which is excreted in the urine.

For a review of the degradation of methionine to cysteine in relation to homocystinuria, see D. A. Roe, *Br. J. Derm.*, 1969, *81, Suppl.* 2, 49.

The biological half-life of methionine was reported to be 50 days.— W. A. Ritschel, *Drug Intell. & clin. Pharm.*, 1970, *4*, 332.

For a review of the genetic background to homocystinuria and the involvement of pyridoxine, vitamin B_{12}, and folic acid metabolism, see C. R. Scriver, in *Treatment of Inborn Errors of Metabolism*, J.W.T. Seakins *et al.* (Ed.), London, Churchill Livingstone, 1973, p. 127.

Uses. Methionine is an amino acid which is an essential constituent of the diet (see p.47) and has a lipotropic action similar to that of choline (p.1651). There is however no acceptable evidence that supplementation of an adequate diet with lipotropic agents facilitates recovery from liver disease.
Methionine has been given in doses of 200 mg three or four times daily to lower the pH of the urine and thus reduce odour and irritation due to ammoniacal urine.
Methionine is used in the treatment of paracetamol poisoning. It enhances the synthesis of glutathione necessary for the detoxification of the toxic metabolite of paracetamol. The usual dose is 2.5 g every 4 hours for 4 doses starting less than 10 hours after ingestion of the paracetamol. It has also been given intravenously. A suggested oral dose for children aged 3 years is 1 g every 4 hours for 4 doses.
The literature relating to the use of methionine in paracetamol poisoning is, in general, imprecise as to the form of methionine used. In the UK the doses quoted above refer to racemethionine.
It is also used as a dietary supplement as is L-methionine which is also used in amino-acid solutions for parenteral use.

Paracetamol poisoning. None of 15 patients with paracetamol poisoning treated with methionine (L) intravenously within 10 hours (5 g initially followed by infusion to a total of 20 g in 20 hours) died or developed acute renal failure; in 12 liver damage was absent or trivial. In 5 treated within 10 to 12 hours liver-function tests were only mildly disturbed.— L. F. Prescott *et al.*, *Lancet*, 1976, *2*, 109.

Methionine provided a simpler alternative to cysteamine in the treatment of paracetamol overdose and could be started more quickly than cysteamine which required the measurement of blood concentrations. However, methionine might not always prevent liver damage since paracetamol-induced glutathione removal might be greater than the methionine-induced increase in the rate of glutathione synthesis. The technique involving methionine included gastric lavage and the administration of methionine 2.5 g by mouth or intravenous injection and repeated every 4 hours to a total dose of 10 g.— A. E. M. McLean (letter), *Lancet*, 1976, *2*, 362. See also P. Crome *et al.* (preliminary communication), *ibid.*, 829.

For children aged 11 to 13 years poisoned with paracetamol the adult dose of methionine (2.5 g four-hourly to a total of 10 g) was suggested.— T. J. Meredith *et al.*, *Br. med. J.*, 1978, *2*, 478.

All of 96 patients with potentially severe paracetamol poisoning survived after treatment with methionine by mouth within 10 hours, though 7 suffered severe liver damage. Of 36 treated after 10 hours 17 suffered severe liver damage and 2 died. Acetylcysteine might be preferable in the few patients with intractable vomiting.— J. A. Vale *et al.* (letter), *Br. med. J.*, 1979, *2*, 1435.
See also under Paracetamol, p.269.

Preparations

Racemethionine Capsules *(U.S.P.).* Capsules containing racemethionine. Protect from light.

Racemethionine Tablets *(U.S.P.).* Tablets containing racemethionine. Protect from light.

Proprietary Preparations

Meonine *(Wyeth, UK).* A brand of methionine [isomer not specified].

Other Proprietary Names of Methionine or Racemethionine

Antamon *(S.Afr.)*; Lobamine *(Fr.)*; Methnine *(Austral.)*; Monile, Ninol *(both Canad.)*; Pedameth, Uracid, Uranap *(all USA)*.

Preparations containing methionine were formerly marketed in Great Britain under the proprietary names Litrison (*Roche*) and Unihepa (*Unigreg*).

607-f

Methyl Cysteine Hydrochloride. Mecysteine Hydrochloride. Methyl L-2-amino-3-mercaptopropionate hydrochloride.

$C_4H_9NO_2S,HCl=171.6$.

CAS — 2485-62-3 (methyl cysteine); 18598-63-5 (hydrochloride).

White crystals. **Soluble** in water, alcohol, and warm methyl alcohol; practically insoluble in acetone and ether.

Adverse Effects. Nausea and heartburn have occasionally been reported.

Uses. Methyl cysteine hydrochloride has been used in the treatment of disorders of the respiratory tract associated with excessive mucus.
The suggested dose is 200 mg twice or thrice daily. It has also been administered as an aerosol.

Bronchitis. Eighty-two men with chronic bronchitis were given two 100-mg tablets of methyl cysteine hydrochloride thrice daily for a month and compared with 82 chronic bronchitics taking placebo tablets. Those taking methyl cysteine showed a significant reduction in cough and sputum compared with the controls, but there was no significant reduction in dyspnoea.— K. N. V. Palmer *et al.*, *Br. med. J.*, 1962, *1*, 280.

In a placebo-controlled study of 30 patients with chronic obstructive bronchitis methyl cysteine hydrochloride 1.2 g taken daily for one week, then 800 mg daily for a further week followed by 600 mg daily for 4 weeks, reduced the frequency and severity of cough, and changed the consistency of sputum with a resultant easing of expectoration and increase in volume of sputum expectorated. There was no significant reduction in dyspnoea.— M. Aylward *et al.*, *Curr. med. Res. Opinion*, 1978, *5*, 461.

Further references: B. Mann *et al.*, *Br. J. Dis. Chest*, 1963, *57*, 192.

Proprietary Preparations

Visclair *(Sinclair, UK).* Methyl cysteine hydrochloride, available as tablets of 100 mg.

Other Proprietary Names

Acthiol J *(Fr., Switz.)*; Actiol *(Ital.)*; Daiace, Ethitanin *(both ethylcysteine hydrochloride) (both Jap.)*.

608-d

Ornithine. L-Ornithine; α,δ-Diaminovaleric Acid. L-5-Aminonorvaline; L-2,5-Diaminovaleric acid.
$C_5H_{12}N_2O_2=132.2$.

CAS — 70-26-8.

Microcrystals. M.p. 140°. Freely **soluble** in water and alcohol; sparingly soluble in ether. Aqueous solutions are alkaline.

Uses. Ornithine is an amino acid. The aspartate, hydrochloride, and α-ketoglutarate, have been used in the treatment of hyperammonaemia.

References: H. Leonhardt and H. J. Bungert, *Medsche Klin.*, 1972, *67*, 1052; D. Henglein-Ottermann, *Therapie Gegenw.*, 1976, *115*, 1504.

Proprietary Names of Ornithine Aspartate
Hepa-Merz *(Merz, Ger.)*; Hepato-Spartan *(Craveri, Arg.)*.

Proprietary Names of Ornithine Ketoglutarate
Ornicetil *(Logeais, Fr.; Nordmark-Werke, Ger.; Semar, Spain; Logeais, Switz.)*.

609-n

Peptone *(B.P.C. 1949)*. A mixture of proteoses, peptones, and amino acids, prepared from blood fibrin and other proteins by peptic digestion or other processes.

Pharmacopoeias. In *Arg.*, *Port.*, and *Span.*

A light yellowish-brown powder or granules with a meat-like but not putrid odour.
Freely **soluble** in water; practically insoluble in alcohol, chloroform, and ether. A 1% solution in water has a pH of 6.5 to 7. Solutions for injection are **sterilised** by autoclaving or by filtration. **Store** in airtight containers.
Other varieties of peptone for nutritional or bacteriological purposes may be made by the peptic or tryptic digestion of fibrin or other proteins such as lean beef and casein.

Uses. Peptone was formerly used for nonspecific desensitisation in allergic conditions such as asthma, hay fever, and urticaria.

610-k

Phenylalanine *(U.S.P.)*. L-Phenylalanine; α-Aminohydrocinnamic acid. L-2-Amino-3-phenylpropionic acid.
$C_9H_{11}NO_2$=165.2.

CAS — 63-91-2.

Pharmacopoeias. In *Jap.* and *U.S.*

A white odourless crystalline powder with a slightly bitter taste. M.p. about 283° with decomposition. **Soluble** about 1 in 35 of water; very slightly soluble in alcohol, methyl alcohol, and dilute mineral acids; practically insoluble in ether. A solution in water is laevorotatory. A 1% solution in water has a pH of 5.4 to 6. **Protect** from light.

Uses. Phenylalanine is an essential amino acid, normally metabolised to tyrosine. The enzyme required for this metabolism is lacking in children with phenylketonuria, in whom accumulating phenylalanine is converted to phenylpyruvic acid which is excreted in the urine. Prevention of mental retardation in such children is achieved by feeding diets low in phenylalanine from birth so that the blood concentration is maintained between 15 and 40 mg per litre. For preparations used in the treatment of phenylketonuria, see p.63.

In 23 patients with endogenous depression not responsive to treatment with usual antidepressants, DL- or D-phenylalanine 50 or 100 mg daily for 15 days was effective in 17. Side-effects of headache and vertigo occurred in 6 patients.— E. Fischer *et al.*, *Arzneimittel-Forsch.*, 1975, *25*, 132. See also H. Beckmann and E. Ludolph, *ibid.*, 1978, *28*, 1283.

The management of phenylketonuria in pregnancy.— G. M. Komrower *et al.*, *Br. med. J.*, 1979, *1*, 1383. Some case reports.— K. B. Nielsen *et al.* (letter), *Lancet*, 1979, *1*, 1245; N. R. M. Buist *et al.* (letter), *ibid.*, 1979, *2*, 589.

Parkinsonism. Tremor and rigidity in 7 of 8 patients with parkinsonism were exacerbated when DL-phenylalanine 1.6 to 12.6 g daily was given by mouth.— G. C. Cotzias *et al.*, *New Engl. J. Med.*, 1967, *276*, 374.

In 13 patients with parkinsonism the absorption and excretion of phenylalanine, given intravenously or by mouth, did not differ from absorption and excretion in controls.— A. Granerus *et al.*, *Br. med. J.*, 1971, *4*, 262.

Rigidity, walking disability, speech difficulty, and psychic depression greatly improved in 15 patients with parkinsonism after receiving D-phenylalanine 200 to 500 mg daily for 4 weeks.— B. Heller *et al.*, *Arzneimittel-Forsch.*, 1976, *26*, 577.

Proprietary Names of D-Phenylalanine
Sabiden *(Szabó, Arg.)*.

611-a

Potassium Aspartate. Potassium aminosuccinate hemihydrate.
$C_4H_6KNO_4,½H_2O$=180.2.

CAS — 7259-25-8 (hemihydrate).

Uses. A mixture of equal parts of potassium aspartate and magnesium aspartate has been claimed to be of value in the management of fatigue, heart conditions, and liver disorders but the claims are not supported by adequate evidence.
Up to 2 g of the mixture has been given daily in divided doses. It may occasionally cause nausea, abdominal discomfort, and diarrhoea, and should not be given to patients with renal insufficiency.

Studies of 50 patients undergoing extracorporeal blood perfusion showed that disturbances of potassium and sodium balance induced by dilution with 5.25% dextrose infusion could be diminished or abolished by the infusion of a potassium and magnesium aspartate solution.— E. Struck *et al.*, *Arzneimittel-Forsch.*, 1969, *19*, 113.

Proprietary Names of Potassium and Magnesium Aspartate
Aspara *(Jap.)*; Panangin *(Gedeon Richter, Hung.)*; Trommcardin *(Trommsdorff, Ger.)*; Trophicard *(Köhler, Ger.)*.

Proprietary Names of other Aspartates
Potenciator (arginine aspartate) *(Valderrama, Spain)*; Sargenor (arginine aspartate) *(Sarget, Fr.)*.

612-t

Potassium Glutamate. Monopotassium L-Glutamate. Potassium hydrogen L-(+)-2-aminoglutarate monohydrate.
$C_5H_8KNO_4,H_2O$=203.2.

CAS — 19473-49-5 (anhydrous); 6382-01-0 (monohydrate).

A white, practically odourless, hygroscopic, crystalline powder. Each g represents approximately 4.9 mmol (4.9 mEq) of potassium. Freely **soluble** in water; slightly soluble in alcohol. A 2% solution in water has a pH of 6.7 to 7.3. **Store** in airtight containers.

Uses. Potassium glutamate has uses similar to those of sodium glutamate (see p.59), and both salts have been used together in injections to reduce the risk of sodium toxicity. Large doses may cause the adverse effects described under Potassium Salts (p.628). Potassium glutamate is also used as a flavouring agent in sodium-free condiments.

613-x

Proline *(U.S.P.)*. L-Proline. L-Pyrrolidine-2-carboxylic acid.
$C_5H_9NO_2$=115.1.

CAS — 147-85-3.

Pharmacopoeias. In *U.S.*

Odourless white crystals or crystalline powder with a slightly sweet taste. Freely **soluble** in water and dehydrated alcohol; practically insoluble in butyl alcohol, ether, and isopropyl alcohol. A solution in water is laevorotatory. **Protect** from light.

Uses. Proline is an amino acid occurring in many proteins, particularly gelatin. It is used as a dietary supplement.

614-r

Protein Hydrolysate Injection *(U.S.P.)*.

Protein Hydrolysates (Intravenous).

CAS — 9015-54-7.

A sterile solution of amino acids and short-chain peptides which represent the approximate nutritive equivalent of the casein, lactalbumin, plasma, fibrin, or other suitable protein from which it is derived by acid, enzymatic, or other method of hydrolysis. It may be modified by partial removal and restoration or addition of one or more amino acids and it may contain alcohol, dextrose, or other carbohydrate suitable for intravenous infusion. Not less than 50% of the total nitrogen present is in the form of α-amino nitrogen. pH 4 to 7. It is a yellowish to reddish-amber transparent liquid. **Store** at a temperature not exceeding 40°.
The label includes the name of the protein from which it has been derived. If it contains not more than 30 mg of sodium per 100 ml it may be labelled Protein Hydrolysate Injection, Low Sodium, or by a similar title.

CAUTION. *Solutions of protein hydrolysates are excellent media for microbial growth. Once a sealed container is opened the contents should be used forthwith.*

Casein hydrolysate. The amino acids present in casein hydrolysate were stable at temperatures from 8° to 47° for 12 weeks. Levoglutamide added to the casein hydrolysate preparation was unstable in aqueous solution but preparations containing levoglutamide could possibly be stored at low temperatures as degradation was relatively slow at 8°. Cysteine was converted to cystine very rapidly.— J. E. Friend *et al.*, *Am. J. Hosp. Pharm.*, 1972, *29*, 743. Ammonia and cystine contents increased during storage of sterile aqueous 5% solutions of casein hydrolysate due to the instability of levoglutamide and cysteic acid. Freeze-drying increased the stability of levoglutamide, but not of cysteic acid or of tyrosine. All other substances tested, including levoglutamide, remained stable in the freeze-dried preparation for up to 12 weeks at temperatures up to 47°.— *idem*, 835. See also L. Monnens *et al.* (letter), *Lancet*, 1973, *1*, 1116.

The concentrations of dextrose and amino acids and pH are fairly stable after mixing 8.5% amino-acid solutions with 50% dextrose solutions, or casein hydrolysate 10% with dextrose 50%, and also during storage at 4° and room temperature for 14 days. Nevertheless, solutions should be used as soon as possible after mixing or refrigerated until used.—D. A. Rowlands *et al.*, *Am. J. Hosp. Pharm.*, 1973, *30*, 436.

Incompatibility. Protein hydrolysate was incompatible with chlortetracycline hydrochloride, pentobarbitone sodium, and sodium dehydrocholate; a haze or precipitate occurred within 1 to 6 hours with sulphafurazole diethanolamine and within 6 to 24 hours with chlorothiazide sodium.— W. D. Kirkland *et al.*, *Am. J. Hosp. Pharm.*, 1961, *18*, 694.

Protein hydrolysate was incompatible with chlortetracycline, nitrofurantoin sodium, novobiocin sodium, pentobarbitone sodium, and thiopentone sodium.— J. A. Patel and G. L. Phillips, *Am. J. Hosp. Pharm.*, 1966, *23*, 409.

A haze or precipitate occurred within 1 to 6 hours when protein hydrolysate was mixed with oxytetracycline hydrochloride 500 mg per litre.— E. A. Parker, *Am. J. Hosp. Pharm.*, 1970, *27*, 327.

Protein hydrolysate is also stated to be incompatible with conjugated oestrogens.

Adverse Effects. Protein hydrolysate injections may cause nausea, vomiting, occasional skin rashes, vasodilatation, abdominal pain, oedema at the site of injection, phlebitis, thrombosis, and convulsions. Technique should be rigorously controlled to reduce the risk of infection.

The effect of total parenteral nutrition with casein or fibrin hydrolysates for 5 to 150 days was studied in 23 infants aged 2 to 135 days. Complications included septicaemia in 3, hyperosmolarity in 3, and transient metabolic acidosis in 7. Severe osteoporosis occurred in 2 who had received treatment for more than 30 days. Blood-ammonia studies in 8 receiving protein hydrolysate 2.2 to 4.3 g per kg body-weight daily showed 7 with elevated concentrations and of these 4 also had abnormal liver function; this disappeared in 3 when treatment was discontinued. Abnormalities of liver or liver function were seen in 4 of 9 children who were not hyperammonaemic. It was suggested that parenteral nutrition with protein hydrolysates should be initiated with only 1 to 1.5 g per kg per day or with preparations with low ammonia concentrations.— J. D. Johnson *et al.*, *J. Pediat.*, 1972, *81*, 154.

Metabolic acidosis was noted in babies who received parenteral nutritional mixtures containing synthetic amino acids, although it was not observed in those who received protein hydrolysate solutions.— W. C. Heird *et al.*, *New Engl. J. Med.*, 1972, *287*, 943. See also *ibid.*, 982.

Coma occurred in 4 neonates when the infusion-rate of casein hydrolysate was increased beyond 4 g per kg body-weight daily.— R. J. Touloukian, *J. Pediat.*, 1975, *86*, 270.

Conjugated hyperbilirubinaemia in 5 premature infants given protein hydrolysate intravenously.— J. Bernstein *et al.*, *J. Pediat.*, 1977, *90*, 361.

Precautions. Protein hydrolysate injections should not be given in the presence of irreversible liver damage and in severe uraemia where no facilities exist for dialysis.

The electrolyte and acid-base balance should be monitored and care should be taken to avoid excessive volumes of fluid.

Uses. Protein hydrolysate injection is used, with carbohydrates or other sources of energy, as a source of nitrogen in total parenteral nutrition (see p.48).

Dosage must be assessed according to the needs of the individual patient. Some advantages have been claimed (in terms of positive nitrogen balance) for hydrolysates as compared with amino acids. At best these differences are marginal.

Hyperalimentation with casein hydrolysates or amino acids with 23% dextrose and containing 5 g per litre of utilisable nitrogen reduced plasma concentrations of cholesterol and low- and high-density lipoproteins in 3 patients with severe familial hypercholesterolaemia.— H. Torsvik *et al.*, *Lancet*, 1975, *1*, 601.

Protein loss during dialysis. The mean fall of serum-protein concentrations after peritoneal dialysis was reduced from 5.5 to 1 g per litre by adding casein hydrolysate solution to the dialysing fluid. Patients were given 45 litres of dialysing fluid to which 25 ml of Aminosol-Glucose was added to each litre. No adverse reaction occurred during dialysis.— J. Gjessing (preliminary communication), *Lancet*, 1968, *2*, 812.

615-f

Protein Hydrolysates (Oral). A preparation of amino acids and short-chain peptides obtained by the hydrolysis, usually enzymatic, of casein or other suitable protein.

Protein hydrolysate preparations for oral use have been used, usually with added carbohydrate and fat, to supplement the diet in certain conditions requiring a very high protein intake and in patients intolerant of normal diet.

A protein hydrolysate preparation for oral use was formerly marketed in Great Britain under the proprietary name Aminosol Powder (*KabiVitrum*).

616-d

Serine *(U.S.P.).* L-Serine; β-Hydroxyalanine. L-2-Amino-3-hydroxypropionic acid.

$C_3H_7NO_3$=105.1.

CAS — 56-45-1.

A white odourless crystalline powder with a sweet taste. M.p. about 228° with decomposition. **Soluble** in water; practically insoluble in dehydrated alcohol and ether. A solution in hydrochloric acid is dextrorotatory.

Uses. Serine is an amino acid present in many foods. Serine and DL-serine are used as dietary supplements.

617-n

Sodium Glutamate.

Natrii Glutamas; Monosodium Glutamate; Chinese Seasoning; MSG. Sodium hydrogen L-(+)-2-aminoglutarate monohydrate.

$C_5H_8NNaO_4,H_2O$=187.1.

CAS — 142-47-2 (anhydrous).

Pharmacopoeias. In *It.* and *Pol.*

A white or almost white crystalline powder with a slight peptone-like odour and a meat-like taste. Sodium glutamate 32 g is approximately equivalent to anhydrous sodium glutamate 29 g or glutamic acid 25 g. Each g represents 5.3 mmol (5.3 mEq) of sodium. Freely **soluble** in water; sparingly soluble in alcohol. A 5% solution in water has a pH of 6.7 to 7.2. Solutions are **sterilised** by autoclaving. **Store** in airtight containers.

Adverse Effects. The large doses of sodium glutamate required for the treatment of hepatic encephalopathy may result in dangerous alkalosis and hypokalaemia owing to excessive intake of sodium and it is therefore important to keep a close control on the electrolyte balance during therapy. Too rapid administration of the injection should be avoided as it may give rise to salivation, flushing, and vomiting.

Flushing, headache, and chest pain may occur in hypersensitive persons taking sodium glutamate by mouth.

For background toxicological information, see *Fd Add. Ser. Wld Hlth Org. No. 5*, 1974.

Sodium glutamate-induced shuddering attacks in children might be associated with essential tremor.— F. Andermann *et al.* (letter), *New Engl. J. Med.*, 1976, *295*, 174.

A mother and son who experienced acute reactions to sodium glutamate also had chronic psychiatric symptoms which disappeared when they ate food free from sodium glutamate.— A. D. Colman (letter), *New Engl. J. Med.*, 1978, *299*, 902. Criticism.— R. A. Kenney (letter), *ibid.*, 1979, *300*, 503; R. E. Cristol (letter), *ibid.*, 504.

Flushing syndrome. Sodium glutamate had been held responsible for the 'Chinese restaurant syndrome' which was characterised by onset 15 to 25 minutes after a meal, duration of 45 minutes, and a fluctuating intensity. A burning sensation at the back of the neck, followed by burning over the forearms and anterior thorax, a feeling of infra-orbital pressure and variable substernal discomfort was reported by sensitive persons after sodium glutamate 5 g. There was no erythema or pruritus, and no evidence of muscular contraction. Other symptoms, syncope, tachycardia, lachrymation, fasciculation, and nausea, were attributable to accompanying anxiety. Equivalent doses of sodium, as chloride, or of glutamic acid failed to induce the reaction, which was not prevented by diphenhydramine.— H. H. Schaumburg and R. Byck (letter), *New Engl. J. Med.*, 1968, *279*, 105. See also R. H. M. Kwok (letter), *ibid.*, *278*, 796; H. H. Schaumburg *et al.*, *Science*, 1969, *163*, 826.

Studies in 24 volunteers, one-half of whom were given 3 g of sodium glutamate in a meal, indicated that sodium glutamate did not cause the Chinese restaurant syndrome.— P. L. Morselli and S. Garattini, *Nature*, 1970, *227*, 611.

Of 77 subjects, 25 reported untoward symptoms after drinking a preparation containing sodium glutamate 5 g compared with 11 when given placebo. The symptoms were similar to some of those previously reported but symptoms typical of the Chinese restaurant syndrome were not seen.— R. A. Kenney and C. S. Tidball, *Am. J. clin. Nutr.*, 1972, *25*, 140.

A study in 55 subjects casting doubt on the role of sodium glutamate in inducing the symptoms associated with the 'Chinese restaurant syndrome' (facial pressure, chest pain, and a burning sensation, particularly of the head and upper trunk). Although reactions to sodium glutamate were significant, they were not dose-related, and women were no more susceptible than men.— M. E. Gore and P. R. Salmon (letter), *Lancet*, 1980, *1*, 251.

Precautions. Injections of sodium glutamate should be given with caution to patients with hepatic cirrhosis, impaired renal function, or liver disease not associated with hyperammonaemia. Care is necessary where there is a danger of severe electrolyte imbalance.

The adverse effects of sodium glutamate were enhanced in a patient taking phenytoin, possibly as a result of the inhibition of folic acid absorption by phenytoin.— A. R. M. Upton and H. S. Barrows (letter), *New Engl. J. Med.*, 1972, *286*, 893.

Little if any of a 6-g dose of sodium glutamate was concentrated in breast milk.— L. D. Stegink *et al.*, *Proc. Soc. exp. Biol. Med.*, 1972, *140*, 836.

Sodium glutamate was less 'salty' than sodium chloride with equivalent sodium content. This could lead to excessive sodium intake in those whose sodium intake should be restricted.— L. M. Bartoshuk *et al.* (letter), *J. Am. med. Ass.*, 1974, *230*, 670. Criticisms.— A. G. Ebert (letter), *ibid.*, 1975, *233*, 224; J. Reaume (letter), *ibid.* A reply.— L. M. Bartoshuk *et al.* (letter), *ibid.*, 225.

Uses. Sodium glutamate has been used in the treatment of hyperammonaemia in conditions such as hepatic encephalopathy. It has been given to adults in a dose of 32 g in 0.5 to 1 litre of dextrose intravenous infusion 5 or 10% by intravenous infusion over a period of 1 to 4 hours. This dose has been repeated after 8 to 12 hours. Administration of 32 g of sodium glutamate also means that the patient has been given 171 mmol (171 mEq) of sodium.

Sodium glutamate is widely used as a flavour enhancer and seasoning for foods and imparts a salty meaty flavour. It is used as a flavouring agent in some pharmaceutical preparations, such as oral preparations of liver and of protein hydrolysates.

Estimated acceptable daily intake for adults, and children aged over 12 weeks: up to 120 mg, as glutamic acid, additional to glutamic acid from all natural dietary sources, per kg body-weight.— Seventeenth Report of the FAO/WHO Expert Committee on Food Additives, *Tech. Rep. Ser. Wld Hlth Org. No. 539*, 1974.

618-h

Sorbitol *(B.P.).*

Sorbite; D-Sorbitol; Sorbol. D-Glucitol.

$C_6H_{14}O_6$=182.2.

CAS — 50-70-4.

Pharmacopoeias. In *Aust.*, *Belg.*, *Br.*, *Cz.*, *Ger.*, *Hung.*, *It.*, *Jap.*, *Roum.*, and *Swiss.* Also in *U.S.N.F.*

A white, slightly hygroscopic, odourless, microcrystalline powder, granules, or flakes with a sweet taste. The *B.P.* specifies not less than 98% and not more than the equivalent of 101% of D-glucitol, calculated on the anhydrous basis; the *U.S.N.F.* specifies 91 to 100.5% of $C_6H_{14}O_6$ calculated on the anhydrous basis and permits small amounts of other polyhydric alcohols. M.p. about 95°. **Soluble** 1 in 0.5 of water and 1 in 25 of alcohol; practically insoluble in chloroform and ether; slightly soluble in acetic acid and in methyl alcohol; very slightly soluble in acetone. A 20% solution in water is clear. A 10% solution has a pH of about 6.7. A 5.48% solution of sorbitol hemihydrate is iso-osmotic with serum. Solutions for injection are **sterilised** by autoclaving. **Incompatible** with oxidising agents. **Store** in airtight containers.

619-m

Sorbitol for Parenteral Use *(B.P.).*

D-Sorbitol.

$C_6H_{14}O_6$=182.2.

Pharmacopoeias. In *Br.*

A white, slightly hygroscopic, odourless, microcrystalline powder. **Solubility, Sterilisation, Incompatibility**, and **Storage** as for Sorbitol, p.59.

A summary of the properties and uses of sorbitol with typical formulas for vehicles and preparations.— G. E. Schumacher, *Am. J. Hosp. Pharm.*, 1967, *24*, 378.

Palatability. Of various combinations of syrup, sorbitol solution, and artificial sweeteners tested, the following unmedicated vehicles were judged to have equivalent palatability: sucrose 40%, sucrose 30% with sorbitol 20%, sucrose 15% with sorbitol 40%, and sodium cyclamate 0.8% with saccharin sodium 0.08%. In medicated preparations such as guaiphenesin 2% syrup, a vehicle of sorbitol 40% and sucrose 15% was preferred.— G. E. Schumacher, *Am. J. Hosp. Pharm.*, 1968, *25*, 154.

Adverse Effects and Precautions. Excessive amounts of sorbitol may cause flatulence, abdominal distension, and diarrhoea when taken by mouth. The rapid infusion of large amounts of sorbitol may cause nausea and vomiting and increased serum concentrations of uric acid. Epigastric, substernal, and abdominal pain may occur. Prolonged infusion may cause thrombophlebitis. Lactic acidosis may occur. Utilisation of sorbitol given intravenously may be impaired in patients with severe liver insufficiency and give rise to diuresis and possible aggravation of electrolyte deficiencies. Sorbitol should be infused with care in diabetic patients.

For background toxicological information, see *Fd Add. Ser. Wld Hlth Org. No. 5*, 1974.

There were 17 instances of upper abdominal pain, hypertension, and vomiting during peritoneal dialysis in 7 patients when a dialysate containing sorbitol was used. Some patients became comatose. These side-effects did not occur when dextrose was employed in place of sorbitol.— E. Quelhorst *et al.*, *Dt. med. Wschr.*, 1975, *100*, 1431.

Infusion of sorbitol could cause raised blood concentrations of lactate. The Australian Drug Evaluation Committee had recommended that simple solutions of sorbitol be banned from the Australian market and that combination solutions be permitted only if the concentration of sorbitol, or sorbitol plus laevulose if both were present, did not exceed 5%.— *Med. J. Aust.*, 1976, *1*, 582.

Fatal liver and renal toxicity occurred in a woman with laevulose intolerance given an infusion of sorbitol.— M. -J. Schulte and W. Lenz (letter), *Lancet*, 1977, *2*, 188.

Absorption and Fate. Sorbitol is slowly absorbed from the gastro-intestinal tract. In the body, part is converted, mainly in the liver, to laevulose and then to glucose; negligible amounts of glucose appear in the blood, except in diabetic patients in whom blood-glucose concentrations may be slightly increased. About 3% of a 35-g dose of sorbitol appears in urine after administration by mouth; at least 75% is metabolised to carbon dioxide. At normal infusion-rates, about 5% of a dose of intravenously injected sorbitol appears in urine.

When sorbitol was administered to 16 surgical patients the average loss of total carbohydrate in the urine in 24 hours was only about 6% of the administered dose of sorbitol, even when 30% solutions were infused rapidly. The percentage of the dose excreted as sorbitol was 4.5%, as laevulose 0.45%, and as glucose 0.35%. Sorbitol did not produce hyperglycaemia and appeared to be metabolised like laevulose.— P. A. Bye, *Br. J. Surg.*, 1969, *56*, 653.

Uses. Sorbitol is about one-half as sweet as sucrose. It provides about 17 kJ (4 kcal) per g. A 30% solution may be employed similarly to dextrose by intravenous infusion at a rate not exceeding 2 ml per minute in conditions associated with carbohydrate insufficiency. A 50% solution has been injected intravenously to promote diuresis and to prevent or treat cerebral oedema or to reduce intra-ocular pressure. Sorbitol has been given by rapid intravenous injection in doses of 20 ml of a 50% solution for the prophylaxis and treatment of postoperative paralytic ileus. The dose may be repeated after 2 hours. Sorbitol has been given by mouth as a laxative in a dosage of 5 to 15 g daily in divided doses; doses of 30 to 50 g have been given to induce purging. Sorbitol has been tried in place of dextrose in peritoneal dialysis solutions.

Sorbitol Solution is used as a sweetening agent and substitute for glycerol in pharmaceutical preparations. It has about one-half the sweetening power of simple syrup. When added to syrups containing sucrose it reduces the tendency to deposit crystals on storage; for this purpose, about 20% to 30% of Sorbitol Solution is sufficient. Though its solubility is decreased in the presence of alcohol, Sorbitol Solution can usually be employed in elixirs and other preparations containing up to 40% of alcohol.

Sorbitol Solution is used as a humectant in pharmaceutical and cosmetic creams and is an ingredient of some toothpastes. It is also used as a plasticiser in the manufacture of gelatin capsules. Sorbitol may be used, in a daily dose of up to about 30 g, by diabetics in place of sucrose.

In patients with acute viral hepatitis the half-life of sorbitol was 48.5 minutes compared with 23.8 minutes in controls.— D. Brachtel *et al.*, *Klin. Wschr.*, 1974, *52*, 101.

The Food Standards Committee considered that sorbitol was an undesirable ingredient for general use in soft drinks since some individuals had a low gastric tolerance for sorbitol. It was recommended that its use in soft drinks be limited to those intended for consumption by diabetics.— *Review of the Soft Drinks Regulations 1964 (as amended)*, FSC/REP/65, Ministry of Agriculture, Fisheries and Food, London, HM Stationery Office, 1976. Long-term *animal* feeding studies using sorbitol 20% in the diet showed unwanted effects and further toxicological studies are required.— Twenty-second Report of Joint FAO/WHO Expert Committee on Food Additives, *Tech. Rep. Ser. Wld Hlth Org. No. 631*, 1978.

Preparations

Sorbitol Intravenous Infusion *(B.P.)*. Sorbitol Injection. A sterile solution of sorbitol for parenteral use in Water for Injections. Sterilised by autoclaving.

A 30% solution provides 4710 kJ (1125 kcal) per litre and should be administered through a plastic catheter.

Sorbitol Solution *(U.S.P.)*. An aqueous solution containing not less than 64% w/w of sorbitol. A clear, colourless, syrupy liquid with a sweet taste. Specific gravity not less than 1.285. It is neutral to litmus. Store in airtight containers.

Sorbitol Solution (70 per cent) *(B.P.)*. Sorbitol Solution; Sorbitol Liquid. A clear colourless, odourless, viscous liquid with a sweet taste, containing 68 to 72% w/w of hexitols expressed as D-glucitol. Relative density not less than 1.29. Miscible with water, glycerol, and propylene glycol; soluble in alcohol; very slightly soluble in most other organic solvents. A similar solution is described in several pharmacopoeias.

It is available in 'crystallising' and 'non-crystallising' grades, the latter usually containing a small proportion of related products which help to retard crystallisation of the sorbitol under normal conditions of storage. Store in airtight containers.

Proprietary Preparations

Howsorb 1 *(Laporte, UK)*. A brand of crystallising grade Sorbitol Solution. **Howsorb 2** is a non-crystallising grade of Sorbitol Solution.

Klyx *(Ferring, UK: Nordic, UK)*. An enema containing sorbitol 25% and docusate sodium 0.1%, with methyl and propyl hydroxybenzoates 0.12%, available in plastic bottles of 120 and 240 ml and fitted with a rectal nozzle.

Sorbex RP *(Hefti, Switz.: Steetley Trading, UK)*. A brand of sorbitol. **Sorbex RS**. A brand of Sorbitol Solution.

Sorbitol EGIC *(Egic, Fr.: Servier, UK)*. Sorbitol, available as an infusion solution containing 30%.

Sorbitol Powder *(Laporte, UK)*. A brand of sorbitol.

Other Proprietary Names

Cinecolex R-X *(Spain)*; Sorbilande *(Austral., Ital.)*; Sorbostyl *(Fr., Switz.)*; Syn MD *(Belg., Switz.)*.

660-b

Sucrose *(B.P., Eur. P., U.S.N.F.)*. Refined Sugar; Saccharose; Saccharum; Sucrosum; Sucre; Zucker; Azúcar; Sacarosa. β-D-Fructofuranosyl-α-D-glucopyranoside.

$C_{12}H_{22}O_{11}$=342.3.

CAS — 57-50-1.

Pharmacopoeias. In all pharmacopoeias examined except *Braz., Int., Rus.*, and *U.S.*, but in *U.S.N.F. U.S.N.F.* also includes Compressible Sugar, which contains sucrose 95 to 98% and may contain starch, malto-dextrin, or invert sugar, and a suitable lubricant; and Confectioner's Sugar, which contains sucrose not less than 95% with maize starch, in fine powder.

Colourless, odourless crystals, crystalline masses, or white crystalline powder, with a sweet taste, obtained from the juice of the sugar-cane, *Saccharum officinarum* (Gramineae), white-rooted varieties of sugar-beet, *Beta vulgaris* (Chenopodiaceae), and other sources. It absorbs insignificant amounts of moisture at 25° at relative humidities up to about 85% but under damper conditions it absorbs substantial amounts.

Soluble 2 in 1 of water and 1 in 370 of alcohol; freely soluble in alcohol (70%); sparingly soluble in dehydrated alcohol; practically insoluble in chloroform and ether. A solution in water is dextrorotatory and neutral to litmus. A 9.25% solution in water is iso-osmotic with serum. Solutions are **sterilised** by autoclaving or by filtration.

Growth of micro-organisms is usually inhibited in solutions with a concentration of sucrose above 65% w/w, but at this strength crystallisation may occur.

Adverse Effects. Intolerance to sucrose has been reported, particularly in children, due to deficiency of sucrase and isomaltase; intolerance may occur in patients intolerant of laevulose. Sucrose consumption increases the incidence of dental caries. Renal tubular damage may be caused by repeated intravenous injections of sucrose.

A hypothesis linking the intake of sucrose with dental caries, dyspepsia, seborrhoeic dermatitis, myopia, protein deficiency, diabetes, ischaemic heart disease, and gout.— J. Yudkin, *Nature*, 1972, *239*, 197.

Precautions. Sucrose should be administered with care to patients with diabetes mellitus. It is contra-indicated in patients with the glucose-galactose malabsorption syndrome, laevulose intolerance, or sucrase deficiency.

Absorption and Fate. Sucrose is hydrolysed in the small intestine by the enzyme sucrase to dextrose and laevulose, which are then absorbed. Sucrose is excreted unchanged in the urine when given intravenously.

In healthy subjects, oral administration of 50 g of disaccharide caused an increase in blood-glucose concentration of at least 200 μg per ml above fasting values, but in patients with disaccharidase deficiency the increase was usually less.— G. Neale, *J. clin. Path.*, 1971, *24*, *Suppl.* 5, 22.

Uses. Sucrose is used as a sweetening agent and demulcent. If the sweetness of sucrose is taken as 100, laevulose has a value of about 173, dextrose 74, maltose 32, galactose 32, and lactose 16. Syrups prepared from concentrated solutions of sucrose form the basis of many linctuses. Sucrose is also used as a lozenge basis. It is commonly used as household sugar.

A number of reports have suggested that sucrose can replace dextrose in oral electrolyte solutions for use in cholera and infantile diarrhoea (see under Sodium Chloride, p.637.

Sucrose as a sweetening agent.— A. J. Vleitos, in *Symposium: Sweeteners*, G.E. Inglett (Ed.), Westport, AVI, 1974, p. 63.

The application of icing sugar to control the smell of malignant ulcers of the breast.— R. H. Thomlinson (letter), *Lancet*, 1980, *2*, 707.

Diarrhoea. Reports of and references to the use of sucrose in oral electrolyte solutions.— P. A. Moenginah *et al.* (letter), *Lancet*, 1975, *2*, 323; D. L. Palmer *et al.*, *New Engl. J. Med.*, 1977, *297*, 1107; M. Field, *ibid.*, 1121; G. I. Sandle *et al.* (letter), *ibid.*, 1978, *298*, 797; D. L. Palmer *et al.* (letter), *ibid.*, 798; A. Chatterjee *et al.*, *Lancet*, 1977, *1*, 1333; N. Hirschhorn and D. R. Nalin (letter), *ibid.*, *2*, 1230; P. Hutchins *et al.* (letter), *ibid.*, 1978, *1*, 1211; D. R. Nalin *et al.*, *ibid.*, *2*, 277; D. A. Sack *et al.*, *ibid.*, 280; *ibid.*, 300; *ibid.*, 1979, *1*, 939.

Hiccups. Administration of a teaspoon of dry granulated sugar resulted in the immediate cessation of hiccups in 19 of 20 patients who had had hiccups for up to 6 weeks.— E. G. Engleman *et al.* (letter), *New Engl. J. Med.*, 1971, *285*, 1489.

Preparations

Paediatric Simple Linctus *(B.P.)*. Simple Linctus Paediatric. Simple linctus 1.25 ml, syrup to 5 ml. Store at a temperature not exceeding 25°. When a dose less than 5 ml is prescribed, the linctus should be diluted to 5 ml with syrup. Such dilutions must be used within 2 weeks of preparation. *Dose.* Children, 5 to 10 ml.

Simple Basis for Lozenges *(B.P.C. 1973)*. For 100 lozenges: sucrose in fine powder 100 g, acacia in fine powder 7 g, water q.s.

Simple Linctus *(A.P.F.)*. Citric acid monohydrate 125 mg, concentrated anise water 0.05 ml, concentrated chloroform water 0.15 ml, amaranth solution 0.1 ml, syrup to 5 ml. *Dose.* 5 to 10 ml.

Simple Linctus *(B.P.)*. Citric acid monohydrate 125 mg, concentrated anise water 0.05 ml, chloroform spirit 0.3 ml, amaranth solution 0.075 ml, syrup to 5 ml. Store at a temperature not exceeding 25°. When a dose less than 5 ml is prescribed, the linctus should be diluted to 5 ml with syrup. Such dilutions must be used within 2 weeks of preparation. *Dose.* 5 ml.

Sucrose Eye-drops *(Moorfields Eye Hosp.)*. Sucrose 10 to 30, phenylmercuric nitrate 0.002, Water for Injections to 100. For reduction of corneal oedema.

Syrup *(B.P.)*. Syr.; Simple Syrup. Sucrose 66.7% w/w in water. Wt per ml 1.315 to 1.333 g. It may contain one or more suitable antimicrobial preservatives. Syrup should not be exposed to undue fluctuations in temperature.

A similar syrup is included in most pharmacopoeias.

There was evidence of physical incompatibility (turbidity or precipitation) when the following of the *B.P.C. 1973* preparations were prepared with or diluted with syrup preserved with 0.05% of a combination of hydroxybenzoate esters (Nipastat) or with syrup preserved with methyl hydroxybenzoate 0.03% and propyl hydroxybenzoate 0.015%: Paediatric Belladonna and Ephedrine Mixture, Paediatric Belladonna and Ipecacuanha Mixture, Ferrous Sulphate Mixture, Paediatric Ferrous Sulphate Mixture, Paediatric Ipecacuanha Mixture, Methadone Linctus, Noscapine Linctus, Paediatric Opiate Ipecacuanha Mixture, Paediatric Opiate Squill Linctus, Potassium Citrate Mixture, and Sodium Citrate Mixture. Incompatibility for Cloxacillin Elixir had not been established.— Pharm. Soc. Lab. Rep. P/79/2, 1979. A similar conclusion in respect of Methadone Mixture 1 mg/1 ml (*D.T.F.*).— Pharm. Soc. Lab. Rep. P/80/1, 1980.

Syrup *(U.S.N.F.)*. Sucrose 85% w/v in water. Store, preferably in a cool place, in airtight containers.

661-v

Invert Sugar

CAS — 8013-17-0.

An equimolecular mixture of dextrose and laevulose, prepared by the action of dilute mineral acid on sucrose. Invert sugar forms in simple syrup on keeping. Very **soluble** in water forming solutions with a pH of 3.5 to 6.

Adverse Effects and Precautions. As for Laevulose, p.54.

A discussion of allergic reactions due to contaminants in sucrose and invert sugar infusions.— G. B. West, *Chemist Drugg.*, 1976, *205*, 217.

Polysaccharide contaminants of the dextran type were isolated from 2 batches of sucrose, in quantities of 100 ppm and 10 ppm respectively. Both gave positive immunological reactions with antiserum; it was possible that they were responsible for the anaphylactic reactions occasionally seen after intravenous administration of invert sugar solutions.— A. Berge *et al.*, *Acta pharm. suec.*, 1976, *13*, 459. See also J. K. Wold and T. Heen, *ibid.*, 1978, *15*, 51.

Thrombophlebitis. A 10% solution of invert sugar buffered to pH 6.8 caused a significantly lower incidence of thrombophlebitis than a solution of the same strength with a pH between 3.5 and 4.5 following the concurrent intravenous injection of 500-ml quantities in 76 patients. Only 2 instances of thrombophlebitis occurred with the buffered solution but 12 occurred with the other. Sodium acid phosphate 52 mg and sodium phosphate 59.4 mg dissolved in Water for Injections 1 ml was added immediately before infusion to buffer the solution pH to 6.8.— G. Elfving and K. Saikku, *Lancet*, 1966, *1*, 953.

A controlled study indicated that the incidence of thrombophlebitis after the intravenous infusion of 10% invert sugar solution was 28.2% while that following the infusion of 5% dextrose solution was 26.4%. Infusions of both solutions were given to 110 patients in either 500- or 1000-ml volumes.— G. Elfving *et al.* (letter), *Lancet*, 1966, *2*, 226.

Uses. Invert sugar is given by intravenous infusion as a 10% solution and has uses similar to those of dextrose (p.51) and laevulose (p.55).

Invert Syrup, when mixed in suitable proportions with syrup, prevents the deposition of crystals of sucrose under most conditions of storage.

Preparations

Infundibile Invertosi 10% *(Nord. P.)*. Sucrose 9.5 g, 0.1M hydrochloric acid 400 mg, Water for Injections to 100 ml. Sterilised by autoclaving at 110° for 1 hour.

Invert Syrup *(B.P.)*. A clear, colourless to pale straw-coloured, odourless, syrupy liquid with a sweet taste containing not less than 67% w/w of invert sugars. It is prepared by hydrolysing a 66.7% solution of sucrose with a suitable mineral acid, and neutralising the solution with, for example, calcium carbonate or sodium carbonate. The degree of inversion is at least 95%. pH 5 to 6. Wt per ml 1.338 to 1.344 g. It contains not more than 70 ppm of sulphur dioxide. Miscible with water forming a clear solution; partly soluble in alcohol. Store at 35 to 45°.

NOTE. Invert Sugar Solution and Invert Sugar Syrup as defined by The Specified Sugar Products Regulations 1976 (SI 1976: No. 509) consist of aqueous solutions of sucrose which have been partially inverted by hydrolysis; they contain not less than 62% of dry matter of which, respectively, 3 to 50% and more than 50% consist of invert sugar.

Proprietary Preparations

Travert *(Travenol, UK)*. Invert sugar, available as a 10% solution in sodium chloride injection or in Water for Injections. For intravenous use. Each litre provides approximately 1600 kJ (375 kcal).

Other Proprietary Names

Emetrol *(Spain, USA)*; Inverdex, Invertos *(both Swed.)*; Invertose *(Denm., Norw.)*; Invert-Oso *(Ital.)*.

A preparation containing invert sugar was also formerly marketed in Great Britain under the proprietary name Emetrol (*Rorer, USA: Pharmax*).

662-g

Threonine *(U.S.P.)*. L-Threonine; β-Methylserine. L-2-Amino-3-hydroxybutyric acid.

$C_4H_9NO_3$=119.1.

CAS — 72-19-5.

Pharmacopoeias. In *Jap.* and *U.S.*

A white odourless crystalline powder with a slightly sweet taste. M.p. about 256° with decomposition. Freely **soluble** in water; practically insoluble in dehydrated alcohol, chloroform, and ether. A solution in water is laevorotatory. A 1% solution in water has a pH of about 6.

Uses. Threonine is an amino acid which is an essential constituent of the diet. It is used as a dietary supplement.

663-q

Treacle. Theriaca.

The uncrystallisable residue from sugar refining.

Uses. Treacle is an ingredient of Chloroform and Morphine Tincture. A 50% solution of treacle in hot milk in doses of about 125 to 500 ml has been used as an enema.

664-p

Tryptophan *(U.S.P.)*. L-Tryptophan. L-2-Amino-3-(indol-3-yl)propionic acid.

$C_{11}H_{12}N_2O_2$=204.2.

CAS — 73-22-3.

Pharmacopoeias. In *Cz.*, *Jap.*, and *U.S.*

White to slightly yellowish-white odourless crystals or crystalline powder with a slightly bitter taste. **Soluble** 1 in about 100 of water; very slightly soluble in alcohol; practically insoluble in chloroform and ether; soluble in hot alcohol and solutions of dilute acids and alkali hydroxides. A solution in water is laevorotatory. A 1% solution in water has a pH of 5.5 to 7. **Protect** from light.

Adverse Effects. Nausea, anorexia, and drowsiness have been reported.

A report of sexual disinhibition in 4 male patients under treatment with preparations containing tryptophan.— G. P. Egan and G. E. M. Hammad (letter), *Br. med. J.*, 1976, *2*, 701. See also R. P. Hullin and T. Jerram (letter), *ibid.*, 1010. There was no change in sexual motivation in patients with multiple sclerosis given tryptophan 1.5 to 2 g daily.— M. T. Hyyppä (letter), *ibid.*, 1073. Sexual disinhibition in patients taking tryptophan had been seen in 1962 and was not confined to psychiatric patients.— I. Oswald (letter), *ibid.*, 1559. Hypersexuality has not been seen in over 500 patients; it might have been due to concomitant administration with phenothiazines.— A. D. Broadhurst and B. Rao (letter), *ibid.*, 1977, *1*, 51.

Precautions. The concomitant administration of tryptophan and a monoamine oxidase inhibitor may provoke a reaction likened to inebriation and may enhance the effects of the monoamine oxidase inhibitor (see under Phenelzine Sulphate p.128). If concomitant administration is desired the initial dose of tryptophan should be 500 mg daily, gradually increased after one week. Such treatment should be initiated in hospital.

Absorption and Fate. Tryptophan is readily absorbed from the gastro-intestinal tract. Tryptophan is extensively bound to serum albumin. It is metabolised to serotonin and other metabolites, including kynurenine derivatives, and excreted in the urine. Pyridoxine and ascorbic acid appear to be concerned in its metabolism.

The biological half-life of tryptophan was reported to be 15.8 hours.— W. A. Ritschel, *Drug Intell. & clin. Pharm.*, 1970, *4*, 332.

A comparison of the urinary metabolites of tryptophan in depressed and non-depressed patients did not indicate any increased excretion by the kynurenine route rather than the serotonin route in depressed patients.— A. Frazer *et al.*, *Archs gen. Psychiat.*, 1973, *29*, 528.

In healthy subjects concurrent administration of pyridoxine and ascorbic acid with tryptophan caused no significant increase in serum-tryptophan concentrations compared with administration of tryptophan alone.— G. Ashley *et al.*, *J. Pharm. Pharmac.*, 1976, *28*, *Suppl.*, 39P.

Uses. Tryptophan is an amino acid which is an essential constituent of the diet.

Tryptophan is a precursor of serotonin. Because serotonin is involved in depression, tryptophan has been used in treatment. Pyridoxine and ascorbic acid are considered to be involved in the metabolism of tryptophan to serotonin and are often given concomitantly. A dose of 1 g of tryptophan thrice daily may be adequate in mild or moderate depression, with 2 g thrice daily for severe depression. The efficacy of treatment is not universally accepted.

Tryptophan and DL-tryptophan are used as dietary supplements.

A loading dose of tryptophan caused striking increases in plasma-insulin concentrations in 13 patients when given 2 hours after a meal but in 6 fasting patients it had little or no effect.— B. Ajdukiewicz *et al.* (letter), *Lancet*, 1968, *1*, 92.

In a crossover study in 20 patients ECT seizures were significantly shortened in patients given tryptophan 6 g on the day before and 3 g four hours before ECT. The threshold to induce seizures was not affected.— H. Raotma, *Acta psychiat. scand.*, 1978, *57*, 253.

Depression. Tryptophan 6 to 12 g daily for 10 to 34 days caused a marked increase in serotonin concentration of platelets in 8 depressed patients.— D. L. Murphy, *Am. J. Psychiat.*, 1972, *129*, 141, per *Int. pharm. Abstr.*, 1973, *10*, 260.

Tryptophan 3 to 6 g daily was as effective as imipramine 150 to 225 mg daily in acute depression.— N. S. Kline and B. K. Shah, *Curr. ther. Res.*, 1973, *15*, 484. Similar reports: K. Jensen *et al.* (letter), *lancet*, 1975, *2*, 920; B. Rao and A. D. Broadhurst (letter), *Br. med. J.*, 1976, *1*, 460.

In an MRC study of 40 severely depressed patients tryptophan 6 g daily for 2 weeks then 8 g daily for 2 weeks given with pyridoxine 100 mg daily was compared with ECT. After the first 2 weeks there was no difference in response between ECT and tryptophan but at 4 weeks there was a significantly greater response to ECT. It was considered that tryptophan was not a suitable alternative to ECT.— R. N. Herrington *et al.*, *Lancet*, 1974, *2*, 731.

In a comparative study of 25 patients with unipolar depression 12 were treated with tryptophan 3 g daily in 2 divided doses with nicotinamide 250 mg four times daily and 13 with ECT twice weekly for at least 4 weeks. There was significantly greater improvement with tryptophan after 21 days than with ECT although by the 28th day improvement in the 2 groups was almost identical.— D. A. MacSweeney (letter), *Lancet*, 1975, *2*, 510.

Absence of benefit from tryptophan, in doses up to 16 g daily, in a small double-blind study in patients with depression.— J. Mendels *et al.*, *Archs gen. Psychiat.*, 1975, *32*, 22.

In 14 patients with depression there was no significant difference between those treated with tryptophan 9 g daily and those given also pyridoxine hydrochloride 90 mg and ascorbic acid 180 mg daily. Those given vitamins showed marginally greater improvement.— A. Coppen (letter), *Lancet*, 1976, *1*, 90.

Allopurinol with tryptophan was tried in the treatment of depression in 8 male patients since allopurinol might increase brain concentrations of tryptophan by blocking appropriate liver enzyme activity. Five patients gained remission of symptoms and 2 showed some improvement.— B. Shopsin (letter), *Lancet*, 1976, *1*, 1189.

The efficacy of tryptophan with nicotinamide (given to reduce liver breakdown of tryptophan) decreased when the dose was increased above 4 g with 1 g daily. Concomitant treatment with imipramine might be helpful in bipolar depression.— G. Chouinard *et al.* (letter), *Br. med. J.*, 1978, *1*, 1422.

Further references: A. Coppen *et al.*, *Lancet*, 1967, *2*, 1178; *Drug & Ther. Bull.*, 1972, *10*, 75; C. K. Rao (letter), *Br. J. Psychiat.*, 1972, *120*, 127; A. Coppen *et al.*, *Archs gen. Psychiat.*, 1972, *26*, 234; S. N. Young and T. L. Sourkes (letter), *Lancet*, 1974, *2*, 897; *Br. med. J.*, 1976, *1*, 242.

Effect on sleep. In 5 of 16 healthy young men, the delay in the onset of rapid-eye-movement sleep was reduced to less than 45 minutes when 5 to 10 g of tryptophan was given on retiring.— I. Oswald *et al.*, *Br. J. Psychiat.*, 1966, *112*, 391.

Rapid-eye-movement (REM) sleep decreased while delta-wave sleep and non-REM sleep increased in 5 healthy persons given tryptophan 7.5 g for 10 consecutive nights. Total sleep increased in all but 1 of 7 patients with insomnia given tryptophan. Tryptophan produced significant increases in non-REM sleep and decreases in REM sleep when given with fenclonine to block the metabolism of tryptophan to serotonin in 4 patients. It seemed that tryptophan produced its sleep effects through a non-serotonin mechanism.— R. J. Wyatt *et al.*, *Lancet*, 1970, *2*, 842.

Studies in 6 patients failed to show that tryptophan 7.5 g had any effect on the disturbed sleep pattern which had been induced by substituting a placebo for normal hypnotics.— V. Březinová *et al.* (letter), *Lancet*, 1972, *2*, 1086. See also M. H. Greenwood *et al.*, *Clin. Pharmac. Ther.*, 1974, *16*, 455.

Tryptophan showed promise as a non-addictive hypnotic.— E. L. Hartmann, *Archs intern. Med.*, 1977, *137*, 272.

A review of the use of tryptophan as a hypnotic.— *Med. Lett.*, 1977, *19*, 108.

Further references: A. N. Nicholson and B. M. Stone, *Br. J. clin. Pharmac.*, 1979, *7*, 418P.

Migraine. Tryptophan 500 mg every 6 hours gave useful reduction in migraine symptoms in 4 of 8 patients.— P. Kangasniemi *et al.*, *Headache*, 1978, *18*, 161.

Pain. In a double-blind crossover study involving 5 patients with intractable pain, tolerance to the pain relief obtained by central grey stimulation (electrical stimulation of grey matter) was reversed in 4 by concurrent administration of tryptophan 750 mg four times daily. The fifth patient experienced acute gastric pain on ingestion of tryptophan and did not continue the study.— Y. Hosobuchi (letter), *Lancet*, 1978, *2*, 47.

Psychosis. In a double-blind study in 5 patients with mania, tryptophan was slightly superior to chlorpromazine.— A. J. Prange *et al.*, *Archs gen. Psychiat.*, 1974, *30*, 56.

Absence of benefit in 10 patients with mania.— C. A. Chambers and G. J. Naylor, *Br. J. Psychiat.*, 1978, *132*, 555.

Rheumatic disorders. Some patients with rheumatoid arthritis given tryptophan as an antidepressant had reduced rheumatic symptoms, with recurrence when tryptophan was withdrawn.— A. D. Broadhurst (letter), *Br. med. J.*, 1977, *2*, 456.

Proprietary Preparations

Optimax *(E. Merck, UK)*. Tablets each containing tryptophan 500 mg, pyridoxine hydrochloride 5 mg, and ascorbic acid 10 mg. For depression. *Dose.* 2 to 4 tablets thrice daily. **Optimax Powder** contains twice the above amounts in each sachet. Optimax tablets are also available without vitamins.

Pacitron *(Berk Pharmaceuticals, UK)*. Tryptophan, available as tablets of 500 mg.

Other Proprietary Names

Trofan, Tryptacin *(both USA)*.

665-s

Tyrosine *(U.S.P.)*. L-Tyrosine. L-2-Amino-3-(4-hydroxyphenyl)propionic acid.
$C_9H_{11}NO_3$=181.2.

CAS — 60-18-4.

Pharmacopoeias. In *U.S.*

Odourless, tasteless, colourless crystals or white crystalline powder. **Soluble** 1 in about 230 of water at 25°; much less soluble in cold water; practically insoluble in alcohol and ether; soluble in dilute mineral acids and in alkaline solutions. A solution in hydrochloric acid is laevorotatory.

Uses. Tyrosine is an amino acid present in many foods. About 70 to 75% of the daily requirement of phenylalanine may be met by tyrosine. Tyrosine is concerned in the biosynthesis of adrenaline, melanin, and thyroid hormones. It is used as a dietary supplement.

Possible use in depression.— I. K. Goldberg (letter), *Lancet*, 1980, *2*, 364; A. J. Gelenberg and R. J. Wurtman (letter), *ibid.*, 863. See also J. A. Hoskins (letter), *ibid.*, 597.

666-w

Valine *(U.S.P.)*. L-Valine; α-Aminoisovaleric acid. L-2-Amino-3-methylbutyric acid.
$C_5H_{11}NO_2$=117.1.

CAS — 72-18-4.

Pharmacopoeias. In *Jap.* and *U.S.*

A white odourless crystalline powder with a slightly sweet taste and a bitter after-taste. **Soluble** in water; practically insoluble in alcohol, acetone, and ether. A solution in hydrochloric acid is dextrorotatory. A 5% solution in water has a pH of 5.5 to 7.

Uses. Valine is an amino acid which is an essential constitutent of the diet. It is used as a dietary supplement.

667-e

Xylitol. Xylit.

$C_5H_{12}O_5$=152.1.

CAS — 87-99-0; 16277-71-7(D).

Pharmacopoeias. In *Jap.*

A polyhydric alcohol related to the pentose sugar, xylose (p.526). A white, odourless, hygroscopic, crystalline powder with a sweet taste. M.p. 92° to 95°. **Soluble** in water and alcohol; sparingly soluble in methyl alcohol. **Store** in airtight containers.

Adverse Effects. Large amounts taken by mouth may cause diarrhoea. Hyperuricaemia, changes in liver-function tests, and acidosis (including lactic acidosis) have occurred after intravenous infusion.

Tolerance of xylitol given by mouth in doses up to 220 g daily.— U. C. Dubach *et al.*, *Schweiz. med. Wschr.*, 1969, *99*, 190.

Doses of 1.22 to 3.13 g per kg body-weight of xylitol given intravenously to volunteers as 5 or 10% solutions produced hyperuricaemia. Doses of 2.3 to 2.9 g per kg produced both hyperuricaemia and hyperuricosuria, and in some subjects hyperbilirubinaemia.— J. F. Donahoe and R. J. Powers (letter), *New Engl. J. Med.*, 1970, *282*, 690.

Diuresis of more than 200 ml per hour in 7 patients followed by oliguria in 5 of these, with azotaemia in 3, occurred among 22 patients who had received xylitol by intravenous infusion. Acidosis was noted in 8 patients, changes in liver-function tests with elevated serum bilirubin and serum aspartate aminotransferase (SGOT) concentrations in 4, hyperuricaemia in 2, cerebral disturbances in 5, and deposition of crystals, probably calcium oxalate, in kidney tissue in 5 and in the brain in one. The average dose in affected patients was 490 mg per kg body-weight hourly for about 40 hours.— D. W. Thomas *et al.*, *Med. J. Aust.*, 1972, *1*, 1238. Diuresis and lactic acidosis were observed in a 46-year-old man given xylitol, 1 g per kg body-weight per hour by intravenous infusion for 7 hours.— *idem*, 1246.

Infusion of 25 or 100 g of xylitol caused elevations of serum uric acid, but within the normal range; 2 infusions per day caused elevations above the normal range. Total bilirubin concentrations were elevated within the normal range. Side-effects in some patients included light-headedness, nausea, vomiting, diarrhoea, weakness, and subdiaphragmatic and right upper quadrant pain. The study of xylitol intravenously had been discontinued in USA.— J. F. Donahoe and R. J. Powers, *J. clin. Pharmac.*, 1974, *14*, 255.

Uses. Xylitol is used as a food additive; about 20% of ingested xylitol is absorbed.

Xylitol has been tried as a substitute for dextrose in intravenous nutrition but generally abandoned as conferring no advantages.

Xylitol or dextrose was given by intravenous infusion to 11 patients with uraemia and to 10 volunteers. In both groups, xylitol was rapidly cleared from the blood and urinary excretion was minimal. It stimulated the release of insulin but to a lesser extent than dextrose. Xylitol might be a useful nutritional agent in uraemia and other disorders characterised by carbohydrate intolerance and insulin resistance.— I. M. Spitz *et al.*, *Metabolism*, 1970, *19*, 24. See also S. Yamagata *et al.*, *Lancet*, 1965, *2*, 918.

Xylitol was metabolised in the liver to D-xylulose and then to fructose-6-phosphate without the aid of insulin. However, for utilisation and storage of the glucose so formed insulin was needed.— E. R. Froesch and U. Keller, in *Parenteral Nutrition*, A.W. Wilkinson (Ed.), London, Churchill Livingstone, 1972, p. 105.

The effects of high-dose (1 g per kg body-weight per hour) infusion of dextrose, laevulose, and xylitol.— H. Förster and D. Zagel, *Dt. med. Wschr.*, 1974, *99*, 1300.

The effects of infusions of dextrose, laevulose, and xylitol—250 mg per kg body-weight over 48 hours.— H. Förster *et al.*, *Dt. med. Wschr.*, 1974, *99*, 1723.

Xylitol used instead of sugar in the diet might reduce the incidence of dental caries. There was no evidence that xylitol in chewing-gum led to a lower incidence of caries than not chewing gum at all.— *Med. Lett.*, 1977, *19*, 79.

The available evidence on the oral administration of xylitol had not indicated adverse effects such as had been seen in *animal* studies. Trials in progress for the prevention of dental caries, using up to 5 g daily per child, should continue. Up to 20 g daily might be given to children aged 8 to 13, subject to dental and clinical supervision.— *Bull. Wld Hlth Org.*, 1979, *57*, 213.

Preparations

Xylitol Injection *(Jap. P.)*. A sterile solution of xylitol in Water for Injections. pH 4.5 to 7.5.

Proprietary Names

Eutrit, Klinit, Kylit, Newtol, Xyranit *(all Jap.)*.

668-l

Proprietary Amino-acid Preparations

Included below are miscellaneous amino-acid preparations for intravenous or oral administration as well as milk foods. Amino-acid preparations that are suitable for adults are not automatically suitable for infants since they may not contain all the amino acids essential for growth.

NOTE. One kcal is equivalent to 4.184 kJ.

Some Proprietary Amino-acid Preparations for Intravenous Administration

Aminofusin L600 *(Pfrimmer, Ger.: E. Merck, UK)*. A solution containing in each litre alanine 6 g, arginine 4 g, glutamic acid 9 g, glycine 10 g, histidine 1 g, isoleucine 1.55 g, leucine 2.2 g, lysine hydrochloride 2.5 g, methionine[L] 2.1 g, phenylalanine 2.2 g, proline 7 g, threonine 1 g, tryptophan 450 mg, and valine 1.5 g, with sorbitol 100 g, ascorbic acid 400 mg, inositol 500 mg, nicotinamide 60 mg, pyridoxine hydrochloride 40 mg, and riboflavine sodium phosphate 2.5 mg, providing 2500 kJ and the following ions: sodium 40 mmol, potassium 30 mmol, magnesium 5 mmol, and chloride 14 mmol. **Aminofusin L1000** contains in addition alcohol 52.8 g per litre and provides 4200 kJ. **Aminofusin L Forte** contains in each litre alanine 12 g, arginine 8 g, glutamic acid 18 g, glycine 20 g, histidine 2 g, isoleucine 3.1 g, leucine 4.4 g, lysine hydrochloride 5 g, methionine[L] 4.2 g, phenylalanine 4.4 g, proline 14 g, threonine 2 g, tryptophan 900 mg, and valine 3 g, with inositol 500 mg, nicotinamide 60 mg, pyridoxine hydrochloride 40 mg, and riboflavine sodium phosphate 2.5 mg, providing 1700 kJ and the following ions: sodium 40 mmol, potassium 30 mmol, magnesium 5 mmol, and chloride 27 mmol. For use with energy from other sources in intravenous nutrition.

Aminoplex 5 *(Geistlich, UK)*. A solution containing in each litre alanine 4.03 g, arginine 3.7 g, glutamic acid 800 mg, glycine 1.77 g, histidine 890 mg, isoleucine 1.53 g, leucine 2.33 g, lysine hydrochloride 2.74 g, L-malic acid 1.85 g, methionine[L] 1.93 g, L-ornithine-L-aspartate 800 mg, phenylalanine 2.77 g, proline 4.83 g, serine 970 mg, threonine 1.29 g, tryptophan 560 mg, and valine 1.8 g, with alcohol 50 g and sorbitol 125 g, providing 4200 kJ and the following ions: sodium 35 mmol, potassium 28 mmol, magnesium 4 mmol, chloride 43 mmol, and acetate 28 mmol. A balanced food for intravenous nutrition. **Aminoplex 12**. A solution containing in each litre alanine 10 g, arginine 9.2 g, glutamic acid 2 g, glycine 4.4 g, histidine 2.2 g, isoleucine 3.8 g, leucine 5.8 g, lysine hydrochloride 6.8 g, L-malic acid 4.6 g, methionine[L] 4.8 g, L-ornithine-L-aspartate 2 g, phenylalanine 6.88 g, proline 12 g, serine 2.4 g, threonine 3.2 g, tryptophan 1.4 g, and valine 4.48 g, providing 12.44 g of nitrogen and the following ions: sodium 35 mmol, potassium 30 mmol, magnesium 2.5 mmol, chloride 67.2 mmol, and acetate 5 mmol. For use with energy from other sources in intravenous nutrition. **Aminoplex 14**. A solution containing in each litre alanine 14.8 g, arginine 9.2 g, glycine 12 g, histidine 2.8 g, isoleucine 3.2 g, leucine 4.4 g, lysine hydrochloride 8.49 g, L-malic acid 5.36 g, methionine[L] 6.4 g, L-ornithine-L-aspartate 2 g, phenylalanine 4.4 g, proline 4 g, threonine 3.2 g, tryptophan 1.6 g, and valine 5.2 g, with nicotinamide 50 mg and pyridoxine hydrochloride 30 mg, providing 1400 kJ and the following ions: sodium 35 mmol, potassium 30 mmol, and chloride 81 mmol. For use with energy from other sources in intravenous nutrition.

FreAmine II *(Boots, UK)*. A solution containing in each litre alanine 6 g, arginine 3.1 g, glycine 17 g, histidine 2.4 g, isoleucine 5.9 g, leucine 7.7 g, lysine acetate equivalent to lysine 6.2 g, methionine 4.5 g, phenylalanine 4.8 g, proline 9.5 g, serine 5 g, threonine 3.4 g, tryptophan 1.3 g, and valine 5.6 g, with cysteine hydrochloride less than 200 mg, providing 12.5 g of nitrogen and the following ions: sodium 10 mmol and phosphate 10 mmol; available in infusion bottles of 500 ml. **FreAmine II Hyperalimentation Kit (40% Dextrose)**. Kit consisting of one 500-ml bottle of FreAmine II and one 1000-ml bottle containing 500 ml of dextrose injection 40%. A similar kit containing dextrose injection 50% is also available.

Perifusin *(E. Merck, UK)*. A solution containing in each litre alanine 3.96 g, arginine 2.64 g, glutamic acid 5.94 g, glycine 6.6 g, histidine 660 mg, isoleucine 1.06 g, leucine 1.45 g, lysine hydrochloride 1.65 g, L-malic acid 3 g, methionine[L] 1.39 g, phenylalanine 1.45 g, proline 4.62 g, threonine 660 mg, tryptophan 330 mg, and valine 990 mg, providing 550 kJ and the following electrolytes: sodium 40 mmol, potassium 30 mmol, magnesium 5 mmol, chloride 9 mmol, and acetate 10 mmol.

Comment on Perifusin.— *Drug & Ther. Bull.*, 1981, *19*, 57.

Pluritene *(Lipha, UK)*. A solution containing in each litre arginine hydrochloride 6 g, glycine 6 g, histidine hydrochloride 2 g, isoleucine 5.85 g, leucine 6.25 g, lysine hydrochloride 8 g, methionine[L] 10 g, phenylalanine 9.6 g, threonine 5 g, tryptophan 2.5 g, and valine 7.2 g, with sorbitol 40 g, providing 1900 kJ and sodium 15 mmol. For use with energy from other sources in intravenous nutrition.

Synthamin 7S (known in *USA* as Travasol) *(Travenol, UK)*. A solution containing in each litre alanine 8.29 g, arginine 4.14 g, glycine 8.29 g, histidine 1.75 g, isoleucine 1.91 g, leucine 2.47 g, lysine (as hydrochloride) 2.31 g, methionine[L] 2.31 g, phenylalanine 2.47 g, proline 1.67 g, threonine 1.67 g, tryptophan 720 mg, tyrosine 160 mg, valine 1.84 g, with sorbitol 150 g, providing 6.7 g of nitrogen and 2500 kJ (non-protein) and the following ions: sodium 38 mmol, potassium 30 mmol, magnesium 2.5 mmol, chloride 35 mmol, acetate 60 mmol, and phosphate 15 mmol. **Synthamin 9**. A solution containing in each litre alanine 11.4 g, arginine 5.7 g, glycine 11.4 g, histidine 2.41 g, isoleucine 2.63 g, leucine 3.4 g, lysine (as hydrochloride) 3.18 g, methionine[L] 3.18 g, phenylalanine 3.4 g, proline 2.3 g, threonine 2.3 g, tryptophan 990 mg, tyrosine 220 mg, and valine 2.52 g, providing 9.26 g of nitrogen and the following ions: sodium 73 mmol, potassium 60 mmol, magnesium 5 mmol, chloride 70 mmol, acetate 100 mmol, and phosphate 30 mmol. **Synthamin 14**. A solution containing in each litre alanine 17.6 g, arginine 8.8 g, glycine 17.6 g, histidine 3.72 g, isoleucine 4.06 g, leucine 5.26 g, lysine (as hydrochloride) 4.92 g, methionine[L] 4.92 g, phenylalanine 5.26 g, proline 3.56 g, threonine 3.56 g, tryptophan 1.52 g, tyrosine 340 mg, and valine 3.9 g, providing 14.3 g of nitrogen and ions as in Synthamin 9, except acetate 130 mmol. **Synthamin 17**. A solution containing in each litre alanine 20.8 g, arginine 10.4 g, glycine 20.8 g, histidine 4.4 g, isoleucine 4.8 g, leucine 6.2 g, lysine (as hydrochloride) 5.8 g, methionine[L] 5.8 g, phenylalanine 6.2 g, proline 4.2 g, threonine 4.2 g, tryptophan 1.8 g, tyrosine 400 mg, and valine 4.6 g, providing 16.9 g of nitrogen and ions as in Synthamin 9, except acetate 150 mmol. **Synthamin 14** and **17 Without Electrolytes** have the same amino-acid composition, and provide acetate 68 mmol and chloride 34 mmol (Synthamin 14), and acetate 82 mmol and chloride 40 mmol (Synthamin 17).

Vamin N *(KabiVitrum, UK)*. A solution containing in each litre alanine 3 g, arginine 3.3 g, aspartic acid 4.1 g, cysteine and/or cystine 1.4 g, glutamic acid 9 g, glycine 2.1 g, histidine 2.4 g, isoleucine 3.9 g, leucine 5.3 g, lysine 3.9 g, methionine[L] 1.9 g, phenylalanine 5.5 g, proline 8.1 g, serine 7.5 g, threonine 3 g, tryptophan 1 g, tyrosine 500 mg, and valine 4.3 g, providing 1000 kJ and the following ions: sodium 50 mmol, potassium 20 mmol, calcium 2.5 mmol, magnesium 1.5 mmol, and chloride 55 mmol. **Vamin Fructose**. A similar solution containing in addition laevulose 10%, providing 2700 kJ per litre. **Vamin Glucose**. A similar solution to Vamin N containing in addition dextrose 10%, providing 2700 kJ per litre. For intravenous nutrition.

Preparations of amino acids were formerly marketed in Great Britain under the proprietary names Aminosol (*KabiVitrum*), Travasol (*Travenol*), and Trophysan (*Égic, Fr.: Servier*).

Some Proprietary Dietary and Nutritive Preparations

Aglutella Gentili *(G.F. Dietary Supplies, UK)*. A range of low-protein, gluten-free pasta and semolina containing in each 100 g carbohydrate 86.8 g, with fat and protein not more than 500 mg, and low sodium and potassium content. For use in phenylketonuria, renal failure, liver failure, and gluten enteropathy.

Aglutella Azeta Wafers *(G.F. Dietary Supplies, UK)*. Low-protein, gluten-free wafers containing in each 100 g protein 500 mg, carbohydrate 71.75 g, fat 25.5 g, and phenylalanine not more than 12 mg. For use in phenylketonuria, renal failure, and liver failure.

al 110 *(Nestlé, UK)*. A powder containing fat 21%, dextrose 51.1%, and protein 22.2%, with added vitamins and minerals. Lactose content not more than 0.5%. For use in conditions associated with intolerance to lactose and other disaccharides.

Albumaid *(Scientific Hospital Supplies, UK)*. A range of amino-acid preparations, including **Albumaid Complete**, free from carbohydrate and fat; **Albumaid Cystine Low**, containing in each 100 g cystine not more than 40 mg and methionine not more than 200 mg; **Albumaid Histidine Low**, free from histidine; **Albumaid Methionine Low**, containing methionine not more than 40 mg per 100 g;**Albumaid RVHB**, free from methionine; **Albumaid XP**, containing phenylalanine not more than 10 mg per 100 g; **Albumaid XP Concentrate**, containing phenylalanine not more than 25 mg per 100 g and free from carbohydrate; and **Albumaid Phenylalanine/Tyrosine Low**, containing in each 100 g phenylalanine not more than 10 mg and tyrosine not more than 10 mg. For the dietary control of metabolic disorders.

The use of Caloreen and Albumaid by nasogastric tube.— A. M. J. Woolfson *et al.*, *Postgrad. med. J.*, 1976, *52*, 678.

Allergilac *(Cow & Gate, UK)*. A dried milk powder with reduced lactalbumin and added lactic acid and vitamins A and D, containing fat 16%, casein 25.8%, lactalbumin 1%, lactose 43.4%, mineral salts 8%, and lactic acid 2.8%. For use in certain milk protein allergies.

Aminex *(Cow & Gate, UK)*. A low-protein food in the form of biscuits; each 100 g contains protein 1 g and phenylalanine not more than 21 mg; it is free from sucrose. For use in phenylketonuria and other conditions requiring a low protein diet or restriction on the intake of a specific amino acid.

Aminogran *(Allen & Hanburys, UK)*. A food supplement comprising a mixture of all essential amino acids except phenylalanine, and a separate mixture of mineral salts. It is given, with vitamin supplements, and in conjunction with a diet of controlled phenylalanine content, in phenylketonuria.

For a comparison of Aminogran with Cymogran and Minafen in infants with phenylketonuria, see Minafen, below.

Aminutrin *(Geistlich, UK)*. An amino-acid powder, for preparation with liquid before use, providing the equivalent of 11.7 g of protein in each 15-g sachet. For use as a protein source in oral or gastric tube feeding.

Aproten *(Farmitalia Carlo Erba, UK)*. A range of dietetic products free from gluten and with a low protein, potassium, and sodium content.

Bi-Aglut Gluten-free Biscuits *(Farmitalia Carlo Erba, UK)*. Ingredients: starch, sugar, eggs, skimmed milk solids, and flavourings. For use in coeliac disease.

Calonutrin *(Geistlich, UK)*. Each 100-g sachet contains glucose approximately 24 g, maltose approximately 9 g, and polysaccharides approximately 67 g. For use as an energy source in oral or gastric tube feeding.

Cantabread *(Cantassium Co., UK)*. A gluten-free mix for preparing bread.

Casilan *(Farley, UK)*. A whole protein powder containing all essential amino acids. Contains 90% of protein; sodium content is less than 0.1%. For providing extra protein in case of inadequate protein intake or abnormal protein loss.

Clinifeed *(Roussel, UK)*. A range of gluten-free complete liquid foods prepared from maltodextrin, sucrose, whey proteins, egg yolk, milk, chicken meat, maize oil, and soya oil, with vitamins, minerals, and flavouring. For oral or nasogastric feeding.

Complan *(Farley, UK)*. A complete food prepared from skimmed milk, maltodextrin, vegetable oil, and sucrose, with vitamins and minerals.

Cymogran *(Allen & Hanburys, UK)*. A dried food of low phenylalanine content (not more than 10 mg per 100 g). It is prepared from hydrolysed casein with added amino acids, fat, carbohydrate, and minerals. It is given, with vitamin supplements, and in conjunction with a diet of controlled phenylalanine content, in phenylketonuria.

For a comparison of Cymogran with Aminogran and Minafen in infants with phenylketonuria, see Minafen, below.

Dialamine *(Scientific Hospital Supplies, UK)*. A liquid containing amino acids 30 g in each 100 g, ascorbic acid, minerals, and trace elements. For use as an oral amino-acid supplement together with energy from other sources.

dp Cookies *(G.F. Dietary Supplies, UK)*. Low-protein biscuits. For phenylketonuria, renal failure, and liver failure.

Edosol *(Cow & Gate, UK)*. A powder containing in each 100 g fat 28.1 g, protein 27.8 g, carbohydrates 37.8 g, and mineral salts 4.5 g, and providing sodium not more than 30 mg. For use as a 12.5% solution, with additional vitamins, to replace milk in low-sodium diets.

Energen Starch Reduced Bran Crispbread *(RHM Foods, UK)*. Prepared from wheat gluten, wheat bran, and wheat flour, with added sodium chloride. For use in conditions requiring a high-residue diet.

Ensure Plus *(Abbott, UK)*. A complete liquid food containing in each 100 ml carbohydrate (corn syrup solids and sucrose) 20 g, protein (casein and soya protein isolate) 5.5 g, and corn oil 5.3 g, with added vitamins and minerals. Free from lactose and gluten. A low-residue diet.

Farley's Gluten-free Biscuits *(Farley, UK)*. Ingredients: soya flour, sugar, hydrogenated vegetable oil, cornflour, skim milk solids, salt, and flavouring. For use in coeliac disease.

Flexical *(Bristol-Myers Pharmaceuticals, UK)*. A synthetic food powder prepared from hydrolysed casein, amino acids, modified tapioca starch, corn syrup solids, fractionated coconut oil, and soya oil, with added vitamins, minerals, and trace elements; containing protein 9.9%, fat 15%, and carbohydrate 67.3%. A complete low-residue diet to replace parenteral feeding and for use in disorders of the gastro-intestinal tract.

A favourable report of the early postoperative use, by duodenal tube, of an elemental diet (Flexical).— S. Sagar *et al.*, *Br. med. J.*, 1979, *1*, 293.

Forceval Protein *(Unigreg, UK: Vestric, UK)*. A dispersible powder containing calcium caseinate 60% and carbohydrates 30%, with vitamins and minerals, and providing protein not less than 55%, fat not more than 1%, and sodium not more than 0.12%. Protein, vitamin, and mineral supplement.

Formula HF(2) *(Cow & Gate, UK)*. A powder prepared from amino acids, glucose syrup, vegetable fat, wheat starch, minerals, and vitamins, and containing fat 26%, carbohydrates 39.9%, and protein 25%; it is free from histidine. For the dietary treatment of histidinaemia.

Formula MCT(1) *(Cow & Gate, UK)*. A synthetic food prepared from protein, glucose syrup, and a mixture of medium-chain triglycerides, and containing fat 28%, protein 25.6%, and carbohydrates 40.6%. For the dietary treatment of certain fat malabsorption syndromes.

Formula S Soya Food *(Cow & Gate, UK)*. A milk substitute powder prepared from soya protein isolate, glucose syrup, and vegetable oil, with added vitamins and minerals, containing carbohydrate 54%, fat 24%, and protein 16%. For patients allergic to milk protein or lactose.

Fosfor *(Consolidated Chemicals, UK).* Phosphorylcolamine (2-aminoethyl phosphate, $C_2H_8NO_4P=141.1$), a synthetic amino acid, available as **Injection** containing 25% of the sodium salt in ampoules of 10 ml and as **Syrup** containing 5%. For neurasthenic and depressed conditions, acute and chronic hepatitis, for use in postoperative convalescence, and for parenteral feeding. *Dose.* 20 ml of syrup thrice daily; by intravenous injection, 20 ml daily or on alternate days; for a course of up to 20 injections. (Also available as Fosfor in *Spain*).

Galactomin Formula 17 *(Cow & Gate, UK).* A powder containing in each 100 g fat 22.3 g, protein 22.3 g, carbohydrates 50.2 g, and mineral salts 3 g. For use as a 12.5% solution, with additional vitamins, to replace milk in galactosaemia. **Galactomin Formula 18, Reduced Fat** is a modification of Galactomin with a reduced fat content (14.4%). **Galactomin, Fructose Formula 19** is a modification of Galactomin with a reduced fat content (14.4%) and with laevulose as the sole carbohydrate. For the dietary treatment of glucose-galactose intolerance.

A review: *Drug & Ther. Bull.*, 1971, *9*, 53.

Glutenex *(Cow & Gate, UK).* A gluten-free diet in the form of biscuits; free from milk products. For patients suffering from coeliac disease and other disorders of the digestive tract.

Isocal *(Bristol-Myers Pharmaceuticals, UK).* A synthetic liquid food prepared from soya protein isolate, caseinate solids, triglycerides of medium-chain fatty acids, soya oil, and glucose oligosaccharides, with added vitamins, minerals, and trace elements, providing protein 13%, fat 37%, and carbohydrate 50%. A complete low-residue diet for use in disorders of the gastro-intestinal tract.

Juvela *(G.F. Dietary Supplies, UK).* A mix for preparing bread and cakes, available in gluten-free and protein-free formulas.

NOTE. The name Juvela is also applied to a preparation of Alpha Tocopheryl Acetate, see p.1664.

Komplexogran *(Keimdiät, Ger.: Thomson & Joseph, UK).* A powder prepared from skimmed milk, cereal germ oil, wheat-germ extract, lecithin, and extract of dates. For use as an additive in pharmaceutical, dietary, and cosmetic preparations.

Locasol *(Cow & Gate, UK).* A powder containing in each 100 g fat 23.3 g, protein 21.4 g, carbohydrates 51.6 g, and mineral salts 1.8 g, and providing calcium not more than 48 mg. For use as a 12.5% solution, with vitamin supplements, to replace milk in low-calcium diets.

Lofenalac *(Bristol-Myers Pharmaceuticals, UK).* A complete food containing the equivalent of 15% of protein, fat 18%, carbohydrate 59%, vitamins, mineral salts, and phenylalanine not more than 80 mg per 100 g. Free of lactose and gluten. For use in phenylketonuria.

Maxipro HBV *(Scientific Hospital Supplies, UK).* A protein supplement prepared from whey protein isolate with added amino acids and minerals.

Metabolic Mineral Mixture *(Scientific Hospital Supplies, UK).* A mixture of mineral salts for dietary supplementation in disorders of carbohydrate and amino-acid metabolism.

Minafen *(Cow & Gate, UK).* A powder containing in each 100 g protein hydrolysate 16 g (equivalent to 12.5 g protein), carbohydrate 48 g, fat 31 g, and not more than 20 mg of phenylalanine. For use as a 12.5% or stronger solution, with additional vitamins, in phenylketonuria.

A comparison of 3 feeding regimens using Aminogran, Cymogran, and Minafen in 15 neonates with phenylketonuria. The treatment of choice was Minafen, given until the infants were twice their birth-weight, gradually replaced by Aminogran at 8 to 10 months of age.— I. Smith *et al.*, *Archs Dis. Childh.*, 1975, *50*, 864.

MSUD Aid *(Scientific Hospital Supplies, UK).* A food supplement containing all essential amino acids except isoleucine, leucine, and valine. It is given, with vitamin and mineral supplements, in the dietary control of maple-syrup-urine disease.

Nutramigen *(Bristol-Myers Pharmaceuticals, UK).* A gluten-free food prepared from hydrolysed casein, sucrose, starch, and maize oil, with added vitamins and minerals; containing protein 15%, fat 18%, and carbohydrate 59%. For use in conditions of intolerance to intact proteins, in galactosaemia, and in lactose intolerance.

Nutranel *(Nutricia, Neth.: Roussel, UK).* A complete food, prepared as powder, containing in each 100 g, carbohydrate (maltodextrin with a small amount of lactose) 74.3 g, protein (whey protein hydrolysate) 15.8 g, fat (maize oil and medium-chain triglycerides) 4 g, with added vitamins and minerals. A low-residue diet.

PK Aid I and II *(Scientific Hospital Supplies, UK).* Food supplements providing all essential amino acids except phenylalanine. Given, with vitamin and mineral supplements, in the dietary control of phenylketonuria in children over 2 years of age.

Portagen *(Bristol-Myers Pharmaceuticals, UK).* A complete food, supplied as powder for preparation with water before use, prepared from sodium caseinate, corn syrup solids, sucrose, medium-chain triglycerides, and corn oil, with added vitamins and minerals, containing carbohydrate 54.3%, fat 22.5%, and protein 16.5%. For use in conditions associated with malabsorption of fats, and lactose intolerance.

Pregestimil *(Bristol-Myers Pharmaceuticals, UK).* A gluten-free powder prepared from hydrolysed casein, amino acids, corn syrup solids, modified tapioca starch, maize oil, and medium-chain triglycerides, with added vitamins and minerals. It contains no lactose or sucrose. For infants and young children with disaccharide intolerance, sensitivity to intact proteins, or other disorders of the gastro-intestinal tract.

A review: *Drug & Ther. Bull.*, 1973, *11*, 37.

Prosobee *(Bristol-Myers Pharmaceuticals, UK).* A concentrated liquid milk substitute prepared from soya protein isolate, soya oil, corn syrup solids, and coconut oil, with added minerals and vitamins, containing protein 4%, fat 7.2%, and carbohydrate 13.8%. **Prosobee Powder.** A complete food prepared from similar ingredients, providing protein 15.6%, fat 28%, and carbohydrate 51.6%. Lactose-free and gluten-free. For patients allergic to milk or with galactosaemia.

Rite-Diet Gluten-Free Products *(Welfare Foods, UK).* A range of foods free from wheat and rye gluten. For use in coeliac disease and other disorders of the digestive tract.

Rite-Diet Protein-Free Products *(Welfare Foods, UK).* A range of foods stated to be very low in protein. For use in phenylketonuria and other disorders of amino-acid metabolism, and chronic renal failure.

Separated Milk Food *(Cow & Gate, UK).* A dried milk powder containing fat 0.8%, protein 35.5%, lactose 52.8%, and mineral salts 7.9%. For use in fat intolerance and coeliac disease.

Triosorbon MCT *(Pfrimmer, Ger.: E. Merck, UK).* A synthetic food for preparation with liquid before use, providing in each 85-g sachet protein 19 g, fat 19.2 g, and carbohydrate 56 g, with added vitamins and minerals. A low-residue diet for use in disorders of the gastro-intestinal tract.

Tyrosinaid *(Scientific Hospital Supplies, UK).* An amino-acid powder free from phenylalanine and tyrosine. For tyrosinosis and tyrosinaemia.

Velactin *(Wander, UK).* A powdered milk substitute of vegetable origin, free from lactose, supplemented with vitamins and minerals and containing protein 12%, fat 19.5%, and carbohydrate 62%; to replace milk in the diet of infants, children, and adults allergic to milk, and as a basic feed pending the identification of specific allergens.

Verkade Gluten-free Biscuits *(G.F. Dietary Supplies, UK).* Ingredients: corn starch, vegetable fat, eggs, milk solids, salt, and flavourings. For use in coeliac disease.

Vivonex *(Norwich-Eaton, UK).* A synthetic food, supplied as powder for preparation with water before use, providing in each 80-g sachet amino acids 6.18 g, simple sugars 69 g, and safflower oil 435 mg, with added vitamins and minerals. A complete low-residue diet to replace parenteral feeding and for use in disorders of the gastro-intestinal tract. **Vivonex HN.** A similar preparation, providing in each 80-g sachet amino acids 13.31 g, simple sugars 63.3 g, and safflower oil 261 mg, with added vitamins and minerals. A complete low-residue diet to replace parenteral feeding when a high-nitrogen intake is required. Separate flavour sachets are available for use with both preparations.

Replacement of the usual diet with an elemental diet (Vivonex) in 6 patients with bile acid-induced diarrhoea reduced faecal weight, frequency, and bile acid excretion.— L. M. Nelson *et al.*, *Gut*, 1977, *18*, 792.

The long-term nocturnal use of Vivonex HN in a girl with cystic fibrosis.— J. A. Bradley *et al.*, *Br. med. J.*, 1979, *1*, 167.

A report of essential fatty acid deficiency in a woman with Crohn's disease who had taken 6 packets of Vivonex daily as her only nutrition.— M. J. G. Farthing *et al.* (letter), *Lancet*, 1980, *2*, 1088.

Wysoy *(Wyeth, UK).* A milk substitute powder prepared from soya protein isolate, corn syrup solids, sucrose, vegetable oils, destearinated beef fat, and coconut oil, with added vitamins and minerals, containing fat 48%, carbohydrate 39%, and protein 13%. **Wysoy Ready-to-Feed** is the ready-prepared liquid presentation. Lactose-free. For patients allergic to milk protein or lactose or with galactosaemia.

Dietary and nutritive preparations were formerly marketed in Great Britain under the proprietary names Azeta (*G.F. Supplies*), Eledon (*Nestlé*), Formula LPLS(1), Formula LPT(1), Formula LPTM(2), Himaizol, and Prosol (all *Cow & Gate*),Kidnamin (*KabiVitrum*), Nefranutrin (*Geistlich*), Sobee (*Mead Johnson*), and Supro (*Eucomark*).

Some Proprietary Milk Foods

The Department of Health had recommended that National Dried Milk and certain other milk foods should not be used for feeding infants under 6 months of age. Recommended proprietary milk foods included Babymilk Plus, C & GV Formula, Cow & Gate Premium Babyfood, Ostermilk Complete Formula, SMA, and Gold Cap SMA; those not recommended included Babymilk 2 and Ostermilk Two.— *Pharm. J.*, 1976, *1*, 107.

Carnation *(Carnation Foods, UK).* Evaporated full-cream milk with added vitamin D. For infant feeding, 1 part is diluted with 2 parts or more of water; sucrose may be added.

Milumil *(Milupa, UK).* A modified dried milk food containing carbohydrate 60%, fat 22%, and protein 13.3%, with added vitamins and minerals.

Nenatal *(Nutricia, Neth.: Cow & Gate, UK).* A prepared milk food containing carbohydrate (lactose, glucose, and maltodextrin) 7.4%, fat (mostly maize oil and medium-chain triglycerides) 4.5%, and protein 1.8%, with added vitamins and minerals. For administration to low birth-weight infants until their nutritional requirements become the same as those of full-term infants.

Osterfeed *(Farley, UK).* A modified milk food powder containing carbohydrate (lactose) 54%, fat 29%, and protein 11%, with added vitamins and minerals. **Osterfeed Ready-to-Feed** is the ready-prepared liquid presentation.

Ostermilk Complete Formula *(Farley, UK).* A modified milk food powder containing carbohydrate (lactose and maltodextrin) 62%, fat 19%, and protein 12%, with added vitamins and minerals. **Ostermilk Ready-to-Feed** is the ready-prepared liquid presentation. **Ostermilk Two Improved Formula** is a modified milk powder containing carbohydrate 61%, fat 18%, protein 13%, with added mineral salts and vitamins.

Plus *(Cow & Gate, UK).* A modified dried milk food with added lactose, vegetable oil, vitamins, and minerals, providing when prepared carbohydrate (lactose) 6.9%, fat 3.5%, and protein 1.9%.

Prematalac *(Cow & Gate, UK).* A ready-prepared modified milk food prepared from demineralised whey, skimmed milk, butterfat, and vegetable oils, with added vitamins and minerals, providing carbohydrate (lactose) 6.6%, fat 5%, and protein 2.4%. For low birth-weight infants, both premature and small for gestational age. Not intended for domiciliary use.

Premium Babyfood *(Cow & Gate, UK).* A modified dried milk food with added lactose, vegetable oils, vitamins, and minerals, providing when prepared carbohydrate (lactose) 7.2%, fat 3.8%, and protein 1.5%.

SMA *(Wyeth, UK).* A milk powder providing, when prepared, protein 1.5%, lactose 7%, and animal and vegetable fat 3.5 to 4%, with vitamins and minerals. **Gold Cap SMA.** A milk food providing, when prepared, protein 1.5%, lactose 7.2%, and fat 3.6%, with added vitamins and minerals; available as concentrated or ready-to-feed liquid, and as powder.

The incidence of metabolic acidosis among 103 breast-fed 6-day-old infants was 4.9% compared with 41% in 61 fed on SMA. A pH-adjusted milk formula was desirable when breast milk was not available for preventing and treating neonatal metabolic acidosis.— A. Moore *et al.*, *Br. med. J.*, 1977, *1*, 129. See also H. M. Berger *et al.*, *Archs Dis. Childh.*, 1978, *53*, 926.

A milk food was formerly marketed in Great Britain under the proprietary name Lactogen (*Nestlé*). Some other milk foods were also marketed under the proprietary names C & GV Formula, Frailac, St. Ivel Milk, and Trufood (all *Cow & Gate*).

Anorectics

1470-g

Anorectic agents are substances that suppress appetite or the sensation of hunger. However, the weight-loss achieved by using anorectics is hardly dramatic and they must be considered only as an adjuvant to other treatments, particularly as an aid to acceptance of a reduced energy intake. Generally they should be given only for short periods as tolerance frequently develops.
The anorectic agents are mainly sympathomimetic agents and many have a pronounced stimulant effect upon the central nervous system. The increased metabolic stimulation characteristic of sympathomimetic action is considered to play little part in the action of anorectic agents; their action depends mainly upon suppression of appetite, mediated possibly through the hypothalamus.
The use of anorectic agents with bulk-forming agents such as methylcellulose, diuretics, or sedatives is unnecessary.
Other drugs with a stimulant effect upon the central nervous system are described in the section on Central and Respiratory Stimulants, p.360.

Reviews and comments on obesity and its treatment.— J. R. Bennett and M. Baddeley, *Br. med. J.*, 1976, *2*, 1052; D. Craddock, *Drugs*, 1976, *11*, 378; J. F. Munro, *Prescribers' J.*, 1979, *19*, 106 and 142; *idem*, *Int. J. Obesity*, 1979, *3*, 171; J. G. Douglas and J. F. Munro, *Drugs*, 1981, *21*, 362.

1471-q

Benzphetamine Hydrochloride. (+)-*N*-Benzyl-*N*α-dimethylphenethylamine hydrochloride.
$C_{17}H_{21}N,HCl=275.8$.

CAS — 156-08-1 (benzphetamine); 5411-22-3 (hydrochloride).

A white to off-white odourless crystalline powder. M.p. about 155°. Freely **soluble** in water, alcohol, and chloroform; slightly soluble in ether. **Protect** from light.

Adverse Effects. As for Dexamphetamine Sulphate, p.361.

Treatment of Adverse Effects. Marked hypertension, excitement, or convulsions may be treated as described under Dexamphetamine Sulphate, p.362.

Precautions. As for Dexamphetamine Sulphate, p.362.

Absorption and Fate. Benzphetamine is readily absorbed from the gastro-intestinal tract.

Uses. Benzphetamine hydrochloride is a sympathomimetic agent used as an anorectic in the treatment of obesity. The usual initial dose is 25 to 50 mg in mid-morning, subsequently adjusted, according to requirements, to a dose of 25 to 50 mg once to thrice daily.

Proprietary Names
Didrex *(Upjohn, USA)*; Inapétyl *(Upjohn, Fr.)*.

Benzphetamine hydrochloride was formerly marketed in Great Britain under the proprietary name Didrex (*Upjohn*).

1472-p

Chlorphentermine Hydrochloride. S62. 4-Chloro-αα-dimethylphenethylamine hydrochloride.
$C_{10}H_{14}ClN,HCl=220.1$.

CAS — 461-78-9 (chlorphentermine); 151-06-4 (hydrochloride).

A white or off-white odourless powder with a bitter taste. M.p. about 234°. **Soluble** in water and alcohol; sparingly soluble in chloroform; practically insoluble in ether. A 1% solution in water has a pH of 5 to 6.

Adverse Effects. As for Dexamphetamine Sulphate, p.361.
Chlorphentermine is reported to cause fewer side-effects due to stimulation of the central nervous system than dexamphetamine and drowsiness may occur.

Treatment of Adverse Effects. Marked hypertension, excitement, or convulsions may be treated as described under Dexamphetamine Sulphate, p.362.

Precautions. Chlorphentermine should be used with care in patients with cardiovascular disease, glaucoma, hypertension, or hyperthyroidism, and in patients of unstable personality.
Chlorphentermine should not be given to patients being treated with a monoamine oxidase inhibitor or within 14 days of stopping such treatment (see Precautions for Phenelzine Sulphate, p.128).
The response to insulin and antidiabetic agents may vary in diabetic patients receiving anorectic agents.

Though the use of chlorphentermine had been banned in Sweden and W. Germany, the Committee on Safety of Drugs had no evidence suggesting danger to health from its use. The Committee had requested that doctors report any occurrences of pulmonary hypertension following the use of anorectics.— *Chemist Drugg.*, 1969, *191*, 485.

Pulmonary blood pressure was increased by 50 to 75% in *rats* treated for several weeks with chlorphentermine.— H. Lullmann *et al.*, *Arzneimittel-Forsch.*, 1972, *22*, 2096.

Absorption and Fate. Chlorphentermine is absorbed from the gastro-intestinal tract. It has a biological half-life of about 40 hours, part being excreted unchanged in the urine.

References.— H. W. Jun *et al.*, *Can. J. pharm. Sci.*, 1969, *4*, 27; H. W. Jun and E. J. Triggs, *J. pharm. Sci.*, 1970, *59*, 306; A. H. Beckett and P. M. Bélanger (letter), *J. Pharm. Pharmac.*, 1974, *26*, 205; A. H. Beckett and P. M. Bélanger, *Br. J. clin. Pharmac.*, 1977, *4*, 193.

Uses. Chlorphentermine hydrochloride is a sympathomimetic agent used as an anorectic in the treatment of obesity. It is claimed to have little stimulant effect on the central nervous system. Usual doses are the equivalent of 65 mg of chlorphentermine base after breakfast.

Proprietary Names
Apsedon *(Lensa, Spain)*; Desopimon *(EGYT, Hung.)*; Pre-Sate *(Warner, Austral.*; *Parke, Davis, Canad.*; *Warner, S.Afr.*; *Parke, Davis, USA)*.

Chlorphentermine hydrochloride was formerly marketed in Great Britain under the proprietary name Lucofen SA (*Warner*).

1473-s

Clobenzorex Hydrochloride. SD 271-12. (+)-*N*-(2-Chlorobenzyl)-α-methylphenethylamine hydrochloride.
$C_{16}H_{18}ClN,HCl=296.2$.

CAS — 13364-32-4 (clobenzorex); 5843-53-8 (hydrochloride).

A white crystalline powder. M.p. 182° to 183°. **Soluble** in water and alcohol; slightly soluble in chloroform and methyl alcohol.

Uses. Clobenzorex hydrochloride is a sympathomimetic agent used as an anorectic in the treatment of obesity. It has been given in usual doses of 30 mg twice daily before meals.

Proprietary Names
Dinintel *(Diamant, Fr.)*; Rexigen *(Marxer, Arg.)*.

1474-w

Clortermine Hydrochloride. Su-10568. 2-Chloro-αα-dimethylphenethylamine hydrochloride.
$C_{10}H_{14}ClN,HCl=220.1$.

CAS — 10389-73-8 (clortermine); 10389-72-7 (hydrochloride).

Adverse Effects. As for Dexamphetamine Sulphate, p.361.

Treatment of Adverse Effects. Marked hypertension, excitement, or convulsions may be treated as described under Dexamphetamine Sulphate, p.362.

Precautions. As for Chlorphentermine Hydrochloride (above).
The response to insulin and oral antidiabetic agents may vary in diabetic patients receiving anorectic agents.

Absorption and Fate. Clortermine is absorbed from the gastro-intestinal tract.
The half-life of clortermine hydrochloride was 9 to 24 hours.— *Med. Lett.*, 1974, *16*, 54.

Uses. Clortermine hydrochloride is a sympathomimetic agent used as an anorectic in the treatment of obesity. It is the ortho isomer of chlorphentermine hydrochloride. The usual dose is 50 mg given mid-morning.
An evaluation of clortermine hydrochloride.— M. H. M. Dykes, *J. Am. med. Ass.*, 1974, *230*, 270.

Proprietary Names
Voranil *(USV Pharmaceutical Corp., USA)*.

1475-e

Diethylpropion Hydrochloride *(B.P., U.S.P.)*. Amfepramone Hydrochloride; Anfepramona Clorhidrato. 2-Diethylaminopropiophenone hydrochloride.
$C_{13}H_{19}NO,HCl=241.8$.

CAS — 90-84-6 (diethylpropion); 134-80-5 (hydrochloride).

Pharmacopoeias. In *Br.* and *U.S.*

A white to off-white fine crystalline powder, odourless or with a slight characteristic odour and a slightly bitter taste. The *B.P.* permits the addition of 1% of tartaric acid as a stabilising agent. M.p. about 175° with decomposition. **Soluble** 1 in 0.5 of water, 1 in 3 of alcohol, and 1 in 3 of chloroform; practically insoluble in ether. **Store** at a temperature not exceeding 25°. Protect from light.

Adverse Effects. As for Dexamphetamine Sulphate, p.361.
Cardiovascular effects may be less than with dexamphetamine. Diethylpropion hydrochloride may produce dependence of the amphetamine type (see p.361). Many instances of abuse have been reported.

Abuse. Reports of the abuse of diethylpropion.— L. J. Clein and D. R. Benady, *Br. med. J.*, 1962, *2*, 456; E. V. Kuenssberg (letter), *ibid.*, 729; J. Caplan, *Can. med. Ass. J.*, 1963, *88*, 943; H. S. Jones, *Med. J. Aust.*, 1968, *1*, 267; J. H. Willis (letter), *Lancet*, 1976, *1*, 37.

Effects on the endocrine system. Gynaecomastia developed in 2 men taking diethylpropion.— J. F. Bridgman and J. M. H. Buckler (letter), *Br. med. J.*, 1974, *3*, 520.

Effects on mental state. A schizophrenia-like reaction associated with diethylpropion in one patient.— B. H. Fookes (letter), *Lancet*, 1976, *2*, 1206.

Auditory delusions of 4 weeks' duration were reported to have commenced in a 48-year-old woman 2 months after she had started taking diethylpropion 25 mg thrice daily for the treatment of moderate obesity. She recovered after treatment with trifluoperazine.— B. F. Hoffman (letter), *Can. med. Ass. J.*, 1977, *116*, 351.

A report on 7 patients who had psychiatric disorders associated with the use of diethylpropion hydrochloride.— M. W. P. Carney and M. Harris, *Practitioner*, 1979, *223*, 549.

Sleep disturbances. No evidence of dependence or of alteration in normal sleep patterns was found in 340 obese adults and children treated with diethylpropion for at least 1 year.— G. M. Kneebone (letter), *Med. J. Aust.*, 1968, *2*, 246.

For a comparison of the effects of fenfluramine and diethylpropion on sleep, see Fenfluramine Hydrochloride, p.66.

Treatment of Adverse Effects. Marked hypertension, excitement, or convulsions may be treated as described under Dexamphetamine Sulphate, p.362.

Precautions. As for Dexamphetamine Sulphate, p.362.
The response to insulin and antidiabetic agents

may vary in diabetic patients receiving anorectic agents.

Absorption and Fate. Diethylpropion is readily absorbed from the gastro-intestinal tract and is excreted in the urine. Many metabolites have been reported.

Removal of the *N*-ethyl groups and reduction of the keto group gave rise to the main basic aromatic non-hydroxylated metabolites of diethylpropion hydrochloride.— F. Banci *et al.*, *Arzneimittel-Forsch.*, 1971, *21*, 1616. See also E. C. Schreiber *et al.*, *J. Pharmac. exp. Ther.*, 1968, *159*, 372; B. Testa, *Acta pharm. suec.*, 1973, *10*, 441; B. Testa and A. H. Beckett, *Pharm. Acta Helv.*, 1974, *49*, 21.

Uses. Diethylpropion hydrochloride is a sympathomimetic agent used as an anorectic in the treatment of obesity.

The usual dose is 25 mg thrice daily 1 hour before meals and at night if necessary, or 75 mg, as a sustained-release preparation, in mid-morning.

Preparations

Diethylpropion Hydrochloride Tablets *(U.S.P.)*. Tablets containing diethylpropion hydrochloride.

Proprietary Preparations

Apisate *(Wyeth, UK)*. Sustained-release tablets each containing diethylpropion hydrochloride 75 mg, thiamine hydrochloride 5 mg, riboflavine 4 mg, pyridoxine hydrochloride 2 mg, and nicotinamide 30 mg. For obesity. *Dose.* 1 tablet daily before breakfast or mid-afternoon, increased if necessary to 1 tablet twice daily.

Tenuate Dospan *(Merrell, UK)*. Sustained-release tablets each containing diethylpropion hydrochloride 75 mg. (Also available as Tenuate Dospan in *Austral.*, *Belg.*, *Canad.*, *Fr.*, *Ital.*, *S.Afr.*, *USA*.

Diethylpropion hydrochloride was also formerly marketed in Great Britain under the proprietary name Tenuate (*Merrell*).

Other Proprietary Names

Arg.— Alipid, Brendalit, Controlgras, Keramik, Nulobes, Redicres, Sinapet; *Belg.*—Dietil Retard, Menutil, Prefamone, Regenon; *Canad.*— Dietec, D.I.P., Nobensine-75, Regibon; *Denm.*— Dobesin, Regenon; *Fr.*— Moderatan Diffucap, Préfamone; *Ger.*—Regenon retard; *Ital.*—Linea, Magrene, Regenon; *Neth.*—Frekentine; *Spain*—Delgamer, Lipomin; *Swed.*—Danylen; *Switz.*—Adiposan, Adipyn, Lineal-Rivo, Préfamone, Regenon; *USA*—Tepanil.

NOTE. The name Lineal is also applied to Fenproporex (see p.68) and the name Tepanil is also applied to phenylpropanolamine hydrochloride (see p.26).

1477-y

Difemetorex Hydrochloride. Diphemethoxidine Hydrochloride; Ba 18189. 2-(2-Diphenylmethylpiperidino)ethanol hydrochloride.

$C_{20}H_{25}NO,HCl=331.9$.

CAS — 13862-07-2 (difemetorex); 20269-19-6 (hydrochloride).

Uses. Difemetorex hydrochloride has been used as an anorectic in the treatment of obesity. It was formerly given in usual doses of 5 mg before breakfast and 2.5 mg before the midday meal.

1476-l

Dimepropion Hydrochloride. Métamfépramone Hydrochloride; Metamfepyramone Hydrochloride. 2-Dimethylaminopropiophenone hydrochloride.

$C_{11}H_{15}NO,HCl=213.7$.

CAS — 15351-09-4 (dimepropion); 10105-90-5 (hydrochloride).

Uses. Dimepropion hydrochloride is a sympathomimetic agent which has been used as an anorectic in the treatment of obesity. It is the dimethyl analogue of diethylpropion. It was formerly given in usual doses of 50 mg twice daily before meals.

1478-j

Fenfluramine Hydrochloride *(B.P.)*. S 768.

N-Ethyl-α-methyl-3-trifluoromethylphenethylamine hydrochloride.

$C_{12}H_{16}F_3N,HCl=267.7$.

CAS — 458-24-2 (fenfluramine); 404-82-0 (hydrochloride).

Pharmacopoeias. In *Br.*

A white odourless crystalline powder with a slightly bitter taste. M.p. 168° to 172°. **Soluble** 1 in 20 of water and 1 in 10 of alcohol and chloroform; practically insoluble in ether.

Adverse Effects. Fenfluramine hydrochloride may often cause nausea, diarrhoea, headache, dizziness, and sedation. Other side-effects reported include dry mouth, flatulence, abdominal discomfort, constipation, fatigue, reduction or lightening of sleep, increase of depression, nightmare, palpitations, shivering, fluid retention, urinary frequency, impotence, skin rash, alopecia, and haemolytic anaemia.

After overdosage fenfluramine has caused vomiting, mydriasis and nystagmus, tremors, rigidity, hyperpyrexia, sweating, hyperreflexia, rapid respiration, tachycardia, facial flushing, hypertension, cardiac arrhythmias, convulsions, unconsciousness, and death from cardiac arrest. Many of these symptoms are typical of the effects of large doses of amphetamines. Abuse for euphoric effect has been reported, and reports of the occurrence of depression after the withdrawal of fenfluramine suggest the possibility of dependence of the amphetamine type (see Dexamphetamine Sulphate, p.361).

Abuse. Of 448 South African young men called up for military service and with a positive history of drug abuse 115 were users of fenfluramine, 38 experimentally, 26 occasionally, and 51 regularly. The frequency of abuse of fenfluramine was exceeded only by that of cannabis, amphetamines, and lysergide. The dose of fenfluramine ranged from 80 to 500 mg, usually 120 to 200 mg. The psychotomimetic state consisted of euphoria, relaxation, and inane laughter, usually with alterations of perception (visual, temperature), derealisation, and depersonalisation. In some cases depression and fear of impending doom occurred at the end of the state.— A. Levin, *Postgrad. med. J.*, 1975, *51, Suppl.* 1, 186. See also *idem* (letter), *Br. med. J.*, 1973, *2*, 49.

Further references.— H. P. Rosenvinge (letter), *Br. med. J.*, 1975, *1*, 735; G. L. Dare and R. D. Goldney, *Med. J. Aust.*, 1976, *2*, 537.

Effects on the blood. A 46-year-old obese woman, who had taken fenfluramine on 2 earlier occasions, developed haemolytic anaemia on the third occasion. She had taken no other drugs.— A. M. Nussey (letter), *Br. med. J.*, 1973, *1*, 177.

Effects on growth. In some children dietary restriction and concomitant administration of fenfluramine might lead to a reduction in linear growth velocity, even in the absence of weight loss.— P. H. W. Rayner and J. M. Court, *Postgrad. med. J.*, 1975, *51, Suppl.* 1, 120. See also W. R. Sulaiman and R. H. Johnson, *Br. med. J.*, 1973, *2*, 329; D. L. F. Dunleavy *et al.* (letter), *ibid.*, 1973, *3*, 48; E. M. E. Poskitt and P. H. W. Rayner (letter), *ibid.*, 348.

Effects on mental state. In a double-blind crossover trial involving 30 obese psychiatric patients it was noted that anxiety was reduced in 10 of the 17 anxious patients, but depression was increased in 5 of the 11 depressed patients when they were taking fenfluramine.— R. Gaind, *Br. J. Psychiat.*, 1969, *115*, 963.

In a double-blind study in 50 young nurses significantly more subjects felt stimulated and euphoric after fenfluramine 40 or 60 mg than after a placebo.— M. -A. Gagnon *et al.*, *Clin. Pharmac. Ther.*, 1974, *15*, 205.

Brief case histories of 3 patients in whom fenfluramine might have been responsible for precipitating psychosis—paranoid schizophrenia; hyperactivity; and homicidal suicidal tendencies with auditory hallucinations.— P. J. Shannon *et al.* (letter), *Br. med. J.*, 1974, *3*, 576.

In 8 subjects given, in a blind crossover study, fenfluramine 60, 120, or 240 mg, or dexamphetamine 20 or 40 mg, fenfluramine had little effect on blood pressure or temperature but caused dose-related pupillary dilatation. Three subjects taking 240 mg of fenfluramine experienced visual and olfactory hallucinations, alterations of mood, distorted time sense, fleeting paranoia, and sexual ideation.— J. D. Griffith *et al.*, *Clin. Pharmac. Ther.*, 1974, *15*, 207.

Sleep disturbances. When given at bedtime diethylpropion caused frequent awakenings, suppression and delay of paradoxical sleep (associated with dreaming and rapid eye movement), and frequent shifts into and increased time in stage 1 sleep (drowsiness), while fenfluramine only caused frequent shifts into stage 1 sleep and increase of time spent in it.— I. Oswald *et al.*, *Br. med. J.*, 1968, *1*, 796.

No evidence of dependence or of alteration in normal sleep patterns was found in 340 obese adults and children treated with fenfluramine for at least 1 year.— G. M. Kneebone (letter), *Med. J. Aust.*, 1968, *2*, 246.

Repeated nightmares occurred in a woman who took more than one 20-mg tablet of fenfluramine daily.— M. Y. Alvi (letter), *Br. med. J.*, 1969, *4*, 237.

Thirteen of 15 patients taking fenfluramine and no other drugs experienced an increase in dreaming while taking fenfluramine; the effect was dose-related. Five patients experienced terrifying dreams. The presence or absence of ascorbic acid in the diet had no effect.— A. Mullen *et al.*, *Br. med. J.*, 1977, *1*, 70. See also A. Mullen and C. W. M. Wilson (letter), *Lancet*, 1974, *2*, 594. Comment that although fenfluramine may cause increased dreaming in some patients, the clinical significance of this finding is small.— D. B. Campbell and C. Reuter, *Servier* (letter), *Br. med. J.*, 1977, *1*, 293.

Further references.— G. Ellis (letter), *Br. med. J.*, 1969, *4*, 558 (extreme sleepiness and lethargy).

Effects on the uterus. Of 50 patients treated with fenfluramine 40 mg thrice daily 4 complained of menorrhagia.— C. Wakes-Miller, *S. Afr. med. J.*, 1971, *Suppl.* (June 19), 16.

Extrapyramidal effects. A patient with a history of drug abuse manifested facial dyskinesia after taking fenfluramine.— S. Brandon (letter), *Br. med. J.*, 1969, *4*, 557.

See also under Overdosage (below).

Overdosage. Three 16-year-old girls ingested 400, 600, and 800 mg respectively of fenfluramine. They did not lose consciousness but developed symptoms including dilated pupils non-reactive to light, rotary nystagmus, hyperreflexia, jaw tremor, rapid respiration, and burning sensation in the epigastrium. They suffered sleep disturbances similar to those of mild amphetamine intoxication, with later rebound abnormalities.— I. Riley *et al.*, *Lancet*, 1969, *2*, 1162.

From a study of 30 subjects who had taken overdoses of fenfluramine it appeared that mild overdosage (200 to 400 mg) caused agitation, tremor, mydriasis, tachycardia, and hypertension; severe overdosage (400 to 800 mg) caused vomiting, convulsions, facial flushing, hyperpyrexia, unconsciousness, respiratory depression, and cardiac arrhythmias including ventricular fibrillation. Treatment should include the monitoring of plasma concentrations, ECG control, diazepam, treatment of hyperpyrexia, and anti-arrhythmic agents including propranolol if needed.— D. B. Campbell, *S. Afr. med. J.*, 1971, *Suppl.* (June 19), 51.

Extrapyramidal symptoms in 2 children following fenfluramine overdosage.— J. M. Darmady, *Archs Dis. Childh.*, 1974, *49*, 328.

Further references.— A. P. Haines and P. J. Shoenberg (letter), *Br. med. J.*, 1972, *1*, 632; J. Wolfsdorf and K. S. Kanarek, *S. Afr. med. J.*, 1972, *46*, 651; J. C. Veltri and A. R. Temple, *J. Pediat.*, 1975, *87*, 119; K. E. von Muhlendahl and E. G. Krienke, *Clin. Toxicol.*, 1979, *14*, 97.

Treatment of Adverse Effects. In general the management of overdosage with fenfluramine involves supportive and symptomatic therapy.

In severe overdosage the stomach should be emptied by aspiration and lavage. Diazepam may be given to control convulsions.

The ECG should be monitored and a beta-adrenoceptor blocking agent may be required to control cardiac arrhythmias.Measures should be taken to control increased body temperature.

It has been suggested that acidification of the urine may enhance the elimination of fenfluramine, but for comments on the hazards of procedures such as forced acid diuresis, see below, and under Dexamphetamine Sulphate, p.362.

A report of death in a 5-year-old child after ingestion of 20 long-acting capsules of fenfluramine (a total of 1.2 g). Following gastric lavage she suffered a tonic-clonic convulsion which was treated immediately with diazepam 5 mg intravenously. Convulsions ceased after 2 minutes and she became limp and pulseless, with fixed, dilated pupils; despite intensive resuscitative efforts she died about 3 hours after ingestion. An ipecacuanha emetic preparation might be preferable to gastric lavage in fenfluramine poisoning.— H. Simpson and I. McKinlay, *Br. med. J.*, 1975, *4*, 462.

The use of diazepam in the management of fenfluramine poisoning of 2 children.— J. M. Darmady, *Archs Dis. Childh.*, 1974, *49*, 328.

Diuresis. Forced diuresis has a limited application in the management of drug overdosage to those few drugs that are excreted to a significant extent unchanged in the urine. Forced acid diuresis has been used for poisoning by basic drugs such as fenfluramine but symptomatic treatment is usually adequate and is probably much safer. Forced diuresis should never be undertaken lightly. It is potentially lethal in elderly patients and in those with cardiac and renal disease.

Other complications include electrolyte and acid-base disturbances, water intoxication, and cerebral oedema.— L. F. Prescott, Limitations of haemodialysis and forced diuresis, in *The Poisoned Patient: the role of the Laboratory*, Ciba Foundation Symposium 26, Oxford, Elsevier, 1974, p. 269. See also J. A. Vale, *Prescribers' J.*, 1978, *18*, 67; J. A. Vale and R. Goulding, *ibid.*, 163.

Precautions. Fenfluramine hydrochloride should not be given to patients with depression or a history of depression or to patients being treated with a monoamine oxidase inhibitor or within 14 days of stopping such treatment (see Precautions for Phenelzine Sulphate, p.128). As fenfluramine causes drowsiness in some patients, care is necessary, until the effects of the drug can be determined, in patients who take charge of motor vehicles or operate machinery. It may enhance the effects of antihypertensive and hypoglycaemic agents.

Studies on the effect of fenfluramine on performance.— P. Turner, *S. Afr. med. J.*, 1971, *Suppl.* (June 19), 13; C. C. Brown *et al.*, *J. clin. Pharmac.*, 1974, *14*, 369.

Interactions. Drowsiness and acute confusional episodes occurred in 2 patients who took fenfluramine while already taking phenelzine and chlordiazepoxide and chlordiazepoxide alone, respectively.— S. Brandon (letter), *Br. med. J.*, 1969, *4*, 557.

A study in obese hypertensive patients indicating that, unlike amphetamines, fenfluramine enhances rather than diminishes the effect of antihypertensive agents. Results of long-term observations in patients given fenfluramine indicated some long-term fall in blood pressure in 6 taking diuretics, 1 taking rauwolfia, 3 taking methyldopa, and 3 taking guanethidine; virtually no change in blood pressure occurred in 2 taking diuretics or nothing, 2 taking bethanidine, 2 taking beta-blockers, and 1 taking debrisoquine. One patient taking guanethidine and bethanidine had an initial fall followed by a moderate rise but the relationship of this rise to the fenfluramine therapy was doubtful. These findings confirmed the results of a short-term study in 38 patients which indicated that the addition of fenfluramine could induce quite a considerable fall in the blood pressure of patients taking guanethidine, bethanidine, methyldopa, rauwolfia, and diuretics or nothing; this fall was not noted in the group of patients taking debrisoquine.— F. O. Simpson and H. J. Waal-Manning, *S. Afr. med. J.*, 1971, *Suppl.* (June 19), 47.

For the effect of fenfluramine on amitriptyline, see Amitriptyline Hydrochloride, p.113.

Interference with diagnostic tests. Fenfluramine could interfere chemically with estimations for hydrocortisone in the blood to produce erroneous raised results.— *Drug & Ther. Bull.*, 1972, *10*, 69.

Withdrawal. A 46-year-old woman with a history of 'absences' and of a convulsion 5 months earlier showed bizarre behaviour and impaired mental function with EEG changes 24 hours after abruptly ceasing to take fenfluramine; she returned to normal 4 days later after treatment with diazepam, phenytoin, and phenobarbitone. Minor EEG changes in 2 of 18 patients, without epilepsy, after the abrupt withdrawal of fenfluramine were of uncertain significance.— D. L. Davidson *et al.*, *Postgrad. med. J.*, 1975, *51*, *Suppl.* 1, 174.

Depression occurred in 3 patients following withdrawal of fenfluramine.— T. Harding (letter), *Br. J. Psychiat.*, 1972, *121*, 338. See also J. M. Steel and M. Briggs, *Br. med. J.*, 1972, *3*, 26 (depression on withdrawal in a double-blind study).

Absorption and Fate. Fenfluramine is readily and completely absorbed from the gastro-intestinal tract but is subject to extensive first-pass metabolism. It is excreted in the urine in the form of unchanged drug and metabolites. The rate of excretion is influenced by urinary pH and urinary flow, being somewhat increased in acid urine.

Paths of metabolism of fenfluramine include *N*-de-ethylation to form norfenfluramine, an active metabolite, followed by deamination to *m*-trifluoromethylbenzoic acid which is conjugated with glycine to form *m*-trifluoromethylhippuric acid. The plasma half-life of fenfluramine is reported to range from about 11 to 30 hours. It is widely distributed throughout the body and is reported to be taken up by the red blood cells, concentrations reaching 40% higher than those in plasma.

Absorption and plasma concentrations. In 6 male subjects given fenfluramine hydrochloride 60 mg in solution, peak plasma concentrations were achieved in 2 to 4 hours and remained constant for a further 4 to 6 hours. The mean peak concentration in 5 subjects was 63 ng per ml and in the sixth (weighing 121 kg) the peak concentration was 24 ng per ml. Norfenfluramine was detectable in the plasma within 2 hours of ingestion of fenfluramine, and reached a mean peak concentration of about 16 ng per ml within 4 to 6 hours. The half-life of fenfluramine ranged from 13.8 to 30.1 hours.In 6 subjects given fenfluramine hydrochloride 20 mg every 8 hours (as tablets) for 9 to 14 days a plateau plasma-fenfluramine concentration of 40 to 120 ng per ml was achieved in 3 to 4 days.— D. B. Campbell, *Br. J. Pharmac.*, 1971, *43*, 465P.

In 41 obese women given fenfluramine for 20 weeks in increasing doses to the limit of toleration (with a maximum of 160 mg daily) there was no correlation between dose and weight loss, but there was a significant correlation between plasma-fenfluramine concentrations and weight loss, those with a concentration of up to 99 ng per ml (mean 78) losing a mean of 2.1 kg, 100 to 199 ng per ml (mean 148) losing a mean of 5.1 kg, 200 to 299 ng per ml (mean 239) losing a mean of 8.8 kg. Dreaming occurred in 22 of the 41 patients and was correlated with the plasma-fenfluramine concentration.— J. A. Innes *et al.*, *Br. med. J.*, 1977, *2*, 1322.

Further references.— S. Caccia *et al.*, *Eur. J. Drug Metab. Pharmacokinet.*, 1979, *4*, 129.

Excretion. Urinary recovery of fenfluramine and its major metabolite norfenfluramine was similar following oral or intravenous administration, showing that the drug was completely absorbed from the intestine. Rate of excretion was controlled by urinary pH. About 60% of the fenfluramine was de-ethylated to norfenfluramine.— A. H. Beckett and L. G. Brookes, *J. Pharm. Pharmac.*, 1967, *19*, *Suppl.*, 42S.

Metabolism. Fenfluramine was absorbed, and excreted in urine as fenfluramine, de-ethylated fenfluramine, and *m*-trifluoromethylhippuric acid (66 to 93% of dose), the 3 compounds accounting for 79 to 100% of the dose. A peak blood concentration of 29 µg per litre of blood was reached after 3 hours in 2 subjects, and concentrations were still above 10 µg per litre after 6 hours.— R. B. Bruce and W. R. Maynard, *J. pharm. Sci.*, 1968, *57*, 1173.

First-pass metabolism. When administered by mouth fenfluramine was significantly *N*-dealkylated in the intestine as well as in the liver.— A. H. Beckett and J. A. Salmon, *J. Pharm. Pharmac.*, 1972, *24*, 108.

Uses. Fenfluramine hydrochloride is a sympathomimetic agent used as an anorectic in the treatment of obesity. It is reported to have no stimulant effect upon the central nervous system in the usual therapeutic doses.

The usual initial dose is 20 mg twice daily for the first week, increased by 20 mg each week to a total daily dose of 60 mg for mildly obese patients and 80 mg for moderately obese patients. The dose may be increased to 120 mg daily for severely obese patients. When treatment ceases, the dosage should be gradually reduced.

It is also given as sustained-release capsules of 60 mg, one or two being taken before breakfast.

A suggested dose for children aged 6 to 10 years is 20 mg daily and for those aged 10 to 12 years 40 mg daily.

In maturity-onset diabetes it is recommended that the dosage be adjusted to the needs of the individual patient and may vary between 80 and 120 mg daily.

Action. A detailed review of the action and uses of fenfluramine.— R. M. Pinder *et al.*, *Drugs*, 1975, *10*, 241.

Further reviews, comments, and reports of seminars and symposia.— *S. Afr. med. J.*, 1971, *Suppl.* (June 19);; N. Sapeika, *Practitioner*, 1972, *208*, 660; *Med. Lett.*, 1973, *15*, 33; M. H. M. Dykes, *J. Am. med. Ass.*, 1974, *230*, 270; *Postgrad. med. J.*, 1975, *51*, *Suppl.* 1, 1–189; *Can. med. Ass. J.*, 1978, *119*, 1436; *Curr. med. Res. Opinion*, 1979, *6*, *Suppl.* 1.

Some studies and comments on the mode of action of fenfluramine.— W. J. H. Butterfield and M. J. Whichelow (letter), *Lancet*, 1968, *2*, 109 (increased uptake by muscle); G. L. S. Pawan, *Lancet*, 1969, *1*, 498 (fat-mobilising effect); B. K. Anand and J. E. Blundell, *S. Afr. med. J.*, 1971, *Suppl.* (June 19), 53 (effect on hypothalamus); P. Ghalioungui, *S. Afr. med. J.*, 1971, *Suppl.* (June 19), 34 (effect on the hypothalamus); D. P. Bliss *et al.*, *Postgrad. med. J.*, 1972, *48*, 409 (improved glucose tolerance and reductions in fasting blood-cholesterol and β-lipoprotein concentrations); J. S. Garrow *et al.*, *Lancet*, 1972, *2*, 559 (no evidence of a 'glycoliptic' effect); R. D. Lele *et al.*, *Br. J. clin. Pract.*, 1972, *26*, 79 (metabolic effect); J. R. W. Dykes, *Postgrad. med. J.*, 1973, *49*, 314 and 318 (effect on glucose tolerance and insulin secretion); M. J. Kirby and P. Turner, *Br. J. clin. Pharmac.*, 1974, *1*, 340P (increased uptake of glucose into muscle in presence of insulin); E. Evans *et al.*, *Postgrad. med. J.*, 1975, *51*, *Suppl.* 1, 115 (no evidence of a reduction in fat absorption); L. J. Hipkin and J. C. Davis (letter), *Lancet*, 1976, *1*, 754 (possible calorie-wasting effect); M. J. Kirby and P. Turner, *Lancet*, 1976, *1*, 566 (increased peripheral utilisation of energy substrates); D. R. Mottram and D. Wadhwani, *Br. J. Pharmac.*, 1977, *59*, 615 (indirect sympathomimetic amine in *animals*); R. Ranquin and H. M. Brems, *Curr. med. Res. Opinion*, 1977, *5*, 341 (effect on glucose tolerance, insulin response, and serum cholesterol and triglyceride concentrations); J. J. Wurtman and R. J. Wurtman, *Science*, 1977, *198*, 1178 (sparing of protein consumption while suppressing calorie intake in *animals*); C. E. de la Vega *et al.*, *Clin. Pharmac. Ther.*, 1977, *21*, 216 (anti-adrenergic action); M. S. Sian and A. J. H. Rains, *Postgrad. med. J.*, 1979, *55*, 180 (possible enhanced catabolism of cholesterol).

Administration in renal failure. Twenty-five patients who had undergone renal transplantation, some of whom were obese and some hyperlipidaemic, were treated with fenfluramine for 6-week periods. Weight loss did not affect the cushingoid facial appearance. Of 16 patients with hypercholesterolaemia 11 showed a fall, with a mean fall (for the 16) of 440 µg per ml; triglyceride concentrations showed no consistent fall, but there was reversion from type IIb hyperlipidaemia towards normal in several patients. Allograft function was not affected.— S. A. Tomlinson *et al.*, *Postgrad. med. J.*, 1975, *51*, *Suppl.* 1, 166.

Alcohol and drug withdrawal. *Alcohol.* In a double-blind 12-month study completed by 27 chronic alcoholic patients significantly fewer lapses on biochemical but not on clinical criteria occurred in those given fenfluramine 120 mg daily compared with those given fenfluramine 60 mg daily or a placebo.— N. Krasner *et al.*, *Br. J. Psychiat.*, 1976, *128*, 346. See also D. J. Spencer, *J. Alcoholism*, 1972, *7*, 89.

Amphetamines. Four of 6 patients dependent on amphetamines were successfully transferred to fenfluramine 120 to 180 mg daily and were able to discontinue treatment. Hypotension was disturbing.— H. S. Jones, *S. Afr. med. J.*, 1971, *Suppl.* (June 19), 31.

Diabetes. Fenfluramine infused into the forearm increased glucose uptake by skeletal muscle for at least 60 minutes; after about 90 minutes free fatty acids were released and the effect on glucose uptake was abolished. The short-term effect of fenfluramine in lowering blood-glucose concentrations could be utilised in patients with diabetes mellitus particularly to prevent the postabsorption rise in blood sugar in patients marginally controlled on diet or sulphonylureas.— J. R. Turtle and J. A. Burgess, *Diabetes*, 1973, *22*, 858. Fenfluramine 40 mg thrice daily taken by 10 obese hospitalised patients with diabetes mellitus who also received a controlled diet produced a moderate but significant reduction in blood-glucose concentration in a single-blind, crossover study. After 7 days' treatment the blood-glucose and insulin response to an intravenous glucose load were similar for fenfluramine and placebo. The hypoglycaemic effect of fenfluramine might be due to increased glucose uptake in skeletal muscle. However, this hypoglycaemic effect was considered to be less than that seen with the sulphonylureas and biguanides in obese diabetics and was of limited clinical importance in such patients.— S. Larsen *et al.*, *Br. J. clin. Pharmac.*, 1977, *4*, 529.

See also above under Action.

Lipodystrophic diabetes. A girl with congenital generalised lipodystrophy who developed manifest insulin-resistant diabetes at 11 years of age responded to treatment with fenfluramine 60 mg twice daily. Voracious hunger and profuse perspiration were reduced, serum lipids became normal, blood glucose fell, and sensitivity to exogenous insulin increased.— D. Trygstad *et al.*, *Int. J. Obes.*, 1977, *1*, 287.

Mania. In a controlled pilot study 4 patients in the manic phase of manic-depression improved when given fenfluramine in doses of up to 180 mg daily for 2 weeks. The improvement was more noticeable in mood than behaviour. One patient recovered fully but the other 3 relapsed when taken off fenfluramine and given placebo or no further medication.— J. B. Pearce (letter), *Lancet*, 1973, *1*, 427.

Obesity. Results of a controlled study comparing behaviour therapy, pharmacotherapy, and the two together in the treatment of obesity, indicated that addition of pharmacotherapy, although providing initially improved weight loss, apparently compromised the long-term effects of behaviour therapy. Of 80 obese women who completed the study, 32 received behaviour therapy, 25 received pharmacotherapy with fenfluramine up to 120 mg daily, and 23 received both treatments together. All 3 groups lost significantly more weight than 10 control women assigned to waiting list control (who gained weight), and 8 assigned to a doctor's office regimen designed to resemble conventional management of obesity, including medication with fenfluramine, reducing diets, instructions for exercise, and advice and encouragement (who lost weight). In the treatment groups women given either fenfluramine alone or with behaviour therapy, lost significantly more weight than those who received behaviour therapy alone. A striking reversal of the results was found, however, one year after the end of treatment, since behaviour-therapy patients regained far less weight than pharmacotherapy and combined treatment patients; although they had weighed significantly more than the other 2 groups at the end of treatment, one year later they weighed less. Of 14 obese men in the study, the pattern in 6 who received pharmacotherapy was indistinguishable from that for the women in the pharmacotherapy group. Two-thirds of the patients were hypertensive (one-third receiving medication), and analysis of blood pressure data indicated a striking reduction in blood pressure, which was particularly large among hypertensive patients, due solely to weight loss. There was no evidence of the influence of fenfluramine on blood pressure that has sometimes been reported.— A. J. Stunkard *et al.*, *Lancet*, 1980, *2*, 1045.

Parkinsonism. Absence of effect of fenfluramine in patients with parkinsonism.— B. L. Beasley *et al.*, *Archs Neurol.*, 1977, *34*, 255.

Skin disorders. In some patients taking fenfluramine, pigmented naevi had faded and some had disappeared.— D. W. Bartlett (letter), *Br. med. J.*, 1972, *3*, 115.

Encouraging results were noted in 16 of 20 patients with chronic psoriasis who completed a double-blind crossover study of fenfluramine 40 to 80 mg daily.— T. Russell and C. Reuter, *Practitioner*, 1975, *214*, 114. See also E. Stewart (letter), *Med. J. Aust.*, 1973, *2*, 869.

Preparations

Fenfluramine Tablets *(B.P.)*. Tablets containing fenfluramine hydrochloride. They are film-or sugar-coated.

Ponderax *(Servier, UK)*. Fenfluramine hydrochloride, available as tablets of 20 and 40 mg. (Also available as Ponderax in *Austral., Ger., S.Afr.*). **Ponderax Pacaps.** Sustained-release capsules each containing fenfluramine hydrochloride 60 mg. (Also available as Ponderax Pacaps in *Austral., S.Afr.*).

Other Proprietary Names

Arg.— Acino, Obedrex, Ponderal; *Belg.*— Ponderal; *Canad.*—Ponderal, Pondimin; *Denm.*—Ponderal; *Fr.*—Ponderal; *Ital.*—Dima-fen, Ponderal; *Neth.*—Kataline, Ponderal; *Spain*—Ponderal; *Switz.*—Adipomin, Ponflural; *USA*—Pondimin.

1479-z

Fenproporex. *N*-2-Cyanoethylamphetamine. (±)-3-(α-Methylphenethylamino)propionitrile.
$C_{12}H_{16}N_2$=188.3.

CAS — 15686-61-0.

Pharmacopoeias. In *Braz.* as the hydrochloride.

Fenproporex is a sympathomimetic agent used as an anorectic in the treatment of obesity.

It has been given as the hydrochloride in usual doses equivalent to 10 mg of fenproporex base, generally twice daily before meals. Fenproporex has also been given as the diphenylacetate as a sustained-release preparation in usual doses equivalent to 20 mg of fenproporex base daily.

In order to establish whether metabolism to amphetamine and hence stimulant side-effects were absent with fenproporex, the absorption and metabolism were studied. It was found that after a dose by mouth fenproporex was rapidly *N*-dealkylated to amphetamine, probably in the intestine or during the first pass through the liver, the metabolism being virtually complete within 4 hours. In acid urine peak excretion of amphetamine occurred between 1 and 4 hours and 5 to 9% of a dose was detected as unchanged fenproporex in the urine.— A. H. Beckett *et al.*, *J. Pharm. Pharmac.*, 1972, *24*, 194.

A study indicating that usual therapeutic doses of fenproporex slightly interfere with colour vision.— J. Laroche and C. Laroche, *Annls pharm. fr.*, 1972, *30*, 433.

Proprietary Names

Antiobes Retard (hydrochloride) *(Frumtost, Spain)*; Appetitzügler (hydrochloride) *(Sagitta, Ger.)*; Dicel *(Lasa, Spain)*; Gacilin (hydrochloride) *(Andromaco, Arg.)*; Grasmin (resinate) *(Infale, Spain)*; Lineal *(Roussel, Arg.)*; Perphoxen (hydrochloride) *(Bottu, Switz.)*; Perphoxene (hydrochloride) *(Bottu, Belg.)*; Solvolip *(Knoll, Arg.)*; Tegisec *(Roussel-Amor Gil, Spain)*.

NOTE. The name Lineal is also applied to Diethylpropion Hydrochloride (see p.66)..

1480-p

Furfenorex Cyclamate. SD 271-5; Furfenorex Cyclohexylsulphamate; Furfurylmethylamphetamine Cyclamate. (+)-*N*-Methyl-*N*-(α-methylphenethyl)furfurylamine *N*-cyclohexylsulphamate.
$C_{15}H_{19}NO,C_6H_{13}NO_3S$=408.6.

CAS — 3776-93-0 (furfenorex); 3776-92-9 (cyclamate).

Uses. Furfenorex cyclamate is a sympathomimetic agent used as an anorectic in the treatment of obesity. It has been given in usual doses of 40 mg twice or thrice daily before meals.

Proprietary Names

Frugal *(Bagó, Arg.)*; Frugalan *(Diamant, Fr.; Farmabion, Spain)*.

1481-s

Levophacetoperane Hydrochloride. RP8228; Ro-1284; Phacetoperane Hydrochloride. (−)-*threo*-α-Phenyl-α-(2-piperidyl)methyl acetate hydrochloride.
$C_{14}H_{19}NO_2,HCl$=269.8.

CAS — 24558-01-8 (levophacetoperane); 23257-56-9 (hydrochloride).

Uses. Levophacetoperane hydrochloride is an amphetamine congener used as an anorectic in the treatment of obesity. It has been given in usual doses equivalent to 5 to 15 mg of levophacetoperane base before meals. It has also been advocated for use as an antidepressant in the treatment of mild to moderate depression.

Proprietary Names

Lidepran *(Rhône-Poulenc, Canad.)*.

1482-w

Mazindol *(U.S.P.)*. 42-548; AN 448. 5-(4-Chlorophenyl)-2,5-dihydro-3*H*-imidazo[2,1-*a*]isoindol-5-ol.

$C_{16}H_{13}ClN_2O$=284.7.

CAS — 22232-71-9.

Pharmacopoeias. In *U.S.*

Store in airtight containers.

Adverse Effects. As for Dexamphetamine Sulphate, p.361. The possibility that dependence of the amphetamine type might develop should be borne in mind.

Treatment of Adverse Effects. Marked hypertension, excitement, or convulsions may be treated as described under Dexamphetamine Sulphate, p.362.

Precautions. As for Dexamphetamine Sulphate, p.362. It has been recommended that mazindol should not be administered with other sympathomimetic substances. The response to insulin and oral antidiabetic agents may vary in diabetic patients receiving anorectic agents.

Mazindol 2 mg daily was given for 6 weeks to 18 obese patients with maturity-onset diabetes. Of 4 patients who were insulin-dependent 2 required an adjustment of dose when weight was lost but no patient receiving oral hypoglycaemic agents needed a change of dose.— M. Sanders and H. Breidahl, *Med. J. Aust.*, 1976, *2*, 576.

Interactions. A patient already taking methyldopa and flurazepam suffered 'violent tremors and cyanosis' after taking mazindol.— W. P. Maclay and M. G. Wallace, *Practitioner*, 1977, *218*, 431.

For the effect of mazindol on bethanidine, see Bethanidine Sulphate, p.136.

For the effect of mazindol on lithium, see Lithium Carbonate, p.1539.

Absorption and Fate. Mazindol is readily absorbed from the gastro-intestinal tract and is excreted in the urine, partly unchanged and partly as metabolites.

Mazindol has an estimated half-life of 12 to 24 hours.— *Med. Lett.*, 1974, *16*, 54.

Uses. Mazindol is a sympathomimetic agent used as an anorectic in the treatment of obesity. The usual dose is 2 mg after breakfast. Doses of 1 mg thrice daily 1 hour before meals have also been given.

Action. Reviews and comments on the actions and uses of mazindol.— M. H. M. Dykes, *J. Am. med. Ass.*, 1974, *230*, 270; *Drug & Ther. Bull.*, 1974, *12*, 101; *Med. Lett.*, 1974, *16*, 54.

Some studies and comments on the mode of action of mazindol.— K. G. Charlton and M. F. Sugrue, *Br. J. Pharmac.*, 1976, *58*, 271P (similar neurochemical profile to dexamphetamine in *animals*); M. J. Kirby and P. Turner, *Lancet*, 1976, *1*, 566 (increased peripheral utilisation of energy substrates); Z. L. Kruk and M. R. Zarrindast, *Br. J. Pharmac.*, 1976, *58*, 367 (dopaminergic mechanism).

Narcolepsy. Beneficial results in narcolepsy in 32 of 34 patients with the narcolepsy syndrome receiving mazindol 3 to 8 mg daily for 1 year. Cataplexy and sleep paralysis did not respond. There were no mean changes in appetite or weight.— J. D. Parkes and M. Schachter, *Acta neurol. scand.*, 1979, *60*, 250.

Preparations

Mazindol Tablets *(U.S.P.)*. Tablets containing mazindol. Store at a temperature not exceeding 25° in airtight containers.

Teronac *(Wander, UK)*. Mazindol, available as scored tablets of 2 mg. (Also available as Teronac in *Ger., Neth., S.Afr., Spain, Switz.*).

Other Proprietary Names

Afilan, Dimagrir, Magrilan (all *Arg.*); Mazildene *(Ital.)*; Samonter *(Arg.)*; Sanorex *(Austral., Canad., USA)*.

1483-e

Mefenorex Hydrochloride. Ro-4-5282. *N*-(3-Chloropropyl)-α-methylphenethylamine hydrochloride.
$C_{12}H_{18}ClN,HCl=248.2$.

CAS — 17243-57-1 (mefenorex); 5586-87-8 (hydrochloride).

Uses. Mefenorex hydrochloride is a sympathomimetic agent used as an anorectic in the treatment of obesity. It has been given in usual doses equivalent to 40 mg of mefenorex base once or twice daily before meals.

Proprietary Names
Doracil *(Gador, Arg.)*; Pondinil *(Roche, Belg.; Roche, Fr.; Roche, Spain; Sauter, Switz.)*; Pondinol *(Roche, Arg.)*; Rondimen *(Homburg, Ger.)*.

1484-l

Pentorex Tartrate. Phenpentermine Tartrate. ααβ-Trimethylphenethylamine hydrogen tartrate.
$C_{11}H_{17}N,C_4H_6O_6=313.3$.

CAS — 434-43-5 (pentorex); 22876-60-4 (tartrate).

Uses. Pentorex tartrate is a sympathomimetic agent used as an anorectic in the treatment of obesity. It has been given in usual doses of 10 mg twice daily before meals.

Proprietary Names
Liprodène *(Anphar-Rolland, Fr.)*; Modatrop *(Nordmark-Werke, Ger.; Nordmark, Switz.)*.

1485-y

Phenbutrazate Hydrochloride. Fenbutrazate Hydrochloride; R 381. 2-(3-Methyl-2-phenylmorpholino)ethyl 2-phenylbutyrate hydrochloride.
$C_{23}H_{29}NO_3,HCl=403.9$.

CAS — 4378-36-3 (phenbutrazate); 6474-85-7 (hydrochloride).

A fine white crystalline powder. Slightly **soluble** in water; soluble in alcohol and acetone; practically insoluble in ether. A saturated solution in water has a pH of 6.2.

Uses. Phenbutrazate hydrochloride is used in conjunction with phenmetrazine theoclate as an anorectic agent.

1486-j

Phendimetrazine Tartrate. Phendimetrazine Acid Tartrate; Phendimetrazine Bitartrate. (+)-3,4-Dimethyl-2-phenylmorpholine hydrogen tartrate.
$C_{12}H_{17}NO,C_4H_6O_6=341.4$.

CAS — 634-03-7 (phendimetrazine); 50-58-8 (tartrate).

A white odourless powder with a bitter taste. Freely **soluble** in water; very slightly soluble in alcohol; practically insoluble in chloroform and ether.

Adverse Effects. As for Dexamphetamine Sulphate, p.361. Other adverse effects occasionally reported include glossitis, stomatitis, and cystitis.

Treatment of Adverse Effects. Marked hypertension, excitement, or convulsions may be treated as described under Dexamphetamine Sulphate, p.362.

Precautions. As for Dexamphetamine Sulphate, p.362. The response to insulin and oral antidiabetic agents may vary in diabetic patients receiving anorectic agents.

Uses. Phendimetrazine tartrate is a sympathomimetic agent used as an anorectic in the treatment of obesity. The usual dose is 35 mg twice or thrice daily 1 hour before meals. In some cases a dose of 17.5 mg may be adequate and the maximum recommended dose is 70 mg thrice daily. Single daily doses of 105 mg have been given in a controlled release formulation.

Proprietary Names
Anorex *(Dunhall, USA)*; Antapentan *(hydrochloride) (Gerot, Belg.; Gerot, Switz.)*; Bacarate *(Tutag, USA)*; Bontril PDM *(Carnrick, USA)*; Melfiat *(Reid-Provident, USA)*; Obesan-X *(SCS, S.Afr.)*; Obex *(Rio, S.Afr.)*; Phenazine *(base) (Legere, USA)*; Plegine *(Ayerst, Ital.; Ayerst, USA)*; Prelu-2 *(Boehringer Ingelheim, USA)*; Statobex *(Lemmon, USA)*; Trimstat *(Laser, USA)*; Trimtabs *(Mayrand, USA)*; Wehless *(Hauck, USA)*.

NOTE. The name Anorex was also formerly applied to phenmetrazine hydrochloride.

1487-z

Phenmetrazine Hydrochloride *(U.S.P., B.P. 1973)*. Phenmetrazine Hydrochlor.; Oxazimédrine. (±)-*trans*-3-Methyl-2-phenylmorpholine hydrochloride.
$C_{11}H_{15}NO,HCl=213.7$.

CAS — 134-49-6 (phenmetrazine); 1707-14-8 (hydrochloride).

Pharmacopoeias. In *U.S. Cz.* specifies the dextro isomer (Dexphenmetrazinium Chloratum).

A white or off-white odourless crystalline powder with a slightly bitter taste. M.p. 172° to 182° with a range of not more than 3°. **Soluble** 1 in 0.4 of water, 1 in 2 of alcohol, and 1 in 2 of chloroform; slightly soluble in ether. A 2.5% solution in water has a pH of 4.5 to 5.5. **Store** in airtight containers.

Dependence and Adverse Effects. As for Dexamphetamine Sulphate, p.361.

Marked prostration resembling septic shock, disseminated intravascular coagulation, rhabdomyolysis with myoglobinuria and uraemia appeared to be associated with the intravenous abuse of phenmetrazine or methylamphetamine in 5 patients. From 4 to 11 litres of sodium chloride injection were required in the first 24 hours to maintain blood pressure and urine output suggesting that shock resulted from massive loss of intravascular volume into necrotic muscle.— W. C. Kendrick *et al.*, *Ann. intern. Med.*, 1977, *86*, 381.

Abuse and dependence. Reports of the abuse of and dependence on phenmetrazine.— J. Evans, *Lancet*, 1959, *2*, 152; M. Silverman, *Br. med. J.*, 1959, *1*, 696; I. Oswald and V. R. Thacore, *ibid.*, 1963, *2*, 427; E. Vencovský and S. Nevole, *Čslká Psychiat.*, 1965, *61*, 411; G. Rylander, *Läkartidningen*, 1966, *63*, 4973; E. Negulici and D. Christodorescu (letter), *Br. med. J.*, 1968, *3*, 316.

Treatment of Adverse Effects. Marked hypertension, excitement, or convulsions may be treated as described under Dexamphetamine Sulphate, p.362.

Precautions. As for Dexamphetamine Sulphate, p.362. The response to insulin and oral antidiabetic agents may vary in patients receiving anorectic agents.

Pregnancy and the neonate. Evaluation of anorectic agents prescribed, during the years 1959-66, to about 2000 pregnant women provided no evidence that the use of phenmetrazine is associated with the production of severe congenital anomalies.— L. Milkovich and B. J. van den Berg, *Am. J. Obstet. Gynec.*, 1977, *129*, 637. See also A. Notter and M. F. Delande, *Gynécol. Obstét.*, 1962, *61*, 359.

Individual reports of malformations in exposed infants.— W. Lenz (letter), *Lancet*, 1962, *2*, 1332 (diaphragmatic defects); P. D. Moss (letter), *Br. med. J.*, 1962, *2*, 1610 (limb deformities); P. D. Powell and J. M. Johnstone (letter), *Br. med. J.*, 1962, *2*, 1327 (diaphragmatic defects).

Absorption and Fate. Phenmetrazine hydrochloride is readily absorbed from the gastro-intestinal tract. The half-life of phenmetrazine in the circulation has been reported to be about 8 hours.

Phenmetrazine was well absorbed from the gastro-intestinal tract and had a serum half-life of about 8 hours; average peak concentrations were obtained about 2 hours after ingestion. A single dose of a sustained-release preparation (Preludin Endurets) containing phenmetrazine 75 mg yielded blood concentrations at 8 and 12 hours after ingestion comparable to those obtained with the same dose of phenmetrazine hydrochloride, but with the advantage of not producing such untoward effects as sweating and nervousness.— G. P. Quinn *et al.*, *Clin. Pharmac. Ther.*, 1967, *8*, 369.

Further references.— R. B. Franklin *et al.*, *Drug Metab. & Disposit.*, 1977, *5*, 223.

Uses. Phenmetrazine hydrochloride is a sympathomimetic agent used as an anorectic in the treatment of obesity.

It is reported to have less stimulant action on the central nervous system than amphetamine. The usual dose is 12.5 to 25 mg twice or thrice daily 1 hour before meals. It is also given once daily as sustained-release tablets of 50 or 75 mg.

Diabetes insipidus. Two patients with diabetes insipidus experienced a decrease in thirst and a reduction in polyuria after treatment with phenmetrazine.— J. F. Aloia (letter), *Lancet*, 1973, *2*, 501.

Preparations

Phenmetrazine Hydrochloride Tablets *(U.S.P.)*. Tablets containing phenmetrazine hydrochloride. Store in airtight containers.

Phenmetrazine Tablets *(B.P. 1973)*. Phenmetrazine Tab. Tablets containing phenmetrazine hydrochloride.

Proprietary Names
Preludin *(Boehringer Ingelheim, USA)*.

Phenmetrazine hydrochloride was formerly marketed in Great Britain under the proprietary name Preludin (*Boehringer Ingelheim*).

1488-c

Phenmetrazine Theoclate. R 382. 3-Methyl-2-phenylmorpholine 8-chlorotheophyllinate.
$C_{11}H_{15}NO,C_7H_7ClN_4O_2=391.9$.

CAS — 13931-75-4.

A white powder. **Soluble** in water and alcohol; slightly soluble in acetone and ether. A saturated solution in water has a pH of about 6.7.

Uses. Phenmetrazine theoclate has the actions and uses of phenmetrazine hydrochloride (above).

A preparation containing phenmetrazine theoclate and phenbutrazate hydrochloride was formerly marketed in Great Britain under the proprietary name Filon (*Berk Pharmaceuticals*).

1489-k

Phentermine. αα-Dimethylphenethylamine.
$C_{10}H_{15}N=149.2$.

CAS — 122-09-8.

A colourless oily liquid with a amine-like odour. Slightly **soluble** in water; soluble in alcohol, chloroform, and ether.

Adverse Effects. As for Dexamphetamine Sulphate, p.361. The incidence of side-effects is reported to be lower with phentermine than with dexamphetamine.

Effects on the eyes. A study indicating that usual therapeutic doses of phentermine interfere with colour vision.— J. Laroche and C. Laroche, *Annls pharm. fr.*, 1972, *30*, 433.

Effects on mental state. Symptoms of delusion in a 20-year-old woman referred for psychiatric treatment developed 1 month after she started taking phentermine, 30 mg daily in 'diet pills'. She recovered after treatment with trifluoperazine.— B. F. Hoffman (letter), *Can. med. Ass. J.*, 1977, *116*, 351.

Further references.— R. T. Rubin, *Am. J. Psychiat.*, 1964, *120*, 1124.

Pulmonary hypertension. Pulmonary hypertension in a patient associated with the use of phentermine.— L. Heuer *et al.*, *Chir. Praxis*, 1978, *23*, 497.

Treatment of Adverse Effects. Marked hypertension, excitement, or convulsions may be treated as described under Dexamphetamine Sulphate, p.362.

Precautions. As for Dexamphetamine Sulphate, p.362. It has been recommended that phentermine should be used with caution in patients receiving other sympathomimetic substances. The response to insulin and oral antidiabetic agents may vary in patients receiving anorectic agents.

Absorption and Fate. Phentermine is readily absorbed from the gastro-intestinal tract and is excreted in the urine, partly unchanged and partly as metabolites.

Uses. Phentermine is a sympathomimetic agent used as an anorectic in the treatment of obesity.

Phentermine is usually given as a complex with an ion-exchange resin for sustained release. The usual dose is 15 to 30 mg at breakfast. A suggested dose for children aged 6 to 12 years is 15 mg at breakfast.

Proprietary Preparations

Duromine *(Carnegie, UK).* Phentermine, available as capsules of 15 and 30 mg as an ion-exchange resin complex for sustained release. (Also available as Duromine in *Austral., S.Afr.*).

Ionamin *(Lipha, UK).* Phentermine, available as capsules of 15 and 30 mg as an ion-exchange resin complex for sustained release. (Also available as Ionamin in *Canad., USA*).

Other Proprietary Names

Arg.—Omnibex; *Denm.*—Mirapront; *Fr.*—Linyl; *Ital.*—Lipopill, Mirapront; *Neth.*—Mirapront; *Spain*—Mirapront; *Switz.*—Adipex Neu, Ionamine, Phentermyl.

1490-w

Phentermine Hydrochloride. αα-Dimethylphenethylamine hydrochloride.

$C_{10}H_{15}N,HCl=185.7$.

CAS — 1197-21-3.

A white crystalline powder. Very **soluble** in water, alcohol, and chloroform; practically insoluble in ether.

Uses. Phentermine hydrochloride is a sympathomimetic agent used like phentermine (above) as an anorectic in the treatment of obesity. The usual dose is about 30 mg after breakfast.

Proprietary Names

Adipex-P *(Lemmon, USA)*; Bellapront *(Boehringer, Arg.)*; Fastin *(Beecham, Canad.; Beecham, USA)*; Minobese *(Harvard, S.Afr.)*; Panbesy *(Biothera-Asperal, Belg.)*; Pronidin *(Trianon, Canad.)*; Teramine *(Legere, USA)*.

Antacids and some other Gastro-intestinal Agents

670-g

Antacids are used to anticipate and relieve pain in the symptomatic management of gastric and duodenal ulcers and reflux oesophagitis by neutralising hydrochloric acid in the gastric secretion, but there is no evidence that they significantly affect the rate of healing of ulcers. Antacids are also used as domestic remedies in conditions affecting the stomach which may not necessarily be related to hyperacidity.

Antacids do not reduce the volume of hydrochloric acid secreted and may increase it, but by increasing the gastric pH they diminish the activity of pepsin in the gastric secretion. Increase in gastric pH stimulates the liberation of gastrin from cells of the antral mucosa. Gastrin is one of a number of peptides present in the gastro-intestinal tract, others include secretin, pancreozymin, glucagon, and somatostatin, which are discussed in various sections of *Martindale* depending on their actions and uses.

Adsorbents, such as attapulgite, activated charcoal, and kaolin, are used in the treatment of gastro-intestinal disorders and because they are adsorbent for many drugs they have been used in the treatment of acute poisoning. Polymeric adsorbents are of use for the recovery and concentration of water-soluble amino acids, polypeptides, proteins, and steroids during manufacturing processes. Polymeric adsorbents and activated charcoal have been used in haemoperfusion systems for the treatment of poisoning. Other substances described in this section include carbenoxolone sodium and bran.

Care is necessary when giving drugs to patients receiving antacids. Gastro-intestinal absorption can be reduced by adsorption on insoluble antacids or changes in gastric emptying time and the effects of a drug may be diminished or enhanced by alterations in the intestinal pH or by the formation of complexes.

In addition to the drugs described in this section, calcium phosphate (see p.623), and some bismuth salts (see p.927) have been used as antacids. Sodium bicarbonate (see p.634) is a commonly used antacid; though highly effective it can cause systemic alkalosis.

Drugs used in the treatment of peptic ulcers include the anticholinergic agents (see p.289), and the histamine-H_2 antagonists, particularly cimetidine (see p.1300), which now has a major role.

Reviews of antacid therapy: D. W. Piper and J. Kang, *Drugs*, 1979, *17*, 124; T. Morris and J. Rhodes, *Gut*, 1979, *20*, 538; M. M. Sundle, *Prescribers' J.*, 1979, *19*, 125; I. N. Marks, *Drugs*, 1980, *20*, 283; *Drug & Ther. Bull.*, 1980, *18*, 17; M. P. Dutro and A. B. Amerson (letter), *New Engl. J. Med.*, 1980, *302*, 967; *Br. med. J.*, 1981, *282*, 1495; D. C. Stolinsky (letter), *New Engl. J. Med.*, 1981, *305*, 166 (sugar and saccharin content).

References to the neutralising capacity of antacids: J. S. Fordtran, *New Engl. J. Med.*, 1973, *288*, 924; M. Gibaldi *et al.*, *Clin. Pharmac. Ther.*, 1974, *16*, 520 (effect on urinary pH); R. E. Barry and J. Ford, *Gut*, 1977, *18*, A969; *idem*, *Br. med. J.*, 1978, *1*, 413; A. W. Harcus, *Reckitt & Colman* (letter), *Br. med. J.*, 1978, *1*, 787; J. R. B. J. Brouwers and G. N. J. Tytgat, *J. Pharm. Pharmac.*, 1978, *30*, 148.

Heartburn of pregnancy. In a double-blind study in pregnant patients with heartburn there was no significant difference in the response to an acid or an alkaline mixture, suggesting that heartburn might be due to acid reflux or bile regurgitation. Treatment after meals and at night for 7 days was suggested with an acid mixture to be replaced, if not effective, by an alkaline mixture. The experimental mixtures consisted of dilute hydrochloric acid 0.1 ml in 10 ml, or sodium bicarbonate 500 mg in 10 ml.— R. D. Atlay *et al.*, *Br. med. J.*, 1978, *2*, 919.

Reflux oesophagitis. Reviews of reflux oesophagitis and its treatment: *Med. Lett.*, 1980, *22*, 26; P. I. Reed, *Practitioner*, 1980, *224*, 357.

Steatorrhoea. Concurrent administration of antacids did not further improve fat absorption in 6 patients with advanced pancreatic insufficiency compared with administration of pancreatin alone.— P. T. Regan *et al.*, *New Engl. J. Med.*, 1977, *297*, 854.

Ulcer, gastric and duodenal. In a double-blind study, of 36 patients with duodenal ulcer who took 7 daily doses of an antacid preparation containing either magnesium hydroxide and aluminium hydroxide or aluminium hydroxide alone (in the event of diarrhoea), either preparation providing approximately 144 mEq of neutralising capacity, the ulcer healed in 28 in 28 days, compared with 17 cures in 38 placebo-treated patients. These results indicated that high-dose antacid therapy accelerated duodenal ulcer healing. Symptoms, which were found to be a poor indication of ulcer status, were not relieved by the antacids; supplementary antacid tablets (providing approximately 6.2 mEq of neutralising capacity) which could be taken as needed for the relief of ulcer pain were not taken significantly more frequently by the placebo group than by the treated group.— W. L. Peterson *et al.*, *New Engl. J. Med.*, 1977, *297*, 341. Comment.— *Lancet*, 1977, *2*, 1012.

Comment on the potential adverse effects of duodenal ulcer treatment with large amounts of antacids, and the view that, set against their lack of clear advantages over specific ulcer-healing drugs, antacids cannot be recommended for the healing of duodenal ulcers.— *Br. med. J.*, 1981, *282*, 1495.

Further references: D. Hollander and J. Harlan, *J. Am. med. Ass.*, 1973, *226*, 1181 (duodenal and gastric); T. Morris and J. Rhodes, *Gut*, 1979, *20*, 538 (duodenal and gastric); I. N. Marks, *S. Afr. med. J.*, 1979, *55*, 331 (duodenal and gastric); S. K. Lam *et al.*, *Gastroenterology*, 1979, *76*, 315 (duodenal).

For further studies on the role of gastric pH in ulcer therapy, see Cimetidine, p.1300.

Symptomatic relief. A double-blind study in 10 patients showed that a locally prepared liquid preparation containing aluminium hydroxide and magnesium trisilicate was no better than a placebo containing carboxymethylcellulose 9% in providing acute relief of spontaneous duodenal ulcer pain.— R. A. L. Sturdevant *et al.*, *Gastroenterology*, 1977, *72*, 1. In a single-blind crossover study in 10 patients with duodenal ulcer, administration of an antacid gave complete relief of pain on 95% of occasions compared with relief on 43% of occasions after a saline placebo. Antacid gave some degree of relief in all patients but placebo was without effect in 24% of patients.— S. H. Lorber *et al.*, *Gastroenterology*, 1978, *74*, 1058.

Further references: R. L. Powell *et al.*, *J. clin. Pharmac.*, 1971, *11*, 296 and 288; S. J. Rune and A. Zachariassen, *Scand. J. Gastroenterol.*, 1980, *15*, *Suppl.* 58, 41.

Ulceration, stress-induced. Adequate dosage with antacids was advocated as prophylactic treatment for stress-associated gastro-intestinal bleeding in patients with trauma, burns, sepsis, or with acute respiratory failure.— *Br. med. J.*, 1978, *1*, 531.

In a randomised controlled study with 100 critically ill patients in danger of developing stress ulceration, prophylactic antacid treatment decreased the incidence of acute gastro-intestinal bleeding; 2 of 51 treated patients bled compared with 12 of 49 controls. Antacid was given every hour and the dose adjusted to keep the gastric contents above pH 3.5. Side-effects included diarrhoea in 10, gross regurgitation in 2, and elevated serum-magnesium concentrations in 3 patients. Patients with one or more of the recognised risk factors (respiratory failure, sepsis, peritonitis, jaundice, renal failure, hypotension, trauma, operative procedures, and burns) should be given antacids prophylactically to prevent acute bleeding.— P. R. Hastings *et al.*, *New Engl. J. Med.*, 1978, *298*, 1041. Comments and criticisms.— P. B. Gregory and B. W. Brown (letter), *ibid.*, *299*, 830; W. F. Cathcart-Rake and A. Hurwitz (letter), *ibid.*, 831; J. Weinreb (letter), *ibid.* Reply.— J. J. Skillman *et al.* (letter), *ibid.* In a randomised study of 75 critically ill patients, cimetidine was less effective than antacid in providing adequate prophylaxis against acute gastro-intestinal bleeding. Of 38 patients given cimetidine intravenously 7 had evidence of upper gastro-intestinal tract bleeding compared with none of 37 given antacid. Bleeding stopped in 4 patients on cimetidine when antacids were also given.— H. -J. Priebe *et al.*, *New Engl. J. Med.*, 1980, *302*, 426. Comments and criticisms.— R. Menguy, *ibid.*, 461; J. G. Spenney and B. I. Hirschowitz (letter), *ibid.*, *303*, 108; D. S. Bloom (letter), *ibid.*; J. K. Siepler *et al.* (letter), *ibid.*; H. L. Bonkowsky (letter), *ibid.*, 109; J. P. Roberts and R. P. Saik (letter), *ibid.* Reply.— H. -J. Priebe *et al.* (letter), *ibid.*

For further studies on the role of gastric pH in stress-induced gastro-intestinal ulceration, see Cimetidine (Ulceration, stress-induced), p.1306.

Use in surgery. See under Magnesium Trisilicate, p.83.

712-d

Alexitol Sodium. Sodium poly(hydroxyaluminium) carbonate-hexitol complex.

CAS — 66813-51-2.

Alexitol is an antacid used similarly to aluminium hydroxide. The usual dose is 360 to 720 mg, as required.

Proprietary Preparations

Actal (known in some countries as Actonalt and Talakt) *(WinPharm, UK)*. Alexitol sodium, available as **Suspension** containing 360 mg in each 5 ml and as **Tablets** of 360 mg.

671-q

Aluminium Glycinate *(B.P.)*. Dihydroxyaluminum Aminoacetate *(U.S.P.)*; Basic Aluminium Glycinate. (Glycinato-*N,O*)dihydroxyaluminium hydrate.

$C_2H_6AlNO_4(+xH_2O) = 135.1$.

CAS — 13682-92-3 (anhydrous); 41354-48-7 (hydrate).

Pharmacopoeias. In *Br.* and *U.S.*

A white or almost white odourless powder with a faintly sweet taste. The *B.P.* specifies 34.5 to 38.5% of Al_2O_3 and 9.9 to 10.8% of nitrogen, calculated on the dried substance, and not more than 12% loss of weight on drying. The *U.S.P.* specifies 35.5 to 38.5% of Al_2O_3 and permits small amounts of aluminium oxide and glycine and not more than 14.5% loss on drying.

Practically **insoluble** in water and organic solvents; soluble in dilute mineral acids and solutions of alkali hydroxides. A 4% suspension in water has a pH of 6.5 to 7.5. **Store** in airtight containers.

Uses. Aluminium glycinate is an antacid which is used similarly to aluminium hydroxide mixture (see p.72). It is given in doses of 0.5 to 2 g.

Preparations

Dihydroxyaluminum Aminoacetate Magma *(U.S.P.)*. A white viscous suspension of aluminium glycinate yielding an amount of Al_2O_3 equivalent to 28.5 to 35% w/w of the labelled amount of $C_2H_6AlNO_4$. Store in airtight containers. Protect from freezing.

Dihydroxyaluminum Aminoacetate Tablets *(U.S.P.)*. Tablets containing aluminium glycinate yielding an amount of Al_2O_3 equivalent to 28.5 to 35% of the labelled amount of $C_2H_6AlNO_4$.

Prodexin *(Bencard, UK)*. Tablets each containing aluminium glycinate 900 mg and magnesium carbonate 100 mg. Antacid. *Dose.* 1 or more tablets to be sucked or chewed every hour.

Other Proprietary Names

Alcap *(Ital.)*; Rinveral *(Spain)*; Robalate *(Canad., USA)*.

Aluminium glycinate was also formerly marketed in Great Britain under the proprietary name Robalate (*Robins*). A preparation containing aluminium glycinate was also formerly marketed in Great Britain under the proprietary name Glycinal (*Medo-Chemicals*).

672-p

Aluminium Hydroxide Mixture *(B.P.)*.

Aluminium Hydroxide Gel; Alum. Hydrox. Gel; Aluminum Hydroxide Gel *(U.S.P.)*; Gelat. Alumin. Hydrox.; Colloidal Aluminium Hydroxide.

CAS — 21645-51-2 [Al(OH)₃].

Pharmacopoeias. In *Arg*., *Belg*., *Br*., *Braz*., *Cz*., *Ind*., *Mex*., *Turk*., and *U.S*.

The *B.P.* describes an aqueous suspension of hydrated aluminium oxide together with varying quantities of basic aluminium carbonate, containing 3.5 to 4.4% w/w of Al_2O_3 (=102.0). It contains peppermint oil 0.015% v/v as a flavouring agent; saccharin sodium may be added as a sweetening agent. It is a white suspension from which small amounts of clear liquid may separate on standing. It may exhibit thixotropic properties. A 50% dilution in water has a pH of not more than 7.5. **Store** at a temperature not exceeding 30° and avoid freezing.

The *U.S.P.* describes a suspension of aluminium hydroxide and hydrated oxide; it may contain varying amounts of basic aluminium carbonate and bicarbonate; it contains the equivalent of 3.6 to 4.4% w/w of Al_2O_3. It may contain peppermint oil, glycerol, sorbitol, sucrose, saccharin, or other suitable flavouring agents, and suitable antimicrobial agents. pH 5.5 to 8. **Store** in airtight containers and avoid freezing.

The viscosity of aluminium hydroxide mixture increased as the solid ingredients were washed. Washing also resulted in elution of chloride ions and decreased electrophoretic mobility.— R. H. Green and S. L. Hem, *J. pharm. Sci.*, 1974, *63*, 635.

Carbonate ions were an integral part of the structure of reactive aluminium hydroxide mixture and had a stabilising effect.— J. L. White and S. L. Hem (letter), *J. pharm. Sci.*, 1975, *64*, 468.

Aluminium hydroxide mixture became less reactive on ageing. Addition of water caused a sharp loss of reactivity directly related to the degree of dilution and was probably caused by a change in equilibrium between stabilising ions in the gel structure and in solution. When diluted with dioxan or the mother liquor there was no change in reactivity.— N. J. Kerkhof *et al.*, *J. pharm. Sci.*, 1975, *64*, 940.

Adverse Effects. Aluminium hydroxide mixture in common with other aluminium compounds is astringent and may cause nausea, vomiting, and constipation. Large doses can cause intestinal obstruction. Excessive doses, or even normal doses in patients with low-phosphate diets, may lead to phosphate depletion accompanied by increased resorption and urinary excretion of calcium with the risk of renal rickets in the young or osteomalacia in older patients. Increases in plasma-concentrations of aluminium are a toxic hazard of aluminium hydroxide mixture given to patients with poor renal function, or to those on dialysis, and encephalopathy and dementia have occurred.

Three patients with acute renal failure developed intestinal obstruction due to desiccated deposits of aluminium hydroxide during treatment with an aluminium suspension.— C. M. Townsend *et al.*, *New Engl. J. Med.*, 1973, *288*, 1058.

Two patients, 1 of whom had sustained extensive burns and 1 who had renal failure, developed intestinal obstruction from medicated bezoars of aluminium hydroxide mixture. Although this was considered to be a rare complication patients who were most at risk were those who were inactive, subject to dehydration, and who ingested large amounts of aluminium hydroxide mixture.— M. D. Korenman *et al.*, *J. Am. med. Ass.*, 1978, *240*, 54.

Similar reports of intestinal obstruction occurring in children: J. K. Hurley, *J. Pediat.*, 1978, *92*, 592; A. Portuguez-Malavasi and J. V. Aranada, *Pediatrics*, 1979, *63*, 679.

Theoretical considerations and studies in *rats* suggested that the bile-salt-binding property of aluminium hydroxide might indirectly promote cancer of the colon by increasing the delivery of bile salts to the large intestine.— J. P. Cruse *et al.* (letter), *Lancet*, 1978, *1*, 1261. Data on men with gastrectomy or peptic ulcer did not support the view that aluminium hydroxide can increase the risk for colorectal cancer.— A. Nomura *et al.* (letter), *ibid.*, 1978, *2*, 785. A report of *animal* studies which provide reassurance that aluminium hydroxide (Aludrox) does not promote colon cancer.— P. Cruse *et al.* (letter), *Lancet*, 1980, *2*, 1030.

Dialysis encephalopathy. The aluminium content of muscle and bone was higher in uraemic patients on long-term dialysis than in controls and there was significant correlation between muscle aluminium content and duration of dialysis. The aluminium content of brain grey matter was higher in uraemic patients who had had dialysis and whose death was due to encephalopathy of unknown cause than in uraemic dialysis patients who had died from other causes. Dialysis patients received aluminium hydroxide mixtures to control phosphorus concentrations and it was suggested that the encephalopathy syndrome might be due to aluminium toxicity.— A. C. Alfrey *et al.*, *New Engl. J. Med.*, 1976, *294*, 184. Comment.— W. H. Diamant and J. G. Gambertoglio (letter), *ibid.*, *294*, 1129. See also D. J. Selkoe (letter), *ibid.*; V. V. Rozas *et al.* (letter), *ibid.*, 1130; G. M. Berlyne (letter), *ibid.*; V. Parsons (letter), *ibid.*; A. C. Alfrey and W. D. Kaehny (letter), *ibid.*, 1131; D. D. Ulmer (letter), *ibid.*

Haemodialysis encephalopathy or dialysis dementia was considered to be associated with phosphate depletion due either to the dialysis or to the excessive use of compounds known to be phosphate binders like aluminium hydroxide. Withdrawal of aluminium hydroxide produced no benefit in 4 patients but withdrawal of aluminium hydroxide plus the administration of phosphate supplements in 3 patients improved symptoms and stopped the encephalopathy. No new cases of haemodialysis encephalopathy had been seen since the use of phosphate binders was virtually halted.— A. M. Pierides *et al.* (letter), *Lancet*, 1976, *1*, 1234. Dialysis dementia in 6 patients was attributed to aluminium contamination of the dialysate.— J. A. Flendrig *et al.* (letter), *ibid.*, 1235.

Aluminium in joint tissues of a dialysis patient taking aluminium hydroxide.— P. Netter *et al.* (letter), *Lancet*, 1981, *1*, 1056.

Further references: *Lancet*, 1976, *1*, 349; J. P. Masselot *et al.* (letter), *Lancet*, 1978, *2*, 1386.

For a discussion of the role of aluminium ions in water, rather than aluminium hydroxide, in dialysis encephalopathy, see under Aluminium, p.926.

Effects on calcium and phosphate metabolism. Hyperplastic changes in parathyroid glands which might progress to parathyroid tumour could follow ingestion of excessive quantities of aluminium hydroxide.— J. Shafar (letter), *Br. med. J.*, 1969, *3*, 530.

A 49-year-old woman developed osteomalacia due to phosphate depletion caused by excessive intake of aluminium hydroxide—she had taken about 20 g daily for some months.— C. E. Dent and C. S. Winter, *Br. med. J.*, 1974, *1*, 551. See also K. L. Insogna *et al.*, *J. Am. med. Ass.*, 1980, *244*, 2544.

A 26-year-old woman on haemodialysis developed hypophosphataemia, osteomalacia, and myopathy. The condition regressed when aluminium hydroxide was withdrawn and phosphates were given; vitamin D was not required.— L. R. I. Baker *et al.*, *Br. med. J.*, 1974, *3*, 150.

Reversible congestive cardiomyopathy was associated with hypophosphataemia in 3 patients who had consumed large quantities of aluminium hydroxide mixture.— J. R. Darsee and D. O. Nutter, *Ann. intern. Med.*, 1978, *89*, 867.

Further references: H. M. Shields, *Gastroenterology*, 1978, *75*, 1137.

Precautions. Aluminium hydroxide mixture interferes with or reduces the absorption of a number of other drugs including anticholinergic agents, barbiturates, digoxin, quinine, quinidine, warfarin, tetracyclines, and vitamins. For references to the effects of aluminium hydroxide and other antacid preparations on drug absorption, see under the individual drug monographs.

The effects of aluminium hydroxide mixture on phosphate should always be carefully considered.

Aluminium hydroxide could cause white discoloration of the faeces.— J. Karlstrand, *J. Am. pharm. Ass.*, 1977, *NS17*, 735.

Absorption and Fate. The insoluble aluminium compounds that constitute aluminium hydroxide mixture are slowly but perhaps incompletely converted to aluminium chloride in the stomach. Some absorption of soluble aluminium salts occurs from the gastro-intestinal tract with some excretion in the urine. Some unabsorbed aluminium hydroxide combines with phosphates present in the gut to form insoluble aluminium phosphates and some forms carbonates and salts of fatty acids; all these salts are excreted in the faeces.

Patients with chronic renal failure absorbed up to 17% of the administered dose of aluminium when given aluminium hydroxide mixture 75 to 150 ml daily.— R. R. Bailey (letter), *Lancet*, 1972, *2*, 276.

An increase in urine pH occurred within 24 hours of the administration of a magnesium and aluminium hydroxides suspension (Maalox) 15 ml four times daily to 8 healthy males. After 6 days the antacid was withdrawn but the effect on urine pH persisted for a further 24 hours.— M. Gibaldi *et al.*, *J. pharm. Sci.*, 1975, *64*, 2003.

Studies of the absorption of aluminium hydroxide, aluminium carbonate, aluminium glycinate, and aluminium phosphate by healthy subjects demonstrated that although the gastro-intestinal tract was a formidable barrier to entry of aluminium it was not impervious. Following ingestion of the first 3 compounds plasma-aluminium concentrations rose significantly and urinary excretion rose markedly. Absorption of aluminium phosphate (virtually insoluble at acid pH but slightly more soluble than aluminium hydroxide in alkaline pH) was insignificant which correlated with the hypothesis that aluminium absorption occurred largely in the acid milieu of the proximal duodenum or stomach and very little if at all in the rest of the gastro-intestinal tract.— W. D. Kaehny *et al.*, *New Engl. J. Med.*, 1977, *296*, 1389.

Uses. Aluminium hydroxide mixture is a slow-acting antacid. It is used to provide symptomatic relief in gastric and duodenal ulcer and in reflux oesophagitis, and is used in the treatment of hyperchlorhydria. It may be administered in doses of 7.5 to 15 ml every 2 to 4 hours or more frequently in water or milk, or tablets containing the dried ingredients may be sucked or chewed. Aluminium hydroxide mixture diluted with 2 to 3 parts of water may be given by intragastric drip at a rate of 15 to 20 drops a minute throughout the day.

Aluminium hydroxide mixture is used in a daily dose of up to 100 ml to reduce the absorption of phosphates and hence reduce blood-phosphate concentrations to below 2.0 mmol per litre or 60 µg per ml in patients with bone disorders associated with chronic renal failure (but see above under Adverse Effects). It is also given in the management of urinary phosphatic calculi in doses of 40 ml after meals and at bedtime.

Aluminium hydroxide is also used as an adjuvant in adsorbed vaccines to increase their potency and reduce the incidence of undesirable reactions either by delaying the release of antigen or by altering tissue reactivity.

The constipating effect of aluminium hydroxide mixture may be counteracted by the addition of magnesium hydroxide or trisilicate.

Aluminium hydroxide in allergen injections acted by modifying tissue reactivity rather than by delaying the release of antigen from the tissues.— L. Guibert *et al.*, *Revue fr. Allerg.*, 1971, *11*, 123.

Diarrhoea. Aluminium hydroxide mixture 30 to 40 ml given first thing in the morning and at night or sometimes thrice daily controlled choleraic diarrhoea in 8 patients. This treatment probably acted by bile acid binding to the unabsorbed aluminium ion.— A. Sali *et al.*, *Lancet*, 1977, *2*, 1051.

A further report of the use of aluminium hydroxide in the management of bile-salt diarrhoea.— *Gut*, 1977, *18*, A419.

Ectopic calcification. A 9-year-old boy with extensive ectopic calcifications in the soft tissues was treated with aluminium hydroxide mixture, 15 ml four times daily. The treatment induced a deficiency of phosphate and led to a decrease in the ectopic calcification over a period of 18 months.— J. R. Nassim and C. K. Connolly, *Archs Dis. Childh.*, 1970, *45*, 118.

Further references: G. M. Berlyne and A. B. Shaw, *Lancet*, 1967, *1*, 4; G. Mozaffarian *et al.*, *Ann. intern. Med.*, 1972, *77*, 741.

Paget's disease. Relief of pain, occurred after 20 to 70 days in 8 of 9 patients with painful Paget's disease of the bone who were treated for 200 days with a combination of aluminium hydroxide, calcium by mouth, a thiazide diuretic, and a low-phosphate diet. The mean plasma concentration of alkaline phosphatase was reduced gradually after 1 month and the reduction maintained; the mean plasma calcium content was increased.— R. A. Evans, *Aust. N.Z. J. Med.*, 1977, *7*, 259. Comment.— *Lancet*, 1978, *1*, 915.

Renal failure. A recommendation that aluminium hydroxide mixture be used in the management of renal osteodystrophy so as to maintain serum concentrations of phosphorus between 46 and 61 μg per ml and to allow a more liberal diet. Over-enthusiastic treatment with aluminium hydroxide mixture was probably more harmful than no treatment.— D. J. Hosking, *Br. med. J.*, 1977, *2*, 110. See also A. C. Kennedy, *Br. med. J.*, 1977, *2*, 506; *Drug & Ther. Bull.*, 1978, *16*, 61.

Ulcer, gastric and duodenal. For reports and studies on the role of antacid therapy, including aluminium hydroxide, in gastric and duodenal ulcer, see p.71.

Use with ostomies. A report of the application of aluminium hydroxide mixture as a protective barrier between the skin and the ostomy appliance and as a treatment for associated burns.— J. Karlstrand, *J. Am. pharm. Ass.*, 1977, *NS17*, 735.

673-s

Dried Aluminium Hydroxide *(B.P.)*. Dried Aluminium Hydroxide Gel; Dried Aluminum Hydroxide Gel *(U.S.P.)*; Al. Hydrox. Coll.; Dried Alum. Hydrox. Gel; Gelat. Alumin. Hydrox. Sicc.; Aluminium Hydrate Powder; Aluminium Hydroxide Powder; Hydrous Oxide of Aluminium; Algedratum Des-Acidans; Argilla Alba; Argilla pura.

Pharmacopoeias. In *Arg., Aust., Br., Hung., Ind., Jap., Mex., Neth., Pol., Port., Rus., Swiss, Turk.*, and *U.S.* (Most with not less than 50% Al_2O_3.).

A fine, white, odourless, tasteless, amorphous powder with some aggregates. The *B.P.* specifies that it consists largely of hydrated aluminium oxide and contains not less than 47% of Al_2O_3. The *U.S.P.* specifies 50 to 57.5% of Al_2O_3 in the form of hydrated oxide and permits varying quantities of basic aluminium carbonate and bicarbonate. Heating to a temperature much in excess of 30° results in gradual dehydration and loss of therapeutic value. Its neutralising activity may be reduced by tabletting. At relative humidities between about 15 and 70%, the equilibrium moisture contents at 25° are between about 17 and 20%, but at relative humidities above 75% it absorbs substantial amounts of moisture.

Practically **insoluble** in water and alcohol; soluble in dilute mineral acids and in excess of caustic alkali solutions. A 4% suspension in water has a pH of not more than 10. **Store** at a temperature not exceeding 25° in airtight containers.

Inactivation. Sodium citrate or tartrate inhibited neutralisation of gastric acid by dried aluminium hydroxide. A water-soluble complex was formed and hydrogen ions liberated. This effect, with flocculation, retarded the speed of neutralisation.— M. Gibaldi and D. Mufson, *J. pharm. Sci.*, 1967, *56*, 46.

Uses. Dried aluminium hydroxide has the same action and uses as aluminium hydroxide mixture and may be administered as capsules and tablets. It is given in a usual dose of 0.5 to 1 g, repeated in accordance with the patient's needs.

Preparations

Mixtures

Aluminium Hydroxide and Belladonna Mixture *(A.P.F.)*. Belladonna tincture 0.5 ml, concentrated chloroform water 0.2 ml, citric acid monohydrate 100 mg, aluminium hydroxide mixture to 10 ml. It should be freshly prepared and used within 14 days. *Dose.* 10 ml.

Aluminium Hydroxide and Belladonna Mixture *(B.P.C. 1973)*. Belladonna tincture 0.5 ml, chloroform spirit 0.25 ml, aluminium hydroxide mixture to 5 ml. It should be recently prepared. *Dose.* 5 ml, suitably diluted.

Adsorption of hyoscyamine was not detected, so it was concluded that stabilisation was due to the viscosity of the mixture.— S. A. H. Khalil and S. El-Masry, *J. Pharm. Pharmac.*, 1978, *30*, 664.

Aluminium Hydroxide and Kaolin Mixture *(A.P.F.)*. Aluminium Hydroxide Gel with Kaolin. Light kaolin or light kaolin (natural) 2 g, sodium citrate 10 mg, concentrated chloroform water 0.2 ml, aluminium hydroxide mixture to 10 ml. *Dose.* Initial, 15 ml; repeated, 5 to 10 ml.

Aluminium Hydroxide and Kaolin Mixture CF *(A.P.F.)*. Aluminium Hydroxide Gel with Kaolin for Children. Light kaolin or light kaolin (natural) 1 g, sodium citrate 5 mg, concentrated chloroform water 0.1 ml, aluminium hydroxide mixture to 5 ml. *Dose.* 5 to 10 ml.

A reminder that the essential consequence of acute diarrhoea is dehydration, and the fundamental treatment is rehydration.— W. A. M. Cutting and W. C. Marshall (letter), *Lancet*, 1979, *2*, 1022.

Aluminium Hydroxide and Phenobarbitone Mixture *(A.P.F.)*. Phenobarbitone sodium 20 mg, water 0.1 ml, concentrated chloroform water 0.2 ml, aluminium hydroxide mixture to 10 ml. *Dose.* 10 ml.

Aluminium Hydroxide, Phenobarbitone and Belladonna Mixture *(A.P.F.)*. Phenobarbitone sodium 20 mg, water 0.1 ml, citric acid monohydrate 150 mg, belladonna tincture 0.5 ml, concentrated chloroform water 0.2 ml, aluminium hydroxide mixture to 10 ml. It should be freshly prepared and used within 14 days. *Dose.* 10 ml.

Pastes

Aluminium Hydroxide Topical Paste *(Adelaide Child. Hosp.)*. Aluminium hydroxide in fine powder 2.4 g, tragacanth powder 4.8 g, glycerol 32 ml, hydroxybenzoates spirits 4 ml, water 66 ml. Shelf-life 6 months. Applied 3 to 4 times daily to stomal ulcers to protect from urine.

Powders

Aluminium and Magnesium Trisilicate Powder *(A.P.F.)*. Dried aluminium hydroxide 10 g, magnesium trisilicate 50 g, and light kaolin or light kaolin (natural) 40 g. *Dose.* 2 to 5 g.

Suspensions

Alumina and Magnesia Oral Suspension *(U.S.P.)*. A mixture containing aluminium oxide (Al_2O_3), as aluminium hydroxide and hydrated aluminium oxide, and magnesium hydroxide. It contains the equivalent of 3.1 to 4% w/w of aluminium oxide, 1.4 to 2.2% w/w of magnesium hydroxide, and 4.5 to 6.2% w/w of combined aluminium oxide and magnesium hydroxide; it may contain a flavouring agent, and suitable antimicrobial agents. pH 7.3 to 7.9. Store in airtight containers. Avoid freezing.

See also Magnesia and Alumina Oral Suspension, p.82.

Alumina and Magnesium Trisilicate Oral Suspension *(U.S.P.)*. Potency is expressed in terms of aluminium oxide (Al_2O_3) and magnesium oxide (MgO). Store in airtight containers.

Tablets

Alumina and Magnesia Tablets *(U.S.P.)*. Tablets containing aluminium hydroxide and magnesium hydroxide.

See also Magnesia and Alumina Tablets, p.83.

Aluminium Hydroxide Tablets *(B.P.)*. Alum. Hydrox. Tab. Each contains 500 mg of dried aluminium hydroxide, flavoured with sucrose and peppermint oil. Store at a temperature not exceeding 25° in airtight containers. *Dose.* 1 or 2 tablets; they should be chewed before swallowing.

Dried Aluminum Hydroxide Gel Tablets *(U.S.P.)*. Tablets containing Al_2O_3 equivalent to 62 to 72% of the labelled amount of aluminium hydroxide.

Proprietary Preparations

For other preparations containing aluminium hydroxide, see Silicones, p.1069.

Abacid Plus *(Ticen, Eire)*. Suspension containing in each 5 ml dried aluminium hydroxide 200 mg, magnesium trisilicate 100 mg, dimethicone 20 mg, and dicyclomine hydrochloride 2.5 mg. For hyperacidity and flatulence. *Dose*: 5 to 10 ml.

Actonorm Gel *(Wallace Mfg Chem., UK: Farillon, UK)*. Contains in each 5 ml dried aluminium hydroxide 220 mg, magnesium hydroxide 100 mg, activated dimethicone 25 mg, and peppermint oil 0.00075 ml. **Actonorm-Sed Gel** contains, in addition, belladonna tincture 0.15 ml in each 5 ml. For hyperacidity and gastric disorders. *Dose.* Actonorm Gel: 5 to 20 ml after meals; Actonorm-Sed Gel: 10 ml four times daily, after meals and at bedtime.

Alu-cap *(Riker, UK)*. Dried aluminium hydroxide, available as capsules of 475 mg.

Aludrox Gel *(Wyeth, UK)*. A brand of aluminium hydroxide mixture. **Aludrox Tablets.** Scored tablets each containing 750 mg of an aluminium hydroxide-sucrose mixture providing the equivalent of 375 mg of $Al(OH)_3$.

NOTE. In Austral. and USA the name Aludrox is applied to a preparation also containing magnesium hydroxide.

Aludrox SA *(Wyeth, UK)*. Suspension containing in each 5 ml aluminium hydroxide mixture 4.75 ml, magnesium hydroxide 100 mg, and ambutonium bromide 2.5 mg. For peptic ulceration. *Dose.* 5 to 10 ml 3 or 4 times daily between meals and at bedtime.

Aluhyde *(Sinclair, UK)*. Tablets each containing dried aluminium hydroxide 245 mg, magnesium trisilicate 245 mg, and belladonna liquid extract 7.8 mg. For peptic ulcer and hyperacidity. *Dose.* 2 tablets, with water, after meals.

Gastrocote Tablets *(MCP Pharmaceuticals, UK)*. Each contains dried aluminium hydroxide 80 mg, magnesium trisilicate 40 mg, sodium bicarbonate 70 mg, and alginic acid 200 mg. For gastric reflux. *Dose.* 1 to 3 tablets, thoroughly chewed, after each meal and at bedtime.

Gaviscon *(Reckitt & Colman Pharmaceuticals, UK)*. **Granules** containing in each 5-g sachet dried aluminium hydroxide 208 mg, magnesium trisilicate 52 mg, alginic acid 481 mg, sodium alginate 521 mg, and sodium bicarbonate 177 mg, with sucrose and mannitol, and **Tablets** each containing dried aluminium hydroxide 100 mg, magnesium trisilicate 25 mg, alginic acid 500 mg, and sodium bicarbonate 170 mg, with sucrose and mannitol. For hiatus hernia and conditions associated with gastric reflux. *Dose.* The contents of 1 sachet or 1 or 2 tablets, thoroughly chewed, after meals and at bedtime.

Infant Gaviscon *(Reckitt & Colman Pharmaceuticals, UK)*. Powder containing in each 2-g sachet dried aluminium hydroxide 200 mg, magnesium trisilicate 50 mg, alginic acid 924 mg, and sodium bicarbonate 340 mg, in a basis containing mannitol and silicon dioxide. Each 2-g sachet contains sodium 4 mmol (4 mEq). For gastric regurgitation and gastric reflux. *Dose.* The contents of ½ to 1 sachet mixed with each milk feed or mixed with water and taken after each meal.

NOTE. In view of its high sodium content this preparation should not be used in premature infants or in situations where excess water-loss is likely, such as fever or high room-temperature; some sources have recommended that it should be avoided altogether in children less than 6 months of age.

See also Liquid Gaviscon, p.635..

Gelusil *(General Diagnostics, UK)*. **Suspension** containing in each 5 ml dried aluminium hydroxide 310 mg and magnesium trisilicate 620 mg (suggested diluent, water) and **Tablets** each containing dried aluminium hydroxide 250 mg and magnesium trisilicate 500 mg. For gastric hyperacidity. *Dose.* 5 to 10 ml of suspension or 1 or 2 tablets, chewed, after meals, or when necessary.

Kolanticon Gel *(Merrell, UK)*. Contains in each 10 ml dried aluminium hydroxide 400 mg, dicyclomine hydrochloride 5 mg, light magnesium oxide 200 mg, and activated dimethicone 40 mg. For hyperacidity, spasm, and flatulence. *Dose.* 10 to 20 ml every 4 hours.

Kolantyl *(Merrell, UK)*. **Gel** containing in each 5 ml dried aluminium hydroxide 200 mg, dicyclomine hydrochloride 2.5 mg, and light magnesium oxide 100 mg and **Tablets** each containing dried aluminium hydroxide 240 mg, dicyclomine hydrochloride 5 mg, magnesium hydroxide 144 mg, magnesium trisilicate 90 mg, and dextrose monohydrate 1.124 g. For peptic ulcer and hyperacidity. *Dose.* 10 to 20 ml of gel, or 1 or 2 tablets to be chewed or sucked, every 4 hours.

NOTE. In the USA the name Kolantyl is applied to preparations containing aluminium hydroxide and magnesium hydroxide.

Maalox *(Rorer, UK)*. **Suspension** containing in each 5 ml dried aluminium hydroxide 220 mg and magnesium hydroxide 195 mg. **Tablets** each containing dried aluminium hydroxide 400 mg and magnesium hydroxide 400 mg. Antacid. *Dose.* 10 to 20 ml of suspension, or 1 or 2 tablets, chewed, 20 to 60 minutes after meals and at bedtime.

Maalox Plus *(Rorer, UK)*. **Suspension** containing in each 5 ml dried aluminium hydroxide 220 mg, magnesium hydroxide 195 mg, and activated dimethicone 25 mg. **Tablets** each containing dried aluminium hydroxide 200 mg, magnesium hydroxide 200 mg, and activated dimethicone 25 mg. Antacid. *Dose.* 10 to 20 ml of suspension, or 2 to 4 tablets, 4 times daily.

Mucaine (known in some countries as Mucoxin, Mutesa, Muthesa, Oxaine, and Tepilta) *(Wyeth, UK)*. A suspension containing in each 5 ml aluminium hydroxide mixture 4.75 ml, oxethazaine 10 mg, and magnesium hydroxide 100 mg. For oesophagitis and heartburn. *Dose.* 5 to 10 ml three or four times daily 15 minutes before meals and at bedtime; to be taken without a drink.

Neutrolactis *(Wander, UK)*. Tablets each containing dried aluminium hydroxide 140 mg, magnesium trisilicate 200 mg, calcium carbonate 280 mg, and high-protein milk solids 1.5 g. For peptic ulcer and dyspepsia. *Dose.* 1 or 2 tablets to be chewed or sucked every 2 hours.

Topal *(Concept Pharmaceuticals, UK).* Tablets each containing dried aluminium hydroxide 30 mg, light magnesium carbonate 40 mg, and alginic acid 200 mg, with sucrose and lactose. For conditions associated with gastric reflux. *Dose.* 1 to 3 tablets, chewed, 4 times daily between meals and at bedtime.

Other Proprietary Names

Arg.— Aldrox; *Austral.*— Adagel, Alusorb, Alu-Tab, Amphojel, Amphotabs, Basaljel, Gelox, Minajel; *Belg.*— Aldrox; *Canad.*— Amphojel, Basaljel; *Ger.*— Palliacol; *Ital.*— Gamma-gel; *Neth.*— Aluminox; *Norw.*— Allulose; *S.Afr.*— Alumag, Amphojel; *Spain*— Alugelibys, Pepsamar, Uldecan; *Switz.*— Gastracol; *USA*— Alternagel, Amphojel, Dialume.

NOTE. The name Basaljel is also used for basic aluminium carbonate.

Preparations containing aluminium hydroxide were also formerly marketed in Great Britain under the proprietary names Alubarb (*Norton*), Ascon (*Cox-Continental*), Antidiar (see also under Ethacridine Lactate) (*Armour*), and Gelusil Lac (*Warner*).

Proprietary Preparations of Some Other Aluminium Compounds

Droxalin *(Sterling Health).* Tablets each containing polyhydroxyaluminium sodium carbonate 162 mg and magnesium trisilicate 162 mg. For hyperacidity and peptic ulcer. *Dose.* 1 or 2 tablets to be chewed as required.

Unemul *(Universal Emulsifiers, UK: Blagden, UK).* An emulsifying and suspending agent consisting of an inert gelatinous hydrated aluminium oxide, almost insoluble in acids and alkalis.

It normally produces oil-in-water emulsions but, with auxiliary emulsifiers, it may be used for water-in-oil emulsions; also used as a suspending agent. The simplest method of using Unemul as an emulsifying agent is to mix it with the water, add the oil and shake, then pass through a homogeniser.

Other Proprietary Names of Some Other Aluminium Compounds

Basaljel *(basic aluminium carbonate) (USA)*; Lithiagel *(aluminium hydrocarbonate) (Fr.)*; Rocgel *(aluminium oxide) (Fr.)*.

NOTE. The name Basaljel is also used for aluminium hydroxide.

An antacid preparation containing aluminium compounds was formerly marketed in Great Britain under the proprietary name Alcin (*Reckitt & Colman*).

674-w

Aluminium Hydroxide-Magnesium Carbonate Co-dried Gel.

F-MA 11. A co-precipitate of aluminium hydroxide and magnesium carbonate carefully dried to contain a critical proportion of water for high antacid activity.

A white, odourless, tasteless, fine, free-flowing powder, containing the equivalent of 40 to 43% Al_2O_3 and 6 to 9% MgO. A 4% suspension in water has a pH of 8.5 to 9.5.

Uses. Aluminium hydroxide-magnesium carbonate co-dried gel is used for the same purposes as dried aluminium hydroxide in doses of up to 1 g but is reported to retain its acid-neutralising capacity and speed of neutralisation of acid better than dried aluminium hydroxide during storage.

Proprietary Preparations

Gastalar *(Armour, UK).* Chewable tablets each containing aluminium hydroxide-magnesium carbonate-sorbitol co-dried gel 500 mg. For dyspepsia and hyperacidity. *Dose.* 1 or 2 tablets to be chewed as required.

Gastrils *(Ernest Jackson, UK).* Pastilles each containing aluminium hydroxide-magnesium carbonate co-dried gel 500 mg, with carbohydrate 1.75 g. For hyperacidity and peptic ulcer. *Dose.* 1 or 2 pastilles to be sucked as required.

Other Proprietary Names

Acinorm *(Denm.)*; Allulose *(Norw.)*; Dijene *(Austral.)*.

Aluminium hydroxide-magnesium carbonate co-dried gel was also formerly marketed in Great Britain under the proprietary name Almacarb (*Duncan, Flockhart*).

675-e

Aluminium Phosphate Mixture *(B.P.)*.

Aluminium Phosphate Gel; Aluminum Phosphate Gel *(U.S.P.)*; Alum. Phos. Gel.

CAS — 7784-30-7 ($AlPO_4$).

Pharmacopoeias. In *Br.* (containing 7 to 8% $AlPO_4$), *Mex.* (3.8 to 4.5% $AlPO_4$), and *U.S.* (4 to 5% $AlPO_4$).

The *B.P.* describes an aqueous suspension of aluminium orthophosphate containing 7 to 8% w/w of $AlPO_4$ (=122.0). It contains peppermint oil 0.01% v/v as a flavouring agent; saccharin sodium may be added as a sweetening agent. It is a white viscous suspension from which small amounts of clear liquid may separate on standing. A 50% dilution in water has a pH of 5 to 6. **Store** at a temperature not exceeding 30° and avoid freezing.

The *U.S.P.* describes an aqueous suspension containing 4 to 5% w/w of $AlPO_4$; it may contain up to 0.5% of sodium benzoate, benzoic acid, or other suitable agent as a preservative. pH 6 to 7.2. **Store** in airtight containers.

676-l

Dried Aluminium Phosphate *(B.P.)*.

Dried Aluminium Phosphate Gel; Dried Alum. Phos. Gel.

Pharmacopoeias. In *Br.*

An odourless, tasteless, white powder containing some friable aggregates. It consists largely of hydrated aluminium orthophosphate and contains not less than 80% of $AlPO_4$ (=122.0). Practically **insoluble** in water, alcohol, and solutions of alkali hydroxides; soluble in dilute mineral acids. A 4% suspension in water has a pH of 5.5 to 6.5. **Store** at a temperature not exceeding 30°.

Uses. Aluminium phosphate mixture is a slow-acting antacid used similarly to Aluminium Hydroxide Mixture (see p.72). Unlike aluminium hydroxide, it does not interfere with phosphate absorption and is used when a high-phosphorus diet cannot be maintained or if there is diarrhoea or a deficiency of pancreatic juice. It is also used as an adjuvant in adsorbed vaccines.

The mixture is given in doses of 5 to 15 ml and dried aluminium phosphate in doses of 400 to 800 mg.

Effect on strontium absorption. In 7 patients a preparation of aluminium phosphate mixture, containing between 3.8% and 4.5% of aluminium phosphate, reduced strontium-85 absorption by more than 86% when given in doses of 100 to 300 ml. A dose of 100 ml was as effective as larger doses.— H. Spencer *et al.* (letter), *Lancet*, 1967, *2*, 156.

Preparations

Aluminium Phosphate Tablets *(B.P.).* Alum. Phos. Tab. Each contains dried aluminium phosphate equivalent to 360 to 440 mg of $AlPO_4$ and is flavoured with peppermint oil. Store at a temperature not exceeding 30°. *Dose.* 1 or 2 tablets; they should be chewed before swallowing.

Synergel *(Biothérax, Fr.: Servier, UK).* A mixture containing aluminium phosphate mixture 55% with pectin and agar, in sachets of 20 g. For dyspepsia. *Dose.* The contents of 1 sachet twice or thrice daily.

Other Proprietary Names

Fosfalugel *(Denm., Norw.)*; Fosfidral *(Ital.)*; Fosfoalugel *(Spain)*; Phosphaljel*(USA)*; Phosphalugel *(Belg., Fr., Ger., Switz.)*; Phosphalutab *(Ger.)*.

Aluminium phosphate mixture was also formerly marketed in Great Britain under the proprietary name Aluphos Gel (*Fisons*).

677-y

Aluminium Sodium Silicate. Sodium Aluminium Silicate.

CAS — 1344-00-9.

A white powder.

Uses. Aluminium sodium silicate is used as an antacid. Almasilate, which is the artificial form of aluminium magnesium silicate hydrate, is reported to possess antacid properties.

Proprietary Preparations

Neutradonna *(Nicholas, UK).* **Powder** containing in each g aluminium sodium silicate 989.6 mg and belladonna alkaloids (calculated as hyoscyamine) 75 µg and **Tablets** each containing aluminium sodium silicate 650 mg and belladonna alkaloids (calculated as hyoscyamine) 48 µg. For dyspepsia and peptic ulcer. *Dose.* 1 or 2 level teaspoonfuls of powder, or 2 or 3 tablets, 3 or 4 times daily.

Other Proprietary Names

Neutralon *(Austral., Spain)*.

A preparation containing aluminium sodium silicate was also formerly marketed in Great Britain under the proprietary name Neutradonna Sed (*Nicholas*).

678-j

Amixetrine Hydrochloride. 1-[2-(4-Methylbutoxy)-2-phenylethyl]pyrrolidine hydrochloride.
$C_{17}H_{27}NO,HCl$=297.9.

CAS — 24622-72-8 (amixetrine); 24622-52-4 (hydrochloride).

Uses. Amixetrine hydrochloride is reported to have anti-inflammatory and antispasmodic effects; it has been given in doses of 50 mg thrice daily in the treatment of oesophagitis, gastric and duodenal ulcers, and colitis.

Urinary excretion in *animals* and man.— M. Constantin *et al.*, *Arzneimittel-Forsch.*, 1976, *26*, 80.

Pharmacokinetics of amixetrine in the *dog*.— M. Constantin and J. F. Pognat, *Arzneimittel-Forsch.*, 1978, *28*, 646.

679-z

Activated Attapulgite *(B.P., B.P. Vet.)*.

Attapulgite Attivata.

CAS — 1337-76-4 (attapulgite).

Pharmacopoeias. In *Br.* and *It.*

A purified native aluminium magnesium silicate belonging to the palygorskite-sepiolite group of mineral clays, heated to increase the adsorptive capacity. A light cream- or buff-coloured, very fine powder, free or almost free from gritty particles.

Practically **insoluble** in water, organic solvents, and in solutions of the alkali hydroxides. A 5% suspension in water has a pH of 7.5 to 9.

Store in airtight containers.

It is available in 2 grades: regular activated attapulgite, which is processed to minimise colloidal properties while maintaining optimum adsorptive activity, and colloidal activated attapulgite which is processed to develop maximum colloidal properties. The average particle size of the regular grade is 2.9 µm and of the colloidal grade 0.14 µm. Activated attapulgite has a surface area many times greater than that of kaolin.

Precautions. As for Light Kaolin p.81.

Uses. Activated attapulgite is highly absorbent and adsorbent and is employed both for these properties and as a suspending and emulsifying agent. It is, however, difficult to form stable emulsions with activated attapulgite as the sole emulsifying agent. Suspensions are thixotropic.

Activated attapulgite may be used to adsorb some alkaloids, bacteria, dyes, odours, toxins and viruses. It is stated to be non-toxic and has been used in mixtures for the same purposes as light kaolin. It may also be used as a basis for dusting-powders and greaseless ointments and in the preparation of tablets.

In preparing mixtures of attapulgite to be taken by mouth, a mixture of regular grade (10%) and colloidal grade (3%) is often employed, sometimes with the addition of pectin. The usual daily dose range of activated attapulgite is 9 to 12 g.

Activated attapulgite was about 5 times as effective as kaolin in adsorbing diphtheria toxin and in the colloidal form was about 7 times as active.— M. Barr and E. S. Arnista, *J. Am. pharm. Ass., scient. Edn*, 1957, *46*, 493.

Aqueous suspensions of both grades of activated attapulgite exhibited maximum viscosities between pH 6 and pH 8.5; the suspensions were thixotropic, this property being greater in suspensions prepared from the colloidal grade. It was capable of neutralising acid over a wide pH range, the regular grade being slightly superior to the colloidal grade in this respect.— M. Barr, *Drug Cosmet. Ind.*, 1960, *86*, 340.

Under the conditions of the *B.P.C. 1973* adsorption tests for charcoal, activated attapulgite adsorbed only 3.5% of its weight of phenazone and 37.9% of its weight of chloroform vapour. It was superior to kaolin, but not as effective as charcoal.— S. C. Barker and W. J. Horgan (letter), *Pharm. J.*, 1967, *2*, 414.

Activated attapulgite was less effective than activated charcoal in reducing the absorption of pentobarbitone, sodium salicylate, or an organophosphorus pesticide from the *animal* gastro-intestinal tract.— J. P. Atkinson and D. L. Azarnoff, *Clin. Toxicol.*, 1971, *4*, 31.

Proprietary Preparations

Attasorb *(Lawrence Industries, UK)*. A range of industrial grades of activated attapulgite.

Pharmasorb *(Lawrence Industries, UK)*. Activated attapulgite, available in regular and colloidal grades for pharmaceutical use.

Other Proprietary Names

Actapulgite *(Belg., Fr.)*; Rheaban *(USA)*.

Preparations containing activated attapulgite were formerly marketed in Great Britain under the proprietary names Atasorb and Atasorb N (both *Lilly*).

681-s

Bran. The fibrous outer layers of cereal grains, usually wheat, consisting of the pericarp, testa, and aleurone layer. It contains celluloses, polysaccharides or hemicelluloses, protein, fat, minerals, and moisture and may contain part of the germ or embryo.

It comprises about 12% of the weight of the grain and is a byproduct of flour milling. It is available in various grades.

A review of the importance of fibre. Nutritionalists restricted the term fibre to filamentous material in plant food. The term 'dietary fibre' had been introduced to provide a practical term to cover all structures of the plant cell-wall that were not digested by human alimentary enzymes. Dietary fibre was composed of the unavailable carbohydrates, i.e. cellulose and other plant cell-wall polysaccharides (hemicelluloses), and also lignins. The constituents of dietary fibre were not given in any food tables and hypotheses concerning the role of dietary fibre in health and disease had to be provisionally evaluated in terms of the crude fibre content. In most Western-type diets the content of dietary fibre (DF) was about 4 to 8 times the crude fibre (CF). The term crude fibre signified a heterogeneous residue remaining after a plant foodstuff had been treated successively with dilute acid and dilute alkali under conditions specified in the Fertilisers and Feeding Stuff Regulations.— H. C. Trowell, *Chemist Drugg.*, 1975, *204*, 692.

Dietary fibre might be defined as the plant polysaccharides and lignin resistant to hydrolysis by the digestive enzymes of man.— H. Trowell *et al.* (letter), *Lancet*, 1976, *1*, 967. In order to avoid the limitation imposed by defining dietary fibre as plant material it could be called edible fibre and defined as polysaccharides, related polymers, and lignin resistant to hydrolysis by the digestive enzymes of man. This would include animal aminopolysaccharides in the diet of Eskimos.— E. W. Godding (letter), *Lancet*, 1976, *1*, 1129.

Wheat bran contained about 4% of 'crude fibre' and 30 to 35% of unavailable carbohydrate. The addition to the diet of 15 g or more of bran daily was the simplest and least expensive way of producing a high residue diet and all forms of processed bran in Britain were considered roughly equivalent.— *Br. med. J.*, 1976, *1*, 1461.

The term 'plantix' has been coined and used to describe non-fibrous plant polymers such as cellulose, hemicelluloses, and pectins which are resistant to human digestion and are frequently included as dietary fibre.— G. A. Spiller (letter), *Lancet*, 1977, *1*, 198.

Adverse Effects. Large quantities of bran may temporarily increase flatulence and distension, and intestinal obstruction may occur rarely. Interference with iron and calcium absorption has been reported; calcium phosphate may be added to bran to neutralise phytic acid present, and so avoid interference with calcium absorption.

Acute gingivitis occurred in a patient after about 6 weeks of ingesting untreated bran with his breakfast cereal. Debridement revealed large amounts of bran particles in periodontal fissures.— M. Glasby (letter), *Lancet*, 1976, *2*, 1087.

Fibre and not phytate might be mainly responsible for the unavailability of zinc, iron, and possibly calcium in wholemeal bread; zinc bound to starch or protein was released by the action of digestive enzymes while that bound to fibre might remain unavailable.— J. G. Reinhold *et al.*, Binding of Zinc to Fibre and other Solids of Wholemeal Bread, in *Trace Elements in Human Health and Disease*, Vol. I, A.S. Prasad and D. Oberleas (Ed.), London, Academic Press, 1976, 163. See also P. J. R. Shah *et al.*, *Br. med. J.*, 1980, *281*, 426.

High fibre intake may lead to enough wastage of vitamin D to produce rickets.— J. G. Reinhold (letter), *Lancet*, 1976, *2*, 1132.

The possible effects of dietary fibre on calcium availability.— W. P. T. James *et al.* (preliminary communication), *Lancet*, 1978, *1*, 638.

Intestinal obstruction occurred in a 53-year-old woman after the prolonged ingestion of excessive amounts of unprocessed bran.— J. Y. Kang and W. F. Doe, *Br. med. J.*, 1979, *1*, 1249.

Precautions. Bran is contra-indicated in patients with intestinal obstruction. Bran should not be eaten dry because of the possibility of oesophageal obstruction. The absorption of digoxin may be decreased if bran is given concurrently. By lowering the transit time through the gut the absorption of other drugs could also be affected.

Bran may be contra-indicated in some patients with ulcerative colitis or regional ileitis.— *Med. Lett.*, 1975, *17*, 93.

A comment on the risk of bezoar formation in diabetic patients with neuropathy receiving a fibre-rich dietary regimen.— B. Canivet *et al.* (letter), *Lancet*, 1980, *2*, 862.

Uses. Bran's main use is as a source of indigestible dietary fibre in the treatment of disorders of the gastro-intestinal tract such as constipation and diverticular disease of the colon. Its use has also been suggested in the prophylaxis and treatment of other disorders. It is used as the basis for some breakfast cereals.

Reviews and discussions on dietary fibre: N. S. Painter, *Postgrad. med. J.*, 1974, *50*, 629; P. F. Heywood, *Med. J. Aust.*, 1975, *2*, 179; *Med. Lett.*, 1975, *17*, 93; E. W. Godding, *Pharm. J.*, 1975, *2*, 34; *J. Am. med. Ass.*, 1976, *235*, 182; K. W. Heaton, *Prescribers' J.*, 1976, *16*, 76; A. I. Mendeloff, *New Engl. J. Med.*, 1977, *297*, 811; H. C. Trowell, *Practitioner*, 1977, *219*, 350; R. M. Kay and M. A. Eastwood, *J. Am. med. Ass.*, 1977, *238*, 1715; E. W. Pomare, *Drugs*, 1977, *14*, 213; *Lancet*, 1977, *2*, 337; *Drug & Ther. Bull.*, 1981, *19*, 29.

Serum concentrations of iron and ionised calcium decreased after administration of bran; in elderly people serum concentrations of iron and ionised calcium were often abnormally low.— I. Persson *et al.* (letter), *Lancet*, 1976, *1*, 643.

The colonic response to dietary fibre from carrot, cabbage, apple, bran, and guar gum.— J. H. Cummings *et al.*, *Lancet*, 1978, *1*, 5.

Choice of bran. The hydrophilic properties of fine bran (all finer than 1 mm) and coarse bran (all coarser than 1 mm) were assessed in 14 patients with diverticular disease or constipation who took 10 g twice daily over a period of 4 weeks. Coarse bran held markedly more water, and significantly lowered colonic motility and transit time; after milling both brans to the same particle size the advantageous properties of the coarse bran were lost. It was concluded that the water-holding capacity of coarse bran was a function of particle size and that these 2 factors were related to motility changes.— W. O. Kirwan *et al.*, *Br. med. J.*, 1974, *4*, 187.

It had been suggested that wholemeal bread was a better source of dietary fibre than unprocessed bran. Phytic acid in bran combined with essential minerals to form insoluble complexes, but it was hydrolysed during bread making.— E. W. Godding, *Pharm. J.*, 1975, *2*, 34.

There was no evidence to indicate that All Bran was more effective than raw, unprocessed miller's bran. A comparative controlled study in 10 healthy subjects suggested that the cooking-malting process reduced the weight for weight laxative effect of wheat bran although in practice the processed varieties might be easier to take in effective amounts because of their greater palatability.— J. B. Wyman *et al.* (letter), *Br. med. J.*, 1976, *2*, 944.

In 21 healthy subjects given bran 20 g daily there was a significantly greater increase in stool weight when the bran was of large particle size, compared to milling it finely.— A. J. M. Brodribb and C. Groves, *Gut*, 1978, *19*, 60.

Diverticular disease. For a discussion on the use of bran in the treatment of diverticular disease of the colon, see T. P. Almy and D. A. Howell, *New Engl. J. Med.*, 1980, *302*, 324.

There was significant subjective symptomatic relief in 9 patients with diverticular disease after 3 months' treatment with bran supplying about 6.7 g of dietary fibre daily compared with a placebo supplying about 0.6 g daily given to 9 similar patients. It was considered that it took several months for a high-fibre diet to produce its maximum effect.— A. J. M. Brodribb, *Lancet*, 1977, *1*, 664.

The effects of bran, ispaghula, and lactulose on colonic function were compared in 31 patients with diverticular disease. Treatment continued for 4 weeks with coarse cereal bran 20 g daily (7 patients), ispaghula as Fybogel, 2 sachets daily (14), and lactulose 20 to 40 ml daily (10). All preparations increased stool weight but only ispaghula had a significant effect. Bran reduced transit time and generally reduced colonic motility before and after food. Ispaghula increased basal motility but, like lactulose, had no significant effect on food-stimulated motility. Although all of the preparations relieved symptoms, bran remained the treatment of choice since it added to stool weight and lowered intraluminal pressure.— M. A. Eastwood *et al.*, *Gut*, 1978, *19*, 1144.

In a comparative study of 264 non-vegetarians with an average dietary fibre intake of 21.4 g daily and 56 vegetarians with a significantly higher average daily intake of 41.5 g diverticular disease was significantly more common in the non-vegetarians. Further studies within the groups suggested that fibre of cereal origin is the most important component of dietary fibre for protection against diverticular disease.— J. S. S. Gear *et al.*, *Lancet*, 1979, *1*, 511.

In a double-blind 4-month crossover study in 58 patients with symptomatic diverticular disease treated with bran (Energen bran crispbread) or ispaghula (Fybogel), only constipation was significantly affected.— M. H. Ornstein *et al.*, *Br. med. J.*, 1981, *282*, 1353.

Further references: A. J. M. Brodribb and D. M. Humphreys, *Br. med. J.*, 1976, *1*, 424 and 428; J. Søltoft *et al.*, *Lancet*, 1976, *1*, 270; A. P. Manning and K. W. Heaton (letter), *ibid.*, 588; J. Weinreich (letter), *ibid.*, 810; I. Taylor and H. L. Duthie, *Br. med. J.*, 1976, *1*, 988; A. Herxheimer (letter), *Br. med. J.*, 1976, *1*, 1341; I. Taylor and H. L. Duthie (letter), *ibid.*; *Lancet*, 1979, *1*, 1175.

Effect on blood sugar. A discussion of the hypoglycaemic effect of bran.— S. Vaisrub, *J. Am. med. Ass.*, 1978, *240*, 379.

A review of dietary fibre and its possible use in the management of diabetes.— D. J. A. Jenkins, *Lancet*, 1979, *2*, 1287. Criticisms.— J. I. Mann and H. C. R. Simpson (letter), *ibid.*, 1980, *1*, 44.

In a study of 8 insulin-dependent diabetic patients who received a diet with either 3 or 20 g of added crude fibre for 10 days, mean plasma-glucose concentrations were about 169 mg per ml on the low-fibre diet and about 121 mg on the high-fibre diet. Seven of the 8 patients had lower mean plasma-glucose concentrations on the high-fibre diet.— P. M. Miranda and D. L. Horwitz, *Ann. intern. Med.*, 1978, *88*, 482.

Further references: *Lancet*, 1981, *1*, 423.

Effect on colonic cancer. A possible protective effect of dietary fibre against colonic cancer.— The International Agency for Research on Cancer Intestinal Microecology Group, *Lancet*, 1977, *2*, 207.

The administration of increased dietary fibre to *rats* (in

the form of bran) reduced the incidence of induced colonic cancer. This reduction could not be accounted for by reduction of calorific intake alone.— D. Fleiszer *et al.*, *Lancet*, 1978, *2*, 552. Criticism of the design of the study.— S. M. Brown and H. L. Falk (letter), *ibid.*, 1252. The protective effect of bran could have been due, at least in part, to its lower energy value.— K. W. Heaton and R. C. N. Williamson (letter), *ibid.*, 784. Further criticism.— J. P. Cruse *et al.* (letter), *ibid.*, 843.

In a controlled study administration of bran failed to protect *rats* against the development of, or mortality associated with, experimental colonic cancer. The case for a protective effect of bran in both human and *animal* cancer is not proven.— J. P. Cruse *et al.*, *Lancet*, 1978, *2*, 1278. The relevance of the *animal* model to human carcinogenesis is questionable.— R. G. Newcombe (letter), *ibid.*, 1979, *1*, 108. Further criticisms.— M. C. Thorne (letter), *ibid.*; A. B. Lowenfels (letter), *ibid.*; T. J. Crofts (letter), *ibid.* Reply.— P. Cruse *et al.*, *ibid.*, 376.

Effect on lipids and bile. A review of dietary fibre and its possible use in the management of hyperlipidaemia.— D. J. A. Jenkins, *Lancet*, 1979, *2*, 1287.

Alteration of bile-salt metabolism by dietary fibre.— E. W. Pomare and K. W. Heaton, *Br. med. J.*, 1973, *4*, 262. See also K. W. Heaton and A. C. B. Wicks, *Gut*, 1977, *18*, A951; D. L. Topping and D. G. Oakenfull (letter), *Lancet*, 1981, *2*, 39; M. Eastwood (letter), *ibid.*, 150.

There was a reduction in serum-cholesterol and serum-iron concentrations in 14 elderly subjects given 20 g of bran daily for 6 weeks.— I. Persson *et al.* (letter), *Lancet*, 1975, *2*, 1208. Criticism.— A. S. Truswell and R. M. Kay (letter), *ibid.*, 1976, *1*, 367.

In 7 patients with type IV hyperlipoproteinaemia the addition of bran 50 g daily to the diet had no effect on serum concentrations of cholesterol or triglycerides.— W. F. Bremner *et al.*, *Br. med. J.*, 1975, *3*, 574. No effect in 8 patients.— P. M. Brooks *et al.*, *Med. J. Aust.*, 1976, *2*, 753. No effect in 12 subjects.— T. L. Raymond *et al.*, *J. clin. Invest.*, 1977, *60*, 1429.

A study in 16 subjects of the effect of taking 50 g to about 120 g of wheat bran daily for up to 6 months showed no significant changes in serum-triglyceride concentrations except in the 6 patients with previous myocardial infarctions, in whom increases in serum cholesterol concentrations correlated with amount of bran intake. An increased consumption of milk was noted in 11 of the 16 subjects.— J. Rhodes *et al.*, *Curr. med. Res. Opinion*, 1977, *5*, 310.

Bran did not increase serum concentrations of high-density lipoproteins in a study of 16 subjects.— M. Dixon (letter), *Br. med. J.*, 1978, *1*, 578.

Studies in 22 patients with diverticular disease fed either a high-fibre or control diet suggested that administration of bran decreased cholesterol synthesis; this correlated with a decrease in faecal bile acids.— S. Tarpila *et al.*, *Gut*, 1978, *19*, 137.

Administration of metronidazole to 11 healthy men to inhibit colonic anaerobic bacterial activity and so depress biliary deoxycholate concentrations, caused a concomitant reduction in biliary cholesterol concentrations in 10 of the 11 subjects; withdrawal led to increased biliary cholesterol concentrations in all 11. It was thus considered that dietary measures, such as high-fibre dietary regimens, which reduce the return of newly formed deoxycholate to the liver and hence also depress biliary cholesterol concentrations, might also reduce the risk of gall-stones developing.— T. S. Low-Beer and S. Nutter, *Lancet*, 1978, *2*, 1063.

In a controlled study, administration of bran (500 mg per kg body-weight daily) for 4 or 8 weeks did not significantly alter cholesterol saturation of bile in healthy subjects. Results of the study did not support the hypothesis of decreased degradation of bile acid in fibre-rich diets.— G. P. Van Berge Henegouwen *et al.*, *Gut*, 1979, *20*, A930.

Hypercalciuria. A significant reduction in urinary calcium occurred in 22 of 30 patients with idiopathic hypercalciuria treated with unprocessed bran.— P. J. R. Shah *et al.*, *Br. med. J.*, 1980, *281*, 426.

Irritable bowel syndrome. In a controlled study of 24 patients with the irritable bowel syndrome a diet high in wheat fibre which provided about 20 g of bran daily produced significant improvement. The frequency and intensity of pain and colonic motor activity were reduced while bowel habit improved. Wholemeal bread was considered to provide the most pleasant method of administering wheat fibre.— A. P. Manning *et al.*, *Lancet*, 1977, *2*, 417.

Further references.— *Lancet*, 1978, *2*, 557.

Pre-operative use. Twenty-one women given a bran-enriched dietary regimen for 10 days before elective gynaecological surgery passed both gas and faeces earlier after the operation than did 21 similar control women given a normal dietary regimen.— O. Sculati *et al.* (letter), *Lancet*, 1980, *1*, 1252. See also J. -P. Manshande *et al.* (letter), *ibid.*, *2*, 476.

Ulcerative colitis. A study in about 40 patients with ulcerative colitis provided no evidence that a high-fibre diet (wholemeal bread, vegetables, and bran) was of value in preventing relapse when sulphasalazine was withdrawn.— P. S. Davies and J. Rhodes, *Br. med. J.*, 1978, *1*, 1524.

Proprietary Preparations

Fybranta *(Norgine, UK)*. Tablets each containing bran 2 g and calcium phosphate 100 mg. Dietary fibre supplement. *Dose.* 6 to 12 tablets daily in divided doses; to be chewed, and swallowed with liquid. (Also available as Fybranta in *Fr., USA*).

Fybranta tablets were much more expensive than ordinary bran and implied that treatment was a medical rather than a dietary matter. Nevertheless, if an individual found it impossible to take bran, Fybranta was a useful alternative.— *Drug & Ther. Bull.*, 1975, *14*, 63.

HC5 *(William Davies, UK)*. Cereal containing bran 1 part and wheatgerm 2 parts, with malt 8.5%, cocoa 4.25%, and sodium chloride 2.125%. Dietary fibre supplement. *Dose.* 2 heaped tablespoonfuls twice daily, mixed with liquid or added to food.

Proctofibe *(Cassenne, UK)*. Tablets each containing bran 375 mg and fibrous extract of citrus 94 mg. Dietary fibre supplement. *Dose.* 4 to 12 tablets daily in divided doses, taken with water.

682-w

Calcium Carbonate *(B.P., Eur. P.)*. Calc. Carb.; Calcii Carbonas; Precipitated Calcium Carbonate *(U.S.P.)*; Precipitated Chalk; Calcium Carbonicum; Creta Preparada.

$CaCO_3$=100.1.

CAS — 471-34-1.

Pharmacopoeias. In all pharmacopoeias examined except *Chin.*, *Int.*, and *Rus.*
Jap. includes *Fossilia Ossis Mastodi*, the ossified bone of large mammals, consisting mainly of calcium carbonate.

A white, odourless, tasteless, microcrystalline powder. Grades of different densities are available in commerce. It absorbs insignificant amounts of moisture at 25° at relative humidities up to about 90%. Each g represents 9.99 mmol (19.98 mEq) of calcium.

Practically **insoluble** in water; slightly soluble in water containing carbon dioxide or ammonium salts; practically insoluble in alcohol; soluble with effervescence in dilute mineral acids. **Sterilised** by maintaining the whole in a closed container at a temperature not less than 160° for 1 hour.

Adverse Effects. Calcium carbonate, like other calcium salts, may cause constipation. Flatulence from released carbon dioxide is not usually a serious problem though eructation may occur in some patients. Hypercalcaemia can occur as can alkalosis following the regular use of calcium carbonate. Similar effects, with renal dysfunction, metastatic calcification, nausea, but absence of hypercalciuria (the milk-alkali syndrome), have developed in some patients taking calcium carbonate with large quantities of milk or cream in the treatment of peptic ulcer.

Hypercalcaemia. Twenty-eight patients with peptic ulceration were given 500 mg per kg body-weight of calcium carbonate daily in hourly doses for 3 weeks, with a ward diet, but no extra milk. Symptoms of hypercalcaemia or alkalosis developed in 5 patients within 3 days and in 1 within 3 weeks with serum-calcium concentrations of up to 177 µg per ml. All symptoms disappeared within 2 days after withdrawal of calcium. The other 22 patients were unaffected. If calcium carbonate was used in such doses, it was necessary to determine serum-calcium concentrations weekly.— J. N. Stiel *et al.*, *Gastroenterology*, 1967, *53*, 900.

Hypercalcaemia occurred in 3 patients on maintenance haemodialysis when given calcium carbonate 3.2 to 6.4 g daily.— D. S. Ginsburg *et al.*, *Lancet*, 1973, *1*, 1271.

Acute hypercalcaemia occurred in 1 patient and recurrent nephrolithiasis in another 2, after the ingestion of calcium carbonate 7 to 15 g daily and sodium bicarbonate 20 to 30 g daily for many years.— R. H. Robson and R. C. Heading, *Postgrad. med. J.*, 1978, *54*, 36.

Further references: R. Makim *et al.*, *Can. med. Ass. J.*, 1979, *121*, 591.

Treatment of Adverse Effects. Hypercalcaemia and alkalosis respond to reduction in dosage of calcium carbonate. In the milk-alkali syndrome, fluid and electrolyte losses should also be replaced. See also under Calcium Salts, p.619.

Precautions. When calcium carbonate is used in large doses, serum-calcium concentrations and kidney function should be determined weekly or at the first sign of hypercalcaemia. Calcium salts (see p.620) may enhance the cardiac effects of digitalis glycosides. Calcium carbonate may interfere with the absorption of tetracycline given concomitantly.

Absorption and Fate. Calcium carbonate is converted to calcium chloride by gastric acid. Some of the calcium is absorbed from the intestines but about 80% is reconverted to insoluble calcium salts such as the carbonate and stearate, and excreted.

Single doses of 1 to 12 g of calcium carbonate briefly raised the blood-calcium concentration of normal subjects to low hypercalcaemic levels. About 16.6% of a 2-g dose of calcium carbonate was absorbed equally in normal subjects and patients with acute milk-alkali syndrome. There was no significant difference in the absorption of calcium from 500 mg of calcium gluconate or 800 mg of the carbonate. Calcium was not absorbed from the carbonate in 4 patients with achlorhydria.— P. Ivanovich *et al.*, *Ann. intern. Med.*, 1967, *66*, 917.

Uses. Calcium carbonate relieves the pain of gastric or duodenal ulcer. It is liable to have a constipating effect which may be counteracted by giving magnesium compounds concomitantly. Calcium carbonate is used, as chalk, in the treatment of diarrhoea. It is also used as a polishing agent in tooth-powders.

A preparation of a native calcium carbonate (Calcarea Carbonica; Calc. Carb.) is used in homoeopathic medicine.

Osteoporosis. A study of 60 healthy postmenopausal women showed their treatment for 2 years with calcium carbonate 2.6 g daily was not as effective in reducing bone loss as treatment with conjugated oestrogens 0.625 mg given with methyltestosterone 5 mg both daily for 21 days per month. However, calcium carbonate was safer for prophylactic use.— R. R. Recker *et al.*, *Ann. intern. Med.*, 1977, *87*, 649. Criticism.— M. L. Stilphen (letter), *ibid.*, 1978, *89*, 149. A reply.— R. R. Recker (letter), *ibid.*

For further reference to calcium salts in osteoporosis, see under Calcium Salts, p.621.

Renal failure. Doses of 20 g daily of calcium carbonate may be required to correct the calcium malabsorption of renal failure. Any induced hypercalcaemia can be readily reversed by reducing calcium intake. This treatment may not prevent metastatic calcification particularly in the presence of hyperphosphataemia; the risk of metastatic calcification may be less with aluminium hydroxide. Calcium supplements of about 1 g daily may be required to maintain calcium balance in patients with chronic renal failure who may have poor dietary intake of calcium.— D. J. Hosking, *Br. med. J.*, 1977, *2*, 110.

Ulcer, gastric and duodenal. For reports and studies on the role of antacid therapy in gastric and duodenal ulcer, see p.71.

Preparations

Calcium and Kaolin Mixture CF *(A.P.F.)*. Calcium and Kaolin Mixture for Children. Calcium carbonate 500 mg, light kaolin or light kaolin (natural) 1 g, alum 5 mg, concentrated chloroform water 0.1 ml, water to 5 ml. *Dose.* 5 ml.

A reminder that the essential consequence of acute diarrhoea is dehydration, and the fundamental treatment is rehydration.— W. A. M. Cutting and W. C. Marshall (letter), *Lancet*, 1979, *2*, 1022.

Calcium Carbonate Mixture Compound *(A.P.F.)*. Calcium carbonate 1 g, magnesium hydroxide mixture 3 ml, syrup 1 ml, concentrated chloroform water 0.25 ml, water to 10 ml. *Dose.* 10 ml.

Calcium Carbonate Tablets *(U.S.P.).* Tablets containing calcium carbonate.

Camphorated Chalk *(B.P.C. 1949).* Cret. Camph.; Creta cum Camphora. Camphor in calcium carbonate. It loses camphor readily and should be stored in well-closed containers; when freshly prepared it should contain not less than 9% of camphor; after storage, not less than 5%. Used as a dentifrice.

Compound Calcium Carbonate Powder *(B.P.C. 1973).* Calcium carbonate 37.5 g, sodium bicarbonate 37.5 g, light kaolin or light kaolin (natural) 12.5 g, heavy magnesium carbonate 12.5 g. *Dose.* 1 to 5 g. See also Compound Magnesium Carbonate Powder, p.82.

Paediatric Compound Calcium Carbonate Mixture *(B.P.C. 1973).* Calcium carbonate, light magnesium carbonate, and sodium bicarbonate, of each 50 mg, aromatic cardamom tincture 0.05 ml, syrup 0.5 ml, double-strength chloroform water 2.5 ml, water to 5 ml. It should be recently prepared. *Dose.* Children, up to 1 year, 5 ml; 1 to 5 years, 10 ml.

Tooth powder. Calcium carbonate 935 g, hard soap 50 g, saccharin sodium 2 g, peppermint oil 4 ml, cinnamon oil 2 ml, and methyl salicylate 8 ml. This powder was included in *U.S.N.F.XI* (1960) under the title NF Dentifrice.

Proprietary Preparations

Titralac *(Riker, UK).* Tablets each containing calcium carbonate 420 mg and glycine 180 mg. For hyperacidity. *Dose.* 1 or 2 tablets to be chewed, sucked, or swallowed whole as required.

Other Proprietary Names

Austral.— Cal-tab, Spar-Cal; *Fr.*— Calcilève, Carbonate De Chaux Adrian; *USA*— Alka-2, Equilet, Os-Cal 500.

683-e

Calcium Silicate. A naturally occurring mineral, the most common forms being calcium metasilicate ($CaSiO_3$ = 116.2), calcium diorthosilicate (Ca_2SiO_4 = 172.2), and calcium trisilicate (Ca_3SiO_5 = 228.3). It is usually found in hydrated forms containing various amounts of water of crystallisation. Commercial calcium silicate is prepared synthetically.

CAS — 1344-95-2; 10101-39-0 ($CaSiO_3$); 10034-77-2 (Ca_2SiO_4); 12168-85-3 (Ca_3SiO_5).

Pharmacopoeias. In *U.S.N.F.* which describes a compound of calcium oxide and silicon dioxide containing not less than 25% of CaO and not less than 45% of SiO_2.

A white or slightly cream-coloured, free-flowing powder. Practically **insoluble** in water; with mineral acids it forms a siliceous gel. A 5% aqueous suspension has a pH of 8.4 to 10.2.

Uses. Calcium silicate is used as an antacid.

Proprietary Names

Sil-Ca *(Centrallab., Denm.).*

685-y

Carbenoxolone Sodium *(B.P.).*

Disodium Enoxolone Succinate. The disodium salt of 3β-(3-carboxypropionyloxy)-11-oxo-olean-12-en-30-oic acid.

$C_{34}H_{48}Na_2O_7$=614.7.

CAS — 5697-56-3 (carbenoxolone); 7421-40-1 (disodium salt).

Pharmacopoeias. In *Br.*

A white or pale cream-coloured hygroscopic powder with a slightly sweet taste and a persistent soapy after-taste. It contains not more than 4% of water.

Soluble 1 in 6 of water and 1 in 30 of alcohol; practically insoluble in chloroform and ether. A solution in methyl alcohol and sodium carbonate solution is dextrorotatory. A 10% solution in water has a pH of 7.9 to 8.7. **Store** in airtight containers.

CAUTION. *Carbenoxolone sodium powder is irritating to nasal membranes.*

Adverse Effects. Carbenoxolone sodium may produce sodium and water retention, leading to oedema, alkalosis, hypertension, hypokalaemia, and impaired glucose tolerance. Renal failure has developed in some patients. Heartburn on swallowing the tablets, myoglobinuria, and myasthenia have been reported.

A short review of the toxic effects of carbenoxolone sodium.— *Med. Lett.*, 1975, *17*, 67.

A patient died following the development of polyarteritis nodosa during a 5-week course of treatment with carbenoxolone sodium.— J. Sloan and J. A. Weaver, *Ir. J. med. Sci.*, 1968, *1*, (Nov.), 505.

Three to 7 hours after ingestion of a preparation of carbenoxolone sodium (Duogastrone), a loud noise like a pistol shot occurred in a 40-year-old woman with a duodenal ulcer.— C. C. Evans and J. B. Ridyard (letter), *Br. med. J.*, 1969, *1*, 120.

Changes in liver function occurred in 5 patients after 6 successive courses of carbenoxolone: return to normal function occurred 5 to 35 days after discontinuation of the medicament.— F. Laubenthal, *Dt. med. Wschr.*, 1972, *97*, 1351.

After 1 month's treatment with carbenoxolone for duodenal ulcer, a 39-year-old woman was found to have mycosis of the duodenal bulb. Whitish pseudomembranes adhering to the duodenal mucosa had not been present the month before; laboratory cultures indicated a growth of mycetes of the *Penicillium* spp. Owing to persistence of the ulcer cimetidine was given. After a month she still had epigastric pain, nausea, and vomiting but no ulcer was found on endoscopy although the whitish pseudomembranes were still present, and again grew *Penicillium* spp. She was given nystatin instead of cimetidine after which both endoscopic and laboratory findings were negative for mycosis and she was symptom-free. If a patient treated with carbenoxolone or cimetidine is still complaining of symptoms resembling those of peptic ulcer at the end of treatment, the possibility of duodenal mycosis should be explored.— L. Lombardo *et al.* (letter), *Lancet*, 1979, *1*, 607.

Hypokalaemia. An account of 8 patients with serious side-effects due to carbenoxolone therapy. Side-effects of carbenoxolone due to electrolyte disturbances were frequent, particularly in the elderly, and the varied clinical presentations were of importance although not well recognised. Headache, oedema, breathlessness, cardiac failure, angina, hypertension, and epilepsy had all been reported in association with sodium retention. Hypokalaemia most commonly presented with muscular weakness, and peripheral paraesthesias might be reported. The effect of hypokalaemia in patients with ischaemic heart disease receiving digoxin was potentially very serious.— G. J. Davies *et al.*, *Br. med. J.*, 1974, *3*, 400.

A report of 3 patients who developed hypokalaemia, weakness, and arreflexia simulating the Guillain-Barré syndrome after taking carbenoxolone. Wrong diagnosis might result in worsened hypokalaemia due to steroid treatment.— A. Royston and B. J. Prout, *Br. med. J.*, 1976, *2*, 150.

Further reports of hypokalaemia associated with carbenoxolone: A. G. G. Turpie and T. J. Thomson, *Gut*, 1965, *6*, 591; A. Muir *et al.* (letter), *Br. med. J.*, 1969, *2*, 512; J. H. Baron (letter), *ibid.*, 1969, *3*, 476; P. C. Barnes and J. H. C. Leonard, *Postgrad. med. J.*, 1971, *47*, 813.

Muscle damage. Muscular pain in a man receiving carbenoxolone sodium 100 mg thrice daily, appeared to be related to the treatment: prompt and sustained remission followed the withdrawal of carbenoxolone. The clinical features and electromyograms were suggestive of myositis.— T. N. Morgan *et al.* (letter), *Br. med. J.*, 1966, *2*, 48.

A 61-year-old man given carbenoxolone 300 mg daily and chlorthalidone every other day, without potassium supplement, developed hypokalaemic alkalosis associated with acute tubular necrosis and muscle necrosis.— C. Descamps *et al.*, *Br. med. J.*, 1977, *1*, 272. Criticism.— C. J. Edmonds (letter), *ibid.*, 775. A reply.— C. Descamps *et al.*, *ibid.*

Renal damage. Carbenoxolone (200 mg daily for 5 years) might have been the precipitating factor in a patient who had acute renal failure; she had a long history of analgesic abuse and had hypertension and urinary infection, and had been treated with gentamicin.— B. Hurley (letter), *Br. med. J.*, 1977, *1*, 1472.

Total body-potassium depletion and renal tubular dysfunction developed in a 64-year-old patient who had received carbenoxolone sodium 50 mg four times daily for 8 weeks.— R. J. Dickinson and R. Swaminathan, *Postgrad. med. J.*, 1978, *54*, 836.

Treatment of Adverse Effects. Symptoms of sodium and water retention may be relieved by a restricted sodium diet or by the concomitant administration of a thiazide diuretic such as chlorothiazide, with potassium supplements.

For the treatment of hypertension and hypokalaemia developing in patients receiving carbenoxolone, see W. Sircus, *Prescribers' J.*, 1972, *12*, 1.

Precautions. Carbenoxolone sodium should be used with caution in the elderly and in patients with cardiac disease, hypertension, or impaired hepatic or renal function. It should not be given with digitalis unless serum-electrolyte concentrations are measured at weekly intervals and measures are taken to avoid hypokalaemia.

The effects of corticosteroids are enhanced by carbenoxolone. Although spironolactone relieves sodium and water retention, it should not be used with carbenoxolone as it antagonises the healing properties of carbenoxolone.

Carbenoxolone was to be avoided in peptic ulceration in the elderly because of the tendency to produce hypokalaemia.— D. E. Hyams, *Br. med. J.*, 1974, *1*, 150.

A comparative study of healthy adults and geriatric patients suggested that protein binding of carbenoxolone was reduced in the elderly, and was associated with lower plasma albumin concentrations; the half-life of carbenoxolone was longer in the elderly subjects. These two factors would contribute to the higher incidence of carbenoxolone side-effects in the elderly.— M. J. Hayes *et al.*, *Gut*, 1977, *18*, 1054.

Interactions. Spironolactone blocked the side-effects of carbenoxolone in patients with gastric ulcer but also reduced the healing of the ulcers.— R. Doll *et al.*, *Gut*, 1968, *9*, 42.

Carbenoxolone was absorbed only from acid gastric juice and should not be taken with antacids or anticholinergic agents. Because of the risk of severe hypokalaemia, blood pressure and serum potassium should be determined every 7 to 10 days and carbenoxolone stopped if serum potassium fell.— *Med. J. Aust.*, 1972, *2*, 401.

For a report that carbenoxolone is not affected by concurrent antacid administration after the first few days, see under Absorption and Fate, below.

Absorption and Fate. Carbenoxolone sodium is absorbed from the gastro-intestinal tract; the main site of absorption is the stomach; absorption is reduced if the gastric pH is above 2. Maximum plasma concentrations are obtained 1 hour after administration in a fasting state but may be delayed for several hours if the dose is taken after food; a second peak appears 2 or 3 hours later probably due to enterohepatic cycling of metabolites. It is bound to proteins in the circulation.

Carbenoxolone is mainly excreted in the faeces via the bile.

Carbenoxolone was as readily absorbed from a positioned-release capsule as from tablets.— W. E. Lindup *et al.*, *Gut*, 1970, *11*, 555.

The absorption of carbenoxolone in 15 patients with gastric ulcer (as Biogastrone) and 8 patients with duodenal ulcer (as Duogastrone) was not affected by concurrent antacid administration after the first few days of treatment. There was no significant difference in serum-carbenoxolone concentration when Biogastrone tablets were taken before or after meals. Serum concentrations were higher in older patients and side-effects could be correlated with them although ulcer healing could not. This suggests that the ulcer-healing effect of carbenoxolone is topical whereas the metabolic effects are systemic.— J. H. Baron *et al.*, *Gut*, 1978, *19*, 330.

Excretion. Following administration by mouth of ^{14}C-carbenoxolone to 3 patients, the radioactivity was excreted as follows: 70 to 81% in the faeces, 10 to 19% in the respiratory carbon dioxide, and 0.2 to 1% in the urine. The biliary metabolites consisted of glucuronide and sulphate conjugates of carbenoxolone.— O. Craig *et al.*, *Practitioner*, 1967, *199*, 109. See also D. V. Parke *et al.*, *Clin. Sci.*, 1972, *43*, 393.

Carbenoxolone 200 mg, administered to patients with gastric ulcer, was rapidly absorbed from the stomach and produced blood concentrations of 20 to 30 µg per ml after 1 to 2 and 3 to 6 hours. About 20% of the dose was excreted in the bile and only about 2% in the urine.— H. D. Downer *et al.*, *J. Pharm. Pharmac.*, 1970, *22*, 479.

Protein binding. At therapeutic concentrations in plasma (10 to 100 µg per ml) carbenoxolone was more than 99% bound to plasma protein; without this binding character the capacity of carbenoxolone for uncoupling of oxidative phosphorylation would prevent its use in man.— W. Sircus, *Gut*, 1972, *13*, 816.

Uses. Carbenoxolone sodium is a derivative of enoxolone with marked anti-inflammatory actions. It appears to act locally on the stomach possibly by stimulating the production of protective mucus, the composition of which may be altered. It is used in the treatment of peptic, mainly gastric ulcers, where it accelerates the rate of healing; this effect is obtained in ambulant patients and is as effective as bed-rest.

The suggested dose in gastric ulcer is 100 mg thrice daily for one week followed by 50 mg thrice daily. Doses should be taken after meals or, if heartburn occurs, with milk. Similarly the dose in duodenal ulcer is 50 mg in a capsule for release in the duodenum, swallowed whole with liquid 4 times daily 15 to 30 minutes before meals; antacids may be given (but see Precautions) and anticholinergics should be discontinued. Potassium salts should generally be given concomitantly with carbenoxolone. Carbenoxolone sodium is also used as a gel in the treatment of ulcers of the mouth.

Detailed reviews of carbenoxolone sodium.— W. Sircus, *Gut*, 1972, *13*, 816; R. M. Pinder *et al.*, *Drugs*, 1976, *11*, 245–307.

A metabolic study for 17 days of a woman with gastric ulcer suggested that the mineralocorticoid effects of carbenoxolone sodium were due to an aldosterone-like action. In the presence of sodium depletion, aldosterone secretion was possibly suppressed through hypokalaemia. The side-effects of carbenoxolone sodium were related to its mineralocorticoid effects and could be prevented by the simultaneous administration of spironolactone, though at the cost of loss of therapeutic effect in ulcer healing.— J. H. Baron *et al.*, *Br. med. J.*, 1969, *2*, 793.

Ulcer, gastric and duodenal. The role of carbenoxolone sodium in the treatment of peptic ulcer.— D. W. Piper and T. R. Heap, *Drugs*, 1972, *3*, 366; D. W. Piper *et al.*, *ibid.*, 1975, *10*, 56; M. J. S. Langman, *ibid.*, 1977, *14*, 105; *idem, Practitioner*, 1979, *223*, 500; I. N. Marks, *Drugs*, 1980, *20*, 283; *Scand. J. Gastroenterol.*, 1980, *15, Suppl.* 65.

In 16 studies in 5 volunteers carbenoxolone had no significant effect on the diffusion of hydrogen ions through the gastric mucosa following the instillation of taurocholic acid. The mechanism of action of carbenoxolone was unlikely to be that of preventing hydrogen-ion diffusion after the reflux of bile.— K. J. Ivey and C. Gray, *Gastroenterology*, 1973, *64*, 1101.

Carbenoxolone reduced the secretion of pepsins in 7 of 9 patients with peptic ulcer.— V. Walker and W. H. Taylor (letter), *Lancet*, 1975, *1*, 1335.

Treatment with carbenoxolone for 4 weeks did not significantly alter basal or peak acid output in patients with gastric or duodenal ulcer.— J. H. Baron, *Gut*, 1977, *18*, 721.

Duodenal ulcer. In a double-blind controlled trial, carbenoxolone sodium as positioned-release capsules in a dose of 200 mg daily was more effective in healing duodenal ulcers than a placebo. Symptomatic improvement and endoscopic evidence of healing occurred in 11 of 16 and 4 of 18 in the treatment and placebo groups respectively after 12 weeks. Serum-carbenoxolone concentrations varied widely and were above 20 µg per ml in the elderly and in those with healed ulcers. The most severe side-effects occurred in 3 patients with serum concentrations of 82, 82, and 55 µg per ml, in whom diuretics and potassium supplements were required.— W. A. Davies and P. I. Reed, *Gut*, 1977, *18*, 78.

In a double-blind multicentre study involving 119 patients there was healing of duodenal ulcers in 75% of patients given carbenoxolone 50 mg four times daily for 6 weeks compared with 48% in patients given a placebo. Analgesics were taken more frequently by patients given carbenoxolone.— A. Archambault *et al.*, *Can. med. Ass. J.*, 1977, *117*, 1155.

The effect of 3 months of maintenance treatment with cimetidine, 400 mg given at bedtime, was compared with carbenoxolone, 150 mg given daily, in 55 patients whose duodenal ulcers had healed after an initial course of cimetidine. Carbenoxolone significantly enhanced mucus secretion, whereas in the cimetidine group no mucus recovery was found. Relapse occurred within 6 months of healing in 13 of the patients taking cimetidine and in 6 taking carbenoxolone.— M. Guslandi *et al.*, *Scand. J. Gastroenterol.*, 1980, *15*, 369.

References to the effective use of carbenoxolone sodium in the treatment of duodenal ulcer: B. O. Amure, *Gut*, 1970, *11*, 171; *Br. J. clin. Pract.*, 1973, *27*, 50; *Gut*, 1977, *18*, 717; G. S. Nagy, *Gastroenterology*, 1978, *74*, 7.

References to carbenoxolone sodium being no more effective than a placebo in the treatment of duodenal ulcer: J. M. Cliff and G. J. Milton-Thompson, *Gut*, 1970, *11*, 167; P. Brown *et al.*, *Gut*, 1972, *13*, 324; *Br. J. clin. Pract.*, 1973, *27*, 140.

Gastric ulcer. In 18 patients with gastric ulcer or gastritis the aspirin-induced gastric potential difference was significantly depressed after treatment with carbenoxolone; this supported the hypothesis that carbenoxolone protected the gastric mucosa against damage by aspirin.— A. Hossenbocus and D. G. Colin-Jones, *Gut*, 1974, *15*, 335.

The increase in immunoreactive secretin observed in 14 patients with rheumatoid arthritis when given carbenoxolone might explain the effect of carbenoxolone on gastric ulcer.— P. J. Rooney *et al.*, *Lancet*, 1974, *1*, 592.

A study in healthy subjects and patients with gastric ulcer suggested that carbenoxolone reduced the increased rate of epithelial cell turnover associated with gastric ulcer, so encouraging healing.— W. Domschke *et al.*, *Gut*, 1977, *18*, 817.

Of 54 patients with endoscopically proven gastric ulcer 27 were randomly allocated to receive cimetidine 200 mg four times daily for 6 weeks while the remainder received carbenoxolone sodium 100 mg thrice daily for a week then 50 mg thrice daily for 5 weeks. Pain was reduced within one week in patients taking cimetidine and within 2 weeks in patients taking carbenoxolone. Ulcers healed in 78% and 52% respectively of patients. Side-effects were minimal with cimetidine but 44% of patients taking carbenoxolone experienced hypokalaemia or oedema.— S. J. La Brooy *et al.*, *Br. med. J.*, 1979, *1*, 1308. See also M. Petrillo *et al.*, *Curr. ther. Res.*, 1979, *26*, 990.

Further references to carbenoxolone and gastric ulcer: R. Doll *et al.*, *Gut*, 1968, *9*, 42; R. D. Montgomery *et al.*, *Practitioner*, 1969, *202*, 398; J. B. Cocking and J. N. MacCaig, *Gut*, 1969, *10*, 219; J. A. C. Wilson, *Br. J. clin. Pract.*, 1972, *26*, 563; W. -P. Fung *et al.*, *Lancet*, 1974, *2*, 10.

Ulcer, oral and oesophageal. Bioral Gel, containing 2% of carbenoxolone sodium, produced a helpful response in large and painful recurrent mouth ulcers in a middle-aged man. Pain and discomfort disappeared promptly and healing was speeded considerably.— O. W. Samuel, *Practitioner*, 1967, *199*, 220.

A report of the effective use of carbenoxolone sodium together with cimetidine for the treatment of Barrett's ulcer of the oesophagus.— W. G. Thompson and R. Barr, *Gastroenterology*, 1977, *73*, 808.

A double-blind comparison of treatment with a combination of carbenoxolone and alginate and antacid (Pyrogastrone) or alginate and antacid alone in 37 patients with reflux oesophagitis. Symptomatic relief after 4 weeks was similar with both preparations but after 8 weeks healing and relief of symptoms was significantly better with the combined preparation of carbenoxolone with alginate antacid.— P. I. Reed and W. A. Davies, *Gut*, 1978, *19*, A985. The same conclusions.— P. I. Reed and W. A. Davies, *Am. J. dig. Dis.*, 1978, *23*, 161. Comment on carbenoxolone in reflux oesophagitis.— *Drug & Ther. Bull.*, 1979, *17*, 63.

Topical carbenoxolone for orofacial herpes simplex infections.— D. E. Poswillo and G. J. Roberts (letter), *Lancet*, 1981, *2*, 143.

Ulcer, venereal. In a double-blind study in 50 patients with non-specific balanitis carbenoxolone gel applied topically was as effective as hydrocortisone cream. In some patients with acute or subacute ulcers carbenoxolone was the more effective.— G. W. Csonka and M. Murray, *Br. J. vener. Dis.*, 1971, *47*, 179.

Preparations

Carbenoxolone Tablets *(B.P.).* Tablets containing carbenoxolone sodium; peppermint oil may be added as a flavouring agent.

Proprietary Preparations

Biogastrone *(Winthrop, UK).* Carbenoxolone sodium, available as scored tablets of 50 mg. (Also available as Biogastrone in *Austral., Belg., Canad., Ger., Jap., Neth., S.Afr., Switz.*).

Bioral Gel *(Winthrop, UK).* Contains carbenoxolone sodium 2% in a basis which adheres firmly to the wet mucosal surface. For mouth ulcers. To be applied thickly to the lesions after meals and at bedtime. (Also available as Bioral in *Austral., S.Afr.*).

Duogastrone *(Winthrop, UK).* Carbenoxolone sodium, available as capsules of 50 mg; the capsules are designed to release their contents in the pyloric antrum. For duodenal ulcer. (Also available as Duogastrone in *Austral., Belg., Canad., Fr., S.Afr., Switz.*).

Pyrogastrone *(Winthrop, UK).* Tablets each containing carbenoxolone sodium 20 mg, dried aluminium hydroxide 240 mg, and magnesium trisilicate 60 mg, in a basis containing sodium bicarbonate and alginic acid. For hiatus hernia and conditions associated with gastric reflux. *Dose.* 1 tablet, thoroughly chewed, thrice daily after meals and 2 at bedtime.

Other Proprietary Names

Gastrausil *(Ital.)*; Neogel *(Ger.)*; Sanodin *(Spain)*; Sustac (see also Glyceryl Trinitrate) *(Arg.)*; Terulcon *(Belg.)*; Ulcus-Tablinen *(Ger.)*.

713-n

Chalk *(B.P., B.P. Vet.).* Creta; Creta Praeparta; Prepared Chalk; Drop Chalk.

$CaCO_3$=100.1.

CAS — 13397-25-6.

Pharmacopoeias. In *Br.*

A native calcium carbonate purified by elutriation. It consists of the calcareous shells and detritus of various cretaceous fossil foraminifera such as *Globigerina* and *Textularia*, together with minute disks or rings, and contains when dried not less than 97% of $CaCO_3$.

White or greyish-white, odourless, tasteless, amorphous, earthy, friable masses, usually conical in form, or powder.

Practically **insoluble** in water; slightly soluble in water containing carbon dioxide; practically insoluble in alcohol; soluble in mineral acids with effervescence.

Uses. Chalk is an antacid and has the same actions and uses as calcium carbonate (see p.76). It is used with other compounds in the treatment of diarrhoea and as an antacid. The usual dose of chalk is about 1 to 3 g.

Preparations

Aromatic Chalk Powder *(B.P.C. 1973).* Pulvis Cretae Aromaticus. Chalk 25 g, cinnamon 10 g, nutmeg 8 g, clove 4 g, cardamom seed 3 g, and sucrose 50 g. Store in airtight containers. *Dose.* 0.5 to 5 g.

Aromatic Chalk with Opium Mixture *(B.P.).* Mistura Cretae Aromatica cum Opio; Mist. Cret. Aromat. c. Opio; Chalk and Opium Mixture. Chalk 325 mg, sucrose 650 mg, tragacanth 20 mg, opium tincture, catechu tincture, and aromatic ammonia solution, of each 0.5 ml, compound cardamom tincture 1 ml, double-strength chloroform water 5 ml, water to 10 ml. It contains 5 mg of anhydrous morphine in 10 ml. It should be recently prepared.
Dose. 10 to 20 ml.

Aromatic Chalk with Opium Powder *(B.P.C. 1973).* Pulvis Cretae Aromaticus cum Opio. Powdered opium 2.5% in aromatic chalk powder. It contains about 2.5 mg of anhydrous morphine in 1 g. Store in airtight containers. *Dose.* 0.5 to 5 g.

Chalk and Kaolin Mixture *(A.P.F.).* Mist. Cret. et Kaolin. Chalk 1.5 g, light kaolin or light kaolin (natural) 2.5 g, alum 10 mg, concentrated chloroform water 0.25 ml, water to 10 ml. *Dose.* 10 to 20 ml.

Chalk Mixture *(B.P.C. 1954).* Aromatic chalk powder 1.029 g, chalk 1.029 g, tragacanth 34.5 mg, cinnamon water to 15 ml. *Dose.* 15 to 30 ml.

Paediatric Chalk Mixture *(B.P.).* Mistura Cretae pro Infantibus; Chalk Mixture Paediatric. Chalk 100 mg, tragacanth 10 mg, syrup 0.5 ml, concentrated cinnamon water 0.02 ml, double-strength chloroform water 2.5 ml, water to 5 ml. It should be recently prepared.
Dose. Children up to 1 year, 5 ml; 1 to 5 years, 10 ml.

A reminder that the essential consequence of acute diarrhoea is dehydration, and the fundamental treatment is rehydration.— W. A. M. Cutting and W. C. Marshall (letter), *Lancet*, 1979, *2*, 1022.

A preparation containing chalk was formerly marketed in Great Britain under the proprietary name Triscal (*Nicholas*).

686-j

Activated Charcoal *(B.P., Eur. P.)*. Decolorising Charcoal; Carbo; Carbo Activatus; Charcoal; Medicinal Charcoal; Charbon Activé; Adsorbent Charcoal; Medizinische Kohle; Carbone Attivo.

CAS — 16291-96-6 (charcoal).

Pharmacopoeias. In all pharmacopoeias examined except *Int. It. P.* also includes Carbone Vegetale.

A very fine, odourless, tasteless, black powder, free from grittiness. The *B.P.* describes material prepared from vegetable matter such as sawdust, peat, cellulose residues, and coconut shells by carbonisation processes intended to confer a high adsorbing power. The *U.S.P.* describes the residue from the destructive distillation of various organic materials, treated to increase its adsorptive power. It loses not more than 15% of its weight on drying.

The *B.P.* specifies that it adsorbs from solution not less than 40% of its weight of phenazone. The *U.S.P.* has tests for adsorptive power in respect of alkaloids and dyes. Practically **insoluble** in all usual solvents. **Store** in airtight containers.

Commercial varieties of charcoal differ widely in their characteristics, depending largely on the method of manufacture. The adsorptive power of charcoal depends on the total available surface area, which may include external and internal surfaces. Charcoals showing high adsorptive power for gases may be relatively inactive in liquid-phase systems and charcoals showing high adsorptive power in liquid media may be relatively inactive for gases.

Adverse Effects. Activated charcoal appears to be nontoxic when given by mouth, although regular ingestion may affect the normal gastro-intestinal absorption pattern.

Haemoperfusion with activated charcoal has produced various adverse effects including platelet damage and aggregation, charcoal embolism, thrombocytopenia, haemorrhage, and hypotension; these effects are reduced when charcoal particles coated with an acrylic hydrogel are used. Activated charcoal should not be given with an emetic.

Activated charcoal could cause black discoloration of the faeces.— J. Karlstrand, *J. Am. pharm. Ass.*, 1977, *NS17*, 735.

Precautions. Activated charcoal diminishes the action of ipecacuanha and other emetics when given concomitantly by mouth. It is of no value in the treatment of poisoning by strong acids or alkalis and its adsorptive capacity is too low to be of use in poisoning with ferrous sulphate and other iron salts, cyanides, tolbutamide and other sulphonylureas, malathion, and dicophane.

The availability of an antidote to a poison renders the use of activated charcoal unnecessary. Moreover, certain substances used orally as antidotes, such as methionine and acetylcysteine, may themselves be adsorbed by activated charcoal.— *Br. med., J.*, 1980, *280*, 692.

Uses. Activated charcoal is an adsorbent for many drugs including aspirin, paracetamol, barbiturates, and tricyclic antidepressants. It is used to remove drugs from the gastro-intestinal tract by oral administration or from the blood by haemoperfusion.

In the oral treatment of poisoning activated charcoal is given usually as a thick slurry following gastric aspiration and lavage. Repeat doses may be of value for drugs which undergo enterohepatic recycling. A recommended dose is 5 to 10 g initially given as a suspension in about 100 ml of water, followed by a further 5 to 10 g twenty minutes later and repeated at intervals of 15 to 20 minutes until a total maximum of 50 g has been given. Activated charcoal may also be given before gastric lavage but should not delay or replace it. Correlation of adsorptive capacity with dose suggests that activated charcoal might be best employed in removing drugs such as the tricyclic antidepressants that are toxic in small amounts. Mixtures such as 'universal antidote' which contain tannic acid with activated charcoal should not be used.

In the haemoperfusion treatment of poisoning coated granules of activated charcoal should be used; a coating of an acrylic hydrogel reduces the hazards of this technique which is effective in removing drugs such as the barbiturates from the blood stream. Response would be expected to be slow with drugs that are widely distributed throughout the tissues.

Activated charcoal has been used as an intestinal marker and as a deodorant for foul-smelling wounds and ulcers. It has also been tried in the treatment of flatulence.

Technical grades of activated charcoal are used as purifying and decolorising agents, for the removal of residual gases in low-pressure apparatus, and in respirators as a protection against toxic gases.

Charcoal (Carbo vegetabilis; Carbo veg.) is used in homoeopathic medicine.

The use of activated charcoal in a quick test for hepatitis B antigen.— S. Polak (letter), *Lancet*, 1974, *1*, 406.

Adsorptive capacity. A review of the use of activated charcoal as an adsorbent in acute poisoning. *In vitro* studies have indicated that *aspirin, chlorpheniramine, colchicine, dexamphetamine, dextropropoxyphene, iodine, phenol, phenytoin,* and *primaquine* are very efficiently adsorbed, and *chloroquine, chlorpromazine, dichlorophenoxyacetic acid, glutethimide, mepacrine, meprobamate, methyl salicylate, quinidine,* and *quinine* are efficiently adsorbed.— J. W. Hayden and E. G. Comstock, *Clin. Toxicol.*, 1975, *8*, 515.

In a randomised study in 5 healthy subjects the absorption of *phenobarbitone* 200 mg, *carbamazepine* 400 mg, or *phenylbutazone* 200 mg was reduced to less than 3%, less than 5%, and 2% respectively (of control values) when activated charcoal 50 g was given within 5 minutes. The effect was greatly reduced when the charcoal was given after 1 hour. When charcoal 50 g was given after 10 hours, with further 17-g doses at 14, 24, 36, and 48 hours the mean half-life of phenobarbitone was reduced from 110 to 19.8 hours, that of carbamazepine from 32 to 17.6 hours, and that of phenylbutazone from 51.5 to 36.7 hours, judged to be due to prevention of absorption after recycling. While the effect might be changed after massive overdosage charcoal was considered to shorten the period of intoxication caused by any drug with a long half-life and extensive enterohepatic or enteroenteric cycle.— P. J. Neuvonen and E. Elonen, *Br. med. J.*, 1980, *280*, 762.

Adsorptive capacity. Further references: A. H. Andersen, *Acta pharmac. tox.*, 1946, *2*, 69 (*mercuric chloride, salicylic acid, phenobarbitone*); D. L. Sorby *et al.*, *J. pharm. Sci.*, 1966, *55*, 785 (*phenothiazines*); D. M. C. de Saintonge and A. Herxheimer, *Eur. J. clin. Pharmac.*, 1971, *4*, 52 (*propantheline*); G. Levy and T. Tsuchiya, *Clin. Pharmac. Ther.*, 1972, *13*, 317 (*aspirin*); T. Tsuchiya and G. Levy, *J. pharm. Sci.*, 1972, *61*, 586 (*aspirin, salicylamide, phenylpropanolamine*); T. Tsuchiya and G. Levy, *J. pharm. Sci.*, 1972, *61*, 624 (preference for powder over tablets); P. J. Neuvonen *et al.*, *Eur. J. clin. Pharmac.*, 1978, *13*, 213 (*digoxin, phenytoin, aspirin*); R. A. Braithwaite *et al.*, *Br. J. clin. Pharmac.*, 1978, *5*, 369P (*tricyclic antidepressants*); C. Sintek *et al.*, *J. Pediat.*, 1979, *94*, 314 (*theophylline*); P. J. Neuvonen *et al.*, *Clin. Pharmac. Ther.*, 1980, *27*, 275 (*dapsone*).

For reference to the relative efficacy of activated charcoal and Amberlite resins in adsorbing polar and non-polar drugs, see p.85.

Charcoal cloth. A noticeable reduction in wound odour occurred in 24 of 26 patients with chronic stasis leg ulcers and in all of 13 patients with suppurating postoperative wounds, following application of a charcoal cloth. The cloth was also found to adsorb bacteria. There was no conclusive evidence that the material facilitated wound healing, although wound cleansing was noted in 31 patients. No adverse reactions to the material were noted although care was needed in the choice of the outer envelope. The dressings did not adhere to the wounds and were removed without trauma.— R. Beckett *et al.* (letter), *Lancet*, 1980, *2*, 594.

Further references: *Lancet*, 1980, *1*, 271; *Chem. in Br.*, 1980, *16*, 172.

Diarrhoea. A study of 204 patients with acute non-specific diarrhoea indicated that treatment with kaolin and pectin, diphenoxylate and atropine, or activated charcoal was no more effective than a controlled diet in reducing the frequency or looseness of stools.— K. Alestig *et al.*, *Practitioner*, 1979, *222*, 859.

Effect of flavouring and suspending agents. A 20% suspension of activated charcoal in water reduced the absorption of aspirin 1 g, taken immediately before, by 65%, but a 20% suspension in equal parts of ice cream and water decreased absorption by only 42%. Although more palatable to children the ice-cream mixture should not be used.— G. Levy *et al.*, *Am. J. Hosp. Pharm.*, 1975, *32*, 289.

Studies *in vitro* indicated that the addition of jams to activated charcoal did not significantly decrease the adsorptive capacity of the charcoal for aspirin whereas the addition of syrup or milk did reduce adsorption.— R. De Neve, *Am. J. Hosp. Pharm.*, 1976, *33*, 965.

The formulation of activated charcoal with carmellose resulted in a decrease of the adsorptive capacity of activated charcoal for aspirin compared to a simple aqueous slurry of activated charcoal.— L. K. Mathur *et al.*, *Am. J. Hosp. Pharm.*, 1976, *33*, 717. Criticism.— M. Manes (letter), *ibid.*, 1120. Reply.— L. K. Mathur *et al.* (letter), *ibid.*, 1122.

An *in vitro* study showed saccharin to be a suitable sweetening agent for inclusion in activated charcoal preparations; it did not significantly alter the adsorptive capacity.— D. O. Cooney, *Am. J. Hosp. Pharm.*, 1977, *34*, 1342.

In a crossover study in 8 healthy subjects activated charcoal formulations containing sorbitol, carmellose sodium, starch, and chocolate syrup were statistically equivalent to a plain activated charcoal slurry in reducing the amount of aspirin absorbed after administration by mouth. These preparations were more palatable than the plain slurry. A formulation employing liquid paraffin emulsion did not effectively inhibit aspirin absorption.— E. C. Scholtz *et al.*, *Am. J. Hosp. Pharm.*, 1978, *35*, 1355. See also M. Mayersohn *et al.*, *Clin. Toxicol.*, 1977, *11*, 561.

Hepatic failure. A brief review and discussion on the use of haemoperfusion with activated charcoal in the treatment of fulminant hepatic failure.— I. M. Murray-Lyon and P. N. Trewby, Hepatic failure, in *Recent Advances in Intensive Therapy*, No. 1, I.M. Ledingham (Ed.), London, Churchill Livingstone, 1977, 125. See also D. B. A. Silk and R. Williams, *Br. J. Hosp. Med.*, 1979, *22*, 437.

A favourable report on the use of haemoperfusion with activated charcoal in the treatment of 22 patients with fulminant hepatic failure.— B. G. Gazzard *et al.*, *Lancet*, 1974, *1*, 1301.

Hiccup. Patients with intractable hiccup were recommended to chew tablets of activated charcoal. The aim of this treatment was to remove swallowed air from the stomach.— S. Goldwater, *Br. med. J.*, 1977, *2*, 708.

Pruritus. Pruritus associated with cholestasis was alleviated in all of 8 patients after 2 plasma perfusions through glass beads coated with activated charcoal *U.S.P.* Each patient underwent 2 or 3 perfusions involving a total of 957 to 6100 ml of plasma. The duration of relief lasted for 24 hours to 5 months and did not correlate with the amount of bile acids removed. The prolonged relief obtained by some patients suggested that a pruritogen other than bile acids may also have been removed since it was calculated that bile-acid concentrations would return to preperfusion concentrations within 3 to 5 days.— B. H. Lauterburg *et al.*, *Lancet*, 1980, *2*, 53.

In a double-blind crossover study, administration of activated charcoal 6 g daily for 8 weeks was more effective than placebo in relieving generalised pruritus in 11 patients undergoing maintenance haemodialysis.— J. A. Pederson *et al.*, *Ann. intern. Med.*, 1980, *93*, 446.

Thyroid storm. Charcoal haemoperfusion using activated charcoal was of value in 2 of 3 patients with thyroid storm.— J. Herrmann *et al.* (letter), *Lancet*, 1977, *1*, 248.

Treatment of poisoning. Comment on the role of activated charcoal with special reference to the effervescent form, Medicoal, in the treatment of acute poisoning. Its use does *not* replace gastric aspiration and lavage, and its main role is in overdosage with drugs like amitriptyline where a small weight of drug can cause serious toxicity.— *Drug & Ther. Bull.*, 1979, *17*, 7.

Further reviews of the use of activated charcoal in the treatment of acute poisoning: *Med. Lett.*, 1979, *21*, 70 (oral); S. Pond *et al.*, *Clin. Pharmacokinet.*, 1979, *4*, 329 (haemoperfusion).

Reports and studies on the use of haemoperfusion with activated charcoal in the management of poisoning.— J. A. Vale *et al.*, *Br. med. J.*, 1975, *1*, 5 (barbiturate, glutethimide, methyl salicylate); E. A. Luzhnikov *et al.* (letter), *Lancet*, 1977, *1*, 38 (parathion-methyl); M. C. Gelfand *et al.*, *Trans. Am. Soc. artif. internal Organs*, 1977, *23*, 599 (paraquat); E. F. Nielsen (letter), *Lancet*, 1978, *1*, 506 (chlordane); B. M. Iversen *et al.* (letter), *Lancet*, 1978, *1*, 388 (nortriptyline); J. A. Diaz-Buxo *et al.*, *Trans. Am. Soc. artif. internal Organs*, 1978, *24*, 699 (amitriptyline); H. -J. Gilfrich *et al.* (letter), *Lancet*, 1978, *1*, 505 (digitoxin); J. P. Wauters *et al.*, *Br. med. J.*, 1978, *2*, 1465 (*Amanita phalloides*); S. M. Ehlers *et al.*, *J. Am. med. Ass.*, 1978, *240*, 474 (theophylline); A. Koffler *et al.*, *Archs intern. Med.*, 1978, *138*, 1691; H. -J. Gilfrich *et al.*, *Vet. hum. Toxicol.*, 1979, *21*, *Suppl.*, 18 (digitoxin); S. E. Warren and D. D. Fanestil, *J. Am. med. Ass.*, 1979, *242*, 2100; *ibid.*, 2106 (digoxin); B. M. Iversen *et al.*, *Clin. Toxicol.*, 1979, *15*, 139 (barbiturates); S. M. Mauer *et al.*, *J. Pediat.*, 1980, *96*, 136 (chloramphenicol); T. M. S. Chang *et al.*, *Pediatrics*, 1980, *65*, 811 (theophylline); S. Okonek *et al.* (letter), *Lancet*, 1980, *2*, 589 (paraquat); S. Vesconi *et al.* (letter), *Lancet*, 1980, *2*, 854 (*Amanita phalloides*).

Reports and studies on the use of activated charcoal by mouth in the management of poisoning.— P. Crome *et al.*, *Lancet*, 1977, *2*, 1203 (nortriptyline).

See also above under Adsorptive Capacity.

Use in ostomies. Activated charcoal tablets have been used in ostomy pouches to reduce odour.— J. Karlstrand, *J. Am. pharm. Ass.*, 1977, *NS17*, 735.

Preparations

Universal Antidote. Activated charcoal 2, tannic acid 1, and magnesium oxide 1.

Proprietary Preparations

Carbellon *(Medo Chemicals, UK)*. Tablets each containing activated charcoal 100 mg, belladonna dry extract 6 mg, magnesium hydroxide 100 mg, and peppermint oil 0.003 ml. For indigestion, flatulence, and dyspepsia. *Dose.* 2 to 4 tablets thrice daily; children, 1 tablet.

Darco G-60 *(Atlas, UK)*. A brand of activated charcoal.

Haemocol *(Smith & Nephew Pharmaceuticals, UK)*. A single-use unit for haemoperfusion comprising a column containing activated charcoal granules 300 g, coated with an acrylic hydrogel. **Haemocol 100** contains 100 g of adsorbent.

Medicoal *(Leo, Swed.: Lundbeck, UK)*. Each sachet contains activated charcoal 5 g in an effervescent basis. For preparing a suspension in water for use in the treatment of poisoning.

Other Proprietary Names

Charcocaps, Charcotabs (both *USA*); Intosan *(Switz.)*; Kolsuspension *(Swed.)*; Kullsuspensjon *(Norw.)*; Medikol *(Swed.)*; Norit Medicinaal *(Neth.)*.

A preparation containing activated charcoal was also formerly marketed in Great Britain under the proprietary name Carbomucil (*Norgine*).

687-z

Animal Charcoal. Carbo Animalis; Purified Animal Charcoal.

Pharmacopoeias. In *Port.* and *Span.*

An odourless, tasteless black powder prepared by boiling crude animal charcoal with hydrochloric acid, washing thoroughly, drying, and reheating. Crude animal charcoal is the material prepared by heating bones with a limited access of air and consists chiefly of calcium phosphate and other inorganic constituents of bone and about one-tenth of its weight of carbon.

Uses. Animal charcoal has been used as a decolorising agent and adsorbent, but activated charcoal is usually preferred for these purposes.

688-c

Chlorbenzoxamine Hydrochloride. 1-[2-(2-Chlorobenzhydryloxy)ethyl]-4-(2-methylbenzyl)piperazine dihydrochloride dihydrate.
$C_{27}H_{31}ClN_2O,2HCl,2H_2O=544.0$.

CAS — 522-18-9 (chlorbenzoxamine); 5576-62-5 (hydrochloride, anhydrous).

Uses. Chlorbenzoxamine hydrochloride has been used in the treatment of gastric and duodenal ulcers in doses of up to 180 mg daily.

Proprietary Names

Antiulcera Master *(Coli, Ital.)*; Gastomax *(Brocchieri, Ital.)*; Libratar *(UCB, Arg.; UCB, Denm.; UCB, Ger.; UCB, Ital.; IBYS, Spain)*.

689-k

Dihydroxyaluminum Sodium Carbonate *(U.S.P.)*. Dihydroxaluminiumnatriumkarbonat; Aluminium Sodium Carbonate Hydroxide. Sodium (carbonato)dihydroxyaluminate(1-).
$CH_2AlNaO_5=144.0$.

CAS — 12011-77-7; 16482-55-6.

Pharmacopoeias. In *Nord.* and *U.S.*

A fine white odourless powder. It loses not more than 14.5% of its weight on drying. Practically **insoluble** in water and organic solvents; soluble in dilute mineral acids with the evolution of carbon dioxide. A 4% suspension in water has a pH of 9.9 to 10.2. **Store** in airtight containers.

Uses. Dihydroxyaluminum sodium carbonate is an antacid that has been used in doses of 300 to 600 mg for the relief of gastric hyperacidity.

Preparations

Dihydroxyaluminum Sodium Carbonate Tablets *(U.S.P.)*. Tablets containing dihydroxyaluminum sodium carbonate. Potency is expressed in terms of anhydrous material. The tablets should be chewed before swallowing.

Proprietary Names

Kompensan *(Pfizer, Ger.; Roerig, Switz.)*; Minicid *(Pharmacia, Norw.; Pharmacia, Swed.)*; Noacid *(Pharmacia, Denm.)*.

690-w

Gefarnate. Geranyl Farnesylacetate. A mixture of stereoisomers of 3,7-dimethylocta-2,6-dienyl 5,9,13-trimethyltetradeca-4,8,12-trienoate.
$C_{27}H_{44}O_2=400.6$.

CAS — 51-77-4.

A slightly yellowish liquid with a faint terpene-like odour. Practically **insoluble** in water, glycerol, and propylene glycol; soluble in alcohol, acetone, ether, and fixed oils.

Adverse Effects. Urticarial rashes may occur.

Uses. Gefarnate has been used in doses of 50 mg four times daily before meals in the treatment of gastric and duodenal ulcers; higher doses have been given. It has also been given by intramuscular injection.

In 11 patients with gastric ulcer given carbenoxolone 100 mg thrice daily for 4 weeks the mean reduction in ulcer size was 75.6% compared with 37% in 11 given gefarnate 50 mg four times daily (62% if one patient in whom the ulcer doubled in size was excluded). In 12 patients given gefarnate 100 mg four times daily the reduction in ulcer size was 69.3% compared with 80.8% in a second group of 11 given carbenoxolone. In 12 patients given gefarnate 200 mg four times daily the reduction in ulcer size was 47.6% compared with 85.3% in a third group of 11 given carbenoxolone. Overall the reductions in ulcer size for gefarnate and carbenoxolone were 51.7% and 80.6% respectively. Twelve patients taking carbenoxolone needed diuretics compared with only 2 of those taking gefarnate, which might have a limited place in the treatment of gastric ulcers in the elderly or in those prone to fluid retention.— M. J. S. Langman *et al.*, *Br. med. J.*, 1973, *3*, 84.

In a double-blind trial of gefarnate for the treatment of duodenal ulcer 56 patients were treated for a minimum of 6 months and 43 completed 1 year's continuous treatment. Gefarnate was given in doses of 50 mg thrice daily for 6 weeks followed by 50 mg twice daily or a placebo; 29 received gefarnate and 27 placebo. Gefarnate was shown to be slightly more effective in reducing symptoms.— C. R. Newman and D. A. Montgomery, *Br. J. clin. Pract.*, 1973, *27*, 85.

In a double-blind study 23 ambulant patients with chronic gastric ulcer who were treated with gefarnate 50 mg four times daily for 5 weeks obtained a mean percentage reduction in ulcer size of 70.4%, whereas 22 who received placebo had a mean reduction of only 27.8%.— P. B. Newcomb *et al.*, *Practitioner*, 1976, *217*, 435.

Follow-up studies in patients with chronic gastric ulcer given gefarnate 200 or 400 mg thrice daily for 1 year showed that 8 of 11 men were cured in a mean of 33 months compared with 3 of 11 given a placebo. Gefarnate was less effective than a placebo for the 10 women studied. No side-effects were reported.— S. C. Truelove and M. Rocca, *Curr. med. Res. Opinion*, 1976, *4*, 218.

After 4 weeks of treatment for gastric ulcer, 7 of 10 patients treated with cimetidine 1 g daily were healed compared with 1 of 9 treated with gefarnate 250 mg daily; after 6 weeks, 8 and 2 patients respectively were healed. Pain relief was greater and consumption of antacids lower in patients receiving cimetidine.— M. Cambielli *et al.*, *Acta ther.*, 1978, *4*, 207.

Proprietary Names

Andoin *(ICN, Spain)*; Alsanate, Arsanyl, Dixnalate, Gefalon, Gefarnate C, Gefulcer, Matorozin, Polyl, Salanil, Terpanil, Zackal, Zenowal (all *Jap.*); Farnesil *(AGIPS, Ital.)*; Farnisol *(FIRMA, Ital.)*; Gefarnil *(Labohain, Belg.; De Angeli, Ital.; De Angeli, S.Afr.; Almirall, Spain; de Angeli, Switz.)*; Gefarol *(Iti, Ital.)*; Nolesil *(Geyfarm, Ital.)*; Ulco *(Usafarma, Ital.)*; Ulcofarm *(Ausonia, Ital.)*; Ulcotrofina *(Ripari-Gero, Ital.)*; Vagogernil *(Benvegna, Ital.)*.

Gefarnate was formerly marketed in Great Britain under the proprietary name Gefarnil (*WB Pharmaceuticals*).

691-e

Hydrotalcite. Aluminium magnesium hydroxide carbonate hydrate.
$Mg_6Al_2(OH)_{16}CO_3,4H_2O=604.0$.

CAS — 12304-65-3.

A white, odourless, tasteless, crystalline powder. Practically **insoluble** in water. **Store** in airtight containers.

Adverse Effects and Precautions. Diarrhoea and vomiting have been reported. Hydrotalcite might affect the absorption of tetracyclines.

Uses. Hydrotalcite is used as an antacid and is claimed to maintain the pH between 3 and 5 for over 2 hours. It has been given in doses of 1 g between meals and at bedtime.

References: B. P. Collins *et al.*, *Clin. Trials J.*, 1973, *10*, 103; A. C. Playle *et al.*, *Pharm. Acta Helv.*, 1974, *49*, 298; *Drug & Ther. Bull.*, 1975, *13*, 71; D. Mendelsohn and L. Mendelsohn, *S. Afr. med. J.*, 1975, *49*, 1011; A. F. Llewellyn *et al.*, *Pharm. Acta Helv.*, 1977, *52*, 1; A. M. Hoare *et al.*, *Br. J. Surg.*, 1977, *64*, 849; K. J. Watters *et al.*, *Curr. med. Res. Opinion*, 1979, *6*, 85.

Proprietary Preparations

Altacite *(Roussel, UK)*. Hydrotalcite, available as **Suspension** containing 500 mg in each 5 ml and as **Tablets** of 500 mg. (Also available as Altacite in *Canad.*, *S.Afr.*). **Altacite Plus. Suspension** containing in each 5 ml hydrotalcite 500 mg and activated dimethicone 125 mg and **Tablets** each containing hydrotalcite 500 mg and activated dimethicone 250 mg. For hyperacidity and flatulence. *Dose.* 10 ml of suspension or 2 tablets, chewed or crushed, between meals and at bedtime.

Other Proprietary Names

Altacet *(Swed.)*; Hi-Ti, Nacid (both *Jap.*); Talcid *(Ger.)*; Ultacit *(Neth.)*.

692-l

Heavy Kaolin *(B.P., Eur. P.).* Kaolinum Ponderosum; China Clay; Argilla Alba; Bol Blanc; Bolus Alba; Weisser Ton; Arcilla Blanca; Caolin; Tierra Silicea Purificada; Caulim.

Pharmacopoeias. In *Arg., Aust., Belg., Br., Chin., Eur., Fr., Ger., Hung., Ind., It., Jap., Mex., Neth., Nord., Pol., Port., Rus., Span., Swiss,* and *U.S.*

A purified native hydrated aluminium silicate of variable composition. A fine white or greyish-white unctuous powder, odourless and almost tasteless; when mixed with hot water it has an odour of clay. Practically **insoluble** in water, organic solvents, mineral acids, and solutions of alkali hydroxides. **Sterilised** by maintaining the whole at a temperature not less than 160° for not less than 1 hour.

NOTE. The *B.P.* directs that when Kaolin or Light Kaolin is prescribed or demanded, Light Kaolin must be dispensed or supplied unless it has been ascertained that Light Kaolin (Natural) is required.

Adverse Effects.

Kaolinosis. A report of 24 patients with disease of the lung due to inhalation of kaolin dust. Twenty-two were men engaged in extraction of the material and 2 were women working with the pure substance in a chemical factory. X-ray examination in 4 showed very heavy lung markings, emphysema (often at the bases), and nodular pneumoconiosis.— A. Granata, *Folia med., Napoli,* 1957, *40,* 329, per *Abstr. Wld Med.,* 1957, *22,* 412.

Uses. Heavy kaolin is used in the preparation of kaolin poultice, which is applied with the intention of reducing inflammation and alleviating pain.

Preparations

Kaolin Poultice *(B.P.).* Cataplasma Kaolini *(F.N. Belg.).* Heavy kaolin 52.7%, boric acid 4.5%, with glycerol, methyl salicylate, peppermint oil, and thymol. Store in containers which minimise absorption, diffusion, or evaporation.

K/L One-minute Kaolin Poultice *(K/L Pharmaceutical, UK).* A brand of Kaolin Poultice *B.P.,* in single-use foiled pouches.

693-y

Light Kaolin *(B.P., B.P. Vet.).* Kaolinum Leve.

Pharmacopoeias. In *Br.* and *Ind.* But see under Heavy Kaolin as most pharmacopoeias do not differentiate between the light and heavy varieties.
Jap. P. also includes a natural and synthetic aluminium silicate.

A native hydrated aluminium silicate, freed from most of its impurities by elutriation, and dried. It contains a suitable dispersing agent. The particle size is controlled by limit tests. A light, white, odourless, almost tasteless powder free from gritty particles. When 2 g is triturated with 2 ml of water, the resulting mixture flows. At relative humidities between about 15 and 65%, the equilibrium moisture contents are about 1% at 25°, but small amounts of moisture are absorbed above about 75% relative humidity. Practically **insoluble** in water, mineral acids, and solutions of alkali hydroxides. **Sterilised** by maintaining the whole at a temperature not less than 160° for not less than 1 hour.

694-j

Light Kaolin (Natural) *(B.P.).*

Pharmacopoeias. In *Br. U.S.* includes Kaolin, a native hydrated aluminium silicate, powdered and freed from gritty particles by elutriation.

Light Kaolin (Natural) is Light Kaolin which does not contain a dispersing agent. When 2 g is triturated with 2 ml of water the resulting mixture does not flow.

NOTE. The *B.P.* directs that when Kaolin or Light Kaolin is prescribed or demanded, Light Kaolin must be dispensed or supplied unless it is ascertained that Light Kaolin (Natural) is required.

Adverse Effects and Precautions. The adsorbent properties of kaolin and other clays may influence the gastro-intestinal absorption of other drugs. The absorption of lincomycin has been reported to be significantly reduced by kaolin.

Under the conditions of the *B.P.C. 1963* adsorption tests for charcoal, light kaolin adsorbed no phenazone and only 5.4% of its weight of chloroform vapour, and was by comparison a poor adsorbent; activated attapulgite was appreciably more adsorbent.— S. C. Barker and W. J. Horgan (letter), *Pharm. J.,* 1967, *2,* 414.

A report of defibrination syndrome in a 34-year-old man who injected himself with 30 ml of a preparation containing kaolin (Donnagel).— S. B. Lanse and S. Farzan (letter), *Archs intern. Med.,* 1979, *139,* 251.

For a report of the adsorption of atropine by kaolin, see Atropine Sulphate, p.292.

For reference to decreased absorption of digoxin following concurrent administration of kaolin, see Digoxin, p.533.

Uses. Light kaolin is adsorbent, and when given by mouth adsorbs toxic and other substances from the alimentary tract and increases the bulk of the faeces. It is employed in the symptomatic treatment of gastro-intestinal conditions associated with diarrhoea. It is administered as a suspension in doses of 15 to 75 g.

Externally, it is used as a dusting-powder and as an ingredient of toilet-powders. Kaolin is liable to be heavily contaminated with bacteria, including *Bacillus anthracis, Clostridum tetani,* and *Cl. welchii.* When used in dusting-powders, it should be sterilised. Other uses of light kaolin are for clarification purposes and as the basis of disinfectant powders.

Light Kaolin (Natural) is used for the same purposes as light kaolin.

Gastro-enteritis. Kaolin has no part to play in the treatment of infantile gastro-enteritis.— M. D. Holdaway, *Drugs,* 1977, *14,* 383.

A study of 204 patients with acute non-specific diarrhoea indicated that treatment with kaolin and pectin, diphenoxylate and atropine, or activated charcoal was no more effective than a controlled diet in reducing the frequency or looseness of stools.— K. Alestig *et al., Practitioner,* 1979, *222,* 859.

Preparations

Dusting-powders

Kaolin Dusting-powder Compound *(A.P.F.).* Conspers. Kaolin. Co. Light kaolin 25, zinc oxide 25, and purified talc 50. Sterilise by heating at a temperature not lower than 160° in a closed container for not less than 2 hours.

Emulsions

Liquid Paraffin and Kaolin Emulsion *(B.P.C. 1949).* Emuls. Paraff. Liq. et Kaolin. Light kaolin 2.812 g, liquid paraffin 3.75 ml, acacia 514 mg, tragacanth 68.6 mg, benzoic acid 45 mg, chloroform water to 15 ml. *Dose.* 15 to 60 ml.

Mixtures

Kaolin and Morphine Mixture *(B.P.).* Mistura Kaolini et Morphinae; Mist. Kaolin. et Morph.; Mistura Kaolini Sedativa. Light kaolin or light kaolin (natural) 2 g, sodium bicarbonate 500 mg, chloroform and morphine tincture 0.4 ml, water to 10 ml. It contains 700 µg of anhydrous morphine in 10 ml. It should be recently prepared, unless the kaolin has been sterilised.
Dose. 10 ml.

Stability of morphine in Kaolin and Morphine Mixture (*B.P.*).— K. Helliwell and P. Game, *Pharm. J.,* 1981, *2,* 128.

Kaolin and Opium Mixture *(A.P.F.).* Mist. Kaolin. et Opii. Light kaolin or light kaolin (natural) 2.5 g, alum 10 mg, opium tincture 0.5 ml, concentrated chloroform water 0.25 ml, water to 10 ml. *Dose.* 10 to 20 ml.

Kaolin Mixture *(B.P.).* Mistura Kaolini Alkalina. Light kaolin or light kaolin (natural) 2 g, light magnesium carbonate and sodium bicarbonate, of each 500 mg, concentrated peppermint emulsion 0.25 ml, double-strength chloroform water 5 ml, water to 10 ml. It should be recently prepared, unless the kaolin has been sterilised.
Dose. 10 to 20 ml.

Paediatric Kaolin Mixture *(B.P.).* Kaolin Mixture Paediatric. Light kaolin or light kaolin (natural) 1 g, raspberry syrup 1 ml, benzoic acid solution 0.1 ml, amaranth solution 0.05 ml, double-strength chloroform water 2.5 ml, water to 5 ml. It should be recently prepared, unless the kaolin has been sterilised.
Dose. Children up to 1 year, 5 ml; 1 to 5 years, 10 ml.

A reminder that the essential consequence of acute diarrhoea is dehydration, and the fundamental treatment is rehydration.— W. A. M. Cutting and W. C. Marshall (letter), *Lancet,* 1979, *2,* 1022.

Powders

Compound Kaolin Powder *(B.P.C. 1963).* Pulv. Kaolin. Co. Light kaolin 3, heavy magnesium carbonate 2, and sodium bicarbonate 1. *Dose.* 2 to 8 g.
A.P.F. has light kaolin or light kaolin (natural) 55, heavy magnesium carbonate 30, sodium bicarbonate 15, and peppermint oil 0.2. *Dose.* 2 to 5 g.

Proprietary Preparations

Kaopectate *(Upjohn, UK).* A suspension containing kaolin 1.03 g in each 5 ml, with pectin (suggested diluent, water). For diarrhoea. *Dose.* 30 to 120 ml.

Kaylene *(Dendron, UK).* A brand of light kaolin. **Kaylene-Ol** is an emulsion containing light kaolin 7.5% with liquid paraffin 22.5% for use as an evacuant and adsorbent. *Dose.* 10 ml or more thrice daily before meals.

KLN Suspension *(Ashe, UK).* Contains in each 5 ml kaolin 1.15 g, pectin 57.5 mg, peppermint oil 1.15 mg, and sodium citrate 17.25 mg. For diarrhoea in children. *Dose.* 6 to 12 months, 5 ml; 1 to 3 years, 10 ml; 3 to 10 years, 20 ml.

A reminder that the essential consequence of acute diarrhoea is dehydration, and the fundamental treatment is rehydration.— W. A. M. Cutting and W. C. Marshall (letter), *lancet,* 1979, *2,* 1022.

695-z

Magaldrate *(U.S.P.).* Hydrated Magnesium Aluminate; Monalium Hydrate; AY 5710. Tetrakis(hydroxymagnesium)decahydroxydialuminate dihydrate. $Al_2H_{14}Mg_4O_{14},2H_2O=425.3$.

CAS — 1317-26-6.

Pharmacopoeias. In *Braz.* and *U.S.*

A white odourless crystalline powder containing the equivalent of 29 to 40% MgO and 18 to 26% Al_2O_3. It loses not more than 10% of its weight on drying. Practically **insoluble** in water and alcohol; soluble in dilute mineral acids.

Uses. Magaldrate is an antacid that has been used in doses of about 400 to 800 mg for the relief of gastric hyperacidity.

References: I. N. Marks, *S. Afr. med. J.,* 1979, *55,* 331.

Preparations

Magaldrate Oral Suspension *(U.S.P.).* A suspension containing magaldrate. Store in airtight containers.

Magaldrate Tablets *(U.S.P.).* Tablets containing magaldrate. The label states whether they are to be swallowed or chewed.

Proprietary Names

Riopan *(Ayerst, Canad.; Ayerst, Ital.; Ayerst, USA; Tosse, Ger.);* Riopone *(Ayerst, S.Afr.).*

696-c

Magnesium Carbonate *(U.S.P.).* Magnesium Subcarbonicum; Magnesium Carbonicum; Magnesium Carbonicum Hydroxydatum; Basisches Magnesiumcarbonat; Magnesia Alba.

CAS — 546-93-0 ($MgCO_3$); 23389-33-5 (normal, hydrate); 39409-82-0 (basic, hydrate).

Pharmacopoeias. In *Arg., Aust., Belg., Cz., Hung., It., Jug., Mex., Pol., Port., Roum., Rus., Span., Turk.,* and *U.S.*

The light or heavy variety of magnesium carbonate. A basic hydrated magnesium carbonate or a normal hydrated magnesium carbonate containing the equivalent of 40 to 43.5% MgO.

697-k

Heavy Magnesium Carbonate *(B.P., Eur. P.)*. Heavy Mag. Carb.; Magnesii Carbonas Ponderosus; Mag. Carb. Pond.; Magnesii Subcarbonas Ponderosus; Heavy Magnesium Subcarbonate.

Pharmacopoeias. In *Br., Braz., Chin., Eur., Fr., Ger., Ind., Jap., Neth., Nord.,* and *Swiss.* Most pharmacopoeias include a single monograph which permits both the heavy and light varieties—see Magnesium Carbonate (*U.S.P.*).

A hydrated basic magnesium carbonate of varying composition corresponding approximately to the formula $3MgCO_3,Mg(OH)_2,4H_2O$ and containing the equivalent of 40 to 45% MgO. A white odourless tasteless powder. 15 g occupies a volume of about 30 ml. Each g represents about 10.5 mmol (21 mEq) of magnesium. At relative humidities from about 15 to 65%, the equilibrium moisture contents at 25° are about 1%, but at relative humidities above about 75% the powder absorbs small amounts of moisture. Practically **insoluble** in water and in alcohol; soluble, with effervescence, in dilute acids. **Store** in airtight containers.

Uses. The uses and medicinal properties of heavy magnesium carbonate are the same as those of the light variety. Because of its smaller bulk it is usually administered, in association with other antacids, as powders or tablets.

Preparations

Compound Magnesium Carbonate Powder *(B.P.C. 1973).* Pulv. Mag. Carb. Co. Heavy magnesium carbonate 4, calcium carbonate 4, sodium bicarbonate 3, and light kaolin or light kaolin (natural) 1. *Dose.* 1 to 5 g.
See also Compound Calcium Carbonate Powder, p.77.

Compound Magnesium Carbonate Tablets *(B.P.C. 1973).* Each contains heavy magnesium carbonate 200 mg, calcium carbonate 200 mg, sodium bicarbonate 120 mg, light kaolin or light kaolin (natural) 60 mg, ginger 60 mg, and peppermint oil 0.006 ml. *Dose.* 1 or 2 tablets; they should be chewed before swallowing.

Magnesium and Calcium Carbonate Powder *(A.P.F.).* Pulv. Antacid. Heavy magnesium carbonate 25, calcium carbonate 25, magnesium trisilicate 50, peppermint oil 0.2. *Dose.* 2 to 5 g.

698-a

Light Magnesium Carbonate *(B.P., B.P. Vet., Eur. P.)*. Light Mag. Carb.; Magnesii Carbonas Levis; Mag. Carb. Lev.; Magnesii Subcarbonas Levis; Magnesium Carbonate; Magnesium Carbonicum Hydroxydatum; Magnesii Subcarbonas.

Pharmacopoeias. In *Br., Braz., Eur., Fr., Ger., Ind., Jap., Neth., Nord.,* and *Swiss.* Most pharmacopoeias include a single monograph which permits both the light and heavy varieties—see Magnesium Carbonate (*U.S.P.*)

A hydrated basic magnesium carbonate of varying composition corresponding approximately to the formula $3MgCO_3,Mg(OH)_2,3H_2O$ and containing the equivalent of 40 to 45% MgO. A very light, white, odourless, tasteless powder. 15 g occupies a volume of about 180 ml. Each g represents about 10.5 mmol (21 mEq) of magnesium. Practically **insoluble** in water and in alcohol; soluble, with effervescence, in dilute acids. **Store** in airtight containers.

Adverse Effects and Precautions. Magnesium carbonate in common with other magnesium salts can cause diarrhoea; mucosal irritation and absorption of magnesium may occur if there is gastro-intestinal atony or obstruction. The release of carbon dioxide in the stomach may cause discomfort. If renal function is impaired hypermagnesaemia may result producing the adverse effects described under Magnesium Salts, p.625.
Magnesium carbonate in common with other magnesium salts may interfere with the absorption of tetracyclines when these are taken concomitantly.

Treatment of Adverse Effects. The adverse effects of systemic magnesium poisoning are treated by the intravenous administration of calcium salts as described under Magnesium Salts, p.625.

Absorption and Fate. Magnesium carbonate is converted to magnesium chloride and carbon dioxide in the stomach. In the intestine, magnesium salts act as saline laxatives; they are more soluble at intestinal pH than calcium salts. Any absorbed magnesium is usually excreted rapidly in the urine.

Uses. Magnesium carbonate is a weak antacid and a mild laxative; the neutralising value of magnesium carbonate is about half that of magnesium oxide. It is given as an antacid in doses of 0.25 to 1 g, repeated in accordance with the patient's needs. Doses of 2 to 5 g are given as a laxative.
Antacids based on magnesium salts are frequently given in combination with aluminium-containing antacids to reduce the constipating effect of the latter compounds.
Light magnesium carbonate is the more suitable form for the preparation of mixtures, and the heavy carbonate for powders and tablets.
Light magnesium carbonate is used for dispersing volatile oils in inhalations having an aqueous vehicle.

Ulcer, gastric and duodenal. For reports and studies on the role of antacid therapy in gastric and duodenal ulcer, see p.71.

Preparations

Aromatic Magnesium Carbonate Mixture *(B.P.).* Magnesium Carbonate Aromatic Mixture; Mistura Carminativa; Mist. Carminat. Light magnesium carbonate 300 mg, sodium bicarbonate 500 mg, aromatic cardamom tincture 0.3 ml, double-strength chloroform water 5 ml, water to 10 ml. It should be recently prepared.
Dose. 10 to 20 ml.

Magnesium Carbonate Mixture *(B.P.C. 1973).* Light magnesium carbonate 500 mg, sodium bicarbonate 800 mg, concentrated peppermint emulsion 0.25 ml, double-strength chloroform water 5 ml, water to 10 ml. It should be recently prepared. *Dose.* 10 to 20 ml.

Proprietary Preparations

APP Stomach Powder *(Consolidated Chemicals, UK).* Contains magnesium carbonate 37%, magnesium trisilicate 19.98%, dried aluminium hydroxide 3%, bismuth carbonate 2%, calcium carbonate 37.82%, papaverine hydrochloride 0.1%, and homatropine methobromide 0.1%. **APP Stomach Tablets.** Each contains magnesium carbonate 180 mg, magnesium trisilicate 107.5 mg, dried aluminium hydroxide 15 mg, bismuth carbonate 12.5 mg, calcium carbonate 180.5 mg, papaverine hydrochloride 3 mg, and homatropine methobromide 1.5 mg. For peptic ulcer and other conditions associated with hypersecretion and spasm. *Dose.* 1 teaspoonful of powder or 1 or 2 tablets 4 times daily with milk.

Actonorm Powder *(Wallace Mfg Chem., UK: Farillon, UK).* Contains magnesium carbonate 30%, dried aluminium hydroxide 5%, atropine sulphate 0.01%, calcium carbonate 14.5%, diastase 1%, kaolin 5%, magnesium trisilicate 5%, pancreatin 1%, papaverine hydrochloride 0.04%, peppermint oil 0.05%, sodium bicarbonate 37.3%, and thiamine hydrochloride 0.1%. **Actonorm Tablets.** Each contains magnesium carbonate 225 mg, dried aluminium hydroxide 25 mg, atropine sulphate 50 µg, calcium carbonate 109 mg, diastase 5 mg, kaolin 75 mg, magnesium trisilicate 50 mg, pancreatin 5 mg, papaverine hydrochloride 200 µg, peppermint oil 250 µg, and thiamine hydrochloride 500 µg. For hyperacidity and gastric disorders. *Dose.* 1 level teaspoonful of powder, in water or milk, or 1 or 2 tablets, thrice daily and on retiring.

Other Proprietary Names

Palmicol *(Ger.).*

699-t

Magnesium Hydroxide *(B.P., U.S.P.)*. Mag. Hydrox.; Magnesii Hydroxydum; Magnesium Hydrate.

$Mg(OH)_2=58.32$.

CAS — 1309-42-8.

Pharmacopoeias. In *Arg., Br., Span.,* and *U.S.*

A white, amorphous, odourless or almost odourless, tasteless powder. It slowly absorbs carbon dioxide on exposure to air. Each g represents about 17 mmol (34 mEq) of magnesium. Practically **insoluble** in water, alcohol, chloroform, and ether; soluble in dilute acids. **Store** in airtight containers.

Adverse Effects and Precautions. As for Magnesium Carbonate (above), but without the side-effects associated with carbon dioxide release.

For a report of magnesium hydroxide increasing plasma-dicoumarol concentrations, see Dicoumarol, p.771.

For the effect of magnesium hydroxide on cimetidine, see Cimetidine, p.1303.

For reference to decreased absorption of digoxin following concurrent administration of magnesium hydroxide, see Digoxin, p.533.

Uses. Magnesium hydroxide is used as an antacid in doses of 500 to 750 mg; owing to the formation of magnesium chloride in the stomach, it also acts as a mild saline laxative for which it is given in doses of 2 to 4 g.

In a small controlled study it was found that when magnesium hydroxide, in a dose equivalent to 1 g of elemental magnesium, was given to patients with an adequate dietary intake of calcium, sustained increases occurred in the concentrations of calcium and magnesium in serum and urine. Faecal losses of both elements were reduced. It appeared that intestinal absorption of both calcium and magnesium was enhanced and the amounts retained in the body were increased. Excretion of phosphate in urine was decreased and a reduction of absorption of dietary phosphate occurred.— A. M. Briscoe and C. Ragan, *Am. J. clin. Nutr.*, 1966, *19*, 296.

Nine patients with primary hyperoxaluria were treated with Magnesium Hydroxide Mixture and/or phosphate in an attempt to increase urine solubility of oxalate. Both patients treated with phosphate appeared to benefit. Of 8 treated with magnesium hydroxide 2 had improved, 3 ceased to deteriorate, and 3 showed only minor evidence of increased calcification.— C. E. Dent and T. C. B. Stamp, *Archs Dis. Childh.*, 1970, *45*, 735.

For a report of the reversal of metabolic acidosis by magnesium hydroxide in conjunction with sodium polystyrene sulphonate, see Sodium Polystyrene Sulphonate, p.870.

For reports and studies on the role of antacid therapy, including magnesium hydroxide, in gastric and duodenal ulcers, see p.71.

For a report of the ineffectiveness of magnesium hydroxide in preventing gastro-intestinal haemorrhage in patients with gastric erosions associated with fulminant hepatic failure, see Cimetidine, p.1304.

Preparations

Lotions

Magnesium Hydroxide and Phenol Lotion *(St. Mark's Hosp.).* Phenol 3.571 g, zinc oxide 7.142 g, calamine 3.571 g, glycerol 7.142 ml, rose water 12.5 ml, magnesium hydroxide mixture to 100 ml.

Mixtures and Suspensions

Magnesia and Alumina Oral Suspension *(U.S.P.).* A mixture containing 2.9 to 4.2% w/w of magnesium hydroxide $Mg(OH)_2$, the equivalent of 2 to 2.4% w/w of aluminium oxide (Al_2O_3) as aluminium hydroxide and hydrated aluminium oxide, and 4.9 to 6.6% w/w of combined magnesium hydroxide and aluminium oxide; it may contain flavouring agents and suitable antimicrobial agents. pH 7.3 to 8.5.
See also Alumina and Magnesia Oral Suspension, p.73.

Magnesium Hydroxide Mixture *(B.P.).* Mag. Hydrox. Mixt.; Cream of Magnesia. An aqueous suspension of hydrated magnesium oxide containing the equivalent of 7.45 to 8.35% w/w of $Mg(OH)_2$; the equivalent of about 550 mg of MgO in 10 ml. It should not be stored in a cold place.
Dose. 5 to 10 ml, repeated in accordance with the patient's needs as an antacid; 25 to 50 ml as a laxative.

A similar preparation is included in several pharmacopoeias.

Milk of Magnesia *(U.S.P.)*. A suspension containing magnesium hydroxide 7 to 8.5% w/w; it may contain 0.1% of citric acid and up to 0.05% of one or more essential oils for flavouring. Store at a temperature not exceeding 35° in airtight containers; avoid freezing.

NOTE. In Great Britain the name Milk of Magnesia is a trade-mark (see p.1782).

In some other countries Phillips' Milk of Magnesia is a trade-mark.

Tablets

Magnesia and Alumina Tablets *(U.S.P.)*. Tablets containing magnesium hydroxide and aluminium hydroxide.

See also Alumina and Magnesia Tablets, p.73.

Magnesia Tablets *(U.S.P.)*. Tablets containing magnesium hydroxide.

Proprietary Preparations

Aquamag *(Chemical & Insulating Co., UK)*. A paste containing approximately 28% w/w of magnesium hydroxide in aqueous suspension which can be readily diluted to an 8% w/v suspension.

Other Proprietary Names

Chlorumagène *(Fr., Switz.)*.

700-t

Magnesium Oxide *(U.S.P.)*. Mag. Oxid.; Magnesia Usta; Magnesium Oxydatum; Magnesia Calcinada; Gebrannte Magnesia.

$MgO = 40.30$.

CAS — 1309-48-4.

Pharmacopoeias. In *Aust., Belg., Cz., It., Jug., Mex., Pol., Port., Roum., Rus., Span., Turk.*, and *U.S.*

A very bulky white powder known as light magnesium oxide (5 g occupies about 40 to 50 ml) or a relatively dense white powder known as heavy magnesium oxide (5 g occupies about 10 to 20 ml). **Store** in airtight containers.

701-x

Heavy Magnesium Oxide *(B.P.)*. Heavy Mag. Oxide; Magnesii Oxidum Ponderosum; Mag. Oxid. Pond.; Heavy Magnesia; Magnesia Ponderosa.

$MgO = 40.30$.

Pharmacopoeias. In *Arg., Br., Chin., Ind., Jap., Neth., Nord.*, and *Swiss*. Many pharmacopoeias include a single monograph which permits both the heavy and light varieties—see Magnesium Oxide (above).

A fine white odourless powder with a slightly alkaline taste. 15 g occupies a volume of about 30 ml. Each g represents 24.8 mmol (49.6 mEq) of magnesium. Practically **insoluble** in water and alcohol; soluble in dilute acids. On exposure to air it absorbs moisture and carbon dioxide; it does not form a gelatinous mass when allowed to stand in contact with water (see Light Magnesium Oxide). **Store** in airtight containers.

Uses. The properties of heavy magnesium oxide are the same as those of the light variety but because of its smaller bulk it is more convenient for use in powders and tablets.

702-r

Light Magnesium Oxide *(B.P., Eur. P.)*. Light Mag. Ox.; Magnesii Oxidum Leve; Mag. Oxid. Lev.; Light Magnesia; Magnesia Levis; Magnésie Calcinée.

$MgO = 40.30$.

Pharmacopoeias. In *Arg., Br., Eur., Fr., Ger., Hung., Ind., It., Jap., Neth., Nord.*, and *Swiss*. Many pharmacopoeias include a single monograph which permits both the light and heavy varieties—see Magnesium Oxide (above).

A very light, fine, white, odourless, amorphous powder with a slightly alkaline taste. 20 g occupies a volume of not less than 150 ml. Each g represents 24.8 mmol (49.6 mEq) of magnesium. Practically **insoluble** in water and in alcohol; soluble in dilute acids with slight effervescence. On exposure to air it rapidly absorbs moisture and carbon dioxide. It forms a gelatinous mass on standing for about 30 minutes with 15 times its weight of water. **Store** in airtight containers.

Adverse Effects and Precautions. As for Light Magnesium Carbonate, p.82.

Uses. Light magnesium oxide is a potent antacid and a mild laxative. Its neutralising value is more than twice that of magnesium carbonate and about 4 times that of sodium bicarbonate. The usual dose as an antacid is 250 to 500 mg, repeated in accordance with the needs of the patient. The usual laxative dose is 2 to 5 g.

When prescribed in mixtures, light magnesium oxide should be used but for powders heavy magnesium oxide is preferable.

Light magnesium oxide is also used in dentifrices.

Renal calculus. Of 36 patients with histories of recurring calcium oxalate renal stone formation given magnesium oxide 200 mg and pyridoxine 10 mg daily for 5 years or more, 30 had shown no or decreased recurrence of stone formation. After 1 year on this regimen, a marked increase in their capacity to maintain calcium oxalate in solution in the urine was observed in 45 of 51 patients.— S. N. Gershoff and E. L. Prien, *Am. J. clin. Nutr.*, 1967, *20*, 393.

Ulcer, gastric and duodenal. For reports and studies on the role of antacid therapy in gastric and duodenal ulcer, see p.71.

Proprietary Names

Oxabid *(Pharmacare, USA)*.

703-f

Magnesium Phosphate *(U.S.P., B.P.C. 1949)*. Mag. Phosph.; Tribasic Magnesium Phosphate; Trimagnesium Phosphate.

$Mg_3(PO_4)_2,5H_2O = 352.9$.

CAS — 7757-87-1 (anhydrous); 10233-87-1 (pentahydrate).

Pharmacopoeias. In *U.S.*

A white odourless tasteless powder. Practically **insoluble** in water; readily soluble in dilute mineral acids.

Uses. Magnesium phosphate is an antacid and mild laxative that has been used in doses of 1 to 4 g; it resembles magnesium trisilicate in action.

704-d

Magnesium Trisilicate *(B.P., Eur. P., U.S.P.)*. Mag. Trisil.; Magnesii Trisilicas; Magnesium Trisilicate Powder; Magnesium Trisilicate Oral Powder; Magnesium Silicate.

CAS — 14987-04-3 (anhydrous); 39365-87-2 (hydrate).

Pharmacopoeias. In *Arg., Aust., Br., Braz., Chin., Eur., Fr., Ger., Hung., Ind., Jap., Jug., Mex., Neth., Nord., Rus., Span., Swiss, Turk.*, and *U.S.*

A hydrated magnesium silicate corresponding approximately to the formula $2MgO,3SiO_2$, with water of crystallisation. An odourless, tasteless, slightly hygroscopic, white powder free from gritty particles. The *B.P.* specifies that it loses 20 to 30% of its weight on ignition and contains not less than 29% MgO and not less than the equivalent of 65% of SiO_2 after ignition. The *U.S.P.* specifies that it contains not less than 20% of MgO and not less than 45% of SiO_2. At relative humidities between about 15 and 65%, the equilibrium moisture content at 25° is about 17 to 23%, and about 24 and 30% at relative humidities from about 75 to 95%.

Practically **insoluble** in water and alcohol. It reacts slowly with dilute mineral acids with the formation of the magnesium salt of the acid and the separation of colloidal silica. **Store** in airtight containers.

With tap water as the vehicle, bacterial contamination of magnesium trisilicate mixtures remained within acceptable limits over a 28-day period provided that clean working conditions had been observed during manufacture. Mixtures needing a longer shelf-life than 28 days required a preservative: inclusion of methyl and propyl hydroxybenzoates gave better protection than benzoic acid or chloroform.— D. Fearnley and K. A. Ellwal, *J. Hosp. Pharm.*, 1972, *30*, 263.

A study on the effect of storage time and excipients on the acid-neutralising capacity of magnesium trisilicate.— S. A. H. Khalil and S. S. El-Gamal, *Mfg Chem.*, 1978, *49* (Mar.), 71.

Loss of chloroform from Magnesium Trisilicate Mixture *B.P.* under simulated conditions of use.— R. Purkiss, *J. clin. Pharm.*, 1978, *2*, 163.

Chloroform at concentrations greater than 125 µg per ml was effective in preserving magnesium trisilicate mixture against the growth of micro-organisms, present initially at low contamination levels, for 13 to 27 months. High levels of contamination developed in unpreserved mixture after only 1 month's storage but contamination was low in refrigerated samples.— D. W. Carrington and C. S. Terry, *Pharm. J.*, 1980, *1*, 566.

Adverse Effects and Precautions. As for Light Magnesium Carbonate, p.82. Development of a siliceous calculus has followed the prolonged use of magnesium trisilicate.

Interactions. Dimethicone did not affect the *in vitro* absorption of digoxin but magnesium trisilicate reduced absorption by 99.5%.— J. C. McElnay *et al.* (letter,), *Br. med. J.*, 1978, *1*, 1554. See also under Digoxin, p.533.

For the effect of antacids on corticosteroid bioavailability, see Corticosteroids, p.450.

Renal calculus. A 68-year-old man with a history of renal calculus passed a 300-mg stone which was found to consist chiefly of silicon dioxide. He had been taking the equivalent of 2 g of magnesium trisilicate daily for many years.— A. M. Joekes *et al.*, *Br. med. J.*, 1973, *1*, 146.

Absorption and Fate. Magnesium chloride and hydrated silica gel are formed during neutralisation. About 5% of the magnesium is absorbed and traces of the liberated silica may be absorbed and excreted in the urine.

Uses. Magnesium trisilicate is antacid and adsorbent. The antacid action is exerted slowly, so that it does not give such rapid symptomatic relief as the alkali carbonates, bicarbonates, and oxides. However, the action is prolonged and the compound is of value in the management of gastric and duodenal ulcer. The usual dose is 0.5 to 2 g repeated in accordance with the patient's needs.

It does not generally give rise to alkalosis. The hydrated silica gel formed in the presence of gastric acid also possesses adsorbent properties, though inferior in this respect to the original compound.

A dose of 1.6 g of magnesium trisilicate given to patients with gastric ulcer 30 minutes after a test meal had no significant effect on gastric pH or peptic activity.— S. G. F. Matts *et al.*, *Br. med. J.*, 1965, *1*, 753.

Ulcer, gastric and duodenal. For reports and studies on the role of antacid therapy in gastric and duodenal ulcer, see p.71.

Use in surgery. Antacids were recommended before surgery especially in obstetrics to raise the pH of any stomach contents. Aspiration would not be prevented but the dangers might be reduced by the aspirate being of reduced acidity and the acid-aspiration syndrome might be prevented. In obstetrics a dose of 15 ml of Magnesium Trisilicate Mixture was recommended by J.S. Crawford (*Practitioner*, 1974, *212*, 677; see also J.D. Holdsworth *et al.* (letter), *Br. J. Anaesth.*, 1977, *49*, 520); this should be given every 2 hours from the time of admission until completion of the third stage of labour. Associated with this is the application of cricoid pressure before induction. There have been several reports of the acid-aspiration syndrome occurring in patients given antacids (G. Taylor, *Br. J. Anaesth.*, 1975, *47*, 615; G.A.H. Heaney and H.D. Jones (letter), *ibid.*, 1979, *51*, 266; R.M. Whittington *et al.*, *Lancet*,

1979, *2*, 228). Although some of the patients had not been treated according to the above recommendations there was a plea that the technique should be reappraised (R.M. Whittington *et al.* (letter), *Lancet*, 1979, *2*, 630). There was also evidence in *dogs* that aspiration of the antacid might not be without its own dangers (C.P. Gibbs *et al.*, *Anesthesiology*, 1979, *51*, 380).

Preparations

Granules

Granulatum Magnesii Silicatis *(Nord. P.)*. Granules containing 60% of magnesium trisilicate in a chocolate basis.

Mixtures

Magnesium Trisilicate and Belladonna Mixture *(B.P.C. 1973)*. Belladonna tincture 0.5 ml, magnesium trisilicate mixture to 10 ml. It must be freshly prepared. *Dose*. 10 to 20 ml.

Atropine and hyoscine were adsorbed on to magnesium trisilicate in the *B.P.C. 1973* mixture and were only eluted by gastric acid below pH 2, a condition unlikely to be fulfilled after taking the mixture.— S. El-Masry and S. A. H. Khalil, *J. Pharm. Pharmac.*, 1974, *26*, 243. At room temperature the time for 10% decomposition of hyoscyamine was 21.2 days.— S. A. H. Khalil and S. El-Masry, *J. Pharm. Pharmac.*, 1978, *30*, 664.

Magnesium Trisilicate Mixture *(A.P.F.)*. Magnesium trisilicate 1 g, calcium carbonate 500 mg, light magnesium carbonate 500 mg, concentrated peppermint water 0.25 ml, concentrated chloroform water 0.25 ml, water to 10 ml. *Dose*. 10 to 20 ml.

Magnesium Trisilicate Mixture *(B.P.)*. Mist. Mag. Trisil.; Compound Magnesium Trisilicate Mixture; Mist. Mag. Trisil. Co. Magnesium trisilicate, light magnesium carbonate, and sodium bicarbonate, of each 500 mg, concentrated peppermint emulsion 0.25 ml, double-strength chloroform water 5 ml, water to 10 ml. It should be recently prepared.
Dose. 10 to 20 ml.

Powders

Compound Magnesium Trisilicate Oral Powder *(B.P.)*. Compound Magnesium Trisilicate Powder; Magnesium Trisilicate Compound Powder. Equal parts of magnesium trisilicate, heavy magnesium carbonate, chalk, and sodium bicarbonate.
Dose. 1 to 5 g.

Magnesium Trisilicate and Belladonna Powder *(A.P.F.)*. Pulv. Mag. Trisil. et Bellad. Magnesium trisilicate 99.2 g and belladonna dry extract 800 mg. *Dose*. 2 to 4 g.

Tablets

Compound Magnesium Trisilicate Tablets *(B.P.)*. Magnesium Trisilicate Compound Tablets; Aluminium Hydroxide and Magnesium Trisilicate Tablets. Each contains magnesium trisilicate 250 mg, dried aluminium hydroxide 120 mg, and peppermint oil 0.003 ml. They should be chewed then swallowed.
Dose. 1 or 2 tablets.

Tablettae Magnibellini *(Dan. Disp.)*. Tablets each containing magnesium trisilicate 500 mg and belladonna extract (*Nord. P.*, containing 1.4% alkaloids) 1.5 mg.

Proprietary Preparations

Alka-Donna *(Carlton Laboratories, UK)*. Tablets each containing magnesium trisilicate 500 mg, dried aluminium hydroxide 250 mg, and belladonna dry extract 8 mg. **Alka-Donna P.** Tablets containing, in addition, phenobarbitone 8 mg. **Alka-Donna Suspension.** Contains in each 5 ml magnesium trisilicate 342.5 mg, aluminium hydroxide mixture 2.15 ml, and belladonna tincture 0.2 ml. For gastric disorders and peptic ulcer. **Alka-Donna P Suspension.** Contains, in addition, phenobarbitone 8 mg in each 5 ml. *Dose*. 1 or 2 tablets, sucked slowly, or 5 to 10 ml of suspension thrice daily.

Magsorbent *(Dendron, UK)*. A brand of magnesium trisilicate powder.

Nulacin *(Bencard, UK)*. Tablets prepared from whole milk combined with dextrins and maltose, together with magnesium trisilicate 230 mg, magnesium oxide 130 mg, calcium carbonate 130 mg, magnesium carbonate 30 mg, and peppermint oil. For peptic ulceration and hyperacidity. *Dose*. 1 or more tablets to be sucked or chewed as required.

A report of dental decay in 2 caries-free patients associated with their use of Nulacin tablets taken freely as required.— M. R. Y. Dyer (letter), *Br. dent.J.*, 1978, *144*, 100.

Some other proprietary preparations containing magnesium trisilicate are described under Dried Aluminium Hydroxide, p.73..

Other Proprietary Names

Gastrobin *(Ger.)*; Magnesiumsilikat *(Denm.)*; rolo *(Ger.)*; Silimag *(Spain)*; Trisil *(Austral.)*.

Magnesium trisilicate was also formerly marketed in Great Britain under the proprietary name Trisillac (*Philip Harris*).

705-n

Proglumide.

Xylamide; CR 242; W 5219. (±)-4-Benzamido-*NN*-dipropylglutaramic acid.
$C_{18}H_{26}N_2O_4$=334.4.

CAS — 6620-60-6.

Uses. Proglumide has an inhibitory effect on gastric secretion. Proglumide is reported to be a gastrin-receptor antagonist. It is used in the treatment of gastric or duodenal ulcer and gastritis in doses of 0.8 to 1.2 g of proglumide daily before meals; it is also given by intramuscular or by slow intravenous injection.

Studies of the absorption and excretion of proglumide after oral, intramuscular, and intravenous administration to *rats* and man.— A. L. Rovati and G. Picciola, *Boll. chim.-farm.*, 1971, *110*, 595.

A double-blind trial in 30 patients with gastric or duodenal ulcers; proglumide 1.2 g daily and cimetidine 1.2 g daily for 28 successive days were considered to be equally effective in reducing clinical symptoms and gastric secretion. But cimetidine alone was reported to be associated with marked hypertrophy and hyperplasia of the antral mucosa. Both drugs caused slight increases in plasma-creatinine concentrations.— M. Galeone *et al.*, *Curr. med. Res. Opinion*, 1978, *5*, 376.

In a double-blind trial for up to 28 days completed by 32 of 33 patients with rheumatological disease, the addition of proglumide 150 mg to each 25-mg dose of indomethacin did not significantly affect the therapeutic effectiveness of indomethacin, but greatly increased its gastric tolerability; of 16 patients receiving indomethacin with a placebo, 14 suffered some gastric upset after the third day of treatment and this upset increased on subsequent days. Patients receiving proglumide had decreased urinary pepsinogen and no gastric upsets.— V. Pipitone, *Curr. med. Res. Opinion*, 1976, *4*, 267.

In 16 patients with gastric ulcer undergoing a 4-week double-blind study, ulcers disappeared, as assessed by endoscopy, in 6 of 8 receiving proglumide 1.2 g daily and in 2 of 8 receiving magnesium trisilicate 1.32 g daily. No significant difference between the effect of proglumide and magnesium trisilicate was observed in 35 patients with duodenal ulcer. Proglumide had no effect on serum-gastrin concentration or on basal or maximally stimulated acid secretion.— S. E. Miederer *et al.*, *Dt. med. Wschr.*, 1979, *104*, 313.

Proglumide and other Gastrin-receptor Antagonists, J. Weiss and S.E. Miederer (Ed.), Oxford, Excerpta Medica, 1979.

Proprietary Names

Gastridine *(Bernabó, Arg.)*; Gastrotopic *(Perga, Spain)*; Milid *(Opfermann, Ger.*; *Rotta, Ital.*; *Ethimed, S.Afr.*; *Max Ritter, Switz.)*; Milide *(Fournier Frères, Fr.*; *Farma-Lepori, Spain)*; Promid *(Jap.)*; Snol *(Inexfa, Spain)*; Triulco *(Santos, Spain)*; Xyla-Ulco *(Miluy, Spain)*.

706-h

Sodium Amylosulphate.

Sodium Amylopectin Sulphate; SN 263. The sodium salt of the sulphated form of amylopectin derived from potatoes, *Solanum tuberosum* (Solanaceae).

CAS — 9010-01-9.

Uses. Sodium amylosulphate inhibits the activity of pepsin and has been used for the treatment of gastric and duodenal ulcer.

In a double-blind study in 75 patients with duodenal ulcer, recurrences were 75, 39, 16, and 13% respectively in those given placebo, propantheline, sodium amylosulphate, and propantheline with sodium amylosulphate.— D. C. H. Sun and M. L. Ryan, *Gastroenterology*, 1970, *58*, 756. See also D. S. Zimmon *et al.*, *ibid.*, 1969, *56*, 19.

In a double-blind study in 65 male patients, treatment for 48 weeks with sodium amylosulphate 500 mg 6 times daily with concomitant propantheline therapy was no more effective than sodium amylosulphate or propantheline alone or placebo in controlling the symptoms of duodenal ulceration. Radiological assessment of ulcer healing also failed to show any superiority.— J. B. Cocking, *Gastroenterology*, 1972, *62*, 6.

In a double-blind study sodium amylosulphate was shown to be no better than placebo treatment for duodenal ulcer.— J. H. Baron *et al.*, *Gut*, 1977, *18*, 723.

Brief discussions: D. W. Piper and T. R. Heap, *Drugs*, 1972, *3*, 366; D. W. Piper *et al.*, *ibid.*, 1975, *10*, 56. See also M. J. S. Langman, *Br. med. J.*, 1969, *4*, 100.

Proprietary Names

Depepsen *(Searle, UK)*.

707-m

Sucralfate.

Sucrose hydrogen sulphate basic aluminium salt; Sucrose octakis(hydrogen sulphate) aluminium complex.

CAS — 54182-58-0.

A white powder. Practically **insoluble** in water and most organic solvents; soluble in acids and alkalis.

Adverse Effects. Constipation is the most frequently reported adverse effect though other gastro-intestinal effects may occur.

Uses. Sucralfate is used in the treatment of gastric and duodenal ulcers. The recommended dose is 1 g four times daily.

A review of the use of sucralfate in the treatment of peptic ulcers.— I. N. Marks, *Drugs*, 1980, *20*, 283. See also I. N. Marks *et al.* (letter), *Br. med. J.*, 1980, *281*, 1281; J. Rhodes (letter), *ibid.*; *Proceedings of the Sucralfate Symposium, Hamburg 1980*, Munich, Urban & Schwarzenberg, 1980.

In a double-blind study in 28 patients with gastric ulcer, treatment with sucralfate 1.5 g thrice daily for 4 weeks was considered better than a placebo but the results did not confirm its value in healing gastric ulcer. During the study there was no significant difference in incidence of pain, vomiting, or antacid consumption between the 2 groups.— J. F. Mayberry *et al.*, *Br. J. clin. Pract.*, 1978, *32*, 291.

Studies in *rats* indicated that, apart from its antipeptic effect, sucralfate formed an adherent and protective chemical complex with proteins at the site of ulceration. This layer limited the back diffusion of hydrogen ions.— R. Nagashima and T. Hirano, *Arzneimittel-Forsch.*, 1980, *30*, 80. See also R. Nagashima *et al.*, *ibid.*, 84 and 88.

In an 18-month controlled study, the rate of ulcer recurrence in 167 patients with previously healed gastric ulcers was reduced in those who received 6 months of treatment with sucralfate and an antacid compared with those who only received the antacid.— T. Miyake *et al.*, *Dig. Dis. Scis*, 1980, *25*, 1.

In a controlled study 112 patients with duodenal or gastric ulcers were treated with cimetidine 1 g or sucralfate 4 g daily in divided doses. In the group with duodenal ulcers 24 of 29 patients receiving sucralfate had healed after 6 weeks of therapy compared with 20 of 28 who received cimetidine; after 12 weeks, 29 and 24 patients respectively healed. In patients with gastric ulcers 17 of 27 receiving sucralfate had healed after 6 weeks compared with 21 of 28 receiving cimetidine and after 12 weeks healing had occurred in 20 and 25 patients respectively.— I. N. Marks *et al.*, *S. Afr. med. J.*, 1980, *57*, 567.

After 6 weeks of treatment, 24 of 30 patients receiving sucralfate, 1 g four times daily, showed evidence of healing of duodenal ulcers (18 complete, 6 partial) compared with 15 of 29 who received placebo (7 complete, 8 partial). After 12 weeks there was evidence of healing in 25 (23 complete, 2 partial) and 16 (12 complete, 4 partial) respectively. However, there was no significant difference between the groups when compared for healing of small ulcers.— M. G. Moshal *et al.*, *S. Afr. med. J.*, 1980, *57*, 742.

Proprietary Preparations

Antepsin *(Ayerst, UK)*. Sucralfate, available as scored tablets of 1 g. (Also available as Antepsin in *Arg.*, *Ital.*).

Other Proprietary Names

Sulcrate *(Canad.)*; Ulcerban *(USA)*; Ulcerlmin *(Jap.)*; Ulsanic *(S.Afr.)*.

708-b

Sucralox. Manalox AS. A polymerised complex of sucrose and aluminium hydroxide.

CAS — 12040-73-2.

A white to cream-coloured powder, containing about 49% of Al_2O_3 and 29% of sucrose.

Uses. Sucralox is an antacid used in doses of 0.5 to 1 g for the treatment of gastric hyperacidity and associated conditions.

A preparation containing sucralox was formerly marketed in Great Britain under the proprietary name Alusac (*Calmic*).

709-v

Urogastrone. An inhibitory factor of gastric secretion derived from human urine.

CAS — 9010-53-1.

Uses. Urogastrone may be of use in the treatment of duodenal and gastric ulcer and related disorders.

The 2 closely related water-soluble polypeptides β- and γ-urogastrone, isolated from male and female urine, were found to consist of 52 amino-acid residues in the same sequence, with β-urogastrone possessing an additional terminal arginine residue. Human epidermal growth factor, recently isolated from the urine of pregnant women, was considered to be synonymous with β-urogastrone.— H. Gregory (letter), *Nature*, 1975, *257*, 325.

In 12 healthy subjects the infusion of highly purified urogastrone inhibited gastric acid and intrinsic factor secretion but had a less marked effect on the gastric output of pepsin. Plasma-gastrin concentrations were not significantly affected. A dose of 250 ng per kg over 1 hour appeared to be optimal for further evaluation. Two subjects receiving 500 ng per kg experienced severe headache.— J. B. Elder *et al.*, *Gut*, 1975, *16*, 887.

In 4 patients with the Zollinger-Ellison syndrome the administration of urogastrone 250 ng per kg body-weight over 1 hour reduced gastric acid output by 50 to 82%; the concentration of intrinsic factor and pepsin in gastric juice rose by 60 to 300%, and the peak plasma-gastrin concentration by 127 to 164%. Ulcer pain was relieved 30 to 60 minutes after the start of the infusion.— J. B. Elder *et al.*, *Lancet*, 1975, *2*, 424.

Urogastrone-like immunoreactivity has been localised to cells of the duodenal and submandibular glands.— P. U. Heitz *et al.*, *Gut*, 1978, *19*, 408.

Proprietary Names
Supergastrone (*STIP, Ital.*).

710-r

Zolimidine. 2-(4-Methylsulphonylphenyl)imidazo-[1,2-*a*]pyridine.
$C_{14}H_{12}N_2O_2S$=272.3.

CAS — 1222-57-7.

Uses. Zolimidine is used in the treatment of gastric and duodenal ulcers and associated disorders. The usual dose is 600 to 800 mg daily; it is also used as suppositories.

Comparison with carbenoxolone.— S. Kenwright *et al.*, *Clin. Trials J.*, 1974, *11*, 51.

Further references: E. Camarri *et al.*, *Arzneimittel-Forsch.*, 1972, *22*, 768; L. Celli *et al.*, *Curr. ther. Res.*, 1975, *18*, 105; E. Schraven and D. Trottnow, *Arzneimittel-Forsch.*, 1976, *26*, 213; R. Chermat *et al.*, *Thérapie*, 1977, *32*, 643.

Proprietary Names
Gastronilo (*Aristegui, Spain*); U.G.D. (*Szabó, Arg.*); Solimidin (*Selvi, Ital.*).

711-f

Proprietary Preparations of Some Polymeric Adsorbents

Included below are preparations of polymeric adsorbents not described in this chapter

Amberlite XAD (*Rohm & Haas, UK*). A range of polystyrene (XAD-1, -2, and -4) or acrylic ester (XAD-7 and -8) adsorbents available in grades of different polarities and surface characteristics.

Treatment of poisoning. A review of the pharmacokinetics of haemoperfusion for drug overdose including the use of Amberlite resins. Amberlite resins have a more specific adsorptive capacity for non-polar organic molecules than activated charcoal and in clinical studies they have usually achieved the greatest clearance of non-polar drugs. However, polar drugs such as salicylates, methotrexate, and water soluble metabolites of polar or non-polar drugs may be removed more efficiently by activated charcoal.— S. Pond *et al.*, *Clin. Pharmacokinet.*, 1979, *4*, 329.

Amberlite XAD-2 haemoperfusion systems might be superior to haemodialysis in the treatment of drug intoxication with various barbiturates, glutethimide, and ethchlorvynol.— J. L. Rosenbaum, *Clin. Toxicol.*, 1972, *5*, 331.

Haemoperfusion, using Amberlite XAD-4, was successful in the treatment of 10 patients after poisoning with barbiturates, glutethimide, and tricyclic antidepressants but was ineffective in one patient with chloroquine poisoning.— J. A. P. Trafford *et al.*, *Br. med. J.*, 1977, *2*, 1453. Haemoperfusion had limited value in poisoning by tricyclic antidepressants.— G. N. Volans *et al.* (letter), *Br. med. J.*, 1978, *1*, 174; O. M. Bakke *et al.* (letter), *ibid.*

See also under Amitriptyline Hydrochloride, p.112.

A report of the successful use of haemoperfusion using an Amberlite XAD-4 column for acute digoxin poisoning in a 40-year-old man.— G. H. Gleeson *et al.* (letter), *J. Am. med. Ass.*, 1978, *240*, 2731. Two further reports of the management of digoxin toxicity with haemoperfusion using a macroreticular styrene divinylbenzene copolymer column for 1 patient and a cellulose coated activated charcoal column in another.— J. W. Smiley, *ibid.*, 2736. See also M. C. Gelfand, *ibid.*, 2761.

Haemoperfusion for 4 hours using an Amberlite XAD-4 column transiently reduced plasma-methotrexate concentrations in a woman with metastatic breast carcinoma with signs of methotrexate toxicity. Studies *in vitro* showed that haemoperfusion with uncoated charcoal was more effective than Amberlite XAD-4.— T. P. Gibson *et al.*, *Clin. Pharmac. Ther.*, 1978, *23*, 351.

Anthelmintics and Schistosomicides

750-g

Anthelmintics are used to treat helminth or worm infections. Schistosomicides are used to treat those helminth infections known as schistosomiasis or bilharziasis caused by the flukes of the genus *Schistosoma.*

The worms that cause infection in man generally fall either into the phylum Platyhelminthes, which includes the cestodes or tapeworms and the trematodes or flukes, or into the phylum Nematoda which includes the nematodes or roundworms.

Cestodes are flat segmented worms and include
**Diphyllobothrium latum*—broad fish tapeworm
Hymenolepis nana—dwarf tapeworm
**Taenia saginata*—beef tapeworm
**Taenia solium*—pork tapeworm
Echinococcus granulosus and *E. multilocularis*—causing hydatid disease.

The larvae of *Taenia solium* cause cysticercosis.

Trematodes (flukes) are generally flat, leaf-shaped, unsegmented worms and include
Fasciola hepatica—liver fluke
Fasciolopsis buski—intestinal fluke
Heterophyes heterophyes—dwarf fluke
Opisthorchis sinensis = *Clonorchis sinensis*—Chinese liver fluke
Paragonimus westermani—Oriental lung fluke
Schistosoma haematobium
Schistosoma intercalatum
Schistosoma japonicum
Schistosoma mansoni.

Nematodes are round unsegmented worms; those chiefly infecting the intestine include
Ancylostoma duodenale—Old World hookworm
**Ascaris lumbricoides*—roundworm
Capillaria philippinensis
**Enterobius vermicularis* = *Oxyuris vermicularis*—threadworm, pinworm
Necator americanus—New World hookworm
Strongyloides stercoralis—sometimes called threadworm in USA
Ternidens deminutus=*Ternidens diminutus*—false hookworm
Trichostrongylus spp.
**Trichuris trichiura* = *Trichocephalus trichiurus*—whipworm

Nematodes chiefly infecting the tissues include the filarial worms
Brugia malayi—causing elephantiasis
Loa loa—eye worm
Onchocerca volvulus—causing river blindness (onchocerciasis)
Wuchereria bancrofti—causing elephantiasis
Dracunculus medinensis —guinea-worm
**Toxocara canis* and *T. cati*
**Trichinella spiralis.*

*NOTE. Infections due to the helminths marked with an asterisk may occur in Great Britain and other temperate climates; infections due to the other helminths are generally limited to tropical or localised areas, but may occur in travellers who have visited those areas.

The principal drugs of this section are listed below following the worm against which they may be effective. The probable drugs of choice are listed first; others are listed alphabetically as 'also used.'

Diphyllobothrium latum—niclosamide; also used, dichlorophen, male fern
Hymenolepis nana—niclosamide; also used dichlorophen, hexylresorcinol
Taenia saginata—niclosamide; also used, dichlorophen, male fern, mebendazole
Taenia solium—niclosamide; also used, male fern, mebendazole
Echinococcus spp.—mebendazole
Fasciolopsis buski—hexylresorcinol, tetrachloroethylene
Heterophyes heterophyes—tetrachloroethylene
Opisthorchis sinensis—hexachloroparaxylene
Schistosoma haematobium—niridazole; also used, antimony sodium (or potassium) tartrate, hycanthone, lucanthone, stibocaptate, stibophen
Schistosoma japonicum—antimony sodium (or potassium) tartrate; also used, niridazole, stibocaptate, stibophen
Schistosoma mansoni—niridazole or stibocaptate or stibophen; also used, antimony sodium (or potassium) tartrate, hycanthone, lucanthone, oxamniquine
Ancylostoma duodenale—mebendazole or pyrantel; also used, bephenium, bitoscanate, levamisole, tetrachloroethylene, thiabendazole
Ascaris lumbricoides—pyrantel or mebendazole or piperazine; also used bephenium, levamisole, tetramisole, thiabendazole
Brugia malayi—diethylcarbamazine
Capillaria philippinensis—mebendazole, thiabendazole
Dracunculus medinensis—niridazole; also used, mebendazole, thiabendazole
Enterobius vermicularis—pyrantel, mebendazole, or viprynium; also used, piperazine, thiabendazole
Loa loa—diethylcarbamazine
Necator americanus—mebendazole or pyrantel; also used, bitoscanate, levamisole, tetrachloroethylene, thiabendazole
Onchocerca volvulus—diethylcarbamazine
Strongyloides stercoralis—thiabendazole; also used, levamisole, viprynium
Ternidens deminutus—bephenium, pyrantel, thiabendazole
Toxocara spp.—diethylcarbamazine
Trichinella spiralis—thiabendazole; also used, mebendazole
Trichostrongylus spp.—thiabendazole; also used, bephenium, pyrantel
Trichuris trichiura—mebendazole; also used oxantel, thiabendazole
Wuchereria bancrofti—diethylcarbamazine

For the use of paromomycin in tapeworm infections, metronidazole in guinea-worm infections, bithionol in trematode infections, chloroquine in clonorchiasis, and metriphonate in schistosomiasis, see the respective monographs.

The pentavalent antimony compounds such as sodium stibogluconate that are included in this section possess antiprotozoal activity and are used in the treatment of visceral leishmaniasis (kala-azar) caused by the protozoon *Leishmania donovani* and in the treatment of cutaneous leishmaniasis (oriental sore), a form due to *L. tropica.* Other drugs used in the treatment of leishmaniasis are hydroxystilbamidine isethionate (p.725) and pentamidine isethionate (p.982).

Reviews of anthelmintics: A. Davis, *Drug Treatment in Intestinal Helminthiases*, Geneva, World Health Organization, 1973; *Med. Lett.*, 1974, *16*, 6 and 11; *Drug & Ther. Bull.*, 1975, *13*, 65; D. Botero R., *Prog. Drug Res.*, 1975, *19*, 28; B. J. Vakil and N. J. Dalal, *ibid.*, 166; A. M. Geddes, *Adv. Med. Topics Ther.*, 1976, *2*, 1; M. J. Miller, *Prog. Drug Res.*, 1976, *20*, 433; H. M. Gilles, *Br. med. J.*, 1976, *2*, 1314; M. Katz, *Drugs*, 1977, *13*, 124; D. S. Blumenthal, *New Engl. J. Med.*, 1977, *297*, 1437; A. Gatherer, *Practitioner*, 1977, *219*, 871; J. M. Foy, *Pharm. J.*, 1977, *1*, 320; H. Van den Bossche, *Nature*, 1978, *273*, 626; *Pediatrics*, 1978, *62*, 251; *Med. Lett.*, 1979, *21*, 105; K. M. Goel, *Prescribers' J.*, 1980, *20*, 107.

For reviews of the treatment and control of schistosomiasis, see C. Wilcocks, *Abstr. Wld Med.*, 1967, *41*, 325; P. Jordan, *Br. med. Bull.*, 1972, *28*, 55; *Br. med. J.*, 1972, *1*, 128; H. Most, *New Engl. J. Med.*, 1972, *287*, 698; *Med. Lett.*, 1974, *16*, 5; N. O. Crossland, *Adv. Drug Res.*, 1977, *12*, 53; A. A. Mahmoud, *New Engl. J. Med.*, 1977, *297*, 1329 (Criticism H. Most (letter), *ibid.*, 1978, *298*, 850 and a reply A.A.F. Mahmoud (letter), *ibid.*); Scientific Working Group on Schistosomiasis, *Bull. Wld Hlth Org.*, 1978, *56*, 361; H. Van den Bossche, *Nature*, 1978, *273*, 626; *Med. Lett.*, 1979, *21*, 105; Epidemiology and Control of Schistosomiasis, Report of a WHO Expert Committee, *Tech. Rep. Ser. Wld Hlth Org. No. 643*, 1980.

A report of a symposium on schistosomiasis with special reference to long-term toxicity.— *J. Toxic. environ. Hlth*, 1975, *1*, 173–351.

751-q

Alantolactone. Alant Camphor; Elecampane Camphor; Inula Camphor; Helenin.
(3a*R*,5*S*,8a*S*,9a*R*)-3a,5,6,7,8,8a,9,9a-Octahydro-5,8a-dimethyl-3-methylenenaphtho[2,3-*b*]furan-2(3*H*)-one.
$C_{15}H_{20}O_2$=232.3.

CAS — 546-43-0.

A terpene obtained from the roots of *Inula helenium* (Compositae). Crystals. M.p. 78° to 79°. Practically **insoluble** in water; freely soluble in alcohol, chloroform, ether, and oils.

Adverse Effects. Contact dermatitis has been reported.

Uses. Alantolactone has been given by mouth or rectally in the treatment of roundworm (*Ascaris*), threadworm, hookworm, and whipworm infection. The usual dose was 300 mg daily, usually for 2 courses, each of 5 days, separated by 10 days; children, 50 to 200 mg daily.

752-p

Albendazole. SKF 62979. Methyl 5-propylthio-1*H*-benzimidazol-2-ylcarbamate.
$C_{12}H_{15}N_3O_2S$=265.3.

CAS — 54965-21-8.

Uses. Albendazole is a benzimidazole anthelmintic structurally related to thiabendazole (see p.107). It is used in veterinary practice.

Manufacturers
Smith Kline & French, UK.

753-s

Amphotalide. M & B 2948A; RP 6171. *N*-[5-(4-Aminophenoxy)pentyl]phthalimide.
$C_{19}H_{20}N_2O_3$=324.4.

CAS — 1673-06-9.

A yellow, odourless, tasteless, microcrystalline powder. Very slightly **soluble** in water.

Adverse Effects. Gastro-intestinal disturbances and temporary visual disturbance.

Uses. Amphotalide was formerly used in the treatment of schistosomiasis, particularly infections due to *Schistosoma haematobium.*

754-w

Antimony Lithium Thiomalate.
Anthiolimine.

Corresponds approximately to the formula $C_{12}H_9Li_6O_{12}S_3Sb,9H_2O$=766.9.

CAS — 305-97-5 (anhydrous).

A hygroscopic powder containing about 16% of antimony. A 6% solution of antimony lithium thiomalate contains in 1 ml the equivalent of about 10 mg of antimony. Very **soluble** in water; very slightly soluble in alcohol and ether.

Adverse Effects. As for Antimony Sodium Tartrate, p.87. It is claimed to be less likely to cause coughing and vomiting.

Uses. Antimony lithium thiomalate has been used similarly to antimony sodium tartrate in the treatment of schistosomiasis. The average initial dose for adults was 1 ml of a 6% solution intramuscularly increased by 1 ml, at subsequent injections, according to tolerance until a dose of 4 ml was reached. The dose was maintained at this level until a total of 40 to 60 ml had been given. Injections were usually given on alternate days.

Children could be given up to 2.5 to 3 mg (0.04 to 0.05 ml) of antimony lithium thiomalate per kg body-weight.

Antimony lithium thiomalate was formerly marketed in certain countries as Anthiomaline (*May & Baker*).

755-e

Antimony Potassium Tartrate *(B.P.C. 1973).*

Antim. Pot. Tart.; Potassium Antimonyltartrate; Tartar Emetic; Kalii Stibyli Tartras; Stibii et Kalii Tartras, Tartarus Stibiatus; Brechweinstein.

CAS — 11071-15-1 ($C_8H_4K_2O_{12}Sb_2$); 28300-74-5 ($C_8H_4K_2O_{12}Sb_2,3H_2O$).

NOTE. The structure for antimony potassium tartrate is variously represented. *B.P.C. 1973* gave $C_4H_4KO_7Sb$ (= 324.9) and *U.S.P.* gives $C_8H_4K_2O_{12}Sb_2,3H_2O$ (= 667.9).

Pharmacopoeias. In *Nord.* (as *B.P.C. 1973*). In *Aust., Chin., It., Mex., Pol., Port., and Span.* (as *B.P.C. 1973*; all with ½H_2O). In *Braz.* (as *U.S.P.*) and *U.S.* (both with $3H_2O$).

Odourless or almost odourless colourless crystals or white granular powder. It may occur as the hemihydrate with about 2.7% moisture, but it effloresces in dry air. The salt becomes anhydrous at 100° and does not readily rehydrate on exposure to the atmosphere.

Soluble 1 in 13 of water, 1 in 3 of boiling water, and 1 in 20 of glycerol; practically insoluble in alcohol, chloroform, and ether. Solutions in water are acid to litmus. Solutions are **sterilised** by autoclaving or by filtration. **Incompatible** with acids and alkalis, salts of heavy metals, albumin, soap, and tannins. **Store** in airtight containers.

Antimony Potassium Tartrate Injection and Antimony Sodium Tartrate Injection could be sterilised by autoclaving or filtration without an increase in toxicity. Injections stored at room temperature, at 4°, or at 40° showed no increase in toxicity after storage for at least 12 months.— G. F. Somers and T. D. Whittet, *Pharm. J.*, 1958, *2*, 494.

Adverse Effects and Precautions. As for Antimony Sodium Tartrate, below.

Uses. Antimony potassium tartrate has the actions and uses of antimony sodium tartrate (see below) but it is less soluble and more irritant than the sodium salt which is therefore more suitable for intravenous injection.

Schistosomiasis. Antimony potassium tartrate was the drug used at centres providing treatment for schistosomiasis in Egypt. Twelve intravenous injections of a 6% solution were given at weekly intervals. Centres reported that 26 to 100% of the patients who received the treatment were cured. Pain and nausea occurred after the injections.— M. Farooq, *Chronicle Wld Hlth Org.*, 1967, *21*, 175.

No deterioration of the heart condition was observed in 40 Egyptian children with rheumatic valvular lesions who responded well to a course of 14 injections of antimony potassium tartrate as a 6% solution for the treatment of schistosomiasis due mainly to *S. haematobium*.— Z. H. Abdin and M. A. M. Abul-Fadl, *J. Egypt. med. Ass.*, 1972, *55*, 779, per *Trop. Dis. Bull.*, 1973, *70*, 983.

Preparations

Antimony Potassium Tartrate Injection *(B.P. 1963).* Antim. Pot. Tart. Inj.; Potassium Antimonyltartrate Injection. A sterile solution in Water for Injections.

820-b

Antimony Sodium Dimethylcysteine Tartrate.

NAP; Antimony Sodium Penicillamine Tartrate.

CAS — 34755-53-8.

NOTE. The synonym NAP has also been used for nandrolone phenylpropionate.

A crystalline solid prepared by the chelation of antimony sodium tartrate with penicillamine. It can be made with varying amounts of antimony but usually contains about 14.5% of Sb. **Soluble** in water.

Uses. Antimony sodium dimethylcysteine tartrate is a derivative of antimony sodium tartrate claimed to be better tolerated. It is used in the mass treatment of schistosomiasis due to *Schistosoma japonicum* and *S. mansoni* in doses of 400 mg by intramuscular injection daily for 5 days.

Of 101 patients examined up to 3 months after treatment on 5 consecutive days with daily intramuscular injections of antimony sodium dimethylcysteine tartrate, 95 were free from infection with *S. mansoni*. Side-effects prevented full treatment in 4 patients. Other patients experienced mild side-effects including nausea, vomiting, fever, myalgia, and skin rashes.— M. R. Pedrique *et al.*, *Ann. trop. Med. Parasit.*, 1970, *64*, 255, per *Trop. Dis. Bull.*, 1971, *68*, 68.

Antimony sodium dimethylcysteine tartrate, prepared to contain 14.5% of antimony, given as 5 intramuscular injections of 400 mg daily, cured 9 of 10 patients infected with *S. japonicum*. Side-effects were moderately severe and included myocardial ischaemia which persisted for 77 days in 1 patient.— A. T. Santos *et al.*, *J. Philipp. med. Ass.*, 1970, *46*, 254, per *Trop. Dis. Bull.*, 1971, *68*, 844. A similar report in 400 patients infected with *S. mansoni*. The dose was better tolerated than equivalent doses of antimony sodium tartrate.— M. R. Pedrique and N. Ercoli, *Bull. Wld Hlth Org.*, 1971, *45*, 411.

756-l

Antimony Sodium Tartrate *(B.P.).*

Antim. Sod. Tart.; Sodium Antimonyltartrate; Stibium Natrium Tartaricum.

$C_4H_4NaO_7Sb$=308.8.

CAS — 34521-09-0.

Pharmacopoeias. In *Br.* and *Ind.*

Colourless and transparent, or whitish, odourless, hygroscopic scales or powder with a sweetish taste. It loses not more than 6% of its weight when dried.

Soluble 1 in 1.5 of water; practically insoluble in alcohol. A 7.9% solution is iso-osmotic with serum. Solutions are **sterilised** by autoclaving or by filtration. **Incompatible** with acids and alkalis, salts of heavy metals, albumin, soap, and tannins. **Store** in airtight containers.

Antimony Potassium Tartrate Injection and Antimony Sodium Tartrate Injection could be sterilised by autoclaving or filtration without an increase in toxicity. Injections stored at room temperature, at 4°, or at 40° showed no increase in toxicity after storage for at least 12 months.— G. F. Somers and T. D. Whittet, *Pharm. J.*, 1958, *2*, 494.

Adverse Effects. Antimony sodium tartrate and other trivalent antimony compounds are cardiotoxic and their administration is usually accompanied by changes in the ECG, such as flattening or inversion of the T-wave; bradycardia, hypotension, and cardiac arrhythmias may develop. Collapse and sudden deaths due to anaphylactic-type reactions have occurred. Large doses of antimony compounds given by mouth have an emetic action and therapeutic doses given intravenously cause nausea, vomiting, cough, abdominal pain, and diarrhoea.

Other side-effects include anorexia, chest, muscle, and joint pains, pruritus, skin rashes, dizziness, and oedema. Renal and hepatic damage occur rarely and haemolytic anaemia has been reported. Trivalent antimony compounds are generally more toxic than pentavalent antimony compounds.

Continuous treatment with small doses of antimony may give rise to symptoms of subacute poisoning similar to those of chronic arsenical poisoning.

Sudden death or cardiovascular collapse due to idiosyncrasy might occur at any time during treatment with antimony potassium tartrate. Reversible ECG changes occurred in every patient and appeared to be more pronounced in Africans and Asians than in Europeans. The ECG returned to normal within about 2 months after treatment with antimony was stopped. These changes were also seen, but to a lesser degree, in patients treated with other trivalent antimony compounds. The damage appeared to be to the myocardium.— *Br. med. J.*, 1961, *1*, 1665.

Of 26 patients with schistosomiasis or mucocutaneous leishmaniasis who received trivalent antimony compounds, the ECG remained normal in 3; 20 showed diffuse alterations in ventricular repolarisation, 16 developed a prolonged Q-T interval, and 6 cardiac ischaemia. Of 10 patients who received pentavalent antimony compounds, 3 remained unaffected and the corresponding numbers of patients who experienced side-effects were 6, 7, and 2 or 3 respectively.— F. C. De Lacerda *et al.*, *Revta Inst. Med. trop. S Paulo*, 1965, *7*, 210, per *Trop. Dis. Bull.*, 1966, *63*, 175.

Hyperventilation, obstructive ventilatory defect, and uneven ventilation were observed in patients who were given antimony potassium tartrate, sodium antimonylgluconate, stibocaptate, stibophen, and niridazole. The effects which were more marked in patients with associated chest disease lasted about a month.— A. Mousa *et al.*, *J. Egypt. med. Ass.*, 1968, *51*, 765, per *Trop. Dis. Bull.*, 1970, *67*, 299.

The pharmacology and toxicology of antimony.— K. L. Stemmer, *Pharmac. Ther.*, 1976, *1*, 157.

Treatment of Adverse Effects. If antimony compounds have been ingested, empty the stomach by aspiration and lavage. In severe poisoning, treatment with dimercaprol may be of benefit.

To minimise the undesirable effects on the liver of antimony therapy, 15 patients with schistosomal cirrhosis were given concurrently 30 mg of prednisone daily. The liver damage and dysfunction were not increased by the antimony treatment.— A. Zaky *et al.*, *J. trop. Med. Hyg.*, 1963, *66*, 188, per *Trop. Dis. Bull.*, 1964, *61*, 54.

Precautions. Antimony therapy is contra-indicated in pneumonia, myocarditis, hepatitis, and nephritis. Intravenous injections should be administered very slowly and stopped if coughing, vomiting, or substernal pain occurs. Antimony sodium tartrate can cause severe pain and tissue necrosis and is therefore not given by intramuscular or subcutaneous injection; extravasation should be avoided during intravenous administration.

Ascaris infection, rheumatoid arthritis, and diseases of the digestive and nervous systems were contra-indications to therapy with antimony.— J. R. da Silva, *Revta bras. Malar. Doenç. trop.*, 1959, *11*, 425, per *Trop. Dis. Bull.*, 1962, *59*, 367.

Absorption and Fate. Antimony sodium tartrate is poorly absorbed from the gastro-intestinal tract. Like most trivalent compounds of antimony it is slowly excreted in the urine and bile; antimony accumulates in the body during treatment and persists for several months afterwards. Trivalent antimony has a greater affinity for cell proteins than for plasma proteins.

Insufficient absorption coupled with emetic action made it difficult to achieve therapeutic effects with antimony compounds given by mouth without marked intestinal side-effects. When given parenterally they produced high but transient concentrations in the blood and very high and more sustained concentrations in organs such as the liver and the kidney. Since concentrations of antimony in the blood were rarely, if ever, maintained long enough to have an effect on schistosomes it was possible that antimony might be concentrated by the parasite, particularly the female parasite.— *Chronicle Wld Hlth Org.*, 1966, *20*, 92.

In 7 patients who had received antimony compounds 6 months to 2 years previously, average concentrations of antimony in blood and urine in ng per 100 ml were: 6 months after treatment 23 and 109.4; after 1 year 6.7 and 27.6; and after 2 years 8.6 and 23.2. By comparison with concentrations in the blood and urine of persons who had not had antimony treatment, it was concluded that antimony persisted in the body for over a year and in some persons for 2 years.— M. M. Mansour *et al.* (letter), *Nature*, 1967, *214*, 819.

Uses. Antimony sodium tartrate is toxic to the parasites of schistosomiasis and leishmaniasis. It inhibits phosphofructokinase which regulates the main source of energy of schistosomes. *Schistosoma haematobium* is considered most susceptible followed by *S. mansoni* then *S. japonicum*.

In schistosomiasis, intravenous injections are given every other day, usually as a 6% solution. The initial dose contains 30 mg, the second and third doses 60 and 90 mg respectively, and subsequent doses 120 mg up to a total of not less than 1.2 g. The patient should be kept in bed. A more intensive course of daily doses is sometimes given.

In the treatment of leishmaniasis, antimony sodium tartrate has been largely replaced by less irritant and less toxic pentavalent antimony compounds as well as by hydroxystilbamidine or pentamidine isethionate.

Antimony sodium tartrate has also been given intravenously in the treatment of lymphogranuloma inguinale but a tetracycline or sulphonamide is to be preferred. Antimony sodium tartrate was formerly used as an emetic and reflex expectorant.

Schistosomiasis. One hundred and sixty men with urinary schistosomiasis were treated with either antimony sodium tartrate intravenously, stibocaptate intramuscularly, or sodium antimonylgluconate intravenously. Doses were adjusted so that each patient received an equivalent amount of antimony daily for 15 days, increasing from about 10 to 40 mg in days 1 to 4 and continuing at this dosage until a total of about 530 mg had been given. Comparable high cure-rates were obtained with antimony sodium tartrate and stibocaptate; sodium antimonylgluconate was slightly less effective. Of 63 patients who failed to complete the treatment because of the severity of side-effects, 35 received antimony sodium tartrate and 26 received stibocaptate. Acute vascular collapse occurred in 3 patients treated with antimony sodium tartrate; 1 attack occurred immediately after the first injection.— A. Davis, *Bull. Wld Hlth Org.*, 1968, *38*, 197.

Seventeen Egyptian subjects, aged 8 to 27 years, infected with *S. haematobium* were given twice-weekly intravenous injections of antimony sodium tartrate (30 mg per 15 kg body-weight) for 12 doses. By the twelfth week of the follow-up 14 had ceased to pass live eggs in the urine—a cure rate of 82%.— Z. Farid *et al.*, *Br. med. J.*, 1968, *3*, 713.

Preparations

Antimony Sodium Tartrate Injection *(B.P., Ind. P.)*. Antim. Sod. Tart. Inj.; Sodium Antimonyltartrate Injection. A sterile solution in Water for Injections. Sterilised by autoclaving.

757-y

Antimony Sodium Thioglycollate.

Sodium Antimonylthioglycollate; Stibii et Natrii Thioglycollas. $C_4H_4NaO_4S_2Sb$=324.9.

CAS — 539-54-8.

A white or pink powder which is odourless or has a faint mercaptan-like odour. It is discoloured by exposure to light. **Soluble** in water; practically insoluble in alcohol. Solutions are **sterilised** by autoclaving or by filtration. **Protect** from light.

Uses. Antimony sodium thioglycollate has been employed in the treatment of leishmaniasis and granuloma inguinale due to *Leishmania donovani*. It has been stated to be less toxic and less irritating than antimony potassium tartrate. It was given in doses of 50 to 100 mg subcutaneously or intramuscularly every 3 or 4 days.

758-j

Areca *(B.P.C. 1949)*.

Arecae Semen; Areca Nuts; Betel Nuts; Noix d'Arec; Arekasame.

Pharmacopoeias. In *Aust.*, *Chin.*, and *Jap.*

The dried ripe seeds of *Areca catechu* (Palmae) containing not less than 0.25% of alkaloids calculated as arecoline.

Uses. Areca was formerly employed in doses of 1 to 4 g for tapeworm infection.

It has sialagogue properties and is used in eastern countries as a masticatory (see also Betel, p.672) but an increased incidence of oral leucoplakia and oral carcinoma has been reported in persons in the habit of chewing areca.

A review of areca.— K. N. Arjungi, *Arzneimittel-Forsch.*, 1976, *26*, 951.

In addition to arecoline, areca contained smaller amounts of the related alkaloid guvacoline and the amino acids arecaidine and guvacine. Guvacine and, to a lesser extent, arecaidine were competitive inhibitors of γ-aminobutyric acid uptake *in vitro*.— G. A. R. Johnston *et al.* (letter), *Nature*, 1975, *258*, 627.

Increased oral cancer associated with the chewing of 'quids' composed of areca, lime, and, occasionally, tobacco leaf, might be associated with the arecaidine content.— J. Ashby *et al.* (letter), *Lancet*, 1979, *1*, 112. Criticisms.— B. G. Burton-Bradley (letter), *ibid.*, *2*, 903.

759-z

Arecoline Hydrobromide *(B.P.C. 1949, B. Vet. C. 1965)*.

Methyl 1,2,5,6-tetrahydro-1-methylnicotinate hydrobromide.
$C_8H_{13}NO_2$,HBr=236.1.

CAS — 63-75-2 (arecoline); 300-08-3 (hydrobromide).

Pharmacopoeias. In *Arg.*, *Hung.*, *Nord.*, *Pol.*, *Port.*, *Span.*, and *Swiss*.

A white odourless crystalline powder with a bitter taste. **Soluble** 1 in 1 of water and 1 in 10 of alcohol; very slightly soluble in chloroform and ether. A 3.88% solution in water is iso-osmotic with serum. Solutions may be **sterilised** by autoclaving, by filtration, or by heating with a bactericide. **Store** in airtight containers. Protect from light.

Uses. Arecoline is an alkaloid present in Areca (see above); it has a parasympathomimetic action similar to that of pilocarpine. It has been used in veterinary medicine as a purgative and taenifuge. It is not taenicidal.

760-p

Arecoline-acetarsol *(B. Vet. C. 1965)*.

Drocarbil. Arecoline 3-acetamido-4-hydroxyphenylarsonate.
$C_8H_{13}NO_2$,$C_8H_{10}AsNO_5$=430.3.

CAS — 900-77-6.

A white or very pale yellow, almost odourless, somewhat glistening powder. Solutions in water and alcohol decompose. **Store** in airtight containers. Protect from light.

Uses. Arecoline-acetarsol is a veterinary anthelmintic which has been used in the treatment of tapeworm infection in small domestic animals.

761-s

Ascaridole.

Ascaridol. 1-Isopropyl-4-methyl-2,3-dioxabicyclo[2.2.2]oct-5-ene.
$C_{10}H_{16}O_2$=168.2.

CAS — 512-85-6.

The active principle of chenopodium oil. It is an unstable liquid which is liable to explode when heated or when treated with organic acids.

Uses. Ascaridole has the same actions and uses as chenopodium oil (see p.90). It has been administered as capsules in doses of up to 600 mg daily.

762-w

Bephenium Hydroxynaphthoate *(B.P., B.P. Vet., U.S.P.)*.

Naphthammonum. Benzyldimethyl(2-phenoxyethyl)ammonium 3-hydroxy-2-naphthoate.
$C_{28}H_{29}NO_4$=443.5.

CAS — 7181-73-9 (bephenium); 3818-50-6 (hydroxynaphthoate).

Pharmacopoeias. In *Br.*, *Braz.*, *Chin.*, *Rus.*, and *U.S.*

A yellow to greenish-yellow odourless or almost odourless crystalline powder with a bitter taste. M.p. 168° to 173° with decomposition.

Practically **insoluble** in water; soluble 1 in 50 of alcohol. **Store** in airtight containers.

Adverse Effects. Nausea, diarrhoea, vomiting, headache, and vertigo have occasionally been reported.

Absorption and Fate. Only a small fraction of a dose of bephenium hydroxynaphthoate is absorbed from the gastro-intestinal tract.

Uses. Bephenium hydroxynaphthoate is an effective anthelmintic against hookworms of the species *Ancylostoma duodenale*, roundworms (*Ascaris*), and species of *Trichostrongylus*. It is less effective against hookworms of the species *Necator americanus* and whipworms.

A single 5-g dose of granules, equivalent to 2.5 g of base, is usually effective in removing hookworms of the species *Ancylostoma duodenale* and roundworms (*Ascaris*). The dose should be given, suspended in water or other suitable liquid, on an empty stomach and food withheld for 1 hour afterwards. Purgation is not necessary. In the presence of severe infection, treatment may be repeated after 3 days. For *Necator americanus*, 2 doses on each of 3 successive days, may be needed to remove all the worms.

Children weighing less than 10 kg or under 2 years old may be given the equivalent of 1.25 g of bephenium daily.

Hookworm (*Necator*). Resistance to bephenium hydroxynaphthoate by *Necator americanus* was demonstrated in 1 patient in Ghana who received 9 doses over 45 days. Poor response to bephenium and to other anthelmintics was shown by 4 other patients.— J. O. O. Commey and D. R. W. Haddock, *Ghana med. J.*, 1970, *9*, 94, per *Trop. Dis. Bull.*, 1971, *68*, 733. See also W. A. Chinery *et al.*, *Ann. trop. Med. Parasit.*, 1973, *67*, 75, per *Trop. Dis. Bull.*, 1973, *70*, 665.

For further reports of the use of bephenium hydroxynaphthoate, see Pyrantel Embonate, p.104.

Ternidens deminutus. A single dose of bephenium was effective in clearing infection by *Ternidens deminutus* in 28 of 32 Rhodesian patients. A second dose was required by 4 patients.— J. M. Goldsmid, *J. trop. Med. Hyg.*, 1971, *74*, 19, per *Trop. Dis. Bull.*, 1971, *68*, 732.

Trichostrongylus. Bephenium hydroxynaphthoate in a single dose, equivalent to 2.5 g base, was effective in eliminating *Trichostrongylus colubriformis* from the faeces of 30 of 49 patients; 6 patients required a second dose 1 to 2 months later.— M. Cotin *et al.*, *Harefuah*, 1972, *83*, 54, per *Trop. Dis. Bull.*, 1973, *70*, 62.

Preparations

Bephenium Granules *(B.P.C. 1973)*. Contains bephenium hydroxynaphthoate with starch and other pharmaceutical adjuvants; each 5 g of granules contains the equivalent of 2.5 g of bephenium base.

Bephenium Hydroxynaphthoate for Oral Suspension *(U.S.P.)*. A mixture of bephenium hydroxynaphthoate and starch. Potency is expressed in terms of the equivalent amount of bephenium. A suspension in water is neutral to litmus. Store in airtight containers.

Alcopar *(Wellcome, UK)*. Bephenium hydroxynaphthoate in dispersible granules, available in 5-g sachets each containing the equivalent of 2.5 g of bephenium base. (Also available as Alcopar in *Fr.*, *Ger.*, *S.Afr.*; available as Alcopara in *USA*).

763-e

Betanaphthol *(B.P. 1948)*.

Naphthol; β-Naftol. Naphth-2-ol.
$C_{10}H_8O$=144.2.

CAS — 135-19-3.

Pharmacopoeias. In *Aust.*, *Cz.*, *Hung.*, *Jug.*, *Nord.*, *Pol.*, *Port.*, *Span.*, and *Swiss*.

White or almost white crystalline leaflets or powder with a faint phenolic odour and a sharp taste. Stable in air but darkens on exposure to light. M.p. 121° to 123°. **Soluble** 1 in 1000 of water, 1 in 2 of alcohol, and 1 in 1.5 of ether; soluble in chloroform, glycerol, olive oil, soft paraffin, and solutions of alkali hydroxides. A saturated solution in water is neutral to litmus. **Incompatible** with camphor, menthol, phenazone, and phenol. **Protect** from light.

Adverse Effects. Symptoms of overdosage include vomiting, diarrhoea, haemolysis, lens opacitics, oliguria, and convulsions. Nephritis has followed absorption from intact skin.

Uses. Betanaphthol was formerly used as an anthelmintic in hookworm and tapeworm infections, but it has been superseded by less toxic and more efficient drugs. It is excreted chiefly as the glucuronide and gives a reddish tint to the urine.

Betanaphthol has a potent parasiticidal effect and has been used as an ointment (up to 10%) in the treatment of scabies, ringworm, and other skin diseases.

The absorption of betanaphthol from a paste containing 20%, with sulphur and soft soap, ranged from 5 to 41% of the amount applied to 10 patients. It was recommended that betanaphthol paste be applied to areas not larger than 150 cm^2, only to patients capable of metabolising betanaphthol, and be left on the skin for not more than 1 hour twice daily. A high output of urine was necessary, preferably alkaline, and treatment should not be given during pregnancy.— H. G. W. M. Hemels, *Br. J. Derm.*, 1972, *87*, 614.

764-l

Bitoscanate.
Hoechst 16842. Phenylene-1,4-bisisothiocyanate.
$C_8H_4N_2S_2$=192.3.

CAS — 4044-65-9.

A yellowish-white, almost odourless, tasteless, crystalline powder. Practically **insoluble** in water; soluble in alcohol and chloroform.

Adverse Effects. Transient mild to moderate side-effects may occur in up to half of the patients treated. They include nausea and vomiting, anorexia, abdominal pain, diarrhoea, headache, and dizziness.

Absorption and Fate. Bitoscanate is partly absorbed from the gastro-intestinal tract and slowly excreted; a half-life of 26 days has been reported.

Uses. Bitoscanate is an anthelmintic used in the treatment of hookworms (*Ancylostoma duodenale* and *Necator americanus*). It has been given in 3 doses of 100 mg at 12-hourly intervals or as a single dose of 150 mg. It is recommended that 8 weeks should elapse before a course is repeated.

Hookworm infection (due mainly to *Ancylostoma duodenale*) in 30 children was treated with bitoscanate; children aged 5 to 10 years received 2 doses of 50 mg at 12-hourly intervals and older children received 2 doses of 100 mg. Hookworms were cleared from 26 children and the egg count was greatly reduced in the remaining 4. Side-effects (nausea in 3 patients, vomiting in 5, diarrhoea in 2, and anorexia in 1) did not necessitate discontinuation of treatment.— B. Bhandari and L. N. Shrimali, *J. trop. Med. Hyg.*, 1969, *72*, 164.

In a survey of 1395 patients with mixed infection treated with bitoscanate the cure-rate for those with hookworms was highest for patients aged 10 to 14 years who received the total adult dose of 300 mg. Bitoscanate was effective also against giardiasis and against the dwarf tapeworm *Hymenolepis nana*.— G. S. Mutalik *et al.*, *Ann. trop. Med. Parasit.*, 1970, *64*, 79, per *Trop. Dis. Bull.*, 1971, *68*, 890.

Bitoscanate in single doses of 50 mg for children under 9 years of age, of 100 mg for ages 10 to 14, and of 150 mg for older patients was effective in the treatment of 50 patients infected with *Necator americanus*. Vomiting some time after dosage by 12 patients did not reduce the effect of the drug.— D. R. O'Holohan and J. Hugoe-Matthews, *S.E. Asian J. trop. Med. publ. Hlth*, 1972, *3*, 403, per *Trop. Dis. Bull.*, 1973, *70*, 474.

In a survey including 1714 persons, a single dose of bitoscanate 150 mg was considered to be of value for large-scale eradication of hookworms (*Ancylostoma* and *Necator*).— J. Holz *et al.*, *S.E. Asian J. trop. Med. publ. Hlth*, 1972, *3*, 99, per *Trop. Dis. Bull.*, 1972, *69*, 938.

Further references: G. S. Mutalik and R. B. Gulati, *Clin. Pharmac. Ther.*, 1969, *10*, 635; S. C. Johnson, *J. trop. Med. Hyg.*, 1971, *74*, 133, per *Trop. Dis. Bull.*, 1972, *69*, 653; D. R. O'Holohan *et al.*, *S.E. Asian J. trop. Med. publ. Hlth*, 1971, *2*, 51, per *Trop. Dis. Bull.*, 1972, *69*, 653; J. M. Goldsmid and R. J. MacCabe, *Cent. Afr. J. Med.*, 1972, *18*, 227, per *Trop. Dis. Bull.*, 1974, *71*, 173; S. Chitrathorn *et al.*, *S.E. Asian J. trop. Med. publ. Hlth*, 1972, *3*, 103, per *Trop. Dis. Bull.*, 1972, *69*, 938; K. M. Patel and C. L. M. Olweny, *E. Afr. med. J.*, 1972, *49*, 270, per *Trop. Dis. Bull.*, 1972, *69*, 1283; F. Biagi, *Prog. Drug Res.*, 1975, *19*, 23; S. Johnson, *ibid.*, 70; G. S. Mutalik *et al.*, *ibid.*, 81; M. R. Samuel, *ibid.*, 96.

765-y

Bromonaphthol. 1-Bromonaphth-2-ol.
$C_{10}H_7BrO$=223.1.

CAS — 34369-04-5 (1-bromonaphthol).

White needle-shaped crystals with a naphthol-like, slightly bitter taste. Sparingly **soluble** in water; soluble in most organic solvents.

Adverse Effects. Side-effects include nausea, abdominal pain, loss of appetite, dizziness, and headache.

Uses. Bromonaphthol is used in the treatment of hookworm infections (*Ancylostoma* and *Necator*) and also appears to be effective against whipworms. It has been given with water in doses of 1 to 3 g in the evening with the same dose being repeated the following morning.

For a comparison of bromonaphthol and pyrantel embonate in the treatment of hookworm (*Necator*) infection, see Pyrantel Embonate, p.104.

Proprietary Names
Wormin *(Toyama, Jap.).*

766-j

Cambendazole. MK 905. Isopropyl 2-(thiazol-4-yl)-1*H*-benzimidazol-5-ylcarbamate.
$C_{14}H_{14}N_4O_2S$=302.4.

CAS — 26097-80-3.

Uses. Cambendazole is a benzimidazole anthelmintic structurally related to thiabendazole (see p.107); it has been used in strongyloid worm infections. It is also used in veterinary practice.

Cambendazole was teratogenic in *rats*.— P. Delatour and Y. Richard, *Thérapie*, 1976, *31*, 505.

Success-rates of 95 to 100% against *Strongyloides stercoralis* after single doses of 5 mg per kg body-weight: L. D. Rodrigues *et al.*, *Revta Inst. Med. trop. S Paulo*, 1977, *19*, 57, per *Trop. Dis. Bull.*, 1977, *74*, 848; V. A. Neto *et al.*, *Revta Inst. Med. trop. S Paulo*, 1978, *20*, 161, per *Trop. Dis. Bull.*, 1978, *75*, 898; M. C. Baranski *et al.*, *Revta Inst. Med. trop. S Paulo*, 1978, *20*, 213, per *Trop. Dis. Bull.*, 1979, *76*, 95.

Manufacturers
Merck Sharp & Dohme, UK.

767-z

Carbon Tetrachloride
(B.P. Vet., B.P.C. 1959). Carboneum Tetrachloratum Medicinale. Tetrachloromethane.
CCl_4=153.8.

CAS — 56-23-5.

Pharmacopoeias. In *Arg., Aust., Belg., Cz., Fr., Hung., Mex., Nord., Pol., Span.,* and *Turk.* Also in *U.S.N.F.*

A heavy, clear, colourless, volatile liquid with a chloroform-like odour and a burning taste; it is non-inflammable but in contact with a flame it decomposes and gives rise to toxic products, including phosgene, with an acrid odour. Wt per ml 1.592 to 1.595 g. B.p. 76° to 78°.

Soluble 1 in 1500 of water; soluble in fixed and volatile oils; miscible with dehydrated alcohol, chloroform, ether, and light petroleum. It is slowly decomposed by light and by various metals if moisture is present. **Store** at a temperature not exceeding 30° in airtight containers. Protect from light.

Adverse Effects. Even small doses of carbon tetrachloride may cause drowsiness, giddiness, headache, mental confusion, nausea, and vomiting. Occasionally, more severe symptoms may follow 1 or 2 weeks later, especially cellular necrosis of the kidneys and liver with uraemia, oliguria, and convulsions. Central nervous system depression and respiratory failure may precede death. Adverse effects are more likely to occur in alcoholics.

Inhalation of concentrations of 1000 ppm of the vapour even for short periods may give rise to acute toxic reactions including dizziness, stupor, and loss of consciousness, and may result in death from respiratory or cardiac failure. Exposure to high concentrations may also result in delayed systemic poisoning characterised by epigastric pain, vomiting, and albuminuria. Continued exposure to concentrations of even less than 100 ppm may give rise to chronic poisoning leading to acute nephritis, jaundice, toxic hepatitis, or aplastic anaemia. Similar toxic effects may also be caused by absorption of liquid carbon tetrachloride through the skin.

Dependence on carbon tetrachloride has been reported.

Maximum permissible atmospheric concentration 10 ppm.

For toxicological data, see 1971 Evaluations of some Pesticide Residues in Food, *Pestic. Residue Ser. Wld Hlth Org. No. 1*, 1972.

Extrapyramidal symptoms responsive to levodopa occurred in a 40-year-old man exposed for about 3 months to carbon tetrachloride vapour.— E. Melamed and S. Lavy (letter), *Lancet*, 1977, *1*, 1015.

Radiographic findings in carbon tetrachloride poisoning.— F. M. Bagnasco *et al.*, *N.Y. St. J. Med.*, 1978, *78*, 646.

Treatment of Adverse Effects. If the vapour has been inhaled remove the patient to the fresh air. Remove clothing contaminated by liquid and wash the skin. In severe overdosage by mouth the stomach should be emptied by aspiration and lavage; give a purgative such as sodium sulphate 30 g in 250 ml of water.

Alleviate shock and assist respiration. Fluids should be given cautiously to maintain renal flow. Haemodialysis may be needed if renal function is impaired. Oils, fats, alcohol, and sympathomimetic agents should be avoided.

Five patients poisoned by carbon tetrachloride (by inhalation or injection) developed acute renal failure, which was sufficiently severe in 4 to warrant haemodialysis. All 5 eventually regained full renal function. Since 1953, of 120 cases of carbon tetrachloride poisoning with renal failure, 44 had been treated by dialysis, the mortality-rate being 17%. Between 1939 and 1953, of 74 similar cases, the overall mortality-rate was 36%.— V. K. Nielsen and J. Larsen, *Acta med. scand.*, 1965, *178*, 363, per *Abstr. Wld Med.*, 1966, *39*, 262. See also W. C. Alston, *J. clin. Path.*, 1970, *23*, 249.

For the symptoms and treatment of poisoning with carbon tetrachloride, see *Poisonous Chemicals used on Farms and Gardens*, London, Department of Health and Social Security, 1969.

Experiments in *rats* indicated that cysteine had a very promising role in the treatment of carbon tetrachloride poisoning; this might be enhanced by its use with more specific antidotes.— E. C. de Ferreyra *et al.*, *Toxic. appl. Pharmac.*, 1974, *27*, 558.

Precautions. Carbon tetrachloride should not be given to patients taking phenobarbitone or other inducers of hepatic enzymes, nor for about 10 days after such treatment.

Absorption and Fate. Carbon tetrachloride is readily absorbed after inhalation. It is also absorbed from the gastro-intestinal tract and through the skin.

Carbon tetrachloride is slowly excreted from the body via the lungs, urine, and faeces.

Uses. Carbon tetrachloride was formerly used in man as an anthelmintic against tapeworms and hookworms in single doses of 2 to 4 ml but it has been superseded by equally effective and less toxic agents. It is used as an anthelmintic in veterinary practice, and has been used for the fumigation of cereals.

It is widely employed in industry as a solvent and degreaser. It was formerly used in certain types of fire extinguisher. It was formerly widely used as an industrial and domestic dry cleaner but it has been largely replaced for this purpose by less toxic cleaners such as trichloroethane and tetrachloroethylene. It should only be used under conditions of adequate ventilation.

Carbon tetrachloride was a simple and effective agent for the destruction of wasps' nests; it was rapidly effective against larvae and adult wasps; 150 to 300 ml were poured or injected, at dusk, into the nest entrance, which was then blocked.— Wasps, *Advis. Leafl. Ministry of Agriculture Fisheries and Food, No. 451*, London, HM Stationery Office, 1965.

768-c

Chenopodium Oil *(B.P.C. 1959)*. Oil of American Wormseed; Aetheroleum Chenopodii; Wurmsamenöl; Esencia de Quenopodio Vermifuga.

CAS — 8006-99-3.

Pharmacopoeias. In *Arg., Ind., It., Mex., Port., Span.*, and *Turk.*

Distilled with steam from the fresh flowering and fruiting plants, excluding roots, of *Chenopodium ambrosioides* var. *anthelminticum.* It contains not less than 65% w/w of ascaridole.

A colourless or pale yellow liquid with a characteristic unpleasant odour and a bitter burning taste. Wt per ml 0.955 to 0.975 g. **Soluble** 1 in 10 of alcohol (70%). **Store** in a cool place in airtight containers. Protect from light.

NOTE. Chenopodium oil may explode when heated.

Adverse Effects. Chenopodium oil may produce headache, vertigo, tinnitus, nausea, vomiting, temporary deafness, and kidney and liver damage. There have been numerous fatalities. Cumulative effects may be produced by small doses given several days apart.

Epidermal necrolysis. Toxic epidermal necrolysis had been reported after the ingestion of chenopodium.— B. Potter *et al.*, *Archs Derm.*, 1960, *82*, 903.

Precautions. It is contra-indicated in pregnancy and in patients with impaired kidney or liver function. It is inadvisable to use it in children, the elderly, or the debilitated.

Uses. Chenopodium oil is an anthelmintic which has been used for the expulsion of roundworms (*Ascaris*) and hookworms but it has been largely superseded for this purpose by less toxic compounds. The usual dose was 0.6 ml, in a capsule, on an empty stomach, followed 2 hours later by a similar dose, and 2 hours after this by a saline purgative.

It was recommended that chenopodium herb be prohibited for use as a flavouring agent.— *Report on the Review of Flavourings in Food*, FAC/REP/22, London, HM Stationery Office, 1976.

769-k

Cucurbita *(B.P.C. 1934)*. Melon Pumpkin Seeds; Pepo; Semence de Courge; Kürbissame; Abóbora.

Pharmacopoeias. In *Port.* which permits other species of *Cucurbita.*

The fresh seeds of *Cucurbita maxima* (Cucurbitaceae).

Uses. Cucurbita has been used for the expulsion of tapeworms (*Taenia*).

After administration of a saline purge, the seeds (deprived of testa and tegmen, and bruised) mixed with water or milk to a creamy consistence are given as a single dose; after several hours, a purgative dose of castor oil is given. Doses of 100 to 400 g or more have been used.

770-w

Desaspidin. 3′-[(5-Butyryl-2,4-dihydroxy-3,3-dimethyl-6-oxocyclohexa-1,4-dien-1-yl)methyl]-2′,6′-dihydroxy-4′-methoxybutyrophenone.

$C_{24}H_{30}O_8$=446.5.

CAS — 114-43-2.

A phloroglucinol derivative obtained from the Finnish broad buckler-fern, *Dryopteris austriaca* (Polypodiaceae). It has also been found in the American aspidium, or marginal fern, *D. marginalis*, but *not* in Swiss and Austrian samples of *D. austriaca.*

Uses. Desaspidin has been used as an anthelmintic in a dose of 200 mg against the fish tapeworm, *Diphyllobothrium latum.*

771-e

Dichlorophen *(B.P., B.P. Vet.)*. Di-phenthane-70; G 4. 2,2′-Methylenebis(4-chlorophenol).

$C_{13}H_{10}Cl_2O_2$=269.1.

CAS — 97-23-4.

Pharmacopoeias. In *Aust.* and *Br.*

A white or slightly cream-coloured powder with a not more than slightly phenolic odour and a saline and phenolic taste. M.p. about 175°. Practically **insoluble** in water; soluble 1 in 1 of alcohol and 1 in less than 1 of ether.

Adverse Effects. Dichlorophen may cause nausea, vomiting, gastro-intestinal colic, and diarrhoea. In some patients it has produced an urticarial rash. Jaundice has occurred after a large dose.

Of 100 patients with allergic contact dermatitis, 2 gave positive reactions to patch testing with dichlorophen 1% in soft paraffin.— A. A. Fisher *et al.*, *Archs Derm.*, 1971, *104*, 286.

Further references: W. F. Schorr, *Archs Derm.*, 1970, *102*, 515; *Med. J. Aust.*, 1973, *1*, 35.

Treatment of Adverse Effects. In gross overdosage gastric lavage should be followed by symptomatic treatment.

Precautions. Dichlorophen is contra-indicated in the presence of impaired liver function and in conditions in which purgation is undesirable, such as during the last few months of pregnancy, in acute fevers, or in severe heart disease.

Alkalis and alcoholic beverages should be avoided during treatment with dichlorophen.

Uses. Dichlorophen is an anthelmintic used in the treatment of infection by tapeworms (*Diphyllobothrium latum* and *Taenia saginata*) and dwarf tapeworm (*Hymenolepis nana*). It has also been used in the treatment of infection by the pork tapeworm (*T. solium*) when suitable measures were taken against any cysticercosis, see below.

It has a direct lethal action on the tapeworm. After the tapeworm has been killed, the segments are partially digested in the intestine and the scolex is therefore generally unrecognisable.

The usual dose for adults is 6 g and for children 2 to 4 g on each of 2 or 3 successive days. Alternatively, 2 to 3 g may be given thrice in 24 hours with 1 to 2 g thrice in 24 hours for children. A single dose of 9 g has been used in mass treatment.

Dichlorophen is best given in the morning on an empty stomach as the dose is usually followed in 2 to 3 hours by intestinal colic and the passing of a few loose stools. Vomiting occurs occasionally and there is the theoretical possibility that segments or ova regurgitated into the stomach could cause cysticercosis if used for *T. solium.* This risk may be reduced by giving an anti-emetic before treatment and a purgative after treatment to clear the colon.

Dichlorophen is used against tapeworms in animals, in animal ringworm, as a fungicide, and as a germicide in soaps. The use of dichlorophen in cosmetics and toiletries is restricted under the Cosmetic Products Regulations 1978 (SI 1978: No. 1354).

A review of antimicrobial agents, including dichlorophen, used in cosmetics.— I. R. Gucklhorn, *Mfg Chem.*, 1970, *41* (Nov.), 48.

For the use of dichlorophen to reduce bacterial contamination (especially *Pseudomonas aeruginosa*) in diving chambers during saturation dives (prolonged periods without decompression), see S. R. Alcock, *J. Hyg., Camb.*, 1977, *78*, 395.

Dichlorophen 1.5 to 4 g, or niclosamide 70 to 150 mg per kg body-weight, was given as a single dose to 29 children under 14 years of age who were passing eggs of *Fasciolopsis buski* in faeces. The mean reductions in the egg count obtained after treatment were 83.3% for dichlorophen and 48.5% for niclosamide. Repeat treatment with dichlorophen completely eradicated the infection but repeat treatment with niclosamide did not improve the results.— M. Idris *et al.*, *J. trop. Med. Hyg.*, 1980, *83*, 71.

Preparations

Dichlorophen Tablets *(B.P.)*. Tablets containing dichlorophen.

Proprietary Names

Anthiphen *(May & Baker, S.Afr.)*; Ovis *(Warner, Ger.)*; Plath-Lyse *(Génévrier, Fr.)*; Wespuril *(Spitzner, Ger.)*.

Dichlorophen was formerly marketed in Great Britain under the proprietary name Anthiphen (*May & Baker*).

772-l

Diethylcarbamazine Citrate *(B.P., B.P. Vet., U.S.P.)*. Diethylcarbam. Cit.; RP 3799; Diethylcarbamazini Citras; Ditrazini Citras; Diethylcarbamazine Acid Citrate. *NN*-Diethyl-4-methylpiperazine-1-carboxamide dihydrogen citrate.

$C_{10}H_{21}N_3O,C_6H_8O_7$=391.4.

CAS — 90-89-1 (diethylcarbamazine); 1642-54-2 (citrate).

Pharmacopoeias. In *Arg., Br., Braz., Chin., Cz., Fr., Ind., Int., Jap., Nord., Rus.*, and *U.S.*

A white, crystalline, slightly hygroscopic powder, odourless or with a slight odour and a bitter acid taste. M.p. 136° to 141°.

Very **soluble** in water; soluble 1 in 35 of alcohol; practically insoluble in acetone, chloroform, and ether. A 6.29% w/v solution is iso-osmotic with serum. Solutions for injection are **sterilised** by autoclaving or filtration. **Store** in airtight containers. Solutions should be protected from light.

A solution of diethylcarbamazine in water iso-osmotic with serum (6.29%) caused 100% haemolysis of erythrocytes cultured in it for 45 minutes. The solution turned dark brown.— E. R. Hammarlund and K. Pedersen-Bjergaard, *J. pharm. Sci.*, 1961, *50*, 24.

Adverse Effects. Anorexia, nausea and vomiting, headache, dizziness, and drowsiness occur but are seldom severe enough to cause discontinuance of treatment. Allergic reactions can occur due to release of foreign proteins in the tissues by the death of microfilariae, larvae, or adult worms, and are especially prominent in onchocerciasis and in *Brugia malayi* infections. Encephalitis and retinal haemorrhage may occur in patients with loaiasis and is probably due to massive lysis of microfilariae.

In patients, especially children, with heavy roundworm (*Ascaris*) infection, acute abdominal symptoms may occur.

Of 291 986 persons in Bombay State who were given mass treatment with diethylcarbamazine, 29% complained of reactions; these were less severe in children.— T. B. Patel and P. D. Paranjpey, *Indian J. Malar.*, 1958, *12*, 171, per *Trop. Dis. Bull.*, 1959, *56*, 751.

A child developed acute respiratory distress within 30 minutes of taking 12.5 mg of diethylcarbamazine for *Onchocerca volvulus* infection, despite the prophylactic use of betamethasone.— H. Fuglsang and J. Anderson (letter), *Trans. R. Soc. trop. Med. Hyg.*, 1974, *68*, 72.

Mobilisation of microfilariae of *Onchocerca volvulus* into the CSF during treatment with diethylcarbamazine caused severe vertigo in 6 patients and a parkinsonian condition in 1.— B. O. L. Duke *et al.*, *Tropenmed.*

Parasit., 1976, *27*, 123, per *Trop. Dis. Bull.*, 1977, *74*, 84.

Multiple reactions occurred in 9 Nigerian patients with severe untreated onchocerciasis given diethylcarbamazine 100 mg. Individual susceptibility could not be predicted. Treatment should start in hospital or at least patients should remain recumbent for 48 hours.— A. D. M. Bryceson *et al.*, *Br. med. J.*, 1977, *1*, 742.

A discussion on inflammatory reactions in onchocerciasis, including the reactions to diethylcarbamazine citrate and other filaricidal drugs.— P. M. Henson *et al.*, *Bull. Wld Hlth Org.*, 1979, *57*, 667.

Effects on the eyes. For comments on the severe adverse effects on the eyes associated with the destruction of ocular microfilariae, see under Uses (Onchocerciasis), below.

Effects on the kidneys. A report of significant proteinuria in patients with moderate onchocerciasis receiving diethylcarbamazine topically or by mouth for periods of 4 to 6 months.— B. M. Greene *et al.* (letter), *Lancet*, 1980, *1*, 254. Similar findings.— J. L. Ngu *et al.* (letter), *ibid.*, 710.

Fatality. Seven patients, whose general condition was poor, lapsed into irreversible coma after being given diethylcarbamazine, 225 to 900 mg in 3 to 8 days, for onchocerciasis. Death followed 1 to 4 days later.— A. P. Oomen (letter), *Trans. R. Soc. trop. Med. Hyg.*, 1969, *63*, 548.

Treatment of Adverse Effects. The allergic reactions occurring during treatment with diethylcarbamazine citrate may be diminished by the concomitant administration of antihistamines or corticosteroids.

In acute overdosage the stomach should be emptied by aspiration and lavage and the patient treated symptomatically.

Precautions. Diethylcarbamazine should be used cautiously in reduced dosage for the mass treatment of populations where onchocerciasis is common, because allergic reactions may involve the eyes and require the administration of corticosteroids. Special care should also be taken in using diethylcarbamazine in areas where both onchocerciasis and loaiasis occur.

In patients taking diethylcarbamazine citrate, the sensitivity of filarial skin tests using extracts of *Wuchereria bancrofti* was reduced.— J. C. Katiyar *et al.* (letter), *Trans. R. Soc. trop. Med. Hyg.*, 1974, *68*, 169. Similar results with skin tests using *Brugia malayi*.— P. K. Murthy *et al.*, *Indian J. med. Res.*, 1978, *68*, 428, per *Trop. Dis. Bull.*, 1979, *76*, 1029.

The use of diethylcarbamazine 2 mg per kg body-weight as a provocative day test for the detection of microfilariae of nocturnally periodic *Wuchereria bancrofti* in the blood, was not suitable in the presence of onchocerciasis or loaiasis.— J. E. McMahon *et al.*, *Bull. Wld Hlth Org.*, 1979, *57*, 759.

Absorption and Fate. Diethylcarbamazine citrate is readily absorbed from the gastro-intestinal tract and is excreted mainly as metabolites in the urine.

References.— G. H. Rée *et al.*, *Trans. R. Soc. trop. Med. Hyg.*, 1977, *71*, 542.

Uses. Diethylcarbamazine citrate is used in the treatment of filariasis, particularly when due to *Wuchereria bancrofti* or *Loa loa*. It is also used in onchocerciasis and *Brugia malayi* infections, but with care because of the more prominent risk of allergic reactions.

It has been used successfully in the treatment of tropical eosinophilia and it is sometimes of value in the early stages of elephantiasis if there is still evidence of microfilarial infection. It has been used in the treatment of roundworm (*Ascaris*) infection.

In the treatment of *W. bancrofti* infections with diethylcarbamazine the number of microfilariae in peripheral blood is rapidly reduced. In some patients microfilariae do not recur, suggesting a lethal or sterilising effect on adult female worms. Local reactions, sometimes with abscess formation, sometimes appear at the sites which commonly harbour adult worms.

In loaiasis, both microfilariae and adult worms are killed. In onchocerciasis, the microfilariae are killed but the adult worms are not significantly affected.

Diethylcarbamazine citrate is usually administered by mouth as tablets. In the treatment of filarial infections due to *W. bancrofti*, *B. malayi*, *O. volvulus*, and *Loa loa* the usual dose of diethylcarbamazine citrate is 6 mg per kg body-weight daily in 3 divided doses for 3 weeks. In order to reduce the incidence and severity of allergic reactions due to the destruction of microfilariae, particularly in the treatment of onchocerciasis and malayan filariasis an initial dosage of 1 mg per kg daily in divided doses is recommended, gradually increased to 6 mg per kg daily over 3 days or longer. Similar doses are recommended for children.

In onchocerciasis a course of suramin may be given to kill the adult worms, followed by a further short course of diethylcarbamazine citrate. For further details, see under Onchocerciasis, below.

In the prophylaxis of bancroftian and malayan filariasis a dose of 50 mg monthly is recommended, and in the prophylaxis of loaiasis a dose of 4 mg per kg body-weight for 3 successive days each month is recommended.

In tropical eosinophilia, 6 to 12 mg per kg daily for 5 to 10 days has been employed.

Diethylcarbamazine citrate has also been given by intramuscular injection.

Diethylcarbamazine base ($C_{10}H_{21}N_3O$ = 199.3) is used in veterinary practice.

No significant advances had been made in the treatment of filariasis in recent years and diethylcarbamazine was still the only drug used in mass treatment. Results had been good in Polynesia but disappointing in India. For individuals diethylcarbamazine citrate, 4 to 6 mg per kg body-weight daily in single or divided doses after meals for 14 to 21 days was commonly used. For mass treatment of *Brugia malayi* a total of at least 36 mg per kg should be given to at least 80% of a population and for *W. bancrofti* 72 mg per kg. The addition of diethylcarbamazine to salt or school drinks had not been tried on a large scale. Mass treatment could not be used in areas where *Loa loa* or *Onchocerca volvulus* were common because individual reactions could be severe; initial doses should be reduced and given with corticosteroids. Infection with *Dipetalonema streptocerca* in West Africa could be treated with diethylcarbamazine citrate 200 mg daily.— Third Report of a WHO Expert Committee on Filariasis, *Tech. Rep. Ser. Wld Hlth Org. No. 542*, 1974.

Twelve single doses of 6 mg per kg body-weight were used to treat bancroftian filariasis. Administration at weekly intervals was preferable to a daily or alternate day schedule.— R. M. Sundaram *et al.*, *J. Commun. Dis.*, 1974, *6*, 290, per *Trop. Dis. Bull.*, 1975, *72*, 737.

A report of declining infection with malayan filariasis in a Korean community in which infected persons were treated yearly with diethylcarbamazine for 4 years.— B. S. Seo and K. I. Whang, *Korean J. Parasit.*, 1974, *12*, 21, per *Trop. Dis. Bull.*, 1975, *72*, 458.

It was considered that subperiodic *Wuchereria bancrofti* filariasis might not respond to diethylcarbamazine in the same manner as the nocturnally periodic type.— P. F. Weller and E. A. Ottesen, *Trans. R. Soc. trop. Med. Hyg.*, 1978, *72*, 31.

Reduction of carrier-rates in patients infected with *W. bancrofti*, following single doses of diethylcarbamazine (400 mg for men, 300 mg for women) given at yearly intervals for 3 years.— J. Laigret *et al.*, *Bull. Wld Hlth Org.*, 1978, *56*, 985.

From the results of a study of filariasis control using diethylcarbamazine it was considered that daily doses of 6 mg per kg body-weight given for 12 days was the best regimen for large-scale control.— C. K. Rao *et al.*, *J. Commun. Dis.*, 1978, *10*, 194, per *Trop. Dis. Bull.*, 1980, *77*, 131.

Diethylcarbamazine had no microfilaricidal action against *Mansonella ozzardi* in 8 subjects studied.— C. F. Bartholomew *et al.*, *Trans. R. Soc. trop. Med. Hyg.*, 1978, *72*, 423.

The microfilaria rate of *Brugia timori* was drastically reduced in an Indonesian population after mass treatment with a total of diethylcarbamazine 50 mg per kg body-weight given over 9 days followed by selective re-treatment for 4 days 1 year later.— F. Partono *et al.*, *Trans. R. Soc. trop. Med. Hyg.*, 1979, *73*, 536.

A discussion on filariasis. Diethylcarbamazine remains the treatment of choice but is not easy to administer because of the necessity for repeated doses and the serious side reactions such as lymphangitis, lymphadenitis, and fever, which occur in many people when the adult worms are killed.— G. S. Nelson, *New Engl. J. Med.*, 1979, *300*, 1136.

Asthma. A daily dose of diethylcarbamazine citrate, 10 mg per kg body-weight, was given to 15 asthmatic patients whose condition had been intractable with other treatment and improvement followed in 14 patients within 24 hours. One complained of nausea and vomiting, which were overcome without loss of efficacy by reducing the daily dose to 7 mg per kg. It was suggested that diethylcarbamazine might with advantage replace corticosteroids in some asthmatic patients.— M. S. Mallén, *Ann. Allergy*, 1965, *23*, 534.

No elucidation of any mode of action in bronchial asthma was found in studies of the effects of diethylcarbamazine on smooth muscle *in vitro*.— A. K. Abaitey and J. R. Parratt, *J. Pharm. Pharmac.*, 1977, *29*, 428.

Onchocerciasis. In 9 patients with onchocerciasis, the instillation 4 times daily of diethylcarbamazine 3% eye-drops tended to reduce the number of microfilariae in the anterior chamber and led to an invasion of the cornea by microfilariae. Three patients with heavy infection developed anterior uveitis; itching, conjunctival injection, lid swelling, and skin eruptions were also observed.— J. Anderson and H. Fuglsang, *Trans. R. Soc. trop. Med. Hyg.*, 1973, *67*, 710.

Mass therapy with diethylcarbamazine for onchocerciasis in a hyperendemic zone caused only slight decrease in the prevalence of the infection but appreciable reduction in the intensity of the infection. The original plan, to give 25 mg twice daily gradually increased to 200 mg twice daily followed by maintenance dosage with 50 mg weekly, was abandoned owing to severe side-effects with about 20 subjects suffering a severe toxic and allergic reaction. Self-medication was then taken at an amended dose of 25 mg in the first week and 50 mg weekly thereafter.— A. Rougemont *et al.*, *Bull. Wld Hlth Org.*, 1976, *54*, 403.

In a follow-up study of 100 patients in London with onchocerciasis, treatment with a single course of diethylcarbamazine in doses increased to 9 mg per kg body-weight daily for 3 weeks gave apparent cures in 48% of patients. The remainder of patients required further courses of treatment.— G. H. Rée, *Br. J. Derm.*, 1977, *97*, 551.

In a study of 54 heavily infected patients with ocular onchocerciasis a successful treatment regimen with reduced side-effects consisted of diethylcarbamazine citrate 25 mg on day 1, slowly increasing to 150 to 200 mg twice daily on days 8 to 14, betamethasone 1.5 mg twice daily for 2 days prior to starting diethylcarbamazine and during the increasing dosage, followed by suramin normally 1 g weekly for 3 to 5 weeks. Young or underweight patients had the dosages adjusted.— J. Anderson and H. Fuglsang, *Br. J. Ophthal.*, 1978, *62*, 450. If such a complex regimen proves safe and effective, there would be considerable logistic difficulties in delivering this treatment to large populations.— A. C. Bird *et al.*, *ibid.*, 1980, *64*, 191.

In onchocerciasis, diethylcarbamazine citrate caused transient mobilisation of microfilariae into the blood, CSF, sputum, and urine. In the cornea microfilariae were killed, after an initial reaction, in 24 to 48 hours; disappearance from the anterior chamber might take a few days longer. Rare increases in intra-ocular pressure could be controlled by acetazolamide. Established posterior lesions were not responsive. Treatment usually lasted 1 to 3 weeks; weekly maintenance doses of 50 to 200 mg were effective but because of skin reactions were not usually acceptable. A 1- to 2-week course of diethylcarbamazine was best followed with 4 to 7 weekly injections of suramin and then, after 1 to 4 weeks, with a further 3- to 7-day course of diethylcarbamazine. Careful medical supervision was essential.— B. Thylefors, *Bull. Wld Hlth Org.*, 1978, *56*, 63.

Beneficial results in onchocerciasis using topical diethylcarbamazine applied as a 1 or 2% lotion.— M. E. Langham *et al.*, *Tropenmed. Parasit.*, 1978, *29*, 156. Administration of diethylcarbamazine citrate to 18 men with onchocerciasis who were moderately to heavily infected, eliminated or considerably reduced microfilariae from skin snips, but was associated with a high incidence of posterior segment changes and associated visual field defects. Follow-up is required to determine whether these field defects are transient or permanent.— A. C. Bird *et al.* (letter), *Lancet*, 1979, *2*, 46. In patients heavily infected with *Onchocerca volvulus*, daily application of a lotion containing diethylcarbamazine citrate 1% did not result in the dramatic reduction of microfilarial counts found by A.C. Bird *et al.* in similarly infected patients from the same area given standard oral doses; in less heavily infected patients the response was variable and only rarely were microfilariae eliminated from the skin snips. Side-effects included severe skin reactions in the area of application, and systemic reactions in the heavily infected patients that were more severe and prolonged than in those recorded by A.C. Bird *et al.* following standard doses by mouth. Microfilaricidal effects were not, however, seen in the eyes of even those with heavily parasitised corneas in whom lotion had been applied to the whole body, including the face. Therefore, although the results of M.E. Langham *et al.* cannot be confirmed, in view of the findings of A.C. Bird *et al.*, further assessment of alternative therapy with diethylcarbamazine citrate is justified.— D. B. A. Hutchinson *et al.* (letter), *ibid.* Results of a double-blind comparative 6-month study in 20 men with moderately severe infection with *Onchocerca volvulus* and no significant visual impairment, comparing oral and topical diethylcarbamazine therapy. Ten of the men received diethylcarbamazine citrate as tablets in a dose of 50 mg on the first day, 50 mg thrice daily for the following 7 days, 50 mg thrice daily on one day a week for the next 2 months, and 100 mg twice daily on one day a week thereafter. The other 10 men had daily applications of 15 ml of a lotion containing diethylcarbamazine citrate 2%, for 8 days, and weekly applications thereafter. Those receiving active tablets also had placebo lotion and those receiving active lotion also had placebo tablets. Mean microfilarial skin-snip counts fell in both groups but the count in the tablet group fell more rapidly and to a lower value. Side-effects included lymphadenopathy in all patients, and skin rashes which were more common and more severe in those receiving the lotion; proteinuria was noted in some patients, and pruritus occurred in 9 of the patients receiving lotion and 4 receiving tablets; ocular reactions were at least as frequent following topical therapy. It was concluded that weekly diethylcarbamazine suppresses microfiliarial counts, as measured by skin-snip tests, and that long-term oral diethylcarbamazine given weekly might prevent the ocular complications of onchocerciasis, but that the means of avoiding the side-effects with long-term therapy must be achieved before a mass programme can be implemented. Oral diethylcarbamazine is more effective and produces fewer and milder side-effects than topical diethylcarbamazine when both are given weekly.— H. R. Taylor *et al.*, *Lancet*, 1980, *1*, 943. A view based on experience on this and another study, and with reference to studies by other workers, that the oral use of diethylcarbamazine may lead to serious visual damage in onchocerciasis patients, whereas, using topical diethylcarbamazine to eliminate microfilariae from the skin there is a net movement from the eye; thus ocular tissues are protected from the damage resulting from death of microfilariae in the eye.— M. E. Langham (letter), *ibid.*, 977. Comment on the use of diethylcarbamazine citrate lotion for onchocerciasis.— *Lancet*, 1980, *2*, 1232.

The only rational management of onchocerciasis avoiding the use of suramin is to give an initial intensive course of treatment with diethylcarbamazine followed by weekly doses. The initial course will kill almost all the microfilariae, but the adult worms will stay alive; therefore, in order to keep the microfilarial density in the skin low, without the need to give suramin, diethylcarbamazine is given weekly. Normally, a weekly dose of 200 mg is quite sufficient; it should be continued for 10 years.— D. Bell (letter), *Br. med. J.*, 1979, *1*, 1213.

Further references: J. Sowa and S. C. I. Sowa, *Ann. trop. Med. Parasit.*, 1978, *72*, 79 (in children), per *Trop. Dis. Bull.*, 1978, *75*, 1119.

For a favourable report of mebendazole compared with diethylcarbamazine in onchocerciasis, see Mebendazole, p.99.

Toxocariasis. Treatment of infection due to *Toxocara canis* and *T. cati* with diethylcarbamazine citrate, 3 mg per kg body-weight daily for 21 days could provide symptomatic improvement.— *Lancet*, 1972, *1*, 730. See also P. M. Schantz and L. T. Glickman, *New Engl. J. Med.*, 1978, *298*, 436.

Diethylcarbamazine, 3 mg per kg body-weight thrice daily for 21 days was used successfully in 21 patients with eye infections due to *Toxocara canis* or *T. cati*, which without such diagnosis would have been confused with the presence of retinoblastoma requiring removal of the affected eye.— A. W. Woodruff, *Trans. R. Soc. trop. Med. Hyg.*, 1973, *67*, 755.

Tropical eosinophilia. Diethylcarbamazine citrate, 5 mg per kg body-weight daily by mouth for 7 days, or 3 mg per kg intramuscularly then 6 mg per kg on the 3rd and 5th days, was compared with carbarsone, 250 mg thrice daily for 10 days, in patients with tropical pulmonary eosinophilia. Response occurred in 8 to 10 days in 15 of 18 given injections, in up to 14 days in 10 of 16 given diethylcarbamazine by mouth, and in 8 of 16 given carbarsone.— R. N. Dutta and S. C. Kapoor, *Armed Forces med. J. India*, 1970, *26*, 175, per *Trop. Dis. Bull.*, 1971, *68*, 887.

Preparations

Diethylcarbamazine Citrate Tablets *(U.S.P.)*. Tablets containing diethylcarbamazine citrate. Store in airtight containers.

Diethylcarbamazine Tablets *(B.P.)*. Diethylcarbam. Tab. Tablets containing diethylcarbamazine citrate.

Proprietary Preparations

Banocide *(Wellcome, UK)*. Diethylcarbamazine citrate, available as scored tablets of 50 mg.

Hetrazan *(Lederle, UK)*. Diethylcarbamazine citrate, available as scored tablets of 50 mg. (Also available as Hetrazan in *Austral., Ger., Neth., Switz., USA*).

Other Proprietary Names

Notézine *(Fr.)*.

773-y

Diphenan *(B.P. 1953)*. Carbaurine. 4-Benzylphenyl carbamate.
$C_{14}H_{13}NO_2$=227.3.

CAS — 101-71-3.

A white, odourless, tasteless, crystalline powder. Practically **insoluble** in water; sparingly soluble in alcohol.

Uses. Diphenan was formerly used as an anthelmintic for the expulsion of threadworms (*Enterobius*).

774-j

Diphezyl. Difezil. (3-Acetyl-5-chloro-2-hydroxybenzyl)dimethyl(2-phenoxyethyl)ammonium 3-hydroxy-2-naphthoate.
$C_{30}H_{30}ClNO_6$=536.0.

CAS — 34987-38-7.

Uses. Diphezyl has been tried as an anthelmintic for hookworm and whipworm infections.

References: A. I. Krotov *et al.*, *Medskaya Parazit.*, 1969, *38*, 80, per *Trop. Dis. Bull.*, 1969, *66*, 594; G. M. Maruashvili *et al.*, *Medskaya Parazit.*, 1969, *38*, 197, per *Trop. Dis. Bull.*, 1970, *67*, 196; N. V. Grinenko *et al.*, *Medskaya Parazit.*, 1969, *38*, 613, per *Trop. Dis. Bull.*, 1970, *67*, 327.

775-z

Dithiazanine Iodide. 3,3′-Diethylthiadicarbocyanine Iodide. 3-Ethyl-2-[5-(3-ethylbenzothiazol-2(3*H*)-ylidene)penta-1,3-dienyl]benzothiazolium iodide.
$C_{23}H_{23}IN_2S_2$=518.5.

CAS — 7187-55-5 (dithiazanine); 514-73-8 (iodide).

A dark greenish crystalline powder. Practically **insoluble** in water and ether; very slightly soluble in alcohol and methyl alcohol. **Store** in airtight containers.

Adverse Effects. These include nausea, vomiting, diarrhoea, oedema, and fever. It is considered a toxic anthelmintic.

Uses. Dithiazanine iodide is an anthelmintic that has been used against whipworms and strongyloid worms in doses of 100 to 200 mg. It stains the stools a bluish-green colour.

Proprietary Names

Ossiurene *(AMSA, Ital.)*.

776-c

Dymanthine Hydrochloride. Dimantine Hydrochloride; GS 1339. *NN*-Dimethyloctadecylamine hydrochloride.
$C_{20}H_{43}N,HCl$=334.0.

CAS — 124-28-7 (dymanthine); 1613-17-8 (hydrochloride).

Adverse Effects. These include nausea, vomiting, diarrhoea, headache, vertigo, and sleep disturbances.

Uses. Dymanthine hydrochloride is an anthelmintic reported to be effective against hookworm (*Ancylostoma* and *Necator*), roundworms (*Ascaris*), dwarf tapeworms, threadworms (*Enterobius*), and whipworms. The citrate and embonate have also been used.

References: J. E. Lynch and J. E. Margison, *Curr. ther. Res.*, 1963, *5*, 279; S. K. Sama *et al.*, *Am. J. trop. Med. Hyg.*, 1967, *16*, 170, per *Trop. Dis. Bull.*, 1968, *65*, 158; L. J. Llanozas Herrera, *Acta méd. venez.*, 1967, *14*, 179, per *Trop. Dis. Bull.*, 1968, *65*, 439.

777-k

Embelia *(B.P.C. 1934)*. Vidang.

CAS — 550-24-3 (embelic acid).

Pharmacopoeias. In *Ind.*

The dried fruits of *Embelia ribes* and *E. robusta* (= *E. tsjeriamcottam*) (Myrsinaceae), containing about 2.5% of embelic acid (embelin). **Store** in a cool dry place.

Uses. Embelia has been used in India and other eastern countries in doses of 4 to 16 g for the expulsion of tapeworms. As it is only slightly laxative, it should be followed by a purgative.

778-a

Fenbendazole. Hoe 881V. Methyl 5-phenylthio-1*H*-benzimidazol-2-ylcarbamate.
$C_{15}H_{13}N_3O_2S$=299.3.

CAS — 43210-67-9.

Uses. Fenbendazole is a benzimidazole anthelmintic structurally related to thiabendazole (see p.107). It is also used in veterinary practice.

Fenbendazole in doses of 1 to 1.5 g was effective in roundworm (*Ascaris*) infection and, in doses of 1.5 g, in whipworm (*Trichuris*) infection; it was not effective in *Necator* infection.— K. Bruch and J. Haas, *Ann. trop. Med. Parasit.*, 1976, *70*, 205, per *Trop. Dis. Bull.*, 1976, *73*, 936.

Fenbendazole was not teratogenic in *rats*, but the mitotic index was increased.— P. Delatour and Y. Richard, *Thérapie*, 1976, *31*, 505.

Fenbendazole 100 mg given every 12 hours for 3 days was effective for the treatment of infection with *Trichuris trichiura, Necator americanus,* and *Ascaris lumbricoides* but was ineffective for the treatment of *Strongyloides stercoralis*.— C. Sánchez-Carrillo and F. Beltrán-Hernández, *Salud públ. Méx.*, 1977, *19*, 691, per *Trop. Dis. Bull.*, 1979, *76*, 676.

Manufacturers

Hoechst, UK.

779-t

Furapromidium. F 30066. *N*-Isopropyl-3-(5-nitro-2-furyl)acrylamide.
$C_{10}H_{12}N_2O_4$=224.2.

CAS — 1951-56-0.

Pharmacopoeias. In *Chin.*

Adverse Effects. These include gastro-intestinal disturbances, dizziness, weakness, muscular spasm, and mild psychiatric changes.

Uses. Furapromidium is a schistosomicide reported to be effective against *Schistosoma japonicum* and in the treatment of clonorchiasis. F 30069, an analogue of furapromidium, has been tried in schistosomiasis.

For reports on the uses of furapromidium and of F 30069, see H. H. Lei *et al.*, *Chin. med. J.*, 1963, *82*, 90; J. K. Hsü *et al.*, *ibid.*, 92; H. C. Chou *et al.*, *ibid.*, 1965, *84*, 591; C. N. Wang *et al.*, *ibid.*, 672.

Concomitant use, in *Schistosoma japonicum*, with metriphonate suppositories to mobilise flukes to the liver for attack there by furapromidium.— Shanghai Furapromidium Research Coordinating Group, *Chin. med. J.*, 1977, *3*, 103, per *Trop. Dis. Bull.*, 1977, *74*, 933.

A report of 2 patients with clonorchiasis successfully treated with hexachloroparaxylene with furapromidium.— X. Zhipiao *et al.*, *Chin. med. J.*, 1979, *92*, 423, per *Trop. Dis. Bull.*, 1980, *77*, 64.

780-l

Hexachloroethane *(B. Vet. C. 1965).*
C_2Cl_6=236.7.

CAS — 67-72-1.

Pharmacopoeias. In *Aust., Cz.,* and *Nord.*

Colourless or nearly colourless, almost tasteless crystals or crystalline powder with a camphoraceous odour. Practically **insoluble** in water; soluble 1 in 20 of alcohol; very soluble in ether and tetrachloroethylene.

Uses. Hexachloroethane has been used in veterinary medicine as an anthelmintic in liver-fluke (*Fasciola*) infection. It is also active against *Haemonchus* worms in the stomach, but it is ineffective against intestinal helminths, including tapeworms.

781-y

Hexachloroparaxylene. Chloxyle; Hexachloroparaxylol. 1,4-Bis(trichloromethyl)benzene.
$C_8H_4Cl_6$=312.8.

CAS — 68-36-0.

A white tasteless crystalline solid with a slight aromatic odour. M.p. 107° to 111°. Practically **insoluble** in water; soluble in alcohol, acetone, chloroform, ether, light petroleum, and fixed vegetable oils.

Adverse Effects. Adverse effects reported during the use of hexachloroparaxylene include cardiac arrhythmias, gastro-intestinal disturbances, haemolysis, and visual hallucinations.

A review of 37 patients with hexachloroparaxylene-induced haemolysis, most of whom appeared to have an underlying blood disorder. All the patients had received hexachloroparaxylene 50 mg per kg body-weight daily for 7 to 10 days. Haemolysis occurred during treatment in 27 patients and within one month of treatment in the other 10. One patient had received one course of treatment without adverse effect but developed haemolysis after a second course.— J. Liu *et al., Chin. med. J.,* 1979, *92,* 286.

Uses. Hexachloroparaxylene has been used in China and the USSR as an anthelmintic. It has been reported to be effective against *Opisthorchis sinensis.*

Excellent results, with no significant side-effects, had been achieved in patients with clonorchiasis given hexachloroparaxylene 30 mg per kg body-weight daily for 10 days, or every other day for 10 doses.— W. H. Jopling (letter), *Br. med. J.,* 1975, *3,* 767. See also *idem,* 1978, *1,* 1346.

Other references: N. M. Komarova and T. N. Sadkova, *Medskaya Parazit.,* 1971, *40,* 397; Z. S. Yaldygian *et al., ibid.,* 401, per *Trop. Dis. Bull.,* 1971, *68,* 1352; *Br. med. J.,* 1973, *2,* 543; N. N. Ozeretskovskaya *et al., Medskaya Parazit.,* 1973, *42,* 581, per *Trop. Dis. Bull.,* 1974, *71,* 168.

782-j

Hexylresorcinol *(B.P., U.S.P.).* Hexylresorc.; Esilresorcina. 4-Hexylbenzene-1,3-diol.

$C_{12}H_{18}O_2$=194.3.

CAS — 136-77-6.

Pharmacopoeias. In *Arg., Aust., Br., Braz., It., Mex., Nord., Swiss,* and *U.S.*

White or yellowish-white, acicular crystals, crystalline plates, or crystalline powder with a pungent odour and a sharp, astringent, numbing taste. It acquires a brownish-pink tint on exposure to light and air. M.p. 62° to 68°.
Soluble 1 in 2000 of water; freely soluble in alcohol, chloroform, ether, glycerol, methyl alcohol, and fixed oils; very slightly soluble in light petroleum. **Incompatible** with alkalis and oxidising agents.
Store in airtight containers. Protect from light.

CAUTION. *Hexylresorcinol is irritating to the oral mucosa, to the respiratory tract, and to the skin; alcoholic solutions have vesicant properties.*

Adverse Effects. High concentrations of hexylresorcinol are irritant and corrosive.

Precautions. Hexylresorcinol should be given with care to patients with peptic ulcer or inflammation of the gastro-intestinal tract.

Absorption and Fate. Hexylresorcinol is partially absorbed from the gastro-intestinal tract; about 30% of a dose by mouth is rapidly excreted in the urine, the remainder in the faeces.

Uses. Hexylresorcinol is an anthelmintic active against roundworms (*Ascaris*) and dwarf tapeworms. It is also active against hookworms (*Ancylostoma* and *Necator*), threadworms (*Enterobius*), whipworms (*Trichuris*), and the giant intestinal fluke (*Fasciolopsis buski*). It has been generally superseded by newer drugs. Hexylresorcinol is administered by mouth as a single dose of 1 g for an adult. A dose of 100 mg per year of age, up to 10 years, has been suggested for children. A saline purgative should be given 2 hours after the dose and no food should be allowed for 5 hours. The treatment may be repeated after 3 to 7 days, if necessary.
For the expulsion of hookworms, 3 courses of treatment at intervals of 3 days may be necessary.
For the expulsion of dwarf tapeworms, treatment may be given weekly for 3 weeks to ensure that auto-infection does not occur. In the treatment of whipworm infection hexylresorcinol has also been used as a 0.2 to 0.4% retention enema suspended in 500 to 700 ml of water with either tragacanth or kaolin and retained for at least 30 minutes. The enema may be used on 2 successive days. Prior protection of the anal area with soft paraffin is necessary to prevent skin damage.
Hexylresorcinol has disinfectant properties and is active in both acid and alkaline media.
Externally, a 0.1% solution of hexylresorcinol in a 30% solution of glycerol in water was formerly used as a disinfectant for the skin and mucous membranes, for the treatment of superficial wounds and abrasions and, diluted with water, as a gargle or spray. Lozenges of hexylresorcinol have been used in the treatment of throat infections.
Hexylresorcinol has been used as a spermicide in contraceptive creams and pessaries.

Hexylresorcinol is considered to be the drug of choice in the treatment of *Fasciolopsis buski* infections. The recommended single dose for adults and children of 13 years of age is 1 g. Paediatric doses are: one to 7 years, 400 mg; 8 years, 500 mg; 9 years, 600 mg; 10 years, 700 mg; 11 years, 800 mg; 12 years, 900 mg.— *Med. Lett.,* 1979, *21,* 105.

Preparations

Hexylresorcinol Pills *(U.S.P.).* Pills with a rupture-resistant coating that is dispersible in the digestive tract.

Proprietary Names

Oxana *(Biologici Italia, Ital.).*

783-z

Hycanthone Mesylate. Win 24933; Hydroxylucanthone Methanesulphonate. 1-(2-Diethylaminoethylamino)-4-hydroxymethylthioxanthen-9-one methanesulphonate.

$C_{20}H_{24}N_2O_2S,CH_3SO_3H$=452.6.

CAS — 3105-97-3 (hycanthone); 23255-93-8 (mesylate).

Pharmacopoeias. In *Braz.*

A yellow to orange, odourless, crystalline powder with a bitter taste. Hycanthone mesylate 1.27 g is approximately equivalent to 1 g of hycanthone. Very **soluble** in water; freely soluble in alcohol; slightly soluble in chloroform; practically insoluble in ether; soluble in methyl alcohol; very slightly soluble in acetone. A 10% solution in water is stable for at least 24 hours after preparation. **Store** in airtight containers. Protect from light.

Adverse Effects. Nausea and vomiting often occur a few hours after injection, and local induration often occurs at the injection site with tenderness persisting for several days. Abdominal discomfort, headache, dizziness, and myalgia may occur. There have been reports of liver damage, including necrosis; fatalities have occurred. ECG changes, apparently of little clinical significance, have occurred.

When hycanthone was given in a dose of 2 or 3 mg per kg body-weight twice daily for 5 days to 52 patients with *S. mansoni* infections the commonest side-effects were nausea, vomiting, anorexia, vertigo, and headache. Flattening of the S-T segment and the T-wave occurred in the ECG of 13 of 23 patients 1 to 4 weeks after therapy and slight impairment of hepatic function occurred in 3 of 20 patients examined in the first week after treatment.— N. Katz *et al., Am. J. trop. Med. Hyg.,* 1968, *17,* 743, per *Trop. Dis. Bull.,* 1969, *66,* 1134.

In a preliminary study in 39 patients with schistosomiasis who were given a single intramuscular injection of hycanthone 3 mg per kg body-weight, 51% had considerable fall in blood pressure without ECG changes, 43% vomited, 23% had headache, and 15% had giddiness. Symptoms developed after about 3 to 6 hours and lasted until next day. Transaminase values were raised in all of 16 patients studied and markedly raised in 9. A very anaemic boy developed jaundice after 2 days and died.— I. D. Mar *et al., Bull. Soc. méd. Afr. noire Langue franç.,* 1972, *17,* 90, per *Trop. Dis. Bull.,* 1973, *70,* 54.

Psychotic disturbance which responded to treatment was reported in a patient infected with *S. mansoni* following administration of hycanthone 3 mg per kg body-weight by intramuscular injection.— M. P. T. Ferraz *et al., Revta paul. Med.,* 1973, *81,* 275, per *Trop. Dis. Bull.,* 1974, *71,* 164.

ECG changes, of little clinical significance, in 56 of 80 patients given a single dose of hycanthone 2.5 mg per kg body-weight intramuscularly.— L. Takaoka *et al., Revta Inst. Med. trop. S Paulo,* 1976, *18,* 378, per *Trop. Dis. Bull.,* 1977, *74,* 415.

Hepatotoxicity. Toxic hepatitis in 2 patients given hycanthone 2.5 or 3 mg per kg body-weight; massive necrosis of hepatocytes in a patient who died after 4 mg per kg; acute pancreatitis in a patient who died after 2 mg per kg; icterus and cirrhosis in 2 patients after doses of 2.5 and 4 mg per kg.— C. S. Gonçalves *et al., Revta Ass. méd. bras.,* 1977, *23,* 305, per *Trop. Dis. Bull.,* 1978, *75,* 371.

Fatal necrosis of liver cells occurred in 3 children aged 8 to 10 years old, given hycanthone 2.9 to 3.3 mg per kg body-weight intramuscularly for the treatment of schistosomiasis. An 11-year-old patient had abnormally high liver function tests after treatment with 3 mg per kg; a liver biopsy specimen appeared normal but chronic persistent hepatitis was evident 1 year later.— C. Cohen, *Gastroenterology,* 1978, *75,* 103.

Further reports of hepatitis or signs of liver damage: A. S. Cunha *et al., Revta Inst. Med. trop. S Paulo,* 1971, *13,* 213 (1 of 120 patients), per *Trop. Dis. Bull.,* 1971, *68,* 1349; Z. Farid *et al., Br. med. J.,* 1972, *2,* 88 (2 patients); R. P. Marinho *et al., Revta Inst. Med. trop. S Paulo,* 1974, *16,* 54 (one fatality), per *Trop. Dis. Bull.,* 1974, *71,* 1038; R. P. Marinho *et al., Revta Inst. Med. trop. S Paulo,* 1974, *16,* 354 (one fatality), per *Trop. Dis. Bull.,* 1975, *72,* 821; K. Tshiani *et al., Méd. Afr. noire,* 1978, *25,* 85 (2 fatalities), per *Trop. Dis. Bull.,* 1979, *76,* 365.

Absence of liver toxicity in 2723 patients given hycanthone 1 to 3 mg per kg body-weight; 92 received a second dose.— J. A. Cook and P. Jordan, *Ann. trop. Med. Parasit.,* 1976, *70,* 109, per *Trop. Dis. Bull.,* 1976, *73,* 760.

Teratogenic effects. Teratogenic effects occurred in *mice* given hycanthone mesylate 35 or 50 mg per kg body-weight.— J. A. Moore (letter), *Nature,* 1972, *239,* 107.

Hycanthone, 25 or 50 mg per kg body-weight, was toxic to the embryo and teratogenic in *mice* when given in early pregnancy.— S. M. Sieber and R. H. Adamson, *J. Toxic. environ. Hlth,* 1975, *1,* 309.

See also under Precautions.

Precautions. Hycanthone is contra-indicated during pregnancy and in patients with hepatic disease, serious bacterial infection, acute febrile states, or a history of sensitivity to lucanthone or other related drugs.

Phenothiazines and other drugs liable to affect liver function should not be given before or with hycanthone.

Although carcinogenic effect had been shown for hycanthone in cell culture and in *mice* with *S. mansoni* infection, this had not been confirmed by other workers. Until the risks were resolved, hycanthone should not be administered to children or patients with a long life expectancy.— *Med. Lett.*, 1974, *16*, 62.

Hycanthone had been reported to inhibit aldehyde oxidase and to have some antineoplastic activity in *rats*.— S. Archer, *Prog. Drug Res.*, 1974, *18*, 15. Evidence that hycanthone was an alkylating agent.— J. L. Miller and P. B. Hulbert, *J. Pharm. Pharmac.*, 1976, *28*, *Suppl.*, 18P. A study of the strong non-covalent binding of hycanthone to DNA.— M. Jahangir *et al.*, *J. Pharm. Pharmac.*, 1977, *29*, *Suppl.*, 78P.

Hepatorenal failure in 2 patients given hycanthone in doses above 3.5 mg per kg body-weight, with a phenothiazine. Recovery after intensive treatment including haemodialysis and exchange transfusion.— J. C. Kallmeyer *et al.*, *S. Afr. med. J.*, 1977, *51*, 109, per *Trop. Dis. Bull.*, 1977, *74*, 416.

Hycanthone has only a limited genetic effect, if any, on mammalian germinal tissue; however, it proved mutagenic in mammalian somatic cells and induced chromosomal alterations in each system used. In a limited evaluation in 13 patients there was no evidence of chromosome abnormalities found in circulating lymphocytes following a dose of 2.5 mg per kg body-weight. Data available from carcinogenicity studies in *animals* do not permit a definite judgement on the tumorigenic potential of hycanthone.— Epidemiology and Control of Schistosomiasis, Report of a WHO Expert Committee, *Tech. Rep. Ser. Wld Hlth Org. No. 643*, 1980.

For reports of teratogenesis in *mice*, see under Adverse Effects, above.

Further references: D. Clive *et al.*, *Mutat. Res.*, 1972, *14*, 262 (mutagenicity); R. P. Batzinger and E. Beuding, *J. Pharmac. exp. Ther.*, 1977, *200*, 1 (mutagenicity).

Absorption and Fate. Hycanthone mesylate is readily absorbed after intramuscular injection and is rapidly excreted in the bile as conjugated metabolites. Several metabolites are also found in the urine.

Uses. Hycanthone, an active metabolite of lucanthone, is used as a schistosomicide in the individual or mass treatment of infection with *Schistosoma haematobium* and *S. mansoni*. It is given as the mesylate by deep intramuscular injection as a single dose containing the equivalent of 3 mg of hycanthone per kg body-weight, up to a maximum of 200 mg. The injection may be repeated after 1 to 3 months.

There is some experimental evidence of hycanthone possessing antineoplastic activity.

Experimentally induced resistance of *S. mansoni* to hycanthone.— W. B. Jansma *et al.*, *Am. J. trop. Med. Hyg.*, 1977, *26*, 926, per *Trop. Dis. Bull.*, 1978, *75*, 213.

Schistosomiasis. Hycanthone was administered by mouth or by intramuscular injection to 97 patients infected with *S. haematobium* or *S. mansoni*. By mouth the dose was 2.5 mg per kg body-weight daily for 3 or 4 days, and the intramuscular dose was 3 or 3.5 mg per kg, to a maximum of 200 mg, as a single injection. The treatment was as effective as other schistosomicides and there was little difference in the efficacy of the different dosages and routes of administration employed. Six women who were pregnant during the trial gave birth to normal infants.— V. de V. Clarke *et al.*, *Cent. Afr. J. Med.*, 1969, *15*, 1, per *Abstr. Wld Med.*, 1969, *43*, 662.

When hycanthone was given in various dosage regimens (as enteric coated tablets or intramuscularly as the mesylate or sulphamate) to patients infected with *S. mansoni*, clinical improvement occurred in most patients a few weeks after treatment. Side-effects, mainly headache and gastro-intestinal symptoms, were more marked when treatment was given by mouth than when given intramuscularly and necessitated withdrawal of treatment in 6 of 86 patients treated by mouth. The most satisfactory regimen was 2 or 3 mg per kg body-weight of hycanthone mesylate as a single intramuscular injection, which cured 49 of 52 patients, with minimal side-effects.— N. Katz *et al.*, *Am. J. trop. Med. Hyg.*, 1969, *18*, 924.

In a trial involving 113 patients with schistosomiasis mainly due to *S. haematobium*, hycanthone 2.5 to 3.5 mg per kg body-weight given as a single intramuscular injection was considered to be more useful for mass treatment for schistosomiasis and caused fewer side-effects than hycanthone 2.5 mg per kg given daily by mouth for 3 or 4 days or lucanthone 20 mg per kg daily by mouth for 3 days. The cure-rate was about 77%.— D. H. Greenfield and D. M. Du Toit, *Cent. Afr. J. Med.*, 1970, *16*, 265, per *Trop. Dis. Bull.*, 1971, *68*, 833.

In a trial involving 173 children with schistosomiasis due to *S. mansoni*,94% of those given single doses of hycanthone by injection were free from infection 1 month later and 73% free 3 months later. The corresponding results after treatment with niridazole 25 mg per kg body-weight by mouth daily for 5 days were 84 and 27% compared with 34 and 22% respectively among children given a placebo.— P. H. Rees *et al.*, *E. Afr. med. J.*, 1970, *47*, 634, per *Trop. Dis. Bull.*, 1974, *71*, 163.

Of 433 patients with *S. mansoni* infection treated with a single injection of hycanthone 3 mg per kg body-weight 190 were followed for 2 years. Egg excretion was reduced by 98% at 1 year and 87% at 2 years; viable eggs were not detected in 86% of patients at 1 year and 76% at 2 years. Patients older than 15 years responded less well than younger patients.— J. A. Cook *et al.*, *Am. J. trop. Med. Hyg.*, 1974, *23*, 910, per *Trop. Dis. Bull.*, 1975, *72*, 356.

Based on experience in treating 540 patients with *S. mansoni* infection with hycanthone in doses of 3, 2.5, 2, 1.5, or 1 mg per kg body-weight, a dose of 1.5 to 2 mg per kg was recommended for mass treatment.— J. A. Cook *et al.*, *Am. J. trop. Med. Hyg.*, 1976, *25*, 602, per *Trop. Dis. Bull.*, 1977, *74*, 238.

Hycanthone in a dose of 1.5 mg per kg body-weight, half the usual dose, reduced the egg output by 96% and produced a cure-rate of 32% at 4 months in 56 patients infected with *Schistosoma mansoni* without producing major side-effects. A dose of 750 µg per kg reduced the egg output by 80% in 55 patients with a cure-rate of about 8% but a dose of 375 µg per kg had no effect on egg output. Since *Schistosoma mansoni* does not multiply within the human host, morbidity could be improved significantly by reducing and not necessarily eradicating the infection. The smaller doses thus required would be less toxic and cheaper than standard doses.— K. S. Warren *et al.*, *Lancet*, 1978, *1*, 352.

Mass treatment with hycanthone 0.75 mg or 1.5 mg per kg body-weight, failed to control schistosomiasis due to *S. mansoni* in a study in Zaire, probably due to reinfection.— A. M. Polderman and J. P. Manshande, *Lancet*, 1981, *1*, 27.

Further references.— V. Buaiz *et al.*, *Revta Ass. med. bras.*, 1976, *22*, 171, per *Trop. Dis. Bull.*, 1976, *73*, 1063; Z. R. Sotomayor *et al.*, *J. trop. Med. Hyg.*, 1976, *79*, 18, per *Trop. Dis. Bull.*, 1976, *73*, 760.

For other reports and references, see Martindale 27th Edn, p. 1374.

Typhoid fever. Hycanthone 3 to 3.5 mg per kg body-weight by intramuscular injection as a single dose was effective in the treatment of 5 patients with chronic typhoid fever associated with schistosomiasis due to *S. mansoni*. Fever disappeared within 7 to 10 days and blood cultures quickly became free from *Salmonella typhi* in 4 patients, and more slowly in the 5th. All patients were freed from schistosomes.— V. Macêdo *et al.*, *Gazeta med. Bahia*, 1970, *70*, 194, per *Abstr. Hyg.*, 1972, *47*, 910.

Further references: R. P. Marinho and J. Neves, *Revta Inst. Med. trop. S Paulo*, 1974, *16*, 70, per *Trop. Dis. Bull.*, 1974, *71*, 927.

Proprietary Preparations

Etrenol *(Winthrop, UK)*. Hycanthone mesylate (supplied as powder for preparing injections), available in vials containing the equivalent of 200 mg of hycanthone. (Also available as Etrenol in *S.Afr.*).

784-c

Iodothymol. Thymolan. 6-Iodothymol.
$C_{10}H_{13}IO=276.1$.

CAS — 2364-44-5.

NOTE. The name iodothymol has also been applied to thymol iodide (see p.577).

Uses. Iodothymol is an anthelmintic which has been used in the treatment of hookworm infections.

785-k

Kainic Acid. Digenic Acid. 2-(2-Carboxy-4-isopropenylpyrrolidin-3-yl)acetic acid monohydrate.
$C_{10}H_{15}NO_4,H_2O=231.2$.

CAS — 487-79-6 (anhydrous).

Pharmacopoeias. In *Jap.*

White odourless crystals or crystalline powder with an acid taste obtained from the dried red alga *Digenea simplex*. M.p. about 252° with decomposition. Sparingly **soluble** in water; very slightly soluble in alcohol and glacial acetic acid; practically insoluble in chloroform; slightly soluble in methyl alcohol; soluble in dilute hydrochloric acid and in solutions of alkali hydroxides. A 1% solution in water has a pH of 2.8 to 3.5. **Store** in airtight containers.

Uses. Kainic acid is an anthelmintic used in roundworm (*Ascaris*) infection, in single doses of 5 to 20 mg. It has been used to enhance the effects of santonin.

Proprietary Names

Digenin *(Jap.)*.

786-a

Kamala *(B.P.C. 1934)*. Glandulae Rottlerae; Camala.

CAS — 12624-07-6.

Pharmacopoeias. In *Aust.* and *Port.*

The trichomes and glands from the fruits of *Mallotus philippinensis* (Euphorbiaceae). An odourless, tasteless, fine, mobile, dull reddish-brown powder of heterogeneous nature which floats when sprinkled on water; with chloroform, ether, or solutions of caustic alkalis, a reddish-brown solution is obtained.

Uses. Kamala produces purgation and has been used in doses of 2 to 8 g in the treatment of tapeworm infection. It has been given in honey or gruel or as a draught, suspended in water; the dose should be preceded by the administration of sodium bicarbonate thrice daily for 48 hours.

787-t

Kousso *(B.P.C. 1949)*. Cusso; Brayera; Cousso; Flos Koso; Kosoblüte.

Pharmacopoeias. In *Port.* and *Span.*

The dried panicles of the fertilised pistillate flowers of *Brayera anthelmintica* (=*Hagenia abyssinica*) (Rosaceae). **Protect** from light.

Uses. Kousso has been used in a dose of 8 to 16 g as an anthelmintic, particularly for the expulsion of tapeworms, but there is little evidence that it dislodges the heads.

788-x

Levamisole Hydrochloride *(B.P., B.P. Vet.)*.

l-Tetramisole Hydrochloride; ICI 59623; NSC 177023; R 12564; RP 20605. (−)-(*S*)-2,3,5,6-Tetrahydro-6-phenylimidazo[2,1-*b*]thiazole hydrochloride.
$C_{11}H_{12}N_2S,HCl=240.8$.

CAS — 14769-73-4 (levamisole); 16595-80-5 (hydrochloride).

Pharmacopoeias. In *Br.* and *Chin.*

A white to pale cream-coloured, odourless or almost odourless, crystalline powder. Levamisole hydrochloride 1.18 g is approximately equivalent to 1 g of levamisole. **Soluble** 1 in 2 of water and 1 in 5 of methyl alcohol; practically insoluble in ether. A solution in water is laevorotatory. Solutions for injections are **sterilised** by filtration.

Adverse Effects. Side-effects after the use of levamisole include nausea, vomiting, abdominal pain, taste disturbances, fatigue, headache, confusion, insomnia, dizziness, fever, an influenza-like syndrome, arthralgia, muscle pain, hypotension, vasculitis, and skin rash. Proteinuria has occasionally occurred. Neutropenia and thrombocytopenia have occurred; there have been a number of reports of agranulocytosis, usually reversible, occurring particularly in patients with rheumatic disorders or malignant disease.

Of 30 patients treated with levamisole 2 developed a severe febrile reaction and 3 severe but transient neutropenia. All 5 had levamisole withdrawn.— F. T. Christiansen *et al.* (letter), *Lancet*, 1977, *1*, 1111.

Side-effects due to levamisole and severe enough to stop treatment in 15 of 69 cancer patients included a flu-like reaction, gastro-intestinal effects, urticarial rash, central effects, and in 1 patient reversible agranulocytosis with sepsis. Levamisole had been given by mouth in a dose of 2.5 mg per kg body-weight daily for 2 days a week for between 8 and 52 weeks.— D. R. Parkinson *et al.*, *Lancet*, 1977, *1*, 1129.

The febrile reactions to levamisole might be associated with the restoration to activity of the cellular immune system associated with induction of fibrinolysis. Exacerbation of underlying infection in 30 patients given levamisole was associated with restoration of T-lymphocytic activity. Side-effects occurred in 128 of 301 patients (43%), agranulocytosis occurring in 5. A very severe reaction occurred in 1 patient who was also taking a monoamine oxidase inhibitor.— R. D. Thornes (letter), *Lancet*, 1977, *2*, 90. Fever, chills, and confusion occurred in a patient given levamisole and recurred with loss of consciousness on challenge. Clinical and laboratory findings indicated allergy.— I. Yust *et al.* (letter), *ibid.*, 457.

In one patient with skin rash caused by levamisole examination of skin biopsy material showed deposits of immunoglobulin and complement indicating that levamisole could cause immediate-type as well as Arthus-type hypersensitivity reactions.— L. Secher *et al.* (letter), *Lancet*, 1977, *2*, 932.

Headache occurred on 3 isolated occasions in one patient following single doses of levamisole 150 mg. On the first occasion the headache was slight but on the other 2 she experienced severe headache, vomiting, cramps or spastic contractions of the muscles of the extremities, and fever. Chest pain occurred on the 2nd occasion and motor aphasia on the 3rd.— J. A. Sigidin and N. V. Bunchuk (letter), *Lancet*, 1977, *2*, 980.

A report of high fever, skin rash, and seizures associated with the use of levamisole in 3 children with juvenile rheumatoid arthritis. Symptoms could have been associated with severe viral infections with levamisole acting as a predisposing factor.— A. M. Prieur *et al.*, *J. Pediat.*, 1978, *93*, 304.

A 54-year-old woman with rheumatoid arthritis developed a severe hypogammaglobulinaemia during treatment with levamisole 150 mg daily. She had received prednisone 10 to 15 mg daily as treatment but this was discontinued when levamisole alleviated her condition. The hypogammaglobulinaemia improved when levamisole was withdrawn but she had a relapse of rheumatoid arthritis 20 months later.— H. Berghs *et al.*, *Ann. Allergy*, 1978, *41*, 342.

From a study of 20 patients with rheumatoid arthritis, 9 of whom developed skin reactions while receiving treatment with levamisole, it appeared that levamisole was able to elicit atopic responses to allergens through stimulation of T-lymphocytes.— L. Hodinka *et al.*, *Int. Archs Allergy appl. Immun.*, 1979, *58*, 362.

A report of lichenoid skin eruptions in 2 patients treated with levamisole for rheumatoid arthritis. Although the rash subsided in both patients when levamisole was discontinued, one patient had severe scarring alopecia of the scalp and widespread atrophic and hyperpigmented lesions over his skin a year later.— J. D. Kirby *et al.*, *J. R. Soc. Med.*, 1980, *73*, 208.

A 39-year-old male complained of giddiness and collapsed 5 hours after receiving a single dose of levamisole 150 mg given as part of treatment for periodic *Brugia malayi*. He became agitated, violent, and then went into fits. His fits were controlled with chlorpromazine and the patient fully recovered after withdrawal of levamisole.— J. W. Mak and V. Zaman, *Trans. R. Soc. trop. Med. Hyg.*, 1980, *74*, 285.

Arthritis. Two of 8 patients with Crohn's disease developed severe arthritis after treatment for 3 and 5 months with levamisole, probably by unmasking latent mechanisms of joint damage.— A. W. Segal *et al.*, *Br. med. J.*, 1977, *2*, 555.

Arthralgia occurred on 2 occasions in a 67-year-old woman with Behçet's syndrome after being given levamisole.— P. Siklos (letter), *Br. med. J.*, 1977, *2*, 773.

Blood disorders. *Agranulocytosis.* Levamisole caused reversible agranulocytosis perhaps by acting as a hapten on the leucocyte membrane. The frequency was highest, at about 3%, in patients with severe rheumatic diseases. The onset of agranulocytosis was unpredictable and had developed as long as 2 years after treatment had started. Regular blood examinations were recommended in patients with rheumatic diseases and in all patients with typical early symptoms of sudden fever, shivering, and infection. Corticosteroids and blood transfusions should be avoided.— M. Rosenthal *et al.* (letter), *Lancet*, 1977, *1*, 904. Corticosteroid therapy should be considered if agranulocytosis due to levamisole was prolonged.— W. V. Epstein *et al.* (letter), *Lancet*, 1977, *2*, 245.

A high incidence of agranulocytosis was noted in patients suffering from breast cancer treated with levamisole. Of 174 patients whose therapy included levamisole 17 developed agranulocytosis.— L. Teerenhovi *et al.* (letter), *Lancet*, 1978, *2*, 151. See also S. Retsas *et al.* (letter), *ibid.*, 324.

Case reports of agranulocytosis with levamisole: I. A. Williams (letter), *Lancet*, 1976, *1*, 1080 (one patient); O. Ruuskanen *et al.* (letter), *ibid.*, *2*, 958 (2 children); H. Graber *et al.* (letter), *ibid.*, 1248 (one patient); R. Clara and J. Germanes (letter), *ibid.*, 1977, *1*, 47 (2 patients, one fatality); R. Vanholder and W. Van Hove (letter), *ibid.*, 100 (one patient); K. L. Schmidt and C. Mueller-Eckhardt (letter), *ibid.*, *2*, 85 (2 patients); E. M. Veys *et al.* (letter), *ibid.*, 764; C. C. Benz *et al.*, *Br. J. Derm.*, 1977, *97*, 87 (one patient); E. M. Veys *et al.* (letter), *Lancet*, 1978, *1*, 148 (3 patients); C. L. Vogel *et al.*, *Cancer Treat. Rep.*, 1978, *62*, 1587 (6 patients).

Leucopenia. Neutropenia occurred in 3 of 5 children receiving maintenance therapy for acute lymphoblastic leukaemia when levamisole was added to their regimen. Levamisole was considered to enhance the potential myelodepressant effect of antineoplastic therapy.— M. L. N. Willoughby *et al.* (letter), *Lancet*, 1977, *1*, 657. See also M. Rosenthal *et al.* (letter), *ibid.*, 1976, *1*, 369.

Further reports: G. T. Williams *et al.*, *Ann. rheum. Dis.*, 1978, *37*, 366; S. I. Drew *et al.*, *ibid.*, 1980, *39*, 59.

Thrombocytopenia. Thrombocytopenia occurred on 2 occasions in a 59-year-old woman given levamisole for rheumatoid arthritis, the platelet count reverting to normal when levamisole was withdrawn.— A. F. El-Ghobarey and H. A. Capell, *Br. med. J.*, 1977, *2*, 555.

Further reports: K. L. Schmidt and C. Mueller-Eckhardt (letter), *Lancet*, 1977, *2*, 85.

Kidney damage. Beta-*N*-acetylglucosaminidase (NAG) excretion, a marker of renal tubular (but not glomerular) damage, was decreased in patients with rheumatoid arthritis given levamisole 150 mg daily, indicating absence of tubular damage.— P. A. Dieppe *et al.*, *Br. med. J.*, 1978, *2*, 664.

Reversible levamisole-induced nephropathy developed in a man with rheumatoid arthritis who had had several episodes of a severely itching rash during levamisole therapy but who did not appear to be hypersensitive to levamisole on testing.— T. M. Hansen *et al.* (letter), *Lancet*, 1978, *2*, 737.

Photosensitivity. A photosensitive erythematous papular rash developed in a patient after 2 months' therapy with levamisole 50 mg twice daily.— M. M. Ferguson and D. G. Macdonald (letter), *Br. dent. J.*, 1978, *144*, 29.

Vasculitis. A cutaneous leucocytoclastic vasculitis developed in a 65-year-old woman taking levamisole 150 mg daily for 2 months for rheumatoid arthritis; the condition regressed when levamisole was withdrawn.— D. G. Macfarlane and P. A. Bacon, *Br. med. J.*, 1978, *1*, 407.

A report of cutaneous necrotising vasculitis in a 59-year-old woman who had taken levamisole 150 mg daily on 3 days a week for 3 months.— M. A. Scheinberg *et al.*, *Br. med. J.*, 1978, *1*, 408.

Treatment of Adverse Effects. In severe overdosage the stomach should be emptied by aspiration and lavage. Further treatment is symptomatic.

Precautions. The use of levamisole should be avoided in patients with advanced liver or kidney disease, and in patients with pre-existing blood disorders.

The appearance of side-effects in 9 of 10 patients with rheumatoid arthritis and Sjögren's syndrome while being treated with levamisole led to abandonment of the study. Patients were given 50 mg daily in the first week, 100 mg daily in the 2nd week, and 150 mg daily in the 3rd week; an erythematous maculopapular pruritic eruption occurred in the 3rd or 4th week in 7 patients; other symptoms occurring were increase in articular pain and swelling, muscle weakness or pain, an influenza-like illness, confusion, and insomnia. Symptoms recurred in 5 patients given challenge doses. Levamisole should be given with caution, if at all, in patients with Sjögren's symdrome.— G. Balint *et al.*, *Br. med. J.*, 1977, *2*, 1386.

The presence of HLA B27 in seropositive rheumatoid arthritis is an important predisposing factor to the development of agranulocytosis during treatment with levamisole; it is recommended that the use of levamisole in this group should be avoided. Although the incidence of agranulocytosis did not appear to be reduced by any of the treatment schemes used, the use of a single dose per week, with blood counts 10 hours after drug intake, allowed high risk patients to be detected early.— H. Mielants and E. M. Veys, *J. Rheumatol.*, 1978, *5*, *Suppl.* 4, 77.

Absorption and Fate. Levamisole is readily absorbed from the gastro-intestinal tract. Peak blood concentrations of about 500 ng per ml are reached within 2 hours of a dose of 150 mg. The plasma half-life is about 4 hours. Levamisole is extensively metabolised in the liver and elimination is virtually complete, via the urine and faeces, in 2 days. Levamisole appears in breast milk.

References: J. G. Adams, *J. Rheumatol.*, 1978, *5*, *Suppl.* 4, 137.

Uses. Levamisole hydrochloride is the laevo-isomer of tetramisole hydrochloride. It is used as an anthelmintic and for its effects on the immune system.

Levamisole is effective in the treatment of roundworm (*Ascaris*) infection and is considered to paralyse *Ascaris* muscle by inhibition of succinate dehydrogenase. It is also active against hookworms (*Ancylostoma* and *Necator*) and has shown some effect against strongyloids (*Strongyloides*).

The usual dose in ascariasis is the equivalent of 120 to 150 mg of levamisole as a single dose. Children have been given 3 mg per kg body-weight as a single dose. In hookworm infection, doses of 2.5 to 5 mg per kg daily have been given for 2 or 3 days.

Levamisole affects the immune response. The term 'immunostimulant' has often been used; it is appropriate only in so far as restoration of a depressed response is concerned; stimulation above normal levels does not seem to occur. Levamisole influences host defences by modulating cell-mediated immune responses. It restores polymorphonuclear, macrophage, or T-cell functions. Levamisole has been used for a wide variety of disorders involving the immune response, including infections of mucous membranes and the respiratory tract, virus infections, rheumatic disorders, and as an adjunct in patients with malignant disease. A dose of 2.5 mg per kg on one day a week has been recommended in rheumatoid arthritis.

A review of the development and uses of levamisole.— P. A. J. Janssen, *Janssen, Belg.*, *Prog. Drug Res.*, 1976, *20*, 347. See also W. K. Amery, *Janssen, Belg.* (letter), *Br. med. J.*, 1977, *1*, 573; J. Symoens and M. Rosenthal, *Janssen, Belg.*, *J. reticuloendoth. Soc.*, 1977, *21*, 175.

Discussions of the effect of levamisole on the immune response: *Lancet*, 1975, *1*, 151; M. Biniaminov and B. Ramot (letter), *ibid.*, 464; D. G. Hopper *et al.* (letter), *ibid.*, 574; G. Versijp *et al.* (letter), *ibid.*, 798; J. Symoens (letter), *ibid.*, 867; H. Verhaegen *et al.* (letter), *ibid.*, 978; G. W. Fischer *et al.* (letter), *ibid.*, 1137; S. H. Chan and M. J. Simons (letter), *ibid.*, 1246; M. Rosenthal (letter), *ibid.*, 1977, *2*, 665; L. F. Skinnider and M. Rieder (letter), *ibid.*, 932; M. Kondo *et al.* (letter), *New Engl. J. Med.*, 1978, *298*, 1146; G. Renoux, *Drugs*, 1980, *20*, 89.

There was partial improvement in a patient with angio-immunoblastic lymphadenopathy treated with levamisole 150 mg daily for 3 days each week over 6 weeks.— J. -C. Bensa *et al.* (letter), *Lancet*, 1976, *1*, 1081.

A beneficial response to levamisole in a child with the Wiskott-Aldrich syndrome.— G. Fontan *et al.* (letter), *Lancet*, 1976, *2*, 1247.

Levamisole increased the T-cell concentration in 7 patients with HBs-positive chronic active liver disease, and might accelerate lysis of infected hepatocytes.— R. G. Chadwick *et al.*, *Gut*, 1977, *18*, A979.

Favourable reports of the use of levamisole in diseases

characterised by neutropenia or neutrophil dysfunction: A. Rebora *et al.*, *Br. J. Derm.*, 1978, *99*, 569 (Buckley's syndrome); S. J. Proctor *et al.*, *Postgrad. med. J.*, 1979, *55*, 279 (cyclical neutropenia); A. Rebora *et al.*, *Br. J. Derm.*, 1980, *102*, 49.

A discussion calling for caution in the use of levamisole as an 'immunostimulant'.— *Lancet*, 1979, *2*, 291. Criticisms.— W. K. Amery, *Janssen, Belg.* (letter), *ibid.*, 528.

Favourable results were obtained in 7 children with minimal lesion nephrotic syndrome using levamisole 1.5 to 3.9 mg per kg body-weight given twice weekly for 1 to 6 months.— P. Tanphaichitr *et al.*, *J. Pediat.*, 1980, *96*, 490.

A 21-year-old man with widespread recurrent pyoderma resistant to antimicrobial therapy for 3 years was found to have cellular immunodeficiency. Levamisole 150 mg was given on 2 consecutive days per week and after 6 weeks all lesions had cleared. Treatment was continued for a total of 12 weeks.— D. Djawari and O. P. Hornstein, *Dermatologica*, 1980, *161*, 116.

A review of levamisole in the treatment of viral infections.— A. S. Russell, *Drugs*, 1980, *20*, 117.

A review of levamisole in the treatment of parasitic infections.— M. J. Miller, *Drugs*, 1980, *20*, 122.

Arthritis. Reviews of levamisole in the treatment of rheumatic diseases: E. C. Huskisson and J. G. Adams, *Drugs*, 1980, *20*, 100; G. L. Craig and W. W. Buchanan, *ibid.*, 453.

For the proceedings of an international symposium on levamisole in rheumatoid arthritis, see *J. Rheumatol.*, 1978, *5*, *Suppl.* 4, 1–153.

In a double-blind study of levamisole 150 mg daily and a placebo in 28 patients with rheumatoid arthritis, levamisole produced no benefit and might have had a deleterious effect.— Y. Dinai and M. Pras (letter), *Lancet*, 1975, *2*, 556.

Studies of the effect of levamisole on hyaluronic acid produced by cultured human synovial fibroblasts suggested that the beneficial effect in rheumatoid arthritis might not be due only to its action on the immune system; in some concentrations it might inhibit pathological accumulation of hyaluronic acid in inflamed joints.— M. Yaron *et al.* (letter), *Lancet*, 1976, *1*, 369.

In a controlled study in patients with definite or classical rheumatoid arthritis on an optimum anti-inflammatory regimen 12 patients received levamisole 50 mg thrice daily for 6 months (reduced in 3 patients with rash to 150 mg daily for 2 days a week), 12 received penicillamine 250 mg daily gradually increased to 1 g daily, and 10 received a placebo. After 6 months levamisole and penicillamine produced significant improvement in pain, morning stiffness, proximal interphalangeal joint circumference, ESR, latex titre, and IgG concentration, and a significant reduction in technetium index. Side-effects from levamisole included nausea, skin rash, mouth ulcers, minor taste disturbances, and tremor. An increased responsiveness to tuberculin and the absence, in *animals*, of anti-inflammatory effect suggested that levamisole had a specific, probably immunostimulant, effect in rheumatoid arthritis.— E. C. Huskisson *et al.*, *Lancet*, 1976, *1*, 393.

Levamisole did not appear to benefit patients with psoriatic arthritis.— M. Rosenthal and U. Trabert (letter), *New Engl. J. Med.*, 1976, *295*, 1204.

Subjective and objective improvement occurred in 7 of 9 patients with rheumatoid arthritis, in a patient with Reiter's syndrome, and subjective improvement in 7 and objective improvement in 4 of 13 patients with ankylosing spondylitis, after treatment with levamisole 150 mg daily for 4 weeks, then 3 days a week; non-steroidal anti-inflammatory agents were permitted. Clinical improvement was accompanied by immunological changes in only a few patients.— M. Rosenthal *et al.*, *Scand. J. Rheumatol.*, 1976, *5*, 216.

In a controlled crossover study 37 patients with seronegative spondylarthritis were treated in turn for 12 weeks either with a placebo or levamisole 150 mg daily for 3 days a week. Nine patients withdrew because of side-effects, the only serious one being transient agranulocytosis with pneumonia in one patient. In the remaining 28 patients improvement in joint inflammation, low-back flexibility, and morning stiffness was associated with levamisole.— K. M. Goebel *et al.*, *Lancet*, 1977, *2*, 214.

Levamisole given to 27 patients with rheumatoid arthritis was associated with an increase in cold lymphocytotoxic antibodies.— J. D. Browning *et al.* (letter), *Lancet*, 1977, *2*, 820.

Although a significant increase in blood cell phagocyte activity was found in 11 of 15 rheumatoid arthritic patients following 6 weeks of levamisole therapy, no such increase was found in synovial fluid cells of 5 of these patients, and increased phagocytosis did not correlate with clinical improvement.— K. M. Wynne *et al.*, *Ann. rheum. Dis.*, 1977, *36*, 482.

In a 6-month, double-blind, placebo-controlled study involving 363 patients with rheumatoid arthritis, 2 regimens of levamisole 150 mg daily given on 3 or 7 consecutive days each week were shown to be active and equally effective in the treatment of rheumatoid arthritis. Adverse reactions occurred in about 50% of the patients who received levamisole compared with 30% of those who received placebo, the excess 20% of side-effects in the levamisole-treated patients being caused by severe idiosyncratic reactions (agranulocytosis, severe rash, severe febrile or influenza-like illness, and severe mouth ulceration).— Multicentre Study Group, *Lancet*, 1978, *2*, 1007. In a further study involving 87 similar patients once weekly doses of 50 or 150 mg were compared. The efficacy to side-effect ratio obtained with 150 mg once weekly was considered to be better than that previously obtained (*Lancet*, 1978, *2*, 1007) with 150 mg given on 3 or 7 consecutive days each week. Although the incidence of idiosyncratic reactions was reduced with the 50-mg dose so was efficacy. It was proposed that in the treatment of rheumatoid arthritis levamisole should be given as a single 150-mg dose once weekly at bedtime. This regimen also allowed for haematological control to detect agranulocytosis at an early stage; blood counts should be performed every fortnight on the morning following treatment.— *idem*, *J. Rheumatol.*, 1978, *5*, *Suppl.* 4, 5. See also E. M. Veys *et al.*, *ibid.*, 1981, *8*, 45.

Further references.— Y. Schuermans (letter), *Lancet*, 1975, *1*, 111; E. M. Veys *et al.* (letter), *ibid.*, 1976, *1*, 808; D'A. Laidlaw, *Med. J. Aust.*, 1976, *2*, 382; *ibid.*, 400; E. M. Veys and H. Mielants, *J. Rheumatol.*, 1977, *4*, 27; L. A. Runge *et al.*, *Arthritis Rheum.*, 1977, *20*, 1445; J. Scott *et al.*, *Ann. rheum. Dis.*, 1978, *37*, 259; T. Di Perri *et al.*, *Eur. J. Rheumatol. Inflamm.*, 1978, *1*, 155; A. F. El-Ghobarey *et al.*, *Q. J. Med.*, 1978, *47*, 385; L. A. Runge *et al.*, *Ann. rheum. Dis.*, 1979, *38*, 122; P. Franchimont *et al.*, *Scand. J. Rheumatol.*, 1979, *8*, 43; *idem*, *Eur. J. Rheumatol. Inflamm.*, 1979, *2*, 243; B. Miller *et al.*, *Arthritis Rheum.*, 1980, *23*, 172; P. L. Kinsella *et al.*, *J. Rheumatol.*, 1980, *7*, 288.

Brucellosis. Levamisole added to antibiotic therapy in a dose of 150 mg daily for 1 week then 150 mg daily for 3 consecutive days each week reversed the immunodepression in 8 patients with brucellosis and eradicated symptoms.— M. Renoux and G. Renoux (letter), *Lancet*, 1977, *1*, 372. Favourable results in 10 patients.— M. Raptpoulou-Gigi *et al.*, *J. Immunopharmac.*, 1980, *2*, 85.

Crohn's disease. Eight patients with Crohn's disease had remissions induced within 14 days of starting a protein-free diet. Levamisole 50 mg (25 mg in one patient) every 8 hours for 3 consecutive days every 2 weeks was started and after the 2nd course a normal diet was resumed. Seven patients remained in remission. Arthritis occurred in 2 patients but resolved when levamisole was discontinued; one of these patients remained in remission, the other had a recurrence of Crohn's disease when arthritis developed.— A. W. Segal *et al.* (preliminary communication), *Lancet*, 1977, *2*, 382.

Absence of response of Crohn's disease to levamisole in a double-blind study against placebo in 21 patients.— E. Wesdorp *et al.*, *Gut*, 1977, *18*, A971. See also E. T. Swarbrick and D. P. O'Donoghue (letter), *Lancet*, 1979, *1*, 392.

Filaria. In 10 patients with *Brugia malayi* infection given levamisole 120 mg as a single dose (40 mg for a child) and 17 given similar doses for 3 days microfilarial counts dropped, but often returned to previous values by the end of a week.— D. R. O'Holohan and V. Zaman, *J. trop. Med. Hyg.*, 1974, *77*, 113, per *Trop. Dis. Bull.*, 1974, *71*, 1047.

The microfilarial count in 27 carriers of *Wuchereria bancrofti* fell by 98.5% after a course of levamisole gradually increased over 4 days to 3 mg per kg body-weight and then given daily for 8 days. At follow-up 45 days later the reduction was 93.1%. A second course was desirable. For mass treatment a shorter course followed by a single monthly dose was suggested.— J. -P. Moreau *et al.*, *Méd. trop. Marseille*, 1975, *35*, 451.

Levamisole 3 mg per kg body-weight given for 8 days followed by mebendazole 6 mg per kg daily for 10 days was more effective in permanently reducing microfilariae rate and density in patients infected with *W. bancrofti* than levamisole given alone. However, diethylcarbamazine was more effective than either treatment regimen.— M. V. V. L. Narasimham *et al.*, *S.E. Asian J. trop. med. publ. Hlth*, 1978, *9*, 571.

Levamisole 3% in drops was microfilaricidal when applied to an eye of each of 4 patients with ocular onchocerciasis, and was comparable to diethylcarbamazine citrate 0.03%. Lower dilutions of levamisole of 0.01 and 0.3% were ineffective.— B. R. Jones *et al.*, *Br. J. Ophthal.*, 1978, *62*, 440.

In a study involving 78 patients infected with *W. bancrofti* or *B. malayi* the optimum dosage regimen for treatment with levamisole appeared to be 100 mg initially followed by 100 mg twice daily for 10 days. This regimen was at least as effective as diethylcarbamazine 2 mg per kg body-weight given thrice daily for 21 days.— J. W. Mak and V. Zaman, *Trans. R. Soc. trop. Med. Hyg.*, 1980, *74*, 285.

For reports of the use of levamisole with mebendazole in the treatment of infections due to *Dipetalonema perstans*, see Mebendazole, p.98.

For disappointing results with levamisole in onchocerciasis, see Mebendazole, p.99.

Hepatitis. A controlled study in 50 patients indicated that levamisole, given in a dose of 150 mg daily for 3 consecutive days during the second and third week of the acute disease, might be beneficial in viral hepatitis type B.— A. Pár (letter), *Lancet*, 1977, *1*, 702. See also R. G. Chadwick *et al.*, *Gut*, 1977, *18*, A979.

Although levamisole improved the immunological status of 5 children with chronic persistent hepatitis, it had no effect on the disease; a dose of 2 mg per kg body-weight daily on 3 consecutive days per week was given for 4 weeks and patients were followed up for 5 months.— M. Masi *et al.* (letter), *Archs Dis. Childh.*, 1978, *53*, 764.

Herpes. Levamisole 100 mg taken at the first sign of an outbreak of herpes simplex, then 100 mg on each of the next 2 mornings, was no more beneficial than a placebo in a 6-month study of 28 subjects with frequent cutaneous lesions.— K. A. Mehr and L. Albano (letter), *Lancet*, 1977, *2*, 773.

In a double-blind crossover study in 40 adults with intractable herpes genitalis levamisole, 50 mg thrice daily on 2 days a week for 6 months, was no more effective than a placebo.— S. M. Bierman, *Cutis*, 1978, *21*, 352.

Rapid relief of pain with subsequent clearance of lesions was achieved in 8 patients with acute herpes genitalis after treatment with levamisole 50 mg thrice daily for 4 days, the course being repeated after 10 to 14 days. Six patients with recurrent herpes genitalis and 1 with infection of the buttock also benefited from treatment with 150 mg daily for 2 days a week for 4 to 8 weeks.— J. Adno, *S. Afr. med. J.*, 1978, *53*, 547.

In a double-blind study in 99 patients with herpes labialis there was no significant difference in the severity or duration of lesions during treatment with levamisole, about 2.5 mg per kg body-weight, daily on 2 days a week for 6 months, compared with a placebo.— A. S. Russell *et al.*, *J. infect. Dis.*, 1978, *137*, 597.

A study of 42 patients who were observed for 4 to 12 months indicated that levamisole should not be used in the management of recurrent herpes simplex labialis because it might increase lesion frequency while producing only a mild reduction in lesion severity.— S. L. Spruance *et al.*, *Antimicrob. Ag. Chemother.*, 1979, *15*, 662.

A neonate suffering from convulsions and skin lesions due to disseminated herpes simplex infection was given levamisole 6 mg on alternate days starting from day 16 of life. Skin lesions and convulsions disappeared completely on day 38 and the patient was discharged at the age of 50 days receiving 7 mg twice weekly. An attempt to reduce the dose to once weekly was unsuccessful and later the dose had to be increased to 15 mg twice weekly. Treatment was discontinued at the age of 20 months and the patient was in good health at 29 months except for a slight motor deficit.— A. Constantopoulos *et al.*, *Dermatologica*, 1980, *160*, 121.

Further references: T. -W. Chang and N. Fiumara, *Antimicrob. Ag. Chemother.*, 1978, *13*, 809; D. G. Jose and C. C. J. Minty, *Med. J. Aust.*, 1980, *2*, 390; E. Hernandez-Perez, *Dermatologica*, 1980, *160*, 118.

Hookworm (*Ancylostoma* and *Necator*). A group of 41 patients with hookworm infection were given levamisole in a single dose of 5 mg per kg body-weight; another 9 patients received a second dose of levamisole 2 days after the first. All patients were shown to be cured 7 days after treatment. No serious side-effects were seen with this dose of levamisole.— G. Al-Saffar *et al.* (letter), *Trans. R. Soc. trop. Med. Hyg.*, 1971, *65*, 836.

Levamisole 150 mg twice daily for 4 days cured 92% of 50 patients infected with hookworms, mostly *Ancylostoma*. Levamisole, 3 mg per kg body-weight repeated after 12 hours cured only 63% of 60 other patients. Tetramisole was much less effective when given either as a single dose of 3 mg per kg, or as 3 doses of 150 mg each at 10-day intervals.— D. Banerjee *et al.*, *Indian J. med. Res.*, 1972, *60*, 834, per *Trop. Dis. Bull.*, 1973, *70*, 265.

Leishmaniasis. Treatment with levamisole produced complete healing in 6 to 8 weeks in 11 of 12 patients with chronic cutaneous leishmaniasis. The usual dose was 150 mg daily for 2 consecutive days per week for as long as it took the lesions to heal.— P. G. Butler, *J. trop. Med. Hyg.*, 1978, *81*, 221.

Lupus erythematosus. Significant clinical benefit, with reduction of steroid dosage, was achieved in 15 of 16 patients with systemic lupus erythematosus treated with levamisole. The dose was 150 mg daily for 3 days every 2 weeks increased to 3 days every week if needed, for about 7 to 20 months. A controlled study was needed.— B. L. Gordon and R. Yanagihara, *Ann. Allergy*, 1977, *39*, 227. A controlled study indicating that levamisole was ineffective.— T. Hadidi *et al.*, *Arthritis Rheum.*, 1981, *24*, 60.

Further references: P. H. Feng *et al.*, *Singapore med. J.*, 1978, *19*, 120; K. Ogawa *et al.*, *Ann. Allergy*, 1979, *43*, 187.

Malignant neoplasms. A review of 20 studies on the use of levamisole in the treatment of malignant disease. Levamisole is not a remission-inducing agent since it does not act on cancer cells and its use alone has no rationale. However, it can be of use as adjuvant therapy in patients at risk of recurrent disease after they have undergone effective primary antineoplastic therapy. Appropriate dosage based on body-weight or body surface area, early treatment after completion of primary treatment, and neoplasm responsiveness to primary therapy appear to be important determinants of therapeutic effectiveness with levamisole. It was recommended that levamisole should be given intermittently avoiding concomitant administration with cytotoxic agents in order to avoid bone marrow damage. Further data were required before it could be determined if levamisole was more effective than BCG vaccine or *Corynebacterium parvum*.— F. Spreafico, *Drugs*, 1980, *20*, 105.

In 111 patients who had undergone surgery for bronchial carcinoma and who were followed for a year there were 10 recurrences (7 deaths) in 51 who had received levamisole 50 mg thrice daily for 3 days before surgery and then 3 days each fortnight, compared with 23 recurrences (12 deaths) in 60 given a placebo. Though the difference was not significant the results in favour of levamisole were considered promising. Levamisole was considered to prevent, at least in part, the immunosuppression due to surgery.—Study Group for Bronchogenic Carcinoma, *Br. med. J.*, 1975, *3*, 461.

Levamisole 150 mg on 3 consecutive days on alternate weeks administered after radiotherapy to 20 women with inoperable breast cancer significantly prolonged the disease-free period (25 months) and survival (90% alive at 30 months) compared with placebo in 23 women (disease-free period of 9 months and survival of 35% at 30 months). Effective levamisole treatment was associated with an increase in skin reactivity.— A. J. Rojas *et al.*, *Lancet*, 1976, *1*, 211.

In 18 patients receiving chemotherapy for neoplastic disease the use of levamisole 150 mg daily every third day between courses of antineoplastic agents permitted shorter intervals between such courses, the use of longer courses, and reduced haemorrhage and infection.— J. C. Lods *et al.* (letter), *Lancet*, 1976, *1*, 548. See also P. Dujardin *et al.*, *Thérapie*, 1976, *31*, 733.

In 31 patients with advanced cancer given levamisole 150 mg thrice weekly survival was related to increased T-cell reactivity.— G. Renoux and M. Renoux, *Nouv. Presse méd.*, 1976, *5*, 67.

The immunocompetence of patients with cancer treated with levamisole.— S. A. Wilkins *et al.*, *Cancer*, 1977, *39*, 487.

In a 2-year placebo-controlled study adjuvant treatment with levamisole in patients with resectable lung cancer prolonged the disease-free interval and survival time after surgery. Levamisole was given in a dosage of 50 mg thrice daily for 3 consecutive days before surgery and repeated every 2 weeks but this dose appeared to be sufficient only for patients weighing 70 kg or less. It was recommended that in future studies the daily dose should be adjusted to patient's weight or surface area; a daily dose of 2.5 mg per kg body-weight or 100 mg per m^2 body-surface given in 2 or 3 divided doses was suggested.— W. K. Amery, *Cancer Treat. Rep.*, 1978, *62*, 1677.

Evidence that adjuvant therapy with levamisole increases the breast-cancer recurrence rate in patients with histologically positive lymph-nodes but without distant metastasis. On the basis of these observations the use of adjuvant therapy with levamisole cannot be recommended in such patients.—Executive Committee of the Danish Breast Cancer Cooperative Group (preliminary report), *Lancet*, 1980, *2*, 824. Criticisms.— H. M. Anthony (letter), *ibid.*, 1133; W. K. Amery, *Janssen, Belg.* (letter), *ibid.*

The final report of a randomised double-blind controlled study of levamisole as adjuvant therapy in 203 patients with malignant melanoma treated surgically, concluded that levamisole is of no benefit when compared with placebo. However, a trend towards a longer time to visceral recurrence and improved survival in patients with stage I melanoma treated with levamisole was considered to warrant further study.— L. E. Spitler and R. Sagebiel, *New Engl. J. Med.*, 1980, *303*, 1143. Comment.— W. D. Terry, *ibid.*, 1174.

Further studies and reports of the use of levamisole in the treatment of malignant neoplasms: H. W. C. Ward (letter), *Lancet*, 1976, *1*, 394; J. L. Marx, *Science*, 1976, *191*, 57; G. Sanchez and A. G. Mira (letter), *New Engl. J. Med.*, 1977, *296*, 1412 (lymphocytic leukaemia); H. J. Wanebo *et al.*, *Cancer Treat. Rep.*, 1978, *62*, 1663 (head and neck); R. L. Gonzalez *et al.*, *ibid.*, 1703 (melanoma); H. Miwa and K. Orita, *Acta med. Okayama*, 1978, *32*, 363 (gastric); G. N. Hortobagyi *et al.*, *Cancer*, 1979, *43*, 1112 (breast); S. W. Hall *et al.*, *ibid.*, 1195 (melanoma); A. J. Olivari *et al.*, *Cancer Treat. Rep.*, 1979, *63*, 983 (head and neck); P. Klefström, *ibid.*, 1980, *64*, 65 (breast).

Hodgkin's disease. A beneficial immunostimulatory effect was noted in 4 patients in remission from Hodgkin's disease who received levamisole 150 mg daily by mouth for 3 consecutive days every 2 weeks.— E. Berényi *et al.* (letter), *New Engl. J. Med.*, 1977, *296*, 941. See also B. Ramot *et al.*, *New Engl. J. Med.*, 1976, *294*, 809; R. H. Phillips *et al.*, *Br. med. J.*, 1977, *1*, 1447.

Respiratory-tract infections. In a double-blind study in 70 children with recurrent upper respiratory-tract infections levamisole twice daily for 2 days each week for 6 months significantly reduced the incidence, duration, and severity of infection. Doses were: up to 15 kg body-weight, 12.5 mg twice daily; 15 to 29 kg, 25 mg; 30 kg or more, 50 mg. A minimum dose of 1.25 mg per kg twice daily appeared to be necessary.— M. Van Eygen *et al.*, *Lancet*, 1976, *1*, 382.

Further studies with favourable results: F. De Loore *et al.*, *Curr. med. Res. Opinion*, 1979, *6*, 142; M. Van Eygen *et al.*, *Eur. J. Pediat.*, 1979, *131*, 147.

Roundworm (*Ascaris*). From a review of studies comparing the anthelmintics used for the treatment of roundworm infection, levamisole hydrochloride 150 mg as a single dose appeared to be the drug of choice; it might lead to toxic effects if obstruction in the intestine prevented expulsion of the dead worms and permitted absorption of disintegration products.— B. J. Vakil and N. J. Dalal, *Prog. Drug Res.*, 1975, *19*, 166.

A cure-rate of 92% was achieved in 453 children with roundworm (*Ascaris*) infection treated with a single dose of levamisole compared with 66% in 461 treated with piperazine citrate 150 mg per kg body-weight with a maximum of 3.5 g. The dose of levamisole was: 10 to 20 kg, 50 mg; 20 to 40 kg, 100 mg; over 40 kg, 150 mg. Levamisole was considered suitable for mass treatment.— M. J. Miller *et al.*, *Sth. med. J.*, 1978, *71*, 137.

Further references.— N. D. W. Lionel *et al.*, *Br. med. J.*, 1969, *4*, 340; B. J. Vakil *et al.*, *Trans. R. Soc. trop. Med. Hyg.*, 1972, *66*, 250; M. Moens *et al.*, *Am. J. trop. Med. Hyg.*, 1978, *27*, 897; H. F. Nagaty *et al.*, *J. trop. Med. Hyg.*, 1978, *81*, 195, per *Trop. Dis. Bull.*, 1979, *76*, 676.

Toxoplasmosis. A decrease in antitoxoplasma antibody titres and an increase in T-lymphocyte percentage counts was found in 5 patients with toxoplasmosis given levamisole 150 mg daily for 3 days every 14 days for 2 months; 2 patients were also given co-trimoxazole daily for 30 days. Clinical improvement was observed in all patients on examination 30 days after commencement of treatment.— M. Fegies and J. Guerrero, *Trans. R. Soc. trop. Med. Hyg.*, 1977, *71*, 178.

Tropical eosinophilia. A 52-year-old woman with tropical eosinophilia was treated with levamisole 120 mg every other day for 12 days. She showed marked improvement with the disappearance of rhonchi and dyspnoea. No side-effects occurred.— V. Zaman and W. P. Fung (letter), *Trans. R. Soc. trop. Med. Hyg.*, 1973, *67*, 144.

Tuberculosis. Studies indicating that levamisole might be useful as an adjunct to standard antituberculosis therapy in the treatment of pulmonary tuberculosis: D. Tanphaichitra, *Bull. int. Un. Tuberc.*, 1979, *54*, 166; N. Y. Yaseen *et al.*, *J. Infect.*, 1980, *2*, 125.

Ulcers. In a double-blind study of patients with chronic leg ulcers 30 patients received levamisole 100 to 250 mg daily in divided doses for 2 consecutive days per week for up to 20 weeks and 29 received placebo. The number of patients cured taking levamisole became significantly greater than those taking placebo after 8 weeks. Treatment was discontinued in 2 patients taking levamisole and in 8 taking placebo because there was no healing. At the end of the study all the remaining patients taking levamisole were healed compared with 76% of those taking placebo.— J. Morias *et al.*, *Arzneimittel-Forsch.*, 1979, *29*, 1050.

Aphthous ulcers. A review of levamisole in the treatment of recurrent aphthous stomatitis.— M. F. Miller, *Drugs*, 1980, *20*, 131.

In a collaborative study 25 of 82 patients with aphthous ulcers became free of lesions within a month of receiving levamisole 150 mg daily for 3 days each fortnight; the lesions were less severe in a further 25 patients. Of 25 patients with recurrent herpes infection 24 responded.— J. Symoens and J. Brugmans (letter), *Br. med. J.*, 1974, *4*, 592.

In a double-blind crossover study of 47 patients with recurrent aphthous and herpetiform ulceration, levamisole 50 mg thrice daily for 2 days every week for 8 weeks eradicated or reduced ulceration in 30; in 7 patients the response was evident only during the period of levamisole administration.— T. Lehner *et al.*, *Lancet*, 1976, *2*, 926.

Treatment with levamisole 150 mg daily for 3 days in 15 for 4 months cured 6 of 15 patients with recurrent aphthous stomatitis present for a mean of 9.5 years and seven patients showed great improvement, with very few outbreaks and smaller lesions.— C. A. de Q. Carvalho *et al.* (letter), *Trans. R. Soc. trop. Med. Hyg.*, 1976, *70*, 355.

In 3 studies in 124 patients with long-standing recurrent aphthous stomatitis significant benefit was obtained after treatment with levamisole 150 mg daily for 3 days in each 2 weeks or when new episodes occurred.— J. De Meyer *et al.*, *Br. med. J.*, 1977, *1*, 671.

For the proceedings of a workshop on aphthous stomatitis and Behçet's syndrome including the use of levamisole, see *J. Oral Path.*, 1978, *7*, 341–440. Results from 5 double-blind studies indicated that levamisole was not effective in the treatment of aphthous ulcers or Behçet's syndrome, although some patients in each study had responded well to treatment. However, it was recommended that further studies should be performed on patients with severe recurrent oral ulceration using high and low dosage regimens.— E. A. Graykowski *et al.*, *ibid.*, 439.

Levamisole was not considered to be of any help in the treatment of Behçet's disease.— J. J. H. Gilkes, *Practitioner*, 1978, *221*, 822.

Further references.— H. Verhaegen *et al.* (letter), *Lancet*, 1973, *2*, 842; H. Verhaegen *et al.*, *Postgrad. med. J.*, 1976, *52*, 511.

Warts. After treatment with levamisole 50 to 150 mg thrice weekly every 2 weeks for up to 3 months, multiple warts resistant to conventional treatment regressed in 9 of 10 children.— P. Helin and M. Bergh (letter), *New Engl. J. Med.*, 1975, *291*, 1311.

Three of 8 patients had complete regression of warts and 2 others had considerable improvement after treatment with levamisole hydrochloride 150 mg on 2 consecutive days each week for 7 months.— J. D. Sutton (letter), *Archs Derm.*, 1977, *113*, 521.

In a 6-week double-blind study in 49 patients with common warts and 50 with venereal warts (condylomata acuminata) there was no greater wart regression in those given levamisole 150 mg on 3 consecutive days every other week than in those given a placebo.— M. Schou and P. Helin, *Acta derm.-vener., Stockh.*, 1977, *57*, 449.

Proprietary Preparations

Ketrax (Available only in certain countries) *(ICI Pharmaceuticals, UK)*. Levamisole hydrochloride, available as **Syrup** containing in each 5 ml the equivalent of 40 mg levamisole and as **Tablets** each containing the equivalent of 40 mg levamisole.

Other Proprietary Names

Decaris *(Denm., Hung.)*; Ergamisol *(Belg., Ital., S.Afr.)*; Meglum *(Arg.)*; Solaskil *(Fr.)*; Stimamizol *(Arg.)*.

789-r

Lucanthone Hydrochloride *(B.P. 1968)*. Lucanth. Hydrochlor.; Lucanthoni Hydrochloridum; BW 57-233; NSC 14574. 1-(2-Diethylaminoethylamino)-4-methylthioxanthen-9-one hydrochloride.
$C_{20}H_{24}N_2OS,HCl=376.9$.

CAS — 479-50-5 (lucanthone); 548-57-2 (hydrochloride).

Pharmacopoeias. In *Int.* and *Turk.*

A yellowish-orange crystalline powder with a very slight odour and a bitter taste followed by a prolonged burning sensation. M.p. 195° to 198°. It readily stains the skin.
Soluble 1 in 110 of water, 1 in 85 of alcohol, and 1 in 20 of chloroform; practically insoluble in acetone and ether.

Adverse Effects. Nausea, vomiting, anorexia, headache, depression, dizziness, and epigastric or abdominal pain are common side-effects and are often severe enough to warrant discontinuance of treatment. Convulsions and psychotic reactions may also occur; the incidence of serious side-effects is greater in adults than in children. The local human tolerance variation is quite marked, however, and people with dark skins have been stated to tolerate the drug better than those with lighter skins.
Liver damage which may be severe and occasionally fatal has occurred in patients given hycanthone, an active metabolite of lucanthone.

Precautions. Lucanthone hydrochloride may cause yellow discoloration of the skin.
It would be advisable to consider the precautions given for hycanthone (see p.93).

Absorption and Fate. Lucanthone is readily absorbed from the gastro-intestinal tract. It is metabolised in the body and only 10% is excreted unchanged in the urine. Hycanthone is an active metabolite.

Uses. Lucanthone hydrochloride is a schistosomicide used especially in the treatment of *Schistosoma haematobium* infections. It is less effective against *S. mansoni* and is of little value against *S. japonicum*. In *S. haematobium* infections it produces rapid clinical improvement with cessation of haematuria and disappearance of viable ova from the urine.
Many dosage schedules have been used; an intensive 3-day course has been found effective, the usual dosage for an adult being 1 g by mouth morning and evening for 3 days, followed by a similar course 1 month later. The total amount of lucanthone hydrochloride to be given in 1 course of treatment has been variously stated as 60 to 200 mg per kg body-weight. Smaller doses can be given weekly or monthly to reduce the egg output in infected populations.

Schistosomiasis. In a pilot study, lucanthone hydrochloride 500 mg twice weekly for 5 weeks and then once weekly for 5 weeks produced a greater reduction in egg output than 500 mg taken once weekly for 10 weeks in 41 patients with schistosomiasis.— J. E. McMahon, *Trans. R. Soc. trop. Med. Hyg.*, 1970, *64*, 433. A non-intensive dose regimen such as this might be useful in seriously ill persons when it was necessary to avoid drug reactions.— J. E. McMahon (letter), *ibid.*, 460.

For other reports see Martindale 27th Edn, p. 1375.

Preparations

Lucanthone Tablets *(B.P. 1968)*. Lucanth. Tab. Tablets containing lucanthone hydrochloride.

Lucanthone hydrochloride was formerly marketed in Great Britain under the proprietary name Nilodin (*Wellcome*).

790-j

Male Fern *(B.P. 1973)*. Filix Mas; Aspidium; Rhizoma Filicis Maris; Fougère Mâle; Farnwurzel; Helecho Macho; Feto Macho; Felce Maschio.

Pharmacopoeias. In *Arg., Aust., Fr., Ind., Int., It., Mex., Nord., Port., Roum., Rus., Span., Swiss,* and *Turk.*
Int. and *Mex.* allow also *D. marginalis. Ind.* specifies *D. odontoloma, D. marginata, D. chrysocoma, D. ramosa,* and *D. sarbigera.*

The rhizome, frond-bases, and apical bud of *Dryopteris filix-mas* agg. (Polypodiaceae), collected late in the autumn, divested of the roots and dead portions and carefully dried, retaining the internal green colour. It contains not less than 1.5% of filicin. During storage the green colour of the interior gradually disappears, often after a lapse of 6 months, and such material is unfit for medicinal use. **Store** in airtight containers. Protect from light.
Filicin is the mixture of ether-soluble substances obtained from male fern. Its activity is chiefly due to flavaspidic acid, a phloroglucinol derivative.

Adverse Effects. Male fern is highly toxic but poorly absorbed; severe toxicity may occur if its absorption is increased, for example in the presence of fatty foods. Adverse effects include headache, nausea and vomiting, severe abdominal cramp, diarrhoea, dyspnoea, albuminuria, and bilirubinaemia. Other adverse effects include dizziness, tremors, convulsions, xanthopsia, optic neuropathy, blindness (possibly permanent), stimulation of uterine muscle, respiratory failure, cardiac arrhythmias, and cardiac failure. Fatalities have occurred.

Treatment of Adverse Effects. In severe overdosage empty the stomach by aspiration and lavage. Give a purgative such as sodium sulphate, 30 g in 250 ml of water, followed by demulcent drinks, but *avoid* oils and fats. Convulsions may be controlled by the intravenous injection of diazepam 5 to 10 mg or a short-acting barbiturate such as thiopentone sodium. Respiration may require assistance.

Precautions. Male fern should not be given to infants, the elderly, or the debilitated, or during pregnancy. It should not be given to patients with anaemia, gastro-intestinal ulceration, or impaired cardiac, hepatic, or renal function.
Since the absorption and toxic effects of male fern may be increased in the presence of oils or fats, these should not be given concomitantly.

Absorption and Fate. Filicin is variably absorbed from the gastro-intestinal tract and partly excreted unchanged in the urine.

Uses. Male fern is an effective anthelmintic for the expulsion of tapeworms *Diphyllobothrium latum, Taenia saginata,* and *T. solium*; it has been largely replaced by other less toxic agents. It is administered as Male Fern Extract, in a draught; the draught may be given by duodenal tube.
The patient should be given a semi-fluid diet preferably for 2 days before the extract is administered and a saline purgative each evening. The extract should be given on the morning of the third day to the fasting patient in 1 dose of 3 to 6 ml or in several equal portions at half-hourly intervals, followed 2 hours after the last portion by a saline purgative.
Treatment may have to be repeated on several occasions but an interval of 7 to 10 days should elapse between treatments.

It was recommended by the Food Additives and Contaminants Committee that male fern rhizome be prohibited for use in foods as a flavouring agent.— *Report on the Review of Flavourings in Food*, FAC/REP/22, Ministry of Agriculture, Fisheries and Food, London, HM Stationery Office, 1976.

Preparations

Male Fern Extract *(B.P. 1973)*. Ext. Filic.; Aspidium Oleoresin; Male Fern Oleoresin; Extractum Filicis Maris Tenue; Extractum Filicis Aethereum. A thick greenish-brown liquid, often containing a granular sediment. Wt per ml not less than 0.995 g. Prepared by ether extraction of male fern and adjusted with arachis oil or other suitable official fixed oil to contain 21 to 23% w/w of filicin. It should be thoroughly stirred before use. Store in airtight containers. Protect from light. *Dose.* 3 to 6 ml. A similar extract is included in *Int. P.* and many other pharmacopoeias, the specified filicin content varies from 17 to 28% w/w.

Male Fern Extract Capsules *(B.P. 1958)*. Caps. Ext. Filic. Capsules containing male fern extract.

Male Fern Extract Draught *(B.P.C. 1973)*. Male Fern Draught; Haustus Filicis. Male fern extract 4 g, acacia 4 g, water to 50 ml. It should be recently prepared. *Dose.* 50 ml.

791-z

Mebendazole *(U.S.P.)*. R 17635. Methyl 5-benzoyl-1*H*-benzimidazol-2-ylcarbamate.
$C_{16}H_{13}N_3O_3=295.3$.

CAS — 31431-39-7.

Pharmacopoeias. In *U.S.*

A white to slightly yellow amorphous powder. M.p. about 290°. Practically **insoluble** in water, alcohol, chloroform, ether, and dilute mineral acids; freely soluble in formic acid.

Adverse Effects and Precautions. Nausea, vomiting, abdominal pain, and diarrhoea may occasionally occur.
Mebendazole is teratogenic in *rats* and should not be given to pregnant women.

Two of over 100 patients, treated with mebendazole in normal doses for 3 days, complained of slight headache and dizziness. There were no reports of gastro-inestinal side-effects or of skin rashes.— S. K. K. Seah, *Can. med. Ass. J.*, 1976, *115*, 777.

Adverse effects experienced during treatment with mebendazole have included, gastro-intestinal disturbances, pruritus, dizziness, drowsiness, headache, abnormalities in liver-function tests, eosinophilia, lowered haemoglobin concentrations, leucopenia, haematuria, and casts. No serious or life-threatening reactions have been reported.— T. C. Beard *et al.*, *Med. J. Aust.*, 1978, *1*, 633.

Respiratory symptoms with cough and fever had been reported in 8 of 133 Kenyan patients receiving mebendazole for hydatid disease. Glomerulonephritis, histologically confirmed in 6, was possibly a result of immune complexes liberated into the circulation.— *Br. med. J.*, 1979, *2*, 563.

Pyrexia. Fever in 2 patients given mebendazole for hydatid cysts possibly represented drug-induced tissue necrosis in the cysts.— I. M. Murray-Lyon and K. W. Reynolds, *Br. med. J.*, 1979, *2*, 1111. Criticism. There is no good evidence in man that mebendazole penetrates intact, established cysts in sufficient concentrations to produce destruction.— D. R. Osborne (letter), *ibid.*, 1980, *280*, 183.

Pyrexia in one patient receiving mebendazole 100 mg twice daily for 3 days was probably due to a different mechanism than that in patients with hydatid cysts since it only occurred while the patient was taking mebendazole.— A. Harris (letter), *Br. med. J.*, 1979, *2*, 1365.

Absorption and Fate. Mebendazole is not significantly absorbed from the gastro-intestinal tract; only about 2% of a dose is excreted unchanged or as a metabolite in the urine.

After administration of mebendazole 1.5 g by mouth to 3 fasting subjects, plasma concentrations did not exceed 17 nmol per litre but when given with food peak plasma concentrations reached 91 to 142 nmol per litre within 2 to 4 hours. Plasma half-lives ranged from 1.5 to 5.5 hours. In one patient with echinococcosis and cholestasis who received a similar dose the peak plasma concentration was 379 nmol per litre 4 hours after administration and the plasma half-life was 8 hours. In patients on long-term treatment, increases in plasma concentrations after a dose of mebendazole showed great intra-individual variations.— G. J. Münst *et al.*, *Eur. J. clin. Pharmac.*, 1980, *17*, 375.

Further references: A. Bryceson (letter), *Br. med. J.*, 1980, *280*, 796.

Uses. Mebendazole is an anthelmintic effective against threadworms (*Enterobius*), roundworms (*Ascaris*), whipworms (*Trichuris*), and hookworms (*Ancylostoma* and *Necator*). It is also used in the treatment of capillariasis and is possibly effective against tapeworms; it is not consistently effective against strongyloid worms.
The usual dose for adults and children aged 2 years or over with threadworm infection is 100 mg as a single dose, repeated if necessary after 2 to 3 weeks; for hookworm, roundworm, and whipworm infections the usual dose is 100 mg twice daily for 3 days.

A short review of the use of mebendazole.— *Med. Lett.*, 1975, *17*, 37.

The anthelmintic action of mebendazole was considered to be due to its inhibition of glucose uptake by nematodes.— U. K. Sheth, *Prog. Drug Res.*, 1975, *19*, 147.

Favourable results or cure were obtained in 2 patients infected with microfilariae of *Dipetalonema perstans* treated with mebendazole 400 mg twice daily for 14 days followed by a second treatment with mebendazole 100 mg twice daily and levamisole 50 mg daily for 14 days.— J. M. Goldsmid and S. Rogers, *Cent. Afr. J. Med.*, 1979, *25*, 51, per *Trop. Dis. Bull.*, 1979, *76*, 1129.

Three of 4 patients infected with microfilariae resembling *Dipetalonema perstans* were successfully treated with mebendazole 100 mg thrice daily and levamisole 100 mg twice daily for 10 days.— H. C. Bernberg *et al.*, *Trans. R. Soc. trop. Med. Hyg.*, 1979, *73*, 233.

For a study of a regimen consisting of levamisole and mebendazole used in the treatment of *W. bancrofti* infection, see Levamisole, p.96.

Capillaria infections. Mebendazole, in doses of 400 mg daily for 20 or 30 days, was considered to be very effective in the treatment of intestinal capillariasis.— C. N. Singson *et al.*, *Am. J. trop. Med. Hyg.*, 1975, *24*, 932.

Guinea-worm. In 12 patients with guinea-worm infection given mebendazole 200 mg four times daily for 6 days (repeated if necessary) there was rapid relief of pain and inflammation, and the worm was fragmented and extruded.— A. Z. Shafei, *J. trop. Med. Hyg.*, 1976, *79*, 197. An unfavourable report.— O. O. Kale, *Am. J. trop. Med. Hyg.*, 1975, *24*, 600.

Hookworm (*Ancylostoma*). Of 53 patients examined 50 were freed from infection with hookworm by treatment with mebendazole 200 mg twice daily for 4 days. No side-effects were reported.— D. Banerjee *et al.*, *Indian J. med. Res.*, 1972, *60*, 562, per *Trop. Dis. Bull.*, 1973, *70*, 363.

Hookworm (*Necator*). From a review of studies comparing anthelmintics used in the treatment of hookworm infection, mebendazole 200 mg twice daily for 4 days was recommended for use in necatoriasis.— B. J. Vakil and N. J. Dalal, *Prog. Drug Res.*, 1975, *19*, 166.

For a comparative study of the use of mebendazole and pyrantel embonate in the treatment of *Necator americanus* infection, see Pyrantel Embonate, p.104.

Hydatid disease. Discussions on the use of mebendazole in the treatment of hydatid disease: T. C. Beard *et al.*, *Med. J. Aust.*, 1978, *1*, 633; *Br. med. J.*, 1979, *2*, 563.

Complete regression of intrahepatic cysts was achieved in 4 patients with hepatic hydatid disease treated with mebendazole in increasing doses up to 400 to 600 mg thrice daily for 21 to 30 days, courses being repeated to a total of nine.— A. Bekhti *et al.*, *Br. med. J.*, 1977, *2*, 1047. Further studies of the use of high doses of mebendazole in the treatment of hydatid disease: T. C. Beard (letter), *Med. J. Aust.*, 1976, *2*, 230; H. T. Goodman (letter), *ibid.*, 662; J. F. Wilson *et al.*, *Am. Rev. resp. Dis.*, 1978, *118*, 747, per *Abstr. Hyg.*, 1978, *53*, 1495; J. Starke, *Dt. med. Wschr.*, 1979, *104*, 1132; R. Ammann *et al.*, *Schweiz. med. Wschr.*, 1979, *109*, 148; H. J. S. Kayser, *S. Afr. med. J.*, 1980, *58*, 560.

Although there is some evidence that after high doses by mouth mebendazole can be detected in plasma in low concentrations, it is not reasonable to treat hydatid disease which requires significant blood and cyst fluid concentrations, by mouth with a drug developed specifically to be poorly absorbed from the gastro-intestinal tract. Alternative compounds and routes of administration are to be studied.— A. L. Macnair, *Janssen* (letter), *Br. med. J.*, 1980, *280*, 1055.

Mixed infections. In a series of investigations involving 602 patients aged 7 to 17 years, mebendazole 200 mg twice daily for 4 days was considered more effective than levamisole, and gave complete cures to patients infected with roundworms and threadworms, was 84.2 to 100% effective against hookworms, 96 to 100% effective against whipworms, but was ineffective against *Strongyloides stercoralis*. No side-effects were reported.— G. Chaia and A. S. Cunha, *Folha med.*, 1971, *63*, 843, per *Trop. Dis. Bull.*, 1972, *69*, 922.

Mebendazole 100 mg twice daily for 3 days given to 58 children aged 3 to 15 years, eradicated roundworm and threadworm infections and over 92% of hookworm and whipworm infections without causing side-effects.— G. Chaia *et al.*, *Folha med.*, 1972, *64*, 139, per *Trop. Dis. Bull.*, 1972, *69*, 922.

Whipworm was eradicated from 37 children given mebendazole 100 mg daily for 6 days. Mebendazole 100 mg twice daily for 3 days eradicated hookworm (*Necator*) from 49 children and cured 85 to 95% of those also infected with whipworm.— G. Chaia *et al.*, *Revta Inst. Med. trop. S Paulo*, 1973, *15*, 239, per *Trop. Dis. Bull.*, 1974, *71*, 64.

Complete eradication of roundworms, almost complete eradication of hookworms (*Ancylostoma*), and 96.8 to 99% cure of whipworm infection followed the treatment of 225 patients with mebendazole 200 mg daily for 3 or 4 days. No significant relapses occurred during the 3 months following treatment, and practically no side-effects were observed.— J. Vandepitte *et al.*, *Bull. Soc. Path. exot.*, 1973, *66*, 165, per *Trop. Dis. Bull.*, 1974, *71*, 69.

Mebendazole 100 mg 30 minutes before breakfast and again 3 hours after food at night, given for 3 consecutive days to 48 patients aged 4 to 14 years who had mixed infections, eradicated roundworms and whipworms, and cured 97.5% of patients with hookworm infection. There were also 5 apparent cures in patients harbouring tapeworms.— D. W. C. Souza *et al.*, *Revta Inst. Med. trop. S Paulo*, 1973, *15*, 30, per *Trop. Dis. Bull.*, 1974, *71*, 264.

After treatment of 85 children with mebendazole 100 mg twice daily for 3 days the overall cure-rate for ascaris infection was 100%, for trichuris 94%, for hookworm 82%, and for hymenolepis 39%. Infection with *Giardia lamblia* cysts was eliminated in 10 of 25 children.— J. G. P. Hutchison *et al.*, *Br. med. J.*, 1975, *2*, 309. Similar results in 91 children and adults treated with mebendazole 50 to 100 mg twice daily for 3 days.— S. K. K. Seah, *Can. med. Ass. J.*, 1976, *115*, 777.

Success-rates of 98.5% against threadworm, 100% against roundworm (*Ascaris*), 100% against whipworm, and 54.5% against dwarf tapeworm in 68 children treated with mebendazole plus thiabendazole.— H. Schenone *et al.*, *Boln chil. Parasit.*, 1975, *30*, 89, per *Trop. Dis. Bull.*, 1976, *73*, 322.

Success-rates of 87.2% against roundworm (*Ascaris*) and 86% against hookworm (*Ancylostoma*) in 143 patients treated with mebendazole 100 mg twice daily for 3 days.— K. C. Singhal *et al.*, *J. Ass. Physns India*, 1975, *23*, 903, per *Trop. Dis. Bull.*, 1976, *73*, 936.

Mebendazole 100 mg twice daily for 3 days and pyrantel in the same dosage were equally effective in 117 patients against roundworm (*Ascaris*) and hookworm infection; mebendazole had a success-rate of 71.4% against whipworm and 66.6% against *Strongyloides*.— N. Islam and N. A. Chowdhury, *S.E. Asian J. trop. med. publ. Hlth*, 1976, *7*, 81, per *Trop. Dis. Bull.*, 1977, *74*, 231.

Reduced incidence of roundworm (*Ascaris*), hookworm, and whipworm after mass treatment with mebendazole 200 mg daily for 3 or 4 days.— T. C. Banzon *et al.*, *J. Philipp. med. Ass.*, 1976, *52*, 239, per *Trop. Dis. Bull.*, 1977, *74*, 246. See also J. C. Bina *et al.*, *Revta Inst. Med. trop. S Paulo*, 1977, *19*, 47, per *Trop. Dis. Bull.*, 1977, *74*, 744.

Mebendazole 100 mg twice daily for 3 days or 200 mg twice daily for 2 days followed by 100 mg twice daily for 2 days was given to 255 patients with moderate to severe infections with intestinal nematodes. Cure-rates for the high-dose regimen were 100% against ascariasis, 93.3% against hookworm, 96.7% against whipworm, and 80% for strongyloidiasis. Cure-rates of 100, 86.7, 73.3, and 46.7% were obtained with the low-dose regimen.— A. Z. Shafei, *Niger. med. J.*, 1978, *8*, 340.

Further references.— E. Klein, *Dt. med. Wschr.*, 1972, *97*, 1215, per *Trop. Dis. Bull.*, 1972, *69*, 1160; J. Vandepitte and D. Thienpont (letter), *Br. med. J.*, 1972, *4*, 549; D. W. C. Souza *et al.*, *Revta Soc. bras. Med. trop.*, 1973, *7*, 237, per *Trop. Dis. Bull.*, 1974, *71*, 512; A. P. Chavarria *et al.*, *Am. J. trop. Med. Hyg.*, 1973, *22*, 592, per *Trop. Dis. Bull.*, 1974, *71*, 511; O. Devay, *Revta patol. trop.*, 1974, *3*, 43, per *Trop. Dis. Bull.*, 1974, *71*, 1152; H. Schenone *et al.*, *Boln chil. Parasit.*, 1974, *29*, 2, per *Trop. Dis. Bull.*, 1975, *72*, 69; F. Partono *et al.*, *S.E. Asian J. trop. med. publ. Hlth*, 1974, *5*, 258, per *Trop. Dis. Bull.*, 1975, *72*, 151; B. J. Vakil *et al.*, *J. trop. Med. Hyg.*, 1975, *78*, 154, per *Trop. Dis. Bull.*, 1976, *73*, 151; B. S. Seo *et al.*, *Korean J. Parasit.*, 1977, *15*, 11, per *Trop. Dis. Bull.*, 1978, *75*, 381.

Onchocerciasis. Evidence that mebendazole may be a useful alternative to diethylcarbamazine in onchocerciasis. In a double-blind study in 40 male patients with onchocerciasis, the following 4 drug regimens were employed: mebendazole 1 g twice daily for 28 days, levamisole 150 mg weekly for 5 weeks, the mebendazole and levamisole regimens together, or diethylcarbamazine citrate 100 mg twice daily for 28 days. Diethylcarbamazine produced the more rapid fall in skin counts but on follow-up at 6 months those receiving mebendazole alone or with levamisole showed similar or slightly greater reductions. Examination of adult worms in nodules excised at 2 months showed changes suggestive of an interruption of embryogenesis in those receiving the mebendazole-containing regimens only. Levamisole alone had no significant effect on microfilariae counts. Despite corticosteroid administration during the initial stages of diethylcarbamazine therapy, more systemic side-effects occurred in the diethylcarbamazine group; ocular complications were also more common and more severe in those receiving diethylcarbamazine.— A. R. Rivas-Alcalá *et al.*, *Lancet*, 1981, *2*, 485. Twelve-month follow-up.— *idem*, 1043.

Tapeworm (*Taenia*). Mebendazole 200 mg twice daily for 4 days cured 90% of patients infected with tapeworms, in a trial involving 31 patients. Treatment for shorter periods or with smaller doses was much less effective.— N. Katz and F. Zicker, *Revta Soc. bras. Med. trop.*, 1973, *7*, 225, per *Trop. Dis. Bull.*, 1974, *71*, 519.

Cure of 10 patients with *Taenia saginata* or *T. solium* infection with mebendazole 600 mg daily for 3 days.— A. P. Chavarria *et al.*, *Am. J. trop. Med. Hyg.*, 1977, *26*, 118, per *Trop. Dis. Bull.*, 1977, *74*, 846. See also P. V. Arambulo *et al.*, *Acta trop.*, 1978, *35*, 281, per *Trop. Dis. Bull.*, 1979, *76*, 490.

Threadworm. In a study in 702 persons (mainly children), most of whom had threadworm (*Enterobius*) infection, treatment with mebendazole 75 mg as a single dose for children and 100 to 200 mg for adults resulted in cure-rates of 92 and 88% respectively of those affected. There were no side-effects even after larger doses.— J. P. Brugmans *et al.*, *J. Am. med. Ass.*, 1971, *217*, 313. See also E. Fierlafijn and O. F. Vanparijs, *Trop. geogr. Med.*, 1973, *25*, 242, per *Trop. Dis. Bull.*, 1974, *71*, 522.

Trichinella. Mebendazole was shown to be highly effective, well tolerated, and to be superior to corticosteroids in the treatment of trichinellosis caused by *Trichinella spiralis*.— N. N. Ozeretskovskaya *et al.*, *Medskaya Parazit.*, 1978, *47*, 43, per *Abstr. Hyg.*, 1979, *54*, 129.

Mebendazole is considered to be an alternative to thiabendazole in the treatment of *Trichinella spiralis* infections. The recommended adult dose is 200 to 400 mg thrice daily for 3 days then 400 to 500 mg thrice daily for 10 days.— *Med. Lett.*, 1979, *21*, 105.

Whipworm. Mebendazole 100 mg twice daily for 3 days was given to 107 children with trichuriasis, 88 of whom also had concomitant ascariasis. Egg reduction-rates of 97.6 and 99.5% and cure-rates of 68.2 and 98.8% were obtained for *Trichuris trichiura* and *Ascaris lumbricoides* respectively.— M. S. Wolfe and J. M. Wershing, *J. Am. med. Ass.*, 1974, *230*, 1408.

Mebendazole 100 mg twice daily for 3 days administered to 35 patients with trichuriasis produced a cure-rate of 69%. It was ineffective when given as a single dose of 300 mg. In 74 patients with enterobiasis 71 were cured after a single dose of 100 mg.— M. J. Miller *et al.*, *J. Am. med. Ass.*, 1974, *230*, 1412.

Cure-rates of 53.3, 64.3, and 66.7% were achieved at 6 weeks in patients with *Trichuris trichiura* infection after treatment for 2, 3, or 4 days respectively with mebendazole 100 mg twice daily.— R. G. Sargent *et al.*, *Am. J. trop. Med. Hyg.*, 1974, *23*, 375, per *Trop. Dis. Bull.*, 1974, *71*, 940.

Apparent cure was achieved in 48 of 50 children with *Trichuris trichiura* infection given mebendazole 100 mg twice daily for 3 days.— S. Maqbool *et al.*, *J. Pediat.*, 1975, *86*, 463, per *Abstr. Hyg.*, 1975, *50*, 711.

Mebendazole appeared to be more effective than tetramisole or thiabendazole during comparative studies of the treatment of trichuriasis.— B. J. Vakil and N. J. Dalal, *Prog. Drug Res.*, 1975, *19*, 166.

Mebendazole 100 mg twice daily given for 3 consecutive days to 49 patients with trichuriasis produced an 82% cure-rate and an egg reduction of 87%.— M. G. Blechman, *Curr. ther. Res.*, 1975, *18*, 800.

In 60 patients with *Trichuris trichiura* infection treatment with mebendazole 100 mg twice daily for 3 or 4 days produced clearance-rates of 65.6 and 89.3% respectively.— R. G. Sargent *et al.*, *Sth. med. J.*, 1975, *68*, 38, per *Int. pharm. Abstr.*, 1976, *13*, 26.

Further references.— F. M. Paul and V. Zaman, *Singapore med. J.*, 1975, *16*, 11, per *Trop. Dis. Bull.*, 1975, *72*, 1084; M. S. Shiratsuchi *et al.*, *Revta Inst. Med. trop. S Paulo*, 1975, *17*, 206, per *Trop. Dis. Bull.*, 1975, *72*, 1084; N. D. W. Lionel *et al.*, *J. trop. Med. Hyg.*, 1975, *78*, 75, per *Trop. Dis. Bull.*, 1975, *72*, 1084; I. Nagalingam *et al.*, *Am. J. trop. Med. Hyg.*, 1976, *25*, 568, per *Trop. Dis. Bull.*, 1977, *74*, 249; J. N. Scragg and E. M. Proctor, *Am. J. trop. Med. Hyg.*, 1977, *26*, 198.

Preparations

Mebendazole Tablets *(U.S.P.)*. Tablets containing mebendazole.

Vermox *(Janssen, UK)*. Mebendazole, available as **Suspension** containing 100 mg in each 5 ml and as scored chewable **Tablets** of 100 mg. (Also available as Vermox in *Austral., Belg., Canad., Ger., Ital., Neth., NZ, S.Afr., Switz., USA*).

Other Proprietary Names
Mebendacin *(Spain)*; Mebutar, Nemasole *(both Arg.)*.

792-c

Meglumine Antimonate. Antimony Meglumine; RP 2168; Protostib. 1-Deoxy-1-methylamino-D-glucitol antimonate.
$C_7H_{18}NO_8Sb$=366.0.

CAS — 6284-40-8 (meglumine); 133-51-7 (antimonate).

A white powder. **Soluble** 1 in 3 of water; practically insoluble in alcohol.

Uses. Meglumine antimonate has the actions and uses of antimony sodium tartrate (see p.87) and has been used in the treatment of cutaneous leishmaniasis and kala-azar in doses of 100 mg per kg body-weight, by deep intramuscular injection daily for 10 to 12 days and repeated if required after an interval of 4 to 6 weeks.

A report of agranulocytosis occurring in a 23-month-old child during treatment of visceral leishmaniasis with meglumine antimonate. The child had received intramuscularly 20 mg per kg body-weight for 2 days, 40 mg per kg for 2 days, and 60 mg per kg for 3 days.— P. Bourée and O. Dulac, *Archs fr. Pédiat.*, 1977, *34*, 659.

Proprietary Names
Glucantim *(Farmitalia, Ital.)*; Glucantime *(Specia, Fr.; Rhodia, Spain)*.

793-k

Niclosamide *(B.P., B.P. Vet.)*. Bayer 2353; Phenasale. 2′,5-Dichloro-4′-nitrosalicylanilide; 5-Chloro-*N*-(2-chloro-4-nitrophenyl)-2-hydroxybenzamide.

$C_{13}H_8Cl_2N_2O_4$=327.1.

CAS — 50-65-7.

Pharmacopoeias. In *Br.* and *Nord.*, *Jug.* and *Nord.* include the monohydrate.

A cream-coloured odourless or almost odourless tasteless powder. M.p. about 228°. Practically **insoluble** in water; soluble 1 in 150 of alcohol, 1 in 400 of chloroform, and 1 in 350 of ether; soluble in acetone. **Protect** from light.

Adverse Effects. Nausea and gastro-intestinal pain and discomfort may occur occasionally.

The toxic actions of niclosamide were due to its ability to uncouple oxidative phosphorylation. However, its mammalian toxicity was low and it was considered that the consumption of the very small concentrations likely to be present in water after niclosamide had been used as a molluscicide would not present any human hazard.— Safe Use of Pesticides, Twentieth Report of the WHO Expert Committee on Insecticides, *Tech. Rep. Ser. Wld Hlth Org. No. 513*, 1973.

Absorption and Fate. Niclosamide is not significantly absorbed from the gastro-intestinal tract.

Uses. Niclosamide is an anthelmintic which is active against most tapeworms, including the beef tapeworm (*Taenia saginata*), the pork tapeworm (*T. solium*), the fish tapeworm (*Diphyllobothrium latum*), and the dwarf tapeworm (*Hymenolepis nana*).

Niclosamide is administered in tablets, which must be chewed thoroughly before swallowing and washed down with the minimum amount of water. For infections with beef, pork, and fish tapeworms the patient should abstain from solid food from the evening before treatment. The next morning a dose of 1 g is given on an empty stomach, followed 1 hour later by another dose of 1 g, or a single 2-g dose may be given. A meal may be taken 2 hours thereafter.

A brisk purgative is recommended 2 hours after the last dose to expel the killed worms and to minimise the possibility of the migration of ova of *T. solium* into the stomach, with the consequent risk of cysticercosis. An anti-emetic may be given before treatment to reduce this risk.

In dwarf-tapeworm infections an initial dose of 2 g is given after food and followed by 1 g daily for 6 days. The course may be repeated after 1 month. Higher doses may be required.

Children aged 2 to 6 years are given half the above doses and children under 2 years of age given one-quarter the above doses.

After treatment with niclosamide, portions of the worm are voided in a partially digested form and the scolex is rarely identifiable.

Niclosamide has been given in conjunction with dichlorophen.

The ethanolamine salt of niclosamide has been used as a molluscicide.

Niclosamide 43 to 160 mg per kg body-weight given as a single morning dose or in 2 consecutive morning doses to 27 children infected with the intestinal fluke *Fasciolopsis buski* reduced the egg concentration by 41%. Tetrachloroethylene 0.08 to 0.14 ml per kg as a single dose reduced the eggs by 97% in 13 children. Side-effects were mild with niclosamide but numerous and severe with tetrachloroethylene.— P. Suntharasamai *et al.*, *S.E. Asian J. trop. med. publ. Hlth*, 1974, *5*, 556, per *Trop. Dis. Bull.*, 1975, *72*, 733.

For a comparison of niclosamide with dichlorophen in the treatment of *Fasciolopsis buski* infection, see Dichlorophen, p.90.

Dog tapeworm. Seven children, aged under 2 years, were treated with niclosamide for infection with dog tapeworm (*Dipylidium caninum*); in 6 the worm was expelled complete with scolex and in the seventh there was no sign of the worm in a 4-month follow-up.— R. Belmar, *Boln chil. Parasit.*, 1963, *18*, 63, per *Trop. Dis. Bull.*, 1964, *61*, 939. Success in 43 patients.— W. E. Jones, *Am. J. trop. Med. Hyg.*, 1979, *28*, 300, per *Trop. Dis. Bull.*, 1980, *77*, 487.

Mesocestoides infections. Niclosamide 1 g was used successfully in the treatment of infection by a tapeworm (*Mesocestoides*) in a 2-year-old child for whom treatment with other drugs was ineffective.— N. N. Gleason *et al.*, *Am. J. trop. Med. Hyg.*, 1973, *22*, 757, per *Trop. Dis. Bull.*, 1974, *71*, 386.

For other references to the use of niclosamide for the elimination of tapeworms, see Martindale 27th Edn, p. 107.

Use as molluscicide. For reports, see P. Jordan *et al.*, *Bull. Wld Hlth Org.*, 1978, *56*, 139; K. Y. Chu, *ibid.*, 313.

Preparations

Niclosamide Tablets *(B.P.)*. Tablets containing niclosamide with sweetening and flavouring agents. The tablets should be chewed then swallowed. Protect from light.

Yomesan *(Bayer, UK)*. Niclosamide, available as chewable tablets of 500 mg. (Also available as Yomesan in *Arg., Austral., Canad., Denm., Ger., Ital., Neth., S.Afr., Switz.*).

Other Proprietary Names
Cestocida *(Spain)*; Sulqui *(Arg.)*; Trédémine *(Fr.)*.

794-a

Niridazole. Ba-32644. 1-(5-Nitrothiazol-2-yl)imidazolidin-2-one.

$C_6H_6N_4O_3S$=214.2.

CAS — 61-57-4.

A yellow, odourless, tasteless, crystalline powder. Practically **insoluble** in water and most organic solvents. Unstable in alkaline solutions.

Adverse Effects. Common side-effects include anorexia, nausea, vomiting, diarrhoea, dizziness, headache, and abdominal pain. Insomnia, minor cardiac arrhythmias, anxiety, confusion, and hallucinations occur less frequently. Convulsions are rare but serious and treatment should be stopped. Allergic reactions and paraesthesia have been reported. Haemolysis may occur in persons with a deficiency of glucose-6-phosphate dehydrogenase.

A 17-month-old child in Tanzania who was given 3 doses of niridazole (total of no more than 1 g) for *S. mansoni* infection developed convulsions and died. Severe schistosomal liver damage appeared to be a predisposing cause of death and possibly the convulsions resulted from failure of the liver to metabolise niridazole.— N. G. Nicholson and J. E. McMahon (letter), *Br. med. J.*, 1966, *2*, 1261.

Treatment with niridazole, 30 mg per kg body-weight daily for 5 days, had to be interrupted in 16 of 20 patients and discontinued in 4 because of side-effects. Headache, vomiting, dizziness, muscle pain, and weakness on the second and third days of treatment were reported. The addition of promethazine 25 mg twice daily failed to affect the incidence of side-effects in 10 patients. Aspirin 600 mg twice daily given in conjunction with niridazole 25 mg per kg body-weight daily to 25 patients appeared to reduce the intensity and frequency of headaches.— J. E. McMahon, *Trans. R. Soc. trop. Med. Hyg.*, 1967, *61*, 648.

Of 221 patients with *S. mansoni* infection treated with niridazole 40 mg per kg body-weight daily it was necessary to discontinue treatment in 7 because of toxicity, and severe side-effects occurred in 15. Convulsions occurred in 2 patients, hallucinations in 14, and haematemesis in 2. Severe side-effects occurred mainly in those patients with the hepatosplenic form of the infection.— C. A. Argento *et al.*, *Revta bras. Malar. Doenç. trop.*, 1967, *19*, 455, per *Trop. Dis. Bull.*, 1968, *65*, 1008.

In 40 patients with *Schistosoma* infections treated with niridazole, side-effects in order of frequency were loss of weight, headache, painful eyes, dizziness, loss of appetite, nausea and giddiness, psychic alterations, and painful muscles, bones, and joints. Disorders of cardiac rhythm and urticarial exanthema occurred rarely. Acute psychosis occurred in 1 patient.— W. Mohr and C. Roth, *Z. Tropenmed. Parasit.*, 1968, *19*, 263, per *Trop. Dis. Bull.*, 1969, *66*, 1288.

Side-effects of allergic conjunctivitis and pellagra-like dermatitis occurred in 2 and 5 patients respectively during hospital treatment with niridazole. Niridazole might interfere with nicotinamide metabolism.— S. Bassily *et al.* (letter), *Trans. R. Soc. trop. Med. Hyg.*, 1973, *67*, 312.

In addition to 2 cases already reported, at least 10 patients developed pulmonary reactions after treatment with niridazole by mouth; on occasion the reaction had been relieved only by the intravenous injection of 100 mg of hydrocortisone sodium succinate.— Z. Farid *et al.* (letter), *Br. med. J.*, 1973, *2*, 661.

Carcinogenicity. Niridazole was shown to be a potent carcinogen in *mice*.— H. K. Urman *et al.*, *Cancer Letts*, 1975, *1*, 69.

Cardiac arrhythmias. ECG changes caused by niridazole were less frequent and less severe than those caused by antimony compounds.— J. A. F. Da Silva *et al.*, *Hospital, Rio de J.*, 1967, *72*, 1455, per *Trop. Dis. Bull.*, 1968, *65*, 1130.

Mutagenicity. Studies have revealed that niridazole exerts a mutagenic effect on the male germinal epithelium and have indicated a cytotoxic action on spermatogonia, spermatids, and spermatozoa in *mice*. However, there was no evidence of mutagenic effects on somatic cells in various mammalian systems.— Epidemiology and control of schistosomiasis, Report of a WHO Expert Committee, *Tech. Rep. Ser. Wld Hlth Org. No. 643*, 1980.

Neuropsychiatric disturbances. Psychotic symptoms unresponsive to phenobarbitone or chlorpromazine occurred in 7 of 12 patients with hepatosplenic schistosomiasis and 2 of 5 with intestinal schistosomiasis during treatment with niridazole 21 to 31 mg per kg body-weight daily.— R. F. Zyngier *et al.*, *Hospital, Rio de J.*, 1967, *72*, 1469, per *Trop. Dis. Bull.*, 1968, *65*, 1130.

In 20 patients with schistosomiasis given divided doses of 25 mg per kg body-weight of niridazole daily for 7 days, confusion, hallucinations, and headaches were the main neuropsychiatric symptoms and EEG changes were noted in 8 patients.— J. C. Davidson, *Trans. R. Soc. trop. Med. Hyg.*, 1969, *63*, 579.

A young woman committed suicide while being treated with niridazole. Retrospective study showed neuropsychiatric symptoms (including convulsions and suicide) in 7 of 72 patients treated.— S. P. Calloway, *Med. J. Zambia*, 1976, *10*, 70, per *Trop. Dis. Bull.*, 1977, *74*, 237.

Precautions. Niridazole should not be given to patients with epilepsy, severe heart disease, or a history of mental disturbance. It should not be given to patients being treated with isoniazid. Care is necessary in patients with impaired liver function or with liver damage due to heavy infection with *Schistosoma mansoni*.

The urine of patients taking niridazole might be coloured a deep brown.

Absorption and Fate. Niridazole is slowly absorbed from the gastro-intestinal tract over 10 to 15 hours and peak concentrations appear in the blood after about 6 hours. It is rapidly metabolised in the liver and metabolites are present in much greater concentrations than unchanged drug in peripheral blood. Niridazole and its metabolites are widely distributed in the tissues; the metabolites are bound to plasma proteins. Dark brown metabolites are excreted in the urine and bile. The schistosomicidal activity is due to the unchanged niridazole in the blood which amounts to about 1.5% of the dose; high concentrations are reached in the portal vein. About half of a dose is excreted in the urine within 48 hours: the remainder is excreted in the bile.

In patients with advanced schistosomiasis and portal-systemic shunts, the blood concentrations of niridazole were higher and caused more side-effects than in patients with mild disease.— J. W. Faigle, *Acta pharmac. tox.*, 1971, *29*, 233, per *Int. pharm. Abstr.*, 1973, *10*, 32.

Uses. Niridazole is a schistosomicide; it accumulates in the eggs and germ cells of adult schistosomes and is particularly active against *S. haematobium*. It is also used in the treatment of amoebiasis and in infections with guinea-worm (*Dracunculus medinensis*).

In schistosomiasis it is given in a daily dose of 25 mg per kg body-weight, up to a maximum of 1.5 g, in 2 divided doses. In *S. haematobium* infection treatment is usually given for 7 days and for *S. mansoni* infection for 10 days. Children may be given up to 35 mg per kg daily in divided doses; treatment for 5 days is often adequate for *S. haematobium* infection. Patients with hepatosplenic schistosomiasis should be treated in hospital.

In amoebiasis, a dose of 500 mg twice or thrice daily has been given for 7 to 10 days.

In guinea-worm infections courses of treatment similar to those for schistosomiasis are given for 7 to 10 days.

For reports of 45 papers dealing with the pharmacology and clinical uses of niridazole and other compounds used in the treatment of schistosomiasis, see *Ann. N.Y. Acad. Sci.*, 1969, *160*, 427–946, per *Trop. Dis. Bull.*, 1970, *67*, 299.

In 11 patients with schistosomiasis given niridazole for 7 days serum-uric acid concentrations had decreased by a mean of 44% at the end of the therapy and in a further group of 7 patients given niridazole a 30 to 50% decrease in serum-uric acid concentrations occurred which was still reduced 4 days after discontinuing treatment. It was concluded that niridazole had uricosuric properties.— M. Weintraub *et al.*, *Clin. Pharmac. Ther.*, 1977, *22*, 568.

Amoebiasis. In a study involving 100 patients, niridazole in a dosage of 500 mg twice or thrice daily (approximating to 25 mg per kg body-weight daily) for 10 days was an effective directly-acting amoebicide. Of 50 patients with acute amoebic dysentery, 40 had healed ulcers and were free from amoebae, 5 were free from amoebae but ulcers still remained, and 5 failed to respond. Of 25 patients with amoebic liver abscess, all were apparently cured within 38 days of commencing treatment but 2 subsequently relapsed. Of 25 patients treated concurrently with niridazole and dehydroemetine, 1.5 mg per kg daily, 24 were cured. Minor side-effects included headache, anorexia, nausea, and vomiting in 9 patients. Other side-effects included abdominal pain and peripheral oedema in a malnourished patient, confusional states commencing between the eighth and tenth days of treatment in 4 patients, and tachycardia in 6 patients. ECG studies indicated T-wave inversion or flattening in 53 of 75 patients who had niridazole alone and T-wave changes in 22 of the 25 patients who had niridazole and dehydroemetine. Niridazole was considered to be more effective than emetine preparations.— S. J. Powell *et al.*, *Lancet*, 1966, *2*, 20.

Niridazole 500 mg twice daily for 7 days was effective in the treatment of amoebiasis in 20 of 22 patients treated, but 1 patient relapsed 5 weeks after treatment.— T. K. Saha and J. N. Mandal, *J. Indian med. Ass.*, 1970, *55*, 127, per *Trop. Dis. Bull.*, 1971, *68*, 707.

For another report of the treatment of amoebiasis with niridazole, see Emetine Hydrochloride, p.979.

Guinea worm. Complete healing of lesions occurred in 51 of 56 patients infected with guinea worm and treated with niridazole 25 mg per kg body-weight daily for 10 days. In 47 of them lesions healed within 20 days and in the remainder within 30 days. Twenty-eight of 62 patients given a placebo obtained complete healing of lesions but in 25 of these it took 1 to 2 months for healing to occur. A number of patients were considered to have stopped treatment because of red discoloration of the urine.— M. L. Kothari, *Trans. R. Soc. trop. Med. Hyg.*, 1969, *63*, 608. See also *idem*, *Am. J. trop. Med. Hyg.*, 1968, *17*, 864, per *Trop. Dis. Bull.*, 1970, *67*, 197.

Niridazole 25 mg per kg body-weight daily for 10 days given to 28 patients and metronidazole 40 mg per kg given to 26 patients daily for 3 days were both more effective in reducing the time taken for the expulsion of guinea worms and for the healing of ulcers than procaine penicillin and yeast tablets used in the treatment of 23 control patients. Both drugs also provided rapid relief of pain, but there were fewer parasitic relapses among patients given niridazole.— O. O. Kale, *Ann. trop. Med. Parasit.*, 1974, *68*, 91, per *Trop. Dis. Bull.*, 1974, *71*, 834.

Immunosuppressant activity. Serum from 2 patients (group 1) with schistosomiasis given niridazole 1.5 g daily for 7 days had an inhibitory effect, on the 6th day, on the one-way mixed lymphocyte reaction, comparable with that of serum from 5 patients (group 2) with kidney transplants, given azathioprine 100 to 150 mg daily and prednisolone 40 to 150 mg daily for the first 2 weeks after transplantation. In 7 patients (group 3) with kidney transplants given azathioprine and prednisolone, and niridazole 1.5 g on alternate days, the inhibitory effect appeared to be additive. Inhibition reached a maximum of about 70% at day 7 in group 1; about 60% at day 7 and about 100% at day 13 in group 2; and about 80% at day 1 and 90% at day 5 in group 3; in group 3 inhibition by serum from 6 of the 7 patients was about 100% on day 1. The results suggested that niridazole should be added to the usual immunosuppressant regimen after graft procedures.— B. M. Jones *et al.*, *Br. med. J.*, 1977, *2*, 792.

Further references: L. T. Webster *et al.*, *New Engl. J. Med.*, 1975, *292*, 1144.

Onchocerciasis. Niridazole 25 mg per kg body-weight daily for 7 to 10 days appeared to have some microfilaricidal action when given to 95 patients being treated for onchocerciasis. Treatment in conjunction with diethylcarbamazine citrate was also tried in 63 other patients but 12.7% of these had positive skin tests after treatment.— R. William-Olsson, *Acta trop.*, 1970, *27*, 173, per *Trop. Dis. Bull.*, 1971, *68*, 856.

Schistosomiasis (*S. haematobium*). Mass treatment with niridazole 25 mg per kg body-weight for 5 days reduced the incidence of infection with *S. haematobium* in a Moroccan village from over 50% to 8.3% 15 months later. Niridazole tolerance was good in all but 2 of 659 patients treated.— B. Nejjai, *Maroc méd.*, 1970, *50*, 453, per *Trop. Dis. Bull.*, 1971, *68*, 830. See also J. Roux *et al.*, *Medna trop.*, 1975, *35*, 377, per *Trop. Dis. Bull.*, 1976, *73*, 422.

Schistosomiasis (*S. japonicum*). Of 19 patients with *S. japonicum* infections who were treated with niridazole in a daily dose of 15 mg per kg body-weight for 5 to 7 days, 5 remained free of *Schistosoma* eggs for 1 year after treatment compared with 21 of 43 who received 20 mg per kg daily. Side-effects were not reduced when an antihistamine was given in conjunction with niridazole but they were reduced when a sedative was given.— M. Yokogawa *et al.*, *Jap. J. Parasit.*, 1968, *17*, 471, per *Trop. Dis. Bull.*, 1969, *66*, 560.

The cure-rate 6 months after treatment of 72 patients with schistosomiasis due to *S. japonicum* who were treated with niridazole ranged from 48.3 to 84.8% while the reduction in egg production was between 96.3 and 98.9%. Transient psychiatric disturbances were reported in some patients.— A. T. Santos *et al.*, *J. Philipp. med. Ass.*, 1971, *47*, 203, per *Trop. Dis. Bull.*, 1971, *68*, 1349.

Further references: F. S. Sy, *J. Philipp. med. Ass.*, 1977, *53*, 151, per *Trop. Dis. Bull.*, 1978, *75*, 553.

Schistosomiasis (*S. mansoni*). Niridazole was considered the drug of choice for the treatment of intestinal schistosomiasis.— Z. Farid *et al.*, *Trans. R. Soc. trop. Med. Hyg.*, 1972, *66*, 119.

Schistosomal intestinal polyps disappeared in 12 patients and were reduced in number in 5 of 17 patients treated with niridazole 25 mg per kg body-weight for 10 days.— Z. Farid *et al.*, *J. trop. Med. Hyg.*, 1974, *77*, 65, per *Trop. Dis. Bull.*, 1974, *71*, 1037.

For further reports of the use of niridazole in the treatment of schistosomiasis, see Martindale 27th Edn, p. 1376.

Proprietary Preparations

Ambilhar *(Ciba, UK)*. Niridazole, available as tablets of 100 and 500 mg. (Also available as Ambilhar in *Fr.*, *S.Afr.*, *Switz.*).

795-t

Oxamniquine.

UK-4271. 1,2,3,4-Tetrahydro-2-isopropylaminomethyl-7-nitro-6-quinolylmethanol.

$C_{14}H_{21}N_3O_3$=279.3.

CAS — 21738-42-1.

Pharmacopoeias. In *Braz.*

A light orange crystalline powder. M.p. 151° to 152°. **Soluble** 1 in about 3300 of water at 27°; soluble in acetone, chloroform, and methyl alcohol.

Adverse Effects. Pain at the injection site, which may be accompanied by induration and fever, frequently occurs within 48 hours of a deep intramuscular injection and lasts for about 2 to 7 days.

Other side-effects include abdominal and muscular pains, headache, dizziness, somnolence, nausea, diarrhoea, skin eruptions, and insomnia. A reddish discoloration of urine, probably due to a metabolite, has been reported. Minor changes in the ECG have occurred as have increases in liver-function test values, possibly representing slight liver toxicity.

Oxamniquine 7.5 mg per kg body-weight given by intramuscular injection to 104 patients aged between 5 and 43 years caused pain lasting from 1 to 16 days at the injection site within 12 to 24 hours. Headache was reported in 5 patients, dizziness and skin eruptions in 3, fever, nausea, and diarrhoea in 2, and abdominal and muscular pains in 1 patient. A large increase in plasma-creatine phosphokinase concentration occurred in 1 patient with smaller increases in some others. Small increases in serum aspartate aminotransferase (SGOT) and serum alanine aminotransferase (SGPT) were reported with indication of liver toxicity in 2 patients. Observed changes in ECG had no clinical significance. Of 71 patients followed up, 11 treated within the first 6 months after infection and 55 with chronic schistosomiasis were cured; 4 patients relapsed and 1 became reinfected.— N. Katz *et al.*, *Revta Inst. Med. trop. S Paulo*, 1973, *15*, *Suppl.* 1, 35. See also J. R. Coura *et al.*, *ibid.*, 41.

Absence of chromosome aberrations.— M. V. Monsalve *et al.*, *J. Toxic. environ. Hlth*, 1976, *1*, 1023, per *Trop. Dis. Bull.*, 1977, *74*, 238.

A patient with a history of epilepsy had a grand mal seizure 2 hours after his second dose of oxamniquine 15 mg per kg body-weight which he was receiving twice daily for schistosomiasis. Two further patients had transient EEG changes while receiving oxamniquine therapy.— J. S. Keystone, *Am. J. trop. Med. Hyg.*, 1978, *27*, 360.

Of 106 patients treated in Egypt with oxamniquine for schistosomiasis 40 developed a characteristic fever 1 to 3 days after the completion of the course and lasting 2 to 5 days.— G. I. Higashi and Z. Farid, *Br. med. J.*, 1979, *2*, 830. Comment.— P. Jordan (letter), *Br. med. J.*, 1979, *2*, 1366.

Uses. Oxamniquine has schistosomicidal activity against *Schistosoma mansoni*. It causes worms to shift from the mesenteric veins to the liver where they are destroyed. Single doses of 7.5 mg per kg body-weight by deep intramuscular injection have been effective in a number of studies, but doses of up to 30 mg per kg have been required, possibly due to varying sensitivity of *S. mansoni* in different countries and to other local factors.

Oxamniquine has no significant effect against *S. haematobium*.

Oxamniquine is often given by mouth; a common dose is 15 mg per kg given as a single dose or given twice daily for 2 days; children appear to need proportionately slightly higher doses than adults.

Schistosomiasis. Reports of studies and discussions on the treatment of schistosomiasis with oxamniquine: *Revta Inst. Med. trop. S Paulo*, 1973, *15*, *Suppl.* 1,

1–175; Epidemiology and Control of Schistosomiasis, Report of a WHO Expert Committee, *Tech. Rep. Ser. Wld Hlth Org. No. 643*, 1980.

Negative stools at 1 month in 21 of 24 children with *S. mansoni* infection, many of whom had significant liver enlargement, after treatment for 2 days with oxamniquine 800 mg per m^2 body-surface daily. Only 6 of 25 children with *S. haematobium* infection were cured.— J. H. M. Axton and P. A. Garnett, *S. Afr. med. J.*, 1976, *50*, 1051, per *Trop. Dis. Bull.*, 1976, *73*, 1063.

S. mansoni infection was treated in 200 children or young adults with oxamniquine by mouth in a dosage varying from a single dose of 10 mg per kg body-weight to a total of 60 mg per kg in 4 doses over 2 days. With the latter dose regimen, which was recommended as standard treatment, a cure-rate of 70% was achieved.— V. de V. Clarke *et al.*, *S. Afr. med. J.*, 1976, *50*, 1867, per *Trop. Dis. Bull.*, 1977, *74*, 617.

Cure-rates of 96.1%, 67.5%, and 95% respectively were achieved in patients with *S. mansoni* infection given single doses of oxamniquine: 7.5 mg per kg body-weight intramuscularly; 10 mg per kg by mouth; and 15 mg per kg by mouth.— R. J. Pedro *et al.*, *Revta Inst. Med. trop. S Paulo*, 1977, *19*, 130, per *Trop. Dis. Bull.*, 1977, *74*, 1038.

A cure-rate of 73.7% was achieved in 19 children with *S. mansoni* infection given a single oral dose of oxamniquine 20 mg per kg body-weight; 62.2% in 47 given two doses of 10 mg per kg; and 82.4% in 154 adults given a single dose of 15 mg per kg. Side-effects were dizziness, drowsiness, and headache.— N. Katz *et al.*, *Am. J. trop. Med. Hyg.*, 1977, *26*, 234, per *Trop. Dis. Bull.*, 1977, *74*, 1038.

A cure-rate of 95% was achieved at 6 months (in those available for follow-up) in 73 patients with *Schistosoma mansoni* infection given oxamniquine 60 mg per kg body-weight (15 mg per kg twice daily for 2 days) by mouth, compared with 79% in 37 given 40 mg per kg (20 mg per kg daily for 2 days) and 69% in 66 given 30 mg per kg (15 mg per kg twice daily for 1 day). Egg counts were significantly reduced by all dose regimens; the lowest dose could therefore be used when low cost was necessary. Dizziness was the most common side-effect; other minor effects were headache, malaise, vertigo, pruritus, abdominal pain, and diarrhoea. A reddish colouration of the urine was probably due to a metabolite. Eosinophilia occurred in some patients, and a transient rise in serum alanine aminotransferase (SGPT) values.— A. H. S. Omer, *Br. med. J.*, 1978, *2*, 163 and 469.

Oxamniquine 10 mg per kg body-weight given twice daily on 2 successive days was effective and safe for the treatment of schistosomal polyposis of the colon in 20 patients followed-up for 6 months. The polyps resolved in 5 patients and were greatly reduced in size in the other 15.— H. H. Abaza *et al.*, *Trans. R. Soc. trop. Med. Hyg.*, 1978, *72*, 602.

Eight of 11 patients with advanced hepatosplenic schistosomiasis were free from infection with *S. mansoni* and clinically improved after receiving oxamniquine 20 mg per kg body-weight for 3 consecutive days.— Z. Farid *et al.*, *Trans. R. Soc. trop. Med. Hyg.*, 1980, *74*, 400. See also *idem*, *Ann. trop. Med. Parasit.*, 1979, *73*, 501, per *Trop. Dis. Bull.*, 1980, *77*, 676.

A cure was obtained in 5 of 11 patients with the toxaemic form of *S. mansoni* infection after receiving a single dose of oxamniquine 20 mg per kg body-weight given by mouth.— J. R. Lambertucci *et al.*, *Am. J. trop. Med. Hyg.*, 1980, *29*, 50.

Further references: A. L. C. Domingues and A. Coutinho, *Revta Inst. Med. trop. S Paulo*, 1975, *17*, 164, per *Trop. Dis. Bull.*, 1976, *73*, 66; L. C. Silva *et al.*, *Revta Inst. Med. trop. S Paulo*, 1975, *17*, 307, per *Trop. Dis. Bull.*, 1976, *73*, 601; M. Koura *et al.*, *J. Egypt. med. Ass.*, 1975, *58*, 287, per *Trop. Dis. Bull.*, 1976, *73*, 1064; M. Z. Rouquayrol *et al.*, *Revta Soc. bras. Med. trop.*, 1976, *10*, 91, per *Trop. Dis. Bull.*, 1978, *75*, 123; J. E. McMahon, *Ann. trop. Med. Parasit.*, 1976, *70*, 121, per *Trop. Dis. Bull.*, 1976, *73*, 761; N. Katz *et al.*, *Revta Inst. Med. trop. S Paulo*, 1976, *18*, 371, per *Trop. Dis. Bull.*, 1977, *74*, 618; A. Prata *et al.*, *Revta Soc. bras. Med. trop.*, 1976, *10*, 127, per *Trop. Dis. Bull.*, 1978, *75*, 372; J. P. Nozais, *Méd. Afr. noire*, 1978, *25*, 265, per *Trop. Dis. Bull.*, 1978, *75*, 1204; R. J. Pitchford and M. Lewis, *S. Afr. med. J.*, 1978, *53*, 677, per *Trop. Dis. Bull.*, 1979, *76*, 86; A. Z. Shafei, *J. trop. Med. Hyg.*, 1979, *82*, 18, per *Trop. Dis. Bull.*, 1979, *76*, 1019; V. M. Eyakuze *et al.*, *E. Afr. med. J.*, 1979, *56*, 22, per *Trop. Dis. Bull.*, 1980, *77*, 480; F. M. Raposo de Almeida *et al.*, *Revta Ass. méd. bras.*, 1979, *25*, 101, per *Trop. Dis. Bull.*, 1980, *77*, 582.

Resistance. A report of 10 patients with hepato-intestinal schistosomiasis due to *S. mansoni* which was resistant to treatment with hycanthone and oxamniquine.— R. X. Guimarães *et al.*, *Revta Ass. méd. bras.*, 1979, *25*, 48, per *Trop. Dis. Bull.*, 1980, *77*, 582.

Proprietary Names

Mansil *(Pfizer, Braz.)*; Vancil *(Pfizer, USA)*; Vansil *(Pfizer, S.Afr.)* *(also available in some other African countries)*.

796-x

Oxantel Embonate.

Oxantel Pamoate; CP-14445-16. (*E*)-3-[2-(1,4,5,6-Tetrahydro-1-methylpyrimidin-2-yl)vinyl]phenol 4,4′-methylenebis(3-hydroxy-2-naphthoate).

$C_{13}H_{16}N_2O,C_{23}H_{16}O_6=604.7$.

CAS — 36531-26-7 (oxantel); 68813-55-8 (embonate).

A pale yellow crystalline powder. Oxantel embonate 2.8 g is approximately equivalent to 1 g of oxantel. Practically **insoluble** in water.

Adverse Effects. Nausea, vomiting, abdominal pain, and diarrhoea may occasionally occur.

Absorption and Fate. Oxantel embonate is only slightly absorbed from the gastro-intestinal tract. Urinary excretion indicates that up to 8% of a therapeutic dose may be absorbed.

Uses. An anthelmintic effective against whipworm (*Trichuris*) infection. For mild or moderate infection a single dose equivalent to 10 to 20 mg of oxantel per kg body-weight may be given, repeated if necessary after 10 to 14 days. Patients with diarrhoea may be given the dose on 2 consecutive days. In severe infection the dose may be given once or twice daily for up to 5 days. For children weighing less than 6.25 kg the total dose should not exceed 20 mg per kg.

It has also been given with pyrantel to treat mixed infection with roundworm (*Ascaris*), hookworm, and threadworm.

Cure-rates of 65, 88, and 100% were achieved in groups of about 35 children with *Trichuris* infection treated respectively with oxantel (base) 10 mg per kg body-weight as a single dose, 15 mg per kg as a single dose, and 10 mg per kg daily for 3 days.— V. Zaman and N. N. Sabapathy, *S.E. Asian J. trop. med. publ. Hlth*, 1975, *6*, 103, per *Trop. Dis. Bull.*, 1976, *73*, 85.

A good clinical response was achieved in 17 of 25 children with *Trichuris trichiura* infection given oxantel 10 mg per kg body-weight twice daily for 3 days, and in the remaining 8 after a second course; eggs were still present in the faeces of 17 patients at the end of treatment.— E. L. Lee *et al.*, *Am. J. trop. Med. Hyg.*, 1976, *25*, 563, per *Trop. Dis. Bull.*, 1977, *74*, 249.

Trichuris trichiura was eliminated from 20 of 26 children and adults given oxantel 10 mg per kg body-weight as a single dose, from 23 of 25 given 15 mg per kg, and from 10 of 10 given 20 mg per kg.— E. G. Garcia, *Am. J. trop. Med. Hyg.*, 1976, *25*, 914. Another favourable report in whipworm infection.— F. M. Paul and V. Zaman, *Singapore med. J.*, 1976, *17*, 219, per *Trop. Dis. Bull.*, 1977, *74*, 634.

Use with pyrantel. For reports of the use of oxantel with pyrantel to eliminate or reduce mixed infection with other nematodes, see H. J. Rim *et al.*, *Korean J. Parasit.*, 1975, *13*, 97, per *Trop. Dis. Bull.*, 1976, *73*, 753; E. Farahmandian *et al.*, *Iran. J. publ. Hlth*, 1977, *6*, 46, per *Trop. Dis. Bull.*, 1978, *75*, 1096; S. H. Lee *et al.*, *Korean J. Parasit.*, 1977, *15*, 121, per *Trop. Dis. Bull.*, 1978, *75*, 1112; O. O. Kale, *Curr. ther. Res.*, 1977, *22*, 802; E. D. Garcia, *Drugs*, 1978, *15*, *Suppl.* 1, 70; A. S. Dissamaike, *ibid.*, 73; B. D. Cabrera and F. S. Sy, *ibid.*, 78; P. P. Chanco and J. Y. Vidad, *ibid.*, 87; S. -H. Lee and J. -K. Lim, *ibid.*, 94; J. K. Lim, *ibid.*, 99; I. Farahmandian *et al.*, *Curr. ther. Res.*, 1979, *26*, 114.

Manufacturers

Pfizer, USA.

797-r

Pelletierine Tannate *(B.P. 1948)*. Punicine Tannate.

Pharmacopoeias. In *Arg.*

A mixture of the tannates of the alkaloids obtained from the bark of the root and stems of the pomegranate, *Punica granatum* (Punicaceae). *Arg. P.* allows other varieties.

It is a light yellow, odourless, amorphous powder with an astringent taste. **Soluble** 1 in 700 of water and 1 in 80 of alcohol; practically insoluble in chloroform.

Adverse Effects. Pelletierine tannate may cause headache, vertigo, drowsiness, diplopia, nausea, vomiting, diarrhoea, and colic; overdosage may cause twitching, convulsions, respiratory failure, paralysis, temporary blindness, and death.

Precautions. Pelletierine tannate is contra-indicated in pregnancy.

Uses. Pelletierine tannate has a specific action on tapeworms but is ineffective against other intestinal parasites. Its highly toxic nature prohibits its use in all but healthy adults and it is now seldom used. It was used in a dose of 120 to 500 mg.

798-f

Phenothiazine *(B. Vet. C. 1965)*.

$C_{12}H_9NS=199.3$.

CAS — 92-84-2.

Pharmacopoeias. In *Arg.*, *Aust.*, *Cz.*, *It.*, and *Nord.*

An olive-green or greyish-green tasteless crystalline or amorphous powder with a characteristic odour. It is slowly oxidised in air and darkens on exposure to light. It is not wetted by water. M.p. about 184°.

Practically **insoluble** in water; soluble 1 in 60 of alcohol, 1 in 5 of acetone, and 1 in 20 of chloroform. **Protect** from light.

Uses. Phenothiazine is too toxic for use in human medicine. It has been used as an anthelmintic in veterinary medicine.

Many derivatives of phenothiazine are used in human medicine, particularly as antihistamines and tranquillisers.

799-d

Piperazine Adipate *(B.P., B.P. Vet., Eur. P.)*.

Piperaz. Adip.; Piperazini Adipas; Piperazinum Adipicum.

$C_4H_{10}N_2,C_6H_{10}O_4=232.3$.

CAS — 110-85-0 (piperazine); 142-88-1 (adipate).

Pharmacopoeias. In *Aust.*, *Br.*, *Cz.*, *Eur.*, *Fr.*, *Ger.*, *Int.*, *It.*, *Jap.*, *Jug.*, *Neth.*, *Nord.*, *Pol.*, *Roum.*, *Rus.*, and *Turk.*

A white odourless crystalline powder with a slightly acid taste. M.p. about 250° with decomposition. Piperazine adipate 120 mg is approximately equivalent to 100 mg of piperazine hydrate. **Soluble** 1 in 18 of water; practically insoluble in alcohol, chloroform, ether, and acetone. A 5% solution in water has a pH of 5 to 6. **Store** in airtight containers. Protect from light.

800-d

Piperazine Calcium Edetate.

Piperazine Calcium Edathamil.

$C_4H_{10}N_2,C_{10}H_{14}CaN_2O_8=416.4$.

CAS — 12002-30-1.

A chelate compound produced by reacting edetic acid with calcium carbonate and piperazine. Piperazine calcium edetate 214 mg is approximately equivalent to 100 mg of piperazine hydrate. Freely **soluble** in water; very slightly soluble in alcohol and chloroform; practically insoluble in ether.

801-n

Piperazine Citrate *(B.P., B.P. Vet., Eur. P.)*.

Piperazini Citras; Hydrous Tripiperazine Dicitrate.

$(C_4H_{10}N_2)_3,2C_6H_8O_7, xH_2O=642.7$.

CAS — 144-29-6 (anhydrous); 41372-10-5 (hydrate).

Pharmacopoeias. In *Br., Chin., Eur., Fr., Ger., Ind., Int., Neth., Turk.*, and *U.S.*

A fine, white, odourless or almost odourless, crystalline or granular powder with an acid taste. It contains 10 to 14% of water. M.p. about 190°. Piperazine citrate 125 mg is approximately equivalent to 100 mg of piperazine hydrate. **Soluble** 1 in 1.5 of water; practically insoluble in alcohol and ether. A 5% solution in water has a pH of 5 to 6. **Store** in airtight containers. Protect from light.

802-h

Piperazine Hydrate *(B.P., Eur. P.)*.

Piperazine; Piperazini Hydras; Piperazidine; Diethylenediamine; Hexahydropyrazine. Piperazine hexahydrate.

$C_4H_{10}N_2,6H_2O=194.2$.

CAS — 142-63-2.

Pharmacopoeias. In *Br., Cz., Eur., Fr., Ger., Jug., Neth., Pol., Port., Roum., Span.*, and *Swiss. Braz.* and *U.S.* include anhydrous piperazine ($C_4H_{10}N_2$ = 86.14).

Colourless glassy deliquescent crystals with a faint characteristic odour and a saline taste. M.p. about 43°. It absorbs carbon dioxide from the air.

The dosage of the salts of piperazine is usually expressed in terms of piperazine hydrate; 100 mg of piperazine hydrate is approximately equivalent to 120 mg of piperazine adipate, to 214 mg of piperazine calcium edetate, to 125 mg of piperazine citrate, and to 104 mg of piperazine phosphate.

Soluble 1 in 3 of water and 1 in 1 of alcohol; very slightly soluble in ether. A 5% solution in water is alkaline to litmus. **Incompatible** with alkaloidal salts and salts of copper and iron. **Store** in airtight containers. Protect from light.

A decrease in the content of piperazine in syrups on storage was attributed to interaction with laevulose and dextrose formed by hydrolysis of sucrose. A syrup prepared with sorbitol lost no potency when stored at 25° for 14 months.— A. Nielsen and P. Reimer, *Arch. Pharm. Chemi, scient. Edn*, 1975, *3*, 73.

803-m

Piperazine Phosphate *(B.P., B.P. Vet., U.S.P.)*.

Piperazini Phosphas.

$C_4H_{10}N_2,H_3PO_4,H_2O=202.1$.

CAS — 14538-56-8 (anhydrous); 18534-18-4 (monohydrate).

Pharmacopoeias. In *Br., Chin., Int.*, and *U.S.*

A white odourless or almost odourless crystalline powder with a slightly acid taste. Piperazine phosphate 104 mg is approximately equivalent to 100 mg of piperazine hydrate. **Soluble** 1 in 60 to 65 of water; practically insoluble in alcohol, chloroform, and ether; soluble in dilute hydrochloric acid. A 1% solution in water has a pH of 6 to 6.5. **Store** in airtight containers. Protect from light.

Adverse Effects. Serious adverse effects are rare with piperazine and are generally evidence of overdosage or impaired excretion. Nausea, vomiting, diarrhoea, abdominal pain, headache, paraesthesia, and urticaria occasionally occur and usually disappear rapidly when treatment is stopped. Severe neurotoxicity has been reported with symptoms including somnolence, vertigo, nystagmus, muscular incoordination and weakness, ataxia, myoclonic contractions, choreiform movements, tremor, convulsions, and loss of reflexes.

Cataract formation and hypersensitivity or allergy have been reported rarely.

A 4-year-old African boy developed haemolytic anaemia. He, but no other member of the family, had a deficiency of glucose-6-phosphate dehydrogenase. No cause for the haemolysis was found except that 2 days previously he had taken Pripsen (piperazine and senna).— N. Buchanan *et al.* (letter), *Br. med. J.*, 1971, *2*, 110.

A reaction resembling viral hepatitis occurred on 2 occasions in a 25-year-old woman after the administration of piperazine; it appeared to be a hypersensitivity reaction.— A. N. Hamlyn *et al.*, *Gastroenterology*, 1976, *70*, 1144, per *J. Am. med. Ass.*, 1976, *236*, 1183.

Miosis, disturbance of accommodation, and paralytic strabismus had been reported during treatment with piperazine usually in excessively high doses.— *Med. Lett.*, 1976, *18*, 63.

A 55-year-old man, with a history of eczema and respiratory symptoms due to occupational exposure to piperazine, developed pruritus and respiratory symptoms on patch testing with piperazine.— S. Fregert, *Contact Dermatitis*, 1976, *2*, 61.

Treatment of Adverse Effects. In severe poisoning empty the stomach by aspiration and lavage. Convulsions may be controlled by the intravenous injection of diazepam 5 to 10 mg or a short-acting barbiturate such as thiopentone sodium.

Precautions. Piperazine is contra-indicated in patients with liver disease or epilepsy and should be given with care to patients with latent epilepsy, neurological disturbances, or impaired renal function.

Interactions. Enhancement of the effect of chlorpromazine by piperazine was clinically significant only when high concentrations of piperazine were reached in the body.— G. Sturman, *Br. J. Pharmac.*, 1974, *50*, 153.

Absorption and Fate. Piperazine hydrate is readily absorbed from the gastro-intestinal tract and is excreted in the urine, partly as metabolites. The rate at which different individuals excrete piperazine has been reported to vary widely.

Following the administration of piperazine citrate by mouth, between 15 and 75% was recovered from the urine. Urinary excretion was maximal between 2 and 6 hours and nearly completed in 24 hours.— S. Hanna and A. Tang, *J. pharm. Sci.*, 1973, *62*, 2024.

Uses. Piperazine is an anthelmintic effective against roundworms (*Ascaris*) and threadworms (*Enterobius*) but it has no significant effect on hookworms, tapeworms, or whipworms.

In roundworms, piperazine produces reversible muscle paralysis which takes at least 5 hours to develop; the worms are then easily dislodged from their position by the movement of the gut and are expelled in the faeces. Since activity of the worms is not stimulated, there is little danger of blockage of the intestines or the bile duct, even in heavily infected patients. Piperazine affects all stages of the parasite in the gut but appears to have little or no effect on larvae in the tissues.

Little is known about the mode of action of piperazine on threadworms.

Piperazine is usually administered as the adipate, citrate, or phosphate, or as the chelated compound with calcium edetate, but dosage is usually stated in terms of the hexahydrate, piperazine hydrate. The fumarate, stearate, and tartrate have also been used.

For the treatment of roundworms (*Ascaris*) infection, a single dose with the evening meal is usually sufficient to paralyse the worms which are passed with the next stool. The dose for adults is the equivalent of 4 g of piperazine hydrate as a single dose or on two successive days. Children should be given the equivalent of 120 mg per kg body-weight up to a maximum of 4 g; some authorities suggest the equivalent of 75 mg per kg.

If the patient has normal bowel movements, a purgative is not necessary; if the patient is constipated, a saline purgative should be given on the morning after the dose of piperazine so that the worms are expelled before the effect of the drug wears off. To eradicate infections in endemic areas, the whole population may need to be treated at 2- to 3-monthly intervals for several months.

For elimination of threadworms, treatment should be continued for 7 days. Adults and children over 12 years of age should receive the equivalent of 2 g of the hydrate daily in 2 or 3 divided doses, children of 6 to 12 the equivalent of 1.5 g daily, with 250 mg per year of age for those up to 6 years. A second course after a 7-day interval may be required.

Piperazine hydrate has been given in conjunction with thiabendazole to combat mixed infection with roundworm, hookworm, strongyloid, and threadworm, and some good results have been claimed.

Piperazine has been used as suppositories as adjuvant treatment.

A possible mode of action of piperazine.— J. L. Phillips *et al.*, *Br. J. Pharmac.*, 1975, *54*, 219P.

Mixed infections. Piperazine hydrate 60 mg per kg body-weight given with thiabendazole 15 mg per kg to 82 patients on 3 successive days eliminated hookworm infection in 50%, roundworm in 41%, and whipworm in 26%. Reductions in egg-counts were also found in other patients.— L. Camillo-Coura *et al.*, *Revta Soc. bras. Med. trop.*, 1971, *5*, 103, per *Trop. Dis. Bull.*, 1972, *69*, 116.

Piperazine hydrate, 750 mg together with thiabendazole 375 mg given daily in 2 doses for 5 days to 405 children aged 4 to 14 years who had mixed infections, eliminated strongyloid and threadworm, and cured 91.7% of those with roundworm and 90.6% of those with hookworm infection. Complaints of gastro-intestinal disturbances, giddiness, and headache were made by 15 patients and treatment was interrupted for 1 patient.— J. L. Fernandes and E. Garcia, *Revta Soc. bras. Med. trop.*, 1971, *5*, 155, per *Trop. Dis. Bull.*, 1972, *69*, 115. See also F. F. Filho *et al.*, *Revta Soc. bras. Med. trop.*, 1971, *5*, 209, per *Trop. Dis. Bull.*, 1972, *69*, 32.

Tyloxapol, in a total dose of 20 mg for children under 6 years old and up to 60 mg for older children, given with piperazine 140 mg per kg body-weight was considered to reduce the duration of the successful treatment of patients with roundworm or threadworm infections to 2 days. No troublesome side-effects were reported.— E. G. Garcia and N. L. Jueco, *Acta med. philipp.*, 1971, *7*, 107, per *Trop. Dis. Bull.*, 1972, *69*, 529.

Roundworm (*Ascaris*). A simplified dose schedule for Piperazine Citrate Elixir in the mass treatment of roundworm infection: 5 to 10 ml (equivalent to piperazine hydrate 0.75 to 1.5 g) for patients from 5 to 9 kg body-weight; 15 ml for patients from 10 to 14 kg; 20 ml for patients from 15 to 19 kg; 30 ml for patients over 20 kg.— Report of a WHO Expert Committee on Control of Ascariasis, *Tech. Rep. Ser. Wld Hlth Org. No. 379*, 1967.

For a comparison of levamisole and piperazine in roundworm (*Ascaris*) infection, see Levamisole Hydrochloride, p.97.

Threadworms. Whole-gut perfusion with a technique involving piperazine dissolved in an iso-osmotic electrolyte solution apparently cured a woman with a 29-year history of recurrent threadworm infection.— P. Woo *et al.*, *Br. med. J.*, 1976, *1*, 433.

Preparations of Piperazine and its Salts

Elixirs

Piperazine Citrate Elixir *(B.P.)*. Piperazine citrate 937.5 mg, peppermint spirit 0.025 ml, green S and tartrazine solution 0.075 ml, glycerol 0.5 ml, syrup 2.5 ml, water to 5 ml. It contains in 5 ml the equivalent of about 750 mg of piperazine hydrate. Store at a temperature not exceeding 25°. Protect from light. When a dose less than, or not a multiple of, 5 ml is prescribed, the elixir should be diluted to 5 ml, or a multiple, with syrup. Such dilutions should be freshly prepared and not used more than 2 weeks after issue.

Ind. P. includes a similar elixir with 900 mg of piperazine citrate in 5 ml, flavoured with orange oil.

Dose. In threadworm infection, daily, adults and children over 12 years of age, 15 ml; children, 9 to 24 months, 2.5 ml; 2 to 3 years, 5 ml; 4 to 6 years, 7.5 ml;

7 to 12 years, 10 ml. In roundworm (*Ascaris*) infection, up to 30 ml, according to the patient's age, as a single dose.

Piperazine Elixir *(A.P.F.)*. Piperazine hydrate 500 mg, citric acid monohydrate 375 mg, syrup 2.5 ml, glycerol 0.5 ml, green solution *(A.P.F.)* 0.1 ml, concentrated chloroform water 0.1 ml, concentrated peppermint water 0.05 ml, water to 5 ml. *Dose.* In threadworm infection, 10 to 20 ml daily in divided doses; in roundworm (*Ascaris*) infection, 45 ml as a single dose. Children, in threadworm infection 0.4 ml per kg body-weight daily in divided doses; in roundworm infection 1.2 ml per kg up to 40 ml for a single dose. Store in a cool place. Protect from light.

Syrups

Piperazine Citrate Syrup *(U.S.P.)*. A syrup prepared from piperazine citrate or from piperazine to which an equivalent amount of citric acid has been added. Potency is expressed in terms of the equivalent amount of piperazine hydrate. Store in airtight containers.

Tablets

Piperazine Adipate Tablets *(B.P. 1973)*. Tablets containing piperazine adipate.

Piperazine Citrate Tablets *(U.S.P.)*. Tablets containing piperazine citrate. Potency is expressed in terms of the equivalent amount of piperazine hydrate. Store in airtight containers.

Piperazine Phosphate Tablets *(B.P.)*. Tablets containing piperazine phosphate.

Piperazine Phosphate Tablets *(U.S.P.)*. Tablets containing piperazine phosphate. Store in airtight containers.

Proprietary Preparations of Piperazine and its Salts

Antepar Elixir *(Wellcome, UK)*. Contains in each 5 ml piperazine citrate and piperazine hydrate together equivalent to 750 mg of piperazine hydrate (suggested diluent, syrup). Antepar syrup in USA and Canada contains piperazine citrate.

Antepar Tablets *(Wellcome, UK)*. Each contains piperazine phosphate equivalent to 500 mg of piperazine hydrate. Antepar tablets in USA contain piperazine citrate.

Ascalix *(Wallace Mfg Chem., UK: Farillon, UK)*. Syrups containing piperazine citrate equivalent to piperazine hydrate, 750 mg in each 5 ml, or 4 g in 20 ml, or 4 g in 30 ml.

Helmezine Elixir *(Allen & Hanburys, UK)*. (Available only in certain countries). An elixir containing in each 4 ml piperazine citrate 550 mg.

Helmezine Tablets *(Allen & Hanburys, UK)*. (Available only in certain countries). Piperazine phosphate, available as tablets of 260 mg.

Pripsen *(Westminster, Reckitt & Colman Pharmaceuticals, UK)*. Powder available as 10-g sachets each containing piperazine phosphate 4 g and standardised senna equivalent to 15.3 mg of sennosides calculated as sennoside B. For roundworm and threadworm infections. *Dose.* Adults and children over 6 years, the contents of 1 sachet; children, 3 months to 1 year and 1 to 6 years, one-third and two-thirds of the adult dose respectively; stirred into a small glass of water or milk. The dose may be repeated after an interval of 14 days.

Other Proprietary Names

Arg.— Piperacina Midy, Piperazine Midy, Uvilon *(all hydrate)*; *Austral.*— Divermex *(adipate)*; *Belg.*— Adiver *(adipate)*, Citrazine *(citrate)*; *Canad.*— Entacyl *(adipate)*; *Eire*— Citrazine *(citrate)*; *Fr.*— Antelmina *(hydrate)*, Nématorazine *('sébacate')*, Pipérazine Adrian *(hydrate)*, Pipérazine Fermé *(citrate)*, Pipérazine Midy *(hydrate)*, Pipérol Fort *(citrate)*; *Ger.*— Eraverm *(hydrate)*, Tasnon *(hydrate or phosphate)*, Vermicompren *(adipate)*; *Ital.*— Adipalit *(adipate)*, Antelmina *(hydrate)*, Diatesurico , Ismiverm *(adipate)*, Oxiustip *(adipate or hydrate)*, Piperiod *(hydrate)*, Uvilon *(hydrate)*; *Jap.*— Pipenin *(citrate or adipate)*; *Norw.*— Oxurasin *(adipate)*; *Pol.*— Antivermine *(adipate)*, Piperasol *(hydrate)*; *Spain*— Ascarinex, Bioxurin, Jarabe Neox, Lombrikal Piperazina *(all citrate)*, Lombrimade *(adipate)*, Vermenter *(hydrate)*; *Switz.*— Escovermin *(adipate or anhydrous)*, Helmizin *(citrate)*, Oxyvermin *(hydrate)*, Piperverm *(hydrate)*, Wurmex *(adipate or hydrate)*, Wurmsirup Siegfried *(citrate)*.

Piperazine adipate was also formerly marketed in Great Britain under the proprietary name Entacyl (*Duncan, Flockhart*).

804-b

Pomegranate Bark. Pomegranate Root Bark *(B.P.C. 1934)*; Granati Cortex; Granatum; Pomegranate; Grenadier; Granatrinde; Granado; Melograno; Romeira.

Pharmacopoeias. In *Port.* and *Span.*

NOTE. Pomegranate Rind, the dried pericarp separated from the fruit of the pomegranate, contains gallotannic acid but no alkaloids.

The dried bark of the stem and root of *Punica granatum* (Punicaceae) containing about 0.4 to 0.9% of alkaloids (see Pelletierine Tannate, p.102).

Uses. Pomegranate bark has been used for the expulsion of tapeworms as a 1 in 5 decoction in doses of 60 ml every 2 hours for 4 doses, the treatment being preceded and followed by the administration of a purgative.

It was recommended by the Food Additives and Contaminants Committee that pomegranate root be prohibited for use in foods as a flavouring agent.— *Report on the Review of Flavourings in Food*, FAC/REP/22, Ministry of Agriculture Fisheries and Food, London, HM Stationery Office, 1976.

805-v

Pyrantel Embonate.

CP-10423-16; Pyrantel Pamoate *(U.S.P.)*; Pirantel Pamoate. 1,4,5,6-Tetrahydro-1-methyl-2-[(*E*)-2-(2-thienyl)vinyl]-pyrimidine 4,4′-methylenebis(3-hydroxy-2-naphthoate).

$C_{11}H_{14}N_2S,C_{23}H_{16}O_6$=594.7.

CAS — 15686-83-6 (pyrantel); 22204-24-6 (embonate).

Pharmacopoeias. In *Chin.* and *U.S.*

A yellow to tan-coloured, odourless, tasteless, crystalline powder. Pyrantel embonate 2.9 g is approximately equivalent to 1 g of pyrantel. Practically **insoluble** in water, alcohol, and methyl alcohol; soluble in dimethyl sulphoxide; slightly soluble in dimethylformamide. **Protect** from light.

Adverse Effects. Mild and transient side-effects include nausea and vomiting, anorexia, abdominal pain and discomfort, diarrhoea, headache, fever, dizziness, and elevation of serum aspartate aminotransferase (SGOT) values. Drowsiness, insomnia, and skin rashes have also been reported.

Precautions. It should be used with caution in patients with impaired liver function. The anthelmintic effect of pyrantel may be antagonised by piperazine.

Absorption and Fate. A small proportion of a dose of pyrantel embonate is absorbed from the gastro-intestinal tract. Up to about 7% is excreted as unchanged drug and metabolites in the urine but over half of the dose is excreted in the faeces.

Uses. Pyrantel embonate is an anthelmintic effective against roundworms (*Ascaris*), threadworms (*Enterobius*), and hookworms (*Ancylostoma*); it is possibly less effective against *Necator*. It paralyses roundworms which are then dislodged by peristaltic activity.

The usual single dose for roundworms and threadworms is the equivalent of 10 mg of pyrantel per kg body-weight. For hookworm infection, the dose may be given on 3 consecutive days; up to 20 mg per kg may be given as a single dose and repeated daily for 1 or 2 days if necessary.

Pyrantel is used concomitantly with oxantel when infection includes whipworms.

For reviews, see R. Greenwood, *Drug Intell. & clin. Pharm.*, 1972, *6*, 226; *Med. Lett.*, 1972, *14*, 49; C. L. Bishop, *Can. pharm. J.*, 1977, *110*, 207.

Hookworm (*Ancylostoma* and *Necator*). Pyrantel as embonate in single doses of 10 to 100 mg per kg body-weight eliminated hookworms in all of 59 patients treated for *Ancylostoma* or *Necator* infection. Nausea and vomiting occurred in 2 patients given 75 and 100 mg per kg respectively.— K. N. Pandey *et al.*, *Br. med. J.*, 1971, *4*, 399.

In a study in 322 patients with hookworm (*Necator*) infection patients were given pyrantel as embonate 10 mg per kg body-weight as a single dose (group A), pyrantel as embonate 20 mg per kg (group B), or bromonaphthol 8 g as a single dose (group C). In group A the cure-rates were 92.3 to 46.2% dependent upon the degree of infection; in group B, 90.6 to 59.4%; and in group C, 92 to 84.4%. Those with heavy infections were less responsive.— A. Sato *et al.*, *Jap. J. Parasit.*, 1973, *22*, 331, per *Trop. Dis. Bull.*, 1974, *71*, 832.

In a study in 105 patients pyrantel as embonate, 10 mg per kg body-weight for 3 days, was more effective than bephenium hydroxynaphthoate or tetrachloroethylene in the treatment of hookworm (*Necator*) infection.— D. Botero and A. Castano, *Am. J. trop. Med. Hyg.*, 1973, *22*, 45, per *Int. pharm. Abstr.*, 1974, *11*, 540.

A cure-rate of 42% was achieved in children with hookworm (*Necator*) infection treated with pyrantel as embonate 10 mg per kg body-weight as a single dose, compared with 28% for bephenium hydroxynaphthoate, 27% for levamisole, and nil for bitoscanate. Cure-rates for roundworm (*Ascaris*) infection were 90, 74, 86, and 24% respectively.— S. W. Chege *et al.*, *E. Afr. med. J.*, 1974, *51*, 60, per *Trop. Dis. Bull.*, 1975, *72*, 78.

Of 72 patients with hookworm (*Necator americanus*) infections, 20 were treated with mebendazole 100 mg thrice daily for 2 days, 22 received tetrachloroethylene 0.1 ml per kg body-weight as a single dose, and 30 received pyrantel embonate 20 mg per kg daily for 2 days. Cure-rates were 70, 77.3, and 36.7% respectively.— S. Migasena *et al.*, *Ann. trop. Med. Parasit.*, 1978, *72*, 199, per *Trop. Dis. Bull.*, 1979, *76*, 98.

Mixed infections. Of 43 children with threadworm infection given a single dose of 10 mg per kg body-weight of pyrantel as the embonate, 36 were cured, and all 79 children with ascariasis were cleared of infection after a single dose of 8.5 to 10 mg per kg body-weight. In the same dosage range pyrantel embonate proved very effective against *Trichostrongylus orientalis* and hookworms, and moderately effective against *Trichuris trichiura*. Side-effects were mild and transient.— H. J. Rim and J. K. Lim, *Trans. R. Soc. trop. Med. Hyg.*, 1972, *66*, 170.

Pyrantel as embonate in doses of 750 mg for adults, 500 mg for children aged 11 to 18 years, and 250 mg for children aged 6 to 10 years, given as a single dose after breakfast in the treatment of mixed infections, cleared roundworms from 67 of 68 patients, *Ancylostoma duodenale* from 57 of 72, and *Trichostrongylus* from all of 23 in 21 days, without untoward side-effects.— W. J. Bell and S. Nassif, *J. Egypt. med. Ass.*, 1972, *55*, 111, per *Trop. Dis. Bull.*, 1973, *70*, 351.

In 175 patients the cure-rate against *A. duodenale* infection of a single dose of pyrantel embonate equivalent to 10 mg base per kg body-weight, followed by a purge 3 hours later, was 96% compared with 92% for bephenium hydroxynaphthoate. For roundworm and *Trichostrongylus* infections the corresponding results were 90.2% and 45.4% respectively with pyrantel and 52.9% and 56% with bephenium.— I. Farahmandian *et al.*, *J. trop. Med. Hyg.*, 1972, *75*, 205, per *Trop. Dis. Bull.*, 1973, *70*, 473.

Cure-rates of 92.6% against roundworm (*Ascaris*) infection, 85.7% against hookworm, and 19.4% against whipworms in 117 patients given pyrantel as embonate 100 mg twice daily for 3 days.— N. Islam and N. A. Chowdhury, *S.E. Asian J. trop. med. publ. Hlth*, 1976, *7*, 81, per *Trop. Dis. Bull.*, 1977, *74*, 231.

Further references: O. O. Kale, *Afr. J. Med. med. Sci.*, 1977, *6*, 89, per *Trop. Dis. Bull.*, 1978, *75*, 670.

Roundworm (*Ascaris*). Pyrantel as embonate, 10 mg per kg body-weight by mouth as a single dose, produced negative egg counts after 3 weeks in 56 of 63 patients (88.9%) with ascariasis. Side-effects were mild and transient.— A. Kobayashi *et al.*, *Jap. J. Parasit.*, 1970, *19*, 296, per *Trop. Dis. Bull.*, 1971, *68*, 340.

Stool samples were free of ova at 1 and 4 weeks in all of 205 patients with roundworm (*Ascaris*) infection after treatment with a single dose of pyrantel as embonate 10 mg per kg body-weight.— E. Ghadarian *et al.*, *J. trop. Med. Hyg.*, 1972, *75*, 195, per *Trop. Dis. Bull.*, 1973, *70*, 471.

In a study involving 30 children aged 3 to 12 years, pyrantel as embonate in a single dose of 10 mg per kg body-weight was as effective as 20 mg per kg and slightly more effective than piperazine citrate 120 mg per kg in the treatment of roundworm infection, but it caused mild abdominal pain and diarrhoea in some children.— M. A. Haleem *et al.*, *J. Pakistan med. Ass.*, 1972, *22*, 276, per *Trop. Dis. Bull.*, 1973, *70*, 769.

Cure-rates of 76.2, 85, and 92.3% were achieved in 54 patients with roundworm (*Ascaris*) infection given pyrantel as embonate 10 mg per kg body-weight as a single dose daily for 1, 2, or 3 days. Only 3 of 11 patients with *Trichuris* infection were cured.— S. K. K. Seah, *S.E. Asian J. trop. med. publ. Hlth*, 1973, *4*, 534, per *Trop. Dis. Bull.*, 1974, *71*, 832.

Reduction of the incidence of ascariasis from 84.4% to 33.9%, 8.7%, 7.5%, and 0.5% after 4 treatments, at 3-monthly intervals, with pyrantel as embonate 5 mg per kg body-weight as single doses.— B. D. Cabrera *et al.*, *S.E. Asian J. trop. med. publ. Hlth*, 1975, *6*, 510, per *Trop. Dis. Bull.*, 1976, *73*, 951.

Cure-rates of 95% or better had been obtained in the mass treatment of ascariasis using pyrantel embonate in doses of 2.5 to 5 mg per kg body-weight.— S. Kojima *et al.*, *Jap. J. Parasit.*, 1978, *27*, 151, per *Trop. Dis. Bull.*, 1979, *76*, 583.

Ternidens. Pyrantel as embonate in a single dose of 20 mg per kg body-weight given to 10 patients with *Ternidens deminutus* infection cured 9 and cleared the infection in 2 further patients who were given the reduced dose of 10 mg per kg.— J. M. Goldsmid and C. R. Saunders (letter), *Trans. R. Soc. trop. Med. Hyg.*, 1972, *66*, 375.

Threadworm. Sixty-nine children in an institution were given pyrantel as embonate, 10 mg per kg body-weight in a single dose by mouth as a 5% suspension, to control threadworm infection. *Enterobius vermicularis* infection had been diagnosed in 28 of the children. Immediately after treatment only 1 child was infected; after 3 months 5 children showed signs of infection. Six children had diarrhoea and/or vomiting on the day after treatment and 6 had some elevation of serum aspartate aminotransferase (SGOT) values.— T. S. Bumbalo *et al.*, *Am. J. trop. Med. Hyg.*, 1969, *18*, 50, per *Trop. Dis. Bull.*, 1970, *67*, 193.

Pyrantel embonate in a single dose of 10 mg base per kg body-weight was considered to be as effective as viprynium embonate, equivalent to 5 mg base per kg, in the mass treatment of 95 patients infected with threadworms and to have a lower incidence of side-effects, which were mild and transient with both drugs.— M. Yokogawa *et al.*, *Jap. J. Parasit.*, 1970, *19*, 593, per *Trop. Dis. Bull.*, 1971, *68*, 966. A similar report.— M. C. Baranski *et al.*, *Revta Inst. Med. trop. S Paulo*, 1971, *13*, 422, per *Trop. Dis. Bull.*, 1972, *69*, 528.

In a study of 200 Egyptian schoolboys infected with threadworms, pyrantel 250 mg for those aged 5 to 10 years and 500 mg for older boys was effective in 79% compared with viprynium 5 mg per kg body-weight which was effective in 60%. The response to pyrantel was quicker than to viprynium. Relapse-rates were 62% for pyrantel and 48% for viprynium.— S. Nassif *et al.*, *J. trop. Med. Hyg.*, 1974, *77*, 270, per *Trop. Dis. Bull.*, 1975, *72*, 557.

Trichostrongylus infections. Pyrantel 10 mg per kg body-weight as embonate given as a single dose before breakfast to adults and children infected with *Trichostrongylus orientalis* cured 88.4% of 552 persons who attended for follow-up examination. Mild transient side-effects were reported in 22% of about 600 patients treated.— T. Yamaguchi *et al.*, *Jap. J. Parasit.*, 1975, *24*, 93, per *Trop. Dis. Bull.*, 1975, *72*, 1079.

Preparations

Pyrantel Pamoate Oral Suspension *(U.S.P.)*. A suspension of pyrantel embonate in a suitable aqueous vehicle. Potency is expressed in terms of the equivalent amount of pyrantel. pH 4.5 to 6. Store in airtight containers. Protect from light.

Proprietary Names

Antiminth *(Roerig, USA)*; Aut *(Elea, Arg.)*; Cobantril *(Pfizer, Switz.)*; Combantrin *(Pfizer, Arg.; G.P. Laboratories, Austral.; Pfizer, Belg.; Pfizer, Canad.; Pfizer, Fr.; Pfizer, Ital.; Pfizer, Neth.; Pfizer, S.Afr.)*; Helmex *(Pfizer, Ger.)*; Lombriareu *(Areu, Spain)*; Trilombrin *(Pfizer, Spain)*.

806-g

Santonica *(B.P.C. 1934)*. Wormseed; Wormwood Flowers; Semen Contra; Semen Cinae; Flos Cinae; Zitwerblüte.

Pharmacopoeias. In *Aust.*, *Rus.*, and *Span.*

The dried unexpanded flowerheads of *Artemisia cina* and other species of *Artemisia* (Compositae) containing not less than 2% of santonin.

Uses. Santonica is used as a source of santonin.

807-q

Santonin *(B.P. 1963)*. Santoninum.
(3*S*,3a*S*,5a*S*,9b*S*)-3a,5,5a,9b-Tetrahydro-3,5a,9-trimethylnaphtho[1,2-*b*]furan-2,8(3*H*,4*H*)-dione.
$C_{15}H_{18}O_3$=246.3.

CAS — 481-06-1.

Pharmacopoeias. In *Arg.*, *Aust.*, *Chin.*, *Ind.*, *Int.*, *It.*, *Jap.*, *Mex.*, *Nord.*, *Port.*, *Rus.*, *Span.*, *Swiss*, and *Turk.*

A crystalline lactone obtained from the dried unexpanded flowerheads of *Artemisia cina* and other species of *Artemisia* (Compositae). It occurs as colourless odourless crystals or white crystalline powder with a slightly bitter taste. It becomes yellow on exposure to light. M.p. about 173°.

Practically **insoluble** in water; slightly soluble in hot water; soluble 1 in 50 of alcohol and 1 in 3 of chloroform; slightly soluble in ether, castor oil, and solutions of alkalis. **Store** in airtight containers. Protect from light.

Adverse Effects. Poisoning affects vision, white objects looking green, blue, or yellow (xanthopsia). It may also cause headache, vertigo, nausea, vomiting, apathy, profuse sweating, and diarrhoea. Large doses may give rise to epileptiform convulsions followed by coma. Disorders of hearing and haematuria may also occur. Death may occur from respiratory failure.

Uses. Santonin was formerly used as an anthelmintic in the treatment of roundworm (*Ascaris*) infection in doses of 60 to 200 mg daily for 3 days; it has been superseded by other less toxic anthelmintics. An oxidation product of the absorbed santonin colours acid urine bright yellow or orange and alkaline urine purplish-red.

The potential toxicity of santonin might be reduced by administering it with kainic acid, since lower doses of santonin could then be used to give the same effect. There was clinical evidence that the 2 drugs together were appreciably more effective than either used alone in the treatment of ascariasis.— Report of a WHO Expert Committee on Control of Ascariasis, *Tech. Rep. Ser. Wld Hlth Org. No. 379*, 1967.

808-p

Sodium Antimonylgluconate *(B.P. 1968)*.

Sod. Antimonylgluc.; Antimonyl Sodium Gluconate; Stibii Natrii Gluconas.

CAS — 12550-17-3.

Pharmacopoeias. In *Chin.*

A white, almost odourless, amorphous powder, containing 34 to 39% of total antimony, of which not less than 95% consists of trivalent antimony. It loses 6 to 10% of its weight on drying.

Soluble in water; practically insoluble in organic solvents. A 5% solution in water has a pH of 5.5 to 6.5. Aqueous solutions deteriorate on storage and should be used immediately after preparation. Solutions for injection are prepared by dissolving the sterile powder in Water for Injections immediately before use. **Store** in airtight containers.

Gamma-irradiation of sodium antimonylgluconate at 250 000 Gy caused the development of a caramel-like odour and a buff colour and solutions became pale buff and opalescent; the total antimony content was not affected but there was evidence of some change in the concentration of trivalent antimony.— *The Use of Gamma Radiation Sources for the Sterilisation of Pharmaceutical Products*, London, ABPI, 1960.

Adverse Effects. As for Antimony Sodium Tartrate, p.87, but the side-effects are less severe.

Uses. Sodium antimonylgluconate has the actions and uses of antimony sodium tartrate (see p.87) and is used in the treatment of schistosomiasis.

For an adult of 70 kg or more the usual dosage is 190 mg daily by slow intravenous injection in 4 or 5 ml of Water for Injections. This dose is given for 6 consecutive days, or the same total dose may be given over 4 days.

Preparations

Sodium Antimonylgluconate Injection *(B.P. 1968)*. Sod. Antimonylgluc. Inj. A sterile solution of sodium antimonylgluconate in Water for Injections prepared by dissolving, immediately before use, the sterile contents of a sealed container in the requisite amount of Water for Injections. The sealed container may also contain a suitable buffering agent.

Sodium antimonylgluconate was formerly marketed in Great Britain under the proprietary name Triostam (*Wellcome*).

809-s

Sodium Stibogluconate *(B.P.)*.

Sod. Stibogluc.; Sodium Antimony Gluconate; Stibogluconat-Natrium.

CAS — 16037-91-5.

Pharmacopoeias. In *Br.* and *Ind.*

A pentavalent antimony derivative of indefinite composition containing, when dried, 30 to 34% of antimony. It has been represented by the formula $C_6H_9Na_2O_9Sb$ but usually there are less than 2 atoms of Na for each atom of Sb.

It is a colourless odourless mostly amorphous powder. It loses 10 to 15% of its weight when dried.

Very **soluble** in water; practically insoluble in alcohol and ether. A solution in water is dextrorotatory. A solution containing 10% of antimony has a pH of 5 to 5.6 after autoclaving. Solutions are **sterilised** by autoclaving or by filtration. **Store** in airtight containers. Protect from light.

Adverse Effects. As for Antimony Sodium Tartrate, p.87, but the side-effects are less severe.

Absorption and Fate. In common with other pentavalent antimony compounds sodium stibogluconate is not bound by red blood cells but remains in the plasma and is rapidly excreted by the kidney. Small amounts may be reduced to trivalent antimony in the liver.

A study of the renal excretion of sodium stibogluconate in healthy subjects and in patients with kala-azar. Preliminary observations failed to demonstrate antimony in the faeces during a course of sodium stibogluconate. Following intravenous administration sodium stibogluconate appeared to be confined to the extracellular fluid compartment, and was rapidly excreted in a manner similar to that of inulin (over 95% being excreted in the urine in the first 6 hours), hence it is probably not metabolised. Following intramuscular injection blood concentrations were lower and more sustained, but over 80% was excreted in the first 6 hours. It thus appears that the fears of cumulative toxicity following sodium stibogluconate administration may be unfounded. On the basis of these results prolonged courses of sodium stibogluconate have been given to patients not responding to 30-day courses; in one instance the course was continued for 176 days. No side-effects attributable to sodium stibogluconate were seen in these extended courses.— P. H. Rees *et al.*, *Lancet*, 1980, *2*, 226.

Uses. Sodium stibogluconate is given by intravenous or intramuscular injection of a 33% solution (equivalent to 10% of total antimony) in the treatment of visceral leishmaniasis (kala-azar). A course of treatment consists of 6 to 10 daily injections, each of 6 ml, repeated if necessary on 2 occasions after 10-day intervals; a longer course of 30 daily injections may be necessary in some areas. Children may be given 0.1 ml per kg body-weight daily for 21 days or 0.25 ml per kg daily for 12 to 14 days with a maximum daily dose of 6 ml. It is also employed in a similar dose for the treatment of cutaneous leishmaniasis (oriental sore); alternatively the 33% solution may be infiltrated round the edges of the lesions in a dosage of not more than 2 ml at any one time.

In American mucocutaneous leishmaniasis 6 ml is given daily for 10 days, the course being repeated, if necessary, on 2 occasions at monthly intervals.

Intravenous injections should be given slowly.

Leishmaniasis. Pentavalent antimony given as sodium stibogluconate 0.1 ml of a 34% solution per kg body-weight daily for at least 14 days, given preferably by intravenous injection, was recommended for the treatment of cutaneous leishmaniasis. The patient's cardiac rhythm and blood pressure should be monitored for the first hour after intravenous injection, and the treatment interrupted for any vomiting or arrhythmias.— A. Bryceson, *Br. J. Derm.*, 1976, *94*, 223.

Further references.— F. Kern and J. K. Pedersen, *J. Am. med. Ass.*, 1973, *226*, 872; Z. A. Sebai *et al.*, *J. Egypt. publ. Hlth Ass.*, 1975, *50*, 59, per *Trop. Dis. Bull.*, 1977, *74*, 609; M. J. Miller, *Prog. Drug Res.*, 1976, *20*, 433; S. Ghosn, *Curr. med. Res. Opinion*, 1979, *6*, 280.

Preparations

Sodium Stibogluconate Injection *(B.P.)*. Sod. Stibogluc. Inj. A sterile solution of sodium stibogluconate in Water for Injections, containing 10% w/v of total antimony; 6 ml contains the equivalent of 600 mg of total antimony or 2 g of sodium stibogluconate. Sterilised by autoclaving. pH 5 to 5.6. Protect from light. *Ind. P.* includes a similar preparation.

Pentostam *(Wellcome, UK)*. A brand of Sodium Stibogluconate Injection, available in rubber-capped bottles of 100 ml.

810-h

Stibocaptate.

Antimony Sodium Dimercaptosuccinate; Ro 4-1544/6; Sb-58; TWSb/6. Antimony sodium *meso*-2,3-dimercaptosuccinate. The formula varies from $C_{12}H_{11}NaO_{12}S_6Sb_2$ = 806.1 to $C_{12}H_6Na_6O_{12}S_6Sb_2$ = 916.0.

CAS — 3064-61-7 ($C_{12}H_6Na_6O_{12}S_6Sb_2$).

A white to yellowish-white, practically odourless, crystalline solid. The commercial product contains 25 to 26% of trivalent antimony. **Soluble** 1 in 4 of water, 1 in 50 of alcohol, and 1 in about 1000 of acetone. A 10% solution in water has a pH of about 5.2. Solutions in water are unstable and should be used within 24 hours of their preparation.

Adverse Effects. As for Antimony Sodium Tartrate, p.87. Side-effects are usually less severe.

During treatment of 250 patients with stibocaptate, side-effects were: pain at the injection site in all patients, nausea and vomiting in 70%, and diarrhoea, lassitude, substernal pain and extrasystoles, collapse, abdominal pain, and a metallic taste each in a few.— A. Awkati, *Trans. R. Soc. trop. Med. Hyg.*, 1969, *63*, 576.

Uses. Stibocaptate is used in the treatment of schistosomiasis, particularly against infection due to *Schistosoma haematobium*. It is less active against *S. mansoni* and *S. japonicum*. It appears to have certain advantages over antimony sodium tartrate: it can be given by intramuscular injection and is relatively well tolerated.

The total dose usually employed is 30 to 50 mg per kg body-weight, with a maximum of 2.5 g in 5 divided doses administered intramuscularly, as a 10% solution, at weekly or twice-weekly intervals; in children under 20 kg, a total dose of 40 to 60 mg per kg body-weight may be given. The higher doses are appropriate in infections due to *S. mansoni* or *S. japonicum*. If the doses are given at shorter intervals (daily or every 2 days), side-effects are frequently severe and may necessitate discontinuance of treatment. Monthly doses have been given for 5 or 6 months in suppressive therapy.

Stibocaptate may also be administered, at the same dosage, by slow intravenous injection, but the incidence of toxic reactions is greater than when the intramuscular route is employed. Antimony potassium dimercaptosuccinate (TWSb) and antimony magnesium dimercaptosuccinate (TWSb/1) have therapeutic activity similar to that of stibocaptate.

Schistosomiasis. Two years after 127 children had been treated with daily or weekly regimens of stibocaptate for *S. haematobium* infections, 18 of 71 who had been cured were probably re-infected. Over the 2 years, egg deposition in the tissues was considerably reduced, so that the patients benefited from the treatment even if they were not cured.— P. Jordan, *Trans. R. Soc. trop. Med. Hyg.*, 1968, *62*, 413.

Infection with *S. haematobium* in 234 Zanzibar schoolchildren was treated by monthly intramuscular injections of stibocaptate, between June 1964 and Dec. 1966. In 149 of the 162 still at school at the time of examination, 40.3% were voiding viable eggs of *S. haematobium* in the urine, but in much reduced numbers. X-rays showed little change in the urological lesions, and bladder calcification was not reversed by treatment. The urological state of some children improved but that of others remained unchanged or deteriorated.— G. Macdonald and D. M. Forsyth, *Trans. R. Soc. trop. Med. Hyg.*, 1968, *62*, 766. Monthly intramuscular injections of stibocaptate, 10 mg per kg body-weight, had no unpleasant side-effects apart from pain at the injection site. An injection every 3 months might be equally effective. Results would almost certainly have been better if children of pre-school age had also been treated.— G. Macdonald *et al.*, *ibid.*, *775*.

For other reports of the use of stibocaptate in the treatment of schistosomiasis, see Martindale 27th Edn, p. 1378.

Proprietary Preparations

Astiban *(Roche, UK)*. Stibocaptate, available as powder for preparing injections, in ampoules of 500 mg. (Also available as Astiban in *Switz.*).

811-m

Stibophen *(B.P. 1968)*.

Stibophenum; Fouadin; Estibofeno. Bis[4,5-dihydroxybenzene-1,3-disulphonato(4−)-O^4,O^5]antimonate(5−) pentasodium heptahydrate.

$C_{12}H_4Na_5O_{16}S_4Sb,7H_2O$ = 895.2.

CAS — 15489-16-4 (heptahydrate).

Pharmacopoeias. In *Ind.*, *Int.*, *It.*, *Jug.*, and *Turk.*

A white, odourless, fine, somewhat glistening, crystalline powder. **Soluble** 1 in 1 of water; practically insoluble in alcohol, acetone, chloroform, ether, and light petroleum. A 5% solution in water has a pH of 6 to 7. A neutral solution in water readily becomes oxidised in air, acquiring a yellowish tint which deepens to lemon-yellow; the formation of the yellow colour may be retarded by the addition of acid. Solutions are **sterilised** by autoclaving. **Store** in airtight containers and avoid contact with iron and iron compounds. Protect from light.

When stored for a long time, stibophen could undergo molecular dissociation with enhanced toxicity.— A. Halawani *et al.*, *Lancet*, 1956, *1*, 190.

Gamma-irradiation of Stibophen Injection at 200 000 Gy caused a black precipitate in full ampoules, a brown discoloration in half-filled ampoules with air above the solution, and a black precipitate in half-filled ampoules where the air was displaced by nitrogen.— *The Use of Gamma Radiation Sources for the Sterilisation of Pharmaceutical Products*, London, ABPI, 1960.

Adverse Effects. As for Antimony Sodium Tartrate, p.87. Stibophen is less toxic than antimony sodium tartrate but adverse effects such as nausea and vomiting, bradycardia, and epigastric pain may occasionally occur and, if the course of treatment is prolonged, some damage to the heart and liver may result. Haemolytic anaemia and sulphaemoglobinuria have been reported following stibophen therapy.

Two patients developed haemolytic anaemia after intramuscular injections of stibophen, and 1 died. Reference was made to 6 other similar cases, 4 of them fatal. Generally, these patients had received previous courses of stibophen and after an injection in a repeat course they experienced allergic shock and developed haemolytic anaemia.— M. V. Torregrosa *et al.*, *J. Am. med. Ass.*, 1963, *186*, 598.

Further references: M. Saif, *J. Egypt. med. Ass.*, 1957, *40*, 849, per *Trop. Dis. Bull.*, 1958, *55*, 778; W. O'Brien, *Trans. R. Soc. trop. Med. Hyg.*, 1959, *53*, 482.

Uses. Stibophen is used principally in the treatment of schistosomiasis. It is less toxic, but also less effective than antimony sodium tartrate or sodium antimonylgluconate.

For *Schistosoma haematobium* infection, about 100 mg of stibophen is given by intramuscular or intravenous injection on the first day, about 200 mg on the second day, and 300 mg on the third and every other day to a total of 2.4 to 4.5 g. The smaller quantity is often sufficient to cause the disappearance of the ova of the parasite from the urine, but if viable ova are still present, further injections must be given. In *S. japonicum* infection more intensive treatment may be necessary. In *S. mansoni* infections the liver is frequently damaged, and large doses of antimony should be avoided, if possible, in patients with impaired liver function. Stibophen is usually given intramuscularly.

Injections of stibophen have also been used in the treatment of erythema nodosum leprosum.

Leishmaniasis. Three courses each of 25 intramuscular injections of stibophen 17.2 mg given on alternate days with 3 weeks between courses was effective for the treatment of 10 patients with cutaneous lesions which developed between 1 and 17 years after the original kala-azar infection with *Leishmania donovani*, and in whose skin Leishman-Donovan bodies were found.— H. S. Girgla *et al.*, *Br. J. Derm.*, 1977, *97*, 307.

A 6-year-old boy with leishmaniasis (kala-azar) contracted in Yugoslavia responded to treatment with stibophen.— H. Löhr and H. Wolf, *Dt. med. Wschr.*, 1978, *103*, 424.

Preparations

Stibophen Injection *(B.P. 1968)*. Stibophen Inj. A sterile solution of stibophen 6.4% and sodium acid phosphate 0.25% in Water for Injections. pH 5 to 6. Protect from light. It contains about 300 mg of stibophen in 5 ml.

Similar injections are included in some other pharmacopoeias.

Proprietary Names

Fantorin *(Glaxo, Ind.)*.

812-b

Stilbazium Iodide.

BW 61-32. 1-Ethyl-2,6-bis[4-(pyrrolidin-1-yl)styryl]pyridinium iodide.

$C_{31}H_{36}IN_3$ = 577.6.

CAS — 3784-99-4 (iodide).

Adverse Effects. Side-effects include nausea and vomiting.

Uses. Stilbazium iodide is an anthelmintic reported to be effective against roundworms (*Ascaris*), threadworms (*Enterobius*), and, to some extent, whipworms. Doses of 10 mg per kg body-weight have been given once or twice daily for up to 3 days. It stains the stools red.

813-v

Tetrachloroethylene *(B.P.)*.

Tetrachloroethylenum; Perchloroethylene.

C_2Cl_4 = 165.8.

CAS — 127-18-4.

Pharmacopoeias. In *Arg.*, *Aust.*, *Br.*, *Braz.*, *Fr.*, *Ind.*, *Int.*, *It.*, *Nord.*, *Turk.*, and *U.S.*

Arg., *Aust.*, and *U.S.* specify 0.5 to 1% w/w of alcohol. *Nord.* specifies either 0.5% of alcohol or 0.01% of thymol. *Int.* and *It.* specify 0.5% alcohol or may also contain 0.01% thymol.

A colourless, heavy, mobile liquid with a characteristic ethereal odour; it contains thymol 0.01% w/w as a preservative. Wt per ml 1.62 to 1.626 g. B.p. 118° to 122°.

Practically **insoluble** in water; soluble in alcohol; miscible with chloroform, ether, light petroleum, and most fixed and volatile oils. It is slowly decomposed by light and by various metals in the presence of moisture. **Store** in airtight containers. Protect from light.

Adverse Effects and Treatment. As for Carbon Tetrachloride, p.89. Symptoms are less severe.

Dependence of the barbiturate-alcohol type may follow habitual inhalation of small quantities of tetrachloroethylene vapour. Maximum permissible atmospheric concentration 100 ppm.

Toxic epidermal necrolysis had been reported after the ingestion of tetrachloroethylene.— B. Potter *et al.*, *Archs Derm.*, 1960, *82*, 903.

A 68-year-old launderette worker was anaesthetised and suffered erythema and 30% superficial burns after spilling a container of tetrachloroethylene over his clothes. The defatting property of tetrachloroethylene would lead to cracking of damaged skin.— B. Morgan (letter), *Br. med. J.*, 1969, *2*, 513.

A 25-year-old man became unconscious after exposure to the vapour of tetrachloroethylene which he was using for cleansing the interior of a tank. He recovered consciousness within 30 minutes of removal from the tank and his subsequent clinical progress was uneventful except for fatigue when resuming work about 3 days later. Elevated serum aspartate aminotransferase (SGOT) and urobilinogen concentrations were indicative of slight liver damage. There was no specific treatment for tetrachloroethylene poisoning. Sympathomimetic drugs should not be used to counter hypotension because of the danger of inducing ventricular fibrillation.— R. D. Stewart, *J. Am. med. Ass.*, 1969, *208*, 1490. A similar report.— L. K. Lackore and H. M. Perkins, *ibid.*, 1970, *211*, 1846. A 21-year-old man who had been exposed to fumes of tetrachloroethylene developed acute pulmonary oedema and become comatose. He received isoprenaline 800 µg in one litre of dextrose injection intravenously, frusemide 40 mg, aminophylline 250 mg, and dexamethasone 10 mg intravenously. Oxygen was administered. After 6 hours improvement was noted. No evidence of liver or kidney damage was seen.— R. Patel *et al.* (letter), *J. Am. med. Ass.*, 1973, *223*, 1510.

Intoxication resembling drunkenness in a 62-year-old factory worker exposed to tetrachloroethylene 500 ppm in his work.— J. K. McMullen (letter), *Br. med. J.*, 1976, *2*, 1563.

Disorders resembling vinyl chloride disease (coldness, stiffness, burning pain, and discoloration of the hands on exposure to cold; sclerotic changes of the hands, forearms, and face; an immune complex vasculitis) had occurred after exposure to tetrachloroethylene.— N. Rowell, *Practitioner*, 1977, *219*, 820.

Precautions. Some authorities consider that tetrachloroethylene should not be given to patients also with roundworm (*Ascaris*) infection, since by stimulating the worms it may initiate migration within the bowel; treatment for roundworms should therefore precede tetrachloroethylene therapy. It should not be administered to alcoholics or to patients with impaired liver function, severe debility or anaemia, or inflammation or ulceration of the gastro-intestinal tract.

Purgatives may enhance the toxic effects of tetrachloroethylene.

Absorption and Fate. Tetrachloroethylene is slightly absorbed from the gastro-intestinal tract; absorption is increased in the presence of alcohol and oils. It is absorbed following inhalation. It is excreted in expired air.

Obstructive jaundice in a 6-week old infant was considered to be caused by tetrachloroethylene in the breast milk of her mother who was exposed at intervals to vapours from a dry-cleaning plant.— P. C. Bagnell and H. A. Ellenberger, *Can. med. Ass. J.*, 1977, *117*, 1047.

Uses. Tetrachloroethylene is an effective anthelmintic against hookworms (*Ancylostoma* and *Necator*) and intestinal flukes (*Heterophyes*) but it is of little value against threadworms (*Enterobius*) and is ineffective against roundworms (*Ascaris*) and liver flukes. It may be given as a draught or in gelatin capsules.

The usual single dose is 0.1 to 0.12 ml per kg body-weight to a maximum of 5 ml for adults, and 0.1 ml per kg to a maximum of 4 ml for children. Treatment may be repeated after 4 to 7 days. Alternate-day treatment or treatment on 3 consecutive days has also been given. During treatment, it is advisable to keep the patient in bed for 4 hours; fats and alcohol should be avoided for 24 hours before and after treatment. The use of purgatives is unnecessary and undesirable.

Tetrachloroethylene is widely used as a solvent in industry.

Tetrachloroethylene, 0.1 ml per kg body-weight on 3 successive mornings, effectively treated hookworm infection in 15 children with kwashiorkor. There were no signs of liver toxicity.— S. Balmer *et al.*, *J. trop. Pediat.*, 1970, *16*, 20, per *Trop. Dis. Bull.*, 1970, *67*, 1273.

Treatment with tetrachloroethylene in 4 doses at 6-weekly intervals followed by yearly doses for 4 years reduced the prevalence of hookworm in workers in a coffee plantation in Costa Rica from 56% to 8%. Mild side-effects were observed in 40% of the 600 persons treated.— J. C. Swartzwelder *et al.*, *Revta Biol. trop.*, 1972, *20*, 295, per *Trop. Dis. Bull.*, 1973, *70*, 880.

For a comparison of tetrachloroethylene with niclosamide in *Fasciolopsis buski* infection, see Niclosamide, p.100.

For comparison of tetrachloroethylene with mebendazole and pyrantel embonate in *Necator americanus* infections, see Pyrantel Embonate, p.104.

Preparations

Tetrachloroethylene Capsules *(U.S.P., B.P. 1973).* Capsules containing tetrachloroethylene. Store in a cool place. Protect from light.

Tetrachloroethylene Draught *(B.N.F. 1966).* Tetrachloroethylene 2.5 ml, acacia 2 g, peppermint emulsion 0.3 ml, chloroform water to 50 ml. *Dose.* 50 to 100 ml. It should be recently prepared.

NOTE. The physical stability of emulsions of tetrachloroethylene can be enhanced by diluting the tetrachloroethylene with arachis oil before emulsification. This practice may be harmful because the oil increases the absorption, and thus the toxicity, of the drug.

Perklone *(ICI Mond, UK).* A brand of tetrachloroethylene for dry-cleaning purposes.

814-g

Tetramisole Hydrochloride *(B.P. Vet.).*

ICI 50627; McN-JR 8299; R 8299. (±)-2,3,5,6-Tetrahydro-6-phenylimidazo[2,1-*b*]thiazole hydrochloride.

$C_{11}H_{12}N_2S,HCl=240.8$.

CAS — 5036-02-2 (tetramisole); 5086-74-8 (hydrochloride).

Pharmacopoeias. In *Nord.*

A white to pale cream-coloured, odourless or almost odourless, crystalline powder with a bitter taste.

Soluble 1 in 5 of water, 1 in 50 of alcohol, 1 in 3000 of chloroform, and 1 in 10 of methyl alcohol; very slightly soluble in ether; practically insoluble in acetone. Solutions are most stable buffered at pH 3 in the presence of sodium metabisulphite and disodium edetate.

Adverse Effects. Tetramisole may cause nausea, vomiting, abdominal pain, headache, and vertigo. Somnolence has been reported. See also under Levamisole Hydrochloride, p.94.

A report of transient optic neuritis in one patient with hookworm and roundworm infection given tetramisole 150 mg as a single dose.— B. S. Bomb *et al.*, *Trans. R. Soc. trop. Med. Hyg.*, 1979, *73*, 110.

Uses. Tetramisole hydrochloride is the racemic form of levamisole hydrochloride (see p.94). It is effective in roundworm (*Ascaris*) infection; single doses of 2.5 to 5 mg per kg body-weight have usually been employed. It has also been used as the cyclamate.

It is used as an anthelmintic in veterinary practice.

Tetramisole was reported to cause a marked increase in the muscular tone in roundworms followed by irreversible paralysis and death. It might also inhibit fumarate reductase.— U. K. Sheth, *Prog. Drug Res.*, 1975, *19*, 147.

Hookworm. A single dose of tetramisole (80 to 120 mg) was given to 37 Egyptian farmers with hookworm and roundworm infections. All 14 patients with roundworm infection and 27 of 29 patients with hookworm infection were cured. Severe anaemia did not interfere with tetramisole therapy.— Z. Farid *et al.* (letter), *Trans. R. Soc. trop. Med. Hyg.*, 1973, *67*, 425.

Roundworm. Tetramisole 3 mg per kg body-weight cured 44 of the 46 patients infected with roundworms whose progress was followed for at least 2 of the examinations made after 7, 14, and 21 days. Mild side-effects, including nausea, vomiting, headache, and abdominal pain, lasted less than 24 hours and were reported in 8 patients.— O. Prakash *et al.*, *Indian J. med. Res.*, 1970, *58*, 1578, per *Trop. Dis. Bull.*, 1972, *69*, 530.

Periodic deworming with tetramisole 50 mg daily for 2 days, repeated twice at 4-monthly intervals, reduced the frequency of roundworm infection but did not eradicate it in 74 children receiving food supplements and living in a roundworm-infected area when compared with 80 similar control children. However, the nutritional status of the treated children improved.— M. C. Gupta *et al.*, *Lancet*, 1977, *2*, 108.

815-q

Thenium Closylate *(B.P. Vet.).* Dimethyl(2-phenoxyethyl)(2-thenyl)ammonium 4-chlorobenzenesulphonate.

$C_{21}H_{24}ClNO_4S_2=454.0$.

CAS — 16776-64-0 (thenium); 4304-40-9 (closylate).

A white, odourless or almost odourless, crystalline powder with a slightly bitter taste. M.p. 156° to 162°.

Soluble 1 in 200 of water, 1 in 25 of alcohol, and 1 in 35 of chloroform; readily soluble in hot water, any excess forming an oily layer.

Uses. Thenium closylate is a veterinary anthelmintic used for the treatment of canine hookworm infections; it is generally used in conjunction with piperazine.

816-p

Thiabendazole *(B.P., B.P. Vet., U.S.P.).*

Tiabendazole; MK 360. 2-(Thiazol-4-yl)-1*H*-benzimidazole.

$C_{10}H_7N_3S=201.3$.

CAS — 148-79-8.

Pharmacopoeias. In *Br., Braz., Nord.,* and *U.S.*

A white or cream-coloured, odourless or almost odourless, tasteless powder. M.p. 296° to 303°.

Practically **insoluble** in water; soluble 1 in 150 of alcohol, 1 in 300 of chloroform, and 1 in 2000 of ether; slightly soluble in acetone; soluble in dilute mineral acids.

Adverse Effects. Side-effects tend to occur 3 to 4 hours after ingestion and include anorexia, nausea, vomiting, epigastric distress, and vertigo. Other adverse effects occurring occasionally include pruritus, skin rashes, diarrhoea, headache, fatigue, drowsiness, hyperglycaemia, disturbance of colour vision (xanthopsia), leucopenia, and bradycardia and hypotension. Fever, chills, and lymphadenopathy have been reported and possibly represent allergic response to dead parasites. Crystalluria, which promptly subsided on discontinuation of treatment, has also been reported. Erythema multiforme has occurred rarely.

Two patients who had suffered with long-standing urticaria and diarrhoea developed muscle aches on exercise 3 weeks after being given a single dose of 3 g of thiabendazole. The aches persisted for 10 weeks and were severe and at times incapacitating.— W. J. Cunliffe and S. Shuster (letter), *Lancet*, 1967, *1*, 579.

An acute psychiatric reaction (paranoia, delusion, agitation, and violence) occurred in a woman after 2 days' treatment with thiabendazole, 1.5 g twice daily.— R. H. Lloyd-Mostyn (letter), *Br. med. J.*, 1968, *3*, 557.

For toxicological data, see 1971 and 1972 Evaluations of some Pesticide Residues in Food, *Pestic. Residue Ser. Wld Hlth Org. Nos 1*, 1972 and *2*, 1973, respectively..

Persistent cholestasis associated with nausea, pruritus, and a generalised rash occurred in a 32-year-old woman after treatment with thiabendazole.— R. Jalota and J. W. Freston, *Am. J. trop. Med. Hyg.*, 1974, *23*, 676, per *Trop. Dis. Bull.*, 1974, *71*, 1142.

When thiabendazole 80.8 mg per kg body-weight was given daily for 4 days to 8 pregnant *rats* the incidence of embryonic death was 6.1%; there were no external anomalies.— P. Delatour and Y. Richard, *Thérapie*, 1976, *31*, 505.

A 29-year-old woman developed bullous erythema multiforme and toxic epidermal necrolysis 14 days after receiving thiabendazole 1.8 g in 2 divided doses for the treatment of whipworm (*Trichuris*) infection.— H. M.

Robinson and C. S. Samorodin, *Archs Derm.*, 1976, *112*, 1757.

Precautions. Thiabendazole is contra-indicated in patients with a history of hypersensitivity and should be discontinued at the first sign of hypersensitivity. It should be used with caution in patients with hepatic or renal impairment. Thiabendazole causes drowsiness in some patients and those receiving it should not take charge of vehicles or machinery where loss of attention could cause accidents.

Interactions. For a reference to the possible inactivation of thiabendazole by a corticosteroid, see J. H. Seabury *et al.*, *Am. J. trop. Med. Hyg.*, 1971, *20*, 209, per H. A. Reimann, *Postgrad. med. J.*, 1972, *48*, 363.

For the effect of thiabendazole on serum concentrations of theophylline during treatment with aminophylline, see Aminophylline, p.343.

Residues in the diet. Maximum acceptable daily intake of thiabendazole in the diet: 50 µg per kg body-weight.— Report of the 1972 Joint FAO/WHO Meeting on Pesticide Residues in Food, *Tech. Rep. Ser. Wld Hlth Org. No. 525*, 1973.

Absorption and Fate. Thiabendazole is readily absorbed from the gastro-intestinal tract and reaches peak concentrations in the plasma after 1 to 2 hours. It is metabolised to the 5-hydroxy derivative and excreted in the urine as conjugates; about 90% is recovered in the urine within 48 hours of ingestion. Absorption may occur from preparations applied to the skin or eyes.

References: D. J. Tocco *et al.*, *Toxic. appl. Pharmac.*, 1966, *9*, 31.

Uses. Thiabendazole is an anthelmintic which is effective against threadworms (*Enterobius*), strongyloid worms (*Strongyloides stercoralis*), creeping eruption, and *Trichostrongylus* worms. It is moderately effective against hookworms (*Ancylostoma* and *Necator*) and roundworms (*Ascaris*) and has useful activity against whipworms (*Trichuris*). It has also been used in the treatment of acute trichinella infection and in capillariasis. It is the treatment of choice of most authorities in creeping eruption and in strongyloid infection, and despite its limited effectiveness, is often used in whipworm infection. It is useful in mixed infections. Thiabendazole also has some antifungal activity.

The usual dose is 25 mg per kg body-weight after the evening meal and 25 mg per kg after breakfast the following morning, to a maximum daily dose of 3 g, on 2 or 3 consecutive days, according to the severity of the infection. Up to 4 days' treatment may be required for acute trichinella infection. In threadworm infection, a dose of 25 mg per kg body-weight evening and morning, repeated after 7 or 14 days, has commonly been used.

In mass treatments, a single dose of 50 mg per kg body-weight, preferably at night after a full meal, has proved effective, but the incidence of toxic reactions is higher than when 2 doses of 25 mg per kg are given.

Dietary restrictions are unnecessary during treatment with thiabendazole.

In creeping eruption (*larva migrans*), a cream containing up to 15% in a water-soluble basis or a 10% suspension has been applied topically.

Some patients may excrete a metabolite of thiabendazole which imparts an odour to the urine similar to that which may occur after ingestion of asparagus.

Under the Preservatives in Food Regulations 1979 (SI 1979: No. 752) and Preservatives in Food (Scotland) Regulations 1979 [SI 1979: No. 1073 (S.96)], bananas may contain up to 3 mg per kg and citrus fruit up to 10 mg per kg of thiabendazole.

Thiabendazole is widely used in veterinary practice.

For a report of a symposium on the actions and uses of thiabendazole, see *Tex. Rep. Biol. Med.*, 1969, *27*, 533, per *Trop. Dis. Bull.*, 1971, *68*, 208.

Thiabendazole had analgesic, antipyretic, and anti-inflammatory effects in *rats*.— W. C. Campbell (letter), *J. Am. med. Ass.*, 1971, *216*, 2143.

Thiabendazole, applied topically, was an effective antifungal agent and cleared ringworm lesions as rapidly as systemically administered griseofulvin. Its action was enhanced in alcoholic media, and reduced by macrogols.— F. Battistini *et al.*, *Archs Derm.*, 1974, *109*, 695, per *J. Am. med. Ass.*, 1974, *228*, 1183.

Thiabendazole inhibited the fumarate reductase metabolism of helminths.— U. K. Sheth, *Prog. Drug Res.*, 1975, *19*, 147.

Gapeworm (*Syngamus*) infection in a 34-year-old woman responded to treatment with thiabendazole.— G. A. C. Grell *et al.*, *Br. med. J.*, 1978, *2*, 1464.

A patient with keratitis due to *Aspergillus flavus* was successfully treated with thiabendazole eye-drops. After approximately 14 days' treatment with a 4% suspension instilled every 2 hours, smear and culture of corneal scrapings yielded no fungal growth.— M. P. Upadhyay *et al.*, *Br. J. Ophthal.*, 1980, *64*, 30. See also *Br. med. J.*, 1977, *1*, 667.

Capillaria. From a study in 28 patients thiabendazole, 25 mg per kg body-weight given daily for up to 30 days, was considered more effective than bithionol, 2.4 g daily for 12 days, or bephenium 5 g daily for 14 days, in the treatment of infection due to *Capillaria philippinensis*. Relapses occurred in 6 of 16 given courses of treatment for less than 11 days.— G. E. Whalen *et al.*, *Am. J. trop. Med. Hyg.*, 1971, *20*, 95, per *Trop. Dis. Bull.*, 1974, *71*, 284.

Intestinal capillariasis caused by *C. philippinensis* could be treated with fluid and electrolyte replacement, a nutritious diet, and thiabendazole 25 mg per kg body-weight daily over a period of several weeks.— R. H. Watten *et al.*, *Trans. R. Soc. trop. Med. Hyg.*, 1972, *66*, 828. See also G. E. Whalen *et al.*, *Lancet*, 1969, *1*, 13.

Chromomycosis. Of 14 patients with chromomycosis given thiabendazole 2 to 3 g daily 3 appeared to be cured, 9 were improved, and 2 unchanged. Cultures were usually negative and clinical improvement was noted within a few months. Treatment was continued for up to 8 months. A dose of 2 g daily was well tolerated. One patient experienced noticeable improvement in 3 months after twice-daily topical application of thiabendazole in dimethyl sulphoxide.— A. E. Solano, *Medna Cutánea*, 1966, *1*, 277, per *Trop. Dis. Bull.*, 1968, *65*, 1047.

A cure-rate of 36.4% was achieved in 22 patients with chromomycosis treated with thiabendazole alone or with surgery, only 1 patient having a recurrence during a 4-year follow-up period after stopping treatment. Six patients developed hypersensitivity to thiabendazole.— M. A. Bayles (letter), *Br. J. Derm.*, 1974, *91*, 715.

Creeping eruption. In 50 patients with creeping eruption, a cure-rate of 28% was achieved in 3.5 days, 42% in 7 days, and 94% in 14 days after the application, 5 or 6 times daily, of thiabendazole suspension (about 14%).— D. A. Whiting, *S. Afr. med. J.*, 1976, *50*, 253, per *Trop. Dis. Bull.*, 1976, *73*, 684.

Earlier favourable reports of the use of 10 to 15% suspensions, with or without corticosteroid creams or occlusive dressings.— W. H. Eyster, *Archs Derm.*, 1967, *95*, 620, per *Trop. Dis. Bull.*, 1968, *65*, 294; C. M. Davis and R. M. Israel, *Archs Derm.*, 1968, *97*, 325, per *J. Am. med. Ass.*, 1968, *203* (Mar. 25), A188; F. Battistini, *Tex. Rep. Biol. Med.*, 1969, *27*, 645, per *J. Am. med. Ass.*, 1969, *210*, 1959.

Further references.— J. L. Bada, *Medna trop.*, 1971, *47*, 124, per *Trop. Dis. Bull.*, 1972, *69*, 654; E. M. Escandon, *Int. J. Derm.*, 1971, *10*, 192, per *Trop. Dis. Bull.*, 1972, *69*, 300; R. J. A. Aur *et al.*, *Am. J. Dis. Child.*, 1971, *121*, 226, per *Trop. Dis. Bull.*, 1971, *68*, 1231; P. S. E. G. Harland *et al.* (letter), *Br. med. J.*, 1977, *2*, 772.

Guinea worm. Thiabendazole was used to treat 750 patients with dracunculosis in doses of 50, 75, and 100 mg per kg body-weight once or twice daily during the 1st, 2nd, and 3rd day respectively. Cure by elimination, encystment, or devitalisation of the worms occurred within 5 to 20 days.— G. Raffier, *Bull. Soc. Path. exot.*, 1969, *62*, 581, per *Trop. Dis. Bull.*, 1970, *67*, 323. See also *idem*, *Méd. trop.*, 1967, *27*, 673, per *Trop. Dis. Bull.*, 1968, *65*, 1276.

Favourable results in 50 patients with guinea-worm infection given thiabendazole 50 mg per kg body-weight on 2 successive days.— R. K. Bhargava *et al.*, *J. Ass. Physns India*, 1975, *23*, 763, per *Trop. Dis. Bull.*, 1976, *73*, 687.

Further references: S. C. Sastry *et al.*, *J. trop. Med. Hyg.*, 1978, *81*, 32, per *Trop. Dis. Bull.*, 1979, *76*, 273.

Hookworm (*Necator*). Treatment with thiabendazole, 25 mg per kg body-weight twice daily for 2 days, was effective in 82.9% of patients with hookworm infection (*N. americanus*); side-effects occurred in 46.8% but were not persistent. Bephenium, in a single dose of 100 mg per kg, cured 40% of patients and produced severe side-effects in 48%.— M. K. Irgasheva *et al.*, *Medskaya Parazit.*, 1970, *39*, 414, per *Trop. Dis. Bull.*, 1970, *67*, 1501.

Mixed infections. Thiabendazole, in a dose of 500 mg daily for 3 days, was used in the treatment of schoolchildren. There was an initial cure-rate of 51% for those with roundworms (*Ascaris*) and 92% for strongyloid infection. Nine of 10 children with threadworms were also cured.— G. Chaia and A. S. Cunha, *Revta Inst. Med. trop. S Paulo*, 1970, *12*, 152, per *Trop. Dis. Bull.*, 1971, *68*, 121.

In the treatment of 200 patients with mixed infections of *Necator americanus*, strongyloid worms, and other intestinal infections, there was no evidence to show that the action of thiabendazole, 50 mg per kg body-weight, was enhanced by giving it in conjunction with levamisole 5 mg per kg.— M. Gentilini *et al.*, *Bull. Soc. Path. exot.*, 1971, *64*, 891, per *Trop. Dis. Bull.*, 1973, *70*, 61.

Thiabendazole 50 mg per kg body-weight and viprynium embonate 10 mg per kg daily in divided doses for 3 days failed to reduce the incidence of infection with *Trichuris trichiura* and *Hymenolepis nana* in 40 aboriginal children, but did eliminate *Ascaris lumbricoides* from 3 children and *Strongyloides stercoralis* from 2. Six children complained of nausea or dizziness.— J. E. Stuart and J. S. Welch, *Med. J. Aust.*, 1973, *2*, 1017.

Further references.— N. N. Ozertskovskaya *et al.*, *Medskaya Parazit.*, 1971, *40*, 346, per *Trop. Dis. Bull.*, 1971, *68*, 1227; C. Gateff *et al.*, *Annls Soc. belge Méd. trop.*, 1972, *52*, 103, per *Trop. Dis. Bull.*, 1972, *69*, 1275; O. O. Kale, *Afr. J. Med. med. Sci.*, 1977, *6*, 89, per *Trop. Dis. Bull.*, 1978, *75*, 670.

For the concomitant use of thiabendazole and mebendazole, see Mebendazole, p.99.

Ovicidal action. A report of the minimum concentrations of thiabendazole in nightsoil required to inhibit the subsequent development of, or to kill, the eggs of *Ascaris* and *Trichuris* at varying temperatures and after varying periods of exposure.— H. Kutsumi and Y. Komiya, *Jap. J. med. Sci. Biol.*, 1969, *22*, 51, per *Trop. Dis. Bull.*, 1970, *67*, 184.

Roundworm. A single dose of thiabendazole 50 mg per kg body-weight cleared *Ascaris* infection in 15 of 60 patients and reduced the mean egg count by 80.2%.— A. Sanati *et al.*, *Méd. trop.*, 1970, *30*, 522, per *Trop. Dis. Bull.*, 1971, *68*, 968.

Scabies. Scabies in 19 patients was cured by the application of a 5% ointment of thiabendazole for 5 days or, for larger lesions, 10 days.— F. Biagi and R. Delgado-y-Garnica, *Int. J. Derm.*, 1974, *13*, 102, per *Abstr. Hyg.*, 1974, *49*, 565.

Of 40 patients with scabies 32 had a satisfactory response after topical treatment with thiabendazole 10% suspension; 6 needed a second course of treatment, and 2 received triamcinolone.— E. Hernăndez-Pérez, *Archs Derm.*, 1976, *112*, 1400.

Strongyloid. Two patients with linear urticaria caused by strongyloidiasis were each given a single dose of 3 g of thiabendazole, but the treatment was unsuccessful. Side-effects included albuminuria, nausea, vomiting, severe diarrhoea, and incapacitating muscle pain on exercise. Serum-aldolase values were elevated, suggesting muscle damage.— W. J. Cunliffe and L. G. E. Silva, *Br. J. Derm.*, 1968, *80*, 108.

Of 174 patients with strongyloidiasis, over 90% were cured after treatment with thiabendazole in doses of either 25 mg per kg body-weight daily for 2 days or 15 mg per kg twice daily for 2 days.— J. Thomas *et al.*, *Méd. Afr. noire*, 1969, *16*, 216, per *Trop. Dis. Bull.*, 1970, *67*, 434.

Successful use in experimental infection with *Strongyloides fülleborni* in 1 patient.— S. Pampiglione and M. L. Ricciardi, *Lancet*, 1972, *1*, 663. See also M. E. Ament, *J. Pediat.*, 1972, *81*, 685, per *Int. pharm. Abstr.*, 1973, *10*, 591.

For the use of high total doses of thiabendazole (up to 40 g over 15 days) in strongyloid hyperinfection in malignant lymphoma, see M. Adam *et al.*, *Br. med. J.*, 1973, *1*, 264.

Of 602 ex-prisoners of war, 88 had strongyloid infection 23 to 33 years after repatriation; creeping eruption was common and gastro-intestinal symptoms rare. Treatment with thiabendazole 25 mg per kg body-weight twice daily for 3 days was generally effective.— G. V. Gill and D. R. Bell, *Br. med. J.*, 1979, *2*, 572.

The persistence of strongyloidiasis in ex-prisoners of war. Such patients should probably be given thiabendazole before being given immunosuppressant drugs.— D. I. Grove, *Br. med. J.*, 1980, *280*, 598.

Further references: R. R. Behar, *Revta cub. Med. trop.*, 1971, *23*, 141, per *Trop. Dis. Bull.*, 1972, *69*, 309; G. V. Gill *et al.*, *Br. med. J.*, 1977, *1*, 1007.

Ternidens deminutus. Of 21 patients infected with *Ternidens deminutus* 19 were cured following treatment with 2 doses of thiabendazole 25 mg per kg body-weight given on consecutive days with an interval of 12 hours. In 2 other patients there was a 50% reduction in egg count.— J. M. Goldsmid, *S. Afr. med. J.*, 1972, *46*, 1046, per *Trop. Dis. Bull.*, 1973, *70*, 264.

Toxocara. A Negro infant with visceral larva migrans, believed to be due to *Toxocara*, was successfully treated with thiabendazole, 25 mg per kg body-weight twice daily for 7 days and, after relapse, for 4 weeks.— J. D. Nelson *et al.*, *Am. J. trop. Med. Hyg.*, 1966, *15*, 930, per *Trop. Dis. Bull.*, 1967, *64*, 1233.

Trichinella. In an epidemic of trichinella infection, 23 patients were treated with thiabendazole 50 mg per kg body-weight daily up to a maximum daily dose of 3 g and a maximum total of 30 g. Signs and symptoms promptly regressed and muscle biopsy, which had previously demonstrated living larvae in 16 patients, revealed larvae in 1 patient who had had inadequate treatment. Side-effects occurred in 14 patients and necessitated discontinuation of treatment in 4.— H. H. Hennekeuser *et al.*, *Dt. med. Wschr.*, 1968, *93*, 867, per *J. Am. med. Ass.*, 1968, *204* (May 27), A199.

Three patients with trichinella infection due to eating infected black-bear meat were successfully treated with thiabendazole.— P. S. Clark *et al.*, *Ann. intern. Med.*, 1972, *76*, 951.

Thiabendazole was effective in trichinella infection but should always be given in conjunction with a corticosteroid because of the risk of a Herxheimer-type reaction.— *J. Am. med. Ass.*, 1974, *228*, 735.

Further references: A. J. Casali and E. A. Costa, *Boln chil. Parasit.*, 1977, *32*, 66, per *Trop. Dis. Bull.*, 1978, *75*, 800.

Trichostrongylus. Thiabendazole, 25 mg per kg body-weight twice daily for 2 to 3 days, was effective in clearing mild *Trichostrongylus* infection in 3 patients.— E. K. Markell, *New Engl. J. Med.*, 1968, *278*, 831.

Tropical eosinophilia. Thiabendazole 2 g initially followed by 1 g daily for 7 days reduced the incidence of blood eosinophils and improved the condition of a 23-year-old man who developed eosinophilia associated with bronchial symptoms after infection with a nematode parasite, probably *Syngamus*.— C. Junod *et al.*, *Bull. Soc. Path. exot.*, 1970, *63*, 483, per *Trop. Dis. Bull.*, 1971, *68*, 1092.

Preparations

Thiabendazole Eye-drops. Thiabendazole 4 g, hydroxyethylcellulose 1 g, benzalkonium chloride 20 mg, disodium edetate 50 mg, sorbitol solution 1 ml, water to 100 ml. Sterile thiabendazole is added aseptically to the previously sterilised eye-drop vehicle. For *Fusarium* and *Aspergillus* infection of the eye.—A. Baker, *J. Hosp. Pharm.*, 1972, *30*, 45.

Thiabendazole Oral Suspension *(U.S.P.)*. A suspension containing thiabendazole. pH 3.4 to 4.2. Store in airtight containers.

Thiabendazole Tablets *(B.P.)*. Tablets containing thiabendazole. They may contain suitable flavouring and sweetening agents. They should be chewed before swallowing.

Proprietary Preparations

Mintezol *(Merck Sharp & Dohme, UK)*. Thiabendazole, available as chewable tablets of 500 mg. (Also available as Mintezol in *Austral., Canad., S.Afr., Switz.*).

Other Proprietary Names

Foldan *(Arg.)*; Minzolum *(Ger.)*; Triasox *(Spain)*.

817-s

Triclofenol Piperazine.

CI 416; Piperazine Trichlorophenate. Piperazine bis(2,4,5-trichlorophenolate). $C_4H_{10}N_2,2C_6H_3Cl_3O=481.0$.

CAS — 5714-82-9.

Uses. Triclofenol piperazine is an anthelmintic acting against roundworms (*Ascaris*) and hookworms (*Ancylostoma* and *Necator*). It was formerly used as capsules in single doses of 50 mg per kg body-weight repeated on 2 or more successive days, preferably on an empty stomach.

818-w

Urea Stibamine.

Carbostibamide.

CAS — 1340-35-8.

Pharmacopoeias. In *Ind.*

A pale greyish, pale brownish, or pinkish amorphous powder containing 38 to 42% of antimony. Its chemical structure is not defined.

Soluble in water; practically insoluble in most organic solvents. It is unstable in air. **Store** below 30° in sealed containers from which the air has been evacuated or replaced by an inert gas. It should not be used if it has become darker or if the colour is significantly changed. Injections are prepared by dissolving, immediately before use, the sterile contents of a sealed container in the requisite amount of Water for Injections.

Uses. Urea stibamine has the actions of antimony sodium tartrate (see p.87). It is used in the treatment of leishmaniasis, particularly in India, and has been employed in filariasis and schistosomiasis. It is given by intravenous injection, in doses of 100 to 200 mg on alternate days. The total recommended dose is 3 g for adults, and 650 mg for infants.

Of 2 patients in north-west India given urea stibamine 200 mg daily intravenously for the treatment of kala-azar one died after receiving 1.6 g and the other responded to the full course of 3 g.— S. R. Naik *et al.*, *Trans. R. Soc. trop. Med. Hyg.*, 1979, *73*, 61.

819-e

Viprynium Embonate *(B.P.)*.

Viprynium Pamoate; Pyrvinium Embonate; Pyrvinium Pamoate *(U.S.P.)*. Bis{6-Dimethylamino-2-[2-(2,5-dimethyl-1-phenylpyrrol-3-yl)vinyl]-1-methylquinolinium} 4,4′-methylenebis(3-hydroxy-2-naphthoate).

$C_{52}H_{56}N_6,C_{23}H_{14}O_6=1151.4$.

CAS — 3546-41-6 (embonate).

Pharmacopoeias. In *Br., Braz., Cz.,* and *U.S.*

A bright orange or orange-red to almost black, almost odourless, tasteless, crystalline powder. M.p. about 206° with decomposition. It loses not more than 6% of its weight on drying. Viprynium embonate 7.5 mg is approximately equivalent to 5 mg of viprynium.

Practically **insoluble** in water and ether; very slightly soluble in alcohol and methyl alcohol; soluble 1 in 1000 of chloroform and 1 in 330 of methoxyethanol; freely soluble in glacial acetic acid. **Store** in airtight containers. Protect from light.

Adverse Effects. Viprynium occasionally causes nausea, vomiting, and diarrhoea. Allergic reactions and photosensitivity have been reported.

A 5-year-old boy developed a severe allergic reaction 8 hours after taking a single dose of 100 mg of viprynium embonate.— K. B. Desser and M. Baden, *Am. J. Dis. Child.*, 1969, *117*, 589, per *J. Am. med. Ass.*, 1969, *208*, 1037.

Erythema multiforme. Viprynium had been implicated in the Stevens-Johnson syndrome.— D. B. Coursin, *J. Am. med. Ass.*, 1966, *198*, 113.

Absorption and Fate. Viprynium embonate is not significantly absorbed from the gastro-intestinal tract.

No evidence of systemic absorption was noted following administration of viprynium embonate to 12 healthy subjects. Minute concentrations of drug, but not metabolites, were noted in the liver and plasma of *rats* after high doses.— T. C. Smith *et al.*, *Clin. Pharmac. Ther.*, 1976, *19*, 802.

Uses. Viprynium is an effective anthelmintic in the treatment of threadworm (*Enterobius*) infection. It has also been found of value in some cases of strongyloidiasis. It is not active against roundworm (*Ascaris*) infection.

Viprynium embonate is administered by mouth in a single dose equivalent to 5 mg of viprynium base per kg body-weight. One or two subsequent doses at intervals of 2 to 3 weeks may sometimes be necessary.

Viprynium stains the stools bright red and may stain clothing if vomiting occurs.

Viprynium interfered with the absorption of glucose by helminths.— U. K. Sheth, *Prog. Drug Res.*, 1975, *19*, 147.

Strongyloid. The stools of 8 of 10 Japanese patients heavily infected with strongyloid worms were negative 15 days after treatment with 5 mg per kg body-weight of viprynium embonate daily for 5 days. Four patients were observed for 65 to 216 days; small numbers of larvae reappeared in 2, and 1 with a pulmonary lesion relapsed.— H. Tanaka *et al.*, *Jap. J. Parasit.*, 1965, *14*, 20, per *Trop. Dis. Bull.*, 1965, *62*, 1026.

Threadworm. *For reports of the use of viprynium embonate in threadworm infection, see Martindale 27th Edn, p. 115.*

Preparations

Pyrvinium Pamoate Oral Suspension *(U.S.P.)*. Contains viprynium embonate equivalent to 0.9 to 1.1 g of viprynium in each 100 ml. pH 6 to 8. Store in airtight containers. Protect from light.

Pyrvinium Pamoate Tablets *(U.S.P.)*. Tablets containing viprynium embonate. Potency is expressed in terms of the equivalent amount of viprynium. Store in airtight containers. Protect from light.

Viprynium Mixture *(B.P.)*. Viprynium Suspension. A suspension of viprynium embonate in a suitable flavoured vehicle. pH 7.5 to 8. Potency is expressed in terms of the equivalent amount of viprynium. Protect from light. When a dose less than or not a multiple of 5 ml is prescribed, the mixture should be diluted to 5 ml, or a multiple, with syrup. Such dilutions must be freshly prepared and not used more than 2 weeks after issue.

Viprynium Tablets *(B.P.)*. Viprynium Embonate Tablets. Tablets containing viprynium embonate. They are film-coated or sugar-coated. Potency is expressed in terms of the equivalent amount of viprynium.

Proprietary Names

Molevac *(Parke, Davis, Ger.; Parke, Davis, Switz.)*; Neo-Oxypaat *(Katwijk, Neth.)*; Oxialum *(Wolner, Spain)*; Pamovin *(Frosst, Canad.)*; Pamoxan *(Uriach, Spain)*; Polyquil *(Parke, Davis, Spain)*; Povan *(Parke, Davis, USA)*; Povanyl *(Parke, Davis, Fr.)*; Pyr-Pam *(ICN, Canad.)*; Pyrvin *(Benzon, Denm.)*; Tru *(Elea, Arg.)*; Vanquin *(Parke, Davis, Austral.; Parcor, Belg.; Parke, Davis, Canad.; Parke, Davis, Denm.; Parke, Davis, Ital.; Parke, Davis, Neth.; Parke, Davis, Norw.)*; Vermitiber *(Tiber, Ital.)*.

Viprynium embonate was formerly marketed in Great Britain under the proprietary name Vanquin (*Parke, Davis*).

Antidepressants

2500-b

The main drugs used in the treatment of depression are classified into 2 groups according to whether they inhibit monoamine oxidase or whether they are similar to phenothiazine but the mechanisms that account for their antidepressant activity are not clear.

Most of the *monoamine oxidase inhibitors* are hydrazine derivatives and include: phenelzine, p.128, iproniazid, p.122, isocarboxazid, p.122, mebanazine, p.123, and nialamide, p.125. Tranylcypromine (p.131) is a nonhydrazine monoamine oxidase inhibitor. Pargyline, which is used mainly in the treatment of hypertension and is described under Antihypertensive Agents (p.156) is also not a hydrazine derivative.

The actions and uses of monoamine oxidase inhibiting antidepressants (MAOI) are described under Phenelzine Sulphate (p.128).

The second group of drugs described in this chapter causes changes in the electroencephalogram similar to those produced by the phenothiazines. Some of them have marked sedative actions and some possess tranquillising properties. These drugs are mainly dibenzazepine or dibenzocycloheptene derivatives and because of their structures are commonly known as the *tricyclic antidepressants*, although it has been suggested that they might be more accurately classified according to their effect on biogenic amine re-uptake; they include: amitriptyline, p.110, butriptyline, p.115, clomipramine, p.115, desipramine, p.116, dibenzepin, p.117, dothiepin, p.118, doxepin, p.118, imipramine, p.119, nortriptyline, p.126, opipramol, p.128, protriptyline, p.130, and trimipramine, p.133. Iprindole (p.121) has a different tricyclic structure; maprotiline (p.122) and mianserin (p.123) have a *tetracyclic* structure; tofenacin (p.131), trazodone (p.132), and viloxazine (p.133) have different structures; each has uses similar to those of the classical tricyclic antidepressants, but some have fewer side-effects.

The actions and uses of tricyclic antidepressants are described under Amitriptyline Hydrochloride (p.110).

The monoamine oxidase inhibitors are generally considered to be less effective than the tricyclic antidepressants and, as the hazards associated with their use can be great, the tricyclic compounds are often preferred.

Drugs formerly used in the treatment of depression include stimulants such as dexamphetamine, methylphenidate, and pipradrol which are described under Central and Respiratory Stimulants (p.360) but these are no longer advocated. Tranquillisers such as diazepam (p.1523) are often used in anxiety associated with depression and lithium carbonate (see p.1540) has been found to be of value in the management of depressive states.

Reviews of antidepressants: P. S. J. Spencer, *Br. J. clin. Pharmac.*, 1977, *4*, 57S; M. Lader, *ibid.*, 135S; *Br. med. J.*, 1978, *1*, 128; T. Silverstone, *Prescribers' J.*, 1978, *18*, 133; *Drug & Ther. Bull.*, 1980, *18*, 73; *Med. Lett.*, 1980, *22*, 77; L. E. Hollister, *Drugs*, 1981, *22*, 129.

A review of the adverse effects of antidepressant drugs.— B. Blackwell, *Drugs*, 1981, *21*, 201.

Comment on the biochemical classification of depression.— *Lancet*, 1979, *1*, 1279.

Reports, studies, and comments on the potential role of a modified dexamethasone test to predict the status of depression: I. K. Goldberg (letter), *Lancet*, 1980, *1*, 376; W. A. Brown *et al.* (letter), *ibid.*, 928; M. S. Gold *et al.* (letter), *ibid.*, 1190; I. K. Goldberg (letter), *ibid.*, *2*, 92; F. Holsboer *et al.* (letter), *ibid.*, 706; R. Shulman (letter), *ibid.*, 1085.

Reports, studies, and comments on the role of electroconvulsive therapy in depressive illness: D. Avery and G. Winokur, *Archs gen. Psychiat.*, 1976, *33*, 1029; J. Davidson *et al.*, *ibid.*, 1978, *35*, 639; *Br. J. Psychiat.*, 1977, *131*, 261; *Lancet*, 1977, *2*, 593; D. G. Grahame-Smith *et al.*, *ibid.*, 1978, *1*, 254; C. P. L. Freeman *et al.*, *ibid.*, 738; G. R. Cutter (letter), *ibid.*, 1151; T. J. Crow *et al.* (letter), *ibid.*; C. P. L. Freeman (letter), *ibid.*, 1305; *ibid.*, 1979, *2*, 888; M. G. Revill (letter), *ibid.*, 1022; M. Fink (letter), *ibid.*, 1303; P. K. Bridges (letter), *ibid.*, 1980, *1*, 152; E. C. Johnstone *et al.*, *ibid.*, *2*, 1317; H. Bourne (letter), *ibid.*, 1981, *1*, 98; R. J. Russell (letter), *ibid.*; P. Aylett (letter), *ibid.*; M. G. Sandifer (letter), *ibid.*; G. A. MacGregor (letter), *ibid.*; J. L. T. Birley (letter), *ibid.*, 222; C. -N. Chen (letter), *ibid.*; K. Callender and G. Jones (letter), *ibid.*, 283; D. Gordon (letter), *ibid.*, 284; R. H. Lenox and L. A. Weaver (letter), *ibid.*, 841; B. N. Gangadhar *et al.* (letter), *ibid.*, 842; R. Maggs (letter), *ibid.*; E. C. Johnstone *et al.* (letter), *ibid.*; T. R. P. Price (letter), *New Engl. J. Med.*, 1981, *304*, 53; G. Jones and K. Callender (letter), *Lancet*, 1981, *1*, 500; J. Pippard and L. Ellam, *Electroconvulsive Treatment in Great Britain, 1980*, Gaskell (Royal College of Psychiatrists), London, 1981; *Lancet*, 1981, *2*, 1207.

2501-v

Amitriptyline Embonate *(B.P.)*.

$(C_{20}H_{23}N)_2,C_{23}H_{16}O_6$=943.2.

CAS — 50-48-6 (amitriptyline); 17086-03-2 (embonate).

Pharmacopoeias. In *Br.* and *Nord.*

A pale yellow to brownish-yellow odourless or almost odourless powder. M.p. about 140°. Amitriptyline embonate 1.5 g is approximately equivalent to 1 g of amitriptyline hydrochloride and 0.88 g of amitriptyline. Practically **insoluble** in water; soluble 1 in 120 of alcohol, 1 in 6 of acetone, and 1 in 8 of chloroform. **Protect** from light.

2502-g

Amitriptyline Hydrochloride *(B.P., U.S.P.)*.

Cloridrato de Amitriptilina. 3-(10,11-Dihydro-5*H*-dibenzo[*a,d*]cyclohepten-5-ylidene)-*NN*-dimethylpropylamine hydrochloride.

$C_{20}H_{23}N,HCl$=313.9.

CAS — 549-18-8.

Pharmacopoeias. In *Br., Braz., Cz., Jap., Nord.*, and *U.S.*

Odourless or almost odourless, colourless crystals or white or almost white powder, with a bitter, burning taste, followed by a sensation of numbness. M.p. 195° to 199°.

Soluble 1 in 1 of water, 1 in 1.5 of alcohol, 1 in 56 of acetone, 1 in 1.2 of chloroform, and 1 in 1 of methyl alcohol; practically insoluble in ether. A 1% solution in water has a pH of 4.5 to 6. Solutions are **sterilised** by filtration. **Store** in airtight containers. Protect from light.

Stability. Decomposition occurred when solutions of amitriptyline hydrochloride in water or phosphate buffers were autoclaved at 115° to 116° for 30 minutes in the presence of excess oxygen.— R. P. Enever *et al.*, *J. pharm. Sci.*, 1975, *64*, 1497. The decomposition of amitriptyline as the hydrochloride in buffered aqueous solution was accelerated by metal ions particularly from amber glass ampoules. Disodium edetate 0.1% significantly reduced the decomposition rate of these amitriptyline solutions but propyl gallate and hydroquinone were less effective. Sodium metabisulphite produced an initial lowering of amitriptyline concentration and subsequently an acceleration of decomposition.— R. P. Enever *et al.*, *J. pharm. Sci.*, 1977, *66*, 1087.

Solutions of amitriptyline hydrochloride in water are stable for at least 8 weeks at room temperature if protected from light either by storage in a cupboard or in amber containers. Decomposition to ketone and, to a lesser extent, other unidentified products was found to occur on exposure to light.— J. Buckles and V. Walters, *J. clin. Pharm.*, 1976, *1*, 107.

The photochemical stability of *cis* and *trans* isomers of tricyclic neuroleptic drugs.— A. Li Wan Po and W. J. Irwin, *J. Pharm. Pharmac.*, 1980, *32*, 25.

Adverse Effects. Many side-effects of amitriptyline and the other tricyclic antidepressants are caused by their anticholinergic actions. These include dry mouth, sour or metallic taste, constipation occasionally leading to paralytic ileus, urinary retention, blurred vision and changes in accommodation, palpitations, and tachycardia.

Other adverse effects of tricyclic antidepressants include drowsiness (but sometimes nervousness and insomnia may occur), tremor, orthostatic hypotension, occasionally hypertension, dizziness, sweating, weakness and fatigue, ataxia, epileptiform seizures, occasional extrapyramidal symptoms including speech difficulties, and gastric irritation with nausea and vomiting. Susceptible patients may swing from depression to hypomania, and delirium may occur, particularly in the elderly. Weight loss may occur and also weight gain, sometimes with inappropriate appetite (carbohydrate craving). Allergic skin reactions and photosensitisation have been reported and, rarely, jaundice and blood disorders, including eosinophilia, bone-marrow depression, thrombocytopenia, and agranulocytosis.

The tricyclic antidepressants have an adverse effect on the myocardium and can cause conduction defects and cardiac arrhythmias; an increased risk of sudden death has been suspected in cardiac patients receiving tricyclic antidepressants.

Endocrine effects associated with tricyclic antidepressant therapy include changes in libido, impotence, gynaecomastia and breast enlargement, and galactorrhoea. Changes in blood sugar concentrations may also occur, and, very occasionally, inappropriate secretion of antidiuretic hormone.

Symptoms of overdosage are excitement and restlessness with marked anticholinergic effects, including dryness of the mouth, dilated pupils, tachycardia, urinary retention, and absent bowel sounds. Severe symptoms include convulsions and myoclonus, hypotension, and respiratory and cardiac depression, with life-threatening cardiac arrhythmias that may recur some days after apparent recovery.

The incidence of toxic effects in 260 patients treated with tricyclic antidepressants was 15.4%, which included drowsiness in 16, disorientation and agitation in 8, autonomic disturbance in 7, psychoses and hallucinations in 4, exacerbation of depression and headache 1 of each, and extrapyramidal signs in 3. There was no difference in cardiovascular complications attributed to the treatment between 80 of these patients with cardiovascular disease and 3994 other patients who were also monitored.—Report from Boston Collaborative Drug Surveillance Program, *Lancet*, 1972, *1*, 529.

See also under Effects on the Heart (below).

Abuse. Comment on the high incidence of amitriptyline abuse among drug-dependent patients.— R. Cantor (letter), *J. Am. med. Ass.*, 1979, *241*, 2378.

Child abuse. After a second hospital admission with lethargy, tachycardia, abdominal distension, and absent bowel sounds, an infant was found to have amitriptyline and nortriptyline in his urine and gastric aspirate.— F. A. Simon (letter), *J. Pediat.*, 1980, *96*, 785.

Diabetogenic effect. Occasional instances of diabetes mellitus, aggravation of existing diabetes, abnormal glucose tolerance, glycosuria, and hyperglycaemia have been reported after the use of antidepressants, such as amitriptyline.— *Br. med. J.*, 1980, *281*, 596.

Effects on the blood. *Agranulocytosis.* A woman taking between 75 and 150 mg of amitriptyline daily developed agranulocytosis which was probably attributable to the drug.— J. E. Gault (letter), *Lancet*, 1963, *2*, 44.

Aplastic anaemia. Amitriptyline had been reported to cause aplastic anaemia.— R. H. Girdwood, *Drugs*, 1976, *11*, 394.

Thrombocytopenia. Thrombocytopenia which developed in a 73-year-old woman after treatment with doxepin hydrochloride recurred when she was given amitriptyline.— D. D. Nixon (letter), *J. Am. med. Ass.*, 1972, *220*, 418.

Effects on the endocrine system. Inappropriate secretion of antidiuretic hormone developed in 1 patient who had received amitriptyline hydrochloride 50 mg thrice daily for 6 weeks.— D. Beckstrom *et al.* (letter), *J. Am. med. Ass.*, 1979, *241*, 133.

Effects on the eyes. Increased intra-ocular pressure had been reported to occur, especially during treatment with amitriptyline and with imipramine, and occasionally was accompanied by narrow-angle glaucoma.— *Med. Lett.*, 1976, *18*, 63.

Individual reports of adverse effects of amitriptyline on the eyes: D. J. Goode, *Am. J. Psychiat.*, 1977, *134*, 1043 (increased palpebral aperture resembling exophthalmos); M. S. Smith (letter), *Ann. intern. Med.*, 1979, *91*, 793 (ophthalmoplegia).

Effects on the gastro-intestinal tract. During the past 13 years the Committee have been notified of cases of ileus, probably resulting from the anticholinergic effects of tricyclic antidepressants. Various tricyclics were taken by different patients, there being no suggestion that any one is especially liable to cause ileus. Fortunately the complication appears to be rare.— Committee on Safety of Medicines, *Current Problems No. 3*, Feb., 1978. See also D. C. McNeill (letter), *Br. med. J.*, 1966, *1*, 1360; A. J. Cass, *ibid.*, 1978, *2*, 932.

Effects on the heart. The cardiovascular effects of tricyclic antidepressants can in part be explained by the known pharmacology of the drugs. Many tricyclics inhibit the neuronal re-uptake of noradrenaline and thus facilitate sympathetic transmission. Their atropine-like (anticholinergic) action increases the speed of diastolic repolarisation of the sino-atrial node, and hence the frequency of discharge, and it encourages ectopic impulse formation. Impaired conduction in the specialised conducting system of the ventricles is probably caused by a direct effect on the conducting-cell membrane. In addition to direct effects on the heart, tricyclic drugs can cause postural hypotension, but the mechanism for this is obscure. Weight gain, arising from increased carbohydrate intake and water retention, may also contribute to cardiac embarrassment. A rough estimation from available evidence has indicated that almost all patients have some postural hypotension and three-quarters experience dizziness at some time. Most patients have slight tachycardia and minor ECG changes (notably a lengthened P-R interval); 10% have impaired atrioventricular conduction. Patients with pre-existing cardiac disease are more likely to develop these complications and the elderly appear especially vulnerable.— *Drug & Ther. Bull.*, 1979, *17*, 13. See also D. S. Robinson and E. Barker, *J. Am. med. Ass.*, 1976, *236*, 2089.

Individual reports and studies on the adverse effects of tricyclic antidepressants on the heart: D. C. Moir *et al.*, *Lancet*, 1972, *2*, 561; D. C. Moir, *Am. Heart J.*, 1973, *86*, 841; G. D. Burrows *et al.*, *Br. J. Psychiat.*, 1976, *129*, 335; N. O. Fowler *et al.*, *Am. J. Cardiol.*, 1976, *37*, 223; D. Burckhardt *et al.*, *J. Am. med. Ass.*, 1978, *239*, 213; E. A. Raeder *et al.*, *Br. med. J.*, 1978, *2*, 666; T. C. Brown and A. Leversha, *Clin. Toxicol.*, 1979, *14*, 253; C. D. Burgess *et al.*, *Postgrad. med. J.*, 1979, *55*, 704.

Effects on the liver. A report of 3 cases of jaundice, one mild, one fatal, and one severe but leading to good recovery, in patients given amitriptyline. In 2 of the patients other drugs had been taken but they were considered to be less likely to be responsible.— D. H. Morgan, *Br. J. Psychiat.*, 1969, *115*, 105.

Further references to adverse effects of amitriptyline on the liver: R. W. Biagi and B. N. Bapat, *Br. J. Psychiat.*, 1967, *113*, 1113 (intrahepatic obstructive jaundice); J. Yon and S. Anuras, *J. Am. med. Ass.*, 1975, *232*, 833 (hepatitis); B. N. Anderson and I. R. Henrikson, *J. clin. Psychiat.*, 1978, *39*, 730 (eosinophilia and jaundice).

Effects on mental state. Amitriptyline in a dose of 150 mg daily with diazepam 20 mg daily produced visual hallucinations in a 50-year-old woman with depressive neurosis.— G. J. O'Connell *et al.* (letter), *Can. med. Ass. J.*, 1972, *106*, 115.

Both short-term memory and performance in learning tasks were impaired in 20 healthy subjects who took amitriptyline 25 mg thrice daily for 2 weeks in a double-blind crossover study; the effect was enhanced by alcohol. There was no impairment following mianserin 10 mg thrice daily and no enhanced effects after alcohol. Amitriptyline alone or either drug together with alcohol produced a significant decrease in ability in critical flicker fusion tests. Drowsiness was reported by 14 subjects who took mianserin and by 10 who took amitriptyline.— R. Liljequist *et al.*, *Br. J. clin. Pharmac.*, 1978, *5*, 149.

Further references: J. C. Nelson *et al.*, *Am. J. Psychiat.*, 1979, *136*, 574 (exacerbation of psychosis).

Effects on sexual function. While taking amitriptyline 200 mg daily a 22-year-old man failed to ejaculate during orgasm. Within one day of discontinuing amitriptyline he was again able to ejaculate at orgasm.— J. E. Nininger, *Am. J. Psychiat.*, 1978, *135*, 750.

Effects on speech. See under Extrapyramidal Effects (below).

Effects on the skin. Skin reactions to antidepressant drugs are rarely severe. Allergic reactions usually occur between 14 and 60 days after the start of medication.— F. Quitkin, *J. Am. med. Ass.*, 1979, *241*, 1625.

Comment on photosensitivity reactions from drugs, and mention that tricyclic antidepressants may cause photosensitivity.— *Med. Lett.*, 1980, *22*, 64.

Epileptogenic effect. The Boston Collaborative Drug Surveillance Program monitored consecutively 32 812 medical inpatients. Drug-induced convulsions occurred in 1 of 60 patients given amitriptyline and perphenazine.— J. Porter and H. Jick, *Lancet*, 1977, *1*, 587.

Analysis of the number of cases of convulsions associated with antidepressants reported to the Committee on Safety of Medicines up to November 1979. Although cause and effect is difficult to prove, the number of seizures reported in patients on amitriptyline and imipramine is small, although they have been marketed for a long time and have a large share of the market. In contrast, many cases (112) have been associated with maprotiline, which has been marketed in Britain for only a few years (3.6% share of the market). Mianserin has been associated with 30 reports (5.8% share of the market).— J. G. Edwards (letter), *Lancet*, 1979, *2*, 1368. Comment.— M. R. Trimble (letter), *ibid.*, 1980, *1*, 307.

A study suggesting that the overall incidence of seizures during tricyclic treatment is approximately 1% and among non-epileptic patients is perhaps 0.5%.— M. R. Lowry and F. J. Dunner, *Am. J. Psychiat.*, 1980, *137*, 1461.

Individual reports of epileptic fits in patients receiving amitriptyline: T. A. Betts *et al.*, *Lancet*, 1968, *1*, 390; A. W. J. Houghton (letter), *ibid.*, 1971, *1*, 138; T. Ives and R. Heath (letter), *Drug Intell. & clin. Pharm.*, 1980, *14*, 378.

Extrapyramidal effects. The Boston Collaborative Drug Surveillance Program monitored consecutively 32 812 medical inpatients. Drug-induced extrapyramidal symptoms occurred in 2 of 668 patients given a tricyclic antidepressant.— J. Porter and H. Jick, *Lancet*, 1977, *1*, 587.

Individual reports of extrapyramidal effects associated with tricyclic antidepressant therapy: W. E. Fann *et al.*, *Br. J. Psychiat.*, 1976, *128*, 490 (dyskinesias in 2 patients); S. Lippman *et al.*, *Am. J. Psychiat.*, 1977, *134*, 90 (myoclonus in one patient).

Dysarthria. A 48-year-old woman developed dysarthria on the fourth day of treatment with amitriptyline 25 to 50 mg thrice daily; the condition regressed when the drug was withdrawn.— S. E. Quader, *Br. med. J.*, 1977, *2*, 97. Dysarthria is not uncommon in patients taking tricyclic antidepressants in doses of 300 to 450 mg daily.— M. Saunders (letter), *ibid.*, 317.

Tardive dyskinesia. Cases of tardive dyskinesia have been associated with treatment with tricyclic antidepressants.— Committee on Safety of Medicines, *Current Problems Series No. 4*, Apr., 1979.

Hypotension. For a comment on the incidence of postural hypotension in patients taking tricyclic antidepressants, see under Effects on the Heart (above).

Overdosage. A study of 153 cases of poisoning by tricyclic antidepressants. Emphasis is placed on the importance of being especially prepared to cope immediately with cardiac complications.— C. Thorstrand, *Acta med. scand.*, 1976, *199*, 337. A report on 20 cases of low-dose amitriptyline overdosage (estimated range 0.5 to 1.35 g). It was concluded that severe toxic reactions may occur in approximately 25% of patients ingesting 0.5 to 1 g of amitriptyline.— J. P. O'Brien, *Am. J. Psychiat.*, 1977, *134*, 66. In 150 patients who had taken estimated overdoses of 0.3 to 3 g of amitriptyline, sinus tachycardia occurred in 62%, and a tendency to hypotension was noted in patients who had taken larger amounts. Serious cardiotoxicity was not considered to be as common as it appears from the literature and side-effects did not closely correlate with the amount of drug taken.— J. H. Siddiqui *et al.*, *Curr. ther. Res.*, 1977, *22*, 321. An analysis of tricyclic antidepressant poisoning in 489 patients. No statistically significant differences could be demonstrated between the toxicity of individual antidepressants. Overdose of amitriptyline-like drugs resulted in a significantly higher incidence of coma than overdose of imipramine and its analogues, but information on the amounts of drug ingested was insufficient to indicate whether amitriptyline and its congeners are intrinsically more toxic or whether patients ingesting amitriptyline-like drugs ingest larger quantities.— P. Crome and B. Newman, *Postgrad. med. J.*, 1979, *55*, 528.

Further references to analyses of series of patients with tricyclic antidepressant poisoning: R. Woodhead, *Clin. Toxicol.*, 1979, *14*, 499 (100 patients; frequency of cardiac arrhythmias).

Plasma concentrations and clinical features of amitriptyline overdosage in 28 patients where the presence of significant amounts of other drugs was excluded. Patients with plasma amitriptyline plus nortriptyline concentrations above 1 μg per ml had a higher incidence of severe complications than those with lower plasma-drug concentrations. All patients with plasma amitriptyline plus nortriptyline concentrations above 1.3 μg per ml developed one or more serious complications. Measurement of plasma concentrations of amitriptyline and other tricyclic antidepressants is potentially useful where diagnosis is difficult because of unusual symptoms or uncertain patient history, and in severe poisoning to indicate the likely duration of toxic effects. In interpreting the results for an individual patient, attention should be paid to the timing of the blood sample, the possible effects of other drugs, and preceding events such as respiratory arrest.— R. A. Braithwaite *et al.*, *Br. J. clin. Pharmac.*, 1979, *8*, 388P. See also P. Crome and R. A. Braithwaite, *Archs Dis. Childh.*, 1978, *53*, 902 (children).

Some other studies attempting to correlate plasma concentrations of tricyclic antidepressants with symptoms: C. Hallstrom and L. Gifford, *Postgrad. med. J.*, 1976, *52*, 687; D. G. Spiker and J. T. Biggs, *J. Am. med. Ass.*, 1976, *236*, 1711; J. T. Biggs *et al.*, *ibid.*, 1977, *238*, 135; J. M. Petit *et al.*, *Clin. Pharmac. Ther.*, 1977, *21*, 47; J. M. Petit and J. T. Biggs, *Pediatrics*, 1977, *59*, 283; D. N. Bailey *et al.*, *Am. J. Psychiat.*, 1978, *135*, 1325.

Individual reports of overdosage with tricyclic antidepressants: A. Marshall and K. Moore, *Br. med. J.*, 1973, *1*, 716 (delayed onset of the adult respiratory distress syndrome); F. D. Lindström *et al.*, *Acta med. scand.*, 1977, *202*, 203 (adult respiratory distress syndrome with non-bacterial thrombotic endocarditis); D. J. Comyn, *S. Afr. med. J.*, 1979, *55*, 1055 (absence of characteristic cardiac symptoms in a patient who also took a beta-blocker); D. Herschthal and M. J. Robinson, *Archs Derm.*, 1979, *115*, 499 (skin blisters and sweat gland necrosis in a woman who also took clorazepate); J. B. Marshall (letter), *J. Am. med. Ass.*, 1980, *244*, 1900 (no cardiac arrhythmias other than sinus tachycardia, despite massive dose).

Peripheral neuropathy. A 50-year-old woman developed paraesthesia over the whole of the left side of the body and face after treatment with amitriptyline, 20 mg thrice daily for 2 weeks. The symptoms gradually subsided and did not recur when treatment with amitriptyline was resumed.— B. Blackwell (letter), *Lancet*, 1968, *1*, 426. See also C. L. Brechter (letter), *ibid.*, 590; D. D. Brown, *Practitioner*, 1968, *200*, 288; J. P. Casarino, *N.Y. St. J. Med.*, 1977, *77*, 2124.

Sudden death. Sudden deaths and hypertensive episodes during acute emotional crises (presumably accompanied by high concentrations of circulating endogenous catecholamines) have occurred in patients receiving tricyclic antidepressants.— A. J. Boakes, *Br. J. clin. Pharmac.*, 1974, *1*, 9.

Weight gain. Weight gain and a craving for carbohydrates were associated with amitriptyline in 51 female patients with depression.— E. S. Paykel *et al.*, *Br. J. Psychiat.*, 1973, *123*, 501. See also J. H. Brown and J. D. Brown (letter), *Can. med. Ass. J.*, 1967, *97*, 1361; *Br. med. J.*, 1974, *1*, 168.

A study of glucose tolerance in 6 healthy subjects given amitriptyline 50 mg twice daily for 28 days showed that they had no significant weight gains or increased blood-insulin concentrations during this period although 2 subjects reported an increase in appetite.— B. R. S. Nakra *et al.*, *Curr. med. Res. Opinion*, 1977, *4*, 602.

Comment on excessive weight gain associated with the long-term use of amitriptyline and thioridazine for chronic pain.— A. K. Pfister (letter), *J. Am. med. Ass.*, 1978, *239*, 1959.

Treatment of Adverse Effects. The stomach should be emptied by aspiration and lavage. The use of activated charcoal as an adjunct to gastric lavage has been recommended. Supportive therapy alone may then suffice for patients who are not severely poisoned (for general guidelines to the symptomatic therapy of drug overdosage, see Phenobarbitone, p.812).

In particular the patient should be monitored for cardiac arrhythmias and anti-arrhythmic measures instituted as necessary; the risk of cardiac arrhythmias continues even after apparent recovery. Propranolol has been used in cardiac arrhythmias associated with tricyclic antidepressant poisoning, but digoxin is not recommended. Some of the cardiac effects respond to cautious administration of physostigmine salicylate (see p.1043) but its routine use is not recommended. Infusions of sodium bicarbonate have also been suggested but it is not clear if they are of value in the absence of metabolic acidosis.

Convulsions are also a prominent symptom in tricyclic antidepressant overdosage; they can be managed by giving diazepam intravenously. Physostigmine (not neostigmine) may also be used to control convulsions but caution must be exercised, since among its other adverse effects it can also induce convulsions. Paraldehyde and inhalation anaesthetics have also been recommended for the management of convulsions. Phenobarbitone may be required although barbiturates are not generally advocated since they exacerbate respiratory depression. Forced diuresis, peritoneal dialysis, and haemodialysis are not of value in tricyclic antidepressant poisoning. Some workers have had promising results with charcoal haemoperfusion in very severely poisoned patients but this remains controversial (see below).

In about 7½ years 44 children with amitriptyline poisoning and 16 with imipramine poisoning had been admitted to one hospital. Symptoms of mild poisoning included drowsiness, restlessness, flushing of the face, hallucinations, vomiting, mydriasis, and sinus tachycardia; symptoms of moderate poisoning included ataxia, convulsions, dysarthria, nystagmus, a positive Babinski reflex, and systolic hypertension; 3 children with severe poisoning had coma, convulsions, hypotension, ECG abnormalities, and cardiorespiratory arrest and needed assisted respiration. Ventricular premature systoles in the 3 severely poisoned children were controlled by lignocaine 0.5 to 1 mg per minute intravenously; ventricular tachycardia in 2 was treated with procainamide 700 mg and propranolol 2 mg respectively. Convulsions in 8 patients responded to diazepam 200 µg per kg intravenously. Gastric lavage should be performed and all children with tricyclic antidepressant poisoning should be monitored under ECG control for 24 hours because of the danger of arrhythmias.— K. M. Goel and R. A. Shanks, *Br. med. J.*, 1974, *1*, 261. Comment on the dangers of tricyclic antidepressant poisoning in children.— *Lancet*, 1979, *2*, 511.

Of 21 patients treated with physostigmine salicylate in 2-mg doses intravenously, repeated if required, for tricyclic antidepressant overdosage, untoward effects occurred in 4 patients and included bradycardia, hypersalivation, convulsions, and cerebrovascular accident. Although physostigmine salicylate reversed many of the effects of tricyclic antidepressant overdosage its routine use in patients free of complications was not recommended.— R. W. Newton, *J. Am. med. Ass.*, 1975, *231*, 941. For further comments on the use of physostigmine to reverse tricyclic antidepressant poisoning, see Physostigmine Salicylate, p.1043.

The treatment of severe overdosage with tricyclic antidepressants should include treatment of metabolic acidosis and hypokalaemia with, respectively, alkali and potassium given intravenously, in massive doses if needed.— S. Farquharson (letter), *Br. med. J.*, 1972, *1*, 378. Of 12 children with cardiac arrhythmias caused by tricyclic antidepressant poisoning, 9 promptly reverted to sinus rhythm after being given only sodium bicarbonate 0.5 to 2 mmol per kg body-weight intravenously.— T. C. K. Brown, *Med. J. Aust.*, 1976, *2*, 382. See also M. Gaultier (letter), *Lancet*, 1976, *2*, 1258; T. C. K. Brown (letter), *ibid.*, 1977, *1*, 375.

Activated charcoal. Studies *in vitro* indicated that the adsorptive capacity of 1 g of activated charcoal (Norit-A) was: amitriptyline 125 mg, nortriptyline 130 mg, imipramine 163 mg, desipramine 166 mg, and protriptyline 163 mg; 1 g of Medicoal, which contains approximately half its own weight of activated charcoal, had an adsorptive capacity of: amitriptyline 282 mg and nortriptyline 318 mg. Studies in 6 healthy subjects indicated that Medicoal markedly reduced peak plasma concentrations of therapeutic doses of nortriptyline (75 mg); the reductions were greater after multiple doses of charcoal. Activated charcoal may be of value in the treatment of tricyclic overdose to reduce both peak plasma concentrations and availability.— R. A. Braithwaite *et al.*, *Br. J. clin. Pharmac.*, 1978, *5*, 369P. Comment on the role of activated charcoal with special reference to the effervescent form, Medicoal, in the treatment of acute poisoning. Its use categorically does not replace gastric aspiration and lavage, and its main role is in overdosage with drugs like amitriptyline where a small weight of drug can cause serious toxicity.— *Drug & Ther. Bull.*, 1979, *17*, 7.

See also under Activated Charcoal, p.79.

Dialysis and haemoperfusion. Dialysis and haemoperfusion are of little value in patients who have ingested drugs such as the tricyclic antidepressants which have a very large volume of distribution. The plasma contains only a very small proportion of the total amount of drug in the body and the rate of transfer from tissues to plasma may be very slow. Moreover, the amount removed by these procedures would be negligible compared to hepatic elimination.— J. A. Vale and R. Goulding, *Prescribers' J.*, 1979, *19*, 163. Although at any one time only a very small part of a tricyclic antidepressant ingested is found in the plasma pool, major adverse effects correlate with the concentration of tricyclic antidepressant in plasma. If the plasma concentration can be kept beneath a critical value the prognosis may, therefore be improved. A 56-year-old man who had ingested about 2 g of amitriptyline had a beneficial response to haemoperfusion through XAD-4 Amberlite resin.— R. S. Pedersen (letter), *Lancet*, 1980, *1*, 154. Mention of 4 patients with tricyclic antidepressant poisoning who responded to Amberlite haemoperfusion.— A. Heath *et al.* (letter), *ibid.*, 155. One indication for the use of resin (not charcoal) haemoperfusion is severe tricyclic intoxication.— A. Trafford *et al.* (letter), *ibid.* Studies in *dogs*, infused with toxic doses of nortriptyline, have not demonstrated any beneficial effect of charcoal haemoperfusion in terms of either quantities of drug removed or reduction of cardiotoxicity.— P. Crome and B. Widdop (letter), *ibid.*, 306.

Further references to studies on the merits of dialysis and haemoperfusion in amitriptyline overdosage: J. A. Diaz-Buxo *et al.*, *Trans. Am. Soc. artif. internal Organs*, 1978, *24*, 699 (beneficial results); R. S. Pedersen *et al.* (letter), *Lancet*, 1978, *1*, 719 (beneficial results in 2 patients with amitriptyline overdosage and one with doxepin overdosage).

Precautions. Amitriptyline and other tricyclic antidepressants should be used with caution in patients with cardiovascular disease and should be avoided in the immediate recovery phase after myocardial infarction. Tricyclic antidepressants should also be used with caution in patients with hyperthyroidism or with impaired liver function, and in those with a history of epilepsy, glaucoma, urinary retention, prostatic hypertrophy, or constipation.

Psychosis may be activated in schizophrenic patients and manic-depressive patients may switch to a manic phase; patients with suicidal tendencies should be carefully supervised during treatment. Blood-sugar concentrations may be altered in diabetic patients.

Despite occasional reports of their use together (see p.114), tricyclic antidepressants should not generally be given to patients receiving monoamine oxidase inhibitors or for at least 14 days after their discontinuation; severe hypertensive reactions have been reported. Similarly, several days should elapse between withdrawing a tricyclic antidepressant and starting a monoamine oxidase inhibitor.

The effects of the direct-acting sympathomimetic agents adrenaline and noradrenaline are enhanced by tricyclic antidepressants and local anaesthetics containing these vasoconstrictors should be used with great caution. The interaction is liable to be considerably more hazardous if these agents are injected intravenously. It has been recommended that, where possible, tricyclic antidepressants should be stopped some days before elective surgery.

Care is necessary in patients taking barbiturates, anticholinergic drugs such as atropine, or alcohol. The effects of guanethidine, clonidine, and some other antihypertensive agents may be diminished by tricyclic antidepressants. The effects of tricyclic antidepressants are enhanced by thyroid preparations.

Elderly patients and children under 5 years of age can be especially sensitive to the side-effects of tricyclic antidepressants; reduced dosage should be used.

Drowsiness is often experienced at the start of tricyclic antidepressant therapy and patients should be advised not to take charge of vehicles or other machinery during this period.

Comment on antidepressant therapy and driving. Although sedative properties vary from one antidepressant to another it is not an either/or phenomenon, and large interindividual variation in the degree of sedation is evident with any antidepressant. Patients with clear depressive symptoms are poor drivers, irrespective of their treatment. In mildly depressed patients there may be some risk in traffic in the initial phase of antidepressant therapy, but only if sedation occurs. Treatment should begin with small doses in order to reduce sedation in the initial phase of treatment.— T. Seppala *et al.*, *Drugs*, 1979, *17*, 389.

Dementia. The quiet demented patient may be wrongly diagnosed as a depressive or may, in fact, be suffering from both conditions, since awareness of mental deterioration can lead to reactive depression. Tricyclic antidepressants can make dementia worse and should be used with caution in these cases.— A. Stedeford, *Br. J. Hosp. Med.*, 1978, *20*, 694.

Epilepsy. For an estimate of the incidence of seizures in patients receiving tricyclic antidepressant therapy see under Adverse Effects (Epileptogenic Effect).

Glaucoma. In patients with chronic simple glaucoma tricyclic antidepressants and other anticholinergic drugs could cause a small rise in intra-ocular pressure; this was usually overcome by adequate treatment of the glaucoma. Patients with closed-angle glaucoma treated by peripheral iridectomy or those using miotics were not at risk; in patients with premonitory symptoms of closed-angle glaucoma tricyclic antidepressants might precipitate acute glaucoma.— *Drug & Ther. Bull.*, 1975, *13*, 7.

Interactions. The administration of anthelmintic *piperazine* preparations to patients who were receiving tricyclic antidepressants produced transient neurological and psychiatric disturbances.— H. Helmchen and H. Hippius, *Arzneimittel-Forsch.*, 1966, *16*, 244.

The amount of amitriptyline hydrochloride not bound to plasma proteins was 3.6%. This value was increased in the presence of *phenytoin*.— O. Borgå *et al.*, *Biochem. Pharmac.*, 1969, *18*, 2135. For a comment on the significance of tricyclic antidepressants and protein binding, see under Absorption and Fate (Protein Binding). For the effect of tricyclic antidepressants on *phenytoin*, see Phenytoin, p.1239. See also under Nortriptyline Hydrochloride, p.127.

A 44-year-old woman who had been treated with amitriptyline, 75 mg daily for 4 weeks, developed a hypotensive crisis during surgery for which she had been given *quinalbarbitone*, *atropine*, *halothane*, and *thiamylal*. A few days after amitriptyline was discontinued, she suffered no untoward effects when the operation was repeated using the same anaesthetic agents. It was suggested that amitriptyline treatment should be discontinued about 1 week before surgery.— J. M. Rhoads and D. E. McCollum (letter), *Lancet*, 1969, *2*, 741.

A 49-year-old woman given amitriptyline 75 mg daily for depression developed a toxic psychosis 4 days after she started treatment with *furazolidone*, 300 mg daily. She developed blurred vision and profuse perspiration followed by alternating chills and hot flushes, restlessness, motor hyperactivity, persecutory delusions, auditory hallucinations, and visual illusions. These symptoms cleared 24 hours after stopping furazolidone. She was also taking *conjugated oestrogens* and *diphenoxylate* and *atropine*. Furazolidone was a monoamine oxidase inhibitor.— R. M. Aderhold and C. E. Muniz (letter), *J. Am. med. Ass.*, 1970, *213*, 2080.

Concurrent administration of *hydrocortisone* and of *testosterone* decreased the elimination of nortriptyline in *dogs*.— C. von Bahr *et al.*, *Eur. J. Pharmac.*, 1970, *9*, 106. For various adverse reactions in women given *ethinyloestradiol* in addition to tricyclic antidepressant therapy, and paranoid reactions in men given *methyltestosterone*, see Imipramine Hydrochloride, p.120.

In 12 psychiatric patients, plasma concentrations of amitriptyline were not altered by the concomitant administration of *chlordiazepoxide*, *diazepam*, *nitrazepam*, or *oxazepam*. In a smaller group of patients, plasma concentrations of amitriptyline were lowered when *amylobarbitone* was given concomitantly.— G. Silverman and R. Braithwaite (letter), *Br. med. J.*, 1972, *4*, 111. See also *idem*, 1973, *3*, 18. In 5 subjects the half-life and plasma concentration of amitriptyline increased when *diazepam* was given concomitantly.— R. Dugal *et al., Curr. ther. Res.*, 1975, *18*, 679. See also under Nortriptyline Hydrochloride, p.127.

Preliminary results from a study of 45 depressed patients indicated that tricyclic antidepressants might be enhanced by *lithium*.— O. Lingjaerde (letter), *Lancet*, 1973, *2*, 1260. A woman developed epileptic seizures on addition of *lithium* to her amitriptyline therapy.— J. G. Solomon, *Postgrad. Med.*, 1979, *66*, 145.

In 3 subjects given amitriptyline 50 mg thrice daily till a steady plasma-amitriptyline concentration had been reached, those concentrations rose when *fenfluramine* up to 60 mg daily was added to their treatment, and fell slowly over 1 to 2 weeks when fenfluramine was withdrawn.— L. Gunne *et al., Postgrad. med. J.*, 1975, *51*, *Suppl.* 1, 117.

A study of the impairment of skills related to driving in healthy subjects receiving *alcohol* during amitriptyline, doxepin, nortriptyline, clomipramine, or placebo administration. It seemed that concurrent ingestion of doxepin or amitriptyline might be especially dangerous to driving.— T. Seppälä *et al., Clin. Pharmac. Ther.*, 1975, *17*, 515. See also A. A. Landauer *et al., Science*, 1969, *163*, 1467.

For the effect of amitriptyline and other tricyclic antidepressants on *direct-acting sympathomimetics*, see Adrenaline, p.3, Noradrenaline, p.21, and Phenylephrine, p.24; on *indirect-acting sympathomimetics*, see Ephedrine, p.11; on *anticoagulants*, see Dicoumarol, p.771 and Warfarin Sodium, p.776; on *antipsychotic agents*, see Chlorpromazine, p.1512 and Thioridazine, p.1560.

For the effect of *fenclonine* on a tricyclic antidepressant, see Imipramine Hydrochloride, p.120.

For evidence of *folate* deficiency in patients taking long-term tricyclic antidepressant therapy, see Chlorpromazine, p.1512.

Myasthenia gravis. Amitriptyline has not been implicated clinically, but experimentally it interferes with neuromuscular transmission, and should be used with caution in patients with myasthenia.— Z. Argov and F. L. Mastaglia, *New Engl. J. Med.*, 1979, *301*, 409.

Porphyria. Amitriptyline probably does not precipitate acute porphyria.— *Drug & Ther. Bull.*, 1976, *14*, 55.

Pregnancy and the neonate. In a study in 836 infants with congenital malformations there was no significant difference in the maternal usage of tricyclic antidepressants during the first trimester of pregnancy compared with the use in 836 controls.— G. Greenberg *et al., Br. med. J.*, 1977, *2*, 853. See also D. L. Crombie *et al.* (letter), *Br. med. J.*, 1972, *1*, 745; E. V. Kuenssberg and J. D. E. Knox (letter), *Br. med. J.*, 1972, *2*, 292.

Lactation. Concentrations of amitriptyline and nortriptyline were roughly comparable in milk and in serum in a 36-year-old patient who had taken amitriptyline, usually 100 mg daily throughout pregnancy and who continued with this dose while breast-feeding. Concentrations were not detected in the infant's serum.— T. F. Bader and K. Newman, *Am. J. Psychiat.*, 1980, *137*, 855. See also E. Eschenhof and J. Rider, *Arzneimittel-Forsch.*, 1969, *19*, 957.

Withdrawal. On withdrawal of amitriptyline an 8-year-old boy developed nausea, vomiting, and abdominal cramps. He developed dehydration, ketonuria, and acidosis. He required intravenous fluids and electrolytes and for 2 weeks after discharge from hospital continued to vomit whenever he ate solid foods.— C. T. Gualtieri and J. Staye, *Am. J. Psychiat.*, 1979, *136*, 457.

Absorption and Fate. Amitriptyline is readily absorbed from the gastro-intestinal tract, peak plasma concentrations occurring within about 6 hours of oral administration. Since amitriptyline slows gastro-intestinal transit time, absorption can, however, be delayed, particularly in overdosage.

Amitriptyline is extensively demethylated in the liver to its primary active metabolite, nortriptyline. Paths of metabolism of both amitriptyline and nortriptyline include hydroxylation (possibly to active metabolites), *N*-oxidation, and conjugation with glucuronic acid. Amitriptyline is excreted in the urine, mainly in the form of its metabolites, either free or in conjugated form.

Amitriptyline and nortriptyline are widely distributed throughout the body and are extensively bound to plasma and tissue protein. Amitriptyline has been estimated to have a half-life ranging from 9 to 25 hours, which may be considerably extended in overdosage. Plasma concentrations of amitriptyline and nortriptyline vary very widely between individuals and no simple correlation with therapeutic response has been established.

Amitriptyline and nortriptyline cross the placental barrier and are excreted in breast milk (see under Precautions).

Eight fasted subjects were given a single 50-mg dose of amitriptyline hydrochloride and urine was collected regularly for up to 180 hours. The approximate total excretion in the urine was amitriptyline 5%, 10-hydroxyamitriptyline 28%, nortriptyline and desmethylnortriptyline 6%, 10-hydroxynortriptyline 41%, and amitriptyline *N*-oxide 1%, 90% of the *N*-oxide being excreted during the first 12 hours.— G. Santagostino *et al., J. pharm. Sci.*, 1974, *63*, 1690. Evidence of wide interindividual differences in the demethylation of amitriptyline.— D. E. Rollins *et al., Clin. Pharmac. Ther.*, 1980, *28*, 121.

Following the intravenous infusion of amitriptyline hydrochloride equivalent to amitriptyline 15 mg to 4 healthy subjects the mean calculated biological half-life was about 17 hours (range about 15 to 19 hours).— A. Jørgensen and V. Hansen, *Eur. J. clin. Pharmac.*, 1976, *10*, 337. See also A. Jørgensen and P. Staehr, *J. Pharm. Pharmac.*, 1976, *28*, 62 (range of 9.0 to 25.3 hours for amitriptyline half-life following discontinuation of a sustained-release preparation in 8 patients).

Investigation of the half-life of amitriptyline following administration of 25 mg by mouth to 9 healthy subjects and using an improved thin-layer chromatographic method for amitriptyline estimation. The mean plasma half-life was determined as 14.00 hours (range 9.23 to 20.54 hours) or 12.86 hours (range 8.35 to 16.90 hours) according to the method of calculation used.— H. J. Rogers *et al.* (letter), *Br. J. clin. Pharmac.*, 1978, *6*, 181.

Plasma concentrations. A warning that spuriously low plasma concentrations of imipramine, amitriptyline, and doxepin and their metabolites desipramine, nortriptyline, and desmethyldoxepin have resulted from the collection of blood samples in Vacutainer tubes.— R. C. Veith and C. Perera (letter), *New Engl. J. Med.*, 1979, *300*, 504.

Studies and comments on assay techniques for estimation of tricyclic antidepressants: H. B. Hucker and S. C. Stauffer, *J. pharm. Sci.*, 1974, *63*, 296; S. Dawling and R. A. Braithwaite, *J. Chromat.*, 1978, *146*, 449; R. G. Jenkins and R. O. Friedel, *J. pharm. Sci.*, 1978, *67*, 17; V. E. Ziegler *et al., ibid.*, 554; S. Jones and P. Turner (letter), *Br. med. J.*, 1979, *1*, 1217.

Reviews of the therapeutic relevance of plasma concentrations of tricyclic antidepressants: *Br. med. J.*, 1978, *2*, 783; S. C. Risch *et al., J. clin. Psychiat.*, 1979, *40*, 4 and 58; J. Amsterdam *et al., Am. J. Psychiat.*, 1980, *137*, 653; G. Tognoni *et al., Clin. Pharmacokinet.*, 1980, *5*, 105.

There was no correlation between clinical response or side-effects and amitriptyline or nortriptyline steady-state plasma concentrations in a WHO collaborative study of 54 patients with primary depression treated in hospital with amitriptyline.— A. Coppen *et al., Lancet*, 1978, *1*, 63. Comment on similar results.— G. D. Burrows *et al.* (letter), *ibid.*, 497. Criticisms and reply.— K. Reed (letter), *ibid.*, 565; R. Draper and A. Darragh (letter), *ibid.*, 776; A. Coppen *et al.* (letter), *ibid.* Further criticism expressing, in particular, concern that the WHO depressed population may be atypical.— W. Z. Potter and F. K. Goodwin (letter), *ibid.*, 1049. Reply.— A. Coppen *et al.* (letter), *ibid.*, 1050. Results of a study in 49 patients who received amitriptyline were in general agreement that there was no significant relationship between plasma concentrations and clinical effects. It is agreed that the evidence does not support routine monitoring of plasma concentrations of tricyclic antidepressants.— D. S. Robinson and A. Nies (letter), *ibid.*, *2*, 100.

In a study of 28 patients with endogenous depression no correlation was found between percentage improvement and plasma-amitriptyline concentrations, doubtful correlation was found between improvement and plasma-nortriptyline concentrations, and no correlation between improvement and the sum of the amitriptyline and nortriptyline concentrations. Correlation was, however, observed between higher rates of demethylation from amitriptyline to nortriptyline, and improvement.— G. Jungkunz and H. J. Kuss (letter), *Lancet*, 1978, *2*, 1263. On re-examination of data from a study involving 34 patients no significant correlation was found, but the trend was opposite.— A. Coppen and V. A. R. Rao (letter), *ibid.*, 1979, *1*, 49.

In 65 patients with endogenous depression given amitriptyline 150 mg at night for 6 weeks the mean change in the Hamilton score was 72% in those with amitriptyline plus nortriptyline concentrations in the range 80 to 200 ng per ml, compared with 42% in those below or above that range.— S. A. Montgomery *et al., Br. med. J.*, 1979, *1*, 230. Criticism, including comment on the problems of studies attempting to correlate plasma concentrations and clinical response.— T. R. Norman *et al.* (letter), *ibid.*, 894. Reply.— S. A. Montgomery *et al.* (letter), *ibid.*, 1711.

Further reports, studies, and comments on the relevance of plasma concentrations of amitriptyline and nortriptyline, and on factors, such as age, sex, and race, which might influence this: V. E. Ziegler *et al., Clin. Pharmac. Ther.*, 1976, *19*, 795 (therapeutic concentration); D. J. Kupfer *et al., Clin. Pharmac. Ther.*, 1977, *22*, 904 (therapeutic concentration); A. Nies *et al., Am. J. Psychiat.*, 1977, *134*, 790 (age); V. E. Ziegler *et al., Archs gen. Psychiat.*, 1977, *34*, 607 (therapeutic concentration); V. E. Ziegler *et al., Br. J. Psychiat.*, 1977, *131*, 168 (therapeutic concentration); V. E. Ziegler and J. T. Biggs, *J. Am. med. Ass.*, 1977, *238*, 2167; A. Rifkin *et al.* (letter), *ibid.*, 1978, *239*, 1845 (age, sex, smoking, and race); S. Vandel *et al., Eur. J. clin. Pharmac.*, 1978, *14*, 185 (therapeutic concentration).

Protein binding. Comment on the serious technical problems in the determination of plasma protein binding of antidepressant drugs, the difficulty in generalising from one drug to another, and the need to put into perspective the significance of individual differences. Such differences may represent an additional source of variability, but are relatively less important than the 20- to 30-fold interindividual differences in total plasma concentrations that are commonly observed with antidepressants.— R. A. Braithwaite, *Postgrad. med. J.*, 1980, *56*, *Suppl.* 1, 107.

Uses. Amitriptyline is a tricyclic antidepressant. It has marked anticholinergic and sedative properties, and prevents the re-uptake (and hence the inactivation) of noradrenaline and serotonin at nerve terminals. Its mode of action in depression is not fully understood.

Amitriptyline and other tricyclic antidepressants are used in the treatment of depression, particularly endogenous depression; they are less effective in reactive depression. Associated anxiety may respond to the sedative action of tricyclics, but concomitant administration of an anxiolytic, such as a benzodiazepine (see Diazepam, p.1523) may also be necessary. The sedative action of tricyclics is not delayed. Since up to a month may elapse before an antidepressant response is obtained, severely suicidal patients may require electroconvulsive therapy initially. Where considered essential, in refractory cases, concomitant electroconvulsive therapy may be given.

Amitriptyline is usually given as the hydrochloride, by mouth, in doses of 75 mg daily initially, gradually increased if necessary, to 150 mg daily, the additional doses being given in the late afternoon or evening. Therapy may also be initiated with a single dose of 50 to 100 mg at night increased by 25 or 50 mg as necessary to a total of 150 mg daily. Maintenance doses are usually 50 to 100 mg daily and therapy should be continued for at least several months before being gradually withdrawn. Hospital in-patients may be given amitriptyline hydrochloride in doses of up to 200 mg daily and, occasionally, up to 300 mg daily.

Adolescent or elderly patients often have reduced tolerance to tricyclic antidepressants and amitriptyline hydrochloride 50 mg daily may be adequate, given either as divided doses or as a single dose, preferably at night.

In the initial stages of treatment, if administration by mouth is impracticable or inadvisable, 20 to 30 mg of the hydrochloride may be given by intravenous or intramuscular injection 4 times daily, but oral administration should be substituted as soon as possible; in some countries only the intramuscular route is recommended. Amitriptyline may also be given as a syrup by mouth in the form of the embonate.

Amitriptyline is also given for the treatment of nocturnal enuresis in children. The use of tricyclic antidepressants for nocturnal enuresis in children is controversial, not least in view of the hazards of accidental overdosage. In particular, tricyclic antidepressant therapy is not suitable for younger children (for further comment, see below under Enuresis). Doses that have been suggested are 10 to 20 mg at bedtime for children aged 6 to 10 years, and 25 to 50 mg at bedtime for children over 11 years of age.

Action. A review of the pharmacology of tricyclic antidepressants.— A. S. Horn, *Postgrad. med. J.*, 1980, *56*, *Suppl.* 1, 9.

Reports, studies, and comments on the mode of action of tricyclic antidepressants: J. L. Sullivan *et al.*, *Am. J. Psychiat.*, 1977, *134*, 188 (inhibition of platelet MAO); J. P. Green and S. Maayani, *Nature*, 1977, *269*, 163 (central histamine H_2-receptor inhibition); D. F. Horrobin, *Headache*, 1977, *17*, 113 (prostaglandin inhibition in migraine); P. D. Kanof and P. Greengard, *Nature*, 1978, *272*, 329; *Lancet*, 1978, *1*, 808; J. W. Black (letter), *ibid.*, *2*, 53 (all 3 references deal with central histamine H_2-receptor inhibition); E. Richelson, *Nature*, 1978, *274*, 176; *Mayo Clin. Proc.*, 1979, *54*, 669 (both references deal with histamine receptor antagonism); P. C. Whybrow and A. J. Prange (letter), *Lancet*, 1980, *1*, 1037 (involvement in the hypothalamic-pituitary-thyroid axis).

Administration. Although it is always best to use the smallest effective dose of tricyclic antidepressant, it is poor practice to settle for an inadequate result without having tried the whole dosage range.— L. E. Hollister, *Drugs*, 1977, *14*, 161. See also M. A. Schuckit and J. P. Feighner, *Am. J. Psychiat.*, 1972, *128*, 1456 (safety of high-dose therapy); A. Coppen and S. Montgomery (letter), *Br. med. J.*, 1975, *1*, 91 (effective dosage); H. Kramer and G. Spring, *Dis. nerv. Syst.*, 1977, *38*, 641 (inadequacy of dosage).

A means of predicting tricyclic antidepressant dosage requirements following administration of a single dose.— Braithwaite R.A. *et al.*, *Postgrad. med. J.*, 1980, *56*, *Suppl.* 1, 112.

Administration in the elderly. There is a dosage problem with tricyclics in old age, as plasma concentrations have shown up to 10-fold variation on comparable dosage. The golden rule is to start with a very low dose and increase only very gradually, watching for adverse effects as well as the expected therapeutic response.— J. Williamson, *Practitioner*, 1978, *220*, 749.

Administration in renal failure. Amitriptyline can be given in usual doses to patients with renal failure. Concentrations of amitriptyline are not affected by haemodialysis or peritoneal dialysis.— W. M. Bennett *et al.*, *Ann. intern. Med.*, 1977, *86*, 754. See also *idem*, 1980, *93*, 286. Symptoms of encephalopathy developed in a patient on maintenance haemodialysis when given amitriptyline. Similar symptoms had occurred when he was taking flurazepam.— L. Taclob and M. Needle, *Lancet*, 1976, *2*, 704.

Anorexia nervosa. Six patients with anorexia nervosa improved when treated with amitriptyline 75 to 150 mg daily. Weight gain started between the 6th and 12th day. There was also improvement in mood and a parkinsonian-like disorder present in 4 patients.— H. L. Needleman and D. Waber (letter), *Lancet*, 1976, *2*, 580. Amitriptyline therapy was associated with the production of obesity in a woman with anorexia nervosa. Because of the phobic fear of obesity in many anorectic patients, this is a potentially significant side-effect of amitriptyline for this condition.— K. S. Kendler, *Am. J. Psychiat.*, 1978, *135*, 1107.

Anxiety. A discussion on whether antidepressants, such as amitriptyline, have a role in the treatment of anxiety.— *Lancet*, 1980, *2*, 897. See also E. C. Johnstone *et al.*, *Psychol. Med.*, 1980, *10*, 321.

Asthma. Amitriptyline has been used in intractable asthma.— D. C. Webb-Johnson and J. L. Andrews, *New Engl. J. Med.*, 1977, *297*, 758.

Behaviour disorders. In the mentally handicapped, tricyclic antidepressants occasionally help in behaviour disorders that are not obviously depressive in origin. Bed wetting, a frequent problem in mentally handicapped children, may also improve with this treatment.— *Drug & Ther. Bull.*, 1978, *16*, 93.

While the antidepressants have been shown to be of some value in hyperkinetic children, their response is generally less regular and less marked than that of the stimulants and side-effects are more troublesome. Dosage is a controversial issue, since, when used in the hyperkinetic syndrome, it has been considerably higher than that used in enuresis; these higher doses can produce much more serious side-effects, notably seizures and cardiotoxic effects. The use of tricyclic antidepressants in paediatric pharmacotherapy should be regarded as still being exploratory and requiring close medical supervision. Current use for enuresis is particularly indefensible since cures are rare, tolerance and escape from suppression of enuresis the rule, and minor side-effects common.— J. S. Werry, *Drugs*, 1979, *18*, 392. See also under Imipramine Hydrochloride, p.121.

Depression. A review of tricyclic antidepressants. Tricyclic antidepressants closely resemble the phenothiazines chemically and, to a lesser extent, pharmacologically, and they possess varying degrees of 3 major pharmacological actions. First, they are sedatives, not stimulants, and the sedation resembles that induced by phenothiazines rather than that induced by benzodiazepines. Second, they have both peripheral and central anticholinergic action. Third, they block the 'amine pump', an active transport system located in the presynaptic nerve ending that recaptures released amine neurotransmitters. Evidence from clinical studies strongly suggests that tricyclic antidepressants are specifically useful only in endogenous depression, which explains why it has often been difficult to demonstrate their efficacy, compared with placebo treatment, in heterogeneous groups of depressed patients. Since the diagnosis of endogenous depression may be uncertain in individual patients, on balance it is probably better to treat too many patients with tricyclics than to miss treating those who may benefit.— L. E. Hollister, *New Engl. J. Med.*, 1978, *299*, 1106. Comments.— G. W. Vogel (letter), *ibid.*, 1979, *300*, 504; M. Callaham (letter), *ibid.*, 505. Reply.— L. E. Hollister (letter), *ibid.*

A discussion on depressive symptoms in schizophrenia. The value of antidepressants even for schizophrenics with definite depression has yet to be firmly substantiated. Until adequate studies have been carried out, good clinical practice should use a trial-and-error approach on individual patients with depressive symptoms.— *Br. med. J.*, 1980, *280*, 1037.

Evidence that patients with familial pure depressive disease and a Newcastle scale score in the 4 to 8 range, may be the only group to show a substantial improvement with amitriptyline.— P. Milln and A. Coppen (letter), *Lancet*, 1980, *1*, 763.

For a comment on the clinical impression that many patients with reactive or neurotic depression may respond to smaller dosages of tricyclic antidepressants, see Iprindole Hydrochloride, p.122.

Assessments of studies into tricyclic antidepressant therapy in depressive illness: J. B. Morris and A. T. Beck, *Archs gen. Psychiat.*, 1974, *30*, 667 (review of research); S. C. Rogers and P. M. Clay, *Br. J. Psychiat.*, 1975, *127*, 599 (statistical review of controlled trials of imipramine and placebo).

Individual reports on tricyclic antidepressant therapy in depression: *Int. Drug Ther. Newslett.*, 1976, *11*, 21 (with bethanechol to counter side-effects); D. E. Sternberg and M. E. Jarvick, *Archs gen. Psychiat.*, 1976, *33*, 219 (improvement in depressive memory deficit with tricyclic therapy); V. E. Ziegler *et al.*, *Br. J. Psychiat.*, 1977, *131*, 168 (once-daily administration); C. M. Banki and M. Vojnik, *Eur. J. clin. Pharmac.*, 1978, *13*, 259 (amitriptyline infusion to hasten effect); A. J. Gelenberg and G. L. Klerman, *J. nerv. ment. Dis.*, 1978, *166*, 365 (with lithium in patient with 48-hour recurrent depression); D. de Maio and A. Levi-Minzi, *Br. J. Psychiat.*, 1979, *135*, 73 (once-daily administration); C. C. Weise *et al.*, *Archs gen. Psychiat.*, 1980, *37*, 555 (once-daily administration).

Reports and comments on the merits and hazards of using tricyclic antidepressants and monoamine oxidase inhibitors concomitantly: D. R. Gander (letter), *Br. med. J.*, 1965, *1*, 521; *idem*, *Lancet*, 1965, *2*, 107; M. Schuckit *et al.*, *Archs gen. Psychiat.*, 1971, *24*, 509; *Br. med. J.*, 1976, *2*, 69; D. G. Spiker and D. D. Pugh, *Archs gen. Psychiat.*, 1976, *33*, 828; R. S. Goldberg and W. E. Thornton, *J. clin. Pharmac.*, 1978, *18*, 143.

For further comments on the hazards of giving tricyclic antidepressants with monoamine oxidase inhibitors, see under Precautions, above. See also under Phenelzine Sulphate Precautions, p.129.

For the use of liothyronine as a adjunct to tricyclic antidepressant therapy in depression, see Liothyronine, p.1501.

Enuresis. A definition of childhood nocturnal enuresis as involuntary nocturnal micturition in children over 5 years of age, and a review of its treatment. The first treatment, especially in the younger child, should be explanation, reassurance, and support to the family. A waking device should next be tried, especially in children over 8 years of age. Tricyclic antidepressants are the only effective drugs but as relapse usually occurs on discontinuation, they should be reserved for instances when the alarm has proved impracticable. These drugs are unsuitable for children less than 5 years of age.— *Drug & Ther. Bull.*, 1977, *15*, 26. Comment on the hazards of tricyclic antidepressant overdosage in children, with particular reference to the dangers associated with pleasant-tasting elixirs. Young children should not be given antidepressant treatment for enuresis. If such treatment is prescribed the child should be old enough to take tablets.— *Br. med. J.*, 1979, *1*, 705. See also *Lancet*, 1979, *2*, 511.

Studies of amitriptyline in nocturnal enuresis: A. F. Poussaint *et al.*, *Clin. Pharmac. Ther.*, 1966, *7*, 21; W. I. Forsythe *et al.*, *Br. J. clin. Pract.*, 1972, *26*, 116.

For a comment that the use of antidepressants for enuresis is indefensible, see Behaviour Disorders, above.

Headache. Amitriptyline, 10 to 25 mg thrice daily, was one of a number of drugs found to be effective in the treatment of chronic tension headache in 280 patients.— J. W. Lance and D. A. Curran, *Lancet*, 1964, *1*, 1236. See also *Lancet*, 1964, *2*, 1067 and 1343. See also under Pain, below.

A study demonstrating that amitriptyline is effective in the prophylaxis of migraine. The antimigraine response seems to be relatively independent of the antidepressant activity. Overall experience suggests that only a small percentage of patients who have not responded to 100 mg daily will respond to higher doses.— J. R. Couch and R. S. Hassanein, *Archs Neurol., Chicago*, 1979, *36*, 695. See also J. D. Gomersall and A. Stuart, *J. Neurol. Neurosurg. Psychiat.*, 1973, *36*, 684; J. R. Couch *et al.*, *Neurology, Minneap.*, 1976, *26*, 121.

Nausea. Antidepressants are considered useful for relief of nausea with vegetative depression and without organic cause.— D. W. Swanson *et al.*, *Mayo Clin. Proc.*, 1976, *51*, 257.

Pain. Beneficial results with fluphenazine, amitriptyline, or the two together in diabetic neuropathy.— J. L. Davis *et al.*, *J. Am. med. Ass.*, 1977, *238*, 2291. Doubts as to efficacy and concern about possible adverse effects.— L. F. Romain (letter), *ibid.*, *239*, 1037; W. W. Weddington (letter), *ibid.* Further references: G. N. Gade *et al.*, *J. Am. med. Ass.*, 1980, *243*, 1160 (diabetic neuropathic cachexia).

A study of amitriptyline and clomipramine in the management of severe pain. The greatest success for both drugs was found in the treatment of trigeminal neuralgia, relatively successful treatment was found for the tension headache group, and only moderate success was found in the control of postherpetic pain.— R. L. Carasso *et al.*, *Int. J. Neurosci.*, 1979, *9*, 191. See also A. Taub, *J. Neurosurg.*, 1973, *39*, 235 (postherpetic neuralgia); M. Mehta, *Anaesthesia*, 1978, *33*, 258 (postherpetic neuralgia).

Further references to the use of amitriptyline in pain: M. A. Tyber, *Can. med. Ass. J.*, 1974, *111*, 137 (painful shoulder syndrome); D. S. Shimm *et al.*, *J. Am. med. Ass.*, 1979, *241*, 2408 (chronic cancer pain).

Phobias. Comment on the limited value of antidepressants in agoraphobia.— *Lancet*, 1979, *2*, 679.

Preparations

Injections

Amitriptyline Hydrochloride Injection *(U.S.P.)*. A sterile solution of amitriptyline hydrochloride in Water for Injections. pH 4 to 6.

Amitriptyline Injection *(B.P. 1973)*. A sterile solution of amitriptyline hydrochloride in Water for Injections; it may contain dextrose and a suitable buffering agent. pH 4 to 6.

Mixtures

Amitriptyline Embonate Mixture *(B.P.)*. Amitriptyline Mixture; Amitriptyline Syrup. A suspension of amitriptyline embonate in a suitable flavoured vehicle which may be coloured. Potency is expressed in terms of the equivalent amount of amitriptyline. pH 5 to 7. When a dose less than, or not a multiple of, 5 ml is prescribed, the mixture should be diluted to 5 ml, or a multiple, with syrup. Such dilutions must be freshly prepared and not used more than 2 weeks after issue.

Tablets

Amitriptyline Hydrochloride Tablets *(U.S.P.)*. Tablets containing amitriptyline hydrochloride.

Amitriptyline Tablets *(B.P.)*. Tablets containing amitriptyline hydrochloride. The tablets are film-coated or sugar-coated.

Chlordiazepoxide and Amitriptyline Hydrochloride Tablets *(U.S.P.)*. Tablets containing chlordiazepoxide and amitriptyline hydrochloride. The potency of amitriptyline is expressed in terms of the equivalent amount of amitriptyline. The *U.S.P.* requires 85% dissolution of chlordiazepoxide and of amitriptyline in 30 minutes. Store in airtight containers. Protect from light.

Proprietary Preparations

Domical *(Berk Pharmaceuticals, UK).* Amitriptyline hydrochloride, available as tablets of 10, 25, and 50 mg.

Elavil *(DDSA Pharmaceuticals, UK).* Amitriptyline hydrochloride, available as film-coated tablets of 10 and 25 mg. (Also available as Elavil in *Austral., Canad., Fr., USA*).

Lentizol *(Warner, UK).* Amitriptyline hydrochloride, available as sustained-release capsules of 25 and 50 mg.

Limbitrol 10 (known in some countries as Limbatril) *(Roche, UK).* Capsules each containing amitriptyline hydrochloride equivalent to amitriptyline 25 mg and chlordiazepoxide 10 mg. For depression with anxiety. *Dose.* 3 to 9 capsules daily. **Limbitrol 5.** Capsules each containing half the above amounts.

Saroten *(Warner, UK).* Amitriptyline hydrochloride, available as tablets of 10 and 25 mg. (Also available as Saroten in *Austral., Denm., Ger., S.Afr., Swed.*).

Triptafen-DA *(Allen & Hanburys, UK).* Tablets each containing amitriptyline hydrochloride 25 mg and perphenazine 2 mg. For depression with associated anxiety. *Dose.* 1 tablet thrice daily and additionally 1 at night if necessary. **Triptafen-Minor.** Tablets each containing amitriptyline hydrochloride 10 mg and perphenazine 2 mg.

Triptafen-Forte *(Allen & Hanburys, UK).* Tablets each containing amitriptyline hydrochloride 25 mg and perphenazine 4 mg. For psychotic disorders with depressive overlay. *Dose.* According to the patient's needs, usually not more than 6 tablets daily.

Tryptizol *(Morson, UK).* Amitriptyline hydrochloride, available as **Injection** containing 10 mg per ml, in vials of 10 ml and as **Tablets** of 10, 25, and 50 mg. **Tryptizol 75.** Sustained-release capsules each containing amitriptyline hydrochloride 75 mg.

Tryptizol Syrup contains in each 5 ml amitriptyline embonate equivalent to 10 mg of amitriptyline base (suggested diluent, syrup). (Also available as Tryptizol in *Belg., Denm., Ger., Neth., Norw., Spain, Swed., Switz.*).

Other Proprietary Names

Arg.—Tryptanol, Uxen; *Austral.*—Laroxyl, Tryptanol; *Belg.*—Laroxyl, Redomex; *Canad.*—Amiline, Deprex (see also under Dibenzepin Hydrochloride), Levate, Meravil, Novotriptyn; *Fr.*—Laroxyl; *Ger.*—Laroxyl; *Hung.*—Teperin; *Ital.*—Adepril, Amilit, Amitriptol, Laroxyl, Triptizol; *Jap.*—Annolytin, Miketorin; *Neth.*—Sarotex; *Norw.*—Sarotex; *S.Afr.*—Amilent, Trepiline, Tryptanol; *Swed.*—Larozyl; *Switz.*—Laroxyl; *USA*—Amavil, Amitid, Amitril, Endep, SK-Amitriptyline.

2503-q

Amoxapine.

CL 67772. 2-Chloro-11-(piperazin-1-yl)dibenz[*b,f*][1,4]oxazepine.
$C_{17}H_{16}ClN_3O$=313.8.

CAS — 14028-44-5.

Adverse Effects and Treatment. As for Amitriptyline Hydrochloride, p.110.

Analysis of side-effects in 30 patients given amoxapine for depression compared with 31 given amitriptyline for depression. Treatment had to be discontinued because of side-effects in 4 patients in the amoxapine group and in 3 patients in the amitriptyline group. The 5 most common side-effects in the amoxapine group were: constipation (10 patients), impotence and loss of libido (8 patients), drowsiness (8 patients), dryness of mouth (6 patients), and dizziness and lightheadedness (4 patients), whereas the 5 most common side-effects in the amitriptyline group were dryness of mouth (17 patients), drowsiness (15 patients), blurred vision (5 patients), dizziness and lightheadedness (5 patients), and confusion and disorientation (4 patients).— L. J. Hekimian *et al., J. clin. Psychiat.*, 1978, *39*, 633.

Effects on the endocrine system. Evidence of galactorrhoea and increased 24-hour prolactin secretion, suggesting that amoxapine may have a dopamine-blocking effect, and hence may be an effective antipsychotic agent as well as an antidepressant.— A. J. Gelenberg *et al., J. Am. med. Ass.*, 1979, *242*, 1900. See also K. Jaffe and S. Zisook, *J. clin. Psychiat.*, 1978, *39*, 821.

Precautions. As for Amitriptyline Hydrochloride, p.112.

For a general comment on antidepressant therapy and driving, see Amitriptyline Hydrochloride, p.112.

Absorption and Fate. Amoxapine is readily absorbed from the gastro-intestinal tract. Since amoxapine slows gastro-intestinal transit time, absorption can, however, be delayed, particularly in overdosage.

Amoxapine bears a close chemical relationship to loxapine and is similarly metabolised by hydroxylation. It is excreted in the urine, mainly as its metabolites in conjugated form.

Amoxapine has been reported to have a half-life of 8 hours and its major metabolite, 8-hydroxyamoxapine has been reported to have a half-life of 30 hours. Amoxapine is extensively bound to plasma proteins.

Absorption and fate studies of amoxapine and loxapine.— T. B. Cooper and R. G. Kelly, *J. pharm. Sci.*, 1979, *68*, 216.

Uses. Amoxapine is a tricyclic antidepressant with actions and uses similar to those of amitriptyline (p.113). It is the *N*-desmethyl derivative of loxapine (p.1544).

In the treatment of depression amoxapine is given in doses of 50 mg thrice daily initially, gradually increased to 100 mg thrice daily as necessary. Higher doses of up to 600 mg daily may be required in severely depressed hospital patients. Once-daily dosage regimens, usually given at night, are suitable for amoxapine up to 300 mg daily; divided-dosage regimens are recommended for doses above 300 mg daily.

Action. Antidepressant and neuroleptic actions of amoxapine in *animals*.— E. N. Greenblatt *et al., Archs int. Pharmacodyn. Thér.*, 1978, *233*, 107.

For a comment on the possible antipsychotic profile of amoxapine see under Adverse Effects (Effects on the Endocrine System).

Depression. For a general review of the role of tricyclic antidepressants in depression, see Amitriptyline Hydrochloride, p.114.

References to amoxapine in depression: A. Yamhura and A. Villalobos, *Curr. ther. Res.*, 1977, *21*, 502; A. Åberg and G. Holmberg, *ibid.*, *22*, 304; L. F. Fabre *et al., ibid.*, 611; I. C. Wilson *et al., ibid.*, 620; L. J. Hekimian *et al., J. clin. Psychiat.*, 1978, *39*, 633; V. N. Bagadin *et al., Curr. med. Res.*, 1979, *26*, 417; K. Fruensgaard *et al., Acta psychiat. scand.*, 1979, *59*, 502; J. M. C. Holden *et al., Curr. med. Res. Opinion*, 1979, *6*, 338; B. B. Sethi *et al., Curr. ther. Res.*, 1979, *25*, 726; A. Kiev and L. Okerson, *Clin. Trials J.*, 1979, *16*, 68; R. M. Steinbook *et al., Curr. ther. Res.*, 1979, *26*, 490; R. Takahashi *et al., J. int. med. Res.*, 1979, *7*, 7; H. S. Kaumeier and H. J. Haase, *Int. J. clin. Pharmac. Biopharm.*, 1980, *18*, 177; *Med. Lett.*, 1981, *23*, 39.

Proprietary Names

Demolox *(Lederle, S.Afr.).*

2504-p

Benmoxin.

Benmoxine; Benmoxinum. 2′-(α-Methylbenzyl)benzohydrazide.
$C_{15}H_{16}N_2O$=240.3.

CAS — 7654-03-7.

Crystals. M.p. 93° to 94°.

Uses. Benmoxin is a monoamine oxidase inhibitor with actions and uses similar to those of phenelzine (p.128). It has been given in doses of 50 to 75 mg daily (in 2 divided doses morning and midday).

Proprietary Names

Neuralex *(Millot-Solac, Fr.).*

2505-s

Butriptyline Hydrochloride.

AY 62014. (±)-3-(10,11-Dihydro-5*H*-dibenzo[*a,d*]cyclohepten-5-yl)-2,*N*,*N*-trimethylpropylamine hydrochloride.
$C_{21}H_{27}N,HCl$=329.9.

CAS — 35941-65-2 (butriptyline); 5585-73-9 (hydrochloride).

A white crystalline powder. M.p. about 186°. **Soluble** in water, alcohol, and chloroform; practically insoluble in ether.

Adverse Effects, Treatment, and Precautions. As for Amitriptyline Hydrochloride, p.110.

For a general comment on antidepressant therapy and driving, see Amitriptyline Hydrochloride, p.112.

Uses. Butriptyline hydrochloride is a tricyclic antidepressant. In the treatment of depression it is given by mouth as the hydrochloride in doses equivalent to butriptyline 25 mg thrice daily initially, gradually increased to a maximum of 100 to 150 mg daily as necessary.

In 2 male volunteers butriptyline 50 mg given by mouth was readily absorbed. Plasma concentrations were variable and the rate of excretion slow, with 57 and 78% being excreted within 7 days.— B. D. Cameron *et al., Arzneimittel-Forsch.*, 1974, *24*, 93. Butriptyline 50 mg thrice daily for 22 days was an effective antidepressant in 10 patients with a primary depressive illness. Plasma-butriptyline concentrations ranged from 35 to 295 ng per ml (mean 139.4 ng per ml) during treatment but were not related to a clinical response.— G. D. Burrows *et al., Med. J. Aust.*, 1977, *2*, 604.

Butriptyline was shown to differ from other tricyclic antidepressants in not inhibiting the pressor effect of tyramine. There was no marked anticholinergic activity in human subjects.— K. Ghose *et al.* (letter), *Br. J. clin. Pharmac.*, 1977, *4*, 91.

Comment on the inappropriate use of butriptyline as an anti-anginal agent.— B. L. Remakus *et al.* (letter), *New Engl. J. Med.*, 1981, *304*, 1543.

Depression. References to butriptyline in depression: A. P. Kapadia and S. M. Smith, *Curr. med. Res. Opinion*, 1976, *4*, 278; E. Suy, *Acta ther.*, 1976, *2*, 345; N. H. Brodie *et al., Practitioner*, 1978, *221*, 128.

For a general review of the role of tricyclic antidepressants in depression, see Amitriptyline Hydrochloride, p.114.

Proprietary Preparations

Evadyne *(Ayerst, UK).* Butriptyline hydrochloride, available as tablets each containing the equivalent of 25 or 50 mg of butriptyline. (Also available as Evadyne in *Belg., Neth., S.Afr.*).

Other Proprietary Names

Centrolyse *(Arg.)*; Evadene *(Ital.).*

2506-w

Caroxazone.

FI 6654. 2-(3,4-Dihydro-2-oxo-2*H*-1,3-benzoxazin-3-yl)acetamide.
$C_{10}H_{10}N_2O_3$=206.2.

CAS — 18464-39-6.

Adverse Effects, Treatment, and Precautions. As for Amitriptyline Hydrochloride, p.110.

For a general comment on antidepressant therapy and driving, see Amitriptyline Hydrochloride, p.112.

Uses. Caroxazone is an antidepressant with general properties similar to those of amitriptyline (p.113). In the treatment of depression it has been given by mouth in doses of 100 to 200 mg thrice daily.

Metabolic studies of caroxazone.— L. Bernardi *et al., Arzneimittel-Forsch.*, 1979, *29*, 1412.

Depression. In a 3-week double-blind study of 40 patients with neurotic or anxious-neurotic depression caroxazone 100 mg to 200 mg thrice daily was as effective in relieving symptoms as amitriptyline 25 to 50 mg thrice daily. The incidence of side-effects was similar for both drugs.— S. Cecchini *et al., J. int. med. Res.*, 1978, *6*, 388. See also L. Conti *et al., Curr. ther. Res.*, 1980, *27*, 458.

2507-e

Clomipramine Hydrochloride.

Chlorimipramine Hydrochloride; Monochlorimipramine Hydrochloride; G 34586. 3-(3-Chloro-10,11-dihydro-5*H*-dibenz[*b,f*]azepin-5-yl)-*NN*-dimethylpropylamine hydrochloride.
$C_{19}H_{23}ClN_2,HCl$=351.3.

CAS — 303-49-1 (clomipramine); 17321-77-6 (hydrochloride).

Pharmacopoeias. In *Nord.*

An odourless or almost odourless white crystalline powder with a bitter burning taste and numbing after-taste. M.p. about 192°. **Soluble** 1 in 8 of water, 1 in 5 of alcohol, 1 in 3 of chloroform, and 1 in 100 of ether.

Adverse Effects, Treatment, and Precautions. As for Amitriptyline Hydrochloride, p.110.

Orthostatic hypotension may occur during intravenous infusion of clomipramine hydrochloride.

For a general comment on antidepressant therapy and driving, see Amitriptyline Hydrochloride, p.112.

Effects on the blood. Agranulocytosis in a 37-year-old woman given clomipramine for 26 days; 3 other cases had been reported to the manufacturers.— R. L. Souhami *et al., Postgrad. med. J.*, 1976, *52*, 472.

Effects on the endocrine system. A report of dilutional hyponatraemia due to inappropriate secretion of antidiuretic hormone in a 57-year-old woman, possibly associated with the administration of clomipramine hydrochloride.— M. Garson, *Practitioner*, 1979, *222*, 411.

Effects on sexual function. For delayed ejaculation as an adverse effect of clomipramine, see under Narcolepsy (below). See also Premature Ejaculation (below) for the use of this effect.

Epileptogenic effect. A 31-year-old woman with severe depression was treated with clomipramine by intravenous infusion; she was given 25 mg on the first day, gradually increased over 14 days to 250 mg. On the fifteenth day, after receiving 170 mg in 47 minutes, she developed severe epileptic convulsions and cardiac arrest. She was resuscitated and later given clomipramine by mouth.— G. Singh (letter), *Br. med. J.*, 1972, *3*, 698.

Hypertension. Hypertension developed in 3 of 6 patients who were treated with clomipramine.— I. Hessov (letter), *Br. med. J.*, 1971, *1*, 406.

Pregnancy and the neonate. Withdrawal symptoms in a neonate whose mother received clomipramine throughout pregnancy. Phenobarbitone controlled the symptoms and may have also induced the hepatic conjugating enzymes needed to metabolise clomipramine.— A. Ben Musa and C. S. Smith (letter), *Archs Dis. Childh.*, 1979, *54*, 405.

Withdrawal. For a report of neonatal clomipramine withdrawal, see under Pregnancy and the Neonate, above.

Absorption and Fate. Clomipramine is readily absorbed from the gastro-intestinal tract, and extensively demethylated by first-pass metabolism in the liver to its primary active metabolite, desmethylclomipramine. Since clomipramine slows gastro-intestinal transit time, absorption can, however, be delayed, particularly in overdosage.

Paths of metabolism of both clomipramine and desmethylclomipramine include hydroxylation, *N*-oxidation, and conjugation. Clomipramine is excreted in the urine, mainly in the form of its metabolites, either free or in conjugated form.

Clomipramine and desmethylclomipramine are widely distributed throughout the body and are extensively bound to plasma and tissue protein. Clomipramine has been estimated to have a plasma half-life ranging from 17 to 28 hours, which may be considerably extended in overdosage; that of desmethylclomipramine is longer.

Maximum plasma concentrations of clomipramine were achieved in 5 healthy subjects 2 to 5 hours after oral administration of 100-mg tablets. The plasma half-lives were estimated to range from 17 to 28 hours.— H. G. M. Westenberg *et al., Postgrad. med. J.*, 1977, *53*, *Suppl.* 4, 124. Clomipramine was estimated to have a half-life ranging from 22 to 84 hours in 10 depressed subjects. The plasma concentration of desmethylclomipramine continued to increase after that of clomipramine had begun to fall, indicating that its half-life is longer than that of the parent compound.— S. Dawling *et al., ibid.*, 1980, *56*, *Suppl.* 1, 115.

Further references: L. D. Corte, *Br. J. Psychiat.*, 1979, *134*, 390 (mean half-life of about 22 hours).

Plasma concentrations. In a study involving 50 depressed in-patients in 2 hospital units (one in England and one in Italy) no significant correlation was found between clinical response and plasma-clomipramine concentrations. In the Italian group, however, clinical improvement appeared to be associated with plasma concentrations of the metabolite, desmethylclomipramine, of over 240 ng per ml.— L. D. Corte *et al., Br. J. Psychiat.*, 1979, *134*, 390.

Further reports, studies, and comments on the relevance of plasma concentrations of clomipramine, and into factors, such as age, sex, and race, which might influence this: R. B. Jones and D. K. Luscombe, *Br. J. Pharmac.*, 1976, *57*, 430P (single dose and steady state plasma concentrations); S. J. Dencker and A. Nagy, *Acta psychiat. scand.*, 1979, *59*, 326 (once-daily administration); L. Träskman *et al., Clin. Pharmac. Ther.*, 1979, *26*, 600 (biochemical subgroup of responders); D. K. Luscombe and V. John, *Postgrad. med. J.*, 1980, *56*, *Suppl.* 1, 99 (smoking and age).

Uses. Clomipramine is a tricyclic antidepressant with actions and uses similar to those of amitriptyline (p.113).

In the treatment of depression, clomipramine is given by mouth as the hydrochloride in doses of 30 to 50 mg daily; higher doses of up to 75 mg or more daily may be required in more severely depressed patients; in obsessional and phobic states it is recommended that the dosage be started at 25 mg daily and gradually increased to 100 to 150 mg daily. A suggested initial dose for the elderly is 10 mg daily. Clomipramine may be given in divided doses throughout the day, but since it has a prolonged half-life, once-daily dosage regimens are also suitable, usually given at night.

In the initial stages of treatment, if administration by mouth is impracticable or inadvisable, up to 150 mg or more of the hydrochloride may be given daily in divided doses by intramuscular injection, but oral administration should be substituted as soon as possible. Clomipramine hydrochloride may also be given by intravenous infusion in initial doses of 25 to 50 mg diluted to 200 to 500 ml with sodium chloride injection or dextrose injection and infused over 2 hours to assess tolerance; the dose may then be increased by 25 mg daily until an optimum therapeutic dose is achieved; this is usually about 100 mg daily, although more may be required. As the initial dose is gradually increased the volume of infusion fluid may be decreased to a minimum of 125 ml, and the duration of infusion decreased to a minimum of 45 minutes. Infusions are usually given for 7 to 10 days, but more prolonged treatment may be required in severely depressed and obsessional and phobic patients. Although regular daily infusions are preferable, oral therapy using double the intravenous dose may be substituted on occasion, for example, at weekends. When a satisfactory response to intravenous infusion has been obtained it should be gradually decreased and oral therapy substituted, initially giving double the maximum intravenous dose by mouth and subsequently adjusting to a satisfactory maintenance dose if necessary. Patients must be carefully supervised during intravenous infusion of clomipramine hydrochloride and the blood pressure carefully monitored owing to the risk of orthostatic hypotension.

Reviews and symposia on clomipramine: *Postgrad. med. J.*, 1976, *52*, *Suppl.* 3, 1–120; *ibid.*, 1977, *53*, *Suppl.* 4, 1–215; *ibid.*, 1980, *56*, *Suppl.* 1, 1–143; *J. int. med. Res.*, 1977, *5*, *Suppl.* 1, 1–163.

Action. Evidence of marked inhibition of serotonin uptake by clomipramine and less marked inhibition of dopamine uptake.— P. Turner and R. S. B. Ehsanullah, *Postgrad. med. J.*, 1977, *53*, *Suppl.* 4, 14. Clomipramine was about ten times more potent than amitriptyline in inhibiting uptake of serotonin by platelets.— O. Lingjaerde, *Eur. J. clin. Pharmac.*, 1979, *15*, 335.

For general references to the possible mode of action of tricyclic antidepressants, see Amitriptyline Hydrochloride, p.114.

Administration. Once-daily clomipramine administration.— D. S. P. Schubert and S. I. Miller, *J. nerv. ment. Dis.*, 1978, *166*, 875.

See also under Absorption and Fate, Plasma Concentrations.

Anorexia nervosa. A double-blind placebo-controlled study in which 8 female anorectic hospital in-patients were given clomipramine 50 mg at night while 8 similar in-patients were given placebo. Treatment was otherwise identical. All gained weight.— J. H. Lacey and A. H. Crisp, *Postgrad. med. J.*, 1980, *56*, *Suppl.* 1, 79.

Depression. For a general review of the role of tricyclic antidepressants in depression, see Amitriptyline Hydrochloride, p.114.

Narcolepsy. Comment on the excellent response of patients with cataplexy to clomipramine and clonazepam. Although neither drug improved narcolepsy, sleep paralysis was usually abolished. In most of 75 patients, the frequency of attacks of cataplexy was totally or markedly reduced with clomipramine 10 to 150 mg daily for 4 to 7 years. Side-effects, which occurred in 18 patients, were: weight gain of 5 to 25 kg (14), rash with photosensitivity (1), nausea (1), and reduction in libido with delayed ejaculation (5). An excellent or good response to clonazepam 0.5 to 2 mg daily was obtained in 10 of 14 of the patients who had responded poorly to clomipramine (6) or who had unacceptable side-effects (8); 4 had no response. Side-effects in those given clonazepam were increased narcolepsy in one patient and nightmares in another.— J. D. Parkes and M. Schachter (letter), *Lancet*, 1979, *2*, 1085. See also M. Schachter and J. D. Parkes, *J. Neurol. Neurosurg. Psychiat.*, 1980, *43*, 171. Severe hypermotility during sleep in a narcoleptic patient given clomipramine.— E. Bental *et al., Israel J. med. Scis*, 1979, *15*, 607.

Pain. For references to the use of clomipramine in trigeminal neuralgia, postherpetic pain, and tension headache, see Amitriptyline Hydrochloride, p.114.

Phobias. References to clomipramine in the management of phobias and obsessive neuroses: D. Waxman (letter), *Br. med. J.*, 1974, *4*, 721; N. Capstick (letter), *ibid.*, 720; J. A. Yaryura-Tobias *et al., Curr. ther. Res.*, 1976, *20*, 541; J. Ananth *et al., ibid.*, 1979, *25*, 703; *J. int. med. Res.*, 1977, *5*, *Suppl.* 5, 1–128.

Premature ejaculation. Beneficial results with clomipramine in premature ejaculation.— H. Eaton, *J. int. med. Res.*, 1973, *1*, 432.

For mention of delayed ejaculation in patients given clomipramine, see under Narcolepsy, above.

Proprietary Preparations

Anafranil *(Geigy, UK).* Clomipramine hydrochloride, available as **Capsules** of 10, 25, and 50 mg; as **Injection** containing 12.5 mg per ml, in ampoules of 2 and 8 ml; and as **Syrup** containing 25 mg in each 5 ml [suggested diluent, water (for dilutions containing more than 15 mg in 5 ml) or equal parts of syrup and freshly prepared tragacanth mucilage (for dilutions containing less than 15 mg in 5 ml)]. (Also available as Anafranil in *Arg., Belg., Canad., Denm., Fr., Ger., Ital., Neth., Norw., NZ, S.Afr., Spain, Swed., Switz.*).

2508-l

Clorgyline Hydrochloride. Clorgiline Hydrochloride; M & B 9302. *N*-[3-(2,4-Dichlorophenoxy)propyl]-*N*-methylprop-2-ynylamine hydrochloride.
$C_{13}H_{15}Cl_2NO,HCl=308.6$.

CAS — 17780-72-2 (clorgyline); 17780-75-5 (hydrochloride).

A white crystalline powder. M.p. 102° to 103°. Very **soluble** in water; soluble in chloroform.

Uses. Clorgyline hydrochloride is a monoamine oxidase inhibitor. It has been tried in the treatment of depression in doses of 10 to 30 mg daily.

Raised plasma-prolactin concentrations in patients receiving clorgyline.— S. L. Slater *et al.* (preliminary communication), *Lancet*, 1977, *2*, 275.

In a comparative trial with imipramine in 92 patients, clorgyline 15 mg twice daily was found to be an effective antidepressant. Side-effects were similar to those of imipramine.— D. Wheatley, *Br. J. Psychiat.*, 1970, *117*, 573. See also J. A. Herd, *Clin. Trials J.*, 1969, *6*, 219.

Manufacturers
May & Baker, UK.

2509-y

Desipramine Hydrochloride *(B.P., Eur. P., U.S.P.).* Desmethylimipramine Hydrochloride; EX 4355; G 35020; JB 8181. 3-(10,11-Dihydro-5*H*-dibenz[*b,f*]azepin-5-yl)-*N*-methylpropylamine

hydrochloride.
$C_{18}H_{22}N_2,HCl = 302.8$.

CAS — 50-47-5 (desipramine); 58-28-6 (hydrochloride).

Pharmacopoeias. In *Br., Eur., Fr., Ger., Jug., Neth.,* and *U.S.*

A white or almost white, odourless or almost odourless, crystalline powder with a bitter slightly numbing taste. M.p. about 214°.
Soluble 1 in 20 of water, 1 in 20 of alcohol, and 1 in about 4 of chloroform; practically insoluble in ether; freely soluble in methyl alcohol. A 8% solution in water has a pH of 4.5 to 5.7. Solutions are **sterilised** by autoclaving or by filtration. **Store** in airtight containers. Protect from light.

Adverse Effects and Treatment. As for Amitriptyline Hydrochloride, p.110.
The anticholinergic and sedative actions of desipramine are reported to be less marked than those of amitriptyline.

Allergy. An 80-year-old woman with no known history of allergy or liver disease, who had received imipramine, 50 mg daily, and ethchlorvynol for about 2 weeks, developed an allergic reaction due to imipramine. Imipramine was replaced with desipramine 100 to 150 mg daily for about 5 days. Pruritus developed, and 25 days later jaundice supervened. Exfoliative dermatitis simulating the Stevens-Johnson syndrome was associated with mucous membrane desquamation and eosinophilia. Autopsy revealed hepatic necrosis.— W. J. Powell *et al., J. Am. med. Ass.,* 1968, *206,* 643. See also D. R. Jones and T. R. Maloney, *Am. J. Psychiat.,* 1980, *137,* 115.

Effects on the blood. Desipramine hydrochloride was considered to be the most likely cause for the development of neutropenia in a 76-year-old woman being treated for depression. She had concomitantly been treated with amylobarbitone sodium, digoxin, and ferrous sulphate. Prior to treatment with desipramine she had been taking chlordiazepoxide and phenelzine. Leucopenia became evident during the third week of treatment with desipramine and though treatment was stopped her condition gradually progressed to agranulocytosis. She died due to a pulmonary embolism.— J. L. Crammer and A. Elkes (letter), *Lancet,* 1967, *1,* 105.

Effects on the endocrine system. Inappropriate antidiuresis and dilutional hyponatraemia in a man given desipramine.— S. K. Dhar *et al.* (letter), *Archs intern. Med.,* 1978, *138,* 1750.

Effects on the heart. Studies of ECG changes in patients given desipramine.— M. V. Rudorfer and R. C. Young, *Am. J. Psychiat.,* 1980, *137,* 984; R. C. Veith *et al., Clin. Pharmac. Ther.,* 1980, *27,* 796.

Overdosage. A 14-month-old boy who took 100 to 200 mg of desipramine developed status epilepticus, hypotension, and hyperpyrexia which damaged the brain permanently and the child made only a partial recovery. A delay of about 15 hours before treatment was initiated could have been responsible for this.— W. R. Edwards (letter), *Br. med. J.,* 1967, *4,* 358. Convulsions and grand mal seizures occurred in a 3-year-old child about 20 minutes after she had taken desipramine 100 mg.— S. G. Jue, *Drug Intell. & clin. Pharm.,* 1976, *10,* 52.

Precautions. As for Amitriptyline Hydrochloride, p.112.

For a general comment on antidepressant therapy and driving, see Amitriptyline Hydrochloride, p.112.

Interactions. Hypertension occurred during an operation under *trichloroethylene* anaesthesia in a woman who had been taking desipramine and thioridazine.— J. V. Farman (letter), *Lancet,* 1966, *2,* 436. See also K. M. F. Murray and S. E. Smith (letter), *ibid.,* 591; J. V. Farman (letter), *ibid.,* 702.

The amount of desipramine not bound to plasma proteins was about 10%. This value was increased in the presence of *aspirin, phenacetin, phenazone, amitriptyline, nortriptyline, meprobamate,* and *phenytoin,* but not by *lithium carbonate, phenobarbitone,* or *protriptyline.*— O. Borgå *et al., Biochem. Pharmac.,* 1969, *18,* 2135. For a comment on the significance of tricyclic antidepressants and protein binding, see under Absorption and Fate for Imipramine (Protein Binding), p.120.

Hyperpyrexia and shock in a patient taking desipramine hydrochloride and *tranylcypromine sulphate.*— W. N. Rom and E. J. Benner, *Calif. Med.,* 1972, *117,* 65.

For the effect of desipramine on *butaperazine,* see Butaperazine Maleate, p.1506. For the effect of desipramine on *clonidine,* see Clonidine Hydrochloride, p.140. For the effect of desipramine on *methyldopa,* see Methyldopa, p.153.

Phaeochromocytoma. Phaeochromocytoma unmasked in one patient by desipramine therapy.— M. R. Achong and P. M. Keane, *Ann. intern. Med.,* 1981, *94,* 358.

Pregnancy and the neonate. For reference to the excretion of desipramine in human breast milk, see Imipramine Hydrochloride, p.120.

Withdrawal. Over a period of 12 years a man gradually increased his dose of desipramine from 75 mg daily to 1 g daily. He was admitted to hospital and the desipramine was successfully withdrawn at a rate of 100 mg daily over a period of 10 days with the aid of placebo medication. Surprisingly, no active medication became necessary during withdrawal. Withdrawal symptoms included nervousness, soreness in shoulders and back, headache, poor sleep, and vivid dreams. During the month after withdrawal all symptoms gradually disappeared and he was discharged on a placebo regimen. The majority of the desipramine was rapidly excreted as the 2-hydroxy conjugate suggesting that the long-term high dosage of desipramine may have led to the induction of hydroxylating enzyme. Adverse electrocardiographic effects were rapidly reversed on withdrawal, and EEG effects also showed reversibility.— G. M. Brown *et al., Archs gen. Psychiat.,* 1978, *35,* 1261.

Neonatal withdrawal. Symptoms considered to be due to drug withdrawal were observed in a neonate whose mother had taken desipramine throughout pregnancy.— P. A. C. Webster (letter), *Lancet,* 1973, *2,* 318.

Absorption and Fate. Desipramine is the principal active metabolite of imipramine. For an account of its metabolism, see Imipramine Hydrochloride, p.120.
Desipramine has been reported to have a longer plasma half-life than imipramine.

In 2 patients with depression given desipramine 100 mg daily for at least 2 weeks, mean serial steady-state plasma-desipramine concentrations of 55.9 and 62.4 ng per ml respectively occurred. In another 2 patients receiving desipramine 150 and 200 mg daily the plasma concentrations were 105.2 and 217.7 ng per ml respectively.— V. E. Ziegler *et al., J. pharm. Sci.,* 1978, *67,* 554.

Studies of plasma concentrations of desipramine and clinical response: R. Khalid *et al., Psychopharmac. Bull.,* 1978, *14,* 43; J. Amsterdam *et al., J. clin. Psychiat.,* 1979, *40,* 141 (inadequate plasma concentration with standard dose); M. V. Rudorfer and R. C. Young, *Clin. Pharmac. Ther.,* 1980, *28,* 703 (anticholinergic effects and plasma concentrations).

Uses. Desipramine is a tricyclic antidepressant with actions and uses similar to those of amitriptyline (p.113). It is the principal active metabolite of imipramine (p.119) and, like imipramine, has less marked sedative properties than amitriptyline. In the treatment of depression, desipramine is given by mouth as the hydrochloride in doses of 25 mg thrice daily initially, gradually increased to 50 mg three or four times daily; higher doses of up to 300 mg daily may be required in severely depressed hospital patients. A suggested initial dose for adolescents and the elderly is 25 to 50 mg daily, gradually increased to 100 mg daily if necessary. Since desipramine has a prolonged half-life, once-daily dosage regimens are also suitable.

Administration in renal failure. Desipramine can be given in usual doses to patients with renal failure. Concentrations of desipramine were not affected by haemodialysis or peritoneal dialysis.— W. M. Bennett *et al., Ann. intern. Med.,* 1977, *86,* 754. See also *idem,* 1980, *93,* 286.

Depression. For a general review of the role of tricyclic antidepressants in depression, see Amitriptyline Hydrochloride, p.114.

Parkinsonism. In 39 patients with parkinsonism, treatment for 3 weeks with desipramine, 25 mg daily initially increasing to 100 mg daily over 7 days, gave good results in 10 of 20 patients, in comparison with 3 of 19 patients who received a placebo. Side-effects, including nausea and giddiness, occurred in 6 patients given desipramine and necessitated withdrawal of treatment in 4.— L. Laitinen, *Acta neurol. scand.,* 1969, *45,* 109.

Preparations

Desipramine Hydrochloride Capsules *(U.S.P.).* Capsules containing desipramine hydrochloride. Store in airtight containers.

Desipramine Hydrochloride Tablets *(U.S.P.).* Tablets containing desipramine hydrochloride. Store in airtight containers.

Desipramine Tablets *(B.P.).* Tablets containing desipramine hydrochloride. The tablets are sugar-coated.

Proprietary Preparations

Pertofran *(Geigy, UK).* Desipramine hydrochloride, available as tablets of 25 mg. (Also available as Pertofran in *Austral., Denm., Fr., Ger., Neth., S.Afr., Switz.*).

Other Proprietary Names

Nebril (as hydrochloride and dibudinate) *(Arg.)*; Norpramin *(Canad., USA)*; Nortimil *(Ital.)*; Pertofrana *(Spain)*; Pertofrane *(Canad., USA)*; Pertofrin *(Swed.)*; Sertofren *(Norw.)*.

2510-g

Dibenzepin Hydrochloride.

HF 1927. 10-(2-Dimethylaminoethyl)-5,10-dihydro-5-methyl-11*H*-dibenzo[*b,e*][1,4]diazepin-11-one hydrochloride.
$C_{18}H_{21}N_3O,HCl = 331.8$.

CAS — 4498-32-2 (dibenzepin); 315-80-0 (hydrochloride).

A colourless, odourless, fine crystalline powder with a bitter taste. M.p. about 237°. **Soluble** 1 in 16 of water; soluble in alcohol and chloroform. A solution in water has a pH of 4 to 5.

Adverse Effects, Treatment, and Precautions. As for Amitriptyline Hydrochloride, p.110.

For a general comment on antidepressant therapy and driving, see Amitriptyline Hydrochloride, p.112.

Effects on mental state. Two weeks after starting therapy with dibenzepin a 63-year-old depressed man developed a 48-hour affective cycle, depressed days alternating with days of normal to cheerful mood. He became depressed again on stopping dibenzepin and when it was re-instituted a more attenuated less regular cycling pattern began to develop. Dibenzepin therapy was stopped and he subsequently responded to ECT therapy.— B. Lerer *et al., Br. J. Psychiat.,* 1980, *137,* 183.

Absorption and Fate. Dibenzepin is readily absorbed from the gastro-intestinal tract and extensively metabolised to its primary active demethylated metabolite. Since dibenzepin slows gastro-intestinal transit time absorption can, however, be delayed, particularly in overdosage. Dibenzepin is excreted in the urine, mainly in the form of its metabolites either free or in conjugated form; appreciable amounts are also excreted in the faeces.

The elimination half-life of dibenzepin and its major demethylation metabolite after administration of 8 mg per kg body-weight to 12 patients was about 4 hours. Unlike imipramine a steady plasma concentration could not be achieved with these doses. There was a correlation between age of the patient and plasma concentrations.— R. Gauch and J. Modestin, *Arzneimittel-Forsch.,* 1973, *23,* 687. See also H. Lehner *et al., ibid.,* 1967, *17,* 185 (metabolism).

Plasma concentrations. In a preliminary report of a study of dibenzepin there was a positive linear correlation between the median plasma concentration of dibenzepin and the rate of response, and between the median plasma concentration and age.— J. Modestin (letter), *Lancet,* 1972, *1,* 634.

Uses. Dibenzepin hydrochloride is a tricyclic antidepressant with actions and uses similar to those of amitriptyline (p.113).
In the treatment of depression dibenzepin hydrochloride is given by mouth in doses of 80 mg thrice daily initially, gradually increased to 160 mg thrice daily; higher doses of up to 560 mg daily in divided doses may be required. Maintenance doses of 320 to 400 mg daily in divided doses may be adequate. Elderly patients should be given reduced doses.
Dibenzepin has also been given by intravenous infusion.

Action. The pharmacology of dibenzepin.— M. Rehavi *et al., Psychopharmacology,* 1977, *54,* 35.

Depression. In the treatment of patients with moderate to severe depression, there was no significant difference in effectiveness and the rate of onset of effect between dibenzepin, 160 mg thrice daily, and imipramine, 50 mg thrice daily. Similar side-effects occurred to the same degree after both treatments; mainly a marked decrease in restlessness and an increase in dryness of the mouth.— J. M. Fielding, *Med. J. Aust.,* 1969, *1,* 614. See also H. Heimann *et al., Arzneimittel-Forsch.,* 1964, *14,* 553 (high-dose therapy); J. Collard *et al., Arzneimittel-Forsch.,* 1973, *23,* 537 (prolonged action preparation).

Beneficial results using high-dose intravenous infusion of dibenzepin to obtain rapid alleviation of depression.— M. Assael and N. Kauly, *Pharmatherapeutica,* 1979, *2,* 239.

For a general review of the role of tricyclic antidepressants in depression, see Amitriptyline Hydrochloride, p.114.

Proprietary Names

Ecatril *(Sandoz, Fr.)*; Deprex *(Novo, Belg.; Novo, Denm.; Novo, Norw.)* (see also under Amitriptyline Hydrochloride); Noveril *(Sandoz, Austral.; Wander, Belg.; Sandoz, Fr.; Wander, Ger.; Sandoz, Ital.; Wander, S.Afr.; Sandoz, Spain; Wander, Switz.).*

Dibenzepin hydrochloride was formerly marketed in Great Britain under the proprietary name Noveril (*Wander*).

2511-q

Dimetacrine Tartrate. SD 709; Dimetacrine Hydrogen Tartrate; Dimetacrine Bitartrate; Dimethacrine Tartrate. 3-(9,9-Dimethylacridan-10-yl)-*NN*-dimethylpropylamine hydrogen tartrate.
$C_{20}H_{26}N_2,C_4H_6O_6$=444.5.

CAS — 4757-55-5(dimetacrine); 3759-07-7(tartrate).

A white crystalline powder. M.p. 154° to 158°. **Soluble** in water; slightly soluble in alcohol; practically insoluble in ether and chloroform. A 2% solution in water has a pH of 3 to 3.5.

Adverse Effects, Treatment, and Precautions. As for Amitriptyline Hydrochloride, p.110.

Uses. Dimetacrine is a tricyclic antidepressant with general properties similar to those of amitriptyline (p.113). It has been given as the tartrate in usual doses of 75 to 300 mg daily.

References to dimetacrine in depression: U. Jahn and G. Häusler, *Wien. klin. Wschr.,* 1966, *78,* 21; S. Taen and W. Poldinger, *Schweiz. med. Wschr.,* 1966, *96,* 1616; F. S. Abuzzahab, *Int. J. clin. Pharmac.,* 1973, *8,* 244.

Proprietary Names

Istonil *(Siegfried, Belg.; Siegfried, Ger.)*; Linostil *(ACF, Neth.).*

2512-p

Dothiepin Hydrochloride *(B.P.).*

Dosulepin Hydrochloride; Dosulepinium Chloratum. 3-(Dibenzo[*b,e*]thiepin-11(6*H*)-ylidene)-*NN*-dimethylpropylamine hydrochloride.
$C_{19}H_{21}NS,HCl$=331.9.

CAS — 113-53-1 (dothiepin); 897-15-4 (hydrochloride).

Pharmacopoeias. In *Br.* and *Cz.*

A white to faintly yellow almost odourless crystalline powder. It consists chiefly of the *trans*-isomer. M.p. about 224° with decomposition. **Soluble** 1 in 2 of water, 1 in 8 of alcohol, and 1 in 2 of chloroform; practically insoluble in ether. **Protect** from light.

Adverse Effects and Treatment. As for Amitriptyline Hydrochloride, p.110.

A placebo-controlled study in healthy subjects suggesting that dothiepin reduces salivary-rate less than imipramine.— U. K. Sheth *et al., Br. J. clin. Pharmac.,* 1979, *8,* 475.

Extrapyramidal effects. A 54-year-old man developed slurred speech, shaking of the hands, and incoordination after taking dothiepin 25 mg; the syndrome recurred after each of several subsequent doses.— D. D. Brown, *J. R. Coll. gen. Pract.,* 1972, *22,* 65. A 42-year-old woman developed dysarthria on the third day of treatment with dothiepin 25 mg thrice daily; the condition regressed when the drug was withdrawn.— S. E. Quader, *Br. med. J.,* 1977, *2,* 97.

Precautions. As for Amitriptyline Hydrochloride, p.112.

For a general comment on antidepressant therapy and driving, see Amitriptyline Hydrochloride, p.112.

Pregnancy and the neonate. A dothiepin concentration of 11 ng per ml was found in the milk of a woman taking dothiepin hydrochloride 25 mg thrice daily and whose serum concentration of dothiepin measured at the same time was 33 ng per ml.— J. A. Rees *et al., Practitioner,* 1976, *217,* 686.

Absorption and Fate. Dothiepin is readily absorbed from the gastro-intestinal tract, and extensively demethylated by first-pass metabolism in the liver to its primary active metabolite, desmethyldothiepin (also termed northiaden). Since dothiepin slows gastro-intestinal transit time absorption can, however, be delayed, particularly in overdosage.

Paths of metabolism also include *S*-oxidation. Dothiepin is excreted in the urine, mainly in the form of its metabolites; appreciable amounts are also excreted in the faeces. A half-life of about 50 hours has been reported for dothiepin and its metabolites.

Dothiepin is excreted in breast milk (see under Precautions).

Metabolism of dothiepin in *animals* and man, including tentative identification of hydroxylated dothiepin in *rat* urine.— E. L. Crampton *et al., Br. J. Pharmac.,* 1978, *64,* 405P.

Plasma concentrations. Studies of steady-state serum concentrations in 5 healthy subjects following administration of dothiepin 25 mg thrice daily or 75 mg at night.— B. R. S. Nakra *et al., J. int. med. Res.,* 1977, *5,* 391. See also J. Mendlewicz *et al., Br. J. Psychiat.,* 1980, *136,* 154 (serum concentrations and clinical response).

Uses. Dothiepin hydrochloride is a tricyclic antidepressant with actions and uses similar to those of amitriptyline (p.113). Like amitriptyline, it also has sedative properties.

In the treatment of depression, dothiepin hydrochloride is given by mouth in doses of 25 mg thrice daily initially, gradually increased to 50 mg thrice daily if necessary; higher doses of up to 225 mg daily have been given in severely depressed hospital patients. Since dothiepin has a prolonged half-life, once-daily dosage regimens are also suitable, usually given at night.

Depression. For a general review of the role of tricyclic antidepressants in depression, see Amitriptyline Hydrochloride, p.114.

Preparations

Dothiepin Capsules *(B.P.).* Capsules containing dothiepin hydrochloride. Store at a temperature not exceeding 30°.

Prothiaden *(Boots, UK).* Dothiepin hydrochloride, available as **Capsules** of 25 mg and as **Tablets** of 75 mg. (Also available as Prothiaden in *Austral., Cz., Fr., S.Afr.*).

2513-s

Doxepin Hydrochloride *(B.P., U.S.P.).*

P 3693A. A mixture of the *cis* and *trans* isomers of 3-(dibenz[*b,e*]oxepin-11(6*H*)-ylidene)-*NN*-dimethylpropylamine hydrochloride.
$C_{19}H_{21}NO,HCl$=315.8.

CAS — 1668-19-5(doxepin); 1229-29-4(hydrochloride).

Pharmacopoeias. In *Br., Nord.,* and *U.S.*

A white crystalline powder with a slight amine-like odour. M.p. 185° to 191°. Doxepin hydrochloride 113 mg is approximately equivalent to 100 mg of doxepin. **Soluble** 1 in 1.5 of water, 1 in 1 of alcohol, and 1 in 2 of chloroform; very slightly soluble in ether. An aqueous solution has a slightly acid reaction. **Protect** from light.

Adverse Effects. As for Amitriptyline Hydrochloride, p.110.

Effects on the blood. A 73-year-old woman developed thrombocytopenia when treated for a depressive reaction with doxepin hydrochloride. Thrombocytopenia recurred when the patient was exposed to amitriptyline, a structurally related compound.— D. D. Nixon (letter), *J. Am. med. Ass.,* 1972, *220,* 418.

Effects on the heart. Comparison of the cardiovascular toxicities of imipramine, amitriptyline, and doxepin.— T. C. Brown and A. Leversha, *Clin. Toxicol.,* 1979, *14,* 253.

Overdosage. A 4-year-old child collapsed for no apparent reason after a morning of normal activity and was taken comatose to her local physician. A grand mal seizure ensued which progressed to status epilepticus during her transfer to hospital. Although the parents had not suspected an overdose, doxepin poisoning was established by recovery of a portion of a capsule from the patient's oesophagus. The child recovered with treatment and did not develop cardiac arrhythmias at any time.— D. C. Walter *et al.* (letter), *Am. J. Dis. Child.,* 1980, *134,* 202.

Weight gain. Patients taking doxepin appeared to gain weight despite poor appetite.— A. A. Khan (letter), *Br. med. J.,* 1974, *3,* 350. Weight gain occurred in 7 of 23 patients given doxepin for tension headache.— T. J. Mørland *et al., Headache,* 1979, *19,* 382.

Treatment of Adverse Effects. As for Amitriptyline Hydrochloride, p.111.

Dialysis and haemoperfusion. For reference to the use of charcoal haemoperfusion in doxepin overdosage, see Amitriptyline Hydrochloride p.112.

Precautions. As for Amitriptyline Hydrochloride, p.112.

Results of a study in depressed subjects indicated that doxepin may have some harmful effects on psychomotor skills related to driving. The effects of doxepin were most conspicuous in the acute phase of treatment up to the seventh day, but gradually waned after that.— T. Seppälä *et al., Ann. clin. Res.,* 1978, *10,* 214. See also under Interactions (below).

The effect of chlordiazepoxide and doxepin on cognitive performance was studied in 72 hospitalised psychoneurotic patients. Performance in control subjects and in doxepin treated subjects was enhanced by high motivation. This effect was reversed in the chlordiazepoxide group.— V. Pishkin *et al., Curr. ther. Res.,* 1979, *25,* 165.

For a general comment on antidepressant therapy and driving, see Amitriptyline Hydrochloride, p.112.

Interactions. A study of the impairment of skills related to driving in healthy subjects receiving *alcohol* during amitriptyline, doxepin, nortriptyline, clomipramine, or placebo administration. It seemed that concurrent ingestion of doxepin or amitriptyline might be especially dangerous to driving.— T. Seppälä *et al., Clin. Pharmac. Ther.,* 1975, *17,* 515. Further references: G. Milner and A. A. Landauer, *Med. J. Aust.,* 1973, *1,* 837.

Withdrawal. A 42-year-old man was admitted to hospital with depression and given doxepin 75 mg daily gradually increased to 150 mg daily for 2 weeks. His depression did not respond and he complained of the sedative effects, therefore doxepin was abruptly withdrawn. Two days later he began to wander aimlessly about the ward, at times undressed, and became confused and disorientated as to time. The EEG was consistent with the diagnosis of delirium. His mental state cleared within 7 days. The patient was also taking disulfiram which may have played a role in the reaction.— A. B. Santos and L. McCurdy, *Am. J. Psychiat.,* 1980, *137,* 239.

Absorption and Fate. Doxepin is readily absorbed from the gastro-intestinal tract, and extensively demethylated by first-pass metabolism in the liver, to its primary active metabolite, desmethyldoxepin. Since doxepin slows gastro-intestinal transit time absorption can, however, be delayed, particularly in overdosage.

Paths of metabolism of both doxepin and desmethyldoxepin include hydroxylation, *N*-oxidation, and conjugation with glucuronic acid. Doxepin is excreted in the urine, mainly in the form of its metabolites, either free or in conjugated form.

Doxepin and desmethyldoxepin are widely distributed throughout the body and are extensively bound to plasma and tissue protein. Doxepin has been estimated to have a plasma half-life ranging from 8 to 24 hours, which may be considerably extended in overdosage; that of desmethyldoxepin is longer.

Doxepin crosses the blood-brain barrier and the placental barrier.

Details of the metabolism of doxepin.— Y. Kimura *et al.*, *Pharmacometrics*, 1972, *6*, 955. See also L. J. Dusci and L. P. Hackett, *J. Chromat.*, 1971, *61*, 231.

A study of the pharmacokinetics of doxepin in 7 healthy subjects, following oral administration of 75 mg. Peak plasma concentrations of doxepin were reached within 4 hours of administration, and the distribution followed first-order kinetics and was biphasic with a distribution and an elimination phase. Doxepin was extensively metabolised to desmethyldoxepin during the first pass through the liver. The elimination half-life of doxepin ranged from 8.2 to 24.5 hours and that of desmethyldoxepin from 33.2 to 80.7 hours.— V. E. Ziegler *et al.*, *Clin. Pharmac. Ther.*, 1978, *23*, 573.

Plasma concentrations. In 5 patients with depression receiving doxepin 75 to 300 mg daily plasma concentrations of 17 to 122 ng per ml of doxepin and 24 to 118 ng per ml of desmethyldoxepin were detected 8 to 10 hours after the last dose.— R. G. Jenkins and R. O. Friedel, *J. pharm. Sci.*, 1978, *67*, 17. In 4 patients with depression given doxepin 100 mg daily for at least 2 weeks mean serial steady-state plasma-doxepin concentrations were 13.7, 9.2, 15.3, and 145.8 ng per ml respectively with corresponding desmethyldoxepin concentrations of 15.7, 21.2, 23.1, and 93.7 ng per ml.— V. E. Ziegler *et al.*, *ibid.*, 554. Plasma concentrations of *cis*-doxepin, *trans*-doxepin, *cis*-desmethyldoxepin, and *trans*-desmethyldoxepin were about 2.5, 15, 10, and 5 ng per ml respectively in a patient given doxepin 75 mg daily for 2 weeks and about 5, 58, 44, and 46 ng per ml respectively in another patient receiving doxepin 200 mg daily. A considerable fraction appeared as *cis*-desmethyldoxepin as the administered doxepin contained only approximately 15% of the *cis*-isomer.— M. T. Rosseel *et al.*, *ibid.*, 802.

Further reports, studies, and comments on the relevance of plasma concentrations of doxepin and desmethyldoxepin, and on factors, such as age, sex, and race, which might influence this: J. T. Biggs *et al.*, *J. clin. Psychiat.*, 1978, *39*, 740 (correlation with regimens).

Uses. Doxepin is a tricyclic antidepressant with actions and uses similar to those of amitriptyline (p.113). Like amitriptyline it has marked sedative properties.

In the treatment of depression doxepin is given by mouth as the hydrochloride in doses equivalent to doxepin 25 mg thrice daily initially, gradually increased to 50 mg thrice daily as necessary. Higher doses of up to 300 mg daily may be required, particularly in severely depressed hospital patients; mildly affected patients may respond to as little as 10 mg thrice daily. Since doxepin has a prolonged half-life, once-daily dosage regimens are also suitable, usually given at night.

Reviews and symposia on doxepin: R. M. Pinder *et al.*, *Drugs*, 1977, *13*, 161; *Curr. med. Res. Opinion*, 1980, *6*, *Suppl.* 9, 1–59.

Administration in the elderly. In elderly patients doxepin treatment should begin with a low dose of 25 to 50 mg daily, but some depressed elderly subjects need and can tolerate 150 or even 300 mg daily if the dose is gradually increased.— R. M. Pinder *et al.*, *Drugs*, 1977, *13*, 161.

Anxiety. A discussion on whether antidepressants have a role in the treatment of anxiety.— *Lancet*, 1980, *2*, 897. See also E. C. Johnstone *et al.*, *Psychol. Med.*, 1980, *10*, 321.

Depression. For a general review of the role of tricyclic antidepressants in depression, see Amitriptyline Hydrochloride, p.114.

Drug and alcohol abuse. A report on 2 separate methadone detoxification regimens used in a thousand diamorphine addicts. Adjunct use of doxepin appeared to provide the patients with some degree of emotional stability which increased their ability to resist the psychic craving for diamorphine.— R. G. Dufficy, *Milit. Med.*, 1973, *138*, 748.

Headache. After 4 weeks of treatment with placebo, doxepin hydrochloride 10 mg, diazepam 2 mg, or amitriptyline 10 mg, given to 80 patients three or four times daily, the majority of patients with psychogenic headache with anxiety and depression were helped by the active treatment, with doxepin and amitriptyline being the most effective. At 8 weeks only doxepin continued to give significant improvement.— A. Okasha *et al.*, *Br. J. Psychiat.*, 1973, *122*, 181. See also T. J. Mørland *et al.*, *Headache*, 1979, *19*, 382.

Preparations

Doxepin Capsules *(B.P.)*. Capsules containing doxepin hydrochloride. Potency is expressed in terms of the equivalent amount of doxepin. Store at a temperature not exceeding 30°.

Doxepin Hydrochloride Capsules *(U.S.P.)*. Capsules containing doxepin hydrochloride. Potency is expressed in terms of the equivalent amount of doxepin. The *U.S.P.* requires 80% dissolution in 30 minutes.

Doxepin Hydrochloride Oral Solution *(U.S.P.)*. A solution containing doxepin hydrochloride. Potency is expressed in terms of the equivalent amount of doxepin. pH 4 to 7. Store in airtight containers. Protect from light. To be diluted with water or other suitable fluid immediately before ingestion.

Proprietary Preparations

Sinequan *(Pfizer, UK)*. Doxepin hydrochloride, available as capsules each containing the equivalent of 10, 25, 50, or 75 mg of doxepin. (Also available as Sinequan in *Austral.*, *Belg.*, *Canad.*, *Fr.*, *Ital.*, *Neth.*, *Norw.*, *S.Afr.*, *Spain*, *USA*).

Other Proprietary Names

Adapin *(USA)*; Aponal *(Ger.)*; Novoxapin *(Spain)*; Quitaxon *(Austral.*, *Belg.*, *Denm.*, *Fr.*, *Neth.*, *S.Afr.)*; Sinquan *(Denm.*, *Ger.*, *Switz.)*; Spectra *(Ind.)*; Toruan *(Spain)*.

2514-w

Imipramine.

3-(10,11-Dihydro-5*H*-dibenz[*b*,*f*]-azepin-5-yl)-*NN*-dimethylpropylamine.

$C_{19}H_{24}N_2$=280.4.

CAS — 50-49-7.

Imipramine 0.88 g is approximately equivalent to 1 g of imipramine hydrochloride.

2515-e

Imipramine Embonate.

Imipramine Pamoate.

$(C_{19}H_{24}N_2)_2,C_{23}H_{16}O_6$=949.2.

CAS — 10075-24-8.

A yellow odourless tasteless powder. Imipramine embonate 1.5 g is approximately equivalent to 1 g of imipramine hydrochloride. Practically **insoluble** in water; soluble in alcohol, chloroform, ether, and acetone.

2516-l

Imipramine Hydrochloride *(B.P., Eur. P., U.S.P.)*.

Imipram. Hydrochlor.; Imipramini Chloridum; Imipramini Hydrochloridum; Imizine.

$C_{19}H_{24}N_2,HCl$=316.9.

CAS — 113-52-0.

Pharmacopoeias. In *Belg.*, *Br.*, *Braz.*, *Cz.*, *Eur.*, *Fr.*, *Ger.*, *It.*, *Jap.*, *Neth.*, *Nord.*, *Roum.*, *Rus.*, *Swiss*, and *U.S.*

A white or slightly yellow, odourless or almost odourless, crystalline powder with a burning taste, followed by a sensation of numbness. M.p. 170° to 174°. **Soluble** 1 in 2 of water, 1 in 1.5 of alcohol, 1 in 1.5 of chloroform, and 1 in 15 of acetone; practically insoluble in ether. A 10% solution in water has a pH of 4.2 to 5.2. Solutions for injection are **sterilised** by autoclaving or by filtration. Aqueous solutions are stable when protected from oxygen and light. The powder absorbs insignificant amounts of moisture at 23° at relative humidities up to 60%; under damper conditions it absorbs significant amounts. **Store** in airtight containers. Protect from light.

Adverse Effects. As for Amitriptyline Hydrochloride, p.110.

Abuse. A report of a 7-year-old child who was repeatedly given toxic doses of imipramine by his mother.— J. B. G. Watson *et al.*, *Archs Dis. Childh.*, 1979, *54*, 143.

Cytogenetic effects. Addition of imipramine to leucocyte cultures obtained from healthy subjects. Imipramine concentrations corresponding to therapeutic plasma concentrations had no effect on mitotic index regardless of the length of exposure.— T. K. Fu *et al.*, *Archs gen. Psychiat.*, 1977, *34*, 728.

Effects on the blood. Agranulocytosis in a 39-year-old woman after taking imipramine for a few weeks; she had previously been receiving amitriptyline. Review of the literature suggests that agranulocytosis associated with tricyclic use is a rare, idiosyncratic condition resulting from a direct toxic effect rather than an allergic mechanism and particularly affecting the elderly from 4 to 8 weeks after starting treatment.— R. S. Albertini and T. M. Penders, *J. clin. Psychiat.*, 1978, *39*, 483.

Effects on the ears. Tinnitus in 4 patients given imipramine. Reduction in dosage was usually sufficient to control the tinnitus.— J. Racy and E. A. Ward-Racy, *Am. J. Psychiat.*, 1980, *137*, 854.

Effects on the heart. A study of the electrocardiographic effects of therapeutic doses of imipramine in 44 depressed patients. Imipramine prolonged the P-R, Q-R-S, and Q-Tc intervals, increased the heart-rate, and lowered T-wave amplitude during the 4 weeks of treatment. No patients developed high-grade atrioventricular block or severe intraventricular conduction abnormalities, and imipramine had a potent anti-arrhythmic action in patients recovering from depression.— E. -G. V. Giardina *et al.*, *Circulation*, 1979, *60*, 1045.

Effects on the liver. A woman taking imipramine in association with many other psychotropic drugs had abnormalities of liver function. On withdrawal of all drug therapy her liver function returned towards normal, but 48 hours after receiving a 50-mg dose of imipramine hydrochloride by mouth there was a sharp rise in hepatic enzymes.— G. A. Weaver *et al.*, *Am. J. dig. Dis.*, 1977, *22*, 551.

Effects on the skin. A brief review of cutaneous side-effects of imipramine.— J. Almeyda, *Br. J. Derm.*, 1971, *84*, 298.

Epileptogenic effect. Seizures in a psychotic preschool child given imipramine. The child was thought to be seizure prone.— T. A. Petti and M. Campbell, *Am. J. Psychiat.*, 1975, *132*, 538.

For the use of imipramine with increased anticonvulsant therapy in the management of resistant petit mal, see under Uses, Epilepsy.

Hypertension. A report of reversible mild hypertension in a woman taking imipramine 100 to 150 mg daily.— I. Hessov (letter), *Lancet*, 1970, *1*, 84.

Further references: C. R. Lake *et al.*, *Clin. Pharmac. Ther.*, 1979, *26*, 647 (hypertensive effect in children).

Hypotension. A retrospective study of 148 patients who had been treated with imipramine hydrochloride indicated that 29 (just under 20%) had side-effects usually associated with orthostatic hypotension, serious enough to require different treatment. In a prospective study of 44 patients, the best predictor of orthostatic hypotension during treatment was the degree of orthostatic hypotension before treatment. No correlation was found with age, pre-existing heart disease, or the plasma concentrations of imipramine and desmethylimipramine. Nevertheless, it was considered that the potential seriousness of these effects would increase with increasing age and pre-existing heart disease. It is considered that the commonest and most serious cardiovascular effect of imipramine is orthostatic hypotension.— A. H. Glassman *et al.*, *Lancet*, 1979, *1*, 468. See also J. R. Hayes *et al.*, *Mayo Clin. Proc.*, 1977, *52*, 509.

Overdosage. Death of a 4-year-old child after the ingestion of imipramine 450 mg, as syrup, prescribed for enuresis.— A. J. Cronin *et al.*, *Br. med. J.*, 1979, *1*, 722. Young children should not be given antidepressant treatment for enuresis. If such treatment is prescribed the child should be old enough to take tablets.— *ibid.*, 705.

Treatment of Adverse Effects. As for Amitriptyline Hydrochloride, p.111.

Cardiac arrhythmias in a child who had taken an overdose of imipramine were controlled with hypertonic sodium chloride and lignocaine infusions.— P. Dolara and F. Franconi, *Clin. Toxicol.*, 1977, *10*, 395.

Dialysis and haemoperfusion. A 2-year-old child who had taken imipramine 23 mg per kg body-weight and a 4-year-old child who had taken 20 mg per kg were deeply comatose, with convulsions and ECG abnormalities, but regained consciousness within 4 to 5 hours after haemodialysis.— H. W. Asbach and H. W. Schuler (letter), *Br. med. J.*, 1974, *2*, 386. Criticism.— H. Matthew (letter), *ibid.*, 726. Further comment claiming the usefulness of haemodialysis in imipramine poisoning.— H. W. Asbach and H. W. Schuler (letter), *ibid.*, 1974, *3*, 524.

Data supporting the use of charcoal haemoperfusion in imipramine poisoning.— H. W. Asbach *et al.*, *Clin. Toxicol.*, 1977, *11*, 211.

Precautions. As for Amitriptyline Hydrochloride, p.112.

For a general comment on antidepressant therapy and driving, see Amitriptyline Hydrochloride, p.112.

Gilles de la Tourette's syndrome. For exacerbation of Gilles de la Tourette's disease by imipramine, see Methylphenidate Hydrochloride, p.366.

Interactions. The amount of imipramine not bound to plasma proteins was 4.2%. This value was increased to 10.3% in the presence of *phenytoin*.— O. Borgå *et al.*, *Biochem. Pharmac.*, 1969, *18*, 2135. For a comment on the significance of tricyclic antidepressants and protein binding, see under Absorption and Fate (Protein Binding), p.120. For the effect of imipramine on phenytoin, see Phenytoin, p.1239.

The urinary excretion of radioactive imipramine was decreased by 25 to 50% when *perphenazine* 20 to 48 mg per day, *haloperidol* 12 to 20 mg per day, or *chlorpromazine* 300 mg per day, was given concomitantly. *Flupenthixol* or *biperiden* had no similar effect. Clinical signs of the interactions had not been reported.— L. F. Gram and K. F. Overø, *Br. med. J.*, 1972, *1*, 463.

Ethinyloestradiol given in doses of 50 µg together with imipramine 150 mg to 5 depressed patients, induced severe lethargy in all 5, hypotension in 4, coarse tremor in 2, and mild depersonalisation in 2. However, in a further trial in 30 women using doses of 25 µg and 50 µg of ethinyloestradiol with imipramine, patients on the lower dose of oestrogen and imipramine showed greater improvement than those taking the higher dose of oestrogen and imipramine or than those taking imipramine alone.— *J. Am. med. Ass.*, 1972, *219*, 143. See also R. C. Khurana (letter), *ibid.*, *222*, 702; S. M. Somani and R. C. Khurana (letter), *ibid.*, 1973, *223*, 560. Of 5 men with depression given imipramine and *methyltestosterone* 15 mg daily, 4 showed a paranoid response which regressed when methyltestosterone was withdrawn.— I. C. Wilson *et al.*, *Am. J. Psychiat.*, 1974, *131*, 21.

The antidepressant effect of imipramine was reversed by *fenclonine*.— B. Shopsin *et al.*, *Archs gen. Psychiat.*, 1976, *33*, 811.

In a study in 4 subjects who received imipramine 25 mg three times daily for 3 weeks and *amylobarbitone* 200 mg nightly for the last 10 days of this period, plasma steady-state concentrations of imipramine fell from 31.5 to 6.3 ng per ml, while those of desmethylimipramine rose from 19.2 to 23.0 ng per ml. It was considered that the antidepressant effect of imipramine might be reduced in patients taking barbiturate hypnotics.— D. S. Hewich *et al.*, *Br. J. clin. Pharmac.*, 1977, *4*, 399P.

For the effect of imipramine on *phenylephrine*, see Phenylephrine Hydrochloride, p.24. For the effect of imipramine on *thyroxine*, see Thyroxine Sodium, p.1502.

Phaeochromocytoma. A 36-year-old pregnant woman with an undetected phaeochromocytoma was given imipramine 25 mg every 8 hours for depression. About 6 hours after the fourth dose she experienced 3 grand mal seizures.— J. S. Kaufmann (letter), *J. Am. med. Ass.*, 1974, *229*, 1282.

In an 11-year-old girl imipramine 50 mg caused hypertension, tachycardia, and profuse sweating; the same dose 2 months earlier had had similar effects. She was later shown to have a phaeochromocytoma.— J. Mok and I. Swann, *Archs Dis. Childh.*, 1978, *53*, 676.

Pregnancy and the neonate. In a study in 836 infants with congenital malformations there was no significant difference in the maternal usage of tricyclic antidepressants during the first trimester of pregnancy compared with the use in 836 controls.— G. Greenberg *et al.*, *Br. med. J.*, 1977, *2*, 853. See also M. Sim (letter), *Br. med. J.*, 1972, *2*, 45; G. S. Rachelefsky *et al.* (letter), *Lancet*, 1972, *1*, 838; P. Banister *et al.* (letter), *ibid;* E. V. Kuensberg and J. D. E. Knox (letter), *Br. med. J.*, 1972, *2*, 292; J. Idänpään-Heikkilä and L. Saxén, *Lancet*, 1973, *2*, 282.

Individual reports and comments on congenital malformations in the infants of mothers given imipramine during pregnancy: A. J. Barson (letter), *Br. med. J.*, 1972, *2*, 45; W. G. McBride (letter), *Med. J. Aust.*, 1972, *1*, 492; A. W. Morrow (letter), *ibid.*, 658.

For withdrawal symptoms in the infants of mothers given imipramine, see under Withdrawal (below).

Lactation. Concentrations of imipramine and desipramine in the milk of a lactating woman taking imipramine 200 mg at night were similar to those in her plasma.— R. Sovner and P. J. Orsulak, *Am. J. Psychiat.*, 1979, *136*, 451.

Withdrawal. Three patients taking imipramine 300 to 450 mg daily in divided doses developed an akathisia-like syndrome with acute anxiety and motor restlessness when their medication was abruptly withdrawn.— G. L. Sathananthan and S. Gershon, *Am. J. Psychiat.*, 1973, *130*, 1286.

Withdrawal symptoms of nausea and dizziness after single missed doses of imipramine.— S. L. Stern and J. Mendels, *J. clin. Psychiat.*, 1980, *41*, 66.

Neonatal withdrawal. Withdrawal symptoms were observed in 3 neonates whose mothers had taken imipramine during pregnancy.— E. Eggermont (letter), *Lancet*, 1973, *2*, 680. See also *idem* (letter), *Archs Dis. Childh.*, 1980, *55*, 81.

Absorption and Fate. Imipramine is readily absorbed from the gastro-intestinal tract, and extensively demethylated by first-pass metabolism in the liver, to its primary active metabolite, desipramine. Since imipramine slows gastro-intestinal transit time absorption can, however, be delayed, particularly in overdosage.

Paths of metabolism of both imipramine and desipramine include hydroxylation, *N*-oxidation, and conjugation with glucuronic acid. Imipramine is excreted in the urine, mainly in the form of its metabolites, either free or in conjugated form.

Imipramine and desipramine are widely distributed throughout the body and are extensively bound to plasma and tissue protein. Imipramine has been estimated to have a half-life ranging from 8 to 19 hours, which may be considerably extended in overdosage. Plasma concentrations of imipramine and desipramine vary very widely between individuals but some correlation with therapeutic response has been established.

Imipramine and desipramine cross the blood-brain barrier and placental barrier and are excreted in breast milk (see under Precautions).

There was decreased absorption of imipramine from the gastro-intestinal tract when gastric juice pH was between 3.5 and 6.— R. Fischbach, *Arzneimittel-Forsch.*, 1975, *25*, 123. Following administration of imipramine to 3 patients who had undergone catheterisation of the portal vein absorption appeared to be complete within 80 minutes of ingestion. Demethylation of imipramine did not seem to occur in the intestinal wall but there was evidence of an enterohepatic circulation of imipramine and desipramine.— H. Dencker *et al.*, *Clin. Pharmac. Ther.*, 1976, *19*, 584.

A study in 4 subjects indicating that imipramine is fully absorbed from the gastro-intestinal tract, but that there is striking intersubject variation in first-pass metabolism to desipramine. Half-lives were estimated to range from 8 to 16 hours, but these estimates were considered to be relatively inaccurate due to the short half-lives and few measurements; the plasma curve after intravenous administration appeared to be biphasic with an initial α-phase lasting for 3 to 8 hours. There was no clear correlation between first-pass metabolism, plasma half-life, and apparent clearance. Imipramine, desipramine, imipramine-*N*-oxide, 2-hydroxyimipramine, 2-hydroxydesipramine, imipramine-2-*O*-glucuronide, desipramine-2-*O*-glucuronide, and some unknown metabolites were identified in the urine of 3 of the subjects.— L. F. Gram and J. Christiansen, *Clin. Pharmac. Ther.*, 1975, *17*, 555. See also L. F. Gram *et al.*, *ibid.*, 1971, *12*, 239 (excretion in acid urine); G. L. Sathananthan and S. Gershon, *ibid.*, 1974, *15*, 218 (CSF concentrations).

Investigation of the half-life of imipramine and desipramine in 23 patients who had been taking imipramine, usually in a dose of 50 mg thrice daily for a minimum of 21 days, and with special reference to the effect of age. Patients over 65 years of age had longer imipramine and desipramine plasma half-lives (24 hours versus 19 hours for imipramine and 76 hours versus 34 hours for desipramine).— D. S. Robinson and A. Nies, *Clin. Pharmac. Ther.*, 1977, *21*, 116.

Plasma concentrations. A warning that spuriously low plasma concentrations of imipramine, amitriptyline, and doxepin and their metabolites desipramine, nortriptyline, and desmethyldoxepin have resulted from the collection of blood samples in Vacutainer tubes.— R. C. Veith and C. Perera (letter), *New Engl. J. Med.*, 1979, *300*, 504.

Studies and comments on assay techniques for estimation of tricyclic antidepressants: H. B. Hucker and S. C. Stauffer, *J. pharm. Sci.*, 1974, *63*, 296; S. Dawling and R. A. Braithwaite, *J. Chromat.*, 1978, *146*, 449; R. G. Jenkins and R. O. Friedel, *J. pharm. Sci.*, 1978, *67*, 17; V. E. Ziegler *et al.*, *ibid.*, 554; S. Jones and P. Turner (letter), *Br. med. J.*, 1979, *1*, 1217.

Reviews of the therapeutic relevance of plasma concentrations of tricyclic antidepressants: *Br. med. J.*, 1978, *2*, 783; S. C. Risch *et al.*, *J. clin. Psychiat.*, 1979, *40*, 4 and 58; J. Amsterdam *et al.*, *Am. J. Psychiat.*, 1980, *137*, 653; G. Tognoni *et al.*, *Clin. Pharmacokinet.*, 1980, *5*, 105.

Eleven of 12 patients who responded satisfactorily to antidepressant therapy with imipramine had plasma-imipramine concentrations of 45 ng per ml or more and plasma-desipramine concentrations of more than 75 ng per ml, whereas 12 patients who did not respond satisfactorily had concentrations of one or both below these levels. Both imipramine and its metabolite desipramine appeared to be required for the antidepressant action of imipramine.— L. F. Gram *et al.*, *Clin. Pharmac. Ther.*, 1976, *19*, 318. See also *idem*, *Psychopharmacology*, 1977, *54*, 255; N. Reisby *et al.*, *ibid.*, 263.

In 60 patients with depression given imipramine hydrochloride 3.5 mg per kg body-weight daily for 4 weeks plasma concentrations of imipramine and the metabolite desipramine ranged from 50 to 1050 ng per ml. Except for those with delusional unipolar depression clinical response correlated with plasma concentration. Response-rates of 29, 64, and 93% respectively occurred with concentrations below 150 ng per ml, 150 to 225 ng per ml, and above 225 ng per ml.— A. H. Glassman *et al.*, *Archs gen. Psychiat.*, 1977, *34*, 197.

Further reports, studies, and comments on the relevance of plasma concentrations of imipramine and desipramine, and on factors, such as age, sex, and race, which might influence this: G. L. Sathananthan *et al.*, *Archs gen. Psychiat.*, 1976, *33*, 1109 (CSF concentrations); J. F. Giudicelli and J. P. Tillement, *Clin. Pharmacokinet.*, 1977, *2*, 157 (sex; review); A. Nies *et al.*, *Am. J. Psychiat.*, 1977, *134*, 790 (age); W. J. Jusko, *J. Pharmacokinet. Biopharm.*, 1978, *6*, 7 (smoking).

Protein binding. Comment on the serious technical problems in the determination of plasma protein binding of antidepressant drugs, the difficulty in generalising from one drug to another, and the need to put into perspective the significance of individual differences. Such differences may represent an additional source of variability, but are relatively less important than the 20- to 30-fold interindividual differences in total plasma concentrations that are commonly observed with antidepressants.— R. A. Braithwaite, *Postgrad. med. J.*, 1980, *56*, *Suppl.* 1, 107.

Individual studies on the binding of imipramine to plasma and tissue proteins: K. M. Piafsky and O. Borgå, *Clin. Pharmac. Ther.*, 1977, *22*, 545 (correlation with plasma α_1-acid glycoprotein concentration); A. Danon and Z. Chen, *Clin. Pharmac. Ther.*, 1979, *25*, 316 (influence of hyperlipoproteinaemia).

Uses. Imipramine is a tricyclic antidepressant with actions and uses similar to those of amitriptyline (p.113). It has less marked sedative properties.

In the treatment of depression, imipramine is given by mouth as the hydrochloride in doses of 25 mg thrice daily initially, gradually increased to 50 mg three or four times daily as necessary; higher doses of up to 300 mg daily may be required in severely depressed hospital patients. A suggested initial dose for adolescents and the elderly is 10 mg thrice daily. Since imipramine has a prolonged half-life, once-daily dosage regimens are also suitable, usually given at night. In the initial stages of treatment, if administration by mouth is impracticable or inadvisable, up to 100 to 150 mg of the hydrochloride may be given daily in divided doses by intramuscular injection, but oral administration should be substituted as soon as possible. In addition to the hydrochloride, imipramine is available as the embonate for oral administration, as capsules in strengths suitable for adults only.

Imipramine is also given for the treatment of nocturnal enuresis in children. Suggested doses are 25 mg at bedtime for children aged 6 to 12 years and 50 mg at bedtime for children aged over 12 years. The use of tricyclic antidepressants for nocturnal enuresis in children is controversial, not least in view of the hazards of accidental overdosage. In particular, tricyclic antidepressant therapy is not suitable for younger children; for further comment, see under Amitriptyline Hydrochloride (Enuresis), p.114.

Administration. Although it is always best to use the smallest effective dose of tricyclic antidepressant, it is poor practice to settle for an inadequate result without having tried the whole dosage range.— L. E. Hollister, *Drugs*, 1977, *14*, 161. See also G. M. Simpson *et al.*, *Archs gen. Psychiat.*, 1976, *33*, 1093 (imipramine 300 mg daily).

A possible means of predicting imipramine and desipramine dosage requirements following administration of a single dose.— D. J. Brunswick *et al.*, *Clin. Pharmac. Ther.*, 1979, *25*, 605. See also R. A. Braithwaite *et al.*, *Postgrad. med. J.*, 1980, *56*, *Suppl.* 1, 112.

Administration in renal failure. Imipramine can be given in usual doses to patients with renal failure. Concentrations of imipramine were not affected by haemodialysis or peritoneal dialysis.— W. M. Bennett *et al.*, *Ann. intern. Med.*, 1977, *86*, 754. See also *idem*, 1980, *93*, 286.

Anorexia nervosa. Two patients with features of secondary anorexia nervosa and depression had a good response to imipramine and intensive individual psychotherapy.— J. H. White and N. L. Schnaultz, *Dis. nerv. Syst.*, 1977, *38*, 567.

Arthritis. In a double-blind crossover trial, treatment with 25 mg of imipramine thrice daily for 3 weeks improved symptoms in 15 of 22 patients with arthritis. In 7, function and grip were improved. The only side-effects were dizziness in 3 and dry mouth in 4 patients.— W. A. M. Scott, *Practitioner*, 1969, *202*, 802. A study demonstrating that imipramine only improves rheumatic symptoms in patients who are also psychiatrically ill with depression.— P. D. Fowler *et al.*, *Curr. med. Res. Opinion*, 1977, *5*, 241.

Behaviour disorders. Of 19 schoolboys with hyperactivity who completed an 8-week course of treatment with imipramine, 14 were judged to be much improved though they tended to relapse when treatment was withdrawn; the initial dose was 50 mg daily, later increased to 100 to 200 mg daily. About three-quarters of the boys experienced weight loss.— J. Waizer *et al.*, *Am. J. Psychiat.*, 1974, *131*, 587. See also J. L. Rapoport *et al.*, *Archs gen. Psychiat.*, 1974, *30*, 789.

For comments on the hazards and limitations of tricyclic antidepressant therapy in behaviour disorders, see Amitriptyline Hydrochloride, p.114.

Cardiac disorders. A decrease in both atrial and ventricular premature depolarisations occurred in each of 2 patients treated with imipramine for depression and cardiac arrhythmias.— J. T. Bigger *et al.*, *New Engl. J. Med.*, 1977, *296*, 206.

Evidence that imipramine has a potent anti-arrhythmic action in patients recovering from depression.— E. -G. V. Giardina *et al.*, *Circulation*, 1979, *60*, 1045.

Cramps. A patient (the writer) was free from night cramps when taking imipramine 10 mg three or four times daily.— H. B. Lee (letter), *Br. med. J.*, 1976, *2*, 1259.

Depression. For a general review of the role of tricyclic antidepressants in depression, see Amitriptyline Hydrochloride, p.114.

For the use of liothyronine as an adjunct to tricyclic antidepressant therapy in depression, see Liothyronine, p.1501.

Enuresis. In a controlled trial in children aged up to 15 years, pad-and-bell conditioning proved the best deterrent to bed-wetting. Imipramine initially produced a significantly better response than placebo but there was a considerable relapse-rate with gradual withdrawal of the drug.— N. McConaghy, *Med. J. Aust.*, 1969, *2*, 237.

From the results of a double-blind crossover study with 125 children it appeared that the optimum dose of imipramine for the treatment of enuresis was 0.9 to 1.5 mg per kg body-weight.— C. Maxwell and J. Seldrup, *Arzneimittel-Forsch.*, 1971, *21*, 1352. See also *idem*, *Practitioner*, 1971, *207*, 809.

Further references to imipramine in nocturnal enuresis: D. Schaffer *et al.*, *Archs Dis. Childh.*, 1968, *43*, 665; G. I. Martin, *Am. J. Dis. Child.*, 1971, *122*, 42; A. C. Diokno *et al.*, *J. Urol.*, 1972, *107*, 42; A. T. Cole and F. A. Fried, *ibid.*, 44; A. Kales *et al.*, *Pediatrics*, 1977, *60*, 431; P. M. Bindelglas and G. Dee, *Am. J. Psychiat.*, 1978, *135*, 1549 (absence of long-term toxicity); O. S. Jorgensen *et al.*, *Clin. Pharmacokinet.*, 1980, *5*, 386 (plasma-imipramine concentrations in nocturnal enuresis).

For comments on the hazards and limitations of tricyclic antidepressant therapy in noctural enuresis, see Amitriptyline Hydrochloride, p.114.

Epilepsy. Imipramine hydrochloride produced a good response in 15 of 20 patients with petit mal or minor motor seizures resistant to standard therapy. Six of the patients continued to show a good response for more than 1 year. Imipramine exacerbated grand mal or psychomotor seizures in 5 patients, necessitating an increase in their dose of phenytoin or primidone.— G. F. Fromm *et al.*, *Archs Neurol., Chicago*, 1972, *27*, 198.

Narcolepsy. Imipramine 25 mg together with methylphenidate 5 or 10 mg thrice daily effectively controlled sleep attacks and catalepsy in 45 patients and produced less side-effects than amphetamines alone.— V. Zarcone, *New Engl. J. Med.*, 1973, *288*, 1156. See also Y. Hishikawa *et al.*, *J. neurol. Sci.*, 1966, *3*, 453; C. Guilleminault *et al.*, *Archs Neurol., Chicago*, 1974, *30*, 90.

Parkinsonism. Imipramine or amitriptyline 10 to 25 mg four times daily improved akinesia and rigidity as well as depressive symptoms especially when given with antiparkinsonian agents.— M. D. Yahr and R. C. Duvoisin, *New Engl. J. Med.*, 1972, *287*, 20.

Phobias. Imipramine 10 to 300 mg daily (mean 180 mg) for 26 weeks with behaviour therapy or supportive psychotherapy was significantly superior to a placebo with behaviour therapy in the treatment of 71 patients with mixed phobias or agoraphobia. In 40 patients with simple phobias no significant difference was found between imipramine and a placebo.— C. M. Zitrin *et al.*, *Archs gen. Psychiat.*, 1978, *35*, 307. See also R. P. Snaith (letter), *Br. J. Psychiat.*, 1972, *121*, 238.

Rhinitis. Of 41 patients with vasomotor rhinitis who took part in a double-blind study of imipramine, 6 needed only 1 course of treatment (1 was taking placebo). Of the 35 who completed 2 courses, 19 preferred imipramine and 9 preferred placebo.— E. H. M. Foxen, *Br. J. clin. Pract.*, 1972, *26*, 363.

Sexual disorders. Administration of imipramine was associated with an ejaculate of normal volume and consistency, containing motile spermatozoa, in a man with aspermia following retroperitoneal lymph node dissection.— M. E. Kelly and M. A. Needle, *Urology*, 1979, *13*, 414.

Preparations

Imipramine Hydrochloride Injection *(U.S.P.)*. A sterile solution of imipramine hydrochloride, 11.5 to 13.5 mg per ml, in Water for Injections. pH 4 to 5.

Imipramine Hydrochloride Tablets *(U.S.P.)*. Tablets containing imipramine hydrochloride. Store in airtight containers.

Imipramine Tablets *(B.P.)*. Tablets containing imipramine hydrochloride. The tablets are sugar-coated.

Solutio Imizini 1.25% pro Injectionibus *(Rus. P.)*. Imipramine Hydrochloride Injection. Imipramine hydrochloride 1.25 g, sodium chloride 600 mg, ascorbic acid 200 mg, sodium metabisulphite 100 mg, exsiccated sodium sulphite 100 mg, Water for Injections to 100 ml; in ampoules of 2 ml. pH 3.7 to 4.5. Store in a cool place. Protect from light.

Proprietary Preparations

Berkomine *(Berk Pharmaceuticals, UK)*. Imipramine hydrochloride available as tablets of 10 mg.

Praminil *(DDSA Pharmaceuticals, UK)*. Imipramine hydrochloride, available as tablets of 10 and 25 mg.

Tofranil *(Geigy, UK)*. Imipramine hydrochloride, available as tablets of 10 and 25 mg. **Tofranil Syrup**. Contains in each 5 ml imipramine (as a resin complex) equivalent to 25 mg imipramine hydrochloride (suggested diluent, as for Anafranil, p.116). (Also available as Tofranil in *Arg., Austral., Belg., Canad., Denm., Fr., Ger., Ital., Neth., Norw., S.Afr., Spain, Switz., USA*).

Other Proprietary Names

Austral.—Imiprin, Iramil, Melipramine, Prodepress, Somipra; *Canad.*—Impril, Novopramine; *Denm.*—Deprinol; *Ital.*—Dynaprin, Surplix; *Jap.*—Chimoreptin, Eferanol, Imidol; *S.Afr.*—Panpramine; *USA*—Antipress, Imavate, Janimine, Presamine, SK-Pramine, W.D.D.

Imipramine hydrochloride was also formerly marketed in Great Britain under the proprietary names Dimipressin (*R.P. Drugs*), Norpramine (*Norton*), Oppanyl (*Oppenheimer*), and in Eire under the proprietary name Tiziramine (*Ticen, Eire*).

2517-y

Imipramine Oxide Hydrochloride. Imipraminoxide Hydrochloride; Imipraminoxidi Chloridum; Imipramine *N*-Oxide Hydrochloride. 3-(10,11-Dihydro-5*H*-dibenz-[*b,f*]azepin-5-yl)-*NN*-dimethylpropylamine *N*-oxide hydrochloride.

$C_{19}H_{24}N_2O,HCl = 332.9$.

CAS — 19864-71-2.

Pharmacopoeias. In *Nord.*

A white or off-white odourless hygroscopic crystalline powder with a bitter taste. **Soluble** 1 in 80 of water, 1 in 12 of alcohol, and 1 in 5 of chloroform; practically insoluble in ether. **Protect** from light.

Uses. Imipramine oxide hydrochloride is an antidepressant with actions and uses similar to those of imipramine hydrochloride. It is given in doses of 25 to 50 mg thrice daily.

Proprietary Names

Elepsin *(Andromaco, Arg.)*; Imiprex *(Dumex, Denm.; Dumex, Norw.)*.

2518-j

Iprindole Hydrochloride.

Pramindole Hydrochloride; Wy-3263. 3-(6,7,8,9,10,11-Hexahydro-5*H*-cyclo-oct[*b*]indol-5-yl)-*NN*-dimethylpropylamine hydrochloride.

$C_{19}H_{28}N_2,HCl = 320.9$.

CAS — 5560-72-5 (iprindole); 17993-64-5 (hydrochloride).

A white or off-white odourless powder. M.p. about 144°. Iprindole hydrochloride 16.9 mg is approximately equivalent to 15 mg of iprindole. **Soluble** in water, alcohol, and chloroform.

Adverse Effects and Treatment. As for Amitriptyline Hydrochloride, p.110.

Side-effects such as dry mouth, blurred vision, difficulty in micturition, and sweating occur less frequently with iprindole than with imipramine, and are usually less severe, as are cardiovascular effects.

Jaundice or bilirubinuria has been reported with iprindole, usually during the first 14 days of treatment.

Effects on the liver. Reversible liver damage was reported in 21 patients, 15 of whom were jaundiced, within 4 to 21 days of starting treatment with iprindole and signs of hypersensitivity reactions were present in some patients.— A. B. Ajdukiewicz *et al.*, *Gut*, 1971, *12*, 705. See also P. J. W. Young (letter), *Br. med. J.*, 1970, *1*, 367; D. F. Harrison and I. M. Stanley (letter), *ibid.*, 1970, *4*, 368; *Drug & Ther. Bull.*, 1971, *9*, 10.

Precautions. As for Amitriptyline Hydrochloride, p.112. It should not be given to patients with impaired liver function or a history of liver disease.

For a general comment on antidepressant therapy and driving, see Amitriptyline Hydrochloride, p.112.

Interactions. Iprindole had no effect on the blood-pressure responses to tyramine or noradrenaline in 5 patients.— W. E. Fann *et al.*, *Archs gen. Psychiat.*, 1972, *26*, 158.

Absorption and Fate. Iprindole is readily absorbed from the gastro-intestinal tract and extensively metabolised. It has a prolonged half-life and is excreted in the urine mainly in the form of metabolites.

Uses. Iprindole hydrochloride has actions and uses similar to those of the tricyclic antidepressants such as amitriptyline (p.113), but it only has weak anticholinergic effects.

The initial dose in mild depression and in the

elderly is the equivalent of 15 mg of iprindole thrice daily. In moderate to severe depression, the initial dose is the equivalent of 30 mg of iprindole thrice daily, which may be increased up to 60 mg thrice daily. The usual maintenance dose is the equivalent of 30 mg of iprindole thrice daily.

Depression. A critical review of the clinical and pharmacological profiles of iprindole and mianserin. Whereas iprindole is a relatively weak re-uptake inhibitor for both noradrenaline and serotonin, mianserin shows at least modest potency in inhibiting noradrenaline uptake. Evidence is as yet insufficient to prove the superiority of iprindole over placebo in the treatment of endogenous depression, but it was found superior to placebo in all 3 studies conducted in out-patients with neurotic or reactive depression. Although it has generally been reported that response to standard tricyclics is associated with the presence of endogenous patterns, clinicians have noted that many reactive or neurotic patients seem to respond to smaller dosages of these drugs, an observation that is perhaps analogous to the response of the neurotically depressed patients to iprindole.— A. P. Zis and F. K. Goodwin, *Archs gen. Psychiat.*, 1979, *36*, 1097.

Proprietary Preparations

Prondol *(Wyeth, UK).* Iprindole hydrochloride, available as tablets each containing the equivalent of 15 or 30 mg of iprindole.

2519-z

Iproclozide. PC 603. 2-(4-Chlorophenoxy)-2′-isopropylacetohydrazide.
$C_{11}H_{15}ClN_2O_2$=242.7.

CAS — 3544-35-2.

Uses. Iproclozide is a monoamine oxidase inhibitor with actions and uses similar to those of phenelzine (p.128). In the treatment of depression it has been given in doses of 5 to 10 mg thrice daily. It has also been used in angina pectoris.

Reference: A. Barrillon *et al.*, *Thérapie*, 1970, *25*, 349.

Interactions. Three patients died from fulminant hepatitis after receiving iproclozide in association with microsomal enzyme inducers (butobarbitone, meprobamate, and phenobarbitone). It was speculated that, like isoniazid, iproclozide could be transformed into a hepatotoxic metabolite, and that this might be enhanced by microsomal enzyme induction.— D. Pessayre *et al.*, *Gastroenterology*, 1978, *75*, 492.

Proprietary Names

Sursum *(Coirre, Belg.; Ibsa, Switz.).*

2520-p

Iproniazid Phosphate. 2′-Isopropylisonicotinohydrazide phosphate.
$C_9H_{13}N_3O,H_3PO_4$=277.2.

CAS — 54-92-2 (iproniazid); 305-33-9 (phosphate).

A white or almost white crystalline powder. Iproniazid phosphate 155 mg is approximately equivalent to 100 mg of iproniazid. **Soluble** 1 in 5 of water and 1 in 90 of alcohol; practically insoluble in chloroform and ether.

Adverse Effects, Treatment, and Precautions. As for Phenelzine Sulphate, p.128.

Effects on the liver. Surveys had shown that the incidence of liver damage was 1 in 4000 and the mortality was 1 in 10 000 of patients treated with iproniazid. Hepatotoxicity was associated only with those antidepressants which were hydrazine derivatives.— W. L. Rees, *Prescribers' J.*, 1967, *7*, 13. Role of metabolism in the hepatotoxicity of isoniazid and iproniazid.— J. A. Timbrell, *Drug Metab. Rev.*, 1979, *10*, 125.

Interactions. Reactions have occurred in patients taking iproniazid and *pethidine*.— C. Papp and S. Benaim, *Br. med. J.*, 1958, *2*, 1070; J. C. Shee, *ibid.*, 1960, *2*, 507. Reaction with iproniazid and *noradrenaline*.— L. Mond and I. Mack, *Am. Heart J.*, 1960, *59*, 134.

Absorption and Fate. Iproniazid is readily absorbed from the gastro-intestinal tract and excreted in the urine mainly in the form of metabolites.

Data following administration of a single dose of iproniazid 50 mg in one subject permitted calculation of a plasma half-life of 8.8 hours which agrees well with results of B.A. Koechlin *et al.* (*J. Pharmac. exp. Ther.*, 1962, *138*, 11) who revealed 2 components with half-lives of about 10 and 20 hours respectively; comparison with these results demonstrates the first component to have been free iproniazid.— R. M. de Sagher *et al.*, *J. pharm. Sci.*, 1976, *65*, 878.

Uses. Iproniazid is a monoamine oxidase inhibitor with actions and uses similar to those of phenelzine (p.130). In the treatment of depression iproniazid is given as the phosphate in doses of 100 to 150 mg daily. Once a response has been obtained the dosage may be gradually reduced for maintenance therapy; some patients may respond to 25 to 50 mg daily.

Iproniazid, which is the isopropyl derivative of isoniazid, was developed for use in tuberculosis but owing to its toxicity it is no longer used for this purpose.

Proprietary Preparations

Marsilid *(Roche, UK).* Iproniazid phosphate, available as scored tablets each containing the equivalent of 25 or 50 mg of iproniazid. (Also available as Marsilid in *Austral., Belg., Fr., Spain*).

2521-s

Isocarboxazid *(U.S.P., B.P. 1973).* Ro 50831. 2′-Benzyl-5-methylisoxazole-3-carbohydrazide.
$C_{12}H_{13}N_3O_2$=231.3.

CAS — 59-63-2.

Pharmacopoeias. In *U.S.*

A white or creamy-white, tasteless, crystalline powder with a faint characteristic odour. M.p. 105° to 108°. Slightly **soluble** in water; soluble 1 in 150 of alcohol, 1 in 3 of chloroform, and 1 in 50 of ether.

Adverse Effects, Treatment, and Precautions. As for Phenelzine Sulphate, p.128.

For a general comment on antidepressant therapy and driving, see Amitriptyline Hydrochloride, p.112.

A 61-year-old man with a history of depressive psychosis developed massive oedema within 2 weeks of being given isocarboxazid 20 to 30 mg daily with amitriptyline and chlordiazepoxide. Isocarboxazid was withdrawn and the oedema responded to treatment with frusemide.— S. K. Pathak (letter), *Br. med. J.*, 1977, *1*, 1220.

Absorption and Fate. Isocarboxazid is readily absorbed from the gastro-intestinal tract and excreted in the urine mainly in the form of metabolites.

Data following administration of isocarboxazid in man.— B. A. Koechlin *et al.*, *J. Pharmac. exp. Ther.*, 1962, *138*, 11.

Uses. Isocarboxazid is a monoamine oxidase inhibitor with actions and uses similar to those of phenelzine (p.130).

In the treatment of depression isocarboxazid is given in doses of 30 mg daily. Once a response has been obtained the dosage may be gradually reduced to a maintenance of 10 to 20 mg daily.

Depression. A report of the successful use of isocarboxazid with lithium carbonate in 3 severely depressed patients.— H. Zall, *Am. J. Psychiat.*, 1971, *127*, 1400.

Hyperoxaluria. Urine-oxalate and glycolate concentrations fell in a child with hyperglycolic hyperoxaluria given isocarboxazid 0.2 to 1.2 mg per kg body-weight daily.— E. Bourke *et al.*, *Ann. intern. Med.*, 1972, *76*, 279.

Isocarboxazid 20 mg daily had no effect on the excretion of oxalate by a patient with hyperoxaluria.— B. Koch *et al.*, *Can. med. Ass. J.*, 1972, *106*, 1323.

Parkinsonism. Isocarboxazid 10 mg thrice daily had a mild beneficial effect in selected patients with parkinsonism, possibly due to its effect on depression and on dopamine.— M. D. Yahr and R. C. Duvoisin, *New Engl. J. Med.*, 1972, *287*, 20.

Preparations

Isocarboxazid Tablets *(B.P. 1973).* Tablets containing isocarboxazid.

Isocarboxazid Tablets *(U.S.P.).* Tablets containing isocarboxazid. Protect from light.

Marplan *(Roche, UK).* Isocarboxazid, available as scored tablets of 10 mg. (Also available as Marplan in *Austral., Belg., Canad., Denm., Fr., Ital., Switz., USA*).

2522-w

Lofepramine Hydrochloride. Lopramine Hydrochloride; Leo 640. 4′-Chloro-2-[3-(10,11-dihydro-5*H*-dibenz[*b,f*]azepin-5-yl)-*N*-methylpropylamino]acetophenone hydrochloride.
$C_{26}H_{27}ClN_2O,HCl$=455.4.

CAS — 23047-25-8 (lofepramine); 26786-32-3 (hydrochloride).

Adverse Effects, Treatment, and Precautions. As for Amitriptyline Hydrochloride, p.110.

For a general comment on antidepressant therapy and driving, see Amitriptyline Hydrochloride, p.112.

Absorption and Fate. Lofepramine is readily absorbed from the gastro-intestinal tract, and extensively demethylated by first-pass metabolism in the liver to its primary metabolite, desipramine. Since lofepramine slows gastro-intestinal transit time absorption can, however, be delayed, particularly in overdosage. Paths of metabolism also include *N*-oxidation, hydroxylation, and conjugation. Lofepramine is excreted in the urine, mainly in the form of its metabolites.

Metabolism of lofepramine.— G. P. Forshell *et al.*, *Eur. J. clin. Pharmac.*, 1976, *9*, 291. A further study in *animals*.— G. P. Forshell, *Xenobiotica*, 1975, *5*, 73. See also K. Matsubayashi *et al.*, *J. Chromatogr. biomed. Appl.*, 1977, *143*, 571.

Uses. Lofepramine hydrochloride is a tricyclic antidepressant with actions and uses similar to those of amitriptyline (p.113). One of its metabolites is reported to be desipramine (p.116). Like imipramine and desipramine, it has less marked sedative properties than amitriptyline.

In the treatment of depression lofepramine is given in doses of 70 to 210 mg daily.

Pharmacology of lofepramine in *animals*.— E. Eriksoo and O. Rohte, *Arzneimittel-Forsch.*, 1970, *20*, 1561.

Depression. Studies of lofepramine in depression.— S. Wright and L. Herrmann, *Arzneimittel-Forsch.*, 1976, *26*, 1167; E. Lehmann and H. Hopes, *ibid.*, 1977, *27*, 1100; B. Siwers *et al.*, *Acta psychiat. scand.*, 1977, *55*, 21.

For a general review of the role of tricyclic antidepressants in depression, see Amitriptyline Hydrochloride, p.114.

Proprietary Names

Gamonil *(E. Merck, Ger.)*; Tymelyt *(Leo, Swed.).*

2524-l

Maprotiline Hydrochloride. Ba-34276. 3-(9,10-Dihydro-9,10-ethanoanthracen-9-yl)-*N*-methylpropylamine hydrochloride.

$C_{20}H_{23}N,HCl$=313.9.

CAS — 10262-69-8 (maprotiline); 10347-81-6 (hydrochloride).

A white odourless crystalline powder. **Soluble** in water and some organic solvents.

Adverse Effects, Treatment, and Precautions. As for Amitriptyline Hydrochloride, p.110.

Maprotiline administered to 25 healthy subjects in single or repeated doses produced side-effects (tiredness, dry mouth) similar to those caused by tricyclic antidepressants.— N. Matussek and M. Aarons, *Arzneimittel-Forsch.*, 1974, *24*, 1107.

For a general comment on antidepressant therapy and driving, see Amitriptyline Hydrochloride, p.112.

Allergy. Urticaria and severe granulocytopenia in one patient were associated with maprotiline hydrochloride.— N. M. Johnson *et al.* (letter), *Lancet*, 1976, *2*, 1357.

Effects on the blood. For a reference to granulocytopenia in a patient taking maprotiline, see under Allergy, above.

Epileptogenic effect. A grand mal seizure occurred in 3 women taking maprotiline 75 to 150 mg at night; no further seizures occurred when maprotiline was withdrawn and no other cause was detected.— G. A. A. Shepherd and F. Kerr, *Br. med. J.*, 1978, *1*, 1523. A 20-year-old nurse experienced 2 grand mal seizures 7 days after her dose of maprotiline was increased from 75 mg at night (for 2 weeks) to 300 mg at night.— M. J. Hall and R. I. Russell (letter), *ibid.*, *2*, 961. Comment; epileptic seizures are rare when the dose is below 150 mg.— D. Burley *et al.*, *Ciba* (letter), *ibid.*, 1230.

Comment on antidepressant therapy and the seizure threshold. It is interesting that 3 of the 4 patients were taking the contraceptive pill.— M. Trimble (letter), *ibid.*, 1430.

For details of the number of reports of epilepsy associated with maprotiline therapy in proportion to its share of the antidepressant market, see Amitriptyline Hydrochloride (Epileptogenic Effect), p.111.

Further reports and comments on convulsions associated with maprotiline.— *Committee on Safety of Medicines, Current Problems Series No. 2,* Aug., 1976; P. Marks *et al., Postgrad. med. J.*, 1979, *55,* 742.

Overdosage. Six patients with maprotiline overdosage had some or all of the features typical of tricyclic poisoning, including unconsciousness, convulsions, urinary retention, and delirium. All recovered with supportive treatment. Physostigmine might be of value in severely ill patients; haemodialysis, forced diuresis, or haemoperfusion were unlikely to be of value.— J. Park and A. T. Proudfoot, *Br. med. J.*, 1977, *1,* 1573. Experience with 41 cases of maprotiline overdosage has suggested that, unlike mianserin, the clinical features of maprotiline poisoning resemble those of the more conventional tricyclic antidepressants.— P. Crome and B. Newman (letter), *ibid.*, *2,* 260.

Absorption and Fate. Maprotiline is slowly but completely absorbed from the gastro-intestinal tract. Since maprotiline slows gastro-intestinal transit-time absorption may be further delayed in overdosage. Maprotiline is extensively demethylated to its principal active metabolite, desmethylmaprotiline; paths of metabolism of both maprotiline and desmethylmaprotiline include *N*-oxidation, aliphatic and aromatic hydroxylation, and the formation of aromatic methoxy derivatives. In addition to desmethylmaprotiline, maprotiline-*N*-oxide is also reported to be pharmacologically active. Maprotiline is excreted in the urine, mainly in the form of its metabolites, either in free or in conjugated form; appreciable amounts are also excreted in the faeces.

Maprotiline is widely distributed throughout the body and is extensively bound to plasma protein. It has been estimated to have a very prolonged plasma half-life of about 2 days. Maprotiline is excreted in breast milk.

A study indicating that maprotiline is completely absorbed after administration by mouth. About two-thirds was excreted in the urine and about one-third in the faeces.— W. Riess *et al., Boll. chim.-farm.*, 1973, *112,* 677.

A comparison of the bioavailability and kinetics of one 50 mg tablet of maprotiline hydrochloride and 50 mg of radioactively labelled maprotiline hydrochloride in solution following simultaneous administration. Peak plasma concentrations were achieved after about 8 to 24 hours and the terminal half-life ranged from 36 to 108 hours.— D. Alkalay *et al., Clin. Pharmac. Ther.*, 1980, *27,* 697.

Further references.— W. Riess *et al., J. int. med. Res.*, 1975, *3, Suppl.* 2, 16.

Plasma concentrations. A study of the relation between clinical efficacy and serum concentrations after repeated intravenous and oral administration of maprotiline to depressed patients.— R. Fischbach, *Arzneimittel-Forsch.*, 1979, *29,* 352.

Uses. Maprotiline is a *tetracyclic* antidepressant with structural similarities to the tricyclic antidepressants. It is used similarly to amitriptyline (p.113) in the treatment of depression. Like amitriptyline, it also has marked sedative properties.

In the treatment of depression maprotiline is given by mouth as the hydrochloride in doses of 25 mg thrice daily, gradually increased to a maximum of 50 mg thrice daily if necessary. The dosage should be adjusted after 1 or 2 weeks according to response. Because of the prolonged half-life of maprotiline the total daily dose may also be given as a single dose, usually at night. A suggested initial dose for elderly or other susceptible patients is 10 mg thrice daily (or 30 mg at night).

Reviews and symposia on maprotiline.— *J. int. med. Res.*, 1977, *5, Suppl.* 4;; R. M. Pinder *et al., Drugs*, 1977, *13,* 321.

Cardiac disorders. In 9 patients with cardiac arrhythmias treatment with maprotiline reduced the incidence of ventricular premature beats, reduced the severity of arrhythmias, and reduced the incidence of exercise-induced ventricular premature beats.— E. A. Raeder *et al., Br. med. J.*, 1979, *2,* 102.

Depression. In a 3-week multicentre study in 10 000 patients with depressive illness, maprotiline 75 mg at night was effective in 85% of the 7250 patients completing the study. Of those withdrawing 1343 did so because of side-effects with drowsiness as the main complaint.— W. A. Forrest, *Ciba, J. int. med. Res.*, 1977, *5,* 42.

Further studies of maprotiline in depression.— N. E. Kay and B. Davies, *Med. J. Aust.*, 1974, *1,* 704; A. Kessell and N. F. Holt, *ibid.*, 1975, *1,* 773; B. Lauritsen, *J. int. med. Res.*, 1975, *3, Suppl.* 2, 61; J. E. Murphy, *ibid.*, 97; H. E. Lehmann *et al., Curr. ther. Res.*, 1976, *19,* 463; A. N. Singh *et al., ibid.*, 451; G. Molnar, *Can. psychiat. Ass. J.*, 1977, *22,* 19; J. T. Silverstone *et al., Practitioner*, 1977, *218,* 279; H. O'Hara, *ibid.*, 1978, *221,* 419; E. Väisänen *et al., Acta psychiat. scand.*, 1978, *57,* 193; J. N. Logue *et al., J. clin. Pharmac.*, 1979, *19,* 64; D. H. Mielke *et al., Curr. ther. Res.*, 1979, *25,* 738.

Proprietary Preparations

Ludiomil *(Ciba, UK).* Maprotiline hydrochloride, available as tablets of 10, 25, 50, and 75 mg. (Also available as Ludiomil in *Arg., Belg., Canad., Denm., Fr., Ger., Ital., Neth., S.Afr., Spain, Swed., Switz.*). Maprotiline mesylate is also available as Ludiomil in some countries.

2525-y

Mebanazine. ICI 31397. α-Methylbenzylhydrazine.
$C_8H_{12}N_2$=136.2.

CAS — 65-64-5.

Practically **insoluble** in water, alcohol, and ether. **Incompatible** with alkalis.

Adverse Effects, Treatment, and Precautions. As for Phenelzine Sulphate, p.128.

Interactions. Enhancement of the hypoglycaemic effect of chlorpropamide and tolbutamide on concomitant administration of mebanazine.— L. Wickström and K. Pettersson, *Lancet*, 1964, *2,* 995.

A reaction in a woman, who was taking mebanazine, after eating *Canadian Cheddar cheese.*— E. H. J. Cotter (letter), *Br. med. J.*, 1967, *4,* 552.

Reaction in a man, receiving mebanazine together with dexamphetamine, after taking *Cheddar cheese* and *spirits.*— G. Simpson (letter), *Br. med. J.*, 1969, *2,* 635.

Uses. Mebanazine is a monoamine oxidase inhibitor with actions and uses similar to those of phenelzine (p.130). In the treatment of depression it has been given in doses of 5 to 30 mg daily.

Mebanazine was formerly marketed in Great Britain under the proprietary name Actomol (*I.C.I. Pharmaceuticals*).

2526-j

Melitracen Hydrochloride. N7001; U-24973A. 3-(9,10-Dihydro-10,10-dimethyl-9-anthrylidene)-*NN*-dimethylpropylamine hydrochloride.
$C_{21}H_{25}N,HCl$=327.9.

CAS — 5118-29-6 (melitracen); 10563-70-9 (hydrochloride).

Adverse Effects, Treatment, and Precautions. As for Amitriptyline Hydrochloride, p.110.

For a general comment on antidepressant therapy and driving, see Amitriptyline Hydrochloride, p.112.

Overdosage. Melitracen poisoning without ECG changes.— C. Martini and F. Fici, *Int. J. clin. Pharmac. Biopharm.*, 1978, *16,* 129.

Uses. Melitracen is a tricyclic antidepressant with actions and uses similar to those of amitriptyline (p.113). In the treatment of depression it is given as the hydrochloride in usual doses equivalent to melitracen 25 to 50 mg thrice daily. It has also been given intramuscularly as the mesylate.

Depression. A double-blind study in 31 patients indicated that melitracen and imipramine were equally effective in the treatment of depression.— G. Francesconi *et al., Curr. ther. Res.*, 1976, *20,* 529.

Further references.— D. Biros *et al., Curr. ther. Res.*, 1969, *11,* 289.

For a general review of the role of tricyclic antidepressants in depression, see Amitriptyline Hydrochloride, p.114.

Proprietary Names

Dixeran *(Lundbeck, Belg.; Lundbeck, Switz.)*; Melixeran *(Lusofarmaco, Ital.)*; Trausabun *(Promonta, Ger.; Byk, Neth.).*

2527-z

Mianserin Hydrochloride. Org GB 94.
1,2,3,4,10,14b-Hexahydro-2-methyldibenzo[*c,f*]-pyrazino[1,2-*a*]azepine hydrochloride.
$C_{18}H_{20}N_2,HCl$=300.8.

CAS — 24219-97-4 (mianserin); 21535-47-7 (hydrochloride).

Adverse Effects. Adverse effects associated with mianserin include drowsiness. Changes in blood sugar concentrations may occur, and susceptible patients may swing from depression to mania. Other side-effects reported include weight changes and blood disorders.

Symptoms of overdosage are mainly drowsiness, coma, hypertension or hypotension, tachycardia or bradycardia, dilated or constricted pupils, vomiting, and dizziness and ataxia have also been reported. Unlike amitriptyline, convulsions and life-threatening cardiac arrhythmias do not appear to have been a problem.

A study in depressed patients indicating that mianserin and amitriptyline in oral antidepressant doses have markedly different autonomic actions. Their influence on salivary volume demonstrated that amitriptyline possessed significant anticholinergic properties while mianserin appeared to be free of such an action. The fall in salivary volume was only marked in the first week of amitriptyline treatment and in the mianserin group there was a significant increase in salivary volume; this may have been related to the improvement in clinical state being associated with an increase in salivary flow.— K. Ghose *et al., Psychopharmacology*, 1976, *49,* 201.

A study indicating that in healthy males, mianserin up to 60 mg daily seems to lack the anticholinergic effects and postural hypotension associated with amitriptyline treatment.— H. Kopera, *Br. J. clin. Pharmac.*, 1978, *5, Suppl.* 1, 29S.

In a comparative study with diazepam in depressed patients, significantly greater instances of tachycardia in the first 2 weeks, and dry mouth and constipation throughout the trial, were seen with mianserin treatment. Baseline data were not determined, which may have enhanced the apparent incidence of drug-related side-effects.— W. Hamouz *et al., Curr. med. Res. Opinion*, 1980, *6, Suppl.* 7, 72. Of 192 out-patients in a general psychiatric practice treated with mianserin in doses of up to 130 mg daily the main side-effect was moderate drowsiness during the first 2 to 3 days, reported by almost all patients taking 30 mg or more daily, but this decreased after 7 days. No definite relationship was noted between dose levels and side-effects, and no anticholinergic or cardiotoxic effects were reported. Fourteen patients withdrew from the study because of the sudden development of severe restlessness, 9 because of severe drowsiness, 2 because of severe anxious dreaming, and 1 because of severe nausea. Most patients reported increased appetite, and 17 women and 2 men had a remarkable increase in body-weight.— H. Hopman, *ibid.*, 107.

A study in 5 depressed subjects indicated that mianserin administration was followed by a significant increase in salivary flow and decrease in pupillary diameter. These preliminary findings are consistent with other reports on mianserin reflecting not only a lack of anticholinergic activity, but also in the case of salivary flow, a possible increase in cholinergic activity.— W. H. Wilson *et al., J. clin. Psychiat.*, 1980, *41,* 63.

Diabetogenic effect. Raised blood sugar concentrations in 22 of 28 patients given mianserin 30 mg as a single dose at bedtime.— R. V. Magnus, *Br. J. clin. Pract.*, 1979, *33,* 251.

Effects on the blood. A 49-year-old alcoholic woman taking thyroxine developed agranulocytosis 5 weeks after starting to take mianserin 20 mg thrice daily; mianserin was considered responsible. The Committee on Safety of Medicines had received 4 reports of blood dyscrasia related to treatment with mianserin including one of leucopenia in a patient who had taken only mianserin.— D. A. Curson and A. S. Hale, *Br. med. J.*, 1979, *1*, 378. See also A. M. McHarg and J. F. McHarg (letter), *ibid.*, 623.

Effects on the heart. A study of the cardiovascular effects of amitriptyline, mianserin, zimelidine, and nomifensine in depressed patients. Whereas amitriptyline was shown to have a direct action the changes brought about by mianserin were probably due to effects on the peripheral circulation. Mianserin and zimelidine appeared to be safer antidepressants than amitriptyline and should be preferred to the latter, especially in patients with known heart disease and perhaps in the elderly. Nomifensine was studied in an inadequate number of patients to clarify its place, but it too seems to be safer than amitriptyline.— C. D. Burgess *et al.*, *Postgrad. med. J.*, 1979, *55*, 704. See also H. Kopera *et al.*, *Int. J. clin. Pharmac. Biopharm.*, 1980, *18*, 104.

Effects on mental state. Three hours after taking her initial dose of mianserin 10 mg, a 32-year-old woman collapsed with an apparently exaggerated central sedative response, and recovered about 14 hours later unaware of any lapse in time; she had been admitted after taking paracetamol 6 g following a bereavement and was receiving a small dose of diazepam.— A. E. Tulloch (letter), *Lancet*, 1978, *1*, 1097. Criticism. The evidence incriminating mianserin was tenuous.— W. L. Shaw, *Organon* (letter), *Lancet*, 1978, *2*, 45.

For the absence of impairment of short-term memory and performance by mianserin, see Amitriptyline, p.111. For reference to mania in subjects with bipolar affective illness given mianserin, see under Precautions, below.

Effects on the skin. Toxic epidermal necrolysis in a 34-year-old woman might have been associated with mianserin.— P. Randell (letter), *Med. J. Aust.*, 1979, *2*, 653.

Epileptogenic effect. An epileptic fit in a 60-year-old woman with a long history of depressive illness may have been associated with mianserin therapy. She had been taking mianserin 30 mg daily for 6 weeks before the seizure occurred and had discontinued lorazepam 2.5 mg thrice daily 3 days before the seizure. Since lorazepam has anticonvulsant properties it is considered that had she not been taking this concomitantly the seizure might have occurred sooner. Fourteen other cases of convulsions associated with mianserin treatment have been reported to the Committee on Safety of Medicines. Although further evidence is needed before mianserin can be considered definitely epileptogenic, caution is needed when prescribing it for patients with a history of seizures.— P. Tyrer *et al.* (letter), *Lancet*, 1979, *2*, 798. The seizure may have been caused by withdrawal of lorazepam rather than administration of mianserin.— T. R. Einarson (letter), *ibid.*, 1980, *1*, 151. Reply. Although lorazepam withdrawal must have been a contributory cause, it is unlikely to be the sole explanation.— P. Tyrer (letter), *ibid.*

A 22-year-old woman who had been receiving flupenthixol decanoate 40 mg intramuscularly every 3 weeks for about 3 months, together with benzhexol 2 mg thrice daily, was also given mianserin 10 mg thrice daily. Ten days later she had a major epileptic seizure. All her drugs were withdrawn and the EEG changes found were considered to be due to drugs.— W. I. Mikhail (letter), *Lancet*, 1979, *2*, 969.

For details of the number of reports of epilepsy associated with mianserin therapy in proportion to its share of the antidepressant market, see Amitriptyline Hydrochloride (Epileptogenic Effect), p.111.

Hypotension. Comments on the lower incidence of postural hypotension associated with mianserin in comparison with the tricyclic antidepressants.— P. Pichot *et al.*, *Br. J. clin. Pharmac.*, 1978, *5*, *Suppl.* 1, 87S. See also C. B. Pull *et al.*, *Curr. med. Res. Opinion*, 1980, *6*, *Suppl.* 7, 81; R. De Buck, *ibid.*, 88.

Overdosage. A 53-year-old woman who took at least 600 mg of mianserin with 20 tablets of a carbromal-like hypnotic and 250 ml of alcohol 40% had a plasma-mianserin concentration of 780 ng per ml when measured about 5 hours after ingestion. She was unconscious, with initial hypotension and tachycardia. No debris was recovered during gastric lavage. Haemodialysis for 6 hours was not considered to have been useful. There were no significant changes in the ECG. The patient recovered consciousness 17 hours after ingestion.— F. H. J. Jansen, *Organon* (letter), *Br. med. J.*, 1977, *2*, 896. A 39-year-old woman ingested mianserin hydrochloride 580 mg, diazepam 35 mg, and nitrazepam 30 mg; she induced vomiting shortly afterwards. On admission to hospital she was drowsy and had a dry mouth. Blood pressure was 115/95 mmHg and heart-rate was 90 per minute. ECG showed first-degree heart block persisting for 14 hours by which time the concentration of mianserin in serum had fallen from 439 ng per ml to a therapeutic level; QRS and S-T complexes and the Q-T interval were not affected.— S. D. R. Green and P. Kendall-Taylor, *ibid.*, 1190. Experience with 44 patients confirmed that mianserin in overdosage did not cause the severe complications seen with tricyclic antidepressants.— P. Crome *et al.* (letter), *Br. med. J.*, 1978, *1*, 859.

Symptoms in 42 patients who had taken an overdose of mianserin alone included drowsiness (16), coma (2), hypertension (4), sinus tachycardia (3), bradycardia (2), vomiting (3), dizziness and ataxia (1), constricted pupils (1), dilated pupils (1), and hypotension (1).— W. L. Shaw, *Curr. med. Res. Opinion*, 1980, *6*, *Suppl.* 7, 44.

Weight gain. Weight gain associated with unusual craving for bread and butter, chocolate, and bread respectively, was noted in 3 patients given mianserin for depression.— B. Harris and M. Harper (letter), *Lancet*, 1980, *1*, 590. Three women who, despite vigorous dieting efforts, had gained 6 to 20 kg above their normal weight on amitriptyline, regained their former weights on transfer to mianserin. Carbohydrate craving disappeared and weight loss began (in 2 cases associated with dieting) within one to two weeks.— W. Williams (letter), *Med. J. Aust.*, 1980, *1*, 132.

For mention of a high incidence of weight gain in women given mianserin, see above.

Treatment of Adverse Effects. The stomach should be emptied by aspiration and lavage. The use of activated charcoal as an adjunct to gastric lavage may be of value. Supportive therapy alone may then suffice (for general guidelines to the symptomatic therapy of drug overdosage, see Phenobarbitone, p.812).

The absence of anticholinergic effects in mianserin overdosage suggests that physostigmine or other cholinesterase inhibitors should not be used in therapy.— P. Crome and B. Newman (letter), *Br. med. J.*, 1977, *2*, 260.

Precautions. Although mianserin does not have the cardiotoxicity of the tricyclic antidepressants, it should be used with caution in patients with cardiovascular disorders, such as ischaemic heart disease. It should similarly be used with caution in patients with epilepsy, and hepatic or renal insufficiency. Manic depressive patients may switch to a manic phase during mianserin therapy, and patients with suicidal tendencies should be carefully supervised during treatment. Blood sugar concentrations may be altered in diabetic patients.

Unlike the tricyclic antidepressants, mianserin is considered unlikely to interact with monoamine oxidase inhibitors, but until more is known it is recommended that it should not be given to patients receiving monoamine oxidase inhibitors or for at least 14 days after their discontinuation. Similarly, mianserin does not appear to diminish the effects of antihypertensive agents such as guanethidine and bethanidine; some interaction may, however, occur with clonidine and, in general, blood pressure should be monitored when mianserin is prescribed with antihypertensive therapy. The sedative effects of mianserin may be enhanced by concurrent administration with alcohol, and concomitant administration with barbiturates is not recommended.

Drowsiness is often experienced at the start of mianserin antidepressant therapy and patients liable to take charge of vehicles or other machinery should be warned that their judgement may be impaired.

Single doses of mianserin hydrochloride 10 or 20 mg significantly prolonged reaction time in 8 healthy subjects, and patients should be warned of possible sedation when first starting treatment.— P. Crome and B. Newman, *J. int. med. Res.*, 1978, *6*, 430. See also K. J. Hofner, *Clin. Ther.*, 1978, *1*, 280; M. J. Mattila *et al.*, *Br. J. clin. Pharmac.*, 1978, *5*, *Suppl.* 1, 53S.

For a general comment on antidepressant therapy and driving, see Amitriptyline Hydrochloride, p.112.

Interactions. Mianserin 20 mg administered thrice daily for 2 to 4 weeks to 5 patients with endogenous or neurotic depression produced little or no change in pressor response to doses of *noradrenaline*. It was considered that adrenergic interactions with mianserin 20 mg thrice daily would be negligible.— K. Ghose (letter), *Br. J. clin. Pharmac.*, 1977, *4*, 712. See also A. J. Coppen and K. Ghose, *Arzneimittel-Forsch.*, 1976, *26*, 1166; K. Ghose *et al.*, *Psychopharmacology*, 1976, *49*, 201. A study in *rats* demonstrating interference of mianserin with *noradrenaline* uptake.— I. Cavero *et al.*, *Br. J. Pharmac.*, 1979, *66*, 132P.

In a double-blind crossover study, 6 moderately depressed hypertensive patients being treated with *bethanidine* were also given mianserin or placebo. No significant changes occurred in blood pressures, indicating that mianserin had no significant effect on the antihypertensive action of bethanidine.— A. Coppen *et al.*, *Br. J. clin. Pharmac.*, 1978, *5*, *Suppl.* 1, 13S. In an open study in 3 depressed hypertensive patients mianserin did not antagonise the antihypertensive action of *propranolol* or *propranolol and hydralazine*. In a double-blind study compared with desipramine, mianserin did not antagonise the antihypertensive action of either *guanethidine* or *bethanidine*.— C. D. Burgess *et al.*, *ibid.*, 21S.

Reduced plasma concentrations of mianserin and desmethylmianserin in 6 patients also receiving anti-epileptic therapy.— S. Nawishy *et al.* (letter), *Lancet*, 1981, *2*, 871.

For the effect of mianserin on *clonidine*, see Clonidine Hydrochloride, p.139.

Mania. Evidence that mianserin may be capable of inducing mania in susceptible subjects with bipolar affective illness. Within a 3-month trial period 6 of 10 such patients became manic while receiving mianserin 20 mg thrice daily. Since this has been previously described with other groups of antidepressants it may be a general property of antidepressants. Three other patients in the study left in the first few days due to drowsiness in 2 and insomnia in the third.— A. Coppen *et al.*, *Int. Pharmacopsychiat.*, 1977, *12*, 95.

Absorption and Fate. Mianserin is readily absorbed from the gastro-intestinal tract, but its bioavailability is reduced to about 70% by extensive first-pass metabolism in the liver.

Paths of metabolism of mianserin include aromatic hydroxylation, *N*-oxidation, and *N*-demethylation.

Mianserin is excreted in the urine, almost entirely as its metabolites, either free or in conjugated form; some is also found in the faeces.

Mianserin is widely distributed throughout the body and is extensively bound to plasma proteins. It has been found to have a biphasic plasma half-life with the duration of the terminal phase ranging from 6 to 39 hours. Although plasma concentrations of mianserin vary widely between individuals there are some indications of a correlation with therapeutic response.

Mianserin crosses the blood-brain barrier. Studies *in vitro* and in *animals* have suggested that only small amounts cross the placenta and are excreted in breast milk.

Peak plasma concentrations of mianserin were generally obtained about 2 hours after oral administration to 4 healthy subjects. Estimations of the β-phase plasma half-life ranged from 7.7 to 19.2 hours with a median of 10.0 hours, but it was considered that this may have been a considerable underestimation.— M. Fink *et al.*, *Psychopharmacology*, 1977, *54*, 249.

A short summary of data from a pharmacokinetic study in 4 male and 4 female subjects given mianserin 20 mg by mouth. Peak plasma concentrations were achieved after 1.1 to 3.1 hours, slightly slower absorption and a slightly lower peak occurring in the females. The plasma half-life was bi-exponential with an initial rapid phase ranging from 0.5 to 2.6 hours and a slower phase ranging from 6 to 39 hours. The volumes of distribution for female subjects were significantly higher than for males.— H. Jansen, *Br. J. clin. Pharmac.*, 1978, *5*, *Suppl.* 1, 96S and 97S.

Plasma concentrations. Results of a double-blind controlled study in 26 depressed in-patients and 24 depressed out-patients showed no significant difference between the response to mianserin 60 mg given as a single dose at night or daily in 3 divided doses. There appeared to be a range of plasma concentrations within which an optimum therapeutic response was obtained, with an upper limit of 70 ng per ml. Variation in plasma concentrations achieved increased with age, suggesting that a lower dose may be more appropriate in the older group. The highly significant clinical disadvantage associated with higher plasma concentrations of mianserin indicated that a daily dose of 60 mg may be higher than necessary.— S. Montgomery *et al.*, *Br. J. clin. Pharmac.*, 1978, *5, Suppl.* 1, 71S.

Uses. Mianserin is a *tetracyclic* antidepressant. It does not appear to have significant anticholinergic properties, but has a marked sedative action. Unlike amitriptyline, it does not prevent the peripheral re-uptake of noradrenaline; it blocks presynaptic alpha-adrenoceptors and increases the turnover of brain noradrenaline. It has little effect on central serotonin uptake but has been shown to increase peripheral serotonin uptake in depressed subjects. It has antihistamine properties. Although many of the effects of mianserin differ from those of amitriptyline, its activity in depression is similar. Like amitriptyline, its mode of action in depression is not fully understood. In the treatment of depression mianserin is given by mouth as the hydrochloride in doses of 30 mg daily initially, increased to 60 mg daily if necessary after the first week. The daily dosage may be divided throughout the day or given as a single dose at night. Divided daily dosages of up to 200 mg have been given, but some sources have suggested that there is a ceiling above which the therapeutic response deteriorates.

Reviews, comments and symposia on mianserin.— *Br. J. clin. Pharmac.*, 1978, *5, Suppl.* 1, 55S–99S; R. N. Brogden *et al.*, *Drugs*, 1978, *16*, 273; A. P. Zis and F. K. Goodwin, *Archs gen. Psychiat.*, 1979, *36*, 1097; *Curr. med. Res. Opinion*, 1980, *6, Suppl.* 7, 1–151.

Action. Some studies into the mode of action of mianserin.— W. J. van der Burg *et al.*, *J. med. Chem.*, 1970, *13*, 35 (antiserotonin potency); P. A. Baumann and L. Maître, *Archs Pharmac.*, 1977, *300*, 31 (brain presynaptic alpha-receptor blockade); I. Goodlet *et al.*, *Br. J. Pharmac.*, 1977, *61*, 307 (absence of monoamine oxidase uptake); R. D. Robson *et al.*, *Eur. J. Pharmac.*, 1978, *47*, 431 (clonidine antagonism); A. Coppen *et al.*, *Br. J. clin. Pharmac.*, 1978, *5, Suppl.* 1, 13S (peripheral noradrenaline and serotonin uptake).

For general comments on the possible mode of action of antidepressants, see Amitriptyline Hydrochloride, p.114.

Administration. In a 6-week double-blind study of 90 depressed patients, mianserin 30 mg as a single dose at night was as effective as mianserin 10 mg thrice daily in relieving symptoms; both dosage regimens were significantly more effective than placebo. The incidence of drowsiness was initially higher in patients receiving mianserin at night.— R. V. Magnus, *Br. J. clin. Pract.*, 1979, *33*, 251.

See also under Absorption and Fate (above).

Depression. In a 6-week trial in 39 patients with primary depressive illness mianserin 20 mg thrice daily was as effective as amitriptyline 150 mg daily. Patients with reactive or endogenous depression responded equally well to mianserin.— A. J. Coppen and K. Ghose, *Arzneimittel-Forsch.*, 1976, *26*, 1166. See also A. J. Coppen *et al.*, *Br. J. Psychiat.*, 1976, *129*, 342.

A 6-week double-blind controlled study in 46 moderately to severely depressed hospital patients to assess the antidepressant action of mianserin; diazepam was used as the control drug. Mianserin was given initially in doses of 30 mg daily, gradually increased to 120 mg daily if necessary; when the code was broken it was found that, of 24 patients given mianserin, 18 had reached 90 to 120 mg daily. After one week of administration mianserin led to a significantly greater reduction in scores than diazepam, and a significantly larger number of those failing to improve and withdrawn from the trial were in the diazepam group. There was a tendency for those with 'endogenous' depression to respond better to mianserin than those with 'reactive' depression, but this could not be established statistically. On the other hand, symptoms of 'retarded' depression yielded significantly more readily to mianserin than symptoms of an 'anxious' depression. Mianserin also seemed to be as effective as diazepam in controlling anxiety symptoms.— G. F. M. Russell *et al.*, *Br. J. clin. Pharmac.*, 1978, *5, Suppl.* 1, 57S.

Results of a 2-week placebo-controlled study in 39 depressed in-patients confirmed that mianserin is an antidepressant. An improved sleep pattern in patients given mianserin may have been secondary to the improvement in the depressive illness, but was more likely to have been the effect of the hypnotic sedative properties of the drug, since it began from the first night of the trial.— A. H. W. Smith *et al.*, *ibid.*, 67S.

Experience in a general psychiatric practice using mianserin in doses of up to 130 mg daily in 192 out-patients. Approximately 80% of the involutional, endogenous, agitated, and reactive patients improved within the first 2 weeks, but mianserin appeared to be less successful in patients with neurotic depression. Patients receiving the highest dosages did not show more side-effects than those given less than 60 mg daily, and this applied even to the elderly patients treated.— H. Hopman, *Curr. med. Res. Opinion*, 1980, *6, Suppl.* 7, 107.

For a suggestion that clinical disadvantage may be associated with high doses of mianserin, and also that reduced doses may be more appropriate for the elderly, see under Absorption and Fate, Plasma Concentrations (above).

Phobias. Of 8 patients with severe primary obsessional illnesses treated with mianserin in a dose increasing to 20 mg thrice daily for 4 weeks, 2 were unchanged, 3 slightly improved, 2 moderately improved, and 1 greatly improved.— E. Väisänen *et al.*, *J. int. med. Res.*, 1977, *5*, 289.

Proprietary Preparations

Bolvidon *(Organon, UK).* Mianserin hydrochloride, available as tablets of 10, 20, and 30 mg.

Norval *(Bencard, UK).* Mianserin hydrochloride, available as tablets of 10, 20, and 30 mg.

NOTE. The name Norval was formerly applied to a preparation containing docusate sodium.

Other Proprietary Names

Lantanon *(Ital., S.Afr.)*; Lerivon *(Belg.)*; Tolvin *(Ger.)*; Tolvon *(Austral., Denm., Switz.)*.

2528-c

Nialamide *(B.P. 1973).* 2′-(2-Benzylcarbamoylethyl)isonicotinohydrazide.
$C_{16}H_{18}N_4O_2$=298.3.

CAS — 51-12-7.

A white, almost odourless, crystalline powder with a bitter taste. M.p. 151° to 153°. **Soluble** 1 in 400 of water, 1 in 40 of alcohol, 1 in 150 of chloroform, and 1 in 10 of methyl alcohol. **Store** in airtight containers. Protect from light.

Adverse Effects, Treatment, and Precautions. As for Phenelzine Sulphate, p.128.

Uses. Nialamide is a monoamine oxidase inhibitor with actions and uses similar to those of phenelzine (p.130). In the treatment of depression it has been given in doses of 75 to 150 mg daily. It has also been given in angina pectoris.

Preparations

Nialamide Tablets *(B.P. 1973).* Tablets containing nialamide. Protect from light.

Proprietary Names

Niamid *(Roerig, Belg.*; *Pfizer, Denm.*; *Pfizer, Spain)*; Niamide *(Pfizer, Fr.)*.

Nialamide was formerly marketed in Great Britain under the proprietary name Niamid (*Pfizer*).

2529-k

Nomifensine Maleate. 36-984; Hoe 984.

8-Amino-1,2,3,4-tetrahydro-2-methyl-4-phenylisoquinoline hydrogen maleate.
$C_{16}H_{18}N_2,C_4H_4O_4$=354.4.

CAS — 24526-64-5 (nomifensine); 32795-47-4 (maleate).

A white or slightly yellowish odourless powder. **Soluble** in dimethylformamide and methyl alcohol.

Adverse Effects. Side-effects associated with nomifensine include restlessness, insomnia, nausea, headache, dry mouth, tachycardia and palpitations, and dizziness. Fever, haemolytic anaemia, nightmares, paranoid symptoms, and drowsiness have also been reported. Susceptible patients may swing from depression to hypomania. Unlike amitriptyline, convulsions and life-threatening cardiac arrhythmias have not been a problem in overdosage.

In a comparative study of nomifensine and amitriptyline in 30 depressed patients the most frequent side-effect was drowsiness in the nomifensine group and dry mouth in the amitriptyline group. Side-effects in those patients who took nomifensine included drowsiness (the most common effect), dry mouth (9 patients), dizziness/weakness (8 patients), weight gain (5 patients), headache (4 patients), insomnia (3 patients), and hypotension (3 patients). One of the 15 patients in the nomifensine group had to discontinue therapy owing to high fever, rigor, nausea and vomiting, abnormal haematological findings (white blood cell count of 2,500), and abnormal liver function; another discontinued therapy because of intercurrent infection, the symptoms of which included frequency of micturition, dysuria, and haematuria. Five of the 15 patients in the amitriptyline group suffered constipation but none in the nomifensine group did. As therapy continued beyond the first week the relative incidence of side-effects decreased more in the nomifensine group.— J. Ananth and N. Van den Steen, *Curr. ther. Res.*, 1978, *23*, 213.

Further references.— A. Forrest *et al.*, *Br. J. clin. Pharmac.*, 1977, *4, Suppl.* 2, 215S (similar incidence of side-effects with nomifensine and imipramine); P. Grof *et al.*, *ibid.*, 221S (in contrast to those of amitriptyline, nomifensine side-effects primarily related to the depression); H. A. McClelland *et al.*, *ibid.*, 233S (similar incidence but lower severity of side-effects compared with amitriptyline).

Effects on the blood. Immune haemolytic anaemia and acute renal failure in a 50-year-old woman were associated with ingestion of nomifensine.— F. Bournerias and B. Habibi (letter), *Lancet*, 1979, *2*, 95.

Effects on the heart. Nomifensine in doses of up to 200 mg daily had no significant cardiac effects in 8 ambulant patients. Electrophysiological study of cardiac conduction in *guinea-pig* atrial preparations indicated that nomifensine has significantly less effect on cardiac activity than amitriptyline and doxepin.— G. D. Burrows *et al.*, *Med. J. Aust.*, 1978, *1*, 341. See also C. D. Burgess *et al.*, *Postgrad. med. J.*, 1979, *55*, 704.

Effects on mental state. A comparative study in healthy subjects indicated that nomifensine showed none of the subjectively pleasant effects associated with taking amphetamine.— K. Taeuber *et al.*, *Int. J. clin. Pharmac. Biopharm.*, 1979, *17*, 32.

Effects on the skin. Dermatitis in 2 of 10 patients given nomifensine for depression.— J. C. Pecknold *et al.*, *Int. J. clin. Pharmac. Biopharm.*, 1975, *11*, 304.

Epileptogenic effect. A study in photosensitive baboons suggesting that nomifensine has less epileptogenic potential than imipramine, clomipramine, and maprotiline.— M. R. Trimble *et al.*, *Br. J. clin. Pharmac.*, 1977, *4, Suppl.* 2, 101S.

Overdosage. Apart from a brief sinus tachycardia there were no untoward effects in one patient considered to have taken 1.5 g of nomifensine. The plasma-nomifensine concentration on admission to hospital was 2.780 µg per ml and the following morning 1.915 µg per ml.— S. Montgomery *et al.* (letter), *Lancet*, 1978, *1*, 828. While receiving treatment for depression a 43-year-old woman took nomifensine 3.5 g, nitrazepam 20 mg, and chlorpromazine 200 mg. On admission to hospital 4 hours later she was alert but her speech was slurred. Throughout her hospital stay she exhibited no cardiovascular, ECG, or neurological abnormality. It thus appeared that nomifensine is relatively free from cardiovascular side-effects.— J. K. Vohra *et al.* (letter), *ibid.*, 1978, *2*, 902. Details of 26 adult patients with suspected overdose with nomifensine alone or in association with other drugs, reinforced the impression that nomifensine has a low incidence of serious adverse reactions, particularly of cardiotoxicity and convulsions, when taken in overdose.— S. Dawling *et al.* (letter), *ibid.*, 1979, *1*, 56.

A report of acute haemolysis and renal failure requiring dialysis in a woman after an overdose of nomifensine and (possibly) nitrazepam and chlordiazepoxide.— L. F. Prescott *et al.*, *Br. med. J.*, 1980, *281*, 1392.

Treatment of Adverse Effects. The stomach should be emptied by aspiration and lavage. The use of activated charcoal as an adjunct to gastric lavage may be of value. Supportive therapy alone may then suffice (for general guidelines to the symptomatic therapy of drug overdosage, see Phenobarbitone, p.812).

Precautions. Nomifensine should be used with caution in patients with ischaemic heart disease. Nomifensine should be used with neuroleptics in depressed schizophrenic patients since psychosis may be activated. Manic depressive patients may switch to a manic phase and patients with suicidal tendencies should be carefully supervised during treatment. It has been recommended that nomifensine should be given in reduced doses to patients with impaired renal function and should be avoided in those with a glomerular filtration rate below 25 ml per minute. Like tricyclic antidepressants (see amitriptyline hydrochloride, p.112) nomifensine should not be given to patients receiving monoamine oxidase inhibitors or for at least 14 days after their discontinuation. Nomifensine may also interact with direct- and indirect-acting sympathomimetic agents in a pattern similar to that of amitriptyline, and may similarly diminish the effects of guanethidine and some other antihypertensive agents. It has been suggested that nomifensine should be discontinued 48 hours before elective surgery.

Although drowsiness is not considered to be an important side-effect of nomifensine, which may have an alerting effect, nevertheless patients liable to take charge of vehicles or other machinery should be warned that their judgement may be impaired, particularly at the start of therapy.

Absence of effect of single doses of nomifensine on psychomotor performance in healthy subjects.— M. -Y. Chan *et al.*, *Br. J. clin. Pharmac.*, 1980, *9*, 247. See also D. Bente *et al.*, *Arzneimittel-Forsch.*, 1976, *26*, 1120; I. Hindmarch and A. C. Parrott, *Br. J. clin. Pharmac.*, 1977, *4*, *Suppl.* 2, 167S; I. Hindmarch, *ibid.*, 175S.

For a general comment on antidepressant therapy and driving, see Amitriptyline Hydrochloride, p.112.

Interactions. A study in 3 healthy subjects suggesting that a single dose of nomifensine causes less reduction in the tyramine pressor response than an equivalent single dose of desipramine.— J. McEwen, *Br. J. clin. Pharmac.*, 1977, *4*, *Suppl.* 2, 157S.

No evidence of interaction between single doses of *clobazam* and nomifensine in healthy subjects.— W. Rupp *et al.*, *Br. J. clin. Pharmac.*, 1977, *4*, *Suppl.* 2, 143S.

Single doses of nomifensine did not appear to enhance the effect of *alcohol* in healthy subjects.— K. Taeuber, *Br. J. clin. Pharmac.*, 1977, *4*, *Suppl.* 2, 147S.

Reduced plasma concentrations of nomifensine in 6 patients also receiving anti-epileptic therapy.— S. Nawishy *et al.* (letter), *Lancet*, 1981, *2*, 871.

Absorption and Fate. Nomifensine is readily absorbed from the gastro-intestinal tract, and almost entirely excreted in the urine; only very small amounts have been detected in the faeces. Over two-thirds is excreted in the urine as the glucuronide conjugate of nomifensine and this is converted to nomifensine in acid pH. The remainder is metabolised to 4′-hydroxynomifensine (which appears to be pharmacologically active), 3′-methoxy-4′-hydroxynomifensine, and 3′-hydroxy-4′-methoxynomifensine. Other metabolites account for less than 1% of a dose.

Nomifensine is widely distributed throughout the body and is fairly extensively bound to plasma proteins. Unlike the tricyclic antidepressants it has a short plasma half-life of only about 2 hours, with only traces still detectable in the plasma 24 hours after administration.

From a study in 4 healthy subjects and from comparisons made with previous studies it was concluded that nomifensine is rapidly absorbed after oral administration. Peak plasma concentrations were achieved about 1.5 hours after dosage and the conjugate was cleared with a half-life of 1 to 2 hours.— J. Chamberlain and H. M. Hill, *Br. J. clin. Pharmac.*, 1977, *4*, *Suppl.* 2, 117S. Peak plasma concentrations of nomifensine were achieved within 1.5 to 2 hours of oral administration in healthy subjects and the plasma half-life was 1.5 to 2 hours.— W. Heptner *et al.*, *ibid.*, 123S. See also L. Vereczkey *et al.*, *Psychopharmacologia*, 1975, *45*, 225 (half-life of about 4 hours).

In 3 healthy male subjects given radioactively labelled nomifensine maleate 25 mg by mouth the peak serum radioactivity occurred 2 hours after administration. Approximately 60% was bound to serum proteins when the serum-nomifensine concentration was between 0.1 and 10 µg per ml. Serum nomifensine was present mainly as an acid-labile conjugate and was mainly excreted in the urine as a conjugate.— W. Heptner *et al.*, *Arzneimittel-Forsch.*, 1978, *28*, 58.

Isolation and identification of the conjugates of nomifensine in human urine. About 30% were conjugates of its metabolites and nearly the entire remainder was nomifensine present in conjugated form as *N*-glucuronide, which could be converted to unchanged nomifensine after acid hydrolysis.— I. Hornke *et al.*, *Br. J. clin. Pharmac.*, 1980, *9*, 255. Kinetics and metabolism of nomifensine in *animals*.— H. -M. Kellner *et al.*, *ibid.*, 1977, *4*, *Suppl.* 2, 109S.

Plasma concentrations. Studies indicated that the concentration of free nomifensine in plasma at room temperature increased with time although the total nomifensine concentration remained constant. This phenomenon was not observed in samples stored at −20°. This finding raises questions about the reliability of previously published data and could offer some explanation for the reported poor agreement between various analytical methods. For pharmacokinetic studies, where both free and conjugated nomifensine concentrations are required, plasma samples must be frozen immediately after collection to prevent hydrolysis. Failure to observe these rigorous sample handling conditions will render any plasma-drug concentration data invalid.— S. Dawling and R. Braithwaite, *J. Pharm. Pharmac.*, 1980, *32*, 304.

Uses. Nomifensine is a tetrahydroisoquinoline antidepressant. It does not have marked anticholinergic or sedative properties. It prevents the re-uptake (and hence the inactivation) of dopamine as well as that of noradrenaline, but has relatively little effect on serotonin. Its mode of action in depression is not fully understood. In the treatment of depression nomifensine is given by mouth as the maleate in doses of 50 mg twice or thrice daily initially adjusted according to response after 7 to 10 days; in some patients 200 mg daily may be required. A suggested initial dose for the elderly and other subjects known to be sensitive to the effects of psychotropic drugs is 25 mg thrice daily.

Reviews and symposia on nomifensine.— *Br. J. clin. Pharmac.*, 1977, *4*, *Suppl.* 2, 57S–248S; *Drug & Ther. Bull.*, 1978, *16*, 43; R. N. Brogden *et al.*, *Drugs*, 1979, *18*, 1.

Action. Nomifensine may release dopamine from stores, and is a potent inhibitor of dopamine and noradrenaline uptake in the brain. Pharmacologically, therefore, nomifensine slots in between the amphetamines and the secondary amine tricyclics.— P. S. J. Spencer, *Br. J. clin. Pharmac.*, 1977, *4*, *Suppl.* 2, 57S.

Administration. Widespread clinical usage has confirmed that nomifensine is a non-sedative drug. It is therefore not suitable for administration as a single evening dose and we recommend that the last dose is given no later than 5 p.m. In certain patients co-prescription of a hypnotic may be desirable.— W. Bogie, *Hoechst* (letter), *Pharm. J.*, 1979, *2*, 73.

Administration in renal failure. Results suggesting that nomifensine is retained in the plasma of patients with impaired renal function. In this respect nomifensine seems to be different from the tricyclic compounds but similar to lithium. Nomifensine is probably not eliminated by non-renal routes, nor is it dialysable. It is suggested that nomifensine should not be given to patients with a glomerular filtration rate of less than 25 ml per minute.— S. Ringoir *et al.*, *Br. J. clin. Pharmac.*, 1977, *4*, *Suppl.* 2, 129S. Comments, including the view that reduced doses could be given at normal time intervals or normal doses at less frequent intervals, in patients with diminished creatinine clearance, but exceeding 50 ml per minute. A suggestion that the free base but not the conjugate might be dialysable.— *ibid.*, 133S and 134S.

Depression. Marked clinical improvement occurred in 7 of 8 patients with depression given nomifensine 100 to 200 mg daily for 3 weeks. No significant cardiological side-effects were seen in any patient. In 5 of the patients receiving 100 mg daily a mean plasma-total nomifensine concentration of 176 ng per ml occurred after 3 weeks.— G. D. Burrows *et al.*, *Med. J. Aust.*, 1978, *1*, 341.

For a comment on the problems in determining plasma concentrations of nomifensine, see under Absorption and Fate, Plasma Concentrations (above).

Further references to nomifensine in depression.— A. Forrest *et al.*, *Br. J. clin. Pharmac.*, 1977, *4*, *Suppl.* 2, 215S (comparison with imipramine); P. Grof *et al.*, *ibid.*, 221S (comparison with amitriptyline); H. A. McClelland *et al.*, *ibid.*, 233S (comparison with amitriptyline); J. Moizeszowicz and S. Subirá, *J. clin. Pharmac.*, 1977, *17*, 81 (comparison with viloxazine in the elderly); M. M. Amin *et al.*, *Psychopharmac. Bull.*, 1978, *14*, 37 (comparison with imipramine); J. Ananth and N. Van der Steen, *Curr. ther. Res.*, 1978, *23*, 213 (comparison with amitriptyline).

Diagnostic use. A single administration of nomifensine 200 mg by mouth, an antidepressant drug which blocks dopamine re-uptake, permits a clear-cut differentiation between individuals with and without pituitary microadenomas. More than 70 patients with hyperprolactinaemia have been successfully treated in this way.— E. E. Müller *et al.* (letter), *Lancet*, 1979, *2*, 257. A note of caution as to the value of nomifensine as a diagnostic tool in the investigation of hyperprolactinaemic states.— M. J. Dunne *et al.* (letter), *ibid.*, 1243.

Further references to the diagnostic use of nomifensine in pituitary adenoma.— A. R. Genazzani *et al.*, *Acta endocr., Copenh.*, 1980, *93*, 139.

Parkinsonism. Evidence of moderate benefit with nomifensine in doses of up to 200 mg daily in Parkinson's disease. Of 29 patients in the study, 3 were previously untreated and 26 continued their levodopa and/or other antiparkinsonian therapy. Moderate improvement was noted in tremor, facial expression, and finger flexion. The young fared better than the elderly and side-effects were fairly frequent, the most common being involuntary movements similar to those associated with levodopa therapy, and generally occurring in those concomitantly receiving levodopa. Six patients complained of insomnia, 5 of nausea, and 5 of headaches. One woman experienced dramatic motor phenomena when her dose reached 200 mg daily; a man on 200 mg daily suffered from agitation, restlessness, confusion, and episodes of deep rapid breathing, most marked about 20 minutes after his divided dose; another woman felt unwell, 'fumbly' and unable to walk about an hour after a dose; and another man experienced involuntary movements 30 minutes after taking a dose.— D. M. Park *et al.*, *Br. J. clin. Pharmac.*, 1977, *4*, *Suppl.* 2, 185S. See also P. F. Teychenne *et al.*, *J. Neurol. Neurosurg. Psychiat.*, 1976, *39*, 1219.

Addition of nomifensine 150 mg daily did not benefit 8 patients who failed or ceased to respond to levodopa, or who had developed the 'on-off' phenomenon. Three of the 8 patients reported slight subjective improvement in disability, but this was not confirmed objectively. Depression in 2 pathologically depressed patients was not cured. There were no side-effects other than low lumbar backache during treatment which was reversible on discontinuation.— P. Bedard *et al.*, *Br. J. clin. Pharmac.*, 1977, *4*, *Suppl.* 2, 187S.

Proprietary Preparations

Merital *(Hoechst, UK)*. Nomifensine maleate, available as capsules of 25 and 50 mg. (Also available as Merital in *S.Afr.*).

Other Proprietary Names

Alival *(Belg., Denm., Fr., Ger., Neth., Switz.)*; Anametrin *(Port.)*; Hostalival *(Arg.)*; Merival *(Thai.)*; Psicronizer *(Ital.)*.

2530-w

Nortriptyline Hydrochloride. B.P., U.S.P.;

3-(10,11-Dihydro-5*H*-dibenzo [*a,d*]cyclohepten-5-ylidene)-*N*-methylpropylamine hydrochloride.
$C_{19}H_{21}N,HCl = 299.8$.

CAS — 72-69-5 (nortriptyline); 894-71-3 (hydrochloride).

Pharmacopoeias. In *Br.*, *Cz.*, *Nord.*, and *U.S.*

A white or off-white powder with a slight characteristic odour and a burning bitter taste followed by a sensation of numbness. M.p. 215° to 220° with a range of not more than 3°. Nortriptyline hydrochloride 22.8 mg is approximately equivalent to 20 mg of nortriptyline.

Soluble 1 in 50 of water, 1 in 10 of alcohol, and 1 in 5 of chloroform; sparingly soluble in methyl alcohol; practically insoluble in ether and most other organic solvents. A 1% solution in water has a pH of about 5. **Store** in airtight containers. Protect from light.

Adverse Effects. As for Amitriptyline Hydrochloride, p.110.

Effects on the heart. Reports on ECG changes associated with therapeutic doses of nortriptyline.— V. E. Ziegler *et al.*, *Am. J. Psychiat.*, 1977, *134*, 441; D. J. E. Taylor and R. A. Braithwaite, *Br. Heart J.*, 1978, *40*, 1005.

Pregnancy and the neonate. For studies indicating absence of teratogenicity of tricyclic antidepressants, see Amitriptyline Hydrochloride, p.113.

Individual reports of malformations in the infants of women receiving nortriptyline.— G. M. Bourke (letter), *Lancet*, 1974, *1*, 98.

The neonate. Urinary retention in a newborn infant was attributed to maternal ingestion of nortriptyline 25 mg four times daily.— W. T. Shearer *et al.*, *J. Pediat.*, 1972, *81*, 570.

Treatment of Adverse Effects. As for Amitriptyline Hydrochloride, p.111.

Activated charcoal. In 6 healthy volunteers given nortriptyline 75 mg peak plasma concentrations of nortriptyline were reduced by 77% when a sachet of activated charcoal (Medicoal) was given 30 minutes later, by 37% when given 2 hours later, and by 19% when given 4 hours later. Medicoal might be useful in the treatment of poisoning by tricyclic antidepressants when given in addition to gastric lavage.— S. Dawling *et al.*, *Eur. J. clin. Pharmac.*, 1978, *14*, 445. See also P. Crome *et al.*, *Lancet*, 1977, *2*, 1203.

See also Amitriptyline Hydrochloride, p.112.

Dialysis and haemoperfusion. Charcoal haemoperfusion did not remove significant amounts of nortriptyline in one patient being treated for nortriptyline poisoning.— B. M. Iversen *et al.* (letter), *Lancet*, 1978, *1*, 388. Evidence of benefit in tricyclic poisoning.— R. S. Pedersen *et al.* (letter), *ibid.*, 719. See also *idem*., 1980, *1*, 154.

For further discussion on the merits of charcoal haemoperfusion, see Amitriptyline Hydrochloride, p.112.

Precautions. As for Amitriptyline Hydrochloride, p.112.

For a general comment on antidepressant therapy and driving, see Amitriptyline Hydrochloride, p.112.

Interactions. Studies in *rats* indicated that nortriptyline inhibited the activity of hepatic microsomal drug-metabolising enzymes.— E. S. Vesell *et al.*, *New Engl. J. Med.*, 1970, *283*, 1484.

When *perphenazine* was given concomitantly with nortriptyline the urinary excretion of nortriptyline was decreased, plasma concentrations of nortriptyline were increased and plasma concentrations of metabolites of nortriptyline were decreased. Clinical signs of the interaction have not been reported.— L. F. Gram and K. F. Overø, *Br. med. J.*, 1972, *1*, 463.

In 9 patients taking nortriptyline there was no evidence of variation in the plasma concentrations of nortriptyline when the benzodiazepines *chlordiazepoxide, diazepam, nitrazepam*, or *oxazepam* were added to their treatment.— G. Silverman and R. A. Braithwaite, *Br. med. J.*, 1973, *3*, 18.

Six epileptic patients stabilised on *anticonvulsant* therapy for at least 3 months were given nortriptyline 25 mg thrice daily for 4 weeks and blood estimations carried out during each week. Blood concentrations of nortriptyline were significantly lower in these patients than in other groups. Suitable adjustment should be made to dosage to allow for the effects of induction of hepatic enzymes.— R. A. Braithwaite *et al.* (letter), *Br. J. clin. Pharmac.*, 1975, *2*, 469. See also under Amitriptyline Hydrochloride, p.112.

For the effect of nortriptyline on *dicoumarol*, see Dicoumarol, p.771.

Pregnancy and the neonate. The plasma half-lives of nortriptyline were 17 and 56 hours respectively in a mother who had taken an overdose on the day before delivery and in the child. High concentrations of the metabolite 10-hydroxynortriptyline were found in the infant's urine during the first and fourth days of life.— F. Sjöqvist *et al.*, *J. Pediat.*, 1972, *80*, 496.

Absorption and Fate. Nortriptyline is the principal active metabolite of amitriptyline. For an account of its metabolism, see Amitriptyline Hydrochloride, p.113.

Nortriptyline has been reported to have a longer plasma half-life than that of amitriptyline.

There was a significant first-pass effect after administration of nortriptyline by mouth, with rapid appearance of 10-hydroxynortriptyline.— G. Alvan *et al.*, *Eur. J. clin. Pharmac.*, 1977, *11*, 219. See also G. Alvan, *Clin. Pharmacokinet.*, 1978, *3*, 155.

Comment on slow hydroxylators of nortriptyline and a report of a woman who could not tolerate more than 20 mg at night.— L. Bertilisson *et al.* (letter), *Lancet*, 1981, *1*, 560.

Plasma concentrations. A study of plasma-nortriptyline concentrations and therapeutic response in 18 depressed out-patients supported the finding that the antidepressant effect of nortriptyline deteriorates at higher plasma concentrations. After 6 weeks of treatment 9 patients with mean plasma-nortriptyline concentrations between 50 and 139 ng per ml had a response that was significantly better than 9 whose mean concentrations were between 140 and 260 ng per ml. The lower limit of the therapeutic range was not tested.— V. E. Ziegler *et al.*, *Clin. Pharmac. Ther.*, 1976, *20*, 458. See also F. Kragh-Sorensen *et al.*, *Psychopharmacologia*, 1976, *45*, 305. In 18 patients with moderate to severe endogenous depression given nortriptyline 100 mg each night for 4 weeks those with steady-state plasma-nortriptyline concentrations below 200 ng per ml and a fast clearance of nortriptyline showed a significantly better clinical response than those with concentrations above this value and slower clearance rates.— S. Montgomery *et al.*, *Clin. Pharmac. Ther.*, 1978, *23*, 309.

In 3 patients with depression given nortriptyline 100 mg daily for at least 2 weeks mean serial steady-state plasma-nortriptyline concentrations of 65.1, 74.3, and 125.6 ng per ml respectively occurred. In a fourth patient receiving 150 mg of the drug daily a mean steady-state plasma-nortriptyline concentration of 150.7 ng per ml occurred.— V. E. Ziegler *et al.*, *J. pharm. Sci.*, 1978, *67*, 554.

Further reports, studies, and comments on the relevance of plasma concentrations of nortriptyline, and on factors, such as age, sex, and race, which might influence this.— G. D. Burrows *et al.*, *Psychol. Med.*, 1977, *7*, 87 (clinical response); A. C. Carr and R. P. Hobson (letter), *Br. med. J.*, 1977, *2*, 1151 (age); J. F. Giudicelli and J. P. Tillement, *Clin. Pharmacokinet.*, 1977, *2*, 157 (sex; review); T. R. Norman *et al.*, *Clin. Pharmac. Ther.*, 1977, *21*, 453 (smoking); V. E. Ziegler *et al.*, *Am. J. Psychiat.*, 1977, *134*, 441 (cardiac effects); S. Nakano and L. E. Hollister, *Clin. Pharmac. Ther.*, 1978, *23*, 199 (circadian rhythm); B. Sørensen *et al.*, *Psychopharmacology*, 1978, *59*, 35 (practical significance); R. A. Braithwaite *et al.*, *Br. J. clin. Pharmac.*, 1980, *9*, 306P (age); S. Dawling *et al.*, *Clin. Pharmacokinet.*, 1980, *5*, 394 (age); P. Kragh-Sørensen and N. -E. Larsen, *Clin. Pharmac. Ther.*, 1980, *28*, 796 (age); K. Reed *et al.*, *Am. J. Psychiat.*, 1980, *137*, 986 (age).

Uses. Nortriptyline is a tricyclic antidepressant with actions and uses similar to those of amitriptyline (p.113). It is the principal active metabolite of amitriptyline.

In the treatment of depression nortriptyline is given by mouth as the hydrochloride in doses equivalent to nortriptyline 10 mg three or four times daily initially, gradually increased to 25 mg four times daily as necessary. A suggested initial dose for adolescents and the elderly is 10 mg thrice daily. Inappropriately high plasma concentrations of nortriptyline have been associated with deterioration in antidepressent response. Since nortriptyline has a prolonged half-life, once-daily dosage regimens are also suitable, usually given at night.

Administration. Effective plasma-nortriptyline concentrations were considered to lie within the range 50 to 150 ng per ml; higher concentrations were less effective. Eleven of 14 depressed patients with nortriptyline concentrations in this range responded to treatment compared with 2 of 22 with higher concentrations. Routine measurement of plasma concentrations was recommended.— S. A. Montgomery *et al.*, *Br. med. J.*, 1977, *2*, 166. In a study of 20 patients with endogenous depression, plasma concentrations of nortriptyline were determined 24, 48, and 72 hours after a single 100 mg dose. The patients were then given 100 mg at night and the steady-state plasma concentrations determined after 4 weeks. Good correlation was obtained between the steady-state plasma concentrations and the 24- and 48-hour plasma concentrations, and it was suggested that these determinations could be used to adjust individual dosage requirements so that steady-state plasma concentrations are in the optimum range for therapeutic effect (50 to 200 ng per ml).— S. A. Montgomery *et al.*, *Clin. Pharmacokinet.*, 1979, *14*, 129. See also under Absorption and Fate (Plasma Concentrations).

A means of predicting nortriptyline dosage requirements following administration of a single dose.— R. A. Braithwaite *et al.*, *Clin. Pharmac. Ther.*, 1978, *23*, 303. See also *idem*., *Postgrad. med. J.*, 1980, *56*, *Suppl.* 1, 112.

Studies and comments on once-daily administration of nortriptyline.— V. E. Ziegler *et al.*, *Archs gen. Psychiat.*, 1977, *34*, 613; I. H. Stevenson and A. A. Schiff (letter), *Br. med. J.*, 1977, *2*, 579; J. L. Nielsen, *Neuropsychobiology*, 1980, *6*, 48; J. H. Pedersen and J. L. Sørensen, *ibid.*, 42.

Administration in renal failure. Nortriptyline can be given in usual doses to patients with renal failure. Concentrations of nortriptyline were not affected by haemodialysis or peritoneal dialysis.— W. M. Bennett *et al.*, *Ann. intern. Med.*, 1977, *86*, 754. See also *idem*., 1980, *93*, 286.

Depression. For a general review of the role of tricyclic antidepressants in depression, see Amitriptyline Hydrochloride, p.114.

Nausea and vomiting. The incidence, severity, and duration of nausea and vomiting was reduced in patients with breast cancer receiving antineoplastic agents when they were given fluphenazine 1.5 mg and nortriptyline 30 mg daily for 5 days. Fluphenazine alone, cyclizine, metoclopramide, or placebo were not effective.— C. Morran *et al.*, *Br. med. J.*, 1979, *1*, 1323.

Urticaria. Nortriptyline 25 mg thrice daily was given to 12 patients with urticarial wheals or dermographism for 4 weeks and a placebo was given for a further 4 weeks. Ten patients improved when taking nortriptyline, but not when taking the placebo. There was dramatic improvement in 3 of 4 with dermographism. Maintenance with nortriptyline was necessary for continued control of urticaria.— W. N. Morley, *Br. J. clin. Pract.*, 1969, *23*, 305.

Preparations

Nortriptyline Capsules *(B.P.).* Capsules containing nortriptyline hydrochloride. Potency is expressed in terms of the equivalent amount of nortriptyline. Store at a temperature not exceeding 30°.

Nortriptyline Hydrochloride Capsules *(U.S.P.).* Capsules containing nortriptyline hydrochloride. Potency is expressed in terms of the equivalent amount of nortriptyline. The *U.S.P.* requires 85% dissolution in 30 minutes. Store in airtight containers.

Nortriptyline Hydrochloride Oral Solution *(U.S.P.).* Nortriptyline Hydrochloride Solution. A solution containing nortriptyline hydrochloride, with alcohol 3 to 5%. Potency is expressed in terms of the equivalent amount of nortriptyline. pH 2.5 to 4. Store in airtight containers. Protect from light.

Nortriptyline Tablets *(B.P.).* Nortriptyline Hydrochloride Tablets. Tablets containing nortriptyline hydrochloride. They are film-coated. Potency is expressed in terms of the equivalent amount of nortriptyline.

Proprietary Preparations

Allegron *(Dista, UK).* Nortriptyline hydrochloride, available as tablets each containing the equivalent of 10 mg (unscored) and 25 mg (scored) of nortriptyline. (Also available as Allegron in *Austral., Belg.*).

Aventyl *(Lilly, UK).* Nortriptyline hydrochloride, available as **Liquid** containing in each 5 ml the equivalent of 10 mg of nortriptyline (suggested diluent, syrup) and as **Capsules** each containing the equivalent of 10 or 25 mg of nortriptyline. (Also available as Aventyl in *Austral., Canad., S.Afr., USA*).

Motipress *(Squibb, UK).* Tablets each containing nortriptyline hydrochloride equivalent to 30 mg of nortriptyline and fluphenazine hydrochloride 1.5 mg. For anxiety states and depression. *Dose.* 1 tablet daily, before retiring.

Motival *(Squibb, UK).* Tablets each containing nortriptyline hydrochloride equivalent to nortriptyline 10 mg and fluphenazine hydrochloride 500 μg. For anxiety states and depression. *Dose.* 1 tablet 2 to 4 times daily.

Other Proprietary Names

Arg.—Ateben, Kareon; *Austral.*—Nortab; *Belg.*—Nortrilen; *Denm.*—Sensival; *Fr.*—Altilev, Psychostyl; *Ger.*—Nortrilen; *Ital.*—Noritren, Vividyl; *Jap.*—Sensival; *Norw.*—Noritren; *S.Afr.*—Nortrilin; *Spain*— Martimil, Paxtibi; *Swed.*—Noritren, Sensaval; *Switz.*—Nortrilen, Sensival; *USA*—Pamelor.

2531-e

Noxiptyline Hydrochloride. Bay 1521; Dibenzoxine Hydrochloride; Noxiptiline Hydrochloride. 10,11-Dihydro-5*H*-dibenzo[*a,d*]cyclohepten-5-one *O*-(2-dimethylaminoethyl)oxime hydrochloride.
$C_{19}H_{22}N_2O,HCl=330.9$.

CAS — 3362-45-6 (noxiptyline); 4985-15-3 (hydrochloride).

A white crystalline powder.

Adverse Effects, Treatment, and Precautions. As for Amitriptyline Hydrochloride, p.110.

For a general comment on antidepressant therapy and driving, see Amitriptyline Hydrochloride, p.112.

Uses. Noxiptyline is a tricyclic antidepressant with actions and uses similar to those of amitriptyline (p.113).

In the treatment of depression noxiptyline has been given by mouth as the hydrochloride in doses of 10 to 150 mg daily; in hospital patients up to 200 mg daily has been given. In the initial stages of treatment if administration by mouth has been impracticable or inadvisable 25 to 50 mg of the hydrochloride has been given intramuscularly once or twice daily.

Nornoxiptyline has also been tried as an antidepressant.

References to noxiptyline: K. Heinrich and G. Herrman, *Arzneimittel-Forsch.*, 1971, *21*, 602; U. Spiegelberg *et al.*, *ibid.*, 609; E. Schmid-Claudy and R. Schmid-Claudy, *ibid.*, 628; J. Angst *et al.*, *ibid.*, 635; P. Berner *et al.*, *ibid.*, 638; D. Bente *et al.*, *ibid.*, 1973, *23*, 247; D. Bente *et al.*, *ibid.*, 1974, *24*, 205.

References to noxiptyline and nornoxiptyline: L. Rosenberg, *Arzneimittel-Forsch.*, 1971, *21*, 207.

Proprietary Names

Agedal *(Dolorgiet, Ger.*; *Bayer, Ital.)*; Nogédal *(Thérаplix, Fr.)*.

2532-l

Opipramol Hydrochloride. G 33040. 2-{4-[3-(5*H*-Dibenz[*b,f*]azepin-5-yl)propyl]piperazin-1-yl}ethanol dihydrochloride.

$C_{23}H_{29}N_3O,2HCl=436.4$.

CAS — 315-72-0 (opipramol); 909-39-7 (hydrochloride).

A light yellow, crystalline powder which develops a reddish tinge on prolonged exposure to light. M.p. about 210° with decomposition.

Very **soluble** in water; soluble in alcohol; practically insoluble in acetone.

Adverse Effects, Treatment, and Precautions. As for Amitriptyline Hydrochloride, p.110.

For a general comment on antidepressant therapy and driving, see Amitriptyline Hydrochloride, p.112.

Overdosage. Sudden and unexpected death occurred in a child weighing 9 kg about 18 hours after ingestion of 1 g of opipramol, despite an apparent recovery from the initial coma. Of 18 reported instances of overdosage with opipramol, 6 had been fatal and 4 of these had been attributed to sudden cardiac arrest.— C. A. Fuge (letter), *Br. med. J.*, 1967, *4*, 108.

Uses. Opipramol is a tricyclic antidepressant with general properties similar to those of amitriptyline (p.113). Opipramol hydrochloride has been given in doses of 150 to 300 mg daily, either in divided doses throughout the day or with the major part given at night.

Proprietary Names

Ensidon *(Geigy, Swed.)*; Insidon *(Geigy, Austral.*; *Geigy, Belg.*; *Geigy, Denm.*; *Geigy, Eire*; *Geigy, Fr.*; *Geigy, Ger.*; *Geigy, Ital.*; *Geigy, Neth.*; *Geigy, Norw.*; *Ciba-Geigy, Switz.)*; Nisidana *(Padro, Spain)*.

Opipramol hydrochloride was formerly marketed in Great Britain under the proprietary name Insidon *(Geigy)*.

2533-y

Phenelzine Sulphate *(B.P.)*. Phenelzine Sulfate *(U.S.P.)*. Phenethylhydrazine hydrogen sulphate.

$C_8H_{12}N_2,H_2SO_4=234.3$.

CAS — 51-71-8 (phenelzine); 156-51-4 (sulphate).

Pharmacopoeias. In *Br.* and *U.S.*

A white or yellowish-white powder or pearly platelets with a pungent odour and a characteristic taste. M.p. 164° to 168°. Phenelzine 15 mg is approximately equivalent to 25 mg of phenelzine sulphate. **Soluble** 1 in 7 of water; practically insoluble in alcohol, chloroform, and ether. A 1% solution has a pH of 1.4 to 1.9. **Store** in a cool place in airtight containers. Protect from light.

Adverse Effects. Adverse effects commonly associated with phenelzine and other monoamine oxidase inhibitors include postural hypotension and attacks of dizziness. Other common side-effects include drowsiness, weakness and fatigue, dryness of mouth, constipation and other gastro-intestinal disturbances (including nausea and vomiting), and oedema. Agitation and tremors, insomnia and restless sleep, blurred vision, difficulty in micturition, convulsions, skin rashes, leucopenia, sexual disturbances, and weight gain with inappropriate appetite may also occur. Psychotic episodes, with hypomanic behaviour, confusion, and hallucinations, may be induced in susceptible persons. Jaundice has been reported and, on rare occasions, fatal progressive hepatocellular necrosis. Peripheral neuropathies associated with the hydrazine derivatives may be due to pyridoxine deficiency.

Symptoms of overdosage may not occur for some hours after ingestion. They include agitation with hyperactivity and hallucinations, tachycardia, hypertension sometimes with severe headache (hypotension may also develop), hyperreflexia and spasticity, profuse sweating and hyperthermia (hypothermia may also develop), dilated pupils, urinary retention, coma, convulsions, and signs of peripheral collapse.

Severe hypertensive reactions, sometimes fatal, may occur if a monoamine oxidase inhibitor is given simultaneously with some other drugs or cheese and certain other foods (see Precautions). These reactions are characterised by severe headache, a rapid and sometimes prolonged rise in blood pressure followed by intracranial haemorrhage or acute cardiac failure.

Concern about an apparent increase in the prescribing of monoamine oxidase inhibitors. In the year ended September 1977, 35 of 119 clients who contacted the St Albans Drug Information and Advisory Service with drug problems, had crises arising out of the use of monoamine oxidase inhibitors; at least 4 of these crises were fatal. Problems also occurred with the action of the monoamine oxidase inhibitors themselves; these included withdrawal symptoms with some.— S. P. Wright (letter), *Lancet*, 1978, *1*, 284.

Effects on the blood. Phenelzine has been reported to cause aplastic anaemia.— R. H. Girdwood, *Drugs*, 1976, *11*, 394.

Effects on the endocrine system. Galactorrhoea occurred in a woman taking phenelzine 30 mg thrice daily for 3 months.— M. Segal and R. F. Heys (letter), *Br. med. J.*, 1969, *4*, 236. See also H. Arroyo, *Presse méd.*, 1966, *74*, 1764.

For the elevation of plasma-prolactin concentration by monoamine oxidase inhibitors, see Clorgyline Hydrochloride, p.116.

Effects on the liver. Jaundice developed in 4 patients on 6 occasions following the administration of monoamine oxidase inhibitors. The drugs implicated were as follows: phenelzine 6.3 g over 5 months; pheniprazine, 2.5 g over 7 months, 560 mg over 60 days, 1.5 g—no time stated; nialamide 1.6 g over 3 weeks; iproniazid—no dose or time stated.— C. D. Holdsworth *et al.*, *Lancet*, 1961, *2*, 621.

A mention of 2 patients with hepatic failure, progressing to encephalopathy, attributed to a hypersensitivity reaction after administration of monoamine oxidase inhibitors.— S. P. Wilkinson *et al.*, *Br. med. J.*, 1974, *1*, 186.

Angiosarcoma of the liver in a 64-year-old woman who had taken phenelzine for 6 years was possibly drug-related; such a relationship had been reported in *mice*.— T. K. Daneshmend *et al.*, *Br. med. J.*, 1979, *1*, 1679.

Phenelzine is a substituted hydrazine; for a review of the hepatotoxicity of another substituted phenylhydrazine, see Isoniazid, p.1572.

Effects on mental state. Psychosis developed in a chronically depressed 30-year-old woman after she had received phenelzine for 21 days and regressed within 48 hours of stopping phenelzine.— L. M. Sheehy and J. S. Maxmen, *Am. J. Psychiat.*, 1978, *135*, 1422.

Effects on sexual function. Reversible ejaculatory impairment in one man receiving phenelzine and orgasmic and ejaculatory incompetence in a second.— M. S. Rapp, *Am. J. Psychiat.*, 1979, *136*, 1200. Orgasmic inhibition in a woman receiving phenelzine.— J. L. Barton, *ibid.*, 1616.

Spermatogenesis. A review of drugs associated with male infertility. Monoamine oxidase inhibitors produce an initial transient increase in the sperm count, but this is followed by a profound drop almost to azoospermic levels, with a high percentage of abnormal cells. These antidepressants (including phenelzine, isocarboxazid, and tranylcypromine) may also cause impotence, and should not therefore be used in sexually active men who want children.— B. H. Stewart, *Drug Ther.*, 1975, *156*, 42.

Lupus. A reversible lupus-like reaction developed in a 66-year-old woman who had been taking phenelzine sulphate for 8 months.— C. Swartz, *J. Am. med. Ass.*, 1978, *239*, 2693.

Weight gain. In patients receiving monoamine oxidase inhibitors for phobias, a troublesome problem was excessive weight gain due to a craving for carbohydrates produced by the antidepressants.— D. Kelly *et al.*, *Br. J. Psychiat.*, 1970, *116*, 387.

Treatment of Adverse Effects. The stomach should be emptied by aspiration and lavage. Supportive therapy should be instituted (for general guidelines to the symptomatic therapy of drug overdosage, see Phenobarbitone, p.812), special care being taken with any drug therapy, in view of the many hazards of monoamine oxidase inhibitor interactions. In particular, metaraminol and other sympathomimetic agents are not suitable for the treatment of hypotension, which should be managed with intravenous fluids and, in severe shock, intravenous hydrocortisone.

Chlorpromazine is indicated for restlessness and agitation, and also to combat hyperthermia unresponsive to mechanical cooling. Morphine, pethidine and other narcotic analgesics should be avoided.

Hypertensive crises associated with monoamine oxidase inhibitor overdosage or with a food or drug interaction, should be treated urgently with slow intravenous injection of phentolamine mesylate 5 to 10 mg, repeated as necessary, or followed by an intravenous infusion of phenoxybenzamine 100 mg in 200 ml of 5% dextrose solution, given over 90 minutes. Pentolinium has also been recommended, and chlorpromazine or tolazoline may be of value if more effective treatments are not available. It has been suggested that haemodialysis may be of value in very severely poisoned patients.

The acute effects of monoamine oxidase inhibitor overdosage may be followed by the delayed effects of monoamine oxidase inhibition which do not develop until several days later.

Precautions. Phenelzine and other monoamine oxidase inhibitors should not be given to patients with liver disease or blood dyscrasias, or, because of their effects on blood pressure, to patients with cerebrovascular disease or phaeochromocytoma. They should be avoided or only used with great caution in patients with cardiovascular disease; masking of pain may occur in those with angina pectoris. Monoamine oxidase inhibitors should similarly be avoided or used with great caution in elderly or agitated patients or those with diminished renal function, who may be particularly susceptible to their adverse effects. They should be given with caution in epileptic patients since they may influence the incidence of seizures and affect anticonvulsant requirements; they may also affect insulin requirements in diabetic subjects.

Monoamine oxidase inhibitors may activate psychosis in susceptible patients and manic-depressive patients may switch to a manic phase; patients with suicidal tendencies should be carefully supervised during treatment.

Monoamine oxidase inhibitors have a prolonged action so patients should not take any of the foods or drugs known to cause reactions (see below) for at least 14 days after stopping treatment. A similar drug-free period should elapse before any patient undergoes surgery since it may involve the use of agents which can interact with monoamine oxidase inhibitors. Patients should carry cards giving details of their monoamine oxidase inhibitor therapy; they and their relatives should be fully conversant with the implications of food and drug interactions and the precautions to be taken.

Patients liable to take charge of vehicles or other machinery should be warned that monoamine oxidase inhibitors may modify behaviour and state of alertness.

For a general comment on antidepressant therapy and driving, see Amitriptyline Hydrochloride, p.112.

Interference with diagnostic tests. Abnormally low values of urinary 4-hydroxy-3-methoxymandelic acid and abnormally high values of urinary metadrenaline found in patients given monoamine oxidase inhibitors could affect adrenal medullary tests for phaeochromocytoma.— *Adverse Drug React. Bull.*, 1972, June, 104. See also *Drug & Ther. Bull.*, 1972, *10*, 69.

Pregnancy and the neonate. The use of monoamine oxidase inhibitors, including isocarboxazid, should be avoided during the first trimester of pregnancy unless absolutely necessary. There was no evidence of teratogenicity but they might be incompatible with drugs used during the management of labour or abortion, and their use might cause anxiety in mothers concerned about possible damage to their unborn children.— *Br. med. J.*, 1976, *1*, 1524.

In a study in 836 infants with congenital malformations there was no significant difference in the maternal usage of monoamine oxidase inhibitors during the first trimester of pregnancy compared with the use in 836 controls.— G. Greenberg *et al.*, *Br. med. J.*, 1977, *2*, 853.

Withdrawal. A patient experienced severe headache and intense cold after stopping phenelzine; another patient experienced cold. A possible similarity to the 'cold turkey' phenomenon of opiate withdrawal was suggested.— B. Pitt (letter), *Br. med. J.*, 1974, *2*, 332. Some monoamine oxidase inhibitors produce withdrawal symptoms.— S. P. Wright (letter), *Lancet*, 1978, *1*, 284.

Reactions to foods rich in pressor amines can occur in patients being treated with monoamine oxidase inhibitors, producing hypertensive crises due to the inhibition of the metabolism of the amines and enhancement of their pressor activity. Cheese, especially Cheddar cheese, hydrolysed protein extracts such as Marmite which contain tyramine, and broad bean pods which contain levodopa have caused such reactions. Game and alcoholic beverages such as Chianti which contain tyramine may also cause reactions. Any protein-containing food subject to hydrolysis and fermentation or spoilage could contain tyramine derived from tyrosine. Foods such as liver or pickled herrings that have been improperly stored may cause reactions. It is recommended that patients should be warned not to eat any of these foods while being treated with a monoamine oxidase inhibitor.

Interactions with foods. A discussion of the interactions between monoamine oxidase inhibitors and foodstuffs and drugs with indications of those combinations which are prohibited and those for which careful control is necessary. It has been estimated that 10 mg of tyramine needs to be ingested to produce a reaction. Headache without rise in blood pressure has been attributed to histamine, the metabolism of which is also inhibited by MAOIs.— A. J. Boakes, *Prescribers' J.*, 1971, *11*, 109. See also I. H. Stockley, *Pharm. J.*, 1973, *1*, 590; *Med. Lett.*, 1976, *18*, 32.

A review of interactions between monoamine oxidase inhibitors, amines, and foodstuffs with a detailed analysis of the amine content of many foods.— E. Marley and B. Blackwell, in *Advances in Pharmacology and Chemotherapy*, S. Garattini *et al.* (Eds), Vol. 8, London, Academic Press, 1970, pp. 185–239.

Evidence that phenelzine is a weak inhibitor of hepatic microsomal mixed function oxidase, which may provide an important source of interaction in some patients.— S. E. Smith *et al.*, *Br. J. clin. Pharmac.*, 1980, *9*, 21.

For reports of interactions with serotonin, see below, under Reactions to other Drugs (Interactions).

Analysis of various cheeses and other foods and beverages showed that tyramine was present in greatest amounts in (New York State) *Cheddar cheese*, 1.416 mg per g. As little as 20 g of Cheddar cheese eaten by patients treated with the monoamine oxidase inhibitor pargyline could induce a pressor response. *Chianti wine*, in which 25.4 µg of tyramine per ml was found, could easily provoke symptoms if taken in amounts sufficient to produce mild alcoholic intoxication.— D. Horwitz *et al.*, *J. Am. med. Ass.*, 1964, *188*, 1108. A further study on the analysis and significance of tyramine in 28 varieties of *cheeses*, 15 varieties of *wines* and *beers*, and in several other foodstuffs. Many of the cheeses studied contained a large amount of tyramine (up to 2.1 mg per gram); the concentration of tyramine varied widely in different varieties of Cheddar cheese and other varieties of cheese. For the alcoholic drinks, 2 varieties of Chianti and most of the beers contained appreciable amounts of tyramine. Three of the 5 yeast extracts contained very large amounts of tyramine (up to 2.2 mg per gram); moreover, yeast extracts are reported to contain large amounts of histamine which can release catecholamines from the adrenal medulla, thus causing a secondary pressor response. Although histamine is easily metabolised in the body by histaminase or inactivated by methylation, these enzymes are also inactivated by MAO inhibitors.— N. P. Sen, *J. Food Sci.*, 1969, *34*, 22. The histamine content of a number of *wines*.— E. R. Trethewie (letter), *Med. J. Aust.*, 1979, *1*, 94.

Isolated reports have implicated a number of foods such as *pickled herrings, yogurt, soya sauce, nuts, high protein foods* such as *Complan*, and tinned and packet *soups* in MAOI interactions, and in some of these the adverse effects may have been due to tyramine from degraded protein formed during storage. *Banana peel* contained significant amounts of tyramine, 65 µg per g, and small amounts were present in *raspberries* and *avocados;* there was little evidence that over-ripe fruits might be dangerous although headache had been reported following the consumption of rotten bananas. *Fresh cream* and *chocolate* were not likely to provoke reactions.— M. M. Stewart, *Adverse Drug React. Bull.*, 1976, Jun., 200. Analysis of the tyramine content of some *canned* and *packet soups*. Calculations gave concentrations of less than 2 and 4 mg per pint (approximately 570 ml) for the chicken and pea soups respectively and less than 4 mg per can for the liquid variety. Therefore it seems highly unlikely that a reaction to these particular soups would occur even if the contents were consumed at one time.— R. W. Daisley and H. V. Gudka, *J. Pharm. Pharmac.*, 1980, *32*, 77.

A 33-year-old woman taking phenelzine developed a severe headache after drinking a *cola beverage*. Her headache recurred and she had a slight blood-pressure rise on again drinking the cola beverage. The interaction was considered to be due to the caffeine content of the drink and it is suggested that patients maintained on monoamine oxidase inhibitors should at least limit the amount of cola beverages they imbibe.— G. E. Pakes (letter), *Am. J. Hosp. Pharm.*, 1979, *36*, 736.

References to reactions with various foods.— J. V. Hodge *et al.* (letter), *Lancet*, 1964, *1*, 1108 (*broad beans* with their *pods*); D. J. Blomley (letter), *ibid.*, *2*, 1181 (*broad beans* with their *pods*); M. Harper, *ibid.*, 312 (*Bovril*); B. Blackwell *et al.* (letter), *ibid.*, 1964, *1*, 722 (*Marmite*); B. Blackwell, *ibid.*, 1963, *2*, 849 (*Cheddar cheese*); A. A. Boulton *et al.*, *Can. med. Ass. J.*, 1970, *102*, 1394 (*stale liver*); A. Comfort (letter), *Lancet*, 1981, *2*, 472 (New Zealand prickly spinach).

For further reports of reactions to foods during treatment with a monoamine oxidase inhibitor, see Mebanazine (p.123) and Tranylcypromine Sulphate (p.132).

Reactions to other drugs are very likely in patients treated with monoamine oxidase inhibitors.

Severe hypertensive reactions due to enhancement of pressor activity have followed the administration of sympathomimetic agents such as amphetamine, ephedrine, levodopa, phenylephrine, and phenylpropanolamine. Reactions may also follow the use of anorectic agents and stimulants with sympathomimetic activity such as fenfluramine and methylphenidate. Adrenaline and noradrenaline in the usual doses of local anaesthetic solutions are no longer considered likely to cause hypertensive reactions in patients taking monoamine oxidase inhibitors unless they already have cardiovascular disease. Monoamine oxidase inhibitors also inhibit other drug-metabolising enzymes; they may enhance the effects of barbiturates and possibly other hypnotics, insulin and other hypoglycaemic agents, and possibly anticholinergic agents. Alcohol metabolism may be altered and its effects enhanced. Antihypertensive agents including guanethidine, reserpine, and methyldopa should be given with caution; hypotensive and hypertensive reactions have been suggested with different agents; the hypotensive effects of thiazide diuretics may be enhanced.

Severe reactions have been reported in patients receiving tricyclic antidepressants such as amitriptyline while being treated with a monoamine oxidase inhibitor, though drugs from both groups have occasionally been used together. The administration of pethidine and other narcotic analgesics to patients taking a monoamine oxidase inhibitor has also been associated with very severe reactions. Interactions can also occur between monoamine oxidase inhibitors themselves.

Interactions with drugs. A discussion of the interactions between monoamine oxidase inhibitors and other drugs and foodstuffs with indications of those combinations which were prohibited and those for which careful control was necessary.— A. J. Boakes, *Prescribers' J.*, 1971, *11*, 109. See also I. H. Stockley, *Pharm. J.*, 1973, *1*, 590; *ibid.*, *2*, 95.

An industrial chemist experienced a severe reaction to his first dose of phenelzine, presumably because his amine detoxification systems were saturated. He used *amine compounds* as vapours in his industrial research.— L. D. Gardner (letter), *Br. med. J.*, 1979, *1*, 1218.

Antidiabetic agents. Sensitivity to the hypoglycaemic action of *insulin* was increased in 6 patients with depression after treatment with phenelzine, 45 mg daily, or mebanazine, 20 mg daily. In 5 diabetics poorly controlled with *sulphonylurea* treatment, tolerance to glucose was improved when mebanazine 20 mg daily was given for 5 weeks.— P. I. Adnitt, *Diabetes*, 1968, *17*, 628.

Antihypertensive agents. Studies in *animals* suggested that hyperexcitability could occur if a patient was given a monoamine oxidase inhibitor and then either *reserpine* or *methyldopa*, but no reaction would occur if the treatments were given in the reverse order.— S. Natarajan (letter), *Lancet*, 1964, *1*, 1330.

For the effect of monoamine oxidase inhibitors on *guanethidine*, see Guanethidine Monosulphate, p.146.

Benzodiazepines. Massive oedema in a 64-year-old man who had taken various antidepressant drugs for 5 years and occurring 16 weeks after taking phenelzine might have been evidence of interaction between the phenelzine and a *benzodiazepine*.— A. Goonewardene and P. J. Toghill, *Br. med. J.*, 1977, *1*, 879. Phenelzine alone is capable of producing severe oedema in elderly patients who are on a high dosage as was the case with the patient reported.— D. L. F. Dunleavy (letter), *ibid.*, 1353.

Muscle relaxants. A preliminary report suggesting that low serum pseudocholinesterase concentrations in 4 patients might have been due to phenelzine. One of the patients developed apnoea following modified ECT with *suxethonium bromide*.— P. O. Bodley *et al.*, *Br. med. J.*, 1969, *3*, 510.

Narcotic agents. A woman who had been taking phenelzine collapsed when given 100 mg of *pethidine* by intramuscular injection. She developed hypotension, generalised rigidity, nystagmus, and fever, and died 8 hours later.— N. C. R. W. Reid and D. Jones (letter), *Br. med. J.*, 1962, *1*, 408.

For further reports of severe interactions with *pethidine*, see Pethidine Hydrochloride, p.1026.

As only a small percentage of patients who were taking monoamine oxidase inhibitors showed a profound reaction if they were given either an analgesic or pressor drug, it was suggested that a sensitivity test be carried out before operation. The test for sensitivity to analgesics was carried out as follows: blood pressure, pulse, respiration, and general state of awareness were noted, and then either 5 mg of pethidine or 500 µg of morphine was given intramuscularly. The vital signs and any change in the level of consciousness were recorded every 5 minutes for 20 minutes and then every 10 minutes for the remainder of the first hour. If there had been no change, the test was repeated similarly either with pethidine in increasing doses every hour (10, 20, then 40 mg) or with morphine in similarly increasing doses every hour (1, 2, then 4 mg). It was unnecessary to continue the tests beyond these 4 hours as any sensitivity response would be apparent by that time.— H. C. Churchill-Davidson (letter), *Br. med. J.*, 1965, *1*, 520. Fifteen volunteers who had been treated with monoamine oxidase inhibiting drugs for not less than 3 weeks, received in random order on 3 successive days, graded doses of 5 to 40 mg of *pethidine*, 0.5 to 4 mg of *morphine*, and a placebo, under double-blind conditions. The maximum alteration in blood pressure was 35 mmHg and in heart-rate 28 beats per minute. It was judged that all subjects reacted normally. Patients who required morphine whilst undergoing MAOI therapy should be subjected to a sensitivity test.— C. D. G. Evans-Prosser, *Br. J. Anaesth.*, 1968, *40*, 279.

The ingestion of a cough preparation containing *dextromethorphan* was probably the cause of death in a 26-year-old woman who had been treated with phenelzine 15 mg four times daily.— N. Rivers and B. Horner (letter), *Can. med. Ass. J.*, 1970, *103*, 85.

Neuroleptics. Enhancement of the effects of *droperidol* by phenelzine occurred in a 61-year-old man who had taken phenelzine 45 mg daily and perphenazine 6 mg daily for 5 months. Four days after the drugs had been discontinued, 20 mg of droperidol was given by mouth as premedication but the operation was postponed as he became cyanosed and generally unwell and his blood pressure fell to 75/60 mmHg. The blood pressure gradually returned to normal and 11 days later the operation was performed.— G. N. Penlington (letter), *Br. med. J.*, 1966, *1*, 483.

Serotonin and tryptophan. When *tryptophan* was given by mouth in doses of 20 and 50 mg per kg body-weight concomitantly with a monoamine oxidase inhibitor, a reaction likened to inebriation persisted for several hours. Hyperreflexia and clonus had also occurred. The same dose of tryptophan given alone had produced no objective or subjective reaction.— A. Sjoerdsma *et al.*, *J. Pharmac. exp. Ther.*, 1959, *126*, 217. In a small controlled trial, tryptophan in a single daily dose of 5 to 7 g given in conjunction with pyridoxine hydrochloride in a dose of 100 mg daily was found to be as effective as ECT in the treatment of patients with severe depression. The effectiveness of the regimen appeared to be improved when tranylcypromine 30 mg daily, potassium 97 mmol daily in divided doses, and carbohydrate supplements were given concurrently.— A. Coppen *et al.* (preliminary communication), *Lancet*, 1967, *2*, 1178. Further references.— D. L. Murphy *et al.*, *J. nerv. ment. Dis.*, 1977, *164*, 129.

Sympathomimetics, direct-acting. A review of reactions to monoamine oxidase inhibitors when given in conjunction with other drugs with special reference to dental drugs. It was concluded that *adrenaline* and *noradrenaline*, which were metabolised by catechol-*O*-methyltransferase, were only slightly enhanced by monoamine oxidase inhibitors. In the small amounts injected with local anaesthetics it was not likely that a reaction would occur, and omission of the vasoconstrictor could lead to more serious effects.— J. Glover, *Br. dent. J.*, 1967, *123*, 315. In 4 volunteers pretreated with monoamine oxidase inhibitors (phenelzine 15 mg thrice daily or tranylcypromine 10 mg thrice daily) for 7 days the pressor effect of *phenylephrine* was significantly enhanced but there was no significant change in the response to *adrenaline, noradrenaline,* or *isoprenaline*. Isoprenaline-induced tachycardia was significantly reduced. It was unlikely that patients taking monoamine oxidase inhibitors would be seriously at risk if given noradrenaline in local anaesthetic solutions.— A. J. Boakes *et al.*, *Br. med. J.*, 1973, *1*, 311. The Committee on Safety of Medicines stated that there was no hazard to patients given local anaesthetics when they were taking monoamine oxidase inhibitors unless they were suffering from cardiovascular disease and were given local anaesthetics containing adrenaline.— *Pharm. J.*, 1973, *1*, 510.

Sympathomimetics, indirect-acting. Two women, each of whom took 1 Procol tablet (containing 50 mg of *phenylpropanolamine hydrochloride* and 2.5 mg of *isopropamide iodide*), developed severe throbbing headache, in 1 patient followed by unconsciousness and status epilepticus. One woman was taking phenelzine 15 mg thrice daily and the other mebanazine 5 mg thrice daily.— C. M. Tonks and A. T. Lloyd (letter), *Br. med. J.*, 1965, *1*, 589.

A 30-year-old woman died about 3 hours after the start of a hypertensive episode which was precipitated by 20 mg of *dexamphetamine sulphate* taken in addition to her usual treatment with phenelzine 15 mg thrice daily, and trifluoperazine 2 mg at night.— J. T. A. Lloyd and D. R. H. Walker (letter), *Br. med. J.*, 1965, *2*, 168.

A 58-year-old hypertensive man given pargyline hydrochloride in a total daily dose increased from 25 to 75 mg became hypotensive within 5 weeks of starting this treatment. He was given for this a single intramuscular injection of 4 mg of *metaraminol*, a sympathomimetic amine, which precipitated within 10 minutes a hypertensive crisis with systolic blood pressure above 300 mmHg.— A. R. Horler and N. A. Wynne, *Br. med. J.*, 1965, *2*, 460.

In experiments in 4 normal subjects, a sympathomimetic agent was given before, during, and usually after a course of phenelzine or tranylcypromine. *Noradrenaline* intravenously was not inactivated or enhanced whereas *ephedrine* given orally or intravenously was substantially enhanced. *Phenylephrine* was only moderately enhanced when given intravenously but a dangerous enhancement occurred after oral administration.— J. Elis *et al.*, *Br. med. J.*, 1967, *2*, 75.

A 38-year-old woman who had been taking phenelzine sulphate 15 mg thrice daily for 3 months developed a hypertensive crisis 15 minutes after she took a tablet containing *phenylpropanolamine* 32 mg.— A. M. S. Mason and R. M. Buckle (letter), *Br. med. J.*, 1969, *1*, 845. A similar report.— P. M. Humberstone (letter), *ibid.*, 846.

Absorption and Fate. Phenelzine is readily absorbed from the gastro-intestinal tract and is excreted in the urine almost entirely in the form of metabolites.

Although many of the actions of phenelzine are rapid in onset, several days elapse before maximum blockade of monoamine oxidase. Phenelzine itself blocks monoamine oxidase irreversibly but the blockade produced by some other monoamine oxidase inhibitors is reversible. The significance of monoamine oxidase inhibition in relation to the lifting of depression is not clear, but the adverse interactions liable to occur as a result of monoamine oxidase inhibition remain a hazard for about 14 days after discontinuation of the drug, i.e. until fresh supplies of the enzyme have been generated in the body.

Acetylation. Detection of small amounts of unmetabolised phenelzine in urine, the proportion being lower in rapid acetylators, these differences being consistent with acetylation being a major route of elimination of phenelzine.— B. Caddy *et al.*, *Br. J. clin. Pharmac.*, 1976, *3*, 633. See also *idem*, 1978, *6*, 185.

The response of 30 patients with depressive neurosis, 15 with anxiety neurosis, and 15 with phobic anxiety, to phenelzine administration did not correspond to their acetylator status. Significantly greater improvement was, however, noted in patients whose initial dose was increased to 90 mg daily compared to those whose initial dose was only increased to 45 mg daily.— P. Tyrer and M. Gardner (letter), *Lancet*, 1978, *2*, 994. Criticism. They are related but the association is not striking.— W. J. Tilstone and E. C. Johnstone (letter), *ibid.*, 1151. Further reference.— P. Tyrer *et al.*, *Br. J. Psychiat.*, 1980, *136*, 359.

Comment on studies attempting to correlate the presumed acetylator status and clinical response with reference to phenelzine. The present evidence does not support either the hypothesis that phenelzine undergoes polymorphic acetylation, or that acetylator phenotype is a determinant of the drug's clinical effects.— G. L. Sanders and M. D. Rawlins, *Br. J. clin. Pharmac.*, 1979, *7*, 451. See also E. F. Marshall *et al.*, *Br. J. clin. Pharmac.*, 1978, *6*, 247.

Uses. Phenelzine is a hydrazine derivative and a monoamine oxidase inhibitor. Its mode of action in depression is not fully understood.

Phenelzine and other monoamine oxidase inhibitors are used in the treatment of depression, particularly reactive depression; they are probably less effective in endogenous depression. Associated anxiety may also respond, but concomitant administration of an anxiolytic, such as a benzodiazepine (see Diazepam, p.1523) may also be necessary. Since up to a month may elapse before an antidepressant response is obtained, severely ill patients may require electroconvulsive therapy initially. After a response has been obtained maintenance therapy may need to be continued for several months to avoid relapse on withdrawal. In view of the serious food and drug interactions that are liable to occur in patients given monoamine oxidase inhibitors this form of therapy is usually reserved for depressed or phobic patients who have not responded to other forms of therapy. Monoamine oxidase inhibitor therapy is not indicated for children and, where possible, should also be avoided in the elderly. Moreover, it is not suitable for patients considered unable to adhere to the strict dietary requirements necessary for its safe usage.

Phenelzine is given as the sulphate in doses equivalent to phenelzine 15 mg thrice daily; if no response has been obtained after 2 weeks the dosage may be increased to 15 mg four times daily; severely depressed hospital patients may be given up to 30 mg thrice daily. Once a response has been obtained the dosage may be gradually reduced for maintenance therapy; some patients may continue to respond to 15 mg on alternate days.

Some monoamine oxidase inhibitors, including phenelzine, were formerly used in the treatment of angina pectoris.

Depression. A review of the clinical pharmacology of phenelzine. Drugs such as phenelzine have been found to be effective in nonendogenous depression and phobic disorders. A significant association has been found between high levels of monoamine oxidase inhibition, clinical improvement, and dosage. The most prudent starting dose of phenelzine would appear to be 1 mg per kg body-weight daily (phenelzine 60 to 75 mg daily).— D. S. Robinson *et al.*, *Archs gen. Psychiat.*, 1978, *35*, 629.

A review of data from double-blind, placebo-controlled studies of the monoamine oxidase inhibitors indicates that phenelzine is clearly effective in neurotic or atypical depressives, but its effect in endogenous depressives is inconclusive. Similar conclusions are warranted for tranylcypromine, although fewer studies have been carried out. The implications of fast acetylation, selective MAO inhibitors, types MAO_A and MAO_B, and measures of platelet MAO inhibition are also discussed.— F. Quitkin *et al.*, *Archs gen. Psychiat.*, 1979, *36*, 749.

For references to reports and comments on the merits and hazards of using tricyclic antidepressants and monoamine oxidase inhibitors concurrently, see Amitriptyline Hydrochloride, p.114.

For further comments on the hazards of giving tricyclic antidepressants with monoamine oxidase inhibitors, see under Precautions, above. See also under Amitriptyline Hydrochloride, Precautions, p.112.

For studies attempting to correlate dosage and acetylator status of phenelzine with clinical response, see under Absorption and Fate (Acetylation).

Hypotension. For studies and comments on the merits and hazards of phenelzine and other monoamine oxidase inhibitors in the management of orthostatic hypotension, see Tyramine Hydrochloride, p.526.

Narcolepsy. Seven patients with narcolepsy related to frequent attacks of REM sleep were given phenelzine in a dose of 60 to 90 mg daily. The amount of REM sleep was suppressed for long periods while the patient had less frequent attacks of catalepsy, sleep paralysis, and hallucinations.— R. J. Wyatt *et al.*, *New Engl. J. Med.*, 1971, *285*, 987.

Phobia. For comments on the role of monoamine oxidase inhibitors in the management of phobic states, see under Depression, above.

Skin disorders. The use of phenelzine in neurodermatitis.— S. Friedman *et al.*, *J. nerv. ment. Dis.*, 1978, *166*, 349.

Preparations

Phenelzine Sulfate Tablets *(U.S.P.)*. Tablets containing phenelzine sulphate. Potency is expressed in terms of the equivalent amount of phenelzine. Store in a cool place in airtight containers. Protect from light.

Phenelzine Tablets *(B.P.)*. Phenelzine Sulphate Tablets. Tablets containing phenelzine sulphate. They are sugar-coated. Potency is expressed in terms of the equivalent amount of phenelzine.

Nardil *(Warner, UK)*. Phenelzine sulphate, available as tablets each containing the equivalent of 15 mg of phenelzine. (Also available as Nardil in *Austral., Canad., Ital., USA*).

Other Proprietary Names

Nardelzine *(Belg., Spain)*.

2534-j

Protriptyline Hydrochloride *(B.P., U.S.P.)*.

MK-240. 3-(5*H*-Dibenzo[*a,d*]cyclohepten-5-yl)-*N*-methylpropylamine hydrochloride.

$C_{19}H_{21}N,HCl=299.8$.

CAS — 438-60-8 (protriptyline); 1225-55-4 (hydrochloride).

Pharmacopoeias. In *Br.* and *U.S.*

A white to yellowish odourless or almost odourless powder with a bitter taste. M.p. about 168°.

Soluble 1 in 2 of water, 1 in 3.5 of alcohol, and 1 in 2.5 of chloroform; practically insoluble in ether. A 1% solution in water has a pH of 5 to 6.5.

Adverse Effects, Treatment, and Precautions. As for Amitriptyline Hydrochloride, p.110.

Anxiety, agitation, tachycardia, and hypotension may occur more frequently.

For a general comment on antidepressant therapy and driving, see Amitriptyline Hydrochloride, p.112.

Interactions. The amount of protriptyline not bound to plasma proteins was 7.8%. This value was increased from 8.2 to 10.9% in the presence of phenytoin.— O. Borgå *et al.*, *Biochem. Pharmac.* 1969, *18*, 2135.

For a comment on the significance of tricyclic antidepressants and protein binding see under Absorption and Fate (Protein Binding), p.131.

Absorption and Fate. Protriptyline is well but slowly absorbed after oral administration, peak plasma concentrations being achieved after several hours. Since protriptyline slows gastro-intestinal transit-time, absorption can be further delayed in overdosage.

Paths of metabolism of protriptyline include *N*-oxidation, and hydroxylation and conjugation with glucuronic acid. Protriptyline is excreted in the urine, mainly in the form of its metabolites, either free or in conjugated form.

Protriptyline is widely distributed throughout the body and extensively bound to plasma and tissue protein. Protriptyline has been estimated to have a very prolonged half-life ranging from 55 to 124 hours, which may be further prolonged in overdosage. Plasma concentrations of protriptyline vary very widely but some correlation with therapeutic response has been established.

Two normal subjects received protriptyline labelled with carbon-14 after a 12-hour fast. Plasma radioactivity was at a maximum 8 to 12 hours after ingestion and then gradually declined. Significant plasma concentrations of radioactivity were present 37 days after ingestion. The cumulative urinary excretion during the first 16 days accounted for approximately 50% of the protriptyline. Very little of the drug was excreted in the faeces.— K. D. Charalampous and P. C. Johnson, *J. clin. Pharmac.*, 1967, *7*, 93. The biotransformation of protriptyline in *pigs*, *dogs* and man. Oxidative metabolism and conjugation was noted in all 3, but a primary amine resulting from *N*-demethylation was found to be operative only in *dogs*.— S. F. Sisenwine *et al.*, *J. Pharmac. exp. Ther.*, 1970, *175*, 51. Following administration of protriptyline to *rats* the 10,11-epoxide was isolated in the urine.— V. Rovei *et al.*, *J. pharm. Sci.*, 1976, *65*, 810.

The steady-state plasma half-life of protriptyline estimated in 9 depressed patients was 78 to 198 hours. In 5 healthy subjects given a single 30-mg dose of protriptyline hydrochloride, the plasma half-life was 55 to 124 hours.— J. P. Moody *et al.*, *Eur. J. clin. Pharmac.*, 1977, *11*, 51. A study of the pharmacokinetics of protriptyline in 8 healthy subjects following oral administration of protriptyline hydrochloride 30 mg. It was confirmed that protriptyline is slowly absorbed, highly tissue bound, and slowly metabolised. The estimated first-pass metabolism through the liver was only 10 to 25%. Peak plasma concentrations were achieved 6 to 12 hours after the oral dose, and plasma half-lives ranged from 53.6 to 91.7 hours.— V. E. Ziegler *et al.*, *Clin. Pharmac. Ther.*, 1978, *23*, 580.

Plasma concentrations. In a study completed by 21 depressed patients, 8 of 9 whose plasma-protriptyline concentrations were above 70 ng per ml at 4 weeks responded to therapy whereas only 5 of 12 whose concentrations were below this did so. An upper limit of therapeutic response was not demonstrated but since concentrations of 167 ng per ml appeared to be well tolerated, a therapeutic range of plasma-protriptyline concentrations of 70 to 170 ng per ml was proposed. As expected from the long half-life, the mean plasma concentration did not reach its maximum until the fourth week and concentrations in 3 patients were still rising at this time. From this study and that of S.F. Whyte *et al.*(*Br. J. Psychiat.*, 1976, *128*, 384) it appeared that concentrations within the therapeutic range would most often be achieved with doses of 20 to 40 mg daily.— Biggs. J.T. and V. E. Ziegler, *Clin. Pharmac. Ther.*, 1977, *22*, 269.

Mean serial steady-state plasma-protriptyline concentrations of 111.6, 144.3, and 164.2 ng per ml occurred in 3 patients with depression given protriptyline 20, 30, or 40 mg daily respectively for at least 2 weeks.— V. E. Ziegler *et al.*, *J. pharm. Sci.*, 1978, *67*, 554.

Protein binding. Comment on the serious technical problem in the determination of plasma protein binding of antidepressant drugs, the difficulty in generalising from one drug to another, and the need to put into perspective the significance of individual differences. Such differences may represent an additional source of variability, but are relatively less important than the 20- to 30-fold interindividual differences in total plasma concentrations that are commonly observed with antidepressants.— R. A. Braithwaite, *Postgrad. med. J.*, 1980, *56*, *Suppl.* 1, 107.

Uses. Protriptyline is a tricyclic antidepressant with actions and uses similar to those of amitriptyline (p.113). It has considerably less marked sedative properties, and may have a stimulant effect; concomitant administration of a tranquilliser may be necessary, particularly in the early stages of therapy.

In the treatment of depression, protriptyline is given by mouth as the hydrochloride in doses of 5 to 10 mg three or four times daily; it has been suggested that dosage increases should be added to the morning dose first, and if insomnia occurs the last dose should be given no later than mid-afternoon; higher doses of up to 60 mg daily may be required in severely depressed hospital patients. A suggested initial dose for adolescents and the elderly is 5 mg thrice daily; close monitoring of the cardiovascular system is required if the dose exceeds a total of 20 mg daily in elderly subjects. Since protriptyline has a prolonged half-life, once-daily dosage regimens are also suitable and, since protriptyline is very slowly absorbed, it has been suggested that this dose could be given at night (rather than in the morning) to provide maximum plasma concentrations, and the concomitant alerting effect of protriptyline, the following morning.

Administration. Comment on the important clinical implications of the unusually long half-life of protriptyline. The two to three weeks required to reach steady-state, together with the well-documented delay between the onset of tricyclic antidepressant treatment and recovery from depression, can be a source of confusion. Adequate therapeutic doses, if not given the required time to reach steady state, may be considered ineffective, and a potentially toxic dose may be well tolerated initially, until the plasma concentration increases to a toxic range. Loading doses, if well tolerated, may be useful, and divided daily doses are rarely necessary. Although protriptyline is most often prescribed in the morning or afternoon because of its non-sedating or even stimulating properties, since it is slowly absorbed with peak plasma concentrations reached 8 to 9 hours after the oral dose, bedtime administration would appear to be effective in providing morning stimulation.— V. E. Ziegler *et al.*, *Clin. Pharmac. Ther.*, 1978, *23*, 580.

Depression. For a general review of the role of tricyclic antidepressants in depression, see Amitriptyline Hydrochloride, p.114.

Diabetes insipidus. A 13-year-old boy with sleep apnoea and cataplexy who also suffered from chronic diabetes insipidus was given protriptyline to control his sleep-related symptoms. An unexpected result was the apparent reversal of his chronic diabetes insipidus.— R. W. Clark *et al.*, *Sth. med. J.*, 1978, *71*, 1567.

For reference to inappropriate secretion of antidiuretic hormone in patients given tricyclic antidepressants, see Amitriptyline Hydrochloride, Effects on the Endocrine System, p.111, and Clomipramine Hydrochloride, Effects on the Endocrine System, p.116.

Glaucoma. Protriptyline hydrochloride 0.05% administered topically 6 times daily maintained the intra-ocular pressure below 20 mmHg for more than 1 year in 6 of 24 patients with primary open-angle glaucoma.— Y. Kitazawa, *Am. J. Ophthal.*, 1972, *74*, 588.

For reference to increased intra-ocular pressure in patients given tricyclic antidepressant therapy, see Amitriptyline Hydrochloride, Adverse Effects, p.110, and Precautions, p.112.

Narcolepsy. Although it was found to have relatively poor REM sleep-suppressing properties, protriptyline 10 to 20 mg at bedtime had a beneficial effect in 5 patients with the narcolepsy-cataplexy syndrome and hypersomnia. Several patients noted a tendency for the drug to induce vivid dreaming, particularly in the first 2 weeks of therapy and in one patient the dreaming was sufficiently unpleasant for him to stop therapy.— H. S. Schmidt *et al.*, *Am. J. Psychiat.*, 1977, *134*, 183. See also R. W. Clark *et al.*, *Neurology, Minneap.*, 1979, *29*, 1287.

Preparations

Protriptyline Hydrochloride Tablets *(U.S.P.)*. Tablets containing protriptyline hydrochloride. Store in airtight containers.

Protriptyline Tablets *(B.P.)*. Tablets containing protriptyline hydrochloride. They are film-coated.

Concordin-5 *(Merck Sharp & Dohme, UK)*. Protriptyline hydrochloride, available as tablets of 5 mg. **Concordin-10**. Protriptyline hydrochloride, available as tablets of 10 mg. (Also available as Concordin in *Arg.*, *Austral.*, *Belg.*, *Denm.*, *Ital.*, *Neth.*, *Swed.*).

Other Proprietary Names

Concordine *(Fr.)*; Maximed *(Ger.)*; Triptil *(Austral.*, *Canad.)*; Vivactil *(USA)*.

NOTE. The name Vivactil is also applied to a vitamin/amino acid preparation.

2535-z

Safrazine Hydrochloride. 1-Methyl-3-(3,4-methylenedioxyphenyl)propylhydrazine hydrochloride. $C_{11}H_{16}N_2O_2,HCl=244.7$.

CAS — 33419-68-0 (safrazine); 27849-94-1 (hydrochloride).

A white to pale yellow crystalline powder. M.p. about 120°. Freely **soluble** in water and methyl alcohol; sparingly soluble in alcohol; practically insoluble in chloroform and ether.

Uses. Safrazine is a monoamine oxidase inhibitor with actions and uses similar to those of phenelzine (p.128). In the treatment of depression it has been given as the hydrochloride.

Proprietary Names

Safra *(Ono, Jap.)*.

2536-c

Tofenacin Hydrochloride. BS 7331 (Tofenacin); Desmethylorphenadrine Hydrochloride. *N*-Methyl-2-(2-methylbenzhydryloxy)ethylamine hydrochloride. $C_{17}H_{21}NO,HCl=291.8$.

CAS — 15301-93-6 (tofenacin); 10488-36-5 (hydrochloride).

A white to off-white crystalline powder. M.p. 143° to 147°. **Soluble** about 1 in 3 of water, 1 in 8 of alcohol, 1 in 425 of acetone, 1 in 3 of chloroform, and 1 in 2 of methyl alcohol; practically insoluble in ether. A 5% solution in water has a pH of 4.8 to 5.6. **Store** in airtight containers. Protect from light.

Adverse Effects, Treatment, and Precautions. As for Atropine, p.289.

Tofenacin has been contra-indicated with monoamine oxidase inhibitors or within 14 days of discontinuing such therapy.

Uses. Tofenacin is a derivative of orphenadrine (see p.307). It is given as the hydrochloride in doses of 80 mg up to thrice daily in the treatment of mild to moderate depression in the elderly.

Proprietary Preparations

Elamol *(Brocades, UK)*. Tofenacin hydrochloride, available as capsules of 80 mg.

Other Proprietary Names

Tofacine *(Belg.)*.

2537-k

Tranylcypromine Sulphate. B.P.; Tranylcypromine Sulfate *(U.S.P.)*; Tranilcipromina (base); Transamine Sulphate; SKF 385. (±)-*trans*-2-Phenylcyclopropylamine sulphate. $(C_9H_{11}N)_2,H_2SO_4=364.5$.

CAS — 155-09-9 (tranylcypromine); 13492-01-8 (sulphate).

Pharmacopoeias. In *Br.* and *U.S.*

A white or almost white crystalline powder with an acid taste; odourless or with a faint odour of cinnamaldehyde. Tranylcypromine sulphate 13.7 mg is approximately equivalent to 10 mg of tranylcypromine.

Soluble 1 in 20 to 25 of water and 1 in 2000 of ether; very slightly soluble in alcohol; practically insoluble in chloroform. **Store** in airtight containers.

Adverse Effects. As for Phenelzine Sulphate, p.128.

Insomnia is a common side-effect if tranylcypromine is given in the evening.

Hypertensive reactions are more likely to occur with tranylcypromine than with phenelzine or other antidepressants derived from hydrazine, but severe liver damage occurs less frequently.

Abuse. An unstable patient became dependent on tranylcypromine sulphate and needed twenty 10-mg tablets daily.— J. LeGassicke (letter), *Lancet*, 1963, *1*, 270. See also J. Mielczarek and J. Johnson (letter), *Lancet*, 1963, *1*, 388; O. Ben-Arie and G. C. W. George, *Br. J. Psychiat.*, 1979, *135*, 273.

Effects on the heart. An alcoholic patient had left-sided chest pain, relieved by glyceryl trinitrate, on several occasions after starting treatment with tranylcypromine and diazepam, each 30 mg daily.— J. D. Wilson (letter), *Br. med. J.*, 1974, *3*, 580.

Overdosage. A 62-year-old woman who had taken 20 Parstelin tablets developed hyperpyrexia, increased muscle tone with generally hyperactive reflexes, and much increased heart-rate and respiration-rate. Severe hypotension occurred with respiratory failure and she died 10 hours later. Before her death she had developed a haematological disorder with prolonged bleeding and clotting times and spontaneous haemorrhaging.— J. A. Mawdsley (letter), *Med. J. Aust.*, 1968, *2*, 292.

Treatment of Adverse Effects. As for Phenelzine Sulphate, p.128.

A 27-year-old pregnant woman who took tranylcypromine 500 mg developed hypertension, tachycardia, and pyrexia; she became cyanosed, and her muscles went into tonic spasm. Her stomach was emptied and she was given chlorpromazine 100 mg intramuscularly with little effect. Her pyrexia persisted despite artificial cooling. Chlorpromazine 70 mg was given intravenously over 3 hours and her temperature dropped from 41.1° to 38.9°. Despite cardiac arrests and pulmonary oedema she recovered, but the foetus was aborted.— J. C. Robertson, *Postgrad. med. J.*, 1972, *48*, 64.

Practolol 10 mg was given intravenously to a patient with symptoms of beta-adrenergic overactivity following the ingestion of 20 to 30 tablets of tranylcypromine 10 mg. A second dose was given after 2 hours. All signs of overactivity rapidly subsided.— J. T. Shepherd and B. Whiting (letter), *Lancet*, 1974, *2*, 1021.

Haemodialysis. A 15-year-old girl who had taken 350 mg of tranylcypromine sulphate was successfully treated by haemodialysis.— B. J. Matter *et al.*, *Archs intern. Med.*, 1965, *116*, 18.

Precautions. As for Phenelzine Sulphate, p.128.

For a general comment on antidepressant therapy and driving, see Amitriptyline Hydrochloride, p.112.

Interactions with food. A report of a hypertensive reaction caused by *pickled herrings* in a patient during tranylcypromine treatment.— W. F. Nuessle *et al.*, *J. Am. med. Ass.*, 1965, *192*, 726.

Six serious hypertensive episodes and 4 moderately severe reactions occurred in patients who ate *chicken livers* during treatment with tranylcypromine. Chicken livers were found to contain about 100 µg of tyramine per g.— D. L. Hedberg *et al.*, *Am. J. Psychiat.*, 1966, *122*, 933.

Of patients in the Maudsley Hospital prescribed monoamine oxidase inhibitors for depression between January 1963 and June 1964, 4.3% experienced sudden hypertensive attacks. The incidence of attacks was 5 times greater with tranylcypromine than with phenelzine. Because over one-half the patients studied ate cheese with impunity during treatment with monoamine oxidase inhibitors it would be wrong to infer that no connection existed; variables could occur in the patient or in the patient's food or treatment which could affect the immunity or susceptibility. Prolonged treatment could predispose to hypertension when amines were taken in food.— B. Blackwell *et al.*, *Br. J. Psychiat.*, 1967, *113*, 349.

A severe reaction occurred in one patient receiving treatment with tranylcypromine and following the ingestion of 4 heaped tablespoonfuls of Iranian *caviar*. Russian caviar was found to contain 680 µg of tyramine per g. If the tyramine content of the two types of caviar was similar, the patient probably took about 60 mg of tyramine.— P. Isaac *et al.*, *Lancet*, 1977, *2*, 816.

A systematic study of 98 patients receiving tranylcypromine revealed that only one-third of the patients adhered strictly to the dietary recommendations, while over one-third acknowledged substantial non-compliance. The 11.2% incidence of hypertensive reactions did not differ significantly from that reported during the time before dietary restrictions, although there were no serious complications. Cheeses and liqueurs (Drambuie, Kalua, and Creme de Cacao) were the most common precipitants of the reactions.— J. F. Neil *et al.*, *J. clin. Psychiat.*, 1979, *40*, 33.

Interactions with drugs. Severe occipital headache, shortness of breath, wheezing, and coughing developed in a woman who consumed about 84 ml of *alcoholic beverages* during treatment with tranylcypromine, 10 mg four times daily. A man receiving tranylcypromine 10 mg thrice daily and *methylphenidate hydrochloride* 10 mg thrice daily experienced severe occipital headache, hyperventilation, nausea, abdominal cramps, weakness, and paraesthesia of extremities.— M. Sherman *et al.*, *Am. J. Psychiat.*, 1964, *120*, 1019.

A rapid and dramatic rise in blood pressure followed the administration of 50 mg of *phenylpropanolamine* to a healthy adult who had been taking tranylcypromine 30 mg daily.— M. F. Cuthbert *et al.*, *Br. med. J.*, 1969, *1*, 404.

A 19-year-old youth ingested a multiple overdose of tranylcypromine 250 mg, *trifluoperazine* 25 mg, and about 100 mg of *protriptyline*, and ate 2 *cheese* rolls. He became agitated with fever and very high systolic pressure. Hypertension was successfully treated with phentolamine until an infusion of phenoxybenzamine could be assembled.— A. V. Simmons *et al.*, *Lancet*, 1970, *1*, 214.

Hyperpyrexia and shock occurred in a patient taking tranylcypromine sulphate and *desipramine hydrochloride*.— W. N. Rom and E. J. Benner, *Calif. Med.*, 1972, *117*, 65.

The antidepressant effect of tranylcypromine (and imipramine) was reversed by *fenclonine*.— B. Shopsin *et al.*, *Archs gen. Psychiat.*, 1976, *33*, 811.

For reference to a toxic reaction in *rats* pretreated with *disulfiram* following concurrent administration of tranylcypromine, see Disulfiram, p.579.

Absorption and Fate. Tranylcypromine is readily absorbed from the gastro-intestinal tract and excreted in the urine mainly in the form of metabolites.

In 2 healthy subjects given tranylcypromine 20 mg by mouth a peak plasma concentration of about 25 ng per ml occurred 2.5 hours after administration.— A. Lang *et al.*, *Arzneimittel-Forsch.*, 1978, *28*, 575. Determination and comparison of the plasma and urine concentrations in subjects given the stereo-isomers of tranylcypromine.— *idem*, 1979, *29*, 154.

Uses. Tranylcypromine is a nonhydrazine monoamine oxidase inhibitor with actions and uses similar to those of phenelzine (p.130). Unlike phenelzine, it does not induce irreversible inhibition of monoamine oxidase, the activity of which is reported to recover within 3 to 5 days of withdrawing tranylcypromine.

Tranylcypromine is given as the sulphate in doses equivalent to tranylcypromine 10 mg in the morning and 10 mg at midday; if no response has been obtained after a week the midday dose may be increased to 20 mg; a dosage of 30 mg daily should only be exceeded with caution. Once a response has been obtained the dosage may be gradually reduced for maintenance; some patients may continue to respond to 10 mg daily.

Depression. Four patients with delusional thinking and depression obtained a dramatic response to therapy with tranylcypromine. Treatment with tricyclics had been unsuccessful in 3 of the patients and a tricyclic and a phenothiazine had been unsuccessful in the fourth.— J. Lieb and C. Collins, *J. nerv. ment. Dis.*, 1978, *166*, 805.

For general comments on the treatment of depression with monoamine oxidase inhibitors, see Phenelzine Sulphate, p.130.

Hypotension. For studies and comments on the merits and hazards of tranylcypromine and other monoamine oxidase inhibitors in the management of orthostatic hypotension, see Tyramine Hydrochloride, p.526. See also Fludrocortisone, p.470 and Levodopa, p.888.

Multiple sclerosis. Two patients with multiple sclerosis benefited in their physical symptoms from treatment with tranylcypromine 10 to 20 mg daily; 2 other patients did not benefit. A larger trial is recommended.— R. M. Whittington (letter), *Br. med. J.*, 1976, *2*, 371.

Parkinsonism. Tranylcypromine 10 mg thrice daily had a mild beneficial effect in selected patients with parkinsonism, possibly due to its effect on depression and on dopamine.— M. D. Yahr and R. C. Duvoisin, *New Engl. J. Med.*, 1972, *287*, 20.

Preparations

Tranylcypromine Sulfate Tablets *(U.S.P.)*. Tablets containing tranylcypromine sulphate. Potency is expressed in terms of the equivalent amount of tranylcypromine. Protect from light.

Tranylcypromine Tablets *(B.P.)*. Tranylcypromine Sulphate Tablets. Tablets containing tranylcypromine sulphate. They are sugar-coated. Potency is expressed in terms of the equivalent amount of tranylcypromine.

Proprietary Preparations

Parnate *(Smith Kline & French, UK)*. Tranylcypromine sulphate, available as tablets each containing the equivalent of 10 mg of tranylcypromine. (Also available as Parnate in *Austral., Canad., Ger., S.Afr., Spain, USA*).

Parstelin *(Smith Kline & French, UK)*. Tablets each containing tranylcypromine sulphate equivalent to tranylcypromine 10 mg and trifluoperazine hydrochloride equivalent to trifluoperazine 1 mg. For depression with anxiety. *Dose.* 1 to 3 tablets daily.

Other Proprietary Names

Tylciprine *(Fr.)*.

2541-y

Trazodone Hydrochloride. AF-1161. 2-{3-[4-(3-Chlorophenyl)piperazin-1-yl]propyl}-1,2,4-triazolo[4,3-*a*]pyridin-3(2*H*)-one hydrochloride.

$C_{19}H_{22}ClN_5O,HCl = 408.3$.

CAS — 19794-93-5 (trazodone); 25332-39-2 (hydrochloride).

White odourless crystals with a bitter taste. M.p. about 225°. Sparingly **soluble** in water, alcohol, and methyl alcohol; soluble in chloroform.

Adverse Effects. Adverse effects associated with trazodone include drowsiness. Other side-effects occasionally reported include dizziness, headache, nausea and vomiting, weakness, weight changes, tremor, dry mouth, bradycardia or tachycardia, postural hypotension, constipation, diarrhoea, blurred vision, restlessness, confusional states, insomnia, and skin rash.

Analysis of side-effects in a placebo-controlled study in which 17 depressed patients received trazodone and 18 received imipramine. Drowsiness was the most frequent side-effect in the trazodone group (12 patients), whereas anticholinergic effects such as dry mouth (16 patients), bowel movement disturbances (11 patients), and visual disturbances (10 patients) predominated in the imipramine group. Few side-effects of any type were reported in the placebo group. Side-effects were considered clinically significant in 5 trazodone-treated patients; they included a drugged feeling, drowsiness, lethargy, dizziness, decreased blood pressure, nausea, headache, and an increase in psychomotor retardation. Because of a lack of anticholinergic activity, trazodone does not commonly produce many of the side-effects characteristic of tricyclic antidepressants. Also the data suggests decreased potential for significant cardiovascular side-effects for trazodone.— J. P. Feighner, *J. clin. Psychiat.*, 1980, *41*, 250.

Treatment of Adverse Effects. The stomach should be emptied by aspiration and lavage. The use of activated charcoal as an adjunct to gastric lavage may be of value. Supportive therapy alone may then suffice (for general guidelines to the symptomatic therapy of drug overdosage, see Phenobarbitone, p.812.

Precautions. Although trazodone does not have the cardiotoxicity of the tricyclic antidepressants,

it should be used with caution in patients with cardiovascular disorders, such as ischaemic heart disease. It should similarly be used with caution in patients with epilepsy and hepatic or renal insufficiency. Patients with suicidal tendencies should be carefully supervised during treatment.
Unlike the tricyclic antidepressants, trazodone is considered unlikely to interact with monoamine oxidase inhibitors, but until more is known it is recommended that it should not be given to patients receiving monoamine oxidase inhibitors or for at least 14 days after their discontinuation. Similarly, trazodone is unlikely to diminish the effects of antihypertensive agents, such as guanethidine; some interaction may, however, occur with clonidine and, in general, blood pressure should be monitored when trazodone is prescribed with antihypertensive therapy. The sedative effects of trazodone may be enhanced by concurrent administration with alcohol or other central nervous system depressants.
Drowsiness is often experienced at the start of trazodone antidepressant therapy and patients liable to take charge of vehicles or other machinery should be warned that their judgement may be impaired.

For a general comment on antidepressant therapy and driving, see Amitriptyline Hydrochloride, p.112.

Interactions. Evidence that trazodone 50 mg thrice daily has no effect on the blood pressure response to *tyramine* and may slightly decrease sensitivity to *noradrenaline*.— P. Larochelle *et al.*, *Clin. Pharmac. Ther.*, 1979, *26*, 24.

Absorption and Fate. Trazodone is absorbed from the gastro-intestinal tract and extensively metabolised. Paths of metabolism of trazodone include *N*-oxidation and hydroxylation. Trazodone is excreted in the urine almost entirely in the form of its metabolites, either in free or in conjugated form.

The metabolism of trazodone.— L. Baiocchi *et al.*, *Arzneimittel-Forsch.*, 1974, *24*, 1699.

Plasma concentrations. A study of trazodone blood concentrations and therapeutic responsiveness.— S. Putzolu *et al.*, *Psychopharmac. Bull.*, 1976, *12*, 41.

Uses. Trazodone is a triazolopyridine antidepressant. It does not appear to have very significant anticholinergic properties, but has a marked sedative action. Unlike amitriptyline, it does not prevent the peripheral re-uptake of noradrenaline. It has been shown to be a selective inhibitor of central serotonin uptake and to decrease peripheral serotonin uptake. It also appears to increase the turnover of brain dopamine. The mode of action of trazodone in depression is not fully understood.
In the treatment of depression trazodone is given by mouth as the hydrochloride in doses of 100 or 150 mg daily initially, increased to 200 or 300 mg daily respectively after the first week. The daily dosage may be divided throughout the day after food or given as a single dose at night. Divided daily dosages of up to 600 mg may be given in exceptionally severe depression.

A review of the actions and uses of trazodone.— R. N. Brogden *et al.*, *Drugs*, 1981, *21*, 401.

Action. The pharmacology of trazodone from a psychological point of view.— B. Silvestrini and R. Lisciani, *Curr. ther. Res.*, 1973, *15*, 749. Selective inhibition of serotonin uptake by trazodone.— E. Stefanini *et al.*, *Life Sci.*, 1976, *18*, 1459. The effect of trazodone on brain dopamine metabolism.— *idem*, *J. Pharm. Pharmac.*, 1976, *28*, 925.

Administration in the elderly. In a double-blind controlled study in 60 depressed geriatric patients trazodone in an initial dose of 100 mg increased to 400 mg daily was as effective as imipramine in an initial dose of 50 mg increased to 200 mg daily and both antidepressants were more effective than placebo in relieving depression. Trazodone was much better tolerated with fewer side-effects, and may therefore possess an advantage for antidepressant treatment of certain patients in the older age groups.— R. Gerner *et al.*, *J. clin. Psychiat.*, 1980, *41*, 216.

Further references: N. P. V. Nair *et al.*, *Curr. ther. Res.*, 1973, *15*, 769.

Administration in renal failure. Trazodone 25 mg thrice daily produced similar plasma concentrations of trazodone after 1, 4, and 12 days of dosage in 10 patients with normal renal function and 12 with renal impairment.— B. Catanese *et al.*, *Boll. chim.-farm.*, 1978, *117*, 424.

Alcohol and drug dependence. Trazodone 3 mg per kg body-weight given intravenously daily in 2 divided doses for 5 days followed by 1.5 mg per kg daily in 3 doses by mouth for 6 days prevented the withdrawal syndrome in 63 diamorphine addicts. Freedom from dependence without additional treatment 1 year later was reported for 4 of 22 patients who had returned home and for 19 of 41 in a 'therapeutics community'.— S. Fedeli *et al.*, *Boll. chim.-farm.*, 1979, *118*, 368.

Depression. A review of clinical studies since 1967 showed that trazodone had a marked antidepressant effect. It had considerable tranquillising activity. It had no marked antipsychotic effect. Doses had varied widely but were usually in the range 75 to 600 mg daily. Doses of 50 mg had been successfully used intramuscularly or intravenously for premedication before surgery and other procedures. Tolerance had been good; side-effects reported included gastric discomfort, dry mouth, headache, dizziness, fatigue, drowsiness, insomnia, and slight hypotension.— R. U. Udabe, *Curr. ther. Res.*, 1973, *15*, 755.

A double-blind placebo-controlled study comparing trazodone with imipramine in depressed subjects. Seven of 17 patients in the trazodone group, 9 of 18 in the imipramine group, and 7 of 10 in the placebo group left the study prematurely because of lack of efficacy or the appearance of significant side-effects. Trazodone appeared to have a relatively rapid onset of action. It remains to be seen whether this advantage of trazodone materialises in actual clinical practice.— J. P. Feighner, *J. clin. Psychiat.*, 1980, *41*, 250. See also J. J. Kellams *et al.*, *ibid.*, 1979, *40*, 390.

Further studies of trazodone in depression.— A. N. Singh *et al.*, *Curr. ther. Res.*, 1978, *23*, 485 (with phenothiazines, in schizophrenia); L. F. Fabre *et al.*, *Curr. ther. Res.*, 1979, *25*, 827 (comparison with imipramine); S. Gershon and R. Newton, *J. clin. Psychiat.*, 1980, *41*, 100 (comparison with imipramine).

Proprietary Preparations

Molipaxin *(Roussel, UK)*. Trazodone hydrochloride, available as capsules of 50 and 100 mg.

Other Proprietary Names

Manegan *(Arg.)*; Thombran *(Ger.)*; Trittico *(Ital., Switz.)*.

2538-a

Trimipramine. IL 6001; RP 7162; Trimeprimine. 3-(10,11-Dihydro-5*H*-dibenz[*b,f*]azepin-5-yl)-2,*N*,*N*-trimethylpropylamine.

$C_{20}H_{26}N_2$=294.4.

CAS — 739-71-9.

A pale yellowish-white waxy solid. M.p. about 45°. Practically **insoluble** in water; readily soluble in alcohol.

2539-t

Trimipramine Maleate *(B.P., Eur. P.)*. Trimipramini Maleas. Trimipramine hydrogen maleate.

$C_{20}H_{26}N_2,C_4H_4O_4$=410.5.

CAS — 521-78-8.

Pharmacopoeias. In *Br.*, *Eur.*, *Fr.*, *Ger.*, *It.*, and *Neth.*

A white odourless or almost odourless crystalline powder with a bitter numbing taste. M.p. 140° to 144°. Trimipramine maleate 34.9 mg is approximately equivalent to 25 mg of trimipramine. Slightly **soluble** in water and alcohol; freely soluble in chloroform; practically insoluble in ether. **Protect** from light.

Adverse Effects, Treatment, and Precautions. As for Amitriptyline Hydrochloride, p.110.

For a general comment on antidepressant therapy and driving, see Amitriptyline Hydrochloride, p.112.

Absorption and Fate. Trimipramine is readily absorbed after oral administration and excreted in the urine mainly in the form of its metabolites. It is extensively bound to plasma proteins.

Determination of trimipramine in serum.— P. Hartvig *et al.*, *Analyt. Chem.*, 1976, *48*, 390.

Uses. Trimipramine is a tricyclic antidepressant with actions and uses similar to those of amitriptyline (p.113). Like amitriptyline, it has marked sedative properties. In the treatment of depression, trimipramine is given by mouth as the maleate in doses equivalent to 75 mg of trimipramine daily initially, gradually increased to 150 mg daily as necessary; higher doses of up to 250 to 300 mg daily may be required in severely depressed hospital patients; a dosage in excess of 200 mg daily is not recommended for maintenance therapy. A suggested initial dose for adolescents and the elderly is 50 mg daily, gradually increased to 100 mg daily as necessary. Trimipramine may be given in divided doses during the day, but since it has a prolonged half-life, once-daily dosage regimens are also suitable, usually given at night.
Trimipramine has been given intramuscularly as the mesylate in doses equivalent to trimipramine 25 to 50 mg every 6 to 8 hours.

Reviews of trimipramine: *Med. Lett.*, 1980, *22*, 16; E. C. Settle and F. J. Ayd, *J. clin. Psychiat.*, 1980, *41*, 266.

Depression. In a double-blind study in 125 patients with mild or moderate depression treatment for 6 weeks with trimipramine (mean dose in the last 3 weeks 106 mg daily at night) was more effective than phenelzine (45 mg daily in divided doses) or isocarboxazid (32 mg daily in divided doses) or phenelzine or isocarboxazid plus trimipramine (approximately similar doses). Most patients were also taking diazepam or nitrazepam. The results were at variance with the clinical impression that combined treatment was often more effective.— J. P. R. Young *et al.*, *Br. med. J.*, 1979, *2*, 1315. For a recommendation that tricyclic antidepressants should not be given concurrently with monoamine oxidase inhibitors, see Amitriptyline Hydrochloride, Precautions, p.112.

For a general review of the role of tricyclic antidepressants in depression, see Amitriptyline Hydrochloride, p.114.

Enuresis. In a controlled study in 186 children, trimipramine was no more effective than a placebo in the treatment of enuresis.— W. I. Forsythe *et al.*, *Br. J. clin. Pract.*, 1972, *26*, 119.

Gastro-intestinal disorders. Trimipramine has been found effective in Norway in both duodenal and gastric ulcer.— *Br. med. J.*, 1980, *281*, 95.

References to trimipramine in the management of duodenal and gastric ulcer: S. Wetterhus *et al.*, *Scand. J. Gastroenterol.*, 1979, *14*, *Suppl.*, 124; K. Valnes *et al.*, *ibid.*, 1980, *15*, *Suppl.*, 65 and 71.

Preparations

Trimipramine Tablets *(B.P.)*. Tablets containing trimipramine maleate. They are compression-coated. Potency is expressed in terms of the equivalent amount of trimipramine.

Surmontil *(May & Baker, UK)*. Trimipramine maleate, available as **Capsules** each containing the equivalent of 50 mg of trimipramine and as **Tablets** containing the equivalent of 10 or 25 mg of trimipramine. (Also available as Surmontil in *Arg.*, *Austral.*, *Belg.*, *Canad.*, *Denm.*, *Fr.*, *Ital.*, *Neth.*, *Norw.*, *S.Afr.*, *Spain*, *Switz.*, *USA*). Trimipramine mesylate and trimipramine embonate are also available in some countries as Surmontil.

Other Proprietary Names

Stangyl *(as maleate and mesylate)* *(Ger.)*.

2540-l

Viloxazine Hydrochloride. ICI 58834. 2-(2-Ethoxyphenoxymethyl)morpholine hydrochloride.

$C_{13}H_{19}NO_3,HCl$=273.8.

CAS — 46817-91-8 (viloxazine); 35604-67-2 (hydrochloride).

Adverse Effects. Nausea is commonly associated with viloxazine therapy, and vomiting and headache may also occur. Viloxazine has been associated with fewer anticholinergic side effects such as dry mouth, disturbance of accommodation, tachycardia, constipation, and difficulty with micturition than the tricyclic antidepressants. Susceptible patients may swing from depression to mania. Exacerbation of anxiety, agitation, drowsiness, confusion, ataxia, dizziness, insomnia, nightmares, tremor, paraesthesia, sweating, musculo-skeletal pain, mild hypertension, skin rashes, convulsions, and jaundice with elevated transaminases have also been reported.

Symptoms of overdosage have included drowsiness or coma, decreased reflexes, miosis, and hypotension. Tachycardia has occurred but, unlike amitriptyline, life-threatening cardiac arrhythmias do not appear to have been a problem.

In 5 double-blind crossover studies, each in 6 healthy subjects, designed to compare the effects of viloxazine hydrochloride equivalent to 100 mg of viloxazine, imipramine hydrochloride 50 mg, or placebo, on heart-rate, blood pressure, forced expiratory volume in 1 second, reaction time, critical flicker frequency, salivary flow-rate, pupil size, palpebral fissure height, and the effect of alcohol, the significant effects of viloxazine were: increased heart-rate at 4 hours, increased standing diastolic blood pressure at 7 hours, a postural fall in blood pressure at 7 hours, reduction in critical flicker frequency at 5 hours. Clinically no significant effects on heart-rate or blood pressure had occurred in 770 treated patients.— P. F. C. Bayliss and S. M. Duncan, *Br. J. clin. Pharmac.*, 1974, *1*, 431.

Epileptogenic effect. A 50-year-old man had 3 grand mal seizures and hallucinations on the sixth day of treatment with viloxazine 100 mg thrice daily. He had earlier been taking benzodiazepines which had been withdrawn when he started viloxazine.— J. G. Edwards, *Br. med. J.*, 1977, *2*, 96.

For comments on the incidence of convulsions on withdrawal of benzodiazepines, see Diazepam, p.1519.

Headache. During an open study of viloxazine, 15 of 30 patients complained of headache, in some cases accompanied by nausea. Six of these patients had a migraine-like syndrome although only one had a history of migraine.— T. R. E. Barnes *et al.* (letter), *Lancet*, 1979, *2*, 1368.

Overdosage. A report of 12 patients who took overdoses of viloxazine. Gastric lavage was carried out in most patients. None of the 12 died. Another patient who took a large overdose received no treatment and died.— R. D. Brosnan *et al.*, *I.C.I. Pharmaceuticals*, *J. int. med. Res.*, 1976, *4*, 83.

Weight changes. Mention of a tendency to weight loss associated with viloxazine therapy.— D. Nugent, *Clin. Trials J.*, 1979, *16*, 13.

Treatment of Adverse Effects. The stomach should be emptied by aspiration and lavage. The use of activated charcoal as an adjunct to gastric lavage may be of value. Supportive therapy alone may then suffice (for general guidelines to the symptomatic therapy of drug overdosage, see Phenobarbitone, p.812).

Precautions. Although viloxazine appears to be less cardiotoxic than the tricyclic antidepressants, it should be used with caution in patients with cardiovascular disease and should be avoided in the immediate recovery phase after myocardial infarction. Viloxazine should also be avoided or used with caution in patients with impaired liver function or a history of peptic ulcer; caution is also necessary in patients with epilepsy or renal insufficiency. Manic depressive patients may switch to a manic phase during viloxazine therapy, and patients with suicidal tendencies should be carefully supervised during treatment.

Viloxazine should not be given to patients receiving monoamine oxidase inhibitors or for at least 14 days after their discontinuation. Viloxazine may diminish the effects of antihypertensive agents, such as guanethidine and bethanidine; some interaction may also occur with clonidine and, in general, blood pressure should be monitored when viloxazine is prescribed with antihypertensive therapy. Blood concentrations of phenytoin may be increased in patients concurrently given viloxazine and phenytoin dosage reduction may be necessary. Since viloxazine appears to have some influence on brain dopamine metabolism viloxazine should be given with caution to patients receiving levodopa. The central nervous system depressant action of alcohol may be enhanced by concurrent administration of viloxazine.

Withdrawal of viloxazine may occasionally be associated with malaise, headache, and vomiting.

Impaired alertness may be experienced at the start of viloxazine antidepressant therapy and patients liable to take charge of vehicles or other machinery should be warned that their judgement may be impaired.

Viloxazine hydrochloride 50 mg thrice daily or imipramine 25 mg thrice daily had no significant effect on the performance of 40 healthy subjects in the Stroop Colour-Word test compared with placebo or no treatment at all. After 7 doses there was a slight worsening of performance with imipramine and a slight improvement with viloxazine.— P. G. Harvey *et al.*, *Br. J. clin. Pharmac.*, 1978, *5*, 305. See also D. Bente *et al.*, *Arzneimittel-Forsch.*, 1978, *28*, 1308.

For a general comment on antidepressant therapy and driving, see Amitriptyline Hydrochloride, p.112.

Interactions. In a double-blind study in 12 subjects viloxazine 100 mg caused a significant increase in heart-rate evident 4 hours after the dose, but there was no evidence of an anticholinergic effect. In doses of 300 mg daily it had no effect on the adrenergic system as assessed by the tyramine pressor response. There was no evidence of marked central sedation or stimulation.— P. Turner *et al.*, *J. int. med. Res.*, 1975, *3*, *Suppl.* 3, 41. In 2 subjects viloxazine 100 mg twice daily for 7 days had affected sleep patterns in a manner similar to that caused by other antidepressants and amphetamine.— I. Oswald, *ibid.*

The assessment of interactions between tyramine and viloxazine in an open study in 5 healthy subjects and a series of double-blind studies in 6 healthy subjects. Viloxazine was found to be similar to imipramine in so far as it reduces the pressor response to tyramine, but under the conditions of the study the effect is clearly much lower than with imipramine.— K. Ghose *et al.* (letter), *Br. J. clin. Pharmac.*, 1976, *3*, 668.

Absorption and Fate. Viloxazine is readily absorbed from the gastro-intestinal tract and extensively metabolised. The principal paths of metabolism of viloxazine include hydroxylation and conjugation. Viloxazine is excreted in the urine, mainly in the form of its metabolites, either free or in conjugated form.

Unlike the tricyclic antidepressants, viloxazine has a short plasma half-life of about 2 to 5 hours.

Viloxazine crosses the blood-brain barrier.

In 4 studies viloxazine hydrochloride was rapidly and almost totally absorbed after administration by mouth, only 2% being found in the faeces. It was rapidly eliminated by the kidneys and the half-life in the blood was in the range of 2 to 5 hours with maximal blood concentrations occurring 1 to 4 hours after administration by mouth. Maximum blood concentrations over the range studied were proportional to the dose administered by mouth.— P. F. C. Bayliss and D. E. Case, *Br. J. clin. Pharmac.*, 1975, *2*, 209.

The metabolism of viloxazine in healthy subjects. Half-lives in 2 subjects were 4.0 and 4.2 hours.— D. E. Case and P. R. Reeves, *Xenobiotica*, 1975, *5*, 113. *Animal studies of the metabolism of viloxazine*.— D. E. Case *et al.*, *ibid.*, 81.

Plasma concentrations. Details of a plasma concentration assay of viloxazine. There was apparently no accumulation over a period of time, and no evidence that the drug induces or inhibits its own metabolism.— D. E. Case, *J. int. med. Res.*, 1975, *3*, *Suppl.* 3, 47.

Relationship between blood and CSF concentrations of viloxazine.— O. Elwan and H. K. Adam, *Eur. J. clin. Pharmac.*, 1980, *17*, 179.

Uses. Viloxazine is an oxazine antidepressant and chemically distinct from the tricyclic and tetracyclic antidepressants. It does not have marked anticholinergic or sedative properties and may have some stimulant action. Its properties include inhibitory effects on the re-uptake (and hence the inactivation) of biogenic amines in the central nervous system. Its mode of action in depression is not fully understood.

In the treatment of depression viloxazine is given by mouth as the hydrochloride in doses equivalent to viloxazine 50 mg thrice daily initially, gradually increased to 100 mg thrice daily if necessary. The last dose of the day should not be given later than 6 p.m. A maximum total daily dose of 400 mg should not be exceeded. A suggested initial dose for the elderly is 100 mg daily cautiously increased if necessary.

Reviews and symposia on viloxazine: *Drug & Ther. Bull.*, 1975, *13*, 39; *J. int. med. Res.*, 1975, *3*, *Suppl.* 3, 1–125; R. M. Pinder *et al.*, *Drugs*, 1977, *13*, 401.

Action. Viloxazine has some of the properties of an amphetamine-like central stimulant but it differs in several important respects.— R. M. Pinder *et al.*, *Drugs*, 1977, *13*, 401.

Administration in the elderly. Beneficial results with viloxazine 100 to 200 mg daily in a placebo-controlled double-blind study involving 21 depressed elderly subjects considered unsuitable for tricyclic antidepressant therapy because of cardiac disease, tendency to urinary retention, or a history of confusion following tricyclic use. No significant difference was noted between active and placebo groups after one week, but after a further 2 weeks, patient improvements were greater in the viloxazine group. Four patients were withdrawn from the viloxazine group (one following increased anxiety, one because of nausea and vomiting, and 2 for non-medical reasons). One other patient in the viloxazine group suffered nausea and vertigo, but generally it was well tolerated, possibly because of the relatively low dosages employed.— L. Von Knorring, *J. int. med. Res.*, 1980, *8*, 18.

Depression. Four of 9 depressed patients given viloxazine showed rapid improvement in their depression during the first week.— F. J. Bereen (letter), *Lancet*, 1973, *1*, 379.

A placebo-controlled study in 29 patients with moderate or severe depression suggested that viloxazine 100 mg thrice daily for 1 week was less effective than the placebo. The reported rapid initial response to viloxazine could be a placebo response.— J. G. Edwards, *Br. med. J.*, 1977, *2*, 1327. See also *idem*, *Curr. med. Res. Opinion*, 1977, *5*, 226.

Viloxazine 50 mg thrice daily compared favourably with imipramine 25 mg thrice daily in 50 patients with depression participating in a double-blind study. Viloxazine gave better results in patients over 50 years of age with fewer side-effects such as vegetative dysfunction, vertigo, and weight increase. However more initial fatigue reactions, slight sleep disturbances, and 3 transient hypertensive reactions occurred in the viloxazine treated group.— L. Floru *et al.*, *Arzneimittel-Forsch.*, 1976, *26*, 1170.

In a 4-week sequential trial involving 11 pairs of patients with moderately severe depression there was no significant difference between the effects of viloxazine 100 mg thrice daily and imipramine 50 mg thrice daily. Fewer side-effects were reported by the patients receiving viloxazine.— B. Davies *et al.*, *Med. J. Aust.*, 1977, *1*, 521.

Further studies of viloxazine in the treatment of depression.— G. Sedman, *Curr. med. Res. Opinion*, 1977, *5*, 217 (comparison with amitriptyline); L. G. Kiloh *et al.*, *Aust. N.Z. J. Psychiat.*, 1979, *13*, 357 (comparison with amitriptyline); P. Santonastaso *et al.*, *Acta psychiat. scand.*, 1979, *60*, 137 (comparison with imipramine); O. Elwan, *J. int. med. Res.*, 1980, *8*, 7 (comparison with imipramine).

Proprietary Preparations

Vivalan *(ICI Pharmaceuticals, UK)*. Viloxazine hydrochloride, available as film-coated tablets each containing the equivalent of 50 mg of viloxazine. (Also available as Vivalan in *Belg.*, *Fr.*, *Ger.*).

Other Proprietary Names

Vicilan *(Arg., Ital.)*; Vivarint *(Spain)*.

Antihypertensive Agents

850-w

Blood pressure is expressed in terms of the arterial systolic and diastolic pressures. Since many factors influence blood pressure it is not possible to define normality or abnormality precisely using only the figures for systolic and diastolic pressures. An arbitrary definition of normal adult blood pressure provided by the World Health Organization (WHO) is a systolic pressure equal to or below 140 mmHg (18.7 kPa) together with a diastolic (fifth Korotkoff phase) pressure equal to or below 90 mmHg (12.0 kPa). Hypertension in adults is also arbitrarily defined by WHO as a systolic pressure equal to or greater than 160 mmHg (21.3 kPa) and a diastolic pressure (fifth phase) equal to or greater than 95 mmHg (12.7 kPa). Blood pressure is still expressed in mmHg and this is the unit used throughout *Martindale*. The SI unit, the kilopascal (kPa), has not been generally accepted for expressing blood pressure.

Life expectancy is reduced in patients with elevated blood pressure. Evidence has accumulated that reduction of elevated blood pressure reduces the risks of morbidity and mortality.

The drugs used in the treatment of hypertension belong to groups with distinct pharmacological actions, though the precise mode of action of some of them is not as yet fully understood. Major drugs used in the treatment of hypertension are diuretics (see Diuretics, p.581) and beta-adrenoceptor blocking agents (see Propranolol and other Beta-adrenoceptor Blocking Agents, p.1324). Those described in this section may be broadly classified as:

1. adrenergic neurone blocking agents which interfere with postganglionic sympathetic nervous transmission but are without effect on the parasympathetic nervous system; they include the guanidium antihypertensive agents:
bethanidine, p.136, bretylium, p.137, debrisoquine, p.142, guanethidine, p.145, guanoclor, p.147, guanoxan, p.148;
2. rauwolfia alkaloids and related compounds which have central and peripheral depressant actions; they include:
deserpidine, p.142, methoserpidine, p.151, rescinnamine, p.162, reserpine, p.163, syrosingopine, p.168;
3. ganglion-blocking agents which interfere with nervous transmission of both sympathetic and parasympathetic ganglia (their troublesome side-effects are due largely to parasympathetic blockade); they include:
hexamethonium, p.148, mecamylamine, p.151, pempidine, p.157, pentolinium, p.157, trimetaphan, p.169;
4. alpha-adrenoceptor blocking agents; they include:
phenoxybenzamine, p.158, phentolamine, p.159, and also indoramin, p.150, prazosin, p.160;
5. enzyme inhibitors such as methyldopa (p.151) which probably acts centrally, the monoamine oxidase inhibitor, pargyline (p.156), and captopril (p.138).

Other drugs used in the treatment of hypertension and described in this section include clonidine hydrochloride (p.139) which has been reported to have a predominantly central effect, hydralazine (p.148), minoxidil (p.155), and diazoxide (p.142) which appear to have a predominantly peripheral effect, sodium nitroprusside (p.166), and the veratrum alkaloids, alkavervir (p.136) and protoveratrines A and B (p.162).

Salt restriction was an effective method of reducing blood pressure in 31 patients with a diastolic blood pressure between 90 and 105 mmHg. The response was not quite as good as with antihypertensive therapy but was sufficient in many patients to bring the blood pressure within the usual range. Restricting the salt intake to 70 mmol daily should be assessed as a treatment for this degree of hypertension before drug therapy is instituted.— T. Morgan *et al.*, *Lancet*, 1978, *1*, 227. Discussion and comment.— *Lancet*, 1978, *1*, 1136; P. Kincaid-Smith, *Drugs*, 1978, *16*, 172.

A report of significant reduction in blood pressure associated with weight loss without dietary salt restriction in overweight patients with uncomplicated essential hypertension.— E. Reisin *et al.*, *New Engl. J. Med.*, 1978, *298*, 1. Comment.— L. Tobian, *ibid.*, 46.

Lowering blood pressure by salt restriction.— *Lancet*, 1980, *2*, 459.

Further references: C. R. P. George and A. M. Burke, *Postgrad. med. J.*, 1980, *56*, 18; *Br. med. J.*, 1981, *282*, 1993.

Choice of Antihypertensive Agent. The choice of antihypertensive agent is largely dependent on the degree of hypertension and the acceptance of the treatment by the patient. Treatment with more than one antihypertensive agent may be of benefit and such regimens may enhance the antihypertensive effect and reduce the individual side-effects. Initial treatment of severe hypertension should not reduce diastolic pressure too rapidly since autoregulation is impaired.

Of 380 selected men with mild or moderate hypertension, whose initial diastolic blood pressure averaged 90 to 114 mmHg after 3 days' bed-rest, 194 were given a placebo and 186 received either hydrochlorothiazide and reserpine, or hydralazine. When assessed by life-table analysis, antihypertensive therapy had reduced the risk of developing a morbid event within 5 years from 55 to 18%. Treatment was most effective in preventing hypertensive complications and least effective in preventing atherosclerotic complications, particularly those associated with coronary artery disease. Treatment of patients with moderate hypertension was beneficial.— Veterans Administration Cooperative Study Group on Antihypertensive Agents, *J. Am. med. Ass.*, 1970, *213*, 1143. There was little, if any, factual evidence from Britain regarding the long-term beneficial effects of treating mild hypertension (diastolic pressure less than 100 mmHg) with antihypertensive agents.— W. O'Brien, *ibid.*, 1974, *229*, 693.

A multicentre single-blind pilot study had been completed of the value of treating mild or moderate hypertension (diastolic pressure of 90 to 109 mmHg) in men and women aged 35 to 64 years; 1849 patients entered the study; 972 had been observed for more than a year, 629 for more than 2 years, and 219 for more than 3 years. Basic treatment was with bendrofluazide 5 mg twice daily (supplemented when necessary by propranolol or methyldopa) or propranolol up to 240 mg daily (supplemented when necessary by bendrofluazide or guanethidine). The difference in mean blood pressure, after 2 years, between treated patients and controls (13 to 17 mmHg systolic, 6 to 8 mmHg diastolic) was less than expected because the fall in blood pressure in the controls was greater and more prolonged than expected. Compliance was considered satisfactory and no serious reactions were reported. A full-scale trial to cover 90 000 person-years was justified and feasible and the study continued.—Report of MRC Working Party on Mild to Moderate Hypertension, *Br. med. J.*, 1977, *1*, 1437.

A report of the Joint National Committee on detection, evaluation, and treatment of high blood pressure.— *J. Am. med. Ass.*, 1977, *237*, 255.

Analysis of the incidence of coronary heart disease in 1026 men with hypertension indicated that therapy in 635 reduced the total number of myocardial infarctions and deaths from coronary heart disease. Antihypertensive therapy seemed to prevent or postpone coronary heart disease.— G. Berglund *et al.*, *Lancet*, 1978, *1*, 1.

Reduced mortality in 635 men treated with antihypertensive agents and followed for 4.3 years.— L. Wilhelmsen *et al.*, *Br. J. clin. Pharmac.*, 1979, *7*, *Suppl.* 2, 261S.

Reduced mortality over 5 years in a study involving more than 10 000 people.— Hypertension Detection and Follow-up Program Cooperative Group, *J. Am. med. Ass.*, 1979, *242*, 2562. Criticism.— W. S. Peart and W. E. Miall (letter), *Lancet*, 1980, *1*, 104.

Results of the Australian National Blood Pressure Study indicated that antihypertensive treatment reduces mortality and morbidity in subjects found by population screening to have mild, symptomless hypertension.— Report by the Management Committee, *Lancet*, 1980, *1*, 1261. Comment.— *ibid.*, 1283.

Discussions.— J. M. Walker and D. G. Beevers, *Drugs*, 1979, *18*, 312; *Br. med. J.*, 1980, *280*, 1062; A. S. Relman, *New Engl. J. Med.*, 1980, *302*, 293.

A 5-year follow-up of the treatment of hypertension showing the beneficial effects of treatment.— J. A. P. Trafford *et al.*, *Br. med. J.*, 1981, *282*, 1111. Criticism.— P. L. Drury (letter), *ibid.*, 1470.

An interim analysis on trials of the treatment of mild hypertension.— WHO/ISH Mild Hypertension Liaison Committee, *Lancet*, 1982, *1*, 149.

Further reports and studies on the merits of antihypertensive therapy: K. L. Stuart *et al.*, *Br. med. J.*, 1972, *2*, 21; D. G. Beevers *et al.*, *Lancet*, 1973, *1*, 1407; Hypertension-Stroke Cooperative Study Group, *J. Am. med. Ass.*, 1974, *229*, 409; W. B. Stason and M. C. Weinstein, *New Engl. J. Med.*, 1977, *296*, 732; R. Fein, *ibid.*, 751; M. H. Alderman, *ibid.*, 753; T. W. Anderson, *Lancet*, 1978, *2*, 1139; A. Helgeland, *Am. J. Med.*, 1980, *69*, 725; N. M. Kaplan, *Am. Heart J.*, 1981, *101*, 867; M. Moser, *ibid.*, 465.

General reviews of antihypertensive agents and therapy: J. C. Gilbert, *Br. med. J.*, 1976, *2*, 31; J. C. Petrie, *Br. med. J.*, 1976, *2*, 289 and 359; *Br. med. J.*, 1976, *2*, 1025; *Drugs*, 1976, *11*, *Suppl.* 1;; M. Wilhelm and G. DeStevens, *Prog. Drug Res.*, 1976, *20*, 197 to 259; *Br. med. J.*, 1977, *1*, 1429; C. T. Dollery, *A. Rev. Pharmac. & Toxic.*, 1977, *17*, 311; M. Hamilton, *Adv. Med. Topics Ther.*, 1977, *3*, 180; L. J. Beilin, *ibid.*, 189; *Lancet*, 1977, *1*, 1243; *Med. Lett.*, 1977, *19*, 21; M. G. Myers, *Can. med. Ass. J.*, 1977, *116*, 173; A. J. Smith, *Adv. Med. Topics Ther.*, 1977, *3*, 202; G. L. Wollam *et al.*, *Drugs*, 1977, *14*, 420; *Arterial Hypertension*, Report of a WHO Expert Committee, *Tech. Rep. Ser. Wld Hlth Org. No. 628*, 1978; G. E. Bauer and S. N. Hunyor, *Drugs*, 1978, *15*, 80; *Br. med. J.*, 1978, *2*, 75; R. W. Gifford and R. C. Tarazi, *Ann. intern. Med.*, 1978, *88*, 661; R. M. Pearson and C. W. H. Havard, *Br. J. Hosp. Med.*, 1978, *20*, 447; E. Z. Rabin, *Can. med. Ass. J.*, 1978, *118*, 941; F. O. Simpson, *Br. med. J.*, 1978, *2*, 882; *Lancet*, 1979, *1*, 1066; *Drug & Ther. Bull.*, 1979, *17*, 57; *Drug & Ther. Bull.*, 1979, *17*, 61; *Ann. intern. Med.*, 1980, *93*, 771 (resistant hypertension); L. E. Ramsay, *Prescribers' J.*, 1980, *20*, 115 (resistant hypertension); M. H. Alderman, *Am. J. Med.*, 1980, *69*, 653; A. Helgeland, *Am. J. Med.*, 1980, *69*, 725; L. T. Bannan *et al.*, *Br. med. J.*, 1980, *281*, 1053, 1120, and 1200; F. O. Simpson, *Drugs*, 1980, *20*, 69; *Archs intern. Med.*, 1980, *140*, 1280 (The Joint National Committee on Detection, Evaluation, and Treatment of High Blood Pressure).

Adverse effects. Reports and comments on adverse effects associated with antihypertensive therapy: S. K. Robinson, *J. clin. Pharmac.*, 1972, *12*, 123 (general); J. Almeyda and A. Levantine, *Br. J. Derm.*, 1973, *88*, 313 (cutaneous); M. A. Riddiough, *Am. J. Hosp. Pharm.*, 1977, *34*, 465 (general); J. E. Crook and A. S. Nies, *Drugs*, 1978, *15*, 72 (interactions); *Med. Lett.*, 1978, *20*, 15 (postural hypotension); P. Turner, *Prescribers' J.*, 1978, *18*, 94 (impotence); *Br. med. J.*, 1979, *2*, 883 (impotence); F. V. Costa *et al.*, *Int. J. clin. Pharmac. Biopharm.*, 1979, *17*, 405 (general); P. J. Lewis, *Prescribers' J.*, 1979, *19*, 94 (interactions); *Lancet*, 1979, *2*, 510 (hazards of too rapid reduction of blood pressure); *Br. med. J.*, 1979, *2*, 228 (hazards of too rapid reduction of blood pressure).

Hypertension in children. A report of hypertension and its management in 100 children.— D. G. Gill *et al.*, *Archs Dis. Childh.*, 1976, *51*, 951.

Further references: *Br. med. J.*, 1977, *2*, 76; *Pediatrics*, 1977, *59*, *Suppl.*, 808; L. G. McLain, *J. Am. med. Ass.*, 1978, *239*, 755.

Hypertension in the elderly. Elderly patients with signs and symptoms of hypertension are likely to benefit from antihypertensive treatment, but in other elderly patients the advantages of treatment are not clear and must be weighed against unwanted drug effects.— *Drug & Ther. Bull.*, 1978, *16*, 75.

Report of a major decline in the incidence of stroke, especially in the elderly, in the population of Rochester, Minnesota during the period of 1945 to 1974.— W. M. Garraway *et al.*, *New Engl. J. Med.*, 1979, *300*, 449. Comment.— R. I. Levy, *ibid.*, 490.

Further references: G. Jackson *et al.*, *Lancet*, 1976, *2*, 1317; M. H. Alderman *et al.* (letter), *ibid.*, 1977, *1*, 259; R. H. Briant, *Drugs*, 1977, *13*, 225; F. I. Caird, *Prescribers' J.*, 1977, *17*, 52; R. E. Vestal, *Drugs*, 1978, *16*, 358; J. J. Hammond and W. M. Kirkendall, *Geriat-*

rics, 1979, *34*, 27; *Lancet*, 1980, *1*, 1396; K. O'Malley and E. O'Brien, *New Engl. J. Med.*, 1980, *302*, 1397.

Hypertension in pregnancy. A discussion of the management of hypertension in pregnancy.— J. M. Roberts and D. L. Perloff, *Am. J. Obstet. Gynec.*, 1977, *127*, 316.

Further references: R. A. Bear and N. Erenrich, *Can. med. Ass. J.*, 1978, *118*, 936; G. V. P. Chamberlain *et al.*, *Br. med. J.*, 1978, *1*, 626 and 847; D. C. Dukes, *Practitioner*, 1978, *220*, 285; E. D. M. Gallery *et al.*, *Med. J. Aust.*, 1978, *1*, 540; D. D. Mathews *et al.*, *Br. med. J.*, 1978, *2*, 623; C. A. Michael, *Drugs*, 1978, *15*, 317; *Br. med. J.*, 1980, *280*, 1483.

Antihypertensive Therapy during Anaesthesia. Unwanted hypotension may occur during anaesthesia in patients being treated with some antihypertensive agents; this should be prevented or corrected by means of light anaesthesia, careful replacement of blood loss, maintenance of the patient in a slight head-down position, and avoidance of bradycardia. Awareness by the anaesthetist of the type of antihypertensive agent being taken is of the greatest importance.

In some surgical procedures it may be desirable to induce hypotension (hypotensive anaesthesia); an antihypertensive agent such as sodium nitroprusside (see p.167)may be used for this purpose.

A study of 7 normotensive patients, 7 untreated hypertensive patients, and 15 patients under treatment with a variety of antihypertensive agents including bethanidine, guanethidine, methyldopa, reserpine, and thiazide diuretics, demonstrated that untreated high arterial pressure constituted a serious risk to patients undergoing anaesthesia and surgery, and that withdrawal of antihypertensive therapy before anaesthesia was not only unnecessary but potentially dangerous, both during the pre-operative period and during anaesthesia.— C. Prys-Roberts *et al.*, *Br. J. Anaesth.*, 1971, *43*, 122. See also *idem*, 531; P. Foëx *et al.*, *ibid.*, 644. Further study indicated that patients with high arterial pressures, whether due to lack of treatment, withdrawal of treatment, or inadequate treatment should have their blood pressure stabilised before receiving elective anaesthesia and surgery.— C. Prys-Roberts *et al.*, *ibid.*, 1972, *44*, 335.

Comment on anaesthesia in the hypertensive patient.— *Lancet*, 1979, *2*, 400.

A recommendation that in hypertensive patients who are to undergo anaesthesia all antihypertensives, including beta-adrenoceptor blocking agents and catecholamine-depleting drugs, should be continued until the night before operation.— W. T. Edwards (letter), *New Engl. J. Med.*, 1979, *301*, 158.

851-e

Alkavervir. A mixture of alkaloids obtained from green veratrum and standardised for total antihypertensive effect.

CAS — 8002-39-9 (see also under Veratrum, Green).

A light yellow powder with a strong sternutatory action. Practically **insoluble** in water; freely soluble in alcohol.

Adverse Effects. Side-effects include gastro-intestinal disturbances, dizziness, headache, weakness, paraesthesia, and fatigue; blurred vision has been reported.

Overdosage gives rise to substernal and epigastric burning, severe nausea and vomiting, cold sweats, respiratory depression, postural hypotension, and extreme bradycardia or cardiac arrhythmias.

Treatment of Adverse Effects. If alkavervir has been swallowed, the stomach should be emptied by aspiration and lavage with warm water. Excessive hypotension with bradycardia or cardiac arrhythmias may be treated by injection of atropine sulphate 500 µg intramuscularly. The patient should be placed in the supine position with the feet raised.

Precautions. Alkavervir should be used with caution in patients with angina pectoris, cardiac arrhythmia, cardiac infarction, or impaired kidney function. It should not be used in patients with phaeochromocytoma or aortic coarctation. Hypotension may occur during anaesthesia in patients being treated with alkavervir (see p.136).

Concurrent administration of digitalis with alkavervir may cause excessive bradycardia and cardiac arrhythmias.

The hypotensive effects of alkavervir may be enhanced by concomitant administration of thiazide diuretics; they may be antagonised by pressor agents such as adrenaline or amphetamine. Quinidine is contra-indicated in patients receiving alkavervir.

Uses. Alkavervir causes a fall in blood pressure, bradycardia, and peripheral vasodilatation probably by inhibition of the vasomotor centre and stimulation of the vagus. Alkavervir has been used in the treatment of hypertension but as the margin between the therapeutic dosage and the dosage causing toxic effects is very narrow it is no longer recommended for routine use. The usual dose is from 9 to 15 mg daily, in 3 doses at intervals of 6 to 8 hours.

Proprietary Preparations

Thiaver *(Riker, UK)*. Scored tablets each containing alkavervir 4 mg and epithiazide 4 mg. For hypertension. *Dose.* 1 tablet twice or thrice daily.

Veriloid *(Riker, UK)*. Alkavervir, available as scored tablets of 2 mg.

A preparation containing alkavervir was formerly marketed in Great Britain under the proprietary name Veriloid-VP (*Riker*).

852-l

Alseroxylon. Selected alkaloid hydrochlorides of *Rauwolfia serpentina*.

CAS — 8001-95-4.

A reddish-brown amorphous powder with a characteristic odour.

Adverse Effects, Treatment, and Precautions. As for Reserpine, p.163.

Uses. Alseroxylon has actions and uses similar to those described under reserpine (see p.164). For the treatment of hypertension it is given in initial doses of 1 to 4 mg daily, and maintenance doses of 1 to 2 mg daily. Doses of up to 8 mg daily have also been recommended.

Proprietary Preparations

Pentoxylon *(Riker, UK)*. Tablets each containing alseroxylon 1 mg and pentaerythritol tetranitrate 10 mg. For angina pectoris. *Dose.* 1 or 2 tablets 4 times daily between meals.

Rauwiloid *(Riker, UK)*. Alseroxylon, available as tablets of 2 mg. (Also available as Rauwiloid in *Austral.*, *Norw.*).

Rauwiloid + Veriloid *(Riker, UK)*. Tablets each containing alseroxylon 1 mg and alkavervir 3 mg. For moderate to severe hypertension. *Dose.* Initial, 1 tablet thrice daily; maintenance, 1 to 2 tablets 4 times daily.

Other Proprietary Names

Angioserpina, Iposalfa, Rauwan, Ra-Valeas (all *Ital.*).

853-y

Azamethonium Bromide. Pentamethazene Bromide; Pentaminum. 2,2′-Methyliminobis(diethyldimethylammonium) dibromide.

$C_{13}H_{33}Br_2N_3$=391.2.

CAS — 60-30-0 (azamethonium); 306-53-6 (dibromide).

Pharmacopoeias. In *Rus.*

A white or yellowish-white hygroscopic crystalline powder with a faint odour. M.p. about 213°. **Soluble** in water and alcohol; practically insoluble in ether. Store in airtight containers.

Uses. Azamethonium bromide is a ganglion-blocking agent that has been used in the treatment of hypertension. The doses given in the *Rus. P.* are: intramuscularly, max. single, 150 mg; max. in 24 hours, 450 mg.

A clinical comparison showed azamethonium bromide to be qualitatively similar to hexamethonium bromide. Before tolerance developed, approximately equal falls of blood pressure were induced by subcutaneous injections of 15 mg of hexamethonium and 17 mg of azamethonium bromide. After tolerance had developed azamethonium was usually much less effective than hexamethonium.— F. H. Smirk, *Lancet*, 1952, *2*, 1002. See also A. G. Baikie and J. R. Smith, *ibid.*, 1952, *1*, 1144.

Preparations

Solutio Pentamini 5% pro Injectionibus *(Rus. P.)*. Azamethonium Bromide Injection. A sterile 5% solution of azamethonium bromide in Water for Injections; in ampoules of 1 or 2 ml. pH 6 to 7.5.

854-j

Bethanidine Sulphate *(B.P.)*. Betanidini Sulfas. 1-Benzyl-2,3-dimethylguanidine sulphate. $(C_{10}H_{15}N_3)_2,H_2SO_4$=452.6.

CAS — 55-73-2 (bethanidine); 114-85-2 (sulphate).

Pharmacopoeias. In *Br.* and *Nord.*

A white odourless powder with a bitter taste. M.p. about 285°. **Soluble** 1 in 1 of water and 1 in 30 of alcohol; practically insoluble in ether.

Adverse Effects, Treatment, and Precautions. As for Guanethidine Monosulphate, p.145.

With bethanidine sulphate parotid pain does not occur, and diarrhoea is rare. Transient sweating and headache may occur.

Interactions. *Sympathomimetics.* In a 46-year-old hypertensive woman receiving bethanidine sulphate 20 mg by mouth daily in divided doses, administration of a sustained-release capsule containing *phenylpropanolamine* thrice at 12-hourly intervals caused a rise in blood pressure which was resistant or partially resistant to treatment with diazoxide and trimetaphan camsylate. The hypertension was controlled by administration of methyldopa intravenously, and subsequently by mouth.— J. R. Misage and R. H. McDonald, *Br. med. J.*, 1970, *4*, 347.

In a patient taking bethanidine 30 mg thrice daily a single 2-mg dose of *mazindol* was sufficient to reverse completely the antihypertensive effect of bethanidine.— A. J. Boakes (letter), *Br. J. clin. Pharmac.*, 1977, *4*, 486.

Tricyclic antidepressants. In 3 patients whose blood pressure was controlled with bethanidine, the concomitant administration of *desipramine* 30 minutes before bethanidine antagonised the antihypertensive effect. An average of 5 days elapsed after discontinuation of desipramine before the effect of bethanidine reappeared. *Protriptyline* had a similar antagonistic effect.— J. R. Mitchell *et al.*, *J. Am. med. Ass.*, 1967, *202*, 973.

Further references: C. Skinner *et al.*, *Lancet*, 1969, *2*, 564; D. Shen *et al.*, *Clin. Pharmac. Ther.*, 1975, *17*, 363.

Withdrawal. Serious rebound hypertension was not associated with the abrupt withdrawal of bethanidine therapy.— M. J. Kendall, *Prescribers' J.*, 1978, *18*, 25.

Absorption and Fate. Bethanidine is rapidly but incompletely absorbed from the gastro-intestinal tract. It is excreted unchanged in the urine.

A study of the pharmacokinetics of bethanidine in 3 hypertensive subjects following intravenous and oral administration. Bethanidine was incompletely absorbed from the gastro-intestinal tract. It was excreted unchanged in the urine by active transport, and despite high renal clearance had an apparent half-life for the terminal urinary excretion phase of about 7 to 11 hours; this may be explained by a large apparent volume of distribution, suggesting that it is extensively bound to tissues, though not to plasma albumin.— D. Shen *et al.*, *Clin. Pharmac. Ther.*, 1975, *17*, 363. A study in 3 healthy subjects demonstrating time-dependent change in the renal clearance of bethanidine. Peak blood concentrations were achieved 2 to 4 hours after oral administration of 10 mg, suggesting rapid absorption. The postabsorption decline of blood concentration was noticeably slower than the corresponding decline in urinary excretion rate, suggesting a lack of constancy in the renal clearance of bethanidine.— A. N. Chremos *et al.*, *J. pharm. Sci.*, 1976, *65*, 140.

Further references: C. N. Corder *et al.*, *J. pharm. Sci.*, 1975, *64*, 785; L. G. Dring *et al.*, *Br. J. clin. Pharmac.*, 1977, *4*, 390P; C. N. Corder, *J. clin. Pharmac.*, 1978, *18*, 249; C. N. Corder, *J. clin. Pharmac.*, 1979, *19*, 428.

Uses. Bethanidine is an antihypertensive agent with actions similar to those of guanethidine monosulphate (see p.146), but without guanethidine's action on tissue noradrenaline. It also has a more rapid onset, together with a shorter duration of action, than guanethidine.

Bethanidine is used in the treatment of moderate and severe hypertension or for the treatment of mild hypertension in patients where other drugs have proved inadequate. It reduces the standing blood pressure but has a less marked effect on the supine blood pressure. It may provide a useful alternative to guanethidine when diarrhoea is a troublesome side-effect.

The usual initial dose of bethanidine sulphate is 10 mg thrice daily. The dosage is then increased by 5 mg thrice daily at brief intervals according to the response of the patient. The maintenance dose varies from 20 to 200 mg daily. To reduce side-effects smaller doses of bethanidine may be given in conjunction with a thiazide diuretic.

In hypertensive heart disease, hypertensive crises, or malignant hypertension, an initial dose of 20 mg of bethanidine sulphate may be given and increased by 10 to 20 mg every 4 to 6 hours.

Hypertension. Satisfactory control of blood pressure was obtained in 51 of 70 patients with hypertension treated with bethanidine for 6 months to 2 years. Symptoms of postural hypotension were experienced by 31 patients. The daily dose of bethanidine ranged from 10 to 120 mg. An oral diuretic was added to bethanidine treatment in 28 patients because of difficulty in controlling blood pressure, side-effects, or fluid retention. No striking differences in the results of treatment with guanethidine, methyldopa, debrisoquine, and bethanidine were seen in patients with hypertensive disease of comparative severity.— J. Bath *et al.*, *Br. med. J.*, 1967, *4*, 519.

Further reports of bethanidine in hypertension: E. Montuschi and P. T. Pickens, *Lancet*, 1962, *2*, 897; H. Smirk, *ibid.*, 1963, *1*, 743; A. W. Johnston *et al.*, *ibid.*, 1964, *2*, 659; R. W. Gifford, *J. Am. med. Ass.*, 1965, *193*, 901; R. F. O'Shea, *Med. J. Aust.*, 1966, *1*, 55; S. Talbot *et al.* (letter), *Br. med. J.*, 1975, *2*, 278.

For a comparison of the effects of bethanidine and guanethidine in hypertension, see Guanethidine Monosulphate, p.147.

In pregnancy. Hypertension of pregnancy was usually mild and on the rare occasions when drug treatment was necessary a diuretic supplemented by a small dose of bethanidine or methyldopa could be used. Reserpine was useful but if used up to the time of delivery might have some effects on the infant; it should be withdrawn some days before the expected date of delivery.— I. M. Noble, *Practitioner*, 1974, *212*, 657.

Hyperthyroidism. Bethanidine or guanethidine eye-drops were effective in treating pathological lid retraction. Bethanidine gave a more rapid response than guanethidine.— A. J. Gay *et al.*, *Archs Ophthal., N.Y.*, 1967, *77*, 341.

Tetanus. For a report of bethanidine being used in conjunction with propranolol to control symptoms of sympathetic overactivity occurring during intensive treatment of tetanus with intermittent positive-pressure respiration, see Propranolol Hydrochloride, p.1334.

Preparations

Bethanidine Tablets *(B.P.)*. Tablets containing bethanidine sulphate.

Esbatal *(Calmic, UK)*. Bethanidine sulphate, available as scored tablets of 10 and 50 mg. (Also available as Esbatal in *Arg.*, *Austral.*, *Belg.*, *Ital.*, *Neth.*, *Norw.*, *S.Afr.*, *Swed.*).

Other Proprietary Names

Batel *(Spain)*; Benzoxine, Betaling, Hypersin *(all Jap.)*; Esbaloid *(Canad.)*; Eusmanid *(Aust.)*; Regulin *(Denm., Norw.)*.

855-z

Bretylium Tosylate. Bretylium Tosilate.

(2-Bromobenzyl)ethyldimethylammonium toluene-4-sulphonate.

$C_{11}H_{17}BrN,C_7H_7O_3S=414.4$.

CAS — 59-41-6 (bretylium); 61-75-6 (tosylate).

Pharmacopoeias. In *Chin.*

A white crystalline powder. M.p. about 98°. Freely **soluble** in water and alcohol; practically insoluble in ether.

Adverse Effects, Treatment, and Precautions. As for Guanethidine Monosulphate, p.145.

Transient noradrenaline release on parenteral administration of bretylium may enhance the toxicity of digitalis; therapy with the 2 drugs should not be initiated concurrently.

Intramuscular injection may cause tissue necrosis, and rapid intravenous injection may cause severe nausea and vomiting.

Seven patients with recent cardiac infarction, 3 with and 4 without left ventricular failure, received bretylium tosylate 5 to 10 mg per kg body-weight intravenously. Initial transient tachycardia, hypertension and late sustained bradycardia, hypotension with decreased vascular resistance, and increased calf blood flow and venous capacitance occurred in all 7 patients. Bretylium should be used cautiously in patients with hypotension as it might cause a significant reduction in arterial pressure.— K. Chatterjee *et al.*, *J. Am. med. Ass.*, 1973, *223*, 757.

Absorption and Fate. Bretylium tosylate is rapidly but incompletely absorbed from the gastro-intestinal tract. It is not metabolised in the body and is largely excreted in the urine.

An average plasma-bretylium concentration of 1.31 µg per ml was detected in 4 subjects 30 minutes after being given 300 mg of bretylium tosylate by intramuscular injection and was found to decrease gradually over 24 hours when the half-life increased from 1 to 5.5 hours. Between 70 and 80% of the dose was excreted in the urine as unchanged bretylium during this period and another 8 to 9% during the next 3 days.— R. Kuntzman *et al.*, *Clin. Pharmac. Ther.*, 1970, *11*, 829.

Further references: J. L. Anderson *et al.*, *Clin. Pharmac. Ther.*, 1980, *28*, 468.

Uses. Bretylium tosylate is a quaternary ammonium antihypertensive agent with actions similar to those of guanethidine monosulphate (see p.146) but without guanethidine's action on tissue noradrenaline; it is also less liable to induce noradrenaline release following intravenous injection. Because of a lack of uniformity in its effects, and because tolerance frequently occurs, it has been superseded by other drugs in the treatment of hypertension. The suggested dose of bretylium tosylate by mouth was 100 mg thrice daily on the first day, and 200 mg thrice daily on the second. An increase of 100 mg per dose could then be made if necessary up to a maximum of 400 mg thrice daily.

Bretylium tosylate is also a class III anti-arrhythmic agent (for details see Quinidine and some other Anti-arrhythmic Agents, p.1370). It is given parenterally under electrocardiographic monitoring to control ventricular arrhythmias resistant to standard treatment; a delay of up to 2 hours may occur before the onset of the anti-arrhythmic activity therefore it should only be used if the arrhythmia is resistant to more rapidly acting agents. The patient should be supine or closely observed for postural hypotension. A suggested dose by intramuscular injection is 5 to 10 mg per kg body-weight as a 5% (50 mg per ml) solution, repeated in 1 to 2 hours if the arrhythmia persists, and subsequently given every 6 to 8 hours for up to about 3 to 5 days. Some sources do not recommend doses over 5 mg per kg. The site of injection should be varied on repeated injection and not more than 5 ml should be given into any one site.

Since bretylium tosylate causes nausea and vomiting on rapid intravenous injection, some sources do not recommend its administration by this route. Moreover, there is disagreement as to whether the anti-arrhythmic effect is achieved any more rapidly after intravenous administration. In immediately life-threatening ventricular arrhythmias, however, a suggested dose is 5 mg per kg as a 5% (50 mg per ml) solution by rapid intravenous injection, in association with other resuscitative measures and cardioversion, increased to 10 mg per kg if the ventricular fibrillation persists, and repeated at intervals of 15 to 30 minutes until a total dose of not more than 30 mg per kg has been given. In less urgent situations to avoid severe nausea and vomiting it has been recommended that bretylium injection should be diluted to not more than 1% (10 mg per ml) with dextrose injection or sodium chloride injection and given by slow intravenous injection over a period greater than 8 minutes, in a suggested dose of 5 to 10 mg per kg every 6 hours for up to about 3 to 5 days. A constant intravenous infusion dose of 1 to 2 mg per minute has also been recommended for a similar duration of time.

Administration in renal failure. Preliminary data from 3 subjects, one healthy and 2 with renal disease, indicate that bretylium accumulates with progressive renal impairment and is removed by haemodialysis. Appropriate adjustment of dosage should be made.— J. Adir *et al.* (letter), *New Engl. J. Med.*, 1979, *300*, 1390.

Further references: W. M. Bennett *et al.*, *Ann. intern. Med.*, 1980, *93*, 286.

Cardiac arrhythmias. A detailed review of the actions and uses of bretylium in cardiac arrhythmias. The onset of anti-arrhythmic effect is fastest after intravenous bolus injection; by this route it can facilitate cardioversion and suppress recurrent ventricular fibrillation within minutes. After intramuscular administration the onset of anti-arrhythmic action may be delayed by 20 minutes to an hour. In some patients the full anti-arrhythmic effects of bretylium require several hours to develop. Anti-arrhythmic effects of a single dose last for 6 to 12 hours.— J. Koch-Weser, *New Engl. J. Med.*, 1979, *300*, 473.

Comment on the anti-arrhythmic properties of bretylium tosylate. Hypotension can be a troublesome side-effect. Another problem is that against some ventricular arrhythmias it takes 20 to 40 minutes to act, though against ventricular fibrillation it acts very quickly.— L. H. Opie, *Lancet*, 1980, *1*, 861.

Further reviews: J. L. Anderson *et al.*, *Drugs*, 1978, *15*, 271; *Med. Lett.*, 1978, *20*, 105; R. H. Heissenbuttel and J. T. Bigger, *Ann. intern. Med.*, 1979, *91*, 229.

Therapeutic use. Bretylium suppressed cardiac arrhythmias within 5 minutes to several hours in 27 of 30 patients, many of whom had not responded to other treatment. The intramuscular route was preferred and a dose of 5 mg per kg body-weight was consistently effective with 2 to 3 mg per kg every 8 to 12 hours for maintenance. For intravenous use, bretylium was given in dextrose injection over 5 minutes.— M. B. Bacaner, *Am. J. Cardiol.*, 1968, *21*, 530.

Of 25 patients with life-threatening ventricular arrhythmias resistant to lignocaine and other anti-arrhythmic agents, 5 with right ventricular tachycardia responded well to bretylium but 11 of 20 with left ventricular tachycardia did not.— H. C. Cohen *et al.*, *Circulation*, 1973, *47*, 331, per *J. Am. med. Ass.*, 1973, *223*, 1558.

Twenty-seven patients with cardiac arrest and ventricular fibrillation were unresponsive to external cardiac massage, lignocaine, DC shock, and 1 or more of the following: propranolol, procainamide, and phenytoin. Bretylium tosylate 5 mg per kg body-weight intravenously was given with continued standard resuscitative technique, usually including further DC shock. Conversion to some form of stable rhythm occurred in 20 patients and these were given further doses of bretylium intramuscularly every 6 to 8 hours for 48 hours; 12 survived to leave hospital.— D. A. Holder *et al.*, *Circulation*, 1977, *55*, 541.

Further references: J. G. Bernstein and J. Koch-Weser, *Circulation*, 1972, *45*, 1024; G. Sanna and R. Arcidiacono, *Am. J. Cardiol.*, 1973, *32*, 982.

Prophylactic use. Prophylactic treatment with bretylium tosylate, 300 mg intramuscularly every 6 hours for 5 days, was compared with a placebo in 100 patients with recent acute cardiac infarction. Of 63 patients given bretylium, treatment was stopped because of hypotension in 21 and nausea and vomiting in 4. Significant arrhythmias occurred in 8 of the treated and 16 of the control patients but there was no significant effect on ventricular arrhythmias. There was insufficient clinical benefit to justify the prophylactic use of bretylium in cardiac infarction.— S. H. Taylor *et al.*, *Br. Heart J.*, 1970, *32*, 326, per *Abstr. Wld Med.*, 1970, *44*, 898.

Bretylium tosylate was as effective as lignocaine in preventing arrhythmias following acute cardiac infarction. However, there was significant supine hypotension in 7 of 16 patients given bretylium tosylate and it was considered to be contra-indicated for routine use and for the prophylaxis of arrhythmias following acute cardiac infarction.— K. Luomanmäki *et al.*, *Archs intern. Med.*, 1975, *135*, 515.

Further references: A. R. Castaneda and M. B. Bacaner, *Am. J. Cardiol.*, 1970, *25*, 461; H. W. Day and M. B. Bacaner, *ibid.*, 1971, *27*, 177.

Proprietary Preparations

Bretylate *(Wellcome, UK).* Bretylium tosylate, available as an injection containing 50 mg per ml, in ampoules of 2 ml. (Also available as Bretylate in *Austral., Belg., Canad., Fr., Neth.*).

Other Proprietary Names

Bretylol *(USA).*

856-c

Captopril.

SQ 14225. 1-[(2*S*)-3-Mercapto-2-methylpropionyl]-L-proline.

$C_9H_{15}NO_3S$=217.3.

CAS — 62571-86-2.

Adverse Effects. Skin rash, an allergic reaction, pruritus, and taste disturbance (sometimes associated with weight loss) may occur. Proteinuria has occurred, with the nephrotic syndrome and renal failure in some patients. Leucopenia and agranulocytosis have been reported. Blood-potassium concentrations may be raised. Other adverse effects reported with captopril include stomatosis resembling aphthous ulcers, gastric irritation and abdominal pain, a precipitous fall in blood pressure, tachycardia (in volume-depleted patients), paraesthesias of the hands, a serum-sickness-like syndrome, cough, bronchospasm, and lymphadenopathy.

A fall in plasma-sodium concentration occurred in 5 men with congestive heart failure during treatment with captopril.— M. G. Nicholls *et al., Br. med. J.*, 1980, *281*, 909.

Ischaemic complications of captopril.— K. M. Baker *et al., Hypertension*, 1980, *2*, 73.

Allergy. A report of an allergic reaction, resembling serum sickness, in a patient taking captopril.— S. J. Hoorntje *et al.* (letter), *Lancet*, 1979, *2*, 1297.

Eosinophilia in 7 of 20 patients treated with captopril for one year.— J. G. Kayanakis *et al.* (letter), *Lancet*, 1980, *2*, 923.

Aphthous ulcers. A report of severe aphthous ulcers in a woman taking captopril. The ulcers resolved when captopril was withdrawn and recurred when captopril was given again.— Y. K. Seedat (letter), *Lancet*, 1979, *2*, 1297.

Effects on the blood. Reports of leucopenia and agranulocytosis.— P. van Brummelen *et al.* (letter), *Lancet*, 1980, *1*, 150; F. W. Amann *et al.* (letter), *ibid.*; J. Staessen *et al.* (letter), *ibid.*, 926; F. Elijovisch and L. R. Krakoff (letter), *ibid.*, 927; C. R. W. Edwards *et al.* (letter), *ibid.*, 1981, *1*, 723; A. El Matri *et al., Br. med. J.*, 1981, *283*, 277; T. Forslund *et al.* (letter), *Lancet*, 1981, *1*, 166.

Effects on the heart. Hyperkinetic circulation associated with captopril therapy.— F. M. Fouad *et al.* (letter), *New Engl. J. Med.*, 1981, *305*, 405.

Effects on the kidneys. Reports of proteinuria.— D. B. Case *et al., J. Am. med. Ass.*, 1980, *244*, 346; C. Rosendorf *et al., S. Afr. med. J.*, 1980, *58*, 172.

Reports of the nephrotic syndrome.— E. J. L. Prins *et al.* (letter), *Lancet*, 1979, *2*, 306; Y. K. Seedat *et al., S. Afr. med. J.*, 1980, *57*, 390.

Reports of membranous glomerulopathy.— S. J. Hoorntje *et al., Lancet*, 1980, *1*, 1212.

Reports of renal failure.— P. R. Farrow and R. Wilkinson, *Br. med. J.*, 1979, *1*, 1680; R. R. Bailey *et al., N.Z. med. J.*, 1980, *92*, 31 (irreversible); A. Grossman *et al.* (letter), *Lancet*, 1980, *1*, 712 (with disproportionate hyperkalaemia).

Increased serum-creatinine concentration.— K. Woodhouse *et al., Br. med. J.*, 1979, *2*, 1146.

Effects on the skin. Captopril-induced skin eruptions.— J. K. Wilkin *et al., Archs Derm.*, 1980, *116*, 902.

Pemphigus erythematosus in one patient.— P. S. Parfrey *et al., Br. med. J.*, 1980, *281*, 194.

Pregnancy and the neonate. Administration of captopril to *sheep* and *rabbits* in doses analogous to those suitable for man, was associated with an increase in stillbirths.— F. B. Pipkin *et al.* (letter), *Lancet*, 1980, *1*, 1256.

Taste disturbance. Taste disturbance in 3 of 16 patients taking captopril.— J. J. McNeil, *Br. med. J.*, 1979, *2*, 1555. See also P. H. Vlasses and R. K. Ferguson (letter), *Lancet*, 1979, *2*, 526.

Treatment of Adverse Effects. Volume expansion with an intravenous infusion of sodium chloride injection has been recommended for the treatment of hypotension.

Precautions. There may be a severe initial fall in blood pressure in sodium-depleted patients.

The urine should be monitored for signs of proteinuria; regular blood counts should be made during the initial stages of treatment special caution being recommended in patients with systemic lupus erythematosus and other auto-immune collagen disorders.

Since raised serum-potassium concentrations may develop potassium-sparing diuretics or potassium supplements should be used with caution.

Hypotension after a 25-mg dose of captopril in one patient; captopril should be given with caution in the hyponatraemic hypertensive syndrome.— A. B. Atkinson *et al.* (letter), *Lancet*, 1979, *1*, 557.

Interactions. Neuropathy in 2 patients receiving captopril in association with cimetidine.— A. B. Atkinson *et al.* (letter), *Lancet*, 1980, *2*, 36.

Patients receiving captopril give false-positive reactions with the alkaline-nitroprusside test for urinary ketones.— S. E. Warren (letter), *New Engl. J. Med.*, 1980, *303*, 1003.

Leucopenia in a patient given captopril with azathioprine which resolved when either drug was given alone.— E. J. Kirchertz *et al.* (letter), *Lancet*, 1981, *1*, 1363.

Pregnancy and the neonate. A study indicating that only very small amounts of captopril enter breast milk. Since the kidneys of neonates are immature, however, more accumulation may occur than in adults.— R. G. Devlin and P. M. Fleiss, *J. clin. Pharmac.*, 1981, *21*, 110.

Absorption and Fate. Captopril is readily absorbed from the gastro-intestinal tract. It is about 30% bound to plasma proteins. Transfer to breast milk is minimal. It is largely excreted in the urine as unchanged drug, as disulphide, and as other metabolites.

Excretion in breast milk.— R. G. Devlin and P. M. Fleiss, *Clin. Pharmac. Ther.*, 1980, *27*, 250.

Metabolism.— K. J. Kripalani *et al., Clin. Pharmac. Ther.*, 1980, *27*, 636.

Further references: D. N. McKinstry and K. J. Kripalani, *Clin. Pharmac. Ther.*, 1980, *27*, 270.

Uses. Captopril inhibits the enzyme (angiotensin converting enzyme; kininase II) involved in the conversion of angiotensin I to angiotensin II; it is active when given by mouth.

Captopril is used in the treatment of severe hypertension where other therapy has failed. The usual initial dose is 25 mg thrice daily gradually increased to a recommended maximum of 150 mg thrice daily; larger doses have been given. Proportionately smaller doses are needed in patients with impaired renal function. Captopril should be taken an hour before meals. Captopril is commonly given in conjunction with a thiazide or loop diuretic.

Captopril has also been used in the treatment of congestive heart failure; smaller doses than those used in hypertension have sometimes been effective.

A suggested dose of captopril for children is 1 mg per kg body-weight daily initially, gradually increased to a maximum of 6 mg per kg daily, in 3 divided doses.

Reviews and discussion.— A. B. Atkinson and J. I. S. Robertson, *Lancet*, 1979, *2*, 836; *Br. med. J.*, 1980, *281*, 630; R. C. Heel *et al., Drugs*, 1980, *20*, 409; *Med. Lett.*, 1980, *22*, 39; *Lancet*, 1980, *2*, 129; D. G. Vidt *et al., New Engl. J. Med.*, 1982, *306*, 214.

Action. Urinary kallikrein excretion was reduced in 11 patients receiving captopril for essential hypertension. This decrease may reflect accumulation of bradykinin (or other kinins) in the blood, which may inhibit kallikrein production in the kidney by negative feedback. The potent vasodilator properties of bradykinin probably contribute to the hypotensive effect of captopril.— B. E. Karlberg *et al.* (letter), *Lancet*, 1980, *1*, 150. Criticism of the assumption of a negative feedback.— R. J. Cunningham and B. H. Brouhard (letter), *ibid.*, 832; M. Marin-Grez *et al.* (letter), *ibid.*, 1033.

Further references: S. A. Atlas *et al., Hypertension*, 1979, *1*, 274; J. R. Luderer *et al., Clin. Pharmac. Ther.*, 1980, *27*, 268; P. Lijnen *et al., Clin. Pharmac. Ther.*, 1980, *28*, 310; A. Maruyama *et al., Clin. Pharmac. Ther.*, 1980, *28*, 316; S. L. Swartz *et al., Clin. Pharmac. Ther.*, 1980, *28*, 499.

Administration in renal failure. In 15 patients with renal failure the concentration of unchanged captopril in blood was decreased and that of metabolites was increased. There was a linear relationship between individual overall elimination-rate constants and endogenous creatinine clearance.— A. J. Rommel *et al., Clin. Pharmac. Ther.*, 1980, *27*, 282.

See also under Hypertension, below.

Bartter's syndrome. Beneficial results with captopril in 3 patients with Bartter's syndrome characterised by hypokalaemia, hyper-reninaemia, and (usually) low blood pressure.— M. Aurell and A. Rudin (letter), *New Engl. J. Med.*, 1981, *304*, 1609.

Cardiac disease. Favourable reports of the use of captopril in congestive heart failure.— R. Davis *et al., New Engl. J. Med.*, 1979, *301*, 117; V. J. Dzau *et al., New Engl. J. Med.*, 1980, *302*, 1373; R. Ader *et al., Circulation*, 1980, *61*, 931; D. N. Sharpe *et al., Lancet*, 1980, *2*, 1154 (small initial doses); A. H. Maslowski *et al., Lancet*, 1981, *1*, 71.

Further references: J. N. Cohn, *New Engl. J. Med.*, 1980, *302*, 1414.

Hypertension. Of 68 patients with moderate to severe essential hypertension treated with captopril, 32 were controlled (supine diastolic blood pressure not more than 90 mmHg) and 20 had a reduction of at least 10% in blood pressure; of 43 with renovascular hypertension the corresponding responses occurred in 27 and 9; of 13 with chronic renal failure 8 and 2 responded; and of 3 with primary aldosteronism one was controlled and one had a partial response; about 30% of patients needed a diuretic and/or low-sodium diet to achieve maximum effect. The initial dose of captopril was 10 or 25 mg increased up to 600 mg (originally 1000 mg) daily as required. The results of treatment of 476 patients treated by captopril, and/or propranolol or hydrochlorothiazide are reported.— A. C. Jenkins and D. N. McKinstry, *Med. J. Aust.*, 1979, *2*, *Suppl.* (Oct. 20), 32.

Successful use in a child with refractory malignant hypertension.— S. E. Oberfield *et al., J. Pediat.*, 1979, *95*, 641.

In 15 patients with moderate essential hypertension blood pressure fell from a mean of 178/112 mmHg to a mean of 158/103 mmHg after the first 25-mg dose of captopril and to 150/97 mmHg after treatment for 4 weeks with doses gradually increased to 150 mg thrice daily. The fall in blood pressure was significantly correlated with the initial plasma-renin activity.— G. A. MacGregor *et al., Br. med. J.*, 1979, *2*, 1106.

The effect of captopril on blood pressure in an anephric woman depended on the state of sodium balance.— A. J. Man in't Veld *et al., Br. med. J.*, 1979, *2*, 1110.

Captopril was used to treat essential or renovascular hypertension, or hypertension associated with renal failure, in 22 patients. Initial doses were 10 to 25 mg by mouth, increasing to a maximum of 200 mg twice daily, for approximately 3 weeks. The 25-mg and 200-mg doses produced a similar degree of lowering of blood pressure, but the effect was more prolonged with 200-mg doses. Treatment was continued successfully in 17 patients for up to 7 months, additional diuretic therapy being required in 4 patients, 3 of whom had hypertension associated with chronic renal failure. No side-effects were noted.— H. R. Brunner *et al., Ann. intern. Med.*, 1979, *90*, 19. See also *idem, Br. J. clin. Pharmac.*, 1979, *7*, *Suppl.* 2, 205S.

In 7 anephric patients captopril caused a reduction in blood pressure one hour after dialysis (fluid depletion) but not 2 days after dialysis (fluid repletion). The plasma concentration of renin was low. Captopril might be of value in patients with low renin concentrations.— A. J. Man in't Veld *et al., Br. med. J.*, 1980, *280*, 288.

In 5 anephric patients captopril 50 mg failed to reduce blood pressure; blood pressure rose in 3 patients. The hypotensive effect of captopril appeared to depend on an active renal renin-angiotensin system.— B. R. Leslie *et al., Br. med. J.*, 1980, *280*, 1067.

Eleven patients with severe hypertension unresponsive to previous therapy achieved sustained control of blood pressure following administration of captopril, in an initial dose of 6.25 mg or 25 mg gradually increased to 450 mg daily divided into 3 doses, together with frusemide 40 mg to 2 g daily (10 patients) or hydrochlorothiazide 100 mg daily (1 patient). Side-effects included temporary loss of taste in 2 patients, tachycardia at rest which was controlled by concomitant propranolol administration in one patient, and the nephrotic syndrome in one patient.— A. B. Atkinson *et al.*, *Lancet*, 1980, *2*, 105.

Control of refractory high blood pressure in 10 patients using captopril and frusemide. There appears to be a biphasic or possibly triphasic response in the fall in blood pressure, with an initial (introduction) phase characterised by a transient fall after each dose; then there is a smoother fall over a period of days, and finally there is a further reduction of blood pressure over several months.— N. J. White *et al.*, *Lancet*, 1980, *2*, 108.

Comparison with hydrochlorothiazide.— J. J. McNeil *et al.*, *Med. J. Aust.*, 1979, *2*, *Suppl.* (Oct. 20), 22; D. N. Sharpe, *ibid.*, 24.

Comparison with propranolol.— D. H. Friedlander, *Med. J. Aust.*, 1979, *2*, *Suppl.* (Oct. 20), 30; Y. K. Seedat, *S. Afr. med. J.*, 1979, *56*, 983; C. M. Huang *et al.*, *Clin. Pharmac. Ther.*, 1980, *27*, 258.

Further references: D. B. Case, *Prog. cardiovasc. Dis.*, 1978, *21*, 195; M. Aurell *et al.* (letter), *Lancet*, 1979, *2*, 149; D. H. Friedlander, *N.Z. med. J.*, 1979, *90*, 146; J. M. Sullivan *et al.*, *Hypertension*, 1979, *1*, 397; C. I. Johnston *et al.*, *Lancet*, 1979, *2*, 493; R. K. Ferguson *et al.*, *Am. Heart J.*, 1980, *99*, 579; H. R. Brunner *et al.*, *Hypertension*, 1980, *2*, 558; D. W. Johns *et al.*, *Hypertension*, 1980, *2*, 567; J. H. Laragh *et al.*, *Hypertension*, 1980, *2*, 586; A. Friedman *et al.*, *J. Pediat.*, 1980, *97*, 664; D. B. Case *et al.*, *J. cardiovasc. Pharmac.*, 1980, *2*, 339; M. H. Weinberger, *Clin. Pharmac. Ther.*, 1980, *27*, 293.

Oedema. In a 32-year-old woman with idiopathic oedema, all symptoms disappeared during treatment with captopril and resumed rapidly when placebo was given.— A. Mimran and R. Targhetta (letter), *New Engl. J. Med.*, 1979, *301*, 1289.

Scleroderma. A report of the dramatic reversal by captopril of vascular and renal crises in 2 patients with scleroderma.— J. A. Lopez-Ovejero *et al.*, *New Engl. J. Med.*, 1979, *300*, 1417.

Proprietary Preparations

Capoten *(Squibb, UK)*. Captopril, available as tablets of 25 mg and scored tablets of 50 and 100 mg.

Other Proprietary Names

Lopirin *(Switz.)*.

857-k

Clonidine Hydrochloride *(B.P.)*. St 155; 2-(2,6-Dichloroanilino)-2-imidazoline Hydrochloride; 2-(2,6-Dichlorophenylamino)-2-imidazoline Hydrochloride. 2,6-Dichloro-*N*-(imidazolidin-2-ylidene)aniline hydrochloride. $C_9H_9Cl_2N_3,HCl = 266.6$.

CAS — 4205-90-7 (clonidine); 4205-91-8 (hydrochloride).

Pharmacopoeias. In *Br.* and *Chin.*

A white or almost white, odourless or almost odourless, crystalline powder with a bitter taste. M.p. about 313°. **Soluble** 1 in 13 of water, 1 in 25 of alcohol, 1 in 38 of dehydrated alcohol, and 1 in 250 of chloroform; practically insoluble in ether. A 5% solution in water has a pH of 4 to 5. **Protect** from light.

Adverse Effects. Drowsiness and dryness of mouth commonly occur during the initial stages of therapy. Anxiety, angio-oedema, parotid pain, instances of a syndrome resembling Raynaud's phenomenon, and generalised pruritus have been reported. Depression, dizziness, oedema, constipation, nausea, weight gain as well as anorexia, bradycardia and electrocardiographic abnormalities, euphoria, headache, ocular irritation, slight orthostatic hypotension, gynaecomastia, occasional impotence, difficult micturition, paraesthesia, nocturnal unrest, skin rash, weakness, and transient hyperglycaemia after high doses may occur. Facial pallor may follow injection of clonidine.

Effects on the eyes. The rare occurrence of miosis had been reported during treatment with clonidine.— *Med. Lett.*, 1976, *18*, 63.

Out of 215 reports to the World Health Organization describing 337 events associated with clonidine, only 7 ocular effects are listed: abnormal vision (4), conjunctivitis, eye abnormality, and papilloedema.— *Aust. Prescriber*, 1976, *1*, 79.

Effects on the gastro-intestinal tract. A 26-year-old male renal transplant recipient suffered pseudo-obstruction of the bowel while receiving clonidine therapy. He recovered after withdrawal of clonidine despite continuing to take other antihypertensive agents. An informal survey of other patients taking clonidine revealed that constipation was common.— R. Bear and K. Steer, *Br. med. J.*, 1976, *1*, 197. A further report.— G. E. Bauer and K. J. Hellestrand (letter), *ibid.*, 769.

Effects on the heart. A report on 2 patients with hypertension, that clonidine hydrochloride might have been associated with a cardiac conduction defect.— L. E. Kibler and P. C. Gazes, *J. Am. med. Ass.*, 1977, *238*, 1930. A further report of the development of atroventricular dissociation in 1 patient who had received clonidine hydrochloride up to 200 µg every 8 hours for 10 days.— P. Abiuso and G. Abelow (letter), *ibid.*, 1978, *240*, 108.

Further references: P. L. Williams *et al.*, *Chest*, 1977, *72*, 784.

Effects on mental state. A 74-year-old man taking debrisoquine, bendrofluazide, and clonidine developed dementia, characterised by amnesia, unsteadiness of gait, drowsiness, aggressiveness, and urinary incontinence, 5 months after starting to take clonidine. He improved markedly a week after clonidine was withdrawn.— P. Lavin and C. P. Alexander (letter), *Br. med. J.*, 1975, *1*, 628.

Acute paranoid reactions associated with treatment for hypertension with clonidine were reported on 2 occasions with an interval of 18 months in a 54-year-old man. The reactions included delusions and auditory hallucinations and cleared on withdrawal of clonidine.— M. D. Enoch and G. E. M. Hammad, *Curr. med. Res. Opinion*, 1977, *4*, 670.

Sleep patterns. The duration of REM sleep was reduced from 107.9 to 10.3 minutes and was abolished completely in 2 subjects in a study of 5 healthy subjects given 300 µg of a slow-release preparation of clonidine before retiring. Systolic blood pressure was also significantly reduced.— C. T. Dollery *et al.*, *Br. J. clin. Pharmac.*, 1977, *4*, 634P.

Further references: A. Autret *et al.*, *Eur. J. clin. Pharmac.*, 1977, *12*, 319.

Effects on sexual function. The incidence of impotence in 59 hypertensive patients given clonidine was 24%; the incidence during a control period was 8%.— G. Onesti *et al.*, *Am. J. Cardiol.*, 1971, *28*, 74.

Hypotension. Severe hypotension developed in 3 patients who, on the discontinuation of sodium nitroprusside infusion, were given clonidine hydrochloride 100 µg by mouth. The fall in blood pressure was not observed until 45 to 135 minutes after the infusion was stopped when it would have been expected that the vasodilating effect of the sodium nitroprusside was dissipated.— I. M. Cohen *et al.* (letter), *Ann. intern. Med.*, 1976, *85*, 205.

Treatment of Adverse Effects. If overdosage occurs the stomach should be emptied by aspiration and lavage. Severe hypotension may respond to placing the patient in the supine position with the feet raised. The effects of gross overdosage may respond to infusion of plasma.

Hypertension due to sudden withdrawal of clonidine therapy may be treated by re-introduction of clonidine or by the administration of alpha-adrenergic blocking agents such as phentolamine.

Analysis by the National Poisons Information Service of poisoning by clonidine in 133 children and 37 adults revealed the following percentage incidence of signs and symptoms: impaired consciousness 85 and 78% respectively, pallor 27 and 16%, bradycardia 24 and 49%, cardiac arrhythmias 5 and 0%, cardiac arrest 0 and 3%, hypotension 21 and 32%, depressed respiration 15 and 5%, apnoea 2 and 0%, miosis 14 and 8%, unreactive pupils 5 and 0%, hypotonia 11 and 5%, irritability 11 and 3%, hyporeflexia 4 and 3%, extensor plantar reflex 3 and 0%, hypertension 2 and 11%, dry mouth 2 and 11%. There were no deaths but clinical features were often severe. Supportive measures were usually adequate but atropine was often needed for severe and persistent bradycardia. Forced diuresis was not advised because hypotension could be enhanced and there was no evidence that excretion of clonidine was increased. The role of alpha-blockers was limited and unproven.— B. Stein and G. N. Volans, *Br. med. J.*, 1978, *2*, 667.

Individual reports. A patient took an estimated dose of 4.8 mg of clonidine hydrochloride with an unknown amount of alcohol. Three hours later on admission to hospital he was alert but dizzy on standing. Supine blood pressure was 110/78 mmHg, on standing this fell to 50/30 mmHg; pulse-rates were 78 and 98 per minute respectively. Maintenance fluids were given intravenously and by the 13th hour his blood pressure was at his pre-admission value; a dose of 0.4 mg of clonidine was given on the second day. There was no rebound hypertension.— M. A. Moore and P. Phillipi (letter), *Lancet*, 1976, *2*, 694.

A hypertensive crisis, in a patient who had been withdrawn from propranolol, clonidine, and bendrofluazide, believed to be associated with the withdrawal of clonidine, was relieved by a single intravenous bolus injection of labetalol 150 mg.— E. A. Rosei *et al.*, *Br. J. clin. Pharmac.*, 1976, *3*, *Suppl.* 3, 809. See also J. J. Brown *et al.* (letter), *Br. med. J.*, 1976, *1*, 1341.

Two children, a boy aged 3.6 years and a girl aged 2.5 years, took between them 20 to 25 tablets of clonidine 25 µg three hours before arriving at hospital. The girl was unsteady, pale with peripheral vasoconstriction, and her conscious level fluctuated. There were episodes of bradycardia. Treatment consisted of gastric lavage and atropine 200 µg given intravenously on 5 occasions whenever the pulse-rate persisted at a low value. Four seizures occurred in the first 8 hours. The boy had less severe effects and no seizures. Neither child became hypotensive or hypothermic.— R. MacFaul and G. Miller (letter), *Lancet*, 1977, *1*, 1266.

Hypotension associated with clonidine poisoning in a 2½-year-old child did not respond to intravenous administration of tolazoline 5 mg. A second 5-mg injection given 15 minutes later temporarily raised the blood pressure. A rapid rise in the blood pressure occurred after a third injection of 5 mg another 15 minutes later. Tolazoline reversed all the symptoms of clonidine overdosage in this child, with the exception of bradycardia, which persisted for 16 hours.— J. E. Mendoza and M. Medalie, *Clin. Pediat.*, 1979, *18*, 123.

Recovery of 2 patients from a thousand-fold clonidine overdose.— J. A. O. Rotellar *et al.* (letter), *Lancet*, 1981, *1*, 1312.

Further reports and comments: L. Hansson and S. N. Hunyor, *Clin. Sci. & mol. Med.*, 1973, *45*, *Suppl.* 1, 181s; S. N. Hunyor *et al.*, *Br. med. J.*, 1973, *2*, 209; L. Hansson *et al.*, *Am. Heart J.*, 1973, *85*, 605; S. N. Hunyor *et al.*, *Br. med. J.*, 1975, *4*, 23; L. M. H. Wing *et al.* (letter), *ibid.*, 408; G. S. Pai and D. P. Lipsitz, *Pediatrics*, 1976, *58*, 749; R. E. Patnode *et al.* (letter), *J. Pediat.*, 1977, *90*, 848.

Precautions. Clonidine should be used with caution in patients with cerebral, or coronary insufficiency, Raynaud's disease or thromboangiitis obliterans, or with a history of depression. The hypotensive effect may be antagonised by tricyclic antidepressants, and enhanced by thiazide diuretics. Clonidine causes drowsiness and patients should not drive or operate machinery where loss of attention could be dangerous. The effects of other central nervous system depressants may be enhanced.

Withdrawal of clonidine therapy should be gradual as sudden discontinuation may cause agitation and a hypertensive crisis. Because of this possibility it has been suggested that patients should be warned of the possibility of a reaction 8 to 24 hours after withdrawal, and should carry a reserve supply of tablets.

Although hypotension may occur during anaesthesia in clonidine-treated patients (see p.136) clonidine should not be withdrawn, indeed if necessary it should be given intravenously during the operation to avoid the risk of rebound hypertension. Intravenous injections of clonidine should be given slowly to avoid a possible transient pressor effect especially in patients already receiving other antihypertensive agents such as guanethidine or reserpine.

Interactions. *Animal* studies demonstrating antagonism by yohimbine, piperoxan, and mianserin, of some cardiovascular and behavioural effects of clonidine.— R. D. Robson *et al.*, *Eur. J. Pharmac.*, 1978, *47*, 431.

Beta-adrenoceptor blockers. The concomitant administration of high doses of clonidine with high doses of propranolol had been associated with the development of nightmares, delusions, and marked drowsiness; 5 patients with impaired renal function had become semicomatose for periods of 2 to 5 days. Rapid recovery followed withdrawal of clonidine.— P. Kincaid-Smith *et al.*, *Med. J. Aust.*, 1975, *1*, 327.

In 6 of 10 patients with hypertension associated with recent cerebral damage or with uncomplicated hypertension, concurrent administration of clonidine and sotalol caused increased blood pressure compared with administration of sotalol or clonidine alone. Concurrent administration of clonidine and beta-adrenoceptor blocking agents should be avoided until the interaction had been investigated.— H. Saarimaa, *Br. med. J.*, 1976, *1*, 810.

A report of clonidine withdrawal symptoms and the suggestion that they may have been enhanced by beta-adrenoceptor blockade.— R. R. Bailey and T. J. Neale, *Br. med. J.*, 1976, *1*, 942.

Further references: A. L. Harris (letter), *New Engl. J. Med.*, 1976, *294*, 845; W. A. Pettinger (letter), *ibid.*

Phenothiazines. In *cats* the antihypertensive action of clonidine was antagonised by prior intra-arterial administration of the phenothiazine derivatives chlorpromazine, promazine, promethazine, thiethylperazine, and thioridazine, also of chlorprothixene, and to a limited extent haloperidol. Similar results were observed in *rats* after prior intravenous administration of phenothiazine derivatives and also of piperoxan. The benzodiazepines chlordiazepoxide, diazepam, and flurazepam, and also pimozide, had virtually no effect on response to clonidine in *cats*.— P. A. van Zwieten, *J. Pharm. Pharmac.*, 1977, *29*, 229.

For the effect of clonidine on fluphenazine, see Fluphenazine, p.1530.

Tricyclic antidepressants. In 4 of 5 hypertensive patients who had been treated for at least 2 years with clonidine and a diuretic, blood pressure rose when desipramine 75 mg daily was added to their treatment. The effect was not usually evident before 24 hours.— R. H. Briant *et al.*, *Br. med. J.*, 1973, *1*, 522. A similar rise in blood pressure occurred in a patient with urinary incontinence given imipramine 25 mg daily in addition to clonidine; control of blood pressure was re-established when imipramine was withdrawn.— D. E. Coffler (letter), *Drug Intell. & clin. Pharm.*, 1976, *10*, 114.

Animal studies on the interaction between clonidine and tricyclic antidepressants.— A. J. Draper *et al.*, *J. Pharm. Pharmac.*, 1976, *28*, 34P; N. K. Dadkar *et al.*, *J. Pharm. Pharmac.*, 1978, *30*, 58.

Pregnancy and the neonate. The infants of 5 women given clonidine intravenously to control hypertensive crisis in labour were not affected in any way.— P. W. Leighton and H. Tighe (letter), *Med. J. Aust.*, 1974, *2*, 680.

Further references: C. I. Johnston and D. R. Aickin, *Med. J. Aust.*, 1971, *2*, 132.

Resistance. Two patients, with high plasma-clonidine concentrations of 26.2 and 14.4 ng per ml respectively after large doses of clonidine, were resistant to the antihypertensive effect of the drug. Seven or 8 months after withdrawal of clonidine an antihypertensive effect was obtained after doses of 300 µg, with plasma concentrations of 1.4 and 0.9 ng per ml respectively. While there was tolerance to the central sedative effects of clonidine the resistance was attributed primarily to the predominance of peripheral alpha-receptor stimulation at high concentrations.— L. M. H. Wing *et al.*, *Br. med. J.*, 1977, *1*, 136.

Withdrawal. Reviews of clonidine withdrawal and hypertension: *Drug & Ther. Bull.*, 1977, *15*, 99.

A patient from whom clonidine was suddenly withdrawn had intractable vomiting; clonidine was reinstituted and later withdrawn slowly without incident.— J. A. C. Hopkirk *et al.* (letter), *Br. med. J.*, 1975, *3*, 435.

The intentionally abrupt withdrawal of clonidine produced within 36 hours a rapid rise in blood pressure towards pretreatment values in 6 of 7 hypertensive patients. The effect appeared to be dose-dependent; the 6 susceptible patients had been taking 0.45 to 5.4 mg daily while the patient who had not responded had been taking 0.15 mg daily without it having any effect on his blood pressure. Three of these patients had to be withdrawn from the study because of the severity of their rebound. These patients had also been taking propranolol up to 3 days before the study. Subjective symptoms occurred after 20 hours and lasted for 10 hours or more; they included headache, sweating, insomnia, flushing, agitation, tremor, emotional upset, and in 1 patient nausea and vomiting. Plasma-noradrenaline concentrations were elevated in the 6 patients on clonidine withdrawal.— J. L. Reid *et al.*, *Lancet*, 1977, *1*, 1171. Three similar cases.— M. J. Reza (letter), *ibid.*, 1977, *2*, 89.

In a double-blind crossover study involving 20 patients with mild to moderate hypertension abrupt withdrawal of clonidine did not lead to withdrawal symptoms or a generalised rebound or overshoot in blood pressure.— T. L. Whitsett *et al.*, *Am. J. Cardiol.*, 1978, *41*, 1285.

Further reports and comments: J. Webster *et al.* (letter), *Lancet*, 1974, *2*, 1381; F. P. Stelzer *et al.* (letter), *New Engl. J. Med.*, 1976, *294*, 1182; J. C. Frolich (letter), *ibid.*, *295*, 1261; A. D. Goldberg *et al.*, *Postgrad. med. J.*, 1976, *52*, *Suppl.* 7, 128; S. W. Hoobler and T. Kashima, *Mayo Clin. Proc.*, 1977, *52*, 395; F. G. Strauss *et al.*, *J. Am. med. Ass.*, 1977, *238*, 1734; M. A. Weber (letter), *ibid.*, 1978, *239*, 833; R. Vanholder *et al.*, *Br. med. J.*, 1977, *1*, 1138; J. S. Yudkin (letter), *Lancet*, 1977, *1*, 546.

Reports of acute postoperative clonidine withdrawal symptoms: J. B. Brodsky and J. J. Bravo, *Anesthesiology*, 1976, *44*, 519; W. I. Brenner and A. N. Lieberman, *Ann. thorac. Surg.*, 1977, *24*, 80; H. M. Spotnitz, *ibid.*, 1978, *25*, 179; F. E. Husserl *et al.*, *Sth. med. J.*, 1978, *71*, 496.

Absorption and Fate. Clonidine is absorbed from the gastro-intestinal tract. Peak plasma concentrations are observed 1½ to 3 hours after administration, declining with a half-life up to about 12 hours. About 50% of the dose absorbed is excreted in the urine as unchanged clonidine.

Following administration of clonidine hydrochloride 300 µg by intravenous route to 5 healthy normotensive subjects distribution appeared to follow a two-compartment model with the half-life of the alpha phase ranging from 2.2 to 28.7 minutes and the beta phase from 6.9 to 11.1 hours. Following administration by mouth of the same dose the bioavailability varied from 70.6 to 81.5% and the terminal half-life from 5.2 to 13.0 hours with plasma concentrations reaching a mean maximum of about 1.35 ng per ml at 1 hour. Although the onset of effect was more rapid following intravenous administration the degree of hypotension was similar, as was the time of maximum effect (1.5 to 2 hours) by either route. From 40 to 50% of the bioavailable dose was excreted in the urine as unchanged drug in the first 24 hours with a further 5 to 10% in the next 48 hours; renal clearance was variable but apparently unrelated to pH and exceeded the calculated glomerular filtration rate in some subjects, suggesting tubular secretion.— D. S. Davies *et al.*, *Clin. Pharmac. Ther.*, 1977, *21*, 593.

Further references: C. T. Dollery *et al.*, *Clin. Pharmac. Ther.*, 1976, *19*, 11; L. M. H. Wing *et al.*, *Eur. J. clin. Pharmac.*, 1977, *12*, 463; A. Keränen *et al.*, *ibid.*, 1978, *13*, 97; L. -C. Chu *et al.*, *J. pharm. Sci.*, 1979, *68*, 72.

Uses. Clonidine is an antihypertensive agent which appears to act centrally by stimulating alpha-adrenergic receptors and producing a reduction in sympathetic tone. It also acts peripherally, partly by blocking alpha-adrenergic receptors and partly by reducing vascular reactivity. When given by mouth, its effects appear in about 30 minutes, reaching a maximum after 2 to 4 hours and lasting about 6 to 8 hours.

Clonidine hydrochloride is used in the treatment of all grades of hypertension. Tolerance to clonidine has been reported.

The usual initial dose of clonidine hydrochloride is 50 to 100 µg thrice daily increased every second or third day according to the response of the patient; the usual maintenance dose is 0.3 to 1.2 mg daily but doses of up to 1.8 mg or more daily may be required. To reduce side-effects, a smaller dose of clonidine may be given in conjunction with a thiazide diuretic.

Clonidine hydrochloride may be given by slow intravenous injection, usually in doses of 150 to 300 µg. The effect usually appears within 10 minutes, but transient hypertension may precede hypotension. The effect reaches a maximum about 30 to 60 minutes after administration and the duration is about 3 to 7 hours; up to 750 µg may be given intravenously over 24 hours, and higher daily doses have been reported.

Clonidine hydrochloride is also used in lower doses for the prophylaxis of migraine or recurrent vascular headaches and in the treatment of menopausal flushing. The dose is 50 µg twice daily increased, if there is no remission after 2 weeks, to 75 µg twice daily.

An account of the pharmacology of clonidine.— R. Laverty, *Br. med. Bull.*, 1973, *29*, 152.

A depressor response to carotid sinus nerve stimulation in a patient during high-dose clonidine therapy suggested that the hypotensive effect of clonidine was mediated in part by its facilitation of the baroreceptor reflex.— M. G. Myers, *Br. med. J.*, 1977, *2*, 802.

Administration of clonidine 300 µg to 6 tetraplegic subjects had no hypotensive effect whereas similar administration to 5 healthy control subjects caused a fall in blood pressure. This supported *animal* studies indicating that the hypotensive effect of clonidine is predominantly centrally mediated.— J. L. Reid *et al.*, *Clin. Pharmac. Ther.*, 1977, *21*, 375.

Studies on the effect of clonidine on aldosterone, renin, and growth hormone: B. De Wurstemberger and E. Gysling, *Can. med. Ass. J.*, 1976, *115*, 1107 (renin); M. A. Weber *et al.*, *Am. J. Cardiol.*, 1976, *38*, 825 (renin and aldosterone); S. A. Atlas *et al.*, *Lancet*, 1977, *2*, 785 (renin); C. Ferrari *et al.* (letter), *Br. med. J.*, 1977, *2*, 123 (growth hormone); B. E. Karlberg *et al.*, *Curr. ther. Res.*, 1977, *21*, 10 (renin-angiotensin-aldosterone system).

References to *animal* studies on the action of clonidine: R. Bloch *et al.*, *Thérapie*, 1974, *29*, 251; A. J. Draper *et al.*, *J. Pharm. Pharmac.*, 1977, *29*, 175; P. Zandberg and W. De Jong, *ibid.*, 697; T. W. Stone and D. A. Taylor, *Br. J. Pharmac.*, 1978, *64*, 369.

Relief of diabetic gustatory sweating by clonidine.— H. U. Janka *et al.*, *Ann. intern. Med.*, 1979, *91*, 130.

The effects of clonidine on hormone and substrate responses to hypoglycaemia.— S. A. Metz and J. B. Halter, *Clin. Pharmac. Ther.*, 1980, *28*, 441.

Administration in renal failure. The normal half-life of clonidine was 6 to 23 hours. The dose should be reduced to 50 to 75% in patients with a glomerular filtration-rate of less than 10 ml per minute.— W. M. Bennett *et al.*, *Ann. intern. Med.*, 1980, *93*, 286.

Further references: J. S. Cheigh, *Am. J. Med.*, 1977, *62*, 555.

See also under Absorption and Fate.

Dysmenorrhoea. In all of 15 women with severe dysmenorrhoea relief of pain was obtained by administration of clonidine 25 µg thrice daily for 14 days before and during the period.— L. K. Levens (letter), *Br. med. J.*, 1974, *1*, 577.

Epilepsy. Clonidine 0.2 to 0.4 mg per day reduced basal concentrations of catecholamines in a patient suffering from autonomic epilepsy with a seizure focus in the temporal lobe. Clonidine also reduced the concentrations of catecholamines during the attacks and abolished the associated flushing of the skin without any effect on other symptoms. Treatment with carbamazepine 200 to 600 mg per day controlled all the epileptic manifestations in the patient.— S. A. Metz *et al.*, *Ann. intern. Med.*, 1978, *88*, 189.

Gilles de la Tourette's syndrome. Eight children with Tourette's syndrome, either uncontrolled by haloperidol or in whom it produced unacceptable side-effects, obtained control of their symptoms following administration of small doses of clonidine. In 7 of the children control of motor and phonic tics, compulsive actions, and other behavioural symptoms was obtained with doses of 50 to 150 µg daily; in a 14-year-old girl weighing 90 kg dramatic improvement followed doses of up to 600 µg daily. Some of the children have now taken clonidine for up to one year with continued relief of symptoms.— D. J. Cohen *et al.*, *Lancet*, 1979, *2*, 551. Absence of benefit in one patient with a 30-year history of Tourette syndrome studied under double-blind conditions.— M. W. Dysken *et al.* (letter), *Lancet*, 1980, *2*, 926. Another favourable report in one patient.— I. G. McKeith *et al.* (letter), *Lancet*, 1981, *1*, 270.

Glaucoma. In a study in 21 patients with open-angle glaucoma, clonidine 0.125% and 0.25% as eye-drops was effective in lowering intra-ocular pressure. Pupil diameter was unchanged in most patients after clonidine. There was a slight fall in both diastolic and systolic blood pressure.— R. Harrison and C. S. Kaufmann, *Archs Ophthal., N.Y.*, 1977, *95*, 1368.

Further references: O. K. Graupner and A. E. Muller, *Zentralbl. Pharm. Pharmakother. Laboratoriums-Diagn.*, 1972, *111*, 227, per *Int. pharm. Abstr.*, 1973, *10*, 412.

Growth hormone stimulation test. A study in 18 healthy children and adolescents, and 7 patients with hypopituitarism, indicated that oral administration of clonidine 150 µg per m^2 body-surface may provide a sensitive and reliable test for the evaluation of growth hormone reserves in children and adolescents.— I. Gil-Ad *et al.*, *Lancet*, 1979, *2*, 278. See also C. Ferrari *et al.* (letter), *ibid.*, 796; C. Barbieri *et al.*, *Clin. Sci.*, 1980, *58*, 135.

Hypertension. In 7 patients with hypertension, clonidine reduced the mean supine arterial pressure by 17% and diminished cardiac output similarly. The fall in arterial pressure was 33% with the patients in the tilted position and was associated with a significant reduction in the peripheral vascular resistance. Renal plasma flow and glomerular filtration were unaffected by clonidine, but urinary excretion of sodium and chloride was halved.— G. Onesti *et al.*, *Circulation*, 1969, *39*, 219.

In an uncontrolled trial 153 patients with hypertension were treated with clonidine, 75 µg twice or thrice daily initially, increasing at regular intervals according to response. A good therapeutic response occurred in 99 patients, a fair response in 24, and a poor response in 15. Sedation was the most troublesome side-effect and resulted in treatment failure in 15 patients. Other side-effects were dryness of mouth, constipation, and Raynaud's phenomenon. Two patients experienced withdrawal reactions within 48 hours of ceasing clonidine therapy.— J. Raftos *et al.*, *Med. J. Aust.*, 1973, *1*, 786.

A study in 12 hypertensive hospital in-patients supported the view that clonidine given alone is an effective antihypertensive agent. Although thrice daily dosage gave better blood pressure control, patients preferred a large single dose at night since it provided a good night's sleep and considerably reduced daytime drowsiness. Twice daily dosage was only studied in 2 of the patients but blood pressure control was better than with either thrice or once daily dosage.— A. K. Jain *et al.*, *Clin. Pharmac. Ther.*, 1977, *21*, 382.

Owing to the risks of rebound hypertension on withdrawal clonidine could not be recommended as a drug of first choice for treating hypertension.— *Drug & Ther. Bull.*, 1977, *15*, 99.

Clonidine in hypertension: a 6-year review.— A. A. H. Lawson and M. Keston, *Curr. med. Res. Opinion*, 1979, *6*, 168.

Comparison with other antihypertensive agents. In a double-blind crossover study 41 patients with moderate to severe hypertension who were receiving chlorthalidone daily were also given clonidine hydrochloride 450 µg daily or methyldopa 750 mg daily, in 3 divided doses, for 3 months.Each regimen was significantly more effective than chlorthalidone alone, and side-effects were similar and minor both in type and frequency. Drowsiness occurred more commonly with clonidine and dizziness with methyldopa.— W. J. Mroczek *et al.*, *Ann. intern. Med.*, 1972, *76*, 875. See also *idem*, *Am. J. Cardiol.*, 1972, *30*, 536.

Clonidine and propranolol were equipotent in reducing blood pressure, in a double-blind crossover study on 32 patients with moderate hypertension. Clonidine was reported to have more initial side-effects than propranolol.— P. R. Wilkinson and E. B. Raftery, *Br. J. clin. Pharmac.*, 1977, *4*, 289.

Further references: Y. K. Seedat *et al.* (letter), *Lancet*, 1969, *2*, 591; *idem*, *S. Afr. med. J.*, 1970, *44*, 300 (methyldopa); A. Amery *et al.*, *Br. med. J.*, 1970, *4*, 392 (methyldopa); M. R. Putzeys and S. W. Hoobler, *Am. Heart J.*, 1972, *83*, 464 (methyldopa); W. A. Pettinger *et al.*, *Clin. Pharmac. Ther.*, 1977, *22*, 164 (propranolol); W. M. Kirkendall *et al.*, *J. Am. med. Ass.*, 1978, *240*, 2553 (prazosin).

Enhancement of effect. Studies on the concurrent administration of clonidine with other antihypertensive agents: M. C. Igloe, *Curr. ther. Res.*, 1973, *15*, 559 (chlorthalidone); W. J. Mroczek *et al.*, *Curr. ther. Res.*, 1975, *17*, 47 (chlorthalidone); A. H. Griep, *Curr. ther. Res.*, 1978, *24*, 1 (chlorthalidone); W. J. Mroczek and M. E. Davidov, *Curr. ther. Res.*, 1978, *23*, 294 (chlorthalidone and hydralazine); M. A. Weber *et al.*, *J. clin. Pharmac.*, 1978, *18*, 233 (propranolol).

Parenteral routes. Clonidine given intravenously was found to be an effective antihypertensive agent in 13 patients with stable hypertension but was ineffective in 7 patients with accelerated hypertension. The pressor phase noted in all 20 patients after administration of clonidine was transitory and of small magnitude in those with stable hypertension but was greater and of longer duration in the others. Since the major need for a parenteral antihypertensive agent was in the treatment of crises the value of clonidine by the intravenous route was considered limited.— W. J. Mroczek *et al.*, *Clin. Pharmac. Ther.*, 1973, *14*, 847.

In hypertensive crises of pregnancy clonidine was given in doses of 150 to 300 µg intravenously up to a maximum of 600 µg. Satisfactory control of blood pressure was achieved in 13 minutes in 6 patients and 50 minutes in the seventh. Patients became very pale after administration of clonidine and developed pin-point pupils. Drowsiness was a prominent side-effect. The infants of women given clonidine were not affected in any way.— P. W. Leighton and H. Tighe (letter), *Med. J. Aust.*, 1974, *2*, 680.

Intravenous administration of clonidine using a cumulative regimen was studied in 8 hypertensive patients. The first dose of clonidine was 25 µg, then increments of 12.5 µg were given every 15 minutes until the blood pressure was within normal range or to a maximum single dose of 100 µg. Advantages over the single-dose method were that severe hypotension was avoided and an adequate hypotensive response was regularly obtained.— M. Velasco *et al.*, *Clin. Pharmac. Ther.*, 1976, *20*, 31. See also *idem*, *Curr. ther. Res.*, 1975, *18*, 769.

Clonidine 150 µg by intramuscular injection reduced mean blood pressure by more than 20 mmHg in 13 of 16 hypertensive patients. The fall in blood pressure occurred within 5 to 10 minutes and was maximum at 75 minutes. In 6 patients a dose of 300 µg produced a more rapid and greater fall in blood pressure.— R. M. Graham *et al.*, *Aust. N.Z. J. Med.*, 1977, *7*, 131.

Intravenous injections of clonidine ranging from 75 to 275 µg were given to 13 hypertensive patients. A dose-dependent decrease in blood pressure occurred and was significantly related to plasma concentrations of clonidine. The peak hypotensive effect was seen 0.5 to 1 hour after injection. Plasma half-lives ranged from 7.4 to 11.4 hours.— M. Frisk-Holmberg *et al.*, *Br. J. clin. Pharmac.*, 1978, *6*, 227.

Further references: A. L. Muir *et al.*, *Lancet*, 1969, *2*, 181; A. P. Niarchos and A. K. Baksi, *Postgrad. med. J.*, 1973, *49*, 908; S. N. Anavekar and C. I. Johnston, *Med. J. Aust.*, 1974, *1*, 829; A. P. Niarchos, *J. clin. Pharmac.*, 1978, *18*, 220.

Mania. Provisional study of clonidine in mania.— R. Jouvent *et al.*, *Am. J. Psychiat.*, 1980, *137*, 1275.

Menopausal symptoms. In a double-blind crossover study in general practice, clonidine 25 to 75 µg twice daily was significantly more effective than a placebo in reducing the number of menopausal hot flushes in 86 patients. In general, side-effects occurred as often with the placebo as with clonidine but leg pain and ankle oedema were noted in 3 patients taking clonidine.— J. R. Clayden *et al.*, *Br. med. J.*, 1974, *1*, 409. See also *idem* (letter), *Lancet*, 1972, *2*, 1361; C. W. L. Williams (letter), *ibid.*, 1973, *1*, 1388.

Migraine. Reviews and discussions on clonidine in migraine: *Med. Lett.*, 1976, *18*, 55; E. S. Johnson, *Postgrad. med. J.*, 1978, *54*, 231.

In a controlled study of 42 patients with migraine, clonidine 50 µg twice daily for one or two 8-week sessions reduced the number of severe attacks of migraine significantly in 24 patients. A further 8 patients with a history of consistent and very frequent attacks showed no such reduction. Follow-up treatment with 100 to 150 µg daily for 1 year in 27 patients led to significant further improvement and 3 of 5 of the patients with very frequent attacks who were included in the follow-up study demonstrated a reduction in symptoms.— J. Shafar *et al.*, *Lancet*, 1972, *1*, 403. Criticism.— S. Nurick (letter), *Lancet*, 1972, *1*, 901. A reply.— P. A. Pollard *et al.* (letter), *Lancet*, 1972, *1*, 1242.

Clonidine was reported to have aborted migraine attacks in 7 of 20 patients when given in the early stages; another 5 gained much relief and 8 had no benefit. No patient took their usual migraine-relieving therapy.— E. Poźniak-Patewicz (letter), *Lancet*, 1976, *2*, 968.

During a double-blind crossover study completed by 70 of 96 patients with migraine, clonidine 150 µg daily in divided doses for 6 months was not more effective than a placebo in reducing frequency of headaches but the severity and duration of long-lasting headaches may have been decreased. The effect of clonidine may have persisted after withdrawal in some patients when placebo was substituted for clonidine for the second 6-month period of study.— E. I. Adam *et al.*, *J. R. Coll. gen. Pract.*, 1978, *28*, 587.

Further conflicting reports on the merits of clonidine in migraine: K. W. G. Heathfield and J. D. Raiman, *Practitioner*, 1972, *208*, 644; M. C. Wall and M. Wilkinson (letter), *Lancet*, 1973, *2*, 510; J. Munro (letter), *Med. J. Aust.*, 1975, *2*, 108; G. J. R. Clarke, *Clin. Trials J.*, 1976, *13*, 137; T. Kallanranta *et al.*, *Headache*, 1977, *17*, 169; K. Mondrup and C. E. Møller, *Acta neurol. scand.*, 1977, *56*, 405; R. H. Wicks (letter), *Med. J. Aust.*, 1977, *1*, 41.

Narcotic addiction. Discussion of the use of clonidine in the management of opiate withdrawal symptoms.— *Med. Lett.*, 1979, *21*, 100; *Lancet*, 1980, *2*, 349.

Possible mechanism of action.— J. Watkins *et al.*, *Clin. Pharmac. Ther.*, 1980, *28*, 605; T. W. Uhde *et al.* (letter), *Lancet*, 1980, *2*, 1375.

In a double-blind placebo-controlled study both subjective and objective methadone-withdrawal symptoms were dramatically controlled in 11 addicts by administration of clonidine 5 µg per kg body-weight by mouth. On discharge from hospital control of symptoms was successfully maintained by 9 of 10 patients with the same dose taken twice daily. The tenth discontinued clonidine and experienced withdrawal symptoms for which she took diamorphine.— M. S. Gold *et al.*, *Lancet*, 1978, *2*, 599.

Studies in *rats* indicated that although clonidine initially suppressed all the major symptoms of morphine withdrawal it also produced effects that were indicative of psychosis. Moreover, as the effect of clonidine wore off some rebound effects occurred with more intense clinical irritability and hyperaesthesia than before its administration.— J. J. Lipman and P. S. J. Spencer (letter), *Lancet*, 1978, *2*, 521.

Experience with a 10-day clonidine regimen in 88 out-patients, to alleviate withdrawal symptoms following abrupt termination of chronic methadone or diamorphine use. No single clonidine dose is best for all patients, but for most a clonidine dosage regimen of 100 or 200 µg every 4 to 6 hours, with a larger dose at bedtime, provides adequate relief of withdrawal symptoms with few or no side-effects. Most patients require additional night sedation to alleviate insomnia.— A. M. Washton *et al.* (letter), *Lancet*, 1980, *1*, 1078.

Details of the successful use of clonidine in acute opiate withdrawal, including mention of the use of clonidine 17 µg per kg body-weight daily to detoxify 100 patients from chronic methadone addiction.— M. S. Gold *et al.* (letter), *Lancet*, 1980, *2*, 1078.

Clonidine may not be superior to methadone detoxification, although it might still be very useful as a rapid detoxification treatment, or when methadone detoxification is inappropriate, unsuccessful, or unavailable.— A. M. Washton and R. B. Resnick (letter), *Lancet*, 1980, *2*, 1297. Criticism.— M. S. Gold *et al.* (letter), *ibid.*, 1981, *1*, 621.

Further references: M. S. Gold *et al.*, *Am. J. Psychiat.*, 1979, *136*, 100; C. E. Riordan and H. D. Kleber, *Lancet*, 1980, *1*, 1079; M. S. Gold *et al.*, *J. Am. med. Ass.*, 1980, *243*, 343.

Rosacea. In a double-blind crossover study in 17 patients with rosacea and facial erythema and flushing clonidine 50 µg twice daily was without marked effect though 5 patients had some relief from flushing; 4 patients had an exacerbation of the pustular element. Topical application of a 2% cream to 20 patients was not of value.— W. J. Cunliffe *et al.* (letter), *Br. med. J.*, 1977, *1*, 105.

Further references: W. J. Cunliffe *et al.*, *Br. J. Derm.*, 1975, *93*, *Suppl.* 11, 11.

Schizophrenia. Treatment with clonidine in doses of 0.9 to 2.1 mg produced pronounced sedative and hypotensive effects in 9 patients with chronic schizophrenia and agitation, anxiety, and overactivity. The dose was slowly increased to this level, and treatment lasted 12 weeks. There was a mild initial improvement in behaviour, but no antipsychotic activity or control of overactivity was observed.— G. M. Simpson *et al.*, *J. clin. Pharmac.*, 1967, *7*, 221. See also A. A. Sugerman, *ibid.*, 226.

Preparations

Clonidine Hydrochloride Injection *(B.P.).* Clonidine Hydrochlor. Inj.; Clonidine Injection. A sterile solution of clonidine hydrochloride in Water for Injections. Sterilised by autoclaving. pH 4 to 7.

Clonidine Hydrochloride Tablets *(B.P.).* Clonidine Hydrochlor. Tab.; Clonidine Tablets. Tablets containing clonidine hydrochloride; they may be sugar-coated.

Proprietary Preparations

Catapres *(Boehringer Ingelheim, UK).* Clonidine hydrochloride, available as 1-ml **Ampoules** of injection containing 150 µg per ml and as **Tablets** of 100 and 300 µg. For hypertension. **Catapres PL Perlongets.** Sustained-release capsules each containing clonidine hydrochloride 250 µg. *Dose.* 1 capsule daily increased, if necessary, to 2 or 3 capsules daily. (Also available as Catapres in *Austral., Canad., Jap., S.Afr., USA).*

Dixarit *(WB Pharmaceuticals, UK: Boehringer Ingelheim, UK).* Clonidine hydrochloride, available as tablets of 25 µg. For migraine. *Dose.* 2 tablets twice daily increased, if necessary, to 3 tablets twice daily. (Also available as Dixarit in *Austral., Belg., Neth., S.Afr.*).

Other Proprietary Names

Catapresan *(Arg., Denm., Ger., Ital., Neth., Norw., Spain, Swed., Switz.)*; Catapressan *(Belg., Fr.)*; Clonilou *(Spain)*; Drylon *(Norw.)*; Hyposyn *(Denm.)*; Ipotensium *(Ital.)*; Isoglaucon *(Ger., Ital., Switz.)*; Tensinova *(Spain).*

858-a

Cryptenamine Acetates. The acetate salts of alkaloids derived from an extract of green veratrum.

Uses. Cryptenamine acetates has the actions and uses of Alkavervir, p.136. It has been given intravenously (diluted) or intramuscularly for the management of eclampsia and hypertensive crises; the equivalent of cryptenamine 1 mg diluted with 20 ml of dextrose injection was infused intravenously at the rate of about 1 ml per minute, regulated according to the blood pressure.

Proprietary Names
Unitensen Aqueous Injection *(Wallace, USA).*

859-t

Cryptenamine Tannates. The tannate salts of alkaloids derived from an extract of green veratrum.

CAS — 1405-40-9.

A brown amorphous powder. Slightly **soluble** in water; soluble in alcohol.

Uses. Cryptenamine tannates has the actions and uses of Alkavervir, p.136. For the control of moderate to severe hypertension, an initial dose equivalent to cryptenamine 2 mg is given twice daily by mouth. For patients in hospital, this dose may be increased gradually each day until the blood pressure is reduced to the desired level. For out-patients, the dose should not be increased more frequently than once weekly. Usual dose range 4 to 12 mg daily. If the total daily dose exceeds 4 mg it should be given in 3 divided doses.

Hypertension. Cryptenamine 2 mg with methyclothiazide 2.5 mg four times daily was effective in lowering blood pressure in a double-blind study of 18 patients with essential hypertension.— C. C. Kennedy *et al., J. pharm. Sci.*, 1971, *60,* 1139. See also B. M. Cohen, *Curr. ther. Res.*, 1966, *8,* 424.

Proprietary Names
Unitensen Tablets *(Wallace, USA).*

860-l

Debrisoquine Sulphate *(B.P.).* Ro 5-3307/1; Isocaramidine Sulphate. 1,2,3,4-Tetrahydroisoquinoline-2-carboxamidine sulphate.

$(C_{10}H_{13}N_3)_2,H_2SO_4=448.5$.

CAS — 1131-64-2 (debrisoquine); 581-88-4 (sulphate).

Pharmacopoeias. In *Br.*

A white odourless or almost odourless crystalline powder with a bitter taste. Debrisoquine sulphate 12.8 mg is approximately equivalent to 10 mg of debrisoquine. M.p. about 274° with decomposition. **Soluble** 1 in 40 of water; very slightly soluble in alcohol; practically insoluble in chloroform and ether. **Protect** from light.

Adverse Effects, Treatment, and Precautions. As for Guanethidine Monosulphate, p.145.

With debrisoquine sulphate diarrhoea is rare. Sweating and headache may occur.

The metabolism of debrisoquine is subject to genetic polymorphism and non-metabolisers may show a marked response to doses that have little or no effect in metabolisers.

Tolerance and side-effects during long-term treatment of hypertension with debrisoquine sulphate.— W. B. Jackson, *Aust. N.Z. J. Med.*, 1972, *4,* 357.

Markedly prolonged ischaemia developed at the site of subcutaneous injection of lignocaine and adrenaline in an elderly woman who had been receiving debrisoquine for 10 years.— A. J. French and Y. V. Patel (letter), *Lancet*, 1980, *2,* 484.

Interactions. Debrisoquine could interfere biologically with laboratory estimations for vanilmandelic acid in the urine to produce erroneous lowered results.— *Drug & Ther. Bull.*, 1972, *10,* 69.

Amines in food. A woman with hypertension who had commenced debrisoquine therapy 1 week previously suffered a rise in blood pressure from 140/95 to 195/165 mmHg, after ingesting 50 g of Gruyère cheese.— A. Amery and W. Deloof (letter), *Lancet*, 1970, *2,* 613.

Sympathetic neurone monoamine oxidase was inhibited by debrisoquine as shown by pressor responses to tyramine intravenously but non-neuronal monoamine oxidase was not inhibited as shown by unaltered tryptamine and tyramine excretion, and a minimal increase in sensitivity to tyramine by mouth.— W. A. Pettinger and W. D. Horst, *Ann. N.Y. Acad. Sci.*, 1971, *179,* 310.

Narcotic analgesics. For reference to a toxic reaction in *rabbits* pretreated with debrisoquine and subsequently given pethidine, see Pethidine Hydrochloride, p.1026.

Sympathomimetics. For an account of the enhancement of the effect of phenylephrine by debrisoquine, see Phenylephrine Hydrochloride, p.24.

Tricyclic antidepressants. In 2 patients with essential hypertension, antihypertensive therapy with debrisoquine was antagonised by the concurrent administration of *imipramine* 100 mg daily and *amitriptyline* 150 mg daily respectively, for depression.— C. Skinner *et al., Lancet*, 1969, *2,* 564.

Absorption and Fate. Debrisoquine is rapidly absorbed from the gastro-intestinal tract. Its metabolism is subject to genetic polymorphism.

Three of 94 healthy subjects had a defect in the metabolism of debrisoquine to active 4-hydroxydebrisoquine and were classified as non-metabolisers. Study of the families of the 3 non-metabolisers indicated that the incomplete acyclic 4-hydroxylation of debrisoquine was an autosomal recessive trait.— A. Mahgoub *et al., Lancet*, 1977, *2,* 584. Similar findings in 51 patients.— G. T. Tucker *et al.* (letter), *ibid.*, 718.

In 12 patients taking debrisoquine 40 mg daily recovery of the drug from the urine varied from 8.6 to 80.2% of the dose while that of 4-hydroxydebrisoquine (largely inactive) was nil to 29.7%. In 11 patients the fall in standing systolic blood pressure varied from 0.3 to 44.4 mmHg. A poor response was associated with extensive metabolism of the drug and was overcome by increasing the dose rather than by adding other antihypertensive agents.— J. H. Silas *et al., Br. med. J.*, 1977, *1,* 422.

Pre-systemic metabolism of debrisoquine to its metabolite 4-hydroxydebrisoquine occurred in 15 patients with hypertension and 4 healthy subjects. Results indicated that debrisoquine or its metabolite could inhibit this metabolism and therefore increases in the dose of debrisoquine could produce disproportionate decreases in blood pressure. The estimated half-life of elimination for debrisoquine and 4-hydroxydebrisoquine ranged from 11.5 to 26 hours and from 5.8 to 14.5 hours respectively. A further study of one healthy subject indicated that debrisoquine was actively taken up by platelets and that this was responsible for its long half-life.— J. H. Silas *et al., Br. J. clin. Pharmac.*, 1978, *5,* 27. See also *idem*, 1980, *9,* 419 and 427.

Further references: J. R. Idle *et al., Life Sci.*, 1978, *22,* 979.

Uses. Debrisoquine sulphate is an antihypertensive agent with actions similar to those of guanethidine monosulphate (see p.146), but without guanethidine's action on tissue noradrenaline. When administered by mouth, debrisoquine is reported to act within about 4 to 10 hours and to have effects lasting for 9 to 24 hours. When given intravenously a rise in blood pressure precedes its hypotensive effects.

Debrisoquine is used in the treatment of moderate and severe hypertension or for the treatment of mild hypertension in patients where other drugs have proved inadequate. It reduces the standing blood pressure but has a less marked effect on the supine blood pressure.

The usual initial dose is the equivalent of 10 mg of debrisoquine once or twice daily. The daily dose is then increased by 10 to 20 mg, according to the severity of the condition, every 3 or 4 days. The usual maintenance dose is 40 to 120 mg daily, but up to 300 mg or more daily may be given. To reduce side-effects smaller doses of debrisoquine may be given in conjunction with a thiazide diuretic.

For reviews, with references, of the pharmacology and clinical uses of debrisoquine, see W. I. Cranston, *Practitioner*, 1967, *198,* 723; *Br. med. J.*, 1968, *1,* 166.

A report on 229 hypertensive patients taking bethanidine, debrisoquine, or guanethidine, sometimes in association with a diuretic. Blood pressure was more effectively controlled by debrisoquine or guanethidine than by bethanidine. Symptoms of orthostatic or exertional hypotension were significantly more frequent in those taking guanethidine. Diarrhoea occurred in 23% on guanethidine, 4% on bethanidine, and 1% on debrisoquine.— S. Talbot *et al.* (letter), *Br. med. J.*, 1975, *2,* 278.

Further references: A. H. Kitchin and R. W. D. Turner, *Br. med. J.*, 1966, *2,* 728; E. S. Orgain and A. Kern, *Archs intern. Med.*, 1970, *125,* 255; A. Heffernan *et al., Br. med. J.*, 1971, *1,* 75; F. C. Adi *et al., ibid.*, 1975, *1,* 482; L. Belleau *et al., Curr. ther. Res.*, 1977, *22,* 134.

Preparations

Debrisoquine Tablets *(B.P.).* Tablets containing debrisoquine sulphate. Potency is expressed in terms of the equivalent amount of debrisoquine.

Declinax *(Roche, UK).* Debrisoquine sulphate, available as scored tablets each containing the equivalent of 10 or 20 mg of debrisoquine. (Also available as Declinax in *Arg., Austral., Belg., Canad., S.Afr., Switz.*).

Other Proprietary Names

Equitonil *(Arg.).*

861-y

Deserpidine. 11-Demethoxyreserpine. Methyl 11-demethoxy-18-*O*-(3,4,5-trimethoxybenzoyl)reserpate.
$C_{32}H_{38}N_2O_8=578.7$.

CAS — 131-01-1.

An ester alkaloid isolated from the root of *Rauwolfia canescens.*

Adverse Effects, Treatment, and Precautions. As for Reserpine, p.163.

Uses. Deserpidine has actions and uses similar to those described under reserpine (see p.164). In the treatment of hypertension some sources have recommended an initial dose of 0.75 to 1 mg daily subsequently reduced to a maintenance dose of about 250 µg daily, while others have recommended an initial dose of 250 µg daily subsequently increased, if necessary, up to 250 µg four times daily; intervals of 10 to 14 days are recommended between dosage adjustments.

In psychiatric conditions the average initial dose is reported to be 500 µg daily with a range of 0.1 to 1 mg; doses of 2 to 3 mg daily were formerly given.

For a report on the use of deserpidine with methyclothiazide in the treatment of hypertension, see Methyclothiazide, p.607.

Proprietary Preparations

Harmonyl *(Abbott, UK).* Deserpidine, available as scored tablets of 250 µg. (Also available as Harmonyl in *Belg., USA*).

862-j

Diazoxide *(B.P., U.S.P.).* SRG 95213. 7-Chloro-3-methyl-2*H*-1,2,4-benzothiadiazine 1,1-dioxide.

$C_8H_7ClN_2O_2S=230.7$.

CAS — 364-98-7.

Pharmacopoeias. In *Br.* and *U.S.*

A white or creamy-white odourless crystalline powder. Practically **insoluble** in water, chloroform, and ether; soluble 1 in 250 of alcohol; very soluble in solutions of alkali hydroxides; freely soluble in dimethylformamide. Solutions of the sodium salt are **sterilised** by autoclaving or by filtration.

Adverse Effects. In addition to inappropriate hypotension and hyperglycaemia, side-effects frequently include oedema (with precipitation of congestive heart failure) and hypertrichosis (especially in children); nausea is also common in the initial stages of therapy. Other side-effects are anorexia, vomiting, headache, flushing, hyperuricaemia, hypotension, palpitations, tachycardia, and electrocardiograph changes. Cardiac arrhythmias, skin rashes, extrapyramidal effects, leucopenia, and thrombocytopenia have been reported. There have been rare reports of cataracts. Hyperglycaemia is usually temporary after diazoxide, but persistent hyperglycaemia has occasionally occurred.

If given during parturition, diazoxide may delay delivery unless oxytocin is given concomitantly. Alopecia has been reported in infants born to mothers taking diazoxide. Diazoxide may cause a burning sensation in the vein used for injection; extravasation of the alkaline solution is painful.

Side-effects of diazoxide in childhood hypoglycaemia included advancement of bone-age and depression of immunoglobulin.— L. Kollée and L. Monnens (letter), *Lancet*, 1978, *1*, 668.

The high incidence of neurological complications reported by J.G.G. Ledingham and B. Rajagopalan (*Q.J. Med.*, 1979 *48*, 25) may have been due to an unusually aggressive protocol rather than diazoxide itself.— T. Thien *et al.* (letter), *Lancet*, 1979, *2*, 847.

Allergy. After being treated for 7 days with diazoxide, 300 mg four times daily, for hypoglycaemic attacks secondary to a partial gastrectomy, a 41-year-old woman developed oedema and a generalised erythematous rash and had a temperature of 38.7°. The addition of hydrochlorothiazide produced a marked diuresis but the fever and rash persisted and subsided gradually only when treatments were stopped. Leucopenia and thrombocytopenia were noted during diazoxide therapy and also followed challenge doses. The patient tolerated hydrochlorothiazide.— J. K. Wales and F. Wolff (letter), *Lancet*, 1967, *1*, 53.

A 51-year-old man developed thrombocytopenia and a skin eruption after treatment for 8 days with diazoxide 500 mg daily, with other drugs. The eruption disappeared 4 days after stopping diazoxide and reappeared when diazoxide was again given.— P. Kuan (letter), *Br. med. J.*, 1973, *1*, 114.

Effects on the blood. A 26-year-old man with hypertension developed reversible haemolytic anaemia when treated with diazoxide by mouth on 3 separate occasions. Total amounts of diazoxide received on each occasion were 11.2 g over 37 days, 9.9 g over 84 days, and 3 g over 15 days, respectively.— R. A. Best and H. M. Clink, *Postgrad. med. J.*, 1975, *51*, 402.

See also under Allergy (above).

Effects on the heart. A 9-year-old girl given diazoxide 20 mg per kg body-weight for 6 months developed cardiomegaly possibly attributable to diazoxide.— W. J. Appleyard, *Proc. R. Soc. Med.*, 1968, *61*, 1257.

Heart block (2:1) lasting for a minute occurred in a 6-month-old child with the haemolytic-uraemic syndrome and congestive heart failure given diazoxide 37.5 mg by venous catheter into the right atrium. She subsequently tolerated 20 mg intravenously without arrhythmia.— S. M. Mauer and B. L. Mirkin, *J. Pediat.*, 1972, *80*, 657.

Diazoxide 200 to 300 mg given as an intravenous bolus over 5 to 10 seconds to 14 patients with hypertensive crisis produced significant ST or T changes in the ECG. Angina-like chest symptoms occurred in 6 patients, 5 of whom also had ECG irregularities and in 1 of these patients there were signs of myocardial infarction. The ECG changes were associated with a greater fall in blood pressure. Alternative therapy should be considered for hypertensive emergencies in patients with a history of angina pectoris or myocardial infarction.— S. A. Kanada *et al.*, *Ann. intern. Med.*, 1976, *84*, 696.

Further references: W. J. Mroczek and W. R. Lee (letter), *ibid.*, *85*, 529; J. M. Falko (letter), *ibid.*, 1977, *86*, 111.

Effects on the kidneys. After treatment with diazoxide, 300 mg daily for 2 days then 600 mg daily for 3 days, a 58-year-old woman with hypoglycaemia, due to an extra-pancreatic tumour, developed oliguria and gross fluid retention which failed to respond to a diuretic. She became anuric and died despite intravenous administration of frusemide, mannitol, soluble insulin, and the removal of 2 litres of fluid by peritoneal dialysis.— G. H. Robb, *Postgrad. med. J.*, 1969, *45*, 43.

Effects on the nervous system. In 6 patients with severe hypertension, extrapyramidal symptoms developed 2 to 42 days after the start of treatment with diazoxide 200 to 400 mg daily, sometimes in association with methyldopa or propranolol. In 1 patient the symptoms occurred simultaneously with a high peak of free diazoxide in serum (calculated as 9% of total serum diazoxide). Such symptoms had been seen in 15 patients with mean serum-diazoxide concentrations of 98.8 µg per ml compared with 55 µg per ml in 56 patients not so affected.— D. Neary *et al.*, *Br. med. J.*, 1973, *3*, 474.

In a study of 100 hypertensive patients receiving diazoxide, the incidence of extrapyramidal symptoms was 15%.— J. E. F. Pohl, *Am. Heart J.*, 1975, *89*, 401.

Effects on the skin. A patient who had taken diazoxide 150 mg four times daily for 3 months developed hypertrichosis and a lichenoid eruption affecting her face, neck, and arms.— R. S. Wells, *Proc. R. Soc. Med.*, 1973, *66*, 326.

See also under Allergy (above).

Hyperglycaemia. Diabetic ketoacidosis induced by diazoxide in one patient.— S. J. Updike and A. R. Harrington, *New Engl. J. Med.*, 1969, *280*, 768. See also A. Drash *et al.*, *Diabetes*, 1966, *15*, 319.

A report of a severe, non-ketotic, hyperglycaemic, hyperosmolar state which developed very rapidly in a patient given diazoxide.— B. D. W. Harrison *et al.* (letter), *Lancet*, 1972, *2*, 599.

Further references: M. Lancaster-Smith *et al.*, *Postgrad. med. J.*, 1974, *50*, 175.

Hypotension. Severe hypotension occurred in 4 patients treated with diazoxide. All had received hydralazine in conjunction with diazoxide and 2 had previously received potential catecholamine-depleting agents. It was suggested that diazoxide should be administered with caution to patients being treated with other potential vasodilatory or catecholamine-depleting agents.— W. L. Henrich *et al.*, *J. Am. med. Ass.*, 1977, *237*, 264. A further report of hypotension, with unexpected bradycardia, in a patient treated with diazoxide and hydralazine.— S. Mizroch and M. Yurasek (letter), *ibid.*, 2471.

Further references: W. A. Tansey *et al.* (letter), *J. Am. med. Ass.*, 1973, *225*, 749; G. K. Kumar *et al.*, *ibid.*, 1976, *235*, 275; G. P. Romberg and R. E. Lordon (letter), *ibid.*, 1977, *238*, 1025.

Pancreatitis. Ten patients with severe hypertension and renal failure were treated with diazoxide in a last attempt to avert nephrectomy; 1 patient developed acute pancreatitis and another diabetic ketoacidosis. Both patients recovered from these ill effects when diazoxide was withdrawn.— M. De Broe *et al.* (letter), *Lancet*, 1972, *1*, 1397. See also M. M. Mussche *et al.*, *Clin. Nephrol.*, 1975, *4*, 99.

Voice changes. In addition to marked hypertrichosis, 2 children who had received diazoxide for several years, were noted to have unusually deep (low-pitched) voices.— R. J. West (letter), *Br. med. J.*, 1978, *2*, 506.

Treatment of Adverse Effects. Severe hypotension can be controlled with infusions of electrolytes or sympathomimetics such as noradrenaline. Severe hyperglycaemia may be corrected by giving appropriate hypoglycaemic therapy. Antiparkinsonian agents, such as procyclidine, have been given to control extrapyramidal effects; antinauseants may be given for nausea. Diazoxide can be removed from the body by dialysis but recovery is relatively low owing to extensive protein binding.

Precautions. Diazoxide should be used with care in patients with impaired cardiac or cerebral circulation. During prolonged therapy blood-glucose concentrations should be monitored and the blood should be examined regularly for signs of leucopenia and thrombocytopenia, and, in children, bone and psychological maturation and growth should be regularly assessed. The hyperglycaemic and hypotensive actions of diazoxide may be enhanced by diuretics.

Interactions. Phenothiazines. A report of chlorpromazine enhancing the hyperglycaemic effect of diazoxide in a 2-year-old child.— A. Aynsley-Green and R. Illig (letter), *Lancet*, 1975, *2*, 658.

Phenytoin. For the effect of diazoxide on phenytoin, see Phenytoin p.1240.

Warfarin. For the effect of diazoxide, *in vitro*, in displacing warfarin from albumin binding sites, see Warfarin Sodium, p.779.

Pregnancy and the neonate. In *sheep* and *goats* diazoxide crossed the placenta and reached high concentrations in foetal blood. Destruction of pancreatic islet cells was found in aborted foetuses and in neonates who died on the fifth day after delivery.— B. M. Boulos *et al.*, *J. clin. Pharmac.*, 1971, *11*, 206.

In 4 mothers given diazoxide for 5 days before delivery the plasma concentration of diazoxide at delivery was 11 to 43 µg per ml. Diazoxide was present in cord blood at delivery and fell little in the infants in the first 24 hours (5 to 26 µg per ml). Diazoxide was slowly excreted by the infants during the first week of life. There was no effect on blood pressure in the infants. Two, whose mothers were diabetics, had impaired glucose tolerance. All had some degree of alopecia and 1 had hypertrichosis lanuginosa. One had retarded ossification of the wrist at 1 year.— R. D. G. Milner and S. K. Chouksey, *Archs Dis. Childh.*, 1972, *47*, 537.

For a report of severe depression among infants born to mothers given both diazoxide and chlormethiazole edisylate for the treatment of toxaemia of pregnancy, see Chlormethiazole Edisylate, p.798.

See also under Uses (below).

Absorption and Fate. Diazoxide is readily absorbed from the gastro-intestinal tract and extensively bound to plasma proteins. Its plasma half-life has been estimated to range from about 20 to 70 hours but to be shorter for children. The plasma half-life greatly exceeds the duration of vascular activity. Diazoxide is partly metabolised in the liver and is excreted in the urine both unchanged and in the form of metabolites; only small amounts are recovered from the faeces. It crosses the placenta and the blood-brain barrier.

A review of the metabolism and disposition of diazoxide.— P. G. Dayton *et al.*, *Drug Metab. & Disposit.*, 1975, *3*, 226. See also J. Koch-Weser, *New Engl. J. Med.*, 1976, *294*, 1271.

Estimations of the half-life of diazoxide.— B. Calesnick *et al.*, *J. pharm. Sci.*, 1965, *54*, 1277; S. Symchowicz *et al.*, *ibid.*, 1967, *56*, 912; E. M. Sellers and J. Koch-Weser, *New Engl. J. Med.*, 1969, *281*, 1141; A. W. Pruitt and P. G. Dayton, *Eur. J. clin. Pharmac.*, 1971, *4*, 59; A. W. Pruitt *et al.*, *Clin. Pharmac. Ther.*, 1973, *14*, 73; W. Sadee *et al.*, *J. Pharmacokinet. Biopharm.*, 1973, *1*, 295; A. W. Pruitt *et al.*, *J. Pharmac. exp. Ther.*, 1974, *188*, 248.

Studies in 4 hypertensive subjects indicated that diazoxide is well absorbed from the gastro-intestinal tract, the extent of absorption being related to the dissolution rate.— B. Calesnick *et al.*, *J. pharm. Sci.*, 1965, *54*, 1277.

A finding in severely hypertensive patients that metabolism may become the main route of elimination of diazoxide.— W. Sadee *et al.*, *J. Pharmacokinet. Biopharm.*, 1973, *1*, 295. Metabolism of diazoxide in man and *animals*.— A. W. Pruitt *et al.*, *J. Pharmac. exp. Ther.*, 1974, *188*, 248.

In children. In a child with hypoglycaemia the concentration of diazoxide in the CSF was 17 µg per ml while the concentration in blood was 118 µg per ml.— A. W. Pruitt *et al.*, *Pharmacologist*, 1971, *13*, 196.

A pharmacokinetic study of diazoxide in 4 children with hypoglycaemia revealed a plasma half-life of 9.5 to 24 hours which is considerably shorter than that in adults.— A. W. Pruitt *et al.*, *Clin. Pharmac. Ther.*, 1973, *14*, 73.

Protein binding. About 90% of a usual therapeutic dose of diazoxide was bound to plasma proteins. Repeated administration for a sustained hypotensive effect caused the accumulation of bound inactive diazoxide so that plasma concentration did not correlate well with intensity of hypotension. To achieve maximum hypotensive effect the drug must be given by rapid intravenous injection.— E. M. Sellers and J. Koch-Weser, *New Engl. J. Med.*, 1969, *281*, 1141. Evidence of decreased protein binding in uraemia.— K. O'Malley *et al.*, *Clin. Pharmac. Ther.*, 1975, *18*, 53.

Uses. Diazoxide increases the concentration of glucose in the plasma; it inhibits the secretion of insulin by the beta cells of the pancreas, increases the release of catecholamines, and may increase the hepatic output of glucose. When administered intravenously, it produces a fall in blood pressure by a vasodilator effect on the arterioles.

Diazoxide is used in the treatment of intractable hypoglycaemia such as idiopathic hypoglycaemia of infancy or the hypoglycaemia resulting from inoperable tumours of the pancreas. Initially, 5 mg per kg body-weight daily is administered in 2 or 3 divided doses by mouth, then the dosage is adjusted according to the needs of the patient. Doses of up to 1 g daily have been used. In children with leucine-sensitive hypoglycaemia a suggested dose is 15 to 20 mg per kg daily. Frusemide or ethacrynic acid should be given concomitantly to reduce fluid retention.

Diazoxide is used intravenously for the treatment of severe hypertensive crises. Rapid bolus injection of 300 mg within 30 seconds produces a fall in blood pressure within 5 minutes and the effect usually lasts 4 to 6 hours, but may vary considerably. Up to 4 doses may be given in 24 hours if required. Diazoxide 0.4 to 1 g daily in 2 or 3 divided doses has also been given by mouth. A suggested dose for hypertension in children is 5 mg per kg body-weight intravenously.

A detailed review of diazoxide including its mechanism of action, clinical use and indications, metabolism, and side-effects.— J. Koch-Weser, *New Engl. J. Med.*, 1976, *294*, 1271.

Diazoxide and tolmesoxide produced similar dose-dependent increases in arterial blood flow and dilatation of preconstricted veins in a study of healthy subjects. Both drugs were about 10 000 times less potent than prazosin, glyceryl trinitrate, or sodium nitroprusside as venodilators and 1000 times less potent as arterial dilators.— J. G. Collier *et al.*, *Br. J. clin. Pharmac.*, 1978, *5*, 35.

Administration in children. Experience with 16 children given diazoxide showed that many responded to doses smaller than the usual 5 mg per kg body-weight; the desired response could be achieved by repeated small injections.— R. C. Boerth and W. R. Long, *Circulation*, 1977, *56*, 1062.

Administration in renal failure. Marked decrease in binding of diazoxide to plasma proteins was found to occur in patients with uraemia. A retrospective study in which blood urea nitrogen was found to be positively correlated with the hypotensive effect of diazoxide in hypertensive patients suggested that this finding had clinical relevance.— K. O'Malley *et al.*, *Clin. Pharmac. Ther.*, 1975, *18*, 53. See also R. M. Pearson and A. M. Breckenridge, *Br. J. clin. Pharmac.*, 1976, *3*, 169.

Diazoxide can be removed from the body by peritoneal dialysis or haemodialysis, but dialysance is relatively low because of extensive binding to serum albumin.— J. Koch-Weser, *New Engl. J. Med.*, 1976, *294*, 1271.

The pharmacokinetics of diazoxide with particular reference to the influence of renal failure. Excessive reduction of blood pressure with diazoxide may be anticipated in patients with renal failure and could be avoided by giving doses smaller than those usually employed.— R. M. Pearson, *Clin. Pharmacokinet.*, 1977, *2*, 198.

Further references: E. C. Kohaut *et al.*, *J. Pediat.*, 1975, *87*, 795; M. M. Mussche *et al.*, *Clin. Nephrol.*, 1975, *4*, 99.

Diabetes insipidus. Urine volume, free water clearance, and sodium excretion were reduced in 3 patients with vasopressin-deficient diabetes insipidus and 1 with nephrogenic diabetes insipidus after the intravenous injection of diazoxide.— J. E. F. Pohl *et al.*, *Clin. Sci.*, 1972, *42*, 145.

Diabetes mellitus. Improved insulin secretion in diabetes mellitus after treatment with diazoxide.— R. H. Greenwood *et al.*, *Lancet*, 1976, *1*, 444.

Hypertension. In 20 patients with hypertension following cardiac infarction the rapid injection of diazoxide 300 mg into an infusion line reduced the mean initial pressure of 194/122 mmHg by a mean of 58/40 mmHg; 7 patients received a second injection. The maximum effect occurred within 5 minutes on 20 occasions and within 1 minute on 12 of these, and often lasted more than 24 hours. No patient developed severe hypotension. The appearance however of ECG changes suggestive of increased myocardial ischaemia, without clinical signs of deterioration, suggested the need for caution.— K. P. O'Brien *et al.*, *Br. med. J.*, 1975, *4*, 74.

The failure of two 300-mg doses of diazoxide adequately to reduce severe hypertension in a 53-year-old woman and the success of a third dose after the bed had been tilted 10° foot down suggested the possible importance of posture.— M. C. Bateson (letter), *Br. med. J.*, 1976, *2*, 698.

Intravenous injection of diazoxide 25 or 50 mg, followed by increments of 25 mg every ten minutes to a total dose of 200 mg, reduced the blood pressure of hypertensive patients to normal limits without the excessive hypotension which had occurred in some patients after a single bolus injection.— M. Velasco *et al.*, *Curr. ther. Res.*, 1976, *19*, 185. See also C. V. S. Ram, *Am. J. Cardiol.*, 1979, *43*, 627.

The effects of diazoxide, 15 mg per minute by intravenous infusion, in patients with chronic hypertension and with hypertensive crisis.— T. A. Thien *et al.*, *Clin. Pharmac. Ther.*, 1979, *25*, 795.

Further references: M. Nellen, *S.Afr. med. J.*, 1970, *44*, 106; W. J. Mroczek *et al.*, *New Engl. J. Med.*, 1971, *285*, 603; P. N. McLaine and K. N. Drummond, *J. Pediat.*, 1971, *79*, 829; J. E. F. Pohl and H. Thurston, *Br. med. J.*, 1971, *4*, 142; W. R. Lee *et al.*, *Clin. Pharmac. Ther.*, 1975, *18*, 154; E. B. Pedersen *et al.*, *Dan. med. Bull.*, 1975, *22*, 211; I. Cullhed and H. Aberg, *Läkartidningen*, 1976, *73*, 140; W. J. McDonald *et al.*, *Am. J. Cardiol.*, 1977, *40*, 409; D. G. Vidt and R. W. Gifford, *Clin. Pharmac. Ther.*, 1977, *21*, 120.

Hypertension, pulmonary. Symptoms were completely resolved in a 19-year-old girl with primary pulmonary hypertension when she took diazoxide 300 mg daily. Relief was still maintained after 6 months of treatment.— W. P. Klinke and J. A. L. Gilbert, *New Engl. J. Med.*, 1980, *302*, 91. Comment.— J. T. Reeves, *ibid.*, 112. Diazoxide may be effective in only a minority of patients with primary pulmonary hypertension. Important dose-limiting side-effects occurred in 5 of 7 patients.— L. Cotter and M. Honey (letter), *New Engl. J. Med.*, 1980, *302*, 1260.

Remission of primary pulmonary hypertension in one patient during treatment with diazoxide.— D. R. Hall and M. C. Petch, *Br. med. J.*, 1981, *282*, 1118.

Hypoglycaemia. A review of the use of diazoxide in the treatment of hypoglycaemia. It would be useful in the treatment of hypoglycaemia due to hyperinsulinism, especially in infants and children, but should not be used for functional hypoglycaemia.— *Med. Lett.*, 1978, *20*, 110.

Two girls, aged 10 and 11 months, 1 with idiopathic infantile hypoglycaemia and 1 with leucine-sensitive hypoglyaemia, were given 6 and 8.5 mg per kg body-weight daily respectively of diazoxide in 3 divided doses. The daily dose was doubled in the first after 4 days and raised to 14 mg per kg in the second patient after 7 days. The blood glucose concentration rose to normal or near-normal levels in both children, but fell if medication was discontinued. Transient vomiting occurred early in treatment, and mild hirsutism appeared later.— T. R. Mereu *et al.*, *New Engl. J. Med.*, 1966, *275*, 1455.

Treatment with diazoxide and chlorothiazide in a 3-year-old child with idiopathic leucine-sensitive hypoglycaemia appeared to reduce the serum-insulin response to leucine and glucose.— D. B. Grant *et al.*, *Br. med. J.*, 1966, *2*, 1494.

Further references: R. M. Ehrlich and J. M. Martin, *Am. J. Dis. Child.*, 1969, *117*, 411; J. Spencer-Peet *et al.*, *Q. J. Med.*, 1971, *40*, 95; J. Kühnau and W. Martin, *Dt. med. Wschr.*, 1972, *97*, 1870; M. W. Moncrieff *et al.*, *Postgrad. med. J.*, 1977, *53*, 159.

Chlorpropamide-induced hypoglycaemia. Diazoxide was effective in controlling hypoglycaemia in a 9-year-old boy who had ingested about 5 g of chlorpropamide, about 5 g of methyldopa, and about 3 g of chlorothiazide. Infusions of dextrose failed to control hypoglycaemia.— R. F. Jacobs *et al.*, *J. Pediat.*, 1978, *93*, 801.

Further references: S. F. Johnson *et al.*, *Am. J. Med.*, 1977, *63*, 799.

Toxaemia of pregnancy. The administration by mouth of diazoxide to 4 pregnant women with toxaemia controlled hypertension unresponsive to other treatments and permitted the pregnancies to be prolonged for up to 10 weeks. In each instance a healthy child was delivered. Hyperglycaemia in 1 patient was readily controlled with tolbutamide and 2 dependent on insulin required slight increases in their insulin dosage.— J. E. F. Pohl *et al.*, *Br. med. J.*, 1972, *2*, 568.

Diazoxide 300 mg was given by rapid intravenous injection to 1 eclamptic and 13 pre-eclamptic obstetric patients without causing hyperglycaemia or profound hypotension. The mean duration of action was 7.5 hours and 4 patients required more than 1 injection. Of 10 women given diazoxide before delivery 9 produced healthy infants, and the foetus in 1 died before the administration of diazoxide. Side-effects included nausea, dry mouth, tachycardia, and reduced uterine activity.— J. C. Pennington and R. H. Picker, *Med. J. Aust.*, 1972, *2*, 1051.

Another report of diazoxide being used in eclampsia or pre-eclampsia.— J. A. Morris *et al.*, *Obstet. Gynec.*, 1977, *49*, 675.

Severe criticism of recommendations to use diazoxide in toxaemia of pregnancy. The use of diazoxide is neither necessary nor generally reasonable (except in the most unusual circumstances) when a viable foetus is present and alive.— R. P. Perkins (letter), *J. Am. med. Ass.*, 1977, *238*, 2143. See also R. P. Perkins, *Am. J. Obstet. Gynec.*, 1976, *126*, 296.

It is potentially extremely dangerous to administer a bolus dose of diazoxide 300 mg as this may result in severe hypotension and so produce foetal death. Incremental doses can be given every 5 minutes until the blood pressure is normal. A suitable regimen is 50 mg followed at intervals of 5 minutes by 100 mg, 75 mg, 75 mg and 50 mg.— D. J. Tiller *et al.*, *Med. J. Aust.*, 1978, *1*, 32.

Recommendation for a treatment regimen for diazoxide in the treatment of severe pre-eclamptic hypertension: an indwelling intravenous catheter is inserted and doses of diazoxide 30 mg are injected at intervals of 60 seconds up to a dose of 300 mg; this total is seldom required. Blood pressure is measured at intervals of one minute and the diazoxide stopped when the desired blood pressure has been reached. Simultaneous administration of a diuretic, such as frusemide, may be required, and if the patient is already on methyldopa a smaller dose of diazoxide will be needed.— M. C. Macnaughton, *Prescribers' J.*, 1979, *19*, 52.

Preparations

Diazoxide Injection *(B.P.)*. A sterile solution of diazoxide in Water for Injections, prepared with the aid of sodium hydroxide. pH 11.2 to 11.9. Sterilised by autoclaving. Protect from light.

Diazoxide Injection *(U.S.P.)*. A sterile solution of diazoxide in Water for Injections prepared with the aid of sodium hydroxide. pH 11.2 to 11.9. Protect from light.

Diazoxide Tablets *(B.P.)*. Tablets containing diazoxide; they are sugar-coated.

Proprietary Preparations

Eudemine Injection *(Allen & Hanburys, UK)*. Contains diazoxide 300 mg in each 20 ml in aqueous solution (pH 11.6), in ampoules of 20 ml. Protect from light. For intravenous injection; do not dilute with infusion solutions.

Eudemine Tablets *(Allen & Hanburys, UK)*. Each contains diazoxide 50 mg.

Other Proprietary Names

Hyperstat *(Arg., Austral., Belg., Canad., Denm., Fr., Ital., Neth., Norw., S.Afr., Spain, Swed., Switz., USA)*; Hypertonalum *(Ger.)*; Proglicem *(Fr., Ger., Ital., Neth., S.Afr.)*; Proglycem *(USA)*.

863-z

Dicolinium Iodide. Dicolinum. 2-[2-(Diethylmethylammonio)ethoxycarbonyl]-1,1,6-trimethylpiperidinium diiodide.

$C_{16}H_{34}I_2N_2O_2$=540.3.

CAS — 382-82-1.

Pharmacopoeias. In *Rus.*

A white or creamy-white, odourless or almost odourless, hygroscopic, crystalline powder. M.p. about 212° with decomposition. Freely **soluble** in water; soluble in alcohol; practically insoluble in acetone and ether. **Store** in airtight containers. Protect from light.

Uses. Dicolinium iodide is a ganglion-blocking agent that has been used in the treatment of hypertension. The doses given in the *Rus. P.* are: by mouth, max. single dose 300 mg, max. in 24 hours 1 g; intramuscularly or subcutaneously, max. single dose 30 mg, max. in 24 hours 100 mg.

Preparations

Dragée Dicolini *(Rus. P.)*. Tablets each containing 50 mg of dicolinium iodide.

Solutio Dicolini 1% pro Injectionibus *(Rus. P.)*. Dicolinium Iodide Injection. Dicolinium iodide 1 g, sodium citrate 250 mg, Water for Injections to 100 ml; in ampoules of 2 ml. pH 4.2 to 4.9. Sterilised with steam at 100° for 30 minutes. Protect from light.

864-c

Dihydralazine Sulphate. Dihydralazinum Sulfuricum; Dihydrallazine Sulphate. 1,4-Dihydrazinophthalazine sulphate.

$C_8H_{10}N_6,H_2SO_4$=288.3.

CAS — 484-23-1 (dihydralazine); 7327-87-9 (sulphate).

Pharmacopoeias. In *Chin.* and *Cz. Roum. P.* specifies the dihydrate.

A white to slightly yellow, odourless, crystalline powder with a bitter taste. Slightly **soluble** in water; practically insoluble in alcohol, chloroform, and methyl alcohol. **Protect** from light.

Uses. Dihydralazine sulphate is an antihypertensive agent with action and uses similar to those of hydralazine (see p.148). It has been given in doses of 12.5 to 150 mg daily in divided doses. The mesylate is given by injection.

Association with hepatic damage: M. Knoblauch *et al.*, *Schweiz. med. Wschr.*, 1977, *107*, 651; R. Enat *et al.*, *ibid.*, 657.

Use in hypertension of pregnancy: R. Lammintausta, *Int. J. clin. Pharmac. Biopharm.*, 1978, *16*, 581.

Proprietary Names

Nepresol (as sulphate or mesylate) *(Ciba, Belg.; Ciba, Denm.; Ciba, Ger.; Ciba, Ital.; Ciba, Neth.; Ciba, Norw.; Ciba, S.Afr.; Ciba-Geigy, Switz.)*; Népressol *(Ciba, Fr.)*.

865-k

Guanabenz Acetate. Wy-8678. 1-(2,6-Dichlorobenzylideneamino)guanidine acetate.
$C_8H_8Cl_2N_4,C_2H_4O_2=291.1$.

CAS — 5051-62-7 (guanabenz); 23256-50-0 (acetate).

Analytical studies showed guanabenz acetate to be the *E*-isomer.— C. M. Shearer and N. J. DeAngelis, *J. pharm. Sci.*, 1979, *68*, 1010.

Adverse Effects. Drowsiness and dry mouth occur commonly. Dizziness, headache, a bitter taste, gastro-intestinal symptoms, blurred vision, sweating, urinary frequency, palpitations, nervousness, transient chest pain, numbness and cramps of hands, and skin rash have also been reported.

Withdrawal. Three of 4 hypertensive patients receiving guanabenz 48 mg daily developed a withdrawal syndrome of sympathetic overactivity within 16 to 48 hours of its abrupt discontinuation. None of 20 other patients, who had been receiving doses of 32 mg daily or less, developed the withdrawal syndrome. Guanabenz therapy should not be discontinued abruptly and, where possible, the dosage should be limited to less than 48 mg daily.— C. V. S. Ram *et al.*, *J. clin. Pharmac.*, 1979, *19*, 148.

Uses. Although, like guanethidine, guanabenz has an adrenergic neurone blocking action, *animal* studies have indicated that its main mode of action is central. It has been given in doses of 8 to 64 mg daily in the treatment of hypertension.

A report of *animal* studies suggesting that guanabenz acts primarily at sites which regulate the basal level of sympathetic outflow.— T. Baum and A. T. Shropshire, *Eur. J. Pharmac.*, 1976, *37*, 31.

Further references: T. Baum *et al.*, *J. Pharm. exp. Ther.*, 1970, *171*, 276.

Metabolism.— R. H. Meacham *et al.*, *Clin. Pharmac. Ther.*, 1980, *27*, 44.

Hypertension. A placebo-controlled study completed by 42 mainly black, female patients with mild to moderate hypertension indicated that guanabenz 4 to 16 mg twice daily (usually 16 mg twice daily) reduced blood pressure in most, significantly more than placebo; standing blood pressure was reduced more than supine. Main side-effects were drowsiness and dry mouth but dizziness, headache, a bitter taste, gastro-intestinal symptoms, blurred vision, sweating, urinary frequency, palpitations, nervousness, restlessness at night, transient chest pain, numbness and cramps of hands, shivering fingers, choking sensation in throat, and skin rash were also reported; guanabenz was discontinued in one patient due to disorientation.— F. G. McMahon *et al.*, *Clin. Pharmac. Ther.*, 1977, *21*, 272.

In a 6-month double-blind study in 36 patients with essential hypertension guanabenz 32 to 64 mg daily was as effective as methyldopa 1 to 2 g daily. Side-effects were similar with both drugs and were limited to mild sedation, dizziness, and dry mouth in a few patients.— B. R. Walker *et al.*, *Clin. Pharmac. Ther.*, 1977, *22*, 868.

Comparison with clonidine.— Y. Kluyskens and J. Snoeck, *Curr. med. Res. Opinion*, 1980, *6*, 638.

Comparison with methyldopa.— P. Hirvonen *et al.*, *Curr. ther. Res.*, 1980, *27*, 197.

Further references: D. T. Nash, *J. clin. Pharmac.*, 1973, *13*, 416; P. Bosanac *et al.*, *ibid.*, 1976, *16*, 631; R. S. Shah *et al.*, *Clin. Pharmac. Ther.*, 1976, *19*, 732; W. P. Leary *et al.*, *S. Afr. med. J.*, 1979, *55*, 83.

Proprietary Names

Rexitene *(LPB, Ital.)*.

866-a

Guanacline Sulphate.
Cyclazenin Sulphate; B 1464; FBA 1464. 1-[2-(1,2,3,6-Tetrahydro-4-methylpyrid-1-yl)ethyl]guanidine sulphate dihydrate.
$C_9H_{18}N_4,H_2SO_4,2H_2O=316.4$.

CAS — 1463-28-1 (guanacline); 1562-71-6 (sulphate, anhydrous); 23389-32-4 (sulphate, dihydrate).

Adverse Effects, Treatment, and Precautions. As for Guanethidine Monosulphate, p.145. Severe postural hypotension and parotid pain, which persisted for periods of 3 weeks to several years after discontinuing the drug, have been reported.

Reports of toxic effects.— K. D. Bock and V. Heimsoth, *Dt. med. Wschr.*, 1969, *94*, 256; Y. K. Seedat and E. I. Vawda (letter), *Br. med. J.*, 1970, *2*, 50; M. L. M. Parker, *Eur. J. clin. Pharmac.*, 1975, *8*, 131.

Uses. Guanacline sulphate is an antihypertensive agent with actions similar to those of guanethidine monosulphate (see p.146). It has been given in doses of 30 to 360 mg daily.

Hypertension. Clinical trials in hypertension: G. V. Hall and G. Michell, *Med. J. Aust.*, 1968, *1*, 1047; G. Jerums *et al.*, *ibid.*, 1968, *2*, 466; M. L. M. Parker and M. Bullen, *ibid.*, 1969, *1*, 159.

Manufacturers

Bayer, Ger.

867-t

Guanadrel Sulphate. CL 1388R; U 28288D. 1-(Cyclohexanespiro-2′-[1′,3′]dioxolan-4′-ylmethyl)guanidine sulphate; 1-(1,4-Dioxaspiro[4.5]dec-2-ylmethyl)guanidine sulphate.
$(C_{10}H_{19}N_3O_2)_2,H_2SO_4=524.6$.

CAS — 40580-59-4 (guanadrel); 22195-34-2 (sulphate).

Adverse Effects, Treatment, and Precautions. As for Guanethidine Monosulphate, p.145.

Uses. Guanadrel sulphate is an antihypertensive agent with actions similar to those of guanethidine monosulphate (see p.146) but with a shorter half-life. It has been given in doses of up to 400 mg daily in the treatment of hypertension.

References: D. K. Bloomfield and J. L. Cangiano, *Curr. ther. Res.*, 1969, *11*, 727 and 736; *idem, Clin. Pharmac. Ther.*, 1970, *11*, 200; A. V. Pascual and S. Julius, *Curr. ther. Res.*, 1972, *14*, 333; L. Hansson *et al.*, *Clin. Pharmac. Ther.*, 1973, *14*, 204; S. G. Chrysant and E. D. Frohlich, *Curr. ther. Res.*, 1976, *19*, 379; F. G. McMahon *et al.*, *Clin. Pharmac. Ther.*, 1977, *21*, 110; W. J. Mroczek, *ibid.*, 1980, *27*, 272.

868-x

Guancydine.
CL 2422; Guancidine. 2-Cyano-1-*tert*-pentylguanidine.
$C_7H_{14}N_4=154.2$.

CAS — 1113-10-6.

A white crystalline solid. M.p. about 156°.

Adverse Effects. Oedema and tachycardia are common. Anxiety, palpitations, faintness, paraesthesia, headache, vomiting, constipation, urinary retention, and gynaecomastia have also been reported.

Uses. Guancydine is an antihypertensive agent. It is a guanidine derivative like guanethidine but its antihypertensive action differs from that of guanethidine.

A review of the pharmacology of guancydine.— *Drugs of the Future*, 1978, *3*, 291.

Hypertension. Guancydine given to hypertensive patients in doses of 250, 500, and 625 mg reduced their blood pressure but increased the heart-rate and caused fluid retention. The tachycardia was potentiated by the additional use of quinethazone and suppressed by reserpine; when all 3 drugs were given together there was a slight increase in heart-rate and no fluid retention.— J. Hammer *et al.*, *Clin. Pharmac. Ther.*, 1971, *12*, 78.

The hypotensive effect of a single oral dose of guancydine 500 to 750 mg lasted for about 6 to 7 hours, and was accompanied by a decrease in platelet adhesiveness, activation of fibrinolysis, and an increase in venous blood oxygenation. Guancydine decreased urinary excretion of water and electrolytes and should be administered with caution to patients with impaired renal function.— S. Hărăguş *et al.*, *Cor Vasa*, 1977, *19*, 214.

Further studies: C. Werning *et al.*, *Dt. med. Wschr.*, 1970, *95*, 1756; J. Stenberg *et al.*, *Eur. J. clin. Pharmac.*, 1971, *3*, 63; H. Villarreal *et al.*, *Clin. Pharmac. Ther.*, 1971, *12*, 838; C. Russo and M. Mendlowitz, *ibid.*, 1972, *13*, 875; D. W. Clark and L. I. Goldberg, *Ann. intern. Med.*, 1972, *76*, 579; H. Villarreal *et al.*, *Mayo Clin. Proc.*, 1977, *52*, 383.

Manufacturers

Lederle, USA.

869-r

Guanethidine Monosulphate *(B.P.)*.
Guanethidine Sulphate. 1-[2-(Perhydroazocin-1-yl)ethyl]guanidine monosulphate.
$C_{10}H_{22}N_4,H_2SO_4=296.4$.

CAS — 55-65-2 (guanethidine); 645-43-2 (monosulphate).

Pharmacopoeias. In *Br.*, *Cz.*, *Jap.*, *Jug.*, and *Nord.* *Braz.*, *Turk.*, and *U.S.* include the hemisulphate, $(C_{10}H_{22}N_4)_2,H_2SO_4$.

A colourless, almost odourless, crystalline powder. M.p. about 250° with decomposition. **Soluble** 1 in 1.5 of water; practically insoluble in alcohol, chloroform, and ether. A 2% solution in water has a pH of 4.7 to 5.5. Solutions for injection are **sterilised** by autoclaving or by filtration. **Store** in airtight containers. Protect from light.

NOTE. Guanethidine hemisulphate was first isolated in the USA and all investigations into its pharmacology, toxicology, and clinical uses were made with this salt and submitted to the authorities in that country. In Europe, including the UK, guanethidine monosulphate, which was developed and investigated later, was preferred because of its greater stability and ease of formulation.— A. B. Tattersall, *Ciba*, *Personal Communication*, 1965.

Adverse Effects. The commonest side-effects occurring during the initial stages of therapy with guanethidine are severe postural and exertional hypotension and diarrhoea. Dizziness, syncope, muscle weakness, and lassitude are liable to occur, especially in the morning. Other frequent side-effects are bradycardia, dyspnoea, failure of ejaculation, fatigue, and oedema. Increased uraemia may occur in patients with poor renal function or in patients who already have an elevated blood concentration of urea nitrogen.

Nausea, vomiting, occasional headache, nasal congestion, parotid tenderness, blurring of vision, chest pain, myalgia, muscle tremor, hair loss, asthma, dermatitis, depression, disturbed micturition, impotence, paraesthesia, aggravation of intermittent claudication, and exacerbation of peptic ulcer have also been reported. It has been reported that guanethidine may possibly cause anaemia, leucopenia, and thrombocytopenia.

When guanethidine is used as eye-drops, common side-effects are conjunctival congestion and miosis. Burning sensations, nasal congestion, ptosis, and superficial punctate keratitis have also occurred.

Symptoms resembling polyarteritis nodosa were reported in 3 patients during treatment of hypertension with guanethidine.— H. A. Dewar and M. J. T. Peaston, *Br. med. J.*, 1964, *2*, 609.

An account of guanethidine therapy following experience with its use in over 250 patients. The most frequent side-effects are dizziness and weakness. Diarrhoea, bloating, gas pains, and indigestion also occur. Other side-effects are failure of normal ejaculation and orthostatic hypotension.— M. Moser, *Am. Heart J.*, 1969, *77*, 423.

Forty-four of 134 patients with hypertension treated continuously with guanethidine for at least a year developed fluid retention, mostly within the first 6 months.— A. J. Smith, *Circulation*, 1965, *31*, 485. Oedema during treatment with guanethidine was attributed to sodium retention.— M. I. Salomon (letter), *New Engl. J. Med.*, 1967, *276*, 639.

Conjunctival congestion and miosis occurred in each of 81 patients treated with guanethidine eye-drops. Other side-effects included a burning sensation in 14 patients, exacerbation of superficial ocular infection in 2, local sensitivity in 3, nasal congestion in 2, uni-ocular ptosis in 4, and superficial punctate keratitis in 3.— J. S. Cant and D. R. H. Lewis, *Br. J. Ophthal.*, 1969, *53*, 239.

Severe abdominal pain occurred in 2 patients who were being treated with guanethidine eye-drops; pain was not uncommon when larger doses were given by mouth.— A. N. Bowden and F. C. Rose, *Br. J. Ophthal.*, 1969, *53*, 246.

Urine retention was associated with guanethidine in 1 patient.— M. C. Bateson *et al.* (letter), *Lancet*, 1973, *1*, 1394.

Side-effects in 28 men with hypertension during treatment with guanethidine were postural hypotension (13), diarrhoea (8), nasal congestion (14), and fatigue (10). Some impairment of sexual function occurred in the majority of men but all regained normal function after withdrawal of the drug, regardless of the duration of therapy which ranged from 1 month to nearly 12 years.— G. E. Bauer *et al.*, *Med. J. Aust.*, 1973, *1*, 930.

The incidence of impotence associated with even low doses of guanethidine was considered to be greater than published studies indicated.— *Med. Lett.*, 1977, *19*, 81.

Treatment of Adverse Effects. If overdosage occurs the stomach should be emptied by aspiration and lavage. Withdrawal of guanethidine or reduction in dosage reverses many side-effects. Diarrhoea may be controlled by reducing dosage or giving codeine phosphate, or anticholinergic agents, such as propantheline bromide. In emergency surgery, atropine may be used to prevent excessive bradycardia. Severe hypotension may respond to placing the patient in the supine position with the feet raised. The effects of gross overdosage may be treated by the infusion of plasma or by the slow intravenous injection of low doses of pressor agents such as angiotensin, noradrenaline, or phenylephrine (but see Precautions). The patient must be observed for several days.

Precautions. Guanethidine should not be given to patients with phaeochromocytoma as it may cause a rise in blood pressure. It should be used with caution in patients with renal, cerebral, or coronary insufficiency, or with a history of peptic ulceration. Exercise and heat may increase the hypotensive effect of guanethidine. Hypotension may occur during anaesthesia in patients being treated with guanethidine (see p.136); hypertension may also occur, due to hypersensitivity to catecholamine release during operative stress; large doses of atropine should be given before induction of anaesthesia to prevent excessive bradycardia.

Patients taking guanethidine are sensitive to adrenaline, amphetamine, and other sympathomimetic agents. The hypotensive effects may also be antagonised by tricyclic antidepressants, monoamine oxidase inhibitors, and phenothiazine derivatives and related antipsychotic agents. It has been reported that oral contraceptives may reduce the hypotensive action of guanethidine. Concurrent administration of digitalis with guanethidine may cause excessive bradycardia. The hypotensive effects of guanethidine may be enhanced by thiazide diuretics and levodopa. Alcohol may cause orthostatic hypotension in patients taking guanethidine.

An unpleasant taste has been reported following instillation of guanethidine eye-drops.

The intra-arterial blood pressure, pulse, and ECG were monitored continuously in 11 hypertensive patients being treated only with adrenergic neurone blocking agents (guanethidine, bethanidine, or debrisoquine). All experienced large sudden variations in blood pressure and all had severe postural hypotension. Three had ECG evidence of myocardial dysfunction during hypotensive episodes and 1 experienced right-sided weakness during exertion. It was considered that adrenergic neurone blocking agents might predispose patients to cerebral or myocardial infarction by alternately raising and lowering perfusion pressure in vessels damaged by atheromatous disease.— A. D. Goldberg and E. B. Raftery, *Lancet*, 1976, *2*, 1052.

Interactions. Mechanism of the selective blockade of adrenergic neurones by guanethidine and related agents and its antagonism by drugs.— J. R. Mitchell and J. A. Oates, *J. Pharmac. exp. Ther.*, 1970, *172*, 100.

Antihistamines. Mepyramine both prevented and reversed the blocking action of guanethidine on the cold pressor response. Caution should be exercised in the concomitant administration of the drugs.— B. S. Verma and O. D. Gulati, *Proc. Congr. Int. Dermatol.*, 1968, *13* (2), 1053.

Antipsychotic agents. In a pilot study in 4 patients with hypertension who were treated with guanethidine, *chlorpromazine* was shown to reverse its hypotensive effect. *Haloperidol* and *thiothixene* also seemed to reverse the effects of guanethidine. It was suggested that an alternative antihypertensive agent be used if patients were already taking antipsychotic agents.— D. S. Janowsky *et al.*, *J. Am. med. Ass.*, 1972, *220*, 1288. See also W. E. Fann *et al.* (letter), *Lancet*, 1971, *2*, 436.

Cocaine. For reference to the risk of interaction with cocaine, see under Cocaine Hydrochloride, p.915.

Dantrolene. For reference to a possible interaction between adrenergic neurone blocking agents and dantrolene, see Dantrolene Sodium, p.989.

Insulin. A striking increase in insulin requirements was noticed when guanethidine was discontinued in a 43-year-old diabetic woman. She had been taking bendrofluazide 5 mg daily for 6 months.— K. K. Gupta and C. A. Lillicrap (letter), *Br. med. J.*, 1968, *2*, 697. See also K. K. Gupta (letter), *ibid.*, 1968, *3*, 679.

When guanethidine 10 mg four times daily was administered to healthy persons the plasma-insulin concentrations were significantly lower following the intravenous injection of glucose 25 g than before guanethidine administration while the rate of glucose disappearance increased slightly. It was suggested that the sensitivity of tissues to endogenous insulin was enhanced during treatment with guanethidine.— P. C. Kansal *et al.*, *Curr. ther. Res.*, 1971, *13*, 517.

Monoamine oxidase inhibitors. Studies involving the reversal of adrenergic neurone blocking agents by monoamine oxidase inhibitors: M. D. Day, *Br. J. Pharmac. Chemother.*, 1962, *18*, 421; O. D. Gulati *et al.*, *Clin. Pharmac. Ther.*, 1966, *7*, 510.

Phenylbutazone. Since phenylbutazone promotes sodium and water retention it might diminish the hypotensive activity of guanethidine.— R. M. Pearson and C. W. H. Havard, *Br. J. Hosp. Med.*, 1974, *12*, 812.

Sympathomimetics. Dexamphetamine, 10 mg by mouth, and *methylamphetamine*, 30 mg intramuscularly, totally reversed the adrenergic blocking action of guanethidine, as shown by the cold-pressor test, and antagonised its antihypertensive effect in patients receiving 25 to 35 mg of guanethidine daily. *Methylphenidate*, 20 mg by mouth, had a similar but less marked effect. *Ephedrine*, 90 mg by mouth, increased blood pressure but did not affect the cold-pressor response.— O. D. Gulati *et al.*, *Clin. Pharmac. Ther.*, 1966, *7*, 510. The antihypertensive effect of guanethidine given to 5 patients in doses of 15 to 20 mg twice daily was reduced by *dexamphetamine* 10 mg. No effect was seen when tripelennamine, prochlorperazine, or amitriptyline was given, but the antihypertensive action of guanethidine was enhanced by methyldopa.— K. F. Ober and R. I. H. Wang, *ibid.*, 1973, *14*, 190. Investigations in *dogs* indicated that whereas *dexamphetamine* could reverse the acute effects of guanethidine, it exerted little or no effect after 8 months of guanethidine administration.— B. S. Jandhyala *et al.*, *J. pharm. Sci.*, 1974, *63*, 1497.

Methylphenidate, given in a dose of 5 mg twice daily, provoked ventricular tachycardia during antihypertensive therapy with guanethidine 25 mg daily. Sinus rhythm returned after treatment with procainamide.— B. S. Deshmankar and J. A. Lewis, *Can. med. Ass. J.*, 1967, *97*, 1166.

Tricyclic antidepressants. In 5 patients whose blood pressure was controlled with guanethidine, the concomitant administration of *desipramine* 30 minutes before guanethidine antagonised the antihypertensive effect. An average of 5 days elapsed after discontinuation of desipramine before the effect of guanethidine reappeared. *Protriptyline* had a similar antagonistic effect.— J. R. Mitchell *et al.*, *J. Am. med. Ass.*, 1967, *202*, 973. See also J. A. Oates, *ibid.*, 1969, *208*, 1898.

A 47-year-old hypertensive Negro man, who had been adequately maintained on 75 mg daily of guanethidine sulphate, was given *amitriptyline* 25 mg thrice daily to treat depression. The dose of guanethidine was subsequently increased to 300 mg daily to control the blood pressure. When amitriptyline was discontinued he was adequately controlled with 87.5 mg daily of guanethidine. During subsequent investigations the effects of guanethidine were again eliminated after 5 days of amitriptyline 150 mg daily. The hypotensive effect of guanethidine did not return until 18 days after amitriptyline had been discontinued.— J. F. Meyer *et al.*, *J. Am. med. Ass.*, 1970, *213*, 1487.

Doxepin in doses of 200 to 300 mg daily antagonised the antihypertensive effects of guanethidine and bethanidine.— W. E. Fann *et al.*, *Psychopharmacologia*, 1971, *22*, 111. See also J. A. Oates *et al.*, *Psychosomatics*, 1969, *10*, 12; J. R. Mitchell *et al.*, *J. clin. Invest.*, 1970, *49*, 1596.

Withdrawal. Serious rebound hypertension was not associated with the abrupt withdrawal of guanethidine therapy.— M. J. Kendall, *Prescribers' J.*, 1978, *18*, 25.

Absorption and Fate. Guanethidine is incompletely absorbed from the gastro-intestinal tract. It is partially metabolised in the liver, and is excreted in the urine as metabolites and unchanged guanethidine. It has a half-life of several days. Guanethidine is actively transported into adrenergic neurones; it probably does not penetrate the blood-brain barrier. It is not bound to plasma proteins.

In a study of 2 patients given tritiated guanethidine, 50% of a dose given by intramuscular injection was excreted mostly in the urine in the first 2 or 3 days as guanethidine and 2 metabolites considered to be guanethidine *N*-oxide and2-(6-carboxyhexylamino)ethylguanidine. Thereafter the dose was excreted with a half-life of 9 to 10 days. When a dose of 50 mg was given by mouth, the plasma-guanethidine concentration rose to 6.5 ng per ml at 1 hour and was still at this figure at 12 hours with a peak of 8.6 ng per ml at 3 hours. By 24 hours the plasma concentration fell to 3.3 ng per ml. Plasma-metabolite concentrations were much higher for the first 24 hours, reaching a peak at 2 to 4 hours. The renal and hepatic clearance of guanethidine and its metabolites was high.— C. McMartin *et al.*, *Clin. Pharmac. Ther.*, 1970, *11*, 423.

In an investigation of variations in dosage requirements of guanethidine, urine samples from 6 patients with hypertension controlled by guanethidine sulphate 40 to 200 mg daily were studied. The mean amount of guanethidine absorbed daily varied from 6.4 to 29.9 mg calculated as 3% to 27% of the dose and inter-individual differences in absorption were found. It was considered that other factors apart from absorption also played a part in the need for dosage variations.— C. McMartin and P. Simpson, *Clin. Pharmac. Ther.*, 1971, *12*, 73.

Pharmacokinetics of guanethidine during chronic oral therapy.— J. H. Hengstmann and F. C. Falkner, *Eur. J. clin. Pharmac.*, 1979, *15*, 121.

Pregnancy and the neonate. Guanethidine given to a lactating mother in therapeutic doses was excreted in the milk in negligible quantities, and had no hypotensive effect on the child.— B. E. Takyi, *J. Hosp. Pharm.*, 1970, *28*, 317.

Uses. Guanethidine is an antihypertensive agent which acts by selectively inhibiting transmission in post-ganglionic adrenergic nerves. It is believed to act mainly by preventing the release of noradrenaline at nerve endings; it causes the depletion of noradrenaline stores in peripheral sympathetic nerve terminals and, unlike other common adrenergic neurone blocking agents, also causes significant depletion of tissue noradrenaline. It does not prevent the secretion of catecholamines by the adrenal medulla. It has similar effects to ganglion-blocking agents, but there is no parasympathetic blockade.

When administered by mouth its maximal effects take 2 to 3 days or longer to appear and persist for 7 to 10 days after treatment has been stopped. It causes an initial reduction in cardiac output (which may be subsequently compensated by increased stroke volume despite continued bradycardia) but its main hypotensive effect is to cause peripheral vasodilatation; it reduces the vasoconstriction which normally results from standing up and which is the result of reflex sympathetic nervous activity.

Guanethidine is used in the treatment of moderate and severe hypertension, or for mild hypertension when other drugs have proved inadequate. In the majority of patients it reduces the standing blood pressure but has a less marked effect on the supine blood pressure. Tolerance to guanethidine has occurred in some patients; this may

be countered by intensive diuretic therapy.
The usual initial dose of guanethidine monosulphate is 10 to 20 mg daily. This is increased by increments of 10 mg every 7 days according to the response of the patient. The usual maintenance dose varies from 30 to 100 mg daily as a single dose but up to 300 mg daily may be given. Children have been given 200 μg per kg body-weight daily with increments of 200 μg per kg every 7 to 10 days until a satisfactory response is achieved; a dose of about 1.5 mg per kg daily may be required.
To reduce side-effects smaller doses of guanethidine may be given in conjunction with a thiazide diuretic, which should also reduce the oedema that sometimes occurs with guanethidine therapy.
Guanethidine has been given intramuscularly in the treatment of hypertensive crises, including toxaemia of pregnancy, but more suitable agents are available. An intramuscular dose of 10 to 20 mg is reported to produce a fall in blood pressure within 30 minutes, reaching a maximum in 1 to 2 hours and lasting for 4 to 6 hours. Intravenously, guanethidine produces an initial hypertensive effect.
Eye-drops containing guanethidine 5% are used in the treatment of lid retraction which may accompany thyrotoxicosis and in the treatment of glaucoma.

A review of the mechanisms of action of some antihypertensive drugs, including guanethidine, bethanidine, bretylium, and debrisoquine.— R. Laverty, *Br. med. Bull.*, 1973, *29*, 152.

The use of guanethidine by mouth to prevent autonomic hyperreflexia in 200 patients with spinal cord injury.— B. T. Brown *et al.*, *J. Urol.*, 1979, *122*, 55.

Further references: W. A. Pettinger and W. D. Horst, *Ann. N.Y. Acad. Sci.*, 1971, *179*, 310.

Adie's syndrome. Of 6 patients with unilateral Adie's syndrome, 2 who were treated with guanethidine eye-drops 5% had a spontaneous recovery of light reflexes.— V. J. Marmion (letter), *Br. med. J.*, 1969, *2*, 450.

Administration in renal failure. The interval between guanethidine doses should be extended from 24 up to 36 hours in patients with a glomerular filtration rate of less than 10 ml per minute.— W. M. Bennett *et al.*, *Ann. intern. Med.*, 1980, *93*, 286.

Glaucoma. Solutions of 1, 2, 3, 4, and 5% guanethidine were found to produce a fall in intra-ocular pressure. Despite twice daily instillation, this was not maintained and within a month little hypotensive effect remained. Instillation of 5% guanethidine solutions concurrently with 1% adrenaline gave a more prolonged fall in intra-ocular pressure.— G. D. Paterson and G. Paterson, *Br. J. Ophthal.*, 1972, *56*, 288.

Over a mean period of 11 months in a group of 29 patients with raised intra-ocular pressure which was difficult to control, treatment with eye-drops of guanethidine 5% and neutral adrenaline 0.25 or 0.5% controlled the pressure in 25 affected eyes and these patients continued treatment. Treatment was considered ineffective in the other 24 affected eyes.— J. A. Roth, *Br. J. Ophthal.*, 1973, *57*, 507.

In a study involving 100 patients with glaucoma, eye-drops containing adrenaline 0.05 to 0.5% with guanethidine 1% gave a beneficial clinical response without causing the side-effects associated with these drugs.— S. Nagasubramanian *et al.*, *Trans. ophthal. Soc. U.K.*, 1976, *96*, 179.

Further references: L. Bonomi and P. Di Comite, *Archs Ophthal., N.Y.*, 1967, *78*, 337; J. A. Castrén *et al.*, *Ophthalmologica, Basel*, 1968, *155*, 194; K. B. Mills and A. E. Ridgway, *Br. J. Ophthal.*, 1978, *62*, 320; J. Romano and G. Patterson, *ibid.*, 1979, *63*, 52; P. F. J. Hoyng and C. L. Dake, *ibid.*, 1979, *63*, 56; D. E. P. Jones *et al.*, *ibid.*, 1979, *63*, 813.

Hypertension. A review of guanethidine therapy.— R. L. Woosley and A. S. Nies, *New Engl. J. Med.*, 1976, *295*, 1053.

Guanethidine and oxprenolol given together were shown to have an additive effect in reducing blood pressure in 9 patients with essential hypertension.— R. M. Pearson *et al.*, *Br. med. J.*, 1976, *1*, 933. Criticism of the use of guanethidine in patients with mild hypertension.— W. D. Alexander (letter), *ibid.*, 1341.

In a double-blind multicentre study in 108 patients with hypertension (diastolic pressure 100 to 129 mmHg) taking hydrochlorothiazide, a mean reduction of 18.4 mmHg was achieved after treatment for 5 to 6 months with guanethidine in individual optimum doses (range 7.5 to 150 mg daily) and a reduction of 13.6 mmHg after treatment with bethanidine (range 12.6 to 350 mg daily); the difference was significant. A reduction of diastolic pressure to less than 90 mmHg was achieved in 68.8% of those taking guanethidine and 45.5% of those taking bethanidine; the difference was significant.— Veterans Administration Cooperative Study Group on Antihypertensive Agents, *Circulation*, 1977, *55*, 519.

Results of a study in 4 hypertensive subjects indicated that single large doses of guanethidine of 100 mg by mouth do not release enough catecholamine to cause cardiovascular effects so that large loading doses of guanethidine should be safe even in patients with ischaemic heart disease or dissecting aneurysm of the aorta.— I. E. Walter and A. S. Nies, *Clin. Pharmac. Ther.*, 1977, *21*, 706. See also R. G. McAllister, *J. clin. Pharmac.*, 1975, *15*, 771.

Further references: A. W. D. Leishman and G. Sandler, *Lancet*, 1965, *1*, 668; A. W. D. Leishman and G. Sandler, *Angiology*, 1967, *18*, 705; P. R. Levine *et al.*, *Archs intern. Med.*, 1968, *21*, 305; E. L. Tarpley, *Curr. ther. Res.*, 1974, *16*, 1187; I. E. Walter *et al.*, *Clin. Pharmac. Ther.*, 1975, *18*, 571; R. H. Barnes and L. G. Eichner, *Curr. ther. Res.*, 1978, *24*, 786.

Hyperthyroidism. For the use of guanethidine in hyperthyroidism, see S. S. Waldstein *et al.*, *J. Am. med. Ass.*, 1964, *189*, 609.

Thyroid storm. For a report of guanethidine being added to the regimen of treatment of patients with thyroid storm, see E. L. Mazzaferri and T. G. Skillman, *Archs intern. Med.*, 1969, *124*, 684.

Thyrotoxic eye changes. In a double-blind crossover trial in 22 euthyroid patients (15 previously thyrotoxic and 7 suffering from Graves' disease) treatment with 5% eye-drops of guanethidine in buffered methylcellulose solution produced a significant long-term decrease in the palpebral aperture with improvement in lid retraction of 1 mm or greater and a reduction in intra-ocular pressure, but no improvement in exophthalmos.— N. E. F. Cartlidge *et al.*, *Br. med. J.*, 1969, *4*, 645.

Further references: J. S. Cant *et al.*, *Br. J. Ophthal.*, 1969, *53*, 233; A. N. Bowden and F. C. Rose, *ibid.*, 246; E. R. Asregadoo, *Archs Ophthal., N.Y.*, 1970, *84*, 21.

Porphyria. For 9 years guanethidine 75 or 100 mg daily had provided successful symptomatic relief in a patient with acute intermittent porphyria.— P. Wahlberg (letter), *Br. med. J.*, 1973, *3*, 544.

Regional sympathetic blockade. A technique for producing regional sympathetic blockade by injecting guanethidine 10 to 20 mg with 500 units of heparin for the upper extremities and 20 mg with 1000 units of heparin for the lower extremities after applying a tourniquet.— J. G. Hannington-Kiff, *Lancet*, 1974, *1*, 1019.

Comment on the mode of action of guanethidine in the relief of causalgia.— *Lancet*, 1978, *2*, 462.

Relief of causalgia in 10 patients by regional intravenous block using guanethidine.— J. G. Hannington-Kiff, *Br. med. J.*, 1979, *2*, 367.

Further references: J. G. Hannington-Kiff, *Lancet*, 1977, *1*, 1132; N. N. S. Kay *et al.*, *Br. med. J.*, 1977, *1*, 1575.

The use of sympathetic block using guanethidine for the relief of pain due to lesions of the central nervous system.— L. Loh *et al.*, *Br. med. J.*, 1981, *282*, 1026.

Amputations. The use of guanethidine sympathetic block for replacing a severed thumb.— K. H. Davies, *Br. med. J.*, 1976, *1*, 876.

Scleroderma. Five patients with scleroderma given guanethidine 30 to 50 mg daily for 4 to 6 weeks had a varied improvement in skin blood flow as measured by an increased clearance of xenon-133 which had been administered intracutaneously in sodium chloride injection.— E. C. Leroy *et al.*, *J. clin. Invest.*, 1971, *50*, 930.

Tachycardia. Guanethidine, 20 to 50 mg daily, was given to 5 patients, aged 31 to 66 years, with attacks of paroxysmal tachycardia occurring at least twice weekly. In all 5 patients complete relief was obtained but on discontinuing guanethidine attacks recurred.— H. J. Cragnolino (letter), *Lancet*, 1965, *1*, 606.

Further references: G. L. Jackson, *New Engl. J. Med.*, 1963, *269*, 518.

Preparations

Guanethidine Sulfate Tablets *(U.S.P.)*. Tablets containing guanethidine hemisulphate.

Guanethidine Tablets *(B.P.)*. Tablets containing guanethidine monosulphate. Protect from light.

Proprietary Preparations

Ganda 1+0.2 *(Smith & Nephew Pharmaceuticals, UK)*. Eye-drops containing guanethidine monosulphate 1% and adrenaline 0.2% in a buffered iso-osmotic solution. **Ganda 3+0.5** contains guanethidine monosulphate 3% and adrenaline 0.5%. **Ganda 5+0.5** contains guanethidine monosulphate 5% and adrenaline 0.5%. **Ganda 5+1** contains guanethidine monosulphate 5% and adrenaline 1%. For reducing intra-ocular pressure in primary and secondary glaucoma. *Admininistration.* 1 drop once or twice daily.

Ismelin *(Ciba, UK)*. Guanethidine monosulphate, available in 1-ml **Ampoules** of an injection containing 10 mg per ml and as scored **Tablets** of 10 and 25 mg. (Also available, monosulphate or hemisulphate, as Ismelin in *Austral., Canad., Denm., Ger., Ital., Neth., Norw., S. Afr., Spain, Switz., USA*).

Ismelin Eye Drops *(Zyma, UK)*. Contain guanethidine monosulphate 5%.

Other Proprietary Names

*(*Monosulphate or hemisulphate*)* Antipres, Antipres-M *(*both *Austral.)*; Dopom, Ipotidina, Visutensil *(*all *Ital.)*; Ismeline *(Belg.)*; Isméline *(Fr.)*; Solo-ethidine *(S.Afr.)*.

A preparation containing guanethidine monosulphate was formerly marketed in Great Britain under the proprietary name Ismelin-Navidrex-K *(Ciba)*.

870-j

Guanoclor Sulphate. 1-[2-(2,6-Dichlorophenoxy)ethylamino]guanidine sulphate.
$(C_9H_{12}Cl_2N_4O)_2,H_2SO_4=624.3$.

CAS — 5001-32-1 (guanoclor); 551-48-4 (sulphate).

A white crystalline powder. M.p. about 208°. **Soluble** 1 in about 400 of water.

Adverse Effects, Treatment, and Precautions. As for Guanethidine Monosulphate, p.145.
Headache and sweating may occur. Increased blood urea concentrations have been reported and occasionally elevations of serum aspartate and alanine aminotransferases have occurred.
Guanoclor should be administered with caution to patients with impaired liver function.

Uses. Guanoclor sulphate is an antihypertensive agent with actions similar to those of guanethidine monosulphate (see p.146), but it has also been reported to cause depletion of catecholamines in the central nervous system and inhibition of the enzymic conversion of dopamine to noradrenaline. It is reported to begin to act within 24 hours of administration, exerting a maximum effect in 48 hours. It has a more marked effect on the standing than on the supine blood pressure.
The initial dose for patients in hospital is 10 mg twice daily, increased by increments of 10 mg twice daily at intervals of 2 to 3 days according to the patient's response. For out-patients it is advisable to start with a dose of 5 mg twice daily, increasing by increments of 10 mg daily at intervals of not less than a week. If no response has been obtained with a dose of 40 mg daily, the daily dose can be increased by 20 mg at intervals of not less than a week. The average maintenance dose is 10 to 120 mg daily. Up to 200 mg or more has been given daily.
To reduce side-effects, a smaller dose of guanoclor sulphate may be given in conjunction with a thiazide diuretic.

Hypertension. A fall in blood pressure occurred within 2 to 5 days of treatment in all 33 patients with hypertension given guanoclor in doses of 20 to 240 mg daily for about 6 months. Side-effects included muscle pains, ankle swelling, raised blood-urea and SGOT values, and a raised ESR. Guanoclor was given for up to 15 months without the development of tolerance.— J. V. Hodge, *Br. med. J.*, 1966, *2*, 981.

Further reports: T. D. V. Lawrie *et al.*, *Br. med. J.*, 1964, *1*, 402; R. Sinniah and P. B. B. Gatenby, *Ir. J. med. Sci.*, 1965, *6*, 111; T. D. V. Lawrie, *Practitioner*, 1967, *199*, 239; J. Mackinnon and L. M. El Baz, *Br. J. clin. Pract.*, 1971, *25*, 135.

For a reference to guanoclor being withdrawn from a double-blind trial due to severe side-effects, see Methyldopa, p.154.

Proprietary Preparations

Vatensol *(Pfizer, UK)*. Guanoclor sulphate, available as scored tablets of 10 and 40 mg.

871-z

Guanoxan Sulphate. 1-(1,4-Benzodioxan-2-ylmethyl)guanidine sulphate.
$(C_{10}H_{13}N_3O_2)_2,H_2SO_4$=512.5.

CAS — 2165-19-7 (guanoxan); 5714-04-5 (sulphate).

A white crystalline powder. M.p. about 206°. **Soluble** 1 in 50 of water.

Adverse Effects and Treatment. As for Guanethidine Monosulphate, p.145. Liver damage has followed treatment with guanoxan.

A syndrome resembling systemic lupus erythematosus was associated with administration of guanoxan in a 60-year-old man.— P. L. Boardman *et al.* (letter), *Br. med. J.*, 1967, *1*, 111.

Of 96 patients treated with guanoxan, 26 had some derangement of liver function, severe in 10; four of these developed jaundice and 1 of the 4 patients died with chronic hepatic necrosis. Systemic lupus erythematosus was also observed in 1 patient.— S. G. Cotton and E. Montuschi (letter), *Br. med. J.*, 1967, *3*, 174. See also E. D. Frohlich *et al.*, *Clin. Pharmac. Ther.*, 1966, *7*, 599.

Precautions. As for Guanethidine Monosulphate, p.146. Guanoxan should not be given to patients with impaired liver function. It is advisable to perform liver-function tests before commencing treatment with guanoxan and to repeat them at regular intervals.

Uses. Guanoxan sulphate is an antihypertensive agent with actions similar to those of guanethidine monosulphate (see p.146), but it has also been reported to cause depletion of catecholamines in the central nervous system. In view of reports of hepatotoxicity it is only recommended for patients with severe hypertension that has failed to respond to conventional therapy. It is reported to begin to act within 24 hours of administration, exerting a maximum effect in 48 hours. It has a more marked effect on the standing than on the supine blood pressure.

The suggested dosage for patients in hospital is an initial dose of 10 mg twice daily, increased by increments of 10 mg twice daily at intervals of 2 to 3 days according to the patient's response. For out-patients it is advisable to start with a dose of 5 mg twice daily, increasing by increments of 5 to 10 mg daily at weekly intervals. The average maintenance dose is about 10 to 50 mg daily. Up to 120 mg or more has been given daily.

To reduce side-effects a smaller dose of guanoxan may be given in conjunction with a thiazide diuretic.

Three subjects characterised as extensive metabolisers of debrisoquine showed greater metabolic activity for guanoxan than did 2 patients characterised phenotypically as poor metabolisers of debrisoquine.— R. L. Smith *et al.* (letter), *Lancet*, 1978, *1*, 943. See also T. P. Sloan *et al.*, *Br. med. J.*, 1978, *2*, 655.

Hypertension. No difference was found between guanoxan and guanethidine in antihypertensive efficacy in a double-blind crossover trial involving 52 patients with essential hypertension. With both drugs the urinary excretion of noradrenaline was reduced.— J. Ruedy and R. O. Davies, *Clin. Pharmac. Ther.*, 1967, *8*, 38.

Further references: S. G. Sheps *et al.*, *Mayo Clin. Proc.*, 1966, *41*, 577; M. A. Özen *et al.*, *Curr. ther. Res.*, 1966, *8*, 385; G. Persson *et al.*, *Acta med. scand.*, 1967, *182*, 567.

Guanoxan sulphate was formerly marketed in Great Britain under the proprietary name Envacar (*Pfizer*).

872-c

Hexamethonium Benzenesulphonate. Benzohexonium; Hexonium B. *NN'*-Hexamethylenebis(trimethylammonium) di(benzenesulphonate).
$C_{12}H_{30}N_2,2C_6H_5O_3S$=516.7.

Pharmacopoeias. In *Rus.*

A white or creamy-white microcrystalline powder with a faint characteristic odour. Freely **soluble** in water; sparingly soluble in alcohol; practically insoluble in acetone and ether.

Uses. Hexamethonium benzenesulphonate has actions and uses similar to those of hexamethonium bromide; 14 mg of hexamethonium benzenesulphonate is approximately equivalent to 10 mg of hexamethonium bromide. The doses given in the *Rus. P.* are: max. single dose by subcutaneous injection 75 mg, and max. in 24 hours 300 mg; max. single dose by mouth 300 mg, and max. in 24 hours 900 mg.

Rus. P. includes an injection (2.5% in Water for Injections) and tablets (100 and 250 mg).

873-k

Hexamethonium Bromide *(B.P.C. 1968).*

Hexamethonii Bromidum; Hexonium Bromide. *NN'*-Hexamethylenebis(trimethylammonium) dibromide.
$C_{12}H_{30}Br_2N_2$=362.2.

CAS — 60-26-4 (hexamethonium); 55-97-0 (dibromide).

Pharmacopoeias. In *Fr.*

A white or creamy-white, almost odourless, hygroscopic powder with a saline taste. It loses not more than 10% of its weight on drying at 105°. M.p. about 280°, with decomposition. **Soluble** 1 in less than 1 of water and 1 in 60 of alcohol; practically insoluble in acetone, chloroform, and ether. A 4.99% solution is iso-osmotic with serum. Solutions are **sterilised** by autoclaving or by filtration. **Incompatible** with phenylmercuric nitrate. **Store** in airtight containers.

Adverse Effects, Treatment, and Precautions. As for Pempidine Tartrate, p.157.

There is a possible danger of bromism from the continued ingestion of hexamethonium bromide, particularly in patients on a low sodium diet.

Absorption and Fate. Hexamethonium bromide is incompletely and erratically absorbed from the gastro-intestinal tract, and the absorbed material is mainly excreted unchanged in the urine. In the body it is largely confined to the extracellular fluid; there is little penetration of the blood-brain barrier.

The biological half-life of hexamethonium was 1.5 hours.— W. A. Ritschel, *Drug Intell. & clin. Pharm.*, 1970, *4*, 332.

Pregnancy and the neonate. Hexamethonium crossed the placenta.— N. Morris, *Lancet*, 1953, *1*, 322.

Further references: J. Hallum and W. Hatchuel, *Archs Dis. Childh.*, 1954, *29*, 354.

Uses. Hexamethonium bromide is a quaternary ammonium ganglion-blocking agent with actions similar to those of pempidine tartrate (see p.157).

Hexamethonium bromide has been given subcutaneously or intramuscularly in an initial dose of 5 to 15 mg, but tolerance develops quickly and doses of up to 500 mg daily have been required. Administration every 4 to 6 hours has usually been necessary.

Hyphaemia. Two young boys with traumatic hyphaemia and secondary glaucoma were effectively treated with hexamethonium bromide, 37.5 mg intravenously, to prevent further haemorrhage during and after surgical removal of clotted blood from the anterior chamber of the eye. A second injection of 25 mg was given after surgery.— J. G. Moore and P. M. E. Youngman, *Br. J. Ophthal.*, 1968, *52*, 172.

Hexamethonium bromide was formerly marketed in Great Britain under the proprietary name Vegolysen (*May & Baker*).

874-a

Hexamethonium Chloride *(B.P.C. 1954).* Hexonium Chloride. *NN'*-Hexamethylenebis(trimethylammonium) dichloride.
$C_{12}H_{30}Cl_2N_2$=273.3.

CAS — 60-25-3.

Pharmacopoeias. In *Braz.*

A white crystalline hygroscopic powder with a slight odour. Very **soluble** in water; soluble in alcohol; practically insoluble in chloroform and ether. A 3.3% solution is iso-osmotic with serum.

Uses. Hexamethonium chloride has actions and uses similar to those of hexamethonium bromide; 8 mg is approximately equivalent to 10 mg of hexamethonium bromide.

A beneficial effect of hexamethonium chloride in chronic intractable congestive heart failure.— G. E. Burch *et al.*, *Am. Heart J.*, 1976, *91*, 735.

875-t

Hexamethonium Iodide *(B.P.C. 1954).* Hexonium Iodide. *NN'*-Hexamethylenebis(trimethylammonium) di-iodide.
$C_{12}H_{30}I_2N_2$=456.2.

CAS — 870-62-2.

A white, odourless, slightly hygroscopic, crystalline powder with a saline taste. **Soluble** 1 in 2 of water; practically insoluble in alcohol.

Uses. Hexamethonium iodide has actions and uses similar to those of hexamethonium bromide; 13 mg is approximately equivalent to 10 mg of hexamethonium bromide.

Proprietary Names

Gastrometonio *(Fabo, Ital.).*

876-x

Hexamethonium Tartrate *(B.P. 1963).* Hexamethonii Tartras; Hexamethonium Acid Tartrate; Hexamethonium Bitartrate. *NN'*-Hexamethylenebis(trimethylammonium) bis(hydrogen tartrate).
$C_{20}H_{40}N_2O_{12}$=500.5.

CAS — 2079-78-9.

Pharmacopoeias. In *Int.* and *Turk.*

A white or creamy-white, almost odourless, hygroscopic powder with an acid taste. M.p. about 186° with decomposition. **Soluble** 1 in 0.7 of water and 1 in 500 of alcohol. A solution in water is acid to litmus. A 5.68% solution is iso-osmotic with serum.

Uses. Hexamethonium tartrate has actions and uses similar to those of hexamethonium bromide; 14 mg of hexamethonium tartrate is approximately equivalent to 10 mg of hexamethonium bromide.

877-r

Hydracarbazine. 6-Hydrazinopyridazine-3-carboxamide.

$C_5H_7N_5O$=153.1.

CAS — 3614-47-9.

Uses. Hydracarbazine is a derivative of hydralazine (p.148) that has been used with pempidine (p.157) in the treatment of hypertension. It has been given in doses of 1.5 to 6 mg daily.

878-f

Hydralazine Hydrochloride *(U.S.P., B.P. 1963).*

Apressinum; Hydralazini Hydrochloridum; Hydrallazine Hydrochloride; Cloridrato de Hidralazina. 1-Hydrazinophthalazine hydrochloride.
$C_8H_8N_4,HCl$=196.6.

CAS — 86-54-4 (hydralazine); 304-20-1 (hydrochloride).

Pharmacopoeias. In *Braz.*, *Int.*, *Jap.*, *Nord.*, *Rus.*, and *U.S.*

A white to off-white odourless crystalline powder with a bitter saline taste. M.p. about 275° with decomposition. **Soluble** 1 in 25 of water and 1 in 500 of alcohol; very slightly soluble in ether. A 2% solution in water has a pH of 3 to 4. Administration in solutions of dextrose is inadvisable. **Store** in airtight containers.

Incompatibility. A yellow colour was produced when hydralazine hydrochloride 80 mg per litre was mixed with aminophylline 1 g per litre, ampicillin sodium 2 g per litre, sodium calciumedetate 4 g per litre, hydrocortisone sodium succinate 400 mg per litre, or mephentermine sulphate 120 mg per litre in dextrose injection. A yellow colour with a precipitate, which developed over 3 hours, occurred when hydralazine hydrochloride was mixed with ethamivan 2 g per litre, phenobarbitone sodium 800 mg per litre, or sulphadiazine sodium 4 g per litre in dextrose injection, and with chlorothiazide 2 g per litre, methohexitone sodium 2 g per litre, or sulphadimidine sodium 4 g per litre in dextrose injection or sodium chloride injection.— B. B. Riley, *J. Hosp. Pharm.*, 1970, *28*, 228.

A comment that hydralazine infused from any glass container appears to be ineffective but that the use of plastic containers is satisfactory.— R. P. Perkins (letter), *J. Am. med. Ass.*, 1977, *238*, 2143.

For a report of an incompatibility with ethacrynic acid, see Ethacrynic Acid, p.594.

Adverse Effects. Toxic effects occur frequently with hydralazine, particularly tachycardia, palpitations, angina pectoris, severe headache, anorexia, nausea, vomiting, diarrhoea, and postural hypotension.

Side-effects which occur less frequently are blood disorders, conjunctivitis, lachrymation, chills, fever, vertigo, flushing, dyspnoea, malaise, muscle cramps, nasal congestion, peripheral neuritis with numbness and tingling of the extremities, and urticaria. Occasionally, hepatitis, oedema, pruritus, skin rashes, urinary retention, paralytic ileus, depression, anxiety, and tremor occur.

A more serious toxic reaction which may occur following the prolonged use of large doses is a condition resembling either early rheumatoid arthritis or systemic lupus erythematosus. It is rare with doses less than 200 mg daily. The rheumatic condition usually disappears when the drug is withdrawn; the severe erythematous condition may be controlled with corticosteroids.

Death of a 72-year-old woman, associated with massive intestinal bleeding and mucosal ulcers resulting from necrotising vasculitis and fibrinoid degeneration. The patient had been taking hydralazine for hypertension in doses of 100 mg daily for 2 years.— G. Bendersky and C. Ramirez, *J. Am. med. Ass.*, 1960, *170*, 1789.

In a modified 'repeated-insult' patch test, 10% hydralazine was found to produce extreme sensitisation of the skin.— A. M. Kligman, *J. invest. Derm.*, 1966, *47*, 393.

Paradoxical hypertension in an 18-year-old woman following administration of hydralazine on 3 occasions.— D. B. Webb and J. P. White, *Br. med. J.*, 1980, *280*, 1582.

Effects on the blood. A 63-year-old man developed Coombs' positive haemolysis while receiving hydralazine 25 mg daily for mild hypertension. The Coombs' test was negative 11 weeks after withdrawal of hydralazine therapy which had continued for about 3 years.— A. A. Orenstein *et al.*, *Ann. intern. Med.*, 1977, *86*, 450.

Effects on the kidneys. Acute haemorrhagic glomerulonephritis was reported to be associated with treatment with hydralazine.— R. Muehrke and R. Kark, *Lancet*, 1966, *1*, 1148.

Effects on the liver. Hydralazine could cause hepatic granuloma.— K. G. Tolman, *Med. J. Aust.*, 1977, *2*, 655.

A report of hepatitis occurring as part of a hypersensitivity reaction to hydralazine.— H. S. Forster (letter), *New Engl. J. Med.*, 1980, *302*, 1362. See also E. Bartoli *et al.*, *Archs intern. Med.*, 1979, *139*, 698.

Asymptomatic disturbance of liver function associated with hydralazine.— D. B. Barnett *et al.*, *Br. med. J.*, 1980, *280*, 1165.

Obstructive jaundice, pancytopenia, and hydralazine.— G. W. Stewart *et al.* (letter), *Lancet*, 1981, *1*, 1207.

Effects on the nervous system. Peripheral neuropathy occurs rarely, if at all, when doses of hydralazine in the range of 100 to 200 mg daily are used.— D. Burley and J. Steen, *Ciba* (letter), *Br. med. J.*, 1979, *1*, 1082.

Headache. Of 5 patients who complained of severe headache after receiving a single dose of hydralazine 75 mg by mouth 4 were slow acetylators.— A. S. P. Hua *et al.*, *Med. J. Aust.*, 1978, *1*, 45.

Hypotension. Reports of severe hypotension in patients receiving diazoxide and hydralazine.— W. L. Henrich *et al.*, *J. Am. med. Ass.*, 1977, *237*, 264; G. P. Romberg and R. E. Lordon (letter), *ibid.*, *238*, 1025.

Lupus erythematosus. The histories were studied of 50 patients who had rheumatic, febrile, or cutaneous reactions when given hydralazine, and they were followed up for 6 months to 9 years. Previous histories suggesting a diathesis of systemic lupus erythematosus were found in 74% compared with 13% of 100 hypertensive patients studied as controls.— D. Alarcón-Segovia *et al.*, *New Engl. J. Med.*, 1965, *272*, 462.

Fourteen of 32 patients with hypertension treated with hydralazine for 1 to 144 months developed a syndrome resembling systemic lupus erythematosus or rheumatoid arthritis. The titre of antinuclear antibodies in the blood of these patients varied inversely with the interval that had elapsed since their last exposure to hydralazine, and sometimes remained significant long (up to 9 years) after the last dose of drug. Four of 15 control patients who failed to show any toxic reactions to hydralazine nevertheless possessed antinuclear antibodies. The occurrence of antibodies was not related to the total dose of drug or to the duration of treatment. Caucasian women were more liable to develop systemic lupus erythematosus than were men, and Negroes were found to be immune.— J. J. Condemi *et al.*, *New Engl. J. Med.*, 1967, *276*, 486.

The lupus erythematosus-like reaction to hydralazine was more likely to occur in subjects who were slow acetylators.— H. M. Perry *et al.*, *Proc. cent. Soc. clin. Res.*, 1967, *40*, 81.

A report of the successful use of hydralazine in 7 hypertensive patients with systemic lupus erythematosus, receiving concomitant immunosuppressive therapy.— M. J. Reza *et al.*, *Arthritis Rheum.*, 1975, *18*, 335.

A retrospective analysis of patients treated with hydralazine indicated that 6 of 200 had developed a lupus-like syndrome. All these 6 patients were slow acetylators and had not received more than 200 mg of hydralazine daily.— R. F. Bing *et al.*, *Br. med. J.*, 1980, *281*, 353.

A report of hydralazine-induced lupus erythematosus-like syndrome in a 49-year-old woman. The patient was a rapid acetylator of sulphadimidine but investigations with hydralazine were characteristic of the slow acetylator phenotype.— S. J. Harland *et al.*, *Br. med. J.*, 1980, *281*, 273.

Further references: B. H. Hahn *et al.*, *Ann. intern. Med.*, 1972, *76*, 365; H. M. Perry, *Am. J. Med.*, 1973, *54*, 58; J. J. Irias, *Am. J. Dis. Child.*, 1975, *129*, 862.

See also under Absorption and Fate.

Retroperitoneal fibrosis. Mention of retroperitoneal fibrosis as a side-effect of hydralazine.— J. R. Curtis, *Br. med. J.*, 1977, *2*, 375.

Vasculitis. Hydralazine-induced cutaneous vasculitis in 2 patients.— R. M. Bernstein *et al.*, *Br. med. J.*, 1980, *280*, 156. See also A. Peacock and D. Weatherall, *ibid.*, 1981, *282*, 1121; A. Y. Finlay *et al.* (letter), *ibid.*, 1703.

Treatment of Adverse Effects. If overdosage occurs the stomach should be emptied by aspiration and lavage. Withdrawal of hydralazine or reduction of the dosage causes the reversal of many side-effects. Severe hypotension may respond to placing the patient in the supine position with the feet raised. The effects of gross overdosage may be treated by the infusion of plasma or by the slow intravenous injection of minimal doses of pressor agents such as angiotensin or noradrenaline. Peripheral neuritis has been reported to be alleviated by pyridoxine.

Reversal of hydralazine-induced peripheral neuropathy by pyridoxine in 2 patients.— N. H. Raskin and R. A. Fishman, *New Engl. J. Med.*, 1965, *273*, 1182.

Further references: J. Cawano and L. J. Davis, *Drug Intell. & clin. Pharm.*, 1978, *12*, 112 and 297.

Precautions. Hydralazine is contra-indicated in patients with tachycardia and should be used with caution in patients with a history of coronary disease. Patients who are slow acetylators of hydralazine require lower doses than those who are fast acetylators. Hypotension may occur during anaesthesia in patients being treated with hydralazine (see p.136).

Hydralazine is teratogenic in some species of *animals* and should therefore be avoided during the first half of pregnancy.

Adrenaline should not be given to antagonise the hypotensive effects of hydralazine since it enhances the cardiac-accelerating effects. Caution should be observed if hydralazine is administered concurrently with monoamine oxidase inhibitors or tricyclic antidepressants. The hypotensive effects of hydralazine may be enhanced by thiazide diuretics and by beta-adrenoceptor blocking agents which may also diminish the cardiac-accelerating effects.

Interactions. Hydralazine hydrochloride affected the estimation of urinary 17-oxo-steroids and 17-oxogenic-steroids.— *Adverse Drug React. Bull.*, 1972, June, 104.

Severe hypotension with diazoxide and hydralazine.— W. L. Henrich *et al.*, *J. Am. med. Ass.*, 1977, *237*, 264; G. P. Romberg and R. E. Lordon (letter), *ibid.*, *238*, 1025.

Absorption and Fate. Hydralazine is rapidly absorbed from the gastro-intestinal tract and peak concentrations have been reported to occur in the plasma after about one hour. It is metabolised by hydroxylation of the ring system and conjugation with glucuronic acid, and by *N*-acetylation.

In a detailed review of studies on the clinical pharmacokinetics of hydralazine, T. Talseth (*Clin. Pharmacokinet.*, 1977, *2*, 317) has emphasised their limitations, which include problems with the analytical procedures and the instability of hydralazine, as well as the paucity of studies in patients as against healthy subjects.

Hydralazine has been estimated by S.B. Zak *et al.* (*J. pharm. Sci.*, 1974, *63*, 225) to be rapidly absorbed from the gastro-intestinal tract with peak plasma concentrations usually occurring within an hour of taking the commercial tablets; recoveries of 3 to 12% in the faeces may reflect lack of absorption or biliary excretion.

Hydralazine is subject to polymorphic *N*-acetylation (D.A.P. Evans and T.A. White, *J. lab. clin. Med.*, 1964, *63*, 394) and significant first-pass metabolism involving the *N*-acetylation process, which may be capacity limited, affects fast acetylators considerably more than slow acetylators. The difference between fast and slow acetylators does not remain so marked in relation to the terminal elimination half-life of hydralazine, which has been estimated as ranging from less than 1 to nearly 8 hours (M.M. Reidenberg *et al.*, *Clin. Pharmac. Ther.*, 1973, *14*, 970; T. Talseth, *Eur. J. clin. Pharmac.*, 1976, *10*, 183 and 395; and others). This may be because both monomorphic and polymorphic *N*-acetylation of hydralazine takes place, with the polymorphic type becoming of relatively minor importance when equilibrium distribution of the drug has occurred.

Hydralazine has been reported by J.M. Lesser *et al.* (*Drug Metab. & Disposit.*, 1974, *2*, 351) to be about 87% bound to plasma proteins, but as the figures are obtained from equilibrium dialysis due consideration must be paid to the instability of the drug.

Although hydralazine accumulates in renal failure (M.M. Reidenberg *et al.*, *Clin. Pharmac. Ther.*, 1973, *14*, 970; T. Talseth, *Eur. J. clin. Pharmac.*, 1976, *10*, 311) it has been variously reported that up to only 11 to 14% of hydralazine is excreted unchanged in the urine and often considerably less (T. Talseth, *Eur. J. clin. Pharmac.*, 1976, *10*, 395; S.B. Zak *et al.*, *J. pharm. Sci.*, 1974, *63*, 225; and earlier studies). Possible explanations are that unchanged drug in urine has been underestimated or that hydralazine metabolism is impaired in uraemia.

Although some workers (A.J. Jounela *et al.*, *Acta med. scand.*, 1975, *197*, 303; R. Zacest and J. Koch-Weser, *Clin. Pharmac. Ther.*, 1972, *13*, 420) have correlated the hypotensive effect of hydralazine with the serum concentrations, others (T. Talseth *et al.*, *Curr. ther. Res.*, 1977, *21*, 157) have been unable to do so. Moreover, the duration of hypotensive effect has been shown to exceed considerably that predicted from the rate of elimination (K. O'Malley *et al.*, *Clin. Pharmac. Ther.*, 1975, *18*, 581). Possible explanations are the accumulation of hydralazine at its sites of action in the arterial walls (D. Moore-Jones and H.M. Perry, *Proc. Soc. exp. Biol. Med.*, 1966, *122*, 576) or the existence of active metabolites (K. Barron *et al.*, *Br. J. Pharmac.*, 1977, *61*, 345; K.D. Haegele *et al.*, *Br. J. clin. Pharmac.*, 1978, *5*, 489; P.A. Reece *et al.*, *J. pharm. Sci.*, 1978, *67*, 1150).

Concurrent intake of food has been found by A. Melander *et al.* (*Clin. Pharmac. Ther.*, 1977, *22*, 104) to enhance considerably the bioavailability of hydralazine (see also A. Melander, *Clin. Pharmacokinet.*, 1978, *3*, 337).

Further references.— J. Wagner *et al.*, *Arzneimittel-Forsch.*, 1977, *27*, 2388 (metabolism in healthy subjects); D. W. Schneck *et al.*, *Clin. Pharmac. Ther.*, 1978, *24*, 714 (acetylation; lack of influence of procainamide); D. D. Shen *et al.*, *J. Pharmacokinet. Biopharm.*, 1980, *8*, 53 (pharmacokinetics); T. M. Ludden *et al.*, *Clin. Pharmac. Ther.*, 1980, *27*, 268 (pharmacokinetics in hypertensive subjects using improved technique); P. A. Reece *et al.*, *Clin. Pharmac. Ther.*, 1980, *27*, 280 (3-methyl-1,2,4-triazolo[3,4-*a*]phthalazine metabolite); A. M. M. Shepherd *et al.*, *Clin. Pharmac.*

Ther., 1980, *27*, 286 (specific assay technique in hypertensive patients); W. E. Wagner *et al.*, *Clin. Pharmac. Ther.*, 1980, *27*, 291 (hypertensive patients); J. A. Timbrell *et al.*, *Clin. Pharmac. Ther.*, 1980, *28*, 350 (polymorphic acetylation); T. M. Ludden *et al.*, *Clin. Pharmac. Ther.*, 1980, *28*, 736 (hypertensive patients); P. A. Reece *et al.*, *Clin. Pharmac. Ther.*, 1980, *28*, 769 (slow and fast acetylators); A. M. M. Shepherd *et al.*, *Clin. Pharmac. Ther.*, 1980, *28*, 804 (kinetics).

Further reviews: Z. H. Israili and P. G. Dayton, *Drug Metab. Rev.*, 1977, *6*, 283.

Metabolic studies on slow-release preparations of hydralazine: T. Talseth *et al.*, *Curr. ther. Res.*, 1977, *21*, 157.

Pregnancy and the neonate. Transient thrombocytopenia in 3 neonates was associated with hydralazine taken by their mothers for some months before delivery.— E. Widerlöv *et al.* (letter), *New Engl. J. Med.*, 1980, *303*, 1235.

Uses. Hydralazine is an antihypertensive agent which acts predominantly by causing direct peripheral vasodilatation. Hydralazine tends to improve renal, uterine, and cerebral blood flow and its effect on diastolic pressure is more marked than on systolic pressure. It has a more marked action on the standing than the supine blood pressure and is used for the treatment of moderate to severe hypertension usually in conjunction with a beta-adrenoceptor blocking agent and a thiazide diuretic.

The usual initial dose of hydralazine hydrochloride by mouth is 25 mg twice or thrice daily increased according to the patient's response, to a maximum of 200 mg daily in divided doses.

Hydralazine hydrochloride is also given by intramuscular injection, slow intravenous injection, or by intravenous infusion in a dose of 20 to 40 mg for hypertensive emergencies such as pre-eclampsia, the dose being repeated as necessary. A maximum fall in blood pressure is usually obtained within 10 to 80 minutes.

A suggested initial dose for children is 187.5 µg per kg body-weight by mouth 4 times daily, and 425 µg per kg intramuscularly or intravenously 4 times daily. Some sources use a slightly higher initial dose by mouth of 250 µg per kg four times daily.

Findings that administration of the same daily dosage of hydralazine in 2 doses rather than 4 gives equally effective blood pressure control and may increase patient compliance.— K. O'Malley *et al.*, *Clin. Pharmac. Ther.*, 1975, *18*, 581. The dose of hydralazine in a fast acetylator is about 50% greater than in a slow acetylator to achieve the same concentration and effect. In fast acetylators the dose can be increased to 300 mg daily instead of the usual 200 mg daily.— *Lancet*, 1977, *1*, 342. A study of the kinetics of hydralazine elimination in 2 slow acetylators and 2 rapid acetylators emphasised the need to assess acetylator phenotype of patients when evaluating the therapeutic response to hydralazine, especially at doses above 25 mg.— T. Talseth, *Clin. Pharmac. Ther.*, 1977, *21*, 715. Studies in 5 healthy subjects indicated that 2 to 3 times as much hydralazine entered the general circulation when it was taken with food than when it was taken on an empty stomach.— A. Melander *et al.*, *Clin. Pharmac. Ther.*, 1977, *22*, 104. Evidence that food has little influence on hydralazine absorption.— R. J. Walden *et al.*, *Eur. J. clin. Pharmac.*, 1981, *20*, 53.

Administration in renal failure. A study of elimination rates and steady-state concentrations of hydralazine in 13 patients with impaired renal function.— T. Talseth, *Eur. J. clin. Pharmac.*, 1976, *10*, 311.

Hydralazine was reported to be 87% bound to plasma proteins. The normal half-life was 2.4 to 4.5 hours. The interval between doses should be extended from 8 hours (fast acetylators) and 12 hours (slow acetylators) to 8 to 16 hours (fast acetylators) and 12 to 24 hours (slow acetylators) in patients with a glomerular filtration-rate of less than 10 ml per minute. Concentrations of hydralazine were not affected by haemodialysis or peritoneal dialysis.— W. M. Bennett *et al.*, *Ann. intern. Med.*, 1980, *93*, 286.

Heart disease. In a study involving 16 patients with congestive heart failure hydralazine 50 to 100 mg by mouth resulted in increased cardiac output, a reduction in arterial and pulmonary arterial pressure, and a slight rise in heart-rate. Hydralazine may be useful in the treatment of chronic left ventricular failure and preliminary studies have suggested enhancement of this effect by nitroprusside.— J. A. Franciosa *et al.*, *Ann. intern. Med.*, 1977, *86*, 388.

Sustained beneficial haemodynamic effects of hydralazine in patients with chronic heart failure.— K. Chatterjee *et al.*, *Ann. intern. Med.*, 1980, *92*, 600.

Improved renal function in patients with congestive heart failure treated with hydralazine.— G. L. Pierpont *et al.*, *Circulation*, 1980, *61*, 323.

The need for individual adjustment of dose.— M. Packer *et al.*, *Clin. Pharmac. Ther.*, 1980, *27*, 337.

Further references: T. LeJemtel *et al.*, *Circulation*, 1977, *56*, *Suppl.3*, 9; K. Chatterjee *et al.*, *Am. J. Med.*, 1978, *65*, 134; J. Mehta *et al.*, *Br. Heart J.*, 1978, *40*, 845; G. L. Pierpont *et al.*, *Chest*, 1978, *73*, 8; L. H. Opie, *Lancet*, 1980, *1*, 966.

Hypertension. Reviews of hydralazine in hypertension: J. Koch-Weser, *New Engl. J. Med.*, 1976, *295*, 320; *Lancet*, 1977, *1*, 342.

A study on the use of hydralazine in the differential diagnosis of hypertension.— H. Ueda *et al.*, *Archs intern. Med.*, 1968, *122*, 387. A study suggesting that the use of hydralazine as a diagnostic test might be hazardous in ischaemic heart disease.— D. K. Falch and N. Norman, *Acta med. scand.*, 1978, *203*, 433.

In a double-blind study in 450 patients with mild hypertension propranolol, alone or in combination with hydrochlorothiazide and hydralazine was compared with reserpine with hydrochlorothiazide. Reduction of diastolic blood pressures to below 90 mmHg and a reduction of at least 5 mmHg from the initial blood pressure after 6 months' treatment was achieved in 92% of patients taking propranolol with hydrochlorothiazide and hydralazine, 88% taking reserpine and hydrochlorothiazide, 81% taking propranolol and hydrochlorothiazide, 72% taking propranolol and hydralazine, and 52% taking propranolol alone. No regimen had any advantage over any other with relation to side-effects.— Veterans Administration Cooperative Study Group on Antihypertensive Agents, *J. Am. med. Ass.*, 1977, *237*, 2303. See also *idem*, 1970, *213*, 1143.

Further references: T. B. Gottlieb *et al.*, *Circulation*, 1972, *45*, 571; R. Zacest *et al.*, *New Engl. J. Med.*, 1972, *286*, 617; A. J. Jounela *et al.*, *Acta med. scand.*, 1975, *197*, 303; K. O'Malley *et al.*, *Clin. Pharmac. Ther.*, 1975, *18*, 581; H. M. Perry *et al.*, *J. chron. Dis.*, 1977, *30*, 519; J. F. Winchester *et al.*, *Br. J. clin. Pharmac.*, 1976, *3*, 863; M. Gutkin *et al.*, *J. clin. Pharmac.*, 1977, *17*, 509; M. Hansen *et al.*, *Acta med. scand.*, 1977, *202*, 385; M. Velasco and J. L. McNay, *Mayo Clin. Proc.*, 1977, *52*, 430; R. G. Wilcox and J. R. A. Mitchell, *Br. med. J.*, 1977, *2*, 547; W. A. Forrest, *Br. J. clin. Pract.*, 1978, *32*, 326; S. Kalowski *et al.*, *Med. J. Aust.*, 1979, *2*, 439.

In pregnancy. Reviews of hydralazine in the management of toxaemia: R. P. Perkins, *Obstet. Gynec.*, 1977, *49*, 498; B. M. Hibbard and M. Rosen, *Br. J. Anaesth.*, 1977, *49*, 3.

An account of the standardised treatment of 154 consecutive cases of eclampsia, treated over a period of 20 years, using magnesium sulphate, in association with hydralazine if necessary to control diastolic pressures exceeding 110 mmHg, and intravenous fluid therapy. The hydralazine dosage regimen was: if the diastolic blood pressure exceeded 110 mmHg a test dose of hydralazine 5 mg was injected intravenously as a bolus and the blood pressure monitored every 5 minutes; if the diastolic pressure was not lowered to about 100 mmHg in 20 minutes a dose of 10 mg was administered similarly, continuing to monitor the blood pressure; this dose was repeated until the diastolic blood pressure had been lowered to about 100 mmHg. The desired effect was almost always achieved with 5 to 20 mg of hydralazine. Hydralazine was repeated whenever the diastolic blood pressure exceeded 110 mmHg.— J. A. Pritchard and S. A. Pritchard, *Am. J. Obstet. Gynec.*, 1975, *123*, 543. Mention of the use of infusion rather than bolus intravenous injection of hydralazine.— R. R. De Alvarez, *ibid.*, 550.

Further references: D. N. Joyce and V. G. Kenyon, *J. Obstet. Gynaec. Br. Commonw.*, 1972, *79*, 250.

Hypertension, Pulmonary. Hydralazine by mouth induced a persistent improvement in haemodynamic function at rest in 4 patients with primary pulmonary hypertension and in 3 of the patients who were also studied during exercise. Treatment was continued and improvement was maintained 3 to 6 months later. Pulmonary arteriolar dilatation appeared to be the most likely explanation for the beneficial effect of hydralazine.— L. J. Rubin and R. H. Peter, *New Engl. J. Med.*, 1980, *302*, 69. Comment.— J. T. Reeves, *ibid.*, 112. Criticism.— S. Rich (letter), *ibid.*, 1980, *302*, 1260.

Preparations

Hydralazine Hydrochloride Injection *(U.S.P.)*. A sterile solution of hydralazine hydrochloride in Water for Injections. pH 3.4 to 4.4.

Hydralazine Hydrochloride Tablets *(U.S.P.)*. Tablets containing hydrazaline hydrochloride. Store in airtight containers. Protect from light.

Hydrallazine Tablets *(B.P. 1963)*. Tablets containing hydralazine hydrochloride.

Proprietary Preparations

Apresoline *(Ciba, UK)*. Hydralazine hydrochloride, available as powder for preparing injections in **Ampoules** of 20 mg and as **Tablets** of 25 mg and 50 mg. (Also available as Apresoline in *Austral., Canad., Neth., USA*).

Other Proprietary Names

Aprelazine *(Jap.)*; Apresolin *(Denm., Norw., Swed.)*; Apresolina *(Spain)*; Dralzine *(USA)*; Hyperazin *(Jap.)*; Hyperex *(S.Afr.)*; Ipolina *(Ital.)*.

879-d

Indoramin. Wy-21901. *N*-[1-(2-Indol-3-ylethyl)-4-piperidyl]benzamide.

$C_{22}H_{25}N_3O = 347.5$.

CAS — 26844-12-2.

Adverse Effects and Precautions. Adverse effects reported for indoramin include sedation, dry mouth, nasal congestion, dizziness, depression, weight gain (almost certainly due to fluid retention), failure of ejaculation, and skin rash.

As an alpha-adrenoceptor blocking agent indoramin would be expected to have a cardiac-accelerating action, but this has not been reported with therapeutic doses, possibly owing to its other pharmacological properties.

Indoramin should be avoided in patients with heart failure; it has been recommended that incipient heart failure should be controlled with diuretics and digitalis before giving indoramin, and that caution should be observed in patients with hepatic or renal insufficiency, or Parkinson's disease.

Animal studies have indicated that, in addition to sedation and hypotension, hypothermia and (in some species) convulsions may occur on overdosage.

A clinical evaluation of indoramin showed that it was an effective antihypertensive agent, but its use was limited by severe side-effects including sedation, fluid retention, and failure of ejaculation.— P. J. Lewis *et al.*, *Eur. J. clin. Pharmac.*, 1973, *6*, 211.

Effects on sexual function. Failure of ejaculation in 6 of 9 men taking indoramin for migraine.— B. Pentland *et al.*, *Br. med. J.*, 1981, *282*, 1433. See also B. A. Gould *et al.* (letter), *ibid.*, 1796.

Interactions. Indoramin might be of value in hypertensive patients, especially those requiring tricyclic antidepressants; there were no changes in blood pressure in 4 patients on indoramin when they were given desipramine.— C. de B. White *et al.*, *Postgrad. med. J.*, 1974, *50*, 729.

Treatment of Adverse Effects. If overdosage occurs the stomach should be emptied by aspiration and lavage. Severe hypotension may respond to placing the patient in the supine position with the head raised.

It has been recommended that the patient should be monitored for hypothermia and convulsions, in addition to hypotension.

Absorption and Fate. Indoramin is readily absorbed from the gastro-intestinal tract, and very extensively metabolised into active metabolites.

Following administration of indoramin 40 or 60 mg by mouth as a single dose and labelled with carbon-14 to 4 hypertensive and 3 healthy subjects, the drug was well absorbed and quickly and almost completely metabolised. About 35 and 47% of the drug appeared in the urine and faeces respectively. The peak plasma concentration of indoramin and its metabolites occurred 1 to 2 hours after administration. Indoramin was about 92% bound to plasma protein. Results following oral and intravenous administration suggested that the drug underwent significant first-pass metabolsim either in the gut wall or in the liver; no difference was found in the pharmacological activity of indoramin and its metabolites.— G. H. Draffan *et al.*, *Br. J. clin. Pharmac.*, 1976, *3*, 489.

Uses. Indoramin is an antihypertensive agent which is reported to act, at least in part, by post-synaptic alpha-adrenoceptor antagonism; it is also reported to have membrane-stabilising properties.

In the treatment of hypertension indoramin is given as

the hydrochloride in initial doses equivalent to 25 mg of the base twice daily, increased in steps of 25 or 50 mg at intervals of 2 weeks to a maximum of 200 mg daily in 2 or 3 divided doses. It reduces both standing and supine blood pressure.

A review of the actions and uses of alpha- and beta-adrenoceptor blocking agents including indoramin.— D. G. McDevitt, *Drugs*, 1979, *17*, 267.

Comment on the mode of action of indoramin. In addition to its action as a post-synaptic alpha-receptor antagonist, *animal* studies have indicated that indoramin has a centrally mediated hypotensive action. Part of its antihypertensive action may involve a central mechanism.— D. W. J. Clark (letter), *Pharm. J.*, 1981, *2*, 102.

Studies on the mode of action of indoramin: A. J. Boakes *et al.*, *Br. J. Pharmac.*, 1972, *44*, 378P; R. B. Royds *et al.*, *Clin. Pharmac. Ther.*, 1972, *13*, 380; D. H. Variava and P. Turner, *J. Pharm. Pharmac.*, 1973, *25*, 629.

Animal studies. B. J. Alps *et al.*, *Br. J. Pharmac.*, 1972, *44*, 52; S. Rashid and B. J. Alps, *J. Pharm. Pharmac.*, 1973, *25*, 700; J. M. Elliott and D. W. J. Clark, *Eur. J. Pharmac.*, 1977, *45*, 13; J. L. Black, *Br. J. Pharmac.*, 1978, *62*, 374P.

Asthma. In 11 patients indoramin 20 to 70 mg prevented exercise-induced bronchoconstriction.— S. Bianco *et al.*, *Br. med. J.*, 1974, *4*, 18. Comment.— K. N. V. Palmer *et al.* (letter), *ibid.*, 409. Criticism.— S. Godfrey (letter), *ibid.*, 469.

A study indicating that indoramin has no place in the treatment of mild bronchial asthma.— A. J. Dyson *et al.*, *Br. J. Dis. Chest*, 1980, *74*, 403.

Further references: F. J. Prime (letter), *Br. med. J.*, 1974, *4*, 770; G. T. Dixon *et al.* (letter), *ibid.*; J. P. Seale *et al.*, *Scand. J. resp. Dis.*, 1976, *57*, 261; I. A. Campbell and A. J. Dyson, *Br. J. Dis. Chest*, 1977, *71*, 105; J. L. Black *et al.*, *Scand. J. resp. Dis.*, 1978, *59*, 307; J. A. Utting, *Br. J. Dis. Chest*, 1979, *73*, 317.

Enuresis. In a study in 14 children, indoramin 10 or 20 mg taken 30 minutes before bedtime was ineffective in the treatment of enuresis.— D. Shaffer *et al.*, *Develop. Med. Child Neurology*, 1978, *20*, 183.

Hypertension. A double-blind study evaluated indoramin against a placebo in 39 patients with mild to moderate hypertension. Doses of indoramin started at 100 mg daily in divided doses during the first week, with weekly increases if required to 200 mg daily. Three patients showing no response to indoramin after 2 to 3 weeks were withdrawn and 36 completed a 4-week study, with 16 patients receiving indoramin. In these patients a significantly greater fall in diastolic blood pressure, both standing and lying, was reported than in patients on the placebo. Heart-rates, haematological and biochemical tests, and ECG states were all unaffected by indoramin. Side-effects included tiredness in 6 patients, dry mouth (2), and weight increase (2).— J. Ramirez, *Curr. med. Res. Opinion*, 1976, *4*, 177.

Further reports: R. B. Royds, *Br. J. Pharmac.*, 1972, *44*, 379P; C. T. Dollery *et al.*, *ibid.*, *46*, 542P; P. J. Lewis *et al.* (letter), *Lancet*, 1972, *1*, 1232; G. S. Stokes *et al.*, *Clin. Pharmac. Ther.*, 1979, *25*, 783; A. J. Marshall *et al.*, *Br. J. clin. Pharmac.*, 1980, *10*, 217.

Migraine. In 31 patients with migraine the intravenous dose of tyramine needed to raise systolic blood pressure by 30 mmHg was significantly less (mean 3.8 mg) than in 27 controls (mean 6 mg). In 22 patients given indoramin 30 or 60 mg daily for a month the dose of tyramine required to raise the blood pressure was significantly increased. Of 13 patients 6 experienced a migraine attack after intravenous tyramine during a control period compared with 1 of 13 while taking indoramin.— K. Ghose *et al.*, *Br. med. J.*, 1977, *1*, 1191.

Further references: G. Wainscott *et al.* (letter), *Lancet*, 1975, *2*, 32.

Raynaud's disease. Preliminary findings from a double-blind controlled study in 13 patients with digital artery disease suggested that indoramin 90 mg daily had a beneficial effect on digital blood flow and that further studies were indicated.— P. Robson *et al.* (letter), *Br. J. clin. Pharmac.*, 1978, *6*, 88.

In a double-blind crossover study in 11 patients with acrocyanosis, finger blood flow, measured 1 to 2 hours after medication, was increased in 8 after treatment for 6 weeks with indoramin 50 mg thrice daily. Mean finger blood flow (for the 11) increased from 4.11 to 6.12 ml per minute per 100 g.— D. L. Clement, *Eur. J. clin. Pharmac.*, 1978, *14*, 331.

Further references: R. B. Royds and J. D. F. Lockhart, *Br. J. clin. Pharmac.*, 1974, *1*, 13.

Proprietary Preparations

Baratol *(Wyeth, UK)*. Indoramin hydrochloride, available as tablets each containing the equivalent of 25 mg of indoramin and as scored tablets each containing the equivalent of 50 mg.

880-c

Mecamylamine Hydrochloride *(U.S.P., B.P. 1968)*.

Mecamylamini Hydrochloridum; Mecamylamini Chloridum. *N*-Methyl-2,3,3-trimethylbicyclo[2.2.1]hept-2-ylamine hydrochloride.

$C_{11}H_{21}N,HCl$=203.8.

CAS — 60-40-2 (mecamylamine); 826-39-1(hydrochloride).

Pharmacopoeias. In *Ind.*, *Int.*, *Turk.*, and *U.S.*

A white odourless or almost odourless crystalline powder with a slightly bitter taste. M.p. about 245° with decomposition. **Soluble** 1 in 5 of water, 1 in 12 of alcohol, 1 in 10 of glycerol, and 1 in 30 of isopropyl alcohol; freely soluble in chloroform; practically insoluble in ether. **Store** in airtight containers.

Adverse Effects, Treatment, and Precautions. As for Pempidine Tartrate, p.157. The administration of mecamylamine may cause tremor, convulsions, and mental aberrations.

Mecamylamine had induced intra-alveolar fibrinous oedema which could be converted to fibrous tissue with consequent impairment of ventilation.— P. D. B. Davies, *Br. J. Dis. Chest*, 1969, *63*, 57.

Interactions. Ambenonium. Mecamylamine must not be used with ambenonium because of the resultant non-depolarising neuromuscular blocking effect.— E. M. Mahoney *et al.*, *New Engl. J. Med.*, 1959, *260*, 1065.

Absorption and Fate. Mecamylamine hydrochloride is almost completely absorbed from the gastro-intestinal tract. It diffuses into the tissues, with high concentrations in the liver and kidney. It also diffuses across the placenta and the blood-brain barrier. It is excreted unchanged and fairly slowly in the urine, the rate being diminished in alkaline urine.

References: K. D. Allanby and J. R. Trounce, *Br. med. J.*, 1957, *2*, 1219.

Uses. Mecamylamine hydrochloride is a ganglion-blocking agent with actions and uses similar to those of pempidine tartrate (see p.157). The usual initial dosage is 2.5 mg twice daily, gradually increased, usually by increments of 2.5 mg at intervals of not less than 2 days, until a satisfactory response is obtained. Tolerance may develop.

Preparations

Mecamylamine Hydrochloride Tablets *(U.S.P.)*. Tablets containing mecamylamine hydrochloride.

Mecamylamine Tablets *(B.P. 1968)*. Mecamylam. Tab. Tablets containing mecamylamine hydrochloride.

Inversine *(Merck Sharp & Dohme, UK)*. Mecamylamine hydrochloride, available as scored tablets of 2.5 and 10 mg.

Other Proprietary Names

Mevasine*(Austral., Neth.)*.

881-k

Methoserpidine *(B.P.)*.

Methoserp.; 10-Methoxydeserpidine. Methyl 11-demethoxy-10-methoxy-18-*O*-(3,4,5-trimethoxybenzoyl)reserpate.

$C_{33}H_{40}N_2O_9$=608.7.

CAS — 865-04-3.

Pharmacopoeias. In *Br.*

A cream-coloured, odourless, tasteless, hygroscopic, microcrystalline powder. M.p. about 171° with decomposition. It darkens on exposure to light. Practically **insoluble** in water; soluble 1 in 60 of alcohol, 1 in 5 of chloroform, and 1 in 8 of dioxan. A solution in dioxan is laevoratatory. **Store** in airtight containers. Protect from light.

Adverse Effects, Treatment, and Precautions. As for Reserpine, p.163.

Of 119 patients treated with methoserpidine, 22 developed mental depression, usually after 3 to 6 months' treatment.— W. R. Layland *et al.* (letter), *Br. med. J.*, 1962, *1*, 639. See also R. Berlin (letter), *Lancet*, 1965, *2*, 497.

Epidermal necrolysis. Methoserpidine might have been responsible for a case of toxic epidermal necrolysis.— A. Lyell, *Br. J. Derm.*, 1967, *79*, 662.

Uses. Methoserpidine has actions and uses similar to those described under reserpine (see p.164).

In the treatment of mild or moderate hypertension the initial dose is 10 mg thrice daily for at least a week. The daily dose of 30 mg is then adjusted by increments or decrements of 5 to 10 mg weekly according to the response of the patient. The maintenance dose varies from 15 to 50 mg daily in divided doses. Some sources have recommended a daily maintenance dose of 10 to 20 mg.

Hypertension. References to the use of methoserpidine in hypertension: T. M. Forrester and G. G. Shirriffs, *Lancet*, 1967, *1*, 141.

Preparations

Methoserpidine Tablets *(B.P.)*. Methoserp. Tab. Tablets containing methoserpidine. Protect from light.

Decaserpyl *(Roussel, UK)*. Methoserpidine, available as scored tablets of 5 and 10 mg. (Also available as Decaserpyl in *Belg.*, *Fr.*).

Decaserpyl Plus *(Roussel, UK)*. Scored tablets each containing methoserpidine 10 mg and benzthiazide 20 mg. For moderate to severe hypertension. *Dose.* Initial, 1 tablet thrice daily for 2 weeks; maintenance, 1 to 5 tablets daily.

882-a

Methyldopa *(B.P., U.S.P.)*.

Alpha-methyldopa; MK 351; Methyldopum Hydratum; Metildopa. (−)-3-(3,4-Dihydroxyphenyl)-2-methyl-L-alanine sesquihydrate; (−)-2-Amino-2-(3,4-dihydroxybenzyl)propionic acid sesquihydrate.

$C_{10}H_{13}NO_4,1\frac{1}{2}H_2O$=238.2.

CAS — 555-30-6 (anhydrous); 41372-08-1 (sesquihydrate).

Pharmacopoeias. In *Br.*, *Braz.*, *Cz.*, *Jap.*, *Jug.*, *Neth.*, *Nord.*, and *US*

Colourless or almost colourless crystals or a white to yellowish-white odourless, almost tasteless, fine powder which may contain friable lumps. M.p. about 310°. Methyldopa 1.13 g is approximately equivalent to 1 g of anhydrous methyldopa.

Soluble 1 in 100 of water, 1 in 400 of alcohol, and 1 in 0.5 of dilute hydrochloric acid; practically insoluble in chloroform and ether. A solution in water containing aluminium chloride is laevorotatory. **Store** in airtight containers. Protect from light.

Adverse Effects. The most common side-effect of methyldopa is drowsiness.

Other side-effects include depression, psychic effects, nightmares, nausea, dryness of the mouth, nasal stuffiness, gastro-intestinal upsets, diarrhoea, constipation, fever, dizziness, light-headedness, disorders of sexual function, and, more rarely, headache, black tongue, breast enlargement, lactation, oedema, pancreatitis and salivary gland inflammation, paraesthesia, Bell's palsy, parkinsonism, skin rash, weakness, arthralgia, myalgia, uraemia, and aggravation of angina pectoris. There may be bradycardia and postural hypotension. Involuntary choreoathetotic movements have occurred in patients with severe bilateral cerebrovascular disease.

Thrombocytopenia, leucopenia, granulocytopenia, and haemolytic anaemia have also been reported. A positive response to the direct Coombs' test may occur frequently, usually without evidence of haemolysis. Liver damage with jaundice and fever may occur within the first few weeks of therapy; liver damage may also develop after long-term administration. A condition resembling systemic lupus erythematosus has been reported.

Methyldopa may occasionally cause urine to darken because of the breakdown of the drug or its metabolites.

During 1966–75 the Swedish Adverse Drug Reaction Committee received 308 reports of reactions to methyldopa including fever in 166, haemolysis in 67, hepatic effects in 29, allergic reactions in 23, gastro-intestinal symptoms in 17, and effects on the nervous system in 13. It was suggested that methyldopa should not be used as the drug of first choice in the treatment of benign hypertension.— A. -K. Furhoff, *Acta med. scand.*, 1978, *203*, 425.

A Boston Collaborative Drug Surveillance Program survey revealed that adverse reactions to methyldopa were reported by 149 of 1067 patients receiving methyldopa for hypertension. Most frequent side-effects were hypotension in 110, drowsiness in 26, depression in 5, and extrapyramidal signs and gastro-intestinal upsets in 4 each. Headaches, skin reactions, haemolytic anaemia, drug fever, bradycardia, and increase in blood-urea nitrogen occurred in 2 each, and altered liver function and disturbance in libido in 1 each. The findings suggested that methyldopa therapy should be commenced cautiously especially in younger patients, in the non-obese, and in those with impaired renal function.— D. H. Lawson *et al.*, *Am. Heart J.*, 1978, *96*, 572.

A report of asthma developing in a 27-year-old woman working in a factory where methyldopa tablets were manufactured. In a provocation test her FEV_1 fell by 30% eleven hours after exposure for 30 minutes to methyldopa dust.— M. G. Harries *et al.*, *Br. med. J.*, 1979, *1*, 1461.

Effects on the blood. Auto-immune haemolysis and agranulocytosis occurred in a 71-year-old man after treatment with methyldopa, 2 g daily, for 16 months. These effects were unlikely to have been due to chlorpropamide which had also been taken in the preceding 6 months.— K. G. A. Clark, *Br. med. J.*, 1967, *4*, 94. See also G. P. Hallwright, *N.Z. med. J.*, 1961, *60*, 567; R. Greene and A. W. Spence (letter), *Br. med. J.*, 1967, *4*, 618.

Two patients developed thrombocytopenia, which reverted to normal on withdrawal of methyldopa. One patient also developed transient leucopenia.— A. ten Pas *et al.* (letter), *Can. med. Ass. J.*, 1966, *95*, 322. See also S. M. Manohitharajah *et al.*, *Br. med. J.*, 1971, *1*, 494; G. J. Marcus *et al.*, *Am. J. clin. Path.*, 1975, *64*, 113.

A 67-year-old woman who had received methyldopa 750 mg daily for 2 years developed acute aplastic anaemia and died.— N. G. Durgé *et al.* (letter), *Lancet*, 1968, *1*, 695. See also J. M. Murdoch *et al.* (letter), *Lancet*, 1968, *1*, 207.

Haemolytic anaemia. In an analysis of 1395 patients from 14 publications S.M. Worlledge (*Semin. Hematol.*, 1969, *6*, 181) reported that the overall incidence of a positive direct antiglobulin test (positive Coombs' test) was 15% in patients taking methyldopa and that the cumulative incidence of the development of overt haemolysis was 0.8%, with a variation of 0 to 5% in the different groups; most of the patients whose red cells gave positive direct antiglobulin tests were not anaemic and showed no evidence of increased haemolysis. Haemolytic anemia had been diagnosed as early as 18 weeks and as late as 4 years after the start of treatment with methyldopa; it was clinically and haematologically identical to 'idiopathic' auto-immune haemolytic anaemia. Once methyldopa had been withdrawn the positive direct antiglobulin test usually became negative within 1 month to 2 years according to the initial strength of the positive test; most patients who developed overt haemolytic anaemia recovered fairly rapidly although some had died and a few had required corticosteroid therapy. In most recorded cases there did not appear to be any correlation between the rate of recovery and the total dose of methyldopa or the length of treatment, though K.C. Carstairs *et al.* (*Lancet*, 1966, *2*, 133) reported that the incidence of positive tests was dose dependent, and A. Breckenridge *et al.* (*ibid.*, 1967, *2*, 1265) reported that the direct antiglobulin test did not become positive until after 4 months' treatment in a patient who restarted methyldopa after recovery from a positive test as a result of a prior course and was still negative in a further 2 patients after 6 months. A lower incidence of positive tests in non-white patients has been reported by some authors but this may result from environmental and dietary factors as much as from genetic differences. A. Breckenridge *et al.*(*Lancet*, 1967, *2*, 1265) also found antinuclear factor in the serum of 15% of patients taking methyldopa, but no correlation was found between the incidence of antinuclear factor and positive direct antiglobulin tests. For further references see under Lupus Erythematosus. See also S. M. Worlledge, in *Blood Disorders due to Drugs and Other Agents*, R.H. Girdwood (Ed.), Amsterdam, Excerpta Medica, 1973.

Effects on the gastro-intestinal tract. Methyldopa produced severe colitis and hepatitis in a man on 2 occasions. Fever, rash, and eosinophilia were also present. Symptoms disappeared after discontinuing methyldopa.— H. L. Bonkowksy and J. Brisbane, *J. Am. med. Ass.*, 1976, *236*, 1602.

Reversible malabsorption in a 58-year-old man, with partial villous atrophy, inflammatory infiltrate of the mucosa, and giant-cell granuloma, was related to treatment with methyldopa.— J. M. Shneerson and B. G. Gazzard, *Br. med. J.*, 1977, *2*, 1456.

Comment on reports of acute colitis associated with the use of methyldopa.— C. F. Graham *et al.* (letter), *New Engl. J. Med.*, 1981, *304*, 1044.

Effects on the heart. Five hypertensive patients being treated with methyldopa died suddenly. Autopsy revealed myocarditis in all and hepatitis in 4. Inflammatory changes were consistent with hypersensitivity. All patients had received or were receiving diuretics. Methyldopa was suspected of causing the hypersensitivity reactions.— F. G. Mullick and H. A. McAllister, *J. Am. med. Ass.*, 1977, *237*, 1699. See also *ibid.*, *238*, 399.

A report of syncope associated with carotid sinus hypersensitivity possibly enhanced by methyldopa.— R. Bauernfeind *et al.*, *Ann. intern. Med.*, 1978, *88*, 214. See also P. A. Alfino *et al.* (letter), *New Engl. J. Med.*, 1981, *305*, 344.

Effects on the kidneys. Bilateral renal calculi occurred in 2 women after taking methyldopa 750 mg and 2 g daily for 10 and 8 years respectively. Both patients had urine which darkened on standing.— K. H. Murphy, *Med. J. Aust.*, 1976, *2*, 20. In a retrospective study of 54 patients with hypertension and renal calculi and a control group without calculi no significant difference in the use of methyldopa was found.— L. E. Ramsay, *ibid.*, 1977, *2*, 495.

The effects of methyldopa on renal haemodynamics and tubular function.— M. Grabie *et al.*, *Clin. Pharmac. Ther.*, 1980, *27*, 522.

Effects on the liver. A report of 6 cases of hepatitis in patients taking methyldopa and a review of 77 cases from the literature.— J. S. Rodman *et al.*, *Am. J. Med.*, 1976, *60*, 941.

Further reviews: L. G. Cacace and M. Cohen, *Drug Intell. & clin. Pharm.*, 1976, *10*, 144; *Lancet*, 1976, *2*, 299; E. Thomas *et al.*, *Am. J. Gastroent.*, *N.Y.*, 1977, *68*, 125.

Of 20 patients with liver damage due to methyldopa most developed jaundice 3 to 16 weeks after starting treatment; the total dose did not usually exceed about 65 g. Four patients had recurrences of jaundice after a second course of treatment. Of the 20 cases 14 presented as hepatitis syndromes, 2 as cholestasis, 2 as active chronic hepatitis, 1 as cirrhosis without clinical evidence of liver disease, and 1 as fulminant hepatic failure; the last 2 patients died.— P. J. Toghill *et al.*, *Br. med. J.*, 1974, *3*, 545.

A 49-year-old woman developed granulomatous hepatitis after taking methyldopa 250 mg twice daily for only 2 days; her condition quickly improved when methyldopa was stopped and recurred when methyldopa was resumed.— A. C. Miller and W. M. Reid, *J. Am. med. Ass.*, 1976, *235*, 2001.

Oxidation of methyldopa by cytochrome-P-450-generated superoxide anion may result in a highly reactive semi-quinone or quinone causing liver damage.— E. Dybing *et al.*, *Mol. Pharmac.*, 1976, *12*, 911.

In an analysis of 36 patients with liver damage due to methyldopa, hepatic injury tended to occur in 2 phases—acute and chronic. Acute liver damage developed within weeks of starting treatment with methyldopa, was usually characterised by jaundice, and was considered to be an allergic reaction to methyldopa metabolites. The chronic form usually occurred at least a year after starting methyldopa, and was thought to be due to increasing damage to liver microsomes and accumulation of fat in the liver. Recovery after withdrawal of methyldopa was directly related to duration of exposure and degree of liver damage. There was also a suggestion of genetic predisposition, as acute methyldopa-induced liver damage occurred in 4 members of a family.— E. A. Sotaniemi *et al.*, *Eur. J. clin. Pharmac.*, 1977, *12*, 429.

Association of biliary carcinoma with methyldopa.— G. Brodén and L. Bengtsson, *Acta chir. scand.*, 1980, *Suppl.* 500, 7.

Further references: E. R. Williams and M. A. Khan, *J. Ther.*, 1967, *1* (6), 5; R. Wyburn-Mason and C. Anastassiades (letter), *Br. med. J.*, 1969, *1*, 780; R. P. Brouillard and O. Barrett (letter), *J. Am. med. Ass.*, 1973, *224*, 904; O. U. Rehman *et al.*, *ibid.*, 1390; A. M. Hoyumpa and A. M. Connell, *Am. J. dig. Dis.*, 1973, *18*, 213; B. I. Hoffbrand *et al.*, *Br. med. J.*, 1974, *2*, 559; W. C. Maddrey and J. K. Boitnott, *Gastroenterology*, 1975, *68*, 351; *idem*, 1976, *70*, 149; L. Sataline and D. Lowell (letter), *ibid.*, 148; S. L. Hyer and A. J. Knell, *Br. med. J.*, 1977, *1*, 879; A. R. Puppala and F. U. Steinheber, *Am. J. Gastroent.*, *N.Y.*, 1977, *68*, 578; J. Seggie *et al.*, *S. Afr. med. J.*, 1979, *55*, 75.

Effects on mental state. Depression as a side-effect of treatment with methyldopa was well established and a history of depression continued to be a contra-indication to its use.— D. Pariente (letter), *Br. med. J.*, 1973, *4*, 110.

In 2000 patients treated with methyldopa depression had occurred in a considerable number of patients.— H. A. Fleming (letter), *Br. med. J.*, 1973, *4*, 232. A rebuttal of the association.— C. J. Bulpitt and C. T. Dollery (letter), *ibid.*

Effects on the nervous system. Two patients taking methyldopa for hypertension developed reversible parkinsonism after 3 to 4 weeks of a stabilising dose of 2 g daily.— R. R. Strang, *Can. med. Ass. J.*, 1966, *95*, 928. See also B. M. Groden, *Br. med. J.*, 1963, *1*, 1001; M. J. T. Peaston, *ibid.*, 1964, *2*, 168.

Methyldopa, 1 g daily increased after 22 days to 1.5 g daily for hypertension, caused involuntary choreoathetotic movements resembling those of Huntington's chorea in a 59-year-old man with cerebrovascular disease. He recovered when methyldopa therapy was withdrawn.— A. Yamadori and M. C. Albert (letter), *New Engl. J. Med.*, 1972, *286*, 610.

Effects on sexual function. Seven of 27 men, aged 43 to 64 years, had some disorder of sexual function a few days after starting to take methyldopa 0.5 to 2 g daily; there were no similar effects in 22 comparable patients treated with a thiazide.— R. J. Newman and H. R. Salerno (letter), *Br. med. J.*, 1974, *4*, 106.

In 30 men taking methyldopa the incidence of failure of erection was 7% (volunteered) or 53% after specific questioning.— W. D. Alexander and J. I. Evans (letter), *Br. med. J.*, 1975, *2*, 501.

Effects on the skin. A report on 16 patients who developed eczema whilst taking methyldopa. The lesions cleared only when methyldopa was stopped, and challenge doses in 8 patients produced a recurrence.— R. Church, *Br. J. Derm.*, 1974, *91*, 373.

A review of 17 patients who had persistent oral ulceration while taking methyldopa. Relief and healing occurred after methyldopa was withdrawn but took several months in some patients.— K. D. Hay and P. C. Reade, *Br. dent. J.*, 1978, *145*, 195.

Further references: C. J. Stevenson (letter), *Br. J. Derm.*, 1971, *85*, 600; J. N. Burry and J. Kirk (letter), *Br. J. Derm.*, 1974, *91*, 475; P. J. A. Holt and A. Navaratnam, *Br. med. J.*, 1974, *3*, 234.

Fever. Hyperpyrexia, antinuclear factors, LE cells, and ocular disturbances occurred in a 65-year-old female given methyldopa 250 mg thrice daily. After withdrawal the temperature returned to normal but a challenge dose provoked another fever. All tests appeared normal 2 months later.— W. Chan, *Med. J. Aust.*, 1977, *2*, 14.

In a comparative study, 5 hypertensive patients who developed febrile reactions in association with methyldopa were found to metabolise it to a lesser extent than 5 hypertensive patients, who did not develop febrile reactions, and 4 healthy subjects.— K. Valnes *et al.*, *Acta med. scand.*, 1978, *204*, 21.

Further references: G. E. Glontz and S. Saslaw, *Archs intern. Med.*, 1968, *122*, 445; E. B. Pugsley (letter), *Can. med. Ass. J.*, 1972, *106*, 1064; W. A. Parker (letter), *J. Am. med. Ass.*, 1974, *228*, 1097.

Galactorrhoea. Lactation had been observed in 5 of 15 women with hypertension undergoing prolonged treatment with methyldopa.— W. A. Pettinger *et al.*, *Br. med. J.*, 1963, *1*, 1460. A similar report.— R. A. Vaidya *et al.*, *Metabolism*, 1970, *19*, 1068.

Joint pain. A patient developed excruciating pain in his joints on the thirteenth day of treatment with methyldopa. Administration of salicylates and indomethacin did not produce relief, but within 12 hours of withdrawal of methyldopa he had only a slight residual ache in 1 shoulder.— P. C. Marendy (letter), *Med. J. Aust.*, 1967, *2*, 708.

A 59-year-old man developed arthralgia, nodular skin lesions, and fever after 2 to 4 months on methyldopa 250 mg four times daily. These effects were reversed on withdrawal of the drug.— J. D. Wells *et al.* (letter), *Ann. intern. Med.*, 1974, *81*, 701. See also under Fever.

Lupus erythematosus. The incidence of antinuclear antibodies was 13% in 269 hypertensive patients taking methyldopa (irrespective of other medication), compared with 3.8% in 448 hypertensive patients not taking methyldopa. Apart from the occasional case of methyldopa-induced lupus, however, patients did not appear to be at risk.— J. D. Wilson *et al.*, *Br. med. J.*, 1978, *1*, 14 (See also A. Breckenridge *et al.*, *Lancet*, 1967, *2*,

1265, under Effects on the Blood).

Further references: M. Eliastam and A. W. Holmes, *Am. J. dig. Dis.*, 1971, *16*, 1014; H. M. Perry *et al.*, *J. Lab. clin. Med.*, 1971, *78*, 905.

Retroperitoneal fibrosis. A 60-year-old patient developed retroperitoneal fibrosis and a positive direct Coombs' test associated with methyldopa given in a daily dose of 750 [mg] with bendrofluazide 2.5 mg for about 5 years.— B. M. Iversen *et al.*, *Lancet*, 1975, *2*, 302. See also J. J. Flynn and J. A. Greco (letter), *New Engl. J. Med.*, 1976, *295*, 112. Reply.— C. A. Olsson (letter), *ibid.*

Treatment of Adverse Effects. Withdrawal of methyldopa or reduction in dosage causes the reversal of many side-effects. If overdosage occurs the stomach should be emptied by aspiration and lavage. Treatment is largely symptomatic, but if necessary, intravenous infusions may be given to promote urinary excretion, and pressor agents such as metaraminol or noradrenaline given cautiously. Methyldopa is dialysable.

Precautions. Methyldopa should be used with caution in patients with impaired kidney or liver function or with a history of liver disease or mental depression. It should not be given to patients with acute liver disease or phaeochromocytoma.

It is advisable to make blood counts and to perform liver-function tests at intervals during the first 6 to 12 weeks of treatment or if the patient develops an unexplained fever.

Positive Coombs' tests in a patient taking methyldopa may indicate an incompatible cross-match when transfusion is required and an indirect Coombs' test should be carried out.

Hypotension may occur during anaesthesia in patients being treated with methyldopa (see p.136). Methyldopa has been reported to aggravate porphyria. The hypotensive effects may be diminished by sympathomimetics, tricyclic antidepressants, phenothiazine derivatives, and monoamine oxidase inhibitors. The hypotensive effects of methyldopa are enhanced by thiazide diuretics and levodopa.

Interactions. Methyldopa could cause chemical interference in laboratory tests for catecholamines, blood, or urine creatinine and uric acid.— *Med. Lett.*, 1971, *13*, 82. Methyldopa did not interfere with the determination of serum-uric acid concentration by the phosphotungstate method.— R. E. Small *et al.*, *Am. J. Hosp. Pharm.*, 1976, *33*, 556. Interference by methyldopa in the Watson-Schwartz test could be expected in patients receiving more than 750 mg of methyldopa daily.— C. A. Pierach *et al.* (letter), *New Engl. J. Med.*, 1977, *296*, 577.

The presence of methyldopa in the serum interfered with measurements of SGOT by the Babson method.— M. Pearson *et al.*, *Med. J. Aust.*, 1972, *2*, 84.

Alpha-adrenoceptor antagonists. Urinary incontinence on concomitent administration of methyldopa and phenoxybenzamine.— P. G. Fernandez *et al.*, *Can. med. Ass. J.*, 1981, *124*, 174.

Antipsychotic agents. A woman with systemic lupus erythematosus taking trifluoperazine up to 15 mg daily and prednisone up to 120 mg daily was given methyldopa up to 2 g and triamterene for high blood pressure. Her blood pressure rose further to 200/140 mmHg. After discontinuation of trifluoperazine blood pressure returned to 160/100 mmHg.— F. B. Westervelt and N. O. Atuk (letter), *J. Am. med. Ass.*, 1974, *227*, 557.

Two patients with essential hypertension who had been receiving methyldopa for 3 years and 18 months respectively developed symptoms of dementia within days of concurrent administration of haloperidol for anxiety. In both patients the symptoms resolved rapidly on discontinuation of haloperidol.— W. E. Thornton, *New Engl. J. Med.*, 1976, *294*, 1222. See also I. Nadel and M. Wallach, *Br. J. Psychiat.*, 1979, *135*, 484.

Decarboxylase inhibitors. Concurrent administration of methyldopa with the peripheral decarboxylase inhibitor, carbidopa, to hypertensive subjects only affected blood pressure by a small, albeit significant, amount providing further evidence for a central mode of action of methyldopa.— F. Kersting *et al.*, *Clin. Pharmac. Ther.*, 1977, *21*, 547.

The hypotensive effect of methyldopa was not altered by concurrent administration of benserazide, a decarboxylase inhibitor, although the metabolism of methyldopa was inhibited.— G. Planz *et al.*, *Eur. J. clin. Pharmac.*, 1977, *12*, 241.

Lithium carbonate. For reference to the development of lithium toxicity on concurrent administration of methyldopa, see Lithium Carbonate, p.1539.

Monoamine oxidase inhibitors. A 55-year-old woman experienced visual hallucinations for 2 weeks during the administration of pargyline 100 mg daily and methyldopa 250 to 500 mg daily. No further hallucinations occurred after the drugs were withdrawn. It appeared probable that the hallucinations involved a cerebral action of the drugs, either methyldopa alone or the combination with pargyline.— E. S. Paykel (letter), *Br. med. J.*, 1966, *1*, 803.

Further references: J. M. van Rossum, *Lancet*, 1963, *1*, 950.

Phenobarbitone. Evidence of enhancement of methyldopa metabolism by phenobarbitone.— A. Káldor *et al.*, *Br. med. J.*, 1971, *3*, 518. See also *idem*, *Int. J. clin. Pharmac. Biopharm.*, 1975, *11*, 10.

In 5 patients taking methyldopa 0.75 to 1.5 g daily in 3 divided doses, the administration of phenobarbitone 100 mg daily for 7 days caused no appreciable alteration in the serum concentration of methyldopa and its metabolite α-methyldopa-*O*-sulphate.— M. Kristensen *et al.* (letter), *Br. med. J.*, 1973, *1*, 49.

Propranolol. A patient receiving methyldopa and hydralazine developed a hypertensive response to propranolol following its intravenous administration to lower his pulse-rate after a cerebrovascular incident. A study in *dogs* indicated that propranolol can enhance the pressor action of alpha-methylnoradrenaline, a metabolite of methyldopa. It is postulated that the patient released large amounts of catecholamines, including alpha-methylnoradrenaline due to the stress of the cerebrovascular incident, the vasconstrictor effects of which had been enhanced by beta-blockade. The interaction did not occur in 2 patients receiving methyldopa who were normotensive and at rest.— A. S. Nies and D. G. Shand, *Clin. Pharmac. Ther.*, 1973, *14*, 823.

Sympathomimetics. A patient who was already taking methyldopa and flurazepam suffered 'violent tremors and cyanosis' after taking *mazindol*.— W. P. Maclay and M. G. Wallace, *Practitioner*, 1977, *218*, 431.

A 31-year-old man whose hypertension was well controlled with methyldopa and oxprenolol suffered a severe hypertensive episode when he took a preparation for a cold containing *phenylpropanolamine*.— E. H. McLaren, *Br. med. J.*, 1976, *2*, 283.

Tricyclic antidepressants. A 50-year-old man, who had renal defects, became agitated and had fine tremors in the hands and palpitations during treatment with methyldopa and amitriptyline. His heart-rate was 148 beats per minute and his blood pressure 170/110 mmHg. Both blood pressure and heart-rate decreased 1 week after stopping therapy.— A. G. White (letter), *Lancet*, 1965, *2*, 441.

In a double-blind crossover study in 5 subjects, pretreatment for 4 days with desipramine 75 mg daily had no significant effect on the hypotensive action of methyldopa 750 mg.— J. L. Reid *et al.*, *Eur. J. clin. Pharmac.*, 1979, *16*, 75.

Further references: A. K. Kale and R. S. Satoskar, *Eur. J. Pharmac.*, 1970, *9*, 120; H. W. van Spanning and P. A. van Zwieten, *Int. J. clin. Pharmac. Biopharm.*, 1975, *11*, 65.

Leukaemia. Thrombocytopenia with a bleeding tendency and a positive Coombs' test developed in a hypertensive 68-year-old woman with chronic lymphocytic leukaemia, following several years of therapy with methyldopa. Her symptoms resolved on withdrawal of methyldopa. Since asymptomatic patients with this condition were not generally treated, the possibility of methyldopa-induced symptoms should be considered before instituting cytotoxic therapy.— O. Shalev and M. Brezis (letter), *New Engl. J. Med.*, 1977, *297*, 1471.

Pregnancy and the neonate. Findings of slightly reduced head circumference in infants born to women who received methyldopa within the 16th to 20th weeks of pregnancy.— V. A. Moar *et al.*, *Br. J. Obstet. Gynaec.*, 1978, *85*, 933. Follow-up has demonstrated no association between smaller head size at birth and mental retardation.— M. Ounsted *et al.* (letter), *Lancet*, 1980, *1*, 705.

Reduced blood pressure in the infants of mothers given methyldopa.— A. Whitelaw, *Br. med. J.*, 1981, *283*, 471.

For a report of meconium ileus in 3 newborn infants whose mothers had received methyldopa, see Frusemide, p.600.

Withdrawal. Rebound hypertension was reported in a 65-year-old man who omitted taking methyldopa for 48 hours after taking a maintenance dose of 1.5 g daily for 6 months. He responded to treatment with a bolus injection of diazoxide 300 mg, methyldopa 250 mg thrice daily, and propranolol.— A. C. Burden and C. P. T. Alexander, *Br. med. J.*, 1976, *1*, 1056.

Further references: J. N. Scott and D. G. McDevitt, *ibid.*, 1976, *2*, 367; D. B. Frewin and R. K. Penhall, *Med. J. Aust.*, 1977, *1*, 659.

Absorption and Fate. Methyldopa is incompletely absorbed from the gastro-intestinal tract. It is partly conjugated, mainly to the O-sulphate, and is excreted by the kidneys. Elimination follows a biphasic pattern. Plasma protein binding is reported to be minimal. It crosses the placenta and small amounts appear in breast milk.

A study of the pharmacokinetics of methyldopa in 5 healthy subjects. Methyldopa appeared to be distributed into an extravascular compartment, and differences between radioactive and chemical estimations suggested the presence of an unidentified metabolite. Excretion was entirely renal and there was no evidence of enterohepatic recycling. Most of an intravenous dose was excreted within the first 4 hours as unchanged methyldopa and unidentified metabolite, and urinary recovery was virtually complete within 48 hours. Elimination was biphasic with a radioactively determined half-life of 0.74 to 1.10 hours for the α-phase and 8.0 to 65.0 hours for the β-phase. Less than half an orally administered dose was absorbed and some of this was conjugated in the gut before absorption, this conjugate being detected in the urine only following oral administration. Peak plasma concentrations were obtained about 2 hours after oral administration.— Ø. Stenbaek *et al.*, *Eur. J. clin. Pharmac.*, 1977, *12*, 117.

Metabolic disposition of methyldopa in hypertensive and renal-insufficient children.— R. F. O'Dea and B. L. Mirkin, *Clin. Pharmac. Ther.*, 1980, *27*, 37.

Further references: W. Y. W. Au *et al.*, *Biochem. J.*, 1972, *129*, 1; J. A. Saavedra *et al.*, *Eur. J. clin. Pharmac.*, 1975, *8*, 381; K. C. Kwan *et al.*, *J. Pharmac. exp. Ther.*, 1976, *198*, 264.

Pregnancy and the neonate. Results of a preliminary study conducted around the time of delivery in 12 women who had received methyldopa 0.75 to 2 g daily for at least 4 weeks up to the time of delivery. Concentrations of both free and conjugated methyldopa were similar in maternal and foetal plasma but in the amniotic fluid total concentrations and the proportion of conjugated drug were generally higher than in the plasma. Milk samples collected from 3 women between 30 and 60 hours after delivery contained very small amounts of methyldopa, most of which was conjugated.— H. M. R. Jones and A. J. Cummings (letter), *Br. J. clin. Pharmac.*, 1978, *6*, 432.

Uses. Methyldopa is an antihypertensive agent which may act centrally by stimulating alpha-adrenergic receptors. It inhibits the decarboxylation of dopa to dopamine but this action does not appear to be responsible for its hypotensive effect. It is suggested that a metabolite, alpha-methylnoradrenaline, may act as a false transmitter in the central nervous system. Methyldopa reduces the tissue concentrations of dopamine, noradrenaline, adrenaline, and serotonin.

When administered by mouth its effects may appear after about 2 hours and reach a maximum in 6 to 8 hours, although the maximum hypotensive effect may not occur until the second day of treatment; some effect is still usually apparent until 48 hours after a dose.

Methyldopa is used in the treatment of moderate to severe hypertension. It reduces the standing blood pressure and also reduces the supine blood pressure.

The usual initial dose by mouth is the equivalent of 250 mg of anhydrous methyldopa twice or thrice daily for 2 days; this is then adjusted by small increments or decrements not more frequently than every other day according to the response of the patient. Although higher doses have been given it is generally considered that no advantage can be gained by giving doses larger than 3 g daily. The usual maintenance dosage is the equivalent of 0.5 to 2 g of anhydrous methyldopa daily.

To reduce side-effects smaller doses of methyldopa may be given in conjunction with a thiazide diuretic, which would also reduce the oedema that sometimes occurs with methyldopa therapy. Tolerance may develop.

A suggested initial dose for children is 10 mg per kg body-weight daily in 2 to 4 divided doses, increased as necessary to a maximum of 65 mg per kg daily.

For hypertensive crises, methyldopa has been given intravenously as methyldopate hydrochloride (see below).

For discussions of the pharmacology of methyldopa, see R. Laverty, *Br. med. Bull.*, 1973, *29*, 152; D. Robertson and A. S. Nies, *Recent Adv. clin. Pharmac.*, 1978, *1*, 55 to 92; E. D. Frohlich, *Archs intern. Med.*, 1980, *140*, 954.

In 7 hypertensive patients given a single dose of 0.75 or 1 g of methyldopa serum-prolactin concentrations rose from a mean of 9.9 µg per litre to a mean of 23 µg per litre. Seven patients who had taken methyldopa for a mean of 13.4 months had similarly elevated serum-prolactin concentrations. The importance of the changes was difficult to assess. In 11 patients given methyldopa for 2 to 3 weeks the growth-hormone concentration in serum during insulin hypoglycaemia was significantly increased, but this was not evident in 10 patients treated for a mean of 13.4 months. This probably represented the substitution of endogenous catecholamines with metabolites of methyldopa in the brain.— J. Steiner *et al.*, *Br. med. J.*, 1976, *1*, 1186. Absence of effect on growth-hormone concentrations.— E. K. G. Syvälahti (letter), *ibid.*, 1976, *2*, 110.

Animal studies on the actions of methyldopa: P. R. Blower *et al.*, *J. Pharm. Pharmac.*, 1976, *28*, 437; A. Scriabine *et al.*, *A. Rev. Pharmac. & Toxic.*, 1976, *16*, 113; A. J. Ingenito and L. Procita, *J. clin. Pharmac.*, 1977, *17*, 95.

Administration in renal failure. About 60% of a dose of methyldopa was removed by peritoneal or haemodialysis in 5 patients with chronic uraemia.— B. K. Yeh *et al.*, *Proc. Soc. exp. Biol. Med.*, 1970, *135*, 840.

A study in 6 hypertensive subjects with advanced renal disease and 7 with essential hypertension and normal or only slightly reduced renal function, indicated that those with renal disease were more sensitive to the hypotensive effect of methyldopa. This did not appear to be associated with accumulation of unconjugated methyldopa.— Ø. Stenbaek *et al.*, *Acta med. scand.*, 1972, *191*, 333.

Methyldopa was reported not to be bound to plasma proteins. The interval between doses should be extended from 6 hours to 9 to 18 hours in patients with a glomerular filtration-rate of 10 to 50 ml per minute, and to 12 to 24 hours in those with a glomerular filtration-rate of less than 10 ml per minute.— W. M. Bennett *et al.*, *Ann. intern. Med.*, 1980, *93*, 286.

Further references: S. Mohammed *et al.*, *Am. Heart J.*, 1968, *76*, 21; *idem*, *Circulation Res.*, 1969, *25*, 543.

Carcinoid syndrome. A man with a carcinoid lesion and metastases experienced relief from his diarrhoea and skin flushing when he was treated with methyldopa in doses rising gradually to 6 g daily by mouth and then reduced to a maintenance of 2 g daily. Another man gained no such relief; a woman found the nausea and vomiting attributable to methyldopa worse than the symptoms arising from her carcinoid lesions.— G. I. Nicholson *et al.*, *Br. med. J.*, 1962, *2*, 961.

Dyskinesias. Methyldopa 250 mg thrice daily for 2 weeks or a placebo was added to the usual neuroleptic medication of 15 psychogeriatric patients with severe dyskinesias. Tremor, rigidity, and dystonic spasms were significantly relieved but oro-facial dyskinesias, akinesia, and akathisia were not.— M. Viukari and M. Linnoila, *Curr. ther. Res.*, 1975, *18*, 417.

Further references: O. Tzavellas *et al.*, *Dt. med. Wschr.*, 1967, *92*, 1065; A. Villeneuve and Z. Böszörményi, *Lancet*, 1970, *1*, 353; H. Kazamatsuri and J. O. Cole, *Archs gen. Psychiat.*, 1972, *27*, 824.

Hypertension. A total of 100 patients with hypertension were treated for periods of 6 to 36 months with methyldopa in an average dose of 1.3 g daily. Thirty-four patients also took chlorthalidone, usually in a dose of 50 mg daily. The reduction in blood pressure was good in 49, fair in 36, and poor in 15 patients. Tolerance occurred in only 3 patients. Side-effects occurred in 72 patients, the commonest being drowsiness, listlessness, dryness of the mouth, nasal congestion, and oedema. In a comparison between 37 patients treated with methyldopa and 66 treated with guanethidine, the 2 drugs appeared to be equally effective in controlling blood pressure. Side-effects were fewer and milder with methyldopa.— P. Johnson *et al.*, *Br. med. J.*, 1966, *1*, 133.

In a double-blind trial in 40 patients with moderate or severe hypertension, a satisfactory response without side-effects or with slight side-effects was obtained in 34 patients with methyldopa, 25 with guanoxan, and 20 with guanethidine. The average daily doses were 1 g of methyldopa, 30 mg of guanoxan, and 33 mg of guanethidine and each drug was given for an average of 3½ months. Severe side-effects necessitated early withdrawal of guanoclor from the trial.— V. Vejlsgaard *et al.*, *Br. med. J.*, 1967, *2*, 598.

A comparison of bethanidine, guanethidine, and methyldopa in the treatment of hypertension in 30 patients showed that methyldopa resulted in the best control of blood pressure, but 20% of patients could not tolerate it.— B. N. C. Prichard *et al.*, *Br. med. J.*, 1968, *1*, 135.

The effect of methyldopa on cardiac output in hypertensive patients.— M. E. Safar *et al.*, *Clin. Pharmac. Ther.*, 1979, *25*, 266.

Further references: W. M. Smith *et al.*, *Ann. intern. Med.*, 1966, *65*, 657; F. G. McMahon, *J. Am. med. Ass.*, 1975, *231*, 155; M. Hansen *et al.*, *Acta med. scand.*, 1977, *202*, 385; J. W. Hollifield and P. E. Slaton, *Curr. ther. Res.*, 1978, *24*, 818; J. G. Kleinman *et al.*, *Curr. ther. Res.*, 1979, *26*, 247.

Effect on plasma renin. In a study of 40 hypertensive patients classified as having high, normal, or low plasma-renin activity, the fall in blood pressure following administration of methyldopa was similar in all groups, and appeared to be independent of the renin system.— H. Gavras *et al.*, *J. clin. Pharmac.*, 1977, *17*, 372.

In pregnancy. In a controlled study of 242 women with early or late hypertension of pregnancy, 117 were treated with methyldopa together if necessary with other drugs such as hydralazine and compared with 125 untreated controls. There was 1 pregnancy loss in the treated group compared with 9 in the control. Two infants lost had congenital abnormalities, one in the control group and the other with an absent left kidney being that in the treated group. Treatment was effective in reducing the hypertension and had no ill effect on foetal growth or birthweight. Methyldopa was considered safe for mother and foetus when used in special units with careful antenatal management for chronic maternal hypertension.— C. W. G. Redman *et al.*, *Lancet*, 1976, *2*, 753. See also *idem*, *Br. J. Obstet. Gynaec.*, 1977, *84*, 419.

Further references: H. M. Leather *et al.*, *Lancet*, 1968, *2*, 488.

Single bedtime dosage. In a preliminary double-blind crossover study of 14 hypertensive patients adequately controlled by methyldopa, the daily amount required was found to be as efficacious when given as a single dose at bedtime as when given as a thrice daily regimen. A further 3 patients were dropped from the study: 1 owing to non-compliance, 1 owing to altered liver-function values, and 1 owing to an intolerable swimming sensation in her head and insomnia on taking what proved to be methyldopa 750 mg at night.— J. M. Wright *et al.*, *Clin. Pharmac. Ther.*, 1976, *20*, 733.

Parkinsonism. In 18 patients with parkinsonism methyldopa 250 mg as a single dose or levodopa in a mean daily dose of 1.5 g had no effect on standing systolic blood pressure. When the 2 drugs were given concomitantly systolic pressure fell by a mean of about 13 mmHg. Methyldopa could be given, in hospital, to hypertensive patients taking levodopa.— F. B. Gibberd and E. Small, *Br. med. J.*, 1973, *2*, 90.

For reports of methyldopa being used in conjunction with levodopa in the treatment of parkinsonism, see Levodopa, p.887.

Raynaud's syndrome. Methyldopa, 1 to 2 g daily, prevented episodes of Raynaud's syndrome in 11 of 15 patients with primary Raynaud's disease, 17 of 22 with associated scleroderma, and in 3 with systemic lupus erythematosus. Two patients with cryoglobulinaemia were not improved.— D. P. Varadi and A. M. Lawrence, *Archs intern. Med.*, 1969, *124*, 13, per *Abstr. Wld Med.*, 1970, *44*, 189.

Stroke. Methyldopa significantly increased cerebral blood flow and significantly reduced the cerebral metabolic-rate and the blood pressure in 13 patients with hypertension who had had a stroke.— J. S. Meyer *et al.*, *Neurology, Minneap.*, 1968, *18*, 772, per *J. Am. med. Ass.*, 1968, *205* (Sept. 2), A148.

Preparations

Methyldopa Tablets *(B.P.)*. Tablets containing methyldopa. They are film-coated. Potency is expressed in terms of the equivalent amount of anhydrous methyldopa. Protect from light.

Methyldopa Tablets *(U.S.P.)*. Tablets containing methyldopa. Potency is expressed in terms of the equivalent amount of anhydrous methyldopa.

Proprietary Preparations

Aldomet *(Merck Sharp & Dohme, UK)*. Methyldopa, available as tablets each containing the equivalent of 125, 250, or 500 mg of anhydrous methyldopa. (Also available as Aldomet in *Arg., Austral., Canad., Denm., Fr., Ital., Neth., Norw., S.Afr., Spain, Swed., Switz., USA*).

Co-Caps Methyldopa *(DDSA Pharmaceuticals, UK)*. Capsules each containing the equivalent of 250 mg of anhydrous methyldopa.

Dopamet *(Berk Pharmaceuticals, UK)*. Methyldopa, available as tablets each containing the equivalent of 125, 250, or 500 mg of anhydrous methyldopa. (Also available as Dopamet in *Canad., Denm., Norw., Swed., Switz.*).

Hydromet (known in Canada and USA as Aldoril) *(Merck Sharp & Dohme, UK)*. Tablets each containing the equivalent of anhydrous methyldopa 250 mg and hydrochlorothiazide 15 mg. For hypertension. *Dose*. Initial, 1 tablet twice daily, the dose to be adjusted at intervals of at least 2 days until adequate response is achieved (usually not more than 8 tablets daily).

Medomet *(DDSA Pharmaceuticals, UK)*. Methyldopa, available as tablets each containing the equivalent of 250 mg of anhydrous methyldopa.

Other Proprietary Names

Aldometil *(Ger.)*; Alphamex *(S.Afr.)*; Baypresol *(Spain)*; Dopegyt *(Hung.)*; Grospisk, Medopa, Methoplain *(all Jap.)*; Hy-po-tone *(S.Afr.)*; Medimet-250 *(Canad.)*; Medopal *(Norw.)*; Medopren *(Ital.)*; Novomedopa *(Canad.)*; Presinol *(Belg., Ger., Ital.)*; Sembrina *(Ger., Ital., Neth., Switz.)*; Hyperpax (racemic) *(Denm., Neth., Norw., Switz.)*; Hyperpaxa (racemic) *(Swed.)*; Mulfasin (racemic) *(Neth.)*.

883-t

Methyldopate Hydrochloride *(B.P., U.S.P.)*.

Cloridrato de Metildopato. The hydrochloride of the ethyl ester of anhydrous methyldopa; Ethyl (−)-2-amino-2-(3,4-dihydroxybenzyl)propionate hydrochloride.

$C_{12}H_{17}NO_4,HCl = 275.7$.

CAS — 2544-09-4 (methyldopate); 2508-79-4 (hydrochloride).

Pharmacopoeias. In *Br.*, *Braz.*, and *U.S.*

A white or almost white, odourless or almost odourless, crystalline powder. **Soluble** 1 in 1 of water, 1 in 3 of alcohol, and 1 in 2 of methyl alcohol; slightly soluble in chloroform; practically insoluble in ether. A solution in hydrochloric acid is laevorotatory. A 1% solution in water has a pH of 3 to 5. A 4.28% solution is iso-osmotic with serum. Solutions for injection are **sterilised** by filtration. **Protect** from light.

Incompatibility. A haze developed over 3 hours when methyldopate hydrochloride 1 g per litre was mixed with amphotericin 200 mg per litre in dextrose injection; crystals were produced with methohexitone sodium 200 mg per litre in sodium chloride injection, but a haze developed when they were mixed in dextrose injection. A crystalline precipitate occurred with tetracycline hydrochloride 1 g per litre in dextrose injection, and with sulphadiazine sodium 4 g per litre in dextrose injection or sodium chloride injection.— B. B. Riley, *J. Hosp. Pharm.*, 1970, *28*, 228.

Adverse Effects, Treatment, and Precautions. As for Methyldopa (above).

Hypertensive response. An intravenous injection of 250 mg of methyldopa failed to lower the blood pressure of a young man with hypertension. One hour after a second similar dose his blood pressure rose by 25/30 mmHg and 1½ hours after a dose of 500 mg a further increase of 25/40 mmHg occurred.— R. J. Levine and B. S. Strauch, *New Engl. J. Med.*, 1966, *275*, 946.

Further references: W. Feldman *et al.*, *Pediatrics*, 1967, *39*, 780, per *J. Am. med. Ass.*, 1967, *200* (May 15), A207.

Uses. Methyldopate hydrochloride has the actions described under methyldopa (see p.153) and has been administered by intravenous infusion in the treatment of hypertensive crises. The hypotensive effect may be obtained within 4 to 6 hours and last for 10 to 16 hours. A paradoxical pressor response may occasionally occur.

The usual dose is 250 to 500 mg in 100 ml of dextrose injection administered over 30 to 60 minutes every 6 hours. It is suggested that the dose should not exceed 1 g every 6 hours. A suggested dose for children is 5 to 10 mg per kg body-weight every 6 hours.

Absorption. A study in 7 hypertensive subjects indicated that there were considerable pharmacokinetic differences between methyldopa administered intravenously and methyldopate hydrochloride administered intravenously. Results after administration by mouth suggested that sulphate conjugation took place during absorption from the gastro-intestinal tract.— J. A. Saavedra *et al.*, *Eur. J. clin. Pharmac.*, 1975, *8*, 381.

Preparations

Methyldopate Injection *(B.P.)*. A sterile solution of methyldopate hydrochloride in Water for Injections containing suitable stabilising agents. Sterilised by filtration. It may contain some methyldopa. pH 3.5 to 4.2. Protect from light.

Methyldopate Hydrochloride Injection *(U.S.P.)*. A sterile solution in Water for Injections, containing 47.5 to 55 mg of methyldopate hydrochloride in each ml. pH 3 to 4.2.

Aldomet Injection *(Merck Sharp & Dohme, UK)*. Contains methyldopate hydrochloride 50 mg per ml, in ampoules of 5 ml.

884-x

Minoxidil. U-10858; Minoxidilum. 2,6-Diamino-4-piperidinopyrimidine 1-oxide.

$C_9H_{15}N_5O$=209.3.

CAS — 38304-91-5.

A white or off-white crystalline solid. M.p. about 225° with decomposition. **Soluble** 1 in about 500 of water; readily soluble in alcohol and propylene glycol; practically insoluble in acetone, chloroform, and ethyl acetate.

Adverse Effects, Treatment, and Precautions. Adverse effects commonly include hypertrichosis, fluid retension, and reflex tachycardia. Pericardial effusion may also occur. Nausea, ECG changes, gynaecomastia, polymenorrhoea, conjunctival redness, pruritus, exacerbation of systemic lupus, depressed platelet count, and weight gain have been reported.

The cardiac accelerating effects of minoxidil may be controlled by concurrent administration of propranolol and the fluid retention by concurrent administration of diuretics. Minoxidil is dialysable. Depilatories have been employed topically to treat hypertrichosis.

Minoxidil is contra-indicated in phaeochromocytoma.

Animal studies on the toxicology of minoxidil: R. G. Carlson and E. S. Feenstra, *Toxic. appl. Pharmac.*, 1977, *39*, 1; E. H. Herman *et al.*, *ibid.*, 1979, *47*, 493.

A satisfactory response to minoxidil was achieved in 4 of 5 patients with essential hypertension, 5 of 6 with hypertension and renal failure, and in 3 with renal artery stenosis. ST-segment depression and T-wave inversion, indicative of ischaemia, occurred in 3 patients, hypertrichosis was common, 2 women experienced polymenorrhoea, and 1 patient had exacerbation of systemic lupus. Minoxidil should be reserved for patients unresponsive to other drugs.— P. Larochelle *et al.*, *Eur. J. clin. Pharmac.*, 1978, *14*, 1.

Thrombocytopenia associated with the use of minoxidil.— S. J. Peitzman and C. Martin (letter), *Ann. intern. Med.*, 1980, *92*, 874.

A 2-year-old boy estimated to have taken 20 tablets of minoxidil 5 mg suffered no symptoms other than reflex tachycardia.— C. Isles *et al.* (letter), *Lancet*, 1981, *1*, 97.

Effects on the eyes. Redness of the conjunctiva occurred in 2 patients taking minoxidil, one of whom complained of mild itching of the eyes.— Y. M. Traub *et al.*, *Israel J. med. Scis*, 1975, *11*, 991.

Effects on the heart. Cardiotoxicity associated with long-term administration of high doses of minoxidil to *dogs*.— D. W. DuCharme *et al.*, *J. Pharmac. exp. Ther.*, 1973, *184*, 662.

Pericardial effusions occurred in 7 of 18 patients given minoxidil for refractory hypertension; 6 of the 7 were symptom-free. Of the 7, four were on dialysis for terminal renal failure and 1 had moderate renal insufficiency. A review of the manufacturer's records on 1760 patients showed that 53 patients developed pericardial effusions of whom 36 had renal impairment or some other cause for their pericarditis. Effusion disappeared spontaneously without treatment in 5 of the remaining 17 patients despite their continuing minoxidil. Of 18 affected patients on haemodialysis 7 developed fatal tamponade. It was considered that pericardial effusions in patients without renal impairment might be part of the general fluid retention associated with minoxidil; their incidence might be reduced by controlling fluid weight gain.— A. Marquez-Julio and P. R. Uldall (letter), *Lancet*, 1977, *2*, 816. Pericardial effusion associated with minoxidil in a patient without renal impairment.— W. M. Bennett (letter), *ibid.*, 1356.

Further references: M. J. Reichgott, *Clin. Pharmac. Ther.*, 1981, *30*, 64.

Effects on the skin and hair. A report of hair colour changes in 3 patients taking minoxidil. The dark hair of 2 patients became 'pepper and salt' and the completely white hair of a third patient became yellowish.— Y. M. Traub *et al.*, *Israel J. med. Scis*, 1975, *11*, 991.

Hypertrichosis, with associated pruritus in 3 patients.— R. E. Mutterperl *et al.*, *J. clin. Pharmac.*, 1976, *16*, 499.

A cream containing calcium thioglycollate was used successfully at intervals of from 2 to 4 weeks to control the hypertrichosis occurring in 5 women during treatment with minoxidil for serious hypertension not responsive to other drugs.— R. M. Earhart *et al.*, *Sth. med. J.*, 1977, *70*, 442.

A bullous eruption associated with minoxidil.— T. Rosenthal *et al.*, *Archs intern. Med.*, 1978, *138*, 1856.

Glucose tolerance. Glucose tolerance tests in 10 of 18 patients given minoxidil indicated that it has no adverse effect on carbohydrate metabolism.— A. Marquez-Julio *et al.*, *Proc. Eur. Dialysis Transplant Ass.*, 1977, *14*, 501.

Pulmonary hypertension. In 7 patients with severe hypertension treated with propranolol, hydrochlorothiazide, and minoxidil no increase in mean pulmonary artery pressure occurred over 2 months. In patients with pre-existing pulmonary hypertension, chronic congestive heart failure, or significant renal impairment, care should be exercised lest the enhanced cardiac output cause an increase in pulmonary artery pressure.— P. E. Klotman *et al.*, *Circulation*, 1977, *55*, 394.

Further references: J. M. Atkins *et al.*, *Am. J. Cardiol.*, 1977, *39*, 802.

Withdrawal. Rebound hypertension on minoxidil withdrawal.— S. P. Makker and B. Moorthy, *J. Pediat.*, 1980, *96*, 762.

Absorption and Fate. Minoxidil is readily absorbed from the gastro-intestinal tract, and is excreted in the urine mainly in the form of metabolites. Its duration of action is longer than would be predicted from its plasma half-life of only about 4 hours, possibly owing to accumulation at its site of action.

In a study in 7 patients with hypertension given minoxidil 6 or 3 mg, the plasma half-life was 4.2 hours, peak serum concentrations occurring at one hour. Recovery in the urine (97±2%) and faeces (3±1%) was complete and over 80% was recovered from the urine in the first 24 hours. Three metabolites were found but only a glucuronide conjugate was identified. Minoxidil was not bound to plasma proteins and appeared to be excreted by the kidney, mainly by filtration. Despite the rapid excretion the hypotensive action could exceed 24 hours.— T. B. Gottlieb *et al.*, *Clin. Pharmac. Ther.*, 1972, *13*, 436.

Minoxidil has a long half-life varying from 1 to 4 days in hypertensive patients.— W. A. Pettinger and H. C. Mitchell, *New Engl. J. Med.*, 1973, *289*, 167.

Metabolism in *animals*.— R. C. Thomas *et al.*, *J. pharm. Sci.*, 1975, *64*, 1360; R. C. Thomas and H. Harpootlian, *ibid.*, 1366.

Uses. Minoxidil is an antihypertensive agent which acts predominantly by causing direct peripheral vasodilatation. It is usually administered concurrently with other antihypertensive agents for the treatment of severe hypertension unresponsive to standard therapy. An initial dose of 5 mg daily is gradually increased to 50 mg daily according to the patient's response; in exceptional circumstances up to 100 mg daily has been given. The daily dose may be given as a single dose or in 2 divided doses. Beta-adrenoceptor blocking agents are used to diminish the cardiac-accelerating effects, and diuretics to control oedema. For children 12 years of age or under, the recommended initial dose is 200 µg per kg body-weight daily, increased in steps of 100 to 200 µg per kg at intervals of not less than 3 days, until control of blood pressure has been achieved or a maximum of 1 mg per kg daily has been reached.

A study of the pharmacodynamics of minoxidil as a guide for individual dosage regimens in hypertension. Only in the most severe case did dosing frequency exceed twice daily while in milder hypertension a daily single dose was adequate.— D. Shen *et al.*, *Clin. Pharmac. Ther.*, 1975, *17*, 593.

Administration in renal failure. Minoxidil 10 to 40 mg daily and propranolol had controlled blood pressure for periods of 5 to 32 months in 8 patients who were receiving long-term haemodialysis. Three of the 8 recovered sufficient renal function to allow discontinuation of dialysis. Hirsutism and sodium retention developed in all patients.— F. C. Luft *et al.*, *J. Am. med. Ass.*, 1978, *240*, 1985. See also H. C. Mitchell *et al.*, *Ann. intern. Med.*, 1980, *93*, 676.

Minoxidil was reported not to be bound to plasma proteins. The normal half-life was 2.8 to 4.2 hours which did not reflect extensive tissue binding; the half-life 'for blood pressure' was 12 to 24 hours. It could be given in usual doses to patients in renal failure.— W. M. Bennett *et al.*, *Ann. intern. Med.*, 1980, *93*, 286.

Heart disease. Beneficial haemodynamic effects of minoxidil in patients with congestive heart failure.— J. A. Franciosa *et al.*, *Clin. Pharmac. Ther.*, 1980, *27*, 254.

Hypertension. Reviews: *Br. med. J.*, 1973, *4*, 185; P. J. Cannon, *New Engl. J. Med.*, 1978, *299*, 886; M. E. Kosman, *J. Am. med. Ass.*, 1980, *244*, 73; *Med. Lett.*, 1980, *22*, 21; W. A. Pettinger, *New Engl. J. Med.*, 1980, *303*, 922.

In 17 patients who were partially or totally refractory to conventional antihypertensive therapy, minoxidil was given initially in a single daily dose of 2.5 to 5 mg, and gradually increased to a maximum of 60 mg daily or until a satisfactory response was obtained. Propranolol hydrochloride was given to combat reflex tachycardia and treatment included diuretics and salt restriction. Initial control was excellent in 16 but 3 developed secondary resistance. One patient did not response to minoxidil. The main side-effects were fluid retention in 8, hypertrichosis in 10, accompanied in some patients by a coarsening of facial features. Renal function stabilised or improved in several patients, and urine output increased in the 3 patients undergoing haemodialysis.— P. K. Mehta *et al.*, *J. Am. med. Ass.*, 1975, *233*, 249.

Minoxidil to a maximum dose of 40 mg daily in conjunction with diuretic therapy and propranolol to control induced tachycardia, increased cardiac output, stimulation of renin release, and sodium and fluid retention, was more effective than standard therapy in a study of 30 patients with resistant hypertension. Angina at rest occurred in 2 patients given minoxidil despite doses of 600 to 800 mg daily of propranolol but disappeared with higher doses of propranolol. Hemiparesis occurred in one patient on minoxidil and was controlled by dexamethasone. Severe generalised fluid retention with cardiomegaly and pulmonary oedema occurred in 3 patients, 2 of whom responded to increases in diuretic therapy while continuing on minoxidil, the third withdrawing from the study; all but 1 patient on minoxidil required frusemide in a mean dose of 353 mg daily. Generalised hypertrichosis occurred in all patients but was considered acceptable.— H. J. Dargie *et al.*, *Lancet*, 1977, *2*, 515. An emphasis on the risks of heart disease occurring with minoxidil.— G. B. Ambrosio (letter), *ibid.*, 1087.

Severe hypertension in 44 patients unresponsive to or intolerant of other agents was treated with minoxidil 2.5 mg daily on the first day increased up to 60 mg daily if needed; a beta-adrenoceptor blocking agent was used to control tachycardia and a diuretic was given for sodium retention. Eleven patients needed additional antihypertensive agents. Mean blood pressure was reduced from 221/134 to 162/98 mmHg. Hirsutism occurred consistently, 3 men had gynaecomastia, and the platelet count was depressed in 2 patients. In 22 patients with impaired renal function there was not further impairment. There were 5 deaths and although 2 were due to myocardial infarction minoxidil was not implicated. ECG abnormalities indicating further anterolateral ischaemia occurred in 1 patient but resolved when minoxidil was discontinued. In one of the patients who died there was no necropsy evidence of the cardiotoxic effect on the right atrium reported in *dogs*.— B. L. Devine *et al.*, *Br. med. J.*, 1977, *2*, 667.

In 8 patients with high blood pressure despite treatment with chlorthalidone, spironolactone, a beta-adrenoceptor blocking agent, and dihydralazine, blood pressure was controlled when dihydralazine was replaced with minoxidil in increasing doses up to 2.5 to 27.5 (mean 12.5) mg daily. In 6 patients remaining in the study the beta-blocking agent was reduced and withdrawn, with no change in blood pressure or heart-rate in 3 and only slight changes in the other 3. Beta-blockers, probably necessary in the early stages of treatment with minoxidil, might be unnecesssary in some patients after prolonged treatment.— H. R. Brunner *et al.*, *Br. med. J.*, 1978, *2*, 385.

Further references: E. Gilmore *et al.*, *New Engl. J. Med.*, 1970, *282*, 521; T. B. Gottlieb *et al.*, *Circulation*, 1972, *45*, 571; C. J. Limas and E. D. Freis, *Am. J. Cardiol.*, 1973, *31*, 355; W. A. Pettinger and H. C. Mitchell, *New Engl. J. Med.*, 1973, *289*, 167; J. Koch-Weser, *ibid.*, 213; D. P. Redmond *et al.*, *Clin. Pharmac. Ther.*, 1974, *15*, 217; J. C. Dormois *et al.*, *Am. Heart J.*, 1975, *90*, 360; K. O'Malley and J. L. McNay, *Clin. Pharmac. Ther.*, 1975, *18*, 39; J. R. Ryan *et al.*, *Curr. ther. Res.*, 1975, *17*, 55; R. L. Wilburn *et al.*, *Circulation*, 1975, *52*, 706; R. G. Jacomb and F. J. Brunnberg, *Clin. Sci. & mol. Med.*, 1976, *51*, 579s; O. L. Pedersen, *Acta Cardiol.*, 1977, *32*, 283; R. K. Bryan *et al.*, *Am. J. Cardiol.*, 1977, *39*, 796; K. Chatterjee *et al.*, *Ann. intern. Med.*, 1977, *85*, 467; D. Höffler and H. G. Demers, *Dt. med. Wschr.*, 1977, *102*, 1766; T. Nawar *et al.*, *Can. med. Ass. J.*, 1977, *117*, 1178; H. C. Mitchell and W. A. Pettinger, *J. Am. med. Ass.*, 1978, *239*, 2131; G. W. Keusch *et al.*, *Nephron*, 1978, *21*, 1.

Renal scleroderma. Malignant hypertension associated with oliguric renal failure in a 39-year-old man with scleroderma was successfully controlled when minoxidil 5 mg twice daily was given, although hydralazine 400 mg and propranolol 480 mg daily had been ineffective. After management of renal failure with haemodialysis for 6 months, renal function spontaneously improved. Dialysis was discontinued and blood pressure controlled with minoxidil 40 mg, propranolol 320 mg, and frusemide 400 mg daily. Nephrectomy had previously been advocated in this situation since antihypertensive therapy had frequently been reported to be ineffective and the renal failure in scleroderma considered irreversible.— P. D. Mitnick and P. U. Feig, *New Engl. J. Med.*, 1978, *299*, 871.

Further references: J. H. Felts *et al.* (letter), *J. Am. med. Ass.*, 1978, *239*, 1494.

Hypertension in children. Minoxidil was effective in the treatment of severe refractory hypertension which developed in a 10-year-old girl after renal transplantation.— S. P. Makker, *J. Pediat.*, 1975, *86*, 621.

A report on the successful use of minoxidil in 6 children with severe hypertension.— A. J. Pennisi *et al.*, *J. Pediat.*, 1977, *90*, 813.

Further references: A. R. Sinaiko and B. L. Mirkin, *J. Pediat.*, 1977, *91*, 138.

Proprietary Preparations

Loniten *(Upjohn, UK)*. Minoxidil, available as scored tablets of 2.5, 5, or 10 mg. (Also available as Loniten in *Austral.*, *USA*).

885-r

Mistletoe *(B.P.C. 1934)*. Viscum; Visci Caulis; Gui; Tallo de muérdago.

Pharmacopoeias. In *Span.*

The dried, evergreen, dioecious semi-parasite, *Viscum album* (Lorantheaceae), which grows on the branches of deciduous trees, chiefly apple, poplar, and plum. It occurs as a mixture of broken stems and leaves and occasional fruits.

Mistletoe has a vasodilator action and was formerly used for lowering blood pressure. Its action was reported usually to be delayed with a maximum effect reached 3 to 4 days after the commencement of treatment. It has also been used in hysteria and chorea. It was administered as a soft extract or as an infusion or tincture (1 in 8; *dose*: 0.3 to 0.6 ml). Ingestion of the berries and other parts has been reported to cause nausea, vomiting, diarrhoea, and bradycardia.

Hepatitis due to the ingestion of a herbal remedy containing mistletoe.— J. Harvey and D. G. Colin-Jones, *Br. med. J.*, 1981, *282*, 186.

Proprietary Preparations

Iscador *(Society for Cancer Research, Switz.: Weleda, UK)*. Preparations of mistletoe, claimed to be of use in cancer.

Lack of any substantial basis for expecting Iscador to be of value in treating cancer.— *Br. med. J.*, 1978, *2*, 49.

Other Proprietary Names

Mistel-Pflanzensaft *(Ger.)*; Plenosol *(Ger.)*; Viscyat Bürger *(Ger.)*.

886-f

Pargyline Hydrochloride *(U.S.P.)*. *N*-Methyl-*N*-prop-2-ynylbenzylamine hydrochloride.

$C_{11}H_{13}N,HCl = 195.7$.

CAS — 555-57-7 (pargyline); 306-07-0 (hydrochloride).

Pharmacopoeias. In *U.S.*

A white or almost white crystalline powder with a slight odour. M.p. 158° to 162°; sublimation occurs when kept at raised temperatures.

Soluble 1 in 0.6 of water, 1 in 5 of alcohol, and 1 in about 7 of chloroform; very slightly soluble in acetone. Aqueous solutions are unstable. A 3.18% solution is iso-osmotic with serum. **Store** in airtight containers.

Adverse Effects. The toxic effects of pargyline are similar to those described for monoamine oxidase inhibitors and include nausea, vomiting, constipation, dryness of the mouth, headache, arthralgia, sweating, insomnia, nightmares, disorientation, agitation, hallucinations, paranoid delusions, postural hypotension, dizziness, palpitations, increased appetite, oedema, weight gain, difficulty in micturition, impotence and delayed ejaculation, skin rash, and purpura; muscle twitching, acute extrapyramidal syndrome and, very rarely, fever, have been reported. There have been reports of congestive heart failure in patients with reduced cardiac reserve.

Severe toxic reactions may occur if pargyline is taken simultaneously with certain other drugs or with cheese, yeast extract, and certain other foods—see under Precautions, below and under Precautions for Phenelzine Sulphate, p.128.

Effects on mental state. Out of 33 patients who were given pargyline hydrochloride for hypertension, 3 developed hallucinations and paranoid delusions, and a further patient developed disorientation.— A. I. Sutnick *et al.*, *J. Am. med. Ass.*, 1964, *188*, 610.

For reference to recovery from a state of depression and mental deterioration on withdrawal of long-term pargyline therapy see under Interactions (below).

Overdosage. About 15 hours after ingesting 150 or 175 mg of pargyline hydrochloride, a 2½-year-old child was anorectic, sleepless, lethargic, and mentally confused. Her eyes rolled, her teeth chattered, her speech was slurred, and she staggered. She complained of abdominal pain. Both pupils were dilated and responded only sluggishly to light; the accommodation reflex was absent and the eye movements hyperactive. After a day in hospital the child went into a short coma with Babinski reflexes and opisthotonos. Her subsequent behaviour alternated between extreme agitation and lethargy. — D. Lipkin and T. Kushnick, *J. Am. med. Ass.*, 1967, *201*, 57.

Treatment of Adverse Effects. If overdosage occurs the stomach should be emptied by aspiration and lavage. Mania or hyperexcitement may be treated with chlorpromazine, 25 mg intramuscularly or intravenously. Severe hypotension may respond to placing the patient in the supine position with the feet raised; the effects of gross overdosage may be treated by the infusion of plasma. Hypertension may be treated with alpha-adrenoceptor blocking agents such as phentolamine mesylate or phenoxybenzamine hydrochloride. Chlorpromazine or tolazoline have also been suggested as emergency treatment.

Advice on antihypertensive drugs and anaesthesia, together with inclusion of a reference table suggesting that noradrenaline, used with extreme caution, may be a suitable pressor agent in patients receiving monoamine oxidase inhibitors such as pargyline. There is also a warning that monoamine oxidase inhibitors, which preserve noradrenaline stores, dangerously potentiate the indirect-acting vasopressors, and that potentiation of the action of adrenaline or noradrenaline is unusual in the presence of monoamine oxidase inhibitors, but will occur under certain conditions, and great care should be taken until more information is available.— H. R. Dingle, *Anaesthesia*, 1966, *21*, 151.

Precautions. Pargyline should be given with caution to patients with impaired hepatic or renal function or to patients suffering from Cushing's syndrome or parkinsonism. It should not be given to patients with malignant hypertension, advanced renal failure, hyperthyroidism or an excitable personality, phaeochromocytoma, or schizophrenia. The hypotensive effect of pargyline may be increased during febrile illnesses. Pargyline may induce hypoglycaemia in some patients. Hypotension may occur during anaesthesia in patients being treated with pargyline or within 14 days of cessation of treatment with pargyline.

See also under Precautions for Phenelzine Sulphate, p.128, particularly with reference to other drugs and items of diet contra-indicated during therapy with monoamine oxidase inhibitors. Pargyline should not be given concomitantly with methyldopa or dopamine. Guanethidine or reserpine or other antihypertensive agents which may cause hypertensive reactions due to sudden release of catecholamines should not be given parenterally to patients taking pargyline or for at least 14 days after cessation of treatment with pargyline. The hypotensive effects of pargyline may be enhanced by thiazide diuretics. It has been reported that the nerve-blocking effects of local anaesthetics such as lignocaine may be diminished by prolonged administration of pargyline.

Hypoglycaemia. In a study in 18 hypertensive diabetics, in whom the fasting blood sugar was raised during treatment with methyclothiazide, pargyline was shown to have a definite hypoglycaemic effect.— B. J. Kravitz and J. C. Hutchison, *Curr. ther. Res.*, 1968, *10*, 18.

Interactions. A 70-year-old woman with hypertension who had been treated for 6 months with pargyline, 10 mg twice daily increased to 25 mg twice daily ate Swiss cheese and 20 minutes later suddenly experienced near syncope with excruciating pounding headache. Profuse sweating and nausea followed. Treatment included the withdrawal of the monoamine oxidase inhibitor and the administration of phentolamine mesylate.— E. W. Beasley (letter), *Lancet*, 1964, *2*, 586. Similar reports: J. W. Leonard *et al.* (letter), *Lancet*, 1964, *1*, 883; F. S. Glazener *et al.*, *J. Am. med. Ass.*, 1964, *188*, 754; J. C. Hutchison (letter), *Lancet*, 1964, *2*, 151.

A man taking 25 mg of pargyline hydrochloride every morning and 30 to 60 g of Cheddar cheese every evening experienced particularly horrifying nightmares which ceased on withdrawal of the cheese from his diet.— J. C. Shee (letter), *Br. med. J.*, 1964, *1*, 1441.

A hypertensive reaction occurred following the ingestion of chocolate by a patient who had been treated with pargyline.— D. M. Krikler and B. Lewis (letter), *Lancet*, 1965, *1*, 1166.

Methyldopa. A woman receiving pargyline developed vivid hallucinations on concomitant administration of methyldopa.— E. S. Paykel (letter), *Br. med. J.*, 1966, *1*, 803.

Pethidine. For severe effects occurring when pargyline and pethidine were given concomitantly, see Pethidine Hydrochloride, p.1026.

Sympathomimetics. A 58-year-old hypertensive man given pargyline hydrochloride in a total daily dose increased from 25 to 75 mg became hypotensive within 5 weeks of starting this treatment. He was then given a single intramuscular injection of 4 mg of *metaraminol*, a sympathomimetic amine, which precipitated within 10 minutes a hypertensive crisis with systolic blood pressure above 300 mmHg.— A. R. Horler and N. A. Wynne, *Br. med. J.*, 1965, *2*, 460.

A 62-year-old woman who had taken pargyline 25 mg daily for 10 years, discontinued the drug 3 weeks before a surgical operation but, nevertheless, overreacted to an intravenous injection of methylamphetamine 3 mg given for hypotension. Following this incident she did not restart pargyline therapy and it was noted that her previous state of progressive mental deterioration and long-standing depression had been reversed within 3 months.— M. J. Cousins and J. R. Maltby, *Br. J. Anaesth.*, 1971, *43*, 803.

Absorption and Fate. Pargyline is absorbed from the gastro-intestinal tract. In *rats* about 90% of a dose has been reported to be excreted in the urine within 24 hours.

N-Methylbenzylamine was a metabolite of pargyline in man.— R. Pirisino *et al.*, *Br. J. clin. Pharmac.*, 1979, *7*, 595.

Uses. Pargyline hydrochloride is a monoamine oxidase inhibitor which is occasionally used in the treatment of resistant hypertension and it has been claimed to have a beneficial effect on the mood of the patient. It has a more marked effect on the standing than the supine blood pressure. Its effects take place slowly and last for some time after the drug has been withdrawn.

The usual initial dose is 25 mg daily gradually increased as necessary by 10-mg increments at intervals of not less than 7 days. The usual maintenance dose may be 25 or 50 mg daily; doses of more than 200 mg daily should not generally be exceeded. To reduce side-effects smaller doses of pargyline may be given in conjunction with a thiazide diuretic, which would also reduce the oedema that sometimes occurs with pargyline.

Plasma-prolactin concentrations were moderately but consistently increased in 10 depressed patients during the administration of pargyline 75 to 150 mg daily or clorgyline 20 to 40 mg daily. This effect was considered to be directly due to the monoamine oxidase inhibitor.— S. L. Slater *et al.* (preliminary communication), *Lancet*, 1977, *2*, 275.

Glaucoma. Eye-drops of pargyline hydrochloride 0.5% substantially lowered intra-ocular pressure in patients with chronic open-angle glaucoma and absolute glaucoma.— K. S. Mehra *et al.*, *Archs Ophthal., N.Y.*, 1974, *92*, 453.

Hypertension. Pargyline hydrochloride was given to 19 patients with hypertension in doses of 12.5 to 25 mg initially, increased by 25 to 50 mg daily at intervals of 1 or 2 weeks until a satisfactory response occurred or a maximum dose of 200 mg daily was reached. All the patients had a satisfactory initial hypotensive response, but it was maintained in only 8 patients for periods of 6 months or 2 years. Eleven patients became refractory and 4 of them developed fluid retention and 1 a psychotic episode.— J. H. Esbenshade *et al.*, *Am. J. med. Sci.*, 1966, *251*, 81.

Pargyline was of particular value in patients who had been depressed on other therapy, but its use should be limited because of its dangers as a monoamine oxidase inhibitor.— R. G. Lewis and A. Young, *Med. J. Aust.*, 1967, *1*, 339.

Further references: A. N. Brest *et al.*, *Am. Heart J.*, 1964, *68*, 621; B. F. Levy, *Curr. ther. Res.*, 1966, *8*, 343; A. I. Sutnick *et al.*, *Vasc. Dis.*, 1966, *3*, 145; H. J. Hamm, *ibid.*, 378; M. C. Holt, *Br. J. clin. Pract.*, 1967, *21*, 447; R. Sannerstedt, *Acta med. scand.*, 1967, *181*, 699; J. C. Hutchison, *Curr. ther. Res.*, 1968, *10*, 128; F. W. Fletcher, *ibid.*, 394; J. Buch, *Clin. Med.*, 1969, *76* (Jan.), 26.

Preparations

Pargyline Hydrochloride Tablets *(U.S.P.)*. Tablets containing pargyline hydrochloride.

Eutonyl *(Abbott, UK)*. Filmtabs (film-coated tablets) each containing pargyline hydrochloride 25 mg. (Also available as Eutonyl in *USA*).

Other Proprietary Names

Eudatine *(Belg.)*.

887-d

Pempidine Tartrate *(B.P. 1968)*. 1,2,2,6,6-Pentamethylpiperidine hydrogen tartrate.

$C_{10}H_{21}N,C_4H_6O_6$=305.4.

CAS — 79-55-0 (pempidine); 546-48-5 (tartrate).

A white odourless or almost odourless, crystalline powder with a bitter acid taste. M.p. about 160°. **Soluble** 1 in 2 of water and 1 in 14 of alcohol; very slightly soluble in acetone; practically insoluble in chloroform and ether. **Store** in airtight containers.

Adverse Effects. Treatment with pempidine tartrate is associated with the effects of ganglionic blockade, most commonly postural hypotension, increased or sometimes decreased heart-rate, blurring of vision, constipation, and dryness of the mouth. Nausea, difficulty in micturition, drowsiness, occasional diarrhoea, and impotence may also occur. Paralytic ileus is a serious hazard of long-term therapy.

Ganglion-blocking agents induced interstitial pulmonary fibrosis.— E. C. Rosenow, *Ann. intern. Med.*, 1972, *77*, 977.

Treatment of Adverse Effects. Neostigmine has been given to relieve the constipation associated with pempidine therapy.

If overdosage occurs the stomach should be emptied by aspiration and lavage. Patients with severe hypotension should be placed in the supine position with the feet raised. The effects of gross overdosage may be treated by the infusion of plasma or by the cautious intravenous infusion of metaraminol.

Precautions. Pempidine should not be used in patients with pyloric stenosis. It should be used with caution in patients with cerebral or coronary vascular disease or impaired renal function.

Hypotension may occur during anaesthesia in patients being treated with pempidine (see p.136).

Patients taking pempidine are sensitive to adrenaline, amphetamine, and other sympathomimetic agents. The effects of pempidine may be enhanced if alkalis are taken concomitantly in amounts sufficient to increase the urinary pH.

Absorption and Fate. Pempidine is rapidly and completely absorbed from the gastro-intestinal tract, and peak concentrations appear in the plasma after about 2 hours. It is not significantly bound to plasma proteins. Most of a dose is excreted in the urine in 24 hours. Excretion is reduced in alkaline urine.

References: M. Harington *et al.*, *Lancet*, 1958, *2*, 6; C. T. Dollery *et al.*, *Br. med. J.*, 1960, *1*, 521.

Uses. Pempidine is a tertiary amine ganglion-blocking agent which inhibits the transmission of nerve impulses in both sympathetic and parasympathetic ganglia. The sympathetic block produces peripheral vasodilatation which causes increased blood flow, raised skin temperature, and reduced blood pressure. The parasympathetic block diminishes movement of the gastro-intestinal tract and bladder, reduces gastric and salivary secretion, and produces disturbance of visual accommodation.

Pempidine has been used in the treatment of severe or malignant hypertension, but has largely been superseded by drugs that do not produce the effects of parasympathetic blockade. The usual initial dosage is 2.5 mg of pempidine tartrate by mouth 3 or 4 times a day, adjusted by increments or decrements of 2.5 mg until an effective hypotensive dose is reached. The usual maintenance dose is 10 to 80 mg daily in 4 divided doses. Tolerance to pempidine rarely develops.

Reports of the use of pempidine in hypertension: A. Kitchin *et al.*, *Lancet*, 1961, *1*, 143; C. T. Dollery (letter), *ibid.*, 336; F. J. T. Croll *et al.*, *Med. J. Aust.*, 1961, *2*, 98.

Preparations

Pempidine Tablets *(B.P. 1968)*. Tablets containing pempidine tartrate. Store in airtight containers.

Pempidine tartrate was formerly marketed in Great Britain under the proprietary name Perolysen *(May & Baker)*.

888-n

Pempidine Tosylate. Pempidine Tosilate; Pirilenum. 1,2,2,6,6-Pentamethylpiperidine toluene-4-sulphonate.

$C_{10}H_{21}N,C_7H_8O_3S$=327.5.

Pharmacopoeias. In *Rus.*

A white or creamy-white, odourless or almost odourless, crystalline powder. M.p. about 158°. Freely **soluble** in water and alcohol; sparingly soluble in acetone; practically insoluble in ether.

Uses. Pempidine tosylate has the actions and uses of pempidine tartrate (above). The doses given in the *Rus. P.* are: max. single, 10 mg: max. in 24 hours, 30 mg.

889-h

Pentamethonium Bromide. Dibromure de Pentaméthonium. *NN'*-Pentamethylenebis(trimethylammonium) dibromide.

$C_{11}H_{28}Br_2N_2$=348.2.

CAS — 2365-25-5 (pentamethonium); 541-20-8 (dibromide).

Uses. A quarternary ammonium ganglion-blocking agent which has been used similarly to pentamethonium iodide in doses of 0.2 to 1.2 g daily in divided doses.

Proprietary Names

Penthonium *(Delagrange, Fr.)*.

890-a

Pentamethonium Iodide *(B.P.C. 1954)*. *NN'*-Pentamethylenebis(trimethylammonium) di-iodide.

$C_{11}H_{28}I_2N_2$=442.2.

CAS — 5282-80-4.

Uses. Pentamethonium iodide is a quaternary ammonium ganglion-blocking agent which has similar actions to pempidine tartrate. It has been used in the treatment of hypertension and as an aid to the reduction of bleeding during surgical operations.

For a brief discussion of the effects of pentamethonium iodide, see A. P. Adams, *Br. J. Anaesth.*, 1975, *47*, 777.

891-t

Pentolinium Tartrate *(B.P.)*. Pentolonium Tartrate; Tartrate de Pyrroplégium; Pentapyrrolidinium Bitartrate; Pentolinio Tartrato. *NN'*-Pentamethylenebis(1-methylpyrrolidinium) bis(hydrogen tartrate).

$C_{23}H_{42}N_2O_{12}$=538.6.

CAS — 144-44-5 (pentolinium); 52-62-0 (tartrate).

Pharmacopoeias. In *Br.* and *It.*

A white or almost white, odourless powder with an acid taste. M.p. about 206° with decomposition. **Soluble** 1 in 0.4 of water and 1 in 800 of alcohol; practically insoluble in chloroform and ether. A 10% solution in water has a pH of 3.4 to 3.7. Solutions are **sterilised** by autoclaving or by filtration. **Store** in a cool place in airtight containers.

Adverse Effects, Treatment, and Precautions. As for Pempidine Tartrate, p.157.

Fatal pulmonary changes in a woman given anti-hypertensive therapy which included pentolinium.— T. Hilden *et al.*, *Lancet*, 1958, *2*, 830.

Absorption and Fate. Pentolinium tartrate is incompletely and irregularly absorbed from the gastro-intestinal tract.

Uses. Pentolinium tartrate is a quaternary ammonium ganglion-blocking agent with actions similar to those of pempidine tartrate (see p.157). There is a lack of uniformity in its effects when administered by mouth.

Pentolinium tartrate is given to produce controlled hypotension in patients undergoing surgical procedures. Doses of 2.5 to 25 mg have been recommended and should be given intravenously; elderly or hypertensive patients should be given reduced doses.

In the treatment of hypertension subcutaneous administration was usually started with a dose of 1 to 2.5 mg, repeated at 12-hourly intervals and increased by increments of 0.5 to 1 mg to an effective dose. The development of tolerance over 10 to 12 weeks necessitated increasing the dose, usually to a range of 20 to 100 mg daily, given in divided doses every 6 or 8 hours. Pentolinium was given intravenously in similar initial doses every 5 minutes in acute emergencies.

Subcutaneous injections of 2 mg have been used in the emergency treatment of eclampsia and up to 2 mg, repeated as necessary, in the treatment of hypertensive encephalopathy.

By mouth, the dose was 10 to 20 mg every 12 hours, gradually increased according to the response of the patient by increments of not more than 20 mg. The usual maintenance dose varied from 100 to 900 mg daily.

Failure of pentolinium to reduce plasma-catecholamine concentrations as a test for the diagnosis of phaeochromocytoma.— M. J. Brown *et al.*, *Lancet*, 1981, *1*, 174.

Controlled hypotension. A brief discussion of the use of pentolinium in controlled hypotension during surgery.— G. E. H. Enderby, *Postgrad. med. J.*, 1974, *50*, 572.

Satisfactory haemostasis was achieved on 84% of 700 occasions in which controlled hypotension for middle-ear surgery, in patients aged 20 to 66 years, was achieved by the use of thiopentone-halothane-nitrous oxide anaesthesia with pentolinium. The following doses of pentolinium appeared to be satisfactory: aged 20 to 40 years, 25 mg; 41 to 50 years, 15 mg; 51 to 60 years, 10 mg; over 60 years, 5 mg.— A. R. Kerr, *Br. J. Anaesth.*, 1977, *49*, 447.

Further references: J. E. Eckenhoff and J. C. Rich, *Anesth. Analg. curr. Res.*, 1966, *45*, 21; A. R. Kerr (letter), *Br. med. J.*, 1969, *3*, 473; T. H. Mallory (letter), *J. Am. med. Ass.*, 1973, *224*, 248; N. R. Fahmy and M. B. Laver, *Anesthesiology*, 1976, *44*, 6.

In paraplegic subjects. The prophylactic effect of pentolinium was assessed in quadriplegic or paraplegic patients who were liable to develop autonomic hyperreflexia, with marked increases in arterial pressure, during surgical procedures on the urinary tract, colon or rectum. Mean systolic arterial pressure was significantly less in 6 patients given pentolinium tartrate 10 to 15 mg intravenously about 10 minutes before the procedure compared with 10 controls who only received the drug during the procedure when systolic pressure exceeded 140 mmHg.— J. W. Basta *et al.*, *Br. J. Anaesth.*, 1977, *49*, 1087.

Reports of the use of pentolinium tartrate in the treatment of hypertension: A. Agrest and S. W. Hoobler, *J. Am. med. Ass.*, 1955, *157*, 999; D. W. Ashby *et al.*, *Lancet*, 1955, *1*, 224; C. W. C. Bain *et al.*, *Br. med. J.*, 1955, *1*, 817; H. T. N. Sears *et al.*, *Br. med. J.*, 1959, *1*, 462.

Preparations

Pentolinium Injection *(B.P.)*. A sterile solution of pentolinium tartrate in Water for Injections, adjusted to pH 6.5 (limits: pH 6 to 7) by the addition of sodium hydroxide, but when issued in containers sealed so as to permit the withdrawal of successive doses on different occasions and containing chlorbutol as the bactericide, the pH is not less than 4. Sterilised by autoclaving.

Pentolinium Tablets *(B.P.C. 1968)*. Tablets containing pentolinium tartrate. Store in a cool place in airtight containers.

Proprietary Names

Ansolysen *(May & Baker, Austral.; May & Baker, S.Afr.)*; Pentio *(Estedi, Spain)*.

Pentolinium tartrate was formerly marketed in Great Britain under the proprietary name Ansolysen (*May & Baker*).

892-x

Phenoxybenzamine Hydrochloride *(B.P., U.S.P.)*.

Phenoxybenz. Hydrochlor.; SKF 688A. *N*-(2-Chloroethyl)-*N*-(1-methyl-2-phenoxyethyl)benzylamine hydrochloride.
$C_{18}H_{22}ClNO,HCl=340.3$.

CAS — 59-96-1 (phenoxybenzamine); 63-92-3 (hydrochloride).

Pharmacopoeias. In *Br.* and *U.S.*

A white or almost white, odourless or almost odourless, almost tasteless, crystalline powder. M.p. 136° to 141°.

Soluble 1 in 25 of water, 1 in 9 of alcohol, and 1 in 9 of chloroform; soluble in propylene glycol; practically insoluble in ether. Neutral and alkaline solutions are unstable. **Store** in airtight containers. Protect from light.

CAUTION. *Phenoxybenzamine should not be allowed to come into contact with eyes or skin, as it may cause irritation.*

Adverse Effects. Phenoxybenzamine may cause orthostatic hypotension and tachycardia which may be of sufficient severity to militate against its use.

Other side-effects include nasal congestion, dryness of the mouth, miosis, drowsiness, sedation, and inhibition of ejaculation. Gastro-intestinal effects are usually slight.

Local pain, skin and tissue changes, widespread oedema and urticaria, and malaise occurred in 2 patients given 50 µg of sterile phenoxybenzamine intradermally as a 0.1% solution.— S. L. Alexander *et al.* (letter), *Lancet*, 1973, *1*, 317.

Respiratory effects. Phenoxybenzamine 1 mg per kg body-weight in 200 ml of dextrose injection was infused intravenously in ½ to 2 hours or more after standard treatment for hypotension secondary to cardiac infarction had failed in 7 patients suffering from shock and associated symptoms. Marked circulatory improvement became evident in 2 patients and was maximal after 6 hours. Six patients showed severe adverse respiratory effects including the development of wheezing, rales, and rhonchi associated with the appearance or worsening of pulmonary oedema. In 3 patients who received rapid infusions, the wheezing and expiratory difficulty were very pronounced, and suggestive of bronchospasm. Only 1 of the 7 patients survived. Phenoxybenzamine should be used with caution in cardiac infarction, and the rate of administration probably should not exceed 500 µg per minute.— J. F. Riordan and G. Walter, *Br. med. J.*, 1969, *1*, 155. Untoward delay in giving phenoxybenzamine might explain its lack of success in treating cardiogenic shock. Several patients received phenoxybenzamine for, or to prevent, pulmonary oedema, the moist lungs in each case clearing completely where digoxin and frusemide had failed.— D. A. L. Watt *et al.* (letter), *ibid.*, 507. Administration of phenoxybenzamine was contra-indicated when the central venous pressure was low.— N. M. Lamont and K. Posel (letter), *ibid.*, *3*, 116.

Treatment of Adverse Effects. If overdosage occurs the stomach should be emptied by aspiration and lavage. Severe hypotension may respond to placing the patient in the supine position with the feet raised, and to the infusion of plasma. Infusion of noradrenaline has been advocated to attempt to overcome the effects of alpha-blockade, but adrenaline is contra-indicated since it also stimulates beta-receptors causing increased tachycardia and vasodilatation and an overall further drop in blood pressure.

The effects of overdosage with phenoxybenzamine may be very prolonged.

Precautions. Phenoxybenzamine should be given with care to patients with congestive heart failure, coronary or cerebral arteriosclerosis, or renal impairment. It should not be given in any conditions in which a fall in blood pressure would be dangerous.

Exercise, heat, a large meal, and alcohol may increase the hypotensive effect of phenoxybenzamine. Since phenoxybenzamine only blocks alpha-receptors, leaving the beta-receptors unopposed, concomitant administration of drugs, such as adrenaline, which also stimulate beta-receptors, may enhance the cardiac-accelerating and hypotensive action of phenoxybenzamine.

When given intravenously, phenoxybenzamine hydrochloride should always be diluted and given by infusion. Intravenous fluids must always be given beforehand to ensure an adequate circulating blood volume and to prevent a precipitous fall in blood pressure (see also under Uses). Care must be taken to avoid extravasation of the infusion as it may be irritating to muscle tissue.

Absorption and Fate. Phenoxybenzamine is incompletely absorbed from the gastro-intestinal tract. The maximum effect is attained in about 1 hour after an intravenous dose. Most is excreted in the urine and bile within 24 hours, but small amounts remain in the body for several days. It has a prolonged action probably owing to stable covalent bonding.

Uses. Phenoxybenzamine is a powerful alpha-adrenoceptor blocking agent with a prolonged duration of action. A single large dose of phenoxybenzamine can cause postural hypotension for 3 days or longer. It has been used in the treatment of peripheral vascular disorders due to vasospasm. The usual initial dose of phenoxybenzamine hydrochloride is 10 mg daily, increased at intervals of at least 4 days, according to the patient's response, to 60 mg daily in divided doses.

It is also used to control the hypertension caused by phaeochromocytoma; for this purpose doses of up to as much as 200 mg daily have been required. In the operative management of phaeochromocytoma phenoxybenzamine may be given by intravenous infusion on 3 days before operation and, if necessary, before induction of anaesthesia (E.J. Ross *et al.*, *Br. med. J.*, 1967, *1*, 191).

Phenoxybenzamine is occasionally used, as an adjunct to other antihypertensive agents, in the treatment of some other forms of hypertension.

Phenoxybenzamine hydrochloride has been given intravenously in the treatment of shock. It should be given under continuous supervision in a dose of 1 mg per kg body-weight in 200 to 500 ml of Sodium Chloride Intravenous Infusion over a period of at least 1 hour as an adjunct to more specific treatment. It reduces vasoconstriction and increases tissue perfusion. It is essential to administer blood and other volume expanders rapidly beforehand to ensure adequate circulating volume and prevent a precipitous fall in blood pressure as a result of alpha-adrenoceptor blockade.

Phenoxybenzamine has also been used in the treatment of pulmonary oedema and as an adjunct in the management of urinary retention as a result of a neurogenic bladder or prostatic hypertrophy.

The mechanism of the prolonged adrenoceptor blockade produced by phenoxybenzamine.— M. Nickerson, *Archs int. Pharmacodyn.*, 1962, *140*, 237.

Studies in 31 healthy persons showed that intravenous infusions of phenoxybenzamine caused a slight but consistent early rise in resting blood-glucose concentrations and substantial hyperglycaemia during starvation. The rate of fat mobilisation was significantly enhanced.— E. J. Pinter *et al.* (letter), *Lancet*, 1967, *2*, 101.

Phenoxybenzamine, given by infusion to 7 healthy men, caused a reduction in arterial blood pressure and peripheral resistance and a gradual increase in cardiac output. The rate of secretion of aldosterone generally increased, and urine flow and sodium excretion generally decreased.— J. J. Skillman *et al.*, *Surgery, St Louis*, 1968, *64*, 368.

Adrenaline overdosage. For a report recommending the use of phenoxybenzamine and propranolol in the treatment of adrenaline overdosage, see Adrenaline, p.3.

Anorexia nervosa. A 21-year-old woman with anorexia nervosa gained weight during administration of phenoxybenzamine in doses of 10 to 30 mg daily by mouth. Propranolol had no beneficial effect.— D. E. Redmond *et al.* (letter), *Lancet*, 1976, *2*, 307.

Cerebral artery spasm. Following operations for the treatment of cerebral arterial aneurysms, phenoxybenzamine in doses of up to 10 mg was injected into the carotid artery of 23 patients for the prevention or treatment of cerebral artery spasm. A rapid improvement in neurological symptoms occurred in 3 patients with marked neurological disability. In other patients in whom the treatment was prophylactic and given at the time of immediate postoperative arteriogram no deterioration occurred during the first 36 hours after injection.— B. H. Cummins and H. B. Griffith, *Br.*

med. J., 1971, *1*, 382.

Fabry disease. A patient with angiokeratoma corporis diffusum (Fabry disease), an inherited disorder of glycolipid metabolism, obtained remission of psychotic signs and symptoms after administration of phenoxybenzamine hydrochloride 10 mg four times a day.— E. H. Liston *et al.*, *Archs gen. Psychiat.*, 1973, *29*, 402.

Fat embolism. Five patients in deep coma after fat embolism following road accidents recovered after a regimen which included vasodilatation with phenoxybenzamine, intermittent positive-pressure ventilation, and hypothermia.— A. G. Larson, *Lancet*, 1968, *2*, 250.

Hyperreflexia. Autonomic hyperreflexia in 2 patients, one of them quadriplegic and the other paraplegic, was relieved indefinitely by administration of phenoxybenzamine hydrochloride 50 and 30 mg respectively, twice daily by mouth for 3 days.— G. W. Sizemore and W. W. Winternitz, *New Engl. J. Med.*, 1970, *282*, 795.

Hypertension. Concomitant administration of propranolol and phenoxybenzamine, controlled supine blood pressure in 14 and upright blood pressure in 17 of 19 patients with hypertension. There was partial inhibition of ejaculation in 3 of 6 of the men.— N. D. Vlachakis and M. Mendlowitz, *Am. Heart J.*, 1976, *92*, 750.

Further references: G. Sandler *et al.*, *Circulation*, 1968, *38*, 542; N. D. Vlachakis and M. Mendlowitz, *J. clin. Pharmac.*, 1976, *16*, 352.

Phaeochromocytoma. In the operative management of phaeochromocytoma phenoxybenzamine should be given in a dose of 100 mg intravenously on each of 3 days before operation to control blood pressure and to enable the blood volume to re-expand. A further dose of 50 mg seemed desirable on the morning of the operation. Phenoxybenzamine produced better control of blood pressure than phentolamine in the patients studied.— E. J. Ross *et al.*, *Br. med. J.*, 1967, *1*, 191. For full details of the regimen, see Propranolol Hydrochloride, p.1334.

Further references: H. Sack *et al.*, *Dt. med. Wschr.*, 1968, *93*, 151; J. R. Crout and B. R. Brown, *Anesthesiology*, 1969, *30*, 29; M. I. Griffith *et al.*, *J. Am. med. Ass.*, 1974, *229*, 437; T. Himathongkam *et al.*, *J. Am. med. Ass.*, 1974, *230*, 1692.

Prinzmetal's angina. Phenoxybenzamine 20 to 30 mg daily abolished episodes of chest pain in a 62-year-old man with Prinzmetal's angina. Chest pain recurred when dosage was reduced to 10 mg daily. The patient remained symptom-free on a dose of 20 mg daily for a one-year follow-up period.— S. Thanavaro *et al.*, *Sth. med. J.*, 1979, *72*, 221.

Raynaud's disease. Treatment with phenoxybenzamine, while antineoplastic treatment was discontinued, improved the condition of the fingers in a man who developed Raynaud's phenomenon when given bleomycin and vinblastine. The antineoplastic treatment was later reintroduced with no effect on the fingers.— D. P. Chernicoff *et al.*, *Cancer Treat. Rep.*, 1978, *62*, 570.

Renal failure. In a study in 31 patients undergoing cardiac surgery, phenoxybenzamine appeared to be effective in preventing postoperative renal ischaemia; it inhibited the effects of adrenaline and noradrenaline upon the renal vasculature.— R. A. Indeglia *et al.*, *J. thorac. cardiovasc. Surg.*, 1966, *51*, 244.

Two patients with renal failure due to *Plasmodium falciparum* malaria and who were passing hypertonic urine of low sodium content had an increased output of urine after the infusion of phenoxybenzamine. Two further patients with urine of the same osmolarity as their plasma, higher sodium content, and with more limited creatinine clearance, failed to respond.— V. Sitprija, *Aust. N.Z.J. Med.*, 1971, *1*, 44.

Pretreatment of the donor with phenoxybenzamine appeared to increase the tolerance of the kidney to warm and cold ischaemia times during preservation. This might reduce the incidence of acute renal necrosis after transplantation.— W. A. Sterling *et al.* (letter), *Lancet*, 1975, *1*, 108.

Shock. To decrease peripheral resistance and lower central venous pressure in the treatment of shock, intravenous phenoxybenzamine in a dose of 1 mg per kg body-weight was considered to be one of the most effective drugs available. The same therapy was considered to be the treatment of choice for patients with pulmonary oedema who had not responded to digitalis.— R. C. Lillehei, 26th Annual Meeting of the Society of University Surgeons, 1965, per *Surgery, St Louis*, 1965, *58*, 213.

Five young patients with septic shock were unresponsive to adequate fluid therapy and showed signs of sympathetic overactivity such as pallor, cold extremities, weak pulse, and decreased capillary filling. Administration of phenoxybenzamine hydrochloride, 1 mg per kg body-weight in 200 ml of Sodium Chloride Intravenous Infusion in 2 hours, led to dramatic improvement and relief of symptoms. Urinary output returned to normal and there was no rise in arterial pressure, but central venous pressure dropped. Cardiac function was directly affected and improved tissue perfusion.— R. W. Anderson *et al.*, *Ann. Surg.*, 1967, *165*, 341, per *Can. med. Ass. J.*, 1967, *97* (Oct. 7), 6.

Further references: *Lancet*, 1966, *1*, 645; J. Freeman, *Med. J. Aust.*, 1969, *2*, 1151.

Urinary disorders. Following diagnosis using phentolamine intravenously, phenoxybenzamine, in a usual dose of 10 mg twice or thrice daily by mouth, improved urinary function in 10 of 18 neurological patients, with neurogenic bladder dysfunction considered to be due to uncoordinated sympathetic activity during voiding. Two children in the study received 2.5 mg daily increased to 5 mg in one.— S. A. Awad *et al.*, *Br. J. Urol.*, 1978, *50*, 336.

Further references: P. F. Boreham *et al.*, *Br. J. Surg.*, 1977, *64*, 756.

Preparations

Phenoxybenzamine Capsules *(B.P.)*. Capsules containing phenoxybenzamine hydrochloride. Store at a temperature not exceeding 30°.

Phenoxybenzamine Hydrochloride Capsules *(U.S.P.)*. Capsules containing phenoxybenzamine hydrochloride.

Dibenyline *(Smith Kline & French, UK)*. Phenoxybenzamine hydrochloride, available as **Capsules** of 10 mg and as **Injection Concentrate** containing 50 mg per ml, in ampoules of 2 ml. (Also available as Dibenyline in *Austral.*, *Neth.*).

Other Proprietary Names

Dibenzyline *(USA)*; Dibenzyran *(Ger.)*.

893-r

Phentolamine Hydrochloride *(U.S.P., B.P. 1963)*.

Phentolam. Hydrochlor.; Phentolamini Hydrochloridum; Phentolaminium Chloride; Cloridrato de Fentolamina. 3-[*N*-(2-Imidazolin-2-ylmethyl)-*p*-toluidino]phenol hydrochloride.
$C_{17}H_{19}N_3O,HCl=317.8$.

CAS — 50-60-2 (phentolamine); 73-05-2 (hydrochloride).

Pharmacopoeias. In *Arg.*, *Braz.*, *Int.*, and *U.S.*

A white or faintly cream-coloured odourless crystalline powder with a bitter taste. M.p. about 240°.

Soluble 1 in 50 of water and 1 in about 120 of alcohol; very slightly soluble in chloroform and ether. Solutions in water have a pH of about 5 and foam on shaking. **Incompatible** with iron. **Store** in airtight containers. Protect from light.

894-f

Phentolamine Mesylate *(B.P., U.S.P.)*.

Phentolamine Mesilate; Phentolamine Methanesulphonate; Phentolamini Mesylas. 3-[*N*-(2-Imidazolin-2-ylmethyl)-*p*-toluidino]phenol methanesulphonate.
$C_{17}H_{19}N_3O,CH_3SO_3H=377.5$.

CAS — 65-28-1.

Pharmacopoeias. In *Arg.*, *Br.*, *Int.*, *Turk.*, and *U.S.*

A white or off-white slightly hygroscopic, odourless, crystalline powder with a bitter taste. M.p. 177° to 181°.

Soluble 1 in 1 of water, 1 in 5 of alcohol, and 1 in 700 of chloroform. Solutions in water have a pH of about 5 and slowly deteriorate on storage. An 8.23% solution is iso-osmotic with serum. Solutions are **sterilised** by filtration and distributed into containers the air in which is replaced by nitrogen or other suitable gas. **Incompatible** with iron. **Store** in airtight containers. Protect from light.

Adverse Effects. Phentolamine may cause hypotension and severe tachycardia with anginal pain, particularly when given parenterally. Nausea, vomiting, and diarrhoea may also occur. Other side-effects include weakness, dizziness, flushing, sweating, apprehension, palpitation, and nasal stuffiness.

Hypotension. Reports of the death of a 21-year-old pregnant woman following administration of phentolamine mesylate for the diagnosis of a phaeochromocytoma (the presence of which was confirmed at autopsy). The patient developed profound vasomotor shock immediately after administration of the drug.— C. B. Roland, *J. Am. med. Ass.*, 1959, *171*, 1806.

Further references: D. A. Emanuel *et al.*, *J. Am. med. Ass.*, 1956, *161*, 436.

Treatment of Adverse Effects. As for Phenoxybenzamine Hydrochloride, p.158.

Phentolamine has a more rapid onset of action than phenoxybenzamine; its effect is much less prolonged.

Precautions. Phentolamine should not generally be given to patients with angina pectoris or coronary artery disease.

Interactions. *Ethambutol.* A 46-year-old woman taking streptomycin, ethambutol, and rifampicin gave a false positive reaction to a phentolamine test for phaeochromocytoma. The reaction became negative when medication was withdrawn and positive again on 2 occasions when ethambutol was given.— R. Gabriel, *Br. med. J.*, 1972, *3*, 332.

Absorption and Fate. The bioavailability of phentolamine following oral administration is lower than following intravenous administration.

Phentolamine 40 mg by mouth produced its maximum effect about 30 minutes after administration and had a duration of action of 3 to 6 hours. Slow-release formulations of phentolamine 100 or 200 mg produced their maximum effect after 4 hours and had a duration of action of about 12 hours for the 100-mg dose and between 12 and 24 hours for the 200-mg dose.— B. Pfister and P. Imhof, *Br. J. clin. Pharmac.*, 1978, *5*, 175.

Uses. Phentolamine is an alpha-adrenoceptor blocking agent which also has a generalised direct vasodilator effect on all muscular walled vessels. It is given by intravenous or intramuscular injection.

Phentolamine mesylate 5 to 10 mg by intravenous injection is of value in the treatment of hypertension due to overdosage with sympathomimetic agents with alpha-adrenergic activity such as noradrenaline; it may also be used in association with a beta-adrenoceptor blocking agent, such as propranolol, in overdosage with sympathomimetics with mixed alpha- and beta-adrenergic activity, such as adrenaline. It may also be given in the treatment of hypertensive crises occurring in patients taking monoamine oxidase inhibitors or in patients with rebound hypertension as a result of clonidine withdrawal (see p.139). Speed is essential for successful treatment.

Phentolamine may be of value as an adjunct in the treatment of shock or heart failure and has been given in doses of 1 to 2 mg of the mesylate per minute by intravenous infusion for up to 3 hours. More recently a dose of 5 to 60 mg given over a period of 10 to 30 minutes at an infusion-rate of 0.1 to 2 mg per minute has been recommended for acute left ventricular failure (cardiogenic shock), particularly following myocardial infarction. If necessary 5 mg may be given over the first minute. The infusion-rate should be reduced if the systolic pressure falls below 100 mmHg.

In surgery for removal of a phaeochromocytoma, to prevent the hypertensive crisis due to emotional stress, anaesthesia, or manipulation of the tumour, phentolamine mesylate 5 mg is given intravenously, a few minutes, or intramuscularly, about half-an-hour, before surgery. During surgery this dose may be repeated intravenously as necessary.

Phentolamine has been given by mouth as the hydrochloride prior to surgery for the control of hypertension in patients with phaeochromocytoma. The usual dose is 50 mg four to six times daily.

Phentolamine mesylate has been employed for the differential diagnosis of phaeochromocytoma but it has been superseded by estimations of catecholamines in blood and urine. If the patient had a phaeochromocytoma, injection of the drug was usually followed by a fall of more than 35 mmHg in the systolic pressure and of more than 25 mmHg in the diastolic pressure. This occurred within 2 minutes after intravenous injection and within 20 minutes after intramuscular injection. The pressure returned to pre-injection levels within 10 to 15 minutes after intravenous injection and within 3 or 4 hours after intramuscular injection. The test is not without risk.

A false positive response could be given by patients with uraemia or who have received sedatives or narcotics during the 24 hours before the test. False negative responses could be given if the tumour was not secreting sufficient pressor substances to raise the blood pressure significantly, or if the condition was complicated by essential hypertension. The usual dose was 5 mg by intravenous or intramuscular injection for adults. A suggested dose for children was 100 µg per kg body-weight intravenously.

A detailed account of the pharmacology and clinical uses of phentolamine.— L. Gould and C. V. R. Reddy, *Am. Heart J.*, 1976, *92*, 397.

Further references: M. Zahir and L. Gould, *J. clin. Pharmac.*, 1971, *11*, 197; P. J. Logsdon *et al.*, *J. Allergy & clin. Immunol.*, 1973, *52*, 148; J. Zener and D. C. Harrison, *Cardiovasc. Res.*, 1973, *7*, 748; B. Pfister and P. R. Imhof, *Ciba-Geigy, Switz.*, *Eur. J. clin. Pharmac.*, 1977, *11*, 7; D. A. Richards *et al.*, *Br. J. clin. Pharmac.*, 1978, *5*, 507.

Asthma. In a study of 6 patients with asthma phentolamine alone had no bronchodilator action but it enhanced the bronchodilation produced by isoprenaline. This effect could be due to alpha-adrenoceptor blockade by phentolamine leaving the effect of isoprenaline beta-adrenoceptors unopposed.— A. Geumei *et al.* (letter), *Br. J. clin. Pharmac.*, 1975, *2*, 539.

Variable response among 68 asthmatic patients given phentolamine 5 mg per ml by inhalation.— S. L. Spector (letter), *New Engl. J. Med.*, 1979, *301*, 388.

Further references: P. J. Logsdon *et al.* (letter), *Lancet*, 1972, *2*, 232; K. R. Patel and J. W. Kerr (letter), *ibid.*, 1975, *1*, 348; G. N. Gross *et al.*, *Chest*, 1974, *66*, 397.

Blood-sugar concentrations. A 15-year-old boy in an acute diabetic state with a blood-sugar concentration of 3.55 mg per ml was given phentolamine 1 mg intravenously followed by 8 mg over the next 4 hours. His blood sugar fell over a period of hours.— L. Cegrell (letter), *Lancet*, 1972, *2*, 1421.

A study in patients undergoing elective surgery indicated that stress-induced suppression of insulin secretion is blocked by phentolamine.— K. Nakao and M. Miyata, *Eur. J. clin. Invest.*, 1977, *7*, 41.

Cardiac disorders. Phentolamine 50 mg four times a day by mouth, increased if necessary to 400 mg daily, abolished premature ventricular contractions in 15 of 21 episodes in 18 patients and reduced their frequency in a further 5 episodes.— L. Gould *et al.*, *Br. Heart J.*, 1971, *33*, 101.

Phentolamine given by continuous intravenous injection at a rate of 300 µg per minute to 10 patients with chronic pulmonary heart disease effectively reduced the mean pulmonary artery pressure and pulmonary vascular resistance.— L. Gould *et al.*, *J. clin. Pharmac.*, 1972, *12*, 153. Phentolamine administered intravenously in a dose of 300 µg per minute for 15 minutes to 30 patients with supraventricular premature beats was effective in reducing or abolishing them in 22. No side-effects were noted.— *idem*, 356.

In 6 patients with chronic hypertension and 5 with acute hypertension following cardiac infarction, the infusion of phentolamine at an initial rate of 750 µg per minute reduced the elevated left ventricular filling pressure and reduced arterial pressure and systemic resistance. Myocardial oxygen requirements were reduced in those with acute hypertension.— D. T. Kelly *et al.*, *Circulation*, 1973, *47*, 729.

In a double-blind study on 39 patients who had suffered an acute cardiac infarction in the previous 24 hours, phentolamine 200 mg daily gave effective prophylaxis against arrhythmias.— L. Gould *et al.*, *J. clin. Pharmac.*, 1975, *15*, 191.

A slight improvement in cardiac function and decrease in pulmonary congestion was seen in 45 patients with severe heart failure given sustained-release phentolamine in addition to digitalis and diuretics. In a further 34 patients with less severe heart failure phentolamine increased the exercise tolerance.— A. J. Georgopoulos *et al.*, *Eur. J. clin. Pharmac.*, 1978, *13*, 325.

Further references: J. -F. Enrico *et al.*, *Schweiz. med. Wschr.*, 1971, *101*, 325; R. Haider and S. P. Singh (letter), *Br. med. J.*, 1970, *4*, 307; D. M. Krikler (letter), *ibid.*, 558; P. A. Majid *et al.*, *ibid.*, 328; *idem*, *Lancet*, 1971, *2*, 719; P. Walinsky *et al.*, *Am. J. Cardiol.*, 1974, *33*, 37; R. J. Henning *et al.*, *Am. J. Med.*, 1977, *63*, 568.

Hypertension. When 10 hypertensive patients taking oxprenolol and cyclopenthiazide and not maximally controlled were given phentolamine 60 or 120 mg daily in a double-blind study no further significant lowering of blood pressure occurred.— J. F. Winchester *et al.*, *Br. J. clin. Pharmac.*, 1976, *3*, 863.

Phaeochromocytoma. A woman with phaeochromocytoma who had refused operation had taken phentolamine hydrochloride continuously for about 9 years. The dose was 25 mg every 3 hours during waking hours, the first dose being taken between 4 and 5 a.m. Antihypertensive drugs were also given.— J. E. Bellas, *J. Am. med. Ass.*, 1963, *185*, 601.

Though phentolamine and histamine tests were valuable specialised diagnostic tests for phaeochromocytoma, for purposes of primary screening the advantages of simplicity and reliability lay with methoxycatecholamine determinations. This latter method, while no more expensive, was also highly accurate and safe.— J. R. Crout (letter), *J. Am. med. Ass.*, 1966, *198*, 90. See also G. Spergel *et al.*, *ibid.*, 1970, *211*, 266; *ibid.*, 292. Similar reports: S. H. Taylor *et al.*, *Circulation*, 1965, *31*, 741; D. E. Santos *et al.*, *Archs intern. Med.*, 1966, *117*, 752.

Experience in 1 patient suggested that phentolamine might be useful in the localisation of phaeochromocytoma since localised pain was experienced following rapid injection.— J. P. Simmonds *et al.* (letter), *Lancet*, 1974, *2*, 1452.

Shock. Four patients with septic shock experienced immediate and marked benefit after treatment with phentolamine, which appeared to increase tissue perfusion.— E. Jacob *et al.*, *Harefuah*, 1972, *83*, 189, per *J. Am. med. Ass.*, 1972, *222*, 727.

Preparations of Phentolamine Salts

Phentolamine Hydrochloride Tablets *(U.S.P.)*. Phentolamine Tablets *(B.P. 1963)*. Tablets containing phentolamine hydrochloride.

Phentolamine Injection *(B.P.)*. Phentolamine Mesylate Injection. A sterile solution of phentolamine mesylate in Water for Injections containing anhydrous dextrose and sodium metabisulphite. pH 3.5 to 5. Protect from light.

Phentolamine Mesylate for Injection *(U.S.P.)*. Sterile phentolamine mesylate or a sterile mixture of phentolamine mesylate with a suitable buffer or diluents. A freshly prepared 1% solution has a pH of 4.5 to 6.5.

Proprietary Preparations

Rogitine *(Ciba, UK)*. Phentolamine mesylate, available as an injection containing 10 mg per ml, in ampoules of 1 ml and 5 ml. (Also available as Rogitine in *Canad.*, *NZ*).

Other Proprietary Names

(hydrochloride or mesylate) Regitin *(Denm., Ger., Ital., Norw., Swed., Switz.)*; Regitina *(Arg.)*; Regitine *(Austral., Belg., Neth., S.Afr., USA)*.

918-j

Piperoxan Hydrochloride *(B.P.C. 1963)*. Piperoxane Hydrochloride; Benzodioxane Hydrochloride; Compound 933F; Fourneau 933. 2-Piperidinomethyl-1,4-benzodioxan hydrochloride.
$C_{14}H_{19}NO_2$,HCl=269.8.

CAS — 59-39-2 (piperoxan); 135-87-5 (hydrochloride).

A white odourless crystalline powder with a bitter acid taste. **Soluble** 1 in 3.5 of water and 1 in 12 of alcohol; soluble in chloroform; very slightly soluble in ether. A 1% solution in water has a pH of about 5. Solutions are **sterilised** by autoclaving or by filtration.

Piperoxan hydrochloride is an alpha-adrenoceptor blocking agent with actions and uses similar to those of phentolamine mesylate (p.159). It was formerly used for the diagnosis of phaeochromocytoma and for the control of hypertension during the surgical removal of the tumour. It was given in doses of 10 to 20 mg intravenously.

Animal prolactin evidence for antipsychotic activity of piperoxan.— M. S. Gold *et al.* (letter), *Lancet*, 1977, *2*, 96.

For the effect of piperoxan on clonidine, see Clonidine Hydrochloride, p.140.

895-d

Potassium Thiocyanate *(B.P.C. 1954)*. Kalium Rhodanatum; Potassium Sulphocyanate; Potassium Sulphocyanide; Potassium Rhodanate; Potassium Rhodanide. KCNS=97.18.

CAS — 333-20-0.

Pharmacopoeias. In *Aust.*, *Chin.*, and *Hung.*

Colourless odourless deliquescent crystals with a saline taste. **Soluble** 1 in 0.5 of water, 1 in 10 of alcohol, and 1 in 15 of dehydrated alcohol. A 10% solution in water is not alkaline to bromothymol blue. When dissolved in its own weight of water the temperature drops about 30°. **Incompatible** with copper, iron, mercury, and silver salts.

The apparent reduction in thiocyanate content of an aqueous solution of potassium thiocyanate on autoclaving was not excessive. However it might be advisable to consider filtration as a method of sterilisation.— Pharm. Soc. Lab. Rep. P/76/9, 1976.

Uses. Potassium thiocyanate was formerly used in doses of 50 to 300 mg thrice daily to treat hypertension. It was superseded by less toxic and more efficient hypotensive agents, but the hypotensive action of thiocyanate has subsequently been developed in the use of sodium nitroprusside (p.166).

896-n

Prazosin Hydrochloride. CP 12,299-1;

Furazosin Hydrochloride. 1-(4-Amino-6,7-dimethoxyquinazolin-2-yl)-4-(2-furoyl)piperazine hydrochloride.
$C_{19}H_{21}N_5O_4$,HCl=419.9.

CAS — 19216-56-9(prazosin); 19237-84-4 (hydrochloride).

A white to tan-coloured powder. M.p. about 264° with decomposition.

Adverse Effects. Sudden collapse may follow the initial dose of prazosin.

Side-effects commonly include nasal congestion, dryness of mouth, depression, diarrhoea, drowsiness, headache, postural hypotension, lethargy, nausea, nervousness, oedema, chest pain, and palpitations. Constipation, dyspnoea, urinary frequency, blurred vision, paraesthesia, reddened sclera, tinnitus, skin rashes, pruritus, diaphoresis, syncope, tachycardia, impotence, and vomiting may also occur. Paroxysmal tachycardia and vivid dreams have occurred in association with prazosin.

Of 8 patients treated with prazosin 7 developed severe side-effects: severe hypotension (2), postural hypotension (2), tachycardia (2), and palpitations (1); other side-effects included weakness, dizziness, light-headedness, and diarrhoea.— M. J. Bendall *et al.*, *Br. med. J.*, 1975, *2*, 727.

One patient developed 'flu-like' symptoms and arthritis 10 weeks after starting treatment with prazosin; the symptoms recurred when prazosin was given again.— S. A. Cairns and S. C. Jordan, *Br. med. J.*, 1976, *2*, 1424.

Persistent painful erection in 2 men taking prazosin.— A. K. Bhalla *et al.*, *Br. med. J.*, 1979, *2*, 1039.

Hypothermia, recurring on challenge, in a woman given prazosin.— P. W. de Leeuw and W. H. Birkenhäger, *Br. med. J.*, 1980, *281*, 1181.

Metabolic effects.— C. Barbieri *et al.*, *Clin. Pharmac. Ther.*, 1980, *27*, 313. See also P. Leren *et al.*, *Lancet*, 1980, *2*, 4.

Antinuclear factor. Antinuclear factor, without systemic lupus erythematosus, was detected in 19 of 57 patients treated with prazosin.— A. J. Marshall *et al.*, *Br. med. J.*, 1979, *1*, 165. The incidence of antinuclear factor was 9.8% in 132 hypertensive patients taking prazosin compared with 11.6% in 1087 patients taking other antihypertensive agents.— J. D. Wilson *et al.* (letter), *ibid.*,

553. None of 42 patients converted from negative to positive in antinuclear factor tests while under long-term prazosin treatment.— A. Melkild and P. I. Gaarder (letter), *ibid.*, 620. The association between prazosin and antinuclear factor was not proved.— B. Ø. Kristensen (letter), *ibid.*, 621.

First-dose collapse. The Committee on Safety of Medicines reported that sudden collapse with loss of consciousness for periods of time ranging from a few minutes to an hour occurred in over 1% of patients treated with prazosin, usually within 30 to 90 minutes of receiving the initial 2-mg dose.— *Pharm. J.*, 1975, *1*, 228. Reports of the reaction continued to be received. Symptoms had included urinary incontinence, blurred vision, abdominal pain, sweating, giddiness, and pallor; some patients had required admission to hospital. There had been a few reports of serious reactions after a period of uneventful treatment.—Committee on Safety of Medicines, *Current Problems Series No. 1*, Sept 1975.

Three of 10 hypertensive subjects who completed a double-blind crossover study of prazosin suffered postural hypotension 1 to 2 hours after the first dose. The effect was noted with doses as low as 250 to 500 µg, particularly when patients were also taking a beta-adrenoceptor blocking agent or an adrenergic neurone blocking agent such as debrisoquine. During prazosin therapy there was evidence of slight weight gain but fluid retention was not noted.— P. Bolli *et al.*, *Clin. Pharmac. Ther.*, 1976, *20*, 138.

Studies *in vitro* with visceral and peripheral arteries showed evidence of competitive alpha-adrenoceptor antagonism with prazosin 40 and 80 nmol per litre in the visceral but not the peripheral arteries. This might explain the cardiovascular collapse produced by prazosin; selective blockade of visceral sympathetic activity could produce pooling of blood in the viscera with the redistribution of blood volume leading to an acute hypovolaemic state and cardiovascular collapse.— R. F. W. Moulds and R. A. Jauernig (letter), *Lancet*, 1977, *1*, 200. Experience with prazosin alone or with other agents in 25 hypertensive patients appeared to confirm these findings. Orthostatic faintness that was not temporary occurred in 19 and 8 collapsed.— T. Thien *et al.* (letter), *ibid.*, 363.

Further references: R. Gabriel *et al.* (letter), *Lancet*, 1975, *1*, 1095; Y. K. Seedat *et al.* (letter), *Br. med. J.*, 1975, *3*, 305; C. Rosendorff, *ibid.*, 1976, *2*, 508; A. S. Turner (letter), *ibid.*, 1257; R. M. Graham *et al.*, *ibid.*, 1293; G. S. Stokes *et al.*, *ibid.*, 1977, *1*, 1507.

Urinary incontinence. Urinary incontinence in a 58-year-old woman was probably due to prazosin which appeared to cause alpha-adrenoceptor blockade.— T. Thien *et al.*, *Br. med. J.*, 1978, *1*, 622.

Treatment of Adverse Effects. If overdosage occurs the stomach should be emptied by aspiration and lavage. Severe hypotension may respond to placing the patient in the supine position with the feet raised. The effects of gross overdosage may be treated by the cautious intravenous infusion of a pressor agent such as metaraminol.

A 19-year-old man who had taken 200 mg of prazosin had a pulse-rate of 110 per minute and blood pressure of 120/80 mmHg after 90 minutes. Emesis was induced. Over the next 2 hours his pulse-rate rose to 140 per minute. He recovered after bed-rest for 36 hours with no serious after-effects.— W. J. McClean (letter), *Med. J. Aust.*, 1976, *1*, 592.

Precautions. Adrenaline should not be given to antagonise the hypotensive effects of prazosin in overdosage since it may enhance any cardiac-accelerating effects which may occur; the hypotensive effects of prazosin are enhanced by thiazide diuretics.

Prazosin gradually increased to a dose of 4 mg thrice daily for 2 weeks was given to 10 patients with severe congestive heart failure. It was then abruptly withdrawn and the heart condition of 3 deteriorated markedly. Prazosin, and possibly other vasodilators, must be used with extreme caution in patients with chronic heart failure.— S. P. Hanley *et al.*, *Lancet*, 1980, *1*, 735. Severe criticism.— J. E. F. Pohl and A. C. Burden (letter), *ibid.*, 1032.

Interactions. A patient who was taking chlorpromazine and amitriptyline developed acute agitation on receiving prazosin. The symptoms settled rapidly when prazosin was discontinued.— P. Bolli and F. O. Simpson (letter), *Br. med. J.*, 1974, *1*, 637.

The hypotensive effect of prazosin was prolonged if glyceryl trinitrate was given concurrently.— J. Raftos, *Drugs*, 1976, *11*, 55.

Reduction of prazosin-induced hypotension by indomethacin in 4 of 9 subjects.— P. Rubin *et al.*, *Br. J. clin. Pharmac.*, 1980, *10*, 33.

Absorption and Fate. Prazosin is readily absorbed from the gastro-intestinal tract and excreted mainly in the form of metabolites. Less than 10% is excreted unchanged in the urine. Its duration of action is longer than would be predicted from its relatively short plasma half-life of about 4 hours.

In a study of 10 healthy subjects who received prazosin 5 mg by mouth after fasting overnight, peak plasma concentrations of about 23 ng per ml were reached after 2 or 3 hours. There was some variation in absorption-rate: 2 subjects achieved peak concentrations after 1 hour, 1 after 4 hours, and 1 after 5 hours. There was less variation in the elimination-rate, the mean plasma half-life being 3.8 hours. Prazosin had a marked effect on standing blood pressure without affecting supine blood pressure—subjects felt faint during the first 3 or 4 hours and 2 subjects felt too faint for nearly 6 and 10 hours respectively to allow standing blood pressure to be recorded.— A. J. Wood *et al.* (letter), *Br. J. clin. Pharmac.*, 1976, *3*, 199.

Further references: J. A. Taylor *et al.*, *Xenobiotica*, 1977, *7*, 357; D. N. Bateman *et al.*, *Eur. J. clin. Pharmac.*, 1979, *16*, 177; D. T. Lowenthal *et al.*, *Clin. Pharmac. Ther.*, 1980, *27*, 779; N. P. Chau *et al.*, *ibid.*, 1980, *28*, 6; M. K. Dynon *et al.*, *Clin. Pharmacokinet.*, 1980, *5*, 583.

Protein binding. Prazosin was weakly bound to bovine serum albumin *in vitro* and was considered unlikely to interfere with the protein binding of other drugs in usual doses.— A. Crispino and F. Di Carlo, *Farmaco, Edn prat.*, 1978, *33*, 22.

Prazosin was extensively bound to plasma proteins; in 14 healthy subjects the mean free fraction was 0.051; this was increased to 0.064, 0.077, and 0.064 respectively in patients with cirrhosis, chronic renal failure, and congestive heart failure. The free fraction was not affected by propranolol.— P. Rubin and T. Blaschke, *Br. J. clin. Pharmac.*, 1980, *9*, 177.

An extensive review of the clinical pharmacokinetics of prazosin. The binding of prazosin to plasma proteins (97%) was reported not to be affected by propranolol, phenytoin, methyldopa, dicoumarol, phenobarbitone, polythiazide, or chlordiazepoxide.— P. Jaillon, *Clin. Pharmacokinet.*, 1980, *5*, 365.

Uses. Prazosin is an antihypertensive agent the mode of action of which is unclear; some sources claim that it causes peripheral arteriolar vasodilatation whereas others consider it to act by selective blockade of post-synaptic alpha-adrenoceptors. It reduces both standing and supine blood pressure.

Prazosin is used in the treatment of all grades of hypertension. To lessen the risk of collapse which may occur in some patients after the first dose (see Adverse Effects) the usual initial dose of prazosin hydrochloride is 500 µg twice or thrice daily for at least 3 days, the starting dose being given in the evening; if tolerated the dose may then be increased to 1 mg thrice daily, and thereafter gradually increased, according to the patient's response, to a usual maximum of 20 mg daily in divided doses. Although sources in Great Britain recommend 20 mg as a maximum daily dose, sources in the USA report that a few patients may obtain benefit from up to 40 mg daily in divided doses. To reduce side-effects smaller doses of prazosin may be given in conjunction with a thiazide diuretic.

Prazosin is used in the treatment of congestive heart failure; tolerance may develop.

Prazosin possesses specificity for postsynaptic alpha-adrenoceptors; this explains why its administration, unlike that of conventional alpha-adrenoceptor blocking agents, does not provoke tachycardia, tolerance, and renin release.— D. Cambridge *et al.*, *Br. J. Pharmac.*, 1977, *59*, 514P. See also C. V. S. Ram *et al.*, *Clin. Pharmac. Ther.*, 1981, *29*, 719.

A detailed review of prazosin, including comments on pharmacological studies on those properties which are of clinical significance, such as selective postsynaptic alpha-adrenoceptor blockade, and those which are unlikely to be of clinical significance at therapeutic doses, such as phosphodiesterase and dopamine beta-hydroxylase inhibition.— R. M. Graham and W. A. Pettinger, *New Engl. J. Med.*, 1979, *300*, 232.

For references to further reviews see under Hypertension (below).

Further references.— P. C. Rubin and T. F. Blaschke, *Br. J. clin. Pharmac.*, 1980, *10*, 23; *Curr. med. Res. Opinion*, 1980, *6*, *Supp.* 9, 1.

Administration in renal failure. Prazosin 2 to 6 mg daily added to the existing antihypertensive regimen of 7 patients with chronic renal failure and 5 patients with renal transplants who were also suffering from renal failure was an effective antihypertensive agent. One patient developed severe postural hypotension after receiving 1 mg thrice daily for 1 week; subsequently all patients with chronic renal failure were started on a dose of 1 mg twice daily. Since only 3 to 4% of a dose of prazosin was excreted in the urine in 24 hours increased sensitivity in renal failure was unlikely to be due to accumulation. One patient developed an erythema nodosum-like skin eruption after receiving prazosin for about 5 weeks but this was probably associated with concomitant propranolol therapy.— J. R. Curtis and F. J. ABateman, *Br. med. J.*, 1975, *4*, 432. See also J. M. Hayes *et al.* (letter), *ibid.*, 1974, *4*, 108.

Prazosin could be given in usual doses to patients with renal failure.— W. M. Bennett *et al.*, *Ann. intern. Med.*, 1980, *93*, 286.

Asthma. Bronchodilator effect in 2 subjects with asthma.— G. E. Marlin *et al.* (letter), *Lancet*, 1981, *1*, 225. Comment.— P. Barnes (letter), *ibid.*, 391.

Cardiac disease. A preliminary study in 10 patients with severe ischaemic cardiomyopathy and heart failure indicated that prazosin 2 to 7 mg by mouth had a beneficial effect on congestive heart failure by producing a relatively prolonged reduction in both cardiac preload and impedance.— R. R. Miller *et al.*, *New Engl. J. Med.*, 1977, *297*, 303. Comment.— E. Braunwald, *ibid.*, 331.

Studies of the use of prazosin in congestive heart failure, and reports of the development of tolerance.— M. Packer *et al.*, *Am. J. Cardiol.*, 1979, *44*, 310; U. Elkayam *et al.*, *Am. J. Cardiol.*, 1979, *44*, 540; C. E. Desch *et al.*, *Am. J. Cardiol.*, 1979, *44*, 1178; S. B. Arnold *et al.*, *Ann. intern. Med.*, 1979, *91*, 345; S. A. Goldman *et al.*, *Am. J. Med.*, 1980, *68*, 36; W. S. Colucci *et al.*, *Am. J. Cardiol.*, 1980, *45*, 337; J. Mehta *et al.*, *Br. Heart J.*, 1980, *43*, 556; D. H. Fitchett *et al.*, *Br. Heart J.*, 1980, *44*, 215; O. Bertel, *Cardiology*, 1980, *65*, *Suppl.* 1, 70; S. A. Rubin *et al.*, *Circulation*, 1980, *61*, 543; R. T. Dillon *et al.*, *J. Pediat.*, 1980, *96*, 623; U. Elkayam *et al.*, *Clin. Pharmac. Ther.*, 1981, *30*, 23.

Further references: N. A. Awan *et al.*, *Clin. Pharmac. Ther.*, 1977, *22*, 79; *idem*, *Circulation*, 1977, *56*, 346; N. A. Awan *et al.*, *Am. J. Med.*, 1978, *65*, 146; W. S. Aronow and D. T. Danahy, *ibid.*, 155; J. Mehta *et al.*, *Am. J. Cardiol.*, 1978, *41*, 925; W. S. Aronow *et al.*, *Circulation*, 1979, *59*, 344; S. A. Rubin *et al.*, *Am. J. Cardiol.*, 1979, *43*, 810.

Hypertension. Reviews of prazosin in hypertension: R. N. Brogden *et al.*, *Drugs*, 1977, *14*, 163; *Med. J. Aust.*, 1977, *2*, *Suppl.*1, 1-53; *Med. Lett.*, 1977, *19*, 1; P. E. Groth and B. Lee, *Drug Intell. & clin. Pharm.*, 1978, *12*, 22; *Aust. J. Pharm.*, 1979, *60*, 29; R. M. Graham and W. A. Pettinger, *New Engl. J. Med.*, 1979, *300*, 232.

A summary of clinical experience, as submitted to the FDA, in more than 1000 patients treated with prazosin yielded the following information: the antihypertensive effect was due to a fall in total peripheral resistance without significant tachycardia or effect on cardiac output; renal haemodynamics were not compromised; prazosin might be used in patients with impaired renal function. Antihypertensive activity was comparable with that of methyldopa or thiazide diuretics; the effect of prazosin was enhanced by thiazides. Side-effects, possibly drug-related, in 934 patients included blurred vision (36), dry mouth (42), constipation (21), postural dizziness (138), oedema (41), palpitations (54), dyspnoea (20), syncope (13), tachycardia (2), headache (79), depression (23), drowsiness (77), nervousness (24), vertigo (22), nasal congestion (37), sweating (9), nausea (49), vomiting (15), diarrhoea (15), urinary frequency (37), impotence (6), skin rash (10), pruritus (8), lack of energy (70), weakness (66), insomnia (2), and malaise (2). More than 50% of patients experienced no side-effects; less than 9% had to discontinue treatment. There was a low incidence of abnormalities in laboratory estimation of blood, hepatic, renal, metabolic, and electrolyte values.— N. E. Pitts, *Prazosin*, Proceedings of a Symposium, Amsterdam, Excerpta Medica, 1974, p. 149.

A study suggesting that prazosin may be effective if given twice daily.— A. S. P. Hua *et al.*, *Med. J. Aust.*, 1978, *1*, 45. Correspondence: R. Zacest and C. L. Wilson (letter), *ibid.*, 443; P. Kincaid-Smith (letter), *ibid.*, 444.

Of 35 patients with renal or essential hypertension who started therapy with prazosin and were followed up for up to 19 months, 11 ceased treatment within 3 months and a further 7 withdrew in the next 16 months. Withdrawal was because of postural hypotension (8), poor control of blood pressure (6), or myocardial infarction (1). Control of blood pressure had been obtained in 17 patients. Three patients developed angina while on prazosin and one with dubious chest pain developed definite angina. It was suggested that prazosin should not be used as initial treatment of hypertension and that it might be of use when other agents had failed or were contra-indicated.— L. E. Ramsay, *Practitioner*, 1979, *222*, 127.

Further references: A. S. P. Hua *et al.*, *Med. J. Aust.*, 1976, *1*, 559; J. M. Hayes *et al.*, *ibid.*, 562; M. C. Koshy *et al.*, *Circulation*, 1977, *55*, 533; A. J. Marshall *et al.*, *Lancet*, 1977, *1*, 271; Y. K. Seedat *et al.*, *Curr. med. Res. Opinion*, 1977, *4*, 627; A. S. Turner *et al.*, *N.Z. med. J.*, 1977, *86*, 282 and 286; M. S. Kochar *et al.*, *Clin. Pharmac. Ther.*, 1979, *25*, 143.

Comparative studies of prazosin with other antihypertensive agents: G. S. Stokes and M. A. Weber, *Br. med. J.*, 1974, *2*, 298 (methyldopa and propranolol); W. J. Mroczek and F. A. Finnerty, *Prazosin*, Proceedings of a Symposium, Amsterdam, Excerpta Medica, 1974, p. 92 (methyldopa); H. Adriaensen and R. Vryens, *Practitioner*, 1975, *214*, 268 (methyldopa); A. Hua and P. Kincaid-Smith (letter), *Br. med. J.*, 1974, *3*, 804 (hydralazine); K. Rasmussen and H. A. Jensen (letter), *ibid.*, 1975, *4*, 346 (hydralazine); A. S. P. Hua *et al.*, *Med. J. Aust.*, 1977, *2*, 5 (hydralazine); W. F. Bradley *et al.*, *Curr. ther. Res.*, 1977, *21*, 28 (methyldopa); A. Schirger and S. G. Sheps, *J. Am. med. Ass.*, 1977, *237*, 989 (hydrochlorothiazide); W. M. Kirkendall *et al.*, *ibid.*, 1978, *240*, 2553 (clonidine); G. S. Stokes *et al.*, *Clin. Pharmac. Ther.*, 1979, *25*, 783 (indoramin).

Raynaud's disease. Raynaud's phenomenon in a 66-year-old woman with mild essential hypertension improved after therapy with prazosin.— B. R. Appleby (letter), *Med. J. Aust.*, 1978, *2*, 437.

Prazosin produced a degree of dilatation of preconstricted veins which was about 17 times greater than the increase it produced in arterial blood flow in a study of healthy subjects. Increases in arterial blood flow were dose-dependent. Prazosin had a similar potency as a venodilator and dilator of arteries to glyceryl trinitrate and sodium nitroprusside, and was 10 000 times more potent as a venodilator and 1000 times more potent as a dilator of arteries than tolmesoxide and diazoxide.— J. G. Collier *et al.*, *Br. J. clin. Pharmac.*, 1978, *5*, 35.

The successful use of prazosin hydrochloride 2 mg daily for the treatment of Raynaud's disease in 1 patient.— R. Waldo, *J. Am. med. Ass.*, 1979, *241*, 1037.

Comments on the use of prazosin in peripheral vascular disease.— W. N. Beaucher (letter), *New Engl. J. Med.*, 1979, *301*, 159; J. D. Coffman (letter), *New Engl. J. Med.*, 1979, *301*, 159.

Proprietary Preparations

Hypovase *(Pfizer, UK)*. Prazosin hydrochloride, available as tablets of 500 µg and as scored tablets of 1, 2, and 5 mg.

Other Proprietary Names

Minipres *(Arg.)*; Minipress *(Austral., Belg., Canad., Ger., Ital., Neth., S.Afr., Switz., USA)*; Peripress *(Denm., Norw., Swed.)*.

Prazosin hydrochloride was also formerly marketed in Great Britain under the proprietary name Sinetens (*Farmitalia Carlo Erba*).

916-l

Protoveratrine A. Protoverine 6,7-diacetate 3(*S*)-(2-hydroxy-2-methylbutyrate) 15(*R*)-(2-methylbutyrate).
$C_{41}H_{63}NO_{14}$=793.5.

CAS — 143-57-7.

An alkaloid from white veratrum, *Veratrum album* (Liliaceae).

917-y

Protoveratrine B. Protoverine 6,7-diacetate 3(*S*)-(2,3-dihydroxy-2-methylbutyrate) 15(*R*)-(2-methylbutyrate).
$C_{41}H_{63}NO_{15}$=809.9.

CAS — 124-97-0.

An alkaloid from white veratrum.

897-h

Protoveratrines A and B

CAS — 8053-18-7.

A white, odourless, slightly bitter, crystalline powder with a strong sternutatory action. Practically **insoluble** in water and light petroleum; soluble in chloroform; very slightly soluble in ether. A saturated solution in water has a pH of 6.5 to 7.3. Solutions of pH 4 to 6 are stable, but in alkaline and alcoholic solutions it is rapidly decomposed.

Adverse Effects, Treatment, and Precautions. As for Alkavervir, p.136.

Uses. Protoveratrines A and B have been used for the same purposes as alkavervir (see p.136). The 2 alkaloids possess the same action but protoveratrine B is less active than protoveratrine A. For the management of pre-eclampsia and eclampsia 100 to 400 µg was given intramuscularly at intervals of 1 to 6 hours if necessary. A solution prepared by adding 100 to 500 µg to 1 litre of Dextrose Intravenous Infusion was administered by intravenous infusion at a rate of 30 drops per minute. Doses of 0.25 to 1 mg were given by mouth every 2 to 4 hours according to the patient's response.
Doses of 500 µg by mouth after meals and at bedtime were given in the treatment of hypertension. The average effective dose was from 0.4 to 1.5 mg four times daily.

Proprietary Names
Pro-Amid (protoveratrine A) *(Amid, USA)*.

Protoveratrines A and B were formerly marketed in Great Britain under the proprietary name Puroverine (*Sandoz*).

898-m

Rauwolfia Serpentina *(B.P.C. 1973, U.S.P.)*. Rauwolfia; Rauvolfia; Chotachand; Rauwolfiae Radix; Rauwolfiawurzel.

CAS — 8063-17-0 (rauwolfia).

Pharmacopoeias. In *Fr.* and *Ger.* (not less than 1% of alkaloids); in *Ind.* (not less than 0.8% of alkaloids); and *U.S.* (not less than 0.15%).
Ind. specifies dried roots with bark intact, collected in autumn from plants 3 to 4 years old.

The dried roots of *Rauwolfia serpentina* (Apocynaceae). It contains not less than 0.15% of reserpine-like alkaloids.
Rauwolfia serpentina contains numerous alkaloids, the most active as hypotensive agents being the ester alkaloids, reserpine and rescinnamine. Other alkaloids present have structures related to reserpic acid, but are not esterified, and include ajmaline (rauwolfine), ajmalinine, ajmalicine, isoajmaline (isorauwolfine), serpentine, rauwolfinine, and sarpagine. **Store** at 15° to 30°.

Adverse Effects, Treatment, and Precautions. As for Reserpine, p.163.

Uses. The actions of rauwolfia serpentina are those of its alkaloids and it is used for the same purposes as reserpine, p.164. It is administered by mouth as the powdered whole root, in initial doses of 200 mg daily in 2 divided doses for 1 to 3 weeks, and maintenance doses of 50 to 300 mg daily.
The crude drug has been used in India for centuries in the treatment of insomnia and certain forms of mental illness, in doses up to 1 to 2 g.

Preparations

Powdered Rauwolfia Serpentina *(U.S.P.)*. Rauwolfia serpentina reduced to a fine or very fine powder and adjusted to contain 0.15 to 0.2% of reserpine-rescinnamine group alkaloids, calculated as reserpine. Store at 15° to 30°.

Rauwolfia Dry Extract *(Ind. P.)*. Dry Rauwolfia Extract. Prepared by percolation with alcohol (90%); the percolate is evaporated at not more than 60° under reduced pressure to a soft extract, starch is added, and the product dried; it is standardised to contain 4% w/w of the total alkaloids of rauwolfia. *Dose.* 15 to 60 mg.

Rauwolfia Liquid Extract *(Ind. P.)*. Liquid Rauwolfia Extract. Prepared by percolation with alcohol (90%) and standardised to contain 1% w/v of the total alkaloids of rauwolfia. *Dose.* 0.2 to 0.5 ml.

Rauwolfia Serpentina Tablets *(U.S.P.)*. Tablets containing powdered rauwolfia serpentina. Store in airtight containers. Protect from light.

Proprietary Preparations

Hypercal *(Carlton Laboratories, UK)*. A mixture of selected alkaloids of rauwolfia serpentina including reserpine and rescinnamine, available as tablets of 2 mg. For hypertension. **Hypercal-B.** Tablets containing, in addition, amylobarbitone 15 mg. *Dose.* Hypercal: 1 tablet night and morning or 2 tablets at night; Hypercal-B: 1 or 2 tablets at night.

Raudixin *(Squibb, UK)*. Rauwolfia serpentina, available as tablets of 50 mg. (Also available as Raudixin in *Austral., Canad., USA*).

Rautrax *(Squibb, UK)*. Tablets each containing rauwolfia serpentina 50 mg, hydroflumethiazide 50 mg, and potassium chloride 625 mg (potassium 8.4 mmol; 8.4 mEq). For hypertension. *Dose.* Initial, 1 to 3 tablets daily; maintenance, 1 tablet daily.

Other Proprietary Names
Bagoserfia *(Arg.)*; Rauval *(USA)*; Rauwolfinetas *(Spain)*; Rawlina *(Austral.)*; Rivadescin *(Ger., Switz.)*; Serenol *(Austral.)*; Serpetin *(Jap.)*; Tensowolfia *(Spain)*.

Rauwolfia serpentina was also formerly marketed in Great Britain under the proprietary names Hypertane and Hypertensan (both *Medo-Chemicals*). Preparations containing rauwolfia serpentina were formerly marketed in Great Britain under the proprietary names Hypertane Compound, Hypertane Forte (both *Medo-Chemicals*), Mio-Pressin (*Smith Kline & French*), and Rautrax sine K (*Squibb*).

899-b

Rauwolfia Vomitoria *(B.P.C. 1973)*. African Rauwolfia; Rauwolfia Africana.

CAS — 8063-17-0 (rauwolfia).

The dried roots of *Rauwolfia vomitoria* (Apocynaceae). It contains not less than 0.2% of reserpine-like alkaloids.

Rauwolfia vomitoria is used for the production of reserpine.

900-b

Rescinnamine. Methyl 18-*O*-(3,4,5-trimethoxycinnamoyl)reserpate.
$C_{35}H_{42}N_2O_9$=634.7.

CAS — 24815-24-5.

A white or pale buff- to cream-coloured, odourless, crystalline powder. It slowly darkens on exposure to light but more rapidly when in solution. M.p. about 226°. Practically **insoluble** in water; soluble in alcohol, acetic acid, and chloroform. **Store** in airtight containers. Protect from light.

Uses. Rescinnamine has actions and uses similar to those described under reserpine (see below). For the treatment of hypertension it is given in initial doses of 0.25 to 1 mg daily for up to 14 days, and maintenance doses of 250 to 500 µg daily.

Proprietary Names
Anaprel *(Eutherapie, Belg.)*; Cartric *(Jap.)*; Cinnasil *(Amfre-Grant, USA)*; Moderil *(Pfizer, USA)*; Rescimin *(Torlan, Spain)*.

Rescinnamine was formerly marketed in Great Britain under the proprietary name Anaprel 500 (*Servier*).

901-v

Reserpine *(B.P., B.P. Vet., Eur. P.).* Reserpinum. Methyl 11,17α-dimethoxy-18β-(3,4,5-trimethoxybenzoyloxy)-3β,20α-yohimbane-16β-carboxylate; Methyl 18-*O*-(3,4,5-trimethoxybenzoyl)reserpate.

$C_{33}H_{40}N_2O_9$=608.7.

CAS — 50-55-5.

Pharmacopoeias. In *Arg., Aust., Belg., Br., Braz., Cz., Eur., Fr., Ger., Hung., Ind., Int., It., Jap., Jug., Neth., Nord., Pol., Roum., Rus., Swiss, Turk.,* and *U.S.*

An alkaloid obtained from the roots of certain species of *Rauwolfia* (Apocynaceae), mainly *Rauwolfia serpentina* and *R. vomitoria,* or by synthesis. The material obtained from natural sources may contain closely related alkaloids.

It occurs as odourless, almost tasteless, fine, white or pale buff to slightly yellow-coloured cyrstals or crystalline powder. M.p. about 270° with decomposition. It darkens slowly on exposure to light but more rapidly when in solution.

Practically **insoluble** in water and ether; soluble 1 in 2000 of alcohol, 1 in 90 of acetone, 1 in 6 of chloroform, and 1 in 2000 of methyl alcohol; freely soluble in acetic acid. A solution in chloroform is laevorotatory. Solutions may be **sterilised** by filtration. **Store** in airtight containers. Protect from light.

Reserpine and its preparations discoloured rapidly when exposed to light but loss in potency was usually small. Solutions in benzene or chloroform were very sensitive to light, losing potency almost as soon as exposed.— A. F. Leyden *et al., J. Am. pharm. Ass., scient. Edn,* 1956, *45,* 771.

Butylated hydroxyanisole, hydroquinone, nordihydroguaiaretic acid, and propyl gallate were shown to prevent oxidation of reserpine during preparation of tablets. The antioxidants did not prevent deterioration of the tablets when stored in daylight.— O. Weis-Fogh, *Arch. Pharm. Chemi,* 1958, *65,* 859.

Preparations of reserpine must be protected from light during manufacture and storage, and from oxidation by the exclusion of free oxygen or by the addition of an antioxidant other than sodium metabisulphite.— O. Weis-Fogh, *Pharm. Acta Helv.,* 1960, *35,* 442, per *Am. J. Hosp. Pharm.,* 1960, *17,* 772. See also A. F. Asker *et al., Pharmazie,* 1971, *26,* 90, per *Pharm. J.,* 1971, *2,* 32.

For a report of an incompatibility with ethacrynic acid, see Ethacrynic Acid, p.594.

Adverse Effects. Side-effects commonly include nasal congestion, dryness of mouth, depression, drowsiness, lethargy, nightmares, diarrhoea, gastro-intestinal upsets, and vertigo; dyspnoea, pruritus, and skin rashes sometimes occur and a few patients show an increase in appetite and weight.

Higher doses may cause flushing, cardiac arrhythmias, an angina-like syndrome, bradycardia, severe depression which may lead to suicide, and occasionally a parkinsonian-like syndrome.

Paradoxical anxiety, blurred vision, breast engorgement and galactorrhoea, gynaecomastia, disturbance of ejaculation, impotence, epistaxis, headache, difficulty in micturition, sodium retention, oedema, peptic ulceration, and purpura have also been reported. Intramuscular or intravenous injection may cause duodenal ulcers and postural hypotension.

Several reports have suggested that there might be an association between the ingestion of reserpine and the development of neoplasms of the breast (see below) but other surveys have failed to confirm the association.

Excessive bleeding after prostatectomy occurred in 5 of 7 patients taking reserpine but in only 3 of 125 similar patients not taking reserpine. Excessive bleeding in patients taking reserpine was possibly the result of a decrease in reflex vasoconstriction.— D. J. Card and M. Schiff, *J. Urol.,* 1972, *107,* 97.

For a report of a carcinoid syndrome developing in 7 thyrotoxic patients given reserpine, see Hyperthyroidism under Uses.

Bronchospasm. An intramuscular injection of reserpine 1.25 mg given to a middle-aged woman reduced her blood pressure from 180/140 to 130/110 mmHg within 2 hours, but aggravated dyspnoea and induced marked bronchospasm.— J. R. Wise (letter), *New Engl. J. Med.,* 1969, *281,* 563.

Effects on the blood. Thrombocytopenia had been associated with treatment with reserpine; there was a potential hazard to the foetus when reserpine was given to the mother.— M. G. Wilson, *Am. J. Obstet. Gynec.,* 1962, *83,* 818.

Effects on the endocrine system. In a study in 15 women who had taken reserpine for 2 months to 23 years, serum-prolactin concentrations were significantly higher during reserpine treatment than 6 weeks after discontinuing reserpine. Fourteen women were postmenopausal. Only 1 of those took conjugated oestrogen and serum-prolactin concentrations did not fall after discontinuing reserpine in this patient. In 3 men serum concentrations of luteinising hormone were lower after reserpine was discontinued.— P. A. Lee *et al., J. Am. med. Ass.,* 1976, *235,* 2316.

Effects on the eyes. A study indicating that reserpine in usual therapeutic doses interferes slightly with colour vision.— J. Laroche and C. Laroche, *Annls pharm. fr.,* 1972, *30,* 433.

Miosis, lachrymation, and conjunctival hyperaemia were reported to have occurred occasionally during treatment with reserpine.— *Med. Lett.,* 1976, *18,* 63.

Effects on the gastro-intestinal tract. Peripheral vasodilatation occurred in 2 of 12 patients with scleroderma and Raynaud's disease immediately after being given reserpine 1 mg intra-arterially and was followed within 2 hours by an episode of haematemesis.— E. Sharon *et al.* (letter), *Ann. intern. Med.,* 1972, *77,* 479. Comment.— J. T. Willerson, *ibid.*

Effects on mental state. Seventy-seven depressive episodes occurred in 63 of 270 hypertensive patients given continuous treatment with various extracts of rauwolfia. The average period of time between the start of treatment and onset of depression was 6.7 months. Fifty-one of the episodes occurred in patients receiving reserpine in dosages of 750 µg or more daily.— E. Bolte *et al., Can. med. Ass. J.,* 1959, *80,* 291. See also *Med. Lett.,* 1976, *18,* 19.

Lupus erythematosus. Two patients with systemic lupus erythematosus had received prolonged reserpine therapy.— I. Rivero *et al., Arthritis Rheum.,* 1963, *6,* 293.

Neoplasms of the breast. Reviews of reserpine and the risk of breast cancer: *Lancet,* 1974, *2,* 701; *Br. med. J.,* 1974, *4,* 121; H. Jick, *J. Am. med. Ass.,* 1975, *233,* 896.

Of 150 women with newly diagnosed breast cancer 11 (7.3%) had taken preparations containing reserpine, and 10 of these were over 50 years of age. Among 600 matched medical controls 13 (2.2%) had taken reserpine preparations; identical figures were obtained with 600 surgical controls. The rate of exposure to other antihypertensive agents was similar in all groups. The risk ratio for breast cancer among patients taking reserpine relative to the 2 control groups was 3.5. There was a suggestion that reserpine use might be associated with neoplasms of the brain, uterus, pancreas, skin, and kidney.— Report from the Boston Collaborative Drug Surveillance Program, *Lancet,* 1974, *2,* 669.

When a group of 708 patients with breast cancer was examined together with 1430 control patients with other neoplasms the relative risk of breast cancer in patients taking rauwolfia derivatives was 2. This risk increased to the statistically significant figure of 3.9 when patients with neoplasms that might be associated with rauwolfia derivatives were removed from the control group.— B. Armstrong *et al., Lancet,* 1974, *2,* 672. See also *idem,* 1976, *2,* 8.

Analysis of 438 women with breast cancer and 438 controls showed that 53 in the cancer group (all over 50 years of age) had taken reserpine compared with 31 in the control group. In 68 matched pairs, where only 1 member of the pair was taking reserpine, the drug was used by 45 of the cancer patients and by 23 of the control subjects. The risk ratio for breast cancer between users of reserpine and non-users was 2.— O. P. Heinonen *et al., Lancet,* 1974, *2,* 675. In criticising the 3 studies on the risk of breast cancer from rauwolfia derivatives it was considered that the control groups were not truly representative of the use of reserpine, that with patients over the age of 60 the probability of hypertension increased with the probability of breast cancer so that the carcinogenicity of reserpine was illusory, and that there was an imbalance in the age groups.— H. Immich (letter), *ibid.,* 774. Further criticisms: R. D. Mann *et al.* (letter), *ibid.,* 966; C. Siegel and E. Laska (letter), *ibid.* Replies: Boston Collaborative Drug Surveillance Program Research Group (letter), *ibid.,* 1315; O. P. Heinonen and S. Shapiro (letter), *ibid.,* 1316.

There appeared to be no association between hypertension and breast cancer among the 1111 women who developed and died of breast cancer during the American Cancer Society's large-scale prospective study.— L. Garfinkel and E. C. Hammond (letter), *Lancet,* 1974, *2,* 1381.

In a study of 111 cases of breast cancer occurring in an affluent retirement community, matched in each case with 4 controls from the same community, the risk ratio for correlation with use of rauwolfia alkaloids was low and was no higher than that for the use of other drugs.— T. M. Mack *et al., New Engl. J. Med.,* 1975, *292,* 1366.

A study of 450 women with breast cancer and 475 controls with cholelithiasis in Minnesota showed no association between rauwolfia alkaloids and breast cancer.— W. M. O'Fallon *et al., Lancet,* 1975, *2,* 292. A similar report.— E. M. Laska *et al., ibid.,* 296. See also *ibid.,* 312; W. M. O'Fallon and D. R. Larbarthe (letter), *ibid.,* 773; A. Aromaa *et al.* (letter), *ibid.,* 1976, *2,* 518.

A study was carried out in 164 women with breast cancer compared with matched controls. Neither reserpine, methyldopa, nor thiazides were found to be significantly associated with breast cancer.— A. M. Lilienfeld *et al., Johns Hopkins med. J.,* 1976, *139,* 41.

Results of a multicentre study in 995 patients with breast cancer failed to substantiate an association with previous administration of rauwolfia derivatives.— L. J. Christopher *et al., Eur. J. clin. Pharmac.,* 1977, *11,* 409. See also *idem* (letter), *Lancet,* 1977, *1,* 140.

Preliminary results from a study comparing 181 women found to have breast cancer with 307 women with a benign breast disorder and 101 with other conditions requiring surgery did not support the hypothesis that reserpine was associated with breast cancer.— H. Kewitz *et al., Eur. J. clin. Pharmac.,* 1977, *11,* 79.

Absence of an association in about 2000 women.— D. R. Labarthe and M. O'Fallon, *J. Am. med. Ass.,* 1980, *243,* 2304.

Treatment of Adverse Effects. Withdrawal of reserpine or reduction of the dosage causes the reversal of many side-effects. If overdosage occurs the stomach should be emptied by aspiration and lavage. Severe hypotension may respond to placing the patient in the supine position with the feet raised. The effects of gross overdosage may be treated by the cautious infusion of plasma or injection of noradrenaline, phenylephrine, or metaraminol. If there is marked bradycardia, especially with cardiac arrhythmias, vagal blocking agents such as atropine sulphate may be injected together with other appropriate measures. The patient must be observed for at least 72 hours.

A child who took over 1 g of crystalline reserpine survived, apparently without much difficulty.— L. E. Hollister, *Clin. Pharmac. Ther.,* 1966, *7,* 142.

Three children, aged 2½ to 4 years, ingested large doses of reserpine; 2 had taken at least 25 mg between them. Coma, with hypothermia and bradycardia developed, and the urinary excretion of catecholamines rose markedly in 2 children, but 1 had hypertension and tachycardia. Each was treated successfully by gastric lavage, saline enemas, the application of heat during the hypothermic phase, and fluid maintenance for the first 36 hours.— J. M. H. Loggie *et al., Clin. Pharmac. Ther.,* 1967, *8,* 692.

Precautions. Reserpine should not be used in patients with a history of mental depression, with active gastric or duodenal ulcer, or with ulcerative colitis.

It should be used with caution in debilitated patients, and in the presence of cardiac arrhythmias, cardiac infarction, severe cardiac damage, gall-stones, epilepsy, or allergic conditions such as bronchial asthma.

If used in conjunction with electroconvulsive therapy an interval of at least 7 days should be allowed to elapse between the last dose of reserpine and the commencement of the shock treatment.

Hypotension may occur during anaesthesia in patients being treated with reserpine (see p.136) and it has been recommended that sufficient doses of atropine should be given before induction of anaesthesia to prevent excessive bradycardia.

Patients taking reserpine are sensitive to adrenaline and other direct-acting sympathomimetic agents which should not be given except to antagonise reserpine. The hypotensive effects may also be antagonised by indirect-acting sympathomimetic agents such as ephedrine and by tricyclic antidepressants. The hypotensive effects of reserpine are enhanced by thiazide diuretics and may be enhanced by monoamine oxidase inhibitors which should be given with extreme caution since reserpine may cause mania in patients receiving monoamine oxidase inhibitors. Concurrent administration of digitalis or quinidine may cause cardiac arrhythmias.

Interactions. The administration of reserpine could interfere with measurements of urinary 17-hydroxycorticosteroids.— J. M. Rosenberg and I. S. Kampa, *Drug Intell. & clin. Pharm.*, 1973, *7*, 33.

Reserpine might interfere with fluorimetric estimations of urinary catecholamines.— J. Millhouse, *Adverse Drug React. Bull.*, 1974, Dec., 164.

Pregnancy and the neonate. Infant and maternal mortality were reduced by the use of reserpine for toxaemia and hypertension in 2400 pregnant mothers. There was a fair incidence of resultant nasal congestion in the babies delivered but it was stated that serious complications could be avoided by not allowing the affected infants to assume the supine position, by the use of nasal vasoconstrictors, and by duly advising the nursery personnel.— F. A. Finnerty, *J. Am. med. Ass.*, 1956, *160*, 997. See also I. S. Budnick *et al.*, *Am. J. Dis. Child.*, 1955, *90*, 286.

Animal studies indicated that reserpine given during the second part of gestation led to comparable depletion of catecholamine stores in both foetus and mother.— K. Adamsons and I. Joelsson, *Am. J. Obstet. Gynec.*, 1966, *96*, 437.

Reserpine had been shown to interfere with cell proliferation in the developing brain of newborn *rats*.— P. D. Lewis *et al.* (preliminary communication), *Lancet*, 1977, *1*, 399. Further references to *animal* studies: A. S. Goldman and W. C. Yakovac, *Proc. Soc. exp. Biol. Med.*, 1965, *118*, 857.

Two infants developed hypothermia that was associated with maternal ingestion of reserpine.— D. Anagnostakis and N. Matsaniotis (letter), *Lancet*, 1974, *2*, 471.

Reserpine was useful in hypertension of pregnancy but should be withdrawn some days before the expected date of delivery.— I. M. Noble, *Practitioner*, 1974, *212*, 657.

A study of the effect of maternally administered drugs on bilirubin concentrations in 1107 consecutively born infants. Maternally ingested reserpine lowered the infants' serum bilirubin concentrations.— J. H. Drew and W. H. Kitchen, *J. Pediat.*, 1976, *89*, 657.

Of 50 282 children born to mothers monitored by the Collaborative Perinatal Project 48 were found to have been exposed to rauwolfia alkaloids, and possibly other drugs, at some time during the first 4 months of the pregnancy. The findings that 4 of these children were malformed indicated that the teratogenic potential of reserpine and related agents ought to be investigated further.—O. P. Heinonen *et al.*, *Birth Defects and Drugs in Pregnancy*, Littleton MA, Publishing Sciences Group, 1977, p. 371.

Further references: D. E. Sobel, *Archs gen. Psychiat.*, 1960, *2*, 606.

Absorption and Fate. Reserpine is absorbed from the gastro-intestinal tract. About 6% has been reported to be excreted in the urine in the first 24 hours and about 8% in the first 4 days, mainly as the metabolite trimethoxybenzoic acid. Over 60% is excreted in the faeces in the first 4 days, mainly unchanged. Reserpine crosses the placental barrier and also appears in breast milk.

In 6 volunteers, radioactive reserpine, 250 µg in water by mouth, gave peak concentrations in 2 hours ranging from 1.4 to 1.8 ng per ml in whole blood to 1.5 to 3 ng per ml in plasma. Urinary excretion averaged approximately 6% of the dose in 24 hours and 8% in 4 days; the main excretory product was trimethoxybenzoic acid. The plasma half-lives of reserpine were 4.5 and 271 hours. Radioactivity was also detectable in the plasma, urine, and faeces after 11 to 12 days. Radioactivity in the faeces was mainly due to unchanged reserpine.— A. R. Maass *et al.*, *Clin. Pharmac. Ther.*, 1969, *10*, 366.

The biological fate of reserpine.— R. E. Stitzel, *Pharmac. Rev.*, 1977, *28*, 179.

Uses. Reserpine has central depressant and sedative actions and a primarily peripheral antihypertensive effect accompanied by bradycardia. It causes depletion of noradrenaline stores in peripheral sympathetic nerve terminals and depletion of catecholamine and serotonin stores in the brain, heart, and many other organs. When given by mouth its action is slow in onset and continues for many days after withdrawal of treatment. It has a cumulative effect. Tolerance does not develop.

In the treatment of hypertension, reserpine is of most value in patients with mild labile hypertension associated with tachycardia. In patients with severe long-established hypertension, it is best used in conjunction with more potent antihypertensive drugs. The usual dosage for adults is 250 to 500 µg daily for about 2 weeks, then reduced to the lowest dose necessary to maintain the response. A daily dose of about 250 µg is usually adequate and 500 µg should not normally be exceeded. To reduce side-effects smaller doses of reserpine may be given in conjunction with a thiazide diuretic.

When given parenterally the effect usually begins 1 to 4 hours after intravenous or intramuscular injection. The effect is variable. Although reserpine, 2.5 mg every 4 to 8 hours for 4 doses, has been given intramuscularly in hypertensive crisis, more effective drugs are available. In the USA, doses of 0.5 to 1 mg intramuscularly, followed by 2 to 4 mg every 3 hours, if necessary, have been suggested in hypertensive crisis.

Reserpine has been used as a sedative in anxiety states and chronic psychoses in daily doses of 0.1 to 1 mg or more, but for these purposes it has largely been replaced by safer and more effective agents.

A suggested dose for children is 20 µg per kg body-weight daily in divided doses.

Administration in renal failure. The effect of renal failure on the excretion and metabolism of tritiated reserpine was studied in 15 patients. Plasma concentrations and urinary and faecal excretion of the drug were studied for 7 days following a single intramuscular injection. Correlation was found between the urinary excretion of total radioactivity, plasma half-life, and creatinine clearance but none between faecal excretion and degree of renal impairment. It was concluded that the metabolism of reserpine was not altered by renal failure and dosage reduction was unnecessary.— T. T. Zsotér *et al.*, *Clin. Pharmac. Ther.*, 1973, *14*, 325.

Reserpine was reported to be 40% bound to plasma proteins. The normal terminal half-life of 50 to 170 hours was increased to 87 to 320 hours in end-stage renal failure. It could be given in usual doses to patients with renal failure. Concentrations of reserpine were not affected by haemodialysis or peritoneal dialysis.— W. M. Bennett *et al.*, *Ann. intern. Med.*, 1980, *93*, 286.

Dyskinesia. Good control of severe generalised phenothiazine-induced dyskinesias, which persisted after discontinuation of the phenothiazine treatment, was obtained in 5 elderly mental patients by administration of reserpine in doses of 0.5 to 5 mg daily.— S. Sato *et al.*, *Dis. nerv. Syst.*, 1971, *32*, 680. See also H. A. Peters *et al.* (letter), *New Engl. J. Med.*, 1972, *286*, 106; R. C. Duvoisin (letter), *ibid.*, 611.

Further references: A. Villeneuve and Z. Böszörményi (letter), *Lancet*, 1970, *1*, 353.

Frostbite. A report on the beneficial effect of reserpine given by intra-arterial injection in the treatment of frostbite injuries in 5 patients.— J. M. Porter *et al.*, *Am. J. Surg.*, 1976, *132*, 625.

Heart disease. For reports of the effects of reserpine on cardiac function, see S. I. Cohen *et al.*, *Circulation*, 1968, *37*, 738; A. Kaldor and P. Juvancz, *Br. med. J.*, 1969, *2*, 486; B. Trappler *et al.* (letter), *S. Afr. med. J.*, 1977, *52*, 750 (myocardial infarction).

Hypertension. In a double-blind study in 450 patients with mild hypertension propranolol, alone or in combination with hydrochlorothiazide and hydralazine was compared with reserpine with hydrochlorothiazide. Reduction of diastolic blood pressures to below 90 mmHg and a reduction of at least 5 mmHg from the initial blood pressure after 6 months' treatment was achieved in 92% of patients taking propranolol with hydrochlorothiazide and hydralazine, 88% taking reserpine and hydrochlorothiazide, 81% taking propranolol and hydrochlorothiazide, 72% taking propranolol and hydralazine, and 52% taking propranolol alone. No regimen had any advantage over any other with relation to side-effects.— Veterans Administration Cooperative Study Group on Antihypertensive Agents, *J. Am. med. Ass.*, 1977, *237*, 2303.

Further references: H. Ausubel and M. L. Levine, *Curr. ther. Res.*, 1967, *9*, 29; D. K. Bloomfield and J. L. Cangiano, *ibid.*, 1969, *11*, 351; W. E. Gibb *et al.*, *Lancet*, 1970, *2*, 275; A. T. Carty (letter), *ibid.*, 421; F. M. Gonzalez and K. H. Muller-Ehrenberg, *Clin. Med.*, 1971, *78* (Mar.), 16; J. I. Haft *et al.*, *Chest*, 1972, *62*, 188; M. Velasco *et al.*, *Curr. ther. Res.*, 1975, *18*, 395; N. A. David *et al.*, *ibid.*, 741.

Hyperthyroidism. A report of aggravation of the clinical state of 7 thyrotoxic patients following administration of reserpine. They developed a carcinoid syndrome characterised by an erythematous flush of face and trunk, diarrhoea, increased tremor, nausea, fatigue, nervousness and, in one case, bronchial asthma. Three of 4 control subjects developed some of these symptoms.— M. Blumenthal *et al.*, *Archs intern. Med.*, 1965, *116*, 819.

Reserpine was given intramuscularly, in a dose of 1 to 5 mg initially and in a total dose of 70 to 300 µg per kg body-weight in the first 24 hours, to 7 patients during 8 episodes of thyrotoxic crisis. All the patients survived, and hyperthermia, tachycardia, tachypnoea, and psychological aberrations improved in 4 to 8 hours. Diarrhoea occurred in 2 patients and transient cutaneous blush in 1 patient. Hypotension did not occur.— P. T. Dillon *et al.*, *New Engl. J. Med.*, 1970, *283*, 1020.

In a double-blind trial in 15 hyperthyroid patients, the effects of 10 days' treatment with reserpine 250 µg twice daily were compared with those of a placebo. Reserpine was found to have no effect on thyroid metabolism, but pulse-rate, finger tremor, and hyperkinetic movements were signficantly reduced.— J. S. Cheah, *Med. J. Aust.*, 1972, *1*, 322.

In 15 patients ECG changes due to hyperthyroidism were not corrected by adrenergic blockade with reserpine or propranolol. Heart-rate was slowed but did not return to normal.— P. C. Teoh and J. S. Cheah, *Med. J. Aust.*, 1973, *2*, 116. See also C. H. Lee and J. S. Cheah, *ibid.*, 1974, *1*, 794.

Further references: S. H. Ingbar, *New Engl. J. Med.*, 1966, *274*, 1252; A. Zarate *et al.*, *Clin. Med.*, 1966, *73* (Feb.), 19; S. R. Newmark *et al.*, *J. Am. med. Ass.*, 1974, *230*, 592.

Migraine. A double-blind controlled crossover trial of the prophylaxis of migraine in 28 patients had shown that reserpine was significantly more effective in reducing the frequency of attacks (by 50% or more) than a placebo.— R. Grahame (letter), *Lancet*, 1970, *2*, 832.

Further references: F. Fog-Møller *et al.*, *Headache*, 1976, *15*, 275; G. Nattero *et al.*, *ibid.*, 279.

Raynaud's syndrome. Good or excellent responses were obtained by two-thirds of 102 patients with Raynaud's syndrome who received intra-arterial injections of reserpine 1 to 1.5 mg in 2.5 ml of sodium chloride injection. Benefit continued in some patients for many months while others obtained remissions with monthly injections; there was no important difference in response between patients with Raynaud's disease and those with Raynaud's phenomenon. Side-effects were not directly related to dosage suggesting that the reserpine remained in the injected extremity.— J. P. Tindall *et al.*, *Archs Derm.*, 1974, *110*, 233.

No difference in efficacy was demonstrated between reserpine or control in a randomised double-blind crossover study comparing intra-arterial injections of reserpine 1 mg in 0.4 ml of vehicle against sodium chloride injection 0.4 ml in 12 patients with severe Raynaud's phenomenon.— R. C. Siegel and J. F. Fries, *Archs intern. Med.*, 1974, *134*, 515. A similar study.— I. J. McFadyen *et al.*, *Archs intern. Med.*, 1973, *132*, 526.

Improvement occurred in a woman with calcinosis circumscripta and Raynaud's phenomenon after a single intra-arterial injection of reserpine 2 mg and probenecid 2 g daily by mouth.— D. Meyers, *Med. J. Aust.*, 1976, *2*, 457.

A review of the treatment of peripheral vascular disease including a brief account of reserpine therapy. Reserpine 0.25 to 1 mg daily produces remarkable amelioration of symptoms in about 50% of patients with Raynaud's phenomenon. The author had given reserpine by intra-arterial injection only in the most severe cases and had found no difference from oral therapy.— J. D. Coffman, *New Engl. J. Med.*, 1979, *300*, 713.

Intra-arterial injection of reserpine 1 mg in 2 ml of saline given slowly over 1 minute increased basal skin blood flow in 7 patients with systemic sclerosis and severe Raynaud's phenomenon accompanied by peripheral ischaemia and ulceration. The effect usually lasted 1 to 3 weeks. Repeat injections of reserpine in 5 of the patients with ulcers of the fingers resulted in healing in 4 and the pain experienced by the other 2 patients was relieved by a single injection.— K. H. Nilsen and M. I. V. Jayson, *Br. med. J.*, 1980, *280*, 1408.

Further references: J. Rösch *et al.*, *Circulation*, 1977, *55*, 807; B. A. Nobin *et al.*, *Ann. Surg.*, 1978, *187*, 12.

Rodenticide. Brief account of the Golden Jubilee (1926–76) report of the Universities Federation for Animal Welfare commenting on the use of reserpine as a rodenticide to control *mice*.— *Practitioner*, 1976, *217*, 695.

Preparations

Reserpine and Hydrochlorothiazide Tablets *(U.S.P.)*. Tablets containing reserpine and hydrochlorothiazide. Store in airtight containers. Protect from light.

Reserpine Elixir *(U.S.P.)*. An elixir containing reserpine and alcohol 11 to 13%. Store in airtight containers. Protect from light.

Reserpine, Hydralazine Hydrochloride, and Hydrochlorothiazide Tablets *(U.S.P.)*. Tablets containing, unless otherwise specified, reserpine 100 µg, hydralazine hydrochloride 25 mg, and hydrochlorothiazide 15 mg. Store in airtight containers. Protect from light.

Reserpine Injection *(U.S.P.)*. A sterile solution of reserpine in Water for Injections, prepared with the aid of a suitable acid. It contains suitable antoxidants. pH 3 to 4. Protect from light.

Reserpine Injection. Reserpine 250 mg, benzyl alcohol 2 ml, anhydrous citric acid 250 mg, polysorbate '80' 10 ml, Water for Injections to 100 ml. Dissolve the reserpine and citric acid in the benzyl alcohol by warming slightly, add the polysorbate 80 and Water for Injections and filter. Sterilise by filtration as discoloration occurs when autoclaved.—A.F. Leyden *et al.*, *J. Am. pharm. Ass., scient. Edn*, 1956, *45*, 771.

Reserpine Tablets *(B.P.)*. Tablets containing reserpine. Protect from light.

Reserpine Tablets *(U.S.P.)*. Tablets containing reserpine. Store in airtight containers. Protect from light.

Proprietary Preparations

Abicol Tablets *(Boots, UK)*. Each contains reserpine 150 µg and bendrofluazide 2.5 mg. For hypertension. *Dose.* ½ to 1 tablet morning and evening.

Seominal (known in some countries as Serpentinum and Theominal RS) *(Winthrop, UK)*. Tablets each containing reserpine 200 µg, phenobarbitone 10 mg, and theobromine 325 mg. For hypertension. *Dose.* 1 tablet twice daily.

Serpasil *(Ciba, UK)*. Reserpine, available as tablets of 100 µg and as scored tablets of 250 µg. (Also available as Serpasil in *Austral., Belg., Fr., Ger., Ital., S.Afr., Switz., USA*).

Serpasil-Esidrex *(Ciba, UK)*. Tablets each containing reserpine 150 µg and hydrochlorothiazide 10 mg. For hypertension. **Serpasil-Esidrex K.** Tablets containing in addition potassium chloride 600 mg (potassium 8.1 mmol; 8.1 mEq) in a slow-release wax core. *Dose.* 2 to 3 tablets daily.

Other Proprietary Names

Arg.— Sedaraupin, Serpasol; *Canad.*— Neo-Serp, Reserfia, Reserpanca; *Ger.*— Sedaraupin; *Spain*— Rausan, Rauwita, Resedril, Rese-Lar, Serpasol, Serpresan; *Switz.*— Mephaserpin; *USA*— Lemiserp, Rau-Sed, Resercen, Reserpoid, Sandril, Serpate, SK-Reserpine, Vio-Serpine.

NOTES. The name Protensin has been applied to a proprietary preparation containing hydroflumethiazide, reserpine, and protoveratrine. This name has also been applied to a preparation containing chlordiazepoxide.

Reserpine was also formerly marketed in Great Britain under the proprietary name Reserpine Dellipsoids D29 (*Pilsworth*). A preparation containing reserpine was formerly marketed in Great Britain under the proprietary name Tensanyl (*Leo*).

902-g

Saralasin Acetate.

The acetate of 1-Sar-8-Ala-angiotensin; P-113. The hydrated acetate of Sar-Arg-Val-Tyr-Val-His-Pro-Ala; [1-(*N*-Methylglycine),5-L-valine,8-L-alanine]-angiotensin II acetate hydrate.

$C_{42}H_{65}N_{13}O_{10}$, xCH$_3$COOH, xH$_2$O.

CAS — 34273-10-4 (saralasin); 39698-78-7 (acetate, hydrate).

The acetate of an octapeptide differing from angiotensin only in the terminal amino-acid residues.

Adverse Effects, Treatment, and Precautions. Infusion of saralasin acetate has been followed by severe hypotension. Acute hypertensive episodes have also occurred and it has been recommended that phentolamine should be available when using saralasin for diagnosis in hypertensive patients. Patients receiving vasodilators or drugs which stimulate the renin-angiotensin system, or who have been depleted of sodium and water, have an enhanced response to saralasin infusion.

A study in 3 healthy subjects indicated that saralasin had agonist and antagonist activity depending on angiotensin II concentration and sodium intake. It was advised that when using saralasin acetate to test for angiotensin II-mediated hypertension it was important to use an incremental dose as the agonist activity of larger doses could mask its hypotensive action.— G. A. MacGregor and P. M. Dawes, *Br. J. clin. Pharmac.*, 1976, *3*, 483. See also *idem* (letter), *Lancet*, 1975, *2*, 923.

In a study involving 6 hypertensive subjects, haemodynamic changes during the first few minutes of saralasin infusion closely resembled those caused by noradrenaline infusion.— N. D. Vlachakis *et al.*, *Am. Heart J.*, 1978, *95*, 78.

See also under Hypertension (below).

Hypertension. Rebound hypertension, controlled by propranolol, occurred in 4 sodium-depleted hypertensive patients within 3 hours of infusion of saralasin acetate.— H. J. Keim *et al.*, *New Engl. J. Med.*, 1976, *295*, 1175.

Saralasin could lead to a potentially hazardous initial rise in blood pressure when plasma-renin activity was low.— W. H. L. Hoefnagels and T. Thien (letter), *Br. med. J.*, 1976, *2*, 1196.

Phaeochromocytoma. A precipitate increase in arterial pressure indicative of catecholamine release occurred in a patient with phaeochromocytoma and neurofibromatosis during the infusion of saralasin 1.3 mg per minute.— F. G. Dunn *et al.*, *New Engl. J. Med.*, 1976, *295*, 605. In 12 hypertensive patients infusion of saralasin caused a significant increase of noradrenaline, but in a patient with phaeochromocytoma, infusion of about 20 µg per kg per minute had reduced blood pressure to normal. Pressor response is not invariable in patients with phaeochromocytoma.— A. Röckel *et al.* (letter), *ibid.*, 1977, *296*, 50. Speculation on the reasons for the difference. Since saralasin can increase circulating concentrations of catecholamines, phentolamine should always be available when using saralasin for diagnostic purposes in hypertensive patients.— E. D. Frohlich *et al.* (letter), *ibid.*, 51. Further comment. A significant increase in plasma- noradrenaline concentrations without change in plasma-adrenaline concentrations had followed infusion of saralasin 1 µg per kg body-weight per minute in 14 healthy subjects.— B. McGrath *et al.* (letter), *ibid.*, 880.

Hypotension. Hypotension with premature ventricular contractions occurred during saralasin infusion in a patient under treatment with other potent hypotensive drugs.— W. A. Pettinger and K. Keeton, *Lancet*, 1975, *1*, 1387. Comment.— G. A. MacGregor (letter), *ibid.*, 1975, *2*, 181.

Serious hypotension developed in a woman with angiotensin-dependent hypertension when she was given a second infusion of saralasin 10 µg per kg body-weight per minute after vigorous volume depletion with hydrochlorothiazide, amiloride, and frusemide.— R. Beckerhoff *et al.*, *Br. med. J.*, 1976, *2*, 849. Comment.— G. A. MacGregor (letter), *ibid.*, 1323.

Infusion of saralasin 10 µg per kg body-weight per minute, induced a severe hypotensive response in a 57-year-old man with renovascular hypertension, who had discontinued guanethidine 3 weeks previously. The response could have been due to his very high plasma-renin values, induced by sodium-depleting therapy in preparation for the test. Infusion of saralasin should be preferred to bolus injection, and the initial rate of infusion should be lower than 10 µg per kg per minute.— R. Fagard *et al.* (letter), *Lancet*, 1976, *1*, 1136.

Interactions. To avoid excessive hypotension, caution was necessary in titrating saralasin infusion for patients receiving vasodilators. Minoxidil and hydralazine, which cause elevated renin activity, should be avoided in patients receiving saralasin to investigate the renin dependency of hypertension.— W. A. Pettinger *et al.*, *Clin. Pharmac. Ther.*, 1975, *17*, 146.

Diuretic-induced sodium depletion before saralasin testing elicits stimulation of renin secretion and participation of the angiotensin component in the maintenance of elevated blood pressure.— H. Gavras *et al.*, *New Engl. J. Med.*, 1976, *295*, 1278. Comment on the practical aspects of diuretic therapy in the saralasin test.— R. E. Keenan *et al.* (letter), *ibid.*, 1977, *297*, 52 (See also under Uses).

Absorption and Fate. Saralasin is rapidly inactivated in the body. When given by infusion it has a pharmacological half-life of about 8 minutes and a biochemical half-life of about 3 minutes. It crosses the blood-brain barrier.

Radioimmunoassay and pharmacokinetics of saralasin in *rats* and in hypertensive patients. In hypertensive patients responding to saralasin, the mean pharmacological half-life was 8.2 minutes and the mean biochemical half-life was 3.2 minutes.— W. A. Pettinger *et al.*, *Clin. Pharmac. Ther.*, 1975, *17*, 146.

Further references: W. A. Pettinger *et al.*, *Pharmacologist*, 1974, *16*, 295.

Uses. Saralasin acetate is a competitive antagonist of angiotensin II and thus blocks its pressor action; it permits the identification of patients in whom hypertension is maintained by angiotensin. It also has therapeutic application in the control of severe hypertension. It is usually given as an infusion in a dose of 10 µg per kg body-weight per minute but to avoid the risk of hypotensive or hypertensive reactions some sources have recommended much slower initial rates of infusion. It has been estimated that a constant response will usually be obtained within about 20 minutes. Doses of 20 µg per kg per minute have also been used.

A detailed account of the structure, properties and actions of saralasin acetate.— *Drugs of the Future*, 1978, *3*, 675.

Further reviews and comments: *Br. med. J.*, 1975, *3*, 59; *New Engl. J. Med.*, 1975, *292*, 695; L. S. Marks *et al.*, *Ann. intern. Med.*, 1977, *87*, 176; E. Haber, *New Engl. J. Med.*, 1978, *298*, 1023.

The effect of angiotensin II blockade by saralasin in 6 healthy subjects.— H. Ibsen *et al.*, *Eur. J. clin. Pharmac.*, 1978, *14*, 171.

Further studies on the action of saralasin and the role of the renin-angiotensin system in hypertension: H. Gavras *et al.*, *New Engl. J. Med.*, 1976, *295*, 1278; G. G. Geyskes *et al.*, *Lancet*, 1976, *1*, 1049.

Administration. Excessive hypotension during saralasin infusion tests in patients receiving multiple antihypertensive therapy can be avoided by careful adjustment of the rate of infusion, which should be started at a maximum of 100 ng per kg body-weight per minute, and by measuring the standing blood pressures. Such patients should, however, be excluded from screening programmes looking for angiotensin II-dependent hypertensive patients not only because of the risk of hypotension but because of the risk of false-positive results.— G. A. MacGregor (letter), *Lancet*, 1975, *2*, 181. The fall in blood pressure that may occur with saralasin infusion can be controlled by starting at infusion rates of, for example, 50 to 250 ng per kg per minute and increasing progressively.— *idem* (letter), *Br. med. J.*, 1976, *2*, 1323.

Comments on the practical application of saralasin in the estimation of angiotensin II-dependent hypertension. A study was carried out involving 342 patients, mildly depleted of sodium by administration of frusemide 80 mg the night before the test, and studied in the supine position. Of those expected to exhibit a depressor saralasin response 95% did so, and of those expected to exhibit a neutral or pressor response, 87% did so.— R. E. Keenan *et al.* (letter), *New Engl. J. Med.*, 1977, *297*, 52. Comment.— D. B. Case and J. H. Laragh (letter), *ibid.*, 52.

The saralasin infusion test should be considered the primary screening procedure for the detection of angiotensin-dependent hypertension because of its specificity and relatively infrequent false negatives.— J. G. McAfee *et al.*, *J. nucl. Med.*, 1977, *18*, 669.

Saralasin was ineffective in 2 patients in predicting the response to surgery for renovascular hypertension.— R. D. Thomas *et al.*, *Lancet*, 1977, *1*, 724.

A study in 15 patients with hypertension who were undergoing haemodialysis indicated that those patients who responded to an infusion of saralasin with a fall in blood pressure would be expected to have an improvement in their hypertension after bilateral nephrectomy, while those who did not respond would not be expected to benefit from nephrectomy.— M. D. Lifschitz *et al.*, *Ann. intern. Med.*, 1978, *88*, 23. See also J. Tuma *et al.*, *Schweiz. med. Wschr.*, 1977, *107*, 704; S. L. Linas *et al.*, *New Engl. J. Med.*, 1978, *298*, 1440.

Further references: H. R. Brunner *et al.*, *Lancet*, 1973, *2*, 1045; A. J. M. Donker and F. H. H. Leenen, *ibid.*, 1974, *2*, 1535; L. S. Marks *et al.*, *Lancet*, 1975, *2*, 784; D. H. P. Streeten *et al.*, *New Engl. J. Med.*, 1975, *292*, 657; J. H. Laragh, *ibid.*, 695; L. Baer *et al.*, *Ann. intern. Med.*, 1977, *86*, 257; I. Arlart and J. Rosenthal, *Dt. med. Wschr.*, 1978, *103*, 1790; D. B. Case and J. H. Laragh, *Ann. intern. Med.*, 1979, *91*, 153; G. Bönner *et al.*, *Dt. med. Wschr.*, 1979, *104*, 432; *Kidney Int.*, 1979, *15*, *Suppl.* 9;; G. H. Anderson *et al.*, *Lancet*, 1980, *2*, 821.

Therapeutic uses. A patient with intractable congestive cardiac failure secondary to reno-vascular hypertension and severe coronary artery disease received saralasin acetate by infusion at a rate of 10 µg per kg body-weight per minute for 35 minutes. Cardiac output was almost doubled, left ventricular stroke work increased, while systemic and pulmonary vascular resistance decreased. Inhibition of angiotensin appeared to be the treatment of choice for this patient.— H. Gavras *et al.*, *J. Am. med. Ass.*, 1977, *238*, 880.

Proprietary Names

Sarenin *(Röhm, Ger.; Norwich-Eaton, USA)*.

903-q

Sodium Nitroprusside *(B.P., U.S.P.)*.

Sodium Nitroferricyanide; Disodium (*OC*-6-22)-Pentakis(cyano-*C*)nitrosylferrate Dihydrate. Sodium nitrosylpentacyanoferrate(III) dihydrate. $Na_2Fe(CN)_5NO, 2H_2O$=298.0.

CAS — 14402-89-2 (anhydrous); 13755-38-9 (dihydrate).

Pharmacopoeias. In *Br.* and *U.S.*; *U.S.* also includes Sterile Sodium Nitroprusside.

Reddish-brown odourless or almost odourless crystals or powder. Freely **soluble** in water; slightly soluble in alcohol; very slightly soluble in chloroform. Aqueous solutions slowly decompose. Solutions for injection are prepared immediately before use, by the addition of the requisite amount of dextrose injection to the sterile contents of a container and dilution in further dextrose injection. Solutions may also be **sterilised** by filtration.

Store in airtight containers. Protect from light.

CAUTION. *Solutions of sodium nitroprusside must be protected from light during infusion by wrapping the container with aluminium foil or some other opaque material. Solutions discoloured by reaction of nitroprusside with organic and inorganic materials should be discarded. Solutions should not be used more than 4 hours after preparation.*

Stability in solution. The pH of a solution of sodium nitroprusside in water was 4.5 to 5 and its colour darkened from orange-yellow on standing. Sodium nitroprusside was more stable in acid solutions and less stable in alkaline solutions. A 2% aqueous control solution of sodium nitroprusside of pH 4.7 did not discolour or precipitate for 13 days. By comparison, the addition of sodium metabisulphite, pH 9 buffer, or hydroxybenzoates reduced stability; 20% alcohol or propylene glycol had no effect, while other hydroxy compounds increased stability, to up to 51 days in the case of 50% glycerol. Sodium citrate 5% increased stability to more than 800 days. Other salts with anionic chelating potential such as sodium acetate or phosphate were also effective. Solutions containing sodium nitroprusside 2% and sodium citrate 5% were unchanged in colour and clarity after autoclaving for 60 minutes at 121°, but loss of potency was not determined.— G. E. Schumacher, *Am. J. Hosp. Pharm.*, 1966, *23*, 532.

Solutions of sodium nitroprusside 100 mg in 250 ml of 5% dextrose solution decomposed with the formation of a pale blue-green precipitate when autoclaved at 115° for 30 minutes. Using as a criterion the absence of a perceptible colour change and/or the formation of a precipitate, 2% solutions in various vehicles were stable for 12 months if stored in a refrigerator or in the dark, but decomposed rapidly if stored in the light, especially at high pH. Solutions in 1% nitric acid were stable in the light, even in clear glass containers, for 12 months. Autoclaving, or storage in partially-filled containers, did not appear to affect the rate of decomposition, but sterilisation by filtration was recommended until these findings were confirmed by chemical analysis.— R. G. Challen (letter), *Australas. J. Pharm.*, 1967, *48*, S110.

Spectrophotometry was considered a more sensitive indication of decomposition of sodium nitroprusside solutions than colour changes. There were negligible changes in absorbance for up to 6 months when solutions were stored at 25° in the dark, in aqueous solution, or in the presence of sodium citrate, citric acid, acetic acid, or acetate buffer (pH 4.6). There was less deterioration after heating at 115° than after exposure to light.— R. A. Anderson and W. Rae, *Aust. J. pharm. Sci.*, 1972, *1*, 45.

A study of the degradation of 1% aqueous solutions of sodium nitroprusside demonstrated that light was essential for the change in colour from straw to orange which was independent of pH, whereas further degradation leading to the appearance of a blue precipitate required an acid pH. The appearance of a blue coloration should be taken to indicate that injections were unfit for use.— R. E. Hargrave, *J. Hosp. Pharm.*, 1974, *32*, 188.

Sodium nitroprusside solutions for injection could be made using Water for Injections providing it did not contain any preservatives. Such solutions could then be added to the dextrose infusion.— R. B. Vrabel and A. B. Amerson, *Am. J. Hosp. Pharm.*, 1975, *32*, 140.

Preparation of a stable solution of sodium nitroprusside containing citric acid and sterilisable by autoclaving.— A. C. Van Loenen and W. Hofs-Kemper, *Pharm. Weekbl. Ned., scient. Edn*, 1979, *1*, 52.

Further references: F. A. Finnerty, *J. Am. med. Ass.*, 1974, *229*, 1479; C. J. Vesey and G. A. Batistoni, *J. clin. Pharm.*, 1977, *2*, 105.

Adverse Effects. Intravenous infusion of sodium nitroprusside may produce anorexia, nausea and vomiting, apprehension, headache, dizziness, disorientation, restlessness, perspiration, palpitations, retrosternal discomfort, abdominal pain, muscle weakness, and muscle twitching, but these effects may be reduced by slowing the rate of infusion. Plasma concentrations of cyanide and thiocyanate may be raised and hypothyroidism, methaemoglobinaemia, phlebitis, irreversible hypotension, and metabolic acidosis have also been reported.

A discussion of the hazards of sodium nitroprusside infusions, of precautions to be observed, and of treatment of potential cyanide poisoning.— *Br. med. J.*, 1978, *2*, 784.

Further references: L. Greiss *et al.*, *Can. Anaesth. Soc. J.*, 1976, *23*, 480; *Med. Lett.*, 1976, *18*, 68.

Acidosis. Death attributed to sodium nitroprusside occurred in a 20-year-old man following anaesthesia during which he had received 750 mg of sodium nitroprusside. There was severe acidosis and hyperkalaemia but no chemical evidence of cyanide toxicity.— A. J. Merrifield and M. D. Blundell (letter), *Br. J. Anaesth.*, 1974, *46*, 324. Severe metabolic acidosis occurred on 1 of more than 600 occasions when sodium nitroprusside was used to induce hypotension during anaesthesia.— W. R. MacRae and M. Owen, *ibid.*, 795.

A 66-year-old woman developed lactic acidosis after receiving an infusion of sodium nitroprusside for 28 hours (total dose 490 mg). The infusion was discontinued and the patient recovered. Lactic acidosis could occur during the use of high doses of sodium nitroprusside for prolonged periods.— S. H. Humphrey and D. A. Nash, *Ann. intern. Med.*, 1978, *88*, 58.

Cyanide poisoning. A patient died of cyanide poisoning during an operation for which he had received 400 mg (10 mg per kg body-weight) of sodium nitroprusside to induce hypotension.— D. W. Davies *et al.*, *Can. Anaesth. Soc. J.*, 1975, *22*, 547.

Until a method is devised for measuring free cyanide in the blood as opposed to total cyanide (including that fraction complexed with methaemoglobin), blood-cyanide concentrations following the administration of nitroprusside must be regarded as inappropriately high.— R. P. Smith and H. Kruszyna (letter), *Br. J. Anaesth.*, 1976, *48*, 396.

Further references: J. D. Michenfelder and J. H. Tinker, *Anesthesiology*, 1977, *47*, 441.

Effects on the blood. *Aplastic anaemia.* Thiocyanates had been reported to cause aplastic anaemia.— R. H. Girdwood, *Drugs*, 1976, *11*, 394.

Methaemoglobinaemia. Methaemoglobinaemia developed in a man whilst he was receiving sodium nitroprusside in a total dose of 321 mg over 4 days after extensive cardiac infarction. On cessation of the sodium nitroprusside the infarction spread and the patient died 3 days later.— P. J. Bower and J. N. Peterson, *New Engl. J. Med.*, 1975, *293*, 865.

Reaction of haemoglobin and nitroprusside could produce cyanmethaemoglobin.— M. A. Posner (letter), *New Engl. J. Med.*, 1976, *294*, 166. See also R. P. Smith and R. A. Carleton (letter), *ibid.*, 502.

Platelets. Platelet counts decreased in 7 of 8 patients with congestive heart failure 1 to 6 hours after intravenous infusion of nitroprusside was started. The counts began to return to normal 24 hours after the infusion was stopped.— P. Mehta *et al.* (letter), *New Engl. J. Med.*, 1978, *299*, 1134.

Further references: A. Saxon and H. E. Kattlove, *Blood*, 1976, *47*, 957; A. Saxon (letter), *New Engl. J. Med.*, 1976, *295*, 281.

Hypotension. A 50-kg patient, who had received about 13 mg of nitroprusside over 90 minutes, developed irreversible hypotension and died 2 hours after nitroprusside infusion was stopped. It was suggested that hypotension and death was probably due to cyanide toxicity and that hydroxocobalamin should be administered prophylactically to all patients receiving nitroprusside even in small doses.— J. Montoliu *et al.* (letter), *Am. Heart J.*, 1979, *97*, 541.

Hypothyroidism. Continuous intravenous infusion of sodium nitroprusside, in a total dose of 3.9 g given over 21 days, was effective in controlling blood pressure in a 35-year-old woman with accelerated hypertension, but the patient developed hypothyroidism, with a serum-thiocyanate concentration of 95 µg per ml which receded when the nitroprusside was discontinued and the patient was treated with peritoneal dialysis. It was suggested that the abnormality of thyroid function was mainly due to inhibition of iodide-concentrating capacity by thiocyanate derived from the nitroprusside, though the latter ion could have contributed.— D. S. Nourok *et al.*, *Am. J. med. Sci.*, 1964, *248*, 129.

Increase in intracranial pressure. Intracranial pressure rose significantly while the mean blood pressure was 90 or 80% of initial values in 14 normocapnic patients given an infusion of sodium nitroprusside to produce controlled hypotension prior to neurosurgery; values reverted towards normal at mean blood pressures of 70% of controls. A similar but insignificant trend occurred in 5 hypocapnic patients. The effect was considered to be due to vasodilatation increasing cerebral blood flow. Surgery was rendered difficult in some patients.— J. M. Turner *et al.*, *Br. J. Anaesth.*, 1977, *49*, 419.

Phlebitis. Acute transient phlebitis following sodium nitroprusside administration.— R. Miller and D. C. C. Stark (letter), *Anesthesiology*, 1978, *49*, 372.

Treatment of Adverse Effects. Side-effects due to excessive hypotension may be treated by slowing or discontinuing the infusion. Hypothyroidism with plasma-thiocyanate concentrations over 100 µg per ml has been treated with peritoneal dialysis.

For details of the treatment of cyanide poisoning see Hydrocyanic Acid, p.790. Raised erythrocyte-cyanide concentrations have been lowered by the administration of hydroxocobalamin intravenously.

Following infusion of sodium nitroprusside solution for a prolonged period erythrocyte-cyanide concentrations rose in a patient suffering from a dissecting aneurysm with malignant hypertension. A sharp reduction in the erythrocyte-cyanide concentration was obtained after intravenous administration of hydroxocobalamin 5 mg, despite continued administration of sodium nitroprusside.— C. J. Vesey *et al.*, *Br. med. J.*, 1974, *2*, 140.

In a study involving 14 patients requiring nitroprusside hypotensive anaesthesia, blood-cyanide concentrations of those who concomitantly received an intravenous infusion of hydroxocobalamin 100 mg in 100 ml of dextrose injection at a rate of 12.5 mg per 30 minutes throughout the duration of nitroprusside administration, were significantly decreased compared with those who received nitroprusside alone. They received a total of 87.5 to 100 mg of hydroxocobalamin and no significant adverse effects were noted other than transient pink discoloration of mucous membranes and urine.— J. E. Cottrell *et al.*, *New Engl. J. Med.*, 1978, *298*, 809.

Dialysis. Thiocyanate intoxication can be corrected with haemodialysis.— J. F. Winchester *et al.*, *Trans. Am. Soc. artif. internal Organs*, 1977, *23*, 762.

Precautions. Sodium nitroprusside should not be used in the presence of compensatory hypertension as in arteriovenous shunt or aortic coarctation. It should be used with caution in elderly patients and in those with impaired renal or hepatic function or with hypothyroidism or hypothermia. It has been suggested that sodium nitroprusside should not be used in patients with low plasma-cobalamin concentrations or Leber's optic atrophy. The use of hydroxocobalamin before and during administration of sodium nitroprusside, has been advocated.

In controlled hypotension, renal or hepatic failure were serious contra-indications to the use of sodium nitroprusside.— I. R. Verner, *Postgrad. med. J.*, 1974, *50*, 584.

In a study in 26 anaesthetised patients sodium nitroprusside, infused throughout surgery, produced a marked reversible reduction in oxygen tension whether ventilation was spontaneous or artificial.— J. A. W. Wildsmith *et al.*, *Br. J. Anaesth.*, 1975, *47*, 1205.

Detailed recommendations for the safe use of sodium nitroprusside.— P. Cole, *Anaesthesia*, 1978, *33*, 473.

Pregnancy and the neonate. Sodium nitroprusside was successfully used during surgery for a cerebral aneurysm in a 25-year-old woman who was 7 months pregnant. A healthy baby was delivered 2 months later and at 2 years the child's development was normal.— Y. Donchin *et al.*, *Br. J. Anaesth.*, 1978, *50*, 849.

Tachyphylaxis. A report of tachyphylaxis to sodium nitroprusside, associated with high plasma concentrations of cyanide but in the absence of metabolic acidosis, in 3 patients undergoing hypotensive anaesthesia.— J. E. Cottrell *et al.*, *Anesthesiology*, 1978, *49*, 141.

Further references: L. Amaranath and W. F. Kellermeyer, *Anesthesiology*, 1976, *44*, 345.

Withdrawal. Rebound haemodynamic changes produced a profound but transient deterioration in cardiac performance 10 to 30 minutes after the discontinuation of an infusion of sodium nitroprusside in 20 patients.— M. Packer *et al.*, *New Engl. J. Med.*, 1979, *301*, 1193.

Rebound hypertension after withdrawal of sodium nitroprusside during surgery.— H. J. Khambatta *et al.*, *Anesthesiology*, 1979, *51*, 127. See also J. E. Cottrell *et al.*, *Clin. Pharmac. Ther.*, 1980, *27*, 32.

Absorption and Fate. Sodium nitroprusside is converted in the body to cyanide which is metabolised in the liver to thiocyanate by the enzyme rhodanase and slowly excreted in the urine.

In 17 patients given sodium nitroprusside solution (100 μg per ml) as an infusion to induce hypotension during anaesthesia, plasma-thiocyanate concentrations were unchanged, but plasma-cyanide concentrations rose to more than 4 times their initial value. In 2 further patients given sodium nitroprusside for longer periods for hypertension, both thiocyanate and cyanide concentrations were affected. Patients undergoing nitroprusside therapy should be given hydroxocobalamin concomitantly.— C. J. Vesey *et al.*, *Br. med. J.*, 1974, *2*, 140.

Infusion of a total dose of sodium nitroprusside 1.5 mg per kg body-weight over 2 hours would produce a plasma-cyanide concentration of about 3 μmol per litre, the level at which histotoxic hypoxia occurred in *dogs*. The above dose should not therefore be exceeded.— C. J. Vesey *et al.* (letter), *Br. med. J.*, 1975, *3*, 229.

Metabolic studies in children.— D. W. Davies *et al.*, *Can. Anaesth. Soc. J.*, 1975, *22*, 553.

Further references: K. Bödigheimer *et al.*, *Dt. med. Wschr.*, 1979, *104*, 939.

Uses. Sodium nitroprusside is a short-acting hypotensive agent. It produces peripheral vasodilatation and reduces peripheral resistance by a direct action on blood vessels and may be used in the treatment of hypertensive crises. It may also be used to produce controlled hypotension during general anaesthesia. It has also been used in congestive heart failure and other cardiac disorders. Its effects appear within a few seconds of intravenous infusion.

It is given by continuous infusion of a 0.005 or 0.01% solution in dextrose injection, usually at a rate of 0.5 to 8 μg per kg body-weight per minute, under close supervision; 0.02% solutions have sometimes been used. The average dose required to maintain the blood pressure 30 to 40% below the pretreatment diastolic blood pressure is 3 μg per kg per minute. The maximum recommended rate is about 10 μg per kg per minute, and infusions should be stopped after 10 minutes if there is no response. It is only suitable for administration in the form of an infusion and care should be taken to prevent extravasation. Tachyphylaxis is rare and infusions may be continued for several days provided that the blood-thiocyanate concentration does not exceed 100 μg per ml. Alternative oral therapy should be introduced as soon as possible.

For the induction of hypotension during anaesthesia a maximum dose of 1.5 μg per kg body-weight per minute is recommended.

Sodium nitroprusside is also used in Rothera's test for the detection of acetone and acetoacetic acid in urine.

A review of the pharmacology, toxicology, and therapeutic indications of sodium nitroprusside.— J. H. Tinker and J. D. Michenfelder, *Anesthesiology*, 1976, *45*, 340. See also R. F. Palmer and K. C. Lasseter, *New Engl. J. Med.*, 1975, *292*, 294; P. Cole, *Anaesthesia*, 1978, *33*, 473; J. N. Cohn and L. P. Burke, *Ann. intern. Med.*, 1979, *91*, 752.

There was evidence of cyanide toxicity when sodium nitroprusside was infused at doses not exceeding a maximum total of 1.5 mg per kg body-weight. It was recommended that for short infusions the dose of sodium nitroprusside should not exceed 500 μg per kg.— D. Aitken *et al.*, *Can. Anaesth. Soc. J.*, 1977, *24*, 651.

Further references: J. Krapez and P. Cole (letter), *Br. med. J.*, 1978, *2*, 1088; P. Daggett and I. Verner (letter), *ibid.*

Administration in renal failure. The successful use of sodium nitroprusside in a patient with renovascular hypertension and left ventricular failure, and during corrective surgery.— G. I. Russell *et al.*, *Br. med. J.*, 1978, *2*, 14.

The normal half-life of sodium nitroprusside was less than 10 minutes. It could be given in usual doses to patients in renal failure. In patients with a glomerular filtration-rate of less than 10 ml per minute it was necessary to monitor plasma-thiocyanate concentrations to ensure they did not rise above 100 μg per ml. Concentrations of sodium nitroprusside were affected by haemodialysis and peritoneal dialysis.— W. M. Bennett *et al.*, *Ann. intern. Med.*, 1980, *93*, 286.

See also under Precautions.

Cardiac diseases. A study indicating that the primary direct action of sodium nitroprusside in coronary disease is vasodilatation of the coronary artery.— B. K. Yeh *et al.*, *Am. Heart J.*, 1977, *93*, 610.

The use of sodium nitroprusside and adrenaline in heart surgery.— G. Benzing *et al.*, *Ann. thorac. Surg.*, 1979, *27*, 523.

Acute dissecting aneurysms. Following worsening of 2 patients' conditions, and *animal* studies, the use of propranolol and nitroprusside to treat dissecting aneurysms of the aorta had been temporarily abandoned. Trimetaphan remained the drug of choice.— R. F. Palmer and K. C. Lasseter (letter), *New Engl. J. Med.*, 1976, *294*, 1403. Sodium nitroprusside was still the agent of choice.— J. N. Cohn (letter), *ibid.*, *295*, 567.

The successful use of sodium nitroprusside over 22 days in a patient with dissecting aortic aneurysm.— K. Hillman and J. Krapez, *Br. med. J.*, 1978, *2*, 799.

Heart failure. In 18 patients with heart failure unresponsive to digitalis and diuretics, breathing was improved in 14 by the intravenous infusion of sodium nitroprusside. Mean arterial pressure (for the 18) fell from 99 to 83 mmHg; left ventricular filling pressure fell from 32.2 to 17.2 mmHg; diastolic pressure fell by about 15 mmHg; and cardiac output increased from 2.98 to 5.2 litres per minute. In 5 patients studied, urine volume and sodium excretion increased. Sodium nitroprusside was given initially at a rate of 15 μg per minute and increased to a mean of 40 μg per minute (range 25 to 120 μg). The effect lasted only so long as the infusion continued; it had been given for up to 72 hours.— N. H. Guiha *et al.*, *New Engl. J. Med.*, 1974, *291*, 587.

In 9 patients with chronic congestive heart failure the concomitant infusion of sodium nitroprusside 40 to 100 μg (mean 68 μg) per minute and dopamine 5 to 7 μg per kg body-weight per minute was judged to be superior to either agent used alone. Sodium nitroprusside reduced left ventricular end-diastolic pressure and dopamine increased cardiac index; the maintenance of arterial pressure by dopamine permitted the use of sodium nitroprusside in patients with mild or moderate hypotension.— R. R. Miller *et al.*, *Circulation*, 1977, *55*, 881.

The use of sodium nitroprusside and ephedrine in heart failure.— J. A. Franciosa and J. N. Cohn, *Am. J. Cardiol.*, 1979, *43*, 79.

Further references: C. W. Harshaw *et al.*, *Ann. intern. Med.*, 1975, *83*, 312; K. Chatterjee, *ibid.*, 421; E. B. Stinson *et al.*, *J. thorac. cardiovasc. Surg.*, 1977, *73*, 523; P. K. Shah, *Am. Heart J.*, 1977, *93*, 403; S. Mookherjee *et al.*, *J. clin. Pharmac.*, 1978, *18*, 67; S. A. Lukes *et al.*, *Br. Heart J.*, 1979, *41*, 187.

Myocardial infarction. Intravenous infusions of sodium nitroprusside in a mean dose of 79 μg per minute (range 30 to 150 μg) given to 15 patients with acute cardiac infarction reduced the left ventricular filling pressure by approximately 50% with only a slight fall in the mean arterial pressure and no change in the heart-rate. Cardiac output consistently rose in patients with clinical signs of left ventricular failure and a low control cardiac index. There was a fall in pressure-time per minute which, together with the reduction in left ventricular filling pressure, suggested a fall in myocardial oxygen consumption. Subjective improvement was reported by most patients during infusion.— J. A. Franciosa *et al.*, *Lancet*, 1972, *1*, 650.

Twenty-seven patients with acute myocardial infarctions received intravenous infusions of sodium nitroprusside 10 to 200 μg per minute for 24 to 72 hours. At 12 hours after the onset of treatment mean arterial pressure had fallen by 19%, end-diastolic pressure in the pulmonary artery by 33%, and total peripheral resistance by 32%, whereas stroke volume and cardiac index had risen by 12 and 17% respectively. Although the mortality-rate due to cardiogenic shock was reduced to 25% a number of unexpected deaths after the fourth day, mainly due to arrhythmias, raised the total mortality-rate to 50%.— W. Kupper *et al.*, *Dt. med. Wschr.*, 1977, *102*, 548.

Concomitant use of sodium nitroprusside and salbutamol.— M. B. Fowler *et al.*, *Br. med. J.*, 1980, *280*, 435.

Further references: W. Baedeker *et al.*, *Dt. med. Wschr.*, 1977, *102*, 1751; V. Kötter *et al.*, *Br. Heart J.*, 1977, *39*, 1196; T. Mann *et al.*, *Circulation*, 1977, *56*, *Suppl.* 3, 33; N. A. Awan *et al.*, *ibid.*, 38; R. R. Miller *et al.*, *Am. J. Med.*, 1978, *65*, 167.

Controlled hypotension. Reviews of sodium nitroprusside in controlled hypotension: W. Fitch, *Br. J. Anaesth.*, 1977, *49*, 399; *Br. med. J.*, 1978, *2*, 784.

From haemodynamic studies on 5 patients, sodium nitroprusside, 50 μg per ml given by intravenous infusion during anaesthesia induced by thiopentone and maintained by nitrous oxide and halothane, was found to produce an increase in cardiac output, and was considered to be the drug of choice where controlled hypotension during anaesthesia was required.— J. A. W. Wildsmith *et al.*, *Br. J. Anaesth.*, 1973, *45*, 71.

Sodium nitroprusside, as a 0.01% intravenous infusion, was used to induce controlled hypotension in 20 patients undergoing cerebral surgery. Mean arterial pressure was rapidly reduced by 42% for periods of 17 to 93 minutes. This was associated with a 45% decrease in central venous pressure and an 11% increase in pulse-rate. Cerebrovascular resistance was decreased by 40% but, in the group as a whole, there was no significant decrease in cerebral blood flow or change in the cerebral metabolic rate for oxygen.— D. P. G. Griffiths *et al.*, *Br. J. Anaesth.*, 1974, *46*, 671.

In 12 patients undergoing plastic surgery the dose range of sodium nitroprusside by infusion required to achieve controlled hypotension was wide, and in 6 patients it was difficult to maintain stable blood pressure.— J. B. Hester, *Postgrad. med. J.*, 1974, *50*, 582.

In 26 patients receiving sodium nitroprusside infusion for hypotensive surgery increases in the concentration of cyanide in plasma and red blood-cells were correlated with the total dose; 98% of cyanide in the blood was in the red blood-cells; there were minimal changes in the concentration of thiocyanate in plasma. The concentration of cyanide in plasma was considered the critical factor in cyanide poisoning. The logarithm of the cyanide concentration in expired air was linearly related to the concentration in plasma. The total dose of sodium nitroprusside should be limited to 1.5 mg per kg body-weight over the duration of surgery; if the dose were greater or if administration was prolonged monitoring of plasma-cyanide concentrations was recommended; this could be done directly or the measurement of cyanide in expired air could be considered.— C. J. Vesey *et al.*, *Br. J. Anaesth.*, 1976, *48*, 651.

Further references: A. P. Adams, *Br. J. Anaesth.*, 1975, *47*, 777; N. W. Lawson *et al.*, *Anesth. Analg. curr. Res.*, 1976, *55*, 654; W. A. L. Rawlinson *et al.*, *Br. J. Anaesth.*, 1978, *50*, 937; J. A. W. Wildsmith *et al.*, *Br. J. Anaesth.*, 1979, *51*, 875; G. Barbier-Böhm *et al.*, *Br. J. Anaesth.*, 1980, *52*, 1039; J. A. Stirt *et al.*, *ibid.*, 1045.

Ergotamine poisoning. For the use of sodium nitroprusside in the treatment of cyanosis of the extremities due to ergotamine overdosage, see Ergotamine Tartrate, p.665.

Hypertension. When given by mouth to 16 hypertensive patients (9 with malignant and 7 with severe essential hypertension), sodium nitroprusside exhibited a slow, moderate hypotensive action in 9 cases. The effect was indistinguishable from that produced by sodium thiocyanate.— I. H. Page *et al.*, *Circulation*, 1955, *11*, 188.

A detailed account of the treatment of malignant hypertension in 7 patients by administration of sodium nitroprusside intravenously with the use of a constant infusion pump for periods lasting 1 to 12 days. The patients' blood pressures had not been controlled by various regimens using methyldopa, hydralazine, frusemide, and reserpine; 1 patient was resistant to diazoxide. The average blood pressure before treatment was 240/132 mmHg and the diastolic blood pressure was reduced to 90 to 100 mmHg within 5 minutes of sodium nitroprusside infusion. There were no marked toxic effects and it was considered that sodium nitroprusside could be a very effective agent in the treatment of hypertensive emergencies when diazoxide was unavailable, ineffective, or associated with unacceptable side-effects.— D. J. Ahearn *et al.*, *Archs intern. Med.*, 1974, *133*, 187.

Further references: M. K. Mani, *Br. med. J.*, 1971, *3*, 407; I. Tuzel *et al.*, *Curr. ther. Res.*, 1975, *17*, 95; *Med. Lett.*, 1975, *17*, 82.

Hypertension in children. An 11-year-old girl with refractory malignant hypertension received a continuous infusion of sodium nitroprusside for 28 days without evidence of toxicity.— J. R. Luderer *et al.*, *J. Pediat.*, 1977, *91*, 490.

Further references: G. Gordillo-Paniagua *et al.*, *J. Pediat.*, 1975, *87*, 799.

Phaeochromocytoma. Sodium nitroprusside was successfully used by infusion to prevent and control hypertensive episodes during arteriography and surgery in patients with phaeochromocytoma; 2 case reports were presented. The total dose should not exceed 500 µg per kg body-weight and the infusion-rate should not exceed 800 µg per minute; preparatory adrenoceptor blockade permitted doses to be kept within these limits.— P. Daggett *et al.*, *Br. med. J.*, 1978, *2*, 311. Comment on the dosage.— J. Krapez and P. Cole (letter), *ibid.*, 1088. Reply.— P. Daggett and I. Verner (letter), *ibid.*

Further references: D. S. Nourok *et al.*, *J. Am. med. Ass.*, 1963, *183*, 841; A. Lipson *et al.*, *ibid.*, 1978, *239*, 427.

Pyrexia. The intravenous infusion of sodium nitroprusside to induce peripheral vasodilatation was successfully used to treat extreme pyrexia in a 55-year-old man in whom conventional treatment had failed.— M. R. Katlic *et al.* (letter), *New Engl. J. Med.*, 1978, *299*, 154.

Respiratory distress syndrome. The successful use of sodium nitroprusside in a neonate with the idiopathic respiratory distress syndrome.— T. R. Abbott *et al.*, *Br. med. J.*, 1978, *1*, 1113.

Further references.— D. W. Beverley *et al.* (letter), *Archs Dis. Childh.*, 1979, *54*, 403.

Test for isoniazid. Details of a test using an alkaline sodium nitroprusside solution and acetic acid as reagents for detecting the presence of isoniazid and acetylisoniazid in urine.— K. V. N. Rao *et al.*, *Tubercle*, 1967, *48*, 45.

Preparations

Diagnostic Nitroprusside Tablets *(D.T.F.).* Rothera's Tablets. Each contains sodium nitroprusside 1 mg, anhydrous glycine 9 mg, anhydrous sodium phosphate 94 mg, anhydrous sodium borate 73 mg, lactose 20 mg, starch 2.5 mg, and magnesium stearate 500 µg; they are supplied with a colour chart.

Sterile Sodium Nitroprusside *(U.S.P.).* Sodium nitroprusside suitable for parenteral use. Protect from light.

Proprietary Preparations

Acetest *(Ames, UK).* A proprietary brand of Diagnostic Nitroprusside Tablets—see p.527.

Nipride *(Roche, UK).* Sodium nitroprusside, available as powder for preparing infusions, in ampoules of 50 mg; supplied with 2-ml ampoules of dextrose injection. (Also available as Nipride in *Austral., Canad., Denm., Ger., Neth., Switz., USA*).

Other Proprietary Names

Hypoten *(S. Afr.)*; Nipruss *(Ger., Neth., Switz.)*.

904-p

Sphaerophysine Benzoate. Spherophysine Benzoate. 1-[4-(3-Methylbut-1-enylamino)butyl]guanidine dibenzoate.

$C_{10}H_{22}N_4,2C_6H_5COOH$=442.6.

CAS — 1369-80-8 (sphaerophysine); 2233-20-7 (dibenzoate).

NOTE. Sphaerophysine benzoate has also been described as the structural isomer, *N*-(4-aminobutyl)-*N*-(3-methylbut-2-enyl)guanidine dibenzoate.

Pharmacopoeias. In *Rus.*

The benzoate of sphaerophysine, an alkaloid isolated from *Sphaerophysa salsula* (Leguminosae). It occurs as a white odourless crystalline powder with a bitter taste. M.p. about 152°.

Soluble 1 in 2 of water and 1 in 4 of alcohol; practically insoluble in chloroform and ether; freely soluble in solutions of alkali hydroxides and carbonates.

Uses. A ganglion-blocking agent that has been used in the USSR in the treatment of hypertension. It is administered by mouth. The doses given in the *Rus. P.* are: max. single 50 mg; max. in 24 hours 100 mg.

905-s

Syrosingopine. Methyl Carbethoxysyringoyl Reserpate. Methyl 18-*O*-(4-ethoxycarbonyloxy-3,5-dimethoxybenzoyl)reserpate.

$C_{35}H_{42}N_2O_{11}$=666.7.

CAS — 84-36-6.

A white or slightly yellowish, odourless, crystalline powder. Practically **insoluble** in water; freely soluble in chloroform and acetic acid; slightly soluble in ether and methyl alcohol. **Store** in airtight containers. Protect from light.

Uses. Syrosingopine has actions and uses similar to those described under reserpine (see p.163) but both its peripheral and its central effects are less pronounced. For the treatment of hypertension it has been given in initial doses of 1 to 2 mg daily, and maintenance doses of 0.5 to 3 mg daily.

Proprietary Names

Hipotensor Zambe Alfa *(Zambeletti, Spain)*; Neoreserpan *(Panthox & Burck, Ital.)*; Novoserpina *(Ghimas, Ital.)*; Raunova *(Zambeletti, Ital.)*; Aurugopin, Londomin, Seniramin, Siringina, Siroshuten, Syrogopin *(all Jap.)*.

906-w

Teprotide. BPP_{9a}; SQ 20881; L-Pyroglutamyl-L-tryptophyl-L-prolyl-L-arginyl-L-prolyl-L-glutaminyl-L-isoleucyl-L-prolyl-L-proline; 2-L-Tryptophan-3-de-L-leucine-4-de-L-proline-8-L-glutaminebradykinin potentiator B. 5-OxoPro-Trp-Pro-Arg-Pro-Gln-Ile-Pro-Pro.

$C_{53}H_{76}N_{14}O_{12}$=1101.3.

CAS — 35115-60-7.

Teprotide is a synthetic nonapeptide initially found in the venom of the pit-viper, *Bothrops jararaca.*

Teprotide inhibits the enzyme responsible for converting the inactive angiotensin I into active angiotensin II and thus blocks the pressor action of angiotensin II; it also prevents the degradation of bradykinin. It is used as an investigational tool in hypertension and also has therapeutic application. It has been given intravenously, intramuscularly, and subcutaneously in doses of 125 to 500 µg per kg body-weight every 8 hours to control resistant hypertension.

Severe hypotension in a patient with renovascular hypertension given teprotide.— D. W. Duhme *et al.* (letter), *Lancet*, 1974, *1*, 408. There was no excessive hypotension in 23 hypertensive patients given teprotide in doses of 0.5 to 5.4 mg. It was considered that serious hypotension would only coincide with severe volume or sodium depletion and/or blockade of sympathetic activity.— H. Gavras *et al.* (letter), *ibid.*, *2*, 353.

Action. A detailed account of the structure, properties, and actions of teprotide.— *Drugs of the Future*, 1978, *3*, 62.

Teprotide, 125 to 500 µg per kg body-weight intravenously, blocked the pressor effect of angiotensin I in 5 healthy subjects.— J. G. Collier *et al.*, *Lancet*, 1973, *1*, 72.

A study of 9 healthy subjects and 6 patients with essential hypertension demonstrated that teprotide had the desirable property of increasing renal blood flow in addition to reducing blood pressure. Its effects were more pronounced in the hypertensive subjects. The mode of action was unclear and might involve both renin-angiotensin and kallikrein-bradykinin systems.— G. H. Williams and N. K. Hollenberg, *New Engl. J. Med.*, 1977, *297*, 184. See also N. K. Hollenberg *et al.*, *New Engl. J. Med.*, 1979, *301*, 9. Criticism.— M. D. Bianchi and M. Fernandes (letter), *ibid.*, 1980, *302*, 179.

Teprotide 1 mg per kg body-weight was administered intravenously to 18 patients with hypertensive emergencies. Diastolic blood pressure decreased more than 15 mmHg within 20 minutes in 5 patients, who were considered to have renin-dependent hypertension, and were subsequently treated with propranolol. Decrease in diastolic blood pressure was less than 10 mmHg in 8 patients who were considered to have non-renin-dependent hypertension and were then treated with frusemide and other diuretics and a low-sodium diet. An intermediate response occurred in the other patients who were then treated with combination therapy. Teprotide was considered a useful diagnostic agent for determining renin-dependency of hypertension in a particular patient prior to treatment of hypertension.— C. P. Tifft *et al.*, *Ann. intern. Med.*, 1979, *90*, 43. See also D. B. Case and J. H. Laragh, *Ann. intern. Med.*, 1979, *91*, 153.

Haemodynamics.— T. R. Vrobel and J. N. Cohn, *Am. J. Cardiol.*, 1980, *45*, 331; D. P. Faxon *et al.*, *Circulation*, 1980, *61*, 925; A. P. Niarchos *et al.*, *Clin. Pharmac. Ther.*, 1980, *28*, 592.

Further references: D. B. Case *et al.*, *New Engl. J. Med.*, 1977, *296*, 641; G. H. Williams, *ibid.*, 684.

Therapeutic use. Reviews of renin inhibitors including teprotide.— E. Haber, *New Engl. J. Med.*, 1978, *298*, 1023; *Lancet*, 1978, *2*, 663; *Br. med. J.*, 1980, *281*, 630.

The successful use for several months of teprotide, initially intravenously, then intramuscularly and subcutaneously to control high-renin hypertension in a 19-year-old woman after renal transplantation. She received doses of 125 to 250 µg per kg body-weight every 8 hours.— M. J. Vandenburg *et al.*, *Br. med. J.*, 1978, *2*, 866.

Further references: H. Gavras *et al.*, *New Engl. J. Med.*, 1974, *291*, 817.

Manufacturers

Squibb, UK.

907-e

Tetraethylammonium Bromide *(B.P.C. 1954).* TEAB; Tetramone Bromide; Tetrylammonium Bromide.

$C_8H_{20}BrN$=210.2.

CAS — 71-91-0.

Colourless or almost colourless crystals or white crystalline powder. **Soluble** 1 in less than 1 of water, 1 in 1 of alcohol (90%), and 1 in 4 of chloroform. A 10% solution in water has a pH of 5 to 7. A 3.17% solution is iso-osmotic with serum. Solutions are **sterilised** by heating with a bactericide or by filtration; phenylmercuric nitrate should not be used as the bactericide.

Uses. Tetraethylammonium bromide is a quaternary ammonium ganglion-blocking agent. It has been given in doses of 100 to 500 mg intravenously in the treatment of hypertension but is now seldom employed.

915-e

Tetraethylammonium Chloride.

$C_8H_{20}ClN$=165.7.

CAS — 56-34-8.

908-l

Tetraethylammonium Chloride Solution *(B.P.C. 1954).*

A colourless, or nearly colourless, aqueous solution containing 50% w/v of tetraethylammonium chloride. When diluted with 4 times its volume of water it has a pH of 5 to 7. A 2.67% solution is iso-osmotic with serum. It is **sterilised** by heating with a bactericide or by filtration;

phenylmercuric nitrate should not be used as the bactericide. Benzethonium chloride 0.005% is a suitable preservative for solutions of tetraethylammonium chloride. **Store** in airtight containers.

Uses. Tetraethylammonium chloride is a quaternary ganglion-blocking agent. The solution has been given intravenously in doses of 0.2 to 1 ml in the treatment of hypertension but it is now seldom employed.

909-y

Tolonidine Nitrate. ST 375. 2-(2-Chloro-*p*-toluidino)-2-imidazoline nitrate.
$C_{10}H_{12}ClN_3,HNO_3$=272.7.

CAS — 4201-22-3 (tolonidine); 57524-15-9 (nitrate).

Uses. Tolonidine nitrate is an antihypertensive agent with the actions and uses of clonidine (see p.139). It is given in doses of 500 μg at night for the first week, 250 μg in the morning and 500 μg at night for the second week, and subsequently increased from the third week according to the patient's response. Maintenance doses are usually between 0.75 and 1.5 mg daily. It has been recommended that tolonidine should not be administered concurrently with guanethidine.

Pharmacology in *animals*.— D. Cosnier *et al.*, *Arzneimittel-Forsch.*, 1975, *25*, 1557, 1802, and 1926.

Proprietary Names
Euctan *(Delalande, Fr.)*.

910-g

Trimazosin Hydrochloride. CP-19106-1. 2-Hydroxy-2-methylpropyl 4-(4-amino-6,7,8-trimethoxyquinazolin-2-yl)piperazine-1-carboxylate hydrochloride monohydrate.
$C_{20}H_{29}N_5O_6,HCl,H_2O$=490.0.

CAS — 35795-16-5 (trimazosin); 35795-17-6 (hydrochloride, anhydrous); 53746-46-6 (hydrochloride, monohydrate).

White crystals. M.p. about 167°.

Adverse Effects, Treatment, and Precautions. Side-effects reported include headache, sedation, tachycardia, and dizziness.

Uses. Trimazosin is an antihypertensive agent which acts by causing direct peripheral vasodilatation. It has been given in doses of 25 to 300 mg thrice daily.

A review of the actions and uses of trimazosin. *Animal* studies indicate that it causes a peripheral vasodilatation by a specific action on arterioles, probably due to a direct effect on smooth muscle, because there was no evidence of any interference with adrenergic mechanisms.— *Drugs of the Future*, 1978, *3*, 325.

Cardiac disease. Haemodynamics.— J. R. Orlando *et al.*, *Clin. Pharmac. Ther.*, 1978, *24*, 531.

In a study of patients with chronic cardiac failure of varying cause and severity, trimazosin produced symptomatic improvement and a sustained increase in exercise tolerance and aerobic capacity.— K. T. Weber *et al.*, *New Eng. J. Med.*, 1980, *303*, 242.

Hypertension. Trimazosin 25 to 300 mg taken thrice daily was considered to be as effective as methyldopa 125 to 750 mg taken thrice daily and more effective than placebo, in lowering both supine and standing systolic and diastolic blood pressure in a double-blind study of 57 patients with hypertension. Side-effects occurred in 2 of 20 patients who took trimazosin, in 7 of 18 who took methyldopa, and in 2 of 19 who took placebo. Side-effects for trimazosin included moderate headache and mild sedation.— W. S. Aronow *et al.*, *Curr. ther. Res.*, 1978, *23*, 448.

Further references: D. De Guia *et al.*, *Curr. ther. Res.*, 1973, *15*, 339; N. D. Vlachakis *et al.*, *ibid.*, 1975, *17*, 564; W. S. Aronow *et al.*, *Am. J. Cardiol.*, 1977, *40*, 789; *idem*, *Clin. Pharmac. Ther.*, 1977, *22*, 425; W. S. Aronow and D. T. Danahy, *Am. J. Med.*, 1978, *65*, 155.

Manufacturers
Pfizer, USA.

911-q

Trimetaphan Camsylate *(B.P. 1968)*.

Trimetaphan Camphorsulphonate; Trimetaphan Camsilate; Trimethaphan Camsylate *(U.S.P)*; Trimetaphani Camsylas; Méthioplégium. 1,3-Dibenzylperhydro-2-oxoimidazo[4,5-*c*]thieno[1,2-*a*]thiolium (+)-camphor-10-sulphonate; 4,6-Dibenzyl-1-thionia-4,6-diazatricyclo[6,3,0,0^{3,7}]undecan-5-one (+)-camphor-10-sulphonate.
$C_{22}H_{25}N_2OS,C_{10}H_{15}O_4S$=596.8.

CAS — 7187-66-8(trimetaphan); 68-91-7(camsylate).

Pharmacopoeias. In *Int.* and *U.S.*

Colourless crystals or white crystalline powder, odourless or with a slight odour and with a bitter taste. M.p. about 232° with decomposition. **Soluble** 1 in less than 5 of water and 1 in 2 of alcohol; freely soluble in chloroform; practically insoluble in ether. A solution in water is dextrorotatory. A 1% solution in water has a pH of 5 to 6. **Incompatible** with thiopentone sodium, sodium thiamylal, gallamine triethiodide, iodides, bromides, and strongly alkaline solutions. **Store** below 8° in airtight containers.

Incompatibility. A haze developed over 3 hours when trimetaphan camsylate 1 g per litre was mixed with tubocurarine chloride 60 mg per litre in dextrose injection.— B. B. Riley, *J. Hosp. Pharm.*, 1970, *28*, 228.

Adverse Effects, Treatment, and Precautions. As for Pempidine Tartrate, p.157.

Trimetaphan may induce pupillary dilatation. Trimetaphan should be avoided in patients with severe cerebral or coronary vascular disease, and should only be used with extreme caution in those with impaired hepatic or renal function, degenerative disease of the central nervous system, Addison's disease, and diabetes. Owing to a histamine-liberating effect it should be used with caution in allergic subjects. Trimetaphan should also be used with caution in patients being treated with other antihypertensive agents, drugs which depress cardiac function, muscle relaxants, and in those taking corticosteroids.

Respiratory arrest in association with large doses of trimetaphan camsylate.— R. C. Dale and E. T. Schroeder, *Archs intern. Med.*, 1976, *136*, 816.

Uses. Trimetaphan is a ganglion-blocking agent with similar actions to pempidine tartrate (see p.157) but with a very brief duration of action. It is used with postural tilting for inducing controlled hypotension during surgical procedures. It acts rapidly to produce a hypotensive response which persists for 10 to 30 minutes according to the amount given.

Trimetaphan camsylate is administered by the slow intravenous infusion of a freshly prepared solution in sodium chloride injection or sodium chloride and dextrose injection, the usual strength of solution being 1 mg per ml. The infusion is started at the rate of 3 to 4 mg per minute and then adjusted according to the response of the patient. Similar doses have been recommended for children. A double-strength infusion may be required, particularly in children, to prevent overloading the circulation. It may also be given intermittently by intravenous injection. A frequent check on the blood pressure is essential and this should be allowed to rise before wound closure.

Adrenaline should not be infiltrated locally at the site of incision when trimetaphan is being given since control of blood pressure may be lost.

Trimetaphan has also been used for the emergency treatment of hypertensive crises, especially in association with pulmonary oedema.

Controlled hypotension. Discussions on the use of trimetaphan in controlled hypotension during surgery.— G. E. H. Enderby, *Postgrad. med. J.*, 1974, *50*, 572; A. P. Adams, *Br. J. Anaesth.*, 1975, *47*, 777.

Induced hypotension with trimetaphan camsylate to control life-threatening haemorrhage.— R. W. Hopkins *et al.*, *Archs Surg., Chicago*, 1967, *95*, 517.

Trimetaphan, 500 μg per ml given by intravenous infusion to 10 patients to induce hypotension during surgery, had no serious effect on cardiac output with patients in the horizontal position. The fall in blood pressure was frequently prolonged for up to 30 minutes after administration of trimetaphan was discontinued.— D. B. Scott *et al.*, *Br. J. Anaesth.*, 1972, *44*, 523.

There was no significant change in mean intracranial pressure in 21 patients given trimetaphan for controlled hypotension prior to neurosurgery, but 2 patients had individual increases of 5.7 and 9.3 mmHg.— J. M. Turner *et al.*, *Br. J. Anaesth.*, 1977, *49*, 419.

Cardiac disorders. The use of trimetaphan therapy to reduce the predicted infarct size following myocardial infarction.— W. E. Shell and B. E. Sobel, *New Engl. J. Med.*, 1974, *291*, 481.

Trimetaphan remains the drug of choice for the medical treatment of acute dissecting aneurysm.— R. F. Palmer and K. C. Lasseter (letter), *New Engl. J. Med.*, 1976, *294*, 1403.

Preparations

Trimetaphan Injection *(B.P. 1968)*. A sterile solution of trimetaphan camsylate in Water for Injections, prepared by dissolving the sterile contents of a sealed container in the requisite amount of Water for Injections.

Trimethaphan Camsylate Injection *(U.S.P.)*. A sterile solution of trimetaphan camsylate in Water for Injections. pH 4.9 to 5.6. Store at 2° to 8°. Avoid freezing. To be diluted before use.

Arfonad *(Roche, UK)*. Trimetaphan camsylate, available as an injection containing 50 mg per ml, in ampoules of 5 ml. Store in a refrigerator. (Also available as Arfonad in *Austral., Belg., Canad., Fr., Ital., Jap., Neth., S.Afr., Swed., USA*).

912-p

Trimethidinium Methosulphate. 1,3,8,8-Tetramethyl-3-(3-trimethylammoniopropyl)-3-azoniabicyclo-[3.2.1]octane bis(methylsulphate).
$C_{17}H_{36}N_2,2CH_3SO_4$=490.7.

CAS — 2624-50-2(trimethidinium); 14149-43-0 (methosulphate).

A white hygroscopic powder which may have a slight camphoraceous odour. M.p. 194° to 202°. Very **soluble** in water and alcohol; very slightly soluble in acetone; practically insoluble in ether. A 2% solution in water has a pH of 4 to 6.5. **Store** in airtight containers.

Uses. Trimethidinium methosulphate is a quaternary ammonium ganglion-blocking agent with actions and uses similar to those of pempidine tartrate (see p.157). The initial dose is 20 mg before breakfast and supper, increased by increments of 20 mg every 3 days until a satisfactory response is obtained. Maintenance doses have varied from 20 to 300 mg daily.

913-s

Green Veratrum. Green Hellebore *(B.P.C. 1954)*; American Hellebore; American Veratrum; Green Hellebore Rhizome; Veratrum Viride; Veratro Verde. The dried rhizome and roots of *Veratrum viride* (Liliaceae).

CAS — 8002-39-9 (see also under Alkavervir).

Uses. The action of green veratrum is due to its many alkaloidal constituents. It lowers the blood pressure and slows the heart-rate. It has been used in hypertension, especially that associated with the toxaemias of pregnancy. It is employed as a source of alkavervir (see p.136) and has been administered as a tincture (1 in 10; *dose:* 0.3 to 2 ml).

Veratrum alkaloids had been superseded in the UK as antihypertensive agents because of their lack of efficacy and their toxicity; tolerance was also a problem.— A. M. Breckenridge, *Practitioner*, 1979, *223*, 742.

Proprietary Names
Vera-67 *(Mallard, USA)*.

914-w

White Veratrum *(B.P.C. 1934)*. White Hellebore; European Hellebore; White Hellebore Rhizome; Veratrum Album.

Pharmacopoeias. In *Cz., Hung.*, and *Swiss*, with not less than 1% of total alkaloids.

The dried rhizome and roots of *Veratrum album* (Liliaceae). The alkaloidal constituents are similar to those of green veratrum.

Uses. White veratrum is employed as a source of the alkaloids protoveratrines A and B (see p.162).

Antineoplastic Agents and Immunosuppressants

1800-p

Antineoplastic agents (also known as cytotoxic agents) are used in the treatment of malignant disease when surgery or radiotherapy is not possible or has proved ineffective, as an adjunct to surgery or radiotherapy, or, as in leukaemia, as the initial treatment. Therapy with antineoplastic agents is notably successful in a few malignant conditions and may be used to palliate symptoms and prolong life in others.

The two main groups of drugs used in the treatment of malignant disease are the alkylating agents and the antimetabolites. Nitrogen mustards, ethyleneimine compounds, and alkyl sulphonates, are the main *alkylating agents* and those described in this section include: busulphan (p.193), chlorambucil (p.195), cyclophosphamide (p.199), ethoglucid (p.208), hexamethylmelamine (p.211), melphalan (p.213), mitobronitol (p.220), mitolactol (p.221), mustine (p.222), pipobroman (p.224), thiotepa (p.228), and treosulfan (p.229).

Other compounds with an alkylating action include the nitrosoureas, carmustine (p.195), lomustine (p.212), semustine (p.225), streptozocin (p.226), and chlorozotocin (p.196). Cisplatin (p.197) and dacarbazine (p.204) appear to act similarly.

All the effective alkylating agents appear to act by alkylating and cross-linking guanine and possibly other bases in deoxyribonucleic acid thus arresting cell division; they are described as cell cycle nonspecific agents. Not only malignant cells are affected but also other actively dividing cells such as those of bone marrow, skin, gastro-intestinal mucosa, and foetal tissues.

The *antimetabolites* combine with the same enzymes as physiologically occurring cellular metabolites but prevent the metabolic process. Usually, the synthesis of nucleic acid is affected by folic acid, purine, or pyrimidine antagonists. They are described as cell cycle specific agents. The antimetabolites described in this section include: azacitidine (p.189), azathioprine (p.190), cytarabine (p.203), floxuridine (p.209), fluorouracil (p.209), mercaptopurine (p.214), methotrexate (p.215), tegafur (p.227), and thioguanine (p.228).

Azathioprine is mainly used as an immunosuppressant, see below.

Several *antibiotics* interfere with nucleic acids and are effective as antineoplastic agents. They are cell cycle nonspecific agents and those described here include: actinomycin D (p.187), bleomycin (p.192), daunorubicin (p.205), doxorubicin (p.205), mithramycin (p.220), mitomycin (p.221), streptozocin (p.226), and zinostatin (p.233).

Although streptozocin is an antibiotic it is usually classed as a nitrosourea (above).

Some plant *alkaloids* are used as antineoplastics and include the following cell cycle stage-specific agents: vinblastine (p.230), vincristine (p.231), and vindesine (p.232).

The antineoplastic agents etoposide (p.208) and teniposide (p.227) are derivatives of podophyllotoxin; mitopodozide (p.222) is derived from podophyllin.

Also described in this section are other agents which act by various routes to affect the growth and proliferation of malignant cells. They include: aminoglutethimide (p.188), colaspase (p.198), hydroxyurea (p.212), mitotane (p.222), nafoxidine (p.223), procarbazine (p.224), razoxane (p.225), and tamoxifen (p.226).

Glucocorticoids (see Corticosteroids, p.451) are used in association with antineoplastic agents in the treatment of malignant disease, especially in acute leukaemias and lymphomas. Other agents used in antineoplastic therapy include sex hormones (p.1401), radiopharmaceuticals (p.1386), and immunostimulants such as BCG vaccine (p.1588).

References: S. K. Carter *et al.*, Chemotherapy of Cancer, London, John Wiley, 1977; M. J. Cline and C. M. Haskell, Cancer Chemotherapy, 3rd Edn, London, Saunders, 1980; R. T. Dorr and W. L. Fritz, Cancer Chemotherapy Handbook, London, Kimpton, 1980.

Adverse Effects with Antineoplastic Agents and Immunosuppressants. The toxicity of the compounds described in this chapter is generally a function of their therapeutic activity. Although they may have differing modes of action, their antineoplastic effect is dependent on a cytotoxic action which is not selective for malignant cells but may affect all rapidly dividing cells. The spectrum of adverse effects occurring with antineoplastic agents is therefore similar, but there may be marked quantitative differences and the speed of onset of adverse effects is variable. However, some adverse effects appear to be specific for individual agents, such as the cardiotoxicity of the anthracyclines, doxorubicin and daunorubicin, and may not be related to their principal effect on dividing cells. Also it may be difficult to attribute many of the adverse effects seen in patients with cancer to a specific agent because of the nature of the disease and the complexity of treatment.

Despite its toxicity, cancer chemotherapy is valuable because in some instances malignant cells are slightly more sensitive than normal cells and in general malignant cells surviving treatment recover less readily than do normal cells surviving treatment. In addition, toxicity may be minimised by careful control of the size and timing of doses of individual antineoplastic agents and by using drugs with different dose-limiting adverse effects in combination chemotherapy regimens.

Adverse effects common to all antineoplastic agents to a varying extent may be divided into acute effects occurring shortly after administration, delayed effects occurring days or weeks after administration, and long-term effects which may not become evident for years. Acute effects include anorexia, nausea and vomiting, allergic reactions, and local irritant effects. Nausea and vomiting are common to most antineoplastic agents, are often central in origin, and may occur, with varying severity, minutes or hours after an injection. Allergic reactions include skin rashes, pruritus, and erythema, often of areas previously irradiated, as well as symptoms such as fever, headache, hypotension, malaise, and weakness; anaphylaxis has also been reported. Many antineoplastic agents have vesicant or irritant effects on the skin and mucous membranes and may cause thrombophlebitis when injected intravenously.

Delayed or long-term adverse effects may result from the action of antineoplastic agents on rapidly dividing normal cells in the bone marrow, lymphoreticular tissue, gastro-intestinal mucosa, skin, gonads, and foetus. The most common serious effect is probably bone-marrow depression with leucopenia, anaemia, and thrombocytopenia and bleeding, as well as an immunosuppressant effect involving both antibody and cell-mediated immunity. The attendant increased risks of infection and haemorrhage can be life-threatening although the severity of myelosuppression varies for individual agents and may occur days or weeks after administration. Some agents, including the nitrosoureas carmustine, lomustine, and semustine, may cause cumulative delayed bone-marrow depression leading to prolonged severe pancytopenia. Adverse effects on the gastro-intestinal tract have included stomatitis, mouth ulcers, oesophagitis, abdominal pain, haemorrhage, diarrhoea, and intestinal ulceration and perforation. The active cells of the hair follicles are susceptible to most antineoplastic agents, but especially cyclophosphamide and doxorubicin, and reversible alopecia may occur. Wound healing may be delayed.

Antineoplastic chemotherapy may have long-term effects on the gonads with suppression of ovarian and testicular function resulting in amenorrhoea and the inhibition of spermatogenesis. Gynaecomastia has been reported. The majority of antineoplastic agents are potentially mutagenic and teratogenic. An apparent increase in the incidence of second malignancies in patients who have previously received successful cancer chemotherapy may reflect the increased numbers of patients achieving long-term remissions from their primary disease. This carcinogenic effect has been linked with the ability of antineoplastic agents to induce mutations and with the effects of prolonged immunosuppression.

Other adverse effects occurring with antineoplastic agents include hyperuricaemia and acute renal failure due to uric acid nephropathy which may result from the lysis of large numbers of cells and the breakdown of nucleoproteins. Hyperphosphataemia and other disturbances of electrolyte balance have also been reported. Pigmentation of the skin and nails occurs with several antineoplastic agents and may occasionally be part of an Addisonian syndrome. Jaundice and abnormal liver-function tests may sometimes be a manifestation of the disease rather than its treatment. With some agents pulmonary or neurotoxic effects are dose-limiting.

Reviews of the adverse effects of antineoplastic agents.— M. H. Cullen, *Prescribers' J.*, 1979, *19*, 42.

Adrenal suppression. For references to the controversy surrounding adrenal suppression in patients receiving corticosteroids and cytotoxic therapy, see Corticosteroids, p.446.

Carcinogenicity. Antineoplastic agents, including the alkylating agents, which are known to have a radiomimetic action, nitrosoureas, and procarbazine have been shown to be carcinogenic (S.M. Sieber and R.H. Adamson, *Adv. Cancer Res.*, 1975, *22*, 57) and many are mutagenic. There have now been numerous reports of second cancers, particularly leukaemias, lymphomas, and squamous cell carcinomas, occurring after a latent period of about 4 years following the initiation of cancer chemotherapy. However, it may be difficult to apportion blame since patients will have often received radiotherapy as well as chemotherapy with a number of antineoplastic agents. Immunosuppressant drugs such as azathioprine and cyclophosphamide impair antibody production and the cellular immune response and might compromise host resistance (*Lancet*, 1977, *1*, 519); their use, especially over prolonged periods, has been associated with an increasing incidence of neoplasms which may occur months or years after the start of treatment. As a result the use of antineoplastic agents, in particular alkylating agents such as cyclophosphamide, is being seriously questioned in patients with non-malignant diseases. It has been suggested (R. Althouse *et al.*, *Br. med. J.*, 1979, *1*, 1630) that over a period of 10 years, 5 to 15% of patients given alkylating agents will develop cancer.

Studies on the incidence of malignancies associated with antineoplastic therapy. In a survey of second-cancers in 5455 patients with ovarian cancer from 1970 through 1975, fifteen cases of leukaemia were reported compared with an expected 1.62. The excess of leukaemia was due to 13 cases of nonlymphocytic leukaemia, a figure 21 times greater than expected, and was associated with administration of alkylating agents although this effect might have been enhanced by radiation exposure.— R. R. Reimer *et al.*, *New Engl. J. Med.*, 1977, *297*, 177. Of 579 patients with Hodgkin's disease who were treated with radiotherapy, chemotherapy, or both, 5, given radiotherapy and chemotherapy with MOPP, subsequently developed diffuse histiocytic or undifferentiated non-Hodgkin's lymphomas. As previously reported by C.N. Coleman *et al.* (*New Engl. J. Med.*, 1977, *297*, 1249) 6 further patients in the group developed acute myelocytic leukaemia. At 10 years the actuarial risk of non-Hodgkin's lymphoma for the entire group was 4.4% compared with a risk of acute leukaemia of 2%. In those patients who received radiotherapy and chemotherapy the risks were calculated to be 15.2% and 3.9%

respectively at 10 years compared with 1.3% and 2.3% at 7 years.— J. G. Krikorian *et al.*, *New Engl. J. Med.*, 1979, *300*, 452. In 764 patients with Hodgkin's disease treated with radiotherapy, chemotherapy, or both, the incidence of second solid tumours within 10 years was 7.3% and that of acute non-lymphoblastic leukaemia (ANLL) was 2.4%. Solid tumours occurred only in patients given radiotherapy, and ANLL only in patients who had MOPP or modified MOPP regimens. Radiotherapy and treatment with doxorubicin, bleomycin, vinblastine, and dacarbazine (ABVD) has not been associated with second tumours or ANLL. A high incidence (5.4%) of leukaemia after radiotherapy and MOPP called for weighing benefit against risk.— P. Valagussa *et al.*, *Br. med. J.*, 1980, *280*, 216. A suggestion that doxorubicin might be acting similarly to actinomycin D (G.J. D'Angio *et al.*, *Cancer*, 1976, *37*, *Suppl.* 2, 1177) in protecting against radiation-associated cancers, although doxorubicin might not be protective when alkylating agents are present.— G. J. D'Angio (letter), *ibid.*, 1452.

Reviews and reports of carcinogenicity associated with antineoplastic therapy: *Lancet*, 1977, *1*, 519 (a discussion on leukaemia linked with therapy); R. S. Brody *et al.*, *Cancer*, 1977, *40*, 1917; G. G. Caldwell, *Cancer*, 1977, *40*, 1952; B. A. Chabner, *New Engl. J. Med.*, 1977, *297*, 213 (comment on second neoplasms as a complication of cancer chemotherapy); J. D. Khandekar *et al.*, *Archs intern. Med.*, 1977, *137*, 355 (acute leukaemia has been reported in a total of 11 patients who had received prolonged chemotherapy for ovarian carcinoma); D. Schmähl, *Cancer*, 1977, *40*, 1927; S. M. Sieber and R. H. Adamson, *Cancer*, 1977, *40*, 1950; R. K. Woodruff *et al.*, *Lancet*, 1977, *2*, 900 (Hodgkin's disease developed in 3 patients during maintenance treatment for acute lymphoblastic leukaemia in remission); *Br. med. J.*, 1978, *1*, 334; D. C. Crafts *et al.*, *Cancer Treat. Rep.*, 1978, *62*, 177; M. B. Spaulding *et al.* (letter), *New Engl. J. Med.*, 1979, *301*, 384; F. Cavalli *et al.* (letter), *New Engl. J. Med.*, 1980, *302*, 1478; C. G. Geary, *Br. J. Hosp. Med.*, 1980, *24*, 538.

Individual reports of second malignancies associated with antineoplastic therapy: ***Busulphan*** H. Stott *et al.*, *Br. med. J.*, 1977, *2*, 1513 (leukaemia after treatment of bronchial carcinoma).

Chlorambucil. G. A. M. Castro *et al.* (letter), *New Engl. J. Med.*, 1973, *289*, 103 (acute myeloblastic leukaemia after treatment of chronic lymphocytic leukaemia); T. Hague *et al.*, *Am. J. med. Sci.*, 1976, *272*, 225 (acute myelogenous leukaemia after treatment of ovarian carcinoma); R. R. Reimer *et al.*, *New Engl. J. Med.*, 1977, *297*, 177 (leukaemia after treatment of ovarian carcinoma); Y. Carcassone *et al.*, *Cancer Treat. Rep.*, 1978, *62*, 1110 (acute leukaemia); P. D. Berk *et al.*, *New Engl. J. Med.*, 1981, *304*, 441 (leukaemia after treatment of polycythaemia vera).

Cyclophosphamide. C. G. S. Smit and L. Meyler (letter), *Lancet*, 1970, *2*, 671 (acute myeloid leukaemia after treatment of adenocarcinoma); P. Gutjahr and J. Spranger (letter), *J. Pediat.*, 1975, *87*, 1004 (acute leukaemia after radiotherapy and cyclophosphamide following the removal of a rhabdomyosarcoma); R. L. Wall and K. P. Clausen, *New Engl. J. Med.*, 1975, *293*, 271 (squamous cell carcinoma of the bladder after treatment of myeloma and Hodgkin's disease); J. G. Erskine *et al.*, *Br. med. J.*, 1977, *2*, 1329 (chronic granulocytic leukaemia after treatment of lymphoma); R. R. Reimer *et al.*, *New Engl. J. Med.*, 1977, *297*, 177 (leukaemia after treatment of ovarian cancer); W. V. Fairchild *et al.*, *J. Urol.*, 1979, *122*, 163 (bladder cancer); G. A. McLoughlin *et al.*, *Br. med. J.*, 1980, *280*, 524 (squamous cell carcinoma of the stomach).

Doxorubicin. R. R. Reimer and C. W. Groppe (letter), *Ann. intern. Med.*, 1979, *90*, 989 (acute leukaemia after treatment of endometrial carcinoma with radiotherapy, doxorubicin, and cyclophosphamide).

Fluorouracil. A. G. Finley (letter), *Med. J. Aust.*, 1973, *1*, 815 (squamous carcinoma after the topical use of fluorouracil).

Melphalan. R. A. Kyle *et al.*, *Archs intern. Med.*, 1975, *135*, 185 (acute myelomonocytic leukaemia after treatment of multiple myeloma); S. M. Sieber and R. H. Adamson (letter), *Br. med. J.*, 1975, *2*, 557 (a brief review of acute leukaemia after treatment of multiple myeloma); R. Bell *et al.*, *J. Am. med. Ass.*, 1976, *236*, 1609 (carcinoma of the breast after treatment of multiple myeloma); I. E. Burton *et al.*, *Br. med. J.*, 1976, *1*, 20 (acute leukaemia after treatment of melanoma); N. A. Buskard *et al.*, *Can. med. Ass. J.*, 1977, *117*, 788 (plasma cell leukaemia after treatment with radiotherapy and melphalan following removal of an ovarian carcinoma); R. R. Reimer *et al.*, *New Engl. J. Med.*, 1977, *297*, 177 (leukaemia following treatment of ovarian cancer); N. Einhorn, *Cancer*, 1978, *41*, 444 (acute leukaemia following treatment of ovarian carcinoma); M. R. Shetty and R. Freel, *Gynecol. Oncol.*, 1979, *7*, 264 (acute myelomonocytic leukaemia following treatment of ovarian cancer); R. Stegman and R. Alexanian, *Ann. intern. Med.*, 1979, *90*, 780 (the incidence of solid tumour development was not significantly greater in 628 patients with multiple myeloma who had been treated with melphalan and prednisolone than in a control population).

Mustine hydrochloride. P. H. Kravitz and C. J. McDonald, *Acta derm.-vener., Stockh.*, 1978, *58*, 421 (squamous cell carcinoma following the topical use of mustine in mycosis fungoides).

Semustine. R. J. Cohen (letter), *New Engl. J. Med.*, 1980, *302*, 120 (leukaemia).

Thiotepa W. S. A. Allan (letter), *Lancet*, 1970, *2*, 775 (acute myeloblastic leukaemia after treatment following removal of cystic ovarian tumour); D. H. Garfield (letter), *Lancet*, 1970, *2*, 1037 (erythromegakaryocytic leukaemia); M. Perlman and R. Walker (letter), *J. Am. med. Ass.*, 1973, *224*, 250 (acute myelogenous leukaemia following treatment of breast cancer); T. Hague *et al.*, *Am. J. med. Sci.*, 1976, *272*, 225 (acute myelogenous leukaemia following treatment of ovarian carcinoma); *New Engl. J. Med.*, 1977, *297*, 102 (acute myelogenous leukaemia following treatment of transitional-cell carcinoma of the bladder); R. R. Reimer *et al.*, *New Engl. J. Med.*, 1977, *297*, 177 (leukaemia following treatment of ovarian cancer).

Trofosfamide E. Petri and J. E. Altwein, *Dt. med. Wschr.*, 1978, *103*, 30 (bladder carcinoma after treatment of Hodgkin's disease).

Uramustine. R. R. Reimer *et al.*, *New Engl. J. Med.*, 1977, *297*, 177 (leukaemia after treatment of ovarian cancer).

A discussion on the role of immunosuppression in the development of malignant neoplasms. Skin cancers and lymphomas have been reported to account for about two thirds of all malignancies in transplant patients reported to the Denver Transplant Tumour Registry (I. Penn, *Transplant Proc.*, 1975, *7*, 323). Skin cancers in renal transplant patients occur primarily on areas exposed to the sun and the risk of developing them increases with the length of immunosuppression. The majority of these skin cancers are squamous cell carcinomas and in immunosuppressed patients the progression of solar keratoses to squamous cell carcinomas appears to be accelerated. Immunosuppressants may also act as co-carcinogens with u.v. light in the induction of skin cancers but the potentiation of viral oncogenesis by immunosuppression seems an unlikely explanation for these cancers. Undue exposure to the sun should be avoided in patients receiving long-term immunosuppressant therapy and the skin should be examined regularly.— J. C. Maize, *J. Am. med. Ass.*, 1977, *237*, 1857. A 4-year study of 133 patients receiving immunosuppressants, not in association with organ transplantation, indicated that there was no substantial risk of cancer.— G. R. Symington *et al.*, *Aust. N.Z. J. Med.*, 1977, *7*, 368. In 3823 patients who had undergone renal transplantation and were taking azathioprine, cyclophosphamide, or chlorambucil the incidence of deaths from non-Hodgkin's lymphoma was 26 times that expected, with a 10-fold increase in squamous-cell skin cancer. The incidence of non-Hodgkin's lymphoma and squamous-cell skin cancer were increased about 60-fold and 23-fold respectively. In 1349 patients without transplants who had taken the immunosuppressants for at least 12 weeks for non-malignant conditions the incidence of the 2 neoplasms was significantly increased but to a lesser degree. Other rare neoplasms, including mesenchymal tumours, were increased in transplant and non-transplant patients. There was no evidence that common [other] neoplasms were increased.— L. J. Kinlen *et al.*, *Br. med. J.*, 1979, *2*, 1461.

Individual reports of cancers developing in association with immunosuppressant therapy for non-malignant conditions: *Azathioprine* N. Manny *et al.* (letter), *Br. med. J.*, 1972, *2*, 291 (malignant melanoma after prednisone and azathioprine); I. Sneddon and J. M. Wishart (letter), *Br. med. J.*, 1972, *4*, 235 (cutaneous lymphomatous vulval ulcer); L. McAdam *et al.*, *Arthritis Rheum.*, 1974, *17*, 92 (adenocarcinoma of the lung); E. Alexson and K. D. Brandt, *Am. J. med. Sci.*, 1977, *273*, 335 (acute leukaemia); J. S. Ghosh (letter), *Postgrad. med. J.*, 1977, *53*, 420 (acute myeloid leukaemia); I. T. Gilmore *et al.*, *Postgrad. med. J.*, 1977, *53*, 173 (acute myeloid leukaemia); D. J. Hodgkinson and T. J. Williams, *Gynecol. Oncol.*, 1977, *5*, 308 (endometrial malignancy); J. Scharf *et al.*, *J. Am. med. Ass.*, 1977, *237*, 152 (transitional-cell carcinoma of the bladder); H. O. Jauregui, *Archs Derm.*, 1978, *114*, 1052 (lymphomatoid granulomatosis after prednisone and azathioprine); A. N. Krutchik *et al.* (letter), *J. Am. med. Ass.*, 1978, *239*, 107 (breast cancer after azathioprine and prednisolone); R. G. Norfleet and C. E. Sampson, *Am. J. Gastroent., N.Y.*, 1978, *70*, 383 (cervical carcinoma after prednisone and azathioprine); J. J. Vismans *et al.*, *Acta med. scand.*, 1980, *207*, 315 (subacute myelomonocytic leukaemia after prednisone and azathioprine); F. M. Younis *et al.* (letter), *Lancet*, 1980, *2*, 1141 (malignant melanoma developing from a pigmented mole after treatment with azathioprine and prednisolone).

Chlorambucil I. J. Forbes, *Med. J. Aust.*, 1972, *1*, 918 (erythromyeloid leukaemia); S. Cameron (letter), *New Engl. J. Med.*, 1977, *296*, 1065 (leukaemia); Y. Lebranchu *et al.* (letter), *Lancet*, 1980, *1*, 649 (acute leukaemia).

Cyclophosphamide. B. N. Bashour *et al.*, *J. Pediat.*, 1973, *82*, 292 (cervical tumour after prednisone and cyclophosphamide); M. M. Roberts and R. Bell, *Lancet*, 1976, *2*, 768 (acute myeloid leukaemia); J. Chang and C. G. Geary (letter), *Lancet*, 1977, *1*, 97 (acute myeloblastic leukaemia after prednisolone and cyclophosphamide); P. A. Knowlson (letter), *Lancet*, 1977, *2*, 457; J. S. Marks and C. L. Scholtz, *Postgrad. med. J.*, 1977, *53*, 48 (pleural sarcoma); H. C. Puri and R. A. Campbell (letter), *Lancet*, 1977, *1*, 1306 (tumours of the breast and cervix); M. C. Hochberg and L. E. Shulman, *Johns Hopkins med. J.*, 1978, *142*, 211 (leukaemia).

Melphalan. R. A. Kyle *et al.*, *Blood*, 1974, *44*, 333 (acute leukaemia); R. F. K. De Bock and M. E. Peetermans (letter), *Lancet*, 1977, *1*, 1208 (leukaemia).

Methotrexate R. Keeleter *et al.*, *Dt. med. Wschr.*, 1972, *97*, 514 (lymphoreticular hyperplasia); C. A. D. Ringrose, *Am. J. Obstet. Gynec.*, 1974, *119*, 1132 (cervical carcinoma); P. L. Bailin *et al.*, *J. Am. med. Ass.*, 1975, *232*, 359 (a 7-year follow-up study of 205 patients who had received methotrexate for psoriasis).

Effects on chromosomes . Chromosomal aberrations associated with antineoplastic agents have been found in studies in vitro and on examination of the blood cells and bone marrow of patients given antineoplastic therapy: W. Bell *et al.*, *Blood*, 1966, *27*, 771 (cytarabine); I. Hansteen (letter), *Lancet*, 1969, *2*, 744 (demecolcine); R. S. Bornstein *et al.*, *Cancer Res.*, 1971, *31*, 2004 (bleomycin); P. J. Balson, *Adverse Drug React. Bull.*, 1972, Dec., 116 (azaserine, cyclophosphamide, daunorubicin, methotrexate, mitomycin, and rufocromomycin); E. Gebhart *et al.*, *Dt. med. Wschr.*, 1974, *99*, 52 (busulphan); S. F. Tolchin *et al.*, *Arthritis Rheum.*, 1974, *17*, 375 (cyclophosphamide); B. R. Reeves *et al.*, *Br. med. J.*, 1975, *4*, 22 (chlorambucil); B. K. Vig and R. Lewis, *Mutat. Res.*, 1978, *55*, 121 (bleomycin); N. Tatsumi and Y. Wada (letter), *New Engl. J. Med.*, 1979, *300*, 44 (vinblastine).

See also under Effects on Reproductive Potential (below).

Effects on the bladder. Cyclophosphamide (see p.199) is the antineoplastic agent most frequently associated with adverse effects on the bladder, but see also Busulphan, p.194, and Chlorambucil, p.195.

Effects on the blood. *Bone-marrow depression.* The formation and development of blood cells takes place in the bone-marrow. Myeloid cells are produced by cell division and maturation from the 3 major cell lines of bone marrow, erythroblastic, granulocytic, and megakaryocytic, from which red cells, white cells, and platelets are derived. The development of each of these cell-types takes about a week but their half-lives in the circulation are very different. Red cells circulate for about 120 days and platelets for 8 to 10 days; the half-life of granulocytes is about 7 hours.

Bone-marrow depression or myelosuppression, is common to the majority of antineoplastic agents and is the single most important dose-limiting adverse effect. Involvement of all cellular elements may result in pancytopenia. However, depression is often selective and in any event white cells and platelets tend to be affected before red cells since they have a more rapid turnover in the circulation. The most usual manifestation of bone-marrow depression is leucopenia, followed by thrombocytopenia and anaemia; anaemia may be characterised by falling haemoglobin concentrations and megaloblastic changes in the bone marrow. The degree and duration of myelosuppression varies greatly with different antineoplastic agents and they may be graded according to the severity of their effect on leucocyte and platelet counts and according to the time of onset, nadir, and recovery time of their depressive effect. The cytotoxic effect on haematopoietic cells, relative to that on other normal or malignant cells, varies for different agents. Marrow aplasia is generally transient and may last from 5 to 10 days but with agents such as busulphan it may be prolonged or even permanent; nitrosoureas such as carmustine are known to have a cumulative delayed myelosuppressive effect. A few agents such as bleomycin, mitotane, and tamoxifen do not appear to be myelosuppressive in therapeutic doses and suppression may be relatively mild with colaspase and vincristine. Specific differences in their effects on bone marrow are discussed under the individual antineoplastic agents.

See also under Effects on Immune Response (below).

Some individual reports on the adverse effects of antineoplastic agents and immunosuppresants on the blood and bone marrow: H. M. Yonet *et al.*, *Am. J. med. Sci.*, 1967, *254*, 48 (haemolytic anaemia due to cyclophosphamide); R. W. Monto *et al.*, *Cancer Res.*, 1969, *29*, 697 (thrombocytopenia and coagulation defects with mithramycin); M. Swanson, *Drug Intell. & clin. Pharm.*, 1973, *7*, 6 (haemolytic anaemia with chlorambucil); S. Spier *et al.*, *Br. J. Derm.*, 1973, *89*, 199 (macrocytosis with hydroxyurea); J. H. Klippel and J. L. Decker, *J. Am. med. Ass.*, 1974, *229*, 180 (increased erythrocyte mean corpuscular volume, haemoglobin loss, and megaloblastic erythropoiesis with cyclophosphamide or azathioprine); H. M. Pinedo *et al.* (letter), *Br. med. J.*, 1974, *3*, 525 (myelofibrosis with procarbazine); H. -P. Lohrmann *et al.*, *Br. J. Haemat.*, 1978, *40*, 369 (residual bone-marrow damage after treatment with cyclophosphamide and doxorubicin); S. D. Gisser and K. B. Chung, *Am. J. Med.*, 1979, *67*, 151 (fatal myelofibrosis with chlorambucil).

For reports of lithium reducing the incidence and degree of neutropenia and decreasing the risk of infection in patients receiving cancer chemotherapy, see Lithium Carbonate, p.1541.

Effects on bones and joints. A report of osteonecrosis in 7 patients receiving combined chemotherapy for Hodgkin's disease. The corticosteroid component might be implicated.— A. R. Timothy *et al.* (letter), *Lancet*, 1978, *1*, 154. Further reports: R. Obrist *et al.* (letter), *Lancet*, 1978, *1*, 1316 (aseptic bone necrosis in a patient given cyclophosphamide, methotrexate, and fluorouracil); B. W. Hancock *et al.*, *Postgrad. med. J.*, 1978, *54*, 545 (avascular necrosis of the bone associated with antineoplastic agents and corticosteroids in 2 patients).

Effects on electrolytes. Hyperphosphataemia (due to drug-induced release of phosphorus from destroyed malignant lymphoblasts) and acute renal failure in a patient given antineoplastic agents for lymphoma.— A. Kanfer *et al.*, *Br. med. J.*, 1979, *1*, 1320.

For a report of cardiac arrest due to hyperkalaemia and hyperuricaemia following chemotherapy for leukaemia, see Effects on the Heart (below).

Effects on the gastro-intestinal tract. Reports of adverse effects on the gastro-intestinal mucosa: N. M. Matolo *et al.*, *Am. J. Surg.*, 1976, *132*, 753 (intestinal necrosis and perforation associated with immunosuppressants); J. M. Merrill *et al.*, *Lancet*, 1976, *1*, 1105 (inflammatory anorectal lesions associated with radiotherapy and combined chemotherapy for lung cancer); L. Lubitz and H. Ekert (letter), *Lancet*, 1979, *2*, 532 (severe, but reversible, changes in the duodenal mucosa and profuse diarrhoea associated with high-dose cytotoxic chemotherapy).

A Mallory-Weiss tear of the gastric mucosa occurred in one patient following nausea and vomiting leading to violent retching induced by combined cancer chemotherapy.— R. E. Enck (letter), *Lancet*, 1977, *2*, 927.

Effects on growth. Growth-hormone secretion was reduced by chemotherapy and radiotherapy in a study of 9 children with acute lymphoblastic leukaemia. There appeared to be a gradual recovery of secretion after cessation of CNS prophylaxis.— G. Schiliro *et al.* (letter), *Lancet*, 1976, *2*, 1031. From a study of 14 children treated for brain tumours, it appears that poor growth in such children occurs irrespective of whether radiation-induced growth-hormone deficiency develops and that while chemotherapy is continued treatment with growth hormone will not necessarily be effective.— S. M. Shalet *et al.*, *Archs Dis. Childh.*, 1978, *53*, 491.

Effects on the heart. Cardiotoxicity resulting from antineoplastic chemotherapy has generally been limited to the anthracycline antibiotics daunorubicin (see p.205) and doxorubicin (see p.206) although fatalities have been reported with high doses of cyclophosphamide and with fluorouracil.

Cardiac arrest due to hyperkalaemia in association with hyperuricaemia following successful chemotherapy for acute lymphoblastic leukaemia with a large tumour burden and despite allopurinol cover. Haemodialysis was required to clear the uric acid and the patient survived.— D. Wilson *et al.*, *Cancer*, 1977, *39*, 2290.

Effects on immune response. Lymphocytes are produced by lymphoid tissue in the bone marrow and at other sites, including the thymus, and are involved in humoral and cell-mediated immunity. The majority of agents described in this chapter have a depressant effect on bone marrow (see Effects on the Blood, above) and many have immunosuppressant properties although the degree of suppression varies considerably and may depend on the dose and schedule of administration used. Immunosuppression decreases the patient's resistance to infection and has also been implicated in the development of malignancies (see Carcinogenicity, above).

For a discussion on the effects of immunosuppressant therapy on the immune response and the infections associated with it, see Corticosteroids, p.447.

The lymphocytopenia produced by mustine with vinblastine, procarbazine and prednisolone (MVPP) in patients with Hodgkin's disease was not prolonged nor selective, affecting both T and B lymphocytes.— A. Clay *et al.*, *Br. J. clin. Pharmac.*, 1977, *4*, 475.

Immunisation of 53 patients with Hodgkin's disease and 10 controls, using dodecavalent pneumococcal vaccine, indicated that antibody response was profoundly impaired in patients who had received intensive radiotherapy and/or chemotherapy. Impairment persisted for at least 4 years after the completion of intensive therapy.— G. R. Siber *et al.*, *New Engl. J. Med.*, 1978, *299*, 442. Further references to abnormal immune responses associated with antineoplastic chemotherapy: H. S. Chung *et al.*, *J. Pediat.*, 1977, *90*, 548; P. Kechijian *et al.*, *Ann. intern. Med.*, 1979, *91*, 868 (an inflammatory exacerbation of seborrhoeic keratosis during therapy with cytarabine).

Individual reports of infections associated with antineoplastic and immunosuppressant chemotherapy: J. Ruskin and J. S. Remington, *J. Am. med. Ass.*, 1967, *202*, 1070 (*Pneumocystis carinii* pneumonia); R. K. Park *et al.*, *Archs Derm.*, 1967, *95*, 345 (persistent varicella, severe herpes simplex infection, and fatal disseminated histoplasmosis); K. N. Drummond (letter), *Br. med. J.*, 1969, *2*, 576 (cyclophosphamide should not be used in patients who have not had varicella); S. R. Meadow *et al.*, *Lancet*, 1969, *2*, 876 (measles and fatal giant-cell pneumonia); J. D. Smith and J. M. Knox, *Br. J. Derm.*, 1971, *84*, 590 (tuberculosis); T. C. Northfield and C. I. Roberts, *Gut*, 1972, *13*, 124 (abdominal abscess in a patient with Crohn's disease); M. Adam *et al.*, *Br. med. J.*, 1973, *1*, 264 (strongyloidiasis); C. R. Pullan *et al.*, *Br. med. J.*, 1976, *1*, 1562 (giant-cell pneumonia and fatal measles encephalopathy); W. J. Stone *et al.*, *Am. J. Med.*, 1977, *63*, 511 (herpesvirus hominis infection); M. J. Lewis *et al.*, *Br. med. J.*, 1978, *1*, 330 (measles presenting atypically as giant-cell pneumonia or as methotrexate pneumonia); G. Schieferstein *et al.*, *Dt. med. Wschr.*, 1978, *103*, 1521 (herpesvirus hominis infection); J. B. S. Coulter *et al.*, *Archs Dis. Childh.*, 1979, *54*, 640 (fatal subacute sclerosing panencephalitis following the contraction of measles); O. B. Eden and J. Santos, *Archs Dis. Childh.*, 1979, *54*, 557 (rhinopulmonary mucormycosis); S. B. Lucas *et al.* (letter), *Lancet*, 1979, *2*, 1372 (bizarre disseminated parasitic infection due to the dwarf tapeworm *Hymenolepis nana*); R. Ashford *et al.* (letter), *Lancet*, 1980, *1*, 1037 (malaria).

See also under Activation of Infection (below).

Effects on the kidneys. Nephropathies associated with antineoplastic agents and immunosuppressants include: inappropriate secretion of antidiuretic hormone with the vinca alkaloids and cyclophosphamide; acute interstitial nephritis with azathioprine and mercaptopurine; and acute tubular necrosis with cisplatin, doxorubicin, and methotrexate.— J. R. Curtis, *Br. J. Hosp. Med.*, 1980, *24*, 29.

For a report of acute renal failure associated with hyperphosphataemia, see Effects on Electrolytes (above).

See also Effects on the Bladder (above).

Effects on the liver. Agents that are clearly hepatotoxic include methotrexate, mercaptopurine, and azathioprine whereas cyclophosphamide, chlorambucil, and melphalan have rarely been associated with liver damage.— D. L. Sweet and J. E. Ultmann, *J. Am. med. Ass.*, 1977, *238*, 2307. A review of antineoplastic agents and the liver.— D. B. Ménard *et al.*, *Gastroenterology*, 1980, *78*, 142.

Hepatic dysfunction was reported in 13 patients who had received daunorubicin 180 to 450 mg per m^2 body-surface. Eleven of the patients had also received thioguanine, cytarabine, or vincristine or combinations of these antineoplastic agents. A study in *rabbits* suggested that doxorubicin might modify the metabolism of mercaptopurine and thereby increase blood-mercaptopurine concentrations (F. Pannuti *et al.*, *Riv. Patol. Clin.*, 1974, *29*, 169). A previous study by R.A. Minow *et al.* (*Cancer*, 1976, *38*, 1524) indicated that the hepatotoxicity of mercaptopurine might be enhanced by doxorubicin in leukaemic patients. It is therefore suggested that a similar interaction could be involved in the possible hepatotoxicity of daunorubicin, thioguanine, cytarabine and other antineoplastic agents.— J. S. Penta *et al.* (letter), *Ann. intern. Med.*, 1977, *87*, 247.

Effects on mental state. Increased psychiatric morbidity in women given cyclophosphamide, methotrexate, and fluorouracil after mastectomy compared with those given melphalan or receiving no chemotherapy after surgery.— C. P. Maguire *et al.*, *Br. med. J.*, 1980, *281*, 1179.

Effects on the nervous system. A review of the neurotoxicity of antineoplastic agents including colaspase, fluorouracil, methotrexate, mustine, procarbazine, and the vinca alkaloids.— H. D. Weiss *et al.*, *New Engl. J. Med.*, 1974, *291*, 75 and 127. Clinical syndromes of drug-induced neuropathy which have been associated with the use of antineoplastic agents include sensory neuropathy with procarbazine, paraesthesia with cytarabine, sensorimotor neuropathy with vincristine and chlorambucil, and localised neuropathies with mustine and ethoglucid.— Z. Argov and F. L. Mastaglia, *Br. med. J.*, 1979, *1*, 663.

Peripheral neuropathy with vincristine is dose-limiting and is discussed on p.231. The intrathecal administration of methotrexate (p.216), and occasionally cytarabine, may be associated with damage to the central nervous system.

Effects on reproductive potential. *Chromosomes.* The mutagenic effects of antineoplastic agents may not be seen for many years after successful chemotherapy has been completed. Follow-up studies in adults who received radiotherapy and chemotherapy for cancer in childhood (F.P. Li and N. Jaffe, *Lancet*, 1974, *2*, 707; H.A. Holmes and F.F. Holmes, *Clin. Pediat.*, 1975, *14*, 819) showed no increase in abortions, stillbirths, cancer, or major chronic disease in their offspring.— *Br. med. J.*, 1978, *2*, 785. A view that an adequate assessment of the risk of genetic damage following treatment is not yet possible.— R. L. Schilsky *et al.*, *Ann. intern. Med.*, 1980, *93*, 109. Evidence of little hazard.— J. Blatt *et al.*, *Am. J. Med.*, 1980, *69*, 828.

Congenital defects in the offspring of men given immunosuppressant therapy: M. B. Tallent *et al.* (letter), *J. Am. med. Ass.*, 1970, *211*, 1854 (radiotherapy, azathioprine, prednisone).

Reports of congenital malformations in the offspring of men previously given antineoplastic agents: J. A. Russell *et al.*, *Br. med. J.*, 1976, *1*, 1508 (the 2 men were fertile 3 and 7 months after chemotherapy ceased).

Reports of normal offspring fathered by men previously treated with antineoplastic agents: T. Kroner and A. Tschumi, *Br. med. J.*, 1977, *1*, 1322 (after treatment including methotrexate and mercaptopurine); A. Shani *et al.* (letter), *Lancet*, 1979, *2*, 637 (a normal foetus at abortion following vinblastine, bleomycin, and actinomycin D 6 months before conception); J. S. Lilleyman (letter), *Lancet*, 1979, *2*, 1125 (after receiving cytarabine from 14 to 16 years of age).

Analysis of the reproductive performance of 314 women successfully treated for gestational trophoblastic tumours indicated that a significant number are able to conceive, and that an increased incidence of abnormal pregnancies or foetal abnormalities after chemotherapy is not evident. It is advised that conception should be delayed for a year from the cessation of chemotherapy, which may permit mature ova, damaged by exposure to cytotoxic agents, to be eliminated.— P. A. M. Walden and K. D. Bagshawe (letter), *Lancet*, 1979, *2*, 1241. See also S. A. Johnson *et al.* (letter), *Lancet*, 1979, *2*, 93.

Further references: S. J. Horning *et al.*, *New Engl. J. Med.*, 1981, *304*, 1377 (female reproductive potential after treatment for Hodgkin's disease).

For references to chromosomal aberrations with antineoplastic agents, see Carcinogenicity (above).

See also under Pregnancy and the Neonate.

Gonads. The germinal epithelium of the gonads may be damaged, sometimes irreversibly, by antineoplastic or immunosuppressant chemotherapy, although radiotherapy may also be implicated.

With the successful treatment of malignant diseases such as acute lymphoblastic leukaemia, Hodgkin's disease, choriocarcinoma, and testicular cancer the long-term effects of antineoplastic agents on gonadal function have become more important. Although prospective studies are lacking and there is little information on newer agents such as bleomycin and cisplatin, it appears that testicular germinal epithelium in adult men is sensitive to alkylating agents, in particular chlorambucil or cyclophosphamide, in a progressive dose-related fashion. Combination chemotherapy may produce more long-lasting azoospermia and H.P. Roeser *et al.* (*Aust. N.Z. J. Med.*, 1978, *8*, 250) have suggested that the use of procarbazine in combination treatment regimens may be associated with more lasting testicular damage than when alkylating agents alone are used. Testicular biopsy has shown complete germinal aplasia and clinically there may be a marked decrease of testicular volume, severe oligospermia or azoospermia, and infertility. Abnormal serum-testosterone concentrations have not been noted in adults. Recovery of spermatogenesis is unpredictable but may be related to the total dose administered and to the time of therapy. Similarly to the testis, the ovary can be damaged by alkylating agents but little information is available for other antineoplastic agents. At biopsy ovarian fibrosis, follicle destruction, the arrest of follicular maturation, and the absence of ova have been noted. The occurrence and persistence of amenorrhoea may be related to the total dose of drug and the age of the patient; younger patients may tolerate higher total doses before amenorrhoea becomes irreversible. Reports suggest that at least 50% of women treated with combination chemotherapy will become amenorrhoeic due to primary ovarian failure.

Conflicting reports in boys suggest differences in the sensitivity of the prepubertal, pubertal, and adult testis to alkylating agents. The prepubertal testis may be more resistant to germinal epithelial injury but it appears that a threshold dose exists above which damage will occur. Combination chemotherapy may have profound effects on both the Leydig cells and germinal epithelium in pubertal boys; gynaecomastia may be the clinical manifestation of the endocrine dysfunction. Although profound ovarian dysfunction has not been reported in young girls given antineoplastic agents, the effects of combination chemotherapy on the prepubertal and pubertal ovary requires further evaluation.— R. L. Schilsky *et al.*, *Ann. intern. Med.*, 1980, *93*, 109. See also L. M. Glode *et al.*, *Lancet*, 1981, *1*, 1132 (possible protection); J. L. Graner (letter), *ibid.*, *2*, 41 (comment).

The effect of chemotherapy and irradiation on the gonads of children with cancer.— *Br. med. J.*, 1978, *2*, 785. Gynaecomastia occurred in 9 of 13 pubertal boys (11 to 16 years) an average of 28 months after the onset of combination chemotherapy for Hodgkin's disease with mustine, vincristine, procarbazine, and prednisone. Increased plasma concentrations of FSH and LH, low plasma-testosterone concentrations, and the results of testicular biopsies in 6 boys confirmed that germ-cell depletion had occurred.— R. J. Sherins *et al.*, *New Engl. J. Med.*, 1978, *299*, 12. Cyclophosphamide and cytarabine were associated with a significant depression of the tubular fertility index in 44 boys; in some the effects might prove irreversible.— M. Lendon *et al.*, *Lancet*, 1978, *2*, 439.

Normal testicular function in boys after chemotherapy for acute lymphoblastic leukaemia.— J. Blatt *et al.*, *New Engl. J. Med.*, 1981, *304*, 1121.

Reduced function, not severe enough to suggest infertility, in men treated during childhood with a single course of cyclophosphamide for nephrotic syndrome.— R. S. Trompeter *et al.*, *Lancet*, 1981, *1*, 1177.

Further references: L. G. Sobrinko *et al.*, *Am. J. Obstet. Gynec.*, 1971, *109*, 135; R. M. Chapman *et al.*, *J. Am. med. Ass.*, 1979, *242*, 1882 (ovarian failure); A. Y. Rostom and W. F. White (letter), *Lancet*, 1979, *1*, 555 (azoospermia; amenorrhoea); M. L. Steckman (letter), *New Engl. J. Med.*, 1980, *303*, 817.

For individual reports of the effects of antineoplastic agents on gonadal function, see Chlorambucil, p.196; Cyclophosphamide, p.199; Methotrexate, p.216; Vinblastine, p.230; Vincristine, p.231.

See also Pregnancy and the Neonate.

Sexual function. A retrospective study on fertility and gonadal function was carried out on 74 men aged 17 to 72 years who had received cyclical combination chemotherapy consisting of mustine, vinblastine, procarbazine, and prednisolone, to treat Hodgkin's disease; 8 of the men had also received doxorubicin, bleomycin, and dacarbazine. Results of a questionnaire indicated that 40 of 54 men noted a decrease in libido and sexual performance during therapy which persisted in 25 on completion of therapy. Semen analysis of 64 of the men revealed that all were azoospermic 1 to 14 months after stopping therapy; of those investigated later only 5 produced samples containing viable motile sperm, but 1 had become azoospermic in subsequent investigation. The wives of 2 of the 4 patients had become pregnant and one had given birth to a normal infant. Hormone estimations indicated that median follicle-stimulating hormone concentrations were consistently raised, median luteinising-hormone concentrations were around the upper limit of normal, and median testosterone concentrations were consistently normal; the range of prolactin concentrations was wide but median values were mainly within normal limits. The data obtained did not support the suggestion by H.P. Roeser *et al.* (*Aust. N.Z. J. Med.*, 1978, *8*, 250) that declining follicle-stimulating hormone concentrations may indicate return of spermatogenesis. No relationship was noted between depressed libido and testosterone concentrations. It was concluded that patients receiving such therapy should be warned about possible changes in sexual activity and its possible effect on personal relationships, and since infertility is certain with recovery unlikely, such patients should be offered sperm-storage facilities and advice on contraceptive practice.— R. M. Chapman *et al.*, *Lancet*, 1979, *1*, 285.

A 23-year-old man fathered a normal child while receiving maintenance chemotherapy for acute leukaemia. By the time of conception he had received 16 g of cytarabine, 10.2 g of thioguanine, and 1.1 g of daunorubicin.— J. H. Matthews and J. K. Wood (letter), *New Engl. J. Med.*, 1980, *303*, 1235. Fatherhood in 2 men who had been azoospermic for years after chemotherapy for Hodgkin's disease.— S. Stricker *et al.* (letter), *ibid.*, 1981, *304*, 1175.

See also Pregnancy and the Neonate.

Effects on respiratory function. Interstitial pneumonitis and pulmonary fibrosis have been reported with the alkylating agents, busulphan, chlorambucil, cyclophosphamide, melphalan, and uramustine; the nitrosoureas, carmustine and semustine; the antineoplastic antibiotics, bleomycin, mitomycin, and zinostatin; the antimetabolites, mercaptopurine and methotrexate; and with procarbazine. Pulmonary toxicity occurs frequently with bleomycin and, with more awareness of the problem, is being diagnosed and reported more often with other agents. Symptoms include tachypnoea, dyspnoea, and nonproductive cough. Chest X-rays show interstitial infiltrates which are usually bilateral, and pulmonary-function tests show hypoxaemia and ventilation-perfusion dysfunction. Other causes of pneumonitis such as infection should be ruled out; the surest method of diagnosis is lung biopsy. However, the only effective control is to stop the offending treatment at the first hint of pulmonary toxicity. Once pneumonitis becomes apparent clinically it is often fatal and treatment with corticosteroids is generally ineffective. There may be enhanced toxicity when more than one drug is used concomitantly and when a drug is used in association with thoracic irradiation or with high oxygen concentrations in inspired air. Further studies are needed to define risk factors, dose relationships, and methods of control or prevention of pulmonary toxicity.— R. B. Weiss and F. M. Muggia, *Am. J. Med.*, 1980, *68*, 259.

Individual reports of adverse effects on respiratory function with antineoplastic chemotherapy: P. Schulman *et al.*, *Chest*, 1979, *75*, 194 (pneumothorax).

The pulmonary toxicity of antineoplastic agents is also discussed under the individual monographs.

Effects on the skin. *Alopecia.* In contrast to hair loss due to other types of drug, alopecia caused by antineoplastic agents may be an early sign of toxicity occurring a few days after treatment. These agents can all cause anagen effluvium, an increased shedding of hair in the growth phase, but cyclophosphamide is more likely to cause hair loss than others.— *Drug & Ther. Bull.*, 1978, *16*, 77.

Photosensitivity. Dacarbazine, fluorouracil, methotrexate, and vinblastine may all cause photosensitivity reactions.— *Med. Lett.*, 1980, *22*, 64.

Pigmentation. Cancer chemotherapy has been associated with pigmentation of the skin, especially in the interphalangeal and palmar creases, and of the nails and nail-beds, with pigmented banding of the nails. Hyperpigmentation has been reported in black patients.

Assay of serum concentrations of melanocyte-stimulating hormone in 2 black patients did not attribute the pigmentary changes induced by doxorubicin to an action on this hormone. A direct effect on the melanocytes might be the cause.— M. C. Kew *et al.* (letter), *Lancet*, 1977, *1*, 811. See also S. Arakawa *et al.*, *Archs Dis. Childh.*, 1978, *53*, 249.

Individual reports of pigmentation with antineoplastic agents: B. M. Harrison and C. B. S. Wood (letter), *Br. med. J.*, 1972, *2*, 352 (cyclophosphamide); I. S. Cohen *et al.*, *Archs Derm.*, 1973, *107*, 553 (bleomycin); C. B. Pratt and E. C. Shanks (letter), *J. Am. med. Ass.*, 1974, *228*, 460 (doxorubicin); J. A. Romankiewicz, *Am. J. Hosp. Pharm.*, 1974, *31*, 1074 (cyclophosphamide); G. Moore; D. Meiselbough (letter), *Lancet*, 1975, *2*, 128 (fluorouracil); C. St. J. O'Doherty (letter), *Lancet*, 1975, *2*, 365 (mustine); D. J. Stoner and T. G. Baumgartner (letter), *Lancet*, 1975, *2*, 128 (cyclophosphamide); W. J. Hrushesky (letter), *J. Am. med. Ass.*, 1976, *236*, 138 (fluorouracil); D. W. Nixon, *Archs intern. Med.*, 1976, *136*, 1117; I. P. Law (letter), *Archs Derm.*, 1977, *113*, 379 (doxorubicin); D. Morris *et al.*, *Cancer Treat. Rep.*, 1977, *61*, 499 (doxorubicin); N. M. Price, *Archs Derm.*, 1977, *113*, 1387 (mustine used topically); M. R. Shetty, *Cancer Treat. Rep.*, 1977, *61*, 501 (bleomycin); M. de Marinis *et al.* (letter), *Ann. intern. Med.*, 1978, *89*, 516 (daunorubicin and cytarabine).

Effects on zinc concentrations. Following induction of remission from acute myelogenous leukaemia with various chemotherapeutic agents, a 12-year-old girl suffered zinc deficiency after treatment of relapse with methotrexate, mercaptopurine and prednisone. Since prednisone (which was associated with lowered serum-zinc concentrations) had been discontinued a month before the appearance of symptoms, the zinc deficiency might have been associated with chemotherapy.— E. A. Cutler *et al.* (letter), *New Engl. J. Med.*, 1977, *297*, 168.

Gynaecomastia. Gynaecomastia may occur when the testis is damaged by infections, physical agents, or chemical agents such as antineoplastic drugs.— A. P. Forbes, *New Engl. J. Med.*, 1978, *299*, 42.

Reports of gynaecomastia in men receiving antineoplastic agents: R. H. Smith and O. Barrett, *Calif. Med.*, 1967, *107*, 347 (vincristine); A. E. Schorer *et al.*, *Cancer Treat. Rep.*, 1978, *62*, 574 (carmustine).

See also Effects on Reproductive Potential, Gonads.

Local irritant effects. Findings indicating that a third of all antineoplastic agents administered intravenously are associated with the development of thrombophlebitis. A change of solvent, pH, or volume of vehicle has sometimes reduced the risk.— J. E. Henney *et al.*, *Drug Intell. & clin. Pharm.*, 1977, *11*, 266.

Pregnancy and the neonate. Most of the agents discussed in this chapter are potentially teratogenic. Congenital abnormalities appear to be particularly common when alkylating agents or antimetabolites are given to the mother during the first trimester of pregnancy. See also under Precautions for Antineoplastic Agents (below).

First trimester. Individual reports of congenital malformations in the babies and foetuses of mothers given antineoplastic agents during the first trimester of pregnancy: *Busulphan.*— J. Sokal and E. Lessmann, *J. Am. med. Ass.*, 1960, *172*, 1765 (with mercaptopurine); A. Abramovici *et al.*, *Teratology*, 1978, *18*, 241. *Chlorambucil.*— D. Shotton and I. W. Monie, *J. Am. med. Ass.*, 1963, *186*, 74. *Cyclophosphamide.*— L. H. Greenberg and K. R. Tanak, *J. Am. med. Ass.*, 1964, *188*, 423. *Cytarabine.*— V. M. Wagner *et al.* (letter), *Lancet*, 1980, *2*, 98. *Fluorouracil.*— J. D. Stephens *et al.*, *Am. J. Obstet. Gynec.*, 1980, *137*, 747. *Methotrexate.*— H. R. Powell and H. Ekert, *Med. J. Aust.*, 1971, *2*, 1076.

Treatment of the Adverse Effects of Antineoplastic Agents. Control of nausea and vomiting may be attempted by giving phenothiazines such as perphenazine (p.1551), prochlorperazine (p.1555), promethazine (p.1296), or thiethylperazine (p.1558), before antineoplastic agents are administered. In bone-marrow depression, transfusions of blood or platelets are given to diminish the risk of life-threatening haemorrhage. Granulocyte transfusions and injections of antibiotics may be necessary to combat infection in the neutropenic patient. Hyperuricaemia is avoided by the addition of allopurinol to treatment schedules and measures such as alkalinisation of the urine and hydration may also be adopted.

Techniques attempting to prevent the occurrence of alopecia have met with varying success. Scalp tourniquets and ice-packs (see Doxorubicin, p.206) have been used to minimise concentrations of antineoplastic agents in the scalp after intravenous injection. However, such methods may allow the development of a cancer-cell sanctuary and should not be used in patients with leukaemia or other conditions with circulating malignant cells. The treatment of extravasation is controversial and the only specific antidote reported is that for mustine (see p.223). Warm moist soaks or ice-packs have been applied and a corticosteroid may sometimes be instilled into the affected area.

See under Adrenaline (p.4) for the treatment of anaphylaxis.

Hypertransfusion in 27 children before treatment with large doses of immunosuppressants did not appear to be of any benefit in protecting the children against myelodepression.— L. Helson *et al.* (letter), *Lancet*, 1976, *2*, 1033.

A scalp tourniquet placed immediately below the hairline 5 minutes before the intravenous injection of doxorubicin, cyclophosphamide, vincristine, or teniposide and maintained in position for a further 20 minutes reduced the frequency and extent of alopecia in 37 patients when compared with 31 controls. Five patients could not tolerate the tourniquet.— A. Pesce *et al.* (letter), *New Engl. J. Med.*, 1978, *298*, 1204.

Precautions for Antineoplastic Agents. These agents should only be used as immunosuppressants in life-threatening situations. Immunosuppression and bone-marrow depression are features of the majority of the agents described in this chapter and their use is associated with an increased risk of infections caused by pathogenic bacteria or opportunistic micro-organisms including fungi, viruses, and protozoa, and a reduced capacity to cope with them. Those agents which are immunosuppressant should not be given to patients with acute infections and should be withdrawn if infection develops; the appropriate precautions described under Corticosteroids, p.449, should be observed. Special care is necessary in debilitated patients. There is also a risk that prolonged immunosuppression may stimulate the development of neoplasms (see Carcinogenicity, above).

Blood counts and measurement of haemoglobin concentrations should be carried out routinely to help predict the onset of bone-marrow depression and antineoplastic agents should be given with extreme caution when the marrow is already depressed following radiotherapy or therapy with other antineoplastic agents.

Although positive evidence of teratogenicity in humans is not available for all antineoplastic agents, it is considered that they are best avoided during pregnancy, especially during the first trimester, and should not be used in mothers who are breast-feeding.

Many antineoplastic drugs, particularly the alkylating agents, are vesicant or irritant. They must be handled with great care and contact with skin and eyes avoided; they should not be inhaled. Care must be taken to avoid extravasation since severe pain and tissue damage may ensue.

Thrombophlebitis has followed the intravenous administration of some antineoplastic agents.

See under Treatment of Adverse Effects for the caution required when attempting to prevent alopecia.

Bronchiectasis occurred in 5 children taking antineoplastic agents during remission of acute lymphoblastic leukaemia. Chest X-ray should be a routine part of follow-up.— P. J. Kearney *et al.*, *Br. med. J.*, 1977, *2*, 857.

Activation of infection. Fulminant and fatal acute hepatitis type B developed in 3 patients after the withdrawal of antineoplastic therapy. HB_sAg was detected in each patient at least 6 months before the hepatitis appeared and it was considered that immunosuppression permitted diffuse infection of the hepatocytes without the normal response; withdrawal of the immunosuppressants instigated the rapid destruction of the infected hepatocytes with consequent liver damage. All patients about to receive cytotoxic therapy should be screened for hepatitis B antigen and those at risk should be closely observed for alterations in liver function so that immediate treatment with corticosteroids could be started at the first sign of acute hepatitis.— R. M. Galbraith *et al.*, *Lancet*, 1975, *2*, 528.

Humoral studies indicated that aggressive therapy with chemical agents and radiation enhanced the risk of post-splenectomy septicaemia in patients with Hodgkin's disease.— S. A. Weitzman *et al.*, *New Engl. J. Med.*, 1977, *297*, 245.

A report on 11 patients receiving immunosuppressant therapy who developed tuberculosis. Three of 4 patients who died did so directly as a result of the tuberculosis, 3 patients were critically ill at the time of diagnosis but recovered with antitubercular therapy, and the other 4 had advanced cavitated pulmonary disease with miliary spread in one. All patients should have a tuberculin skin test and chest and abdominal radiographs before long-term immunosuppressant therapy is started. Isoniazid chemoprophylaxis in a dose of 300 mg daily continued for as long as the immunosuppressant therapy is prescribed, is recommended in patients with a grade III or IV positive skin test, or with old healed calcified lesions on chest X-ray, or calcified abdominal glands on abdominal films. In all patients regular clinical, bacteriological, and radiological review is essential. The risk seems to be highest in patients receiving more than 10 mg of prednisolone daily particularly in association with additional immunosuppressant agents.— J. W. Millar and N. W. Horne, *Lancet*, 1979, *1*, 1176. See also under Corticosteroids, p.450.

Although cytomegalovirus antibody titre increased in 35 of 39 patients soon after renal transplantation, virus excretion was rare and there were no late cases of cytomegalovirus disease.— E. S. Spencer and H. Z. Andersen, *Br. med. J.*, 1979, *2*, 829.

See also under Effects on Immune Response, above.

Hazards of handling antineoplastic agents. Most antineoplastic agents can cause local toxic or allergic reactions if handled without due care. The potential risks of carcinogenicity and mutagenicity should also be borne in mind and although there is little evidence on which to base any recommendations, caution is advised when handling these drugs. The manufacturers generally advise that contact with injection solutions should be avoided by wearing gloves and eye protection and, where appropriate, a mask to prevent inhalation of powder. However, K. Thomson and H.I. Mikkelsen (*Contact Dermatitis*, 1975, *1*, 268) reported that rubber or polyethylene gloves allowed penetration of mustine and that only polyvinyl chloride gloves provided any protection. A procedure for dealing with spillage of cytotoxic drugs includes the placing of spilled materials together with the mopping-up material in two sealed polythene bags and incinerating. Contaminated areas should be washed with copious amounts of water while exposed areas of skin should be washed with soap and water, the cleaning materials being disposed of as above. Only massive spillage is considered likely to be a health hazard. The manufacturers' recommendation for disposal of unwanted injections is usually to flush the drug through the drainage system with copious amounts of water.— R. S. Knowles and J. E. Virden, *Br. med. J.*, 1980, *281*, 589. See also *Pharm. J.*, 1977, *2*, 335.

Findings of mutagenic activity in the urine of the personnel handling, as well as the patients receiving, cytostatic drugs.— K. Falck *et al.* (letter), *Lancet*, 1979, *1*, 1250. No differences were observed in the immune function of 10 nurses working in an oncology unit and 10 matched control subjects. These observations indicate that the occupational handling of anticancer drugs is not likely to be a health hazard.— O. Lassila *et al.* (letter), *ibid.*, 1980, *2*, 482. Lack of mutagenic activity in urine of pharmacists admixing antitumour drugs.— N. Staiano *et al.* (letter), *ibid.*, 1981, *1*, 615.

Interactions. *With drugs.* Absorption of other drugs given in association with antineoplastic agents may be impaired as a result of damage to the gastro-intestinal mucosa.

A review of interactions with antineoplastic agents.— R. D. Warren and R. A. Bender, *Cancer Treat. Rep.*, 1977, *61*, 1231.

Thrombocytopenia and neutropenia leading to death occurred in a patient after his sixth course of cytarabine and daunorubicin for the control of myeloblastic leukaemia, together with sulphadimidine and pyrimethamine treatment for toxoplasmosis.— M. S. Rose *et al.* (letter), *Lancet*, 1973, *1*, 600. Since pyrimethamine could cause normal resting marrow cells to enter their reproductive cycle, both normal and malignant cells would have been susceptible to the antineoplastic agents. Pyrimethamine and trimethoprim, which would have the same effect, should not be given between courses of antineoplastic agents.— L. A. Price and P. K. Bondy (letter), *ibid.*, 727. See also F. H. J. Claas *et al.*, *Br. med. J.*, 1979, *2*, 898.

The use of some antineoplastic agents in conjunction with glucocorticoids could block the antitumour activity of the glucocorticoid.— M. E. Lippman and E. B. Thompson (letter), *Lancet*, 1973, *1*, 1198.

A report of antineoplastic antibiotics enhancing or diminishing the activity of antimicrobial agents *in vitro* against strains of *Staphylococcus aureus*.— J. Y. Jacobs *et al.*, *Antimicrob. Ag. Chemother.*, 1979, *15*, 580. See also J. Michel *et al.*, *ibid.*, *16*, 761 (against Gram-negative bacteria).

With radiation. Interactions with radiotherapy include enhanced pulmonary toxicity of antineoplastic agents (see Effects on Respiratory Function, above), an apparent enhanced toxicity of radiotherapy with doxorubicin (A. Horwich *et al.*, *Lancet*, 1975, *2*, 561), and enhanced susceptibility to radiation in patients receiving actinomycin D or doxorubicin (T.L. Phillips, *Cancer*, 1977, *39*, 987).

A recall phenomenon, in which latent radiation effects were reactivated in a previously irradiated field, was observed in 2 children treated with doxorubicin and was similar to that seen with actinomycin D.— S. S. Donaldson *et al.* (letter), *Ann. intern. Med.*, 1974, *81*, 407. See also J. Burdon *et al.* (letter), *J. Am. med. Ass.*, 1978, *239*, 931.

Local irritant effect. The following antineoplastic agents are considered to be potent vesicants and if infiltration occurs during intravenous administration they may cause erythema, pain, and inflammation and sometimes necrosis and tissue sloughing: actinomycin D, chlorozotocin, dacarbazine, daunorubicin, doxorubicin, mitomycin, mustine, streptozocin, vinblastine, and vincristine.— M. Summerfield *et al.* (letter), *Am. J. Hosp. Pharm.*, 1979, *36*, 1470.

Severe ulceration of the dorsum of the hand and forearm has followed a single large extravasation of an antineoplastic agent given intravenously. All possible precautions should be taken to prevent this occurring with the drug being introduced into a fast-flowing drip under constant supervision. The drip should be stopped immediately if extravasation occurs and an attempt made to aspirate as much of the drug as possible. Tissue damage may be minimised by an injection of hyaluronidase and the application of warmth to the affected site. The ulcers may be extremely resistant to therapy but excision is not necessarily effective and conservative management should be persevered with. This includes frequent moist antiseptic dressings, elevation of the affected limbs, and antibiotic therapy if there is evidence of cellulitis.— L. A. Chait and M. I. Dinner, *S. Afr. med. J.*, 1975, *49*, 1935.

Pregnancy and the neonate. Most antineoplastic agents cross the placenta and may cause abortion or foetal abnormalities when given during the first trimester of pregnancy; therapeutic abortion should be recommended when these agents are essential in early pregnancy. There is still some risk in the second trimester but the foetus should be relatively safe in the third trimester. The alkylating agents and procarbazine are best avoided at all stages of pregnancy.— *Lancet*, 1977, *1*, 1041. A warning that neuroblasts probably multiply in the brain to achieve virtually their adult number during the second trimester; antineoplastic therapy at this time may be responsible for subsequent mental retardation in the offspring.— J. Dobbing (letter), *ibid.*, 1155.

An apparently normal infant girl was born to a woman in whom acute leukaemia was diagnosed when she was 16 weeks pregnant, and who was treated with a regimen involving doxorubicin, vincristine, prednisolone, colaspase, cyclophosphamide, mercaptopurine, and methotrexate.— M. Khurshid and M. Saleem (letter), *Lancet*, 1978, *2*, 534.

A preliminary analysis of reproduction in 37 women with Hodgkin's disease. Of 17 pregnancies occurring before therapy there were 11 normal infants, 3 elective abortions, 1 spontaneous abortion, 1 stillbirth, and 1 minor malformed infant. Of 14 pregnancies where therapy was given at conception or during pregnancy, there were 4 normal infants, 5 elective abortions, 1 spontaneous abortion, and 4 malformed offspring. Of 44 pregnancies after therapy there were 23 normal infants, 4 elective abortions, 6 premature or small-for-gestational-age infants, 4 spontaneous abortions, 2 stillbirths, and 5 malformed offpsring (one which may have been related to maternal kyphoscoliosis). In contrast to the third group the second group yielded fewer normal live births and more major malformations.— E. A. McKeen *et al.* (letter), *Lancet*, 1979, *2*, 590.

See also Adverse Effects of Antineoplastic Agents (above).

Choice of Antineoplastic Agent. Antineoplastic agents are used for the primary treatment of choriocarcinoma, leukaemia, myeloma, and other conditions where surgery or radiotherapy is impracticable. Permanent remissions are possible in choriocarcinoma and in acute lymphoblastic leukaemia. Chemotherapy alone or with surgery and/or radiotherapy may also be effective in Burkitt's lymphoma, Hodgkin's disease, retinoblastoma, some tumours of the testis, and Wilms' tumour; survival may be prolonged in other conditions including histiocytic lymphoma, acute myeloid leukaemia, sarcomas, and carcinomas of the breast and lung. In advanced malignant disease chemotherapy is widely used and produces varying degrees of remission or palliation.

Adjuvant chemotherapy is given following surgery and/or radiotherapy in diseases such as breast cancer in an attempt to eradicate micrometastases since a single malignant cell is capable of multiplying and eventually killing the patient. Surgery and radiotherapy only remove localised and regional malignancy and a tumour may often be microscopically disseminated at diagnosis.

Immunotherapy with non-specific immunostimulants such as BCG vaccine (p.1588), *Corynebacterium parvum* (p.1698), and levamisole (p.95) has been tried as a adjunct to the treatment of cancer in an attempt to stimulate the patient's own defences against his disease.

Most of the antineoplastic agents are very toxic and should only be used where there is a reasonable chance of success. In most cases treatment is best carried out in hospitals experienced in the treatment of malignant disease.

Antineoplastic agents do not all act at the same sites and at the same stages in the mitotic cycle. Treatment with several agents together or in sequence, with breaks in the treatment to allow for recovery of normal cell function, is usually more effective than treatment with a single agent. The likelihood of resistance to a particular agent may also be reduced. Also, since not all agents have the same toxicity, combination therapy can give a lower spread of side-effects rather than the crippling toxicity that can occur with high doses of some single agents.

Reviews of antineoplastic agents: R. A. Bender *et al., Drugs*, 1978, *16*, 46; M. Sainsbury, *Chem. in Br.*, 1979, *15*, 127 (naturally occurring plant products); R. C. Young *et al., New Engl. J. Med.*, 1981, *305*, 139 (anthracycline antineoplastic agents, including daunorubicin and doxorubicin).

General reviews of the treatment of cancer with antineoplastic agents: H. Bush, *Br. J. Hosp. Med.*, 1978, *20*, 260 (adjuvant chemotherapy); H. M. Maurer, *New Engl. J. Med.*, 1978, *299*, 1345 (childhood malignancies); P. M. Jones, *Practitioner*, 1979, *222*, 221 (childhood malignancies); T. J. McElwain, *Practitioner*, 1979, *222*, 203; R. B. Weiss and V. T. DeVita, *Ann. intern. Med.*, 1979, *91*, 251 (carcinoma of the breast and colon, osteosarcoma, and melanoma); *Med. Lett.*, 1980, *22*, 101; S. K. Carter, *Drugs*, 1980, *20*, 375.

An evaluation of an *in vitro* tissue-culture test predicting the positive human response to antineoplastic agents.— H. L. Holmes and J. M. Little, *Lancet*, 1974, *2*, 985. See also S. E. Salmon *et al., New Engl. J. Med.*, 1978, *298*, 1321; E. Frei and H. Lazarus, *ibid.*, 1358.

Action. By using a mouse leukaemia as a model it was possible to predict the kinetics of leukaemic cell generation and the rate of cell kill that would need to be achieved by chemotherapy to produce lasting clinical remissions in acute childhood leukaemia. A single remaining leukaemic cell, doubling itself every 4 days, could reproduce in 164 days to give the cell population of about 2.5×10^{12} necessary for a clear-cut relapse. The effectiveness of various treatments could be assessed by determining the time from cessation of treatment to time of relapse. A complete kill of the leukaemic cells could lead to permanent remission, but the doses necessary should be tolerable.— C. G. Zubrod, *Proc. R. Soc. Med.*, 1965, *58*, 988.

A comparison of the sensitivity of normal haematopoietic and transplanted lymphoma colony-forming cells to antineoplastic agents and the classification of these agents according to their response.— W. R. Bruce *et al., J. natn. Cancer Inst.*, 1966, *37*, 233. Discussion of the importance of the Bruce model for reducing the toxicity of cancer combination schedules.— L. A. Price and B. T. Hill (letter), *Lancet*, 1976, *2*, 1195. Criticism.— M. H. N. Tattersall and J. S. Tobias (letter), *ibid.*, 1977, *1*, 141. An answer.— L. A. Price and B. T. Hill (letter), *ibid.*, 306.

A discussion of the concepts for systemic treatment of micrometastases to achieve a total tumour cell kill, a probable requirement for the cure of at least some tumours. Micrometastases containing up to 10^6 viable tumour cells are generally undetectable and therefore unsuitable for surgery or radiotherapy. The fraction of viable cells undergoing active cell replication is inversely related to population size and micrometastases should be more sensitive to cell cycle specific agents than the primary tumour. First-order cell kill kinetics characterise effective drug kill of tumour cells and when micrometastases are likely, drug treatment should be started as soon after the end of radiotherapy or surgery as possible, using cell cycle specific agents (antimetabolites) or cell cycle stage-specific agents (cytarabine, hydroxyurea, vinblastine, and vincristine). Cell cycle nonspecific agents (alkylating agents and antibiotics) have steep dose-response curves and the relatively high doses required prolong normal cell recovery times. Combination chemotherapy aimed at avoiding or controlling the selection of drug-resistant tumour cells is important.— F. M. Schabel, *Cancer*, 1975, *35*, 15.

A review of tumour cell kinetics and response to treatment. Growth rates of solid tumours affect response to therapy and tumours may be classified into 3 groups according to cell-population doubling time. The minimum detectable body burden of tumour in man is of the order of 1×10^9 cells, equivalent to about 1 g of tissue, and represents about 30 doublings. The lethal body tumour burden is reached when the tumour cell mass approaches or exceeds 1×10^{12} cells, equivalent to about 1 kg and representing 40 doublings. Ewing's sarcoma, testicular carcinoma, and non-Hodgkin's lymphomas (primarily histiocytic lymphoma) have mean doubling times that are shorter than 30 days; Hodgkin's disease, osteogenic sarcoma, and fibrosarcoma have intermediate growth rates with mean doubling times ranging from 30 to 70 days. Adenocarcinoma, squamous cell and small cell carcinomas of the lung, adenocarcinoma of the colon, and advanced breast cancer have mean doubling times which exceed 70 days. Doubling time distributions for individual tumour types are quite wide, adenocarcinoma of the lung has a reported doubling time of 15 to 960 days. Correlations between tumour doubling time and patient survival patterns suggest that the rate of tumour cell proliferation is a major determinant of therapeutic response; median survival is not considered the best measure of therapeutic effectiveness. The relationship between a cytotoxic drug and a tumour cell population can be described as a first-order kinetic process; a given dose or course of therapy kills a given fraction of the cell population rather than a number of cells. Thus, treatment of rapidly growing tumours produces a high initial fractional cell kill with frequent clinical complete responses and perhaps eradication of the last tumour cell in many patients. Rapidly growing tumours in advanced stages will undergo growth retardation on treatment but with a critical reduction in fractional cell kill. Fractional cell kills are also small in slowly growing tumours explaining the partial responses and shallow complete responses to treatment. In the treatment of slowly growing tumours the fractional tumour cell kills achieved at maximum tolerated therapeutic intensity were not sufficient to produce high complete response rates or durable responses without associated toxicity from long-term therapy. Clinical studies based on cell kinetic principles would improve therapeutic results in patients with responsive tumours but protocols for the treatment of patients with slowly growing tumours require reappraisal.— S. E. Shackney *et al., Ann. intern. Med.*, 1978, *89*, 107.

Further references to cell kinetics and the treatment of neoplastic diseases: C. Focan (letter), *Lancet*, 1976, *2*, 638; R. B. Livingston and J. S. Hart, *A. Rev. Pharmac. & Toxic.*, 1977, *17*, 529; E. Mihich and G. B. Grindey, *Cancer*, 1977, *40*, 534; E. Frei, *ibid.*, 569; C. A. Nichol, *Cancer*, 1977, *40*, 519.

Administration. Apart from the routine methods of administration special techniques have been designed to improve effectiveness. Antineoplastic agents may be injected directly into the tumour or body cavity or they may be administered by isolated regional perfusion or intra-arterial infusion. Isolated regional perfusion entails isolation of a tumour and its blood supply in an extracorporeal circulation so that the antineoplastic agent can be given in sufficiently high dosage to destroy the tumour. This is more easily carried out in the limbs, but in tumours of the abdomen or pelvis there is a risk of leakage and an alternative is to employ continuous intra-arterial infusion into an artery as close as possible to the tumour.

Comment on dosage and the pharmacokinetics of cytotoxic drugs.— J. R. Trounce, *Br. J. clin. Pharmac.*, 1979, *8*, 205.

For references to the use of carriers for antineoplastic agents, see G. Gregoriadis, in *Drug Carriers in Biology and Medicine*, G. Gregoriadis (Ed.), London, Academic Press, 1979, p. 287 (liposomes); W. T. Shier, *ibid.*, p. 43 (lectins); A. Trouet *et al., ibid.*, p. 87 (deoxyribonucleic acid).

Blood disorders, non-malignant. Polycythaemia vera. Polycythaemia vera is a chronic myeloproliferative disorder in which red cell count, packed cell volume, and haemoglobin are increased. It may be treated by venesection, chemotherapy, or radiotherapy. Busulphan or chlorambucil are the drugs most commonly used but neither appears to be very satisfactory. Treatment with phosphorus-32 remains the method of choice, especially in older patients and those with severe disease.— S. M. Lewis, *Br. J. Hosp. Med.*, 1976, *16*, 125.

In a prospective randomised study of 431 patients with polycythaemia vera, chlorambucil offered no advantage over phosphorus-32 and was associated with a significant increase in the incidence of acute leukaemia when compared with phlebotomy or phosphorus-32. The use of chlorambucil for the long-term management of polycythaemia vera has been discontinued.— P. D. Berk *et al., New Engl. J. Med.*, 1981, *304*, 441 (Polycythaemia Vera Study Group).

Burkitt's lymphoma. Despite previously disappointing results in the treatment of Burkitt's lymphoma in non-endemic areas, the survival rate in 54 multicentre American patients treated with regimens involving cyclophosphamide, vincristine, and methotrexate, or cyclophosphamide, vincristine, methotrexate, and prednisolone, was similar to results obtained in Africa. Youth and a low tumour load were both favourable prognostic factors. Other factors, including the efficacy of methotrexate intrathecally in preventing CNS recurrence, could not be evaluated but the results of this and other studies suggested several approaches such as high-dose chemotherapy, removal of tumour bulk soon after the initial induction course, and immunological approaches, which might improve the prognosis for the high-risk patients.— J. L. Ziegler, *New Engl. J. Med.*, 1977, *297*, 75.

A 10-year follow-up of 192 Ugandan patients with Burkitt's lymphoma treated with various regimens containing high doses of cyclophosphamide (cyclophosphamide, methotrexate, vincristine, and cytarabine) at the Lymphoma Treatment Centre in Kampala between 1967 and 1973. The results demonstrated that, at a conservative estimate, approximately 50% of patients with Burkitt's lymphoma can achieve long-term survival and are cured after complete remission has been induced by chemotherapy. Contrary to clinical experience in undifferentiated lymphoma outside Africa, meningeal lymphoma was curable. Another unusual feature was the high survival-rate in those who relapsed. None of the treatment regimens was clearly superior when clinical stage at presentation was taken into account.— J. L. Ziegler *et al., Lancet*, 1979, *2*, 936.

A review of Burkitt's lymphoma.— J. L. Ziegler, *New Engl. J. Med.*, 1981, *305*, 735.

Earlier reports on the use of antineoplastic agents in the treatment of Burkitt's lymphoma: D. Burkitt, *Cancer*, 1966, *19*, 1131 (vincristine), per *Abstr. Wld Med.*, 1967, *41*, 120; P. Clifford, *E.Afr. med. J.*, 1966, *43*, 179 (cyclophosphamide, melphalan, or orthomerphalan); R. H. Morrow *et al., Br. med. J.*, 1967, *4*, 323 (cyclophosphamide, mercaptopurine, mustine, methotrexate, vincristine); E. H. Williams, *Br. J. Cancer*, 1971, *25*, 37 (cyclophosphamide; intrathecal methotrexate), per *Trop. Dis. Bull.*, 1972, *69*, 62; J. L. Ziegler and A. Z. Bluming, *Br. med. J.*, 1971, *3*, 508 (intrathecal methotrexate or cytarabine).

Carcinoid syndrome. Reference to the use of antineoplastic agents in patients with carcinoid syndrome who fail to respond to conventional treatment. Fluorouracil has been the agent most widely used. A. Solomon *et al.* (*Cancer Treat. Rep.*, 1976, *60*, 273) reported doxorubicin in association with cyclophosphamide and methotrexate to be effective in one patient.— *Br. med. J.*, 1978, *1*, 1572. See also S. S. Legha *et al., Cancer Treat. Rep.*, 1977, *61*, 1699.

A report of the successful use of tamoxifen in carcinoid syndrome resistant to chemotherapy.— G. P. Stathopoulos *et al.* (letter), *New Engl. J. Med.*, 1981, *305*, 52.

Choriocarcinoma. Chemotherapy with methotrexate is the treatment of choice in patients with gestational choriocarcinoma. Treatment is continued for 4 to 6 weeks after all evidence of disease has disappeared. A high proportion of patients are cured. Actinomycin D may be tried if methotrexate proves ineffective; chlorambucil and cyclophosphamide are also active.— Report of a WHO Expert Committee on Chemotherapy of Solid Tumours, *Tech. Rep. Ser. Wld Hlth Org. No. 605*, 1977, p. 47.

Individual reports of the treatment of choriocarcinoma and other trophoblastic tumours: K. D. Bagshawe *et al., Br. med. J.*, 1969, *3*, 733 (methotrexate and mercaptopurine or methotrexate and folinic acid in invasive hydatidiform mole or choriocarcinoma); J. A. Wider *et al., New Engl. J. Med.*, 1969, *280*, 1439 (methotrexate, chlorambucil, and actinomycin D in persistent primary carcinoma and choriocarcinoma); D. P. Goldstein, *Obstet. Gynec.*, 1971, *38*, 817 (methotrexate or actinomycin D in the prevention of trophoblastic disease in women with molar pregnancy); *idem*, 1974, *43*, 475 (actinomycin D in molar pregnancy); *idem*, 1976, *48*, 321 (methotrexate and folinic acid rescue in nonmetastatic gestational trophoblastic neoplasms); *idem*, 1978, *51*, 93 (methotrexate and folinic acid rescue); A. P. Weetman and L. K. Borysiewicz, *Br. med. J.*, 1980, *281*, 585 (successful chemotherapy of disseminated choriocarcinoma in a man with Klinefelter's syndrome).

Fibromatosis. References to the use of antineoplastic agents in the treatment of fibromatosis: R. Stein, *J. Pediat.*, 1977, *90*, 482 (vincristine, actinomycin D, and cyclophosphamide in fibromatosis of the neck); R. J. Hutchinson *et al.*, *Pediatrics*, 1979, *63*, 157 (vincristine, actinomycin D, and cyclophosphamide in abdominal fibromatosis).

Histiocytosis X. The term histiocytosis X refers to a group of rare syndromes, Letterer-Siwe disease, Hand-Schüller-Christian disease, and eosinophilic granuloma, that share certain histopathological features, namely granulomatous formation with infiltration and proliferation of histiocytes. The clinical manifestations can range from a solitary eosinophilic granuloma in the medullary cavity of bone to acute disseminated fulminant disease. The standard treatment of chemotherapy or radiotherapy or both is similar to that used in the treatment of cancer.— M. E. Osband *et al.*, *New Engl. J. Med.*, 1981, *304*, 146.

Reports of chemotherapy in the treatment of histiocytosis X: K. A. Starling *et al.*, *Am. J. Dis. Child.*, 1972, *123*, 105 (cyclophosphamide, vinblastine, and vincristine used singly or sequentially); M. Alexander and J. R. Daniels, *Cancer*, 1977, *39*, 1011 (cyclophosphamide, doxorubicin, vincristine and prednisone); D. M. Komp *et al.*, *Cancer Treat. Rep.*, 1977, *61*, 855 (MOPP-type regimen).

Hodgkin's disease and other lymphomas. A brief discussion on lymphomas including the phenomenon of premalignant change and conditions associated with an increased risk of lymphoreticular neoplasms.— *Lancet*, 1979, *1*, 306.

The role of radiotherapy and chemotherapy in the treatment of lymphomas such as Hodgkin's disease and non-Hodgkin's lymphomas, especially Burkitt's lymphoma and intestinal lymphoma.— B. Ramot and I. Ben-Bassat, *Bull. Wld Hlth Org.*, 1979, *57*, 857.

Progress and setbacks in the understanding of Hodgkin's disease.— *Lancet*, 1981, *1*, 924.

Hodgkin's disease. The localised stages of Hodgkin's disease are usually treated by total nodal irradiation. Chemotherapy is the treatment of choice for advanced disease and a variety of agents have been used. The commonest treatment remains combination chemotherapy with mustine, vincristine, procarbazine, and prednisone (MOPP) introduced by V.T. DeVita *et al.* (*Ann. intern. Med.*, 1970, *73*, 881). Mustine 6 mg per m² body-surface and vincristine 1.4 mg per m² are given intravenously on days 1 and 8 and procarbazine 100 mg per m² and prednisone 40 mg per m² are taken by mouth on days 1 to 14, courses being repeated every 4 weeks; the schedule may be modified. Vinblastine 6 mg per m² has been substituted for vincristine (MVPP). Other regimens, including doxorubicin, bleomycin, vinblastine, and dacarbazine (ABVD) have been used to treat patients resistant to MOPP. Combined modality treatment with radiotherapy and chemotherapy may be tried when results with one or the other are disappointing but the added hazards must be considered.

Reviews on the management of Hodgkin's disease: C. W. Berard *et al.*, *Ann. intern. Med.*, 1976, *85*, 351; T. J. McElwain, *Adv. Med. Topics Ther.*, 1976, *2*, 65; I. E. Smith and T. J. McElwain, *Archs Dis. Childh.*, 1977, *52*, 725; R. C. Young *et al.*, *Curr. Probl. Cancer*, 1977, *1*, 1; A. C. Aisenberg, *New Engl. J. Med.*, 1978, *299*, 1228 (staging and treatment); S. A. Rosenberg, *ibid.*, 1246; *Lancet*, 1978, *2*, 875 (staging laparotomy); J. F. Desforges *et al.*, *New Engl. J. Med.*, 1979, *301*, 1212; R. A. Streuli and J. E. Ultmann, *Ann. intern. Med.*, 1980, *92*, 693; C. J. Williams, *Br. med. J.*, 1980, *280*, 1310 (changing priorities).

Radiotherapy is accepted as the best treatment for the early stages of Hodgkin's disease classified as stages I and II. With advanced or stage IV disease chemotherapy is best. As the optimum therapy of stage III Hodgkin's disease was not definite, a prospective multi-centre study was carried out by the British National Lymphoma Investigation over 5 years in 117 patients with stage IIIA disease. When the stage of the disease was assessed with the aid of laparotomy, total nodal irradiation was more effective than combined chemotherapy with a MOPP schedule modified slightly by giving procarbazine for only 10 days of each course and prednisone with all courses. When the disease was staged without diagnostic laparotomy there was no significant difference in response to chemotherapy or total nodal irradiation; this result might be explained by the patients having a more advanced disease than expected with areas being affected outside the irradiation field. Adjuvant chemotherapy might still have a useful role even in patients with stage IIIA disease classified with the aid of laparotomy.— *Lancet*, 1976, *2*, 991. From long-term follow up of 198 patients with advanced Hodgkin's disease, who were treated with MOPP, the disease appears to be curable by chemotherapy. Complete remission was achieved by 159 patients (80%) and 63% of these have remained free of disease 10 years after the end of treatment.— V. T. DeVita *et al.*, *Ann. intern. Med.*, 1980, *92*, 587.

In 49 patients with stage IV Hodgkin's disease a remission-rate of 80% was achieved by treatment with mustine, vincristine, procarbazine, and prednisone (MOPP), compared with 44% in 41 patients for whom prednisone was omitted (MOP).—Report by the British National Lymphoma Investigation, *Br. med. J.*, 1975, *3*, 413. In a retrospective study in 211 patients with Hodgkin's disease there was no significant difference between those treated with the MOPP regimen and those in whom prednisone was omitted; complete remission-rates were 81.5 and 77.8% respectively.— C. Jacobs *et al.*, *Br. med. J.*, 1976, *2*, 1469. Investigation of tumour glucocorticoid receptors and glucocorticoid sensitivity *in vitro* may allow selection of patients with lymphoma who should receive glucocorticoids as part of combination chemotherapy.— C. D. Bloomfield *et al.*, *Lancet*, 1980, *1*, 952.

Preliminary results from a comparative study of 45 patients with advanced Hodgkin's disease indicated that combination chemotherapy with MOPP or ABVD produced similar remission-rates. The ABVD regimen was given monthly for a total of 6 treatments and consisted of doxorubicin 25 mg per m² body-surface, bleomycin 10 mg per m², and vinblastine 6 mg per m², all given intravenously on days 1 and 14, and dacarbazine 150 mg per m² given intravenously on the first 5 days of each cycle; no treatment was given from day 15 to 28. MOPP was administered according to the schedule of V.T. DeVita *et al.* (*Ann. intern. Med.*, 1970, *73*, 881). There appeared to be no cross-resistance between the 2 treatment regimens. It is stressed that, because of the potentially severe toxicity of both doxorubicin and bleomycin, ABVD should only be used in Hodgkin's disease resistant to MOPP.— G. Bonadonna *et al.*, *Cancer*, 1975, *36*, 252. See also G. Bonadonna *et al.*, *Cancer Treat. Rep.*, 1977, *61*, 769. One complete and 14 partial remissions were obtained in 24 patients with Hodgkin's disease resistant to MOPP and treated with a schedule of doxorubicin, bleomycin, dacarbazine, and vinblastine (ABDV). The effectiveness of ABDV appeared to be less than that with bleomycin, lomustine, and vinblastine.— D. C. Case *et al.*, *Cancer*, 1977, *39*, 1382. Findings from a study of the ABVD regimen in 41 patients with Hodgkin's disease, resistant to MVPP at induction or at relapse, indicate that there is cross-resistance between the 2 regimens and that patients whose disease progresses through MVPP achieve little benefit from ABVD. Patients were given doxorubicin 25 mg per m² body-surface, bleomycin 10 mg per m², vincristine 1.5 mg per m², if previously given MVPP, or vinblastine 6 mg per m², if previously given MOPP, and dacarbazine 350 mg per m². A complete response was achieved in 3 patients (7%), a partial response in 23 (56%), and no apparent response in 15 (37%).— S. B. Sutcliffe *et al.*, *Cancer Chemother. Pharmac.*, 1979, *2*, 209.

A schedule (CVB) of lomustine (C), vinblastine or vincristine (V), and bleomycin (B) was used to treat 39 patients with advanced Hodgkin's disease resistant to standard combination schedules. The regimen consisted of lomustine 100 mg per m² body-surface on day 1 of a 28-day cycle, vinblastine 6 mg per m² intravenously on days 1 and 8 or, where vinblastine had been included in the primary therapy, vincristine 1.4 mg per m² on days 1 and 8, and bleomycin 15 mg intramuscularly on days 1 and 8. Ten patients achieved a complete and 23 a partial remission. The mean number of courses to produce a complete remission was 2.— J. M. Goldman and A. A. Dawson, *Lancet*, 1975, *2*, 1224.

A 21-day cyclic regimen of cyclophosphamide, vinblastine, procarbazine, and prednisone (CVPP) was evaluated in 50 patients with advanced Hodgkin's disease. Complete remission occurred in 31 patients; there were 13 in the 23 patients with no previous therapy, 15 in the 19 who had received major radiotherapy, and 3 in 8 who had received both chemotherapy and radiotherapy. Maintenance therapy had no significant effect but there were fewer relapses and remissions lasted longer in patients who received more than 6 courses of induction therapy. This regimen was similar to MOPP but had less toxicity.— C. H. Diggs *et al.*, *Cancer*, 1977, *39*, 1949.

Complete remissions after treatment with the MVPP regimen were achieved more often (76%) in 49 patients with advanced Hodgkin's disease who had no prior chemotherapy and in 42 patients who had received prior radiotherapy (90%) than in 42 who had received earlier single-agent chemotherapy (40%).— S. B. Sutcliffe *et al.*, *Br. med. J.*, 1978, *1*, 679.

As irradiation produces excellent disease-free survival in many patients with Hodgkin's disease care should be exercised in the routine use of adjuvant chemotherapy.— A. R. Timothy *et al.*, *Br. med. J.*, 1978, *1*, 1246. A report of the successful use of combination chemotherapy in patients with stage I or stage II Hodgkin's disease. Although the study only involved 14 patients, it suggests rates of complete remission and survival comparable with, perhaps better than, those achieved with radiotherapy alone.— F. Lauria *et al.* (letter), *Lancet*, 1979, *2*, 1072.

Of 108 patients in remission from Hodgkin's disease after 6 courses of MVPP, 53 were treated with 10 maintenance courses of MVPP over 3.5 years while 55 received similar courses without mustine and prednisone (VP). During follow-up for nearly 5 years after randomisation 10 of those given maintenance MVPP and 6 of those given maintenance VP had died; the difference was not significant. The 2-drug maintenance could be given without hospital admission; there was a tendency for those relapsing after VP to survive longer; 2 patients who died of leukaemia had received MVPP. If patients were given maintenance therapy the 2-drug regimen seemed preferable.—MRC's Working Party on Lymphomas *Br. med. J.*, 1979, *1*, 1105.

Results in 118 patients with Hodgkin's disease treated with chlorambucil, vinblastine, procarbazine, and prednisolone (ChlVPP) were similar to those usually achieved with schedules including mustine and side-effects were fewer. Chlorambucil 6 mg per m² body-surface daily was given by mouth for 14 days and the remaining drugs were given as in the MVPP regimen (see above).— S. B. Kaye *et al.*, *Br. J. Cancer*, 1979, *39*, 168.

Alternative chemotherapy should be used in patients with Hodgkin's disease who developed progressive disease during MOPP therapy or relapse shortly after therapy is completed.— R. I. Fisher *et al.*, *Ann. intern. Med.*, 1979, *90*, 761.

Administration of a polyvalent pneumococcal vaccine is recommended for all patients with Hodgkin's disease, to be given before or after splenectomy, but before specific immunosuppressive therapy is started.— J. E. Addiego *et al.*, *Lancet*, 1980, *2*, 450.

Further reports of the treatment of Hodgkin's disease: J. L. Ziegler *et al.*, *Lancet*, 1972, *2*, 679; C. L. M. Olweny *et al.* (letter), *ibid.*, 1974, *2*, 1397 (MOPP in children); E. Frei *et al.*, *Ann. intern. Med.*, 1973, *79*, 376 (MOPP; no overall survival benefit in patients given maintenance treatment); J. K. Luce *et al.*, *Archs intern. Med.*, 1973, *131*, 391 (MOPP); T. J. McElwain, *Br. J. Hosp. Med.*, 1973, *9*, 451 (MVPP); L. Stutzman and O. Glidewell, *J. Am. med. Ass.*, 1973, *225*, 1202 (MOPP compared with vincristine and procarbazine alternating with vinblastine, chlorambucil, and prednisone); R. C. Young *et al.*, *Lancet*, 1973, *1*, 1339 (MOPP; maintenance with carmustine had no significant effect); C. D. Bloomfield *et al.*, *Cancer*, 1976, *38*, 42 (cyclophosphamide, vinblastine, procarbazine, prednisone; CVPP); D. T. Harrison and P. E. Neiman, *Cancer Treat. Rep.*, 1977, *61*, 789 (carmustine alone or with vincristine, procarbazine, and prednisone); H. P. Roeser *et al.*, *Med. J. Aust.*, 1977, *2*, 821 (modified MOPP); V. Vinciguerra *et al.*, *J. Am. med. Ass.*, 1977, *237*, 33 (bleomycin, vinblastine, doxorubicin, and streptozocin; /BVDS/); S. D. Williams and L. H. Einhorn, *J. Am. med. Ass.*, 1977, *238*, 1659 (lomustine and doxorubicin, sometimes with bleomycin); J. Armata *et al.*, *Acta paediat. scand.*, 1978, *67*, 269 (MVPP and radiotherapy); H. J. Weh *et al.*, *Dt. med. Wschr.*, 1978, *103*, 1825 (combined chemotherapy and radiotherapy in Stage IV disease); M. Morgenfeld *et al.*, *Cancer*, 1979, *43*, 1579 (CVPP alone and with lomustine); P. H. Wiernik *et al.*, *Am. J. Med.*, 1979, *67*, 183 (combined modality treatment of disease confined to lymph nodes); M. R. Cooper *et al.*, *Cancer*, 1980, *46*, 654 (lomustine, vinblastine, prednisone, procarbazine); J. A. Green *et al.*, *Br. J. clin. Pharmac.*, 1980, *9*, 511 (measurement of the intensity of chemotherapy received compared to the calculated planned doses); J. M. Goldman and A. A. Dawson (letter), *Lancet*, 1981, *2*, 252 (outcome for advanced resistant disease).

Reports of individual antineoplastic agents used in Hodgkin's disease: J. E. Kurnick, *Chest*, 1977, *72*, 798 (bleomycin in resistant disease); H. H. Hansen *et al.*, *Cancer*, 1981, *7*, 7 (lomustine).

Non-Hodgkin's lymphomas. A discussion on lymphomas other than Hodgkin's disease with reference to histopathological classification. Careful staging is important and affects both treatment and prognosis.— D. Crowther and G. Blackledge, *Adv. Med.*, 1977, *13*, 68.

The non-Hodgkin's lymphomas are relatively common tumours and are highly responsive to therapy. Patients with localised *lymphocytic lymphomas* are given radiotherapy; those with stage III and IV disease are probably not curable but T. Anderson *et al.* (*Cancer*

Treat. Rep., 1977, *61*, 1057) have shown a low risk of recurrence after complete remission in patients given cyclophosphamide, vincristine, procarbazine, and prednisone (C-MOPP). Cyclical treatment with cyclophosphamide, vincristine, and prednisone (CVP) has also induced remissions (C.M. Bagley *et al.*, *Ann. intern. Med.*, 1972, *76*, 227). Chlorambucil may be given alone, continuously or intermittently, when the disease progresses slowly. Low-dose whole-body irradiation has been used as an alternative to chemotherapy in patients with stage III and IV disease. Patients with localised *histiocytic lymphomas* may be cured by surgery and radiotherapy; Stage II disease requires combined modality treatment and combination chemotherapy with regimens such as C-MOPP or cyclophosphamide, doxorubicin, vincristine, and prednisone (CHOP), as used by the Southwest Oncology Group (E.M. McElvey *et al.*, *Cancer*, 1976, *38*, 1484), should improve the cure-rate. All patients with stage III and IV histiocytic lymphomas should receive combination chemotherapy. *Lymphoblastic lymphomas* are rare and the disease merges clinically and morphologically with acute lymphoblastic leukaemia of poor prognosis. The chemotherapy schedules used for unfavourable acute leukaemia in children (S.B. Murphy, *Cancer Treat. Rep.*, 1977, *61*, 1161) or adult lymphoblastic leukaemia are indicated.— S. A. Rosenberg, *New Engl. J. Med.*, 1979, *301*, 924.

Further reviews on the management of non-Hodgkin's lymphoma: C. W. Berard *et al.*, *Ann. intern. Med.*, 1976, *85*, 351; D. L. Sweet *et al.*, *Ann. intern. Med.*, 1976, *85*, 521; S. B. Murphy, *New Engl. J. Med.*, 1978, *299*, 1446 (children).

Combination chemotherapy with six 4-week cycles of mustine 6 mg per m^2 body-surface or cyclophosphamide 650 mg per m^2 and vincristine 1.4 mg per m^2 on days 1 and 8, procarbazine 100 mg per m^2 by mouth daily for the first 14 days and prednisone 40 mg per m^2 by mouth daily for the first 14 days of cycles 1 and 4 (MOPP and C-MOPP) were used to treat 27 patients with diffuse histiocytic lymphomas. A complete remission was achieved in 11 and a partial response in 8; a response-rate of 70%. Ten of the 11 patients in complete remission remained free of disease for at least 26 months and might be considered to be cured. The 16 who gained a partial or negative response died with a median survival-time of 5 months.— V. T. DeVita *et al.*, *Lancet*, 1975, *1*, 248.

In a study of 56 patients with advanced diffuse histiocytic lymphoma, complete response-rates and survival curves were very similar with MOPP, C-MOPP, or BACOP chemotherapy regimens. The BACOP regimen consisted of: cyclophosphamide 650 mg per m^2 body-surface, doxorubicin 25 mg per m^2, and vincristine 1.4 mg per m^2 all given intravenously on days 1 and 8; bleomycin 5 mg per m^2 given intravenously on days 15 and 22; and prednisone 60 mg per m^2 taken by mouth on days 15 to 29; the cycle was then repeated. All patients were treated for a minimum of 6 cycles or 2 cycles following remission. No maintenance therapy was given. Mean survival for the group was 11.4 months with 38% alive at 5 years. Of the 56 patients, 26 (46%) had complete remissions with 82% of these still alive at 3 years, 21 (38%) had partial remissions with a median survival of 7.6 months, and 9 patients had no response and a median survival of 3.2 months.— R. I. Fisher *et al.*, *Am. J. Med.*, 1977, *63*, 177. See also P. S. Schein *et al.*, *Ann. intern. Med.*, 1976, *85*, 417.

Diffuse histiocytic lymphoma was treated with at least 6 courses of a combination chemotherapy schedule (COPP) of cyclophosphamide 1 to 1.5 g per m^2 body-surface (maximum 2.5 g) on day 1, vincristine sulphate 1.4 mg per m^2 (maximum 2 mg) on days 1, 8 and 15, prednisone 100 mg by mouth on days 1 to 4, and procarbazine hydrochloride 150 mg by mouth on days 21 to 31. Median survival was 52 weeks for 7 patients with partial remission and more than 129 weeks for 8 patients with complete remissions. Relapse occurred in 5 of the 8 complete responders though for 3 of these remission was re-induced.— B. H. Weinerman *et al.*, *J. Am. med. Ass.*, 1977, *237*, 2403.

Complete remissions were achieved in 4 of 31 patients with non-Hodgkin's lymphoma, of favourable histological type, treated with chlorambucil, and in 13 of 35 treated with the CVP regimen; the joint incidence of complete and good partial remissions was not significantly different. Neither regimen of treatment was considered to give a satisfactory response. The regimens were: chlorambucil 10 mg daily for 6 weeks, rest 2 weeks, then three 15-day cycles of chlorambucil 10 mg daily with 15-day intervals; CVP: cyclophosphamide 400 mg per m^2 body-surface for 5 days, vincristine 1.4 mg per m^2 to a maximum of 2 mg intravenously on day 1, and prednisolone 100 mg per m^2 daily for 5 days, 6 cycles being given at 21-day intervals.— T. A. Lister *et al.*, *Br. med. J.*, 1978, *1*, 533.

A proposal that initial systemic chemotherapy is more effective than initial radiotherapy in the treatment of localised diffuse histiocytic lymphoma. Confirmation of this and the role of adjuvant radiotherapy must be tested in larger numbers of patients.— T. P. Miller and S. E. Jones, *Lancet*, 1979, *1*, 358.

Complete remission was achieved in 23 of 42 patients with advanced diffuse histiocytic lymphoma given combination sequential chemotherapy with cyclophosphamide, vincristine, methotrexate with folinic acid rescue, and cytarabine (COMLA).— D. L. Sweet *et al.*, *Ann. intern. Med.*, 1980, *92*, 785. The current standard therapy for this disease is cyclophosphamide, doxorubicin, vincristine, and prednisone (CHOP). Alternatives include cyclophosphamide, prednisone, vincristine, and bleomycin (CPOB) or C-MOPP.— S. A. Grossman (letter), *ibid.*, *93*, 640. See also D. L. Sweet (letter), *ibid.*, 641. Further mention of treatment schedules for advanced diffuse histiocytic lymphoma including C-MOPP, BACOP, CHOP, HOP (doxorubicin, vincristine, and prednisone), and COMLA.— B. A. Mason (letter), *ibid.* See also D. L. Sweet (letter), *ibid.*, 642.

Further references to the management of non-Hodgkin's lymphomas: T. Pick *et al.*, *J. Pediat.*, 1974, *84*, 96 (radiotherapy and cyclophosphamide in lympho-epithelioma); R. S. Stein *et al.*, *Ann. intern. Med.*, 1974, *81*, 601 (vincristine and prednisone or COPP); H. P. Roeser *et al.*, *Br. J. Haemat.*, 1975, *30*, 233 (CVP); R. E. Lenhard *et al.*, *Cancer*, 1976, *38*, 1052 (COP or CO, cyclophosphamide and vincristine); C. S. Portlock and S. A. Rosenberg, *Cancer*, 1976, *37*, 1275 (CVP); S. Monfardini *et al.*, *Med. Pediat. Oncol.*, 1977, *3*, 67 (CVP compared with doxorubicin, bleomycin and prednisone; ABP); F. -J. Tigges *et al.*, *Dt. med. Wschr.*, 1977, *102*, 1537 (C-MOPP); B. J. Kennedy *et al.*, *Cancer*, 1978, *41*, 23 (CVP); S. R. Newcom and M. E. Kadin, *Lancet*, 1979, *1*, 462 (angio-immunoblastic lymphadenopathy).

See also under Burkitt's Lymphoma (above) and Mycosis Fungoides (below).

Leukaemia, acute. Reviews on the treatment of acute leukaemia: K. P. Cotter, *Practitioner*, 1977, *218*, 250 (in adolescents); *Br. med. J.*, 1978, *1*, 321 (possible long-term effects in children); *Ann. intern. Med.*, 1979, *91*, 758; *Br. med. J.*, 1981, *283*, 1205 (in adults).

References to the management of infections in patients with acute leukaemia: *Lancet*, 1977, *1*, 1294; *Lancet*, 1978, *2*, 769; R. G. Strauss *et al.*, *New Engl. J. Med.*, 1981, *305*, 597 (granulocyte transfusions; risks outweigh benefit). See also under Neomycin Sulphate, p.1190.

Results in 33 patients with acute lymphoblastic or myeloblastic leukaemia who underwent high-dose chemotherapy and total-body irradiation followed by allogeneic bone-marrow transplantation indicated that such treatment could produce long-term remissions if performed during complete or partial remission. Suitable candidates for treatment are adults with all forms of acute leukaemia; children with acute myeloblastic leukaemia or T-cell acute lymphoblastic leukaemia during first complete remission, in 'good' partial remission, or 'early' relapse; and children and adolescents with acute lymphoblastic leukaemia during second complete remission.— K. G. Blume, *New Engl. J. Med.*, 1980, *302*, 1041. A technique for the removal of bone marrow from leukaemic patients in remission, treatment with antileukaemic antibodies, and storage in liquid nitrogen for use after intensive combination chemotherapy and high doses of radiation therapy, when the patient has a leukaemic relapse. Of 2 patients treated one died of heart failure but evidence of take was found, and the other achieved complete remission.— B. Netzel *et al.*, *Lancet*, 1980, *1*, 1330. See also *Ann. intern. Med.*, 1977, *86*, 155 (preparation for bone-marrow transplantation with a regimen consisting of thioguanine, cyclophosphamide, cytarabine, daunorubicin, and total-body irradiation: SCARI); K. A. Dicke *et al.*, *Lancet*, 1979, *1*, 514 (autologous marrow transplantation); R. L. Powles *et al.*, *Lancet*, 1980, *1*, 1047; R. F. Webb (letter), *ibid.*, 1413 (bone-marrow transplantation in acute myelogenous leukaemia).

Further reports on the management of acute leukaemia: Second Report to the MRC of the Working Party on the Evaluation of Different Methods of Therapy in Leukaemia, *Br. med. J.*, 1966, *1*, 1383; G. P. Bodey *et al.*, *J. Am. med. Ass.*, 1976, *235*, 1021 (late intensification therapy); D. M. Komp *et al.*, *Cancer*, 1976, *37*, 1243; G. Mathé *et al.* (letter), *Lancet*, 1976, *1*, 1130; A. S. D. Spiers *et al.*, *Cancer*, 1977, *40*, 20 (thioguanine, daunorubicin, cytarabine, methotrexate, prednisolone, cyclophosphamide, vincristine, and colaspase: TRAMPCOL); M. P. Sullivan *et al.*, *Blood*, 1977, *50*, 471 (combination intrathecal therapy for meningeal leukaemia); *Lancet*, 1978, *2*, 823 (chromosomes and leukaemia); H. M. Golomb *et al.*, *New Engl. J. Med.*, 1978, *299*, 613 (prognostic value of chromosome-banding studies); W. N. Hittelman *et al.*, *New Engl. J. Med.*, 1980, *303*, 479 (prediction of relapse using the premature chromosome condensation technique); *Br. med. J.*, 1980, *281*, 959 (possible role of viruses in childhood leukaemia).

Some earlier references defining the following regimens for acute leukaemias: CART (cytarabine, colaspase, daunorubicin, and thioguanine); CAMP (cyclophosphamide, methotrexate, mercaptopurine, and prednisolone); OAP (vincristine, cytarabine, and prednisone); COAP (cyclophosphamide and OAP); DOAP (daunorubicin and OAP); POMP (mercaptopurine, vincristine, methotrexate, and prednisone); VAMP (vincristine, methotrexate, mercaptopurine, and prednisolone); L 2 (prednisone, vincristine, and daunorubicin for induction; cytarabine, thioguanine, colaspase and carmustine for consolidation; and thioguanine, cyclophosphamide, hydroxyurea, daunorubicin, methotrexate, carmustine, cytarabine, and vincristine for maintenance.— N. V. Khvatova *et al.*, *Terap. Arkh.*, 1971, *43*, 3, per *Abstr. Wld Med.*, 1971, *45*, 755; A. S. DSpiers, *Clins Haemat.*, 1972, *1*, 127; V. Rodriguez *et al.*, *Cancer*, 1973, *32*, 69, per *J. Am. med. Ass.*, 1973; *226*, 377; M. Haghbin *et al.*, *Cancer*, 1974, *33*, 1491, per *J. Am. med. Ass.*, 1974, *229*, 1825; J. U. Gutterman *et al.*, *lancet*, 1974, *2*, 1405.

For reference to the treatment of an erythroleukaemia, Di Guglielmo's disease, see Daunorubicin Hydrochloride, p.205.

Acute lymphoblastic leukaemia. Cooperative studies on large numbers of patients have shown that acute lymphoblastic leukaemia is best treated with cyclic or sequential regimens. Such treatment may produce severe toxic effects and should be carried out in special centres equipped to reduce the risk of infection. Several regimens have been shown to be effective, especially in children.

Treatment of acute lymphoblastic leukaemia may be divided into several stages: induction, consolidation, CNS prophylaxis, maintenance, and intensification. Usually a remission is induced with vincristine 1.5 mg per m^2 body-surface weekly by intravenous injection and prednisone 40 mg per m^2 daily by mouth, sometimes with colaspase or with daunorubicin or doxorubicin for refractory patients. Consolidation involves the continuation of this intensive therapy after the achievement of complete remission. It is common practice to protect the patient from meningeal leukaemia by CNS prophylaxis with cranial irradiation and methotrexate administered intrathecally. Maintenance of remission is generally with methotrexate and mercaptopurine, sometimes with the addition of cyclophosphamide. Intensification therapy or periodic re-induction involves the intermittent use of the initial induction regimen during the maintenance phase.

Unlike the disease in adults, acute lymphoblastic leukaemia of childhood has been demonstrated to be curable (J. Simone *et al.*, *Cancer*, 1972, *30*, 1488). Immunological subtyping of adults with acute lymphoblastic leukaemia appears to be important prognostically, as has been previously shown in children (J.M. Chessels *et al.*, *Lancet*, 1977, *2*, 1307), and might help identify those who would benefit from more aggressive therapy.— J. D. Bitran (letter), *New Engl. J. Med.*, 1978, *299*, 1317; *ibid.*, 1979, *300*, 148. Differences in response to treatment in children and adults appear to be related to the differing proportions of leukaemia subgroups. The incidence of common acute lymphoblastic leukaemia (ALL) is higher in children. Adults with common ALL have a prognosis superior to that of adults with null-cell ALL, T-cell ALL, or B-cell ALL and results with chemotherapy can approach those in children with common ALL.— M. F. Greaves and T. A. Lister (letter), *New Engl. J. Med.*, 1981, *304*, 119.

Of 80 children with acute lymphoblastic leukaemia in whom remission had been achieved by the use of multiple antineoplastic agents, 26 had CNS relapses within 71 weeks of the end of the first 12-week period. This compared with 1 of 75 who had received irradiation of the cranium followed by injection intrathecally of part of the methotrexate from the usual continuing multiple therapy. Total relapse and deaths in the 2 groups were 32 and 18 respectively. Children less than 10 years old appeared to benefit more than older children. There were 4 deaths in remission in the irradiated group and haematological relapses were more common. The overall results confirmed the value of prophylaxis against CNS relapse.—Report to the MRC by the Leukaemia Committee and the Working Party on Leukaemia in Childhood, *Br. med. J.*, 1973, *2*, 381. Of 43 patients who received twelve 12-week maintenance courses 28 (65%) remained in unbroken remission 5 to 6 years after starting treatment compared with 19 of 39 (49%) receiving 6 maintenance courses. Treatment for 19 months was therefore too short. There were more relapses in boys than in girls. There was tendency for bone-marrow relapses to be less in older patients and surprisingly in those with high initial leucocyte counts, although if patients with high initial counts survived in remission for 2 years they were considered to do as well as those with low initial counts.—Report to the MRC by the Working Party on Leukaemia in Childhood, *Br. med. J.*, 1977, *2*, 495. In a multicentre study in 284 children and persons under 20 with acute lymphoblastic leukaemia (UKALL II) girls benefited more than boys, due in part to a high incidence of testicular relapse when chemotherapy ceased. A schedule of high-dose spinal irradiation was less effective than schedules with some or no spinal irradiation but with methotrexate intrathecally. There was no evidence that cyclophosphamide 600 mg per m^2 body-surface every 12 weeks was beneficial; it was possibly deleterious. Twelve 12-week courses after the 12-week induction phase were no more effective than eight 12-week courses.— Report to the MRC by the Working Party on Leukaemia in Childhood, *Br. med. J.*, 1978, *2*, 787.

From results of a toxicity study by the Southwest Oncology Group it was concluded that methotrexate and cytarabine, either in combination or in sequence, were unsuitable for maintaining remission in acute lymphocytic leukaemia in children. There was a high incidence of nausea and vomiting, associated particularly with cytarabine injection.— R. Nitschke *et al.*, *J. clin. Pharmac.*, 1978, *18*, 131.

A remission-rate of 71% was achieved in 51 adults with acute lymphoblastic leukaemia treated by the OPAL regimen, followed by CNS treatment or prophylaxis, and by maintenance treatment with mercaptopurine, cyclophosphamide, and methotrexate. Of the 35 experiencing remission 18 continued in remission after 12 to 52 months. Factors adversely affecting the duration of remission were: the extent of disease at presentation, clinical hepatomegaly or splenomegaly or both, a high initial peripheral blood blast-cell count, and Burkitt-like leukaemia. The OPAL regimen consisted of doxorubicin 30 mg per m^2 body-surface and vincristine 1.4 mg per m^2 intravenously on days 0, 14, 28, and 42 with 2 further doses if needed, prednisolone 40 mg daily, and colaspase 10 000 units per m^2 intravenously on days 0 to 14. Complete remission was achieved in all 16 patients who received at least 2 courses of doxorubicin and vincristine, after the interval had been extended from 7 to 14 days.— T. A. Lister *et al.*, *Br. med. J.*, 1978, *1*, 199.

A study of relapses in 53 children with acute lymphoblastic leukaemia.— M. A. Cornbleet and J. M. Chessells, *Br. med. J.*, 1978, *2*, 104. Eighteen of 39 patients with refractory acute leukaemia achieved remissions after intensive treatment with methotrexate and colaspase. Excluding 5 early deaths due to complications of previous treatment, remissions were achieved in 13 of 19 with acute lymphoblastic leukaemia, 3 of 5 with acute undifferentiated leukaemia, and 2 of 10 with acute myeloblastic leukaemia. The median duration of remission was 20 weeks and of survival in responders 45 weeks. The regimen was considered relatively non-toxic and suitable for use in outpatients. After an initial dose of methotrexate 50 to 80 mg per m^2 body-surface intravenously, colaspase 40 000 units per m^2 was given intravenously 3 hours later; 7 to 14 days later methotrexate was given in doses increased (at each course) by 40 mg per m^2 to the limit of tolerance; colaspase was given 24 hours later in doses of 40 000 units per m^2 (reduced in later patients to 20 000 units per m^2). Colaspase was considered to act as 'rescue' providing relative protection from methotrexate toxicity.— B. -S. Yap *et al.*, *Br. med. J.*, 1978, *2*, 791. Remission of disease was obtained in 48 of 69 children with recurrent acute lymphoblastic leukaemia after induction with a regimen consisting of colaspase, vincristine and prednisone. No significant improvement was obtained when cyclophosphamide was added to this regimen.— F. H. Kung *et al.*, *Cancer*, 1978, *41*, 428.

Of 639 children with acute lymphocytic leukaemia who were treated with prednisone and vincristine, sometimes combined with daunorubicin or colaspase or both, sometimes with prophylactic cranial irradiation, with or without associated intrathecal methotrexate, 278 had all treatment stopped, usually after 2½ years of complete remission. Relapses occurred in 55 of these children, in 41 of them during the first year after therapy was stopped, and they were more frequent in boys than girls. There have been no relapses in the 79 patients who have remained in complete remission for at least 4 years after treatment was stopped. The long-term prognosis for patients who relapse off therapy is poor, the median survival after relapse being only 2 years. In a study of 282 of the 639 children the relapse-rate was 10% in those who had been treated with 2 drugs compared with 25% in those given 3 or 4. A working definition of cure in acute lymphocytic leukaemia could be that of remaining in complete remission for at least 4 years after the cessation of all antileukaemic therapy. Acute lymphocytic leukaemia appears curable in over one-third of all newly-diagnosed patients given treatment for about 2½ years.— S. L. George *et al.*, *New Engl. J. Med.*, 1979, *300*, 269.

A report of successful marrow transplantation in a patient with acute lymphoblastic leukaemia. Although donor and recipient were not related they were phenotypically HLA-A, HLA-B, HLA-D, and HLA-DR identical.— J. A. Hansen *et al.*, *New Engl. J. Med.*, 1980, *303*, 565. Benefit of marrow transplantation over chemotherapy.— F. L. Johnson *et al.*, *ibid.*, 1981, *305*, 846.

Late marrow recurrences in childhood acute lymphoblastic leukaemia.— J. M. Chessells and F. Breatnach, *Br. med. J.*, 1981, *283*, 749.

Differences in prognosis for boys and girls with acute lymphoblastic leukaemia.— H. Sather *et al.*, *Lancet*, 1981, *1*, 739.

Role of CNS prophylaxis.— M. E. Nesbit *et al.*, *Lancet*, 1981, *1*, 1386.

Further references to the treatment of acute lymphoblastic leukaemia: *New Engl. J. Med.*, 1972, *287*, 769 (acute leukaemia Group B: treatment schedules and survival expectancy); T. S. Gee *et al.*, *Cancer*, 1976, *37*, 1256 (adults and children); H. Grobe *et al.*, *Dt. med. Wschr.*, 1977, *102*, 49 (children); J. S. Malpas, *Br. J. Hosp. Med.*, 1977, *17*, 444 (children); G. Mathé *et al.*, *Nouv. Presse méd.*, 1977, *6*, 2401 (children); J. A. Ortega *et al.*, *Cancer Res.*, 1977, *37*, 535 (children); M. E. Nesbit *et al.*, *J. Pediat.*, 1979, *95*, 727 (children); R. Sibbald and D. Catovsky, *Br. J. Haemat.*, 1979, *42*, 488 (prolymphocytic leukaemia).

Acute myeloid leukaemia. Acute myeloid leukaemia (used here to include the terms acute myeloblastic, acute myelogenous, or acute nonlymphocytic leukaemia) is less responsive to chemotherapy than the acute lymphoblastic disease, but the introduction of complex cyclic and sequential regimens has improved the response.

A review of the management of adult acute myelogenous leukaemia. Induction of complete remission is generally achieved by giving thioguanine and cytarabine in courses of 5 to 7 days with daily intravenous injections of daunorubicin or doxorubicin for 1 to 3 days; cytarabine is often given as a continuous intravenous infusion. Remission-rates of 62 to 85% have been reported using one or two such courses. Most patients subsequently relapse although a few have survived for up to 10 years without further treatment. The majority have some residual leukaemic cells and in theory further consolidation therapy with high doses of the drugs used for induction or maintenance therapy with lower doses of these or other drugs should improve results. Only a few controlled studies of maintenance therapy have been reported and the results are conflicting. On balance, some form of maintenance chemotherapy for 1 to 2 years seems reasonable. Unfortunately the median duration of remission has generally been short and reported median survivals of 10 to 21 months remain disappointing. Immunotherapy with leukaemic cells or agents such as BCG has sometimes prolonged survival but its place in the treatment of acute myelogenous leukaemia remains controversial. CNS prophylaxis with cranial irradiation and intrathecal methotrexate or cytarabine is not recommended routinely because of the low incidence of meningeal infiltration when compared with acute lymphoblastic leukaemia and the relatively short survival of most patients with acute myelogenous leukaemia. Preliminary results with bone-marrow transplantation suggest that a cure is possible for those patients who reach remission and have an HLA-matched sibling donor. For patients without suitable donors other methods of treatment, including further intensive chemotherapy after about 12 months' remission and autotransplantation of bone marrow collected during remission, are being studied.— J. A. Whittaker, *Br. med. J.*, 1980, *281*, 960. See also R. P. Gale, *New Engl. J. Med.*, 1979, *300*, 1189; C. D. Bloomfield, *Ann. intern. Med.*, 1980, *93*, 133.

A schedule of cytarabine, thioguanine, and daunorubicin with allopurinol cover (TAD) given for up to three 7-day cycles at intervals of 14 to 21 days induced complete remissions in 22 patients and a partial remission in 1 out of a group of 28 adults with acute myeloid leukaemia. Doses consisted of cytarabine 100 mg per m^2 body-surface by intravenous infusion over 30 minutes and thioguanine 100 mg per m^2 every 12 hours for 7 days [it is implied that cytarabine is also given every 12 hours for 7 days]. Daunorubicin 60 mg per m^2 was injected intravenously on days 5, 6, and 7. Consolidation therapy was 2 cycles at 21-day intervals of cytarabine and thioguanine every 12 hours for 5 days followed by one injection of daunorubicin. Prophylaxis against CNS involvement was given during this phase and consisted of cranial irradiation and 5 doses of cytarabine 100 mg per m^2 injected intrathecally. Maintenance of remission was with either monthly cycles of 5 days' treatment with cytarabine and thioguanine alternating with one dose of daunorubicin or this therapy plus *Corynebacterium parvum* and irradiated leukaemic blast-cells. No difference was found between either maintenance schedule, the median duration of remission for the whole group being 280 days and the median survival in those achieving remission being 375 days. Just over half the patients were alive at 1 year. However, median survival after relapse was brief at 95 days. Most patients experienced profound bone-marrow depression and 5 showed signs of altered liver function. An addendum lists 6 further patients all of whom achieved complete remissions with TAD.— R. P. Gale and M. J. Cline, *Lancet*, 1977, *1*, 497. Of 40 patients with acute myeloid leukaemia treated with daunorubicin 50 mg per m^2 on day 1 and cytarabine 100 mg per m^2 every 12 hours and thioguanine 100 mg per m^2 every 12 hours on days 1 to 5 (DAT), 34 entered complete remission. The median duration of survival has been 104 weeks and the median duration of remission 61 weeks. A second remission following a relapse was obtained in 45%.— J. K. H. Rees and F. G. J. Hayhoe (letter), *Lancet*, 1978, *1*, 1360.

Intensive chemotherapy produced complete remissions in 24 of 40 adult patients with acute nonlymphocytic leukaemia (mainly myelogenous) and all 24 were then given weekly maintenance therapy with thioguanine 2 mg per kg body-weight by mouth on 4 successive days followed on the 5th day by an intramuscular injection of cytarabine 1.5 mg per kg. The median duration of complete remission was 16.5 months with a range of 3 to more than 56 months and was considered to compare well with a duration of about 12 months with other more toxic and complicated maintenance schedules and with the usual duration of about 3 months for patients receiving no maintenance. In spite of side-effects which included alterations in liver function, depression of bone-marrow, and gastro-intestinal upset, maintenance therapy was well tolerated.— B. A. Peterson and C. D. Bloomfield, *Lancet*, 1977, *2*, 158.

Of 25 patients with acute myeloid leukaemia 15 achieved complete remission and 5 partial remission after treatment with up to 6 courses of TRAP (thioguanine, daunorubicin, cytarabine, and prednisolone). Maintenance was intensive with cycles of 2 courses of modified COAP (cyclophosphamide, vincristine, cytarabine, and prednisolone), 3 courses of TRAP, 2 courses of modified POMP (prednisolone, vincristine, methotrexate, and mercaptopurine), and 3 courses of TRAP. Remissions had lasted 28 to 208 (median 66) weeks and survival 32 to 249 (median 102) weeks. The TRAP programme could be regarded only as palliative.— A. S. D. Spiers *et al.*, *Br. med. J.*, 1977, *2*, 544. A modification of this regimen.— P. Stavem *et al.* (letter), *Br. med. J.*, 1977, *2*, 831.

A report of encouraging results obtained with a protocol directed at the problem of relapse from complete remission in children and adults with acute myelogenous leukaemia. The protocol was designed to reduce and, if possible, eradicate the leukaemic clone of cells and includes the following features: early and late intensification of chemotherapy during remission, the sequencing of different chemotherapy combinations during remission, and the use of high-dose continuous infusions of cytarabine during remission to provide therapeutic concentrations of drug in the CSF. Chemotherapy was given in 2 phases to 83 previously untreated patients with acute myelogenous leukaemia. In the first phase remission was induced with 2 courses of vincristine, doxorubicin, prednisolone, and cytarabine. Patients with complete remission were then given intensive sequential combination chemotherapy for 14 months. In this second phase, therapy was divided into 4 sequences, the first and last being designated as early intensification and late intensification, each sequence being given four times at intervals of 3 to 4 weeks. The following drugs were given in sequence: doxorubicin and cytarabine; doxorubicin and azacitidine; vincristine, methylprednisolone, mercaptopurine, and methotrexate; and cytarabine. Cytarabine was given in a dose of 200 mg per m^2 body-surface daily by continuous intravenous infusion. Complete remissions were achieved by 58 patients (70%) and the median duration of complete remission is projected to be 23 months. Overall there have been 22 relapses, and 2 deaths and 5 withdrawals during remission. Of the 22 patients who have completed treatment the median follow-up after stopping therapy has been 11 months and only 4 had relapsed. The durability of complete remission appears to be independent of age.— H. J. Weinstein *et al.*, *New Engl. J. Med.*, 1980, *303*, 473. See also M. M. Bern *et al.* (letter), *ibid.*, 1981, *305*, 642.

Further references to the treatment of acute myeloid leukaemia: B. D. Clarkson, *Cancer*, 1972, *30*, 1572 (the L6 protocol: induction and consolidation with cytarabine and thioguanine; maintenance with vincristine, methotrexate, carmustine, thioguanine, cyclophosphamide, hydroxyurea, and daunorubicin, given in order); J. A. Levi *et al.*, *Ann. intern. Med.*, 1972, *76*, 397 (hydroxyurea, thioguanine, cytarabine in non-lymphatic leukaemias); D. S. Rosenthal and W. C. Moloney, *New Engl. J. Med.*, 1972, *286*, 1176 (vincristine, cytarabine, daunorubicin); D. Crowther *et al.*, *Br. med. J.*, 1973, *1*, 131 (induction with daunorubicin and cytarabine; maintenance by chemotherapy and or immunotherapy); C. B. Freeman *et al.*, *Br. med. J.*, 1973, *4*, 571 (induction with daunorubicin and cytarabine; cytoreduction with cyclophosphamide and thioguanine; some also received immunotherapy); W. Paolino *et al.*, *Br. med. J.*, 1973, *3*, 567 (TRAP); F. Cavalli *et al.* (letter), *Br. med. J.*, 1975, *4*, 227 (etoposide in relapsed patients); P. Jacobs *et al.* (letter), *Br. med. J.*, 1975, *1*, 396 (cytarabine, etoposide, and doxorubicin); F. Cavalli *et al.*, *Schweiz. med. Wschr.*, 1976, *106*, 1265; J. Gmür *et al.*, *Schweiz. med. Wschr.*, 1976, *106*, 205 (daunorubicin in acute promyelocytic leukaemia); P. A. Pizzo *et al.*, *J. Pediat.*, 1976, *88*, 125; D. A. G. Galton *et al.* (letter), *Lancet*, 1977, *2*, 973 (role of immunotherapy); D. A. Van Echo *et al.*, *Cancer Treat. Rep.*, 1977, *61*, 1599 (vinblastine, azacitidine, and etoposide); A. J. Collins *et al.*, *Archs intern. Med.*, 1978, *138*, 1677 (daunorubicin and prednisone in acute promyelocytic leukaemia); M. J. Pippard *et al.*, *Br. med. J.*, 1979, *1*, 227 (CNS prophylaxis); E. J. Saponara *et al.*, *Archs intern. Med.*, 1979, *139*, 1277 (cytarabine and thioguanine); R. L. Powles *et al.*, *Lancet*, 1980, *1*, 1047 (survival and remission-rates higher with bone-marrow transplantations than with chemotherapy); J. G. Watson *et al.*, *Lancet*, 1981, *2*, 957 (marrow transplantation); J. A. Whittaker *et al.*, *Br. med. J.*, 1981, *282*, 692 (role of immunotherapy).

For a report of large doses of hydroxyurea being given prior to combination chemotherapy in patients with acute non-lymphocytic leukaemia, see Hydroxyurea, p.212.

Leukaemia, chronic. In chronic lymphatic and myeloid leukaemias in adults, useful palliative effects may be obtained with drugs such as chlorambucil and busulphan respectively.

Chronic lymphatic leukaemia. Comment on the use of radiotherapy for chronic lymphatic leukaemia.— *Lancet*, 1979, *1*, 82.

Chronic myeloid leukaemia. Chronic granulocytic or myeloid leukaemia represents less than one quarter of adult leukaemias and is associated with a chromosome abnormality, the Philadelphia chromosome (Ph^1). A terminal blastic phase generally develops; in a minority of patients this may be lymphoblastic and brief remissions have been obtained with vincristine and prednisone. Reconstitution of the bone marrow with cytogenetically normal cells may be successful if undertaken during the chronic phase of the disease.— G. P. Canellos, *New Engl. J. Med.*, 1979, *300*, 360. A report of successful marrow transplantation following vigorous chemotherapy and radiotherapy in 4 patients with chronic granulocytic leukaemia. Dimethylbusulphan 5 mg per kg body-weight was given intravenously in 10% dimethyl sulphoxide on day 1 and cyclophosphamide 60 mg per kg daily intravenously on days 2 and 3. Total-body irradiation on day 7 preceded the intravenous infusion of bone marrow from each patient's identical twin. The patients remained haematologically and clinically normal 22 to 31 months after transplantation, their marrow having been successfully repopulated by normal marrow stem cells.— A. Fefer *et al.*, *New Engl. J. Med.*, 1979, *300*, 333.

Details of a chemotherapeutic regimen for 12 previously untreated patients with Ph^1-positive chronic myeloid leukaemia, with the aim of bringing about karyotypic conversion, which is associated with improved prognosis. A change in karyotypic status was achieved in 7 of the 12 patients; no patient died as a result of therapy. An initial 6 courses of chemotherapy at intervals of 2 to 3 weeks consisted of: doxorubicin initially 30 mg per m^2 body-surface intravenously increased to 60 mg per m^2 after the first 2 patients, and vincristine 1.5 mg per m^2 (max. 2 mg intravenously), on day 1; cytarabine 30 mg per m^2 as a 12-hourly infusion on days 1 to 7 for the first 2 patients, increased to 50 mg per m^2 for further patients, and subsequently to 100 mg per m^2 for the last 2 patients, and thioguanine 80 mg per m^2 orally also on days 1 to 7, increased to twice daily for the last 2 patients. After 6 courses, more conventional drugs were given in a 3-month cycle.— J. C. Sharp *et al.*, *Lancet*, 1979, *1*, 1370.

A review of the treatment of chronic myelogenous leukaemia.— H. P. Koeffler and D. W. Golde, *New Engl. J. Med.*, 1981, *304*, 1201 and 1269.

Further references to the treatment of chronic myeloid leukaemia: R. P. Herrmann *et al.*, *Med. J. Aust.*, 1972, *1*, 789 (alternating courses of uramustine and busulphan); A. D. S. Spiers *et al.*, *Br. med. J.*, 1974, *3*, 77 (treatment of patients with chronic granulocytic leukaemia in acute transformation using thioguanine, daunorubicin, cytarabine, methotrexate, prednisolone, cyclophosphamide, vincristine, and colaspase: TRAMPCO(L)); A. D. Spiers *et al.*, *Lancet*, 1975, *1*, 829 (primary treatment with thioguanine, with or without allopurinol); *Br. med. J.*, 1977, *2*, 1303 (lymphoid blast crisis); T. Hauch *et al.*, *Blood*, 1978, *51*, 571 (treatment with melphalan).

See also under Busulphan, p.194.

Malignant effusions. Malignant pleural or peritoneal effusion is a complication of many forms of cancer. In general, when a tumour responds to systemic chemotherapy so too does the effusion. In patients with refractory tumours, effusions may be treated after complete drainage by inducing sclerosis by instillation of talc, mepacrine, or alkylating agents such as mustine or thiotepa. More recently tetracycline or bleomycin have been reported to be effective in most patients and at present they represent the least toxic choice. Instillation of doxorubicin also appears to be effective.— *Lancet*, 1981, *1*, 198. See also A. Leff *et al.*, *Ann. intern. Med.*, 1978, *88*, 532; R. S. Stein (letter), *ibid.*, *89*, 139.

Malignant neoplasms. Report of a WHO Expert Committee on Chemotherapy of Solid Tumours, *Tech. Rep. Ser. Wld Hlth Org. No. 605*, 1977. Controversies in WHO tumour classification and an appeal for uniformity.— L. Kreyberg and W. F. Whimster, *Br. med. J.*, 1978, *2*, 1203.

Further reviews on the treatment of solid tumours: J. S. Malpas, *Adv. Med.*, 1977, *13*, 43 (children); N. M. Bleehen and C. R. Wiltshire, *Br. J. Hosp. Med.*, 1978, *19*, 354; J. A. Levi, *Med. J. Aust.*, 1978, *1*, 15.

Further references to the use of antineoplastic agents in the treatment of miscellaneous malignant neoplasms: J. D. Bearden *et al.*, *Cancer*, 1977, *39*, 21 (cyclophosphamide, vincristine, methotrexate, fluorouracil, and prednisone: COMF-P); D. J. Higby *et al.*, *Cancer Treat. Rep.*, 1977, *61*, 869 (doxorubicin with cisplatin or cyclophosphamide); D. Longacre *et al.*, *Cancer Treat. Rep.*, 1977, *61*, 919 (hexamethylmelamine, vincristine, and methotrexate); R. C. Mills *et al.*, *Cancer Treat. Rep.*, 1977, *61*, 477 (doxorubicin and cisplatin); C. G. Schmidt and R. Becher, *Dt. med. Wschr.*, 1979, *104*, 872 (cisplatin and ifosfamide in metastasing melanoblastoma); R. L. Woods and J. F. Stewart, *Postgrad. med. J.*, 1980, *56*, 272 (cyclophosphamide and cisplatin in metastatic basal-cell carcinoma); R. L. Woods *et al.*, *New Engl. J. Med.*, 1980, *303*, 87 (doxorubicin and mitomycin in metastatic adenocarcinomas).

Malignant neoplasms of the adrenal cortex. See under Mitotane, p.222.

Malignant neoplasms of the bladder. The chemotherapy of bladder carcinoma has not been intensively studied. Overall response-rates of 35% and 27% have been reported for fluorouracil and doxorubicin respectively but, because of discouraging results in a placebo-controlled study, fluorouracil cannot be recommended for primary treatment. The intracavitary instillation of thiotepa appears to be beneficial in the treatment of small multiple superficial papillary tumours and has been used prophylactically in patients with multiple tumour recurrences. Other drugs with some activity in bladder cancer include mitomycin, teniposide, and cisplatin.— Report of a WHO Expert Committee on Chemotherapy of Solid Tumours, *Tech. Rep. Ser. Wld Hlth Org. No. 605*, 1977, p. 49.

A discussion on the management of superficial bladder cancer by the instillation of antineoplastic agents. A review of 5 studies indicated complete regression in about 60% of patients and partial regression in 30% when ethoglucid was instilled; a controlled study is needed to confirm its apparent superiority over thiotepa. Other drugs that have been used topically include doxorubicin, bleomycin, mitomycin, and teniposide.— A. Morales, *Can. med. Ass. J.*, 1980, *122*, 1133.

Further reviews on chemotherapy in cancer of the bladder: *Br. med. J.*, 1977, *2*, 1562; J. B. de Kernion, *Cancer Res.*, 1977, *37*, 2271.

Ten patients with metastatic transitional cell carcinoma from the bladder and two with carcinoma from the renal pelvis were treated for 2 days every 21 days. Cyclophosphamide 650 mg per m^2 body-surface and doxorubicin hydrochloride 50 mg per m^2 were given by intravenous infusion on day 1 and cisplatin 100 mg per m^2 intravenously on day 2. If the cumulative dosage of doxorubicin hydrochloride reached 550 mg per m^2, cyclophosphamide dosage was increased to 1 g per m^2 as the doxorubicin hydrochloride was withdrawn. Of the 10 patients with metastatic bladder carcinoma 1 achieved a complete response and 8 a partial response and 1 of the patients with carcinoma from the renal pelvis had a partial response. Almost all patients experienced a range of toxic effects including alopecia, nausea and vomiting, and anaemia.— J. J. Sternberg *et al.*, *J. Am. med. Ass.*, 1977, *238*, 2282.

Further references to the chemotherapy of bladder cancer: N. H. Slack *et al.*, *J. surg. Oncol.*, 1977, *9*, 393, per *J. Am. med. Ass.*, 1977, *238*, 2436; A. Yagoda, *Cancer Res.*, 1977, *37*, 2775, per *Int. pharm. Abstr.*, 1978, *15*, 163; B. Richards *et al.* (letter), *Br. med. J.*, 1978, *2*, 200 (adjuvant chemotherapy with doxorubicin and fluorouracil).

Malignant neoplasms of the bone. Osteosarcoma, chondrosarcoma, and fibrosarcoma are the 3 basic types of primary malignant tumour of bone. Others such as Ewing's tumour and malignant myeloma arise in the marrow rather than the bone itself.— R. Sweetnam, *Br. J. Hosp. Med.*, 1980, *24*, 452.

Four patients with stage IV lymphoma presenting in bone achieved a complete remission with a regimen of bleomycin, doxorubicin, cyclophosphamide, vincristine, and prednisone (BACOP); 2 of the patients had also received radiotherapy. All 4 were still in remission at 11 to 32 months. Of 4 other patients who received cyclophosphamide, vincristine, procarbazine, and prednisone (C-MOPP) one, who had also received radiotherapy, achieved complete remission and was alive and well 24 months after diagnosis. The other 3 gained partial remissions and survived for 8 to 20 months.— R. R. Reimer *et al.*, *Ann. intern. Med.*, 1977, *87*, 50.

See also under Sarcoma (below).

Malignant neoplasms of the brain. Glioblastoma multiforme constitutes 31 to 64% of all the gliomas and is the major CNS malignancy for which new antineoplastic agents are being tested. Cerebral oedema surrounding the tumour can have the same effect as the expanding tumour mass and survival may be prolonged if increased intracranial pressure is alleviated by surgical decompression or the use of corticosteroids (see under Dexamethasone, p.466). Regional chemotherapy with methotrexate has been attempted in order to overcome the blood-brain barrier and lipid-soluble antineoplastic agents are sought. The nitrosoureas are highly lipid-soluble and are probably the only drugs that are genuinely active; a response-rate of 46% with definite prolongation of survival has been reported with carmustine and similar results have been seen with lomustine and semustine. Preliminary results suggest that procarbazine and teniposide may also be active against glioblastoma. There have been few attempts at combination chemotherapy because of the limited number of active agents available.— Report of a WHO Expert Committee on Chemotherapy of Solid Tumours, *Tech. Rep. Ser. Wld Hlth Org. No. 605*, 1977, p. 66.

Tumour reduction occurred initially with radiotherapy and then with combination chemotherapy in a patient with a tumour in the pineal region. The schedule consisted of doxorubicin 100 mg and vincristine 2 mg intravenously on day 1 and bleomycin 30 mg intravenously on days 1 to 3. This was repeated every 3 to 4 weeks depending on the blood picture.— N. de Tribolet and L. Barrelet (letter), *Lancet*, 1977, *2*, 1228 and 1372.

Further reports and reviews on the treatment of malignant neoplasms of the brain: P. Pouillart *et al.*, *Nouv. Presse méd.*, 1975, *4*, 721 (teniposide, lomustine); R. Brisman *et al.*, *Archs Neurol., Chicago*, 1976, *33*, 745 (adjuvant therapy with nitrosoureas); C. B. Wilson *et al.*, *Archs Neurol., Chicago*, 1976, *33*, 739; J. B. Posner, *Semin. Oncol.*, 1977, *4*, 81 (CNS metastases); C. B. Wilson *et al.*, *Curr. Probl. Cancer*, 1977, *1*, 1; D. C. Crafts *et al.*, *J. Neurosurg.*, 1978, *49*, 589 (combination chemotherapy with procarbazine, lomustine, and vincristine in recurrent medulloblastoma); S. B. Kaye *et al.*, *Br. med. J.*, 1979, *1*, 233.

For a study of the relative benefits of radiotherapy and nitrosoureas in the postsurgical treatment of malignant glioma, see Carmustine, p.195.

Malignant neoplasms of the breast. A detailed review of the treatment of primary and metastatic breast carcinoma. Most patients in the USA are still treated initially with mastectomy and are given hormonal therapy at relapse. Radiotherapy is also used in association with, and sometimes without, surgery. Few if any patients are cured after metastases have been found but survival can be prolonged and symptoms of advanced disease relieved for up to 10 years by hormonal therapy, chemotherapy, or a combination of the two. Conventional endocrine therapy includes the administration of oestrogens or endocrine ablation by oophorectomy, adrenalectomy, or hypophysectomy. Highest response-rates to stilboestrol or ethinyloestradiol are seen in patients more than 5 years beyond the menopause but there is almost no response in the first postmenopausal year. Oophorectomy is used in premenopausal women or those immediately postmenopausal; patients under 35 years and those in the first postmenopausal year have a lower response-rate. Adrenalectomy and hypophysectomy are thought to be effective after the menopause or after oophorectomy by removing persistent low concentrations of oestrogen available to the growing breast tumour; results are similar with either procedure. Mean duration of remission appears to be 9 to 10 months after oestrogen therapy or oophorectomy and 12 to 14 months after major endocrine ablation. Androgens, such as fluoxymesterone, progestogens, and corticosteroids are generally reserved as second-line therapy. All forms of endocrine therapy, especially oestrogens, may cause a transient 'flare' or rapid progression of the disease at the start of treatment; hypercalcaemia may be life-threatening.— I. C. Henderson and G. P. Canellos, *New Engl. J. Med.*, 1980, *302*, 17. Response to endocrine therapy can be correlated with the presence of oestrogen receptors in the tumour which in turn are associated with a more slow-growing disease. Despite conflicting reports, patients seem likely to benefit from antineoplastic agents regardless of receptor status. Combination chemotherapy now has an established role in the treatment of advanced disease. Many antineoplastic agents are active against carcinoma of the breast and those most commonly used are doxorubicin, cyclophosphamide, methotrexate, thiotepa, fluorouracil, melphalan, chlorambucil, and vincristine. The agents most frequently used alone, in various combinations, and sequentially, are cyclophosphamide (C), doxorubicin (A), methotrexate (M), and fluorouracil (F); prednisone (P) is also used in combination regimens. They do not appear to be cross-resistant. No one combination of drugs has a clear advantage and the more recent use of regimens including the very active agent doxorubicin has not generally improved response-rates achieved with CMF or CMF-P. Tumour regression occurs in 50 to 75% of patients treated with combination chemotherapy but the complete response-rate is almost always below 20%. The median duration of survival is 14 to 18 months after initiation of treatment. The use of adjuvant chemotherapy immediately following mastectomy is controversial and of no proven value in postmenopausal women or those with negative axillary nodes; it has prolonged remissions and survival in some patients. Immunotherapy has been used in association with chemotherapy but results are inconclusive. Other forms of therapy for breast cancer include the use of tamoxifen, mainly in postmenopausal patients, and 'medical' adrenalectomy with aminoglutethimide in advanced disease.— *idem*, 78. See also Report of a WHO Expert Committee on Chemotherapy of Solid Tumours, *Tech. Rep. Ser. Wld Hlth Org. No. 605*, 1977, p. 26.

Further reviews on the treatment of breast cancer: *Br. med. J.*, 1976, *2*, 832; *Br. med. J.*, 1977, *1*, 336 and 361; *Drug & Ther. Bull.*, 1977, *15*, 49; R. C. Young *et al.*, *Ann. intern. Med.*, 1977, *86*, 784; T. E. Davis and P. P. Carbone, *Drugs*, 1978, *16*, 441; D. A. Decker *et al.*, *J. Am. med. Ass.*, 1979, *242*, 2075; S. K. Carter and R. D. Rubens, *Lancet*, 1981, *2*, 795.

A report on the epidemiology and aetiology of breast cancer.— A. B. Miller and R. D. Bulbrook, *New Engl. J. Med.*, 1980, *303*, 1246.

A discussion on screening for breast cancer.— A. P. M. Forrest and M. M. Roberts, *Br. J. Hosp. Med.*, 1980, *23*, 8. See also *Lancet*, 1979, *2*, 1224; *ibid.*, 1981, *2*, 785.

Further references to the treatment of breast cancer: G. Bonadonna *et al.*, *New Engl. J. Med.*, 1976, *294*, 405 (CMF); C. Brambilla *et al.*, *Br. med. J.*, 1976, *1*, 801 (CMF versus doxorubicin and vincristine); J. G. Murray *et al.*, *Br. med. J.*, 1978, *1*, 408 (melphalan/methotrexate, fluorouracil); J. A. Russell *et al.*, *Cancer*, 1978, *41*, 396 (vincristine, doxorubicin, prednisolone); C. A. Hubay *et al.*, *Surgery, St. Louis*, 1980, *87*, 494.

Early breast cancer. A statement by the British Breast Group on the systemic chemotherapy of early breast cancer stressing the importance of local control of the disease. They advised that chemotherapy should not be used electively in primary operable disease until more information is available.— *Br. med. J.*, 1976, *2*, 861. Further discussion on the best treatment of early breast cancer, including reference to the use of systemic adjuvant chemotherapy which has so far been reserved for patients with stage II disease.— *Lancet*, 1978, *2*, 717. The view that the precise role of chemotherapy remains in doubt.— *Lancet*, 1981, *1*, 761. For studies see under Adjuvant Chemotherapy of Breast Cancer, p. 182.

Advanced breast cancer. Advanced breast cancer refers to stages of the disease not curable by conventional surgical methods and may be described by the Manchester clinical classification of stage III, indicating locally advanced disease, and stage IV, when distant metastases are present. Stage III is conventionally treated by radiotherapy and adjuvant systemic chemotherapy is also being investigated. Patients with stage IV disease have a limited life expectancy and the sequence of therapy for such patients depends on their menopausal status. Perimenopausal women within 5 years of their last menstrual period tend to respond poorly to any therapy. Remission-rates of about 30% have been reported with endocrine manoeuvres and similar results have been achieved, perhaps at the cost of greater toxicity, with single antineoplastic agents such as cyclophosphamide. More recently, combination chemotherapy with 3 or more antineoplastic agents has produced remission-rates of 50 to 80% without additive toxicity. In the UK simple endocrine manoeuvres are usually adopted first and combination chemotherapy only used when these have failed whereas in the USA the aggressive chemotherapy regimens tend to be favoured. Response to endocrine manipulation can be predicted according to the presence or absence of oestradiol receptors in tumours. The following treatment strategy is proposed when the receptor status of the patient is known: when receptors are present, premenopausal women are oophorectomised and postmenopausal women given tamoxifen; subsequent relapse is treated with endocrine ablation and after further relapse combination chemotherapy is given. All women who are receptor-negative are given combination chemotherapy immediately. When receptor status is not known a similar strategy may be adopted, according to the response achieved with oophorectomy and tamoxifen in premenopausal and postmenopausal women respectively.— M. Baum, *Br. J. Hosp. Med.*, 1980, *23*, 32.

Results comparable with those obtained by more toxic regimens were achieved in 42 patients with advanced breast cancer (all had undergone mastectomy and most had had radiotherapy or hormone treatment) by giving intensive therapy over 24 hours, repeated usually every 3 weeks. Of the 42 patients 28 responded, with a mean response lasting more than 24 weeks and mean survival of 52 weeks. The regimen consisted of vincristine sulphate 1 mg per m^2 body-surface area, cyclophosphamide 600 mg per m^2, and fluorouracil 500 mg per m^2, followed by an infusion of methotrexate 100 mg per m^2 over 16 hours; four hours after the end of the infusion calcium folinate 21 mg was given twice (4 hours apart), then 6 mg six-hourly for 4 injections.— J. H. Goldie and L. A. Price, *Br. med. J.*, 1977, *2*, 1064.

In a randomised study in women with recurrent or metastatic breast cancer 22 of 45 given cytotoxic agents (doxorubicin, cyclophosphamide, fluorouracil, and vincristine) achieved objective responses compared with 10 of 47 given endocrine treatment. Only in postmenopausal patients with predominantly soft-tissue disease was endocrine treatment as effective as cytotoxic agents.— T. Priestman *et al.*, *Br. med. J.*, 1977, *1*, 1248. There was no significant difference in overall survival between the 2 groups, but a strong clinical impression that patients with rapidly progressive disease, particularly premenopausal, would have benefited from the immediate action of the cytotoxic agents.— *idem*, 1978, *2*, 1673. See also W. Mattson (letter), *Br. med. J.*, 1977, *2*, 122.

A schedule of cyclophosphamide 500 mg per m^2 body-surface, doxorubicin 50 mg per m^2, and fluorouracil 500 mg per m^2 (CAF) all given intravenously on day 1 of a 21-day cycle was more effective but more toxic than a 5-drug regimen consisting of cyclophosphamide, methotrexate, fluorouracil, vincristine, and prednisone (CMFVP) in a study of 113 patients with metastatic or recurrent breast cancer. Twelve of 59 patients in the CAF group gained complete and 26 partial remission while corresponding figures in the CMFVP group were 3 and 17 respectively. Half the patients given CAF had granulocytopenia, most had nausea and vomiting, and all developed alopecia.— R. V. Smalley *et al.*, *Cancer*, 1977, *40*, 625.

Of 619 patients with metastatic breast cancer 116 achieved complete remission following combined chemotherapy but these responses were usually of short duration and only one-third of these patients remained in remission beyond 24 months. The tendency for relapse to occur in previously involved sites and the temporary nature of the complete remissions suggested that the fractional tumour cell-kill with currently available chemotherapy is small and that many patients with complete response still have a substantial subclinical tumour burden. As most patients relapsed while they were still receiving maintenance therapy it appeared that their tumours had developed resistance. Combined treatment with oophorectomy and chemotherapy resulted in the longest remissions.— S. S. Legha *et al.*, *Ann. intern. Med.*, 1979, *91*, 847. A report of failure of chemotherapy to prolong survival in a group of patients with metastatic breast cancer; survival may even have been shortened in some patients. Nevertheless, survival probably is prolonged in others therefore studies are needed to identify those who may benefit.— T. J. Powles *et al.*, *Lancet*, 1980, *1*, 580.

Two of 3 patients with grossly advanced cancer (stage III disease) involving virtually the whole of the breast, skin, and underlying muscle, obtained total regression of tumour and involved nodes following a regimen of intra-arterial infusion chemotherapy as basal treatment before radiotherapy. The third patient (who received the latter part of her treatment intravenously) obtained a considerable response, but there was a residual small lump in both breast and axilla, and mastectomy was therefore performed. A fourth patient with a stage IV breast carcinoma who also had evidence of liver metastases was treated in a similar manner and also obtained local tumour regression; although she still requires treatment for metastatic disease there is no evidence of residual carcinoma in the breast or axilla 12 months after treatment. Three of the patients have now had no evidence of residual local tumour 1, 2, and 4½ years after presentation (the fourth having had a mastectomy). One of the patients subsequently developed carcinoma in the opposite breast and chose the regimen of intra-arterial chemotherapy followed by radiotherapy, rather than mastectomy. Although the series is small the results are such that it is believed that further studies are mandatory and should include not only those with large inoperable tumours, but also patients with less advanced disease who refuse mastectomy. An additional advantage of the intra-arterial regimen may be that some of the inevitable escape into the general circulation could be valuable for those who may have micrometastases; follow-up radiotherapy is considered necessary to eradicate residual breast disease, and follow-up adjuvant chemotherapy to reduce the risk of overt metastases developing. The chemotherapeutic regimen was as follows: day 1, fluorouracil 400 mg per m^2 body-surface intra-arterially and hydroxyurea 1.4 g per m^2 by mouth; day 2, vincristine 700 µg per m^2 intra-arterially; day 3, doxorubicin 15 mg per m^2 intra-arterially; day 4, methotrexate 30 mg per m^2 intra-arterially; days 5 and 6, folinic acid 6 mg intramuscularly every 8 hours. The cycle was then repeated; cyclophosphamide 100 mg was given daily by mouth; the intra-arterial agents were infused over 24 hours in one litre of physiological saline containing heparin 10 000 units. The fourth patient also received the following intra-arterial regimen 2 weeks later: fluorouracil 500 mg for 8 hours, doxorubicin 15 mg for 5 minutes, vinblastine 5 mg for 5 minutes, methotrexate 30 mg for 5 minutes, and mitomycin 3 mg for 5 minutes; during infusion of the last 4 agents a cuff was inflated around the upper arm above arterial pressure to ensure maximal flow into the breast and axillary regions, and a 5-minute rest with the cuff deflated was allowed between each infusion.— F. O. Stephens *et al.*, *Lancet*, 1980, *2*, 435. Similar beneficial results in 5 of 6 patients given 1 to 6 courses of mitomycin in the internal mammary artery.— W. Mattsson *et al.* (letter), *ibid.*, 925.

Further references to the chemotherapy of advanced breast cancer: G. P. Canellos *et al.*, *Br. med. J.*, 1974, *1*, 218; *idem*, 1975, *1*, 37; *idem*, *Ann. intern. Med.*, 1976, *84*, 389 (cyclophosphamide, methotrexate, fluorouracil, prednisone); G. A. Edelstyn *et al.*, *Lancet*, 1975, *2*, 209; *idem*, 1977, *1*, 592 (cyclophosphamide, methotrexate, fluorouracil, vincristine); G. A. Edelstyn and K. D. MacRae (letter), *Lancet*, 1975, *2*, 1095; *idem*, 1976, *1*, 649 (doxorubicin and other agents); S. E. Jones *et al.*, *Cancer*, 1975, *36*, 90 (doxorubicin and cyclophosphamide); B. Hoogstraten *et al.*, *Cancer*, 1976, *38*, 13 (cyclophosphamide, methotrexate, fluorouracil, vincristine, and prednisone, compared with doxorubicin); C. A. Presant *et al.*, *Cancer*, 1976, *37*, 620 (carmustine, cyclophosphamide, doxorubicin); R. V. Smalley *et al.*, *Cancer Res.*, 1976, *36*, 3911 (combination versus sequential chemotherapy); P. J. Dady *et al.*, *Br. med. J.*, 1977, *1*, 554 (vincristine, doxorubicin, prednisolone); C. M. Haskell, *Med. Clins N. Am.*, 1977, *61*, 967 (a discussion including mention of immunotherapy); H. B. Muss *et al.*, *Archs intern. Med.*, 1977, *137*, 1711 (a comparison of cyclophosphamide, methotrexate, and fluorouracil, with or without vincristine and prednisone); J. A. Russell *et al.*, *Br. med. J.*, 1977, *2*, 1390; D. C. Tormey *et al.*, *Cancer Res.*, 1977, *37*, 529 (doxorubicin and mitolactol); J. Aisner, *Am. J. med. Sci.*, 1978, *275*, 5 (a review); C. H. Collis, *Br. J. clin. Pract.*, 1978, *32*, 139 (sequential combination chemotherapy); S. L. George and B. Hoogstraten, *J. natn. Cancer Inst.*, 1978, *60*, 731 (prognostic factors); M. De Lena *et al.*, *Cancer Chemother. Pharmac.*, 1978, *1*, 53 (chemotherapy with radiotherapy); T. Nemoto *et al.*, *Cancer*, 1978, *41*, 2073 (cyclophosphamide, fluorouracil, and prednisone compared with adrenalectomy and doxorubicin); O. H. Pearson *et al.*, *Cancer Res.*, 1978, *38*, 4323 (the role of pituitary hormones); D. P. D'Souza *et al.*, *J. Ir. med. Ass.*, 1978, *71*, 607 (chemotherapy in association with warfarin, levamisole, and BCG); G. Stolzenbach and D. von Domarus, *Dt. med. Wschr.*, 1978, *103*, 864 (cyclophosphamide, methotrexate, and prednisone); B. Tranum *et al.*, *Cancer*, 1978, *41*, 2078 (doxorubicin, cyclophosphamide, methotrexate, fluorouracil); R. T. Chlebowski *et al.*, *Cancer Res.*, 1979, *39*, 4503 (combination versus sequential chemotherapy); K. D. Swenerton *et al.*, *Cancer Res.*, 1979, *39*, 1552 (prognostic factors).

Adjuvant chemotherapy of breast cancer. The use of antineoplastic agents after primary therapy of breast cancer is called adjuvant chemotherapy, its purpose being to eradicate occult metastatic disease which would otherwise be fatal. Efficacy of treatment must be balanced against toxicity and the basic measure of therapeutic benefit is patient survival with an acceptable quality of life. Primary breast cancer is a heterogeneous disease with varying potentials for metastatic relapse and response to adjunctive chemotherapy. The 3 critical variables which form the basis of planning for clinical studies are involvement of axillary lymph nodes, menopausal state, and oestrogen-receptor levels. Comparative studies must allow long-term follow-up and must take account of acute and remote toxicity. Adjuvant chemotherapy studies reported so far have used radical or modified radical mastectomy for primary therapy; future studies may use less radical surgery but the impact of this on chemotherapy remains to be determined. Adjuvant chemotherapy using combination regimens of agents with known activity in advanced breast cancer and given at full dosage, now appears to be indicated for premenopausal patients with histological evidence of lymph node metastases who have undergone mastectomy. The use of adjuvant radiotherapy in association with chemotherapy has had no additional beneficial effect in patients with stage II disease. Oestrogen-receptor activity is an essential factor for classification and should be measured routinely in all patients with breast cancer. No hormonal manipulation has been established sufficiently to make hormonal alterations, alone or with chemotherapy, a standard form of adjuvant therapy. Nevertheless recent data regarding potential benefits for hormonal treatment in patients with significant oestrogen-receptor activity are encouraging. Patients with stage I disease, without lymph node involvement, have a good prognosis after local therapy and the 5-year disease-free survival without adjuvant chemotherapy may be at least 80%; the routine use of adjuvant chemotherapy in these patients cannot be recommended. Preliminary results in postmenopausal women with positive axillary nodes suggest that adjuvant chemotherapy may be beneficial and those with tumours containing oestrogen receptors may benefit from hormonal treatment in association with antineoplastic agents used at full dosage.—Summary of an NIH Consensus Statement *Br. med. J.*, 1980, *281*, 724; *New Engl. J. Med.*, 1980, *303*, 831.

Various combinations of antineoplastic agents are being tried in adjuvant chemotherapy of breast cancer but 5-year results are so far only available for the CMF regimen: cyclophosphamide 100 mg per m^2 body-surface by mouth on days 1 to 14, with methotrexate 40 mg per m^2 and fluorouracil 600 mg per m^2 both given intravenously on days 1 and 8, the course being repeated every 28 days for 1 year. A total relapse-free survival-rate of about 63% has been achieved with CMF following radical mastectomy compared with 48% in patients who only received surgery. CMF only had a significant effect in premenopausal patients but this might be attributed to the use of lower doses in older patients since other studies have not noted this difference in response. The single most important prognostic factor for the development of metastases is the status of axillary lymph nodes.— G. Bonadonna, *Br. J. Hosp. Med.*, 1980, *23*, 40. Adequate analysis of adjuvant studies will take many years of follow-up. Two studies provide most of the information currently available. In the National Surgical Adjuvant Breast Study Project melphalan has been compared with placebo after radical mastectomy and only appeared to be superior in premenopausal women with 1 to 3 positive axillary nodes. The other study is that reported by G. Bonadonna and P. Valagussa (*New Engl. J. Med.*, 1981, *304*, 10). There is little evidence at present to support the use of adjuvant chemotherapy in patients with negative nodes; the great majority of such patients will have a 5-year relapse-free interval with local therapy only.— S. K. Carter, *ibid.*, 45.

Further reviews on adjuvant chemotherapy in breast cancer: *Br. med. J.*, 1976, *1*, 1035; *J. Am. med. Ass.*, 1977, *237*, 2697; C. M. Haskell, *Ann. intern. Med.*, 1977, *86*, 68; G. G. Jamieson and J. Ludbrook, *Archs Surg.*, 1977, *112*, 119; B. A. Chabner *et al.*, *J. Am. med. Ass.*, 1978, *239*, 2373; M. Rozencweig *et al.*, *New Engl. J. Med.*, 1978, *299*, 1363.

Combined chemotherapy with cyclophosphamide 300 mg, vincristine 0.65 mg and fluorouracil 500 mg on day one and the same doses of cyclophosphamide and vincristine with methotrexate 37.5 mg on day 8 and repeated after a 3-week gap for 6 months was assessed in early breast cancer (stage II) after conventional primary treatment. At 3 months 2 of 117 control patients had recurrences compared with 0 of 114 treated patients; at 6 months corresponding figures were 6 of 102 and 3 of 97 and at 15 months 3 of 30 and 0 of 38.—Multicentre Breast Cancer Chemotherapy Group, *Lancet*, 1977, *2*, 396. Comment.— D. J. Leaper *et al.* (letter), *ibid.*, 660. At 30 months, recurrence rates were just under 50% in the control group and just over 30% in the treatment group. In view of the advantage of chemotherapy it was considered no longer ethical to continue with a no-chemotherapy control group and recruitment to this study was terminated. In the present study the 2-day chemotherapy regimen is being compared with a 1-day regimen involving vincristine, fluorouracil, methotrexate, and chlorambucil. A third stage of the study involves tamoxifen, patients being re-randomised after 6 months of chemotherapy to 6 months of tamoxifen or no further therapy.— G. A. Edelstyn *et al.* (letter), *ibid.*, 1978, *2*, 1092.

Adjuvant chemotherapy with cyclophosphamide, fluorouracil, and prednisone (CFP) with or without radiotherapy was more effective than melphalan in preventing recurrences of breast cancer in a study of 166 women who had undergone mastectomy. Premenopausal women achieved greater benefit. Chemotherapy was given every 6 weeks for 10 courses and doses were: cyclophosphamide 150 mg per m^2 body-surface, fluorouracil 300 mg per m^2 both given for 5 successive days by rapid intravenous infusion, prednisone 30 mg by mouth daily for 7 days, and melphalan 6 mg per m^2 by mouth daily for 5 days.— D. L. Ahmann *et al.*, *Lancet*, 1978, *1*, 893.

The preliminary announcement of a study to compare the benefits of adjuvant chemotherapy with a short course of cyclophosphamide or a long course of anti-oestrogen therapy in patients with early breast cancer.— *Lancet*, 1980, *2*, 602.

Retrospective findings in women with primary breast cancer given postoperative adjuvant chemotherapy with CMF, and those with advanced breast cancer treated similarly, indicate that benefit occurs only when full or nearly full doses are administered. The menopausal status of the patient did not appear to be an important prognostic factor. It is suggested that in future CMF should be given with intermittent intravenous cyclophosphamide to ensure an optimal peak concentration.— G. Bonadonna and P. Valagussa, *New Engl. J. Med.*, 1981, *304*, 10. See also A. Rossi *et al.*, *Br. med. J.*, 1981, *282*, 1427.

Addition of tamoxifen to chemotherapy for primary breast cancer.— B. Fisher *et al.*, *New Engl. J. Med.*, 1981, *305*, 1.

Further references to the adjuvant chemotherapy of breast cancer: B. Fisher *et al.*, *New Engl. J. Med.*, 1975, *292*, 117; D. L. Ahmann *et al.*, *New Engl. J. Med.*, 1977, *297*, 356; F. C. Sparks, *Ann. intern. Med.*, 1977, *86*, 74; R. Nissen-Meyer *et al.*, *Cancer*, 1978, *41*, 2088; A. M. Buzdar *et al.*, *J. Am. med. Ass.*, 1979, *242*, 1509; J. A. Caprini *et al.*, *J. Am. med. Ass.*, 1980, *244*, 243.

Hormonal therapy of breast cancer. Reviews: S. S. Legha *et al.*, *Ann. intern. Med.*, 1978, *88*, 69; B. A. Stoll, *Practitioner*, 1979, *222*, 211.

A controlled study of oestrogen use in postmenopausal patients with breast cancer.— R. K. Ross *et al.*, *J. Am. med. Ass.*, 1980, *243*, 1635. See also P. Meier and R. L. Landau, *ibid.*, 1658.

A report on the role of steroid receptors in breast cancer confirming that the presence of oestrogen receptors is generally predictive of a response to endocrine therapy and recommending that all primary tumours should be assayed for receptors. Since not all tumours containing oestrogen receptors respond to endocrine therapy, quantitative determinations of receptors present in tumour cytosol and the presence of progesterone receptors may enable a more accurate prediction of response to therapy to be made. After an assessment of conflicting results it was concluded that there is so far no clear evidence that response to antineoplastic agents correlates with the presence or absence of receptors.— *New Engl. J. Med.*, 1979, *301*, 1011 (Consensus Development Committee, National Institute of Health, USA). See also *Br. med. J.*, 1980, *281*, 694.

A retrospective study of 143 patients with advanced breast cancer confirmed that those with tumours rich in oestrogen receptors achieved a better response to hormonal therapy than those low in receptors. Contrary to the results reported by M.E. Lippman *et al.*, (*New Engl. J. Med.*, 1978, *298*, 1223), the response-rate to chemotherapy was also significantly higher in receptor-rich tumours; 24 of 28 patients with such tumours responded compared to only 13 of 36 with receptor-poor tumours.— D. T. Kiang *et al.*, *New Engl. J. Med.*, 1978, *299*, 1330.

Further references to oestrogen receptors and their significance in endocrine therapy for breast cancer: J. C. Heuson *et al.*, *Cancer*, 1977, *39*, 1971; D. T. Kiang and B. J. Kennedy, *J. Am. med. Ass.*, 1977, *238*, 32; S. G. Korenman, *Ann. intern. Med.*, 1977, *86*, 68; J. C. Allegra *et al.*, *Cancer Res.*, 1978, *38*, 4299; M. E. Lippman and J. C. Allegra, *New Engl. J. Med.*, 1978, *299*, 930; *J. Am. med. Ass.*, 1979, *242*, 1714 and 1716; J. A. Eisman *et al.*, *Lancet*, 1979, *2*, 1335 (a 1,25-dihydroxyvitamin D receptor in a cloned human breast cancer cell line); R. C. Coombes *et al.*, *Lancet*, 1980, *1*, 296; *ibid.*, 298.

See also under Sex Hormones, p.1401.

Malignant neoplasms of the male breast. A report of the treatment of 18 male patients with advanced breast cancer, using single- or multiple-drug regimens.— H. -Y. Yap *et al.*, *J. Am. med. Ass.*, 1980, *243*, 1739.

Tamoxifen treatment before orchiectomy in advanced breast cancer in men.— R. Becher *et al.* (letter), *New Engl. J. Med.*, 1981, *305*, 169.

Malignant neoplasms of the bronchus and lung. Lung cancer consists of a mixture of histological cell types. Squamous cell lesions are the most common and often remain localised although mortality is still high and they are relatively unresponsive to chemotherapy. Small cell anaplastic or oat cell carcinoma is usually widely disseminated at diagnosis and is relatively responsive to chemotherapy. Therapy is usually palliative but single antineoplastic agents have produced a reasonable response-rate against each cell type; significant improvement in survival times has not however been seen. Combination chemotherapy has only been superior to single agent therapy in small cell carcinomas; cyclophosphamide and lomustine, with or without methotrexate, have been used in various regimens. Studies combining alkylating agents with radiotherapy have given variable results; radiotherapy alone may benefit patients with limited disease. There is no evidence that adjuvant chemotherapy is beneficial following surgery.— Report of a WHO Expert Committee on Chemotherapy of Solid Tumours, *Tech. Rep. Ser. Wld Hlth Org. No 605*, 1977, p. 30.

A review on chemotherapy for lung cancer. Combination chemotherapy with mustine, vinblastine, procarbazine, and prednisolone (A.H. Laing *et al.*, *Lancet*, 1975, *1*, 129), as in Hodgkin's disease, was found to be inappropriate in small cell lung cancer and inferior to cyclophosphamide, doxorubicin, and methotrexate. The MRC's study (MRC Lung Cancer Working Party, *Br. J. Cancer*, 1979, *40*, 1) has shown beneficial results with these last 3 agents used together with vincristine and lomustine, chemotherapy being added to mediastinal radiotherapy. Other studies have found that chemotherapy alone is equal to or better than chemotherapy with radiotherapy. The brain is an important site of relapse and prophylactic cranial irradiation is being used, in association with chemotherapy and mediastinal irradiation, with beneficial results; F.A. Greco *et al.* (*Am. J. Med.*, 1979, *66*, 625) have reported a median survival of over 19 months. Optimal induction regimens are still awaited and may incorporate newer agents such as cisplatin, ifosfamide, etoposide, and hexamethylmelamine.— *Br. med. J.*, 1979, *2*, 815. The most frequently used combination chemotherapy regimen for small cell lung cancer is cyclophosphamide given in association with either doxorubicin and vincristine, or methotrexate and vincristine, or methotrexate and lomustine.— F. A. Greco and R. K. Oldham, *New Engl. J. Med.*, 1979, *301*, 355. See also *Lancet*, 1980, *1*, 77. Critical comments: G. M. Mead *et al.* (letter), *ibid.*, 252; R. K. Oldham and F. A. Greco (letter), *ibid.*, 478.

Further reviews on the chemotherapy of lung cancer: H. Stott *et al.*, *Br. J. Cancer*, 1976, *34*, 167 (adjuvant chemotherapy); *Br. med. J.*, 1977, *1*, 187 (adjuvant chemotherapy); P. A. Bunn *et al.*, *Cancer Treat. Rep.*, 1977, *61*, 333 (small cell carcinoma), per *Int. pharm. Abstr.*, 1977, *14*, 1096; H. H. Hansen, *Med. Clins N. Am.*, 1977, *61*, 979 (pleural mesothelioma), per S. S. Legha and F. M. Muggia, *Ann. intern. Med.*, 1977, *87*, 613; S. S. Legha *et al.*, *Cancer*, 1977, *39*, 1415 (adjuvant chemotherapy); E. D. Gilby, *Br. med. J.*, 1978, *1*, 1331; R. B. Weiss, *Ann. intern. Med.*, 1978, *88*, 522 (small cell carcinoma); K. H. Antman, *New Engl. J.*

Med., 1980, *303*, 200 (malignant mesothelioma).

The use of tumour-specific antibody with chemotherapy was considered to be beneficial, although not significantly so, in a study of 92 patients with bronchial carcinoma.— C. E. Newman *et al.*, *Lancet*, 1977, *2*, 163.

Combination chemotherapy with methotrexate 30 to 40 mg per m^2 body-surface, doxorubicin hydrochloride 30 to 40 mg per m^2, and cyclophosphamide 400 mg per m^2, all given intravenously, together with lomustine 30 mg per m^2 by mouth (MACC), all given on day 1 and repeated every 3 weeks, produced an overall objective response-rate of 52% in 83 patients with advanced lung cancer. Response-rates for the different histological types were: small cell anaplastic carcinoma, 87%; adenocarcinoma, 58%; squamous cell carcinoma, 36%; and large cell anaplastic carcinoma, 35%.— A. P. Chahinian *et al.*, *Cancer*, 1979, *43*, 1590.

Further studies of combination chemotherapy in advanced lung cancer: H. H. Hansen *et al.*, *Cancer*, 1976, *38*, 2201; M. J. Straus, *Cancer*, 1976, *38*, 2232; T. S. Herman *et al.*, *Cancer Treat. Rep.*, 1977, *61*, 875; S. Seeber *et al.*, *Dt. med. Wschr.*, 1977, *102*, 147; T. H. M. Stewart *et al.*, *Can. J. Surg.*, 1977, *20*, 370 (immunochemotherapy); J. D. Bitran *et al.*, *J. Am. med. Ass.*, 1978, *240*, 2743 (cyclophosphamide, doxorubicin, methotrexate, and procarbazine; CAMP; in non-small cell carcinoma); T. P. Butler *et al.*, *Cancer*, 1979, *43*, 1183; H. Takita *et al.*, *Cancer Treat. Rep.*, 1979, *63*, 29 (cisplatin, doxorubicin, cyclophosphamide, lomustine, and vincristine in non-small cell carcinoma).

Reports of beneficial results with various treatment schedules in patients with *small cell anaplastic carcinoma of the lung:* cyclophosphamide 250 to 500 mg per m^2 body-surface, doxorubicin 1 mg per kg body-weight, and vincristine 1 mg per m^2 all given intravenously on day 1, together with methotrexate 1 g by infusion followed by folinic acid rescue. Courses were repeated every 3 weeks.— J. G. W. Burdon *et al.*, *Med. J. Aust.*, 1978, *1*, 353. Cyclophosphamide 1 g per m^2, doxorubicin 40 mg per m^2, and vincristine 1 mg per m^2, given intravenously and repeated every 21 days for 6 cycles. Patients with limited disease were given prophylactic brain irradiation and most received monthly cycles of hexamethylmelamine and etoposide during remission.— F. A. Greco *et al.*, *Br. med. J.*, 1978, *2*, 10. A 4-week cycle of lomustine 70 mg per m^2 by mouth and cyclophosphamide 700 mg per m^2 intravenously on day 1, methotrexate 20 mg per m^2 by mouth on days 18 and 21, and vincristine 1.3 mg per m^2 intravenously weekly for the first cycle and on day 1 of ensuing cycles. There was a 78% objective response with this regimen and a 75% response when the regimen was given without vincristine.— H. H. Hansen *et al.*, *Ann. intern. Med.*, 1978, *89*, 177 and 726. Cyclophosphamide 750 mg per m^2, doxorubicin 50 mg per m^2, and vincristine 1 mg given intravenously on day 1. Doses of cyclophosphamide and doxorubicin were repeated 3 weeks later and then withdrawn until radiotherapy to the tumour and brain had been completed. Vincristine was given weekly for 12 weeks and cyclophosphamide and doxorubicin were then resumed and given every 3 weeks until a total dose of 450 mg per m^2 of doxorubicin had been given. Cyclophosphamide was continued at 1 g per m^2 every 4 weeks and methotrexate 30 mg per m^2 given 3 weeks after each dose of cyclophosphamide.— R. B. Livingston *et al*, *Ann. intern. Med.*, 1978, *88*, 194.

Further references to the chemotherapy of *small cell lung cancer:* L. H. Einhorn *et al.*, *J. Am. med. Ass.*, 1976, *235*, 1225 (doxorubicin, bleomycin, cyclophosphamide, and vincristine); R. C. Kane *et al.*, *J. Am. med. Ass.*, 1976, *235*, 1717 (lomustine, methotrexate, and cyclophosphamide in patients with vena caval obstruction); M. H. Cohen *et al.*, *Cancer Treat. Rep.*, 1977, *61*, 349; M. H. Cohen *et al.*, *Cancer Treat. Rep.*, 1977, *61*, 485 (vincristine, doxorubicin, and procarbazine); E. D. Gilby *et al.*, *Cancer*, 1977, *39*, 1959 (cyclophosphamide, vincristine, doxorubicin, methotrexate, and prednisolone; COPAM); P. Y. Holoye *et al.*, *J. Am. med. Ass.*, 1977, *237*, 1221 (cyclophosphamide, vincristine, and doxorubicin); L. Israel *et al.*, *Cancer Treat. Rep.*, 1977, *61*, 343 (immunochemotherapy); H. I. Saiontz *et al.*, 481 1977 (cyclophosphamide, doxorubicin, and dacarbazine).

Reports of combination chemotherapy in patients with squamous cell carcinoma of the lung: R. B. Livingston *et al.*, *Cancer*, 1976, *37*, 1237 (bleomycin, doxorubicin, lomustine, vincristine, and mustine; BACON); P. Pouillart *et al.* (letter), *Lancet*, 1976, *1*, 751 (doxorubicin, vincristine, lomustine, and fluorouracil); G. P. Bodey *et al.*, *Cancer*, 1977, *39*, 1026 (cyclophosphamide or cyclophosphamide, vincristine, semustine, and bleomycin; COMB); L. Hyde *et al.*, *Chest*, 1978, *73*, 603.

Malignant neoplasms of the cervix. Both radiotherapy and surgery are effective therapy for carcinoma of the cervix. Chemotherapy has usually been limited to short palliative courses of a single antineoplastic agent in patients with recurrences following extensive radiotherapy, although following other forms of treatment makes chemotherapy difficult. Cyclophosphamide, fluorouracil, and methotrexate are all active and bleomycin, doxorubicin, hexamethylmelamine, and vincristine have some activity. These agents have been used in several combination regimens with no apparent advantage so far.— Report of a WHO Expert Committee on Chemotherapy of Solid Tumours, *Tech. Rep. Ser. Wld Hlth Org. No. 605*, 1977, p. 43.

Complete remission of disease was obtained in 12 of 15 patients with squamous cell type of metastatic cervical carcinoma and partial remission in 2 after treatment with bleomycin 5 mg daily for one week and an injection of mitomycin 10 mg once a week, both on alternate weeks for 2 to 5 courses. Four of the complete responders had recurrence after 4.5 months, and 3 subsequently died; this was attributed to either an inadequate number of courses for initial treatment or lack of further therapy.— T. Miyamoto *et al.*, *Cancer*, 1978, *41*, 403.

Further references to the chemotherapy of cervical cancer: J. F. Conroy *et al.*, *Cancer*, 1976, *37*, 660 (bleomycin with methotrexate); M. Haid *et al.*, *Obstet. Gynec.*, 1977, *50*, 103 (doxorubicin with methotrexate); T. G. Day *et al.*, *Am. J. Obstet. Gynec.*, 1978, *132*, 545 (doxorubicin with semustine).

Malignant neoplasms of the endometrium. The majority of patients with localised endometrial carcinoma are treated by surgery or radiotherapy with a 75% cure-rate in favourable cases. Chemotherapy has mainly been used in the management of invasive adenocarcinoma of the endometrium. Progestational agents are generally given and achieve a regression-rate of about 30% in advanced disease. Experience with antineoplastic agents is meagre but a response-rate of 23% has been reported with fluorouracil. Responses have also been achieved with cyclophosphamide or doxorubicin but not with chlorambucil.— Report of a WHO Expert Committee on Chemotherapy of Solid Tumours, *Tech. Rep. Ser. Wld Hlth Org. No. 605*, 1977, p. 45. In patients with endometrial cancer whose aortic lymph nodes are involved a treatment regimen including cyclophosphamide, doxorubicin, fluorouracil, and megestrol acetate has been found useful.— S. B. Gusberg, *New Engl. J. Med.*, 1980, *302*, 729.

Of 8 patients with advanced metastatic endometrial adenocarcinoma 3 achieved complete remissions (lasting 4.5, 10, and more than 12 months) and 2 achieved partial remissions after treatment with cyclophosphamide 500 mg per m^2 body-surface in association with doxorubicin 37.5 mg per m^2 intravenously every 3 weeks; 12 or more courses had been given.— F. M. Muggia *et al.*, *Am. J. Obstet. Gynec.*, 1977, *128*, 314.

Further references to the chemotherapy of advanced endometrial adenocarcinomas: H. W. Bruckner and G. Deppe, *Obstet. Gynec.*, 1977, *50*, *Suppl.* 1, 10S (doxorubicin, cyclophosphamide, fluorouracil, and medroxyprogesterone acetate).

See also under Sex Hormones, p.1401.

Malignant neoplasms of the eye. See Retinoblastoma (below).

Malignant neoplasms of the gastro-intestinal tract. The major sites of cancer in the gastro-intestinal tract are the stomach, colon, rectum, and oesophagus in decreasing order of incidence. Fluorouracil and mitomycin are commonly used to treat gastric cancer and carmustine, the other nitrosoureas, and doxorubicin have shown activity. Combination chemotherapy regimens used have included mitomycin, fluorouracil, and cytarabine (MFC); fluorouracil and carmustine or semustine; and mitomycin with fluorouracil given by mouth or tegafur given by mouth or by rectum. So far there is no evidence that adjuvant chemotherapy following surgery should be used routinely. Fluorouracil is the standard treatment for advanced colorectal cancer; mitomycin and the nitrosoureas have also been used. Combinations of these agents have not generally proved beneficial. Bleomycin is the only agent with any marked activity in cancer of the oesophagus; response-rates of about 30% have been reported but the duration of response is extremely short.— Report of a WHO Expert Committee on Chemotherapy of Solid Tumours, *Tech. Rep. Ser. Wld Hlth Org. No. 605*, 1977, p. 32. See also J. M. Heal and P. S. Schein, *Med. Clins N. Am.*, 1977, *61*, 991; C. G. Moertel, *New Engl. J. Med.*, 1978, *299*, 1049; T. J. Priestman, *J.R. Soc. Med.*, 1978, *71*, 195; G. R. Giles and J. de Mello, *Br. J. Hosp. Med.*, 1981, *25*, 15.

The 5-year survival-rate for gastric carcinoma is only 5 to 15%. Combination chemotherapy with fluorouracil and a nitrosourea has been tried in advanced disease in an attempt to improve response-rates and slightly more encouraging results have been achieved with regimens containing doxorubicin. J.A. Levi *et al.*(*Br. med. J.*, 1979, *2*, 1471) reported complete remission in 2 and partial remission in 16 of 35 patients treated cyclically with fluorouracil, doxorubicin, and carmustine. Partial remissions were achieved by 26 of 62 similar patients given fluorouracil, doxorubicin, and mitomycin (FAM) intravenously in 8-week cycles of fluorouracil 600 mg per m^2 body-surface on days 1, 8, 29, and 36; doxorubicin 30 mg per m^2 on days 1 and 29; and mitomycin 10 mg per m^2 on day 1 (J.S. Macdonald *et al.*, *Ann. intern. Med.*, 1980, *93*, 533). In both studies median survival in responders was increased by about 8 months when compared with non-responders.— *Lancet*, 1980, *2*, 1174. Comment.— R. J. Keehn and G. A. Higgins (letter), *ibid.*, 1981, *1*, 323. See also S. K. Carter and R. L. Comis, *J. natn. Cancer Inst.*, 1977, *58*, 567.

There is at present no effective drug against cancer of the large bowel although several agents have some activity. Fluorouracil and semustine are the most active and mitomycin, razoxane, cyclophosphamide, and methotrexate are decreasingly effective; the vinca alkaloids have no appreciable activity when used alone. Combination regimens have not been shown to extend survival.— R. J. Nicholls, *Br. J. Hosp. Med.*, 1980, *24*, 309. See also *Br. med. J.*, 1976, *2*, 342.

Further references to the chemotherapy of gastro-intestinal cancer: T. Buroker *et al.*, *Cancer Treat. Rep.*, 1977, *61*, 463 (tegafur with mitomycin or semustine); W. Queisser *et al.*, *Dt. med. Wschr.*, 1979, *104*, 1231 (carmustine with fluorouracil or tegafur).

Further references to the chemotherapy of gastric cancer: J. L. Franz and A. B. Cruz, *J. surg. Oncol.*, 1977, *9*, 131 (adjuvant chemotherapy); R. D. Kingston *et al.*, *Clin. Oncol.*, 1978, *4*, 55 (fluorouracil and semustine); M. O. Rake *et al.*, *Gut*, 1979, *20*, 797 (vincristine, methotrexate, cyclophosphamide, fluorouracil, and mitomycin).

Further references to the chemotherapy of colorectal cancer: A. A. Epenetos *et al.*, *Br. med. J.*, 1980, *281*, 587 (lack of effect with semustine and fluorouracil with vincristine or mitomycin).

Further references to the chemotherapy of oesophageal cancer: A. Y. Rostom *et al.* (letter), *Lancet*, 1980, *2*, 912 (methotrexate, bleomycin, fluorouracil, and vincristine); R. B. Buchanan and R. E. Lea (letter), *ibid.*, 1134 (vincristine, bleomycin, and methotrexate).

Malignant neoplasms of the head and neck. Tumours of the head and neck are a heterogeneous group of lesions involving the upper digestive tract and air passages, the majority being squamous cell carcinomas of the oral cavity, pharynx, larynx, and sinuses. Methotrexate has been the drug studied most extensively and an overall response-rate of 40% has been reported. The response-rate with bleomycin is only 30% but its relative lack of toxicity to bone marrow makes it a candidate for use with other agents. Cyclophosphamide, fluorouracil, hydroxyurea, doxorubicin, and mitolactol also have some activity and many combination regimens are being investigated. Administration by intra-arterial infusion appears to offer no advantage over the systemic route. The role of chemotherapy in association with radiotherapy and/or surgery has not yet been evaluated.— Report of a WHO Expert Committee on Chemotherapy of Solid Tumours, *Tech. Rep. Ser. Wld Hlth Org. No. 605*, 1977, p. 54.

Further references to the chemotherapy of tumours of the head and neck: L. A. Price *et al.*, *Br. med. J.*, 1975, *3*, 10 (vincristine, doxorubicin, bleomycin, methotrexate, fluorouracil, hydroxyurea, and mercaptopurine); H. R. Grant, *J. Lar. Otol.*, 1976, *90*, 433; G. Stathopoulos *et al.*, *Br. J. clin. Pract.*, 1976, *30*, 188 (bleomycin, cyclophosphamide, methotrexate, and fluorouracil injected intravenously every 2 to 4 weeks); A. Biörklund *et al.*, *J. Lar. Otol.*, 1979, *93*, 1105; P. Clifford, *J. Lar. Otol.*, 1979, *93*, 1151; A. D. O'Connor *et al.*, *Clin. Otolaryngol.*, 1979, *4*, 329 (vincristine, bleomycin, and methotrexate in association with radiotherapy); W. K. Hong *et al.*, *Cancer*, 1979, *44*, 19 (cisplatin and bleomycin); R. L. Woods *et al.*, *Br. med. J.*, 1981, *282*, 600 (high-dose methotrexate).

For reference to the possible antineoplastic activity of tetracyclines in tumours of the head and neck, see Tetracycline Hydrochloride, p.1221.

Malignant neoplasms of the kidney. See Wilms' Tumour (below), and under Sex Hormones, p.1401.

Malignant neoplasms of the liver. The 5-year survival-rate for liver cell carcinoma is generally quite poor and radiotherapy is not an effective palliative. Fluorouracil, sometimes in association with carmustine, has been used and doxorubicin is also reported to be active.— Report of a WHO Expert Committee on Chemotherapy of

Solid Tumours, *Tech. Rep. Ser. Wld Hlth Org. No. 605,* 1977, p. 39.

Quadruple chemotherapy alone using fluorouracil, cyclophosphamide, methotrexate, and vincristine was more effective than radiotherapy followed by the same chemotherapy in a study of 18 patients with hepatocellular carcinoma.— A. M. G. Cochrane *et al., Cancer,* 1977, *40,* 609.

The palliative role of hepatic arterial infusion and arterial occlusion in colorectal carcinoma metastatic to the liver.— Y. Z. Patt *et al., Lancet,* 1981, *1,* 349.

Malignant neoplasms of the nerves. Combined therapy with cyclophosphamide, vincristine, doxorubicin, and dacarbazine (cyVADIC) produced complete remissions in 2 patients with metastic malignant schwannoma.— R. L. Goldman *et al., Cancer,* 1977, *39,* 1955.

See also under Neuroblastoma (below).

Malignant neoplasms of the ovary. Ovarian cancer spreads early beyond the primary site and most patients need systemic therapy. Remissions have been achieved in about one third of patients with various alkylating agents including chlorambucil, thiotepa, cyclophosphamide, or melphalan. The choice of alkylating agent is determined mainly by convenience and side-effects; intraperitoneal administration has no proven advantage. Median survival is reported to be only 17 to 22 months in responders compared with 6 to 13 months in non-responders. Similar response-rates have been seen with other antineoplastic agents such as fluorouracil, methotrexate, hexamethylmelamine, doxorubicin, ifosfamide, and cisplatin, but toxicity is generally more severe. Combination chemotherapy has not greatly improved on remission-rates or survival times. Objective remissions have been reported in about one third of patients with advanced ovarian cancer after a course of progestogen. Oestrogen and progesterone receptors are said to be present in 40 to 50% of ovarian cancers and may help to predict those tumours susceptible to endocrine therapy. Patients generally relapse quickly when maintenance therapy is stopped. Plasma concentrations of CEA (carcinoembryonic antigen), in mucinous cystadenocarcinoma, or alpha-fetoprotein, in some types of germ-cell tumour, may be useful as indicators of tumour burden.— *Lancet,* 1980, *2,* 1010.

Further reviews on the treatment of ovarian cancer: Report of a WHO Expert Committee on Chemotherapy of Solid Tumours, *Tech. Rep. Ser. Wld Hlth Org. No. 605,* 1977, p. 40; C. N. Hudson, *Br. J. Hosp. Med.,* 1978, *20,* 568; H. J. Solomon, *Med. J. Aust.,* 1978, *2,* 241; *Br. med. J.,* 1979, *1,* 1034; *Br. med. J.,* 1979, *2,* 687.

Confirmation of the value of estimations of human chorionic gonadotrophin and alpha-fetoprotein in monitoring the treatment of ovarian teratomas.— E. S. Newlands *et al.* (letter), *Br. med. J.,* 1979, *1,* 1213. A very accurate *in vitro* clonogenic assay for predicting response of ovarian cancer to chemotherapy.— D. S. Alberts *et al., Lancet,* 1980, *2,* 340.

In a prospective randomised study of patients with advanced ovarian adenocarcinoma, 39 were given melphalan 200 µg per kg body-weight by mouth daily for 5 days and the course repeated every 4 to 5 weeks depending on bone-marrow recovery. A further 41 patients received combination chemotherapy, each cycle consisting of fluorouracil 600 mg per m^2 body-surface and methotrexate 40 mg per m^2 both given intravenously on days 1 and 8, cyclophosphamide and hexamethylmelamine both given at 150 mg per m^2 by mouth from day 1 to 14, followed by 2 treatment-free weeks. This intermittent treatment was continued in all patients for 6 months when they were re-assessed and additional cycles of treatment given to those with residual disease. Of those studied for longer than 7 months, 30 of 40 patients on combination chemotherapy responded to treatment and 13 had complete remission. This response-rate was significantly greater than that of the melphalan group in which only 20 of 37 patients responded and 6 had complete remissions. Survival-rate was also significantly better in the combination chemotherapy group with an overall median survival of 29 months compared with 17 months for those given melphalan. Side-effects were more frequent in the group given combination chemotherapy.— R. C. Young *et al., New Engl. J. Med.,* 1978, *299,* 1261.

Further references to the use of chemotherapy in ovarian cancer: A. Kessinger *et al., Obstet. Gynec.,* 1976, *48,* 134; P. E. Schwartz and J. P. Smith, *Am. J. Obstet. Gynec.,* 1976, *125,* 402; G. M. De Palo *et al., Cancer Treat. Rep.,* 1977, *61,* 355 (doxorubicin with or without melphalan); F. Cavalli *et al., Dt. med. Wschr.,* 1978, *103,* 927 (doxorubicin and cisplatin); S. L. Curry *et al., Am. J. Obstet. Gynec.,* 1978, *131,* 845; S. B. Lele *et al., Obstet. Gynec.,* 1978, *51,* 101; W. T. Creasman *et al., Obstet. Gynec.,* 1979, *53,* 226; S. E. Vogl *et al., J. Am. med. Ass.,* 1979, *241,* 1908 (hexamethylmelamine and cisplatin, with or without doxorubicin); G. H. Barker and E. Wiltshaw, *Lancet,* 1981, *1,* 747 (cisplatin and chlorambucil, with or without doxorubicin).

See also under Treosulfan, p.229.

Malignant neoplasms of the pancreas. Surgery offers the only possibility of cure in adenocarcinoma of the pancreas and although chemotherapy has had a palliative effect in some patients in general it has not been successful. Fluorouracil has a reported overall response-rate of 38% which is probably an overestimate and similar results have been achieved with mitomycin. About half of patients with islet cell carcinoma of the pancreas have responded to streptozocin. Survival gains with fluorouracil in association with carmustine have not been significant but beneficial results have been achieved with fluorouracil in association with radiotherapy when compared with radiotherapy alone.— Report of a WHO Expert Committee on Chemotherapy of Solid Tumours, *Tech. Rep. Ser. Wld Hlth Org. No. 605,* 1977, p. 36. See also G. R. Giles and J. de Mello, *Br. J. Hosp. Med.,* 1981, *25,* 15.

Further references to the use of chemotherapy in pancreatic carcinoma: C. G. Moertel *et al., Cancer Treat. Rep.,* 1976, *60,* 1659 (semustine); P. S. Schein *et al., Cancer,* 1978, *42,* 19 (doxorubicin, methotrexate, and actinomycin D); R. L. Stephens *et al., Archs intern. Med.,* 1978, *138,* 115 (carmustine and fluorouracil, with or without spironolactone); C. N. Mallinson *et al., Br. med. J.,* 1980, *281,* 1589 (cyclophosphamide, fluorouracil, vincristine, and methotrexate followed by fluorouracil and mitomycin); K. Reynolds and T. Allen-Mersh (letter), *Br. med. J.,* 1981, *282,* 142 (fluorouracil, doxorubicin, chlorambucil, and mitomycin).

Malignant neoplasms of the prostate. The treatment of prostatic adenocarcinoma at each stage of the disease, from local tumour to extensive bony metastases, is still controversial. It includes local therapy with surgery and radiotherapy and systemic treatment using hormone manipulation with oestrogens, anti-androgens, orchidectomy, adrenalectomy, and hypophysectomy, or chemotherapy with antineoplastic agents. There have been a number of studies in hormone-resistant patients using single antineoplastic agents and combination regimens. Of the agents tested cyclophosphamide has been studied most extensively; it is superior to secondary hormonal manoeuvres once orchidectomy or oestrogens have failed and is slightly more active than fluorouracil. Doxorubicin has an objective response-rate of about 25% and dacarbazine appears promising. Estramustine has been used in patients previously given extensive radiotherapy. Cisplatin may prove to be the most active single agent. Combination chemotherapy has not shown definite superiority over single agent so far. The use of acid phosphatase as a tumour marker has been of limited prognostic value but may be improved by new methods of assay.— F. M. Torti and S. K. Carter, *Ann. intern. Med.,* 1980, *92,* 681. The measurement of androgen receptors in prostatic tissue may help predict therapeutic response in prostatic carcinoma.— L. A. Klein, *New Engl. J. Med.,* 1979, *300,* 824. Further reviews: *Br. med. J.,* 1977, *2,* 781; *ibid.,* 1979, *2,* 752; J. G. Smart, *Practitioner,* 1979, *223,* 312; *Br. med. J.,* 1980, *280,* 883.

A report of beneficial results in 5 patients with carcinoma of the prostate given combination chemotherapy with fluorouracil, cyclophosphamide, vincristine, methotrexate, and prednisone. After induction of remission, maintenance therapy was continued with prednisone, stilboestrol, and cyclophosphamide.— M. Petersen and J. D. Taylor (letter), *Med. J. Aust.,* 1978, *1,* 340.

Further references: D. P. Ewing and W. Woods (letter), *Med. J. Aust.,* 1978, *2,* 32.

See also under Sex Hormones, p.1401.

Malignant neoplasms of the skin. The most common skin cancers are basal cell carcinomas and squamous cell carcinomas and topical treatment with fluorouracil is used. Bleomycin has also been given systemically. Kaposi's sarcoma is predominantly a cutaneous tumour but may involve many other tissues. It is responsive to chemotherapy and has been treated with actinomycin D, alone or with vincristine; dacarbazine has also been used.— Report of a WHO Expert Committee on Chemotherapy of Solid Tumours, *Tech. Rep. Ser. Wld Hlth Org. No. 605,* 1977, p. 57.

See also under Melanoma (below).

Malignant neoplasms of the testis. Testicular tumours vary in their response to treatment; seminomas are particularly responsive to radiotherapy while embryonal carcinomas and teratomas are more responsive to chemotherapy. Antineoplastic agents have been used in the treatment of primary tumours and metastatic disease and in adjuvant chemotherapy at all stages. Testicular tumours are responsive to a wide range of agents including vinblastine (52%), actinomycin D (52%), bleomycin (42%), melphalan (57%), doxorubicin (20%), cisplatin, and mithramycin. Combination therapy with bleomycin and vinblastine led to overall response-rates of nearly 100% and prolonged remissions. The addition of other agents, such as cisplatin has produced very high response-rates but the schedules are highly toxic.— Report of a WHO Expert Committee on Chemotherapy of Solid Tumours, *Tech. Rep. Ser. Wld Hlth Org. No. 605,* 1977, p. 51. Improvements in the management of teratomas are due to better staging of the disease, the introduction of tumour markers (alpha-fetoprotein and beta subunit human chorionic gonadotrophin), and the use of highly active combination chemotherapy, with or without surgery, for patients with bulky or metastatic disease. Complete remission has been achieved with chemotherapy in 75% of patients with extensive disease.— *Br. med. J.,* 1979, *1,* 840. A review on combination chemotherapy regimens for testicular tumours. Bleomycin, vinblastine, and cisplatin form the basis of a number of regimens including those in which actinomycin D (VAB II), actinomycin D and cyclophosphamide (VAB III), or actinomycin D, cyclophosphamide, and doxorubicin (VAB IV) have been added.— R. Anderson *et al., Ann. intern. Med.,* 1979, *90,* 373. See also E. E. Fraley *et al., New Engl. J. Med.,* 1979, *301,* 1420; G. Morgan and A. Freedman, *Med. J. Aust.,* 1979, *1,* 122; *Lancet,* 1980, *2,* 1175.

Of 40 patients with disseminated testicular non-seminoma treated with a regimen comprising cisplatin, vinblastine, and bleomycin, 24 obtained complete remission, 11 achieved partial remission, 3 died of toxicity (agranulocytic sepsis, myocardial infarction, and lung fibrosis), and 2 did not respond. Of the patients who achieved complete remission 22 have maintained this for 5 to 30 months. In view of the small numbers of patients with this often curable condition and the relatively high proportion of severe complications they should be treated in centres specialised in the complicated management required. The regimen used was as follows: after prehydration with a litre of saline, cisplatin 20 mg per m^2 body-surface in 300 ml of mannitol 15% was infused over 2 hours for 5 consecutive days, 3 to 4 cycles being given, with the next cycle starting on day 22 of the previous cycle; during each treatment cycle, diuresis was maintained by at least 4 litres of saline per 24 hours; vinblastine 200 µg per kg body-weight daily was given as an intravenous bolus on days 1 and 2; bleomycin 30 units intravenously was given as a 15-minute infusion 6 hours after the vinblastine on day 2 of each cycle, and also at weekly intervals between cycles until a total dose of 360 units had been given; after the remission-induction chemotherapy complete responders were maintained on vinblastine 300 µg per kg body-weight intravenously, alternating with vinblastine 200 µg per kg intravenously plus cisplatin 50 mg per m^2 body-surface at 3-week intervals for 2 years. In addition to the toxic effects from which 3 patients died the following were noted: inability to taste, possibly due to zinc deficiency (7 patients), foul taste (9 patients), body odour (7 patients), transient hoarseness (3 patients); all patients suffered nausea and vomiting which seems to respond to metoclopramide; clinical neurotoxicity occurred in 27 patients but it was uncertain whether this was related to vinblastine or cisplatin; 2 patients became allergic to cisplatin during maintenance therapy.— G. Stoter *et al., lancet,* 1979, *1,* 941.

Confirmation that metastatic teratoma of the testis may be curable. A chemotherapeutic regimen has been used which includes cisplatin together with lower doses of vinblastine and bleomycin than those used by M.L. Samuels *et al.* (*Cancer,* 1975, *36,* 318) which are considered unacceptably toxic. This has been given to 27 patients and complete remission was achieved in 18 for at least 3 months; 13 had remained alive and disease-free for a median of 8 months. The regimen consists of vinblastine 6 mg per m^2 body-surface intravenously on days 1 and 2, bleomycin 10 mg per m^2 intramuscularly every 12 hours on days 2 to 4, and cisplatin 15 mg per m^2 intravenously in 500 ml of saline daily on days 2 to 6, the patient drinking 2 litres of fluid before the infusion. The courses are repeated monthly to a maximum of 4 courses and followed by irradiation. Six courses of maintenance chemotherapy are then given consisting of vinblastine 6 mg per m^2, actinomycin D 1.2 mg per m^2, and methotrexate 50 mg per m^2 given as a single intravenous push in the out-patient clinic.— P. Wilkinson *et al.* (letter), *Lancet,* 1979, *1,* 1185.

Preliminary results of an approach to the management of malignant teratoma of the testis involving the use of radiotherapy to manage early-stage disease, with chemotherapy on relapse only, or in patients with advanced disease. All of 28 men with early-stage disease treated between January 1976 and March 1978 were alive and disease-free. Three of 56 patients with advanced-stage disease given chemotherapy with vinblastine and bleomycin died of complications attributable to chemotherapy. Chemotherapy should be avoided in patients for whom the prognosis is good, and in advanced disease should be used by clinicians experienced in managing the attendant iatrogenic problems. In the chemotherapy group those with limited lung disease did well whereas those with bulky lung metastases did poorly.— M. J. Peckham *et al.*, *Lancet*, 1979, *2*, 267.

Further references to the use of chemotherapy in the treatment of testicular tumours: L. H. Einhorn and J. Donohue, *Ann. intern. Med.*, 1977, *87*, 293 (cisplatin, vinblastine, bleomycin, with BCG therapy); O. Klepp *et al.*, *Cancer*, 1977, *40*, 638 (vincristine, doxorubicin, cyclophosphamide, actinomycin D, medroxyprogesterone acetate; VACAM); L. H. Einhorn, *Cancer Treat. Rep.*, 1979, *63*, 1659 (cisplatin, bleomycin, vinblastine, with or without doxorubicin); G. J. Bosl *et al.*, *Am. J. Med.*, 1980, *68*, 492 (vinblastine, bleomycin, cisplatin); L. H. Einhorn *et al.*, *New Engl. J. Med.*, 1981, *305*, 727 (role of maintenance therapy); N. J. Vogelzang *et al.*, *Ann. intern. Med.*, 1981, *95*, 288 (Raynaud's phenomenon as an adverse effect of chemotherapy).

Malignant neoplasms of the thyroid. Iodine-131 is the mainstay of treatment following thyroidectomy in thyroid cancer and doxorubicin and cyclophosphamide are the only drugs known to produce occasional regressions.— Report of a WHO Expert Committee on Chemotherapy of Solid Tumours, *Tech. Rep. Ser. Wld Hlth Org. No. 605*, 1977, p. 57.

Nine of 14 patients with advanced anaplastic thyroid carcinoma unresponsive to surgery, external radiotherapy, and radioactive iodine derived some benefit from chemotherapy with doxorubicin, vincristine, and bleomycin (ABC). After some modification the regimen given to 8 patients was: doxorubicin 60 mg per m^2 body-surface in association with vincristine 2 mg, both given intravenously, followed 4 to 6 hours later by 30 mg of bleomycin given intramuscularly, the cycle being repeated every 3 to 4 weeks.— M. Sokal and C. L. Harmer, *Clin. Oncol.*, 1978, *4*, 3.

Melanoma. Surgery is usually curative in superficial melanoma but of all cancers originating in the skin, it has the greatest potential for dissemination with a propensity to metastasise to the brain. Chemotherapy is used in advanced disease. Dacarbazine is the agent most extensively studied in malignant melanoma and an overall remission-rate of 5% has been consistently observed. The nitrosoureas have also been used and semustine appears to be as effective as dacarbazine. Antimetabolites have been consistently inactive; actinomycin D may have some activity. Melphalan is widely used for isolated perfusion but the alkylating agents are not very active when given systemically. Initial high response-rates reported with hydroxyurea have not been substantiated. Vincristine has low activity but has been used widely in combination regimens. A variety of regimens has been tested but none can definitely be recommended. Immunotherapy is also being tried.— Report of a WHO Expert Committee on Chemotherapy of Solid Tumours, *Tech. Rep. Ser. Wld Hlth Org. No. 605*, 1977, p. 59. Vindesine has achieved objective response-rates in advanced malignant melanoma similar to those seen with dacarbazine and is far better tolerated. Beneficial results are possible with dexamethasone, cranial irradiation, and combination chemotherapy including lomustine in patients with cerebral metastases.— S. Retsas, *Practitioner*, 1980, *224*, 1019. See also J. D. Everall and P. M. Dowd, *Lancet*, 1977, *2*, 286; J. L. Lichtenfeld, *Med. Clins N. Am.*, 1977, *61*, 1013; G. W. Milton, *Med. J. Aust.*, 1978, *1*, 17.

A brief review of the status of immunotherapy of melanoma and other cancers.— W. D. Terry, *New Engl. J. Med.*, 1980, *303*, 1174. There was an extension in expected median survival in 6 patients with malignant melanoma treated with antineoplastic chemotherapy together with tumour-directed anti-melanoma immunoglobulin prepared for each patient. In one of the 6 the immunoglobulin was linked covalently to melphalan to provide a stable antibody-drug complex or conjugate. Three of 4 patients with mycosis fungoides responded beneficially to similar treatment. Treatment was withdrawn in the fourth because of a temporary fall in blood pressure. There were no other adverse effects from the immunoglobulin which was given in total doses of up to about 6 g for periods of several months.— J. D. Everall *et al.* (letter), *Lancet*, 1977, *1*, 1105.

Results from combination chemotherapy for malignant melanoma were no better than results from dacarbazine alone.— E. M. McKelvey *et al.*, *Cancer*, 1977, *39*, 1 and 5.

Further references to the treatment of malignant melanoma: S. M. Cohen *et al.*, *Cancer*, 1972, *29*, 1489 (carmustine, dacarbazine, and vincristine); M. E. Costanza *et al.*, *Cancer*, 1972, *30*, 1457 (dacarbazine with or without carmustine); E. T. Krementz and R. F. Ryan, *Ann. Surg.*, 1972, *175*, 900 (regional perfusion); J. U. Gutterman *et al.*, *New Engl. J. Med.*, 1974, *291*, 592 (dacarbazine with or without BCG vaccine); M. J. Byrne, *Cancer*, 1976, *38*, 1922 (cyclophosphamide and vincristine with or without procarbazine); G. De Wasch *et al.*, *Cancer Treat. Rep.*, 1976, *60*, 1273 (lomustine, vincristine, and bleomycin); L. H. Einhorn and B. Furnas, *Cancer Treat. Rep.*, 1977, *61*, 881 (dacarbazine, vincristine, and semustine); T. Ghose *et al.*, *J. natn. Cancer Inst.*, 1977, *58*, 845 (immunochemotherapy with chlorambucil-bound antimelanoma globulins); W. C. Wood *et al.*, *Surgery, St Louis*, 1978, *83*, 677 (adjuvant therapy with dacarbazine and BCG vaccine); *Am. Pharm.*, 1978, *NS18* (Jan.), 32 (dacarbazine, actinomycin D, and *Corynebacterium parvum* vaccine).

Mesothelioma. Discussions on malignant mesothelioma and its treatment.— S. S. Legha and F. M. Muggia, *Ann. intern. Med.*, 1977, *87*, 613; K. H. Antman, *New Engl. J. Med.*, 1980, *303*, 200.

See also under Sarcoma (below).

Mycosis fungoides. A brief report on treatment protocols for mycosis fungoides from the Dutch Mycosis Fungoides Study Group. Topical application of mustine is one of the alternatives in early stages of the disease. In more advanced stages combination chemotherapy with cyclophosphamide, vincristine, and prednisone (COP) or with mustine, vincristine, procarbazine, and prednisone (MOPP) is used, often in association with topical treatment.— L. Hamminga and W. A. van Vloten, *Br. J. Derm.*, 1980, *102*, 477.

Myeloma. Standard treatment for myeloma has been melphalan given by mouth, either continuously or intermittently with prednisone. Objective responses have been produced in 40 to 50% of patients, with a median survival for all patients of about 2 years. Better understanding of the disease and prognostic factors has resulted in an improved response to treatment. In addition to melphalan and prednisone other antineoplastic agents have been used singly and in combination for the treatment of myeloma. D.C. Case *et al.* (*Am. J. Med.*, 1977, *63*, 897) have reported improved survival with vincristine, carmustine, cyclophosphamide, melphalan, and prednisone (M-2 protocol). The Southwest Oncology Group (R. Alexanian *et al.*, *Cancer*, 1977, *40*, 2765) have also reported an improved response to combinations of vincristine with alkylating agents and prednisone, with or without doxorubicin. Encouraging results have been achieved with melphalan given intravenously, compared with the oral route (O.R. McIntyre *et al.*, *Blood*, 1978, *52, Suppl.* 1, 274). About 60% of patients now receiving treatment with various combination regimens will achieve an estimated 75% or greater reduction in myeloma cell burden. Acute monomyelogenous leukaemia may occur in 2 to 6% of patients, usually after prolonged treatment and R. Alexanian *et al.*(*Blood*, 1978, *51*, 1005) have suggested that all treatment should be stopped after 12 months, if a 75% or greater reduction in tumour cell mass has occurred.— O. R. McIntyre, *New Engl. J. Med.*, 1979, *301*, 193.

In a study of 364 patients with plasma cell myeloma, response-rate and survival were no better with a treatment regimen of melphalan, cyclophosphamide, and carmustine given concurrently or alternately, together with prednisone, than with melphalan and prednisone taken alone. Acute leukaemia developed in 14 patients with no significant difference between treatment groups; the incidence was greater than expected for all age groups and the risk of developing leukaemia had increased rapidly to 17.4% at 50 months.— D. E. Bergsagel *et al.*, *New Engl. J. Med.*, 1979, *301*, 743. With the M-2 protocol [melphalan, cyclophosphamide, carmustine, prednisone, and vincristine] median survival was 50 months compared with the 24 months achieved by D.E. Bergsagel *et al.*— D. C. Case (letter), *ibid.*, 1980, *302*, 407.

R. Alexanian *et al.* (*Blood*, 1978, *51*, 1005) have identified groups of patients most likely to remain stable when therapy for myeloma is withdrawn. The present study demonstrated that 56 of 127 patients with multiple myeloma entered a stable plateau phase which seems to be an indolent state when cells resistant to initial induction are essentially dormant and one would predict that intensive therapy during this period would not be especially fruitful. These findings provide the basis for a more rational approach to intensive initial induction therapy and the type and duration of maintenance therapy.— B. G. M. Durie *et al.*, *Lancet*, 1980, *2*, 65.

Further references to the treatment of myeloma: S. L. Rivers and M. E. Patno, *J. Am. med. Ass.*, 1969, *207*, 1328 (cyclophosphamide or melphalan); R. Alexanian *et al.*, *Cancer*, 1972, *30*, 382 (melphalan, procarbazine, and prednisone); D. E. Bergsagel *et al.*, *Can. med. Ass. J.*, 1972, *107*, 851 (cyclophosphamide in patients resistant to melphalan); R. P. George *et al.*, *Cancer*, 1972, *29*, 1597 (intermittent combination chemotherapy); L. Azam and I. W. Delamore, *Br. med. J.*, 1974, *4*, 560 (carmustine, melphalan, cyclophosphamide, prednisolone); D. S. Alberts *et al.*, *Cancer Treat. Rep.*, 1977, *61*, 381; *Br. med. J.*, 1978, *1*, 1653; J. S. Malpas and D. Parker (letter), *Br. med. J.*, 1978, *2*, 563 (a view that drugs other than melphalan, cyclophosphamide, and prednisolone should not yet be used routinely for myeloma).

Neuroblastoma. Neuroblastoma is the most common extracranial malignancy in infants and children. Active antineoplastic agents include cyclophosphamide, doxorubicin, dacarbazine, and vincristine. Combination chemotherapy with cyclophosphamide and vincristine gives a response-rate of about 50% in advanced disease; the remissions are relatively short-lived.— Report of a WHO Expert Committee on Chemotherapy of Solid Tumours, *Tech. Rep. Ser. Wld Hlth Org. No. 605*, 1977, p. 71.

References to the chemotherapy of neuroblastoma: A. E. Evans *et al.*, *J. Am. med. Ass.*, 1969, *207*, 1325 (cyclophosphamide and vincristine); A. Sawitsky, *Am. J. Dis. Child.*, 1970, *119*, 308 (cyclophosphamide and vincristine); S. Leikin *et al.*, *Cancer Chemother. Rep.*, 1975, *59*, 1015 (doxorubicin and dacarbazine); G. A. Hayes *et al.*, *Cancer Res.*, 1977, *37*, 3766 (cyclophosphamide and doxorubicin); J. Ninane *et al.*, *Archs Dis. Childh.*, 1981, *56*, 544 (role of doxorubicin).

Retinoblastoma. Retinoblastoma is a rare and highly malignant childhood tumour of the eye which may remain localised for a long period and then rapidly metastasise. Small tumours are treated by radiotherapy but larger ones, especially those with seeding within the eye, may be treated by intra-arterial chemotherapy followed by radiotherapy. In metastatic disease alternating weekly courses of vincristine and cyclophosphamide have usually been given.— Report of a WHO Expert Committee on Chemotherapy of Solid Tumours, *Tech. Rep. Ser. Wld Hlth Org. No. 605*, 1977, p. 73.

Treatment for malignant meningitis due to retinoblastoma should include cranial and spinal irradiation, methotrexate intrathecally, and appropriate systemic alkylating agents. One of 6 children treated was surviving apparently clear of disease.— C. E. Stannard *et al.*, *Br. J. Ophthal.*, 1975, *59*, 362.

Sarcoma. *Bone sarcoma.* Osteogenic and Ewing's sarcoma are the commonest malignant bone tumours and occur most frequently in childhood. Until recently 80% of patients with osteogenic sarcoma developed pulmonary metastases irrespective of treatment to the primary tumour. Following surgery, adjuvant chemotherapy with high doses of methotrexate with folinic acid rescue, doxorubicin and combinations of these drugs with other agents has been successful in prolonging disease-free survival. Where pulmonary metastases are already present or where aggressive chemotherapy regimens are ineffective or inappropriate, methotrexate or razoxane may be used with radiotherapy. Aggressive chemotherapy and radiotherapy are beginning to alter the poor prognosis in Ewing's sarcoma. Vincristine, cyclophosphamide, actinomycin D, doxorubicin, or razoxane with radiotherapy have been more promising than radiotherapy alone. Since micrometastases are nearly always present at diagnosis chemotherapy is essential, one of the most effective regimens being vincristine, cyclophosphamide, doxorubicin, and actinomycin D.— Report of a WHO Expert Committee on Chemotherapy of Solid Tumours, *Tech. Rep. Ser. Wld Hlth Org. No. 605*, 1977, p. 65.

An MRC randomised study of adjuvant chemotherapy in *osteosarcoma* is comparing 2 protocols involving vincristine, doxorubicin, and methotrexate with folinic acid rescue, to start within 2 weeks of amputation and to be continued for 1 year. Although long-term results are not yet known the development of lung metastases is certainly delayed by adjuvant chemotherapy.— R. Sweetnam, *Br. J. Hosp. Med.*, 1980, *24*, 452.

Further references to the chemotherapy of *osteosarcoma:* W. W. Sutow *et al.*, *J. clin. Pharmac.*, 1975, *15*, 530 (vincristine, actinomycin D, and cyclophosphamide); W. W. Sutow *et al.*, *Cancer*, 1975, *36*, 1598 (cyclophosphamide, vincristine, melphalan, and doxorubicin); N. Jaffe *et al.*, *Br. med. J.*, 1976, *2*, 1039 (vincristine, methotrexate, and folinic acid); K. Winkler *et al.*, *Dt. med. Wschr.*, 1977, *102*, 1831 (methotrexate, doxorubicin, and cyclophosphamide).

A retrospective analysis of 22 patients with *Ewing's sarcoma.* Of 14 patients with localised Ewing's sarcoma

9 survived without recurrence for 12 to over 59 months after radiotherapy followed by combined chemotherapy consisting of doxorubicin (later replaced by methotrexate), cyclophosphamide, vincristine, and in some cases dacarbazine. Of a further 8 patients with extensive metastases given chemotherapy followed by radiotherapy or surgery as indicated, a full clinical remission was achieved in 5 lasting in 3 for more than 18, 40, and 44 months respectively.— S. Seeber *et al.*, *Dt. med. Wschr.*, 1979, *104*, 804. Haemopoietic recovery in Ewing's sarcoma after intensive combination therapy and autologous marrow transfusions.— R. A. Abrams *et al.*, *Lancet*, 1980, *2*, 385.

Further references to the chemotherapy of Ewing's sarcoma: G. Rosen *et al.*, *Cancer*, 1974, *33*, 384 (actinomycin D, doxorubicin, vincristine, and cyclophosphamide).

Kaposi's sarcoma. See under Malignant Neoplasms of the Skin (above).

Soft-tissue sarcoma. Soft-tissue sarcomas are a group of tumours consisting of a variety of malignancies derived from mesenchymal tissue. A 68% 5-year response-rate has been reported in children with *embryonal rhabdomyosarcoma* given intensive radiotherapy, chemotherapy with vincristine, actinomycin D, and cyclophosphamide, and resection of gross tumours where possible. In adults the tumour is far less sensitive and until the advent of doxorubicin no single antineoplastic agent showed any useful activity in adult soft-tissue sarcomas. Greater response-rates have been obtained by using doxorubicin in association with dacarbazine, cyclophosphamide, and vincristine; most types of soft-tissue sarcomas respond to this combination regimen but chondrosarcomas and mesotheliomas do poorly. Soft-tissue sarcomas are often very bulky and may be reduced pre-operatively by intensive chemotherapy, with or without radiotherapy.— Report of a WHO Expert Committee on Chemotherapy of Solid Tumours, *Tech. Rep. Ser. Wld Hlth Org. No. 605*, 1977, p. 63.

Preliminary beneficial results reported with the combined forms of treatment of soft-tissue sarcomas include the following non-randomised studies: surgery, postoperative radiotherapy, and adjuvant chemotherapy with doxorubicin, cyclophosphamide, and methotrexate (S.A. Rosenberg *et al.*, *Surgery, St Louis*, 1978, *84*, 62); radiotherapy and intra-arterial doxorubicin with local resection, some patients also receiving chemotherapy postoperatively, with or without immunotherapy (D.L. Morton *et al.*, *Ann. Surg.*, 1976, *184*, 268); concomitant radiotherapy and intra-arterial doxorubicin (C.P. Karakousis, *et al.*, *N.Y. St. J. Med.*, 1979, *79*, 328). Randomised studies of adjuvant chemotherapy are in progress in Europe and the USA. Results of chemotherapy for metastatic soft-tissue sarcomas have been less encouraging. Adjuvant immunotherapy has been used but without convincing benefit so far.— *Br. med. J.*, 1979, *2*, 562.

Of 11 children with *rhabdomyosarcoma* treated with surgery, radiotherapy, and chemotherapy (vincristine 1.5 mg per m², actinomycin D 600 µg per m², and cyclophosphamide 300 mg per m², all being given weekly for 6 courses if the blood count permitted, and subsequently every 2 weeks or more depending on the patient's condition) 8 were still alive 4 to 36 months after diagnosis compared with only 2 of 17 in an earlier group treated with surgery and radiotherapy alone. The improvement shown was probably due to chemotherapy and more extensive radiotherapy. No deaths and no undue short-or long-term toxicity had occurred as a result of the drugs used.— J. S. Malpas *et al.*, *Br. med. J.*, 1976, *1*, 247.

Further references to the treatment of rhabdomyosarcoma: A. A. Razek *et al.*, *Cancer*, 1977, *39*, 2415; M. Tefft *et al.*, *Cancer*, 1977, *39*, 665.

In a comparative study involving 3 chemotherapeutic regimens in 75 assessable patients with soft-tissue sarcoma, no regimen was obviously better than any other. The response-rate did not necessarily correlate with survival and it was considered that there was an urgent need for further study so that a more rational approach to therapy could be developed. The regimens compared were: methotrexate alone; methotrexate with folinic acid rescue, cyclophosphamide, vincristine, and actinomycin D (MDS regimen); and methotrexate, with folinic acid rescue, doxorubicin, and dacarbazine (STS-I regimen).— S. Subramanian and E. Wiltshaw, *Lancet*, 1978, *1*, 683.

Further references to the chemotherapy of sarcomas: J. A. Gottlieb *et al.*, *Cancer*, 1972, *30*, 1632 (doxorubicin and dacarbazine); J. P. Kushner *et al.*, *Cancer*, 1975, *36*, 1577 (doxorubicin and dacarbazine in synovial cell sarcoma); W. A. Blattner *et al.*, *J. Am. med. Ass.*, 1977, *238*, 334 (cyclophosphamide and vincristine in malignant mesenchymoma); M. Schmidt *et al.*, *Dt. med. Wschr.*, 1978, *103*, 1206 (cyclophosphamide, vincristine, doxorubicin, and dacarbazine in advanced disease); F. Azizi *et al.*, *Am. J. Obstet. Gynec.*, 1979, *33*, 379 (vincristine, doxorubicin, and dacarbazine in uterine leiomyosarcomas).

Warts. Venereal warts (Condylamata acuminata) resolved completely after 2 weekly doses of fluorouracil 1 g in a 38-year-old woman with ovarian carcinoma and after one course of cisplatin, vinblastine, and bleomycin in a 19-year-old man with carcinoma of the testis.— D. C. Doll and P. I. Wasserman (letter), *New Engl. J. Med.*, 1979, *301*, 1288.

See also under Fluorouracil, p.211, and Bleomycin Sulphate, p.193.

Wilms' tumour. The childhood malignancy, Wilms' tumour or nephroblastoma is treated by immediate excision followed by radiotherapy. Adjuvant chemotherapy has made a dramatic change in patients at early and late stages of the disease and 60 to 80% of all children now survive for 2 years, a survival that may correlate with cure. In early stages vincristine and actinomycin D are the drugs of choice but more intensive combination chemotherapy is required at late stages; cyclophosphamide and doxorubicin have given encouraging results.— Report of a WHO Expert Committee on Chemotherapy of Solid Tumours, *Tech. Rep. Ser. Wld Hlth Org. No. 605*, 1977, p. 72.

A multicentre study indicated that maintenance chemotherapy with vincristine was marginally more effective than with actinomycin D in preventing recurrence of Wilms' tumour. The study was terminated when results from the US National Wilms' Tumour Study (G.J. D'Angio *et al.*, *Cancer*, 1976, *38*, 633) indicated that combination chemotherapy with vincristine and actinomycin D was more effective than either agent alone.— *Archs Dis. Childh.*, 1978, *53*, 112 (MRC Working Party on Embryonal Tumours in Childhood). The 3-year survival-rate of 98 children was 77% compared with 58% (a significant difference) in 104 eligible for inclusion in the MRC study but not included. All children with Wilms' tumour should be treated according to well-defined protocols which take into account the age of the child and the stage of the disease, and which include a full course of maintenance chemotherapy.— E. L. Lennox *et al.*, *Br. med. J.*, 1979, *2*, 567.

In 79 children under one year of age with nephroblastoma treated surgically, the 3-year survival-rate was higher (though not significantly so) in those also given chemotherapy (usually actinomycin D, vincristine, or both) than in those given surgery only.— C. A. Stiller and E. L. Lennox, *Br. med. J.*, 1980, *281*, 1246.

Use of Immunosuppressants. Antilymphocyte and antithymocyte immunoglobulins, cyclosporin A, and azathioprine are used as immunosuppressants mainly to prolong the survival of organ and tissue transplants. Azathioprine and some of the following antineoplastic agents that possess immunosuppressant properties are also used in a variety of auto-immune disorders including those affecting the skin, kidneys, and joints: actinomycin D (p.187), chlorambucil (p.195), cyclophosphamide (p.199), cytarabine (p.203), daunorubicin (p.205), doxorubicin (p.205), fluorouracil (p.209), hydroxyurea (p.212), melphalan (p.213), mercaptopurine (p.214), methotrexate (p.215), mustine (p.222), razoxane (p.225), and thiotepa (p.228).

These agents may be given in association with corticosteroids (p.451), the other main group of immunosuppressants, to permit a reduction in the dosage of corticosteroids. They are also used in conditions refractory to corticosteroids and other therapy.

Reviews on the actions of immunosuppressants.— J. F. Bach, *Drugs*, 1976, *11*, 1; G. H. Heppner and P. Calabresi, *A. Rev. Pharmac. & Toxic.*, 1976, *16*, 367 (selective suppression of immunity by antineoplastic agents); C. M. Haskell, *A. Rev. Pharmac. & Toxic.*, 1977, *17*, 179 (immunological aspects of antineoplastic agents).

Reviews on the clinical uses of immunosuppressants.— N. L. Gerber and A. D. Steinberg, *Drugs*, 1976, *11*, 14; *idem*, 90.

Amyloidosis. Because of the grave prognosis in monoclonal protein amyloidosis, a trial of antineoplastic agents appears warranted especially when an associated immunocyte dyscrasia can be documented. Antineoplastic agents have also been used to treat reactive amyloidosis associated with collagen vascular diseases.— G. G. Glenner, *New Engl. J. Med.*, 1980, *302*, 1333.

Gastro-intestinal disorders. For the use of immunosuppressants in inflammatory diseases of the bowel, see Azathioprine, p.191.

Hepatic disorders. For reference to the use of immunosuppressants in chronic active hepatitis, see Azathioprine, p.191.

Neurological disorders. ***Multiple sclerosis.*** A brief discussion on intensive immunosuppressant therapy in multiple sclerosis including the use of azathioprine, cyclophosphamide, cytarabine, antilymphocyte immunoglobulin, and corticosteroids.— L. A. Liversedge, *Br. med. Bull.*, 1977, *33*, 78. See also *Br. med. J.*, 1980, *280*, 65.

See also under Corticosteroids, p.456.

Further references to immunosuppressants in the treatment of multiple sclerosis: P. Millac and H. Miller (letter), *Lancet*, 1969, *1*, 783 (cyclophosphamide); V. Wieczorek *et al.*, *Dte GesundhWes.*, 1971, *26*, 1791 (cyclophosphamide with prednisone); D. Silberberg *et al.*, *Archs Neurol., Chicago*, 1973, *28*, 210 (no beneficial effect with azathioprine); E. Frick *et al.*, *Münch. med. Wschr.*, 1974, *116*, 2105 (azathioprine); E. Frick *et al.*, *Münch. med. Wschr.*, 1977, *119*, 1111 (azathioprine; antilymphocyte immunoglobulin); R. E. Gonsette *et al.*, *J. Neurol.*, 1977, *214*, 173 (cyclophosphamide).

Organ and tissue transplantation. In addition to corticosteroids, immunosuppressants used to prolong the survival of transplants include antilymphocyte immunoglobulin, antithymocyte immunoglobulin, azathioprine, cyclophosphamide, and cyclosporin A. (See under individual monographs and under Corticosteroids, p.456).

Renal disorders. For reference to the use of immunosuppressants in the nephrotic syndrome and other renal disorders, see Corticosteroids, p.457.

Rheumatic disorders. Immunosuppressants have been given in refractory rheumatoid arthritis but are not widely used because of their toxicity. Azathioprine is preferred to cyclophosphamide. Chlorambucil has also been used.— F. D. Hart, *Drugs*, 1976, *11*, 451; D. Latt, *Med. J. Aust.*, 1979, *1*, *Suppl.* 3, 21; T. P. Anastassiades, *Can. med. Ass. J.*, 1980, *122*, 405; T. P. Anastassiades *et al.*, *Can. med. Ass. J.*, 1980, *122*, 1223; V. Wright and R. Amos, *Br. med. J.*, 1980, *280*, 964.

Antineoplastic agents are only used in the treatment of juvenile rheumatoid arthritis (Still's disease) in those patients with amyloidosis. Chlorambucil has been most successful in controlling joint symptoms.— B. M. Ansell, *Practitioner*, 1972, *208*, 91.

In a double-blind study of patients with active rheumatoid arthritis, usually of less than 3 years' duration, 44 were treated with azathioprine, 2.5 mg per kg bodyweight daily in 2 or 3 doses, 39 with cyclophosphamide, 1.5 mg per kg daily in 2 or 3 doses, and 38 with sodium aurothiomalate in progressive weekly intramuscular doses up to 50 mg, then 50 mg every 2 to 4 weeks. Treatment lasted up to 72 weeks. Azathioprine and cyclophosphamide were significantly more effective than gold in relation to functional capacity at 6 months, and cyclophosphamide was more effective than azathioprine or gold in relation to the number of affected joints at 18 months; there were no differences in relation to morning stiffness, grip strength, joint size, walking time, or subjective assessment. Corticosteroid requirements tended to fall in patients taking azathioprine or cyclophosphamide. Treatment was withdrawn (at least temporarily) in 14 patients taking azathioprine, 20 taking cyclophosphamide, and 19 taking sodium aurothiomalate.— H. L. F. Currey *et al.*, *Br. med. J.*, 1974, *3*, 763. Criticism of the conclusions.— P. J. Rooney *et al.* (letter), *ibid.*, 1974, *4*, 771.

A discussion on the treatment of arthritis associated with psoriasis, with reference to the use of methotrexate, mercaptopurine, or azathioprine.— *Br. med. J.*, 1978, *1*, 262.

See also under Methotrexate, p.219.

Skin disorders. ***Dermatomyositis.*** Seven young patients with dermatomyositis who had failed to respond to treatment with corticosteroids showed clinical improvement following treatment with methotrexate or cyclophosphamide.— A. El-Ghobarey *et al.*, *Postgrad. med. J.*, 1978, *54*, 516.

See also Methotrexate, p.219.

Pemphigus. Methotrexate or azathioprine act rather slowly and are not suitable for the initial control of pemphigus and pemphigoid. They remain a useful adjunct to maintenance therapy especially when the side-effects of corticosteroids become serious.— J. A. Savin, *Practitioner*, 1977, *219*, 847.

A retrospective review of patients seen between 1968 and 1975 showed that of 57 patients with active bullous pemphigoid and of 51 with active cicatricial pemphigoid a number had been maintained on treatment with antineoplastic agents including azathioprine and cyclophosphamide, usually in conjunction with corticosteroids.— J. R. Person and R. S. Rogers, *Mayo Clin. Proc.*, 1977, *52*, 54.

Psoriasis. A discussion on the treatment of psoriasis including the use of methotrexate, hydroxyurea, razoxane, azathioprine, azaribine, and mustine in patients with very severe disease.— R. H. Champion, *Br. med. J.*, 1981, *282*, 343.

For reference to the treatment of psoriatic arthritis, see Rheumatic Disorders (above).

Wegener's granulomatosis. A study on the angiitides and granulomatous diseases of the lung in 35 patients. These disorders can be classified into Wegener's granulomatosis, lymphomatoid granulomatosis, and benign lymphocytic angiitis and granulomatosis of the lung. They appear to result from a hypersensitivity or immunologically mediated process but respond differently to various immunosuppressant chemotherapeutic regimens. *Wegener's granulomatosis*, a systemic disease characterised by necrotising granulomatous vasculitis of the upper and lower airways, glomerulonephritis, and disseminated small vessel vasculitis, is very sensitive to cyclophosphamide and in most cases long-term remissions and even cures can be achieved. Cyclophosphamide was effective in 7 of 8 patients with Wegener's granulomatosis but azathioprine was of no value in 4 similar patients and the disease progressed in one patient given prednisone. *Lymphomatoid granulomatosis* is characterised by necrotic atypical lymphoreticular infiltrates in the lung and frequent cutaneous and neurological involvement; it may terminate in a malignant lymphomatous process. In advanced disease it is refractory to cyclophosphamide and is usually fatal despite combination chemotherapy. *Benign lymphocytic angiitis and granulomatosis* were formerly included in the previous two categories but have been classified as a separate group because they are mainly limited to the lungs and are consistently responsive to chlorambucil. Azathioprine and cyclophosphamide are also effective but chlorambucil is considered to be less toxic.— H. L. Israel *et al.*, *Ann. intern. Med.*, 1977, *87*, 691. See also A. S. Fanci, *ibid.*, 782.

Further references to the treatment of Wegener's granulomatosis: K. Keczkes, *Br. J. Derm.*, 1976, *94*, 391; L. Abraham-Inpijn, *J. Lar. Otol.*, 1980, *94*, 785; A. J. Pinching *et al.*, *Br. med. J.*, 1980, *281*, 836 (the role of infection in relapse).

See also Vasculitis and Wegener's Granulomatosis; in Cyclophosphamide, p.201.

1801-s

Actinomycin C. Cactinomycin; HBF 386. A mixture of antineoplastic substances with a chromopeptide structure obtained from *Streptomyces chrysomallus*. It is a mixture of actinomycin C_2 (45%), actinomycin C_3 (45%), and actinomycin D (10%).

CAS — 8052-16-2.

Orange-red crystals. Sparingly **soluble** in water, chloroform, and methyl alcohol; practically insoluble in alcohol and ether; soluble in acetone and methylene chloride.

Solutions should be prepared immediately before use but are stable for a few days if stored under sterile conditions in the dark. They should not be mixed with any medicaments other than sodium chloride injection. **Protect** from light.

Actinomycin C has properties similar to those of actinomycin D (see below) and was formerly given intravenously in doses of 200 μg in the treatment of Hodgkin's disease and other malignancies.

Actinomycin C was formerly marketed in Great Britain under the proprietary name Sanamycin (*Bayer*).

1802-w

Actinomycin D. Dactinomycin *(U.S.P.)*; Meractinomycin; NSC 3053; WR 2878.
$C_{62}H_{86}N_{12}O_{16}$=1255.4.
CAS — 50-76-0.

Pharmacopoeias. In *Braz.*, *Chin.*, and *U.S.*

An antineoplastic antibiotic produced by the growth of *Streptomyces chrysomallus* and *S. antibioticus*. It is a bright red, somewhat hygroscopic, crystalline powder. It has a potency of not less than 900 μg per mg, calculated on the dried basis.

Soluble in water at 10°, slightly soluble in water at 37°, freely soluble in alcohol; very slightly soluble in ether. **Store** at a temperature not exceeding 40° in airtight containers. Protect from light.

CAUTION *Actinomycin D is irritant; avoid contact with skin and mucous membranes.*

Adverse Effects, Treatment, and Precautions. For an outline of the adverse effects experienced with antineoplastic agents and immunosuppressants, general guidelines for their treatment, and precautions, see Antineoplastic Agents, p.171, pp.174-5.

Actinomycin D is only given in short courses because of its potential for severe toxicity. Apart from nausea and vomiting adverse effects are often delayed, occurring days or weeks after the completion of a course of treatment. Bone-marrow depression is apparent 1 to 7 days after therapy and may be manifest first as thrombocytopenia; agranulocytosis has been reported. There have been fatalities. Other delayed side-effects include erythema, stomatitis, fever, hypocalcaemia, myalgia, gastro-intestinal effects, and kidney and liver abnormalities. Actinomycin D is very irritant and extravasation results in severe tissue damage.

The effects of radiotherapy are enhanced by actinomycin D and severe reactions may follow the concomitant use of high doses. Erythema and pigmentation of the skin occurs especially in areas previously irradiated. Actinomycin D should not be given to patients with varicella as severe and even fatal reactions may occur. It should be used with care in patients with renal impairment. Its use is best avoided in infants under 1 year who are reported to be highly susceptible to the toxicity of actinomycin D.

Effects on the liver. Abnormalities in liver function and an enlarged liver were associated with actinomycin D and radiotherapy in a 5-year-old child with Wilms' tumour.— S. Jayabose *et al.* (letter), *J. Pediat.*, 1976, *88*, 898.

Effects on the skin. A skin rash appeared in 8 of 9 men on the fifth day of treatment with actinomycin D. Initial facial erythema was followed by papules and pustules by the eighth day, and the rash spread to involve chest, back, and sometimes, the buttocks. Scaling or crusting after 9 or 10 days led to an acneform condition which persisted for several months.— E. H. Epstein and M. A. Lutzner, *New Engl. J. Med.*, 1969, *281*, 1094.

Absorption and Fate. Actinomycin D appears to be only slightly metabolised. It has a prolonged half-life and is slowly excreted in urine and faeces.

In a study of the distribution and excretion of actinomycin D in 3 adult patients with malignant melanoma actinomycin D was found to be slightly metabolised; it was concentrated in nucleated cells, and did not readily penetrate the blood-brain barrier. The slow phase of the plasma disappearance of actinomycin D had a half-life of about 36 hours although results in 1 patient who had received doses on each of the 4 previous days indicated that prior administration of actinomycin D altered drug clearance. Substantial amounts were found in the granulocytes and leucocytes of 1 patient 9 days after administration; this might impair their ability to repair irradiation damage which could explain why marked local reaction to irradiation had been noted in patients receiving radiotherapy several weeks after actinomycin D.— M. H. N. Tattersall *et al.*, *Clin. Pharmac. Ther.*, 1975, *17*, 701.

Uses. Actinomycin D is a highly toxic antibiotic with antineoplastic properties. It inhibits the proliferation of cells by forming a stable complex with DNA and interfering with DNA-dependent RNA synthesis. It may enhance the cytotoxic effects of radiotherapy (but see also Adverse Effects, above). Actinomycin D also has immunosuppressant properties (p.186).

It is used in the treatment of Wilms' tumour, rhabdomyosarcoma, and tumours of the uterus and testis, and also in Ewing's sarcoma, osteogenic sarcoma, Kaposi's sarcoma, and other solid tumours. In Wilms' tumour actinomycin D is given in conjunction with radiotherapy and vincristine. Other agents such as cyclophosphamide and vincristine are used with actinomycin D in the treatment of rhabdomyosarcoma while methotrexate and chlorambucil may be employed with actinomycin D in patients with neoplasms of the testis. Beneficial results have been achieved in patients with choriocarcinoma resistant to methotrexate. See also under Choice of Antineoplastic Agent, p.175.

The usual adult dose is 500 μg intravenously, daily, for a maximum of 5 days and this course may be repeated after several weeks if there are no signs of residual toxic effects. The gap between courses may vary from 2 to 6 weeks.

The usual dose for children is 15 μg per kg body-weight daily for 5 days; alternatively, a total of 2.4 mg per m^2 of body-surface may be given over a period of 7 days.

Great care must be taken to avoid extravasation. An isolation-perfusion technique has also been used.

Malignant neoplasms of the breast. Actinomycin D in a dose of 4 to 5 μg per kg ideal or actual body-weight, whichever was the less, for the first 7 days of radiation therapy then thrice weekly for the rest of the course of radiotherapy was considered to enhance the chance of radiotherapy controlling regional soft-tissue recurrent breast cancer. Results from a randomised study of 32 and a retrospective study of 124 patients showed local control in 60 of 76 patients given actinomycin D plus radiation compared with 48 of 80 given radiotherapy alone.— C. E. Olson *et al.*, *Cancer*, 1977, *39*, 1981.

Organ and tissue transplantation. For the use of actinomycin D for the treatment of graft rejection following cardiac transplantation in 3 patients, see E. B. Stinson *et al.*, *J. Am. med. Ass.*, 1969, *207*, 2233.

Osteitis deformans. Four patients with Paget's disease of bone were treated with actinomycin D to a total dose of 2.5 mg given over 3 to 5 days intravenously in dextrose injection. There was marked clinical improvement in 3. Biochemical tests showed reductions in urinary calcium and hydroxyproline concentrations and in serum alkaline phosphatase.— J. J. Fennelly and J. F. Groarke, *Br. med. J.*, 1971, *1*, 423. A brief discussion of the hypocalcaemic effect of actinomycin D.— G. R. Mundy and L. G. Raisz, *Drugs*, 1974, *8*, 250. Further references: P. J. Somerville and R. A. Evans, *Med. J. Aust.*, 1975, *2*, 13.

Sarcoma. References to the use of actinomycin D in various sarcomas: C. L. Vogel *et al.*, *Cancer*, 1973, *31*, 1382 (with or without vincristine in Kaposi's sarcoma); C. M. McBride, *Archs Surg., Chicago*, 1974, *109*, 304 (with melphalan, by isolated perfusion in soft-tissue sarcomas); R. F. Canalis *et al.*, *Archs Otolar.*, 1976, *102*, 104 (with cyclophosphamide in rhabdomyosarcoma); A. L. Pahor, *J. Lar. Otol.*, 1976, *90*, 585 (rhabdomyosarcoma); E. Caceres and M. E. Moran (letter), *Cancer Treat. Rep.*, 1977, *61*, 498 (metastatic osteogenic sarcoma).

See also under Choice of Antineoplastic Agent, p.185.

Wilms' tumour. From the results of the US National Wilms' Tumour Study it was concluded that combination chemotherapy with vincristine and actinomycin D is more effective than either agent used alone.— G. J. D'Angio *et al.*, *Cancer*, 1976, *38*, 633.

Further references to actinomycin D in the treatment of Wilms' tumour: J. A. Wolff *et al.*, *New Engl. J. Med.*, 1968, *279*, 290; *idem*, 1974, *290*, 84; R. D. T. Jenkin (letter), *Br. med. J.*, 1973, *2*, 485; T. F. Sandeman (letter), *Br. med. J.*, 1973, *2*, 485; R. D. T. Jenkin *et al.*, *Can. med. Ass. J.*, 1976, *115*, 136; T. B. Haddy *et al.*, *J. Pediat.*, 1977, *90*, 784.

See also under Choice of Antineoplastic Agent, p.186.

Preparations

Dactinomycin for Injection *(U.S.P.)*. A sterile mixture of actinomycin D 500 μg and mannitol in each container. Store at a temperature not exceeding 40°. Protect from light. The injection is prepared by the addition of diluent before use. pH of the prepared injection 5.5 to 7. Dactinomycin for Injection may be reconstituted immediately before use with Water for Injections; precipitation may occur if sodium chloride injection or water containing a bacteriostat is used.

Cosmegen, Lyovac *(Merck Sharp & Dohme, UK).* Actinomycin D, available as powder for preparing injections, in vials each containing 500 µg and mannitol 20 mg. (Also available in *Austral., Belg., Canad., Ger., Ital., Neth., Norw., S.Afr., Swed., Switz., USA*).

1803-e

Aminoglutethimide.
Ba 16038. 2-(4-Aminophenyl)-2-ethylglutarimide; 3-(4-Aminophenyl)-3-ethylpiperidine-2,6-dione.
$C_{13}H_{16}N_2O_2$=232.3.

CAS — 125-84-8.

Adverse Effects. Adverse effects reported with aminoglutethimide include skin rashes, lethargy, ataxia, nystagmus, confusion, respiratory depression, gastro-intestinal disturbances, bone-marrow depression, hypothyroidism, and virilisation of female patients.

Lupus. A report of systemic lupus erythematosus induced by aminoglutethimide in one patient.— M. McCraken *et al., Br. med. J.*, 1980, *281*, 1254.

Uses. Aminoglutethimide is an analogue of glutethimide (p.802) and was formerly used for its weak anticonvulsant properties. By its inhibitory action on the adrenal cortex, aminoglutethimide blocks the production of adrenal steroids to produce a state of 'medical' adrenalectomy. It is used in the treatment of metastatic breast cancer in doses of 250 mg four times daily by mouth. Replacement therapy with a corticosteroid must also be given. Aminoglutethimide is used in similar doses in the treatment of Cushing's syndrome.

Results of a pharmacokinetic study in 13 women with metastatic breast carcinoma, who were given aminoglutethimide 1 g and hydrocortisone 40 mg daily over one year, indicated that aminoglutethimide increases its own metabolism which may explain why adverse effects diminish during treatment. In 6 of the patients mean half-lives of aminoglutethimide fell from about 13.3 hours at the start of therapy to about 7.3 hours after 6 to 32 weeks; conversely, mean clearance-rates increased. Serum concentrations of aminoglutethimide in 7 patients were similar throughout treatment with a mean value of 11.5 µg per ml.— F. T. Murray *et al., J. clin. Pharmac.*, 1979, *19*, 704.

Cushing's syndrome. Although drugs have only a limited role in the treatment of Cushing's disease, aminoglutethimide has been used in association with metyrapone before surgery or in patients awaiting the effects of radiotherapy.— C. A. Hardisty and D. S. Munro, *Practitioner*, 1978, *221*, 499.

The successful use of aminoglutethimide in 3 patients with Cushing's syndrome.— R. I. Misbin *et al., J. clin. Pharmac.*, 1976, *16*, 645. See also H. Bricaire and J. P. Luton, *Thérapie*, 1974, *29*, 645.

Malignant neoplasms of the breast. Aminoglutethimide appears promising as a means of endocrine ablation for the treatment of advanced breast cancer. Although the principal site of action is thought to be a block in the adrenal conversion of cholesterol to pregnenolone, R.J. Santen *et al.* (*Lancet*, 1979, *1*, 44) have reported that aminoglutethimide blocks oestrogen production by an extra-adrenal as well as an adrenal mechanism. The response-rate to aminoglutethimide with either dexamethasone or hydrocortisone has been reported in more than 280 patients and varies from 25 to 50% with an average response of 31%.— I. C. Henderson and G. P. Canellos, *New Engl. J. Med.*, 1980, *302*, 78. See also S. S. Legha *et al., Ann. intern. Med.*, 1978, *88*, 69; *J. Am. med. Ass.*, 1980, *244*, 9.

Hydrocortisone is preferred to dexamethasone in combination with aminoglutethimide for the treatment of metastatic breast cancer since the degradation of dexamethasone is enhanced by aminoglutethimide.— *J. Am. med. Ass.*, 1978, *239*, 590.

Administration of aminoglutethimide 250 mg four times daily to 40 oophorectomised or postmenopausal women with metastatic breast carcinoma, to suppress synthesis of adrenal steroid hormones, was at least as effective as surgical adrenalectomy in producing beneficial responses. Of 20 patients who responded, 2 relapsed after 6 months, 1 after 11, and the other 17 were still receiving treatment after 3 to 17 months. In particular, rapid and sometimes dramatic relief of bone pain was obtained in 19 of 36 patients with bony metastases, which confirmed previous experience with adrenalectomy. A response was most common in patients who had previously responded to other forms of endocrine therapy. Cortisone acetate 25 mg twice or thrice daily was given concurrently to prevent symptoms of adrenal insufficiency. Side-effects included itchy, erythematous, maculopapular rashes over the trunk and limbs of 5 patients 8 to 10 days after the start of therapy (2 were withdrawn from the study, in 1 the rash subsided after 3 days despite continuing therapy, and in 2 withdrawal followed by readministration with prednisolone 40 mg daily for the first 4 days permitted continuation of therapy with only transient recurrence), transient somnolence and light-headedness occurred in 9 (mainly elderly) patients, symptoms of adrenal insufficiency occurred in 3 (rapidly responding to parenteral hydrocortisone and subsequently controlled by addition of fludrocortisone 100 µg on alternate days), clinical and biochemical features of inappropriate secretion of antidiuretic hormone occurred in 1 patient (and settled spontaneously when therapy was stopped), and transient nausea occurred in 2 patients; no side-effects occurred in the other 23.— I. E. Smith *et al., Lancet*, 1978, *2*, 646. See also A. P. M. Forrest *et al.* (letter), *ibid.*, 1149; I. E. Smith and T. J. Powles (letter), *ibid.*

A view that aminoglutethimide with dexamethasone is unlikely to have any advantage over corticosteroid therapy alone in the treatment of breast cancer. A maintenance dose of 15 to 20 mg of prednisone daily is usually considered adequate for long-term inhibition of metastatic breast carcinoma and the side-effects are less disabling than those reported with aminoglutethimide.— H. M. Lemon (letter), *Ann. intern. Med.*, 1978, *89*, 422. A contrary view. The superiority of aminoglutethimide over corticosteroid therapy has been demonstrated and aminoglutethimide has been shown to have the same general order of activity as hypophysectomy.— S. S. Legha (letter), *ibid.*, 423.

Aminoglutethimide appeared to be as effective as tamoxifen in a controlled study involving 117 patients with advanced breast cancer.— I. E. Smith *et al., Br. med. J.*, 1981, *283*, 1432.

Further references to aminoglutethimide in the treatment of breast cancer.— C. T. Griffiths *et al., Cancer*, 1973, *32*, 31; R. J. Santen *et al., J. Am. med. Ass.*, 1974, *230*, 1661; R. J. Misbin (letter), *Ann. intern. Med.*, 1977, *86*, 828; S. A. Wells *et al., Ann. Surg.*, 1978, *187*, 475.

See also under Choice of Antineoplastic Agent, p.180.

Malignant neoplasms of the prostate. For the effect of stilboestrol and aminoglutethimide on plasma concentrations of testosterone in patients with prostatic carcinoma, see M. R. G. Robinson and B. S. Thomas, *Br. med. J.*, 1971, *4*, 391.

Pregnancy and the neonate. A 22-year-old woman with Cushing's disease was given aminoglutethimide in doses up to 2.5 g daily throughout the first 21 weeks of pregnancy after which it was discontinued and bilateral adrenalectomy was performed. At term she was delivered of a female infant free of any evidence of masculinisation or congenital abnormalities.— T. J. Hanson *et al.* (letter), *J. Am. med. Ass.*, 1974, *230*, 963.

Proprietary Preparations

Orimeten *(Ciba, UK).* Aminoglutethimide, available as scored tablets of 250 mg.

1804-l

Aminopterin. 4-Aminopteroylglutamate. *N*-{4-[(2,4-Diaminopteridin-6-ylmethyl)amino]benzoyl}-L(+)-glutamic acid.
$C_{19}H_{20}N_8O_5$=440.4.

CAS — 54-62-6.

Yellow crystals or an orange-yellow powder. **Soluble** in aqueous solutions of sodium hydroxide.

Uses. Aminopterin is a folic acid antagonist with the general properties of Methotrexate, p.215. It was formerly used, sometimes as the sodium salt, for the treatment of acute leukaemia in children.

Pregnancy and the neonate. *First trimester.* A 28-year-old woman who ingested aminopterin sodium in the first trimester of pregnancy gave birth to a baby girl at 39 weeks. She had almost no calcification of the skull except at the base, protuberant small eyes, poorly developed orbital ridges, facial asymmetry, and disproportionately short forearms and legs. Bone and mental age were both retarded but she was alive at 4½ years of age.— E. B. Shaw and H. L. Steinbach, *Am. J. Dis. Child.*, 1968, *115*, 477. See also E. B. Shaw, *ibid.*, 1972, *124*, 93.

1824-c

Ancitabine Hydrochloride. Cyclocytidine Hydrochloride; NSC 145688. 2,2′-Anhydro-1-β-D-arabinofuranosylcytosine hydrochloride.
$C_9H_{11}N_3O_4$,HCl=261.7.

CAS — 31698-14-3 (ancitabine); 10212-25-6 (hydrochloride).

Uses. Ancitabine hydrochloride is an antineoplastic agent which is hydrolysed slowly to cytarabine (p.203) *in vivo*. It has been used in acute myeloid leukaemia and other malignant diseases and has been given intravenously or subcutaneously in doses of 200 to 300 mg per m^2 body-surface daily.

Clinical pharmacology of ancitabine.— D. H. W. Ho *et al., Clin. Pharmac. Ther.*, 1975, *17*, 66.

Clinical reports of ancitabine: M. A. Burgess *et al., Cancer Treat. Rep.*, 1977, *61*, 437.

Proprietary Names

Cyclo C *(Jap.).*

1805-y

Antilymphocyte Serum.
ALS; Lymphocytic Antiserum. Native serum prepared by injecting viable lymphoid cells into suitable animals and collecting the sera.

1806-j

Antilymphocyte Immunoglobulin (Horse).
AHLG; ALG; Anti-human Lymphocyte Immunoglobulin; Anti-lymphocytic Globulin; Lymphocytic Antiglobulin. A purified preparation of horse immunoglobulins containing antibodies to human lymphocytes and obtained from antilymphocyte serum.

Adverse Effects. Fever, shivering, nausea, tachycardia, and hypotension can occur shortly after administration. Allergic reactions are common; anaphylaxis may occur. There may be a decrease in the incidence of reactions with antilymphocyte immunoglobulin compared with the serum. As well as lymphocytopenia patients may experience leucopenia and thrombocytopenia. Nephrotoxicity is a hazard with antilymphocyte serum but may be less with the immunoglobulin. Immunosuppressants are capable of stimulating the growth of neoplasms. Intravenous injections may cause thrombophlebitis. Patients with auto-immune disorders are reported to have a higher incidence of side-effects to antilymphocyte immunoglobulin than transplant patients.

Allergy and anaphylaxis. The anaphylactic reaction which developed in 1 patient when given antilymphocyte serum was associated with kinin liberation.— J. Bradley *et al., Lancet*, 1971, *2*, 578.

No severe allergic reactions occurred in 50 renal transplant patients who received antilymphocyte immunoglobulin for 2 weeks after transplantation. Mild fever, chills, and malaise occurred after injection of antilymphocyte immunoglobulin in 5 patients but were of short duration.— W. J. Martin *et al., J. Am. med. Ass.*, 1976, *236*, 1729.

Further references.— J. Ring *et al., Klin. Wschr.*, 1973, *51*, 487.

Precautions. Antilymphocyte immunoglobulin and serum are contra-indicated in hypersensitive patients. Patients should always be tested for hypersensitivity. Care should be exercised in treating patients with acute infections.

Interactions. For a report of increased muscle relaxant requirements in patients given antilymphocyte immunoglobulin, see Azathioprine, p.190.

Uses. Antilymphocyte immunoglobulin and serum produce immunosuppression without greatly affecting the development of immunity to infection and are used mainly to prolong the survival of organ and tissue transplants. They have also been used similarly to azathioprine (see p.190) in the treatment of various auto-immune disorders. See also under Use of Immunosuppressants, p.186.

Following a test dose, antilymphocyte immunoglobulin is administered by intravenous infusion in doses of 10 to 30 mg of immunoglobulin per kg body-weight daily. Doses of 5 to 15 mg per kg daily have been given in auto-immune disorders. The daily dose of antilymphocyte immunoglobulin is diluted in 250 to 500 ml of sodium chloride injection and infused slowly over 1 to 2 hours.

Proceedings of a symposium on antilymphocyte immunoglobulin.— *Postgrad. med. J.*, 1976, *52, Suppl.* 5, 1–148.

A detailed review of the actions and uses of antilymphocyte serum.— F. Spreafico, *Adv. Pharmacol. & Chemother.*, 1972, *10*, 257.

A review of antilymphocyte immunoglobulin.— *Drug & Ther. Bull.*, 1976, *14*, 98.

Blood disorders, non-malignant. *Aplastic anaemia.* Antilymphocyte immunoglobulin with or without allogeneic bone-marrow infusions produced a beneficial response on 17 of 29 patients with severe aplastic anaemia. Serum sickness developed in 20 patients 10 days after immunoglobulin treatment and resolved with prednisone. Doses ranged from 15 mg per kg body-weight daily for 4 or 5 days to 40 mg per kg daily for 4 days. Survival was similar to that achieved with bone-marrow transplantation with cyclophosphamide but bone-marrow recovery was considered to be less complete.— B. Speck *et al.*, *Lancet*, 1977, *2*, 1145. In a study in 50 patients treatment of severe aplastic anaemia with antilymphocyte globulin and norethandrolone, with or without bone-marrow infusion, was more effective than bone-marrow transplantation.— *idem*, *Br. med. J.*, 1981, *282*, 860. See also V. Silingardi and U. Torelli, *Archs intern. Med.*, 1979, *139*, 582.

Enhancement of effect. Studies in *mice, dogs,* and 2 patients demonstrated that antilymphocyte or antithymocyte serum was potentiated by procarbazine.— G. L. Floersheim (letter), *Lancet*, 1973, *2*, 1386.

Gastro-intestinal disorders. Failure of antilymphocyte immunoglobulin in acute ulcerative colitis.— M. F. Heyworth and S. C. Truelove (letter), *Lancet*, 1981, *1*, 1060.

Neurological disorders. *Multiple sclerosis.* Antilymphocyte immunoglobulin 4 to 20 mg per kg body-weight daily by intravenous injection for 7 to 14 days was ineffective and toxic in 4 patients with disseminated sclerosis.— D. J. MacFadyen *et al.*, *Neurology, Minneap.*, 1973, *23*, 592, per *J. Am. med. Ass.*, 1973, *225*, 777.

In a study of 20 patients with multiple sclerosis treated with thoracic-duct drainage or antilymphocyte immunoglobulin 10 to 20 mg per kg body-weight daily intravenously or both, 11 patients showed significant clinical improvement. The best results were achieved with thoracic-duct drainage and antilymphocyte immunoglobulin, 6 of 9 patients improving. Where immune unresponsiveness was induced to normal horse immunoglobulin prior to treatment with antilymphocyte immunoglobulin then the effectiveness of the antiglobulin was significantly improved.— J. Ring *et al.*, *Lancet*, 1974, *2*, 1093. See also F. R. Seiler and H. G. Schwick (letter), *ibid.*, 1975, *1*, 806.

See also under Use of Immunosuppressants, p.186.

Organ and tissue transplantation. *Kidney.* A discussion of the problematic place of antilymphocyte serum in kidney transplantation.— *Lancet*, 1976, *1*, 521. Much of the controversy over the efficacy of antilymphocyte immunoglobulin in renal transplant patients is because it has been used in association with other immunosuppressants. It remains to be established whether antilymphocyte immunoglobulin as part of an immunosuppressant regimen, will be more valuable than combination chemotherapy with chemical immunosuppressants.— R. D. Guttmann, *New Engl. J. Med.*, 1979, *301*, 1038. See also A. A. Bakir and G. Dunea, *Br. med. J.*, 1979, *1*, 914.

From a multicentre randomised study with 179 patients observed for 1 year after receiving kidney transplants, graft survival was better, particularly over the first 3 months among the group of 87 patients given antilymphocyte immunoglobulin 20 mg per kg body-weight intravenously, in saline, over 8 hours daily for up to 10 days after transplant than among 92 patients given conventional treatment. The full 10-day course was not completed by 20 patients who developed thrombocytopenia. A clinically significant decrease in platelet count occurred in about 30% of patients given antilymphocyte immunoglobulin, but this soon returned to normal at the end of treatment.— H. E. Taylor *et al.*, *Can. med. Ass. J.*, 1976, *115*, 1205.

Antilymphocyte immunoglobulin of high potency as assessed by primate skin-graft assay was associated with a higher renal transplant survival over 1 and 2 years in 37 patients than a moderate-potency form given to 34 patients. Immunosuppression following transplantation consisted of azathioprine and prednisone; the immunoglobulin which was of *rabbit* origin was given in a dose of 1.5 mg per kg body-weight daily for the first five days. The difference between the 2 forms of immunoglobulin was attributed to their activity in the first 3 months when the graft rejection and death-rate were higher in the group receiving the moderate-potency form. Immunosuppression with the antilymphocyte immunoglobulin of moderate potency was considered to have no more advantages than azathioprine with prednisone.— F. Thomas *et al.*, *Lancet*, 1977, *2*, 671.

Further references.— A. G. R. Sheil *et al.*, *Lancet*, 1971, *1*, 359; *idem*, 1973, *2*, 227; S. A. Birkeland, *Acta med. scand.*, 1975, *198*, 409.

Skin disorders. There was initial improvement in 2 patients with the advanced Sézary syndrome [a lymphoproliferative disorder characterised by intractable itching erythroderma with Sézary cells (abnormal lymphocytes) in the skin and peripheral blood] when treated with antilymphocyte immunoglobulin. This treatment should only be used when no other was effective since immunosuppression is dangerous in such patients and had contributed to the death of one of the above 2 patients in this report.— A. J. Barrett *et al.*, *Lancet*, 1976, *1*, 940.

Proprietary Preparations

Pressimmune *(Hoechst, UK)*. Antilymphocyte immunoglobulin available as a solution for infusion containing 50 mg of equine immunoglobulin (IgG and IgT) per ml, in vials of 5 and 10 ml.

Other Proprietary Names

Immossar *(Fr.)*; Pressimmun *(Ger.)*.

1807-z

Antithymocyte Serum.

Antithymic Serum; Thymitic Antiserum. Native serum prepared by injecting thymus cells into suitable animals and collecting the sera.

1808-c

Antithymocyte Immunoglobulin.

ATG; ATGAM; Antithymocyte Gammaglobulin; Antithymocyte Globulin; Thymocytic Antiglobulin. A purified preparation of immunoglobulins from antithymocyte serum.

Uses. Antithymocyte immunoglobulin and serum have properties similar to those of antilymphocyte immunoglobulin and serum (above) and are used as immunosuppressants to prolong the survival of organ and tissue transplants. See also under Use of Immunosuppressants, p.186.

Lymphoma. The beneficial effect of antithymocyte immunoglobulin in a patient with mycosis fungoides classified as a T-cell lymphoma.— R. L. Edelson *et al.* (letter), *Lancet*, 1977, *2*, 249. Failure of this treatment in 1 patient.— D. J. Gould *et al.* (letter), *ibid.*, 1365.

A 63-year-old man with a T-cell lymphoma who had not responded to chemotherapy experienced a 75% reduction in adenopathy and complete resolution of skin erythema after 7 daily infusions of antithymocyte serum 825 mg. Despite continuing tumour regression the patient died of an intracerebral haemorrhage, secondary to thrombocytopenia.— R. I. Fisher *et al.*, *Ann. intern. Med.*, 1978, *88*, 799.

Organ and tissue transplantation. *Heart.* From experiments carried out in *rats*, antithymocyte serum appeared to be more effective than antilymphocyte serum in prolonging cardiac homograft survival.— *J. Am. med. Ass.*, 1971, *215*, 1747.

For details of the use of antithymocyte immunoglobulin in the management of heart transplantation, see Corticosteroids, p.456.

Kidney. Treatment with antithymocyte immunoglobulin in renal transplant patients has been associated with an increased incidence of viraemia and clinical cytomegalovirus syndromes (S.H. Cheeseman *et al.*, *New Engl. J. Med.*, 1979, *300*, 1345) and with increased excretion of Epstein-Barr virus (*S.H. Cheeseman et al.*, *Ann. intern. Med.*, 1980, *93*, 39).

Comment on the variable results achieved with antithymocyte immunoglobulin in prolonging the survival of kidney transplants.— *J. Am. med. Ass.*, 1979, *242*, 2266.

Further references.— A. B. Cosimi *et al.*, *Surgery, St Louis*, 1976, *80*, 155.

Skin. Antithymocyte immunoglobulin is the immunosuppressant of choice in patients with burns undergoing skin transplantation.— P. S. Russell and A. B. Cosimi, *New Engl. J. Med.*, 1979, *301*, 470.

Manufacturers

Upjohn, USA.

1809-k

Azacitidine. 5-Azacytidine; Ladakamycin; NSC 102816; U 18496; WR 183027. 4-Amino-1-β-D-ribofuranosyl-1,3,5-triazin-2(1*H*)-one.
$C_8H_{12}N_4O_5$=244.2.

CAS — 320-67-2.

A white powder. Azacitidine is unstable in solution. **Store** in a refrigerator. Solutions for injection are prepared, immediately before use, by dissolving the sterile contents of a sealed container in Water for Injections. Such solutions, containing azacitidine 5 mg per ml and mannitol 5 mg per ml, are reported to have a pH between 6 and 7.5 and may be further diluted in lactated Ringer's solution before infusion.

Stability in solution. A solution of azacitidine maintained at pH 2.5 with a 5- to 10-fold excess of sodium bisulphite (relative to the concentration of azacitidine) was stable for 20 hours at room temperature and for about 4 days at refrigeration temperature. The ready reversibility of the bisulphite-azacitidine addition product to yield azacitidine at neutral pH values indicated that the addition product would act as an azacitidine prodrug in the body.— D. C. Chatterji and J. F. Gallelli, *J. pharm. Sci.*, 1979, *68*, 822.

Adverse Effects, Treatment, and Precautions. For an outline of the adverse effects experienced with antineoplastic agents and immunosuppressants, general guidelines for their treatment, and precautions, see Antineoplastic Agents, p.171, pp.174-5. Nausea and vomiting with azacitidine may be severe, especially after rapid injection.

Reports of adverse effects associated with azacitidine.— H. P. Koeffler and C. M. Haskell, *Cancer Treat. Rep.*, 1978, *62*, 573 (rhabdomyolysis).

Uses. Azacitidine is an antineoplastic agent which acts similarly to cytarabine (p.203). It has been used mainly in the treatment of acute myeloid leukaemia and may be given by continuous intravenous infusion in a dose of 50 to 200 mg per m^2 body-surface daily for 5 days. Azacitidine is unstable in solution and it has been suggested that infusions should be freshly prepared every 3 to 4 hours. It has also been given subcutaneously.

A review on azacitidine.— D. D. Von Hoff *et al.*, *Ann. intern. Med.*, 1976, *85*, 237.

Reports of pharmacokinetic studies on azacitidine.— Z. H. Israili *et al.*, *Cancer Res.*, 1976, *36*, 1453.

Reports of clinical studies on azacitidine.— J. A. Levi and P. H. Wiernik, *Cancer*, 1976, *38*, 36; B. I. Shnider *et al.*, *J. clin. Pharmac.*, 1976, *16*, 205; W. R. Vogler *et al.*, *Blood*, 1976, *48*, 331; G. A. Omura, *Cancer Treat. Rep.*, 1977, *61*, 915.

Manufacturers

Upjohn, USA.

1810-w

Azaribine. Triacetyl Azauridine; CB 304; NSC 67239. 2-β-D-Ribofuranosyl-1,2,4-triazine-3,5(2*H*,4*H*)-dione 2′,3′,5′-triacetate.
$C_{14}H_{17}N_3O_9$=371.3.

CAS — 2169-64-4.

Uses. Azaribine has the general properties of azauridine (p.192). It was formerly used in the treatment of mycosis fungoides and psoriasis but was withdrawn from the market in the USA after reports of serious thrombosis.

For reports of the use of azaribine, see Martindale 27th Edn, p. 123.

1811-e

Azaserine. CI 337; CN 15757; NSC 742; Serynl. L-Serine diazoacetate; L-2-Amino-3-diazoacetoxypropionic acid.

$C_5H_7N_3O_4$=173.1.

CAS — 115-02-6.

Yellow-green crystals. Very **soluble** in water; slightly soluble in alcohol, methyl alcohol, and acetone. M.p. about 157°. An antimicrobial and antifungal substance produced by a strain of *Streptomyces*.

Uses. Azaserine is an inhibitor of enzymic action involving glutamine and has been used as an antineoplastic agent.

A review of the actions and uses of azaserine.— C. C. Cheng and K. -Y. Zee-Cheng, *J. pharm. Sci.*, 1972, *61*, 485.

Azaserine is reported to produce chromosome damage *in vitro*.— P. J. Balson, *Adverse Drug React. Bull.*, 1972, Dec., 116.

Manufacturers
Parke, Davis, USA.

1812-l

Azathioprine *(B.P., U.S.P.)*. BW 57322; NSC 39084. 6-(1-Methyl-4-nitroimidazol-5-ylthio)purine.

$C_9H_7N_7O_2S$=277.3.

CAS — 446-86-6.

Pharmacopoeias. In *Br.*, *Braz.*, and *U.S.*

A pale yellow odourless powder. M.p. about 238° with decomposition. Practically **insoluble** in water; very slightly soluble in alcohol and chloroform; sparingly soluble in dilute mineral acids; soluble in dilute solutions of alkali hydroxides but decomposes in stronger solutions. Solutions of azathioprine sodium for injection are alkaline; they are prepared by dissolving in Water for Injections, immediately before use. **Store** in airtight containers. Protect from light.

Adverse Effects and Treatment. For an outline of the adverse effects experienced with antineoplastic agents and immunosuppressants and general guidelines for their treatment, see Antineoplastic Agents, p.171 and p.174.

Depression of the bone marrow, commonly manifest as leucopenia and less often thrombocytopenia, may be delayed. Other side-effects associated azathioprine include drug fever, liver damage, and pancreatitis. Solutions for injection are very irritant.

Allergy and anaphylaxis. Reports of allergic reactions associated with azathioprine.— M. D. Lockshin and L. J. Kagen (letter), *New Engl. J. Med.*, 1972, *286*, 1321 (meningitic reactions); N. B. Hershfield (letter), *Can. med. Ass. J.*, 1973, *109*, 1082 (polyarthritis and fever); L. J. Brandt, *Ann. intern. Med.*, 1977, *87*, 458 (formication); A. E. Cocco and G. P. Pavlides, *Md St. med. J.*, 1977, *26*, 61 (fever); J. S. Sergent and M. Lockshin (letter), *J. Am. med. Ass.*, 1978, *240*, 529 (meningitic reaction); M. J. G. Farthing *et al.*, *Br. med. J.*, 1980, *280*, 367 (fever, arthralgia, polyneuritis).

Effect on the blood. Splenectomy appeared to reduce the leucopenic effect of azathioprine in 2 renal transplant patients.— J. E. Woods *et al.*, *J. Am. med. Ass.*, 1971, *218*, 1430.

See also Antineoplastic Agents, p.173.

Effects on the liver. Hepatic disease occurring after renal transplantation may possibly result from acute viral hepatitis, exacerbation of chronic hepatitis, or systemic infection, or it may be associated with azathioprine. There is uncertainty as to whether azathioprine damages the liver (see P. Ireland *et al.*, *Archs intern. Med.*, 1973, *132*, 29) but it definitely may cause intrahepatic cholestasis.— *Br. med. J.*, 1979, *1*, 1102. The hepatic side-effects of azathioprine are probably related to the mercaptopurine moiety.— M. Davis *et al.*, *Postgrad. med. J.*, 1980, *56*, 274.

A 27-year-old woman who received azathioprine therapy for 22 months after renal transplantation developed severe jaundice and died of hepatic failure. It is suggested that patients should be maintained only with corticosteroids if the liver function becomes abnormal.— Z. Zarday *et al.*, *J. Am. med. Ass.*, 1972, *222*, 690.

Further reports of adverse effects on the liver associated with azathioprine.— A. T. Marubbio and B. Danielson, *Gastroenterology*, 1975, *69*, 739 (hepatic veno-occlusive disease); J. Freise *et al.*, *Dt. med. Wschr.*, 1976, *101*, 1223 (cholestatic jaundice).

Effects on the pancreas. Reports of pancreatitis associated with azathioprine treatment.— J. R. Nogueira and M. A. Freedman, *Gastroenterology*, 1972, *62*, 1040; D. Paloyan *et al.*, *Am. J. dig. Dis.*, 1977, *22*, 839; I. Hamed *et al.*, *Am. J. med. Sci.*, 1978, *276*, 211; J. N. Isenberg, *J. Pediat.*, 1978, *93*, 1043; L. J. Herskowitz *et al.*, *Archs Derm.*, 1979, *115*, 179; R. A. L. Sturdevant *et al.*, *Gastroenterology*, 1979, *77*, 883.

Effects on respiratory function. After 6 weeks of treatment with azathioprine 100 mg daily a patient with ulcerative colitis developed acute respiratory depression with cough and dyspnoea. Symptoms disappeared when azathioprine was withdrawn.— G. Rubin *et al.*, *Aust. N.Z. J. Med.*, 1972, *2*, 272.

Hypotension. Pronounced hypotension in 2 patients with rheumatoid arthritis given azathioprine.— T. Cunningham *et al.*, *Br. med. J.*, 1981, *283*, 823.

Precautions. For reference to the precautions necessary with antineoplastic agents and immunosuppressants, see Antineoplastic Agents, p.175.

Azathioprine should be used with care in patients with liver damage or a history of liver disease.

The effects of azathioprine are enhanced by allopurinol and the dose of azathioprine should be reduced to about one-quarter when allopurinol is given concomitantly. Reduced doses may be required in patients with impaired renal function.

Interactions. Requirements of non-depolarising muscle relaxants were increased 2 to 4 times in 26 patients given azathioprine or antilymphocyte immunoglobulin prior to surgery; 2 of the patients also received guanethidine. The potency of tubocurarine was reduced by azathioprine and significantly reduced by azathioprine and guanethidine.— K. B. Vetten, *S. Afr. med. J.*, 1973, *47*, 767.

Pregnancy and the neonate. From a detailed analysis of successful pregnancies notified to the European Dialysis and Transplant Association, only 7 of 110 babies born to 97 women with renal transplants had congenital abnormalities, one of them being a congenital cytomegalovirus infection. Abnormalities were trivial in 3 babies. Chromatid breaks were found in 2 of 16 babies who underwent chromosome analysis. Mothers of the 7 babies with abnormalities had taken significantly higher daily doses of azathioprine (a mean of 2.64 mg per kg body-weight) compared with those who had normal babies (a mean of 2.02 mg per kg). There was no significant difference in the daily dose of prednisone. This congenital abnormality-rate is probably not excessive when compared with a reported figure of 2% for all births.—The Registration Committee of the European Dialysis and Transplant Association, *Br. J. Obstet. Gynaec.*, 1980, *87*, 839.

For reports of normal babies born to women who had taken azathioprine during pregnancy, see P. N. Gillibrand, *Proc. R. Soc. Med.*, 1966, *59*, 834; J. J. Kaufman *et al.*, *J. Am. med. Ass.*, 1967, *200*, 338; J. A. Board *et al.*, *Obstet. Gynec.*, 1967, *29*, 318; J. Erkman and J. G. Blythe, *Obstet. Gynec.*, 1972, *40*, 708; E. Sharon *et al.*, *Am. J. Obstet. Gynec.*, 1974, *118*, 25. Despite the lack of evidence for foetal damage associated with azathioprine, it seems prudent to avoid its use in pregnancy if possible.— M. de Swiet, *Prescribers' J.*, 1979, *19*, 59.

Absorption and Fate. Azathioprine is absorbed from the gastro-intestinal tract and is distributed throughout the body. After oral or intravenous administration it disappears rapidly from the circulation and is extensively metabolised to mercaptopurine (see p.214). About 10% of a dose is reported to be split between the sulphur and the purine ring to give 1-methyl-4-nitro-5-thioimidazole. Small amounts of unchanged azathioprine and mercaptopurine are eliminated in the urine.

Rosette-inhibiting activity was detected in the serum 30 minutes after azathioprine administration to healthy subjects and reached a peak at 1 hour. By 4 hours activity had decreased by 50% and by 12 hours, 75%. Azathioprine activity was not affected by renal damage but no activity was found in patients with cirrhosis or acute or chronic hepatitis. Delayed metabolism of azathioprine might account for its toxic effect on the bone marrow.— J. F. Bach *et al.*, *Nouv. Presse méd.*, 1972, *1*, 2293, per *J. Am. med. Ass.*, 1972, *222*, 1458.

Azathioprine has been reported to be 30% bound to plasma proteins, with a normal half-life of 3 hours.— W. M. Bennett *et al.*, *Ann. intern. Med.*, 1980, *93*, 286.

Mean peak immunosuppressive activity as measured by rosette-inhibiting activity occurred in the serum and cerebrospinal fluid 1 and 4 hours respectively after administration of azathioprine 50 mg intravenously to 13 patients. The maximum activity found in the cerebrospinal fluid was about 12.5% of that in serum.— E. Frick, *Arzneimittel-Forsch.*, 1978, *28*, 473.

Reports on assays of azathioprine and its metabolites.— J. L. Maddocks, *Br. J. clin. Pharmac.*, 1979, *8*, 273; L. Fletcher and J. L. Maddocks, *Br. J. clin. Pharmac.*, 1980, *10*, 287.

Further references to pharmacokinetic studies with azathioprine.— V. Schusziarra *et al.*, *Int. J. clin. Pharmac. Biopharm.*, 1976, *14*, 298 (during haemodialysis).

Uses. Azathioprine is an immunosuppressant (see p.186) and antineoplastic agent with similar actions to those of mercaptopurine (p.214), to which it is slowly converted in the body. Its effects are reported to appear within 2 to 4 days of administration although a clinical response may not be seen for at least 2 to 4 weeks. It is given by mouth or by slow intravenous injection as azathioprine sodium, well diluted.

Azathioprine is mainly used as an immunosuppressant for facilitating the survival of organ and tissue transplants. The dose for this purpose varies from 1 to 5 mg per kg body-weight daily and depends partly on whether other drugs, such as a corticosteroid, or radiotherapy are employed at the same time. The dose is usually increased if there is incipient rejection of the graft, but large fluctuations in dosage should be avoided. About one-half the dose may be adequate for maintenance therapy.

It is also used in a wide variety of conditions such as lupus erythematosus, rheumatoid arthritis, renal disorders, chronic active hepatitis, and some severe skin disorders which are considered to be auto-immune in character and for which corticosteroid therapy is often tried. Its use in conjunction with a corticosteroid (see p.451) may allow a lower dose of both drugs to be used, thus reducing side-effects. The usual dose is 1 to 2.5 mg per kg body-weight daily by mouth in adults and children.

Blood counts should be carried out regularly during treatment and azathioprine withdrawn or the dosage reduced at the first indication of bone-marrow depression.

During a study in *rats* it was found that azathioprine may have an antidiabetogenic effect.— A. S. Serra *et al.* (letter), *Lancet*, 1979, *1*, 1292.

Administration in hepatic insufficiency. In 13 patients with severe liver damage, azathioprine 1.5 mg per kg body-weight did not generally increase pretreatment titres of immunosuppressive activity of the serum, measured 1 hour after dosage. Initial low titres were elevated to normal in a further patient during recovery from viral hepatitis. Increasing the dose of azathioprine to 3 mg per kg had no effect when liver function was poor, although titres were dose-dependent.— G. Whelan and S. Sherlock, *Gut*, 1972, *13*, 907.

It was recommended that the dose of azathioprine should be restricted to 75 to 100 mg daily when used with prednisolone in the treatment of active chronic hepatitis.— *Br. med. J.*, 1973, *2*, 193. See also Corticosteroids, p.454 and Prednisolone, p.480.

See also Effects on the Liver (above) and Hepatic Disorders (below).

Administration in renal insufficiency. The interval between doses of azathioprine should be extended from 24 hours to 24 to 36 hours in patients with a glomerular filtration-rate of less than 10 ml per minute. Concentrations of azathioprine are affected by haemodialysis.— W. M. Bennett *et al.*, *Ann. intern. Med.*, 1977, *86*, 754; *idem*, 1980, *93*, 286. See also P. Sharpstone, *Br. med. J.*, 1977, *2*, 36. An opinion that no dose adjustment is needed.— J. S. Cheigh, *Am. J. Med.*, 1977, *62*, 555.

See also under Organ and Tissue Transplantation and Renal Disorders (below).

Blood disorders, non-malignant. *Haemolytic anaemia.* Auto-immune haemolytic anaemia in 3 infants was treated with large doses of corticosteroids with only partial success. Azathioprine 2 to 5 mg per kg body-weight daily was effective in 1 child and allowed reduction of corticosteroid doses in the other 2, with consequent resumption of growth.— W. H. Hitzig and L. Massimo, *Blood*, 1966, *28*, 840, per *J. Am. med. Ass.*, 1967, *199* (Feb. 13), A191. Further references.— D. S. Rosenthal and B. Sack, *J. Am. med. Ass.*, 1971, *216*, 2011; L. E. Böttiger and A. Rausing, *Ann. intern. Med.*, 1972, *76*, 593.

Haemosiderosis. In a 22-year-old man with idiopathic pulmonary haemosiderosis given azathioprine 50 mg and 100 mg on alternate days, haemoptysis ceased and haemoglobin and serum-iron concentrations returned to normal without supplementary doses of iron. Treatment was discontinued after 21 months and the patient had remained asymptomatic.— R. B. Byrd and D. R. Gracey, *J. Am. med. Ass.*, 1973, *226*, 458.

Thrombocytopenic purpura. Of 17 patients with idiopathic thrombocytopenic purpura most of whom had had splenectomy and corticosteroids, 12 obtained remissions after treatment with azathioprine, usually in conjunction with prednisone. The dose of azathioprine was 50 to 250 mg daily and that of prednisone 20 to 30 mg daily, progressively reduced. Duration of treatment ranged from 3 to 38 months and of remissions from 1 to 44 months. In some patients maintenance therapy was not required. Reversible leucopenia was the only side-effect observed.— B. A. Bouroncle and C. A. Doan, *J. Am. med. Ass.*, 1969, *207*, 2049. See also K. M. Goebel and F. D. Goebel, *Chemotherapy, Basle*, 1973, *18*, 112, per *Int. pharm. Abstr.*, 1973, *10*, 697.

Gastro-intestinal disorders, non-malignant. In a double-blind study in 80 patients with *ulcerative colitis*, the addition of azathioprine 2.5 mg per kg body-weight [daily] to initial corticosteroid therapy had no significant effect on acute attacks. When given for maintenance it conveyed no benefit to those presenting with their first attack but was of limited value to those presenting with a relapse.— D. P. Jewell and S. C. Truelove, *Br. med. J.*, 1974, *4*, 627. Doses of 5.25 and 6 mg of azathioprine per kg body-weight daily were required in 2 patients with ulcerative colitis before a remission was achieved.— R. A. Jones (letter), *Lancet*, 1974, *2*, 107. Further references.— J. L. Rosenberg *et al.*, *Gastroenterology*, 1975, *69*, 96; T. C. Northfield, *Drugs*, 1977, *14*, 198; T. C. Northfield, *Prescribers' J.*, 1979, *19*, 80.

A patient with *coeliac disease* inadequately controlled by prednisone in doses as high as 20 mg daily was effectively treated with azathioprine 2 mg per kg body-weight daily. It was possible to reduce the dose of prednisone to 2.5 mg daily.— J. D. Hamilton *et al.*, *Lancet*, 1976, *1*, 1213.

A review on the management of *Crohn's disease* with reference to the use of azathioprine. Despite controlled studies of treatment with corticosteroids, sulphasalazine, and immunosuppressants, a particular regimen can still not be recommended. The design and interpretation of the National Cooperative Crohn's Disease Study (*Gastroenterology*, 1979, *77*, 825–944) have been criticised; azathioprine was found to be ineffective in active disease and in maintaining remission and R.W. Summers *et al.* (*Gastroenterology*, 1979, *77*, 847) stated that there was no justification for its use in Crohn's disease. However, D.P. O'Donoghue *et al.* (*Lancet*, 1978, *2*, 955) found that long-term maintenance treatment with azathioprine 2 mg per kg body-weight daily appeared to reduce the rate of relapse in a highly selected group of patients with Crohn's disease although it was potentially toxic and one patient who had received azathioprine for more than 10 years died of pancytopenia. The fear of adverse effects such as malignancy has limited the use of azathioprine but the report by D.H. Present *et al.* (*New Engl. J. Med.*, 1980, *302*, 981) on the successful use of mercaptopurine (see p.215) has renewed interest in immunosuppressant treatment. In general, immunosuppressants such as azathioprine are perhaps best reserved for patients who need a reduction in corticosteroid dosage or who cannot tolerate sulphasalazine or surgery and need maintenance therapy.— *Br. med. J.*, 1980, *281*, 893. See also *Lancet*, 1980, *2*, 298; M. H. Sleisenger, *New Engl. J. Med.*, 1980, *302*, 1024.

In some patients with *Crohn's disease*, azathioprine exacerbated the condition and also caused joint and skin lesions. Other adverse effects were nausea, vomiting, and pyrexia. The bone-marrow depressant effect of azathioprine might be enhanced if the drug were given together with sulphamethoxazole and trimethoprim. Small doses of azathioprine were recommended for use in patients with associated renal disease.— *Med. J. Aust.*, 1972, *2*, 579.

Further reviews, reports and studies of azathioprine in Crohn's disease.— B. N. Brooke *et al.*, *Lancet*, 1969, *2*, 612; F. A. Jones *et al.* (letter), *ibid.*, 795; J. Rhodes *et al.*, *ibid.*, 1971, *2*, 1273; J. M. T. Willoughby *et al.*, *ibid.*, 944; M. Klein *et al.*, *Gastroenterology*, 1974, *66*, 916; B. N. Brooke *et al.*, *Lancet*, 1976, *1*, 1041; T. C. Northfield, *Drugs*, 1977, *14*, 198; *idem*, *Prescribers' J.*, 1979, *19*, 80.

References to azathioprine in the treatment of general gastro-intestinal disorders.— A. D. Jorge and D. Sanchez, *Gut*, 1973, *14*, 104 (chronic gastritis).

For further references to the management of inflammatory bowel disease, see Corticosteroids, p.453, and Sulphasalazine, p.1483.

Hepatic disorders, non-malignant. Although many immunosuppressants have been tried in the treatment of chronic active hepatitis it is suggested that prednisone 10 mg daily in association with azathioprine 50 mg daily is probably the safest effective regimen. Controlled studies stratified according to disease activity are needed to establish whether the benefits of such treatment always outweigh the risks.— *Lancet*, 1978, *2*, 507. Occasionally immunosuppression might worsen the course of chronic active hepatitis and some encouraging results had been reported with immunostimulation. The routine use of immunosuppressants cannot be recommended.— C. van Ypersele de Strihou and Y. Pirson (letter), *ibid.*, 836. Criticism of the use of azathioprine.— I. G. Toth (letter), *ibid.*, 947.

Further reports of azathioprine used alone or with corticosteroids in hepatic disorders.— I. R. Mackay, *Q.J. Med.*, 1968, *37*, 379 (active chronic auto-immune hepatitis); R. B. Stern *et al.*, *Gut*, 1973, *14*, 419 (active chronic hepatitis); A. J. Czaja and W. H. J. Summerskill, *Med. Clins N. Am.*, 1978, *62*, 71 (chronic hepatitis); T. Gottesman and S. Moeschlin, *Dt. med. Wschr.*, 1978, *103*, 1989 (active chronic hepatitis); J. Crowe *et al.*, *Gastroenterology*, 1980, *78*, 1005 (primary biliary cirrhosis).

See also under Corticosteroids, p.454, and also Administration in Hepatic Insufficiency, above.

Immunosuppression. For reference to the use of azathioprine in association with corticosteroids in a variety of immune disorders, see Corticosteroids, p.451.

Lupus erythematosus. Azathioprine is less toxic than cyclophosphamide and is the immunosuppressant of choice in systemic lupus erythematosus. It is reported to enable lower doses of corticosteroids to be used.— G. R. V. Hughes, *Br. med. J.*, 1979, *2*, 1019. Comment that any therapeutic advantage of immunosuppressants over corticosteroids in systemic lupus erythematosus appears to be countered by their toxicity and that the use of azathioprine and cyclophosphamide should still be considered investigational.— L. E. Shulman, *J. Am. med. Ass.*, 1979, *241*, 23.

Acute exacerbation of systemic lupus erythematosus, resulting in death in 1 patient, occurred in 7 of 9 patients when azathioprine therapy was abruptly discontinued compared with 1 of 7 in a control group who continued azathioprine. Exacerbations started from 21 to 200 days after cessation of the drug and were treated initially with increased doses of prednisone. However the 7 patients required renewal of azathioprine therapy as well as increased doses of the prednisone, which were greater than those at the start of the trial. It was suggested that a gradual withdrawal of azathioprine might be better than an abrupt withdrawal, but the need for close observation during this time was stressed.— E. Sharon *et al.*, *New Engl. J. Med.*, 1973, *288*, 122.

Further reports of azathioprine in the treatment of systemic lupus erythematosus.— N. R. Rowell, *Br. med. J.*, 1969, *2*, 427; J. F. Maher and G. E. Schreiner, *Archs intern. Med.*, 1970, *125*, 293, per *J. Am. med. Ass.*, 1970, *211*, 1394; B. H. Hahn *et al.*, *Ann. intern. Med.*, 1975, *83*, 597; A. J. Fish *et al.*, *Am. J. Med.*, 1977, *62*, 99.

See also Renal Disorders (below) and also under Corticosteroids, p.455.

Muscular disorders, non-malignant. For reference to the use of azathioprine in muscular disorders including myasthenia gravis and polymyositis, see Corticosteroids, p.455.

Neurological disorders, non-malignant. Reports of a beneficial effect of azathioprine in various neurological disorders.— K. N. V. Palmer (letter), *Lancet*, 1966, *1*, 265 (Guillain-Barré syndrome); S. J. Oh, *Archs Neurol., Chicago*, 1978, *35*, 509 (subacute demyelinating polyneuropathy); B. Pentland, *Postgrad. med. J.*, 1980, *56*, 734 (chronic relapsing polyneuropathy).

For reference to azathioprine in the treatment of multiple sclerosis, see Use of Immunosuppressants, p.186, and Corticosteroids, p.456.

Ocular disorders, non-malignant. When azathioprine 1.5 mg per kg body-weight daily was added to the normal treatment of thyrotoxicosis in 109 patients with Graves' disease who were expected to develop malignant exophthalmos because of a positive leucocyte migration test, no clinical signs of exophthalmos developed.— R. Winand and P. Mahieu (letter), *Lancet*, 1973, *1*, 1196.

Further references to the use of azathioprine in ocular disorders.— R. H. Andrasch *et al.*, *Archs Ophthal., N.Y.*, 1978, *96*, 247 (with prednisone in severe chronic uveitis).

Organ and tissue transplantation. *Cornea.* Because repeated corneal grafts in 2 patients became opaque within 4 to 16 weeks despite treatment with corticosteroids, it was assumed that an immune reaction was involved and immunosuppressive drugs were therefore used. Azathioprine was started on the day before operation and daily maintenance doses were continued for 1 to 2 years. Prednisolone was also given in the postoperative period. In both patients the grafts remained clear.— I. R. Mackay *et al.*, *Lancet*, 1967, *2*, 479.

Heart. See Corticosteroids, p.456.

Kidney. For details of a standard maintenance regimen with azathioprine and prednisone in patients with kidney transplants, see Corticosteroids, p.456.

Azathioprine was withdrawn from the immunosuppressive schedules of 22 patients with renal transplants without any significant change in renal function or survival. In 7 of the patients azathioprine was withdrawn because of bone-marrow depression and not restarted; in the remaining 15 it was withdrawn electively after 2 years' treatment. It is doubtful whether azathioprine is necessary for successful renal transplantation.— M. H. R. Sheriff *et al.*, *Lancet*, 1978, *1*, 118. See also Y. Pirson *et al.* (letter), *ibid.*, 506. Of 7 renal transplant patients who were obliged to stop azathioprine therapy prednisolone requirements were slightly increased in 2, decreased in 4, and unchanged in 1.— P. Schmidt *et al.* (letter), *ibid.*, 1978, *2*, 314.

Nerve. Azathioprine 3 mg per kg body-weight daily, or less depending on the white-cell count, was administered to 7 patients following nerve allografts for between 4 and 6 months until there were signs of regeneration. Three of the patients whose nerve damage was due to leprosy also received prednisone 5 mg thrice daily for 2 weeks. All 7 patients recovered some sensation, although only 1 patient whose nerve damage had been due to trauma showed some motor recovery. One further patient who discontinued treatment after 4 weeks showed no improvement and surgical exploration after 9 months showed conversion of the allograft to fibrous tissue.— R. S. Gye *et al.*, *Lancet*, 1972, *1*, 647.

Skin. A combination of tissue typing and immunosuppression prolonged the survival of allografts in 3 children with full-thickness burns of over 70% of the body surface. Azathioprine was given by mouth as follows: 5 to 6 mg per kg body-weight on the day before tissue grafting, then 3 mg per kg for 3 days, and then 1.5 mg per kg thereafter. Treatment was carried out in a controlled environment and wound bacteriology did not differ from that in non-immunised patients in a similar environment.— J. F. Burke *et al.*, *New Engl. J. Med.*, 1974, *290*, 269.

Pregnancy and the neonate. For reports of normal babies born to women who had taken azathioprine during pregnancy, see Precautions, above.

Renal disorders, non-malignant. Azathioprine 2 mg per kg body-weight daily for 8 weeks was ineffective in preventing relapse in a controlled study of 24 children with frequently relapsing corticosteroid-responsive nephrotic syndrome.— T. M. Barratt *et al.*, *Archs Dis. Childh.*, 1977, *52*, 462.

For further reference to the use of azathioprine and other immunosuppressants in renal disorders, see Corticosteroids, p.457.

See also Administration in Renal Insufficiency, above.

Rheumatic disorders, non-malignant. Of 49 patients with severe rheumatoid arthritis, 25 received azathioprine, 2.5 mg per kg body-weight daily, and 24 a placebo, together with prednisolone and paracetamol given in minimum effective doses which were modified monthly according to the clinical response. After 12 months the mean reduction in prednisolone dosage possible without clinical deterioration was 750 µg per day in the placebo group and 4.3 mg per day (36%) in the azathioprine group. Side-effects led to withdrawal of 4 patients from each group, and 2 and 1 patients respectively withdrew because of exacerbation of rheumatoid arthritis. Azathioprine caused a significant depression in the white-cell count in some patients.— M. Mason *et al.*, *Br. med. J.*, 1969, *1*, 420. Follow-up for 30 months showed that there was no further significant decrease in corticosteroid dosage. Only 10 patients were still taking azathioprine; 10 had withdrawn for reasons other than toxicity, the remainder because of toxicity; some who withdrew still needed a smaller dose of corticosteroids 18 months later.— J. Harris *et al.*, *ibid.*, 1971, *4*, 463.

Evidence that the dose of azathioprine must be 2.5 mg per kg body-weight daily for the management of rheumatoid arthritis.— J. Woodland *et al.*, *Ann. rheum. Dis.*, 1981, *40*, 355.

Further references to azathioprine in rheumatic disorders.— W. H. Dodson and J. C. Bennett, *J. clin. Pharmac.*, 1969, *9*, 251; M. B. Urowitz *et al.*, *Arthritis Rheum.*, 1973, *16*, 411; H. Berry *et al.*, *Br. med. J.*, 1976, *1*, 1052 (comparison with penicillamine); K. M. Goebel *et al.*, *Eur. J. clin. Pharmac.*, 1976, *9*, 405; I. L. Dwosh *et al.*, *Arthritis Rheum.*, 1977, *20*, 685 (comparison of azathioprine, gold, and chloroquine); M. I. V. Jayson and D. L. Easty, *Ann. rheum. Dis.*, 1977, *36*, 428 (melting of the cornea associated with rheumatoid arthritis).

See also under Use of Immunosuppressants, p.186.

Skin disorders, non-malignant. Twenty-nine patients with severe psoriasis were treated with azathioprine 100 mg daily, increased after 2 weeks to 200 mg daily (exceptionally 300 mg daily) continued as required and reduced when remission was obtained; 19 patients were judged to have benefited. Cholestasis occurred in 2 patients and portal fibrosis in 8. Regular monitoring of liver function by biopsy was necessary.— A. du Vivier *et al.*, *Br. med. J.*, 1974, *1*, 49.

Further reports of azathioprine in the treatment of various skin disorders.— G. T. Jansen *et al.*, *Archs Derm.*, 1968, *97*, 690 (scleroderma); M. W. Greaves and R. Dawber (letter), *Br. med. J.*, 1970, *2*, 237 (psoriasis); G. A. Hunter and I. J. Forbes, *Br. J. Derm.*, 1972, *87*, 42 (pityriasis); J. G. L. Morrison and E. J. Schulz, *Br. J. Derm.*, 1978, *98*, 203 (eczema).

For reference to the use of azathioprine in pemphigoid, see Corticosteroids, p.459.

Wegener's granulomatosis. Reports of azathioprine in the treatment of Wegener's granulomatosis.— S. R. Kaplan *et al.*, *New Engl. J. Med.*, 1968, *278*, 239 (azathioprine in association with duazomycin in corticosteroid-resistant disease); D. F. N. Harrison, *Br. med. J.*, 1974, *4*, 205 (with prednisone).

See also under Choice of Antineoplastic Agent, p.175.

Preparations

Azathioprine Sodium for Injection *(U.S.P.)*. A sterile solid prepared by freeze-drying an aqueous solution of azathioprine and sodium hydroxide. Potency is expressed in terms of the equivalent amount of azathioprine. The injection is prepared by the addition of diluent before use. Store at 15° to 30°. pH of the solution 9.8 to 11.

Azathioprine Tablets *(B.P., U.S.P.)*. Tablets containing azathioprine. Protect from light.

Imuran *(Wellcome, UK)*. Azathioprine, available as scored tablets of 50 mg.

Imuran Injection *(Wellcome, UK)*. Azathioprine sodium, available as powder for preparing injections, in vials containing the equivalent of 50 mg of azathioprine. (Also available as Imuran in *Arg.*, *Austral.*, *Belg.*, *Canad.*, *Ital.*, *Neth.*, *S.Afr.*, *USA*).

Other Proprietary Names

Azanin *(Jap.)*; Imurek *(Aust., Ger., Switz.)*; Imurel *(Denm., Fr., Norw., Spain, Swed.)*.

1813-y

Azauridine. 6-Azauridine; 6-AzUR; NSC 32074. β-D-Ribofuranosyl-1,2,4-triazine-3,5(2*H*,4*H*)-dione.
$C_8H_{11}N_3O_6$=245.2.

CAS — 54-25-1.

Uses. Azauridine is an antineoplastic agent which acts as an antimetabolite (see p.171) and interferes with pyrimidine biosynthesis to retard the formation of cell nucleic acids. It was formerly tried in the treatment of acute leukaemia.

1814-j

Azetepa. Azatepa; NSC 64826. *PP*-Bis(aziridin-1-yl)-*N*-ethyl-*N*-1,3,4-thiadiazol-2-ylphosphinamide.
$C_8H_{14}N_5OPS$=259.3.

CAS — 125-45-1.

Azetepa is an antineoplastic agent with properties similar to those of thiotepa (p.228). It was formerly given by mouth in doses of 10 to 30 mg daily in the treatment of various malignant conditions.

Manufacturers
Lederle, USA.

1815-z

Bleomycin Sulphate.

The sulphates of a mixture of basic antineoplastic glycopeptide antibiotics, including bleomycin A_2 and B_2, obtained by the growth of *Streptomyces verticillus* or by any other means. It has a mol. wt of about 1400.

CAS — 11056-06-7 (bleomycin); 9041-93-4 (sulphate).

Pharmacopoeias. U.S. includes Sterile Bleomycin Sulphate. *Jap.* includes Bleomycin Hydrochloride.

A cream-coloured amorphous powder. It loses not more than 6% of its weight when dried. Very **soluble** in water. A solution in water containing 10 units per ml has a pH of 4.5 to 6. **Incompatible** with amino acids, aminophylline, ascorbic acid, dexamethasone, frusemide, riboflavine, and agents containing sulphydryl groups.

Units. One unit of bleomycin is approximately equivalent to 1 mg of bleomycin.

Sterile Bleomycin Sulfate (*U.S.P.*) contains 1.5 to 2 units of bleomycin in each mg.

It was noted that a freeze-dried preparation of bleomycin complex A_2/B_2 is now available for standardisation. The material is extremely hygroscopic and potency should be defined on the basis of the number of international units per ampoule. It was suggested that there is a need for an international reference material for bleomycin A_5.— Thirtieth Report of WHO Expert Committee on Biological Standardization, *Tech. Rep. Ser. Wld Hlth Org. No. 638*, 1979.

Adverse Effects and Treatment. For an outline of the adverse effects experienced with antineoplastic agents and immunosuppressants and general guidelines for their treatment, see Antineoplastic Agents, p.171 and p.174.

The most frequent side-effects with bleomycin involve the skin and mucous membranes and include rash, pruritus, vesiculation, hyperkeratosis, nail changes, striae, and stomatitis. There is little depression of the bone marrow. Local reactions, thrombophlebitis, and fever may follow parenteral administration.

The most serious delayed effect is pulmonary toxicity; pneumonitis and fibrosis occurs in about 10% of patients and produces an overall mortality-rate of 1% of patients treated with bleomycin. Acute reactions with hyperpyrexia and cardiorespiratory collapse have been reported in patients with lymphoma.

Allergy and anaphylaxis. The Boston Collaborative Drug Surveillance Program monitored consecutively 32 812 medical inpatients. Drug-induced anaphylaxis occurred in 1 of 54 patients given bleomycin.— J. Porter and H. Jick, *Lancet*, 1977, *1*, 587.

Endotoxin equivalent to 50 ng per ml was found in 2 samples of bleomycin and could account for pyrogen reactions.— D. Fumarola, *Farmaco, Edn prat.*, 1977, *32*, 444.

Individual reports of allergic reactions to bleomycin: B. T. Alcorn, *Can. J. Hosp. Pharm.*, 1980, *33*, 92.

Effects on the ears. Bleomycin may be ototoxic when it is given in high dosage.— J. Ballantyne, *Audiology*, 1973, *12*, 325.

Effects on respiratory function. Pulmonary fibrosis is a well-recognised side-effect of treatment with bleomycin and is usually irreversible; patients receiving cumulative doses of more than 150 mg should be observed carefully. Pulmonary toxicity is enhanced when bleomycin and thoracic irradiation are administered concomitantly (R. Catane *et al.*, *Int. J. Radiat. Oncol. Biol. Phys.*, 1979, *5*, 1513) or sequentially (M.L. Samuels *et al.*, *J. Am. med. Ass.*, 1976, *235*, 1117) and when bleomycin is given in association with high oxygen concentrations (P.L. Goldiner *et al.*, *Br. med. J.*, 1978, *1*, 1664). K. Nygaard *et al.*, (*Cancer*, 1978, *41*, 17) found an increased risk of serious postoperative pulmonary disease in patients treated for oesophageal cancer with bleomycin and radiotherapy followed by surgery and oxygen ventilation postoperatively; 3 of 8 patients so treated died of interstitial pneumonitis and fibrosis within 6 weeks of operation.— R. B. Weiss and F. M. Muggia, *Am. J. Med.*, 1980, *68*, 259.

Three patients developed hypersensitivity pneumonitis after treatment with bleomycin. Since all the patients responded to therapy with prednisone it was suggested that hypersensitivity pneumonitis induced by bleomycin should be regarded as a separate entity from interstitial pneumonitis which seldom responds to treatment with corticosteroids.— P. Y. Holoye *et al.*, *Ann. intern. Med.*, 1978, *88*, 47.

Further reports of pulmonary reactions associated with bleomycin: M. A. Luna *et al.*, *Am. J. clin. Path.*, 1972, *58*, 501; H. F. Krous and W. B. Hamlin, *Archs Path.*, 1973, *95*, 407; S. Adler *et al.* (letter), *J. Am. med. Ass.*, 1976, *235*, 2814; C. Haas *et al.*, *Thérapie*, 1976, *31*, 723; J. R. Iacovino *et al.*, *J. Am. med. Ass.*, 1976, *235*, 1253; A. Burkhardt *et al.*, *Dt. med. Wschr.*, 1977, *102*, 281; F. Frey *et al.*, *Schweiz. med. Wschr.*, 1977, *107*, 1418; W. G. Brown *et al.*, *J. Am. med. Ass.*, 1978, *239*, 2012 (also mitomycin).

Effects on the skin. Linear streaking of the torso and arms appeared over areas of pruritus in 2 patients receiving bleomycin. Streaking could be induced by placing an adhesive dressing on selected skin sites after the drug had been given.— B. B. Lowitz (letter), *New Engl. J. Med.*, 1975, *292*, 1300.

A report of contracture formation associated with the subcutaneous administration of bleomycin.— J. C. Kimball and A. Cangir, *Cancer Treat. Rep.*, 1979, *63*, 552.

Effects on the vascular system. Raynaud's symptoms developed in a patient 3 and 7 months after treatment with bleomycin and radiotherapy.— B. Sundstrup (letter), *Med. J. Aust.*, 1978, *2*, 266. For reports of Raynaud's phenomenon occurring after treatment with bleomycin and vinblastine, see C. Teutsch *et al.*, *Cancer Treat. Rep.*, 1977, *61*, 925; D. P. Chernicoff *et al.*, *ibid.*, 1978, *62*, 570; A. R. Soble, *ibid.*

Precautions. For reference to the precautions necessary with antineoplastic agents and immunosuppressants, see Antineoplastic Agents, p.175.

Bleomycin should be given cautiously to patients with renal impairment. Extreme caution is necessary when treating patients with pulmonary incapacity. Respiratory function should be monitored in all patients. Because of the risk of anaphylaxis patients with lymphomas should receive low doses initially. Elderly patients should also receive low doses. Contact with skin should be avoided.

Mucosal reactions may be enhanced when bleomycin is given in association with radiotherapy and doses may need to be reduced.

In dogs and monkeys bleomycin caused skin lesions at pressure sites. It is therefore desirable to watch pressure sites carefully in patients treated with bleomycin.— J. R. Baker *et al.*, *Toxic. appl. Pharmac.*, 1973, *25*, 190.

Absorption and Fate. Following the intramuscular or intravenous injection of 15 mg bleomycin, peak plasma concentrations of about 1 and 3 µg per ml respectively have been reported. Up to 40% of a dose is excreted unchanged in the urine within 24 hours.

Continuous intravenous infusions of bleomycin 30 mg daily for 4 to 5 days resulted in an average steady state plasma concentration of 146 ng per ml, generally in 24 hours, in 6 cancer patients and initial and terminal half-lives of 1.3 and 8.9 hours respectively were found after the termination of infusions. A similar patient, but with impaired renal function, attained a steady state plasma concentration of about 1 µg per ml and half-lives of 2 and 33 hours respectively. In patients with normal renal function about 60% of the administered dose was eliminated in the urine, probably by glomerular filtration up to 48 hours after infusion. Low concentrations of bleomycin were found in the saliva of 2 patients. Since overall plasma clearance was generally greater than renal clearance a non-renal mechanism is also important in bleomycin elimination.— A. Broughton *et al.*, *Cancer*,

1977, *40,* 2772.

A study of the pharmacokinetics of bleomycin given by intravenous bolus injection to 9 patients with advanced cancer in a mean dose of 15 mg per m^2 body-surface. Eight patients had normal renal function and mean initial and terminal plasma half-lives were 24 minutes and 4 hours respectively; 24-hour urinary excretion accounted for about 45% of the dose in 7 patients. In one patient with moderately severe renal failure (serum creatinine of 1.5 mg per 100 ml) plasma half-lives were 74 and 624 minutes and only 12% of the dose was excreted in the urine in 24 hours.— D. S. Alberts *et al., Cancer Chemother. Pharmac.,* 1978, *1,* 177.

Further references to the pharmacokinetics of bleomycin: T. Hayakawa *et al., J. Neurol. Neurosurg. Psychiat.,* 1976, *39,* 341 (uptake of bleomycin by brain tumours); W. G. Kramer *et al., J. clin. Pharmac.,* 1978, *18,* 346.

Uses. Bleomycin is an antineoplastic antibiotic which binds to DNA and causes strand scissions. It is used in squamous cell carcinomas, including those of the cervix, oesophagus, and head and neck, in Hodgkin's disease and other lymphomas, and in malignant neoplasms of the testis. It is also used in carcinoma of the bladder, lung, and thyroid, and in the treatment of malignant effusions. Bleomycin is often used in association with other antineoplastic agents. In Hodgkin's disease it is given with doxorubicin, vinblastine, and dacarbazine. Treatment schedules of bleomycin, vinblastine, and cisplatin are used in testicular tumours. See also under Choice of Antineoplastic Agent, p.175.

Tumour localisation may be carried out with a complex of bleomycin and indium-111; a complex with cobalt-57 has also been used.

Bleomycin can be administered by subcutaneous, intramuscular, intravenous, and intra-arterial injection. The usual dose is 15 to 60 mg weekly in divided doses or 10 to 20 mg per m^2 body-surface once or twice weekly to a total dose of 300 mg. Elderly patients should receive doses in the lower ranges and even smaller doses should be used in elderly patients with lymphomas. Remissions in Hodgkin's disease have been maintained with a weekly dose of 5 mg. A continuous intravenous infusion of 15 mg per 24 hours for up to 10 days or 30 mg per 24 hours for up to 5 days has also been used in squamous cell carcinoma and testicular tumours.

If intramuscular injections are painful they may be given in a 1% solution of lignocaine.

Reviews of bleomycin: H. Umezawa, *Lloydia,* 1977, *40,* 67; L. E. Goldberg, *Antibiotiki,* 1978, *23,* 648; J. M. Bennett and S. D. Reich, *Ann. intern. Med.,* 1979, *90,* 945.

Action. References to the use of bleomycin as a cell synchronising agent.— S. C. Barranco *et al., Cancer Res.,* 1973, *33,* 882; R. B. Livingston and J. S. Hart, *A. Rev. Pharmac. & Toxic.,* 1977, *17,* 529.

The influence of acronine, bleomycin, and cytarabine, alone and combined with radiation, on the cell cycle.— S. B. Reddy *et al., Arzneimittel-Forsch.,* 1977, *27,* 1549.

The use of penicillamine with bleomycin produced enhanced cytotoxicity in *rodents* without additional toxicity. No toxicity, apart from one case of uncharacteristic leucopenia, occurred in patients. It was considered that chelatable copper might reduce the effectiveness of bleomycin *in vivo* and that removing this copper could have beneficial effects.— A. W. Preece *et al.* (letter), *Lancet,* 1977, *1,* 953. Studies *in vitro* confirmed the hypothesis that bleomycin is more cytotoxic in cells that have been treated with the copper chelator diethyldithiocarbamate.— P. S. Lin *et al.* (letter), *Lancet,* 1979, *1,* 777. Lowering of copper concentrations does not affect the toxicity of bleomycin towards whole cells, therefore an alternate explanation must be found for enhancement of the cytotoxic effect of bleomycin by prior administration of penicillamine.— J. Lunec and A. D. Nunn (letter), *Lancet,* 1979, *2,* 739.

Administration in renal insufficiency. The dose of bleomycin should be reduced to 75% in patients with a glomerular filtration-rate between 10 and 50 ml per minute and to 50% when the rate is less than 10 ml per minute. Bleomycin is not removed by haemodialysis.— W. M. Bennett *et al., Ann. intern. Med.,* 1980, *93,* 286.

Further references: S. T. Crooke *et al.,, Cancer Treat. Rep.,* 1977, *61,* 1631 (effects of variations in renal function on the clinical pharmacology of bleomycin); *idem, Cancer,* 1977, *39,* 1430.

Blood disorders, non-malignant. Autoimmune cytopenia in 2 patients with lymphomas in remission was successfully treated with bleomycin after conventional therapy had failed.— E. A. Phillips *et al.* (letter), *New Engl. J. Med.,* 1980, *302,* 1031.

Hodgkin's disease and other lymphomas. Bleomycin was given to 100 patients, 54 with Hodgkin's disease, 17 with lymphosarcoma, 22 with histiocytic lymphoma, and 7 with mycosis fungoides. The dose was usually 15 mg twice weekly and the total dose averaged 200 mg (range 60 to 810 mg). Complete and partial remissions respectively occurred in the 4 groups as follows: 2 and 14; 1 and 6; 0 and 8; and 1 and 3. Pyrexia occurred in 40 patients, skin lesions of varied appearance in 27, nausea and vomiting in 15, and stomatitis in 9. Alopecia was uncommon. Bone marrow toxicity was low; only 4 patients showed any significant fall in the peripheral blood count.—European Organization for Research on the Treatment of Cancer, Co-operative Group for Leukaemia and Reticulocytosis, *Br. med. J.,* 1972, *1,* 285.

See also Choice of Antineoplastic Agent, p.175.

Malignant effusions. Preliminary results of a multicentre study involving 153 patients indicate that bleomycin is well tolerated and is effective as palliative treatment of malignant effusions. Aspiration of effusions was followed by an intracavitary injection of 30 to 150 mg of bleomycin in 100 ml of physiological saline; the most usual dose was 60 mg. An overall response-rate of 58% was attained in 117 evaluable patients; pleural effusions responding better (63%) than peritoneal effusions (49%). The two most common side-effects were fever (8%) and pain at the the site of injection (10%).— M. J. Ostrowski and G. M. Halsall (letter), *Br. med. J.,* 1980, *281,* 64. See also W. T. Berrill, *ibid.,* 459; M. J. Ostrowski (letter), *ibid.,* 681.

Further reference to bleomycin in the management of malignant effusions: W. Paladine *et al., Cancer,* 1976, *38,* 1903.

See also under Choice of Antineoplastic Agent, p.180.

Malignant neoplasms. Bleomycin was administered to 237 patients with tumours in the visible and actively growing phase. In 25 patients with tumours of the head and neck it was given by arterial perfusion in a daily dose of 10 to 20 mg per m^2 body-surface for 6 to 14 days. The remaining patients received intramuscular or intravenous injections of bleomycin. Bleomycin was more effective than other drugs against squamous cell cancer of the skin, cancer of the penis, vulva, oesophagus, and uterine cervix, melanoma, and mycosis fungoides. Complete regressions occurred in squamous cell cancer of the skin, cancer of the penis, and mycosis fungoides. For choriocarcinoma of the testis and neoplasms of the upper respiratory tract and upper digestive tract, bleomycin was at least as effective as other chemotherapeutic drugs. It was less active than other drugs against breast and ovarian carcinomas.—Clinical Screening Co-operative Group of the European Organization for Research on the Treatment of Cancer, *Br. med. J.,* 1970, *2,* 643.

In a random controlled study of 70 patients with advanced squamous cell carcinoma, 34 patients received bleomycin 30 mg intramuscularly twice weekly to a total of 300 mg where possible and the rest received conventional cytotoxic therapy. No advantage was found for bleomycin over conventional cytotoxic therapy. If bleomycin was to advance the treatment of squamous cell carcinoma it would only be in association with other drugs or with radiotherapy.—Report of MRC Working Party on Bleomycin, *Br. med. J.,* 1976, *1,* 188.

Further references to the use of bleomycin in various malignant neoplasms: K. E. Halnan *et al., Br. med. J.,* 1972, *4,* 635; A. Yagoda *et al., Ann. intern. Med.,* 1972, *77,* 861; M. C. Huntington *et al., Cancer,* 1973, *31,* 153 (intra-arterial infusions); F. O. Stephens, *Med. J. Aust.,* 1973, *1,* 1277; D. R. Hunt (letter), *ibid., 2,* 296; F. O. Stephens, *Med. J. Aust.,* 1974, *2,* 587; V. Shanta and S. Krishnamurthi, *Clin. Radiol.,* 1980, *31,* 617 (bleomycin and radiotherapy in oral cancer).

See also under Malignant Neoplasms, in Choice of Antineoplastic Agent, p.180.

Malignant neoplasms of the bladder. In a 76-year-old man malignant cells were present in the urine after resection of several tumours from the bladder. He was treated weekly with bleomycin, 30 mg in 60 ml saline instilled into the bladder and left for 2 hours. After 8 weeks there were no malignant cells and the patient remained asymptomatic.— N. Sadoughi *et al.* (letter), *J. Am. med. Ass.,* 1973, *226,* 465.

Skin disorders. Bleomycin in a total dose of 315 mg given in single doses of 15 mg by intra-arterial injection, initially 5 times weekly reducing in frequency over 6 weeks was successful in the treatment of a patient with oral florid papillomatosis.— M. Hagedorn *et al., Archs Derm.,* 1978, *114,* 1083.

Bleomycin applied topically produced a complete response in 4 of 7 patients with Paget's disease of the vulva, and a partial response in another. Treatment consisted of twice-daily topical application of an ointment containing bleomycin 3.5% for 2 weeks, a break for 4 to 6 weeks, and then another course. No patient received more than 4 courses. Recurrence in one patient was successfully re-treated with bleomycin. One patient developed hypotension and urticaria and was withdrawn from treatment.— W. G. Watring *et al., Cancer,* 1978, *41,* 10.

Warts. A report of the successful use of intralesional injections of bleomycin in the treatment of warts. An overall cure-rate of more than 99% was achieved when bleomycin was injected into the base of 1052 warts, including mosaic, plantar, common, plane, and eponychial warts. An injection of 0.1 ml of a solution of bleomycin 1 mg per ml in physiological saline was repeated every 4 weeks, if necessary, to a maximum total dose of 2 mg.— P. H. Shumack and M. J. Haddock, *Aust. J. Derm.,* 1979, *20,* 41. See also L. G. Abbott, *Aust. J. Derm.,* 1978, *19,* 69.

Preparations

Sterile Bleomycin Sulfate *(U.S.P.).* Bleomycin sulphate suitable for parenteral use. It contains 1.5 to 2 units of bleomycin per mg. It contains 60 to 70% of bleomycin A_2, 25 to 32% of bleomycin B_2, and not more than 1% of bleomycin B_4; the content of bleomycin A_2 and B_2 is not less than 90% of total bleomycin.

Reconstituted solutions of bleomycin in sodium chloride injection or dextrose injection are reported to be stable for 24 hours at room temperature, or 7 days if refrigerated.

Bleomycin, Lundbeck *(Lundbeck, UK).* Bleomycin sulphate, available in ampoules each containing the equivalent of 15 mg of bleomycin, for preparing injections. (Also available as Bleomycin in *Denm., Norw., Swed., Switz.*).

Other Proprietary Names

Blenoxane *(Austral., Canad., S.Afr., USA)*; Bleo Oil *(Jap.)*; Bleomicina *(Ital., Spain)*; Bléomycine *(Belg., Fr.)*; Bleomycinum *(Ger.)*; Bleo-S *(Jap.)*; Blocamicina *(hydrochloride) (Arg.)*; Verbublen *(Canad.).*

1816-c

Broxuridine. BUDR; NSC 38297. 5-Bromo-2′-deoxyuridine; 5-Bromo-1-(2-deoxy-β-D-ribofuranosyl)pyrimidine-2,4(1*H*,3*H*)-dione.
$C_9H_{11}BrN_2O_5$=307.1.

CAS — 59-14-3.

A white crystalline powder. Sparingly **soluble** in water and methyl alcohol.

Uses. Broxuridine is an antineoplastic agent which acts as an antimetabolite (p.171). It has been given by intra-arterial infusion in association with radiotherapy in the treatment of tumours of the head and neck. Broxuridine has been tried in the treatment of encephalitis.

In 135 patients with brain tumours who were treated with continuous infusions of broxuridine in doses of 1 g daily together with an antimetabolite such as methotrexate and irradiation, the lives of the patients were prolonged and the quality of most lives was much improved.— K. Sano *et al., J. Am. med. Ass.,* 1972, *220,* 1289. See also *J. Am. med. Ass.,* 1966, *196* (May 16), A.45.

Broxuridine was reported to enhance the activity of radiation against cancer cells *in vitro* and in *animals* but clinical value has not been proven.— T. L. Phillips, *Cancer,* 1977, *39,* 987.

Proprietary Names

Radibud *(Takeda, Jap.).*

1817-k

Busulphan *(B.P.).* Busulfan *(U.S.P.)*; Busulfanum; CB 2041; GT 41; NSC 750; WR 19508; Myelosan. Tetramethylene di(methanesulphonate); Butane-1,4-diol di(methanesulphonate).

$C_6H_{14}O_6S_2$=246.3.

CAS — 55-98-1.

Pharmacopoeias. In *Br., Cz., Ind., Int., Jap., Jug., Nord., Rus., Turk.,* and *U.S.*

A white, almost odourless, crystalline powder. M.p. 115° to 118° **Soluble** 1 in 750 of water and 1 in 25 of acetone; slightly soluble in alcohol. **Store** in airtight containers. Protect from light.

CAUION. *Busulphan is irritant; avoid contact with skin and mucous membranes.*

Adverse Effects and Treatment. For an outline of the adverse effects experienced with antineoplastic agents and immunosuppressants and general guidelines for their treatment, see Antineoplastic Agents, p.171 and p.174.

The most important side-effects of busulphan in high dosage are thrombocytopenia and haemorrhage symptoms. Large doses may also cause irreversible bone-marrow depression which may not become apparent for several months after the initiation of therapy. The nadir of granulocytes has been reported at 11 to 30 days with recovery occurring over 24 to 54 days.

Interstitial pulmonary fibrosis, known as 'busulphan lung', and cataract formation can occur on prolonged treatment as can hyperpigmentation which may be part of a syndrome simulating Addison's disease.

Adrenal suppression. A syndrome resembling Addison's disease with hyperpigmentation of the skin, severe weakness, fatigue, anorexia, nausea, and loss of weight has followed prolonged treatment with busulphan but without any evidence of adrenocortical failure.— B. P. Harrold, *Br. med. J.*, 1966, *1*, 463.

Further references.— R. J. Vivacqua *et al., Ann. intern. Med.*, 1967, *67*, 380; Y. Sidi *et al., J. Am. med. Ass.*, 1977, *238*, 1951.

Effects on the bladder. A report of haemorrhagic cystitis associated with the use of busulphan.— R. J. Millard, *Br. J. Urol.*, 1978, *50*, 210.

Effects on the eyes. Busulphan is known to cause cataracts in *animals;* posterior subcapsular lens opacities and early lens changes in patients with chronic granulocytic leukaemia have been associated with the duration of disease and treatment with busulphan.— S. M. Podos and G. P. Canellos, *Am. J. Ophthal.*, 1969, *68*, 500. See also M. P. Ravindranathan *et al., Br. med. J.*, 1972, *1*, 218 (bilateral cataracts in a patient given busulphan for about 4 years); Y. Sidi *et al., J. Am. med. Ass.*, 1977, *238*, 1951 (bilateral cataracts and severe sicca syndrome in a patient given busulphan for 9 years).

Effects on the liver. Jaundice in the terminal phase of chronic granulocytic leukaemia in a 31-year-old man was attributed to busulphan which had been taken for 6 years.— J. C. E. Underwood *et al.* (letter), *Br. med. J.*, 1971, *1*, 556.

Busulphan toxicity involving the liver, with 'busulphan lung', in an elderly man who had taken busulphan for 54 months for myeloid leukaemia, might have been a contributory factor in the development of portal hypertension.— M. D. Foadi *et al., Postgrad. med. J.*, 1977, *53*, 267.

Effects on respiratory function. The syndrome of 'busulphan lung' or fibrosing alveolitis is well established but relatively rare and pulmonary fibrosis has generally been reported in adults after several months or years of treatment. For reviews, see W. A. Burns *et al., Am. Rev. resp. Dis.*, 1970, *101*, 408; H. D. Sostman *et al., Am. J. Med.*, 1977, *62*, 608.

A report of 'busulphan lung' in a 16-month-old child.— M. Pearl, *Am. J. Dis. Child.*, 1977, *131*, 650.

Reversible pulmonary fibrosis occurred in a patient after only 6 weeks of treatment with busulphan. When uramustine was subsequently substituted, pulmonary toxicity occurred again.— D. G. Hankins *et al., Chest*, 1978, *73*, 415.

Further reports of pulmonary toxicity with busulphan.— B. E. Heard and R. A. Cooke, *Thorax*, 1968, *23*, 187; W. A. Littler and C. Ogilvie, *Br. med. J.*, 1970, *4*, 530; H. J. Woodliff and L. R. Finlay-Jones, *Med. J. Aust.*, 1972, *2*, 719; A. Weinberger *et al., J. Am. med. Ass.*, 1975, *231*, 495 (endocardial fibrosis as well as interstitial pulmonary fibrosis); A. R. Soble and H. Perry, *Am. J. Roentg.*, 1977, *128*, 15 (associated with radiotherapy).

Effects on the skin. Itchy, erythematous, maculopapular skin eruptions which occurred in 2 patients receiving allopurinol and busulphan, although characteristic of allopurinol, were found to be associated with busulphan administration.— M. J. Leyden and A. Manoharan (letter), *Lancet*, 1978, *2*, 797.

Pregnancy and the neonate. Reports of a teratogenic effect with busulphan.— I. Diamond *et al., Pediatrics*, 1960, *25*, 85 (mercaptopurine was also taken); J. E. Sokal and E. M. Lessmann, *J. Am. med. Ass.*, 1960, *172*, 1765 (and mercaptopurine); A. Abramovici *et al., Teratology*, 1978, *18*, 241 (myeloschisis in a 6-week-old embryo).

In *rats* busulphan inhibited development of sperm but did not affect the fertility of female *rats*; offspring of pregnant *rats* given busulphan 5 to 6 days before full-term birth were sterile.— R. E. Marsh and W. E. Howard, *Bull. Wld Hlth Org.*, 1973, *48*, 309.

See also Precautions, below.

Precautions. For reference to the precautions necessary with antineoplastic agents and immunosuppressants, see Antineoplastic Agents, p.175.

Since secondary gout occurred in up to 10% of patients with polycythaemia vera given busulphan, allopurinol was recommended for routine prophylaxis.— *Drug & Ther. Bull.*, 1975, *13*, 73.

Pregnancy and the neonate. *Second trimester.* A report of intra-uterine growth retardation of an infant whose mother had been given busulphan from 20 weeks gestation.— S. J. Boros and J. W. Reynolds, *Am. J. Obstet. Gynec.*, 1977, *129*, 111.

See also Adverse Effects, above.

Absorption and Fate. Busulphan is readily absorbed from the gastro-intestinal tract and rapidly disappears from the blood. It is largely excreted in the urine as sulphur-containing metabolites.

Busulphan was rapidly cleared from the plasma at first, then gradually accumulated with repeated dosage. Less then 50% of the total dose was excreted in the urine.— H. Vodopick *et al., J. Lab. clin. Med.*, 1969, *73*, 266, per *J. Am. med. Ass.*, 1969, *207*, 2312.

Busulphan was hydrolysed to 4-methanesulphonyloxybutanol and then cyclised to tetrahydrofuran, but the biological action of busulphan is not considered to be due to the intermediate.— P. W. Feit and N. Rastrup-Anderson, *J. pharm. Sci.*, 1973, *62*, 1007.

Uses. Busulphan is an antineoplastic agent, with an alkylating action unlike that of the nitrogen mustards, and having a selective depressant action on bone marrow. In small doses, it depresses granulocytopoiesis and to a lesser extent thrombocytopoiesis but has little effect on lymphocytes. With larger doses, severe bone-marrow depression eventually ensues.

Because of its selective action, busulphan is used in the treatment of chronic myeloid leukaemia. It provides symptomatic relief with a reduction in spleen size and a general feeling of well-being. The fall in leucocyte count is usually accompanied by a rise in the haemoglobin concentration. True remission is not induced.

Busulphan has been used in patients with polycythaemia vera who are resistant to phosphorus-32.

See also under Choice of Antineoplastic Agent, p.175.

The usual dosage of busulphan in chronic myeloid leukaemia is 4 mg or 60 µg per kg body-weight, whichever is the less, daily by mouth, continued until the white cell count has fallen to between 20 000 and 25 000 per mm^3. It should be discontinued earlier if the platelet count falls below 100 000 per mm^3. Higher doses may be given if the response after 3 weeks is inadequate; 6 to 8 mg daily has been given in refractory cases but this increases the risk of irreversible damage to the bone marrow and calls for special vigilance. Children may be given 60 µg per kg once daily.

Large doses cause a rapid fall in granulocytes but with small doses this may not occur for several weeks. Complete blood counts should be made every week and the trends followed closely; if haemorrhagic tendencies occur or there is a steep fall in the white cell count indicating severe bone-marrow depression, busulphan should be withdrawn until marrow function has returned.

Maintenance treatment with doses of 0.5 to 2 mg daily may be given, especially when remission is shorter than 3 months, the aim being to maintain a white cell count of 10 000 to 15 000 per mm^3. Alternatively treatment may be discontinued until the count reaches 50 000 per mm^3.

Blood disorders, non-malignant. Results of a study involving 268 patients with polycythaemia vera indicated that although the median duration of remission of 48 months in patients receiving busulphan is superior to that of those receiving phosphorus-32 (32 months) the median survival times of the 2 groups did not differ significantly.— G. Mathé (letter), *New Engl. J. Med.*, 1978, *298*, 279. Dosage correction.— N. I. Berlin (letter), *ibid.*, 913.

Further references.— I. Brodsky *et al., Br. J. Haemat.*, 1968, *14*, 351 (polycythaemia vera); J. Levine and P. D. Swanson, *Neurology, Minneap.*, 1968, *18*, 711 (thrombocytosis).

See also under Choice of Antineoplastic Agent, p.175.

Leukaemia. The successful treatment of a 45-year-old man with apparent eosinophilic leukaemia, possibly an unusual sign of hypersensitivity, with busulphan and prednisolone for 16 months. Haematological values had been normal, without treatment, for 3 years.— P. J. Hamilton and A. A. Dawson, *Br. med. J.*, 1977, *1*, 1195.

Leukaemia, chronic myeloid. In a comparative study of treatment for chronic myeloid leukaemia, the results after a minimum follow-up of 3 years indicated that busulphan was superior to radiotherapy in respect of survival and efficacy in restoring and maintaining satisfactory haemoglobin concentrations. Initially, busulphan and radiotherapy were equally effective in reducing the size of the spleen.—Report of the MRC Working Party for Therapeutic Trials in Leukaemia, *Br. med. J.*, 1968, *1*, 201. Preliminary notification of an MRC study to compare a 2-drug regimen of busulphan and thioguanine with standard busulphan therapy in chronic myeloid leukaemia.— *Lancet*, 1980, *1*, 889.

Encouraging results were obtained in 7 patients with chronic granulocytic leukaemia using a regimen involving busulphan 2 mg daily in association with mercaptopurine, 50 mg daily if allopurinol was also given, or 100 mg daily if not. The therapy was well tolerated. Although a precipitous fall in the nucleated-cell count occurred this did not continue once the normal range was reached.— N. C. Allan *et al.* (letter), *Lancet*, 1978, *2*, 523.

See also under Choice of Antineoplastic Agent, p.175.

Pregnancy and the neonate. *First trimester.* An apparently normal baby, apart from transient anaemia and neutropenia and low birth-weight, was born to a woman who received busulphan from the 8th week of pregnancy to term.— M. Dugdale and A. T. Fort, *J. Am. med. Ass.*, 1967, *199*, 131. See also N. Uhl *et al., Dt. med. Wschr.*, 1968, *93*, 1856.

See also under Adverse Effects and Precautions, above.

Preparations

Busulfan Tablets *(U.S.P.).* Tablets containing busulphan.

Busulphan Tablets *(B.P.).* Tablets containing busulphan. They are compression-coated or sugar-coated.

Myleran *(Wellcome, UK).* Busulphan, available as tablets of 0.5 and 2 mg. (Also available as Myleran in *Austral., Belg., Canad., Denm., Ger., Ital., Neth., Norw., S.Afr., Switz., USA*).

Other Proprietary Names

Misulban *(Fr., Ital.).*

1818-a

Carboquone. 2,5-Bis(aziridin-1-yl)-3-(2-hydroxy-1-methoxyethyl)-6-methyl-*p*-benzoquinone carbamate.

$C_{15}H_{19}N_3O_5$=321.3.

CAS — 24279-91-2.

Red to reddish-brown odourless crystals or crystalline powder. M.p. about 202° with decomposition. Practically **insoluble** in water; very slightly soluble in acetone and dehydrated alcohol; slightly soluble in chloroform.

Carboquone is an alkylating agent (see p.171) which has been used in the treatment of malignant diseases.

Proprietary Names

Esquinon *(Sankyo, Jap.).*

1819-t

Carmustine. BCNU; NSC 409962; WR 139021. 1,3-Bis(2-chloroethyl)-1-nitrosourea. $C_5H_9Cl_2N_3O_2$=214.1.

CAS — 154-93-8.

A white powder. M.p. 27°; exposure to this or higher temperatures results in the liquefaction and decomposition of carmustine. **Soluble** 1 in 250 of water and 1 in 2 of alcohol. **Store** at 2° to 8°.

Solutions for injection may be prepared by dissolving 100 mg of carmustine in 3 ml of absolute alcohol and adding 27 ml of Water for Injections to produce a clear colourless solution with a pH of 5.6 to 6.0. When further diluted with sodium chloride injection or dextrose injection the resulting solution is reported to be stable for 48 hours if protected from light and stored at 4°.

Stability in solution. Studies on the stability of carmustine in various solutions.— T. L. Loo *et al.*, *J. pharm. Sci.*, 1966, *55*, 492; P. A. Laskar and J. W. Ayres, *ibid.*, 1977, *66*, 1073; *idem*, 1076.

Adverse Effects and Treatment. For an outline of the adverse effects experienced with antineoplastic agents and immunosuppressants and general guidelines for their treatment, see Antineoplastic Agents, p.171 and p.174. Delayed and cumulative bone-marrow depression is the most frequent and serious side-effect of carmustine. Platelets and leucocytes are affected with nadirs occurring at 4 to 6 weeks after administration; although thrombocytopenia is usually more severe, leucopenia may also be dose-limiting. Other side-effects reported include pulmonary fibrosis, renal and hepatic damage, and optic neuritis. Venous irritation may follow intravenous injection and transient hyperpigmentation has been noted after contact of a solution with the skin.

Effects on the eyes. Optic neuritis has been associated with the concomitant use of carmustine and procarbazine.— R. McLennan and H. RTaylor, *Med. Pediat. Oncol.*, 1978, *4*, 43.

Effects on respiratory function. In an analysis of 794 patients who were treated with carmustine, cyclophosphamide, and prednisone, in combination with other drugs, 9 developed pulmonary fibrosis. Similar symptoms developed in another patient who received carmustine and radiation therapy. Symptoms of pulmonary toxicity developed within 8 months of stopping chemotherapy in all but 1 patient, their severity appearing unrelated to the total dose of carmustine administered (between 400 and 2075 mg per m^2 body-surface). Seven patients died as a result of pulmonary toxicity.— J. R. Durant *et al.*, *Ann. intern. Med.*, 1979, *90*, 191. A view that cyclophosphamide might be responsible in the 9 patients who developed fibrosis.— J. R. Cohn (letter), *ibid.*, 856. See also R. Stillerman (letter), *ibid.*, *91*, 132; J. R. Durant (letter), *ibid.*

A retrospective study of the risk factors associated with the development of pulmonary toxicity in patients treated with carmustine. Symptomatic pulmonary disease developed in 19 of 93 patients with malignant gliomas who were treated with carmustine; 3 of the patients died from their pulmonary disease. A history of lung disease, the total dose of carmustine, and duration of treatment were the most important factors in predicting lung toxicity. The optimum dose and duration of treatment are not yet clear but in the light of this study a cumulative dose of carmustine limited to 1.4 g per m^2 body-surface is recommended and patients are not given carmustine if they have pre-existing symptomatic pulmonary disease or if tests of base-line pulmonary function show a forced vital capacity or a diffusing capacity below 70% of predicted.— P. A. Aronin *et al.*, *New Engl. J. Med.*, 1980, *303*, 183.

Reports of fatal pulmonary fibrosis developing over a relatively short period in patients receiving carmustine as the sole antineoplastic agent.— D. L. Sweet (letter), *Ann. intern. Med.*, 1979, *91*, 132; G. A. Patten *et al.*, *J. Am. med. Ass.*, 1980, *244*, 687.

Precautions. For reference to the precautions necessary with antineoplastic agents and immunosuppressants, see Antineoplastic Agents, p.175.

A suggestion that, if the long-term use of nitrosoureas is being considered, creatinine clearance should be measured periodically and renal size monitored frequently.— W. E. Harmon *et al.* (letter), *New Engl. J. Med.*, 1979, *301*, 662.

For reference to risk factors associated with the pulmonary toxicity of carmustine, see Adverse Effects (above).

Interactions. Concurrent administration of streptozocin with carmustine profoundly enhanced marrow toxicity and the incidence of thrombocytopenia; therapeutic activity was not enhanced. Addition of fluorouracil to the streptozocin and carmustine regimen resulted in a comparable incidence and magnitude of thrombocytopenia to that of the 2-drug regimen, but a somewhat higher incidence of severe leucopenia.— J. J. Lokich *et al.*, *Clin. Pharmac. Ther.*, 1975, *17*, 374.

Reductions in white cell counts and platelet counts well below those normally attributed to treatment with carmustine alone were seen in 6 of 8 patients receiving their first course of carmustine and steroids in association with cimetidine given prophylactically.— R. G. Selker *et al.* (letter), *New Engl. J. Med.*, 1978, *299*, 834. See also D. N. Posnett *et al.*, *Archs intern. Med.*, 1979, *139*, 584.

Absorption and Fate. Carmustine is readily absorbed from the gastro-intestinal tract. It is rapidly metabolised, with an estimated half-life of less than 15 minutes; metabolites have a much longer half-life. Up to 48% of a dose given by mouth may be excreted in the urine within 24 hours; up to 38% of an intravenous dose may be excreted in the same period. Carmustine diffuses very readily into the cerebrospinal fluid, appearing almost immediately after intravenous injection. Very small amounts have been detected in the faeces.

Pharmacology of carmustine in man and *animals*.— V. T. DeVita *et al.*, *Clin. Pharmac. Ther.*, 1967, *8*, 566.

Uses. Carmustine is an antineoplastic agent belonging to the nitrosourea group of compounds, which are considered to function as alkylating agents. It has been used in the treatment of brain tumours, as an adjunct in meningeal leukaemia, and in combination chemotherapy for multiple myeloma, Hodgkin's disease, and other lymphomas. See also under Choice of Antineoplastic Agent, p.175.

Carmustine is given intravenously as a single dose of 200 mg per m^2 body-surface or divided into doses of 100 mg per m^2 given on 2 successive days. Doses are repeated every 6 weeks provided that blood counts have returned to acceptable levels, that is, platelets above 100 000 per mm^3 and leucocytes above 4 000 per mm^3. Subsequent doses must be adjusted according to the haematological response. Reconstituted solutions are further diluted with sodium chloride or dextrose injection and infused over 1 to 2 hours.

A brief review of carmustine.— *Med. Lett.*, 1978, *20*, 79.

Carmustine might enhance the cytotoxic effect of radiotherapy.— T. L. Phillips, *Cancer*, 1977, *39*, 987.

Malignant neoplasms of the brain. A report by M.D. Walker *et al.* (*J. Neurosurg.*, 1978, *49*, 333) concluded that patients with malignant glioma who received radiotherapy, with or without carmustine, had a significantly improved survival over those receiving only carmustine or only supportive care. In the randomised study now reported the relative benefits of radiotherapy and nitrosoureas, after surgery, were investigated further and 4 treatment regimens, semustine alone, radiotherapy alone, carmustine and radiotherapy, and semustine and radiotherapy, were compared in 358 patients. The results confirmed the benefits of radiotherapy in the treatment of malignant glioma and suggested that carmustine remains the drug of choice for chemotherapy. Semustine alone was inferior to regimens that included radiotherapy, as was carmustine previously, and semustine in combination with radiotherapy provided no advantage over carmustine and radiotherapy. Whether nitrosourea combined with radiotherapy is better than radiotherapy alone is not certain. Corticosteroids are virtually mandatory for symptomatic control in patients with malignant brain tumours but an oncolytic effect has not yet been demonstrated; preliminary results of a study of intermittent high-dose methylprednisolone, with or without carmustine, have not shown any survival benefit. On the basis of the results so far it appears best to use radiotherapy in the treatment of malignant glioma and to continue the search for chemotherapy regimens to use in association with radiotherapy.— M. D. Walker *et al.*, *New Engl. J. Med.*, 1980, *303*, 1323.

Mycosis fungoides. Studies of the urinary excretion of carmustine in 5 patients with mycosis fungoides showed that there was greater absorption of a dose of carmustine applied in a methyl alcohol solution to diseased skin than of a similar dose applied to healthy skin.— H. S. Zackheim *et al.*, *Br. J. Derm.*, 1977, *97*, 65. For earlier reports of the use of carmustine, see H. S. Zackheim, *Archs Derm.*, 1972, *106*, 177; H. S. Zackheim and E. H. Epstein, *Archs Derm.*, 1975, *111*, 1564.

Myeloma. Carmustine together with doxorubicin, both given in doses of 30 mg per m^2 body-surface area every 3 to 4 weeks, was considered useful in patients with multiple myeloma who had relapsed after more conventional treatment involving alkylating agents. Of 13 such patients, 7 responded to carmustine and doxorubicin; of these 2 had more than 75% tumour regression which was taken to be a complete remission, and 5 had partial remissions with more than 50% tumour regression.— D. S. Alberts *et al.*, *Lancet*, 1976, *1*, 926. In a study of 364 patients with plasma cell myeloma, response-rate and survival were no better with a treatment regimen of melphalan, cyclophosphamide, and carmustine given concurrently or alternately, together with prednisone, than with melphalan and prednisone taken alone.— D. E. Bergsagel *et al.*, *New Engl. J. Med.*, 1979, *301*, 743.

Further reports of treatment regimens for myeloma.— H. J. Cohen *et al.*, *Blood*, 1979, *54*, 824 (carmustine, cyclophosphamide, and prednisone).

Sarcoma. Carmustine given to 12 patients with Ewing's sarcoma produced a complete remission in 1 for 2.5 years and partial remissions with 50% shrinkage of the tumour in 4 lasting for 2 to 8 months.— J. Palma *et al.*, *Cancer*, 1972, *30*, 909, per *J. Am. med. Ass.*, 1972, *222*, 1699.

Proprietary Preparations

BiCNU *(Bristol-Myers Pharmaceuticals, UK)*. Carmustine, available as powder for preparing injections, in vials of 100 mg, with 3 ml of alcohol diluent. (Also available as BiCNU in *Canad.*, *USA*).

Other Proprietary Names

Nitrumon *(Ital.)*.

1820-l

Chlorambucil *(B.P., U.S.P.)*. CB 1348; NSC 3088; WR 139013, Chlorbutinum, 4-[4-Bis(2-chloroethyl)aminophenyl]butyric acid. $C_{14}H_{19}Cl_2NO_2$=304.2.

CAS — 305-03-3.

Pharmacopoeias. In *Br.*, *Jug.*, *Rus.*, *Turk.*, and *U.S.*

A white or off-white crystalline or granular powder with a slight odour. M.p. 64° to 69°. Practically **insoluble** in water; soluble 1 in 1.5 of alcohol, 1 in 2 of acetone, and 1 in 2.5 of chloroform; soluble in dilute solutions of alkali hydroxides. **Store** in a cool place in airtight containers. Protect from light.

CAUTION. *Chlorambucil is irritant; avoid contact with skin and mucous membranes.*

Adverse Effects and Treatment. For an outline of the adverse effects experienced with antineoplastic agents and immunosuppressants and general guidelines for their treatment, see Antineoplastic Agents, p.171 and p.174.

A reversible progressive lymphocytopenia tends to develop during treatment with chlorambucil. Neutropenia may continue to develop up to 10 days after the last dose. Irreversible bone-marrow depression can occur particularly when the total dosage for the course approaches 6.5 mg per kg body-weight.

Two patients taking chlorambucil developed symptoms suggestive of the syndrome (interstitial fibrosis, cutaneous pigmentation, and adrenal cortical insufficiency) of busulphan toxicity.— M. S. Rose, *Br. med. J.*, 1975, *2*, 123.

Effects on the bladder. Chlorambucil-induced cystitis was reported in a 73-year-old woman given 2 mg daily for over 2 years for the treatment of lymphocytic lymphoma.— D. Daoud *et al.* (letter), *Drug Intell. & clin. Pharm.*, 1977, *11*, 491.

Effects on the nervous system. Neurotoxicity associated with chlorambucil.— R. M. Sandler and M. Gonsalkorale, *Br. med. J.*, 1977, *2*, 1265 (peripheral sensorimotor neuropathy); S. A. Williams *et al.*, *J. Pediat.*, 1978, *93*, 516 (seizures in children); A. Naysmith and R. H. Robson, *Postgrad. med. J.*, 1979, *55*, 806 (focal fits).

Effects on reproductive potential. *Gonads.* Reports of azoospermia in patients treated with chlorambucil.— P. Richter *et al.*, *Cancer*, 1970, *25*, 1026; D. G. Miller, *J. Am. med. Ass.*, 1971, *217*, 1662.

Effects on respiratory function. A 73-year-old woman developed pulmonary fibrosis during treatment with chlorambucil for polycythaemia vera. Resolution of the symptoms occurred on discontinuation of the chlorambucil and treatment with corticosteroids.— S. R. Cole *et al.*, *Cancer*, 1978, *41*, 455.

Interstitial pneumonia in a 67-year-old man was associated with his treatment with chlorambucil which had been given for several years providing an approximate total dose of 7.5 g.— P. Godard *et al.*, *Chest*, 1979, *76*, 471.

Overdosage. A 2-year-old child took a tenfold overdose of chlorambucil. He recovered from moderate pancytopenia.— A. A. Green and J. L. Naiman, *Am. J. Dis. Child.*, 1968, *116*, 190, per *J. Am. med. Ass.*, 1968, *205* (Aug. 26), A113.

Precautions. For reference to the precautions necessary with antineoplastic agents and immunosuppressants, see Antineoplastic Agents, p.175.

Chlorambucil should not be administered for at least 4 weeks after treatment with radiotherapy or other antineoplastic agents unless only low doses of radiation have been given to parts remote from the bone marrow and the neutrophil and platelet counts are not depressed. The dose should be reduced if there is lymphocytic involvement of the bone marrow or if it is hypoplastic.

Absorption and Fate. Chlorambucil is reliably absorbed from the gastro-intestinal tract and is almost completely metabolised.

Preliminary pharmacokinetic data from 6 cancer patients given oral doses ranging from about 0.6 to 1.2 mg per kg body-weight indicate that chlorambucil is rapidly absorbed and cleared from plasma and is almost completely metabolised. Extremely small amounts are excreted in the urine. In 4 patients the mean terminal-phase half-life of chlorambucil was about 92 minutes with peak plasma concentrations of 1.1 µg per ml when the dose was adjusted to 0.6 mg per kg. The major metabolite of chlorambucil, phenylacetic acid mustard, was seen in plasma within 15 minutes of a dose. The mean terminal phase plasma half-life of the metabolite was about 1.6 times greater than that of chlorambucil.— D. S. Alberts *et al.*, *Cancer Treat. Rev.*, 1979, *6*, *Suppl.*, 9.

A pharmacokinetic study of chlorambucil given by mouth or intravenously to cancer patients. Although the intravenous route produced higher concentrations, absorption from the gastro-intestinal tract was consistently rapid and appeared to be complete; peak plasma concentrations were achieved in 40 to 70 minutes. An hour after administration by either route the rate of metabolism was similar and sufficient to make a contribution to the activity of the drug. Two metabolites were detected and one was identified as the β-oxidation product of chlorambucil, 2[4-*N*,*N*,-bis(2-chloroethyl)aminophenyl] acetic acid, also called phenylacetic mustard. This metabolite is known to have an alkylating action in *animals*.— A. McLean *et al.*, *Cancer Treat. Rev.*, 1979, *6*, *Suppl.*, 33.

Uses. Chlorambucil is an antineoplastic agent derived from mustine (p.222) and has a similar mode of action. It acts on lymphocytes and to a lesser extent on neutrophils and platelets. Chlorambucil is most valuable in those conditions associated with the proliferation of white blood cells, especially lymphocytes, and is used in the treatment of chronic lymphocytic leukaemia and lymphomas, including Hodgkin's disease. It is also used in Waldenström's macroglobulinaemia and in carcinoma of the breast, ovary, and testis. Chlorambucil has immunosuppressant properties and has been given in various auto-immune disorders.

See also under Choice of Antineoplastic Agent, p.175.

Chlorambucil is better tolerated than mustine hydrochloride and serious bone-marrow toxicity is not usually a problem with normal doses. Chlorambucil is administered by mouth in an average single dose of 200 µg per kg body-weight daily for 3 to 6 weeks. It is recommended that chlorambucil should be taken before food. If lymphocytic infiltration of the bone marrow is present or if the bone marrow is hypoplastic, the daily dose should not exceed 100 µg per kg.

Clinical improvement is usually evident by the third week. Once a remission has been established the patient may receive continuous maintenance with 30 to 100 µg per kg body-weight daily. However, short interrupted courses appear to be safer and are generally preferred for maintenance. A dose of 100 µg per kg daily may be adequate for the treatment of lymphosarcoma or chronic lymphocytic leukaemia; in Hodgkin's disease, 200 µg per kg daily is usually required.

Total and differential white-cell counts and haemoglobin examinations should be made each week during treatment with chlorambucil. Skin and mucous membranes should be examined for signs of haemorrhage. Many patients develop a slowly progressive lymphocytopenia during treatment but the lymphocyte count usually returns rapidly to normal on discontinuance of therapy. Neutropenia usually develops after the third week of therapy and the neutrophil count may continue to fall for about 10 days after cessation of treatment.

Blood disorders, non-malignant. *Cold-haemagglutinin disease.* Reports of the use of chlorambucil in the treatment of cold-haemagglutinin disease.— E. Hippe *et al.*, *Blood*, 1970, *35*, 68; R. S. Evans *et al.*, *Blood*, 1973, *42*, 463.

Polycythaemia vera. See under Choice of Antineoplastic Agent, p.175.

Leukaemia. The amount of tritiated thymidine incorporated into lymphocytes and the DNA of these cells taken from patients with chronic lymphocytic leukaemia was increased 3 to 5 times when the cells were suspended in a solution containing chlorambucil, and the DNA concentration per cell had increased to approximately 170% of control values.— B. T. Hill (letter), *Lancet*, 1972, *2*, 1318.

Reports of the treatment of leukaemia with chlorambucil.— A. Sawitsky *et al.*, *Blood*, 1977, *50*, 1049 (an intermittent treatment regimen for chronic lymphocytic leukaemia).

Lupus erythematosus. Five women with systemic lupus erythematosus and nephritis and 1 with systemic lupus erythematosus and vasculitis were unresponsive to or intolerant of corticosteroids. Treatment with chlorambucil was started usually with an initial dose of 4 to 6 mg daily, with reduced doses of corticosteroids; chlorambucil was gradually reduced. Treatment lasted for 24 to 64 months. All the women showed favourable biological and clinical improvement. Amenorrhoea in 4 was probably due to chlorambucil. Transient lymphopenia or neutropenia occurred in 2 patients and moderate pancytopenia in 1. The possibility of spontaneous improvement could not be excluded. There had been an earlier report of the unsuccessful use of chlorambucil in 12 patients (B. Amor *et al.*, *Nouv. Presse méd.*, 1972, *1*, 1699).— M. I. Snaith *et al.*, *Br. med. J.*, 1973, *2*, 197.

Lymphomas. *Waldenström's macroglobulinaemia.* Chlorambucil given alone or with corticosteroids appeared to be the drug of choice for the treatment of Waldenström's macroglobulinaemia; melphalan and cyclophosphamide had also been used during a study of 45 patients. The mean survival-time of about 6 years after first symptoms appeared was not affected by anaemia, serum-IgM concentration, or Bence-Jones proteinuria, but was decreased in patients with hypoalbuminaemia, increased blood-nitrogen, or abnormal liver function.— M. Krajny and W. Pruzanski, *Can. med. Ass. J.*, 1976, *114*, 899.

Ocular disorders, non-malignant. Treatment with chlorambucil led to some improvement (improved visual acuity, general condition, or reduction in steroid dosage) in 2 of 3 patients with chronic generalised uveitis, 1 of 3 with uveitis with retinal vasculitis, 3 of 5 with Behçet's disease, temporary improvement in a patient with Vogt-Koyanagi-Harada disease, probable improvement in a patient with sympathetic ophthalmitis, and no improvement in a patient with pars planitis. The dose was usually 5 mg daily initially reduced after several months to every other day usually for about 9 months. Benefit in Behçet's disease was considered the most promising.— W. J. Dinning and E. S. Perkins, *Br. J. Ophthal.*, 1975, *59*, 397. Comment.— *ibid.*, 395.

Further reports of the use of chlorambucil in ocular disorders.— M. I. Abdalla and N. El-D. Bahgat, *Br. J. Ophthal.*, 1973, *57*, 706 (Behçet's syndrome); J. G. Mamo, *Archs Ophthal., N.Y.*, 1976, *94*, 580 (Behçet's disease); D. Tricoulis, *Br. J. Ophthal.*, 1976, *60*, 55 (Behçet's disease); R. H. Andrasch *et al.*, *Archs Ophthal., N.Y.*, 1978, *96*, 247 (severe chronic uveitis).

Renal disorders, non-malignant. For the use of immunosuppressants, including chlorambucil, in the treatment of nephrotic syndrome and similar renal disorders, see Corticosteroids, p.457.

Rheumatic disorders, non-malignant. Chlorambucil 7.5 to 35 mg weekly for 71 to 77 weeks was given to 22 patients with rheumatoid arthritis who were receiving corticosteroid therapy. After 5 years 12 had full remission, 7 partial remission and 3 had died from neoplastic disorders. Corticosteroid therapy was no longer necessary in 12 patients.— P. Thorpe *et al.*, *Med. J. Aust.*, 1976, *2*, 197.

Sarcoidosis. A report of chlorambucil in the treatment of sarcoidosis.— Y. P. Kataria, *Chest*, 1980, *78*, 36.

Skin disorders, non-malignant. A favourable report of the use of chlorambucil 2 to 6 mg daily in association with prednisone 5 to 20 mg daily in 8 patients with Sézary's syndrome. Local application of aqueous solutions of mustine hydrochloride 0.025% led to further improvement in 3 patients.— L. Hamminga *et al.*, *Br. J. Derm.*, 1979, *100*, 291. See also R. K. Winkelmann and J. W. Linman, *Am. J. Med.*, 1973, *55*, 192; R. K. Winkelmann *et al.*, *Mayo Clin. Proc.*, 1974, *49*, 590.

Further reports of the use of chlorambucil in skin disorders.— R. Degos *et al.*, *Dermatologica*, 1967, *135*, 345 (Kaposi's disease); R. I. Rudolph, *Archs Derm.*, 1979, *115*, 1212 (disseminated granuloma annulare).

Wegener's granulomatosis. Complete regression of lesions and relief of symptoms occurred in 2 patients with Wegener's granulomatosis who were treated with chlorambucil only.— S. K. McIlvanie, *J. Am. med. Ass.*, 1966, *197*, 90.

See also under Choice of Antineoplastic Agent, p.175.

Preparations

Chlorambucil Tablets *(B.P.)*. Tablets containing chlorambucil. They are compression-coated or sugar-coated.

Chlorambucil Tablets *(U.S.P.)*. Tablets containing chlorambucil. Protect uncoated tablets from light.

Leukeran *(Wellcome, UK)*. Chlorambucil, available as tablets of 2 and 5 mg. Store at 2° to 8°. (Also available as Leukeran in *Austral.*, *Belg.*, *Canad.*, *Denm.*, *Ger.*, *Ital.*, *Neth.*, *Norw.*, *S.Afr.*, *Switz.*, *USA*).

Other Proprietary Names

Chloraminophène *(Fr.)*.

1821-y

Chlorozotocin. NSC 178248. 2-[3-(2-Chloroethyl)-3-nitrosoureido]-2-deoxy-D-glucopyranose.
$C_9H_{16}ClN_3O_7$=313.7.

CAS — 54749-90-5.

Chlorozotocin is an analogue of the antineoplastic agent streptozocin (p.226) and has been reported not to have a diabetogenic effect.

The pharmacology of single intravenous doses of chlorozotocin.— D. Hoth *et al.*, *Clin. Pharmac. Ther.*, 1978, *23*, 712.

Progressive normochromic normocytic anaemia was noted in a 46-year-old woman who had been given chlorozotocin 120 mg per m^2 body-surface intravenously every 6 weeks during the previous 12 months, for the treatment of bronchoalveolar carcinoma. Therapy was continued for a further 6 months, when a total dose of 2.1 g had been given. Over the following 4 to 6 weeks progressive renal failure developed from which the patient died.— J. J. Baker *et al.* (letter), *New Engl. J. Med.*, 1979, *301*, 662.

Further references to the use of chlorozotocin.— R. J. Gralla and A. Yagoda, *Cancer Treat. Rep.*, 1979, *63*, 1007 (renal cell carcinoma).

Manufacturers

Dome, USA.

1822-j

Cisplatin. *cis*-DDP; DDP; NSC 119875; Cis-platinum; Platinum Diamminodichloride. *cis*-Diamminedichloroplatinum. $(NH_3)_2.PtCl_2$=300.1.

CAS — 15663-27-1.

A white powder. M.p. 207°. **Soluble** 1 in 1000 of water and 1 in 42 of dimethylformamide. **Incompatible** with aluminium. **Store** at 2° to 8°.

Solutions for injection, containing 1 mg per ml, are prepared by dissolving cisplatin in Water for Injections and should be kept at room temperature, protected from light, and used within 20 hours of preparation. They are further diluted before administration (see Uses, below).

Incompatibility. A report of a chemical reaction between cisplatin and sodium bisulfite. Such antoxidants might inactivate cisplatin before administration if they are present in intravenous fluids.— A. A. Hussain *et al.*, *J. pharm. Sci.*, 1980, *69*, 364.

Stability in solution. Studies on the stability of cisplatin in aqueous solution indicated that when reconstituted with sodium chloride injection it was stable for 24 hours at room temperature. It was not necessary to prepare a solution immediately before use provided it was protected from light. If stored at refrigerator temperatures the concentration should be less than 600 µg per ml to prevent precipitation.— R. F. Greene *et al.*, *Am. J. Hosp. Pharm.*, 1979, *36*, 38.

The rate of loss of cisplatin in aqueous parenteral solutions was dependent on the concentration present and was not affected by dextrose or mannitol; cisplatin stability was decreased in the presence of sodium bicarbonate, but enhanced by sodium chloride.— A. A. Hincal *et al.*, *J. parent. Drug Ass.*, 1979, *33*, 107.

Adverse Effects and Treatment. For an outline of the adverse effects experienced with antineoplastic agents and immunosuppressants and general guidelines for their treatment, see Antineoplastic Agents, p.171 and p.174.

Severe nausea and vomiting usually occurs during treatment with cisplatin.

Serious toxic effects on the kidneys, bone marrow, and ears have been reported in about one third of patients given a single dose of cisplatin; the effects are generally dose-related and cumulative. Damage to the renal tubules may be evident during the second week after a dose of cisplatin and renal function must return to normal before further cisplatin is given. Intravenous hydration prior to treatment and the administration of cisplatin by infusion, with the addition of mannitol, have been used in an attempt to reduce nephrotoxicity.

Bone-marrow depression may be severe with higher doses of cisplatin. Nadirs in platelet and leucocyte counts occur between days 18 and 23 and most patients recover by day 39; anaemia is commonly seen.

Ototoxicity may be more severe in children. It can be manifest as tinnitus, loss of hearing in the high frequency range, and occasionally deafness. Other neurological effects reported include peripheral neuropathies and seizures.

Severe allergic reactions and cardiac abnormalities have occurred.

Dexamethasone as an anti-emetic in patients treated with cisplatin.— M. S. Aapro and D. S. Alberts (letter), *New Engl. J. Med.*, 1981, *305*, 520.

Allergy and anaphylaxis. Eight cases of anaphylactic reactions (facial oedema, wheezing, tachycardia, hypotension) had been reported to the National Cancer Institute over the past year. The reactions occurred within a few minutes of the intravenous administration of cisplatin and responded to treatment with adrenaline, corticosteroids, or an antihistamine.— D. D. Von Hoff *et al.* (letter), *Lancet*, 1976, *1*, 90. A report of 3 patients who developed a syndrome of rigors, pyrexia, and tachycardia following infusion of cisplatin. The syndrome was wholly unlike allergic reactions to cisplatin. In one patient it has been prevented by intramuscular injection of hydrocortisone before cisplatin infusions.— R. F. U. Ashford *et al.* (letter), *Lancet*, 1980, *2*, 691.

Effects on the blood. A report of 2 patients with positive responses to the direct antiglobulin test after prolonged treatment with cisplatin 70 mg every 3 weeks. Both patients were rechallenged with a 70-mg dose of cisplatin and one developed overt haemolysis.— E. P. Getaz *et al.*, *New Engl. J. Med.*, 1980, *302*, 334. All of 28 cancer patients treated with a regimen including cisplatin became anaemic and in 13 the anaemia was severe. Underproduction of red blood cells might have been an important pathogenic factor. No positive antiglobulin tests were seen.— M. E. Kuzur and F. A. Greco (letter), *ibid.*, *303*, 110. Comment.— E. P. Getaz *et al.* (letter), *ibid.*

Findings which suggest that cisplatin-induced anaemia probably has 2 mechanisms, the more usual being destruction of the erythroid stem-cell pool and the less usual being haemolysis.— S. A. Rothmann and J. K. Weick (letter), *New Engl. J. Med.*, 1981, *304*, 360.

Effects on the ears. Reports of ototoxicity associated with cisplatin.— L. Helson *et al.*, *Clin. Toxicol.*, 1978, *13*, 469.

Effects on electrolytes. In a retrospective study of 37 patients who had received cisplatin 70 mg per m^2 body-surface by intravenous injection every 3 weeks, 21 patients developed hypomagnesaemia, while receiving cisplatin, which eventually returned to normal in 10 patients, and a further 8 developed hypomagnesaemia after cisplatin was withdrawn. Symptomatic hypomagnesaemia requiring hospitalisation occurred in 2 patients, while inappropriate renal magnesium loss occurred in 4 patients. In a prospective study of a further 7 patients who received a standard liquid diet for 4 days before cisplatin administration, 2 developed hypomagnesaemia.— R. L. Schilsky and T. Anderson, *Ann. intern. Med.*, 1979, *90*, 929. A report of severe hypomagnesaemic-hypocalcaemic tetany with marked hypokalaemia in a woman undergoing cisplatin therapy. The electrolyte losses were replaced and chemotherapy continued satisfactorily.— C. F. Winkler *et al.* (letter), *ibid.*, *91*, 502. A report of tetany in a 23-year-old man receiving cisplatin without concurrent administration of a diuretic. Serum magnesium and calcium concentrations should be monitored in patients receiving cisplatin so that replacement therapy can be started promptly.— R. Stuart-Harris *et al.* (letter), *Lancet*, 1980, *2*, 1303.

Effects on the eyes. Cisplatin was associated with ophthalmic toxicity in 2 patients.— S. Ostrow *et al.*, *Cancer Treat. Rep.*, 1978, *62*, 1591.

Effects on the kidneys. The renal toxicity of cisplatin. A study of 12 patients indicated that the renal lesions consisted of focal acute necrosis in distal tubules and collecting ducts, dilatation of convoluted tubules, and the formation of casts. Mannitol was considered to reduce the renal toxicity since the effects with low doses were the same as those with high doses given with mannitol.— J. C. Gonzalez-Vitale *et al.*, *Cancer*, 1977, *39*, 1362.

Sensitive tests to determine the extent of kidney damage in subjects given cisplatin 20 mg per m^2 body-surface daily for 5 days by rapid intravenous infusion, hydration being maintained with 3 litres of intravenous fluid daily throughout this period. Values indicated that in all but one patient the renal damage was mild. These preliminary results indicate that adequate hydration during cisplatin therapy protects the kidney from severe toxicity.— J. J. Fleming *et al.* (letter), *Lancet*, 1979, *2*, 960.

Further references to nephrotoxicity associated with cisplatin.— N. E. Madias and J. T. Harrington, *Am. J. Med.*, 1978, *65*, 307; B. R. Jones *et al.*, *Clin. Pharmac. Ther.*, 1980, *27*, 557 (methods of evaluating nephrotoxicity).

See also Effects on Electrolytes, above, and Administration in Renal Insufficiency, below.

Effects on the liver. Reports of hepatotoxicity with cisplatin.— F. Cavalli *et al.*, *Cancer Treat. Rep.*, 1978, *62*, 2125.

Effects on the nervous system. A report of peripheral sensorimotor neuropathy of the lower limbs after 5 courses of treatment including cisplatin. The neuropathy resolved over 2 months following withdrawal of chemotherapy.— A. M. Arnold and C. J. Williams (letter), *Br. med. J.*, 1979, *1*, 955.

Precautions. For reference to the precautions necessary with antineoplastic agents and immunosuppressants, see Antineoplastic Agents, p.175. Cisplatin should not be given to patients with a history of hypersensitivity to platinum-containing compounds. It is generally contra-indicated in patients with renal or hearing impairment. Renal function and hearing should be monitored during treatment and adequate hydration and urinary output maintained. The concomitant use of other nephrotoxic or ototoxic drugs should be avoided.

Absorption and Fate. After intravenous administration cisplatin disappears from the plasma in a biphasic manner and half-lives of 25 to 49 minutes and 58 to 73 hours have been reported. The majority of a dose is rapidly bound to plasma protein. Cisplatin is concentrated in the liver, kidneys, and large and small intestines. Penetration into the central nervous system appears to be poor. Excretion is mainly in the urine but is incomplete and prolonged.

Concentrations of platinum were measured in the plasma and urine of 8 cancer patients given an intravenous infusion of cisplatin 70 mg per m^2 body-surface over 1 hour, in conjunction with diuretics. Clearance from plasma was biphasic with calculated half-lives of 23 minutes and 67 hours. Plasma concentrations of platinum after 21 days were higher than expected, which suggests a third excretory phase. Cisplatin is extensively and strongly bound to serum protein and platinum concentrations probably do not reflect accurately the amount of active drug present. By 4 to 5 hours after infusion, non-protein-bound platinum constituted less than 2 to 3% of total serum platinum; biphasic plasma clearance was rapid with half-lives of 8 to 10 minutes and 40 to 45 minutes. Renal excretion appears to be predominantly by glomerular filtration; 17% of the total dose of cisplatin was excreted in the urine in the first 4 hours and 23% in the first 24 hours.— P. E. Gormley *et al.*, *Clin. Pharmac. Ther.*, 1979, *25*, 351.

Further references to pharmacokinetic studies with cisplatin.— C. Jacobs *et al.*, *Cancer*, 1978, *42*, 2135; T. F. Patton *et al.*, *Cancer Treat. Rep.*, 1978, *62*, 1359; G. A. Frick *et al.*, *Cancer Treat. Rep.*, 1979, *63*, 13; K. J. Himmelstein *et al.*, *Clin. Pharmac. Ther.*, 1981, *29*, 658.

Uses. The antineoplastic agent cisplatin is a platinum-containing complex which may act similarly to the alkylating agents (p.171). It also causes immunosuppression which is reported to be followed by an increase in the host immune response and may contribute to the effect of cisplatin against tumours.

Cisplatin is of value in the treatment of metastatic tumours of the testis, usually as a major component of combination chemotherapy regimens. It is also used in metastatic ovarian tumours and has been reported to be active against other solid tumours including those of the bladder, prostate, and head and neck.

See also under Choice of Antineoplastic Agent, p.175.

Cisplatin is administered intravenously, not more frequently than every 3 to 4 weeks. It is given as a single dose of 50 to 120 mg per m^2 body-surface, alternatively 15 to 20 mg per m^2 may be given daily for 5 days. In combination chemotherapy regimens, lower doses ranging from 20 mg per m^2 upwards are given every 3 to 4 weeks.

The reconstituted injection is administered in 2 litres of sodium chloride injection or dextrose and sodium chloride injection and infused over 6 to 8 hours. To aid diuresis and protect the kidneys, 37.5 g of mannitol may be added to the infusion. In order to initiate diuresis the patient is usually hydrated by the infusion of 1 to 2 litres of a suitable fluid for 8 to 12 hours before the administration of cisplatin.

Reviews of cisplatin.— F. K. V. Leh and W. Wolf, *J. pharm. Sci.*, 1976, *65*, 315 (platinum complexes); M. Rozencweig *et al.*, *Ann. intern. Med.*, 1977, *86*, 803; W. Check, *J. Am. med. Ass.*, 1978, *240*, 2521; *Med. Lett.*, 1979, *21*, 33; *Drug & Ther. Bull.*, 1979, *17*, 99; L. H. Einhorn and S. D. Williams, *New Engl. J. Med.*, 1979, *300*, 289; N. O. Hill (letter), *ibid.*, *301*, 47; C. J. Williams and J. M. A. Whitehouse, *Br. med. J.*, 1979, *1*, 1689; D. Osoba, *Can. J. Hosp. Pharm.*, 1980, *33*, 81; *Lancet*, 1982, *1*, 374.

Administration. Reports of preventative measures used during the administration of cisplatin to reduce the risk of nephrotoxicity.— K. K. Chary *et al.*, *Cancer Treat. Rep.*, 1977, *61*, 367 (forced diuresis); D. M. Hayes *et al.*, *Cancer*, 1977, *39*, 1372 (prehydration; mannitol); J. J. Stark and S. B. Howell, *Clin. Pharmac. Ther.*, 1978, *23*, 461 (moderate hydration).

Administration in renal insufficiency. The use of cisplatin should be avoided in patients with a glomerular filtration-rate of less than 10 ml per minute. It is reported to be removed by haemodialysis during the first 3 hours after a dose.— W. M. Bennett *et al.*, *Ann. intern. Med.*, 1980, *93*, 286.

Although cisplatin is nephrotoxic and is not recommended unless the blood urea is below 9 mmol per litre, it was successfully used in a woman with obstructive nephropathy associated with adenocarcinoma sensitive to cisplatin.— D. G. Pickering *et al.* (letter), *Lancet*, 1980, *2*, 588.

Further references.— A. W. Prestayko *et al.*, *Med. pediat. Oncol.*, 1978, *5*, *Suppl.*, 183 (cisplatin in a haemodialysis patient).

See also Adverse Effects and Treatment and Precautions, above.

Antiprotozoal action. Cisplatin had significant activity against *Trypanosoma rhodesiense* infections in *mice*.— K. E. Kinnamon *et al.*, *Antimicrob. Ag. Chemother.*, 1979, *15*, 157.

Malignant neoplasms. Reports on cisplatin in the treatment of various malignant neoplasms.— R. Osieka *et al.*, *Dt. med. Wschr.*, 1976, *101*, 191 (testis); D. J. Higby *et al.*, *Cancer Treat. Rep.*, 1977, *61*, 869; P. Kamalakar *et al.*, *Cancer Treat. Rep.*, 1977, *61*, 835 (children); R. E. Wittes *et al.*, *Cancer Treat. Rep.*, 1977, *61*, 356 (head and neck); A. Yagoda, *Cancer Res.*, 1977, *37*, 2775 (bladder); F. Cavalli *et al.*, *Dt. med. Wschr.*, 1978, *103*, 927 (with doxorubicin in ovarian carcinoma); C. Merrin, *J. Urol.*, 1978, *119*, 493 (bladder); C. Merrin, *J. Urol.*, 1978, *119*, 522 (prostate); H. Y. Yap *et al.*, *Cancer Treat. Rep.*, 1978, *62*, 405 (no benefit in breast cancer); M. Hayat *et al.*, *Nouv. Presse méd.*, 1979, *8*, 1231; C. G. Schmidt and R. Becher, *Dt. med. Wschr.*, 1979, *104*, 872 (melanoblastoma); M. H. N. Tattersall *et al.*, *Med. J. Aust.*, 1980, *1*, 419 (adrenal cortex).

For the use of cisplatin, with bleomycin and vinblastine, in malignant neoplasms of the testis, see Choice of Antineoplastic Agent, p.184.

Proprietary Preparations

Neoplatin *(Bristol-Myers Pharmaceuticals, UK)*. Cisplatin, available as powder for preparing injections in vials of 10 and 50 mg.

Other Proprietary Names

Cisplatyl *(Fr.)*; Platinex *(Ger.)*; Platinol *(Canad., Lux., S.Afr., USA)*.

1823-z

Colaspase.
Asparaginase; L-Asparaginase; L-Asparagine Amidohydrolase; NSC 109229.

CAS — 9015-68-3.

An enzyme obtained from cultures of *Escherichia coli* ATCC 9637. Colaspase has also been obtained from *Erwinia carotovora*. A white or almost white slightly hygroscopic powder. **Soluble** in water; practically insoluble in acetone, chloroform, ether, and methyl alcohol. Aqueous solutions show no significant loss of potency when stored for 7 days at 20° or for 14 days at 5°, but solutions for injection should be used within 24 hours of preparation. **Store** at 2° to 10°.

Assay methods for colaspase.—Asparaginase, in *Pharmaceutical Enzymes*, R. Ruyssen and A. Lauwers (Ed.), Gent, E. Story-Scientia, 1978, p. 181.

Units. One unit of colaspase splits 1 μmol of ammonia from L-asparagine in 1 minute under standard conditions. The purest commercial samples contain about 260 units per mg.

Adverse Effects. Reported side-effects with colaspase include anorexia, nausea and vomiting, pyrexia, weight loss, uraemia, disturbances of the central nervous system, impaired liver function, hyperglycaemia, pancreatitis, and anaphylaxis and other allergic reactions. The bone marrow may be depressed and there may be decreased blood concentrations of fibrinogen and clotting factors. There may be alterations in blood concentrations of lipids and cholesterol. Fatal leucopenia has occasionally occurred. Several of these side-effects are attributable to the protein nature of colaspase; they may also be related to the bacterial source of the enzyme.

There was a higher incidence of side-effects to colaspase derived from *Escherichia coli* than from *Erwinia carotovora*. Allergic reactions were the most frequent and there did not appear to be cross-sensitivity between the 2 forms. The toxicity was probably caused by their protein nature and enzyme activity and not by contaminating endotoxin.— D. A. Rutter (letter), *Lancet*, 1975, *1*, 1293. Endotoxin equivalent to 50 ng per ml was found in 2 samples of colaspase and could account for pyrogen reactions.— D. Fumarola, *Farmaco, Edn prat.*, 1977, *32*, 444.

A report of severe diabetic ketoacidosis, severe pancytopenia, hyperuricaemia, and acute renal failure in a patient receiving colaspase for relapse of acute lymphatic leukaemia.— G. Summerfield and D. Swirsky (letter), *Br. med. J.*, 1978, *2*, 1373.

See also Diabetogenic Effect (below).

Allergy and anaphylaxis. The Boston Collaborative Drug Surveillance Program monitored consecutively 32 812 medical inpatients. Drug-induced anaphylaxis occurred in 2 of 8 patients given colaspase. One patient died.— J. Porter and H. Jick, *Lancet*, 1977, *1*, 587.

Diabetogenic effect. Three of 5 patients who were treated with colaspase developed a diabetic state. Some diabetic signs were still present in 2 of the patients at the end of the study.— S. Gailani *et al.*, *Clin. Pharmac. Ther.*, 1971, *12*, 487.

Further references: J. P. Whitecar *et al.*, *Metabolism*, 1970, *19*, 581; N. Jaffe, *J. Pediat.*, 1972, *81*, 1220; U. Carpentieri and M. T. Baleh, *J. Pediat.*, 1978, *93*, 775.

Effects on the blood. *Bone-marrow depression.* Individual reports of adverse effects with colaspase: M. J. Oehlers *et al.*, *Med. J. Aust.*, 1969, *2*, 907 (fatal leucopenia); N. E. Kay *et al.* (letter), *J. Am. med. Ass.*, 1973, *226*, 673 (megaloblastic changes).

Coagulation defects. A 55-year-old man with acute lymphoblastic leukaemia developed iliofemoral vein thrombosis 3 days after completing a course of colaspase therapy. His plasma antithrombin III concentration was only 56% before heparin therapy began; a month later it was 81%. More detailed observations in a second patient revealed a rapid and dramatic fall in plasma antithrombin III concentration associated with colaspase therapy. Venous thrombosis may be associated with reduced antithrombin concentrations; the rarity of this complication during colaspase therapy may be explained by a concomitant decrease in coagulation factors.— W. R. Pitney *et al.* (letter), *Lancet*, 1980, *1*, 493. The fall in antithrombin III associated with colaspase therapy may be the explanation for reports of pulmonary embolism following colaspase therapy.— E. Vellenga *et al.* (letter), *ibid.*, 649. See also J. Conard *et al.* (letter), *ibid.*, 1091.

Further references: N. K. C. Ramsay *et al.*, *Cancer*, 1977, *40*, 1398.

Effects on the pancreas. Reports of pancreatitis associated with colaspase: M. T. Shaw *et al.* (letter), *Lancet*, 1970, *2*, 721; R. Jain and S. V. Ramanan, *Archs intern. Med.*, 1978, *138*, 1726 (fatal); G. A. Koniver and J. E. Scott, *Delaware med. J.*, 1978, *50*, 330.

Pregnancy and the neonate. Studies in pregnant *rabbits* showed that colaspase had embryotoxic properties.— R. H. Adamson and S. Fabro (letter), *Nature*, 1968, *218*, 1164.

Precautions. For reference to the precautions necessary with antineoplastic agents and immunosuppressants, see Antineoplastic Agents, p.175.

Colaspase is contra-indicated in patients with pancreatitis. It should be given cautiously to patients with impaired liver function. Test doses should always be administered at the start of treatment to check for hypersensitivity, as described below under Uses. Re-treatment with colaspase may be associated with an increased risk of allergic reactions.

A comparison of the myelosuppressant effects of different treatment regimens for acute lymphoblastic leukaemia indicated that neutropenia, and to a lesser extent, thrombocytopenia, were more severe when colaspase was given in addition to prednisolone and vincristine in the induction phase of treatment. Life-threatening infections and deaths were more common in the patients receiving colaspase.— P. G. B. Johnston *et al.*, *Br. med. J.*, 1974, *3*, 81.

Interactions. The anti-tumour effect of colaspase in *mouse* lymphoma was antagonised by the administration of methionine or choline.— A. Khan *et al.* (letter), *Lancet*, 1970, *2*, 1082.

In certain circumstances methotrexate interfered with the action of colaspase.— J. Q. Matthias, *Practitioner*, 1973, *211*, 465.

Interference with diagnostic tests. A report of a transient but dramatic reduction in serum concentrations of thyroxine-binding globulin and a consequent rapid reduction in total thyroxine concentrations within 2 days of patients starting a course of colaspase. Concentrations of the globulin returned to pretreatment values within 4 weeks of the last dose.— M. B. Garnick and P. R. Larsen, *New Engl. J. Med.*, 1979, *301*, 252.

Absorption and Fate. Colaspase is not absorbed from the gastro-intestinal tract. Following intravenous injection the plasma half-life has varied from 8 to 48 hours. About 20% of a given dose may be found in the lymph. There is virtually no diffusion into the CSF. Little is excreted in the urine.

In patients with various neoplastic diseases the biological half-life of colaspase has been reported to be 22 to 48 hours.— J. D. Broome (letter), *Lancet*, 1968, *2*, 980.

In a study of 15 patients with various neoplasms given colaspase the plasma half-life varied from 8 to 30 hours and was not dose-dependent nor was it affected by sex, age, body-surface area, type or extent of disease, or liver or kidney function. When the highest dose of 400 000 units per m^2 body-surface was given, a plasma concentration of 200 units per ml was achieved. Most of the colaspase remained in the plasma, 20% entered the lymph slowly, up to 1% entered the CSF, and only traces were detected in the urine.— D. H. W. Ho *et al.*, *Clin. Pharmac. Ther.*, 1970, *11*, 408.

The plasma half-life of colaspase was about 14 to 22 hours, and there was cumulation following repeated doses. Enzyme activity was detectable 13 to 22 days after injection.— T. Ohnuma *et al.*, *Cancer Res.*, 1970, *30*, 2297, per *Int. pharm. Abstr.*, 1973, *10*, 22.

Uses. Colaspase is an enzyme which acts as an antineoplastic agent by breaking down the amino acid L-asparagine to aspartic acid and ammonia. It interferes with the growth of those malignant cells which, unlike healthy cells, are unable to synthesise L-asparagine for their metabolism.

Colaspase is used mainly for the induction of remissions in children with acute lymphoblastic leukaemia. See also under Choice of Antineoplastic Agent, p.178. It may be given intravenously in a dose of 1000 units per kg body-weight daily for 10 days following treatment with vincristine and prednisone or intramuscularly in a dose of 6000 units per m^2 body-surface given every third day for 9 doses during treatment with vincristine and prednisone. Colaspase is not generally used alone as an induction agent but doses of 200 units per kg daily have been given intravenously for 28 days to adults and children. Children appear to tolerate colaspase better than adults. Although not entirely reliable, a test dose of about 2 units should be given intradermally before treatment with colaspase and the injection site observed for at least an hour for evidence of a positive reaction; desensitisation has been advocated if no alternative antineoplastic treatment is available. The risk of sensitivity reactions may be increased with intermittent courses of treatment. When administered intravenously a solution of colaspase in Water for Injections or sodium chloride injection should be given over not less than 30 minutes through a running infusion of sodium chloride injection or dextrose injection. When given intramuscularly no more than 2 ml of a solution in sodium chloride injection should be injected at a single site.

A brief review of enzymes, including colaspase, as antineoplastic agents.— J. S. Holcenberg and J. Roberts, *A. Rev. Pharmac. & Toxic.*, 1977, *17*, 97.

Action. The concentrations of serum-immunoglobulins increased in 8 children with acute lymphoblastic leukaemia or rheumatoid arthritis after treatment with colaspase. It was suggested that the enzyme acted as an antigen and also possibly produced immunological stimulation or effected the release of immunoglobulins into the blood stream.— G. R. Burgio *et al.* (letter), *Lancet*, 1970, *2*, 1364.

Colaspase prepared from *Erwinia carotovora* had similar

actions to the enzyme produced from *Escherichia coli* and was well tolerated by 4 patients who had experienced anaphylactic reactions from *E. coli* materials.— T. Ohnuma *et al.*, *Cancer*, 1972, *30*, 376, per *Int. pharm. Abstr.*, 1974, *11*, 394.

Administration. Extracorporeal perfusion of blood for 4 hours over plates coated with colaspase reduced serum-asparagine concentrations almost to zero and rendered the lymphocytes unreactive to mitogenic stimulation in human subjects and *baboons*. This technique avoided the toxicity of colaspase.— D. Sampson *et al.*, *J. surg. Oncol.*, 1974, *6*, 39, per *J. Am. med. Ass.*, 1974, *228*, 1185.

Colaspase, from *Erwinia carotovora*, covalently and irreversibly bound to an activated soluble dextran exhibited an increased circulatory half-life in the *rabbit* compared to the half-life of the native enzyme. The results suggested that the major limitations to the use of colaspase (its rapid inactivation and the immunological consequences of repeated injections) may be overcome by its immobilisation with soluble dextran.— R. L. Foster and T. Wileman, *J. Pharm. Pharmac.*, 1979, *31*, *Suppl.*, 37P.

Leukaemia. A brief review of colaspase in induction regimens for acute lymphoblastic leukaemia.— *Med. Lett.*, 1978, *20*, 103.

See also under Choice of Antineoplastic Agent, p.178.

The effects of colaspase in acute lymphoblastic leukaemia could be enhanced by a diet low in protein.— B. Halikowski *et al.* (letter), *Lancet*, 1969, *1*, 423.

For earlier reports of colaspase in the treatment of acute leukaemia, see Martindale 27th Edn, p. 134.

See also under Precautions (above).

Pregnancy and the neonate. *Second trimester.* An apparently normal infant girl was born to a woman in whom acute leukaemia was diagnosed when she was 16 weeks pregnant, and who was treated with a regimen including colaspase.— M. Khurshid and M. Saleem (letter), *Lancet*, 1978, *2*, 534.

Proprietary Names

Crasnitine *(Bayer, Belg.)*; Elspar *(Merck Sharp & Dohme, USA)*; Kidrolase *(Rhône-Poulenc, Canad.; Specia, Fr.)*; Laspar *(Kyowa Hakko Kogyo, S.Afr.)*; Leunase *(May & Baker, Austral.)*.

Colaspase was formerly marketed in Great Britain under the proprietary name Crasnitin (*Bayer*; *May & Baker*).

1825-k

Cyclophosphamide *(B.P., U.S.P.)*. Cyclophospham.; B 518; NSC 26271; WR 138719.

2-[Bis(2-chloroethyl)amino]perhydro-1,3,2-oxazaphosphorine 2-oxide monohydrate.

$C_7H_{15}Cl_2N_2O_2P,H_2O=279.1$.

CAS — 6055-19-2; 50-18-0 (anhydrous).

Pharmacopoeias. In *Br.*, *Braz.*, *Chin.*, *Jap.*, *Jug.*, *Rus.*, *Turk.*, and *U.S.*

A fine, white, odourless or almost odourless, crystalline powder with a slightly bitter taste. M.p. 49.5° to 53°. It liquefies upon loss of its water of crystallisation. It discolours on exposure to light. **Soluble** 1 in 25 of water and 1 in 1 of alcohol; slightly soluble in ether. A freshly prepared 2% solution in water has a pH of 4 to 6. *U.S.P.* requires that a 1% solution should have a pH of 3.9 to 7.1 when determined 30 minutes after preparation. Solutions deteriorate on storage. Aqueous solutions may be kept for a few hours at temperatures up to 25°. At temperatures above 30° hydrolysis occurs with removal of chlorine.

Solutions for injection are prepared by dissolving, immediately before use, the sterile contents of a sealed container in Water for Injections. **Store** at 2° to 32° in airtight containers. Protect from light.

Incompatibility. The calculated rate constant for decomposition of cyclophosphamide in water preserved with benzyl alcohol was significantly larger than the value for cyclophosphamide in sterile Water for Injection.— D. Brooke *et al.*, *Am. J. Hosp. Pharm.*, 1973, *30*, 134.

Stability in solution. Solutions of cyclophosphamide reconstituted with water and diluted to 4 mg per ml with sodium chloride injection lost about 3.5% potency in 24 hours and 11.9% in 1 week when stored at 25°. When protected from light and stored at 5° the loss was 0.55% after 1 week and 1% after 4 weeks.— J. F. Gallelli, *Am. J. Hosp. Pharm.*, 1967, *24*, 425.

The determination of first-order rate constants for the degradation of cyclophosphamide in injection vehicles indicated that solutions lost not more than 1.5% of their potency when stored for up to 6 days at 5° or for up to 8 hours at about 25°.— D. Brooke *et al.*, *Am. J. Hosp. Pharm.*, 1973, *30*, 134.

Warming vials of cyclophosphamide to facilitate dissolution could result in decreased potency.— D. Brooke *et al.*, *Am. J. Hosp. Pharm.*, 1975, *32*, 44.

Adverse Effects and Treatment. For an outline of the adverse effects experienced with antineoplastic agents and immunosuppressants and general guidelines for their treatment, see Antineoplastic Agents, p.171 and p.174.

Cyclophosphamide produces leucopenia and lymphocytopenia. Following single doses, maximum depression of the white cell count may occur in 5 to 10 days with full recovery usually in 3 to 4 weeks. Thrombocytopenia may be less severe than with other alkylating agents.

Alopecia is a frequent side-effect but tends to be reversible. It may develop in about 20% of patients within 3 weeks of starting treatment at normal doses. Most patients will experience alopecia at high doses.

Urinary complications include cystitis which can often be severe and haemorrhagic.

Other occasional side-effects include interstitial pulmonary fibrosis and cardiotoxicity.

Allergy and anaphylaxis. Reports of allergic reactions associated with cyclophosphamide: I. Maxwell (letter), *J. Am. med. Ass.*, 1974, *229*, 137 (hypotension and pulmonary oedema following injection); J. D. Lakin and R. A. Cahill, *J. Allergy & clin. Immunol.*, 1976, *58*, 160 (generalised urticaria); R. K. Karchmer and V. L. Hansen, *J. Am. med. Ass.*, 1977, *237*, 475 (respiratory arrest, hypotension, and rash immediately after infusion); W. E. Ross and B. A. Chabner, *Cancer Treat. Rep.*, 1977, *61*, 495 (in a patient sensitive to mustine); A. N. Krutchik *et al.*, *Archs intern. Med.*, 1978, *138*, 1725 (urticaria; no cross sensitivity to chlorambucil); L. Murti and L. R. Horsman, *J. Pediat.*, 1979, *94*, 844 (anaphylaxis).

Diabetogenic effect. Three women with carcinoma developed diabetes mellitus after treatment with cyclophosphamide for periods of about 5½, 6, and 8 months respectively; none had a family history of diabetes. The dosage ranged from 50 to 200 mg daily.— C. R. Pengelly (letter), *Br. med. J.*, 1965, *1*, 1312.

Effects on the bladder. Sterile haemorrhagic cystitis, believed to be secondary to renal excretion of alkylating metabolites, occurs following high-dose infusions of cyclophosphamide or, more commonly, with prolonged low-dose administration. The cystitis appears to result from chronic inflammation leading to fibrosis and telangiectasia of the bladder epithelium; haemorrhage may be life-threatening if drug administration is continued. Forced diuresis during high-dose infusions of cyclophosphamide has been attempted to minimise the risk of haemorrhagic cystitis but severe impairment of water excretion has been reported, leading to hyponatraemia, weight gain, and inappropriately concentrated urine.— R. A. Bender *et al.*, *Drugs*, 1978, *16*, 46.

In a study of 54 patients with systemic lupus erythematosus or rheumatoid arthritis treated with oral cyclophosphamide, 7 episodes of acute haemorrhagic cystitis were reported, and 2 patients developed carcinoma of the bladder. The use of cyclophosphamide in the treatment of nonmalignant inflammatory rheumatic conditions should be limited.— P. H. Plotz *et al.*, *Ann. intern. Med.*, 1979, *91*, 221.

Limited fluid intake following her daily dose of cyclophosphamide, which had been taken at the evening meal, may have contributed to the development of severe haemorrhagic cystitis in a 17-year-old girl who had taken cyclophosphamide 100 mg daily, gradually reduced to 25 mg daily over 4 years. The drug was withdrawn and haematuria and anaemia slowly resolved during the following 4 months.— M. D. Bischel (letter), *J. Am. med. Ass.*, 1979, *242*, 238.

Haemorrhagic cystitis in 3 men was attributed to treatment with cyclophosphamide which had been discontinued 3 to 6 months earlier.— B. Armstrong *et al.* (letter), *New Engl. J. Med.*, 1979, *300*, 45. See also B. M. Berkson *et al.*, *J. Am. med. Ass.*, 1973, *225*, 605.

Further reports of the adverse effects of cyclophosphamide on the bladder: R. G. Aptekar *et al.*, *Arthritis Rheum.*, 1973, *16*, 461; W. Vahlensieck *et al.*, *Münch. med. Wschr.*, 1974, *116*, 1889; H. J. Lawrence *et al.*, *Cancer*, 1975, *36*, 1572 (occurrence in children); S. S. Seltzer *et al.*, *Urology*, 1978, *11*, 352; F. F. Marshall and H. F. Klinefelter, *Urology*, 1979, *14*, 573.

For the use of mesna to reduce cyclophosphamide-induced bladder toxicity, see Mesna, p.651.

Effects on the eyes. Blurred vision of varying onset and duration occurred in 5 of 29 children after the intravenous administration of cyclophosphamide.— G. Kende *et al.*, *Cancer*, 1979, *44*, 69.

Effects on the gastro-intestinal tract. In 7 children receiving large doses of cyclophosphamide vomiting was controlled by the intravenous infusion over 1 hour every 6 to 8 hours of promethazine hydrochloride, 75 mg per m^2 body-surface per 24 hours.— P. J. Kearney (letter), *Br. med. J.*, 1975, *1*, 95.

Effects on the heart. Reports of cardiotoxicity associated with cyclophosphamide: F. R. Appelbaum *et al.*, *Lancet*, 1976, *1*, 58 (acute and fatal myopericarditis associated with high doses); B. A. Mills and R. W. Roberts, *Cancer*, 1979, *43*, 2223 (fatal cardiomyopathy).

Effects on the kidneys. After 38 days' treatment with cyclophosphamide a woman was found to have severe necrosis of the renal tubular epithelium.— V. M. Lopes (letter), *Lancet*, 1967, *1*, 1060.

Cyclophosphamide was associated in 13 of 17 patients with water intolerance characterised by a rise in urine osmolarity, a fall in urine flow, weight gain, and hyponatraemia. All patients with these symptoms had received 50 mg per kg body-weight or more of cyclophosphamide.— R. A. DeFronzo *et al.*, *Ann. intern. Med.*, 1973, *78*, 861.

Effects on the pancreas. Acute haemorrhagic pancreatitis associated with cyclophosphamide.— A. Kobayashi *et al.*, *Am. J. Dis. Child.*, 1973, *125*, 726.

Effects on reproductive potential. *Gonads.* Reduced sperm-counts were observed in patients 3 weeks after treatment with cyclophosphamide 50 to 100 mg daily. Azoospermia could develop after 4 months but was always present after 6. Only 3 of 11 patients studied for 3 to 19 months after stopping treatment had mature spermatozoa and the counts were very low. There was no spermatogenesis in 6 patients who were still being treated or who had just stopped treatment, although spermatogenesis was seen in 2 patients 12 months and 15 months after stopping cyclophosphamide.— K. F. Fairley *et al.*, *Lancet*, 1972, *1*, 568. Within 6 months of starting treatment with cyclophosphamide 26 men became azoospermic. When cyclophosphamide was withdrawn spermatogenesis returned in 12 patients within 15 to 49 months.— J. D. Buchanan *et al.*, *Lancet*, 1975, *2*, 156. Further references: D. G. Miller, *J. Am. med. Ass.*, 1971, *217*, 1662; D. A. Blake *et al.*, *Johns Hopkins med. J.*, 1976, *139*, 20.

The occurrence of pregnancy in patients taking cyclophosphamide and the return to normal menstruation in other women after discontinuing treatment suggested that ovarian tissue was less sensitive to cyclophosphamide than testicular germinal epithelium.— J. S. Cameron and C. S. Ogg (letter), *Lancet*, 1972, *1*, 1174. Of 22 women with glomerulonephritis or rheumatoid arthritis receiving cyclophosphamide usually in a dose of 50 to 100 mg daily, 17 developed definite or probable ovarian failure. One patient regained normal ovarian function after stopping cyclophosphamide.— G. L. Warne *et al.*, *New Engl. J. Med.*, 1973, *289*, 1159. Further references: P. R. Uldall *et al.* (letter), *Lancet*, 1972, *1*, 693.

A discussion of the gonadal hazards of cyclophosphamide when given to children with the idiopathic nephrotic syndrome.— G. C. Arneil (letter), *Lancet*, 1972, *2*, 1259. Further references to the effect of cyclophosphamide on gonadal function in children: C. L. Berry *et al.* (letter), *Lancet*, 1972, *2*, 1033; G. W. DeGroot *et al.*, *J. Pediat.*, 1974, *84*, 123; A. J. Pennisi *et al.*, *Am. J. Dis. Child.*, 1975, *129*, 315; J. N. Etteldorf *et al.*, *J. Pediat.*, 1976, *88*, 206; R. T. Kirkland *et al.*, *J. Pediat.*, 1976, *89*, 941; R. D. Lentz *et al.*, *J. Pediat.*, 1977, *91*, 385; A. Parram *et al.*, *J. Pediat.*, 1978, *92*, 117; C. A. Alfiler, *Aust. paediat. J.*, 1979, *15*, 120; A. C. Hsu *et al.*, *Fert. Steril.*, 1979, *31*, 173; R. S. Trompeter *et al.*, *Lancet*, 1981, *1*, 1177.

Effects on respiratory function. Cyclophosphamide is known to occasionally produce pneumonitis and pulmonary fibrosis. In one report by C.S. Alvarado *et al.* (*J. Pediat.*, 1978, *92*, 443) 2 children developed hypoxaemia and pulmonary fibrosis 4 and 6 years respectively after they had stopped taking cyclophosphamide.— R. B. Weiss and F. M. Muggia, *Am. J. Med.*, 1980, *68*, 259.

Individual reports of pulmonary toxicity associated with

cyclophosphamide: G. J. Mark *et al.*, *Thorax*, 1978, *33*, 89 (pneumonitis); J. I. Spector *et al.*, *J. Am. med. Ass.*, 1979, *242*, 2852 (interstitial pneumonitis); J. I. Spector *et al.* (letter), *J. Am. med. Ass.*, 1980, *243*, 1133 (interstitial pneumonitis).

Effects on the thyroid. Adverse effects on the thyroid associated with cyclophosphamide.— I. R. McDougall *et al.*, *Br. med. J.*, 1971, *4*, 275 (thyrotoxicosis); V. J. Coffey (letter), *Br. med. J.*, 1971, *4*, 682 (myxoedema).

Pregnancy and the neonate. *First trimester.* A woman treated with cyclophosphamide throughout her pregnancy gave birth prematurely to a baby with bilateral inguinal hernias and without both big toes.— L. H. Greenberg and K. R. Tanaka, *J. Am. med. Ass.*, 1964, *188*, 423.

Precautions. For reference to the precautions necessary with antineoplastic agents and immunosuppressants, see Antineoplastic Agents, p.175.

Cyclophosphamide should not be given to patients with haemorrhagic cystitis. It should be given with care to those with diabetes mellitus. Reduced doses should be employed in patients with renal or hepatic failure. Liberal fluid intake and frequent micturition are advised to reduce the risk of cystitis.

Since cyclophosphamide must undergo metabolism before it is active, interactions are possible with drugs which either inhibit or stimulate the enzymes responsible.

There was a rapid deterioration in renal function in 2 of 6 patients with systemic lupus erythematosus and nephritis who had cyclophosphamide withdrawn from their therapy.— R. G. Aptekar *et al.* (letter), *New Engl. J. Med.*, 1972, *286*, 1159.

Interactions. *Allopurinol.* The incidence of bone-marrow depression in 95 patients with neoplastic diseases other than leukaemia who received cyclophosphamide or other cytotoxic drugs was 12.6%. There was a significantly higher incidence of bone-marrow depression (33.8%) in 65 patients who also received allopurinol.— Boston Collaborative Drug Surveillance Program, *J. Am. med. Ass.*, 1974, *227*, 1036. Further references: J. Witten *et al.*, *Acta pharmac. tox.*, 1980, *46*, 392.

Antibacterial agents. Administration of chloramphenicol prior to cyclophosphamide prolonged the mean cyclophosphamide serum half-life from 7.5 to 11.5 hours and reduced the peak activity in all of 5 subjects. Administration of sulphaphenazole prior to cyclophosphamide significantly inhibited the rate of biotransformation of cyclophosphamide in 2 of 7 subjects and enhanced it in 2; it remained unchanged in 3.— O. K. Faber *et al.*, *Br. J. clin. Pharmac.*, 1975, *2*, 281.

Barbiturates. Prior administration of the insecticide chlordane to *rats* induced enzyme stimulation in liver microsomes so that the cytotoxic effects of cyclophosphamide were increased. Phenobarbitone could have the same effect.— R. L. Dixon, *J. pharm. Sci.*, 1968, *57*, 1351. Although patients receiving cyclophosphamide developed higher peak plasma concentrations of active cyclophosphamide metabolites when given enzyme-inducing agents such as barbiturates, the active metabolites also disappeared rapidly.— C. M. Bagley *et al.*, *Cancer Res.*, 1973, *33*, 226. Further references: J. Y. Jao *et al.*, *Cancer Res.*, 1972, *32*, 2761.

Corticosteroids. A suggestion that since corticosteroids appear to inhibit the enzyme systems which activate cyclophosphamide, doses should be reduced when concomitant treatment with corticosteroids is withdrawn.— S. R. Kaplan and P. Calabresi, *New Engl. J. Med.*, 1973, *289*, 952. Doubts about this conclusion. Single doses of prednisone have been found to inhibit the activation of cyclophosphamide but after longer-term treatment the rate of activation has increased.— O. K. Faber and H. T. Mouridsen (letter), *ibid.*, 1974, *291*, 211.

Insulin. Cyclophosphamide should be given with caution to patients with diabetes mellitus because it can depress blood-sugar concentrations, necessitating a reduction in maintenance doses of insulin or oral hypoglycaemic agents. It was suggested that cyclophosphamide could prevent abnormal binding of endogenous insulin to serum, and of exogenous insulin to antibodies.— H. U. Kruger, *Medsche Klin.*, 1966, *37*, 1462.

Suxamethonium. Cyclophosphamide might depress the concentrations of pseudocholinesterase and thereby potentiate the action of suxamethonium.— J. A. G. Horton, *Adverse Drug React. Bull.*, 1975, Feb., 168. References: I. R. Walker *et al.*, *Aust. N.Z. J. Med.*, 1972, *2*, 247.

Absorption and Fate. Cyclophosphamide may be incompletely absorbed from the gastro-intestinal tract. It rapidly disappears from the plasma and peak concentrations occur about 1 hour after a dose is taken by mouth. Cyclophosphamide has to undergo metabolism in the liver before it is active. Irritant metabolites are excreted in the urine together with unchanged drug.

A review of the clinical pharmacokinetics of cyclophosphamide. It undergoes a complicated process of metabolic activation yielding compounds with a wide range of cytotoxic potential. The primary metabolites are 4-hydroxycyclophosphamide, which may be oxidised to the non-cytotoxic compound 4-ketocyclophosphamide, and aldophosphamide, which may be converted to the toxic metabolites phosphoramide mustard and acrolein or oxidised to non-cytotoxic carboxyphosphamide, which is converted to nornitrogen mustard, an active alkylating agent at acid pH. Although very little cyclophosphamide is bound to protein, more than 50% of metabolites have been reported protein-bound. Only 5 to 25% of an administered dose is recovered unchanged in the urine.— L. B. Grochow and M. Colvin, *Clin. Pharmacokinet.*, 1979, *4*, 380.

In 11 patients (9 African) most of whom had Burkitt's lymphoma, the half-life of cyclophosphamide after an intravenous dose of 5 mg per kg body-weight was 3 to 6.5 hours. In 9 of the patients urinary recovery of cyclophosphamide and its metabolites in 48 hours was 36.5 to 99.3% (usually between 60 and 80%); about 64% of the excreted material was as metabolites. In 7 patients (6 African) given 40 mg per kg the half-life was 3.5 to 6.8 hours except in 1 patient (12.5 hours); in 6 patients urinary recovery in 48 hours was 36 to 65%, about 60% being present as metabolites.— R. H. Adamson, *Ann. N.Y. Acad. Sci.*, 1971, *179*, 432.

In a comparison of the pharmacokinetics of cyclophosphamide following oral and intravenous doses in 7 cancer patients, plasma half-lives ranged from 1.32 to 6.0 hours after oral administration compared with 5.97 to 12.37 hours after intravenous injection. Systemic availability after oral use indicated a relatively modest first-pass hepatic metabolism although on average the plasma alkylating activity produced by an oral dose of cyclophosphamide was 3.5 times that with an intravenous dose; this difference might reflect a differing pattern of metabolites, depending on the route of administration.— F. D. Juma *et al.*, *Br. J. clin. Pharmac.*, 1979, *8*, 209.

Further references: C. M. Bagley *et al.*, *Cancer Res.*, 1973, *33*, 226; H. T. Mouridsen *et al.*, *Acta pharmac. tox.*, 1976, *38*, 508 (pharmacokinetics of cyclophosphamide following treatment with methotrexate); M. D'Incalci *et al.*, *Eur. J. Drug Metab. Pharmacokinet.*, 1979, *4*, 83 (pharmacokinetics after prolonged treatment); G. Edwards *et al.*, *Br. J. clin. Pharmac.*, 1980, *10*, 281.

Diffusion. Cyclophosphamide was identified in the blood, cerebrospinal fluid, milk, saliva, sweat, synovial fluid, and urine of patients receiving cyclophosphamide for malignant disease or for rheumatoid arthritis.— J. H. Duncan *et al.*, *Toxic. appl. Pharmac.*, 1973, *24*, 317.

Pregnancy and the neonate. Reports of the excretion of cyclophosphamide in breast milk: P. H. Wiernik and J. H. Duncan (letter), *Lancet*, 1971, *1*, 912; D. Amato and J. S. Niblett (letter), *Med. J. Aust.*, 1977, *1*, 383.

Uses. Cyclophosphamide is an antineoplastic agent which is converted in the body to an active alkylating metabolite with properties similar to those of mustine (p.223). It also possesses marked immunosuppressant properties.

Cyclophosphamide is widely used, often in combination with other agents, in the treatment of a variety of malignant diseases including Burkitt's lymphoma, Hodgkin's disease and other lymphomas, acute and chronic lymphoblastic leukaemia, acute myeloid leukaemia, multiple myeloma, and mycosis fungoides. It is also used in the treatment of various solid tumours such as carcinoma of the breast, cervix, lung, and ovary; neuroblastoma; retinoblastoma; and sarcomas. The immunosuppressant properties of cyclophosphamide are used in Wegener's granulomatosis and in prolonging the survival of homografts, such as in kidney transplantation. It has also been used in the management of auto-immune disorders such as systemic lupus erythematosus, the nephrotic syndrome, and rheumatoid arthritis.

See also under Choice of Antineoplastic Agent, p.175.

Cyclophosphamide is given by mouth or intravenous injection; it is not a tissue irritant or vesicant. The dosage given depends on the malignant disease being treated, the condition of the patient including the state of the bone marrow, and the concomitant use of radiotherapy or other chemotherapy. Regimens used include: cyclophosphamide 2 to 6 mg per kg body-weight daily as a single intravenous dose or in divided doses by mouth; 10 to 15 mg per kg weekly as a single intravenous dose; 20 to 40 mg per kg (1 to 1.5 g per m^2 body-surface) as a single intravenous dose every 10 to 20 days; and 60 to 80 mg per kg as a single intravenous dose every 3 to 4 weeks. Even higher doses have been used. Children have been given initial doses of 2 to 8 mg per kg daily by intravenous injection or by mouth and maintenance doses of 2 to 5 mg per kg twice weekly by mouth.

A daily dose of 3 mg per kg body-weight has been used in children with the nephrotic syndrome in whom corticosteroids have been unsuccessful.

In the *B.P.* the potency of Cyclophosphamide Injection is expressed in terms of the equivalent amount of anhydrous cyclophosphamide whereas the potency of Cyclophosphamide Tablets is given in terms of the monohydrate; the *U.S.P.* expresses potency in terms of anhydrous cyclophosphamide for both injection and tablets.

Cyclophosphamide has also been given intraperitoneally, intrapleurally, and intra-arterially, and by local perfusion (but see Absorption and Fate). A liquid preparation of cyclophosphamide for oral use may be prepared using the powder for injection.

Regular blood counts are essential during therapy with cyclophosphamide and in general treatment should be withdrawn or delayed if the leucocyte count is below 4000 per mm^3 or the platelet count below 100 000 per mm^3.

Ringberg-Klinik regimen. Patients with rapidly progressive malignant growth and metastases who had not responded to immunotherapy with pyrogens, vaccines, desensitising agents, or serum activators were given cyclophosphamide in high doses of 50 to 80 mg per kg body-weight. The dose was sometimes repeated but might reduce the immune response so that subsequent immunotherapy was less effective.— J. Issels, *Clin. Trials J.*, 1970, *7*, 357. The doses of cyclophosphamide given by Issels were administered intravenously within 5 minutes and produced vomiting, loss of hair, and very low white cell counts in most patients. Some impressive remissions were obtained. However, his general method of 'immuno-therapy' was judged to have no effect on tumour growth and there was no evidence that it contributed significantly to the patients' survival.— Joint Co-Ordinating Committee on Cancer Research, *A Report on the Treatment of Cancer at the Ringberg-Clinic, Rottach Egern, Bavaria*, London, Department of Health and Social Security, HM Stationery Office, 1971.

Acceleration of bone-marrow recovery. Bone-marrow recovery of 7 patients who received cyclophosphamide 500 mg intravenously one week before a high dose of melphalan (140 mg per m^2) was more rapid than that of 4 controls who received smaller doses of melphalan (60 to 125 mg per m^2) without previous cyclophosphamide therapy. The role of cyclophosphamide priming to accelerate bone-marrow recovery after high doses of alkylating agents appears to merit further study.— D. W. Hedley *et al.*, *Lancet*, 1978, *2*, 966.

Administration in renal insufficiency. Doses of cyclophosphamide should be halved and the interval between doses extended from 12 hours to 18 to 24 hours in patients with a glomerular filtration-rate of less than 10 ml per minute. Concentrations of cyclophosphamide are affected by haemodialysis.— W. M. Bennett *et al.*, *Ann. intern. Med.*, 1980, *93*, 286.

A study indicating that significant amounts of cyclophosphamide are removed by dialysis.— L. H. Wang *et al.*, *Clin. Pharmac. Ther.*, 1981, *29*, 365.

Further references: J. S. Cheigh, *Am. J. Med.*, 1977, *62*, 555; P. Sharpstone, *Br. med. J.*, 1977, *2*, 36; J. Kroener and M. Green, *Am. J. Med.*, 1978, *64*, 725; R. A. V. Milsted and M. Jarman, *Br. med. J.*, 1978, *1*, 820; M. R. Bending and R. E. Finch (letter), *ibid.*,

1145.

See also under Renal Disorders (below).

Blood disorders, non-malignant. *Aplastic anaemia.* Two of 6 patients with aplastic anaemia resistant to anabolic steroids had obtained a beneficial response to cyclophosphamide therapy with almost complete remission after 5 months of therapy.— J. Pizzuto *et al.* (letter), *New Engl. J. Med.*, 1978, *298*, 164. See also D. T. Baran *et al.*, *New Engl. J. Med.*, 1976, *295*, 1522.

Haemophilia. Reports on the use of cyclophosphamide in patients with haemophilia: I. M. Nilsson *et al.*, *Ann. intern. Med.*, 1973, *78*, 91; R. S. Stein (letter), *Ann. intern. Med.*, 1974, *81*, 706.

Thrombocytopenic purpura. Beneficial results with cyclophosphamide in patients with thrombocytopenic purpura.— R. K. Laros and J. A. Penner, *J. Am. med. Ass.*, 1971, *215*, 445; B. Weinerman *et al.*, *Can. med. Ass. J.*, 1974, *111*, 1100.

Enhancement of effect. Enhancement of the effect of cyclophosphamide by vitamin A in *mice*.— L. Nathanson *et al.*, *J. clin. Pharmac.*, 1969, *9*, 359.

There was an additive effect on *mouse* tumours when cyclophosphamide was given with thymidine or adenosine.— H. Osswald, *Arzneimittel-Forsch.*, 1972, *22*, 1184.

See also under Precautions.

Hepatic disorders, non-malignant. In a study of 20 patients with active chronic hepatitis moderate disease responded more favourably to cyclophosphamide; in advanced disease corticosteroids were preferable. The dose of cyclophosphamide was 200 mg daily by intravenous injection to a total of 5 to 6 g; after an interval of 1 to 3 months 100 to 150 mg daily by mouth or intravenous injection to a total of 4 to 5 g; after a further interval of 1 to 3 months 100 to 150 mg daily to a total of 4 to 5 g.— R. Naccarato *et al.*, *Postgrad. med. J.*, 1974, *50*, 16. A small controlled study did not suggest that cyclophosphamide was of value in hepatitis-B-negative active chronic hepatitis.— I. T. Gilmore *et al.*, *Br. med. J.*, 1979, *1*, 1120. See also under Azathioprine, p.191.

Immunosuppression. A warning of the carcinogenic potential of cyclophosphamide. In future cyclophosphamide will not be recommended for use in non-malignant diseases except in life-threatening situations.— P. A. Knowlson, *WB Pharmaceuticals* (letter), *Lancet*, 1977, *2*, 457.

A study on the immunosuppressant properties of cyclophosphamide.— F. L. Shand, *Int. J. Immunopharmac.*, 1979, *1*, 165.

Various references to the use of cyclophosphamide, with or without corticosteroids, as an immunosuppressant: W. F. Doe *et al.*, *Gut*, 1972, *13*, 947 (alpha-chain disease); O. N. Manousos *et al.*, *Br. med. J.*, 1974, *2*, 409 (alpha-chain disease); P. J. Gill *et al.*, *Am. J. med. Sci.*, 1977, *273*, 213 (red cell aplasia); H. Fowler *et al.* (letter), *Lancet*, 1979, *2*, 1193 (severe progressive polyneuropathy after influenza vaccination); *Lancet*, 1980, *1*, 187 (auto-immune sensorineural hearing loss).

See also under side-headings for non-malignant disorders, and under Use of Immunosuppressants, p.186.

Lupus erythematosus. Since 1965, cyclophosphamide had been used in the treatment of 42 patients (37 female, 5 male) with systemic lupus erythematosus. Prednisolone, 15 to 60 mg daily, was given initially. Cyclophosphamide 400 mg was given intravenously once a week, then 100 mg by mouth 4 times a week; some patients continued to take small doses of prednisolone. Treatment had continued for 6 to 84 months and in some patients was no longer required; 16 patients had complete clinical and biochemical remissions and 12 had minimal residual clinical and biochemical involvement. Side-effects included alopecia (8 patients), herpes zoster (5), tuberculous infections (2), fungous infections (2), haematuria (1), leucopenia (1), and menstrual disturbances (14).— P. H. Feng *et al.*, *Br. med. J.*, 1973, *2*, 450.

See also under Azathioprine, p.191.

Malignant effusions. The intrapleural administration of cyclophosphamide for pleural effusions is ineffective since cyclophosphamide required activation in the liver. It is unsuitable for regional use.— K. L. Sutton, *Postgrad. med. J.*, 1973, *49*, 729.

Malignant neoplasms. A view that cyclophosphamide may alter tumour cell antigenicity and, in so doing, set into motion an immune response directed against the previously tolerated cancer cells.— R. H. Wander and H. R. Hilgard (letter), *Lancet*, 1980, *2*, 1077.

References to cyclophosphamide in the treatment of various malignant neoplasms: M. Fox, *Br. J. Urol.*, 1965, *37*, 399 (urinary tract); D. G. Decker *et al.*, *Am. J. Obstet. Gynec.*, 1967, *97*, 656 (ovary); J. P. Smith *et al.*, *Am. J. Obstet. Gynec.*, 1967, *97*, 800 (cervix).

See also under Choice of Antineoplastic Agent, p.180.

Malignant neoplasms of the breast. Prolonged treatment with cyclophosphamide for 4 to 6 months following mastectomy in 46 women with breast cancer produced a better 10-year survival-rate than no chemotherapy or a single injection of cyclophosphamide or thiotepa at surgery in an earlier group of 167 women. Comparison of 5-year survival-rates with a later group who had received no chemotherapy or a single injection at surgery also showed better results for prolonged treatment in patients classified as axillary-node negative. The cyclophosphamide schedule produced a high incidence of alopecia.— I. A. Donovan *et al.* (letter), *Lancet*, 1976, *1*, 42.

Cyclophosphamide appeared to induce primary ovarian failure which might explain its activity in breast cancer.— H. Koyama *et al.*, *Cancer*, 1977, *39*, 1403.

See also under Choice of Antineoplastic Agent, p.180.

Malignant neoplasms of the bronchus and lung. In a 3-year-study of 466 patients with operable pulmonary carcinoma the survival rate of those treated postoperatively with cyclophosphamide was no greater than that of a control group which did not receive cytostatic medication.— E. A. C. Buyze and F. A. Nelemans, *Arzneimittel-Forsch.*, 1973, *23*, 860. Combined chemotherapy with cyclophosphamide, vincristine, semustine, and bleomycin (COMB) was no better than cyclophosphamide alone in advanced squamous carcinoma of the lung. Partial responses occurred in 1 of 20 in the combined group and 1 of 27 in the cyclophosphamide group.— G. P. Bodey *et al.*, *Cancer*, 1977, *39*, 1026.

See also under Choice of Antineoplastic Agent, p.182.

Muscular disorders, non-malignant. Two patients with severe myasthenia gravis, which was not controlled by anticholinesterase drugs or improved after each patient had had a thymoma removed, were given cyclophosphamide intravenously in a dose of 200 mg daily for 20 or 30 days. After a short period there was a continuous slow improvement which was maintained for 2 years in 1 patient. The other patient had 2 relapses which responded to further cyclophosphamide.— K. Nouza and V. Smat, *Revue fr. Étud. clin. biol.*, 1968, *13*, 161, per *Abstr. Wld Med.*, 1968, *42*, 797.

See also under Corticosteroids, p.455.

Ocular disorders, non-malignant. The symptoms of Graves' ophthalmopathy were improved in 2 patients by treatment with cyclophosphamide 150 mg daily for 15 months and 85 mg daily for 5 months by mouth. Similar symptoms improved in another patient receiving cyclophosphamide 700 mg intravenously each month for 12 months to treat ovarian carcinoma.— S. T. Bigos *et al.*, *Ann. intern. Med.*, 1979, *90*, 921.

Organ and tissue transplantation. The successful use of cyclophosphamide in bone-marrow transplantation.—The Royal Marsden Hospital Bone-Marrow Transplantation Team, *Lancet*, 1977, *2*, 742.

A discussion of the use of cyclophosphamide and corticosteroids in large doses, given to kidney donors, to improve transplant survival.— *Br. med. J.*, 1977, *2*, 1172. See also under Corticosteroids, p.456.

Further references: T. E. Starzl *et al.*, *Surgery Gynec. Obstet.*, 1971, *133*, 981; E. D. Thomas *et al.*, *Lancet*, 1972, *1*, 284 (cyclophosphamide and methotrexate in marrow transplantation); H. Zincke *et al.*, *Mayo Clin. Proc.*, 1976, *51*, 693 (cyclophosphamide or procarbazine in kidney transplantation).

Pregnancy and the neonate. *First trimester.* See Adverse Effects, above.

Second trimester. Reports of apparently normal infants born to women given cyclophosphamide in the second trimester of pregnancy: M. J. Lacher and W. Geller, *J. Am. med. Ass.*, 1966, *195*, 486; M. Khurshid and M. Saleem (letter), *Lancet*, 1978, *2*, 534.

Third trimester. Cyclophosphamide apparently had no effect on the foetus when given to a woman in the last trimester of pregnancy.— J. A. Hardin, *Obstet. Gynec.*, 1972, *39*, 850. See also J. I. Durodola, *J. natn. med. Ass.*, 1979, *71*, 165.

Renal disorders, non-malignant. Cyclophosphamide 3 mg per kg body-weight was compared with azathioprine 2.5 to 3 mg per kg in the treatment of 24 Nigerian children with the nephrotic syndrome mainly associated with quartan malaria and generally considered to be corticosteroid-resistant. Both drugs were given daily for 12 weeks and 12 additional patients acted as controls. Complete clinical remission occurred in 2 children treated with cyclophosphamide, and considerable improvement in 6, but there was a high incidence of adverse effects and the 5-year survival-rate was not improved. Complete clinical remission occurred in 2 children treated with azathioprine, but there was increased mortality due to renal failure. No remissions were noted in the control group. It was recommended that cyclophosphamide could be used to treat West African children with a short history of nephrotic syndrome and relatively mild histological lesions, and that azathioprine was contra-indicated.— A. Adeniyi *et al.*, *Archs Dis. Childh.*, 1979, *54*, 204.

For further reference to the use of cyclophosphamide in renal disorders, see Corticosteroids, p.457.

Rheumatic disorders, non-malignant. In 2 patients with Felty's syndrome [a syndrome including rheumatoid arthritis] the granulocytopenia responded to cyclophosphamide therapy in doses of 100 mg daily (subsequently reduced to 50 mg daily in 1 patient).— K. B. Wiesner *et al.* (letter), *New Engl. J. Med.*, 1977, *296*, 1172.

Comparisons of high-dose and low-dose cyclophosphamide regimens in patients with rheumatoid arthritis.— H. J. Williams *et al.*, *Clin. Pharmac. Ther.*, 1979, *25*, 253; H. J. Williams *et al.*, *Arthritis Rheum.*, 1980, *23*, 521.

Further references to cyclophosphamide in rheumatoid arthritis: I. Stojanovic *et al.*, *Scand. J. Rheumatol.*, 1978, *7*, 1; N. D. Hall *et al.*, *Agents and Actions*, 1979, *9*, 97.

For earlier references to cyclophosphamide in the treatment of rheumatic disorders, see Martindale 27th Edn, p. 140.

Skin disorders, non-malignant. Reports on the use of cyclophosphamide in the treatment of severe skin diseases: A. Medved and I. Maxwell, *Can. med. Ass. J.*, 1974, *111*, 245 (pemphigus vulgaris and bullous pemphigoid); J. S. Pasricha *et al.*, *Br. J. Derm.*, 1975, *93*, 573 (pemphigus); H. J. Brody and D. J. Pirozzi, *Archs Derm.*, 1977, *113*, 1598 (benign mucous membrane pemphigoid); R. J. Martin *et al.*, *Milit. Med.*, 1977, *142*, 158 (panniculitis); M. J. Fellner *et al.*, *Archs Derm.*, 1978, *114*, 889 (pemphigus vulgaris); J. G. L. Morrison and E. J. Schulz, *Br. J. Derm.*, 1978, *98*, 203 (eczema); *J. Am. med. Ass.*, 1979, *241*, 2475 (ichythyosis linearis circumflexa and poikiloderma congenitale).

Vasculitis. Systemic vasculitis is often associated with immunopathogenic mechanisms and is characterised by inflammation and necrosis of blood vessels. It is the major and primary manifestation of a number of syndromes as well as being a relatively minor component of other primary disease processes. Attempts have been made to classify diseases in the spectrum of vasculitis and they include the polyarteritis nodosa group of systemic necrotising vasculitis, hypersensitivity vasculitis, and Wegener's granulomatosis. There may be considerable overlap, especially between classic polyarteritis nodosa and systemic necrotising vasculitis. Several of these serious systemic syndromes are now proving responsive to chronic low-dose treatment with cyclophosphamide.— A. S. Fauci *et al.*, *Ann. intern. Med.*, 1978, *89*, 660.

Complete, sometimes dramatic, remissions were achieved in 13 of 16 patients with severe systemic necrotising vasculitis when they took cyclophosphamide 2 mg per kg body-weight daily, and in one patient who took the same dose of azathioprine; 3 patients died although 2 were in remission. Within 2 weeks of starting treatment with cyclophosphamide, the corticosteroid regimens which 16 patients had been on previously were tapered; 6 remained on alternate-day therapy and corticosteroids were eventually stopped in 7. The cyclophosphamide dose was continually titrated and readjusted to maintain the total neutrophil count at not less than 1000 to 1500 per mm^3. There were no relapses during treatment with cyclophosphamide and remissions ranged from 2 to 61 months.— A. S. Fauci *et al.*, *New Engl. J. Med.*, 1979, *301*, 235. Comment.— B. Zweiman, *ibid.*, 266.

Further references to the use of cyclophosphamide in patients with vasculitis: S. Tuma *et al.*, *J. Am. med. Ass.*, 1976, *235*, 280 (acute periarteritis nodosa in the kidney); A. S. Fauci *et al.*, *Am. J. Med.*, 1978, *64*, 890 (advanced polyarteritis nodosa); T. Abel *et al.*, *Ann. intern. Med.*, 1980, *93*, 407 (rheumatoid vasculitis); *Lancet*, 1980, *2*, 407.

See also under Wegener's Granulomatosis (below).

Wegener's granulomatosis. Reports of the successful use of cyclophosphamide in patients with Wegener's granulomatosis: B. F. Haynes and A. S. Fauci, *New Engl. J. Med.*, 1978, *299*, 764; L. Abraham-Inpijn, *J. Lar. Otol.*, 1980, *94*, 785; H. L. Harrison *et al.*, *J. Am. med. Ass.*, 1980, *244*, 1599; T. I. Steinman *et al.*, *Am. J. Med.*, 1980, *68*, 458.

See also under Use of Immunosuppressants, p.187, and under Vasculitis (above).

Preparations

Cyclophosphamide for Injection *(U.S.P.)*. A sterile mixture of cyclophosphamide and sodium chloride. The injection is prepared by the addition of diluent before use. Potency is expressed in terms of the equivalent amount of anhydrous cyclophosphamide. Store at 2° to 32°. A 3.3% solution has a pH of 3.9 to 6.7 determined 30 minutes after its preparation.

Cyclophosphamide Injection *(B.P.)*. A sterile solution of cyclophosphamide in Water for Injections containing sodium chloride, prepared by dissolving, immediately before use, the sterile contents of a sealed container (Cyclophosphamide for Injection) in the requisite amount of Water for Injections. The sealed container contains a mixture of cyclophosphamide 100 parts and sodium chloride 45 parts by wt. Potency is expressed in terms of the equivalent amount of anhydrous cyclophosphamide.

Cyclophosphamide Tablets *(B.P.)*. Tablets containing cyclophosphamide (monohydrate). They are sugar-coated or compression-coated.

Cyclophosphamide Tablets *(U.S.P.)*. Tablets containing cyclophosphamide. Potency is expressed in terms of the equivalent amount of anhydrous cyclophosphamide. Store at 2° to 32° in airtight containers.

Proprietary Preparations

Cyclophosphamide *(Farmitalia Carlo Erba, UK)*. Available as **Tablets** of 50 mg, and as powder (with sodium chloride) for preparing injections, in **Vials** containing 0.1, 0.2, 0.5, and 1 g.

Endoxana *(WB Pharmaceuticals, UK: Boehringer Ingelheim, UK)*. Cyclophosphamide, available as **Tablets** of 10 and 50 mg, and as powder (with sodium chloride 45 mg for each 100 mg of cyclophosphamide) for preparing injections, in **Vials** each containing the equivalent of 0.1, 0.2, 0.5, or 1 g of anhydrous cyclophosphamide.

Other Proprietary Names

Cytoxan *(Canad., USA)*; Endoxan *(Belg., Denm., Ger., Neth., S.Afr.)*; Endoxan-Asta *(Arg., Austral., Fr., Ital., Switz.)*; Enduxan *(Braz.)*; Genoxal *(Spain)*; Procytox *(Canad.)*; Sendoxan *(Norw., Swed.)*.

1882-m

Cyclosporin A.

A metabolite of the fungi *Cylindrocarpon lucidum* Booth and *Trichoderma polysporum*. Cyclosporin A is a cyclic polypeptide consisting of 11 amino acids and with a molecular weight of 1203.

CAS — 59865-13-3.

Practically **insoluble** in water; soluble in alcohol and fixed oils.

Adverse Effects and Treatment. Nephrotoxicity is a major adverse effect of cyclosporin A but may be avoided by adequate hydration and mannitol diuresis. Treatment with cyclosporin A may be associated with the development of lymphomas, a 10% incidence has been reported in one study of transplant patients. Other adverse effects include gastro-intestinal disturbances, transient hepatotoxicity, hirsutism, rashes, gum hypertrophy, angio-oedema, and mild tremor.

Carcinogenicity. A report by R.Y. Calne *et al.* (*Lancet*, 1979, *2*, 1033 and 1202) of the disturbing occurrence of 3 lymphomas, one in a patient receiving only cyclosporin A, in a study of 34 transplant patients over only 15 months was followed by a similar report in *primate* allograft recipients whose postoperative treatment included cyclosporin A (C.P. Bieber *et al.*, *Lancet*, 1980, *1*, 43). An Epstein-Barr-virus related lymphoma similar to a Burkitt's lymphoma has occurred in a renal transplant patient given long-term cyclosporin A therapy (D.H. Crawford *et al.*, *Lancet*, 1980, *1*, 1355); this group (*idem*, 1981, *1*, 10) have also presented evidence *in vitro* that renal transplant patients receiving cyclosporin A cannot mount a cytotoxic response to Epstein-Barr-virus infected B cells. Nevertheless P. Jacobs and E.C. Gordon-Smith (*Lancet*, 1980, *2*, 1296) consider that the case for cyclosporin A being responsible for the development of lymphoma is not proved. In an attempt to put the incidence of lymphoma in perspective R.Y. Calne *et al.* (*Br. med. J.*, 1980, *280*, 43) stress that a high incidence has been reported with the use of all immunosuppressants, that transplant patients are suffering from lethal diseases, and that cyclosporin A has enabled previously hopeless patients to receive transplants. Further studies may enable the dose to be reduced so that sufficient immunosuppression is achieved without a high incidence of lymphoma.

A report of 2 women patients who developed benign breast lumps following treatment with cyclosporin A.— K. Rolles and R. Y. Calne (letter), *Lancet*, 1980, *2*, 795.

Effects on the kidneys. The management of nephrotoxicity associated with cyclosporin A.— G. B. G. Klintmalm *et al.*, *Lancet*, 1981, *1*, 470.

Precautions. For reference to the precautions necessary with immunosuppressants, see Antineoplastic Agents, p.175.

A warning that the commercially prepared drinking solution providing cyclosporin A 10 mg per kg body-weight daily for *animal* studies may be more potent than the olive oil solution providing 10 mg per kg daily. Dosages calculated using the olive oil solution should not be extrapolated.— W. P. Homan *et al.* (letter), *Lancet*, 1979, *2*, 421.

Uses. Cyclosporin A is a powerful immunosuppressant (p.186) with relatively little effect on the bone marrow; it is used to prolong the survival of organ and tissue transplants. It has been given by mouth or intramuscularly in doses usually ranging from 10 to 25 mg per kg body-weight daily.

Action. A suggestion, based on findings in *mice*, that cyclosporin A may have an antileukaemic activity.— W. Kreis (letter), *Lancet*, 1980, *1*, 1033.

A study indicating that cyclosporin A is a unique immunosuppressant acting on the regulatory balance of the immune system.— G. Routhier *et al.*, *Lancet*, 1980, *2*, 1223.

Experimental studies on the action of cyclosporin A: J. F. Borel *et al.*, *Agents and Actions*, 1976, *6*, 468; J. F. Borel, *Immunology*, 1976, *31*, 631; J. F. Borel *et al.*, *Immunology*, 1977, *32*, 1017; J. F. Borel *et al.*, *Eur. J. Rheumat. Inflam.*, 1978, *1*, 237; R. Y. Calne, *Clin. exp. Immun.*, 1979, *35*, 1.

Administration in hepatic insufficiency. The pharmacodynamics of cyclosporin A are not yet known but it is thought to be excreted in the bile and abnormalities of liver function probably interfere with absorption and excretion of the drug.— R. Y. Calne *et al.*, *Lancet*, 1979, *2*, 1033 and 1202.

Administration in renal insufficiency. See Organ and Tissue Transplantation, Kidney (below).

Lupus erythematosus. Of 5 patients with systemic lupus erythematosus, who were given a total of 6 courses of cyclosporin A in liquid form at a dose of 10 mg per kg body-weight daily, only 2 patients, both with severe arthralgia, benefited and no patient could tolerate the drug for longer than 7 weeks. Side-effects included nausea, vomiting, a burning sensation in the skin, increasing alopecia, renal toxicity, and angio-oedema. The angio-oedema occurred in 3 patients, began about 2 weeks after the start of treatment, and persisted for up to 2 weeks after treatment was stopped.— D. A. Isenberg *et al.* (letter), *New Engl. J. Med.*, 1980, *303*, 754.

Organ and tissue transplantation. Reviews of cyclosporin A: *Lancet*, 1979, *2*, 779; *J. Am. med. Ass.*, 1979, *242*, 2265; P. J. Tutschka, *Blut*, 1979, *39*, 81.

A study indicating that in *rabbits* cyclosporin A is a donor specific, not a tissue specific, immunosuppressive agent.— C. J. Green *et al.*, *Lancet*, 1979, *2*, 123.

Bone marrow. A report of encouraging results with cyclosporin A for the prevention of graft-versus-host disease in 23 patients who received allogeneic bone-marrow transplantation; 21 had acute leukaemia, 1 had chronic granulocytic leukaemia, and 1 had aplastic anaemia. Cyclosporin A was given intramuscularly in a dose of 12.5 mg per kg body-weight every 12 hours for 24 hours before the infusion of marrow, and continued for 5 days, half this dose was then given by mouth in a specially prepared 'drink solution'. Three patients whose cyclosporin A was stopped owing to the development of rashes, developed graft-versus-host disease, although 2 had previously been biopsy-negative. It was subsequently decided not to stop cyclosporin A therapy just for rashes. Thirteen of the remaining 20 patients are alive and well after a median follow-up of 7 months (maximum 13 months), and no second malignancies have been detected. Only one of the 20 patients developed acute graft-versus-host disease compared with 11 of 26 patients in an unpublished series given methotrexate. Side-effects of cyclosporin A included raised serum creatinine and urea concentrations, although histological examination of some kidneys revealed unimportant changes; other side-effects included abnormal body hair and nail growth, mild tremors, a 'flat affect', and anorexia; cyclosporin A may have contributed to a raised serum bilirubin in some patients; thrombocytopenia and mild anaemia, associated with a hypocellular and dysplastic marrow, in some patients, may have been associated with other drug therapy and, in some instances renal dysfunction, but a direct marrow-depressant effect of cyclosporin A could not be excluded.— R. L. Powles *et al.*, *Lancet*, 1980, *1*, 327.

Cornea. Administration of cyclosporin A considerably prolonged the survival of vascularised corneal grafts in *rabbits*.— D. J. Coster *et al.* (letter), *Lancet*, 1979, *2*, 688. See also W. F. I. Shepherd *et al.*, *Br. J. Ophthal.*, 1980, *64*, 148; *ibid.*, 145.

Heart. References to the use of cyclosporin A in prolonging the survival of heart transplants in *animals:* R. Y. Calne *et al.*, *Lancet*, 1978, *1*, 1183; S. W. Jamieson *et al.* (letter), *Lancet*, 1979, *1*, 545.

Kidney. A report of continuing experience with cyclosporin A as the only initial immunosuppressant in transplant recipients, in doses of 10, 17, or 25 mg per kg body-weight daily. Of 32 patients with renal failure, all of whom had received previous blood transfusions, 31 received first allografts and one a second allograft, and one received a pancreas from the kidney donor; 2 patients were orthotopically transplanted with livers, and one of these received a heterotopic pancreatic allograft. Most patients had 2 or more mismatches. Following the earlier evidence of nephrotoxicity this was avoided in 19 by peri-operative hydration and mannitol diuresis, which has now become standard policy. Life is still being supported by 26 renal allografts, 3 of these more than a year after transplantation, and the pancreases and livers are also still functioning. Of 16 patients treated with cyclosporin A alone, 2 developed self-limiting viral infections, one developed cytomegalovirus infection and immunosuppression was changed, one allograft became infected with bacteria and was removed, and one patient required resection of a gastroduodenal lymphoma. Five of 6 given corticosteroids and a cyclophosphamide derivative, died of sepsis and one of these was found at necropsy to have a jejunal lymphoma. One of 11 patients given additional corticosteroids, died of sepsis and pulmonary lymphoma; of the remaining 10, one had severe herpes simplex infection, and one required a colostomy for a perforated sigmoid diverticulum. Other side-effects were abnormalities of liver function early after operation, which tended to resolve as the dose of cyclosporin A was reduced; most had increased hair growth on the face and body, and most with their own teeth developed gum hypertrophy which tended to get better with time; mild tremor was common in the postoperative phase and resolved with time, in 3 it was severe. None of the 26 patients with life-supporting renal allografts has entirely normal kidney function, the worst function, as a group, being in those still receiving additional corticosteroids. On several occasions an improvement in renal function has been noted as the dose of cyclosporin A was reduced; most patients surviving more than 6 months are receiving 10 to 12 mg per kg daily, although one is receiving only 1.6 mg per kg daily; evidence of rejection was shown in 2 grafts on dosage reduction. The optimum dosage of cyclosporin A has not yet been clarified but an initial dose of 10 mg per kg daily may be too little and 25 mg per kg too much. Better results are being obtained with 17 mg per kg daily, slowly reduced to 10 mg per kg daily; it has only been reluctantly reduced to below this dose, and has not been stopped in any of the currently surviving patients. If possible, it is most important to avoid adding other immunosuppressants in view of the high incidence of side-effects in patients treated with additional drugs. The occurrence of 3 lymphomas, one in a patient receiving only cyclosporin A, occurring in this trial of 34 patients extending over only 15 months is disturbing, and has led to a reluctance to speculate about the future of cyclosporin A. In man, cyclosporin A appears to be the most powerful immunosuppressant used in the management of patients with cadaveric renal allografts, and advantages include its steroid-sparing properties, its relative lack of bone-marrow toxicity, and its patient acceptability.— R. Y. Calne *et al.*, *Lancet*, 1979, *2*, 1033 and 1202.

Further references: P. A. Keown *et al.*, *Lancet*, 1981, *1*, 686.

In a pilot study of prednisone in association with cyclosporin A in cadaveric renal transplantation, patients received 12 to 14 mg per kg body-weight of cyclosporin A pre-operatively and daily postoperatively without adjustment of dosage for graft function. Three of 15 patients were oliguric from one to 13 days postoperatively and required dialysis. All of these patients were discharged by the 21st postoperative day with resolving acute tubular necrosis and a mean serum creatinine of 1.7 mg per 100 ml.— J. J. Rynasiewicz *et al.* (letter), *Lancet*, 1981, *1*, 276.

Liver. Liver transplantation with the use of cyclosporin A and prednisone.— T. E. Starzl *et al.*, *New Engl. J. Med.*, 1981, *305*, 266.

See also under Kidney, above.

Pancreas. References to *animal* studies with cyclosporin A in pancreatic transplantation: J. F. W. Garvey *et al.* (letter), *Lancet*, 1979, *1*, 971; P. McMaster *et al.*, *Br. med. J.*, 1980, *280*, 444.

Skin disorders, non-malignant. *Psoriasis.* Preliminary results suggesting that the skin lesions of psoriasis can be beneficially affected by cyclosporin A. Psoriatic plaques almost disappeared 5 days after the start of treatment with cyclosporin A 900 mg daily then 450 mg daily in a 64-year-old woman with widespread psoriasis and progressive psoriatic arthropathy. A beneficial effect was also seen in 3 similar patients, with less severe joint changes, given 300 to 450 mg daily for about a week. The lesions gradually returned in all patients about 2 weeks after stopping cyclosporin A.— W. Mueller and B. Herrmann (letter), *New Engl. J. Med.*, 1979, *301*, 555.

Manufacturers
Sandoz, Switz.

1826-a

Cytarabine *(B.P., U.S.P.).* Arabinosylcytosine; Ara-C; Cytosine Arabinoside; NSC 63878 *(hydrochloride)*; U 19 920; WR 28453. 1-β-D-Arabinofuranosylcytosine; 4-Amino-1-β-D-arabinofuranosylpyrimidin-2(1*H*)-one.
$C_9H_{13}N_3O_5$=243.2.

CAS — 147-94-4.

Pharmacopoeias. In *Br.*, *Chin.*, and *U.S. U.S.P.* also includes Sterile Cytarabine.

An odourless white to off-white crystalline powder. **Soluble** 1 in 10 of water and 1 in 1000 of alcohol and chloroform. A 1% solution in water is dextrorotatory and has a pH of 4 to 6. An 8.92% solution in water is iso-osmotic with serum. **Store** in a cool place. Protect from light.

For details of the use of cytarabine in solutions for intrathecal administration, see Methotrexate, p.215.

Incompatibility. The u.v. absorption spectrum of cytarabine was slightly altered, suggesting incompatibility, when a dilute solution in dextrose injection was mixed with a solution of fluorouracil; the spectrum of fluorouracil was not affected.— M. P. McRae and J. C. King, *Am. J. Hosp. Pharm.*, 1976, *33*, 1010.

Stability in solution. An aqueous solution of cytarabine should maintain 90% potency for 6 months at 25° in a 0.06M phosphate buffer pH 6.9. Solutions were much less stable at acid and alkaline pH.— R. E. Notari, *J. pharm. Sci.*, 1972, *61*, 1189. See also *idem*, 1967, *56*, 804.

Cytarabine 5 mg per ml was stable for 7 days at room temperature and at 30° in Elliott's B solution, sodium chloride injection, and Lactated Ringer's Injection (*U.S.P.*).— J. C. Cradock *et al.*, *Am. J. Hosp. Pharm.*, 1978, *35*, 402.

Adverse Effects and Treatment. For an outline of the adverse effects experienced with antineoplastic agents and immunosuppressants and general guidelines for their treatment, see Antineoplastic Agents, p.171 and p.174.

The nadir of granulocytopenia may occur 12 to 14 days after starting treatment with cytarabine, with recovery in about 3 weeks; striking megaloblastic changes have also been reported. Nausea and vomiting is more severe when cytarabine is given rapidly. Other side-effects reported include neurotoxicity, renal dysfunction, abnormal liver-function tests, and a 'flu-like' syndrome.

Corneal ulceration has followed local application in the eye. There may be pain at injection sites and thrombophlebitis has occurred.

Deoxycytidine was reported to antagonise the toxic as well as some antitumour effects of cytarabine.— V. M. Buchman *et al.* (letter), *Lancet*, 1977, *1*, 1061.

Allergy and anaphylaxis. Reports of allergic reactions associated with cytarabine: T. A. Bensinger *et al.* (letter), *J. Am. med. Ass.*, 1974, *229*, 1578 (fever, prevented by diphenhydramine); A. L. Rassiga *et al.*, *Archs intern. Med.*, 1980, *140*, 425 (anaphylaxis and successful desensitisation).

Effects on the nervous system. Two patients developed sensory peripheral neuropathy after receiving a total of 4 g and 600 mg respectively of cytarabine.— J. A. Russell and R. L. Powles (letter), *Br. med. J.*, 1974, *4*, 652.

Reactions to intrathecal injections of cytarabine: A. M. Marmont and E. E. Damasio (letter), *Br. med. J.*, 1973, *4*, 47 (nerve damage causing dysphagia, aphonia, and diplopia); R. H. A. Campbell *et al.*, *Archs Dis. Childh.*, 1977, *52*, 850 (arachnoiditis); L. Wolff *et al.*, *Cancer*, 1979, *43*, 83 (paraplegia). See also Methotrexate, p.216.

Effects on the vascular system. A fatal Budd-Chiari-like illness or toxic veno-occlusive disease of the liver developed in 2 adult male patients during treatment with thioguanine. Both patients had also received cytarabine. There were 4 further reports of veno-occlusive disease of the liver in children with acute myelogenous leukaemia during maintenance therapy with thioguanine and daunorubicin; all had been previously treated with cytarabine.— P. F. Griner *et al.*, *Ann. intern. Med.*, 1976, *85*, 578.

Precautions. For reference to the precautions necessary with antineoplastic agents and immunosuppressants, see Antineoplastic Agents, p.175.

Cytarabine should be given with care to patients with impaired liver function.

A single dose of cytarabine and thioguanine resulted in profound hyperphosphataemia, hypocalcaemia, cardiac arrest, and death when given to a patient with acute myelofibrosis and severe hypercalcaemia, who was also receiving mithramycin.— J. A. Libnoch *et al.*, *Am. J. Med.*, 1977, *62*, 432.

Interactions. Flucytosine has been reported to be competitively inhibited by cytarabine.— R. Y. Cartwright, *Br. med. J.*, 1978, *2*, 108.

For a report of antagonism between methotrexate and cytarabine in *mice*, see Methotrexate, p.217.

For a study indicating that cytarabine reduced the activity of gentamicin and amikacin *in vitro* against some Gram-negative organisms, see Gentamicin, p.1168.

Pregnancy and the neonate. *First trimester.* A report of limb and ear deformities in the infant of a woman given cytarabine at the estimated time of conception and at an estimated 4 to 8 weeks after conception.— V. M. Wagner *et al.* (letter), *Lancet*, 1980, *2*, 98. Of 20 cases reported, including 3 women who conceived while taking cytarabine and 2 who received it at 10 to 12 weeks after conception, no congenital abnormalities were noted in any of the 17 normal infants, 5 therapeutic abortions, and one stillbirth (following pre-eclamptic toxaemia).— G. Morgenstern (letter), *ibid.*, 259.

Absorption and Fate. Cytarabine is not effective by mouth, less than 20% of a dose is absorbed from the gastro-intestinal tract. After intravenous injection it disappears rapidly from the plasma. It is converted to an active form by phosphorylation and is rapidly deaminated, mainly in the liver and the kidneys, to inactive 1-β-D-arabinofuranosyluracil (uracil arabinoside). The majority of an intravenous dose is excreted in the urine as the inactive metabolite within 24 hours.

There is only moderate diffusion of cytarabine across the blood-brain barrier but, because of low deaminase activity in the cerebrospinal fluid, concentrations achieved after continuous intravenous infusion or intrathecal injection are maintained for longer in the CSF than are those in plasma.

Single doses of 47 mg to 3 g per m^2 body-surface of tritiated cytarabine given intravenously to 8 patients produced total plasma concentrations which decreased in a biphasic pattern with a mean half-life for the 1st phase of 12 minutes and for the 2nd of 111 minutes. Most of the activity was accounted for by cytarabine and uracil arabinoside; after the 1st phase over 80% of the radioactivity in the plasma and urine was due to uracil arabinoside. Red blood cell and liver concentrations were detected in patients and higher red blood cell concentrations occurred in patients with solid tumours. A dose of 112 mg per m^2 daily given by constant infusion produced a steady plasma concentration of 50 to 100 ng per ml. When 400 mg per m^2 was given, the plasma concentration increased to nearly 500 ng per ml and 1 patient maintained a steady CSF concentration of 200 ng per ml. The intrathecal administration of 50 mg per m^2 to 1 patient produced a CSF concentration which decreased exponentially with a half-life of 2 hours; after 7 hours only 10% was in the form of uracil arabinoside. Following parenteral administration between 70 and 84% of the dose was excreted in the urine within 24 hours, 7 to 8% as cytarabine, but in 3 patients given their dose by mouth only 14% was excreted in 24 hours and less than 3% was as cytarabine.— D. H. W. Ho and E. Frei, *Clin. Pharmac. Ther.*, 1971, *12*, 944. A study of the pharmacokinetics of cytarabine following bolus intravenous injections in 14 patients with acute myeloid leukaemia. Following the initial half-life phase of about 1 to 2 minutes, the plasma half-life of the second phase was 6.6 to 18.9 minutes which agreed with R.L. Momparler *et al.* (*Cancer Res.*, 1972, *32*, 408) and B.C. Baguley and E.M. Falkenhaug (*Eur. J. Cancer*, 1975, *11*, 43) and suggested that the mean initial phase of 12 minutes found by D.H.W. Ho and E. Frei (*Clin. Pharmac. Ther.*, 1971, *12*, 944) might correspond to the second phase with their second-phase finding of 111 minutes possibly indicating a third phase of about 2 hours. Variations in elimination or degradation might be important in predicting the results of chemotherapy since a complete remission was obtained in 9 of the patients with an average second-phase half-life of 15.1 minutes whereas therapy failed in the other 5 whose average was 9.6 minutes. Push injections with an increased dose or continuous infusions might improve the results in patients with a short half-life.— R. van Prooijen *et al.*, *Clin. Pharmac. Ther.*, 1977, *21*, 744. A further study in which most patients showed a biphasic or triphasic decline in plasma concentrations with terminal half-lives ranging from 7 to 107 minutes. The pharmacokinetics of cytarabine varied markedly from patient to patient and a wide range of plasma concentrations was associated with therapeutic response. Unless plasma concentrations can be related to tissue concentrations of active metabolites, individualisation of therapy will remain difficult.— A. L. Harris *et al.*, *Br. J. clin. Pharmac.*, 1979, *8*, 219.

Further references to the absorption and fate of cytarabine: W. Kreis *et al.*, *Cancer Treat. Rep.*, 1977, *61*, 723.

Uses. Cytarabine, a pyrimidine nucleoside analogue, is an antineoplastic agent which inhibits the synthesis of deoxyribonucleic acid. It also has antiviral and immunosuppressant properties.

Cytarabine is used mainly in the treatment of leukaemia, especially acute myeloid leukaemia in adults when it is usually given in association with thioguanine and doxorubicin or daunorubicin (see p.179). The usual dose in leukaemia in adults and children is up to 2 mg per kg body-weight intravenously daily for 10 days; if after 10 days a response and adverse effects are not evident, the dose may be increased to 4 mg per kg daily. Alternatively 0.5 to 1 mg per kg may be infused daily in 1 to 24 hours for 10 days then 2 mg per kg daily. It may also be given intermittently in doses of 3 to 5 mg per kg daily by intravenous injection for 5 consecutive days repeated after an interval of 2 to 9 days. For maintenance, 1 mg per kg may be given intravenously or subcutaneously once or twice weekly.

In leukaemic meningitis cytarabine has been given intrathecally, often in a dose of 30 mg per m^2 body-surface every 4 days; it has also been used prophylactically.

Cytarabine has also been used in the treatment of herpes infection in doses of 100 mg per m^2 body-surface daily by intravenous injection or 2 to 4 mg per kg body-weight daily for about 5 days. Doses of 10 mg per m^2 have also been given intrathecally for encephalitis.

White cell and platelet counts should be determined regularly during treatment with cytarabine and therapy should be stopped immediately if the count falls rapidly or to low values.

Administration in renal insufficiency. Cytarabine could be given in usual doses to patients with renal failure.— W. M. Bennett *et al.*, *Ann. intern. Med.*, 1977, *86*, 754. See also *idem*, 1980, *93*, 286.

Infections. Cytarabine has been used in the treatment of a number of viral infections including herpes, cytomegalovirus, and smallpox. In general, controlled studies have not substantiated earlier reports of beneficial results and in some cases cytarabine appears to have potentiated infections, particularly in immunosuppressed patients.

A review of the mechanism of the lethal action of cytarabine on viruses indicated that it was due to its conversion to its aranucleoside triphosphate that appeared to act by relatively specific inhibition of DNA synthesis and possibly by incorporation into cell or virus DNA.— S. S. Cohen, *Cancer*, 1977, *40*, 509. The antiviral activity of derivatives of cytarabine.— K. Sato *et al.*, *Antimicrob. Ag. Chemother.*, 1977, *11*, 191; S. Nishiyama *et al.*, *ibid.*, 198.

Double-blind studies which failed to demonstrate a beneficial effect with cytarabine in patients with herpes zoster: C. M. Davis *et al.*, *J. Am. med. Ass.*, 1973, *224*, 122; D. A. Stevens *et al.*, *New Engl. J. Med.*, 1973, *289*, 873; S. C. Schimpff *et al.*, *J. infect. Dis.*, 1974, *130*, 673, per *Abstr. Hyg.*, 1975, *50*, 295; R. F. Betts *et al.*, *Ann. intern. Med.*, 1975, *82*, 778; C. E. Orfanos *et al.*, *Dt. med. Wschr.*, 1977, *102*, 312. Reports of beneficial effects from uncontrolled studies: W. Hryniuk *et al.*, *J. Am. med. Ass.*, 1972, *219*, 715; I. E. Fortuny *et al.* (letter), *Lancet*, 1973, *1*, 38; T. C. Hall *et al.*, *Postgrad. med. J.*, 1973, *49*, 429; L. E. Pierce and R. B. Jenkins, *Archs Ophthal., N.Y.*, 1973, *89*, 21; M. Baron and H. L. Wechsler, *Archs Derm.*, 1975, *111*, 910; S. Kernbaum (letter), *Br. med. J.*, 1976, *1*, 224; R. K. Laha *et al.*, *Can. med. Ass. J.*, 1976, *115*, 236 (herpes simplex encephalitis); S. N. Chatterjee *et al.*, *Am. J. Surg.*, 1977, *133*, 719; R. E. DuBois, *Sth. med. J.*, 1978, *71*, 909. Further references: B. E. Juel-Jensen, *Practitioner*, 1974, *213*, 508 (genital herpes).

Leukaemia. A brief review of studies using cytarabine as a cell synchronising agent, in the treatment of acute myelogenous leukaemia.— R. B. Livingston and J. S. Hart, *A. Rev. Pharmac. & Toxic.*, 1977, *17*, 529. The activity of doxorubicin and daunorubicin both of which act by inhibiting DNA synthesis had been enhanced by cytarabine possibly synchronising the leukaemic cell phase. Giving cytarabine over days 1 to 3 and doxorubicin on day 5 to 32 to adult patients with untreated acute nonlymphoid leukaemia did not increase the expected remission-rate although this had been reported when daunorubicin and doxorubicin were given sequentially on days 6 and 7. Further studies would be required to evaluate the value of synchronisation.— J. A. Whittaker *et al.* (letter), *Lancet*, 1977, *2*, 557. Further references to the effects of cytarabine on the cell cycle: P. J. Burke *et al.*, *Cancer Res.*, 1977, *37*, 2138; S. B. Reddy *et al.*, *Arzneimittel-Forsch.*, 1977, *27*, 1549; A. A. MacKinney and B. Flynn, *Am. J. Hematol.*, 1978, *5*, 93.

The degree to which cytarabine suppressed incorporation of tritiated thymidine into the leukaemic cell could be used to predict a remission of acute leukaemia in adults after intensive therapy. A complete or partial remission occurred in 13 of 14 patients with suppression to 15% or less of control counts compared with 2 of 12 patients not suppressed to that value.— P. C. Raich, *Lancet*, 1978, *1*, 74.

References to cytarabine in the management of *meningeal leukaemia*: P. R. Band *et al.*, *Cancer*, 1973, *32*, 744; M. Masi *et al.*, *Minerva paediat.*, 1975, *27*, 1624; M. Haghbin, *Cancer Treat. Rep.*, 1977, *61*, 661.

See also under Effects on the Nervous System in Adverse Effects (above).

Intravenous administration of cytarabine provided dramatic relief of severe bone pain and acute arthritis, without haematological remission, in a 60-year-old man with chronic myelomonocytic leukaemia.— D. Douer *et al.*, *Ann. rheum. Dis.*, 1977, *36*, 192.

See also under Choice of Antineoplastic Agent, p.180.

Neurological disorders, non-malignant. Disappointing results in 4 patients with multiple sclerosis given 4 intrathecal injections of cytarabine 40 mg in water at intervals of 5 days.— M. Gore *et al.* (letter), *Lancet*, 1979, *2*, 204.

Further references: R. Buckman and E. Wiltshaw, *Br. J. Haemat.*, 1976, *34*, 153 (the successful use of cytarabine in a patient with progressive multifocal leucoencephalopathy).

Pregnancy and the neonate. *First trimester.* See Precautions, above.

Second trimester. Treatment with cytarabine and thioguanine was effective in a woman with acute myelocytic leukaemia who first received therapy in the 26th week of pregnancy. She delivered a normal infant at term.— P. C. Raich and L. B. Curet, *Cancer*, 1975, *36*, 861, per *J. Am. med. Ass.*, 1975, *234*, 1280.

Third trimester. Reports on normal babies born to women given cytarabine during the 3rd trimester of pregnancy: B. G. M. Durie and H. R. Giles, *Archs intern. Med.*, 1977, *137*, 90.

Preparations

Cytarabine Injection *(B.P.)*. A sterile solution of cytarabine in Water for Injections containing 0.9% of benzyl alcohol. It is prepared by dissolving the contents of a sealed container (Cytarabine for Injection) in the requisite amount of solvent. pH of a 2% solution 4 to 6. Use within 48 hours of preparation.

Sterile Cytarabine *(U.S.P.)*. Cytarabine suitable for parenteral use. A 1% solution in water has a pH of 4 to 6.

When reconstituted with Bacteriostatic Water for Injection, solutions of sterile cytarabine are stable at room temperature for 48 hours.

Cytosar *(Upjohn, UK)*. Cytarabine, available in vials of 100 mg, with 5 ml of solvent (Water for Injections containing benzyl alcohol 0.9%). (Also available as Cytosar in *Belg., Canad., Denm., Jap., Neth., Norw., S.Afr., Swed., Switz.*).

Other Proprietary Names

Alexan *(Belg., Ger., Neth., Spain, Switz.)*; Arabitin *(Jap.)*; Aracytin *(Arg., Ital.)*; Aracytine *(Fr.)*; Cytosar-U *(Austral., USA)*; Iretin *(Jap.)*; Udicil *(Ger.)*.

1827-t

Dacarbazine. DIC; DTIC; NSC 45388; WR 139007; Imidazole Carboxamide. 5-(3,3-Dimethyl-1-triazeno)imidazole-4-carboxamide.

$C_6H_{10}N_6O$=182.2.

CAS — 4342-03-4.

A white to ivory-coloured solid. M.p. 204° to 207°. **Store** at 2° to 8°. Protect from light.

Solutions for injection are prepared by dissolving the sterile contents of a sealed container in Water for Injections. Such solutions, containing the equivalent of dacarbazine 10 mg per ml, have a pH of 3 to 4 and are stable for up to 8 hours at room temperature or for 72 hours at 4°. If further diluted with sodium chloride injection or dextrose injection the resulting solution is stable for up to 8 hours at room temperature or 24 hours at 4°. A colour change of the reconstituted solution from pale yellow to pink indicates decomposition.

CAUTION. *Dacarbazine is irritant; avoid contact with skin and mucous membranes.*

Stability in solution. Solutions of pure dacarbazine are sensitive to light and rapidly photolyse to 5-diazoimidazole-4-carboxamide and then to 2-azahypoxanthine, both of which are biologically active. Photodegradation of the commercial product, which when reconstituted contains dacarbazine citrate and mannitol, differs significantly from that of pure dacarbazine. A dilute aqueous solution of DTIC-Dome 1 mg in 100 ml is completely transformed within one minute to 5-diazoimidazole-4-carboxamide in direct sunlight and after 30 minutes 5-hydroxyimidazole-4-carboxamide, not 2-azahypoxanthine, has been identified. A concentrated aqueous solution of DTIC-Dome 100 mg in 50 ml evolves gas and turns red when exposed to sunlight. Dacarbazine should be protected from light at all times.— M. F. G. Stevens and L. Peatey, *J. Pharm. Pharmac.*, 1978, *30*, *Suppl.*, 47P.

The stability of dacarbazine solutions in the presence of a range of cytotoxic agents was monitored by ultra violet and visible spectrometry both in the dark and in ambient laboratory light. No detectable interaction occurred with actinomycin D, bleomycin, carmustine, cyclophosphamide, cytarabine, doxorubicin, fluorouracil, lomustine, methotrexate, or vinblastine. The only notable chemical change was the photo-decomposition of dacarbazine itself.— J. K. Horton and M. F. G. Stevens, *J. Pharm. Pharmac.*, 1979, *31*, *Suppl.*, 64P.

See also under Adverse Effects, below.

Adverse Effects, Treatment, and Precautions. For an outline of the adverse effects experienced with antineoplastic agents and immunosuppressants, general guidelines for their treatment and precautions, see Antineoplastic Agents, p.171, pp.174-5.

Leucopenia and thrombocytopenia with dacarbazine may be severe and the maximum effect may not be seen for 3 to 4 weeks. Anorexia, nausea, and vomiting are very common. Other side-effects include an influenza-like syndrome and facial flushing and paraesthesia. Extravasation produces pain and tissue damage.

Local venous pain and systemic side-effects such as nausea, vomiting, and hepatic toxicity after injection of dacarbazine might be due to photodegradation products. After reconstituting and rapidly injecting the drug at a concentration of 100 mg in 10 ml in a room lit only with a red photographic light, 3 patients received a total of 14 injections with no pain or only minor discomfort during the first few seconds. Nausea and vomiting also seemed to be reduced.— G. M. Baird and M. L. N. Willoughby (letter), *Lancet*, 1978, *2*, 681.

Allergy and anaphylaxis. Eosinophilia, associated with the injection of dacarbazine in a 65-year-old woman, appeared to represent an idiosyncratic-allergic drug reaction.— M. A. Movsesian and J. M. Merrill (letter), *Ann. intern. Med.*, 1980, *93*, 642.

Effects on the liver. Fatal hepatic vascular lesions associated with dacarbazine.— M. A. Greenstone *et al.*, *Br. med. J.*, 1981, *282*, 1744.

Interactions. A report that BCG injected into *rats* reduced the activity of liver enzymes which metabolise dacarbazine.— T. L. Loo *et al.*, *Cancer Treat. Rep.*, 1976, *60*, 149.

Pregnancy and the neonate. Studies in *rats* and *rabbits* indicated that dacarbazine was toxic to mother and foetus; a marginal effect on spermatozoal integrity was also noted.— D. J. Thompson *et al.*, *Toxic. appl. Pharmac.*, 1975, *33*, 281.

Absorption and Fate. Dacarbazine is poorly absorbed from the gastro-intestinal tract. Following intravenous injection it is rapidly distributed with an initial plasma half-life of about 20 minutes; the terminal half-life is reported to be about 5 hours. Only about 5% is bound to protein. Penetration into the cerebrospinal fluid is poor. Dacarbazine is extensively metabolised in the liver; the major active metabolite appears to be 5-aminoimidazole-4-carboxamide. About half of a dose is excreted unchanged in the urine by tubular secretion.

References: T. L. Loo *et al.*, *Cancer Res.*, 1968, *28*, 2448; G. E. Housholder and T. L. Loo, *J. Pharmac. exp. Ther.*, 1971, *179*, 386; T. L. Loo *et al.*, *Cancer Treat. Rep.*, 1976, *60*, 149.

Uses. Decarbazine is an antineoplastic agent which may function as an alkylating agent (see p.171) after it has been activated in the liver. It has minimal immunosuppressant activity. Decarbazine is used mainly in the treatment of malignant melanoma and has also been given to patients with sarcomas and Hodgkin's disease, usually in association with other drugs. See also under Choice of Antineoplastic Agent, p.175.

It is given intravenously in doses of 2 to 4.5 mg per kg body-weight daily for 10 days and repeated after intervals of 4 weeks or 250 mg per m^2 body-surface daily for 5 days and repeated after intervals of 3 weeks. Injections may be given over one minute. In an attempt to prevent pain along the injected vein the reconstituted solution has been further diluted with dextrose injection or sodium chloride injection and given by infusion.

Antiprotozoal action. Dacarbazine had significant activity against *Trypanosoma rhodesiense* infections in *mice*.— K. E. Kinnamon *et al.*, *Antimicrob. Ag. Chemother.*, 1979, *15*, 157.

Malignant neoplasms of the pancreas. Reports of the successful use of dacarbazine in the treatment of malignant glucagonoma: G. M. Strauss *et al.*, *Ann. intern. Med.*, 1979, *90*, 57; S. P. Marynick *et al.*, *Ann. intern. Med.*, 1980, *93*, 453.

Melanoma. Although dacarbazine is considered the best drug available for the treatment of metastatic malignant melanoma, it is not very effective and combination treatment regimens are being sought.— *Drug & Ther. Bull.*, 1976, *14*, 39. See also under Choice of Antineoplastic Agent, p.185.

Further references to the use of dacarbazine in malignant melanoma: L. Nathanson *et al.*, *Clin. Pharmac. Ther.*, 1971, *12*, 955; L. H. Einhorn *et al.*, *Cancer*, 1973, *32*, 749 (intra-arterial); G. P. Susens *et al.* (letter), *Ann. intern. Med.*, 1976, *84*, 175; P. B. McCulloch *et al.*, *Can. med. Ass. J.*, 1977, *117*, 33 (dacarbazine 850 mg per m^2 body-surface, given as a single injection to patients also receiving BCG vaccine).

Proprietary Preparations

DTIC-Dome *(Dome/Hollister-Stier, UK).* Dacarbazine, available as powder for preparing injections, in vials of 100 and 200 mg, with mannitol and citric acid. (Also available as DTIC-Dome in *Canad., Ital., Neth., NZ, S.Afr., Swed., USA*).

Other Proprietary Names

Deticene *(Fr., Ital., Neth.).*

1828-x

Daunorubicin Hydrochloride *(U.S.P.).*

Daunomycin Hydrochloride; Rubidomycin Hydrochloride; NDC 0082-4155; NSC 82151; RP 13057 (daunorubicin). (1*S*,3*S*)-3-Acetyl-1,2,3,4,6,11-hexahydro-3,5,12-trihydroxy-10-methoxy-6,11-dioxonaphthacen-1-yl 3-amino-2,3,6-trideoxy-α-L-lyxopyranoside hydrochloride.

$C_{27}H_{29}NO_{10}$,HCl=564.0.

CAS — 20830-81-3 (daunorubicin); 23541-50-6 (hydrochloride).

Pharmacopoeias. In *Chin.* and *U.S.*

The hydrochloride of an antineoplastic anthracycline antibiotic produced by *Streptomyces coeruleorubidus* or *S. peucetius.* An orange-red hygroscopic microcrystalline powder. M.p. about 210° with decomposition. **Soluble** in water and methyl alcohol. A 0.5% solution has a pH of 4.5 to 6.5. Solutions for injection are freshly prepared aseptically but may be kept for up to 48 hours at room temperature protected from light. **Store** at a temperature not exceeding 40° in airtight containers. Protect from light. Daunorubicin has been reported to be **incompatible** with heparin sodium.

For the preparation and physical properties of daunorubicin, see G. L. Tong *et al., J. pharm. Sci.,* 1967, *56,* 1691; R. Despois *et al., Arzneimittel-Forsch.,* 1967, *17,* 934; R. Maral *et al., ibid.,* 939.

Adverse Effects, Treatment, and Precautions. As for Doxorubicin, p.206.

Severe cardiotoxicity is likely when the total dose of daunorubicin exceeds 550 mg per m^2 body-surface.

Transient red discoloration of the urine may occur.

Effects on the heart. The overall incidence of cardiotoxicity in a review of 5613 children and adults given daunorubicin was 1.96%; congestive heart failure occurred in 65 patients and ECG changes only in 45.— D. D. Von Hoff *et al., Am. J. Med.,* 1977, *62,* 200.

Absorption and Fate. After intravenous injection, daunorubicin is concentrated in the liver, lungs, kidneys, spleen, and heart. It is metabolised mainly in the liver and excreted in the bile. About 5 to 18% is excreted unchanged in the urine within 24 hours and 12 to 29% within 7 days. About 20% of a dose has been recovered from the faeces within 7 days.

A biphasic plasma-daunorubicin disappearance pattern of an initial rapid fall in plasma concentration followed by a prolonged elimination was observed in 11 patients with solid tumours given daunorubicin 80 or 120 mg per m^2 body-surface intravenously; the short plasma half-life was about 45 minutes and the long plasma half-life about 55 hours. Daunorubicin imparted a reddish colour to the urine for the first few days and over 7 days 12 to 13% of the dose was estimated by fluorescence studies to be excreted in the urine. In a patient given tritiated daunorubicin about 20% of the radioactivity was found in the lyophilised faeces collected over 7 days. Highest tissue concentrations were found in the kidneys, liver, lungs, and spleen. Because of the prolonged half-life it was recommended that daunorubicin be given as a single large dose rather than in repeated doses.— D. S. Alberts *et al., Clin. Pharmac. Ther.,* 1971, *12,* 96.

Daunorubicin given in a dose of 180 mg per m^2 body-surface to 8 patients was rapidly and extensively metabolised. Two metabolites, daunorubicinol (also cytotoxic) and one not identified were detected in the plasma. These 2 metabolites were also found in the urine together with another unidentified metabolite.— D. H. Huffman *et al., Clin. Pharmac. Ther.,* 1972, *13,* 895. See also D. H. Huffman and N. R. Bachur, *Blood,* 1972, *39,* 637.

A radioimmunoassay technique for determining doxorubicin and daunorubicin concentrations and comparison with fluorescence assay.— N. R. Bachur *et al., Clin. Pharmac. Ther.,* 1977, *21,* 70.

Further references: S. Takanashi and N. R. Bachur, *J. Pharmac. exp. Ther.,* 1975, *195,* 41; H. Loveless *et al., Cancer Res.,* 1978, *38,* 593 (metabolism).

Uses. Daunorubicin is an antineoplastic antibiotic closely related to doxorubicin (p.205). It forms a stable complex with DNA and interferes with the synthesis of nucleic acids. Daunorubicin also has antibacterial, antiviral, and immunosuppressant properties. It is used with other antineoplastic agents to induce remissions in acute leukaemia. Daunorubicin is given in association with vincristine and prednisone in acute lymphoblastic leukaemia and with cytarabine and thioguanine in acute myeloblastic leukaemia. See also under Choice of Antineoplastic Agent, p.178. It has also been used in neuroblastoma.

In treatment regimens for acute myeloblastic leukaemia, daunorubicin is given in doses of 45 to 60 mg per m^2 body-surface daily for 3 days by injecting a solution in sodium chloride injection into a fast-running infusion of sodium chloride. A dose of 25 mg per m^2 has been given intravenously once a week in acute lymphoblastic leukaemia. The maximum total dose should not exceed 550 mg per m^2; in some patients it may be advisable to limit the total dose to about 450 mg per m^2.

Blood counts should be determined daily during treatment as daunorubicin has a rapid effect on bone-marrow function. Electrocardiogram examination should be made at regular intervals to detect signs of cardiotoxicity.

A brief review of daunorubicin.— *Med. Lett.,* 1980, *22,* 34.

A discussion of the possible use of daunorubicin complexed with deoxyribonucleic acid as an antineoplastic agent.— *Nature,* 1972, *239,* 194. See also A. Trouet *et al., Nature New Biol.,* 1972, *239,* 110.

Histiocytosis X. An 8-month-old baby with symptoms of Letterer-Siwe's disease responded dramatically after a 5-day course of daunorubicin, 1 mg per kg body-weight daily. A second course was given 2 weeks later.— G. Segni *et al.* (letter), *Lancet,* 1968, *2,* 461.

Leukaemia, acute. For reference to the use of daunorubicin with other agents in the treatment of acute lymphoblastic leukaemia and acute myeloblastic leukaemia, see Choice of Antineoplastic Agent, p.178.

Di Guglielmo's disease. Nine patients with Di Guglielmo's syndrome, an erythroleukaemia considered resistant to chemotherapy, were treated with daunorubicin 1 mg per kg body-weight daily by rapid intravenous infusion for 5 days. Prednisone was taken concomitantly at a dose of 60 mg daily, continued at 40 mg daily until the platelet count exceeded 100 000 per mm^3, then tailed off. Four patients obtained complete remission and 3 patients partial remission 3 to 8 weeks afterthe start of therapy; all patients with no prior treatment responded. The duration of remission was from 2 to 16 months with a median duration of survival of 12 months. Maintenance therapy was instituted with other cytotoxic agents; following relapse only 1 patient responded to daunorubicin and prednisone. After daunorubicin injection 1 patient demonstrated cardiotoxicity and another developed recurrent thrombophlebitis without extravasation, otherwise therapy was well tolerated.— C. D. Bloomfield *et al., Ann. intern. Med.,* 1974, *81,* 746.

Preparations

Daunorubicin Hydrochloride for Injection *(U.S.P.).* A sterile mixture of daunorubicin hydrochloride and mannitol. Potency is expressed in terms of the equivalent amount of daunorubicin. A solution, prepared as directed on the label, has a pH of 4.5 to 6.5. Protect from light.

Proprietary Names

Cerubidin *(May & Baker, Austral.; Rhone-Poulenc, Denm.; Rhône-Poulenc, Norw.; May & Baker, S.Afr.; Leo, Swed.);* Cerubidine *(Specia, Belg.; Rhône-Poulenc, Canad.; Specia, Fr.; Specia, Neth.; Specia, Switz.; Ives, USA);* Daunoblastin *(Farmitalia, Ger.);* Daunoblastina *(Farmitalia, Ital.).*

Daunorubicin hydrochloride was formerly marketed in Great Britain under the proprietary name Cerubidin *(May & Baker).*

1829-r

Demecolcine. Colchamine; Omaine. *N*-Deacetyl-*N*-methylcolchicine; 6,7-Dihydro-1,2,3,10-tetramethoxy-7-methylamino-5*H*-benzo[*a*]heptalen-9-one.

$C_{21}H_{25}NO_5$=371.4.

CAS — 477-30-5.

An alkaloid isolated from colchicum corm. It occurs as a pale yellow crystalline powder. **Soluble** 1 in 50 of water.

Adverse Effects, Treatment, and Precautions. For an outline of the adverse effects experienced with antineoplastic agents and immunosuppressants, general guidelines for their treatment, and precautions, see Antineoplastic Agents, p.171, pp.174-5.

Demecolcine has a depressant effect on the bone-marrow and this has occasionally been severe and even fatal. Topical preparations should not be applied to mucous membranes.

Demecolcine ointment caused normal skin to react with hyperaemia, oedema, and weeping.— N. V. Musin, *Trudÿ Kirgiz, nauchno-issled. Inst.,* 1964, *1,* 128, per *Int. pharm. Abstr.,* 1966, *3,* 1544.

Uses. Demecolcine is an antineoplastic agent with antimitotic properties. It has been used for the treatment of malignant neoplasms of the skin as an ointment containing 0.5% of which not more than 1.5 g should be applied at a time; a 0.1% ointment has also been used.

For reports on the use of demecolcine in malignant neoplasms of the skin, see Martindale 27th Edn, p. 145.

1830-j

Dichlorodiethylsulphide. Mustard Gas; Sulfur Mustard; Yellow Cross Liquid. Bis(2-chloroethyl)sulphide.

$C_4H_8Cl_2S$=159.1.

CAS — 505-60-2.

An oily liquid. B.p. about 217°. Sp. gr. 1.274. Very sparingly **soluble** in water; soluble in alcohol and other organic solvents.

Dichlorodiethylsulphide has even more severe vesicant and irritant properties than its nitrogen analogue, mustine (p.223). It was formerly used topically in the treatment of psoriasis.

1831-z

Doxorubicin Hydrochloride *(U.S.P.).*

Adriamycin Hydrochloride; FI 106 (doxorubicin); FI 6804 (doxorubicin); NSC 123127 (doxorubicin); 14-Hydroxydaunorubicin Hydrochloride. (1*S*,3*S*)-3-Glycoloyl-1,2,3,4,6,11-hexahydro-3,5,12-trihydroxy-10-methoxy-6,11-dioxonaphthacen-1-yl 3-amino-2,3,6-trideoxy-α-L-lyxopyranoside hydrochloride.

$C_{27}H_{29}NO_{11}$, HCl=580.0.

CAS — 23214-92-8 (doxorubicin); 25316-40-9 (hydrochloride).

Pharmacopoeias. In *U.S.*

An antineoplastic antibiotic isolated from *Streptomyces peucetius* var. *caesius.* It has a potency of 900 to 1100 μg per mg, calculated on the dried basis.

An orange-red hygroscopic crystalline powder. **Soluble** in water and methyl alcohol; practically insoluble in chloroform, ether, and other organic solvents. A 0.5% solution in water has a pH of 3.8 to 6.5. **Incompatible** with heparin. It may be incompatible with aminophylline, cephalothin sodium, dexamethasone, fluorouracil, or hydrocortisone. **Store** at a temperature not exceeding 40° in airtight containers. Protect from light.

CAUTION. *Doxorubicin hydrochloride is irritant; avoid contact with skin and mucous membranes.*

Stability in solution. The stability of refrigerated and frozen solutions of doxorubicin hydrochloride.— D. M. Hoffman *et al., Am. J. Hosp. Pharm.*, 1979, *36*, 1536.

Studies indicating that doxorubicin in solution is photodegradable and that at concentrations lower than 500 µg per ml appreciable loss of biochemical activity occurs if exposure to light is not prevented. However as higher concentrations (2 mg per ml) are usually prepared for administration to patients with cancer special precautions do not appear to be necessary to protect freshly prepared solutions from light during intravenous administration.— N. Tavoloni *et al., J. Pharm. Pharmac.*, 1980, *32*, 860.

Adverse Effects. For an outline of the adverse effects experienced with antineoplastic agents, see Antineoplastic Agents, p.171.

Doxorubicin causes pronounced bone-marrow depression with leucopenia at a maximum 10 to 15 days after administration and blood counts returning to normal after about 21 days. Severe cardiotoxicity is likely when the total dose of doxorubicin exceeds 550 mg per m^2 body-surface. Doxorubicin is very irritant and thrombophlebitis has been reported following injection. Alopecia occurs in the majority of patients. The urine may be coloured red.

Allergy and anaphylaxis. Reports of allergic reactions associated with doxorubicin: A. H. G. Paterson, *Cancer Treat. Rep.*, 1978, *62*, 1269; L. Souhami and R. Feld, *J. Am. med. Ass.*, 1978, *240*, 1624 (possible allergic skin rashes occurring near the site of intravenous injection); D. J. Arnold and C. T. Stafford, *Cancer Treat. Rep.*, 1979, *63*, 150 (systemic allergic reaction); E. Fallah-Sohy and A. T. Figueredo (letter), *J. Am. med. Ass.*, 1979, *241*, 1108 (generalised urticaria); J. E. Maldonado (letter), *New Engl. J. Med.*, 1979, *301*, 386 (angioneurotic oedema).

Effects on the gastro-intestinal tract. Oesophagitis, sometimes progressing to oesophageal strictures, has occurred in patients receiving radiotherapy and doxorubicin; doxorubicin may enhance the toxic effect of the radiotherapy.— A. Horwich *et al.* (letter), *Lancet*, 1975, *2*, 561; F. A. Greco *et al., Ann. intern. Med.*, 1976, *85*, 294.

Effects on the heart. The anthracycline antibiotics, doxorubicin and daunorubicin, have a unique chronic effect on the heart. Cardiotoxicity is manifested both by acute transient ECG changes, usually benign arrhythmias only rarely of clinical consequence, and a late irreversible cardiomyopathy which, until it was recognised, resulted in an abrupt onset of congestive heart failure which was usually fatal. The majority of patients probably have some degree of cardiac damage after treatment with doxorubicin but when administration is routinely stopped after a cumulative dose of 450 mg per m^2 body-surface the incidence of congestive heart failure is low.— I. C. Henderson and E. Frei, *New Engl. J. Med.*, 1979, *300*, 310.

The therapeutic potential of doxorubicin has been limited by its cardiotoxicity since congestive heart failure has been related to the cumulative dose administered and discontinuation of doxorubicin therapy has been advised once a total dose of 550 mg per m^2 body-surface is reached. Unfortunately this precludes the administration of doxorubicin to patients who might derive further benefit from it. A number of monitoring methods have been advocated for the early detection of congestive heart failure and these include: serial measurements of voltage on ECGs, cardiac enzymes, systolic time intervals, QRS-Korotkoff intervals, and echocardiograms, more recently transvenous cardiac biopsies and radionuclide cineangiography have shown promise. Reported risk factors for doxorubicin-induced heart failure include previous radiotherapy to the mediastinum, concomitant use of cyclophosphamide, advanced age, and previous cardiovascular disease. In a retrospective study of 3941 patients given doxorubicin, total dose, dosage schedule, and age were independent risk factors for developing heart failure. Of these patients congestive heart failure occurred in 88 (2.2%) and was fatal in 38. Toxicity was noted at a mean of 33 days after the last dose; the mean total dose of doxorubicin in those developing heart failure was 364 mg per m^2 compared with 237 mg per m^2 in those who did not. There was a continuum of increasing risk of heart failure as the cumulative dose increased although the risk was accelerated above a dose of about 550 mg per m^2. A weekly dosage schedule was associated with a significantly lower incidence of congestive heart failure than dosage every 3 weeks. The risk generally increased with age although children (under 15 years) might be at greater risk. In this study performance status, sex, race or tumour type were not risk factors; no conclusions could be reached on previous cardiac disease, previous radiotherapy, or the concomitant use of other antineoplastic agents, as risk factors.— D. D. Von Hoff *et al., Ann. intern. Med.*, 1979, *91*, 710.

Recommendations for the prevention of cardiotoxicity during treatment with doxorubicin: (1) if the absolute QRS voltage of the 6 limb leads of the ECG decreased by 30% or more during therapy, doxorubicin should be discontinued. (2) No matter what the ECG reading might be the cumulative dose should not exceed 550 mg per m^2 body-surface in most patients. (3) As cyclophosphamide and radiotherapy to the heart appeared to enhance the cardiotoxicity of doxorubicin, the cumulative dose in such cases should not exceed 450 mg per m^2. (4) The dose should also be limited to 450 mg per m^2 where it has to be used in patients with associated heart disease that might increase cardiac work-load. (5) There should be early diagnosis of cardiotoxicity with prompt withdrawal of doxorubicin.— R. A. Minow *et al., Cancer*, 1977, *39*, 1397. In studies on 33 patients, doxorubicin produced dose-related myocardial degeneration which began before abnormalities in left ventricular function could be detected clinically. Heart failure occurred at cumulative doses ranging from 330 to 545 mg per m^2.— M. R. Bristow *et al., Ann. intern. Med.*, 1978, *88*, 168.

Further studies on the monitoring of cardiac function in patients receiving doxorubicin: A. K. Chacko *et al., J. nucl. Med.*, 1977, *18*, 680 (myocardial scanning with technetium-99m); J. Alexander *et al., New Engl. J. Med.*, 1979, *300*, 278 (noninvasive quantitative radionuclide angiocardiography); S. A. D. Al-Ismail and J. A. Whittaker (letter), *Lancet*, 1978, *1*, 1315 (systolic time interval); M. A. Friedman *et al., J. Am. med. Ass.*, 1978, *240*, 1603 (endomyocardial biopsy); G. W. Morgan *et al.* (letter), *Lancet*, 1978, *1*, 1315 (a radionucleotide method); S. A. D. Al-Ismail and J. A. Whittaker, *Br. med. J.*, 1979, *1*, 1392 (systolic time interval).

Individual reports of cardiotoxicity in children given cumulative doses of doxorubicin below 500 mg per m^2 body-surface: M. A. Gerber *et al., J. Pediat.*, 1975, *87*, 629 (fatal result after 350 mg per m^2 and irradiation); J. Merrill *et al.* (letter), *Ann. intern. Med.*, 1975, *82*, 122 (enhanced by radiotherapy); A. C. Gilladoga *et al., Cancer*, 1976, *37*, 1070 (also daunorubicin); R. P. Rieker and R. B. Patterson (letter), *J. Pediat.*, 1976, *89*, 517 (after 270 mg per m^2 of doxorubicin and 120 mg per m^2 of daunorubicin); B. Kaduk and G. Seiler, *Dt. med. Wschr.*, 1977, *102*, 1813 (fatal result after 470 mg per m^2); M. N. Prout *et al., Cancer*, 1977, *39*, 62 (after 350 and 400 mg per m^2); U. Fuhrmann *et al., Dt. med. Wschr.*, 1978, *103*, 387 (the cumulative dose of doxorubicin should not exceed 500 mg per m^2 in children without risk factors); C. B. Pratt *et al., Cancer Treat. Rep.*, 1978, *62*, 1381 (children under 10 years more susceptible).

Reports of possible risk factors for doxorubicin cardiotoxicity: A. U. Buzdar *et al., Cancer Treat. Rep.*, 1978, *62*, 1005 (enhanced cardiotoxicity with mitomycin); P. Bhanot *et al., J. Pediat.*, 1979, *95*, 561 (enhanced cardiotoxicity after hepatic irradiation); J. S. Gottdiener *et al., Ann. intern. Med.*, 1981, *94*, 430 (long-term cardiotoxicity below 550 mg per m^2 or less).

Ventricular arrhythmia occurred during infusion of doxorubicin in a 21-year-old man.— T. M. Cosgriff (letter), *Ann. intern. Med.*, 1980, *92*, 434. Experimental data suggest that doxorubicin-associated dysrhythmias may be commoner than presently appreciated.— R. A. Levandowski (letter), *ibid.*, 866.

Further references: J. E. Byfield, *Cancer Treat. Rep.*, 1977, *61*, 497 (mechanism of doxorubicin-induced cardiotoxicity).

Effects on the kidneys. Renal failure in a 78-year-old man was associated with administration of doxorubicin.— J. F. Burke *et al., Archs intern. Med.*, 1977, *137*, 385.

See also under Mitomycin, p.221.

Effects on the nervous system. A report of hypertensive encephalopathy following doxorubicin.— A. H. G. Paterson, *Cancer Treat. Rep.*, 1978, *62*, 1269.

Doxorubicin was neurotoxic when perfused through the cerebrospinal fluid spaces in *rhesus monkeys*. Its intrathecal use is not recommended.— P. C. Merker *et al., Toxic. appl. Pharmac.*, 1978, *44*, 191.

Effects on the skin. A patient who received doxorubicin 400 µg per kg body-weight intravenously for 6 doses in 10 days followed by twice weekly doses for 13 weeks, developed stomatitis a week after the loading-dose course, followed by alopecia. Soreness of the palms and feet, onycholysis, plantar callus formation, and epidermolysis developed in the following weeks. After doxorubicin was discontinued the soreness subsided and the general condition of his hands and feet improved.— F. B. Manalo *et al., J. Am. med. Ass.*, 1975, *233*, 56.

Treatment of Adverse Effects. For general guidelines, see Antineoplastic Agents, p.174.

Digoxin appeared to have a protective effect against doxorubicin cardiotoxicity. ECG abnormalities were present in 5 of 6 patients who had received doxorubicin in a dose of at least 400 mg per m^2 body-surface area but not (apart from abnormalities due to digoxin) in 16 given digoxin 250 µg daily starting 7 days before doxorubicin. The incidence of muscle weakness fell from 58 to 8%. Ouabain appeared to have some protective value but its short half-life made digoxin preferable. Oxytetracycline, with a structure similar to that of doxorubicin, had been used empirically in treatment in 2 patients.— D. Guthrie and A. L. Gibson, *Br. med. J.*, 1977, *2*, 1447. A randomised study of the possible protective effect of digoxin against doxorubicin cardiotoxicity is needed.— C. J. Williams, *ibid.*, 1978, *1*, 176.

Extravasation following the inadvertent administration of doxorubicin hydrochloride subcutaneously into the forearm was treated with immediate infiltration into the same area of 5 ml of an 8.4% solution of sodium bicarbonate followed by dexamethasone 4 mg.— J. I. Zweig and B. Kabakow (letter), *J. Am. med. Ass.*, 1978, *239*, 2116.

Hypothermia of the scalp provided good protection against alopecia throughout all cycles of treatment in 20 of 33 cancer patients who were receiving chemotherapy with doxorubicin by intravenous injection. Ice-packs were applied to the scalp 5 minutes before each injection of doxorubicin and were left in place for 35 minutes. The protective effect of hypothermia was inversely related to the dose of doxorubicin. It was considered later that the ice should be applied for 10 minutes before injection; the technique should not be used in leukaemias or other neoplastic diseases in which numerous tumour stem cells may be present in the scalp.— J. C. Dean *et al., New Engl. J. Med.*, 1979, *301*, 1427. Ice-packs held in place for 20 minutes before and after injection of doxorubicin prevented alopecia in 2 patients despite almost total loss of hair in the pubic and axillary regions.— A. R. Timothy *et al.* (letter), *Lancet*, 1980, *1*, 663. See also G. A. Edelstyn *et al.* (letter), *Lancet*, 1977, *2*, 253.

A report on the treatment of doxorubicin-induced cardiomyopathy including the use of prazosin.— G. C. Carlon *et al., Chest*, 1980, *77*, 570.

Precautions. For reference to the precautions necessary with antineoplastic agents and immunosuppressants, see Antineoplastic Agents, p.175.

Doxorubicin is generally contra-indicated in patients with heart disease. Doses should not be repeated when there is bone-marrow depression or ulceration of the mouth. It should be given with great care in reduced doses to elderly patients and to those with hepatic impairment. Extravasation results in severe tissue damage and doxorubicin should not be given by intramuscular or subcutaneous injection. The adverse effects of irradiation may be enhanced by doxorubicin and skin reactions previously induced by radiotherapy may recur.

Interactions. Side-effects due to doxorubicin were increased when doxorubicin and streptozocin were given together. Streptozocin apparently caused enough liver damage to slow down the metabolism of doxorubicin.— P. Chang *et al., J. Am. med. Ass.*, 1976, *236*, 913. Results of a study involving 31 evaluable patients indicated that administration of doxorubicin with streptozocin had no advantage over administration of doxorubicin alone.— P. Chang and P. H. Wiernik, *Clin. Pharmac. Ther.*, 1976, *20*, 605. Administration with streptozocin increased the side-effects of doxorubicin.— *idem*, 611.

The toxicity of doxorubicin was enhanced in a patient with osteogenic sarcoma when it was given after methotrexate rather than before.— J. H. Robertson *et al., Br. med. J.*, 1976, *1*, 23.

Absorption and Fate. After intravenous injection doxorubicin is rapidly cleared from the blood and is widely distributed. It is metabolised in the liver and mainly excreted in the bile; about 40% of a dose has been recovered from the bile or faeces within 7 days. Only about 5% of a dose is excreted in the urine within 5 days.

A radioimmunoassay technique for determining doxorubicin and daunorubicin concentrations and comparison with fluorescence assay.— N. R. Bachur *et al.*, *Clin. Pharmac. Ther.*, 1977, *21*, 70.

A brief discussion on the pharmacokinetics of doxorubicin. Plasma clearance has been reported to be triphasic (N.R. Bachur *et al.*, *Clin. Pharmac. Ther.*, 1977, *21*, 70; R.S. Benjamin *et al.*, *Cancer Res.*, 1977, *37*, 1416) with mean half-lives of 12 minutes, 3.3 hours, and 29.6 hours. Doxorubicin is rapidly extracted from plasma by the liver and undergoes extensive metabolism (S. Takanashi and N.R. Bachur, *Drug Metab. & Disposit.*, 1976, *4*, 79). Metabolites, including adriamycinol, appear rapidly in plasma and disappear in a biphasic and triphasic manner.— R. A. Bender *et al.*, *Drugs*, 1978, *16*, 46.

A study in cancer patients with or without hepatomas, who were treated with doxorubicin, indicated that plasma profiles of doxorubicin were similar. Formation and elimination of the major active metabolite, adriamycinol, appeared to be impaired in hepatoma patients.— K. K. Chan *et al.*, *Cancer Res.*, 1980, *40*, 1263.

Further references to the pharmacokinetics of doxorubicin: R. S. Benjamin *et al.*, *Cancer*, 1974, *33*, 19 (biphasic plasma clearance); C. E. Riggs *et al.*, *Clin. Pharmac. Ther.*, 1977, *22*, 234 (biliary disposition); M. Kummen *et al.*, *Acta pharmac. tox.*, 1978, *42*, 212 (free and DNA-complexed doxorubicin); H. Lovless *et al.*, *Cancer Res.*, 1978, *38*, 593 (metabolism).

Pregnancy and the neonate. Neither doxorubicin nor its major metabolite, adriamycinol, were found in the amniotic fluid of a pregnant women who required treatment with doxorubicin at 20 weeks' gestation. This suggests that doxorubicin is not transferred transplacentally to the foetus at this age.— J. Roboz *et al.* (letter), *Lancet*, 1979, *2*, 1382.

Uses. Doxorubicin is an antineoplastic antibiotic which appears to act by forming a stable complex with DNA and interfering with the synthesis of nucleic acids. It also has immunosuppressant properties. It has uses similar to those of daunorubicin (p.205), but it is effective against a wider range of tumours. Doxorubicin is used, often in association with other antineoplastic agents, in the treatment of acute leukaemia, lymphomas, sarcomas, neuroblastoma, Wilm's tumour, and malignant neoplasms of the bladder, breast, lung, and thyroid. It is also used in other tumours including those of the cervix, liver, ovary, and testis. Doxorubicin is given with vincristine and prednisone to induce remissions in acute lymphoblastic leukaemia and with cytarabine and thioguanine in acute myeloblastic leukaemia. See also under Choice of Antineoplastic Agent, p.178.

Doxorubicin hydrochloride is given in a dose of 60 to 75 mg per m^2 body-surface or 1.2 to 2.4 mg per kg body-weight as a single dose every 3 weeks. It is administered by injecting a solution in Water for Injections or sodium chloride injection into a fast-running infusion of sodium chloride or dextrose injection. Alternatively, the dose may be divided equally over 3 successive days and repeated every 3 weeks. Doses may need to be reduced to 30 to 40 mg per m^2 if doxorubicin is given with other antineoplastic agents. The maximum total dose should not exceed 550 mg per m^2; in some patients it may be advisable to limit the total dose to about 450 mg per m^2.

Doxorubicin has also been given by intra-arterial injection. Great care must be taken to avoid extravasation. In the treatment of non-invasive tumours, solutions containing 50 mg of doxorubicin hydrochloride in 100 ml of physiological saline have been instilled into the bladder.

Doses should be halved in patients with moderate liver dysfunction; those with severe impairment should be given a quarter of the usual dose.

Blood counts should be made routinely during treatment with doxorubicin and electrocardiograms should be examined at regular intervals for early signs of cardiotoxicity.

Doxorubicin octanoate has been studied in *animals*.

Action. Doxorubicin enhanced the cytotoxic effect of radiotherapy.— T. L. Phillips, *Cancer*, 1977, *39*, 987. See also Precautions, above.

Doxorubicin is reported to be active against methotrexate-resistant cells.— B. T. Hill and K. Hellmann (letter), *Lancet*, 1977, *1*, 47.

The activity of doxorubicin and daunorubicin both of which act by inhibiting DNA synthesis had been enhanced by cytarabine possibly synchronising the leukaemic cell phase. Giving cytarabine over days 1 to 3 and doxorubicin on day 5 to 32 adult patients with untreated acute nonlymphoid leukaemia did not increase the expected remission-rate although this had been reported when daunorubicin and doxorubicin were given sequentially on days 6 and 7. Further studies are required to evaluate the value of synchronisation.— J. A. Whittaker *et al.* (letter), *Lancet*, 1977, *2*, 557.

Administration. Because of the dosage limit of 550 mg per m^2 body-surface of doxorubicin a dose-response study was carried out in 818 patients to find out means of prolonging the period of administration. Individual doses of 75 mg per m^2 could be used for induction in good-risk patients with sarcomas. Other good-risk patients could receive 60 mg per m^2 unless rapid remission is required. Poor-risk patients should receive 25 mg per m^2 for 3 or 4 doses for remission induction unless treatment is for breast cancer when 50 mg per m^2 could be given. Irreversible congestive heart failure could occur with doses of 240 mg per m^2 and appropriate precautions should be taken to detect any cardiotoxicity when the dose exceeds this figure.— R. M. O'Bryan *et al.*, *Cancer*, 1977, *39*, 1940.

Doxorubicin is reported to be neurotoxic in animals. It should not be given by intrathecal injection.— P. C. Merker *et al.*, *Toxic. appl. Pharmac.*, 1978, *44*, 191.

Administration in children. Doxorubicin was given in low doses of 10 or 20 mg per m^2 body-surface weekly or biweekly to a maximum of 500 mg per m^2 for remission maintenance in solid tumours in 6 children. Three children were disease-free over 1 year later. This schedule was considered to avoid the serious toxicity of doxorubicin.— E. V. Hvizdala *et al.*, *Cancer*, 1977, *39*, 2411.

Administration in hepatic insufficiency. For references to the impaired metabolism of doxorubicin in patients with hepatoma, see Absorption and Fate (above).

Administration in renal insufficiency. Doxorubicin can be given in usual doses to patients in renal failure.— W. M. Bennett *et al.*, *Ann. intern. Med.*, 1977, *86*, 754. See also *idem*, 1980, *93*, 286.

Hodgkin's disease and other lymphomas. Doxorubicin given alone in a dose of 60 to 75 mg per m^2 body-surface intravenously every 3 weeks produced 5 complete and 4 partial remissions lasting a median of more than 7 months in 18 patients with Hodgkin's disease or other lymphomas that had become resistant to extensive chemotherapy. Combined treatment with doxorubicin, cytarabine, vincristine, and prednisone produced 4 complete and 4 partial remissions with a median duration of 2.5 months in 16 patients resistant to other treatment or with extensive bone-marrow involvement. A combination of doxorubicin with cyclophosphamide, vincristine, and prednisone produced 7 complete and 2 partial remissions with a median duration of more than 8 months in a group of 9 patients who had minimal or no previous chemotherapy.— J. A. Gottlieb *et al.*, *Cancer Res.*, 1973, *33*, 3024, per *Int. pharm. Abstr.*, 1974, *11*, 542.

See also under Choice of Antineoplastic Agent, p.177.

Leukaemia, acute. Nine patients aged 9 to 58 years with acute myelogenous leukaemia resistant to daunorubicin were given doxorubicin 1.5 to 2 mg per kg body-weight daily for 1 to 3 days as a single rapid intravenous injection at the end of a 24-hour infusion of cytarabine 10 mg per kg. One of the patients was given a second course 14 days after the first. Four patients went into remission, although 1 relapsed after 2 months; the other 3 remained in remission after 4 to 5 months. Side-effects were common and sometimes persisted for 2 or 3 days. They included oral ulceration, pharyngitis, and gastro-intestinal symptoms. All patients developed alopecia and all had severe bone-marrow depression. It was considered that the high doses of doxorubicin accounted for the beneficial results; high doses were employed since it had been suggested that cross-resistance might occur between doxorubicin and daunorubicin.— I. E. Smith and T. J. McElwain (letter), *Lancet*, 1974, *2*, 161.

Further references: H. E. Wilson *et al.*, *Cancer Treat. Rep.*, 1977, *61*, 905.

For reference to the use of doxorubicin with other agents in the treatment of acute lymphoblastic leukaemia and in acute and chronic myeloid leukaemia, see Choice of Antineoplastic Agent, p.178.

Malignant effusions. Doxorubicin 30 mg in 30 to 100 ml of physiological saline had been injected intracavitarily, after diagnostic or therapeutic aspiration of the malignant effusion, in 12 patients; probably at least 500 ml of residual effusion remained at the time of drug administration in all cases. Doxorubicin appears to be a safe, and sometimes effective, local treatment for malignant disease.— M. H. N. Tattersall *et al.* (letter), *Lancet*, 1979, *1*, 390. Caution is needed in interpreting the absolute value of topical doxorubicin or other chemotherapeutic agents. Three untreated patients had been noted to have satisfactory results in terms of effusions which might have been ascribed to therapy had it been given. Results from an initial 14 patients in a controlled study had shown no systemic or topical toxicity probably because a dose of only 10 mg in 15 ml of saline is being used.— S. D. Desai and A. Figueredo (letter), *ibid.*, 872. See also R. F. Kefford *et al.*, *Med. J. Aust.*, 1980, *2*, 447.

See also Choice of Antineoplastic Agent, p.175.

Malignant neoplasms. Some reports of the use of doxorubicin in the treatment of malignant neoplasms: S. Di Pietro *et al.*, *J. surg. Oncol.*, 1973, *5*, 421 (intra-arterial infusion especially in tumours of the head and neck); E. P. Cortes *et al.*, *Cancer*, 1974, *34*, 518 (lung); C. B. Pratt and E. C. Shanks, *Am. J. Dis. Child.*, 1974, *127*, 534; S. H. Weinstein and J. D. Schmidt, *Urology*, 1976, *8*, 336 (advanced transitional cell carcinoma); M. D. Banks *et al.*, *J. Urol.*, 1977, *118*, 757 (by instillation in bladder tumours); A. Yagoda *et al.*, *Cancer*, 1977, *39*, 279 (urinary tract).

For the use of doxorubicin in combination chemotherapy regimens see Malignant Neoplasms in Choice of Antineoplastic Agent, p.180.

Malignant neoplasms of the liver. In 44 patients with hepatocellular carcinoma considered unfit for surgery, 8 of whom were judged to have a good prognosis and 36 a poor prognosis, doxorubicin 60 mg per m^2 diluted with dextrose injection was given by slow intravenous injection every 3 weeks to a maximum total of 550 mg per m^2. An objective response was obtained in 14 (32%) of the patients, 3 of whom were in the good prognosis and 11 in the poor prognosis group. Of the 14 responders 5 were considered to have achieved complete clinical remission with continuing survival periods of up to 2 years. A fall in serum-alpha-fetoprotein was predictive of a good response. Side-effects were strikingly mild compared with quadruple chemotherapy or infusion of drugs through the hepatic artery.— P. J. Johnson *et al.*, *Lancet*, 1978, *1*, 1006. Although experience in 11 patients had shown that doxorubicin could be beneficial, no complete remission had been obtained; a controlled series was required.— J. Vilaseca *et al.* (letter), *ibid.*, 1367. Further references: C. L. Vogel *et al.*, *Cancer*, 1977, *39*, 1923.

Malignant neoplasms of the thyroid. Eleven of 30 patients with malignant neoplasm of the thyroid refractory to surgery or radiotherapy achieved partial remission with doxorubicin after an average of 3 courses at a starting dose of 75 mg per m^2 of body-surface. Doxorubicin-induced cardiomyopathy, fatal in 1 case, developed in 3 patients who had received a total dose of doxorubicin in excess of 550 mg per m^2.— J. A. Gottlieb and C. S. Hill, *New Engl. J. Med.*, 1974, *290*, 193.

In 21 patients with metastasising thyroid carcinoma given chemotherapy, 2 achieved full remission and 5 partial remission. Treatment consisted of doxorubicin 75 mg per m^2 body-surface intravenously every 3 weeks (to a total dose of 550 mg per m^2) and bleomycin 30 mg intramuscularly every week (to a total dose of 360 mg).— G. Benker *et al.*, *Dt. med. Wschr.*, 1977, *102*, 1908.

Further references: A. G. Katsas (letter), *New Engl. J. Med.*, 1980, *302*, 467.

Melanoma. A study in 44 patients with disseminated malignant melanoma indicated that doxorubicin was without beneficial effect in this condition.— D. L. Ahmann *et al.*, *Clin. Pharmac. Ther.*, 1976, *19*, 821.

Mycosis fungoides. Doxorubicin was considered effective in the induction treatment of mycosis fungoides. Thirteen patients received 60 mg per m^2 body-surface intravenously every 21 days and 3 gained complete and 5 partial remissions. Maintenance consisted of methotrexate 15 mg per m^2 twice a week by intramuscular injection and cyclophosphamide 750 mg per m^2 intravenously every 3 weeks.— J. A. Levi *et al.*, *Cancer*, 1977, *39*, 1967.

Myeloma. For a report of doxorubicin with carmustine being used in patients with refractory multiple myeloma, see Carmustine, p.195.

Pregnancy and the neonate. Two women given doxorubicin from the 22nd and 24th weeks of pregnancy respectively were delivered of apparently healthy infants. Doxorubicin given in late pregnancy does not appear to be a serious hazard to the foetus.— J. S. Tobias *et al.*

(letter), *Lancet*, 1980, *1*, 776 and 836. See also M. Khurshid and M. Saleem (letter), *Lancet*, 1978, *2*, 534.

Sarcoma. Twenty-four patients with osteogenic sarcoma were treated with doxorubicin to a maximum cumulative dose of 540 mg per m² body-surface, starting about 8 weeks after surgery. Of these, 13 remained free of pulmonary metastases or local recurrences for from 9 to more than 40 months.— E. P. Cortes *et al.*, *New Engl. J. Med.*, 1974, *291*, 998.

See also under Choice of Antineoplastic Agent, p.185.

Preparations

Doxorubicin Hydrochloride for Injection *(U.S.P.)*. A sterile mixture of doxorubicin hydrochloride and lactose. The injection is prepared by the addition of diluent before use. Protect from light.

Doxorubicin Hydrochloride for Injection may be reconstituted by shaking with sodium chloride injection. The resulting solution is reported to be stable for 24 hours at room temperature or 48 hours when stored between 2° and 8°, when protected from light.

Adriamycin *(Farmitalia Carlo Erba, UK)*. Doxorubicin hydrochloride, available as powder for preparing injections in vials of 10 and 50 mg. (Also available as Adriamycin in *Canad., Swed., USA*).

The name Adriamicina has been used for methacycline hydrochloride.

Other Proprietary Names

Adriblastin *(Ger., Switz.)*; Adriblastina *(Arg., Belg., Ital., Neth., S.Afr.)*; Adriblastine *(Fr.)*; Farmiblastina *(Spain)*.

1832-c

Estramustine Sodium Phosphate.

Ro 21-8837/001; NSC 89199 (estramustine phosphate). Estra-1,3,5(10)-triene-3,17β-diol 3-[bis(2-chloroethyl)carbamate] 17-(disodium phosphate).

$C_{23}H_{30}Cl_2NNa_2O_6P=564.4$.

CAS — 2998-57-4 (estramustine); 4891-15-0 (phosphate); 52205-73-9 (sodium phosphate).

Adverse Effects, Treatment, and Precautions. As for Mustine Hydrochloride, p.223. Side-effects related to the oestrogenic activity of estramustine, such as gynaecomastia and cardiovascular effects, may also occur.

It is contra-indicated in patients with peptic ulceration and severe hepatic or cardiac disease.

Absorption and Fate. About 75% of a dose of estramustine sodium phosphate is absorbed from the gastro-intestinal tract. It is concentrated in prostatic tissue. The phosphate moiety appears to be lost in the gastro-intestinal tract, liver, and phosphatase-rich tissue such as the prostate. Following breakage of the carbamate linkage the oestrogenic and alkylating moieties are excreted independently.

A study on the absorption and fate of estramustine sodium phosphate in patients with carcinoma of the prostate.— G. P. Forshell *et al.*, *Investve Urol.*, 1976, *14*, 128.

Uses. Estramustine is a combination of oestradiol and normustine and has weaker oestrogenic activity than oestradiol and weaker antineoplastic activity than mustine (p.222) and most other alkylating agents. Estramustine phosphate is given by mouth as the disodium salt in the treatment of advanced prostatic carcinoma; it has been used with meglumine by injection.

The usual initial dosage by mouth is the equivalent of 560 mg of estramustine phosphate daily, with meals; the dose may later be adjusted to between 140 mg and 1.4 g daily according to the response and gastro-intestinal tolerance. The equivalent of 150 to 450 mg of estramustine phosphate has been given daily by slow intravenous injection for about 3 weeks, followed by maintenance doses of 150 to 300 mg on 2 days a week.

Malignant neoplasms of the prostate. Reports on estramustine in the treatment of carcinoma of the prostate: G. Leander, *Läkartidningen*, 1973, *70*, 2237; A. Mittelman *et al.*, *Cancer Chemother. Rep.*, 1975, *59*, 219; A. Mittelman *et al.*, *J. Urol.*, 1976, *115*, 409; T. Nilsson and G. Jonsson, *J. Urol.*, 1976, *115*, 168; R. Catane *et al.* (letter), *J. Am. med. Ass.*, 1977, *237*, 2471; A. Mittelman *et al.*, *Cancer Treat. Rep.*, 1977, *61*, 307; R. Nagel and C. -P. Kolln, *Br. J. Urol.*, 1977, *49*, 73; D. D. Von Hoff *et al.*, *J. Urol.*, 1977, *117*, 464; W. Leistenschneider and R. Nagel, *Eur. Urol.*, 1980, *6*, 111.

See also under Choice of Antineoplastic Agent, p.184.

Proprietary Preparations

Estracyt *(Lundbeck, UK)*. Estramustine sodium phosphate, available as capsules each containing the equivalent of 140 mg of estramustine phosphate. Store at 2° to 8°. (Also available as Estracyt in *Denm., Ger., Neth., Norw., S.Afr., Spain, Swed., Switz.*).

Other Proprietary Names

Emcyt *(Canad.)*.

1833-k

Ethoglucid.

Etoglucid; ICI 32,865; Triethyleneglycol Diglycidyl Ether. 1,2:15,16-Diepoxy-4,7,10,13-tetraoxahexadecane.

$C_{12}H_{22}O_6=262.3$.

CAS — 1954-28-5.

A clear colourless slightly viscous liquid. Sp. gr. 1.13. **Miscible** with water giving neutral solutions. The liquid should be stored in a cool place but above 10°. It is unstable in the presence of air. Only freshly prepared solutions should be used. Concentrated solutions of ethoglucid react with plastics; glass syringes should be used for such solutions.

CAUTION. *Ethoglucid is irritant; avoid contact with skin and mucous membranes.*

Stability of ethoglucid in plastic disposable syringes.— M. G. Lee (letter), *Pharm. J.*, 1981, *2*, 651.

Adverse Effects and Treatment. For an outline of the adverse effects experienced with antineoplastic agents and immunosuppressants and general guidelines for their treatment, see Antineoplastic Agents, p.171 and p.174.

Following injection of ethoglucid, transient hypotension, local pain and discomfort, and oedema can occur. Convulsions have been reported with large doses. Haematological depression reaches a maximum about 14 days after injection.

Systemic effects may be less severe with intracavitary instillation of ethoglucid but local irritant effects occur.

Precautions. For reference to the precautions necessary with antineoplastic agents and immunosuppressants, see Antineoplastic Agents, p.175.

Ethoglucid should be used with care in patients with impaired liver function. It should not be used when regional oedema might be dangerous.

Absorption and Fate. Ethoglucid is rapidly removed from the blood following intravenous injection and is localised in most tissues. It diffuses into the cerebrospinal fluid. It is rapidly metabolised in the liver and only a very small proportion is excreted unchanged in the urine.

Uses. Ethoglucid is an antineoplastic agent which acts by alkylation (see p.171). It must be diluted before administration and is used mainly for the treatment of non-invasive tumours of the bladder by the instillation of a solution containing 1 or 2% v/v of ethoglucid in water or sodium chloride solution. The patient's fluid intake should be restricted beforehand.

Intra-arterial injections of 3 to 12 g, diluted to a 10 to 20% solution, have been given and appear to be more effective than intravenous injections but local oedema may sometimes occur. A similar solution has occasionally been used intravenously. The maximum intravenous dose of ethoglucid varies from 200 to 250 mg per kg body-weight according to the condition of the patient, given as a single dose or in divided doses, and repeated every 3 to 5 weeks. Care should be taken to avoid extravasation.

Intracavitary injections of 3 to 18 g have also been given to patients with malignant effusions of the pleura and peritoneum.

Proprietary Preparations

Epodyl *(ICI Pharmaceuticals, UK)*. Ethoglucid, available in ampoules of 1 ml. (Also available as Epodyl in *Neth., S.Afr.*).

1834-a

Etoposide.

EPEG; NSC 141540; VP 16-213. 4′-*O*-Demethyl-1-*O*-(4,6-*O*-ethylidene-β-D-glucopyranosyl)epipodophyllotoxin; 9-(4,6-*O*-Ethylidene-β-D-glucopyranosyloxy)-5,8,8a,9-tetrahydro-5-(4-hydroxy-3,5-dimethoxyphenyl)-2*H*-isobenzofuro[5,6-*f*][1,3]benzodioxol-6(5a*H*)-one.

$C_{29}H_{32}O_{13}=588.6$.

CAS — 33419-42-0.

NOTE. The trivial name epipodophyllotoxin has occasionally been used incorrectly for this derivative.

A white to yellow-brown crystalline powder. M.p. about 221°. Poorly **soluble** in water; soluble in organic solvents.

Adverse Effects, Treatment, and Precautions. For an outline of the adverse effects experienced with antineoplastic agents and immunosuppressants, general guidelines for their treatment, and precautions, see Antineoplastic Agents, p.171, pp.174-5.

Mention of peripheral neuropathy associated with the use of etoposide.— A. M. Arnold and C. J. Williams (letter), *Br. med. J.*, 1979, *1*, 955.

Uses. Etoposide is an antineoplastic agent with antimitotic properties; it is a semi-synthetic derivative of podophyllotoxin. It is given by intravenous infusion as a solution in sodium chloride injection in doses of 60 to 120 mg per m² body-surface daily for 5 days in the treatment of solid tumours of the lung and testis. Double the intravenous dose may be given by mouth.

The concentration of the intravenous infusion must not be more than 250 µg per ml and the infusion should be given over a period of not less than 30 minutes; hypotension may follow excessively rapid infusion. Care must be taken to avoid extravasation.

Nine cancer patients were given radioactively-labelled etoposide in a dose of 220 or 290 mg per m² body-surface by intravenous infusion over 1 hour in 500 ml of dextrose injection. Plasma decay was biphasic and there was poor penetration into the cerebrospinal fluid. Two-thirds of urinary activity appeared as unchanged drug but less than 50% of the administered dose was found in the urine. Recovery of drug in the faeces was very erratic and ranged from below 1.5% to about 16% of the dose.— P. J. Creaven and L. M. Allen, *Clin. Pharmac. Ther.*, 1975, *18*, 221. See also F. R. Pelsor *et al.*, *J. pharm. Sci.*, 1978, *67*, 1106.

A review of etoposide and comparison with teniposide failed to reveal any significant differences between the two.— M. Rozencweig *et al.*, *Cancer*, 1977, *40*, 334.

Further reviews of etoposide: A. M. Arnold, *Cancer Chemother. Pharmac.*, 1979, *3*, 71; B. F. Issell and S. T. Crooke, *Cancer Treat. Rev.*, 1979, *6*, 107; A. M. Arnold and J. M. A. Whitehouse, *Lancet*, 1981, *2*, 912.

Two of 4 patients with acute 'monocytoid' leukaemia and 2 of 4 with acute 'myelomonocytoid' leukaemia had apparently complete remissions after treatment with etoposide 50 mg per m² body-surface daily for 5 days, the course being repeated at intervals of 5 to 25 days. Treatment was less effective in other types of acute leukaemia, Hodgkin's disease, histiocytic lymphoma, and lymphosarcoma. Pronounced regression of melanoma and carcinoma of the bladder, breast, kidney, oesophagus, or thyroid was achieved in some patients. Treatment was given intravenously to 200 patients and, in twice the dosage, by mouth to 50 patients. Leucopenia occurred in 40 patients, thrombocytopenia in 17, and pancytopenia in 16. Other side-effects included nausea, vomiting, anorexia, alopecia, headache, hypertension, and fever, but treatment had to be discontinued in only 9 of the 250 patients.—European Organization for Research on the Treatment of Cancer, Clinical Screening Group, *Br. med. J.*, 1973, *3*, 199.

Etoposide was given to 20 patients with acute myelogenous leukaemia who had failed to respond to conventional therapy; 18 patients received 50 mg per m² body-surface daily for 5 days by intravenous injection (diluted to 50 ml with sodium chloride injection) and the course was repeated every 2 weeks if there was a response. Complete remissions of 8 months and 10 weeks were achieved in 2 patients and a partial remission in a further patient. Continuous 24-hour infusion of 200 to 250 mg per m² in 3 litres of dextrose injection was unsuccessful in 4 patients. The drug was well tolerated, with transient nausea in 5 patients and reversible alopecia in 1; bone-marrow toxicity was rarely severe. It was considered that better results might be achieved by increasing the dose or by using etoposide in combination chemotherapy.— J. E. Smith *et al.*, *Postgrad. med. J.*, 1976, *52*, 66. See also under Choice of Antineoplastic Agent, p.180.

Further reports of etoposide in the treatment of various

malignant disorders: P. Jacobs and H. S. King (letter), *Lancet*, 1975, *2*, 129 (histiocytic lymphoma); W. F. Jungi *et al.*, *Schweiz. med. Wschr.*, 1975, *105*, 1365 (small cell carcinoma of the lung); E. S. Newlands and K. D. Bagshawe (letter), *Lancet*, 1977, *2*, 87 (teratoma and choriocarcinoma); F. Cavalli *et al.* (letter), *Lancet*, 1977, *2*, 362 (teratoma; etoposide 180 mg per m^2 body-surface given daily for 3 days in patients with hepatomas); M. H. Cohen *et al.*, *Cancer Treat. Rep.*, 1977, *61*, 489 (small cell bronchogenic carcinoma); M. Hansen *et al.*, *Cancer*, 1977, *40*, 633 (small cell carcinoma of the lung); N. I. Nissen *et al.*, *Cancer*, 1980, *45*, 232 (large-scale study in advanced neoplastic disease).

Proprietary Preparations

Vepesid Capsules *(Bristol-Myers Pharmaceuticals, UK).* Each contains etoposide 100 mg.

Vepesid Injection *(Bristol-Myers Pharmaceuticals, UK).* Etoposide, available as a solution containing 20 mg per ml, in ampoules of 5 ml. Protect from light.

1835-t

Floxuridine *(U.S.P.).* 5-FUDR; 5-Fluoro-2′-deoxyuridine; 5-Fluorouracil Deoxyriboside; NSC 27640; WR 138720. 2′-Deoxy-5-fluorouridine; 1-(2-Deoxy-β-D-ribofuranosyl)-5-fluoropyrimidine-2,4(1*H*,3*H*)-dione.

$C_9H_{11}FN_2O_5$=246.2.

CAS — 50-91-9.

Pharmacopoeias. In *U.S.* which also includes Sterile Floxuridine.

A white to off-white odourless powder. M.p. 149° to 153°. **Soluble** 1 in 3 of water, 1 in 12 of alcohol, 1 in 43 of isopropyl alcohol, and 1 in 7 of methyl alcohol; practically insoluble in chloroform, ether, and light petroleum. A 1% solution in water is dextrorotatory. A 2% solution in water has a pH of 4 to 5.5. An 8.47% solution in water is iso-osmotic with serum. **Store** in airtight containers. Protect from light.

An aqueous solution of floxuridine iso-osmotic with serum (8.47%) caused 3% haemolysis of erythrocytes cultured in it for 45 minutes.— C. Sapp *et al.*, *J. pharm. Sci.*, 1975, *64*, 1884.

Adverse Effects, Treatment, and Precautions. As for Fluorouracil, p.209. Local reactions, including erythema and stomatitis, are more common than systemic effects following intra-arterial infusion. There have also been signs of liver dysfunction.

Absorption and Fate. It is poorly absorbed from the gastro-intestinal tract and it is usually given by injection. Floxuridine is metabolised to fluorouracil following rapid injection. When given by slow intra-arterial infusion it is reported to be converted to active floxuridine monophosphate.

For a review of the absorption and fate of floxuridine, see V. T. Oliverio and C. G. Zubrod, *A. Rev. Pharmac.*, 1965, *5*, 335.

Further references: W. D. Ensminger *et al.*, *Cancer Res.*, 1978, *38*, 3784 (hepatic arterial infusions).

Uses. Floxuridine is an antineoplastic agent which acts as an antimetabolite similarly to fluorouracil. When it is administered by rapid injection it acts as fluorouracil, but when infused slowly, usually intra-arterially, it is converted to floxuridine monophosphate which is reported to be a more active inhibitor of DNA synthesis.

Floxuridine is used in the palliative treatment of malignant neoplasms of the liver and gastro-intestinal tract. Doses of 100 to 600 μg per kg body-weight daily are given by continuous arterial infusion, usually with the aid of an infusion pump. It used to be given by intravenous injection in doses of 30 mg per kg body-weight daily for up to 5 days, followed by a lower maintenance dose. White cell and platelet counts should be carried out regularly during therapy and treatment should be stopped if the white cell count falls rapidly or falls to below 3 500 per mm^3, if the platelet count falls below 100 000 per mm^3, or if adverse effects occur.

Antiprotozoal action. Floxuridine had significant activity against *Trypanosoma rhodesiense* infections in *mice.*— K. E. Kinnamon *et al.*, *Antimicrob. Ag. Chemother.*, 1979, *15*, 157.

Malignant neoplasms. Comparative studies of the efficacy of floxuridine and fluorouracil given intravenously in carcinoma of the bowel have not shown that floxuridine has any advantage over fluorouracil.— C. G. Moertel and R. J. Reitemeier (letter), *J. Am. med. Ass.*, 1967, *201*, 780.

Further references to the use of floxuridine in the treatment of malignant neoplasms: M. Fiorentino and E. Finotto (letter), *Br. med. J.*, 1967, *4*, 294 (intravenous infusion); R. C. DeConti *et al.*, *Cancer*, 1973, *31*, 894 (intravenous infusion in breast and gastro-intestinal carcinomas); R. W. Dwight *et al.*, *J. surg. Oncol.*, 1973, *5*, 243 (lack of beneficial effect as an adjuvant to surgery); B. Cady and R. A. Oberfield, *Am. J. Surg.*, 1974, *127*, 220 (hepatic intra-arterial infusions).

Preparations

Sterile Floxuridine *(U.S.P.).* Sterile floxuridine suitable for intra-arterial infusion. A 2% solution in water has a pH of 4 to 5.5. Reconstituted solutions should be stored at 2° to 8° for not more than 2 weeks.

Proprietary Names

FUDR *(Roche, USA).*

1836-x

Fluorouracil *(U.S.P.).* 5-Fluorouracil; 5-FU; Ro 2-9757; NSC 19893; WR 69596. 5-Fluoropyrimidine-2,4(1*H*,3*H*)-dione.

$C_4H_3FN_2O_2$=130.1.

CAS — 51-21-8.

Pharmacopoeias. In *Braz.*, *Chin.*, and *U.S.*

A white to almost white, almost odourless, crystalline powder. It decomposes at about 282°. Sparingly **soluble** in water; slightly soluble in alcohol; practically insoluble in chloroform and ether. Solutions discolour on storage. **Store** in airtight containers. Protect from light.

CAUTION. *Fluorouracil is irritant; avoid contact with skin and mucous membranes.*

Incompatibility. For a report of incompatibility between methotrexate sodium and fluorouracil, see Methotrexate, p.215.

Adverse Effects and Treatment. For an outline of the adverse effects experienced with antineoplastic agents and immunosuppressants and general guidelines for their treatment, see Antineoplastic Agents, p.171 and p.174.

The toxic effects of fluorouracil may be severe and sometimes fatal. Leucopenia is the main dose-limiting effect and the occurrence of stomatitis or severe diarrhoea are early signs that treatment should be stopped. Depression of the white-cell count is greatest after 7 to 20 days and counts may return to normal after about 30 days. Thrombocytopenia is usually at a maximum 7 to 17 days after the first dose. Reducing the rate of injection to a slow infusion over 2 to 8 hours can decrease the toxicity but this may be less effective than administration by rapid injection.

Local inflammatory and photosensitivity reactions have occurred following topical use.

Allergy and anaphylaxis. Of 35 patients without previous exposure to fluorouracil one showed asymptomatic macular erythema after intracutaneous testing with fluorouracil and none of 12 reacted to epicutaneous testing. Of 35 patients with previous exposure to fluorouracil 6 reacted to intracutaneous and epicutaneous testing; pruritus was intense; 2 had widespread reactions and 2 local flare; 5 of the 6 had had 2 earlier courses of fluorouracil; of the remaining 29 two showed asymptomatic erythema.— D. K. Goette and R. B. Odom, *Archs Derm.*, 1977, *113*, 1058.

Individual reports of allergic reactions associated with fluorouracil: T. Bernstein (letter), *New Engl. J. Med.*, 1977, *297*, 337 (a severe skin reaction after intravenous injection of fluorouracil following previous topical use); E. F. Omura (letter), *ibid.*, 946 (doubt about the allergic nature of the reaction); D. K. Goette *et al.*, *Archs Derm.*, 1977, *113*, 196 (allergic contact dermatitis); H. A. Schlang and R. Curtin (letter), *J. Am. med. Ass.*, 1977, *238*, 1722 (a skin rash on an irradiated area).

Effects on the eyes. Of 46 patients receiving fluorouracil, 250 mg to 1.1 g weekly by intravenous injection, 16 complained of eye symptoms; these included excessive watering of the eyes in 14, excessive nasal discharge in 8, irritation of the eyes in 7, reddening of the eyes in 5, blurring of vision in 2, matter in the eyes in 2, and blood in the nose in 2. These side-effects disappeared 1 or 2 weeks after the drug was discontinued.— J. Hamersley *et al.* (letter), *J. Am. med. Ass.*, 1973, *225*, 747. Excessive watering of the eyes was associated with fluorouracil in 6 patients, one of whom had symptoms consistent with fibrosis of the tear duct. Only one patient improved when fluorouracil was discontinued.— D. J. Haidak *et al.*, *Ann. intern. Med.*, 1978, *88*, 657. Fluorouracil can be detected in the tear fluid and may produce local irritation of the tear duct.— N. Christophidis *et al.* (letter), *ibid.*, *89*, 574. See also N. Christophidis *et al.*, *Aust. N.Z. J. Med.*, 1979, *9*, 143.

A report of oculomotor disturbances associated with fluorouracil.— W. W. Bixenman *et al.*, *Am. J. Ophthal.*, 1977, *83*, 789.

Effects on the gastro-intestinal tract. A 49-year-old man with malignant neoplasm of the liver was treated with fluorouracil 250 mg daily by intra-arterial infusion with complete resolution of the neoplasm for 4½ years, but with gross scarring which led to the formation of gastro-oesophageal varices and eventual fatal haemorrhage.— J. M. Anderson *et al.*, *Br. med. J.*, 1972, *3*, 454.

Further references: T. Narsete *et al.*, *Ann. Surg.*, 1977, *186*, 734 (gastric ulceration associated with the intra-hepatic infusion of fluorouracil).

Effects on the heart. Four patients without a history of myocardial infarction, angina pectoris, or hypertension developed severe chest pain after 2nd or 3rd doses of fluorouracil; the ECG was altered in 3. The cause was not known, but earlier ventricular irradiation, possibly inducing small-vessel thrombosis, might have been a contributory factor.— A. Pottage *et al.*, *Br. med. J.*, 1978, *1*, 547.

Further reports of cardiotoxicity associated with fluorouracil: M. E. Carpenter (letter), *Br. med. J.*, 1972, *2*, 595 (tachycardia, controlled by quinidine given immediately before fluorouracil); R. G. Dent and I. McColl (letter), *Lancet*, 1975, *1*, 347 (angina pectoris); D. L. Stevenson *et al.* (letter), *Lancet*, 1977, *2*, 406 (chest pain, tachycardia, breathlessness, and pulmonary oedema; protection with prednisolone and glyceryl trinitrate was generally effective); M. Soukop *et al.* (letter), *Br. med. J.*, 1978, *1*, 1422 (severe chest pain and fatal myocardial infarction).

Effects on the kidneys. For a report of a haemolytic-uraemic state associated with long-term therapy with mitomycin and fluorouracil, see Mitomycin, p.221.

Effects on mental state. A 70-year-old man and an 80-year-old woman experienced severe mental confusion after starting weekly therapy with fluorouracil. The total dose of fluorouracil was 8 g and 3 g respectively. Both showed marked improvement after withdrawal of fluorouracil.— E. S. Greenwald (letter), *J. Am. med. Ass.*, 1976, *235*, 248.

Effects on the nervous system. A brief discussion on cerebral ataxia associated with fluorouracil. Although in general fewer than 1% of patients receiving fluorouracil will have manifestations of cerebellar dysfunction, the incidence increases when high doses or intensive daily treatment regimens are used. It is important to differentiate between this reversible and rarely serious neurotoxicity and metastatic involvement of the cerebellum.— H. D. Weiss *et al.*, *New Engl. J. Med.*, 1974, *291*, 75.

Effects on the skin. Fluorouracil might temporarily exacerbate chloasma and rosacea when applied to the skin. Exposure to sunlight increases discomfort at the reactive stage of treatment.— W. M. Sams, *Archs Derm.*, 1968, *97*, 14.

Pellagra reported in patients receiving treatment with fluorouracil was considered to be due to inhibition of endogenous nadide synthesis; fluorouracil had also been shown to inhibit the conversion of tryptophan into nicotinic acid.— J. D. Stratigos and A. Katsambas, *Br. J. Derm.*, 1977, *96*, 99.

Precautions. For reference to the precautions necessary with antineoplastic agents and immunosuppressants, see Antineoplastic Agents, p.175.

Interactions. Experimental studies indicating that methotrexate might inhibit the antitumour effect of fluorouracil or floxuridine.— T. H. Maugh, *Science*, 1976, *194*, 310; S. Waxman and H. Bruckner (letter), *ibid.*,

1112; J. R. Bertino (letter), *ibid.*, 1113; A. Goldin (letter), *ibid.*, 1115.

Interference with diagnostic tests. Serum concentrations of total thyroxine and total tri-iodothyronine rose in 15 patients with mammary carcinoma during treatment with fluorouracil; the patients remained clinically euthyroid.— L. V. A. M. Beex *et al.* (letter), *Lancet*, 1976, *1*, 866.

Absorption and Fate. Absorption of fluorouracil from the gastro-intestinal tract is unpredictable and fluorouracil is usually given intravenously. Little is absorbed when fluorouracil is applied to healthy skin but up to 20% of a dose applied to diseased skin may be excreted in the urine over 24 hours. It is also absorbed to a small extent through serous membranes.

After intravenous injection fluorouracil is cleared rapidly from plasma. It is distributed throughout body tissues and fluids including the cerebrospinal fluid and malignant effusions, and disappears from the plasma within about 3 hours. Fluorouracil is converted to active nucleotide metabolites within the target cell itself. About 15% of an intravenous dose is excreted unchanged in the urine within 6 hours. The remainder is inactivated primarily in the liver and is catabolised similarly to endogenous uracil. A large amount is excreted as respiratory carbon dioxide; urea is also produced.

A review of the pharmacokinetic features of fluorouracil and their interrelationship with biochemical kinetics in monitoring therapy. The elimination half-life of fluorouracil from plasma is about 10 minutes and plasma concentrations cannot be detected 2 hours after an intravenous dose. Nevertheless, the activity of fluorouracil may persist for several days following a single intravenous injection. Studies in *animals* have shown that the active metabolite 5-fluoro-2′-deoxyuridine 5′-monophosphate (FdUMP) remains in tissues over several days and a terminal elimination half-life for fluorouracil of 20 hours has been reported in *rats* by C. Finn and W. Sadee (*Cancer Chemother. Rep.*, 1975, *59*, 279). Erratic concentrations of fluorouracil have followed oral administration with peak plasma concentrations between 0.8 and 40 μg per ml 10 minutes to 2 hours after a dose of 15 mg per kg body-weight. The active fluorouracil nucleotides are trapped within the cell because of their high polarity and direct measurements of metabolites in target and host tissues appear to be necessary to obtain a link between drug concentrations and response. Preferential uptake of FdUMP has been reported in a number of experimental and human tumour systems but this alone may not be a good indicator of tumour response.— W. Sadee and C. G. Wong, *Clin. Pharmacokinet.*, 1977, *2*, 437.

Peak plasma concentrations ranged from 24 to 125 μg per ml with an elimination half-life of 10 to 30 minutes following the intravenous bolus injection of fluorouracil in 12 cancer patients. Doses ranged from 9 to 16 mg per kg body-weight. When the same dose was given by mouth to these patients plasma concentrations were below 10 μg per ml and bioavailability ranged from 0 to about 75% but was usually increased markedly if the dose was doubled. No correlation was found between liver abnormalities and bioavailability. Plasma concentrations ranged from 0 to 8 μg per ml in 6 patients given fluorouracil 20 to 30 mg per kg body-weight daily by slow intravenous infusion on 5 consecutive days. In 4 patients fluorouracil could not be detected in the plasma after rectal administration by enema in 100 ml of saline.— N. Christophidis *et al.*, *Clin. Pharmacokinet.*, 1978, *3*, 330.

Plasma concentrations of fluorouracil after oral and intravenous administration in cancer patients.— R. E. Finch *et al.*, *Br. J. clin. Pharmac.*, 1979, *7*, 613. See also *J. Am. med. Ass.*, 1974, *229*, 1109.

Further references to pharmacokinetic studies of fluorouracil: H. S. Shukla *et al.*, *Gut*, 1976, *17*, 402; D. S. Sitar *et al.*, *Cancer Res.*, 1977, *37*, 3981; W. D. Ensminger *et al.*, *Cancer Res.*, 1978, *38*, 3784 (hepatic arterial infusions); W. E. MacMillan *et al.*, *Cancer Res.*, 1978, *38*, 3479; J. M. Collins *et al.*, *Clin. Pharmac. Ther.*, 1980, *28*, 235.

Uses. Fluorouracil, a pyrimidine analogue, is an antineoplastic agent which acts as an antimetabolite to uracil. After intracellular conversion to the active deoxynucleotide it interferes with the synthesis of DNA by blocking the conversion of deoxyuridylic acid to thymidylic acid by the cellular enzyme thymidylate synthetase. It can also interfere with RNA synthesis. It also has immunosuppressant properties. Fluorouracil is used in the palliation of inoperable malignant neoplasms, especially those of the gastro-intestinal tract, breast, liver, and pancreas. It is often used with cyclophosphamide and methotrexate in the combination chemotherapy of breast cancer. See also Choice of Antineoplastic Agent, p.180.

Therapeutic doses are close to toxic levels and fatalities have occurred. Initial treatment should always be given in hospital.

A usual dose by intravenous injection is 12 mg per kg body-weight daily to a maximum of 1 g daily for 3 or 4 days. If there is no evidence of toxicity, this is followed after 1 day by 6 mg per kg on alternate days for 3 or 4 further doses. An alternative schedule is to give 15 mg per kg intravenously once a week throughout the course. Maintenance is usually with 5 to 15 mg per kg weekly. Fluorouracil may also be given by intravenous infusion, 15 mg per kg daily, to a maximum of 1 g daily, being infused in 500 ml of dextrose injection over 4 hours and repeated on successive days until toxicity occurs or a total of 12 to 15 g has been given. The course may be repeated after 4 to 6 weeks. It is also given by intra-arterial infusion and by mouth.

The white cell count should be determined daily during treatment with fluorouracil and therapy stopped immediately if the count falls rapidly or falls to below 3500 per mm^3, if the platelet count falls below 100 000 per mm^3, or if adverse effects occur.

Fluorouracil is used topically in the treatment of solar or actinic keratoses and other tumours of the skin including Bowen's disease and superficial basal cell carcinomas, usually as a 5% cream or ointment or as a 1 to 5% solution in propylene glycol.

Administration. A brief discussion on the relative merits of different dosage schedules for fluorouracil, using the intravenous or oral route.— B. I. Shnider (letter), *J. Am. med. Ass.*, 1977, *238*, 1070.

See also E. M. Jacobs *et al.*, *Cancer*, 1968, *22*, 1233; J. Horton *et al.*, *Ann. intern. Med.*, 1970, *73*, 897; E. M. Jacobs *et al.*, *Cancer*, 1971, *27*, 1302; J. R. Bateman *et al.*, *Cancer*, 1971, *28*, 907; H. S. Shukla *et al.*, *Am. J. Surg.*, 1977, *133*, 346 (intramural, intraluminal, and intravenous routes).

A study in 13 cancer patients suggested that allopurinol modulates the toxicity of fluorouracil, permitting a two-fold increase in dosage, without hindering tumour response.— R. M. Fox *et al.* (letter), *Lancet*, 1979, *1*, 677. Co-administration of allopurinol with fluorouracil would preferentially protect tumour cells, not normal cells, from fluorouracil toxicity. The patients may have responded because the high doses of fluorouracil used may have overcome allopurinol protection of colon tumour cells.— G. Tisman and S. J. G. Wu (letter), *ibid.*, 1353.

Administration in renal insufficiency. Fluorouracil could be given in usual doses to patients with renal failure. Concentrations of fluorouracil are affected by haemodialysis.— W. M. Bennett *et al.*, *Ann. intern. Med.*, 1977, *86*, 754. See also *idem*, 1980, *93*, 286.

Carcinoid syndrome. Fluorouracil produced frequent but relatively brief remissions in a study of 94 patients with the malignant carcinoid syndrome.— Z. Davis *et al.*, *Surgery Gynec. Obstet.*, 1973, *137*, 637, per *J. Am. med. Ass.*, 1974, *227*, 702.

Enhancement of effect. In *mice* the antitumour activity of fluorouracil and floxuridine was enhanced in the presence of 2-deoxyuridine.— J. Jato and J. J. Windheuser, *J. pharm. Sci.*, 1973, *62*, 1975.

Laryngeal papillomas. Comment on the role of fluorouracil in the adjuvant treatment of laryngeal papillomas.— *Lancet*, 1981, *1*, 367.

Malignant neoplasms. Fluorouracil is commonly used for the treatment of malignant neoplasms at the following sites. Primary approach: breast (combination chemotherapy with cyclophosphamide, methotrexate, and fluorouracil, with or without vincristine and prednisone), stomach, large bowel, pancreas, liver, skin (topical); secondary approach: endometrium, bladder. Activity has also been reported in cancer of the ovary, cervix, and head and neck.— Report of a WHO Expert Committee on Chemotherapy of Solid Tumours, *Tech. Rep. Ser. Wld Hlth Org. No. 605*, 1977.

Individual reports on fluorouracil in the treatment of various malignant neoplasms: G. R. Prout *et al.*, *Cancer*, 1968, *22*, 926 (bladder); J. J. Kaufman, *Archs Surg., Chicago*, 1969, *99*, 477 (bladder); F. F. Gollin *et al.*, *Am. J. Roentg.*, 1972, *114*, 83 (head and neck); J. P. Smith *et al.*, *Am. J. Roentg.*, 1972, *114*, 110 (cervix); J. E. Nevin *et al.*, *Cancer*, 1973, *31*, 138 (bladder and prostate); T. E. Carson *et al.*, *Obstet. Gynec.*, 1976, *47*, 59S (vulva, topical use); J. P. Forney *et al.*, *Am. J. Obstet. Gynec.*, 1977, *127*, 801 (no benefit from topical use on vulvar carcinoma); K. E. Briscoe *et al.*, *J. Am. med. Ass.*, 1978, *240*, 51 (intra-arterial hyperthermic perfusion with melphalan in metastatic sweat gland carcinoma); M. S. Piver *et al.*, *Am. J. Obstet. Gynec.*, 1979, *135*, 377 (topical use on the vagina).

The effect of fluorouracil in conjunction with vinblastine in 75 patients with solid tumours. Drug toxicity was significantly reduced. The response of tumours of the gastro-intestinal tract was similar to that produced by fluorouracil alone.— M. Al-Sarraf *et al.*, *Oncology*, 1972, *26*, 99, per *J. Am. med. Ass.*, 1972, *220*, 1030.

Malignant neoplasms of the breast. See under Choice of Antineoplastic Agent, p.180.

Malignant neoplasms of the gastro-intestinal tract. Fluorouracil is the single agent most extensively studied for the treatment of stomach cancer. The usual loading dose is now 13.5 mg per kg body-weight daily by intravenous injection for 5 days, followed by half-doses until toxicity occurs, then weekly maintenance schedules. Combination chemotherapy has been more successful in stomach cancer than other gastro-intestinal neoplasms. The standard single agent for therapy of advanced large bowel cancer is fluorouracil; an overall response-rate of 20% has been observed. A loading course schedule is the commonest approach, oral administration cannot be recommended for routine use. Fluorouracil as an adjuvant to surgery has not been significantly successful.— Report of a WHO Expert Committee on Chemotherapy of Solid Tumours, *Tech. Rep. Ser. Wld Hlth Org. No. 605*, 1977, p. 32.

Despite efforts to increase the therapeutic index of the fluorinated pyrimidines, fluorouracil and floxuridine, in gastro-intestinal cancer, there is no firm evidence that they contribute to the overall survival of patients, regardless of the stage of the disease at which they are used; only 15 to 20% of patients will achieve objective responses. Reports suggest that, for fluorouracil, the oral route of administration is considerably inferior to the intravenous route, the weekly schedule is inferior to the loading course, and treatment with a nontoxic dose is inferior to that with doses producing mild or moderate adverse effects. Administration of fluorouracil or floxuridine by continuous intravenous infusion appears to offer no advantage over rapid intravenous injection and there is no evidence that hepatic-artery infusion techniques contribute to the survival of patients with gastro-intestinal carcinoma and metastases limited to the liver. Fluorouracil and floxuridine appear to be equivalent in therapeutic effect; tegafur offers no apparent advantage.— C. G. Moertel, *New Engl. J. Med.*, 1978, *299*, 1049. Regression-rates of 33 to 38% have resulted from a flexible 3-phase fluorouracil regimen (F.J. Ansfield *et al.*, *Cancer*, 1977, *39*, 34) consisting of a loading course, titration to mild toxicity, and sustained weekly maintenance therapy thereafter.— F. J. Ansfield and E. M. Greenspan (letter), *ibid.*, 1979, *301*, 328. In 20 years of clinical study, fluorouracil alone has not been shown to improve survival but beneficial results with radiotherapy and fluorouracil have been reported in pancreatic carcinoma (Gastrointestinal Tumor Study Group, *Ann. Surg.*, 1979, *189*, 205) and a probable gain in survival after treatment of advanced gastric carcinoma with doxorubicin and fluorouracil has been suggested (C.G. Moertel *et al.*, *Proc. Am. Ass. Cancer Res. Am. Soc. clin. Oncol.*, 1979, *20*, 288).— C. G. Moertel (letter), *ibid.*, 329.

Further references to the use of fluorouracil in the management of malignant neoplasms of the gastro-intestinal tract: C. G. Moertel *et al.*, *Lancet*, 1969, *2*, 865; G. Falkson and H. C. Falkson, *ibid.*, 1252; F. Richards *et al.*, *Cancer*, 1975, *36*, 1589; M. C. Li and S. T. Ross, *J. Am. med. Ass.*, 1976, *235*, 2825 (adjuvant chemotherapy after colorectal surgery). See also C. G. Moertel (letter), *ibid.*, *236*, 1935; M. C. Li (letter), *ibid.*, 1977, *237*, 872; B. Ecanow *et al.* (letter), *ibid.*, *238*, 481; T. C. Lo *et al.*, *Am. J. Roentg.*, 1976, *126*, 229 (with radiotherapy in carcinoma of the oral cavity and oropharynx); T. B. Grage *et al.*, *Am. J. Surg.*, 1977, *133*, 59 (adjuvant chemotherapy after colorectal surgery); I. Taylor *et al.*, *Br. med. J.*, 1977, *2*, 1320 (adjuvant chemotherapy using portal perfusion after resection of colorectal cancer); A. Barrett *et al.* (letter), *Lancet*, 1978, *2*, 101 (disappointing results with fluorouracil and semustine in colorectal cancer); P. Huck, *Practitioner*, 1979, *222*, 689 (poor results in carcinoma of the rectum).

See also under Malignant Neoplasms of the Liver and of the Pancreas, below, and Choice of Antineoplastic Agent, pp.183-4.

Malignant neoplasms of the liver. Although there is considerable enthusiasm in the USA for the administration of fluorinated pyrimidines by hepatic-artery infusion in liver cell carcinoma, an advantage over traditional systemic chemotherapy has not been established. Responses have been observed with fluorouracil in association with carmustine.— Report of a WHO Expert Committee on Chemotherapy of Solid Tumours, *Tech. Rep. Ser. Wld Hlth Org. No. 605*, 1977, p. 39.

There were objective responses in 15 of 23 patients with primary or metastatic liver carcinoma treated with fluorouracil and mitomycin, both given by intrahepatic arterial infusion. The activity of each agent might be enhanced by the other.— N. C. Misra *et al.*, *Cancer*, 1977, *39*, 1425.

Six of 12 patients with unresectable hepatoma gained an objective response with increased survival when treated with fluorouracil by mouth in a dose of 15 mg per kg body-weight weekly.— P. S. Kennedy *et al.*, *Cancer*, 1977, *39*, 1930. No beneficial results were achieved in 21 similar patients given the same dose either by mouth or intravenously. In some patients the dose was increased to 20 mg per kg weekly or decreased to 12 mg per kg weekly.— J. S. Link *et al.*, *ibid.*, 1936.

Portal perfusion of fluorouracil after resection of colorectal cancer appeared to limit the development of liver metastases. Fluorouracil 1 g in dextrose injection was given by continuous infusion daily for 7 days into the obliterated umbilical vein.— I. Taylor *et al.*, *Br. med. J.*, 1977, *2*, 1320.

Further references to fluorouracil in the treatment of malignant neoplasms of the liver: F. J. Ansfield *et al.*, *Cancer*, 1971, *28*, 1147 (intra-arterial infusions); R. N. Tandon *et al.*, *Surgery, St Louis*, 1973, *73*, 118 (intra-arterial infusions); M. A. Goodman and A. M. J. Laden, *Med. J. Aust.*, 1977, *1*, 220 (constant intra-arterial infusion for 26 days, followed by 3 courses of fluorouracil given intravenously).

Malignant neoplasms of the pancreas. Fluorouracil has been the most thoroughly studied drug in the palliative treatment of adenocarcinoma of the pancreas. Analysis of the literature gives an overall response-rate of 38% but this may be an overestimate. The standard loading course schedule of treatment has generally been used. Combination chemotherapy with fluorouracil and carmustine has not improved survival significantly.— Report of a WHO Expert Committee on Chemotherapy of Solid Tumours, *Tech. Rep. Ser. Wld Hlth Org. No. 605*, 1977, p. 36.

Further references to the use of fluorouracil in pancreatic carcinoma: J. J. Lokich and J. R. Brooks, *Ann. Surg.*, 1973, *177*, 13; W. R. Waddell, *Surgery, St Louis*, 1973, *74*, 420; H. M. Lemon *et al.*, *Cancer*, 1973, *31*, 17.

For a report of a beneficial response to streptozocin and fluorouracil in advanced islet-cell carcinoma, see Streptozocin, p.226.

Malignant neoplasms of the skin. Topical chemotherapy with fluorouracil is the treatment of choice for actinic keratosis and is highly effective for the management of multiple superficial basal cell carcinomas and squamous cell carcinomas *in situ* when extensive involvement of the body surface precludes the use of other treatment modalities. Palliation of recurrent tumours of the skin has been possible in about 50% of patients. Cutaneous side-effects are relatively insignificant and readily reversible; topical chemotherapy does not cause systemic toxicity. Local treatment with fluorouracil is usually not indicated with nodular invasive lesions of basal cell or squamous cell carcinomas.— Report of a WHO Expert Committee on Chemotherapy of Solid Tumours, *Tech. Rep. Ser. Wld Hlth Org. No. 605*, 1977, p. 57.

Individual reports of the topical use of fluorouracil in various malignant skin diseases: F. E. Anderson *et al.*, *Med. J. Aust.*, 1969, *2*, 385; F. Serri (Ed.), *Dermatologica*, 1970, *140*, *Suppl.* 1, 1–134; D. K. Goette *et al.*, *J. Am. med. Ass.*, 1975, *232*, 934 (erythroplasia of Queyrat); R. B. Amon and P. E. Goodkin (letter), *New Engl. J. Med.*, 1976, *295*, 677; H. A. Haynes (letter), *ibid.*, 678 (possible use in basal-cell-naevus syndrome).

Actinic (solar) keratoses. A collodion-based varnish containing fluorouracil 5% and salicylic acid 5, 8, or 10% was used in the treatment of solar keratoses in 20 patients, 6 of whom had been previously treated with fluorouracil ointment 5%. The varnish adhered to the skin for 2 to 3 weeks and lesions were therefore treated only every 3 weeks. Those on the face required 1 to 5 applications and those of 2 patients on the hands 7 and 9. There was no dermatitis or photosensitisation. The varnish appeared to be superior to the ointment except where a rapid response was required or the lesions were very numerous.— J. C. A. Goncalves, *Br. J. Derm.*, 1975, *92*, 85. The morning application of tretinoin 0.1% and the evening application of fluorouracil cream 5% eradicated all keratoses on the forearms and hands of 20 patients. Tretinoin was discontinued after 8 to 14 days when inflammation developed. Fluorouracil cream alone was effective against keratoses of the face, some of the forearms, but ineffective against those on the hands.— T. A. Robinson and A. M. Kligman, *Br. J. Derm.*, 1975, *92*, 703.

Further references: J. C. Belisario, *Med. J. Aust.*, 1969, *2*, 1136; A. C. Williams, *Ann. Surg.*, 1971, *173*, 864; T. Breza *et al.*, *Archs Derm.*, 1976, *112*, 1256.

Basal cell carcinoma. Following experience gained in treating 103 patients, the topical treatment of invasive basal cell carcinoma of the face with fluorouracil was not recommended since it often produced the appearance of control by superficial inhibition of the tumour while the deeper extensions continued to grow.— F. E. Mohs *et al.*, *Archs Derm.*, 1978, *114*, 1021.

Further references: *J. Am. med. Ass.*, 1968, *203* (Mar. 25), A31; H. L. Stoll, *J. invest. Derm.*, 1969, *52*, 304; *J. Am. med. Ass.*, 1974, *228*, 209.

See also under Skin Disorders, Non-malignant, below.

Skin disorders, non-malignant. Reports of beneficial results with fluorouracil applied topically in the treatment of various skin disorders: P. C. H. Newbold, *Br. J. Derm.*, 1972, *86*, 87 (psoriasis; 1% or 5% fluorouracil in propylene glycol); T. Tsuji and T. Sugai, *Archs Derm.*, 1972, *105*, 208 (psoriasis; 5% fluorouracil ointment and polyethylene occlusion); T. Fredriksson, *Archs Derm.*, 1974, *110*, 735 (psoriasis); F. K. Bagatell (letter), *Archs Derm.*, 1977, *113*, 378 (onychomycosis, 1% fluorouracil in propylene glycol); E. Epstein, *Archs Derm.*, 1977, *113*, 906 (keratosis of the lip, 5% fluorouracil solution); H. F. Haberman *et al.*, *Can. med. Ass. J.*, 1978, *118*, 161 (scrotal skin lesions of extramammary Paget's disease, 1% fluorouracil cream); H. P. Lebandter and R. F. Ryan (letter), *New Engl. J. Med.*, 1978, *298*, 913 (Gorlin's syndrome, fluorouracil cream); R. B. Odom and D. K. Goette, *Archs Derm.*, 1978, *114*, 1779 (keratoacanthomas, intralesional injections of fluorouracil); P. D. Wilson and F. A. Ive, *Dermatologica*, 1980, *160*, 337 (hyperkeratosis lenticularis perstans, 5% fluorouracil cream).

See also under Malignant Neoplasms of the Skin, above.

Warts. The value of topical fluorouracil in the treatment of warts is limited. Cure-rates are no better than those achieved with simpler substances.— M. H. Bunney, *Drugs*, 1977, *13*, 445.

Further references: J. C. A. Goncalves, *Br. J. Derm.*, 1975, *92*, 89; M. W. Hursthouse, *Br. J. Derm.*, 1975, *92*, 93.

Preparations

Fluorouracil Cream *(U.S.P.)*. A cream containing fluorouracil. It may contain sodium hydroxide to adjust the pH. Store at 15° to 30° in airtight containers.

Fluorouracil Injection *(U.S.P.)*. A sterile solution in Water for Injections, prepared with the aid of sodium hydroxide. It contains 45 to 55 mg of fluorouracil in each ml. pH 8.6 to 9. Store at 15° to 30°. Avoid freezing; protect from light. If a precipitate forms, redissolve by warming to 60°, with shaking, and cool.

Fluorouracil Topical Solution *(U.S.P.)*. A solution of fluorouracil. It may contain sodium hydroxide to adjust the pH. Store at 15° to 30° in airtight containers.

Proprietary Preparations

Efudix *(Roche, UK)*. Fluorouracil, available as a cream containing 5%. (Also available as Efudix in *Austral.*, *Belg.*, *Fr.*, *Ger.*, *Ital.*, *Jap.*, *Neth.*, *S.Afr.*, *Spain*, *Switz.*).

Fluoro-uracil *(Roche, UK)*. Fluorouracil sodium, available as **Capsules** each containing the equivalent of fluorouracil 250 mg, and as a solution containing the equivalent of fluorouracil 25 mg per ml, in **Ampoules** of 10 ml. (Also available as Fluoro-uracil in *Austral.*, *Belg.*, *Neth.*).

Other Proprietary Names

Arg.—Fluorouracilo; *Austral.*—Fluoroplex; *Canad.*—Adrucil, Efudex, Fluoroplex; *Fr.*—Fluoro-Uracile; *Ger.*—Effluderm; *Jap.*—Arumel, Carzonal, FU, Timazin, ULUP; *USA*—Adrucil, Efudex, Fluoroplex.

1837-r

Guanazole. NSC 1895. 3,5-Diamino-1*H*-1,2,4-triazole. $C_2H_5N_5$=99.10.

CAS — 1455-77-2.

Uses. Guanazole is an antineoplastic agent (p.171) which has been used in the treatment of acute leukaemia.

Pharmacokinetic studies of guanazole: N. Gerber *et al.*, *Clin. Pharmac. Ther.*, 1973, *14*, 264; C. Dave *et al.*, *Clin. Pharmac. Ther.*, 1975, *17*, 36.

Guanazole given by continuous intravenous infusion to 44 adults with acute leukaemia in doses of 7.5 g increased if necessary to 30 g per m² body-surface daily for 5 days and repeated at 14-day intervals for further 5-day courses in doses modified according to the presence of blast-cells, produced a complete remission in 4, partial remission in 2, and some haematological improvement in 4 patients; 16 died during the study and in 4 of these guanazole was a contributing factor. Significant leucopenia occurred in 35 and thrombocytopenia in 43 patients. Other side-effects included stomatitis, rash, myalgia, vomiting, and fever.— J. S. Hewlett *et al.*, *Clin. Pharmac. Ther.*, 1973, *14*, 271.

References to guanazole in the treatment of acute myeloid leukaemia: D. Yakar *et al.*, *Cancer Res.*, 1973, *33*, 972; J. A. Levi and P. H. Wiernik, *Cancer*, 1976, *38*, 36 (comparison with azacitidine).

Manufacturers

National Institutes of Health, USA.

1838-f

Hexamethylmelamine.

NSC 13875; WR 95704. 2,4,6-Tris(dimethylamino)-1,3,5-triazine. $C_9H_{18}N_6$=210.3.

CAS — 645-05-6.

M.p. about 172°. Slightly **soluble** in water; freely soluble in chloroform; soluble in ether.

Adverse Effects, Treatment, and Precautions. For an outline of the adverse effects experienced with antineoplastic agents and immunosuppressants, general guidelines for their treatment, and precautions, see Antineoplastic Agents, p.171, pp.174-5.

Neurological reactions have been reported with hexamethylmelamine.

Absorption and Fate. Variable absorption of hexamethylmelamine has been reported from the gastro-intestinal tract. It is demethylated in the body to pentamethylmelamine and other metabolites.

References: G. T. Bryan *et al.*, *Clin. Pharmac. Ther.*, 1968, *9*, 777; M. M. Ames *et al.*, *Cancer Res.*, 1979, *39*, 5016.

Uses. Hexamethylmelamine is an antineoplastic agent structurally similar to tretamine (p.229) although its mode of action may not be attributed to alkylation only. It has been given by mouth in the treatment of ovarian carcinoma and other solid tumours in doses ranging from 4 to 12 mg per kg body-weight daily.

Some references to the use of hexamethylmelamine: J. Louis *et al.*, *Clin. Pharmac. Ther.*, 1967, *8*, 55; J. G. de la Garza *et al.*, *Cancer*, 1968, *22*, 571; W. L. Wilson *et al.*, *Cancer*, 1970, *25*, 568, per *J. Am. med. Ass.*, 1970, *212*, 652; D. C. Stolinsky *et al.*, *Cancer*, 1972, *30*, 654; P. G. Dyment *et al.*, *J. clin. Pharmac.*, 1973, *13*, 111; S. S. Legha *et al.*, *Cancer*, 1976, *38*, 27; J. T. Wharton *et al.*, *Am. J. Obstet. Gynec.*, 1979, *133*, 833 (ovarian carcinoma).

For reference to the use of hexamethylmelamine in the combination chemotherapy of advanced ovarian adenocarcinoma, see Choice of Antineoplastic Agent, p.184.

Proprietary Names

Hexastat *(Bellon, Fr.)*.

1839-d

Hydroxyurea *(B.P., U.S.P.).* Hydroxycarbamide; NSC 32065; SQ 1089; WR 83799. HO.NH.CO.NH_2=76.05.

CAS — 127-07-1.

Pharmacopoeias. In *Br.* and *U.S.*

A white to off-white, odourless or almost odourless, tasteless, crystalline powder. It is hygroscopic and decomposes in the presence of moisture. M.p. above 133° with decomposition. Freely **soluble** in water and hot alcohol; slightly soluble in alcohol. **Store** in airtight containers.

Adverse Effects and Treatment. For an outline of the adverse effects experienced with antineoplastic agents and immunosuppressants and general guidelines for their treatment, see Antineoplastic Agents, p.171 and p.174.

Bone-marrow suppression, including megaloblastic changes, is the main adverse effect of hydroxyurea. The erythema caused by irradiation may be exacerbated by hydroxyurea. Other side-effects reported have included impairment of renal function, pulmonary oedema, and neurological reactions such as headache, dizziness, drowsiness, disorientation, hallucinations, and convulsions.

Precautions. For reference to the precautions necessary with antineoplastic agents and immunosuppressants, see Antineoplastic Agents, p.175.

Hydroxyurea should be used with caution in patients with impaired renal function. Patients should not drive or operate hazardous machinery if drowsiness occurs.

Absorption and Fate. Hydroxyurea is readily absorbed from the gastro-intestinal tract and distributed throughout the body. Peak plasma concentrations are reached in 2 hours and hydroxyurea is rapidly excreted in the urine; about 80% of a dose of 7 to 30 mg per kg body-weight is excreted in the urine within 12 hours.

References to pharmacokinetic studies of hydroxyurea: H. Sauer *et al.*, *Klin. Wschr.*, 1976, *54*, 203.

Uses. Hydroxyurea is an antineoplastic agent which may act by inhibition of deoxyribonucleic acid synthesis. It also has some immunosuppressant activity. Hydroxyurea is used in the treatment of chronic myeloid leukaemia though busulphan is usually preferred. It has also been used in the treatment of malignant melanoma and inoperable tumours of the ovary. Beneficial results have been obtained with radiotherapy and hydroxyurea in squamous cell carcinomas of the head and neck. See also under Choice of Antineoplastic Agent, p.183.

It is given by mouth in a single dose of 20 to 30 mg per kg body-weight daily or in a single dose of 80 mg per kg every third day.

The haemoglobin concentration, white cell and platelet counts, and hepatic and renal function should be determined repeatedly during treatment. Treatment should be interrupted if the white cell count drops to 3000 per mm^3 or the platelet count to 100 000 per mm^3.

A review of hydroxyurea and related substances.— G. Zinner, *Pharm. Ztg, Berl.*, 1978, *123*, 919, per *Int. pharm. Abstr.*, 1978, *15*, 1032.

Blood disorders, non-malignant. For a report of beneficial results with hydroxyurea in patients with corticosteroid-resistant hypereosinophilia, see Corticosteroids, p.453.

Leukaemia. Chronic myeloid leukaemia in 43 patients was treated with hydroxyurea 1.5 to 2.5 g daily followed by maintenance doses of 500 mg daily. Apparent complete remission was achieved in 1 patient and partial remission in 39. Leucophaeresis was performed in 36 patients; treatment was deliberately withdrawn in order to permit a rise in the white-cell count to about 60 000 per mm^3 as a source of donor cells for treating agranulocytosis. Eighteen patients also underwent splenectomy. Leucophaeresis was not considered to have affected the patients adversely; survival-times were comparable with those obtained by conventional treatments.— L. Schwarzenberg *et al.*, *Br. med. J.*, 1973, *1*, 700.

The results of a retrospective study in 87 patients with acute non-lymphocytic leukaemia indicated that large doses of hydroxyurea prior to combination chemotherapy were of great value in achieving a rapid lowering of the leucocyte count and reducing the hazard of cerebral haemorrhage arising from extreme leucocytosis. Doses of either 3 g per m^2 body-surface or 6 g per m^2 had been given on 2 occasions 24 hours apart and subsequent induction chemotherapy begun 4 days after the first dose of hydroxyurea.— J. Berg *et al.*, *Med. J. Aust.*, 1979, *1*, 480. See also F. M. Grund *et al.*, *Archs intern. Med.*, 1977, *137*, 1246.

See also under Choice of Antineoplastic Agent, p.180.

Malignant neoplasms. Reports on the use of hydroxyurea in the treatment of various malignant neoplasms: H. B. Nevinny and T. C. Hall, *J. clin. Pharmac.*, 1968, *8*, 352 (metastatic renal carcinoma); I. M. Ariel, *Cancer*, 1970, *25*, 705; H. Lipshutz and H. J. Lerner, *Am. J. Surg.*, 1973, *126*, 519 (with radiotherapy in carcinoma of the head and neck); H. J. Lerner and T. R. Malloy, *Urology*, 1977, *10*, 35 (with chlorotrianisene in carcinoma of the prostate); M. S. Piver *et al.*, *Am. J. Obstet. Gynec.*, 1977, *129*, 379 (as a radiation sensitiser in carcinoma of the uterine cervix).

Skin disorders, non-malignant. Sixteen patients with disabling psoriasis were treated with hydroxyurea 0.5 to 1.5 g daily for 6 to 28 weeks with continuation of their previous topical treatment; 14 had excellent or good responses. However, treatment was discontinued in 5 because of side-effects, which included anaemia in 10 patients, leucopenia in 5, hyperpigmentation in 7, fatigue (probably due to anaemia) in 7, and slight reduction in creatinine clearance in 4. There was no evidence of hepatotoxicity. It was considered that methotrexate was safer and as effective, and hydroxyurea should only be used if methotrexate had failed or was contra-indicated by liver damage.— M. G. C. Dahl and J. S. Comaish, *Br. med. J.*, 1972, *4*, 585.

Preparations

Hydroxyurea Capsules *(B.P.).* Capsules containing hydroxyurea. Store at a temperature not exceeding 30°.

Hydroxyurea Capsules *(U.S.P.).* Capsules containing hydroxyurea. Store in airtight containers.

Hydrea *(Squibb, UK).* Hydroxyurea, available as capsules of 500 mg. (Also available as Hydrea in *Austral.*, *Belg.*, *Canad.*, *Fr.*, *Ital.*, *Neth.*, *USA*).

Other Proprietary Names

Litalir *(Ger.)*; Onco-Carbide *(Spain)*.

1840-c

Ifosfamide. Iphosphamide; Isophosphamide; MJF 9325; NSC 109724; Z 4942. 3-(2-Chloroethyl)-2-(2-chloroethylamino)perhydro-1,3,2-oxazaphosphorine 2-oxide.

$C_7H_{15}Cl_2N_2O_2P$=261.1.

CAS — 3778-73-2.

For the physical properties, including stability and storage, of ifosfamide, see L. A. Trissel *et al.*, *Drug Intell. & clin. Pharm.*, 1979, *13*, 340.

Adverse Effects, Treatment, and Precautions. As for Cyclophosphamide, p.199. Toxic effects on the urinary tract may be more severe with ifosfamide. About 10% of patients are reported to experience central nervous system side-effects, especially confusion and lethargy.

For the use of mesna to reduce ifosfamide-induced bladder toxicity, See Mesna, p.651.

Absorption and Fate. The pharmacokinetics of ifosfamide are similar to those of cyclophosphamide (p.200). Ifosfamide must be metabolised in the liver before it is active.

References to the absorption and fate of ifosfamide: P. J. Creaven *et al.*, *Clin. Pharmac. Ther.*, 1974, *16*, 77; L. M. Allen and P. J. Creaven, *Clin. Pharmac. Ther.*, 1975, *17*, 492; L. M. Allen *et al.*, *Cancer Treat. Rep.*, 1976, *60*, 451; R. L. Nelson *et al.*, *Clin. Pharmac. Ther.*, 1976, *19*, 365.

Uses. Ifosfamide is used similarly to cyclophosphamide (p.200) in the treatment of malignant diseases.

Ifosfamide is given intravenously in courses of single daily doses over 3 to 10 days to a total dose for each course of 8 to 10 g per m^2 body-surface. Courses may be repeated after 2 to 4 weeks, depending on the blood count. Large single doses are reported to be less effective and more toxic than when the same dose is given over several days. Before injection, solutions are diluted to less than 4% and injected directly into the vein; alternatively ifosfamide may be infused in dextrose and sodium chloride over 30 minutes to 2 hours.

References to the use of ifosfamide: V. Rodriguez *et al.*, *Cancer Res.*, 1976, *36*, 2945 (dose fractionation); J. Schnitker *et al.*, *Arzneimittel-Forsch.*, 1976, *26*, 1783; R. E. Rentschler *et al.*, *Cancer Res.*, 1978, *38*, 2209; C. G. Schmidt and R. Becher, *Dt. med. Wschr.*, 1979, *104*, 872 (melanoblastoma).

Proprietary Preparations

Mitoxana *(WB Pharmaceuticals, UK: Boehringer Ingelheim, UK).* Ifosfamide, available as powder for preparing injections, in vials of 0.5, 1, or 2 g. Store below 30°. Protect from light.

Solutions for injection, prepared by dissolving ifosfamide in Water for Injections, should be used within 2 hours of preparation.

Other Proprietary Names

Holoxan *(Fr., Ger., Neth.)*.

1841-k

Lomustine. CCNU; NSC 79037; RB 1509; WR 139017. 1-(2-Chloroethyl)-3-cyclohexyl-1-nitrosourea.

$C_9H_{16}ClN_3O_2$=233.7.

CAS — 13010-47-4.

A yellow crystalline powder. M.p. about 89°. Practically **insoluble** in water; soluble in alcohol. Solutions in alcohol are stable for 7 days at 0°.

A vehicle for lomustine consisting of 10% alcohol and 5% polyethoxylated vegetable oil (Emulphor EL620) in saline solution was found to be suitable for intravenous administration in *rabbits*. The distribution with this vehicle was similar to that with an alcohol-propylene glycol (1:4) and an alcohol-fat emulsion vehicle.— C. L. Litterst *et al.*, *J. pharm. Sci.*, 1974, *63*, 1718.

Adverse Effects, Treatment, and Precautions. As for Carmustine, p.195, although bone-marrow depression may be even more delayed with lomustine. Neurological reactions such as confusion and lethargy have been reported.

Interactions. Theophylline. Leucopenia and thrombocytopenia in a 45-year-old woman are believed to have been secondary to an interaction between theophylline and lomustine.— P. M. Zeltzer and S. A. Feig (letter), *Lancet*, 1979, *2*, 960.

Absorption and Fate. Lomustine is absorbed from the gastro-intestinal tract and is rapidly metabolised; metabolites have a prolonged plasma half-life reported to range from 16 to 48 hours. Active metabolites readily appear in the cerebrospinal fluid. About half a dose is excreted as metabolites in the urine within 24 hours but less than 75% is excreted within 4 days. About 60% of the cyclohexyl moiety of lomustine is reported to be bound to plasma proteins.

Uses. Lomustine is a nitrosourea with actions and uses similar to those of carmustine (p.195). It has been used in the treatment of brain tumours and Hodgkin's disease, and also lung cancer, malignant melanoma, and various solid tumours.

Lomustine is given by mouth to adults and children as a single dose of 130 mg per m^2 body-surface. A dose of 100 mg per m^2 should be given to patients with compromised bone-marrow function. Providing blood counts have returned to acceptable levels, that is, platelets above 100 000 per mm^3 and leucocytes above 4000 per mm^3, doses may be repeated every 6 weeks.

A brief review of lomustine.— *Med. Lett.*, 1976, *18*, 102.

Reports of treatment with lomustine: A. B. Cruz *et al.*,

Cancer, 1976, *38*, 1069, per *J. Am. med. Ass.*, 1977, *237*, 75.

Hodgkin's disease. The Acute Leukaemia Group B demonstrated that lomustine was superior to carmustine in the treatment of Hodgkin's disease resistant to alkylating agents, vinca alkaloids, procarbazine, and prednisolone.— S. K. Carter and M. A. Goldsmith (letter), *Lancet*, 1973, *1*, 264.

Malignant neoplasms of the brain. References to the use of lomustine in patients with malignant brain tumours: M. L. Rosenblum *et al.*, *J. Neurosurg.*, 1973, *39*, 306; H. W. C. Ward (letter), *Br. med. J.*, 1974, *1*, 642 (children with medulloblastoma); F. H. Hochberg *et al.*, *J. Am. med. Ass.*, 1979, *241*, 1016.

Malignant neoplasms of the bronchus and lung. References to the use of lomustine: H. Takita and A. Brugarolas, *J. natn. Cancer Inst.*, 1973, *50*, 49; G. J. Vosika, *J. Am. med. Ass.*, 1979, *241*, 594 (prolonged survival in a patient with large cell carcinoma of the lung).

Malignant neoplasms of the kidney. Lomustine produced an objective remission lasting from 3 to 6 months in 4 of 20 patients with renal cell carcinoma.— A. Mittelman *et al.*, *J. Am. med. Ass.*, 1973, *225*, 32.

Skin disorders. A report of the topical use of lomustine in the treatment of psoriasis.— G. L. Peck *et al.*, *Archs Derm.*, 1972, *106*, 172.

Proprietary Preparations

CCNU Lundbeck *(Lundbeck, UK)*. Lomustine, available as capsules of 40 mg. Store in airtight containers. Protect from light.

CeeNU *(Bristol-Myers Pharmaceuticals, UK)*. Lomustine, available as capsules of 10, 40, and 100 mg. (Also available as CeeNU in *Canad.*, *USA*).

Other Proprietary Names

Belustine *(Fr., Ital.)*; Cecenu *(Belg., Neth.)*; Lucostine *(Denm., Swed.)*.

1842-a

Mannomustine Hydrochloride *(B.P.C. 1973)*. BCM; Mannitol Mustard. 1,6-Bis(2-chloroethylamino)-1,6-dideoxy-D-mannitol dihydrochloride.

$C_{10}H_{22}Cl_2N_2O_4,2HCl = 378.1$.

CAS — 576-68-1 (mannomustine); 551-74-6 (hydrochloride).

A white, odourless or almost odourless, crystalline powder. M.p. 241°, with decomposition. **Soluble** 1 in 2 of water; slightly soluble in alcohol; practically insoluble in dehydrated alcohol, chloroform, and ether. A 2.5% solution in water has a pH of 2 to 3.5.

Uses. Mannomustine is an antineoplastic agent with the general properties of Mustine, p.222. It has been used in the treatment of various malignant diseases but other alkylating agents such as cyclophosphamide are preferred.

Mannomustine hydrochloride has been administered by intravenous injection in doses of 50 to 100 mg daily or on alternate days, as a 0.5 to 1% solution in sodium chloride injection; it has also been given as an intravenous infusion in doses of 100 to 200 mg in 1 or 2 litres of fluid on alternate days. Total doses of up to 2 g have been given over 24 hours.

Mannomustine hydrochloride has also been given by mouth, in maintenance doses of 100 to 150 mg weekly; these are discontinued if the white cell count falls below 3000 per mm^3.

Frequent blood counts are essential during therapy and for up to 6 weeks after its cessation.

Preparations

Mannomustine Injection *(B.P.C. 1973)*. Mannomustine Hydrochloride Injection. A sterile solution of mannomustine hydrochloride prepared by dissolving, shortly before use, the sterile contents of a sealed container in sodium chloride injection. The injection deteriorates on storage and it must be used within 24 hours of preparation.

Proprietary Names

Degranol *(Landerlan, Spain)*.

Mannomustine hydrochloride was formerly marketed in Great Britain under the proprietary name Degranol *(Sinclair)*.

1843-t

Melphalan *(B.P., U.S.P.)*. Phenylalanine Nitrogen Mustard; CB 3025; NSC 8806; PAM; WR 19813. 4-Bis(2-chloroethyl)amino-L-phenylalanine.

$C_{13}H_{18}Cl_2N_2O_2 = 305.2$.

CAS — 148-82-3.

NOTE. Merphalan (CB 3007; NSC 14210) is the racemic form of melphalan; Medphalan (CB 3026; NSC 35051) is the D-isomer of melphalan.

Pharmacopoeias. In *Br.* and *U.S.* Sarcolysini Hydrochloridum (*Int. P.*) and Sarcolysinum (*Rus. P.*) are the hydrochlorides of merphalan. *Chin. P.* includes Betamerphalanum, Formylmerphalanum, and Methoxymerphalanum.

A white to buff-coloured powder, odourless or with a faint odour. M.p. about 177° to 180°, with decomposition. It loses not more than 7% of its weight on drying.

Practically **insoluble** in water, chloroform, and ether; slightly soluble in alcohol; soluble in dilute mineral acids; soluble 1 in 150 of methyl alcohol. A solution in methyl alcohol is laevorotatory. **Store** at a temperature not exceeding 25° in airtight containers. Protect from light.

Stability in solution. Melphalan had a half-life of 12.5 hours in physiological saline at 20° and of 1.8 hours at 37°.— F. E. Weale, *Lancet*, 1964, *1*, 23.

Melphalan 30 µg per ml was completely hydrolysed in aqueous solution at 37° after 8 hours. The presence of bovine serum albumin reduced the rate of hydrolysis. It was suggested that solutions for parenteral administration should be prepared immediately prior to use and kept cold or prepared from diluent containing albumin.— S. Y. Chang *et al.*, *J. pharm. Sci.*, 1978, *67*, 682.

Further references: D. E. Pegg *et al.* (letter), *Lancet*, 1964, *1*, 332; S. Y. Chang *et al.*, *J. Pharm. Pharmac.*, 1979, *31*, 853.

Adverse Effects and Treatment. For an outline of the adverse effects experienced with antineoplastic agents and immunosuppressants and general guidelines for their treatment, see Antineoplastic Agents, p.171 and p.174.

The onset of neutropenia and thrombocytopenia is variable; maximum bone-marrow depression has been reported 2 to 3 weeks after starting treatment with melphalan but has also occurred after only 5 days. Recovery may be prolonged.

Adverse effects resulting from regional perfusion include oedema, neurotoxicity, and vesiculation of the skin.

Allergy and anaphylaxis. Reports of allergic reactions associated with melphalan: M. W. Skehan and A. M. Bernath (letter), *J. Am. med. Ass.*, 1978, *240*, 2733 (vasculitis); G. G. Cornwell *et al.*, *Cancer Treat. Rep.*, 1979, *63*, 399.

Effects on respiratory function. Although pulmonary toxicity with melphalan seems rare it may sometimes have gone unrecognised.— R. B. Weiss and F. M. Muggia, *Am. J. Med.*, 1980, *68*, 259.

Reports of pulmonary toxicity with melphalan.— P. P. Major *et al.*, *Can. med. Ass. J.*, 1980, *123*, 197 (interstitial pneumonitis and lung fibrosis); B. T. Westerfield *et al.*, *Am. J. Med.*, 1980, *68*, 767.

Precautions. For reference to the precautions necessary with antineoplastic agents and immunosuppressants, see Antineoplastic Agents, p.175.

When melphalan is given to patients with impaired renal function, urea concentrations should be monitored.

Interference with diagnostic tests. Melphalan could produce a false positive response to the Coombs' test.— P. D. Hansten, *Am. J. Hosp. Pharm.*, 1971, *28*, 629.

Absorption and Fate. Absorption of melphalan from the gastro-intestinal tract is reported to be variable.

In a study involving 9 cancer patients, melphalan rapidly disappeared from the plasma after the intravenous injection of 600 µg per kg body-weight. Composite plasma α-half-life was 7.7 minutes and β-half-life was 107.6 minutes. The mean 24-hour urinary excretion of melphalan was 13% of the administered dose. The results differ from those reported by M.H.N. Tattersall *et al.* (*Eur. J. Cancer*, 1978, *14*, 507). In 2 patients given labelled melphalan, monohydroxy and dihydroxy melphalan products made up a large portion of the drug found in plasma and urine samples up to 24 hours after administration.— D. S. Alberts *et al.*, *Clin. Pharmac. Ther.*, 1979, *26*, 73. A further study in 14 cancer patients given single doses of 600 µg per kg by mouth or intravenously. The systemic availability of melphalan given as tablets or oral solution was extremely variable, the first appearance in plasma ranging from a few minutes to 6 hours after a dose. In one patient melphalan did not appear in the plasma or urine. Monohydroxy and dihydroxy derivatives were detected in the plasma within 30 minutes of an oral dose. Spontaneous degradation rather than enzymatic metabolism may be the major determinant of plasma half-life. The mean plasma terminal phase half-life for 12 patients given melphalan by mouth was 90 minutes and mean 24-hour urinary excretion was 10.9% of the total dose; the mean peak plasma concentration was 280 ng per ml (range 70 to 630 ng per ml). In 5 of the patients half-lives after administration of melphalan by mouth were similar to those achieved after intravenous injection but the mean area under the plasma concentration time curve was less than 60% of that after an intravenous dose; 24-hour urinary excretion was 28% of the oral dose and 56.4% of the intravenous dose. It is considered that variability in the bioavailability of oral melphalan might help to explain the variability in response to treatment and, if there is no evidence of myelosuppression or antitumour effect after increased dosage, melphalan should be given intravenously or replaced by another alkylating agent.— D. S. Alberts *et al.*, *Clin. Pharmac. Ther.*, 1979, *26*, 737.

Further references: S. Y. Chang *et al.*, *J. pharm. Sci.*, 1978, *67*, 679; S. Y. Chang *et al.*, *J. pharm. Sci.*, 1978, *67*, 682 (peak plasma concentration of about 1 µg per ml after intravenous bolus injection of melphalan 600 µg per kg); D. W. Hedley *et al.*, *Lancet*, 1978, *2*, 966 (a concentration of melphalan in CSF only about one-tenth of that in blood, after an intravenous dose).

Uses. Melphalan is an antineoplastic agent derived from mustine (p.222) and has a similar mode of action. It is used mainly in the treatment of multiple myeloma. Melphalan is also given to patients with carcinoma of the breast and ovary and has been administered by intra-arterial regional perfusion for malignant melanoma and soft-tissue sarcomas. It has immunosuppressant properties and has been used in the treatment of auto-immune disorders. Melphalan is usually given by mouth; it is also administered intravenously.

See also under Choice of Antineoplastic Agent, p.175.

Suggested doses for the treatment of multiple myeloma depend on whether continuous or intermittent therapy is used. Numerous regimens have been tried and there is still controversy as to the best schedule. Examples of oral dosage regimens for melphalan are: 150 µg per kg body-weight daily for 7 days followed by a rest period of about 3 weeks and continuing witl. maintenance doses of 50 µg per kg daily or less, when the leucocyte and platelet counts are rising; or 250 µg per kg daily for 4 consecutive days and repeated after a rest period of up to 6 weeks or followed by maintenance doses of 2 to 4 mg daily; or melphalan 150 µg per kg daily and prednisone 40 mg daily, both given for 4 days and repeated every 6 weeks.

In the treatment of breast cancer, suggested doses of melphalan are 200 to 300 µg per kg daily or 6 mg per m^2 body-surface daily for 4 to 6 days, repeated every 3 to 6 weeks.

Melphalan should not be given if the platelet counts falls below 75 000 per mm^3 or the neutrophil count below 2000 per mm^3. During administration of melphalan, frequent blood counts are essential, especially during continuous administration. It should not be given with radiotherapy or if the neutrophil count has recently been depressed by chemotherapy or radiotherapy.

Melphalan is also given intravenously as a single dose of 1 mg per kg, repeated in 8 weeks if the platelet and neutrophil counts are normal. It may be infused in sodium chloride injection over not more than 8 hours or injected into the tubing of a fast-running drip. The intra-arterial perfusion method of administration involves giving a dose of 70 to 100 mg to the part of the body affected by the tumour, isolated from the rest of the body. In some patients it may be possible to repeat this dose twice.

Acceleration of bone-marrow recovery. For reference to the accelerating effect of cyclophosphamide priming on bone-marrow recovery following high doses of melphalan, see Cyclophosphamide, p.200.

Administration in renal insufficiency. Melphalan may be given in normal doses to patients with renal failure.— W. M. Bennett *et al.*, *Ann. intern. Med.*, 1980, *93*, 286. But see Precautions (above).

Amyloidosis. A discussion on the treatment of primary amyloidosis with reference to the use of melphalan.— *Lancet*, 1978, *2*, 1187.

Individual reports of the control of primary amyloidosis: N. F. Jones *et al.*, *Lancet*, 1972, *2*, 616 (melphalan 2 mg daily); H. J. Cohen *et al.*, *Ann. intern. Med.*, 1975, *82*, 466 (remission of severe nephrotic syndrome, attributed to primary amyloidosis, maintained with melphalan 6 mg weekly and prednisone and fluoxymesterone daily); J. Corkery *et al.* (letter), *Lancet*, 1978, *2*, 425 (melphalan, penicillamine, and prednisone).

Blood disorders, non-malignant. *Polycythaemia vera.* References to the use of melphalan in the treatment of polycythaemia vera: S. I. de Vries, *Ned. Tijdschr. Geneesk.*, 1973, *117*, 331, per *J. Am. med. Ass.*, 1973, *224*, 1211; J. Horowitz and N. Mani, *Harefuah*, 1974, *87*, 351.

Gastro-intestinal disorders, non-malignant. Remission of symptoms of alpha-chain disease accompanied by gains in weight were achieved in 2 patients given melphalan, 10 mg daily for 1 week every 6 weeks. For 1 patient prednisone 40 mg daily was also given intermittently and the other patient received tetracycline 500 mg twice daily.— W. F. Doe *et al.*, *Gut*, 1972, *13*, 947.

A 62-year-old man with malabsorption syndrome and steatorrhoea with IgG(λ)M components in the blood and IgG deposits in the intestinal wall responded well to treatment with courses of melphalan and prednisone given for 4 days a month for 6 months, and repeated as required.— E. J. Prokipchuk and W. Pruzanski, *Can. med. Ass. J.*, 1976, *114*, 922.

Lupus erythematosus. A report of melphalan and methotrexate in the treatment of systemic lupus erythematosus.— F. Clément, *Schweiz. med. Wschr.*, 1973, *103*, 1369.

Melanoma. A group of 150 patients with melanoma of the limbs were treated with cytotoxic drugs and examined periodically for a year. The drugs most frequently employed for regional perfusion in conjunction with a tourniquet were melphalan and thiotepa. The usual total dosage for a leg was 60 mg of melphalan and 25 mg of thiotepa or 75 mg and 35 mg respectively. The usual total dosage for an arm was 45 mg of melphalan and 15 mg of thiotepa or 60 mg and 25 mg respectively. Tumours were eradicated in 64 patients, with or without excision, but in 17 there was no effect. The other 69 patients died and in 61 of these death was due to progression of the melanoma. Complications were related to wound healing. Toxic effects included leucopenia and thrombocytopenia in 17 patients, oedema in 12, and neurotoxicity in 12.— O. Creech and E. T. Krementz, *J. Am. med. Ass.*, 1964, *188*, 855.

Further references to the regional perfusion of melphalan in malignant melanoma: J. S. Stehlin *et al.*, *Surgery Gynec. Obstet.*, 1975, *140*, 339 (hyperthermic perfusion); P. C. Weaver *et al.*, *Clin. Oncol.*, 1975, *1*, 45; E. V. Sugarbaker and C. M. McBride, *Cancer*, 1976, *37*, 188; J. A. Hansson *et al.*, *Acta chir. scand.*, 1977, *143*, 33; H. S. Koops *et al.*, *Am. J. Surg.*, 1977, *133*, 221.

See also under Choice of Antineoplastic Agent, p.185.

Myeloma. Reports and studies of melphalan in the treatment of multiple myeloma: R. Alexanian *et al.*, *J. Am. med. Ass.*, 1969, *208*, 1680 (melphalan and prednisone); L. H. Rodriguez *et al.*, *Ann. intern. Med.*, 1972, *76*, 551; J. Brook *et al.*, *Archs intern. Med.*, 1973, *131*, 545; G. Costa *et al.*, *Am. J. Med.*, 1973, *54*, 589 (melphalan and prednisone); Southwest Oncology Group Study, *Archs intern. Med.*, 1975, *135*, 147 (an evaluation of various schedules); Southeastern Cancer Study Group, *Archs intern. Med.*, 1975, *135*, 157; M. Yalon *et al.*, *Harefuah*, 1977, *92*, 296 (intermittent low-dose melphalan and prednisone); R. Alexanian *et al.*, *Blood*, 1978, *51*, 1005; A. D. Mehta, *Br. J. clin. Pract.*, 1978, *32*, 358.

A brief review of acute leukaemia associated with melphalan, especially when used in multiple myeloma. Since the Southwest Oncology Study Group had reported that continuing therapy for myeloma beyond 1 year with a schedule incorporating melphalan was of no major value, maintenance with melphalan could be abandoned or reduced in duration.— S. M. Sieber and R. H. Adamson (letter), *Br. med. J.*, 1975, *2*, 557.

See also under Choice of Antineoplastic Agent, p.185.

Preparations

Melphalan Injection *(B.P.)*. A sterile solution of melphalan hydrochloride prepared immediately before use by completely dissolving the contents of a sealed container (Melphalan for Injection) containing melphalan in the required amount of alcohol (96%) containing 2% of hydrogen chloride, and diluting the resulting solution with the requisite amount of a solution containing potassium phosphate 1.2% dissolved in a solution of propylene glycol 60% v/v in Water for Injections. A 1% injection has a pH of 6 to 7. It deteriorates on storage. Potency is expressed in terms of the equivalent amount of anhydrous melphalan.

Melphalan Tablets *(B.P.)*. Compression-coated or film-coated tablets containing melphalan. Store at a temperature not exeeding 25°.

Melphalan Tablets *(U.S.P.)*. Tablets containing melphalan. Protect from light.

Proprietary Preparations

Alkeran *(Wellcome, UK)*. Melphalan, available as **Tablets** of 2 and 5 mg, and as **Injection** in vials each containing the equivalent of 100 mg of anhydrous melphalan, supplied with 1-ml ampoules of sterile solvent and 9-ml ampoules of sterile diluent. The pH of the final solution is about 7; it should be injected within 15 to 30 minutes of preparation. (Also available as Alkeran in *Austral., Belg., Canad., Denm., Fr., Ger., Ital., Neth., Norw., Swed., Switz., USA*).

Other Proprietary Names

Alkerana *(Arg.)*.

1844-x

Mercaptopurine *(B.P., U.S.P.)*.

Mercaptopur.; Mercaptopurinum; 6MP; NSC 755; WR 2785. 6-Mercaptopurine monohydrate; Purine-6-thiol monohydrate.

$C_5H_4N_4S,H_2O$=170.2.

CAS — 6112-76-1; 50-44-2 (anhydrous).

Pharmacopoeias. In *Br., Cz., Int., Jap., Jug., Nord., Rus., Turk.*, and *U.S.*

A yellow, odourless or almost odourless, almost tasteless, crystalline powder. M.p. above 308°, with decomposition. It darkens on exposure to air and light.

Practically **insoluble** in water, acetone, chloroform, and ether; soluble 1 in 950 of alcohol; soluble in hot alcohol and in solutions of alkali hydroxides; slightly soluble in M sulphuric acid. **Store** in airtight containers. Protect from light.

A 1% solution of mercaptopurine sodium in Water for Injections is reported to have a pH of 10 to 11.

Mercaptopurine underwent dehydration at about 125°.— S. Niazi, *J. pharm. Sci.*, 1978, *67*, 488.

Stability in solution. When reconstituted with water, 500 mg to 50 ml, then diluted to 150 ml with dextrose injection or sodium chloride injection, mercaptopurine, as the sodium salt, was stable for up to 7 days at 5°.— J. F. Gallelli, *Am. J. Hosp. Pharm.*, 1967, *24*, 425.

Adverse Effects and Treatment. For an outline of the adverse effects experienced with antineoplastic agents and immunosuppressants and general guidelines for their treatment, see Antineoplastic Agents, p.171 and p.174.

Bone-marrow depression with mercaptopurine may be delayed; hypoplasia may occur. Mercaptopurine is less toxic to the gastro-intestinal tract than the folic acid antagonists. Jaundice and hepatotoxicity have been reported. Crystalluria with haematuria has been observed rarely.

Effects on respiratory function. See Antineoplastic Agents, p.174.

Effects on the skin. Pellagra reported in patients receiving treatment with mercaptopurine could have occurred because of inhibition of endogenous nadide synthesis.— J. D. Stratigos and A. Katsambas, *Br. J. Derm.*, 1977, *96*, 99.

Effects on the vascular system. Portal hypertension, with oesophageal varices and severe haematemesis, was associated with mercaptopurine 50 mg daily in a 6-year-old girl.— A. D. Lascari *et al.*, *New Engl. J. Med.*, 1968, *279*, 303.

Precautions. For reference to the precautions necessary with antineoplastic agents and immunosuppressants, see Antineoplastic Agents, p.175.

Mercaptopurine should be used with care in patients with hepatic or renal damage or biliary stasis. The effects of mercaptopurine are enhanced by allopurinol and the dose of mercaptopurine should be reduced to about one-quarter when allopurinol is given concomitantly.

Interactions. *Allopurinol.* In a study of the effect of allopurinol in patients receiving mercaptopurine, the production of 6-thiouric acid was almost completely inhibited but the pharmacokinetics of mercaptopurine did not appear to have been altered.— J. J. Coffey *et al.*, *Cancer Res.*, 1972, *32*, 1283.

Anticoagulants. For a report of mercaptopurine diminishing the activity of warfarin, see Warfarin Sodium, p.777.

Pregnancy and the neonate. *First trimester.* When given mercaptopurine during pregnancy, 7 women produced normal infants and so did 3 women on busulphan, but 1 woman given both mercaptopurine and busulphan in the first trimester produced an infant with multiple deformities.— J. Sokal and E. Lessmann, *J. Am. med. Ass.*, 1960, *172*, 1765. A woman who was receiving treatment with mercaptopurine, 50 mg twice daily for acute myeloblastic leukaemia, became pregnant and while continuing treatment with mercaptopurine and prednisone gave birth at 32 weeks to an infant with no malformations but with an abnormal blood picture similar to microangiopathic haemolytic anaemia. This gradually improved and he made good progress.— J. B. McConnell and R. Bhoola, *Postgrad. med. J.*, 1973, *49*, 211.

Absorption and Fate. Mercaptopurine is readily absorbed from the gastro-intestinal tract. It is distributed throughout the body water and diffuses into the cerebrospinal fluid though not in therapeutic concentrations. Plasma half-lives ranging from about 10 to 90 minutes have been reported after intravenous injection. Mercaptopurine is activated in the body by intracellular conversion to nucleotide forms. It is rapidly and extensively degraded in the liver to a variety of oxidised and methylated products including 6-thiouric acid, sulphates, and other metabolites; xanthine oxidase plays an important role in this catabolism. After the oral or intravenous administration of mercaptopurine metabolites are excreted rapidly in the urine. About half of an oral dose has been recovered in the urine within 24 hours, up to 8% as unchanged mercaptopurine. A small proportion is excreted for up to 17 days.

Studies on the absorption, distribution, metabolism, and excretion of mercaptopurine in children and adults.— T. L. Loo *et al.*, *Clin. Pharmac. Ther.*, 1968, *9*, 180.

Rapid degradation *in vivo* and acquired resistance are two major obstacles to the successful use of mercaptopurine. Its derivative, azathioprine, is slowly metabolised to mercaptopurine.— W. J. Cook and C. E. Bugg, *J. pharm. Sci.*, 1975, *64*, 221.

Uses. Mercaptopurine is an antineoplastic agent which acts as an antimetabolite (p.171). It is an analogue of the natural purines, hypoxanthine and adenine. After the intracellular conversion of mercaptopurine to active nucleotides, including thioinosinic acid, it interferes with nucleic acid synthesis. It also has immunosuppressant properties.

Mercaptopurine is used, usually with other agents, in the treatment of leukaemia. It induces remissions in acute lymphoblastic and myeloblastic leukaemias but other agents are generally preferred and mercaptopurine is chiefly employed in maintenance programmes. It may also be effective in chronic myeloid leukaemia. For details of treatment schedules, see Choice of

Antineoplastic Agent, p.178. There is cross-resistance between mercaptopurine and thioguanine (p.228). Mercaptopurine is administered by mouth. The usual initial dose for children and adults is 2.5 mg per kg body-weight daily but the dosage varies according to individual response and tolerance. In maintenance schedules the dose may vary from 50 to 90 mg per m^2 body-surface daily. If there is no clinical improvement and no evidence of white cell depression after 4 weeks, the dose may be cautiously increased up to 5 mg per kg daily. Blood counts should be taken at least once a week and if there is a steep fall in the white cell count or severe bone-marrow depression the drug should be withdrawn immediately. Therapy may be resumed carefully if the white cell count remains constant for 2 or 3 days or rises.

It has been administered intravenously as mercaptopurine sodium.

Administration. Crystalluria and haematuria were noted in a group of children who were receiving mercaptopurine in high doses (500 to 1250 mg per m^2 body-surface). It was suggested that by prolonging the period of administration over 4 to 5 hours and by maintaining a urine flow of more than 300 ml per hour, high doses of the drug could be administered without crystalluria from the unchanged drug.— M. J. Duttera *et al.*, *New Engl. J. Med.*, 1972, *287*, 292.

Administration in hepatic insufficiency. Side-effects which occurred in 8 patients with active chronic hepatitis who were treated with mercaptopurine in daily doses of from 50 to 125 mg included anaemia, hepatic coma, jaundice, leucopenia, and thrombocytopenia. Hepatic coma and jaundice occurred in 4 and 6 patients respectively after only 2 to 3 weeks' treatment. It was suggested that the initial dose in chronic hepatitis should be 25 mg daily increased by small increments if no toxic effects occurred.— W. P. Fung and S. P. Mistilis, *Gut*, 1967, *8*, 198.

Gastro-intestinal disorders, non-malignant. *Crohn's disease.* The results of a 2-year randomised double-blind crossover study indicated that mercaptopurine was more effective than placebo in the treatment of patients with chronic Crohn's disease in whom conventional treatment had failed. The mean initial dose of mercaptopurine was 1.5 mg per kg body-weight, subsequently adjusted according to blood counts. The crossover study was completed by 39 patients and of those who improved 26 (67%) had been taking mercaptopurine during their better year and 3 (8%) had been taking placebo. Mercaptopurine was also more effective than placebo in the 33 patients who completed 2 full years of the study without crossover and was more effective in closing fistulas. Treatment with corticosteroids could be discontinued or reduced and clinical improvement maintained in 28 of 44 patients (64%) during mercaptopurine therapy compared with only 6 of 39 patients (15%) during placebo therapy. The onset of improvement with mercaptopurine was often delayed; the mean time of response was 3.1 months with a range of 2 weeks to 9 months. Treatment with mercaptopurine was stopped in 7 of 68 patients because of reversible adverse effects; the majority of patients had mild leucopenia at some time but only 2 had substantial bone-marrow depression.— D. H. Present *et al.*, *New Engl. J. Med.*, 1980, *302*, 981. Correction.— *ibid.*, *303*, 537. Comment.— M. H. Sleisenger, *ibid.*, 1024.

See also under Azathioprine, p.191.

Ulcerative colitis. References to mercaptopurine in the treatment of ulcerative colitis: R. H. D. Bean, *Br. med. J.*, 1966, *1*, 1081; B. I. Korelitz *et al.*, *Am. J. dig. Dis.*, 1973, *18*, 317.

Hepatic disorders, non-malignant. The value of mercaptopurine in the treatment of chronic hepatitis and chronic ulcerative colitis was controversial; it should not be used except under rigid control.— *J. Am. med. Ass.*, 1969, *207*, 1617. Treatment with mercaptopurine had a beneficial effect on 30 patients with chronic active hepatitis who had no signs of cirrhosis. Ten patients with cirrhosis had no response to this treatment.— L. Demeulenaere and L. Van Waes (letter), *Lancet*, 1973, *1*, 1124.

See also under Administration in Hepatic Insufficiency (above).

Immunosuppression. Mercaptopurine has generally been replaced by azathioprine (p.190) in the treatment of immune disorders.

References to the use of mercaptopurine as an immunosuppressant in various disorders: K. Lorenz, *Arch. Kinderheilk.*, 1966, *175*, 8 (rheumatoid arthritis); M. H. N. Tattersall, *Br. med. J.*, 1967, *3*, 93 (thrombocytopenic purpura); J. F. Maher, *Br. med. J.*, 1970, *2*, 645 (nephrotic syndrome); J. Baum *et al.*, *Arthritis Rheum.*, 1973, *16*, 139 (psoriatic arthritis).

See also under Gastro-intestinal Disorders and Hepatic Disorders, above.

Leukaemia. For a report of beneficial results and reduced side-effects using mercaptopurine in association with busulphan to treat chronic granulocytic leukaemia, see Busulphan, p.194.

See also under Choice of Antineoplastic Agent, p.178.

Pregnancy and the neonate. *First trimester.* See Precautions, above.

Second trimester. An apparently normal infant girl was born to a woman in whom acute leukaemia was diagnosed when she was 16 weeks pregnant, and who was treated with a regimen including mercaptopurine.— M. Khurshid and M. Saleem (letter), *Lancet*, 1978, *2*, 534.

Preparations

Mercaptopurine Tablets *(B.P.)*. Tablets containing mercaptopurine. Protect from light.

Mercaptopurine Tablets *(U.S.P.)*. Tablets containing mercaptopurine.

Puri-Nethol *(Wellcome, UK)*. Mercaptopurine, available as scored tablets of 50 mg. (Also available as Puri-Nethol in *Austral., Belg., Canad., Denm., Fr., Ger., Ital., Neth., Norw., S.Afr., Switz., USA*).

1845-r

Methotrexate *(B.P., Eur. P., U.S.P.)*.

Methotrexatum; Amethopterin; α-Methopterin; NSC 740; WR 19039; 4-Amino-10-methylfolic Acid; 4-Amino-10-methylpteroyl-L-glutamic Acid. *N*-{4-[(2,4-Diaminopteridin-6-ylmethyl)methylamino]benzoyl}-L(+)-glutamic acid.

$C_{20}H_{22}N_8O_5$=454.4.

CAS — 59-05-2.

Pharmacopoeias. In *Br., Braz., Chin., Eur., Fr., Ger., It., Jap., Neth.*, and *U.S.*

A mixture of 4-amino-10-methylfolic acid and related substances. The *B.P.* and *Eur. P.* specify not less than 85% of $C_{20}H_{22}N_8O_5$, calculated on the anhydrous basis, and not more than 8% loss on drying; the *U.S.P.* specifies not less than 94% of $C_{20}H_{22}N_8O_5$, calculated on the anhydrous basis , and not more than 12% loss on drying. A yellow to orange-brown crystalline powder. M.p. 182° to 189°.

Practically **insoluble** in water, alcohol, chloroform, and ether; very soluble in dilute solutions of alkali hydroxides and carbonates; slightly soluble in 6M hydrochloric acid. Solutions are **sterilised** by filtration. **Store** in airtight containers. Protect from light.

CAUTION. *Methotrexate is irritant; avoid contact with skin and mucous membranes.*

The pH and osmolarity of solutions of methotrexate and cytarabine for intrathecal administration made with an artifical spinal fluid (Elliott's B solution) were closer to the physiological normal than those made with Sodium Chloride Injection *U.S.P.* or Bacteriostatic Water for Injection *U.S.P.*— M. J. Duttera *et al.* (letter), *Lancet*, 1972, *1*, 540.

Incompatibility. The u.v. spectra of fluorouracil and methotrexate were altered, suggesting incompatibility, when dilute solutions in dextrose injection were mixed. The spectrum of methotrexate sodium was slightly altered when a dilute solution in dextrose injection was mixed with a solution of cytarabine; the spectrum of cytarabine was not affected.— M. P. McRae and J. C. King, *Am. J. Hosp. Pharm.*, 1976, *33*, 1010. A suggestion that the alteration of the u.v. absorption spectra was only pH dependent and therefore did not indicate true incompatibility.— R. A. Morrison *et al.* (letter), *ibid.*, 1978, *35*, 15. It is nevertheless inadvisable to mix fluorouracil and methotrexate.— J. C. King (letter), *ibid.*, 18.

Purity. A report on the separation and identification of impurities in parenteral methotrexate preparations.— C. E. Hignite *et al.*, *Cancer Treat. Rep.*, 1978, *62*, 13.

Stability in solution. Methotrexate 2.5 mg per ml was stable for 7 days at room temperature and at 30° in Elliott's B solution, sodium chloride injection, or lactated Ringer's injection.— J. C. Cradock *et al.*, *Am. J. Hosp. Pharm.*, 1978, *35*, 402.

The stability of methotrexate at a concentration of 750 µg per ml was determined in an intravenous preparation containing dextrose 5% with sodium bicarbonate 0.05 mmol (0.05 mEq) per ml. When stored at 4° to 5° and protected from light there was a mean decrease in the methotrexate concentration of 1.4% after 72 hours, and 6.1% after one week. The mean decrease in methotrexate concentrations in the preparations stored at room temperature and exposed to light were 6.2 and 14.9% respectively, while the mean decrease in 24 hours was 4.2%.— A. Humphreys *et al.*, *Aust. J. Hosp. Pharm.*, 1978, *8*, 66.

There were no significant differences in the potency of methotrexate or the pH values of solutions, measured over a 30-hour period at 20° and 28°, when methotrexate was added to sodium chloride injection in plastic packs (Polyfusor, *Boots*; Viaflex, *Travenol*) or glass bottles. Leaching of plasticiser or similar compounds was not observed.— M. Roach (letter), *Pharm. J.*, 1979, *2*, 557.

Further references: D. C. Chatterji and J. F. Gallelli, *J. pharm. Sci.*, 1978, *67*, 526.

Adverse Effects. For an outline of the adverse effects experienced with antineoplastic agents and immunosuppressants, see Antineoplastic Agents, p.171.

Early signs of toxicity with methotrexate include leucopenia, thrombocytopenia, ulceration of the mouth, and gastro-intestinal effects; stomatitis or diarrhoea are signs that treatment should be interrupted, otherwise haemorrhagic enteritis and intestinal perforation may follow. Bone-marrow depression may occur abruptly; megaloblastic anaemia has been reported. Methotrexate is immunosuppressant and hypogammaglobulinaemia may occur. Liver damage has been reported, especially in patients with psoriasis given long-term treatment with relatively small doses of methotrexate; it may occur in the absence of other signs of methotrexate toxicity. Kidney damage, osteoporosis, and pulmonary and neurotoxic reactions have also developed. Fatalities have occurred.

Neurotoxic reactions are especially associated with the intrathecal use of methotrexate. Teratogenic effects and foetal deaths have been reported.

Reports and reviews of toxicity associated with methotrexate: E. C. Cadman *et al.*, *Archs intern. Med.*, 1976, *136*, 1321; M. Nesbit *et al.*, *Cancer*, 1976, *37*, 1048 (hepatic, pulmonary, and skeletal systems); H. Chan *et al.*, *Cancer Treat. Rep.*, 1977, *61*, 797 (prognostic factors for recovery from toxicity); D. D. Von Hoff *et al.*, *Cancer Treat. Rep.*, 1977, *61*, 745 (high-dose methotrexate); T. E. Hoffman and W. Watson, *Cutis*, 1978, *21*, 68 (in psoriasis); A. Nyfors, *Dan. med. Bull.*, 1978, *25*, 208 (in psoriasis).

In 7 patients under treatment with methotrexate for psoriasis, folate activity in lymphocytes (assessed by measuring the incorporation of ^{14}C-formate into serine) was reduced to about half of that in controls. The serum concentration of cyanocobalamin was reduced below normal in 3 patients; reduction was related to length of treatment.— J. Ellegaard *et al.*, *Br. J. Derm.*, 1972, *87*, 248.

Allergy and anaphylaxis. Reports of allergic reactions associated with methotrexate: P. Lanzkowsky *et al.* (letter), *Am. J. Dis. Child.*, 1976, *130*, 675 (vasculitis associated with high doses of methotrexate and resolved during treatment with corticosteroids); A. D. Lascari *et al.*, *Cancer*, 1977, *40*, 1393 (fatal angioneurotic oedema of the lung after an oral dose given 7 days after the last of 4 intrathecal injections); N. H. Goldberg *et al.*, *Cancer*, 1978, *41*, 52 (sudden cardiovascular collapse after high doses of methotrexate given in association with intracutaneous BCG); I. Gluck-Kuyt and L. E. Irwin, *Cancer Treat. Rep.*, 1979, *63*, 797 (anaphylaxis without prior BCG therapy).

Carcinogenicity. A view that there is no justification for describing methotrexate as carcinogenic.— C. Turnbull and M. Roach, *Lederle* (letter), *Br. med. J.*, 1980, *281*, 808. But see also under Antineoplastic Agents, p.171.

Effects on bones and joints. References: S. O'Regan *et al.*, *Am. J. Dis. Child.*, 1973, *126*, 489 (osteoporosis).

Effects on the gastro-intestinal tract. In a study in 18 children with acute lymphoblastic leukaemia, absorption of D-xylose was reduced in 14 who had been taking methotrexate, compared with 4 studied before methotrexate was given; in those who had taken methotrexate within the last 7 days the reduction in absorption was significant. Reduction in absorption was progressive and related to the total cumulative dose of methotrexate.— A. W. Craft *et al., Br. med. J.*, 1977, *2*, 1511. A suggestion that once-weekly treatment might be too frequent.— A. W. Craft and W. Aherne, *Archs Dis. Childh.*, 1978, *53*, 262.

Severe methotrexate enteropathy (presenting as chronic diarrhoea and anorexia) in a 6-year-old leukaemic child was considered to be due to enterohepatic recycling. Abnormal gut toxicity may be related to abnormally efficient biliary excretion of methotrexate.— G. M. Baird and J. F. B. Dossetor (letter), *Lancet*, 1981, *1*, 164. Comment.— C. R. Pinkerton and J. F. T. Glasgow (letter), *ibid.*, 996.

Effects on the kidneys. A patient who had been receiving intramuscular injections of methotrexate 25 mg every 2 or 3 weeks for 10 months developed albuminuria, and, though methotrexate was discontinued, died with uraemic fits 1 month later.— A. W. McKenzie and C. V. E. Aitken (letter), *Br. J. Derm.*, 1967, *79*, 122.

Effects on the liver. The liver fibrosis and cirrhosis reported in psoriatic patients treated with methotrexate (J. Almeyda *et al., Br. J. Derm.*, 1971, *85*, 302; M.G.C. Dahl *et al., Br. med., J.*, 1971, *1*, 625) appeared to be more prevalent in subjects given frequent small doses of methotrexate than in those given intermittent large doses and was also related to the duration of treatment (M.G.C. Dahl *et al., Br. med. J.*, 1972, *1*, 654). G. Weinstein *et al.* (*Archs Derm.*, 1973, *108*, 36) also found increased liver damage in psoriatic patients given daily doses of methotrexate and daily administration has since been abandoned in favour of weekly doses. A. Nyfors and H. Poulsen (*Acta path. microbiol. scand., A, Path.*, 1976, *84*, 262) carried out liver biopsies in psoriatic patients receiving weekly doses of up to 25 mg of methotrexate and found the incidence of portal fibrosis to be 5.6% and that of cirrhosis 6.8%; the incidence of liver damage increased rapidly beyond a cumulative dose of 2 to 4 g (A. Nyfors, *Acta path. microbiol. scand., A, Path.*, 1977, *85*, 511). Liver-function tests alone do not allow an adequate assessment of possible liver damage and biopsies should be performed at least once a year in patients on long-term methotrexate therapy. Although a comprehensive assessment of the hepatotoxicity of high-dose regimens of methotrexate is not yet possible, mild transient reversible elevations of serum bilirubin and aminotransferases appear to be quite frequent. Portal fibrosis has been found in children on long-term maintenance therapy with high-dose methotrexate (S. McIntosh *et al., J. Pediat.*, 1977, *90*, 1019). Patients on high-dose regimens are not as frequently subjected to hepatotoxicity as might be expected and it is suggested that the duration of exposure to supra-threshold concentrations of methotrexate determines the incidence of hepatotoxicity.— D. B. Ménard *et al., Gastroenterology*, 1980, *78*, 143.

An evaluation of the hepatotoxicity of methotrexate, given in a weekly divided dose regimen comprising 3 oral doses of 2.5 to 5 mg at 12-hour intervals over 24 hours, in the maintenance therapy of psoriasis. Fibrosis of the liver necessitating withdrawal of methotrexate developed in 11 of 43 patients given an average cumulative dose of 1.25 g. Significant risk factors in these severely psoriatic patients were age and duration of therapy. It is not clear whether this dosage schedule is more toxic than a single weekly dose of 25 mg, but in any event serial liver biopsies are considered necessary every 12 to 18 months throughout a course of treatment with methotrexate.— J. K. Robinson *et al., Archs Derm.*, 1980, *116*, 413. See also H. Zachariae *et al., Br. J. Derm.*, 1980, *102*, 407.

Further reports of liver damage in psoriatic patients given methotrexate: H. M. Palmer, *Practitioner*, 1973, *211*, 324 (no correlation with duration of therapy or cumulative dose); B. J. Pondurgiel *et al., Mayo Clin. Proc.*, 1973, *48*, 787; H. Tobias and R. Auerbach, *Archs intern. Med.*, 1973, *132*, 391; H. Zachariae and H. Sogaard, *Dermatologica*, 1973, *146*, 149 (liver damage might have been associated with the psoriasis).

Effects on the nervous system. *Intrathecal methotrexate.* Neurological side-effects in acute, subacute, or chronic forms have been associated with the intrathecal administration of methotrexate and preservative-free solutions have been advocated in an attempt to eliminate this neurotoxicity.

Five of 25 patients with acute leukaemia receiving preservative-free methotrexate by intrathecal injection developed severe neurotoxicity. The average age (25.8 years) of those with toxicity was significantly greater than that of the non-toxic group (9.4 years). Also 4 of the 10 patients with meningeal leukaemia developed toxicity compared with only 1 of 15 who were treated prophylactically. Toxicity was associated with high cerebrospinal-fluid concentrations of methotrexate. It was suggested that doses given intrathecally for the treatment of meningeal leukaemia should be lower than those normally used for prophylaxis.— W. A. Bleyer *et al., New Engl. J. Med.*, 1973, *289*, 770.

Neurological disorders related to methotrexate treatment developed in 17 of 333 children with acute lymphoblastic leukaemia. In most children the reactions were associated with intrathecal administration. Complications included arachnoiditis, convulsions, progressive intellectual impairment, and coma and occurred more frequently in children who had had previous CNS leukaemia. It was considered that viral infections and methotrexate provided the greatest neurological hazards to children with leukaemia.— R. H. A. Campbell *et al., Archs Dis. Childh.*, 1977, *52*, 850. Prophylactic CNS irradiation and methotrexate given intrathecally as part of the leukaemia treatment regimen produced both EEG and biochemical signs of brain dysfunction or injury when 8 children so treated were compared with controls. However, such treatment should not be withheld at least until other safer and effective methods are developed.— S. Similä *et al.* (letter), *Lancet*, 1977, *1*, 1000. In 27 children who had received irradiation and intrathecal methotrexate for acute lymphoblastic leukaemia there was no evidence, from CAT scans, of brain damage.— R. E. Day *et al., Br. med. J.*, 1978, *2*, 1752. Findings of abnormal computed tomography scans in 17 of 32 asymptomatic patients with acute lymphocytic leukaemia who had received prophylactic cranial irradiation in association with intrathecal methotrexate or cytarabine, were considered possibly to represent preclinical evidence of treatment-related CNS toxicity. Reappraisal of CNS prophylaxis should be considered.— N. Peylan-Ramu *et al., New Engl. J. Med.*, 1978, *298*, 815. Pathological changes in the brain were detected in many children with acute lymphoblastic leukaemia and non-Hodgkin's lymphoma before treatment.— P. Gutjahr and K. Kretzschmar, *Dt. med. Wschr.*, 1979, *104*, 1068. Damage linked with cranial irradiation.— A. T. Meadows *et al., Lancet*, 1981, *2*, 1015.

Further references to neurotoxicity with intrathecal methotrexate: K. D. Bagshawe *et al.* (letter), *Lancet*, 1969, *2*, 1258 (also cytarabine); H. E. M. Kay *et al.* (letter), *Lancet*, 1971, *2*, 542 (dementia); S. McIntosh and G. T. Aspnes, *Pediatrics*, 1973, *52*, 612 (meningoencephalopathy); P. D. Lewis *et al.* (letter), *Br. med. J.*, 1974, *4*, 42 (also cytarabine); S. Mueller *et al., J. Pediat.*, 1976, *88*, 650 (cerebral calcifications); P. A. Pizzo *et al., J. Pediat.*, 1976, *88*, 131 (dementia with intraventricular therapy); K. D. Waters (letter), *Lancet*, 1978, *2*, 46 (leucoencephalopathy); S. Weiss and Y. Kahn, *Acta haemat.*, 1978, *60*, 59 (paraplegia).

Effects on reproductive potential. *Gonads.* Oligospermia occurred in a man treated for psoriasis with methotrexate.— A. Sussman and J. M. Leonard, *Archs Derm.*, 1980, *116*, 215.

Effects on respiratory function. A review of pneumonitis associated with methotrexate. Both allergic and cytotoxic effects have been implicated in methotrexate-induced pulmonary disease.— H. D. Sostman *et al., Medicine, Baltimore*, 1976, *55*, 371. Methotrexate produces a more transient, treatable, and less often fatal pulmonary reaction than many other antineoplastic agents and the onset does not appear to be dose-related. A reversible hypersensitivity reaction sometimes occurs rather than a direct effect on alveolar epithelium with irreversible fibrosis. Pneumonitis has been reported after oral, intravenous, or intrathecal administration; symptoms have sometimes been resolved by corticosteroids.— R. B. Weiss and F. M. Muggia, *Am. J. Med.*, 1980, *68*, 259.

Seven patients developed severe pulmonary complications during maintenance treatment with methotrexate. The complications appeared 12 to 100 days after commencing treatment and were characterised by cough, malaise, pyrexia, dyspnoea, and cyanosis. Bilateral, diffuse, interstitial pulmonary infiltrates were seen on X-ray examination. Pulmonary complications have been reported in 38 of 93 other patients treated intermittently with methotrexate.— A. M. Clarysse, *J. Am. med. Ass.*, 1969, *209*, 1861.

Further reports of pulmonary reactions with methotrexate: K. M. Robbins *et al., J. Pediat.*, 1973, *82*, 84; P. A. M. Walden *et al., Br. med. J.*, 1977, *2*, 867 (pleuritis in 20 of 317 patients given methotrexate intramuscularly); R. L. Kaplan and D. H. Waite, *Archs Derm.*, 1978, *114*, 1800 (progressive interstitial lung disease with long-term methotrexate); C. W. M. Bedrossian *et al., Sth. med. J.*, 1979, *72*, 313 (pneumonitis).

Overdosage. Two children who ingested unknown amounts of methotrexate were treated with a folinic acid preparation. Serum concentrations of serum aspartate aminotransferase (SGOT) and lactate dehydrogenase increased but there were no other signs of toxicity. Methotrexate was slowly excreted and concentrations were still measurable in the plasma after 13 days.— A. W. Pruitt *et al., J. Pediat.*, 1974, *85*, 686, per *J. Am. med. Ass.*, 1975, *232*, 211.

Pregnancy and the neonate. *First trimester.* Congenital malformations, mainly affecting the skull bones, occurred in an infant whose mother had been given methotrexate early in her pregnancy for psoriasis.— H. R. Powell and H. Ekert, *Med. J. Aust.*, 1971, *2*, 1076. See also A. Milunsky *et al., J. Pediat.*, 1968, *72*, 790; J. Warkany, *Teratology*, 1978, *17*, 353.

Treatment of Adverse Effects. For general guidelines, see Antineoplastic Agents, p.174.

Folinic acid neutralises the immediate toxic effects of methotrexate on the bone marrow and is given by mouth, intramuscularly, by intravenous bolus injection, or by infusion as calcium folinate. When overdosage is suspected the dose of calcium folinate should be at least as high as that of methotrexate and should be administered within the first hour; further doses are given as required. When average doses of methotrexate have an adverse effect, the equivalent of 6 to 12 mg of folinic acid may be given intramuscularly every 6 hours for 4 doses. See also under Calcium Folinate, p.1648.

Folinic acid may also be given in association with high-dose methotrexate regimens to prevent damage to normal tissue and this is discussed in the Uses section below.

A 4-year-old girl was given 10 times the usual dose of methotrexate intrathecally. Folinic acid was immediately given and continued for 48 hours. No neurological or other effects occurred.— B. C. Lampkin *et al., Cancer*, 1967, *20*, 1780, per *Int. pharm. Abstr.*, 1968, *5*, 461. Administration of folinic acid did not counteract all the side-effects of high-dose methotrexate therapy. Levodopa and 5-hydroxytryptophan might alleviate the CNS symptoms.— R. G. H. Cotton (letter), *Lancet*, 1978, *2*, 484. The folate derivative 5-methyltetrahydrofolic acid might be a more suitable antidote.— R. J. Leeming and J. A. Blair (letter), *ibid.*, 737.

Two patients who developed bilateral pulmonary infiltrates after treatment with methotrexate responded promptly to treatment with prednisone. Radiological examination showed complete resolution of the infiltrates.— I. R. Schwartz and M. K. Kajani (letter), *J. Am. med. Ass.*, 1969, *210*, 1924.

In *mice*, thymidine prevented methotrexate toxicity without inhibiting its antitumour effect.— M. H. N. Tattersall *et al.* (letter), *Nature*, 1975, *253*, 198. References to the clinical use of thymidine: W. D. Ensminger and E. Frei, *Cancer Res.*, 1977, *37*, 1857; S. B. Howell *et al., Cancer Res.*, 1978, *38*, 325.

Results in 2 patients indicated that peritoneal dialysis or haemodialysis are of no major benefit in patients with high plasma-methotrexate concentrations and mild or moderate renal failure. In total anuria methotrexate may be removed over several days by haemodialysis if no other therapeutic options are available.— K. R. Hande *et al.* (letter), *Ann. intern. Med.*, 1977, *87*, 495. Haemoperfusion for 4 hours using an Amberlite XAD-4 column transiently reduced plasma-methotrexate concentration in a woman with metastatic breast carcinoma with signs of methotrexate toxicity. Studies *in vitro* showed that haemoperfusion with uncoated charcoal was more effective than Amberlite XAD-4.— T. P. Gibson *et al., Clin. Pharmac. Ther.*, 1978, *23*, 351. See also I. Djerassi *et al., Cancer Treat. Rep.*, 1977, *61*, 751 (charcoal filters or haemodialysis).

Further references: A. I. Pavlotsky *et al., Cancer Treat. Rep.*, 1977, *61*, 895 (selective protection of gastro-intestinal tract).

Precautions. For reference to the precautions necessary with antineoplastic agents and immunosuppressants, see Antineoplastic Agents, p.175.

Methotrexate should be used with great care in patients with hepatic or renal impairment. It should also be used cautiously in alcoholics or those with ulcerative disorders of the gastro-intestinal tract. With high-dose regimens, plasma concentrations of methotrexate and urinary excretion should be monitored. Precipitation of methotrexate or its metabolites in the renal tubules may be prevented by alkalinisation of the urine using sodium bicarbonate, maintaining an adequate urine flow, and the withholding of therapy until pleural or ascitic effusions, which may act as a depot for methotrexate, have been drained.

The effects of methotrexate may be enhanced by concurrent administration of aminobenzoic acid, chloramphenicol, phenylbutazone, phenytoin, probenecid, salicylates, sulphonamides, and tetracyclines.

Interactions. With drugs. When methotrexate was given 6 hours before cytarabine to *mice* inoculated with lymphoma cells, no antitumour effect was seen. Both compounds were shown to increase survival if given separately, together, or if cytarabine was given 6 hours before methotrexate.— M. H. N. Tattersall *et al.* (letter), *Lancet*, 1972, *2*, 1378.

Neither methotrexate 5 mg per kg body-weight intraperitoneally nor *phenobarbitone* 100 mg per kg produced alopecia when given separately to *rats*, but when given together alopecia was observed.— T. K. Basu *et al.* (letter), *Lancet*, 1973, *2*, 331.

Studies *in vitro* suggested that the cellular uptake of methotrexate and therefore its antimetabolic effect might be reduced by 50% in the presence of some corticosteroids.— S. Waxman and H. Bruckner (letter), *Science*, 1976, *194*, 1112.

In 4 patients the excretion of methotrexate was delayed when *probenecid* was given concomitantly; the serum-methotrexate concentration 24 hours after a single intravenous dose was 4 times that in 4 patients given methotrexate without probenecid; serum-methotrexate concentrations at 24 hours were comparable with those achieved after 20-hour or 24-hour infusion. Elimination of the drugs in the urine within 12 hours was 58% and 83% respectively.— G. W. Aherne *et al.*, *Br. med. J.*, 1978, *1*, 1097. See also R. E. Kates *et al.*, *Biochem. Pharmac.*, 1976, *25*, 1485.

For references to methotrexate inhibiting the effect of *fluorouracil* or *floxuridine*, see Fluorouracil, p.209.

With radiation. Analysis of neutrophil counts for 18 months in children with acute lymphoblastic leukaemia, some of whom were given CNS irradiation, showed that methotrexate was the main agent associated with severe neutropenia. Methotrexate-induced neutropenia was significantly greater in patients given CNS irradiation and was considered to have contributed to 3 of 5 deaths during remission.—Report to the MRC of the Working Party on Leukaemia in Childhood, *Br. med. J.*, 1975, *3*, 563.

Comment on intrathecal methotrexate as a cause of encephalopathy and its possible exacerbation by irradiation.— M. C. -van Daele and W. van de Casseye (letter), *Lancet*, 1978, *2*, 834. See also A. T. Meadows *et al.*, *Lancet*, 1981, *2*, 1015.

Pregnancy and the neonate. An infant born to a woman who had conceived within 6 months of completing treatment with methotrexate, had desquamating fibrosing alveolitis. The rarity of this pulmonary disorder, particularly in childhood, and the fact that methotrexate can be retained in the tissues of both animals and man, suggest that it may have been a causative factor.— P. A. M. Walden and K. D. Bagshawe (letter), *Lancet*, 1979, *2*, 1241.

See also Adverse Effects, above, and Absorption and Fate and Uses, below.

Absorption and Fate. When given in low doses, methotrexate is rapidly absorbed from the gastro-intestinal tract to give plasma concentrations equivalent to those obtained by intravenous administration. Higher doses are less well absorbed. It is distributed mainly in the extracellular spaces but a proportion penetrates cell membranes and is strongly bound to dihydrofolate reductase. Only small amounts of methotrexate diffuse into the cerebrospinal fluid but higher concentrations are achieved with high doses. About 50% is bound to plasma proteins. Biphasic and triphasic clearance from plasma has been reported. The majority of a dose is excreted unchanged in the urine within 24 hours and up to 15% may appear in the bile although because of reabsorption less may be excreted in the faeces. Bound methotrexate may be retained in the body for many months.

A review of the clinical pharmacokinetics of methotrexate. Following intramuscular injection of methotrexate absorption is rapid and complete and more sustained serum concentrations are achieved than those following rapid intravenous administration. Gastro-intestinal absorption is dose-dependent, peak serum concentrations occurring 1 to 2 hours after doses below 30 mg per m^2 body-surface. A slowing in the rate of absorption has been noted during a 6-week course of therapy in some patients. Absorption has been reduced to 50 to 70% at doses above 80 mg per m^2. Although earlier studies suggested that methotrexate was not metabolised, nearly a third of an oral dose may be excreted in the urine as metabolites as a result of the action of intestinal bacteria prior to absorption. A major metabolite is 4-amino-4-deoxy-N^{10}-methylpteroic acid. Only 6% of an intravenous dose is excreted as metabolites. Plasma clearance of methotrexate is reported to be biphasic or triphasic. Following the intravenous administration of 30 mg per m^2 of methotrexate to cancer patients D.H. Huffman *et al.*(*Clin. Pharmac. Ther.*, 1973, *14*, 572) found that plasma disappearance was triphasic with mean half-lives of 0.75, 3.49, and 26.99 hours respectively; there was considerable variation between patients and terminal half-lives ranged from 6 to 69 hours. R.G. Stoller *et al.* (*Cancer Chemother. Rep.*, 1975, *6*, 19) reported a biphasic decline in plasma concentrations after high-dose infusion of methotrexate with mean half-lives of about 2 and 10 hours. Although plasma concentrations are roughly proportional to dose, methotrexate elimination may be saturable at very high doses.

Methotrexate is transported across cellular membranes by a carrier-mediated active-type process. With high doses the carrier route becomes saturated and passive diffusion becomes more important. Being highly ionised at physiological pH little methotrexate penetrates the blood-brain barrier in general but persisting and high concentrations in the CSF can be achieved with high-dose intravenous infusions, at the cost of increased systemic toxicity. After the intrathecal injection of methotrexate, a half-life in CSF of 12 to 18 hours was reported by W.A. Bleyer *et al.* (*New Engl. J. Med.*, 1973, *289*, 770). W.R. Shapiro *et al.* (*New Engl. J. Med.*, 1975, *293*, 161) found considerable variation in peak intraventricular concentrations after the administration of methotrexate by lumbar puncture; more consistent concentrations were achieved with an indwelling intraventricular-subcutaneous reservoir. S.A. Jacobs *et al.* (*J. clin. Invest.*, 1976, *57*, 534) have reported significant quantities of 7-hydroxy methotrexate in the urine of patients given high doses of methotrexate with 24-hour excretion ranging from 1 to 11% of the dose. This metabolite is a less effective inhibitor of dihydrofolate reductase than methotrexate and is also less soluble; it may contribute to renal toxicity during high-dose therapy. Up to 9% of an intravenous dose of methotrexate has been recovered in the faeces after secretion in the bile; enterohepatic circulation might explain the long terminal elimination half-life of methotrexate. About 80% of a dose is excreted in the urine by glomerular filtration and active renal tubular secretion. Intratubular precipitation of methotrexate is possible with high doses. A peak concentration in urine of 5 mg per ml has been reported in patients receiving high doses. This exceeds the saturation concentration of methotrexate at low urinary pHs and routine administration of fluid and/or bicarbonate is therefore recommended. Renal function and plasma concentrations of methotrexate should be monitored for impending toxicity. Very low concentrations of methotrexate have been found in breast milk and saliva. Methotrexate may be contaminated with byproducts of its synthesis or with degradation products and these impurities may be confused with methotrexate metabolites.— D. D. Shen and D. L. Azarnoff, *Clin. Pharmacokinet.*, 1978, *3*, 1. See also W. A. Bleyer, *Cancer*, 1978, *41*, 36.

Plasma concentrations of methotrexate following intrathecal administration of 12 mg per m^2 body-surface to 2 patients were considerably higher after 24 hours than those following oral administration of the same dose after 24 hours. Further study in 1 of the patients showed no difference in the pharmacokinetic behaviour of methotrexate given by mouth or intravenously.— S. A. Jacobs *et al.* (letter), *Lancet*, 1975, *1*, 465. An assessment of changes in the transfer-rate of methotrexate from spinal fluid to plasma in adults and children receiving intrathecal injections. Two patterns were identified: the 'slow' type in which plasma concentrations reached a rather low maximum followed by a relatively slow decline and the 'fast' type in which plasma concentrations increased rapidly to a high value followed by a relatively rapid biphasic decline. The incidence of 'fast' type increased progressively with the number of intrathecal injections and might be attributed to facilitated leakage from the spinal fluid possibly resulting from damage caused by repeated injections, the effects of radiotherapy, or altered circulation of the spinal fluid. Therapeutic efficacy in the CNS is likely to be less for the 'fast' type whereas systemic toxicity is expected to be higher in the 'slow' type.— J. Lankelma *et al.*, *Clin. Pharmacokinet.*, 1980, *5*, 465.

A study involving 78 cancer patients with normal BUN and serum creatinine values given 395 infusions of high-dose methotrexate (50 to 250 mg per kg body-weight over a period of 6 hours). Following 375 of the infusions plasma-methotrexate concentrations after 48 hours fell below 9×10^{-7}M [mol per litre] and were not associated with subsequent toxicity. Owing either to subsequent rapid reduction in blood concentrations or to supplementary high-dose folinic acid given to 4 of them, no subsequent toxicity occurred in 6 patients where the concentrations were still above 9×10^{-7}M [mol per litre] after 48 hours. A seventh patient whose concentration remained above 9×10^{-7}M [mol per litre] after 48 hours without subsequent rapid clearance received supplementary high-dose folinic acid and suffered only moderate leucopenia but in 6 similar patients who did not receive supplementary high-dose folinic acid therapy serious myelosuppression occurred. Measurement of plasma-methotrexate concentrations 48 hours after infusion could identify patients at high risk of toxicity and administration of supplementary high doses of folinic acid might prevent toxicity.— R. G. Stoller *et al.*, *New Engl. J. Med.*, 1977, *297*, 630.

The prolonged administration of methotrexate might lead to a change from a fast to a slow pattern of absorption with lower peak blood concentrations.— A. W. Craft and W. Aherne, *Archs Dis. Childh.*, 1978, *53*, 262.

Further references to the absorption and fate of methotrexate: H. V. Dubin and E. R. Harrell (letter), *J. Am. med. Ass.*, 1969, *210*, 1104 (slow and rapid absorption patterns); D. G. Johns *et al.*, *Am. J. Obstet. Gynec.*, 1972, *112*, 978 (secretion in milk); S. Salasoo *et al.*, *Med. J. Aust.*, 1976, *1*, 777 and 826 (high-dose); Y. Wang *et al.*, *Clin. Chem.*, 1976, *22*, 1053 (concentrations in blood, urine, and CSF after high doses); W. A. Bleyer and R. L. Dedrick, *Cancer Treat. Rep.*, 1977, *61*, 703 (intrathecal methotrexate); W. A. Bleyer, *Cancer Treat. Rep.*, 1977, *61*, 1419 (intrathecal); A. H. Calvert *et al.*, *Cancer Treat. Rep.*, 1977, *61*, 1647; W. H. Isacoff *et al.*, *Cancer Treat. Rep.*, 1977, *61*, 1665 (high-dose methotrexate with folinic acid rescue); S. A. Jacobs *et al.*, *Cancer Treat. Rep.*, 1977, *61*, 651 (dose-dependent metabolism); J. R. Taylor and K. M. Halprin, *Archs Derm.*, 1977, *113*, 588 (binding to albumin); D. Bratlid and P. J. Moe, *Eur. J. clin. Pharmac.*, 1978, *14*, 143 (pharmacokinetics in children); B. A. Chabner *et al.*, *Drug Metab. Rev.*, 1978, *8*, 107 (disposition in cancer patients); Y. M. Wang *et al.*, *Med. pediat. Oncol.*, 1978, *4*, 221 (children); K. Boomla *et al.*, *Br. J. Derm.*, 1979, *101*, 109 (concentrations in plasma and skin exudates in patients with psoriasis); R. C. Donehower *et al.*, *Clin. Pharmac. Ther.*, 1979, *26*, 63 (2,4-diamino-N^{10}-methylpteroic acid, a contaminant of methotrexate, is probably also a metabolite in high-dose therapy); S. B. Howell *et al.*, *Clin. Pharmac. Ther.*, 1979, *26*, 641 (the failure of probenecid to alter the clearance of methotrexate from the CSF); W. H. Steele *et al.*, *Eur. J. clin. Pharmac.*, 1979, *15*, 363 (binding in vitro); W. H. Steele *et al.*, *Br. J. clin. Pharmac.*, 1979, *7*, 207 (concentrations in serum, tears, and saliva); J. R. Lawrence *et al.*, *Eur. J. clin. Pharmac.*, 1980, *17*, 371 (dose-dependent elimination after intravenous injection); S. M. Wigginton *et al.*, *Arthritis Rheum.*, 1980, *23*, 119 (intra-articular injections).

Uses. Methotrexate is an antineoplastic agent which acts as an antimetabolite (p.171) of folic acid. It also has immunosuppressant properties. Within the cell, folic acid is reduced to dihydrofolic and then tetrahydrofolic acid. Methotrexate competitively inhibits the enzyme dihydrofolate reductase and prevents the formation of tetrahydrofolate which is necessary for purine and pyrimidine synthesis and consequently the formation of DNA and RNA. High doses of methotrexate have been used in an effort to increase intracellular concentrations of methotrexate. Folinic acid, the 5-formyl derivative of tetrahydrofolic acid is given after high doses to bypass the block in tetrahydrofolate production in normal cells and prevent the adverse effects of methotrexate. A suggested schedule for this *folinic acid rescue* is described under Calcium Folinate, p.1648. The nucleoside thymidine has also been used as a methotrexate antagonist (see also under Treatment of Adverse Effects, above). Methotrexate, in very high doses, followed by folinic acid rescue, is being investigated in a number of malignant diseases.

Methotrexate is used in the management of acute

lymphoblastic leukaemia. It is seldom used for the induction of remission but is employed in maintenance programmes and in the prophylaxis and treatment of meningeal leukaemia. It is effective in the treatment of choriocarcinoma and other trophoblastic tumours and is used, often in association with other antineoplastic agents, in the treatment of a variety of malignant diseases including lymphosarcoma, Burkitt's lymphoma, osteogenic sarcoma, and tumours of the bladder, brain, breast, cervix, head and neck, lung, ovary, and testis. See also under Choice of Antineoplastic Agent, p.175.

Methotrexate is of value in the treatment of psoriasis but because of the risks associated with this use, it should only be given when the disease is severe and has not responded to other forms of treatment. It has been used as an immunosuppressant (see p.186) in other non-malignant diseases.

Methotrexate may be given by mouth, or by injection as methotrexate sodium.

A common dose for maintenance therapy of acute lymphoblastic leukaemia is 20 mg per m^2 body-surface weekly, by mouth or intravenously, with other agents such as mercaptopurine. Meningeal leukaemia may be treated by the intrathecal injection of 12 mg per m^2 body-surface, to a maximum of 15 mg, once or twice weekly. Similar doses are given prophylactically to patients with lymphoblastic leukaemia, often in association with cranial irradiation. Methotrexate in intravenous doses of about 500 mg per m^2, followed by folinic acid rescue, may also produce effective concentrations in the CSF.

Choriocarcinoma has been treated with doses of 15 to 30 mg daily by mouth or intramuscularly for 5 days, at intervals of 1 to 2 weeks, for 3 to 5 courses. Alternatively 0.25 to 1 mg per kg body-weight up to a maximum of 60 mg has been given intramuscularly every 48 hours for 4 doses, followed by folinic acid rescue, and repeated at intervals of 7 days. Combination chemotherapy may be necessary in patients with metastases. A range of doses of methotrexate has been used in the management of solid tumours. Very high doses have been given by intravenous infusion, followed by folinic acid, in patients with osteogenic sarcoma and carcinoma of the lung and of the head and neck.

Methotrexate has been given by mouth, intramuscularly, and intravenously in the treatment of psoriasis. Single weekly doses of 10 to 25 mg may be given by mouth or injection. Alternatively 2.5 mg has been administered by mouth every 12 hours for 3 doses or every 8 hours for 4 doses each week or 2.5 mg may be given daily by mouth for 5 days out of 7.

It is essential that examinations of blood and tests of renal and liver function should be made before, during, and after each course of treatment with methotrexate. If there is a severe fall in the white cell or platelet counts, methotrexate should be withdrawn.

Reviews of methotrexate: W. A. Bleyer, *Cancer Treat. Rev.*, 1977, *4*, 87; *idem*, *Cancer*, 1978, *41*, 36.

Action. Methotrexate caused a reduction in the free intracellular pool of thymidylate triphosphate in phytohaemagglutinin-transformed human lymphocytes and a rise in the concentration of deoxyadenosine triphosphate.— A. V. Hoffbrand and E. Tripp, *Br. med. J.*, 1972, *2*, 140. See also M. H. N. Tattersall (letter), *ibid.*, 408.

Administration. A brief review of the use of methotrexate in association with calcium folinate rescue.— J. F. Bender *et al.*, *Am. J. Hosp. Pharm.*, 1977, *34*, 961. See also R. D. Lauper (letter), *ibid.*, 1978, *35*, 377. Criticism of the use of high-dose methotrexate therapy.— W. E. Evans and R. H. Taylor (letter), *ibid.*, 1978, *35*, 779.

A report of experience with high doses of methotrexate given by mouth to outpatients for a variety of malignant diseases. Methotrexate 25 mg was given as tablets every hour for 16 hours and folinic acid rescue started at 24 hours. Tolerance was good and there was evidence that blood concentrations of methotrexate were similar to those achieved with infusions.— R. Bell *et al.* (letter), *Br. med. J.*, 1978, *1*, 857. Since absorption of high doses of methotrexate has been reported to be protracted and incomplete, with plasma concentrations less than a tenth of those achieved after intravenous administration, the cytotoxic efficacy of this dose is open to question.— G. W. R. Hill and M. Roach, *Lederle* (letter), *ibid.*, 1140. A pharmacokinetic study in 5 patients and experience in 14 patients showed that high doses of methotrexate (800 mg in a day), as part of a multiple chemotherapeutic regimen, could be given by mouth; 50 mg was given each hour for 16 hours, with folinic acid rescue starting 8 hours after the last dose. Bioavailability was 82 to 91% and tolerance was good.— N. Christophidis *et al.*, *Br. med. J.*, 1979, *1*, 298. Further references to the use of high-dose methotrexate and folinic acid rescue: I. Djerassi *et al.*, *Cancer Treat. Rep.*, 1977, *61*, 749; R. G. Stoller *et al.*, *Cancer Res.*, 1979, *39*, 908; E. Frei *et al.*, *Am. J. Med.*, 1980, *68*, 370.

See also Treatment of Adverse Effects (above).

To sustain a plasma-methotrexate concentration of about 1×10^{-4}M as recommended by S. Salasoo *et al.* (*Med. J. Aust.*, 1976, *1*, 777) throughout intravenous infusion, 10 cancer patients were given methotrexate over 6 hours as follows: 33% of the total dose during the first 30 minutes, 17% during the next 30 minutes, and the remainder over 5 hours. Total doses ranged from 1.5 to 3.5 g (20 to 50 mg per kg body-weight). Folinic acid rescue was started 2 to 24 hours after the end of infusions. Of 14 infusions given, 12 resulted in a mean concentration of about 1.5×10^{-4}M at 30 minutes, gradually falling to about 1×10^{-4}M at 6 hours. The other 2 infusions in 1 patient produced a mean concentration of about 5×10^{-4}M and were associated with the development of bone-marrow depression.— J. W. Paxton *et al.* (letter), *Br. J. clin. Pharmac.*, 1978, *6*, 551.

Studies of methotrexate-induced malabsorption in children with acute lymphoblastic leukaemia indicated that prolonged administration may lead to slower absorption and lower peak blood concentrations and that once-weekly dosage may be too frequent.— A. W. Craft and W. Aherne, *Archs Dis. Childh.* 1978, *53*, 262. A study in 10 similar children indicated that methotrexate absorption is delayed by food, particularly milk. Peak plasma-methotrexate concentrations were reduced. For maximum absorption it is therefore recommended that methotrexate should not be taken at meal times.— C. R. Pinkerton *et al.*, *Lancet*, 1980, *2*, 944. Xylose absorption studies should not be used to predict methotrexate absorption.— *idem*, 1981, *282*, 1276.

Further references: J. Marty *et al.*, *Clin. exp. Pharmac. Physiol.*, 1979, *6*, 649 (comparison of oral and intravenous high-dose methotrexate therapy).

Administration in the elderly. A reduction in dosage should be considered when methotrexate is given to elderly patients.— J. P. Kampmann and J. E. M. Hansen, in *Drugs and the Elderly* J. Crooks; I.H. Stevenson (Ed.), London, Macmillan Press, 1979, p. 77.

Administration in renal insufficiency. Doses of methotrexate should be reduced to 75% of normal in patients with a glomerular filtration-rate (GFR) of 10 to 50 ml per minute, and to 50% in those with a GFR of less than 10 ml per minute.— W. M. Bennett *et al.*, *Ann. intern. Med.*, 1977, *86*, 754. See also *idem*, 1980, *93*, 286.

Burkitt's lymphoma. For reference to methotrexate in the treatment of Burkitt's lymphoma, see Choice of Antineoplastic Agent, p.176.

Choriocarcinoma. For reference to methotrexate in the treatment of choriocarcinoma, see Choice of Antineoplastic Agent, p.176.

Immunosuppression. For the use of methotrexate as an immunosuppressant see under the headings for non-malignant disorders in this section and under Use of Immunosuppressants, p.186.

References to the use of methotrexate in various immune disorders: G. A. Farber *et al.*, *J. Am. med. Ass.*, 1967, *200*, 171 (Reiter's disease); M. Lazar *et al.*, *Am. J. Ophthal.*, 1969, *67*, 383 (uveitis); F. D. B. Haas, *Ned. Tijdschr. Geneesk.*, 1976, *120*, 611 (Reiter's disease).

Infections. A consideration of the use of methotrexate in the treatment of malaria.— A. B. G. Laing (letter), *Trans. R. Soc. trop. Med. Hyg.*, 1972, *66*, 518.

Leukaemia, acute. References to the use of high-dose methotrexate therapy in patients with acute lymphoblastic leukaemia: J. J. Wang *et al.*, *Cancer Res.*, 1976, *36*, 1441; A. I. Freeman *et al.*, *Cancer Treat. Rep.*, 1977, *61*, 727; P. J. Moe and M. Seip, *Acta paediat. scand.*, 1978, *67*, 265.

High-dose methotrexate therapy with folinic acid rescue has been reported to have limited effectiveness in patients with acute myelogenous leukaemia.— R. P. Gale, *New Engl. J. Med.*, 1979, *300*, 1189. See also J. R. Bertino *et al.*, *Cancer Treat. Rep.*, 1977, *61*, 667.

See Choice of Antineoplastic Agent, p.178, for the use of methotrexate with other agents in the treatment of acute lymphoblastic leukaemia.

Meningeal leukaemia. No neurological complications were observed in 59 children with acute lymphoblastic leukaemia when treated with a single dose of methotrexate 10 µg per kg given intrathecally daily or every 2 to 3 days. This dose was considered to be as effective as the higher intrathecal doses of 150 to 500 µg per kg used by others.— F. Mollica *et al.* (letter), *Lancet*, 1971, *2*, 771. No serious neurological complication followed the use of methotrexate given intrathecally in a dose of 12 mg per m^2 to 45 children, therapeutically at intervals of 1 week or prophylactically every 90 days.— E. S. Baum and C. P. Holton (letter), *Lancet*, 1972, *1*, 380.

Although it has not been shown that intraventricular administration of methotrexate is clinically superior to lumbar puncture the number of episodes of recurrent meningeal leukaemia was reduced by use of the reservoir method.— W. R. Shapiro *et al.*, *New Engl. J. Med.*, 1975, *293*, 161.

A study indicating that there was considerably less variability in the concentrations of methotrexate achieved in CSF when a constant intrathecal dose of 12 mg was given rather than a dose of 12 mg per m^2 body-surface.— W. A. Bleyer, *Cancer Treat. Rep.*, 1977, *61*, 1419.

A retrospective comparison of methods of CNS prophylaxis in childhood leukaemia. The results strongly suggest that prophylactic cranial irradiation, administered shortly after bone-marrow remission is achieved, should remain an integral component of management for many children with acute lymphoblastic leukaemia.— D. M. Green *et al.*, *Lancet*, 1980, *1*, 1398. Comment.— M. E. Nesbit *et al.* (letter), *ibid.*, 1981, *1*, 322.

Further references to the use of intrathecal methotrexate in the treatment and prophylaxis of CNS leukaemia: D. Bramlet *et al.*, *Neurology, Minneap.*, 1976, *26*, 287 (meningeal carcinomatosis); F. S. Muriel *et al.*, *Br. J. Haemat.*, 1976, *34*, 119; M. A. Gribbin *et al.*, *Archs Dis. Childh.*, 1977, *52*, 673; M. Haghbin, *Cancer Treat. Rep.*, 1977, *61*, 661.

See also under Effects on the Nervous System in Adverse Effects (above).

Lupus erythematosus. A report of methotrexate and melphalan in the treatment of systemic lupus erythematosus.— F. Clement, *Schweiz. med. Wschr.*, 1973, *103*, 1369.

Lymphoma, non-Hodgkin's. A 69-year-old woman with cutaneous lymphosarcoma and symptomatic hypercalcaemia was given a continuous intravenous infusion of methotrexate, 5 mg in 1 litre of dextrose injection daily, until haematological toxicity was observed. The clinical condition of the patient improved immediately, with regression of the tumour mass and suppression of hypercalcaemia. Administration of methotrexate by mouth was ineffective.— W. J. Dube *et al.*, *J. Am. med. Ass.*, 1968, *203*, 359.

Reports of high-dose methotrexate therapy and folinic acid rescue in various non-Hodgkin's lymphomas: I. Djerassi and J. S. Kim, *Cancer*, 1976, *38*, 1043 (lymphosarcoma and histiocytic lymphoma); A. T. Skarin *et al.*, *Blood*, 1977, *50*, 1039.

Malignant neoplasms. For reports on the use of methotrexate with other agents in the treatment of various malignant neoplasms, see Choice of Antineoplastic Agent, p.180.

Some individual reports of methotrexate in the treatment of malignant neoplasms: J. K. Wyatt and L. N. McAninch, *Can. J. Surg.*, 1967, *10*, 421 (embryonal carcinoma of the testis); C. C. Altman *et al.*, *J. Urol.*, 1972, *108*, 271 (bladder); M. A. Broquet *et al.*, *Schweiz. med. Wschr.*, 1974, *104*, 18 (oropharyngeal-laryngeal squamous cell carcinoma); J. W. M. Vegers *et al.*, *Archs Otolar.*, 1979, *105*, 192 (squamous cell carcinoma of the buccal mucosa).

Malignant neoplasms of the brain. The identification of dihydrofolate reductase in tumours of the central nervous system provided a biochemical rationale for the use of antifolate compounds such as methotrexate in these tumours.— H. T. Abelson *et al.*, *Lancet*, 1978, *1*, 184.

High-dose methotrexate therapy consisting of a 4-hour intravenous infusion of 300 mg per kg body-weight of methotrexate followed by calcium folinate 9 mg by mouth 2 hours after the end of infusion and continued every 6 hours for 12 doses was administered to a 9-year-old boy with pontine glioma. This was repeated at intervals of 2 to 4 weeks using a dose of 500 mg per kg of methotrexate and 6 mg of calcium folinate. Adverse effects were mild nausea, stomatitis, and leucopenia. The patient's condition was improved by chemotherapy but 4 weeks after the last treatment he experienced a clinical relapse which did not respond to further methotrexate.— G. Rosen *et al.*, *J. Am. med. Ass.*, 1974, *230*, 1149. See also *idem*, *Cancer Treat. Rep.*, 1977, *61*, 681.

Further references to the use of high-dose methotrexate in the management of brain tumours: I. Djerassi *et al.*, *Cancer Treat. Rep.*, 1977, *61*, 691; W. R. Shapiro, *Cancer Treat. Rep.*, 1977, *61*, 753.

Malignant neoplasms of the bronchus and lung. Methotrexate in high doses (600 µg per kg body-weight twice weekly by intramuscular injection) and in low doses (200 µg per kg) given similarly was compared with a placebo in 227 patients with lung cancer. Tumour regression was dose-related and most obvious in epidermoid carcinoma. The incidence of overall tumour regression when it could be measured was 10 of 48 patients on the high dose, 4 of 37 on low dose, and 2 of 34 on placebo.— O. Selawry *et al.*, *Cancer*, 1977, *40*, 4.

Therapy with high doses of methotrexate with folinic acid rescue was considered to be potentially useful in the treatment of squamous cell carcinoma of the lung. A response or stabilisation of disease occurred in 6 of 13 patients after treatment but tumour response was poor.— K. Tornyos and H. Faust, *Cancer*, 1978, *41*, 400.

Further references: I. Djerassi, *Cancer*, 1972, *30*, 22; R. Bean, *Med. J. Aust.*, 1973, *2*, 737.

Malignant neoplasms of the head and neck. Methotrexate has been the drug most extensively studied in cancer of the head and neck and has been given by intra-arterial infusion or systemically, by mouth or intravenously, with or without folinic acid rescue. All these approaches have shown significant antitumour activity but none is clearly superior. In view of the toxicity of intra-arterial infusion the use of this route is questionable. Systemic methotrexate has been given mainly by intermittent weekly or twice-weekly intravenous injections; monthly courses of a 5-day loading dose programme of oral or intravenous administration have been less successful in reducing tumour size. Other schedules have included intravenous injection every 2 weeks and 1 to 3 mg per kg body-weight over 24 hours by continuous infusion, sometimes with folinic acid rescue.— Report of a WHO Expert Committee on Chemotherapy of Solid Tumours, *Tech. Rep. Ser. Wld Hlth Org. No. 605*, 1977, p. 54.

In a clinical study 38 patients with squamous cell carcinomas of upper-respiratory and digestive passages and the skin were treated with methotrexate. The dose of 30 mg per m^2 body-surface was given intravenously in 20 ml of saline weekly. The average dose was 50 mg weekly and this was increased to 100 mg if no response occurred. Complete healing occurred in 10 patients, 7 improved, and there was no effect in 16. No patient treated previously by radiotherapy or surgery showed complete healing.— G. F. Adler, *Med. J. Aust.*, 1973, *1*, 747.

Further reports of methotrexate in the treatment of malignant neoplasms of the head and neck: R. C. Donaldson, *Am. J. Surg.*, 1973, *126*, 507 (with BCG and isoniazid); N. Arlen, *Am. J. Surg.*, 1976, *132*, 536 (with radiotherapy); R. Papac *et al.*, *Cancer Res.*, 1978, *38*, 3150 (with or without BCG); S. G. Taylor *et al.*, *Archs Otolar.*, 1978, *104*, 647 (with folinic acid).

Organ and tissue transplantation. References to the use of methotrexate as an immunosuppressant in patients given bone-marrow transplants: E. D. Thomas *et al.*, *Lancet*, 1972, *1*, 284 (with cyclophosphamide); E. D. Thomas *et al.*, *New Engl. J. Med.*, 1975, *292*, 832.

Pregnancy and the neonate. *First trimester*. See Adverse Effects, above.

Second trimester. An apparently normal infant girl was born to a woman in whom acute leukaemia was diagnosed when she was 16 weeks pregnant, and who was treated with a regimen including methotrexate.— M. Khurshid and M. Saleem (letter), *Lancet*, 1978, *2*, 534.

Rheumatic disorders, non-malignant. Methotrexate is of potential value in the treatment of the most severe cases of psoriatic arthritis although toxicity constitutes a major threat. A single weekly dose is advisable and some authorities recommend liver biopsies before treatment and at yearly intervals while therapy continues. Intra-articular methotrexate may be of value and is less toxic than administration by mouth.— D. H. Loebl *et al.*, *J. Am. med. Ass.*, 1979, *242*, 2447. See also *Br. med. J.*, 1978, *1*, 262.

Following the beneficial result achieved with methotrexate 2.5 mg injected into each knee in a patient with persistent bilateral knee effusions due to chronic psoriatic arthropathy, 11 other patients with persistent knee effusions were also treated with intra-articular injections of methotrexate and 9 gained complete relief from inflammation or marked improvement.— G. H. Hall and Head A.C. (letter), *Lancet*, 1975, *2*, 409. Methotrexate 5 mg given by intra-articular injection with hydrocortisone 50 mg was no more effective than hydrocortisone alone in a study of 12 patients with chronic synovitis of the knee in rheumatoid arthritis.— J. S. Marks *et al.* (letter), *Lancet*, 1976, *2*, 857. See also G. H. Hall *et al.*, *Ann. rheum. Dis.*, 1978, *37*, 351.

Sarcoidosis. In the treatment of sarcoidosis methotrexate 25 mg once weekly initially, reduced gradually if improvement occurred, cleared cutaneous lesions in 12 of 16 patients and uveal lesions in 3 of the 4 patients in whom the eyes were also involved. The effect on hilar node, lung, and other sarcoidosis lesions was less certain.— N. K. Veien and H. Brodthagen, *Br. J. Derm.*, 1977, *97*, 213. Methotrexate should only be used if corticosteroids are contra-indicated.— B. L. Fanburg, *Am. J. Hosp. Pharm.*, 1979, *36*, 351.

Sarcoma. Methotrexate plus folinic acid as adjuvant therapy to surgery or radiation appeared to reduce the incidence of pulmonary metastases in patients with osteogenic sarcoma. Of 20 patients treated 19 were surviving after follow-up periods of 2 to 23 months. Treatment consisted of vincristine 2 mg per m^2 body-surface followed by methotrexate, initially 1.5 g per m^2 increasing to a maximum of 7.5 g per m^2 over 6 hours. Folinic acid 9 to 15 mg per m^2 was given by intramuscular injection every 6 hours for 12 doses starting 2 hours after the end of methotrexate infusion. This schedule was repeated at 2-weekly intervals.— N. Jaffe *et al.*, *New Engl. J. Med.*, 1974, *291*, 994. Improvement in the survival of patients with primary osteosarcomas was not related to postoperative adjuvant chemotherapy with vincristine and high doses of methotrexate.— J. H. Edmonson *et al.* (letter), *New Engl. J. Med.*, 1980, *303*, 642.

See also under Choice of Antineoplastic Agent, p.185.

Skin disorders, non-malignant. A review on methotrexate and its use in the treatment of various skin disorders. Methotrexate remains the drug of choice in the treatment of severe psoriasis although it may ultimately be replaced by photochemotherapy (see Methoxsalen, p.498). It has also been effective in mycosis fungoides, a cutaneous and systemic lymphoma, and has been used, sometimes with other immunosuppressants in disorders such as pemphigus, pityriasis, and polymyositis-dermatomyositis. Its lack of effect when used topically might be due to inadequate percutaneous penetration.— G. D. Weinstein, *Ann. intern. Med.*, 1977, *86*, 199.

References to the use of methotrexate in various skin disorders: R. L. Jetton and C. S. Eby, *Pediatrics*, 1971, *47*, 911 (no effect on epidermolytic hyperkeratosis); R. L. Cornelison *et al.*, *Archs Derm.*, 1972, *106*, 507 (pityriasis lichenoides et varioliformis acuta); W. F. Lever, *Archs Derm.*, 1972, *106*, 491 (pemphigus vulgaris); J. L. Kestel and D. S. Blair (letter), *Archs Derm.*, 1973, *108*, 723 (kerato-acanthoma).

Dermatomyositis. The current treatment of choice for corticosteroid-resistant polymyositis and dermatomyositis is probably methotrexate in association with a corticosteroid according to the method of A.L. Metzger *et al.* (*Ann. intern. Med.*, 1974, *81*, 182) in which methotrexate in an initial dose of 10 to 15 mg; increased gradually if tolerated to 500 to 800 µg per kg body-weight, was given weekly by intravenous injection together with prednisone, continued for about 6.5 months, and then decreased to twice monthly or monthly. Methotrexate toxicity has been relatively mild and always reversible and a substantial corticosteroid-sparing effect becomes apparent when muscle enzymes are normal. Two patients who had received methotrexate intravenously in a total dose of over 2 g did develop mild hepatotoxicity.— W. F. Durward (letter), *Br. med. J.*, 1976, *1*, 1341.

Five children with dermatomyositis that had not responded to corticosteroids were treated additionally with methotrexate (2 also received azathioprine). Four of the children were considered to be well after treatment with doses of up to 75 mg every 2 weeks and had received no treatment for up to 7 years. The fifth patient still had profound muscle weakness and rash and continued treatment with methotrexate 350 mg intravenously biweekly with folinic acid cover and prednisone 25 mg on alternate mornings.— J. C. Jacobs, *Pediatrics*, 1977, *59*, 212.

Further references to methotrexate in dermatomyositis: A. N. Malaviya *et al.*, *Lancet*, 1968, *2*, 485; R. Schrago and P. A. Miescher, *Schweiz. med. Wschr.*, 1974, *104*, 1311 (azathioprine, mercaptopurine, methotrexate, and sometimes prednisone); A. El-Ghobarey *et al.*, *Postgrad. med. J.*, 1978, *54*, 516.

Psoriasis. A retrospective study of 50 patients with chronic intractable psoriasis showed that 82% had benefited from treatment with methotrexate for periods of up to 15 years, without significant side-effects. Although serial biopsies indicated that methotrexate commonly caused liver changes at an average dose of 15 mg weekly, only 3 patients developed cirrhosis of the liver. Treatment was withdrawn in 6 further patients because of other side-effects.— L. G. Millard *et al.*, *Br. J. Derm.*, 1979, *101*, *Suppl.* 17, 14.

Further references to methotrexate in the treatment of psoriasis: H. Baker, *Br. J. Derm.*, 1970, *82*, 65; R. O. Noojin *et al.*, *Archs Derm.*, 1970, *101*, 646; H. Baker (letter), *Br. med. J.*, 1972, *1*, 506; H. H. Roenigk *et al.*, *Archs Derm.*, 1973, *108*, 35; G. C. Sauer, *Archs Derm.*, 1973, *107*, 369 (with hydroxyurea); C. Kennedy and H. Baker (letter), *Br. J. Derm.*, 1976, *94*, 702; R. J. Taylor and K. M. Halprin, *Br. J. Derm.*, 1977, *96*, 167; K. Weismann, *Acta derm.-vener.*, *Stockh.*, 1977, *57*, 185; A. E. Newburger *et al.*, *J. invest. Derm.*, 1978, *70*, 183.

For comment on the use of methotrexate in pustular psoriasis, see Corticosteroids, p.459.

See also under Rheumatic Disorders, Non-malignant (above) and under Effects on the Liver in Adverse Effects.

Wegener's granulomatosis. Two patients gained a remission from Wegener's granulomatosis when treated with methotrexate by mouth in weekly doses of 50 mg reduced to 25 or 15 mg.— R. L. Capizzi and J. R. Bertino, *Ann. intern. Med.*, 1971, *74*, 74.

Preparations

Methotrexate Injection *(B.P.)*. A sterile solution of methotrexate in Water for Injections containing sodium hydroxide. Sterilised by filtration. pH 8 to 9. When intended for intrathecal use it contains no preservative. Protect from light.

Methotrexate Sodium Injection *(U.S.P.)*. A sterile solution of methotrexate in Water for Injections prepared with the aid of sodium hydroxide. Potency is expressed in terms of methotrexate. pH 8 to 9. Protect from light.

Methotrexate Syrup. A liquid formulation of methotrexate to be taken by mouth and containing 10 mg in 5 ml may be prepared by adding 23 ml of vehicle to the contents of an ampoule of methotrexate injection containing 50 mg in 2 ml. The recommended vehicle contains syrup 25 g, sodium bicarbonate 2 g, and chloroform water to 100 ml. This formulation is stable for 3 months at room temperature.— M. Roach, *Lederle, Personal Communication*, 1978.

Methotrexate Tablets *(B.P.)*. Tablets containing methotrexate.

Methotrexate Tablets *(U.S.P.)*. Tablets containing methotrexate.

Proprietary Preparations

Emtexate *(Pharmachemie, Neth.: Nordic, UK)*. Vials each containing methotrexate sodium equivalent to methotrexate 0.5 and 1 g, free from preservatives; for preparing injection solutions of approximately pH 8.4. (Also available as Emtexate in *Ger.*, *Switz.*).

Emtexate PF *(Pharmachemie, Neth.: Nordic, UK)*. Methotrexate sodium, available as a solution (free from preservatives) containing the equivalent of methotrexate 2.5 or 25 mg per ml, in ampoules of 2 ml, adjusted to pH 7.5 to 8.8.

Methotrexate Injection *(Lederle, UK)*. Methotrexate sodium (not less than 94% purity), available as a solution (free from preservatives) containing the equivalent of methotrexate 2.5 or 25 mg per ml in ampoules of 1 or 2 ml, and 25 mg per ml in ampoules of 10 ml, with sodium chloride, and adjusted to approximately pH 8.5.

Methotrexate Powder for Injection 50 mg *(Lederle, UK)*. Vials each containing methotrexate sodium (not less than 94% purity) equivalent to methotrexate 50 mg, with sodium chloride, and methyl and propyl hydroxybenzoates; for preparing solutions of approximately pH 8.4 for injection. **Methotrexate Powder for Injection 500 mg**. Vials each containing methotrexate sodium equivalent to methotrexate 500 mg, free from preservatives.

Methotrexate Tablets *(Lederle, UK)*. Methotrexate (not less than 94% purity), available as scored tablets of 2.5 mg and tablets of 10 mg. (Also available as Methotrexate, tablets and injection, in *Austral.*, *Fr.*, *Switz.*, *USA*).

Other Proprietary Names
Emthexate *(Neth.)*; Ledertrexate *(Belg., Fr., Neth.)*; Methotrexat *(Ger.)*; Metotrexato *(Arg.)*; Mexate *(USA)*.

1846-f

Mithramycin *(U.S.P.)*. A2371; NSC 24559; PA 144; Aureolic Acid.

$C_{52}H_{76}O_{24}$=1085.2.

CAS — 18378-89-7.

Pharmacopoeias. In *U.S.*

An antineoplastic antibiotic produced by the growth of *Streptomyces argillaceus*, *S. plicatus* and *S. tanashiensis*. It is a yellow, odourless, hygroscopic, crystalline powder, containing not less than 90% of the activity of mithramycin, calculated on the dry basis. It loses not more than 8% of its weight when dried. Slightly **soluble** in water and methyl alcohol; very slightly soluble in alcohol; freely soluble in ethyl acetate. A 0.05% solution in water has a pH of 4.5 to 5.5. Solutions for injection are prepared by dissolving, immediately before use, the sterile contents of a sealed container in Water for Injections. **Store** at 2° to 8° in airtight containers. Protect from light.

Stability in solution. A solution of mithramycin 2.5 mg diluted with 1 litre of dextrose injection was stable for 4 to 6 hours at room temperature.— B. E. Kirschenbaum and C. J. Latiolais, *Am. J. Hosp. Pharm.*, 1976, *33*, 767.

Adverse Effects and Treatment. For an outline of the adverse effects experienced with antineoplastic agents and immunosuppressants and general guidelines for their treatment, see Antineoplastic Agents, p.171 and p.174. Gastro-intestinal effects are common during treatment with mithramycin. Other side-effects include fever, malaise, weakness, headache, depression, skin rashes, facial flushing, and reduced serum concentrations of calcium, phosphorus, and potassium. The main adverse effects are epistaxis and haematemesis leading to a bleeding syndrome, bone-marrow depression, manifest especially as thrombocytopenia, and reversible impairment of hepatic and renal function. Deaths have resulted from treatment.

Extravasation of mithramycin solutions may cause local irritation, cellulitis, phlebitis, and thrombosis.

Effects on the skin. Toxic epidermal necrolysis occurring in a 22-year-old man was attributed to treatment with mithramycin.— D. Purpora *et al.* (letter), *New Engl. J. Med.*, 1978, *299*, 1412.

Precautions. For reference to the precautions necessary with antineoplastic agents and immunosuppressants, see Antineoplastic Agents, p.175.

Mithramycin should only be given with great care to patients with impaired hepatic or renal function. It should not be administered to patients with depressed bone-marrow function or coagulation disorders.

Uses. Mithramycin is a highly toxic antibiotic with antineoplastic and hypocalcaemic properties. It may act by inhibiting synthesis of ribonucleic acid.

It is used in the treatment of inoperable metastatic neoplasms of the testis which cannot be treated by radiotherapy. The usual dose is 25 to 30 µg per kg body-weight daily by slow intravenous infusion over 4 to 6 hours in a litre of dextrose injection or sodium chloride injection for not more than 10 doses. Individual daily doses should not exceed 30 µg per kg. Doses have also been given on alternate days. Courses may be repeated at monthly intervals.

It is also used for the symptomatic treatment of hypercalcaemia and hypercalciuria. The usual dose is 25 µg per kg daily by slow intravenous infusion for 3 or 4 days. To achieve calcium balance further doses may be given at intervals of a week or more.

Platelet and white cell counts, bleeding time, prothrombin time, and hepatic and renal function should be determined frequently during treatment and for several days after, and treatment stopped if there is any sudden change.

Mithramycin was successfully used to reverse the hypoglycaemia which occurred in a 59-year-old woman with metastatic islet-cell carcinoma. After the first dose of 1 mg, given intravenously, serum-insulin concentration was rapidly reduced. A further 4 doses for mild episodes of hypoglycaemia were well tolerated.— D. T. Kiang *et al.*, *New Engl. J. Med.*, 1978, *299*, 134.

Administration in renal insufficiency. Doses of mithramycin should be reduced to 75% in patients with a glomerular filtration-rate of 10 to 50 ml per minute and to 50% when the rate is less than 10 ml per minute.— W. M. Bennett *et al.*, *Ann. intern. Med.*, 1980, *93*, 286. See also P. Veyssier *et al.*, *Nouv. Presse méd.*, 1976, *5*, 585.

Hypercalcaemia. A review of the management of hypercalcaemic crisis secondary to hyperparathyroidism or malignancy. Mithramycin is a potent hypocalcaemic agent which acts by a direct inhibition of bone resorption. V.G. Schweitzer *et al.* (*Archs Surg.*, 1978, *113*, 373) consider it to be the drug of choice when hypercalcaemia cannot be controlled by saline and frusemide. A dose of 25 µg per kg body-weight by intravenous bolus injection or infusion over 3 hours is usually effective in 12 to 36 hours and the hypocalcaemic response may persist for 3 to 7 days. Adverse effects are usually only encountered with repeated doses.— *Lancet*, 1978, *2*, 617. A review of hypercalcaemia and neoplastic disease.— T. M. Murray *et al.*, *Can. med. Ass. J.*, 1978, *119*, 915.

In a study in 16 patients with malignant disease, mithramycin given in a dosage of 25 µg per kg body-weight in 0.45% saline by continuous infusion for 8 days was shown to have a consistent hypocalcaemic effect leading to a fall in the urinary excretion of calcium despite a sustained calcium intake. Urinary output of hydroxyproline also fell under treatment with mithramycin. These results suggested mithramycin blocked the peripheral action of parathyroid hormone on gut and bone, either by direct action or by making the patient vitamin-D-resistant.— V. Parsons *et al.*, *Br. med. J.*, 1967, *1*, 474. Further studies of the hypocalcaemic effects of mithramycin: W. J. Dubé and R. A. Oberfield, *Lahey Clin. Bull.*, 1970, *19*, 85; D. T. Kiang *et al.*, *J. clin. Endocr. Metab.*, 1979, *48*, 341.

Pre-operative administration of mithramycin 25 µg per kg body-weight intravenously lowered the severely raised serum-calcium concentrations in a woman with Paget's disease and superimposed primary hyperparathyroidism, permitting safe operative treatment of the hyperparathyroidism.— J. D. Veldhuis (letter), *Lancet*, 1978, *1*, 1152.

Reports on the use of mithramycin in the treatment of cancer patients with hypercalcaemia: C. P. Perlia *et al.*, *Cancer*, 1970, *25*, 389; R. E. Slayton *et al.*, *Clin. Pharmac. Ther.*, 1971, *12*, 833; F. B. Stapleton *et al.*, *J. Pediat.*, 1976, *89*, 1029; H. J. Senn and P. Peyer, *Dt. med. Wschr.*, 1978, *103*, 101.

Malignant neoplasms of the testis. There were complete remissions in 2 and partial remission in 1 of 11 patients with progressive embryonal cancer who were given mithramycin in five daily doses of 30 µg per kg body-weight in a fast intravenous infusion, repeated at intervals of 4 to 8 weeks. There were partial remissions in 2 of 3 who developed severe haemorrhage when given daily doses of 50 µg per kg.— C. R. Koons *et al.*, *Bull. Johns Hopkins Hosp.*, 1966, *118*, 462. Further references: G. J. Hill *et al.*, *Cancer*, 1972, *30*, 900.

See also under Choice of Antineoplastic Agent, p.184.

Myeloma. Mithramycin 15 µg per kg body-weight daily by intravenous infusion for 4 days of benefit in 2 patients with osteolytic myelomatosis.— T. C. B. Stamp *et al.*, *Lancet*, 1975, *1*, 719.

Osteitis deformans. A review of the treatment of Paget's disease of bone. As well as relieving pain, therapy with mithramycin, calcitonin, or diphosphonates, returns increased osteoclastic bone resorption, osteoblastic activity, raised urinary excretion of hydroxyproline, and high plasma-alkaline-phosphatase activity towards normal. Nevertheless, Paget's disease of bone is still incurable and rebound may occur, especially with mithramycin. Drawbacks to the use of mithramycin include the necessity for administration by slow intravenous infusion and effects on the liver and kidneys.— *Lancet*, 1978, *1*, 914. Mithramycin is not selectively toxic to osteoclasts but would interfere with the metabolism of most active cells and therapy is usually accompanied by serious adverse effects. The main aim of specific therapy for Paget's disease should be to prevent complications and not to relieve pain, since the pain usually responds to analgesics.— R. Hamdy (letter), *ibid.*, 1267. The effect of mithramycin is short-lived and there seems little justification for its use when more effective and less toxic agents are available except possibly in patients with Paget's disease of bone resistant to combined treatment with calcitonin and diphosphonate.— H. K. Ibbertson *et al.*, *Drugs*, 1979, *18*, 33.

Further conflicting views on the use of mithramycin for Paget's disease of bone. A.S. Russell (*Lancet*, 1980, *1*, 884) has reported the successful use of low doses of mithramycin for the pain of Paget's disease. Doses of about 10 µg per kg body-weight were given daily by intravenous injection for 10 days and complete relief of pain was achieved by 4 or 5 days. Although this regimen was reported to be safe, I.M.A. Evans and J.C. Stevenson (*ibid.*, 1093) have criticised the use of such a potentially toxic drug when there is a safe alternative in calcitonin. C. Nagant de Deuxchaisnes *et al.*(*ibid.*, 1193) consider that, unlike calcitonin, it has not been proved that mithramycin can strengthen bone and control the disease process while relieving pain. The toxicity of mithramycin necessitates extensive monitoring of the patient during treatment and calcitonin is considered preferable.

Mithramycin was given to 13 out-patients with disseminated Paget's disease of bone in 1 of 3 regimens. A dose of 15 or 25 µg per kg body-weight was given as an intravenous bolus injection in 5 ml of water on 5 consecutive days each week for 4 weeks, or once a week for up to 14 months, or twice weekly for up to 5 months. All patients experienced improvement of symptoms and a decrease in serum alkaline phosphatase concentration. In several patients the disease was in remission 8 months after therapy. Hepatotoxicity seemed related to dose and frequency of administration.— D. Lebbin *et al.*, *Ann. intern. Med.*, 1974, *81*, 635.

Further references to mithramycin in the treatment of Paget's disease of bone: J. M. Aitken and R. Lindsay (letter), *Lancet*, 1973, *1*, 1177; W. G. Ryan (letter), *Lancet*, 1973, *1*, 1319; A. G. Hadjipavlou *et al.*, *J. Bone Jt Surg.*, 1977, *59*, 1045; W. G. Ryan, *Clin. Orthop.*, 1977, *127*, 106; A. S. Russell *et al.*, *Arthritis Rheum.*, 1979, *22*, 215; W. G. Ryan *et al.* (letter), *Ann. intern. Med.*, 1980, *92*, 129.

Sarcoma. Two of 5 patients with progressive metastatic Ewing's sarcoma had excellent regression of their tumours following treatment with mithramycin. One patient remained tumour-free after more than 7 years.— S. Kofman *et al.*, *Cancer*, 1973, *31*, 889, per *Int. pharm. Abstr.*, 1974, *11*, 391.

Preparations

Mithramycin for Injection *(U.S.P.)*. A sterile dry mixture of mithramycin and mannitol; each pack contains 2.5 mg of mithramycin. It may contain a suitable buffer. A solution prepared as directed has a pH of 5 to 7.5. Store at 2° to 8°. Protect from light.

Mithracin *(Pfizer, UK)*. Vials each containing mithramycin 2.5 mg, with mannitol 100 mg and sodium phosphate, as powder for preparing a solution containing 500 µg per ml by the addition of 4.9 ml of Water for Injections, for intravenous infusion. (Also available as Mithracin in *Austral., Norw., USA*).

Other Proprietary Names
Mithracine *(Fr.)*.

1847-d

Mitobronitol *(B.P.)*. Dibromomannitol; DBM; NSC 94100; R 54; WR 220057. 1,6-Dibromo-1,6-dideoxy-D-mannitol.

$C_6H_{12}Br_2O_4$=308.0.

CAS — 488-41-5.

Pharmacopoeias. In *Br.* and *Chin.*

A white or almost white odourless crystalline solid. M.p. 178°. **Soluble** 1 in 500 of water, 1 in 200 of alcohol, and 1 in 135 of acetone; soluble in dimethylformamide and hot methyl alcohol; practically insoluble in chloroform. It is slowly hydrolysed in acid solutions. **Protect** from light.

Adverse Effects, Treatment, and Precautions. For an outline of the adverse effects experienced with antineoplastic agents and immunosuppressants, general guidelines for their treatment, and precautions, see Antineoplastic Agents, p.171, pp.174-5.

Bone-marrow depression during treatment with mitobronitol may be severe.

Effects on the eyes. A report of an association between mitobronitol and cataract.— S. M. Podos and G. P. Canellos, *Am. J. Ophthal.*, 1969, *68*, 500.

Absorption and Fate. Mitobronitol is readily absorbed from the gastro-intestinal tract and is excreted through the liver into the bile with reabsorption in the small intestine. It is eliminated in the urine, partly as bromine-containing metabolites. Mitobronitol in the plasma is mainly bound to albumin and only slowly loses its alkylating activity.

Uses. Mitobronitol is an antineoplastic agent which appears to act as an alkylating agent and has similar properties to those of busulphan (p.194). It has been used in the treatment of chronic myeloid leukaemia.

The usual dose is 250 mg daily until the white cell count falls to 20 000 per mm^3 when a maintenance dosage of about 125 mg daily or on alternate days is given, adjusted according to the white cell count. Frequent examination of the blood should be performed during treatment.

Leukaemia, chronic. The use of mitobronitol in chronic myelocytic leukaemia.— C. Tomov *et al.*, *Therapia hung.*, 1976, *24*, 56.

Preparations

Mitobronitol Tablets *(B.P.).* Tablets containing mitobronitol. Protect from light.

Myelobromol *(Sinclair, UK).* Mitobronitol, available as tablets of 125 mg. (Also available as Myelobromol in *Ger., Switz.*).

Other Proprietary Names

Myebrol *(Jap.)*.

1848-n

Mitoguazone. Methylglyoxal Bisguanylhydrazone; Methyl GAG. 1,1′-[(Methylethanediylidene)dinitrilo]-diguanidine.

$C_5H_{12}N_8$=184.2.

CAS — 459-86-9.

Uses. Mitoguazone is an antineoplastic agent (p.171) which has been used as the hydrochloride or acetate in the treatment of acute myeloblastic leukaemia. It has been given by intravenous infusion in doses of about 150 mg per m^2 body-surface daily.

For a short review of the adverse effects, absorption and fate, and use of mitoguazone, see V. T. Oliverio and C. G. Zubrod, *A. Rev. Pharmac.*, 1965, *5*, 335.

Proprietary Names

Méthyl-GAG *(Riom, Fr.)*.

1849-h

Mitolactol. Dibromodulcitol; DBD; NSC 104800; WR 138743. 1,6-Dibromo-1,6-dideoxy-D-galactitol.

$C_6H_{12}Br_2O_4$=308.0.

CAS — 10318-26-0.

A white crystalline powder. M.p. 186° to 190°. **Soluble** 1 in about 3000 of water; practically insoluble in organic solvents.

Adverse Effects, Treatment, and Precautions. For an outline of the adverse effects experienced with antineoplastic agents and immunosuppressants, general guidelines for their treatment, and precautions, see Antineoplastic Agents, p.171, pp.174-5.

Myelosuppression is the most significant adverse effect of mitolactol.

Uses. Mitolactol is an antineoplastic agent which may act by alkylation (p.171). It has been given by mouth in the treatment of metastatic breast carcinoma, squamous cell carcinoma of the head and neck, malignant melanoma, and other solid tumours. Doses of 2.5 to 3.5 mg per kg body-weight daily have been given. Blood counts should be taken regularly during treatment and mitolactol withdrawn if bone-marrow depression occurs.

Reviews of mitolactol: I. Gonda, *Gyógyszerészet*, 1976, *20*, 178, per *Int. pharm. Abstr.*, 1977, *14*, 274; N. E. Mischler *et al.*, *Cancer Treat. Rev.*, 1979, *6*, 191.

Mitolactol is rapidly absorbed from the gastro-intestinal tract. Following a dose of 15 mg per kg body-weight it has been detected in the blood in 15 minutes with peak plasma concentrations achieved in 1 hour. It is widely distributed in the body and is firmly bound to red blood cells; it diffuses into the cerebrospinal fluid and into pleural and ascitic fluid. Mitolactol is rapidly hydrolysed to monobromodulcitol and various diepoxides; within 2 hours of a dose less than 5% is reported to be unchanged. Renal excretion is the only known route of elimination and 70 to 80% of a dose is present in the urine within 48 hours as unchanged drug and metabolites, some of which have alkylating activity. Dianhydrogalactitol is the most stable of the diepoxihexitol derivatives and has the most pronounced biological effect.— N. E. Mischler *et al.*, *Cancer Treat. Rev.*, 1979, *6*, 191. See also M. A. Belej *et al.*, *Clin. Pharmac. Ther.*, 1972, *13*, 563.

Reports on the use of mitolactol in various malignant disorders: G. Perényi *et al.*, *Therapia hung.*, 1977, *25*, 16 (squamous cell pulmonary cancer); D. C. Tormey *et al.*, *Cancer Res.*, 1977, *37*, 529 (with doxorubicin in metastatic breast carcinoma); R. E. Bellet *et al.*, *Cancer Treat. Rep.*, 1978, *62*, 2095 (malignant melanoma); J. K. Luce, *Cancer Treat. Rep.*, 1978, *62*, 2009 (malignant melanoma).

Proprietary Names

Elobromol *(Chinoin, Hung.)*.

1850-a

Mitomycin *(U.S.P.).* Mitomycin C; Mitomycin X; NSC 26980; 7-Amino-9α-methoxymitosane. 6-Amino-1,1a,2,8,8a,8b-hexahydro-8-hydroxymethyl-8a-methoxy-5-methylazirino[2′,3′:3,4]-pyrrolo[1,2-*a*]indole-4,7-dione carbamate.

$C_{15}H_{18}N_4O_5$=334.3.

CAS — 50-07-7.

Pharmacopoeias. In *Jap.* and *U.S.*

An antineoplastic antibiotic produced by the growth of *Streptomyces caespitosus.* It has a potency of not less than 900 µg per mg. It occurs as a blue-violet crystalline powder. **Soluble** in water, acetone, methyl alcohol, butyl acetate, and cyclohexanone; sparingly soluble in ether. A 0.5% solution in water has a pH of 6 to 8. Stable for at least 2 years at room temperature. Solutions in water are most stable at pH 6 to 9. The colour of solutions varies with pH. **Store** in airtight containers. Protect from light.

A discussion on the structural relationship of mitomycin A and B with antibacterial activity and of mitomycin C with antitumour activity.— A. Andreani and G. Mungiovino, *Boll. chim.-farm.*, 1979, *118*, 192, per *Int. pharm. Abstr.*, 1980, *17*, 126.

A conjugate of mitomycin with dextran was a potential high molecular weight pro-drug of mitomycin.— T. Kojima *et al.*, *J. Pharm. Pharmac.*, 1980, *32*, 30.

Adverse Effects, Treatment, and Precautions. For an outline of the adverse effects experienced with antineoplastic agents and immunosuppressants, general guidelines for their treatment, and precautions, see Antineoplastic Agents, p.171, pp.174-5.

The main adverse effect of mitomycin is delayed cumulative bone-marrow suppression. Profound leucopenia and thrombocytopenia occurs after about 4 weeks with recovery in about 8 weeks. Blood counts may not recover in about one-quarter of patients. Fatalities have been reported. Other serious adverse-effects include renal damage and pulmonary reactions. Local tissue necrosis occurs if the solution escapes from the vein.

Mitomycin is contra-indicated in patients with impaired renal function.

Effects on the kidneys. Evidence that long-term therapy with mitomycin and fluorouracil is hazardous, in that it appears to produce a low-grade haemolytic-uraemic state. Attempts to correct this by compatible blood transfusions in 2 patients led to exacerbation of the haemolytic process, with schistocytes in the peripheral blood, rapidly progressive renal failure, and death. Treatment with corticosteroids, antiplatelet drugs, and fresh frozen plasma had no significant effect in the patient in whom these were tried. The therapeutic regimen of mitomycin with fluorouracil should be terminated at the first sign of intravascular haemolysis, persistent proteinuria, and rising serum-urea concentrations.— B. G. Jones *et al.*, *Lancet*, 1980, *1*, 1275. Dose correction, and report of a patient who had a rash while on chemotherapy, followed, 2 months after his last dose of mitomycin, by nephritis, renal insufficiency, haemolysis, and severe hypertension.— D. A. Karlin and J. R. Stroehlein (letter), *ibid.*, *2*, 534. Chronic haemolysis and progressive renal impairment following a prolonged course of fluorouracil, doxorubicin, and mitomycin. This patient also deteriorated clinically following red cell transfusion. Limited success was obtained after one plasmaphaeresis (the platelet count increased, but the azotaemia and anaemia got worse) but the patient died before the efficacy could be adequately assessed.— K. D. Lempert (letter), *ibid.*, *2*, 369. Haemolysis and renal failure in a woman treated with mitomycin without fluorouracil. Once again, the symptoms got worse with blood transfusion, and there was a latency period of about 4 months after the last mitomycin treatment.— K. W. Rumpf *et al.* (letter), *ibid.*, *2*, 1037.

Further references: K. Liu *et al.*, *Cancer*, 1971, *28*, 1314.

Effects on respiratory function. Reports of pulmonary reactions associated with mitomycin: J. W. L. Fielding *et al.*, *Br. med. J.*, 1978, *2*, 602; *ibid.*, 1979, *2*, 551 (interstitial fibrosis); E. S. Orwoll *et al.*, *Ann. intern. Med.*, 1978, *89*, 352 (interstitial pneumonia); A. T. Andrews *et al.* (letter), *ibid.*, 1979, *90*, 127 (interstitial pneumonia); K. W. Rumpf *et al.* (letter), *Lancet*, 1980, *2*, 1037 (pulmonary fibrosis).

Interactions. For a report of mitomycin possibly enhancing the cardiotoxicity of doxorubicin, see A. U. Buzdar *et al.*, *Cancer Treat. Rep.*, 1978, *62*, 1005.

Absorption and Fate. Mitomycin disappears rapidly from the blood after intravenous injection. It is widely distributed but does not appear to cross the blood-brain barrier. Mitomycin is metabolised mainly in the liver; up to 10% of a dose is excreted unchanged in the urine.

Uses. Mitomycin is a highly toxic antibiotic with antineoplastic properties. It acts as an alkylating agent (p.171) after activation *in vivo* and also suppresses the synthesis of nucleic acids.

Mitomycin is used, often with other antineoplastic agents, in the palliative treatment of gastric, pancreatic, and colorectal adenocarcinomas. It has also been given to patients with other solid tumours including those of the bladder and breast. The usual dose is 10 to 20 mg per m^2 body-surface given as a single dose through a running intravenous infusion and repeated every 6 to 8 weeks. Alternatively it may be given intravenously in divided doses of 2 mg per m^2 daily for 5 days, repeated after 2 days for a further 5 days. Subsequent doses are adjusted according to the effect on bone marrow and treatment should not be repeated until the leucocyte count is above 3000 per mm^3 and the platelet count above 75 000 per mm^3.

Mitomycin is also used as a bladder instillation: 4 to 10 mg is instilled daily in the prevention of recurrent bladder tumours and 10 to 40 mg is instilled in the treatment of bladder tumours.

Action. A discussion on the mechanism of action of mitomycin.— H. W. Moore, *Science*, 1977, *197*, 527.

Administration. The use of arterial infusion of mitomycin microencapsulated with ethylcellulose in 2 patients with renal cell carcinoma. These preliminary results suggest that arterial infusion of mitomycin microcapsules is effective in cancer patients with an invasive primary lesion or a localised metastatic lesion where selective catheterisation is possible.— T. Kato *et al.* (letter), *Lancet*, 1979, *2*, 479.

Malignant neoplasms. A randomised study of 2 combination chemotherapy regimens in patients with metastatic adenocarcinomas of unknown primary site suggested that treatment with doxorubicin and mitomycin may be useful.— R. L. Woods *et al.*, *New Engl. J. Med.*, 1980, *303*, 87.

Malignant neoplasms of the breast. A complete or partial response was obtained in 13 of 48 patients who had malignant neoplasms of the breast refractory to hormonal and/or combination chemotherapy after treatment with megestrol acetate 40 mg four times daily and mitomycin 20 mg per m^2 body-surface intravenously every 4 to 6 weeks. The mean survival-time for patients who responded to treatment was 7 months compared with 2 months in non-responders. The myelosuppressive toxicity of mitomycin was cumulative and therefore smaller doses were given in subsequent courses at increasing intervals.— A. U. Buzdar *et al.*, *Cancer*, 1978, *41*, 392.

A report of beneficial results in 5 of 6 patients with locally recurrent breast cancer not responding to radiotherapy, endocrine treatment, or systemic chemotherapy, when they were given 1 to 6 courses of mitomycin in the internal mammary artery.— W. Mattsson *et al.* (letter), *Lancet*, 1980, *2*, 925.

See also Choice of Antineoplastic Agent, p.180.

Malignant neoplasms of the gastro-intestinal tract. Mitomycin is the drug most commonly used to treat gastric cancer in Japan and is second to fluorouracil in the USA. The response-rate is about 30% with durations of response ranging from 1 to 3 months. Combination chemotherapy regimens including mitomycin appear to be more successful. Mitomycin is also capable of inducing regressions in colorectal cancer but toxicity limits its usefulness.— Report of a WHO Expert Committee on Chemotherapy of Solid Tumours, *Tech. Rep. Ser. Wld Hlth Org. No. 605*, 1977, p. 32.

Further references: C. G. Moertel *et al.*, *J. Am. med. Ass.*, 1968, *204*, 1045 (mitomycin in advanced gastro-intestinal cancer); T. Nakajima *et al.*, *Int. J. clin. Pharmac. Biopharm.*, 1978, *16*, 209 (adjuvant chemotherapy of gastric cancer with mitomycin).

For the use of mitomycin with other agents in the treatment of gastric cancer, see Choice of Antineoplastic Agent, p.183.

Malignant neoplasms of the liver. For beneficial results with fluorouracil and mitomycin, given by intra-arterial infusion in carcinoma of the liver, see Fluorouracil, p.211.

Malignant neoplasms of the pancreas. After fluorouracil, mitomycin is the most extensively used drug in pancreatic cancer and response-rates for the two drugs are similar. There is a risk of delayed toxicity to the bone marrow with mitomycin.— Report of a WHO Expert Committee on Chemotherapy of Solid Tumours, *Tech. Rep. Ser. Wld Hlth Org. No. 605*, 1977, p. 36.

Preparations

Mitomycin for Injection *(U.S.P.)*. A dry mixture of mitomycin and mannitol. A solution prepared as directed has a pH of 6 to 8. Protect from light.
Mitomycin for Injection may be reconstituted by shaking with Water for Injections and allowing to stand if necessary; a blue-grey solution is produced. Reconstituted solutions are reported to be stable for 14 days if refrigerated or 7 days at room temperature, protected from light. Such solutions may be further diluted for administration by intravenous infusion and are reported to be stable for 3 hours in dextrose injection, 12 hours in sodium chloride injection, or 24 hours in sodium lactate injection at room temperature.

Mitomycin-C *(Kyowa, Jap.: Martindale Pharmaceuticals, UK)*. Mitomycin, available as powder, for preparing injections, in vials containing 2 and 10 mg, with sodium chloride. (Also available as Mitomycin-C in *Austral.*).

Other Proprietary Names

Amétycine *(Fr.)*; Mitomycine *(Belg.)*; Mutamycin *(Canad., USA)*.

1851-t

Mitopodozide.

SPI. 2′-Ethylpodophyllohydrazide; 2′-Ethyl-1,2,3,4-tetrahydro-4-hydroxy-3-hydroxymethyl-6,7-methylenedioxy-1-(3,4,5-trimethoxyphenyl)-2-naphthohydrazide.
$C_{24}H_{30}N_2O_8$=474.5.

CAS — 1508-45-8.

An amorphous powder.

Uses. Mitopodozide is an antineoplastic agent derived from podophyllin and has properties similar to those of etoposide (p.208). It has been given intravenously and has been applied locally, in the treatment of malignant neoplasms. Doses of 200 mg have been administered by slow intravenous injection and up to 1 g has been given by infusion.
A glucoside derivative of mitopodozide has been given by mouth.

Proprietary Names
Proresid *(Sandoz, Ger.)*.

1852-x

Mitotane

(U.S.P.). CB313; NSC 38721; WR 13045; *o,p′*DDD; Ortho-para-prime DDD. 1,1-Dichloro-2-(2-chlorophenyl)-2-(4-chlorophenyl)ethane.
$C_{14}H_{10}Cl_4$=320.0.

CAS — 53-19-0.

Pharmacopoeias. In *U.S.*

A white crystalline powder with a slight aromatic odour. M.p. 75° to 81°. Practically **insoluble** in water; soluble in alcohol, ether, light petroleum, and in fixed oils. **Store** in airtight containers. Protect from light.

Adverse Effects. Almost all patients given mitotane experience anorexia, nausea, and vomiting and about 40% suffer some central toxicity with dizziness, sedation, lethargy, and vertigo. Permanent brain damage may develop with prolonged dosage. Ocular side-effects may occur with blurred vision, diplopia, lenticular opacities, and retinopathy. Other side-effects include allergic reactions, diarrhoea, skin rashes, renal impairment, haemorrhagic cystitis, flushing, hypertension, and orthostatic hypotension.

Precautions. Mitotane inhibits the adrenal cortex and adrenal insufficiency may develop during treatment. In trauma or shock corticosteroids should be given systemically. It should be given with care to patients with liver disease and its use should be avoided during pregnancy. Patients should not take charge of vehicles or machinery where loss of attention may lead to accidents. Behavioural and neurological assessments should be carried out regularly.

Interactions. Administration of mitotane up to 3 g daily to a 65-year-old patient with Cushing's syndrome appeared to be ineffective and did not produce the side-effects usually associated with mitotane whilst the patient was also receiving treatment with spironolactone.— J. Wortsman and N. G. Soler, *J. Am. med. Ass.*, 1977, *238*, 2527.

Absorption and Fate. Up to 40% of a dose of mitotane is absorbed from the gastro-intestinal tract. After daily doses of 5 to 15 g, concentrations in the blood of 7 to 90 µg per ml of unchanged drug and 29 to 54 µg per ml of metabolite have been reported. Mitotane has been detected in the blood 10 weeks after stopping treatment. It is widely distributed and appears to be stored mainly in fatty tissues. From 10 to 25% of a dose has been recovered in the urine as a water-soluble metabolite. About 60% of a dose is excreted unchanged in the faeces.

Metabolism of mitotane was shown to involve hydroxylation and oxidation.— V. D. Reif *et al.*, *J. pharm. Sci.*, 1974, *63*, 1730.

Uses. Mitotane is an antineoplastic agent with a selective inhibitory action on adrenal cortex activity. It is given in the treatment of inoperable adrenocortical tumours and has also been used in patients with Cushing's syndrome.
The usual initial dosage is 9 to 10 g daily by mouth in 3 or 4 divided doses, adjusted to the maximum tolerated dose which may range from 2 to 16 g daily. Patients are treated in hospital until a stable dosage is determined.

Mitotane had a uricosuric action in a 34-year-old woman with Cushing's syndrome.— G. Reach *et al.* (letter), *Lancet*, 1978, *1*, 1269. See also B. Zumoff, *Am. J. med. Sci.*, 1979, *278*, 145.

Cushing's syndrome. Mitotane 4 to 12 g daily was given for an average of 8 months (range 3 to 34 months) to 62 patients with Cushing's syndrome. Cobalt irradiation of the pituitary was also carried out in 16 of the patients before or during treatment with mitotane. Remissions were achieved in 38 of the 46 patients who received only mitotane and in all of the 16 who also received irradiation. Relapses occurred in 20 of the 38 an average of 17 months later and further treatment was required; in 14 patients Cushing's syndrome was still controlled 6 to 80 months later. Overall, the syndrome had been controlled in 63% of the patients and surgery avoided so far. Nausea, vomiting, and anorexia were common side-effects and occasionally treatment had to be interrupted; 2 patients experienced hypersialorrhoea. A rash in one patient disappeared when the dose was reduced. Chloasma occurred in a non-pregnant patient. A few patients experienced drowsiness but severe cerebral effects in 4, including cerebral atrophy and cerebral thrombosis, might not have been related to the use of mitotane. Serum-cholesterol concentrations were elevated but returned to basal values on withdrawal of the drug; alkaline phosphatase concentrations also increased. Gynaecomastia in 8 of 16 male patients was reversed when mitotane was discontinued but gonadal function did not appear to be disturbed in either sex.— J. P. Luton *et al.*, *New Engl. J. Med.*, 1979, *300*, 459. Criticism of the use of mitotane and the view that trans-sphenoidal resection of pituitary adenomas is the treatment of choice for Cushing's disease.— P. R. Cooper and W. A. Shucart (letter), *ibid.*, *301*, 48. In some cases the alternative of adrenalectomy or mitotane may still be the therapeutic choice.— H. Bricaire *et al.* (letter), *ibid.*, 49.

Remission was achieved in 29 of 36 patients with Cushing's disease who were given low doses of mitotane in association with irradiation of the pituitary. Remission was maintained after treatment was discontinued in 17 patients. Initial doses of 4 g daily in divided doses were gradually reduced during the first 3 to 4 months to 1.5 to 2 g daily. After sustained suppression of cortisol concentrations for many months and with remission of the disease, the dose was decreased to as low as 500 mg twice weekly in some patients. The longest duration of treatment at these low doses was 7 years.— D. E. Schteingart *et al.*, *Ann. intern. Med.*, 1980, *92*, 613. Criticism.— A. Sacerdote *et al.* (letter), *ibid.*, 1981, *94*, 141. Reply.— D. E. Schteingart (letter), *ibid.*

Further references to the use of mitotane in Cushing's syndrome: T. E. Temple *et al.*, *New Engl. J. Med.*, 1969, *281*, 801; A. Golik *et al.*, *Harefuah*, 1975, *89*, 563; Z. Dickerman *et al.*, *Israel J. med. Scis*, 1979, *15*, 455.

Malignant neoplasms of the adrenal cortex. Mitotane was given to 115 patients with inoperable malignant neoplasms of the adrenal cortex. Dosage ranged from about 2 g daily up to the maximum tolerated dose of 16 g. Tumour regression was measurable in 32 patients and ranged from 1 to 36 months. Overall clinical improvement occurred in 54 of 100 patients who could be evaluated.— J. A. Lubitz *et al.*, *J. Am. med. Ass.*, 1973, *223*, 1109.

Further references to the use of mitotane in adrenocortical carcinoma: A. M. Hutter and D. E. Kayhoe, *Am. J. Med.*, 1966, *41*, 581; R. D. M. Scott, *Postgrad. med. J.*, 1975, *51*, 35 (Cushing's syndrome due to adrenocortical carcinoma); J. Takamatsu *et al.* (letter), *New Engl. J. Med.*, 1981, *305*, 957 (effect on pituitary).

Preparations

Mitotane Tablets *(U.S.P.)*. Tablets containing mitotane. Store in airtight containers. Protect from light.

Proprietary Names

Lysodren *(Bristol, Canad.; Bristol, USA)*.

1853-r

Mustine Hydrochloride

(B.P.). Chlormethine Hydrochloride; Chlorethazine Hydrochloride; Chlormethini Hydrochloridum; Mechlorethamine Hydrochloride *(U.S.P.)*; Nitrogen Mustard; HN2; NSC 762; WR 147650. *NN*-Bis(2-chloroethyl)methylamine hydrochloride; 2,2′-Dichloro-*N*-methyldiethylamine hydrochloride.
$C_5H_{11}Cl_2N,HCl$=192.5.

CAS — 51-75-2 (mustine); 55-86-7 (hydrochloride).

Pharmacopoeias. In *Br.*, *Chin.*, *Fr.*, *Jug.*, and *U.S.*

A white or almost white, hygroscopic, vesicant, crystalline powder or mass. M.p. 108° to 111°. Very **soluble** in water. A 0.2% solution in water has a pH of 3 to 5. Solutions lose their activity very rapidly. Solutions for injections are prepared by dissolving, immediately before use, the sterile contents of a sealed container in Water for Injections or sodium chloride injection. Unused solutions may be neutralised by mixing with an equal volume of a solution containing sodium thiosulphate 5% and sodium bicarbonate 5% and allowing to stand for 45 minutes; apparatus used in the preparation of mustine hydrochloride solutions may be treated similarly.

Store in a cool place in airtight containers.

CAUTION. *Mustine hydrochloride is a strong vesicant; avoid contact with skin and mucous membranes.*

Adverse Effects. For an outline of the adverse effects experienced with antineoplastic agents and immunosuppressants, see Antineoplastic Agents, p.171.

Mustine hydrochloride is extremely toxic and its use is invariably accompanied by side-effects. Severe nausea and vomiting may commence within an hour of injection of the drug and last for some hours. It causes varying degrees of bone-marrow depression depending on the dose. When the total dose for a single course exceeds 400 µg per kg body-weight there is a risk of severe and possibly fatal depression with anaemia, lymphocytopenia, granulocytopenia, and thrombocytopenia with consequent haemorrhage. Depression of lymphocytes may be apparent within 24 hours of the administration of mustine hydrochloride and maximum suppression of granulocytes and platelets occurs within 7 to 21 days; haematological recovery may be adequate after 4 weeks.

Tinnitus, vertigo, and deafness have been reported. Skin reactions to mustine hydrochloride include maculopapular rashes. There is a high incidence of hypersensitivity when topical preparations are used in conditions such as psoriasis. Mustine hydrochloride has a powerful vesicant action on the skin and mucous membranes and great care must be taken to avoid contact with the eyes. Extravasation of the injection causes severe irritation and even sloughing. Thrombophlebitis is a potential hazard of mustine if it is not sufficiently diluted.

Allergy and anaphylaxis. Severe urticarial reactions occurred in two patients 2.5 years and 1 year respectively after commencing topical whole body applications of mustine hydrochloride for the treatment of mycosis fungoides.— E. Grunnet, *Br. J. Derm.*, 1976, *94*, 101. See also D. Daughters *et al.*, *Archs Derm.*, 1973, *107*, 429 (urticarial and anaphylactoid reactions).

Effects on the ears. For reports of ototoxicity associated with mustine hydrochloride, see J. Ballantyne, *J. Lar. Otol.*, 1972, *84*, 967; *idem*, *Audiology*, 1973, *12*, 325.

Effects on the nervous system. Cerebral toxicity has been reported in a patient given mustine.— N. C. Bethlenfalvay and J. J. Bergin, *Cancer*, 1969, *29*, 366.

Effects on the skin. A report of erythema multiforme associated with mustine.— M. J. Brauer *et al.*, *Archs intern. Med.*, 1967, *120*, 499.

Local irritant effects. Fatal necrosis of the aorta was associated with the infusion of mustine hydrochloride into the bronchial artery of a 33-year-old woman.— R. J. Steckel *et al.*, *J. Am. med. Ass.*, 1967, *199*, 936.

Treatment of Adverse Effects. For general guidelines, see Antineoplastic Agents, p.174.

The administration of anti-emetics and sedation before injection of mustine hydrochloride may help to control severe nausea and vomiting.

If extravasation occurs during injection, the involved area should be infiltrated with a 3% solution of sodium thiosulphate, followed by the application of an ice compress intermittently for 6 to 12 hours. A 1% lignocaine solution may also be infiltrated.

Precautions. For reference to the precautions necessary with antineoplastic agents and immunosuppressants, see Antineoplastic Agents, p.175.

Absorption and Fate. Mustine is only partially absorbed from serous surfaces. Following intravenous injection, it is rapidly converted to a reactive ethyleneimmonium ion. It usually disappears from the blood in a few minutes. A very small proportion is excreted unchanged in the urine.

Uses. Mustine belongs to the group of antineoplastic drugs described as alkylating agents (see p.171). It also possesses immunosuppressant properties.

Mustine hydrochloride is used in the treatment of Hodgkin's disease, usually in conjunction with a vinca alkaloid, procarbazine, and prednisone. It may also be used in other lymphomas and in carcinoma of the lung and other solid tumours. In mycosis fungoides with extensive skin involvement, very dilute solutions of mustine have been applied topically.

See also under Choice of Antineoplastic Agent, p.175.

Single doses of mustine hydrochloride of 400 µg per kg body-weight or a course of 4 daily doses of 100 µg per kg are usually given by intravenous injection in a strength of 1 mg per ml in sodium chloride injection. Rapid injection into the tubing of a fast running intravenous infusion of sodium chloride injection or dextrose injection may reduce, but not abolish, the incidence of thrombophlebitis. A solution of 1 mg in 50 ml of sodium chloride injection has been infused slowly. Doses of 6 mg per m^2 body-surface are used in the combination schedules for Hodgkin's disease. The response should be assessed by the trend of the blood counts. Treatment with mustine may be repeated when the bone-marrow function has recovered.

Intracavitary injections of 200 to 400 µg per kg have been given in the treatment of malignant, especially pleural, effusions.

Gastro-intestinal disorders. The use of ribbon gauze soaked in a solution of mustine hydrochloride in the local treatment of a rectoperineal fistula and an associated benign tumour.— *J. Am. med. Ass.*, 1974, *228*, 209.

Malignant effusions. Nineteen patients with malignant effusions were treated with mustine. After paracentesis to remove as much fluid as possible, most patients received a single dose of 20 mg of mustine hydrochloride dissolved in 20 ml of sodium chloride injection and injected directly into the cavity. This was followed by 50 ml of sodium chloride injection. Improvement was shown in 11 patients. In 6 patients no further paracentesis was required up to the time of death which averaged 6.6 months later. The injection of mustine was preceded half an hour before by an intramuscular injection of 50 mg of chlorpromazine but many patients still had nausea and sickness.— V. B. Levison, *Br. med. J.*, 1961, *1*, 1143. Instillation of a freshly prepared solution of mustine 20 mg in 200 ml of physiological saline, into a nearly empty space, is the preferred method for the control of malignant pleural effusions in lung cancer.— M. L. Sutton, *Postgrad. med. J.*, 1973, *49*, 729.

See also under Choice of Antineoplastic Agent, p.180.

Mycosis fungoides. Whole-body application of mustine, with intralesional injections in many patients, produced complete remissions in 114 of 166 patients with mycosis fungoides followed for at least 6 months; in 14 remissions had lasted more than 3 years. Delayed hypersensitivity reactions were reduced by a prior series of small intravenous doses of mustine to induce immunologic tolerance.— E. C. Vonderheid *et al.*, *Archs Derm.*, 1977, *113*, 454. Intravenous injections of 200 µg of mustine hydrochloride weekly for 5 weeks failed to prevent the development of sensitisation to subsequently applied topical mustine hydrochloride.— S. Leshaw *et al.*, *Archs Derm.*, 1977, *113*, 1406. Contact sensitivity to mustine hydrochloride in 5 patients with mycosis fungoides was suppressed after PUVA treatment (see under Methoxsalen) and in 1 patient permitted re-treatment with mustine.— G. Volden *et al.*, *Br. med. J.*, 1978, *2*, 865. Mycosis fungoides completely cleared in a patient after 4 weeks' treatment with a 0.02% solution of mustine applied daily and PUVA therapy thrice weekly. However, at 5 weeks she developed severe contact dermatitis.— A. du Vivier and D. Vollum (letter), *Br. med. J.*, 1978, *2*, 1300. Epithelial neoplasms other than actinic keratoses were found in 14 of 202 patients with mycosis fungoides who had received topical treatment with mustine hydrochloride and had been followed for up to 9 years. From preliminary observations these neoplasms were considered to be easily treated and application of mustine was still recommended as a not inappropriate treatment for a condition requiring early treatment, while still limited to the skin.— A. du Vivier *et al.*, *Br. J. Derm.*, 1978, *99*, 61.

Further references: N. M. Price *et al.*, *Br. J. Derm.*, 1977, *97*, 547; A. du Vivier and D. I. Vollum, *Br. J. Derm.*, 1980, *102*, 319 (photochemotherapy and topical mustine).

Skin disorders, non-malignant. Reports of the topical use of mustine hydrochloride in the treatment of various skin disorders: E. Epstein and A. R. Ugel, *Archs Derm.*, 1970, *102*, 504 (psoriasis); S. Mandy *et al.*, *Archs Derm.*, 1971, *103*, 272 (psoriasis; 0.02% freshly prepared solution); H. S. Zackheim *et al.*, *Archs Derm.*, 1972, *105*, 702 (psoriasis); D. M. Pariser *et al.*, *Archs Derm.*, 1976, *112*, 1113 (psoriasis); J. F. Dolezal and S. T. Thomson, *Archs Derm.*, 1978, *114*, 85 (histiocytosis X); A. Notowicz *et al.* (letter), *Archs Derm.*, 1978, *114*, 129 (acrodermatitis); H. Zachariae, *Br. J. Derm.*, 1979, *100*, 433 (histiocytosis X in infants; 0.025% solution increased gradually to a 0.1% solution).

See also under Mycosis Fungoides, above.

Preparations

Mechlorethamine Hydrochloride for Injection *(U.S.P.).* A sterile mixture of mustine hydrochloride with sodium chloride or other suitable diluent. A 2% solution has a pH of 3 to 5.

Mustine Injection *(B.P.).* Mustine Hydrochloride Injection. A sterile solution of mustine hydrochloride in Water for Injections, prepared by dissolving, immediately before use, the sterile contents of a sealed container (Mustine Hydrochloride for Injection) in the requisite amount of Water for Injections. The solution decomposes rapidly.

Mustine Hydrochloride *(Boots, UK).* Mustine hydrochloride, available in vials of 10 mg of powder for preparing injections.

Other Proprietary Names

Caryolysine *(Fr.)*; Cloramin *(Ital.)*; Erasol *(Denm.)*; Mustargen *(Canad., USA).*

1854-f

Nafoxidine Hydrochloride. Naphoxidine Hydrochloride; NSC 70735; U-11100A; WR 220110. 1-{2-[4-(3,4-Dihydro-6-methoxy-2-phenyl-1-naphthyl)phenoxy]ethyl}pyrrolidine hydrochloride.
$C_{29}H_{31}NO_2,HCl=462.0$.

CAS — 1845-11-0 (nafoxidine); 1847-63-8 (hydrochloride).

Adverse Effects and Precautions. Side-effects include skin reactions, photosensitivity, and alopecia. Cataract has been reported. It is recommended that patients should avoid exposure to strong sunlight and should wear sunglasses.

Pregnancy and the neonate. Single doses of nafoxidine given to neonatal *rats* caused multiple abnormalities in the development of the females, similar to those found in masculinised female *rats*.— J. H. Clark and S. McCormack, *Science*, 1977, *197*, 164.

Uses. Nafoxidine hydrochloride is an oestrogen antagonist with actions similar to those of tamoxifen citrate (p.226). It has been used in the treatment of breast cancer in doses of 60 mg thrice daily by mouth.

Malignant neoplasms of the breast. Nafoxidine has achieved a mean response-rate of 31% in about 200 patients with advanced breast cancer, results similar to those seen with oestrogens. Patients responding to earlier hormonal therapy are more likely to respond to nafoxidine as are those with tumours having oestrogen receptors (E. Engelsman *et al.*, *Br. med. J.*, 1973, *2*, 750). Remission rates of 31% and 14% for nafoxidine and ethinyloestradiol respectively were reported by J.C. Heuson *et al.* (*Br. med. J.*, 1975, *2*, 711) in postmenopausal women; the superiority of nafoxidine may have been related to better patient tolerance and therefore compliance.— S. S. Legha *et al.*, *Ann. intern. Med.*, 1978, *88*, 69.

Complete tumour regression was achieved in 7 and partial regression (at least 50% reduction in at least some sites) in 11 of 48 patients with advanced neoplasm of the breast; all but 1 of the patients were postmenopausal, most had widespread metastases, and most were unresponsive to or had relapsed from earlier endocrine control. The initial dose of nafoxidine was 90 mg thrice daily, reduced after response to 60 mg thrice daily; treatment was given for 1 to 36 months. Remissions had lasted for 6 months in 17 patients (for 1 to 3 years in 8). Side-effects were dryness of the skin, cutaneous photosensitivity, increased alopecia, reduction of hair pigmentation, and (in 1 patient) bilateral cataract. There was no evidence of untoward effect on the gastro-intestinal or cardiovascular systems, or on thyroid or adrenal function.— H. J. G. Bloom and E. Boesen, *Br. med. J.*, 1974, *2*, 7.

While ethinyloestradiol given to 4 postmenopausal women with advanced breast cancer increased prolactin secretion, nafoxidine given to 6 similar women did not.— M. L'Hermite *et al.* (letter), *Br. med. J.*, 1974, *1*, 390. Comment on the postulated mechanism of action of nafoxidine related to its lack of effect on prolactin.— B. A. Stoll (letter), *ibid.*, 1974, *2*, 447. Objective remissions lasting for a mean of 9 months were achieved in 7 of 36 postmenopausal patients with advanced breast cancer treated with nafoxidine, but in none of 40 treated with levodopa 750 mg daily for a week, then 1.5 g daily.— E. Engelsman *et al.*, *ibid.*, 1975, *2*, 714.

Three patients with breast cancer metastases were given nafoxidine and 2 responded but all 3 failed to respond to subsequent oestrogen therapy. Anti-oestrogens might best be used after oestrogen therapy.— E. Engelsman *et al.* (letter), *Lancet*, 1974, *2*, 171.

Manufacturers
Upjohn, USA.

1855-d

Nitromin. Mustine *N*-Oxide. *NN*-Bis(2-chloroethyl)methylamine *N*-oxide hydrochloride; 2,2′-Dichloro-*N*-methyldiethylamine *N*-oxide hydrochloride.
$C_5H_{11}Cl_2NO,HCl=208.5$.

CAS — 302-70-5.

White odourless crystals or crystalline powder. **Soluble** in water and alcohol; slightly soluble in ether. Discoloured solutions should not be used. **Store** in a cool place. Protect from light.

Uses. Nitromin is converted in solution to an active alkylating form with properties similar to those of mustine (p.222) and was formerly given by mouth or intravenously in a dose of about 1 mg per kg body-weight daily.

1856-n

Novembichine. Novoembichin. *NN*-Bis(2-chloroethyl)-2-chloropropylamine hydrochloride.
$C_7H_{14}Cl_3N,HCl=255.0$.

CAS — 1936-40-9.

Pharmacopoeias. In *Rus.*

A white crystalline powder. M.p. 69° to 71°. **Soluble** in water and alcohol; practically insoluble in ether.

Uses. Novembichine is an antineoplastic agent with properties similar to those of mustine (p.222). It has been used in a maximum dose of 10 mg intravenously, not more frequently than once every 2 days.

1857-h

Pipobroman *(U.S.P.).* A 8103; NSC 25154.

1,4-Bis(3-bromopropionyl)piperazine.
$C_{10}H_{16}Br_2N_2O_2=356.1$.

CAS — 54-91-1.

Pharmacopoeias. In *U.S.*

A white or almost white, crystalline powder with a slightly sharp fruity odour. M.p. 101° to 105°. **Soluble** 1 in 230 of water, 1 in 35 of alcohol, 1 in 4.8 of chloroform, and 1 in 530 of ether; soluble in acetone.

Adverse Effects, Treatment, and Precautions. For an outline of the adverse effects experienced with antineoplastic agents and immunosuppressants, general guidelines for their treatment, and precautions, see Antineoplastic Agents, p.171, pp.174-5.

Uses. Pipobroman is an antineoplastic agent which appears to act by alkylation (see p.171). It has been used in the treatment of polycythaemia vera, particularly in patients resistant to conventional therapy, and in chronic myeloid leukaemia resistant to busulphan and radiotherapy.

The usual dose initially is 1 to 1.5 mg per kg body-weight daily, according to the patient's response, increased to 3 mg per kg, if necessary. Maintenance dosage is 100 to 200 µg per kg daily for polycythaemia vera and from 7 to 175 mg daily in chronic myeloid leukaemia.

In the initial stages of treatment, white cell counts should be determined on alternate days and complete blood counts once or twice weekly. Doses should be discontinued if the white cell count is below 3,000 per mm^3 or the platelet count below 150,000 per mm^3.

Preparations

Pipobroman Tablets *(U.S.P.).* Tablets containing pipobroman.

Proprietary Names
Amedel *(Jap.)*; Vercite 25 *(Abbott, Ital.)*; Vercyte *(Abbott, Belg.; Abbott, Canad.; Abbott, Fr.; Abbott, USA).*

1858-m

Piposulfan. A 20968; NSC 47774. 1,4-Bis[3-(methylsulphonyloxy)propionyl]piperazine; 1,4-Bis(3-hydroxypropionyl)piperazine dimethanesulphonate.
$C_{12}H_{22}N_2O_8S_2=386.4$.

CAS — 2608-24-4.

Uses. Piposulfan is an antineoplastic agent chemically related to pipobroman. It has been given in doses of 1 mg per kg body-weight daily.

References: N. A. Nelson *et al.*, *Clin. Pharmac. Ther.*, 1967, *8*, 385; M. Schmidt and K. Havemann, *Dt. med. Wschr.*, 1970, *95*, 1166.

Manufacturers
Abbott, USA.

1859-b

Prednimustine. Leo 1031; NSC 134087. 11β,17,21-Trihydroxypregna-1,4-diene-3,20-dione 21-(4-{4-[bis(2-chloroethyl)amino]phenyl}butyrate).
$C_{35}H_{45}Cl_2NO_6=646.6$.

CAS — 29069-24-7.

A white odourless crystalline powder. Practically **insoluble** in water; soluble in alcohol, acetone, chloroform, and methyl alcohol.

Uses. Prednimustine is the chlorambucil ester of prednisolone, and has been used in the treatment of various malignant diseases including chronic lymphocytic leukaemia, non-Hodgkin's lymphomas, and carcinoma of the ovary and prostate.

It has been given by mouth in doses of 200 mg daily for 5 consecutive days, repeated after an interval of at least 9 days. Prednimustine has also been given continuously in a dose of 20 to 30 mg daily.

References to the use of prednimustine: C. W. Aungst *et al.*, *J. surg. Oncol.*, 1975, *7*, 457 (chronic lymphocytic leukaemia and lymphosarcoma); L. Brandt *et al.*, *Acta med. scand.*, 1975, *197*, 317 (chronic lymphocytic leukaemia); I. Könyves *et al.*, *Eur. J. Cancer*, 1975, *11*, 841 (absorption and fate); T. R. Moller *et al.*, *Acta med. scand.*, 1975, *197*, 323 (lymphoproliferative disorders); R. Catane *et al.*, *Br. J. Urol.*, 1978, *50*, 29 (prostatic carcinoma); W. Mattsson *et al.*, *Cancer*, 1978, *41*, 112 (lymphocytic and lymphocytic-histiocytic lymphomas).

Proprietary Names
Stéréocyt *(Bellon, Fr.).*

1860-x

Procarbazine Hydrochloride *(U.S.P.).* Ro 4-6467; NSC 77213; Ibenzmethyzin.

N-Isopropyl-α-(2-methylhydrazino)-*p*-toluamide hydrochloride.
$C_{12}H_{19}N_3O,HCl=257.8$.

CAS — 671-16-9 (procarbazine); 366-70-1 (hydrochloride).

Pharmacopoeias. In *Braz.* and *U.S.*

A white to pale yellow crystalline powder with a slight odour. M.p. about 223° with decomposition. Procarbazine hydrochloride 116 mg is approximately equivalent to 100 mg of procarbazine. Freely **soluble** in water; soluble in methyl alcohol; sparingly soluble in alcohol; slightly soluble in chloroform; practically insoluble in ether. Solutions in water are unstable and acid to litmus. **Store** in airtight containers. Protect from light.

A study on the degradation products of procarbazine hydrochloride in capsules.— G. L. Burce and J. P. Boehlert, *J. pharm. Sci.*, 1978, *67*, 424.

Adverse Effects and Treatment. For an outline of the adverse effects experienced with antineoplastic agents and immunosuppressants and general guidelines for their treatment, see Antineoplastic Agents, p.171 and p.174.

The most common adverse effects associated with procarbazine are anorexia, nausea, and vomiting (although patients may soon become tolerant), and bone-marrow depression. Leucopenia and thrombocytopenia may be delayed and recovery protracted. Haemolysis and bleeding tendencies have been reported. Neurotoxicity is also common, with central effects such as somnolence, depression, agitation, psychoses, and dizziness, and peripheral neuropathies including paraesthesias and decreased reflexes. Tremors, convulsions, and coma have occasionally occurred. Other side-effects reported with procarbazine include a 'flu-like' syndrome, pulmonary and skin reactions, tachycardia, hypotension, ocular defects such as blurred vision and papilloedema, and impaired liver function.

Allergy and anaphylaxis. Reports of allergic reactions associated with procarbazine: J. J. Lokich and W. C. Moloney, *Clin. Pharmac. Ther.*, 1972, *13*, 573 (rash and pneumonitis); M. M. Glovsky *et al.*, *J. Allergy & clin. Immunol.*, 1976, *57*, 134 (angio-oedema and urticaria); M. D. Ecker *et al.*, *Am. J. Roentg.*, 1978, *131*, 527 (a reaction including shortness of breath and productive cough).

Effects on the liver. A suggestion that ingestion of substituted hydrazines, such as procarbazine, may have a role in the development of hepatic angiosarcoma.— T. K. Daneshmend and J. W. B. Bradfield (letter), *Lancet*, 1979, *2*, 1249.

Effects on respiratory function. See Allergy and Anaphylaxis (above) and under Antineoplastic Agents, p.174.

Precautions. For reference to the precautions necessary with antineoplastic agents and immunosuppressants, see Antineoplastic Agents, p.175.

Procarbazine should be used with caution in patients with impaired liver or kidney function.

It is stated that procarbazine is a weak monoamine oxidase inhibitor and therefore that reactions with other drugs and food, although very rare, must be borne in mind—for details of such reactions see under Phenelzine Sulphate, p.128. Depression of the central nervous system may be enhanced when procarbazine is given with antihistamines, hypnotics, narcotic analgesics, and phenothiazines; reduced doses of chlorpromazine should be used to control nausea and vomiting. A disulfiram-like reaction has been reported with alcohol and the effects of antihypertensive agents may be enhanced.

Interactions. Reports of interactions attributed to the monoamine oxidase inhibiting properties of procarbazine: A. M. Mann and J. L. Hutchison, *Can. med. Ass. J.*, 1967, *97*, 1350 (with local anaesthetic); J. Bichel (letter), *Lancet*, 1968, *2*, 877 (with cheese).

For a report of antilymphocyte serum being potentiated by procarbazine, see Antilymphocyte Serum, p.189.

Pregnancy and the neonate. Reference to a theoretical risk of induction of the foetal-alcohol syndrome following concurrent ingestion of procarbazine and alcohol during pregnancy.— P. M. Dunn *et al.* (letter), *Lancet*, 1979, *2*, 144.

First trimester. Although it is carcinogenic and teratogenic in *animals*, a woman given procarbazine during the first 5½ weeks of pregnancy gave birth to a normal infant; several small haemangiomas were stable.— J. H. Wells *et al.*, *J. Am. med. Ass.*, 1968, *205*, 935.

Absorption and Fate. Procarbazine is readily absorbed from the gastro-intestinal tract and peak plasma concentrations have been reported within 30 to 60 minutes. If diffuses into the cerebrospinal fluid. A plasma half-life of about 10 minutes has been reported. Procarbazine is rapidly metabolised and only about 5% is excreted unchanged in the urine. The remainder is oxidised to *N*-isopropylterephthalamic acid and excreted in the urine, about 25 to 42% of a dose being excreted in 24 hours. During oxidative breakdown in the body hydrogen peroxide and hydroxyl radicals are formed which may account for the drug's activity.

Uses. Procarbazine hydrochloride is an antineoplastic agent which appears to inhibit protein and nucleic acid synthesis and suppress mitosis. It is unrelated to the other antineoplastic agents and it may be effective when other agents have become ineffective. Procarbazine also has some immunosuppressant activity.

Its main use is the treatment of Hodgkin's disease when it is usually given in association with other drugs such as mustine, one of the vinca alkaloids, and prednisone. Procarbazine has also been used in the treatment of other lymphomas and in malignant neoplasms of the brain and lung. See also under Choice of Antineoplastic Agent, p.175. To reduce nausea and vomiting, the usual initial dose is the equivalent of 50 mg of procarbazine daily, increased daily by 50 mg to 250 or 300 mg daily in divided doses. This dose is continued until a response is obtained or until the white cell or platelet counts fall below 4000 or 100 000 per mm^3 respectively, or there are other signs of toxicity. A maintenance dose of 50 to 150 mg daily is given until signs of bone-marrow depression occur. In children, initial daily doses of the equivalent of 50 mg have been suggested, increased to 100 mg per m^2 body-surface, then adjusted according to the white cell and platelet response.

In the combination regimens procarbazine is given to adults and children in doses of 100 mg per m^2 body-surface on days 1 to 14 of each 4- or 6-week cycle.

The haematological status of the patient should be determined every 3 or 4 days and hepatic and renal function determined weekly.

Blood disorders, non-malignant. References to the use of procarbazine in non-malignant blood disorders: H. Martin and J. C. Schubert, *Dt. med. Wschr.*, 1966, *91*, 55 (polycythaemia vera); P. Mitrou *et al.*, *Dt. med. Wschr.*, 1972, *97*, 1864 (Waldenström's macroglobulinaemia).

Genito-urinary disorders, non-malignant. A report on the use of procarbazine in patients with Peyronie's disease (induration of the corpora cavernosa of the penis).— J. Chesney, *Br. J. Urol.*, 1975, *47*, 209.

Hodgkin's disease and other lymphomas. Procarbazine was given to 22 patients with stage III or IVB Hodgkin's disease resistant to the vinca alkaloids and the alkylating agents in initial doses of 50 to 100 mg increased to 200 or 300 mg daily. There were 13 beneficial responses, all evident within 3 weeks. The average duration of response was 13 weeks.— R. C. DeConti, *J. Am. med. Ass.*, 1971, *215*, 927.

See also under Choice of Antineoplastic Agent, p.177.

Malignant neoplasms of the brain. It was reported that of 16 patients with glial tumours who received procarbazine for 30 days in doses of 150 mg per m^2 body-surface daily, 8 responded to treatment and survived to receive a second course 30 days later. Four of these patients showed excellent improvement with a reduction in the size of the tumours.— *J. Am. med. Ass.*, 1972, *220*, 1291.

See also under Choice of Antineoplastic Agent, p.180.

Organ and tissue transplantation. A comparison of cyclophosphamide and procarbazine in the preparation of kidneys for transplantation.— H. Zincke *et al.*, *Mayo Clin. Proc.*, 1976, *51*, 693.

Preparations

Procarbazine Hydrochloride Capsules *(U.S.P.)*. Capsules containing procarbazine hydrochloride. Potency is expressed in terms of the equivalent amount of procarbazine. Store in airtight containers. Protect from light.

Natulan *(Roche, UK)*. Procarbazine hydrochloride, available as capsules each containing the equivalent of 50 mg of procarbazine. (Also available as Natulan in *Arg., Austral., Belg., Canad., Fr., Ger., Ital., Neth., Norw., S.Afr., Switz.*).

Other Proprietary Names

Matulane *(USA)*; Natulanar *(Denm., Swed.)*.

1861-r

Razoxane.
ICI 59 118; ICRF 159; NSC 129943. (±)-4,4′-Propylenebis(piperazine-2,6-dione).

$C_{11}H_{16}N_4O_4 = 268.3$.

CAS — 21416-87-5.

A white to off-white crystalline powder. M.p. 223°. Slightly **soluble** in water. **Store** in airtight containers. Protect from light.

Adverse Effects, Treatment, and Precautions. For an outline of the adverse effects experienced with antineoplastic agents and immunosuppressants, general guidelines for their treatment, and precautions, see Antineoplastic Agents, p.171, pp.174-5.

The adverse effects of radiotherapy may be enhanced by the concomitant use of razoxane.

Absorption and Fate. Absorption of razoxane from the gastro-intestinal tract is reported to be variable.

Two patients given razoxane 3 g per m^2 body-surface by mouth achieved a peak plasma concentration of about 3.8 µg per ml 2 hours after administration. Absorption by mouth was slow and bioavailability limited when compared with intravenous administration in *animals*.— W. Sadée *et al.*, *J. pharm. Sci.*, 1975, *64*, 998.

From a study of dosage schedules for 12 patients, there appeared to be limited absorption of razoxane when it was given in a single large dose. Administration of divided doses is recommended.— P. J. Creaven *et al.*, *J. Pharm. Pharmac.*, 1975, *27*, 914.

Uses. Razoxane is an antineoplastic agent with inhibitory activity during the pre-mitotic and early mitotic phases of cell growth. It also has some immunosuppressant activity. It is used in association with radiotherapy in the treatment of sarcomas. Razoxane has also been tried in other malignant diseases including leukaemias and some solid tumours. It is given by mouth in a dose of 125 mg twice daily. The white cell count should be monitored during treatment.

Reviews of razoxane: M. T. Bakowski, *Cancer Treat. Rev.*, 1976, *3*, 95; *Drug & Ther. Bull.*, 1978, *16*, 7.

Action. Razoxane was even more effective *in vitro* against methotrexate-resistant than against methotrexate-sensitive lymphoblasts. Cytotoxicity increased to a dose of 10 µg per ml when the effect levelled off.— B. T. Hill and K. Hellmann (letter), *Lancet*, 1977, *1*, 47.

Leukaemia. Experience with 15 patients indicated that razoxane 125 mg three or four times daily with cytarabine intravenously was not a satisfactory treatment for acute myeloid leukaemia. In 2 patients with chronic granulocytic leukaemia in acute blast transformation, results were encouraging.— M. Bhavnani *et al.*, *Br. med. J.*, 1978, *2*, 801. Seven patients with acute myeloid leukaemia had been treated with this regimen; 6 achieved good partial remissions and 4 were alive and well after 10, 14, 26, and 32 weeks.— D. Shaw and G. R. Tudhope (letter), *ibid.*, 1089. Complete remissions had occurred in 7 of 27 patients and partial remissions in 10.— K. Hellmann (letter), *ibid.*, 1161. Razoxane was ineffective in 3 patients.— D. Obeid and P. Cotter (letter), *ibid.*

Sarcoma. Complete or partial regression was obtained in 15 of 19 patients with soft-tissue sarcomas who received razoxane and radiotherapy compared with 8 of 14 who received radiotherapy alone. Leucopenia occurred in 9 patients who received razoxane and in none of those who had radiotherapy alone. Prolonged treatment with razoxane in 13 patients after the completion of radiotherapy did not improve the initial response or recurrence-rate.— K. Hellmann *et al.*, *Cancer*, 1978, *41*, 100.

See also under Choice of Antineoplastic Agent, p.185.

Skin disorders, non-malignant. *Psoriasis.* A report of the beneficial effect of razoxane in 35 patients with severe psoriasis, 9 of whom had previously been treated unsuccessfully with methotrexate. Razoxane was given intermittently in doses of 125 or 250 mg thrice daily, generally on 2 or 3 consecutive days each week or occasionally each fortnight. Some response to treatment was seen in all patients with cutaneous psoriasis and regression to mild or minimal residual disease occurred in 31 of 32 patients. In the patient not adequately controlled, dosage had been reduced because of adverse effects. Patients with arthropathy also benefited. Razoxane was given for up to 2 years in patients with severe disease. Dose-dependent bone-marrow depression was the principal adverse effect and was more conspicuous than that seen with methotrexate, although in general razoxane was considered to be better tolerated. Treatment was only withdrawn in 2 patients. Hepatotoxicity was not seen.— D. J. Atherton *et al.*, *Br. J. Derm.*, 1980, *102*, 307.

Proprietary Preparations

Razoxin *(ICI Pharmaceuticals, UK)*. Razoxane, available as tablets of 125 mg.

1862-f

Rufocromomycin. Streptonigrin; Flomycin; NSC 45383; RP 5278. 5-Amino-6-(7-amino-5,8-dihydro-6-methoxy-5,8-dioxo-2-quinolyl)-4-(2-hydroxy-3,4-dimethoxyphenyl)-3-methylpyridine-2-carboxylic acid.

$C_{25}H_{22}N_4O_8 = 506.5$.

CAS — 3930-19-6.

An antineoplastic antibiotic produced by the growth of *Streptomyces flocculus* or *S. rufochromogenus*.

Rufocromomycin has the general properties of antineoplastic agents (p.171) and has been used in various malignant diseases. It has been given by mouth and by intravenous infusion.

1863-d

Semustine. Methyl-CCNU; Methyl Lomustine; NSC 95441; WR 220076. 1-(2-Chloroethyl)-3-(4-methylcyclohexyl)-1-nitrosourea.

$C_{10}H_{18}ClN_3O_2 = 247.7$.

CAS — 13909-09-6.

Store at 2° to 8° in airtight containers.

Adverse Effects, Treatment, and Precautions. As for Carmustine, p.195.

Severe and prolonged bone-marrow suppression, requiring withdrawal of semustine, has been reported.

Effects on the kidneys. In a retrospective study, from two centres, of 17 children with brain tumours given semustine after radiotherapy, all 6 who had received a total dose of 1500 mg per m^2 body-surface over at least 17 months had severe renal damage. During treatment there was no evidence by blood urea nitrogen or creatinine determinations that the patients were losing renal function. A decrease in kidney size occurred in 2 patients who received lower total doses. The use of semustine should be limited to lower doses given for short periods until its toxicity is clarified.— W. E. Harmon *et al.*, *New Engl. J. Med.*, 1979, *300*, 1200. In a retrospective review of 857 patients treated with semustine over the past 6 years, there were only 4 patients with delayed renal insufficiency that was considered to have been related possibly to semustine.— W. C. Nichols and C. G. Moertel (letter), *ibid.*, *301*, 1181.

Uses. Semustine is a nitrosourea with actions and uses similar to those of carmustine (p.195) and lomustine (p.212). It has been given by mouth in single doses of 200 mg per m^2 body-surface, repeated every 6 weeks if blood counts recover adequately.

References to the use of semustine: R. C. Young *et al.*, *Cancer*, 1973, *31*, 1164; K. Tornyos *et al.*, *Cancer Treat. Rep.*, 1977, *61*, 785 (resistant multiple myeloma); D. E. Lehane *et al.*, *Cancer Treat. Rep.*, 1977, *61*, 889 (with methotrexate in advanced malignancies); A. Barrett *et al.* (letter), *Lancet*, 1978, *2*, 101 (disappointing results with semustine and fluorouracil in colorectal cancer).

Administration in renal insufficiency. Nephrotoxicity has been associated with total doses of semustine above 1200 mg per m^2 body-surface. Its use should be avoided in patients with a glomerular filtration-rate below 10 ml per minute.— W. M. Bennett *et al.*, *Ann. intern. Med.*, 1980, *93*, 286.

Manufacturers

National Institutes of Health, USA.

1864-n

Streptozocin. NSC 85998; U 9889; WR 139502; Streptozotocin. 2-Deoxy-2-(3-methyl-3-nitrosoureido)-D-glucopyranose.

$C_8H_{15}N_3O_7$=265.2.

CAS — 18883-66-4.

An antineoplastic antibiotic produced by the growth of a *Streptomyces achromogenes* variant or by synthesis. Very **soluble** in water; soluble in alcohol. **Store** at 2° to 8°.

A buffered solution for injection is reported to be stable for 48 hours at room temperature and may be diluted with sodium chloride or dextrose injection.

Adverse Effects and Treatment. For an outline of the adverse effects experienced with antineoplastic agents and immunosuppressants and general guidelines for their treatment, see Antineoplastic Agents, p.171 and p.174.

Nephrotoxicity is common with streptozocin and may be severe. Fatal irreversible renal failure has been reported. Other side-effects include severe nausea and vomiting and alterations in liver function.

Streptozocin may affect glucose metabolism. A diabetogenic effect has been reported in some patients; hypoglycaemia attributed to the release of insulin from damaged cells has also occurred.

Lactic acidosis developed in a patient being treated with streptozocin for carcinoma of the lung.— R. G. Narins *et al.*, *Am. J. med. Sci.*, 1973, *265*, 455.

Diabetogenic effect. A review of the diabetogenic activity of streptozocin.— C. C. Rerup, *Pharmac. Rev.*, 1970, *22*, 485.

Precautions. For reference to the precautions necessary with antineoplastic agents and immunosuppressants, see Antineoplastic Agents, p.175.

Streptozocin should be used with extreme care in patients with renal or hepatic impairment.

Interactions. A suggestion that, since phenytoin appeared to protect the beta cells of the pancreas from the cytotoxic effects of streptozocin, its concomitant use with streptozocin should be avoided in patients being treated for pancreatic tumours.— L. Koranyi and L. Gero (letter), *Br. med. J.*, 1979, *1*, 127.

For a report that streptozocin enhanced the adverse effects of carmustine and brought no therapeutic benefit, see Carmustine, p.195.

Uses. Streptozocin is an antineoplastic agent belonging to the nitrosoureas (see Carmustine, p.195) and is used mainly in the treatment of islet-cell tumours of the pancreas. It has been tried in the carcinoid syndrome and other tumours. The usual recommended dose has been 1 g per m^2 body-surface weekly for 4 weeks by intravenous injection. Renal and hepatic function tests should be performed routinely during treatment.

See also under Choice of Antineoplastic Agent, p.175.

Reviews of the actions and uses of streptozocin: C. C. Cheng and K. -Y. Zee-Cheng, *J. pharm. Sci.*, 1972, *61*, 485; B. Rudas, *Arzneimittel-Forsch.*, 1972, *22*, 830; *Lancet*, 1973, *2*, 1063.

Studies in cancer patients given a single intravenous dose of streptozocin 1.5 g per m^2 body-surface suggested that the plasma half-life was about 40 minutes, and the elimination half-life about 13 minutes.— A. B. Adolphe *et al.*, *J. clin. Pharmac.*, 1977, *17*, 379.

Antiprotozoal action. Streptozocin had significant activity against *Trypanosoma rhodesiense* infections in *mice*.— K. E. Kinnamon *et al.*, *Antimicrob. Ag. Chemother.*, 1979, *15*, 157.

Pancreatic disorders. *Adenocarcinoma.* Complete or partial remission was obtained in 10 of 23 patients with advanced adenocarcinoma of the pancreas after treatment with a regimen consisting of streptozocin, mitomycin, and fluorouracil (SMF). The mean survival time of those patients who responded to treatment was 7.5 months compared with 3 months in 8 non-responders (5 patients showed disease stabilisation). Seven patients developed proteinuria and other side-effects included myelosuppression.— R. G. Wiggans *et al.*, *Cancer*, 1978, *41*, 387.

Islet-cell carcinoma. A randomised comparative study confirmed the therapeutic activity of streptozocin in a substantial proportion of patients with advanced islet-cell carcinoma and demonstrated an enhanced response when it was used with fluorouracil. Five-day courses of streptozocin 500 mg per m^2 body-surface daily alone or in association with fluorouracil 400 mg per m^2 daily, both by intravenous injection, were given to 84 patients and repeated every 6 weeks if they improved or remained stable. The dosage of fluorouracil was subsequently reduced if severe leucopenia or thrombocytopenia was present and that of streptozocin was reduced if there was severe nausea and vomiting or any evidence of renal toxicity; streptozocin was discontinued and treatment continued with fluorouracil alone if toxicity persisted. The overall response-rate was 63% in patients given the combined treatment compared with 36% in those given only streptozocin whereas complete response-rates were 33% and 12% respectively. Median survival-times were 26 months for fluorouracil and streptozocin compared with 16.5 months for streptozocin alone; the difference was not statistically significant. The intensive-course regimen of streptozocin with fluorouracil produced a period of more severe nausea and vomiting in many patients but this might be preferable to the constant state of nausea that frequently results from weekly treatment.— C. G. Moertel *et al.*, *New Engl. J. Med.*, 1980, *303*, 1189.

Further references: L. E. Broder and S. K. Carter, *Ann. intern. Med.*, 1973, *79*, 108; P. Schein *et al.*, *Archs intern. Med.*, 1973, *132*, 555.

Non-beta islet-cell carcinoma. Two patients with the pancreatic-cholera syndrome and non-beta islet-cell neoplasms responded to 3 to 5 intra-arterial doses of streptozocin 1.5 g per m^2 body-surface at intervals of 5 to 6 days. Stool volume and the number of hepatic metastases decreased and serum-potassium concentrations returned to normal.— C. R. Kahn *et al.*, *New Engl. J. Med.*, 1975, *292*, 941. See also *Lancet*, 1975, *1*, 1327.

Beneficial results with streptozocin in a patient with a glucagon-secreting tumour.— D. N. Danforth *et al.*, *New Engl. J. Med.*, 1976, *295*, 242.

Zollinger-Ellison syndrome. A patient with the Zollinger-Ellison syndrome, severe weight loss, liver metastases, severe uncontrollable gastro-intestinal bleeding and abdominal pain, and diabetes, achieved control of the bleeding within 24 hours of an intravenous injection of streptozocin 2 g. Regular treatment with 2 to 4 g intravenously every 2 to 3 weeks to a total of 66 g over 12 months produced weight gain, relief of pain, and regression of metastases. Streptozocin was withdrawn and the patient had remained well for almost 2 years despite an increase in serum-gastrin concentration.— L. Sadoff and D. Franklin (letter), *Lancet*, 1975, *2*, 504. Two patients with gastrinoma and liver metastases did not respond to streptozocin.— C. B. H. Lamers and J. H. M. van Tongeren (letter), *ibid.*, 1150. A 38-year-old woman with metastatic gastrinoma who failed to respond to intravenous streptozocin achieved a partial remission of symptoms following 2 intra-arterial injections of streptozocin 4 g into the coeliac axis; she had remained well for 3 years.— J. R. Hayes *et al.*, *Gut*, 1976, *17*, 285.

Further references: F. Stadil *et al.*, *New Engl. J. Med.*, 1976, *294*, 1440; B. W. Ruffner, *Archs intern. Med.*, 1976, *136*, 1032, per *J. Am. med. Ass.*, 1976, *236*, 1410.

Manufacturers

Upjohn, UK.

1865-h

Tamoxifen Citrate. ICI 46 474. (*Z*)-2-[4-(1,2-Diphenylbut-1-enyl)phenoxy]-*NN*-dimethylethylamine citrate.

$C_{26}H_{29}NO,C_6H_8O_7$=563.6.

CAS — 10540-29-1 (tamoxifen); 54965-24-1 (citrate).

Tamoxifen citrate 15.2 mg is approximately equivalent to 10 mg of tamoxifen.

Adverse Effects and Precautions. Adverse effects with tamoxifen include hot flushes, oedema, vaginal bleeding, pruritus vulvae, gastro-intestinal upsets, dizziness, rashes, hypercalcaemia, and tumour pain. Transient thrombocytopenia and leucopenia have been reported. There have also been reports of headache, depression, fatigue, confusion, leg cramps, alopecia, and dry skin. Tamoxifen should not be given during pregnancy and should be used with caution in women with functioning ovaries.

No deaths had been attributed to tamoxifen in more than 10 000 patient-years. Review of 12 studies showed that only 27 of 988 patients withdrew from tamoxifen therapy because of side-effects, few of which were life-threatening or even severe. The most frequent side-effects were gastro-intestinal toxicity in 11, dizziness in 6, rash in 3, and hypercalcaemia in 2. Tamoxifen was neither mutagenic nor teratogenic in *animals*.— J. S. Patterson and M. Baum (letter), *Lancet*, 1978, *1*, 105.

Tamoxifen 20 mg per day might have induced lactation in a 31-year-old woman.— G. R. Favis *et al.* (letter), *Ann. intern. Med.*, 1979, *90*, 993.

Effects on the blood. *Coagulation defects.* One patient died from pulmonary embolism after 10 days of treatment with tamoxifen.— H. J. Lerner *et al.*, *Cancer Treat. Rep.*, 1976, *60*, 1431.

Administration of tamoxifen to 4 women with metastatic breast cancer was associated with the development of deep-vein thrombophlebitis.— K. Nevasaari *et al.* (letter), *Lancet*, 1978, *2*, 946. Tamoxifen should be prescribed with caution in patients with factors predisposing to thrombo-embolism.— A. Hendrick and V. P. Subramanian (letter), *J. Am. med. Ass.*, 1980, *243*, 514.

Effects on electrolytes. Hypercalcaemia in 4 of 26 patients with breast cancer and bone metastases treated with tamoxifen; the hypercalcaemia might represent tumour response.— A. H. Villalon *et al.*, *Br. med. J.*, 1979, *2*, 1329. There is no firm evidence to suggest that hypercalcaemia is indicative of tumour response.— G. J. G. Rees (letter), *ibid.*, 1590. See also M. J. Minton *et al.* (letter), *ibid.*, 1980, *280*, 186.

A report of life-threatening hypercalcaemia in 2 women given tamoxifen for metastatic breast carcinoma. One was treated with fluid replacement, frusemide, and mithramycin, and recovered within 48 hours, and the other responded to rehydration, diuretics, and corticosteroids, returning to normal within 72 hours. Tamoxifen was reintroduced, together with prednisolone in one, who was able to continue the tamoxifen after the prednisolone had been stopped; the other had a second episode of hypercalcaemia. Tamoxifen-induced hypercalcaemia should be treated by stopping tamoxifen, rehydration, corticosteroids, and, if necessary, mithramycin. Tamoxifen should be reintroduced under initial corticosteroid cover with careful monitoring of serum-calcium concentrations.— D. Spooner and B. D. Evans (letter), *Lancet*, 1979, *2*, 413.

Incidence and management of tamoxifen-induced hypercalcaemia.— S. S. Legha *et al.*, *Cancer*, 1981, *47*, 2803.

Further reports of hypercalcaemia associated with tamoxifen: B. Henningsen and H. Amberger, *Dt. med. Wschr.*, 1977, *102*, 713; M. J. Minton *et al.* (letter), *Lancet*, 1978, *1*, 396; M. Valencic *et al.*, *Mt Sinai J. Med.*, 1979, *46*, 396; S. D. Lane *et al.* (letter), *Ann. intern. Med.*, 1980, *92*, 572.

See also under Malignant Neoplasms of the Breast (below).

Effects on the eyes. Four patients treated with tamoxifen have developed retinopathy.— M. I. Kaiser-Kupfer and M. E. Lippman, *Cancer Treat. Rep.*, 1978, *62*, 315.

Absorption and Fate. Peak plasma concentrations of tamoxifen occur several hours after an oral dose. Plasma clearance is reported to be biphasic and the terminal half-life may be longer than 7 days. It is excreted slowly in the faeces with only small amounts appearing in the urine.

The absorption, metabolism, and excretion of tamoxifen was studied in 4 women who took a radioactively-labelled dose of 300 µg per kg body-weight. Peak serum concentrations of 0.06 to 0.14 µg per ml were achieved 4 to 7 hours after the dose with only 20 to 30% of the radioactivity present as tamoxifen. After initial half-lives of 7 to 14 hours serum concentrations decayed with secondary half-lives greater than 7 days. Most of the radioactivity was excreted slowly in the faeces, mainly as conjugates; unchanged drug and hydroxylated metabolites accounted for less than 30%. Two weeks after the dose only 65% could be accounted for although radioactivity was still detectable in the blood. Enterohepatic circulation was considered responsible for prolongation of blood concentrations and the presence of some of the hydroxylated metabolites in faeces.— J. M. Fromson *et al.*, *Xenobiotica*, 1973, *3*, 711.

Monohydroxytamoxifen, a metabolite of tamoxifen, is reported by V.C. Jordan *et al.* (*J. Endocr.*, 1977, *75*, 305) to be a more potent oestrogen antagonist than the parent drug.— V. C. Jordan and K. E. Naylor, *Br. J.

Pharmac., 1978, *64*, 376P.

Further references: J. M. Fromson and D. S. Sharp, *J. Obstet. Gynaec. Br. Commonw.*, 1974, *81*, 321 (uptake by uterine tissue).

Uses. Tamoxifen citrate is an oestrogen antagonist with actions similar to those of clomiphene citrate (p.1407). It is used as an alternative to androgens and oestrogens in the management of breast cancer in doses equivalent to 10 to 20 mg of tamoxifen twice daily (or 20 to 40 mg daily) by mouth.

Tamoxifen citrate is also used to stimulate ovulation in infertility. The usual dose is the equivalent of tamoxifen 10 mg twice daily on days 2, 3, 4, and 5 of the menstrual cycle, increased if necessary in subsequent cycles to 40 mg twice daily; alternatively single daily doses of 20 to 80 mg may be employed on the same days.

Gynaecomastia. Relief of gynaecomastia in 3 men (2 with lung cancer) after treatment with tamoxifen.— D. B. Jefferys, *Br. med. J.*, 1979, *1*, 1119. See also D. Fairlamb and E. Boesen, *Postgrad. med. J.*, 1977, *53*, 269.

Infertility. Tamoxifen has less intrinsic oestrogenic activity than clomiphene and may prove of value in the treatment of infertility.— D. T. Baird, *Prescribers' J.*, 1979, *19*, 99. See also *idem*, *Br. med. Bull.*, 1979, *35*, 193 (female infertility).

In a clinical study 10 mg of tamoxifen was given twice daily for 5 days. If ovulation did not occur a new course was commenced after 45 days and the daily dose doubled up to a maximum of 40 mg twice daily. In 24 women given a total of 106 treatment cycles, ovulation was presumed to have occurred in 17, and 8 became pregnant.— D. C. Macourt, *Med. J. Aust.*, 1974, *1*, 631.

Further references: A. Klopper and M. Hall, *Br. med. J.*, 1971, *1*, 152; J. G. Williamson and J. D. Ellis, *J. Obstet. Gynaec. Br. Commonw.*, 1973, *80*, 844; A. Vermeulen and F. Comhaire, *Fert. Steril.*, 1978, *29*, 320 (effects of tamoxifen in normal and oligospermic men).

Malignant neoplasms of the breast. A review of tamoxifen in the management of patients with breast cancer indicates that tamoxifen is at least as effective as standard treatment with oestrogens or androgens in postmenopausal women and is better tolerated. Similar response-rates were also reported by T. Priestman *et al.* (*Br. med. J.*, 1977, *1*, 1248) when tamoxifen was compared with a regimen of doxorubicin, cyclophosphamide, fluorouracil, and vincristine in patients more than 5 years postmenopausal and with soft-tissue involvement. However tamoxifen was less effective than cytotoxic therapy in patients less than 5 years past the menopause. The highest response-rates with tamoxifen are likely to be in women more than 5 years postmenopausal and with tumours containing oestrogen receptors. The relative effectiveness of tamoxifen in premenopausal women has not yet been clearly evaluated.— R. C. Heel *et al.*, *Drugs*, 1978, *16*, 1. Tamoxifen is replacing oestrogen therapy with stilboestrol as the initial treatment of breast cancer in postmenopausal women. Regression in tumour size of more than 50% has been reported in 30 to 40% of patients. The mean duration of response with oestrogens or anti-oestrogens is 1 to 2 years.— B. A. Stoll, *Practitioner*, 1979, *222*, 211. See also *Med. Lett.*, 1978, *20*, 41; M. Spino, *Can. J. Hosp. Pharm.*, 1978, *31*, 139; I. C. Henderson and G. P. Canellos, *New Engl. J. Med.*, 1980, *302*, 78.

In 45 postmenopausal women with recurrent breast cancer, tamoxifen 20 mg twice daily produced no effect on the luteinising-hormone or follicle-stimulating-hormone response to gonadorelin or on androgen concentrations. Oestradiol concentrations rose in patients who did not respond to treatment. Clinically 18 patients benefited. Response is likely in those in whom the prolactin concentration is within the normal range and the prolactin response to protirelin not excessive. Response might possibly be improved if prolactin production is controlled by bromocriptine.— K. J. Willis *et al.*, *Br. med. J.*, 1977, *1*, 425.

'Tamoxifen flare', a worsening of skeletal pain, occurred within the first few weeks of treatment with tamoxifen citrate in 6 of 23 patients with breast cancer, but later subsided although treatment was continued.— D. Plotkin *et al.*, *J. Am. med. Ass.*, 1978, *240*, 2644. Comments.— D. J. Arnold *et al.* (letter), *J. Am. med. Ass.*, 1979, *241*, 2506; J. D. Veldhuis and R. J. Santen (letter), *ibid.*

Greater caution might be required during the early weeks of treatment with tamoxifen citrate especially in patients with metastatic osteolytic disease because of the possibility of the development of hypercalcaemia.— J. D. Veldhuis (letter), *Ann. intern. Med.*, 1978, *88*, 574. A worldwide review of published reports yielded 36 patients who had developed hypercalcaemia while receiving tamoxifen, an occurrence-rate of less than 0.1%, whereas the incidence of spontaneous hypercalcaemia in advanced breast cancer has been reported to be as high as 14%. The hypercalcaemia occurring on initiation of tamoxifen therapy appears to be directly related to the presence of bone metastases and seems to be transient in most cases where therapy is continued or reintroduced.— J. S. Patterson *et al.*, *ICI* (letter), *ibid.*, *89*, 1013. See also R. Taetle *et al.* (letter), *ibid.*, 287; K. I. Pritchard *et al.* (letter), *ibid.*, 423. See also Adverse Effects (above).

In a study of 22 premenopausal women with metastatic breast cancer, tamoxifen 20 mg twice daily produced a partial response in 7 that had lasted from 10 to 36 weeks; 2 patients remained stable, 1 had a mixed response, and in 12 treatment failed. Three of the 22 patients experienced amenorrhoea whilst taking tamoxifen.— K. I. Pritchard *et al.* (letter), *Ann. intern. Med.*, 1978, *89*, 721.

No significant difference in efficacy was demonstrated between treatment with stilboestrol or tamoxifen in 143 postmenopausal women with advanced breast cancer. However, since tamoxifen was less toxic it appears to be the hormonal agent of choice in such patients.— J. N. Ingle *et al.*, *New Engl. J. Med.*, 1981, *304*, 16.

Further reports of tamoxifen in the treatment of breast cancer: H. W. C. Ward, *Br. med. J.*, 1973, *1*, 13; *idem* (letter), 1974, *2*, 500; E. Ferrazzi *et al.* (letter), *Br. med. J.*, 1977, *1*, 1351; B. Henningsen and H. Amberger, *Dt. med. Wschr.*, 1977, *102*, 713; D. T. Kiang and B. J. Kennedy, *Ann. intern. Med.*, 1977, *87*, 687; H. W. C. Ward *et al.*, *Clin. Oncol.*, 1978, *4*, 11; S. S. Legha *et al.*, *J. Am. med. Ass.*, 1979, *242*, 49 and 1754; I. Ricciardi and A. Ianniruberto, *Obstet. Gynec.*, 1979, *54*, 80.

See also under Choice of Antineoplastic Agent, p.180.

Malignant neoplasms of the male breast. The efficacy of tamoxifen in the treatment of carcinoma of the male breast cannot be ascertained until 20 to 30 patients have been treated. However, since similar response-rates are achieved with stilboestrol in men and women, results with tamoxifen are also expected to be similar.— G. G. Ribeiro (letter), *Br. med. J.*, 1978, *2*, 570.

Beneficial responses to tamoxifen in men with breast cancer.— R. Abele *et al.* (letter), *Br. med. J.*, 1978, *1*, 1697; D. B. Jefferys and J. Efthimiou (letter), *ibid.*; B. M. J. Cantwell *et al.* (letter), *Lancet*, 1978, *2*, 582; J. Aisner *et al.*, *Archs intern. Med.*, 1979, *139*, 480. A lack of response in 2 further patients.— D. A. L. Morgan and A. Hong (letter), *Br. med. J.*, 1978, *2*, 206.

Malignant neoplasms of the endometrium. In a pilot study of tamoxifen 10 mg twice daily for the treatment of advanced endometrial carcinoma, 4 of 7 patients responded.— K. D. Swenerton *et al.* (letter), *New Engl. J. Med.*, 1979, *301*, 105.

Malignant neoplasms of the prostate. A report of encouraging results with tamoxifen in drug-resistant advanced prostatic carcinoma.— M. O. El-Arini (letter), *Lancet*, 1979, *2*, 588. See also A. Kóczé and J. Székely (letter), *Lancet*, 1980, *1*, 539.

Melanoma. Four of 26 patients with advanced malignant melanoma had an objective response to treatment with tamoxifen 20 to 40 mg daily. The 4 who responded all had soft-tissue disease. Adverse effects were generally mild although some men reported decreased sexual performance and one woman had moderate alopecia.— R. A. Nesbit *et al.* (letter), *New Engl. J. Med.*, 1979, *301*, 1241. See also R. O. Mirimanoff *et al.* (letter), *Lancet*, 1981, *1*, 1368. Comment.— C. M. Furnival *et al.* (letter), *ibid.*, *2*, 374.

Pregnancy and the neonate. A report of tamoxifen being used to suppress puerperal lactation.— A. Masala *et al.*, *Br. J. Obstet. Gynaec.*, 1978, *85*, 134.

Proprietary Preparations

Nolvadex *(ICI Pharmaceuticals, UK)*. Tamoxifen citrate, available as tablets each containing the equivalent of 10 mg of tamoxifen. **Nolvadex-D.** Tablets each containing tamoxifen citrate equivalent to tamoxifen 20 mg. Protect from light. (Also available as Nolvadex in *Arg., Austral., Belg., Canad., Denm., Fr., Ger., Ital., Neth., Norw., S.Afr., Spain, Swed., Switz., USA*).

Other Proprietary Names

Istubol *(Chile)*; Zitazonium *(Hung.)*.

1866-m

Tegafur. Ftorafur; FT-207; MJF 12264; NSC 148958; WR 220066. 5-Fluoro-1-(tetrahydro-2-furyl)uracil; 5-Fluoro-1-(tetrahydro-2-furyl)pyrimidine-2,4(1*H*,3*H*)-dione.

$C_8H_9FN_2O_3$=200.2.

CAS — 17902-23-7.

Colourless crystals. M.p. about 166°. Readily **soluble** in hot water and alcohol; practically insoluble in ether.

Adverse Effects, Treatment, and Precautions. As for fluorouracil (p.209). Bone-marrow depression may be less severe with tegafur.

References: C. R. Smart *et al.*, *Cancer*, 1975, *36*, 103.

Absorption and Fate. Tegafur is metabolised slowly to fluorouracil in the body.

References to the absorption and fate of tegafur: S. W. Hall *et al.*, *Cancer Treat. Rep.*, 1977, *61*, 1495; E. B. Hills *et al.*, *J. pharm. Sci.*, 1977, *66*, 1497; J. A. Benvenuto *et al.*, *Cancer Res.*, 1978, *38*, 3867; T. L. Loo *et al.*, *Drug Metab. Rev.*, 1978, *8*, 137.

Uses. Tegafur is an antineoplastic agent which appears to act by the release of fluorouracil (p.209) in the body. It has been used in the management of malignant neoplasms of the breast and gastro-intestinal tract. Doses of 1 to 3 g per m^2 body-surface daily for 5 days have been administered intravenously every 2 to 4 weeks. Tegafur has also been given by mouth.

Clinical reports of tegafur: M. Valdivieso *et al.*, *Cancer Res.*, 1976, *36*, 1821.

Proprietary Names

Ftorafur *(Grünenthal, Ger.)*; Coparogin, Exonal, Fental, FH, Franroze, Fulaid, Fulfeel, Fultol-P, Furafuluor, Furofutran, Futraful, Futraful Zupo, Futraful Zupo-S, Helpa, Icalus, Lamar, Lifril, Lunacin, Neberk, Nitobanil, Pharmic, Richina, Riol, Sinoflurol, Tefsiel-C *(all Jap.)*.

1867-b

Teniposide. PTG; NSC 122819; VM 26; 4-*O*-Demethyl-1-*O*-(4,6-*O*-2-thenylidene-β-D-glucopyranosyl)epipodophyllotoxin. 5,8,8a,9-Tetrahydro-5-(4-hydroxy-3,5-dimethoxyphenyl)-9-(4,6-*O*-2-thenylidene-β-D-glucopyranosyloxy)-2*H*-isobenzofuro[5,6-*f*][1,3]benzodioxol-6(5a*H*)-one.

$C_{32}H_{32}O_{13}S$=656.7.

CAS — 29767-20-2.

A semi-synthetic derivative of podophyllotoxin reported to be practically **insoluble** in water.

Uses. Teniposide is an antineoplastic agent with the general properties of etoposide (p.208). It has been given in the treatment of lymphomas and solid tumours of the bladder and brain. Doses of 30 mg per m^2 body-surface have been administered daily for 5 days by intravenous infusion.

A dose of 67 mg per m^2 body-surface of radioactively-labelled teniposide was administered by intravenous infusion in 300 ml of sodium chloride injection over 30 minutes to 6 cancer patients. Plasma decay was triphasic with terminal half-lives ranging from 11 to 38.5 hours. Penetration into the cerebrospinal fluid was generally poor and protein binding was high. Over 72 hours urinary recovery of radioactivity was about 44% of the administered dose and metabolite accounted for 79% of this. Recovery of drug in the faeces ranged from 0 to 10%.— P. J. Creaven and L. M. Allen, *Clin. Pharmac. Ther.*, 1975, *18*, 227.

References to the use of teniposide: *Br. med. J.*, 1972, *2*, 744 (European Organization for Research on the Treatment of Cancer, Co-operative Group for Leukaemias and Haematosarcomas); J. L. Misset *et al.*, *Nouv. Presse méd.*, 1975, *4*, 3117 (lymphomas); M. Pavone-Macaluso *et al.*, *Eur. Urol.*, 1976, *2*, 138 (bladder cancer).

Adverse effects. Acute intravascular haemolysis and renal failure due to teniposide-related antibody.— B. Habibi *et al.* (letter), *Lancet*, 1981, *1*, 1423.

Proprietary Names

Véhem *(Sandoz, Fr.)*; Vumon *(Bristol, Swed.*; *Bristol, Switz.)*.

1868-v

Thioguanine *(B.P., U.S.P.).* 6-TG; 6-Thioguanine; Tioguanine; NSC 752; WR 1141. 2-Aminopurine-6(1*H*)-thione; 2-Amino-6-mercaptopurine; 2-Aminopurine-6-thiol.
$C_5H_5N_5S$=167.2.

CAS — 154-42-7 (anhydrous); 5580-03-0 (hemihydrate).

Pharmacopoeias. In *Br. Braz.* and *U.S.* permit anhydrous or hemihydrate.

A pale yellow, odourless or almost odourless, crystalline powder. Practically **insoluble** in water, alcohol, and chloroform; freely soluble in dilute solutions of alkali hydroxides. **Store** in airtight containers.

Adverse Effects, Treatment, and Precautions. As for Mercaptopurine, p.214.
In some patients, gastro-intestinal reactions are reported to be less frequent than with mercaptopurine. Normal doses of thioguanine may be employed when it is used with allopurinol.

For a report of a fatal result when thioguanine and cytarabine were given to a patient with myelofibrosis and hypercalcaemia, see Cytarabine, p.203.

Effects on the vascular system. For a report of veno-occlusive disease of the liver occurring during treatment with thioguanine, see Cytarabine, p.203.

Absorption and Fate. Thioguanine is incompletely and variably absorbed from the gastro-intestinal tract. It is rapidly activated in the body by intracellular conversion to its nucleotide thioguanylic acid. Very little thioguanine has been detected circulating in the blood but the half-life of the nucleotide derivatives in the tissues is prolonged. Thioguanine is inactivated by methylation to aminomethylthiopurine and by deamination to thioxanthine; unlike mercaptopurine (p.214) inactivation is independent of xanthine oxidase. About 40% of a dose has been reported to be excreted in the urine within 24 hours as metabolites including aminomethylthiopurine thiouric acid, and sulphate; only negligible amounts of thioguanine have been detected.

A study of the absorption and fate of thioguanine in 24 cancer patients given thioguanine by mouth and intravenously as the sodium salt. After an intravenous dose plasma half-lives of 25 to 240 minutes (a median of 80 minutes) were achieved and about 77% of the dose (range 41 to 81%) was excreted in the urine in 24 hours, entirely as metabolites after 2 hours. After oral doses only metabolites were detected in the urine; 24 to 46% of a dose was excreted in 24 hours. Blood concentrations and incorporation into bone-marrow DNA were dependent on the dose and primarily on the state of the bone marrow. Incorporation into DNA of the bone marrow was slight after one dose but after 5 daily doses thioguanine had almost replaced guanine in the DNA indicating that most cells were stimulated to enter DNA synthesis during that time.— G. A. LePage and J. P. Whitecar, *Cancer Res.*, 1971, *31,* 1627.

Uses. Thioguanine is an analogue of the naturally occurring purine, guanine, and is an antineoplastic agent with actions and uses similar to those of mercaptopurine (see p.214). It appears to cause fewer gastro-intestinal reactions but cross-resistance exists between it and mercaptopurine so that patients who do not respond to one are unlikely to respond to the other.
Thioguanine is given by mouth with other agents, usually cytarabine and daunorubicin or doxorubicin, in the induction and maintenance of remissions in acute myeloid leukaemia, especially in adults. It has also been used in acute lymphoblastic leukaemia and chronic myeloid leukemia.
A dose of 2 to 2.5 mg per kg body-weight daily increased after 4 weeks, if there is no response or toxicity allows, to 3 mg per kg daily may be given to adults and children. A commonly used dose in induction regimens has been 100 mg per m^2 body-surface every 12 hours for up to 10 days. A dose of 2 mg per kg daily is often used for maintenance and up to 10 mg per kg has been given intermittently with other agents. Blood counts should be made daily during induction and when thioguanine is given with other antineoplastic agents, or weekly when given on its own for maintenance. Therapy should be withdrawn at the first sign of severe bone-marrow depression.
It has been administered intravenously as thioguanine sodium.

For reports on the use of thioguanine in the treatment of leukaemia, see Choice of Antineoplastic Agent, p.178.

Preparations

Thioguanine Tablets *(B.P.).* Tablets containing thioguanine.

Thioguanine Tablets *(U.S.P.).* Tablets containing thioguanine. Potency is expressed in terms of anhydrous thioguanine. Store in airtight containers.

Lanvis *(Wellcome, UK).* Thioguanine, available as scored tablets of 40 mg. (Also available as Lanvis in *Austral., Belg., Canad., Neth., Switz.*).

1869-g

Thiotepa *(B.P., U.S.P.).* Triethylene Thiophosphoramide; Thiophosphamide; TESPA; TSPA; NSC 6396; WR 45312. Phosphorothioic tri(ethyleneamide); Tris(aziridin-1-yl)phosphine sulphide.
$C_6H_{12}N_3PS$=189.2.

CAS — 52-24-4.

Pharmacopoeias. In *Br., Chin., Jap., Rus.,* and *U.S.*

Fine white crystalline flakes with a faint odour. M.p. 52° to 57°. **Soluble** 1 in 8 of water, 1 in 2 of alcohol, 1 in 2 of chloroform, and 1 in about 4 of ether. A 5.67% solution in water is iso-osmotic with serum. **Store** at 2° to 10° in airtight containers. At higher temperatures it polymerises and becomes inactive. Protect from light.

CAUTION. *Thiotepa is irritant; avoid contact with skin and mucous membranes.*

An aqueous solution of thiotepa iso-osmotic with serum (5.67%) caused 10% haemolysis of erthrocytes cultured in it for 45 minutes.— C. Sapp *et al., J. pharm. Sci.*, 1975, *64,* 1884.

Adverse Effects, Treatment, and Precautions. For an outline of the adverse effects experienced with antineoplastic agents and immunosuppressants, general guidelines for their treatment, and precautions, see Antineoplastic Agents, p.171, pp.174-5.
Thiotepa is very toxic to the haemopoietic system; maximum depression of the bone marrow may occur up to 30 days after therapy has been discontinued and irreversible hypoplastic anaemia may occur. The relation between dosage and toxicity is highly variable and extreme caution is always required.

Effects on the blood. Ten of 25 consecutive patients given instillations of thiotepa into the bladder had at least one episode of acute dose-related myelosuppression, occurring most often within the first 3 months of treatment. One of the 25, and 4 further patients developed chronic myelosuppression. Thrombocytopenia was the most common abnormality. The 2 forms of myelosuppression were not related and there was no way of predicting which patients will develop chronic myelosuppression. A treatment schedule averaging 90 mg of thiotepa monthly during the first 3 months, reduced to 45 mg monthly over longer periods, is recommended.— D. Hollister and M. Coleman, *J. Am. med. Ass.*, 1980, *244,* 2065.

Effects on the kidneys. A 76-year-old man developed ureteral obstruction and renal failure after topical treatment with thiotepa following bladder resection.— P. F. Schellhammer, *J. Urol.*, 1973, *110,* 498.

Absorption and Fate. The absorption of thiotepa from the gastro-intestinal tract is incomplete and unreliable; variable absorption also occurs from intramuscular injection sites. Absorption through serous membranes such as the bladder and pleura occurs to some extent. Only traces of unchanged thiotepa and triethylene phosphoramide are excreted in the urine, together with a large proportion of metabolites.

References: L. B. Mellett *et al., J. Lab. clin. Med.*, 1962, *60,* 818.

Uses. Thiotepa is an ethyleneimine compound whose antineoplastic effect is related to its alkylating action (see p.171). It has a spectrum of activity similar to that of mustine (p.223) but has generally been replaced by cyclophosphamide (p.200). It is not a vesicant and may be given by all parenteral routes, as well as directly into tumour masses. Thiotepa may be used in the palliation of carcinoma of the breast and ovary and has been given in the treatment of various lymphomas. Instillations of thiotepa are used in the treatment of superficial tumours of the bladder and in the control of malignant effusions. It has been given intrathecally to patients with malignant meningeal disease. Thiotepa has some immunosuppressant activity.
See also under Choice of Antineoplastic Agent, p.175.
Thiotepa is given in a variety of dosage schedules. In general, initial doses to suit the individual patient are followed by maintenance doses given at intervals of one to 4 weeks. Blood counts are recommended before administration and if there is leucopenia the dose should be reduced. Thiotepa should not be given if the white cell count falls below 3000 per mm^3 or the platelet count below 150 000 per mm^3. Up to 60 mg in single or divided doses may be given by intramuscular injection or by instillation in adults and children over 12 years; similar doses have been injected into tumours. Alternatively, 200 µg per kg body-weight daily for 3 to 5 days, followed by a maintenance dose of 200 µg per kg every one to 3 weeks, has been suggested. Intravenous doses of up to 30 mg may be given every one to 4 weeks. A solution containing 1 mg of thiotepa per ml has been injected intrathecally in doses of up to 10 mg.
Following dehydration for 8 to 12 hours, up to 60 mg of thiotepa in 60 ml of sterile water may be instilled into the bladder, where it is retained for 2 hours if possible, and the instillation repeated weekly for 4 weeks; single-dose instillations of 90 mg in 100 ml of sterile water have been used prophylactically as an adjunct to surgery. Malignant effusions may be treated by the instillation of 10 to 30 mg of thiotepa in 20 to 60 ml of sterile water, following aspiration.
Thiotepa for local use has been mixed with solutions of procaine and adrenaline.

Insect chemosterilisation. For the chemosterilisation of *Aedes aegypti* with thiotepa, see E. F. Knipling *et al., Bull. Wld Hlth Org.*, 1968, *38,* 421. Reference to the use of thiotepa in the sterilisation of mosquitoes.— V. P. Sharma (letter), *Nature*, 1976, *261,* 135.

Malignant effusions. For a comparison of thiotepa and mepacrine in the treatment of pleural effusions, see Mepacrine Hydrochloride, p.400.

See also under Choice of Antineoplastic Agent, p.180.

Malignant neoplasms. Reports of the use of thiotepa in various malignant neoplasms: A. R. Lyons and G. A. Edelstyn, *Br. J. Cancer*, 1965, *19,* 490 (breast); R. J. Veenema, *J. Am. med. Ass.*, 1968, *206,* 2725 (bladder); J. Magell (letter), *Lancet*, 1969, *2,* 846 (ovary); B. Fisher *et al., Surgery Gynec. Obstet.*, 1975, *140,* 528 (breast); P. H. Gutin *et al., Cancer Treat. Rep.*, 1977, *61,* 885 (intrathecal use in malignant meningeal disease); G. R. Prout, *Cancer Res.*, 1977, *37,* 2916 (bladder).

Ocular disorders, non-malignant. Following the surgical removal of a pterygium, the recurrence-rate of 50% could be reduced to less than 1% by the use of eyedrops of thiotepa 0.05% every 3 hours during the waking period for 6 to 8 weeks.— J. M. Whaites (letter), *Br. med. J.*, 1970, *2,* 669. See also E. R. Asregadoo, *Am. J. Ophthal.*, 1972, *74,* 960.

Rheumatic disorders, non-malignant. References to the use of intra-articular injections of thiotepa in rheumatic disorders: H. L. F. Currey, *Ann. rheum. Dis.*, 1965, *24,* 382; M. Langkilde and I. Rossell, *Acta rheum. scand.*, 1967, *13,* 92 (comparison with azetepa and osmium tetroxide); M. R. Ellison and A. E. Flatt, *Arthritis Rheum.*, 1971, *14*, 212.

Skin disorders, non-malignant. Fourteen patients with severe psoriasis unresponsive to other treatment were treated by the application once daily of thiotepa 0.4% in yellow soft paraffin containing 20% of wool fat; occlusive dressings were applied for 8 hours. Total clearing of the lesions occurred in 11 patients in an average of 19 days. The treatment caused a tolerable burning sensation for a few days. Irritation of surrounding skin was prevented by the application of macrogol 1500 containing 10% of propylene glycol. Two patients with involvement of 15 and 20% of the body-surface discontinued treatment because of leucopenia.— G. Heydenreich, *Br. J. Derm.*, 1971, *85*, 182.

Preparations

Thiotepa for Injection *(U.S.P.)*. A sterile mixture of thiotepa 1 part, sodium chloride 5.33 parts, and sodium bicarbonate 3.33 parts. A 0.75% solution has a pH of 7 to 8.2. Store at 2° to 8°. Protect from light.

Thiotepa Injection *(B.P.)*. A sterile solution of thiotepa with sodium chloride and sodium bicarbonate in Water for Injections. It is prepared by dissolving the sterile contents of a sealed container (Thiotepa for Injection) in Water for Injections. A 0.75% injection has a pH of 7 to 8.2. Store at 2° to 8°. Under these conditions, the solution may be expected to retain its potency for 5 days. If solid particles separate, the solution should not be used.

Thiotepa *(Lederle, UK)*. Vials each containing thiotepa 15 mg with sodium chloride 80 mg and sodium bicarbonate 50 mg for solution before use. (Also available as Thiotepa in *Austral., Canad., Denm., Fr.*).

Other Proprietary Names

Ledertepa *(Belg., Neth.)*; Onco Tiotepa *(Spain)*; Tifosyl *(Norw., Swed.)*.

1870-f

Tioinosine. Thioinosine. 9-β-D-Ribofuranosyl-9*H*-purine-6-thiol.
$C_{10}H_{12}N_4O_4S$=284.3.

CAS — 574-25-4.

White or pale yellow powder or crystals, practically odourless and with a bitter taste. M.p. about 211° with decomposition. Freely **soluble** in water; practically insoluble in acetone, alcohol, chloroform, ether, and glacial acetic acid; very slightly soluble in methyl alcohol; sparingly soluble in dilute sodium hydroxide solution. A saturated aqueous solution has a slightly acid reaction.

Uses. Tioinosine is the riboside of mercaptopurine (see p.214) and has similar properties. It has been used in the treatment of acute and chronic myeloid leukaemia in doses of 1 to 6 mg per kg body-weight daily.

References: S. Shimano *et al.*, *Curr. ther. Res.*, 1974, *16*, 15.

Proprietary Names
Thioinosie *(Morishita, Jap.)*.

1871-d

Treosulfan.

Dihydroxybusulphan; NSC 39069. L-Threitol 1,4-dimethanesulphonate.
$C_6H_{14}O_8S_2$=278.3.

CAS — 299-75-2.

A white odourless crystalline powder. M.p. about 102°. **Soluble** 1 in about 14 of water; 1 in about 8 of acetone; 1 in about 200 of alcohol; and 1 in about 2000 of chloroform.

Adverse Effects, Treatment, and Precautions. For an outline of the adverse effects experienced with antineoplastic agents and immunosuppressants, general guidelines for their treatment, and precautions, see Antineoplastic Agents, p.171, pp.174-5.

Adrenal suppression. A 58-year-old woman developed adrenal failure following treatment with a total of 60 g of treosulfan given over 6 weeks.— J. Prior and I. White (letter), *Lancet*, 1978, *2*, 1207. Transient marrow depression similar to that seen with chlorambucil occurred in 70 patients given treosulfan 1 g daily for 28 days every second month, but there was no hepatic toxicity or nephrotoxicity. Other side-effects included mild pigmentation in 3 patients and minimal alopecia in one, but no evidence of adrenal insufficiency was noted.— J. J. Fennelly (letter), *Lancet*, 1979, *1*, 106.

Uses. Treosulfan is an antineoplastic agent which is reported to act by alkylation (see p.171) after conversion *in vivo* via the monoepoxide to L-diepoxybutane. It is used palliatively or as an adjunct to surgery in the treatment of ovarian cancer.

Treosulfan 1 g daily is given by mouth in 4 divided doses for one month followed by one month without treatment. The cycle is then repeated, the dose being adjusted if necessary according to the effect on bone marrow. Lower doses should be used if treatment with other antineoplastic drugs or radiotherapy is being given concomitantly. Treosulfan may also be given intravenously in doses of 5 to 15 g every one to three weeks.

References to treosulfan in the management of ovarian cancer: J. Fennelly, *Br. J. Obstet. Gynaec.*, 1977, *84*, 300.

Proprietary Preparations

Treosulfan Leo *(Leo, UK)*. Treosulfan, available as **Capsules** of 250 mg and as intravenous **Injection** (supplied as powder for solution in Water for Injections before use) in infusion bottles of 5 g. (Also available as Treosulfan Leo in *Neth.*).

1872-n

Tretamine *(B.P.C. 1968)*. Tretaminum; Triethylenemelamine; Triethanomelamine; TEM; NSC 9706. 2,4,6-Tris(aziridin-1-yl)-1,3,5-triazine.
$C_9H_{12}N_6$=204.2.

CAS — 51-18-3.

Pharmacopoeias. In *Jug.*

A white or almost white crystalline powder which is odourless or has a slight fish-like odour. M.p. about 160°; it melts to a clear liquid which polymerises vigorously.

Soluble 1 in 3 of water, 1 in 15 of alcohol, 1 in 4 of chloroform, and 1 in 200 of ether; soluble in acetone and carbon tetrachloride. A 1% solution in water is clear. It is relatively stable in alkaline solution but is rapidly decomposed in acid solution. Solutions should be freshly prepared. **Store** below 8° in airtight containers. Protect from light.

CAUTION. *Tretamine is irritant; avoid contact with skin and mucous membranes.*

Adverse Effects, Treatment, and Precautions. For an outline of the adverse effects experienced with antineoplastic agents and immunosuppressants, general guidelines for their treatment, and precautions, see Antineoplastic Agents, p.171, pp.174-5.

Tretamine is a potent bone-marrow depressant with a delayed effect which may not be apparent for 2 weeks or more.

Uses. Similarly to thiotepa (p.228), tretamine is an ethyleneimine compound with antineoplastic properties related to its alkylating action. Tretamine is variably absorbed from the gastro-intestinal tract and was formerly given by mouth in the palliative treatment of retinoblastoma, chronic leukaemias, and lymphomas. Doses of 2.5 to 5 mg twice weekly or 50 to 100 µg per kg body-weight weekly have been given.

1873-h

Triaziquone. Bayer 3231; NSC 29215; Triethyleneiminobenzoquinone. Tris(aziridin-1-yl)-*p*-benzoquinone.
$C_{12}H_{13}N_3O_2$=231.3.

CAS — 68-76-8.

Small violet acicular crystals. M.p. about 162°. **Soluble** in cold water, acetone, methyl alcohol, and warm acetic acid. Unstable in the presence of acids, alkalis, and reducing agents. Solutions should be prepared immediately before injection. **Store** in a cool place. Protect from light.

Adverse Effects, Treatment, and Precautions. For an outline of the adverse effects experienced with antineoplastic agents and immunosuppressants, general guidelines for their treatment, and precautions, see Antineoplastic Agents, p.171, pp.174-5.

Triaziquone is irritant and care should be taken to avoid extravasation during injection.

Uses. Triaziquone is an antineoplastic agent which acts by alkylation (see p.171). It also has immunosuppressant properties. Triaziquone was formerly used in the treatment of ovarian cancer. It has been given in a dose of 200 µg intravenously on alternate days to a total of 3 to 5 mg, followed by maintenance treatment with 0.5 to 1.5 mg weekly given by mouth.

Triaziquone was formerly marketed in Great Britain under the proprietary name Trenimon *(Bayer)*.

1874-m

Trimustine Hydrochloride. Trichlormethine Hydrochloride. Tris(2-chloroethyl)amine hydrochloride; 2,2′,2″-Trichlorotriethylamine hydrochloride.
$C_6H_{12}Cl_3N,HCl$=241.0.

CAS — 555-77-1 (trimustine); 817-09-4 (hydrochloride).

A crystalline powder. **Soluble** in water and alcohol. Aqueous solutions deteriorate rapidly.

Trimustine is an antineoplastic agent with actions and uses similar to those of mustine hydrochloride (p.222).

1875-b

Trofosfamide. Trophosphamide; Trilophosphamide; NSC 109723; Z 4828. 3-(2-Chloroethyl)-2-[bis(2-chloroethyl)amino]perhydro-1,3,2-oxazaphosphorine-2-oxide.
$C_9H_{18}Cl_3N_2O_2P$=323.6.

CAS — 22089-22-1.

White odourless crystals. M.p. 51° to 53°. Slightly **soluble** in water; very readily soluble in chloroform and methyl alcohol; soluble in ether.

Uses. Trofosfamide has the general properties of cyclophosphamide (p.199). Doses of 50 to 400 mg daily have been given by mouth in the treatment of malignant diseases.

References to the use of trofosfamide: P. Drings *et al.*, *Dt. med. Wschr.*, 1970, *95*, 491; G. Falkson and H. C. Falkson, *S. Afr. med. J.*, 1978, *53*, 886.

Proprietary Names
Ixoten *(Asta, Ger.; Schering, Ital.; Asta, Neth.; Noristan, S.Afr.)*.

1876-v

Uramustine.

Uracil Mustard *(U.S.P.)*; NSC 34462; U 8344. 5-Bis(2-chloroethyl)aminouracil; 5-[Bis(2-chloroethyl)amino]pyrimidine-2,4(1*H*,3*H*)-dione.
$C_8H_{11}Cl_2N_3O_2$=252.1.

CAS — 66-75-1.

Pharmacopoeias. In *U.S.*

An off-white odourless crystalline powder. M.p. about 200° with decomposition. Very slightly **soluble** in water; soluble 1 in 150 of alcohol; slightly soluble in acetone; practically insoluble in chloroform. Unstable in the presence of water. **Store** in airtight containers.

CAUTION. *Uramustine is irritant; avoid contact with skin and mucous membranes.*

Adverse Effects, Treatment, and Precautions. For an outline of the adverse effects experienced with antineoplastic agents and immunosuppressants, general guidelines for their treatment, and precautions, see Antineoplastic Agents, p.171, pp.174-5.

Maximum depression of the bone marrow may not occur until 2 to 4 weeks after uramustine has been discontinued and if the total dosage approaches 1 mg per kg body-weight, the cumulative damage to the bone marrow may be irreversible.

Effects on respiratory function. For a report of pulmonary fibrosis occurring with uramustine, see Busulphan, p.194.

Uses. Uramustine is an antineoplastic agent derived from mustine (p.222) and has a similar mode of action. It has been given by mouth in the treatment of chronic lymphocytic leukaemia and malignant lymphomas and has occasionally been used in mycosis fungoides, polycythaemia vera, thrombocytosis, and as an adjunct in carcinoma of the ovary and lung.

A suggested dosage is 1 to 2 mg daily until a clinical response or bone-marrow depression occurs. When the bone marrow recovers or the patient deteriorates treatment is reinstituted with 1 mg daily for 3 weeks, followed by 1 week's rest, and then repeated courses for several months. Another scheme of administration is to give 3 to 5 mg daily for 7 days, followed by 1 mg daily for 3 weeks out of 4. Further reduction to 1 mg once or twice weekly may be possible. The total dose in the first week should not be more than 500 µg per kg body-weight. Total and differential white-cell counts, platelet counts, and haemoglobin examinations should be made once or twice weekly and the dosage adjusted according to the patient's response.

Blood disorders, non-malignant. A report of uramustine being used to treat 8 patients with polycythaemia vera and 6 with essential thrombocytosis.— H. K. Shamasunder *et al.*, *J. Am. med. Ass.*, 1980, *244*, 1454.

Preparations

Uracil Mustard Capsules *(U.S.P.).* Capsules containing uramustine. Store in airtight containers.

Uramustine was formerly marketed in Great Britain as Uracil Mustard (*Upjohn*).

1877-g

Urethane *(B.P. 1963).* Urethanum; Urethan.; Ethylurethane. Ethyl carbamate.
$NH_2.CO.O.C_2H_5$=89.09.

CAS — 51-79-6.

Pharmacopoeias. In *Arg.*, *Aust.*, *Belg.*, *Hung.*, *Ind.*, *Int.*, *Mex.*, *Nord.*, *Pol.*, *Port.*, *Roum.*, *Span.*, and *Turk.*

Colourless crystals or white granular powder with a cooling, saline, slightly bitter taste; odourless or with a slight odour. M.p. 48° to 50°.

Soluble 1 in 1.5 of water, 1 in 1 of alcohol, 1 in 1 of chloroform, 1 in 2 of ether, 1 in 3 of glycerol, 1 in 35 of olive oil, and in other fixed oils. Solutions in water are neutral to litmus. A 2.93% solution is iso-osmotic with serum. Solutions are **sterilised** by autoclaving or by filtration. **Incompatible** with alkalis and acids. It liquefies with benzoic acid, chloral hydrate, camphor, menthol, resorcinol, salicylic acid, and thymol. **Store** in a cool place.

An aqueous solution of urethane iso-osmotic with serum (2.93%) caused 100% haemolysis of erythrocytes cultured in it for 45 minutes.— E. R. Hammarlund and K. Pedersen-Bjergaard, *J. pharm. Sci.*, 1961, *50*, 24.

Adverse Effects and Treatment. For an outline of the adverse effects experienced with antineoplastic agents and immunosuppressants and general guidelines for their treatment, see Antineoplastic Agents, p.171 and p.174.

Bone-marrow depression, anorexia, nausea, vomiting, drowsiness, and dizziness are common side-effects of urethane therapy.

Precautions. For reference to the precautions necessary with antineoplastic agents and immunosuppressants, see Antineoplastic Agents, p.175.

Urethane has been shown to alter the sedative properties of barbiturates.

Absorption and Fate. Urethane is readily absorbed from the gastro-intestinal tract and is metabolised in the body to alcohol, ammonia, and carbon dioxide.

Uses. Urethane is an antineoplastic agent which was formerly used in the treatment of chronic myeloid leukaemia. It is also a mild hypnotic and has been employed as an anaesthetic for small animals.

1878-q

Vinblastine Sulphate *(B.P.).* Vinblastine Sulfate *(U.S.P.)*; Vincaleucoblastine Sulphate; Vincaleukoblastine Sulphate; LE 29060; NSC 49842. The sulphate of an alkaloid, vincaleukoblastine, extracted from *Vinca rosea* (*Catharanthus roseus*) (Apocynaceae).
$C_{46}H_{58}N_4O_9,H_2SO_4$=909.1.

CAS — 865-21-4 (vinblastine); 143-67-9 (sulphate).

Pharmacopoeias. In *Br.*, *Chin.*, and *U.S.* which also includes Sterile Vinblastine Sulfate.

A white to slightly yellow, odourless, very hygroscopic, amorphous or crystalline powder. It loses not more than 17% of its weight on drying.

Soluble 1 in 10 of water, 1 in 1200 of alcohol, and 1 in 50 of chloroform; soluble in methyl alcohol; practically insoluble in ether. A solution in methyl alcohol is laevorotatory. A 0.15% solution in water has a pH of 3.5 to 5 and a 0.3% solution is clear. **Store** at 2° to 10° in airtight containers. Protect from light.

Adverse Effects and Treatment. For an outline of the adverse effects experienced with antineoplastic agents and immonusuppressants and general guidelines for their treatment, see Antineoplastic Agents, p.171 and p.174.

Bone-marrow depression, especially leucopenia, is the most common adverse effect with vinblastine and tends to be dose-limiting. Maximum depression occurs 4 to 10 days after administration with recovery in 1 to 3 weeks. Gastro-intestinal effects are reported to occur less frequently than with the alkylating agents and respond to treatment with anti-emetics.

Neurological effects that can also involve the autonomic nervous system include malaise, headache, depression, psychoses, paraesthesia, neuromyopathy, loss of deep tendon relfexes, peripheral neuritis, constipation and adynamic ileus, parotid gland pain, and convulsions. Overdosage has caused permanent damage to the central nervous system.

Vinblastine is irritant to the skin and mucous membranes.

Effects on the heart. Myocardial infarction in a 37-year-old man was apparently caused by vinblastine injection.— J. L. Lejonc *et al.* (letter), *Lancet*, 1980, *2*, 692. See also A. L. Harris and C. Wong (letter), *ibid.*, 1981, *1*, 787.

Effects on the kidneys. Inappropriate secretion of antidiuretic hormone in 4 patients was considered to be associated with high-dose vinblastine therapy.— S. J. Ginsberg *et al.* (letter), *New Engl. J. Med.*, 1977, *296*, 941.

See also under Overdosage, below.

Effects on the nervous system. Experiments in *rats* indicated that vinblastine given intravenously destroyed adrenergic nerve terminals.— I. Hanbauer *et al.*, *Br. J. Pharmac.*, 1974, *50*, 219.

For reports of ocular changes, salivary gland pain, constipation, and severe abdominal pain occurring in patients treated with vinblastine sulphate, see Vincristine Sulphate, p.231.

Effects on reproductive potential. *Gonads.* Vinblastine impaired fertility in the male *rat*.— R. A. Cooke *et al.*, *Br. J. Pharmac.*, 1978, *63*, 677.

Effects on respiratory function. Pulmonary oedema occurred in a 64-year-old woman 2 hours after the intravenous administration of vinblastine.— R. H. Israel and J. P. Olson (letter), *J. Am. med. Ass.*, 1978, *240*, 1585.

Effects on the skin. Dermatitis of the hands associated with exposure to sunlight occurred on numerous occasions in a 34-year-old man with Hodgkin's disease after injections of vinblastine sulphate.— T. S. Breza *et al.*, *Archs Derm.*, 1975, *111*, 1168.

Effects on the vascular system. A report of Raynaud's phenomenon in a man receiving vinblastine.— H. Rothberg, *Cancer Treat. Rep.*, 1978, *62*, 569.

For similar reports after treatment with bleomycin and vinblastine, see Bleomycin Sulphate, p.192.

Local irritant effect. Corneal changes were apparent in a doctor 24 hours after he had accidentally sprayed his face with a solution of vinblastine sulphate. Over the next 8 days he experienced increasing blepharospasm, photophobia, epiphora, swelling of the eyelids, and a fall in visual acuity. Topical treatment with corticosteroids was required and subepithelial corneal changes persisted.— B. F. McLendon and A. J. Bron, *Br. J. Ophthal.*, 1978, *62*, 97.

Overdosage. Inappropriate secretion of antidiuretic hormone in a 3-year-old boy on maintenance treatment with vinblastine, 3 mg every 14 days, was probably due to the accidental injection of a 30-mg dose. He recovered following exchange transfusions, administration of enemas, and treatment with antibiotics and anti-hypertensives.— S. C. Winter and G. S. Arbus (letter), *Can. med. Ass. J.*, 1977, *117*, 1134.

Precautions. For reference to the precautions necessary with antineoplastic agents and immunosuppressants, see Antineoplastic Agents, p.175.

When injecting vinblastine sulphate care should be taken to avoid extravasation which may be followed by local pain, cellulitis, phlebitis, and venous thrombosis.

Interactions. *With radiation.* Pain, erythema, and oedema developed on the face and neck of an 11-year-old boy on the day following treatment with vinblastine. The reaction lasted about 2 weeks. The affected area had been irradiated 2 months earlier.— B. C. Lampkin (letter), *Lancet*, 1969, *1*, 891.

Absorption and Fate. Vinblastine is not reliably absorbed from the gastro-intestinal tract and it is usually given intravenously. It rapidly disappears from the blood but penetrates only poorly into the cerebrospinal fluid. It is excreted in the bile and in the urine.

In a pharmacokinetic study in 3 patients, elimination after intravenous injection was triphasic with mean half-lives of 3.9, 53, and 1173 minutes, respectively. Vinblastine was metabolised to active deacetylvinblastine, probably in the liver. An intravenous dose of vinblastine, radioactively labelled in the indole aromatic ring rather than the less stable preparation used in earlier studies which was labelled at the 4-acetyl position, was given to one patient. Total amounts of radioactivity excreted in urine and faeces differed from the data previously obtained with 4-acetyl-[^{3}H]vinblastine; only 13.6% of the total radioactive dose was excreted in the urine in 72 hours compared with 18.7 to 23.3% when vinblastine labelled at the 4-acetyl position was used and 9.9% was excreted in the faeces in 72 hours compared with 25 to 41% with vinblastine labelled at the 4-acetyl position. About 73% of the radioactivity was still in the body after 6 days.— R. J. Owellen *et al.*, *Cancer Res.*, 1977, *37*, 2597.

See also under Vindesine Sulphate, p.232.

Uses. Vinblastine sulphate is an antineoplastic agent which acts by arresting mitosis at the metaphase and inhibits RNA synthesis; it may also interfere with amino acid metabolism. It also has some immunosuppressant activity. Cross-resistance with vincristine has not been reported.

Vinblastine sulphate is mainly used, in association with other antineoplastic agents, in the treatment of Hodgkin's disease and other lymphomas. It is also of use in the treatment of some inoperable malignant neoplasms including those of the breast and testis and in neuroblastoma and choriocarcinoma. In the treatment of Hodgkin's disease it is often given with mustine, procarbazine, and prednisone (MVPP), or with doxorubicin, bleomycin, and dacarbazine (ABVD). In carcinoma of the testis vinblastine is given with bleomycin and cisplatin. See also under Choice of Antineoplastic Agent, p.184.

Vinblastine sulphate is given by intravenous injection as a solution containing 1 mg per ml in sodium chloride injection. Care should be taken to avoid extravasation. The suggested dosage scheme is as follows: weekly injections starting with 100 µg per kg body-weight raised by increments of 50 µg per kg to a maximum weekly dose of 500 µg per kg or until the white cell count has fallen to 3000 per mm^3. A maintenance dose is then given every 7 to 14 days and should be one increment smaller than the maximum dose that the patient is able to tolerate without serious leucopenia occurring; weekly doses of 150 to 200 µg per kg are often adequate. A maintenance dose of 10 mg has also been given once or twice a month. Children may be given vinblastine sulphate in an initial dose of 2.5 mg per m^2 body-surface intravenously, increased by 1.25 mg per m^2 weekly to a maximum weekly dose of 7.5 mg per m^2.

White cell counts should be made before each injection and a repeat dose should never be given unless the count has risen to 4000 per mm^3. Generally, older patients require smaller doses and leukaemic children tolerate higher doses.

Vinblastine sulphate has been given by continuous intra-arterial infusion and by injection into body cavities.

The proceedings of symposia on the vinca alkaloids in the chemotherapy of malignant disease.— W.I.H. Shedden (Ed.), Basingstoke, Eli Lilly and Co. Ltd., 1968; *idem*, 1971; *idem*, 1972.

Action. A discussion on the antimitotic actions of the vinca alkaloids.— F. E. Samson, *A. Rev. Pharmac. & Toxic.*, 1976, *16*, 143.

Administration in renal insufficiency. Vinblastine can be given in usual doses to patients with impaired renal function.— W. M. Bennett *et al.*, *Ann. intern. Med.*, 1980, *93*, 286.

Blood disorders, non-malignant. *Thrombocytopenic purpura.* Infusions of vinblastine, bound to platelets by incubation, were given to 11 patients with refractory idiopathic thrombocytopenic purpura in an attempt to achieve selective delivery of large amounts of the drug to the macrophages. All patients had been treated previously with vinca alkaloids by conventional injection but responses had been short-lived. Six patients achieved complete remission, which was maintained for at least 5 months in 3 of them, and 3 achieved partial remission. Side-effects were reversible and included neutropenia, mild confusion, alopecia, jaw pain, and burning tongue.— Y. S. Ahn *et al.*, *New Engl. J. Med.*, 1978, *298*, 1101. Comment.— W. F. Rosse, *ibid.*, 1139.

References to thrombocytosis (raised platelet counts) occurring during treatment with vinblastine.— J. H. Robertson and G. M. McCarthy, *Lancet*, 1969, *2*, 353; G. D. Soppitt and J. R. A. Mitchell (letter), *ibid.*, 539; Y. F. Hwang *et al.* (letter), *ibid.*, 1075.

Further references to the use of vinblastine in patients with thrombocytopenic purpura.— A. M. Marmont *et al.* (letter), *Lancet*, 1971, *2*, 94 (resistant to azathioprine and prednisone).

See also under Vincristine Sulphate (below).

Enhancement of effect. The action of vinblastine against Ehrlich carcinoma was increased when thymidine was given 15 hours afterwards.— H. Osswald, *Arzneimittel-Forsch.*, 1972, *22*, 1421.

Histiocytosis X. A 54-year-old man with histiocytosis X, unresponsive to other treatment, had complete rectal occlusion due to extensive tumefactions which responded to treatment with vinblastine sulphate, 150 µg per kg body-weight intravenously in 5 weekly doses. Improvement was noted within 3 weeks and resolution was complete in 5 weeks. Additional courses were necessary because of recurrence.— F. S. Tennant (letter), *J. Am. med. Ass.*, 1969, *210*, 2284.

Hodgkin's disease and other lymphomas. For reports of the use of vinblastine with other agents in the treatment of lymphomas, see Choice of Antineoplastic Agent, p.177.

Malignant neoplasms. References to the use of vinblastine in various malignant neoplasms.— W. A. Crosbie *et al.*, *Br. J. Dis. Chest*, 1966, *60*, 28 (lung); E. S. Kondi *et al.*, *Cancer*, 1972, *30*, 1169 (bone); C. Merrin *et al.*, *J. Urol.*, 1975, *113*, 21 (renal cell carcinoma, with lomustine or semustine).

For reports on the use of vinblastine with bleomycin and cisplatin in malignant neoplasms of the testis, see Choice of Antineoplastic Agent, p.184.

For a report of the treatment of solid tumours with fluorouracil and vinblastine, see Fluorouracil, p.210.

Pregnancy and the neonate. A woman treated with vinblastine for Hodgkin's disease from the fifth month of pregnancy onwards gave birth to a normal infant.— M. J. Lacher (letter), *Lancet*, 1964, *1*, 1390. A similar report.— J. J. Nordlund *et al.*, *Ann. intern. Med.*, 1968, *69*, 581.

Preparations

Sterile Vinblastine Sulfate *(U.S.P.)*. Vinblastine sulphate suitable for parenteral use.

Vinblastine Injection *(B.P.)*. A sterile solution of vinblastine sulphate prepared by dissolving the contents of a sealed container (Vinblastine Sulphate for Injection) in the requisite quantity of Water for Injections. Potency is expressed in terms of the equivalent amount of anhydrous vinblastine sulphate. Store at 2° to 10° and use within 4 days; if antimicrobial preservatives are included the injection may be stored for 30 days.

Velbe (known in USA as Velban) *(Lilly, UK)*. Vinblastine sulphate, available in vials of 10 mg, supplied with 10-ml vials of solvent containing sodium chloride 0.9% and benzyl alcohol 0.9%. (Also available as Velbe in *Arg., Austral., Belg., Canad., Denm., Fr., Ger., Ital., Neth., Norw., S.Afr., Switz.*).

Vinblastine Sulphate *(Lederle, UK)*. Available in vials of 10 mg, with 10-ml vials of solvent containing sodium chloride 0.9% and benzyl alcohol 2%.

1879-p

Vincristine Sulphate *(B.P.)*.

Vincristine Sulfate *(U.S.P.)*; Leurocristine Sulphate; NSC 67574. The sulphate of an alkaloid, 22-oxovincaleukoblastine, obtained from *Vinca rosea* (*Catharanthus roseus*) (Apocynaceae).

$C_{46}H_{56}N_4O_{10},H_2SO_4$=923.0.

CAS — 57-22-7 (vincristine); 2068-78-2 (sulphate).

Pharmacopoeias. In *Br.*, *Braz.*, *Chin.*, and *U.S.*

A white to slightly yellow, odourless, very hygroscopic, amorphous or crystalline powder. It loses not more than 12% of its weight on drying. **Soluble** 1 in 2 of water, 1 in 600 of alcohol, and 1 in 30 of chloroform; soluble in methyl alcohol; practically insoluble in ether. A 0.1% solution in water has a pH of 3.5 to 4.5. **Store** at 2° to 10° in airtight containers. Protect from light.

Stability. Based on information supplied by the manufacturers vincristine sulphate for injection was stable for several months at a temperature not exceeding 25°.— R. R. Wolfert and R. M. Cox, *Am. J. Hosp. Pharm.*, 1975, *32*, 585.

Adverse Effects and Treatment. As for Vinblastine Sulphate, p.230.

Bone-marrow depression occurs less commonly than with vinblastine but neurological and neuromuscular effects are more severe with vincristine and are dose limiting. Walking may be impaired and the neurological effects may not be reversed for several months after the drug is discontinued. Convulsions, often with hypertension, have occurred. There may be constipation and abdominal pain. Acute uric acid nephropathy has occurred and alopecia is common.

Adverse effects occur less frequently when the weekly dosage is kept below 100 µg per kg body-weight.

Severe adverse effects due to vincristine but unrelated to dose occurred in 4 children, 2 of whom died during the acute toxicity phase.— M. J. O'Callaghan and H. Ekert, *Archs Dis. Childh.*, 1976, *51*, 289.

Effects on the eyes. A report of bilateral optic atrophy and blindness in a patient given vincristine.— A. S. Awidi (letter), *Ann. intern. Med.*, 1980, *93*, 781.

Effects on the gastro-intestinal tract. In 6 patients with vincristine-induced constipation of 7 to 12 days' duration administration of lactulose (50% w/w solution) in doses of up to 25 ml thrice daily produced bowel movement within 1 or 2 days. In 2 patients given lactulose immediately after vincristine therapy constipation did not occur.— A. C. Harris and J. M. Jackson, *Med. J. Aust.*, 1977, *2*, 573.

Effects on the heart. Myocardial infarction associated with vincristine in one patient.— G. Somers *et al.* (letter), *Lancet*, 1976, *2*, 690.

Effects on the kidneys. Increased plasma-antidiuretic hormone concentrations and increased urinary-antidiuretic hormone excretion has been observed during vincristine therapy.— A. M. Moses and M. Miller, *New Engl. J. Med.*, 1974, *291*, 1234. See also R. G. Nicholson and W. Feldman, *Can. med. Ass. J.*, 1972, *106*, 356; G. L. Robertson *et al.*, *Archs intern. Med.*, 1973, *132*, 717.

Effects on the nervous system. Peripheral neuropathy occurs in the majority of patients receiving vincristine and is related to dose and duration of treatment. The earliest sign of neuropathy is depression of the Achilles tendon reflex followed by paraesthesias in the fingers and toes. Muscle pain, weakness, and sensory impairment develop if the drug is continued and further use frequently produces severe generalised motor weakness and occasionally quadriparesis. Recovery commences on withdrawal of vincristine but depressed deep-tendon reflexes return slowly if at all and in most patients minor symptoms such as numbness and tingling of the fingers and toes persist for several months. Apart from peripheral and autonomic neuropathies and the hyponatraemia associated with inappropriate secretion of antidiuretic hormone, vincristine appeared to have no definite effect on mental changes, orthostatic hypotension, and the exacerbation of existing neurological disorders.— S. Rosenthal and S. Kaufman, *Ann. intern. Med.*, 1974, *80*, 733. The incidence of vincristine-induced neuropathy (presenting other than as areflexia) was 61% in 23 patients with lymphoma compared with 14% in 37 patients without lymphoma. Patients with lymphoma should be carefully observed and vincristine withdrawn if progressive neuropathy develops.— S. M. Watkins and J. P. Griffin, *Br. med. J.*, 1978, *1*, 610. Sex might be a factor in the incidence of vincristine-induced neuropathy; 18 of the 23 patients with lymphoma were male whereas 23 of the 37 without lymphoma were female.— M. G. Mott (letter), *ibid.*, 1145.

Three patients being treated with vincristine and 2 patients with vinblastine experienced discomfort, amounting to pain, behind the angle of the jaw immediately prior to a meal. The discomfort was usually experienced on the second or third day of treatment and could continue sporadically for a day or two. It was of brief duration. Severe constipation, in 2 instances followed by severe abdominal pain, had also followed treatment with vinca alkaloids.— M. S. Rose (letter), *Lancet*, 1967, *1*, 213. See also L. L. de Veber (letter), *ibid.*, 503.

Twenty of 40 leukaemic patients treated with vincristine sulphate (18) or vinblastine sulphate (2) showed ocular signs of toxicity (ptosis, other ocular muscle paresis, and 5th and 7th nerve involvement) within 2 weeks to 11 months of commencement of therapy. In 15 cases the ocular changes improved or disappeared when the dose was reduced or the drug withdrawn.— D. M. Albert *et al.*, *Archs Ophthal., N.Y.*, 1967, *78*, 709.

Laryngeal nerve paralysis, causing hoarseness or cough, occurred in 3 patients treated with vincristine; the condition regressed when treatment was withdrawn. The side-effect should be recognised because the symptoms might be considered to be due to mediastinal lymphadenopathy in patients with lymphoma.— J. A. Whittaker and I. P. Griffith, *Br. med. J.*, 1977, *1*, 1251.

Further reports of neurotoxicity with vincristine.— B. A. Mubashir and J. B. Bart (letter), *New Engl. J. Med.*, 1972, *287*, 517 (severe neuropathy and quadriplegia after the first dose of 2 mg); J. A. Whittaker *et al.*, *Br. med. J.*, 1973, *4*, 335 (coma 3 to 10 days after a single dose); R. H. Wheeler and M. Votaw (letter), *Ann. intern. Med.*, 1974, *81*, 709 (quadriparesis); L. P. Levitt and D. Prager, *Neurology, Minneap.*, 1975, *25*, 894 (mononeuropathy); J. M. Mueller and M. J. Flaherty, *Sth. med. J.*, 1978, *71*, 1310 (quadriparesis); R. C. Chisholm and S. B. Curry, *Sth. med. J.*, 1978, *71*, 1364 (dysphagia).

See also under Effects on the Eyes (above).

Effects on reproductive potential. *Gonads.* Vincristine impaired fertility in the male *rat*.— R. A. Cooke *et al.*, *Br. J. Pharmac.*, 1978, *63*, 677.

Overdosage. Reports of overdosage with vincristine.— I. A. Kaufman *et al.*, *J. Pediat.*, 1976, *89*, 671; M. Casteels-Vann Daele *et al.* (letter), *J. Pediat.*, 1977, *90*, 1042.

Treatment. Folinic acid was reported to protect *mice* from the lethal effects of vincristine. It was suggested that folinic acid might be of use in the treatment of vincristine toxicity if it were administered using the same regimen as that for the treatment of the toxicity of high doses of methotrexate.— R. W. Dyke, *Lilly, USA* (letter), *J. Pediat.*, 1977, *91*, 356. Large doses of folinic acid were used in an unsuccessful attempt to treat a 7-year-old girl given vincristine 13.5 mg. There was no response to therapy and she died 68 hours after the accident.— I. A. Kaufman *et al.* (letter), *ibid.*, 357. Folinic acid appeared to shorten the course of toxicity in a 14-year-old boy accidentally given vincristine sulphate 10 mg. Folinic acid 15 mg every 3 hours for 24 doses was begun 48 hours after the vincristine.— O. C. Grush and S. K. Morgan, *Clin. Toxicol.*, 1979, *14*, 71.

Precautions. For reference to the precautions necessary with antineoplastic agents and immunosuppressants, see Antineoplastic Agents, p.175.

Because severe constipation and impaction of faeces often occur with vincristine, enemas or purgatives may be necessary. Care should be taken to avoid extravasation during injection as this may cause cellulitis and phlebitis.

The warning has been given that intrathecal administration of vincristine is usually fatal.

Administration of vincristine for Hodgkin's disease unmasked myotonia dystrophia in a 25-year-old patient. Caution should be exercised when giving vincristine to patients with pre-existing neurological dysfunction.— J. C. Michalak and N. J. Dibella (letter), *New Engl. J. Med.*, 1976, *295*, 283. See also P. L. Weiden and S. E. Wright (letter), *New Engl. J. Med.*, 1972, *286*, 1369 (paraplegia and death in a patient with a pre-existing neuropathy).

Absorption and Fate. Vincristine is not reliably absorbed from the gastro-intestinal tract. After intravenous injection it disappears rapidly from the blood and is excreted in the bile; some also appears in the urine.

Following intravenous administration of radioactively labelled vincristine 2 mg over a period of 1 minute to 4 patients, clearance from the blood appeared to be triphasic with mean half-lives of 0.85, 7.4, and 164 minutes; the initial 2 phases probably represented distribution and binding to formed elements in the blood which was over 50% in 2 patients studied. Elimination of over 80% of the injected dose was recorded in 72 hours, the main route being faecal which accounted for nearly 70% (with over a third in the first 24 hours, indicating that biliary secretion might be rapid and play a major role in elimination, as had already been suggested by *animal* studies); only about 12% was excreted in the 72-hour urine (with over a half of this in the first 3 hours). It was estimated that about 34% of the vincristine dose was excreted as metabolites, indicating extensive metabolism.— R. A. Bender *et al.*, *Clin. Pharmac. Ther.*, 1977, *22*, 430. Results from a patient with pancreatic carcinoma and a T-tube in his common bile duct strongly suggest that biliary secretion is the major route by which vincristine is excreted. After an intravenous injection of 8 µg per kg body-weight of radioactively-labelled vincristine, radioactivity appeared rapidly in the bile with peak excretion occurring 2 to 4 hours after injection. During the first 24 hours the equivalent of 21.7% of the administered dose was excreted in the bile and 76.4% of the cumulative 72-hour biliary excretion. Over the 3-day study period excretion of vincristine and its products into urine, bile, and faeces was 26.2%, 28.4%, and 2.6% respectively of the administered dose. Urinary excretion was greater than reported previously (above) and might be related to differences between neoplastic diseases and other patient variations. Products of vincristine appeared rapidly in the bile and accounted for 53.5% of administered radioactivity during the first 2 hours. It could not be determined whether they were metabolites or decomposition products.— D. V. Jackson *et al.*, *ibid.*, 1978, *24*, 101.

See also under Vindesine Sulphate (below).

Uses. Vincristine sulphate is an antineoplastic agent which may act similarly to vinblastine (above) by arresting mitosis at the metaphase. It also has some immunosuppressant activity. Cross-resistance with vinblastine has not been reported.

It is used principally in combination chemotherapy regimens for acute leukaemia and Hodgkin's disease and other lymphomas, including Burkitt's lymphoma. It is also used in the treatment of Wilm's tumour, neuroblastoma, retinoblastoma, and sarcomas, and in tumours of the breast, brain, and lung. Remissions are induced in acute lymphoblastic leukaemia with vincristine in association with prednisone alone or with daunorubicin (or doxorubicin) or colaspase. In Hodgkin's disease, vincristine is given with mustine, procarbazine, and prednisone (MOPP) and similar regimens have been used in other lymphomas. See also under Choice of Antineoplastic Agent, p.177.

Vincristine sulphate is administered by intravenous injection and solutions containing 0.01 to 1 mg per ml in sodium chloride injection have been used. Care should be taken to avoid extravasation.

In acute leukaemia the weekly dose of vincristine sulphate for children is 1.5 to 2 mg per m^2 body-surface or 50 µg per kg body-weight increasing by weekly increments of 25 µg per kg to a maximum of 150 µg per kg. Adults may be given about 1.4 mg per m^2 or 25 to 75 µg per kg weekly. For other malignancies 25 µg per kg may be given weekly and reduced to 5 to 10 µg per kg for maintenance.

White cell counts should be carried out before giving each dose.

For references to the use of vincristine with other agents in the treatment of a wide variety of malignant diseases, see Choice of Antineoplastic Agent, p.175.

Action. The cytotoxic effects of vincristine on normal and leukaemic lymphocytes differed. It was considered that the antineoplastic effect of vincristine might not be dependent on metaphase arrest.— R. Schrek, *Am. J. clin. Path.*, 1974, *62*, 1, per *J. Am. med. Ass.*, 1974, *230*, 768.

Administration in renal insufficiency. Vincristine can be given in usual doses to patients with renal failure.— W. M. Bennett *et al.*, *Ann. intern. Med.*, 1977, *86*, 754. See also *idem*, 1980, *93*, 286.

Blood disorders, non-malignant. *Thrombocytopenic purpura.* A discussion on idiopathic thrombocytopenic purpura refractory to treatment with corticosteroids and splenectomy. The immunosuppressants azathioprine and cyclophosphamide have been used in the treatment of such patients but since the successful use of vincristine by Y.S. Ahn *et al.* (*New Engl. J. Med.*, 1974, *291*, 376), who administered 2 mg to adults and 1 mg to children every 7 to 10 days for 3 doses, vincristine has taken its place as a valuable immunosuppressant in this disorder. More recently Y.S. Ahn *et al.* (*New Engl. J. Med.*, 1978, *298*, 1101) have given vinblastine (see p.231), bound to platelets, to patients with refractory idiopathic thrombocytopenic purpura in an attempt to deliver the drug to the macrophages where it will presumably be most effective.— W. F. Rosse, *New Engl. J. Med.*, 1978, *298*, 1139.

A report of thrombocytosis (raised platelet counts) occurring during treatment with vincristine in a woman with lymphadenopathy.— J. H. Robertson and G. M. McCarthy, *Lancet*, 1969, *2*, 353.

A follow-up study of 8 of 10 patients with refractory auto-immune thrombocytopenia who were treated with a series of 1 to 6 intravenous injections of vincristine. Of the 4 patients with idiopathic thrombocytopenia, followed up for an average of 3.5 years, 2 responded completely to treatment, 1 responded partially, and 1 did not respond. All 3 patients with collagen vascular disorders, followed up for about 3 years, were complete responders. One patient with drug-induced thrombocytopenia, followed up for 2.5 years, also responded completely. The continued use of vincristine in refractory immune thrombocytopenia appears to be justified.— G. M. Rogers and C. A. Ries (letter), *New Engl. J. Med.*, 1980, *303*, 585.

Further references to vincristine in the treatment of thrombocytopenic purpura.— I. E. Burton *et al.*, *Br. med. J.*, 1976, *2*, 918; C. A. Ries (letter), *New Engl. J. Med.*, 1976, *295*, 1136; J. A. Penner *et al.* (letter), *ibid.*, 1977, *296*, 286; G. Hicsönmez and Ş. Özsoylu (letter), *ibid.*, 454; L. Massimo *et al.* (letter), *New Engl. J. Med.*, 1977, *297*, 397; Y. Tangun and T. Atamer (letter), *ibid.*, 894; N. Abramson (letter), *New Engl. J. Med.*, 1978, *298*, 971.

Leukaemia. For reference to the use of vincristine with other agents in acute lymphoblastic leukaemia, acute myeloid leukaemia, and chronic myeloid leukaemia, see Choice of Antineoplastic Agent, p.180.

Muscular disorders, non-malignant. Vincristine, 1 or 2 mg weekly to total doses of 6 to 10 mg intravenously, was reported to be of some benefit in an uncontrolled study of 14 patients with severe spasticity.— H. -J. Freund and K. Kendel, *Dt. med. Wschr.*, 1971, *27*, 1155, per *Abstr. Wld Med.*, 1971, *45*, 867.

Pregnancy and the neonate. Reports of normal babies born to mothers given vincristine during pregnancy.— B. G. M. Durie and H. R. Giles, *Archs intern. Med.*, 1977, *137*, 90 (3rd trimester); M. Khurshid and M. Saleem (letter), *Lancet*, 1978, *2*, 534 (2nd trimester).

Wilms' tumour. From the results of the US National Wilms' Tumour Study it was concluded that combination chemotherapy with vincristine and actinomycin D is more effective than either agent used alone.— G. J. D'Angio *et al.*, *Cancer*, 1976, *38*, 633.

See also under Choice of Antineoplastic Agent, p.186.

Further references to vincristine in the treatment of Wilms' tumour.— M. P. Sullivan *et al.*, *J. Am. med. Ass.*, 1967, *202*, 381; T. J. Vietti *et al.*, *Cancer*, 1970, *25*, 12; T. B. Haddy *et al.*, *J. Pediat.*, 1977, *90*, 784 (actinomycin D and vincristine in diffuse nephroblastomatosis).

Preparations

Vincristine Injection *(B.P.)*. A sterile solution containing a mixture of 1 part of vincristine sulphate and 10 parts of lactose in Water for Injections. It is prepared by dissolving the sterile contents of a sealed container (Vincristine Sulphate for Injection) in the requisite amount of Water for Injections. Potency is expressed in terms of the equivalent amount of anhydrous vincristine sulphate. Store at 2° to 10° and use within 24 hours: if antimicrobial preservatives are included the injection may be stored for 14 days.

Vincristine Sulfate for Injection *(U.S.P.)*. A sterile mixture of vincristine sulphate with suitable diluents. Store at 2° to 8°.

Oncovin *(Lilly, UK)*. Vincristine sulphate, available in vials each containing 1 mg with lactose 10 mg, 2 mg with lactose 20 mg, or 5 mg with lactose 50 mg, supplied with 10-ml vials of solvent containing sodium chloride 0.9% and benzyl alcohol 0.9%. (Also available as Oncovin in *Arg., Austral., Belg., Canad., Denm., Fr., Neth., Norw., S.Afr., Switz., USA*).

Vincristine Sulphate *(Lederle, UK)*. Available in vials of 1, 2, and 5 mg, with 10-ml vials of solvent containing sodium chloride 0.9% and benzyl alcohol 2%.

Other Proprietary Names

Kyocristine *(Jap.)*; Pericristine *(S.Afr.)*; Vincrisul *(Spain)*.

1880-n

Vindesine Sulphate.

Desacetyl Vinblastine Amide Sulfate; LY 099094; NSC 245467; Compound 112531 *(vindesine)*. 3-Carbamoyl-O^4-deacetyl-3-de(methoxycarbonyl)vincaleukoblastine.

$C_{43}H_{55}N_5O_7,H_2SO_4$=852.0.

CAS — 53643-48-4 (vindesine); 59917-39-4 (sulphate).

A synthetic vinca alkaloid derived from vinblastine sulphate. **Store** in a refrigerator. The pH of a reconstituted solution for injection is reported to range from 4.2 to 4.5 with precipitation occurring in solutions having a pH above 6.

Adverse Effects, Treatment, and Precautions. As for Vinblastine Sulphate, p.230.

The main dose-limiting effect of vindesine is leucopenia. Although neurotoxicity occurs it may be less severe than that seen with vincristine (p.231). Alopecia is the most common side-effect.

Absorption and Fate. The pharmacokinetics of vindesine are similar to those of vincristine (above).

A pharmacokinetic study of vinca alkaloids indicating that vindesine, vinblastine, and vincristine have similar pharmacokinetic properties. After varying intravenous doses, mean elimination half-lives for vindesine in 4 patients were 3.2, 99, and 1213 minutes respectively. Vincristine was only studied for the first 4 hours after a dose and elimination half-lives in 3 patients were 3.4 and 155 minutes; a prolonged third phase was also anticipated. Urinary excretion occurred mainly within 24 hours, a mean of 13.2% of the dose of vindesine being recovered and 9.6% of the dose of vincristine. The remainder of the drugs may be sequestered in the body or eliminated in the bile.— R. J. Owellen *et al.*, *Cancer Res.*, 1977, *37*, 2603.

After the rapid intravenous injection of vindesine in doses of 1 to 3 mg per m^2 body-surface in 5 cancer patients, plasma clearance was triphasic with half-lives of about 2 minutes, 1 hour, and 24 hours. Distribution from plasma to tissues was mainly responsible for the initial rapid clearance.— R. L. Nelson *et al.*, *Cancer Chemother. Pharmac.*, 1979, *2*, 243.

Uses. Vindesine sulphate is an antineoplastic agent derived from vinblastine (p.230) but with a spectrum of activity more similar to that of vincristine (above). It has been used in the treatment of acute lymphoblastic leukaemia resistant to other drugs, in blastic crises of chronic myeloid leukaemia, and in refractory malignant melanoma. See also under Choice of Anti-

neoplastic Agent, p.178.
Vindesine sulphate is given weekly by intravenous injection as a solution containing 1 mg per ml in sodium chloride injection. Care should be taken to avoid extravasation. The usual starting dose for adults is 3 mg per m^2 body-surface which may be raised by increments of 500 µg per m^2 weekly providing that the neutrophil count does not fall below 1500 per mm^3, the platelet count does not fall below 100 000 per mm^3, and acute abdominal pain is not experienced; weekly doses are usually between 3 and 4 mg per m^2. Children may be given 4 mg per m^2 initially, with weekly doses usually ranging between 4 and 5 mg per m^2. Blood counts should be made before each injection.

Proceedings of symposia on vindesine.— *Cancer Chemother. Pharmac.*, 1979, *2*, 229–274; Sixth Vinca Alkaloids Symposium—Vindesine, R.N. Wild (Ed.), Basingstoke, Eli Lilly and Co. Ltd, 1979.

A review of vindesine sulphate.— W. J. Dana, *Drug Intell. & clin. Pharm.*, 1980, *14*, 28.

Proprietary Preparations

Eldisine *(Lilly, UK)*. Vindesine sulphate, available in vials each containing 5 mg with mannitol 25 mg, supplied with 5-ml vials of solvent containing sodium chloride 0.9% and benzyl alcohol 0.9%.
A solution of vindesine sulphate for injection may be stored in a refrigerator for up to 30 days, providing the diluent contains a preservative.

1881-h

Zinostatin. Neocarzinostatin; NSC 157365 *(formerly* NSC 69856*)*. An antineoplastic antibiotic obtained from *Streptomyces carzinostaticus*. It is an acidic polypeptide of 109 amino-acid residues with a molecular weight of about 10 700.

CAS — 9014-02-2.

A white to pale yellowish-white powder. Freely **soluble** in water; practically insoluble in alcohol and acetone. **Store** in airtight containers. Protect from light.

Adverse Effects, Treatment, and Precautions. For an outline of the adverse effects experienced with antineoplastic agents and immunosuppressants, general guidelines for their treatment, and precautions, see Antineoplastic Agents, p.171, pp.174-5.
There have been reports of immediate reactions to injections of zinostatin including fever, chills, rigor, hypertension, and mental confusion.

Uses. Zinostatin is an antibiotic with antineoplastic activity (p.171) and has been used in the treatment of acute leukaemia and malignant neoplasms including those of the stomach and pancreas.

Reviews of zinostatin.— Y. Yagisawa, *Japan med. Gaz.*, 1975, *12* (June 20), 4; B. F. Issell *et al.*, *Cancer Treat. Rev.*, 1979, *6*, 239.

A pharmacokinetic study of zinostatin.— R. L. Comis *et al.*, *Cancer Res.*, 1979, *39*, 757.

References to the clinical use of zinostatin.— H. Maeda *et al.*, *Antimicrob. Ag. Chemother.*, 1977, *11*, 941 (bladder tumours).

Manufacturers
Bristol, USA; Kayaku, Jap.

Aspirin and similar Analgesic and Anti-inflammatory Agents

2600-p

Described in this section are compounds that are used as analgesics in the relief of mild to moderate pain. Some of these compounds may also be antipyretic and others may have anti-inflammatory actions; these anti-inflammatory agents are sometimes known as non-steroidal anti-inflammatory drugs (NSAID).

Aspirin and most other anti-inflammatory and/or analgesic compounds described in this section are considered to act mainly by inhibiting the biosynthesis of prostaglandins. They are often described as peripherally-acting compounds. Antipyretic activity is considered to involve the hypothalamus. Analgesics used for the relief of more severe pain are described in the section on Narcotic Analgesics, p.1001. Other drugs used in the treatment of rheumatoid arthritis and described in other sections include corticosteroids, p.446, penicillamine, p.387, and gold, p.934. Some of the compounds in this section are used in the treatment of acute gout, however, drugs used mainly in the treatment of gout are described under Uricosuric Agents, p.416. The analgesics described here include the following groups:

Aniline derivatives:
paracetamol, p.268, phenacetin, p.271.

Anthranilic acid derivatives:
flufenamic acid, p.254, mefenamic acid, p.262.

Phenylalkanoic acid derivatives and related compounds:
alclofenac, p.244, benoxaprofen, p.247, bufexamac, p.248, diclofenac sodium, p.250, fenclofenac, p.252, fenbufen, p.252, flurbiprofen, p.255, ibuprofen, p.256, ketoprofen, p.261, naproxen, p.264.

Indomethacin and related derivatives:
indomethacin, p.257, sulindac, p.279.

Pyrazole derivatives:
amidopyrine, p.245, azapropazone, p.246, dipyrone, p.251, feprazone, p.254, mofebutazone, p.264, nifenazone, p.267, oxyphenbutazone, p.267, phenazone, p.272, phenylbutazone, p.273.

Salicylic acid derivatives, including:
aloxiprin, p.245, aspirin, p.235, benorylate, p.246, choline salicylate, p.249, diflunisal, p.250, methyl salicylate, p.263, salicylamide, p.277, salicylic acid, p.277, sodium salicylate, p.279.

In studies *in vitro* the concentrations, in µg per ml, of indomethacin, mefenamic acid, phenylbutazone, and aspirin required to achieve 50% inhibition of prostaglandin synthetase were 0.06, 0.17, 2.23, and 6.61 respectively. These values were generally less than the peak plasma concentrations achieved after therapeutic doses, even after allowing for protein binding, and supported the suggestion that anti-inflammatory agents exerted their effect through the inhibition of prostaglandin synthesis. Paracetamol inhibited prostaglandin synthesis only at high concentrations and azathioprine had no effect. The relative inactivity of potent corticosteroid preparations did not necessarily mean that their mode of action was totally different; they might interfere with the transport or release of prostaglandin precursors such as arachidonic acid.— R. Flower *et al.*, *Nature New Biol.*, 1972, *238*, 104.

The role of anti-inflammatory agents in inhibiting prostaglandin synthesis.— E. G. McQueen, *Drugs*, 1973, *6*, 104. See also G. B. West, *Chemist Drugg.*, 1972, *198*, 196; *Nature*, 1972, *240*, 377.

Analgesia. Reviews of analgesics: J. A. Mills, *New Engl. J. Med.*, 1974, *290*, 781 and 1002; F. D. Hart, *Drugs*, 1975, *9*, 321; J. Parkhouse, *ibid.*, *10*, 366; L. Ratoff, *Prescribers' J.*, 1979, *19*, 17; D. L. Savary, *Can. J. Hosp. Pharm.*, 1979, *32*, 6.

A discussion on the treatment of sprains, strains, and bruises.— *Drug & Ther. Bull.*, 1976, *14*, 66.

In cancer. Reviews and discussions on the use of analgesics in the treatment of bone pain in advanced carcinoma.— R. G. Twycross, *Topics Ther.*, 1978, *4*, 94; R. G. Twycross, *Prescribers' J.*, 1978, *18*, 117.

A discussion of the medical management of chronic cancer pain.— D. S. Shimm *et al.*, *J. Am. med. Ass.*, 1979, *241*, 2408.

In dentistry. A review of analgesics used in dentistry.— J. G. Walton and J. W. Thompson, *Br. dent. J.*, 1969, *127*, 472.

Postoperative. A review of the management of postoperative pain with analgesics.— C. L. Knight and M. Mehta, *Br. J. Hosp. Med.*, 1978, *19*, 462.

Dysmenorrhoea. A review of the use of aspirin and other anti-inflammatory agents in the treatment of dysmenorrhoea.— *Med. Lett.*, 1979, *21*, 81. See also *J. Am. med. Ass.*, 1980, *244*, 1885.

Gout. For reviews on the treatment of gout including the use of non-steroidal anti-inflammatory drugs, see R. G. Robinson and A. B. Corrigan, *Drugs*, 1972, *3*, 422; *Br. med. J.*, 1974, *1*, 446; B. T. Emmerson, *Drugs*, 1978, *16*, 158; D. Morgan, *Aust. J. Pharm.*, 1978, *59*, 507 and 758; M. I. V. Jayson, *Prescribers' J.*, 1978, *18*, 111; P. A. Simkin, *Ann. intern. Med.*, 1979, *90*, 812.

Rheumatic disorders. Reviews and discussions on the treatment of rheumatoid arthritis and other rheumatic disorders.— C. J. Smyth, *Postgrad. Med.*, 1972, *51*, 31, per *Drugs*, 1973, *6*, 153; *Br. med. J.*, 1972, *2*, 39; F. D. Hart, *Practitioner*, 1972, *208*, 10; *J. Am. med. Ass.*, 1973, *224*, *Suppl.*, 662–805; A. S. Dixon and D. Henderson, *Prescribers' J.*, 1973, *13*, 41; J. A. Cosh, *Practitioner*, 1974, *213*, 519; D. I. Mason *et al.*, *ibid.*, 1975, *215*, 210; *Drug & Ther. Bull.*, 1975, *13*, 57; T. J. Constable *et al.*, *Lancet*, 1975, *1*, 1176 (systematic approach to the drug treatment of rheumatoid arthritis); *Med. Lett.*, 1976, *18*, 77; F. D. Hart, *Drugs*, 1976, *11*, 451; W. W. Downie and V. Wright, *Practitioner*, 1977, *219*, 463; *Br. med. J.*, 1977, *1*, 1120; *J. int. med. Res.*, 1977, *5*, *Suppl.* 2;; *Drug & Ther. Bull.*, 1977, *15*, 93; *Br. med. J.*, 1977, *2*, 758; J. M. Gumpel, *Br. med. J.*, 1978, *2*, 1068; E. C. Huskisson, *Drugs*, 1978, *15*, 387; *Br. med. J.*, 1978, *1*, 262; A. Klestov, *Med. J. Aust.*, 1979, *1*, *Suppl.* 3, 15; *Br. med. J.*, 1980, *280*, 666; G. L. Craig and W. W. Buchanan, *Drugs*, 1980, *20*, 453; *Med. Lett.*, 1980, *22*, 29; L. S. Simon and J. A. Mills, *New Engl. J. Med.*, 1980, *302*, 1179 and 1237; F. D. Hart, *Prescribers' J.*, 1980, *20*, 123.

Juvenile polyarthritis. For discussions on the treatment of juvenile chronic polyarthritis, see Aspirin, p.242.

Analgesic Abuse. Chronic abuse of analgesics is associated with nephropathy. Patients invariably have a history of regular ingestion of substantial or excessive doses over a period of years. In mild cases the condition is reversible if analgesics are withdrawn; in more severe cases renal function may continue to deteriorate despite the withdrawal of analgesics.

The initial renal lesion is papillary necrosis which is often asymptomatic in its early stages. With continued analgesic use there are secondary atrophic changes in the renal cortex body. Renal complications include renal colic, haematuria, urinary-tract infection, a reduced urine-concentrating ability, sodium loss, ureteric stricture and obstruction, and renal calculi. Other features associated with analgesic abuse include peptic ulceration, gastro-intestinal bleeding, anaemia, and psychiatric disturbances. An abnormally high incidence of transitional cell carcinoma of the renal pelvis and bladder tumours have been reported in patients with analgesic nephropathy.

Phenacetin was originally considered to be the agent responsible for analgesic nephropathy, as it was present in all the various analgesic preparations implicated in the initial clinical reports. The role of phenacetin in analgesic nephropathy is however still uncertain. Phenacetin is rarely taken alone and is usually taken in combination with aspirin, codeine, caffeine, and various other analgesics. Nephropathy has been reported in patients abusing analgesic preparations without phenacetin and less often in patients taking large quantities of single analgesics. The availability of phenacetin-containing preparations has been restricted in many countries. The incidence of analgesic nephropathy following removal of phenacetin from analgesic preparations has declined in some countries but not in others.

The possible role of aspirin in analgesic nephropathy is still uncertain. *Animal* studies have shown that high doses of aspirin alone or in combination can produce renal papillary necrosis. Studies in patients with rheumatoid arthritis have shown that aspirin can cause impairment of renal function but have in general found little evidence that aspirin alone produces analgesic nephropathy.

The mechanism by which analgesics produce nephropathy are not known at present.

In Canada, the incidence of analgesic abuse seemed to be about the same as for narcotic dependence. Addicted persons were generally female and over 40; they took from 25 to more than 100 tablets of aspirin per day, usually for headache. They had been shown to have an extreme fear of pain (E.M. Boyd and S.M.H. Hottenroth, *Toxicol. appl. Pharmac.*, 1968 *12*, 80). It was predicted from *animal* studies that daily ingestion of 25 to 100 tablets of aspirin could eventually produce serious toxic effects in man.— E. M. Boyd, *Can. med. Ass. J.*, 1968, *99*, 790.

A review of phenacetin abuse.— G. Carro-Ciampi, *Toxicology*, 1978, *10*, 311.

Report of a method for the detection of analgesic abuse using Phenistix.— J. M. Duggan and J. E. Dickeson (letter), *Med. J. Aust.*, 1979, *1*, 340.

Nephropathy. Reviews and discussions on analgesic nephropathy.— J. A. Abel, *Clin. Pharmac. Ther.*, 1971, *12*, 583; M. H. Gault, *Can. med. Ass. J.*, 1972, *107*, 756; R. M. Murray, *Practitioner*, 1973, *211*, 639; *Lancet*, 1973, *2*, 1484; *Br. med. J.*, 1973, *3*, 123; *ibid.*, 1974, *1*, 588; R. D. Wagoner, *Postgrad. Med.*, 1976, *60*, 50; R. S. Nanra, *Med. J. Aust.*, 1976, *1*, 745; G. G. Duggin, *Aust. J. pharm. Sci.*, 1977, *6*, 44; P. Kincaid-Smith (Ed.), *Kidney Int.*, 1978, *13*, 1–113; M. Goldberg and T. G. Murray, *New Engl. J. Med.*, 1978, *299*, 716; P. Kincaid-Smith, *Practitioner*, 1978, *220*, 862; L. F. Prescott, *Br. J. clin. Pharmac.*, 1979, *7*, 453; *Br. med. J.*, 1981, *282*, 339.

Renal papillary necrosis occurred in a middle-aged man who ingested 3.7 kg of paracetamol (taken in conjunction with chlormezanone) during 6 months at the rate of 11 to 18 g daily. The lesions first became apparent 7 months after stopping paracetamol.— D. M. Krikler, *Br. med. J.*, 1967, *2*, 615. Of 18 patients who had consumed at least 1 g of paracetamol daily for at least 1 year, with a total consumption of 2.7 to 29.6 kg, none had severe impairment of renal function. Minor impairment of concentrating ability occurred in 6 patients; the incidence and severity of the abnormality was unrelated to the total amount of paracetamol consumed. No significant deterioration in renal function was evident after about 1 year in 13 of the patients who consumed further amounts of paracetamol, mean 2 kg.— O. M. Edwards *et al.*, *Br. med. J.*, 1971, *2*, 87.

There was no association between aspirin intake and nephropathy in a study in 908 patients with rheumatic disorders. Papillary necrosis was present in 4 patients, 3 of whom had taken large quantities of aspirin, phenacetin, and codeine tablets.—New Zealand Rheumatism Association Study *Br. med. J.*, 1974, *1*, 593. Similar findings in 17 patients with rheumatoid arthritis who had taken large amounts of aspirin.— A. F. Macklon *et al.*, *ibid.*, 597.

Interstitial nephritis in 20 of 101 patients was attributed to analgesic abuse, defined as the ingestion of 3 kg or more of aspirin or phenacetin before the onset of uraemia.— T. Murray and M. Goldberg, *Ann. intern. Med.*, 1975, *82*, 453.

Of 403 Australian patients with end-stage renal failure seen in 7 years, 118 were classified as having analgesic nephropathy; this was histologically confirmed in 94.— J. H. Stewart *et al.*, *Br. med. J.*, 1975, *1*, 440.

Macroscopic renal papillary necrosis was present in 30.4% of 23 patients with rheumatoid arthritis at autopsy. Microscopic papillary necrosis was present in 59.1%. Aspirin had been taken by 20 patients; a variety of other anti-inflammatory agents had also been taken.— R. S. Nanra and P. Kincaid-Smith, *Med. J. Aust.*, 1975, *1*, 194.

Results of a retrospective study in 20 patients with rheumatoid arthritis and a prospective study in 8 similar patients and 10 healthy controls indicated that salicylate treatment did cause renal tubular damage but that this resulted in little impairment of function.— H. C. Burry *et al.*, *Br. med. J.*, 1976, *1*, 613.

No reduction in the incidence of analgesic nephropathy was noted in a prospective study of 322 autopsies of adults after phenacetin was removed from a common Australian compound analgesic. Active nephropathy was still seen in patients taking two different compound analgesics not containing phenacetin.— A. Burry and J. Hopkins, *Med. J. Aust.*, 1977, *1*, 879.

In a study of 168 patients with rheumatoid arthritis in Brisbane, those who had taken more than 1 kg of aspirin in the form of compound aspirin and phenacetin preparations had significantly more overt papillary necrosis and higher renal damage scores than those who had taken more than 1 kg of aspirin without phenacetin. There was no justification for allowing phenacetin to remain in compound aspirin preparations.— I. Ferguson *et al.*, *Med. J. Aust.*, 1977, *1*, 950.

Further references to analgesic nephropathy.— E. J. D. Mees *et al.*, *Ned. Tijdschr. Geneesk.*, 1973, *117*, 835; E. Levine and D. Bernard, *S. Afr. med. J.*, 1973, *47*, 2439; R. M. Murray, *Br. J. Addict.*, 1973, *68*, 265; J. Rosner, *Thérapie*, 1974, *29*, 483; S. Ringoir, *ibid.*, 507; A. F. Burry *et al.*, *Med. J. Aust.*, 1974, *1*, 31.

Effects on kidney function. Seven of 10 patients with analgesic nephropathy suffered from sodium loss.— J. R. Cove-Smith and M. S. Knapp, *Lancet*, 1973, *2*, 70.

In a survey of 2933 women, the 56 who had been taking an average of more than 4 analgesic tablets containing aspirin, phenacetin, or paracetamol daily had a higher incidence of symptoms of urinary-tract infection but had no significant changes in plasma urea, plasma creatinine, or blood pressure.— W. E. Waters *et al.*, *Lancet*, 1973, *1*, 341.

Kidney function was assessed in a 4-year study in 623 Swiss women aged 30 to 49 years who were regularly taking analgesics containing phenacetin and in a control group of 621 women not taking such analgesics. There was no significant difference between the 2 groups in the incidence of bacteriuria, haematuria, and proteinuria. There was a higher incidence of loss of urine-concentrating ability in the phenacetin group, 12.9% of them showing possible low urine specific gravity compared with 3.5% in the control group. The significance of this difference was increased when subjects with a high urine concentration of phenacetin metabolite were compared with controls. There was a greater incidence of raised serum-creatinine concentrations in the phenacetin group than in the control group but this was only significant in those subjects with a high urine concentration of phenacetin metabolite; an incidence of 5.4% compared with 0.4% in the control group and 0.4% in those with evidence of low phenacetin intake.— U. C. Dubach *et al.*, *Lancet*, 1975, *1*, 539.

Findings in kidneys damaged by analgesic abuse indicated that the induced papillary necrosis might be due to a narrowing of the pelvic and papillary renal blood vessels.— C. Abrahams, *Lancet*, 1976, *2*, 346.

Beta-*N*-acetyl glucosaminidase (NAG) excretion was a useful marker of renal tubular (but not glomerular) damage. NAG excretion was not increased by standard doses of aspirin, azapropazone, diflunisal, ibuprofen, indomethacin, or naproxen; larger doses of aspirin or diflunisal caused appreciable increase in NAG excretion.— P. A. Dieppe *et al.*, *Br. med. J.*, 1978, *2*, 664.

Findings of microangiopathy and a brown discoloration of the mucosa of the lower urinary tract in patients with a history of the overuse of analgesics.— C. Abrahams (letter), *New Engl. J. Med.*, 1979, *301*, 437.

Fibrosis. Three patients who had taken up to 25 aspirin, phenacetin, and codeine tablets daily for 2 or more years developed analgesic nephropathy with ureteric or periureteric fibrosis without obstruction of the lumen of the ureter. None had taken methysergide. The site of the fibrosis was the same as that affected by retroperitoneal fibrosis and patients with this condition should be questioned concerning their consumption of analgesics.— G. A. MacGregor *et al.*, *Br. med. J.*, 1973, *2*, 271.

Unusual ureteric obstruction occurred in 2 patients with a history of heavy analgesic consumption. Re-examination of the records of 7 patients with retroperitoneal fibrosis showed that 4 had a history of heavy analgesic consumption.– C. T. Lewis *et al.*, *Br. med. J.*, 1975, *2*, 76.

Laxative abuse. Of 10 consecutive patients with analgesic nephropathy 8 were regular takers of laxatives, compared with 4 of 70 patients in a renal clinic, 12 of 200 blood donors, and none of 40 patients with chronic rheumatoid arthritis who had taken large quantities of analgesics for at least 5 years. It was suggested that analgesic nephropathy was more likely in patients who abused both analgesics and laxatives; this could explain why many persons who took large quantities of analgesics failed to develop analgesic nephropathy.— J. S. Wainscoat and R. Finn, *Br. med. J.*, 1974, *4*, 697. Of 150 patients with established phenacetin nephropathy only 3.3% were abusers of laxatives; in 21 further abusers of phenacetin without nephropathy 14.4% were abusers of laxatives.— K. D. Bock and T. Nitzsche (letter), *ibid.*, 1975, *2*, 140. Further doubts of an association with laxatives.— L. Arnold *et al.* (letter), *ibid.*, 141.

Prognosis. Severe papillary damage could be correlated with regular ingestion of phenacetin-containing analgesics in 40 of 42 patients. When more than 4 kg of phenacetin had been taken, the probability of papillary degeneration was 73% and that of death from pyelonephritis with papillary necrosis 37%.— A. F. Burry *et al.*, *Med. J. Aust.*, 1966, *1*, 873.

In a follow-up study of 103 patients with phenacetin nephropathy who had a history of excessive analgesic intake and who were still living from 2 to 10 years after diagnosis, it was found that in about 50% of the patients, substitution of compounds not containing phenacetin for phenacetin mixtures, together with supportive therapy, led to apparent recovery. Return to phenacetin-containing mixtures almost invariably caused a rapid acute episode of necrotising papillitis.— H. H. Pearson, *Med. J. Aust.*, 1967, *2*, 308.

Of 86 patients with renal impairment and a history of analgesic abuse, 22 of 60 had neurological states suggestive of chronic analgesic intoxication and anaemia and peptic ulceration were common. Renal function continued to deteriorate in 23 of 28 patients who persisted in their abuse of compound preparations of phenacetin, but in only 3 of 26 who ceased abuse. Of these 26 patients, 17 showed improved renal function. Most patients had taken compound analgesics of aspirin, phenacetin, and codeine, but 2 patients had taken only aspirin. Renal function continued to deteriorate in some patients after withdrawal of phenacetin from the analgesic preparation.— R. M. Murray *et al.*, *Br. med. J.*, 1971, *1*, 479.

In 17 patients with analgesic nephropathy who continued to take analgesic preparations containing phenacetin, renal function deteriorated in 14 and 9 of them died. In 12 similar patients who continued to take analgesic preparations not containing phenacetin, renal function deteriorated in 9 and 3 of these died. Deterioration was more rapid (a yearly decrease in creatinine clearance of 12.9 ml per minute) in those taking phenacetin than in those not taking phenacetin (4.9 ml per minute).— R. M. Murray, *Br. med. J.*, 1972, *4*, 131.

Further reports on the prognosis in patients with analgesic nephropathy.— D. Bell *et al.*, *Br. med. J.*, 1969, *3*, 378; D. P. E. Kingsley *et al.*, *Br. med. J.*, 1972, *4*, 656; D. Höffler *et al.*, *Dt. med. Wschr.*, 1973, *98*, 2012.

Urinary-tract carcinoma. A short review of the association between analgesic abuse and urinary-tract carcinoma. Patients continue to be at risk even after cessation of analgesic abuse.— T. A. Gonwa *et al.*, *Ann. intern. Med.*, 1979, *90*, 432.

The association between the abuse of phenacetin-containing compounds and tumours of the renal pelvis was believed to be due to the metabolism of phenacetin to 2-hydroxyphenetidine.— U. Bengtsson and L. Angervall (letter), *Lancet*, 1970, *1*, 305.

Reports of urinary-tract carcinoma associated with nephropathy and analgesic abuse: *Br. med. J.*, 1969, *4*, 701; L. Wahlqvist *et al.*, *Nord. Med.*, 1971, *86*, 1156; R. A. Mannion and D. Susmano, *J. Urol.*, 1971, *106*, 692; H. U. Grob, *Helv. chir. Acta*, 1971, *38*, 537; G. Høybye and O. E. Nielsen, *Scand. J. Urol. & Nephrol.*, 1971, *5*, 190; R. Güller and U. C. Dubach, *Helv. med. Acta*, 1972, *36*, 247; W. Leistenschneider and R. Ehmann, *Schweiz. med. Wschr.*, 1973, *103*, 433; *Med. News, Lond.*, 1974, *4* (Jan. 21), 5; P. Rathert *et al.*, *J. Urol.*, 1975, *113*, 653; L. G. Küng, *Schweiz. med. Wschr.*, 1976, *106*, 47; P. Kench, *Med. J. Aust.*, 1977, *2*, 607; J. F. Mahony *et al.*, *Aust. N.Z. J. Med.*, 1977, *7*, 463; F. P. Brunner *et al.*, *Schweiz. med. Wschr.*, 1978, *108*, 1013; V. Moshakis and A. A. Hooper, *Postgrad. med. J.*, 1978, *54*, 285; L. Tomatis (letter), *Science*, 1979, *204*, 129; S. Johansson and L. Angervall, *ibid.*, 130; K. R. Burnett *et al.* (letter), *Ann. intern. Med.*, 1979, *90*, 994; T. A. Gonwa *et al.*, *Ann. intern. Med.*, 1980, *93*, 249.

Renal calculi. Of 266 patients with renal calculi, 45 had a history of heavy consumption (3 or more tablets, powders, or teaspoonfuls of liquid medication per day for more than 1 year) of analgesics—in many cases a mixture of aspirin, phenacetin, and caffeine. It appeared likely that at least some of the patients habituated to analgesics formed calculi because of the calcification of necrotic papillary material.— J. E. Blackman *et al.*, *Br. med. J.*, 1967, *2*, 800.

Testicular atrophy. Few of a group of men admitted to hospital suffering from the abuse of analgesics such as aspirin, paracetamol, and phenacetin had become fathers while taking the analgesics. In *animals*, large doses of the analgesics caused testicular atrophy and inhibition of spermatogenesis E. M. Boyd, *J. clin. Pharmac.*, 1970, *10*, 222. See also D. N. Bateman, *Adverse Drug React. Bull.*, 1980, Dec., 308.

2601-s

Aspirin *(B.P., Eur. P., B.P. Vet., U.S.P.).*

Acetylsalicylic Acid; Acetylsal. Acid; Acidum Acetylsalicylicum; Salicylic Acid Acetate; Polopiryna. *O*-Acetylsalicylic acid; 2-Acetoxybenzoic acid.

$C_9H_8O_4$=180.2.

CAS — 50-78-2.

NOTE. The use of the name Aspirin is limited; in some countries it is a trade-mark.

Pharmacopoeias. In all pharmacopoeias examined.

Colourless or white crystals or white crystalline powder or granules; odourless or almost odourless with a slight acid taste. M.p. about 143°.

Soluble 1 in 300 of water, 1 in 5 to 7 of alcohol, 1 in 17 of chloroform, and 1 in 20 of ether; soluble in solutions of acetates and citrates and, with decomposition, in solutions of alkali hydroxides and carbonates. A solution in water is acid to methyl red. **Incompatible** with free acids, acetanilide, amidopyrine, phenazone, hexamine, iron salts, phenobarbitone sodium, quinine salts, potassium and sodium iodides, and alkali hydroxides, carbonates, and stearates. **Store** in airtight containers.

Aspirin is stable in dry air, but gradually hydrolyses in contact with moisture to acetic and salicylic acids. In solutions with alkalis the hydrolysis proceeds rapidly and the clear solutions formed may consist entirely of acetate and salicylate. Aspirin decomposes rapidly in solutions of ammonium acetate or of the acetates, carbonates, citrates, or hydroxides of the alkali metals. Suspensions of aspirin may be stable for a few days; J.B. Hough and others (*Pharm. J.*, 1969 *1*, 497) have reported 3.2% decomposition to salicylic acid after 7 days at room temperature. Suspensions should be freshly prepared.

A report of 6 polymorphic forms of aspirin and their physical characteristics.— M. P. Summers *et al.* (letter), *J. Pharm. Pharmac.*, 1970, *22*, 615.

Microcrystalline aspirin produced by precipitation from a saturated solution of glycerol was more soluble in water than other crystalline forms; melting points were the same. Between 80 and 90% of microcrystals had dimensions below 10 μm.— A. Affonso and V. R. Naik, *J. pharm. Sci.*, 1971, *60*, 1572.

Acetylsalicylsalicylic acid, which occurred as an impurity in commercial aspirin preparations, could react with amino acids and might cause allergic responses to aspirin.— H. Bundgaard, *J. Pharm. Pharmac.*, 1974, *26*, 18.

Absorption from tablets. The absorption of aspirin from buffered, plain, and soluble tablets.— J. R. Leonards, *Clin. Pharmac. Ther.*, 1963, *4*, 476.

Two aspirin tablet formulations were made either from fine aspirin (80 mesh or finer) or coarse aspirin (all larger than 20 mesh). Under standard conditions plasma-salicylate concentrations were measured in 6 subjects after a 650-mg dose. Absorption was on average about 3 times faster from the tablet made from fine aspirin.— G. Levy *et al.* (letter), *J. pharm. Sci.*, 1967, *56*, 1365.

A study indicated that plasma-salicylate concentrations were more stable after ingestion of sustained-release aspirin tablets than after conventional tablets.— E. H. Wiseman, *Curr. ther. Res.*, 1969, *11*, 681.

Salicylate concentrations in the plasma of 10 subjects were higher during the 2 hours after taking a soluble tablet containing aspirin 660 mg with ascorbic acid 400 mg than after the same dose of aspirin alone. During the first 30 minutes they were 3 to 4 times as high, and after 1 hour more than twice as high.— H. L. Staudacher and H. Müller, *Arzneimittel-Forsch.*, 1969, *19*, 1612.

Incompatibility. Mixtures of aspirin and phenacetin were compatible, but aspirin interacted with paracetamol giving salicylic acid and diacetyl-*p*-aminophenol. This interaction was unaffected by caffeine but accelerated by codeine phosphate and magnesium stearate.— B. G. Boggiano *et al.*, *Aust. J. Pharm.*, 1970, *51*, S14.

Aspirin reacted with homatropine in the absence of water to form acetylhomatropine and free salicylic acid.— E. Shami *et al.*, *J. pharm. Sci.*, 1973, *62*, 1283.

Release from suppositories. Aspirin was rapidly released from macrogol suppository bases and also from bases of polysorbate 61 with glyceryl monolaurate. The rectal doses of aspirin and sodium salicylate were equivalent to the dose by mouth.— E. L. Parrott, *J. pharm. Sci.*, 1971, *60*, 867.

Storage at 4° reduced the decomposition of aspirin in a macrogol suppository basis to less than 4% after 100 days. Decomposition was about 35% after 50 days at 45° and 21% after 100 days at 26°. Addition of 10% acetylated monoglycerides hindered decomposition at 26° to a small extent.— C. W. Whitworth *et al.*, *J. pharm. Sci.*, 1973, *62*, 1372. See also H. W. Jun *et al.*, *ibid.*, 1974, *63*, 133.

Citric acid 5% and tartaric acid 10% hindered the decomposition of aspirin in a macrogol suppository basis. Acetic acid, calcium gluconate, and colloidal silica were less effective.— C. W. Whitworth *et al.*, *J. pharm. Sci.*, 1973, *62*, 1721.

The bioavailability of aspirin from 5 brands of aspirin suppositories was compared in 4 volunteers. In all cases absorption was slow and variable, no more than 40% being absorbed after retention of the suppository for 2 hours. With 4 brands only about 20% of the aspirin was absorbed. Suppositories were not recommended for the administration of aspirin.— M. Gibaldi and B. Grundhofer, *J. pharm. Sci.*, 1975, *64*, 1064.

Solubility. Aspirin was 15 to 20% more soluble and dissolved more rapidly in the presence of glycine.— H. D. C. Rapson *et al.*, *J. Pharm. Pharmac.*, 1959, *11*, 210T.

The solubility of aspirin in water might be more than doubled by the addition of polysorbates (1.2%).— S. S. Ahsan and S. M. Blaug, *Drug Stand.*, 1960, *28*, 95.

Urea increased the solubility of aspirin in water, and also increased the rate of hydrolysis below pH 2.75. It slightly increased the stability of aspirin above pH 2.75.— G. Santopadre and S. Bolton (letter), *J. Pharm. Pharmac.*, 1967, *19*, 550.

Solution-rates. The grade and crystalline form of aspirin used influenced the dissolution-rates of tablets and might be significant *in vivo*.— A. G. Mitchell and D. J. Saville, *J. Pharm. Pharmac.*, 1967, *19*, 729.

Two polymorphic forms of aspirin had appreciably different solution-rates.— R. Tawashi, *Science*, 1968, *160*, 76.

Two commercial samples of aspirin showed different intrinsic dissolution-rates. Crystallographic and solubility determinations failed to reveal any differences. Agitation and temperature effects on intrinsic dissolution-rates showed that the samples had different thermodynamic activities.— A. G. Mitchell and D. J. Saville, *J. Pharm. Pharmac.*, 1969, *21*, 28.

Stability. 50% w/v of crystalline sorbitol had a stabilising action on aspirin suspensions. Solutions buffered to pH 3 were less stable than at pH 2.5. Crystalline sorbitol was found to possess a superior stabilising effect to that produced by glycerol, macrogol 6000, calcium gluconate, and povidone.— S. M. Blaug and J. W. Wesolowski, *J. Am. pharm. Ass., scient. Edn*, 1959, *48*, 691.

Aspirin was degraded in polyethylene glycols in the absence of water to form salicylic acid and acetylated polyethylene glycol.— H. W. Jun *et al.*, *J. pharm. Sci.*, 1972, *61*, 1160. Aspirin was stable at 45°, 26°, and 4° for 30 days in acetylated polyethylene glycol which confirmed that its instability in polyethylene glycol was due to transesterification.— C. W. Whitworth *et al.*, *ibid.*, 1973, *62*, 1184. See also C. W. Whitworth and A. F. Asker, *J. pharm. Sci.*, 1974, *63*, 1790; *idem*, 1975, *64*, 2018.

Stability in dimethicone solutions.— A. F. Asker and C. W. Whitworth, *J. pharm. Sci.*, 1974, *63*, 1630.

Adverse Effects. The most common adverse effects occurring with therapeutic doses of aspirin are gastro-intestinal disturbances such as nausea, dyspepsia, and vomiting. Irritation of the gastric mucosa with erosion, ulceration, haematemesis and melaena may occur; slight blood loss may occur in about 70% of patients with most aspirin preparations, whether buffered, soluble, or plain, and often this is not accompanied by dyspepsia. Slight blood loss is not usually of clinical significance but may cause iron-deficiency anaemia during long-term salicylate therapy.

Some persons, especially asthmatics, exhibit notable sensitivity to aspirin which may provoke various reactions including urticaria and other skin eruptions, angioneurotic oedema, rhinitis, and severe, even fatal, paroxysmal bronchospasm and dyspnoea.

Aspirin increases the bleeding time, decreases platelet adhesiveness, and, in large doses, may cause hypoprothrombinaemia.

Mild chronic salicylate intoxication, or salicylism, usually occurs only after repeated administration of large doses. Symptoms include dizziness, tinnitus, deafness, sweating, nausea and vomiting, headache, and mental confusion, and may be controlled by reducing the dosage. Symptoms of more severe intoxication include hyperventilation, fever, restlessness, ketosis, and respiratory alkalosis and metabolic acidosis. Depression of the central nervous system may lead to coma, cardiovascular collapse, and respiratory failure. In children drowsiness and metabolic acidosis commonly occur; hypoglycaemia may be severe.

The lethal dose of aspirin for an adult is probably in the region of 25 to 30 g but recovery has been achieved by appropriate treatment after the ingestion of twice or thrice this amount. Persons sensitive to aspirin may not tolerate therapeutic doses. Prolonged administration of large doses of aspirin has been associated with renal papillary necrosis (see p.234).

Maximum permissible atmospheric concentration 5 mg per m^3.

Abstracts of reports of toxic effects of salicylate therapy, with an extensive bibliography.— R. H. Moser, *Clin. Pharmac. Ther.*, 1967, *8*, 333.

A review of the toxicity of aspirin and salicylates.— N. W. Blacow, *Pharm. J.*, 1968, *1*, 325.

Aspirin, like corticosteroids, reduced the tensile strength of healing skin and so retarded wound healing.— K. H. Lee, *J. pharm. Sci.*, 1968, *57*, 1042.

Hypouricaemia (serum-urate concentrations of less than 20 µg per ml) in 21 patients could have been due to aspirin.— C. M. Ramsdell and W. N. Kelley, *Ann. intern. Med.*, 1973, *78*, 239.

Aspiration of aspirin caused retardation in 2 young children and death in a third child.— V. J. Roden, *J. Pediat.*, 1973, *83*, 266.

There were 787 reports of adverse reactions to aspirin reported to the Committee on Safety of Medicines between June 1964 and January 1973. These included 95 reports of blood disorders (17 fatal) including thrombocytopenia (26; 2 fatal), aplastic anaemia (13; 7 fatal), and agranulocytosis or pancytopenia (10; 2 fatal), gastro-intestinal haemorrhage (128; 64 fatal). There were 53 reports (26 fatalities) of analgesic nephropathy associated with preparations containing aspirin, phenacetin, and codeine.— M. F. Cuthbert, *Curr. med. Res. Opinion*, 1974, *2*, 600.

In a report from the Boston Collaborative Drug Surveillance Program, adverse reactions attributed to aspirin occurred in 119 of 2391 hospitalised patients who received plain aspirin tablets. Minor gastro-intestinal disturbances occurred in 51 patients, tinnitus in 20, deafness in 8, gastro-intestinal bleeding in 23, and prolonged prothrombin times in 3. Drug fever, leucopenia, and epistaxis occurred in 2 each and sweating, purpura, dyspnoea, stomatitis, hypothermia, metabolic acidosis, and elevated serum concentrations of uric acid in 1 each. Other drugs administered concurrently could have contributed to the adverse reaction in 26 patients. Reactions occurred more often at higher doses and were more common in females.— R. R. Miller and H. Jick, *Am. J. med. Sci.*, 1977, *274*, 271.

Abuse. See under Analgesic Abuse, p.234.

Allergy. Intolerance to aspirin usually occurs in middle-aged adults and is more common in females. Manifestations of the aspirin-intolerance syndrome include vasomotor rhinitis, sinusitis, nasal polyps, bronchial asthma, angioneurotic oedema, urticaria, and eosinophilia. Aspirin-induced prolongation of bleeding time and a tendency for diabetes may exist with it. Hypotension, shock, and syncope may occur. Salicylates other than aspirin are usually well tolerated but cross-reactivity with other analgesics, particularly indomethacin, and with tartrazine may occur. The mechanism underlying aspirin hypersensitivity is not known but an immunological basis seems unlikely.— M. A. Abrishami and J. Thomas, *Ann. Allergy*, 1977, *39*, 28.

Further reviews and discussions on aspirin intolerance including aspirin-induced asthma and urticaria.— M. Samter and R. F. Beers, *Ann. intern. Med.*, 1968, *68*, 975; *Br. med. J.*, 1969, *1*, 6; R. F. Lockey *et al.*, *Ann. intern. Med.*, 1973, *78*, 57; N. Thorne, *Practitioner*, 1973, *211*, 606; *Br. med. J.*, 1973, *3*, 419; *Br. med. J.*, 1974, *3*, 216; *J. Am. med. Ass.*, 1974, *229*, 1704; H. D. Schlumberger *et al.*, *Acta med. scand.*, 1974, *196*, 451; W. A. Parker, *Can. J. Hosp. Pharm.*, 1976, *29*, 64; A. Szczeklik and G. Czerniawska-Mysik (letter), *Lancet*, 1976, *1*, 488; C. Patrono *et al.*, *J. Allergy & clin. Immunol.*, 1978, *62*, 271; *Jap. med. Gaz.*, 1979, *16* (Jan. 20), 10; *Br. med. J.*, 1980, *281*, 958.

In some of 5 aspirin-sensitive patients there was a marked fall in the forced expiratory volume in 1 second after the ingestion of paracetamol 500 mg, indomethacin 25 mg, mefenamic acid 250 mg, and dextropropoxyphene 65 mg. Rhinitis was only seen after challenge with paracetamol, indomethacin, and mefenamic acid. Phenylbutazone had little, if any, effect in precipitating these symptoms.— A. P. Smith, *Br. med. J.*, 1971, *2*, 494. In 11 patients hypersensitive to aspirin, reactions occurred in all when challenged with indomethacin, in 8 of 9 and 7 of 9 challenged respectively with mefenamic and flufenamic acids, and in 4 of 10 challenged with phenylbutazone. There were no reactions to benzydamine, chloroquine, paracetamol, or salicylamide.— A. Szczeklik *et al.*, *Br. med. J.*, 1975, *1*, 67.

In a group of 3781 patients with asthma or rhinitis the incidence of intolerance to aspirin was 2.4%; the incidence in those with asthma was 4.3%. In asthmatics with negative allergy skin tests the incidence was 6.8% compared with 3.5% in those with positive skin tests. Intolerance to aspirin increased with advancing age. Bronchospasm and urticaria were the main signs of intolerance.— F. H. Chafee and G. A. Settipane, *J. Allergy & clin. Immunol.*, 1974, *53*, 193.

Of 131 patients with chronic urticaria, including physical urticarias, 37 showed a reaction to challenge with aspirin by mouth. Only 10 of the 37 had a history of previous reaction to aspirin. Skin reactions included urticaria, angioneurotic oedema, and flushing. Conjunctivitus, nasal congestion, sneezing, rhinorrhoea, cough, dyspnoea, and hoarseness also occurred.— H. M. G. Doeglas, *Br. J. Derm.*, 1975, *93*, 135.

A retrospective study in 445 patients with nasal polyps revealed that 21% had asthma; 2% had polyps, asthma, and aspirin sensitivity; 10% of those with polyps and asthma were sensitive to aspirin; and 6% of all patients were sensitive to aspirin. Asthma developed more often before polypectomy than after. Although it is possible that polypectomy might, on rare occasions, precipitate asthma, it probably does not cause it.— J. R. Moloney, *J. Lar. Otol.*, 1977, *91*, 837.

Further studies in aspirin-sensitive patients with asthma and their reaction to tartrazine.— G. A. Settipane *et al.*, *J. Allergy & clin. Immunol.*, 1974, *53*, 200; G. A. Settipane and R. K. Pudupakkam, *ibid.*, 1975, *56*, 215; P. K. Vedanthan *et al.*, *ibid.*, 1977, *60*, 8; R. W. Weber *et al.*, *ibid.*, 1979, *64*, 32.

Further reports and discussions of urticarial skin reactions and angioneurotic oedema in aspirin-sensitive patients.— J. L. Verbov, *Br. J. clin. Pract.*, 1968, *22*, 229; R. L. Baer and H. Harris, *J. Am. med. Ass.*, 1967, *202*, 710; R. H. Champion *et al.*, *Br. J. Derm.*, 1969, *81*, 588; J. A. Savin, *Br. J. Derm.*, 1970, *83*, 546; A. -M. Ros *et al.*, *Br. J. Derm.*, 1976, *95*, 19.

In children. A review of analgesic sensitivity in children with asthma.— M. Weinberger, *Pediatrics*, 1978, *62*, *Suppl.*, 910.

Further reports on aspirin sensitivity in children with asthma.— J. W. Yunginger *et al.*, *J. Pediat.*, 1973, *82*, 218; C. J. Falliers, *J. Allergy & clin. Immunol.*, 1973, *52*, 141; G. S. Rachelefsky *et al.*, *Pediatrics*, 1975, *56*, 443; P. K. Vedanthan *et al.*, *J. Allergy & clin. Immunol.*, 1977, *60*, 8.

Cerebral oedema. Sudden cerebral oedema in a 5-year-old boy with juvenile rheumatoid arthritis was probably associated with long-term high-dose aspirin therapy. The mechanism was poorly understood but salicylism was known to uncouple oxidative phosphorylation and lower brain-glucose concentrations despite normal blood-glucose concentrations.— P. F. Bray and A. Y. Gardiner (letter), *New Engl. J. Med.*, 1977, *297*, 1235.

Effects on blood. A review of the adverse effects of salicylates on erythrocyte function, with reference to gastro-intestinal haemorrhage and haemolysis, leucocyte function, platelet function, and haemostasis.— B. M. Rothschild, *Clin. Pharmac. Ther.*, 1979, *26*, 145.

Reports of excessive postoperative blood loss attributed to use of aspirin.— H. M. Pinedo *et al.*, *Ann. rheum. Dis.*, 1973, *32*, 66, per *Int. pharm. Abstr.*, 1973, *10*,

760; H. U. Hepsö *et al.*, *Eur. J. clin. Pharmac.*, 1976, *10*, 217; D. W. Davies and D. J. Steward, *Can. Anaesth. Soc. J.*, 1977, *24*, 452; T. McGaul, *J. Dent.*, 1978, *6*, 207; M. Torosian *et al.*, *Ann. intern. Med.*, 1978, *89*, 325; R. N. Rubin (letter), *ibid.*, 1006.

For a report of serious bleeding complications in patients given heparin and aspirin for prophylaxis against deep-vein thrombosis, see Heparin, p.765.

See also Effects on the Gastro-intestinal Tract.

Aplastic anaemia. Reports of aspirin-induced aplastic anaemia.— M. Eldar *et al.* (letter), *S. Afr. med. J.*, 1979, *55*, 318.

Haemolytic anaemia. Aspirin, 4 to 12 g daily, had been reported to cause haemolytic anaemia in certain individuals with a deficiency of glucose-6-phosphate dehydrogenase. The reaction was not considered clinically significant under normal circumstances (e.g. in the absence of infection).— E. Beutler, *Pharmac. Rev.*, 1969, *21*, 73. See also A. Karaklis (letter), *Br. med. J.*, 1981, *283*, 731.

Further reports on the occurrence of aspirin-induced haemolytic anaemia in patients with glucose-6-phosphate dehydrogenase deficiency.— E. R. Burka, *Ann. intern. Med.*, 1966, *64*, 817; B. E. Glader, *J. Pediat.*, 1976, *89*, 1027; T. K. Chan *et al.*, *Br. med. J.*, 1976, *2*, 1227.

Thrombocytopenia. Reports on thrombocytopenia attributed to aspirin.— E. Thiel *et al.*, *Klin. Wschr.*, 1973, *51*, 754; I. H. Scheinberg (letter), *New Engl. J. Med.*, 1979, *300*, 678.

Effects on blood glucose. The hypoglycaemic action of salicylates might be due to suppression of the release of fatty acids from adipose tissue. Plasma-salicylate concentrations of 200 to 300 µg per ml produced maximal hypoglycaemic activity. This effect was not significant in normal persons and salicylate poisoning had been complicated by hyperglycaemia and glycosuria.— V. Fang *et al.*, *J. pharm. Sci.*, 1968, *57*, 2111.

See also under Diabetes (Uses).

Effects on eyes. Transient myopia occurred in a patient following the ingestion of 2.7 g of aspirin.— J. H. Sandford-Smith, *Br. J. Ophthal.*, 1974, *58*, 698.

Aspirin 1.28 g affected colour discrimination in healthy subjects, but the effects were minor.— S. M. Luria *et al.*, *Br. J. clin. Pharmac.*, 1979, *7*, 585.

Effects on the gastro-intestinal tract. There have been numerous clinical reports of gastric erosion, ulceration, and haemorrhage following the ingestion of aspirin. Although there have been numerous fatalities (N. Marshall and J.A. Kuzemko, *Br. med. J.*, 1972, *4*, 612) it has been suggested that the risks of serious gastro-intestinal disturbances might have been overstated (W.D.W. Rees and L.A. Turnberg, *Lancet*, 1980, *1*, 410; D. Coggon and M.J.S. Langman, *Gut*, 1980, *21*, A922). Erosion and ulceration have been confirmed by gastroscopy (D. Edmar, *Acta radiol. Diagnosis*, 1971, *11*, 57, per *Drugs*, 1972, *3*, 443) and by X-ray examination. A high incidence of aspirin consumption has been reported in patients admitted to hospital with serious gastro-intestinal haemorrhage (D.J. Parry and P.H.N. Wood, *Gut*, 1967, *8*, 301; R.I. Russell *et al.*, *Lancet*, 1968, *2*, 603; H.B. Valman *et al.*, *Br. med. J.*, 1968, *4*, 661; M. Levy, *Clin. Pharmac. Ther.*, 1974, *15*, 210), and an association with pre-existing gastric disorders has been suggested (D.J.B. St. John and F.T. McDermott, *Br. med. J.*, 1970, *2*, 450; S.J. Winawer *et al.*, *Archs intern. Med.*, 1971, *127*, 129, per *Clin. Med.*, 1972, *79* (Dec.), 39). Occult blood loss is increased in up to 70% of patients taking aspirin and other salicylates, including aspirin in the form of enteric-coated and buffered formulations (J.T. Scott *et al.*, *Q.J. Med.*, 1961, *30*, 167; D.N. Croft and P.H.N. Wood, *Br. med. J.*, 1967, *1*, 137). The effect appears to be due to local irritation rather than to an effect upon the bleeding time (J.R. Leonards and G. Levy, *J. pharm. Sci.*, 1970, *59*, 1511); the permeability of the gastric mucosa has been reported to be increased (B.M. Smith *et al.*, *New Engl. J. Med.*, 1971, *285*, 716) and the irritant effect has been reported to be increased with large particle size (A.Z. Györy and J.N. Stiel, *Lancet*, 1968, *2*, 300; J.R. Leonards and G. Levy, *J. pharm. Sci.*, 1969, *58*, 1277) and with increased acidity (C. Davidson *et al.*, *Clin. Pharmac. Ther.*, 1966, *7*, 239). The effect is enhanced by the concomitant use of alcohol (K. Goulston and A.R. Cooke, *Br. med. J.*, 1968, *4*, 664; C.H. Morris *et al.* (letter), *J. pharm. Sci.*, 1972, *61*, 81; S.J. Johnston *et al.*, *Br. med. J.*, 1973, *3*, 655; H.S. Murray *et al.*, *ibid.*, 1974, *1*, 19) and is reduced to some extent by the concomitant use of alkalis, and by the use of soluble, buffered, and enteric formulations (V.F. Saldanha and C.W.H. Harvard, *Br. J. clin. Pract.*, 1971, *25*, 169; J.R. Leonards and G. Levy, *Archs intern. Med.*, 1972, *129*, 457, per *Drug Intell. & clin. Pharm.*, 1972, *6*, 366; *Br. med. J.*, 1976, *2*, 6; *ibid.*, 1981, *282*, 91).

The incidence of gastro-intestinal bleeding was monitored in 16 646 hospitalised patients with no predisposing illness by the Boston Collaborative Drug Surveillance Program. Of 2081 who had received aspirin alone, major gastro-intestinal bleeding occurred in 6 (0.3%) and minor gastro-intestinal bleeding in 33 (1.6%).— H. Jick and J. Porter, *Lancet*, 1978, *2*, 87. Comment: M. J. S. Langman (letter), *ibid.*, 633.

Further discussions and reviews of aspirin and its effects on the gastro-intestinal tract.— *Lancet*, 1967, *2*, 460; *Br. med. J.*, 1967, *3*, 810; H. W. Davenport, *New Engl. J. Med.*, 1967, *276*, 1307; *Br. med. J.*, 1970, *2*, 436; A. J. Quick (letter), *Br. med. J.*, 1969, *1*, 315; A. R. Cooke, *Am. J. dig. Dis.*, 1973, *18*, 225; A. H. Gartner, *J. Am. dent. Ass.*, 1976, *93*, 111; E. Shirley, *Proc. R. Soc. Med.*, 1977, *70*, *Suppl.* 7, 4; M. J. S. Langman, *ibid.*, 16; J. S. Goodall, *Chemist Drugg.*, 1977, *208*, 632; M. G. Bramble and C. O. Record, *Drugs*, 1978, *15*, 451; D. Fromm, *Pediatrics*, 1978, *62*, *Suppl.*, 938; J. C. Krantz, *Am. Pharm.*, 1979, *NS19* (July), 51.

Reports of oral and oesophageal injury associated with aspirin use.— Z. Kawashima *et al.*, *J. Am. dent. Ass.*, 1975, *91*, 130; J. G. Williams (letter), *Br. med. J.*, 1979, *2*, 273; V. M. Smith, *Sth. med. J.*, 1978, *71*, *Suppl.* 1, 45.

Reviews and studies of gastro-intestinal damage caused by aspirin compared with other other non-steroidal anti-inflammatory agents.— R. E. Pemberton and L. J. Strand, *Dig. Dis. Sci.*, 1979, *24*, 53; F. L. Lanza *et al.*, *Dig. Dis. Sci.*, 1979, *24*, 823.

Comparative studies of faecal blood losses following aspirin and other anti-inflammatory drugs.— R. M. Rowan *et al.*, *Clin. Trials J.*, 1976, *13*, 60; D. H. Loebl *et al.*, *J. Am. med. Ass.*, 1977, *237*, 976; A. Cohen and H. E. Garber, *Curr. ther. Res.*, 1978, *23*, 187; G. Palme and P. Koeppe, *Arzneimittel-Forsch.*, 1978, *28*, 426; A. Cohen, *J. clin. Pharmac.*, 1979, *19*, 242; S. M. Chernish *et al.*, *Arthritis Rheum.*, 1979, *22*, 376.

Further studies on aspirin-induced gastro-intestinal damage and blood loss.— J. H. Emmanuel and R. D. Montgomery, *Postgrad. med. J.*, 1971, *47*, 227; J. R. Leonards and G. Levy, *Clin. Pharmac. Ther.*, 1973, *14*, 62; J. R. Leonards *et al.*, *New Engl. J. Med.*, 1973, *289*, 1020; K. -J. Hahn *et al.*, *Clin. Pharmac. Ther.*, 1975, *17*, 330; K. M. Cochran *et al.*, *Br. med. J.*, 1975, *1*, 183; G. E. Bergman *et al.*, *J. Pediat.*, 1976, *88*, 501; L. Domellof and B. Sönne, *Läkartidningen*, 1976, *73*, 1521; W. A. Baskin *et al.*, *Ann. intern. Med.*, 1976, *85*, 299; K. D. Rainsford and K. Brune, *Med. J. Aust.*, 1976, *1*, 881; K. J. Ivey *et al.*, *Gastroenterology*, 1979, *76*, 50; J. W. Hoftiezer *et al.*, *Lancet*, 1980, *2*, 609.

See also Effects on Blood.

Gastric ulcer. There was significant correlation between major upper gastro-intestinal bleeding and also benign gastric ulcer and the regular use of aspirin on 4 or more days a week. There was no evidence of an association between the use of aspirin and duodenal ulcer.—A Report from the Boston Collaborative Drug Surveillance Program, *New Engl. J. Med.*, 1974, *290*, 1158.

Further studies which confirmed the association between gastric ulcer and regular aspirin consumption.— B. L. Chapman and J. M. Duggan, *Gut*, 1969, *10*, 443; A. J. Cameron, *Mayo CLin. Proc.*, 1975, *50*, 565; D. W. Piper *et al.*, *Proc. R. Soc. Med.*, 1977, *70*, *Suppl.* 7, 11; G. R. Silvoso *et al.*, *Ann. intern. med.*, 1979, *91*, 517; N. Refsum *et al.*, *Meddr norsk farm. Selsk.*, 1977, *39*, 82, per *Int. pharm. Abstr.*, 1977, *14*, 1080; H. Mielants *et al.*, *J. Rheumatol.*, 1979, *6*, 210.

Effects on hearing. In 52 patients with rheumatoid arthritis, the daily dose of aspirin required to produce tinnitus varied from 3.6 to 10.8 g daily. The average serum-salicylate concentration was 295 µg per ml; tinnitus did not occur at concentrations less than 196 µg per ml. In 15 patients with pre-existing hearing loss tinnitus did not develop despite serum-salicylate concentrations ranging from 311 to 677 µg per ml.— E. Mongan *et al.*, *J. Am. med. Ass.*, 1973, *226*, 142.

The Boston Collaborative Drug Surveillance Program monitored consecutively 32 812 medical inpatients. Drug-induced deafness occurred in a dose-related manner in 32 of 2974 patients given aspirin.— J. Porter and H. Jick, *Lancet*, 1977, *1*, 587.

For reports of reversible and permanent deafness attributed to salicylate therapy, see J. Ballantyne, *J. Lar. Otol.*, 1972, *84*, 967; L. Jardini *et al.*, *Rheumatol. Rehabil.*, 1978, *17*, 233; R. R. Miller, *J. clin. Pharmac.*, 1978, *18*, 468.

Effects on the heart. Administration of aspirin 4 g daily markedly exacerbated anginal attacks in a 66-year-old man with Prinzmetal's variant angina.— K. Miwa *et al.* (letter), *Lancet*, 1979, *2*, 1382.

Effects on the kidneys. Aspirin-induced alterations in renal function were demonstrated in 13 of 23 patients with systemic lupus erythematosus, 4 of 22 with rheumatoid arthritis, and 2 of 3 normal subjects. Changes includes elevation of serum creatinine and blood-urea nitrogen. Aspirin and other non-steroidal anti-inflammatory agents could produce alterations in renal function that might influence the interpretation of clinical data.— R. P. Kimberly and P. H. Plotz, *New Engl. J. Med.*, 1977, *296*, 418. Comment.— P. Kincaid-Smith, *Drugs*, 1977, *14*, 393; *Lancet*, 1977, *1*, 942. Further criticisms and comments.— W. M. Bennett and G. A. Porter (letter), *New Engl. J. Med.*, 1977, *296*, 1168; A. Leonard (letter), *ibid.*; T. F. Ignaczak *et al.* (letter), *ibid.* Reply.— R. P. Kimberly and P. H. Plotz (letter), *ibid.*, 1169.

No significant alterations in renal function were detected in 102 patients with active rheumatoid arthritis treated with aspirin.— B. R. Walker *et al.* (letter), *New Engl. J. Med.*, 1977, *297*, 1405. See also I. L. Nielsen *et al.*, *Br. med. J.*, 1980, *280*, 610.

Renal function in patients with systemic lupus erythematosus was reduced by ibuprofen, naproxen, and fenoprofen as well as aspirin and indomethacin.— R. P. Kimberly *et al.*, *Am. J. Med.*, 1978, *64*, 804.

A further study on the effect of aspirin on renal function in 7 women with systemic lupus erythematosus.— R. P. Kimberly *et al.*, *Ann. intern. Med.*, 1978, *89*, 336. Criticism.— R. S. Muther *et al.* (letter), *ibid.*, 1979, *90*, 274. Reply.— R. P. Kimberley *et al.* (letter), *ibid.*, 275.

See also under Analgesic Abuse, p.234.

Effects on liver. Aspirin-induced hepatotoxicity occurs more frequently in patients with rheumatoid arthritis and other connective tissue disorders than previously recognised. Increased concentrations of serum aminotransferases (SGOT, SGPT) appear to be correlated with salicylate concentrations greater than 250 to 350 µg per ml and with active rheumatoid disease. The effects are reversible on discontinuing aspirin or decreasing the dose. There is no evidence to suggest that children or women are more susceptible.— S. A. Kanada *et al.*, *Am. J. Hosp. Pharm.*, 1978, *35*, 330.

For further reviews and discussions on aspirin-induced hepatotoxicity, see *Br. med. J.*, 1973, *2*, 732; *Lancet*, 1974, *1*, 667; R. R. Babb, *West. J. Med.*, 1978, *129*, 164; C. E. Bryant, *J. Ok. St. med. Ass.*, 1978, *71*, 284.

Further reports of raised serum aminotransferase (SGOT, SGPT) concentrations or other evidence of hepatic dysfunction associated with aspirin.— A. S. Russell *et al.*, *Br. med. J.*, 1971, *2*, 428; T. Iancu (letter), *Br. med. J.*, 1972, *2*, 167; R. R. Rich and J. S. Johnson, *Arthritis Rheum.*, 1973, *16*, 1; H. M. Pinedo *et al.*, *Ann. rheum. Dis.*, 1973, *32*, 66; P. Zucker *et al.*, *Am. J. Dis. Child.*, 1975, *129*, 1433; D. A. Saltzman *et al.*, *Am. J. dig. Dis.*, 1976, *21*, 815; T. Iancu and E. Elian, *Am. J. clin. Path.*, 1976, *66*, 570; W. B. Ricks (letter), *Ann. intern. Med.*, 1976, *84*, 52; T. O'Gorman and R. S. Koff, *Gastroenterology*, 1977, *72*, 726; J. A. Sbarbaro and R. M. Bennett, *Ann. intern. Med.*, 1977, *86*, 183; B. H. Bernstein *et al.*, *Am. J. Dis. Child.*, 1977, *131*, 659; N. Gitlin and J. Grant, *S. Afr. med. J.*, 1977, *51*, 697, per *Drugs*, 1978, *16*, 270; M. H. Ulshen *et al.*, *J. Pediat.*, 1978, *93*, 1034; J. G. Schaller, *Pediatrics*, 1978, *62*, 916; S. A. Kanada *et al.*, *Am. J. Hosp. Pharm.*, 1978, *35*, 330; D. T. D. Bulugahapitiya *et al.* (letter), *Lancet*, 1979, *1*, 1295; A. I. Lazarovits *et al.* (letter), *Ann. intern. Med.*, 1980, *93*, 510.

For reports of hepatotoxicity associated with aspirin in patients with systemic lupus erythematosus or similar disorders, see W. E. Seaman *et al.*, *Ann. intern. Med.*, 1974, *80*, 1; J. D. Wolfe *et al.*, *ibid.*, 74; *ibid.*, 103; R. L. Travers and G. R. V. Hughes, *Br. med. J.*, 1978, *2*, 1532; B. G. Petty *et al.*, *J. Pediat.*, 1978, *93*, 881.

See also under Reye's Syndrome, below.

Effects on the lungs. See under Pulmonary Oedema.

Epidermal necrolysis. Thirteen cases of toxic epidermal necrolysis had been reported associated with the use of aspirin or methyl salicylate.— E. D. Lowney *et al.*, *Archs Derm.*, 1967, *95*, 359.

Overdosage. Reviews of salicylate poisoning.— *Br. med. J.*, 1972, *1*, 263; A. W. Pierce, *Pediatrics*, 1974, *54*, 342; K. J. Bender, *Drug Intell. & clin. Pharm.*, 1975, *9*, 350; L. F. Prescott, *Prescribers' J.*, 1979, *19*, 169.

The onset of symptoms of salicylate poisoning might be delayed for up to 24 hours. All children with suspected salicylate poisoning should be admitted to hospital and kept there at least 24 hours.— I. P. Brown, *Practitioner*, 1973, *211*, 553.

In a study of 73 adults with salicylate poisoning, diagnosis was delayed in those who had ingested salicylate for medical reasons compared with those who took an intentional overdose. Morbidity and mortality-rates were higher when diagnosis was delayed. It was suggested that diagnosis of salicylate intoxication should be considered in patients, and especially elderly patients, with unexplained encephalopathy, tachypnoea, or acid-base abnormalities.— R. J. Anderson *et al.*, *Ann. intern. Med.*, 1976, *85*, 745.

The main physiological effects resulting from acute salicylate poisoning include stimulation of the respiratory centre, uncoupling of oxidative phosphorylation mechanisms, altered glucose metabolism due to inhibition of Krebs cycle enzymes, stimulation of glyconeogenesis, increased tissue glycolysis, and stimulation of lipid metabolism. Other effects include inhibition of amino-acid metabolism and interference with haemostatic mechanisms. The principal manifestations of salicylate poisoning are respiratory alkalosis, metabolic acidosis, altered glucose metabolism, fluid and electrolyte losses, and hypermetabolism. Therapy should be mainly directed to replacement of fluid and electrolyte losses, correction of acidaemia, administration of glucose, prevention of further salicylate absorption, and enhancement of salicylate elimination.— A. R. Temple, *Pediatrics*, 1978, *62, Suppl.*, 873.

Symptoms of mild salicylate poisoning in children include hyperpnoea, lethargy, vomiting, hyperthermia and hypocapnia. Symptoms of moderate poisoning include severe hyperpnoea, marked lethargy or excitability, and compensated metabolic acidosis while symptoms of severe poisoning include coma, uncompensated metabolic acidosis, and possibly convulsions. Inevitable symptoms include vomiting, hyperpnoea, and hyperthermia and salicylate poisoning should always be considered when these occur together in a child.— A. K. Done, *Pediatrics*, 1978, *62*, *Suppl.*, 890.

Asterixis as a manifestation of salicylate toxicity.— R. J. Anderson, *Ann. intern. Med.*, 1981, *95*, 188.

For reference to fatal malignant hyperthermia in a 17-year-old girl who had taken an overdose of aspirin and protizinic acid, see Protizinic Acid, p.276.

Further reports and discussions of salicylate poisoning in children.— *Pharm. J.*, 1964, *1*, 40; J. O. Craig *et al.*, *Br. med. J.*, 1966, *1*, 757; K. Naess (letter), *J. Am. med. Ass.*, 1968, *206*, 2742; I. Mitchell (letter), *Br. med. J.*, 1979, *1*, 1081; S. M. Marcus, *J. med. Soc. New Jers.*, 1979, *76*, 524.

See also Pulmonary Oedema, below.

Acid-base disturbances. Discussions on the acid-base disturbances occurring in salicylate poisoning.— P. D. Dawkins *et al.*, *J. Pharm. Pharmac.*, 1967, *19*, 355; A. T. Proudfoot and S. S. Brown, *Br. med. J.*, 1969, *2*, 547; N. Buchanan and L. Rabinowitz, *J. Pediat.*, 1974, *84*, 391; R. A. Kreisberg, *Ann. intern. med.*, 1980, *92*, 227.

Paracetamol. A comparison of salicylate poisoning and paracetamol poisoning.— B. H. Rumack, *Pediatrics*, 1978, *62, Suppl.*, 943, per *Int. pharm. Abstr.*, 1979, *16*, 403.

A 5½ year old child was initially given aspirin for 7 days but when this failed to control her fever she was given aspirin 300 mg and paracetamol 300 mg alternately every 2 hours (each drug every 4 hours). During the next 12 hours the fever continued and the child had abdominal pains and subsequently vomited. She was comatose and unresponsive to pain on admission to hospital and had signs of cerebral and neurological impairment and liver damage. The child recovered and was ambulatory and discharged 9 days later; she was fully recovered at follow-up after 4 months. The authors concluded that until further study had properly assessed the risk of combined aspirin and paracetamol toxicity, the basis for prescribing such regimens was wholly inadequate. The clinical features of dual intoxication might or might not represent a composite of the toxicity of either drug alone.— R. G. Bickers and R. J. Roberts, *J. Pediat.*, 1979, *94*, 1001.

Pregnancy and the neonate. For a review of the effects of aspirin on the mother and foetus during pregnancy and parturition, see D. G. Corby, *Pediatrics*, 1978, *62*, *Suppl.*, 930.

Regular salicylate takers had an increased frequency of anaemia during pregnancy and of prenatal and postnatal haemorrhage, a slightly longer duration of pregnancy, more complications at delivery, and increased perinatal mortality. Many regular takers were heavy smokers.— E. Collins and G. Turner, *Lancet*, 1975, *2*, 335.

Further reports of increased mortality in newborn infants and mothers associated with aspirin ingestion during pregnancy.— W. A. Bleyer and R. T. Breckenridge, *J. Am. med. Ass.*, 1970, *213*, 2049; R. B. Lewis and J. D. Schulman, *Lancet*, 1973, *2*, 1159; R. R. Haslam *et al.*, *J. Pediat.*, 1974, *84*, 556; G. Turner and E. Collins, *Lancet*, 1975, *2*, 338.

Data analysis of 35 418 women not exposed to aspirin during the first 4 months of pregnancy compared with 5 128 heavily exposed and 9 736 with intermediate exposure suggested that aspirin was not teratogenic.— D. Slone *et al.*, *Lancet*, 1976, *1*, 1373. No significant association between aspirin ingestion and perinatal mortality or birth-weight could be demonstrated by a data analysis of 41 337 women and their offspring.— S. Shapiro *et al.*, *ibid.*, 1375.

Further studies which suggested an association between aspirin ingestion and teratogenicity.— B. S. Sayli *et al.* (letter), *Lancet*, 1966, *1*, 876; I. D. G. Richards, *Br. J. prev. soc. Med.*, 1969, *23*, 218; M. M. Nelson and J. O. Forfar, *Br. med. J.*, 1971, *1*, 523; J. O. Forfar, *Prescribers' J.*, 1973, *13*, 130.

For reports on the adverse effects of maternally-administered indomethacin on the development of neonatal pulmonary vasculature, see Indomethacin, p.258.

Ductus arteriosus closure. Studies in several groups of infants indicated that premature closure of the ductus arteriosus secondary to maternal ingestion of salicylates may be one cause of persistent pulmonary hypertension of the newborn and may explain the absence of right to left ductus shunting in some infants.— R. M. Perkin *et al.*, *J. Pediat.*, 1980, *96*, 721, per *Int. pharm. Abstr.*, 1980, *17*, 894.

Pulmonary oedema. Noncardiogenic pulmonary oedema was the main presenting symptom in a patient suffering from salicylate intoxication. Oedema improved when plasma salicylate concentrations were reduced by forced alkaline diuresis.— J. Heffner *et al.*, *West. J. Med.*, 1979, *130*, 263.

Further reports of pulmonary oedema associated with salicylate intoxication.— P. R. Davis and R. E. Burch (letter), *Ann. intern. Med.*, 1974, *80*, 553; M. G. Tweeddale (letter), *ibid.*, *81*, 710; G. Hrnicek *et al.*, *J. Am. med. Ass.*, 1974, *230*, 866; T. W. Broderick *et al.*, *Am. J. Roentg.*, 1976, *127*, 865; S. C. Sørensen (letter), *Lancet*, 1979, *1*, 1025; C. Thomas (letter), *ibid.*, 1294; A. Kahn and D. Blum (letter), *Lancet*, 1979, *2*, 1131.

Reye's syndrome. Evidence that salicylate may be associated with the development of Reye's syndrome in children with febrile illnesses.— K. M. Starko *et al.*, *Pediatrics*, 1980, *66*, 859. See also J. S. Partin *et al.*, *Lancet*, 1982, *1*, 191. Preliminary findings which do not support the view that there is an association.— B. D. Andresen *et al.* (letter), *ibid.*, 903.

Shock. Shock symptoms associated with the intravenous administration of analgesics containing salicylate and/or compounds of the pyrazolone group.— *Japan med. Gaz.*, 1979, *16* (Feb. 20), 9.

Treatment of Adverse Effects. In acute salicylate overdosage the stomach should be emptied by inducing emesis or by aspiration and lavage. Patients with mild intoxication should be encouraged to drink plenty of fluids. In patients with more severe intoxication (plasma salicylate concentration above 500 µg per ml in adults or 300 µg per ml in children) forced alkaline diuresis may be required and should be continued until the plasma salicylate concentration is less than 350 µg per ml in adults, then intravenous fluids can be stopped and the patient encouraged to take fluids by mouth. Plasma electrolytes, especially potassium, and the acid-base balance should be monitored regularly. Acidaemia must be corrected by infusion of sodium bicarbonate before starting forced diuresis. Details of forced alkaline diuresis are provided under Phenobarbitone, p.812.

In the presence of cardiac or renal impairment or in very severe intoxication, haemodialysis or peritoneal dialysis may be necessary.

Acute allergic reactions to aspirin may be treated, if necessary, by administration of adrenaline, corticosteroids, and an antihistamine.

Studies in 40 patients with moderate or severe salicylate poisoning suggested that an intravenous regimen of forced diuresis using a solution containing sodium chloride 0.225%, sodium bicarbonate 0.315%, potassium chloride 0.15%, and laevulose 2.5% was effective in reducing plasma-salicylate concentrations. The solution was infused at a rate of 2 litres per hour for 3 hours. Treatment with this regimen (forced cocktail diuresis) or forced alkaline diuresis with a regimen of saline, laevulose, and sodium bicarbonate ameliorated symptoms in a few hours; forced water diuresis intravenously (with saline and laevulose) or fluids by mouth required more than 24 hours. All 3 intravenous regimens produced a good diuresis, though it was delayed for up to 2 hours in some patients. Forced alkaline diuresis produced the most rapid fall in plasma-salicylate concentrations but was accompanied by a rise in arterial pH. Excretion of salicylate with the compound solution was less effective but there were no changes in arterial pH or blood-potassium concentrations. Potassium by mouth could be given later to treat delayed falls in plasma concentrations.— A. A. H. Lawson *et al.*, *Q. J. Med.*, 1969, *38*, 31. See also *Lancet*, 1969, *1*, 1038.

Reviews of the treatment of salicylate poisoning.— S. Locket, *Practitioner*, 1973, *211*, 105; A. G. Morgan and A. Polak, *Clin. Sci.*, 1971, *41*, 475; J. B. Hill, *New Engl. J. Med.*, 1973, *288*, 1110; A. W. Pierce, *Pediatrics*, 1974, *54*, 342; A. W. Craft and J. R. Sibert, *Br. J. Hosp. Med.*, 1977, *17*, 469; J. F. Winchester *et al.*, *Trans Am. Soc. artif. internal Organs*, 1977, *23*, 762; A. T. Proudfoot and L. F. Prescott, Poisoning with paraquat, salicylate and paracetamol, in *Recent Advances in Intensive Therapy*, No. 1, I.M. Ledingham (Ed.), London, Churchill Livingstone, 1977, p. 217; A. K. Done, *Pediatrics*, 1978, *62*, *Suppl.*, 890; J. A. Vale and R. Goulding, *Prescribers' J.*, 1979, *19*, 155 and 163.

A brief review of the use of charcoal haemoperfusion in the treatment of salicylate overdosage.— S. Pond *et al.*, *Clin. Pharmacokinet.*, 1979, *4*, 329.

For reports on the value of activated charcoal in the treatment of acute salicylate poisoning.— *J. Am. med. Ass.*, 1969, *209*, 1821; G. Levy and T. Tsuchiya, *Clin. Pharmac. Ther.*, 1972, *13*, 317; M. Mayersohn *et al.*, *Clin. Toxicol.*, 1977, *11*, 561; E. Elonen and P. J. Neuvonen (letter), *Lancet*, 1981, *2*, 536.

See also under Activated Charcoal, p.79.

A report on the protective effect of glucagon against gastric mucosal damage induced by aspirin.— A. Tarnawski *et al.*, *Gastroenterology*, 1978, *74*, 240.

Further reports on the treatment of salicylate poisoning.— G. W. Beveridge *et al.*, *Lancet*, 1964, *1*, 1406; A. A. H. Lawson *et al.*, *Lancet*, 1964, *2*, 260; G. Cumming *et al.*, *Br. med. J.*, 1964, *2*, 1033; I. G. Graber (letter), *ibid.*, 1395; R. L. Summitt and J. N. Etteldorf, *J. Pediat.*, 1964, *64*, 803; R. J. Schlegal *et al.*, *J. Pediat.*, 1966, *69*, 553; K. J. Berg, *Eur. J. clin. Pharmac.*, 1977, *12*, 111.

Precautions. Aspirin should be cautiously employed, if at all, in patients prone to dyspepsia or known to have a lesion of the gastric mucosa. It should not be administered to patients with haemophilia or to those with an intolerance to aspirin (especially aspirin-sensitive asthmatics) and is not recommended for infants under one year of age. Caution is necessary when renal or hepatic function is impaired and, particularly in children, when the patient is dehydrated.

Some of the effects of aspirin on the gastro-intestinal tract are enhanced by alcohol. Aspirin may enhance the activity of coumarin anticoagulants and sulphonylurea hypoglycaemic agents. The haemorrhagic effects of aspirin on the gastric mucosa may be enhanced by anticoagulants. The activity of methotrexate may be markedly enhanced and its toxicity increased by administration with aspirin. Aspirin diminishes the effects of uricosuric agents such as probenecid and sulphinpyrazone. Barbiturates and other sedatives may mask the respiratory symptoms of aspirin overdosage and have been reported to enhance its toxicity.

There was no association between aspirin and gastro-intestinal bleeding in 23 patients on haemodialysis.— G. Remuzzi *et al.* (letter), *Lancet*, 1977, *2*, 359.

For various factors affecting protein binding, see below under Absorption and Fate.

Effects on blood. When aspirin 650 mg was given to healthy persons the bleeding time remained below the upper limit of the normal range, but a dose of 1.3 g caused a small increase in more than 50% of the subjects. Sodium salicylate 1.15 g did not prolong the bleeding time in these subjects. In patients with the Minot-von Willebrand syndrome the bleeding time was significantly prolonged following 650 mg of aspirin.— A. J. Quick, *Am. J. med. Sci.*, 1966, *252*, 265. See also *idem* (letter), *Lancet*, 1966, *2*, 1134.

The bleeding time, measured 2 hours after 1 g of aspirin in capsules, was not significantly prolonged in 21 patients with mild haemophilia, but was greatly prolonged in 8 of 19 others with severe deficiency of factor VIII or IX. Seven patients required transfusions of plasma or concentrated factor VIII to arrest bleeding from the experimental incision.— M. M. Kaneshiro *et al.*, *New Engl. J. Med.*, 1969, *281*, 1039.

In patients with even slightly prolonged bleeding after tooth extraction or other evidence of haemostatic defect the use of aspirin, ibuprofen, indomethacin, meclofenamic acid, and mefenamic acid should be discouraged. Paracetamol or dihydrocodeine tartrate had no effect on platelets and might be given.— *Br. med. J.*, 1974, *3*, 5. See also S. R. Lemkin *et al.*, *Oral Surg.*, 1974, *37*, 498.

See also under Adverse Effects and Uses.

Effects on liver. A report of the effects of aspirin on liver-function tests in patients with rheumatoid arthritis and systemic lupus erythematosus.— W. E. Seaman and P. H. Plotz, *Arthritis Rheum.*, 1976, *19*, 155.

For reports on the hepatotoxic effects of salicylates in patients with rheumatoid arthritis and systemic lupus erythematosus, see under Adverse Effects.

Gout. Salicylates in low doses may increase serum-urate concentrations and lead to the erroneous diagnosis of gout.— A. I. Grayzel *et al.*, *New Engl. J. Med.*, 1961, *265*, 763.

Interactions, drugs. A review of potential drug interactions and adverse effects related to aspirin.— M. Suffness and B. S. Rose, *Drug Intell. & clin. Pharm.*, 1974, *8*, 694.

Antacids. The serum-salicylate concentrations in 3 children with rheumatic fever decreased when an aluminium and magnesium hydroxide antacid was given at the same time as aspirin and increased when the antacid was stopped.— G. Levy *et al.*, *New Engl. J. Med.*, 1975, *293*, 323. See also under Absorption and Fate.

Plasma concentrations of aspirin were highest following administration of unbuffered aspirin tablets, but there was no difference in bioavailability from buffered and unbuffered aspirin tablets. Salicylic acid concentrations in plasma were highest following administration of tablets buffered with magnesium oxide. Absorption was delayed from tablets buffered with aluminium salts.— M. Linnoila and J. Lehtola, *Int. J. clin. Pharmac. Biopharm.*, 1977, *15*, 61.

Antibiotics. Aspirin has been reported to prolong the half-life of benzylpenicillin; to inhibit the serum binding of benzylpenicillin, cloxacillin sodium, dicloxacillin sodium, nafcillin sodium, oxacillin sodium, and phenoxymethylpenicillin.

Ascorbic acid. Platelet- and plasma-ascorbic acid concentrations were significantly reduced in 14 patients with rheumatoid arthritis taking high doses of aspirin with or without corticosteroids, and in 2 patients taking indomethacin. Only plasma concentrations were reduced in 10 patients taking low doses of aspirin or no aspirin. There was no change in either plasma or platelet concentrations in 8 patients taking high doses of aspirin in conjunction with ascorbic acid.— M. A. Sahud and R. J. Cohen, *Lancet*, 1971, *1*, 937. In normal subjects, a therapeutic dose of aspirin inhibited the uptake and storage of ascorbic acid in leucocytes.— H. S. Loh and C. W. M. Wilson, *J. clin. Pharmac.*, 1975, *15*, 36.

Beta-adrenoceptor blocking agents. For the possible adverse effects of non-steroidal anti-inflammatory agents on blood pressure in patients receiving beta-adrenoceptor blocking agents, see under Propranolol, p.1328.

Carbonic anhydrase inhibitors. For reference to possible increased salicylate toxicity in patients also taking carbonic anhydrase inhibitors, see Acetazolamide, p.582.

Corticosteroids. In 4 patients taking salicylates and corticosteroids the serum-salicylate concentration rose when the corticosteroid was withdrawn or the dose reduced. One 5-year-old boy developed salicylism characterised by dyspnoea, lethargy, metabolic acidosis, and a serum-salicylate concentration of 880 μg per ml.— J. R. Klinenberg and F. Miller, *J. Am. med. Ass.*, 1965, *194*, 601.

Concurrent administration of corticosteroids or corticotrophin with aspirin or sodium salicylate was shown to lower the plasma-salicylate concentration.— M. Bardare *et al.*, *Archs Dis. Childh.*, 1978, *53*, 381.

Diclofenac. Pretreatment with diclofenac sodium appeared to enhance renal excretion of salicylate. Acute administration of diclofenac had no effect on plasma-salicylate concentrations. Concurrent administration of aspirin resulted in a significant decrease in plasma concentrations of diclofenac.— F. O. Müller *et al.*, *Int. J. clin. Pharmac. Biopharm.*, 1977, *15*, 397.

Frusemide. For the effect of aspirin on frusemide, see Frusemide, p.597.

Gold. For a tentative suggestion that concurrent administration of gold might enhance aspirin-induced hepatic dysfunction, see J. D. Davis *et al.*, *Clin. Pharmac. Ther.*, 1977, *21*, 52.

Methotrexate. A review of the drug interaction between methotrexate and salicylates.— P. K. Ng, *Can. pharm. J.*, 1979, *112*, 106.

Paracetamol. In a study involving a total of 21 subjects administration of paracetamol with aspirin was noted to increase blood concentrations of unhydrolysed aspirin.— V. F. Cotty *et al.*, *Toxic. appl. Pharmac.*, 1977, *41*, 7.

Spironolactone. For conflicting reports on the effects of concomitant administration of aspirin on the action of spironolactone, see Spironolactone, p.610.

Interactions, tests. Salicylates could interfere with chemical estimations for albumin in the blood and produce erroneous lowered results. Aspirin could interfere with qualitative urine estimations for bilirubin and ketones, and in large doses could lead to false positive results for reducing substances with copper reagent.— *Drug & Ther., Bull.*, 1972, *10*, 69.

In 8 healthy volunteers, clearances of creatinine, inulin, and aminohippuric acid were reduced by 30, 32, and 33% respectively after the intravenous infusion over 40 minutes of aspirin to produce an average blood concentration of 124 μg per ml. Aspirin was given as Aspegic (lysine acetylsalicylate 90% and glycine 10%) 1 g initially, then 1 mg per kg body-weight per minute.— M. Robert *et al.* (letter), *Br. med. J.*, 1972, *2*, 466. See also H. C. Burry and P. A. Dieppe, *Br. med. J.*, 1976, *2*, 16. See also under Effects on the Kidneys, p.237.

Large doses of salicylates might give falsely low results in tests for serum protein-bound iodine.— A. J. J. Wood and J. Crooks, *Prescribers' J.*, 1973, *13*, 94.

Aspirin might interfere with the measurement of serum-uric acid concentrations when the reagent used was phosphotungstic acid.— J. Millhouse, *Adverse Drug. React. Bull.*, 1974, Dec., 164.

For the effect of salicylates on some estimations of blood-theophylline concentrations, see Aminophylline, p.343.

Porphyria. Decreased plasma protein binding of salicylate was shown in patients with cutaneous hepatic porphyria.— W. H. Steele *et al.*, *Eur. J. clin. Pharmac.*, 1978, *13*, 309.

Pregnancy and the neonate. Neonates should not be given salicylates, sulphonamides, or other drugs that could displace bilirubin from serum albumin.— B. B. Brodie, *Proc. R. Soc. Med.*, 1965, *58*, 946.

Salicylates were excreted in breast milk and had caused macular rashes in breast-fed babies.— R. W. Smithells and D. M. Morgan, *Practitioner*, 1970, *204*, 14.

Aspirin appeared in breast milk in moderate amounts and could produce a bleeding tendency either by interfering with the function of the infant's platelets or by decreasing the amount of prothrombin in the blood. The risk was minimal if the mother took the aspirin just after nursing and if the infant had adequate store of vitamin K.— *Med. Lett.*, 1974, *16*, 25.

Aspirin increased the mean injection-abortion interval in nulliparous women undergoing mid-trimester abortion induced with hyperosmolar urea and oxytocin.— J. R. Niebyl *et al.*, *Am. J. Obstet. Gynec.*, 1976, *124*, 607.

For reports of adverse effects of indomethacin and other prostaglandin-synthetase inhibitors on the development of foetal pulmonary vasculature, see under Indomethacin, p.258.

For further reports on the adverse effects of aspirin in pregnancy and parturition, see under Adverse Effects.

Absorption and Fate. Absorption of non-ionised aspirin occurs in the stomach. Acetylsalicylates and salicylates are also readily absorbed from the intestine. Hydrolysis to salicylic acid occurs rapidly in the intestine and in the circulation. Salicylates are extensively bound to plasma proteins; aspirin to a lesser degree. Aspirin and salicylates are rapidly distributed to all body tissues; they appear in milk and cross the placenta. The rate of excretion of aspirin varies with the pH of the urine, increasing as the pH rises and being greatest at pH 7.5 and above. Aspirin is excreted as salicylic acid and as glucuronide conjugates and as salicyluric and gentisic acids.

Reviews of the bioavailability, metabolism, and pharmacokinetics of aspirin.— C. Davison, *Ann. N.Y. Acad. Sci.*, 1971, *179*, 249; M. Mayersohn *et al.*, *J. Am. pharm. Ass.*, 1977, *NS17*, 107; G. Levy, *Pediatrics*, 1978, *62*, *Suppl.*, 867; G. Levy, *Drug Metab. Rev.*, 1979, *9*, 3.

In a study in 104 Caucasian subjects (50 male, 54 female), aspirin-esterase activity in the serum was significantly higher in males than in females. As aspirin-esterase activity was considered to be responsible for about 20% of the metabolism of aspirin, this could explain the higher incidence of side-effects in women than in men.— R. Menguy *et al.* (letter), *Nature*, 1972, *239*, 102.

Saliva and blood concentrations of salicylic acid showed good correlation in 3 subjects given aspirin 650 mg. Significant amounts of salicylic acid appeared in the saliva 30 minutes after administration. Measurement of salivary concentrations of salicylic acid would be of value in the evaluation of aspirin preparations.— G. Graham and M. Rowland, *J. pharm. Sci.*, 1972, *61*, 1219. Retention of some aspirin in the mouth could cause abnormally high saliva concentrations.— W. L. Chiou *et al.* (letter), *J. clin. Pharmac.*, 1976, *16*, 158. A further referernce.— M. Pérez-Mateo *et al.*, *Int. J. clin. Pharmac. Biopharm.*, 1977, *15*, 113.

Absorption. In 6 subjects the administration of 15 ml of magnesium and aluminium hydroxide suspension with 85 ml of water 1 hour prior to and concurrent with the ingestion of enteric-coated aspirin, decreased the time to peak salicylate excretion by an average of 1.7 hours. Average urinary recovery was 90% in each case.— S. Feldman and B. C. Carlstedt (letter), *J. Am. med. Ass.*, 1974, *227*, 660. See also under Precautions.

The rate of absorption of aspirin was increased in 6 achlorhydric patients, reaching a peak plasma level after 1½ hours, compared with 3 hours in 6 controls.— A. Pottage *et al.* (letter), *J. Pharm. Pharmac.*, 1974, *26*, 144.

The rate of absorption of aspirin was reduced by the presence of food but after the first hour there was no difference in plasma salicylate concentrations between fasted and nonfasted subjects.— P. A. Koch *et al.*, *J. pharm. Sci.*, 1978, *67*, 1533.

Further studies of the effects of food on aspirin absorption.— J. H. Wood (letter), *Lancet*, 1967, *2*, 212; A. Melander *et al.*, *Acta med. scand.*, 1977, *202*, 119; C. Bogentoft *et al.*, *Eur. J. clin. Pharmac.*, 1978, *14*, 351.

For a report of reduced aspirin absorption during acute migraine attacks, see under Uses.

Metabolism and excretion. The excretion of salicylates in urine was affected by pH and by corticosteroids. Because both urinary pH and plsama-hydrocortisone concentrations fluctuated throughout the day, changes in the rate of excretion of salicylates were to be expected. Studies in 6 healthy persons by A. Reinberg and others (*Proc. Soc. exp. Biol. Med.*, 1967, *124*, 826) had shown that salicylate excretion followed a diurnal rhythm; the amount of salicylate excreted 4 hours following a dose was greater when the dose was given in the evening than when it was given in the morning. If salicylate excretion was under corticosteroid control, excretion should have been at its highest rate in the morning to coincide with the highest levels of plasma hydrocortisone; it could be assumed that excretion was not significantly dependent on plasma-hydrocortisone levels.— *Lancet*, 1967, *1*, 1265.

The excretion of aspirin could not be completely described by first-order kinetics, and above a dose of 320 mg, elimination was by simultaneous first-order and zero-order processes. The average peak plasma-salicylate concentration after a 1-g dose of aspirin was 51 μg per ml, but after 7 doses of 1 g, given 6-hourly, the average maximum value was 181 μg per ml. The biological half-life of aspirin was 2 to 3 hours after a single small dose, but appeared to be nearer 10 hours after multiple 1-g doses.— A. J. Cummings and B. K. Martin (letter), *J. pharm. Sci.*, 1968, *57*, 891.

An increase in the maintenance dose of salicylate resulted in a more than proportional rise in the plateau concentration of salicylate. This concentration was more slowly reached by repeated large daily doses than by smaller doses. Increases in dosage should be by small increments, allowing time for the new plateau concentration to be reached. The maximum response from the usual therapeutic regimen of salicylate for the treatment of inflammatory disease, 4 g or more daily, would not be expected to occur in less than 1 week.— G. Levy and T. Tsuchiya, *New Engl. J. Med.*, 1972, *287*, 430.

The metabolism and excretion of aspirin follows non-linear dose-dependent kinetics because of a limited capacity for the formation of various metabolites.— G. Levy *et al.*, *Clin. Pharmac. Ther.*, 1972, *13*, 258.

In 60 patients salicylates appeared in the blood 3 to 13 minutes after ingestion and in joint fluid within 11 to 36 minutes. Salicylate concentrations were lower in joint fluid than in blood, and deacetylation progressed more slowly.— A. Soren, *Archs intern. Med.*, 1973, *132*, 668, per *J. Am. med. Ass.*, 1973, *226*, 1027. A similar report.— S. D. Sholkoff *et al.*, *Arthritis Rheum.*, 1967, *10*, 348, per C. Davison, *Ann. N.Y. Acad. Sci.*, 1971, *179*, 249.

The kinetics of salicylate metabolism.— T. Gibson *et*

al., Br. J. clin. Pharmac., 1975, 2, 233; G. Graham et al., Aust. N.Z. J. Med., 1975, 5, 500; L. J. Aarons et al., J. Pharm. Pharmac., 1978, 30, Suppl., 8P.

The bioavailability of aspirin was greater when the dose was given at 6 am compared with 6 pm or 10 pm.— A. Markiewicz and K. Semenowicz, *Int. J. clin. Pharmac. Biopharm.*, 1979, *17*, 409.

Pregnancy and the neonate. Of 272 newborn infants 26 had salicylate concentrations in umbilical blood, at delivery, of 12 to 109 (mean 33) µg per ml. There were no obvious clinical differences between these infants and controls, but the reserve albumin-binding capacity of their sera was depressed.— P. A. Palmisano and G. Cassady, *J. Am. med. Ass.*, 1969, *209*, 556.

Salicylate protein binding in infants and neonates.— A. Windorfer *et al.*, *Eur. J. Pediat.*, 1978, *127*, 163.

For reports on the excretion of salicylates in breast milk, see under Precautions.

Protein binding. A brief review of plasma protein binding of aspirin and salicylate. Salicylate was about 72% bound to plasma proteins at a drug concentration of 50 µg per ml. Although salicylates were not highly protein bound they could have deleterious effects on the binding of other drugs and on endogenous substances.— J. J. Vallner, *J. pharm. Sci.*, 1977, *66*, 447.

Decreased plasma-protein binding of aspirin, salicylic acid, and phenylbutazone had been reported in patients with acute renal failure; this was not entirely due to decreased plasma concentrations of albumin, and these drugs did not bind significantly to other plasma proteins.— F. Andreasen, *Acta pharmac. tox.*, 1973, *32*, 417. See also F. Andreasen, *Acta pharmac. tox.*, 1974, *34*, 284.

Plasma-protein binding of salicylate, given by mouth as sodium acetylsalicylate, was reduced in patients with renal failure and chronic liver disease, and apparently slightly increased in patients with chronic respiratory insufficiency.— M. Pérez-Mateo and S. Erill, *Eur. J. clin. Pharmac.*, 1977, *11*, 225.

Plasma-protein binding was not reduced in patients with chronic alcoholism but was significantly reduced in patients with alcoholic hepatitis or cirrhosis.— S. Boobis and M. J. Brodie, *Br. J. clin. Pharmac.*, 1977, *4*, 629P. See also M. J. Brodie and S. Boobis, *Eur. J. clin. Pharmac.*, 1978, *13*, 435.

Uses. Aspirin has analgesic, anti-inflammatory, and antipyretic actions, and these actions are considered to be due to inhibition of the biosynthesis of prostaglandins. It is used for the relief of the less severe types of pain such as headache, neuritis, myalgias, and toothache; it is relatively ineffective in visceral pain. Aspirin is also used in the treatment of acute and chronic inflammatory disorders such as rheumatoid arthritis.

In the treatment of minor febrile conditions, such as colds or influenza, aspirin is of value for the reduction of temperature and relief of the headache and the joint and muscle pains, but has no effect on the causal infection.

Aspirin is usually taken by mouth. Gastric irritation may be reduced by taking doses after food. Effervescent soluble tablets or enteric-coated tablets may be used. In some instances aspirin may be administered rectally by suppository.

The usual dose of aspirin as an analgesic and antipyretic is 0.3 to 1 g, which may be repeated every 4 hours according to clinical needs, up to a maximum of 4 g daily.

Plasma-salicylate concentrations of 150 to 300 µg per ml are required for optimal anti-inflammatory activity but may produce tinnitus; more serious adverse effects occur at concentrations above 300 µg per ml. Doses need to be adjusted individually to achieve these concentrations. Generally doses of 4 to 8 g daily in divided doses are used for acute rheumatic disorders. Doses of up to 5.4 g daily in divided doses may be sufficient in chronic rheumatic disorders.

Indications for aspirin therapy in young children are very limited and special care is necessary in determining the dosage in children under 2 years of age. Aspirin is not recommended for infants under 1 year of age because of the danger of intoxication and metabolic disturbance. As an analgesic and antipyretic aspirin may be given to children in the following doses: 1 to under 2 years, 75 mg; 2 to under 4 years, 150 mg; 4 to under 6 years, 225 mg; 6 to under 9 years, 300 mg; 9 to under 11 years, 375 mg; 11 to under 12 years, 450 mg. Doses may be repeated at intervals of 4 hours. In rheumatic disorders, doses of 60 to 80 mg per kg body-weight daily are sometimes recommended, but daily doses of up to 125 mg per kg have been given initially in acute conditions.

Aspirin affects platelet function; by blocking synthesis of thromboxane A_2, platelet aggregation is inhibited. High doses may have the opposite effect since they can block the synthesis of prostacyclin which is an inhibitor of platelet aggregation.

Aspirin has been tried in the prevention of myocardial re-infarction but its value remains to be proved. It is also recommended for reducing the risk of some recurrent transient ischaemic attacks, and hence the risk of stroke, in men but not women in doses of 650 mg twice daily or 325 mg four times daily. Again, the value of this treatment is not easy to establish.

Discussions and reviews of the mode of action of aspirin.— H. O. J. Collier, *Nature*, 1969, *223*, 35; J. R. Vane, *Adv. Med. Topics Ther.*, 1975, *1*, 64; J. R. Vane, *J. Allergy & clin. Immunol.*, 1976, *58*, 691; J. Morley, *Proc. R. Soc. Med.*, 1977, *70*, *Suppl.* 7, 32.

Studies on the mode of action of aspirin.— D. Crook and A. J. Collins, *Ann. rheum. Dis.*, 1977, *36*, 459; A. H. Drummond *et al.*, *Br. J. Pharmac.*, 1977, *59*, 661; M. A. Bray and D. Gordon, *Br. J. Pharmac.*, 1978, *63*, 635.

Reviews and discussions of the uses of aspirin and other prostaglandin antagonists.— E. M. Cooperman, *Can. med. Ass. J.*, 1977, *117*, 309; G. R. Fryers, *Chemist Drugg.*, 1977, *208*, 626; T. L. C. Dale, *Chemist Drugg.*, 1977, *208*, 631; *Drug & Ther. Bull.*, 1978, *16*, 51.

For reference to blockade of the chlorpropamide-alcohol flush by aspirin, see Chlorpropamide, p.852.

Administration. There are substantial interindividual differences in the pharmacokinetics of salicylate even when dosage is based on body-weight or surface area. In the treatment of inflammatory disease therefore aspirin dosage should be adjusted on the basis of plasma-salicylate concentrations as well as clinical response.— G. Levy and K. M. Giacomini, *Clin. Pharmac. Ther.*, 1978, *23*, 247.

Further studies on dosage schedules and the achievement of therapeutic plasma-salicylate concentrations.— G. G. Graham *et al.*, *Clin. Pharmac. Ther.*, 1977, *22*, 410; R. L. Talbert *et al.*, *J. clin. Pharmac.*, 1979, *19*, 108.

In children. A suggested dosage schedule for aspirin as an analgesic and antipyretic in children was based on a dose of 10 to 15 mg per kg with a dosage interval of 4 hours.— A. K. Done *et al.*, *J. Pediat.*, 1979, *95*, 617.

For discussions on dosage of salicylates in children with juvenile rheumatoid arthritis, see under Rheumatic Disorders.

Administration in renal failure. Usual short-term analgesic doses can be given to patients with impaired renal function. Plasma-salicylate concentrations should be used as a guide to dosage when high-dosage or long-term therapy is required.— R. J. Anderson *et al.*, *Clinical Use of Drugs in Renal Failure*, Springfield, Thomas, 1976, p. 209.

Aspirin was reported to be 87% bound to plasma proteins. The normal half-life for doses up to 500 mg was 2 to 4.5 hours and was similar in patients with end-stage renal failure. The interval between doses should be extended from 4 hours to 4 to 6 hours in patients with a glomerular filtration-rate (GFR) of 10 to 50 ml per minute; it should be avoided in those with a GFR of less than 10 ml per minute. Concentrations of aspirin were affected by haemodialysis and peritoneal dialysis.— W. M. Bennett *et al.*, *Ann. intern. Med.*, 1980, *93*, 62.

Further references: O. Borgå *et al.*, *Clin. Pharmac. Ther.*, 1976, *20*, 464; E. Rumpel *et al.*, *Dte. Gesundh-Wes.*, 1976, *31*, 2369, per *Int. pharm. Abstr.*, 1977, *14*, 1254.

Administration, rectal. For a report on the rectal use of aspirin postoperatively in children, see under Fever (below).

Analgesia. Plasma concentrations of aspirin and salicyclic acid were serially determined among 20 to 30 subjects for 8 to 12 hours following administration of various dosages and dosage forms of aspirin. The results confirmed that the presence of unhydrolysed aspirin in plasma correlated with the duration of analgesic efficacy. Plasma-salicyclic acid concentrations were of little value in predicting the duration of analgesia but might be of value in predicing the duration of anti-inflammatory activity. Doubling the dose of aspirin doubled peak plasma concentrations but did not significantly prolong the serum concentrations of aspirin. The efficacy of sustained-release preparations of aspirin was dependent upon their formulation.— S. A. Bell *et al.*, *J. new Drugs*, 1966, *6*, 121.

In a double-blind trial involving 80 patients with postoperative or traumatic pain, aspirin 325 mg was no better than placebo for relief of pain but its analgesic effect was markedly increased by the addition of meprobamate 200 mg, although meprobamate had no analgesic effect when given alone.— T. G. Kantor *et al.*, *J. clin. Pharmac.*, 1973, *13*, 152.

In a double-blind study of the relief of mild to moderate pain due to cancer in 100 patients, combinations of aspirin 650 mg plus either codeine 65 mg, oxycodone 9.76 mg, or pentazocine hydrochloride 25 mg produced significantly greater pain relief than aspirin alone. Combinations of aspirin 650 mg plus either dextropropoxyphene napsylate 100 mg, ethoheptazine citrate 75 mg, promazine hydrochloride 25 mg, pentobarbitone sodium 32 mg, or caffeine 65 mg were no more effective than aspirin itself.— C. G. Moertel *et al.*, *J. Am. med. Ass.*, 1974, *229*, 55.

A comparison of the analgesic and antipyretic activity of aspirin and paracetamol in children.— F. H. Lovejoy, *Pediatrics*, 1978, *62*, *Suppl.*, 904.

In cancer. A discussion on the use of aspirin and other non-narcotic analgesics in the treatment of bone pain in advanced cancer.— R. G. Twycross, in *Topics in Therapeutics*, D.W. Vere (Ed.), London, Pitman Medical, 1978, p. 94.

Postoperative. For a study showing that the incidence of postoperative bleeding and swelling due to dental surgery was greater with aspirin than paracetamol, see Paracetamol, p.270.

Postpartum. In a randomised double-blind study of postpartum pain models it was noted that whereas episiotomy pain appeared to be responsive to aspirin and codeine postpartum pain was insensitive to codeine but responsive to aspirin.— S. S. Bloomfield *et al.*, *Clin. Pharmac. Ther.*, 1976, *20*, 499.

Asthma. Aspirin 65 mg was often very effective in preventing the nocturnal wheeze of asthmatics.— C. A. Clarke (letter), *Br. med. J.*, 1969, *1*, 256. Aspirin might have anti-allergic properties, and its use with antihistamines might be prophylactic for some patients with extrinsic asthma.— R. J. Taylor (letter), *ibid.*, 576.

In a 53-year-old asthmatic patient, improvement of forced expiratory volume was marked following test doses of aspirin, mefenamic acid, and ibuprofen, less so with indomethacin, sodium salicylate, and tartrazine. Phenylbutazone produced a deterioration in respiration.— D. Kordansky *et al.*, *Ann. intern. Med.*, 1978, *88*, 508. Another report of a patient whose attacks of bronchial asthma were relieved by aspirin. It was suggested that in these patients, prostaglandins precipitated bronchial obstruction.— A. Szczeklik *et al.*, *Ann. intern. Med.*, 1979, *90*, 126.

Exercise-induced asthma. Aspirin in doses of 1 or 2 g did not prevent the fall in peak expiratory flow-rate after exercise in 5 asthmatic patients. Aspirin as a prostaglandin-synthetase inhibitor was not considered to be of any value in suppressing exercise-induced asthma.— M. Rudolf *et al.* (letter), *Lancet*, 1975, *1*, 450. Similar reports.— A. M. Taveira da Silva and P. Hamosh, *Prostaglandins*, 1976, *11*, 71; E. N. Schachter *et al.* (letter), *Ann. intern. Med.*, 1978, *89*, 287.

For aspirin-induced bronchospasm and other adverse effects, see p.236.

Bartter's syndrome. Aspirin 100 mg per kg body-weight daily given to inhibit prostaglandin synthesis alleviated the symptoms of Bartter's syndrome in a 22-month-old child. Prostaglandins were implicated in the pathogenesis of this syndrome.— L. Norby *et al.*, *Lancet*, 1976, *2*, 604.

Diabetes. Aspirin stimulates insulin and glucagon secretion and increases glucose tolerance in normal and diabetic subjects. Further studies in maturity onset diabetes might be warranted.— P. Micossi *et al.*, *Diabetes*, 1978, *27*, 1196.

A report of the successful treatment of necrobiosis lipoidica diabeticorum with dipyridamole 225 mg and aspirin 1 g daily.— A. Eldor *et al.* (letter), *New Engl. J. Med.*, 1978, *298*, 1033. Necrobiotic skin lesions healed completely within 1 to 3 months in 2 of 3 diabetic patients given aspirin 1.5 to 4.5 g daily. Treatment was unsuccessful in the third patient even when dipyridamole 225 mg daily was given in addition for one month.— B. Fjellner (letter), *ibid.*, *299*, 1366. A report of the successful treatment of necrobiotic lesions with dipyridamole 225 mg daily. From work in *animals*, the proliferation of blood vessels was considered to be induced by dipyridamole and it was thought that this contributed to the healing effect as well as its anti-aggregating effect on platelets.— G. Unge and G. Tornling (letter), *ibid.* Findings from a double-blind comparison in 12 patients that aspirin with dipyridamole is of no benefit in the treatment of necrobiosis lipoidica when compared with placebo.— B. N. Statham *et al.* (letter), *ibid.*, 1980, *303*, 1419.

Diabetic retinopathy. A short discussion on the possibility that aspirin might be of value in the prevention of diabetic retinopathy.— *J. Am. med. Ass.*, 1974, *228*, 1274. See also *J. Am. med. Ass.*, 1978, *239*, 2222.

Diarrhoea. See under Gastro-intestinal Disorders, p.241.

Ductus arteriosus closure. See under Pregnancy and the Neonate, p.242.

Dysmenorrhoea. Discussions on the possible role of prostaglandins in dysmenorrhoea and the use of aspirin and other prostaglandin synthetase inhibitors in its treatment.— C. M. Proudfit, *J. Am. med. Ass.*, 1978, *239*, 1909; *Lancet*, 1980, *1*, 800. See also D. W. T. Roberts, *Br. J. Hosp. Med.*, 1978, *20*, 716.

In a double-blind crossover study in 30 patients with stable dysmenorrhoea aspirin 500 mg or paracetamol 500 mg four times daily for 3 days was no more effective than placebo in the relief of pain; neither active drug increased blood loss.— T. Janbu *et al.*, *Eur. J. clin. Pharmac.*, 1978, *14*, 413.

Effects on blood. Studies in 4 healthy subjects indicated that aspirin or sodium salicylate in doses of 1.8 g had fibrinolytic activity on whole blood. *In vitro* studies suggested that this action of salicylates might be associated with polymorphonuclear leucocytes and distinct from the effect on blood platelets.— L. A. Moroz, *New Engl. J. Med.*, 1977, *296*, 525. Comment.— O. D. Ratnoff, *ibid.*, 566. Criticism.— V. Gurewich and B. Lipinski (letter), *ibid.*, 1299. Reply.— L. A. Moroz (letter), *ibid.*, 1300.

A controlled study involving 102 men did not confirm that aspirin increased plasma-fibrinogen concentrations.— T. W. Meade *et al.* (letter), *Lancet*, 1977, *2*, 1289.

Studies on the effects of aspirin and related analgesics on polymorphonuclear leucocytes.— T. W. Austin and G. Truant, *Can. med. Ass. J.*, 1978, *118*, 493; K. A. Brown and A. J. Collins, *Br. J. Pharmac.*, 1978, *64*, 347.

See also under Myocardial Infarction and Thrombo-embolic Disorders.

Platelet aggregation. Reviews and discussions on the actions and uses of drugs affecting platelet function, including aspirin.— *Br. med. J.*, 1974, *3*, 5; J. C. Delaney (letter), *ibid.*, 412; M. Hamberg *et al.* (letter), *Lancet*, 1974, *2*, 223; P. A. Castaldi, *Drugs*, 1975, *9*, 1; J. F. Mustard and M. A. Packham, *ibid.*, 19; M. Verstraete, *Am. J. Med.*, 1976, *61*, 897; H. J. Weiss, *New Engl. J. Med.*, 1978, *298*, 1344 and 1403; M. Verstraete, *Drugs*, 1978, *15*, 464; J. A. Blakely, *Can. J. Hosp. Pharm.*, 1978, *31*, 11; A. S. Gallus, *Drugs*, 1979, *18*, 439.

In vitro studies on inhibition of platelet aggregation indicated that *indomethacin* had the most powerful action of the compounds studied. The action of *amidopyrine* was equivalent to that of *aspirin* and it was the most potent of the pyrazoline derivatives studied. The activities of *pyrazinobutazone* and its methyl derivative were markedly weaker, and equivalent to those of *phenylbutazone* and *sulphinpyrazone; oxyphenbutazone* and *mofebutazone* were even less active.— J. A. De Muylder and D. Letist, *Acta ther.*, 1977, *3*, 195.

A study in 6 healthy subjects confirmed findings in *animals* that whereas low doses of aspirin prolong bleeding time, high doses do not.— J. O'Grady and S. Moncada (letter), *Lancet*, 1978, *2*, 780. Aspirin in doses up to 1 g prolonged the bleeding time in healthy subjects. The bleeding time returned toward normal at higher doses. It was suggested that if platelet aggregation was dependent on the balance between thromboxane A_2, which promotes aggregation, and prostacyclin, which tends to oppose aggregation, then low doses seem to selectively inhibit thromboxane A_2 while higher doses also inhibit prostacyclin.— S. M. Rajah *et al.* (letter), *ibid.*, 1104. These findings were not confirmed in a crossover study in 21 healthy male subjects when the bleeding time rose strikingly after both low and the high doses of aspirin.— H. C. Godal *et al.* (letter), *ibid.*, 1979, *1*, 1236. Further studies which showed no difference between high and low doses of aspirin.— D. Treacher *et al.* (letter), *ibid.*, 1978, *2*, 1378; A. Girolami *et al.* (letter), *ibid.*, 1979, *2*, 205; F. I. Pareti *et al.* (letter), *ibid.*, 1980, *1*, 371. It seems certain that there will be considerable between-person differences in response to aspirin. The response of each patient may have to be ascertained before treatment.— J. R. O'Brien (letter), *ibid.*, 372.

Further references: R. M. Rowan *et al.*, *Postgrad. med. J.*, 1976, *52*, 71; L. A. Champion *et al.*, *J. Pediat.*, 1976, *89*, 653; T. F. Rohrer *et al.*, *Arzneimittel-Forsch.*, 1977, *27*, 1490; G. R. Buchanan *et al.*, *Am. J. clin. Path.*, 1977, *68*, 355; H. A. Pearson, *Pediatrics*, 1978, *62*, *Suppl.*, 926; A. B. Bikhazi and G. E. Ayyub, *J. pharm. Sci.*, 1978, *67*, 939; M. B. Zucker and K. G. Rothwell, *Curr. ther. Res.*, 1978, *23*, 194; M. Livio *et al.* (letter), *Lancet*, 1978, *1*, 1307; K. A. Jorgensen *et al.* (letter), *Lancet*, 1979, *2*, 302; G. Masotti *et al.*, *Lancet*, 1979, *2*, 1213; E. M. G. Hoogendijk and J. W. ten Cate (letter), *ibid.*, 1980, *1*, 93; P. C. Huijgens *et al.* (letter), *ibid.*, 94; *J. Am. med. Ass.*, 1980, *244*, 1621.

See also under Myocardial Infarction and Thrombo-embolic Disorders.

Polycythaemia. Aspirin 1.2 g daily was successfully used in the treatment of disseminated intravascular coagulation in a 70-year-old woman with polycythaemia vera.— J. M. Levin and T. L. Ostrowski, *J. Am. med. Ass.*, 1974, *229*, 186.

A 44-year-old man with polycythaemia vera and angina due to coronary artery disease was given aspirin 1 g daily. He became free of anginal pain, and haemoglobin levels had not exceeded 16.5 g per 100 ml for 2½ years thus removing the need for phlebotomy.— N. S. Gilbert (letter), *J. Am. med. Ass.*, 1974, *230*, 539.

Relief of ischaemia and other symptoms was obtained by 3 of 5 patients with essential thrombocythaemia after treatment with aspirin 325 mg and dipyridamole 50 mg both 4 times a day. Amaurosis fugax in 1 patient with polycythaemia vera disappeared after the same regimen.— K. K. -Y. Wu, *Ann. intern. Med.*, 1978, *88*, 7.

A report of a patient with polycythaemia vera who developed spontaneous intramuscular haematoma following administration of aspirin.— C. Y. Thomas (letter), *Ann. intern. Med.*, 1978, *88*, 845.

Purpura. Reports of 17 patients with thrombotic thrombocytopenic purpura treated with aspirin usually after corticosteroid treatment and sometimes splenectomy. It appeared that aspirin alone was often unsuccessful and dipyridamole and, in 2 cases, sulphinpyrazone were necessary to effect a rise in platelets.— *Ann. intern. Med.*, 1977, *86*, 102.

Effective treatment of thrombotic thrombocytopenic purpura with aspirin and dipyridamole together with plasmaphaeresis.— T. J. Myers *et al.*, *Ann. intern. Med.*, 1980, *92*, 149.

Further references: J. Amir and S. Krauss, *Blood*, 1973, *42*, 27; E. C. Rossi *et al.*, *J. Am. med. Ass.*, 1974, *228*, 1141.

Effects on the eye. Recurring temporary loss of vision in one eye (amaurosis fugax) was relieved in 2 patients when given aspirin 600 mg daily.— M. J. G. Harrison *et al.*, *Lancet*, 1971, *2*, 743. Further reports: J. Mundall *et al.* (letter), *Lancet*, 1972, *1*, 92; J. Mundall *et al.*, *Neurology, Minneap.*, 1972, *22*, 280.

Aspirin might delay the development of senile cataracts.— *J. Am. med. Ass.*, 1980, *244*, 2593. See also E. Cotlier and Y. R. Sharma (letter), *Lancet*, 1981, *1*, 338.

See also Diabetic Retinopathy under Diabetes and Polycythaemia under Effects on Blood.

Effects on immune response. For a report of the effect of aspirin and sodium salicylate in suppressing lymphocyte transformation and a discussion of the effect on the immune response, see G. Opelz *et al.*, *Lancet*, 1973, *2*, 478. See also C. Loveday and V. Eisen (letter), *ibid.*, 676; L. M. Pachman *et al.* (letter), *ibid.*, 1212; J. J. Twomey *et al.* (letter), *ibid.*, 1974, *1*, 684; J. E. Crout *et al.*, *New Engl. J. Med.*, 1975, *292*, 221; D. E. Snider and C. W. Parker, *J. clin. Invest.*, 1976, *58*, 524.

Administration of sodium salicylate to *rats* promoted survival of heart allografts for longer than either azathioprine or azathioprine with methylprednisolone.— S. W. Jamieson *et al.*, *Lancet*, 1979, *1*, 130.

Effects on neoplasms. Comment on the experimental findings on the role of anti-inflammatory agents in the development and behaviour of experimental tumours.— *Lancet*, 1979, *1*, 420.

Fever. A study of the antipyretic efficacy of aspirin and paracetamol in children.— R. W. Steele *et al.*, *Am. J. Dis. Child.*, 1972, *123*, 204.

In a study in 19 children who had undergone open-heart surgery aspirin 20 to 25 mg per kg body-weight was suggested as an effective rectal dose in postoperative pyrexia.— K. Connolly *et al.*, *Archs Dis. Childh.*, 1979, *54*, 713.

Food intolerance. The prostaglandin-synthetase inhibitors aspirin, ibuprofen, or indomethacin prevented reactions due to food intolerance in 6 patients.— P. D. Buisseret *et al.*, *Lancet*, 1978, *1*, 906.

On over 20 occasions the symptoms of lactose intolerance were prevented in a lactose-intolerant individual by ingestion of aspirin 975 mg, twenty minutes before eating a dairy meal.— J. Lieb (letter), *Lancet*, 1978, *2*, 157. A similar report.— J. Lieb (letter), *J. Am. med. Ass.*, 1980, *243*, 32.

Gastro-intestinal disorders. Soluble aspirin 900 mg was given 4 times daily to 15 women with diarrhoea induced by radiation for cervical cancer. The diarrhoea was abolished in 4 and improved in 8 although in 2 it relapsed despite continued aspirin treatment. Colicky pain was relieved in 3 and nausea in 1 patient.— A. T. Mennie and V. Dalley (letter), *Lancet*, 1973, *1*, 1131.

Aspirin in the buffered form in a dose of 972 mg four times daily was significantly more effective than placebo in alleviating the diarrhoea and other gastro-intestinal side-effects of radiation in a double-blind controlled study of 28 patients.— A. T. Mennie *et al.*, *Lancet*, 1975, *2*, 942. See also *ibid.*, 961. Aspirin should generally be given only after pelvic irradiation had stopped.— R. E. Pounder (letter), *ibid.*, 1044.

Diarrhoea associated with high plasma-prostaglandin concentrations was controlled by soluble aspirin 150 mg four times daily. Indomethacin 12.5 mg four times daily was also effective. When treatment was stopped the diarrhoea returned. Because prolonged treatment with either agent was undesirable treatment was changed to loperamide.— J. A. Dodge *et al.*, *Archs Dis. Childh.*, 1977, *52*, 800.

In a double-blind placebo-controlled study administration of soluble aspirin 25 mg per kg body-weight daily (in 4 divided doses) in addition to standard rehydration therapy, reduced faecal fluid losses and enhanced weight-gain in 31 malnourished infants and children treated in hospital for acute diarrhoea and dehydration, compared with 31 similar infants and children given placebo in addition to standard therapy, and also 20 who received standard therapy without the addition of aspirin or placebo. No side-effects were noted in association with aspirin administration, in particular metabolic acidosis was not a problem and there was no gastro-intestinal bleeding. Aspirin may be useful in reducing fluid loss in childhood diarrhoea, but before it can be widely advocated its side-effects need to be carefully assessed.— V. Burke *et al.*, *Lancet*, 1980, *1*, 1329. Criticism.— D. R. Nalin (letter), *ibid.*, *2*, 793. Reply.— M. Gracey and V. Burke (letter), *ibid.*, 794.

Gout. Aspirin was a potent uricosuric agent when given in a dose of 4 g or more daily, but in smaller doses its effect was anti-uricosuric. Aspirin blocked the uricosuric effect of other drugs.— R. M. Mason, *Prescribers' J.*, 1968, *7*, 125.

Hyperlipidaemia. Because there might be a risk of platelet aggregation in patients with homozygous hypercholesterolaemia undergoing surgery the following regimen was recommended: 500 ml of dextran 70 given intravenously during the operation and daily for 4 or 5 days thereafter. Aspirin 1 g daily and dipyridamole 50 mg thrice daily should then be given until the plasma-cholesterol concentration stopped falling. Children should receive reduced doses and care should be taken with patients in heart failure.— O. Faergeman *et al.* (letter), *Lancet*, 1976, *2*, 1416.

Insect stings. A view that the topical application of soluble aspirin may provide effective treatment for local reactions to stings from wasps and other insects.— R. J. von Witt (letter), *Lancet*, 1980, *2*, 1379.

Kawasaki disease. Aspirin might be useful in preventing sudden death (due to coronary thrombotic occlusion) in patients with Kawasaki disease.— H. Kato *et al.*, *Pediatrics*, 1979, *63*, 175. See also O. H. P. Teixeira *et al.*, *Can. med. Ass. J.*, 1980, *122*, 1013.

Lepra reactions. Aspirin was useful in the management of certain symptoms of lepra reactions because of its antipyretic and analgesic activity.— C. G. S. Iyer *et al.*, *Bull. Wld Hlth Org.*, 1971, *45*, 719.

Lupus erythematosus. Salicylates in doses ranging from 3.6 to 7.2 g per day had probably been under-valued in the treatment of systemic lupus erythematosus when pains and rheumatoid deformities of joints were present.— N. R. Rowell, *Br. med. J.*, 1969, *2*, 427. See also N. F. Rothfield, *Mayo Clin. Proc.*, 1969, *44*, 691.

For reports of hepatotoxicity associated with aspirin in patients with systemic lupus erythematosus, see under Adverse Effects.

Migraine. The use of analgesics in the treatment of migraine.— G. N. Volans, *Adv. Med. Topics Ther.*, 1976, *2*, 156.

A review of migraine and drug absorption. The rate of absorption of aspirin was reduced during migraine compared with the rate in the same patients when headache-free. This was possibly due to gastro-intestinal stasis and a reduced rate of gastric emptying during migraine attacks. Metoclopramide, which reduces gastric emptying time, has been shown to increase the rate of absorption of aspirin during migraine and also to increase the rate of recovery from the attack.— G. N. Volans, *Clin. Pharmacokinet.*, 1978, *3*, 313. See also G. Wainscott *et al.*, *Br. J. clin. Pharmac.*, 1976, *3*, 1015.

Prophylaxis. A controlled study of 57 patients indicated that continuous therapy with prostaglandin-inhibiting analgesics might prevent headache.— A. Bennett *et al.* (letter), *Lancet*, 1978, *1*, 104.

In a double-blind crossover study in 12 migraine sufferers, aspirin prophylaxis with a dose of 650 mg twice daily for 3 months was compared with placebo. Nine of the patients experienced a greater than 50% reduction in headache frequency during the 3 months that they were receiving aspirin.— B. P. O'Neill and J. D. Mann, *Lancet*, 1978, *2*, 1179. See also.— D. J. Dalessio, *J. Am. med. Ass.*, 1978, *239*, 52.

Myocardial infarction. Discussions and reviews on the use of aspirin and other drugs affecting platelet function for the prevention of myocardial infarction.— *Med. Lett.*, 1975, *17*, 25; C. R. Klimt *et al.*, *Thromb. Haemostasis*, 1976, *35*, 49; H. Jick and P. C. Elwood, *Am. Heart J.*, 1976, *91*, 126; J. L. Marx, *Science*, 1977, *196*, 1075; D. A. Chamberlain, *Adv. Med. Topics Ther.*, 1977, *3*, 25; M. Verstraete, *Drugs*, 1978, *15*, 464; J. C. Krantz, *Am. Pharm.*, 1979, *NS19* (Jan.), 14; J. Mehta and P. Mehta, *J. Am. med. Ass.*, 1979, *241*, 2649; *Med. Lett.*, 1980, *22*, 25; J. R. A. Mitchell, *Br. med. J.*, 1980, *280*, 1128; R. J. Jones, *J. Am. med. Ass.*, 1980, *244*, 667; *Lancet*, 1980, *1*, 1172; G. P. McNicol, *ibid.*, *2*, 736.

In a double-blind prospective study in 1529 men a non-significant reducution in mortality was observed in aspirin-treated patients.— Coronary Drug Project Research Group, *J. chron. Dis.*, 1976, *29*, 625.

The incidence of aspirin consumption in 325 patients discharged from hospital with a diagnosis of having suffered acute myocardial infarction was 0.9%, compared with 4.9% in 3807 controls. In a further study the incidence of aspirin consumption in 451 patients with a diagnosis of infarction was 3.5% compared with 7% in 10 091 controls.— Boston Collaborative Drug Surveillance Group, *Br. med. J.*, 1974, *1*, 440. Similar results in a further 333 patients.— H. Jick and O. S. Miettinen, *Br. med. J.*, 1976, *1*, 1057.

In a placebo-controlled double-blind study involving 1682 patients who had had a confirmed myocardial infarction, aspirin 300 mg thrice daily for 1 year reduced total mortality by 17.3% but the result was not considered statistically significant. Admission to the trial occurred within 3 days of the infarction in 25% of patients and within 7 days in 50%. The results, although inconclusive, suggested that women received a smaller benefit from the treatment than men, and that the difference between treatments emerges early and about 3 months after infarction little further difference developed.— P. C. Elwood and P. M. Sweetnam, *Lancet*, 1979, *2*, 1313. See also P. C. Elwood *et al.*, *Br. med. J.*, 1974, *1*, 436; P. C. Elwood (letter), *ibid.*, 1981, *282*, 481.

A multicentre double-blind study, known as the Aspirin Myocardial Infarction Study (AMIS), was carried out in 4524 patients aged between 30 and 69 who had experienced myocardial infarction 8 weeks to 5 years previously. Patients were randomly assigned to receive either placebo or aspirin 500 mg twice daily and were followed for a minimum of 3 years for cardiovascular events. Total mortality for the entire follow-up period was 10.8% in the aspirin group and 9.7% in the placebo group while total mortality for the 3-year follow-up period was 9.6% and 8.8% respectively. The incidence of definite nonfatal myocardial infarction was 6.3% in the aspirin group and 8.1% in the placebo group while the incidence of coronary events (coronary death or definite nonfatal myocardial infarction) was 14.1% and 14.8% respectively. Gastro-intestinal side-effects occurred more frequently in the aspirin group. On the basis of these results, aspirin was not recommended for routine use in patients who have survived myocardial infarction.— Aspirin Myocardial Infarction Study Research Group, *J. Am. med. Ass.*, 1980, *243*, 661.

The Persantine-Aspirin Reinfarction Study (PARIS) involved 2026 patients who had suffered a myocardial infarction within 8 weeks to 60 months; 810 were given dipyridamole 75 mg and aspirin 324 mg thrice daily and 810 were given aspirin 324 mg and placebo thrice daily and 406 were given 2 placebo tablets thrice daily. The average follow-up period was 41 months. There was no significant difference in primary end points of death from all causes, coronary death, and coronary incidence between the 3 groups. However, it was suggested that patients who received either active treatment within six months of infarction might benefit in terms of reduced total and coronary mortality.— Persantine-Aspirin Reinfarction Study Research Group, *Circulation*, 1980, *62*, 449.

Most studies on the use of aspirin following myocardial infarction did not take into account the differential effects of aspirin on different prostaglandins and doses used appeared to be too high to maximise platelet aggregation while minimising prostacyclin inhibition.— F. Prior (letter), *Pharm. J.*, 1980, *1*, 336. Comment on the cardiovascular effects of aspirin; standard doses may not be the best way to achieve an optimal effect. By administering single small doses of aspirin every few days it should be possible to interrupt platelet thromboxane A_2 formation while leaving the prostacyclin-generating capacity of the vessel wall intact.— T. L. Wenger and J. H. Hull, *Wellcome, USA* (letter), *New Engl. J. Med.*, 1980, *303*, 1121. See also L. Wood (letter), *J. Am. med. Ass.*, 1980, *244*, 2414. The AMIS investigators thought that the conclusions in the report were warranted. There seems little reason to believe that a smaller dosage of aspirin would have led to a different result.— J. A. Schoenberger (letter), *ibid.* Aspirin 300 mg and 81 mg inhibited prostacyclin synthesis; 40 mg did not. Doses of 300 mg or 40 mg inhibited platelet thromboxane synthesis.— S. P. Hanley *et al.*, *Lancet*, 1981, *1*, 969.

The International Society and Federation of Cardiology Scientific Councils on Arteriosclerosis, Epidemiology and Prevention, and Rehabilitation accepted the value of dynamic exercise and cessation of smoking in survivors of myocardial infarction; while the value of anti-hyperlipidaemic agents had not been shown, dietary measures to reduce plasma-cholesterol concentrations were recommended; several studies had suggested the value of beta-adrenergic blocking agents; no clear recommendation could be given on the use of platelet-active drugs; it was not unreasonable to give long-term anticoagulant treatment.— *Br. med. J.*, 1981, *282*, 894.

Further studies that provide no evidence that aspirin had a beneficial effect in the prevention of coronary disease or myocardial infarction.— H. A. Isomäki (letter), *Lancet*, 1972, *2*, 831; E. C. Hammond and L. Garfinkel, *Br. med. J.*, 1975, *2*, 269; R. R. Monson and A. P. Hall, *J. chron. Dis.*, 1976, *29*, 459; C. H. Hennekens *et al.*, *Circulation*, 1978, *58*, 35; A. Linos *et al.*, *Mayo Clin. Proc.*, 1978, *53*, 581; E. Walter and C. Staiger (letter), *Lancet*, 1980, *1*, 1131.

See also under Effects on Blood and Thrombo-embolic Disorders.

Osteitis deformans. Clinical improvement in patients with Paget's disease (osteitis deformans) following treatment with aspirin.— P. Galmiche and P. Levy, *Revue Rhum. Mal. ostéo-artic.*, 1967, *34*, 185, per *Abstr. Wld Med.*, 1968, *42*, 231. See also P. F. Maurice *et al.*, *Trans. Ass. Am. Physns.*, 1962, *75*, 208.

Pregnancy and the neonate. Aspirin reduced the excretion of oestriol in 14 pregnant subjects.— J. M. Castellanos *et al.* (letter), *Lancet*, 1975, *1*, 859.

Evidence that ingestion of aspirin during pregnancy might reduce the incidence of pre-eclampsia.— A. J. Crandon and D. M. Isherwood (letter), *Lancet*, 1979, *1*, 1356. The question of the safety of aspirin during pregnancy is more important.— P. C. Buchan and H. N. Macdonald (letter), *ibid.*, *2*, 147.

For reports of increased mortality, in both mother and infant, associated with aspirin ingestion during pregnancy, see under Adverse Effects and Precautions.

Ductus arteriosus closure. Following administration of aspirin 20 mg per kg body-weight every 6 hours for 4 doses to 3 infants, constriction of ductus arteriosus was obtained in 1 and partial constriction in the second; no response was obtained in the third. No side-effects were noted. The variable response to aspirin might have been due to inadequate serum-salicylate concentrations but more dramatic results obtained in other infants with indomethacin could be due to different tissue affinity.— M. A. Heymann *et al.*, *New Engl. J. Med.*, 1976, *295*, 530.

A brief discussion of the use of aspirin and other prostaglandin inhibitors in the treatment of patent ductus arteriosus in infants.— D. R. Lines, *Drugs*, 1977, *13*, 1.

For further reports on the use of prostaglandin-synthetase inhibitors in ductus arteriosus closure in infants, see Indomethacin, p.260.

Rheumatic disorders. The pharmacology of anti-rheumatic drugs and treatment of rheumatic and arthritic disorders.— *Drug Treatment of the Rheumatic Diseases*, F.D. Hart (Ed.), Lancaster, MTP Press, 1978.

Juvenile polyarthritis. The management of children with juvenile chronic polyarthritis, including those with Still's disease and those with rheumatoid arthritis, includes bed rest, suitable exercise, splinting, and surgery as well as drug therapy. Aspirin is the drug of choice and therapy should attempt to achieve salicylate concentrations of 250 to 300 µg per ml. Other non-steroidal anti-inflammatory agents in appropriate doses may be required and gold salts and low-dose penicillamine may be beneficial. Immunosuppressive drugs may be required in secondary amyloidosis and for severely progressive crippling disease. Long-term use of corticosteroids is unjustifiable but alternate-day therapy, intermittent corticotrophin, and intra-articular corticosteroids are sometimes indicated.— E. G. L. Bywaters, *Bull. rheum. Dis.*, 1976, *27*, 882.

In a 15-day study in 19 children with juvenile rheumatoid arthritis who were given aspirin in doses of approximately 100 mg per kg body-weight daily, salicylate intoxication occurred in 7 patients 5 of whom were aged between 11 and 15 years. A dose of 100 mg per kg was considered to be too high for older children weighing more than 40 kg and it was suggested that the daily dose of aspirin should not exceed 3 g per m^2 of body-surface.— A. -L. Mäkelä *et al.*, *Scand. J. Rheumatol.*, 1975, *4*, 250.

Studies in 42 children receiving long-term salicylate therapy for rheumatoid arthritis showed that a given dose produced wide differences in plasma concentration between subjects and in the same subject at different times. In 11 children aspirin 78 to 83.7 mg per kg body-weight daily gave plasma salicylate concentrations of 60 to 240 µg per ml, and in 14 children sodium salicylate 99 to 106 mg per kg produced concentrations of 156 to 306 µg per ml. Concurrent administration of corticosteroids or corticotrophin was shown to lower the plasma salicylate concentration. It was concluded that the optimal dosage of salicylates should be based on the plasma salicylate concentration as well as the clinical response.— M. Bardare *et al.*, *Archs Dis. Childh.*, 1978, *53*, 381.

Further references: J. J. Calabro and J. M. Marchesano, *New Engl. J. Med.*, 1967, *277*, 746; R. A. Doughty *et al.*, *Clin. Pharmac. Ther.*, 1979, *25*, 221.

Rheumatic fever. Aspirin in doses of 100 mg per kg body-weight daily is effective in controlling the fever and joint symptoms of rheumatic fever in patients with no or minimal carditis. In patients with severe carditis or established mitral valve disease, corticosteroids are preferred. Aspirin should be continued in full dosage for 4 to 6 weeks then gradually reduced.— *Drug Treatment of the Rheumatic Diseases*, F.D. Hart (Ed.), Lancaster, MTP Press, 1978, p. 167.

Further references: *Br. med. J.*, 1955, *1*, 555; *Br. med. J.*, 1960, *2*, 1033; Combined Rheumatic Fever Study Group, *New Engl. J. Med.*, 1960, *262*, 895; E. G. L. Bywaters and G. T. Thomas, *Br. med. J.*, 1962, *2*, 221; *New Engl. J. Med.*, 1965, *272*, 63; *Br. med. J.*, 1965, *2*, 607.

Rheumatoid arthritis. For comparative studies on the effectiveness of aspirin and other non-steroidal anti-inflammatory agents in rheumatoid arthritis, see I. Haslock *et al.*, *Br. J. clin. Pract.*, 1975, *29*, 311; R. S. Amos *et al.*, *Br. med. J.*, 1978, *1*, 1396; M. S. Roberts *et al.* (letter), *Med. J. Aust.*, 1979, *1*, 92; W. J. Blechman and B. L. Lechner, *Rheumatol. Rehabil.*, 1979, *18*, 119.

See also above under Juvenile Polyarthritis.

Thrombo-embolic disorders. Reviews and discussions of the use of aspirin and other drugs affecting platelet function in thrombo-embolic disorders.— L. Wood, *Lancet*, 1972, *2*, 532; E. Kopasz, *Therapia hung.*, 1976, *24*, 72; A. S. Gallus and J. Hirsh, *Drugs*, 1976, *12*, 132; M. Pfenninger and U. F. Gruber, *Schweiz. med. Wschr.*, 1977, *107*, 1335; D. Loew, *Proc. R. Soc. Med.*, 1977, *70*, *Suppl.* 7, 28; A. J. Marcus, *New Engl. J. Med.*, 1977, *297*, 1284; H. J. Weiss, *ibid.*, 1978, *298*, 1403; A. G. G. Turpie and J. Hirsh, *Br. med. Bull.*, 1978, *34*, 183; E. C. Tsu, *Am. J. Hosp. Pharm.*, 1978, *35*, 1507; J. A. Blakely, *Can. J. Hosp. Pharm.*, 1978, *31*, 11.

Aspirin with dipyridamole was effective in treating one patient with thrombotic microangiopathy.— M. Giromini *et al.*, *Br. med. J.*, 1972, *2*, 545. Aspirin was effective in the treatment of a patient with microangiopathic haemolytic anaemia and renal failure.— P. C. Raich and M. J. Bozdech, *Am. J. med. Sci.*, 1977, *273*, 227, per *Int. pharm. Abstr.*, 1977, *14*, 1190.

Aspirin combined with anticoagulants offered better protection against arterial thrombo-embolism in patients with aortic ball-valve prostheses than did anticoagulant therapy alone.— J. Dale *et al.*, *Am. Heart J.*, 1977, *94*, 101.

Aspirin 160 mg daily for about 4½ months reduced the incidence of thrombosis in a double-blind study of 44 patients with arteriovenous shunts who were on chronic haemodialysis. Six of 19 patients (32%) taking aspirin had one or more thrombi compared with 18 of 25 (72%) who received placebo. There was no obvious difference between the efficacy of aspirin in men and women.— H. R. Harter *et al.*, *New Engl. J. Med.*, 1979, *301*, 577 and 1404.

Results of a controlled study in 50 patients who had undergone coronary-artery bypass surgery indicated that anticoagulant treatment with warfarin or antiplatelet treatment with aspirin and dipyridamole, starting on the third postoperative day and continuing for 6 months, failed to improve the patency of the grafts.— G. A. Pantely *et al.*, *New Engl. J. Med.*, 1979, *301*, 962. Criticisms.— I. D. Goldberg and M. B. Stemerman (letter), *ibid.*, 1980, *302*, 865; L. Klotz (letter), *ibid.*, 866; H. B. Barner (letter), *ibid.* Reply.— G. A. Pantely *et al.* (letter), *ibid.*

See also under Effects on Blood and Myocardial Infarction.

Postoperative thrombosis. In a double-blind study 44 patients undergoing total hip replacement received aspirin 600 mg twice daily on the day prior to operation and subsequently until completion of radiographic phlebography (after 7 to 10 days) and usually for an additional 2 weeks thereafter; 11 developed a fresh deep-vein thrombosis, compared with 23 of 51 similar patients who received placebo; this difference was significant. Unexpectedly, analysis indicated that the protective effect exerted by aspirin was limited to men since only 4 of 23 developed thrombi compared with 14 of 25 who received placebo, whereas 7 of 21 women did, compared with 9 of 26 on placebo.— W. H. Harris *et al.*, *New Engl. J. Med.*, 1977, *297*, 1246. Different results were obtained in a similarly designed trial when 11 of 37 patients given aspirin and 12 of 34 given placebo developed venous thrombosis.— M. Hume (letter), *ibid.*, 1091.

In a study in 43 evaluated patients, chiefly women, undergoing total knee replacement, aspirin 1.3 g thrice daily and intermittent pneumatic calf and thigh compression each lowered the incidence of postoperative deep-vein thrombosis, when compared with a placebo; aspirin 325 mg thrice daily was not effective.— R. McKenna *et al.*, *Br. med. J.*, 1980, *280*, 514.

Further studies in which aspirin reduced the incidence of postoperative deep-vein thrombosis.— W. H. Harris *et al.*, *J. Bone Jt Surg.*, 1974, *56A*, 1552; M. Hume *et al.*, *Am. J. Surg.*, 1977, *133*, 420.

Further studies in which aspirin did not reduce the incidence of postoperative venous thrombosis.— J. R. O'Brien *et al.* (letter), *Lancet*, 1971, *1*, 399; *Lancet*, 1972, *2*, 441 (Report of the Steering Committee of a Trial Sponsored by the MRC); J. D. Stamatakis *et al.*, *Br. med. J.*, 1978, *1*, 1031; J. D. Schulman *et al.* (letter), *New Engl. J. Med.*, 1978, *299*, 661.

For a report of a reduced incidence of postoperative thrombosis in patients given both aspirin and low-dose heparin, see Heparin, p.768.

For a report of reduced postoperative deep-vein thrombosis among patients given aspirin and dipyridamole, see Dipyridamole, p.1619.

Stroke. Discussions on aspirin in cerebral ischaemia and stroke.— *Br. med. J.*, 1978, *2*, 454; *Lancet*, 1978, *2*, 245; D. J. Dalessio, *J. Am. med. Ass.*, 1978, *239*, 228; B. A. Sandok *et al.*, *Mayo Clin. Proc.*, 1978, *53*, 665; J. P. Mohr, *New Engl. J. Med.*, 1978, *299*, 93; *Drug & Ther. Bull.*, 1978, *16*, 5; W. S. Fields, *Drugs*, 1979, *18*, 150; J. R. A. Mitchell, *Practitioner*, 1979, *223*, 668; *Med. Lett.*, 1980, *22*, 71.

A multicentre comparison of aspirin 650 mg twice daily with placebo showed that aspirin reduced the frequency of carotid transient ischaemic attacks in patients with evidence of cerebral ischaemia. This effect was marked in those patients with a history of multiple attacks. However, the effect was not associated with any significant reduction in cerebral or retinal infarction or death.— W. S. Fields *et al.*, *Stroke*, 1977, *8*, 301. See also *idem*, 1978, *9*, 309.

The prophylactic effect of aspirin and sulphinpyrazone was assessed in a randomised study in 585 patients who had had ischaemic attacks and risked suffering a stroke. There were significantly fewer strokes and deaths in men given aspirin 325 mg four times daily alone, or together with sulphinpyrazone 200 mg four times daily, when compared with patients given sulphinpyrazone alone. There was no synergism between the two drugs. The greatest benefit was seen in men who had not previously had a myocardial infarction. Women did not benefit from this protective effect of aspirin. The failure of sulphinpyrazone to reduce stroke or death contrasted with the findings of the Anturane Reinfarction Trial (*New Engl. J. Med.*, 1978 *298*, 289) when the drug reduced fatalities in patients who had recently suffered a myocardial infarction.— Canadian Cooperative Study Group, *New Engl. J. Med.*, 1978, *299*, 53. Comment.— J. P. Mohr, *ibid.*, 93. A possible modest effect of aspirin alone or in association with sulphinpyrazone was not established.— J. P. Whisnant (letter), *ibid.*, 953. Further criticisms and comment.— J. E. Thompson (letter), *ibid.*, 954; H. H. Trout (letter), *ibid.;* D. J. Glover and E. L. Michelson (letter), *ibid.*. Reply.— D. L. Sackett (letter), *ibid.*, 955.

A small study showed that aspirin afforded no protection against the increased incidence of transient ischaemic attacks when anticoagulants were withdrawn.— J. Jestico *et al.*, *Br. med. J.*, 1978, *1*, 1188.

One patient receiving dipyridamole and aspirin had been free of transient ischaemic attacks when the dose of aspirin was 2 g daily, but these recurred when she had received 1 or 1.5 g daily for some months. Transient ischaemic attacks appeared usually when the blood-salicylate concentration was at or below 100 μmol per litre. The need for increasing doses of aspirin to keep patients free had been noted in other patients and it appears that some patients need higher doses than those commonly recommended on the basis of laboratory tests.— J. -E. Olsson (letter), *Lancet*, 1979, *1*, 830.

Other studies on the benefit of aspirin in patients with transient ischaemic attacks: G. Fassio *et al.*, *J. int. med. Res.*, 1979, *7*, 492 (with dipyridamole); H. J. M. Barnett *et al.*, *Can. med. Ass. J.*, 1980, *122*, 293.

Preparations

Capsules

Aspirin Capsules *(U.S.P.)*. Capsules containing aspirin. The *U.S.P.* requires 80% dissolution in 30 minutes. Store in airtight containers.

Mixtures

APC Mixture *(Roy. Marsden Hosp.)*. Aspirin, Paracetamol, and Caffeine Mixture. Aspirin 300 mg, paracetamol 300 mg, caffeine citrate 150 mg, compound tragacanth powder 250 mg, chloroform water to 10 ml.

Acetylsalicylic Acid Mixture *(B.P.C. 1963)*. Aspirin Mixture. Aspirin 514.5 mg, compound tragacanth powder 343.5 mg, chloroform spirit 0.47 ml, water to 15 ml. *Dose.* 15 to 30 ml.

This mixture deteriorates rapidly and must be freshly prepared.

AMENDED FORMULA. Aspirin 450 mg, compound tragacanth powder 250 mg, chloroform spirit 0.4 ml, water to 10 ml.— *Compendium of Past Formulae 1933 to 1966*, London, The National Pharmaceutical Union, 1969.

Acetylsalicylic Acid Mixture for Infants *(B.P.C. 1963)*. Aspirin Mixture Paediatric; Aspirin Mixture for Infants. Aspirin 146.4 mg, compound tragacanth powder 73.2 mg, raspberry syrup 1 ml, amaranth solution 0.03 ml, water to 4 ml. *Dose.* 4 to 8 ml. This mixture should not be used in children under 1 year of age, see p.240.

This mixture deteriorates rapidly and must be freshly prepared.

AMENDED FORMULA. Aspirin 125 mg, compound tragacanth powder 60 mg, raspberry syrup 1 ml, amaranth solution 0.05 ml, water to 5 ml.—*Compendium of Past Formulae 1933 to 1966*, London, The National Pharmaceutical Union, 1969.

Aspirin Mixture *(A.P.F.)*. Acetylsalicylic Acid Mixture. Aspirin 500 mg, compound tragacanth powder 250 mg, orange syrup 1 ml, concentrated chloroform water 0.25 ml, water to 10 ml. *Dose.* 10 to 20 ml.

The mixture should be freshly prepared.

Aspirin Mixture CF *(A.P.F.)*. Aspirin Mixture for Children. Aspirin 150 mg, compound tragacanth powder 100 mg, raspberry syrup 1 ml, concentrated chloroform water 0.1 ml, water to 5 ml. *Dose.* 5 to 10 ml. This mixture should not be used in children under 1 year of age, see p.240.

The mixture should be freshly prepared.

Sore Throat Mixture. Aspirin 400 mg, potassium citrate 200 mg, codeine phosphate 13.3 mg, benzocaine 40 mg, compound tragacanth powder 200 mg, chloroform water to 10 ml. For sore throats in patients undergoing radiotherapy. *Dose.* 10 ml four times daily; gargle, then swallow.—. N. Johnston *et al.* (letter), *Pharm. J.*, 1979, *1*, 413.

Suppositories

Aspirin Suppositories *(U.S.P.)*. Suppositories containing aspirin. Store in a cool place.

Witepsol suppository bases permitted greater absorption of aspirin than theobroma oil or macrogol bases.— U. Samelius and A. Åström, *Acta pharmac. tox.*, 1958, *14*, 240.

Tablets

Aspirin and Caffeine Tablets *(B.P.)*. Acetylsalicylic Acid and Caffeine Tablets. Each tablet contains aspirin 350 mg and caffeine 30 mg.

Aspirin and Codeine Tablets *(B.P.)*. Acetylsalicylic Acid and Codeine Tablets. Each tablet contains aspirin 400 mg and codeine phosphate 8 mg. Protect from light.

Aspirin, Phenacetin, and Codeine Tablets *(B.P. 1973)*. Aspirin, Phenacetin, and Codeine Tab.; Compound Codeine Tablets; Tab. Codein. Co. Each contains aspirin 250 mg, phenacetin 250 mg, and codeine phosphate 8 mg. Store in a cool place in airtight containers. Protect from light. *Dose.* 1 or 2 tablets.

Aspirin Tablets *(B.P.)*. Acetylsalicylic Acid Tablets. Tablets containing aspirin.
Store in airtight containers.

Aspirin Tablets *(U.S.P.)*. Tablets containing aspirin. The *U.S.P.* requires 80% dissolution in 30 minutes. Tablets containing more than 81 mg contain no added sweetening or flavouring agents. Store in airtight containers.

Aspirin with Ipecacuanha and Opium Tablets *(B.P.C. 1968)*. Acetylsalicylic Acid with Ipecacuanha and Opium Tablets; Tablets of Aspirin and Dover's Powder. Each contains aspirin 150 mg and ipecacuanha and opium powder 150 mg (= 1.5 mg of anhydrous morphine). Store in a cool place in airtight containers. *Dose.* 1 or 2 tablets.

Compound Aspirin Tablets *(B.P.C. 1973)*. Aspirin Compound Tablets; APC Tablets; Aspirin, Phenacetin, and Caffeine Tablets; Compound Tablets of Acetylsalicylic Acid. Each contains aspirin 225 mg, phenacetin 150 mg, and caffeine 30 mg. Store in a cool place in airtight containers. *Dose.* 1 or 2 tablets.

Preparations of Soluble Aspirin

Paediatric Dispersible Aspirin Tablets *(B.P.)*. Paediatric Dispersible Acetylsalicylic Acid Tablets; Paediatric Soluble Aspirin Tablets; Paediatric Soluble Acetylsalicylic Acid Tablets; Tab. Acid. Acetylsal. Sol. pro Inf.; Aspirin Soluble Tablets Paediatric; Soluble Tablets of Acetylsalicylic Acid, Paediatric. Each contains aspirin 75 mg, citric acid 7.5 mg, calcium carbonate 25 mg, and saccharin sodium 750 μg. Store at a temperature not exceeding 25°.

Dispersible Aspirin and Codeine Tablets *(B.P.)*. Dispersible Acetylsalicylic Acid and Codeine Tablets; Soluble Aspirin and Codeine Tablets; Soluble Acetylsalicylic Acid and Codeine Tablets. Each tablet contains aspirin 400 mg, codeine phosphate 8 mg, calcium carbonate 130 mg, citric acid 40 mg, and saccharin sodium 4 mg. Protect from light. *Dose.* 1 or 2 tablets.

Soluble Aspirin, Phenacetin, and Codeine Tablets *(B.P. 1973)*. Sol. Aspirin, Phenacetin, and Codeine Tab.; Soluble Compound Codeine Tablets; Tab. Codein. Co. Sol.; Aspirin, Phenacetin, and Codeine Soluble Tablets. Each contains aspirin 250 mg, phenacetin 250 mg, codeine phosphate 8 mg, calcium carbonate 80 mg, citric acid 26 mg, and saccharin sodium 5 mg. Protect from light. *Dose.* 1 or 2 tablets.

Dispersible Aspirin Tablets *(B.P.)*. Dispersible Acetylsalicylic Acid Tablets; Soluble Aspirin Tablets; Aspirin Soluble Tablets; Soluble Acetylsalicylic Acid Tablets. Each contains aspirin 300 mg, citric acid 30 mg, calcium carbonate 100 mg, and saccharin sodium 3 mg. Store at a temperature not exceeding 25°.

NOTE. The *B.P.* directs that when **Calcium Aspirin Tablets** are prescribed or demanded, Dispersible Aspirin Tablets be dispensed or supplied.

Proprietary Preparations Containing Aspirin

Analgesic Dellipsoids D6 *(Pilsworth, UK)*. Tablets each containing aspirin 250 mg, salicylamide 150 mg, caffeine 15 mg, and quinine salicylate 15 mg. For pain. *Dose.* 1 or 2 tablets 3 or 4 times daily or when necessary.

Anodyne Dellipsoids D4 *(Pilsworth, UK)*. Tablets each containing aspirin 250 mg, codeine phosphate 7.5 mg, salicylamide 150 mg, and phenolphthalein 12.5 mg. Analgesic. *Dose.* 1 or 2 tablets.

Asagran *(Monsanto, UK)*. A granular form of aspirin.

Bayer Aspirin *(Bayer, UK)*. Aspirin, available as tablets of 300 mg. (Also available as Bayer Aspirin in *USA*).

Breoprin *(Sterling Research, UK)*. Aspirin, available as scored tablets of 648 mg; the aspirin is present in a microencapsulated form.

Caprin *(Sinclair, UK)*. Compacted tablets each containing aspirin 324 mg in a basis resistant to acid but which swells in an alkaline medium, for release in the duodenum. The tablets should be swallowed whole before meals.

Hypon *(Calmic, UK).* Tablets each containing aspirin 325 mg, codeine phosphate 5 mg, and caffeine 10 mg. Analgesic and antipyretic. *Dose.* 2 tablets every 4 hours; children, 6 to 12 years, one tablet.

Levius *(Farmitalia Carlo Erba, UK).* Aspirin, available as tablets of 500 mg; the aspirin is present as fine particles microencapsulated in an ethylcellulose film through which the drug is slowly released by dialysis.

A brief evaluation of Levius.— *Drug & Ther. Bull.*, 1972, *10*, 87.

Nu-seals Aspirin *(Lilly, UK).* Aspirin, available as enteric-sealed tablets of 300 and 600 mg.

Paynocil *(Beecham Research, UK).* Scored tablets each containing aspirin 600 mg and glycine 300 mg.

Safapryn *(Pfizer, UK).* Tablets each containing, in an enteric-coated core, aspirin 300 mg and, in an outer layer, paracetamol 250 mg. Analgesic. The tablets should be swallowed whole. **Safapryn-Co.** Tablets containing in addition, in the outer layer, codeine phosphate 8 mg. *Dose.* 1 to 4 tablets of either Safapryn or Safapryn-Co 3 or 4 times daily.

A brief evaluation of Safapryn.— *Drug & Ther. Bull.*, 1972, *10*, 87.

Trancoprin *(Sterling Research, UK).* Scored tablets each containing aspirin 300 mg and chlormezanone 100 mg. For headache, muscle pain, and dysmenorrhoea. *Dose.* 1 or 2 tablets 3 times daily.

Veganin *(Warner, UK).* Scored tablets each containing aspirin 250 mg, codeine phosphate 6.8 mg, and paracetamol 250 mg. Analgesic. *Dose.* 1 or 2 tablets every 3 to 4 hours up to a maximum of 8 in 24 hours; children, 6 to 12 years, half to one tablet every 4 hours up to a maximum of 4 in 24 hours.

Proprietary Preparations Containing Soluble Aspirin

Antoin *(Cox Continental, UK).* Tablets each containing aspirin 400 mg, codeine phosphate 5 mg, caffeine citrate 15 mg, calcium carbonate 130 mg, and citric acid 40 mg. Analgesic. *Dose.* 1 or 2 tablets, dissolved in water, 3 or 4 times daily.

Claradin *(Nicholas, UK).* Scored tablets each containing aspirin 300 mg in an effervescent basis equivalent to sodium bicarbonate 600 mg and citric acid 400 mg. Analgesic and antipyretic.

Codis (known in some countries as Codispril, Codisprina) *(Reckitt & Colman Pharmaceuticals, UK).* Tablets each containing aspirin 500 mg, codeine phosphate 8 mg, calcium carbonate 150 mg, citric acid 50 mg, and saccharin sodium 6 mg. Analgesic. *Dose.* 1 or 2 tablets, dissolved in water, every 4 hours up to a maximum of 8 in 24 hours.

Migravess *(Dome/Hollister-Stier, UK).* Scored tablets each containing aspirin 325 mg, metoclopramide hydrochloride 5 mg, sodium bicarbonate 1.18 g, and citric acid 850 mg. For migraine. *Dose.* 2 tablets, dissolved in water, at the start of an attack, repeated if necessary; maximum dosage 6 tablets in 24 hours; patients, 10 to 15 years, half the adult dose.

Myolgin *(Cox Continental, UK).* Tablets each containing soluble aspirin equivalent to aspirin 200 mg, caffeine citrate 15 mg, codeine phosphate 5 mg, paracetamol 200 mg, citric acid 15 mg, and calcium carbonate 60 mg. For rheumatic and other pain. *Dose.* 1 or 2 tablets, dissolved in water, thrice daily.

Solprin *(Reckitt & Colman Pharmaceuticals, UK).* Tablets each containing aspirin 300 mg, calcium carbonate 100 mg, citric acid 30 mg, and saccharin sodium 3 mg.

Soluble Aspirin and Papaveretum Tablets *(Cox, UK).* Each contains aspirin 500 mg and papaveretum 10 mg, in an effervescent basis. For pain.

Other Proprietary Names of Aspirin, its Salts, and its Complexes

Arg.— AAS, Adiro, Aspirinetas, Bayaspirina, Enteretas, Rhonal; *Austral.*— Bi-prin, Codral Junior, Ecotrin, Elsprin, Novosprin, Prodol, Provoprin, Rhusal, Sedalgin, Solusal, SRA, Winsprin; *Belg.*— Acenterine, Adiro, Aspegic *(*lysine acetylsalicylate*)*, Dispril, Dolean pH 8, Enterosarin, Primaspan, Rhodine, Rhonal, Soparine; *Canad.*— Acetophen, Asadrine C-200, Astrin, Coryphen, Ecotrin, Entrophen, Neopirine-25, Nova-Phase, Novasen, Rhonal, Sal-Adult, Sal-Infant, Supasa, Triaphen-10; *Denm.*— Acetard, Albyl, Albyl-Selters, Globentyl, Idotyl, Kalcatyl, Magnyl, Reumyl; *Fr.*— Aspégic *(*lysine acetylsalicylate*)*, Aspirisucre, Aspisol *(*lysine acetylsalicylate*)*, Catalgine, Claragine, Ivépirine, Juvépirine, Rhonal; *Ger.*— Acetylin, Colfarit, Contrheuma retard, Delgesic *(*lysine acetylsalicylate*)*, Godamed, Halgon, Monobeltin *(*with aluminium acetylsalicylate*)*, Pyracyl *(*magnesium acetylsalicylate*)*, Trineral 600; *Hung.*— Istopirine; *Ital.*— Asatard, Aspegic *(*lysine acetylsalicylate*)*, Cemirit, Dolean pH 8, Domupirina, Endydol, Flectadol *(*lysine acetylsalicylate*)*, Kilios, Longasa, Rectosalyl; *Jap.*— Rhonal, Salitison; *Neth.*— Acenterine, Acetyl, Adiro, Aspegic *(*lysine acetylsalicylate*)*, Chefarine-N, Enterosarine, Rhonal; *Norw.*— Albyl, Dispril, Globentyl, Licyl, Magnyl, Novid; *S.Afr.*— Aquaprin, Aspasol, Aspegic *(*lysine acetylsalicylate*)*; *Spain*— AAS, Adiro, Calmo Yer Analgesico, Casprium Retard, Codalgina Retard, Dolomega *(*lysine acetylsalicylate*)*, Lafena, Mejoral Infantil, Rhonal, Riane *(*arginine acetylsalicylate*)*, Salicilina, Soluspriin *(*lysine acetylsalicylate*)*; *Swed.*— Acetard, Albyl, Albyl-Selters, Apernyl, Bamyl, Bamyl S, Dispril, Magnecyl, Premaspin, Reumyl; *Switz.*—Acentérine, Acetylo, Aspegic *(*lysine acetylsalicylate*)*, Asrivo, Bebesan, Dispril, Dolean pH 8, Enterosarine, Rhonal; *USA*— Aluprin, Ecotrin, Empirin.

Aspirin or soluble aspirin was also formerly marketed in Great Britain under the proprietary names Chu-Pax (*Multipax Laboratories*) and Tasprin-Sol (*Ticen, Eire*). Preparations containing aspirin or soluble aspirin were also formerly marketed under the proprietary names Analgin (*Norton*), Bufferin (*Bristol Laboratories*), Dexocodene (*Medo-Chemicals*), and Tercin and Sol-Tercin (both *Cox-Continental*).

2602-w

Acetaminosalol. Acetyl-*p*-aminosalol; Cétossalol; Phenetsal. 4-Acetamidophenyl salicylate.
$C_{15}H_{13}NO_4$=271.3.

CAS — 118-57-0.

Pharmacopoeias. In *Mex.*, *Port.*, and *Span.*

White, odourless, tasteless, crystalline scales. M.p. about 188°. **Soluble** 1 in 2000 of water, 1 in 160 of alcohol, 1 in 105 of chloroform, and 1 in 105 of ether. **Incompatible** with alkali hydroxides and carbonates, and with hexamine. **Store** in airtight containers. Protect from light.

Uses. Acetaminosalol has antipyretic, anti-inflammatory, and analgesic properties. It has been used in the treatment of rheumatic diseases in doses of 0.3 to 1 g, up to a maximum of 5 g daily.

2603-e

Acetanilide *(B.P.C. 1949).* Antifebrin. *N*-Phenylacetamide.
C_8H_9NO=135.2.

CAS — 103-84-4.

Pharmacopoeias. In *Aust.*, *Hung.*, *Mex.*, *Nord.*, *Port.*, and *Span.*

Odourless, colourless, shining, lamellar crystals, or white crystalline powder, with a pungent taste. M.p. 113° to 115°.

Soluble 1 in 200 of water, 1 in 20 of boiling water, 1 in 3.5 of alcohol, 1 in 8 of chloroform, and 1 in 50 of ether; soluble in acetone and glycerol. A saturated solution in water is neutral to litmus. **Incompatible** with alkalis, nitrous ether spirit, amyl nitrite, and acid solutions of nitrites. Forms liquid mixtures when triturated with aspirin, chloral hydrate, phenazone, phenol, resorcinol, salol, sodium salicylate, and thymol.

Uses. Acetanilide has analgesic and antipyretic actions. It has been replaced by safer analgesics.

2604-l

Acetylcresotinic Acid. *o*-Acetylcresotinic Acid. 2-Acetoxy-3-methylbenzoic acid.
$C_{10}H_{10}O_4$=194.2.

Uses. Acetylcresotinic acid has analgesic, antipyretic, and anti-inflammatory properties and is used in the treatment of rheumatism, usually in doses of up to 4 g daily.

Proprietary Names
Crésopirine *(Lemoine, Fr.).*

2605-y

Alclofenac *(B.P.).* W 7320. (4-Allyloxy-3-chlorophenyl)acetic acid.
$C_{11}H_{11}ClO_3$=226.7.

CAS — 22131-79-9.

Pharmacopoeias. In *Br.*

A white or slightly yellowish-white, odourless or almost odourless, crystalline powder with a pungent taste. M.p. about 91°. Slightly **soluble** in water; soluble 1 in 3 of alcohol, 1 in 4 of chloroform, 1 in 6 of ether.

Adverse Effects. As for Ibuprofen, p.256. Skin rashes are common.

Experimental studies have revealed a mutagenic risk from an alclofenac metabolite.

Alclofenac appeared to be associated with a relatively high incidence of adverse reactions. Out of 230 reports of reactions notified to the Committee on Safety of Medicines 168 were for rash without systemic disturbance, 34 were for rash with systemic disturbance, and 7 were for gastro-intestinal haemorrhage or other symptoms.— D. Mansel-Jones (letter), *Lancet*, 1974, *1*, 97.

Two patients developed widespread cutaneous vasculitis within 5 to 7 days of commencing to take alclofenac 1 g twice or thrice daily. A third patient who developed symptoms 2 days after commencing to take 500 mg thrice daily and who continued to take alclofenac for a week developed a widespread maculopapular eruption and recurrent episodes of purpura, haemoptysis, and haematuria, with evidence of renal involvement.— R. A. Billings *et al.*, *Br. med. J.*, 1974, *4*, 263.

From a study of about 1500 patients who had participated in trials of alclofenac in the UK the incidence of skin rash was 10.3% in those taking tablets and 2.1% in those taking capsules. There might be cross-sensitivity to penicillin, gold salts, or salicylates. Five cases of gastro-intestinal haemorrhage had occurred but the role of alclofenac could not be determined; 5 of 6 anaphylactoid reactions were attributable to alclofenac. Leucopenia had occurred in 2 patients, 1 with Felty's syndrome.— J. F. Hort, *Curr. med. Res. Opinion*, 1975, *3*, 333. See also S. S. Bedi, *Curr. med. Res. Opinion*, 1975, *3*, 309.

Angioneurotic oedema occurred in a 44-year-old woman after taking alclofenac 1 g. She had been taking alclofenac intermittently for osteoarthritis for the previous 18 months, and had noted a rash on one other occasion.— N. G. Kounis, *Br. J. clin. Pract.*, 1975, *29*, 322.

Effects on kidneys. A report of renal papillary necrosis in a 65-year-old woman who had taken aspirin 1.5 kg between 1971 and 1973 and alclofenac 2.2 kg between 1973 and 1975.— R. Gokal and D. R. Matthews, *Br. med. J.*, 1977, *2*, 1517.

Precautions. As for Ibuprofen, p.256. A rise in blood-sugar concentrations has been reported in some diabetic patients given alclofenac. Alclofenac may enhance the effects of oral hypoglycaemic agents, and thyroxine.

Absorption and Fate. Alclofenac appears to be variably absorbed from the gastro-intestinal tract. Peak plasma concentrations are reached 1 to 4 hours after rectal or oral administration. The plasma half-life varies between 1.5 and 5.5 hours. It is excreted in urine mainly as glucuronide and as unchanged drug. Variable amounts are excreted in the faeces.

Studies in man had shown that the main metabolic products of alclofenac were conjugates with glucuronic acid and glycine, with very small amounts of the de-allylated product 4-hydroxy-3-chlorophenylacetic acid and the methylated derivative of 3,4-dihydroxypropyloxy-3-chlorophenylacetic acid.— L. F. Wiggins, *Curr. med. Res. Opinion*, 1975, *3*, 241.

Alclofenac was bound to plasma proteins to the extent of more than 99%. In 10 patients with rheumatoid arthritis given alclofenac 1 g mean peak plasma concentrations of 136 µg per ml occurred at 1 hour and peak synovial fluid concentrations of 32.6 µg per ml at 2 hours. Synovial fluid concentrations then remained fairly constant and at 6 hours exceeded plasma concentrations.— G. M. Thomas *et al.*, *Curr. med. Res. Opinion*, 1975, *3*, 264.

In 32 fasting subjects given a single dose of alclofenac 500 mg as a micronised aqueous suspension mean absorption half-life was 15 minutes and mean elimination half-life 1.5 to 2 hours with the calculated peak plasma concentration occurring at 0.8 hours after administration. In a further 12 subjects given alclofenac shortly before or after a meal the rate but not the extent of alclofenac absorption was significantly decreased. In both groups about 5 to 10% of the administered drug was excreted unchanged in the urine within 24 hours.— L. T. Sennello *et al.*, *Clin. Pharmac. Ther.*, 1978, *23*, 414.

Uses. Alclofenac is a phenylacetic acid derivative which has analgesic, antipyretic, and anti-inflammatory properties and has been used in the treatment of rheumatoid arthritis and other rheumatic disorders in doses of 0.5 to 1 g thrice daily. Alclofenac has also been given by intramuscular injection and as 600-mg suppositories.

Reviews of the actions and uses of alclofenac.— *Drug & Ther. Bull.*, 1972, *10*, 77; R. N. Brogden *et al.*, *Drugs*, 1977, *14*, 241.

Analgesia. In a double-blind study in 221 patients with postoperative pain there was no significant difference between the analgesic effect of paracetamol 1 g plus caffeine 100 mg, glafenine 400 mg, and alclofenac 1 g, all of which were significantly more effective than a placebo.— C. W. R. Phaf *et al.*, *Clin. Trials J.*, 1973, *10*, 125.

Ankylosing spondylitis. In 18 patients with ankylosing spondylitis alclofenac 3 or 4 g daily was as effective as the previous medication (usually indomethacin or phenylbutazone) in 10; morning stiffness increased at 1 month and tended to remain so.— D. Y. Bulgen and B. L. Hazleman, *Curr. med. Res. Opinion*, 1975, *3*, 321.

Rheumatoid arthritis. Studies on the use of alclofenac in rheumatoid arthritis.— M. Aylward and D. B. S. Davies, *Br. J. clin. Pract.*, 1972, *26*, 517; J. van Hoek, *Curr. ther. Res.*, 1970, *12*, 551; M. Aylward, *Br. J. clin. Pract.*, 1973, *27*, 255; M. Aylward *et al.*, *Br. med. J.*, 1975, *2*, 7; M. Aylward, *Curr. med. Res. Opinion*, 1975, *3*, 274; J. Maddock *et al.*, *Curr. med. Res. Opinion*, 1975, *3*, 286; I. Haslock, *ibid.*, 298; S. S. Bedi, *ibid.*, 309; A. G. White and V. M. Martin, *ibid.*, 329; H. Berry *et al.*, *Ann. rheum. Dis.*, 1978, *37*, 93.

Preparations

Alclofenac Capsules *(B.P.)*. Capsules containing alclofenac. Store at a temperature not exceeding 30°.

Proprietary Names

Allopydin *(Jap.)*; Argun *(CEPA, Spain)*; Darkeyfenac *(Cuatrecasas-Darkey, Spain)*; Desinflam *(Sintyal, Arg.)*; Epinal *(Jap.)* (see also under Adrenaline Acid Tartrate); Mervan *(Continental Pharma, Belg.*; *Cooper, Switz.)*; Mirvan *(Labaz, Neth.)*; Prinalgin *(Berk, S.Afr.)*; Vanadian *(Federico Bonet, Spain)*; Zubirol *(Abbott, Arg.)*; Zumaril *(Abbott, Ital.)*.

Alclofenac was formerly marketed in Great Britain under the proprietary name Prinalgin (*Berk Pharmaceuticals*).

2606-j

Aletamine Hydrochloride. NDR 5061 A; Alfetamine Hydrochloride. α-Allylphenethylamine hydrochloride.
$C_{11}H_{15}N,HCl$=197.7.

CAS — 4255-23-6 (aletamine); 4255-24-7 (hydrochloride).

Uses. Aletamine hydrochloride is an analgesic tried in doses of 125 and 250 mg.

References: L. J. Cass and W. S. Frederik, *J. new Drugs*, 1966, *6*, 96; D. W. Nachand *et al.*, *J. clin. Pharmac.*, 1967, *7*, 116.

2607-z

Aloxiprin *(B.P.)*. A polymeric condensation product of aluminium oxide and aspirin.

CAS — 9014-67-9.

Pharmacopoeias. In *Br.* and *Cz.*

A fine white or slightly pink, odourless or almost odourless, tasteless powder. It contains 7.5 to 8.5% of aluminium and 79 to 87.4% of total salicylates. Aloxiprin 600 mg is approximately equivalent to 500 mg of aspirin. Practically **insoluble** in water, alcohol, and ether; soluble 1 in 200 of chloroform. It is hydrolysed rapidly in alkaline media but much less rapidly in acid media.

Adverse Effects, Treatment, and Precautions. As for Aspirin, p.236, p.238.

Aloxiprin appears to be less liable to cause gastric irritation and haemorrhage than aspirin.

Aloxiprin appeared to be associated with less gastro-intestinal bleeding than plain aspirin though the reduction was not uniform in all subjects.— P. H. N. Wood *et al.*, *Br. med. J.*, 1962, *1*, 669.

Absorption and Fate. Aloxiprin is hydrolysed in the gastro-intestinal tract to aspirin, the rate of breakdown being low in the acid conditions of the stomach and greater at the higher pH values of the intestine.

Aspirin from aloxiprin dissolved at an appreciably slower rate than from tablets of aspirin and excretion of salicylate was delayed longer than after the equivalent dose of aspirin, though the total amounts excreted were the same.— A. J. Cummings *et al.*, *J. Pharm. Pharmac.*, 1963, *15*, 56.

Uses. Aloxiprin has actions similar to those of Aspirin, p.240. It is used as an analgesic and anti-inflammatory agent in rheumatic disorders. It is administered as tablets in doses of up to 100 mg per kg body-weight daily in divided doses.

References: Report No. 23 of the General Practitioner Research Group, *Practitioner*, 1962, *188*, 533; P. H. Kendall and W. J. Cahill (preliminary report), *Ann. phys. Med.*, 1967, *9*, 19; J. Geller, *Br. J. clin. Pract.*, 1968, *22*, 392.

For a comparison of aloxiprin and indomethacin given as a single dose at night to patients with rheumatoid arthritis and ankylosing spondylitis, see E. C. Huskisson and F. D. Hart, *Practitioner*, 1972, *208*, 248.

Preparations

Aloxiprin Tablets *(B.P.)*. Tablets containing aloxiprin.

Palaprin Forte *(Nicholas, UK)*. Aloxiprin, available as scored tablets of 600 mg. (Also available as Palaprin Forte in *Austral.*).

Other Proprietary Names

Paloxin *(S.Afr.)*; Rumatral *(Switz.)*; Superpyrin *(Cz.)*.

2608-c

Aluminium Aspirin. Aluminum Aspirin; Aluminum Acetylsalicylate; Aspirin Aluminium. Bis(2-acetoxybenzoato-*O'*)hydroxyaluminium.
$C_{18}H_{15}AlO_9$=402.3.

CAS — 23413-80-1.

Pharmacopoeias. In *Jap.*

A white crystalline powder, odourless or with a slight odour. Practically **insoluble** in water and organic solvents; soluble with decomposition in solutions of alkali carbonates and hydroxides. It is reported to be more stable than aspirin.

Uses. Aluminium aspirin has actions and uses similar to those of Aspirin (see p.235). It has been used in a dose of 670 mg (equivalent to about 600 mg of aspirin) every 4 hours.

Proprietary Preparations

Rumasal *(Marshall's Pharmaceuticals, UK)*. Basic aluminium aspirin, available as tablets of 600 mg (equivalent to 500 mg of aspirin). Rumasal is stated not to be absorbed until it reaches the small intestine, and to be useful where aspirin is indicated but not tolerated.

Other Proprietary Names

Alupir *(Ital.)*; Hyprin *(Jap.)*; Neutracétyl *(Fr.)*.

2609-k

Amidopyrine *(Eur. P., B.P.C. 1954)*. Aminophenazone; Aminopyrine; Aminophenazonum; Amidazofen; Amidopyrine-Pyramidon; Dimethylaminoantipyrine; Dimethylaminophenazone. 4-Dimethylamino-1,5-dimethyl-2-phenyl-4-pyrazolin-3-one.

$C_{13}H_{17}N_3O$=231.3.

CAS — 58-15-1.

Pharmacopoeias. In *Arg., Aust., Belg., Braz., Cz., Eur., Fr., Ger., Hung., Int., It., Jap., Jug., Neth., Nord., Pol., Port., Roum., Rus., Span., Swiss,* and *Turk.*

Small colourless odourless crystals or white crystalline powder with a slightly bitter taste. M.p. about 108°.

Soluble 1 in 20 of water, 1 in 2 of alcohol, 1 in 1 of chloroform, and 1 in 13 of ether. A 5% solution in water has a pH of 7.5 to 9. **Incompatible** with acacia, apomorphine, aspirin, chloral hydrate, iodine, oxidising agents, and tannic acid. **Protect** from light.

Adverse Effects and Precautions. The risk of agranulocytosis in patients taking amidopyrine is sufficiently great to render this drug unsuitable for use. Onset of agranulocytosis may be sudden and unpredictable.

Allergy. Cross-sensitivity occurred between amidopyrine and aspirin in one patient. Amidopyrine produced a life-threatening asthmatic attack on one occasion.— E. Bartoli *et al.* (letter), *Lancet*, 1976, *1*, 1357.

The Boston Collaborative Drug Surveillance Program monitored consecutively 32 812 medical inpatients. Drug-induced anaphylaxis occurred in 1 of 1992 patients given amidopyrine.— J. Porter and H. Jick, *Lancet*, 1977, *1*, 587.

Carcinogenicity. Amidopyrine must be considered a potential carcinogen because it reacted readily with nitrous acid to form dimethylnitrosamine. The reaction was catalysed by thiocyanate present in the saliva particularly in smokers.— E. Boyland and S. A. Walker, *Arzneimittel-Forsch.*, 1974, *24*, 1181. See also *Lancet*, 1979, *1*, 283.

Effects on blood. Agranulocytosis. From 960 patients treated with amidopyrine there were 11 cases of agranulocytosis—an incidence of 1.1%.— Association of Clinical Pathologists, *Lancet*, 1951, *1*, 389.

The AMA Registry of Adverse Reactions recorded 45 cases of agranulocytosis presumed or known to be due to amidopyrine and 25 in which another drug might have been involved in the period 1957–66. A hypersensitivity reaction was probably involved.— *Med. Lett.*, 1973, *15*, 4.

Four patients developed agranulocytosis while taking Chinese herbal medicines for relief of arthritis and back pain. The herbal medicines were found to contain both amidopyrine and phenylbutazone.— C. A. Ries and M. A. Sahud, *J. Am. med. Ass.*, 1975, *231*, 352.

Further reports and discussions of amidopyrine-induced agranulocytosis.— A. J. Barrett *et al.*, *Br. med. J.*, 1976, *2*, 850; R. H. Girdwood, *Practitioner*, 1978, *221*, 293.

Haemolytic anaemia. Amidopyrine had been implicated as a causative agent in immune haemolytic anaemia.— E. Beutler, *Pharmac. Rev.*, 1969, *21*, 73.

Effects on gastro-intestinal tract. Severe gastro-intestinal bleeding occurred in a 9-year-old child following 24 hours' treatment with amidopyrine given in a normal dose.— M. C. -V. Daele and G. de Gaetano, *Acta med. scand.*, 1971, *Suppl.* 525, 287.

Porphyria. Amidopyrine had been reported to precipitate attacks of porphyria.— *Drug & Ther. Bull.*, 1976, *14*, 55.

Absorption and Fate. Amidopyrine is absorbed from the gastro-intestinal tract. It has a half-life of about 1 to 4 hours.

Within 36 hours 60% of a dose of amidopyrine administered rectally was recovered in the urine, mostly as 4-acetylaminoantipyrine.— H. Oehne and E. Schmid, *Arzneimittel-Forsch.*, 1972, *22*, 2115.

The metabolism of amidopyrine.— R. Gradnik and L. Fleischmann, *Pharm. Acta Helv.*, 1973, *48*, 181. Rectal absorption.— L. Fleischmann, *ibid.*, 192.

Protein binding. Amidopyrine was about 13.4% bound to human muscle tissue *in vitro*.— B. Fichtl and H. Kurz, *Eur. J. clin. Pharmac.*, 1978, *14*, 335.

Uses. Amidopyrine has analgesic, anti-inflammatory, and antipyretic actions resembling those of phenazone but owing to the risk of agranulocytosis its use is discouraged. The gentisate has sometimes been used.

Amidopyrine is sometimes used in drug metabolism studies.

Amidopyrine, 648 mg every 4 hours, was effective in reducing fever due to chronic lymphocytic leukaemia and reticulum cell sarcoma in 2 patients.— J. M. Kiely, *Mayo Clin. Proc.*, 1969, *44*, 272.

For reference to the use of amidopyrine in metabolic studies and to the amidopyrine breath test, see G. W. Hepner *et al.*, *J. Am. med. Ass.*, 1976, *236*, 1587; J. Galizzi *et al.*, *Gut*, 1978, *19*, 40.

Preparations

Pyrabitalum *(Jap. P.)*. A mixture of 2 moles of amidopyrine with 1 mole of barbitone. *Jap. P.* also includes a tablet. *Dose.* 300 to 500 mg; max. in 24 hours 3 g.

Proprietary Names
Areumal (as gentisate) *(Ecobi, Ital.)*; Baukal (as hydroxyquinoline sulphonate) (see also under Propyphenazone) *(Bruschettini, Ital.)*; Budirol (as hydroxyquinoline sulphonate) *(Castejon, Spain)*; Depiral C (as ascorbate) *(Conti, Ital.)*; Fenodone (as hydroxyisophthalate) *(Ripari-Gero, Ital.)*; Fever (as hydroxyquinoline sulphonate) *(Courtois, Ital.)*; Ftalazone *(Terapeutico M.R., Ital.)*; Galenopyrin *(Keller, Switz.)*; Glucopirina *(Ganassini, Ital.)*; Hyparon, Inst *(both Jap.)*; Isoftal *(Isola-Ibi, Ital.)*; Katareuma (as hydroxyisophthalate) *(Lafare, Ital.)*; Latepyrine (as ethylamidopyrine carbosalicylate) *(Landerlan, Spain)*; Metapirazone (dinoramidopyrine) *(Jamco, Ital.)*; Netsusarin *(Jap.)*; Nikartrone (as hydroxyisophthalate) *(Pulitzer, Ital.)*; Piramidon *(Hoechst, Spain)*; Pirasco (as ascorbate) *(Aristochimica, Ital.)*; Piraseptolo (as hydroxyquinoline sulphonate) *(Lisapharma, Ital.)*; Piro Rectal *(Madaus Cerafarm, Spain)*; Piroreumal (as hydroxyisophthalate) *(Medosan, Ital.)*; P.S.B.P. (as sulphamidobenzoate) *(Vaillant-Defresne, Fr.)*; Reu-Bon (as hydroxyisophthalate) *(Sierochimica, Ital.)*; Reumanova (as hydroxyisophthalate) *(Gibipharma, Ital.)*; Reumasedina (as hydroxyisophthalate) *(Coli, Ital.)*; Reumoftal (as hydroxyisophthalate) *(Chemil, Ital.)*; Reumo Termina (as ascorbate) *(Made, Ital.)*; Reumotranc (as hydroxyisophthalate) *(Farmalabor, Ital.)*; Revulex (as sulphamidobenzoate) *(Vaillant-Defresne, Switz.)*; Suppnon *(Jap.)*.

2610-w

Azapropazone.
AHR 3018; Mi85; Apazone. 5-Dimethylamino-9-methyl-2-propylpyrazolo-[1,2-*a*][1,2,4]benzotriazine-1,3(2*H*)-dione dihydrate.

$C_{16}H_{20}N_4O_2,2H_2O=336.4$.

CAS — 13539-59-8 (anhydrous).

Adverse Effects. Gastro-intestinal disturbances, allergic skin rashes, headache, vertigo, oedema, and kidney impairment may occur. Gastro-intestinal bleeding and angioneurotic oedema have been reported.

Effects on skin. Two patients developed bullous skin eruptions when treated with azapropazone.— D. J. Barker and J. A. Cotterill (letter), *Lancet*, 1977, *1*, 90. See also D. J. Barker and J. A. Cotterill, *Acta derm.-vener., Stockh.*, 1977, *57*, 461.

Treatment of Adverse Effects. As for Aspirin, p.238.

Precautions. Azapropazone should be given with caution to patients with acute gastritis, impaired renal function, or with gastro-intestinal ulcers. Azapropazone may enhance the activity of coumarin anticoagulants.

Need for reduced dosage in liver failure.— K. -H. Breuing *et al.*, *Eur. J. clin. Pharmac.*, 1981, *20*, 147.

Interactions. Hypoglycaemia induced by azapropazone and tolbutamide interaction.— P. B. Andreasen *et al.*, *Br. J. clin. Pharmac.*, 1981, *12*, 583.

Serious phenytoin toxicity in a woman given concomitant azapropazone.— C. J. C. Roberts *et al.*, *Postgrad. med. J.*, 1981, *57*, 191.

For the enhancement of the effect of warfarin by azapropazone, see under Warfarin Sodium, p.778.

Absorption and Fate. Azapropazone is absorbed from the gastro-intestinal tract and peak plasma concentrations are reached about 5 hours after administration. It is excreted mainly in the urine, partly as unchanged drug.

A metabolite of azapropazone, 6-hydroxyazapropazone, had only a slight anti-inflammatory action in *animals*.— U. Jahn, *Arzneimittel-Forsch.*, 1973, *23*, 666.

Maximum plasma concentrations were reached 4 to 6 hours after administration of azapropazone by mouth. The plasma half-life was about 12 hours and the elimination half-life about 20 hours. About 95% of the dose was excreted in the urine of which 60% was unchanged azapropazone.— L. Klatt and F. W. Koss, *Arzneimittel-Forsch.*, 1973, *23*, 920. Similar conclusions were reached from a study of 6 subjects given a mean dose of azapropazone 8.4 mg per kg body-weight. When azapropazone 300 mg was given thrice daily to these subjects a mean steady plasma concentration of 90 µg per ml was reached after 4 days, compared with a mean of about 45 µg per ml reached after a single dose of 600 mg. Little difference in plasma concentration was noted when the dose was given before or after food.— H. Leach, *Curr. med. Res. Opinion*, 1976, *4*, 35.

In 6 patients given azapropazone 600 mg by mouth peak plasma concentration of 40 to 70 µg per ml occurred about 5 hours after administration.— H. E. Geissler *et al.*, *Arzneimittel-Forsch.*, 1977, *27*, 1713.

Further references.— K. M. Breuing *et al.*, *Arzneimittel-Forsch.*, 1979, *29*, 971.

Protein binding. Azapropazone was about 90% bound to human serum proteins *in vitro* at concentrations of 10 to 15 mg per 100 ml.— U. Jahn *et al.*, *Arzneimittel-Forsch.*, 1973, *23*, 660.

Uses. Azapropazone is a pyrazole derivative which has analgesic, anti-inflammatory, and antipyretic actions. It is used in the treatment of various rheumatic disorders and other musculoskeletal pain. The usual initial dose is 300 mg four times daily; this may be reduced during long-term therapy, according to the response.

In acute gout 2.4 g may be given in divided doses during the first 24 hours, followed by 1.8 g daily until the attack is resolving, then reduced to 1.2 g daily until symptoms have disappeared.

Reviews of the pharmacology and uses of azapropazone.— *Drug & Ther. Bull.*, 1976, *14*, 102; C. J. Jones, *A.H. Robins Co. Ltd.*, *Curr. med. Res. Opinion*, 1976, *4*, 3.

Rheumatic disorders. A short review of the value of azapropazone in the management of rheumatoid conditions.— P. M. Brooks and W. W. Buchanan, *Curr. med. Res. Opinion*, 1976, *4*, 94.

For reports on the use of azapropazone in various rheumatic disorders, see W. Beckschafer, *Arzneimittel-Forsch.*, 1969, *19*, 52; K. Hingorani and J. S. Templeton, *Curr. med. Res. Opinion*, 1975, *3*, 407; P. M. Brooks *et al.*, *ibid.*, 1976, *4*, 50; K. Hingorani, *ibid.*, 57; S. Thune, *ibid.*, 70 and 80; G. Mintz and A. Fraga, *ibid.*, 89; J. A. Hicklin *et al.*, *Practitioner*, 1976, *217*, 799; H. A. Capell *et al.*, *Curr. med. Res. Opinion*, 1976, *4*, 285; D. M. Grennan, *Scott. med. J.*, 1977, *22*, 22.

Proprietary Preparations
Rheumox *(Robins, UK)*. Azapropazone, available as capsules of 300 mg. **Rheumox 600.** Azapropazone, available as scored tablets of 600 mg.

Other Proprietary Names
Cinnamin *(Jap.)*; Pentosol *(Spain)*; Prolix *(S.Afr.)*; Prolixan *(Belg., Denm., Fr., Ger., Hung., Ital., Neth., Switz.)*; Prolixana *(Swed.)*.

2611-e

Benorylate.
Benorilate; Fenasprate; FAW 76; Win 11450. 4-Acetamidophenyl *O*-acetylsalicylate.

$C_{17}H_{15}NO_5=313.3$.

CAS — 5003-48-5.

A white, odourless, tasteless, stable compound. Practically **insoluble** in water; slightly soluble in alcohol; soluble in acetone, chloroform, and lipids.

Benorylate was ground to a particle size of about 5 µm to facilitate absorption.— *Mfg Chem.*, 1972, *43* (Aug.), 35.

Adverse Effects, Treatment, and Precautions. As for Aspirin, p.236, p.238 and Paracetamol, pp.268-9. Benorylate may cause nausea, indigestion, heartburn, and constipation; drowsiness, dizziness, diarrhoea, and skin rashes have also been reported. Some patients have experienced tinnitus and deafness associated with high blood-salicylate concentrations.

Effects on the gastro-intestinal tract. In 15 patients with rheumatic disorders the mean daily blood loss while taking benorylate 4 g twice daily as a suspension was 1.7 ml compared with 5.1 ml when taking soluble aspirin 1.2 g (dissolved in water) four times daily.— D. N. Croft *et al.*, *Br. med. J.*, 1972, *3*, 545. A similar report.— G. Palme and P. Koeppe, *Arzneimittel-Forsch.*, 1978, *28*, 426.

A 67-year-old woman with rheumatoid arthritis receiving benorylate suspension (20%) 5 ml four times daily experienced lower abdominal discomfort within 5 minutes of a dose, persisting for 5 to 10 minutes. When the dose was increased to 8 ml five times daily diarrhoea occurred within a few minutes of each dose. The symptoms ceased when benorylate was withdrawn.— A. J. Marshall and P. Sheridan (letter), *Br. med. J.*, 1973, *1*, 175.

Occult blood was present in the faeces of 4 of 21 patients taking benorylate.— S. G. F. Matts (letter), *Br. med. J.*, 1974, *2*, 52.

Effects on hearing. Eight of 11 patients given benorylate were unable to continue treatment because of loss of hearing, tinnitus, nausea, and disorientation. Some patients developed symptoms after the second dose. None of those who resumed treatment with half the dose [not quoted] were able to continue treatment.— R. E. Hope-Simpson (letter), *Br. med. J.*, 1973, *1*, 296.

Of 20 patients with rheumatoid arthritis given benorylate 4 g twice daily, 11 developed tinnitus and deafness after the second dose; 9 later developed the symptoms after the third dose when given 2 g thrice daily. Mean total plasma-salicylate concentrations were 2.7 mmol per litre.— M. Aylward (letter), *Br. med. J.*, 1973, *2*, 118.

Effects on the liver. Liver necrosis in one patient was attributed to benorylate and penicillamine that had been given for rheumatoid arthritis.— M. Sacher and H. Thaler (letter), *Lancet*, 1977, *1*, 481.

Absorption and Fate. Benorylate is absorbed virtually unchanged from the gastro-intestinal tract, although absorption may be prolonged. Following absorption, benorylate is rapidly metabolised to aspirin and paracetamol. It is excreted mainly as metabolites of salicyclic acid and paracetamol in the urine. A small amount of the administered dose is excreted in the faeces. Benorylate has a longer duration of action than aspirin or paracetamol.

In 9 patients who had previously shown reactions to benorylate, doses of 4 g twice daily gave rise to total salicylate concentrations and free salicylate concentrations significantly higher than those achieved with soluble aspirin 1.2 g four times daily. In 12 further patients total and free salicylate concentrations were comparable after the above doses of benorylate and soluble aspirin. In some individuals benorylate appeared to interfere with the plasma binding of salicylate, but the high total salicylate concentrations in some patients after benorylate remained unexplained.— M. Aylward (letter), *Br. med. J.*, 1973, *3*, 347.

Salicylate absorption was significantly less with benorylate given in a dose providing 1.76 g of salicylic acid than with soluble aspirin equivalent to 1.84 g of salicyclic acid in a study of 7 patients. Excretion was also slower with benorylate, approximately 55% of salicylate being excreted within 48 hours of the above dose compared with about 80% for soluble aspirin.— P. Duckworth and M. Earnshaw, *J. Hosp. Pharm.*, 1975, *33*, 83.

Studies on pharmacokinetics and distribution of benorylate in plasma and synovial fluid.— M. Aylward *et al.*, *Scand. J. Rheumatol.*, 1976, *Suppl.* 13, 9; M. Franke *et al.*, *Scand. J. Rheumatol.*, 1976, *Suppl.* 13, 13.

Uses. Benorylate is the acetylsalicylic acid ester of paracetamol and it has analgesic, anti-inflammatory, and antipyretic properties. It is used in the treatment of rheumatic disorders, in the treatment of mild to moderate pain, and as an antipyretic. In active rheumatoid arthritis 4 g twice daily may be required. In osteoarthritis and other rheumatic conditions 1.5 g thrice daily is usually adequate.

A dose of up to 25 mg per kg body-weight up to 4 times a day has been suggested for use in children. In juvenile chronic polyarthritis the dose of benorylate should be adjusted to produce plasma-salicylate concentrations between 250 and 300 µg per ml.

Reviews of the actions and uses of benorylate.— *Drug & Ther. Bull.*, 1972, *10*, 87; V. Wright, *Scand. J. Rheumatol.*, 1976, *Suppl.* 13, 5.

Administration. The bioavailability of benorylate was not significantly affected when the dose was taken in hot coffee.— N. A. Barrett *et al.*, *Rheumatol. Rehabil.*, 1978, *17*, 23.

Dysmenorrhoea. In a multicentre double-blind study benorylate 1.5 g thrice daily was more effective than placebo in the treatment of 86 women with dysmenorrhoea.— R. Prasad, *Practitioner*, 1980, *224*, 325.

Osteoarthrosis. In a comparative study in 88 patients, benorylate 2 g twice daily was as effective as 4 g twice daily in patients with osteoarthrosis without a significant degree of inflammation. Significantly fewer side-effects were associated with the lower dosage.— E. J. Valtonen, *Scand. J. Rheumatol.*, 1979, *Suppl.* 25, 9.

Further reports on the use of benorylate in the treatment of osteoarthrosis.— D. Kuntz *et al.*, *Scand. J. Rheumatol.*, 1976, *Suppl.* 13, 25; P. J. Cosgrove, *J. int. med. Res.*, 1977, *5*, 120; J. J. Hamill, *ibid.*, 265; B. Y. Marshall, *Clin. Trials J.*, 1978, *15* (3), 73; S. R. Mayhew, *Rheumatol. Rehabil.*, 1978, *17*, 29; P. A. Johnson, *Clin. Trials J.*, 1978, *15* (3), 82; D. Woolf *et al.*, *Practitioner*, 1978, *221*, 791; C. Tranmer, *Rheumatol. Rehabil.*, 1978, *17*, 91.

Rheumatoid arthritis. The effect of benorylate, 4 g twice daily as a suspension, was studied in 35 patients with rheumatoid arthritis and the effects compared with those of soluble aspirin, 1.2 g four times daily, in 34 patients. In each group there was significant improvement in pain, functional grade, and articular index with no significant difference between the 2 treatments.— D. L. Beales *et al.*, *Br. med. J.*, 1972, *2*, 483.

Further studies on the use of benorylate in rheumatoid arthritis and other rheumatic disorders.—Report No. 178 of the General Practitioner Research Group, *Practitioner*, 1973, *210*, 291; V. Wright and I. Haslock (letter), *Br. med. J.*, 1973, *2*, 487; O. Vojtíšek *et al.*, *Arzneimittel-Forsch.*, 1973, *23*, 701; P. N. Sperryn *et al.*, *Ann. rheum. Dis.*, 1973, *32*, 157; M. H. F. Coigley, *Practitioner*, 1975, *215*, 348; K. Hingorani, *Scand. J. Rheumatol.*, 1976, *Suppl.* 13, 29; P. Doury and S. Pattin, *ibid.*, 33.

Juvenile chronic polyarthritis. In 12 children with active Still's disease benorylate 200 mg per kg body-weight daily (approximately twice the recommended analgesic dose) failed to produce adequate salicylate concentrations of 250 to 350 µg per ml in most patients. No side-effects were reported. It was recommended that the initial dose be 200 mg per kg daily, that the dose be adjusted to produce salicylate concentrations of 250 to 300 µg per ml, and that thereafter the dosage be maintained with occasional monitoring of the concentration in the blood.— R. H. Powell and B. M. Ansell, *Br. med. J.*, 1974, *1*, 145.

Proprietary Preparations

Benoral *(Winthrop, UK).* Benorylate, available as **Granules** in sachets each containing 2 g; as **Suspension** containing 2 g in each 5 ml (suggested diluent, syrup); and as **Tablets** of 750 mg. (Also available as Benoral in *Austral.*).

NOTE. Benoral is a proprietary name for benzathine phenoxymethylpenicillin.

Other Proprietary Names

Benortan *(Belg., Denm., Fin., Fr., Ger., Iceland, Neth.,Switz.)*; Benotamol *(Arg.)*; Salipran *(Fr.)*; Winolate *(S.Afr.)*.

2612-l

Benoxaprofen.

Compound 90 459; LRCL 3794. 2-[2-(4-Chlorophenyl)benzoxazol-5-yl]propionic acid.

$C_{16}H_{12}ClNO_3$=301.7.

CAS — 51234-28-7.

A cream solid. M.p. 189° to 190°.

Adverse Effects. Side-effects occurring with benoxaprofen include skin rashes, photosensitivity reactions (in about 10% of patients on long-term therapy), onycholysis, and gastro-intestinal disturbances including peptic ulceration and bleeding. Jaundice has been reported and there have been reports of fatalities mainly involving elderly patients.

Effects on the blood. Neutropenia in a 64-year-old woman with no history of drug sensitivity, appeared to be associated with benoxaprofen. She recovered on discontinuation of the drug.— W. K. Essigman and J. R. B. Williams (letter), *Lancet*, 1980, *2*, 1383.

Effects on the skin. Comment on the type of photosensitivity reaction associated with benoxaprofen.— D. A. Fenton (letter), *Lancet*, 1981, *2*, 1231. See also A. du Vivier (letter), *ibid.*, 1982, *1*, 47.

Severe erythema multiforme associated with benoxaprofen.— A. E. M. Taylor *et al.* (letter), *Br. med. J.*, 1981, *282*, 1433. See also S. H. Morgan and A. R. Behn (letter), *ibid.*, *283*, 144.

Absorption and Fate. Benoxaprofen is readily absorbed from the gastro-intestinal tract. Peak plasma concentrations occur 2 to 6 hours after ingestion. It is about 99% bound to plasma proteins and has a plasma half-life of about 30 to 35 hours. It is excreted in urine mainly as the glucuronide conjugate with small amounts of unchanged drug.

Protein binding. Benoxaprofen was 99.8% bound to human plasma protein *in vitro*. The percent bound did not vary significantly up to concentrations of 120 µg per ml. At therapeutic plasma concentrations benoxaprofen did not displace warfarin, salicylate, prednisolone, or dexamethasone from their binding to plasma proteins.— D. H. Chatfield *et al.*, *Biochem. Pharmac.*, 1978, *27*, 887.

Uses. Benoxaprofen is related to the phenylpropionic acid derivatives and has analgesic, anti-inflammatory, and antipyretic actions. It is used in the treatment of rheumatoid arthritis and osteoarthritis in doses of 600 mg daily. It may be given as a single dose at night or in divided doses twice daily.

Because of reports of adverse reactions and fatalities received in the United Kingdom by the Committee on Safety of Medicines, use of benoxaprofen was severely restricted in August 1982 and the manufacturers halted marketing worldwide.

Studies on the use of benoxaprofen in the treatment of rheumatoid arthritis.— J. R. Lambert and V. Wright, *Curr. med. Res. Opinion*, 1977, *5*, 269; J. Highton and R. Grahame, *Rheumatol., Rehabil.*, 1978, *17*, 259; A. S. Ridolfo *et al.*, *Clin. Pharmac. Ther.*, 1978, *23*, 127; E. C. Huskisson *et al.*, *Rheumatol. Rehabil.*, 1978, *17*, 254; E. C. Huskisson, *Eur. J. Rheumatol. Inflamm.*, 1979, *3*, 29; E. C. Huskisson and J. Scott, *Rheumatol. Rehabil.*, 1979, *18*, 110.

Proprietary Names

Opren *(Dista, UK)*; Oraflex *(Lilly, US)*.

2613-y

Benzydamine Hydrochloride. Benzindamine Hydrochloride; AF 864. 3-(1-Benzyl-1*H*-indazol-3-yloxy)-*NN*-dimethylpropylamine hydrochloride.

$C_{19}H_{23}N_3O,HCl$=345.9.

CAS — 642-72-8 (benzydamine); 132-69-4 (hydrochloride).

Pharmacopoeias. In *Chin.* and *Nord.*

A white odourless crystalline powder with a bitter taste. M.p. about 159°. **Soluble** 1 in 1 of water, 1 in 8 of alcohol, and 1 in 4 of chloroform; practically insoluble in ether.

Adverse Effects. The most common side-effects with benzydamine are gastro-intestinal disturbances. Agitation, anxiety, hallucinations, and convulsions have been reported following overdosage.

Uses. Benzydamine hydrochloride has analgesic, anti-inflammatory, and antipyretic actions. It is used in the management of soft tissue and muscular injuries in doses of 50 mg three to four times a day. It has also been given rectally and applied as a cream or used as a mouth-wash.

In a double-blind study in 50 patients benzydamine, applied topically as a 3% cream, was more effective than placebo in the relief of pain, oedema, and local heat associated with traumatic lesions.— S. Fantato and M. De Gregorio, *Arzneimittel-Forsch.*, 1971, *21*, 1530. A similar report.— D. S. Chatterjee, *J. int. med. Res.*, 1977, *5*, 450.

A mouth-wash containing benzydamine hydrochloride 0.15% was a more effective oral anaesthetic than a mouth-wash containing cetylpyridinium chloride 0.025% or a placebo when used for 1 minute by 87 healthy subjects.— S. Simard-Savoie and D. Forest, *Curr. ther. Res.*, 1978, *23*, 734.

Further references.— D. Cloutier and D. Regoli, *Int. Z. klin. Pharmak.*, 1971, *5*, 297; P. A. Palmisano and E. Rossi, *Arzneimittel-Forsch.*, 1969, *19*, 1180; J. Froom and V. Boisseau, *Curr. ther. Res.*, 1979, *26*, 856.

Proprietary Preparations

Difflam *(Carnegie, UK).* Benzydamine hydrochloride, available as a cream containing 3%. **Difflam Oral Rinse.** A solution containing benzydamine hydrochloride 0.15%.

Other Proprietary Names

Afloben, A-Termadol *(Ital.)*; Bucco-Tantum *(Switz.)*; Enzamin *(Jap.)*; Imotryl *(Fr.)*; Multum *(Ital.)*; Tamas *(Arg.)*; Tantum *(Arg., Austral., Denm., Ger., Ital., Neth., S.Afr., Spain, Switz.)*; Verax *(Ital.)*.

2614-j

Bindazac. Bendazac; AF 983. (1-Benzyl-1*H*-indazol-3-yloxy)acetic acid.

$C_{16}H_{14}N_2O_3$=282.3.

CAS — 20187-55-7.

Adverse Effects. Pruritus, a burning sensation, erythema, vesiculation, and allergic dermatitis have been reported.

Uses. Bindazac has anti-inflammatory actions and is used topically in preparations containing 1 and 3% for the treatment of various skin disorders.

Animal pharmacology.— B. Silvestrini *et al.*, *Arzneimittel-Forsch.*, 1969, *19*, 30.

Clinical evluation.— E. Zar *et al.*, *G. ital. Derm.*, 1970, *45*, 217.

Proprietary Names

Hubersil *(Hubber, Spain)*; Versus *(Angelini, Ital.; Petersen, S.Afr.)*.

2615-z

Sweet Birch Oil *(B.P.C. 1949).* Oleum Betulae; Ol. Betul.; Gaultheria Oil; Wintergreen Oil.

Pharmacopoeias. Arg., *Mex.*, and *U.S.N.F.* allow in addition to synthetic methyl salicylate, the oils obtained from the leaves of *Gaultheria procumbens* (Ericaceae) and the bark of *Betula lenta* (Betulaceae).

Formerly obtained from *Gaultheria procumbens* (Ericaceae), now almost exclusively from *Betula lenta* (Betulaceae). It contains not less than 98% w/w of esters, calculated as methyl salicylate. It is a colourless or pale yellow liquid with the characteristic odour and taste of methyl salicylate. Wt per ml 1.176 to 1.186 g. **Store** in a cool place. Protect from light.

Adverse Effects and Treatment. As for Aspirin, p.236 and p.238.

A 6-year-old boy who was sensitive to aspirin developed generalised pustular psoriasis consequent upon walking in East Pennsylvanian woodland in April. The eruption was traced to inhaling pollen and chewing twigs of *B. lenta* and chewing the leaves of *G. procumbens*, all of which were a source of methyl salicylate.— W. B. Shelley, *J. Am. med. Ass.*, 1964, *189*, 985.

Uses. The properties and uses of sweet birch oil are similar to those of methyl salicylate (see p.263). A dose of 0.3 to 1 ml has been used.

2616-c

Bucloxic Acid. 804CB. 3-(3-Chloro-4-cyclohexylbenzoyl)propionic acid.

$C_{16}H_{19}ClO_3$=294.8.

CAS — 32808-51-8.

Uses. Bucloxic acid has analgesic, anti-inflammatory, and antipyretic properties. It is used, as the calcium salt, in doses equivalent to 400 mg of the acid 2 or 3 times daily.

References: *Arzneimittel-Forsch.*, 1974, *24*, 1359–1444.

Proprietary Names

Esfar (calcium salt) *(Midy, Fr.)*.

2617-k

Bucolome. 5-Butyl-1-cyclohexylbarbituric acid.
$C_{14}H_{22}N_2O_3$=266.3.

CAS — 841-73-6.

An odourless, white or almost white, crystalline powder with a bitter taste. M.p. about 83°. Practically **insoluble** in water; freely soluble in alcohol, acetone, chloroform, and methyl alcohol.

Adverse Effects. Adverse effects occurring with bucolome include dry mouth, stomatitis, gastro-intestinal disorders, headache, drowsiness, ataxia, and, rarely, leucopenia and thrombocytopenia.

Absorption and Fate.
A review of the metabolism of uricosuric agents, including bucolome.— S. Kitazawa, *Yakkyoku*, 1976, *27*, 9, per *Int. pharm. Abstr.*, 1978, *15*, 86.

Uses. Bucolome has analgesic, anti-inflammatory, and antipyretic actions. It is used in the treatment of inflammatory and rheumatic disorders in doses of 0.6 to 1.2 g daily in divided doses. It has also been used in the treatment of gout in doses of 300 to 900 mg daily in divided doses.

Bucolome has been used in 20 neonates with non-haemolytic jaundice and, prophylactically, in 5 premature infants; although a reduction in albumin-bilirubin binding capacity could not be ruled out there did not seem to be any clinical consequences. Until its mechanism of action had been further elucidated it should not be used to treat neonates with hyperbilirubinaemia because of the potential risk of a reduction in albumin-bilirubin binding capacity and because its effect is delayed. Bucolome should only be used prophylactically when the binding capacity can be monitored.— C. Romagnoli *et al.* (letter), *Lancet*, 1978, *1*, 772. See also G. Segni *et al.*, *Archs Dis. Childh.*, 1977, *52*, 549; T. Yamamoto and Y. Adachi (letter), *ibid.*, 1978, *53*, 349; G. Segni *et al.*, *ibid.*

Gout. A report of the efficacy of alternate-day therapy with uricosuric agents, including bucolome.— T. Nishizawa *et al.*, *Rheumatol. Rehabil.*, 1978, *17*, 143.

Thrombo-embolic disorders. For a report on the use of bucolome with warfarin for the prevention of thrombo-embolic complications following mitral valve replacement, see I. Sakashita *et al.*, *Jap. Heart J.*, 1978, *19*, 324.

Proprietary Names
Paramidin *(Jap.)*.

2618-a

Bufexamac. 2-(4-Butoxyphenyl)acetohydroxamic acid.
$C_{12}H_{17}NO_3$=223.3.

CAS — 2438-72-4.

Almost colourless pearly flakes. M.p. 158° to 160° with decomposition.

Adverse Effects. When given by mouth bufexamac may cause gastro-intestinal irritation, particularly in patients with a history of peptic ulcer. Stinging and burning may occur after application of the cream; allergic reactions have been reported.

A report of allergic contact dermatitis with bufexamac.— G. Smeenk, *Dermatologica*, 1973, *147*, 334.

Absorption and Fate.
After administration by mouth of 125 to 500 mg of bufexamac, absorption was rapid and about 75% of the dose was excreted as a conjugate, probably the glucuronide. About 6% was excreted as a conjugate of 4-butoxyphenylacetic acid and less than 1% as free bufexamac or 4-butoxyphenylacetic acid. The peak rate of excretion was after 3 to 6 hours and excretion was complete within 24 hours.— D. R. Borham *et al.*, *J. pharm. Sci.*, 1972, *61*, 164.

Studies *in vitro* and *in vivo* on the penetration of bufexamac from ointment and cream bases into human skin.— H. Schaefer and G. Stüttgen, *Arzneimittel-Forsch.*, 1978, *28*, 1021.

Uses. Bufexamac has analgesic, antipyretic, and anti-inflammatory properties and has been used, in doses of 0.75 to 1.5 g daily, for rheumatic disorders. It has also been used as 1-g suppositories.

As a 5% cream bufexamac is applied topically, in a wide range of dermatoses and in pruritus. It has also been applied for the local treatment of rheumatic and traumatic conditions.

For reviews of the pharmacology and topical use of bufexamac.— *Drug & Ther. Bull.*, 1974, *12*, 102; R. N. Brogden *et al.*, *Drugs*, 1975, *10*, 351; *Drugs Today*, 1976, *12*, 435.

Rheumatic disorders. In a double-blind study in 40 patients with acute periarthritis of the shoulder local infiltration of 20 mg of a 2% suspension of bufexamac was as effective in reducing pain and discomfort as infiltration of 40 mg of triamcinolone acetonide in 4% suspension; 14 patients in each group required a second injection. Both injections caused local pain lasting 1 or 2 days in 13 of 39 patients who returned after the first injection and local irritation among 6 of the 28 receiving second injections. Further local treatment with other drugs was required by 8 patients.— A. Mardjuadi and J. Dequeker, *Curr. med. Res. Opinion*, 1978, *5*, 401.

Osteoarthritis. There was a reduction in pain in the majority of 30 patients with osteoarthritis of the knee who received from 1 to 6 intra-articular injections of bufexamac 20 mg; there was no change in joint size. Reduction in pain, limping and functional incapacity was also considered to be good in 26 of 37 patients with abarticular rheumatism who received a similar dose. Local tenderness after injection occurred on 3 occasions and a further patient had a painful inflammatory reaction in the elbow. In a double-blind study triamcinolone and bufexamac were considered to be of similar efficacy in the treatment of a further 40 patients with abarticular rheumatism. One patient who received bufexamac had a painful reaction after injection. Bufexamac might be a useful alternative to steroid therapy in rheumatology.— M. Wauters, *Curr. ther. Res.*, 1978, *23*, 685.

Rheumatoid arthritis. Bufexamac, 250 mg four times daily by mouth and 1 g as a suppository at night, was compared in a double-blind study with indomethacin, 25 mg thrice daily, in 25 patients with rheumatoid arthritis. Bufexamac appeared to give some relief of symptoms but there was no significant difference between the 2 treatments.— K. Pavelka and F. Wagenhauser, *Curr. ther. Res.*, 1970, *12*, 69.

Twenty-four patients with rheumatoid arthritis were treated with bufexamac, 0.75 to 1.5 g daily (as an enteric-coated preparation) for 1 month. Improvement in morning stiffness and functional activities was more marked than was relief of pain.— B. S. Rose *et al.*, *Curr. ther. Res.*, 1970, *12*, 150.

Skin disorders. In a double-blind study of 83 patients suffering from various skin disorders bufexamac cream 5% was applied to 1 side of the body and betamethasone cream 0.1% or fluocinolone cream 0.025% to the other side. After 4 weeks' treatment no significant difference was found between results obtained with bufexamac and those obtained with betamethasone or fluocinolone, although the recorded results were slightly better for fluocinolone compared with bufexamac.— Report No. 191 of the General Practitioner Research Group, *Practitioner*, 1975, *214*, 689.

Bufexamac 5% and betamethasone valerate 0.1% were equally effective in the treatment of 72 patients with dermatitis. Both were applied as creams twice daily for 2 weeks.— P. Wolf-Jürgensen, *Curr. med. Res. Opinion*, 1979, *5*, 779.

Further favourable reports on the use of bufexamac as cream or ointment in various skin disorders.— J. Van Der Meersch, *Curr. ther. Res.*, 1974, *16*, 904 (psoriasis); J. C. Valle-Jones, *Practitioner*, 1974, *213*, 383.

In a double-blind multicentre study in 193 patients with various forms of dermatitis, bufexamac cream 5% was no more effective than placebo and significantly less effective than creams containing either hydrocortisone 1% or triamcinolone acetonide 0.1%— J. V. Christiansen *et al.*, *Dermatologica*, 1977, *154*, 177.

Proprietary Preparations

Parfenac *(Lederle, UK)*. Bufexamac, available as a cream containing 5% in an aqueous basis. (Also available as Parfenac in *Arg.*, *Austral.*, *Fr.*, *Ger.*, *Switz.*).

Other Proprietary Names
Droxaryl *(Belg., Neth.)*; Flogocid *(Switz.)*; Mofenar *(Spain)*; Norfemac *(Canad.)*; Paraderm *(Austral.)*; Parfenal *(Ital.)*.

Bufexamac was also formerly marketed in Great Britain under the proprietary name Feximac (*Nicholas Laboratories*).

2619-t

Bumadizone Calcium. Calcium 2-(1,2-diphenylhydrazinocarbonyl)hexanoate hemihydrate.
$(C_{19}H_{21}N_2O_3)_2Ca,\frac{1}{2}H_2O$=699.9.

CAS — 3583-64-0 (bumadizone); 34461-73-9 (calcium salt, anhydrous).

Adverse Effects. The commonest side-effects occurring with bumadizone calcium are gastro-intestinal disturbances.

Uses. Bumadizone calcium has analgesic and anti-inflammatory properties and is used in the treatment of rheumatic disorders in doses of 220 mg twice or thrice daily initially and 110 mg twice or thrice daily for maintenance.

Rheumatic disorders. Reports of the efficacy of bumadizone calcium in rheumatoid arthritis and other rheumatic disorders.— M. Widhammer and W. Frenger, *Arzneimittel-Forsch.*, 1973, *23*, 1813; R. Medenica *et al.*, *ibid.*, 1817; L. Solomon and G. Abrams, *S. Afr. med. J.*, 1977, *52*, 391.

Proprietary Names
Bumaflex *(Byk Liprandi, Arg.)*; Eumotol *(Byk Gulden, Ger.; Byk Gulden, Ital.; Byk Gulden, S.Afr.; Byk Gulden, Spain; Byk Gulden, Switz.; Valpan, Fr.)*; Rheumatol *(Tosse, Ger.)*.

2620-l

Calcium Carbaspirin. Calcium Acetylsalicylate Carbamide; Carbasalate Calcium. A 1:1 complex of calcium acetylsalicylate and urea.
$C_{19}H_{18}CaN_2O_9$=458.4.

CAS — 5749-67-7.

A white amorphous powder. **Soluble** 1 in 4.3 of water at 37°.

Uses. Calcium carbaspirin has analgesic, anti-inflammatory, and antipyretic actions and has been used similarly to aspirin (see p.240) in doses equivalent to 300 to 900 mg of aspirin, up to 5 times daily.

Proprietary Names
Alcacyl *(Wander, Switz.)*; Ascal *(ACF, Neth.)*; Calurin *(Dorsey, USA)*; Iromin *(Omegin, Ger.; Schmidgall, Switz.)*.

2621-y

Calcium Succinate.
$C_4H_4CaO_4,3H_2O$=210.2.

CAS — 140-99-8 (anhydrous); 5793-96-4 (trihydrate).

White crystals or granular powder. Slightly **soluble** in water; soluble in dilute acids.

Uses. Calcium succinate has been employed together with aspirin in the treatment of arthritis but it is of doubtful value.

Proprietary Preparations
Rheumalgesia Dellipsoids D5 *(Pilsworth, UK)*. Tablets each containing calcium succinate 250 mg and aspirin 300 mg.

Preparations containing calcium succinate were also formerly marked in Great Britain under the proprietary names Berex and Dolcin (*Clinod Pharmaceuticals*).

2622-j

Carbamoylphenoxyacetic Acid. Salicylamide *O*-acetic acid. (2-Carbamoylphenoxy)acetic acid.
$C_9H_9NO_4$=195.2.

CAS — 25395-22-6.

Crystals. M.p. 221°. **Soluble** in aqueous alkaline solutions.

Uses. Carbamoylphenoxyacetic acid is an analgesic and antipyretic agent used topically as the diethylamine salt in the treatment of rheumatic disorders, neuralgia, and muscular pain. It was formerly given by mouth and (as the sodium salt) parenterally.

Proprietary Names
Akistin *(diethylamine salt) (Hormonchemie, Ger.)*.

2623-z

Chlorthenoxazin. 2-(2-Chloroethyl)-2,3-dihydro-4*H*-1,3-benzoxazin-4-one.
$C_{10}H_{10}ClNO_2$=211.6.

CAS — 132-89-8.

A fine white odourless or almost odourless powder. Practically **insoluble** in water.

Uses. Chlorthenoxazin is a mild analgesic, antipyretic, and anti-inflammatory agent that has been used in the treatment of pain in a dose of 500 mg.

Proprietary Names
Apirogen *(Dessy, Ital.)*; Betix *(Saba, Ital.)*; Ossazin *(Scalari, Ital.)*; Ossazone *(Brocchieri, Ital.)*; Ossipirina *(Radiumfarma, Ital.)*; Oxal *(Saita, Ital.)*; Reugaril *(Farber-Ref, Ital.)*; Reulin *(Isola-Ibi, Ital.)*; Reumital *(Farge, Ital.)*.

2624-c

Choline Magnesium Trisalicylate. A mixture of choline salicylate and magnesium salicylate.

CAS — 64425-90-7.

Uses. Choline magnesium trisalicylate has actions and uses similar to Aspirin, p.235.
It is used in the treatment of rheumatoid disorders in doses equivalent to 1 or 1.5 g of salicylate twice daily. Each unit dose of 500 mg of salicylate is provided by approximately 293 mg of choline salicylate with 362 mg of magnesium salicylate (anhydrous).

A brief review of non-aspirin salicylate drugs concluded that there was insufficient data to judge whether they were as effective as aspirin, or better tolerated, in the treatment of inflammatory disorders.— *Med. Lett.*, 1978, *20*, 100.

The absorption and fate of choline magnesium trisalicylate.— A. Cohen *et al.*, *Curr. ther. Res.*, 1978, *23*, 358; A. Cohen, *ibid.*, 772; *idem*, 1980, *27*, 692.

Blood-loss in the faeces of 10 patients who had taken up to 4.2 g of aspirin daily for 2 weeks was significantly greater than when they took placebo. The blood-loss was not increased in a further 10 patients who took 3 g of salicylate daily for 2 weeks as choline magnesium trisalicylate. Side-effects due to aspirin or choline magnesium trisalicylate were similar.— A. Cohen and H. E. Garber, *Curr. ther. Res.*, 1978, *23*, 187. An absence of effect on platelet aggregation and serotonin release.— M. B. Zucker and K. G. Rothwell, *ibid.*, 194.

Osteoarthrosis. There was no significant difference between the efficacy of choline magnesium trisalicylate equivalent to 1 to 2 g of salicylate or indomethacin 25 to 50 mg both taken twice daily for 7 weeks in a multicentre study completed by 86 patients with osteoarthritis but choline magnesium trisalicylate was more effective in reducing pain of the knee joints and indomethacin more effective in lumbar-spine joints. Side-effects were similar for both drugs and were responsible for withdrawal of 6 of 51 patients who took choline magnesium trisalicylate and 8 of 58 who took indomethacin. Side-effects for choline magnesium trisalicylate were reported to be tinnitus, constipation, gastro-intestinal distress, lightheadedness, headache and rash.— A. Goldenberg *et al.*, *Curr. ther. Res.*, 1978, *24*, 245.

Rheumatoid arthritis. Choline magnesium trisalicylate was comparable with ibuprofen in patients with rheumatoid arthritis except that it produced a greater reduction in swollen joints.— G. E. Ehrlich *et al.*, *Rheumatol. Rehabil.*, 1980, *19*, 30. Similar findings in a comparison with aspirin. Side-effects were greater with aspirin.— W. J. Blechman and B. L. Lechner, *ibid.*, 1979, *18*, 119.

Proprietary Preparations
Trilisate *(Napp, UK)*. Scored tablets each containing choline magnesium trisalicylate equivalent to salicylate 500 mg. (Also available as Trilisate in *USA*).

2625-k

Choline Salicylate. (2-Hydroxyethyl)trimethylammonium salicylate.
$C_{12}H_{19}NO_4$=241.3.

CAS — 2016-36-6.

A white, odourless, crystalline, very hygroscopic powder. M.p. about 50°. A 10% solution in water has a pH of about 6.5.
Very **soluble** in water, alcohol, and acetone; practically insoluble in ether and light petroleum.

Adverse Effects, Treatment, and Precautions. As for Aspirin, p.236, p.238. Choline salicylate is reported to be less irritant to the gastric mucosa.

A 21-month-old boy developed salicylate poisoning after the mother had rubbed the contents of 3 tubes of 'Bonjela' teething ointment on his gums over 48 hours.— A. S. Paynter and F. W. Alexander (letter), *Lancet*, 1979, *2*, 1132.

Uses. Choline salicylate has actions similar to those of aspirin (see p.240). It is used similarly to aspirin in doses of 0.87 to 1.74 g three or four times a day. Children aged 6 to 12 years have been given 210 to 420 mg every 4 hours. It is also used as a local analgesic. A 20% solution is employed in ear affections and an 8.7% gel in lesions of the mouth and nose.

Administration in haemophilia. In 3 patients with haemophilia A and in 10 controls choline salicylate, codeine, dextropropoxyphene, pentazocine, and prednisone, had no appreciable effect on bleeding time. These agents were considered suitable for patients with haemophilia.— R. A. Binder *et al.*, *Am. J. Dis. Child.*, 1974, *127*, 371.

Analgesia. In a trial of 27 patients with acute ear pain, choline salicylate ear-drops (Audax) relieved the pain in a significantly shorter time (18 minutes) than aspirin by mouth (106 minutes). This suggested that the action of the salicylate was peripheral.— H. R. Hewett, *Practitioner*, 1970, *204*, 438. A similar report.— N. Lawrence, *Br. J. clin. Pract.*, 1970, *24*, 478.

Rheumatic disorders. An evaluation of choline salicylate for arthritits.— *Med. Lett.*, 1976, *18*, 119.

Reports on the use of choline salicylate in rheumatic disorders.— G. W. Davis *et al.*, *Am. J. med. Sci.*, 1960, *239*, 273, per *Abstr. Wld Med.*, 1960, *28*, 276; A. D. Everett (letter), *Lancet*, 1961, *2*, 316; S. Miller, *Curr. ther. Res.*, 1979, *26*, 198.

Preparations

Audax *(Napp, UK)*. Ear-drops containing in each ml choline salicylate 200 mg and an ethylene oxide-polyoxypropylene glycol condensate 12.5 mg. For painful conditions of the ear. (Also available as Audax in *Ger.*).

Bonjela *(Lloyds Pharmaceuticals, Reckitt & Colman Pharm., UK)*. A gel containing choline salicylate 8.7%, cetalkonium chloride 0.01%, menthol 0.057%, alcohol 39%, and glycerol 4.6% (all w/w), in a flavoured basis. For lesions of the buccal and nasal mucosa. To be applied with massage 3 or 4 times daily before meals and at bedtime.

Teejel Gel (Moore's) *(Napp, UK)*. A gel for topical application containing choline salicylate 8.7% and cetalkonium chloride 0.01%. For relief of pain from lesions of the buccal mucosa. (Also available as Teejel in *Belg.*).

Other Proprietary Names
Arthropan *(Canad., USA)*; Mundisal *(Norw.)*; Salicol *(Ital.)*; Syrap *(Fr.)*.

2626-a

Cicloprofen. SQ 20824. 2-(Fluoren-2-yl)propionic acid.
$C_{16}H_{14}O_2$=238.3.

CAS — 36950-96-6.

Uses. Cicloprofen is an anti-inflammatory agent. Doses of 50 to 200 mg have been given 4 times daily in pharmacokinetic studies.

References.— T. W. Mischler *et al.*, *J. clin. Pharmac.*, 1975, *15*, 563.

Manufacturers
Squibb, UK.

2627-t

Cinchophen *(B.P. 1953)*. Phenylcinchoninic Acid; Quinophan; Acifenokinolin. 2-Phenylquinoline-4-carboxylic acid.
$C_{16}H_{11}NO_2$=249.3.

CAS — 132-60-5.

Pharmacopoeias. In *Arg.*, *Aust.*, *Braz.*, *Hung.*, *It.*, *Mex.*, *Port.*, *Span.*, and *Swiss.*

White or yellowish, almost odourless crystals or powder with a slightly bitter taste. M.p. 213° to 216°.
Practically **insoluble** in water; soluble 1 in 40 of acetone, 1 in 120 of alcohol, 1 in 400 of chloroform, 1 in 100 of ether; soluble in solutions of alkali hydroxides and carbonates. **Protect** from light.

Adverse Effects. Cinchophen may produce symptoms including vomiting, skin lesions, and angioneurotic oedema. It may also cause severe hepatic symptoms such as acute hepatitis, jaundice, and yellow atrophy of the liver. The symptoms may not be immediately evident and may proceed even when the drug has been discontinued. Toxicity is unrelated to dosage or to previous medication and the fact that cinchophen medication has been given previously without ill effects is not guarantee that the next course of treatment will not cause jaundice.

Uses. Cinchophen possesses analgesic and antipyretic actions similar to those of the salicylates. It was mainly used in doses of 300 to 600 mg, in the treatment of chronic gout but because of its toxcity it has been superseded by other analgesics.

2628-x

Clofezone. ANP 3260. A mixture of clofexamide and phenylbutazone in equimolecular proportions.

CAS — 17449-96-6.

Uses. Clofezone has analgesic and anti-inflammatory properties and is used in the treatment of rheumatism and other inflammatory disorders in doses of 200 to 400 mg thrice daily.

Proprietary Names
Panas *(Jap.)*; Perclusone *(Boehringer, Arg.*; *Anphar-Rolland, Fr.*; *Mack, Illert., Ger.*; *Pierrel, Ital.*; *Mack, Switz.)*; Perclustop *(Uquifa, Spain)*.

2629-r

Clometacin. Clométacine. [3-(4-Chlorobenzoyl)-6-methoxy-2-methylindol-1-yl]acetic acid.
$C_{19}H_{16}ClNO_4$=357.8.

CAS — 25803-14-9.

Adverse Effects.
For a report of hepatitis associated with the use of clometacin, see C. Lenoir *et al.*, *Nouv. Presse méd.*, 1978, *7*, 3035.

Uses. Clometacin is an analgesic structurally related to indomethacin. It is used for the relief of postoperative, traumatic, and rheumatic pain in doses of up to 900 mg daily in divided doses.

Proprietary Names
Dupéran *(Cassenne, Fr.)*.

2630-j

Clonixin. CBA 93626; Sch 10304. 2-(3-Chloro-*o*-toluidino)nicotinic acid.
$C_{13}H_{11}ClN_2O_2$=262.7.

CAS — 17737-65-4.

A colourless or cream-coloured solid with a very bitter taste. M.p. about 234°.

Uses. Clonixin has analgesic and anti-inflammatory actions. It has been used in doses of up to 600 mg.

As an analgesic following surgery or for postpartum patients, clonixin 600 mg by mouth appeared to be as effective as morphine sulphate 10 mg by injection. Minor side-effects included nausea, dizziness, drowsiness, headache, and euphoria.— J. S. Finch and T. J. DeKornfeld, *J. clin. Pharmac.*, 1971, *11*, 371.

Reduced effect, compared with aspirin, on platelet aggregation and bleeding time.— Y. S. Arkel *et al.*, *J. clin. Pharmac.*, 1976, *16*, 30.

In a double-blind study, clonixin 900 mg daily was more effective than placebo and physical therapy in reducing swelling, pain, and tenderness associated with soft-tissue sports injuries.— K. D. Fitch *et al.*, *Aust. J. Sports Med.*, 1977, *9*, 56.

Manufacturers
Schering, USA.

Proprietary Names
Dolalgial (as lysinate) *(Pharmainvesti, Spain)*; Dorixina (as lysinate) *(Roemmers, Arg.)*.

2631-z

Cymene. *p*-Cymene; *p*-Cymol. 4-Isopropyl-1-methylbenzene; 4-Isopropyltoluene.
$C_{10}H_{14}$=134.2.

CAS — 25155-15-1; 99-87-6 (p-cymene).

A colourless transparent liquid with an aromatic odour. B.p. 176° to 177°. Sp. gr. 0.8551. **Insoluble** in water; soluble in alcohol, chloroform, and ether.

Uses. Cymene is a local analgesic applied as a 30% ointment for the relief of pain in lumbago, sciatica, and rheumatic conditions.

Proprietary Names
Dolcymene *(Roland-Marie, Fr.; Semar, Spain)*.

2632-c

Diclofenac Sodium. Diclophenac Sodium; GP 45840. Sodium [2-(2,6-dichloroanilino)phenyl]-acetate.
$C_{14}H_{10}Cl_2NNaO_2$=318.1.

CAS — 15307-86-5 (diclofenac); 15307-79-6 (sodium salt).

Adverse Effects. As for Ibuprofen, p.256.

Adverse reactions were observed in 1564 of 18 992 patients who received diclofenac sodium. Reactions included gastro-intestinal disturbances (1340), oedema (117), skin reactions (103), pruritus (20), dizziness (16), malaise (10), headache (9), drowsiness (9), jaundice (2), and bleeding tendency (1).— *Japan med. Gaz.*, 1978, *15* (July 20), 10.

Lack of any clinical effect from diclofenac on thyroid function.— P. D. Fowler (letter), *Br. med. J.*, 1980, *281*, 1282.

Allergy. All of 11 aspirin-sensitive asthmatic patients developed reactions (rhinorrhoea, tightness of chest, wheezing, dyspnoea) after taking diclofenac in doses of 10 to 25 mg.— A. Szczeklik *et al.*, *Br. med. J.*, 1977, *2*, 231.

Effects on liver. A report of 3 patients in whom hepatic dysfunction occurred during treatment with diclofenac.— *Japan med. Gaz.*, 1976, *13* (Apr. 20), 10.

Effects on muscle. Myoclonus occurred in a man who had taken diclofenac for 4 months and disappeared 48 hours after stopping the drug.— M. Alcalay *et al.*, *Sem. Hôp. Paris*, 1979, *55*, 679.

Precautions. As for Ibuprofen, p.256.

A study in *rats* indicated that diclofenac sodium should be regarded as potentially hazardous for patients with a hereditary hepatic porphyria.— G. H. Blekkenhorst *et al.* (letter), *Lancet*, 1980, *1*, 1367. Criticisms of extrapolating data obtained from *animal* experiments to the treatment of human disease.— M. J. Brodie (letter), *ibid.*, *2*, 86; A. Gorchein (letter), *ibid.*, 152.

Interactions. A study in healthy subjects indicating that diclofenac decreases renal clearance of lithium.— I. W. Reimann and J. C. Frölich, *Clin. Pharmac. Ther.*, 1981, *30*, 348.

Absorption and Fate. Diclofenac is absorbed from the gastro-intestinal tract. Peak plasma concentrations occur about 2 hours after ingestion of enteric-coated tablets. At therapeutic concentrations it is more than 99% bound to plasma proteins. It is metabolised and excreted mainly in the urine. Small amounts are excreted in the bile.

References: P. J. Brombacher *et al.*, *Arzneimittel-Forsch.*, 1977, *27*, 1597; J. V. Willis *et al.*, *Eur. J. clin. Pharmac.*, 1979, *16*, 405.

Uses. Diclofenac sodium is a phenylacetic acid derivative which has analgesic, antipyretic, and anti-inflammatory actions. It is used mainly in the treatment of rheumatoid arthritis and other rheumatic disorders in doses of 25 to 50 mg thrice daily. It has also been given as a suppository.

A review of the actions and uses of diclofenac.— R. N. Brogden *et al.*, *Drugs*, 1980, *20*, 24.

In a 2-week double-blind study in 29 patients with osteoarthritis of the hip or knee, diclofenac 50 mg twice daily was as effective as naproxen 250 mg twice daily in relieving pain and stiffness and more effective in improving hip- or knee-joint movement.— P. Siraux, *J. int. med. Res.*, 1977, *5*, 169.

Further reports on the use of diclofenac sodium in rheumatic disorders.— W. Siegmeth and W. Sieberer, *J. int. med. Res.*, 1978, *6*, 369; W. Siegmeth and P. Placheta, *Schweiz. med. Wschr.*, 1978, *108*, 349; G. J. Abrams *et al.*, *S. Afr. med. J.*, 1978, *53*, 442; B. I. Schubiger *et al.*, *J. int. med. Res.*, 1980, *8*, 167; R. J. Chiswell *et al.*, *Br. J. clin. Pract.*, 1980, *34*, 203; *idem*, 207.

Proprietary Preparations

Voltarol *(Geigy, UK)*. Diclofenac sodium, available as 3-ml **Ampoules** of an injection containing 25 mg per ml; as **Suppositories** each containing 100 mg; and as enteric-coated **Tablets** of 25 and 50 mg.

Other Proprietary Names

Aflamin *(Ital.)*; Blesin, Dichronic, Neriodin, Prophenatin, Seecoren, Sofarin, Tsudohmin (all *Jap.)*; Voltaren *(Arg., Belg., Denm., Ger., Ital., Jap., Neth., Spain, Switz.)*; Voltarène *(Fr.)*.

2633-k

Diethylamine Salicylate *(B.P.)*.
$C_{11}H_{17}NO_3$=211.3.

CAS — 4419-92-5.

Pharmacopoeias. In *Br.*

White or almost white, odourless or almost odourless crystals. M.p. 100° to 102°. **Soluble** 1 in less than 1 of water, 1 in 2 of alcohol, and 1 in 1.5 of chloroform. **Protect** from light. Avoid contact with iron or iron salts.

Uses. Diethylamine salicylate is a topical analgesic used, usually at a concentration of 5 or 10%, in creams for rheumatic and muscular pain.

Preparations

Diethylamine Salicylate Cream *(B.P.)*. A dispersion of diethylamine salicylate in a suitable basis. Store at a temperature not exceeding 25°.

Algesal *(Nicholas, UK)*. Cream containing diethylamine salicylate 10%. For pain in muscles and joints. (Also available as Algesal in *Denm., Ital., Neth., Norw., S.Afr.*).

Aradolene *(Rorer, UK)*. Cream containing diethylamine salicylate 5%, a water-soluble capsicum preparation 0.4%, rectified camphor oil 1.4%, and menthol 2.5%. For rheumatic conditions.

Other Proprietary Names
Almyderm *(Denm.)*.

A preparation containing diethylamine salicylate was formerly marketed in Great Britain under the proprietary name Vascutonex (*Wellcome Consumer Division*).

2634-a

Difenamizole. AP14. 2-Dimethylamino-*N*-(1,3-diphenylpyrazol-5-yl)propionamide.
$C_{20}H_{22}N_4O$=334.4.

CAS — 20170-20-1.

White or yellowish-white, odourless, tasteless crystals or powder. Practically **insoluble** in water; sparingly soluble in alcohol; freely soluble in acetone and chloroform; soluble in ethyl acetate. M.p. about 125°.

Adverse Effects. Gastro-intestinal disturbances are reported to be the most frequent adverse effects occurring with difenamizole.

Hepatitis associated with difenamizole in 1 patient.— S. Imoto *et al.* (letter), *Ann. intern. Med.*, 1979, *91*, 129.

Uses. Difenamizole is an analgesic which is claimed also to have anti-inflammatory, antipyretic, and muscle-relaxing properties. It is used for the relief of the less severe types of pain in a dose of 75 mg thrice daily.

Proprietary Names
Pasalin *(Jap.)*.

2635-t

Diflunisal. MK 647. 5-(2,4-Difluorophenyl)salicylic acid.
$C_{13}H_8F_2O_3$=250.2.

CAS — 22494-42-4.

White crystals. M.p. about 212°. **Soluble** in most organic solvents and in dilute alkalis.

Adverse Effects and Treatment. As for Aspirin, p.236 and p.238. The commonest side-effects occurring with diflunisal are gastro-intestinal disturbances, although the incidence may be slightly less than with aspirin. Peptic ulceration and gastro-intestinal bleeding have been reported. Skin rash, pruritus, dizziness, drowsiness, headache, and tinnitus may also occur.

Effects on blood. A report of an *in vitro* study indicating that diflunisal inhibits platelet aggregation.— D. P. Mikhailidis *et al.* (letter), *Lancet*, 1980, *2*, 215.

Platelet aggregation in patients treated with diflunisal.— M. L. Ghosh and A. Tingle, *Curr. med. Res. Opinion*, 1980, *6*, 510.

Effects on the gastro-intestinal tract. A report of perforated duodenal ulcer after 7 days' treatment with diflunisal.— R. Talbot and H. Rees (letter), *Br. med. J.*, 1978, *2*, 1229.

Severe gastro-intestinal bleeding occurred in a 66-year-old woman following treatment with diflunisal.— A. K. Admani and D. M. N. F. Khaleque (letter), *Lancet*, 1979, *1*, 1247. Reports to the Committee on Safety of Medicines on diflunisal up to Feb 1979, included: gastro-intestinal haemorrhage (9), haematemesis (22), rectal haemorrhage (2), and melaena (13).— *ibid.*

Further reports of gastro-intestinal disturbances, haematemesis, and melaena.— B. Scott (letter), *Br. med. J.*, 1979, *1*, 489; A. M. Mason (letter), *Br. med. J.*, 1979, *1*, 888.

Studies which indicated that patients treated with diflunisal had fewer gastric lesions and less gastro-intestinal bleeding than patients treated with aspirin.— V. M. Tringham and P. Cochrane (letter), *Lancet*, 1979, *1*, 1409; M. Petrillo *et al.*, *ibid.*, 1979, *2*, 638.

Effects on the kidneys. A report of acute interstitial nephritis, presenting as acute oliguric renal failure, erythroderma, and eosinophilia following the use of diflunisal.— L. K. Chan, *Br. med. J.*, 1980, *280*, 84.

Effects on liver. A 64-year-old man developed cholestatic jaundice 5 days after starting to take diflunisal; the condition slowly regressed when diflunisal was withdrawn.— J. S. Warren, *Br. med. J.*, 1978, *2*, 736.

Erythema multiforme. Diflunisal was probably responsible for the Stevens-Johnson syndrome in 2 patients.— J. A. Hunter *et al.* (letter), *Br. med. J.*, 1978, *2*, 1088. Four severe cases of the Stevens-Johnson syndrome in patients taking diflunisal have been reported.— *Pharm. J.*, 1979, *1*, 318.

Overdosage. A 47-year-old woman who took 29 g of diflunisal over 40 minutes, with pseudoephedrine, developed dizziness and blurred vision and became unconscious, recovering spontaneously within 24 hrs.— H. P. Upadhyay and S. K. Gupta (letter), *Br. med. J.*, 1978, *2*, 640.

Treatment. Failure of alkaline diuresis to enhance diflunisal elimination.— M. Balali-Mood and L. F. Prescott, *Br. J. clin. Pharmac.*, 1980, *10*, 163.

Precautions. As for Aspirin, p.238.

Interactions. *Antacids.* Concomitant administration of diflunisal and aluminium hydroxide reduced the bioavailability of diflunisal by about 40%.— R. Verbeeck *et al.*, *Br. J. clin. Pharmac.*, 1979, *7*, 519.

Aspirin. Aspirin 600 mg daily or 300 mg four times daily given in combination with diflunisal 250 mg twice daily had no significant effect on diflunisal plasma concentrations in 14 healthy subjects but aspirin 600 mg four times daily reduced diflunisal plasma concentrations. This was not considered to be clinically important.— P. Schulz *et al.*, *J. int. med. Res.*, 1979, *7*, 61.

Absorption and Fate. Diflunisal is well absorbed from the gastro-intestinal tract and peak plasma concentrations occur about 2 hours after ingestion of a single dose. It is extensively bound to plasma protein and has an elimination half-life of about 11 hrs. It is excreted mainly as glucuronide conjugates in the urine. Less than 5% of a single dose is excreted in the faeces. Diflunisal is excreted in breast milk.

A review of the absorption and fate, actions, and drug interactions of diflunisal.— K. F. Tempero *et al.*, *Br. J. clin. Pharmac.*, 1977, *4*, *Suppl.* 1, 31S.

In single-dose studies in 9 healthy subjects, diflunisal was almost completely absorbed from the gastro-intestinal tract. The major pathway for diflunisal metabolism was conjugation with glucuronic acid and both ester and ether glucuronides were identified. Diflunisal was 98% bound to human plasma protein *in vitro*, and metabolites were not bound to plasma protein.— D. J. Tocco *et al.*, *Drug Metab. & Disposit.*, 1975, *3*, 453.

For reports on the elimination of diflunisal in renal failure, see under Administration in Renal Failure (Uses).

Uses. Diflunisal has analgesic, anti-inflammatory, and antipyretic actions similar to aspirin. It is used as an analgesic in postoperative pain, post-traumatic pain, and in osteoarthritis.

In acute pain an initial dose of 500 mg is given followed by 250 to 500 mg twice daily as required. In the treatment of chronic pain the usual maintenance dose is 250 mg twice daily.

Reviews of the pharmacology, adverse effects, metabolism, and uses of diflunisal.— C. A. Stone *et al.*, *Br. J. clin. Pharmac.*, 1977, *4*, *Suppl.* 1, 19S; S. L. Steelman *et al.*, *Clin. Ther.*, 1978, *1*, *Suppl.* A, 1; *Drugs Today*, 1978, *14*, 269; *Drug & Ther. Bull.*, 1978, *16*, 101; *Chemist Drugg.*, 1978, *209*, 556; R. N. Brogden *et al.*, *Drugs*, 1980, *19*, 84.

Administration in renal failure. Renal excretion of diflunisal was reduced in 17 patients with renal insufficiency compared with 5 healthy subjects. The impaired excretion was associated with increased diflunisal-glucuronide retention in the plasma. The plasma elimination half-life of 10.8 hours obtained in the healthy subjects was progressively prolonged with increasing degrees of renal function impairment.— P. J. De Schepper *et al.*, *Br. J. clin. Pharmac.*, 1977, *4*, 645P. See also R. Verbeeck *et al.*, *ibid.*, 1979, *7*, 273; G. Levy (letter), *ibid.*, 1979, *8*, 601; E. M. Faed (letter), *ibid.*, 1980, *10*, 185.

Influence of chronic renal failure and haemodialysis on diflunisal plasma protein binding.— R. K. Verbeeck and P. J. De Schepper, *Clin. Pharmac. Ther.*, 1980, *27*, 628.

Analgesia. In a multicentre study completed by 1902 patients of whom 967 received diflunisal and 935 received aspirin for treatment of acute pain, mainly due to sprains, strains, and osteoarthritis, diflunisal was considered to be slightly more effective than aspirin and to produce slightly fewer side-effects with significantly less gastro-intestinal side-effects.— E. C. Huskisson, *Practitioner*, 1979, *222*, 415.

Further studies on the use of diflunisal in the treatment of sprains, strains, and fractures.— H. Schlemmer and H. D. Braun, *Dt. med. Wschr.*, 1977, *102*, 1920; I. D. Adams, *Curr. med. Res. Opinion*, 1978, *5*, 580; G. V. Jaffé *et al.*, *ibid.*, 584; J. Barrau, *Clin. ther.*, 1978, *1*, *Suppl.* A, 43, per *Int. pharm. Abstr.*, 1978, *15*, 924; R. Barrington, *Curr. med. Res. Opinion*, 1980, *6*, 630.

Postoperative. In a double-blind study of 150 patients with moderate or severe pain following meniscectomy, diflunisal 500 mg as a single dose was as effective as aspirin 600 mg as a single dose in relieving pain, but doses of 125 mg and 250 mg of diflunisal were not as effective. The duration of action of diflunisal was significantly longer than aspirin.— W. J. Honig *et al.*, *J. int. med. Res.*, 1978, *6*, 172.

Further studies on the efficacy of diflunisal in postoperative pain.— C. Van Winzum and B. Rodda, *Br. J. clin. Pharmac.*, 1977, *4*, *Suppl.* 1, 39S; P. De Vroey *et al.*, *Acta ther.*, 1977, *3*, 205; P. De Vroey, *Clin. Ther.*, 1978, *1*, *Suppl.* A, 30; B. J. Wes, *ibid.*, 34; W. J. Honig, *Curr. med. Res. Opinion*, 1978, *5*, 536; M. E. Buck and D. B. Paintin, *ibid.*, 548; N. Papathéodossiou, *ibid.*, 1979, *6*, 154; J. A. Forbes *et al.*, *Clin. Pharmac. Ther.*, 1980, *27*, 253.

Effects on haemostasis. In 20 healthy subjects, diflunisal 500 mg twice daily for 1 week had only a slight effect on platelet aggregation. Bleeding times were not affected.— C. T. S. Sibinga, *Br. J. clin. Pharmac.*, 1977, *4*, *Suppl.* 1, 37S.

Osteoarthrosis. In two clinical studies involving a total of 810 patients with osteoarthrosis, diflunisal was superior to both aspirin and ibuprofen in overall response as assessed by both patients and investigators. Fewer gastro-intestinal side-effects occurred with diflunisal.— A. Andrew *et al.*, *Br. J. clin. Pharmac.*, 1977, *4*, *Suppl.* 1, 45S.

Further studies on the efficacy of diflunisal in osteoarthritis.— W. K. Essigman *et al.*, *Curr. med. Res. Opinion*, 1978, *5*, 550; B. Bresnihan *et al.*, *ibid.*, 556; J. A. Wojtulewski *et al.*, *ibid.*, 562; M. F. Grayson, *ibid.*, 567; V. J. Cirillo *et al.*, *Clin. Trials J.*, 1978, *15*, 40; I. Bahous *et al.*, *Clin. Ther.*, 1978, *1*, *Suppl.* A, 10; P. Kaklamanis *et al.*, *ibid.*, 20; E. Bautz-Holter, *ibid.*, 25; M. F. Grayson, *Rheumatol. Rehabil.*, 1978, *17*, 265; G. B. W. Tait *et al.*, *N.Z. med. J.*, 1978, *88*, 28; M. F. Grayson, *Curr. med. Res. Opinion*, 1978, *5*, 567; P. A. Dieppe and E. C. Huskisson, *Rheumatol. Rehabil.*, 1979, *18*, 53; W. K. Essigman *et al.*, *Ann. rheum. Dis.*, 1979, *38*, 148; J. G. M. Keet, *J. int. med. Res.*, 1979, *7*, 272.

Proprietary Preparations

Dolobid *(Morson, UK)*. Diflunisal, available as tablets of 250 and 500 mg. (Also available as Dolobid in *Austral.*, *Ital.*).

Other Proprietary Names

Dolisal *(Peru)*; Donobid *(Costa Rica, Denm., Fin.)*; Dopanone *(Greece)*; Dorbid *(Braz.)*; Unisal *(Switz.)*.

2636-x

Diftalone. L-5418. Phthalazino[2,3-*b*]phthalazine-5,12(7*H*,14*H*)-dione.
$C_{16}H_{12}N_2O_2$=264.3.

CAS — 21626-89-1.

Practically **insoluble** in water; soluble in chloroform and ethyl acetate.

Absorption and Fate.

Studies on the absorption, metabolism, and excretion of diftalone.— G. Buniva *et al.*, *Int. J. clin. Pharmac. Biopharm.*, 1977, *15*, 460; L. T. Tenconi *et al.*, *ibid.*, 485; M. S. Benedetti *et al.*, *Arzneimittel-Forsch.*, 1977, *27*, 2364; J. C. Garnham *et al.*, *J. Pharm. Pharmac.*, 1978, *30*, 407.

Uses. Diftalone has analgesic and anti-inflammatory actions. It has been used in the treatment of rheumatoid arthritis and osteoarthrosis. It has been given in initial doses of 1 g daily in divided doses and maintenance doses of 500 to 750 mg daily in divided doses.

Effects on blood. Diftalone 750 mg daily for 7 days decreased platelet adhesiveness in 10 patients with atherosclerosis. Serum-lipid concentrations were not significantly altered.— A. Nicolaescu, *Clin. Trials J.*, 1977, *14*, 89.

Osteoarthrosis. A multicentre 4-week study among 140 selected patients aged 25 to 75 years with osteoarthrosis in knee or hip showed that treatment with diftalone caused significant dose-related improvement. Patients received 1 g daily in divided doses for 1 week, 750 mg daily for 1 week, and 500 mg daily for the following 2 weeks. Most improvement occurred during the first week. Paracetamol was freely available to all patients. Adverse reactions causing withdrawal from treatment occurred in 7 patients and side-effects in 53 others included dizziness, heartburn, nausea, epigastric pain, headache, drowsiness, skin rashes, faintness, and tachycardia.— G. C. Pinheiro, *Curr. med. Res. Opinion*, 1976, *4*, 402.

Further studies on the use of diftalone in osteoarthrosis.— L. Mattara *et al.*, *Clin. Trials J.*, 1977, *14*, 30.

Rheumatoid arthritis. Studies on the use of diftalone in rheumatoid arthritis.— L. Brown *et al.*, *Clin. Trials J.*, 1977, *14*, 50; J. Vachtenheim, *ibid.*, 98; F. Chalem *et al.*, *J. int. med. Res.*, 1977, *5*, 18; P. Sfikakis and D. Charalambopoulos, *Acta ther.*, 1977, *3*, 237; A. Šusta *et al.*, *Clin. Trials J.*, 1977, *14*, 145.

Thyroiditis. A report on the use of diftalone in subacute thyroiditis.— R. Doleček, *J. int. med. Res.*, 1977, *5*, 346.

Proprietary Names

Retilon *(Lepetit, Spain)*.

2637-r

Dipyrocetyl. UCB 5080; Diacetsalicylic Acid. *OO*-Diacetylpyrocatechol-3-carboxylic acid; 2,3-Diacetoxybenzoic acid.
$C_{11}H_{10}O_6$=238.2.

CAS — 486-79-3.

Practically **insoluble** in water; soluble in organic solvents.

Uses. Dipyrocetyl is an acetoxy derivative of aspirin.

Proprietary Names

Movirene *(UCB, S.Afr.)*.

2638-f

Dipyrone. Analginum; Metamizol; Aminopyrine-sulphonate Sodium; Sodium Noramidopyrine Methanesulphonate; Sulpyrine; Methampyrone; Novamidazofen; Natrium Novaminsulfonicum; Noramidazophenum; Noraminophenazonum. Sodium *N*-(2,3-dimethyl-5-oxo-1-phenyl-3-pyrazolin-4-yl)-*N*-methylaminomethanesulphonate monohydrate.
$C_{13}H_{16}N_3NaO_4S,H_2O$=351.4.

CAS — 68-89-3 (anhydrous); 5907-38-0 (monohydrate).

Pharmacopoeias. In *Arg.*, *Aust.*, *Braz.*, *Chin.*, *Ger.*, *Hung.*, *Jap.*, *Jug.*, *Nord.*, *Pol.*, *Roum.*, *Rus.*, *Swiss*, and *Turk.*

A white or yellowish-white odourless crystalline powder with a bitter taste. **Soluble** 1 in 1.5 of water and 1 in 30 of alcohol; very slightly soluble in chloroform; practically insoluble in ether. A 4.65% solution in water is iso-osmotic with serum. Solutions in water turn yellow on standing. Solutions are **sterilised** by autoclaving or by filtration. **Incompatibilities** similar to those of amidopyrine. **Protect** from light.

From a study of the decomposition of dipyrone it was suggested that optimum stability would be obtained if the drug were completely anhydrous and the atmosphere excluded. Improved stability for liquid forms could be achieved by incorporating an antoxidant and storing in an inert atmosphere.— D. D. Dubash and W. E. Moore, *J. pharm. Sci.*, 1972, *61*, 386.

Adverse Effects and Precautions. As for Amidopyrine, p.245.

Allergy. Cross-sensitivity between aspirin and dipyrone occurred in one patient. Dipyrone produced an exacerbation of dyspnoea, cyanosis, and respiratory arrest.— E. Bartoli *et al.* (letter), *Lancet*, 1976, *1*, 1357.

Effects on blood. The AMA Registry of Adverse Reactions recorded 40 cases of agranulocytosis presumed to be due to dipyrone and a further 22 possibly due to the drug in the period 1957–66. A hypersensitivity reaction was probably involved.— *Med. Lett.*, 1973, *15*, 4.

An analysis of blood dyscrasias reported to the Swedish Adverse Drug Reaction Committee for the 5-year period 1966–70 showed that agranulocytosis attributable to dipyrone had been reported on 27 occasions (7 fatal). It was estimated that reported figures represented one-third of the true frequency.— L. E. Bottiger and B. Westerholm, *Br. med. J.*, 1973, *3*, 339.

Precautions. Dipyrone could aggravate haemorrhagic tendencies. Severe hypothermia might result if dipyrone and chlorpromazine were given concomitantly.— *Med. Lett.*, 1973, *15*, 4.

Uses. Dipyrone is the sodium sulphonate of amidopyrine (see p.245) and has similar properties. Its use is justified only in serious or life-threatening situations where no alternative antipyretic is available or suitable. The usual dose is 0.5 to 1 g given up to 3 times daily. It has also been given by subcutaneous, intramuscular, or intravenous injection in doses of 0.5 to 1 g.

References: S. Hady (letter), *Br. med. J.*, 1973, *1*, 744; S. N. Daftary *et al.*, *Curr. med. Res. Opinion*, 1980, *6*, 614; S. Mukherjee and S. Sood, *ibid.*, 619; C. V. Patel *et al.*, *ibid.*, 624.

Preparations

Iniectabile Natrii Novaminsulfonici *(Swiss P.)*. Dipyrone 50 g, sodium thiosulphate 100 mg, Water for Injections to 100 ml; the solution is prepared and the ampoules filled in an atmosphere of nitrogen. Protect from light.

Jap. P. (Sulpyrine Injection) and *Pol. P.* include a similar injection.

Proprietary Names

Adolkin (magnesium analogue) *(Kin, Spain)*; Alginodia *(Upjohn, Arg.)*; Espyre *(Jap.)*; Lagalgin *(Lagap, Switz.)*; Lasain (magnesium analogue) *(Lasa, Spain)*; Metilon *(Jap.)*; Minalgin *(Streuli, Switz.)*; Neo-Melubrina *(Hoechst, Spain)*; Nolotil (magnesium analogue) *(Castejon, Spain)*; Novalgin *(Hoechst, Ger.; Hoechst, Neth.; Winthrop, S.Afr.; Hoechst, Switz.)*; Novalgina *(Hoechst, Arg.)*; Novalgine *(Hoechst, Belg.; Hoechst, Fr.)*; Novaminsulfon *(Drobena, Ger.)*; Novemina *(Lazar, Arg.)*; Reflex Rectal *(Liade, Spain)*; Sulfonovin *(Ibsa, Switz.)*; Tapal *(Sterwin, Spain)*.

2639-d

Ditazole. Diethamphenazole; S 222. 2,2′-[(4,5-Diphenyloxazol-2-yl)imino]diethanol monohydrate.
$C_{19}H_{20}N_2O_3,H_2O$=342.4.

CAS — 18471-20-0 (anhydrous).

Uses. Ditazole is an anti-inflammatory agent with an inhibitory effect on platelet aggregation. It is used in the treatment of phlebitis, thrombosis, and similar disorders in doses of 400 mg twice or thrice daily.

Pharmacology in *animals*.— L. Caprino *et al.*, *Arzneimittel-Forsch.*, 1973, *23*, 1272–87.

Metabolism.— E. Marchetti *et al.*, *Arzneimittel-Forsch.*, 1973, *23*, 1291.

Proprietary Names
Ageroplas *(Serono, Ital.)*.

2640-c

Epirizole. Mepirizole; DA 398. 4-Methoxy-2-(5-methoxy-3-methylpyrazol-1-yl)-6-methylpyrimidine.
$C_{11}H_{14}N_4O_2$=234.3.

CAS — 18694-40-1.

A white or pale yellow crystalline powder with a characteristic odour and a bitter taste. M.p. 90° to 92°. Sparingly **soluble** in water; very soluble in alcohol.

Adverse Effects.
Adverse effects occurred on 1583 occasions in 23 524 patients who received epirizole and included gastro-intestinal disturbances (1372), rash (71), stomatitis (50), dizziness (28), headache (26), oedema of fingers (16), anxiety (6), drowsiness (5), and tinnitus (2).— *Japan med. Gaz.*, 1976, *13* (Mar. 20), 14.

Uses. Epirizole has analgesic, anti-inflammatory, and antipyretic actions. It has been used as an analgesic in doses of 150 to 450 mg daily in 2 to 4 divided doses.

Proprietary Names
Daicon *(Ibi, Ital.)*; Mebron *(Ethimed, S.Afr.)*; Mepiral *(Robert, Spain)*.

2641-k

Etenzamide. Aethoxybenzamidum; Ethenzamide; Ethoxybenzamide; Ethylsalicylamide; HP 209. 2-Ethoxybenzamide.
$C_9H_{11}NO_2$=165.2.

CAS — 938-73-8.

Pharmacopoeias. In *Jap.*

A white or almost white, almost odourless, tasteless, crystalline powder. M.p. 131° to 134°. Practically **insoluble** in cold water; slightly soluble in boiling water and in ether; soluble in alcohol and acetone; freely soluble in chloroform. A saturated solution in water is neutral to litmus.

Uses. Etenzamide has analgesic, anti-inflammatory, and antipyretic actions. It has been given in doses of up to 4 g daily in divided doses.

In a study in 12 patients, gastro-intestinal blood loss was significantly lower after treatment with etenzamide than after treatment with aspirin.— P. Bernades *et al.*, *Thérapie*, 1970, *25*, 715.

Proprietary Names
Lucamid *(Lundbeck, Denm.)*; Trancalgyl *(Innothéra, Fr.)*.

2642-a

Ethosalamide. Salicylamide 2-ethoxyethyl ether. 2-(2-Ethoxyethoxy)benzamide.
$C_{11}H_{15}NO_3$=209.2.

CAS — 15302-15-5.

Uses. Ethosalamide has analgesic and antipyretic properties and has been used, usually in conjunction with paracetamol and caffeine, for less severe types of pain.

A preparation containing ethosalamide was formerly marketed in Great Britain under the proprietary name Antidol (*Lewis*).

2643-t

Ethoxazene Hydrochloride. SN 612; Etoxazene Hydrochloride; *p*-Ethoxychrysoidine Hydrochloride. 4-(4-Ethoxyphenylazo)benzene-1,3-diyldiamine hydrochloride.
$C_{14}H_{16}N_4O,HCl$=292.8.

CAS — 94-10-0 (ethoxazene); 2313-87-3 (hydrochloride).

A reddish powder. Practically **insoluble** in water; soluble in boiling water and in alcohol.

Precautions. Ethoxazene is contra-indicated in patients with severe liver disease, uraemia, or chronic parenchymatous nephritis. It should be used with care in patients with gastro-intestinal disorders. Ethoxazene may colour the urine orange or red.

Uses. Ethoxazene hydrochloride is chemically related to phenazopyridine hydrochloride. It has been used to relieve pain in cystitis, urethritis, and pyelitis in doses of 100 mg thrice daily before meals.

Proprietary Names
Serenium *(Squibb, USA)*.

NOTE. The name Serenium has been applied to a preparation of medazepam.

2644-x

Etofenamate. B 577; TV 485. 2-(2-Hydroxyethoxy)ethyl *N*-(ααα-trifluoro-*m*-tolyl)anthranilate.
$C_{18}H_{18}F_3NO_4$=369.3.

CAS — 30544-47-9.

A pale yellow viscous liquid. Practically **insoluble** in water; miscible with organic solvents.

Uses. Etofenamate has analgesic and anti-inflammatory actions. It is applied topically as a 5% gel for the relief of rheumatic and muscular pain.

Absorption and fate of etofenamate.— H. -D. Dell *et al.*, *Arzneimittel-Forsch.*, 1977, *27*, 1322.

Studies on the use of etofenamate gel.— H. Klug, *Arzneimittel-Forsch.*, 1977, *27*, 1350; E. Waterloh and K. -H. Groth, *ibid.*, 1355; I. Heindl *et al.*, *ibid.*, 1357.

Proprietary Names
Rheumon *(Tropon, Ger.)*.

2645-r

Famprofazone. 4-Isopropyl-1-methyl-5-[*N*-methyl-*N*-(α-methylphenethyl)aminomethyl]-2-phenyl-4-pyrazolin-3-one.
$C_{24}H_{31}N_3O$=377.5.

CAS — 22881-35-2.

Uses. Famprofazone has analgesic and antipyretic properties and is claimed to have mild sympathomimetic properties. It has been used in doses of 25 to 50 mg up to thrice daily, usually in conjunction with other analgesics.

2646-f

Fenbufen. CL 82204. 4-(Biphenyl-4-yl)-4-oxobutyric acid.
$C_{16}H_{14}O_3$=254.3.

CAS — 36330-85-5.

Crystals. M.p. about 180°.

Adverse Effects and Precautions. Effects similar to those experienced with ibuprofen (p.256) may be expected.

Erythema multiforme associated with fenbufen.— A. Peacock and J. Ledingham, *Br. med. J.*, 1981, *283*, 582.

Absorption and Fate. Fenbufen is absorbed from the gastro-intestinal tract. It is metabolised to active metabolites which are reported to have half-lives of 10 hours or more. Excretion is mainly via the urine.

In a healthy subject given a single dose of fenbufen 600 mg the peak serum-fenbufen concentration was 8.69 µg per ml 45 minutes after administration. Major serum metabolites detected were 3-(4-biphenylylhydroxymethyl)propionic acid and 4-biphenylacetic acid which had previously been reported to possess the same spectrum of activity as fenbufen. About 50% of the dose was excreted in the urine within 2 days, the major urinary metabolites being 4′-hydroxy-4-biphenylacetic acid and 3-(4′-hydroxy-4-biphenylylhydroxymethyl)propionic acid.— G. E. Van Lear *et al.*, *J. pharm. Sci.*, 1978, *67*, 1662.

Further references.— G. Cuisinaud *et al.*, *Eur. J. clin. Pharmac.*, 1979, *16*, 59; H. J. Rogers *et al.*, *Clin. Pharmac. Ther.*, 1981, *29*, 74 (in renal insufficiency).

Uses. Fenbufen is a phenylbutyric acid derivative which has analgesic, anti-inflammatory, and antipyretic actions. It is used in the treatment of rheumatoid arthritis and osteoarthrosis in doses of 600 to 900 mg daily. Up to 600 mg may be given as a single daily dose at night.

Reviews of fenbufen: R. N. Brogden *et al.*, *Drugs*, 1981, *21*, 1.

Analgesia. A single dose of fenbufen 800 mg was as effective as aspirin 600 mg for the relief of postoperative pain. A dose of 400 mg also had significant effect.— A. Coutinho *et al.*, *Curr. ther. Res.*, 1976, *19*, 58.

In a double-blind study in 600 patients with pain following surgical removal of an impacted lower wisdom tooth, fenbufen 500 mg was superior to aspirin 750 mg and placebo. Doses were taken every 6 hours for 24 hours. Side-effects were minor and occurred less frequently following treatment with fenbufen.— P. -Å. Henrikson *et al.*, *J. int. med. Res.*, 1979, *7*, 107.

Further studies on the use of fenbufen for the relief of postoperative pain.— A. Sunshine, *J. clin. Pharmac.*, 1975, *15*, 591.

Osteoarthrosis. In a double-blind crossover study in 20 patients with osteoarthritis fenbufen 200 mg thrice daily was significantly more effective than placebo but less effective than indomethacin 25 mg thrice daily. Evidence of hepatotoxicity was detected in 5 patients while taking fenbufen.— R. Buxton *et al.*, *Curr. med. Res. Opinion*, 1978, *5*, 682.

Fenbufen was as effective as aspirin in the treatment of osteoarthrosis.— E. J. Valtonen, *Scand. J. Rheumatol.*, 1979, *Suppl.* 27, 1.

Rheumatoid arthritis. In a 12-week double-blind crossover study in 30 patients with rheumatoid arthritis fenbufen 400 to 600 mg daily was significantly superior to phenylbutazone 150 to 300 mg daily in respect of morning stiffness, grip strength, walking time, and ESR. Side-effects from fenbufen were largely limited to mild drowsiness.— I. de Salcedo *et al.*, *Curr. ther. Res.*, 1975, *18*, 295.

Further studies on the use of fenbufen in rheumatoid arthritis.— F. Chalem *et al.*, *Curr. ther. Res.*, 1977, *22*, 769; F. Ammitzbøll, *Scand. J. Rheumatol.*, 1979, *Suppl.* 23, 5 and 11; S. D. Deodhar and R. Sethi, *Curr. med. Res. Opinion*, 1979, *6*, 263.

Proprietary Preparations
Lederfen *(Lederle, UK)*. Fenbufen, available as **Capsules** and **Tablets** of 300 mg.

Other Proprietary Names
Bufemid *(Braz.)*; Cinopal *(Ital., S.Afr., Switz.)*.

2647-d

Fenclofenac. RX 67 408. [2-(2,4-Dichlorophenoxy)phenyl]acetic acid.
$C_{14}H_{10}Cl_2O_3$=297.1.

CAS — 34645-84-6.

A white to off-white powder. M.p. about 136°. Slightly **soluble** in water (pH 7.4) but less soluble in acid solutions. Freely soluble in most organic solvents.

Adverse Effects. Effects similar to those experienced with ibuprofen (p.256) may be expected.

In an open multicentre study 636 unwanted effects were reported by 229 out of 412 patients. Only 79 patients were withdrawn because of adverse effects and 13 of these subsequently took fenclofenac without further adverse effects. Side-effects were mainly gastro-intestinal disturbances (28.8%), central nervous system effects (27%), and dermatological effects (14.3%). Keratoconjunctivitis sicca and oedema of the legs were reported in a number of patients. Treatment was withdrawn in 4 patients with increased serum aminotransferases, 4 with increased blood-urea-nitrogen, and 1 with decreased platelet count.— R. B. Smith, *Proc. R. Soc. Med.*,

1977, *70, Suppl.* 6, 46.

Effects on the kidneys. A report of nephrotic syndrome in a patient taking fenclofenac.— D. V. Hamilton *et al.* (letter), *Br. med. J.*, 1979, *2*, 391.

Precautions. As for Ibuprofen, p.256.
Fenclofenac also appears to displace thyroid hormones from binding sites. This affects the feedback control mechanism and results in a reduction in total hormone concentration. Thyroid-function tests should therefore be interpreted with caution.

Effects on the thyroid. In a 56-year-old man taking fenclofenac, values for serum thyroxine and free thyroxine index were depressed, but the serum thyrotrophin concentration was normal. This led initially to a false diagnosis of secondary hypothyroidism.— A. J. Isaacs and B. E. Monk (letter), *Lancet*, 1980, *1*, 267. Similar findings in a study of sera from 9 patients under fenclofenac treatment. Although free thyroxine index is an imprecise measure of thyroid function in these patients, both free T_4 and TSH measurements were still capable of functional differentiation.— J. E. M. Midgley and T. A. Wilkins (letter), *ibid.*, *2*, 704.

A report on the effect of fenclofenac 600 mg twice daily on thyroid function in 10 healthy males given it for 28 days. The results indicated that fenclofenac resets the equilibria controlling the concentrations of circulating thyroid hormones and at steady state probably does not interfere with thyroid function. It thus clearly joins the group of drugs which alter readily measurable thyroid indices making interpretation of thyroid function tests difficult.— M. J. Humphrey *et al.*, *Reckitt & Colman* (letter), *Lancet*, 1980, *1*, 487.

Further references: W. A. Ratcliffe *et al.* (letter), *Lancet*, 1980, *1*, 432; B. Taylor *et al.*, *Br. med. J.*, 1980, *281*, 911; W. A. Ratcliffe *et al.* (letter), *ibid.*, 1282; S. J. Capper *et al.*, *Clin. Sci.*, 1980, *59* (Sept.), 26P.

Absorption and Fate. Fenclofenac is absorbed from the gastro-intestinal tract with peak plasma concentrations occurring 2 to 4 hours after ingestion of a single dose. It is metabolised by hydroxylation and conjugation. It is about 96% bound to plasma proteins.

Fenclofenac had a half-life of about 12 hours following administration of a single dose of 100 mg by mouth.— D. C. Atkinson *et al.* (letter), *J. Pharm. Pharmac.*, 1974, *26*, 357.

Uses. Fenclofenac is a phenylacetic acid derivative which has analgesic, anti-inflammatory, and antipyretic actions. It is used in the treatment of rheumatoid arthritis and other rheumatic disorders. It is usually given in doses of 0.6 to 1.2 g daily in 2 divided doses.

A seminar on fenclofenac.— *Proc. R. Soc. Med.*, 1977, *70, Suppl.* 6, 1–52.

References: N. H. Brodie *et al.*, *Br. J. clin. Pract.*, 1980, *34*, 279; H. Berry *et al.*, *Ann. rheum. Dis.*, 1980, *39*, 473.

Proprietary Preparations

Flenac (known in some countries as Feclan, Gidalon) *(Reckitt & Colman Pharmaceuticals, UK)*. Fenclofenac, available as tablets of 300 mg. (Also available as Flenac in *S.Afr.*).

2648-n

Fendosal. HP 129; P 71 0129. 5-(4,5-Dihydro-2-phenyl-3*H*-benz[*e*]indol-3-yl)salicylic acid.
$C_{25}H_{19}NO_3$=381.4.

CAS — 53597-27-6.

Uses. Fendosal has analgesic and anti-inflammatory actions. It has been used as an analgesic in doses of 200 to 400 mg.

Analgesia. *Postpartum.* Fendosal 200 or 400 mg was as effective as aspirin 650 mg in the relief of postpartum uterine pain and had a longer duration of action.— S. M. Bloomfield *et al.*, *Clin. Pharmac. Ther.*, 1978, *23*, 390.

Postoperative. Fendosal 400 mg as a single dose was more effective than a 200-mg dose or aspirin 650 mg (which were equivalent in effect) in patients with moderate to severe postoperative pain. Fendosal 100 mg was not an analgesic dose. The analgesic effect of fendosal appeared to last longer than that of aspirin.— S. A. Cooper *et al.*, *Clin. Pharmac. Ther.*, 1980, *27*, 249.

Proprietary Names

Alnovin *(Hoechst, USA)*.

2649-h

Fenoprofen Calcium *(B.P., U.S.P.)*. 69323; 53858 *(acid)*; Lilly 61169 *(sodium salt)*. Calcium (±)-2-(3-phenoxyphenyl)propionate dihydrate.
$(C_{15}H_{13}O_3)_2Ca,2H_2O$=558.6.

CAS — 31879-05-7 (fenoprofen); 34597-40-5 (calcium salt, anhydrous); 53746-45-5 (calcium salt, dihydrate).

Pharmacopoeias. In *Br.* and *U.S.*

A white or almost white odourless crystalline powder. M.p. 105° to 110°. Fenoprofen calcium (dihydrate) 1.1 g is approximately equivalent to 1 g of fenoprofen. **Soluble** 1 in 400 to 500 of water, 1 in 15 of alcohol, and 1 in 300 of chloroform. **Store** in airtight containers.

Adverse Effects. As for Ibuprofen, p.256. The Stevens-Johnson syndrome (erythema multiforme) has been reported.

Effects on blood. *Agranulocytosis.* Agranulocytosis occurred in a 55-year-old man who had started treatment with fenoprofen 8 weeks previously.— S. D. Simon and M. Kosmin (letter), *New Engl. J. Med.*, 1978, *299*, 490.

A report of pruritus and exfoliative rash following treatment with fenoprofen calcium in 1 patient, and associated with agranulocytosis.— P. J. Treusch *et al.* (letter), *J. Am. med. Ass.*, 1979, *241*, 2700.

Thrombocytopenia. Reports of thrombocytopenia associated with fenoprofen.— R. E. Simpson *et al.* (letter), *New Engl. J. Med.*, 1978, *298*, 629; M. E. Katz and P. Wang (letter), *Ann. intern. Med.*, 1980, *92*, 262.

Effects on the gastro-intestinal tract. The gastro-intestinal blood loss following fenoprofen calcium was significantly less than that following aspirin when both analgesics were given to 8 subjects in therapeutic doses every 6 hours for 4 days.— A. S. Ridolfo *et al.*, *Clin. Pharmac. Ther.*, 1973, *14*, 226. See also S. M. Chernish *et al.*, *Arthritis Rheum.*, 1979, *22*, 376.

Effects on the kidneys. Fenoprofen reduced renal function in 1 patient with systemic lupus erythematosus.— R. P. Kimberly *et al.*, *Am. J. Med.*, 1978, *64*, 804. Severe renal papillary necrosis was associated with administration of fenoprofen calcium (total dose 36 g in 30 days), in a patient with systemic lupus erythematosus and urinary-tract infection.— F. E. Husserl *et al.*, *J. Am. med. Ass.*, 1979, *242*, 1896.

Reversible renal failure and nephrotic syndrome developed in 2 patients who had been taking fenoprofen 1.8 to 2.4 g daily for up to a year. Renal biopsy in one patient revealed prominent interstitial nephritis.— J. H. Brezin *et al.*, *New Engl. J. Med.*, 1979, *301*, 1271.

Further reports of reversible renal failure and nephrotic syndrome.— G. A. Curt *et al.*, *Ann. intern. Med.*, 1980, *92*, 72 (one patient); S. P. Handa (letter), *ibid.*, *93*, 508 (two patients); J. Lorch *et al.* (letter), *ibid.*, 508 (one patient).

Effect on liver. Cholestatic jaundice and hepatitis developed in a 68-year-old woman after treatment with fenoprofen 600 mg four times daily for 7 weeks.— D. J. Stennett *et al.* (letter), *Am. J. Hosp. Pharm.*, 1978, *35*, 901.

Precautions. As for Ibuprofen, p.256. Aspirin is reported to reduce plasma concentrations of fenoprofen.

Interactions, drugs. Investigations in 18 subjects demonstrated that the administration of phenobarbitone might increase the rate of metabolism of fenoprofen.— L. Helleberg *et al.*, *Br. J. clin. Pharmac.*, 1974, *1*, 371.

Porphyria. A study in *rats* indicated that fenoprofen calcium would probably not elicit an acute attack in susceptible porphyric individuals.— G. H. Blekkenhorst *et al.* (letter), *Lancet*, 1980, *1*, 1367. Criticisms of extrapolating data obtained from *animal* experiments to the treatment of human disease.— M. J. Brodie (letter), *ibid.*, *2*, 86; A. Gorchein (letter), *ibid.*, 152.

Absorption and Fate. Fenoprofen is readily absorbed from the gastro-intestinal tract; peak plasma concentrations occur 1 to 2 hours after a dose; the half-life is about 2.5 hours. It is more than 99% bound to plasma proteins. About 95% of a dose is excreted in the urine in 24 hours, chiefly as the glucuronide and the glucuronide of hydroxylated fenoprofen. It has been detected in breast milk. Small amounts (about 2%) are excreted in the faeces.

References: A. Rubin *et al.*, *J. pharm. Sci.*, 1971, *60*, 1797; *idem*, 1972, *61*, 739; *idem*, *Clin. Pharmac. Ther.*, 1972, *13*, 151; J. F. Nash *et al.*, *J. pharm. Sci.*, 1979, *68*, 1087.

Uses. Fenoprofen calcium is a phenylpropionic acid derivative which has analgesic, anti-inflammatory, and antipyretic actions and is used in the treatment of mild to moderate pain and of rheumatic disorders. It may also be used as an antipyretic. The usual dose is the equivalent of 300 to 600 mg of fenoprofen 3 or 4 times a day.

Reviews of the pharmacology, adverse effects, and uses of fenoprofen.— C. M. Gruber, *J. Rheumatol.*, 1976, *3, Suppl.* 2, 8; R. N. Brogden *et al.*, *Drugs*, 1977, *13*, 241; *Aust. J. Pharm.*, 1978, *59*, 590.

Comparative reviews of fenoprofen, naproxen, and tolmetin.— *Med. Lett.*, 1976, *18*, 77; J. R. Lewis, *J. Am. med. Ass.*, 1977, *237*, 1260.

Analgesia. In studies in 270 patients given fenoprofen sodium, dextropropoxyphene hydrochloride, or both, in various dosages, the analgesic effect of fenoprofen was reported to be enhanced by dextropropoxyphene.— A. Sunshine and E. Laska, *Clin. Pharmac. Ther.*, 1971, *12*, 302. Similar results in episiotomy patients.— C. M. Gruber, *J. clin. Pharmac.*, 1976, *16*, 407.

Single doses of fenoprofen 200 mg and paracetamol 500 mg were given separately or together for postoperative pain in a double-blind controlled study involving 240 patients. Of the patients assessed for analgesia 2 hours after the dose, adequate pain relief was achieved in 18 of 47 who received only paracetamol, 23 of 52 who received only fenoprofen, 27 of 45 who received paracetamol and fenoprofen, and 12 of 40 who received placebo. Only paracetamol with fenoprofen produced significantly better analgesia than placebo.— I. T. Davie and N. H. Gordon, *Br. J. Anaesth.*, 1978, *50*, 931.

Further reports on the analgesic efficacy of fenoprofen.— J. E. Murphy *et al.*, *J. int. med. Res.*, 1978, *6*, 375.

A study in 27 patients with 36 affected joints indicated that fenoprofen calcium was effective in the treatment of acute gouty arthritis. Therapy consisted of an initial 800 mg every 6 hours on the first day followed by a variable dose not exceeding 3.2 g daily for up to a further 7 days.— S. Wanasukapunt *et al.*, *Arthritis Rheum.*, 1976, *19*, 933.

Osteoarthrosis. Similar responses with fenoprofen 200 mg to 600 mg as with aspirin 325 mg to 975 mg each given every 6 hours. Only 18 of 30 patients in the study could be evaluated for efficacy.— J. W. Brooke, *J. Rheumatol.*, 1976, *3, Suppl.* 2, 71. A similar study showing fenoprofen to be more effective than aspirin.— *idem*, *Curr. ther. Res.*, 1978, *23*, 538.

Further studies on the use of fenoprofen in osteoarthrosis.— J. A. Wojtulewski *et al.*, *Br. med. J.*, 1974, *2*, 475; W. Standel, *Clin. Trials J.*, 1978, *15*, 24; M. Thompson *et al.*, *Curr. ther. Res.*, 1979, *26*, 779; R. A. Durance *et al.*, *ibid.*, 791.

Rheumatoid arthritis. In a double-blind crossover trial in 60 patients with rheumatoid arthritis there was a significant improvement in pain, duration of morning stiffness, consumption of paracetamol, grip strength, and articular index after treatment with fenoprofen 400 to 600 mg four times a day, compared with placebo. Joint size and joint temperature were not affected. In a further trial comparing the effect of fenoprofen 2.4 g daily in 29 patients with that of aspirin 6 g daily in 31 patients there were only minor differences between the effects of the 2 drugs. Side-effects were significantly less common with fenoprofen which was well tolerated.— E. C. Huskisson *et al.*, *Br. med. J.*, 1974, *1*, 176.

Further studies of the use of fenoprofen in rheumatoid arthritis.— J. F. Fries and M. C. Britton, *Arthritis Rheum.*, 1973, *16*, 629; M. Franke and G. Manz, *Curr. ther. Res.*, 1977, *21*, 43; J. D. Davis *et al.*, *Clin. Pharmac. Ther.*, 1977, *21*, 52; J. E. Himes and I. F. Duff, *J. int. med. Res.*, 1977, *5*, 412; E. Semble *et al.*, *Clin. Pharmac. Ther.*, 1980, *27*, 286.

For comparisons of fenoprofen with naproxen and other nonsteroidal anti-inflammatory drugs in rheumatic disorders, see Naproxen, p.266.

Preparations

Fenoprofen Calcium Capsules *(U.S.P.)*. Capsules containing fenoprofen calcium. Potency is expressed in terms of the equivalent amount of fenoprofen. The *U.S.P.* requires 60% dissolution in 60 minutes and not less than 50% dissolution for any individual capsule.

Fenoprofen Calcium Tablets *(B.P.)*. Tablets containing fenoprofen calcium. They are film-coated. Potency is expressed in terms of the equivalent amount of fenoprofen.

Fenoprofen Calcium Tablets *(U.S.P.)*. Tablets containing fenoprofen calcium. Potency is expressed in terms of the equivalent amount of fenoprofen. The *U.S.P.* requires 60% dissolution in 60 minutes and not less than 50% dissolution for any individual tablet.

Proprietary Preparations

Fenopron *(Dista, UK)*. Fenoprofen calcium, available as tablets each containing the equivalent of 300 or 600 mg of fenoprofen. **Fenopron D.** Dispersible tablets each containing the equivalent of fenoprofen 300 mg. (Also available as Fenopron in *Austral., S.Afr.*).

Progesic *(Lilly, UK)*. Fenoprofen calcium, available as tablets each containing the equivalent of 200 mg of fenoprofen.

Other Proprietary Names

Fepron *(Belg., Ital., Neth.)*; Feprona *(Ger.)*; Nalfon *(Denm., Spain, Switz., USA)*; Nalgésic *(Fr.)*.

2650-a

Feprazone. Prenazone; Phenylprenazone; DA2370. 4-(3-Methylbut-2-enyl)-1,2-diphenylpyrazolidine-3,5-dione. $C_{20}H_{20}N_2O_2$=320.4.

CAS — 30748-29-9.

A white odourless tasteless crystalline powder. M.p. about 156°. Practically **insoluble** in water; slightly soluble in alcohol, ether, and methyl alcohol; very soluble in acetone and chloroform.

Adverse Effects. Gastro-intestinal disturbances, rashes, headache, and tinnitus have been reported.

Effects on blood. Thrombocytopenia and haemolytic anaemia associated with feprazone.— P. M. Bell and C. A. Humphrey, *Br. med. J.*, 1982, *284*, 17.

Precautions. As for Phenylbutazone, p.274. Blood counts should be performed before and during treatment.

Absorption and Fate. Feprazone is absorbed from the gastro-intestinal tract with peak plasma concentrations occurring 4 to 6 hours after ingestion. It has a plasma half-life of about 24 hours.

Uses. Feprazone is a pyrazole derivative which has analgesic, anti-inflammatory, and antipyretic actions. It is used in the treatment of rheumatoid arthritis and osteoarthrosis in doses of 200 to 600 mg daily in divided doses after food.

For a series of papers covering the properties and clinical uses of feprazone, see *Arzneimittel-Forsch.*, 1972, *22*, 171–281.

A study in 4487 patients showed that feprazone was effective in reducing inflammation after dental treatment.— C. Montanari, *Curr. ther. Res.*, 1975, *17*, 166.

Double-blind study of feprazone and phenylbutazone in acute gout.— J. A. Reardon *et al.*, *Curr. med. Res. Opinion*, 1980, *6*, 445.

Osteoarthrosis. In a double-blind crossover study feprazone 600 mg and ibuprofen 1.2 g daily were equally effective in 19 patients with osteoarthrosis.— L. S. Bain *et al.*, *Curr. med. Res. Opinion*, 1977, *4*, 665.

Respiratory disorders. In children with acute inflammation of the respiratory tract, feprazone and aspirin had similar antipyretic activity, and feprazone had slightly greater anti-inflammatory effect.— C. Montanari *et al.*, *Curr. ther. Res.*, 1974, *16*, 1101.

A study on the use of feprazone with bromhexine in paedatric respiratory disorders.— G. Pennacchio and G. Manfredi, *Minerva paediat.*, 1978, *30*, 1265.

Rheumatoid arthritis. In a double-blind crossover study of 14 patients with rheumatoid arthritis, the analgesic and anti-inflammatory activity of feprazone 450 mg daily was indistinguishable from that of indomethacin 75 mg daily. One patient discontinued feprazone because of a maculopapular rash; other side-effects were indigestion (1), dizziness (1), and rash (2).— R. Sturrock *et al.*, *Practitioner*, 1975, *215*, 94.

Further studies on the use of feprazone in rheumatoid arthritis.— P. M. G. Reynolds *et al.*, *Rheumatol. Rehabil.*, 1975, *14*, 67; R. M. Collins *et al.*, *Clin. Trials J.*, 1975, *12*, 25; I. Haslock *et al.*, *Rheumatol. Rehabil.*, 1976, *15*, 81; P. J. Rooney *et al.*, *Curr. med. Res. Opinion*, 1976, *3*, 642.

Proprietary Preparations

Methrazone *(WB Pharmaceuticals, UK: Boehringer Ingelheim, UK)*. Feprazone, available as capsules of 200 mg.

Other Proprietary Names

Arg.— Analud; *Ital.*—Zepelin; *Spain*—Brotazona, Danfenona, Grisona, Naloven, Nilatin, Prenazon, Rangozona, Represil, Tabrien; *Switz.*—Zepelin.

2651-t

Floctafenine. R 4318; RU 15750. 2,3-Dihydroxypropyl *N*-(8-trifluoromethyl-4-quinolyl)anthranilate. $C_{20}H_{17}F_3N_2O_4$=406.4.

CAS — 23779-99-9.

A yellowish-white powder. M.p. 175° to 178°. Slightly **soluble** in water; freely soluble in dimethylformamide and pyridine.

Adverse Effects. Gastro-intestinal disturbances, dizziness, drowsiness, headache, and occasionally tinnitus have been reported with floctafenine.

In a comparative study with aspirin, there was an upward trend in blood loss in 16 healthy subjects given floctafenine 0.2, 0.8, and 1.6 g but this was not significant compared to a control period. Six subjects taking floctafenine complained of 'hot urine' during early morning urination.— I. M. Baird (letter), *Br. J. clin. Pharmac.*, 1976, *3*, 936.

Absorption and Fate. Floctafenine is absorbed from the gastro-intestinal tract. It is metabolised in the liver to floctafenic acid. It is excreted mainly as glucuronide conjugates in the urine and bile.

A study in 1 subject suggested that floctafenic acid was responsible for the analgesic activity of floctafenine.— N. Gerber *et al.*, *Fedn Proc.*, 1976, *35*, 565.

Further studies on the metabolism and excretion of floctafenine.— J. Pottier *et al.*, *Drug Metab. & Disposit.*, 1975, *3*, 133; R. K. Lynn *et al.*, *J. clin. Pharmac.*, 1979, *19*, 20.

Uses. Floctafenine has analgesic and anti-inflammatory actions. It is used in doses of 200 mg as an analgesic for the relief of mild to moderate pain. It is also used in the treatment of rheumatoid arthritis and osteoarthrosis in doses of 200 to 400 mg four times a day.

Analgesia. In a double-blind crossover study in 77 patients after surgery, single doses of floctafenine 200 mg were significantly more effective for pain relief than dextropropoxyphene 130 mg and not significantly different from aspirin 600 mg. Side-effects after floctafenine included vomiting, dizziness, and somnolence.— S. Lipton *et al.*, *Curr. med. Res. Opinion*, 1975, *3*, 175.

In a double-blind crossover study in 40 post-cholecystectomy patients, floctafenine 200 mg was found to have analgesic activity intermediate between that of pethidine 75 mg and dextropropoxyphene 65 mg, all being given as single doses by mouth. Patients reported the fewest side-effects after floctafenine.— M. E. Morris and I. W. D. Henderson, *Clin. Pharmac. Ther.*, 1978, *23*, 383.

Studies on the use of floctafenine as an analgesic.— M. D. Vickers and F. A. Akbar, *J. int. med. Res.*, 1975, *3*, 32; D. M. Lomas *et al.*, *ibid.*, 1976, *4*, 179.

Further studies on the use of floctafenine as an analgesic in postoperative patients.— S. Lipton *et al.*, *Br. J. clin. Pract.*, 1975, *29*, 147; J. K. Stenport, *Curr. ther. Res.*, 1975, *18*, 303; S. Lipton *et al.*, *J. int. med. Res.*, 1975, *3*, 172; J. E. G. Walker and L. W. Kay, *Br. J. clin. Pract.*, 1976, *30*, 43.

Osteoarthrosis. Floctafenine 200 mg and ibuprofen 200 mg each given four times a day produced comparable pain relief in a double-blind crossover study of 30 patients with osteoarthritis.— V. M. Rhind *et al.*, *J. int. med. Res.*, 1978, *6*, 11.

Further references: M. J. Burke *et al.*, *Rheumatol. Rehabil.*, 1976, *15*, 97.

Rheumatoid arthritis. In a 6-week double-blind crossover study, floctafenine 400 mg four times daily and soluble aspirin 1 g four times daily were equally effective in the relief of symptoms in 48 patients with rheumatoid arthritis and were both superior to placebo. There was a significant fall of haemoglobin and greater incidence of positive occult blood during aspirin therapy than with placebo or floctafenine. There was no marked improvement in a further 12 similar patients who received floctafenine 1.6 g daily for 3 months but there was some improvement in 4 of these patients after continuing treatment for a further 3 months.— M. A. Hossain *et al.*, *Rheumatol. Rehabil.*, 1977, *16*, 260.

Further references: E. C. Huskisson and P. J. Scott, *Rheumatol. Rehabil.*, 1977, *16*, 54.

Proprietary Names

Idalon *(Roussel, Neth.)*; Idarac *(Roussel, Arg.; Houde, Belg.; Roussel, Canad.; Diamant, Fr.; Albert-Roussel, Ger.; Roussel Maestretti, Ital.; Roussel, S.Afr.)*.

2652-x

Flufenamic Acid *(B.P.)*. CI 440; INF 1837. *N*-(*ααα*-Trifluoro-*m*-tolyl)anthranilic acid. $C_{14}H_{10}F_3NO_2$=281.2.

CAS — 530-78-9.

Pharmacopoeias. In *Br.*

A pale yellow odourless crystalline powder. Practically **insoluble** in water; soluble 1 in 4 of alcohol, 1 in 7 of chloroform, and 1 in 3 of ether.

Adverse Effects. The commonest side-effects occurring with flufenamic acid are gastro-intestinal disturbances. Skin rash, depression, vertigo, tinnitus, leucopenia, and increased values for serum aminotransferases have occasionally been reported.

Treatment of Adverse Effects and Precautions. As for Mefenamic Acid, p.263.

Absorption and Fate. Flufenamic acid is absorbed from the gastro-intestinal tract and peak plasma concentrations occur about 6 to 8 hours following ingestion. It is extensively bound to plasma proteins. It is metabolised by hydroxylation and conjugation and excreted in the urine and the faeces. It is excreted in bile and enterohepatic circulation has been suggested.

A study in 10 nursing mothers and their infants, in the immediate post-partum period, indicated that only very small amounts of flufenamic acid were excreted into the breast milk and absorbed by the infant.— R. A. Buchanan *et al.*, *Curr. ther. Res.*, 1969, *11*, 533.

Uses. Flufenamic acid is an anthranilic acid derivative which has analgesic, anti-inflammatory, and antipyretic actions. It is used in the treatment of rheumatic disorders. It has also been tried in dysmenorrhoea. The usual dose is 400 to 600 mg daily in divided doses.

Dysmenorrhoea. In 16 women with recurrent severe dysmenorrhoea unresponsive to conventional treatment symptoms were relieved, except for mild nausea in 2 patients and dizziness in 1, in all patients in 31 cycles after the administration of flufenamic acid 125 mg four times daily on the first menstrual day, then thrice daily for 2 or 3 days. The effect was possibly due to inhibition of prostaglandin.— A. Schwartz *et al.*, *Obstet. Gynec.*, 1974, *44*, 709.

In a double-blind crossover study flufenamic acid 200 mg thrice daily produced significant pain relief compared with placebo in 36 of 44 patients with primary dysmenorrhoea; vomiting was reduced in 29 and diarrhoea in 23 patients respectively. Four patients experienced side-effects; dizziness in 2 and mild dyspepsia in 2.— L. Kapadia and M. G. Elder, *Lancet*, 1978, *1*, 348.

For a report of flufenamic acid being more effective than dextropropoxyphene with paracetamol in primary dysmenorrhoea, see Mefenamic Acid, p.263.

Migraine. For a report on the use of flufenamic acid for the symptomatic treatment of migraine, see Y. Vardi *et al.*, *Neurology, Minneap.*, 1976, *26*, 447.

Rheumatoid arthritis. Studies on the use of flufenamic acid in rheumatoid arthritis.— M. E. Fearnley and H. C. Masheter, *Ann. phys. Med.*, 1966, *8*, 204; M. R. Simpson *et al.*, *Ann. phys. Med.*, 1966, *8*, 208; I. C. Cowan and H. C. Masheter, *Clin. Trials J.*, 1966, *3*, 503; O. A. Sydnes, *Acta rheum. scand.*, 1967, *13*, 55, per *Abstr. Wld Med.*, 1968, *42*, 71.

Preparations

Flufenamic Acid Capsules *(B.P.)*. Capsules containing flufenamic acid. Store at a temperature not exceeding 30°.

Meralen *(Merrell, UK)*. Flufenamic acid, available as capsules of 100 mg.

Other Proprietary Names

Alfenamin *(Arg.)*; Ansatin *(Jap.)*; Arlef *(Austral., Belg., Fr., Ger., Ital., S.Afr., Switz.)*; Parlef *(Arg.)*; Sastridex, Surika *(both Ger.)*.

Flufenamic acid was also formerly marketed in Great Britain under the proprietary name Arlef *(Parke, Davis)*.

2653-r

Flurbiprofen. 2-(2-Fluorobiphenyl-4-yl)propionic acid.
$C_{15}H_{13}FO_2$=244.3.
CAS — 5104-49-4.

A colourless crystalline solid. M.p. about 110°. Slightly **soluble** in water; readily soluble in most organic solvents.

Adverse Effects. As for Ibuprofen, p.256.

In 354 patients who had been treated in various centres with flurbiprofen, 83 had gastro-intestinal side-effects, 10 had dermatological side-effects, and 21 had side-effects affecting the CNS. There were 2 reports of thrombocytopenia and 1 of neutropenia; these were of uncertain significance.— J. W. Buckler *et al.*, XIII International Congress of Rheumatology, Japan, 1973, p. 181.

In a long-term study in 1220 patients with rheumatic disorders treated with flurbiprofen, side-effects reported were gastro-intestinal (452), central nervous system (198), skin (75), renal (43), haematological (29), respiratory (45), cardiovascular (28), and miscellaneous (46). Some patients had also received additional drugs. There were no alterations in haematological and biochemical investigations.— F. E. Sheldrake *et al.*, *Curr. med. Res. Opinion*, 1977, *5*, 106.

Precautions. As for Ibuprofen, p.256.

A single dose of ibuprofen 200 mg or flurbiprofen 100 mg did not interfere with the following commercial urine tests: Albustix, Clinitest, Clinistix, Ictotest, Ketostix, Phenistix, or Labstix.— D. A. L. Morgan and D. J. Brown (letter), *Br. J. clin. Pharmac.*, 1977, *4*, 700.

Porphyria. A study in *rats* indicated that flurbiprofen would probably not elicit an acute attack in susceptible porphyric individuals.— G. H. Blekkenhorst *et al.* (letter), *Lancet*, 1980, *1*, 1367. Criticisms of extrapolating data obtained from *animal* experiments to the treatment of human disease.— M. J. Brodie (letter), *ibid.*, *2*, 86; A. Gorchein (letter), *ibid.*, 152.

Absorption and Fate. Flurbiprofen is readily absorbed from the gastro-intestinal tract with peak plasma concentrations occurring about 90 minutes after ingestion. It is reported to be about 99% bound to plasma proteins and to have an elimination half-life of about 3 to 4 hours. It is metabolised mainly by hydroxylation and conjugation and excreted in urine.

In 19 fasting volunteers given flurbiprofen 50 mg mean peak concentrations of about 5.5 µg per ml were achieved in about 1½ hours; the half-life was about 3.9 hours. It was extensively bound (99%) to plasma proteins. Three hydroxylated or methoxylated metabolites were found in the urine. More than 95% of a dose was recovered in the urine in 24 hours including glucuronides of the metabolites.— S. S. Adams *et al.*, XIII International Congress of Rheumatology, Japan, 1973, p. 173.

Further studies on the pharmacokinetics of flurbiprofen.— N. Cardoe *et al.*, *Curr. med. Res. Opinion*, 1975, *3*, *Suppl.* 4, 15; *idem*, 1977, *5*, 21.

Uses. Flurbiprofen is a phenylpropionic acid derivative which has analgesic, anti-inflammatory, and antipyretic actions. It is used in the treatment of rheumatoid arthritis and other rheumatic disorders. The usual dose is 150 to 200 mg daily in divided doses, increased to 300 mg daily in acute conditions.

Reviews on the actions and uses of flurbiprofen: R. N. Brogden *et al.*, *Drugs*, 1979, *18*, 417.

Symposiums on flurbiprofen.— XIII International Congress of Rheumatology, Japan, 1973, pp. 137–187; *Curr. med. Res. Opinion*, 1975, *3*, *Suppl.* 4, 1–52; *ibid.*, 1977, *5*, 1–140.

The anti-inflammatory and pharmacological effects of topically applied flurbiprofen on human skin.— A. K. Black *et al.*, *Br. J. Derm.*, 1979, *101*, *Suppl.* 17, 19.

Administration. Flurbiprofen 100 or 150 mg as a single dose at night was superior to placebo in relief of pain at night, morning stiffness, and sleep disturbance in patients with rheumatoid arthritis.— E. C. Huskisson *et al.*, *Curr. med. Res. Opinion*, 1977, *5*, 85.

A study in 30 patients with ankylosing spondylitis or coxarthrosis showed that twice daily dosage with flurbiprofen was as effective as thrice daily dosage.— P. Doury and S. Pattin, *Curr. med. Res. Opinion*, 1977, *5*, 127.

Ankylosing spondylitis. Flurbiprofen 150 to 200 mg daily showed similar efficacy to phenylbutazone 300 to 400 mg daily in a double-blind trial in 27 patients with ankylosing spondylitis. Subjective assessment of improvement tended to favour phenylbutazone, but was not significant.— H. R. Mena and R. F. Willkens, *Eur. J. clin. Pharmac.*, 1977, *11*, 263.

Further studies on the use of flurbiprofen in ankylosing spondylitis.— A. Calin and R. Grahame, *Br. med. J.*, 1974, *4*, 496; R. D. Sturrock and F. D. Hart, *Ann. Rheum. Dis.*, 1974, *33*, 129; F. D. Hart, *Curr. med. Res. Opinion*, 1975, *3*, *Suppl.* 4, 39; R. Grahame and A. Calin, *Scand. J. Rheumatol.*, 1975, *4*, *Suppl.* 8, S11–22; F. D. Hart, *ibid.*; A. Good and H. Mena, *Curr. med. Res. Opinion*, 1977, *5*, 117.

Blood disorders. Spontaneous platelet aggregation in a patient with polycythaemia rubra vera was unresponsive to aspirin but readily responsive to flurbiprofen.— C. Politis-Tsegos *et al.*, *Br. med. J.*, 1978, *1*, 1323.

Dysmenorrhoea. Beneficial effect and superior to aspirin in dysmenorrhoea.— U. R. Krisna *et al.*, *Br. J. clin. Pharmac.*, 1980, *9*, 605.

Hypotension. Addition of flurbiprofen 50 mg twice daily to fludrocortisone therapy relieved the symptoms of an 18-year-old girl with idiopathic orthostatic hypotension, who had not responded to fludrocortisone 400 µg daily alone.— C. M. Perkins and M. R. Lee (letter), *Lancet*, 1978, *2*, 1058. Similar effects were observed in 5 patients, 4 of whom were also taking fludrocortisone.— S. J. Watt *et al.*, *Clin. Sci.*, 1980, *59* (Sept.), 4P.

Osteoarthrosis. In a double-blind crossover study in 26 patients with osteoarthrosis, flurbiprofen 150 mg daily was as effective as indomethacin 75 mg daily. Side-effects occurred in 3 patients on indomethacin and none on flurbiprofen.— O. Frank, *Curr. med. Res. Opinion*, 1977, *5*, 91.

Further studies on the use of flurbiprofen in the treatment of osteoarthrosis.— O. Kogstad, XIII International Congress of Rheumatology, Japan, 1973, p. 156; E. N. Glick and A. A. J. Goldberg, *ibid.*, p. 178; H. R. Mena *et al.*, *J. int. med. Res.*, 1976, *4*, 152; N. Cardoe, *Curr. med. Res. Opinion*, 1977, *5*, 99; E. C. Huskisson *et al.*, *Eur. J. Rheumatol. Inflamm.*, 1979, *2*, 69.

Rheumatoid arthritis. In a long-term study in 1220 patients with rheumatoid arthritis, osteoarthrosis, and other rheumatic disorders, flurbiprofen in doses of 75 to 400 mg daily was effective in relieving symptoms. Some patients had been followed for up to 5 years and some also received other drugs. Side-effects were responsible for withdrawal from the study in 117 patients who received flurbiprofen alone and 123 who received additional drugs.— F. E. Sheldrake *et al.*, *Curr. med. Res. Opinion*, 1977, *5*, 106.

Further studies on the use of flurbiprofen in rheumatoid arthritis.— P. J. Rooney *et al.*, *Br. J. clin. Pharmac.*, 1978, *5*, 453; D. R. E. Barraclough *et al.*, *Med. J. Aust.*, 1974, *2*, 925; M. Nobunaga *et al.*, *Curr. med. Res. Opinion*, 1975, *3*, *Suppl.* 4, 45; H. A. Capel *et al.* (letter), *Br. J. clin. Pharmac.*, 1977, *4*, 623; H. R. Mena *et al.*, *J. clin. Pharmac.*, 1977, *17*, 56; P. M. Brooks and T. K. Khong, *Curr. med. Res. Opinion*, 1977, *5*, 53; B. L. Hazleman and D. Y. Bulgen, *Curr. med. Res. Opinion*, 1977, *5*, 58; W. Siegmeth, *ibid.*, 64; P. A. Franco *et al.*, *ibid.*, 74; H. H. Kruger, *ibid.*, 77; V. Pipitone *et al.*, *ibid.*, 88.

Thrombo-embolic disorders. For the absence of effect of flurbiprofen in the prophylaxis of deep-vein thrombosis after fracture of the femoral neck, see Heparin, p.768.

Urinary incontinence. In a double-blind crossover study in 30 women with detrusor instability flurbiprofen 50 mg thrice daily significantly relieved frequency, urgency, and urge incontinence.— L. D. Cardozo *et al.*, *Br. med. J.*, 1980, *280*, 281.

Proprietary Preparations

Froben *(Boots, UK)*. Flurbiprofen, available as tablets of 50 and 100 mg. (Also available as Froben in *S.Afr.*, *Switz.*).

Other Proprietary Names

Cebutid *(Fr.)*.

2654-f

Glafenine. Glaphenine. 2,3-Dihydroxypropyl *N*-(7-chloro-4-quinolyl)anthranilate.
$C_{19}H_{17}ClN_2O_4$=372.8.
CAS — 3820-67-5.

A white or slightly yellow crystalline powder. M.p. about 165°. Practically **insoluble** in water; slightly soluble in acetone and chloroform; soluble in dilute acids.

Adverse Effects. Side-effects reported include gastro-intestinal disturbances, headache, drowsiness, fever, and renal failure. Allergic reactions may occur.

Allergy. Reports of anaphylaxis and other allergic reactions occurring with glafenine.— D. Chivrac *et al.*, *Nouv. Presse méd.*, 1974, *3*, 2578; C. Barral and M. Faivre, *ibid.*, 1975, *4*, 2797; J. L. Michaud and L. Doublet, *ibid.*, 1976, *5*, 716; G. J. A. Burgers *et al.*, *Ned. Tijdschr. Geneesk.*, 1976, *120*, 528; R. H. B. Meyboom, *ibid.*, 926.

Effects on the eyes. A study indicating that usual therapeutic doses of glafenine interfere with colour vision.— J. Laroche and C. Laroche, *Annls pharm. fr.*, 1972, *30*, 433.

Effects on the kidneys. Reports of renal failure and interstitial nephritis often following overdosage with glafenine.— M. Gaultier *et al.*, *Nouv. Presse méd.*, 1972, *1*, 3125; D. Chevet *et al.*, *Thérapie*, 1974, *29*, 575; M. Gaultier *et al.*, *ibid.*, 579; J. Mirouze *et al.*, *ibid.*, 587; H. Duplay *et al.*, *ibid.*, 593; J. C. Renier *et al.*, *Nouv. Presse méd.*, 1975, *4*, 670; R. Montagnac *et al.*, *Pharm. Hosp. fr.*, 1978, *46*, 251, per *Int. pharm. Abstr.*, 1980, *17*, 58.

Effects on liver. Acute reversible hepatitis in 2 patients after taking therapeutic doses of glafenine.— R. T. J. M. Ypma *et al.* (letter), *Lancet*, 1978, *2*, 480.

Hepatitis in 5 patients who were taking glafenine.— B. H. Stricker and R. H. B. Meyboom, *Pharm. Weekbl. Ned.*, 1979, *114*, 405, per *Int. pharm. Abstr.*, 1980, *17*, 107.

Absorption and Fate. Glafenine is absorbed from the gastro-intestinal tract with peak plasma concentrations occurring about 1 to 2 hours after ingestion. The half-life is reported to be about 75 minutes. It is metabolised to glafenic acid and excreted in the urine and bile.

Studies on the absorption, metabolism, and excretion of glafenine.— J. Rondelet *et al.*, *Thérapie*, 1966, *21*, 1573; R. Mallein *et al.*, *Thérapie*, 1966, *21*, 1579; *idem*, 1976, *31*, 739.

Uses. Glafenine is an anthranilic acid derivative; it is an analgesic used for the relief of all types of pain. For acute pain 400 mg is given followed by 200 mg as required up to a total of 1 to 1.2 g daily. For less severe pain the initial dose is 200 to 400 mg followed by 200-mg doses up to a total of 600 to 800 mg daily. It has also been given, as the hydrochloride, as 500-mg and 1-g suppositories.

Studies on the analgesic efficacy of glafenine.— J. Ruedy and K. C. Bentley, *Clin. Pharmac. Ther.*, 1970, *11*, 718; J. Ruedy and M. O'Boyle, *J. clin. Pharmac.*, 1971, *11*, 378; D. M. Lithgow and J. Blecher, *S. Afr. med. J.*, 1971, *45*, 203.

For a comparison of the analgesic effect of glafenine, alclofenac, and paracetamol plus caffeine, see Alclofenac, p.245.

Administration in renal failure. A study in 20 subjects indicated that no modification of glafenine dosage was required in renal insufficiency. Further studies were needed on the effects of repeated doses in renal failure.— R. Mallein *et al.*, *Thérapie*, 1976, *31*, 739.

Proprietary Names of Glafenine and Glafenine Hydrochloride

Glifan *(Roussel Maestretti, Ital.)*; Glifanan *(Albert-Roussel, Ger.; Roussel, Arg.; Roussel, Belg.; Roussel, Fr.; Roussel, Neth.; Roussel, S.Afr.; Roussel, Switz.; Roussel-Amor Gil, Spain)*.

2655-d

Glucametacin. 2-{2-[1-(4-Chlorobenzoyl)-5-methoxy-2-methylindol-3-yl]acetamido}-2-deoxy-D-glucose monohydrate.
$C_{25}H_{27}ClN_2O_8,H_2O$=537.0.
CAS — 52443-21-7(anhydrous).

Adverse Effects. Gastro-intestinal disturbances, headache, and dizziness have been reported.

Fewer gastric lesions with glucametacin than with indomethacin.— E. Mirelli *et al.*, *Curr. med. Res. Opinion*, 1978, *5*, 648.

Uses. Glucametacin is a derivative of indomethacin with analgesic, anti-inflammatory, and antipyretic actions. It has been given in doses of 280 to 420 mg daily in divided doses in the treatment of various rheumatic disorders. It has also been administered as 140-mg suppositories.

Studies on the use of glucametacin in rheumatic disorders.— M. Giordano *et al.*, *Arzneimittel-Forsch.*, 1975, *25*, 435; P. Petera *et al.*, *Int. J. clin. Pharmac. Biopharm.*, 1977, *15*, 581; B. Colombo *et al.*, *Clin. Trials J.*, 1978, *15* (3), 66; K. Chlud *et al.*, *Arzneimittel-Forsch.*, 1978, *28*, 1200; A. Romiti *et al.*, *Clin. Trials J.*, 1979, *16*, 108.

Proprietary Names

Teoremac *(Farmades, Ital.)*.

2656-n

Glycol Salicylate. Ethylene Glycol Monosalicylate. 2-Hydroxyethyl salicylate.
$C_9H_{10}O_4$=182.2.

CAS — 87-28-5.

An almost colourless odourless liquid. **Soluble** 1 in about 110 parts of water and 1 in 8 of olive oil; very soluble in alcohol, chloroform, ether, and fixed oils.

Uses. Glycol salicylate is an ingredient of a number of rubefacient creams.

2657-h

Ibuprofen *(B.P., U.S.P.)*. RD 13621. 2-(4-Isobutylphenyl)propionic acid.
$C_{13}H_{18}O_2$=206.3.

CAS — 15687-27-1.

Pharmacopoeias. In *Br.* and *U.S.*

A white or almost white powder or crystals with a characteristic odour and a slight taste. M.p. 75° to 77.5°. Practically **insoluble** in water; soluble 1 in 1.5 of alcohol, 1 in 1 of chloroform, 1 in 2 of ether, and 1 in 1.5 of acetone; soluble in aqueous solutions of alkali hydroxides and carbonates. **Store** in airtight containers.

Adverse Effects. The most frequent adverse effects occurring with ibuprofen are gastro-intestinal disturbances. Peptic ulceration and gastro-intestinal bleeding have been reported. Other side-effects include headache, dizziness, nervousness, skin rash, pruritus, tinnitus, oedema, depression, drowsiness, insomnia, and blurred vision and other ocular reactions. Hypersensitivity reactions, abnormalities of liver function tests, impairment of renal function, agranulocytosis, and thrombocytopenia have occasionally been observed.

There were 388 reports of adverse reactions to ibuprofen reported to the Committee on Safety of Medicines up to January 1974. These included 34 reports of blood disorders (5 fatal) including thrombocytopenia (9; 1 fatal) and agranulocytosis or pancytopenia (6; 2 fatal), gastro-intestinal haemorrhage (37; 6 fatal), and 89 reports involving the CNS including 18 reports of visual abnormalities.— M. F. Cuthbert, *Curr. med. Res. Opinion*, 1974, *2*, 600.

Adverse reactions to ibuprofen reported in Japan included gastro-intestinal haemorrhage (2 cases), hepatic dysfunction (14), blood dyscrasias (2), erythema multiforme (1), and disturbances of vision (2).— *Japan med. Gaz.*, 1977, *14* (Jan. 20), 12.

Reviews. A comparative review of the side-effects of ibuprofen and related anti-inflammatory analgesics.— J. Chabot and L. Auquier, *Thérapie*, 1976, *31*, 343.

Allergy. There had been more reports of bronchospasm, some serious, with ibuprofen than with other non-steroidal anti-inflammatory drugs. It was not possible to assess whether this represented a real difference in incidence.— Committee on Safety of Medicines, *Current Problems Series No. 1*, Sept. 1975.

Studies in 92 patients indicated that ibuprofen was not a suitable substitute for aspirin in patients intolerant to aspirin, butylated hydroxyanisole, or butylated hydroxytoluene if concomitant low iodide tolerance was present or in patients solely intolerant to iodides.— E. W. Fisherman and G. N. Cohen, *Ann. Allergy*, 1976, *37*, 353.

An urticarial rash, laboured breathing, laryngeal oedema, and tightness of the chest occurred in a 53-year-old man after a single dose of ibuprofen 400 mg. The patient had experienced a similar adverse reaction about 7 years previously after a single dose of aspirin.— G. J. Merritt and R. I. Selle, *Am. J. Hosp. Pharm.*, 1978, *35*, 1245.

A patient with systemic lupus erythematosus (SLE) developed a hypersensitivity reaction to ibuprofen, with fever, nausea and vomiting, abdominal pain, and elevated liver-function test values. A similar reaction occurred in a second patient who was found, 2 months later, to have SLE.— M. Sonnenblick and A. S. Abraham, *Br. med. J.*, 1978, *1*, 619.

Aseptic meningitis with nausea, vomiting, fever, rigors, and severe headache was reported in a 21-year-old woman with Raynaud's phenomenon and polyarthritis following administration of ibuprofen. The rapid onset of the symptoms suggested a hypersensitivity reaction.— R. F. Bernstein, *Ann. intern. Med.*, 1980, *92*, 206.

Further reports of hypersensitivity reactions to ibuprofen, including aseptic meningitis, in patients with systemic lupus erythematosus.— B. Mandell *et al.* (letter), *Ann. intern. med.*, 1976, *85*, 209; H. L. Widener and B. H. Littman, *J. Am. med. Ass.*, 1978, *239*, 1062; C. K. Wasner, *J. Rheumatol.*, 1978, *5*, 162; W. R. Finch and M. P. Strottman, *J. Am. med. Ass.*, 1979, *241*, 2616; C. O. Samuelson and H. J. Williams, *West. J. Med.*, 1979, *131*, 57.

See also Erythema Multiforme, below.

Alopecia. Ingestion of ibuprofen was associated with thinning or loss of hair in 16 black patients. These patients also used preparations to straighten hair and it was suggested that ibuprofen might cause fragility or brittleness of the hair so that it breaks at the epidermal level when subjected to the straightening process.— H. C. Meyer (letter), *J. Am. med. Ass.*, 1979, *242*, 142.

Effects on blood. A 33-year-old woman developed bruises on her limbs during the third week of treatment for a painful hip with ibuprofen 600 mg daily. Symptoms cleared on discontinuation of the drug.— T. Ward (letter), *Br. med. J.*, 1969, *4*, 430.

Agranulocytosis and leucopenia leading to death 2 weeks after the cessation of medication was reported in an 82-year-old woman given ibuprofen and paracetamol to replace the long-term use of salicylates for the treatment of rheumatoid arthritis.— C. I. Gryfe and S. Rubenzahl (letter), *Can. med. Ass. J.*, 1976, *114*, 877.

In 2 patients who were taking ibuprofen pre-operatively a significant increase in mediastinal bleeding occurred after coronary by-pass surgery.— M. Torosian *et al.*, *Ann. intern. Med.*, 1978, *89*, 325.

A study in healthy subjects and patients with haemophilia suggested that ibuprofen might be used in haemophiliac patients.— B. A. McIntyre *et al.*, *Clin. Pharmac. Ther.*, 1978, *24*, 616.

Haemolytic anaemia. Immunohaemolytic anaemia in a 69-year-old woman was considered due to ibuprofen; she had taken 400 mg thrice daily for 8 months.— S. Korsager, *Br. med. J.*, 1978, *1*, 79.

Fatal haemolytic anaemia occurred in a man who had been treated with ibuprofen and oxazepam for 10 days before the onset of the acute illness.— J. B. Guidry *et al.*, *J. Am. med. Ass.*, 1979, *242*, 68.

Effects on the eyes. Of 40 patients treated with ibuprofen usually for rheumatoid arthritis, 2 developed toxic amblyopia due to ibuprofen. A further 3 had visual defects possibly related to ibuprofen.— L. M. T. Collum and D. I. Bowen, *Br. J. Ophthal.*, 1971, *55*, 472.

A 57-year-old woman developed toxic amblyopia after treatment for about 5 months with ibuprofen 1.2 g daily.— C. A. L. Palmer (letter), *Br. med. J.*, 1972, *3*, 765.

Visual disturbances were not encountered in 293 patients with rheumatic disorders treated with ibuprofen over a 5-year period. When ocular toxicity occurred it seemed to be early in treatment, rapidly progressive, and reversible.— M. Thompson (letter), *Br. med. J.*, 1972, *4*, 550. Similar findings.— J. W. Melluish *et al.*, *Archs Ophthal., N.Y.*, 1975, *93*, 781; J. Williamson and R. D. Sturrock, *Curr. med. Res. Opinion*, 1976, *4*, 128.

Effects on the gastro-intestinal tract. A 69-year-old man with a duodenal ulcer, but with no complications, developed gastro-intestinal bleeding one week after starting treatment with ibuprofen 200 mg thrice daily. Death due to multiple factors occurred two days after surgery.— D. J. Holdstock (letter), *Lancet*, 1972, *1*, 541.

A study in 34 patients with rheumatoid arthritis suggested that ibuprofen caused less gastro-intestinal blood loss than aspirin.— F. R. Schmid and D. D. Culic, *J. clin. Pharmac.*, 1976, *16*, 418.

Effects on the kidneys. Acute oliguric renal failure in a 65-year-old man was attributed to 6 days' treatment with ibuprofen 400 mg four times daily.— R. D. Brandstetter and D. D. Mar, *Br. med. J.*, 1978, *2*, 1194.

Impairment of renal function has been associated with ingestion of ibuprofen in patients with systemic lupus erythematosus.— R. P. Kimberly *et al.*, *Am. J. Med.*, 1978, *64*, 804; R. P. Kimberly *et al.*, *Arthritis Rheum.*, 1979, *22*, 281.

Further references.— S. N. Novack (letter), *Arthritis Rheum.*, 1975, *18*, 628.

Effects on liver. A 12-year-old girl with juvenile rheumatoid arthritis suffered fever, hepatitis, and lymphocytopenia following treatment with ibuprofen. The symptoms resolved rapidly when ibuprofen was discontinued.— D. A. Stempel and J. J. Miller, *J. Pediat.*, 1977, *90*, 657.

A report of fatal fatty metamorphosis of the liver in a woman with mixed connective tissue disease who was treated with ibuprofen and ampicillin.— J. F. Bravo *et al.* (letter), *Ann. intern. Med.*, 1977, *87*, 200.

See also under Erythema Multiforme, below.

Erythema multiforme. A report of erythema multiforme (Stevens-Johnson syndrome) and toxic hepatitis associated with ingestion of ibuprofen in 1 patient.— P. Sternlieb and R. M. Robinson, *N.Y. St. J. Med.*, 1978, *78*, 1239. At the time of this report there had been reported 17 other cases of ibuprofen-induced hepatotoxicity and 5 cases of serious dermatological problems in the category of erythema multiforme bullosum, including the variant known as Stevens-Johnson syndrome, as well as toxic epidermal necrolysis.— *idem* (letter), *Ann. intern. Med.*, 1980, *92*, 570.

Meningitis. For reports of aseptic meningitis following administration of ibuprofen, see under Allergy.

Overdosage. Depressed consciousness and hypotension after the ingestion by an elderly man of thirty 400-mg tablets of ibuprofen.— D. P. Hunt and R. J. Leigh, *Br. med. J.*, 1980, *281*, 1458. Criticism; the patient had also taken chlorpheniramine. In a study of 55 patients with alleged ibuprofen overdosage, 37 remained symptomless. Only 5 exhibited serious symptoms, of whom one (who had taken a mixed overdose) subsequently died.— H. Court *et al.* (letter), *ibid.*, 1981, *282*, 1073.

Precautions. Ibuprofen should be given with care to patients with bleeding disorders, cardiovascular disease, peptic ulceration or a history of such ulceration, and in those who are receiving coumarin anticoagulants. Patients who are sensitive to aspirin should generally not be given ibuprofen.

Activation of latent tuberculosis in a patient given ibuprofen and indomethacin.— M. Brennan (letter), *Can. med. Ass. J.*, 1980, *122*, 400.

Interactions, drugs. Aspirin. A double-blind study in patients with rheumatoid arthritis revealed only a weak clinical additive effect between aspirin and ibuprofen when both drugs were given together in moderate doses. Aspirin administration produced a significant lowering of ibuprofen concentrations without affecting the elimination half-life. Ibuprofen did not affect salicylate concentrations.— D. M. Grennan *et al.*, *Br. J. clin. Pharmac.*, 1979, *8*, 497.

Interactions, tests. A single dose of ibuprofen 200 mg or flurbiprofen 100 mg did not interfere with the following commercial urine tests: Albustix, Clinistest, Clinistix, Ictotest, Ketostix, Phenistix, or Labstix.— D. A. L. Morgan and D. J. Brown (letter), *Br. J. clin. Pharmac.*, 1977, *4*, 700.

Absorption and Fate. Ibuprofen is absorbed from the gastro-intestinal tract and peak plasma concentrations occur about 1 to 2 hours after ingestion. Ibuprofen is extensively bound to plasma proteins and has a half-life of about 2 hours. It is rapidly excreted in the urine mainly as metabolites and their conjugates. About 1% is excreted in urine as unchanged ibuprofen and about 14% as conjugated ibuprofen.

Peak serum-ibuprofen concentrations of about 11, 15, and 25 μg per ml were achieved in 4, 3, and 5 patients after doses of 200, 300, and 400 mg respectively of ibuprofen.— Y. Ikawa, XIII International Congress of Rheumatology, Japan, 1973.

The plasma half-life of ibuprofen was 1.93 hours. The peak mean plasma concentration of 21.8 μg per ml was observed 1 hour after administration of a single dose of 200 mg by mouth in 20 normal fasting subjects.— D. G. Kaiser and G. J. Vangiessen, *J. pharm. Sci.*, 1974, *63*, 219.

The *d*-isomer was predominant in the plasma and urine after administration of ibuprofen 800 mg (a racemic mixture) to 3 normal fasting subjects. Peak plasma concentrations for the *d*- and *l*-isomers were 25.9 and 22.6 μg per ml 1 hour after administration, and plasma half-lives were 3.34 and 2.01 hours respectively.— G. J. Vangiessen and D. G. Kaiser, *J. pharm. Sci.*, 1975, *64*, 798.

From the administration of single 800-mg doses of the racemic mixture ibuprofen and its enantiomers in 3 healthy subjects it was concluded that: only the (*R*)-(−)-enantiomer was inverted *in vivo* to the (*S*)-(+)-form, both enantiomers were transformed independently to the hydroxy and carboxy metabolites, and the metabolism of ibuprofen to its carboxy metabolite was not stereoselective.— D. G. Kaiser *et al.*, *J. pharm. Sci.*, 1976, *65*, 269.

A mean peak serum concentration of 31.9 μg per ml occurred 30 minutes after administration of ibuprofen 400 mg by mouth as an aqueous solution to 3 healthy fasting subjects. The estimated serum half-life was 1.94 hours.— D. G. Kaiser and R. S. Martin, *J. pharm. Sci.*, 1978, *67*, 627.

Concentrations of ibuprofen in serum and synovial fluid in patients with rheumatoid arthritis.— R. C. Glass and A. J. Swannell, *Br. J. clin. Pharmac.*, 1978, *6*, 453P.

Uses. Ibuprofen is a phenylpropionic acid derivative which has analgesic, anti-inflammatory, and antipyretic actions. It is used in the treatment of rheumatoid arthritis and other musculoskeletal disorders. It has also been used in the treatment of acute gout.

Ibuprofen is usually administered in doses of 0.9 to 2.4 g daily in divided doses. Maintenance doses of 0.6 to 1.2 g daily may be effective in some patients. If gastro-intestinal disturbances occur, ibuprofen should be given with food or milk. A suggested dose for children is 20 mg per kg body-weight daily in divided doses with a maximum of 500 mg for those weighing less than 30 kg.

Ibuprofen aluminium (ibuprofen aluminum; U-18,573G) is under study.

Reviews of the actions and uses and adverse effects of ibuprofen.— E. F. Davies and G. S. Avery, *Drugs*, 1971, *2*, 416; F. D. Hart, *ibid.*, 411; *Med. Lett.*, 1974, *16*, 109; L. J. Davis, *Drug Intell. & clin. Pharm.*, 1975, *9*, 501; J. R. Lewis, *J. Am. med. Ass.*, 1975, *233*, 364; T. G. Kantor, *Ann. intern. Med.*, 1979, *91*, 877.

Ibuprofen significantly reduced protein loss in 40 of 62 patients with *Vibrio cholerae* infection.— S. De *et al.*, *Indian J. med. Res.*, 1974, *62*, 756, per *Trop. Dis. Bull.*, 1975, *72*, 43.

Administration. A study in 32 patients with rheumatoid arthritis indicated that ibuprofen 1.6 g daily was equally effective in 2 or 4 divided doses.— N. E. Brugueras *et al.*, *Clin. Ther.*, 1978, *2*, 13.

Administration in renal failure. The normal half-life of ibuprofen was 2.5 hours. The interval between doses should be extended from 6 hours to 8 hours in patients with a glomerular filtration-rate (GFR) of 10 to 50 ml per minute, and to 12 hours in those with a GFR of less than 10 ml per minute.— W. M. Bennett *et al.*, *Ann. intern. Med.*, 1980, *93*, 286.

Analgesia. In a double-blind study in 80 patients with moderate to very severe episiotomy pain, greater than 50% pain reduction was obtained, over a 6-hour period of evaluation, by 17 of 20 patients who received ibuprofen 300 mg, 17 of 20 patients who received ibuprofen 900 mg, 18 of 20 who received aspirin 900 mg, and 6 of 20 who received placebo.— S. S. Bloomfield *et al.*, *Clin. Pharmac. Ther.*, 1974, *15*, 565.

Ankylosing spondylitis. Ibuprofen 1.2 g daily for at least 2 months was associated with improvement in 27 of 65 patients with ankylosing spondylitis. Subjective improvement only occurred in 5 patients, no change in 17, and deterioration in 16.— J. Nikolić and D. Lukačević, *Scand. J. Rheumatol.*, 1975, *4*, *Suppl.* 8, 20.

Bartter's syndrome. Use of ibuprofen in Bartter's syndrome.— R. J. Cunningham *et al.*, *Pediatrics*, 1979, *63*, 754; G. Lechacz *et al.*, *J. Pediat.*, 1979, *95*, 319.

Dysmenorrhoea. Ibuprofen in the relief of dysmenorrhoea.— D. R. Halbert and L. M. Demers, *J. reprod. Med.*, 1978, *21*, 219; R. M. Larkin *et al.*, *Obstet. Gynec.*, 1979, *54*, 456; W. Y. Chan *et al.*, *Am. J. Obstet. Gynec.*, 1979, *135*, 102.

Gout. Ibuprofen 800 mg thrice daily relieved the symptoms of acute gouty arthritis within 72 hours in a study of 10 patients. On resolution of acute symptoms the dosage of ibuprofen was reduced to 400 mg every 6 hours for an additional 24 to 72 hours. One patient had an acute exacerbation of gout when ibuprofen was discontinued but responded to renewed treatment.— M. C. Schweitz *et al.*, *J. Am. med. Ass.*, 1978, *239*, 34.

Further references.— W. A. Franck and M. M. Brown, *Arthritis Rheum.*, 1976, *19*, 269.

Osteoarthrosis. In a double-blind multicentre study in 232 patients with osteoarthrosis, ibuprofen was as effective as indomethacin and was associated with fewer adverse effects.— G. L. Royer *et al.*, *Curr. ther. Res.*, 1975, *17*, 234.

Further studies on the use of ibuprofen in osteoarthrosis.— L. Mattara *et al.*, *Clin. Trials J.*, 1977, *14*, 30; J. E. Giansiracusa *et al.*, *Sth. med. J.*, 1977, *70*, 49; L. S. Bain *et al.*, *Curr. med. Res. Opinion*, 1977, *4*, 665; C. Tranmer, *Rheumatol. Rehabil.*, 1978, *17*, 91.

Rheumatic disorders. A report of an uncontrolled trial in 201 patients given ibuprofen, 0.4 to 1.8 g daily in divided doses, for the treatment of rheumatic conditions. There were few side-effects.— Report No. 174 of the General Practitioner Research Group, *Practitioner*, 1972, *209*, 229.

Further reports on the use of ibuprofen in rheumatic disorders.— R. P. Saxena and U. Saxena, *Curr. med. Res. Opinion*, 1978, *5*, 484; General Practitioner Research Group, *J. Pharmacother.*, 1979, *2*, 72.

Juvenile polyarthritis. Eight children with moderately active Still's disease, being treated as out-patients, and intolerant of aspirin were given ibuprofen in maximum dosage ranging from 13 to 32 mg per kg body-weight daily. Satisfactory control was achieved in 5 patients and a beneficial result in 1. Of a further 9 children who were more severely affected and were receiving corticosteroids on alternate days, 5 obtained considerable relief of stiffness. A transient rash was noted in 2 patients.— B. M. Ansell, *Practitioner*, 1973, *211*, 659.

Rheumatoid arthritis. In a year-long double-blind multicentre study in 885 patients with rheumatoid arthritis, ibuprofen 0.8 to 1.6 g daily was as effective as aspirin 3 to 6 g daily. Gastro-intestinal side-effects occurred in 17% of patients taking ibuprofen and 31% of those taking aspirin.— W. J. Blechman *et al.*, *J. Am. med. Ass.*, 1975, *233*, 336.

Further reports on the use of ibuprofen in rheumatoid arthritis.— T. M. Chalmers, *Ann. rheum. Dis.*, 1969, *28*, 513; S. Sasaki, *Rheumatol. phys. Med.*, 1970, *Suppl.*, 32; C. D. Brooks *et al.*, *Rheumatol. phys. Med.*, 1970, *Suppl.*, 48; M. Thompson and D. Bell, *ibid.*, 100; A. A. J. Goldberg *et al.*, *Practitioner*, 1971, *207*, 343; J. Dornan and W. J. Reynolds, *Can. med. Ass. J.*, 1974, *110*, 1370; *Curr. med. Res. Opinion*, 1975, *3*, 475–606; A. Calin *et al.*, *J. Rheumatol.*, 1977, *4*, 153; K. Pavelka *et al.*, *J. int. med. Res.*, 1978, *6*, 355; E. J. Valtonen and M. Busson, *Scand. J. Rheumatol.*, 1978, *7*, 183; H. C. Burry and L. Witherington, *N.Z. med. J.*, 1979, *89*, 298; F. Montrone *et al.*, *Rheumatol. Rehabil.*, 1979, *18*, 114; J. P. Molnar and T. E. Moxley, *Curr. ther. Res.*, 1979, *26*, 581; N. H. Brodie *et al.*, *Br. J. clin. Pract.*, 1980, *34*, 279; J. J. Castles and J. L. Skosey, *Curr. ther. Res.*, 1980, *27*, 556.

Preparations

Ibuprofen Tablets *(B.P.).* Tablets containing ibuprofen. The tablets may be film-coated or sugar-coated.

Ibuprofen Tablets *(U.S.P.).* Tablets containing ibuprofen. The *U.S.P.* requires 50% dissolution in 30 minutes.

Proprietary Preparations

Apsifen *(Approved Prescription Services, UK).* Ibuprofen, available as tablets of 200 and 400 mg.

Brufen *(Boots, UK).* Ibuprofen, available as **Syrup** containing 100 mg in each 5 ml and as **Tablets** of 200 and 400 mg. (Also available as Brufen in *Austral.*, *Belg.*, *Denm.*, *Fr.*, *Ger.*, *Ital.*, *Jap.*, *Neth.*, *Norw.*, *S.Afr.*, *Spain*, *Swed.*, *Switz.*).

Ebufac *(DDSA Pharmaceuticals, UK).* Ibuprofen, available as tablets of 200 and 400 mg.

Ibu-Slo *(Rona, UK).* Ibuprofen, available as sustained-release capsules of 300 mg.

Other Proprietary Names

Arg.—Emodin; *Austral.*—Inflam; *Canad.*—Amersol, Motrin; *Ital.*—Algofen, Focus, Rebugen; *Jap.*—Andran, Anflagen, Bluton, Brufanic, Donjust B, Epobron, IB-100, Ibuprocin, Lamidon, Liptan, Mynosedin, Nagifen-D, Napacetin, Nobfelon, Nobgen, Pantrop, Roidenin; *S.Afr.*—Inza; *USA*—Motrin.

2658-m

Indomethacin *(B.P., U.S.P.).* Indometacinum.

[1-(4-Chlorobenzoyl)-5-methoxy-2-methylindol-3-yl]acetic acid.

$C_{19}H_{16}ClNO_4$=357.8.

CAS — 53-86-1.

Pharmacopoeias. In *Br.*, *Braz.*, *Chin.*, *Cz.*, *Jap.*, *Nord.*, and *U.S.*

A white to yellow-tan, odourless or almost odourless, crystalline powder with a faintly astringent taste. Melting point about 158° to 162°. It exhibits polymorphism.

Practically **insoluble** in water; soluble 1 in 50 of alcohol, 1 in 30 of chloroform, and 1 in 40 to 45 of ether; soluble in acetone. Soluble in alkaline solutions but with decomposition. **Protect** from light.

Release from suppository basis. A study *in vitro* indicated that a suppository basis of macrogol gave the highest rate of release of indomethacin.— H. P. M. Kerckhoffs and T. Huizinga, *Pharm. Weekbl. Ned.*, 1967, *102*, 1183, per *Int. pharm. Abstr.*, 1968, *5*, 549.

Adverse Effects. The commonest adverse effects occurring with indomethacin are gastro-intestinal disturbances, headache, and dizziness. Gastro-intestinal ulceration and bleeding may also occur. Other adverse effects include depression, drowsiness, tinnitus, confusion, lightheadedness, insomnia, psychiatric disturbances, syncope, convulsions, coma, peripheral neuropathy, blurred vision and other ocular effects, oedema and weight gain, hypertension, haematuria, skin rashes, pruritus, urticaria, stomatitis, alopecia, and hypersensitivity reactions. Leucopenia, purpura, thrombocytopenia, aplastic anaemia, haemolytic anaemia, agranulocytosis, epistaxis, hyperglycaemia, hyperkalaemia, and vaginal bleeding have been reported. There have been rare reports of renal failure. Hypersensitivity reactions may also occur in aspirin-sensitive patients.

There were 1261 reports of adverse reactions to indomethacin reported to the Committee on Safety of Medicines between June 1964 and January 1973. These included 157 reports of blood disorders (25 fatal) including thrombocytopenia (35; 5 fatal), aplastic anaemia (17; no fatalities), and agranulocytosis or leucopenia (21; 3 fatal), gastro-intestinal haemorrhage (121; 25 fatal), and reports involving the CNS (chiefly headache, giddiness, vertigo, confusion, and visual abnormalities).— M. F. Cuthbert, *Curr. med. Res. Opinion*, 1974, *2*, 600.

Mouth ulcers developed in 3 patients with dentures who were receiving indomethacin for rheumatoid arthritis. The lesions healed after reduction of dosage or discontinuation of indomethacin.— J. Guggenheimer and Y. H. Ismail, *J. Am. dent. Ass.*, 1975, *90*, 632.

Allergy. A fatal asthmatic attack occurred following the use of an indomethacin suppository in an aspirin-sensitive patient.— J. Timperman, *J. forens. Med.*, 1971, *18*, 30.

A patient sensitive to aspirin developed an urticarial reaction 30 minutes after taking his first dose of indomethacin.— J. I. Matthews and D. Stage (letter), *Ann. intern. Med.*, 1974, *80*, 771.

Severe dyspnoea occurred in a 43-year-old woman, with a history of allergy to penicillin and aspirin, after a single dose of indomethacin 50 mg.— N. M. Johnson *et al.* (letter), *Br. med. J.*, 1977, *2*, 1291.

For further reports of adverse reactions to indomethacin in aspirin-sensitive patients, see Aspirin, p.236.

Effects on blood. An analysis of blood dyscrasias reported to the Swedish Adverse Drug Reaction Committee for the 5-year period 1966–70 showed that thrombocytopenia attributable to indomethacin had been reported on 6 occasions. It was estimated that reported figures represented one-third of the true frequency.— L. E. Böttiger and B. Westerholm, *Br. med. J.*, 1973, *3*, 339.

Mention of 8 cases of fatal aplastic anaemia or agranulocytosis in one year probably due to indomethacin.—

W. H. W. Inman, *Br. med. J.*, 1977, *1*, 1500.

Further reports of aplastic anaemia associated with indomethacin.— A. T. Canada and E. R. Burka (letter), *New Engl. J. Med.*, 1968, *278*, 743; G. R. Fredrick and K. R. Tanaka (letter), *ibid.*, *279*, 1290.

Effects on the eyes. Decreased retinal sensitivity occurred in 34 patients who had been taking indomethacin, 22 of whom had presented with ocular complaints. Corneal deposits were observed in 6.— C. A. Burns, *Am. J. Ophthal.*, 1968, *66*, 825.

Five patients with rheumatic disorders developed ocular side-effects after prolonged treatment with indomethacin. The cornea was affected in 2 and the retina in 3. The effects were generally reversed after therapy had been discontinued for 1 year.— G. Palmeris *et al.*, *Ophthalmologica, Basel*, 1972, *164*, 339. There was no greater incidence of retinal malfunction in 18 patients receiving indomethacin than in 10 controls, some with similar diseases. Where abnormalities were present in both groups they were thought to be due to age and the disease.— R. E. Carr and I. M. Siegel, *Am. J. Ophthal.*, 1973, *75*, 302.

A further case of reversible indomethacin-induced retinopathy.— H. E. Henkes *et al.*, *Am. J. Ophthal.*, 1972, *73*, 846.

A study indicating that usual therapeutic doses of indomethacin interfere with colour vision.— J. Laroche and C. Laroche, *Annls pharm. fr.*, 1972, *30*, 433.

Effects on the gastro-intestinal tract. An elderly woman died 3 days after a massive haemorrhage from rectal ulceration following treatment with indomethacin suppositories, 100 mg twice daily, for about 3 weeks. She had previously developed analgesic nephropathy.— J. Walls *et al.* (letter), *Br. med. J.*, 1968, *2*, 52.

Gastric ulcers developed in 10 patients who had taken indomethacin by mouth and sometimes rectally for 2 to 24 months. The ulcers were prepyloric in 6 patients, and in 7 patients they had an appearance falsely suggestive of malignancy. Only 1 patient had had a previous history of gastric ulceration. Withdrawal of indomethacin led to complete healing in 7 patients who had remained symptomless for periods of 4 months to 3 years.— R. T. Taylor *et al.*, *Br. med. J.*, 1968, *4*, 734. See also J. H. Swallow (letter), *ibid.*, 1969, *1*, 783; R. T. Taylor *et al.* (letter), *ibid.*, 1969, *2*, 53.

Rectal bleeding occurred in a 15-year-old boy after several months of treatment with indomethacin 150 mg daily given as suppositories. Bleeding ceased when the indomethacin was withdrawn. Resumption of treatment with 50 mg daily caused very little rectal bleeding.— N. Levy and E. Gaspar (letter), *Lancet*, 1975, *1*, 577.

Two cases of colonic perforation associated with short-term indomethacin therapy.— S. Coutrot *et al.* (letter), *Lancet*, 1978, *2*, 1055.

Of 89 patients admitted to hospital with perforated duodenal ulcer, 11 were taking indomethacin; 8 were women aged over 60. Of 222 women aged over 60 admitted for gall-stones none was recorded as taking indomethacin.— M. R. Thompson, *Br. med. J.*, 1980, *280*, 448. See also *idem* (letter), 1618.

Gastric perforation in a neonate might have been caused by indomethacin given for ductus arteriosus.— A. N. Campbell *et al.* (letter), *Lancet*, 1981, *1*, 1110.

For a report that concomitant administration of dinoprostone reduced faecal blood-loss associated with indomethacin, see C. Johansson *et al.* (letter), *Lancet*, 1979, *1*, 317.

For a report of reduced gastro-intestinal blood loss in patients receiving sodium salicylate and indomethacin, see Sodium Salicylate, p.279.

Effects on hearing. A 79-year-old man who had taken indomethacin 25 mg twice daily for a year developed loss of hearing and tremor.— *J. Am. med. Ass.*, 1973, *226*, 1471.

Effects on the kidneys. Acute renal failure occurred in a woman with congestive heart failure 2 weeks after starting treatment with indomethacin. Renal function improved after indomethacin was withdrawn and deteriorated on rechallenge.— J. J. Walshe and R. C. Venuto, *Ann. intern. Med.*, 1979, *91*, 47.

Irreversible renal failure occurred in 6 children with steroid-resistant nephrosis, but normal renal function, treated with indomethacin.— C. Kleinknecht *et al.* (letter), *New Engl. J. Med.*, 1980, *302*, 691.

Oliguric acute renal failure associated with indomethacin in one patient with no previous kidney impairment.— N. E. Gary *et al.*, *Am. J. Med.*, 1980, *69*, 135.

Further reports of acute renal failure associated with indomethacin therapy in patients with underlying renal disease.— J. L. Bernheim and Z. Korzets (letter), *Ann. intern. Med.*, 1979, *91*, 792; S. Y. Tan *et al.*, *J. Am. med. Ass.*, 1979, *241*, 2732.

See also under Hyperkalaemia, below.

Effects on liver. Toxic hepatitis, possibly due to indomethacin, caused the death of a 12-year-old boy who had been given 100 mg daily for rheumatoid disease.— W. M. Kelsey and M. Scharyj, *J. Am. med. Ass.*, 1967, *199*, 586.

Cholestatic hepatitis with biliverdinaemia developed in a 46-year-old man who had taken indomethacin 75 mg daily for 3 weeks. Symptoms subsided with conservative treatment and withdrawal of indomethacin.— F. F. Fenech *et al.*, *Br. med. J.*, 1967, *3*, 155.

Effects on mental state. A psychotic episode characterised by paranoid delusions and perceptual abnormalities in a 65-year-old woman appeared to be associated with treatment with indomethacin.— M. W. P. Carney, *Br. med. J.*, 1977, *2*, 994.

Effects on the nervous system. Brief case histories of 4 patients who developed peripheral neuropathy while taking indomethacin and in whom the condition slowly regressed when indomethacin was withdrawn.— O. E. Eade *et al.*, *Br. med. J.*, 1975, *2*, 66.

Hyperkalaemia. Indomethacin-induced hyperkalaemia was not necessarily attributable to reduced kaliuresis secondary to hypoaldosteronism. It was suggested that the hyperkalaemia may be produced by a defect in the cellular uptake of potassium rather than through suppression of its renal excretion. This cellular defect may be attributable to hypoaldosteronism *per se* or even possibly to defective pancreatic insulin release.— E. P. MacCarthy and G. S. Stokes (letter), *Ann. intern. Med.*, 1979, *91*,, per 500

Hyporeninaemia ,hypoaldosteronism, and hyperkalaemia were associated with administration of indomethacin in 1 patient with glomerulonephritis.— S. Y. Tan *et al.*, *Ann. intern. Med.*, 1979, *90*, 783.

Severe hyperkalaemia with renal impairment associated in 3 patients with indomethacin therapy.— J. W. Findling *et al.*, *J. Am. med. Ass.*, 1980, *244*, 1127.

Further reports of hyperkalaemia and hyporeninaemia associated with indomethacin.— E. P. MacCarthy *et al.*, *Med. J. Aust.*, 1979, *1*, 550; V. Beroniade *et al.* (letter), *Ann. intern. Med.*, 1979, *91*, 499; P. D. Mitnick *et al.*, *Clin. Pharmac. Ther.*, 1980, *28*, 680.

Hypoaldosteronism. For reports of hypoaldosteronism and hyperkalaemia associated with indomethacin, see under Hyperkalaemia.

Pancreatitis. A 69-year-old man developed acute pancreatitis after 3 months' treatment with indomethacin, 75 mg daily, for osteoarthritis. He was asymptomatic 24 days later.— M. Guerra, *J. Am. med. Ass.*, 1967, *200*, 552.

Pregnancy and the neonate. Clinical symptoms of tachypnoea, cyanosis, retractions, and grunting occurred in 5 of the infants born to 29 mothers who had been treated with indomethacin to prevent premature delivery. Hyaline membrane disease was also present in 1 infant who died. Clinical and laboratory studies suggested the transitory persistence of foetal circulation, possibly resulting from constriction of pulmonary arterioles.— F. F. Rubaltelli *et al.* (letter), *J. Pediat.*, 1979, *94*, 161.

Decrease in glomerular filtration-rate in 7 premature infants given indomethacin for patent ductus arteriosus. The dose was 200 µg per kg body-weight every 24 hours to a maximum of 600 µg per kg.— Z. Catterton *et al.*, *J. Pediat.*, 1980, *96*, 737. Another report of altered renal function.— R. F. Cifuentes *et al.*, *ibid.*, 1979, *95*, 583.

It was suggested that indomethacin given for patent ductus arteriosus closure does not increase the incidence of retinopathy in infants with very low birth weights.— R. S. Procianoy *et al.*, *Archs Dis. Childh.*, 1980, *55*, 362.

No ill effects occurred in the twin infants born to a woman given 1.9 g of indomethacin between the 26th and 35th weeks of pregnancy.— M. J. Johnstone and M. L. Chiswick (letter), *Archs Dis. Childh.*, 1980, *55*, 412.

Further reports on the possible deleterious effects of maternally administered indomethacin on neonatal pulmonary vasculature.— B. M. Goudie and J. F. B. Dossetor (letter), *Lancet*, 1979, *2*, 1187; D. Manchester *et al.*, *Am. J. Obstet. Gynec.*, 1976, *126*, 467; D. L. Levin *et al.*, *J. Pediat.*, 1978, *92*, 478; I. F. Csaba *et al.*, *ibid.*, 484.

Precautions. Indomethacin should be administered with caution to patients with impaired renal function, and to those with bleeding disorders, epilepsy, parkinsonism, or psychiatric disorders. Elderly patients may be specially susceptible to the toxic effects of indomethacin. It should not be given to patients with peptic ulcer or a history of gastro-intestinal lesions or to those who are sensitive to aspirin.

See under Uses for a discussion of indomethacin and similar compounds and their use in pregnancy.

The Canadian Food and Drug Directorate had received several reports that indomethacin had masked symptoms of infection or activated latent bacterial infection in the same way as corticosteroids. Following deaths from intercurrent infection in children treated for rheumatoid arthritis, dermatomyositis, and rheumatic fever, the FDD recommended that indomethacin should not be used in children until the results of further studies became available.— R. A. Chapman, *Can. med. Ass. J.*, 1966, *95*, 1156.

Activation of latent tuberculosis in a patient given ibuprofen and indomethacin.— M. Brennan (letter), *Can. med. Ass. J.*, 1980, *122*, 400.

Further references to masked infection.— L. Solomon (preliminary communication), *Br. med. J.*, 1966, *1*, 961; J. C. Jacobs, *J. Am. med. Ass.*, 1967, *199*, 932; S. H. Block (letter), *ibid.*, 1972, *222*, 1062; *idem*, 1979, *241*, 2786.

Indomethacin could cause green discoloration of the urine and a green discoloration of the faeces due to biliverdinaemia.— R. B. Baran and B. Rowles, *J. Am. pharm. Ass.*, 1973, *NS13*, 139.

Cardiac disorders. A study suggesting that indomethacin should be used with caution in patients with severe coronary artery disease.— P. L. Friedman *et al.*, *New Engl. J. Med.*, 1981, *305*, 1171.

Effects on driving. Administration of indomethacin 50 mg to healthy subjects caused impairment of psychomotor skills related to driving.— M. Linnoila *et al.*, *Br. J. clin. Pharmac.*, 1974, *1*, 477.

Effects on the heart. Indomethacin could aggravate myocardial ischaemia in some patients.— D. Golding (letter), *Br. med. J.*, 1970, *4*, 622.

Interactions. *Antacids.* Studies in 12 healthy subjects suggested that the bioavailability of indomethacin was reduced by administration with an antacid containing aluminium hydroxide—magnesium carbonate and magnesium hydroxide.— R. L. Galeazzi, *Eur. J. clin. Pharmac.*, 1977, *12*, 65.

Aspirin. Chronic administration of aspirin 1.2 g thrice daily reduced mean plasma concentrations of indomethacin by about 20% after single doses and by smaller amounts after multiple doses. After administration of single doses of both drugs together, mean plasma concentrations of indomethacin were reduced by about 8%. Chronic administrataion of indomethacin had no effect on plasma concentrations of salicylate following multiple doses of aspirin.— K. C. Kwan *et al.*, *J. Pharmacokinet. Biopharm.*, 1978, *6*, 451. Similar reports.— R. Jeremy and J. Towson, *Med. J. Aust.*, 1970, *2*, 127; A. Rubin *et al.*, *Arthritis Rheum.*, 1973, *16*, 635.

Studies which did not demonstrate an effect of aspirin on plasma-indomethacin concentrations.— G. D. Champion *et al.*, *Clin. Pharmac. Ther.*, 1972, *13*, 239; P. M. Brooks *et al.*, *Br. med. J.*, 1975, *3*, 69.

Plasma-indomethacin concentrations after rectal administration of indomethacin were not affected by administration of aspirin by mouth.— B. Lindquist *et al.*, *Clin. Pharmac. Ther.*, 1974, *15*, 247.

Increased absorption of indomethacin following pretreatment with, or concomitant administration of, buffered aspirin.— J. C. Garnham *et al.*, *Eur. J. clin. Pharmac.*, 1975, *8*, 107.

Ascorbic acid. For a report of reduced plasma- and platelet-ascorbic acid concentrations in 2 patients with rheumatoid arthritis taking indomethacin, see Aspirin, p.239.

Benzylpenicillin. For a report of indomethacin prolonging the serum half-life of benzylpenicillin, see Benzylpenicillin, p.1107.

Beta-adrenoceptor blocking agents. For an increase in blood pressure in patients taking propranolol or diuretics when given indomethacin, see Propranolol Hydrochloride, p.1328.

Frusemide. Plasma-indomethacin concentrations in 8 patients with rheumatoid arthritis were significantly reduced when frusemide 40 mg by mouth was administered concomitantly.— P. M. Brooks *et al.*, *Br. J. clin. Pharmac.*, 1974, *1*, 485.

Diminished effect of frusemide on concomitant administration of indomethacin or naproxen.— R. Faunch (letter), *Br. med. J.*, 1981, *283*, 989.

See also Frusemide, p.597.

Lithium. For the effect of indomethacin in elevating plasma concentrations of lithium, see Lithium Carbonate, p.1539.

Phenylpropanolamine. For reference to severe hypertension associated with concomitant administration of phenylpropanolamine and indomethacin, see Phenylpropanolamine, p.26.

Probenecid. In 6 subjects the 48-hour urinary excretion of indomethacin was reduced from 30 to 49% to 14% to 39% when probenecid was given concomitantly. The half-life was increased from 10.1 to 17.6 hours.— M. D. Skeith *et al., Clin. Pharmac. Ther.*, 1968, *9,* 89.

Concomitant administration of probenecid to 28 patients with rheumatoid arthritis who were receiving indomethacin by mouth or rectally approximately doubled the blood concentrations of indomethacin and enhanced its effect.— P. M. Brooks *et al., Br. J. clin. Pharmac.*, 1974, *1,* 287.

Probenecid increased plasma concentrations of indomethacin by reducing the non-renal clearance of indomethacin.— N. Baber *et al., Br. J. clin. Pharmac.*, 1978, *5,* 364P. See also *idem, Clin. Pharmac. Ther.*, 1978, *24,* 298.

Pregnancy and the neonate. Convulsions in a breast-fed infant appeared to be associated with ingestion of indomethacin by the mother.— O. Eeg-Olofsson *et al.* (letter), *Lancet*, 1978, *2,* 215.

Porphyria. Indomethacin had been reported to precipitate attacks of porphyria.— *Drug & Ther. Bull.*, 1976, *14,* 55.

A study in *rats* indicated that indomethacin would probably not elicit an acute attack in susceptible porphyric individuals.— G. H. Blekkenhorst *et al.* (letter), *Lancet*, 1980, *1,* 1367. Criticism of extrapolating data obtained from *animal* experiments to the treatment of human disease.— M. J. Brodie (letter), *ibid.*, *2,* 86; A. Gorchein (letter), *ibid.*, 152.

Absorption and Fate. Indomethacin is readily absorbed from the gastro-intestinal tract; peak plasma concentrations are reached ½ to 2 hours after a dose. More than 90% is bound to plasma proteins. It is metabolised in the liver and kidneys and is excreted in the urine, mainly as the glucuronide, and to a much lesser extent in the faeces. Indomethacin is also excreted in milk.

In subjects given radioactive indomethacin 100 mg as a suppository, peak plasma concentrations were reached in 2 or 3 hours. Conjugated indomethacin appeared in the urine in the first hour and small amounts of free indomethacin in the second hour. The bile contained large amounts of conjugated drug.— N. O. Rothermich, *Clin. Pharmac. Ther.*, 1971, *12,* 300.

The elimination of indomethacin from plasma was biphasic and the half-life of the β-phase (terminal plasma half-life) varied between 2.6 and 11.2 hours.— G. Alvan *et al., Clin. Pharmac. Ther.*, 1975, *18,* 364.

In 8 healthy subjects the buccal absorption of indomethacin was reduced from about 25% at pH 5 to about 7% at pH 9. The mean plasma concentrations of indomethacin, after a 50-mg dose, were significantly reduced in 6 subjects by aluminium hydroxide 700 mg as a suspension, and were slightly increased by sodium bicarbonate 1.4 g in solution; the effect of sodium bicarbonate 600 mg as a tablet was similar.— J. C. Garnham *et al., Postgrad. med. J.*, 1977, *53,* 126.

Studies in 8 healthy subjects showed that although the rate of absorption was higher in fasting subjects the total amount of indomethacin absorbed was not affected by the presence of food.— W. W. Wallusch *et al., Int. J. clin. Pharmac. Biopharm.*, 1978, *16,* 40.

Deschlorobenzoylindomethacin and desmethylindomethacin were inactive metabolites of indomethacin.— W. O. A. Thomas *et al., J. Pharm. Pharmac.*, 1979, *31, Suppl.*, 91P.

Pregnancy and the neonate. Nine premature infants with patent ductus arteriosus were given indomethacin in doses of 100, 250, or 300 μg per kg body-weight. Peak plasma concentrations achieved at 4 hours ranged from 27 to 310 ng per ml and plasma half-lives were 11 to 20 hours with the younger infants having slower elimination. More than 98% was protein bound. Absorption by mouth was incomplete.— R. Bhat *et al., J. Pediat.*, 1979, *95,* 313. A brief review of the pharmacokinetics of indomethacin in infants provides similar data; variable prolonged clearance of indomethacin, incomplete oral absorption, and some influence provided by gestational age.— P. L. Morrelli *et al., Clin. Pharmacokinet.*, 1980, *5,* 485.

Evidence of a 20-fold variation in plasma-indomethacin concentrations following a dose in neonates.— A. R. Brash *et al., New Engl. J. Med.*, 1981, *305,* 67.

Further references.— M. A. Evans *et al., Clin. Pharmac. Ther.*, 1979, *26,* 746; M. A. Evans, *J. pharm. Sci.*, 1980, *69,* 219.

Protein binding. Indomethacin and salicylic acid interacted competitively for binding sites on human serum albumin.— D. Hultmark *et al., Acta pharm. suec.*, 1975, *12,* 259.

Uses. Indomethacin has analgesic, anti-inflammatory, and antipyretic actions. It is used in the treatment of rheumatoid arthritis, ankylosing spondylitis, osteoarthritis, and other rheumatic disorders. It is also used in the treatment of acute gout.

The usual initial dose is 25 mg two to four times daily with food, increased, if required, to 150 to 200 mg daily. In acute gout, 50 mg may be given 3 or 4 times daily. To alleviate night pain and morning stiffness, 100 mg may be administered rectally as a suppository on retiring.

Indomethacin has been used to delay pre-term labour but this may be hazardous to the foetus; it is used in newborn infants to close the patent ductus arteriosus (see below under Pregnancy and the Neonate).

A review of the development, pharmacodynamic properties, toxicity, chemistry, metabolism, uses and interactions during use, of indomethacin and of sulindac.— T. -Y. Shen and C. A. Winter, *Adv. Drug Res.*, 1977, *12,* 89.

Actions. Studies on the mode of action of indomethacin as an anti-inflammatory agent.— D. Crook and A. J. Collins, *Ann. rheum. Dis.*, 1977, *36,* 459; D. A. Lewis and H. E. Krygier, *J. pharm. Sci.*, 1977, *66,* 1651; H. S. Kantor and M. Hampton, *Nature*, 1978, *276,* 841.

Administration in renal failure. Indomethacin could be given in usual doses to patients with renal failure.— W. M. Bennett *et al., Ann. intern. Med.*, 1980, *93,* 286. See also G. Stein *et al., Int. J. clin. Pharmac. Biopharm.*, 1977, *15,* 470.

See also under Adverse Effects (Effects on the Kidneys).

Administration, rectal. In 10 patients indomethacin was absorbed satisfactorily from the rectum and the average serum concentration after 100 mg by rectum was 75% of that when given by mouth. Thirty of 40 patients given suppositories obtained a good result, and the clinical effect was similar when the drug was given by mouth or by rectum. Some patients who failed to respond to a daily dosage of 100 to 150 mg were given larger doses, up to 300 mg daily, by supplementing the oral doses with suppositories.— L. P. J. Holt and C. F. Hawkins, *Br. med. J.*, 1965, *1,* 1354.

Further reports on the use of indomethacin suppositories.— D. L. Woolf (letter), *Br. med. J.*, 1965, *1,* 1497; E. C. Huskisson *et al., Ann. rheum. Dis.*, 1970, *29,* 393.

Analgesia. In a short-term double-blind sequential trial in 100 patients with low-back pain, indomethacin was significantly more effective than a placebo in patients with nerve-root pain but no difference was found between the treatments in patients with uncomplicated low-back pain. Indomethacin was given mainly in a dosage of 75 mg daily for 2 days then 100 mg daily for 5 days.— J. H. Jacobs and M. F. Grayson, *Br. med. J.*, 1968, *3,* 158.

Further reports on the use of indomethacin for pain relief.— G. Jaffé, *Curr. med. Res. Opinion*, 1976, *4,* 373; J. G. P. Williams and C. Engler, *Rheumatol. Rehabil.*, 1977, *16,* 265.

Ankylosing spondylitis. A report on the use of indomethacin in ankylosing spondylitis.— T. D. Kinsella *et al., Can. med. Ass. J.*, 1967, *96,* 1454.

Asthma. See under Respiratory Disorders.

Bartter's syndrome. A discussion of the pathophysiology of Bartter's syndrome and the use of prostaglandin synthetase inhibitors.— J. C. McGiff, *Ann. intern. Med.*, 1977, *87,* 369; S. Vaisrub, *J. Am. med. Ass.*, 1978, *239,* 137.

Indomethacin given in a dose of 7.5 mg daily gradually increased over 4 weeks to 20 mg daily in divided doses produced a beneficial response in a 33-month-old child with Bartter's syndrome.— J. M. Littlewood *et al.* (letter), *Lancet*, 1976, *2,* 795. After 1 year indomethacin was replaced by ketoprofen, gradually increased to 60 mg daily, and the improvement was maintained.— *idem, Archs Dis. Childh.*, 1978, *53,* 43.

Indomethacin 1 mg per kg body-weight daily for 4 days followed by 2 mg per kg daily in 2 divided doses for 7 days significantly reduced urinary excretion of kallikrein and immunoreactive prostaglandin E-like material and reduced plasma-renin activity in 2 children with Bartter's syndrome. The sensitivity of both children to saralasin was increased and serum concentrations of potassium were returned to normal. Both children had significant weight gain during therapy with indomethacin.— P. V. Halushka *et al., Ann. intern. Med.*, 1977, *87,* 281.

Further reports on the use of indomethacin in Bartter's syndrome.— L. Zancan *et al.* (letter), *lancet*, 1976, *2,* 1354; A. J. M. Donker *et al., Nephron*, 1977, *19,* 200; R. E. Bowden *et al., J. Am. med. Ass.*, 1978, *239,* 117; T. A. Simatupang *et al., Int. J. clin. Pharmac. Biopharm.*, 1978, *16,* 14; J. P. Rado *et al., Int. J. clin. Pharmac. Biopharm.*, 1978, *16,* 22.

Ductus arteriosus closure. See under Pregnancy and the Neonate.

Dysmenorrhoea. In a double-blind crossover study in 32 patients, indomethacin was significantly more effective than placebo in relieving pain and vomiting associated with primary dysmenorrhoea.— M. G. Elder and L. Kapadia, *Br. J. Obstet. Gynaec.*, 1979, *86,* 645.

Effects on blood. Indomethacin prolonged bleeding time, but coagulation and fibrinolysis were not affected.— G. de Gaetano *et al., Int. J. clin. Pharmac.*, 1971, *5,* 196, per *idem, Br. med. J.*, 1974, *2,* 301.

Indomethacin 50 mg had no significant effect on the bleeding time 2 or 24 hours after ingestion. Platelet aggregation was impaired at 2 hours but not at 24 hours after ingestion. Bleeding times were prolonged in 4 of 5 subjects given multiple doses of indomethacin.— G. R. Buchanan *et al., Am. J. clin. Path.*, 1977, *68,* 355.

Further references.— A. Rane *et al., Clin. Pharmac. Ther.*, 1978, *23,* 658.

Fever. Indomethacin, 25 to 50 mg every 6 to 8 hours, controlled fever due to Hodgkin's disease within 24 hours in all of 9 patients.— H. R. Silberman *et al., J. Am. med. Ass.*, 1965, *194,* 597.

Indomethacin, 50 mg every 4 hours, controlled fever in 3 patients with Hodgkin's disease. A patient with fever due to acute granulocytic leukaemia was given 100 mg every 4 hours; prompt relief was obtained.— J. M. Kieley, *Mayo Clin. Proc.*, 1969, *44,* 272.

Fever and pains were reduced in 4 of 6 patients with glandular fever treated with indomethacin, 50 mg three or four times a day after food.— F. D. Hart (letter), *Br. med. J.*, 1969, *2,* 380.

Gastro-intestinal disorders. Within 11 days of administration of indomethacin, diarrhoea and symptoms of intestinal obstruction began to resolve in a 53-year-old woman with idiopathic intestinal pseudo-obstruction. Indomethacin therapy was continued for 6 months and subsequently withdrawn with no recurrence of her symptoms.— J. R. Luderer *et al., New Engl. J. Med.*, 1976, *295,* 1179.

A 67-year-old woman suffering from the Verner-Morrison syndrome or pancreatic cholera (characterised by profuse watery diarrhoea, metabolic acidosis, and gastric hypersecretion of acid and pepsin) obtained complete remission of her profuse diarrhoea (average 2 to 5 litres daily) following administration of indomethacin 25 mg thrice daily for a week prior to operation for removal of pancreatic tumour. The beneficial effect of indomethacin was considered to be associated with its prostaglandin-inhibiting properties; following removal of the tumour she remained asymptomatic without indomethacin therapy.— B. M. Jaffe *et al., New Engl. J. Med.*, 1977, *297,* 817.

Indomethacin was effective in controlling diarrhoea in 1 patient with irritable bowel syndrome.— J. Rask-Madsen and K. Bukhave, *Gut*, 1978, *19,* A448.

For a further mention of the use of indomethacin in the treatment of diarrhoea, see Aspirin, p.241.

Gout. Twenty-two patients with acute gouty arthritis were given indomethacin, 100 mg by mouth, 4-hourly until most of the pain was relieved, then at 8-hourly intervals with 3 doses of 100 mg, 3 of 75 mg, and 3 of 50 mg. This resulted in rapid relief of pain and subsidence of acute arthritis.— B. T. Emmerson, *Br. med. J.*, 1967, *2,* 272. Patients with gout given these doses of indomethacin were unusually resistant to the side-effects.— I. Haslock (letter), *ibid.*, 1974, *2,* 121.

Hypercalcaemia. A review of hypercalcaemia and neoplastic diseases, with reference to the use of prostaglandin inhibitors for treatment.— T. M. Murray *et al., Can. med. Ass. J.*, 1978, *119,* 915.

Indomethacin 2 mg per kg body-weight daily in 4 to 6 divided doses was given to 5 patients with hypercalcaemia secondary to malignancy. There was a rapid reduction in serum-calcium concentration in 1 patient, a gradual fall in 2, and a slight fall in 1. These decreases might have been due to hydration.— A. Dindogru *et al.* (letter), *Lancet*, 1975, *2*, 365.

Further reports on the use of indomethacin in hypercalcaemia.— H. D. Brereton *et al.*, *New Engl. J. Med.*, 1974, *291*, 83; I. Blum (letter), *Lancet*, 1975, *1*, 866.

Lepra reactions. For favourable reports of the use of indomethacin in lepra reactions, see I. Singh *et al.*, *Lepr. Rev.*, 1968, *39*, 127; A. C. Parikh and R. Ganapati, *ibid.*, 207; A. B. A. Karat *et al.*, *ibid.*, 1969, *40*, 153. An unfavourable report.— G. Thomas *et al.*, *Indian J. med. Sci.*, 1969, *23*, 68.

Migraine. In a double-blind trial in 38 patients with migraine, 19 received indomethacin, 25 mg thrice daily, and 19 patients took placebo capsules. After 1 month's therapy, 7 patients from each group showed a reduction in severity and frequency of migraine attacks. Fifteen patients, mainly those receiving indomethacin, suffered side-effects.— M. Anthony and J. W. Lance, *Med. J. Aust.*, 1968, *1*, 56.

Neoplasms. Indomethacin 100 to 150 mg daily could markedly relieve the pain of bone metastases for 2 to 3 months in some patients with breast cancer.— B. A. Stoll (letter), *Lancet*, 1973, *2*, 384.

See also under Hypercalcaemia.

Ocular disease. If treatment for 3 or 4 days with local steroid therapy did not produce an effect in patients with sclerokeratitis, treatment with daily doses of 100 mg of indomethacin was recommended.— P. G. Watson *et al.*, *Br. J. Ophthal.*, 1968, *52*, 348.

Indomethacin was ineffective in the treatment of chronic cystoid macular oedema.— L. A. Yannuzzi *et al.*, *Am. J. Ophthal.*, 1977, *84*, 517.

Indomethacin eye-drops administered before surgery and for 2 weeks thereafter provided some early protection against aphakic cystoid macular oedema in patients who had undergone cataract extraction. Protection did not extend to 1 to 1½ years after surgery.— K. Miyake *et al.*, *Br. J. Ophthal.*, 1980, *64*, 324.

Orthostatic hypotension. Indomethacin 25 mg thrice daily for the first day subsequently increased to 50 mg thrice daily alleviated symptoms in 4 patients with idiopathic orthostatic hypotension (Shy-Drager syndrome). Administration of propranolol with ephedrine was ineffective, and fludrocortisone was less well tolerated than indomethacin. The mode of action of indomethacin was not known but might be specific since a fifth patient with a different type of orthostatic hypotension did not respond.— M. S. Kochar and H. D. Itskovitz, *Lancet*, 1978, *1*, 1011. Criticism.— R. Bannister *et al.* (letter), *ibid.*, 1312.

In studies in 12 patients with parkinsonism and orthostatic hypotension, indomethacin 50 mg by intravenous infusion over 30 minutes or 50 mg thrice daily by mouth for 6 days, reduced the fall in blood pressure on standing from a mean of 34.8 mmHg to a mean of 9.3 and 17.3 mmHg respectively.— G. Abate *et al.*, *Br. med. J.*, 1979, *2*, 1466. Comment.— I. B. Davies (letter), *ibid.*, 1980, *280*, 181.

Osteoarthrosis. Forty-five patients with osteoarthrosis of the hip were given indomethacin, adjusted to an average optimum dose of 85 mg daily. At intervals over 5 years substitution of a placebo under double-blind conditions showed that indomethacin was effective in relieving symptoms. The optimum dose for relief of pain increased to an average of 155 mg daily in the 12 patients remaining in the fifth year. Reasons for discontinuing treatment included headaches, nausea and vomiting, ataxia, gastro-intestinal haemorrhage, and perforated gastric ulcers. Arthroplasty was considered to give better relief with less hazard in long-term treatment.— R. Hodgkinson and D. Woolf, *Practitoner*, 1973, *210*, 392.

Further reports on the use of indomethacin in the treatment of osteoarthrosis.— E. Zachariae, *Nord. Med.*, 1966, *75*, 384; M. Harth and D. C. Bondy, *Can. med. Ass. J.*, 1969, *101*, 311; D. Woolf *et al.*, *Practitioner*, 1978, *221*, 791.

Osteomyelitis. Indomethacin, 50 to 100 mg daily, or phenylbutazone, 100 to 200 mg daily, was of value in controlling the symptoms of osteitis condensans ilii in 2 patients.— J. D. Soucy *et al.*, *J. Am. med. Ass.*, 1969, *207*, 1145.

Otitis. In a double-blind trial in 50 patients with an acute attack of otitis externa, a 200-mg daily dose of indomethacin, as a suppository, was significantly more effective than a placebo in respect of pain and tenderness O. Densert and N. G. Torealm, *Archs Otolar.*, 1972, *95*, 460, per *J. Am. med. Ass.*, 1972, *220*, 880.

Pericarditis. Of 8 patients with pericarditis due to viral infection who received indomethacin, those whose condition was associated with cardiac infarction responded dramatically. Indomethacin relieved pain, fever, and friction rub, but it was not known whether pleural effusions were ameliorated.— J. T. McGinn (letter), *New Engl. J. Med.*, 1968, *279*, 436. See also J. T. McGinn *et al.*, *N.Y. St. J. Med.*, 1970, *70*, 1783.

Indomethacin given for 3 weeks to 4 months was effective in the treatment of pericarditis associated with haemodialysis. There was rapid improvement in 8 patients within 6 to 24 hours of starting treatment and only 1 required pericardiocentesis.— A. N. W. Minuth *et al.*, *Archs intern. Med.*, 1975, *135*, 807, per *J. Am. med. Ass.*, 1975, *232*, 1293.

Pregnancy and the neonate. Indomethacin was given to 50 women with evidence of premature labour. The initial dose was 100 mg as a suppository, followed by 25 mg by mouth every 6 hours up to 24 hours after contractions ceased. Uterine contractions were stopped completely in 40 women. No adverse effects were noted in the infants and 38 mature and 12 premature infants were born. There were 4 neonatal deaths and 1 stillbirth, all in premature infants weighing less than 2000 g.— H. Zuckerman *et al.*, *Obstet. Gynec.*, 1974, *44*, 787.

Indomethacin halted premature labour in 76% of 98 women for periods of 1 to 12 weeks and 75 infants were born at maturity weighing at least 2.5 kg.— H. Zuckerman *et al.*, *Harefuah*, 1975, *89*, 201, per *J. Am. med. Ass.*, 1975, *234*, 663.

The effects of indomethacin on prostaglandins in labour.— H. Zuckerman *et al.*, *Br. J. Obstet. Gynaec.*, 1977, *84*, 339.

The administration of nonsteroidal anti-inflammatory drugs (NSAID) to pregnant patients can lead to ductal constriction *in utero* and may lead to problems in establishing pulmonary blood flow after birth (see under Adverse Effects). Many obstetricians have changed their policy of using these compounds for delaying pre-term labour. Until more detailed evidence emerges from animal work, pregnancy should be regarded as a contra-indication to administration of NSAID. If there is no other appropriate therapy, then the period of treatment should be kept to a minimum since prolonged exposure seems to increase the hazard.— *Lancet*, 1980, *2*, 185. A view that the hazard of premature closure of the ductus arteriosus by nonsteroidal anti-inflammatory drugs should not rule out their chronic maternal administration in desperate cases of preterm labour.— H. van Kets *et al.* (letter), *ibid.*, 693.

Ductus arteriosus closure. Discussions on the use of indomethacin and other prostaglandin inhibitors in the treatment of patent ductus arteriosus in infants.— A. S. Nadas *et al.*, *New Engl. J. Med.*, 1976, *295*, 563; D. R. Lines, *Drugs*, 1977, *13*, 1; *Lancet*, 1980, *2*, 185; M. L. Chiswick, *Br. med. J.*, 1981, *283*, 1490.

A review of studies on indomethacin in patent ductus arteriosus was carried out with the aim of comparing response with age. In no study in which the average age at initial indomethacin therapy was under 12.5 days, was the response-rate less than 75%, and in no study with average age greater than 12.5 days was it more than 45%. This finding suggests that indomethacin should be used earlier rather than later in the management of patent ductus arteriosus.— J. Firth and D. Pickering (letter), *Lancet*, 1980, *2*, 144. Agreement that results are disappointing after the first 2 weeks of life, but comment on the need for caution in the use of indomethacin.— H. L. Halliday (letter), *ibid.*, 314; E. D. Burnard (letter), *ibid.*, 473.

Indomethacin 100 to 200 µg per kg body-weight was given by mouth or rectally to 50 neonates for closure of the patent ductus. Of the 65 courses employed 32 produced no response, yet the plasma concentrations of indomethacin were no different from those achieved in the 33 courses that produced a response.— B. S. Alpert *et al.*, *J. Pediat.*, 1979, *95*, 578, per *Int. pharm. Abstr.*, 1980, *17*, 463.

Indomethacin was given to 16 preterm infants with intractable cardiac failure for pharmacological ductus closure. Large doses of 2 to 3.75 mg per kg body-weight on 2 consecutive days were effective in 6 infants, smaller doses of 0.1 to 0.3 mg per kg usually once only were effective in 6 of the remaining 10 infants. However, complications included vomiting, severe abdominal distension, melaena, necrotising enterocolitis, and a flare-up of respiratory-tract infections; transient renal insufficiency occurred with the higher doses. This treatment should not be used in infants with any of the above complications; if used, antibiotic cover should be considered and treatment should be carried out in a neonatal intensive-care unit.— E. Harinck *et al.* (letter), *Lancet*, 1977, *2*, 245.

Indomethacin failed to produce permanent closure in 4 premature infants with patent ductus arteriosus. The half-life was over 20 hours, and platelet function was abnormal for several days. Gastro-intestinal bleeding occurred in 1 infant.— Z. Friedman *et al.*, *J. clin. Pharmac.*, 1978, *18*, 272.

Further reports on indomethacin closing the patent ductus arteriosus.— W. F. Friedman *et al.*, *New Engl. J. Med.*, 1976, *295*, 526; M. A. Heymann *et al.*, *ibid.*, 530; M. Heymann and A. Rudolph, *Circulation*, 1977, *56*, *Suppl.* 3, 192; T. A. Merritt *et al.*, *J. Pediat.*, 1978, *93*, 639; H. L. Halliday *et al.*, *Pediatrics*, 1979, *64*, 154; *idem*, *Archs Dis. Childh.*, 1979, *54*, 744; T. A. Merritt *et al.*, *J. Pediat.*, 1979, *95*, 588; H. I. Obeyesekere *et al.*, *Archs Dis. Childh.*, 1980, *55*, 271.

Further studies in which indomethacin failed to close patent ductus arteriosus.— W. A. Neal *et al.*, *J. Pediat.*, 1977, *91*, 621; H. H. Ivey *et al.*, *Br. Heart J.*, 1979, *41*, 304.

Reiter's disease. Daily doses of indomethacin 100 mg were recommended to relieve severe pain in Reiter's disease.— *Br. med. J.*, 1969, *4*, 576.

Renal disorders. Studies and reports of indomethacin in glomerulonephritis.— E. Renner and E. Held, *Arzneimittel-Forsch.*, 1971, *21*, 1849; A. M. Vihert *et al.*, *ibid.*, 1973, *23*, 991; G. de Gaetano *et al.*, *Br. med. J.*, 1974, *2*, 301; M. S. Hoq *et al.*, *ibid.*, 535; I. H. Shehadeh *et al.*, *J. Am. med. Ass.*, 1979, *241*, 1264.

For comment on a possible beneficial role of indomethacin in glomerulonephritis, see Corticosteroids, General, p.457, but for poor results in childhood minimal-change nephrotic syndrome, see E. H. Garin *et al.*, *J. Pediat.*, 1978, *93*, 138.

Renal colic. Indomethacin 50 mg by intravenous injection was significantly more effective than placebo in relieving the pain of acute ureteric colic in a study in 47 patients.— D. Holmlund and J. -G. Sjödin, *J. Urol.*, 1978, *120*, 676.

Respiratory disorders. Pleurisy in 21 patients had been relieved by indomethacin 25 mg twice or thrice daily, sometimes with 50 mg at night.— K. P. Goldman (letter), *Br. med. J.*, 1977, *2*, 1353.

A report of a favourable response to indomethacin in 5 patients with asthma unresponsive to conventional treatment.— M. Hume and V. Eddey, *Scand. J. resp. Dis.*, 1977, *58*, 284.

Rheumatic disorders. A survey, with 108 references, of clinical studies of indomethacin in rheumatic diseases, and of its toxicity.— W. M. O'Brien, *Clin. Pharmac. Ther.*, 1968, *9*, 94.

Rheumatoid arthritis. Studies on the use of indomethacin in rheumatoid arthritis.—Report of Cooperating Clinics Committee of the American Rheumatism Association, *Clin. Pharmac. Ther.*, 1967, *8*, 11; P. Donnelly *et al.*, *Br. med. J.*, 1967, *1*, 69; V. Wright *et al.*, *Ann. rheum. Dis.*, 1969, *28*, 157; E. C. Huskisson and F. D. Hart, *Practitioner*, 1972, *208*, 248; N. Baber *et al.*, *Ann. rheum. Dis.*, 1979, *38*, 128; R. Ekstrand *et al.*, *Eur. J. clin. Pharmac.*, 1980, *17*, 437; S. D. Deodhar and R. Sethi, *Curr. med. Res. Opinion*, 1979, *6*, 263.

The use of indomethacin and diazepam for control of night pain in rheumatoid arthritis.— T. R. L. Bayley and I. Haslock, *J.R. Coll. gen. Pract.*, 1976, *26*, 591; D. Hobkirk *et al.*, *Rheumatol. Rehabil.*, 1977, *16*, 125.

Soft-tissue injuries. Indomethacin was no better than a placebo for the treatment of athletic and minor football injuries.— E. C. Huskisson *et al.*, *Rheumatol. Rehabil.*, 1973, *12*, 159. A similar report.— K. D. Fitch and S. D. Gray, *Med. J. Aust.*, 1974, *1*, 260. See also *Br. med. J.*, 1974, *4*, 488.

Sunburn. A 2.5% indomethacin solution was more effective than a corticosteroid cream in reducing redness and burning of sunburned skin in 8 volunteers when applied 90 minutes after irradiation with ultraviolet light. Areas that had been blanched by the solution became less tanned than the other irradiated areas.— D. S. Snyder and W. H. Eaglestein, *Br. J. Derm.*, 1974, *90*, 91.

Xeroderma. Eight of 9 patients with xeroderma pigmentosum had complete or partial remission following treatment with indomethacin 25 to 100 mg daily, either alone, or in association with prednisolone 250 to 500 micrograms per kg body-weight.— T. Al-Saleem *et al.* (letter), *Lancet*, 1980, *2*, 264.

Preparations

Indomethacin Capsules *(B.P.)*. Capsules containing indomethacin. Store at a temperature not exceeding 30°.

Indomethacin Capsules *(U.S.P.)*. Capsules containing indomethacin. The *U.S.P.* requires 80% dissolution in 15 minutes.

Indomethacin Injection. Administration of a suspension of indomethacin via a nasogastric tube is useful for treating infants with patent ductus arteriosus but the blood levels achieved are not always predictable. To overcome this an injection was formulated to contain 200 µg per ml. The preparation consisted of one ampoule of indomethacin 2 mg dissolved in dehydrated alcohol 1 ml and an ampoule of diluent consisting of sodium chloride injection 4.5 ml with sodium bicarbonate 1 mg. The solution for intravenous injection is prepared by adding 0.5 ml of the indomethacin in dehydrated alcohol to the ampoule of diluent and mixing. The final pH is 7.25 and the alcohol content for a dose of 200 µg per kg body-weight is considered acceptable.—M. Scott, *Pharm. J.*, 1980 *2*, 614.

Indomethacin Mixture *(B.P.C. 1973).* Indomethacin Suspension. A suspension of indomethacin in a suitable coloured flavoured vehicle. It may contain a suitable preservative. pH 4.3 to 4.7. The mixture should not be diluted; where necessary doses should be measured in a graduated pipette. Store in a cool place and avoid freezing.

Indomethacin Suppositories *(B.P.).* Suppositories containing indomethacin in a suitable basis. Store at a temperature not exceeding 30°.

Proprietary Preparations

Artracin *(DDSA Pharmaceuticals, UK).* Indomethacin, available as capsules of 25 and 50 mg.

Imbrilon *(Berk Pharmaceuticals, UK).* Indomethacin, available as **Capsules** of 25 and 50 mg and as **Suppositories** of 100 mg.

Indocid *(Morson, UK).* Indomethacin, available as **Capsules** of 25 and 50 mg; as **Suspension** containing 25 mg in each 5 ml; and as **Suppositories** each containing 100 mg. (Also available as Indocid in *Arg., Austral., Belg., Canad., Denm., Fr., Ital., Neth., Norw., S.Afr., Switz., USA*). **Indocid-R.** Sustained-release capsules each containing indomethacin 75 mg.

Indoflex *(Unimed, UK).* Indomethacin, available as capsules of 25 mg.

Mobilan *(Galen, UK).* Indomethacin, available as capsules of 25 and 50 mg.

Other Proprietary Names

Arg.— Agilex, IM-75; *Austral.*— Rheumacin; *Col.*— Infrocin; *Cz.*— Indren; *Denm.*— Confortid; *Ger.*— Amuno; *Ital.*— Algometacin, Artrobase, Artrocid, Boutycin, Cidalgon, Imet, Indium, Liometacen *(*meglumine salt*)*, Metacen, Metartril, Peralgon, Sadoreum; *Jap.*— Indacin; *Norw.*— Confortid; *S.Afr.*— Arthrexin; *Spain*— Artrinovo, Artrivia, Inacid; *Swed.*— Confortid, Indomee; *Switz.*— Confortid.

Indomethacin was also formerly marketed in Great Britain under the proprietary name Tannex *(Duncan, Flockhart)*.

2659-b

Indoprofen.

Isindone; K 4277. 2-[4-(1-Oxoisoindolin-2-yl)phenyl]propionic acid.
$C_{17}H_{15}NO_3$=281.3.

CAS — 31842-01-0.

Adverse Effects and Precautions. As for Ibuprofen, p.256.

In 8 patients given indoprofen 300 or 600 mg daily for 5 days, faecal blood loss was only slightly increased compared with pre-treatment values.— G. B. Porro *et al.*, *J. int. med. Res.*, 1977, *5*, 155.

Absorption and Fate. Indoprofen is almost completely absorbed from the gastro-intestinal tract with peak plasma concentrations occurring 30 to 120 minutes after ingestion. About 99% is reported to be bound to plasma proteins and it is reported to have a biological half-life of about 2 hours. It is excreted mainly in the urine as the glucuronide with small amounts of other metabolites and unchanged drug. It is excreted in breast milk.

References on the absorption and fate of indoprofen.— L. M. Fuccella *et al.*, *Eur. J. clin. Pharmac.*, 1973, *6*, 256; V. Tamassia *et al.*, *Eur. J. clin. Pharmac.*, 1976, *10*, 257; I. Caruso *et al.*, *Int. J. clin. Pharmac. Biopharm.*, 1977, *15*, 411; D. B. Lakings *et al.*, *J. pharm. Sci.*, 1978, *67*, 831.

Uses. Indoprofen is a phenylpropionic acid derivative which has analgesic and anti-inflammatory actions. It is used for the relief of various types of pain in doses of 100 to 300 mg. It is used in the treatment of rheumatoid arthritis and osteoarthrosis in doses of 600 to 800 mg daily in divided doses.

Analgesia. The analgesic effects of indoprofen.— L. M. Fuccella *et al.*, *Clin. Pharmac. Ther.*, 1975, *17*, 277; V. Ventafridda *et al.*, *ibid.*, 284; S. Pedronetto *et al.*, *J. int. med. Res.*, 1975, *3*, 16; G. Sacchetti *et al.*, *ibid.*, 1978, *6*, 312; G. Martino *et al.*, *Arzneimittel-Forsch.*, 1978, *28*, 1657; A. Chiapuzzo, *J. int. med. Res.*, 1979, *7*, 57; S. A. Cooper *et al.*, *J. clin. Pharmac.*, 1979, *19*, 151; R. Okun *et al.*, *J. clin. Pharmac.*, 1979, *19*, 487; A. D. Cattaneo and D. Roccatagliata, *J. clin. Pharmac.*, 1980, *20*, 475; G. Sacchetti *et al.*, *Br. J. clin. Pharmac.*, 1980, *9*, 165; A. Jain *et al.*, *Clin. Pharmac. Ther.*, 1980, *27*, 260.

Effects on biliary tract. In a single-blind study in 23 patients with T-tubes in the bile-duct following surgery, indoprofen up to 400 mg by intravenous injection did not produce any significant change in biliary pressure in contrast to either morphine or pentazocine. Fewer side-effects occurred with administration of indoprofen. It was considered that indoprofen was appropriate for the treatment of pain due to disorders of the biliary tract.— G. Sacchetti *et al.*, *Clin. Trials J.*, 1978, *15*, 90. See also G. Sacchetti (letter), *Lancet*, 1979, *2*, 425.

Osteoarthrosis. Studies on the use of indoprofen in the treatment of osteoarthrosis.— R. Marcolongo *et al.*, *J. clin. Pharmac.*, 1977, *17*, 48; G. Sacchetti *et al.*, *Curr. ther. Res.*, 1978, *24*, 274; G. C. Saba and G. Orlandi, *ibid.*, 1979, *25*, 260; P. F. Peregalli *et al.*, *Clin. Trials J.*, 1979, *16*, 41; P. F. Innocenti *et al.*, *Curr. med. Res. Opinion*, 1979, *5*, 793; A. Emanueli *et al.*, *ibid.*, *6*, 124.

Rheumatoid arthritis. In a double-blind crossover study in 35 patients with rheumatoid arthritis indoprofen 200 mg four times daily was generally comparable in efficacy to naproxen 250 mg twice daily; patient preference was in favour of indoprofen.— H. Berry *et al.*, *Br. med. J.*, 1978, *1*, 274.

Further studies on the use of indoprofen in rheumatoid arthritis.— E. C. Huskisson and J. Scott, *Rheumatol. Rehabil.*, 1979, *18*, 49; P. Loizzi *et al.*, *Curr. med. Res. Opinion*, 1980, *6*, 598.

Proprietary Names

Flosint *(Montedison, Arg.*; *Carlo Erba, Ital.*; *Chemfarma, S.Afr.).*

2660-x

Isopropylaminophenazone.

Isopyrin. 4-Isopropylamino-1,5-dimethyl-2-phenyl-4-pyrazolin-3-one.
$C_{14}H_{19}N_3O$=245.3.

CAS — 3615-24-5.

NOTE. The name Isopyrin has also been applied to isoniazid.

Uses. Isopropylaminophenazone is an analgesic, anti-inflammatory, and antipyretic agent used with phenylbutazone sodium in veterinary practice.

2661-r

Kebuzone.

Ketophenylbutazone. 4-(3-Oxobutyl)-1,2-diphenylpyrazolidine-3,5-dione.
$C_{19}H_{18}N_2O_3$=322.4.

CAS — 853-34-9.

Pharmacopoeias. In *Cz.*

Kebuzone is an analgesic and anti-inflammatory agent with actions and uses similar to those of phenylbutazone (see p.273). It is used in doses of 0.25 to 1 g daily. It has also been given as suppositories containing 250 mg. Reported adverse effects include kidney and liver damage.

Hypocholesterolaemic effect.— J. Sitar, *Vnitr. Lék.*, 1968, *14*, 228.

Proprietary Names

Chebutan *(Bioindustria, Ital.)*; Chepirol *(Esterfarm, Ital.)*; Chetopir *(Sarm, Ital.)*; Chetosol *(Aristochimica, Ital.)*; Ejor *(Elea, Arg.)*; Gammachetone *(Tiber, Ital.)*; Kétazone *(Beytout, Fr.)*; Ketofen *(Francia Farm., Ital.)*; Neo-Panalgyl *(Ital Suisse, Ital.)*; Neufenil *(Jap.)*.

2662-f

Ketoprofen

(B.P.). RP19583. 2-(3-Benzoylphenyl)propionic acid.
$C_{16}H_{14}O_3$=254.3.

CAS — 22071-15-4.

Pharmacopoeias. In *Br.*

A white or almost white, odourless or almost odourless, crystalline powder. M.p. 93° to 96°. Practically **insoluble** in water; freely soluble in alcohol, chloroform, and ether; soluble in methyl alcohol.

Adverse Effects and Precautions. As for Ibuprofen, p.256.

There were 49 reports of adverse reactions to ketoprofen reported to the Committee on Safety of Medicines up to September 1974. Gastro-intestinal irritation appeared to predominate.— M. F. Cuthbert, *Curr. med. Res. Opinion*, 1974, *2*, 600.

In an open study, ketoprofen caused side-effects requiring withdrawal of treatment in 256 of 4727 patients with rheumatic disorders. Gastro-intestinal effects occurred in 225 patients, including melaena/haematemesis in 7; also central nervous (37 patients), cardiovascular (2), and other side-effects (22). Side-effects not requiring withdrawal occurred in 665 of 4107 patients completing the study.— J. Mason and M. S. Bolton, *Br. J. clin. Pract.*, 1977, *31*, 127.

Allergy. Life-threatening asthma, urticaria, and angioneurotic oedema developed in 2 aspirin-sensitive patients after taking ketoprofen 50 mg by mouth.— P. Frith *et al.* (letter), *Lancet*, 1978, *2*, 847.

Effects on blood. Mention of 1 case of fatal aplastic anaemia or agranulocytosis in one year probably due to ketoprofen.— W. H. W. Inman, *Br. med. J.*, 1977, *1*, 1500.

Effects on the eyes. A 45-year-old Nigerian woman with amyloidosis, twice developed painful swollen eyes with redness, on administration of ketoprofen.— E. M. Umez-Eronini (letter), *Lancet*, 1978, *2*, 737.

Effects on the gastro-intestinal tract. Both ketoprofen and naproxen caused significantly increased gastro-intestinal blood loss compared with drug-free control periods.— B. Magnusson *et al.*, *Scand. J. Rheumatol.*, 1977, *6*, 62.

Intracranial hypertension. A 7-year-old girl with Bartter's syndrome developed symptoms attributable to pseudomotor cerebri after treatment with ketoprofen 20 mg per kg body-weight daily for 15 days. Retention of sodium and water, probably secondary to prostaglandin inhibition, was considered responsible.— D. Larizza *et al.* (letter), *New Engl. J. Med.*, 1979, *300*, 796.

Absorption and Fate. Ketoprofen is readily absorbed from the gastro-intestinal tract; peak plasma concentrations occur ½ to 2 hours after a dose. The plasma half-life is about 1 to 4 hours. Ketoprofen is extensively bound to plasma proteins. It is metabolised mainly by conjugation with glucuronic acid, and is excreted in the urine and to a lesser extent in the faeces.

The peak plasma concentration of ketoprofen following dosage with 100 mg by mouth to healthy subjects occurred 1 hour after administration and effective concentrations were maintained for 4 to 5 hours. Similarly after ketoprofen 50 mg given intramuscularly the peak plasma concentration occurred after 30 minutes, with effective concentrations for the next 2 to 3 hours. Most of the dose was excreted in the urine within the first 6 hours.— G. Sala *et al.*, *Farmaco, Edn prat.*, 1978, *33*, 455.

Uses. Ketoprofen is a phenylpropionic acid derivative which has analgesic, anti-inflammatory, and antipyretic actions and is used in the treatment of rheumatoid arthritis and osteoarthritis. The usual dose is 50 to 100 mg twice daily with food.

An evaluation of ketoprofen.— R. N. Brogden *et al.*, *Drugs*, 1974, *8*, 168. See also *Drug & Ther. Bull.*, 1974, *12*, 25.

Ankylosing spondylitis. Reports on the use of ketoprofen in ankylosing spondylitis.— B. L. Treadwell and J. M. Tweed, *N.Z. med. J.*, 1975, *81*, 411; J. D. Jessop, *Rheumatol. Rehabil.*, 1976, *Suppl.*, 37.

Bartter's syndrome. For the replacement of indomethacin by ketoprofen in the treatment of Bartter's syndrome by prostaglandin synthetase inhibitors, see

Indomethacin, p.259.

Improvement with ketoprofen in an infant with congenital chloride diarrhoea; features of his disorder were similar to those seen with Bartter's syndrome.— A. M. B. Minford and D. G. D. Barr, *Archs Dis. Childh.*, 1980, *55*, 70.

Osteoarthrosis. Significant mean increases in intermalleolar straddle, in hip rotation, and in knee flexion, in addition to analgesic effect were reported in 80 hospital patients with osteoarthrosis, who had taken ketoprofen 200 mg daily at night, with food, for 4 weeks. A further 10 patients had to withdraw from the study because of side-effects including nausea and vomiting in 4 patients and indigestion and headache, each in 2 patients.— J. Goulton, *Br. J. clin. Pract.*, 1979, *33*, 26.

Further studies on the use of ketoprofen in osteoarthrosis.— G. Fava *et al.*, *J. int. med. Res.*, 1977, *5*, 301; R. Franchi *et al.*, *Scand. J. Rheumatol.*, 1979, *Suppl.* 26, 1.

Rheumatic disorders. In a double-blind study in 46 patients with rheumatoid arthritis and 42 with osteoarthritis, ketoprofen 25 mg four times daily was comparable with indomethacin in the same dosage. Side-effects were broadly comparable with those of indomethacin but were less severe. Of the biochemical parameters studied, only hydroxybutyric dehydrogenase concentrations were elevated in some patients taking either ketoprofen or indomethacin; these changes were of doubtful significance.— A. N. Gyory *et al.*, *Br. med. J.*, 1972, *4*, 398.

A multi-centre evaluation of ketoprofen was conducted in 214 patients with rheumatoid arthritis, osteoarthritis, ankylosing spondylitis, and other arthritic conditions. Patients received other anti-inflammatory drugs if required. A total of 131 patients improved while only 35 patients failed to respond or worsened during ketoprofen therapy. Side-effects occurred in 83 patients and included gastro-intestinal disturbances in 55, allergic reactions in 13, and central nervous system reactions in 8. Therapy was discontinued in 44 patients.— M. J. Willans *et al.*, *Curr. ther. Res.*, 1979, *25*, 35.

Further studies on the use of ketoprofen in rheumatic disorders.— R. P. Saxena and U. Saxena, *Curr. med. Res. Opinion*, 1978, *5*, 484.

Rheumatoid arthritis. In a double-blind crossover study in 34 patients with rheumatoid arthritis given ketoprofen 150 mg daily or ibuprofen 1.2 g daily, ketoprofen was superior to ibuprofen in respect of relief of pain and joint circumference. The ESR favoured ibuprofen. There was no significant difference (but a trend in favour of ketoprofen) in respect of morning stiffness, grip strength, and consumption of paracetamol.— S. B. Mills *et al.*, *Br. med. J.*, 1973, *4*, 82.

In a double-blind crossover study, 43 patients with rheumatoid arthritis were given ketoprofen 25 or 33 mg thrice daily or a placebo. Ketoprofen was significantly better than placebo in respect of pain, global assessment, patient preference, and additional consumption of aspirin, but there was no significant difference in respect of functional capacity or morning stiffness. Side-effects were mild.— D. W. Zutshi, *Rheumatol. Rehabil.*, 1973, *12*, 62.

Further studies on the use of ketoprofen in rheumatoid arthritis.— B. J. Cathcart *et al.*, *Ann. rheum. Dis.*, 1973, *32*, 62; J. Chabot *et al.*, *Thérapie*, 1974, *29*, 417; M. Viara *et al.*, *Eur. J. clin. Pharmac.*, 1975, *8*, 205; E. F. El-Ghobarey *et al.*, *Curr. med. Res. Opinion*, 1976, *4*, 432; A. Calin *et al.*, *J. Rheumatol.*, 1977, *4*, 153; D. L. G. Howard, *Curr. ther. Res.*, 1978, *23*, 678; D. L. G. Howard, *J. int. med. Res.*, 1978, *6*, 300; J. Goulton and P. G. Baker, *Curr. med. Res. Opinion*, 1980, *6*, 423.

Preparations

Ketoprofen Capsules *(B.P.)*. Capsules containing ketoprofen. Store at a temperature not exceeding 30°.

Alrheumat *(Bayer, UK)*. Ketoprofen, available as **Capsules** of 50 mg and as **Suppositories** of 100 mg.

Orudis *(May & Baker, UK)*. Ketoprofen, available as **Capsules** of 50 and 100 mg and as **Suppositories** of 100 mg. (Also available as Orudis in *Canad.*, *Denm.*, *Ger.*, *Ital.*, *Jap.*, *S.Afr.*, *Spain*).

Other Proprietary Names

Arg.— Alreumun, Anaus, Kevadon, Lertus, Profenid; *Belg.*— Alrhumat, Rofenid; *Denm.*— Alreumat; *Fr.*— Profénid; *Ger.*— Alrheumun; *Ital.*— Artrosilene (as lysinate), Fastum, Flexen, Iso-K, Kefenid, Ketalgin, Keto, Salient, Sinketol; *Jap.*— Capisten; *Spain*— Remauric; *Switz.*— Alrhumat, Profenid.

2663-d

Lithium Salicylate *(B.P.C. 1949)*. Salicilato de Litio.
$C_7H_5LiO_3$=144.1.

CAS — 552-38-5.

Pharmacopoeias. In *Fr.* and *Span.*

A white or greyish-white, odourless, hygroscopic, crystalline powder with a sweet nauseating taste.

Soluble 1 in 0.7 of water, forming a slightly coloured, slightly acid solution; soluble 1 in 2 of alcohol, and in ether. Solutions are **sterilised** by autoclaving or by filtration. **Incompatible** with acids, alkali carbonates, free ammonia, ferric and quinine salts, and phenazone. **Store** in airtight containers. Protect from light.

Uses. Lithium salicylate has properties resembling those of sodium salicylate (see p.279) and has been used in rheumatism and gout. A 30% solution, usually with the addition of a local anaesthetic, has been used as a sclerosing agent in the injection treatment of varicose veins. Its use cannot be recommended because of the pharmacological effect of the lithium ion.

2664-n

Magnesium Salicylate *(U.S.P.)*.
$C_{14}H_{10}MgO_6,4H_2O$=370.6.

CAS — 18917-89-0 (anhydrous); 6150-94-3; 18917-95-8 (both tetrahydrate).

A white, odourless, efflorescent, crystalline powder. **Soluble** 1 in 13 of water; soluble in alcohol. Aqueous solutions are slightly acid. **Store** in airtight containers.

Uses. Magnesium salicylate has similar actions to aspirin (p.235). It is used in the treatment of rheumatoid arthritis and other rheumatic disorders. The usual dose is 1.8 to 4.8 g of anhydrous magnesium salicylate daily in divided doses.

A brief review of non-aspirin salicylate drugs concluded that there was insufficient data to judge whether they were as effective as aspirin, or better tolerated, in the treatment of inflammatory disorders.— *Med. Lett.*, 1978, *20*, 100.

Preparations

Magnesium Salicylate Tablets *(U.S.P.)*. Tablets containing magnesium salicylate. Potency is expressed in terms of the equivalent amount of anhydrous magnesium salicylate. The *U.S.P.* requires 80% dissolution in 120 minutes. Store in airtight containers.

Proprietary Names

Analate *(Winston, USA)*; Arthrin *(Saron, USA)*; Causalin *(Amfre-Grant, USA)*; Magan *(Adria, USA)*; Mobidin *(Ascher, USA)*; Triact *(Misemer, USA)*.

2717-r

Meclofenamic Acid. CI-583; INF 4668.

N-(2,6-Dichloro-*m*-tolyl)anthranilic acid.
$C_{14}H_{11}Cl_2NO_2$=296.2.

CAS — 644-62-2.

Practically **insoluble** in water.

2665-h

Meclofenamate Sodium.

$C_{14}H_{10}Cl_2NNaO_2$=318.1.

CAS — 6385-02-0.

Sparingly **soluble** in water. A saturated solution in water has a pH of 8.7.

Adverse Effects. Meclofenamate sodium has a high incidence of side-effects. The commonest are gastro-intestinal disturbances including diarrhoea, which may be severe, nausea, vomiting, and abdominal pain. Peptic ulceration and gastro-intestinal bleeding have also been reported. Skin rashes and pruritus may occur.

The commonest adverse effect in 2500 patients who received meclofenamate sodium in double-blind or long-term studies was gastro-intestinal disturbance. Diarrhoea occurred in 11.2% of patients in double-blind studies and 32.8% of patients in long-term studies (up to 3 years). Ulcers were detected in 22 patients during therapy and skin rashes occurred in 4% of patients. Transient increases in serum aminotransferases and BUN occurred in some patients.— S. N. Preston, *Curr. ther. Res.*, 1978, *23*, *Suppl.* 4S, S107.

Precautions. As for Ibuprofen, p.256.

Absorption and Fate. Meclofenamate sodium is readily absorbed when given by mouth; the free acid is absorbed more slowly. Peak plasma concentrations occur ½ to 2 hours after ingestion of the sodium salt. Meclofenamic acid is over 99% bound to plasma proteins. The mean biological half-life of meclofenamate sodium is about 3 hours. It is metabolised by oxidation, hydroxylation, dehalogenation, and conjugation with glucuronic acid and excreted in urine mainly as metabolites. About 20 to 30% is recovered in the faeces.

Studies on the absorption and fate of sodium meclofenamate.— A. J. Glazko *et al.*, *Curr. ther. Res.*, 1978, *23*, *Suppl.* 4S, S22.

Uses. Meclofenamate sodium is an anthranilic acid derivative similar to mefenamic acid. It has analgesic, anti-inflammatory, and antipyretic actions. It is used in the treatment of some rheumatic disorders in doses of 200 to 400 mg daily in divided doses, although it is not recommended for initial treatment because of the high incidence of adverse effects.

The proceedings of a symposium on meclofenamate sodium.— *Curr. ther. Res.*, 1978, *23*, *Suppl.* 4S, S1–S152.

Further references: *Med. Lett.*, 1980, *22*, 111.

Ankylosing spondylitis. Meclofenamate sodium was as effective as indomethacin in a study in 78 patients with ankylosing spondylitis.— R. Eberl, *Curr. ther. Res.*, 1978, *23*, *Suppl.* S4, S126.

Gout. A study on the use of meclofenamate sodium in gout.— J. D. C. Gowans *et al.*, *Curr. ther. Res.*, 1978, *23*, *Suppl.* S4, S138.

Osteoarthrosis. Studies on the use of meclofenamate sodium in osteoarthrosis.— R. Willkens, *Curr. ther. Res.*, 1978, *23*, *Suppl.* 4S, S81; I. Schleyer, *ibid.*, S121.

Rheumatoid arthritis. Studies on the use of meclofenamate sodium in the treatment of rheumatoid arthritis.— J. A. N. Rennie *et al.*, *Curr. med. Res. Opinion*, 1977, *4*, 580; J. Zuckner *et al.*, *Curr. ther. Res.*, 1978, *23*, *Suppl.* 4S, S66; C. V. Multz *et al.*, *ibid.*, S72; R. Wolf, *ibid.*, S113.

Proprietary Names

Meclomen *(Parke, Davis, USA)*.

2666-m

Mefenamic Acid *(B.P.)*. CI 473; INF 3355.

N-(2,3-Xylyl)anthranilic acid.
$C_{15}H_{15}NO_2$=241.3.

CAS — 61-68-7.

Pharmacopoeias. In *Br.*

A white to greyish-white, odourless, tasteless, microcrystalline powder. M.p. about 230° with effervescence.

Practically **insoluble** in water; soluble 1 in 185 of alcohol, 1 in 150 of chloroform, 1 in 80 of ether; soluble in solutions of alkali hydroxides. **Store** in airtight containers.

Formulation of mefenamic acid suppositories.— V. A. Golovkin *et al.*, *Farmatsiya, Mosk.*, 1978, *27*, 16.

Adverse Effects. The commonest adverse effects occurring with mefenamic acid are gastro-intestinal disturbances. Peptic ulceration and gastro-intestinal bleeding have also been reported. Headache, drowsiness, dizziness, nervousness, visual disturbances, and slight elevations in blood-urea-nitrogen have been reported. There may be hypersensitivity reactions. Asthma may be precipitated. Skin rashes occur.Reported haematological effects include haemolytic anaemia, agranulocytosis, pancytopenia, thrombocytopenic purpura, and bone-marrow aplasia.

Therapy should be discontinued if diarrhoea or skin rash occur.

A detailed review of the side-effects of mefenamic acid, flufenamic acid, and niflumic acid. Reports from different workers were very variable but although the side-effects were mainly gastro-intestinal a striking number of skin reactions were noted.— J. Strauss *et al.*, *Thérapie*, 1976, *31*, 325.

Effects on blood. *Haemolytic anaemia.* Three patients who had taken mefenamic acid (1.5 g daily in 2 patients) for 1 to 2 years developed auto-immune haemolytic anaemia during therapy and all recovered completely and rapidly when the drug was withdrawn.— G. L. Scott *et al.*, *Br. med. J.*, 1968, *3*, 534.

A 50-year-old man with rheumatoid arthritis developed haemolytic anaemia while receiving mefenamic acid, prednisone, and sodium aurothiomalate over 3 weeks. The haemolysis was attributed to mefenamic acid, though the possibility that gold had a combined or synergistic effect with mefenamic acid could not be excluded.— J. M. Jackson *et al.* (letter), *Br. med. J.*, 1970, *2*, 297.

A further report of auto-immune haemolytic anaemia induced by mefenamic acid.— J. -J. Farquet *et al.*, *Schweiz. med. Wschr.*, 1978, *108*, 1510.

Effects on the kidneys. Six elderly women who had been prescribed mefenamic acid 1 to 2 g daily for 2 to 6 weeks developed non-oliguric renal failure. Five of the women were admitted to hospital with a history of anorexia, nausea, and diarrhoea, followed by polyuria and dehydration; the sixth had received mefenamic acid after in-patient eye surgery, and had suffered nausea and vomiting, and polyuria. Four of the 6 patients also had rashes. Only one patient was known to have mild chronic renal failure; the remaining 5 had no history of renal disease, but 2 had maturity-onset diabetes well-controlled by diet alone, 2 had taken aspirin for many years, and 2 were taking diuretics; one patient had received tetracycline empirically one day before admission for urinary frequency. All made an uneventful recovery after intravenous fluid and electrolyte replacement, but renal function tests 2 to 4 weeks after admission showed persistent impairment of urinary concentrating ability and creatinine clearance, and at subsequent follow-up only 2 patients regained normal renal function; renal function remaining abnormal for their age in the other 4. Since mefenamic acid does not seem to have any advantage over other analgesics, and diarrhoea is a common side-effect, it is probably best avoided in the elderly and in patients with dehydration or pre-existing renal disease.— C. E. Robertson *et al.*, *Lancet*, 1980, *2*, 232. A report of allergic interstitial nephritis following mefenamic acid ingestion.— V. Venning *et al.* (letter), *ibid.*, 745. A report of a patient who developed glomerulonephritis with widespread vasculitis possibly associated with mefenamic acid.— S. Malik *et al.* (letter), *ibid.*, 746.

Non-oliguric renal failure, recurring on later inadvertent challenge, associated with the use of mefenamic acid.— P. L. Drury *et al.*, *Br. med. J.*, 1981, *282*, 865.

Further references: K. L. Woods and J. Michael (letter), *Br. med. J.*, 1981, *282*, 1471 (interstitial nephritis).

Effects on the gastro-intestinal tract. Reversible steatorrhoea occurred in a 65-year-old man who had been taking mefenamic acid 250 mg thrice daily for about 2 years. Diarrhoea ceased 2 days after stopping mefenamic acid and the faecal fat output was normal 2 weeks later.— J. S. Marks and M. H. Gleeson, *Br. med. J.*, 1975, *4*, 442. Two further cases.— R. G. Chadwick *et al.* (letter), *ibid.*, 1976, *1*, 397.

Effects on liver. Mefenamic acid was associated with hepatitis in 1 patient.— S. Imoto *et al.* (letter), *Ann. intern. Med.*, 1979, *91*, 129.

Overdosage. A report of status epilepticus in a 19-year-old woman 3 hours after the ingestion of mefenamic acid 12.5 g.— R. J. Young (letter), *Br. med. J.*, 1979, *2*, 672.

Single convulsions occurred in 2 adolescent girls who had taken 25 or 50 g of mefenamic acid; plasma concentrations of mefenamic acid were 110 and 72 µg per ml compared with expected therapeutic concentrations of less than 10 µg per ml.— R. H. Robson *et al.* (letter), *Br. med. J.*, 1979, *2*, 1438.

A report on the hazard of convulsions in patients with an overdose of mefenamic acid. Mefenamic acid should probably be avoided in epileptic patients.— M. Balali-Mood *et al.*, *Lancet*, 1981, *1*, 1354. Comment.— R. S. Kingswell, *Warner-Lambert* (letter), *ibid.*, *2*, 307. Reply.— L. F. Prescott *et al.* (letter), *ibid.*, 418.

Treatment of Adverse Effects. In acute poisoning the stomach should be emptied by aspiration and lavage. Activated charcoal has been suggested to reduce the absorption of mefenamic acid.

Precautions. Mefenamic acid is contra-indicated in patients with ulceration or inflammation of the gastro-intestinal tract. It should be used with caution in patients with impaired renal or liver function. It may enhance the effects of the coumarin anticoagulants.

Mefenamic acid has a marked tendency to induce grand mal convulsions in overdosage; some sources have suggested that it should be avoided in epileptic subjects.

In 10 healthy men given mefenamic acid 2 g daily for 28 days, blood-urea-nitrogen values rose; in 2 instances to outside the normal range.— E. L. Holmes and C. E. Moyer, *J. clin. Pharmac.*, 1969, *9*, 228.

Interactions. *Uricosuric agents.* Mefenamic acid and flufenamic acid did not affect the uricosuric action of sulphinpyrazone.— B. A. Latham *et al.*, *Ann. phys. Med.*, 1966, *8*, 242, per *Abstr. Wld Med.*, 1967, *41*, 131.

Pregnancy and the neonate. Mefenamic acid significantly prolonged the instillation-abortion time in patients undergoing hypertonic saline midtrimester abortion. This did not occur with pentazocine.— R. Waltman and V. Tricomi (letter), *Lancet*, 1974, *2*, 468.

Absorption and Fate. Mefenamic acid is absorbed from the gastro-intestinal tract. Peak concentrations in the circulation occur about 2 hours after ingestion. Mefenamic acid is extensively bound to plasma proteins. Approximately 50% of a dose may be recovered in the urine within 48 hours, mainly as conjugated metabolites.

Mefenamic acid given to nursing mothers was found in the breast milk in very small quantities.— R. A. Buchanan *et al.*, *Curr. ther. Res.*, 1968, *10*, 592.

Uses. Mefenamic acid has analgesic, anti-inflammatory and antipyretic actions and is used for the relief of mild to moderate pain in doses of up to 500 mg thrice daily. Conditions treated include rheumatoid arthritis and dysmenorrhoea. A suggested dose for children with Still's disease is 25 mg per kg body-weight daily in divided doses. Mefenamic acid has also been given to children as an antipyretic.

Some authorities suggest that treatment with mefenamic acid should not be continued for longer than 7 days.

An adverse evaluation of mefenamic acid.— *Med. Lett.*, 1972, *14*, 31. See also *ibid.*, 1978, *20*, 104.

Administration in renal failure. Four patients regularly undergoing haemodialysis were given mefenamic acid 500 mg by mouth 2 hours before a dialysis session. The mean drug recovery in the dialysate collected over 3 hours was 1.03 mg (0.2% of the dose).— L. -H. Wang *et al.*, *Clin. Pharmac. Ther.*, 1980, *27*, 292.

Analgesia. The results of a double-blind crossover study in 45 patients with constant pain indicated that mefenamic acid had significant analgesic properties compared with placebo, while flufenamic acid did not produce a significant analgesic effect. Positive tests for the bile in the urine of 6 patients were considered to be due to the presence of drug metabolites rather than to bilirubinuria.— R. M. H. Kater, *Med. J. Aust.*, 1968, *1*, 848.

Mefenamic acid 500 mg was effective in relieving pain due to uterine contractions during suction termination of pregnancy under local anaesthetic.— J. Guillebaud (letter), *Br. med. J.*, 1979, *1*, 1148.

Dysmenorrhoea. Mefenamic acid 250 mg every eight hours was more effective than dextropropoxyphene 32.5 mg with paracetamol 325 mg in a study of 30 patients with primary dysmenorrhoea. Flufenamic acid was also more effective than dextropropoxyphene and paracetamol but it appeared to be less effective than mefenamic acid.— A. B. M. Anderson *et al.*, *Lancet*, 1978, *1*, 345.

Mefenamic acid 250 mg four times a day was more effective than placebo in the treatment of primary dysmenorrhoea in 44 women.— P. W. Budoff, *J. Am. med. Ass.*, 1979, *241*, 2713. Mefenamic acid for dysmenorrhoea in a few patients with intra-uterine contraceptive devices.— *idem* (letter), *242*, 616.

Comment on the expected effect of prostaglandin inhibitors on uterine activity. Any analgesic should be used with caution in women with intra-uterine devices lest perforation, displacement, or infection as causes of pain be overlooked.— R. P. Smith and J. R. Powell (letter), *ibid.*, 1980, *243*, 231.

Further reports on the use of mefenamic acid in the treatment of dysmenorrhoea.— M. O. Pulkkinen and H. -L. Kaihola, *Acta obstet. gynec. scand.*, 1977, *56*, 75.

Menorrhagia. In 6 patients with menorrhagia mean blood loss was reduced from 119 to 60 ml when treated on the days of anticipated heavy loss with mefenamic acid 500 mg thrice daily or (1 patient) flufenamic acid 200 mg thrice daily. A further patient with a mean loss of 158 ml due to an intra-uterine contraceptive device had the loss reduced to 49 and 80 ml on 2 occasions when she took mefenamic acid 500 mg thrice daily for 7 to 10 days starting on the first day of established bleeding.— A. B. M. Anderson *et al.*, *Lancet*, 1976, *1*, 774.

Further reports on the use of mefenamic acid to reduce menstrual blood loss in women with menorrhagia and women using intra-uterine contraceptive devices.— J. Guillebaud *et al.*, *Br. J. Obstet. Gynaec.*, 1978, *85*, 53.

Pyrexia. Studies on the effectiveness of mefenamic acid as an antipyretic in children.— C. F. Weiss *et al.*, *J. Pediat.*, 1968, *72*, 867; S. Similä *et al.*, *Arzneimittel-Forsch.*, 1977, *27*, 687.

Rheumatoid arthritis. In a double-blind crossover study in 60 women with rheumatoid arthritis, mefenamic acid and flufenamic acid appeared to be satisfactory substitutes for aspirin and phenylbutazone. There were no significant differences in efficacy or adverse effects between the 4 drugs. The mean daily dosages used were: aspirin 2.4 g, phenylbutazone 330 mg, mefenamic acid 1.7 g, and flufenamic acid 670 mg.— D. E. Barnardo *et al.*, *Br. med. J.*, 1966, *2*, 342.

Further studies on the use of mefenamic acid in rheumatoid arthritis.— A. Stockman *et al.*, *Med. J. Aust.*, 1976, *2*, 819; R. D. G. Leslie, *J. int. med. Res.*, 1977, *5*, 161; M. E. Mavrikakis *et al.*, *Curr. med. Res. Opinion*, 1977, *4*, 535; M. E. Mavrikakis *et al.*, *Scott. med. J.*, 1978, *23*, 189; W. H. Stephens *et al.*, *Curr. med. Res. Opinion*, 1979, *5*, 754.

Preparations

Mefenamic Acid Capsules *(B.P.)*. Capsules containing mefenamic acid. Store at a temperature not exceeding 30°.

Ponstan *(Parke, Davis, UK)*. Mefenamic acid, available as **Capsules** of 250 mg and as **Paediatric Suspension** containing 50 mg in each 5 ml (suggested diluent, syrup). (Also available as Ponstan in *Austral.*, *Belg.*, *Canad.*, *S.Afr.*, *Switz.*). **Ponstan Forte.** Mefenamic acid, available as tablets of 500 mg.

Other Proprietary Names

Bafameritin-M *(Jap.)*; Bonabol *(Jap.)*; Coslan *(Spain)*; Lysalgo, Mefedolo *(bothItal.)*; Parkemed *(Ger.)*; Parke-Med *(Ital.)*; Ponstel *(USA)*; Ponstil *(Arg.)*; Ponstyl *(Fr.)*; Pontal *(Jap.)*.

2667-b

Methyl Salicylate *(B.P., B.P. Vet., Eur. P.)*.

Methylis Salicylas; Methyl Sal. Methyl 2-hydroxybenzoate.

$C_8H_8O_3$=152.1.

CAS — 119-36-8.

Pharmacopoeias. In *Arg.*, *Aust.*, *Belg.*, *Br.*, *Cz.*, *Fr.*, *Ger.*, *Hung.*, *Ind.*, *It.*, *Jap.*, *Jug.*, *Mex.*, *Neth.*, *Pol.*, *Port.*, *Roum.*, *Rus.*, *Span.*, and *Swiss.* Also in *U.S.N.F.* *Arg.*, *Mex.*, and *U.S.N.F.* allow in addition to synthetic methyl salicylate, the oils obtained from the leaves of *Gaultheria procumbens* (Ericaceae) and the bark of *Betula lenta* (Betulaceae)—see Sweet Birch Oil, p.247. The source of the methyl salicylate must be indicated on the label.

A colourless or pale yellow liquid with a strong persistent characteristic aromatic odour and sweet warm aromatic taste. B.p. about 221° with some decomposition. Relative density 1.182 to 1.187.

Very slightly **soluble** in water; soluble 1 in 10 of alcohol (70%); miscible with alcohol (90%) and with most organic solvents and oils. **Incompatible** with alkalis and iron salts. **Store** in a cool place in airtight containers. Protect from light. Certain plastic containers, such as those made from polystyrene, are unsuitable for liniments or ointments containing methyl salicylate.

NOTE. The *B.P.* directs that methyl salicylate be dispensed or supplied when Oil of Wintergreen, Wintergreen, or Wintergreen Oil is prescribed or demanded; great care, however, must be taken to ensure that these synonyms have not been used inappropriately to describe Methyl Salicylate Liniment, p.264

Adverse Effects and Treatment. As for Aspirin, p.236 and p.238. Doses of as little as 4 ml have caused death in infants.

Acute poisoning occurred in 2 seamen who drank about 90 ml and 30 ml respectively of wintergreen oil. The latter survived but the former died.— J. J. Canselmo, *J. Am. med. Ass.*, 1948, *136*, 651.

A 20-month-old child swallowed about 5 ml of wintergreen oil. Twenty-two hours later he was in a critical condition with poor chances of survival. The blood-salicylate concentration was 727 µg per ml. He recovered following an exchange blood transfusion, which reduced the salicylate concentration by 59%, and intravenous fluids.— J. T. Adams *et al.*, *J. Am. med. Ass.*, 1957, *165*, 1563.

Charcoal haemoperfusion in the successful treatment of poisoning with methyl salicylate.— J. A. Vale *et al.*, *Br. med. J.*, 1975, *1*, 5.

Adsorption. For comment on the *in vitro* adsorption of methyl salicylate by activated charcoal, see p.79.

Allergy. Sensitivity to methyl salicylate, confirmed by patch tests, occurred in 2 patients during the period 1957/66.— J. K. Morgan, *Br. J. clin. Pract.*, 1968, *22*, 261.

Urticaria and angioneurotic oedema occurred on several occasions in an aspirin-sensitive patient following exposure to liniments, toothpaste, and candy containing methyl salicylate.— F. Speer, *Ann. allergy*, 1979, *43*, 36.

Uses. Methyl salicylate has the actions of the salicylates. It is absorbed through the skin and is applied undiluted or in liniments and ointments for the relief of pain in lumbago, sciatica, and rheumatic conditions.

Estimated acceptable daily intake for man: up to 500 µg per kg body-weight.— Eleventh Report of the Joint FAO/WHO Expert Committee on Food Additives, *Tech. Rep. Ser. Wld Hlth Org. No. 383*, 1968.

Preparations

Liniments

Methyl Salicylate Liniment *(B.P., A.P.F.)*. Methyl salicylate 25 ml, arachis oil to 100 ml. Store in non-plastic containers.

Methyl Salicylate Liniment Compound *(A.P.F.)*. Methyl salicylate 25 ml, menthol 4 g, eucalyptus oil 10 ml, arachis oil to 100 ml.

Ointments

Compound Methyl Salicylate Ointment *(B.P.C. 1973)*. Ung. Methyl. Sal. Co.; Unguentum Methylis Salicylatis Compositum Forte; Ung. Betulae Co.; Ung. Analgesicum; Analgesic Balsam. Methyl salicylate 50% w/w, menthol 10% w/w, with cajuput oil and cineole in white beeswax, wool fat, and water. Store in non-plastic containers which prevent evaporation.

Dilute Compound Methyl Salicylate Ointment *(B.P.C. 1949)*. Compound methyl salicylate ointment 25% in hydrous wool fat ointment.

Dilute Methyl Salicylate Ointment *(B.P.C. 1949)*. Ung. Methyl. Salicyl. Dil. Methyl salicylate ointment 25% in hydrous wool fat ointment.

Methyl Salicylate Ointment *(B.P.)*. Strong Methyl Salicylate Ointment. Methyl salicylate 50 g, white beeswax 25 g, hydrous wool fat 25 g. Store at a temperature not exceeding 25° in non-plastic containers.

Unguentum Methylii Salicylici *(F.N. Belg.)*. Methyl salicylate 10% in Unguentum Simplex (*Belg. P.*).

Proprietary Preparations

Balmosa *(Pharmax, UK)*. A non-greasy analgesic cream containing methyl salicylate 4%, menthol 2%, camphor 4%, capsicum oleoresin 0.035%, and sodium iodide 1.2%.

Bengué's Balsam *(Bengué, UK)*. An ointment containing methyl salicylate 20% and menthol 20% in a lanolin basis. Rubefacient for muscular spasm. **Bengué's Balsam SG.** Contains methyl salicylate 15% and menthol 10% in a vanishing cream basis.

Dubam *(Norma, UK: Farillon, UK)*. Ointment containing methyl salicylate 20%, menthol 2%, and cineole 1%. **Dubam Spray Relief.** Contains methyl salicylate 5%, glycol salicylate 5%, and methyl nicotinate 1.6%. For rheumatism, fibrositis, and similar conditions.

A preparation containing methyl salicylate was formerly marketed in Great Britain under the proprietary name Liberol Ointment (*Multipax Laboratories*).

2668-v

Methylcinchophen. Methylum Phenylchinolincarbonicum; Methyl Phenylcinchoninate. Methyl 2-phenylquinoline-4-carboxylate.
$C_{17}H_{13}NO_2$=263.3.

CAS — 4546-48-9.

Pharmacopoeias. In *Aust.* and *Swiss.*

Yellowish tasteless crystals. Practically **insoluble** in water; soluble 1 in 80 of alcohol, and 1 in 6 of ether.

Uses. Methylcinchophen has been used similarly to cinchophen (p.249) in doses of 0.5 to 1 g up to a maximum of 3 g daily.

2669-g

Metiazinic Acid. Methiazinic Acid; RP 16091. (10-Methylphenothiazin-2-yl)acetic acid.
$C_{15}H_{13}NO_2S$=271.3.

CAS — 13993-65-2.

Adverse Effects. Gastro-intestinal disturbances, skin rashes, and dysuria have been reported.

Precautions. Metiazinic acid should be used with caution in patients with peptic ulceration. Reddish-brown discoloration of urine may occur. It may interfere with a number of diagnostic tests on urine and blood.

Uses. Metiazinic acid has analgesic and anti-inflammatory actions and has been used in the treatment of rheumatic disorders in doses of 1 to 2 g daily in divided doses.

References: G. Vignon *et al.*, *Revue Rhum. Mal. ostéo-artic.*, 1969, *36*, 715; S. DeSèze *et al.*, *Revue Rhum. Mal. ostéo-artic.*, 1969, *36*, 709, per *Abstr. Wld Med.*, 1970, *44*, 627; P. Deshayes and J. C. Gogny, *Rhumatologie*, 1970, *22*, 29; W. Siegmeth, *Wien. med. Wschr.*, 1971, *121*, 478.

Proprietary Names

Metian *(Horus, Spain)*; Novartril *(Andromaco, Spain)*; Roimal *(Jap.)*; Soridermal *(Specia, Belg.)*; Soripal *(Specia, Belg.; Specia, Fr.; Farmalabor, Ital.; Specia, Neth.; Rhodia, Spain)*.

2670-f

Mofebutazone. Monophenylbutazone; Monobutazone. 4-Butyl-1-phenylpyrazolidine-3,5-dione.
$C_{13}H_{16}N_2O_2$=232.3.

CAS — 2210-63-1.

Colourless crystals or a white or almost white crystalline powder with a slightly bitter taste. M.p. about 100°. Slightly **soluble** in water; soluble 1 in 4 of alcohol, 1 in 3 of chloroform, and 1 in 125 of ether; soluble in solutions of alkali hydroxides and carbonates. A saturated solution in water is acid to litmus.

Uses. Mofebutazone is a derivative of phenylbutazone (see p.273) with similar actions. A dose of 250 to 500 mg twice daily has been suggested.

A favourable report on the use of mofebutazone in rheumatoid arthritis.— S. Thune, *Acta rheum. scand.*, 1967, *13*, 63.

Mofebutazone was not as effective as phenylbutazone in patients with rheumatoid arthritis.— J. F. L. Woodbury *et al.*, *Can. med. Ass. J.*, 1969, *101*, 801.

Proprietary Names

Chemiartrol *(Gazzini, Ital.)*; Monazone *(Meuse, Belg.)*; Monbutina *(Lafare, Ital.)*; Monoprine *(Sanico, Belg.)*; Reumatox *(Medosan, Ital.)*.

2671-d

Morazone Hydrochloride. 1,5-Dimethyl-4-(3-methyl-2-phenylmorpholinomethyl)-2-phenyl-4-pyrazolin-3-one hydrochloride.
$C_{23}H_{27}N_3O_2$,HCl=413.9.

CAS — 6536-18-1 (morazone); 50321-35-2 (hydrochloride).

Uses. Morazone hydrochloride is an analgesic which has been used, usually in conjunction with other analgesics, in doses of 75 to 150 mg.

Proprietary Names

Rosimon-Neu *(Ravensberg, Ger.)*.

NOTE. Morazone hydrochloride is an ingredient of Delimon, p.277.

2672-n

Naproxen *(B.P., U.S.P.)*. RS-3540. (+)-2-(6-Methoxy-2-naphthyl)propionic acid.
$C_{14}H_{14}O_3$=230.3.

CAS — 22204-53-1.

Pharmacopoeias. In *Br.* and *U.S.*

A white or almost white, odourless or almost odourless, crystalline powder. M.p. about 156°. Practically **insoluble** in water; soluble 1 in 25 of alcohol, 1 in 15 of chloroform, 1 in 40 of ether, and 1 in 20 of methyl alcohol. A solution in chloroform is dextrorotatory. **Store** in airtight containers. Protect from light.

2673-h

Naproxen Sodium. RS 3650.
$C_{14}H_{13}NaO_3$=252.2.

CAS — 26159-34-2.

Naproxen sodium 1.1 g is approximately equivalent to 1 g of naproxen.

Adverse Effects. As for Ibuprofen, p.256.

Inhibition of ejaculation attributed to naproxen in one patient.— N. Wei and J. C. Hood (letter), *Ann. intern. Med.*, 1980, *93*, 933.

Allergy. All of 11 aspirin-sensitive asthmatic patients developed reactions (rhinorrhoea, tightness of chest, wheezing, dyspnoea) after taking naproxen in doses of 40 to 80 mg.— A. Szczeklik *et al.*, *Br. med. J.*, 1977, *2*, 231.

Vasculitis and symptoms of nephritis and paralytic ileus occurred in a woman who had taken naproxen and aspirin for 3 years. Serum IgG, IgA, and IgE and circulating immune complex activity were raised. Symptoms resolved after naproxen and aspirin were discontinued and did not reappear when salicylate was restarted.— D. M. Grennan *et al.*, *N.Z. med. J.*, 1979, *89*, 48.

Effects on blood. Mention of 2 cases of fatal aplastic anaemia or agranulocytosis in one year probably due to naproxen.— W. H. W. Inman, *Br. med. J.*, 1977, *1*, 1500.

Aplastic anaemia in a 47-year-old man might have been caused by naproxen therapy.— R. Arnold and H. Heimpel (letter), *Lancet*, 1980, *1*, 321.

Dose-related prolongation of bleeding time and inhibition of aggregation in healthy subjects given naproxen.— J. J. Bruno *et al.*, *Clin. Pharmac. Ther.*, 1980, *27*, 247. See also J. Nadell *et al.*, *J. clin. Pharmac.*, 1974, *14*, 176.

Effects on the gastro-intestinal tract. There were 52 reports of gastro-intestinal reactions to naproxen reported to the Committee on Safety of Medicines; there were 5 fatalities.— M. F. Cuthbert, *Curr. med. Res. Opinion*, 1974, *2*, 600.

Reports mainly of melaena and sometimes of haematemesis: E. Beck (letter), *Br. med. J.*, 1974, *1*, 572; M. C. Hayes-Allen (letter), *ibid;* F. D. Hart (letter), *ibid.*, *2*, 51; S. G. F. Matts (letter), *ibid.*, 52.

Endoscopic examination of 14 healthy subjects revealed significantly greater gastro-intestinal effects with naproxen 250 mg twice daily than with diclofenac (enteric-coated) 50 mg twice daily. Examination was for gastritis, haemorrhagic lesions, and erosive lesions.— M. Osnes *et al.*, *Clin. Pharmac. Ther.*, 1979, *26*, 399.

Effects on the kidneys. Reversible renal failure and nephrotic syndrome developed in a patient who had been taking naproxen 250 mg twice daily for a year. Renal biopsy revealed prominent interstitial nephritis.— J. H. Brezin *et al.*, *New Engl. J. Med.*, 1979, *301*, 1271. Eight cases of genito-urinary disorders have been reported to the Committee of Safety of Medicines from recipients of at least 1 899 300 prescriptions.— J. H. Brezin (letter), *ibid.*, 1980, *302*, 1092.

Interstitial nephritis and renal insufficiency in an 18-year-old youth with rheumatoid arthritis were attributed to naproxen. Symptoms resolved when naproxen was discontinued.— K. C. Cartwright *et al.*, *Ariz. Med.*, 1979, *36*, 124.

Effects on liver. Approximately 2 months after starting treatment with naproxen 250 mg twice daily a 35-year-old patient developed jaundice which disappeared when treatment was discontinued.— B. H. Bass (letter), *Lancet*, 1974, *1*, 998.

A report of jaundice and an enlarged liver associated with naproxen therapy in a 54-year-old woman. Dramatic improvement with return of liver-function tests to normal occurred within 4 weeks of discontinuation.— I. P. Law and H. Knight (letter), *New Engl. J. Med.*, 1977, *295*, 1201.

Jaundice occurred in a man who had been taking naproxen for one month. Histological findings after liver biopsy were consistent with drug-induced hepatitis.— R. M. M. Victorino *et al.*, *Postgrad. med. J.*, 1980, *56*, 368.

Overdosage. A study of the pharmacokinetics of naproxen following overdosage of healthy subjects with single doses of 1, 2, 3, or 4 g. An increase in the urinary-excretion rate was noted, with acceleration as naproxen-plasma concentrations rose to 100 to 200 µg per ml. Results indicated that the body can apparently handle doses of up to 4 g, without saturating any of its eliminating mechanisms, in a manner similar to doses in the therapeutic range. No side-effects were reported other than mild epigastric pain in 1 subject in the evening after receiving 3 g; clinical laboratory tests were normal.— R. Runkel *et al.*, *Clin. Pharmac. Ther.*, 1976, *20*, 269.

A patient reported to have ingested 25 g of naproxen suffered only mild transient gastro-intestinal distress. The serum concentration of naproxen 15 hours after ingestion was 414 µg per ml.— E. W. Fredell and L. J. Strand (letter), *J. Am. med. Ass.*, 1977, *238*, 938.

Pregnancy and the neonate. Comment on the adverse effects of naproxen on twins and a singleton whose mothers had been given naproxen to delay parturition. The infants had severe hypoxaemia due to persistent pulmonary hypertension, and one of the twins died.— A. R. Wilkinson (letter), *Lancet*, 1980, *2*, 591.

Treatment of Adverse Effects. Following overdosage the stomach should be emptied by inducing emesis or by aspiration and lavage. Activated charcoal has been suggested to reduce the absorption of naproxen. Further treatment is symptomatic.

Precautions. As for Ibuprofen, p.256.

Naproxen may interfere with some tests for 17-ketogenic steroids.

Interactions, drugs. *Antacids.* The absorption of naproxen was altered by antacids. With sodium bicarbonate there was an earlier and increased peak plasma-naproxen concentration, whereas with magnesium oxide and aluminium hydroxide the peak was delayed and lower than with naproxen alone. Combination with a preparation of magnesium and aluminium hydroxides tended to reduce the time to peak plasma-naproxen concentration and to increase slightly the total amount absorbed.— E. J. Segre *et al.* (letter), *New Engl. J. Med.*, 1974, *291*, 582.

Anticoagulants. Studies in healthy subjects showed no evidence of a clinically important alteration of either the pharmacokinetics or anticoagulant activity of racemic warfarin by the usual therapeutic doses of naproxen.— A. Jain *et al.*, *Clin. Pharmac. Ther.*, 1979, *25*, 61. See also J. T. Slattery *et al.*, *ibid.*, 51.

Aspirin. In 6 subjects given naproxen 500 mg and aspirin 1.2 g alone and concomitantly, plasma concentrations of naproxen were reduced when aspirin was given concomitantly; this appeared to be due to increased excretion of naproxen. Preliminary reports of clinical studies suggested that the interaction was not clinically significant.— E. Segre *et al.*, *Scand. J. Rheumatol.*, 1973, *Suppl.* 2, 37.

Diuretics. Diminished effect of frusemide on concomitant administration of indomethacin or naproxen.— R. Faunch (letter), *Br. med. J.*, 1981, *283*, 989.

Probenecid. Probenecid increased plasma concentrations of naproxen and its 6-*O*-desmethyl metabolite in a study of 6 healthy subjects.— R. Runkel *et al.*, *Clin. Pharmac. Ther.*, 1978, *24*, 706.

Porphyria. A study in *rats* indicated that naproxen would probably not elicit an acute attack in susceptible porphyric individuals.— G. H. Blekkenhorst *et al.* (letter), *Lancet*, 1980, *1*, 1367. Criticisms of extrapolating data obtained from *animal* experiments to the treatment of human disease.— M. J. Brodie (letter), *ibid.*, *2*, 86; A. Gorchein (letter), *ibid.*, 152.

Absorption and Fate. Naproxen and naproxen sodium are readily absorbed from the gastro-intestinal tract. Absorption is claimed to be more rapid with the sodium salt. Peak plasma concentrations are attained 2 to 4 hours after ingestion. At therapeutic concentrations naproxen is more than 99% bound to plasma proteins and has a plasma half-life of between 12 and 15 hours. Approximately 95% of a dose is excreted in urine as naproxen and 6-*O*-desmethylnaproxen and their conjugates. Less than 3% of a dose has been recovered in the faeces. Naproxen crosses the placenta and is excreted in breast milk.

A study of the absorption, distribution, metabolism, and excretion of naproxen.— R. Runkel *et al.*, *J. pharm. Sci.*, 1972, *61*, 703.

Absorption of naproxen 300 mg from Carbowax or Witepsol suppository bases was comparable with absorption from the same dose given by mouth.— H. Sevelius *et al.*, *Eur. J. clin. Pharmac.*, 1973, *6*, 22.

In 24 healthy subjects plasma concentrations of naproxen reached a plateau with doses greater than 500 mg twice daily by mouth; this might have been due to accelerated renal clearance.— R. Runkel *et al.*, *Clin. Pharmac. Ther.*, 1974, *15*, 261.

A study of naproxen concentrations in synovial fluid.— S. Javala *et al.*, *Scand. J. Rheumatol.*, 1977, *6*, 155.

Bioavailability of naproxen sodium and its relationship to clinical analgesic effects.— H. Sevelius *et al.*, *Br. J. clin. Pharmac.*, 1980, *10*, 259.

Protein binding. Studies *in vitro* using plasma obtained from healthy subjects showed that a mean of 99.7% of naproxen was bound to plasma proteins but no correlation with α_1-acid glycoprotein or albumin concentration was found.— K. M. Piafsky and O. Borgå, *Clin. Pharmac. Ther.*, 1977, *22*, 545.

Uses. Naproxen is a phenylpropionic acid derivative which has analgesic, anti-inflammatory, and antipyretic actions. Both naproxen and naproxen sodium are used in the treatment of rheumatoid arthritis and other rheumatic or musculoskeletal disorders, dysmenorrhoea, and acute gout. The sodium salt is also recommended as an analgesic for a variety of other painful disorders.

In rheumatic disorders the usual initial dose of naproxen is 250 mg twice daily, adjusted to 500 mg to 1 g daily in 2 divided doses. A dose of 10 mg per kg body-weight daily in 2 divided doses has been used in children over 5 years of age with juvenile rheumatoid arthritis. In acute gout an initial dose of 750 mg followed by 250 mg every 8 hours has been suggested while in dysmenorrhoea 500 mg may be given initially followed by 250 mg every 6 to 8 hours. Rectal administration is sometimes employed.

Naproxen sodium is given similarly in doses of 275 mg, equivalent to about 250 mg of naproxen.

Extensive reviews of the actions and uses of naproxen.— R. N. Brogden *et al.*, *Drugs*, 1975, *9*, 326; *idem*, 1979, *18*, 241.

Proceedings of symposia on naproxen.— *Scand. J. Rheumatol.*, 1973, *Suppl.* 2, 1-181; *Arzneimittel-Forsch.*, 1975, *25*, 278-332; *Eur. J. Rheumatol. Inflamm.*, 1979, *2*, 1-83.

Administration in renal failure. No accumulation of naproxen was seen in a patient undergoing haemodialysis thrice weekly and receiving naproxen 500 mg daily. Dialysis did not clear naproxen and a post-dialysis dose was considered to be unnecessary.— S. S. Weber *et al.*-, *Am. J. Hosp. Pharm.*, 1979, *36*, 1567.

Patients with a glomerular filtration-rate of 10 ml or more per minute could receive naproxen every 12 hours. When the glomerular filtration-rate was less than 10 ml per minute the dose interval should be increased to 18 hours.— W. M. Bennett *et al.*, *Ann. intern. Med.*, 1980, *93*, 286.

A study suggesting that no adjustment of naproxen dosage is needed in renal failure.— M. Anttila *et al.*, *Eur. J. clin. Pharmac.*, 1980, *18*, 263.

Analgesia. In a double-blind study comparing naproxen, codeine sulphate, and aspirin in 230 postpartum women, naproxen 300 or 600 mg or naproxen sodium 275 mg (equivalent to naproxen 250 mg) provided as effective relief of uterine pain as aspirin 650 mg. Onset of action and peak analgesic effect took 2 or more hours to appear following naproxen administration, the analgesia lasting 7 or 8 hours, analgesia was obtained within 1 hour of aspirin administration and continued until the fifth hour. Codeine sulphate 60 mg was noted to be ineffective in this type of pain. Although there was evidence that improved pain relief followed higher naproxen doses this was not significant, possibly owing to a ceiling effect, nor did side-effects of naproxen appear to be dose related.— S. S. Bloomfield *et al.*, *Clin. Pharmac. Ther.*, 1977, *21*, 414.

At evaluation after 7 days of treatment with indomethacin 25 mg or naproxen 250 mg both taken thrice daily, 71 of 95 patients with sports injuries who received naproxen were considered to be cured compared with 45 of 96 similar patients who received indomethacin. Reduction of pain and swelling and increased movement were significantly greater in the naproxen group. Ten patients taking indomethacin and 18 taking naproxen required further treatment. The incidence of adverse effects was similar in both groups, the most common effects being drowsiness, tiredness, dizziness and indigestion.— T. A. Bouchier-Hayes and C. W. Jones, *Practitioner*, 1979, *223*, 706.

Further reports on the analgesic efficacy of naproxen in patients with postoperative pain or musculoskeletal disorders.— J. Ruedy and W. McCullough, *Scand. J. Rheumatol.*, 1973, *Suppl.* 2, 56; D. L. Mahler *et al.*, *Clin. pharmac. Ther.*, 1976, *19*, 18; G. Jaffé, *Curr. med. Res. Opinion*, 1976, *4*, 373; J. G. P. Williams and C. Engler, *Rheumatol. Rehabil.*, 1977, *16*, 265; U. Aromaa and K. Asp, *J. int. med. Res.*, 1978, *6*, 152; G. Sacchetti *et al.*, *ibid.*, 312; G. Martino *et al.*, *Arzneimittel-Forsch.*, 1978, *28*, 1657; D. Wheatley, *Curr. med. Res. Opinion*, 1979, *6*, 229; H. S. Filtzer, *Curr. ther. Res.*, 1980, *27*, 293; H. Sevelius *et al.*, *J. clin. Pharmac.*, 1980, *20*, 480; C. I. Backhouse *et al.*, *Rheumatol. Rehabil.*, 1980, *19*, 113.

Ankylosing spondylitis. In an open study in 36 patients with ankylosing spondylitis 35 found naproxen 250 mg twice daily as effective, after 1 month, as their previous medication; 30 had taken naproxen for 6 months and 22 for at least 12 months. Morning stiffness was relieved and there was a slight increase in spinal flexion.— H. F. H. Hill and A. G. S. Hill, *J. clin. Pharmac.*, 1975, *15*, 355.

In a double-blind crossover study in 20 patients with ankylosing spondylitis, naproxen 500 to 750 mg daily or phenylbutazone 400 to 600 mg daily were given for 5 weeks. Both treatments were found to be equally effective, but the incidence of gastro-intestinal side-effects was higher with phenylbutazone, leading to withdrawal in 1 patient.— F. van Gerwen *et al.*, *Ann. rheum. Dis.*, 1978, *37*, 85.

Further studies on the use of naproxen in ankylosing spondylitis.— B. M. Ansell *et al.*, *Eur. J. Rheumatol. Inflamm.*, 1979, *2*, 45.

Bartter's syndrome. Naproxen given 250 mg thrice daily increased serum-potassium concentrations in a 31-year-old woman with Bartter's syndrome. Plasma-renin activity and urinary-aldosterone concentration were both reduced to normal values.— F. H. Katz and A. I. Bortz (letter), *New Engl. J. Med.*, 1978, *299*, 100.

Dysmenorrhoea. In 2 double-blind studies involving 43 patients with dysmenorrhoea naproxen sodium was significantly more effective than placebo. The permitted dose of naproxen sodium was 550 mg initially then 275 mg every 6 hours for up to 5 days; most patients took the drug for only 3 days.— M. R. Henzl *et al.*, *Am. J. Obstet. Gynec.*, 1977, *127*, 818.

A placebo-controlled study involving 33 women showed naproxen sodium to be effective in alleviating uterine cramping pains caused or aggravated by insertion of an intra-uterine device.— V. Buttram *et al.*, *Am. J. Obstet. Gynec.*, 1979, *134*, 575. See also under Menorrhagia.

Further studies on the use of naproxen or naproxen sodium in dysmenorrhoea.— F. Pauls (letter), *Lancet*, 1978, *2*, 159; F. W. Hanson *et al.*, *Obstet. Gynec.*, 1978, *52*, 583; O. Ylikorkala *et al.* (letter), *Lancet*, 1979, *1*, 278; M. R. Henzl *et al.*, *Am. J. Obstet. Gynec.*, 1979, *135*, 455.

Fever. Comparable antipyretic activity of naproxen and aspirin in children with fever.— T. M. Cashman *et al.*, *J. Pediat.*, 1979, *95*, 626.

Gout. Of 20 patients with acute gout 15 had responded favourably to treatment with naproxen, 600 mg initially followed by 300 mg eight-hourly for 2 to 4 days, or 750 mg initially followed after 8 hours by 500 mg and then by 250 mg eight-hourly for 2 to 3 days.— R. F. Willkens *et al.*, *J. clin. Pharmac.*, 1975, *15*, 363.

Further studies on the use of naproxen in the treatment of acute gout.— P. Cuq, *Scand. J. Rheumatol.*, 1973, *Suppl.* 2, 64; R. A. Sturge *et al.*, *Eur. J. Rheumatol. Inflamm.*, 1979, *2*, 40.

Menorrhagia. Naproxen 500 mg given in the morning and 250 mg in the afternoon for the first 2 days of a menstrual bleed and 250 mg twice daily for up to 7 days reduced the menstrual blood loss in 4 patients with primary menorrhagia. There was also a reduction in 5 patients with a blood loss of more than 80 ml per menstruation whose menorrhagia was associated with an intra-uterine device; there was no reduction in 5 similar women whose blood loss was less than 80 ml per menstruation.— G. Rybo *et al.* (letter), *Lancet*, 1981, *1*, 608.

Osteoarthrosis. A long-term open study was carried out in 145 patients with osteoarthrosis who had shown intolerance to other nonsteroidal anti-inflammatory drugs. Naproxen was given in doses of 250 to 500 mg twice daily for up to 12 months. Reduction of pain and improvement in function were satisfactory in most patients. Therapy was discontinued in 17 patients because of side-effects.— M. Thompson *et al.*, *Eur. J. Rheumatol. Inflamm.*, 1979, *2*, 25.

Further studies on the use of naproxen in osteoarthrosis.— G. Binzus and G. Josenhans, *Scand. J. Rheumatol.*, 1973, *Suppl.* 2, 80; G. M. Cochrane, *ibid.*, 89; T. Kageyama, *ibid.*, 94; C. G. Barnes *et al.*, *J. clin. Pharmac.*, 1975, *15*, 347; W. Blechman *et al.*, *Ann. rheum. Dis.*, 1978, *37*, 80; J. T. Vainio and P. V. Lepistö, *Scand. J. Rheumatol.*, 1978, *Suppl.* 21, 25; A. Car *et al.*, *ibid.*, *Suppl.* 22, 63; S. R. Mayhew, *Rheumatol. Rehabil.*, 1978, *17*, 29; J. W. Melton *et al.*, *J. Rheumatol.*, 1978, *5*, 338.

Rheumatoid arthritis. Discussions on the use of naproxen and other non-steroidal anti-inflammatory agents in the treatment of rheumatoid arthritis.— J. R. Lewis, *J. Am. med. Ass.*, 1977, *237*, 1260; S. Tremblay, *Can. pharm. J.*, 1977, *110*, 315; K. D. Muirden, *Med. J. Aust.*, 1978, *2*, 12.

Over 46 months naproxen had been given to 415 patients, 271 with rheumatoid arthritis, 69 with degenerative joint disease, 10 with gout, and 65 with extra-articular rheumatism or other painful conditions. Most had been in short-term double-blind studies and had then continued treatment for a mean of 152 days (range 4 to 1400 days). Doses ranged from 0.2 to 1 g daily in 2 divided doses with a mean of 632 mg daily. Overall benefit was very good in 46.5% and good in 30.6%. Of 50 patients taking corticosteroids 17 could cease such treatment and 25 reduced the dose by about 60%. Side-effects included headache (40), dizziness (20), nervousness (2), various gastro-intestinal effects, and skin reactions (7). No side-effects were experienced by 83.9% of the patients.— G. Katona, *Scand. J. Rheumatol.*, 1973, *Suppl.* 2, 101.

In a study in 105 patients with rheumatoid arthritis given naproxen 500 mg, fenoprofen 2.4 g, ibuprofen 1.2 g, or ketoprofen 150 mg daily for 2-week periods in rotation, overall effectiveness with the lowest incidence of side-effects favoured naproxen. Fenoprofen was equally effective but caused more side-effects. Ibuprofen was well tolerated but less effective. Ketoprofen had efficacy similar to that of ibuprofen but caused more side-effects. There was wide patient variation and it might be necessary to try all the drugs to find the best for a particular patient.— E. C. Huskisson *et al.*, *Br. med. J.*, 1976, *1*, 1048. Criticism.— A. K. Clarke *et al.* (letter), *ibid.*, 1976, *2*, 472.

Further studies on the use of naproxen in rheumatoid arthritis.— H. Diamond *et al.*, *J. clin. Pharmac.*, 1975, *15*, 335; D. Myhal *et al.*, *ibid.*, 327; P. Helby-Petersen *et al.*, *Scand. J. Rheumatol.*, 1973, *Suppl.* 2, 145; H. F. H. Hill *et al.*, *ibid.*, 176; J. J. B. Flores and S. V. Rojas, *J. clin. Pharmac.*, 1975, *15*, 373; H. Mathies and E. Wolff, *Arzneimittel-Forsch.*, 1975, *25*, 318; S. H. Roth and G. Boost, *J. clin. Pharmac.*, 1975, *15*, 378; H. A. Capell *et al.*, *Curr. med. Res. Opinion*, 1976, *4*, 285; J. J. Castles *et al.*, *Archs intern. Med.*, 1978, *138*, 362; H. Berry *et al.*, *Ann. rheum. Dis.*, 1978, *37*, 370; P. Lee *et al.*, *N.Z. med. J.*, 1978, *87*, 425; F. A. Wollheim *et al.*, *Rheumatol. Rehabil.*, 1978, *Suppl.*, 78; S. Luftschein *et al.*, *J. Rheumatol.*, 1979, *6*, 397; G. Katona *et al.*, *Curr. ther. Res.*, 1979, *25*, 493; A. G. Mowat *et al.*, *Eur. J. Rheumatol. Inflamm.*, 1979, *2*, 19; E. C. Huskisson *et al.*, *ibid.*, 33; H. Berry *et al.*, *ibid.*, 65; J. J. Castles and J. L. Skosey, *Curr. ther. Res.*, 1980, *27*, 556.

Juvenile polyarthritis. Studies in children with juvenile rheumatoid arthritis indicated that naproxen 10 mg per kg body-weight daily was clinically effective and well tolerated. It was associated with fewer side-effects than high-dosage aspirin therapy. In one study significantly prolonged bleeding times were observed in 42% of patients receiving naproxen. The metabolism of naproxen in children was similar to metabolism in adults.— A. -L. Mäkelä, *Scand. J. Rheumatol.*, 1977, *6*, 193.

Further studies on the use of naproxen in juvenile rheumatoid arthritis.— B. M. Ansell *et al.*, *Eur. J. Rheumatol. Inflamm.*, 1979, *2*, 79; H. Moran *et al.*, *Ann. rheum. Dis.*, 1979, *38*, 152.

Preparations

Naproxen Tablets *(B.P.)*. Tablets containing naproxen. Protect from light.

Naproxen Tablets *(U.S.P.)*. Tablets containing naproxen.

Proprietary Preparations of Naproxen and Naproxen Sodium

Naprosyn *(Syntex, UK)*. Naproxen, available as **Suppositories** each containing 500 mg; as **Suspension** containing 25 mg per ml; and as scored **Tablets** of 250 and 500 mg. (Also available as Naprosyn in *Arg., Austral., Canad., Denm., Ger., Ital., Norw., S.Afr., Spain, Swed., Switz., USA*).

Synflex *(Syntex, UK)*. Naproxen sodium, available as capsules of 275 mg.

Other Proprietary Names

Anaprox *(USA)*; Flanax *(Braz., Mex.)*; Floginax, Gibixen, Laser, Leniartril *(all Ital.)*; Naixan *(Jap.)*; Naprosyne *(Belg., Fr., Neth.)*; Proxen *(Ger., Switz.)*; Proxine *(Ital.)*; Xenar *(Ital.)*.

2674-m

Nefopam Hydrochloride.

Benzoxazocine; Fenazoxine; R738. 3,4,5,6-Tetrahydro-5-methyl-1-phenyl-1*H*-2,5-benzoxazocine hydrochloride. $C_{17}H_{19}NO,HCl=289.8$.

CAS — 13669-70-0 (nefopam); 23327-57-3 (hydrochloride).

A white crystalline powder with a bitter taste. M.p. about 252° with decomposition. **Soluble** in water, chloroform, and methyl alcohol.

Adverse Effects. Side-effects occurring with nefopam include nausea, vomiting, sweating, drowsiness, insomnia, dizziness, lightheadedness, nervousness, blurred vision, headache, dry mouth, skin rashes, and tachycardia. Euphoria and convulsions have occasionally been reported. There may be pain at the site of injection.

Nausea of short duration was reported in 5 of 6 healthy male subjects given nefopam 20 mg intramuscularly, but 40 mg caused more severe nausea in 5 subjects, one of whom vomited. Respiration was little affected by the lower dose, and the respiratory depressant effect of nefopam 40 mg was less than that of morphine 5 mg in these subjects. A dose of 80 mg of nefopam given inadvertently to 1 person was considered to have the depressant effect of 4 to 5 mg of morphine.— J. C. Gasser and J. W. Bellville, *Clin. Pharmac. Ther.*, 1975, *18*, 175.

Effects on the gastro-intestinal tract. Insignificant gastro-intestinal blood loss occurred in 19 healthy subjects after administration of nefopam 180 mg daily for 1 week, compared to a marked loss after aspirin 1.8 g daily.— B. J. Baltes, *J. clin. Pharmac.*, 1977, *17*, 120.

Overdosage. An account of a fatal overdose of nefopam, and details of 9 patients who recovered with routine supportive treatment. Treatment should be directed primarily to the prompt removal of ingested drug by gastric lavage, together with control of convulsions and hallucinations; diazepam appears to be effective for this purpose, and beta-adrenergic blockade might help to control the cardiovascular complications.— D. M. Piercy *et al.*, *Br. med. J.*, 1981, *283*, 1508.

Precautions. Nefopam is contra-indicated in patients with a history of convulsive disorders. It should not be used in the treatment of myocardial infarction. It should be used with caution in patients with glaucoma, urinary retention, or impaired hepatic or renal function.

It has been recommended that nefopam should not be given to patients receiving monoamine oxidase inhibitors.

Absorption and Fate. Nefopam is absorbed from the gastro-intestinal tract. Peak plasma concentrations occur 1 to 3 hours after administration by mouth and about 1.5 hours after intramuscular injection. About 73% is bound to plasma proteins. It has an elimination half-life of about 4 hours. It is extensively metabolised and excreted mainly in urine. Less than 5% of a dose is excreted unchanged in the urine. About 8% of a dose is excreted via the faeces.

A peak plasma concentration of 99 ng per ml occurred in a healthy subject 1 hour after receiving nefopam hydrochloride 60 mg.— D. Schuppan *et al.*, *J. pharm. Sci.*, 1978, *67*, 1720.

Uses. Nefopam hydrochloride has analgesic properties. Its mechanism of action is unclear; prostaglandin synthesis is not inhibited. It also has some anticholinergic and sympathomimetic actions. It is used for the relief of acute and chronic pain. The usual dose is 30 to 90 mg thrice daily. It may also be given in doses of 20 mg by intramuscular or intravenous injection, repeated every 6 hours if necessary.

A review of the use and adverse effects of nefopam hydrochloride.— *Drug & Ther. Bull.*, 1979, *17*, 59; R. C. Heel *et al.*, *Drugs*, 1980, *19*, 249.

A study of the muscle-relaxant properties of nefopam.— W. E. Tobin and R. H. Gold, *J. clin. Pharmac.*, 1972, *12*, 230.

A preliminary report of a study in 196 patients which indicated that nefopam administered parenterally or by mouth lowered body temperature.— V. M. Campos, *Curr. ther. Res.*, 1977, *22*, 790.

Haemodynamic studies in 10 patients with coronary heart disease indicated that nefopam had a slight inotropic effect.— K. Hagemann *et al.*, *Dt. med. Wschr.*, 1978, *103*, 1040.

Analgesia. In a double-blind study in 137 patients with muscular or traumatic pain the analgesic effect of 30 and 60 mg of nefopam was somewhat less than that of 300 and 600 mg respectively of aspirin.— F. C. Workmon and L. Winter, *Curr. ther. Res.*, 1974, *16*, 609.

In a study involving 74 patients aged 20 to 76 years, nefopam hydrochloride 20 mg was considered to be almost as effective in analgesic effect as morphine sulphate 12 mg.— A. Sunshine and E. Laska, *Clin. Pharmac. Ther.*, 1975, *18*, 530.

In a double-blind study in 20 patients nefopam hydrochloride 20 mg intramuscularly and pethidine 50 mg were equally effective in the relief of pain. In a further study in 80 patients nefopam hydrochloride 60 mg thrice daily by mouth was more effective than a placebo.— M. M. Gassel *et al.*, *J. clin. Pharmac.*, 1976, *16*, 34.

Nefopam was considered to be of similar efficacy to pentazocine as an analgesic in a multicentre study involving 120 patients.— A. G. Wade and J. Hosie, *Practitioner*, 1979, *223*, 129.

Further studies on the analgesic efficacy of nefopam hydrochloride.— A. Cohen, *Curr. ther. Res.*, 1974, *16*, 184; A. Cohen and C. M. Hernandez, *J. int. med. Res.*, 1976, *4*, 138; A. L. Kolodny and L. Winter, *Curr. ther. Res.*, 1975, *17*, 519; A. Sunshine *et al.*, *Clin. Pharmac. Ther.*, 1978, *24*, 555.

In cancer. Of 34 patients with chronic pain associated with neoplasms, a single intramuscular injection of nefopam hydrochloride 20 mg produced considerable or complete relief of pain in 29 for at least 5 hours. The same dose given thrice daily for 3 weeks gave complete relief of pain in 12 of 15 similar patients, and could be reduced to twice daily in 6 patients after one week. Nefopam 60 mg by mouth thrice daily for 4 weeks gave partial relief of pain in a further 30 patients; the analgesic effect could be detected after 30 minutes. Increased perspiration was the most frequent side-effect.— L. de T. de Boesinghe *et al.*, *Curr. ther. Res.*, 1976, *20*, 59.

Nefopam hydrochloride 60 mg and pentazocine 50 mg were considered to be equally effective analgesics in a double-blind crossover study in 40 patients with cancer. Drowsiness was more pronounced in patients who took pentazocine but other side-effects were similar for both drugs and those most frequently reported included vomiting, gastric distress, dizziness, nausea, and dry mouth.— L. de T. de Boesinghe, *Curr. ther. Res.*, 1978, *24*, 646.

Postoperative. In a double-blind study of postoperative analgesia in 100 patients, nefopam 15 mg and pethidine 50 mg were equally effective with peak analgesia occurring 1 hour after intramuscular injection. Pethidine 100 mg intramuscularly was significantly more effective than nefopam 30 mg which, apart from a more prolonged action, was no more effective than the 15 mg dose and was associated with a higher frequency of side-effects. Nausea and vomiting occurred with both drugs, sweating and tachycardia were more frequent after nefopam, and sedation was more common after pethidine.— I. Tigerstedt *et al.*, *Br. J. Anaesth.*, 1977, *49*, 1133.

Results of a double-blind crossover study comparing morphine sulphate 4 and 8 mg with nefopam hydrochloride 7.5, 15, or 30 mg in 60 post-operative patients indicated that the analgesic potency of nefopam was about one-third that of morphine. Side-effects were similar, except that pain at the injection site and sweating occurred more frequently after nefopam and sedation more frequently after morphine.— W. T. Beaver and G. A. Feise, *J. clin. Pharmac.*, 1977, *17*, 579.

Further studies on the use of nefopam hydrochloride for postoperative analgesia.— R. K. Ferguson and D. M. Turek, *Pharmatherapeutica*, 1977, *1*, 523; D. Trop *et al.*, *Can. Anaesth. Soc. J.*, 1979, *26*, 296; G. Phillips and M. D. A. Vickers, *Br. J. Anaesth.*, 1979, *51*, 961; R. I. H. Wang and E. M. Waite, *J. clin. Pharmac.*, 1979, *19*, 395; S. S. Bloomfield *et al.*, *Clin. Pharmac. Ther.*, 1980, *27*, 502.

Proprietary Preparations

Acupan *(Carnegie, UK)*. Nefopam hydrochloride, available as **Injection** containing 20 mg per ml, in 2-ml ampoules each containing 1 ml, and as **Tablets** of 30 mg. (Also available as Acupan in *Arg.*, *Belg.*, *Switz.*).

Other Proprietary Names

Ajan *(Ger.)*; Sinalgico *(Arg.)*.

2675-b

Neocinchophen. Neocincofeno. Ethyl 6-methyl-2-phenylquinoline-4-carboxylate.

$C_{19}H_{17}NO_2$=291.3.

CAS — 485-34-7.

Pharmacopoeias. In *Arg.*

A white to pale yellow, odourless, tasteless, crystalline powder. M.p. about 75°. Practically **insoluble** in water; soluble in hot alcohol; very soluble in chloroform and ether. **Protect** from light.

Uses. Neocinchophen has been used for the same purposes as cinchophen (see p.249) in doses of 500 mg.

2676-v

Nifenazone. *N*-(2,3-Dimethyl-5-oxo-1-phenyl-3-pyrazolin-4-yl)nicotinamide.

$C_{17}H_{16}N_4O_2$=308.3.

CAS — 2139-47-1.

A pale yellow crystalline powder with a slightly bitter taste. Slightly **soluble** in water and in ether.

Adverse Effects and Precautions. Nausea, dyspepsia, stomatitis, and agranulocytosis have been reported. Nifenazone should be given with caution to patients with peptic ulcer.

Blood dyscrasias in 4 patients being treated with nifenazone had been reported since early in 1964.— Committee on Safety of Drugs, *Adverse Reactions Series No. 3*, Aug. 1965.

Uses. Nifenazone is claimed to have actions similar to those of phenylbutazone. It has been used in doses of 250 to 500 mg twice or thrice daily.

An unfavourable report of the use of nifenazone in rheumatic disorders.— F. D. Hart and P. L. Boardman, *Br. med. J.*, 1964, *1*, 1553.

Proprietary Names

Algotrex *(CT, Ital.)*; Dipiral *(SIRT-BBP, Ital.)*; Dolongan *(SMB, Belg.)*; Neopiran *(Panthox & Burck, Ital.)*; Niapan *(Biosint, Ital.)*; Nicopyron *(Trommsdorff, Ger.)*; Nicoreumal *(SIT, Ital.)*; Niprazina *(ISOM, Ital.)*; Reumatosil *(Saba, Ital.)*; Supermidone *(Salfa, Ital.)*.

Nifenazone was formerly marketed in Great Britain under the proprietary name Thylin (*Sinclair*).

2677-g

Niflumic Acid. UP 83. 2-(ααα-Trifluoro-*m*-toluidino)nicotinic acid.

$C_{13}H_9F_3N_2O_2$=282.2.

CAS — 4394-00-7.

Adverse Effects. Reported adverse effects include gastro-intestinal disturbances, signs of kidney impairment, and headache.

Fluoride associated osteosis with prolonged use of niflumic acid.— A. Prost *et al.*, *Nouv. Presse méd.*, 1978, *7*, 754.

Uses. Niflumic acid has analgesic and anti-inflammatory activity and has been used in rheumatoid disease. It has also been tried in cystalgia, ureteric lithiasis, and urinary frequency. It has been given in doses of 0.5 to 1 g daily.

Clinical study in 60 patients with rheumatoid disease.— A. Verhaeghe *et al.*, *Lille méd.*, 1967, *Suppl.* 12, 1298, per *Abstr. Wld Med.*, 1968, *42*, 635. A similar trial in 70 patients.— J. Gougeon *et al.*, *Thérapie*, 1968, *23*, 951. Niflumic acid was effective in the treatment of osteoarthritis.— J. Moloney *et al.*, *J. Ir. med. Ass.*, 1971, *64*, 605, per *Practitioner*, 1974, *212*, 244.

Clinical study in 25 patients with ureteric lithiasis.— E. Benassayag and J. Thomas, *Thérapie*, 1970, *25*, 1047.

Clinical study in 500 patients with cystalgia and urinary frequency.— E. Benassayag and P. Aboulker, *Thérapie*, 1970, *25*, 1051.

In 30 patients with glomerulonephritis and proteinuria treated for an average of 4 months with niflumic acid 750 mg daily, proteinuria diminished in 73%. Kidney function was not affected by the drug. In the cases of initially increased values, the secretion of fibrinogen degradation products diminished in 70% of the cases.— H. Boeckle *et al.*, *Arzneimittel-Forsch.*, 1975, *25*, 120.

Use of niflumic acid in locomotor disease.— I. Ábrányi and I. Papp, *Therapia hung.*, 1977, *25*, 20; E. Kovács, *ibid.*, 75.

Proprietary Names

Actol *(Heyden, Ger.; Med. y Prod. Quím., Spain)*; Flaminon *(Squibb, Ital.; Squibb, S.Afr.)*; Inflaryl *(Squibb, Belg.; Squibb, Neth.)*; Landruma *(Landerlan, Spain)*; Natik *(Celtia, Arg.)*; Nifluril *(UPSA, Fr.; UPSA, Switz.)*.

2678-q

Oxyphenbutazone *(B.P., U.S.P.)*. G 27202;

Hydroxyphenylbutazone. 4-Butyl-1-(4-hydroxyphenyl)-2-phenylpyrazolidine-3,5-dione monohydrate.

$C_{19}H_{20}N_2O_3,H_2O$=342.4.

CAS — 129-20-4 (anhydrous); 7081-38-1 (monohydrate).

Pharmacopoeias. In *Br.*, *Jap.*, and *U.S.*

A white to yellowish-white, odourless or almost odourless, crystalline powder with a bitter taste. M.p. 85° to 100°.

Practically **insoluble** in water; soluble 1 in 3 of alcohol, 1 in 6 of acetone, 1 in 20 of chloroform, 1 in 20 of ether; soluble in solutions of alkali hydroxides. **Store** in airtight containers.

Adverse Effects. As for Phenylbutazone, p.273.

Sixteen cases of serious complications with 5 deaths in patients given oxyphenbutazone had been reported since early 1964. Toxic effects included liver damage, peptic ulceration, and blood dyscrasias.— Committee on Safety of Drugs, *Adverse Reactions Series No. 3*, Aug. 1965.

There were 421 reports of adverse reactions to oxyphenbutazone reported to the Committee on Safety of Medicines from June 1964 to Jan. 1973. These included 157 reports of blood disorders (74 fatal) including aplastic anaemia (63; 40 fatal), thrombocytopenia (38; 14 fatal), and agranulocytosis or pancytopenia (36; 15 fatal), and gastro-intestinal haemorrhage (16; 5 fatal). The incidence of reports and fatalities was about twice that for phenylbutazone.— M. F. Cuthbert, *Curr. med. Res. Opinion*, 1974, *2*, 600.

Allergy. Oxyphenbutazone was responsible for a fixed drug eruption in 1 patient and was strongly suspected in 2 further cases.— J. A. Savin, *Br. J. Derm.*, 1970, *83*, 546.

A report of contact dermatitis to oxyphenbutazone.— G. Krook, *Contact Dermatitis*, 1975, *1*, 385.

A 52-year-old woman who had received phenylbutazone intermittently for 20 years without any apparent adverse effects developed painful bilateral swelling of the salivary glands, dryness of the mouth, and fever during 5 days treatment with oxyphenbutazone 100 mg thrice daily. Treatment was stopped and saliva flow slowly returned to normal over a period of 8 weeks.— J. H. Chen *et al.*, *J. Am. med. Ass.*, 1977, *238*, 1399.

Effects on blood. An analysis of blood dyscrasias reported to the Swedish Adverse Drug Reaction Committee for the 5-year period 1966–70 showed that thrombocytopenia attributable to oxyphenbutazone had been reported on 2 occasions, aplastic anaemia on 10 occasions (5 fatal), and agranulocytosis on 3 occasions (1 fatal). It was estimated that reported figures represented one-third of the true frequency.— L. E. Böttiger and B. Westerholm, *Br. med. J.*, 1973, *3*, 339.

Aplastic anaemia or agranulocytosis were quoted as underlying or contributory causes of death in 376 death certificates in the year Oct. 1974 to Sept. 1975; adequate medical records were available for 269. Death was probably due to oxyphenbutazone in 11 cases. Mortality was estimated at 3.8 per 100 000 patients.— W. H. W. Inman, *Committee on Safety of Medicines, Br. med. J.*, 1977, *1*, 1500.

Leukaemia. Two fatal cases of acute leukaemia were reported following treatment with oxyphenbutazone in total dosages of 1 g and 1.9 g, respectively.— S. -G. Sjöberg and D. Perers (letter), *Lancet*, 1965, *2*, 441.

Effects on the lungs. A 66-year-old woman who had been taking oxyphenbutazone for nearly 3 years developed a reversible diffuse pulmonary disorder which recurred when given a further challenge course.— D. C. Cameron (letter), *Br. med. J.*, 1975, *2*, 500.

Effects on thyroid. A report of oxyphenbutazone-induced goitre in a 63-year-old woman.— R. J. M. Lane *et al.*, *Postgrad. med. J.*, 1977, *53*, 93.

Epidermal necrolysis. Oxyphenbutazone might have been responsible for 2 cases of toxic epidermal necrolysis.— A. Lyell, *Br. J. Derm.*, 1967, *79*, 662.

Lupus erythematosus. Thrombocytopenia and lupus erythematosus cells were found in a 17-year-old girl after treatment with oxyphenbutazone 100 mg four times daily for 10 days. It was suggested that the patient had developed sensitivity to the drug.— A. J. Handley (letter), *Lancet*, 1971, *1*, 245.

Treatment of Adverse Effects and Precautions. As for Phenylbutazone, p.274.

Interactions, drugs. *Antidiabetic agents* . For the effect of oxyphenbutazone on tolbutamide half-life, see under Tolbutamide, p.860.

Methandienone . Plasma concentrations of oxyphenbutazone were raised by the concomitant administration of methandienone.— M. Weiner *et al.*, *Proc. Soc. exp. Biol. Med.*, 1967, *124*, 1170.

Absorption and Fate. As for Phenylbutazone, p.274.

The biological half-life of oxyphenbutazone was 72 hours.— W. A. Ritschel, *Drug Intell. & clin. Pharm.*, 1970, *4*, 332.

Oxyphenbutazone was reported to have a half-life of 27 to 64 hours.— M. D. Rawlins and T. B. Binns, *Practitioner*, 1975, *214*, 274.

Uses. Oxyphenbutazone is a metabolite of phenylbutazone with similar analgesic, anti-inflammatory, and antipyretic actions and with similar uses (see p.274).

In rheumatic and other musculo-skeletal disorders oxyphenbutazone has the same indications and is used in the same doses as phenylbutazone. It has also been recommended in the management of thrombophlebitis. Blood counts should be made regularly, as indicated for phenylbutazone.

Oxyphenbutazone may also be administered rectally, a suppository containing 250 mg being inserted once or twice daily. Oxyphenbutazone has also been applied topically to the eye.

Inflammation, postoperative. A double-blind study was made on 85 surgical patients of whom 46 were given 400 mg of oxyphenbutazone on the evenings before and after surgery and each morning of the postoperative days. Treatment lasted 3 to 14 days. Effective control of postoperative inflammation and a lessening of pain was obtained in 74% of this group compared with 20% of the controls. An urticarial skin rash developed in 1 patient receiving oxyphenbutazone.— R. Barcelo *et al.*, *Can. med. Ass. J.*, 1963, *88*, 606.

The use of oxyphenbutazone postoperatively in 90 urological patients.— G. Wandschneider and P. Haas, *Wien. med. Wschr.*, 1973, *123*, 210, per *Int. pharm. Abstr.*, 1974, *11*, 146.

For a comparison of oxyphenbutazone and indomethacin treatment following surgery for varicose veins, see K. Jaakkola *et al.*, *Curr. ther. Res.*, 1976, *20*, 134.

Ocular disease. Oxyphenbutazone was effective in the treatment of episcleritis in a comparative trial with prednisolone in 59 patients with episcleritis and scleritis. The doses were: oxyphenbutazone, 600 mg daily for 2 days initially, followed by 400 mg daily for 3 weeks, then progressively withdrawn over a further week; prednisolone 30 mg daily for 2 days, then 20 mg daily for 3 weeks, and then progressively withdrawn. For the first few days prednisolone was more effective, after which improvement due to each agent was roughly equal; after 21 days' treatment, however, patients who received oxyphenbutazone continued to improve rapidly (particularly as to pain and conjunctival and episcleral injection) whereas the prednisolone group deteriorated as treatment was withdrawn.— P. G. Watson *et al.*, *Br. J. Ophthal.*, 1966, *50*, 463.

In a double-blind study in 38 patients with episcleritis there was a significantly greater improvement after 7 days in patients treated with oxyphenbutazone ointment 10% compared with betamethasone ointment 0.1% and placebo. There were no significant differences between the groups after 21 days.— P. G. Watson *et al.*, *Br. J. Ophthal.*, 1973, *57*, 866.

In a controlled study of 26 patients with anterior uveitis, oxyphenbutazone 100 mg four times daily was as effective as hydrocortisone 1% eye-drops given every 4 hours.— P. J. L. Hunter *et al.*, *Br. J. Ophthal.*, 1973, *57*, 892.

Further reports on the use of oxyphenbutazone in inflammatory eye disorders.— V. H. Smith and P. D. Fowler, *Br. J. Ophthal.*, 1966, *50*, 710; D. G. Emery *et al.*, *Practitioner*, 1973, *211*, 809; W. A. I. Rushford *et al.*, *J. int. med. Res.*, 1978, *6*, 141.

Oxyphenbutazone ointment was probably of value in the treatment of episcleritis but there was little evidence that it was useful in the treatment of other external eye diseases. It did not suppress the inflammatory corneal response which produces visual loss in recurrent herpes simplex keratitis. There was no justification for inclusion of chloramphenicol in oxyphenbutazone ointment.— *Drug & Ther. Bull.*, 1979, *17*, 40.

Reiter's disease. Oxyphenbutazone 600 mg daily was recommended to relieve severe pain in Reiter's disease.— *Br. med. J.*, 1969, *4*, 576.

Sarcoidosis. If oxyphenbutazone was to be successful in the treatment of sarcoidosis, it probably needed to be given within 1 year of the diagnosis, in a dose of 100 mg four times a day for 6 months.— D. G. James, *Practitioner*, 1969, *202*, 624. See also D. G. James *et al.*, *Lancet*, 1967, *2*, 526.

Thrombo-embolic disorders. The incidence of deep-vein thrombosis was significantly reduced (from 13 of 23 to 5 of 27) in patients undergoing hip surgery when their legs were bandaged for 14 days postoperatively and they were given oxyphenbutazone 250 mg twice daily as suppositories.— B. Tillberg, *Br. med. J.*, 1976, *1*, 1256.

Beneficial effects were obtained in a multicentre study of patients with superficial thrombophlebitis given oxyphenbutazone 100 mg four times daily.— D. S. Archer and P. D. Fowler, *Practitioner*, 1977, *218*, 712.

Preparations

Oxyphenbutazone Eye Ointment *(B.P.)*. A sterile eye ointment containing oxyphenbutazone.

Oxyphenbutazone Tablets *(B.P.)*. Tablets containing oxyphenbutazone. They are sugar-coated.

Oxyphenbutazone Tablets *(U.S.P.)*. Tablets containing oxyphenbutazone. Store in airtight containers.

Proprietary Preparations

Tandacote *(Geigy, UK)*. Oxyphenbutazone, available as enteric-coated tablets of 100 mg.

Tandalgesic *(Geigy, UK)*. Scored tablets each containing oxyphenbutazone 50 mg and paracetamol 500 mg. For rheumatic pain. *Dose.* 1 or 2 tablets thrice daily, reducing to the minimum required to maintain therapeutic control.

Tanderil *(Geigy, UK)*. Oxyphenbutazone, available as **Suppositories** each containing 250 mg and as **Tablets** of 100 mg. (Also available as Tanderil in *Arg.*, *Austral.*, *Belg.*, *Denm.*, *Fr.*, *Ger.*, *Ital.*, *Neth.*, *Norw.*, *S.Afr.*, *Spain*, *Switz.*).

Tanderil Chloramphenicol Eye Ointment *(Zyma, UK)*. Contains oxyphenbutazone 10% and chloramphenicol 1%, with phenethyl alcohol 0.5%.

Tanderil Eye Ointment *(Zyma, UK)*. Contains oxyphenbutazone 10%.

Other Proprietary Names

Arg.—Butofen (phenyramidol derivative), Naleran; *Canad.*—Oxybutazone, Tandearil; *Denm.*—Rumapax; *Ger.*—Imbun, Phlogase, Phlogistol, Phlogont; *Ital.*—Artroflog, Butaflogin, Butapirone, Butilene, Difmedol (piperazine derivative), Flogistin, Flogitolo, Flogodin, Iridil, Isobutil, Neo-Farmadol, Poliflogil, Piraflogin, Validil; *S.Afr.*—Artzone, Buteril, Fibutrox, Otone; *Spain*—Butolfen, Febutolo (both phenyramidol derivatives), Ipebutona, Oxibutol; *Swed.*—Rheumapax; *Switz.*—Rapostan, Rheumapax; *USA*—Oxalid, Tandearil.

A preparation containing oxyphenbutazone was also formerly marketed in Great Britain under the proprietary name Tanderil-Alka (*Geigy*).

2679-p

Paracetamol *(B.P., Eur. P., B.P. Vet.)*.

Paracetamolum; Acetaminophen *(U.S.P.)*; *N*-Acetyl-*p*-aminophenol. 4′-Hydroxyacetanilide; *N*-(4-Hydroxyphenyl)acetamide.

$C_8H_9NO_2$=151.2.

CAS — 103-90-2.

Pharmacopoeias. In *Belg.*, *Br.*, *Braz.*, *Chin.*, *Eur.*, *Fr.*, *Ger.*, *It.*, *Jap.*, *Jug.*, *Neth.*, *Roum.*, *Rus.*, *Turk.*, and *U.S.*

White odourless crystals or crystalline powder with a bitter taste. M.p. 168° to 172°.

Soluble 1 in 70 of water, 1 in 20 of boiling water, 1 in 7 to 10 of alcohol, 1 in 13 of acetone, 1 in 40 of glycerol, and 1 in 9 of propylene glycol; very slightly soluble in chloroform; practically insoluble in ether; soluble in solutions of alkali hydroxides. A saturated solution in water has a pH of 5.1 to 6.5. **Store** in airtight containers. Protect from light.

A study *in vitro* of paracetamol tablets containing sorbitol indicated that sorbitol did not form an absorbable complex with paracetamol, and improved absorption claimed for such a formulation might be due to its higher dissolution-rate.— V. Walters, *J. Pharm. Pharmac.*, 1968, *20*, *Suppl.*, 228S. See also J. R. Gwilt *et al.*, *ibid.*, 1963, *15*, 445.

Reaction with aspirin. Aspirin acetylated paracetamol to diacetyl-*p*-aminophenol in commercial formulations stored at room temperature. Magnesium stearate was shown to accelerate the reaction and amounts of up to 4 mg of diacetyl-*p*-aminophenol per tablet were found. The compound was considered to have antipyretic activity.— K. T. Koshy *et al.*, *J. pharm. Sci.*, 1967, *56*, 1117. Diacetyl-*p*-aminophenol was not formed in dry mixtures of paracetamol and aspirin. The diacetyl derivative hydrolysed to paracetamol and *p*-aminophenol under humid conditions.— E. Kalatzis, *J. pharm. Sci.*, 1970, *59*, 193.

Further references: B. G. Boggiano *et al.*, *Australas. J. Pharm.*, 1970, *51*, S14.

Stability. Paracetamol was very stable in aqueous solution. The half-life in a solution buffered at pH 6 had been estimated to be 21.8 years; degradation was catalysed by acids and bases and the half-life was 0.73 years at pH 2 and 2.28 years at pH 9. The degradation products were *p*-aminophenol and acetic acid.— K. T. Koshy and J. L. Lach, *J. pharm. Sci.*, 1961, *50*, 113.

Suppository bases. The dissolution and bioavailability of paracetamol from 4 suppository bases was investigated and compared with oral administration in 4 subjects. Paracetamol 120 mg in a basis consisting of macrogol '400' 20 parts and macrogol '4000' 80 parts was more completely absorbed than when administered in glycogelatin, polysorbate, or Massuppol basis.— L. Roller, *Aust. J. Hosp. Pharm.*, 1977, *7*, 97.

Further references.— O. P. Lukash *et al.*, *Farmatsevt. Zh.*, 1975, *30*, 81, per *Int. pharm. Abstr.*, 1977, *14*, 795; P. Seideman *et al.*, *Eur. J. clin. Pharmac.*, 1980, *17*, 465.

Adverse Effects. Side-effects of paracetamol are usually mild, though haematological reactions have been reported. Skin rashes and other allergic reactions occur occasionally.

Symptoms of paracetamol overdosage in the first 24 hours are pallor, nausea, vomiting, anorexia, and abdominal pain. Liver damage may become apparent 12 to 48 hours after ingestion by increases in serum concentrations of aminotransferases and bilirubin and in prothrombin time. Abnormalities of glucose metabolism and metabolic acidosis may occur. In severe poisoning, hepatic failure may progress to encephalopathy, coma, and death. Acute renal failure with acute tubular necrosis may develop even in the absence of severe liver damage. Cardiac arrhythmias have been reported.

Liver damage is likely in adults who have taken 10 g or more of paracetamol. It is considered that excess quantities of a toxic metabolite (usually adequately detoxified by glutathione when normal doses of paracetamol are employed), become irreversibly bound to liver tissue.

Allergy. A report of a fixed drug eruption due to paracetamol.— H. T. H. Wilson, *Br. J. Derm.*, 1975, *92*, 213.

Effects on blood. *Agranulocytosis.* A 78-year-old woman with osteoarthritis who took 2 to 3, and later 4, tablets of paracetamol daily for 6 to 7 months developed agranulocytosis from which she recovered. Paracetamol was considered the provocative agent.— T. W. Lloyd (letter), *Lancet*, 1961, *1*, 114.

Haemolytic anaemia. A report of haemolytic anaemia with episodes of massive haemolysis due to paracetamol in 1 patient.— E. Manor *et al.*, *J. Am. med. Ass.*, 1976, *236*, 2777.

Paracetamol did not cause haemolysis in Chinese patients with glucose-6-phosphate dehydrogenase deficiency.— T. K. Chan *et al.*, *Br. med. J.*, 1976, *2*, 1227.

A 30-year-old man developed thrombocytopenia associated with haemolytic anaemia after taking paracetamol 3 tablets daily for low-back pain during the previous month. His condition resolved spontaneously after a few days but recurred 8 months later after taking 8 tablets of paracetamol.— A. Kornberg and A. Polliack (letter), *Lancet*, 1978, *2*, 1159.

Methaemoglobinaemia. Studies in 160 volunteers indicated that in normal therapeutic doses paracetamol, even when given continuously for up to a week, caused no detectable methaemoglobinaemia.— J. Thomas *et al.* (letter), *Lancet*, 1966, *2*, 1360.

Paracetamol was considered to have been responsible for methaemoglobinaemia in a young woman 6 hours after taking paracetamol tablets. She was free from cyanosis 24 hours later.— D. MacLean *et al.* (letter), *Br. med. J.*, 1968, *4*, 390.

Pancytopenia. For reports of pancytopenia considered to be due to paracetamol, see S. B. Datta (letter), *Br. med. J.*, 1973, *3*, 173; G. K. Webster (letter), *Br. med. J.*, 1973, *3*, 353.

Thrombocytopenia. Reports of thrombocytopenia attributed to paracetamol.— R. C. Heading (letter), *Br. med. J.*, 1968, *3*, 743; E. V. Eisner and N. T. Shahidi, *New Engl. J. Med.*, 1972, *287*, 376; Y. Shoenfeld *et al.* (letter), *ibid.*, 1980, *303*, 47.

Effects on the gastro-intestinal tract. Paracetamol did not appear to produce significant changes in the gastric mucosa.— K. J. Ivey and P. Settree, *Gut*, 1976, *17*, 916; K. J. Ivey *et al.*, *Br. med. J.*, 1978, *1*, 1586.

Effects on the kidneys. For a report of renal papillary necrosis following regular paracetamol ingestion, see Analgesic Abuse, p.234.

For reports of renal failure following paracetamol overdosage, see below.

Effects on the liver. Hepatotoxicity occurred in 2 patients who took up to 5 or 6.5 g of paracetamol daily for several weeks and in 1 patient who took about 3 g of paracetamol and drank 1 pint of vodka daily for several years.— J. D. Barker *et al.*, *Ann. intern. Med.*, 1977, *87*, 299.

A report of liver damage in a 16-year-old woman following ingestion of only 5.85 g of paracetamol.— E. Fernandez and A. C. Fernandez-Brito (letter), *New Engl. J. Med.*, 1977, *296*, 577.

A 59-year-old woman developed liver function abnormalities while taking about 3 g of paracetamol daily for one year for arthritis. The liver function tests returned to normal 5 weeks after withdrawing the paracetamol; the abnormalities recurred on administration of a test dose.— G. K. Johnson and K. G. Tolman, *Ann. intern. Med.*, 1977, *87*, 302.

Further reports of hepatic damage associated with ingestion of therapeutic doses of paracetamol.— D. M.

Rosenberg and F. A. Neelon (letter), *Ann. intern. Med.*, 1977, *88*, 129; D. M. Rosenberg *et al.*, *Sth. med. J.*, 1977, *70*, 660; H. L. Bonkowsky *et al.*, *Lancet*, 1978, *1*, 1016; R. Olsson (letter), *Lancet*, 1978, *2*, 152.

Therapeutic doses of paracetamol were not considered to be implicated in liver damage.— J. Neuberger *et al.*, *J.R. Soc. Med.*, 1980, *73*, 701.

For reports of liver damage following paracetamol overdosage, see below.

Overdosage. Reviews and discussions of paracetamol overdosage.— R. Goulding, *Pediatrics*, 1973, *52*, 883; J. R. Mitchell *et al.*, *Clin. Pharmac. Ther.*, 1974, *16*, 676; *Br. med. J.*, 1975, *1*, 536; O. James *et al.*, *Lancet*, 1975, *2*, 579; *Lancet*, 1975, *2*, 1189; L. F. Prescott, *Adv. Med. Topics Ther.*, 1975, *1*, 21; *Drug & Ther. Bull.*, 1976, *14*, 5; S. Segal *et al.*, *Pediatrics*, 1978, *61*, 108; J. R. Mitchell, *Ann. intern. Med.*, 1977, *87*, 377; L. F. Prescott, *Recent Adv. clin. Pharmac.*, 1978, *1*, 189; M. Black, *Gastroenterology*, 1980, *78*, 382; T. J. Meredith and R. Goulding, *Postgrad. med. J.*, 1980, *56*, 459.

In 41 patients who had ingested overdoses of paracetamol, liver damage was the major complication and occurred in most patients who had ingested more than 15 g. Symptoms of acute overdosage included vomiting, anorexia, nausea, and epigastric pain. Maximum liver damage occurred after 2 to 4 days, the degree of damage being greater the larger the overdose. Jaundice might occur after 2 to 6 days. Profound hypoglycaemia and metabolic acidosis might complicate severe poisoning. One patient died of gastro-intestinal haemorrhage and acute massive necrosis of the liver. Acute tubular necrosis of the kidneys occurred in 1 patient who recovered. The half-life of paracetamol and its metabolites in the circulation was about 4 hours; paracetamol could not be eliminated before it had caused liver damage.— A. T. Proudfoot and N. Wright, *Br. med. J.*, 1970, *3*, 557.

From studies in patients with paracetamol overdosage, it was found that severe hepatic lesions occurred when the plasma-paracetamol concentrations reached more than 300 µg per ml after 4 hours; none occurred in patients with concentrations of less than 120 µg per ml. There was no evidence of liver damage in 11 of 12 patients with plasma concentrations of less than 50 µg per ml at 12 hours, but hepatic necrosis developed in 16 of 18 with concentrations greater than 50 µg. The plasma half-life of unchanged paracetamol was raised from a mean of about 2 hours in 17 healthy adults given therapeutic doses to about 2.9 hours in 13 poisoned patients without liver damage and to about 7.6 hours in 17 patients who developed liver damage.— L. F. Prescott *et al.*, *Lancet*, 1971, *1*, 519.

Biochemical evidence of liver damage was found in 49 of 60 patients admitted to hospital after taking 13 to 100 g of paracetamol. Anorexia, nausea, and vomiting were seen on the first and second days and jaundice on the third or fourth. Serum-bilirubin concentrations of 40 µg or more per ml were observed in 19 patients, 17 of whom developed fulminant hepatic failure with hepatic encephalopathy which led to coma in 15 and death in 12. Gastro-intestinal haemorrhage requiring treatment occurred in 5, transient hypoglycaemia in 4, and renal failure in 6 patients. Liver specimens showed necrosis. Paracetamol overdosage should be treated immediately by gastric lavage, and liver function should be monitored in case the serum-bilirubin concentration should exceed 40 µg per ml during the first 5 days, which would indicate severe liver damage.— R. Clark *et al.*, *Lancet*, 1973, *1*, 66.

In 36 patients with liver damage due to paracetamol overdosage there was a direct relationship between the degree of liver damage and disturbances of coagulation. Minor liver damage caused reduced synthesis of many coagulation factors, but fibrinogen synthesis was increased. Changes indicative of disseminated intravascular coagulation occurred with moderate and severe liver damage.— R. Clark *et al.*, *Gastroenterology*, 1973, *65*, 788.

An analysis of 20 unselected fatal cases of paracetamol overdosage showed that 8 deaths occurred within the first 24 hours and only 2 after 4 days. Liver failure was the cause of death in only 3 patients; other causes included inhalation of vomit or aspiration pneumonia. Kidney damage probably due to severe hypotension was common in those surviving longer than 40 hours.— M. F. Dixon (letter), *Lancet*, 1976, *1*, 35.

In patients with acute paracetamol overdosage, serum-ferritin concentrations correlated closely with pathological changes in the liver.— E. J. Eastham *et al.*, *Br. med. J.*, 1976, *1*, 750.

A 31-year-old woman with a history of heavy alcohol intake developed hepatitis, acute pancreatitis, and renal failure requiring peritoneal dialysis after the ingestion of paracetamol 60 g.— I. T. Gilmore and E. Tourvas, *Br. med. J.*, 1977, *1*, 753. A further case of pancreatitis.— R. A. Coward (letter), *ibid.*, 1086.

Analysis of 160 patients with fulminant hepatic failure due to paracetamol overdosage or other factors showed no relationship between paracetamol and renal failure. This lack of association was confirmed in 190 patients with less severe liver damage. Renal failure when it occurred in any of these patients was related to endotoxaemia.— S. P. Wilkinson *et al.*, *J. clin. Path.*, 1977, *30*, 141. There may be a not infrequent occurrence of acute tubular necrosis with renal failure in patients with relatively mild liver damage without hepatic encephalopathy following paracetamol overdosage. This usually occurred in patients who had taken large quantities of alcohol or other drugs which cause enzyme induction.— L. F. Prescott, in *Side-effects of Drugs Annual 2*, M.N.G. Dukes (Ed.), Oxford, Excerpta Medica, 1978, p. 79.

Paracetamol-induced acute renal failure in the absence of fulminant liver damage.— I. Cobden *et al.*, *Br. med. J.*, 1982, *284*, 21.

Further references to paracetamol overdosage.— L. F. Prescott and N. Wright, *Br. J. Pharmac.*, 1973, *49*, 602; J. A. H. Forrest *et al.*, *Br. med. J.*, 1974, *4*, 499; M. Davis *et al.*, *Q. J. Med.*, 1976, *45*, 181; A. N. Hamlyn *et al.*, *Am. J. dig. Dis.*, 1977, *22*, 605; A. N. Hamlyn *et al.*, *Postgrad. med. J.*, 1978, *54*, 400; J. T. Slattery and G. Levy, *Clin. Pharmac. Ther.*, 1979, *25*, 184; J. Canalese *et al.*, *Br. med. J.*, 1981, *282*, 199.

In children. References: A. G. Nogen and J. E. Bremner, *J. Pediat.*, 1978, *92*, 832.

Treatment of Adverse Effects. Although the likely toxicity of a paracetamol overdose can be assessed by examining the changing pattern of paracetamol blood concentrations, prompt specific treatment is essential. Any patient therefore, who has taken 7.5 g or more of paracetamol and can be treated within 10 hours of ingestion should be given a specific antidote, even if the blood concentrations are not known. There is a risk that the sulphydryl donors used as antidotes may exacerbate any liver damage if given 10 hours after the overdose. Once specific therapy is established then blood concentrations of paracetamol can be monitored. Generally treatment is required if the blood concentration is higher than a line (the '200' line) drawn on log/linear paper joining the points 200 mg per litre at 4 hours and 60 mg per litre at 10 hours. There have been suggestions that treatment may be necessary when lower concentrations of paracetamol are present.

Cysteamine (p.380) is sometimes used by injection as an antidote but acetylcysteine or methionine is now preferred. Acetylcysteine is given by intravenous infusion in an initial dose of 150 mg per kg body-weight over 15 minutes followed by 50 mg per kg over 4 hours and then 100 mg per kg over the next 16 hours. Alternatively methionine 2.5 g may be given by mouth every 4 hours to a total of 4 doses.

Haemoperfusion may be worthwhile if too much time has elapsed since the poisoning to allow use of acetylcysteine or methionine.

Basic measures that may be required include dextrose and blood infusions. Removal of stomach contents by aspiration and lavage forms an early part of treatment and the administration of activated charcoal should be considered.

Reviews and discussions of the treatment of paracetamol overdosage.— *J. int. med. Res.*, 1976, *4*, *Suppl.* 4;; *Br. med. J.*, 1977, *2*, 481; A. T. Proudfoot and L. F. Prescott, Poisoning with paraquat, salicylate and paracetamol, in *Recent Advances in Intensive Therapy*, No. 1, I.M. Ledingham (Ed.), London, Churchill Livingstone, 1977, p. 217; G. J. Merritt and P. U. Joyner, *Drug Intell. & clin. Pharm.*, 1977, *11*, 458; S. Segal *et al.*, *Pediatrics*, 1978, *61*, 108; D. M. Stewart *et al.*, *Clin. Toxicol.*, 1979, *14*, 507; L. F. Prescott, *Prescribers' J.*, 1979, *19*, 169; T. J. Meredith and R. Goulding, *Postgrad. med. J.*, 1980, *56*, 459; *Drug & Ther. Bull.*, 1980, *18*, 81.

In a controlled study in 22 patients with hepatic necrosis due to paracetamol poisoning, 11 were treated by infusions of plasma and 11 by plasma and heparin by constant infusion pump to maintain a blood-heparin equivalent of 5 µg per ml. There was no significant difference in the rate of correction of the coagulation defect or in the clinical outcome.— B. G. Gazzard *et al.*, *Gut*, 1974, *15*, 89.

In a controlled study, charcoal haemoperfusion of 8 patients as an early treatment for paracetamol overdosage appeared to offer no advantage over supportive therapy alone in a further 8 patients and might even have been harmful.— B. G. Gazzard *et al.*, *Br. J. clin. Pharmac.*, 1974, *1*, 271.

Treatment of paracetamol poisoning should be instituted rapidly in patients with alcohol-damaged livers. Treatment with cysteamine given 9.5 hours after paracetamol overdosage to one such patient failed to prevent further liver damage.— C. R. Scott and M. J. Stewart (letter), *Lancet*, 1975, *1*, 452.

A study involving 40 patients at risk of hepatic injury from severe paracetamol overdosage showed that cysteamine and methionine are equally hepatoprotective but that methionine is associated with fewer undesirable side-effects.— A. N. Hamlyn *et al.*, *Gut*, 1980, *21*, A448.

Charcoal haemoperfusion carried out on 8 patients presenting to hospital later than 10 hours after a large paracetamol overdose produced a rapid fall in plasma-paracetamol concentrations and in 4 patients significant amounts of paracetamol were removed. Severe hepatotoxicity developed in 2 patients (fatal in 1); the other 6 suffered only minor disturbances of liver function.— M. Helliwell *et al.* (letter), *Br. med. J.*, 1981, *282*, 473.

Further references.— B. H. Rumack and R. G. Peterson, *Pediatrics*, 1978, *62*, *Suppl.*, 898.

For further reports on the treatment of paracetamol overdosage, see Acetylcysteine, p.645, Cysteamine, p.380, and Methionine, p.57.

Precautions. Paracetamol should be given with care to patients with impaired kidney or liver function.

Paracetamol should also be given with care to patients taking other drugs that affect the liver.

Paracetamol was not metabolised any differently by patients with analgesic nephropathy or with kidney disease not due to analgesics compared with healthy subjects. However there was a slower rate of excretion in those with kidney impairment.— B. H. Thomas *et al.*, *Int. J. clin. Pharmac. Biopharm.*, 1980, *18*, 26, per *Int. pharm. Abstr.*, 1980, *17*, 948.

Interactions, drugs. *Alcohol.* A report of 2 patients in whom paracetamol hepatotoxicity was enhanced by alcohol.— D. J. Emby and B. N. Fraser, *S. Afr. med. J.*, 1977, *51*, 208. See also H. Licht *et al.*, *Ann. intern. Med.*, 1980, *92*, 511; C. J. McClain *et al.*, *J. Am. med. Ass.*, 1980, *244*, 251.

Anticoagulants. See under Warfarin Sodium, p.779.

Anticonvulsants. Phenobarbitone potentiated the hepatotoxicity of paracetamol in a 13-year-old epileptic girl who took an overdose of phenobarbitone and paracetamol.— J. T. Wilson *et al.*, *Am. J. Dis. Child.*, 1978, *132*, 466.

Bioavailability of paracetamol was decreased in epileptic patients possibly because of enhanced first-pass metabolism secondary to enzyme induction.— E. Perucca and A. Richens, *Br. J. clin. Pharmac.*, 1979, *7*, 201.

Aspirin. For a report of paracetamol increasing blood concentrations of aspirin, see Aspirin, p.239.

Chloramphenicol. For a report of paracetamol increasing the half-life of chloramphenicol, see under Chloramphenicol, p.1138.

Desipramine. In 5 of 6 subjects desipramine 75 mg taken 90 minutes before the ingestion of paracetamol 40 mg per kg body-weight delayed and reduced the peak concentration of paracetamol in the blood; in the 6th subject the peak concentration of paracetamol was increased.— R. C. Hall *et al.*, *Postgrad. med. J.*, 1976, *52*, 139.

Doxorubicin. Since doxorubicin as well as paracetamol depleted hepatic glutathione it is likely that there would be an increased risk of liver damage when the two drugs were used together.— P. G. Wells *et al.*, *Toxic. appl. Pharmac.*, 1980, *54*, 197.

Interactions, tests. Paracetamol could interfere with paper chromatographic estimations of urinary amino acids by producing drug spots, and could interfere technically with laboratory estimations for metadrenalines in the urine to produce erroneous raised results.— *Drug & Ther. Bull.*, 1972, *10*, 69.

Paracetamol might interfere with the measurement of serum-uric acid concentrations when the reagent used was phosphotungstic acid.— J. Millhouse, *Adverse Drug React. Bull.*, 1974, Dec., 164.

Contamination of blood samples with heparin led to

false positive results in the colorimetric plasma-paracetamol assay of J.P. Glynn and S.E. Kendall (*Lancet*, 1975, *1*, 1147).— J. Pitts (letter), *Lancet*, 1979, *1*, 213.

Paracetamol interference with Yellow Spring Instruments glucose analyser.— I. Farrance and J. Aldons, *Clin. Chem.*, 1981, *27*, 782. See also M. J. Roddis (letter), *Lancet*, 1981, *2*, 634; J. A. Fleetwood and S. M. A. Robinson (letter), *Br. med. J.*, 1981, *283*, 438.

For the effect of paracetamol on some estimations of blood-theophylline concentrations, see Aminophylline, p.343.

Absorption and Fate. Paracetamol is readily absorbed from the gastro-intestinal tract with peak plasma concentrations occurring about 30 minutes to 2 hours after ingestion. It is metabolised in the liver and excreted in the urine mainly as the glucuronide and sulphate conjugates. Less than 5% is excreted as unchanged paracetamol. The elimination half-life varies from about 1 to 4 hours. Plasma-protein binding is negligible at usual therapeutic concentrations but increases with increasing concentrations.

A minor hydroxylated metabolite which is usually produced in very small amounts by mixed-function oxidases in the liver and which is usually detoxified by conjugation with liver glutathione may accumulate following paracetamol overdosage and cause liver damage.

A review of the absorption and fate and bioavailability of paracetamol.— C. A. Hunt *et al.*, *J. Am. pharm. Ass.*, 1977, *NS17*, 517.

Absorption. A preceding meal of high fat or protein content or a balanced test-meal did not delay significantly the absorption of paracetamol whereas a high carbohydrate meal, especially one with large amounts of pectin, reduced absorption by 60 to 76% in the first 1.5 hours compared with the fasting state.— J. M. Jaffe *et al.*, *J. pharm. Sci.*, 1971, *60*, 1646.

The rate of absorption of paracetamol was reduced by propantheline which delayed gastric emptying and increased by metoclopramide which hastened gastric emptying, but the total amount absorbed was not affected.— J. Nimmo *et al.*, *Br. med. J.*, 1973, *1*, 587.

Peak plasma and saliva concentrations of paracetamol were found in 8 fasting volunteers within 50 minutes of the ingestion of paracetamol 1 g. The concentration reached varied with the formulation of the tablets taken.— J. P. Glynn and W. Bastain (letter), *J. Pharm. Pharmac.*, 1973, *25*, 420.

Studies on the rectal absorption of paracetamol.— S. Keinänen *et al.*, *Eur. J. clin. Pharmac.*, 1977, *12*, 77; J. J. Maron *et al.*, *Curr. ther. Res.*, 1976, *20*, 45; F. Moolenaar *et al.*, *Pharm. Weekbl. Ned., scient. Edn*, 1979, *1*, 25; R. Liedtke *et al.*, *Arzneimittel-Forsch.*, 1979, *29*, 1607.

For the effects of aspirin, caffeine, and codeine on plasma concentrations of paracetamol, see Phenacetin, p.271.

Metabolism and excretion. The excretion-rate of the glucuronide and sulphate metabolites of paracetamol was reduced after the administration of salicylamide, and paracetamol reduced the formation of the sulphate metabolite of salicylamide.— G. Levy and H. Yamada, *J. pharm. Sci.*, 1971, *60*, 215.

A study of paracetamol elimination kinetics in neonates, children, and adults. An adult pattern of metabolism was evident at 12 years of age but no significant differences were noted in the overall rate of elimination among the age groups studied despite the fact that infants and younger children had different major pathways for elimination. A higher percentage of a dose was excreted as the sulphate in neonates and younger children.— R. P. Miller *et al.*, *Clin. Pharmac. Ther.*, 1976, *19*, 284.

Further studies on the effects of age on paracetamol metabolism and excretion.— R. H. Briant *et al.*, *J. Am. Geriat. Soc.*, 1976, *24*, 359; S. N. Alam *et al.*, *Pharmacologist*, 1976, *18*, 231; S. N. Alam *et al.*, *J. Pediat.*, 1977, *90*, 130; B. Fulton *et al.*, *Br. J. clin. Pharmac.*, 1979, *7*, 418P.

Studies on the metabolism of paracetamol after therapeutic doses and following overdosage.— M. Davis *et al.*, *J. int. med. Res.*, 1976, *4*, *Suppl.* 4, 40; D. Howie *et al.*, *J. Pharm. Pharmac.*, 1977, *29*, 235.

A comparison of the pharmacokinetics of paracetamol after administration by intravenous injection and by mouth, suggested that considerable 'first pass' inactivation took place in the gut wall or the liver.— M. D. Rawlins *et al.*, *Eur. J. clin. Pharmac.*, 1977, *11*, 283.

Pharmacokinetics of paracetamol in children.— R. G. Peterson and B. H. Rumack, *Pediatrics*, 1978, *62*, *Suppl.*, 877.

Pregnancy and the neonate. The disposition of paracetamol in the breast milk of 12 nursing mothers.— C. M. Berlin *et al.*, *Pediatric Pharmacol.*, 1980, *1*, 135.

Protein binding. Binding of paracetamol to plasma proteins did not occur with plasma concentrations of less than 60 µg per ml, corresponding to the usual therapeutic concentrations. After toxic doses of paracetamol up to 43% could be bound to plasma proteins.— B. G. Gazzard *et al.*, *J. Pharm. Pharmac.*, 1973, *25*, 964.

Uses. Paracetamol has analgesic and antipyretic actions similar to those of aspirin (see p.240), but it has no useful anti-inflammatory properties. Paracetamol is administered as tablets or as elixir or suppositories. The adult dose is 0.5 to 1 g every 4 hours up to a maximum of 4 g daily. Suggested doses in children are: 3 months to 1 year, 60 to 120 mg; 1 to 6 years, 120 to 250 mg; 7 to 12 years, up to 500 mg. These doses may be given 3 to 4 times daily as required.

Reviews of actions and uses of paracetamol.— J. Koch-Weser, *New Engl. J. Med.*, 1976, *295*, 1297; *Med. Lett.*, 1976, *18*, 73; B. Ameer and D. J. Greenblatt, *Ann. intern. Med.*, 1977, *87*, 202.

Administration in haemophilia. In a controlled study in a small group of patients with haemophilia, the 9 tests carried out on patients given paracetamol 650 mg and the 8 tests on patients given dextropropoxyphene hydrochloride 65 mg showed no prolongation of the bleeding time compared with that measured during 17 tests on patients given placebo. Neither paracetamol nor dextropropoxyphene affected platelet aggregation.— C. K. Kasper and S. I. Rapaport, *Ann. intern. Med.*, 1972, *77*, 189.

A discussion of analgesics for haemophiliacs suggested that paracetamol was the most suitable.— *Lancet*, 1973, *1*, 757.

Administration in hepatic disease. In a single-dose study, the metabolism of paracetamol, as judged by plasma half-life and plasma concentration of metabolites, was not depressed in patients with mild liver disease compared with normal subjects but was significantly impaired in those with severe liver disease. There were no significant differences in the overall 24-hour urinary excretion of paracetamol and its metabolites. There was no evidence that patients with liver disease were at increased risk of hepatotoxicity when given a single therapeutic dose of paracetamol.— J. A. H. Forrest *et al.*, *Eur. J. clin. Pharmac.*, 1979, *15*, 427.

Further references on paracetamol in patients with liver disorders or chronic liver disease.— M. Shamszad *et al.*, *Gastroenterology*, 1975, *69*, 865; A. P. Douglas *et al.*, *Br. J. clin. Pharmac.*, 1976, *3*, 958P; J. A. H. Forrest *et al.*, *Br. med. J.*, 1977, *1*, 1384; A. P. Douglas *et al.*, *Eur. J. clin. Pharmac.*, 1978, *13*, 209; P. B. Andreasen and L. Hutters, *Acta med. scand.*, 1979, *Suppl.* 624, 99.

Administration in renal failure. The normal half-life of paracetamol was about 1.5 to 3.5 hours. In renal failure the interval between doses should be extended from 4 hours to 4 to 6 hours in patients with a glomerular filtration-rate (GFR) above 50 ml per minute, to 6 hours in those with a GFR of 10 to 50 ml per minute, and to 8 hours in those with a GFR of less than 10 ml per minute; metabolites accumulated in patients with a GFR of less than 10 ml per minute. Concentrations of paracetamol were affected by haemodialysis but not by peritoneal dialysis; the half-life was reduced by 50% in dialysis which was the principal route of excretion in anephric patients.— W. M. Bennett *et al.*, *Ann. intern. Med.*, 1980, *92*, 62.

Analgesia. In a double-blind study involving 200 women, paracetamol 650 mg was more effective than dextropropoxyphene 65 mg for relief of pain following episiotomy. No greater benefit was derived by using the 2 drugs concomitantly, and dextropropoxyphene alone was no better than a placebo.— J. H. Hopkinson *et al.*, *J. clin. Pharmac.*, 1973, *13*, 251. An assessment of Distalgesic concluded that the combination of dextropropoxyphene and paracetamol had few advantages, but a number of disadvantages, over paracetamol alone and that it should not be used unless paracetamol had failed to control pain.— *Drug & Ther. Bull.*, 1978, *16*, 71.

In a double-blind crossover study in 32 subjects undergoing removal of bilateral impacted wisdom teeth, paracetamol and aspirin were equally effective in relieving pain, but the incidence of post-operative bleeding and swelling was less after paracetamol. There was no significant benefit in starting drug treatment on the day before operation.— P. Skjelbred *et al.*, *Eur. J. clin. Pharmac.*, 1977, *12*, 257. A further study on the use of paracetamol after oral surgery.— P. Skjelbred and P. Løkken, *ibid.*, 1979, *15*, 27.

Dysmenorrhoea. For an unfavourable report on the use of paracetamol in dysmenorrhoea, see Aspirin, p.241.

Fever. A comparison of the antipyretic activity of aspirin and paracetamol.— F. H. Lovejoy, *Pediatrics*, 1978, *62*, *Suppl.*, 904.

Paracetamol in doses of 15 to 20 mg per kg body-weight was equally effective as an antipyretic when administered by mouth as an elixir or rectally as a suppository to 37 febrile children aged between 3 months and 6 years.— S. Vernon *et al.*, *Archs Dis. Childh.*, 1979, *54*, 469.

Preparations

Acetaminophen Capsules *(U.S.P.)*. Capsules containing paracetamol. Store in airtight containers.

Acetaminophen Elixir *(U.S.P.)*. An elixir containing paracetamol, with alcohol 6.5 to 10.5%. pH 3.8 to 6.1. Store in airtight containers. Avoid continuous excessive cold.

Acetaminophen Oral Suspension *(U.S.P.)*. A suspension of paracetamol in a suitable aqueous vehicle. pH 5.4 to 6.9. Store in airtight containers.

Acetaminophen Tablets *(U.S.P.)*. Tablets containing paracetamol. The *U.S.P.* requires 80% dissolution in 30 minutes. Store in airtight containers.

Paediatric Paracetamol Elixir *(B.P.)*. Elix. Paracetamol pro Inf.; Paracetamol Elixir Paediatric. Paracetamol 120 mg, alcohol 0.5 ml, chloroform spirit 0.1 ml, propylene glycol 0.5 ml, concentrated raspberry juice 0.125 ml, amaranth solution 0.01 ml, invert syrup 1.375 ml, glycerol to 5 ml. Protect from light. The elixir should not be diluted; doses less than 5 ml should be measured in a graduated pipette.

Paracetamol and Opium Mixture *(Bristol Roy. Infirm.)*. Paracetamol 1 g, compound tragacanth powder 200 mg, opium tincture 0.6 ml, chloroform water to 10 ml. It should be freshly prepared.

Paracetamol Suppositories CF *(A.P.F.)*. Paracetamol Suppositories for Children. Suppositories containing paracetamol 120 mg in macrogol 300 and macrogol 4000 (1 part and 4 parts by wt respectively) prepared in a 1-g mould. About 1 g of paracetamol displaces 0.8 g of macrogol basis.

Paracetamol Tablets *(B.P.)*. Tablets containing paracetamol. Protect from light.

Proprietary Preparations

Cafadol *(Typharm, UK)*. Scored tablets each containing paracetamol 500 mg and caffeine 30 mg. Analgesic. *Dose.* 1 or 2 tablets every 4 hours.

Calpol *(Calmic, UK)*. Paracetamol, available as paediatric suspension containing 120 mg in each 5 ml. (Also available as Calpol in *S.Afr.*).

Dimotapp P *(Robins, UK)*. Tablets each containing paracetamol 325 mg, brompheniramine maleate 2 mg, phenylephrine hydrochloride 5 mg, and phenylpropanolamine hydrochloride 5 mg. For sinusitus and rhinitis. *Dose.* 1 to 2 tablets thrice daily; children, 6 to 12 years ½ to 1 tablet.

Dolvan *(Norma, UK: Farillon, UK)*. Tablets each containing paracetamol 300 mg, diphenhydramine hydrochloride 7.5 mg, ephedrine hydrochloride 7.5 mg, and caffeine 30 mg. For colds and influenza. *Dose.* 1 or 2 tablets every 4 hours.

Lobak *(Winthrop, UK)*. Scored tablets each containing paracetamol 450 mg and chlormezanone 100 mg. For muscle pain and dysmenorrhoea. *Dose.* 1 or 2 tablets thrice daily, up to a maximum of 8 daily.

Medised Suspension *(Martindale Pharmaceuticals, UK)*. Contains in each 5 ml paracetamol 120 mg and promethazine hydrochloride 2.5 mg. For symptomatic relief in pain, feverish conditions, and nasal discharge. *Dose.* Children, 3 months to 1 year, 5 ml up to 4 times daily; 1 to 6 years, 10 ml; 6 to 12 years, 20 ml.

Medocodene *(Medo Chemicals, UK)*. Scored tablets each containing paracetamol 500 mg and codeine phosphate 8 mg. For pain. *Dose.* 1 to 2 tablets 3 or 4 times daily; children, 6 to 12 years, ½ to 1 tablet (not more than 4 doses in 24 hours).

Neurodyne Capsules *(Rorer, UK)*. Each contains paracetamol 500 mg and codeine phosphate 8 mg. Analgesic. *Dose.* 1 or 2 capsules every 3 or 4 hours.

Norgesic *(Riker, UK)*. Scored tablets each containing paracetamol 450 mg and orphenadrine citrate 35 mg. For painful muscular conditions. *Dose.* 2 tablets thrice daily.

NOTE. Norgesic (*Riker*, USA) contains orphenadrine citrate 25 mg, aspirin 225 mg, phenacetin 160 mg, and caffeine 30 mg.

Paldesic *(R.P. Drugs, UK)*. Paracetamol, available as **Suspension** and **Syrup** both containing 120 mg in each 5 ml.

Pamol Supps for Babies *(Marshall's Pharmaceuticals, UK)*. Paediatric suppositories each containing paracetamol 200 mg and phenobarbitone 15 mg.

Pamol Tablets *(Marshall's Pharmaceuticals, UK)*. Each containing paracetamol 500 mg.

Panadeine Co *(Winthrop, UK)*. Scored tablets each containing paracetamol 500 mg and codeine phosphate 8 mg in a basis containing sorbitol. For pain. *Dose.* 2 tablets 3 or 4 times daily; children 7 to 12 years, ½ to 1 tablet (not more than 4 doses in 24 hours).

Panadol *(Winthrop, UK)*. Paracetamol, available as **Elixir** containing 120 mg in 5 ml (suggested diluent, syrup) and as **Tablets** of 500 mg. (Also available as Panadol in *Austral., Fin., Neth., Switz.*) **Panadol Caplets.** Paracetamol, available as tablets of 500 mg. **Panadol Soluble**. Paracetamol, available as tablets of 500 mg in an effervescent basis.

Panasorb *(Winthrop, UK)*. Tablets each containing paracetamol 500 mg in a basis containing sorbitol.

Paracodol *(Fisons, UK)*. Effervescent tablets each containing paracetamol 500 mg and codeine phosphate 8 mg with the equivalent (in buffering effect when in solution) of 1.5 g of sodium citrate. Analgesic. *Dose.* 1 or 2 tablets dissolved in water every 4 to 6 hours; children, 5 to 12 years, ½ to 1 tablet, up to a maximum of 3 in 24 hours.

Paradeine *(Scotia, UK)*. Tablets each containing paracetamol 500 mg, codeine phosphate 10 mg, and phenolphthalein 2.5 mg. Analgesic. *Dose.* 1 or 2 tablets every 4 hours.

Parahypon Tablets *(Calmic, UK)*. Scored tablets each containing paracetamol 500 mg, caffeine 10 mg, and codeine phosphate 5 mg. Analgesic and antipyretic. *Dose.* 2 tablets up to 4 times daily; children, 6 to 12 years, 1 to 2 tablets.

Parake *(Galen, UK)*. Tablets each containing paracetamol 500 mg and codeine phosphate 8 mg. For pain. *Dose.* 2 tablets every 4 hours; children, 7 to 12 years, ½ to 1 tablet 3 or 4 times daily.

Paralgin Tablets *(Norton, UK: Vestric, UK)*. Each containing paracetamol 450 mg, codeine phosphate 6 mg, and caffeine 20 mg. Analgesic. *Dose.* 2 tablets every 4 hours.

NOTE. In some countries the name Paralgin is applied to preparations containing only paracetamol.

Paramax Tablets *(Beecham Research, UK)*. Scored tablets each containing paracetamol 500 mg and metoclopramide hydrochloride equivalent to 5 mg of anhydrous metoclopramide hydrochloride. **Paramax Sachets.** Each contains the equivalent of one tablet in an effervescent basis. For migraine. *Dose.* 2 tablets at the start of an attack, repeated at intervals of 4 hours; maximum dosage 6 tablets in 24 hours; patients, 12 to 14 years, 1 tablet; maximum 3 tablets; 15 to 20 years, 1 or 2 tablets; maximum 5 tablets.

Para-seltzer *(Wander, UK)*. Effervescent tablets each containing paracetamol 500 mg and caffeine 20 mg. *Dose.* 1 or 2 tablets dissolved in water every 4 hours; not more than 8 in 24 hours. Children, 6 to 12 years, ½ to 1 tablet.

Pardale *(Martindale Pharmaceuticals, UK)*. Scored tablets each containing paracetamol 400 mg, codeine phosphate 9 mg, and caffeine hydrate 10 mg. For pain. *Dose.* 1 or 2 tablets 3 or 4 times daily.

Paxidal *(Wallace Mfg Chem., UK: Farillon, UK)*. Tablets each containing paracetamol 325 mg, caffeine 65 mg, and meprobamate 135 mg. For pain. *Dose.* 2 tablets thrice daily.

Pharmidone *(Farmitalia Carlo Erba, UK)*. Scored tablets each containing paracetamol 400 mg, codeine phosphate 10 mg, diphenydramine hydrochloride 5 mg, and caffeine 50 mg. For pain. *Dose.* 1 to 2 tablets every 4 hours up to a maximum of 10 in 24 hours.

Propain *(Luitpold-Werk, UK: Farillon, UK)*. Scored tablets each containing paracetamol 400 mg, codeine phosphate 10 mg, diphenydramine hydrochloride 5 mg, and caffeine 50 mg. For pain. *Dose.* 1 or 2 tablets every 4 hours; not more than 10 in 24 hours.

Salzone *(Wallace Mfg Chem., UK: Farillon, UK)*. Paracetamol, available as syrup containing 120 mg in each 5 ml.

Solpadeine *(Winthrop, UK)*. Effervescent tablets each containing paracetamol 500 mg, codeine phosphate 8 mg, and caffeine 30 mg. For pain. *Dose.* 2 tablets dissolved in water 3 or 4 times daily; children, 7 to 12 years, ½ to 1 tablet (not more than 4 doses in 24 hours).

Syndol *(Merrell, UK)*. Scored tablets each containing paracetamol 450 mg, codeine phosphate 10 mg, doxylamine succinate 5 mg, and caffeine 30 mg. For headache. *Dose.* 1 or 2 tablets every 4 to 6 hours.

Ticelgesic *(Ticen, Eire)*. Paracetamol, available as tablets of 500 mg.

Tinol *(Ticen, Eire)*. A syrup containing in each 5 ml paracetamol 120 mg and diphenhydramine hydrochloride 12.5 mg. Analgesic and sedative. *Dose.* Children, 3 months to 1 year, 5 ml; 1 to 6 years, 5 to 10 ml; over 6 years, 15 ml.

Unigesic *(Unimed, UK)*. Capsules each containing paracetamol 500 mg and caffeine 30 mg. For pain. *Dose.* 1 to 2 capsules every 4 hours; children, 8 to 12 years, 1 capsule.

Other Proprietary Names

Arg.—Calip, Custodial, Dirox, Doloral, Fonafor, Tenasfen; *Austral.*—Bramcetamol, Calpon, Ceetamol, Dolamin, Dymadon, Pacemol, Panamax, Paracet, Parasin, Paraspen, Parmol, Placemol, Tempra; *Belg.*—Ben-u-ron, Tempra, Tylenol; *Canad.*—Atasol, Campain, Exdol, Robigesic, Rounox, Tempra, Tivrin, Tylenol; *Denm.*—Panodil; *Eire.*—Cetamol; *Fr.*—Doliprane; *Ger.*—Anaflon, Ben-u-ron, Enelfa; *Iceland*—Panodil; *Ital.*—Acetamol, Nevral, Puernol, Tachipirina; *Neth.*—Kinderfinimal, Paramol; *Norw.*—Panodil, Paracet, Pinex; *S.Afr.*—Ennagesic, Fevamol, Napamol, Paraprom, Pyralen, Repamol, Sedapyren; *Spain*—Gelocatil, Melabon Infantil; *Swed.*—Alvedon, Panodil, Reliv; *Switz.*—Acetalgin, Ben-u-ron, Puernol, Tylenol; *USA*—Acephen, Alba-Temp, Anuphen, Capital, Datril, Dolanex, Febrigesic, Fendon, Korum, Liquiprin, Lyteca, Nebs, Oraphen-PD, Panofen, Phendex, Proval, SK-APAP, Tapar, Tempra, Tylenol, Valadol.

A preparation containing paracetamol was also formerly marketed in Great Britain under the proprietary name Budale (*Dales Pharmaceuticals*, now *Martindale Pharmaceuticals*).

2680-n

Parapropamol. 4′-Hydroxypropionanilide.
$C_9H_{11}NO_2$=165.2.

CAS — 1693-37-4.

Uses. Parapropamol is an analgesic that has been used in the treatment of various types of pain in doses of 1 to 3 g daily.

The analgesic activity of parapropamol was superior to that of aspirin and resembled amidopyrine. It had no anti-inflammatory and antipyretic activity and had no effect on the gastric mucosa.— M. Podesta and D. Aubert, *Boll. chim.-farm.*, 1970, *109*, 528.

Proprietary Names
Solvodol *(Millot-Solac, Fr.)*.

2681-h

Phenacetin *(Eur. P., U.S.P., B.P. 1973)*.

Phenacetinum; Aceto-*p*-phenetidide; Acetophenetidin; Acetylphenetidin; Paracetophenetidin. *p*-Acetophenetidide; 4′-Ethoxyacetanilide; *N*-(4-Ethoxyphenyl)acetamide.
$C_{10}H_{13}NO_2$=179.2.

CAS — 62-44-2.

Pharmacopoeias. In all pharmocopoeias examined except *Br.*

Odourless, white or off-white, glistening, crystalline scales or fine white crystalline powder with a slightly bitter taste. M.p. 134° to 137°. At relative humidities between about 15 and 90% the equilibrium moisture content at 25° is about 2%. **Soluble** 1 in 1300 of water, 1 in 20 of alcohol, and 1 in 20 of chloroform; sparingly soluble in boiling water, freely soluble in boiling alcohol, slightly soluble in ether and glycerol. A saturated solution is neutral to litmus. **Incompatible** with oxidising agents, iodine, and spirit of nitrous ether. It forms liquid mixtures with chloral hydrate, phenol, and many other substances.

Adverse Effects. Phenacetin may cause methaemoglobinaemia, sulphaemoglobinaemia, and haemolytic anaemia.

Prolonged administration of large doses of analgesic mixtures containing phenacetin has been associated with the development of renal papillary necrosis and appears to be associated also with the development of transitional-cell carcinoma of the renal pelvis (see p.234).

Phenacetin could cause yellow discoloration of the urine or brown to black discoloration on standing due to excretion products.— R. B. Baran and B. Rowles, *J. Am. pharm. Ass.*, 1973, *NS13*, 139.

A comparison of the adverse effects of phenacetin and paracetamol.— G. Margetts, *J. int. med. Res.*, 1976, *4, Suppl.* 4, 55.

Effects on blood. Phenacetin had been reported to cause sideroblastic anaemia.— R. H. Girdwood, *Drugs*, 1976, *11*, 394.

Haemolytic anaemia. Phenacetin 3.6 g daily had been reported to cause haemolytic anaemia in certain individuals with a deficiency of glucose-6-phosphate dehydrogenase. The reaction was not considered clinically significant under normal circumstances (e.g. in the absence of infection). Phenacetin had been implicated as a causative agent in immune haemolytic anaemia.— E. Beutler, *Pharmac. Rev.*, 1969, *21*, 73.

Studies in *rats* suggested that *p*-chloroacetanilide (a contaminant) and *p*-phenetidine (a minor metabolite) were responsible for phenacetin-induced haemolytic anaemia.— B. Schnitzer, *Ann. intern. Med.*, 1971, *75*, 320, per *Int. pharm. Abstr.*, 1972, *9*, 42.

Case reports: H. E. Hutchinson *et al.*, *Lancet*, 1962, *2*, 1022; J. Millar *et al.*, *Can. med. Ass. J.*, 1972, *106*, 770.

Sulphaemoglobinaemia. A report of phenacetin-induced sulphaemoglobinaemia.— L. D. Kneezel and C. S. Kitchens, *Johns Hopkins med. J.*, 1976, *139*, 175.

Epidermal necrolysis. Four cases of toxic epidermal necrolysis had been reported associated with the use of phenacetin or acetanilide.— E. D. Lowney *et al.*, *Archs Derm.*, 1967, *95*, 359.

Erythema multiforme. Phenacetin had been implicated in the Stevens-Johnson syndrome.— D. B. Coursin, *J. Am. med. Ass.*, 1966, *198*, 113.

Erythema nodosum. Phenacetin could cause erythema nodosum.— P. F. Naish, *Practitioner*, 1969, *202*, 637.

Treatment of Adverse Effects. As for Paracetamol, p.269. Methaemoglobinaemia may be treated with methylene blue administered intravenously as a 1% solution in a dose of 1 to 4 mg per kg body-weight.

Precautions. Phenacetin should be given with care to patients with impaired kidney or liver function.

Absorption and Fate. Phenacetin is readily absorbed from the gastro-intestinal tract and peak plasma concentrations occur after about an hour. Phenacetin is metabolised in the liver, mainly to paracetamol which is conjugated and excreted as glucuronide and sulphate. Less than 1% of phenacetin is excreted unchanged in the urine. A small amount of phenacetin is de-acetylated to *p*-phenetidine, the precursor of substances believed to be responsible for methaemoglobinaemia.

When phenacetin was given in conjunction with aspirin, caffeine, and codeine to 24 healthy subjects, the urinary excretion of 2-hydroxyphenetidine and plasma-paracetamol concentrations were greater than when phenacetin was given alone. When paracetamol was given in conjunction with aspirin, caffeine, and codeine to the same subjects there was a higher plasma-paracetamol concentration than when paracetamol was given alone. No 2-hydroxyphenetidine was detected in the urine.— B. H. Thomas *et al.*, *Clin. Pharmac. Ther.*, 1972, *13*, 906.

A study on the pharmacokinetics of phenacetin in man.— J. Raaflaub and U. C. Dubach, *Eur. J. clin. Pharmac.*, 1975, *8*, 261.

The detection of conjugates of 3-methylthio-4-hydroxyacetanilide in the urine of subjects given phenacetin or paracetamol.— A. Klutch *et al.*, *Clin. Pharmac. Ther.*, 1978, *24*, 287.

Uses. Phenacetin has analgesic and antipyretic actions similar to those of aspirin. Phenacetin has usually been given with aspirin, caffeine, or codeine in tablets.

2682-m

Phenazone *(B.P., Eur. P.).* Phenazon.; Phenazonum; Antipyrin; Antipyrine *(U.S.P.)*; Azophenum; Analgésine; Fenazona. 1,5-Dimethyl-2-phenyl-4-pyrazolin-3-one.

$C_{11}H_{12}N_2O$=188.2.

CAS — 60-80-0.

Pharmacopoeias. In *Arg., Aust., Belg., Br., Cz., Eur., Fr., Ger., Hung., Int., It., Jap., Mex., Neth., Nord., Pol., Port., Roum., Rus., Span., Swiss, Turk.,* and *U.S.*

Small, colourless, odourless, or almost odourless, crystals or white crystalline powder with a slightly bitter taste. M.p. 110° to 113°.

Soluble 1 in 1 of water, 1 in 1 of alcohol, 1 in 1 of chloroform, and 1 in 50 of ether. A 5% solution in water has a pH of 5.8 to 7. A 6.81% solution is iso-osmotic with serum. Solutions are **sterilised** by autoclaving. **Store** in airtight containers.

Incompatible with nitrites in acid solution, with the cinchona alkaloids, iodides, and tannic acid. It forms liquid mixtures with acetanilide, betanaphthol, camphor, chloral hydrate, sodium salicylate, and many other substances.

A 6.81% solution of phenazone in water, iso-osmotic with serum, caused 100% haemolysis of erythrocytes cultured in it for 45 minutes.— E. R. Hammarlund and K. Pedersen-Bjergaard, *J. pharm. Sci.*, 1961, *50*, 24.

Earlier reports of incompatibility between phenazone and caffeine citrate were investigated. No colour reaction or other signs of incompatibility occurred in solutions containing both substances, though a yellow colour was produced if a trace of an iron salt was added.— *Pharm. J.*, 1961, *2*, 187 (Pharm. Soc. Lab. Rep.).

Adverse Effects. Phenazone is liable to give rise to skin eruptions and in susceptible individuals even small doses may have this effect. Large doses may cause nausea, drowsiness, coma and convulsions.

Phenazone might cause fixed eruptions (eruptions recurring at the same site on re-exposure) and eruptions resembling erythema multiforme.— R. L. Baer and H. Harris, *J. Am. med. Ass.*, 1967, *202*, 710.

Phenazone could cause red discoloration of urine.— E. B. Baran and B. Rowles, *J. Am. pharm. Ass.*, 1973, *NS13*, 139.

Allergy. An immediate allergic reaction to phenazone and a latent leucopenic reaction.— D. Kadar and W. Kalow, *Clin. Pharmac. Ther.*, 1981, *28*, 820.

Effects on blood. Phenazone had been shown to cause haemolytic anaemia in certain individuals with a deficiency of glucose-6-phosphate dehydrogenase.— T. A. J. Prankerd, *Clin. Pharmac. Ther.*, 1963, *4*, 334.

Effects on the kidneys. Recurrent acute renal failure was associated with phenazone in a 32-year-old male patient. A strong positive reaction was obtained in a phenazone skin test.— J. Ortuño and J. Botella, *Lancet*, 1973, *2*, 1473.

Precautions. Phenazone affects the metabolism of some other drugs and its metabolism is affected by other drugs that increase or reduce the activity of liver enzymes.

Phenazone had been reported to precipitate attacks of porphyria.— *Drug & Ther. Bull.*, 1976, *14*, 55.

Phenazone has been reported to increase the plasma concentration of unbound desipramine, see p.117.

Phenazone has been reported to decrease the plasma concentration of warfarin sodium, see p.777.

Absorption and Fate. Phenazone is readily absorbed from the gastro-intestinal tract and is distributed throughout the body fluids. Peak plasma concentrations are usually attained in 1 to 2 hours. Less than 10% is bound to plasma proteins and it has a half-life of about 12 hours. Phenazone is metabolised in the liver; about 30 to 40% is metabolised to 4-hydroxyphenazone which is excreted in the urine as the glucuronide. About 5% is excreted unchanged and about 6% as norphenazone in the urine.

Because phenazone is metabolised primarily in the liver by microsomal mixed-function oxidases, it has been widely used for drug metabolism studies. The half-life of phenazone is decreased by substances which induce liver microsomal enzymes, including barbiturates, phenytoin, rifampicin, and some chlorinated insecticides; it is also decreased by smoking and by hyperthyroidism. Phenazone half-life is increased by substances which inhibit liver microsomal enzymes including oral contraceptives and isoniazid; it is also increased in older subjects and in patients with myxoedema and liver disorders. In addition, phenazone itself induces liver microsomal enzymes and may affect the metabolism of some other drugs.

Uses. Phenazone has analgesic and antipyretic actions. It has been used in doses of 300 to 600 mg. Topically, it has local anaesthetic and styptic actions and solutions containing 5% are used locally as ear drops.

Changes in the half-life of phenazone in the body (antipyrine half-life) have been used as a test for the effect of other drugs on the activity of drug-metabolising enzymes in the liver.

Prophylaxis of neonatal jaundice. In a double-blind study phenazone 300 mg daily was given to 24 women from the thirty-eighth week of pregnancy until delivery of their infants. Neonatal plasma-bilirubin concentrations on the fourth day after birth were reduced by an average of 44% compared with those of the infants of 24 similar women who received placebo.— P. J. Lewis and L. A. Friedman (preliminary communication), *Lancet*, 1979, *1*, 300.

Preparations

Glycerin Otic Solution *(U.S.P.).* A solution of phenazone and benzocaine in glycerol. Store in airtight containers. Protect from light.

Proprietary Preparations

Auralgicin *(Fisons, UK).* Ear-drops containing phenazone 5.5%, ephedrine hydrochloride 1%, benzocaine 1.4%, chlorbutol 1%, and potassium hydroxyquinoline sulphate 0.1% in anhydrous glycerol. For acute otitis media.

Auraltone *(Rorer, UK).* Ear-drops containing phenazone 5% and benzocaine 1% in glycerol. For otitis media.

Sedonan *(Napp, UK).* Ear-drops containing phenazone 5% and chlorbutol 1% in glycerol. For relief of pain in middle- and external-ear conditions.

Preparations containing phenazone were also formerly marketed in Great Britain under the proprietary names Felsol Powders (*Bengué*) and Lanceotic (*Lancet Pharmaceuticals*, now *Kirby-Warrick*).

2683-b

Phenazone and Caffeine Citrate. Migrenin; Antipyrino-Coffeinum Citricum.

Pharmacopoeias. In *Aust., Cz., Hung., Jap.,* and *Swiss.*

A white crystalline powder usually containing phenazone 90%, caffeine 9%, and citric acid monohydrate 1%. **Soluble** 1 in 2 of water. **Store** in airtight containers. Protect from light.

Phenazone and caffeine citrate has been used as an analgesic in doses of 0.3 to 1 g up to a max. of 3 g in 24 hours.

Preparations

Migrenin and Bromovalerylurea Powder *(Jap. P.).* Pulv. Migrenin. et Bromvalerylur. Phenazone and caffeine citrate 30% and bromvaletone 20% with starch or lactose. *Dose.* 1 g.

2684-v

Phenazone Salicylate *(B.P.C. 1949).* Antipyrin Salicylate; Salipyrin.

$C_{11}H_{12}N_2O,C_7H_6O_3$=326.4.

CAS — 520-07-0.

Pharmacopoeias. In *Arg., Aust., Port., Roum.,* and *Span.*

White odourless crystals or crystalline powder with a sweetish bitter taste. M.p. 89° to 92°.

Soluble 1 in 240 of water, 1 in 4 of alcohol, 1 in 1.5 of chloroform, and 1 in 40 of ether; slightly soluble in carbon disulphide. A 0.2% solution in water is acid to litmus. **Incompatible** with iodine and ferric salts.

Phenazone salicylate has analgesic and antipyretic actions and has been used for the relief of the less severe types of pain in doses of 0.3 to 1.2 g.

2685-g

Phenazopyridine Hydrochloride *(U.S.P.).* NC 150; W1655; Chloridrato de Fenazopiridina. 3-Phenylazopyridine-2,6-diyldiamine hydrochloride.

$C_{11}H_{11}N_5$,HCl=249.7.

CAS — 94-78-0 (phenazopyridine); 136-40-3 (hydrochloride).

Pharmacopoeias. In *Braz.* and *U.S.*

A light or dark red to dark violet crystalline powder, odourless or with a slight odour, and with a slightly bitter taste. M.p. about 235° with decomposition.

Soluble 1 in 300 of cold water, 1 in 20 of boiling water, 1 in about 60 of alcohol, 1 in about 330 chloroform, and 1 in 100 of glycerol; very slightly soluble in ether; soluble in glacial acetic acid, ethylene glycol, and propylene glycol. A solution in water is slightly acid.

Incompatible with preparations containing mercury, silver, or sulphur, with mineral acids, chlorides, or iodides, and with solutions containing alcohol, chlorine, or iodine. Phenazopyridine hydrochloride readily forms supersaturated aqueous solutions which deposit slowly on storage; a 1% (supersaturated) solution may be stabilised by the addition of dextrose (10%). **Store** in airtight containers.

REMOVAL OF STAINS. Phenazopyridine stains may be removed from fabric by soaking in a solution of sodium dithionite 0.25%.

Adverse Effects. Phenazopyridine hydrochloride has occasionally caused gastro-intestinal side-effects and abnormalities in liver function. Haemolytic anaemia, methaemoglobinaemia, and acute renal failure have also been reported, generally associated with overdosage or with therapeutic doses in patients with impaired renal function.

Phenazopyridine could cause orange to red discoloration of the faeces.— J. Karlstrand, *J. Am. pharm. Ass.*, 1977, *NS17*, 735.

Effects on blood. *Haemolytic anaemia.* Reports of haemolytic anaemia occurring in patients taking phenazopyridine.— M. S. Greenberg and H. Wong, *New Engl. J. Med.*, 1964, *271*, 431; E. P. Gabor *et al.*, *Can. med. Ass. J.*, 1964, *91*, 756; A. J. Eisinger and R. Jones (letter), *Lancet*, 1969, *1*, 151; H. C. Drysdale and M. D. Hellier (letter), *Br. med. J.*, 1978, *2*, 1021; C. J. T. Bateman (letter), *ibid.*, 1716.

Effects on the kidneys. An 85-year-old woman developed a yellowish-orange pigmentation of the skin and urinary insufficiency after taking phenazopyridine hydrochloride 200 mg by mouth thrice daily. The drug was withdrawn and urinary output was restored the following day.— C. E. Eybel *et al.*, *J. Am. med. Ass.*, 1974, *228*, 1027. A further report of acute renal failure in 2 patients with renal disease treated with large doses of phenazopyridine.— F. A. Alano and G. D. Webster, *Ann. intern. Med.*, 1970, *72*, 89, per *J. Am. med. Ass.* 1970, *211*, 847.

Renal calculi. Vesical calculi composed of pure phenazopyridine were found in the urinary tract of a 67-year-old man who had been taking phenazopyridine hydrochloride 600 mg daily for 2 years.— W. P. Mulvaney *et al.*, *J. Am. med. Ass.*, 1972, *221*, 1511.

Phenazopyridine was deposited on ureteral stones already present in a 55-year-old man with chronic prostatitis who had taken phenazopyridine hydrochloride 200 mg thrice daily for 5 months.— E. D. Crawford and W. P. Mulvaney, *J. Urol.*, 1978, *119*, 280.

Effects on liver. Signs of liver disorder, considered to be a hypersensitivity reaction, occurred on 4 occasions in a woman given phenazopyridine.— B. W. D. Badley, *Br.*

med. J., 1976, *2*, 850.

Further reports of abnormalities of liver function following phenazopyridine.— J. W. Hood and W. N. Toth, *J. Am. med. Ass.*, 1966, *198*, 1366; A. J. Eisinger and R. Jones (letter), *Lancet*, 1969, *1*, 151; S. E. Goldfinger and S. Marx, *New Engl. J. Med.*, 1972, *286*, 1090.

Overdosage. A 13-month-old girl who ingested 2.5 to 3 g of phenazopyridine developed methaemoglobinaemia and haemolytic anaemia, and the haemoglobin concentration fell to 66 mg per ml. She recovered after treatment with methylene blue and blood transfusion.— B. L. Cohen and G. J. Bovasso, *Clin. Pediat.*, 1971, *10*, 537.

After taking phenazopyridine 2.4 g over a 24-hour period for acute loin pain an 18-year-old woman developed methaemoglobinaemia, haemolytic anaemia, and acute renal failure. She was given an intravenous injection of methylene blue 100 mg, with reversal of her methaemoglobinaemia and subsequent recovery.— D. M. Nathan *et al.*, *Archs intern. Med.*, 1977, *137*, 1636.

Further reports of acute renal failure attributed to overdosage with phenazopyridine hydrochloride.— D. A. Feinfeld *et al.*, *J. Am. med. Ass.*, 1978, *240*, 2661; N. Qureshi and R. W. Hedger (letter), *Ann. intern. Med.*, 1979, *90*, 443.

Treatment of Adverse Effects. Methaemoglobinaemia may be treated with methylene blue administered intravenously as a 1% solution in a dose of 1 to 4 mg per kg bodyweight.

Precautions. Phenazopyridine hydrochloride is contra-indicated in glomerulonephritis, severe hepatitis, uraemia, and impaired renal function.

Absorption and Fate. Phenazopyridine hydrochloride is absorbed from the gastro-intestinal tract. It is excreted mainly in the urine; about 40% is excreted as unchanged phenazopyridine.

Following administration of phenazopyridine hydrochloride 200 mg thrice daily to 6 healthy subjects, a mean of about 90% of the dose appeared in the urine within 24 hours, of which 41% was unchanged, 18% was *N*-acetyl-*p*-aminophenol, 24% was *p*-aminophenol, and about 7% was aniline. The amount of aniline released was in excess of the maximal allowable dose of 35 mg daily.— W. J. Johnson and A. Chartrand, *Toxic. appl. Pharmac.*, 1976, *37*, 371.

Uses. Phenazopyridine allays pain and irritability in the urinary tract and is a palliative in cystitis, prostatitis, and urethritis. It is administered as tablets, the usual dose being 200 mg thrice daily before food, and for children over 8 years of age, 100 mg thrice daily. During administration the urine is tinged either orange or red and underclothes are apt to be stained.

Administration in renal failure. The interval between doses should be extended from 8 hours to 8 to 16 hours in patients with a glomerular filtration-rate (GFR) above 50 ml per minute; it should be avoided in those with a GFR of less than 50 ml per minute.— W. M. Bennett *et al.*, *Ann. intern. Med.*, 1980, *93*, 62.

Preparations

Phenazopyridine Hydrochloride Tablets *(U.S.P.)*. Tablets containing phenazopyridine hydrochloride. Store in airtight containers.

Pyridium *(Warner, UK)*. Phenazopyridine hydrochloride, available as tablets of 100 mg. (Also available as Pyridium in *Arg., Austral., Belg., Fr., Ger., Spain, USA*).

Other Proprietary Names

Azodine *(S.Afr.)*; Giracid *(Switz.)*; Phenazo *(Canad.)*; Pyridacil *(Neth., Switz.)*; Uropyridin *(Jap.)*; Uropyrine *(Belg.)*; Vestin *(Spain)*.

2686-q

Phenylbutazone *(B.P., B.P. Vet., Eur. P., U.S.P.)*.

Phenylbutaz.; Phenylbutazonum; Butadione; Fenilbutazona. 4-Butyl-1,2-diphenylpyrazolidine-3,5-dione.

$C_{19}H_{20}N_2O_2=308.4$.

CAS — 50-33-9.

Pharmacopoeias. In *Br., Braz., Cz., Eur., Fr., Ger., Hung., Int., It., Jap., Jug., Neth., Nord., Pol., Port., Roum., Rus., Swiss, Turk.*, and *U.S.*

A fine, white or off-white, odourless or almost odourless, crystalline powder which is tasteless at first but has a slightly bitter after-taste. M.p. 104° to 107°.

Practically **insoluble** in water; soluble 1 in 28 of alcohol, 1 in 1.25 of chloroform, 1 in 15 of ether; soluble aqueous solutions of alkali hydroxides; freely soluble in acetone. **Store** in airtight containers.

Wide bioavailability of brands of phenylbutazone tablets.— R. O. Searl and M. Pernarowski, *Can. med. Ass. J.*, 1967, *96*, 1513; G. R. Van Petten *et al.*, *J. clin. Pharmac.*, 1971, *11*, 177.

Decomposition. From 3 to 21% of decomposition products were found in preparations containing phenylbutazone and aluminium hydroxide, but in 32 of 33 brands of phenylbutazone tablets not more than 0.5% decomposition products were found.— H. D. Beckstead *et al.*, *J. pharm. Sci.*, 1968, *57*, 1952.

Ten per cent decomposition of phenylbutazone in the 3 suppository bases Lasupol G, Witepsol H, and Massupol occurred in 7.9, 154, and 445 days respectively at 20°, and was directly related to the hydroxyl value of the basis.— E. Pawelczyk and M. Zając, *Acta Pol. Pharm.*, 1970, *27*, 113.

Of 14 parenteral preparations of phenylbutazone examined, 12 contained *N*-(2-carboxycaproyl)hydrazobenzol in concentrations between 4 and 11% of the declared phenylbutazone content.— S. L. Ali and T. Strittmatter, *Pharm. Ztg, Berl.*, 1978, *123*, 720.

Adverse Effects. Nausea, vomiting, epigastric distress, oedema due to salt retention, and skin rashes are the most common adverse effects encountered with phenylbutazone. Diarrhoea, vertigo, headache and blurred vision may also occur. More serious reactions include gastric irritation with ulceration and gastro-intestinal bleeding, ulcerative stomatitis, hepatitis, jaundice, haematuria, nephritis, renal failure, and goitre. Salivary gland enlargement, hypersensitivity reactions, and severe generalised reactions including erythema multiforme, (Stevens-Johnson syndrome), toxic epidermal necrolysis, and exfoliative dermatitis have been reported. The most serious adverse effects of phenylbutazone are related to bone-marrow depression and include agranulocytosis and aplastic anaemia. Leucopenia, pancytopenia, haemolytic anaemia, and thrombocytopenia may also occur.

Symptoms of acute overdosage may include nausea, vomiting, epigastric pain, sweating, tinnitus, oedema, acidosis, convulsions, and coma. Impairment of hepatic and renal function, gastro-intestinal ulceration, and bone-marrow depression may also occur. Blood disorders may develop soon after starting treatment or may occur suddenly after prolonged treatment. Blood-cell counts should be performed regularly but should not be relied upon to predict dysplasia. Patients should be told to discontinue the drug at the first signs of toxic effects and to report at once the appearance of symptoms such as fever, sore throat, stomatitis, skin rashes, and weight gain or oedema.Pain, necrosis, and abscesses have been reported at the site of intramuscular injection.

There were 1276 reports of adverse reactions to phenylbutazone reported to the Committee on Safety of Medicines from June 1964 to January 1973. These included 398 reports of blood disorders (204 fatal) including aplastic anaemia (163; 121 fatal), thrombocytopenia (59; 18 fatal), agranulocytosis, leucopenia, or pancytopenia (95; 44 fatal), and gastro-intestinal haemorrhage (104; 27 fatal).— M. F. Cuthbert, *Curr. med. Res. Opinion*, 1974, *2*, 600.

Loss of taste sensitivity associated with phenylbutazone occurred in 3 patients, 2 of whom also received amidopyrine or isopropylaminophenazone.— H. Rollin, *Ann. Otol. Rhinol. Lar.*, 1978, *87*, 37.

Allergy. Reports of lymphadenopathy.— T. G. Plunkett *et al.* (letter), *Lancet*, 1967, *1*, 448; D. W. Littlejohns *et al.*, *Rheumatol. Rehabil.*, 1973, *12*, 57.

A 69-year-old man who had taken phenylbutazone for about 4 weeks developed eosinophilia and physical signs suggestive of pulmonary oedema. The radiological picture later became typical of allergic alveolitis, possibly caused by phenylbutazone.— J. G. B. Thurston *et al.*, *Br. med. J.*, 1976, *2*, 1422.

Effects on blood. An analysis of blood dyscrasias reported to the Swedish Adverse Drug Reaction Committee for the 5-year period 1966–70 showed that thrombocytopenia attributable to phenylbutazone had been reported on 7 occasions (1 fatal), aplastic anaemia on 4 occasions (2 fatal), and agranulocytosis on 5 occasions (2 fatal). It was estimated that reported figures represented one-third of the true frequency.— L. E. Böttiger and B. Westerholm, *Br. med. J.*, 1973, *3*, 339.

Aplastic anaemia or agranulocytosis were quoted as underlying or contributory causes of death in 376 death certificates in the year October 1974 to September 1975; adequate medical records were available for 269. Death was probably due to phenylbutazone in 28 cases. Mortality was estimated at 2.2 per 100 000 patients.— W. H. W. Inman, *Committee on Safety of Medicines, Br. med. J.*, 1977, *1*, 1500.

Aplastic anaemia. Fatal aplastic anaemia occurred in a 20-year-old jockey who had taken 2 g of veterinary phenylbutazone daily for more than 3 days.— R. Ramsey and D. W. Golde, *J. Am. med. Ass.*, 1976, *236*, 1049.

Haemolytic anaemia. Phenylbutazone did not cause haemolysis in Chinese patients with glucose 6-phosphate dehydrogenase deficiency.— T. K. Chan *et al.*, *Br. med. J.* 1976, *2*, 1227.

Leukaemia. The case histories of 5 patients with acute leukaemia who had received treatment with phenylbutazone were given. The association of phenylbutazone with leukaemia was suggested.— H. J. Woodliff and L. Dougan, *Br. med. J.*, 1964, *1*, 744. A similar report in 6 men.— R. H. D. Bean, *ibid.*, 1960, *2*, 1552.

Megaloblastic anaemia. Megaloblastic anaemia occurred in a 36-year-old woman following oral administration of 400 mg of phenylbutazone daily over a period of 5 months. The condition responded to folic acid. A further course of phenylbutazone caused a recurrence of the macrocytosis.— H. N. Robson and J. R. Lawrence, *Br. med. J.*, 1959, *2*, 475.

Pancytopenia. A 77-year-old woman who had taken phenylbutazone for 12 years and quinine sulphate for 3 years developed pancytopenia and platelet antibodies.— A. C. Keat *et al.* (letter), *Br. med. J.*, 1973, *4*, 490.

Thrombocytopenia. Reports of thrombocytopenia in patients receiving phenylbutazone.— K. Dvorák and E. Blazková, *Vnitř. Lék.*, 1965, *11*, 1000, per *Int. pharm. Abstr.* 1966, *3*, 1222; C. Davidson and S. M. Manohitharajah (letter), *Br. med. J.*, 1973, *3*, 545.

Effects on the cardiovascular system. A 64-year-old woman given phenylbutazone 100 mg thrice daily, developed pericarditis and 15 days after the start of treatment her condition was critical. Symptoms did not respond to digoxin or mersalyl but prednisone, in a dosage of 10 mg thrice daily, was life-saving.— J. Shafar, *Br. med. J.*, 1965, *2*, 795.

Four patients with polymyalgic disorders developed temporal arteritis during treatment with phenylbutazone or oxyphenbutazone, and one patient had partial loss of vision in one eye. It appeared that while the drugs were effective in relieving the myalgic pains the disease insidiously progressed. It was suggested that polymyalgia rheumatica and temporal arteritis should not be treated with phenylbutazone or oxyphenbutazone.— B. Wadman and I. Werner, *Lancet*, 1967, *1*, 597.

Effects on chromosomes. Chromosome aberrations in lymphocytes exposed to phenylbutazone.— W. Vormittag and G. Kolarz, *Arzneimittel-Forsch.*, 1979, *29*, 1163.

Effects on the kidneys. A 43-year-old man who had taken 2.2 g of phenylbutazone over 6 days developed acute renal failure with marked acidosis, but recovered after treatment with sodium bicarbonate parenterally.— J. H. Richardson and H. H. Alderfer, *New Engl. J. Med.*, 1963, *268*, 809.

A report of acute interstitial nephritis and renal failure in a patient with a hypersensitivity reaction to phenylbutazone.— G. I. Russell *et al.*, *Br. med. J.*, 1978, *1*, 1322. A similar report.— U. Kuhlmann *et al.*, *Schweiz. med. Wschr.*, 1978, *108*, 494.

Nephrotic syndrome with reversible renal failure in an elderly man given phenylbutazone.— M. Greenstone *et al.*, *Br. med. J.*, 1981, *282*, 950.

See also under Overdosage, below.

Effects on liver. Reports of toxic hepatitis attributed to phenylbutazone.— J. H. Fisher, *Can. med. Ass. J.*, 1960, *83*, 1211; J. M. Muscat-Baron and D. M. Freeman, *Br. J. clin. Pract.*, 1966, *20*, 437; D. J. Maberly and R. M. Greenhalgh, *Br. J. Derm.* 1970, *82*, 618; K. G. Ishak *et al.*, *Am. J. dig. Dis.*, 1977, *22*, 611; T. R. Mayer, *Minn. Med.*, 1979, *62*, 349.

See also under Overdosage, below.

Effects on the thyroid. Three cases of phenylbutazone-induced goitre occurred in 12 years in patients being treated for rheumatoid arthritis.— A. Vermeulen and J. B. van der Schoot, *Ned. Tijdschr. Geneesk.*, 1972, *116*, 369, per *J. Am. med. Ass.* 1972, *220*, 884.

Epidermal necrolysis. Phenylbutazone taken for 7 to 35 days before the eruption, might have been responsible for 6 cases, 2 fatal, of toxic epidermal necrolysis in Britain.— A. Lyell, *Br. J. Derm.*, 1967, *79*, 662.

Three cases of toxic epidermal necrolysis associated with phenylbutazone.— J. Kvasnička *et al.*, *Br. J. Derm.*, 1979, *100*, 551.

Lupus erythematosus. Phenylbutazone was implicated in the development of systemic lupus erythematosus in 2 patients.— M. A. Ogryzlo, *Can. med. Ass. J.*, 1956, *75*, 980.

Overdosage. Hepatic and renal damage in a previously healthy young girl occurring after overdosage with phenylbutazone was possibly associated with abnormal metabolism of the drug.— L. F. Prescott *et al.*, *Br. med. J.*, 1980, *281*, 1106. Another report of overdosage.— J. E. Strong (letter), *ibid.*, 1427.

Treatment of Adverse Effects. Following overdosage the stomach should be emptied by inducing emesis or by aspiration and lavage with sodium bicarbonate solution. Further treatment is symptomatic.

For the effect of activated charcoal on the absorption of phenylbutazone, see Activated Charcoal, p.79.

Precautions. Phenylbutazone is contra-indicated in patients with a history of dyspepsia or gastro-intestinal ulceration or with impaired hepatic or renal function or cardiovascular disease. It is also contra-indicated in patients with thyroid disease or a history of blood disorders or previous reactions.

Reduced doses should be used in elderly patients and courses of treatment should be kept as short as possible. Use with other drugs liable to produce bone-marrow depression should be avoided.

Phenylbutazone enhances the effects of tolbutamide and other sulphonylurea antidiabetic agents and coumarin anticoagulants and may enhance the effects of phenytoin and some sulphonamides.

Phenylbutazone or oxyphenbutazone should not be used unless the urine had been examined for protein and a blood examination had shown that the white-cell and platelet counts were within the normal range.— B. M. Ansell, *Prescribers' J.*, 1969, *8*, 120.

Administration of phenylbutazone 200 mg to healthy subjects caused impairment of psychomotor skills related to driving.— M. Linnoila *et al.*, *Br. J. clin. Pharmac.*, 1974, *1*, 477.

Interactions, drugs. Pretreatment with phenylbutazone increased the metabolism of amidopyrine in 7 subjects. It was suggested that phenylbutazone increased liver microsomal enzyme activity.— W. Chen *et al.*, *Life Sci.*, 1962, *2*, 35.

The plasma half-life of phenylbutazone was reduced from a mean of 78.1 hours to 57.2 hours by pretreatment with drugs which increased liver microsomal enzyme activity. Barbiturates, chlorpheniramine, promethazine, and prednisone induced microsomal activity. The half-life of phenylbutazone might be prolonged in patients with liver disease.— A. J. Levi *et al.*, *Lancet*, 1968, *1*, 1275. Exposure to dicophane lowered the serum half-life of phenylbutazone.— A. Poland *et al.*, *Clin. Pharmac. Ther.*, 1970, *11*, 724.

Allopurinol. Preliminary studies in 6 patients with acute gouty arthritis indicated that allopurinol given with phenylbutazone slightly prolonged the half-life of phenylbutazone, but the effect was not thought to be clinically significant.— D. Horwitz *et al.*, *Eur. J. clin. Pharmac.*, 1978, *12*, 133. See also M. D. Rawlins and S. E. Smith, *Br. J. Pharmac.*, 1973, *48*, 693.

Anticoagulants. For a short discussion of the effect of phenylbutazone on the effects of coumarin anticoagulants, see J. Koch-Weser and E. M. Sellers, *New Engl. J. Med.*, 1971, *285*, 547.

Anticonvulsants. For the effect of phenylbutazone on serum concentrations of phenytoin, see Phenytoin, p.1240.

Antidiabetic agents. For the effect of phenylbutazone in reducing chlorpropamide protein binding, see under Chlorpropamide, p.853.

Aspirin. The uricosuric effects of aspirin were diminished by phenylbutazone.— J. H. Oyer *et al.*, *Am. J. med. Sci.*, 1966, *251*, 1.

Benzylpenicillin. For the effect of phenylbutazone in increaseing benzylpenicillin half-life, see under Benzylpenicillin, p.1107.

Corticosteroids. Hydrocortisone infusion increased the urinary excretion of phenylbutazone metabolites in a study of 3 healthy subjects.— J. Aarbakke *et al.* (letter), *Br. J. clin. Pharmac.*, 1977, *4*, 621.

Digitoxin. For the effect of phenylbutazone in reducing the plasma concentration of digitoxin, see under Digitoxin, p.541.

Methylphenidate. Plasma concentrations of phenylbutazone were increased in 5 patients when methylphenidate 20 mg was given daily for 3 days; in 3 patients the concentration of oxyphenbutazone rose. In 2 of 4 patients given a single 400-mg dose of phenylbutazone the half-life was prolonged by methylphenidate.— P. G. Dayton *et al.*, *Pharmacologist*, 1969, *11*, 272.

Tricyclic antidepressants. The rate of absorption of phenylbutazone was reduced by tricyclic antidepressants.— S. Consolo *et al.*, *Eur. J. Pharmac.*, 1970, *10*, 239.

Interactions, tests. Phenylbutazone, by competing with thyroxine for binding sites on globulin, might give falsely low results in tests for serum protein-bound iodine.— A. J. J. Wood and J. Crooks, *Prescribers' J.*, 1973, *13*, 94.

For the effect of phenylbutazone on some estimations of blood-theophylline concentrations, see Aminophylline, p.343.

Porphyria. It was reported that phenylbutazone might precipitate acute porphyria in genetically susceptible persons.— T. M. French, *J. Hosp. Pharm.*, 1970, *28*, 19.

Absorption and Fate. Phenylbutazone is readily absorbed from the gastro-intestinal tract with peak plasma concentrations occurring about 2 hours after ingestion. Absorption is slow and incomplete following intramuscular administration with peak concentrations occurring after 6 to 10 hours. At therapeutic plasma concentrations phenylbutazone is 98% bound to plasma proteins; at higher concentrations the fraction bound decreases. It is extensively metabolised in the liver by oxidation and by conjugation with glucuronic acid. Oxyphenbutazone and γ-hydroxyphenbutazone are formed by oxidation but only small amounts appear in urine, the remainder being further metabolised. About 1% of a dose is excreted in the urine as unchanged phenylbutazone, and about 10% is excreted in bile, mainly as metabolites. The mean elimination half-life is about 70 hours but it is subject to large variations. Phenylbutazone may cross the placenta and appear in breast milk.

Reviews of the absorption, metabolism, excretion, and bioavailability of phenylbutazone.— A. R. DiSanto *et al.*, *J. Am. pharm. Ass.*, 1976, *NS16*, 365; J. Aarbakke, *Clin. Pharmacokinet.*, 1978, *3*, 369.

The half-life of phenylbutazone in *dogs* was reported to be dependent upon the dose.— P. G. Dayton *et al.*, *J. Pharmac. exp. Ther.*, 1963, *140*, 278. See also P. G. Dayton *et al.*, *ibid.*, 1967, *158*, 305.

In 14 sets of twins, the half-life of phenylbutazone varied from 1.2 to 7.3 days, and was usually between 2.6 and 4 days. Monozygotic twins exhibited very similar phenylbutazone half-lives; greater differences occurred in dizygotic twins. Varying values of the half-life of phenylbutazone appeared to be genetically determined.— E. S. Vesell and J. G. Page, *Science*, 1968, *159*, 1479.

A single dose of radioactive phenylbutazone 400 mg by mouth given to a healthy subject produced a peak plasma concentration of 36 μg per ml after 3 hours with an elimination half-life of 88 hours. Peak plasma-oxyphenbutazone concentration was 5.4 μg per ml after 72 hours and other metabolites were γ-hydroxyphenylbutazone and *p*,γ-dihydroxyphenylbutazone. Excretion was slow, only 88% (61% urinary and 27% faecal) being excreted after 21 days.— W. Dieterle *et al.*, *Arzneimittel-Forsch.*, 1976, *26*, 572.

After a single 600-mg dose of phenylbutazone the main metabolite found in plasma was oxyphenbutazone, but on repeated dosing higher concentrations of the side-chain oxidised metabolite were found, suggesting that side-chain oxidation becomes relatively more important than ring oxidation.— J. Aarbakke *et al.*, *Eur. J. clin. Pharmac.*, 1977, *11*, 359.

A mean peak plasma-phenylbutazone concentration of about 33 μg per ml occurred 3 hours after administration of a single dose of phenylbutazone 300 mg by mouth to 6 healthy subjects. The mean elimination half-life was 68.5 hours.— A. Siuofi *et al.*, *J. pharm. Sci.*, 1978, *67*, 243.

Further references: J. A. Whittaker and D. A. P. Evans, *Br. med. J.*, 1970, *4*, 323; K. K. Midha *et al.*, *J. pharm. Sci.*, 1974, *63*, 1751; *idem*, *67*, 279.

Absorption. In 4 healthy subjects the extent of the absorption of phenylbutazone from tablets was not affected by taking them with milk or with an antacid preparation (Maalox) but the antacid appeared to increase the rate of absorption of phenylbutazone.— J. C. K. Loo *et al.*, *Can. J. pharm. Sci.*, 1977, *12*, 10.

Protein binding. Phenylbutazone was displaced from human albumin by indomethacin, sulphamethoxypyridazine, and tolbutamide.— H. M. Solomon *et al.*, *Biochem. Pharmac.*, 1968, *17*, 143, per E. M. Sellers and J. Koch-Weser, *Ann. N.Y. Acad. Sci.*, 1971, *179*, 213.

About 90% of phenylbutazone was bound to human muscle tissue *in vitro*.— B. Fichtl and H. Kurz, *Eur. J. clin. Pharmac.*, 1978, *14*, 335.

Decreased protein-binding of phenylbutazone had been reported in patients with acute renal failure.— F. Andreasen, *Acta pharmac. tox.*, 1973, *32*, 417.

The binding of phenylbutazone to serum proteins was significantly reduced in patients with alcoholic cirrhosis or hepatitis.— M. J. Brodie and S. Boobis, *Eur. J. clin. Pharmac.*, 1978, *13*, 435.

Uses. Phenylbutazone is a pyrazole derivative which has analgesic, antipyretic, and anti-inflammatory actions, however, because of its toxicity it is not employed as a general analgesic or antipyretic. Although phenylbutazone is effective in almost all rheumatic disorders including ankylosing spondylitis, osteoarthrosis, rheumatoid arthritis, and Reiter's disease, it is generally reserved for use in the treatment of rheumatic disorders where less toxic drugs have failed.

Phenylbutazone has uricosuric actions and in acute gout may be given for several days until symptoms subside. It has also been given for the treatment of superficial thrombophlebitis.

In rheumatic disorders phenylbutazone is given initially in doses of 100 to 200 mg thrice daily with meals. If no improvement occurs within 1 week the drug should be discontinued. When improvement has been obtained the dosage should be reduced to the smallest dose that will provide relief of symptoms. Maintenance dosage should not exceed 400 mg daily and 100 to 200 mg daily may be adequate. Doses of 5 or sometimes 10 mg per kg body-weight daily have been suggested for use in children. Gastric disturbances may be reduced by the concurrent administration of a sodium-free antacid.

A dose of 400 mg initially, followed by 100 mg every 4 hours until articular inflammation subsides has been suggested for the treatment of acute gout.

Blood counts should be made weekly during initial therapy and repeated at frequent intervals if medication is continued over a prolonged period. Irrespective of the blood count, medication should be stopped at the first appearance of toxic symptoms.

Phenylbutazone is sometimes administered by deep intramuscular injection as the sodium salt. As the injection may be painful a local anaesthetic such as lignocaine hydrochloride is usually added to the injection solution.

Phenylbutazone may also be administered rectally, a suppository containing 250 mg being inserted once or twice daily.

Lymphocyte transformation was depressed by phenylbutazone.— G. R. Burgio and A. G. Ugazio (letter), *Lancet*, 1974, *1*, 568.

Symposium on phenylbutazone.— *J. int. med. Res.* 1977, *5*, *Suppl.* 2, 1–120.

Administration in the elderly. After an oral dose of phenylbutazone 6 mg per kg body-weight, the mean plasma half-life in 19 geriatric patients (aged 70 to 100 years, mean 77.6 years) was 104.6 hours compared with

81.2 hours in 18 younger controls (aged 20 to 50 years, mean 26 years).— K. O'Malley *et al.*, *Br. med. J.*, 1971, *3*, 607.

Administration in hepatic disease. After 4 days' treatment with phenylbutazone the ratio between the peak concentrations of phenylbutazone and oxyphenbutazone was similar in 6 patients with cirrhosis of the liver and in 5 controls.— E. F. Hvidberg *et al.*, *Clin. Pharmac. Ther.*, 1974, *15*, 171.

Administration in renal failure. Phenylbutazone could be given in usual doses to patients with a glomerular filtration-rate (GFR) of 10 ml or more per minute; its use should be avoided in those with a GFR of less than 10 ml per minute.— W. M. Bennett *et al.*, *Ann. intern. Med.*, 1980, *93*, 286.

Gout. In acute gout phenylbutazone 600 to 800 mg daily in divided doses was given for 2 to 3 days, followed if necessary by 300 mg daily for 2 to 3 days, 85% or more of acute attacks were relieved in 36 to 48 hours.— *Br. med. J.* 1974, *1*, 446.

Osteoarthrosis. A study on the use of phenylbutazone in osteoarthrosis.— M. S. Pathy, *J. int. med. Res.*, 1978, *6*, 365.

Rheumatoid arthritis. Studies on the use of phenylbutazone in rheumatoid arthritis.— H. Asai and R. Nakamura, *Acta. rheum. scand.*, 1970, *16*, 231; J. R. Golding, *Practitioner*, 1972, *208*, 57; K. -J. Hahn, *Arzneimittel-Forsch.*, 1973, *23*, 851; P. M. Brooks *et al.*, *Br. J. clin. Pharmac.*, 1975, *2*, 437; *J. int. med. Res.*, 1977, *5*, *Suppl.* 2, 40–81.

Thrombophlebitis. For reports on the use of phenylbutazone in thrombophlebitis.— L. R. Kimsey, *J. Am. med. Ass.*, 1960, *172*, 229; R. De Soldenhoff and A. H. M. Ross, *Practitioner*, 1960, *185*, 321.

Puerperal thrombosis. Puerperal venous thrombosis in 160 patients was treated with phenylbutazone 200 mg thrice daily for 3 days and then 100 mg thrice daily for 3 days. Pain was usually relieved within 12 hours and induration resolved within 48 hours. No side-effects were reported.— J. F. O'Sullivan, *Br. J. clin. Pract.*, 1968, *22*, 427.

Preparations

Phenylbutazone Suppositories *(B.P.)*. Phenylbutazone in a suitable suppository basis. Store at a temperature not exceeding 30°.

Phenylbutazone Tablets *(B.P.)*. Tablets containing phenylbutazone. The tablets are sugar-coated or film-coated.

Phenylbutazone Tablets *(U.S.P.)*. Tablets containing phenylbutazone. The *U.S.P.* requires 60% dissolution in 30 minutes. Store in airtight containers.

Proprietary Preparations

Butacote *(Geigy, UK)*. Phenylbutazone, available as enteric-coated tablets of 100 and 200 mg. (Also available as Butacote in *Switz.*).

Butazolidin *(Geigy, UK)*. Phenylbutazone, available as **Tablets** of 100 and 200 mg and as **Suppositories** each containing 250 mg.**Butazolidin Ampoules with Xylocaine.** An injection containing phenylbutazone sodium 200 mg and anhydrous lignocaine hydrochloride 10 mg per ml, in ampoules of 3 ml. (Also available as Butazolidin in *Austral.*, *Canad.*, *Denm.*, *Ger.*, *Neth.*, *Norw.*, *S.Afr.*, *Swed.*, *Switz.*, *USA*).

Butazolidin Alka *(Geigy, UK)*. Tablets each containing phenylbutazone 100 mg, dried aluminium hydroxide 100 mg, and magnesium trisilicate 150 mg. For rheumatic conditions. *Dose.* Initial, 4 to 6 tablets daily in divided doses, with meals; maintenance, 2 or 3 tablets daily.

Butazone *(DDSA Pharmaceuticals, UK)*. Phenylbutazone, available as tablets of 100 and 200 mg. (Also available as Butazone in *Austral.*, *S.Afr.*).

Parazolidin *(Geigy, UK)*. Scored tablets each containing phenylbutazone 50 mg and paracetamol 500 mg. For rheumatic conditions. *Dose.* 1 or 2 tablets twice or thrice daily.

Tibutazone *(Ticen, Eire)*. Phenylbutazone, available as tablets of 100 mg.

Other Proprietary Names

Arg.— Butazolidina; *Austral.*— Butacal, Butalan, Butarex, Butoroid, Butoz, Buzon; *Belg.*— Butazolidine, Glycyl; *Canad.*— Algoverine, Butagesic, Intrabutazone, Malgesic, Nadozone, Neo-Zoline, Phenbutazone; *Denm.*— Artrizin; *Fr.*— Butazolidine; *Ger.*— Praecirheumin, Rheumaphen, Spondyril; *Ital.*— Artropan, Butartril, Butazina, Butazolidina, Diossidone, Fenilbutina *(diethylaminoethyl derivative)*, Kadol, Reumilene *(aminopropyl derivative)*, Ticinil; *Norw.*— Artrizin; *Pol.*— Butapirazol; *S.Afr.*— Butrex, Panazone; *Spain*— Butadiona, Butalgina, Butazolidina, Butial *(benzidamine enolate derivative)*, Fenibutasan, Pirarreumol-P, Sintobutina *(aminopropyl derivative)*, Todalgil; *Switz.*— Butadion, Butaphen, Dibuzon, Elmedal, Mepha-Butazon, Ticinil Calcio *(calcium derivative)*; *USA*— Azolid.

Phenylbutazone was also formerly marketed in Great Britain under the proprietary names Ethibute (*Ethigel*), Flexazone (*Berk Pharmaceuticals*), Oppazone (*Oppenheimer*), and Tetnor (*R.P. Drugs*). A preparation containing phenylbutazone and prednisone was formerly marketed under the proprietary name Delta-Butazolidin (*Geigy*).

2687-p

Phenylbutazone Sodium.

$C_{19}H_{19}N_2NaO_2$=330.4.

CAS — 129-18-0.

Phenylbutazone sodium 1.07 g is approximately equivalent to 1 g of phenylbutazone. A 5.34% solution in water is iso-osmotic with serum. Aqueous solutions prepared by dissolving phenylbutazone in water with the addition of alkali hydroxide are slowly hydrolysed and oxidised by atmospheric oxygen.

Uses. Phenylbutazone sodium is used when it is required to give phenylbutazone by intramuscular injection. Lignocaine hydrochloride is usually added to minimise pain.

2688-s

Phenylbutazone Trimethylgallate.

Phenylbutazone Megallate. 4-Butyl-5-oxo-1,2-diphenyl-3-pyrazolin-3-yl 3,4,5-trimethoxybenzoate.

$C_{29}H_{30}N_2O_6$=502.6.

CAS — 16006-74-9.

Phenylbutazone trimethylgallate 1.63 g is approximately equivalent to 1 g of phenylbutazone.

Uses. Phenylbutazone trimethylgallate is a derivative of phenylbutazone (see p.273) and is used similarly in doses of 320 mg three or four times daily initially, reduced to 320 mg once or twice daily for maintenance.

Proprietary Names

Ditrone *(Hosbon, Spain)*; Mégazone *(Doms, Fr.)*.

2689-w

Phenylsemicarbazide.

Phenicarbazide. 1-Phenylsemicarbazide.

$C_7H_9N_3O$=151.2.

CAS — 103-03-7.

Pharmacopoeias. In *Arg.*, *Belg.*, and *Port.*

White or yellowish-white crystals; **soluble** 1 in 100 of water, 1 in 21 of alcohol, 1 in 90 of chloroform, and 1 in 60 of ether.

Uses. Phenylsemicarbazide is an analgesic which has been used in doses of 250 to 500 mg up to a max. of 1.5 g daily.

Proprietary Preparations

Antipyretic Dellipsoids D26 *(Pilsworth, UK)*. Tablets each containing phenylsemicarbazide 150 mg and sodium benzoate 150 mg.

2690-m

Phenyramidol Hydrochloride.

IN 511. 1-Phenyl-2-(2-pyridylamino)ethanol hydrochloride; α-(2-Pyridylaminomethyl)benzyl alcohol hydrochloride.

$C_{13}H_{14}N_2O,HCl$=250.7.

CAS — 553-69-5 (phenyramidol); 326-43-2 (hydrochloride).

Adverse Effects. Gastro-intestinal disturbances, drowsiness, skin rashes, and fall in blood pressure have been reported.

Precautions. Phenyramidol may enhance the effects of coumarin anticoagulants, hypoglycaemic agents, and phenytoin.

Uses. Phenyramidol hydrochloride has analgesic and muscle relaxant actions. It is used in doses of 400 to 800 mg up to 4 times daily. It has also been given by intragluteal injection.

A review.— N. B. Eddy *et al.*, *Bull. Wld Hlth Org.*, 1969, *40*, 1.

Other references: J. J. Schrogie and H. M. Solomon, *Clin. Pharmac. Ther.*, 1966, *7*, 723; P. E. Siegler *et al.*, *Curr. ther. Res.*, 1967, *9*, 6.

Proprietary Names

Anabloc *(IRBI, Ital.)*; Analexin *(Biotrading, Ital.)*; Aramidol *(ABC, Ital.)*; Cabral *(Kali-Chemie, Ger.)*; Firmalgil *(FIRMA, Ital.)*; Miodar *(ISM, Ital.)*; Vilexin *(Vitrum, Swed.)*.

2691-b

Pipebuzone.

4-Butyl-4-(4-methylpiperazin-1-ylmethyl)-1,2-diphenylpyrazolidine-3,5-dione.

$C_{25}H_{32}N_4O_2$=420.6.

CAS — 27315-91-9.

Uses. Pipebuzone is a piperazine derivative of phenylbutazone and has similar actions to phenylbutazone. It is used in the treatment of rheumatic disorders in doses of 450 to 900 mg daily. It has also been given rectally in doses of 300 to 600 mg daily.

Proprietary Names

Élarzone *(Dausse, Fr.)*.

2692-v

Piroxicam.

CP-16171. 4-Hydroxy-2-methyl-*N*-(2-pyridyl)-2*H*-1,2-benzothiazine-3-carboxamide 1,1-dioxide.

$C_{15}H_{13}N_3O_4S$=331.3.

CAS — 36322-90-4.

Crystals. M.p. 198° to 200°.

Adverse Effects. Gastro-intestinal disturbances are the commonest side-effects occurring with piroxicam. Peptic ulceration and gastro-intestinal bleeding have been reported as have decreased platelet aggregation and prolonged bleeding times. Oedema and changes in liver-function tests have also occurred.

Gastro-intestinal side-effects reported by patients taking piroxicam included epigastric distress, abdominal pain or discomfort, nausea, diarrhoea, flatulence, constipation, indigestion, and vomiting. Central nervous effects included dizziness, headache, drowsiness, and fatigue. Other side-effects reported were oedema and palpitations.— N. E. Pitts and R. R. Proctor, in *Piroxicam*, W.M. O'Brien and E.H. Wiseman (Ed.), London, The Royal Society of Medicine, 1978, p. 97.

Preliminary analysis of side-effects occurring in a study involving 45 patients with rheumatoid arthritis given piroxicam 20 to 40 mg daily showed that 36 reported mostly clinically insignificant side-effects. However in 15 piroxicam had to be discontinued because of new peptic ulcer (13), gastro-intestinal symptoms without ulcer (1), leucopenia (1), abnormal liver function tests (1).— M. Rahman *et al.*, *Clin. Pharmac. Ther.*, 1979, *25*, 243.

Precautions. Piroxicam should be used with caution in patients with a history of gastro-intestinal haemorrhage or ulcers or aspirin sensitivity.

Absorption and Fate. Piroxicam is absorbed from the gastro-intestinal tract. It is metabolised in the liver by hydroxylation and conjugation with glucuronic acid and excreted in the urine. Less than 5% of the dose is excreted unchanged. Piroxicam is extensively bound to plasma proteins (about 99%) and has a long plasma half-life of approximately 35 to 45 hours.

A review of the pharmacokinetics of piroxicam.— E. H. Wiseman, *Eur. J. Rheumatol. Inflamm.*, 1978, *1*, 338.

The pharmacokinetics of piroxicam were studied following single and multiple-doses by mouth. A plasma half-life of about 45 hours was observed. Enterohepatic recirculation of piroxicam was suggested by the presence of multiple peaks in plasma-concentration curves. Absorption and disposition of piroxicam were not affected by concomitant administration of aspirin and antacids.— D. C. Hobbs and T. M. Twomey, *J. clin. Pharmac.*, 1979,

19, 270.

Peak plasma concentrations of piroxicam were delayed following ingestion with food but the total absorption and plasma half-life were not affected.— T. Ishizaki *et al., J. Pharmacokinet. Biopharm.,* 1979, *7,* 369.

Uses. Piroxicam has analgesic, anti-inflammatory, and antipyretic properties and is used in the treatment of rheumatoid arthritis and other rheumatic disorders. It also has uricosuric actions and has been used in the treatment of acute gout.

In rheumatic disorders the usual dose of piroxicam is 20 mg daily in single or divided doses with a range of 10 to 30 mg daily. In acute gout a suggested dose is 40 mg daily for 5 to 7 days.

Symposia: *Piroxicam,* W.M. O'Brien and E.H. Wiseman (Ed.), London, The Royal Society of Medicine, 1978; Proceedings of the IXth European Congress of Rheumatology, New York, Academy Professional Information Services, 1980.

A review of piroxicam.— R. N. Brogden *et al., Drugs,* 1981, *22,* 165.

Analgesia. Piroxicam 20 and 40 mg as a single dose was as effective as aspirin 648 mg and superior to placebo in relieving episiotomy pain in a study in 120 postpartum women.— A. K. Jain *et al., Eur. J. Rheumatol. Inflamm.,* 1978, *1,* 356.

Ankylosing spondylitis. In an uncontrolled study in 57 patients with ankylosing spondylitis, piroxicam was given once daily in doses of 10 to 30 mg for up to 96 weeks. Side-effects occurred in 12 patients and treatment was discontinued temporarily in 2 and permanently in 2 patients because of adverse effects. All clinical features of the disease showed significant improvement. Laboratory tests showed a significant rise in mean blood-urea-nitrogen but treatment was not discontinued in any patient because of these changes.— H. Müller-Fassbender and M. Schattenkirchner, in *Piroxicam,* W.M. O'Brien and E.H. Wiseman (Ed.), London, The Royal Society of Medicine, 1978, p. 83.

Further studies.— I. Radi *et al., Eur. J. Rheumatol. Inflamm.,* 1978, *1,* 349; O. A. Sydnes, *Br. J. clin. Pract.,* 1981, *35,* 40.

Gout. Piroxicam 40 mg once daily for a mean of 5 days produced marked improvement in 8 and moderate improvement in 3 patients with acute gout.— P. Widmark, *Eur. J. Rheumatol. Inflamm.,* 1978, *1,* 346. A similar report.— G. Tausch and R. Eberl, *ibid.,* 365.

A report of the beneficial effect of piroxicam in acute gout. In a multi-centre study involving 29 patients, the majority of whom took single doses of piroxicam 40 mg and then 10 mg four times daily on 4 subsequent days, 12 patients experienced complete relief of painful symptoms. Side-effects were not severe; they included: nausea (4 patients), vomiting (1), epigastric discomfort (1), flatulence (1), diarrhoea (1), dysuria (1), and dry mouth (1).— J. E. Murphy, *J. int. med. Res.,* 1979, *7,* 507.

Osteoarthrosis. In a multicentre study in 1218 patients with osteoarthrosis, piroxicam in doses of 10 to 30 mg daily was generally effective in relieving joint pain and stiffness. Side-effects were reported in 157 patients and were mainly gastro-intestinal (81%). Other side-effects occurring were skin rash, oedema, headache, and insomnia. Treatment was discontinued in 60 patients because of side-effects.— P. Dessain *et al., J. int. med. Res.,* 1979, *7,* 335.

Further reports on the use of piroxicam in osteoarthrosis.— H. Telhag, *Eur. J. Rheumatol. Inflamm.,* 1978, *1,* 352; T. M. Zizic *et al.,* in *Piroxicam,* W.M. O'Brien and E.H. Wiseman (Ed.), London, The Royal Society of Medicine, 1978, p. 71; J. L. Abruzzo *et al., Clin. Pharmac. Ther.,* 1979, *25,* 211; C. H. Hybbinette, *Br. J. clin. Pract.,* 1981, *35,* 30; O. Kogstad, *ibid.,* 45.

Platelet aggregation. In a study in 15 healthy adults, piroxicam decreased platelet aggregation 24 hours after doses of 20 and 40 mg. The effects lasted for up to 2 weeks.— M. Weintraub *et al., Clin. Pharmac. Ther.,* 1978, *23,* 134.

Rheumatoid arthritis. In a study in 41 patients with rheumatoid arthritis there was a significant reduction in joint pain, tenderness, swelling, and limitation of movement following treatment with piroxicam 10 to 40 mg as a single daily dose for up to 2 years. Adverse effects occurred on 30 occasions and 10 patients discontinued treatment because of side-effects.— G. Tausch *et al.,* in *Piroxicam,* W.M. O'Brien and E.H. Wiseman (Ed.), London, The Royal Society of Medicine, 1978, p. 59.

Further studies of piroxicam in rheumatoid arthritis.— J. R. Ward *et al.,* in *Piroxicam,* W.M. O'Brien and E.H. Wiseman (Ed.), London, The Royal Society of Medicine, 1978, p. 31; J. Box *et al., ibid.,* p. 41; J. C. Steigerwald, *ibid.,* p. 47; M. Weintraub *et al., ibid.,* p. 53; P. Mäkisara and P. Nuotio, *ibid.,* p. 65; J. C. Steigerwald, *Eur. J. Rheumatol. Inflamm.,* 1978, *1,* 360; Z. Balogh *et al., Curr. med. Res. Opinion,* 1979, *6,* 148; E. J. Pisko *et al., Curr. ther. Res.,* 1980, *27,* 852; R. Finstad, *Br. J. clin. Pract.,* 1981, *35,* 35.

Proprietary Preparations

Feldene *(Pfizer, UK).* Piroxicam, available as capsules of 10 mg.

2693-g

Pirprofen. Su 21524. 2-[3-Chloro-4-(3-pyrrolin-1-yl)phenyl]propionic acid.

$C_{13}H_{14}ClNO_2$=251.7.

CAS — 31793-07-4.

Adverse Effects. Gastro-intestinal disturbances including gastro-intestinal bleeding, visual and hearing disturbances, and headache have been reported.

Absorption and Fate.

Following administration of pirprofen 100 and 200 mg to 10 subjects on 2 separate occasions pirprofen was rapidly and almost completely absorbed, peak concentrations of 8.9 to 15 μg per ml (average 12 μg per ml) and 14 to 38 μg per ml (average 23 μg per ml) respectively being obtained after an average of about 1 or 2 hours; the apparent elimination half-lives were 5.6 to 10 hours (average 6.8 hours) and 5.9 to 8.2 hours (average 6.5 hours) respectively. In 7 subjects who received pirprofen 1 hour after a substantial meal as well as in the fasting state, peak plasma concentrations were achieved after an average of about 3 hours, the delay not being statistically significant, and the apparent elimination half-lives were 4.7 to 7.7 hours (average 6.3 hours) and 5.9 to 7.8 hours (average 6.9 hours) respectively. In 8 subjects who received 600 mg daily, as 200 mg thrice daily or 150 mg four times daily, average blood concentrations of 11 and 10 μg per ml respectively were found on the morning of the sixth day, 12 hours after the last dose. Absorption and excretion studies following administration of a radioactively labelled dose of 200 mg to 6 subjects indicated that at peak concentrations nearly all the drug in plasma was unchanged; about 80% was excreted in the urine within 24 hours with less than 5% as pirprofen, the major metabolite being the acyl glucuronide; about 8% of the dose was excreted in the faeces.— R. C. Luders *et al., Clin. Pharmac. Ther.,* 1977, *21,* 721.

Further references: M. F. Bartlett *et al., J. clin. Pharmac.,* 1974, *14,* 395; M. B. Maggio-Cavaliere *et al., ibid., 15,* 563.

Uses. Pirprofen is a phenylpropionic acid derivative with anti-inflammatory properties. It is used in the treatment of rheumatic disorders in doses of up to 800 mg daily in divided doses.

Ankylosing spondylitis. Pirprofen, up to 750 mg daily, was as effective as indomethacin, up to 125 mg daily, in a study in 22 patients with ankylosing spondylitis.— A. Calin *et al., Curr. ther. Res.,* 1978, *24,* 838.

Dysmenorrhoea. Pirprofen 200 mg up to thrice daily was effective in relieving mild to moderate pain of dysmenorrhoea in a study of 26 patients.— C. W. Elsner *et al., Clin. Pharmac. Ther.,* 1980, *27,* 25.

Rheumatoid arthritis. Results of a 6-month double-blind study in patients with rheumatoid arthritis indicated that pirprofen 600 mg daily is equivalent to aspirin 3.6 g daily. There was no significant difference in side-effects between the 2 drug regimens. Three of 17 patients in the pirprofen group and 5 of 18 in the aspirin group had positive stool occult blood tests.— R. J. Saykaly *et al., J. clin. Pharmac.,* 1979, *19,* 56.

Further studies on the use of pirprofen in the treatment of rheumatoid arthritis.— J. D. Proctor *et al., Clin. Pharmac. Ther.,* 1974, *16,* 69; J. M. Levin, *Clin. Ther.,* 1978, *1,* 294, per *Int. pharm. Abstr.,* 1978, *15,* 925; H. J. Rowe, *Clin. Ther.,* 1978, *2,* 69; J. D. Davis *et al., Clin. Pharmac. Ther.,* 1979, *25,* 618; R. T. Reid, *J. clin. Pharmac.,* 1980, *20,* 145.

Manufacturers

Ciba-Geigy, UK.

2694-q

Pixifenide. 1-{[4-(1-Hydroxyiminoethyl)phenoxy]-acetyl}piperidine.

$C_{15}H_{20}N_2O_3$=276.3.

CAS — 31224-92-7.

An odourless white powder. M.p. about 170°. Practically **insoluble** in water; slightly soluble in alcohol, chloroform, acetone, and methyl alcohol.

Uses. Pixifenide is an anti-inflammatory agent with analgesic and antipyretic actions. It has been used in the treatment of rheumatic and similar disorders.

2695-p

Propiram Fumarate. FBA 4503; Bay 4503. *N*-(1-Methyl-2-piperidinoethyl)-*N*-(2-pyridyl)propionamide hydrogen fumarate.

$C_{16}H_{25}N_3O,C_4H_4O_4$=391.5.

CAS — 15686-91-6 (propiram); 13717-04-9 (fumarate).

Uses. Propiram fumarate is an analgesic used in doses equivalent to 75 to 150 mg of propiram daily in divided doses. It is also used as suppositories containing the equivalent of 50 mg of propiram.

Studies on the abuse potential of propiram.— D. R. Jasinski *et al., Clin. Pharmac. Ther.,* 1971, *12,* 613.

In studies on the analgesic effects of propiram fumarate in 356 patients undergoing surgery, 90 to 100 mg of propiram was shown to be equal in potency to 10 mg of morphine. Adverse effects were similar with both drugs.— W. H. Forrest *et al., J. clin. Pharmac.,* 1972, *12,* 440.

In an open study in 3000 patients propiram fumarate, 75 to 150 mg daily in divided doses by mouth or 50 to 100 mg daily as suppositories, was considered a highly effective analgesic.— R. Hullmann *et al., Arzneimittel-Forsch.,* 1974, *24,* 718.

For a series of papers covering the properties of propiram fumarate, see *Arzneimittel-Forsch.,* 1974, *24,* 583-722.

Proprietary Names

Algeril *(Bayropharm, Ital.).*

2696-s

Propyphenazone. Isopropylantipyrinum; Isopropylantipyrine. 4-Isopropyl-1,5-dimethyl-2-phenyl-4-pyrazolin-3-one.

$C_{14}H_{18}N_2O$=230.3.

CAS — 479-92-5.

White crystals or white crystalline powder; odourless with a slightly bitter taste. M.p. 101° to 103°. **soluble** 1 in 400 of water; freely soluble in alcohol and chloroform; soluble in ether.

Uses. Propyphenazone is a derivative of phenazone which has been used as an analgesic in doses of 300 to 500 mg. It has also been used, at a concentration of 3% in rubefacient creams.

Proprietary Names

Baukal (see also under Amidopyrine) *(Bruschettini, Ital.).*

A preparation containing propyphenazone was formerly marketed in Great Britain under the proprietary name Saridone (*Roche*).

2697-w

Protizinic Acid. 2-(7-Methoxy-10-methylphenothiazin-2-yl)propionic acid.

$C_{17}H_{17}NO_3S$=315.4.

CAS — 54323-85-2.

Adverse Effects. Gastro-intestinal disturbances, dysuria, and skin rashes have been reported.

Following ingestion of protizinic acid about 8 g and aspirin about 6 g a 17-year-old girl developed fatal malignant hyperthermia. She had no history of myopathy and examination of her parents and siblings revealed no abnormalities. The following 3 causes were considered possible: the overdosage might have triggered a genetic predisposition, the protizinic acid had enhanced aspirin-induced hyperthermia, the effect was due to the neuroleptic effect of massive protizinic acid overdose.— G. Ginies *et al.*, *Thérapie*, 1976, *31*, 755.

Uses. Protizinic acid has analgesic and anti-inflammatory actions. It has been used in the treatment of rheumatic disorders in doses of 400 mg thrice daily.

Proprietary Names
Pirocrid *(Théraplix, Fr.)*.

2698-e

Pyrazinobutazone.

$C_{23}H_{30}N_4O_2$=394.5.

CAS — 4985-25-5.

An equimolecular salt of phenylbutazone and piperazine. M.p. about 140° and, after resolidification, about 180°. Slightly **soluble** in water; soluble in alcohol.

Uses. Pyrazinobutazone has the actions and uses of phenylbutazone (see p.273). It is used in doses of 600 to 900 mg daily in divided doses or 425 mg as a suppository morning and night.

Pharmacokinetics of pyrazinobutazone.— V. v. Bruchhausen *et al.*, *Arzneimittel-Forsch.*, 1978, *28*, 2337.

Proprietary Names
Carudol *(Boehringer Sohn, Arg.; Du Bled, Belg.; Laboratoires Français de Thérapeutique, Fr.; Boehringer Ingelheim, Ital.; Fher, Spain; Wild, Switz.)*; Clavezona *(Finadiet, Arg.)*; Dartranol *(Ester, Spain)*; Ranoroc *(Dieckmann, Ger.)*; Unifalgan *(Unifa, Arg.)*.

2699-l

Salicin *(B.P.C. 1954)*. Salicoside. 2-(Hydroxymethyl)phenyl-β-D-glucopyranoside.

$C_{13}H_{18}O_7$=286.3.

CAS — 138-52-3.

A crystalline β-glucoside obtained from the bark of young shoots of various species of *Salix* and *Populus* especially *S. fragilis* (Salicaceae).

Odourless, colourless crystals or white crystalline powder with a bitter taste. M.p. 199° to 201°. **Soluble** 1 in 30 of water, 1 in 3 of boiling water, and 1 in 80 of alcohol; practically insoluble in chloroform and ether. Solutions in water are neutral to litmus.

Salicin has antipyretic and analgesic actions and has been used similarly to aspirin in doses of 0.3 to 1 g. It often produces skin rashes.

2700-l

Salicylamide. 2-Hydroxybenzamide.

$C_7H_7NO_2$=137.1.

CAS — 65-45-2.

Pharmacopoeias. In *Belg., Hung., Pol., Roum.*, and *Rus.*

A white, almost odourless, crystalline powder. M.p. 139° to 142°. **Soluble** 1 in 500 of water, 1 in 15 of alcohol, 1 in 100 of chloroform, 1 in 35 of ether, and 1 in 20 of propylene glycol; soluble in solutions of alkalis. A saturated solution in water has a pH of 5.2 to 6.0. **Protect** from light.

Adverse Effects and Treatment. As for Aspirin, p.236 and p.238.

Overdosage with salicylamide results in hypotension, depression of the central nervous system, and respiratory arrest.

Gross urticaria in 2 infants followed the use of a teething jelly containing salicylamide 8%.— B. Bentley-Philips (letter), *Br. J. Derm.*, 1968, *80*, 341.

Precautions. As for Aspirin, p.238.

The potential sedative effect had to be considered if salicylamide was given with other sedatives. Salicylamide inhibited the acetylation of sulphonamides, increasing the blood concentration of free sulphonamide. Salicylamide could be given to those allergic to salicylates.— W. H. Barr and R. P. Penna, *Can. pharm. J.*, 1968, *101*, 442.

Simultaneous administration of salicylamide and sodium salicylate in usual doses related in decreased glucuronide formation for both drugs. This could lead to enhanced activity.— G. Levy and J. A. Procknal, *J. pharm. Sci.*, 1968, *57*, 1330.

Absorption and Fate. Salicylamide is readily absorbed from the gastro-intestinal tract and distributed to all body tissues. It is rapidly excreted in the urine, mainly as the glucuronide and sulphate conjugates.

The proportion of a dose of salicylamide excreted as sulphate decreased with increased doses.— G. Levy and T. Matsuzawa, *J. Pharmac. exp. Ther.*, 1967, *156*, 285.

When the dose of salicylamide was increased from 1 g to 2 g the plasma concentration was more than proportionately increased.— W. H. Barr, *Drug Inform. Bull.*, 1969, *3*, 27.

In 9 patients with acute intermittent porphyria and 18 healthy subjects the average half-life of salicylamide was 103 minutes and 72 minutes respectively. This was mainly due to a reduced rate of sulphation and hydroxylation; glucuronidation was not significantly reduced.— C. S. Song *et al.*, *Clin. Pharmac. Ther.*, 1974, *15*, 431.

In a crossover study completed by 5 healthy subjects little or no free salicylamide was found in plasma after usual recommended doses (650 mg). Increased doses gave increased concentrations but peak plasma concentrations were delayed. Higher and earlier peak concentrations were obtained with a solution of sodium salicylamide.— L. Fleckenstein *et al.*, *Clin. Pharmac. Ther.*, 1976, *19*, 451.

The percentage of a dose of salicylamide excreted as sulphate was significantly higher in children than in adults. The glucuronide was the major excretory product in adults.— S. N. Alam *et al.*, *J. Pediat.*, 1977, *90*, 130, per *Int. pharm. Abstr.*, 1977, *14*, 902.

Uses. Salicylamide has some analgesic, anti-inflammatory, and antipyretic properties. Doses of 1.5 to 10 g daily have been given but salicylamide is now little used.

A study of 150 infants and children with pyrexia indicated that aspirin and paracetamol had comparable antipyretic activity but salicylamide was less effective.— A. N. Eden and A. Kaufman, *Am. J. Dis. Child.*, 1967, *114*, 284, per *J. Am. med. Ass.*, 1967, *201* (Sept. 25), A224.

Proprietary Preparations

Delimon Tablets *(Consolidated Chemicals, UK)*. Each contains salicylamide 200 mg, paracetamol 50 mg, and morazone hydrochloride 150 mg. For pain. *Dose.* ½ to 1 tablet several times daily if necessary.

Other Proprietary Names
Amid-Sal *(USA)*; Salamide *(Austral.)*; Salizell *(Ger.)*; Sinedol, Urtosal *(both Ital.)*.

Salicylamide was also formerly marketed in Great Britain under the proprietary name Salimed, and a preparation containing salicylamide was marketed under the name Salimed Compound (both *Medo-Chemicals*).

2701-y

Salicylic Acid *(B.P., Eur. P., U.S.P.)*.

Acidum Salicylicum; Salizylsäure; Acido Ortóxibenzoico. 2-Hydroxybenzoic acid.

$C_7H_6O_3$=138.1.

CAS — 69-72-7.

Pharmacopoeias. In all pharmacopoeias examined.

Colourless feathery crystals or a white crystalline powder with a sweetish acrid taste. It is almost odourless but its dust irritates the nostrils. M.p. 158° to 161°.

Soluble 1 in about 550 of water, 1 in 15 of boiling water, 1 in 3 to 4 of alcohol, 1 in 3 of ether, 1 in 80 of olive or almond oil, 1 in 10 of castor oil, and 1 in 45 of chloroform; soluble also (about 1 in 80) in melted fats and soft paraffin. Borax, ammonium citrate, ammonium acetate, sodium citrate, potassium citrate, and sodium phosphate increase its solubility in water. A solution in water is acid to methyl red. **Incompatible** with iodine, iron salts, and oxidising substances.

Salicylic acid exerted no visible effect on the skin when applied in a zinc oxide paste because it combined with zinc oxide to form zinc salicylate. Salicylic acid exerted its full effects in pastes of titanium dioxide.— H. R. de Vries, *Br. J. Derm.*, 1961, *73*, 371.

Salicylic acid produced a marked increase in viscosity in solutions of surface-active quaternary ammonium compounds; this was probably related to an increase in the size of micelles.— L. S. C. Wan, *J. pharm. Sci.*, 1968, *57*, 1903.

A study of the release and uptake of salicylic acid *in vitro* from ointment bases. Salicylic acid was released most readily from emulsion bases, particularly of the oil-in-water type, and least readily from macrogol ointment.— M. Nakano and N. K. Patel, *J. pharm. Sci.*, 1970, *59*, 985.

Mechanical incorporation of salicylic acid in a cold paraffin basis using a spatula appeared to result in higher rates of salicylic acid diffusion than those encountered with ointments prepared by fusion. This was not affected by drug concentration, surfactants, or the use of a water-in-oil emulsion basis.— C. W. Whitworth and A. F. Asker, *J. pharm. Sci.*, 1974, *63*, 1618.

Adverse Effects. As for Aspirin, p.236.

Salicylic acid is a mild irritant and application of salicylic acid preparations to the skin may cause dermatitis. Symptoms of acute systemic salicylate poisoning have been reported after the application of salicylic acid ointments and solutions to large areas of the body.

Symptoms of salicylism developed in 3 adults, with extensive psoriasis, between the second and fourth day of application 6 times daily of salicylic acid ointment (3 or 6%). The symptoms largely disappeared within 1 day after discontinuing the application of the ointment. Serum concentrations of salicylic acid ranged from 460 to 640 µg per ml. There were 13 deaths from salicylic acid poisoning following application of salicylic acid ointments reported in the literature. Ten of the 13 fatalities occurred in children.— J. F. von Weiss and W. F. Lever, *Archs Derm.*, 1964, *90*, 614.

Two patients died after more than 50% of their body areas had been painted twice with an alcoholic solution of salicylic acid 20.7% for tinea infection. The deaths were preceded by symptoms typical of salicylate poisoning.— C. P. Lindsey, *Med. J. Aust.*, 1968, *1*, 353.

Further reports of salicylate toxicity following topical application of preparations containing salicylic acid.— E. P. Cawley *et al.*, *J. Am. med. Ass.*, 1953, *151*, 372; L. V. Perlman (letter), *New Engl. J. Med.*, 1966, *274*, 164; J. B. Aspinall and K. M. Goel (letter), *Br. med. J.*, 1978, *2*, 1373; M. G. Davies *et al.*, *Br. med. J.*, 1979, *1*, 661; P. A. Soyka and L. F. Soyka (letter), *J. Am. med. Ass.*, 1980, *244*, 660.

Allergy. Of 791 persons with dermatitis or eczema submitted to patch testing with salicylic acid 5% in hydrous wool fat, 2.5% gave a positive reaction. Of 791 persons tested with salicylic acid 5% in wool alcohols ointment, 5.9% gave a positive reaction.— E. Rudzki and D. Kleniewska, *Br. J. Derm.*, 1970, *83*, 543.

Contact sensitivity to salicylic acid was demonstrated in 5 patients who suffered from dermatitis or psoriasis. Four of the patients had previously used salicylic acid lotion. None of the patients was sensitive to aspirin taken by mouth.— E. Rudzki and A. Koslowska, *Contact Dermatitis*, 1976, *2*, 178.

Precautions. Salicylic acid should be used with care on large areas of skin.

Interactions, tests. For a report of salicylic acid interfering with assays for theophylline, see Aminophylline, p.343.

Uses. Salicylic acid has bacteriostatic and fungicidal actions. It is applied externally, usually as a 1 to 5% dusting-powder, lotion, or ointment, for the treatment of chronic ulcers, dandruff, eczema, psoriasis, hyperhydrosis, and parasitic skin diseases. It is also used in conjunction with many other agents, such as benzoic acid, coal tar, resorcinol, and sulphur.

Salicylic acid also has keratolytic properties. Externally it produces slow and painless destruction of the epithelium and it is applied in the form of a paint in a collodion basis (10 to 17%) or as a plaster (20 to 50%) to destroy warts or corns.

A brief review of the properties and uses of salicylic acid.— D. Burrows *et al.*, *Br. J. Derm.*, 1968, *80*, 550.

Onychomycosis. The successful treatment of onychomycosis by boring holes in the affected nail plates, enlarging these with acid, then applying an ointment of precipitated sulphur 3% with salicylic acid 3% in soft paraffin.— J. Brem (letter), *Lancet*, 1977, *2*, 937.

Skin disorders. A double-blind study in 78 patients with psoriasis of the scalp indicated that a lotion containing betamethasone dipropionate with salicylic acid 2% was more effective and produced a more rapid onset of improvement and healing than a lotion containing betamethasone valerate alone.— L. Hillström and L. Pettersson, *Curr. ther. Res.*, 1978, *24*, 46. Betamethasone dipropionate with salicylic acid and flumethasone pivalate with salicylic acid in steroid responsive dermatoses demanding keratolytic penetration.— R. Mattila, *J. int. med. Res.*, 1980, *8*, 247.

Acne. An opinion that salicylic acid, especially in a polar solvent, is an effective comedolytic agent.— H. P. Baden (letter), *New Engl. J. Med.*, 1980, *302*, 1419. There appear to be no controlled studies on the use of salicylic acid in acne.— J. W. Melski and K. A. Arndt (letter), *ibid.*

Warts. In the course of studies assessing the value of treatments for viral warts in a total of 1807 patients, a study of 389 patients in 2 centres showed that against hand warts a mixture of salicylic acid 1 part and lactic acid 1 part in flexible collodion 4 parts (SAL paint) was as effective as liquid nitrogen or as a combination of both treatments, the percentage cures being 67, 69, and 78 respectively. No recurrences of hard warts were reported 6 months after treatment with SAL paints in 46 of 50 patients in a general practice. Other studies indicated that SAL paint cured 45% of patients with mosaic plantar warts and it was no less effective than preparations containing fluorouracil 5%, idoxuridine 5%, a 10% buffered solution of glutaraldehyde, or a paint prepared to contain 40% of an adduct of benzalkonium chloride and bromine (Callusolve 40).— M. H. Bunney *et al.*, *Br. J. Derm.*, 1976, *94*, 667.

Preparations

Collodions

Salicylic Acid Collodion *(B.P.)*. Collod. Acid. Salicyl.; Salicylic Collodion. Salicylic acid 12 g, flexible collodion to 100 ml. Store at a temperature not exceeding 25° in airtight containers.

A.P.F. (Salicylic Acid Paint, Corn Paint), and *F.N. Belg.* have 10% in flexible collodion.

Salicylic Acid Collodion *(U.S.P.)*. Salicylic acid 10 g, flexible collodion *U.S.P.* to 100 ml. Store at 15° to 30° in airtight containers.

Creams

Salicylic Acid and Resorcinol Cream Aqueous *(A.P.F.)*. Salicylic acid 2 g, resorcinol 2 g, aqueous cream to 100 g. Protect from light and avoid contact with metals.

Salicylic Acid and Sulphur Cream Aqueous *(A.P.F.)*. Crem. Acid. Salicyl. et Sulphur. Salicylic acid 2 g, precipitated sulphur 2 g, spike lavender oil 0.5 ml, aqueous cream to 100 g. Avoid contact with metals.

Salicylic Acid and Sulphur Cream *(B.P.)*. Crem. Acid. Salicyl. et Sulph.; Salicylic Acid and Sulphur Application. Salicylic acid 2 g, precipitated sulphur 2 g, aqueous cream to 100 g. Store at a temperature not exceeding 25° in well-closed containers which minimise evaporation and contamination.

Dusting-powders

Conspergens Amyceni *(Dan. Disp.)*. Salicylic acid 5 g, ethyl hydroxybenzoate 5 g, and purified talc 90 g.

Conspergens Salicylicum *(Dan. Disp.)*. Salicylic acid 3 g, potato starch 5 g, wheat starch 5 g, and purified talc 87 g.

Ear-drops

Salicylic Acid Ear Drops *(A.P.F.)*. Aurist. Acid. Salicyl. Salicylic acid 2 g, alcohol 90% 50 ml, freshly boiled and cooled water to 100 ml.

Gels

Salicylic Acid Gel *(U.S.P.)*. Contains salicylic acid in a suitable viscous hydrophilic vehicle; it may contain alcohol. pH of an approximately 10% solution 5 to 8.5. Store at 15° to 30° in airtight containers.

Lotions

Salicylic Acid and Coal Tar Lotion *(A.P.F.)*. Salicylic acid 2 g, coal tar solution 5 ml, castor oil 1 ml, spike lavender oil 0.1 ml, alcohol 90% to 100 ml.

Salicylic Acid and Mercuric Chloride Lotion *(B.P.C. 1973)*. Lotio Acidi Salicylici et Hydrargyri Perchloridi. Salicylic acid 2 g, mercuric chloride 100 mg, castor oil 1 ml, acetone 12.5 ml, alcohol (or industrial methylated spirit) to 100 ml. Store in a cool place in airtight containers. Flammable: keep away from an open flame.

Salicylic Acid and Mercuric Chloride Lotion *(A.P.F.)*. Lot. Acid. Salicyl. Co. Salicylic acid 2 g, mercuric chloride 100 mg, castor oil 1 ml, spike lavender oil 0.1 ml, alcohol 90% to 100 ml.

Salicylic Acid Lotion *(B.P.)*. Lot. Acid. Salicyl. Salicylic acid 2 g, castor oil 1 ml, alcohol (or industrial methylated spirit) to 100 ml. Store in airtight containers. Flammable: keep away from an open flame.

Ointments

Salicylic Acid and Sulphur Emulsifying Ointment *(St. John's Hosp.)*. Salicylic acid 2, precipitated sulphur 2, emulsifying ointment to 100.

Salicylic Acid and Sulphur Ointment *(B.P.C. 1973)*. Ung. Acid. Salicyl. et Sulph. Salicylic acid 3% and precipitated sulphur 3% in oily cream. Store in containers which prevent evaporation.

Salicylic Acid Ointment *(B.P., A.P.F.)*. Salicyl. Acid Oint.; Ung. Acid. Salicyl. Salicylic acid 2% in wool alcohols ointment. Store at a temperature not exceeding 25°.

Plasters

Salicylic Acid Adhesive Plaster *(B.P.)*. Salicylic Acid Self-adhesive Plaster; Salicylic Acid Plaster. Cotton or viscose or cotton and viscose fabric of plain weave, spread evenly with not less than 100 g per m^2 of a self-adhesive plaster mass, which may be made porous or permeable to air, containing 20% or 40% of salicylic acid. The plaster may be perforated and the adhesive surface is covered by a suitable protector; the plaster may be dyed green.

The *B.P.* directs that when no strength is specified, plaster containing 20% of salicylic acid shall be supplied.

Hung. P. and *U.S.P.* include a similar plaster.

Proprietary Preparations

Acnaveen *(Cooper, UK)*. A cleansing bar containing salicylic acid 2% and sulphur 2% in a soapless basis. For acne.

Aspellin *(Rorer, UK)*. A liniment containing methyl and ethyl salicylates equivalent to salicylic acid 0.54%, ammonium salicylate 1%, menthol 1.4%, and camphor 0.6%, in industrial methylated spirit. For rheumatic and similar conditions, and unbroken chilblains.

Duofilm *(Stiefel, UK)*. Liquid containing salicylic acid 16.7% and lactic acid 16.7%, in a collodion basis. For plantar and mosaic warts.

Monphytol *(Laboratories for Applied Biology, UK)*. A paint stated to contain salicylic acid (free and methyl ester) 31%, boric acid 2%, chlorbutol 3%, methyl undecenoate ($C_{12}H_{22}O_2$ = 198.3) 5%, and propyl undecenoate ($C_{14}H_{26}O_2$ = 226.4) 1%. For chronic paronychia and dermatophytoses.

Phytodermine *(May & Baker, UK)*. Powder containing salicylic acid 5% and methyl hydroxybenzoate 5% in a talc basis. For fungous infections of the skin.

Pragmatar *(Smith Kline & French, UK)*. An ointment containing salicylic acid 3%, cetyl alcohol-coal tar distillate 4%, and sulphur 3%, in an oil-in-water basis. For dandruff and common scaly skin disorders.

Salactol *(Dermal Laboratories, UK)*. A paint containing salicylic acid 16.7% w/w and lactic acid 16.7% w/w in flexible collodion. For warts.

Other Proprietary Names

Cornina *(in plaster basis) (Ger.)*; Egocappol *(Austral.)*; Fomac *(USA)*; Guttaplast *(in plaster basis) (Ger.)*; Keralyt *(Canad., USA)*; Salicyl *(Denm.)*; Saligel *(Canad., USA)*; Xseb *(USA)*.

Proprietary Names of Some Other Salicylic Acid Derivatives

Deposal, Tardisal *(Ital.)*; Retarcyl *(Fr.)*; *(all morpholine derivatives)*; Algospray *(Fr.)*; *(picolamine derivative)*; Aspercreme, Mobisyl *(USA)*; Myoflex, Royflex *(Canad.)* *(all triethanolamine derivatives)*.

A preparation containing salicylic acid was also formerly marketed in Great Britain under the proprietary name Sebaveen Shampoo (*Knox Laboratories*).

2702-j

Salsalate. Salicylosalicylic Acid; Sasapyrine; Salicyl Salicylate; Salysal. *O*-(2-Hydroxybenzoyl)salicylic acid.

$C_{14}H_{10}O_5$=258.2.

CAS — 552-94-3.

Odourless colourless crystals or white crystalline powder. Practically **insoluble** in water but gradually hydrolysed by it into 2 molecules of salicylic acid; soluble in alcohol and ether; insoluble in dilute acids.

Adverse Effects, Treatment, and Precautions. As for Aspirin, p.236, p.238.

In a placebo-controlled study involving 20 healthy subjects over 3 weeks, aspirin 1.3 g thrice daily produced significant faecal blood loss when compared with salsalate 1 g thrice daily and with placebo. Salsalate did not produce significant blood loss.— A. Cohen, *J. clin. Pharmac.*, 1979, *19*, 242.

Absorption and Fate. Salsalate is absorbed mainly from the small intestine. Following absorption it is slowly hydrolysed to 2 molecules of free salicylic acid.

Comparative studies on the absorption of salsalate and aspirin.— I. Santillan, *Curr. ther. Res.*, 1978, *23*, 345; I. W. French and C. A. Mildon, *Clin. Ther.*, 1978, *1*, 353, per *Int. pharm. Abstr.*, 1978, *15*, 989.

Comparative study on the absorption and elimination of salsalate and choline magnesium trisalicylate.— A. Cohen, *Curr. ther. Res.*, 1978, *23*, 772.

Uses. Salsalate has analgesic, antipyretic, and anti-inflammatory actions similar to those of aspirin (see p.240). It is used in the treatment of rheumatoid arthritis and other rheumatic disorders in doses up to 1 g three or four times daily with food.

A brief review of non-aspirin salicylate drugs concluded that there was insufficient data to judge whether they were as effective as aspirin, or better tolerated, in the treatment of inflammatory disorders.— *Med. Lett.*, 1978, *20*, 100.

Administration in renal failure. Salsalate could be given in usual doses to patients with renal impairment.— W. M. Bennett *et al.*, *Ann. intern. Med.*, 1980, *93*, 286.

Rheumatic disorders. In a double-blind crossover study 20 patients with osteoarthritis of the hip or knee received a placebo for 1 week followed by salsalate 1 g or aspirin 1.2 g thrice daily for 4 weeks; paracetamol was also taken when required. Salsalate produced similar results to aspirin in 5 clinical assessment criteria and in the number of paracetamol tablets consumed but produced slightly fewer side-effects and significantly less occult blood in the faeces.— S. P. Liyanage and P. K. Tambar, *Curr. med. Res. Opinion*, 1978, *5*, 450.

There was generally a marked improvement in joint pain and morning stiffness in 16 patients with active inflammatory disease, 20 patients with degenerative joint disease and 27 patients with musculoskeletal conditions who took salsalate 1 g thrice daily for 6 weeks; improvement in musculoskeletal pain was less evident. Three of 66 patients discontinued treatment because of side-effects of which the most frequent reported were dyspepsia, increased bowel frequency, nausea or vomiting, drowsiness, and tinnitus.— R. G. Regalado, *Curr. med. Res. Opinion*, 1978, *5*, 454.

In a multicentre study lasting 2 weeks of 102 arthritic patients, salsalate 1 g thrice daily improved symptoms in 67% of the patients. Side-effects included tinnitus in 5 patients, hearing loss in 5, and intestinal bleeding in 2 of 54 patients examined.— O. N. Ré, *J. int. med. Res.*, 1979, *7*, 90.

Proprietary Preparations

Disalcid *(Riker, UK)*. Salsalate, available as capsules of 500 mg. (Also available as Disalcid in *USA*).

Other Proprietary Names

Arcylate *(USA)*; Nobegyl *(Denm.)*.

2703-z

Simetride. 1,4-Bis[(2-methoxy-4-propylphenoxy)acetyl]piperazine.

$C_{28}H_{38}N_2O_6$=498.6.

CAS — 154-82-5.

A white crystalline powder. M.p. about 135°. Practically **insoluble** in water, alcohol, and ether; soluble in chloroform.

Uses. Simetride has analgesic, anti-inflammatory, and antipyretic actions. It has been used as an analgesic.

2704-c

Sodium Gentisate. Natrii Gentisas; Gentisato Sodico. Sodium 2,5-dihydroxybenzoate dihydrate.

$C_7H_5NaO_4,2H_2O$=212.1.

CAS — 490-79-9 (gentisic acid); 4955-90-2 (sodium gentisate, anhydrous).

Pharmacopoeias. In *Cz.* and *Span.*

A white or light grey odourless powder or crystals. **Soluble** 1 in 6 of water and 1 in 16 of alcohol (90%). A 10% solution in water has a pH of 6 to 7.5. **Incompatible** with acids, alkalis, and iron. **Protect** from light.

Sodium gentisate has been employed in acute rheumatic fever and other conditions in which salicylate therapy is indicated, in doses of 5 to 10 g daily.

Two cases of granulocytopenia occurred during treatment of acute rheumatism with sodium gentisate in doses of 10 g daily for 3 or 4 weeks.— R. G. Benians, *Br. med. J.*, 1953, *2*, 1142.

Proprietary Names of Some Related Substances
Gentiazina (piperazine digentisate) *(Lafare, Ital.).*

2705-k

Sodium Salicylate *(B.P., B.P. Vet., Eur. P., U.S.P.).* Sod. Sal.; Sod. Salicyl.; Natrii Salicylas. Sodium 2-hydroxybenzoate.

$C_7H_5NaO_3$=160.1.

CAS — 54-21-7.

Pharmacopoeias. In all pharmacopoeias examined except *Braz.*

Colourless crystals, crystalline flakes, or white or faintly pink powder, odourless or with a faint characteristic odour, and an unpleasant sweetish saline taste. Each g represents approximately 6.25 mmol (6.25 mEq) of sodium.

Soluble 1 in 1 of water, 1 in 11 of alcohol, and 1 in 4 of glycerol; very soluble in boiling water and boiling alcohol; practically insoluble in chloroform and ether. Concentrated aqueous solutions are liable to deposit crystals of the hexahydrate on standing. A 4% solution is neutral or acid to phenol red. A 2.53% solution is iso-osmotic with serum. Solutions are **sterilised** by autoclaving, heating with a bactericide, or by filtration. **Protect** from light.

Incompatible with most acids, free ammonia, solutions of some alkaloids, iron salts, phenazone, and nitrous ether spirit. With alkali bicarbonates, solutions gradually develop a reddish-brown colour which may be retarded by the addition of sodium metabisulphite (0.1%) if the prescriber will authorise the addition. Sodium salicylate forms a deep purple solution with iron salts.

Discoloration. The auto-oxidation of aqueous alkaline sodium salicylate solutions was a photochemical reaction catalysed by copper, iron, and manganese, and dependent on light intensity and concentrations of oxygen and salicylate.— C. B. Beynon and K. C. James, *J. Pharm. Pharmac.*, 1967, *19*, 660.

Incompatibility. Sodium and calcium salicylates interacted with quaternary ammonium surfactants in aqueous solutions and caused a rise in viscosity until a gel was formed at high salicylate concentrations. The effect was enhanced by the presence of other electrolytes.— L. S. C. Wan, *J. pharm. Sci.*, 1967, *56*, 743.

Adverse Effects and Treatment. As for Aspirin, p.236 and p.238.

Retinal haemorrhages were reported in a 60-year-old woman taking sodium salicylate 6 g daily by mouth for 2 months and in a 10-year-old girl taking sodium salicylate, 4 g daily by mouth, for 40 days. In both cases the haemorrhages were gradually resolved after the treatment was stopped.— A. Mortada and I. Abboud, *Br. J. Ophthal.*, 1973, *57*, 199.

Mean gastro-intestinal blood loss was 1.2 ml per day above control values following ingestion of sodium salicylate 3.9 g daily for 7 days compared with 5.6 ml per day when aspirin was taken similarly.— J. R. Leonards and G. Levy, *Clin. Pharmac. Ther.*, 1973, *14*, 62.

In a study in 40 patients with rheumatoid arthritis gastro-intestinal blood loss was less during treatment with indomethacin and sodium salicylate compared with indomethacin alone.— S. Torgyán *et al.*, *Int. J. clin. Pharmac. Biopharm.*, 1978, *16*, 610. See also *idem*, 1979, *17*, 439.

Precautions. As for Aspirin, p.238. Sodium salicylate should be given cautiously to patients on a low-sodium diet; it is contra-indicated in the presence of severe renal disease.

Absorption and Fate. As for Aspirin, p.239. The rate of absorption of sodium salicylate is probably greater than for aspirin and may be reduced by the concomitant administration of alkalis.

Sodium salicylate was rapidly distributed throughout the extracellular fluid of the body and readily penetrated many tissues. In the plasma-salicylate concentrations likely to be achieved in the treatment of acute rheumatic fever and possibly in the treatment of rheumatoid arthritis, inactivation of muscle triosephosphate dehydrogenase might occur.— S. Grisolia *et al.* (letter), *Nature*, 1969, *223*, 79.

In 3 anephric patients and in 3 patients whose kidneys were not functioning, each given sodium salicylate, 580 mg per 1.73 m^2 body-surface, plasma analysis showed that the drug was eliminated as rapidly as in healthy adults.— D. T. Lowenthal *et al.*, *Clin. Pharmac. Ther.*, 1974, *15*, 211.

Pregnancy and the neonate. The foetal distribution of sodium salicylate.— J. Elis *et al.*, *Int. J. clin. Pharmac. Biopharm.*, 1978, *16*, 365.

Uses. Sodium salicylate has analgesic, anti-inflammatory, and antipyretic actions similar to those of aspirin (see p.240). It has been used similarly to aspirin in the treatment of rheumatic and other musculoskeletal disorders, but aspirin is generally preferred. In rheumatic fever doses of 5 to 10 g daily in divided doses have been used. Sodium salicylate has also been administered by intravenous injection.

Diabetes. Intravenous infusion at a constant rate over 2 hours of a solution containing 5 g of sodium salicylate in 300 ml of sodium chloride injection caused significant increases in plasma-insulin concentrations in patients with diabetes mellitus and in healthy controls. Blood-glucose concentrations were decreased and the plasma-insulin response during intravenous glucose-tolerance tests was diminished in the diabetics but was unaffected in the controls.— J. B. Field *et al.*, *Lancet*, 1967, *1*, 1191.

Preparations

Sodium Salicylate Mixture *(A.P.F.).* Sodium salicylate 1 g, liquorice liquid extract 0.25 ml, concentrated chloroform water 0.25 ml, water to 10 ml. *Dose.* 10 to 20 ml.

Sodium Salicylate Mixture *(B.P.).* Sodium salicylate 500 mg, sodium metabisulphite 10 mg, concentrated orange peel infusion 0.5 ml, double-strength chloroform water 5 ml, water to 10 ml. It should be recently prepared.
Dose. 10 to 20 ml.

Strong Sodium Salicylate Mixture *(B.P.).* Sodium salicylate 1 g, sodium metabisulphite 10 mg, concentrated peppermint emulsion 0.25 ml, double-strength chloroform water 5 ml, water to 10 ml. It should be recently prepared.
Dose. 10 to 20 ml.

Tablets

Sodium Salicylate Tablets *(B.P.C. 1963).* Tablets containing sodium salicylate. They should be dissolved in water before administration.

Sodium Salicylate Tablets *(U.S.P.).* Tablets containing sodium salicylate.

Proprietary Preparations

Entrosalyl (Standard) *(Cox Continental, UK).* Enteric-coated tablets each containing sodium salicylate 500 mg.

Other Proprietary Names

Arg.—Enterosalil; *Austral.*—Ancosal, Ensalate, Rhumax; *Fr.*—Entérosalicyl; *Ital.*—Enterosalicyl, Kerasalicyl, Salisod; *Neth.*—Enterosalicyl; *Swed.*—Idocyl; *Switz.*—Saliglutin, Salitine.

2706-a

Sulindac *(U.S.P.).* MK-231. (*Z*)-[5-Fluoro-2-methyl-1-(4-methylsulphinylbenzylidene)inden-3-yl]acetic acid.

$C_{20}H_{17}FO_3S$=356.4.

CAS — 38194-50-2.

Pharmacopoeias. In *U.S.*

A yellow, odourless or almost odourless, tasteless, crystalline powder. M.p. about 182° to 185°. Practically **insoluble** in water and light petroleum; slightly soluble in alcohol, acetone, chloroform, methyl alcohol, and neutral or alkaline aqueous solutions; very slightly soluble in isopropyl alcohol and ethyl acetate.

Adverse Effects. As for Indomethacin, p.257.

A hypertensive reaction with sulindac.— P. A. Easton and A. Koval, *Can. med. Ass. J.*, 1980, *122*, 1273.

Allergy. Hypersensitivity reactions to sulindac.— F. E. Smith and P. J. Lindberg, *J. Am. med. Ass.*, 1980, *244*, 269; I. J. Russell (letter), *Ann. intern. Med* 1980, *92*, 716.

Effects on blood. Aplastic anaemia was associated with sulindac therapy in a 54-year-old man.— J. L. Miller (letter), *Ann. intern. Med.*, 1980, *92*, 129. A similar case.— L. Bennett *et al.* (letter), *ibid.*, 874.

A report of leucopenia and thrombocytopenia, associated with elevation of liver enzymes, in a 37-year-old man taking sulindac.— J. E. Stambaugh *et al.* (letter), *Lancet*, 1980, *2*, 594. Fatal aplastic anaemia in one patient and transitory erythroblastopenia in a second, were associated with sulindac administration.— M. A. Sanz *et al.* (letter), *ibid.*, 802.

Agranulocytosis associated with sulindac administration.— K. R. Romeril *et al.* (letter), *Lancet*, 1981, *2*, 523.

Effects on the gastro-intestinal tract. In a comparative study completed by 39 healthy subjects, aspirin 4.8 g daily caused more gastro-intestinal blood loss than sulindac 400 or 240 mg daily, or placebo.— A. Cohen, *Clin. Pharmac. Ther.*, 1976, *20*, 238.

Effects on the kidneys. The nephrotic syndrome was associated with the use of sulindac in a 57-year-old woman with psoriasis and arthritis.— S. Lomvardias *et al.* (letter), *New Engl. J. Med.*, 1981, *304*, 424.

Effects on liver. Severe but reversible hepatotoxicity developed in an 18-year-old woman about 2 weeks after she had started taking sulindac 200 mg twice daily.— R. J. Anderson (letter), *New Engl. J. Med.*, 1979, *300*, 735. A similar report.— P. B. Wolfe (letter), *Ann. intern. Med.*, 1979, *91*, 656.

Further references: A. K. Dhand *et al.*, *Gastroenterology*, 1981, *80*, 585.

Effects on the lungs. Pneumonitis in a woman given sulindac.— M. Fein (letter), *Ann. intern. Med.*, 1981, *95*, 245.

Effects on mental state. Paranoid psychosis began in a patient 4 hours after the first dose of sulindac, and resolved within 48 hours of the last dose.— R. Kruis and R. Barger (letter), *J. Am. med. Ass.*, 1980, *243*, 1420.

Delirium in one patient associated with sulindac.— T. L. Thornton (letter), *J. Am. med. Ass.*, 1980, *243*, 1630.

Epidermal necrolysis. Toxic epidermal necrolysis occurred in a patient taking sulindac 400 mg daily.— L. Levitt and R. W. Pearson, *J. Am. med. Ass.*, 1980, *243*, 1262.

Pancreatitis. Pancreatitis associated with sulindac in one patient.— J. Goldstein *et al.* (letter), *Ann. intern. Med.*, 1980, *93*, 151. A similar case.— A. D. Siefkin (letter), *Ann. intern. Med.*, 1980, *93*, 932.

Precautions. As for Indomethacin, p.258.

Interactions. *Anticoagulants.* For reference to the possible enhancement of the effect of warfarin by sulindac, see Warfarin, p.779.

Antidiabetic agents. For reference to the absence of any clinically significant interaction with tolbutamide, see Tolbutamide, p.859.

Porphyria. A study in *rats* indicated that sulindac would probably not elicit an acute attack in susceptible porphyric individuals.— G. H. Blekkenhorst *et al.* (letter), *Lancet*, 1980, *1*, 1367. Criticisms of extrapolating data obtained from *anaimal* experiments to the treatment of human disease.— M. J. Brodie (letter), *ibid.*, *2*, 86; A. Gorchein (letter), *ibid.*, 152.

Absorption and Fate. Sulindac is incompletely absorbed from the gastro-intestinal tract. It is metabolised by reversible reduction to the sulphide metabolite, which appears to be the biologically active form, and by irreversible oxidation to the sulphone metabolite. Peak plasma concentrations of the sulphide metabolite are achieved in about 2 to 4 hours. The mean half-life of sulindac is about 7 to 8 hours and of the sulphide metabolite about 16 to 18 hours. About

75% is excreted in the urine mainly as the sulphone metabolite and its glucuronide conjugate, with smaller amounts of sulindac and its glucuronide conjugate. Sulindac and its metabolites are also excreted in bile and undergo extensive enterohepatic circulation.

An account of the pooled results from 5 separate clinical studies involving a total of 56 healthy subjects. Following administration of sulindac 100 to 400 mg by mouth about 90% was absorbed, some being oxidised irreversibly into the sulphone and some reduced reversibly into the sulphide (which appeared to be the biologically active form). The sulphide had an apparent terminal half-life of about 18 hours none being excreted into the urine. In the urine, sulphone and its conjugate constituted nearly 30% of the dose administered whereas sulindac and its glucuronide constituted about 20%; unidentified metabolites were responsible for about 25%. Faecal recovery accounted for about 25% of the dose, this high figure being explained by enterohepatic recycling.— D. E. Duggan *et al.*, *Clin. Pharmac. Ther.*, 1977, *21*, 326. See also *idem*, *Biochem. Pharmac.*, 1978, *27*, 2311.

Studies *in vitro* indicated that sulindac and its principal active metabilite, sulindac sulphide, were both extensively bound to human serum albumin.— M. A. Shams-Eldeen *et al.*, *J. pharm. Sci.*, 1978, *67*, 1077.

Uses. Sulindac is a fluorinated indene with a structural resemblance to indomethacin. It has analgesic, anti-inflammatory, and antipyretic actions. It is used in the treatment of rheumatic and other musculoskeletal disorders. The usual dose is between 100 and 200 mg twice daily taken with food.

Reviews of sulindac.— T. Y. Shen and C. A. Winter, *Adv. Drug Res.*, 1977, *12*, 89; *Lancet*, 1977, *1*, 462; R. N. Brogden *et al.*, *Drugs*, 1978, *16*, 97; *Med. Lett.*, 1979, *21*, 1. Nahata, M *Drug Intell. & clin. Pharm.*, 1979, *13*, 736.

Symposium on sulindac.— *Eur. J. Rheumatol. Inflamm.*, 1978, *1*, 3–68.

Sulindac as an antipyretic.— S. Similä *et al.*, *Curr. ther. Res.*, 1979, *26*, 828.

Administration in renal failure. Dosage reduction of sulindac is not required in patients with renal impairment.— W. M. Bennett *et al.*, *Ann. intern. Med.*, 1980, *93*, 286.

Ankylosing spondylitis. Sulindac and indomethacin had comparable efficacy and tolerance in a double-blind 6-month study of 30 patients with ankylosing spondylitis. The optimum daily dose for sulindac was considered to be 350 mg.— A. Calin and M. Britton, *J. Am. med. Ass.*, 1979, *242*, 1885.

Further reports on the use of sulindac in ankylosing spondylitis.— R. Eberl, *Scand. J. Rheumatol.*, 1975, *4*, *Suppl.* 8, S 04–05; M. Gadomski *et al.*, *ibid.*, S 02–05.

Osteoarthrosis. in a double-blind multicentre study involving 91 patients with osteoarthrosis of the hip, a beneficial response to sulindac was obtained in most of 45 patients receiving sulindac and considered eligible for analysis, compared with 25 patients who received placebo. The optimum dose appeared to be 300 mg daily although some patients obtained a beneficial response for smaller doses.— J. J. Calabro *et al.*, *Clin. Pharmac. Ther.*, 1977, *22*, 358.

Further studies on the use of sulindac in osteoarthrosis.— B. Brackertz and M. Busson, *Br. J. clin. Pract.*, 1978, *32*, 77; M. Thompson *et al.*, *Curr. ther. Res.*, 1979, *26*, 779.

Platelet aggregation. A small double-blind study comparing the effects of sulindac, aspirin, and placebo on platelet aggregation revealed that sulindac had a mild transient inhibitory effect on platelet function.— D. Green *et al.* (letter), *Lancet*, 1977, *1*, 804.

Rheumatoid arthritis. A 10-week double-blind study in 31 patients with rheumatoid arthritis indicated that sulindac 200 mg twice daily was as effective as aspirin 3.6 g daily for the control of pain, but aspirin was better than sulindac in reducing the duration of morning stiffness. Adverse reactions causing withdrawal from the study occurred in 2 patients given sulindac and 4 given aspirin.— P. M. G. Reynolds *et al.*, *Curr. med. Res. Opinion*, 1977, *4*, 485.

Further studies in the use of sulindac in the treatment of rheumatoid arthritis.— T. C. Highton and R. Jeremy, *Scand. J. Rheumatol.*, 1975, *4*, *Suppl.* 8, S 02–06; F. Bachmann and W. Hartl, *Dt. med. Wschr.*, 1977, *102*, 1772; E. C. Huskisson and J. Scott, *Ann. rheum. Dis.*, 1978, *37*, 89; E. C. Huskisson, *Eur. J. Rheumatol. Inflamm.*, 1978, *1*, 12; J. Borrachero del Campo, *Eur. J. Rheumatol. Inflamm.*, 1978, *1*, 16; I. Caruso *et al.*, *ibid.*, 58; H. C. Burry and L. Witherington, *N.Z. med. J.*, 1979, *89*, 298.

Preparations

Sulindac Tablets *(U.S.P.)*. Tablets containing sulindac. The *U.S.P.* specifies 85% dissolution in 30 minutes.

Clinoril *(Merck Sharp & Dohme, UK)*. Sulindac, available as scored tablets of 100 and 200 mg. (Also available as Clinoril in *Arg., Austral., Belg., Canad., Denm., Ital., Neth., S.Afr., Switz., USA*).

Other Proprietary Names

Arthrocine *(Fr.)*; Artribid *(Port.)*; Citireuma *(Ital.)*; Imbaral *(Ger.)*.

2707-t

Suxibuzone. 4-Butyl-4-hydroxymethyl-1,2-diphenylpyrazolidine-3,5-dione hydrogen succinate (ester).
$C_{24}H_{26}N_2O_6$=438.5.

CAS — 27470-51-5.

A white powder with a bitter taste. M.p. about 126°. **Insoluble** in water; soluble in most organic solvents.

Uses. Suxibuzone is a derivative of phenylbutazone (see p.273) and is used similarly in doses of 250 to 300 mg thrice daily.

Proprietary Names

Calibene *(Delalande, Belg.)*; Danalon OM *(Johnson, Arg.)*; Danilon *(Esteve, Spain)*; Flogos *(Gentili, Ital.)*; Solurol *(Delalande, Ger.)*.

2708-x

Thurfyl Salicylate. Tetrahydrofurfuryl salicylate.
$C_{12}H_{14}O_4$=222.2.

CAS — 2217-35-8.

Uses. Thurfyl salicylate is a topical analgesic which has been used at concentrations of 10 to 14%, in creams for rheumatic and muscular pain.

2709-r

Tiaprofenic Acid. FC 3001; RU 15060. 2-(5-Benzoyl-2-thienyl)propionic acid.
$C_{14}H_{12}O_3S$=260.3.

CAS — 33005-95-7.

A white microcrystalline powder. M.p. about 95°. **Soluble** in alcohol and chloroform.

Uses. Tiaprofenic acid is a propionic acid derivative which has anti-inflammatory, analgesic, and antipyretic actions. The usual dose is 600 mg daily initially in divided doses and 300 to 400 mg daily for maintenance.

Absorption and fate of tiaprofenic acid.— J. Pottier *et al.*, *J. pharm. Sci.*, 1977, *66*, 1030.

Proprietary Preparations

Surgam *(Cassenne, UK)*. Tiaprofenic acid, available as tablets of 200 mg. (Also available as Surgam in *Fr.*).

2710-j

Tiaramide Hydrochloride. Tiaperamide Hydrochloride; NTA 194. 5-Chloro-3-{2-[4-(2-hydroxyethyl)piperazin-1-yl]-2-oxoethyl}benzothiazolin-2-one hydrochloride.
$C_{15}H_{18}ClN_3O_3S,HCl$=392.3.

CAS — 32527-55-2 (tiaramide); 35941-71-0 (hydrochloride).

A white odourless crystalline powder with a bitter taste. **Soluble** in water; slightly soluble in alcohol and methyl alcohol; very slightly soluble in glacial acetic acid; practically insoluble in chloroform, ether, and ethyl acetate. A 5% aqueous solution has a pH of about 4.

Uses. Tiaramide hydrochloride is an analgesic and anti-inflammatory agent.

For a series of papers, chiefly relating to *animal* studies, see *Arzneimittel-Forsch.*, 1972, *22*, 711–743.

Toxicity and teratogenicity of tiaramide in *animals*.— N. Watanabe *et al.*, *Arzneimittel-Forsch.*, 1973, *23*, 504.

Metabolism in *animals*.— H. Noguchi *et al.*, *Xenobiotica*, 1977, *7*, 491.

Anti-anaphylactic effect of tiaramide hydrochloride in *animals*.— T. Takashima *et al.*, *Arzneimittel-Forsch.*, 1979, *29*, 903.

Proprietary Names

Solantal *(Fujisawa, Jap.)*.

2711-z

Tinoridine Hydrochloride. Tienoridine Hydrochloride; Y 3642. Ethyl 2-amino-6-benzyl-4,5,6,7-tetrahydrothieno[2,3-*c*]pyridine-3-carboxylate hydrochloride.
$C_{17}H_{20}N_2O_2S,HCl$=352.9.

CAS — 24237-54-5 (tinoridine); 25913-34-2 (hydrochloride).

A yellowish-white or yellow almost odourless powder with a bitter taste. M.p. about 220° with decomposition. Very slightly **soluble** in water, acetone, and ether; slightly soluble in methyl alcohol.

Adverse Effects. Gastro-intestinal disturbances, drowsiness, vertigo, pruritus, urticaria, skin eruptions, and changes in liver function tests may occur.

Uses. Tinoridine hydrochloride has analgesic, anti-inflammatory, and antipyretic actions. It is used for the relief of various types of pain and in the treatment of rheumatic disorders in doses equivalent to 50 to 100 mg of tinoridine thrice daily.

Proprietary Names

Dimaten *(Promeco, Arg.)*; Nonflamin *(Jap.)*.

2712-c

Tolfenamic Acid. *N*-(3-Chloro-*o*-tolyl)anthranilic acid.
$C_{14}H_{12}ClNO_2$=261.7.

CAS — 13710-19-5.

Adverse Effects. Gastro-intestinal disturbances, dysuria, headache, pruritus, sweating, skin rashes, and oedema have been reported.

Uses. Tolfenamic acid is an anthranilic acid derivative which has analgesic, anti-inflammatory, and antipyretic actions. It has been given in doses of 100 to 200 mg in rheumatoid arthritis and as an analgesic.

Analgesia. Tolfenamic acid 100 mg and rimazolium methylsulphate 300 mg were considered to be of similar efficacy when used thrice daily in the treatment of 60 patients with postoperative or post-traumatic pain. Response was considered to be good in 70% of the 30 patients who received tolfenamic acid and side-effects reported included restless legs (1), gastric irritation (1), nausea (1), and fatigue (2).— M. Haataja *et al.*, *Curr. ther. Res.*, 1978, *24*, 284.

Dysmenorrhoea. Results of a double-blind placebo-controlled study involving 122 evaluable women, indicated that adminsitration of tolfenamic acid 200 mg thrice daily for 7 days immediately after insertion of an intra-uterine device and during the next 3 menstrual periods, reduced the incidence of associated cramps and excessive bleeding. Four of the women who received tolfenamic acid experienced dyspepsia and diarrhoea.— O. Ylikorkala *et al.*, *Lancet*, 1978, *2*, 393.

Fever. In an evaluation of antipyretic activity tolfenamic acid was shown to be 8 times more potent than mefenamic acid, and 3 times more potent that flufenamic acid.— S. Keinänen *et al.*, *Eur. J. clin. Pharmac.*, 1978, *13*, 331.

Migraine. In a comparative double-blind, crossover study, 20 women with classic and common migraine took tolfenamic acid 200 mg, ergotamine tartrate 1 mg, aspirin 500 mg, or placebo, followed by an analgesic of choice after 2 hours if required. Tolfenamic acid was as effective as ergotamine tartrate in reducing the intensity and duration of attacks and had fewer side-effects.— H. Hakkarainen *et al.*, *Lancet*, 1979, *2*, 326. Further comment on the importance of gastric factors in the drug therapy of migraine.— J. Parantainen *et al.* (letter), *ibid.*, 1980, *1*, 832.

Rheumatic disorders. Studies on the use of tolfenamic acid in rheumatoid arthritis and other rheumatic disorders.— A. Kajander *et al.*, *Scand. J. Rheumatol.*, 1976, *5*, 158; K. Sørensen and L. V. Christiansen, *ibid.*, 1977,

Suppl. 20;; L. Nyfos, *ibid.*, 1979, *Suppl.* 24, 5; V. Rejholec *et al.*, *ibid.*, 9 and 13.

Proprietary Names
Clotam *(Medica, Fin.)*.

2713-k

Tolmetin Sodium *(U.S.P.)*. McN 2559.

Sodium (1-methyl-5-*p*-toluoylpyrrol-2-yl)acetate dihydrate.
$C_{15}H_{14}NNaO_3,2H_2O=315.3$.

CAS — 26171-23-3 (tolmetin); 35711-34-3 (sodium salt, anhydrous); 64490-92-2 (sodium salt, dihydrate).

Pharmacopoeias. In *U.S.*

Tolmetin sodium 123 mg is approximately equivalent to 100 mg of tolmetin.

Adverse Effects and Precautions. As for Ibuprofen, p.256.

Aseptic meningitis occurred in a patient with systemic lupus erythematosus given tolmetin. She had earlier experienced a similar but milder reaction with ibuprofen.— G. B. Ruppert and W. F. Barth, *J. Am. med. Ass.*, 1981, *245*, 67.

Allergy. Reports of anaphylactic shock in patients taking tolmetin sodium.— C. Restivo and H. E. Paulus, *J. Am. med. Ass.*, 1978, *240*, 246 (2 patients); S. Ahmad (letter), *New Engl. J. Med.*, 1980, *303*, 1417 (1 patient); M. E. Moore and D. P. Goldsmith, *Archs intern. Med.*, 1980, *140*, 1105 (1 patient).

Effects on blood. A fatal case of agranulocytosis in a 52-year-old woman was associated with tolmetin of which she had taken 400 mg thrice daily for 5 weeks. The patient had previously been taking other anti-inflammatory and analgesic drugs for some years.— J. Sakai and M. W. Joseph (letter), *New Engl. J. Med.*, 1978, *298*, 1203.

Effects on the gastro-intestinal tract. In 2 investigations in 30 healthy subjects, 10 subjects received tolmetin 1.2 g daily, 10 received aspirin 3.9 g daily, and 10 received indomethacin 200 mg daily. Aspirin produced a significantly greater mean blood loss than tolmetin or indomethacin, and tolmetin produced about half as much blood loss as indomethacin although this did not reach significance.— J. A. Beirne *et al.*, *Clin. Pharmac. Ther.*, 1974, *16*, 821.

Effects on the kidneys. Interstitial nephritis in a woman given tolmetin.— S. M. Katz *et al.*, *J. Am. med. Ass.*, 1981, *246*, 243.

Interactions, tests. The urine of 5 patients receiving tolmetin gave false positive reactions for protein when tested by the standard sulphosalicylic acid method.— G. E. Ehrlich and G. F. Wortham, *Clin. Pharmac. Ther.*, 1975, *17*, 467.

Absorption and Fate. Tolmetin is almost completely absorbed from the gastro-intestinal tract. Peak plasma concentrations are attained 20 to 60 minutes after ingestion. It is extensively bound to plasma proteins. It has a plasma half-life of about 1 hour and is excreted in the urine as an inactive dicarboxylic acid metabolite and its glucuronide and as tolmetin glucuronide with small amounts of unchanged drug.

The mean half-life of tolmetin in healthy subjects after 400-mg doses was 56 minutes. Absorption and metabolism remained constant after 14 days' treatment with 1.2 g daily. Plasma concentrations were reduced by about 20% when aspirin 3.9 g daily was given concomitantly. Tolmetin was 99% bound to plasma proteins *in vitro;* this figure was reduced to 98% and 96% in the presence respectively of aspirin and salicylic acid.— W. A. Cressman *et al.*, *Clin. Pharmac. Ther.*, 1974, *15*, 203.

A peak plasma concentration of about 32 µg per ml was achieved 1 hour after a 600-mg dose of tolmetin in 1 subject. All of a dose was excreted in the urine within 24 hours but only 2 to 3% as the intact drug. The major metabolite was 5-(*p*-carboxybenzoyl)-1-methylpyrrole-2-acetic acid.— W. A. Cressman *et al.*, *J. pharm. Sci.*, 1975, *64*, 1965.

A study of the absorption and excretion of tolmetin in healthy subjects (dose-response in 6, bioavailability in 18, chronic administration in 12, and chronic administration with aspirin in 11). Tolmetin was absorbed in 10 to 20 minutes, had a plasma half-life of about 60 minutes, and showed a linear dose-plasma concentration response within the therapeutic range. On chronic administration tolmetin did not affect its own metabolism but was displaced from plasma proteins by salicylic acid (administered as aspirin) which was reflected in minor changes in plasma concentrations and pharmacokinetic parameters.— W. A. Cressman *et al.*, *Clin. Pharmac. Ther.*, 1976, *19*, 224.

Protein binding of tolmetin.— M. L. Selley *et al.*, *Clin. Pharmac. Ther.*, 1978, *24*, 694.

Further studies on the absorption and fate of tolmetin.— M. L. Selley *et al.*, *Clin. Pharmac. Ther.*, 1975, *17*, 599; D. D. Sumner *et al.*, *Drug Metab. Disposit.*, 1975, *3*, 283; J. M. Grindel *et al.*, *Clin. Pharmac. Ther.*, 1979, *26*, 122.

Uses. Tolmetin sodium has analgesic, antipyretic, and anti-inflammatory actions. It is used in the treatment of rheumatic and other musculoskeletal disorders in doses equivalent to 600 mg to 1.8 g of tolmetin daily in 3 or 4 divided doses. It should be taken with food or milk.

Tolmetin sodium has been used in the treatment of juvenile chronic polyarthritis in doses of 15 to 30 mg of tolmetin per kg body-weight daily.

A discussion on the use of fenoprofen calcium, naproxen, and tolmetin sodium.— J. R. Lewis, *J. Am. med. Ass.*, 1977, *237*, 1260.

A detailed review of tolmetin and its use in the treatment of rheumatic diseases.— R. N. Brogden *et al.*, *Drugs*, 1978, *15*, 429.

Administration in renal failure. Tolmetin sodium may be given in usual doses to patients with renal impairment.— W. M. Bennett *et al.*, *Ann. intern. med.*, 1980, *93*, 286.

Ankylosing spondylitis. Reports on the use of tolmetin sodium in the treatment of ankylosing spondylitis.— F. Wagenhäuser, *Scand. J. Rheumatol.*, 1975, *4*, *Suppl.* 8, S 10-08; W. Standel, *ibid.*, S 10-09; M. Schattenkirchner and U. Schattenkirchner, *ibid.*, S 10-11; G. Manz, *ibid.*, S 10-10.

Osteoarthrosis. In a 3-month double-blind study in 137 patients with osteoarthritis of the spine, tolmetin sodium was as effective as ibuprofen in reducing the severity of joint symptoms, providing symptomatic relief, and improving functional capacity. Gastro-intestinal symptoms were the main side-effects reported and there was no significant difference in severity or number of side-effects reported between the two groups.— J. J. Cannella *et al.*, *Curr. ther. Res.*, 1979, *25*, 447.

Further studies on the use of tolmetin sodium in the treatment of oestoarthrosis.— R. Rau *et al.*, *Scand. J. Rheumatol.*, 1975, *4*, *Suppl.* 8, S 10-12; F. O. Müller *et al.*, *S.Afr. med. J.*, 1977, *51*, 794; S. P. Liyanage and C. E. Steele, *Curr. med. Res. Opinion*, 1977, *5*, 299; S. Kaplan and R. Salzman, *Curr. ther. Res.*, 1979, *25*, 508; S. Y. Andelman and A. Miyara, *Curr. ther. Res.*, 1979, *26*, 44.

Rheumatoid arthritis. A 6-week study of 24 outpatients with rheumatoid arthritis of up to 17 years' duration indicated that dosage with tolmetin over 1.2 g daily reduced joint pain, walking time over 15 m, and articular index. In a double-blind crossover comparison in a further 22 patients tolmetin 1.4 g daily was as effective as indomethacin 150 mg daily.— M. Aylward *et al.*, *Curr. med. Res. Opinion*, 1976, *4*, 158.

Further studies on the use of tolmetin sodium in the treatment of rheumatoid arthritis.— L. S. Bain *et al.*, *Br. J. clin. Pract.*, 1975, *29*, 208; J. H. Brown *et al.*, *J. clin. Pharmac.*, 1975, *15*, 455; M. Alward *et al.*, *Curr. med. Res. Opinion*, 1977, *4*, 695; N. Cardoe and C. E. Steele, *Curr. med. Res. Opinion*, 1977, *4*, 688; A. M. Freeman *et al.*, *ibid.*, *5*, 262; G. M. Clark *et al.*, *Curr. ther. Res.*, 1977, *21*, 697; J. I. McMillen, *ibid.*, *22*, 266; K. Pavelka and A. Susta, *ibid.*, 1978, *24*, 83; B. M. Ansell *et al.*, *Rheumatol. Rehabil.*, 1978, *17*, 150.

Juvenile polyarthritis. In a double-blind study in 107 children with rheumatoid arthritis, tolmetin sodium was as effective as aspirin in the short-term management of the disease. Tolmetin as the sodium salt was given in doses of 15 to 30 mg per kg body-weight daily with a maximum dose of 1.8 g daily. Adverse effects were similar for both drugs.— J. E. Levinson *et al.*, *J. Pediat.*, 1977, *91*, 799.

Preparations

Tolmetin Sodium Capsules *(U.S.P.)*. Capsules containing tolmetin sodium. Potency is expressed in terms of the equivalent amount of tolmetin. The *U.S.P.* requires 85% dissolution in 30 minutes. Store in airtight containers.

Tolmetin Sodium Tablets *(U.S.P.)*. Tablets containing tolmetin sodium. Potency is expressed in terms of the equivalent amount of tolmetin.

Proprietary Preparations

Tolectin *(Ortho-Cilag, UK)*. Tolmetin sodium, available as scored tablets containing the equivalent of tolmetin 200 mg. **Tolectin DS.** Tolmetin sodium, available as capsules containing the equivalent of tolmetin 400 mg. (Also available as Tolectin in *Belg., Canad., Denm., Ger., Ital., Neth., S.Afr., Switz., USA*).

Other Proprietary Names

Tolmex *(Ital.)*.

2714-a

Tribuzone. Trimetazone; Trimethazone. 4-(4,4-Dimethyl-3-oxopentyl)-1,2-diphenylpyrazolidine-3,5-dione.
$C_{22}H_{24}N_2O_3=364.4$.

CAS — 13221-27-7.

Pharmacopoeias. In *Cz.*

Odourless, tasteless, acicular crystals or white or almost white powder. M.p. 143° to 145°.

Practically **insoluble** in water; soluble in alcohol, acetone, and alkali hydroxides and carbonates; freely soluble in chloroform.

Uses. Tribuzone is an analgesic and anti-inflammatory agent structurally related to phenylbutazone (see p.273). Doses of 250 mg two to four times daily have been employed.

Proprietary Names
Benetazone *(Spofa, Cz.)*.

2715-t

Viminol Hydroxybenzoate. Diviminol Hydroxybenzoate; Z 424 *(base)*. 1-[1-(2-Chlorobenzyl)pyrrol-2-yl]-2-(di-*sec*-butyl)aminoethanol 4-hydroxybenzoate.
$C_{21}H_{31}ClN_2O,C_7H_6O_3=501.1$.

CAS — 21363-18-8 (viminol); 21466-60-4; 23784-10-3 (both hydroxybenzoate).

Uses. Viminol hydroxybenzoate is an analgesic and antipyretic agent used in doses equivalent to 50 to 100 mg of viminol, with a maximum of 400 mg daily.

Studies on the analgesic action of viminol.— P. Procacci *et al.*, *Curr. ther. Res.*, 1969, *11*, 647; L. Martinetti *et al.*, *J. clin. Pharmac.*, 1970, *10*, 390; M. Moroni *et al.*, *Int. J. clin. Pharmac. Biopharm.*, 1978, *16*, 513.

Slight respiratory effect in 8 healthy persons.— G. Ghiringhelli *et al.*, *Curr. ther. Res.*, 1971, *13*, 489.

Antitussive activity of viminol.— G. Sabot *et al.*, *Int. J. clin. Pharmac. Biopharm.*, 1977, *15*, 181.

Proprietary Names
Dividol *(Zambon, Ital.; Zambon, Spain)*; Lenigesial *(Inpharzam, Ger.)*.

2716-x

Zomepirac Sodium. McN-2783-21-98.

Sodium [5-(4-chlorobenzoyl)-1,4-dimethylpyrrol-2-yl]acetate dihydrate.
$C_{15}H_{13}ClNNaO_3,2H_2O=349.7$.

CAS — 33369-31-2 (zomepirac); 64092-48-4 (sodium salt, anhydrous); 64092-49-5 (sodium salt, dihydrate).

Zomepirac sodium 1.2 g is approximately equivalent to 1 g of zomepirac.

Adverse Effects and Precautions. As for Ibuprofen, p.256.

A preliminary report of a multicentre double-blind study of the long-term safety of zomepirac; 405 patients with osteoarthritis given the equivalent of 300 to 400 mg of zomepirac daily, with 107 receiving treatment for at least 1 year, were compared with 202 given aspirin 3 to 4 g daily, with 53 receiving treatment for at least 1 year. There was a greater incidence of lower urinary-tract symptoms in those given zomepirac and a greater incidence of adverse effects on the special senses (mainly tinnitus and hearing loss) in those given aspirin. Other side-effects were similar in both groups with gastro-intestinal affects being the most common. Gastro-intestinal bleeding occurred in 3 given zomepirac and 2 given aspirin. Peptic ulcers occurred in 5 given zomepirac and 4 given aspirin.— S. Honig, *J. clin. Pharmac.*, 1980, *20*, 392.

Allergy. An apparent anaphylactic reaction to zomepirac.— S. A. Samuel (letter), *New Engl. J. Med.*, 1981, *304*, 978.

Porphyria. A study in *rats* indicated that zomepirac sodium would probably not elicit an acute attack in susceptible porphyric subjects.— G. H. Blekkenhorst *et al.* (letter), *Lancet*, 1980, *1*, 1367. Criticisms of extrapolating data from *animal* experiments to the treatment of human disease.— M. J. Brodie (letter), *ibid.*, *2*, 86; A. Gorchein (letter), *ibid.*, 152.

Absorption and Fate. Zomepirac is readily absorbed from the gastro-intestinal tract producting peak plasma concentrations within 1 to 2 hours. It is reported to have a plasma half-life of about 4 hours and to be extensively bound to plasma proteins. It is excreted in the urine, mainly as the glucuronide.

References: L. D. Muschek and J. M. Grindel, *J. clin. Pharmac.*, 1980, *20*, 223; R. K. Nayak *et al.*, *Clin. Pharmac. Ther.*, 1980, *27*, 395.

Uses. Zomepirac sodium is an analgesic structurally very similar to tolmetin sodium. It is used in mild to moderate pain, including that of musculoskeletal disorders, in doses equivalent to 400 to 600 mg of zomepirac daily.

A brief review of zomepirac sodium.— *Med. Lett.*, 1981, *23*, 1.

Absence of withdrawal symptoms with zomepirac.— C. P. O'Brien and F. L. Minn, *J. clin. Pharmac.*, 1980, *20*, 397.

Analgesic effects of zomepirac.— S. A. Cooper and S. Gottlieb, *Clin. Pharmac. Ther.*, 1977, *21*, 101; S. A. Cooper *et al.*, *J. clin. Pharmac.*, 1980, *20*, 98; T. P. Pruss *et al.*, *ibid.*, 216; S. A. Cooper, *ibid.*, 230; W. M. Baird and D. Turek, *ibid.*, 243; S. L. Wallenstein *et al.*, *ibid.*, 250; W. H. Forrest, *ibid.*, 259; J. E. Stambaugh *et al.*, *ibid.*, 261; D. R. Mehlisch *et al.*, *ibid.*, 271; R. H. Messer *et al.*, *ibid.*, 279; T. G. Mayer and G. E. Ruoff, *ibid.*, 285; J. R. deAndrade *et al.*, *ibid.*, 292; S. Diamond, *ibid.*, 298; J. S. Elbaz and A. Bernard, *ibid.*, 303; S. Andelman *et al.*, *ibid.*, 364; J. I. McMillen *et al.*, *ibid.*, 385; S. A. Cooper, *Curr. ther. Res.*, 1980, *28*, 630.

Proprietary Preparations

Zomax *(Ortho-Cilag, UK)*. Zomepirac sodium, available as scored tablets each containing the equivalent of zomepirac 100 mg.

Astringents

290-k

Astringents precipitate proteins and when applied to mucous membranes or to damaged skin they form a superficial protective layer and are not usually absorbed. They harden the skin and check exudative secretions and minor haemorrhage.

291-a

Acetannin *(B.P.C. 1934)*. Acetyltannic Acid; Ácido Diacetilotânico; Diacetyltannin; Tannigen; Tannyl Acetate; Acetilotanino.

CAS — 1397-74-6.

Pharmacopoeias. In *Port.* and *Span.*

A complex mixture of partly acetylated tannic acid derivatives.

It occurs as a yellowish or greyish-white tasteless powder which darkens on exposure to light. It is odourless or has a faint acetous odour.

Very slightly **soluble** in water, alcohol, chloroform, and ether; soluble in acetone, ethyl acetate, and solutions of borax and of sodium phosphate; soluble, with gradual decomposition, in solutions of alkali hydroxides and carbonates. **Incompatible** with alkalis, bismuth compounds, and iron salts. **Store** in airtight containers. Protect from light.

Acetannin is a mild astringent and was formerly used in the treatment of diarrhoea. It has been given in doses of 300 to 600 mg.

292-t

Agaric Acid *(B.P.C. 1934)*. Agaricic Acid; Agaricin; Agaricinic Acid; Laricic Acid. 2-Hexadecylcitric acid sesquihydrate; 2-Hydroxynonadecane-1,2,3-tricarboxylic acid sesquihydrate.

$C_{22}H_{40}O_7,1\frac{1}{2}H_2O$=443.6.

CAS — 666-99-9 (anhydrous); 6034-71-5 (sesquihydrate).

Pharmacopoeias. In *Aust.* and *Port.*

A white, almost odourless and tasteless, microcrystalline powder, obtained from agaric, the dried stroma of the fungus *Polyporus officinalis* (Polyporaceae). Slightly **soluble** in water, chloroform, and ether; soluble 1 in 130 of alcohol.

Agaric acid has been used to control hyperhidrosis; large doses are purgative. It has been given in doses of 5 to 30 mg.

Agaric acid and its tetradecyl homologue norcaperatic acid, isolated from the mushroom*Cantharellus floccosus*, had a delayed action and produced dose-related effects of mydriasis, skeletal muscle weakness, and CNS depression in *rats*. The potentially toxic effects of fungi containing these substances might be related to their similarity to citric acid.— R. A. Carrano and M. H. Malone, *J. pharm. Sci.*, 1967, *56*, 1611.

It was recommended that agaric acid be prohibited for use in foods as a flavouring agent.— *Food Standards Committee Report on Flavouring Agents,* London, HM Stationery Office, 1965.

293-x

Albumin Tannate. Albutannin; Tannalbin; Tannin Albuminate. A compound of tannin with albumin.

CAS — 9006-52-4.

Pharmacopoeias. In *Arg., Aust., Cz., Hung., Jap., Nord., Pol., Port.,* and *Span. Rus. P.* includes Thealbin, a compound of tannins from tea leaves with protein.

A yellowish-white to pale brown, odourless, tasteless powder. Practically **insoluble** in water, alcohol, chloroform, and ether. **Incompatible** with bismuth compounds, oxidising agents, iron salts, and alkali hydroxides and carbonates. **Store** in well-closed containers. Protect from light.

Albumin tannate has been used as an astringent in the treatment of diarrhoea. It is stated to be less likely to cause gastric disturbances than vegetable astringents. It has been given in doses of 0.5 to 1 g.

Preparations

Mixtura Albumini Tannatis *(Dan. Disp.)*. Albumin Tannate Mixture. Contains albumin tannate 20% w/w with acacia mucilage and agar mucilage.

Tablettae Albumini Tannatis *(Nord. P.)*. Albumin Tannate Tablets. Each contains 500 mg of albumin tannate.

Proprietary Names

Tannalbin *(Knoll AG, Austral.; Knoll, Ger.; Knoll, Switz.)*.

294-r

Alum *(B.P., Eur. P.)*. Alumen; Potash Alum; Aluminium Potassium Sulphate; Aluminium Kalium Sulfuricum; Alumbre; Alun; Alaun; Allume; Aluin. Potassium aluminium sulphate dodecahydrate.

$KAl(SO_4)_2,12H_2O$=474.4.

CAS — 7784-24-9.

NOTE. Alum of the *B.P. 1968* was potash alum or ammonia alum, but this was amended in the *Addendum 1971*, in compliance with the requirements of the *Eur. P.*, to potash alum only.

Pharmacopoeias. In all pharmacopoeias examined, except *Braz., Int., Rus.,* and *Turk. U.S.* allows both potash alum (potassium alum) and ammonia alum (ammonium alum).

Colourless, transparent, odourless, crystalline masses or a granular powder with a sweetish astringent taste. When heated it melts and at about 200° loses its water of crystallisation with the formation of the anhydrous salt.

Soluble 1 in 7.5 of water, 1 in 0.3 of boiling water, and 1 in 3 of glycerol; practically insoluble in alcohol. A 10% solution in water has a pH of 3 to 3.5. A 6.35% solution is iso-osmotic with serum. **Incompatible** with borax, alkali hydroxides and carbonates, phosphates, salts of calcium, lead, and mercury, and with tannin. **Store** in airtight containers.

Adverse Effects. Large doses of alum are irritant and may be corrosive; gum necrosis and gastro-intestinal haemorrhage have occurred. Adverse effects on muscle and kidneys have been reported.

Treatment of Adverse Effects. Poisoning with alum should be treated with copious drinks of water and gastric lavage if vomiting has not occurred. Demulcent drinks should be given and shock alleviated if the patient shows signs of collapse.

Uses. Alum precipitates proteins and is a powerful astringent. Alum, either as a solid or as a solution, may be used as a haemostatic for superficial abrasions and cuts and ulcers on the lips. Dilute solutions havc bccn uscd as mouth-washes or gargles.

Local hyperhidrosis may be relieved by bathing the affected parts with a 2% solution of alum. Stronger solutions (5 to 10%) harden the epidermis and are useful in treating soft corns or sore feet; alum in purified talc has been used as a foot powder.

Paediatric Alum and Zinc Dusting-powder (*B.P.C. 1968*) has been employed for application to the umbilical cord; it is not suitable for use as a general dusting-powder.

Alum is also used as a mordant in the dyeing industry.

Treatment of gingival crevices with a saturated solution of alum containing 1% adrenaline acid tartrate and 0.1% sodium metabisulphate [sic] reduced crevicular exudate around crown preparations so that successful dental impressions could be made. This was more effective than mechanical techniques.— C. A. Wilson and W. M. Tay, *Br. dent. J.*, 1977, *142*, 155.

Use in food. the use of potassium aluminium sulphate is permitted in glacé cherries under the Miscellaneous Additives in Food Regulations 1980 (S.I. 1980: No. 1834) for England and Wales and the Miscellaneous Additives in Food (Scotland) Regulations 1980 [SI 1980: No. 1889 (S. 176)].

Preparations

Oculoguttae Aluminis *(Dan. Disp.)*. Alum Eye-drops. Alum (potash) 500 mg, sodium chloride 800 mg, and Water for Injections 98.7 g. Phenylmercuric nitrate 0.001% is a suitable preservative.

Paediatric Alum and Zinc Dusting-powder *(B.P.C. 1968)*. Conspersus Aluminis et Zinci pro Infantibus; Cord Powder. Alum (potash) 1, purified talc 2, zinc oxide 2. Supplied as a sterile powder in suitable envelopes containing 4 g.

Proprietary Preparations

Cordocel *(Wigglesworth, UK)*. A brand of Paediatric Alum and Zinc Dusting-powder. **Cordocel-H.** A sterile powder consisting of Paediatric Alum and Zinc Dusting-powder (*B.P.C. 1968*) with hexachlorophane 0.3%.

295-f

Dried Alum. Burnt Alum; Exsiccated Alum *(B.P.C. 1934)*; Alumen Siccatum; Alumen Ustum; Alun Calciné; Gebrannter Alaun.

$KAl(SO_4)_2$=258.2.

CAS — 10043-67-1.

Pharmacopoeias. In *Arg., Belg., Hung., Jap.,* and *Span.*

Dried alum is made by heating alum until it has lost 45 to 46% of its weight. When heated, alum liquefies at 92° and loses all its water of crystallisation at 200°; if dried above 200°, the product will not dissolve completely owing to formation of oxysulphate.

A white odourless powder or masses with a sweetish astringent taste. **Soluble** slowly, and usually incompletely, 1 in 20 of water; soluble 1 in 2 of boiling water; practically insoluble in alcohol. **Incompatibilities** as for Alum (above). **Store** in airtight containers.

Dried alum has similar properties to Alum, p.283. It is also used for preserving skins and for purifying water.

296-d

Aluminium Acetotartrate. Aluminii Acetotartras; Aluminium Acetico-tartaricum; Essigweinsaure Tonerde. A mixture of aluminium acetate and tartrate approximately equivalent to dialuminium tetra-acetate monotartrate.

$Al_2(CH_3COO)_4 \cdot (C_4H_4O_6)$=438.2.

Pharmacopoeias. In *Nord.* and *Swiss.*

Faintly yellowish translucent crystalline granules or powder with a slight acetic odour and an acid astringent taste, containing about 12.5% of Al. Hygroscopic at relative humidities above about 30%. Slowly **soluble** 1 in 1 of water; practically insoluble in alcohol, chloroform, and ether. A 5% solution in water has a pH of 3.7 to 4.4; a basic salt is precipitated on boiling. **Incompatible** with alkalis, lead salts, phosphates, and tannins. **Store** in airtight containers.

Adverse Effects and Treatment. As for Alum, p.283.

Uses. Aluminium acetotartrate is an astringent. The solution is used as ear-drops, and gauze soaked in a 1 in 10 dilution has been used as a wet dressing for suppurating wounds and dermatitis or as a local application in furunculosis.

Diluted 1 in 20 of water, the solution has been used as an astringent lotion.

An aluminium acetate solution providing 2% acetic acid was instilled into the ear canals of divers operating in conditions liable to produce otitis externa and the solution was allowed to remain in each ear for 5 minutes. Otitis externa did not develop in the divers so treated.— L. Raymond *et al.* (letter), *Br. med. J.*, 1978, *1*, 48.

Preparations containing Aluminium Acetates

Creams

Aluminium Acetate Cream Oily *(A.P.F.).* Burow's Cream. Aluminium acetate solution (*A.P.F.*) 5 ml, zinc oxide 20 g, wool fat 25 g, arachis oil 25 ml, freshly boiled and cooled water 27 ml. Makes 100 g.

Ear-drops

Aluminium Acetate Ear Drops *(A.P.F.).* Aurist. Alumin. Acet. Aluminium acetate solution (*A.P.F.*) 60 ml, freshly boiled and cooled water to 100 ml. The ear-drops should be freshly prepared.

Aluminium Acetate Ear Drops *(B.P.).* Aluminium Acetate Solution; Liquor Aluminii Acetatis; Burow's Solution. A solution of aluminium acetotartrate prepared from aluminium sulphate 22.5 g, acetic acid (33 per cent) 25 ml, calcium carbonate 10 g, and water 75 ml. Allow to stand for not less than 24 hours in a cool place, filter, add tartaric acid 4.5 g, and mix. Store at a temperature not exceeding 25° in well-filled containers. It contains about 13% of aluminium acetate.
Burow's Solution is also used in some countries as a synonym for Aluminium Acetotartrate Solution and for aluminium subacetate solutions.
A.P.F. also describes aluminium acetate solution.

Lotions

Aluminium Acetate Lotion Aqueous *(A.P.F.).* Burow's Lotion. Aluminium acetate solution (*A.P.F.*) 5 ml, freshly boiled and cooled water to 100 ml. It should be freshly prepared and used within 7 days.

Aluminium Acetate Lotion Oily *(A.P.F.).* Burow's Emulsion. Aluminium acetate solution (*A.P.F.*) 25 ml, arachis oil 25 ml, zinc cream oily, to 100 g.

Ointments

Unguentum Aluminii Subacetatis *(Nord. P.).* Aluminium Subacetate Ointment. Aluminium subacetate (8%) solution 20 g, wool fat 40 g, white soft paraffin 40 g.

Pastes

Burow's Paste *(Addenbrooke's Hosp.).* Aluminium Acetate Ear Drops 17, water 10, wool fat 23, compound zinc oxide paste 50.

Solutions

NOTE. Aluminium Acetate Ear Drops *B.P.* have the synonym aluminium acetate solution.

Aluminium Acetotartrate Solution. Solutio Aluminii Aceticotartarici *(Aust. P.)*; Aluminium Aceticum Tartaricum Solutum; Solutio Aluminii Acetici; Liquor Burowi. Prepared from aluminium sulphate 30, acetic acid 30, calcium carbonate 13.5, and water 135. Mix and allow to stand for 3 days with occasional shaking, filter, and to each 100 of filtrate, add 4.5 of tartaric acid and mix. It contains about 10.5% of aluminium acetotartrate. Similar solutions using varying proportions of ingredients are included in *Belg. P., Roum. P., Span. P.*, and *Swiss P.* (all about 10%); *Ger. P.* (6%) and *Hung. P.* (about 4.5%).

Aluminum Acetate Topical Solution *(U.S.P.).* Aluminum Acetate Solution; Burow's Solution. Aluminum subacetate topical solution (*U.S.P.*) 54.5, glacial acetic acid 1.5, water to 100, all by vol.; it may be stabilised by the addition of not more than 0.6% of boric acid. It contains 4.8 to 5.8% of aluminium acetate. pH 3.6 to 4.4. Store in airtight containers.
To be diluted with 10 to 40 vol. of water.
A similar solution is included in *It. P.*

Aluminum Subacetate Topical Solution *(U.S.P.).* Aluminum Subacetate Solution. Aluminium sulphate 14.5 g, acetic acid (36 to 37% w/w) 16 ml, calcium carbonate 7 g, water to 100 ml; it may be stabilised by the addition of not more than 0.9% of boric acid. pH 3.8 to 4.6. Store in airtight containers.
To be diluted with 20 to 40 vol. of water.
Similar solutions are included in *It. P., Jug. P.*, and *Pol. P.* In *Jug.* and *Pol.* the solution is described as Burow's Solution.

Suspensions

Suspensio Siccans *(Hung. P.).* Aluminium acetotartrate (about 4.5%) solution 3 g, boric acid 600 mg, water 21.2 g, polysorbate '20' 200 mg, glycerol 15 g, methylcellulose mucilage (2.5%) 30 g, zinc oxide 15 g, and talc 15 g.

Proprietary Names of Aluminium Acetates

Acid Mantle *(Miles, Canad.; Dorsey, USA)*; Alsol *(Athenstaedt, Ger.)*; Domeboro *(Dome, USA)*; Eddikesur lerjord *(DAK, Denm.)*; Euceta *(Gist-Brocades/Brocatrade, Neth.; Wander, Switz.).*

297-n

Aluminium Chloride. Aluminum Chloride *(U.S.P.)*; Aluminium Chloratum; Cloruro de Aluminio; Cloreto de Aluminio.
$AlCl_3,6H_2O$=241.4.

CAS — 7446-70-0 (anhydrous); 7784-13-6 (hexahydrate).

Pharmacopoeias. In *Arg., Hung., Jug., Swiss*, and *U.S.*

A white or yellowish-white, almost odourless, deliquescent, crystalline powder with a sweet, very astringent taste. **Soluble** 1 in about 1 of water and 1 in 4 of alcohol; soluble in ether and glycerol. Solutions in water are acid to litmus. **Store** in airtight containers.

Adverse Effects. Irritation at the site of application has been reported.

A 23-year-old woman whose unilateral segmental hyperhidrosis had been controlled by weekly occlusive therapy with aluminium chloride 20% in dehydrated alcohol, developed miliaria over the treated area after exertion. The miliaria resolved on discontinuation of treatment but the hyperhidrosis returned.— A. Dworin and A. J. Sober, *Archs Derm.*, 1978, *114*, 770.

Uses. A 6.25 to 20% alcoholic solution of aluminium chloride is used for topical application as an astringent and antiperspirant.

A 30% solution of aluminium chloride produced a rapid response in patients with athlete's foot. This was due mainly to its drying effect.— J. J. Leyden and A. M. Kligman, *Archs Derm.*, 1975, *111*, 1004.

Hyperhidrosis. A solution of aluminium chloride 20% in dehydrated alcohol was effective in relieving axillary hyperhidrosis in 64 of 65 patients. The solution was applied at night to the dry axilla, the axilla being washed with soap and water in the morning. After a week, applications were made only when necessary, usually every 7 to 21 days. Irritation was the only side-effect. Occlusion was not necessary.— K. T. Scholes *et al.*, *Br. med. J.*, 1978, *2*, 84. Disappointing results in 38 patients with axillary hyperhidrosis, waiting for plastic surgery, treated with aluminium chloride 20%; by the end of the sixth month of treatment 26 patients had requested surgery. The results indicated that there is a group of patients with axillary hyperhidrosis who either cannot tolerate aluminium chloride or will not respond to it.— C. R. W. Rayner *et al.*, *Br. med. J.*, 1980, *280*, 1168. Satisfactory results with few complaints of local irritation had been achieved in patients using an aqueous solution of aluminium chloride 20%.— W. F. G. Tucker (letter), *Br. med. J.*, 1980, *281*, 520. Aluminium chloride hydrolyses in aqueous solution to form hydrochloric acid; this is why the injunction to make sure that the site is absolutely dry before the solution is applied must be observed if irritation is to be avoided.— H. Yarrow, *Dermal Laboratories* (letter), *Br. med. J.*, 1980, *281*, 683. Preliminary findings indicating a similar incidence of irritation with alcoholic and aqueous solutions.— G. R. Bailie *et al.*, *Br. med. J.*, 1980, *281*, 1354. Criticism.— H. Yarrow, *Dermal Laboratories* (letter), *Br. med. J.*, 1981, *282*, 150.

Proprietary Preparations

Anhydrol Forte *(Dermal Laboratories, UK).* Aluminium chloride, available as an alcoholic solution containing 20%.

Driclor *(Stiefel, UK).* Aluminium chloride, available as a solution containing 20% in an alcoholic basis.

Other Proprietary Names

Ercoderm *(Denm.)*; Aluwets, Drysol, Xerac AC *(all USA).*

298-h

Aluminium Chlorohydrate. Basic Aluminium Chloride; Aluminium Chlorhydrate; Aluminium Chlorohydroxide; Aluminium Hydroxychloride.
$Al_2(OH)_5Cl(+xH_2O)$.

CAS — 12042-91-0 (anhydrous).

A hygroscopic granular powder; **soluble** in water; practically insoluble in alcohol, glycerol, and propylene glycol. A 20% solution in water has a pH of about 4.4. Avoid contact with metals.

Aluminium chlorohydrate is used as an astringent and antiperspirant in cosmetic products; it is less irritant than more acid aluminium salts.
Aluminum chlorohydrex (aluminum chlorhydroxide alcohol soluble complex; aluminum chlorohydrol propylene glycol complex) is under study as an antiperspirant.

Use in antiperspirant powders.— *Schimmel Briefs*, 1966, No. 375. Use in aerosols.— J. J. Martin *et al.*, *Drug Cosmet. Ind.*, 1966, *99* (Nov.), 54.

A review of antimicrobial agents, including aluminium chlorohydrate, used in cosmetics.— I. R. Gucklhorn, *Mfg Chem.*, 1970, *41* (Feb.), 30.

Use as antiperspirant.— A. B. G. Lansdown, *Soap Perfum. Cosm.*, 1974, *47*, 209. See also H. J. Spoor, *Cutis*, 1974, *13*, 180, per *Drugs*, 1975, *9*, 235.

Preparations

Aluminium Chlorohydrate and Salicylic Acid Dusting Powder *(A.P.F.).* Aluminium chlorohydrate, of commerce, 5 g, salicylic acid 3 g, purified talc, sterilised, 92 g.

Aluminium Chlorohydrate Dusting Powder *(A.P.F.).* Aluminium chlorohydrate, of commerce, 2.5 g, purified talc, sterilised, 97.5 g.

Aluminium Chlorohydrate Paste *(A.P.F.).* Colostomy Paste. Aluminium chlorohydrate, of commerce, 4 g, zinc oxide 20 g, dimethicone '350' 10 g, compound benzoin tincture 12.5 ml, emulsifying ointment to 100 g.

Proprietary Preparations

Chiron Barrier Cream *(Downs, UK).* Contains aluminium chlorohydrate 2% in an emulsified basis. For use as a barrier cream for application round the stoma of colostomy and ileostomy patients.

299-m

Aluminium Formate. Aluminium Triformate.
$Al(CHO_2)_3,3H_2O$=216.1.

CAS — 7360-53-4 (anhydrous).

White crystals. **Soluble** in water.

Aluminium formate is used as an astringent in topical preparations.

Proprietary Names

Ormicet *(Tempelhof, Ger.).*

300-m

Aluminium Subacetate. Aluminii Subacetas; Basic Aluminium Acetate.
$C_4H_7AlO_5$=162.1.

CAS — 142-03-0.

Pharmacopoeias. In *Nord.*

A white light hygroscopic powder with a slight acetic odour. It gradually loses acetic acid, becoming more basic. It contains 12.5 to 18.4% of Al and loses 8 to 17% of water on drying. Sparingly **soluble** in water; practically insoluble in alcohol, chloroform, and ether; soluble in mineral acids and solutions of alkalis. A 2% suspension in water has a pH of 4.3 to 4.9.

Aluminium subacetate has been used as a desiccant and deodorant in powders or with glycerol. Solutions of aluminium subacetate are applied for their astringent properties. Preparations containing aluminium subacetate are described under Aluminium Acetotartrate, p.284.

301-b

Aluminium Sulphate *(B.P., Eur. P.).* Aluminum Sulfate *(U.S.P.)*; Aluminii Sulfas; Aluminium Trisulphate; Aluminium Sulfuricum.
$Al_2(SO_4)_3, xH_2O$=342.1 (anhydrous).

CAS — 10043-01-3 (anhydrous); 17927-65-0 (hydrate).

Pharmacopoeias. In *Aust., Belg., Br., Eur., Fr., Ger., Hung., It., Jug., Neth., Nord., Pol., Port., Roum., Span., Swiss, Turk.*, and *U.S.*

Colourless odourless lustrous crystals or crystalline masses with a sweet astringent taste; efflorescent at relative humidities below about 25%. The *B.P.* specifies 51 to 59% of $Al_2(SO_4)_3$ with a variable quantity of water of crystallisation; the *U.S.P.* specifies 54 to 59% of $Al_2(SO_4)_3$. **Soluble** 1 in 1 of water, yielding a solution which may be opalescent; practically insoluble in alcohol. A 2% solution in water has a pH of 3 to 4. **Incompatible** with calcium and lead salts, phosphates, tannins, alkalis, and alkali carbonates. **Store** in airtight containers.

Adverse Effects and Treatment. As for Alum, p.283.

Uses. Aluminium sulphate has an action similar to that of alum (see p.283) but is more astringent. A saturated solution is employed as a mild caustic. Solutions containing 5 to 10% have been used as local applications to ulcers and to arrest foul discharges from mucous surfaces.

Aluminium sulphate is also used in the preparation of Aluminium Acetate Ear Drops (see p.284).

Proprietary Names

Stingose *(Hamilton, Austral.)*.

302-v

Ammonia Alum. Ammonium aluminium sulphate dodecahydrate.

$NH_4Al(SO_4)_2,12H_2O=453.3$.

CAS — 7784-25-0 (anhydrous); 7784-26-1 (dodecahydrate).

NOTE. Alum of the *B.P. 1968* was potash alum or ammonia alum, but this was amended in the *Addendum 1971*, in compliance with the requirements of the *Eur. P.*, to potash alum only. *U.S.P.* allows both potash alum (potassium alum) and ammonia alum (ammonium alum) under the title alum.

Colourless, transparent, odourless, crystalline masses or a granular powder with a sweetish astringent taste. **Soluble** 1 in 7 of water, 1 in 0.3 of boiling water, and 1 in 3 of glycerol; insoluble in alcohol. **Incompatibilities** and **storage** as for Alum, p.283. Fixed alkalis liberate ammonia from ammonia alum.

Ammonia alum has the actions and uses of alum (see p.283).

303-g

Arnica Flower *(B.P.C. 1949).* Arnicae Flos; Arnica.

Pharmacopoeias. In *Aust., Belg., Braz., Fr., Ger., Pol., Port., Roum., Span.,* and *Swiss.* In some pharmacopoeias the extractive is standardised against quercitin or rutin.

The dried flowerheads of *Arnica montana* (Compositae) containing not less than 15% of alcohol (45%)-soluble extractive. They have an aromatic odour and a slightly bitter taste. **Store** in airtight containers in a cool place. Protect from light.

Adverse Effects. Arnica flower is irritant to mucous membranes and when ingested has produced severe symptoms including gastro-enteritis, nervous disturbances, both tachycardia and bradycardia, and collapse. Tincture of arnica may cause dermatitis when applied to the skin of sensitive persons.

Treatment of Adverse Effects. The stomach should be emptied by aspiration and lavage if the patient has not already vomited. Demulcent drinks such as milk should be given.

Uses. Arnica has been used as a tincture for local application to bruises and sprains where the skin is unbroken and not too tender, but it is of doubtful value. It irritates the stomach and intestines and is not used internally.

The rhizome and root of arnica have also been used for similar purposes.

Arnica is used in homoeopathic medicine.

Preparations

Arnica Flower Tincture *(B.P.C. 1949).* Tinct. Arnic. Flor.; Arnica Tincture. 1 in 10; prepared by percolation with alcohol (45%). Local application may produce severe dermatitis.

Tinctures are included in *Belg. P., Fr. P., Ger. P., Pol. P., Port. P.,* and *Swiss P.*

Aust. P. and *Span. P.* tinctures include arnica flower and arnica rhizome; the alcohol content is 60 to 70%.

304-q

Bael *(B.P.C. 1949).* Bael Fruit; Bela; Bengal Quince; Indian Bael.

Pharmacopoeias. In *Ind.*

The unripe or half-ripe fruit of *Aegle marmelos* (Rutaceae).

Bael is mildly astringent and has been used in India in the treatment of dysentery and diarrhoea as a liquid extract (1 in 1) in doses of 4 to 8 ml.

305-p

Bayberry *(B.P.C. 1949).* Myrica; Bayberry Bark; Candle Berry Bark; Wax Myrtle Bark.

The dried bark of the root of *Myrica cerifera* (Myricaceae). In contains tannic and gallic acids and an acrid astringent resin. **Store** in airtight containers. Protect from light.

Bayberry is astringent and, in large doses, emetic. It has been administered in the form of an infusion or liquid extract; mixed with ginger, capsicum, and clove in varying proportions, it has been used under the name of 'composition powder' as a domestic remedy for colds and chills. It has been given in doses of 0.6 to 4 g.

306-s

Catechu *(B.P., B.P. Vet.).* Gambier; Gambir; Pale Catechu.

CAS — 8001-48-7; 8001-76-1 (black catechu); 154-23-4 [(+)-catechin].

Pharmacopoeias. In *Br.* and *Jap. B.P.* also allows Powdered Catechu. Catechu of *Chin. P., Ind. P.,* and *Port. P.* is Black Catechu from *Acacia catechu* (Leguminosae).

A dried aqueous extract of the leaves and young shoots of *Uncaria gambier* (Rubiaceae) usually occurring as dull pale greyish-brown to dark reddish-brown cubes or pale brown powder; odourless, with a taste at first bitter and very astringent but subsequently sweetish. It contains 7 to 33% of (+)-catechin and 22 to 50% of catechutannic acid with not more than 34% of alcohol-insoluble matter and not more than 33% of water-insoluble matter. It loses not more than 15% of its weight on drying. **Incompatible** with alkaloids, gelatin, and iron salts.

Uses. Catechu is an astringent and is given as an ingredient of Aromatic Chalk with Opium Mixture in the treatment of diarrhoea. It has been given in doses of 0.5 to 1 g. The tincture, diluted 1 in 25, has been used as a gargle.

Preparations

Catechu Tincture *(B.P.).* Tinctura Catechu. Catechu 1 in 5 with cinnamon 1 in 20; prepared by maceration with alcohol (45%).

307-w

Chromium Trioxide *(B.P.C. 1968).* Chromic Acid; Chromic Anhydride; Anhídrido Crómico.

$CrO_3=99.99$.

CAS — 1333-82-0.

Pharmacopoeias. In *Fr., Mex., Nord., Port., Span.,* and *Swiss.*

Odourless, deliquescent, corrosive, dark red crystals or reddish-brown flakes. **Soluble** 2 in 1 of water. **Store** in airtight, glass-stoppered bottles.

CAUTION. *Chromium trioxide is a powerful oxidising agent and is liable to explode in contact with small quantities of alcohol, ether, glycerol, and other organic substances.*

Adverse Effects. Solutions of chromium trioxide are corrosive, acting by oxidation, and solutions stronger than 5% should not be applied to mucous membranes. Repeated contact with chromium and its salts may cause eczematous dermatitis with oedema, particularly in hypersensitive persons and can also cause deep perforating ulcers known as 'chrome holes'. If inhaled, chromic dusts cause rhinitis and painless ulcers which may perforate the nasal septum; inhalation may cause severe lung damage, liver injury, and inflammation of the eyes. There may also be involvement of the central nervous system and increased risk of lung cancer. Hexavalent chromium compounds are more dangerous than di- or trivalent compounds.

Acute symptoms of poisoning from the ingestion of chromium salts include intense thirst, dizziness, abdominal pain with vomiting, anuria or oliguria, and peripheral vascular collapse. Kidney damage may lead to fatal uraemia.

Maximum permissible atmospheric concentration 50 μg per m^3.

In patch testing with a 0.5% solution of potassium dichromate, 28 of 51 workers in direct contact with chrome salts, e.g. printers and electroplaters, gave a positive result; of 97 cement workers, 46 had a positive reaction; of 103 leather workers, 5 were positive; of 64 nickel dermatitis cases, none was positive; 44 control subjects all gave negative results.— D. C. G. Betts, *Trans. a. Rep. St John's Hosp. derm. Soc., Lond.*, 1958, No. 40, p. 40, per *Abstr. Wld Med.*, 1959, *25*, 454.

In a modified 'repeated-insult' patch test, 3% chromium trioxide was found to produce moderate sensitisation of the skin.— A. M. Kligman, *J. invest. Derm.*, 1966, *47*, 393.

Of 4000 patients subjected to patch testing in 5 European clinics, 10.7% of males and 3.6% of females showed positive reactions to chromium.— H. Bandmann *et al.*, *Archs Derm.*, 1972, *106*, 335.

A report of 5 patients with allergic contact dermatitis from chromium or chromate salts.— J. N. Burry and J. Kirk, *Med. J. Aust.*, 1975, *2*, 720.

Treatment of Adverse Effects. Occupational dermatitis may be prevented by the use of protective clothing and the application of barrier creams. Following contact, the exposed skin should be washed with copious amounts of water. Following ingestion of chromium trioxide the stomach should be emptied by aspiration and lavage. The administration of dimercaprol has been suggested. Demulcents such as milk and white of egg delay absorption. If there is evidence of kidney damage care must be taken to maintain fluid and electrolyte balance.

A protective barrier cream containing sodium and calcium edetates and ascorbic acid was used successfully for the prophylaxis and treatment of allergic chromium eczema.— V. Resl and J. Sýkora, *Plzeň. lék. Sb.*, 1966, *26*, 71, per *Int. pharm. Abstr.*, 1967, *4*, 655.

Uses. Chromium trioxide is a powerful oxidising agent and caustic but it is now seldom used in medicine.

A 25 to 100% solution has been applied on a glass rod for the destruction of warts and indolent ulcers, the surrounding tissues being protected with soft paraffin. A 2 to 5% solution was formerly used in the treatment of Vincent's angina, with the warning that stronger solutions were destructive and should not be used.

308-e

Cowberry Leaf. Red Whortleberry Leaf; Vitis Idaeae Folium.

Pharmacopoeias. In *Aust.*, *Pol.*, and *Roum.*

The dried leaves of the cowberry, *Vaccinium vitis-idaea* (Ericaceae).

Cowberry leaf has astringent properties and has been used as a domestic remedy for diarrhoea and also in the treatment of rheumatic conditions.

309-l

Ellagic Acid. Benzoaric Acid. 4,4′,5,5′,6,6′-Hexahydroxydiphenic acid dilactone dihydrate; 2,3,7,8-Tetrahydroxy[1]benzopyrano[5,4,3-*cde*][1]benzopyran-5,10-dione dihydrate.
$C_{14}H_6O_8,2H_2O$=338.2.

CAS — 476-66-4 (anhydrous).

A tannin derivative which occurs free or combined in galls; it has been isolated from the juice of species of *Eucalyptus* (Myrtaceae) or it may be prepared synthetically. Odourless cream-coloured crystals or yellowish powder. M.p. above 360°. Slightly **soluble** in water and alcohol; soluble in alkalis.

Ellagic acid is a haemostatic. A solution has been applied topically to bleeding surfaces and to control capillary oozing.

Effects of ellagic acid on coagulation mechanisms and on traumatic bleeding.— E. E. Cliffton, *Am. J. med. Sci.*, 1967, *254*, 483.

310-v

Gall *(B.P.C. 1963).* Galla; Aleppo Galls; Blue Galls; Galls; Nutgall; Noix de Galle; Galläpfel.

Pharmacopoeias. In *Aust.* and *Pol.*

Excrescences on the twigs of *Quercus infectoria* (Fagaceae), resulting from the stimulus given to the tissues of the young twigs by the development of the larvae of the gall-wasp, *Adleria gallae-tinctoriae*(=*Cynips gallae-tinctoriae*) (Cynipidae). It contains about 50 to 70% of gallotannic acid.

Gall is an astringent and has been used in ointments and suppositories for the treatment of haemorrhoids. It is the main source of tannic acid.

Animal pharmacology.— M. S. Dar *et al.*, *J. pharm. Sci.*, 1976, *65*, 1791.

Preparations

Gall and Opium Ointment *(B.P.C. 1963).* Ung. Gall. et Opii. Gall 18.5 g, powdered opium 7.5 g, and lard 74 g.

Gall Ointment *(B.P.C. 1954).* Ung. Gall.; Nutgall Ointment. Gall 2 and benzoinated lard 8.

311-g

Hamamelis *(B.P.C. 1973).* Hamamelis Leaves; Witch Hazel Leaves; Hamamelidis Folia; Amamelide.

Pharmacopoeias. In *Arg.*, *Belg.*, *It.*, *Port.*, *Roum.*, *Span.*, and *Swiss.*

The dried leaves of *Hamamelis virginiana* (Hamamelidaceae), yielding not less than 20% of alcohol (45%)-soluble extractive. It contains tannins, gallic acid, a bitter principle, and a trace of volatile oil.

Uses. Hamamelis has astringent properties. Its preparations are mainly used in the treatment of haemorrhoids.

Preparations

Hamamelis and Zinc Oxide Suppositories *(B.P.C. 1973).* Suppositories containing hamamelis dry extract and zinc oxide. They are prepared with theobroma oil or other suitable fatty basis. About 1.5 g of hamamelis dry extract and 5 g of zinc oxide each displace 1 g of theobroma oil. Store in a cool place.

Hamamelis Dry Extract *(B.P.C. 1973).* Ext. Hamam. Sicc.; Hamamelis Extract. A dry extract prepared by percolation with alcohol (45%). Store in a cool place in airtight containers.

Hamamelis Liquid Extract *(B.P.C. 1973).* 1 in 1; prepared by percolation with alcohol (45%).

Belg. P. and *It. P.* have a liquid extract, 1 in 1 by weight, prepared by percolation with alcohol (60%) and (45%) respectively. *Arg. P.* uses glycerol and alcohol for percolation. *Swiss P.* uses alcohol.

Hamamelis Ointment *(B.P.C. 1973).* Hamamelis liquid extract 1 g, wool fat 5 g, and yellow soft paraffin 4 g. Store in containers which prevent evaporation. It is employed for haemorrhoids.

Hamamelis Suppositories *(B.P.C. 1973).* Suppositories containing hamamelis dry extract. They are prepared with theobroma oil or other suitable fatty basis. About 1.5 g of hamamelis dry extract displaces 1 g of theobroma oil. Store in a cool place.

312-q

Hamamelis Bark *(B.P.C. 1949).* Hamamelidis Cortex; Witch Hazel Bark.

The dried bark of *Hamamelis virginiana*, containing not less than 20% of alcohol (45%)-soluble extractive.

A local astringent and haemostatic which is usually employed as a tincture. A lotion prepared by diluting the tincture with cold water has been used for bruises, small wounds, and inflammatory swellings, and for the treatment of external haemorrhoids.

Hamamelis bark is used in homoeopathic medicine (under the name of Hamamelis virginica).

Preparations

Hamamelis Tincture *(B.P.C. 1949).* Tinctura Hamamelidis. 1 in 10; prepared by percolation with alcohol (45%).

313-p

Hamamelis Water *(B.P.C. 1973).* Aqua Hamamelidis; Liquor Hamamelidis; Distilled Witch Hazel; Witch Hazel Water; 'Witch Hazel'.

A clear colourless liquid with a characteristic odour and taste, prepared by macerating recently cut and partly dried dormant twigs of *Hamamelis virginiana* in water, distilling, and adding a requisite quantity of alcohol to the distillate. Wt per ml 0.976 to 0.982 g. It contains 13 to 15% v/v of ethyl alcohol and is neutral or slightly acid to litmus.

Uses. Hamamelis water is used as a cooling application to sprains and bruises, as a haemostatic for small superficial wounds, and for minor skin irritation. It is also used in some toilet preparations and, well diluted, as a constituent of eye lotions.

314-s

Hypericum. St. John's Wort; Millepertuis.

CAS — 548-04-9 (hypericin).

Pharmacopoeias. In *Cz.*, *Pol.*, *Roum.*, and *Rus.*

The flowering tops of the common St. John's wort, *Hypericum perforatum* (Hypericaceae).

Hypericum has astringent and diuretic properties and has been used as an infusion (1 in 20).

The herb contains a red pigment, hypericin, which causes photosensitisation; this is of some economic importance in tropical and subtropical countries, where ingestion of the herb has caused considerable losses among cattle and sheep.

Hypericum is used in homoeopathic medicine.

315-w

Kino *(B.P.C. 1949).* East Indian, Malabar, Madras, or Cochin Kino.

CAS — 8052-27-5 (kino); 1407-31-4 (kinotannic acid).

The dried juice from the trunk of *Pterocarpus marsupium* (Leguminosae), containing kinotannic acid 70 to 80%.

Partly **soluble** in cold water and alcohol; more soluble in hot water; practically insoluble in ether. Its solubility decreases with age.

Kino is an astringent and has been employed in the treatment of diarrhoea as the tincture in mixtures with chalk. The tincture has been used in gargles (1 to 16) and mouth-washes.

Preparations

Kino Tincture *(B.P.C. 1949).* Tinctura Kino. 1 in 10; prepared by maceration with a mixture of water, glycerol, and alcohol. It may gelatinise on storage due to the action of enzymes; it is incompatible with mineral acids, with alkalis, and with substances precipitable by the tannin it contains. *Dose.* 2 to 4 ml.

316-e

Myrobalan *(B.P.C. 1934).* Black Chebulic Myrobalans; Small Myrobalan; Jangi Harara.

Pharmacopoeias. In *Ind.*

The dried fruits of *Terminalia chebula* (Combretaceae) containing 20 to 40% of tannin and a greenish oleoresin.

Myrobalan is used in India and the Far East as an equivalent of gall.

317-l

Oak Bark *(B.P.C. 1934).* Quercus; Quercus Cortex; Écorce de Chêne; Eichenrinde.

Pharmacopoeias. In *Aust.*, *Hung.*, *Jug.*, *Nord.*, *Pol.*, *Port.*, *Rus.*, and *Swiss.*

The dried bark from the smaller branches and young stems of the common oak, *Quercus robur* (=*Q. pedunculata*), or the durmast oak, *Q. petraea* (=*Q. sessiliflora*) (Fagaceae). It contains 15 to 20% of quercitannic acid.

Oak bark has astringent properties and was formerly used, in the form of a decoction (about 1 in 15), as a rectal injection for haemorrhoids and as a gargle.

318-y

Potassium Chlorate *(B.P.C. 1973).* Potassii Chloras; Kalium Chloricum.

$KClO_3$=122.5.

CAS — 3811-04-9.

Pharmacopoeias. In *Belg.*, *It.*, *Port.*, *Span.*, and *Swiss.*

Colourless, odourless or almost odourless, crystals or white powder with a cooling saline taste. **Soluble** 1 in 14 of water, 1 in 2 of boiling water, and 1 in 30 of glycerol; almost insoluble in alcohol. A 5% solution in water has a pH of about 7. A 1.88% solution is iso-osmotic with serum.

CAUTION. *Potassium chlorate is unstable and, in contact with organic or readily oxidisable substances such as charcoal, phosphorus, or sulphur it is liable to explode especially if heated or subjected to friction or percussion. It should not be allowed to come into contact with matches or surfaces containing phosphorus compounds. The Council of the Pharmaceutical Society of Great Britain advises pharmacists not to supply materials likely to be used for making fireworks, including chlorates, to children under any circumstances, and recommends that they should be sold only to persons who are, or appear to be, 18 years of age or over.*— see *Pharm. J.*, 1957, *2*, 92; 1970, *1*, 296; 1975, *2*, 459; and 1977, *2*, 392.

Adverse Effects. Symptoms of acute poisoning by potassium chlorate include nausea, vomiting, diarrhoea, abdominal pain, haemolytic anaemia, haemorrhage, methaemoglobinaemia owing to catalytic oxidation, and anuria. There may also be liver damage and central effects with convulsions and coma. Concentrated solutions are irritant to mucous membranes.

Potassium chlorate was considered unsafe for use in food.— Thirteenth Report of the FAO/WHO Expert Committee on Food Additives, *Tech. Rep. Ser. Wld Hlth Org. No. 445,* 1970.

For reports of poisoning by potassium chlorate, see Martindale 27th Edn, p. 219.

Treatment of Adverse Effects. Empty the stomach by lavage and aspiration or by emesis, give demulcents or sweetened drinks, and maintain respiration. Pethidine may be given if required. A 1% solution of sodium thiosulphate may be used for lavage and may also be given by intravenous infusion. Haemodialysis, peritoneal dialysis, or exchange transfusions may be of value in removing chlorate from the blood. Forced diuresis should not be attempted if there is inadequate urine output. Methylene blue is reported by some sources to be ineffective in chlorate-induced methaemoglobinaemia, but others recommend it.

Precautions. Potassium chlorate should not be employed for more than very short periods and not at all in patients with liver or kidney impairment or blood disorders.

Absorption and Fate. Potassium chlorate is absorbed from the gastro-intestinal tract and slowly excreted in the urine.

Uses. Potassium chlorate is a mild astringent and a sialogogue and has been employed in stomatitis, tonsillitis, and other inflammatory conditions of the mouth and pharynx, usually as a mouthwash or gargle. It was formerly given as tablets in a dose of 300 to 600 mg but, as it has no useful antiseptic action, more effective and less toxic agents are now used.

The use of the chlorates of the alkali metals in cosmetics and toiletries is restricted under the Cosmetic Products Regulations 1978 (SI 1978: No. 1354).

Preparations

Potassium Chlorate and Phenol Gargle *(B.P.C. 1973).* Potassium chlorate 3 g, liquefied phenol 1.5 ml, patent blue V (CI No. 42051), food grade of commerce, 1 mg, water to 100 ml. It should be diluted with 10 times its volume of warm water before use. Protect from light.

319-j

Rhatany Root *(B.P., Eur. P.).* Krameria; Krameria Root; Ratanhiae Radix.

Pharmacopoeias. In *Arg., Aust., Belg., Br., Eur., Fr., Ger., Hung., It., Mex., Neth., Port., Roum., Span.,* and *Swiss.*

Arg. and *Mex.* allow both *K. triandra* and *K. argentea; Fr.* and *Span.* allow *K. triandra* and other species.

Br. also describes Powdered Rhatany Root.

The dried root of *Krameria triandra* (Krameriaceae), containing not less than 10% tannins. It is known in commerce as Peruvian rhatany. The root of *K. argentea* is known as Pará rhatany. Preparations of rhatany root are **incompatible** with gelatin and salts of iron. **Protect** from light.

Rhatany root has astringent properties similar to those of tannic acid and was formerly used as a lozenge for sore throats. As a dry extract it was formerly used as a suppository for bleeding or prolapsed haemorrhoids. The tincture, diluted with 12 parts of water, has been used as an astringent gargle and mouth-wash.

Uses and taxonomy.— E. S. Maurer, *Soap Perfum. Cosm.,* 1966, *39,* 164.

In a modified 'repeated-insult' patch test, a 25% extract was found to produce extreme sensitisation of the skin.— A. M. Kligman, *J. invest. Derm.,* 1966, *47,* 393.

Preparations

Krameria Dry Extract *(B.P.C. 1954).* Ext. Kramer. Sicc.; Rhatany Extract. The aqueous percolate evaporated to dryness under reduced pressure. Store in airtight containers in a cool place. *Dose.* 0.3 to 1 g.

A similar extract is included in some other pharmacopoeias.

Krameria Tincture *(B.P.C. 1949).* Rhatany Tincture. 1 in 5; prepared by percolation with alcohol (60%). *Dose.* 2 to 4 ml.

Several other pharmacopoeias include a tincture of this strength.

Syrupus Ratanhiae *(Arg. P.).* Jarabe de Ratania. Rhatany extract, powdered, 3.4 g, distilled water 5 ml, syrup to 100 ml.

320-q

Sambucus *(B.P.C. 1949).* Sambuc.; Elder Flowers; Fleurs de Sureau; Holunderblüten; Sabugueiro.

Pharmacopoeias. In *Aust., Cz., Hung., Pol., Port., Roum.,* and *Swiss.*

Pol. also includes sambucus fruit.

The dried corollas and stamens of the flowers of the elder, *Sambucus nigra* (Caprifoliaceae), together with a proportion of buds, pedicels, and ovaries. It contains about 0.3% of volatile oil. **Store** in airtight containers in a cool place. Protect from light.

Sambucus, in the form of elder-flower water, has been used as a vehicle for eye and skin lotions. Elder-flower ointment, prepared by heating fresh sambucus in melted lard, has been used as a basis for pomades and cosmetic ointments.

Preparations

Elder-flower Water *(B.P.C. 1949).* Aq. Sambuc.; Sambucus Water. Triple elder-flower water 1 vol. and water 2 vol. mixed immediately before use.

Triple Elder-flower Water *(B.P.C. 1949).* Aq. Sambuc. Trip.; Triple Sambucus Water. The undiluted elder-flower water of commerce prepared by distillation from the fresh flowers. It is a saturated aqueous solution of the volatile oil.

321-p

Sodium Chlorate *(B.P.C. 1949).* Sodii Chloras; Natrium Chloricum.

$NaClO_3$=106.4.

CAS — 7775-09-9.

Colourless odourless translucent crystals or white crystalline powder with a cooling saline taste. **Soluble** 1 in 1 of water, 1 in 100 of alcohol, and 1 in 5 of glycerol. **Store** in airtight containers.

CAUTION. As for Potassium Chlorate, p.286.

Investigations had indicated that technically pure sodium chlorate could explode under intense heat in an enclosed place; it had previously been believed that the chemical had to be contaminated by other substances before it would explode.— *Pharm. J.,* 1979, *1,* 325.

Adverse Effects, Treatment, and Precautions. As for Potassium Chlorate (p.286).

For reports of poisoning by sodium chlorate, see Martindale 27th Edn, p. 219.

Uses. Sodium chlorate closely resembles potassium chlorate (p.287) in its properties and has been used for the same purposes. It is mainly used as a weedkiller.

322-s

Tannic Acid *(U.S.P., B.P. 1973).* Tann. Acid; Tannin; Acidum Tannicum; Tanin; Gallotannic Acid.

CAS — 1401-55-4.

Pharmacopoeias. In *Arg., Aust., Belg., Cz., Fr., Hung., Ind., It., Jap., Jug., Mex., Neth., Nord., Pol., Port., Rus., Span., Swiss,* and *U.S.*

A tannin usually obtained from nut-galls, the excrescences produced on the young twigs of *Quercus infectoria* and allied species of *Quercus,* from the seed pods of tara (*Caesalpinia spinosa*), or from the nut-galls or leaves of sumac (any of genus *Rhus*). It corresponds in complexity to at least pentadigalloylglucose, $C_{76}H_{52}O_{46}$.

Commercial grades of tannic acid may contain gallic acid and being less soluble are not suitable for medicinal use.

Yellowish-white or light brown glistening scales, light masses or an impalpable powder, with a characteristic odour and a strongly astringent taste. It loses not more than 12% of its weight when dried.

Soluble 1 in less than 1 of water and of alcohol; very soluble in acetone; slowly soluble 1 in 1 of glycerol; almost insoluble in carbon disulphide, chloroform, ether, fixed oils, and light petroleum. A solution in water is acid to methyl red. Aqueous solutions decompose on keeping. **Incompatible** with acids, alkalis, salts of iron, lead, antimony, and silver, and with albumen, gelatin, gums, and oxidising agents. Tannic acid solution precipitates most alkaloids and many glycosides from solution. **Store** in airtight containers. Protect from light.

Incompatibility. For a report of an incompatibility between tannic acid and surfactants, see Nonionic Surfactants, p.370.

Adverse Effects. There have been reports of fatal liver damage following its use on burns or in barium sulphate enemas. In most of the latter instances the colon had been cleansed with a tannic acid enema before the barium and tannic acid enema. It was initially suggested that the use of tannic acid might continue provided that the concentration did not exceed 1.5%, the enema was not retained, and there had been no inflammation of the mucosa from previous treatment, but it is now no longer advocated.

Gastric irritation, nausea, and vomiting may occur after the administration of large doses by mouth. Kidney damage may also occur owing to the formation of gallic acid.

Absorption and Fate. Tannic acid is absorbed from damaged skin and mucous membranes. It is converted to gallic acid and glucose in the intestine. Gallic acid is not astringent and is largely absorbed. Gallic acid is stated to be degraded in the body and a small proportion is excreted in the urine.

Uses. Tannic acid has been used as an astringent for the mucous membrane of the mouth and throat. Suppositories of tannic acid have been used in the treatment of haemorrhoids.

Tannic acid 0.5 to 1.5% was formerly added to barium sulphate enemas to improve the quality of the pictures in the radiological examination of the colon—but see under Adverse Effects.

It was formerly used as an antidote in certain instances of poisoning but tannic acid's own toxicity makes such a use undesirable. It was also formerly applied to burns but absorption might produce toxicity. Another former use was in the treatment of diarrhoea.

Preparations

Glycerinum cum Acido Tannico *(F.N. Belg.).* Tannic acid 10% w/w in glycerol.

Tannic Acid Glycerin *(B.P.C. 1973).* Glycer. Acid. Tannic. Tannic acid 15% w/w in glycerol. Store in airtight containers.

Tannic Acid Suppositories *(B.P.C. 1954).* Suppositories containing tannic acid in theobroma oil.

Proprietary Preparations

Phytex *(Pharmax, UK).* A paint containing borotannic complex (derived by interaction from tannic acid 61% and boric acid 39%) 9%, salicylic acid 1%, methyl salicylate 0.7%, glacial acetic acid 2%, and benzyl hydroxybenzoate 0.35% in a basis of alcohol and ethyl acetate. For onychomycosis.

Ulcanon *(Wigglesworth, UK).* An application containing tannic acid 5%, sodium benzoate 0.02%, diethyl phthalate 1%, linalyl acetate 0.5%, industrial methylated spirit 70%, and water to 100%. For mouth ulcers.

Other Proprietary Names

Tannosynt (synthetic) *(Ger.).*

323-w

Tilia *(B.P.C. 1949).* Lime Flowers; Fleurs de Tilleul; Lindenblüten; Flor de Tilo.

Pharmacopoeias. In *Arg., Aust., Belg., Cz., Fr., Ger., Hung., Jug., Pol., Port., Roum., Rus., Span.,* and *Swiss.*

The dried inflorescences, with their attached bracts, of the common lime, *Tilia*×*europaea* (Tiliaceae) and certain other species of *Tilia*, collected when the flowers are fully expanded. It contains tannin and a volatile oil. **Store** in airtight containers. Protect from light.

Tilia is mildly astringent and is reputed to have antispasmodic and diaphoretic properties. Lime-flower 'tea' is a traditional domestic remedy.

324-e

Tormentil Rhizome. Erect Cinquefoil; Consolda Vermelha.

Pharmacopoeias. In *Aust., Cz., Jug., Pol.,* and *Port.*

The dried rhizome of the common tormentil, *Potentilla erecta* (Rosaceae). It contains a red colouring principle and about 10 to 15% of tannin.

It has been used both internally and externally as an astringent, usually as a tincture (1 in 5) in doses of 2 to 4 ml.

Atropine and other Anticholinergic Agents

330-s

Anticholinergic agents such as atropine mainly inhibit the responses to stimulation of postganglionic cholinergic (parasympathetic) nerves which innervate exocrine glands and smooth muscle. They are also described as antimuscarinic and as parasympatholytic agents. They prevent acetylcholine from exerting its usual action on the receptor cells; they do not diminish the production of acetylcholine.

The peripheral anticholinergic effects include increase in heart-rate, decreased production of saliva, sweat, and bronchial, lachrymal, nasal, gastric, and intestinal secretions, decreased intestinal motility, and inhibition of micturition.

The ocular effects include dilatation of the pupil, paralysis of ocular accommodation, photophobia, and increased intra-ocular pressure. The central effects consist of stimulation of the medulla and higher cerebral centres, manifested by mild central vagal excitation and respiratory stimulation, and depression of certain motor mechanisms, particularly those associated with the extrapyramidal tract.

The anticholinergic actions of compounds related to atropine are qualitatively similar but differ quantitatively in specificity of action. In particular, the quaternary ammonium compounds are fully ionised in the pH range of body fluids and possess reduced lipid solubility. They thus penetrate cellular barriers less effectively and only pass across the blood-brain barrier or into the eye with difficulty. Accordingly they may display very considerably reduced central and ocular effects when given by oral or parenteral routes while otherwise demonstrating marked peripheral effects. In compounds of this nature gastro-intestinal absorption is also poor so that the oral dose is usually higher than the parenteral dose required to achieve the same effect.

In addition to the alkaloids atropine, hyoscine, and hyoscyamine, and their salts and galenical preparations, a number of synthetic anticholinergic compounds have been developed which may be classified broadly into 3 groups according to whether they are used principally for their antisecretory and antispasmodic effects on the gastro-intestinal tract, for their depressant effects on the tremors and excessive salivation associated with the parkinsonian syndrome, or for their mydriatic and cycloplegic effects on the eye.

The synthetic anticholinergic drugs used mainly for their antisecretory and antispasmodic actions include dicyclomine, p.298, diphemanil, p.299, emepronium, p.299, glycopyrronium, p.300, poldine, p.309, and propantheline, p.310.

The synthetic anticholinergic drugs used mainly for their action on the extrapyramidal motor system include benapryzine, p.294, benzhexol, p.294, benztropine, p.295, biperiden, p.296, chlorphenoxamine, p.297, methixene, p.306, orphenadrine, p.307, and procyclidine, p.309.

The synthetic anticholinergic drugs mainly used in ophthalmic practice include cyclopentolate, p.297 and tropicamide, p.312.

Patients should be warned that such agents will temporarily impair vision; care should also be taken to avoid the accidental ingestion of anticholinergic eye preparations.

A general review of anticholinergic agents.— D. J. Greenblatt and R. I. Shader, *New Engl. J. Med.*, 1973, *288*, 1215.

Anaesthesia. A review of anticholinergic drugs used in anaesthetic practice.— R. K. Mirakhur, *Br. J. Anaesth.*, 1979, *51*, 671.

Asthma. A review of drugs administered by inhalation for the prophylaxis of asthma including anticholinergic agents.— A. J. Woolcock, *Am. Rev. resp. Dis.*, 1977, *115*, 191. See also G. M. Cochrane, *Practitioner*, 1979, *223*, 489.

Gastric and duodenal ulcers. The role of anticholinergic drugs in the treatment of peptic ulcer.— D. W. Piper and T. R. Heap, *Drugs*, 1972, *3*, 366. Further references: D. W. Piper *et al.*, *ibid.*, 1975, *10*, 56; M. J. S. Langman, *ibid.*, 1977, *14*, 105.

Irritable bowel syndrome. A review of the diagnosis and management of the irritable bowel syndrome. Anticholinergic antispasmodic agents could be of value in the treatment of the irritable bowel syndrome but most patients did not require drug therapy.— K. Goulston, *Drugs*, 1973, *6*, 237. Further references: *Lancet*, 1978, *2*, 557.

Parkinsonism. A review of drug therapy in parkinsonism. Adjunct therapy with anticholinergic agents provided additional benefit in more than half the patients obtaining a beneficial effect with levodopa; although there were essentially no pharmacological differences between anticholinergic agents some patients had marked preferences.— J. R. Bianchine, *New Engl. J. Med.*, 1976, *295*, 814. Further references: D. B. Calne and J. L. Reid, *Drugs*, 1972, *4*, 49; *Br. med. J.*, 1972, *1*, 741; *Med. Lett.*, 1979, *21*, 37.

Urinary incontinence. An account of drugs acting on the bladder and urethra, including mention of anticholinergics.— S. L. Stanton, *Br. med. J.*, 1978, *1*, 1607.

331-w

Atropine *(B.P.C. 1973, U.S.P.)*. (±)-Hyoscyamine. (1*R*,3*r*,5*S*)-Tropan-3-yl (±)-tropate. $C_{17}H_{23}NO_3$=289.4.

CAS — 51-55-8.

Pharmacopoeias. In *Ind.*, *Mex.*, *Span.*, *Swiss.*, *Turk.*, and *U.S.*

An alkaloid which may be prepared by racemisation of(−)-hyoscyamine, an alkaloid obtained from *Duboisia* spp. and other solanaceous plants, or prepared by synthesis.

Odourless or almost odourless colourless crystals or white crystalline powder. M.p. 114° to 118°. **Soluble** 1 in 400 of water, 1 in 50 of boiling water, 1 in 3 of alcohol, 1 in 1 of chloroform, 1 in 60 of ether, 1 in 30 of glycerol, and 1 in 40 of olive oil. A saturated solution in water is alkaline to phenolphthalein. **Incompatible** with alkalis, iodine, mercury salts, and tannic acid. **Store** in airtight containers. Protect from light.

For a study of the effect of the addition of water, alcohol, or dimethyl sulphoxide on the diffusion of atropine from different ointment bases, see C. W. Whitworth and R. E. Stephenson, *J. pharm. Sci.*, 1971, *60*, 48.

Adverse Effects. Side-effects of atropine and other anticholinergic agents include dryness of the mouth with difficulty in swallowing, thirst, dilatation of the pupils with loss of accommodation and photophobia, increased intra-ocular pressures, flushing and dryness of the skin, transient bradycardia followed by tachycardia, with palpitations and arrhythmias, and desire to urinate with the inability to do so, as well as reduction in the tone and motility of the gastro-intestinal tract leading to constipation. Occasionally vomiting, giddiness, and staggering may occur. Retrosternal pain may occur due to increased gastric reflux.

Toxic doses cause tachycardia, rapid or stertorous respiration, hyperpyrexia, restlessness, confusion and excitement, and hallucinations passing into delirium. A rash may appear on the face and upper trunk. In severe intoxication depression of the central nervous system may occur with hypertension or with circulatory failure and respiratory depression.

Quaternary ammonium anticholinergic agents, such as atropine methobromide and propantheline bromide, usually have some ganglion-blocking activity so that high doses may cause postural hypotension; in toxic doses non-depolarising neuromuscular block may be produced.

Systemic toxicity may be produced by the instillation of anticholinergic eye-drops, particularly in infants.

There is considerable variation in susceptibility to atropine; recovery has occurred even after 1 g, whereas deaths have been reported from doses of 100 mg or less for adults and 10 mg for children. Hypersensitivity to atropine is not uncommon and occurs as conjunctivitis or a skin rash.

Effects on the eyes. In patients with open-angle glaucoma topical application of atropine caused a prompt rise in ocular pressure. Two 600-µg doses of atropine sulphate administered by mouth did not appreciably affect the ocular pressure.— G. W. Lazenby *et al.*, *Archs Ophthal., N.Y.*, 1968, *80*, 443, per *J. Am. med. Ass.*, 1968, *206*, 906.

A 60-year-old man suffered complete blindness following intravenous injection of atropine 800 µg. After instillation of pilocarpine eye-drops his vision was gradually restored to its original level. Glaucoma was excluded on follow-up and this action of atropine was not fully understood.— J. M. Gooding and M. C. Holcomb, *Anesth. Analg. curr. Res.*, 1977, *56*, 872.

Effects on the gastro-intestinal tract. Chronic constipation with faecal impaction occurred in 8 patients taking drugs with anticholinergic actions or side-effects. The drugs included antiparkinsonian drugs, tricyclic antidepressants, and phenothiazines. The condition usually responded to change of medication, but 3 patients died.— H. Warnes *et al.*, *Can. med. Ass. J.*, 1967, *96*, 1112.

A review of published reports of paralytic ileus occurring during concomitant treatment with antipsychotic agents and anticholinergic agents.— L. C. Wade and G. L. Ellenor, *Drug Intell. & clin. Pharm.*, 1980, *14*, 17.

Effects on the heart. Atropine sulphate to a total of 1 mg per 70 kg body-weight was given in 4 doses at 5-minute intervals to 79 patients aged 6 weeks to 79 years who had no cardiovascular disease and were undergoing elective surgery. Arrhythmias, which were associated with small rather than large doses, occurred in over 20% of patients and more frequently in the young. The cardiac accelerating effect of atropine was decreased in children and in adults over 60 years of age.— P. Dauchot and J. S. Gravenstein, *Clin. Pharmac. Ther.*, 1971, *12*, 274.

Three patients, 2 with acute myocardial infarction, were given atropine sulphate 1 mg intravenously for bradycardia. Tachycardia and ventricular fibrillation occurred in 2 patients and though defibrillation was successful, the patients died from left ventricular failure. The blood pressure of the third patient fell and numerous ectopic beats were recorded. However these effects disappeared within 15 minutes. It was suggested that the initial dose of intravenous atropine sulphate should be 300 to 600 µg in patients with ischaemic heart disease.— R. A. Massumi *et al.*, *New Engl. J. Med.*, 1972, *287*, 336. In 2 patients with myocardial infarction prophylactic administration of atropine sulphate 1 mg and 0.3 mg respectively resulted in tachycardia and an increase in ischaemia.— S. Richman, *J. Am. med. Ass.*, 1974, *228*, 1414.

In a study of 30 patients with acute myocardial infarction and sinus bradycardia, atropine 600 µg given as a bolus injection intravenously increased the heart-rate and arrhythmias. When 300 µg was given as a slow infusion the bradycardia worsened.— N. G. Kounis and R. K. Chopra (letter), *Ann. intern. Med.*, 1974, *81*, 117.

In 2 studies atropine precipitated attacks of angina in patients with coronary disease.— D. Scherf, *Am. Heart J.*, 1973, *86*, 284, per *Int. pharm. Abstr.*, 1974, *11*, 618.

An elderly man with bradycardia and acute myocardial infarction developed ventricular tachycardia and ventricular fibrillation about five minutes after receiving atropine sulphate 500 µg intravenously.— M. J. Cooper and E. G. Abinader, *Am. Heart J.*, 1979, *97*, 225.

Effects on mental state. Acute confusional psychosis, accompanied by myocardial changes, developed in a woman of 33 following the routine administration of atropine sulphate eye-drops (1%) in the treatment of retinal detachment.— J. P. Baker and J. D. Farley, *Br. med. J.*, 1958, *2*, 1390. See also J. Erikssen (letter), *Lancet*, 1969, *1*, 53; E. German and N. Siddiqui (letter), *New Engl. J. Med.*, 1970, *282*, 689.

Association of postoperative delirium with raised serum concentrations of anticholinergic drugs.— L. E. Tune *et al.*, *Lancet*, 1981, *2*, 651.

Effects on sexual function. Atropine was a possible

cause of impotence.— A. J. Cooper, *Postgrad. med. J.*, 1972, *48*, 548. See also *Med. Lett.*, 1977, *19*, 81.

Effects on the skin. Therapeutic use of atropine had occasionally resulted in a violent eczema involving the whole face. Its action as a haptene antigen made it virtually impossible to desensitise to atropine.— J. S. Cant, *Practitioner*, 1969, *202*, 787.

Treatment of Adverse Effects. Empty the stomach by aspiration and lavage. The use of charcoal to prevent absorption, followed by lavage has been suggested. Give a purgative, such as 30 g of sodium sulphate in 250 ml of water.

Physostigmine salicylate has been advocated to control the central and peripheral effects of atropine or hyoscine but is not now generally recommended. Neostigmine methylsulphate only controls the peripheral effects.

Excitement may be controlled by diazepam or a short-acting barbiturate.

Supportive therapy may require oxygen and assisted respiration, ice-bags or alcohol sponges for hyperpyrexia, especially in children, bladder catheterisation, and the administration of fluids.

For comments on the use of physostigmine to reverse anticholinergic poisoning, see Physostigmine Salicylate, p.1043.

Interactions. Use of promethazine to control agitation following atropine poisoning, as advocated by A.L. MacKenzie and J.F.G. Pigott (*Br. J. Anaesth.*, 1971, *43*, 1088) was unwise since promethazine, having anticholinergic properties, might potentiate atropine toxicity.— D. J. Greenblatt and R. I. Shader (letter), *Br. J. Anaesth.*, 1972, *44*, 750.

Test for atropine poisoning. Differentiation between mydriasis due to anticholinergic agents and neurologic mydriasis could be facilitated by instillation of pilocarpine 1% into the affected eye. Pilocarpine would constrict a neurologically dilated pupil but had no effect on the atropinised eye.— R. L. Winslow (letter), *J. Am. med. Ass.*, 1974, *229*, 1863. See also J. L. Pecora (letter), *ibid.*, 1864.

Precautions. Atropine is contra-indicated in patients with prostatic enlargement and should be used with caution in elderly men. It is also contra-indicated in patients suffering from paralytic ileus or pyloric stenosis where its use may lead to obstruction.

Atropine should not be given to patients with closed-angle glaucoma or to patients with a narrow angle between the iris and the cornea, since it may raise intra-ocular pressure. The risk is greater in patients over 40 years of age and when the parenteral route is used. Systemic reactions have followed the absorption of atropine from eye-drops; overdosage is less likely if the eye ointment is used.

Due to the risk of provoking hyperpyrexia atropine should not be given to patients, especially children, when the ambient temperature is high. It should also be used cautiously in patients with fever.

Atropine and other anticholinergic agents should be used with caution in conditions characterised by tachycardia such as thyrotoxicosis, cardiac insufficiency or failure, and in cardiac surgery, where it may further accelerate the heart-rate.

Atropine may cause mental confusion, especially in the elderly. Reduced bronchial secretion associated with the administration of atropine may be associated with the formation of mucous plugs.

In the treatment of parkinsonism, increases in dosage and transfer to other forms of treatment should be gradual and anticholinergic agents should not be withdrawn abruptly. If higher doses provoke severe mental disturbances, the drug should be discontinued, but minor reactions may be controlled by reducing the dose until tolerance has developed.

Persons with Down's syndrome appear to have an increased susceptibility to the actions of atropine, whereas those with albinism may be resistant.

The effects of atropine and other anticholinergic agents may be enhanced by the concomitant administration of other drugs with anticholinergic properties, such as amantadine, some antihistamines, butyrophenones and phenothiazines, and tricyclic antidepressants.

Atropine should be avoided during treatment for urticaria.— P. W. M. Copeman, *Br. J. Hosp. Med.*, 1972, *7*, 339.

The ability of anticholinergics to cause restrosternal pain due to increased oesophageal reflux had to be remembered because it had been confused with ischaemic heart pain.— D. W. Piper and T. R. Heap, *Drugs*, 1972, *3*, 366.

A study of the effect of atropine on performance.— M. Linnoila, *Eur. J. clin. Pharmac.*, 1973, *6*, 107.

Anticholinergic drugs tended to relax the gastro-oesophageal sphincter and were therefore contra-indicated in the management of sliding hiatus hernia.— A. J. Moon, *Practitioner*, 1974, *212*, 346.

Atropine was contra-indicated in the treatment of acute pulmonary oedema complicating acute cardiac infarction.— *J. Am. med. Ass.*, 1974, *227*, 339. See also P. N. Yu and T. Biddle, *ibid.*, 338.

Interactions. *With antipsychotics.* In 9 patients receiving antiparkinsonian therapy in conjunction with antipsychotic agents, symptoms of atropine-like overdosage occurred followed by dyskinesia, visual and tactile hallucinations, and a post-delirious state of increased sleep.— H. Warnes, *Can. psychiat. Ass. J.*, 1967, *12*, 323, per *J. Am. med. Ass.*, 1967, *201* (July 31), A142.

With pralidoxime. The effects of atropine sulphate intramuscularly on heart-rate were significantly delayed when it was mixed with pralidoxime chloride solution 300 mg per ml, whereas there was no delay when atropine sulphate was mixed with pralidoxime chloride 180 mg per ml. Absorption of atropine sulphate appeared to be delayed by solutions of higher osmolarity.— F. R. Sidell, *Clin. Pharmac. Ther.*, 1974, *16*, 711.

Results of a study of 44 healthy subjects indicated that when pralidoxime mesylate and atropine sulphate were given intramuscularly mixed in the same syringe neither drug had a detrimental effect on the absorption of the other. A single injection emergency treatment of organophosphorus poisoning was feasible and possibly desirable.— P. Holland *et al.*, *Br. J. clin. Pharmac.*, 1975, *2*, 333.

With propranolol. Severe bradycardia occurred after the simultaneous administration of atropine and neostigmine, to reverse pancuronium-induced neuromuscular blockade, in a patient on long-term propranolol therapy.— D. H. Sprague, *Anesthesiology*, 1975, *42*, 208.

With suxamethonium. Of 79 patients undergoing caesarean section, 44 received atropine 0.6 to 1 mg and 35 received hyoscine 600 to 800 µg intravenously immediately before induction of anaesthesia, suxamethonium being administered for intubation. The incidence of a rise of 30 mmHg or more in systolic and diastolic blood pressure was 4 to 5 times higher following atropine premedication than with hyoscine.— J. Shah and J. S. Crawford, *Br. J. Anaesth.*, 1969, *41*, 557. Analysis of 197 records of malignant hyperthermia showed that of the 139 patients with rigidity 108 had received atropine or hyoscine with suxamethonium. None of these compounds alone was associated with such a high incidence of rigidity.— W. Kalow and B. A. Britt (letter), *Lancet*, 1973, *2*, 390.

Absorption and Fate. Atropine is readily absorbed from the gastro-intestinal tract and mucous membranes, less readily from the eye and skin; absorption may take place through the lachrymal ducts.

Atropine disappears rapidly from the blood and is distributed throughout the body. It is excreted in the urine, partly as a metabolite. Atropine crosses the placenta and traces appear in milk.

In 2 men who received 2 mg of atropine intramuscularly, between 85% and 88% of the dose was excreted in the urine within 24 hours; about 50% appeared unchanged, and over 33% was excreted as metabolites. Only a trace appeared in the faeces.— R. E. Gosselin *et al.*, *Clin. Pharmac. Ther.*, 1960, *1*, 597.

From studies in 4 subjects given radioactive atropine it appeared that, after the intramuscular injection of 2 mg of atropine, peak activity occurred after 15 to 20 minutes and heart-rate rose (after initial bradycardia in some subjects). Up to 3% might be excreted as carbon dioxide in expired air. Excretion in urine was 77 to 94% in 24 hours, mostly in the first 12 hours. About one-third of excreted radioactivity was unchanged atropine, with significant amounts of, probably, tropine. There appeared to be appreciable subject variability, and possible genetic factors merited study.— S. C. Kalser, *Ann. N.Y. Acad. Sci.*, 1971, *179*, 667. See also S. C. Kalser and P. L. McLain, *Clin. Pharmac. Ther.*, 1970, *11*, 214.

Plasma concentrations of atropine sulphate were determined by radioimmunoassay in 10 patients who received an intravenous or intramuscular injection of atropine sulphate 1 mg. Following intravenous injection there was a rapid reduction of initial plasma concentrations and it was calculated that after 10 minutes less than 5% of the administered dose was present in the circulation. Peak plasma concentrations occurred 30 minutes after intramuscular injection and atropine sulphate was still detectable after 240 minutes. Plasma concentrations after intramuscular and intravenous injection were comparable after one hour.— L. Berghem *et al.*, *Br. J. Anaesth.*, 1980, *52*, 597.

Pregnancy and the neonate. No significant quantities of atropine were found in the milk when the drug was given to lactating women.— B. E. Takyi, *J. Hosp. Pharm.*, 1970, *28*, 317. Atropine might appear in breast milk in concentrations high enough to cause anticholinergic effects in infants.— *Med. Lett.*, 1974, *16*, 27.

A study of the pharmacokinetics of atropine in mother and child in late pregnancy.— G. Barrier *et al.*, *Anesth. Analg. Réanim.*, 1976, *33*, 795.

In a study in 23 women undergoing caesarean section and given radioactive atropine by intravenous injection before delivery, the concentration of radioactivity in the umbilical vein 1 minute after administration was 12% of that in the maternal vein, reaching 93% at 5 minutes. The concentration of atropine in the umbilical artery was about half that in the umbilical vein at 5 minutes; equilibrium was reached at about 30 minutes.— I. Kivalo and S. Saarikoski, *Br. J. Anaesth.*, 1977, *49*, 1017.

Further references: I. Onnen *et al.*, *Eur. J. clin. Pharmac.*, 1979, *15*, 443.

Uses. Atropine is an anticholinergic alkaloid with both central and peripheral actions, see p.289. It first stimulates and then depresses the central nervous system and has antispasmodic actions on smooth muscle.

When given by mouth as the sulphate or methonitrate it reduces smooth-muscle tone and diminishes gastric and intestinal motility; as an adjunct to the treatment of gastric and duodenal ulcers atropine sulphate has been given in initial doses of about 500 µg thrice daily, increased gradually to the maximum the patient could tolerate without excessive side-effects. Atropine sulphate has also been used in aqueous solutions for the treatment of pylorospasm and for the medical treatment of hypertrophic pyloric stenosis in infants, although atropine methonitrate was preferred. Atropine has also been prescribed to mitigate the griping produced by vegetable laxatives, and in the treatment of smooth-muscle spasm in conditions such as renal and biliary colic. It has been used for its antispasmodic effects in bronchial asthma and whooping cough and in the treatment of enuresis.

Atropine reduces secretions, especially salivary, bronchial, and gastric secretions; it also reduces perspiration, but has little effect on the secretion of bile or milk.

Atropine has been used for its depressant action on the central nervous system, especially on certain motor mechanisms, in the symptomatic treatment of idiopathic and postencephalitic parkinsonism. It reduces tremor and muscular rigidity, improves the gait, posture, and speech, and may have a favourable effect on oculogyric crises; it also reduces sialorrhoea. Other anticholinergics such as benzhexol or orphenadrine are now preferred, together with levodopa.

Atropine depresses the vagus and thereby increases the heart-rate although in infancy and old age this effect may be less marked. It acts on partial heart block of vagal origin in young adults but has little effect in older patients with intrinsic heart disease. It has been used to prevent vagal syncope with bradycardia due to an abnormally active carotid sinus reflex, but has no effect on the cerebral (convulsive) form of attack. Bradycardia or asystole due to pilocarpine or choline esters may be overcome by an intramuscular or intravenous injection of 1 to 2 mg of atropine sulphate; considerably higher doses are necessary for the treatment of poisoning due to irreversible anticholinesterases such as organophosphorus insecticides (see Pralidoxime, p.389). Atropine sulphate has been recommended in initial doses of 300 to 600 μg intravenously, subsequently increased according to the response of the patient, in the treatment of the bradycardia of early cardiac infarction.

Atropine is given before the induction of general anaesthesia to diminish the risk of vagal inhibition of the heart and to reduce salivary and bronchial secretions. For premedication prior to anaesthesia 300 to 600 μg of atropine sulphate may be given by subcutaneous or intramuscular injection, usually in conjunction with 10 to 15 mg of morphine sulphate, about an hour before anaesthesia. Alternatively 300 to 600 μg may be given intravenously immediately before induction of anaesthesia.

Suitable paediatric premedication doses of the sulphate are: up to 65 μg subcutaneously for premature infants, 100 μg for full-term infants, 200 μg at 6 months to 1 year, and 10 to 20 μg per kg body-weight for older children, with reduced doses on hot days or for a febrile child. It may be given with thiopentone sodium before electroconvulsive therapy. Atropine sulphate 0.6 to 1.2 mg is given by slow intravenous injection in conjunction with neostigmine methylsulphate to reverse the effects of non-depolarising muscle relaxants (see Neostigmine Methylsulphate, p.1036).

Atropine is used as a cycloplegic and mydriatic. Dilatation of the pupil occurs in half an hour following one local application and lasts for a week or more; marked paralysis of accommodation is obtained in 1 to 3 hours with recovery in 3 to 7 days. It is used in the treatment of iritis to immobilise the ciliary muscle and iris and to prevent or break down adhesions. Atropine may be used as oily eye-drops, or the sulphate or methonitrate may be used in aqueous eye-drops or eye ointments. In some patients atropine may cause conjunctival irritation and for these lachesine chloride may provide a suitable alternative.

Atropine has been used in the form of liniment or belladonna plaster to relieve the pain of muscular rheumatism, sciatica, and neuralgia although there is no rationale for such usage.

Administration in renal failure. Neurological symptoms of drug intoxication were attributed to atropine in 2 patients suffering from renal failure.— G. Richet *et al.*, *Br. med. J.*, 1970, *2*, 394.

Anaesthesia. Increases in heart-rate occurred in 80 patients undergoing anaesthesia when they were given thiopentone, were intubated, or when given atropine 1.2, 1.8, or 3 mg. No difference in heart response was observed between 1.8 and 3 mg of atropine. The tachycardia was reversed by neostigmine 5 mg.— K. Kyei-Mensah, *Br. J. Anaesth.*, 1973, *45*, 507.

Some studies on the value of anticholinergic premedication.— K. M. Leighton and H. D. Sanders, *Can. Anaesth. Soc. J.*, 1976, *23*, 563; M. R. Salem *et al.*, *Anesthesiology*, 1976, *44*, 216.

Administration by mouth. The effects of atropine and hyoscine following oral and intramuscular administration were assessed in 6 healthy adults. Atropine 2 mg or hyoscine 1 mg were considered to be effective as oral premedicants. Inhibition of salivation was adequate but ocular effects were minimal. Tachycardia only occurred with atropine 2 mg. Peak effects were generally seen 2 hours after oral administration compared with 1 hour after intramuscular injection.— R. K. Mirakhur, *Br. J. Anaesth.*, 1978, *50*, 591. See also R. K. Mirakhur *et al.*, *ibid.*, 1979, *51*, 339.

In children. Children under 2 years were more sensitive to atropine than adults; the dose required to produce dry mouth had been shown to be proportional to weight. Doses based on surface area might be excessive in children under the age of 2 years.— G. S. Robinson and V. S. Williams, *Practitioner*, 1970, *204*, 5.

In ECT. Commonly used doses of atropine—650 μg—were only of placebo value in preventing vagal inhibition before ECT.— J. L. Barton (letter), *Br. med. J.*, 1974, *3*, 409. Successful use of 1.2 mg intramuscularly 1 hour before ECT.— P. H. Gosling (letter), *ibid.*

In eye surgery. Experience in 140 children undergoing squint operations confirmed that atropine 10 μg per kg body-weight given intravenously protected patients from the oculocardiac reflex. The incidence of the reflex was 25% with a mean reduction in heart-rate of 2 beats per minute in 20 patients thus treated, compared with 70% and 17 beats per minute in 20 patients given atropine intramuscularly, and 90% and 30 beats per minute in 100 given no atropine.— J. P. Alexander, *Br. J. Ophthal.*, 1975, *59*, 518.

In glaucoma. A single intramuscular dose of up to 600 μg of either atropine sulphate or hyoscine hydrobromide was considered safe for pre-operative treatment in patients with glaucoma. Pilocarpine hydrochloride 1 to 2% or physostigmine salicylate 0.25 to 1% was recommended to be instilled into the conjunctival sac to counteract any potential mydriatic effect of the belladonna drugs and the anaesthetic agent.— H. Schwartz *et al.*, *J. Am. med. Ass.*, 1957, *165*, 144.

Reversal of neuromuscular blockade. For the effects of atropine and neostigmine on heart-rate and rhythm, see V. Rosner *et al.*, *Br. J. Anaesth.*, 1971, *43*, 1066.

Asthma. A review of atropine-like drugs given by inhalation in the treatment of asthma.— *Drug & Ther. Bull.*, 1976, *14*, 85.

A prompt response was noted in a 54-year-old man with severe bronchorrhoea after treatment with atropine sulphate 400 μg by aerosol twice or thrice daily. Daily sputum volume was reduced from 300 to 450 ml to 25 to 75 ml with a dose of 1.2 mg daily.— M. M. Wick and R. H. Ingram, *J. Am. med. Ass.*, 1976, *235*, 1356.

Studies on the merits of atropine as a bronchodilator in asthma: G. J. Cropp, *J. Allergy & clin. Immunol.*, 1975, *55*, 98; D. P. Tashkin *et al.*, *Ann. Allergy*, 1977, *39*, 311; G. Kaik *et al.*, *Int. J. clin. Pharmac. Biopharm.*, 1978, *16*, 1, per *Int. pharm. Abstr.*, 1978, *15*, 770; R. M. Snow *et al.*, *Ann. Allergy*, 1979, *42*, 286.

Cardiac disorders. In the sick sinus syndrome atropine generally produces side-effects which preclude the continued use either of atropine itself or of similar drugs, and it rarely speeds the bradycardia.— *Br. med. J.*, 1973, *2*, 677.

Attacks of Prinzmetal's variant of angina, where chest pain was not induced by effort, were controlled in 1 patient by atropine 600 μg.— H. Yasue *et al.* (letter), *Ann. intern. Med.*, 1974, *80*, 553.

A detailed review of the role of atropine in patients with acute myocardial infarction and sinus bradycardia. Atropine should not be administered routinely to the bradycardic patient and the potential deleterious effects should be weighed against its benefits. A critical reassessment of the role of atropine in myocardial infarction is needed.— P. Dauchot and J. S. Gravenstein, *Anesthesiology*, 1976, *44*, 501.

Some other reports and reviews on atropine in myocardial infarction: *Lancet*, 1972, *2*, 1183; S. W. Webb *et al.*, *Br. med. J.*, 1972, *3*, 89; *J. Am. med. Ass.*, 1974, *227*, *Suppl.*, 852; M. M. Scheinman *et al.*, *Circulation*, 1975, *52*, 627; J. V. Warren and R. P. Lewis, *Am. J. Cardiol.*, 1976, *37*, 68; K. D. Chadda *et al.*, *Am. J. Med.*, 1977, *63*, 503.

Cystic fibrosis. Inhalation of atropine sulphate or isoprenaline hydrochloride decreased airways obstruction and increased flow-rates and specific airways conductance to a greater extent than a saline placebo in children with cystic fibrosis. Although atropine was generally more effective than isoprenaline it was considered that its usefulness was limited by its side-effects.— G. L. Larsen *et al.*, *Am. Rev. resp. Dis.*, 1979, *119*, 399.

Gastro-intestinal disorders. *Atropine suppression test.* In pancreatic tumours the alterations in polypeptide secretion might be the result of alterations in vagal activity. Cholinergic blockade using atropine 15 μg per kg body-weight might eliminate this and permit a useful reference interval for basal polypeptide secretion to be determined. This atropine-suppression test might be helpful in the investigation of patients with watery diarrhoea.— T. W. Schwartz (letter), *Lancet*, 1978, *2*, 326. See also J. M. Kaufman and R. Lubera, *J. Am. med. Ass.*, 1967, *200*, 197.

Pancreatitis. No evidence of benefit from atropine in mild to moderately severe pancreatitis.— J. L. Cameron *et al.*, *Surgery Gynec. Obstet.*, 1979, 148, 206.

Pyloric stenosis. The use of atropine in pyloric stenosis should be abandoned since Ramstedt's operation was curative and safe.— G. C. Robinson and V. S. Williams, *Practitioner*, 1970, *204*, 5.

Hyperhidrosis. Atropine sulphate 500 μg had a beneficial effect in 2 sisters with a new genetic syndrome of cold-induced profuse sweating over the chest and back. Propranolol in doses of up to 160 mg daily, had been ineffective.— E. Sohar *et al.*, *Lancet*, 1978, *2*, 1073.

Neurological disorders. Spontaneous daily and nocturnal attacks of respiratory arrest in a 2-year-old girl were controlled by long-term treatment with atropine sulphate whereas standard anticonvulsants had no effect.— H. Hooshmand, *Neurology, Minneap.*, 1972, *22*, 1217.

Ocular disorders. The possible arrest of myopia by the use of atropine eye-drops.— T. S. -B. Kelly *et al.*, *Br. J. Ophthal.*, 1975, *59*, 529. Comment.— *ibid.*, 527.

Atropine eye-drops 1% often gave great relief from pain in eye injuries; painful iris spasm could be relieved, and the pain of arc eye relieved.— P. A. Gardiner, *Br. med. J.*, 1978, *2*, 1347.

Pulmonary oedema. In most patients with acute pulmonary oedema, a subcutaneous injection of morphine sulphate 15 mg with atropine sulphate 600 μg was sufficient to relieve the attack. A second dose might be needed within 6 hours.— M. S. Segal (letter), *New Engl. J. Med.*, 1966, *275*, 564. Atropine was contra-indicated in the treatment of acute pulmonary oedema complicating acute cardiac infarction.— *J. Am. med. Ass.*, 1974, *227*, 339. See also P. N. Yu and T. Biddle, *ibid.*, 338.

Spider bite. Patients bitten by the black widow spider, *Latrodectus mactans*, responded well to treatment with atropine.— A. Gotlieb (letter), *Lancet*, 1970, *1*, 246.

Preparations

Atropine Oily Eye-drops *(B.P.C. 1954).* Atropine Eye Drops Oily *(A.P.F.)*; Gutt. Atrop. Oleos. Atropine 1% in sterilised castor oil.

Proprietary Names

Atropinol *(Winzer, Ger.)*; Borotropin *(*borate*) (Winzer, Ger.)*.

332-e

Atropine Methobromide *(B.P.).* Methylatropine Bromide *(Eur. P.)*; Atropine Methylbromide; Mydriasine; Methylatropini Bromidum; Methylatropinium Bromatum. (1*R*, 3*r*, 5*S*)-8-Methyl-3-[(±)-tropoyloxy]tropanium bromide.

$C_{18}H_{26}BrNO_3$=384.3.

CAS — 2870-71-5.

Pharmacopoeias. In *Aust.*, *Br.*, *Eur.*, *Fr.*, *Ger.*, *It.*, *Neth.*, *Nord.*, and *Swiss.*

Odourless colourless crystals or a white odourless crystalline powder with a bitter taste. M.p. about 215° with decomposition. **Soluble** 1 in 1 of water, 1 in 20 of alcohol; very slightly soluble in dehydrated alcohol; practically insoluble in chloroform and ether. A 5% aqueous solution has a pH to 6 of 7.5. A 7.03% solution in water is iso-osmotic with serum. Solutions are **sterilised** in the same way as atropine sulphate. **Incompatible** with alkalis, iodine, silver salts, and tannic acid. **Protect** from light.

Adverse Effects, Treatment, and Precautions. As for Atropine, p.289.

Uses. Atropine methobromide is a quaternary ammonium anticholinergic agent with actions and uses similar to those of atropine (see p.290).

Dilatation of the pupil is less persistent than after the use of the sulphate and it has been used as a 0.5 to 2% solution with 1% of cocaine hydrochloride for dilating the pupil in suspected iritis to ascertain whether or not adhesions exist. It has been given in doses of 0.5 to 1 mg, with a maximum of 3 to 4 mg being given in 24 hours.

Studies in 12 women prior to caesarean section showed that atropine methobromide crossed the placenta less readily than the sulphate.— C. B. de Padua and J. S. Gravenstein, *J. Am. med. Ass.*, 1969, *208*, 1022.

Preparations

Tablettae Methylatropini *(Nord. P.).* Tablets each containing atropine methobromide 500 μg.

Proprietary Names

Metylatropin *(DAK, Denm.)*.

333-l

Atropine Methonitrate *(B.P.).*
Methylatropine Nitrate *(Eur. P.)*; Atrop. Methonit.; Methylatropini Nitras; Atropini Methonitras. (1*R*, 3*r*, 5*S*)-8-Methyl-3-[(±)-tropoyloxy]tropanium nitrate.
$C_{18}H_{26}N_2O_6$=366.4.

CAS — 52-88-0.

Pharmacopoeias. In *Aust., Br., Eur., Fr., Ger., Int., It., Neth., Span.,* and *Turk.*

Colourless odourless crystals or a white crystalline powder. M.p. about 167°. **Soluble** 1 in less than 1 of water and 1 in 13 of alcohol; practically insoluble in chloroform and ether. A 5% solution in water has a pH of 6 to 7.5. A 6.52% solution in water is iso-osmotic with serum. Solutions are **sterilised** by filtration.

Aqueous solutions are unstable and should be freshly prepared; they must not be kept for more than 1 week. Stability is enhanced in acid solutions of pH below 6; solutions should be protected from alkalis. Alcoholic solutions are stable for 12 months but precautions are necessary to prevent concentration of the solution due to evaporation of the solvent.

Preservative for eye-drops. Benzalkonium chloride 0.01%, phenylmercuric nitrate 0.002%, or chlorhexidine acetate 0.01% were suitable preservatives for atropine methonitrate eye-drops sterilised by filtration.— Pharm. Soc. Lab. Rep., P/65/5, 1965.

Phenylmercuric borate 0.005% or chlorhexidine gluconate 0.02% were suitable preservatives for atropine methonitrate eye-drops sterilised by filtration.— M. Van Ooteghem, *Pharm. Tijdschr. Belg.*, 1968, *45*, 69.

Adverse Effects, Treatment, and Precautions. As for Atropine, p.289.

Atropine poisoning with high fever (rectal temperature 41.9°) developed in a 2-year-old boy with catarrhal illness who was given atropine methonitrate in a dose of 400 µg with each feed for a week. Atropine and its derivatives should be used with caution especially when there was a pre-existing cause of fever, as in respiratory infections.— M. J. Purcell (letter), *Br. med. J.*, 1966, *1*, 738.

Absorption and Fate. Atropine methonitrate is less readily absorbed than atropine when taken by mouth. It is highly ionised in body fluids.

Uses. Atropine methonitrate is a quaternary ammonium anticholinergic agent with properties similar to those of atropine but it has less effect on the central nervous system and for this reason it is considered to be less toxic than atropine. It also has strong ganglion-blocking activity.

It has been used in the treatment of pylorospasm of infants and congenital hypertrophic pyloric stenosis. It is given in a dose of 200 µg as 0.03 ml (1 drop) of a 0.6% alcoholic solution or as 2 ml of a freshly prepared 0.01% solution half an hour before feeds, up to 7 times during the 24 hours; flushing of the face, dry mouth, excitability, and fever call for immediate reduction of the dose. Care should be taken with alcoholic solutions of atropine methonitrate since concentration through evaporation of the solvent may seriously affect the dose. If the patient responds to this treatment the daily dose can then be increased slowly to a maximum of 600 µg per dose and continued at this level for 2 or 3 weeks after vomiting has ceased, then gradually reduced. It is essential to correct any dehydration or alkalosis before treatment is commenced.

A 0.6% alcoholic solution has also been used in the treatment of whooping cough, 0.06 to 0.4 ml (2 to 12 drops) being given at 4-hourly intervals, according to age and severity of the condition; it has been recommended that up to 0.12 ml (4 drops) may be given 4-hourly at 6 months of age.

Atropine methonitrate has been employed as an ingredient of spray solutions for the relief of asthma and hay fever, e.g. in Compound Adrenaline and Atropine Spray *B.P.* (see p.6).

Anoxic seizures. A report of the successful use of atropine methonitrate in a 2½-year-old child in whom pain-induced reflex anoxic seizures ('white' convulsive breath-holding attacks) nearly proved fatal. Although pain-induced reflex anoxic seizures are generally regarded as alarming but harmless, when total reassurance is difficult, ocular compression-testing suggests that atropine methonitrate at doses of less than 400 µg per kg body-weight daily will suppress the cardiac vagus.— J. B. P. Stephenson (letter), *Lancet*, 1979, *2*, 955.

Pyloric stenosis. For a call to abandon the use of atropine in pyloric stenosis, see under Atropine (above).

Preparations

Atropine Methonitrate Eye-drops *(B.P.C. 1963).* Gutt. Atrop. Methonit. Atropine methonitrate 1 g, sodium chloride 750 mg, solution for eye-drops to 100 ml. They must be freshly prepared by an aseptic technique. Protect from light.

Atropine Methonitrate Mixture CF *(A.P.F.).* Atropine Methonitrate Mixture for Children. Atropine methonitrate 500 µg, lemon syrup 0.5 ml, concentrated chloroform water 0.1 ml, water to 5 ml. It should be freshly prepared and used within 2 weeks. *Dose.* Infants under 6 months, 2 to 5 ml twenty minutes before each feed.

Atropine Methonitrate Nebuliser Solution *(Brompton Hosp.).* Atropine methonitrate 1 g, sodium metabisulphite 100 mg, propylene glycol 5 ml, chlorbutol solution 0.5% w/v to 100 ml. *Dose.* 0.3 ml, diluted to 2 to 3 ml, and inhaled. For intractable asthma and emphysema.

Proprietary Preparations

Eumydrin Drops *(Winthrop, UK).* A 0.6% solution of atropine methonitrate in alcohol (90%) for oral use (dilution not recommended). *Dose.* Initially, 1 to 2 drops. (Also available as Eumydrin in *Austral., S.Afr.*). CAUTION. *This solution may become concentrated through evaporation of the solvent. It should be stored in a cool place in airtight containers. If evaporation occurs during storage the solution should not be used because of risk of overdosage.*

334-y

Atropine Oxide Hydrochloride. Atropine *N*-oxide hydrochloride.
$C_{17}H_{23}NO_4$, HCl=341.8.

CAS — 4438-22-6 (atropine oxide); 4574-60-1 (hydrochloride).

Uses. Atropine oxide hydrochloride has properties similar to those of atropine (see p.289) and is used to alleviate visceral spasms. It has been given in doses of 0.5 to 1 mg twice or thrice daily. It has also been given subcutaneously in doses of 2 mg.

Proprietary Names
Génatropine *(Amido, Fr.).*

335-j

Atropine Sulphate *(B.P., B.P. Vet., Eur. P., U.S.P.).*
Atrop. Sulph.; Atropini Sulfas.
$(C_{17}H_{23}NO_3)_2$, H_2SO_4, H_2O=694.8.

CAS — 55-48-1 (anhydrous); 5908-99-6 (monohydrate).

Pharmacopoeias. In all pharmacopoeias examined except *Chin.*

Odourless colourless crystals or white crystalline powder with a very bitter taste. It effloresces in dry air. M.p. about 190° with decomposition. Atropine sulphate 1.2 mg is approximately equivalent to 1 mg of atropine.

Soluble 1 in less than 1 of water, 1 in 4 or 5 of alcohol, and 1 in 2.5 of glycerol; practically insoluble in chloroform and ether. A 2% solution in water has a pH of 4.5 to 6.2. A 8.85% solution in water is iso-osmotic with serum. Solutions are **sterilised** by autoclaving or by filtration. **Incompatible** with bromides, iodides, alkalis, tannic acid, quinine, and mercury salts. **Store** in airtight containers. Protect from light.

Adsorption. Atropine was adsorbed on to light kaolin in a dilute aqueous suspension at the rate of about 18.8 mg atropine sulphate per g of kaolin.— C. W. Ridout, *Pharm. Acta Helv.*, 1968, *43*, 42. Effect of pH.— *idem*, 177.

Effect of gamma-irradiation. Atropine sulphate was discoloured by gamma-irradiation and its melting-point was progressively depressed from 193.2° to 189.7° as the radiation dose increased. Aqueous solutions of the irradiated material were clear but off-white. Atropine Sulphate Injection (600 µg in 1 ml) was completely inactivated at 25 000 and 250 000 Gy, the colour changing to pale straw; the pH was reduced from 4.3 to 3.15 at 250 000 Gy and a solution containing chlorbutol showed a slight haze.— *The Use of Gamma Radiation Sources for the Sterilisation of Pharmaceutical Products*, London, ABPI, 1960.

An aqueous solution of atropine 0.1% irradiated at 25 000 Gy showed a decrease in pH value and a 39% decrease in atropine content. The addition of a sulphite to the solution and replacement of the atmosphere in the ampoules with nitrogen reduced the loss of atropine to less than 4%.— E. L. Pandula *et al.*, *Radiosterilization of Medical Products*, Vienna, International Atomic Energy Agency, 1967, p. 83. See also E. Pandula and E. Farkas, *Acta pharm. hung.*, 1967, *37*, 78.

Atropine sulphate 0.5% eye ointment was irradiated at 5000, 10 000, and 25 000 Gy. When prepared under clean conditions the irradiated preparations were sterile. There was no significant loss of potency, change in the basis, or evidence of interaction with the gelatin capsules used for packing.— D. J. Trigger and A. D. S. Caldwell, *Pharmax, J. Hosp. Pharm.*, 1968, *25*, 259.

Incompatibility. Methohexitone sodium 5% injection gave a precipitate with atropine sulphate injection; injections should be given in opposite arms.— J. Mokrzycki and G. Phillips (letter), *Br. dent. J.*, 1968, *125*, 432.

Stability in solution. The half-life of atropine in an ophthalmic solution at 120° had been reported to be about 1 hour at pH 6.8 and 60 hours at pH 5 (P. Zvirblis *et al.*, *J. Am. pharm. Ass., scient. Edn*, 1956, *45*, 450 and A.A. Kondritzer and P. Zvirblis, *ibid.*, 1957, *46*, 531). It was therefore very important that only neutral glass or surface-treated soda-glass eye-drop bottles were used.— W. Lund and E. G. John, *Pharm. J.*, 1969, *2*, 217.

Sterilisation of a solution. A solution containing atropine sulphate 50 mg, sodium chloride 625 mg, sodium metabisulphite 100 mg, and chlorbutol 500 mg in water to 100 ml was sterilised by autoclaving at 121° for 7 minutes in 20-ml vials made of borosilicate glass. There was no visible deterioration; assaying before and after sterilisation revealed no significant change in potency; the pH of the solution had decreased from 4.1 to 3.3.— J. T. Murphy and M. J. Stoklosa, *Bull. Am. Soc. Hosp. Pharmsts*, 1952, *9*, 94.

Atropine sulphate has the actions and uses of Atropine, p.289. It is applied topically in eye-drops and eye ointments, and is also administered by mouth in tablets, or injected parenterally in doses of 0.25 to 2 mg daily in single or divided doses (see also under Atropine, p.290).

Preparations

Eye Ointments

Atropine and Cocaine Eye Ointment *(B.P.C. 1968).* Atropine sulphate 1% and cocaine hydrochloride 1% in Eye Ointment Basis. The medicaments are dissolved in the minimum quantity of water and sterilised before incorporation into the melted sterilised basis.

Atropine Eye Ointment *(B.P.).* Atrop. Eye Oint. A sterile eye ointment prepared by incorporating, aseptically, a sterile solution of atropine sulphate, in the smallest quantity of Water for Injections, in Simple Eye Ointment. *A.P.F.* specifies 1%.

Atropine Sulfate Ophthalmic Ointment *(U.S.P.).* A sterile eye ointment containing atropine sulphate in a suitable basis.

Eye-drops

Atropine Eye Drops *(A.P.F.).* Gutt. Atrop. Sulph. Atropine sulphate 1 g, sodium chloride 700 mg, benzalkonium chloride solution 0.02 ml, disodium edetate 50 mg, Water for Injections to 100 ml. Sterilised by autoclaving.

Atropine Eye Drops *(B.P.).* Atropine Sulphate Eye Drops; ATR. A sterile solution of atropine sulphate in water. When intended for use on more than one occasion they also contain phenylmercuric acetate or nitrate 0.002% or benzalkonium chloride 0.01% and should not be used more than one month after first opening the container.

The solution is sterilised by autoclaving or by filtration, or by maintaining at 98° to 100° for 30 minutes; it is adversely affected by alkali.

Atropine Sulfate Ophthalmic Solution *(U.S.P.)*. A sterile aqueous solution of atropine sulphate; it may contain suitable stabilisers and antimicrobial agents. pH 3.5 to 6. Store in airtight containers.

Oculoguttae Atropini *(Nord. P.)*. Atropine sulphate 1 g, boric acid 1.6 g, Water for Injections 97.4 g.

Injections

Atropine Sulfate Injection *(U.S.P.)*. A sterile solution of atropine sulphate in Water for Injections. pH 3 to 6.5.

Atropine Sulphate Injection *(B.P.)*. Atrop. Sulph. Inj.; Atropine Injection. A sterile solution in Water for Injections. The solution may be adjusted to pH 2.8 to 4.5 by the addition of dilute sulphuric acid. Sterilised by autoclaving. Other pharmacopoeias contain similar injections.

Mydricaine Subconjunctival Injection *(A.P.F.)*. Atropine sulphate 1 mg, cocaine hydrochloride 5 mg, adrenaline acid tartrate 100 µg, sodium chloride 1 mg, chlorbutol 300 µg, Water for Injections to 0.3 ml. Filter through sintered glass and sterilise by autoclaving. 0.3 ml of this solution or 0.3 ml of Adrenaline Injection *B.P.* may be mixed with 0.3 to 0.6 ml of Water for Injections or 2% aqueous procaine hydrochloride to prepare a vehicle for benzylpenicillin, polymyxin B sulphate, framycetin, or gentamicin sulphate subconjunctival injections.

Mydricaine Subconjunctival Injection *(Moorfields Eye Hosp.)*. Atropine sulphate 1 mg, procaine hydrochloride 6 mg, adrenaline solution (1 in 1000) 0.12 ml, boric acid 5 mg, sodium metabisulphite 300 µg, Water for Injections to 0.3 ml. *Dose*. Not to exceed 0.3 ml. A similar injection containing half the amounts of atropine sulphate, procaine hydrochloride, and adrenaline solution is prepared for children.

Lamellae

Atropine Lamellae *(B.P.C. 1963)*. Lamellae containing atropine sulphate.

Tablets

Atropine Sulfate Tablets *(U.S.P.)*. Tablets containing atropine sulphate.

Atropine Sulphate Tablets *(B.P.)*. Atrop. Sulph. Tab. Tablets containing atropine sulphate.

Tablettae Atroscopolamini *(Nord. P.)*. Tablets each containing atropine sulphate 400 µg, hyoscine hydrobromide 100 µg, and phenobarbitone 25 mg.

Proprietary Preparations

Alcon Opulets Atropine 1% *(Alcon, UK: Farillon, UK)*. Sterile eye-drops containing atropine sulphate 1%, in single-use disposable applicators.

Isopto Atropine *(Alcon, UK: Farillon, UK)*. Eye-drops containing atropine sulphate 1% with hypromellose 0.5%. (Also available as Isopto Atropine in *Canad., S. Afr.*).

Minims Atropine Sulphate *(Smith & Nephew Pharmaceuticals, UK)*. Sterile eye-drops containing atropine sulphate 1 or 2% in single-use disposable applicators. (Also available as Minims Atropine Sulphate in *Austral., Norw.*).

Mydricaine Formula 1 *(Macarthys, UK)*. Contains atropine sulphate 500 µg, procaine hydrochloride 3 mg, adrenaline solution 0.06 ml, boric acid 5 mg, sodium metabisulphite 300 µg, and Water for Injections to 0.3 ml. For subconjunctival injection. **Formula 2** contains twice the above amounts of atropine sulphate, procaine hydrochloride, and adrenaline solution.

Mydricaine Injection *(Macarthys, UK)*. Atropine sulphate 1 mg, cocaine hydrochloride 5 mg, adrenaline acid tartrate 100 µg, sodium chloride 1 mg, chlorbutol 300 µg, sodium metabisulphite 300 µg, Water for Injections to 0.3 ml.

Other Proprietary Names

Arg.— Cicloplegyl, Midrioftal; *Austral.*— Atropt; *Fr.*— Dosatropine; *Ital.*— Liotropina; *Spain*— Atropina Miro, Sulfatropinol; *Swed.*— Isopto-Atropin.

336-z

Adiphenine Hydrochloride.

Adiphenini Hydrochloridum; Cloridrato de Adifenina; Spasmolytine. 2-Diethylaminoethyl diphenylacetate hydrochloride.

$C_{20}H_{25}NO_2,HCl=347.9$.

CAS — 64-95-9 (adiphenine); 50-42-0 (hydrochloride).

Pharmacopoeias. In *Pol., Port.*, and *Swiss.*

A white odourless crystalline powder with a bitter slightly numbing acid taste. M.p. 112° to 115°. Very **soluble** in water; freely soluble in alcohol and chlorform; practically insoluble in ether. **Incompatible** with alkalis.

Adverse Effects, Treatment, and Precautions. As for Atropine, p.289.

Uses. Adiphenine hydrochloride has been claimed to have weak peripheral effects similar to those of atropine (see p.290) together with a direct antispasmodic action and a local anaesthetic action; it has been used for the symptomatic relief of visceral spasms. It has been given in doses of 75 to 150 mg thrice daily by mouth; it has also been given in doses of 50 mg intramuscularly.

A preparation containing adiphenine hydrochloride was formerly marketed in Great Britain under the proprietary name Neuro-Trasentin (*Ciba*).

337-c

Ambutonium Bromide.

BL 700B; R 100. (3-Carbamoyl-3,3-diphenylpropyl)ethyldimethylammonium bromide.

$C_{20}H_{27}BrN_2O=391.4$.

CAS — 14007-49-9 (ambutonium); 115-51-5 (bromide).

Adverse Effects, Treatment, and Precautions. As for Atropine, p.289.

Uses. Ambutonium bromide is a quaternary ammonium anticholinergic agent with peripheral effects similar to those of atropine (see p.290). It is used as an adjunct to antacids in the treatment of gastric and duodenal ulcer and to relieve visceral spasms. The usual dose is 2.5 to 5 mg.

Ambutonium bromide is an ingredient of Aludrox SA (see p.73).

338-k

Aprofene Hydrochloride.

Aprophenum. 2-Diethylaminoethyl 2,2-diphenylpropionate hydrochloride.

$C_{21}H_{27}NO_2,HCl=361.9$.

CAS — 3563-01-7 (aprofene); 2589-00-6 (hydrochloride).

Pharmacopoeias. In *Rus.*

A white crystalline powder. Freely **soluble** in water, alcohol, and chloroform; sparingly soluble in acetone; practically insoluble in ether. **Store** in airtight containers. Protect from light.

Adverse Effects, Treatment, and Precautions. As for Atropine, p.289.

Uses. Aprofene hydrochloride is an anticholinergic agent with actions and uses similar to those of adiphenine hydrochloride (see above). It has been given in a maximum single dose of 30 mg, with a maximum of 100 mg in 24 hours.

Rus. P. also includes an injection (1% in Water for Injections) and tablets (25 mg).

339-a

Belladonna Herb *(B.P.)*.

Bellad. Leaf; Belladonna Leaf *(Eur. P., U.S.P.)*; Belladonnae Folium; Belladonnae Herba; Belladone; Deadly Nightshade Leaf; Tollkirschenblätter; Hoja de Belladona.

CAS — 8027-38-1 (belladonna).

Pharmacopoeias. In all pharmacopoeias examined except *Jap.* The *B.P.* also describes Powdered Belladonna Herb.

The dried leaves, or leaves and flowering tops of *Atropa belladonna* (Solanaceae). The *B.P.* specifies not less than 0.3% of total alkaloids, calculated as hyoscyamine; the *U.S.P.* specifies not less than 0.35% of alkaloids. It contains (−)-hyoscyamine and small quantities of hyoscine, belladonnine, and other alkaloids. **Store** in a cool dry place. Protect from light.

NOTE. When Belladonna Herb, Belladonna Leaf, or Powdered Belladonna Herb is prescribed, Prepared Belladonna Herb is dispensed.

426-k

Prepared Belladonna Herb *(B.P.)*.

Prep. Bellad.; Prepared Belladonna; Powdered Belladonna; Powdered Belladonna Leaf; Belladonnae Pulvis Normatus *(Eur. P.)*; Belladonnae Herbae Pulvis Standardisatus.

Pharmacopoeias. In *Br., Eur., Fr., Ger., Ind., Int., Neth.*, and *Turk.*

Belladonna herb, reduced to a fine powder and adjusted to contain 0.28 to 0.32% of alkaloids, calculated as hyoscyamine; about 600 µg in 200 mg.

A fine greyish-green powder with a slightly nauseous odour and a slightly bitter taste. **Store** in a cool place in airtight containers. Protect from light.

Stability in mixtures. Atropine in belladonna preparations was unstable at alkaline pH and would quickly be degraded in mixtures with a pH above 7. Such mixtures in the *B.P.C. 1968* [and *1973*] included Aluminium Hydroxide and Belladonna Mixture, Paediatric Belladonna and Ipecacuanha Mixture, Cascara and Belladonna Mixture, and Magnesium Trisilicate and Belladonna Mixture.— Pharm. Soc. Lab. Rep., P/71/9, 1971.

Adverse Effects, Treatment, and Precautions. As for Atropine, p.289.

Abuse. For reports of the abuse of belladonna and stramonium mixtures, see Stramonium, p.311.

Erythema multiforme. Belladonna had been implicated in the Stevens-Johnson syndrome.— D. B. Coursin, *J. Am. med. Ass.*, 1966, *198*, 113.

Uses. Belladonna herb and preparations of belladonna herb have the actions of atropine (see p.290). They are used in the treatment of intestinal and biliary colic and have been prescribed with vegetable laxatives to prevent griping. They have also been used in asthma, whooping cough, and bladder and ureteric spasms. A 1-year-old child may be given 0.15 ml of the tincture.

Belladonna tincture was formerly used for the treatment of enuresis; 0.15 to 0.6 ml, according to age and response, was given in the afternoon and repeated at bedtime.

Belladonna is used in homoeopathic medicine.

Preparations

Extracts

Belladonna Dry Extract *(B.P.)*. Bellad. Dry Ext. An alcoholic (70%) percolate of belladonna herb evaporated to dryness and powdered. It is adjusted to contain 1% of alkaloids, calculated as hyoscyamine; 600 µg in 60 mg. Store in a cool place in small, wide-mouthed, airtight containers.
Dose. 15 to 60 mg.
Most pharmacopoeias include a similar extract and/or a firm (pilular) extract, the specified content of alkaloids varying between 0.5 and 1.5%.

Belladonna Extract *(U.S.P.)*. It is adjusted to contain 1.25% of alkaloids. It may be in the form of a firm extract (Pilular Belladonna Extract) or a dry extract (Powdered Belladonna Extract). Store at a temperature not exceeding 30° in airtight containers.

Belladonna Green Extract *(B.P.C. 1959)*. A soft extract prepared by evaporating an alcoholic percolate of belladonna herb and adjusted to contain 1% of alkaloids. Store in a cool place. *Dose.* 15 to 60 mg.

Glycerins

Belladonna Glycerin *(B.P.C. 1959)*. Belladonna green extract 50 g, triturated to a smooth paste with boiling water 6.25 ml, glycerol to 100 g. It should be stirred thoroughly before use.
It has been applied locally to relieve pain and inflammation.

Mixtures

Belladonna and Alkali Mixture *(B.N.F. 1963)*. Mist. Bellad. Alk. Belladonna tincture 0.4 ml, sodium bicarbonate 1 g, kaolin 600 mg, chloroform water to 15 ml. *Dose.* 15 ml.

Amended formula. Belladonna tincture 0.5 ml, sodium bicarbonate 800 mg, kaolin 500 mg, chloroform water to

10 ml.—*Compendium of Past Formulae 1933 to 1966*, London, The National Pharmaceutical Union, 1969.

Belladonna Mixture CF *(A.P.F.)*. Belladonna Mixture for Children. Belladonna tincture 0.1 ml, orange syrup 1 ml, glycerol 1 ml, benzoic acid solution 0.1 ml, water to 5 ml. *Dose*. Up to 2½ years, 2 to 5 ml daily in divided doses; 2½ to 15 years, 5 to 25 ml daily in divided doses.

Paediatric Belladonna and Ephedrine Mixture *(B.P.C. 1973)*. Belladonna tincture 0.15 ml, potassium iodide 50 mg, ephedrine hydrochloride 7.5 mg, syrup 0.5 ml, liquorice liquid extract 0.15 ml, concentrated anise water 0.1 ml, benzoic acid solution 0.1 ml, water to 5 ml. It should be recently prepared. *Dose*. Children, up to 1 year, 5 ml; 1 to 5 years, 10 ml.

For a report of incompatibility when Paediatric Belladonna and Ephedrine Mixture was prepared with or diluted with syrup preserved with hydroxybenzoates, see under Sucrose, p.61.

Paediatric Belladonna and Ipecacuanha Mixture *(B.P.C. 1973)*. Belladonna tincture 0.15 ml, ipecacuanha tincture 0.1 ml, sodium bicarbonate 100 mg, tolu syrup 1 ml, double-strength chloroform water 2.5 ml, water to 5 ml. It must be freshly prepared. *Dose*. Children, up to 1 year, 5 ml; 1 to 5 years, 10 ml.

For a report of incompatibility when Paediatric Belladonna and Ipecacuanha Mixture was prepared with or diluted with syrup preserved with hydroxybenzoates, see under Sucrose, p.61.

Paediatric Belladonna Mixture *(B.P.C. 1973)*. Belladonna Mixture Paediatric. Belladonna tincture 0.15 ml, syrup 1 ml, glycerol 0.5 ml, benzoic acid solution 0.1 ml, compound orange spirit 0.01 ml, water to 5 ml. It should be recently prepared. *Dose*. Children, up to 1 year, 5 ml; 1 to 5 years, 10 ml.

Tablets

Belladonna and Phenobarbitone Tablets *(B.P.C. 1973)*. Each contains belladonna dry extract 12.5 mg and phenobarbitone 25 mg. Store in airtight containers. Protect from light. *Dose*. 1 tablet.

Belladonna Extract Tablets *(U.S.P.)*. Tablets containing the alkaloids of belladonna leaf. Store in airtight containers. Protect from light.

Tinctures

Belladonna Tincture *(B.P.)*. Bellad. Tinct. Prepared from belladonna herb by alcoholic (70%) percolation and standardised to contain 0.03% of alkaloids calculated as hyoscyamine 600 µg in 2 ml.
Dose. 0.5 to 2 ml.
The *U.S.P.* preparation is similar. Store at a temperature not exceeding 40° in airtight containers. Protect from light.
Similar preparations are included in several pharmacopoeias.

Belladonna tincture in mixtures. Some batches of belladonna tincture gave rise to a greenish deposit or scum of colouring matter when diluted in mixtures; this could be dispersed by the addition of quillaia tincture (approximately 0.5%). Alternatively, cetomacrogol '1000' (1%) might give a clear solution, but it should not be used in the presence of a high concentration of electrolytes since the cetomacrogol might be 'salted out'.—Pharm. Soc. Lab. Rep., *Pharm. J.*, 1961, *2*, 187.

Proprietary Preparations of Belladonna Herb and of Mixed Alkaloids of Belladonna

Bellergal *(Sandoz, UK)*. Tablets each containing 100 µg of the total alkaloids of belladonna leaf, with ergotamine tartrate 300 µg, and phenobarbitone 20 mg. For autonomic disorders. **Bellergal Retard**. Sustained-release tablets each equivalent to 2 Bellergal tablets. *Dose*. Bellergal: 1 to 2 tablets thrice daily. Bellergal Retard: 1 tablet morning and evening.

Bellocarb *(Sinclair, UK)*. Tablets each containing belladonna dry extract 10 mg, magnesium carbonate 300 mg, and magnesium trisilicate 300 mg. Antispasmodic and antacid. *Dose*. 1 or 2 tablets 4 times daily.

Climacteric Dellipsoids D19 *(Pilsworth, UK)*. Tablets each containing belladonna dry extract 10 mg, phenobarbitone 20 mg, and valerian extract (deodorised) 60 mg.

Other Proprietary Names

Atrobel *(Austral.)*; Bellafolin *(Ger., Switz.)*; Bellafolina *(Ital., Spain)*; Bellafit *(Switz.)*; Belap SE *(U.S.A.)*.

Preparations containing belladonna herb or mixed alkaloids of belladonna were also formerly marketed in Great Britain under the proprietary names Belladenal (*Wander*), Donnatal (*Robins*), and Fenobelladine (*Medo-Chemicals*).

340-e

Belladonna Root *(B.P.C. 1973)*. Bellad. Root; Belladonnae Radix; Deadly Nightshade Root.

Pharmacopoeias. In *Arg., Aust., Hung., Ind., Jap., Pol.,* and *Roum. Arg., Pol.,* and *Roum.* specify not less than 0.45%.

The dried root or root and rootstock of *Atropa belladonna*, containing not less than 0.4% of alkaloids, calculated as hyoscyamine. **Store** in a cool dry place.

Adverse Effects, Treatment, and Precautions. As for Atropine, p.289.

Uses. Belladonna root has the same properties as the herb but is used chiefly in preparations for external use. Liniments and plasters have been used as counter-irritants to relieve pain and suppositories have been used to relieve the pain associated with haemorrhoids and anal fistulas. Belladonna plasters were formerly applied to the lactating breast to relieve distension; their use is not advisable. Generally, when belladonna preparations are applied locally the alkaloids are not absorbed sufficiently to produce systemic effects although occasionally toxic effects may occur.

Preparations

Extracts

Belladonna Liquid Extract *(B.P.C. 1973)*. Prepared from belladonna root by percolation with alcohol (80%) and standardised to contain 0.75% of total alkaloids, calculated as hyoscyamine.

Liniments

Belladonna Liniment *(B.P.C. 1968)*. An alcoholic percolate of belladonna root adjusted to contain 0.375% of alkaloids and containing 5% of camphor. Store in a cool place.

Plasters

Belladonna Adhesive Plaster *(B.P.)*. Belladonna Self-adhesive Plaster; Belladonna Plaster. A fabric of plain weave spread with an adhesive plaster mass, which may be made porous or permeable to air, containing about 0.25% of belladonna alkaloids, calculated as hyoscyamine. The fabric may be perforated and the adhesive surface is covered by a suitable protector. It may be dyed flesh-colour.

Severe poisoning, with subsequent recovery, in a 67-year-old woman following continued self-application of belladonna plasters to her back over a period of a month.— S. R. Sims, *Br. med. J.*, 1954, *2*, 1531.

Suppositories

Belladonna Suppositories *(B.P. 1948)*. Suppositories containing belladonna liquid extract.

341-l

Benapryzine Hydrochloride. Benaprizine Hydrochloride; BRL-1288. 2-(*N*-Ethyl-*N*-propylamino)ethyl benzilate hydrochloride.

$C_{21}H_{27}NO_3$, HCl=377.9.

CAS — 22487-42-9 (benapryzine); 3202-55-9 (hydrochloride).

A white or almost white odourless crystalline powder with a bitter taste. M.p. about 166°. **Soluble** 1 in 35 of water, 1 in 56 of dehydrated alcohol, 1 in 120 of acetone, and 1 in 8 of chloroform.

Adverse Effects, Treatment, and Precautions. As for Atropine, p.289.

Anticholinergic antiparkinsonian agents do not control tardive dyskinesia associated with long-term phenothiazine (or other antipsychotic) therapy, and may exacerbate symptoms.

Uses. Benapryzine hydrochloride is an anticholinergic agent with actions and uses similar to those of benzhexol (see p.295). It is used in the symptomatic treatment of arteriosclerotic, idiopathic, and postencephalitic parkinsonism. It may also be used to alleviate the extrapyramidal syndrome induced by drugs such as the phenothiazine derivatives and reserpine (but see also Precautions). The usual dose is 50 mg three or four times daily.

Transition to or from benapryzine therapy should be gradual otherwise symptoms may be aggravated.

For *animal* studies of benapryzine hydrochloride, see B. O. Hughes and B. Spicer, *Br. J. Pharmac.*, 1969, *37*, 501P; G. B. Leslie and G. E. Conway, *Pharmacol. Res. Commun.*, 1970, *2*, 201; G. Clarke *et al.*, *Br. J. Pharmac.*, 1972, *44*, 344P.

Clinical studies: K. R. Hunter and O. P. W. Robinson, *Clin. Trials J.*, 1972, *9* (3), 3; D. J. Vicary *et al.*, *Clin. Trials J.*, 1973, *10* (1), 3.

A brief review.— *Drug & Ther. Bull.*, 1974, *12*, 67.

For reports and comments on the concurrent administration of anticholinergic agents with levodopa in patients with parkinsonism, see under Levodopa, p.887.

Benapryzine hydrochloride was formerly marketed in Great Britain under the proprietary name Brizin (*Beecham Research*).

342-y

Benzhexol Hydrochloride *(B.P.)*. Cyclodolum; Trihexyphenidyli Hydrochloridum; Trihexyphenidyl Hydrochloride *(U.S.P.)*; Trihexyphenidylium Chloride; Cloridrato de Triexilfenidila. 1-Cyclohexyl-1-phenyl-3-piperidinopropan-1-ol hydrochloride.

$C_{20}H_{31}NO$, HCl=337.9.

CAS — 144-11-6 (benzhexol); 52-49-3 (hydrochloride).

Pharmacopoeias. In *Br., Braz., Chin., Cz., Int., Jap., Jug., Nord., Roum., Rus., Turk.,* and *U.S.*

A white or creamy-white, almost odourless, crystalline powder with a bitter, tingling, and numbing taste. M.p. about 250° with decomposition. **Soluble** 1 in 100 of water, 1 in 22 of alcohol, 1 in 15 of chloroform, and 1 in 10 of methyl alcohol; practically insoluble in ether. A saturated solution in water has a pH of 5 to 6. **Store** in airtight containers.

Adverse Effects and Treatment. As for Atropine, p.289. In some patients benzhexol may produce severe mental disturbances and excitement. If minor reactions occur, the dose may be reduced until tolerance has developed, but with more severe reactions, especially psychotic disturbances, administration of the drug should be discontinued.

Abuse. Benzhexol hydrochloride had been abused by young schizophrenic patients. Several patients has presented with an acute brain syndrome after taking excessive amounts.— P. Marriott (letter), *Br. med. J.*, 1976, *1*, 152. See also K. Macvicar, *Am. J. Psychiat.*, 1977, *134*, 809, per *Int. pharm. Abstr.*, 1979, *16*, 504. See also J. S. Rubinstein (letter), *New Engl. J. Med.*, 1978, *299*, 834.

Dyskinesia. A report of 3 patients who were being treated for depression or psychoses with phenothiazines in whom benzhexol provoked or exacerbated tardive dyskinesia.— L. G. Kiloh *et al.*, *Med. J. Aust.*, 1973, *2*, 591.

A report of choreiform movements induced in a 73-year-old man following long-term benzhexol therapy for Parkinsonism.— R. W. Warne and S. S. Gubbay, *Med. J. Aust.*, 1979, *1*, 465.

Glaucoma. Two patients who had been taking benzhexol 15 mg daily for 1 to 2 years each became totally blind in 1 eye due to angle-closure glaucoma. A third patient became practically blind in 1 eye.— Z. Friedman and E. Neumann, *Br. med. J.*, 1972, *1*, 605.

Overdosage. A 34-year-old woman took 300 mg of benzhexol hydrochloride with suicidal intent; 24 hours later she developed a toxic reaction with widely dilated pupils, dry skin, and visual hallucinations. After 3 to 4 days the hallucinations were replaced by illusions; complete recovery occurred after a week, with no special treatment.— J. V. Ananth *et al.* (letter), *Can. med. Ass. J.*, 1970, *103*, 771. See also G. F. Morgenstern, *ibid.*, 1962, *87*, 79.

Psychosis. It had been estimated that 19 to 30% of patients with parkinsonism treated with anticholinergic drugs suffered from depression, confusion, delusions, or hallucinations.— *Br. med. J.*, 1974, *2*, 1.

Precautions. As for Atropine, p.290.
Anticholinergic antiparkinsonian agents do not control tardive dyskinesia associated with long-term phenothiazine (or other antipsychotic) therapy, and may exacerbate symptoms.

Interactions. States of excitement, confusion, and hallucinations were precipitated in 3 elderly patients who took benzhexol 2 mg thrice daily in addition to imipramine or desipramine.— S. C. Rogers (letter), *Br. med. J.*, 1967, *1*, 500.

A patient experienced almost total loss of teeth resulting from extreme dryness of the mouth induced by concomitant administration of benzhexol, imipramine, and diphenhydramine.— J. A. Winer and S. Bahn, *Archs gen. Psychiat.*, 1967, *16*, 239.

The side-effects of benzhexol hydrochloride were enhanced by concomitant administration of amantadine causing nocturnal confusion and hallucinations typical of anticholinergic overdose; reduction of dosage of either amantadine or the anticholinergic agent alleviated the side-effects.— R. S. Schwab *et al.*, *J. Am. med. Ass.*, 1969, *208*, 1168.

For studies of the effect of benzhexol on the plasma concentrations of chlorpromazine, see Chlorpromazine, p.1512.

Absorption and Fate. Benzhexol hydrochloride is absorbed from the gastro-intestinal tract. It disappears rapidly from the tissues.

Uses. Benzhexol hydrochloride is an anticholinergic agent with actions similar to those of atropine (see p.290). It diminishes salivation, increases the heart-rate, dilates the pupils, and reduces spasm of smooth muscle.
Benzhexol is employed mainly in the symptomatic treatment of arteriosclerotic, idiopathic, and postencephalitic parkinsonism; it is also used to alleviate the extrapyramidal syndrome induced by drugs such as phenothiazines and reserpine (but see also Precautions). Rigidity is more readily controlled than tremor and the frequency and duration of oculogyric crises are reduced. It has been used in the treatment of spasmodic torticollis, facial spasms, and other dyskinesias.
Benzhexol hydrochloride is given in 3 or 4 divided doses daily before or with food. The initial dose of 1 or 2 mg daily is gradually increased by 2-mg increments to 6 to 10 mg daily according to the response of the patient; for advanced cases, 12 to 15 mg may be needed daily; higher doses have also been used. As a rule, postencephalitic patients tolerate and require the larger doses; elderly patients may require smaller doses.
Anticholinergic treatment of parkinsonism should never be terminated suddenly and it is usual when changing from one drug to another to withdraw the one in small amounts while gradually increasing the dose of the other.
Benzhexol hydrochloride may be given with other drugs used for the relief of parkinsonism, such as other anticholinergic agents, levodopa, and amantadine; reduced dosage may be needed. In some patients it is possible to withdraw anticholinergic agents after several months without loss of control.

For reports and comments on the concurrent administration of anticholinergic agents with levodopa, in patients with parkinsonism, see Levodopa, p.887.

Administration in renal failure. Benzhexol could be given in usual doses to patients with renal failure.— W. M. Bennett *et al.*, *Ann. intern. Med.*, 1980, *93*, 286.

Preparations

Benzhexol Syrup. Benzhexol hydrochloride 5 mg, lemon spirit 0.03 ml, anhydrous citric acid 10 mg, syrup 2.5 ml, double-strength chloroform water to 5 ml. The benzhexol is dissolved in a suitable amount of the double-strength chloroform water before adding the other ingredients and making up to volume. Such a formulation is stable for 1 month when stored at room temperature.—M. Roach, *Lederle, Personal Communications*, 1978 and 1979.

Benzhexol Tablets *(B.P.).* Tablets containing benzhexol hydrochloride.

Trihexyphenidyl Hydrochloride Elixir *(U.S.P.).* An elixir containing benzhexol hydrochloride 37.2 to 42.8 mg in each 100 ml with 4.5 to 5.5% of alcohol. pH 2 to 3. Store in airtight containers.

Trihexyphenidyl Hydrochloride Tablets *(U.S.P.).* Tablets containing benzhexol hydrochloride. Store in airtight containers.

Proprietary Preparations

Artane *(Lederle, UK).* Benzhexol hydrochloride, available as scored tablets of 2 and 5 mg. **Artane Sustets.** Sustained-release capsules each containing benzhexol hydrochloride 5 mg. (Also available as Artane in *Austral., Belg., Canad., Denm., Fr., Ger., Ital., Neth., Norw., S. Afr., Spain, Swed., Switz., USA*).

Other Proprietary Names

Austral.—Anti-Spas; *Canad.*—Aparkane, Novohexidyl, Trixyl; *Denm.*—Peragit; *Fr.*—Parkinane Retard; *Ital.*—Peragit Gea, Pipanol; *Neth.*—Paralest; *Norw.*—Peragit; *Swed.*—Pargitan; *USA*—Tremin.

343-j

Benzilonium Bromide. 3-Benziloyloxy-1,1-diethylpyrrolidinium bromide.
$C_{22}H_{28}BrNO_3$=434.4.

CAS — 1050-48-2.

A white crystalline powder with an intensely bitter taste. **Soluble** in water.

Adverse Effects, Treatment, and Precautions. As for Atropine, p.289.

Uses. Benzilonium bromide is a quaternary ammonium anticholinergic agent with peripheral effects similar to those of atropine (see p.290). It has been used as an adjunct in the treatment of gastric and duodenal ulcer and to relieve visceral spasms. The usual initial dose is 10 mg by mouth thrice daily, increasing according to the patient's need; a total of more than 60 or 70 mg daily is seldom necessary.

Proprietary Names
Ortyn Retard *(Parke, Davis, Norw.)*; Portyn *(Parke, Davis, Belg.)*; Ulcoban *(Parke, Davis, Denm.*; *Parke, Davis, Swed.).*

Benzilonium bromide was formerly marketed in Great Britain under the proprietary name Portyn (*Parke, Davis*).

344-z

Benztropine Mesylate *(B.P., U.S.P.).*

Benztropine Methanesulphonate; Benzatropine Methanesulfonate. (1*R*,3*r*,5*S*)-3-Benzhydryloxytropane methanesulphonate.
$C_{21}H_{25}NO,CH_4O_3S$=403.5.

CAS — 86-13-5 (benztropine); 132-17-2 (mesylate).

Pharmacopoeias. In *Br., Nord.*, and *U.S.*

A white, odourless, slightly hygroscopic, crystalline powder with a bitter taste. M.p. 141° to 145°.
Soluble 1 in 0.7 of water, 1 in 1.5 of alcohol, and 1 in 2 of chloroform; practically insoluble in ether. Solutions for injection are **sterilised** by autoclaving or by filtration. **Store** in airtight containers. Protect from light.

Adverse Effects and Treatment. As for Atropine, p.289.
In some patients benztropine may produce severe mental disturbances and excitement. If minor reactions occur the dose may be reduced or temporarily withdrawn until tolerance has developed, but with more severe reactions, especially psychotic disturbances, administration of the drug should be discontinued.

Abuse. A report of psychosis in a 17-year-old male following suspected ingestion of an unknown amount of benztropine mesylate and a review of previous reports in the literature of anticholinergic psychosis and its treatment.— P. J. Perry *et al.*, *Am. J. Hosp. Pharm.*, 1978, *35*, 725.

Dyskinesia. Tardive dyskinesia in 3 patients taking antipsychotic drugs was aggravated by the concomitant administration of benztropine.— L. Kiloh *et al.*, *Med. J. Aust.*, 1973, *2*, 591.

Effects on the gastro-intestinal tract. A report of paralytic ileus developing in 2 patients (fatal in one) taking benztropine mesylate and mesoridazine concomitantly.— L. C. Wade and G. L. Ellenor, *Drug Intell. & clin. Pharm.*, 1980, *14*, 17.

Psychosis. Benztropine, administered in daily doses of 12, 6, and 8 mg with perphenazine and imipramine, thioridazine, and chlorpromazine respectively to 3 schizophrenic patients, produced a toxic confusional state and increased psychosis which was alleviated by the injection of physostigmine.— M. K. El-Yousef *et al.* (letter), *J. Am. med. Ass.*, 1972, *220*, 125. The doses of benztropine given to the 3 patients mentioned were much higher than was usual for the treatment of drug-induced parkinsonism and could have contributed to the psychoses which occurred.— M. R. Weinstein and A. Fischer (letter), *ibid.*, 1616.

Precautions. As for Atropine, p.290.
Benztropine causes drowsiness and patients receiving it should not take charge of vehicles or machinery where loss of attention could lead to accidents. Anticholinergic antiparkinsonian agents do not control tardive dyskinesia associated with long-term phenothiazine (or other antipsychotic) therapy, and may exacerbate symptoms.

For a severe criticism of the hazardous practice of concomitantly administering benztropine parenterally with haloperidol in rapid treatment of acute psychosis, see Haloperidol, p.1534.

Interactions. The side-effects of benztropine mesylate were enhanced by concomitant administration of amantadine causing nocturnal confusion and hallucinations typical of anticholinergic overdose; reduction of dosage of either amantadine or the anticholinergic agent alleviated the side-effects.— R. S. Schwab *et al.*, *J. Am. med. Ass.*, 1969, *208*, 1168.

A 45-year-old woman taking chlorpromazine 500 mg, chlorprothixene 200 mg, and benztropine mesylate 6 mg daily, a 25-year-old man taking chlorpromazine 150 mg, trifluoperazine hydrochloride 3 mg, and benztropine 500 µg all four times a day, and a 41-year-old woman treated with haloperidol 2 mg four times a day and benztropine 1 mg twice daily, developed hyperpyrexia attributed to the additive effect of chlorpromazine and benztropine in the first 2 cases and to benztropine in the third. All 3 recovered without incident.— R. J. Westlake and A. Rastegar, *J. Am. med. Ass.*, 1973, *225*, 1250.

Absorption and Fate. Benztropine mesylate is absorbed from the gastro-intestinal tract and has a prolonged duration of action and a cumulative effect.

Uses. Benztropine mesylate is an anticholinergic agent with actions and uses similar to those of benzhexol (see p.295); it also has antihistaminic and local anaesthetic properties. It is used for the symptomatic treatment of arteriosclerotic, idiopathic, and postencephalitic parkinsonism. It may be preferred to benzhexol hydrochloride since, in normal doses, it has sedative effects. It is also used to alleviate the extrapyramidal syndrome induced by drugs such as the phenothiazine derivatives and reserpine (but see also Precautions).
Benztropine mesylate is given by mouth, the usual initial daily dose of 0.5 to 1 mg being gradually increased by 500 µg every 5 to 6 days until the optimum dose for each individual patient is reached. This is usually 2 to 6 mg a day, and may be given as a single dose or in divided doses according to the requirements and tolerance of the patient. In emergency, benztropine mesylate may be injected intramuscularly or intravenously in a dose of 1 to 2 mg; intramuscular administration is reported to produce an effect as quickly as intravenous administration. Transition to or from benztropine therapy should be gradual otherwise symptoms may be aggravated.

Extrapyramidal effects. A 2-week open study comparing amantadine, benztropine, and ethopropazine in 45 psychiatric patients with neuroleptic-induced extrapyramidal signs; although all 3 drugs significantly improved the symptoms they did not completely control them, demonstrating the limitations of available therapy. Toxic psychosis required withdrawal of 1 patient in the benztropine group and 2 in the ethopropazine group; another patient in the ethopropazine group was withdrawn because of epigastric distress.— J. Ananth *et al.*, *Int. J. clin. Pharmac. Biopharm.*, 1975, *11*, 323.

Benztropine did not appear to prevent chlorpromazine-induced extrapyramidal effects; there was an incidence of 9.3% in 86 patients taking chlorpromazine and benztropine compared with 10.6% in 568 patients taking chlorpromazine alone.— C. Swett *et al.*, *Archs gen. Psychiat.*, 1977, *34*, 942. In a 12-week controlled study ethopropazine hydrochloride and benztropine were equally effective in controlling neuroleptic-induced parkinsonian symptoms in 56 schizophrenic patients receiving maintenance treatment with fluphenazine enanthate and both were as effective as previous treatment with procyclidine. However, patients receiving benztropine had a significant increase in tardive dyskinesia compared with procyclidine treatment and they also experienced significantly more anxiety and depression than patients receiving ethopropazine.— G. Chouinard *et al.*, *J. clin. Psychiat.*, 1979, *40*, 147.

See also Precautions (above).

Hyperkinesis. Two of 3 hyperkinetic children improved moderately when given benztropine.— J. S. Carman and L. S. Tucker (letter), *Lancet*, 1973, *2*, 1337.

Parkinsonism. For reports and comments on the concurrent administration of anticholinergic agents with levodopa, in patients with parkinsonism, see under Levodopa, p.887.

Preparations

Benztropine Injection *(B.P.)*. A sterile solution of benztropine mesylate in Water for Injections. Sterilised by autoclaving. pH 5.5 to 6.5.

Benztropine Mesylate Injection *(U.S.P.)*. A sterile solution in Water for Injections. pH 5.5 to 6.5.

Benztropine Mesylate Tablets *(U.S.P.)*. Tablets containing benztropine mesylate.

Benztropine Tablets *(B.P.)*. Tablets containing benztropine mesylate. Store in a cool place in airtight containers. Protect from light.

Proprietary Preparations

Cogentin *(Merck Sharp & Dohme, UK)*. Benztropine mesylate, available as **Injection** containing 1 mg per ml in ampoules of 2 ml, and as scored **Tablets** of 2 mg. (Also available as Cogentin in *Austral.*, *Belg.*, *Canad.*, *Denm.*, *Neth.*, *Norw.*, *Swed.*, *USA*).

Other Proprietary Names

Bensylate *(Canad.)*; Cogentine *(Fr.)*; Cogentinol *(Ger.)*.

345-c

Bevonium Methylsulphate. CG 201; Bevonium Metilsulfate; Bevonum Metylsulfat; Piribenzyl Methyl Sulphate. 2-Benziloyloxymethyl-1,1-dimethylpiperidinium methylsulphate.
$C_{22}H_{28}NO_3,CH_3O_4S$=465.6.

CAS — 33371-53-8 (bevonium); 5205-82-3 (methylsulphate).

A white, odourless, crystalline powder with a bitter taste. M.p. 133° to 136°. Readily **soluble** in water, alcohol, and methyl alcohol; soluble with difficulty in ether and acetone.

Adverse Effects, Treatment, and Precautions. As for Atropine, p.289.

Uses. Bevonium methylsulphate is a quaternary ammonium anticholinergic agent with peripheral effects similar to those of atropine (see p.290). It has been given in the symptomatic treatment of visceral spasms in doses of 50 to 100 mg twice or thrice daily.

Pharmacological and toxicity studies in *animals*.— G. Osterloh *et al.*, *Arzneimittel-Forsch.*, 1966, *16*, 901; R. Beckmann, *ibid.*, 910.

Clinical studies.— H. A. Dittmar and H. Wohlenberg, *Arzneimittel-Forsch.*, 1966, *16*, 919; W. Günther, *ibid.*, 923; B. von Rütte, *ibid.*, 929; F. Jurczok, *ibid.*, 935; H. Appelt, *ibid.*, 936; E. G. Schenck and G. Michael, *ibid.*, 939.

Proprietary Names

Acabel *(Grünenthal, Ger.; Grünenthal, S.Afr.; Sigmatau, Ital.)*; Dalys *(Landó, Arg.)*; Spalgo *(Scharper, Ital.)*.

346-k

Biperiden *(B.P., U.S.P.)*. 1-(Bicyclo[2.2.1]hept-5-en-2-yl)-1-phenyl-3-piperidinopropan-1-ol.
$C_{21}H_{29}NO$=311.5.

CAS — 514-65-8.

Pharmacopoeias. In *Br.* and *U.S.*

A white or almost white, odourless or almost odourless, crystalline powder. M.p. 112° to 116°. Practically **insoluble** in water; soluble 1 in 75 of alcohol, 1 in 2 of chloroform, and 1 in 14 of ether. **Protect** from light.

347-a

Biperiden Hydrochloride *(U.S.P.)*.
$C_{21}H_{29}NO,HCl$=347.9.

CAS — 1235-82-1.

Pharmacopoeias. In *U.S.*

A white, almost odourless, crystalline powder. M.p. about 275° with decomposition.

Slightly **soluble** in water, alcohol, chloroform, and ether; sparingly soluble in methyl alcohol. **Protect** from light.

348-t

Biperiden Lactate.
$C_{21}H_{29}NO,C_3H_6O_3$=401.5.

CAS — 7085-45-2.

Adverse Effects, Treatment, and Precautions. As for Atropine, p.289.

Parenteral administration may be followed by slight transient hypotension.

Biperiden may cause drowsiness and patients should not take charge of vehicles or machinery where loss of attention could cause accidents.

Anticholinergic antiparkinsonian agents do not control tardive dyskinesia associated with long-term phenothiazine (or other antipsychotic) therapy, and may exacerbate symptoms.

Control of lysergide-induced psychosis by administration of chlorpromazine, was lost when biperiden was given concurrently.— L. Tec (letter), *J. Am. med. Ass.*, 1971, *215*, 980.

Uses. Biperiden is an anticholinergic agent with actions and uses similar to those of benzhexol (see p.295). It is used in the symptomatic treatment of arteriosclerotic, idiopathic, and postencephalitic parkinsonism. It may also be used to alleviate the extrapyramidal syndrome induced by drugs such as the phenothiazine derivatives and reserpine (but see also Precautions).

Biperiden is administered by mouth as the hydrochloride and by injection as the lactate.

The initial dose by mouth is 1 mg of the hydrochloride twice daily, gradually increased to 2 mg thrice daily during or after meals. After several days the dose is further increased to find that most suited to the needs of the patient. The optimum maintenance dosage varies from 1 to 4 mg thrice daily.

For a rapid effect in acute drug-induced dystonic reactions biperiden lactate 2 mg may be given intramuscularly and repeated every 30 minutes if needed, or 5 mg may be given by slow intravenous injection; up to 20 mg daily has been given.

Transition to or from biperiden therapy should be gradual, otherwise symptoms may be aggravated.

Extrapyramidal effects. A report of the long-term use of biperiden in the treatment of drug-induced extrapyramidal effects.— N. S. Kline *et al.*, *Curr. ther. Res.*, 1974, *16*, 838. See also Precautions (above).

Parkinsonism. For reports and comments on the concurrent administration of anticholinergic agents with levodopa, in patients with parkinsonism, see under Levodopa, p.887.

Postherpetic neuralgia. A 63-year-old woman with postherpetic neuralgia became completely free of pain 2 days after taking biperiden in a dosage of 2 mg morning and night by mouth. However, she stopped taking the preparation because of side-effects and the pain returned. Biperiden was restarted and despite dizziness the patient took 3 mg daily for 2 weeks with complete relief which persisted after discontinuing biperiden.— G. A. Lang, *Med. J. Aust.*, 1968, *1*, 350.

Preparations

Biperiden Hydrochloride Tablets *(U.S.P.)*. Tablets containing biperiden hydrochloride. Store in airtight containers.

Biperiden Lactate Injection *(B.P., U.S.P.)*. Biperiden Injection. A sterile solution in Water for Injections prepared from biperiden and lactic acid. The solution contains a suitable buffering agent. pH 4.5 to 5.8. Sterilise by autoclaving; protect from light.

Akineton *(Abbott, UK)*. **Ampoules** of 1 ml of an injection containing biperiden lactate 5 mg per ml and scored **Tablets** each containing biperiden hydrochloride 2 mg. (Also available as Akineton in *Arg.*, *Austral.*, *Belg.*, *Canad.*, *Denm.*, *Fr.*, *Ger.*, *Ital.*, *Neth.*, *Norw.*, *S.Afr.*, *Spain*, *Swed.*, *Switz.*, *USA*).

Other Proprietary Names

Akinophyl *(Fr.)*; Tasmolin *(Jap.)*(both hydrochloride).

349-x

Bornaprine Hydrochloride. 3-Diethylaminopropyl 2-phenylbicyclo[2.2.1]heptane-2-carboxylate hydrochloride.
$C_{21}H_{31}NO_2,HCl$=365.9.

CAS — 20448-86-6 (bornaprine); 26908-91-8 (hydrochloride).

An almost white crystalline powder with a faint odour and a bitter taste. M.p. about 149°. **Soluble** in water, alcohol, and chloroform; sparingly soluble in ether.

Uses. Bornaprine hydrochloride is an anticholinergic agent with actions and uses similar to those of benzhexol (see p.294) but it is claimed to be mainly effective against tremor. It is used in initial doses of 2 mg daily gradually increased to 6 to 12 mg daily.

Proprietary Names

Sormodren *(Knoll, Ger.)*.

350-y

Butropium Bromide. (−)-(1*R*,3*r*,5*S*)-8-(4-Butoxybenzyl)-3-[(*S*)-tropoyloxy]tropanium bromide.
$C_{28}H_{38}BrNO_4$=532.5.

CAS — 29025-14-7.

White crystals or crystalline powder with a bitter taste. M.p. about 166°. Slightly **soluble** in water, and in dilute solutions of hydrochloric acid and sodium hydroxide; sparingly soluble in alcohol; soluble in chloroform and dimethylformamide; practically insoluble in acetone and ether; freely soluble in glacial acetic acid.

Adverse Effects, Treatment, and Precautions. As for Atropine, p.289.

A report of 2 patients who suffered shock symptoms and subsequently died after receiving butropium bromide 4 mg intramuscularly.— *Japan med. Gaz.*, 1979, *16* (Jan. 20), 10.

Uses. Butropium bromide is a quaternary ammonium anticholinergic agent with peripheral effects similar to those of atropine (see p.290). It has been used in the symptomatic treatment of visceral spasms in a dose of 10 mg thrice daily by mouth; it has also been given in a dose of 4 mg daily subcutaneously.

Proprietary Names

Coliopan *(Eisai, Jap.)*.

351-j

Buzepide Metiodide. FI 6146; R 661; Diphexamide Iodomethylate; Metazepium Iodide. 1-(3-Carbamoyl-3,3-diphenylpropyl)-1-methylperhydroazepinium iodide.
$C_{23}H_{31}IN_2O$=478.4.

CAS — 15351-05-0.

Crystals. M.p. 212° to 213° with decomposition.

Adverse Effects, Treatment, and Precautions. As for Atropine, p.289.

Uses. Buzepide metiodide is a quaternary ammonium anticholinergic agent with peripheral effects similar to those of atropine (see p.290). It has been given with other compounds for the relief of visceral spasms and of rhinitis.

352-z

Caramiphen Hydrochloride *(B.P. 1968)*. 2-Diethylaminoethyl 1-phenylcyclopentane-1-carboxylate hydrochloride.

$C_{18}H_{27}NO_2,HCl=325.9$.

CAS — 77-22-5 (caramiphen); 125-85-9 (hydrochloride).

White crystals or crystalline powder with a slight characteristic odour and a bitter numbing taste. M.p. 142° to 146°.

Soluble 1 in 4 of water and 1 in 8 of alcohol; practically insoluble in ether. A 5% solution in water has a pH of 4 to 5.

Uses. Caramiphen hydrochloride is a weak anticholinergic agent with actions and uses similar to those of benzhexol (see p.294). It has been used in an initial daily dose of 50 mg, in divided doses; subsequent doses increasing gradually to 300 mg or more daily according to the patient's needs.

Caramiphen has also been used as the edisylate.

Reference: M. E. Farquharson and R. G. Johnston, *Br. J. Pharmac. Chemother.*, 1959, *14*, 559.

Preparations

Caramiphen Tablets *(B.P. 1968)*. Tablets containing caramiphen hydrochloride.

353-c

Chlorphenoxamine Hydrochloride *(U.S.P.)*. 2-(4-Chloro-α-methylbenzhydryloxy)-*NN*-dimethylethylamine hydrochloride.

$C_{18}H_{22}ClNO,HCl=340.3$.

CAS — 77-38-3 (chlorphenoxamine); 562-09-4 (hydrochloride).

Pharmacopoeias. In *U.S.*

A white crystalline powder. M.p. 130° to 135°. **Soluble** 1 in 2 of water, 1 in 1.8 of alcohol, and 1 in 1.5 of chloroform; very soluble in methyl alcohol; soluble in acetone; practically insoluble in ether. **Store** in airtight containers. Protect from light.

Adverse Effects, Treatment, and Precautions. As for Atropine, p.289. See also Adverse Effects of Antihistamines, p.1294.

The use of chlorphenoxamine with caffeine precipitated, or usually exacerbated, ataxia and balance disturbances in about 20% of 60 patients receiving optimum doses for the control of rigidity and tremor in Parkinson's disease.— R. R. Strang, *J. clin. Pharmac.*, 1967, *7*, 214.

Absorption and Fate. Chlorphenoxamine is absorbed from the gastro-intestinal tract and has an onset of action after about 30 minutes and a duration of action of about 4 hours.

Uses. Chlorphenoxamine, a congener of diphenhydramine, has weak anticholinergic actions; it also has antihistaminic, local anaesthetic, and skeletal muscle-relaxant properties. It is used similarly to benzhexol (see p.295) in the symptomatic treatment of arteriosclerotic, idiopathic, and postencephalitic parkinsonism. An initial dose of 50 mg thrice daily after food may be increased to 100 mg three or four times daily according to the response of the patient.

Transition to or from chlorphenoxamine therapy should be gradual, otherwise symptoms may be aggravated.

For reports and comments on the concurrent administration of anticholinergic agents with levodopa, in patients with parkinsonism, see under Levodopa, p.887.

Preparations

Chlorphenoxamine Hydrochloride Tablets *(U.S.P.)*. Tablets containing chlorphenoxamine hydrochloride. Store in airtight containers. Protect from light.

Proprietary Names

Phenoxene *(Dow, Canad.; Dow, USA)*; Systral *(hydrochloride or embonate) (Asta, Belg.; Asta, Denm.; Lucien, Fr.; Asta, Ger.; Asta, Neth.; Asta, Switz.)*; Systraletten *(Asta, Ger.)*.

Chlorphenoxamine hydrochloride was formerly marketed in Great Britain under the proprietary name Clorevan *(Evans Medical)*.

354-k

Clidinium Bromide *(U.S.P.)*. Ro 2-3773. 3-Benziloyloxy-1-methylquinuclidinium bromide.

$C_{22}H_{26}BrNO_3=432.4$.

CAS — 7020-55-5 (clidinium); 3485-62-9 (bromide).

Pharmacopoeias. In *U.S.*

A white or nearly white almost odourless crystalline powder. M.p. about 242°. **Soluble** in water and alcohol; slightly soluble in ether. **Store** in airtight containers. Protect from light.

Adverse Effects, Treatment, and Precautions. As for Atropine, p.289.

Uses. Clidinium bromide is a quaternary ammonium anticholinergic agent with peripheral effects similar to those of atropine (see p.290). It is used in conjunction with chlordiazepoxide in the symptomatic treatment of gastric and duodenal ulcer and other gastro-intestinal disorders. The usual dose of clidinium bromide is 2.5 mg three or four times a day before meals and at bedtime; this may be increased to 5 mg four times a day if necessary.

References: G. McHardy *et al.*, *Gastroenterology*, 1968, *54*, 508, per *J. Am. med. Ass.*, 1968, *204* (May 6), A265; B. O. Amure, *Br. J. clin. Pract.*, 1969, *23*, 290; M. A. Sullivan *et al.*, *New Engl. J. Med.*, 1978, *298*, 878.

Preparations

Clidinium Bromide Capsules *(U.S.P.)*. Capsules containing clidinium bromide. Store in airtight containers. Protect from light.

Libraxin (known in some countries as Librax) *(Roche, UK)*. Tablets each containing clidinium bromide 2.5 mg and chlordiazepoxide 5 mg. For hypermotility, hypersecretion, and emotional factors associated with gastro-intestinal disorders. *Dose.* 1 or 2 tablets 3 or 4 times daily before meals and at bedtime.

Thrombocytopenia occurred in a 32-year-old woman given Librax twice daily for 7 days; the condition regressed within 5 days without specific treatment when Librax was withdrawn.— A. Celada *et al.*, *Br. med. J.*, 1977, *1*, 268.

Other Proprietary Names

Quarzan *(USA)*.

355-a

Cyclopentolate Hydrochloride *(B.P., U.S.P.)*. Cloridrato de Ciclopentolato. 2-Dimethylaminoethyl 2-(1-hydroxycyclopentyl)-2-phenylacetate hydrochloride.

$C_{17}H_{25}NO_3,HCl=327.9$.

CAS — 512-15-2 (cyclopentolate); 5870-29-1 (hydrochloride).

Pharmacopoeias. In *Br.*, *Braz.*, and *U.S.*

A white crystalline powder, odourless or with a characteristic odour. M.p. 135° to 138°. **Soluble** 1 in less than 1 of water and 1 in 5 of alcohol; practically insoluble in ether. A 1% solution in water has a pH of 4.5 to 5.5. Solutions are **sterilised** by filtration. **Store** at a temperature not exceeding 8° in airtight containers.

Adverse Effects, Treatment, and Precautions. As for Atropine, p.289.

Eye-drops of cyclopentolate hydrochloride may cause temporary irritation. Systemic toxicity may occasionally be produced by the instillation of anticholinergic eye-drops, particularly in infants.

Gastro-intestinal toxicity occurred in premature 8-day-old Negro twins 4 hours after the administration of 3 mg (6 drops of a 1% solution) of cyclopentolate eye-drops. Plasma-cyclopentolate concentrations 24 hours after drug administration were 22 μg per ml in twin 1 and 2 μg per ml in twin 2. During the next 2 weeks twin 1 had episodes of vomiting, abdominal distension, apnoea, and convulsions and died from necrotising enterocolitis. Twin 2 had a few episodes of vomiting and distension but recovered in 45 days.— C. R. Bauer *et al.*, *J. Pediat.*, 1973, *92*, 501.

Of 66 patients who received one drop of 2% cyclopentolate eye-drops in each eye, 10 developed systemic toxicity of mild to moderate severity. The manifestations were: physical weakness, nausea, light-headedness, changes in emotional attitude, unprovoked weeping, and loss of equilibrium; tachycardia was always present but changes in blood pressure were insignificant. Nine of the 10 were female and spontaneous recovery occurred within 1 hour to several days. It is recommended that concentrations of cyclopentolate eye-drops above 1% should only be used when absolutely necessary.— K. J. Awan, *Ann. Ophthal.*, 1976, *8*, 695.

Some other reports of toxicity following instillation of cyclopentolate eye-drops: C. W. Simcoe, *Archs Ophthal., N.Y.*, 1962, *67*, 406 (CNS toxicity); H. H. Mark, *J. Am. med. Ass.*, 1963, *186*, 430; W. T. Carpenter, *Archs Ophthal., N.Y.*, 1967, *78*, 445 (incoherence, disorientation, and ataxia); E. W. Adcock, *J. Pediat.*, 1971, *79*, 127 (toxic psychosis and cholinergic postganglionic blockade); J. S. Kennerdell and F. P. Wucher, *Archs Ophthal., N.Y.*, 1972, *87*, 634 (grand mal seizure); K. J. Awan, *Ann. Ophthal.*, 1976, *8*, 803 (mental changes, tachycardia, nausea, inarticulation in speech, and inability to stand erect).

Uses. Cyclopentolate hydrochloride is an anticholinergic agent with actions similar to those of atropine (see p.290). It is used as eye-drops to produce cycloplegia and mydriasis. It acts more quickly than atropine and has a shorter duration of action; the maximum effect is produced in 15 to 60 minutes after instillation of 1 to 2 drops of a 0.5% solution; accommodation recovers within 24 hours but may be hastened if 1 or 2 drops of a 2% solution of pilocarpine nitrate are instilled.

For refraction, 1 drop of a 0.5% solution repeated after about 5 to 15 minutes is usually sufficient, but deeply pigmented eyes may require a 1% solution; children under 6 years of age usually require 1 or 2 drops of a 1% solution, and children aged 6 to 16 years, 1 drop of a 1% solution, but see under Adverse Effects.

A 0.1% solution has been used for mydriasis when cycloplegia is not required.

Studies *in vivo* and *in vitro* showed that the mydriatic activity of the racemate of cyclopentolate hydrochloride was almost entirely due to the laevo-isomer.— S. A. Smith, *Br. J. clin. Pharmac.*, 1976, *3*, 503.

Using a special silicone-rubber-tubing delivery system, single applications of 5-μl amounts of ointment containing cyclopentolate hydrochloride 1 and 2% and tropicamide 1 and 2%, provided mydriasis and/or cycloplegia without producing the ocular stinging and copious lachrymation usually associated with the eye-drops, and without interfering with subsequent eye examinations. Disadvantages were the need to touch the conjunctiva on application, and problems with mass production of the tubing.— M. K. Cable *et al.*, *Archs Ophthal., N.Y.*, 1978, *96*, 84. See also: R. E. Hardberger *et al.*, *ibid.*, 1975, *93*, 42; R. O. Hendrickson and C. Hanna, *Ann. Ophthal.*, 1977, *9*, 333.

Cyclopentolate often gave great relief from pain in eye injuries; painful iris spasm could be relieved.— P. A. Gardiner, *Br. med. J.*, 1978, *2*, 1347.

Preparations

Cyclopentolate Eye Drops *(A.P.F.)*. Cyclopentolate hydrochloride 500 mg, sodium chloride 800 mg, benzalkonium chloride solution 0.02 ml, disodium edetate 50 mg, Water for Injections to 100 ml. Sterilised by filtration. The eye-drops should be recently prepared.

Cyclopentolate Eye Drops *(B.P.)*. CYC. A sterile solution of cyclopentolate hydrochloride in water. When intended for use on more than one occasion they contain benzalkonium chloride 0.01%, may contain boric acid and potassium chloride, and should not be used more than one month after first opening the container.

Cyclopentolate Hydrochloride Ophthalmic Solution *(U.S.P.)*. A sterile aqueous solution of cyclopentolate hydrochloride; it may contain suitable buffers and other additives. pH 3 to 5.5. Store at 15° to 30° in airtight containers.

Proprietary Preparations

Alcon Opulets Cyclopentolate 1% *(Alcon, UK: Farillon, UK).* Sterile eye-drops containing cyclopentolate hydrochloride 1%, in single-use disposable applicators.

Minims Cyclopentolate Hydrochloride *(Smith & Nephew Pharmaceuticals, UK).* Sterile eye-drops containing cyclopentolate hydrochloride 0.5 or 1%, in single-use disposable applicators. (Also available as Minims Cyclopentolate Hydrochloride in *Austral., Norw.*).

Mydrilate *(WB Pharmaceuticals, UK: Boehringer Ingelheim, UK).* Eye-drops containing cyclopentolate hydrochloride 0.5 and 1% in a buffered solution, with benzalkonium chloride 0.01%. (Also available as Mydrilate in *Austral.*).

Other Proprietary Names

Ciclolux *(Ital.)*; Colircusi Ciclopejico *(Spain)*; Colirio Oculos Cicloplegic *(Spain)*; Cyclogyl *(Austral., Canad., Denm., Neth., S.Afr., Swed., Switz., USA)*; Cyclopen *(Austral.)*; Cyclopentol Colircusi *(Belg.)*; Cyplegin *(Jap.)*; Mydplegic *(Canad.)*; Skiacol P.O.S. *(Fr.)*; Zyklolat *(Ger.)*.

356-t

Cycrimine Hydrochloride *(U.S.P.).* Cycriminium Chloride. 1-Cyclopentyl-1-phenyl-3-piperidinopropan-1-ol hydrochloride.

$C_{19}H_{29}NO,HCl=323.9$.

CAS — 77-39-4 (cycrimine); 126-02-3 (hydrochloride).

Pharmacopoeias. In *U.S.*

A white odourless solid with a bitter taste. M.p. about 242° with decomposition. **Soluble** 1 in 175 of water, 1 in 50 of alcohol, and 1 in 35 of chloroform. A 0.5% solution in water has a pH of 5.2 to 5.8. **Store** in airtight containers.

Uses. Cycrimine hydrochloride is an anticholinergic agent with actions and uses similar to those of benzhexol (see p.294). It is given in doses of 1.25 to 5 mg three or four times daily, preferably with food to avoid nausea and anorexia; higher doses have been employed.

Preparations

Cycrimine Hydrochloride Tablets *(U.S.P.).* Tablets containing cycrimine hydrochloride. Store in airtight containers.

Proprietary Names

Pagitan *(Lilly, Arg.)*; Pagitane *(Lilly, Austral.; Lilly, Ital.)*; Pagitane Hydrochloride *(Lilly, USA)*.

357-x

Datura Herb *(B.P.C. 1949).* Datura Leaf; Flos Daturae.

CAS — 8061-05-0 (datura).

Pharmacopoeias. In *Chin.* and *Ind.*

The dried leaves and flowering tops of *Datura metel* and *D. metel* var. *fastuosa* (Solanaceae), containing about 0.25 to 0.55% of hyoscine with only traces of atropine and hyoscyamine.

Uses. Datura herb is used in India for the same purposes as belladonna, hyoscyamus, and stramonium. It has been given as liquid extract (containing 0.25% of alkaloids) in doses of 0.06 to 0.2 ml and as a tincture (containing 0.025% of alkaloids) in doses of 0.3 to 2 ml. Doses of 2 to 16 ml of the tincture have been given in parkinsonism.

358-r

Dexetimide Hydrochloride. R 16470; Dexbenzetimide Hydrochloride. (+)-(*S*)-2-(1-Benzyl-4-piperidyl)-2-phenylglutarimide hydrochloride; (+)-(*S*)-3-(1-Benzyl-4-piperidyl)-3-phenylpiperidine-2,6-dione hydrochloride.

$C_{23}H_{26}N_2O_2,HCl=398.9$.

CAS — 21888-98-2 (dexetimide); 21888-96-0 (hydrochloride).

A white crystalline powder. M.p. 270° to 273°.

Uses. Dexetimide is a long-acting anticholinergic agent with actions similar to those of benzhexol (see p.294). It has been used as the hydrochloride to alleviate neuroleptic-induced parkinsonism in doses equivalent to 0.5 to 1 mg of the base daily given by mouth; lower doses have also been given intramuscularly.

Clinical references: R. De Smedt *et al.*, *J. clin. Pharmac.*, 1970, *10*, 207; H. M. van Praag *et al.*, *Br. med. J.*, 1971, *4*, 710.

Proprietary Names

Tremblex *(Johnson, Arg.; Janssen, Aust.; Janssen, Belg.; Gedeon Richter, Hung.; Janssen, Ital.; Janssen, Neth.; Janssen, Switz.)*.

359-f

Dibutoline Sulphate. (2-Dibutylcarbamoyloxyethyl)ethyldimethylammonium sulphate.

$(C_{15}H_{33}N_2O_2)_2,SO_4=642.9$.

CAS — 21962-82-3 (dibutoline); 532-49-0 (sulphate).

An extremely hygroscopic powder. **Soluble** in water. A 5% solution in water has pH of 6.75 to 7.5. **Sterilise** by filtration. **Store** in airtight containers.

Adverse Effects, Treatment, and Precautions. As for Atropine, p.289.

Uses. Dibutoline sulphate is a quaternary ammonium anticholinergic agent with peripheral effects similar to those of atropine (see p.290). It has been used in ophthalmology as a 5% solution and has been used systemically to relieve visceral spasms but since it is poorly absorbed from the gut it must be given by intramuscular or subcutaneous injection. It has been given in a dose of 25 mg subcutaneously or intramuscularly 3 or 4 times daily.

360-z

Dicyclomine Hydrochloride *(B.P., U.S.P.).*

Cloridrato de Dicicloverina; Dicycloverine Hydrochloride. 2-Diethylaminoethyl bicyclohexyl-1-carboxylate hydrochloride.

$C_{19}H_{35}NO_2,HCl=346.0$.

CAS — 77-19-0 (dicyclomine); 67-92-5 (hydrochloride).

Pharmacopoeias. In *Br.*, *Braz.*, and *U.S.*

A white or almost white, almost odourless, crystalline powder with a bitter numbing taste. M.p. 169° to 174°.

Soluble 1 in 20 of water, 1 in 5 of alcohol, and 1 in 2 of chloroform and glacial acetic acid; practically insoluble in ether. A 1% solution in water has a pH of 5 to 5.5.

Adverse Effects, Treatment, and Precautions. As for Atropine, p.289.

Overdosage. Two children aged 18 and 15 months swallowed about 23 and 30 Debendox tablets respectively. Due to the tablet coating, symptoms did not develop until the tablets had passed into the intestine where they could not be retrieved by gastric lavage or emesis. The first child, who was not admitted for treatment until 9 hours after ingestion, died despite supportive treatment. The second child was admitted to hospital after 2.5 hours and successfully managed with magnesium sulphate by mouth, enemas, colonic wash-outs, and peritoneal dialysis.— S. R. Meadow and G. A. Leeson, *Archs Dis. Childh.*, 1974, *49*, 310.

Recovery of a 3½-year-old boy admitted to hospital 7 hours after taking an unknown amount of Debendox tablets. He was initially treated with pilocarpine 3 mg subcutaneously, chlorpromazine 15 mg intramuscularly, and magnesium hydroxide purgation, followed by more pilocarpine and chlorpromazine after 90 minutes. He then had a generalised convulsion and was sedated with diazepam intravenously, and given intravenous fluids. He subsequently received carbachol intramuscularly for urinary retention and was started on pilocarpine intravenously every half-hour (receiving a total of 24 mg in 12 hours). Despite the purgation no tablets or shells were recovered from the stool. He had fully recovered 24 hours after admission and was discharged with no apparent sequelae. It was noted that pilocarpine appeared to combat the CNS as well as the peripheral effects; the slow intravenous administration of diazepam 4 mg on 2 occasions had no adverse effects.— S. G. Clarkson and A. P. Glanvill (letter), *Br. med. J.*, 1977, *2*, 459.

Pregnancy and the neonate. There have been isolated reports of malformations in infants born to mothers who had taken dicyclomine-containing preparations during the first trimester of pregnancy (D.C. Paterson, *Can. med. Ass. J.*, 1969, *101*, 175; D. Donnai and R. Harris, *Br. med. J.*, 1978, *1*, 691; C.J.G. Menzies, *ibid.*, 925; K. Frith, *ibid.*; S. Mellor, *ibid.*, 1055), but a prospective study by R.W. Smithells and S. Sheppard (*Teratology*, 1978, *17*, 31; see also *Br. med. J.*, 1978, *1*, 1055) of 372 mothers who had started taking a dicyclomine-containing preparation (Debendox) at 6 weeks or earlier, and 1620 who had started at or before 12 weeks, did not provide evidence of a teratogenic effect. However the study has been criticised because the controls could also have taken Debendox (see *Pharm. J.*, 1980, *1*, 235). A retrospective study by S. Shapiro *et al.* (*Am. J. Obstet. Gynec.*, 1977, *128*, 480) did not demonstrate any statistically significant difference between the percentage of malformed children among 1024 children born to mothers who had taken dicyclomine hydrochloride during the first 4 months of pregnancy and 49 258 children not so exposed. Other studies (L. Milkovich and B.J. van den Berg, *Am. J. Obstet. Gynec.*, 1976, *125*, 244; D.W.G. Harron *et al.*, *Br. med. J.*, 1980, *281*, 1379) have also failed to find evidence that dicyclomine-containing preparations were associated with teratogenicity when taken during pregnancy.

The Committee on Safety of Medicines had studied data relating to the teratogenicity of Debendox at the time of the initial reports of abnormalities in babies born to mothers who had taken Debendox during pregnancy and had found no evidence to support a ban of the preparation. It considered that there had been no new evidence since that study.— *Pharm. J.*, 1980, *1*, 109.

Further references: *J. Am. med. Ass.*, 1979, *242*, 2518; D. W. G. Harron *et al.*, *Br. med. J.*, 1980, *281*, 1379; S. M. Barlow and F. M. Sullivan (letter), *ibid.*, *282*, 148; R. G. Shanks *et al.* (letter), *ibid.*, 1972; M. Clarke and D. G. Clayton (letter), *Lancet*, 1981, *1*, 659; J. B. Hall (letter), *ibid.*, *2*, 154; D. M. Fleming *et al.*, *Br. med. J.*, 1981, *283*, 99; J. F. Cordero *et al.*, *J. Am. med. Ass.*, 1981, *245*, 2307; A. A. Mitchell *et al.*, *ibid.*, 2311; H. Jick *et al.*, *ibid.*, *246*, 343; G. T. Gibson *et al.*, *Med. J. Aust.*, 1981, *1*, 410; J. F. Correy and N. M. Newman, *ibid.*, 417.

Uses. Dicyclomine hydrochloride is an anticholinergic agent with peripheral effects similar to but much weaker than those of atropine (see p.290); it also has a direct antispasmodic action and a local anaesthetic action. It is used in biliary, gastro-intestinal, or urinary-tract spasm and is given as an adjunct in the treatment of gastric and duodenal ulcer. For adults and children over 2 years of age a dose of 10 to 20 mg may be given 3 or 4 times a day; for children aged 6 months to 2 years a dose of 5 to 10 mg may be given 3 or 4 times daily, 15 minutes before feeds, to a maximum total daily dose not exceeding 40 mg; for infants aged less than 6 months a dose of 5 mg may be given 3 or 4 times daily, 15 minutes before feeds, to a maximum daily dose not exceeding 20 mg.

It has also been given intramuscularly in a dose of 20 mg every 4 to 6 hours for adults.

Dicyclomine hydrochloride is also given with an antihistamine and pyridoxine for the nausea and vomiting of early pregnancy.

Irritable bowel syndrome. Studies on the use of dicyclomine in the irritable bowel syndrome: S. G. F. Matts, *Br. J. clin. Pract.*, 1967, *21*, 549. Report No. 196 of the General Practitioner Research Group, *Practitioner*, 1976, *217*, 276.

Preparations

Capsules

Dicyclomine Hydrochloride Capsules *(U.S.P.).* Capsules containing dicyclomine hydrochloride.

Elixirs and Syrups

Dicyclomine Elixir *(B.P.).* Dicyclomine Syrup. A solution of dicyclomine hydrochloride in a suitable flavoured vehicle which may be coloured. When a dose less than or not a multiple of 5 ml is prescribed, the elixir should be diluted to 5 ml, or a multiple, with syrup. Such dilutions must be freshly prepared and not used more than 2 weeks after issue. Protect from light.

Dicyclomine Hydrochloride Syrup *(U.S.P.)*. A syrup containing dicyclomine hydrochloride. Store in airtight containers.

Injections

Dicyclomine Hydrochloride Injection *(U.S.P.)*. A sterile iso-osmotic solution of dicyclomine hydrochloride in Water for Injections.

Tablets

Dicyclomine Hydrochloride Tablets *(U.S.P.)*. Tablets containing dicyclomine hydrochloride.

Dicyclomine Tablets *(B.P.)*. Tablets containing dicyclomine hydrochloride.

Proprietary Preparations

Debendox *(Merrell, UK)*. Tablets, coated for delayed action, each containing dicyclomine hydrochloride 10 mg, doxylamine succinate 10 mg, and pyridoxine hydrochloride 10 mg. For nausea and vomiting of pregnancy. *Dose.* 2 tablets at bedtime; in severe nausea, 1 additional tablet on rising and in mid-afternoon.

NOTE. It is anticipated that Debendox will be reformulated in Great Britain to exclude dicyclomine hydrochloride. Debendox was marketed as Bendectin in the USA until 1977, when Bendectin was reformulated without dicylomine hydrochloride.

Merbentyl *(Merrell, UK)*. Dicyclomine hydrochloride, available as **Syrup** containing 10 mg in each 5 ml (suggested diluent, syrup) and as **Tablets** of 10 mg. (Also available as Merbentyl in *Austral., S.Afr.*).

Ovol Colic Drops *(Carter-Wallace, UK: Pharmax, UK)*. Contain in each ml dicyclomine hydrochloride 10 mg and dimethicone 40 mg. For infantile colic.

Other Proprietary Names

Arg.—Babypasmil;*Austral.*—Procyclomin;*Canad.*—Bentylol, Cyclobec, Formulex, Menospasm, Spasmoban, Viscerol;*Ger.*—Atumin;*Ital.*—Ametil, Bentyl;*Jap.*—Icramin, Incron, Mamiesan, Panakiron, Sawamin;*NZ*—Wyovin;*S.Afr.*—Clomin, Colix, Nomocramp;*Spain*—Bentylol;*USA*—Benacol, Bentyl, Or-Tyl, Pasmin.

361-c

Diethazine Hydrochloride *(B.P. 1963)*. Diaethazinum Chloratum; Eazamine Hydrochloride; RP 2987. 10-(2-Diethylaminoethyl)phenothiazine hydrochloride.
$C_{18}H_{22}N_2S,HCl=334.9$.

CAS — 60-91-3 (diethazine); 341-70-8 (hydrochloride).

Pharmacopoeias. In *Cz.*

A white or slightly cream-coloured, almost odourless, crystalline powder with a bitter taste. **Soluble** 1 in 2.5 of water, 1 in 5 of alcohol, and 1 in 2 of chloroform; practically insoluble in ether. **Protect** from light.

Uses. Diethazine hydrochloride is an anticholinergic agent with actions and uses similar to those of ethopropazine hydrochloride (see p.300) but it is more toxic. Granulocytopenia and agranulocytosis have occurred. It has been given in an initial dose of 150 mg daily in divided doses with subsequent doses increasing gradually to 1.5 g daily according to the patient's response.

Preparations

Diethazine Tablets *(B.P. 1963)*. Tablets containing diethazine hydrochloride. The tablets are sugar-coated.

362-k

Difemerine Hydrochloride. UP 57. 2-Dimethylamino-1,1-dimethylethyl benzilate hydrochloride.
$C_{20}H_{25}NO_3,HCl=363.8$.

CAS — 80387-96-8 (difemerine); 70280-88-5 (hydrochloride).

Adverse Effects, Treatment, and Precautions. As for Atropine, p.289.

Uses. Difemerine hydrochloride is an anticholinergic agent with effects similar to those of atropine (see p.290). It has been used in the symptomatic treatment of visceral spasms in doses of 7.5 to 10 mg daily by mouth. It has also been given intramuscularly in doses of 1 to 3 mg daily and rectally in doses of 15 to 30 mg daily.

Proprietary Names

Luostyl *(UPSA, Fr.)*.

363-a

Dihexyverine Hydrochloride. JL 1078; Dihexiverine Hydrochloride. 2-Piperidinoethyl bicyclohexyl-1-carboxylate hydrochloride.
$C_{20}H_{35}NO_2,HCl=358.0$.

CAS — 561-77-3 (dihexyverine); 5588-25-0 (hydrochloride).

Adverse Effects, Treatment, and Precautions. As for Atropine, p.289.

Uses. Dihexyverine hydrochloride is an anticholinergic agent with effects similar to those of atropine (see p.290). It has been given in the symptomatic treatment of visceral spasms in usual doses of 10 to 30 mg thrice daily.

Proprietary Names

Diverine *(Courtois, Ital.)*; Metaspas *(ICN, Canad.)*; Seclin *(Panthox & Burck, Ital.)*; Spasmodex *(Crinex, Fr.)*; Spasmolevel *(Level, Spain)*.

364-t

Diphemanil Methylsulphate.

Diphemanil Methylsulfate *(U.S.P.)*; Diphenmethanil Methylsulphate; Vagophemanil Methylsulphate. 4-Benzhydrylidene-1,1-dimethylpiperidinium methylsulphate.
$C_{20}H_{24}N,CH_3SO_4=389.5$.

CAS — 62-97-5.

Pharmacopoeias. In *U.S.*

A white or almost white, hygroscopic, crystalline powder with a faint characteristic odour and a bitter taste. M.p. 189° to 196°.
Soluble 1 in 33 of water, 1 in 33 of alcohol, and 1 in 33 of chloroform; very slightly soluble in ether. A 1% solution in water has a pH of 4 to 6. **Store** in airtight containers.

Adverse Effects, Treatment, and Precautions. As for Atropine, p.289.

Absorption and Fate. Diphemanil methylsulphate is poorly absorbed from the gastro-intestinal tract. Its effects appear within 1 or 2 hours of a dose being taken, and last approximately 4 hours. It is excreted mainly in the urine and partly as unabsorbed drug in the faeces.

Uses. Diphemanil methylsulphate is a quaternary ammonium anticholinergic agent with peripheral effects similar to those of atropine (see p.290).
It is used as an adjunct in the treatment of gastric and duodenal ulcer, and to relieve visceral spasms. It has also been used in the treatment of excessive sweating.
The usual dose is 100 mg every 4 to 6 hours, increased according to the patient's needs. It has also been given in doses of 15 to 25 mg by subcutaneous or intramuscular injection every 6 hours; the parenteral dose should not exceed 50 mg.
In hyperhidrosis, up to 800 mg daily in divided doses has been given, decreased to the minimum effective dose when sweating is controlled.

Preparations

Diphemanil Methylsulfate Tablets *(U.S.P.)*. Tablets containing diphemanil methylsulphate. The *U.S.P.* requires 80% dissolution in 30 minutes. Store in airtight containers.

Proprietary Names

Prantal *(Essex, Austral.; Cétrane, Fr.; Essex, Ital.; Schering, USA)*; Prentol *(Essex, Spain)*.

365-x

Emepronium Bromide.

Ethyldimethyl(1-methyl-3,3-diphenylpropyl)ammonium bromide.
$C_{20}H_{28}BrN=362.4$.

CAS — 27892-33-7 (emepronium); 3614-30-0 (bromide).

A white crystalline powder. M.p. 201° to 206°.
Soluble in water, alcohol, and chloroform.

Adverse Effects, Treatment, and Precautions. As for Atropine, p.289.
To avoid oesophageal ulceration, tablets of emepronium bromide should always be swallowed with an adequate volume of water, and patients should always be in the sitting or standing position while, and for 10 to 15 minutes after, taking the tablets. Emepronium is contra-indicated in patients with symptoms or signs of oesophageal obstruction or with pre-existing oesophagitis.

Buccal and oesophageal ulceration. Because of the hygroscopic nature of emepronium bromide tablets they should be swallowed with water to prevent any tablet sticking to the oesophageal mucosa with possible risk of ulceration. Patients with difficulties in swallowing tablets should take emepronium bromide tablets as a slurry in water.— Å. Pilbrant, *Kabi, Swed.* (letter), *Lancet*, 1977, *1*, 749.

Reports of buccal or oesophageal ulceration after taking tablets of emepronium bromide: T. M. Strouthidis *et al.*, *Lancet*, 1972, *1*, 72; T. Habeshaw and J. R. Bennett (letter), *ibid.*, 1972, *2*, 1422; J. E. Hale and D. E. Barnardo (letter), *ibid.*, 1973, *1*, 493; H. Kavin (letter), *ibid.*, 1977, *1*, 424; S. Kenwright and A. D. C. Norris (letter), *ibid.*, 548; R. H. Higson (letter), *Br. med. J.*, 1978, *2*, 201; G. J. Huston *et al.*, *Postgrad. med. J.*, 1978, *54*, 331; E. Kobler *et al.*, *Dt. med. Wschr.*, 1978, *103*, 1035; F. J. Collins *et al.*, *Br. med. J.*, 1979, *1*, 1673; R. Hughes (letter), *ibid.*, *2*, 132; R. E. Cowan *et al.* (letter), *ibid;* J. D. R. Rose and G. B. Tobin (letter), *ibid.*, 1980, *280*, 110.

Absorption and Fate. Emepronium bromide is incompletely absorbed from the gastro-intestinal tract and is mainly excreted unchanged in the urine and faeces.

In 4 healthy men given an intramuscular injection of emepronium bromide 25 mg, the maximum serum concentration (about 450 ng per ml) was reached after 15 minutes and the serum half-life was 1½ to 2¼ hours. In subjects given 0.15, 0.6, or 1.2 g of emepronium bromide by mouth, the peak serum concentrations were 8 to 100 ng per ml, 99 to 301 ng per ml, and 174 to 802 ng per ml respectively; only about 1 to 2% of the dose appeared in the urine suggesting that only 2.5 to 5% of the dose had been absorbed.— A. Sundwall *et al.*, *Eur. J. clin. Pharmac.*, 1973, *6*, 191.

Uses. Emepronium bromide is a quaternary ammonium anticholinergic agent with peripheral effects similar to those of atropine (see p.290).
It is mainly used to reduce the muscular tone of the urinary bladder in postoperative vesical tenesmus and in urinary frequency. The usual dose is 200 mg thrice daily. In nocturnal tenesmus, 200 to 400 mg may be given in the evening. It has been given by subcutaneous or intramuscular injection in a dose of 25 mg thrice daily; 25 to 50 mg has been injected during and after cystometric evaluation of bladder function.

Studies and reports on the use of emepronium bromide in bladder spasm and incontinence: G. Johnson and B. Zederfeldt, *Urol. int.*, 1957, *4*, 293; J. C. Brocklehurst *et al.*, *Br. med. J.*, 1969, *2*, 216; A. Ekeland and S. Sander, *Scand. J. Urol. & Nephrol.*, 1976, *10*, 195; J. H. N. Syversen *et al.*, *ibid.*, 201; A. E. S. Ritch *et al.*, *Lancet*, 1977, *1*, 504; R. Neale (letter), *ibid.*, 748.

Proprietary Preparations

Cetiprin *(KabiVitrum, UK)*. Emepronium bromide, available as tablets of 100 mg. (Also available as Cetiprin in *Denm., Neth., Norw., S.Afr., Swed., Switz.*).

Other Proprietary Names

Detrulisin *(Ital.)*; Hexanium *(Spain)*; Uro-Ripirin *(Ger.)*.

366-r

Ethopropazine Hybenzate. Profenamine Hibenzate. 10-(2-Diethylaminopropyl)phenothiazine 2-(4-hydroxybenzoyl)benzoate.
$C_{19}H_{24}N_2S,C_{14}H_{10}O_4$=554.7.
CAS — 522-00-9 (ethopropazine).

A white, odourless, tasteless, crystalline powder. M.p. about 188° with decomposition. Ethopropazine hybenzate 159 mg is approximately equivalent to 100 mg of ethopropazine hydrochloride. Practically **insoluble** in water; slightly soluble in methyl alcohol.

Uses. A tasteless salt of ethopropazine with the actions and uses of ethopropazine hydrochloride (see below). It has been given in an initial dose equivalent to ethopropazine hydrochloride 40 mg daily, gradually increasing to 500 mg daily in divided doses, according to the patient's needs.

Proprietary Names
Parkin *(Jap.)*.

367-f

Ethopropazine Hydrochloride *(B.P. 1973, U.S.P.)*. Profenamini Hydrochloridum; Cloridrato de Profenamina; Profenamine Hydrochloride; Prophenaminum Hydrochloridum; Isothazine Hydrochloride. 10-(2-Diethylaminopropyl)phenothiazine hydrochloride.
$C_{19}H_{24}N_2S,HCl$=348.9.
CAS — 522-00-9 (ethopropazine); 1094-08-2 (hydrochloride).

Pharmacopoeias. In *Braz.*, *Int.*, and *U.S.*

A white or slightly off-white, odourless, crystalline powder with a bitter taste; it darkens in colour on exposure to light. M.p. about 210° with decomposition. **Soluble** 1 in 225 of water, 1 in 35 of alcohol, and 1 in 7 of chloroform; sparingly soluble in acetone; practically insoluble in ether. **Store** in airtight containers. Protect from light.

Incompatibility. Ethopropazine hydrochloride appeared to be decomposed by contact with talc and activated charcoal.— D. L. Sorby and E. M. Plein, *J. pharm. Sci.*, 1961, *50*, 355.

Adverse Effects, Treatment, and Precautions. As for Atropine, p.289.
Ethopropazine may also cause muscle cramps, paraesthesia, drowsiness, and nausea. It bears a structural resemblance to drugs capable of inducing blood disorders and, as with all phenothiazine derivatives, it should be used cautiously in patients with hepatic diseases. Anticholinergic antiparkinsonian agents do not control tardive dyskinesia associated with long-term phenothiazine (or other antipsychotic) therapy, and may exacerbate symptoms.

Uses. Ethopropazine hydrochloride is a phenothiazine derivative with anticholinergic, adrenergic-blocking, slight antihistaminic, local anaesthetic and ganglion-blocking properties. It has been used in the symptomatic treatment of arteriosclerotic, idiopathic, and postencephalitic parkinsonism, and of the extrapyramidal syndrome induced by other phenothiazine compounds or reserpine. It has been used in a usual dose of 50 mg daily initially gradually increased to 500 mg daily in divided doses, according to the response of the patient; higher doses have been given. It has also been tried in the symptomatic treatment of hepatolenticular degeneration and congenital athetosis. Transition to or from ethopropazine therapy should be gradual, otherwise symptoms may be aggravated.

Extrapyramidal effects. A 2-week study comparing amantadine, benztropine, and ethopropazine in 45 psychiatric patients with neuroleptic-induced extrapyramidal signs; although all 3 drugs significantly improved the symptoms they did not completely control them, demonstrating the limitations of available therapy. Toxic psychosis required withdrawal of 1 patient in the benztropine group and 2 in the ethopropazine group; another patient in the ethopropazine group was withdrawn because of epigastric distress.— J. Ananth, *Int. J. clin. Pharmac. Biopharm.*, 1975, *11*, 323.

In a 12-week controlled study ethopropazine hydrochloride and benztropine were equally effective in controlling neuroleptic-induced parkinsonian symptoms in 56 schizophrenic patients receiving maintenance treatment with fluphenazine enanthate and both were as effective as previous treatment with procyclidine. However, patients receiving benztropine had a significant increase in tardive dyskinesia compared with procyclidine treatment and they also experienced significantly more anxiety and depression than patients receiving ethopropazine.— G. Chouinard *et al.*, *J. clin. Psychiat.*, 1979, *40*, 147.

Parkinsonism. For reports and comments on the concurrent administration of anticholinergic agents with levodopa, in patients with parkinsonism, see under Levodopa, p.887.

Pregnancy and the neonate. Teratogenic studies in *rats* and *mice*.— *Japan med. Gaz.*, 1973, *10* (Sept. 20), 5.

Ethopropazine was excreted in the milk of lactating mothers in amounts too small to affect the baby.— J. J. Rowan (letter), *Pharm. J.*, 1976, *2*, 184.

Preparations

Ethopropazine Hydrochloride Tablets *(U.S.P.)*. Tablets containing ethopropazine hydrochloride. Protect from light.

Ethopropazine Tablets *(B.P. 1973)*. Tablets containing ethopropazine hydrochloride. The tablets are sugar-coated.

Proprietary Names
Lysivane *(May & Baker, Austral.)*; Parsidol *(Parke, Davis, USA*; *Sévenet, Fr.)*; Parsitan *(Rhône-Poulenc, Canad.)*; Parsotil *(Rhodia, Spain)*.

Ethopropazine hydrochloride was formerly marketed in Great Britain under the proprietary name Lysivane *(May & Baker)*.

368-d

Ethybenztropine Hydrobromide. Etybenzatropine Hydrobromide; Tropethydryline Hydrobromide; UK 738. (1*R*,3*r*,5*S*)-3-Benzhydryloxy-8-ethylnortropane hydrobromide.
$C_{22}H_{27}NO,HBr$=402.4.
CAS — 524-83-4 (ethybenztropine); 24815-25-6 (hydrobromide).

Ethybenztropine hydrobromide 6.25 mg is approximately equivalent to 5 mg of ethybenztropine.

Uses. Ethybenztropine hydrobromide is an anticholinergic agent with actions and uses similar to those of benzhexol (see p.294). It also has antihistaminic properties. It has been used for the symptomatic treatment of parkinsonism and of the drug-induced extrapyramidal syndrome in doses equivalent to 5 to 30 mg of ethybenztropine daily. The hydrochloride has also been given by injection.

Proprietary Names
Ponalid *(Sandoz, Aust.*; *Sandoz, Spain)*; Ponalide *(Sandoz-Wander, Belg.)*; Ponalide *(hydrochloride) (Sandoz, Fr.)*.

369-n

Eucatropine Hydrochloride *(U.S.P.)*. Eucatropinium Chloride; Clorhidrato de Euftalmina. 1,2,2,6-Tetramethyl-4-piperidyl mandelate hydrochloride.
$C_{17}H_{25}NO_3,HCl$=327.9.
CAS — 100-91-4 (eucatropine); 536-93-6 (hydrochloride).

Pharmacopoeias. In *Arg.*, *Mex.*, and *U.S.*

A white odourless granular powder. M.p. 183° to 186°. Very **soluble** in water; freely soluble in alcohol and chloroform; practically insoluble in ether. Solutions in water are neutral to litmus. **Store** in airtight containers. Protect from light.

Adverse Effects, Treatment, and Precautions. As for Atropine, p.289.

Uses. Eucatropine hydrochloride is an anticholinergic agent with mydriatic properties similar to those of atropine (see p.290). Its action is prompt; maximum dilatation occurs within half an hour and the effect lasts about 2 to 6 hours. There is not much risk of an increase in intra-ocular tension. It has little or no effect on accommodation. For ophthalmoscopic examination, 2 drops of a 2 to 10% solution are instilled into the eye and this is repeated after 5 minutes.

One drop (0.032 ml) of cyclopentolate hydrochloride 0.1 and 0.5%, eucatropine hydrochloride 1, 2, and 5%, homatropine hydrobromide 0.5%, phenylephrine hydrochloride 3%, tropicamide 0.5%, or eucatropine 2% in conjunction with phenylephrine 3% was instilled into the conjunctival sac of 5 healthy subjects and the mydriasis and cycloplegia induced measured. Eucatropine had a short duration of action but had less mydriatic action than all but phenylephrine. When combined with phenylephrine the mydriasis was improved without being prolonged but due to the risk of glaucoma from pupil block during recovery reversal with thymoxamine 0.5% was considered necessary. This combination was considered to be suitable for inspection of the fundus.— S. E. Smith, *Lancet*, 1971, *2*, 837.

Preparations

Eucatropine Hydrochloride Ophthalmic Solution *(U.S.P.)*. A sterile iso-osmotic aqueous solution of eucatropine hydrochloride; it may contain suitable antimicrobial agents. pH 4 to 5. Store in airtight containers.

370-k

Fentonium Bromide. Fentonii Bromidum; Ketoscilium; *N*-(4-Phenylphenacyl)hyoscyaminium Bromide. (−)-(1*R*,3*r*,5*S*)-8-(4-Phenylphenacyl)-3-[(*S*)-tropoyloxy]tropanium bromide.
$C_{31}H_{34}BrNO_4$=564.5.
CAS — 5868-06-4.

Adverse Effects, Treatment, and Precautions. As for Atropine, p.289.

Uses. Fentonium bromide is a quaternary ammonium anticholinergic agent with peripheral effects similar to those of atropine (see p.290). It is used as an adjunct in the treatment of gastric and duodenal ulcer, and to relieve visceral spasms. It has been given in a usual dose of 20 mg three or four times daily.

References: M. Moroni and G. Frigerio, *Curr. ther. Res.*, 1977, *21*, 619; S. Ricciardi and R. Cerqua, *Arzneimittel-Forsch.*, 1977, *27*, 1226; U. Marini *et al.*, *Curr. ther. Res.*, 1980, *27*, 239.

Proprietary Names
Ulcesium *(Inpharzam, Ger.*; *Zambon, Ital.)*.

371-a

Glycopyrronium Bromide.

Glycopyrrolate *(U.S.P.)*; AHR 504. 3-(α-Cyclopentylmandeloyloxy)-1,1-dimethylpyrrolidinium bromide.
$C_{19}H_{28}BrNO_3$=398.3.
CAS — 596-51-0.

Pharmacopoeias. In *Nord.* and *U.S.*

A white odourless crystalline powder with a bitter taste. M.p. 193° to 198°. **Soluble** 1 in about 5 of water and 1 in 10 of alcohol; practically insoluble in chloroform and ether. **Incompatible** with alkalis. **Store** in airtight containers.

The compatibility of glycopyrronium bromide with infusion solutions and additives.— T. S. Ingallinera *et al.*, *Am. J. Hosp. Pharm.*, 1979, *36*, 508.

Adverse Effects, Treatment, and Precautions. As for Atropine, p.289.

Glycopyrronium bromide was given by mouth as a single dose varying from 1 to 6 mg to 12 patients without gastro-intestinal symptoms. In doses up to 4 mg, the drug had no effect on normal bowel movement. With a dose of 6 mg or more there was marked and prolonged depression of bowel motility, accompanied by pupillary dilatation, tachycardia, and a dry mouth; these side-effects were not observed with the smaller doses.— B. Fleshler, *J. new Drugs*, 1962, *2*, 211.

A study of the effect of glycopyrronium bromide on performance.— M. Linnoila, *Eur. J. clin. Pharmac.*, 1973, *6*, 107.

Absorption and Fate. Glycopyrronium bromide is poorly absorbed from the gastro-intestinal tract.

A study of 6 postoperative patients given glycopyrronium bromide 200 μg intravenously showed that 90% of the dose had disappeared from the circulation in 5 minutes and was rapidly excreted in bile and urine, mainly as the free drug.— E. Kaltiala *et al.*, *J. Pharm. Pharmac.*, 1974, *26*, 352.

Uses. Glycopyrronium bromide is a quaternary ammonium anticholinergic agent with peripheral effects similar to those of atropine (see p.290). It is used as an adjunct in the treatment of gastric and duodenal ulcer and to relieve visceral

spasms.
The usual dose is 1 to 4 mg twice or thrice daily. Doses of 100 to 200 μg have been given by subcutaneous, intramuscular, or intravenous injection 3 or 4 times daily.
Glycopyrronium has been used in the control of excessive sweating. Glycopyrronium bromide is also used similarly to atropine in anaesthetic practice. For anaesthetic premedication it is given in doses of 200 to 400 μg intravenously or intramuscularly before the induction of anaesthesia; alternatively, it may be given in a dose of 4 to 5 μg per kg body-weight to a maximum of 400 μg. If necessary, similar doses may be given intravenously during the operation and repeated if required. A suggested dosage for premedication in children is 4 to 8 μg per kg intravenously or intramuscularly to a maximum of 200 μg.
Glycopyrronium bromide is given in conjunction with neostigmine to reverse the effects of non-depolarising muscle relaxants (see Neostigmine Methylsulphate, p.1036). The dose is glycopyrronium bromide 200 μg intravenously per 1 mg of neostigmine (or the equivalent dose of pyridostigmine); alternatively, it may be given in a dose of 10 to 15 μg per kg intravenously with neostigmine 50 μg per kg (or the equivalent dose of pyridostigmine). A suggested dosage for children is 10 μg per kg intravenously with neostigmine 50 μg per kg (or the equivalent dose of pyridostigmine). Glycopyrronium bromide can be administered mixed in the same syringe with the anticholinesterase, and it has been suggested that greater cardiovascular stability results from this method of administration.

Anaesthesia. With a view to evaluating its use for premedication, 6 healthy subjects received glycopyrronium bromide, 100, 200, or 400 μg intramuscularly; 100, 140, or 200 μg intravenously; or 2, 4, or 8 mg by mouth. Administration by any of the 3 routes produced significant antisialic effects and depression of sweat-gland activity. There was little effect on pupillary size, heart-rate, or blood pressure. Absorption of the dose given by mouth was poor, and the onset of its effects was delayed compared with the intravenous or intramuscular routes. Dryness of the mouth was reported to last for up to 24 hours after administration by mouth and for about 8 hours after intravenous or intramuscular administration. Three subjects complained of drowsiness during the study and others reported pain on intramuscular injection of the largest dose.— R. K. Mirakhur *et al.*, *Br. J. clin. Pharmac.*, 1978, *5*, 77.

A double-blind comparison of glycopyrronium bromide 200 μg with atropine 600 μg given intramuscularly as the anticholinergic component of premedication was made in 200 patients undergoing surgery. Although glycopyrronium bromide was associated with a smaller increase in heart-rate, there was no difference between the drugs in respect of cardiac arrhythmia, change in arterial pressure, control of secretions in the upper respiratory-tract, frequency of nausea and vomiting after operation, or the subjective well-being of the patients.— T. D. McCubbin *et al.*, *Br. J. Anaesth.*, 1979, *51*, 885.

Glycopyrronium bromide 200 μg produced less tachycardia, pyrexia, nausea and vomiting, and blurred vision than atropine sulphate 600 μg when used for premedication in a double-blind study in 90 patients undergoing surgery. The sedative effect of glycopyrronium bromide was less than that of hyoscine hydrobromide 400 μg. The antisialogogue actions of the 3 drugs were similar.— A. Sengupta *et al.*, *Br. J. Anaesth.*, 1980, *52*, 513.

Other studies and reports on premedication using glycopyrronium bromide: Y. S. Falick and B. G. Smiler, *Anesthesiology*, 1975, *43*, 472; M. R. Salem *et al.*, *Anesthesiology*, 1976, *44*, 216; R. K. Mirakhur *et al.*, *Br. J. Anaesth.*, 1979, *51*, 339.

Reversal of neuromuscular blockade. Studies in 119 surgical patients suggested that pyridostigmine used with glycopyrronium bromide was effective in reversing neuromuscular blockade due to pancuronium bromide, and produced fewer cardiac effects than neostigmine used with atropine.— L. Gyermek, *Curr. ther. Res.*, 1975, *18*, 377.

Neuromuscular blockade in 20 patients was reversed by atropine 1.2 mg with neostigmine 2.5 mg, and in 20 patients by glycopyrronium 500 μg and neostigmine 2.5 mg. The latter treatment avoided the tachycardia present initially in the atropine group, and the antisialogogue effect of glycopyrronium was considered superior to that of atropine. Transient arrhythmias in the 2 groups were comparable.— R. K. Mirakhur *et al.*, *Br. J. Anaesth.*, 1977, *49*, 825.

Further references: C. H. Klingenmaier *et al.*, *Anesth. Analg. curr. Res.*, 1972, *51*, 468; K. A. Oduro, *Can. Anaesth. Soc. J.*, 1975, *22*, 466; J. W. Dundee *et al.*, *Br. J. clin. Pharmac.*, 1977, *4*, 383P; D. A. Cozanitis *et al.*, *Br. J. Anaesth.*, 1980, *52*, 85.

Brain scanning. Glycopyrronium bromide was considered a useful adjunct in brain scanning using pertechnetate (^{99m}Tc).— R. A. Holmes and C. N. Luth, *J. nucl. Med.*, 1975, *16*, 819.

Gastric and duodenal ulcers. Some studies and reports on glycopyrronium bromide therapy of gastric and duodenal ulcers: D. C. H. Sun, *Am. J. dig. Dis.*, 1964, *9*, 706; M. D. Kaye *et al.*, *Gut*, 1969, *10*, 774; *idem*, 1970, *11*, 559; P. E. Baume *et al.*, *Gastroenterology*, 1972, *63*, 399.

Gout. Glycopyrronium bromide increased the excretion of uric acid in 8 of 19 patients with hyperuricaemia or gout.— A. E. Postlethwaite *et al.*, *Archs intern. Med.*, 1974, *134*, 270.

Hyperhidrosis. Prolonged anhidrosis resulted from iontophoresis of glycopyrronium bromide into palmar and plantar skin but results with axillary treatment were disappointingly transient. Anticholinergic symptoms were usually mild and transient.— E. Abell and K. Morgan, *Br. J. Derm.*, 1974, *91*, 87.

Pregnancy and the neonate. Administration of glycopyrronium intravenously to 20 patients in labour had no significant effect on foetal heart-rate or foetal heart-rate variability. Glycopyrronium appeared to be more suitable than atropine during pregnancy since it did not cross the placental barrier.— T. Abboud *et al.*, *Anesthesiology*, 1980, *53*, S316.

Preparations

Glycopyrrolate Injection *(U.S.P.)*. A sterile solution of glycopyrronium bromide in Water for Injections. pH 2 to 3.

Glycopyrrolate Tablets *(U.S.P.)*. Tablets containing glycopyrronium bromide. Store in airtight containers.

Robinul *(Robins, UK)*. Glycopyrronium bromide, available as scored **Tablets** of 2 mg. **Robinul Injection.** Glycopyrronium bromide, available as a solution containing 200 μg per ml, in ampoules of 1 and 3 ml.

Robinul Powder. Glycopyrronium bromide. For preparing solutions for the iontophoretic treatment of idiopathic hyperhidrosis. (Also available as Robinul in *Austral.*, *Canad.*, *Denm.*, *Ger.*, *Neth.*, *Norw.*, *S.Afr.*, *Switz.*, *USA)*.

Other Proprietary Names

Asécryl *(Fr.)*; Nodapton *(Switz.)*; Robanul *(Spain)*; Tarodyl *(Denm.)*; Tarodyn *(Swed.)*.

372-t

Hexocyclium Methylsulphate.
4-(β-Cyclohexyl-β-hydroxyphenethyl)-1,1-dimethylpiperazinium methylsulphate.
$C_{20}H_{33}N_2O,CH_3O_4S=428.6$.

CAS — 6004-98-4 (hexocyclium); 115-63-9 (methylsulphate).

Adverse Effects, Treatment, and Precautions. As for Atropine, p.289.

Uses. Hexocyclium methylsulphate is a quaternary ammonium anticholinergic agent with peripheral effects similar to those of atropine (see p.290). It is used as an adjunct in the treatment of gastric and duodenal ulcer, and to relieve visceral spasms. It has been given in an initial dose of 100 mg daily in divided doses with a maintenance dose being determined according to the needs and tolerance of the patient.

References: M. H. Alp and A. K. Grant, *Med. J. Aust.*, 1969, *1*, 447; H. Orrego-Matte *et al.*, *Am. J. dig. Dis.*, 1971, *16*, 789, per *Int. pharm. Abstr.*, 1972, *9*, 719.

Proprietary Names

Tral *(Abbott, Ital.*; *Abbott, Switz.*; *Abbott, USA)*; Traline *(Abbott, Fr.*; *Abbott, Ger.)*.

373-x

Homatropine *(B.P.C. 1954)*.
(1*R*,3*r*,5*S*)-Tropan-3-yl (±)-mandelate.
$C_{16}H_{21}NO_3=275.3$.

CAS — 87-00-3.

Almost odourless, small white prismatic crystals or coarse crystalline powder. Practically **insoluble** in water; soluble in alcohol, chloroform, ether, dilute mineral acids, and vegetable oils.

374-r

Homatropine Hydrobromide *(B.P., B.P. Vet., Eur. P., U.S.P.)*.
Homatr. Hydrobrom.; Homatropini Hydrobromidum; Homatropinium Bromide; Homatropinum Bromatum; Bromidrato de Homatropina; Omatropina Bromidrato; Tropyl Mandelate Hydrobromide.
$C_{16}H_{21}NO_3,HBr=356.3$.

CAS — 51-56-9.

Pharmacopoeias. In all pharmacopoeias examined except *Chin.*, *Port.*, and *Roum.*

Colourless odourless crystals or a white crystalline powder with a bitter taste. M.p. 214° to 217° with decomposition.
Soluble 1 in 6 of water and 1 in 60 of alcohol, the solubility increasing rapidly as the temperature rises; soluble 1 in 420 of chloroform; practically insoluble in ether. A 2% solution in water has a pH of 5.5 to 7. A 5.67% solution in water is iso-osmotic with serum. Solutions are **sterilised** by autoclaving or by filtration. **Incompatible** with alkalis, iodides, and iron and silver salts. Store in airtight containers. Protect from light.

An aqueous solution of homatropine hydrobromide iso-osmotic with serum (5.67%) caused 92% haemolysis of erythrocytes cultured in it for 45 minutes.— E. R. Hammarlund and K. Pedersen-Bjergaard, *J. pharm. Sci.*, 1961, *50*, 24.

Decomposition by bacteria. Homatropine hydrobromide was completely decomposed within 24 days after its addition in sterile solution to a culture of *Pseudomonas aeruginosa*.— G. C. Güven and T. Altinhurt, *Eczac. Bült.*, 1967, *9*, 65, per *Int. pharm. Abstr.*, 1967, *4*, 1322.

Hydrolysis. The pH of minimum hydroxide-ion and hydrogen-ion catalysed hydrolysis of homatropine varied from 3.8 at 0° to 3.5 at 100°. A solution containing homatropine hydrobromide 1% and boric acid 1.55% lost 2% of its homatropine content after autoclaving for 20 minutes at 120°; the pH fell from 4.5 to 3.8.— M. H. Krasowska *et al.*, *Dansk Tidsskr. Farm.*, 1968, *42*, 170, per R. J. McBride *et al.*, *Pharm. J.*, 1969, *1*, 96.

Adverse Effects, Treatment, and Precautions. As for Atropine, p.289.
Systemic toxicity may occasionally be produced by the instillation of anticholinergic eye-drops, particularly in infants.

Uses. Homatropine is an anticholinergic agent with effects similar to but much weaker than those of atropine (see p.290). It is used as a mydriatic and is preferred to atropine for diagnostic purposes because its action is more rapid, less prolonged, and is more readily controlled by physostigmine. The effect is exerted in 15 to 30 minutes and passes off in 12 to 24 hours. It is sometimes used with cocaine which enhances its mydriatic action.
Homatropine is not a reliable cycloplegic in children; it does not usually produce complete paralysis of accommodation.
The alkaloid has been used as a 2% solution in castor oil, but more often the hydrobromide in aqueous solution is used, generally in a dose of 1 drop of a 2% solution given three times at 10-minute intervals.

For a study of the effects of homatropine on slowing the heart, see A. H. Hayes and R. A. Katz, *Clin. Pharmac. Ther.*, 1970, *11*, 558.

Mydriasis. A study was made of the mydriatic effects of 4 drugs in the concentrations in which they were used in ophthalmology. Homatropine hydrobromide and phenylephrine hydrochloride produced comparable mydriasis but the effect of homatropine lasted longer. Tropicamide had the shortest latency period and produced the greatest dilatation in the shortest time. Hydroxyamphetamine hydrobromide was the least effective.— H. D. Gambill *et al.*, *Archs Ophthal., N.Y.*, 1967, *77*, 740.

Test for glaucoma. A description of a provocative outflow test for detecting open-angle glaucoma, which utilised 2% homatropine eye-drops and drinking water.— D. A. Leighton *et al.*, *Br. J. Ophthal.*, 1970, *54*, 19.

Preparations

Homatropine Eye Drops *(A.P.F.)*. Gutt. Homatrop. Homatropine hydrobromide 2 g, boric acid 1 g, chlorhexidine acetate 10 mg, Water for Injections to 100 ml. Sterilised by autoclaving.

Homatropine Eye Drops *(B.P.)*. HOM. A sterile solution of homatropine hydrobromide in water. When intended for use on more than one occasion they also contain benzalkonium chloride 0.01% or chlorhexidine acetate 0.01% and should not be used more than one month after first opening the container.

The solution is sterilised by autoclaving or by filtration or, if a preservative is present, by maintaining at 98° to 100° for 30 minutes; it is adversely affected by alkalis.

Homatropine Hydrobromide Ophthalmic Solution *(U.S.P.)*. A sterile, buffered, aqueous solution of homatropine hydrobromide; it may contain suitable antimicrobial agents. pH 2.5 to 5. Store in airtight containers.

Homatropine Lamellae *(B.P. 1953)*. Lamellae containing homatropine hydrobromide.

For eye preparations of homatropine hydrobromide with cocaine, see under Cocaine Hydrochloride, p.916.

Proprietary Preparations

Minims Homatropine Hydrobromide *(Smith & Nephew Pharmaceuticals, UK)*. Sterile eye-drops containing homatropine hydrobromide 2% in single-use disposable applicators. (Also available as Minims Homatropine Hydrobromide in *Austral.*).

Other Proprietary Names

Allergan Homatropine *(Austral.)*; Isopto Homatropine *(Austral., Canad., S.Afr.)*; Homat *(Austral.)*.

Homatropine hydrobromide was also formerly marketed in Great Britain under the proprietary name SMP Homatropine *(Armour)*.

375-f

Homatropine Methobromide.

Brometo de Metil-Homatropina; Homatropine Methylbromide *(U.S.P.)*; Methylhomatropinium Bromide; Methylhomatropinium Bromatum. (1*R*,3*r*,5*S*)-3-[(±)-Mandeloyloxy]-8-methyltropanium bromide.

$C_{16}H_{21}NO_3,CH_3Br$=370.3.

CAS — 80-49-9.

Pharmacopoeias. In *Aust., Braz., Hung.*, and *U.S.*

A white odourless powder with a bitter taste. M.p. about 190°. Very **soluble** in water; freely soluble in alcohol; practically insoluble in acetone and ether. A 1% solution in water has a pH of 4.5 to 6.5. Solutions are **sterilised** by maintaining at 98° to 100° for 30 minutes with a bactericide or by filtration. **Incompatible** with alkalis and iodine. **Store** in airtight containers. Protect from light.

Adverse Effects, Treatment, and Precautions. As for Atropine, p.289.

Uses. Homatropine methobromide is a quaternary ammonium anticholinergic agent with peripheral effects similar to those of atropine (see p.290). It has been used as an adjunct in the treatment of gastric and duodenal ulcer, and to relieve visceral spasms. Usual doses of homatropine methobromide were 3 to 10 mg four times daily.

Preparations

Homatropine Methylbromide Tablets *(U.S.P.)*. Tablets containing homatropine methobromide. Store in airtight containers. Protect from light.

Proprietary Names

Dallapasmo *(Dallas, Arg.)*; Homapin *(Mission Pharmacal, USA)*; Mesopin *(Fulton, Ital.)*; Novatrin *(Ayerst, USA)*; Novatropina *(Chinoin, Ital.; Promesa, Spain)*; Paratropina *(Lazar, Arg.)*; Pasmolona *(Paylos, Arg.)*.

376-d

Hyoscine Butylbromide *(B.P.)*.

Scopolamine Butylbromide; Butylscopolamonii Bromidum; Hyoscine-*N*-Butyl Bromide; Scopolamine *N*-Butyl Bromide. (−)-(1*S*,3*s*,5*R*,6*R*,7*S*)-8-Butyl-6,7-epoxy-3-[(*S*)-tropoyloxy]tropanium bromide.

$C_{21}H_{30}BrNO_4$=440.4.

CAS — 51-34-3 (hyoscine); 149-64-4 (butylbromide).

Pharmacopoeias. In *Br.* and *Roum.*

A white or almost white, odourless or almost odourless, crystalline powder with a bitter taste. M.p. 140° to 144°. **Soluble** 1 in 1 of water, 1 in 50 of alcohol, and 1 in 5 of chloroform; practically insoluble in ether. A 10% solution in water is laevorotatory and has a pH of 5.5 to 6.5. **Protect** from light.

Adverse Effects, Treatment, and Precautions. As for Atropine, p.289.

CAUTION. *Hyoscine may cause drowsiness and dulling of mental alertness. Patients undergoing treatment with hyoscine should not take charge of vehicles, other means of transport, or machinery where loss of attention may lead to accidents. Patients should abstain from alcohol.*

Porphyria. A study in *rats* indicated that hyoscine butylbromide would probably not elicit an acute attack in susceptible porphyric individuals.— G. H. Blekkenhorst *et al.* (letter), *Lancet*, 1980, *1*, 1367. Criticisms of extrapolating data obtained from *animal* experiments to the treatment of human disease.— M. J. Brodie (letter), *ibid.*, *2*, 86; A. Gorchein (letter), *ibid.*, 152. Reply.— G. H. Blekkenhorst and L. Eales (letter), *ibid.*, 1250.

X-ray examination. Administration of hyoscine butylbromide intramuscularly 10 to 15 minutes before radiological examination of the stomach to slow peristaltic movements was recommended only when detailed examination was to be carried out, otherwise deformity of the stomach due to linear and multiple ulcers might be obscured.— T. F. Solanke *et al.*, *Gut*, 1969, *10*, 436.

Absorption and Fate. Hyoscine butylbromide is poorly absorbed from the gastro-intestinal tract.

Absorption and inactivation studies. In 10 experiments in 3 volunteers, hyoscine butylbromide, in single doses of up to 600 mg taken as tablets, appeared to be inactive by mouth; either it remained unabsorbed or it was absorbed more slowly than it was inactivated in the body.— A. Herxheimer and L. Haefeli, *Lancet*, 1966, *2*, 418.

Investigations in 2 healthy subjects indicated that in contrast to propantheline bromide and hyoscine methonitrate, hyoscine butylbromide given intramuscularly produced only transient effects and influenced mainly the near point of ocular accommodation.— J. Möller and A. Rosén, *Acta med. scand.*, 1968, *184*, 201.

After 50 to 100 mg of hyoscine butylbromide was given to 6 male volunteers, by mouth or by intra-intestinal infusion, very little hyoscine butylbromide was absorbed from the upper small intestine and none appeared in the plasma. About 2% and 90% of the dose appeared in the urine and faeces respectively. After intravenous administration of 8 mg to 1 volunteer, 42% was eliminated in the urine and 37% in faeces.— K. Hellström *et al.*, *Scand. J. Gastroenterol.*, 1970, *5*, 585.

When radioactive hyoscine butylbromide was fed to *rats* 6% of the dose was excreted in the bile and 2% in the urine during the 24 hours after administration; 56.6% of the dose was found in the gastro-intestinal tract, half of this in intestinal contents and about 20% absorbed in the walls and lining of the distal small intestine. Following an intraportal injection of hyoscine butylbromide, 42% of the dose was excreted in the bile and 36% in the *rats'* urine within 12 hours of injection.— P. Pentikäinen *et al.*, *J. Pharm. Pharmac.*, 1973, *25*, 371.

Studies in 2 patients showed that hyoscine butylbromide had an enterohepatic circulation.— H. Vapaatalo *et al.*, *J. Pharm. Pharmac.*, 1975, *27*, 542.

Uses. Hyoscine butylbromide is a quaternary ammonium anticholinergic agent the peripheral effects of which are similar to those of atropine (see p.290) but of shorter duration. It is used in conditions associated with visceral spasms.

The usual dose is 20 mg intramuscularly or intravenously, repeated after 30 minutes if necessary. It is also given by mouth in doses of 20 mg four times daily, and has been claimed to be of value in spasmodic dysmenorrhoea.

In studies in 36 healthy persons, subcutaneous injections of hyoscine butylbromide were found to accelerate the heart rapidly and to inhibit salivary secretion; these effects were of short duration. A much slower effect on accommodation was noted: paralysis of accommodation persisted for 1 to 2 hours.— A. Herxheimer and L. Haefeli, *Lancet*, 1966, *2*, 418. A comment.— W. Graubner (letter), *ibid.*, 700. A reply.— A. Herxheimer (letter), *ibid.*

Hyoscine butylbromide had restored sinus rhythm for periods of up to one hour to hearts affected by arrythmias associated with pancuronium and halothane. It had also restored normal cardiac rhythm in 2 cases of nodal bradycardia and hypotension, in 3 cases of multiple ventricular extrasystoles, and in one case of atrioventricular dissociation within one minute of intravenous injection.— E. N. S. Fry (letter), *Br. med. J.*, 1979, *2*, 1075.

Anaesthesia. No oculocardiac reflex occurred in 73 of 74 patients undergoing squint operations who were given hyoscine butylbromide intravenously before surgery.— E. N. S. Fry and B. J. P. Hall-Parker (letter), *Br. J. Ophthal.*, 1975, *59*, 525.

Gastro-intestinal action. In a double-blind study in 7 healthy subjects the effects on gut motility of hyoscine butylbromide following administration by mouth and by intravenous injection were assessed by recording bowel sounds. In 6 subjects, 8 mg of hyoscine butylbromide intravenously reduced bowel sounds for 15 to 30 minutes followed by increased sounds, while 200 mg by mouth had no effect over the succeeding 2½ to 3 hours. In the 7th subject, increased sounds occurred after both oral and intravenous administration.— J. -P. Guignard *et al.*, *Clin. Pharmac. Ther.*, 1968, *9*, 745.

For the effect of hyoscine butylbromide in irritable bowel syndrome, see Ispaghula, p.957.

Further references: E. Schmid *et al.*, *Arzneimittel-Forsch.*, 1968, *18*, 1449; *idem*, 1969, *19*, 998; W. Boriss *et al.*, *Medsche Welt, Stuttg.*, 1971, *22*, 402; A. Miyoshi, *Jap. Archs intern. Med.*, 1973, *20*, 339; E. R. Birke, *Therapiewoche*, 1974, *24*, 1803; H. Sieg, *Z. Gastroent.*, 1974, *12*, 235; E. N. SFry and S. Deshpande (letter), *Br. med. J.*, 1976, *1*, 646; A. Miyoshi *et al.*, *J. int. med. Res.*, 1977, *5*, 223.

X-ray examination. Hyoscine butylbromide, 20 mg by intravenous injection, was administered to 102 patients immediately before X-ray examination of the gastro-intestinal tract. Its antispasmodic properties facilitated the examination of the large intestine and the assessment of achalasia of the cardia and acute peptic ulcer with spasticity.— J. P. Murray, *Br. J. Radiol.*, 1966, *93*, 102, per *Abstr. Wld Med.*, 1966, *40*, 78. See also under Adverse Effects and Precautions, p.302.

The detection of oesophageal varices using barium swallow and parenteral hyoscine butylbromide.— R. Waldram *et al.*, *Clin. Radiol.*, 1977, *28*, 137.

Preparations

Hyoscine Butylbromide Injection *(B.P.)*. A sterile solution of hyoscine butylbromide in Water for Injections. Sterilised by autoclaving. pH 3.7 to 5.5. Protect from light.

Hyoscine Butylbromide Tablets *(B.P.)*. Tablets containing hyoscine butylbromide; they may be sugar-coated.

Buscopan *(Boehringer Ingelheim, UK)*. Hyoscine butylbromide, available as 1-ml **Ampoules** of an injection containing 20 mg per ml and as **Tablets** of 10 mg. (Also available as Buscopan in *Austral., Belg., Canad., Denm., Fr., Ger., Ital., Neth., Norw., S.Afr., Swed., Switz.*).

Other Proprietary Names

Arg.— Buscapina; *Ital.*— Salfalgin, Spasmamina; *Jap.*— Butibol, Butylmido, Diaste-M, Hyospan, Reladan, Scordin-B; *Spain*— Buscapina.

377-n

Hyoscine Hydrobromide *(B.P., B.P. Vet.)*.

Hyoscini Hydrobromidum; Scopolamine Hydrobromide *(U.S.P.)*; Scopolamini Hydrobromidum *(Eur. P.)*; Scopolamine Hydrobromide; Scopolamine Bromhydrate; Ioscina Bromidrato; Bromhidrato de Escopolamina. (−)-(1*S*,3*s*,5*R*,6*R*,7*S*)-6,7-Epoxytropan-3-yl (*S*)-tropate hydrobromide trihydrate.

$C_{17}H_{21}NO_4,HBr,3H_2O$=438.3.

CAS — 114-49-8 (anhydrous); 6533-68-2 (trihydrate).

Pharmacopoeias. In all pharmacopoeias examined except *Braz.*

Odourless, colourless, transparent crystals or white crystalline powder with a somewhat bitter, acrid taste. It is slightly efflorescent in dry air. M.p. about 197° with decomposition, determined on the dried substance.

Soluble 1 in 3.5 of water and 1 in 30 of alcohol; practically insoluble in chloroform and ether. A 5% solution in water has a pH of 4 to 5.5. A 7.85% solution in water is iso-osmotic with serum. Solutions are **sterilised** by autoclaving or by filtration. **Incompatible** with alkalis, iodine, silver salts, and tannic acid. **Store** below 20° in airtight containers. Protect from light.

Incompatibility. A haze has been reported to develop in 1 hour when 10 ml of methohexitone sodium 1% is mixed with 1 ml of solution containing hyoscine hydrobromide 500 µg.

Adverse Effects, Treatment, and Precautions. As for Atropine, p.289. Central stimulation sometimes precedes depression but the main central symptoms are drowsiness leading to coma. The depression may be enhanced by other central depressants administered concomitantly.

CAUTION. *Hyoscine may cause drowsiness and dulling of mental alertness. Patients undergoing treatment with hyoscine should not take charge of vehicles, other means of transport, or machinery where loss of attention may lead to accidents. Patients should abstain from alcohol.*

Reports of confusional states with hallucinations occurring in children given recommended doses of travel-sickness tablets containing hyoscine: G. L. Hindson (letter), *Br. med. J.*, 1958, *2*, 636 (hyoscine); M. E. Bradford (letter), *New Engl. J. Med.*, 1967, *277*, 1209 (hyoscine with meprobamate).

Reports of central and peripheral toxicity following application of hyoscine eye-drops.— S. E. Young *et al.*, *Am. J. Ophthal.*, 1971, *72*, 1136; W. Gopel *et al.*, *Dte GesundhWes.*, 1976, *31*, 927.

For reports and comments on the use of physostigmine to reverse the effects of poisoning by hyoscine and other anticholinergic agents, see Physostigmine Salicylate, p.1043.

Pregnancy and the neonate. A report of hyoscine toxicity in a neonate born to a mother who had received a total of 1.8 mg of hyoscine in divided doses with pethidine and levorphanol prior to delivery. The neonate was lethargic, barrel chested, and had a heart-rate of 200. Symptoms subsided following physostigmine 100 µg given intramuscularly.— R. P. Evens and J. C. Leopold (letter), *Pediatrics*, 1980, *66*, 329.

Absorption and Fate. Hyoscine hydrobromide is readily absorbed from the gastro-intestinal tract. It is almost entirely metabolised in the body. Hyoscine crosses the placental barrier and traces may appear in milk.

In a controlled double-blind study in groups of 8 subjects, measurements were made of saliva flow, heart-rate, pupil diameter, and mental alertness for up to 8 hours after intramuscular injection of 50, 100, 200, and 400 µg of hyoscine hydrobromide. Peak activity was achieved 1 to 2 hours after the dose, with a gradual decline over the 8-hour period.— J. J. Brand, *Br. J. Pharmac. Chemother.*, 1969, *35*, 202.

In 1 subject a peak plasma concentration was achieved about 1 hour after hyoscine 906 µg was taken by mouth. In 2 subjects a total of 4 to 5% of hyoscine was excreted in the urine after a single dose of hyoscine 906 or 800 µg.— W. F. Bayne *et al.*, *J. pharm. Sci.*, 1975, *64*, 288.

Pregnancy and the neonate. No significant quantities of hyoscine were found in milk when the drug was given to lactating women.— B. E. Takyi, *J. Hosp. Pharm.*, 1970, *28*, 317.

See also under Adverse Effects.

Uses. Hyoscine is an anticholinergic agent with central and peripheral actions. The central action differs from that of atropine in that hyoscine produces depression of the cerebral cortex, especially of the motor areas, and acts as a powerful hypnotic; the drowsiness is sometimes preceded by a brief stage of excitement. Unlike atropine, hyoscine usually slows the heart.

Hyoscine hydrobromide has been used with morphine in acute mania and delirium, including delirium tremens. It has also been tried for the relief of withdrawal symptoms in various treatments of morphine dependence.

For pre-operative medication, hyoscine hydrobromide is injected subcutaneously in doses of 400 µg, usually with 10 mg of morphine hydrochloride or sulphate, 20 mg of papaveretum, or 100 mg of pethidine hydrochloride about 45 to 60 minutes before induction of general anaesthesia. This calms the patient, reduces secretions, produces amnesia, diminishes some of the side-effects of the anaesthetic, and assists the induction process.

Hyoscine hydrobromide taken 20 minutes to an hour before a journey is used in doses of 600 µg for the prevention and treatment of motion sickness; further doses of 300 µg may be taken every 6 hours. Children aged 3 to 7 years may be given 75 to 150 µg and those 7 to 12 years, 150 to 300 µg. In intractable hiccup, a dose of 300 µg, repeated if necessary 30 minutes later, may afford relief.

In obstetrics, hyoscine was used in conjunction with morphine or pethidine to produce a condition of amnesia and partial analgesia known as 'twilight sleep'. It has also been used in the symptomatic treatment of idiopathic and postencephalitic parkinsonism.

Hyoscine hydrobromide has been used in the eye for its mydriatic and cycloplegic actions. It has a more rapid onset and shorter duration of action than atropine but is more toxic.

In normal subjects, a rapid intravenous injection of hyoscine hydrobromide, 25 to 200 µg per 70 kg body-weight, decreased the heart-rate by 12 to 15 beats per minute within 10 minutes. Doses of 300 to 600 µg first increased then decreased the heart-rate. Atropine, 200 µg per 70 kg intravenously, given 180 minutes after 300 to 600 µg of hyoscine increased the heart-rate but had no effect when given after lower doses of hyoscine hydrobromide.— J. S. Gravenstein and J. I. Thornby, *Clin. Pharmac. Ther.*, 1969, *10*, 395.

Anaesthesia. In a comparison of the efficacy of drugs commonly used in pre-anaesthetic medication, a double-blind study was made of (1) papaveretum 20 mg with hyoscine 400 µg, (2) pethidine 100 mg with atropine 600 µg, (3) promethazine 50 mg with atropine 600 µg, and (4) hyoscine alone, 400 µg, all given intramuscularly. The majority of patients were neither asleep nor sleepy before operation. Papaveretum with hyoscine produced most sedation and greatest relief of anxiety. Atropine produced greater tachycardia than hyoscine. There was a high incidence of hypotension with the papaveretum-hyoscine and the pethidine-atropine mixtures. Dry throat was commonest after premedication which included hyoscine.— S. A. Feldman, *Anaesthesia*, 1963, *18*, 169.

In 49 patients who had undergone general anaesthesia for an obstetric or gynaecological procedure and who had received hyoscine 800 µg pre-operatively, no incidence of awareness during operation was reported, but 18 of 229 patients who received atropine 0.6 to 1 mg reported awareness, while 2 of 12 patients who received neither reported awareness. When atropine was used, dreams recalled were nearly always described as horrifying and accompanied by a feeling of dizziness, while with the use of hyoscine dreaming was less pronounced and was always pleasant.— J. S. Crawford *et al.* (letter), *Br. med. J.*, 1969, *1*, 508.

A discussion of the use of hyoscine hydrobromide in premedication for hypotensive anaesthesia.— J. G. Goodbody (letter), *Br. med. J.*, 1969, *4*, 368.

A study on the value of anticholinergic premedication.— K. M. Leighton and H. D. Sanders, *Can. Anaesth. Soc. J.*, 1976, *23*, 563.

Administration by mouth. The effects of atropine and hyoscine following oral and intramuscular administration were assessed in 6 healthy adults. Atropine 2 mg or hyoscine 1 mg were considered to be effective as oral premedicants. Inhibition of salivation was adequate but ocular effects were minimal. Tachycardia only occurred with atropine 2 mg. Peak effects were generally seen 2 hours after oral administration compared with 1 hour after intramuscular injection.— R. K. Mirakhur, *Br. J. Anaesth.*, 1978, *50*, 591.

Amnesia. Hyoscine, 600 µg by intravenous injection, produced amnesia in up to 50% of patients studied. The maximum incidence of amnesia occurred at 50 to 80 minutes but effects were still evident in some patients after 120 minutes.— J. W. Dundee and S. K. Pandit, *Br. J. Pharmac.*, 1972, *44*, 140.

Other references to amnesia including comparative studies with diazepam: D. A. Drachman and J. Leavitt, *Archs Neurol., Chicago*, 1974, *30*, 113; M. J. Frumin *et al.*, *Anesthesiology*, 1976, *45*, 406; M. M. Ghoneim and S. P. Mewaldt, *Clin. Pharmac. Ther.*, 1977, *21*, 103.

Epilepsy diagnosis. A dose of 1 mg of hyoscine hybrobromide, injected intravenously, significantly activated the EEG in 45 of 53 patients with psychomotor epilepsy, and was considered superior to the technique of thiopentone narcosis.— C. J. Vas *et al.*, *Electroenceph. clin. Neurophysiol.*, 1967, *22*, 373.

Hyperhidrosis. An account of the topical use of anticholinergic drugs for their antiperspirant action. Esters of hyoscine hydrobromide were found to be much more effective than any other type of compound studied, and this was related to their ability to penetrate intact skin, perhaps 5 to 10% of the amount applied. A 0.025% solution of the benzoyl ester of hyoscine repeatedly applied to a limited area produced 35% reduction of axillary sweating without causing systemic effects, and skin irritation or sensitisation did not occur.— F. S. K. MacMillan *et al.*, *J. invest. Derm.*, 1964, *43*, 363.

Motion sickness. In a study of 26 drugs on thousands of men on transport ships, single doses of hyoscine hydrobromide gave good protection against seasickness but repeated doses were associated with the most distressing side-effects of all the prophylactic drugs used, and provided no protection. Hyoscine was thus of little value in protecting against seasickness of long duration.—Report of a Study by Army, Navy, Air Force Motion Sickness Team, *J. Am. med. Ass.*, 1956, *160*, 755.

Hyoscine hydrobromide in doses equivalent to 100 µg of base protected 75% of susceptible volunteers from motion sickness with minimal side-effects.— J. J. Brand *et al.*, *Br. J. Pharmac. Chemother.*, 1967, *30*, 463.

Beneficial results on motion sickness using transdermally administered hyoscine.— J. E. Shaw *et al.*, *Clin. Pharmac. Ther.*, 1977, *21*, 117. See also N. M. Price *et al.*, *ibid.*, 1981, *29*, 414.

Some other reports and studies: C. D. Wood and A. Graybiel, *Aerospace Med.*, 1968, *39*, 1341; J. J. Brand and P. Whittingham, *Lancet*, 1970, *2*, 232.

Preparations

Eye Ointments

Hyoscine Eye Ointment *(B.P.)*. Oculent. Hyoscin. A sterile eye ointment containing hyoscine hydrobromide in Simple Eye Ointment.

Scopolamine Hydrobromide Ophthalmic Ointment *(U.S.P.)*. A sterile eye ointment containing hyoscine hydrobromide in a suitable basis.

Eye-drops

Hyoscine Eye Drops *(A.P.F.)*. Gutt. Hyoscin. Hyoscine hydrobromide 250 mg, boric acid 1.8 g, chlorhexidine acetate 10 mg, Water for Injections to 100 ml. Sterilised by autoclaving.

Hyoscine Eye Drops *(B.P.)*. HYO. A sterile solution of hyoscine hydrobromide in water. When intended for use on more than one occasion they also contain benzalkonium chloride 0.01% or chlorhexidine acetate 0.01% and should not be used more than one month after first opening the container.

Sterilised by autoclaving or by filtration, or, if containing a bactericide, by maintaining at 98° to 100° for 30 minutes. They are adversely affected by alkalis.

Scopolamine Hydrobromide Ophthalmic Solution *(U.S.P.)*. A sterile buffered aqueous solution of hyoscine hydrobromide. It may contain suitable antimicrobial agents and stabilisers, and additives to increase viscosity. pH 4 to 6. Store in airtight containers.

Injections

Hyoscine Injection *(B.P.)*. Hyoscine Hydrobromide Injection. A sterile solution of hyoscine hydrobromide in Water for Injections. Sterilised by autoclaving. Protect from light.

Scopolamine Hydrobromide Injection *(U.S.P.)*. A sterile solution of hyoscine hydrobromide in Water for Injections. pH 3.5 to 6.5. Protect from light.

Tablets

Hyoscine Tablets *(B.P.)*. Tablets containing hyoscine hydrobromide.

Scopolamine Hydrobromide Tablets *(U.S.P.)*. Tablets containing hyoscine hydrobromide. Store in airtight containers. Protect from light.

Proprietary Preparations

Minims Hyoscine Hydrobromide *(Smith & Nephew Pharmaceuticals, UK)*. Sterile eye-drops containing hyoscine hydrobromide 0.2% in single-use disposable applicators.

Other Proprietary Names
Boro-Scopol (borate) *(Ger.)*; Isopto Hyoscine *(S.Afr.)*; Scopos *(Fr.)*; Skopolamin *(Denm., Norw.)*; Vorigeno *(Spain)*.

378-h

Hyoscine Methobromide *(B.P.)*.
Hyoscine Methylbromide; Epoxymethamine Bromide; Methscopolamine Bromide *(U.S.P.)*; Scopolamine Methylbromide. (−)-(1*S*,3*s*,5*R*,6*R*,7*S*)-6,7-Epoxy-8-methyl-3-[(*S*)-tropoyloxy]tropanium bromide.
$C_{18}H_{24}BrNO_4$=398.3.

CAS — 155-41-9.

Pharmacopoeias. In *Br.* and *U.S.*

White crystals or a white or almost white, odourless or almost odourless crystalline powder with a bitter taste. M.p. about 225° with decomposition. **Soluble** 1 in 3 of water, 1 in 100 of alcohol, and 1 in 40 of methyl alcohol; practically insoluble in acetone and chloroform. A 5% solution in water is laevorotatory and has a pH of 6.5 to 8. **Store** in airtight containers. Protect from light.

Incompatibilities. Solutions of hyoscine methobromide were stable at pH 2 to 6. Solutions at pH 7 and over were decomposed in a few hours. Incompatible with sodium arsenate, arsenite, bicarbonate, glycerophosphate, laurylsulphate, *p*-aminobenzoate, and propionate, with fluorescein sodium, sodium methyl hydroxybenzoate, aluminium hydroxide mixture, and camphorated opium tincture.— J. K. Dale and R. E. Booth, *J. Am. pharm. Ass., pract. Pharm. Edn*, 1955, *16*, 554.

Adverse Effects, Treatment, and Precautions. As for Atropine, p.289.

CAUTION. *Hyoscine may cause drowsiness and dulling of mental alertness. Patients undergoing treatment with hyoscine should not take charge of vehicles, other means of transport, or machinery where loss of attention may lead to accidents. Patients should abstain from alcohol.*

Uses. Hyoscine methobromide is a quaternary ammonium anticholinergic agent with peripheral effects similar to those of atropine (see p.290). It is used as an adjunct in the treatment of gastric and duodenal ulcer, and to relieve visceral spasms. Usual doses of hyoscine methobromide are 2.5 mg thrice daily half an hour before meals and 2.5 to 5 mg at bedtime; doses of 0.25 to 1 mg have been given subcutaneously or intramuscularly every 6 to 8 hours.
Hyoscine methylsulphate has been used for similar purposes.

Hyoscine methobromide appeared to be more reliable than atropine in causing dose-related increments in heart-rate; it could be safely administered in doses of 150 µg or less, intravenously every 5 or 10 minutes until the desired heart-rate had been obtained.— J. B. Neeld *et al.*, *Clin. Pharmac. Ther.*, 1975, *17*, 290.

Preparations

Hyoscine Methobromide Tablets *(B.P.)*. Tablets containing hyoscine methobromide. Protect from light.

Methscopolamine Bromide Injection *(U.S.P.)*. A sterile solution of hyoscine methobromide in Water for Injections. pH 4.5 to 6.

Methscopolamine Bromide Tablets *(U.S.P.)*. Tablets containing hyoscine methobromide. Store in airtight containers.

Proprietary Names
Blocan *(Estedi, Spain)*; Holopon *(Byk, Belg.; Byk Gulden, Ger.)*; Pamine *(Upjohn, Austral.; Upjohn, Canad.; Upjohn, USA)*; Scordin *(Jap.)*.

Hyoscine methobromide was formerly marketed in Great Britain under the proprietary name Pamine (*Upjohn*).

A preparation containing hyoscine methobromide was formerly marketed in Great Britain under the proprietary name Paminal (*Upjohn*).

379-m

Hyoscine Methonitrate *(B.P., Eur. P.)*.
Hyoscine Methylnitrate; Methscopolamine Nitrate; Methylscopolamini Nitras; Methylhyoscini Nitras; Scopolamine Methylnitrate. (−)-(1*S*,3*s*,5*R*,6*R*,7*S*)-6,7-Epoxy-8-methyl-3-[(*S*)-tropoyloxy]tropanium nitrate.
$C_{18}H_{24}N_2O_7$=380.4.

CAS — 6106-46-3.

Pharmacopoeias. In *Br., Eur., Fr., Ger., It., Neth.*, and *Nord.*

Odourless colourless hygroscopic crystals or a white crystalline powder with a bitter taste. M.p. 194° to 199°. **Soluble** 1 in 1.5 of water and 1 in 40 of alcohol; practically insoluble in chloroform and ether. A solution in water is laevorotatory. A 5% solution in water has a pH of 6 to 7. A 6.95% solution in water is iso-osmotic with serum. **Incompatible** with alkalis. Solutions are **sterilised** by autoclaving or by filtration. **Store** in airtight containers. Protect from light.

Uses. Hyoscine methonitrate is a quaternary ammonium anticholinergic agent with the actions and uses of hyoscine methobromide (above). The usual dose is 2 to 4 mg half an hour before meals and at bedtime; the total daily dose should not exceed 12 mg. The parenteral dose is 250 to 500 µg subcutaneously or intramuscularly 3 or 4 times daily. It has been used to treat infantile colic in doses of 60 to 180 µg given 15 minutes before feeds.

Pyloric stenosis. A report of the use of hyoscine methonitrate, in conjunction with gastric lavage and restriction of oral feeding, in the treatment of 16 infants with pyloric stenosis.— L. R. Day, *J. Am. med. Ass.*, 1969, *207*, 949.

Proprietary Names
Skopyl *(Pharmacia, Denm.; Pharmacia, Ger.; Pharmacia, Swed.)*.

Hyoscine methonitrate was formerly marketed in Great Britain under the proprietary name Skopyl (*Pharmacia*).

380-t

Hyoscine Oxide Hydrobromide.
Scopolamine *N*-Oxide Hydrobromide; Scopolamine Aminoxide Hydrobromide. Hyoscine *N*-oxide hydrobromide.
$C_{17}H_{21}NO_5,HBr$=400.3.

CAS — 97-75-6 (hyoscine oxide); 6106-81-6 (hydrobromide).

Uses. Hyoscine oxide hydrobromide has the general properties of hyoscine (see p.302). It has been used, in doses of 1.25 mg thrice daily, in parkinsonism.

Proprietary Names
Génoscopolamine *(Amido, Fr.)*.

381-x

Hyoscyamine *(U.S.P., B.P.C. 1934)*.
l-Hyoscyamine. (−)-1*R*,3*r*,5*S*)Tropan-3-yl (*S*)-tropate.
$C_{17}H_{23}NO_3$=289.4.

CAS — 101-31-5.

Pharmacopoeias. In *U.S.*

An alkaloid obtained from various solanaceous plants, *Hyoscyamus muticus* and *Duboisia myoporoides* being the best sources. It is the laevo-isomer of atropine into which it can be converted by heating or by the action of alkali. A white crystalline powder with a bitter acrid taste. M.p. 106° to 109°. **Soluble** 1 in 280 of water, 1 in 1 of chloroform, and 1 in 48 of ether; freely soluble in alcohol and dilute acids. A 1% solution in diluted alcohol is laevorotatory. A solution in water is alkaline to litmus. **Store** in airtight containers. Protect from light.

For a study on the stability of hyoscyamine in some *B.P.C.* mixtures, see S. A. H. Khalil and S. El-Masry, *J. Pharm. Pharmac.*, 1978, *30*, 664.

Adverse Effects, Treatment, and Precautions. As for Atropine, p.289.

Uses. Hyoscyamine is an anticholinergic agent with actions similar to those of atropine (see p.290) but it is more potent both in its central and its peripheral effects; the dextro-isomer is practically inactive. Hyoscyamine is usually employed as the hydrobromide or the sulphate. It is given in doses of 150 to 300 µg four times daily.

Studies on the effect of hyoscyamine on gastric acidity and salivary flow: G. Dotevall *et al.*, *Gut*, 1967, *8*, 276; M. D. Kaye *et al.*, *ibid.*, 1968, *9*, 590; A. Walan, *Scand. J. Gastroenterol.*, 1969, *4*, 157.

Preparations

Hyoscyamine Tablets *(U.S.P.)*. Tablets containing hyoscyamine. Protect from light.

Proprietary Names
Cystospaz *(Webcon, USA)*.

382-r

Hyoscyamine Hydrobromide *(U.S.P., B.P.C. 1949)*.
Hyoscyamine Bromhydrate; Bromidrato de Hiosciamina.
$C_{17}H_{23}NO_3,HBr$=370.3.

CAS — 306-03-6.

Pharmacopoeias. In *Braz., Span.*, and *U.S.*

White, odourless, prismatic crystals or crystalline powder with a bitter acrid taste. M.p. not less than 149°.
Freely **soluble** in water; soluble 1 in 2.5 of alcohol and 1 in 1.7 of chloroform; very slightly soluble in ether. A 5% solution in water is laevorotatory and has a pH of about 5.4. Solutions are **sterilised** by maintaining at 98° to 100° for 30 minutes with a bactericide or by filtration. **Store** in a cool place in airtight containers. Protect from light.

Uses. Hyoscyamine hydrobromide has the actions and uses of hyoscyamine sulphate and has been given in doses of 300 to 600 µg

---

383-f

Hyoscyamine Sulphate *(B.P., Eur. P., U.S.P.)*.
Hyoscyamini Sulfas; Hyoscyaminium Sulfuricum.
$(C_{17}H_{23}NO_3)_2,H_2SO_4,2H_2O$=712.9.

CAS — 620-61-1 (anhydrous); 6835-16-1 (dihydrate).

Pharmacopoeias. In *Br., Eur., Fr., Ger., It., Neth.*, and *U.S. Swiss* specifies $1H_2O$. Hyoscyamine sulphate (anhydrous) was included in *B.P.C. 1949.*

Odourless colourless needles or a white deliquescent crystalline powder with a bitter acrid taste. M.p. about 203° with decomposition. **Soluble** 2 in 1 of water and 1 in 5 of alcohol; sparingly soluble in dehydrated alcohol; practically insoluble in chloroform and ether. A 5% solution in water is laevorotatory. A 1% solution in water has a pH of about 5.3. Solutions are **sterilised** by maintaining at 98° to 100° for 30 minutes with a bactericide or by filtration. **Incompatibilities** as for Atropine Sulphate, p.292. **Store** in airtight containers. Protect from light.

Adverse Effects, Treatment, and Precautions. As for Atropine, p.289.

Uses. Hyoscyamine sulphate is an anticholinergic agent with actions and uses similar to those of atropine (see p.290). It has been used as an adjunct in the treatment of gastric and duodenal ulcers and to relieve the symptoms of parkinsonism, to quieten mental excitement in delirium tremens and mania, and to prevent motion sickness. Sources in the USA recommend doses of 125 to 250 µg three or four times daily; sources in the UK recommend 400 to 600 µg twice daily, with a maximum dose of 1 mg thrice daily in individual cases. It has also been given by injection.

Preparations

Hyoscyamine Sulfate Tablets *(U.S.P.)*. Tablets containing hyoscyamine sulphate. Store in airtight containers. Protect from light.

Peptard *(Riker, UK)*. Hyoscyamine sulphate, available as sustained-release tablets containing the equivalent of anhydrous hyoscyamine sulphate 200 µg.

Other Proprietary Names
Anaspaz, Cystospaz-M (both *USA*); Egacen *(S.Afr., Switz.)*; Egacene *(Neth.)*; Egazil *(Denm., Norw., Swed.)*; Levsin *(Canad., USA)*; Levsinex *(USA)*.

384-d

Hyoscyamus Leaf *(B.P., Eur. P.)*.
Hyoscy.; Hyoscyamus; Henbane Leaves; Hyoscyami Folium; Hyoscyami Herba; Jusquiame Noire; Bilsenkrautblätter; Giusquiamo; Hojas de Beleno; Meimendro; Banotu.

Pharmacopoeias. In *Arg., Belg., Br., Eur., Fr., Ger., Hung., Ind., Int., It., Mex., Neth., Rus., Span.*, and *Turk. Port.* specifies not less than 0.065% alkaloids, *Roum.* not less than 0.04%, *Swiss* not less than 0.03%. *Br.* also includes Powdered Hyoscyamus Leaf. *Chin.* specifies only the seeds.

The dried leaves, or leaves and flowering tops of *Hyoscyamus niger* (Solanaceae), containing not less than 0.05% of alkaloids calculated as hyoscyamine. The principal alkaloid is hyoscyamine, with smaller amounts of hyoscine and atropine. **Store** in a cool dry place. Protect from light.

428-t

Prepared Hyoscyamus *(B.P., Eur. P.).*

Hyoscyami Pulvis Normatus; Prep. Hyoscy.; Poudre Titrée de Jusquiame.

Pharmacopoeias. In *Br., Eur., Fr., Ger.,* and *Neth.*

Hyoscyamus leaf reduced to a fine powder and adjusted to contain 0.05 to 0.07% of alkaloids calculated as hyoscyamine; about 120 µg in 200 mg. A grey to grey-green powder with a slightly nauseous odour and a slightly bitter taste. **Store** in airtight containers. Protect from light.

Adverse Effects, Treatment, and Precautions. As for Atropine, p.289.

Abuse. Reports of Henbane chewing.— J. M. Sands and R. Sands, *Med. J. Aust.,* 1976, *2,* 55.

Uses. Hyoscyamus leaf and preparations of hyoscyamus have peripheral and central effects similar to those of atropine (see p.290). Hyoscyamus leaf has been used to counteract griping due to strong purgatives and to relieve spasms of the urinary tract.

Preparations

Hyoscyamus Dry Extract *(B.P.).* Hyoscy. Dry Ext.; Ext. Hyoscy. Sicc.; Hyoscyamus Extract. A dry alcoholic extract adjusted to contain 0.3% of alkaloids calculated as hyoscyamine; 180 µg in 60 mg. Store in small wide-mouthed containers.

Hyoscyamus Liquid Extract *(B.P.C. 1973).* An alcoholic percolate adjusted to contain 0.05% of alkaloids, calculated as hyoscyamine; 250 µg in 0.5 ml. *Dose.* 0.2 to 0.5 ml.

Hyoscyamus Tincture *(B.P.).* Hyoscy. Tinct. Prepared from hyoscyamus leaf by percolation with alcohol (70%) and standardised to contain 0.005% of alkaloids, calculated as hyoscyamine; 250 µg in 5 ml.

Oleum Hyoscyami *(Swiss P.).* Hyoscyamus Oil. Hyoscyamus powder 10 g, extracted and dissolved in arachis oil 100 g.

Tinctura Hyoscyami *(Belg. P.).* Teinture de Jusquiame. An alcoholic extract adjusted to contain 0.005% of alkaloids calculated as atropine.

385-n

Hyoscyamus Muticus *(B.P.C. 1949).* Egyptian Henbane; Hyoscyami Mutici Herba; Herbe de Jusquiame d'Egypte; Aegyptisches Bilsenkraut.

Pharmacopoeias. In *Belg.* (not less than 0.75%) and *Int.* (not less than 0.8%).

The dried leaves, flowering tops, and smaller stems of *H. muticus* (Solanaceae), containing not less than 0.6% of alkaloids calculated as hyoscyamine. **Store** in a cool dry place. Protect from light.

Uses. Hyoscyamus muticus is used as a source of hyoscyamine.

386-h

Ipratropium Bromide. Sch 1000.

(1*R*,3*r*,5*S*,8*r*)-8-Isopropyl-3-[(±)-tropoyloxy]tropanium bromide monohydrate.

$C_{20}H_{30}BrNO_3,H_2O$=430.4.

CAS — 22254-24-6 (anhydrous); 66985-17-9 (monohydrate).

A white crystalline substance with a bitter taste. Freely **soluble** in water and alcohol; practically insoluble in chloroform and ether.

Adverse Effects, Treatment, and Precautions. As for Atropine, p.289.

Absorption and Fate. Ipratropium bromide is poorly absorbed from the gastro-intestinal tract. After inhalation some is absorbed from the lungs.

After administration of ipratropium bromide by mouth, intravenously, and by inhalation, cumulative renal excretion was 9.3, 72.1 and 3.2% respectively and faecal excretion was 88.5, 6.3 and 69.4% respectively. The half-life of elimination from plasma was 3.2 to 3.8 hours for all methods of administration.— J. Adlung *et al., Arzneimittel-Forsch.,* 1976, *26,* 1005.

Uses. Ipratropium bromide is a quaternary ammonium anticholinergic agent with peripheral effects similar to those of atropine (see p.290). It is used by inhalation in the treatment of chronic reversible airways obstruction, particularly in chronic bronchitis. The usual dose is 20 or 40 µg (1 or 2 puffs) three or four times daily by inhalation; single doses of up to 80 µg (4 puffs) have been required during the initial stages of treatment. In children aged 6 to 12 years the usual dose is 20 or 40 µg (1 or 2 puffs) thrice daily, and below 6 years the usual dose is 20 µg (1 puff) thrice daily.

Ipratropium bromide given by inhalation is an effective bronchodilator, being at least as effective as inhaled sympathomimetic agents with $beta_2$-adrenoceptor stimulant activity, such as salbutamol, in chronic bronchitis, but somewhat less effective in asthma. The onset of maximum effect with ipratropium bromide is about 1.5 to 2 hours and its duration of action about 4 to 6 hours, suggesting that its use might be more appropriate for prophylaxis than in the treatment of acute bronchospasm. Ipratropium bromide would appear to be indicated primarily in the treatment of airflow obstruction in patients who have failed to respond to $beta_2$-sympathomimetic agents and may be useful in patients who develop side-effects with these agents. Although the use of ipratropium bromide with other bronchodilating agents such as $beta_2$-sympathomimetics or theophylline, or with sodium cromoglycate, has usually showed better response than with single drug therapy further study is required to determine which patients would benefit from combined therapy.— G. E. Pakes *et al., Drugs,* 1980, *20,* 237. See also *Drug & Ther. Bull.,* 1980, *18,* 59.

For the proceedings of a symposium on chronic obstructive airways disease including ipratropium bromide, see *Scand. J. resp. Dis.,* 1979, *Suppl.* 103.

Other reports and studies on ipratropium bromide, including comparisons with other drugs: K. Alanko and H. Poppius (letter), *Br. med. J.,* 1973, *1,* 294; H. Poppius and Y. Salorinne, *ibid.,* 1973, *4,* 134; W. T. Ulmer *et al., Arzneimittel-Forsch.,* 1973, *23,* 468; P. Otto, *ibid.,* 1334; W. Günther and P. L. Kamburoff, *Curr. med. Res. Opinion,* 1974, *2,* 281; C. Emirgil *et al., Curr. ther. Res.,* 1975, *17,* 215; G. R. Petrie and K. N. V. Palmer, *Br. med. J.,* 1975, *1,* 430; *Postgrad. med. J.,* 1975, *51, Suppl.* 7, 1–161; R. -R. Scherberger *et al., Arzneimittel-Forsch.,* 1975, *25,* 1460; B. Simonsson *et al., Scand. J. resp. Dis.,* 1975, *56,* 138; T. Vlagopoulos *et al., J. Allergy & clin. Immunol.,* 1975, *55,* 99; *Arzneimittel-Forsch.,* 1976, *26,* 960–1020; H. Yeager *et al., J. clin. Pharmac.,* 1976, *16,* 198; M. Chan-Yeung, *Chest,* 1977, *71,* 320; P. Chervinsky, *J. Allergy & clin. Immunol.,* 1977, *59,* 22; J. Dry *et al., Thérapie,* 1977, *32,* 181; C. S. May and K. N. V. Palmer (letter), *Br. J. clin. Pharmac.,* 1977, *4,* 491; R. A. Francis *et al., Br. J. Dis. Chest,* 1977, *71,* 173; R. E. Ruffin *et al., J. Allergy & clin. Immunol.,* 1978, *61,* 42; M. T. Lin *et al., Ann. Allergy,* 1978, *40,* 326; I. M. Lightbody *et al., Br. J. Dis. Chest,* 1978, *72,* 181; A. Ahonen *et al., Curr. ther. Res.,* 1978, *24,* 65; G. E. Marlin *et al.* (letter), *Br. J. clin. Pharmac.,* 1978, *6,* 547; D. Pavia *et al., Thorax,* 1979, *34,* 501; G. Schultze-Werninghaus *et al., Dt. med. Wschr.,* 1979, *104,* 1099; P. Ravez *et al., Clin. Trials J.,* 1979, *16,* 147; G. J. Addis *et al., Eur. J. clin. Pharmac.,* 1979, *16,* 97; R. Yeung *et al., Pediatrics,* 1980, *66,* 109; G. V. Jaffé *et al., Practitioner,* 1980, *224,* 433; A. W. Lees *et al., Br. J. clin. Pract.,* 1980, *34,* 340; M. J. Ward *et al., Br. med. J.,* 1981, *282,* 598.

The long-term effect of ipratropium bromide on gastric secretion.— G. Dotevall and A. Walan, *Arzneimittel-Forsch.,* 1978, *28,* 2163.

Proprietary Preparations

Atrovent *(Boehringer Ingelheim, UK).* A pressurised spray for inhalation containing ipratropium bromide and delivering 20 µg in each metered dose, of which 18 µg is available to the patient. (Also available as Atrovent in *Belg., Denm., Ger., Neth., Norw., S.Afr., Swed., Switz.).* **Atrovent Nebuliser Solution** contains 250 µg per ml.

387-m

Isopropamide Iodide *(U.S.P.).* R 79; SKF 4740; Iodeto de Isopropamida. (3-Carbamoyl-3,3-diphenylpropyl)di-isopropylmethylammonium iodide.

$C_{23}H_{33}IN_2O$=480.4.

CAS — 7492-32-2 (isopropamide); 71-81-8 (iodide).

Pharmacopoeias. In *Braz.* and *U.S.*

A white to pale yellow odourless crystalline powder with a bitter taste. M.p. about 181°. Isopropamide iodide 1.36 mg is approximately equivalent to 1 mg of isopropamide. **Soluble** 1 in 50 of water, 1 in 10 of alcohol, and 1 in 5 of chloroform; very slightly soluble in ether. **Protect** from light.

Adverse Effects, Treatment, and Precautions. As for Atropine, p.289.

It is contra-indicated in patients hypersensitive to iodine. Its use interferes with tests of thyroid function.

Uses. Isopropamide is a quaternary ammonium anticholinergic agent with peripheral effects similar to those of atropine (see p.290). It has been used as an adjunct in the treatment of gastric and duodenal ulcer and in the relief of visceral spasms. It is given as isopropamide iodide in doses equivalent to 5 to 10 mg of isopropamide every 12 hours.

Preparations

Isopropamide Iodide Tablets *(U.S.P.).* Tablets containing isopropamide iodide. Potency is expressed in terms of the equivalent amount of isopropamide.

Isopropamide iodide is an ingredient of Eskornade (p.26).

Proprietary Names

Darbid *(Smith Kline & French, Canad.; Smith Kline & French, USA)*; Dipramid *(Valeas, Ital.)*; Priamide *(Janssen, Belg.; Janssen, Denm.; Delalande, Fr.; Janssen, Ger.; Janssen, Neth.)*; Tyrimide *(Smith Kline & French, Austral.).*

Isopropamide iodide was formerly marketed in Great Britain under the proprietary name Tyrimide (*Smith Kline & French*).

388-b

IU7. 1-Methyl-1-(2-bicyclohexylaminoethyl)piperidinium chloride.

$C_{20}H_{39}ClN_2$=343.0.

CAS — 60996-85-2.

Adverse Effects, Treatment, and Precautions. As for Atropine, p.289.

Uses. IU7 is a quaternary ammonium anticholinergic agent used to reduce gastric secretion and motility. It has been given in doses of 20 to 40 mg intramuscularly daily.

389-v

Lachesine Chloride *(B.P.C. 1973).*

Laches. Chlor.; Lachesine; E 3. (2-Benziloyloxyethyl)ethyldimethylammonium chloride.

$C_{20}H_{26}ClNO_3$=363.9.

CAS — 1164-38-1.

A white odourless or almost odourless amorphous powder with a bitter taste. M.p. 212° to 214°. **Soluble** 1 in 3 of water and 1 in 10 of alcohol (90%); very slightly soluble in acetone, chloroform, and ether. Solutions are **sterilised** by autoclaving or by filtration. **Incompatible** in aqueous solution (1% and above) with 0.01% benzalkonium chloride; opalescence may develop in solutions of 2% and above with 0.002% phenylmercuric salts, and with 0.01% chlorhexidine acetate if boiled or autoclaved.

Incompatibility. Lachesine chloride and boric acid produced a white precipitate, and lachesine chloride and benzalkonium chloride a slight precipitate when autoclaved for 15 minutes at 120°.— H. Taylor, *Australas. J. Pharm.*, 1968, *49*, S64.

Adverse Effects, Treatment, and Precautions. As for Atropine, p.289.

Lachesine is not recommended in old people as the subsequent response to miotics is slower than after homatropine.

Systemic toxicity may occasionally be produced by the instillation of anticholinergic eye-drops, particularly in infants.

Uses. Lachesine chloride is a quaternary ammonium anticholinergic agent with cycloplegic and mydriatic properties similar to those of atropine (see p.290). The mydriatic action is slower in onset and less prolonged than that of atropine, reaching its maximum in about an hour and subsiding in 5 or 6 hours. The cycloplegic effect is about midway in duration and extent between those due to homatropine and atropine, but it has been reported to be less reliable than either, especially in children. It has been used as a substitute for atropine or homatropine in patients with hypersensitivity to these drugs. The usual dose is 2 drops of a 1% solution instilled into the eye.

Preparations

Lachesine Eye-drops *(B.P.C. 1973)*. LAC. A sterile solution containing up to 1% of lachesine chloride, with 0.002% of phenylmercuric acetate or nitrate, in water. The solution is sterilised by autoclaving or by filtration or by maintaining at 98° to 100° for 30 minutes; it is adversely affected by alkalis.

390-r

Mepenzolate Bromide *(U.S.P.)*. 3-Benziloyloxy-1,1-dimethylpiperidinium bromide.
$C_{21}H_{26}BrNO_3$=420.3.

CAS — 25990-43-6 (mepenzolate); 76-90-4 (bromide).

Pharmacopoeias. In *U.S.*

A white or light cream-coloured powder. M.p. about 230° with decomposition.

Soluble 1 in 110 of water, 1 in 120 of dehydrated alcohol, 1 in about 630 of chloroform, and 1 in about 8 of methyl alcohol; practically insoluble in ether. **Store** in airtight containers.

Adverse Effects, Treatment, and Precautions. As for Atropine, p.289.

Uses. Mepenzolate bromide is a quaternary ammonium anticholinergic agent with peripheral actions similar to those of atropine (see p.290). It is given in the symptomatic treatment of visceral spasms in doses of 25 to 50 mg three or four times daily.

About 14% of a dose of 25 or 30 mg of mepenzolate bromide was absorbed from the gastro-intestinal tract and excreted in the urine over 4 to 5 days.— H. L. Friedman and R. I. H. Wang, *J. pharm. Sci.*, 1972, *61*, 1663.

Irritable bowel syndrome. References to the use of mepenzolate bromide in spasmodic conditions of the colon: J. A. Riese, *Clin. Med.*, 1969, *76* (Mar.), 32. Report from the General Practitioner Research Group, *Practitioner*, 1974, *212*, 890; R. A. Mountford *et al.*, *Gut*, 1980, *21*, A912.

Pregnancy and the neonate. Mepenzolate bromide has not been detected in the milk of lactating mothers.— T. E. O'Brien, *Am. J. Hosp. Pharm.*, 1974, *31*, 844.

Preparations

Mepenzolate Bromide Syrup *(U.S.P.)*. Mepenzolate Bromide Solution; Mepenzolate Bromide Oral Solution. A syrup containing mepenzolate bromide; it may contain suitable preservatives and stabilising agents. Store in airtight containers. Protect from light.

Mepenzolate Bromide Tablets *(U.S.P.)*. Tablets containing mepenzolate bromide.

Proprietary Preparations

Cantil *(MCP Pharmaceuticals, UK)*. Mepenzolate bromide, available as **Elixir** containing 12.5 mg in each 5 ml (suggested diluent, water) and as **Tablets** of 25 mg. (Also available as Cantil in *Austral., Fr., Swed., USA*).

Cantil with Phenobarbitone *(MCP Pharmaceuticals, UK)*. Tablets each containing mepenzolate bromide 25 mg and phenobarbitone 15 mg. For lower gastro-intestinal spasm, with sedation. *Dose.* 1 to 2 tablets thrice daily with meals, and at bedtime in severe cases.

Other Proprietary Names

Ital.— Cantril, Colibantil, Colum, Gastropidil; *Jap.*— Eftoron, Tralanta.

A preparation containing mepenzolate bromide was also formerly marketed in Great Britain under the proprietary name Neo-cantil (*M.C.P. Pharmaceuticals*).

391-f

Methanthelinium Bromide. Methantheline Bromide *(U.S.P.)*; Bromuro de Metantelina; Brometo de Metantelina; Dixamonum Bromidum. Diethylmethyl[2-(xanthen-9-ylcarbonyloxy)ethyl]ammonium bromide.
$C_{21}H_{26}BrNO_3$=420.3.

CAS — 5818-17-7 (methanthelinium); 53-46-3 (bromide).

Pharmacopoeias. In *Arg., Port.*, and *U.S.* which also includes Sterile Methantheline Bromide.

A white, or almost white, crystalline, almost odourless powder with a very bitter taste. M.p. 171° to 177°. **Soluble** 1 in less than 5 of water, alcohol, and chloroform, and 1 in 390 of acetone; practically insoluble in ether. A solution in water has a pH of about 5. Aqueous solutions hydrolyse slowly.

Uses. Methanthelinium bromide is a quaternary ammonium anticholinergic agent with peripheral effects similar to those of atropine (see p.290). It has been largely replaced in clinical practice by its more potent and less toxic derivative, propantheline bromide (see p.310). Doses of 50 to 100 mg have been given four times daily; it has been given in similar doses by intramuscular or intravenous injection.

Preparations

Methantheline Bromide Tablets *(U.S.P.)*. Tablets containing methanthelinium bromide.

Sterile Methantheline Bromide *(U.S.P.)*. Methanthelinium bromide suitable for parenteral use.

Proprietary Names

Banthine *(Searle, Arg.; Searle, Denm.; Searle, USA)*; Bronerg *(Lancet, Ital.)*; Evogal *(Zambeletti, Ital.)*; Freno-Gastrico *(Spain)*; Probantim *(Lusofarmaco, Ital.)*; Ulcuwas Antiespasmodico *(Wassermann, Spain)*; Vagantin *(Brunnengräber, Ger.)*; Vaxantene *(Boniscontro & Gazzone, Ital.)*; Xantenol *(Janus, Ital.)*.

392-d

Methixene Hydrochloride. Metixene Hydrochloride; SJ 1977. 9-(1-Methyl-3-piperidylmethyl)thioxanthene hydrochloride.
$C_{20}H_{23}NS,HCl$=345.9.

CAS — 4969-02-2 (methixene); 1553-34-0 (hydrochloride).

A white crystalline powder. **Soluble** in water, alcohol, and chloroform. M.p. about 216°.

Adverse Effects, Treatment, and Precautions. As for Atropine, p.289.

Absorption and Fate. Methixene is absorbed from the gastro-intestinal tract and is excreted in the urine, partly unchanged and partly as its isomeric sulphoxides or their metabolites.

Uses. Methixene hydrochloride is an anticholinergic agent with actions similar to those of atropine (see p.290); it also has antihistaminic, direct antispasmodic, and local anaesthetic properties. It is mainly used for the symptomatic treatment of arteriosclerotic, idiopathic, and postencephalitic parkinsonism. Unlike benzhexol and some other anticholinergic antiparkinsonian drugs, it is claimed to be more effective in controlling the tremors than in reducing the rigidity of this syndrome.

The usual dose of methixene hydrochloride is 2.5 mg thrice daily initially, gradually increased according to the response of the patient to a total of 15 to 60 mg daily in divided doses. If rigidity is not sufficiently controlled by methixene another antiparkinsonian drug which acts primarily on rigidity may be given concurrently. Transition to or from methixene therapy should be gradual otherwise symptoms may be aggravated.

In the USA methixene hydrochloride is used as an adjunct in the treatment of gastric and duodenal ulcer, and to relieve visceral spasms. The usual dose is 1 or 2 mg thrice daily.

Epilepsy diagnosis. For a report on the use of methixene administered intravenously as an EEG activating agent in the diagnosis of temporal lobe epilepsy, see C. J. Vas *et al.*, *Epilepsia*, 1967, *8*, 252.

Parkinsonism. In a double-blind study in 13 patients with parkinsonism, objective measurement showed a highly significant reduction or complete abolition of tremor following the intravenous injection of 10 mg of methixene.— S. Clarke *et al.*, *Br. J. Pharmac. Chemother.*, 1966, *26*, 345.

For reports and comments on the concurrent administration of anticholinergic agents with levodopa in patients with parkinsonism, see under Levodopa, p.887.

Proprietary Preparations

Tremonil *(Wander, UK)*. Methixene hydrochloride, available as scored tablets of 5 mg. (Also available as Tremonil in *Austral.*).

Other Proprietary Names

Methyloxan *(Jap.)*; Tremaril *(Belg., Denm., Ital., Neth., S.Afr., Spain, Switz.)*; Tremarit *(Ger.)*; Tremoquil *(Swed.)*; Trest *(USA)*.

393-n

Octatropine Methylbromide. Anisotropine Methobromide; Anisotropine Methylbromide. (1*R*,3*r*,5*S*)-8-Methyl-3-(2-propylvaleryloxy)tropanium bromide.
$C_{17}H_{32}BrNO_2$=362.3.

CAS — 80-50-2.

A white, glistening, odourless, hygroscopic powder with a bitter taste. **Soluble** in water; freely soluble in alcohol and chloroform; slightly soluble in acetone; practically insoluble in ether. A 1% solution in water has a pH of about 6.5. **Store** in airtight containers.

Adverse Effects, Treatment, and Precautions. As for Atropine, p.289.

Uses. Octatropine methylbromide is a quaternary ammonium anticholinergic agent with peripheral actions similar to those of atropine (see p.290). It is used to relieve visceral spasms. Sources in the USA recommend a dose of 50 mg thrice daily; some other countries still recommend 10 mg three or four times daily before meals and at bedtime.

Octatropine methylbromide was excreted in urine. All of an intravenous dose of 5 mg was excreted in an average time of 400 hours. Only about 5% of a dose given by mouth was absorbed from the alimentary tract and the average total excretion time was 80.5 hours following doses of 20 to 25 mg. The multiple peak pattern of excretion suggested that enterohepatic cycling occurred with octatropine and possibly other quaternary drugs.— M. Pfeffer *et al.*, *J. pharm. Sci.*, 1968, *57*, 1375. See also *idem*, 36.

Studies of clinical action in healthy subjects and in patients: J. N. Stiel and C. H. Baxter, *Med. J. Aust.*, 1967, *1*, 1076; J. W. Freston and J. A. Forbes, *J. clin. Pharmac.*, 1977, *17*, 29; J. Bowers *et al.*, *Gastroenterology*, 1977, *72*, 1032; J. H. Bowers *et al.*, *J. clin. Pharmac.*, 1978, *18*, 365; L. Barbara and M. Migliali, *Clin. Trials J.*, 1979, *16*, 140.

Proprietary Names

Valpin *(Endo, Austral.; Endo, Canad.; Crinos, Ital.; Endo, S.Afr.)*; Valpin 50 *(Endo, USA)*; Vapin *(Lacer, Spain)*.

394-h

Orphenadrine Citrate *(B.P., U.S.P.).* Mephenamine Citrate; Orphenadin Citrate.
$C_{18}H_{23}NO,C_6H_8O_7=461.5$.

CAS — 83-98-7 (orphenadrine); 4682-36-4 (citrate).

Pharmacopoeias. In *Br.* and *U.S.*

A white or almost white, almost odourless, crystalline powder with a bitter numbing taste. M.p. 134° to 138°. Orphenadrine citrate 100 mg is approximately equivalent to 66 mg of orphenadrine hydrochloride.
Soluble 1 in 70 of water; slightly soluble in alcohol; very slightly soluble in acetone; practically insoluble in chloroform and ether. **Store** in airtight containers. Protect from light.

395-m

Orphenadrine Hydrochloride *(B.P.).* BS 5930; Mephenamine Hydrochloride; Orphenadin Hydrochloride. *NN*-Dimethyl-2-(2-methylbenzhydryloxy)ethylamine hydrochloride.
$C_{18}H_{23}NO,HCl=305.8$.

CAS — 341-69-5.

Pharmacopoeias. In *Br.*

A white or almost white, odourless, crystalline powder with a bitter numbing taste. M.p. 159° to 162°.
Soluble 1 in 1 of water, 1 in 1 of alcohol, and 1 in 2 of chloroform; practically insoluble in ether. **Store** in airtight containers. Protect from light.

Adverse Effects and Treatment. As for Atropine, p.289. Orphenadrine has been abused for its supposed euphoriant effect.

The following side-effects occurred among 24 patients treated with orphenadrine 100 mg thrice daily for 3 weeks: difficulty in commencing urination (2 patients), dizziness (1 patient), involuntary jerky movements of the limbs (3 patients), nervous (jittery) movements (1 patient), and burning sensation in the throat (5 patients); these symptoms were transient. Bleeding episodes occurred in 2 patients but were possibly coincidental.— G. Onuaguluchi, *Br. med. J.*, 1963, *1*, 443.

A report of orphenadrine-induced intestinal obstruction in a 77-year-old man with parkinsonism.— P. Daggett and S. Z. Ibrahim, *Br. med. J.*, 1976, *1*, 21.

A report of acute urinary retention in a 29-year-old man who took orphenadrine citrate 100 mg three or four times daily for about one week.— *Med. J. Aust.*, 1979, *2*, 374.

Abuse. A 23-year-old schizophrenic man, whose treatment included orphenadrine 100 mg thrice daily, obtained illicit supplies and increased the dose for euphoric effect. On one occasion he had an epileptic convulsion after a 600-mg dose.— M. E. Shariatmadari (letter), *Br. med. J.*, 1975, *3*, 486.

Overdosage. After taking an estimated sixty 50-mg tablets of orphenadrine hydrochloride a 2-year-old boy suffered convulsions which were not controlled by paraldehyde and phenytoin. He was treated with tubocurarine and intermittent positive-pressure ventilation, and eventually made a full recovery. Haemodialysis proved of little value.— J. C. Stoddart *et al.*, *Br. J. Anaesth.*, 1968, *40*, 789.

An account of 2 cases of acute orphenadrine poisoning in children. Both children suffered severe refractory convulsions but recovered fully. Treatment included diazepam and paraldehyde parenterally, and general supportive measures.— D. G. Gill and H. A. Sowerby, *Practitioner*, 1975, *214*, 542.

After apparently recovering from overdosage with an unknown quantity of amitriptyline, orphenadrine, and flurazepam tablets, a 16-year-old girl developed acute dilatation of the stomach. She recovered after gastric aspiration and intravenous infusions of electrolytes. Gastric dilatation might be a late complication of poisoning with drugs with anticholinergic properties.— J. How and R. W. Strachan, *Br. med. J.*, 1976, *1*, 563.

A 25-year-old man who had ingested an estimated 1.2 to 1.5 g of orphenadrine citrate was successfully treated by intravenous injection of physostigmine 1 mg. The patient had been severely mentally agitated but within 5 minutes of injection was alert, orientated and cooperative, and his heart-rate had gone down from 150 beats per minutes to 75. He required no further treatment with physostigmine.— B. D. Synder *et al.* (letter), *New Engl. J. Med.*, 1976, *295*, 1435. Criticism. Since cardiotoxic problems were the direct cause of death in orphenadrine intoxication, and the anticholinergic side-effects of relatively minor importance, the administration of physostigmine was not indicated and could be dangerous. Only after at least 12 hours and when the extent of cardiac involvement had been assessed should administration of physostigmine be considered.— B. Sangster *et al.* (letter), *ibid.*, 1977, *296*, 1006.

A report of reversal of the central anticholinergic syndrome with tacrine hydrochloride: G. Mendelson (letter), *Med. J. Aust.*, 1975, *1*, 839; *idem*, *2*, 906.

Orphenadrine was considered to be a dangerous drug when given in large doses or when overdoses are taken and 3 deaths are reported. Toxic effects can occur rapidly within 2 hours with convulsions, cardiac dysrhythmias, and death; these effects are considered to be very similar to those of tricyclic antidepressants. Eleven patients suffering from the toxic effects of orphenadrine had been admitted to the Regional Poisoning Treatment Centre in Edinburgh in the first 6 months of 1977 and 1 of these patients had died.— W. M. Millar (letter), *Lancet*, 1977, *2*, 566. A further report of fatalities.— B. Sangster *et al.*, *Ned. Tijdschr. Geneesk.*, 1978, *122*, 988.

For a review of the use of physostigmine in anticholinergic poisoning, see under Physostigmine Salicylate, p.1043.

Precautions. As for Atropine, p.290.
Some sources suggest that toxic doses may produce non-depolarising neuromuscular blocking effects.
Anticholinergic antiparkinsonian agents do not control tardive dyskinesia associated with long-term phenothiazine (or other antipsychotic) therapy, and may exacerbate symptoms.

A suggested interaction between orphenadrine and dextropropoxyphene was open to question.— R. E. Pearson and F. J. Salter (letter), *New Engl. J. Med.*, 1970, *282*, 1215. See also W. H. Puckett and J. A. Visconti (letter), *ibid.*, *283*, 544. Criticism.— W. Renforth (letter), *ibid.*, 998.

Absorption and Fate. Orphenadrine is readily absorbed from the gastro-intestinal tract. It is rapidly distributed in tissues and most of a dose is metabolised and excreted in the urine within 3 days. A small proportion is excreted unchanged in the urine.

Studies of the absorption, excretion, and metabolism of orphenadrine citrate in 4 healthy male subjects showed that very low blood concentrations were obtained after either oral or intravenous administration due to rapid distribution into tissue depots. Orphenadrine underwent rapid and extensive metabolism and 60% of a dose was excreted in the urine in 3 days. Only 8% of the dose was excreted unchanged and 8 metabolites were identified in the urine.— T. Ellison *et al.*, *J. Pharmac. exp. Ther.*, 1971, *176*, 284.

Uses. Orphenadrine, which is a congener of diphenhydramine without sharing its soporific effect, is an anticholinergic agent with actions and uses similar to those of benzhexol (see p.295). It also has weak antihistaminic, local anaesthetic, and skeletal muscle-relaxant properties.
Orphenadrine is used as the hydrochloride in the symptomatic treatment of arteriosclerotic, idiopathic, and postencephalitic parkinsonism. It is also used to alleviate the extrapyramidal syndrome induced by drugs such as the phenothiazine derivatives and reserpine (but see also Precautions). The initial dose is 150 mg daily in divided doses gradually increased by 50 mg every 2 or 3 days according to the response of the patient. The usual dose is 150 to 300 mg daily in divided doses but some patients may require a total of up to 400 mg daily. In emergency, orphenadrine hydrochloride may be given intramuscularly in a dose of 20 to 40 mg; up to 120 mg daily in divided doses has been recommended. Transition to or from orphenadrine therapy should be gradual otherwise symptoms may be aggravated.
Orphenadrine is also used as the citrate to relieve pain due to spasm of voluntary muscle. The usual dose of orphenadrine citrate is 100 mg twice or thrice daily by mouth, adjusted according to the patient's response, or 60 mg every 12 hours by intramuscular or slow intravenous injection (over a period of about 5 minutes).

Animal pharmacology studies: U. G. Bijlsma *et al.*, *Archs int. Pharmacodyn. Thér.*, 1956, *106*, 332; G. Cronheim, *J. Pharmac. exp. Ther.*, 1958, *122*, 16A.

Hiccup. Two patients with persistent hiccup were successfully treated with orphenadrine citrate.— A. E. Gibbs, *Practitioner*, 1963, *191*, 646.

Muscular pain. Some reports and studies on the use of preparations containing orphenadrine alone or in association with analgesics, to relieve pain associated with muscle spasm: S. H. Hoddes, *Practitioner*, 1964, *193*, 76; I. M. Levine *et al.*, *Clin. Pharmac. Ther.*, 1967, *8*, 86; J. W. Finch, *Clin. Med.*, 1968, *75* (Mar.), 51; I. W. Birkeland and D. K. Clawson, *Clin. Pharmac. Ther.*, 1968, *9*, 639; T. Tervo *et al.*, *Br. J. clin. Pract.*, 1976, *30*, 62; E. N. S. Fry (letter), *Br. J. Anaesth.*, 1978, *50*, 205; R. H. Gold, *Curr. ther. Res.*, 1978, *23*, 271; R. H. Gold, *Clin. Ther.*, 1978, *1*, 451, per *Int. pharm. Abstr.*, 1979, *16*, 317; L. Winter and A. Post, *J. int. med. Res.*, 1979, *7*, 240; M. S. Mok *et al.*, *Clin. Ther.*, 1979, *2*, 188.

Parkinsonism. A satisfactory response in 15 of 24 patients with postencephalitic parkinsonism and a fair response in 7 followed treatment with orphenadrine hydrochloride, 100 mg thrice daily. Peak activity occurred in about 2 hours. The drug had no effect on the frequency and severity of oculogyric crises.— G. Onuaguluchi, *Br. med. J.*, 1963, *1*, 443.

For reports and comments on the concurrent administration of anticholinergic agents with levodopa, in patients with parkinsonism, see under Levodopa, p.887.

Restless leg syndrome. Orphenadrine was effective in the treatment of restless legs in some patients who could not tolerate diazepam.— L. K. Morgan (letter), *Med. J. Aust.*, 1975, *2*, 753.

Preparations of some Orphenadrine Salts

Orphenadrine Citrate Injection *(U.S.P.).* A sterile solution in Water for Injections prepared with the aid of sodium hydroxide. pH 5 to 6. Protect from light.

Orphenadrine Hydrochloride Tablets *(B.P.).* Tablets containing orphenadrine hydrochloride. They are sugar-coated.

Slow Orphenadrine Citrate Tablets *(B.P.).* Tablets formulated so as to release orphenadrine citrate over several hours.

Proprietary Preparations of some Orphenadrine Salts

Disipal *(Brocades, UK).* Orphenadrine hydrochloride, available as **Injection** containing 20 mg per ml, in ampoules of 2 ml for intramuscular injection, and as **Tablets** of 50 mg. (Also available as Disipal in *Austral.*, *Belg.*, *Canad.*, *Fr.*, *Ital.*, *Neth.*, *Norw.*, *S.Afr.*, *Swed.*, *Switz.*, *USA*).

Norflex *(Riker, UK).* Orphenadrine citrate, available as **Injection** containing 30 mg per ml in ampoules of 2 ml and as long-acting **Tablets** of 100 mg. (Also available as Norflex in *Austral.*, *Belg.*, *Canad.*, *Denm.*, *Ger.*, *S.Afr.*, *Swed.*, *Switz.*, *USA*).

Norgesic. See under Paracetamol p.270.

Other Proprietary Names of some Orphenadrine Salts

Arg.— Distalene *(hydrochloride)*; *Denm.*— Brocadisipal, Lysantin *(both hydrochloride)*; *Ital.*— Euflex *(citrate)*; *S.Afr.*— Orpadrex *(hydrochloride)*; *Spain*— Mefeamina *(hydrochloride)*; *USA*— Tega-Flex, X-Otag *(both citrate)*.

396-b

Oxybutynin Hydrochloride. Oxybutynin Chloride; MJ-4309-1. 4-Diethylaminobut-2-ynyl α-cyclohexylmandelate hydrochloride.
$C_{22}H_{31}NO_3,HCl=394.0$.

CAS — 5633-20-5 (oxybutynin); 1508-65-2 (hydrochloride).

Adverse Effects, Treatment, and Precautions. As for Atropine, p.289.

Hydroureteronephrosis and dilated bladder in a 11-year-old girl given oxybutynin for enuresis. Six months after withdrawing oxybutynin, the hydronephrosis was improved and bladder size reduced.— D. E. Novicki and M. K. Willscher, *Urology*, 1979, *13*, 324.

Uses. Oxybutynin hydrochloride is an anticholinergic agent with effects similar to those of atropine (see p.290). It is given in the symptomatic treatment of visceral spasms in a dose of 5 mg two to four times daily.

References: C. W. Hock, *Curr. ther. Res.*, 1967, *9*, 437; A. C. Diokno and J. Lapides, *J. Urol.*, 1972, *108*, 307.

Proprietary Names
Ditropan *(Marion Laboratories, USA)*.

397-v

Oxyphencyclimine Hydrochloride *(U.S.P., B.P. 1973)*. 1,4,5,6-Tetrahydro-1-methylpyrimidin-2-ylmethyl α-cyclohexylmandelate hydrochloride.
$C_{20}H_{28}N_2O_3$, HCl=380.9.

CAS — 125-53-1 (oxyphencyclimine); 125-52-0 (hydrochloride).

Pharmacopoeias. In *U.S.*

A white odourless crystalline powder with a bitter taste. M.p. about 234°. **Soluble** 1 in 100 of water, 1 in 75 of alcohol, 1 in 20 of methyl alcohol, 1 in 500 of chloroform, and 1 in 3000 of ether. **Store** in airtight containers.

Adverse Effects, Treatment, and Precautions. As for Atropine, p.289.

Uses. Oxyphencyclimine hydrochloride is an anticholinergic agent with effects similar to those of atropine (see p.290). It has a relatively long duration of action. It is used as an adjunct in the treatment of gastric and duodenal ulcer, and to relieve visceral spasms. The usual dose is 5 to 10 mg twice daily but up to 50 mg daily has been given in divided doses.

Preparations

Oxyphencyclimine Hydrochloride Tablets *(U.S.P.)*. Tablets containing oxyphencyclimine hydrochloride. The *U.S.P.* requires 85% dissolution in 15 minutes. Store in airtight containers.

Oxyphencyclimine Tablets *(B.P. 1973)*. Tablets containing oxyphencyclimine hydrochloride.

Proprietary Names
Daricol *(Pfizer, Swed.)*; Daricon *(Pfizer, Austral.; Roerig, Belg.; Pfizer, Denm.; Roerig, Neth.; Pfizer, Norw.; Pfizer, Spain; Beecham, USA)*; Madil *(Nagel, Ital.)*; Manir *(Valpan, Fr.)*; Oximin *(AFI, Norw.)*; Sedomucol *(Asla, Spain)*; Vagogastrin *(Benvegna, Ital.)*.

Oxyphencyclimine hydrochloride was formerly marketed in Great Britain under the proprietary name Daricon (*Pfizer*).

398-g

Oxyphenonium Bromide. Oxphenonii Bromidum; Oxyphenonium Bromatum. 2-(α-Cyclohexylmandeloyloxy)ethyldiethylmethylammonium bromide.
$C_{21}H_{34}BrNO_3$=428.4.

CAS — 14214-84-7 (oxyphenonium); 50-10-2 (bromide).

Pharmacopoeias. In *Cz., Jug.*, and *Pol.*

A white odourless crystalline powder with a bitter taste. M.p. about 190°. Freely **soluble** in water, alcohol, and chloroform. A 1% solution has a pH of about 6. Solutions are **sterilised** by filtration. **Incompatible** with alkalis.

Adverse Effects, Treatment, and Precautions. As for Atropine, p.289.

Uses. Oxyphenonium bromide is a quaternary ammonium anticholinergic agent with peripheral effects similar to those of atropine (see p.290). It is used as an adjunct in the treatment of gastric and duodenal ulcer, and to relieve visceral spasms. The usual dose is 5 to 10 mg four times daily; 1 to 2 mg has been given subcutaneously or intramuscularly every six hours. Smaller doses have also been given by intravenous injection. Oxyphenonium bromide has been used as pre-anaesthetic medication for patients who are sensitive to atropine or hyoscine. A 1% solution has been used as eye-drops for the mydriatic effect.

References: Report No. 37 of the General Practitioner Research Group, *Practitioner*, 1963, *190*, 390; P. Freeling, *ibid.*, 1964, *192*, 797; J. A. Alea and J. T. Aquilina, *Am. J. dig. Dis.*, 1967, *12*, 1122; R. P. Herrmann and M. J. Sulway, *Curr. ther. Res.*, 1973, *15*, 291.

Preparations

Oxyphenonium Eye Drops *(A.P.F.)*. Oxyphenonium bromide 1 g, sodium chloride 700 mg, chlorhexidine acetate 10 mg, Water for Injections to 100 ml. Sterilised by autoclaving.

Proprietary Names
Antrenil *(Ciba, Ital.)*; Antrenyl *(Ciba, Austral.; Ciba, Belg.; Ciba, Ger.; Ciba, Neth.; Ciba, S.Afr.; Ciba, Spain; Ciba-Geigy, Switz.; Ciba, USA)*; Spastrex *(Propan, S.Afr.)*.

Oxyphenonium bromide was formerly marketed in Great Britain under the proprietary name Antrenyl (*Ciba*).

399-q

Oxypyrronium Bromide. LD 3055; Oxipyrroni Bromidum; Hexopyrronium Bromide; Vamelidine. 2-[(α-Cyclohexylmandeloyloxy)methyl]-1,1-dimethylpyrrolidinium bromide.
$C_{21}H_{32}BrNO_3$=426.4.

CAS — 561-43-3.

Adverse Effects, Treatment, and Precautions. As for Atropine, p.289.

Uses. Oxypyrronium bromide is a quaternary ammonium anticholinergic agent with peripheral effects similar to those of atropine (see p.290). It has been used as an adjunct in the treatment of gastric and duodenal ulcer, to relieve visceral spasms, and as an antiperspirant. Doses of 3 to 6 mg have been given daily in 2 or 3 divided doses.

References: R. B. Stoughton *et al.*, *J. invest. Derm.*, 1964, *42*, 151; F. R. Bettley and K. A. Grice, *Br. J. Derm.*, 1965, *77*, 627.

Proprietary Names
Immétropan *(Dausse, Switz.)*.

400-q

Parapenzolate Bromide. 4-Benziloyloxy-1,1-dimethylpiperidinium bromide.
$C_{21}H_{26}BrNO_3$=420.3.

CAS — 5634-41-3.

Adverse Effects, Treatment, and Precautions. As for Atropine, p.289.

Uses. Parapenzolate bromide is a quaternary anticholinergic agent and a structural isomer of mepenzolate bromide (see p.306). It is used as an adjunct in the treatment of gastric and duodenal ulcer and to relieve visceral spasms. A dose of 500 μg has been given twice daily by mouth. Parapenzolate bromide has also been given by injection and rectally.

References: W. P. Fung, *Aust. N.Z. J. Med.*, 1972, *2*, 37.

Proprietary Names
Neupran *(Essex, Arg.)*; Spacine *(Unilabo, Fr.)*; Vagopax *(Essex, Ital.)*.

401-p

Pentapiperide Methylsulphate. Pentapiperium Methylsulphate; Valpipamate Methylsulphate; Pentapiperium Metilsulphate. 1,1-Dimethyl-4-(3-methyl-2-phenylvaleryloxy)piperidinium methylsulphate.
$C_{19}H_{30}NO_2,CH_3O_4S$=415.5.

CAS — 7009-54-3 (pentapiperide); 26372-86-1 (pentapiperium); 7681-80-3 (pentapiperide methylsulphate or pentapiperium methylsulphate).

NOTE. Pentapiperide methylsulphate and pentapiperium methylsulphate are identical but pentapiperide differs from pentapiperium in having one less methyl group.

A white crystalline powder with a bitter taste. M.p. 140° to 148°. Freely **soluble** in water, chloroform, and methyl alcohol; soluble in alcohol.

Adverse Effects, Treatment, and Precautions. As for Atropine, p.289.

Uses. Pentapiperide methylsulphate is a quaternary ammonium anticholinergic agent with peripheral effects similar to those of atropine (see p.290). It is used as an adjunct in the treatment of gastric and duodenal ulcer and to relieve visceral spasms. Doses of 20 to 30 mg are given daily. The hydrogen fumarate has also been used.

References: V. M. Smith *et al.*, *Am. J. Gastroent., N.Y.*, 1963, *39*, 52.

Proprietary Names
Crilin *(Ayerst, Ital.)*; Crylène *(Auclair, Fr.)*.

402-s

Penthienate Methobromide. Penthienate Bromide. 2-[2-Cyclopentyl-2-(2-thienyl)glycoloyloxy]ethyldiethylmethylammonium bromide.
$C_{18}H_{30}BrNO_3S$=420.4.

CAS — 22064-27-3 ($C_{18}H_{30}NO_3S$); 60-44-6 (penthienate methobromide).

A white odourless crystalline powder. M.p. 122° to 128°. **Soluble** in water and alcohol; freely soluble in chloroform; practically insoluble in acetone and ether.

Adverse Effects, Treatment, and Precautions. As for Atropine, p.289.

Uses. Penthienate methobromide is a quaternary ammonium anticholinergic agent with peripheral effects similar to those of atropine (see p.290). It has been used as an adjunct in the treatment of gastric and duodenal ulcer and to relieve visceral spasms. Doses of 2.5 to 10 mg have been given three or four times daily.

Proprietary Preparations

Monodral *(Sterling Research, UK)*. Penthienate methobromide, available as scored tablets of 5 mg. (Also available as Monodral in *Austral., Belg., Norw.*).

403-w

Phenglutarimide Hydrochloride *(B.P. 1963)*. 2-(2-Diethylaminoethyl)-2-phenylglutarimide hydrochloride; 3-(2-Diethylaminoethyl)-3-phenylpiperidine-2,6-dione hydrochloride.
$C_{17}H_{24}N_2O_2$,HCl=324.8.

CAS — 1156-05-4 (phenglutarimide); 1674-96-0 (hydrochloride).

A white odourless crystalline powder with a slightly bitter saline taste. **Soluble** 1 in 1 of water and 1 in 1.5 of alcohol; very slightly soluble in ether. A 1% solution in water has a pH of 4.5 to 5.5.

Uses. Phenglutarimide hydrochloride is an anticholinergic agent with actions and uses similar to those of benzhexol (see p.294). It was formerly used in the treatment of parkinsonism. Doses of 10 to 20 mg have been given daily in divided doses, to a max. of 50 mg daily.

Preparations

Phenglutarimide Tablets *(B.P. 1963)*. Tablets containing phenglutarimide hydrochloride.

Proprietary Names
Aturban *(Ciba-Geigy, Switz.)*.

Phenglutarimide hydrochloride was formerly marketed in Great Britain under the proprietary name Aturbane (*Ciba*).

404-e

Pipenzolate Bromide. Pipenzolate Methobromide. 3-Benziloyloxy-1-ethyl-1-methylpiperidinium bromide.
$C_{22}H_{28}BrNO_3$=434.4.

CAS — 13473-38-6 (pipenzolate); 125-51-9 (bromide).

A white crystalline powder. Freely **soluble** in water. M.p. about 180°.

Adverse Effects, Treatment, and Precautions. As for Atropine, p.289.

Uses. Pipenzolate bromide is a quaternary ammonium anticholinergic agent with peripheral actions similar to those of atropine (see p.290). It is used as an adjunct in the treatment of gastric and duodenal ulcer, and to relieve visceral spasms. The usual dose is 5 mg thrice daily and 5 to 10 mg at bedtime.

Proprietary Preparations

Piptal *(MCP Pharmaceuticals, UK)*. Pipenzolate bromide, available as tablets of 5 mg. (Also available as Piptal in *Austral., Fr., Ital., Switz.*).

Piptalin *(MCP Pharmaceuticals, UK)*. An elixir containing in each 5 ml pipenzolate bromide 4 mg and activated dimethicone 40 mg (suggested diluent, water).

Anticholinergic, antispasmodic, deflatulent. *Dose.* 10 ml three or four times daily before food; infants, 2.5 ml; children, 2.5 to 5 ml.

Other Proprietary Names
Piper *(Ital.)*.

405-l

Piperidolate Hydrochloride *(U.S.P.)*. 1-Ethyl-3-piperidyl diphenylacetate hydrochloride.
$C_{21}H_{25}NO_2,HCl=359.9$.

CAS — 82-98-4 (piperidolate); 129-77-1 (hydrochloride).

A white or cream-coloured powder. M.p. 194° to 198°. **Soluble** 1 in about 18 of water, 1 in about 52 of alcohol, 1 in about 4 of chloroform, and 1 in about 5 of methyl alcohol. **Store** in airtight containers.

Adverse Effects, Treatment, and Precautions. As for Atropine, p.289.

Uses. Piperidolate hydrochloride is an anticholinergic agent with effects similar to those of atropine (see p.290). It is given in the symptomatic treatment of visceral spasms in a dose of 50 mg four times daily.

Preparations

Piperidolate Hydrochloride Tablets *(U.S.P.)*. Tablets containing piperidolate hydrochloride.

Dactil *(MCP Pharmaceuticals, UK)*. Piperidolate hydrochloride, available as tablets of 50 mg. (Also available as Dactil in *Fr., Ger., Ital.*).

406-y

Platyphylline Acid Tartrate. Platyphyllini Hydrotartras; Platyphylline Bitartrate. 1,2-Dihydro-12-hydroxysenecionan-11,16-dione hydrogen tartrate.
$C_{18}H_{27}NO_5,C_4H_6O_6=487.5$.

CAS — 480-78-4 (platyphylline); 1257-59-6 (acid tartrate).

Pharmacopoeias. In *Rus.*

The acid tartrate of platyphylline, an alkaloid occurring in certain ragworts. It is usually obtained from *Senecio platyphyllus* and has also been isolated from *S. adnatus* and *S. hygrophilus.* The acid tartrate occurs as a white crystalline powder, odourless or with a faint characteristic odour and with a bitter taste. M.p. 190° to 195° with decomposition. **Soluble** 1 in 10 of water; very slightly soluble in alcohol; practically insoluble in chloroform and ether; soluble 1 in 42 of boiling alcohol. A 0.2% solution in water has a pH of 3.6 to 4.

Uses. Platyphylline acid tartrate has actions similar to those of atropine (see p.289) and it is used in the USSR for similar purposes. It is less potent than atropine, its mydriatic effects are less prolonged, and its effects on accommodation are less marked. The maximum single dose given by mouth or subcutaneously is 10 mg.

407-j

Poldine Methylsulphate *(B.P.)*.

Poldine Methylsulfate *(U.S.P.)*; Poldine Methosulphate. 2-Benziloyloxymethyl-1,1-dimethylpyrrolidinium methylsulphate.
$C_{21}H_{26}NO_3,CH_3O_4S=451.5$.

CAS — 596-50-9 (poldine); 545-80-2 (methylsulphate).

Pharmacopoeias. In *Br.* and *U.S.*

A white to creamy-white odourless crystalline powder with a bitter taste. M.p. 134° to 142°. **Soluble** 1 in 1 of water, 1 in 20 of alcohol, and 1 in 1000 of chloroform; practically insoluble in ether. A 1% solution in water has a pH of 5 to 7. It is stable in solution below pH 5 but is rapidly hydrolysed in solutions of pH greater than 7. **Store** in airtight containers.

Adverse Effects, Treatment, and Precautions. As for Atropine, p.289.

Side-effects associated with large doses of poldine methylsulphate were dryness of the mouth, slowness in passing urine, blurring of vision, tachycardia, extrasystoles, and less commonly, headache, eructations, and reduced sexual potency.— A. H. Douthwaite *et al., Br. med. J.*, 1961, *1*, 1575.

Absorption and Fate. Poldine methylsulphate is poorly absorbed from the gastro-intestinal tract.

Following repeated administration of poldine methylsulphate by mouth to *rats* nearly 70% of the administered dose was excreted in the faeces unchanged or as metabolites; a proportion of this might have been due to enterohepatic cycling.— P. F. Langley *et al., Biochem. Pharmac.*, 1966, *15*, 1821.

Uses. Poldine methylsulphate is a quaternary ammonium anticholinergic agent with peripheral actions similar to those of atropine (see p.290). It is used as an adjunct in the treatment of gastric and duodenal ulcer, and to relieve visceral spasms. The usual initial dose is 2 to 4 mg four times a day, subsequently adjusted according to the response of the patient. In the treatment of enuresis in children 2 mg has been given at bedtime.

Studies on the effect of poldine on gastric acidity and salivary flow: M. D. Kaye *et al., Gut*, 1968, *9*, 590; F. A. Bieberdorf *et al., Gastroenterology*, 1975, *68*, 50.

Acne. In 10 patients with acne, sebum excretion on the forehead was reduced by the application twice daily of a 5% solution of poldine methylsulphate in alcohol.— M. Cartlidge *et al., Br. J. Derm.*, 1972, *86*, 61.

Endocrine adenoma. Poldine methylsulphate was found to reduce spontaneous gastric hypersecretion in a patient suffering from endocrine adenoma. Poldine was given in gradually increasing doses over a period of 9 days until a dose of 14 mg four times daily was reached.— H. B. Cook and J. E. Lennard-Jones, *lancet*, 1966, *2*, 247.

Gastric and duodenal ulcer. Studies on poldine methylsulphate in gastric and duodenal ulcer: J. E. Lennard-Jones, *Br. med. J.*, 1961, *1*, 1071; A. G. Melrose and I. W. Pinkerton, *ibid.*, 1076; A. H. Douthwaite *et al., ibid.*, 1575; J. N. Hunt and R. C. Wales, *ibid.*, 1966, *2*, 13; J. N. Hunt and T. M. L. Price, *Practitioner*, 1967, *198*, 156.

Hyperhidrosis. Application of poldine methylsulphate 1% under polyethylene occlusion suppressed sweating for 2 to 3 days on some parts of the body. Four to 5 applications of poldine 4% in alcohol suppressed sweating on the forearm for 2 to 3 days. Poldine was less effective on the palms, soles, and axillae. In 3 of 5 subjects with hyperhidrosis of the palms visible sweating was much reduced by poldine 4% under occlusion. Systemic effects from percutaneous absorption were noted in 2 patients with psoriasis, 4 subjects whose palms and periungual regions were painted with poldine 8% and 3 of 7 subjects who were painted on the hand with poldine 4%. The side-effects were noticed 4 to 8 hours after application and lasted 2 to 3 hours after washing off the poldine.— K. A. Grice and F. R. Bettley, *Br. J. Derm.*, 1966, *78*, 458.

For the use of poldine methylsulphate by iontophoresis in the treatment of idiopathic hyperhidrosis, see K. Grice *et al., Br. J. Derm.*, 1972, *86*, 72.

Three patients with unilateral idiopathic hyperhidrosis responded to topical treatment, twice daily, with poldine methylsulphate 5% in talc or alcohol 70%.— W. J. Cunliffe *et al., Br. J. Derm.*, 1972, *86*, 374.

Zollinger-Ellison syndrome. A 73-year-old woman, suffering from the malignant Zollinger-Ellison syndrome with gastrin-containing skin nodules, had diarrhoea, hypokalaemia, and gastric hypersecretion. She was treated with poldine methylsulphate in a dose increasing up to 9 mg four times daily, which markedly decreased gastric secretion and controlled the diarrhoea. Large supplements of potassium by mouth corrected the hypokalaemia. She died about a year later.— D. G. Colin-Jones *et al., Lancet*, 1969, *1*, 492. See also R. S. Lawrie *et al., Lancet*, 1962, *1*, 1002.

Preparations

Poldine Methylsulfate Tablets *(U.S.P.)*. Tablets containing poldine methylsulphate. Store in airtight containers.

Poldine Tablets *(B.P.)*. Tablets containing poldine methylsulphate.

Nacton *(Bencard, UK)*. Poldine methylsulphate, available as scored tablets of 2 mg. **Nacton forte.** Poldine methylsulphate, available as scored tablets of 4 mg.

Other Proprietary Names
Nactate *(Denm., Neth.)*.

A preparation containing poldine methylsulphate was also formerly marketed in Great Britain under the proprietary name Nactisol *(Bencard)*.

408-z

Prampine Methonitrate. Propionyl Atropine Methyl Nitrate; *O*-Propionylatropine Methonitrate. (1*R*,3*r*,5*S*)-8-Methyl-3-(*O*-propionyltropoyloxy)tropanium nitrate.
$C_{21}H_{30}N_2O_7=422.5$.

CAS — 7009-65-6 (prampine); 14319-87-0 (methonitrate).

Adverse Effects, Treatment, and Precautions. As for Atropine, p.289.

Uses. Prampine methonitrate is a quaternary ammonium anticholinergic agent with peripheral effects similar to those of atropine (see p.290). It has been given as an adjunct in the treatment of gastric and duodenal ulcer in a dose of 6 mg three or four times daily.

409-c

Prifinium Bromide. Pyrodifenium Bromide. 3-Diphenylmethylene-1,1-diethyl-2-methylpyrrolidinium bromide.
$C_{22}H_{28}BrN=386.4$.

CAS — 10236-81-4 (prifinium); 4630-95-9 (bromide).

Odourless white crystals or crystalline powder with a bitter taste. M.p. 218°. Very **soluble** in water and methyl alcohol; freely soluble in alcohol and chloroform; slightly soluble in acetone; practically insoluble in ether.

Adverse Effects, Treatment, and Precautions. As for Atropine, p.289.

Uses. Prifinium bromide is a quaternary ammonium anticholinergic agent structurally related to diphemanil methylsulphate (see p.299). It is used as an adjunct in the treatment of gastric and duodenal ulcer and to relieve visceral spasms. Doses of 15 to 30 mg have been given 3 or 4 times daily by mouth; single doses of 60 to 90 mg have also been given. Prifinium bromide has also been administered in a dose of 7.5 mg once daily by subcutaneous, intramuscular, or intravenous injection.

Toxicity studies of prifinium bromide in *animals*.— S. Kumada *et al., Arzneimittel-Forsch.*, 1972, *22*, 706.

Favourable results with the use of prifinium bromide 30 mg thrice daily in the management of irritable bowel syndrome in a double-blind placebo-controlled crossover study in 18 patients.— G. Piai and G. Mazzacca, *Gastroenterology*, 1979, *77*, 500.

Further references: A. Arcangeli *et al., Curr. ther. Res.*, 1979, *25*, 430; W. Silber, *S. Afr. med. J.*, 1979, *56*, 1033.

Proprietary Names
Padrin *(Jap.)*; Riabal *(Gador, Arg.; Logeais, Fr.; Ibi, Ital.; Fujisawa, S.Afr.; Made, Spain)*.

410-s

Procyclidine Hydrochloride *(B.P., U.S.P.)*.

Procyclidini Hydrochloridum. 1-Cyclohexyl-1-phenyl-3-(pyrrolidin-1-yl)propan-1-ol hydrochloride.
$C_{19}H_{29}NO,HCl=323.9$.

CAS — 77-37-2 (procyclidine); 1508-76-5 (hydrochloride).

Pharmacopoeias. In *Br., Int.*, and *U.S.*

A white crystalline powder with a characteristic odour and a bitter taste. M.p. 225° to 227°. **Soluble** 1 in 35 to 40 of water, 1 in 15 of alcohol, and 1 in 6 of chloroform; practically insoluble in acetone and ether. A 1% solution in water has a pH of 4.5 to 6.5. Solutions are **sterilised** by autoclaving or filtration. **Store** in airtight containers. Protect from light.

Adverse Effects, Treatment, and Precautions. As for Atropine, p.289.

Anticholinergic antiparkinsonian agents do not control tardive dyskinesia associated with long-term phenothiazine (or other antipsychotic) therapy, and may exacerbate symptoms.

Absorption and Fate. Procyclidine hydrochloride is absorbed from the gastro-intestinal tract; procyclidine given intravenously acts within 5 to 20 minutes and has a duration of effect of up to 4 hours.

Uses. Procyclidine hydrochloride is an anticholinergic agent with actions and uses similar to those of benzhexol (see p.295). It is mainly used for the symptomatic treatment of arteriosclerotic, idiopathic, and postencephalitic parkinsonism. It may also be used to alleviate the extrapyramidal syndrome induced by drugs such as the phenothiazine derivatives and reserpine (but see also Precautions).

The initial dose of 7.5 mg daily in 3 or 4 divided doses after meals may be increased gradually by 2.5 mg daily until the optimum maintenance dose, usually 20 to 30 mg daily, is reached; daily doses of up to 60 mg have occasionally been required. In emergency, 5 to 10 mg may be given by intramuscular or intravenous injection; a second dose has been given 20 minutes later but the total daily dose by parenteral route must not exceed 20 mg. Transition to or from procyclidine therapy should be gradual otherwise symptoms may be aggravated.

Epilepsy. Procyclidine, 100 to 500 µg per kg body-weight daily up to a maximum of 300 to 700 µg per kg daily, reduced the incidence of seizures in 9 of 11 epileptic children with myoclonic spasms and increased the incidence in 2. It decreased the incidence of seizures in only 1 of a further 4 children with myoclonic spasms complicated by akinetic seizures.— J. G. Millichap *et al.*, *Proc. Soc. exp. Biol. Med.*, 1968, *127*, 1187.

Diagnosis. Results of a controlled study involving epileptic and non-epileptic patients indicated that the ability of procyclidine to provoke subclinical seizure activity in the EEG after intravenous administration may be a useful procedure in the investigation of any patient considered to be suffering from temporal lobe epilepsy. A dose of 20 mg was found to be significantly more effective than 10 mg.— C. J. Vas *et al.*, *Epilepsia*, 1967, *8*, 241.

Parkinsonism. For reports and comments on the concurrent administration of anticholinergic agents with levodopa, in patients with parkinsonism, see under Levodopa, p.887.

Preparations

Procyclidine Hydrochloride Tablets *(U.S.P.)*. Tablets containing procyclidine hydrochloride. Store in airtight containers.

Procyclidine Injection *(B.P.C. 1973)*. Procyclidine Hydrochloride Injection. A sterile solution of procyclidine hydrochloride in Water for Injections. pH 4.5 to 7. Store at a temperature not exceeding 25° and avoid freezing.

Procyclidine Tablets *(B.P.)*. Tablets containing procyclidine hydrochloride.

Proprietary Preparations

Arpicolin Syrup *(R.P. Drugs, UK)*. Contains in each 5 ml procyclidine hydrochloride 2.5 mg.

Kemadrin *(Wellcome, UK)*. Procyclidine hydrochloride, available as **Injection** containing 5 mg per ml in ampoules of 2 ml and as scored **Tablets** of 5 mg. (Also available as Kemadrin in *Austral., Belg., Canad., Denm., Ital., Neth., Norw., S.Afr., Swed., Switz., USA*).

Other Proprietary Names

Kemadren *(Spain)*; Kémadrine *(Fr.)*; Osnervan *(Ger.)*; Procyclid *(Canad.)*.

411-w

Propantheline Bromide *(B.P., U.S.P.)*.

Propanthelini Bromidum; Bromuro de Propantelina. Di-isopropylmethyl[2-(xanthen-9-ylcarbonyloxy)ethyl]ammonium bromide.

$C_{23}H_{30}BrNO_3$=448.4.

CAS — 298-50-0 (propantheline); 50-34-0 (bromide).

Pharmacopoeias. In *Arg., Br., Braz., Chin., Int., Jap., Nord., Turk.*, and *U.S. Nord.* and *U.S.* also include an injectable grade.

A white or yellowish-white odourless powder with a very bitter taste. The dust is irritant to mucous membranes. M.p. 156° to 162° with decomposition. At relative humidities of more than about 50% it is hygroscopic and it is deliquescent above about 90%.

Very **soluble** in water, alcohol, and chloroform; practically insoluble in ether. A solution in water is acid to litmus. **Incompatible** with alkalis. **Store** in airtight containers.

Adverse Effects, Treatment, and Precautions. As for Atropine, p.289.

Toxic doses may produce non-depolarising neuromuscular blocking effects with paralysis of voluntary muscle.

The transit of drugs through the intestine may be slowed by propantheline and other anticholinergic agents, with variable effects on absorption.

Following intravenous administration of propantheline bromide 15 mg as part of a diagnostic procedure, an 80-year-old man with pre-existing heart disease developed supraventricular tachycardia unresponsive to carotid massage or intravenous edrophonium. In older patients or subjects with suspected heart disease, initial doses of propantheline should be given intramuscularly rather than intravenously.— R. Kay *et al.*, *J. Urol.*, 1977, *117*, 813.

Buccal and oesophageal ulceration. Severe buccal mucosal ulceration, which developed in a 95-year-old woman as a result of retaining emepronium bromide tablets in her mouth, recurred on administration of propantheline bromide tablets.— G. J. Huston *et al.*, *Postgrad. med. J.*, 1978, *54*, 331.

Effects on the eyes. Two patients experienced mydriasis following ocular contamination with propantheline bromide that they were both using topically as an antiperspirant.— S. H. Nissen and P. G. Nielsen (letter), *Lancet*, 1977, *2*, 1134.

Effects on sexual function. Impotence followed treatment for about 1 year, with propantheline bromide.— D. Manners (letter), *Med. J. Aust.*, 1966, *2*, 436.

Interactions. Propantheline delayed the absorption of riboflavine from the gastro-intestinal tract by delaying gastric emptying and slowing transit through the small intestine, but total absorption of riboflavine was increased. The administration of anticholinergic drugs could increase the bioavailability of drugs that were not usually completely absorbed.— G. Levy *et al.*, *J. pharm. Sci.*, 1972, *61*, 798. See also J. J. Ashley and G. Levy, *ibid.*, 1973, *62*, 688.

Absorption and Fate. It has been estimated that only about 10% of propantheline is absorbed from the gastro-intestinal tract; some decomposition appears to occur in the small intestine after oral administration. It has a duration of action of about 6 hours and is slowly eliminated, mainly in the urine. There is evidence of enterohepatic cycling.

References: J. Möller and A. Rosén, *Acta med. scand.*, 1968, *184*, 201; M. Pfeffer *et al.*, *J. pharm. Sci.*, 1968, *57*, 1375; B. Beermann *et al.*, *Clin. Pharmac. Ther.*, 1972, *13*, 212; C. W. Vose *et al.*, *Xenobiotica*, 1978, *8*, 745; C. W. Vose *et al.*, *Br. J. clin. Pharmac.*, 1979, *7*, 89.

Pregnancy and the neonate. Propantheline has not been detected in the milk of lactating mothers.— B. E. Takyi, *J. Hosp. Pharm.*, 1970, *28*, 317.

Uses. Propantheline bromide is a quaternary ammonium anticholinergic agent with peripheral effects similar to those of atropine (see p.290). It is used as an adjunct in the treatment of gastric and duodenal ulcer, and to relieve spasm of the gastro-intestinal tract. The usual initial dose is 15 mg thrice daily preferably before meals and 30 mg at bedtime, subsequently adjusted according to the response of the patient. A suggested dose for children is 375 µg per kg body-weight 4 times daily.

It has been used in the treatment of gastritis, acute and chronic pancreatitis, pylorospasm, and biliary and ureteric spasm. For rapid relief of pain, 30 mg dissolved in 10 ml of sodium chloride injection may be injected intravenously.

As an adjunct to X-ray examination of the gastro-intestinal tract or endoscopic examinations, 30 mg has been given intramuscularly immediately before the procedure. In X-ray examination of the biliary tract, 10 to 30 mg has been given intravenously. Because of the poor oral absorption of propantheline bromide, parenteral doses may result in considerably higher plasma concentrations than the equivalent doses given by mouth.

Propantheline has been used in the treatment of enuresis, 15 to 45 mg being given at bedtime.

Propantheline has also been used in the treatment of hyperhidrosis.

In a comparative study of the oral and parenteral routes of administration of propantheline bromide in 40 patients, uniform cessation of peristalsis was obtained with a dose of 10 mg by the intramuscular route, whereas as much as 30 mg was required by mouth to obtain the same effect.— H. Barowsky, *Am. J. Gastroent., N.Y.*, 1955, *23*, 557. In 13 patients weighing 50 to 70 kg the minimum intravenous dose of propantheline bromide required to produce complete cessation of peristalsis was 6 mg.— H. Barowsky *et al.*, *Am. J. dig. Dis.*, 1965, *10*, 506.

Further studies on the effects of propantheline bromide on gastric acidity and motility and some reports on the application of these effects in diagnostic procedures: I. R. Schwartz *et al.*, *Am. J. Gastroent., N.Y.*, 1959, *28*, 518; S. Bank *et al.*, *Lancet*, 1966, *2*, 831; H. M. Goldstein and F. F. Zboralske, *J. Am. med. Ass.*, 1969, *210*, 2086; M. K. Dalinka *et al.*, *Radiology*, 1972, *102*, 281; A. H. Robbins *et al.*, *Am. J. Roentg.*, 1973, *117*, 432; J. T. Ferrucci *et al.*, *J. Can. Ass. Radiol.*, 1974, *25*, 269; R. B. Merlo *et al.*, *Radiology*, 1978, *127*, 61, per *Int. pharm. Abstr.*, 1979, *16*, 1120; H. L. Cooper, *Geriatrics*, 1980, *35*, 43, per *Int. pharm. Abstr.*, 1980, *17*, 944.

Enuresis. Three hundred children, aged 4 to 14 years, with persistent enuresis were treated with propantheline bromide 45 mg, propantheline bromide 45 mg with phenobarbitone 45 mg, or a placebo at bedtime for 2 months and then the dosage was gradually reduced. There was no significant difference between the effectiveness of the 3 regimens in reducing enuresis completely, or for 50% of the treatment period.— I. R. Wallace and W. I. Forsythe, *Br. J. clin. Pract.*, 1969, *23*, 207.

In a retrospective study of 1129 children with enuresis treated between 1952 and 1959 none had been completely relieved while on drug therapy except for 25 of 106 treated with propantheline bromide.— W. I. Forsythe and A. Redmond, *Archs Dis. Childh.*, 1974, *49*, 259.

Gastric and duodenal ulcer. A study involving both high (up to 360 mg daily) and standard (up to 60 mg daily) doses of propantheline bromide led to the conclusion that sustained gastric inactivity was of no value for treating duodenal ulcer in young men.— D. M. Roberts, *Am. J. Gastroent., N.Y.*, 1967, *47*, 124, per *Abstr. Wld Med.*, 1967, *41*, 693.

A study in 9 duodenal ulcer patients indicated that propantheline bromide 15 mg was as effective as near toxic doses (average 48 mg) in suppressing food-stimulated gastric acid secretion; additive inhibition of gastric acid secretion was noted on concurrent administration of propantheline bromide 15 mg and cimetidine 300 mg.— M. Feldman *et al.*, *New Engl. J. Med.*, 1977, *297*, 1427.

Hyperhidrosis. A lotion containing propantheline bromide 5% in a mixture of alcohol and glycerol, pH about 5.5, applied to the skin of 16 men with hyperhidrosis inhibited sweating.— E. A. Knudsen and C. H. K. Meier, *Acta derm.-vener., Stockh.*, 1963, *43*, 154.

In 38 mentally subnormal patients with hyperhidrosis, propantheline applied in 3 metered doses by aerosol reduced excessive sweating of the feet, reduced the severity of macerative keratolysis, and permitted the growth of new skin; erythema was only slightly affected. In general 3 low doses each of 1.85 mg were as effective as 3 doses each of 3.6 mg.— J. C. Frankland and R. H. Seville, *Br. J. Derm.*, 1971, *85*, 577.

Hypoglycaemia. Administration of propantheline 30 mg forty-five minutes before administration of glucose to stimulate insulin-release, prevented hypoglycaemic symptoms in 7 patients with reactive hypoglycaemia. It was considered that anticholinergic agents might be useful adjuncts in the therapy of reactive hypoglycaemia, and that for ordinary meals doses of propantheline as low as 7.5 mg might control the symptoms of reactive hypoglycaemia.— M. A. Permutt *et al.*, *Diabetes*, 1977, *26*,

121.

Inflammatory bowel disease. Anticholinergics might be valuable in reducing abdominal pain and lessening diarrhoea in ulcerative colitis. Propantheline bromide, 15 mg three or four times daily by mouth, was suitable, but should not be given if it was already being used parenterally to assist the retention of a rectal drip; for the latter purpose 15 to 30 mg was sometimes injected intramuscularly shortly before starting the drip. Large doses of anticholinergics might predispose to acute dilatation of the colon, which was dangerous.— S. C. Truelove, *Br. med. J.*, 1968, *2*, 539.

Following massive bowel resection for Crohn's disease, jejunostomy output in the range of 3 to 5 litres daily was dramatically controlled by administration of propantheline 15 mg intramuscularly thrice daily, so that the patient was able to resume her full-time career. Propantheline by mouth was ineffective probably owing to rapid transit and incomplete absorption. Side-effects were severe: dryness of mouth and difficulty in swallowing made eating impossible until 45 minutes after an injection, and dilated pupils with blurred vision, headaches, and tachycardia with palpitations, occurred regularly. Another patient was unable to tolerate the regimen owing to difficulty in micturition.— J. L. Cameron *et al.*, *Johns Hopkins med. J.*, 1976, *138*, 91.

Menetrier's disease. Administration of propantheline bromide gradually increased over a month to 105 mg daily in divided doses and continued for 9 months, corrected the symptoms of Menetrier's disease (a protein-losing gastropathy) in a 28-year-old man, who subsequently remained well without medication. Although spontaneous remission may occur in Menetrier's disease, the propantheline was considered to have had a beneficial effect. Intensive antisecretory therapy should be tried in all such patients before resorting to partial gastrectomy.— R. L. Smith and D. W. Powell, *Gastroenterology*, 1978, *74*, 903.

Ocular disorders. Instillation of a 1% solution of propantheline bromide in the eye caused mydriasis beginning in 10 to 15 minutes, reaching a maximum in about 30 minutes, and lasting 6 to 7 days. It rarely caused cycloplegia. Two patients showing allergy to atropine were not allergic to propantheline bromide.— A. M. Gokhale and S. A. Gokhale, *Br. J. Ophthal.*, 1970, *54*, 683.

Pancreatitis. For reference to the use of propantheline in association with cimetidine in the treatment of pancreatitis, see Cimetidine, p.1305.

Urinary incontinence. Studies and reports on the use of propantheline in urinary incontinence: J. C. Brocklehurst and J. B. Dillane, *Geront. clin.*, 1967, *9*, 182; J. A. Whitehead, *Geriatrics*, 1967, *22*, 154; A. C. Diokno *et al.*, *J. Urol.*, 1972, *107*, 42.

Preparations

Propantheline Bromide Tablets *(U.S.P.)*. Tablets containing propantheline bromide.

Propantheline Tablets *(B.P.)*. Tablets containing propantheline bromide. The tablets are sugar-coated.
Store in airtight containers.

Sterile Propantheline Bromide *(U.S.P.)*. Propantheline bromide suitable for parenteral use.

Proprietary Preparations

Pro-Banthine *(Searle, UK)*. Propantheline bromide, available as tablets of 15 mg. (Also available as Pro-Banthine in *Austral., Belg., Canad., Denm., Neth., Norw., S.Afr., Spain, Switz., USA*. Also available as Probanthine in *Fr.*).

Pro-Banthine with Dartalan *(Searle, UK)*. Tablets each containing propantheline bromide 15 mg and thiopropazate hydrochloride 3 mg. For peptic ulcer and functional dyspepsias associated with anxiety. *Dose.* 3 to 5 tablets daily.

Other Proprietary Names

Austral.— Pantheline; *Canad.*— Banlin, Propanthel; *Denm.*— Ercoril; *Ital.*— Pervagal, Suprantil; *Swed.*— Ercotina; *Switz.*— Mephathelin.

412-e

Propyromazine Bromide. LD 335. 1-Methyl-1-[1-(phenothiazin-10-ylcarbonyl)ethyl]pyrrolidinium bromide.
$C_{20}H_{23}BrN_2OS=419.4$.

CAS — 145-54-0.

Adverse Effects, Treatment, and Precautions. As for Atropine, p.289.

Uses. Propyromazine bromide is a quaternary ammonium anticholinergic agent with peripheral effects similar to those of atropine (see p.290). It is given in the symptomatic treatment of visceral spasms in a dose of 50 mg once to thrice daily by mouth; it is also given in a dose of 20 mg by subcutaneous, intramuscular, or slow intravenous injection.

Proprietary Names
Diaspasmyl *(Diamant, Fr.; Farmabion, Spain)*.

413-l

Stramonium Leaf *(B.P., Eur. P.)*.
Stramonium; Stramonii Folium; Jamestown Weed; Jimson Weed; Thornapple Leaf; Stramonii Herba; Datura; Stramoine; Stechapfelblätter; Hoja de Estramonio; Figueira do Inferno.

Pharmacopoeias. In *Arg., Belg., Br., Braz., Eur., Fr., Ger., Ind., Int., It., Mex., Neth., Pol., Port., Roum., Rus.*, and *Swiss. Aust.* specifies not less than 0.3% of alkaloids; *Hung.* and *Span.* not less than 0.2%. *Br.* also includes Powdered Stramonium Leaf.

The dried leaves and flowering tops of *Datura stramonium* and its varieties (Solanaceae), containing not less than 0.25% of alkaloids calculated as hyoscyamine. The principal alkaloid is hyoscyamine, with smaller amounts of hyoscine and atropine. **Store** in a cool dry place. Protect from light.

414-y

Prepared Stramonium *(B.P., Eur. P.)*.
Stramonii Pulvis Normatus; Prep. Stramon.

CAS — 8063-18-1 (stramonium).

Pharmacopoeias. In *Br., Eur., Fr., Ger.*, and *Neth.*

Stramonium leaf reduced to a fine powder and adjusted to contain 0.25% of alkaloids, calculated as hyoscyamine; 500 µg in 200 mg. A grey to greyish-green powder with a slightly nauseous odour and a bitter taste. **Store** in airtight containers. Protect from light.

Adverse Effects, Treatment, and Precautions. As for Atropine, p.289.

Abuse. In an analysis of 212 cases of stramonium and belladonna abuse, identifiable hallucinatory episodes were obtained by 99 subjects, 5 of whom died as a result of actions provoked by their mental state. Symptoms included hallucinations, amnesia, anxiety, paranoia, disorientation, hyperactivity or aggression, ataxia, dilated pupils, dryness of skin and mucous membranes, flushed skin, hypertension, fever, and tachycardia. Recovery from the acute phase usually occurred within 24 hours although the mydriasis might persist for 7 days. Treatment was best limited to supportive and protective measures.— J. M. Gowdy, *J. Am. med. Ass.*, 1972, *221*, 585. See also K. C. Ullman and R. H. Groh (letter), *ibid.*, 1972, *222*, 361.

A report of 10 cases of stramonium psychosis in teenagers, with disturbance of liver-function tests and cholinesterase activity.— M. M. Robertson and J. E. Morley, *S. Afr. med. J.*, 1974, *48*, 2604.

Reports of poisoning following the abuse of herbal preparations and brews containing *Datura stramonium*, including Potters Asthma Cigarettes: E. A. Harrison and D. H. Morgan (letter), *Br. med. J.*, 1976, *2*, 1195; A. Ballantyne *et al.*, *ibid.*, 1539; A. H. Barnett *et al.*, *ibid.*, 1977, *2*, 1635; R. K. Siegel, *J. Am. med. Ass.*, 1976, *236*, 473; R. W. Henson *et al.* (letter), *Med. J. Aust.*, 1978, *1*, 280; R. G. H. Bethel (letter), *Br. med. J.*, 1978, *2*, 959; R. E. Shervette *et al.*, *Pediatrics*, 1979, *63*, 520, per *Int. pharm. Abstr.*, 1979, *16*, 1160.

Uses. Stramonium leaf and preparations of stramonium have the actions of atropine (see p.290). It is very similar to belladonna (see p.293) and has been given to relieve spasm of the bronchioles in asthma, for which purpose it has been given in tablets or in mixtures. It has also been smoked in cigarettes or burnt in powders and the fumes inhaled but this is only of limited value since the irritation produced by the fumes may aggravate the bronchitis.

Stramonium leaf has also been used to control the salivation and muscular spasm in idiopathic and postencephalitic parkinsonism.

Doses of 30 to 200 mg have been given.

Preparations

Extracts

Stramonium Liquid Extract *(B.P. 1968)*. Stramon. Liq. Ext. An alcoholic extract adjusted to contain 0.25% w/v of alkaloids calculated as hyoscyamine; 500 µg in 0.2 ml. *Dose.* Up to 0.6 ml daily in divided doses.

Mixtures

Compound Lobelia and Stramonium Mixture *(B.P.C. 1973)*. Mist. Lobel. et Stramon. Co.; Mistura Lobeliae Composita. Lobelia ethereal tincture 0.5 ml, stramonium tincture 1 ml, potassium iodide 200 mg, tragacanth mucilage 1 ml, double-strength chloroform water 5 ml, water to 10 ml. It should be recently prepared. *Dose.* 10 ml.

Stramonium and Potassium Iodide Mixture *(B.P.C. 1973)*. Stramonium tincture 1.25 ml, potassium iodide 200 mg, double-strength chloroform water 5 ml, water to 10 ml. It should be recently prepared. *Dose.* 10 ml.

Powders

Species Antiasthmaticae *(Rus. P.)*. Antiasthmatic Powder; Astmatol. Stramonium leaf 6, hyoscyamus 1, and belladonna 2, in coarse powder, with sodium nitrate 1. For bronchial asthma; the powder is burnt and the smoke inhaled.

Port. P. includes a similar powder containing stramonium leaf 4.5, belladonna 3, lobelia 1, potassium nitrate 1.5.

Tinctures

Stramonium Tincture *(B.P.)*. Stramon. Tinct. Prepared from stramonium leaf by percolation with alcohol (45%) and standardised to contain 0.025% of alkaloids calculated as hyoscyamine; 500 µg in 2 ml.

415-j

Stramonium Seed *(B.P.C. 1934)*. Thornapple Seed; Semence de Stramoine; Stechapfelsame.

The seeds of *D. stramonium*, usually containing about 0.2% of alkaloids which consist chiefly of hysocyamine together with small quantities of atropine and hyoscine. Stramonium seed also contains 15 to 30% of fixed oil.

The properties of stramonium seed resemble those of Stramonium Leaf. It has been given in doses of 30 to 200 mg.

Two young children opened the pods of Jimson weed, *Datura stramonium*, and ate the seeds. They became confused, incoherent, ataxic, and stuporose. One developed convulsions. Physical signs included flushing, widely dilated pupils, dryness of the mouth, pyrexia, tachycardia, and exaggerated reflexes. Both children quickly recovered with support and sedation.— C. S. Rosen and M. Lechner, *New Engl. J. Med.*, 1962, *267*, 448.

Of 10 patients with an acute anticholinergic syndrome 2 to 6 hours after ingestion of Jimson seeds (*Datura stramonium*), 6 required admission to hospital because of pronounced hyperthermia and severe neurological derangement. As well as immediate supportive measures the treatment of choice was intravenous injection of physostigmine salicylate 1 to 2 mg repeated at 1- to 2-hour intervals if necessary. No patient required more than three 2-mg doses. Diazepam or hydroxyzine were given intramuscularly for hyperactivity. All patients recovered fully with a rapid return to normal EEG in 2 to 3 days.— J. R. Mikolich *et al.*, *Ann. intern. Med.*, 1975, *83*, 321. It was imperative that emesis was induced in patients who had ingested Jimson weed seeds if anticholinergic signs were present, regardless of the time of ingestion. Belladonna alkaloids in the seeds reduced gut motility and allowed the seeds to remain in the stomach.— R. Levy (letter), *ibid.*, 1976, *84*, 223.

A report of 5 adolescents between 14 and 16 years old who were treated for stramonium poisoning following ingestion of the seeds of *Datura stramonium*. Three were in an acute psychotic state and had symptoms of confusion, agitation, disorientation, hallucinations, tachycardia, dry mouth, dilated pupils not responsive to light, and flushed skin. Treatment was symptomatic.— D. A. Mahler (letter), *J. Am. med. Ass.*, 1975, *231*, 138.

For details and precautions relating to the use of physostigmine in anticholinergic poisoning, see Physostigmine Salicylate, p.1043.

416-z

Sultroponium. A118. (1*R*,3*r*,5*S*)-8-(3-Sulphopropyl)-3-[(±)-tropoyloxy]tropanium inner salt.
$C_{20}H_{29}NO_6S$=411.5.

CAS — 15130-91-3.

Adverse Effects, Treatment, and Precautions. As for Atropine, p.289.

Uses. Sultroponium is a quaternary ammonium anticholinergic agent with peripheral effects similar to those of atropine (see p.290). It is given in the symptomatic treatment of visceral spasms in doses of 15 to 30 mg up to three times daily by mouth; 25 to 75 mg daily has been given rectally as suppositories.

Proprietary Names
Sultroponium B *(Biothérax, Fr.)*.

417-c

Thiphenamil Hydrochloride. Thiphenum; Tifenamil Hydrochloride; Tiphen Hydrochloride. *S*-(2-Diethylaminoethyl) diphenylthioacetate hydrochloride.
$C_{20}H_{25}NOS,HCl$=363.9.

CAS — 82-99-5 (thiphenamil); 548-68-5 (hydrochloride).

Pharmacopoeias. In *Rus.*

A white crystalline powder with a bitter numbing taste. M.p. 124° to 130°. **Soluble** in water and chloroform; freely soluble in alcohol; sparingly soluble in acetone; very slightly soluble in ether. Solutions are **sterilised** by filtration. Aqueous solutions are unstable. **Protect** from light.

A study of the stability of thiphenamil hydrochloride in aqueous solutions.— R. V. Antipkina *et al.*, *Farmatsiya, Mosk.*, 1977, *26*, 58, per *Int. pharm. Abstr.*, 1979, *16*, 264.

Adverse Effects, Treatment, and Precautions. As for Atropine, p.289.

Uses. Thiphenamil hydrochloride has been described as a weak anticholinergic agent with actions similar to those of atropine (see p.290); it also has a direct antispasmodic effect on smooth muscle and a local anaesthetic effect. It is used for the relief of visceral spasms. In the USSR the usual dose is 30 to 100 mg twice or thrice daily to a maximum of 300 mg daily but in the USA the usual dose is 200 mg three or four times daily or initial doses of 400 mg repeated after 4 hours.

Proprietary Names
Trocinate *(Poythress, USA)*.

418-k

Tiemonium Iodide. TE 114. 4-[3-Hydroxy-3-phenyl-3-(2-thienyl)propyl]-4-methylmorpholinium iodide.
$C_{18}H_{24}INO_2S$=445.4.

CAS — 6252-92-2 (tiemonium); 144-12-7 (iodide).

Adverse Effects, Treatment, and Precautions. As for Atropine, p.289. Its use is contra-indicated in patients hypersensitive to iodine.

Uses. Tiemonium iodide is a quaternary ammonium anticholinergic agent with peripheral effects similar to those of atropine (see p.290). It is used as an adjunct in the treatment of gastric and duodenal ulcer, and to relieve visceral spasms. Doses of 50 to 100 mg have been given thrice daily by mouth and 5 to 10 mg has been given by subcutaneous, intramuscular, or intravenous injection. Doses of 20 mg have also been administered rectally as suppositories morning and evening. Tiemonium has also been used as the methylsulphate.

Studies in 9 healthy subjects showed that tiemonium given as either the iodide or the methylsulphate was poorly absorbed, about 8% of either salt being excreted in the urine during the first 24 hours and the remainder within 72 hours; about 70% of the dose was excreted in the faeces.— I. T. Scoular *et al.*, *Curr. med. Res. Opinion*, 1977, *4*, 732.

Proprietary Names
Ottimal (methylsulphate) *(Farnex, Ital.)*; Visceralgin *(Fawns & McAllan, Austral.)*; Visceralgina (iodide) *(Lirca, Ital.)*; Visceralgina Jarabe (methylsulphate) *(Liade, Spain)*; Visceralgine *(Sanders-Probel, Belg.; Provita, Switz.)* Viscéralgine (methylsulphate) *(Riom, Fr.)*.

419-a

Tigloidine Hydrobromide. Tiglylpseudotropeine Hydrobromide. (1*R*,3*s*,5*S*)-3-(3-Methylmethacryloyloxy)tropane hydrobromide.
$C_{13}H_{21}NO_2,HBr$=304.2.

CAS — 495-83-0 (tigloidine); 22846-83-9 (hydrobromide).

Tigloidine was first isolated from *Duboisia myoporoides* (Solanaceae) but is now synthesised. The hydrobromide is a white crystalline solid with a bitter numbing taste. **Soluble** in water.

Adverse Effects, Treatment, and Precautions. As for Atropine, p.289. The anticholinergic side-effects of tigloidine hydrobromide are claimed to be slight but it should be used with caution in glaucoma.

Uses. Tigloidine hydrobromide is chemically similar to atropine. It has been used in the treatment of muscular rigidity and spasticity, particularly when due to lesions of the upper motor neurone. The usual dose is 1 to 2 g daily in 3 divided doses with meals.

For reports on the use of tigloidine in parkinsonism and in spastic paraplegia, see E. M. Trautner and C. M. Noack, *Med. J. Aust.*, 1951, *1*, 751; F. J. O'Rourke *et al.*, *ibid.*, 1960, *1*, 73. For a review, see *Br. med. J.*, 1962, *1*, 253.

Proprietary Preparations
Tiglyssin *(Duncan, Flockhart, UK)*. Tigloidine hydrobromide, available as tablets of 250 mg.

420-e

Tricyclamol Chloride *(B.P. 1968)*. 1-(3-Cyclohexyl-3-hydroxy-3-phenylpropyl)-1-methylpyrrolidinium chloride.
$C_{20}H_{32}ClNO$=337.9.

CAS — 3818-88-0.

A white, almost odourless, crystalline powder with a bitter taste. M.p. 165° to 168°.
Soluble 1 in 3 of water, 1 in 3 of alcohol, and 1 in 25 of chloroform; practically insoluble in ether. A 1% solution in water has a pH of 5 to 7.

Adverse Effects, Treatment, and Precautions. As for Atropine, p.289.

Uses. Tricyclamol chloride is a quaternary ammonium anticholinergic agent with peripheral effects similar to those of atropine (see p.290). It is used as an adjunct in the treatment of gastric and duodenal ulcer, and to relieve visceral spasms. Doses of 50 to 100 mg have been given every 4 to 6 hours and at bedtime.

Preparations
Tricyclamol Tablets *(B.P. 1968)*. Tablets containing tricyclamol chloride.

421-l

Tridihexethyl Chloride *(U.S.P.)*. (3-Cyclohexyl-3-hydroxy-3-phenylpropyl)triethylammonium chloride.
$C_{21}H_{36}ClNO$=354.0.

CAS — 60-49-1 (tridihexethyl); 4310-35-4 (chloride).

Pharmacopoeias. In *U.S.*

A white odourless crystalline powder. M.p. 196° to 202°. **Soluble** 1 in 3 of water and alcohol, 1 in 2 of chloroform; freely soluble in methyl alcohol; practically insoluble in acetone and ether. A 5.62% solution in water is iso-osmotic with serum. **Store** in airtight containers.

Adverse Effects, Treatment, and Precautions. As for Atropine, p.289.

Uses. Tridihexethyl chloride is a quaternary ammonium anticholinergic agent with peripheral effects similar to those of atropine (see p.290). It is used as an adjunct in the treatment of gastric and duodenal ulcer and to relieve visceral spasms. Doses of 25 to 75 mg are given three or four times daily by mouth; 10 to 20 mg has also been administered every 6 hours by subcutaneous, intramuscular, or intravenous injection.

An aqueous solution of tridihexethyl chloride iso-osmotic with serum (5.62%) caused 97% haemolysis of erythrocytes cultured in it for 45 minutes.— C. Sapp *et al.*, *J. pharm. Sci.*, 1975, *64*, 1884.

Preparations
Tridihexethyl Chloride Injection *(U.S.P.)*. A sterile solution in Water for Injections. pH 5 to 7.5.
Tridihexethyl Chloride Tablets *(U.S.P.)*. Tablets containing tridihexethyl chloride. Store in airtight containers.

Proprietary Names
Duoesetil (as iodide) *(Dessy, Ital.)*; Pathilon *(Lederle, USA)*.

422-y

Tropacine Hydrochloride. Tropacinum; Tropatsin; Tropazine. (1*R*,3*r*,5*S*)-Tropan-3-yl diphenylacetate hydrochloride.
$C_{22}H_{25}NO_2$, HCl=371.9.

CAS — 6878-98-4 (tropacine); 548-64-1 (hydrochloride).

Pharmacopoeias. In *Rus.*

A white or creamy-white crystalline powder with a bitter taste. Readily **soluble** in water, alcohol, and chloroform; practically insoluble in ether. M.p. 212° to 216°.

Uses. Tropacine is an anticholinergic agent employed in the USSR chiefly in the treatment of parkinsonism. The maximum dose is 30 mg as a single dose or 100 mg in 24 hours.

423-j

Tropenziline Bromide. MTS 263. (1*R*,3*s*,5*R*)-3-Benziloyloxy-6-methoxy-8-methyltropanium bromide.
$C_{24}H_{30}BrNO_4$=476.4.

CAS — 6732-80-5 (tropenziline); 143-92-0 (bromide).

Adverse Effects, Treatment, and Precautions. As for Atropine, p.289.

Uses. Tropenziline bromide is a quaternary ammonium anticholinergic agent with peripheral effects similar to those of atropine (see p.290). It has been given in the symptomatic treatment of visceral spasms in doses of 20 to 40 mg thrice daily by mouth. Tropenziline bromide has also been given in doses of 10 to 30 mg intramuscularly daily and 10 to 20 mg intravenously daily; it has also been given rectally as suppositories containing 20 mg.

Animal studies.— S. Lecchini *et al.*, *J. Pharm. Pharmac.*, 1969, *21*, 662.

424-z

Tropicamide *(B.P., U.S.P.)*. Bistropamide; Ro 1-7683. *N*-Ethyl-*N*-(4-pyridylmethyl)tropamide.
$C_{17}H_{20}N_2O_2$=284.4.

CAS — 1508-75-4.

Pharmacopoeias. In *Br., Jap.*, and *U.S.*

A white or almost white, odourless or almost odourless, crystalline powder. M.p. 95° to 100°. **Soluble** 1 in 160 of water, 1 in 3.5 of alcohol, and 1 in 2 of chloroform; freely soluble in solutions of strong acids. **Store** in airtight containers. Protect from light.

The cycloplegic effect of tropicamide was enhanced by methylcellulose, and enhanced even more by methylcellulose and cetylpyridinium.— M. J. Mattila *et al.*, *Farmaceutiskt Notisbl.*, 1968, *77*, 205, per *Acta pharm. suec.*, 1969, *6*, 118.

The effect of different ophthalmic vehicles on the activity of tropicamide. Bioavailability of tropicamide generally increased with increasing viscosity of the vehicle.— M. F. Saettone *et al.*, *J. Pharm. Pharmac.*, 1980, *32*, 519.

Adverse Effects, Treatment, and Precautions. As for Atropine, p.289. Systemic toxicity may occasionally be produced by the instillation of anticholinergic eye-drops, particularly in infants.

Uses. Tropicamide is an anticholinergic agent with actions similar to those of atropine (see p.290), but its cycloplegic and mydriatic effects have a more rapid onset and a shorter duration of effect. Two drops of 0.5% solution will produce mydriasis within 15 minutes lasting about 8 hours.

A 1% solution is required to produce cycloplegia, usually by instilling one drop followed by a second drop 5 minutes later. The maximum effects appear within about 20 minutes and only last about 20 minutes so that a third drop is often necessary; complete recovery of accommodation usually occurs within 6 hours. Tropicamide has been reported to be inadequate for cycloplegia in children.

Mydriasis. Reports of ophthalmic uses and comparison with other anticholinergic agents: M. Swerdlow *et al.*, *Anesth. Analg. curr. Res.*, 1959, *38*, 229; H. M. Nano *et al.*, *Am. J. Ophthal.*, 1960, *49*, 958; B. C. Gettes, *ibid.*, 1963, *55*, 84; B. Milder, *Archs Ophthal., N.Y.*, 1961, *66*, 70; H. D. Gambill *et al.*, *ibid.*, 1967, *77*, 740; H. Zauberman and E. Neuman, *Cent. Afr. J. Med.*, 1970, *16*, 8, per *Trop. Dis. Bull.*, 1970, *67*, 1179.

For a favourable reference to the use of tropicamide in an eye ointment rather than in eye-drops, see Cyclopentolate Hydrochloride, p.297.

Test for glaucoma. A series of provocative tests was developed to determine which patients at risk were likely to develop closed-angle glaucoma. Pilocarpine 2% and phenylephrine 10% were instilled alternately thrice at 1-minute intervals and intra-ocular pressure was recorded every 30 minutes. When a significant increase (more than 8 mmHg) occurred the test was terminated by the intravenous injection of acetazolamide 500 mg and the instillation of thymoxamine 0.5%. If after 2 hours the test was negative a further application of pilocarpine and phenylephrine was made. If after 3½ hours the test was negative tropicamide 0.5% was instilled thrice at 1-minute intervals on the next day. Of 119 eyes studied 36 had given negative results to the series of tests; only one developed closed-angle glaucoma when followed for 1 to 7 years.— R. Mapstone, *Br. J. Ophthal.*, 1976, *60*, 115.

Preparations

Tropicamide Ophthalmic Solution *(U.S.P.)*. A sterile aqueous solution of tropicamide containing a suitable antimicrobial agent; it may contain suitable substances to increase its viscosity. pH 4 to 5.8. Store in airtight containers; avoid freezing.

NOTE. The code TRO is permitted in Great Britain for single-dose eye-drops of tropicamide.

Minims Tropicamide *(Smith & Nephew Pharmaceuticals, UK)*. Sterile eye-drops containing tropicamide 0.5 or 1%, in single-use disposable applicators.

Mydriacyl *(Alcon, UK: Farillon, UK)*. Eye-drops containing tropicamide 0.5 or 1% in sterile buffered solution. (Also available as Mydriacyl in *Austral., Canad., Denm., S.Afr., Swed.*).

Other Proprietary Names

Alcon-Mydril *(Arg.)*; Mydrian *(Norw.)*; Mydriaticum *(Belg., Fr., Ger., Neth., Switz.)*; Visumidriatic *(Ital.)*.

425-c

Valethamate Bromide. Diethylmethyl[2-(3-methyl-2-phenylvaleryloxy)ethyl]ammonium bromide.
$C_{19}H_{32}BrNO_2$=386.4.

CAS — 16376-74-2 (valethamate); 90-22-2 (bromide).

A white, almost odourless, crystalline powder. Freely **soluble** in water; very soluble in alcohol; practically insoluble in ether. **Incompatible** with phenobarbitone sodium in solution.

Adverse Effects, Treatment, and Precautions. As for Atropine, p.289.

Uses. Valethamate bromide is a quaternary ammonium anticholinergic agent with peripheral effects similar to those of atropine (see p.290). It has been used as an adjunct in the treatment of gastric and duodenal ulcer, and the relief of visceral spasms. Doses of 10 to 20 mg have been given three or four times daily by mouth; 10 to 20 mg has been given every 4 to 6 hours up to a daily maximum of 60 mg by intramuscular or intravenous injection.

Proprietary Names

Epidosan *(Raffo, Arg.)*; Epidosin *(Kali-Chemie, Ger.; Farmades, Ital.; Kali-Farma, Spain)*; Frenant, Narest *(both Jap.)*.

Balsams and Resins

270-y

Balsams are natural products of varying composition and consist chiefly of resins, gums, essential and volatile oils, and certain aromatic acids (usually cinnamic and benzoic acids).Resins are hard, amorphous, solids or semi-solids which soften on heating and consist of complex mixtures of organic acids and alcohols which are usually aromatic in nature. The term resin was formerly used when referring solely to products of vegetable or animal origin but now includes synthetic products which simulate their properties.

Balsams and resins have been used in the treatment of cough and bronchitis and for their antiseptic and protective properties in various skin conditions. Some balsams and resins are used in the formulation of varnishes, fixatives, and enteric coatings and in perfumery.

Balsams and resins can cause skin sensitisation and since many are chemically related by their content of esters, multiple sensitivities may occur. Many of the ingredients of balsams also occur in spices and essential oils and cross-sensitivity has been reported.

271-j

Ammoniacum *(B.P.C. 1949).* Gummi Resina Ammoniacum.

CAS — 9000-03-7.

Pharmacopoeias. In *Port.* and *Span.*

NOTE. Ammoniacum is strong ammonia solution in *Span. P.*

A gum-resin from the flowering and fruiting stem of *Dorema ammoniacum* and possibly other species of *Dorema* (Umbelliferae). Pale yellow tears or nodular masses with a characteristic odour and acrid taste.

Ammoniacum was formerly used in chronic bronchitis and has been reported to have a mild diuretic action. It has been given in doses of 0.3 to 1 g.

272-z

Asafetida *(B.P.C. 1949).* Gum Asafetida; Devil's Dung; Asant.

CAS — 9000-04-8.

Pharmacopoeias. In *Port.* and *Span.*

An oleo-gum-resin obtained from the living rhizome and root of *Ferula assafoetida, F. foetida, F. rubricaulis,* and probably other species of *Ferula* (Umbelliferae). It is in the form of greyish-white or yellow tears with a garlic-like odour and a bitter acrid taste. **Store** in a cool place.

Asafetida was formerly used in the treatment of flatulence and bronchitis, and for its supposed effect in nervous disorders. It has been given in doses of 0.3 to 1 g.

A report of the use of asafetida in patients with irritable colon.— V. W. Rahlfs and P. Mössinger, *Dt. med. Wschr.*, 1979, *104*, 140.

Preparations

Asafetida Tincture *(B.P.C. 1949).* Tinct. Asafoet. Prepared by macerating asafetida 1 in 5 of alcohol (70%). *Dose.* 2 to 4 ml.

273-c

Siam Benzoin *(B.P., Eur. P.).* Benzoe Tonkinensis.

CAS — 9000-72-0.

Pharmacopoeias. In *Aust., Br., Chin., Eur., Fr., Ger., It., Neth., Span.,* and *Swiss.* Also in many pharmacopoeias under the title benzoin and should not be confused with Sumatra Benzoin.

A balsamic resin from the incised stem of *Styrax tonkinensis* (Styracaceae) and containing about 68% of crystalline coniferyl benzoate together with free benzoic acid, (+)-siaresinolic acid, vanillin, and a small amount of cinnamyl benzoate. Contains not less than 25% of total balsamic acids, calculated as benzoic acid and with reference to the dried material, and not more than 5% of alcohol (90%)-insoluble matter.

Yellowish-white to reddish tears or almond-shaped pieces; when broken the surfaces are whitish and waxy, becoming reddish-brown on storage. It has a pronounced vanillin-like odour and an aromatic slightly acrid taste. It loses not more than 10% of its weight on drying. **Store** at a temperature not exceeding 25°. Protect from light.

Siam benzoin has been used to inhibit the development of rancidity in fats, its action apparently being due to the presence of coniferyl benzoate. It was formerly used in the preparation of benzoinated lard.

274-k

Sumatra Benzoin *(B.P.).* Benzoin; Gum Benzoin; Gum Benjamin; Benzoë; Benjoim.

CAS — 9000-73-1; 9000-05-9 (the first of these numbers is stated to apply to Sumatra benzoin and the second to benzoin).

Pharmacopoeias. In *Br., Jap.,* and *Port.* In *Arg., Belg., Hung., Ind., Mex.,* and *U.S.,* all of which allow both Siam benzoin and Sumatra benzoin.

A balsamic resin from the incised stem of *Styrax benzoin* and of *S. paralleloneurus* (Styracaceae) and containing various esters of benzoic and cinnamic acids together with free acids. It contains not less than 25% of total balsamic acids, calculated as cinnamic acid and with reference to the dried material, and not more than 20% of alcohol (90%)-insoluble matter.

Hard brittle masses of whitish tears embedded in a greyish-brown to reddish-brown translucent matrix, or cream-coloured tears; it has an agreeable balsamic odour and a slightly acrid taste. It loses not more than 10% of its weight on drying. **Store** at a temperature not exceeding 25°. Protect from light.

Adverse Effects. Sumatra benzoin may occasionally cause contact dermatitis.

From patch tests carried out on 413 patients with contact dermatoses, 2 were found to be allergic to compound benzoin tincture.— E. Epstein, *J. Am. med. Ass.*, 1966, *198*, 517.

A 22-year-old man developed acute eczematous contact dermatitis 23 days following the application of benzoin tincture to the skin under a plaster cast. A generalised non-eczematous exanthem appeared within the next 48 hours. Patch tests confirmed sensitisation to benzoin and to other gums and resins.— D. A. Spott and W. B. Shelley, *J. Am. med. Ass.*, 1970, *214*, 1881.

A report of 2 patients with suspected allergy to tincture of benzoin. Both patients had developed eczematous eruptions the first after having the perianal area painted with tincture of benzoin and gentian violet for pruritus ani and the second patient after spraying an area on his leg with a spray containing tincture of benzoin and then covering it with a plaster.— R. J. Coskey (letter), *Archs Derm.*, 1978, *114*, 128.

Uses. Sumatra benzoin is an ingredient of inhalations which are used in the treatment of catarrh of the upper respiratory tract by adding 5 ml of the inhalation to about 500 ml of hot water and inhaling the vapour. Sumatra benzoin is also used in topical preparations for its antiseptic and protective properties.

Preparations

Benzoin Inhalation *(B.P.).* Vap. Benzoin. Prepared by macerating Sumatra benzoin 10 g and prepared storax 5 g with alcohol (or industrial methylated spirit) to 100 ml.

5 ml is added to about 500 ml of hot, not boiling, water and the vapour inhaled.

Benzoin Tincture *(B.P.C. 1973).* Simple Benzoin Tincture. Sumatra benzoin 1 in 10, prepared by maceration with alcohol (90%). It has occasionally been administered internally in chronic bronchitis. It is employed for its local antiseptic, astringent, and protective properties as an ingredient of some skin preparations. *Dose.* 2.5 to 5 ml. Similar tinctures in *Arg. P., Aust. P., Belg. P., Fr. P., Port. P., Span. P.,* and *Swiss P.,* which are 1 in 5.

Compound Benzoin Tincture *(B.P.).* Co. Benz. Tinct.; Tinct. Benz. Co.; Friars' Balsam. Prepared by macerating sumatra benzoin 10%, prepared storax 7.5%, tolu balsam 2.5%, and aloes 2% with alcohol (90%). *Dose.* 2 to 4 ml (*B.P. 1932*). Compound benzoin tincture has occasionally been used internally in chronic bronchitis. It is employed as an inhalation (5 ml to 500 ml of hot water) in bronchitis and acute laryngitis. It is applied undiluted as an antiseptic and styptic to small cuts and to intact skin as a protective dressing under occlusive plasters and bandages. Mixtures with water require the addition of equal parts of mucilages of acacia and tragacanth to suspend the resins, the total amount of mucilage used being one-eighth of the volume of the mixture.

Compound Benzoin Tincture *(U.S.P.).* Prepared by macerating Siam benzoin or Sumatra benzoin 10%, storax *U.S.P.* 8%, tolu balsam 4%, and aloes 2% with alcohol. Store at a temperature not exceeding 40° in airtight containers. Protect from light.

Proprietary Preparations

Benzoin Compound Spray *(Norton, UK: Vestric, UK).* Contains soluble benzoin solids equivalent to benzoin 12.5% and prepared storax 2.5%. For application to the skin under adhesive dressings, and for the treatment of skin fissures and bedsores.

Rikospray Balsam *(Riker, UK).* An aerosol spray solution containing soluble benzoin solids 9% (equivalent to benzoin 12.5%) and prepared storax 2.5% with solvent and propellent. For application to the skin under adhesive plaster dressings in colostomy and ileostomy hygiene, for the prevention of bedsores, and for the treatment of cracked nipples and skin fissures.

Stuart Tinct. Benz. Co. Spray *(Stuart, UK).* A liquid aerosol spray containing compound benzoin tincture 15% with a solvent and propellent. For reducing skin sensitivity to adhesive plasters and for preventing skin irritation in ischaemic areas.

A preparation containing compound benzoin tincture was also formerly marketed in Great Britain under the proprietary name Atmoderm (*Thackray*).

275-a

Canada Balsam *(B.P.C. 1934).* Terebinthina Canadensis; Canada Turpentine; Balsam of Fir.

CAS — 8007-47-4.

The oleoresin from the balsam fir, *Abies balsamea* (Pinaceae). It is a pale yellow viscous liquid with an agreeable odour and a bitter acrid taste; it often exhibits a slight fluorescence. **Soluble** in most organic solvents.

Canada balsam has been used in microscopy as a mounting medium.

276-t

Colophony *(B.P.).* Coloph.; Colophonium; Resin; Rosin *(U.S.P.)*; Resina Pini; Resina Terebinthinae; Colophane.

CAS — 8050-09-7.

Pharmacopoeias. In *Aust., Br., Jap., Nord., Pol., Port., Span., Swiss,* and *U.S.*

The residue left after distilling the volatile oil from the crude oleoresin obtained from various species of *Pinus* (Pinaceae). It contains about 90% of resin acids, of which about a third is abietic acid. The composition varies with source, age, and method of storage, and the acids appear to change on exposure to air. Translucent, pale yellow or brownish-yellow, angular, brittle, readily fusible, glassy masses, with a faint terebinthinate odour and taste.

Practically **insoluble** in water; soluble in alcohol, carbon disulphide, chloroform, ether, some fixed and volatile oils, glacial acetic acid, and dilute solutions of alkali hydroxides; partly soluble in light petroleum. It should be **stored** in the unground condition.

Adverse Effects. Colophony may occasionally cause skin sensitisation.

Of 4000 patients subjected to patch testing in 5 European clinics, 2.9% of males and 3.6% of females showed positive reactions to colophony 20% in soft paraffin.— H. Bandmann *et al.*, *Archs Derm.*, 1972, *106*, 335. See also E. Rudzki and D. Kleniewska, *Br. J. Derm.*, 1970, *83*, 543.

Asthma or respiratory symptoms related to work developed in 21 workers in the electronics industry exposed to solder flux fumes containing colophony. Five of the workers had pre-existing asthma. The median period of exposure before recognised symptoms appeared was 6 years. All the workers had a positive reaction when rechallenged with fumes of heated colophony alone and findings suggested that it was a hypersensitivity reaction.— P. S. Burge *et al.*, *Clin. Allergy*, 1978, *8*, 1.

A discussion on respiratory problems, including colophony-induced asthma, associated with the use of soldering fluxes.— *Lancet*, 1979, *2*, 397.

A report of colophony allergy in 5 wood-workers with positive bronchial challenge tests to the wood dusts with which they worked (oak, makore, mahogany, rosewood, and pine). Also, 4 electronics workers sensitised to colophony from soldering fluxes subsequently had asthmatic attacks induced by walking in pine woods. This might explain why a number of electronics workers with occupational asthma continue to have symptoms after leaving work.— P. S. Burge (letter), *Lancet*, 1979, *2*, 591.

Uses. Colophony is an ingredient of some collodions and plaster-masses and it was formerly extensively used as an ingredient of ointments, as dressings for blisters, and wounds, and as an application for indolent ulcers and boils.

Preparations

Colophony Ointment *(B.P.C. 1959).* Resin Ointment; Yellow Basilicon Ointment. Colophony 26 g, yellow beeswax 26 g, olive oil 26 g, and lard 22 g.

277-x

Galbanum *(B.P.C. 1934).*

CAS — 9000-24-2.

Pharmacopoeias. In *Port.* and *Span.*

A gum-resin obtained from *Ferula galbaniflua* and probably other species of *Ferula* (Umbelliferae) in the form of yellowish-brown or orange-brown, rounded or irregular tears, or in agglutinated tears, or in lumps. It has an aromatic odour and a bitter taste. It contains 5 to 20% of volatile oil, together with resin, gum, moisture, and mineral matter.

Galbanum was formerly used in chronic bronchitis and, with asafetida, in the treatment of nervous disorders. It has been given in doses of 0.3 to 1 g.

278-r

Guaiacum Resin *(B.P.C. 1949).* Guaiac. Res.; Guaiac; Guaiac Resin; Guaiacum; Guajakharz.

CAS — 9000-29-7.

The resin of guaiacum wood. Rounded tears, often covered with a green powder, with an aromatic odour when warmed and a slightly acrid taste. **Soluble** almost completely in alcohol, chloroform, ether, and solutions of caustic alkalis and of chloral hydrate. **Protect** from light in airtight containers.

Guaiacum resin has mild laxative and diuretic actions; it was formerly used in the treatment of rheumatism. It has been given in doses of 0.3 to 1 g. Guaiacum resin is now used in the detection of occult blood in the faeces.

A food grade was specified for use as an antioxidant. Estimated acceptable daily intake: up to 2.5 mg per kg body-weight.— Seventeenth Report of FAO/WHO Expert Committee on Food Additives, *Tech. Rep. Ser. Wld Hlth Org. No. 539*, 1974. For background toxicological information, see *Fd Add. Ser. Wld Hlth Org. No. 5*, 1974..

Test for occult blood in faeces. A brief review of a modified guaiacum-resin test for occult blood in the faeces.— *Med. Lett.*, 1979, *21*, 36.

One drop of a solution containing 2 g of guaiacum resin dissolved in 100 ml of glacial acetic acid was placed on a faecal smear on a filter paper, followed by a drop of hydrogen peroxide solution, 10 volumes. A green-blue colour within 30 seconds was positive, a faint blue colour in 30 seconds was a trace, and no colour was a negative result. The sensitivity of this test was equivalent to the orthotolidine test (orthotolidine 400 mg in glacial acetic acid), and the tablet test (Hematest).— R. H. Wilkinson and W. A. F. Penfold (letter), *Lancet*, 1969, *2*, 847. Comment.— J. Runcie and T. J. Thomson (letter), *ibid.*, 954. See also *ibid.*, 1970, *1*, 819.

The guaiacum resin and 1% orthotolidine tests for occult blood in faeces produced a high number of false positive results in normal infants and normal children eating a meat-containing diet. A modified reduced phenolphthalein test gave no false positives but was insensitive to blood dilutions below 1 in 5000.— A. E. A. Ford-Jones and J. J. Cogswell, *Archs Dis. Childh.*, 1975, *50*, 238.

A transient green discoloration in the guaiacum resin test for occult blood was considered to represent the lower limit of the test's sensitivity rather than a negative result.— K. L. Cohen and E. J. Luminati (letter), *New Engl. J. Med.*, 1978, *299*, 154.

Comments on the value of faecal occult-blood testing as a screening procedure for colonic cancer.— N. Prescott *et al.* (letter), *New Engl. J. Med.*, 1980, *303*, 1306. Reply.— D. Neuhauser (letter), *ibid.*

A study in 157 patients with colorectal tumours indicated that the guaiacum test for occult blood gave a high rate of false negative results.— S. Schewe *et al.*, *Dt. med. Wschr.*, 1979, *104*, 253.

Proprietary Preparations

Haemoccult *(Norwich-Eaton, UK).* A test kit comprising slides impregnated with guaiacum resin and a hydrogen peroxide reagent; for the detection of occult blood in faeces.

Okokit *(Hughes & Hughes, UK).* A test kit comprising tablets containing guaiacum resin, test-papers, and a reagent; for the detection of occult blood in faeces.

279-f

Guaiacum Wood *(B.P.C. 1949).* Guaiaci Lignum; Lignum Vitae; Bois de Gaïac; Guajakholz.

The heartwood of *Guaiacum officinale* and of *G. sanctum* (Zygophyllaceae), containing 18 to 25% of guaiacum resin.

Uses. Guaiacum wood is the source of guaiacum resin, and is an ingredient of compound sarsaparilla decoction.

280-z

Mastic *(B.P.).* Mastiche; Mastix; Almáciga.

CAS — 61789-92-2.

Pharmacopoeias. In *Aust.*, *Br.*, *Port.*, *Span.*, and *Swiss.*

A resinous exudation from certain forms or varieties of *Pistacia lentiscus* (Anacardiaceae). Small, hard, yellowish tears with an aromatic odour and agreeable taste, becoming plastic when chewed. M.p. 105° to 120°.

Practically **insoluble** in water; partly soluble in alcohol and turpentine oil; soluble 2 in 1 of chloroform, 2 in 1 of ether, and in acetone.

Uses. Solutions of mastic in alcohol, chloroform, or ether have been used, applied on cotton wool, as temporary fillings for carious teeth. Compound Mastic Paint has been used as a protective covering for wounds and to hold gauze in position.

Preparations

Compound Mastic Paint *(B.P.).* Pigmentum Mastiches Compositum. Mastic 40 g, castor oil 1.25 ml, equal volumes of acetone and industrial methylated spirit to 100 ml. Store in a cool place in airtight containers. This preparation is inflammable. Keep away from an open flame.

The vehicle of Compound Mastic Paint used to be benzene, nitration grade of commerce, when the synonym benzo-mastic was sometimes used.

Aust. P. and *Swiss P.* include similar preparations.

Microscopic Varnish. Mastic 15 g, caoutchouc 1 g, chloroform 60 ml; macerate and filter.

281-c

Myrrh *(B.P.C. 1973).* Myrrha; Gum Myrrh.

CAS — 9000-45-7.

Pharmacopoeias. In *Aust.*, *Belg.*, *Ger.*, *Port.*, *Span.*, and *Swiss.*

An oleo-gum-resin obtained from the stem of *Commiphora molmol* and possibly other species of *Commiphora* (Burseraceae). Reddish-brown or reddish-yellow tears, with an aromatic odour and a bitter acrid taste. It contains 25 to 40% of resin, 57 to 61% of gum, 7 to 17% of volatile oil, and a bitter principle.

Soluble in water to the extent of about 50% (forms a yellowish emulsion on trituration); partly soluble in alcohol; soluble in alkalis. **Store** in a cool dry place. Protect from light.

Uses. Myrrh is astringent to mucous membranes; the tincture is used in mouth-washes and gargles for ulcers in the mouth and pharynx. It has been used internally as a carminative.

Preparations

Myrrh Tincture *(B.P.C. 1973).* Prepared by macerating myrrh 1 in 5 of alcohol (90%). *Dose.* 2.5 to 5 ml. A similar tincture is included in several pharmacopoeias.

282-k

Peru Balsam *(B.P.C. 1973).* Bals. Peruv.; Peruvian Balsam; Baume du Pérou; Baume du San Salvador.

CAS — 8007-00-9.

Pharmacopoeias. In *Arg.*, *Aust.*, *Belg.*, *Cz.*, *Fr.*, *Ger.*, *Hung.*, *Jug.*, *Mex.*, *Nord.*, *Pol.*, *Port.*, *Roum.*, *Span.*, and *Swiss.*

A balsam exuded from the trunk of *Myroxylon balsamum* var. *pereirae* (Leguminosae). It is a dark brown, viscous liquid with an agreeable balsamic odour and a bitter, acrid, burning taste, containing 49 to 60% of balsamic esters.

Practically **insoluble** in water; miscible 1 in 1 of alcohol (90%), the addition of more alcohol causing turbidity; soluble in chloroform; partly soluble in ether, glacial acetic acid, and light petroleum. Water shaken with the balsam only removes traces of cinnamic acid. Wt per ml 1.14 to 1.17 g. **Protect** from light.

Adverse Effects. Peru balsam may cause skin sensitisation.

Of 4000 patients subjected to patch testing in 5 European clinics, 4.6% of males and 7.6% of females showed positive reactions to Peru balsam 25% in soft paraffin.— H. Bandmann *et al.*, *Archs Derm.*, 1972, *106*, 335. See also E. Rudzki and D. Kleniewska, *Br. J. Derm.*, 1970, *83*, 543.

Uses. Peru balsam has a very mild antiseptic action by virtue of its content of cinnamic and benzoic acids. Diluted with an equal part of castor oil, it has been used as an application to bedsores and chronic ulcers; as an ointment (12.5% in Simple Ointment) it has been used in the treatment of eczema and pruritus. It is an ingredient of some rectal suppositories used for the symptomatic relief of haemorrhoids.

Peru balsam was formerly used in the treatment of scabies.

283-a

Polyvinox. Vinylinum; Polyvinylbutyl Ether; Shostakovsky Balsam. Poly(1-butoxyethylene).

$C_{16}H_{34}O_3,(C_6H_{12}O)_n=2000$ (approx.).

CAS — 25232-87-5.

Pharmacopoeias. In *Rus.*

A pale yellow, viscous liquid with a characteristic odour. Wt per ml about 0.9 g. Practically **insoluble** in water; sparingly soluble in alcohol; very slightly soluble in methyl alcohol; miscible with acetone, chloroform, ether, liquid paraffin, and vegetable oils.

Polyvinox is a synthetic resin, developed in the USSR as a substitute for Peru balsam. It is used in the USSR by external application, either undiluted or as a 20% oily solution or as an ointment, in the treatment of wounds and burns and various skin diseases. It is stated to have a bacteriostatic action and to promote tissue regeneration and epithelialisation. Polyvinox has also been administered by mouth in the treatment of gastric and duodenal ulcers, gastritis, and colitis.

Polyvinox was formerly marketed in Great Britain under the proprietary name Shostakovsky Balsam (*Leopold Charles*).

284-t

Sandarac *(B.P.C. 1949).* Sandaraca; Gum Juniper.

CAS — 9000-57-1.

A resin obtained by incision of the stem of *Tetraclinis articulata* (Cupressaceae). Brittle pale yellow tears, which do not agglomerate when chewed, with a slightly terebinthinate odour and taste. M.p. 130° to 160°. Practically **insoluble** in water; soluble in alcohol, amyl alcohol, and ether; partly soluble in chloroform, carbon disulphide, and turpentine oil.

Sandarac was formerly used in alcoholic solution as a temporary filling for carious teeth. It is used in pill varnishes and in industrial varnishes.

Preparations

Pill Varnish. A solution of sandarac 1 in 2 of alcohol (95%) or, for quicker drying, sandarac 1 in a mixture of alcohol (95%) 1 and ether 1.

285-x

Shellac. U.S.N.F., B.P.C. 1963; Lacca; Lacca in Tabulis.

CAS — 9000-59-3.

Pharmacopoeias. In *Chin.* and *Span. Jap.* includes Purified Shellac and White Shellac (Bleached). Also in *U.S.N.F.*

Shellac is obtained by purification of the resinous secretion of the insect*Laccifer lacca Kerr* (Coccidae). The *U.S.N.F.* describes 4 grades: Orange Shellac is produced by filtration in the molten state or by a hot solvent process, or both; removal of the wax produces Dewaxed Orange Shellac which may be lighter in colour; Regular Bleached (White) Shellac is prepared by dissolving the secretion in aqueous sodium carbonate, bleaching with hypochlorite, and precipitating with sulphuric acid; removal of the wax by filtration during the process produces Refined Bleached Shellac. The bleached shellacs lose not more than 6% of weight on drying.

Practically **insoluble** in water; readily soluble in warm alcohol; very slightly soluble in light petroleum; almost completely soluble in alkali hydroxide solutions and borax solutions.

Uses. Shellac is used with cetostearyl alcohol as an enteric coating for pills and tablets. Bleached shellac, in alcoholic solution, is used as a hair lacquer.

A marked increase in disintegration time occurred with shellac-coated tablets which had aged.— J. G. Wagner *et al.*, *J. Am. pharm. Ass., scient. Edn*, 1960, *49*, 133.

For the experimental use of shellac and stearic acid as a coating for sustained-release tablets, see A. A. Kassem *et al.*, *Mfg Chem.*, 1973, *44* (Mar.), 43.

Addition of 10% w/w of castor oil, theobroma oil, or isopropyl myristate to a shellac-macrogol 4000 tablet coating mixture improved the stability with respect to clumping and fading and improved the disintegration, friability, uniformity of coat, and appearance. The concentration of shellac in the formulation was found to be a controlling factor with regard to disintegration.— P. A. Tuerck and D. E. McVean, *J. pharm. Sci.*, 1973, *62*, 1534.

The disintegration time was unacceptably prolonged in tablets enteric coated with shellac and stored for one year. Cellacephate was more acceptable.— G. T. Luce, *Eastman, USA*, *Mfg Chem.*, 1978, *49* (July), 50.

Lung damage (thesaurosis) from hair-sprays. A chest X-ray survey on 505 hairdressers exposed for varying periods to the inhalation of hair-sprays with shellac or povidone bases, or both, produced no evidence of thesaurosis. A woman hairdresser developed an interstitial pulmonary fibrosis after exposure for 11 years to shellac-based hair lacquer sprays. Reference was made to another case of pulmonary fibrosis reported by E.F. Hirsch and H.B. Russell (*Archs Path.*, 1945, *39*, 281) in a furniture maker due to the inhalation of shellac; they regarded the histological changes as consistent with the inhalation of fatty acids, which constituted at least 60% of shellac. It was probable that thesaurosis occurred only in susceptible or hypersensitive people.— A. I. G. McLaughlin *et al.*, *Food & Cosmet. Toxicol.*, 1963, *1*, 171.

Preparations

Pharmaceutical Glaze *(U.S.N.F.).* A denatured solution containing 20 to 51% of anhydrous shellac, prepared with alcohol (95%) or dehydrated alcohol; it may contain waxes and titanium dioxide as an opaquing agent. Store at a temperature not exceeding 40° (preferably below 25°) in airtight containers.

286-r

Prepared Storax *(B.P.).* Styrax Praeparatus; Liquid Storax; Purified Storax; Balsamum Styrax Liquidus; Styrax Depuratus; Estoraque Líquido.

CAS — 8023-62-9 (storax).

Pharmacopoeias. In *Br.*, *Ind.*, and *Swiss. Port.* and *Span.* specify crude storax.
Storax *U.S.P.* is crude storax from *L. orientalis* (Levant storax) or *L. styraciflua* (American storax).

The purified balsam obtained from the trunk of *Liquidambar orientalis* (Hamamelidaceae). It contains not less than 28.5% of total balsamic acids. It is a brown viscous liquid with an agreeable balsamic odour and taste.

Practically **insoluble** in water; soluble in alcohol (90%), carbon disulphide, chloroform, and glacial acetic acid; partly soluble in ether.

Adverse Effects. Prepared storax may cause skin sensitisation.

Uses. It has actions similar to those of Peru balsam (p.315) and was applied as an ointment in the treatment of scabies and other parasitic skin diseases. It is an ingredient of Compound Benzoin Tincture and of Benzoin Inhalation.

287-f

Tolu Balsam *(B.P., U.S.P.).* Tolu Bals.; Balsamum Tolutanum; Baume de Tolu.

CAS — 9000-64-0.

Pharmacopoeias. In *Arg.*, *Aust.*, *Belg.*, *Br.*, *Fr.*, *Ind.*, *It.*, *Mex.*, *Port.*, *Roum.*, *Span.*, *Swiss*, and *U.S.*

A balsam obtained by incision from the trunk of *Myroxylon balsamum* (=*M. toluiferum*) (Leguminosae). It is a soft, tenacious, brownish-yellow or brown resinous solid when fresh, but it subsequently becomes harder and finally brittle. It has an aromatic and vanilla-like odour and taste. It contains 35 to 50% of total balsamic acids, calculated as cinnamic acid.

Practically **insoluble** in water and light petroleum; soluble in alcohol, chloroform, ether, glacial acetic acid, and solutions of caustic alkalis, but sometimes leaving some insoluble residues; partly soluble in carbon disulphide, the soluble portion consisting chiefly of cinnamic acid. A solution in alcohol (90%) is acid to litmus. **Store** at a temperature not exceeding 40° in airtight containers.

Uses. Tolu balsam is considered to have very mild antiseptic properties and some expectorant action but is mainly used as Tolu Syrup to flavour cough mixtures.

Preparations

Linctuses

Paediatric Compound Tolu Linctus *(B.P.).* Tolu Compound Linctus Paediatric. Citric acid monohydrate 30 mg, invert syrup 1 ml, compound tartrazine solution 0.05 ml, benzaldehyde spirit 0.01 ml, glycerol 1 ml, tolu syrup to 5 ml. Store at a temperature not exceeding 25°. When a dose less than or not a multiple of 5 ml is prescribed the linctus should be diluted to 5 ml, or a multiple, with syrup. Such dilutions must be freshly prepared and not used more than 2 weeks after issue.

Lozenges

Tolu Basis for Lozenges *(B.P.C. 1959).* For 100 lozenges; tolu tincture 2 ml, sucrose 100 g, acacia 7 g, water q.s.

Solutions

Tolu Solution *(B.P.).* Liq. Tolu. Prepared from tolu balsam 5 g, alcohol (90%) 30 ml, sucrose 50 g, and water to 100 ml.

The following formula was proposed for a synthetic tolu solution: cinnamic acid 500 mg, benzoic acid 250 mg, ethyl cinnamate 30 mg, vanillin 10 mg, cinnamon oil 2 mg, sucrose 50 g, alcohol (90%) 30 ml, and water to 100 ml. Synthetic tolu solutions and syrups made to the proposed formulation have proved to be stable for a period in excess of 6 months when kept under ambient temperature conditions.— K. Helliwell and S. Watkins, *Pharm. J.*, 1980, *1*, 103.

Syrups

Tolu Balsam Syrup *(U.S.N.F.).* Tolu Syrup. Tolu balsam tincture 5 ml, triturated with magnesium carbonate 1 g, sucrose 6 g, water 43 ml, and filtered; sucrose 76 g, dissolved in the filtrate, strained, and diluted with water to 100 ml.

Tolu Syrup *(B.P.).* Tolu solution 10 ml, syrup to 100 ml. Store at a temperature not exceeding 30°.

Dilution of a synthetic tolu solution (prepared from cinnamic acid 75 mg, benzoic acid 500 mg, vanillin 2.5 mg, benzyl benzoate 45 mg, benzyl cinnamate 6.25 mg, alcohol (90%) 30 ml, sucrose 50 g, and water to 100 ml) 1 in 10 with unpreserved syrup produced a factitious tolu syrup which was similar in flavour and appearance to the official syrup. Samples of paediatric compound tolu linctus and opiate squill linctus prepared from the factitious syrup were also similar in taste and appearance to the corresponding preparations made with the official syrup. Syrup preserved with hydroxybenzoates might be unsuitable for preparation of the factitious tolu syrup.— Pharm. Soc. Lab. Rep. P/78/4, 1978.

Tinctures

Tolu Balsam Tincture *(U.S.N.F.).* Tolu balsam 20 g, alcohol to 100 ml; prepared by maceration. Store at a temperature not exceeding 40° in airtight containers. Protect from light.

Tolu Tincture *(B.P.C. 1959).* Tinct. Tolu; Tolu Balsam Tincture. 1 in 10 of alcohol (90%). *Belg. P.*, *Fr. P.*, and *Mex. P.* specify 1 in 5. In mixtures the resin must be suspended with mucilage. *Dose.* 2 to 4 ml.

Bitters

520-z

Bitters, usually of vegetable origin, have been traditional remedies for loss of appetite and are still included in many 'tonic' formulations. Mixtures containing bitters are usually taken before meals.

In a Report on the Review of Flavourings in Food, 1976, The Food Additives and Contaminants Committee (FAC/REP/22) recommended that the use of bitters of vegetable origin as flavourings should be controlled by a permitted list system as for other food additives, and that no flavouring should be authorised for use without being included in a published permitted list.

For a review of the use of bitters, see J. D. Kinloch, *Practitioner*, 1971, *206*, 44.

Action of bitters on the stomach. A study of the action of gentian and other bitters on gastric function in a patient after gastrostomy showed that bitters increased gastric function to a variable degree; this action was apparently due to a direct action on the stomach or duodenum and the sensation of bitterness did not appear to contribute significantly to the response though introduction of bitters into the mouth resulted in an immediate salivary response.— S. Wolf and M. Mack, *Drug Stand.*, 1956, *24*, 98.

521-c

Absinthium *(B.P.C. 1934).* Wormwood; Wermutkraut; Absinthii Herba; Assenzio; Losna; Pelin.

CAS — 546-80-5 (α-thujone); 471-15-8 (β-thujone).

Pharmacopoeias. In *Aust.*, *Cz.*, *Ger.*, *Hung.*, *Jug.*, *Pol.*, *Roum.*, and *Swiss.*

The fresh or dried leaves and flowering tops of wormwood, *Artemisia absinthium* (Compositae). Thujone, related to camphor is the major constituent of the essential oil derived from absinthium, and is present also in oils derived from sage, white cedar, and tansy. Absinthium also contains bitter principles including a glycoside. **Protect** from light.

Absinthium has been used as a bitter; usually administered as a tincture or an infusion of absinthium alone or with other bitters; it is also used in small quantities as a flavouring agent in alcoholic beverages. Habitual use or large doses cause absinthism, which is shown by restlessness, vomiting, vertigo, tremors and convulsions.

Thujone was the active principle of *Artemisia absinthium* and was derived from the essential oil absinthol. Its structure was compared to that of tetrahydrocannabinol. It was postulated that thujone and THC interacted with a common receptor in the CNS.— J. del Castillo *et al.* (letter), *Nature*, 1975, *253*, 365.

Analysis of the bitter principles of *Artemisia absinthium*.— G. Schneider and B. Mielke, *Dt. ApothZtg*, 1978, *118*, 469; *idem*, 1979, *119*, 977.

522-k

Andrographis *(B.P.C. 1949).* Kalmegh; Kirayat.

CAS — 5508-58-7 (andrographolide).

Pharmacopoeias. In *Chin.* and *Ind. Chin.* also includes Andrographolide Sodium Bisulphite.

The dried entire plant (*B.P.C. 1949*)or the dried leaves and tender shoots (*Ind. P.*) of *Andrographis paniculata* (Acanthaceae). *Ind. P.* specifies not less than 1% of a bitter principle, andrographolide.

NOTE. *Andrographis paniculata* has sometimes been described as chiretta and should not be confused with Chirata, p.317.

Andrographis is used in Asia as a bitter, usually in the form of a liquid extract.

523-a

Azadirachta. Margosa; Neem.

The dried stem bark, root bark, and leaves of *Azadirachta indica* (=*Melia azadirachta*) (Meliaceae).

Azadirachta is used as a bitter, usually as an infusion or tincture.

An oil expressed from the seeds (neem oil or margosa oil) has been used as a hair tonic and in skin diseases.

Pharmacology.— S. O. Arigbabu and S. G. Don-Pedro, *Afr. J. Pharm. & pharm. Sci.*, 1971, *1*, 181, per *Int. pharm. Abstr.*, 1973, *10*, 115.

The essential oil extracted from *Azadirachta indica* was found to possess antibacterial activity when tested *in vitro*.— S. C. Chaurasia and P. C. Jain, *Indian J. Hosp. Pharm.*, 1978, *15*, 166, per *Int. pharm. Abstr.*, 1979, *16*, 1184.

Severe poisoning in Indian children given margosa oil as a remedy for minor ailments.— D. Sinniah and G. Baskaran, *Lancet*, 1981, *1*, 487.

Proprietary Preparations

Silvose *(Keimdiät, Ger.: Thomson & Joseph, UK).* An extract from the bark of azadirachta. It is claimed to reduce dental caries and inflammation of the mouth when used as an ingredient in dental preparations.

524-t

Berberine Sulphate *(B.P.C. 1949).* Berberine Acid Sulphate; Berberine Bisulphate. 5,6-Dihydro-9,10-dimethoxybenzo[*g*]-1,3-benzodioxolo[5,6-*a*]quinolizinium hydrogen sulphate. $C_{20}H_{18}NO_4,HSO_4$=433.4.

CAS — 2086-83-1 (berberine); 633-66-9 (sulphate).

Pharmacopoeias. Jap. P. includes Berberine Chloride ($C_{20}H_{18}ClNO_4,xH_2O$) and Berberine Tannate.

The acid salt of berberine, a quaternary alkaloid present in hydrastis, in various species of *Berberis*, and in many other plants.

Bright yellow, odourless, acicular crystals or dark yellow powder with a bitter taste. **Soluble** about 1 in 150 of water; slightly soluble in alcohol. Solutions are **sterilised** by autoclaving or by filtration.

Adverse Effects. Large doses of berberine depress respiration and can cause circulatory collapse.

Uses. It is given by mouth as a bitter. It has also been used in the treatment of cholera in doses of up to 150 mg daily. An injection of berberine sulphate has been used in India in the treatment of cutaneous leishmaniasis. A 1% solution of berberine sulphate, together with procaine hydrochloride 1% has been injected subcutaneously around the margins of the lesion once a week for 2 to 5 injections. It is reported to have mild local anaesthetic effects on mucous membranes.

Amoebiasis. Berberine sulphate was shown to be an effective amoebicide *in vitro* against *Entamoeba histolytica* at a concentration of 0.5 to 1 mg per ml; its effectiveness had been confirmed in *animal* studies.— T. V. Subbaiah and A. H. Amin (letter), *Nature*, 1967, *215*, 527.

Cholera and diarrhoea. References to berberine in cholera and diarrhoea: S. C. Lahiri and N. K. Dutta, *J. Indian med. Ass.*, 1967, *48*, 1; D. C. Sharda, *J. Indian med. Ass.*, 1970, *54*, 22; N. K. Dutta *et al.*, *Br. J. Pharmac.*, 1972, *44*, 153; M. Sabir *et al.*, *Indian J. med. Res.*, 1977, *65*, 305, per *Trop. Dis. Bull.*, 1978, *75*, 177.

Trachoma. Berberine in small doses was as effective as sulphadiazine in protecting *chick* embryos from the lethal effects of trachoma organisms injected into yolk sacs.— M. Sabir *et al.*, *Indian J. med. Res.*, 1976, *64*, 1160.

525-x

Calamus *(B.P.C. 1934).* Calamus Rhizome; Sweet Flag Root; Acore Vrai; Kalmus.

CAS — 8015-79-0 (calamus oil).

Pharmacopoeias. In *Aust.*, *Hung.*, *Jug.*, *Pol.*, *Rus.*, and *Swiss.*

Pol. also includes the volatile oil.

The dried rhizome of the sweet flag, *Acorus calamus* (Araceae). It contains 1.5 to 3.5% v/w of a bitter aromatic volatile oil.

A bitter and carminative; it has been used to flavour alcoholic beverages. The volatile oil is used in perfumery.

526-r

Calumba *(B.P.C. 1954).* Calumba Root; Colombo.

Pharmacopoeias. In *Jap.*, *Port.*, and *Span.*

The dried transverse or oblique slices of the root of *Jateorhiza palmata* (=*J. columba*) (Menispermaceae), containing not less than 15% of water-soluble extractive. **Store** in a dry place.

Calumba is a bitter which has been used as a tincture or concentrated infusion in atonic dyspepsia associated with hypochlorhydria and as a flavouring agent in the formulation of liqueurs. It contains no tannin and can be given with iron salts.

527-f

Centaury. Centaurii Minoris Herba; Petite Centaurée; Tausendgüldenkraut.

Pharmacopoeias. In *Aust.*, *Cz.*, *Ger.*, *Hung.*, *Jug.*, *Pol.*, *Roum.*, *Span.*, and *Swiss.*

The dried flowering tops of the common centaury, *Centaurium minus*(=*C. umbellatum; Erythraea centaurium*), and other species of *Centaurium* (Gentianaceae). **Protect** from light.

Centaury is used as a bitter in the form of a liquid extract, infusion, or tincture.

528-d

Chirata *(B.P.C. 1949).* Chirayta; Chiretta; East Indian Balmony.

Pharmacopoeias. In *Ind.*

The dried plant *Swertia chirata* (Gentianaceae) collected when in flower and dried.

NOTE. *Andrographis paniculata* (p.317) has also been described as chiretta and should not be confused with Chirata.

Chirata is a bitter usually administered as a concentrated infusion or as a tincture. It has been used to flavour alcoholic beverages.

The pharmacological effects in *animals* of swertiamarin a secoiridoid glucoside isolated from *Swertia chirata*.— S. K. Bhattacharya *et al.*, *J. pharm. Sci.*, 1976, *65*, 1547.

529-n

Cinchona Bark *(B.P.).* Red Cinchona Bark *(Eur. P.)*; Cinchonae Succirubrae Cortex; Cinchona; Jesuit's Bark; Peruvian Bark; Chinae Cortex; Chinarinde; Quinquinas; Quina; Quinquina Rouge; Quina Vermelha.

Pharmacopoeias. In *Aust.*, *Belg.*, *Br.*, *Braz.*, *Cz.*, *Eur.*, *Fr.*, *Ger.*, *Hung.*, *Ind.*, *It.*, *Jap.*, *Mex.*, *Neth.*, *Nord.*, *Pol.*, *Port.*, *Roum.*, *Span.*, and *Swiss. Arg.* specifies *C. calisaya. Braz.* also includes *C. calisaya* (Quina Amarela). Some pharmacopoeias also permit other species of Cinchona. *Br.* also includes Powdered Cinchona Bark.

The dried bark of *Cinchona succirubra* (=*Cinchona pubescens*) or of its varieties or hybrids, containing not less than 6.5% of total alkaloids, of which not less than 30% and not more than 60% consists of quinine-type alkaloids. Preparations are **incompatible** with alkalis, salicylates and iodides. **Protect** from light.
The dried barks contain varying yields of quinine. Hybrid bark, usually a hybrid between *C. ledgeriana* and *C. succirubra*, forms a large proportion of the bark of commerce and yields a high percentage of quinine.

Adverse Effects, Treatment, and Precautions. As for Quinine, p.404. It may sometimes cause vomiting and if taken over long periods may give rise to symptoms of cinchonism.

Uses. Cinchona bark is a bitter and has astringent properties. To keep the alkaloids in solution, liquid preparations are usually given in acid media but tinctures may be prescribed with ammonium bicarbonate and in these cases acacia mucilage should be added to suspend the alkaloids.

530-k

Cnicus Benedictus. Blessed Thistle; Holy Thistle; Carduus Benedictus; Chardon Bénit; Kardobenediktenkraut; Cardo Santo.

CAS — 24394-09-0 (cnicin).

Pharmacopoeias. In *Aust., Hung., Span.,* and *Swiss.*

The flowering tops of *Cnicus benedictus* (=*Carbenia benedicta; Carduus benedictus*) (Compositae), containing a bitter principle, cnicin, and a volatile oil.

An infusion of cnicus benedictus has been used as a bitter.

531-a

Condurango *(B.P.C. 1934).* Condurango Bark; Eagle-vine Bark.

CAS — 1401-98-5 (condurangin).

Pharmacopoeias. In *Aust., Belg., Jap., Port., Span.,* and *Swiss.*

The dried stem-bark of *Marsdenia condurango* (=*Gonolobus condurango*) (Asclepiadaceae). It contains a poisonous glycoside, or mixture of glycosides, known as condurangin.

Condurango has been used as a bitter and gastric sedative in the form of a liquid alcoholic extract.

532-t

Cusparia *(B.P.C. 1934).* Angostura Bark; Carony Bark; Cusparia Bark.

The bark of *Galipea officinalis* (Rutaceae).

Cusparia is a bitter administered in the form of a concentrated infusion. It is also used for flavouring alcoholic beverages.
It should be noted that 'Angostura Bitters' (*Dr. J.G.B. Siegert & Sons Ltd*) contains gentian and various aromatic ingredients but no cusparia.

533-x

Denatonium Benzoate *(U.S.N.F.).*

Benzyldiethyl(2,6-xylylcarbamoylmethyl)ammonium benzoate.
$C_{28}H_{34}N_2O_3$=446.6.

CAS — 3734-33-6.

Pharmacopoeias. In *U.S.N.F.*

A white odourless crystalline powder with an intensely bitter taste. M.p. 166° to 170°. **Soluble** in water, soluble 1 in about 2 of alcohol, and 1 in about 3 of chloroform; sparingly soluble in acetone; very slightly soluble in ether; slightly soluble in vegetable oils. A 10% solution in water has a pH of 7 to 8. **Store** in airtight containers.

Denatonium benzoate is used where an intensely bitter taste is required for medicinal or industrial purposes and as a partial denaturant for alcohol in toilet preparations. Its taste is readily detectable at a dilution of 1 in 1 million.

Proprietary Preparations

Bitrex *(Macfarlan Smith, UK).* Denatonium benzoate, available as a 0.256% solution; 7.8 ml in 10 litres gives a dilution of 1 in 500 000.

534-r

Gentian *(B.P., Eur. P.).*

Gentian Root; Gentiana; Gentianae Radix; Genziana; Enzianwurzel; Raiz de Genciana.

Pharmacopoeias. In *Arg., Aust., Br., Cz., Eur., Fr., Ger., Hung., It., Jap., Jug., Neth., Nord., Pol., Port., Roum., Span.,* and *Swiss. Br.* also includes Powdered Gentian.
Aust., Cz., and *Hung.* allow also other species of *Gentiana.*
Jap. includes also Japanese Gentian, from *G. scabra. Chin.* specifies *G. scabra* and 3 other species.

The dried partially fermented rhizome and root of*Gentiana lutea* (Gentianaceae), yielding not less than 33% of water-soluble extractive. It contains a glycoside, sugars, and alkaloids. **Incompatible** with iron salts. **Store** in a dry place. Protect from light.

Uses. Gentian is a bitter and is used to stimulate gastric secretion and improve the appetite. It should be given from half to 1 hour before meals. It is usually administered as the compound infusion or compound tincture.

Preparations

Infusions

Compound Gentian Infusion *(B.P.).* Co. Gent. Inf. Concentrated compound gentian infusion 10 ml, water to 100 ml. It should be used within 12 hours of preparation.
Dose. 15 to 40 ml.

Concentrated Compound Gentian Infusion *(B.P.).* Conc. Co. Gent. Inf. Prepared by macerating gentian, dried bitter-orange peel, and dried lemon peel, about 1 in 10 of each, with alcohol (25%).
Dose. 1.5 to 4 ml.

Mixtures

Acid Gentian Mixture *(B.P.C. 1973).* Gentian and Acid Mixture. Concentrated compound gentian infusion 1 ml, dilute hydrochloric acid 0.5 ml, double-strength chloroform water 5 ml, water to 10 ml. It should be recently prepared. *Dose.* 10 to 20 ml.

Acid Gentian Mixture with Nux Vomica *(B.P.C. 1973).* Gentian, Nux Vomica, and Acid Mixture. Nux vomica tincture 0.5 ml, acid gentian mixture to 10 ml. It should be recently prepared. *Dose.* 10 to 20 ml.

Alkaline Gentian Mixture *(B.P.).* Gentian and Alkali Mixture; Mistura Gentianae cum Soda. Concentrated compound gentian infusion 1 ml, sodium bicarbonate 500 mg, double-strength chloroform water 5 ml, water to 10 ml. It should be recently prepared.
A.P.F. (Gentian Mixture Alkaline) has a similar formula with concentrated chloroform water.
Dose. 10 ml.

Alkaline Gentian Mixture with Nux Vomica *(B.P.C. 1973).* Gentian and Alkali Mixture with Nux Vomica; Gentian, Nux Vomica, and Alkali Mixture. Nux vomica tincture 0.5 ml, alkaline gentian mixture to 10 ml. It should be recently prepared. *Dose.* 10 to 20 ml.

Alkaline Gentian Mixture with Phenobarbitone *(B.P.C. 1973).* Gentian and Alkali Mixture with Phenobarbitone; Mist. Gent. Alk. Sed. Phenobarbitone sodium 15 mg, alkaline gentian mixture to 10 ml. It must be freshly prepared. *Dose.* 10 to 20 ml.

Gentian and Rhubarb Mixture *(B.P.C. 1973).* Mistura Gentianae cum Rheo; Gentian Mixture with Rhubarb. Concentrated compound gentian infusion 0.5 ml, compound rhubarb tincture 1 ml, sodium bicarbonate 500 mg, concentrated peppermint emulsion 0.25 ml, double-strength chloroform water 5 ml, water to 10 ml. It should be recently prepared. *Dose.* 10 to 20 ml.

Tinctures

Compound Gentian Tincture *(B.P.C. 1973).* Prepared by macerating gentian 10 g, dried bitter-orange peel 3.75 g, and cardamom seed 1.25 g with alcohol (45%) 100 ml. *Dose.* 2 to 5 ml. Several pharmacopoeias include a simple tincture (1 in 5).

535-f

Lupulus *(B.P.C. 1934).* Hops; Humulus; Strobili Lupuli; Houblon.

The dried strobiles of the hop plant, *Humulus lupulus* (Cannabinaceae). Lupulus preparations are **incompatible** with mineral acids and metallic salts.

Lupulus is a bitter administered as a tincture, as a soft extract, or as a concentrated infusion. It is also used to give a characteristic taste to beer. The oil has been used as a flavouring agent and in perfumes.

536-d

Lupulin

CAS — 8002-59-3 (lupulin oleoresin).

Pharmacopoeias. In *Aust.* and *Pol.*

The glandular trichomes separated from the strobiles of the hop plant, *Humulus lupulus* (Cannabinaceae).

Lupulin is a bitter reported to be mildly sedative.

537-n

Menyanthes. Buckbean; Bogbean; Marsh Trefoil; Folia Trifoli Fibrini; Trèfle d'Eau; Bitterklee.

Pharmacopoeias. In *Aust., Cz., Hung., Pol., Rus.,* and *Swiss.*

The dried leaves of the buckbean, *Menyanthes trifoliata* (Menyanthaceae).

Menyanthes is a bitter, which has been used as a liquid extract, an infusion, or as a tincture.

538-h

Nux Vomica *(B.P.).*

Strychni Semen; Noix Vomique; Brechnuss; Neuz Vómica; Noce Vomica.

CAS — 357-57-3 (brucine, anhydrous).

Pharmacopoeias. In *Arg., Aust., Belg., Br., Cz., Fr., Hung., Ind., It., Jap., Mex., Pol., Port., Roum., Rus., Span.,* and *Swiss.* Many specify not less than 2.5% of total alkaloids, about one-half being strychnine. *Br.* also includes Powdered Nux Vomica.
Port. P. and *Span. P.* also include Ignatia from *Strychnos ignatii.*
Chin. P. specifies *S. pierriana.*

The dried ripe seeds of *Strychnos nux-vomica* (Loganiaceae), containing not less than 1.2% of strychnine.
In addition to strychnine, nux vomica contains the alkaloid brucine ($C_{23}H_{26}N_2O_4,4H_2O$=466.5), together with traces of other alkaloids. About one-half of the total alkaloids present is strychnine, though the proportion is subject to some variation.

Adverse Effects and Treatment. As for Strychnine, p.319.

Uses. Nux vomica has the actions of strychnine (see p.320); brucine may have local anaesthetic properties.
Nux vomica (Nux vom.) is used in homoeopathic medicine. Ignatia is also used in homoeopathic medicine where it is known as Ignatia amara.

Preparations

Elixirs

Nux Vomica Elixir *(B.P.C. 1973).* Elixir Nucis Vomicae. Nux vomica tincture 0.15 ml, compound cardamom tincture 0.5 ml, syrup 2.5 ml, chloroform water to 5 ml. *Dose.* 5 ml.

Extracts

Nux Vomica Dry Extract *(B.P.C. 1963).* Nux Vomica Extract. A defatted alcoholic percolate, evaporated to dryness and adjusted with calcium phosphate to contain 5% of strychnine. Store in a cool place in small, wide-mouth, well-closed containers. *Dose.* 15 to 60 mg.

A similar extract is included in some pharmacopoeias, most of which specify between 8% and 16% of total alkaloids (Extractum Strychni).

Nux Vomica Liquid Extract *(B.P.).* Nux Vom. Liq. Ext. A defatted alcoholic percolate, adjusted to contain 1.425 to 1.575% of strychnine; about 3 mg in 0.2 ml.
Ind. P. and *It. P.* include a similar preparation.
Dose. 0.05 to 0.2 ml.

Mixtures

Acid Nux Vomica Mixture *(B.P.C. 1973).* Mist. Nuc. Vom. Acid; Nux Vomica and Acid Mixture. Nux vomica tincture 0.5 ml, dilute hydrochloric acid 0.5 ml, double-strength chloroform water 5 ml, water to 10 ml. It should be recently prepared. *Dose.* 10 to 20 ml.

Alkaline Nux Vomica Mixture *(B.P.C. 1973).* Nux Vomica and Alkali Mixture. Nux vomica tincture 0.5 ml, sodium bicarbonate 500 mg, double-strength chloroform water 5 ml, water to 10 ml. It should be recently prepared. *Dose.* 10 to 20 ml.

Tinctures

Nux Vomica Tincture *(B.P.).* Nux Vom. Tinct. Nux vomica liquid extract 8.34 ml, alcohol (45%) to 100 ml. It contains 0.119 to 0.131% of strychnine; about 2.5 mg in 2 ml.
Dose. 0.5 to 2 ml.
A similar tincture is included in several other pharmacopoeias; most specify 0.25% of total alkaloids (Tinctura Strychni).

539-m

Quassia *(B.P.C. 1973).* Quassiae Lignum; Bitter Wood; Quassia Wood; Quassiaholz; Leño de Cuasia.

CAS — 76-78-8 (quassin); 76-77-7 (neoquassin).

Pharmacopoeias. In *Fr., Mex., Port.*, and *Span.* All also allow Surinam quassia, *Quassia amara* (Simarubaceae).

The dried stem wood of Jamaica quassia, *Picrasma excelsa* (=*Aeschrion excelsa; Picraena excelsa*) (Simarubaceae), yielding not less than 4% of water-soluble extractive. It contains about 0.2% of the bitter lactone quassin and its hemiacetal neoquassin.

Uses. Quassia is a bitter which is free from tannin and may be prescribed with iron salts. A freshly prepared infusion of quassia (1 to 20 of cold water) has been used as an enema for the expulsion of threadworms, 150 ml being given on 3 successive mornings, together with 15 g of magnesium sulphate by mouth. Infusions of quassia have been used as lotions for pediculosis. Tinctures and extracts have been used as flavouring agents. Extracts of quassia or preparations containing quassin are used to denature alcohol.

Preparations

Enemas

Enem. Quass. pro Infant *(N.F. 1952).* Fresh quassia infusion, undiluted. *Dose.* 150 ml.

Quassia Enema *(B.P.C. 1949).* Fresh quassia infusion, undiluted. *Dose.* 600 ml.

Infusions

Concentrated Quassia Infusion *(B.P.C. 1959).* 1 in 12.5; prepared by maceration with cold water. It contains 21 to 24% v/v of alcohol. *Dose.* 2 to 4 ml.

Fresh Quassia Infusion *(B.P. 1953).* Inf. Quass. Rec. Quassia 1 g and cold water 100 ml, infused in a covered vessel for 15 minutes and strained. It should be used within 12 hours of preparation. *Dose.* 15 to 30 ml.

Quassia Infusion. Prepared by diluting 1 vol. of concentrated quassia infusion to 8 vol. with water. It should be used within 12 hours of preparation. *Dose.* 15 to 30 ml.

Tinctures

Teinture de Quassia *(Fr. P.).* Quassia Tincture. 1 in 5; prepared by percolation with alcohol (60%).

Proprietary Preparations

Quassin Solution 'B' *(Bush Boake Allen, UK).* A standardised solution containing quassin in industrial methylated spirit.

540-t

Quebracho *(B.P.C. 1934).* Quebracho Bark; Aspidosperma; White Quebracho; Quebracho Blanco.

CAS — 1398-11-4 (quebracho); 466-49-9 (aspidospermine); 146-48-5 (yohimbine).

Pharmacopoeias. In *Arg.* and *Span.*

The dried bark of *Aspidosperma quebracho* (Apocynaceae). It contains the alkaloids aspidospermine and yohimbine (=quebrachine) and a considerable quantity of tannin.

Quebracho has been used as a bitter, febrifuge, and antispasmodic, in the form of a liquid extract and tincture. Large doses may cause nausea and vomiting.

541-x

Serpentary *(B.P.C. 1949).* Serpentaria; Serpentary Rhizome; Texan or Virginian Snakeroot.

The dried rhizome and roots of Texan snakeroot, *Aristolochia reticulata*, and of Virginian snakeroot, *A. serpentaria* (Aristolochiaceae).

Serpentary is a bitter employed with mineral acids and with other bitters in dyspepsia. It has been used as a concentrated infusion and as a tincture and it was an ingredient of Compound Cinchona Tincture (*B.P.C. 1949*). The aromatic oil present in *A. serpentaria* is used in some liqueurs.

542-r

Strychnine *(B.P.C. 1959).* Strychnina; Estricnina. Strychnidin-10-one.

$C_{21}H_{22}N_2O_2$=334.4.

CAS — 57-24-9.

Pharmacopoeias. In *Port.* and *Span.*

An alkaloid obtained from nux vomica and the seeds of other species of *Strychnos*. It occurs as odourless translucent colourless crystals or white crystalline powder with a very bitter metallic taste. **Soluble** 1 in 7000 of water, 1 in 250 of alcohol, and 1 in 6 of chloroform; practically insoluble in ether. A saturated solution in water is alkaline to litmus.

543-f

Strychnine Hydrochloride *(B.P.C. 1973).* Strych. Hydrochlor.; Strychninae Hydrochloridum.

$C_{21}H_{22}N_2O_2,HCl,2H_2O$=406.9.

CAS — 1421-86-9 (anhydrous); 6101-04-8 (dihydrate).

Pharmacopoeias. In *Ind.*

Colourless crystals or white crystalline powder with a very bitter taste. It crystallises from aqueous solutions with a slightly variable proportion of water of crystallisation and loses 7 to 9% of its weight when dried. **Soluble** 1 in 40 of water and 1 in 85 of alcohol; practically insoluble in ether. Solutions are **sterilised** by autoclaving or by filtration.

Incompatible with alkali hydroxides and carbonates, aromatic ammonia spirit, bromides and iodides.

544-d

Strychnine Nitrate *(B.P.C. 1934).* Strychninae Nitras; Strychninum Nitricum; Azotato de Estricnina; Nitrato de Estricnina.

$C_{21}H_{22}N_2O_2,HNO_3$=397.4.

CAS — 66-32-0.

Pharmacopoeias. In *Arg., Aust., Belg., Cz., Hung., It., Jug., Nord., Pol., Port., Rus., Span.*, and *Swiss.*

Colourless odourless glistening crystals with a very bitter taste. **Soluble** 1 in 50 of water, 1 in 150 of alcohol, 1 in 110 of chloroform, and 1 in 50 of glycerol; practically insoluble in ether. A solution in water is neutral or slightly acid to methyl red. **Sterilisation** and **incompatibilities** as for Strychnine Hydrochloride.

545-n

Strychnine Oxide Hydrochloride. Strychnine N^6-oxide hydrochloride.

$C_{21}H_{22}N_2O_3,HCl$=386.9.

CAS — 7248-28-4 (strychnine oxide).

546-h

Strychnine Sulphate *(B.P.C. 1959).* Strychninae Sulphas; Strychninum Sulfuricum; Sulfato de Estricnina.

$(C_{21}H_{22}N_2O_2)_2$, $H_2SO_4,5H_2O$=857.0.

CAS — 60-41-3 (anhydrous); 60491-10-3 (pentahydrate).

Pharmacopoeias. In *Arg., Mex., Port., Roum.*, and *Span.*

Odourless colourless crystals or white crystalline powder with a very bitter taste. It is efflorescent in dry air. **Soluble** 1 in 50 of water and 1 in 135 of alcohol; slightly soluble in chloroform; practically insoluble in ether; freely soluble in glycerol. A solution in water is neutral to methyl red.**Sterilisation** and **incompatibilities** as for Strychnine Hydrochloride.

Adverse Effects. The symptoms of poisoning are mainly those arising from stimulation or rather reduction of the normal inhibition of the central nervous system. Early signs occurring within 30 minutes of ingestion include tremors, slight twitching, and stiffness of the face and legs. Painful convulsions develop and may be triggered by minor sensory stimuli. The body becomes arched backwards in hyperextension with the arms and legs extended and the feet turned inward. The jaw is rigidly clamped and contraction of the facial muscles produces a characteristic grinning expression known as 'risus sardonicus'. Contraction of the muscles of the diaphragm, together with spasm of the thoracic and abdominal muscles arrests respiration. The convulsions may recur repeatedly and are followed by a period of relaxation. Death from asphyxia or medullary paralysis usually follows the second to fifth seizure.

The fatal dose by mouth is probably between 50 and 100 mg for adults. Maximum permissible atmospheric concentration (strychnine) 150 μg per m^3.

About 2 hours after taking approximately 200 ml of a tonic containing strychnine, a 21-year-old woman developed muscle stiffness with arching of the back. She felt excited, overactive, and mildly depersonalised for about a day, but recovery was complete within 48 hours.— M. T. Haslam (letter), *Br. med. J.*, 1965, *1*, 1191.

A report of the death of 1-year-old child who ate 10 to 20 Easton's tablets.— National Poisons Information Service, Fifth Annual Report, 1968, per *Br. med. J.*, 1969, *3*, 408.

Fatal toxicity of strychnine was reported in a 2-year-old child who swallowed about 10 tablets each containing strychnine 2 mg.— F. O. Müller, *S. Afr. med. J.*, 1977, *51*, 652.

Treatment of Adverse Effects. The main object of therapy in strychnine poisoning is the prevention or control of convulsions and asphyxia and the immediate treatment is the intravenous injection of diazepam 10 mg, or less for children, and repeated as required. Muscle relaxants such as tubocurarine chloride or suxamethonium chloride may also be given intravenously. When the convulsions are controlled or have been prevented gastric aspiration and lavage with a 0.02% solution of potassium permanganate (*very* pale pink) or with activated charcoal may be employed. Tincture of iodine 0.4% in water has also been given to precipitate an insoluble salt and delay absorption of strychnine. An emetic should not be given. The patient should be kept lying down in a quiet darkened room. If respiratory depression occurs assisted respiration using oxygen should be employed.

The successful use of diazepam given intravenously to children with strychnine poisoning.— G. Jackson *et al.*, *Br. med. J.*, 1971, *3*, 519; Y. Herishanu and H. Landau, *Br. J. Anaesth.*, 1972, *44*, 747. See also B. J. Maron *et al.*, *J. Pediat.*, 1971, *78*, 697.

Peritoneal dialysis. Peritoneal dialysis and forced diuresis were used in conjunction with conventional therapy to treat 2 patients with strychnine poisoning. One patient was completely asymptomatic within 2½ hours of this treatment. The second patient, who had ingested a rodenticide containing 240 mg of strychnine, responded to treatment within 6 hours.— *J. Am. med. Ass.*, 1970, *211*, 388.

Absorption and Fate. Strychnine is readily absorbed from the gastro-intestinal tract. It rapidly leaves the bloodstream; 50% has been reported to enter the tissues in 5 minutes. It is rapidly oxidised, mainly in the liver, but about 20% of a dose is excreted unchanged in the urine.

Uses. Strychnine antagonises the inhibitory action of a number of endogenous substances in the central nervous system.

It has been given in doses of 2 to 8 mg, usually as its salts, as a bitter and analeptic but there is no justification for such uses.

It was recommended that strychnine should only be used as a rodenticide by trained pest control operators in areas to which access by unauthorised persons and useful animals could be prevented completely.— Safe Use of Pesticides, Twentieth Report of the WHO Expert Committee on Insecticides, *Tech. Rep. Ser. Wld Hlth Org. No. 513*, 1973.

NOTE. In the UK the use of strychnine for the killing of animals, except for moles, is prohibited under The Animals (Cruel Poisons) Regulations 1963 (SI 1963; No. 1278). See also The Poison Rules 1978 (SI 1978; No. 1) where provision is made for foxes and rabies.

Nonketotic hyperglycinaemia. A 4-month-old child receiving sodium benzoate to treat nonketotic hyperglycinaemia had a beneficial response to concurrent administration of strychnine 100 µg per kg body-weight daily (in 4 divided doses) subsequently increased to 200 µg per kg daily which was aimed at counteracting the effects of high glycine concentrations within the CNS. This corroborated the result of R. Gitzelmann *et al.* (personal communication) in a similar patient, but caution was recommended since strychnine is a convulsant and might theoretically lower seizure threshold in nonketotic hyperglycinaemia.— L. T. Ch'ien *et al.* (letter), *New Engl. J. Med.*, 1978, *298*, 687. The dose of strychnine used in the treatment of nonketotic hyperglycinaemia was considered inadequate. A similar 6-month-old child has been given strychnine nitrate 300 µg per kg body-weight daily for 6 months, 700 µg per kg daily for 4 months, and 0.9 to 1.1 mg per kg daily since then, by mouth, in 4 divided doses. There have been no untoward side-effects and progress in the child's psychomotor development continues after taking strychnine for 18 months. In 2 similar patients treatment has been less successful.— R. Gitzelmann *et al.* (letter), *ibid.*, 1424.

Further references: D. Arneson *et al.*, *Pediatrics*, 1979, *63*, 369; K. D. MacDermot *et al.*, *ibid.*, 1980, *65*, 61.

Proprietary Names

Movellan (strychnine oxide hydrochloride) (*Asta, Ger.*).

547-m

Taraxacum (*B.P.C. 1949*). Dandelion Root; Taraxacum Root; Pissenlit; Löwenzahnwurzel.

Pharmacopoeias. In *Aust.*, *Hung.*, and *Pol. Chin.* specifies Herb Taraxacum from other species of *Taraxacum*.

The fresh or dried root of the common dandelion, *Taraxacum officinale* (Compositae). **Store** in a cool dry place.

Taraxacum has been used as a bitter and as a mild laxative, usually as a liquid extract or as taraxacum juice.

Blood Preparations

1210-s

Blood is a complex fluid with many functions including the maintenance of hydration of the tissues, maintenance of body temperature, and the transport within the body of gases, ions, nutrients, hormones, enzymes, antibodies, waste products of metabolism, and drugs.

The following figures represent approximate values for adults in normal health:

Blood volume—60 to 80 ml per kg body-weight
Plasma volume—40 to 50 ml per kg
Haematocrit (= packed cell volume)—males, 40 to 54%; females, 37 to 47%
Red cell count—males, 4.5 to 6.5 × 10^6 per mm^3; females, 3.9 to 5.6 × 10^6 per mm^3
Reticulocytes—up to 2%
White cell count—4 to 11 × 10^3 per mm^3
Neutrophils—2 to 7.5 × 10^3 per mm^3
Lymphocytes—1.5 to 3.5 × 10^3 per mm^3
Platelets (thrombocytes)—150 to 400 × 10^3 per mm^3

Precursors in bone marrow of red blood cells include proerythroblasts, erythroblasts, and reticulocytes. Precursors of granulocytes (polymorphonuclear leucocytes—neutrophils, eosinophils, and basophils) include myeloblasts and myelocytes. Precursors of platelets include megakaryocytes.

This chapter is chiefly concerned with the use of blood, or blood products, in the prevention or treatment of disease.

Antisera, usually of animal origin, are described in the section on Vaccines and other Immunological Products (see p.1587).

Haemoglobin: structure, function, and synthesis.— *Br. med. Bull.*, 1976, *32*, 193-287.

Nomenclature for factors of the HLA system.— *Bull. Wld Hlth Org.*, 1978, *56*, 461.

A discussion on haemopoiesis.— P. Quesenberry and L. Levitt, *New Engl. J. Med.*, 1979, *301*, 755, 819, and 868.

The use of stroma-free haemoglobin solutions.— W. J. Rudowski, *Br. J. Hosp. Med.*, 1980, *23*, 389.

Blood Groups. The chief blood group systems are the ABO system and the Rhesus system.

In simple terms red blood cells carry on their surface genetically determined antigens. A person with antigen A, B, A plus B, or neither is classified as group A, B, AB, or O respectively. Such persons will have, in their serum, antibodies to B, A, neither, or both respectively—anti-B(β), anti-A(α), or anti-B plus anti-A ($\alpha + \beta$). Administration of blood containing red cells from a person of group A to a person with anti-A results in agglutination or possibly haemolysis. For the determination of the ABO group the agglutinogens of the red cells and the agglutinins of the serum are determined by testing against known standards.

In the Rhesus system many persons carry an antigen (Rh-positive) which stimulates antibody formation in Rh-negative persons; subsequent exposure to Rh-positive blood causes haemolysis.

Many variants of these systems, and other systems, are recognised.

Viral Hepatitis. Three types of viral hepatitis are recognised. The following nomenclature is recommended:

HAV—hepatitis A virus
Anti-HAV—antibody to hepatitis A virus
HBV—hepatitis B virus (the Dane particle)
HBsAg—hepatitis B surface antigen (Australia antigen)
HBcAg—hepatitis B core antigen
HBeAg—the *e* antigen closely associated with hepatitis B infection
Anti-HBs—antibody to hepatitis B surface antigen
Anti-HBc—antibody to hepatitis B core antigen
Anti-HBe—antibody to the hepatitis B *e* antigen.

Viral hepatitis type A (previously known as infectious hepatitis) is endemic throughout the world, has an incubation period of 3 to 5 weeks, is spread primarily by the faecal-oral route, and is largely controlled by good standards of hygiene. It is rarely transmitted by blood transfusion.

Viral hepatitis type B (previously known as serum hepatitis) has an incubation period of up to 180 days, and is spread largely by the transfusion of blood products and by accidental inoculation with small amounts of blood during surgical procedures, immunisation, drug abuse, acupuncture, and other procedures; it may also be transmitted by intimate personal contact, including transmission to the newborn. Infection with hepatitis B virus leads to the appearance in the serum of hepatitis B surface antigen HBsAg (there are a number of variants of HBsAg), hepatitis B core antigen HBcAg, and hepatitis B *e* antigen which appears to be associated with an unfavourable prognosis and the development of chronic liver disease. There is an association between hepatitis B infection and liver cancer. The persistence of HBsAg in the serum represents a carrier state, the incidence of which is high in some parts of the world.

The occurrence after transfusion of a hepatitis not attributable to hepatitis A virus or hepatitis B virus has led to the recognition of an additional virus or viruses, not yet characterised, and commonly called 'non-A, non-B'; in some areas it is now the most common form of hepatitis after blood transfusion.

The following blood preparations carry the risk of transmitting hepatitis: whole blood; concentrate of red blood cells; dried factor VIII fraction; dried plasma; dried serum; dried fibrinogen; dried fibrinogen for isotopic labelling; and dried thrombin.

Preparations of albumin that have been heated for 10 hours at 60° and preparations of immunoglobulin, made by alcohol fractionation, do not transmit hepatitis type B.

Reviews and discussions.— G. L. Gitnick *et al.*, *Ann. intern. Med.*, 1976, *85*, 488. *Advances in viral hepatitis.*— Report of the WHO Expert Committee on Viral Hepatitis, *Tech. Rep. Ser. Wld Hlth Org. No. 602*, 1977; *Br. med. J.*, 1977, *1*, 985; *Br. med. J.*, 1978, *1*, 942; A. Pollock and A. D. Wright, *Br. dent. J.*, 1978, *144*, 146; A. J. Zuckerman, *Bull. Wld Hlth Org.*, 1978, *56*, 1; *Chronicle Wld Hlth Org.*, 1980, *34*, 495.

To reduce the risk of transmission of hepatitis in renal dialysis units, patients on haemodialysis should be given blood transfusions sparingly. Only blood screened for hepatitis B antigen and antibody should be provided.— *Hepatitis and the Treatment of Chronic Renal Failure*, Report of the Advisory Group 1970–2, London, Dept Hlth Social Security, 1973.

From a study of the hazards of hepatitis B in 362 patients given blood transfusions there appeared to be no hazard to administering blood containing the antibody to hepatitis B antigen.— R. D. Aach *et al.*, *Lancet*, 1974, *2*, 190.

References to the hazard of hepatitis B in anaesthetic practice.— A. P. Waterson, *Br. J. Anaesth.*, 1976, *48*, 21; J. Carstens *et al.*, *Br. J. Anaesth.*, 1977, *49*, 887; L. Strunin, *Br. J. Anaesth.*, 1979, *51*, 913.

Guidelines for the control and prevention of viral hepatitis in general hospitals.— K. J. Breen *et al.*, *Med. J. Aust.*, 1978, *2*, 18.

A discussion of the link between hepatitis B and hepatoma.— *Br. med. J.*, 1978, *2*, 718.

A brief discussion of the transmission of hepatitis B.— *Br. med. J.*, 1979, *2*, 752.

The prevalence of HBsAg, its subtypes, and anti-HBs in various parts of the world.— O. Soběslavský, *Bull. Wld Hlth Org.*, 1980, *58*, 621.

Non-A, non-B hepatitis in 13 of 380 recipients of blood negative for HBsAg.— J. N. Katchaki *et al.*, *Br. med. J.*, 1981, *282*, 107.

Blood-clotting Factors. Roman numerals are used for the designation of those factors which are sufficiently defined as distinct entities by physio-pathological, physical, biochemical, and chemical properties; if considered desirable, a synonymous descriptive term can be used in parentheses following the Roman numeral. The following are the principal terms used:

Factor I (Fibrinogen)
Factor II (Prothrombin)
Factor III (Thromboplastin)
Factor IV (Calcium)
Factor V (Ac-globulin; Labile factor)
Factor VI (Unassigned)
Factor VII (Proconvertin; SPCA)
Factor VIII (Antihaemophilic factor; AHF)
Factor IX (Plasma thromboplastin component; PTC; Christmas factor)
Factor X (Stuart factor)
Factor XI (Plasma thromboplastin antecedent; PTA)
Factor XII (Hageman factor)
Factor XIII (Fibrin stabilising factor; FSF)

The letter 'a' after a factor name denotes the activated form. A number of other factors are also involved in blood clotting.

Hereditary deficiency of all the clotting factors (other than calcium and thromboplastin) has been described; the most important are deficiency of factor VIII causing haemophilia A and von Willebrand's disease, and deficiency of factor IX causing haemophilia B or Christmas disease.

Vitamin K deficiency, treatment with anticoagulants, or liver disease may reduce the concentrations of the vitamin K-dependent factors II, VII, IX, and X.

Preparations used in the treatment of patients with blood-clotting disorders are whole fresh blood, fresh plasma, fibrinogen, factor VIII fraction, and factor IX fraction.

For a report on blood-clotting factors including the diagnosis and treatment of diseases caused by their deficiency, see Inherited Blood Clotting Disorders, *Tech. Rep. Ser. Wld Hlth Org. No. 504*, 1972.

For a report of the genetic nomenclature of coagulation factors incorporating the above roman numeral system and accepted by the International Committee on Thrombosis and Haemostasis, see *Lancet*, 1973, *2*, 891.

It was suggested that factor VIII should be named according to its activity as follows: VIII: C for the coagulant activity, VIIIR:AG for the antigenic activities, and VIIIR:WF for the von Willebrand factor activities.— *J. Am. med. Ass.*, 1975, *234*, 329.

Recommended nomenclature for blood-clotting zymogens and zymogen activation products of the International Committee on Thrombosis and Hemostasis.— C. M. Jackson, *Thromb. Haemostasis*, 1977, *38*, 567.

For detailed reviews covering the field of haemostasis, see *Br. med. Bull.*, 1977, *33*, 183–288.

A review of the use of haemostatic agents including blood products.— G. D. O. Lowe and D. H. Lawson, *Am. J. Hosp. Pharm.*, 1978, *35*, 414.

An account of therapeutic embolisation in the control of haemorrhage, tumours, or vascular malformations.— *Lancet*, 1978, *1*, 1135.

A short review of bleeding disorders.— A. Pollock, *Br. dent. J.*, 1977, *143*, 405.

Units. The expression 'unit of blood' generally represents a volume of about 500 to 540 ml, including anticoagulant. For blood preparations a unit generally refers to the quantity of a blood component obtained from 1 unit of whole blood. Specific units of activity are used for some blood components.

1211-w

Whole Blood *(B.P.).* Human Blood *(Eur. P.)*; Whole Human Blood; Sanguis Humanus.

Whole Blood is sterile blood which has been withdrawn aseptically from human beings and mixed with a suitable anticoagulant (see p.322); the amount of anticoagulant should not exceed 22% of the final volume of the mixture. It contains no added preservative. The blood is obtained from subjects in normal health who are considered to be free from disease transmissible by blood transfusion, are free from syphilitic infection or hepatitis B antigen, and whose blood has a haemoglobin content of not less than 12.5% w/v (females) or 13.3% w/v (males). Whole Blood has a haemoglobin concentration of not less than 9.7% w/v in terms of the Cyanmethaemoglobin Solution for Photometric Haemoglobinometry (BS 3985: 1966).

It is a deep red fluid which separates on standing into a lower layer of sedimented red blood corpuscles and a yellow supernatant plasma free from signs of haemolysis; a layer may be visible between the two, appearing as a whitish film of white cells and platelets.

The label states the ABO group, the Rh group and the nature of specific antisera used in testing, the total volume of fluid, the proportion of blood, and the nature and percentage of anticoagulant and of any other material introduced.

Whole Blood is **stored**, immediately after collection and admixture with the anticoagulant, in sterile containers, sealed to exclude micro-organisms, at a temperature of 4° to 6° and the containers are not opened until immediately before transfusion. It is maintained at this temperature until required for use, except during any period necessary for examination and transport at higher temperatures, any such period to be kept to a minimum, after which the blood must be immediately cooled again to 4° to 6°. It must not be used if there is any visible evidence of deterioration. In order that compatibility and other tests can be carried out, a small quantity of Whole Blood is supplied in a small container attached to each main container.

Whole Blood should be administered with suitable equipment such as that described in Section 3 or Section 4 of *Transfusion Equipment for Medical Use*, BS 2463: 1962.

1212-e

Whole Blood *(U.S.P.).* ACD Whole Blood; CPD Whole Blood; CPDA-1 Whole Blood; Heparin Whole Blood.

Blood which has been withdrawn aseptically from suitable human donors. It contains acid citrate dextrose, citrate phosphate dextrose, citrate phosphate dextrose with adenine, or heparin sodium as an anticoagulant. It may consist of blood from which the antihaemophilic factor has been removed, in which case it is termed 'Modified'.

It is a deep red opaque fluid from which the corpuscles readily settle on standing for 24 to 48 hours leaving a clear yellowish or pinkish supernatant layer of plasma.

The label states among other things the ABO group, the Rh group, the volume of blood, and the quantity and kind of anticoagulant; the ABO group may also be indicated by the use of specified labelling colours.

Store in hermetically-sealed sterile containers at 1° to 6° (with a range of not more than 2°) except during transport when the temperature may be 1° to 10°.

The expiration date is not later than 48 hours after withdrawal (heparin anticoagulant), not later than 21 days after withdrawal (acid citrate dextrose or citrate phosphate dextrose), or not later than 35 days after withdrawal (citrate phosphate dextrose with adenine). In order that various tests can be carried out, a small quantity of Whole Blood is supplied in at least one small container attached to each main container.

Anticoagulants. Various solutions are used to prevent the coagulation of blood *in vitro*.

A solution of sodium citrate is used as an anticoagulant in plasma and blood for fractionation.

Anticoagulant and preservative solutions for the storage of blood contain sodium citrate and citric acid (or sodium acid citrate) with dextrose (Acid Citrate Dextrose; ACD), or sodium citrate, citric acid, and sodium acid phosphate with dextrose (Citrate Phosphate Dextrose; CPD). A number of formulas are used—see under Sodium Citrate, p.640; the varying volume to be used for each 100 ml of blood is specified. Adenine is sometimes added to citrate phosphate dextrose. Heparin is also used as an anticoagulant for stored blood.

Requirements for collection, processing, and quality control of blood and blood products.— *Tech. Rep. Ser. Wld Hlth Org. No. 626,* 1978, 28–93.

The eligibility of patients for blood donation.— *Med. Lett.*, 1980, *22,* 98.

Changes in Stored Blood. During storage, the leucocytes disintegrate in a few hours, most of the platelets and certain clotting factors, particularly factor VIII, disappear in a few days, and prothrombin and complement gradually decrease. Stored Whole Blood is a potentially dangerous fluid, the maintenance of sterility of which depends entirely upon meticulous attention to cleanliness, faultless asepsis, and accurate and constant refrigeration from the time of collection until use. During storage, haemolysis of the red blood corpuscles occurs, and a red colour, which obscures the line of demarcation between the plasma and sediment of corpuscles, may develop in the plasma immediately above the corpuscular layer. Whole Blood which shows these signs of haemolysis should not be used. Haemolysis also results if blood is frozen or heated, and if it becomes infected; infection usually causes rapid and total haemolysis but certain Gram-negative organisms may flourish at 4° to 6° without causing any visible haemolysis.

Blood stored with citrate anticoagulant undergoes several changes, including a lowering of pH and an increase in potassium, citrate, lactate, and pyruvate ions.

The storage temperature of blood should not be lower than 4° since platelet aggregation is strikingly increased below this temperature.— R. A. Oakes *et al.* (letter), *Lancet,* 1978, *2,* 314.

In blood stored in acid-citrate-dextrose solution the erythrocytes rapidly became depleted of 2,3-diphosphoglyceric acid, but a study in 3 patients showed that nearly one-half the loss was restored 4 hours after the blood was transfused.— E. Beutler and L. Wood, *J. Lab. clin. Med.*, 1969, *74,* 300, per *J. Am. med. Ass.*, 1969, *209,* 1939. For reports of recovery of red cell function taking 4 to 7 days after massive transfusions, see A. Doenicke *et al.*, *Br. J. Anaesth.*, 1977, *49,* 681.

For a comprehensive guide to the formation and operation of a blood transfusion service, including the collection, preservation, and distribution of blood, see *Blood Transfusion, A Guide to the Formation and Operation of a Transfusion Service*, C.C. Bowley *et al.* (Ed.), Geneva, World Health Organization, 1971. See also *Notes on Transfusion*, Department of Health and Social Security, London, HM Stationery Office, 1973.

The concentration of 2,3-diphosphoglycerate (DPG) was higher in 52 samples of blood stored in citrate-phosphate-dextrose (CPD) than in 48 samples stored in acid-citrate-dextrose. DPG in high concentrations was associated with rapid release of oxygen; in patients with impaired compensatory ability the use of CPD blood was preferable.— O. Schweizer and W. S. Howland, *Anesth. Analg. curr. Res.*, 1974, *53,* 516, per *J. Am. med. Ass.*, 1974, *230,* 920.

Blood stored in citrate-phosphate-dextrose solution developed microaggregate debris more slowly from donors who had taken aspirin or in the presence of added aspirin, than did blood from donors who had not taken aspirin.— P. J. Arrington and J. J. McNamara, *Surgery, St Louis,* 1974, *76,* 295, per *J. Am. med. Ass.*, 1974, *230,* 1747.

Incubation of stored blood for up to 1 hour at temperatures up to 45° caused no significant haemolysis. At 50° haemolysis occurred and increased linearly with time. Blood stored in acid-citrate-dextrose (ACD) had a lower rate of haemolysis at 50° than that stored in citrate-phosphate-dextrose (CPD), but this did not apply below 45°. Blood stored for 2 weeks in ACD or 3 weeks in CPD did not show significantly higher haemolysis at 50° than blood stored for only 1 day.— C. Chalmers and W. J. Russell, *Br. J. Anaesth.*, 1974, *46,* 742. The osmotic fragility of blood stored in ACD or CPD was unchanged after incubation for one hour at 37° and 46°. There was slight haemolysis at 47° and this was more marked at 48°. Throughout this range of temperatures, blood stored in CPD was consistently more resistent to osmotic stress than that stored in ACD.— J. H. Van der Walt and W. J. Russell, *ibid.*, 1978, *50,* 815.

Chemical and haematological changes were detected in blood stored in citrate-phosphate dextrose infusion. Plasma concentrations of dextrose and bicarbonate fell while concentrations of potassium, lactate, ammonia, haemoglobin, and lactate dehydrogenase increased.— D. N. Bailey and J. R. Bove, *Transfusion, Philad.*, 1975, *15,* 244, per *J. Am. med. Ass.*, 1975, *234,* 352.

The plasma-inorganic-phosphate concentration in blood from 10 healthy subjects fell significantly after incubation for 3 hours at 37°. The concentration in blood from 12 patients with chronic renal failure before dialysis did not change; in blood taken after 3 and 5 hours of dialysis the concentration increased. The difference was not understood.— H. Yatzidis *et al.* (letter), *New Engl. J. Med.*, 1977, *297,* 57.

The activity of carbonic anhydrase in CPD stored blood.— J. Ponte *et al.*, *Br. J. Anaesth.*, 1980, *52,* 867.

Effect of adenine. The addition of adenine to citrated whole blood prolonged the survival of erythrocytes after transfusion so that more than 70% of the infused erythrocytes survived from blood stored for 35 and 42 days. Without adenine, less than 70% of erythrocytes survived transfusion following 35 days' storage but more than 70% survived following 28 days' storage.— C. E. Shields and F. R. Camp, *Transfusion, Philad.*, 1968, *8,* 1, per *J. Am. med. Ass.*, 1968, *203* (Mar. 4), A221.

A mixture of citrate-phosphate-dextrose solution, adenine, and dihydroxyacetone had been shown to be a good blood preservative because at pH 7 dihydroxyacetone maintained the concentration of 2,3-diphosphoglycerate for up to 4 weeks compared with about 1 week for standard preservatives.— *J. Am. med. Ass.*, 1972, *222,* 261.

Mention of the detection in the kidneys of crystals of dihydroxyadenine after massive infusion of acid-citrate-dextrose-adenine blood.— J. R. Curtis, *Prescribers' J.*, 1979, *19,* 29.

Effect of plasticisers. Blood stored in polyvinyl chloride bags at 4° was found to contain a plasticiser, di(2-ethylhexyl) phthalate. The plasticiser was also found in tissue samples taken at autopsy from patients who had received transfusions, although it was not present in those who had not been transfused.— R. J. Jaeger and R. J. Rubin, *New Engl. J. Med.*, 1972, *287,* 1114.

Di(2-ethylhexyl) phthalate (DEHP) was present in all tissue samples taken at autopsy from patients regardless of whether or not they had received blood transfusions.— R. F. Wallin *et al.*, *Bull. parent. Drug Ass.*, 1974, *28,* 278.

A discussion of the possible contamination by plasticiser of blood stored in or run through polyvinyl chloride.— *Br. med. J.*, 1973, *2,* 194.

References to the toxicity, in *animals*, of di(2-ethylhexyl) phthalate.— C. E. Aronson *et al.*, *Toxic. appl. Pharmac.*, 1978, *44,* 155; J. A. Thomas *et al.*, *Toxic. appl. Pharmac.*, 1978, *45,* 1; R. J. Rubin and J. C. F. Chang, *Toxic. appl. Pharmac.*, 1978, *45,* 230; D. E. Moody and J. K. Reddy, *Toxic. appl. Pharmac.*, 1978, *45,* 497.

Adverse Effects. Hepatitis (see p.321) may occur after the transfusion of whole blood. Other infections, including malaria and trypanosomiasis, may be transmitted.

The transfusion of massive volumes of whole blood may overload the circulation and cause pulmonary oedema. Repeated transfusions of blood, as in thalassaemia, may lead to iron overload. Allergic reactions may occur.

The transfusion of incompatible blood causes haemolysis, possibly with renal failure and disseminated intravascular coagulation; haemolytic reactions may occasionally occur where the screening tests have failed to detect antibody.

The effects of the citrate anticoagulant are now considered to be less than earlier reports suggested. Hyperkalaemia may follow the transfusion of stored blood.

See also Changes in Stored Blood, p.322.

Complement-fixing antibodies to cytomegalovirus developed in 30 of 152 patients who had received transfusions with either fresh or stored blood.— A. M. Prince *et al.*, *New Engl. J. Med.*, 1971, *284*, 1125.

An account of common problems in blood transfusion.— F. Nour-Eldin, *Practitioner*, 1976, *216*, 64.

A report of a specific syndrome in thalassaemic patients, involving hypertension, convulsions, and cerebral haemorrhage, following multiple blood transfusions before splenectomy. Of 8 patients who suffered this syndrome 4 developed definite intracranial haemorrhage and 3 died. Vasopressive substances introduced by or related to multiple blood transfusion were considered responsible; host factors might also contribute.— P. Wasi *et al.*, *Lancet*, 1978, *2*, 602.

A man with thalassaemia who had received 404 units of blood triggered a metal detector at an airport security point. His total body-iron concentration was estimated to be over 100 g.— R. T. S. Jim (letter), *Lancet*, 1979, *2*, 1028.

Iron overload after transfusion of thalassaemic patients for less than 4 years.— A. I. Schafer *et al.*, *New Engl. J. Med.*, 1981, *304*, 319.

Immunological reactions to blood and blood products.— P. Hilgard, *Br. J. Anaesth.*, 1979, *51*, 45.

Effects of citrates. For some reports of the effects of citrates in blood, see P. C. Bajpai *et al.*, *Can. med. Ass. J.*, 1967, *96*, 148; K. C. Grigor, *Br. J. Anaesth.*, 1968, *40*, 943; N. Cooper *et al.*, *Archs Surg., Chicago*, 1973, *107*, 756, per *J. Am. med. Ass.*, 1973, *226*, 811; A. Cser and R. D. G. Milner, *Archs Dis. Childh.*, 1974, *49*, 940; R. D. G. Milner and J. S. Woodhead, *Archs Dis. Childh.*, 1975, *50*, 298; J. K. Denlinger *et al.*, *Br. J. Anaesth.*, 1976, *48*, 995.

Fatalities. In about 3.75 years the FDA received 113 reports of transfusion fatalities related to an estimated transfusion of 37 million units (fatality-rate 0.00023%). Hepatitis caused 33 deaths, and 3 deaths occurred in donors. Of the remaining 77 cases, 47 were due to clerical error and 8 to laboratory error; the remainder included anaphylaxis (4), multiple antibodies (5), delayed reactions (3), graft-v-host reaction (1), and respiratory distress syndrome (4).— B. A. Myhre, *J. Am. med. Ass.*, 1980, *244*, 1333.

Comment on transfusion disasters.— *Lancet*, 1981, *2*, 618.

Haemolytic reaction. Acute haemolytic transfusion reactions.— D. Goldfinger, *Transfusion, Philad.*, 1977, *17*, 85.

A haemolytic reaction could develop in patients who had received multiple transfusions of universal donor blood when they were subsequently given a transfusion of blood of their hereditary group. For a discussion of a protocol to prevent this complication, see A. Barnes and T. E. Allen, *J. Am. med. Ass.*, 1968, *204*, 695. See also J. da Costa, *Br. J. Hosp. Med.*, 1973, *9*, 681.

A report of antiglobulin-positive haemolytic anaemia due to a delayed haemolytic transfusion reaction in a patient who had received multiple blood transfusions.— B. J. Boughton and P. R. Galbraith, *Br. med. J.*, 1975, *4*, 430.

Delayed haemolytic reactions, presenting as sickle-cell crisis, in patients with sickle-cell disease after partial exchange transfusion.— W. J. Diamond *et al.*, *Ann. intern. Med.*, 1980, *93*, 231.

Purpura. A 68-year-old woman with no history of blood transfusion, pregnancy, spontaneous bleeding, purpura, or allergy, developed thrombocytopenic purpura following transfusion of whole blood during and after operation for removal of a retroperitoneal liposarcoma. The reaction was believed to be a secondary response. Recovery followed treatment with corticosteroids and packed red cells low in platelet count.— R. J. Nicholls *et al.*, *Br. med. J.*, 1970, *2*, 581.

Treatment of Adverse Effects. Diuretics such as frusemide may be given to control circulatory overload. Allergic responses may be minimised by the administration of an antihistamine. In more severe reactions adrenaline may be required and corticosteroids may be given intravenously. Drugs should not be added to blood.

A 15-year-old girl who had received 3 litres of ABO-incompatible blood was treated with extreme haemodilution, hypothermia, and exchange transfusion. She was asymptomatic 14 days later.— O. A. Seager *et al.*, *J. Am. med. Ass.*, 1974, *229*, 790.

A brief discussion, mentioning antihistamines and corticosteroids, of the prevention of reactions to transfusions in a patient considered, from his history, to be at risk.— *Br. med. J.*, 1977, *2*, 1142.

Precautions. Whole Blood should generally not be transfused unless the ABO and Rh groups of the patient's and the donor's blood have been verified and a compatibility check made between the patient's serum and the donor's red cells.

The Rh group of the recipient should always be determined and ideally all patients should be transfused with blood of homologous Rh groups.

To reduce the possibility of cardiac arrest from cardiac hypothermia when large volumes are used or the blood is transfused rapidly, and to minimise postoperative shivering, stored blood should be carefully warmed to about 37° before transfusion. Dextrose injection should not be administered through the same transfusion equipment as Whole Blood; if necessary, sodium chloride injection may be used to start the transfusion. In open-heart surgery or for exchange transfusion in babies, heparinised blood or very fresh blood, in acid-citrate-dextrose solution, is preferred and the use of stored blood should be avoided.

Drugs should *not* be added to blood.

Analysis of urine collected from 50 donors to commercial blood banks showed drugs present in 15: barbiturates in 1, morphine in 2, nicotine in 2, quinine in 3, and salicylate in 7.— R. J. Coumbis *et al.* (letter), *J. Am. med. Ass.*, 1970, *214*, 596.

Serum samples from 27 of 240 volunteer blood donors had salicylate concentrations ranging from 16 to 136 µg per ml: blood or plasma recipients who were extremely hypersensitive to salicylates might be affected.— W. P. McCann *et al.*, *J. Am. med. Ass.*, 1970, *214*, 753.

For a report of inhibition of agglutination in the ABO blood-group system by phenothiazine derivatives, tricyclic antidepressants, and antihistamines, especially promethazine, thioridazine, thiethylperazine, imipramine, desipramine, and orphenadrine, see B. Tait, *J. Pharm. Pharmac.*, 1970, *22*, 738.

The mean plasma concentrations of lignocaine in 25 samples of outdated donor blood was 0.39 µg per ml and was considered to be derived from the intradermal injection of lignocaine at the time of donation. While the clinical significance was not known it was possible that hypersensitivity reactions to transfused blood might occur because of the widespread use of lignocaine in dental and other procedures.— J. A. G. da Costa *et al.* (letter), *Br. med. J.*, 1973, *1*, 677.

In a study in 41 patients platelet aggregation was significantly lower in those who received 10 or more units of blood compared with those who received less than 10 units.— R. C. Lim *et al.*, *J. Trauma*, 1973, *13*, 577, per *J. Am. med. Ass.*, 1973, *226*, 96.

The use of citrate-phosphate-dextrose anticoagulant appeared to be associated with platelet and white-cell aggregation. The use of large infusions of blood with this anticoagulant appeared to be associated with a high incidence of post-transfusion respiratory insufficiency and miliary lung shadows characteristic of pulmonary vessel occlusion. Acid-citrate-dextrose anticoagulation was to be preferred.— G. Wright and J. M. Sanderson (letter), *Lancet*, 1974, *2*, 173.

A 63-year-old man suffered severe anaphylaxis following transfusion of 2 units of whole blood. Subsequent investigation revealed that one of the donors had a history of allergy, particularly to fish. The patient had eaten fish on 2 occasions on the 2 days before transfusion and it was therefore believed that the non-allergic patient had been passively sensitised by blood from the atopic donor. It was important that atopic subjects should be excluded from donor panels.— R. C. Routledge *et al.*, *Br. med. J.*, 1976, *1*, 434.

Leukostasis was an important cause of early death in patients with high blast counts. Transfusion, increasing viscosity, should be avoided until the blast count was reduced by chemotherapy.— A. L. Harris, *Br. med. J.*, 1978, *1*, 1169.

High concentrations of prostaglandins E and F in the blood used routinely for transfusion of neonates were of possible concern since these prostaglandins have potent cardiovascular effects. Increased concentrations of prostaglandin F might possibly have a role in the syndrome of hypertension, convulsion, and cerebral haemorrhage noted in thalassaemic patients after multiple blood transfusions.— M. D. Mitchell *et al.* (letter), *Lancet*, 1978, *2*, 1382.

For a report of dextrans interfering with direct cross-matching tests, see Dextrans, p.510.

Uses. Whole Blood is used as a source of red cell concentrates, clotting factors, platelets, plasma proteins, and immunoglobulins, each of which has specific indications for use. Because of the risks involved in transfusing Whole Blood and the need for economy in its use, the appropriate blood component should be used whenever possible.

Whole Blood is used to replace blood volume and oxygen-carrying capacity following blood loss during surgery and severe haemorrhage. It is also used to supplement the circulation during cardiac bypass surgery. Fresh whole blood is occasionally used to provide particular labile blood-clotting factors in the treatment of haemophilia.

For the replacement of blood volume Plasma Protein Fraction (see p.335), dextrans (see p.511), and intravenous infusion fluids are preferred. For the replacement of oxygen-capacity a red cell concentrate such as Concentrated Red Blood Cells or Plasma-reduced Blood (see p.325) should be used.

The amount of Whole Blood transfused and the rate at which it is given depend upon the patient's age and general condition, upon the state of his circulatory system, and upon the therapeutic indication for transfusion. The haemoglobin concentration of the blood of the average adult is raised by about 1 g per 100 ml by the transfusion of 540 ml of Whole Blood.

A number of reports have suggested that regular transfusions given for about 3 months before renal transplantation have improved graft survival; reports of the use of transfusions only at the time of surgery are less consistent.

For reviews of blood and blood components and their uses, see R. G. Westphal, *Ann. intern. Med.*, 1972, *76*, 987; *Med. Lett.*, 1972, *14*, 89; P. Schiff, *Med. J. Aust.*, 1973, *1*, 22; R. W. Beal, *Drugs*, 1973, *6*, 127; J. da Costa, *Br. J. Hosp. Med.*, 1973, *9*, 681; *Br. med. J.*, 1974, *3*, 544; *Med. Lett.*, 1975, *17* (Jan.), *Suppl.*, 30; A. Doenicke *et al.*, *Br. J. Anaesth.*, 1977, *49*, 681; S. J. Urbaniak and J. D. Cash, *Br. med. Bull.*, 1977, *33*, 273; E. C. Buchanan, *Am. J. Hosp. Pharm.*, 1977, *34*, 631; Working Party of the Australian Society of Blood Transfusion, *Med. J. Aust.*, 1978, *1*, 96; *Med. Lett.*, 1979, *21*, 93; M. A. Blajchman *et al.*, *Can. med. Ass. J.*, 1979, *121*, 33.

Further details of the use of whole human blood and other blood components, see P. L. Mollison, *Blood Transfusion in Clinical Medicine*, 5th Edn, London, Blackwell Scientific Publications, 1972.

The use of whole blood and blood products in cardiac bypass surgery.— J. K. Roche and J. M. Stengle, *J. Am. med. Ass.*, 1973, *225*, 1516.

The treatment of leprosy reaction by autohaemotherapy.— A. Legrand, *Méd. trop. Marseille*, 1974, *34*, 495.

A review of autologous blood transfusion.— S. M. Brzica *et al.*, *Mayo Clin. Proc.*, 1976, *51*, 723. See also J. M. Hauer and R. B. Dawson (letter), *New Engl. J. Med.*, 1979, *300*, 1276.

Stored blood had reduced concentrations of factor V and VIII and of platelets. Generalised bleeding could occur when more than 5 litres of blood was transfused in 24 hours in an adult; a vicious circle could be established. One unit of fresh blood should be given with each 3 units of stored blood.— M. Verstraete, *Haemostatic Drugs*, The Hague, Martinus Nijhoff, 1977, p. 1.

Exchange transfusion. In a prospective study of the effect and mortality of exchange transfusion, 140 exchange transfusions were performed on 122 infants for hyperbilirubinaemia, haemolytic disease, and glucose-6-phosphate dehydrogenase deficiency. Eight infants deteriorated during transfusion and 2 deaths occurred 2 days after exchange. The clinical status of infants should be monitored during and immediately after the procedure.— K. L. Tan *et al.*, *Med. J. Aust.*, 1976, *1*, 473.

All of 9 infants with group B steptococcal infections survived their septic episodes after receiving blood containing antibodies to their infecting strain. Of 6 infants who received blood without the antibodies, 3 died. A transfusion of 40% or more of the patients' blood-volume was required if the antibody-containing blood was to increase opsonic activity.— A. O. Shigeoka *et al.* (preliminary communication), *Lancet*, 1978, *1*, 636. See also S. E. Courtney *et al.* (letter), *Lancet*, 1979, *2*, 462.

Haemoglobinopathies. The management of thalassaemia major.— B. Modell, *Br. med. Bull.*, 1976, *32*, 270; *Archs Dis. Childh.*, 1977, *52*, 489.

Haemophilia. Fresh whole blood containing 0.3 units of coagulation factors per ml could be used in the treatment of patients with haemophilia A to raise plasma levels of factors VIII to 4 to 6%. Maximum recommended dosage of blood was 15 ml per kg body-weight.— *Tech. Rep. Ser. Wld Hlth Org. No. 504*, 1972.

Pregnancy and the neonate. Discussion of the treatment of anaemia in preterm infants by transfusion of adult blood.— *Lancet*, 1979, *1*, 419. The possible danger of retrolental fibroplasia.— J. D. Baum (letter), *ibid.*, 617.

Over 55 months, 218 intra-uterine transfusions with highly concentrated group O, Rh-negative blood were given to 100 foetuses with erythroblastosis due to Rh iso-immunisation; 48 infants survived and there were no maternal deaths. The initial transfusions were made from the 22nd to 33rd weeks of gestation and were repeated after intervals of 10 to 12 days followed by intervals of 3 to 4 weeks up to a maximum of 4 transfusions. The quantity of blood transfused varied from 40 to 100 ml according to the age of the foetus. Treatment with digoxin might have contributed to the survival of some foetuses with hydrops.— J. M. Bowman *et al.*, *J. Am. med. Ass.*, 1969, *207*, 1101. A similar report.— M. E. Wade *et al.*, *Obstet. Gynec.*, 1969, *34*, 156, per *J. Am. med. Ass.*, 1969, *209*, 2106.

See also under Exchange Transfusion.

Renal transplant survival. Reports of increased renal transplant survival in patients given regular blood transfusions before surgery.— H. Brynger *et al.*, *Proc. Eur. Dialysis Transplant Ass.*, 1977, *14*, 290; P. Schmidt *et al.* (letter), *Lancet*, 1977, *2*, 242; P. R. Uldall *et al.*, *Lancet*, 1977, *2*, 316; R. W. Blamey *et al.*, *Br. med. J.*, 1978, *1*, 138; B. Hulme and M. E. Snell (letter), *Br. med. J.*, 1978, *1*, 361; H. Bühlmann *et al.*, *Dt. med. Wschr.*, 1978, *103*, 293; H. Brynger *et al.* (letter), *Lancet*, 1978, *1*, 1099; F. Vincenti *et al.*, *New Engl. J. Med.*, 1978, *299*, 793; G. Opelz *et al.*, *Lancet*, 1981, *1*, 1223.

A retrospective study of 1360 patients who had received cadaver renal transplants at various centres showed that the beneficial effect of blood transfusions before transplantation was highly significant and proportional to the number of transfusions given. Survival rates at 4 years were 65% in patients who had received more than 20 transfusions compared with 30% in those who had received none. Frozen blood was less effective than whole blood or packed cells.— G. Opelz and P. I. Terasaki, *New Engl. J. Med.*, 1978, *299*, 799.

In 62 patients who had received renal allografts there was no difference in survival-rates, at 3, 6, 12, or 24 months, between those who had received blood transfusions before transplantation and those not transfused.— D. P. S. Sengar and A. Rashid (letter), *Br. med. J.*, 1978, *1*, 988.

Transfusions of blood given before renal transplantation were associated with increased graft survival, the incidence of survival at 1 year being 71% in 31 transfused patients compared with 40% in 25 patients not transfused. Transfusions on the day of surgery produced a better effect than earlier transfusion while additional transfusion after surgery had no beneficial effect on transplant survival.— C. R. Stiller *et al.*, *Lancet*, 1978, *1*, 169. Six of 7 grafts were rejected within one year in 7 patients given their first transfusion at the time of transplantation compared with a survival-rate of 40% at one year in 47 transplant patients not transfused.— J. R. Salaman (letter), *ibid.*, 494. An 18% survival-rate at one year in 33 patients receiving intra-operative transfusions only.— G. G. Persijn and J. J. van Rood (letter), *ibid.* Blood transfusions given at the time of transplantation had no beneficial effect on graft survival in 90 patients followed up for at least 3 months.— J. R. Jeffery *et al.* (letter), *Lancet*, 1978, *1*, 662.

Results of a prospective controlled study in 27 patients who had never had a blood transfusion or been pregnant and who were receiving their first renal allograft, indicated that peroperative blood transfusions improve cadaveric renal allograft survival in non-transfused patients. For 13 patients given 2 units of whole stored blood at transplantation there was a graft survival of 85% at one year, whereas for 14 who were given no blood the graft survival at one year was only 34%. Peroperative transfusion may have as beneficial an effect on graft survival as pre-operative transfusion, without the associated risk of recipient presensitisation.— K. A. Williams *et al.*, *Lancet*, 1980, *1*, 1104.

A discussion on blood transfusions and renal transplantation, including absence of benefit of pre-transplant transfusions in 522 recipients in the UK.— *Lancet*, 1978, *2*, 193.

1213-l

Albumin *(B.P.).* Human Albumin.

A sterile solution of human albumin in water containing a low proportion of salt. It is obtained from pooled liquid plasma from suitable human subjects (see under Whole Blood, p.322) by a suitable fractionation technique, sufficient sodium caprylate or other suitable substances being added to stabilise the protein to heat. Electrophoresis indicates that 96% of the protein present is albumin. It contains no added bactericide or antibiotic. The solution is **sterilised** by filtration and distributed aseptically into containers which are sealed to exclude micro-organisms and maintained at 59.5° to 60.5° for 10 hours to prevent the transmission of viral hepatitis. Finally, the containers are incubated for not less than 14 days at 30° to 32° and examined visually for signs of microbial contamination.

Albumin is a clear amber to deep orange-brown liquid, pH 6.7 to 7.3, containing 15 to 25% of protein, and not more than 0.65 mmol (0.65 mEq) of sodium, 0.05 mmol (0.05 mEq) of potassium, and 0.1 mmol (0.3 mEq) of citrate ions per g of protein. It must not be used if the solution is turbid or contains a deposit. **Store** at 2° to 25°. Protect from light.

NOTE. The expression 'salt-poor' has been used as being equivalent to 'containing a low proportion of salt' (above) but should not be confused with the expression 'salt-poor' previously used in the USA for preparations with a sodium content at least two-thirds that of plasma. Albumin *B.P.* contains not more than 97.5 mmol (97.5 mEq) of sodium (15% protein) or not more than 162.5 mmol (162.5 mEq) of sodium (25% protein) per litre; Albumin Human *U.S.P.* contains 130 to 160 mmol (130 to 160 mEq) of sodium per litre.

1214-y

Dried Albumin *(B.P.).* Dried Human Albumin.

A sterile cream-coloured powder prepared by freeze-drying an aqueous solution of albumin, prepared as above and containing not more than 10% of protein. When dissolved in the amount of Water for Injections stated on the label, it provides a solution of albumin containing 24 to 26% of protein. The requirements for sodium, potassium and citrate ions are as for Albumin.

If, after adding water, a gel forms or solution is incomplete, the preparation must not be used. The solution must be used within 3 hours of being reconstituted. **Store** at 2° to 25° in an atmosphere of nitrogen in sterile containers, sealed to exclude micro-organisms and, as far as possible, moisture. Protect from light. It should be administered with suitable equipment such as that described in Section 3 or Section 4 of *Transfusion Equipment for Medical Use*, BS 2463: 1962.

1215-j

Albumin Human *(U.S.P.).*

A sterile preparation, suitable for intravenous use, of serum albumin obtained by fractionating material (blood, plasma, serum, or placentas) from healthy human donors; it is tested for the absence of hepatitis B surface antigen. Not less than 96% of the total protein is albumin. It may contain sodium acetyltryptophanate with or without sodium caprylate as a stabilising agent; it contains no added antimicrobial agent.

Human Albumin is a clear, moderately viscous, almost odourless, brownish liquid containing 4, 5, 20, or 25% of serum albumin. It contains 130 to 160 mmol (130 to 160 mEq) of sodium per litre. It must not be used if the solution is turbid.

The expiration date is not more than 5 years after release from the manufacturer's cold storage if stored at 2° to 10°, and not more than 3 years after release if stored at a temperature not exceeding 37°. The expiration date is not more than 10 years after manufacture if stored in a hermetically-sealed metal container at 2° to 10°.

Adverse Effects and Precautions. Albumin is a normal constituent of the blood and toxic effects are rare; urticaria, chills, and fever may occur. However, injection solutions containing 15 to 25% of albumin are hyperosmotic and should not be given to dehydrated patients unless additional fluid is given by mouth or by infusion.

Concentrated solutions are contra-indicated in patients with severe anaemia or heart failure and should be given with caution in patients with diminished cardiac reserve because of circulatory overload and pulmonary oedema.

There were 7 anaphylactic reactions in 60 048 infusions of human albumin.— J. Ring and K. Messmer, *Lancet*, 1977, *1*, 466.

Possible adverse effects on respiratory function.— D. W. Weaver *et al.*, *Archs Surg., Chicago*, 1978, *113*, 387, per *J. Am. med. Ass.*, 1978, *239*, 1675. See also M. S. Dahn *et al.*, *Surgery, St Louis*, 1979, *86*, 235, per *J. Am. med. Ass.*, 1980, *243*, 284; C. J. Paton and P. J. Kerry (letter), *Lancet*, 1981, *2*, 747.

Uses. Albumin forms about 55% of the plasma proteins and provides most of the osmotic pressure of plasma. It has a low molecular weight (about 69 000) and is small enough to be excreted in the urine in nephrosis.

Albumin is administered intravenously as a 20 to 25% solution to replace protein lost in conditions such as the nephrotic syndrome and in burns and to compensate for reduced protein synthesis in cirrhosis of the liver. The usual dose is 25 to 75 g daily given at the rate of about 1 ml of 25% solution per minute. It has also been used in ulcerative colitis, eclampsia, cardiovascular surgery, and renal dialysis.

A 5% solution is approximately iso-osmotic with serum and may be administered intravenously as a blood volume expander in hypovolaemia. The usual initial dose is 25 g given at the rate of 2 to 4 ml of a 5% solution per minute but at a higher rate in emergencies and repeated in 15 to 30 minutes if necessary. The 20% or 25% solution may be diluted with a suitable solution.

There is little or no risk of transmitting viral hepatitis type B.

Consideration should be given to the sodium content of the infusion.

Of 13 patients with nephritis 7 failed to respond with adequate weight loss after being treated with a high-protein diet, 500-mg sodium intake, and increasing doses of frusemide, usually with spironolactone, or developed complications rendering an aggressive diuretic policy impossible. Prompt diuresis followed the infusion of 300 ml of 15% low-salt human albumin which could initially be given on alternate days.— A. M. Davison *et al.*, *Br. med. J.*, 1974, *1*, 481.

The chemistry and physiology of human albumin.— J. L. Tullis, *J. Am. med. Ass.*, 1977, *237*, 355 and 460.

The use of albumin was appropriate in shock, burns, adult respiratory distress syndrome, and cardiopulmonary bypass; it was occasionally used in acute liver failure, for the suspension of red blood cells, in ascites, in hypoproteinaemia after surgery, in acute nephrosis, and in renal dialysis; its use in detoxification awaited confirmation; its use was unjustified in undernutrition, chronic nephrosis, and chronic cirrhosis.— J. L. Tullis, *J. Am. med. Ass.*, 1977, *237*, 460.

A study in 12 malnourished children provided no support for the theory that nutritional oedema should be treated with a high-protein dietary regimen or an albumin infusion.— M. H. N. Golden *et al.*, *Lancet*, 1980, *1*, 114.

Dialysis. The addition of albumin 5% to peritoneal dialysing fluid was found to increase the clearance-rate of barbiturates from 6 to 12 ml per minute to 13 to 19 ml per minute in 4 poisoned adults. Two had taken pentobarbitone, 1 quinalbarbitone, and 1 phenobarbitone.— R. E. Gosselin and R. P. Smith, *Clin. Pharmac. Ther.*, 1966, *7*, 279.

Exchange transfusion. Adding albumin 2.5 g to each 100 ml of blood used for exchange transfusion in hyperbilirubinaemic infants increased the amount of bilirubin removed.— A. Comley and B. Wood, *Archs Dis. Childh.*, 1968, *43*, 151, per *Abstr. Wld Med.*, 1968, *42*, 893.

In a study of 20 neonates with jaundice but without haemolytic disease, 7 were given albumin 1.75 g per kg body-weight as a 10% solution 3 hours before transfusion, 7 were transfused without albumin, and 6 were transfused with blood to which albumin 1.5 g per 100 ml had been added. The removal of bilirubin was most efficient in those who had received the albumin-enriched blood and least in the albumin-primed group.— Y. C. Tsao and V. Y. H. Yu, *Archs Dis. Childh.*, 1972, *47*, 250.

Absence of benefit of albumin before exchange transfusion except in infants with low reserve albumin binding capacity.— G. Chan and D. Schiff, *J. Pediat.*, 1976, *88*, 609, per *Int. pharm. Abstr.*, 1976, *13*, 1031.

Kidney perfusion solution. The preservation of cadaveric kidneys for transplantation; with a formula for an albumin perfusion solution.— T. P. Stephenson *et al.*, *Br. med. J.*, 1973, *1*, 379.

The advantages of using machine perfusion with human albumin of cadaver kidneys prior to transplantation.— A. G. R. Sheil *et al.*, *Lancet*, 1975, *2*, 287.

Perfusion of kidneys with albumin provides reliable preservation for up to 50 hours.— R. L. Burleson *et al.*, *Archs Surg., Chicago*, 1978, *113*, 688, per *J. Am. med. Ass.*, 1978, *239*, 2800.

Proprietary Preparations

Albumin Kabi *(KabiVitrum, UK).* Albumin, available for injection as a solution containing 20% of protein. It contains not more than 120 mmol (120 mEq) of sodium ions per litre.

Buminate 20% *(Travenol, UK).* Albumin, available for injection as a solution containing 20% of protein.

Human Albumin 20% *(Immuno, UK).* Albumin, available for injection as a solution containing 20% of protein.

Other Proprietary Names

Albuconn, Albuminar, Albumisol, Albuspan, Albutein, Plasbumin (all *USA*).

1216-z

Antithrombin III. Alpha-2 Globulin; Heparin Cofactor.

There was less variation of potency estimates when the freeze-dried normal plasma preparation was used than when two preparations of purified human antithrombin III were used.— WHO Expert Committee on Biological Standardization, *Tech. Rep. Ser. Wld Hlth Org. No. 638*, 1979.

Units. 0.9 unit of antithrombin III is contained in one ampoule (which contains the freeze-dried residue of 1 ml of normal plasma) of the first International Reference Preparation (1978).

Uses. Antithrombin III is a protein in plasma; it is the major inhibitor of thrombin, it inhibits factor Xa and possibly factors IXa, XIa, and plasmin, and is the cofactor through which heparin (see p.765) exerts its effect. Genetic and acquired deficiency of antithrombin III has been reported and is associated with susceptibility to thrombo-embolic disorders.

A review.— T. W. Barrowcliffe *et al.*, *Br. med. Bull.*, 1978, *34*, 143.

For a brief mention of some conditions associated with changed concentrations of antithrombin III, see M. Brozović, *Br. med. Bull.*, 1977, *33*, 231.

The use of antithrombin-III in 3 patients with disseminated intravascular coagulation.— H. G. Schipper *et al.* (preliminary communication), *Lancet*, 1978, *1*, 854. The use of a pure preparation of antithrombin III for disseminated intravascular coagulation was logical and initial results had been encouraging, but prothrombin complex concentrates should not be used in the setting of disseminated intravascular coagulation until the active ingredients were adequately delineated; normal concentrations of antithrombin III did not always prevent the thrombo-embolic or haemorrhagic side-effects of prothrombin complex concentrate.— P. M. Blatt *et al.* (letter), *Lancet*, 1978, *1*, 1212.

The successful use of antithrombin III in the treatment of a patient with the postpartum haemolytic-uraemic syndrome.— P. Brandt *et al.*, *Br. med. J.*, 1980, *280*, 449.

Manufacturers
KabiVitrum, UK.

1217-c

Concentrated Red Blood Cells *(B.P.).*

NOTE. *B.P. 1980* included Concentrate of Red Blood Cells (Concentrated Human Red Blood Corpuscles; Packed Red Cells; Concentrate of Human Red Blood Cells). This was replaced in the Addendum 1981 by Concentrated Red Blood Cells and Plasma-reduced Blood.

Concentrated Red Blood Cells is Whole Blood from a single donor from which part of the plasma and anticoagulant solution has been removed. It has a packed cell volume greater than 70%. It is prepared from Whole Blood which is preferably not more than 14 days old. It is a dark red fluid which may separate on standing into a sediment of red blood corpuscles and a supernatant layer of yellow plasma. The ABO group and the Rh group of the Whole Blood from which it was made and the nature of the specific antisera used in testing are stated on the label.

Store at 4° to 6° in sterile containers sealed to exclude micro-organisms. It should not be used if there is visible evidence of deterioration.

Red cell concentrates which have been freed from most of their white cells by washing, sedimentation, or centrifugation are also prepared.

Red blood cells from which the plasma, platelets, and leucocytes have been removed, and to which a cryoprotective agent (usually glycerol) has been added, may be stored for long periods at low temperatures (about −65° to −80°). When required for use the red cells are thawed at 37°, washed in a series of solutions, suspended in a suitable vehicle, and used within 24 hours.

1252-t

Plasma-reduced Blood *(B.P.).* Plasma-reduced Whole Blood.

Plasma-reduced Blood is Whole Blood from a single donor from which part of the plasma and anticoagulant solution has been removed. It has a packed cell volume of 60 to 65%. It is prepared from Whole Blood which is preferably not more than 14 days old.

It is a dark red fluid which may separate on standing into a sediment of red blood corpuscles and a supernatant layer of yellow plasma. The ABO group and the Rh group of the Whole Blood from which it was made and the nature of the specific antisera used in testing are stated on the label. **Store** at 4° to 6° in sterile containers sealed to exclude micro-organisms. It should not be used if there is visible evidence of deterioration. It should be administered with suitable equipment such as that described in Section 3 or Section 4 of *Transfusion Equipment for Medical Use*, BS 2463: 1962.

1218-k

Red Blood Cells *(U.S.P.).*

The remaining red blood cells of whole human blood from suitable donors, from which plasma has been removed. It may be prepared by centrifuging or by sedimentation. If intended for extended manufacturer's storage at or below −65° it contains a portion of the plasma sufficient to ensure cell preservation, or a cryophylactic substance.

Store in hermetically-sealed sterile containers at 1° to 6° (with a range of not more than 2°) except during transport when the temperature may be 1° to 10°. A small quantity is supplied in a small container attached to each main container.

The use of closed system plastic packs for blood collection made it unnecessary to enter the container to separate the fractions, and such red cell concentrates could be stored for up to 21 days at 4°. If glass bottles were used the concentrates should be used within 24 hours.— R. W. Beal, *Drugs*, 1973, *6*, 127.

Improved viability, quality, oxygen delivery capacity, and metabolic activity of packed cells was obtained when blood was collected into citrate-phosphate-dextrose anticoagulant with extra dextrose (CP2D) and, after separation of plasma, stored in an adenine-enhanced electrolyte solution. If stored at 4° the cells were viable for 35 days.— V. A. Lovric *et al.*, *Med. J. Aust.*, 1977, *2*, 183.

After collection in citrate-phosphate-dextrose solution and removal of plasma and buffy coat, red blood cells were successfully stored at 4° for 35 days in a simple saline-adenine-glucose medium.— C. F. Högman *et al.*, *New Engl. J. Med.*, 1978, *299*, 1377. Correction.— *ibid.*, 1979, *300*, 512. Comment.— P. J. Schmidt, *ibid.*, 1978, *299*, 1411; W. Schneider and H. Fiedler (letter), *ibid.*, 1979, *300*, 983; E. Beutler (letter), *ibid.*, 984; L. K. Diamond (letter), *ibid.*; G. K. Sherwood *et al.* (letter), *ibid.*

Adverse Effects. As for Whole Blood, p.322.

Some red cell concentrates have a reduced risk of allergic reactions from leucocytes.

Twice-washed red blood-cells provoked an anaphylactic reaction in a patient; after 3 further washings no reaction occurred.— J. Leikola *et al.*, *Blood*, 1973, *42*, 111, per *J. Am. med. Ass.*, 1973, *226*, 95.

Post-transfusion thrombocytopenic purpura occurred in a 43-year-old woman after the infusion of red blood cells; she had earlier had blood transfusions uneventfully.— P. M. Dainer and E. D. Canada, *Br. med. J.*, 1977, *2*, 999.

Hypertension in 2 patients with sickle-cell anaemia and cerebral haemorrhage in one after the infusion of red blood cells.— J. E. Royal and R. A. Seeler (letter), *Lancet*, 1978, *2*, 1207. A similar report in thalassaemia.— S. Yetgin and G. Hicsonmez (letter), *ibid.*, 1979, *1*, 610.

The large-scale use of frozen red cells and washed red cells in a transfusion service had not reduced the incidence of post-transfusion hepatitis.— R. K. Haugen, *New Engl. J. Med.*, 1979, *301*, 393. Criticism.— D. Goldfinger (letter), *ibid.*, 1980, *302*, 581. Further comments.— M. Telischi and R. Hoiberg (letter), *ibid.*, 582; C. L. Lee (letter), *ibid.*

Uses. Transfusions of red blood cells are given for the treatment of severe anaemia without hypovolaemia. As there is a reduced risk of overloading the circulation with salts and plasma proteins it is used in preference to Whole Blood in patients with congestive cardiac failure.

The haemoglobin concentration of the blood of the average adult is raised by about 1 g per 100 ml by the red blood cells obtained from 540 ml of Whole Blood. It is also used for exchange transfusion in babies with haemolytic disease of the newborn.

Discussions of various red blood cell concentrates and their uses.— J. da Costa, *Br. J. Hosp. Med.*, 1973, *9*, 681; R. W. Beal, *Drugs*, 1973, *6*, 127; A. J. Grindon, *J. Am. med. Ass.*, 1976, *235*, 389; H. Chaplin, *New Engl. J. Med.*, 1978, *298*, 679.

Addition of a small volume of iso-osmotic saline (as little as 50 ml) to packed red cells reduced viscosity and allowed more rapid infusion.— M. G. Davey and B. E. Wild (letter), *Med. J. Aust.*, 1973, *2*, 1072.

The risk of a graft-host reaction following intra-uterine transfusions could be avoided by giving red cells. Of 24 infants given transfusions of red cells 12 survived and none of the 12 had any sign of a reaction.— M. G. Davey *et al.* (letter), *Lancet*, 1974, *2*, 778.

The use of saline-washed frozen red blood cells in extracorporeal procedures.— M. Lewis *et al.*, *Ann. thorac. Surg.*, 1975, *19*, 153, per *J. Am. med. Ass.*, 1975, *233*, 192.

The use of frozen red blood cells in neonatal exchange transfusion.— J. Umlas and S. Gootblatt, *Transfusion, Philad.*, 1976, *16*, 636.

The use of red blood cells for enzyme replacement therapy in a child with adenosine deaminase deficiency and severe combined immunodeficiency.— S. H. Polmar *et al.*, *New Engl. J. Med.*, 1976, *295*, 1337. Comments.—

E. Beutler *et al.* (letter), *ibid.*, 1977, *296*, 942; R. C. Harris (letter), *ibid.*, 943.

A discussion on the possible use of neocytes (young red blood cells with potentially increased survival) for transfusion as a means of reducing the frequency of iron overload in patients requiring numerous transfusions.— *J. Am. med. Ass.*, 1979, *242*, 2669.

Anaemia. In a prospective controlled study 13 anaemic, neutropenic children with acute lymphocytic leukaemia were hypertransfused with packed red cells to a haemoglobin concentration of 16 to 18 g per 100 ml whereas 13 similar children were infused where necessary to a haemoglobin concentration of 10 to 12 g per 100 ml. There was a significant increase in the rate of recovery from neutropenia in the hypertransfused group, confirming previous findings (P.J. Smith and H. Ekert, *Lancet*, 1976, *1*, 776) that hypertransfusion is of value in the treatment of childhood lymphocytic leukaemia.— I. R. G. Toogood *et al.*, *Lancet*, 1978, *2*, 862. Comment.— S. Roath (letter), *ibid.*, 1979, *1*, 43.

Haemoglobinopathies. *Sickle-cell disease.* Repeated transfusions of red blood cells during pregnancy may benefit both mothers with sickle-cell haemoglobinopathies and their babies.— *J. Am. med. Ass.*, 1980, *244*, 26.

Renal transplant survival. Studies suggesting that the pretransplant transfusion of frozen washed red cells (frozen blood) had little advantage over the transfusion of whole blood in potential kidney transplant recipients.— R. M. Minchinton *et al.*, *Br. med. J.*, 1980, *281*, 113.

1219-a

Blood Group Specific Substances A, B, and AB. *(U.S.P.).*

A sterile non-anaphylactic iso-osmotic solution of the polysaccharide-amino-acid complexes that are capable of neutralising the anti-A and the anti-B isoagglutinins of group O blood. Substance A is prepared from hog stomach (gastric mucin) and substances B and AB from horse stomach (gastric mucosa). The substances contain no added preservative and have a pH of 6 to 6.8. **Store** in single-dose containers at 2° to 8°.

The substances are used for immunisation of plasma donors for production of *in vitro* diagnostic reagents. The *U.S.P.* directs that the substances should not be given intravenously nor to fertile women. Blood group specific substance B may contain immunogenic A activity.

1220-e

Blood Platelets. Thrombocytes.

Blood platelets may be obtained from whole fresh blood by centrifuging to remove red blood corpuscles and leucocytes, leaving platelet-rich plasma.

Platelet concentrates are obtained by further high-speed centrifuging and the concentrated platelets are suspended in a small volume of plasma. Each unit of platelet concentrate contains about 5 to 7×10^{10} platelets. The concentrate may be **stored** up to 72 hours at 22° with constant agitation provided that strict asepsis is maintained.

1221-l

Platelet Concentrate *(U.S.P.).*

Contains the platelets taken from plasma obtained by whole-blood collection, plasmaphaeresis, or plateletphaeresis from a single suitable human donor. The platelets are suspended in a specified volume (20 to 30 ml, or 30 to 50 ml) of the original plasma. The suspension contains not less than 5.5×10^{10} platelets per unit in not less than 75% of the units tested. pH not less than 6.

Store in hermetically-sealed sterile containers at 20° to 24° (30 to 50 ml volume), or at 1° to 6° (20 to 30 ml volume) except during transport when the temperature may be 1° to 10°.

The expiration time is not more than 72 hours from the time of collection of the source material. Continuous gentle agitation must be maintained if stored at 20° to 24°. The suspension must be used within 4 hours of opening the container.

The bactericidal properties of platelet concentrates.— B. A. Myhre *et al.*, *Transfusion, Philad.*, 1974, *14*, 116, per *J. Am. med. Ass.*, 1974, *228*, 1732.

Aspirin-induced prolonged bleeding time was reduced by a transfusion of platelets stored at 4° for 24 hours and by platelets freeze-preserved with 6% dimethyl sulphoxide and stored at −80° for 24 hours. The life-spans of these platelets were 3 and 8 days respectively. Bleeding time was not reduced by platelets stored at room temperature for 4 hours, or by platelets stored at 22° for 24 hours, or by platelets freeze-preserved with 5% dimethyl sulphoxide and stored at −150° for 24 hours. The life-span of all these platelets was 8 days.— C. R. Valeri, *New Engl. J. Med.*, 1974, *290*, 353.

Gel filtration for the preparation of platelets.— K. M. Fine *et al.*, *Am. J. Path.*, 1976, *84*, 11, per *J. Am. med. Ass.*, 1976, *236*, 2003.

Adverse Effects. See Viral Hepatitis, p.321.

Blood platelets are antigenic, and immunological and allergic reactions have occurred. Many patients receiving repeated transfusions of platelets from random donors become refractory to treatment; the use of HLA histocompatible platelets may allow treatment to be continued. Because platelet preparations contain a small quantity of red cells, Rh immunisation may occur if platelets from an Rh-positive donor are given to an Rh-negative recipient; in such circumstances females of or below childbearing age should be given anti-D immunoglobulin.

There is little risk of overloading the circulation when platelet concentrate is used.

In patients with thrombocytopenia, prolonged bleeding times were corrected in those given platelets from donors who had taken aspirin 36 hours before donation but not in those given platelets from donors who had taken aspirin within 12 hours of donation.— M. J. Stuart *et al.*, *New Engl. J. Med.*, 1972, *287*, 1105.

Platelet transfusions from HLA-typed single donors in sensitised patients.— J. Gmur *et al.*, *Schweiz. med. Wschr.*, 1976, *106*, 1358. See also K. Sintnicolaas *et al.*, *Lancet*, 1981, *1*, 750.

Uses. Blood platelets assist in the clotting process by aggregation to form a platelet thrombus and by participating in the formation of thromboplastin. Transfusions of platelet concentrates, platelet-rich plasma, or fresh whole blood containing platelets are given to patients with thrombocytopenic haemorrhage. Because of their reduced volume platelet concentrates are preferred. They may also be given prophylactically prior to a surgical operation or to reduce the frequency of haemorrhage in thrombocytopenia associated with the chemotherapy of neoplastic disease.

An extensive review of factors influencing platelet function.— J. F. Mustard and M. A. Packham, *Pharmac. Rev.*, 1970, *22*, 97. See also H. J. Weiss, *New Engl. J. Med.*, 1978, *298*, 1344.

For a review of the use of platelets, see *Lancet*, 1972, *1*, 25. See also M. A. Blajchman *et al.*, *Can. med. Ass. J.*, 1979, *121*, 33.

Transfusions of platelets should be given prophylactically if lumbar puncture was essential in patients with coagulation defects.— *Br. med. J.*, 1975, *1*, 3.

Bone-marrow failure. Repeated transfusions of blood platelets or concentrates from 136 units of fresh blood were successfully used in treating a 19-year-old girl with complete bone-marrow aplasia induced by radiation for the treatment of Hodgkin's disease. She was given platelet transfusions, in doses of 3 to 12 units over a period of about 9 weeks, and transfusions of fresh blood.— M. S. Rose, *Lancet*, 1967, *1*, 309.

Dosage. The platelets from 5 to 6 units of blood raised the platelet count by 100 000 per mm³ for 2 to 3 days.— *Lancet*, 1972, *1*, 25.

A peripheral platelet count of less than 20 000 per mm³ was an indication for infusion of platelet concentrate in the treatment of haemorrhage. The usual dose was the platelets concentrated from 4 to 8 units of blood every 3 to 4 days.— P. Schiff, *Med. J. Aust.*, 1973, *1*, 22.

Thrombocytopenia. Platelet-rich red cell concentrate, achieved as a byproduct from whole blood centrifuged so as to produce platelet-poor plasma, was used successfully in the management of thrombocytopenia.— A. E. Shaw (letter), *Lancet*, 1974, *2*, 300.

A study of 29 patients with acute nonlymphoblastic leukaemia indicated that limiting platelet transfusions to serious cases of bleeding with a rapid fall in platelet-count was as effective as routine prophylaxis for bleeding associated with any fall in platelet-count.— J. Solomon *et al.* (letter), *Lancet*, 1978, *1*, 267.

Transfusions of frozen autologous platelets were a valuable adjunct to the management of 25 adult patients with leukaemia, many of whom were alloimmunised. Plateletphaeresis was carried out soon after patients entered remission and multiple donations were well-tolerated. There were no side-effects from the transfusion of residual amounts of dimethyl sulphoxide which was used in the preparation of the frozen platelets.— C. A. Schiffer *et al.*, *New Engl. J. Med.*, 1978, *299*, 7.

1222-y

Bone Marrow. The soft material found in the hollow centre of long bones and in the spaces of other bones. Red and white blood cells and platelets are developed in the bone marrow.

Bone-marrow depression occurs in a variety of diseases, some genetic, or associated with infection, radiation, exposure to chemicals, or drug treatment, particularly with antineoplastic agents.

Bone-marrow transplantation involves the injection, usually after immunosuppression, of material from a suitable HLA-compatible donor and has been used in some immunological deficiencies, in aplastic anaemia, and in leukaemia. The principal risks are infection, graft rejection, and graft-versus-host disease. Autologous transplantation, with frozen material derived from the patient while in remission, has also been used.

Some references: R. Storb *et al.*, *New Engl. J. Med.*, 1977, *296*, 61; *Med. Lett.*, 1978, *20*, 98; R. P. Gale, *New Engl. J. Med.*, 1979, *300*, 1189; *Lancet*, 1980, *2*, 1343; P. L. Weiden *et al.*, *New Engl. J. Med.*, 1981, *304*, 1529.

A preparation of bone marrow and cartilage was formerly marketed in Great Britain under the proprietary name Rumalon (*Robapharm, Switz.: Welbeck*).

1223-j

Dried Factor VIII Fraction *(B.P.).* Dried Human Antihaemophilic Fraction; Dried Human Antihaemophilic Globulin.

Dried Factor VIII Fraction is a sterile dried preparation rich in factor VIII obtained from human plasma from suitable subjects (see under Whole Blood, p.322) by a suitable fractionation technique. The fraction is dissolved in an appropriate liquid, **sterilised** by filtration, distributed in sterile containers, and dried from the frozen state. The air is removed or replaced with nitrogen and the containers are sealed to exclude micro-organisms. No preservative is added.

Dried Factor VIII Fraction is a white powder or friable solid which is completely **soluble**, when warmed to 18° to 22°, within 20 minutes in water. A solution in water has a pH of 6.8 to 7.4. When dissolved in the quantity of Water for Injections stated on the label, the resulting solution contains not less than 6 units per ml and not less than 0.2 unit per mg of protein of which not more than 80% is fibrinogen; the solution contains not more than 200 mmol (200 mEq) of sodium ions per litre and not more than 55 mmol (165 mEq) of citrate ions per litre.

Store below 6° *in vacuo* or in an atmosphere of nitrogen in sterile containers sealed to exclude micro-organisms and, as far as possible, moisture. Protect from light. It should be used as soon as possible after, and not more than 3 hours after, reconstitution. If a gel forms the fraction should not be used. It should be administered with equipment that includes a filter.

1224-z

Antihemophilic Factor *(U.S.P.)*.

CAS — 9001-27-8.

Antihemophilic factor is a sterile freeze-dried powder containing factor VIII fraction prepared from pooled human venous plasma that has been tested for the asbence of hepatitis B surface antigen; it may contain heparin sodium or sodium citrate. It contains not less than 100 units per g of protein.

A white or yellowish powder. **Soluble** in water yielding a yellowish liquid or an opalescent liquid with a slight blue tinge.

Unless otherwise specified, **store** at 2° to 8° in hermetically-sealed containers. It should be used within 4 hours of reconstitution and should be administered with equipment that includes a filter. The expiration date is not later than 2 years from the date of manufacture; during this time it may be stored at room temperature and used within 6 months.

1225-c

Cryoprecipitated Antihemophilic Factor *(U.S.P.)*.

Cryoprecipitated Antihemophilic Factor is a sterile frozen concentrate of human antihaemophilic factor prepared from the cryoprotein fraction, rich in factor VIII, of plasma obtained from suitable whole-blood donors or by plasmaphaeresis. It contains no preservative. It has an average potency of not less than 80 units per container.

A yellow solid. On thawing it becomes a yellow, very viscous, gummy liquid. **Store** at or below −18° in hermetically-sealed containers. Thaw to 20° to 37° before use; store the liquid at room temperature and use within 6 hours of thawing; use within 4 hours of opening the container and administer with equipment that includes a filter. The expiration date is not later than 1 year from the date of collection of the source material.

A thaw-siphon technique for production of cryoprecipitate concentrate of factor VIII provided a higher *in vitro* content of factor VIII reaching 70 to 100%.— E. C. Mason, *Lancet*, 1978, *2*, 15.

A discussion of problems in the manufacture and supply of factor VIII concentrates.— *Br. med. J.*, 1978, *2*, 1450. See also D. E. G. Austen *et al.* (letter), *Lancet*, 1981, *2*, 1167 (manufacturers' labelling discrepancies); T. W. Barrowcliffe and D. P. Thomas (letter), *ibid.*, 1342 (growing improvement in the relationship between measured and labelled potency).

Details of the collection of factor VIII by phaeresis. The yield was approximately 7 times that which would have been obtained from whole blood donation by the same donors and could bring the benefits of reduced donor exposure and thus reduced risk of hepatitis to haemophiliacs, and to patients with fibrinogen deficiency and von Willebrand's disease.— B. C. McLeod *et al.* (preliminary communication), *Lancet*, 1980, *2*, 671.

Units. 1.1 units of blood coagulation factor VIII are contained in 14.02 mg in one ampoule of the second International Standard Preparation (1976). One unit is approximately equivalent to the antihaemophilic activity of 1 ml of pooled plasma.

Adverse Effects and Precautions. The risk of transmission of viral hepatitis type B (see p.321) may be fairly high when fractions from pooled plasma are used, but the risk is lower from single donor pools. Allergic reactions and haemolysis have been reported.

Some haemophiliacs develop antibodies to factor VIII which interfere with effective treatment. Patients undergoing surgery should first be tested for the presence of such antibodies.

In haemophiliacs with endogenous circulating coagulation inhibitors, infusion of antihaemophilic globulin increased the inhibitor titre and its use should, if possible, be avoided.— *Br. med. J.*, 1972, *4*, 628.

Prolongation of bleeding time in patients with haemophilia A treated with antihaemophilic globulin.— A. H. Sutor and C. Jesdinsky-Buscher, *Dt. med. Wschr.*, 1976, *101*, 1715, per *J. Am. med. Ass.*, 1977, *237*, 819.

Adverse reactions occurred in 10 of 53 patients who received an average of 40 000 units of freeze-dried concentrates of factor VIII and in 5 of 17 patients who received the same amount of cryoprecipitate. Effects included anaphylactic or febrile reactions, urticaria, angioedema, nausea, headache, light-headedness and visual disturbances. Antihistamines, prednisone and isoprenaline were routinely supplied to haemophiliacs receiving out-patient therapy.— M. E. Eyster *et al.* (letter), *Ann. intern. Med.*, 1977, *87*, 248. The use of antihistamines could lead to more severe bleeding.— W. G. Hocking, *ibid.*, *88*, 130.

There were signs of disseminated intravascular coagulation in one haemophiliac patient that might have been provoked by the simultaneous administration of cryoprecipitated antihaemophilic factor with a preparation providing factor-VIII-inhibitor bypassing activity.— S. Stenbjerg and J. Jørgensen (letter), *Lancet*, 1977, *1*, 360.

Twenty-five of 47 patients with haemophilia, who had received factor VIII at least once in the preceding year, had persistent abnormalities of liver function. Liver biopsies of 8 of the 25 revealed cirrhosis in 2 and hepatitis in the other 6, two of whom also had granulomas. The high incidence of liver disease was considered to be associated with the introduction of clotting-factor concentrates to treat haemophilia.— F. E. Preston *et al.*, *Lancet*, 1978, *2*, 592. Comment.— J. A. Spero *et al.* (letter), *ibid.*, 937.

Enhancement of factor VIII coagulant activity by desmopressin, facilitating surgery. The effect was lower with successive doses.— G. Lowe *et al.*, *Lancet*, 1977, *2*, 614. See also F. E. Boulton and A. Smith (letter), *Lancet*, 1979, *2*, 535.

Raised serum thyroxine values in a 15-year-old boy with classical haemophilia were associated with injections of cryoprecipitate which he had been receiving for 5 years for the prevention and treatment of haemarthroses.— J. S. D. Winter and P. J. Smail (letter), *Lancet*, 1980, *2*, 652.

Uses. Patients with haemophilia A have a genetic deficiency of factor VIII and are particularly susceptible to bleeding, which is closely related to the concentration of factor VIII. There is also a deficiency of factor VIII in von Willebrand's disease.

Factor VIII fractions are used as infusions during bleeding episodes in the treatment of patients with haemophilia and in the preparation of such patients for dental and surgical procedures. They are much more potent than fresh plasma and their use reduces the hazard of circulatory overload. The effect of a dose lasts from 8 to 24 hours and to control bleeding a quantity sufficient to raise the concentration of factor VIII to 30 to 50% of that in normal plasma is administered twice daily or more often if necessary. A dose of 1 unit per kg body-weight will raise the concentration of factor VIII by up to 2%. Initial doses commonly used range from 10 to 50 units per kg. Further doses are determined by the clinical response and appropriate laboratory tests. Daily doses are used in von Willebrand's disease.

In patients with circulating antibodies treatment is sometimes withheld for minor bleeding in the hope that they will have regressed (anamnestic response) before any severe haemorrhage occurs. Large doses of factor VIII have sometimes been effective. Immunosuppressants have been used with varying degrees of success. A preparation of factor VIII from bovine or porcine sources is sometimes effective. Some patients with antibodies have responded to treatment with factor IX fraction (see p.328).

Reviews and discussions of factor VIII, haemophilia, and von Willebrand's disease.— N. R. Shulman, *Ann. intern. Med.*, 1977, *86*, 598; A. L. Bloom and I. R. Peake, *Br. med. Bull.*, 1977, *33*, 219; C. R. Rizza, *ibid.*, 225; O. D. Ratnoff, *Ann. intern. Med.*, 1978, *88*, 403; E. A. Jaffe, *New Engl. J. Med.*, 1977, *296*, 377.

Antihaemophilic factor VIII concentrates of intermediate purity included those made by the method of Cohn, glycine precipitation, cryoprecipitation, and freeze-drying. Maximum recommended dosage for human freeze-dried concentrates of intermediate purity containing 4 to 10 units per ml was 50 units per kg body-weight. Freeze-dried concentrates of high purity containing 30 units per ml could be used in higher doses. The biological half-life of factor VIII in haemophilia A was 7 to 18 hours and in von Willebrand's disease 18 to 30 hours. Animal antihaemophilic factor of bovine and porcine origin was extremely effective clinically and could be used for periods of 5 to 8 days. However, it was antigenic and could not be used repeatedly in the same patient; maximum recommended dosage of preparations containing 10 to 15 units of coagulation factors per ml was 80 to 100 units per kg body-weight.— Inherited Blood Clotting Disorders, *Tech. Rep. Ser. Wld Hlth Org. No. 504*, 1972.

The half-lives of 2 factor VIII concentrates were determined during therapy in 26 out-patients with haemophilia. In 17 courses of therapy with one the half-life was between 3 and 13 hours with an average of 7.7 hours, and in 19 courses of therapy with the other the half-life was between 1 and 12 hours with an average of 4.8 hours. Clinical responses were good with both products when adequate factor VIII concentrations were achieved.— C. M. Smith *et al.*, *J. Am. med. Ass.*, 1972, *220*, 1352.

Antihaemophilic therapy should be closely controlled by factor VIII assays. For minor bleeding episodes the circulating factor VIII concentration should be kept up to 20 to 30% of normal for several days. After surgery, 30 to 40% of normal should be maintained for at least 10 days. The amount required could be calculated from the patient's plasma volume and factor VIII concentration. The calculated maintenance dose was doubled initially and then repeated 12-hourly.— P. Schiff, *Med. J. Aust.*, 1973, *1*, 22.

Resistance to factor VIII concentrate in a haemophiliac was overcome by the administration of cyclophosphamide and prednisone.— R. S. Stein (letter), *Ann. intern. Med.*, 1974, *81*, 706. See also D. Green, *Blood*, 1971, *37*, 381, per *Int. pharm. Abstr.*, 1972, *9*, 159. Enhancement by azathioprine and prednisone.— J. C. Vera *et al.*, *J. Am. med. Ass.*, 1975, *232*, 1038.

The diagnosis and treatment of haemophilia and related blood disorders.— R. Biggs, Haemophilia and its Related Conditions: a Brief Guide to Diagnosis and Treatment, *MRC Memo. No. 44*, London, HM Stationery Office, 1974.

Discussions of the treatment of haemophilia in the home.— H. Ekert and E. Smibert, *Med. J. Aust.*, 1974, *1*, 803; B. Le Quesne *et al.*, *Lancet*, 1974, *2*, 507; *Br. med. J.*, 1975, *1*, 417; P. Jones *et al.*, *Br. med. J.*, 1978, *1*, 1447; *Lancet*, 1979, *2*, 77.

Failure of a concentrate of antihaemophilic factor to control bleeding in a patient with von Willebrand's disease; cryoprecipitate was effective.— D. Green and E. V. Potter, *Am. J. Med.*, 1976, *60*, 357. See also P. M. Blatt *et al.*, *J. Am. med. Ass.*, 1976, *236*, 2770.

Studies of human factor VIII had indicated that it contained at least 2 biological activities, antihaemophilic factor (AHF) and von Willebrand factor (VWF); determinations of molecular weights which were about 240 000 and 280 000 respectively and aggregation rates were consistent with the conclusion that they were separate proteins.— J. Newman *et al.*, *Nature*, 1976, *263*, 612.

In a study involving 103 subjects with severe haemophilia, factor VIII in a relatively low dose of 7 to 9 units per kg body-weight was often effective in the early control of mild to moderate haemorrhagic episodes.— J. A. Penner *et al.* (letter), *New Engl. J. Med.*, 1977, *297*, 401.

The management, by plasma exchange, of a patient with factor VIII inhibitor.— B. Angelkort and K. H. Stürner, *Dt. med. Wschr.*, 1979, *104*, 182. See also R. T. Wensley *et al.*, *Br. med. J.*, 1980, *281*, 1388.

In a pilot study involving 27 adult haemophiliacs with arthropathy no difference was noted between a mean initial dose of factor VIII concentrate of 7.3 units per kg body-weight used over a first 6-month period to terminate bleeds and a mean initial dose of 5.5 units per kg used over a second 6-month period. The lower dose represented a very considerable saving in this group of patients prone to frequent haemarthroses.— R. I. Harris and J. Stuart, *Lancet*, 1979, *1*, 93.

In a study involving 6 patients with severe haemophilia on home treatment, 108 bleeding-episodes were treated with approximately 400 units of factor VIII (a mean dose of 5.7 units per kg body-weight), and 99 were treated with approximately 200 units (a mean dose of 3 units per kg). In the high-dose group 16 episodes required a second dose, which controlled the bleeding in all cases, whereas in the low-dose group 29 episodes required a second dose and 3 required a third. These results indicated that a mean dose of factor VIII of 5.7 units per kg is significantly more effective in treating bleeds than a mean dose of 3 units per kg.— M. L. Stirling and R. J. Prescott, *Lancet*, 1979, *1*, 813.

Factor-VIII-loaded liposomes given by mouth to a patient with severe haemophilia raised plasma concentrations of factor VIII to therapeutically effective levels. It took longer for therapeutic concentrations to be reached following oral administration than following intravenous administration, but once achieved the concentrations were also maintained for longer (up to 50 hours).— H. C. Hemker *et al.*, *Lancet*, 1980, *1*, 70. Liposomes might be immunological adjuvants.— J. -J. Morgenthaler (letter), *ibid.*, 1980, *1*, 546.

In a double-blind controlled trial in 55 boys with severe haemophilia, doses of factor VIII of 28 units per kg did not appear to offer any advantage over doses of 14 and 7 units per kg in the treatment of haemarthroses that are not frozen. Ankle bleeds of grades 1 and 2 (and by implication grade 0) can safely be given 7 units per kg. Knee bleeds of grades 1 and 2 are adversely affected by lowering the dose of factor VIII from 14 to 7 units per kg; no inference could be drawn about the correct dose for knee bleeds of grade 0. Elbow bleeds of grade 1 and therefore also grade 0 may be treated with 7 units per kg without harm, but grade-2 elbow bleeds seem to need a higher dose.— A. Aronstam *et al.*, *Lancet*, 1980, *1*, 169.

Findings suggesting that infusion of cryoprecipitate shortened the bleeding time and reduced the complications of bleeding in 7 patients with uraemia associated with an abnormal bleeding tendency. Life-threatening bleeding was controlled in 5 patients and major surgery could be safely performed in 6.— P. A. Janson *et al.*, *New Engl. J. Med.*, 1980, *303*, 1318.

For a proposed naming system for factor VIII to cover its various activities, see Blood-clotting Factors, p.321.

Proprietary Preparations

Factorate *(Armour, UK)*. Dried factor VIII fraction for preparing solutions for intravenous use.

Hemofil *(Travenol, UK)*. Dried factor VIII fraction for preparing solutions for intravenous use.

Humanate (formerly known as Koāte) *(Speywood, UK)*. Dried factor VIII fraction for preparing solutions for intravenous use, available in vials containing 250, 500, or 1000 units, and supplied with Water for Injections.

Hyate:C *(Speywood, UK)*. A preparation of porcine antihaemophilic factor, prepared as a powder for solution immediately before use. Each vial contains approximately 500 units (1 unit is equivalent to 1 ml of normal plasma). It may be used in the treatment of patients with a high titre of factor VIII antibodies. Store at −15°. Protect from light.

Advice on the avoidance of reactions to Hyate: C.— P. B. A. Kernoff and E. G. D. Tuddenham (letter), *Br. med. J.*, 1981, *283*, 381.

Kryobulin *(Immuno, UK)*. Dried factor VIII fraction for preparing solutions for intravenous use, available in vials containing 250, 500, and 1000 units.

Other Proprietary Names

Factorate, Hemofil, Humafac, Koāte (all *USA*).

A factor VIII fraction was also formerly marketed in Great Britain under the proprietary name Profilate (*Abbott*).

1226-k

Dried Factor IX Fraction *(B.P.)*. Dried Human Coagulation Fraction (II, IX and X); Dried Human Factor IX Fraction.

Dried Factor IX Fraction is a sterile dried preparation rich in factors II, IX, and X; it may also contain factor VII. It is obtained from human plasma from suitable subjects (see under Whole Blood, p.322) by a suitable fractionation technique. The fraction is dissolved in an appropriate liquid, **sterilised** by filtration, distributed in sterile containers, and dried from the frozen state. The air is removed or replaced with nitrogen and the containers are sealed to exclude micro-organisms.

Dried Factor IX Fraction is a white or slightly coloured powder or friable solid which is completely **soluble** within 10 minutes in water, when warmed to 18° to 22°. When dissolved in the quantity of Water for Injections stated on the label the resulting solution (pH 6.7 to 8) contains not less than 20 units of factor IX per ml, not less than 0.2 unit per mg of protein, not more than 300 mmol (300 mEq) of sodium ions per litre, not more than 60 mmol (180 mEq) of citrate ions per litre, and not more than 50 mmol of phosphate ions per litre. It may contain heparin not more than 0.15 unit per unit of factor IX.

Store below 6° *in vacuo* or in an atmosphere of nitrogen in sterile containers sealed to exclude micro-organisms and, as far as possible, moisture. Protect from light. It should be used as soon as possible after, and not more than 3 hours after, reconstitution. If a gel forms the fraction should not be used.

1227-a

Factor IX Complex *(U.S.P.)*.

Factor IX Complex is a sterile freeze-dried powder consisting of partially purified factor IX fraction, as well as concentrated factor II, VII, and X fractions of venous plasma obtained from healthy human donors. It contains no preservatives.

Store at 2° to 8° in hermetically-sealed containers. The expiration date is not later than 2 years after manufacture. Use within 4 hours after reconstitution and administer with equipment that includes a filter.

Units. 5.62 units of blood coagulation factor IX are contained in 5.92 mg of a freeze-dried concentrate in one ampoule of the first International Standard Preparation (1976).

Adverse Effects and Precautions. These preparations carry a variable but high risk of viral hepatitis type B (see p.321) even when screened for the presence of hepatitis B antigen; they may also cause intravascular clotting in patients with liver disease. Allergic reactions may occur. Overdosage may cause factors II and X to accumulate.

Factor IX fraction should not be given to patients with disseminated intravascular coagulation without prior treatment with heparin, and should be used with care in patients with liver disease.

In 15 patients with Christmas disease and 12 other patients given factor IX concentrate local reactions occurred in 3 patients but none experienced thrombo-embolisms or thrombophlebitis. Hepatitis occurred in 4 patients. Four patients died; 3 of them had impaired hepatic function.— G. L. Grammens and R. T. Breckenridge (letter), *Ann. intern. Med.*, 1974, *80*, 666.

Fatal thrombo-embolism occurred in a patient after the infusion of a coagulation fraction concentrate containing factors II, VII, IX, and X (Proplex). The concentrate contained factors which accelerated the clotting of plasma. It was considered that these concentrates should not be used in patients disposed to thrombosis or with liver disease and that when used, heparin 5 units per ml of reconstituted material should be added.— P. M. Blatt *et al.*, *Ann. intern. Med.*, 1974, *81*, 766. See also *ibid.*, 852.

Factor IX complex was given to 9 patients with fulminant hepatic failure, 4 of whom also received heparin. All 5 patients not receiving heparin died, with major bleeding as the cause of death in 3. Intravascular coagulation was noted in all patients and there was virtually no improvement in factor IX concentrations.— B. G. Gazzard *et al.*, *Gut*, 1974, *15*, 993.

Three patients with underlying liver disease developed disseminated intravascular coagulation whilst being treated with factor IX concentrate.— A. I. Cederbaum *et al.*, *Ann. intern. Med.*, 1976, *84*, 683.

Post-operative factor IX concentrate administration was associated with deep-vein thrombosis in a 63-year-old man with severe Christmas disease.— S. J. Machin and B. R. Miller (letter), *Lancet*, 1978, *1*, 1367.

Four patients who had received factor IX concentrate on account of liver disease developed non-A non-B hepatitis and 3 died; a further 2 patients with heart disease who had received the factor IX concentrate to correct anticoagulation also developed hepatitis.— R. J. Wyke *et al.*, *Lancet*, 1979, *1*, 520.

Uses. Patients with haemophilia B (Christmas disease) have a genetic deficiency of factor IX and are particularly susceptible to bleeding.

Factor IX fraction or concentrate is used for the treatment of bleeding due to deficiencies of factors IX, II, VII, and X, and in the preparation of such patients for surgery.

Doses are administered every 6 to 24 hours depending on the half-life of factor IX in the individual patient to raise the concentration of factor IX to 5 to 10% (minor bleeding), 15 to 30% (moderate bleeding), or over 50% (surgery) of that in normal plasma. A dose of 1 unit per kg body-weight is reported to raise the concentration by 1%. Initial doses commonly used range from 15 to 75 units per kg. Further doses are determined by the clinical response and appropriate laboratory tests.

Factor IX concentrates have been used, with varying degrees of success, in patients with haemophilia A who have developed antibodies to factor VIII. This may be related to their content (probably variable) of activated factors—factor VIII bypassing activity.

The biological half-life of factor IX was 15 to 30 hours, for factor II 2 to 4 days, for factor VII 4 to 6 hours, and for factor X 30 to 70 hours.— Inherited Blood Clotting Disorders, *Tech. Rep. Ser. Wld Hlth Org. No. 504*, 1972.

A prothrombin complex concentrate rich in factor VII was evaluated in 12 patients with liver disorders and prolonged prothrombin times. Infusion of the concentrate produced short-term immediate correction of coagulation without intravascular coagulation. Results returned to preinfusion values within 24 hours.— G. Green *et al.*, *Lancet*, 1975, *1*, 1311.

Christmas disease. A concentrate containing factors II, VII, IX, and X was used to treat 3 patients with haemophilia B, 1 with congenital factor II deficiency, 1 with congenital factor VII deficiency, and 1 with vitamin-K deficiency. The biological half-life of factor II (slow component) was 4 days, and for factor VII was 2 hours for 1 component and 3 hours for the other. The factor IX level dropped rapidly during the first few hours then began to decrease with the biological half-life of 15 to 30 hours.— P. F. Bruning and E. A. Loeliger, *Br. J. Haemat.*, 1971, *21*, 377.

In 2 patients with severe haemophilia B complicated by inhibitors of factor IX, satisfactory haemostasis and suppression of antibody formation required combined treatment with cyclophosphamide and a large enough dose of factor IX to neutralise the inhibitor and increase the concentration of factor IX to at least 50% of normal.— I. M. Nilsson *et al.*, *Ann. intern. Med.*, 1973, *78*, 91.

Factor VIII inhibition. Factor IX complex (Konyne, Proplex) was effective in the treatment of bleeding episodes in 11 haemophilic and 2 non-haemophilic patients with factor VIII inhibitors. Activated prothrombin complex was about 5 times more active than factor IX complex but was not readily available. The fraction in factor IX complex responsible for its effectiveness against factor VIII inhibitors was not known.— P. Kelly and J. A. Penner, *J. Am. med. Ass.*, 1976, *236*, 2061.

Commercial preparations of factor IX complex (Proplex, *Hyland, USA* and Konyne, *Cutter, USA*) are now relatively free of activated factor VIII and IX and no longer achieve a consistent haemostatic response in haemophilic patients with factor VIII antibodies.— J. A. Penner and C. F. Abildgaard (letter), *New Engl. J. Med.*, 1979, *300*, 565.

In a randomised controlled study of 51 patients with haemophilia A, identified as having factor VIII inhibitors, either of 2 commercial prothrombin complex concentrates (Konyne, *Cutter, USA* and Proplex, *Hyland, USA*) were more effective than albumin placebo in the treatment of acute haemarthroses of the elbow, knee, or ankle. In general, the lots of concentrates tested were judged effective in about half of the episodes of acute bleeding and these concentrates are considered appropriate for use in selected patients until a more effective method of treatment is available.— J. MLusher *et al.*, *New Engl. J. Med.*, 1980, *303*, 421. Comment on the thrombotic potential of prothrombin complex concentrates, including reference to the nonactive prothrombin complex concentrates (Konÿne or Proplex) and the activated prothrombin complex concentrates (Autoplex, *Hyland* and Feiba, *Immuno*).— C. F. Abildgaard (letter), *ibid.*, 1981, *304,* 670. Reply.— J. M. Lusher *et al.* (letter), *ibid.*, 671.

A report of experience with the activated factor IX complex Autoplex (*Travenol*) in the treatment of 4 bleeding episodes in 2 patients with factor VIII antibodies. Autoplex appeared to arrest 2 worsening haemarthroses, a minor intra-oral bleeding lesion, and an early haemarthrosis.— A. Aronstam *et al.* (letter), *Lancet,* 1980, *2,* 1294.

Better results with an activated prothrombin complex concentrate (Feiba) than with a nonactivated prothrombin complex concentrate in patients with haemophilia A and antibodies to factor VIII.— L. J. M. Sjamsoedin *et al.*, *New Engl. J. Med.*, 1981, *305,* 717.

Further references to the use of factor IX concentrates in patients with factor VIII antibodies: E. M. Kurczynski and J. A. Penner, *New Engl. J. Med.*, 1974, *291,* 164; T. Exner and K. A. Rickard (letter), *Med. J. Aust.*, 1976, *1,* 720; G. D. O. Lowe *et al.*, *Br. med. J.*, 1976, *2,* 110; D. A. Price *et al.*, *Aust. N.Z. J. Med.*, 1977, *7,* 286, per *J. Am. med. Ass.*, 1977, *238,* 1970; H. H. Brackmann and J. Gormsen (letter), *Lancet*, 1977, *2,* 933; R. T. DeWitt and D. I. Feinstein, *Archs intern. Med.*, 1977, *137,* 1211; H. Rasche *et al.*, *Dt. med. Wschr.*, 1977, *102,* 319; G. R. Buchanan and S. V. Kevy, *Pediatrics,* 1978, *62,* 767, per *Int. pharm. Abstr.*, 1979, *16,* 364; R. H. Yolken and M. W. Hilgartner, *Am. J. Dis. Child.*, 1978, *132,* 287, per *J. Am. med. Ass.*, 1978, *239,* 1340.

Proprietary Preparations

Proplex *(Travenol, UK).* Dried human factor IX complex for preparing solutions for intravenous use, supplied with 30-ml vials of Water for Injections. (Also available as Proplex in *USA*).

Prothromplex *(Immuno, UK).* Dried factor IX fraction for preparing solutions for intravenous use, available in vials containing 500 units, with Water for injections 10 ml.

1228-t

Dried Factor XIII Fraction.

Dried Fibrin-stabilising Factor; Dried FSF. A sterile dried preparation rich in factor XIII.

Store at 4°. Solutions should be used immediately after preparation.

Uses. Factor XIII deficiency is a genetic disorder. Bleeding, particularly umbilical bleeding, is the chief sign and may occur at concentrations below 2% of normal. Because conventional coagulation tests do not detect the abnormality and because the condition responds readily to small infusions of blood or plasma, the condition may easily be missed.

In replacement therapy a quantity, for an adult, equivalent to about 500 ml of fresh plasma may be given every 4 weeks. For the treatment of severe bleeding a dose equivalent to about 500 to 1000 ml of fresh plasma may be given daily until bleeding ceases. In prophylaxis in surgery the latter dose may be given and followed by the equivalent of 500 to 750 ml of fresh plasma daily for 5 days.

Factor XIII deficiency in Henoch-Schönlein's purpura.— P. Henriksson *et al.*, *Acta paediat. scand.*, 1977, *66,* 273.

A lack of factor XIII was demonstrated in a high percentage of patients with acute leukaemia.— H. Zöller, *Arzneimittel-Forsch.*, 1977, *27,* 1500.

Successful treatment of factor XIII deficiency in a neonate with factor XIII concentrate.— J. Francis and P. Todd, *Br. med. J.*, 1978, *2,* 1532.

A discussion of factor XIII deficiency.— *Lancet,* 1980, *1,* 522. Controversy over the prophylactic management of factor XIII deficiency with special reference to Fibrogammin, *Behringwerke*.— P. Stenberg *et al.* (letter), *Lancet,* 1980, *1,* 1136; S. Stenbjerg (letter), *ibid.*, *2,* 257; P. Stenberg *et al.* (letter), *ibid.*

Factor XIII treatment for scleroderma.— F. Delbarre *et al.* (letter), *Lancet,* 1981, *2,* 204.

Proprietary Preparations

Factor XIII Concentrate *(Hoechst, UK).* Available as powder for preparing intravenous injections, in vials each containing Factor XIII activity equivalent to at least 250 ml of fresh cooled citrated plasma, supplied with 4 ml of Water for Injections.

1229-x

Fibrin Foam.

Human Fibrin Foam *(B.P.C. 1973).*

CAS — 9001-31-4.

A dry artificial sterile sponge of human fibrin. It is prepared by clotting with human thrombin a foam of a solution of human fibrinogen. The clotted foam is dried from the frozen state, cut into strips, and **sterilised** by heating at 130° for 3 hours. It is a firm, light, white, spongy material, which is practically **insoluble** in water. **Store** below 25° in sterile containers sealed to exclude micro-organisms and moisture. Protect from light.

Uses. Fibrin Foam is used in conjunction with thrombin as a haemostatic in surgery at sites where bleeding cannot easily be controlled by the commoner methods of haemostasis. A piece of the foam is saturated with a solution of thrombin in sodium chloride injection and placed in contact with the bleeding points. Blood coagulates in contact with the thrombin in the interstices of the foam. Since all the clotting materials are of human origin, they may be left in place when the wound is closed.

Proprietary Preparations of Animal Fibrin

Absele Absorbable Bone Sealant *(Ethicon, UK).* A sterile paste containing stabilised bovine fibrin 17.5%, solubilised bovine collagen 17.5%, dextran '70' 8%, and glycerol 30%. For controlling bleeding from bone during surgery.

Biethium *(Ethicon, UK).* An absorbable prosthesis material with haemostatic properties, formed from stabilised ox fibrin and glycerol; the rate of absorption is controlled by cross-linking with formaldehyde.

1230-y

Dried Fibrinogen *(B.P.).*

Dried Human Fibrinogen; Factor I.

Dried Fibrinogen is a sterile dried preparation of the soluble constituent of liquid human plasma from suitable subjects (see under Whole Blood, p.322) which, on the addition of thrombin, is transformed into fibrin, the insoluble protein which forms the matrix of a clot of human blood. It has a molecular weight of 330 000 to 350 000.

It is prepared by a suitable fractionation technique. The fraction is dissolved in an appropriate liquid, **sterilised** by filtration, distributed in sterile containers, and dried from the frozen state. The air is removed or replaced with nitrogen and the containers are sealed to exclude micro-organisms. It is a white powder or friable solid, **soluble** in water to form an almost colourless slightly turbid liquid which clots on the addition of thrombin. No bactericide or antibiotic is added. **Store** below 25° in an atmosphere of nitrogen in sterile containers sealed to exclude micro-organisms and, as far as possible, moisture. Protect from light.

When Dried Fibrinogen is dissolved in the volume of Water for Injections stated on the label, the resulting solution (pH 7 to 8) contains 1 to 1.5% w/v of fibrinogen, comprising not less than 70% of the total protein present, and not more than 200 mmol (200 mEq) of sodium per litre and not more than 55 mmol (165 mEq) of citrate ions per litre. Dried Fibrinogen is reconstituted, immediately before use, by dissolving the sterile contents of a sealed container in the requisite amount of Water for Injections. It should not be used if a gel forms on reconstitution. It should be administered with suitable equipment such as that described in Section 3 or Section 4 of *Transfusion Equipment for Medical Use,* BS 2463: 1962.

Fibrinogen 200 mg was 'physically incompatible' with metaraminol 20 mg or promazine 100 mg in 100 ml of dextrose injection.— R. D. Dunworth and F. R. Kenna, *Am. J. Hosp. Pharm.*, 1965, *22,* 190.

Purified human fibrinogen could be frozen and refrozen repeatedly without altering its biological properties.— E. Regoeczi and B. A. Stannard, *Biochim. biophys. Acta,* 1969, *181,* 287, per *J. Am. med. Ass.*, 1969, *209,* 302.

Adverse Effects. The use of fibrinogen carries a high risk of transmitting viral hepatitis type B (see p.321).

Uses. Dried Fibrinogen has been used to control haemorrhage associated with low blood-fibrinogen concentration in afibrinogenaemia or hypofibrinogenaemia but the use of plasma or cryoprecipitate is often preferred. It has also been used in disseminated intravascular coagulation (the defibrination syndrome). The usual dose is 2 to 8 g, by slow intravenous infusion, as a 1 to 2% solution.

Fibrinogen has also been used as a solution in conjunction with human thrombin to fix nerve sutures and to assist the adhesion of skin and mucous membrane grafts.

The biological half-life of fibrinogen was reported to be 3 to 5 days.— Inherited Blood Clotting Disorders, *Tech. Rep. Ser. Wld Hlth Org. No. 504,* 1972.

All licences for fibrinogen in the USA had been withdrawn. There were few valid indications and a high incidence of hepatitis B. Cryoprecipitated antihaemophilic factor was an adequate source of fibrinogen.— *FDA Drug Bull.*, 1978, *8,* 15.

A review of diagnosis of deep-vein thrombosis including details of the fibrinogen-uptake test.— N. Browse, *Br. med. Bull.*, 1978, *34,* 163.

Preparations

Dried Fibrinogen for Isotopic Labelling *(B.P.).* Dried Human Fibrinogen for Isotopic Labelling. A sterile dried preparation of fibrinogen prepared from liquid human plasma from suitable donors (see under Whole Blood, p.322) by a suitable fractionation technique. When dissolved in the volume of Water for Injections stated on the label not less than 90% of the total protein consists of clottable protein. It complies with limit tests for plasmin and thrombin activity. The solution should be used immediately after reconstitution. Store at 2° to 8° in an atmosphere of nitrogen in sterile containers sealed to exclude micro-organisms and, as far as possible, moisture. Protect from light.

1231-j

Normal Immunoglobulin Injection *(B.P.).*

Human Normal Immunoglobulin Injection; Human Gamma Globulin; Human Normal Immunoglobulin *(Eur. P.)*; Immunoglobulinum Humanum Normale.

Normal Immunoglobulin Injection is a sterile preparation containing almost all the gamma-G globulins of the source material together with smaller amounts of either other plasma proteins or other globulins of placental origin, depending on the source. It contains the antibodies normally present in adult human subjects.

Normal Immunoglobulin Injection is obtained from the plasma or serum of healthy human subjects or from the normal intact placentas or retroplacental blood from healthy women. It is prepared from pooled material from not fewer than 1000 donors by a suitable fractionation technique known to yield a product that does not transmit infection and that, at a protein concentration of 16%, contains at least 2 antibodies (viral and bacterial, against for example poliomyelitis virus, streptolysin O, staphylococcal alpha-toxin, diphtheria toxin, tetanus toxin) in a concentration at least 10 times that of the original pooled material. No antibiotics are added to plasma, serum, or placentas used for preparation; if added to retroplacental blood the method of preparation should ensure the removal of the antibiotic and its metabolites. Preservatives and stabilising agents may be added in preparing the final bulk material. The gamma-G globulin fraction is dissolved in a suitable liquid, **sterilised** by filtration and distributed in sterile containers which are sealed to exclude micro-organisms.

Normal Immunoglobulin Injection is a clear pale yellow or light brown fluid which may become slightly turbid and in which occasional particles may appear on keeping. pH (of a solution containing 1% of protein) 6.4 to 7.2. It contains 10 to 17% of protein.

Store at 2° to 8°. Protect from light. Under these conditions it may be expected to maintain its potency for not less than 3 years.

It may also be prepared as a freeze-dried white to slightly yellowish powder or a solid friable mass, containing not more than 1% of water; it is completely **soluble** in water. **Store** below 25° under vacuum in an atmosphere of nitrogen in sterile containers, sealed to exclude micro-organisms and, as far as possible, moisture. Protect from light. Under these conditions it may be expected to retain its potency for not less than 5 years. The freeze-dried preparation should be used immediately after reconstitution.

NOTE. The *B.P.* states that when Human Gamma Globulin Injection or Human Gamma-G Immunoglobulin is prescribed or demanded, Normal Immunoglobulin Injection shall be dispensed or supplied.

1232-z

Immune Globulin *(U.S.P.)*. Immune Human Serum Globulin; Immune Serum Globulin (Human).

A sterile solution of globulins that contain many antibodies normally present in human adult blood. It is prepared from pooled material (approximately equal quantities of blood, plasma, serum, or placentas) from not fewer than 1000 donors. It contains 15 to 18% of protein, of which not less than 90% is gamma globulin. It contains glycine as a stabiliser, and a suitable preservative. It contains antibodies against diphtheria, measles, and poliomyelitis.

A transparent or slightly opalescent almost odourless liquid, colourless or brownish in colour because of denatured haemoglobin. A slight granular deposit may develop during storage. **Store** at 2° to 8°. The expiration date is not later than 3 years from release from manufacturer's cold storage.

Adverse Effects. Allergic reactions may occur rarely. Pain and tenderness at the site of intramuscular injection are more common.

Immunoglobulin injections should not be given intravenously, since they had produced tachycardia, respiratory distress, facial flushing, a sensation of pressure in the chest, and pain, particularly in patients with an antibody-deficiency syndrome. Chills, fever, pallor, and malaise might follow the initial reaction. In severe reactions, vomiting and circulatory failure might ensue. When injected intramuscularly, discomfort after large-volume injections was the only common reaction, but occasionally urticaria, angioneurotic oedema, and local inflammation might follow. Shock-like reactions have been extremely rare after intramuscular injection. Prior administration of antihistamines to suspected reactors had reduced the incidence and severity of reactions.— C. A. Janeway and F. S. Rosen, *New Engl. J. Med.*, 1966, *275*, 826.

Many samples of normal immunoglobulin injection contained anti-Rh_0(D) isoagglutinin. This might explain positive direct antihuman globulin tests in many burnt patients.— G. E. Lang and B. Veldhuis, *Am. J. clin. Path.*, 1973, *60*, 205, per *J. Am. med. Ass.*, 1973, *226*, 808.

In 6 patients with IgA deficiency (5 also had hypogammaglobulinaemia) treatment for 3 to 8 years with immunoglobulin did not stimulate the formation of anti-IgA associated with anaphylactic reactions.— J. Koistinen *et al.*, *Br. med. J.*, 1978, *2*, 923.

A technique involving the use of amethocaine, for avoiding the severe pain associated with intramuscular injection of immunoglobulin.— B. Kendrick (letter), *Lancet*, 1979, *2*, 1366.

Normal immunoglobulin injection supplied by the National Blood Transfusion Service contained about 150 mg of IgG per ml and 0.01% of thiomersal; the expiry date was 4 years after manufacture. In 15 samples the thiomersal content varied widely and was reduced with age; in 3 samples near the expiry date no thiomersal was detected. The disappearance of thiomersal was probably due to adsorption on the glass and stopper. In 26 patients with agammaglobulinaemia maintained on normal immunoglobulin injection for 0.5 to 17 years the calculated total dose of thiomersal administered was 8 to 1482 mg. Concentrations of mercury in the urine exceeded 30 µg per litre (the normal upper limit) in 19 patients; there was no overt evidence of mercury toxicity.— M. R. Haeney *et al.*, *Br. med. J.*, 1979, *2*, 12.

Transmission of hepatitis. A report of epidemic hepatitis B following administration of human immunoglobulin. Of 325 persons inoculated, 123 developed jaundice. Batches of the immunoglobulin available for inspection were heavily contaminated.— T. J. John *et al.*, *Lancet*, 1979, *1*, 1074.

Uses. Normal immunoglobulin injection is used for the short-term prevention or modification of some infectious diseases. It is given by intramuscular injection.

For the prevention of viral hepatitis type A (infectious hepatitis) the usual dose is 0.02 to 0.04 ml per kg body-weight; doses of 0.06 to 0.12 ml per kg have been given after massive exposure, with immunity then lasting 4 to 6 months.

For the prevention of rubella in pregnant women exposed to risk the usual dose is 20 ml; it is not recommended for routine prophylaxis. For the prevention of measles the usual dose is 0.2 ml per kg, given within 5 days of exposure; protection lasts about 3 weeks. For the modification of the disease 0.04 ml per kg may be given.

In hypogammaglobulinaemia doses of 1.3 ml per kg (with a maximum of 60 ml) have been given over 48 hours and half this amount repeated every 3 to 4 weeks.

It has been given in doses of up to about 300 ml in the first week after burns, with daily doses of 15 to 30 ml up to the tenth day.

Doses of 0.5 to 1 ml per kg have been given, with antibiotics, in severe bacterial infections, and repeated several times a month.

Preparations of immunoglobulin injection are available (see below) containing high titres of antibody for protection against the erythrocyte factor Rh_0(D), viral hepatitis type B, measles, pertussis, rabies, tetanus, or vaccinia.

For the use of immunoglobulin injection to provide passive protection against arboviruses, see *Arboviruses and Human Disease*, Report of a WHO Scientific Group, *Tech. Rep. Ser. Wld Hlth Org. No. 369*, 1967.

For a review of the uses of human immunoglobulin in premature infants, in antibody-deficiency syndromes, and bacterial and viral infections, see T. M. Pollock, *Br. med. Bull.*, 1969, *25*, 202.

The biological half-life of immunoglobulin was 340 hours.— W. A. Ritschel, *Drug Intell. & clin. Pharm.*, 1970, *4*, 332.

In 5 patients devoid of antibody to *Escherichia coli* there was a reduction in the frequency of their infections after treatment with immunoglobulin injection.— A. D. B. Webster *et al.*, *Br. med. J.*, 1974, *3*, 16.

Gamma globulin from pooled maternal blood sources improved the survival-rates of presensitised kidney transplants.— R. R. Riggio *et al.*, *Lancet*, 1978, *1*, 233.

Immune serum globulins as therapeutic agents.— E. R. Stiehm, *Pediatrics*, 1979, *63*, 301.

The use of immune plasma in Argentine haemorrhagic fever.— J. I. Maiztugui *et al.* (preliminary communication), *Lancet*, 1979, *2*, 1216.

Administration. Immunoglobulin injection should normally be given by intramuscular injection. If it was necessary to give it intravenously it should be diluted with at least 2 volumes of sodium chloride injection and given very slowly.— *Br. med. J.*, 1977, *1*, 521.

Discussion of some formulations of immunoglobulin injection suitable for intravenous use.— *Lancet*, 1979, *2*, 1168.

Slow subcutaneous infusion in 3 patients.— M. Berger *et al.*, *Ann. intern. Med.*, 1980, *93*, 55.

Safety and patient acceptability of intravenous immune globulin in 10% maltose.— H. D. Ochs *et al.*, *Lancet*, 1980, *2*, 1158.

Further references: B. M. Alving and J. S. Finlayson (Ed.), *Immunoglobulins: Characteristics and Uses of Intravenous Preparations*, Washington D.C., US Government Printing Office, 1980.

Agammaglobulinaemia. Immunoglobulin had been used effectively for patients with congenital and acquired agammaglobulinaemia. Invasive bacterial infection was prevented by raising the concentration of immunoglobulin in serum by about 2 g per litre, but in practice initial divided doses of 300 mg per kg body-weight (to raise the serum concentration by 3 g per litre) were used, with monthly supplements of 100 mg per kg.— C. A. Janeway and F. S. Rosen, *New Engl. J. Med.*, 1966, *275*, 826.

After a 10-year study of 176 patients with primary hypogammaglobulinaemia it was suggested that a dose of 25 mg per kg body-weight of human normal immunoglobulin should be given weekly to patients with hypogammaglobulinaemia, but that consideration should be given to increasing the dose to 50 mg per kg in patients who continued to get severe infections. Reactions occurred on 85 occasions in 33 patients; most were mild but a few were severe, and 1 patient died.—Report of a MRC Working-party, *Lancet*, 1969, *1*, 163.

A report of 5 patients with hypogammaglobulinaemia and polyarthritis responsive to gamma globulin.— A. D. B. Webster *et al.*, *Br. med. J.*, 1976, *1*, 1314.

The use, intravenously, of S-sulphonated gammaglobulin in congenital agammaglobulinaemia.— S. Miyazaki *et al.* (letter), *Lancet*, 1978, *1*, 283.

Chicken-pox. Reports favouring the use of zoster immunoglobulin or zoster immune plasma in children at risk from chicken-pox.— H. H. Balfour, *Am. J. Dis. Child.*, 1977, *131*, 693, per *J. Am. med. Ass.*, 1977, *237*, 2865; R. Winsnes, *Acta paediat. scand.*, 1978, *67*, 77, per *Drugs*, 1979, *17*, 507; A. P. Waterson, *Br. med. J.*, 1979, *2*, 564 (treatment within 3 days).

A study indicating that zoster immune globulin is largely ineffective in preventing the development of chicken-pox in high-risk contacts. In most, however, the disease was only mild, indicating that zoster immune globulin may modify its course. High-risk contacts should therefore still be given the immune globulin. All of 11 infants whose mothers had chicken-pox or zoster 5 or more days before delivery had varicella-zoster antibody at birth and none developed chicken-pox, indicating that such infants do not require protection.— E. B. Evans *et al.*, *Lancet*, 1980, *1*, 354. The author writing on behalf of the MRC Working Party on Leukaemia in Childhood considered that zoster immune globulin must be regarded as a life-saver for susceptible children on immunosuppressive therapy.— R. S. Lane *et al.* (letter), *ibid.*, 705.

In a double-blind study in 13 immunocompromised patients, zoster immune globulin was no more effective in the treatment of cutaneous disseminated zoster than placebo.— K. E. Groth *et al.*, *J. Am. med. Ass.*, 1978, *239*, 1877.

Hepatitis, viral type A. Normal immunoglobulin was very effective in preventing infectious hepatitis in schools and other institutions. The incidence of infectious hepatitis and jaundice was 0.9 per 100 among 2050 inoculated subjects and 2.6 per 100 among 2053 controls. No protection was given for the first 2 weeks after injection.—A Report to the Director of the Public Health Laboratory Service, *Br. med. J.*, 1968, *3*, 451.

A single dose of 750 mg of normal immunoglobulin was given to 1079 Voluntary Service Overseas recruits, about a week before departure for work in developing countries, as a prophylactic measure against infectious hepatitis. It provided immunity for 6 months, but was not sufficient for longer periods.— T. M. Pollock *et al.*, *Lancet*, 1969, *1*, 281.

The doses of Immune Serum Globulin *U.S.P.* [XVIII] recommended by the Public Health Service Advisory Committee on Immunization Practices for the prevention of viral hepatitis type A were: 0.022 ml per kg body-weight intramuscularly for prophylaxis or within 6 weeks of contact; 0.11 ml per kg for travellers planning to stay 3 or more months in tropical areas or developing countries, repeated every 4 to 6 months.— *Ann. intern. Med.*, 1972, *77*, 427.

Immunoglobulin was not recommended routinely for travellers using ordinary tourist routes for a proposed stay of less than 3 months. For remote areas the following doses should be given once intramuscularly: up to 23 kg body-weight, 0.5 ml; 23 to 45 kg, 1 ml; more than 45 kg, 2 ml. For a prolonged stay, or in areas where viral hepatitis type A was common or the risk of contamination was greater the doses were 1, 2.5, and 5 ml respectively.— *Br. med. J.*, 1975, *1*, 567.

Immune Serum Globulin (of immune-adherence haemagglutination titre 1:10 000) 0.044 ml per kg body-weight had a significant effect in preventing clinical disease during an outbreak of hepatitis A in a hospital for the mentally retarded.— W. T. Hall and D. L. Madden (letter), *New Engl. J. Med.*, 1977, *296*, 1478.

Studies of batches of immune serum globulin manufactured by 6 USA manufacturers between 1967 and 1977 demonstrated an increase both in the percentage of batches which contained an antibody titre to hepatitis A virus of 1:100 or more, as well as increases in the titres of the antibodies.— L. A. Smallwood *et al.* (letter), *Lancet*, 1980, *2*, 482. See also G. G. Frösner *et al.* (letter), *Lancet*, 1977, *1*, 432.

Lassa fever. The use of Lassa immune serum in Lassa fever.— A. J. Clayton, *Bull. Wld Hlth Org.*, 1977, *55*, 435.

Meningococcal infection. A favourable report of the prophylactic value of gamma globulin.— V. I. Pokrovskii *et al.*, *J. Hyg. Epidem. Microbiol. Immun.*, 1978, *22*, 230, per *Abstr. Hyg.*, 1979, *54*, 433.

Mumps. The radial haemolysis test, if generally available, would identify adult contacts of mumps without antibody and permit the rational use of mumps immune globulin.— P. P. Mortimer, *Br. med. J.*, 1978, *2*, 1523.

Rubella. Reports indicating that normal immunoglobulin was not of value in protecting against rubella.—Report of the Public Health Laboratory Service on Rubella, *Br. med. J.*, 1968, *3*, 203 and 206. Report of the Public Health Laboratory Service Working Party on Rubella, *Br. med. J.*, 1970, *2*, 497.

Immune serum globulin might be used when rubella occurred in a woman who would not consider termination of pregnancy.— Center for Disease Control, *Ann. intern. Med.*, 1978, *88*, 543. See also C. S. Peckham, *Br. med. J.*, 1974, *1*, 259; *ibid.*, 1975, *1*, 566.

In 39 susceptible subjects the antibody response to rubella vaccine was reduced or delayed in those given high-titre rubella immunoglobulin intramuscularly (750 mg protein) simultaneously, compared with those given vaccine only. This protective effect was recommended for those susceptible pregnant women who came into contact with rubella and for whom therapeutic abortion was unacceptable.— G. E. D. Urquhart *et al.*, *Br. med. J.*, 1978, *2*, 1331.

Proprietary Preparations

Gamma Globulin Kabi *(KabiVitrum, UK).* Normal immunoglobulin, available for intramuscular injection as a solution containing 16% of protein in ampoules of 2 and 5 ml.

Other Proprietary Names

Gamastan, Gammagee, Gammar, Immu-G; Immuglobin *(all USA).*

1233-c

Anti-D (Rh_0) Immunoglobulin Injection

(B.P.). Anti-D (Rh_0) Immunoglobulin; Anti-D Immunoglobulin; Anti-Rh_0 (D) Immune Globulin; Rh Immunoglobulin; Rho (D) Immune Globulin (Human). Anti-D (Rh_0) Immunoglobulin Injection is a sterile preparation of the incomplete antibody against the rhesus D antigen of human red blood cells. It may also contain incomplete antibodies against other rhesus antigens and traces of antibodies against the A and B antigens of red blood cells.

It is obtained from pooled liquid plasma from suitable human subjects (see under Whole Blood, p.322) who have been deliberately or naturally immunised against the rhesus D antigen. It is prepared from not less than 50 litres of plasma by a suitable fractionation technique. No bactericide or antibiotic is added during preparation. The separated globulins are dissolved in a suitable liquid which may contain thiomersal 0.01% or other suitable bactericide. If necessary Normal Immunoglobulin Injection may be added to bring the total protein concentration above 3% but not above 17%. The solution is **sterilised** by filtration. It is a clear pale yellow or light brown liquid which may become slightly turbid and in which occasional particles may appear on keeping. pH 6.4 to 7.2. **Store** at 2° to 8° in sterile containers sealed to exclude micro-organisms. Protect from light.

1234-k

Rh_0 (D) Immune Globulin

(U.S.P.). Rh_0 (D) Immune Human Globulin; Rh_0 (D) Immune Globulin (Human). A sterile solution of globulins derived from human blood plasma containing antibody to the erythrocyte factor Rh_0 (D). It contains 10 to 18% of protein, of which not less than 90% is gamma globulin. It contains glycine as a stabilising agent, and a suitable preservative.

An almost odourless, almost colourless, clear or slightly opalescent liquid; a slight granular deposit may develop on storage.

Store at 2° to 8°. The expiration date is not more than 6 months after release from manufacturer's cold storage, or not more than 1 year after manufacture.

Units. 300 units of anti-D immunoglobulin are contained in 14.76 mg of human immunoglobulin, containing 60 µg of anti-D immunoglobulin, in one ampoule of the first International Reference Preparation (1976).

The activity of the first International Reference Preparation of human anti-D immunoglobulin was inadvertently incorrectly calibrated in the original collaborative assay. The activity of 150 international units originally stated to be contained in each ampoule was incorrect though the stated content of 60µg in each ampoule was correct. On the basis of a more recent collaborative assay the activity of the contents of one ampoule was 300 international units.— WHO Expert Committee on Biological Standardization, Thirtieth Report, *Tech. Rep. Ser. Wld Hlth Org. No. 638*, 1979. Collaborative study.— H. H. Gunson *et al.*, *J. clin. Path.*, 1980, *33*, 249.

Adverse Effects and Precautions. Anti-D immunoglobulin should not be administered to rhesus-positive or rhesus-immunised mothers or to infants as it may cause haemolysis.

An injection of anti-D immunoglobulin was given to an infant at the 30th hour of life instead of to the mother. The child developed moderate jaundice which disappeared progressively. In a similar incident in another infant there were no clinical symptoms.— G. Sansone and G. Veneziano (letter), *Lancet*, 1970, *1*, 952.

Uses. Anti-D (Rh_0) immunoglobulin is used to prevent a rhesus-negative mother actively forming antibodies to foetal rhesus-positive red blood cells that may pass into the maternal circulation during childbirth or abortion. In subsequent rhesus-positive children these antibodies could produce haemolytic disease of the newborn. The injection of anti-D immunoglobulin is not effective once the mother has formed anti-D antibodies.

Anti-D immunoglobulin should always be given to rhesus-negative mothers with no anti-D antibodies in their serum and who have delivered rhesus-positive infants. It should be given intramuscularly as soon as possible in a dose of 500 units (100 µg) although a higher dose may be required depending on the amount of transplacental bleeding as assessed by the Kleihauer test. The dose should be given within 60 hours of delivery, but may still be worth while several days later.

Rhesus-negative women having spontaneous or induced abortions should be given 250 units (50 µg) within 60 hours if the duration of pregnancy is 20 weeks or less; if the pregnancy is more advanced 500 units (100 µg) should be given.

There is a risk of sensitisation during pregnancy from threatened abortion, amniocentesis, or external version. Any rhesus-negative woman at risk of transplacental haemorrhage during pregnancy and not known to be sensitised should be given 250 to 500 units (50 to 100 µg) of anti-D immunoglobulin without delay.

Anti-D immunoglobulin is also given after the transfusion of Rh-incompatible blood; up to 50 units (10 µg) may be given for each ml of blood transfused; the dose may be stopped when free antibody is detected in the patient's plasma.

For an extensive review of the preparation, properties, and uses of anti-D immunoglobulin, see Prevention of Rh Sensitization, *Tech. Rep. Ser. Wld Hlth Org. No. 468*, 1971. See also *Memorandum on Haemolytic Disease of the Newborn*, London, HM Stationery Office, 1976.

Further reviews and discussions: M. G. Davey, *Med. J. Aust.*, 1975, *2*, 263; *Br. med. J.*, 1978, *2*, 307; J. Nusbacher and J. R. Bove, *New Engl. J. Med.*, 1980, *303*, 935.

Anti-D immunoglobulin was given, under double-blind conditions, to 1800 Rh-negative women who had born an Rh-positive infant and who were at risk of isoimmunisation; doses of 200, 100, 50, and 20 µg were given respectively to groups of about 450 patients, within 36 hours of delivery. The incidence of positive anti-Rh sera in the mothers 6 months after delivery was 0.22, 0.23, 0.44, and 1.35% respectively in the 4 groups. In 807 patients followed to a second pregnancy with a Rh-positive infant, the incidence of positive anti-Rh sera in the mothers was 1.5, 1.1, 1.5, and 2.9% respectively in the 4 dosage groups. A dose of 20 µg appeared to be suboptimal; a dose of 100 µg appeared to be adequate.—Report to the MRC by the Working Party on the Use of Anti-D Immunoglobulin for the Prevention of Isoimmunization of Rh-negative Women during Pregnancy, *Br. med. J.*, 1974, *2*, 75.

Follow-up of 53 infants born to 40 rhesus-negative mothers in whom anti-D immunoglobulin had failed to provide protection from sensitisation following a rhesus-positive pregnancy suggested that they were less severely affected than would have been expected. Comparison with a series of first-affected cases recorded before anti-D immunoglobulin was available confirmed this.— L. A. D. Tovey and A. E. Robinson, *Br. med. J.*, 1975, *4*, 320.

A discussion on the genetics and function of the Rh system.— M. Stroup, *Mayo Clin. Proc.*, 1977, *52*, 141.

The standard Australian dose of 125 µg of anti-D might not be adequate to prevent sensitisation when the estimated volume of foetal cells in the maternal circulation exceeded 5 ml; this might occur in induced labour, forceps delivery, assisted removal of the placenta, stillbirth, ectopic pregnancy, or operative delivery.— J. U. Barrie (letter), *Med. J. Aust.*, 1977, *2*, 814.

The use of up to 2 mg of anti-D immunoglobulin in women with large transplacental haemorrhages.— P. H. Renton and R. A. Riches (letter), *Br. med. J.*, 1978, *2*, 634.

Anti-D immunoglobulin should be given at the first sign of bleeding in threatened abortion and could be repeated if the patients aborted, or in 2 to 3 weeks.— J. M. Scott *et al.* (letter), *Br. med. J.*, 1978, *2*, 827.

The incidence of iso-immunisation in Rh-negative women was reduced by the routine introduction of antenatal prophylaxis with anti-D immunoglobulin injection at 28 weeks' gestation.— J. M. Pollock, *Can. med. Ass. J.*, 1978, *118*, 627. See also A. Zipursky, *ibid.*, 609; J. M. Bowman *et al.*, *ibid.*, 623.

Because a substantial number of women were immunised during pregnancy, when anti-D given postnatally was ineffective, there was a strong case for an antenatal anti-D programme.— C. Clarke and A. G. W. Whitfield, *Br. med. J.*, 1980, *280*, 903. A contrary view.— G. H. Tovey, *Lancet*, 1980, *2*, 466. See also R. Mitchell *et al.* (letter), *ibid.*, 798.

A case for the antenatal administration of anti-D immunoglobulin to primigravidae.— L. A. D. Tovey and J. M. Taverner, *Lancet*, 1981, *1*, 878.

Further references: A Combined Study from Centres in England and Baltimore, *Br. med. J.*, 1971, *2*, 607; J. C. Woodrow *et al.*, *Br. med. J.*, 1971, *2*, 610; P. A. Hensleigh *et al.*, *Am. J. Obstet. Gynec.*, 1977, *129*, 413; L. A. D. Tovey *et al.*, *Br. med. J.*, 1978, *2*, 106; J. Nusbacher and J. R. Bove, *New Engl. J. Med.*, 1980, *303*, 935; J. M. Bowman (letter), *ibid.*, 1981, *304*, 425; C. Huggins *et al.* (letter), *ibid.*, 426; C. A. Clarke and A. G. W. Whitfield (letter), *ibid.*; J. Nusbacher and J. R. Bove (letter), *ibid.*

Blood transfusion. Three Rh-negative women who were inadvertently transfused with Rh-positive blood were successfully treated with large doses of anti-D immunoglobulin. A suggested dose was not more than 1 mg, in divided doses, for each 40 ml of Rh-positive blood.— J. Eklund and H. R. Nevanlinna, *Br. med. J.*, 1971, *3*, 623.

For transplacental bleeding or mismatched transfusions

exceeding 10 ml of packed red cells, the dose of anti-D immunoglobulin should be calculated on 25 μg for each ml of packed red cells.— P. Schiff, *Med. J. Aust.*, 1973, *1*, 22.

Further references: L. Keith *et al.*, *Am. J. Obstet. Gynec.*, 1976, *125*, 502, per *J. Am. med. Ass.*, 1976, *236*, 1303.

Proprietary Names

Gamulin Rh, HypRho-D, MICRhoGam, RhoGam *(all USA)*.

1235-a

Antihepatitis B Immunoglobulin Injection. Hepatitis B Immune Globulin *(U.S.P.)*.

Antihepatitis B immunoglobulin injection is a sterile solution, free from turbidity, of globulins derived from the plasma of human donors who have high titres of antibodies against hepatitis B surface antigen. It contains 10 to 18% of protein of which not less than 80% is monomeric immunoglobulin G; it contains glycine as a stabilisng agent, and a suitable preservative. pH (of a solution containing 1% of protein) 6.4 to 7.2.

Store at 2° to 8°. The minimum expiration date is not later than one year after manufacture.

Units. 50 units of antihepatitis B immunoglobulin are contained in one ampoule of the first International Reference Preparation (1977).

The US Reference Preparation was a 16.4% protein solution with an anti-HBs titre of 1:100 000 by radioimmunoassay. A dilution of this preparation had been lyophilised from a 9.1 to 9.2% protein solution and was distributed as the WHO Reference Preparation, to which a unitage of 100 units per ml had been assigned. Study of 247 lots of normal immunoglobin manufactured in the USA in 1967–72 showed low titres (radioimmunoassay) of anti-HBs. It had been requested that they should contain anti-HBs in a titre of at least 1:100 and all of 76 lots manufactured in 1979 had such a content.— R. J. Gerety *et al.*, *Bureau of Biologics, FDA* (letter), *New Engl. J. Med.*, 1980, *303*, 529.

Adverse Effects. As for Normal Immunoglobulin Injection, p.330.

Uses. Antihepatitis B immunoglobulin injection is used to provide passive immunity in persons exposed to hepatitis B virus; circulating antibodies persist for about 3 months.

It is used in persons who have been exposed to hepatitis B virus parenterally, by mucous membrane contact, or by oral ingestion. Reports of its value are not unanimous.

The usual dose is 0.06 ml per kg body-weight, given intramuscularly as soon as possible after exposure (preferably within 7 days) and repeated 28 to 30 days after exposure.

It has been used for the control of hepatitis B in dialysis units. Its use in acute fulminant hepatitis B and in the chronic HBsAg carrier state has been discouraging.

Reviews and discussions on the use of antihepatitis B immunoglobulin.— *Morb. Mortal.*, 1977, *26*, 425 and 441, per *Abstr. Hyg.*, 1978, *53*, 726; A. M. Prince, *New Engl. J. Med.*, 1978, *299*, 198; T. -W. Chang and D. R. Snydman, *Drugs*, 1979, *18*, 354; S. Krugman *et al.*, *New Engl. J. Med.*, 1979, *300*, 101.

In 279 patients undergoing cardiac surgery and receiving a mean of 12 blood transfusions there were 24 probable (47 possible) cases of hepatitis and 10 cases of icteric hepatitis. The incidence of post-operative icteric hepatitis was significantly greater in those given a placebo pre-operatively than in those given normal immunoglobulin or normal immunoglobulin with a high titre of hepatitis B antibody; there was no significant difference between the protective effects of the 2 immunoglobulin preparations.— R. G. Knodell *et al.*, *Lancet*, 1976, *1*, 557.

Studies on the infectivity of blood positive for *e* antigen and DNA polymerase indicated that these factors must be considered for the full evaluation of immunoprophylactic measures for hepatitis B.— H. J. Alter *et al.*, *New Engl. J. Med.*, 1976, *295*, 909.

In 2 nurses hepatitis B immune serum globulin, given 7 hours after infection, delayed but did not prevent the appearance of clinical hepatitis 25 to 30 weeks later.— J. P. Wauters and M. Leski, *Br. med. J.*, 1976, *2*, 19. See also G. G. Frösner *et al.* (letter), *Lancet*, 1977, *2*, 1023.

In a controlled double-blind study involving 419 subjects who were accidentally exposed to hepatitis type B, treatment with hepatitis B immunoglobulin 5 ml (anti-HBs titre of 1:100 000 by passive haemagglutination) by intramuscular injection within 7 days of exposure, followed in most cases by a second injection 28 days later, was more effective for the prevention of acute hepatitis than normal immunoglobulin administered similarly. Of the 216 subjects who received hepatitis B immunoglobulin 3 developed acute type B hepatitis, and seroconversion alone occurred in 12. Of 203 subjects who received normal immunoglobulin 12 developed acute type B hepatitis and in 42 seroconversion occurred. The difference between the two treatments was significant and hepatitis B immunoglobulin was considered to be the better therapy for preventing acute hepatitis B infection.— L. B. Seef *et al.*, *Ann. intern. Med.*, 1978, *88*, 285. See also J. H. Hoofnagle *et al.*, *ibid.*, 1979, *91*, 813.

The overall incidence of hepatitis was 12.3%, 10.2%, and 9.8% in 3 groups of workers (totalling 435) after known exposure and who were given normal-titre (1:50 by passive haemagglutination), intermediate-titre (1:5000), or high-titre (1:100 000 to 1:500 000) immunoglobulin. Based upon a total study population of 757 the incidence of hepatitis in the 3 groups was 6.8%, 6.2%, and zero at 4 months, and 8.7%, 7.3%, and 7.2% at 9 months. Re-exposure probably accounted for only 20% of the cases in the high-titre group and it was considered that the immunoglobulin had merely deferred the onset of the disease.— G. F. Grady *et al.*, *J. infect. Dis.*, 1978, *138*, 625.

Of 1000 staff members regularly given hepatitis B immunoglobulin, 23 developed hepatitis; in 21 the interval between injections was 66 to 110 days. Treatment not less than every 2 months was advisable.— D. Kleinknecht *et al.* (letter), *New Engl. J. Med.*, 1978, *299*, 1254.

Studies suggested that hepatitis B immunoglobulin should be given within 2 days after parenteral exposure, and within 7 days after oral ingestion.— S. Krugman (letter), *New Engl. J. Med.*, 1979, *300*, 625.

Hospital workers (322) accidentally exposed to hepatitis B surface antigen (HBsAg) were given 500 mg (5 ml of a solution containing 10% of protein) of an immunoglobulin with a high titre of antibody (HBsAb) to HBsAg (titre of 1:16 000 to 1:32 000 by passive haemagglutination) within 14 days of exposure; 240 were followed for 9 to 12 months. Of the 219 without pre-existing HBsAb, 7 developed hepatitis 16 to 23 weeks after exposure—3 mild, 4 moderately severe—in one patient HBsAg persisted 6 months after the onset of illness. HBsAg was not detected in the serum of any worker without clinical illness. Of 142 samples of sera tested one month after the accident, 140 showed passive HBsAb. Three patients who had received HBsAg-positive transfusions were similarly treated. Two patients who had received renal transplants from the same donor received 1 g of immunoglobulin, repeated in one patient after a month; neither developed hepatitis. The immunoglobulin was considered to be protective.—A Combined Medical Research Council and Public Health Laboratory Service Report, *Lancet*, 1980, *1*, 6.

The use of hepatitis B immunoglobulin for the protection of a patient inadvertently given HBsAg-positive plasma.— M. Telischi *et al.*, *J. Am. med. Ass.*, 1980, *244*, 2312.

Fulminant hepatitis. The administration of hepatitis B immunoglobulin 1.32 g (in later patients 5.28 g) to 53 patients with fulminant type B hepatitis with stage II to IV encephalopathy was no more beneficial than a placebo in a double-blind study.— Acute Hepatic Failure Study Group, *Ann. intern. Med.*, 1977, *86*, 272.

Neonatal hepatitis. A study indicating that administration of hepatitis B immunoglobulin to infants of HBsAg-positive mothers within 48 hours after birth and thereafter monthly for 6 months can prevent a chronic HBsAg carrier state. None of 21 such infants given hepatitis B immunoglobulin, 0.5 ml per kg body-weight within 48 hours after birth and 0.16 ml per kg monthly for 6 months therafter, became HBsAg positive, whereas 5 of 20 untreated children did.— H. W. Reesink *et al.*, *Lancet*, 1979, *2*, 436. Failure of a very similar dosage regimen to prevent the carrier state in a Chinese infant.— E. H. Boxall *et al.* (letter), *ibid.*, 1980, *1*, 419.

Discussion on the prevention of transmission of hepatitis B from mother to infant.— *Lancet*, 1980, *1*, 237.

Use in dialysis units. Hepatitis immune globulin, high-titre (1:500 000 by passive haemagglutination, falling to 1:100 000), medium-titre (1:5000) or normal titre (1:50) was given to 284 patients and 282 staff in renal dialysis units and repeated 4 months later. The incidence of hepatitis B in patients at 8 months was significantly lower in those who received the high-titre material; at 12 months, however, the difference was no longer significant; the effect in staff was broadly similar. The onset of disease was possibly delayed.— A. M. Prince, *J. infect. Dis.*, 1978, *137*, 131.

A favourable report in 10 children.— F. Bläker *et al.*, *Archs Dis. Childh.*, 1977, *52*, 421.

Proprietary Names

H-BIG *(Abbott, USA)*; Hep-B-Gammagee *(Merck Sharp & Dohme, USA)*; HyperHep *(Cutter, USA)*.

1236-t

Antimeasles Immunoglobulin Injection. Human Antimeasles Immunoglobulin; Immunoglobulinum Humanum Antimorbillicum; Human Measles Immunoglobulin *(Eur.P.)*. A preparation containing specific antibodies against the measles virus.

Antimeasles immunoglobulin injection is a liquid or freeze-dried product which may be prepared from a pool of plasma from persons convalescent from or immunised against measles; it contains not less than 50 units of measles antibody per ml, and complies with the requirements for Normal Immunoglobulin Injection (see p.329), except for pool size.

Store at 2° to 10° as for Normal Immunoglobulin Injection (see p.329).

Uses. Antimeasles immunoglobulin injection has been used to prevent or modify measles in susceptible persons who have been exposed to infection. It has been used in children in hospital or with severe or chronic illness. The usual prophylactic dose in adults and children is 0.25 ml per kg body-weight intramuscularly within 6 days after exposure; for modification of an attack the usual dose is 0.05 ml per kg.

1237-x

Antipertussis Immunoglobulin Injection. Pertussis Immune Globulin *(U.S.P.)*; Pertussis Immune Globulin (Human). Antipertussis immunoglobulin injection is a sterile solution of globulins derived from the plasma of adult human donors who have been immunised with pertussis vaccine. It contains glycine as a stabilising agent, and a suitable preservative.

An almost odourless, almost colourless, clear or slightly opalescent liquid; a slight granular deposit may develop on storage.

Store at 2° to 8°. The expiration date is not later than 18 months after release from the manufacturer's cold storage.

Adverse Effects. As for Normal Immunoglobulin Injection, p.330.

Uses. Antipertussis immunoglobulin injection has been given for the passive prophylaxis of pertussis; 1.25 ml is given as soon as possible after exposure and repeated 1 week later.

It has also been given therapeutically—1.25 ml is given initially and repeated every day or two while necessary.

In a controlled double-blind study of 74 children with whooping cough, generally in the first week of the paroxysmal stage, there was no difference in the rate of recovery of patients who received either 2.5 ml of pertussis immune globulin or placebo.— R. Balagtas *et al.*, *J. Pediat.*, 1971, *79*, 203, per *Int. pharm. Abstr.*, 1972, *9*, 890.

Proprietary Names

Hypertussis *(Cutter, USA)*.

1238-r

Antirabies Immunoglobulin Injection *(B.P.)*. Human Antirabies Immunoglobulin Injection; Antirabies Immunoglobulin; Human Rabies Immunoglobulin; Rabies Immune Globulin (Human).

Antirabies immunoglobulin injection is a sterile preparation of human immunoglobulins which specifically neutralises the infectivity of rabies virus. It is obtained from pooled liquid plasma from suitable human subjects (see under Whole Blood, p.322) who have been vaccinated with Rabies Vaccine, by a suitable fractionation technique. No bactericide or antibiotic is added during preparation. The separated globulins are dissolved in a suitable liquid which may contain thiomersal 0.01% or other suitable bactericide. If necessary Normal Immunoglobulin Injection may be added to bring the total protein concentration above 3% but not above 17%. The solution is **sterilised** by filtration. It contains not less than 80 units per ml.

It is a clear pale yellow or light brown liquid which may become slightly turbid and in which occasional particles may appear on keeping. pH 6.4 to 7.2

Store at 2° to 8° in sterile containers sealed to exclude micro-organisms. Protect from light.

1239-f

Rabies Immune Globulin *(U.S.P.)*.

Rabies immune globulin is a sterile solution of globulins derived from plasma or serum, which has been tested for the absence of hepatitis B surface antigen, from selected adult human donors who have been immunised with rabies vaccine and have developed high titres of rabies antibody. It contains 10 to 18% of protein of which not less than 80% is monomeric immunoglobulin G; it contains glycine as a stabilising agent, and a suitable preservative. It contains not less than 110 units per ml.

An almost colourless, almost odourless, slightly opalescent liquid; a slight granular deposit may develop on storage. pH (of a solution containing 1% of protein) 6.4 to 7.2

Store at 2° to 8°. The expiration date is not later than 1 year after release from manufacturer's cold storage.

Units. The unit for antirabies immunoglobulin injection is based on the first International Standard Preparation (1955) of equine antirabies serum; 86.6 units are contained in approximately 86.6 mg in one ampoule.

Adverse Effects. As for Normal Immunoglobulin Injection, p.330.

Uses. Antirabies immunoglobulin injection is used in conjunction with Rabies Vaccine (see p.1604) for prophylaxis in persons who have suffered major bites (multiple bites or bites on the face, head, neck, or finger) or licks of the mucosa by an animal rabid or suspected of being rabid. A single dose of 20 units per kg bodyweight is given intramuscularly and by infiltration around the wound.

Proprietary Names

Hyperab *(Cutter, USA)*.

1240-z

Antitetanus Immunoglobulin Injection.

(B.P.). Human Antitetanus Immunoglobulin Injection; Antitetanus Immunoglobulin; Tetanus Immunoglobulin; Immunoglobulinum Humanum Antitetanicum; Human Tetanus Immunoglobulin *(Eur. P.)*; Human Tetanus Antitoxin.

Antitetanus immunoglobulin injection is a sterile preparation of human immunoglobulins containing specific antibodies against the toxin of *Clostridium tetani*.

It is obtained from pooled liquid plasma of healthy human subjects who have been immunised against tetanus; it contains not less than 50 units of tetanus antitoxin per ml. It is prepared similarly to Normal Immunoglobulin Injection, except that the pooled material may be from fewer than 1000 donors.

It is a clear pale yellow or light brown fluid which may become slightly turbid and in which occasional particles may appear on keeping. pH (of a solution containing 1% of protein) 6.4 to 7.2. It contains 10 to 17% of protein.

Store at 2° to 8°. Protect from light. Under these conditions it may be expected to retain its potency for not less than 3 years. The dried preparation should be stored below 25° under vacuum or in an atmosphere of nitrogen in a sterile container sealed to exclude micro-organisms, and, as far as possible, moisture. Protect from light. Under these conditions it may be expected to retain its potency for not less than 5 years.

1241-c

Tetanus Immune Globulin *(U.S.P.)*.

Tetanus Immune Human Globulin; Tetanus Immune Globulin (Human).

Tetanus Immune Globulin is a sterile solution of globulins derived from the plasma of adult human donors who have been immunised with tetanus vaccine. It contains not less than 50 units of tetanus antitoxin per ml. It contains 10 to 18% of protein of which not less than 90% is gamma globulin; it contains glycine as a stabilising agent, and a suitable preservative.

An almost odourless, almost colourless, clear or slightly opalescent liquid; a slight granular deposit may develop on storage.

Store at 2° to 8°. The expiration date (for material containing a 10% excess of potency) is not later than 3 years from release from manufacturer's cold storage.

Units. The unit for antitetanus immunoglobulin is based on the second International Standard Preparation (1969) of equine tetanus antitoxin; 1400 units (1000 Lf-equivalents for flocculation) are contained in 47 mg in one ampoule.

Adverse Effects and Precautions. There may be transient tenderness and inflammation at the site of injection and local reactions may occur in patients with antibody-deficiency syndromes. Allergic reactions are rare. Antitetanus immunoglobulin may be contra-indicated in patients with a history of reactions to normal immunoglobulin. Antitetanus immunoglobulin should not be injected into the same site or in the same syringe as a tetanus vaccine.

Uses. Antitetanus Immunoglobulin Injection is used to confer passive immunity to tetanus on individuals at risk from wounds who have not received at least 2 previous doses of tetanus vaccine. It is preferred to equine antitoxin. In the usual dose of 250 units intramuscularly it maintains the concentration of immunoglobulin above the protective level of 0.01 unit per ml for about 4 weeks. When more than 24 hours have passed since wounding or in heavily infected wounds the dose is 500 units, irrespective of immunisation history. Unimmunised or incompletely immunised patients should be given a dose of Adsorbed Tetanus Vaccine (p.1609) and active immunisation completed later.

Doses of 30 to 300 units per kg body-weight have been given in the treatment of tetanus.

For recommendations on the use of antitetanus immunoglobulin see *Med. Lett.*, 1973, *15*, 39 and 64; D. W. Fraser, *Ann. intern. Med.*, 1976, *84*, 95.

In the prophylactic treatment of tetanus surgical toilet of the wound was of prime importance for all wounds and was usually sufficient for wounds less than 6 hours old, clean, not penetrating, and with negligible tissue damage. Patients with more serious wounds should be given antitetanus immunoglobulin 250 units intramuscularly unless fully immunised (a complete course or a reinforcing dose within the last 5 years); if such a course or reinforcing dose had been completed within 5 to 10 years a further reinforcing dose of vaccine would suffice. Opportunity should be taken to establish, complete, or reinforce basic immunisation. Antibiotics were generally needed only for the treatment of sepsis.— J. W. G. Smith *et al.*, *Br. med. J.*, 1975, *3*, 453.

In severely burnt patients, protection might be delayed because of loss of antibody into oedema or exudate.— E. J. L. Lowbury *et al.*, *J. Hyg., Camb.*, 1978, *80*, 267, per *Abstr. Hyg.*, 1978, *53*, 686.

Tetanus treatment. Discussion of the use of antitetanus immunoglobulin.— *Lancet*, 1974, *1*, 51. The prophylaxis and treatment of tetanus.— R. S. Edmondson, *Br. J. Hosp. Med.*, 1980, *23*, 596. See also D. Caro and E. Shaw (letter), *Br. med. J.*, 1974, *1*, 389; *ibid.*, 1974, *2*, 553.

Comparability of equine tetanus antitoxin 10 000 units and antitetanus immunoglobulin 500 units in the treatment of tetanus neonatorum in 130 infants.— G. H. McCracken *et al.*, *Lancet*, 1971, *1*, 1146.

In a study of 60 infants with tetanus neonatorum, treatment with antitetanus immunoglobulin 150 units intrathecally, with equine tetanus antitoxin 20,000 units intravenously and 20,000 units intramuscularly, was no more effective in reducing the mortality-rate, days in hospital, and days of sedation than the same doses of tetanus antitoxin given alone.— M. R. Sedaghatian, *Archs Dis. Childh.*, 1979, *54*, 623.

Failure of intracisternal injection of antitetanus immunoglobulin in tetanus.— B. J. Vakil *et al.*, *Trans. R. Soc. trop. Med. Hyg.*, 1979, *73*, 579.

In addition to standard care, 49 patients with mild grade tetanus were given antitetanus immunoglobulin 250 units intrathecally, while 48 similar patients were given 1000 units intramuscularly. Only 3 patients in the intrathecal group progressed to moderate and severe grade, and only 1 died; of those who merely received an intramuscular injection, 15 got worse and 10 died. It was concluded that in patients with tetanus, treated before the onset of spasms, intrathecal human antitetanus immunoglobulin can help arrest the progress of the disease.— P. S. Gupta *et al.*, *Lancet*, 1980, *2*, 439. Comment.— *ibid.*, 464.

Further references: J. M. Adams *et al.*, *Pediatrics*, 1979, *64*, 472.

Proprietary Preparations

Humotet *(Wellcome, UK)*. Antitetanus immunoglobulin injection containing tetanus antitoxin 250 units in each ml, available in vials of 1 ml

Other Proprietary Names

Homo-Tet, Hu-Tet, Hyper-Tet, Immu-Tetanus, Tet-Conn-G *(all USA)*.

1242-k

Antivaccinia Immunoglobulin Injection *(B.P.)*.

Human Antivaccinia Immunoglobulin Injection; Antivaccinia Immunoglobulin; Vaccinia Immunoglobulin; Immunoglobulinum Humanum Antivaccinicum; Human Antivaccinia Immunoglobulin; Human Vaccinia Immunoglobulin *(Eur. P.)*.

Antivaccinia Immunoglobulin injection is a sterile preparation of human immunoglobulins containing specific antibodies against the vaccinia virus. It is obtained from pooled liquid plasma of healthy human subjects who have been recently vaccinated against smallpox; it contains not less than 500 units of vaccinia antibody per ml. It is prepared similarly to Normal Immunoglobulin Injection, except that the pooled material may be from fewer than 1000 donors.

It is a clear pale yellow or light brown fluid which may become slightly turbid and in which occasional particles may appear on keeping. pH (of solution containing 1% of protein) 6.4 to 7.2. It contains 10 to 17% of protein.

Store at 2° to 8°. Protect from light.

NOTE. When Smallpox Immunoglobulin is prescribed or demanded Antivaccinia Immunoglobulin Injection is dispensed or supplied.

1243-a

Vaccinia Immune Globulin *(U.S.P.)*. Vaccinia Immune Human Globulin; Vaccinia Immune Globulin (Human). Vaccinia Immune Globulin is a sterile solution of globulins derived from the plasma of adult human donors who have been immunised with smallpox vaccine. It contains 15 to 18% of protein of which not less than 90% is gamma globulin; it contains glycine as a stabilising agent, and a suitable preservative.

An almost odourless, almost colourless, clear or slightly opalescent liquid; a slight granular deposit may develop on storage.

Store at 2° to 8°. The expiration date is not later than 3 years after issue.

Units. The unit for antivaccinia immunoglobulin injection is based on the first International Standard Preparation (1965) of human antismallpox serum; 1000 units are contained in 84.3 mg in one ampoule.

Uses. Antivaccinia Immunoglobulin Injection is used in the treatment of patients with generalised vaccinia and also those with accidental vaccinia infection endangering the eye. It has been given simultaneously with smallpox vaccine but in the opposite arm when vaccination was required in patients in whom it would normally be contra-indicated. It has also been used to provide passive protection against smallpox when there was not sufficient time to protect contacts.

Auto-infection or infection with smallpox vaccine in children could be treated by immediate intramuscular injection of the specific immunoglobulin and the use each hour of eye-drops of diluted immunoglobulin injection for 36 to 48 hours.— E. C. Cowan, *Practitioner*, 1970, *204*, 72.

Of 431 patients given Antivaccinia Immunoglobulin prophylactically, 427 had no complications, 1 child developed eczema vaccinatum and 3 of 22 pregnant women in the group aborted. Treatment of another 230 patients for complications after vaccination was successful in 206 who improved rapidly within 48 hours; 19 others improved after further treatment, and 5 patients died.— J. C. M. Sharp and W. B. Fletcher, *Lancet*, 1973, *1* 656.

Antivaccinia immunoglobulin should be given, in addition to vaccination, as soon as possible to contacts who had not been traced and vaccinated within 3 days of exposure, to those in whom re-vaccination had not taken, to those never vaccinated, and to those not vaccinated within the previous 5 years. The dose was: under 1 year, 0.5 g; 1 to 6 years, 1 g; 7 years and over, 1.5 g. It should also be given when it was necessary to vaccinate a pregnant woman or a person in whom vaccination would normally be contra-indicated. The dose was: under 1 year, 0.25 g; 1 to 6 years, 0.5 g; 7 to 14 years, 0.75 g; 15 years and over, 1 g.— *Memorandum on the Control of Outbreaks of Smallpox*, Department of Health and Social Security, London, HM Stationery Office, 1975. Antivaccinia immunoglobulin should be given as soon as possible to contacts who had not been traced and vaccinated within 3 days of exposure, to those in whom re-vaccination had not taken, to those never vaccinated and to those not vaccinated within the previous 5 years. The dose was: under 1 year, 2000 units; 1 to 6 years, 4000 units; 7 years and over, 6000 units. It should also be given when it was necessary to vaccinate a pregnant woman or a person in whom vaccination would normally be contra-indicated. The dose was: under 1 year, 2000 units; 1 to 6 years, 4000 units; 7 to 14 years, 6000 units; 15 years and over, 8000 units.— *Memorandum on the Control of Outbreaks of Smallpox*, Scottish Home and Health Department, Edinburgh, HM Stationery Office, 1976..

In 917 patients with adverse reactions to smallpox vaccine and given vaccinial immune globulin the response, when known, was usually good except in erythema multiforme in which 13 of 70 patients had a poor or no response.— B. J. Feery, *Med. J. Aust.*, 1977, *2*, 180.

1244-t

Leucocytes. White blood cells (leucocytes) include granulocytes (neutrophils, eosinophils, and basophils), monocytes, and lymphocytes.

Leucophaeresis involves the preparation, by centrifugation or filtration procedures, of concentrates of granulocytes which are infused into patients (usually leukaemic) with granulocytopenia and infections not responsive to other treatments.

Lymphocytes play a vital role in the immunological response.

Evidence that the risks of prophylactic granulocyte transfusions during remission-induction chemotherapy in acute myelogenous leukaemia outweigh the benefits.— R. G. Strauss *et al.*, *New Engl. J. Med.*, 1981, *305*, 597.

Some references to reports and discussions of leucophaeresis.— D. R. Boggs, *New Engl. J. Med.*, 1974, *290*, 1055; J. P. Isbister and J. C. Biggs, *Med. J. Aust.*, 1976, *1*, 748; *Br. med. J.*, 1976, *2*, 662; J. G. Pole *et al.*, *Archs Dis. Childh.*, 1976, *51*, 521; R. Medenica *et al.*, *Schweiz. med. Wschr.*, 1976, *106*, 1369, per *J. Am. med. Ass.*, 1977, *237*, 82; H. Young *et al.*, *Cancer*, 1977, *40*, 1037; J. E. Curtis *et al.*, *Can. med. Ass. J.*, 1977, *117*, 341; R. H. Herzig *et al.*, *New Engl. J. Med.*, 1977, *296*, 701; J. B. Alavi *et al.*, *ibid.*, 706; D. R. Boggs, *ibid.*, 748; R. A. Clift *et al.*, *New Engl. J. Med.*, 1978, *298*, 1052; J. M. Goldman *et al.*, *Br. med. J.*, 1979, *1*, 1310; J. M. Ford *et al.* (letter), *New Engl. J. Med.*, 1980, *302*, 583; M. S. Rosenshein *et al.*, *New Engl. J. Med.*, 1980, *302*, 1058.

The successful use of leucophaeresis to remove white blood cells and so reduce symptoms caused by associated hyperviscosity in 3 of 6 patients with leukaemia.— F. E. Preston *et al.*, *Br. med. J.*, 1978, *1*, 476.

1253-x

Fresh Frozen Plasma *(B.P.)*. Fresh Frozen Plasma for Infusion.

Fresh Frozen Plasma is prepared from the supernatant fluid which is separated by centrifuging from Whole Blood from a single donor. It contains not less than 50% of the factor VIII activity of the Whole Blood. It is distributed in sterile containers which are immediately sealed and cooled to −30° or below as rapidly as possible and, in any case, within 18 hours of collection.

When thawed it is a light to dark straw-coloured liquid which may be turbid due to the presence of fat. **Store** at a temperature of −30° or below until required for use except for any period (not exceeding 30 minutes) necessary for transportation. The label states the ABO group and the Rh group of the Whole Blood from which it was obtained and the nature of the specific antisera used in testing. It should be used within 3 hours of thawing and should not be refrozen. It should not be used if there is visible evidence of deterioration. It should be administered with suitable equipment such as that described in Section 3 and Section 4 of *Transfusion Equipment for Medical Use*, BS 2463: 1962.

1245-x

Dried Plasma *(B.P.)*. Dried Human Plasma *(Eur. P.)*; Plasma Humanum Cryodesiccatum.

Dried Plasma is prepared from the supernatant fluid which is separated by centrifuging or by standing from Whole Blood from suitable subjects (see under Whole Blood, p.322). Plasma from not more than 12 donors may be pooled. It is distributed in sterile containers and dried from the frozen state. The air is removed or replaced by nitrogen and the containers are sealed.

Dried Plasma is a sterile, pale to deep cream-coloured powder or friable agglomerate, which is completely **soluble** within 10 minutes, in the volume of Water for Injections stated on the label. Such a solution is yellow and is free from visible particles and from haemolysis, and contains not less than 4.5% w/v of protein.

Store below 25° under vacuum or in an atmosphere of nitrogen in sterile containers sealed to exclude micro-organisms and, as far as possible, moisture. Protect from light. It should be used as soon as possible after, and not more than 3 hours after, reconstitution.

When reconstituted, it should be administered with suitable equipment such as that described under Section 3 or Section 4 of *Transfusion Equipment for Medical Use*, BS 2463: 1962.

Adverse Effects. As for Whole Blood, p.322. Plasma prepared from large pools carries a high risk of transmitting viral hepatitis type B (see p.321).

Thrombocytopenic purpura developed in a 77-year-old woman 8 days after receiving 2 units of plasma. A platelet isoantibody was identified and it was probable that the plasma she had received contained platelet fragments. Treatment with corticosteroids was unsuccessful but exchange transfusion with whole blood removed most of the antibody and the platelet count returned to normal.— P. L. Cimo and R. H. Aster, *New Engl. J. Med.*, 1972, *287*, 290.

Pooled plasma had been banned in the USA because of the high risk of transmission of hepatitis.— *Med. Lett.*, 1972, *14*, 89.

Allergic pulmonary oedema after transfusion with fresh frozen plasma.— P. C. O'Connor *et al.*, *Br. med. J.*, 1981, *282*, 379.

Uses. Dried Plasma dissolved in a volume of Water for Injections equivalent to the volume of the liquid plasma from which it was prepared, gives a reconstituted plasma which is mainly used for the restoration of plasma protein or volume in patients suffering from burns, scalds, crush injuries, or peripheral circulatory failure. It is also used in emergencies when Whole Blood is not available or while awaiting the results of compatibility tests.

Fresh plasma or fresh frozen plasma contains useful amounts of clotting factors and is used as a source of factor V for the treatment of parahaemophilia and for the preparation of concentrates of factor VIII fraction (see p.326). It is also used in patients with haemostatic defects caused by liver disease and as a source of pseudocholinesterase for overcoming the prolonged action of suxamethonium chloride in persons deficient in pseudocholinesterase.

Plasma exchange or plasmaphaeresis (the terms are commonly used synonymously) involves the removal of blood, anticoagulation, centrifugation, and the return to the patient of the cellular components suspended in a suitable vehicle such as fresh frozen plasma or plasma protein fraction. There is moderate defibrinogenation and decrease in other clotting factors, and a decrease in concentrations of immunoglobulins and immune complexes.

For a discussion of the uses of plasma, see *Lancet*, 1972, *2*, 1130.

Fresh plasma in a dose of 12 to 15 ml per kg bodyweight could be used to produce a rise of factor IX of 7 to 10%.— *Lancet*, 1973, *2*, 648.

Fresh frozen plasma was suitable for the treatment of intravascular coagulation in haemorrhagic shock when heparin was contra-indicated.— H. J. Hehne *et al.*, *Schweiz. med. Wschr.*, 1976, *106*, 671, per *J. Am. med. Ass.*, 1976, *236*, 523.

A 15-year-old boy suffering acute rejection of a transplanted heart despite standard immunosuppressant therapy improved after receiving a transfusion of 2 units of plasma from a patient whose plasma contained powerful *immunodepressive factors*.— A. S. Coulson *et al.*, *Br. med. J.*, 1976, *1*, 749. See also T. Bednarik *et al.*, *Čslká Farm.*, 1978, *27*, 39, per *Int. pharm. Abstr.*, 1978, *15*, 1123.

A comparison of the value of fresh frozen plasma and plasma protein fraction in patients with massive burns.— J. W. Alexander *et al.*, *J. Trauma*, 1979, *19*, 502.

For a report of an International Commission on Ebola haemorrhagic fever in Zaire, and the use of plasma containing antibodies in the treatment of 2 patients, see *Bull. Wld Hlth Org.*, 1978, *56*, 271. See also *ibid.*, 247.

After receiving a renal transplant a 17-year-old boy became critically ill with cytomegalovirus pneumonitis. Recovery followed administration of a total of 1800 ml of hyperimmune plasma.— B. A. C. Dijkmans *et al.* (letter), *Lancet*, 1979, *1*, 820.

The use of convalescent plasma in the treatment of Lassa fever.— D. J. Grundy *et al.* (letter), *Lancet*, 1980, *2*, 649.

Haemophilia. Fresh human plasma containing 0.6 unit of coagulation factors per ml could be used in the treatment of patients with haemophilia A to raise the plasma level of factor VIII to 15 to 20%. Maximum recommended dosage of plasma was 20 ml per kg bodyweight.— Inherited Blood Clotting Disorders, *Tech. Rep. Ser. Wld Hlth Org. No. 504*, 1972.

Hereditary angioneurotic oedema. Two patients with hereditary angioneurotic oedema improved dramatically after treatment with infusions of 400 ml of fresh frozen plasma.— R. J. Pickering *et al.*, *Lancet*, 1969, *1*, 326.

There were no significant complications in 6 patients with hereditary angioneurotic oedema undergoing dental surgery. Each patient had received infusions of fresh frozen plasma 1 day before surgery.— C. J. Jaffe *et al.*, *J. Allergy & clin. Immunol.*, 1975, *55*, 386, per *J. Am. med. Ass.*, 1975, *233*, 1433.

Liver perfusion solution. The use of plasma in perfusing cadaver livers.— R. Y. Calne and R. Williams, *Br. med. J.*, 1968, *4*, 535. See also J. H. Peacock *et al.*, *ibid.*, 1969, *1*, 349.

Plasma exchange and plasmaphaeresis. Discussions, including reference to its use in Goodpasture's syndrome, haemophilia (high inhibitor titre) hypercholesterolaemia, hyperviscosity syndrome with paraproteinaemia, myasthenia gravis, nephritis, Raynaud's syndrome, rejection of renal transplants, Rh sensitisation, systemic lupus erythematosus, thrombotic thrombocytopenic purpura, and idiopathic thrombocytopenic purpura: *Br. med. J.*, 1978, *1*, 1011 (myasthenia gravis); N. A. Buskard, *Can. med. Ass. J.*, 1978, *119*, 681; A. J. Pinching, *Br. J. Anaesth.*, 1979, *51*, 21; *Lancet*, 1980, *1*, 688 (systemic lupus erythematosus); *Lancet*, 1980, *2*,

241.

Other conditions.— G. Remuzzi *et al.*, *Lancet*, 1978, *2*, 871 (haemolytic-uraemic syndrome); R. P. Brettle *et al.* (letter), *Lancet*, 1978, *2*, 1100 (Guillain-Barré syndrome); P. Dandona *et al.*, *Br. med. J.*, 1979, *1*, 374 (Graves' disease); F. B. Gibberd *et al.*, *Lancet*, 1979, *1*, 575 (heredopathia atactica polyneuritiformis); M. Muggeo, *New Engl. J. Med.*, 1979, *300*, 477 (insulin resistance); S. Eriksson and S. Lindgren (letter), *New Engl. J. Med.*, 1980, *302*, 809 (primary biliary cirrhosis); D. Shaw *et al.*, *Br. med. J* 1980, *281*, 1459 (sweating and pruritus in malignant disease).

Thrombocytopenic purpura. An 18-year-old woman with thrombotic thrombocytopenic purpura resistant to corticosteroids, antiplatelet agents, and splenectomy, responded to exchange transfusions of whole human blood and obtained a dramatic response to plasma infusions. Since she did not respond to infusions of washed red cells and albumin it was considered that the whole human blood transfusions had replaced some deficiency in her plasma rather than removed some toxic substance. The finding that thrombotic thrombocytopenic purpura can be controlled with plasma might pertain to many patients.— J. J. Byrnes and M. Khurana, *New Engl. J. Med.*, 1977, *297*, 1386. The response might have been due to platelets.— R. L. Hanzlick *et al.* (letter), *ibid.*, 1978, *298*, 971. Failure of fresh frozen plasma infusion in the treatment of one patient with thrombotic thrombocytopenic purpura.— J. Ansell *et al.*, *Ann. intern. Med.*, 1978, *89*, 647.

1246-r

Plasma Protein Fraction *(B.P.)*. Human Albumin Fraction (Saline); Human Plasma Protein Fraction.

Plasma Protein Fraction is a sterile solution of the proteins of liquid human plasma, containing albumin and globulins which retain their solubility on heating. It is prepared from pooled liquid plasma from suitable human subjects (see under Whole Blood, p.322) by a suitable fractionation technique, sufficient sodium caprylate or other suitable substances being added to stabilise the protein to heat and sodium chloride to adjust the content of the sodium ions to 130 to 160 mmol (130 to 160 mEq) per litre. It is **sterilised** by filtration and distributed aseptically into containers, which are sealed to exclude micro-organisms and maintained at 59.5° to 60.5° for 10 hours to prevent the transmission of hepatitis. Finally, the containers are incubated for not less than 14 days at 30° to 32° and examined visually for signs of microbial contamination.

Plasma Protein Fraction is an amber liquid which may produce a slight deposit on storage, pH 6.7 to 7.3, containing not less than 4.3% w/v of total protein and not more than 15 mmol (45 mEq) of citrate and not more than 2 mmol (2 mEq) of potassium ions per litre. Electrophoresis indicates that not less than 90% of the protein is albumin, the remainder being globulins; gamma globulin is not detectable. It contains no fibrinogen or antibodies, and contains no added bactericide or antibiotic. It exerts a colloidal osmotic pressure approximately equivalent to that of pooled liquid human plasma containing 5.2% w/v of protein. **Store** at 2° to 25°. Protect from light. It must not be used if the solution is turbid or contains more than a trace of fine deposit.

1247-f

Plasma Protein Fraction *(U.S.P.)*.

Plasma Protein Fraction is a sterile preparation of serum albumin and globulin obtained by fractionating material (blood, plasma, or serum) from healthy human donors, the source material being tested for the absence of hepatitis B surface antigen. It contains sodium acetyltryptophanate with or without sodium caprylate as a stabilising agent; it contains no added antimicrobial agent. It contains 5% of protein; not less than 83% of the total protein is albumin; not more than 17% is alpha and beta globulins; not more than 1% has the electrophoretic properties of gamma globulin. It contains 130 to 160 mmol (130 to 160 mEq) of sodium per litre, and not more than 2 mmol (2 mEq) of potassium per litre. pH 6.7 to 7.3. It must not be used if the solution is turbid.

The minimum expiration date is not more than 5 years after release from the manufacturer's cold storage if stored at 2° to 10°, and not more than 3 years after release if stored at a temperature not exceeding 30°.

1248-d

Dried Plasma Protein Fraction *(B.P.)*. Dried Human Plasma Protein Fraction; Dried Human Albumin Fraction (Saline). Dried Plasma Protein Fraction is a sterile preparation of Plasma Protein Fraction, freeze-dried immediately after heating at 59.5° to 60.5°. When dissolved in the volume of Water for Injections stated on the label the solution provides Plasma Protein Fraction.

Store below 25° in an atmosphere of nitrogen in sterile containers sealed to exclude micro-organisms and, as far as possible, moisture. Protect from light. If after adding water, a gel forms or solution is incomplete, the preparation must not be used. When reconstituted it should be used within 3 hours; it should be administered with suitable equipment such as that described in Section 3 or Section 4 of *Transfusion Equipment for Medical Use,* BS 2463: 1962.

Adverse Effects and Precautions. Toxic effects are uncommon but nausea, vomiting, urticaria, chills, fever, hypotension, and salivation have been reported. Patients should be watched for signs of circulatory overload such as pulmonary oedema or heart failure.

Thirteen different lots of albumin fraction from 1 manufacturer were implicated in 23 reports of hypotension, similar to those reported by J.H.L. Bland *et al.* (*J. Am. med. Ass.*, 1973, *224*, 1721), in patients undergoing surgery. The severity of hypotension ranged from a decrease in mean arterial pressure of 20 mmHg to circulatory collapse and usually occurred within 2 minutes of starting infusion which was given at a rate of 20 to 50 ml per minute. Pre-kallidinogenase activator, present in the fractions, was identified as Hageman-factor (factor XII) fragments and was thought responsible for the hypotension although the severity was related to rate of infusion and condition of the patient as well as to the concentration of activator in the product. Bradykinin and other components of the kallidinogenase-kinin system might also be implicated and until fractions free of these components could be produced they should be used only when blood pressure could be monitored and when rapid expansion of volume was not needed.— B. M. Alving *et al.*, *New Engl. J. Med.*, 1978, *299*, 66. Comment.— R. W. Colman, *ibid.*, 97.

When C_1 esterase-inhibitor concentrate was added to plasma protein solution before its rapid transfusion into 6 patients, their arterial blood pressure fell by only 6% compared with a fall of more than 45% when plasma protein solution alone was transfused into 6 other patients. However, the method is expensive and time-consuming and a practical alternative is needed.— P. van der Starre *et al.* (letter), *New Engl. J. Med.*, 1979, *300*, 1276.

A 26-year-old woman developed acute urticaria after receiving 40 ml of an infusion of a plasma protein preparation (Plasmanate).— R. D. McMillin *et al.*, *Am. J. Surg.*, 1978, *135*, 706.

Metabolic alkalosis developed in 4 patients with limited renal function when they were given preparations of plasma protein fraction.— G. T. Rahilly and T. Berl, *New Engl. J. Med.*, 1979, *301*, 824.

Uses. Plasma Protein Fraction consists mainly of albumin with a small proportion of globulins. It is administered intravenously as a 5% solution to increase the blood volume in patients with hypovolaemia due to surgery or burns, and may be used as a temporary substitute for Whole Blood following severe haemorrhage with monitoring of blood pressure.

It has also been used in the initial treatment of dehydrated infants; the usual dose is 33 ml per kg body-weight, given at a rate of 5 to 10 ml per minute.

It does not contain blood-clotting factors.

Proprietary Preparations

Buminate 5% *(Travenol, UK)*. Plasma protein fraction, available for injection as a solution containing 5% of protein.

Plasma Protein Fraction 4.3% 'Immuno' *(Immuno, UK)*. A brand of Plasma Protein Fraction *B.P.*

Other Proprietary Names

Plasmanate, Plasma-Plex, Plasmatein *(all USA)*.

1249-n

Dried Serum. Dried Human Serum *(B.P. 1973)*.

Dried Serum is prepared by drying a sterile pool of the fluid which separates from human blood from suitable donors (see Whole Blood p.322) which has clotted in the absence of any anticoagulant. To ensure cross-neutralisation of haemagglutinins by soluble blood-group substances, the sera are pooled so that contributions from donors of A, O, and either B or AB groups are represented in approximately the ratio 9:9:2. Not more than 10 separate donations are pooled.

Dried Serum is a sterile, pale to deep cream-coloured powder or friable solid, which is completely **soluble** at 15° to 20°, within 10 minutes, in the volume of Water for Injections stated on the label. Such a solution contains not less than 6.5% w/v of protein.

Store below 25° in an atmosphere of nitrogen in sterile containers sealed to exclude micro-organisms and as far as possible moisture. Protect from light. It should be used immediately after reconstitution. It may be stored for several years in temperate and tropical climates if kept free from moisture.

When reconstituted it should be administered with suitable equipment such as that described in Section 3 or Section 4 of *Transfusion Equipment for Medical Use*, BS 2463: 1962

Adverse Effects. As for Whole Blood, p.322.

Uses. Dried Serum is used for the same purposes as Dried Plasma (see p.334) and it is reconstituted in a similar manner.

1250-k

Dried Thrombin *(B.P.)*. Dried Human Thrombin.

CAS — 9002-04-4.

Dried Thrombin is a preparation of the enzyme which converts human fibrinogen into fibrin. It is prepared from pooled liquid plasma obtained from the blood of suitable human subjects (see under Whole Blood, p.322). The prothrombin fraction is prepared by a suitable fractionation technique; the prothrombin is converted into thrombin in solution by the addition of calcium ions and human thromboplastin; the solution is **sterilised** by filtration and dried from the frozen state. It is a cream-coloured powder which is readily **soluble** in saline solution forming a pale yellow solution which may be cloudy. On adding such a solution to citrated plasma in the absence of added calcium ions, clotting occurs. It contains not less than 10 units per mg of protein.

Store at 2° to 8° under vacuum or in an atmosphere of nitrogen in sterile containers sealed to exclude micro-organisms and, as far as possible, moisture. Protect from light. The reconstituted solution must be used immediately.

Units. 100 units of human thrombin are contained in 8.5 mg (with sucrose) in one ampoule of the first International Standard Preparation (1975).

Adverse Effects. There is a risk of transmission of viral hepatitis type B (see p.321).

Uses. A solution of thrombin in sodium chloride injection, prepared by means of an aseptic technique, is used locally as a haemostatic in conjunction with fibrinogen and fibrin foam. When it is used with fibrinogen, the strength of solution will depend upon the desired rapidity of clotting; when it is used with fibrin foam, a solution containing 30 to 50 units per ml is employed. Solutions of thrombin should not be injected.

A preparation of bovine thrombin is used to control haemorrhage from puncture sites or from capillary oozing in surgery. It is standardised in terms of NIH units—one NIH unit being the amount required to clot 1 ml of a standardised fibrinogen solution in 15 seconds.

Mention of catheterisation of gastric veins and the use of hyperosmotic dextrose and thrombin to sclerose varices.— J. Scott *et al.*, *Gut*, 1976, *17*, 390. See also R. Gunther *et al.*, *Dt. med. Wschr.*, 1976, *101*, 1491.

Thrombin 5000 units in 5 ml applied to surgical wounds in 15 patients who had received heparin prophylaxis for surgery reduced the incidence of wound haematomas; 3 of 15 developed haematomas compared with 24 of 30 control patients.— B. Jasani *et al.* (preliminary communication), *Lancet*, 1977, *2*, 332.

Proprietary Preparations

Thrombostat *(Parke, Davis, UK)*. Thrombin obtained from mammalian plasma, available in vials each containing 5000 NIH units as sterile powder with 5-ml ampoules of diluent. For local application in the control of capillary bleeding.

Preparations of Bovine Thrombin

Thrombin *(U.S.P.)*. A sterile freeze-dried powder containing the protein substance obtained from bovine prothrombin; it contains calcium chloride, sodium chloride, and glycine. Solutions should be used within a few hours after preparation; they must not be injected or allowed to enter large blood vessels. Store at 2° to 8°. The expiration date is not later than 3 years after manufacture or issue.

1251-a

Thromboplastin. Factor III; Thrombokinase. A blood-clotting factor which initiates conversion of prothrombin to thrombin in the formation of the blood clot.

Units. The first International Reference Preparation (1976) for thromboplastin, human, combined consists of ampoules containing a freeze-dried suspension of human brain mixed with bovine factor V, bovine fibrinogen, and calcium chloride (calibration constant = 1.0).

The first International Reference Preparation (1978) for thromboplastin, bovine, combined consists of ampoules containing freeze-dried bovine thromboplastin with bovine plasma, adsorbed with barium sulphate, calcium chloride, and cephalin (calibration constant = 1.0).

The first International Reference Preparation (1978) for thromboplastin, rabbit, plain consists of ampoules containing freeze-dried rabbit brain suspension (calibration constant = 0.6).

These preparations represent respectively National Institute for Biological Standards and Control (NIBSC) preparations 67/40, 68/434, and 70/178.

For proposals for standardisation in the control of oral anticoagulation, including the calibration of thromboplastins, see WHO Expert Committee on Biological Standardization, *Tech. Rep. Ser. Wld Hlth Org. No. 610*, 1977, p. 45.

Doubts were cast on the stability of the international reference preparation by L. Poller *et al.* of the National (UK) Reference Laboratory for Anticoagulant Reagents and Control who advocates the continued use of British Comparative Thromboplastin (*Lancet*, 1977, *2*, 1019). However these doubts were not accepted by the National Institute for Biological Standards and Control in London and the Dutch National Laboratory for Anticoagulant Control [D.R. Bangham and E.A. Loeliger (letter), *Lancet*, 1977, *2*, 1280] nor by WHO [F.T. Perkins (letter), *ibid.*, 1281].

Further references: E. K. Blackburn and N. K. Shinton (letter), *Lancet*, 1978, *1*, 615; K. W. E. Denson (letter), *ibid.*, 1978, *1*, 718; K. F. Yee *et al.* (letter), *ibid.*, 1978, *1*, 1148.

Preparations of thromboplastin have been applied locally as haemostatics. They are also employed in the determination of the prothrombin time for the control of anticoagulant therapy.

Proprietary Preparations

Tachostyptan *(Consolidated Chemicals, UK)*. A preparation containing standardised thromboplastin (derived from brain tissue) 2%, available in ampoules of 5 ml, for intravenous injection. For the control of haemorrhage. *Dose*. Prophylactic, 5 to 10 ml before surgery; treatment, 5 to 10 ml immediately, repeated every 3 or 4 hours until the bleeding is controlled, or the contents of 12 ampoules have been given.

Boric Acid and Borax

260-e

Boric Acid *(B.P., Eur. P., U.S.N.F.).* Acidum Boricum; Boracic Acid; Borsäure; Sal Sedativa de Homberg.
H_3BO_3=61.83.

CAS — 10043-35-3.

Pharmacopoeias. In all pharmacopoeias examined except *Braz., Int., Roum.,* and *U.S.*, but in *U.S.N.F.*

Odourless colourless or white crystals, scales, or white powder with a slightly acid, bitter taste and sweetish after-taste. It is a weak acid and its alkali salts are alkaline. It volatilises in steam. When heated to 100° it loses water and is slowly converted into metaboric acid (HBO_2); tetraboric acid ($H_2B_4O_7$) is formed at 140° and boron trioxide (B_2O_3) at higher temperatures. **Soluble** 1 in 20 of water, 1 in 3.6 of boiling water, 1 in 16 of alcohol, 1 in 4 of glycerol (7 in 10 at 100°); slightly soluble in volatile oils; practically insoluble in ether. A 3.33% solution in water has a pH of 3.8 to 4.8. A 1.9% solution in water is iso-osmotic with serum. Solutions are **sterilised** by autoclaving or by filtration. **Incompatible** with polyvinyl alcohol and tannins.

CAUTION. *The Council of the Pharmaceutical Society of Great Britain advises pharmacists not to sell boric acid as such for use as a dusting-powder. Dusting-powders containing more than 5% of boric acid should be labelled: 'not to be applied to raw or weeping surfaces'.*

An aqueous solution of boric acid iso-osmotic with serum (1.9%) caused 100% haemolysis of erythrocytes cultured in it for 45 minutes.— E. R. Hammarlund and K. Pedersen-Bjergaard, *J. pharm. Sci.*, 1961, *50*, 24.

Solubility in sorbitol. Boric acid was soluble in a 70% solution of sorbitol to the extent of 19% at 25°. This solution could be diluted with water without precipitation of the boric acid.— J. J. Sciarra and D. Elliot, *J. Am. pharm. Ass., scient. Edn,* 1960, *49*, 115.

Adverse Effects. The main symptoms of acute boric acid poisoning are vomiting and diarrhoea, an erythematous rash followed by desquamation, and stimulation of the central nervous system followed by depression. There may be meningeal irritation, and changes in body temperature. There may also be renal damage. Death, resulting from circulatory collapse and shock, may occur within 3 to 5 days. The fatal dose of boric acid by ingestion is about 15 to 20 g in adults and 3 to 6 g in infants.

The slow excretion of boric acid can lead to cumulative toxicity during repeated use. Symptoms of chronic intoxication include anorexia, debility, confusion, dermatitis, menstrual disorders, and alopecia.

Fatalities have occurred most frequently in young children after the accidental ingestion of solutions of boric acid or after the application of boric acid powder to abraded skin. The concentration of boric acid in talcs and products for oral hygiene is limited in countries belonging to the European Economic Community (EEC) to 5 and 0.5% respectively and talcs must be labelled 'not to be used for babies'. In the EEC the concentration of boric acid in other cosmetic products is limited to 3%. Topical preparations of boric acid should not be applied to extensive areas of abraded or damaged skin.

Deaths have resulted from absorption following lavage of body cavaties with solutions of boric acid, and this practice is no longer recommended.

Treatment of Adverse Effects. If the boric acid has been ingested, empty the stomach by emesis or by aspiration and lavage. Give a purgative dose of sodium sulphate. Dehydration should be corrected and, if necessary, the circulation should be maintained with infusions of plasma or suitable electrolyte solutions. Convulsions may be controlled by the intravenous administration of diazepam 5 or 10 mg or, if necessary, thiopentone sodium. Exchange transfusions, peritoneal dialysis, or haemodialysis may be of value.

Absorption and Fate. Boric acid is absorbed from the gastro-intestinal tract, from damaged skin, from wounds, and from mucous membranes. It does not readily penetrate intact skin. About 50% of the amount absorbed is excreted in the urine within 12 hours; the remainder is probably excreted over 3 to 7 days.

Uses. Boric acid possesses weak bacteriostatic and fungistatic properties; it has been superseded by more effective and less toxic disinfectants.

Boric acid is used, usually with borax, as a buffer in eye-drops and was formerly used as a soluble lubricant in solution-tablets. It is not used internally.

The use of boric acid in cosmetics and toiletries is restricted under the Cosmetic Products Regulations 1978 (SI 1978: No. 1354).

For formulas of borate buffers from pH 6.77 to 10.8, see G. E. Schumacher, *Am. J. Hosp. Pharm.*, 1966, *23*, 628.

Boric acid 1.8% equivalent to 500 mg of powdered boric acid per 28 ml bottle, was found to be a suitable preservative for urine samples in transit requiring bacteriological examination. A concentration of 1.8% prevented multiplication of micro-organisms present in urine, though with occasional strains of *Proteus* and *Klebsiella* boric acid appeared to cause a reduction in the number of organisms. By keeping the urine acid, boric acid prevented dissolution of pus cells.— I. A. Porter and J. Brodie, *Br. med. J.*, 1969, *2*, 353. Boric acid appeared to be useful for the preservation of urine specimens but more fundamental work was required before boric acid could be recommended for routine use.— H. H. Johnston *et al.*, in The Bacteriological Examination of Urine: Report of a Workshop on Needs and Methods, *Public Health Laboratory Service Monograph Series No. 10*, P.D. Meers (Ed.), London, HM Stationery Office, 1978.

Preparations

For preparations containing boric acid, see Martindale 27th Edn, p. 273.

261-l

Borax *(B.P., Eur. P.).* Purified Borax; Sodium Borate *(U.S.N.F.)*; Natrii Tetraboras; Sodium Tetraborate; Sodium Biborate or Pyroborate; Natrium Boricum.
$Na_2B_4O_7,10H_2O$=381.4.

CAS — 1330-43-4; 61028-24-8 (both anhydrous); 1303-96-4 (decahydrate).

Pharmacopoeias. In all pharmacopoeias examined except *Roum.* and *U.S.*, but in *U.S.N.F.*

Odourless transparent colourless crystals, crystalline masses, or white crystalline powder with an alkaline taste. It effloresces in dry air.

Soluble 1 in 20 of water, 1 in less than 1 of boiling water and 1 in 1 of glycerol; practically insoluble in alcohol. A 4% solution in water has a pH of 9 to 9.6. A 2.6% solution is iso-osmotic with serum. Solutions are **sterilised** by autoclaving or by filtration. **Incompatible** with alkaloidal salts, mercuric chloride, zinc sulphate, and other metallic salts. In these cases incompatibility may usually be overcome by the addition of glycerol or by replacing half the borax with boric acid. Also incompatible with gums and mineral acids. **Store** in a cool place in airtight containers.

CAUTION. *The Council of the Pharmaceutical Society of Great Britain advises pharmacists not to supply Borax Glycerin or Honey of Borax, even with an appropriate warning, because of the hazards associated with the use of these preparations in infants.*

Adverse Effects and Treatment. As for Boric Acid, p.337.

Uses. Borax has a feeble bacteriostatic action similar to that of boric acid. It is not used internally. Applied externally it is mildly astringent and was formerly used as a gargle or mouthwash in the treatment of aphthous ulcers and stomatitis, as a lotion in bromidrosis and inflammatory conditions of the eye, and as a nasal douche. Borax Glycerin and Honey of Borax were formerly used as paints for the throat and tongue and to alleviate dryness of the mouth but as excessive use may cause toxic effects they should not be used.

It has been used as an emulsifying agent with beeswax in cold creams, and as a mild alkali to remove stains from linen and clothing.

Preparations

For preparations containing borax, see Martindale 27th Edn, p. 273.

Bromides

1020-m

Bromides were formerly used for their sedative and anticonvulsant properties; they have been replaced by more effective and less toxic drugs.

Adverse Effects. During prolonged administration bromide accumulation may occur giving rise to bromide intoxication or bromism. Symptoms include nausea and vomiting, slurred speech, memory impairment, drowsiness, disorientation, irritability, ataxia, dizziness, tremors, hallucinations, mania, stupor, coma, and other manifestations of central nervous system depression. Skin rashes of various types commonly occur. Death after acute poisoning appears to be rare as vomiting follows the ingestion of large doses.

Toxic effects may occur when bromide concentrations in blood are greater than 600 mg per litre (7.5 mmol per litre). A toxic concentration can be reached very rapidly if the intake of chloride is reduced.

For reports and reviews of bromide intoxication and bromide abuse, see G. Bastian, *Arzneimittel-Forsch.*, 1966, *16*, 246; I. Martin, *Med. J. Aust.*, 1967, *1*, 95; R. S. Blume *et al.*, *New Engl. J. Med.*, 1968, *279*, 593; M. W. P. Carney, *Lancet*, 1971, *2*, 523; P. Wilkinson and J. N. Santamaria, *Med. J. Aust.*, 1972, *2*, 318; G. Torosian *et al.*, *Am. J. Hosp. Pharm.*, 1973, *30*, 716; R. J. W. Williams (letter), *Br. med. J.*, 1974, *3*, 629; W. Poser *et al.*, *Dt. med. Wschr.*, 1974, *99*, 2489; R. M. Murray and R. Smith, *Lancet*, 1972, *1*, 73; D. L. Trump and M. C. Hochberg, *Johns Hopkins med. J.*, 1976, *138*, 119; I. Brenner, *Am. J. Psychiat.*, 1978, *135*, 857; R. A. Dominguez, *J. Ky St. med. Ass.*, 1978, *76*, 438; M. A. Raskind *et al.*, *J. Am. Geriat. Soc.*, 1978, *26*, 222.

Treatment of Adverse Effects. In acute poisoning the stomach should be emptied by aspiration and lavage and sodium chloride should be given by intravenous infusion. Dextrose has also been administered and frusemide may be given to aid diuresis. In chronic poisoning, bromide administration is stopped, sodium chloride or ammonium chloride, up to 2 to 3 g three or four times daily, may be given by mouth with adequate amounts of fluid. Diuretics are of value. In severe cases of bromide intoxication or when the usual treatments cannot be used, haemodialysis or peritoneal dialysis may be of value.

A brief review of the treatment of bromide intoxication.— J. F. Winchester *et al.*, *Trans. Am. Soc. artif. internal Organs*, 1977, *23*, 762.

Precautions. Bromides should not be given to patients with impaired renal function, debility, cachexia, or dehydration.

The maximum acceptable daily intake of inorganic bromide derived from bromine-containing fumigants and other sources for man: 1 mg per kg body-weight. The maximum acceptable concentration in raw cereals and wholemeal flour: 50 ppm.— Report of the 1971 Joint FAO/WHO Meeting on Pesticide Residues in Food, *Tech. Rep. Ser. Wld Hlth Org. No. 502*, 1972.

Bromides could interfere technically with chemical estimations for cholesterol in the blood to produce erroneous raised results.— *Drug & Ther. Bull.*, 1972, *10*, 69.

Pregnancy and the neonate. As much as 66 mg per litre of bromide had been recovered in the milk of mothers receiving 5 g daily. The drug could cause drowsiness and skin rashes in infants.— J. A. Knowles, *J. Pediat.*, 1965, *66*, 1068.

Growth retardation in 2 boys was associated with maternal bromide ingestion during pregnancy.— J. M. Opitz *et al.* (letter), *Lancet*, 1972, *1*, 91. Another report.— E. J. R. Rossiter and T. J. Rendle-Short (letter), *ibid.*, 1972, *2*, 705

Neonatal bromide intoxication was associated with the maternal ingestion of a bromide preparation during pregnancy.— J. R. Pleasure and M. G. Blackburn, *Pediatrics*, 1975, *55*, 503.

A further reference.— R. M. Hill and L. Stern, *Drugs*, 1979, *17*, 182.

Absorption and Fate. Bromides replace chloride in extracellular body fluids and have a half-life in the body of about 12 days. They may be detected in the milk of nursing mothers and in the foetus.

Uses. Bromides depress the central nervous system. They were used as sedatives but have been replaced by more effective less toxic agents. Bromides have moderate anticonvulsant activity against generalised tonic clonic seizures but are now rarely used.

There is little justification for the continued use of bromides in medicine.

1021-b

Ammonium Bromide *(B.P.C. 1963)*. Ammon. Brom.; Ammonii Bromidum; Ammonium Bromatum; Brometo de Amônio.

NH_4Br=97.94.

CAS — 12124-97-9.

Pharmacopoeias. In *Arg.*, *Aust.*, *Belg.*, *Chin.*, *Cz.*, *Fr.*, *Hung.*, *Mex.*, *Pol.*, *Port.*, *Roum.*, and *Swiss.*

Colourless, odourless, slightly hygroscopic crystals or white crystalline powder with a saline taste. Each g represents 10.2 mmol (10.2 mEq) of ammonium and of bromide.

Soluble 1 in 1.5 of water and 1 in 20 of alcohol; slightly soluble in ether. **Incompatible** with mineral acids, oxidising substances, mercury and silver salts, many alkaloidal salts, soluble barbiturates, and nitrous ether spirit. **Protect** from light.

Ammonium bromide has actions characteristic of bromides (see above).

1022-v

Bromine *(B.P.C. 1934)*. Bromum.

Br_2=159.8.

CAS — 7726-95-6.

A dark reddish-brown, heavy, mobile liquid which gives off intensely irritating brown fumes. B.p. about 59°. **Soluble** 1 in 30 by wt of water; freely soluble in most organic solvents with gradual decomposition of the solvents.

Adverse Effects. Bromine is intensely irritating and corrosive to mucous membranes and, even in dilute solution, may cause fatal gastro-enteritis if swallowed. Contact with the skin can produce severe burns and inhalation of the vapour causes violent irritation of the respiratory tract and pulmonary oedema. Maximum permissible atmospheric concentration 0.1 ppm.

Treatment of Adverse Effects. Milk, white of egg, and starch mucilage, taken as soon as possible, have been recommended. If bromine vapour has been inhaled, give assisted respiration, if necessary, and oxygen. Splashes on the skin and eyes should be immediately washed off; washing under running water should continue for at least 15 minutes.

Uses. Bromine is used, in the form of an adduct with a quaternary ammonium compound in the treatment of acne and plantar warts.

Proprietary Preparations

Callusolve *(Dermal Laboratories, UK)*. A paint containing 25% of an adduct of benzalkonium chloride and bromine in a non-aqueous volatile solvent. For warts, particularly plantar warts.

Warts. Over one-half of 637 patients were cured of their warts when treated with Callusolve over a period of 2 months. The results were significantly better than the expected 10% rate of spontaneous cure. Mild side-effects and recurrence of warts were reported in 2 cases.— H. Yarrow and S. Hitchcock, *Br. J. clin. Pract.*, 1969, *23*, 395.

1023-g

Bromoform *(B.P.C. 1959)*. Tribromomethane.

$CHBr_3$=252.7.

CAS — 75-25-2.

Pharmacopoeias. In *Arg.*, *Fr.*, *Port.*, and *Span.* (all with 1% w/w of alcohol); in *Belg.* (with 1 to 2% w/w of alcohol); in *It.* (with 1 to 2% v/v of alcohol); in *Roum.* (with 1 to 4% v/w of alcohol); and in *Swiss* (with 1% v/v of alcohol).

A colourless or nearly colourless heavy liquid with an odour resembling that of chloroform and a sweetish taste. It contains about 10 to 13% v/v (=3 to 4% w/w) of ethyl alcohol (*B.P.C. 1959*). Wt per ml about 2.65 g. It is decomposed by air and light but this decomposition is retarded by the presence of alcohol. It is non-inflammable.

Soluble 1 in 800 of water and 1 in 80 of glycerol; miscible with alcohol, ether, and fixed and volatile oils. **Store** in well-filled airtight containers. Protect from light.

Adverse Effects. Symptoms resemble those of chloroform poisoning but are more prolonged.

Maximum permissible atmospheric concentration 0.5 ppm.

Bromoform could cause deep yellow to green discoloration of the urine.— R. B. Baran and B. Rowles, *J. Am. pharm. Ass.*, 1973, *NS13*, 139.

Treatment of Adverse Effects. Empty the stomach by aspiration and lavage and, if necessary, assist respiration. See also under Chloroform, p.745.

Uses. Bromoform has been used in the treatment of whooping cough and mania.

A preparation containing bromoform was formerly marketed in Great Britain under the proprietary name Bromodeine (*Crookes*).

1024-q

Calcium Bromide *(B.P.C. 1949)*. Calcii Bromidum; Calcium Bromatum; Bromure de Calcium; Brometo de Cálcio.

$CaBr_2,2H_2O$=235.9.

CAS — 7789-41-5 (anhydrous).

Pharmacopoeias. In *Arg.*, *Aust.*, *Belg.*, *Fr.*, *Hung.*, *It.*, *Jap.*, *Jug.*, *Mex.*, *Pol.*, *Port.*, *Roum.*, *Span.*, and *Swiss.* Usually described as a hydrated salt with a variable amount of water of crystallisation. In *Hung.* as 33.3% solution. Some pharmacopoeias include an injection (10% $CaBr_2$ in Water for Injections).

A white, odourless, granular, very deliquescent powder with a bitter saline taste. **Soluble** 1 in less than 1 of water and alcohol; practically insoluble in chloroform and ether. Solutions are **sterilised** by autoclaving or by filtration. **Incompatible** with carbonates, phosphates, sulphates, oxidising substances, and many alkaloid salts.

Calcium bromide has actions characteristic of bromides, (see p.338).

1025-p

Dilute Hydrobromic Acid *(B.P.C. 1949)*. Acid. Hydrobrom. Dil.; Verdünnte Bromwasserstoffsäure.

CAS — 10035-10-6 (hydrobromic acid).

A clear colourless odourless liquid with an acid taste, containing 10% w/w of HBr. Wt per ml about 1.073 g. **Store** in glass-stoppered bottles. Protect from light.

Dilute hydrobromic acid was formerly used as a sedative in cough mixtures and in the treatment of tinnitus and vertigo.

1026-s

Potassium Bromide *(B.P., Eur. P.)*. Pot. Brom.; Potassii Bromidum; Kalii Bromidum; Kalium Bromatum; Bromure de Potassium; Brometo de Potássio.

KBr=119.0.

CAS — 7758-02-3.

Pharmacopoeias. In all pharmacopoeias examined except *Braz.* and *U.S.*

Odourless colourless crystals or white crystalline powder with a saline taste. Each g represents 8.4 mmol (8.4 mEq) of potassium and of bromide.
Soluble 1 in 1.6 of water, 1 in 200 of alcohol, and 1 in 5 of glycerol. **Incompatible** with oxidising substances, nitrous ether spirit, mercury and silver salts, and many alkaloidal salts.

Incompatibility. Tablet disintegration tests showed that bromides were incompatible with starch.— F. Kun and K. Katona, *Gyógyszerészet,* 1971, *15,* 263, per *Int. pharm. Abstr.,* 1973, *10,* 112.

Potassium bromide has the general properties characteristic of bromides (see p.338) and of potassium. It has been given in divided doses of up to 6 g daily.

Preparations

For preparations of potassium bromide see Martindale 27th Edn, p. 275.

1027-w

Sodium Bromide *(Eur. P., B.P. 1973).* Sod. Brom.; Sodii Bromidum; Natrii Bromidum; Natrium Bromatum; Bromure de Sodium; Brometo de Sódio.
$NaBr = 102.9$.

CAS — 7647-15-6.

Pharmacopoeias. In all pharmacopoeias examined except *Br., Braz.*, and *U.S.*

Odourless, small, colourless, transparent or opaque crystals or white granular powder with a bitter saline taste. It is deliquescent but does not appear moist until over 20% of water has been absorbed, owing to the formation of the dihydrate, $NaBr,2H_2O$. Each g represents 9.72 mmol (9.72 mEq) of sodium and of bromide.
Soluble 1 in 1.5 of water, 1 in 17 of alcohol, and 1 in 1 of glycerol. Solutions are **sterilised** by autoclaving or by filtration. **Incompatible** with oxidising substances, nitrous ether spirit, mercury and silver salts, and many alkaloidal salts. **Store** in airtight containers.

Sodium bromide has the adverse effects and uses characteristic of bromides (see p.338). A dose of 1 to 6 g daily in divided doses has been used.

Proprietary Names
Sedobrol*(Roche, Belg.).*

1028-e

Strontium Bromide *(B.P.C. 1934).* Stront. Brom.; Strontii Bromidum; Strontium Bromatum; Bromuro de Estroncio.
$SrBr_2,6H_2O = 355.5$.

CAS — 10476-81-0 (anhydrous).

Pharmacopoeias. In *Port., Roum.*, and *Span.*

Colourless odourless transparent crystals with a bitter saline metallic taste. It deliquesces in moist air.
Soluble 2 in 1 of water and 1 in 3 of alcohol; practically insoluble in ether. **Incompatible** with soluble bicarbonates, carbonates, citrates, tartrates, and sulphates, with oxidising substances, soluble barbiturates, and many alkaloidal salts. **Store** in airtight containers.

Strontium bromide has the characteristics of bromides (see p.338) and strontium.

Caffeine and other Xanthines

620-t

The principal xanthines used in medicine are caffeine, theobromine, and theophylline. This group of drugs is of value for its effects on the kidney, smooth muscle, the myocardium, and the central nervous system.

Caffeine and its salts, which are the most active in stimulating the central nervous system, are principally used for this purpose. The diuretic effects of caffeine are less than those of theobromine and theophylline, but the usefulness of theobromine and theophylline is limited by their poor solubility, and more soluble derivatives such as aminophylline are usually employed. Because some theophylline compounds such as aminophylline are highly alkaline and cause irritation, they are not well tolerated. Attempts to overcome this have included the use of enteric coatings for tablets or the use of less alkaline salts of theophylline, such as choline theophyllinate.

The chief usefulness of the xanthines in cardiac conditions is in paroxysmal dyspnoea associated with left heart failure, and for this aminophylline is often employed, followed, if necessary, by digoxin. The bronchodilator effects of such drugs as aminophylline are also of value in asthma, both prophylactically and in the treatment of prolonged attacks. While administration of the xanthines may benefit some patients with angina pectoris, their clinical usefulness in this condition has not been established.

Tolerance to some of the effects of the xanthines, particularly the diuretic effect, may readily develop.

Beverages containing xanthines are very widely used and include coffee, tea, cocoa, and cola drinks.

The xanthine derivative oxpentifylline is described in the section on Vasodilators.

The aetiology of asthma and the use of xanthines in treatment.— A. S. Rebuck, *Drugs*, 1974, *7*, 344 and 370. See also K. M. Piafsky and R. I. Ogilvie, *New Engl. J. Med.*, 1975, *292*, 1218; D. C. Webb-Johnson and J. L. Andrews, *New Engl. J. Med.*, 1977, *297*, 758; G. M. Sterling, *Br. med. J.*, 1978, *1*, 1259; G. M. Cochrane, *Practitioner*, 1979, *223*, 489; A. D. Milner, *Prescribers' J.*, 1980, *20*, 33 (infants and children).

621-x

Caffeine *(B.P., U.S.P.)*. Anhydrous Caffeine; Coffeinum *(Eur. P.)*; Guaranine; Methyltheobromine; Caféine; Théine. 3,7-Dihydro-1,3,7-trimethylpurine-2,6(1*H*)-dione; 1,3,7-Trimethylxanthine; 7-Methyltheophylline.

$C_8H_{10}N_4O_2$=194.2.

CAS — 58-08-2.

Pharmacopoeias. A monograph on Caffeine is included in all pharmacopoeias examined; most also describe the monohydrate, though the use of anhydrous caffeine is usually permitted. Caffeine *U.S.P.* is anhydrous or the monohydrate.

An alkaloid obtained from tea waste, or coffee, or from the dried leaves of *Camellia sinensis* (Theaceae), or prepared synthetically; it is also present in guarana, maté, and kola. It occurs as odourless silky white crystals, usually matted together, or a white crystalline powder, with a bitter taste. It sublimes at about 180°. M.p. 234° to 239°.

When crystallised from water, caffeine contains 1 molecule of water of crystallisation, but it is anhydrous when crystallised from alcohol, chloroform, or ether.

Soluble 1 in 60 of water, 1 in 1 of boiling water, 1 in 130 of alcohol, and 1 in 7 of chloroform; slightly soluble in ether; acids render it more soluble in water, but it is a very weak base, and on concentrating the solution of the salts they are apt to dissociate, and the caffeine crystallises out. It is rendered more soluble in water by the addition of an equal quantity of citric acid, sodium salicylate, or sodium benzoate. Solutions in water are neutral to litmus. **Incompatible** with iodine, silver salts, tannins, and with strong solutions of caustic alkalis. **Store** in airtight containers.

Caffeine extracted from natural sources contained only traces of theobromine and no theophylline, whereas synthetic caffeine contained quantities which could be detected by thin-layer chromatography.— G. Lehmann and P. Martinod, *Arzneimittel-Forsch.*, 1967, *17*, 35.

Caffeine content of beverages. The Food Standards Committee recommended that cola drinks be required to contain not less than 50 and not more than 200 mg of caffeine per litre. Cola drinks containing not more than 5 mg of caffeine per litre should be described as decaffeinated.— *Review of the Soft Drinks Regulations 1964 (as amended)*, FSC/REP/65, Ministry of Agriculture, Fisheries and Food, London, HM Stationery Office, 1976.

European Economic Community regulations direct that the term 'decaffeinated' relates to coffee extracts the anhydrous caffeine content of which does not exceed 0.3% by weight of its coffee-based dry matter content.— *Off. J.E.E.C.*, 1977, *20*, L172, 20.

The approximate caffeine content of various beverages per 6-ounce cup was: brewed coffee 100 to 150 mg, 'instant' coffee 60 to 80 mg, decaffeinated coffee 3 to 5 mg, tea 40 to 100 mg, and cola drinks 17 to 55 mg.— *Med. Lett.*, 1977, *19*, 65.

Analysis of some common soft drinks indicated that no caffeine was detectable in Club Orange, Miwadi Glucose, or Glucoplus. Pepsi Cola contained caffeine 65 µg per ml, Coca Cola contained 110 µg per ml, and Lucozade contained 180 µg per ml.— A. Darragh *et al.* (letter), *Lancet*, 1979, *1*, 1196.

Formation of complexes in solution. Caffeine formed complexes with sulphathiazole, sulphadiazine, aminobenzoic acid, benzocaine, barbitone, and phenobarbitone.— T. Higuchi and J. L. Lach, *J. Am. pharm. Ass., scient. Edn*, 1954, *43*, 349.

Solubility. The solubility of caffeine in water was reduced by the addition of sucrose.— A. N. Paruta and B. B. Sheth, *J. pharm. Sci.*, 1966, *55*, 896.

622-r

Caffeine Hydrate *(B.P., U.S.P.)*. Caffeine Monohydrate *(Eur. P.)*; Coffeinum Monohydricum.

$C_8H_{10}N_4O_2,H_2O$=212.2.

CAS — 5743-12-4.

Pharmacopoeias. As for Caffeine, p.340.

It occurs as odourless silky white crystals, usually matted together, or a white crystalline powder, with a bitter taste. It effloresces in dry air and loses its water of crystallisation when heated, becoming anhydrous at 100°; it sublimes at about 180°. M.p. 234° to 239°.

Soluble 1 in 60 of water and 1 in 110 of alcohol; soluble in chloroform with the separation of water; slightly soluble in ether. Solutions in water are neutral to litmus. **Store** in airtight containers.

Adverse Effects. Side-effects of caffeine include nausea, headache, and insomnia. Excessive consumption of beverages containing caffeine, termed caffeinism, may cause headaches, irritability, and symptoms of anxiety neurosis. Children are more susceptible to excitation than adults.

Large doses may cause restlessness, excitement, muscle tremor, tinnitus, scintillating scotoma, tachycardia, and extrasystoles. Caffeine increases gastric secretions and may cause gastric ulceration. The fatal dose is probably about 10 g.

Caffeine was present in most of the analgesic mixtures associated with nephritis and might add to the nephrotoxicity of phenacetin. Most persons receiving caffeine showed a rise of renal tubular and red blood-cell excretion.— L. F. Prescott, *J. Pharm. Pharmac.*, 1966, *18*, 331.

A few days after hospital admission for severe abdominal symptoms hepatic coma developed in a 35-year-old black, diabetic, alcoholic, male, associated with caffeine accumulation following ingestion of 7 cups of coffee (totalling about 800 mg of caffeine) daily. Whereas the mean plasma half-life of caffeine had been reported by J. Axelrod and J. Reichenthal (*J. Pharmac. exp. Ther.*, 1953, *107*, 519) to be 3.5 hours, the half-life in this patient was about 96 hours. Treatment included reduction of his usual phenytoin dose from 100 mg four times daily to 100 mg twice daily, withdrawal of diazepam 5 mg thrice daily (which had been given to facilitate alcohol withdrawal), and withdrawal of caffeine. The coma resolved over 48 hours.— B. E. Statland *et al.* (letter), *New Engl. J. Med.*, 1976, *295*, 110.

Death in a 34-year-old woman was attributed to the ingestion of an unknown amount of caffeine. A concentration in the blood of about 100 µg per ml was reported with similarly high concentrations in the liver, kidneys, and brain.— J. E. Turner and R. H. Cravey, *Clin. Toxicol.*, 1977, *10*, 341.

Signs of caffeine toxicity occurred in a 23-year-old man with psoriatic erythroderma 3 hours after topical application of about 30 g of caffeine in anhydrous wool alcohols ointment. The serum-caffeine concentrations were 160 and 60 µg per ml 6 and 24 hours respectively after application of the ointment.— H. Ippen and K. Kölmel, *Dt. med. Wschr.*, 1977, *102*, 1851.

Further reports of caffeine toxicity include J. M. Peters, *J. clin. Pharmac.*, 1967, *7*, 131; H. A. Reimann, *J. Am. med. Ass.*, 1967, *202*, 1105; J. R. Harrie (letter), *ibid.*, 1970, *213*, 628; J. F. Greden, *Am. J. Psychiat.*, 1974, *131*, 1089; *Br. med. J.*, 1977, *2*, 284; J. L. Sullivan, *J. Pediat.*, 1977, *90*, 1022 (accidental ingestion in an infant); P. B. Kulkarni and R. D. Dorand, *Pediatrics*, 1979, *64*, 254 (toxicity in a neonate). See also under Prepared Coffee, p.346.

Tolerance. A report of tolerance to caffeine in habitual coffee drinkers.— T. Colton *et al.*, *Clin. Pharmac. Ther.*, 1968, *9*, 31.

Withdrawal. Headache, attributable to caffeine withdrawal, could occur during short-term fasting.— M. A. Shorofsky and N. Lamm, *N.Y. St. J. Med.*, 1977, *77*, 217.

A report of benign fibrocystic disease of the breast regressing after withdrawal of caffeine and other methylxanthines from the diet.— J. P. Minton, *Am. J. Obstet. Gynec.*, 1979, *135*, 157.

Treatment of Adverse Effects. As for Aminophylline (see p.342).

Excessive stimulation of the central nervous system may be controlled by diazepam 5 to 10 mg by mouth or, if necessary, by injection.

Precautions. Caffeine should be given with care to patients with a history of peptic ulceration.

Administration of caffeine 250 mg to 9 healthy non-coffee drinkers who had also abstained from other caffeine-containing beverages for 21 days had a potent stimulating effect on plasma-renin activity and catecholamine secretion. Whether chronic administration of caffeine had similar effects and any association with hypertension remained to be determined.— D. Robertson *et al.*, *New Engl. J. Med.*, 1978, *298*, 181.

Interactions. The effects of caffeine might be enhanced by isoniazid and meprobamate. Meprobamate had been claimed to increase the caffeine concentration in the brain by 55% and to decrease the concentration in kidneys and liver.— J. M. Peters, *J. clin. Pharmac.*, 1967, *7*, 131.

Reference to oral contraceptives impairing the elimination of caffeine.— R. V. Patwardhan *et al.*, *J. Lab. clin. Med.*, 1980, *95*, 603.

Pregnancy and the neonate. A study suggesting that women with a high daily intake of caffeine may have a higher incidence of abortion and prematurity.— P. S. Weathersbee *et al.*, *Postgrad. Med.*, 1977, *62*, 64.

Absorption and Fate. Caffeine is absorbed readily after oral, rectal, or parenteral administration but absorption from the gastro-intestinal tract may be erratic. There is little evidence of accumulation in any particular tissue. Caffeine passes readily into the central nervous system and into saliva; concentrations have also been detected in breast milk.

It is metabolised almost completely and is

excreted in the urine as 1-methyluric acid, 1-methylxanthine, and other metabolites with only about 1% unchanged.

The fate of caffeine in man. The average plasma half-life in 12 men was 3.5 hours.— J. Axelrod and J. Reichenthal, *J. Pharmac. exp. Ther.*, 1953, *107*, 519.

Peak plasma concentrations of 1.5 to 1.8 µg per ml were found in 3 subjects 50 to 75 minutes after a dose of 100 mg of caffeine had been given as coffee.— F. L. Grab and J. A. Reinstein, *J. pharm. Sci.*, 1968, *57*, 1703.

Pregnancy and the neonate. Following the intravenous administration of caffeine to 7 infants of 2½ weeks to 6 months, plasma clearance progressively increased to adult capacity by 3 to 4½ months and exceeded it by 5 to 6 months of age.— J. V. Aranda *et al.*, *Archs Dis. Childh.*, 1979, *54*, 946. Further references: A. Aldridge *et al.*, *Clin. Pharmac. Ther.*, 1979, *25*, 447 (caffeine metabolism in neonates); J. V. Aranda *et al.*, *J. Pediat.*, 1979, *94*, 663 (pharmacokinetics in premature infants); S. M. Somani *et al.*, *J. Pediat.*, 1980, *96*, 1091 (serum and CSF concentrations in premature infants).

Lactation. An hour after taking 150 mg of caffeine as caffeine and sodium benzoate, peak concentrations of caffeine in 5 healthy mothers ranged from 2.39 to 4.05 µg per ml in serum and from 1.4 to 2.4 µg per ml in breast milk.— E. E. Tyrala and W. E. Dodson, *Archs Dis. Childh.*, 1979, *54*, 787.

Uses. Caffeine acts on the central nervous system, on muscle, including cardiac muscle, and on the kidneys. Its action on the central nervous system is mainly on the higher centres and it produces a condition of wakefulness and increased mental activity. Caffeine facilitates the performance of muscular work and increases the total work which can be performed by a muscle. It may stimulate the respiratory centre, increasing the rate and depth of respiration. Its stimulant action on the medullary vasomotor centre is usually compensated by its peripheral vasodilator effect on the arterioles, so that the blood pressure usually remains unchanged.

The diuretic action of caffeine has been accounted for in many ways. It may increase renal blood flow and glomerular filtration rate, but its main action may be due to the reduction of the normal tubular reabsorption. It is less effective as a diuretic than theobromine which has less central stimulating effect and does not cause insomnia. The xanthines are rarely of great value in promoting increased renal function when this is depressed.

Caffeine is claimed to enhance the action of ergotamine and is frequently given with ergotamine in the treatment of migraine.

Caffeine is administered in powder or tablets in doses of 100 to 300 mg. It is frequently included in analgesic preparations with aspirin or codeine. Beverages of coffee, tea, and cola provide active doses of caffeine.

Reviews of the actions of caffeine.— I. B. Syed, *J. Am. pharm. Ass.*, 1976, *NS16*, 568; *Nutr. Rev.*, 1979, *37*, 124.

Slight hyperglycaemia occurred 2 hours after a dose of 250 mg of caffeine; the effect was rather more evident in persons with fewer general symptoms and signs suggestive of disease.— E. Cheraskin and W. M. Ringsdorf (letter), *Lancet*, 1968, *2*, 689. See also E. Cheraskin *et al.*, *ibid.*, 1967, *1*, 1299. Caffeine caused a decrease in blood-sugar concentrations in healthy individuals and an increase in patients with maturity-onset diabetes.— H. Sandberg *et al.*, *J. Am. med. Ass.*, 1969, *208*, 1482.

There was growing evidence that caffeine and theophylline acted by increasing the formation of catecholamines from dopa in the brain.— B. Waldeck (letter), *J. Pharm. Pharmac.*, 1972, *24*, 654.

Caffeine was reported to be a strong prostaglandin antagonist and weak agonist.— M. S. Manku and D. F. Horrobin, *Lancet*, 1976, *2*, 1115.

Comment on the use of caffeine in cocaine substitutes including Cocafine Snuff and Coca Snow Incense.— R. K. Siegel (letter), *New Engl. J. Med.*, 1980, *302*, 817.

Apnoea. Caffeine citrate was given to 17 premature infants with apnoea. The regimen evolved during the study was a loading dose of 20 mg per kg body-weight intravenously followed 2 to 3 days later by maintenance doses of 5 to 10 mg per kg given once or twice daily. The frequency of apnoeic episodes was significantly reduced with complete abolition of apnoea in 6 infants. Plasma half-lives were very prolonged and ranged from 40.7 to 231.0 hours. Controlled trials were necessary to establish the usefulness of caffeine.— J. V. Aranda *et al.*, *J. Pediat.*, 1977, *90*, 467. See also *J. Am. med. Ass.*, 1976, *235*, 693; T. R. Gunn *et al.*, *J. Pediat.*, 1979, *94*, 106.

Dermatitis. In a double-blind study in 28 patients with atopic dermatitis the application for 3 weeks of a 30% caffeine cream produced significantly greater benefit (in terms of erythema, scaling, lichenification, oozing, and excoriation) than a placebo. It was considered that caffeine increased the concentrations of cyclic AMP in the skin.— R. J. Kaplan *et al.* (letter), *Archs Derm.*, 1977, *113*, 107. See also *idem*, 1978, *114*, 60.

Hyperkinetic states. Caffeine might be a suitable alternative to central nervous system stimulants for children with hyperkinetic states.— R. C. Schnackenberg, *Am. J. Psychiat.*, 1973, *130*, 796. See also C. C. Reichard and S. T. Elder, *Am. J. Psychiat.*, 1977, *134*, 144. A contrary view.— C. L. Saccar, *Am. J. Hosp. Pharm.*, 1978, *35*, 544.

Proprietary Names

No Doz *(Bristol, USA)*.

623-f

Caffeine and Sodium Benzoate *(B.P.C. 1954)*. Caffein. et Sod. Benz.; Coffeinum et Natrii Benzoas; Coffeinum-natrium Benzoicum.

CAS — 8000-95-1.

Pharmacopoeias. In *Aust.*, *Cz.*, *Ger.*, *Hung.*, *Int.*, *It.*, *Jap.*, *Jug.*, *Mex.*, *Nord.*, *Pol.*, *Roum.*, *Rus.*, *Swiss*, and *Turk*. The specified caffeine content varies from 38 to 52%.

A mixture of caffeine and sodium benzoate containing 47 to 50% of anhydrous caffeine. It is a white odourless powder with a slightly bitter taste. **Soluble** 1 in about 1.2 of water and 1 in 30 of alcohol; slightly soluble in chloroform. A solution in water has a pH of 6.5 to 8.5. A 3.92% solution in water is iso-osmotic with serum. Solutions are **sterilised** by autoclaving or by filtration. **Incompatible** with mineral acids, iron salts, iodine, salts of heavy metals, and tannin. **Store** in airtight containers. Protect from light.

Because of its ready solubility in water caffeine and sodium benzoate has been employed for administration of caffeine by injection. A 25% solution has been used subcutaneously as a cardiac and respiratory stimulant and as a diuretic in doses of 120 to 300 mg.

Kernicterus. Sodium benzoate in caffeine and sodium benzoate injection could uncouple bilirubin from its albumin binding sites, which might induce kernicterus. Such injections should be administered with caution, if at all, to neonates with raised bilirubin concentrations.— D. Schiff *et al.*, *Pediatrics*, 1971, *48*, 139.

Preparations

Caffeine and Sodium Benzoate Injection *(U.S.P.)*. A sterile solution in Water for Injections; pH 6.5 to 8.5.

A preparation containing caffeine and sodium benzoate was formerly marketed in Great Britain under the proprietary name Elixir Sibec (*Vestric*).

624-d

Caffeine and Sodium Iodide *(B.P.C. 1968)*. Caffein. and Sod. Iod.; Iodocaffeine.

A mixture of caffeine and sodium iodide containing 47 to 50% of anhydrous caffeine. It is a white odourless powder with a bitter saline taste. **Soluble** 1 in 5 of water; partly soluble in alcohol. **Incompatible** with mineral acids, salts of heavy metals, and tannin. **Store** in airtight containers.

Caffeine and sodium iodide has the toxic effects of caffeine (p.340) and of iodine (p.862). It has been used as a cardiac and respiratory stimulant and as a diuretic. It is used for the relief of asthma. Doses of 120 to 600 mg have been given.

Preparations

Caffeine Iodide Elixir *(B.P.C. 1973)*. Caffeine 150 mg, sodium iodide 450 mg, liquorice liquid extract 0.3 ml, chloroform 0.01 ml, decoction prepared from a sufficient quantity of recently ground roasted coffee of commerce and water to 5 ml. *Dose.* 5 ml.

Eupinal *(Cuxson, Gerrard, UK)*. Contains in each 5 ml caffeine 115 mg and ammonium iodide 345 mg in infusion of coffee.

Eupnine Vernade *(Wilcox, UK)*. A solution containing in each 5 ml anhydrous caffeine 155 mg, ammonium iodide 366 mg, liquorice liquid extract 0.0175 ml, cherry-laurel aqueous extract (equivalent to hydrocyanic acid 27 µg) 0.027 ml. *Dose.* 5 ml in water once or twice daily before meals.

625-n

Caffeine and Sodium Salicylate *(B.P.C. 1949)*. Caffein. et Sod. Salicyl.; Coffeinum et Natrii Salicylas; Coffeinum-natrium Salicylicum.

CAS — 8002-85-5.

Pharmacopoeias. In *Aust.* (48 to 52%), *Ger.* (39 to 42%), *Int.* (44 to 46%), *Swiss* (46.8 to 48.6%), and *Turk.* (44 to 46%).

A mixture of caffeine and sodium salicylate containing 47 to 50% of anhydrous caffeine.

A white odourless amorphous powder or granular mass with a bitter saline taste. **Soluble** 1 in 2 of water and 1 in 25 of alcohol. A 5.77% solution in water is iso-osmotic with serum. Solutions are **sterilised** by autoclaving or by filtration. **Incompatible** with mineral acids, iron salts, iodine, salts of heavy metals, and tannin. **Store** in airtight containers. Protect from light.

Caffeine and sodium salicylate was formerly used, by subcutaneous injection as a 50% solution, as a cardiac and respiratory stimulant and as a diuretic.

626-h

Caffeine Citrate *(B.P.C. 1959)*. Caffein. Cit.; Citrated Caffeine; Coffeinum Citricum.
$C_8H_{10}N_4O_2,C_6H_8O_7=386.3$.

CAS — 69-22-7.

Pharmacopoeias. In *Aust.*, *Hung.*, *Ind.*, *Roum.*, and *Span.*

A mixture of caffeine and citric acid containing 47 to 50% of anhydrous caffeine.

A white odourless powder with a bitter acid taste. **Soluble** 1 in 4 of hot water, dissociating on further dilution with the separation of caffeine on cooling which redissolves in about 32 of water; soluble 1 in 25 of alcohol. A solution in water is acid to litmus. **Incompatible** with mixtures containing potassium iodide and nitrous ether spirit, iodine being liberated. Incompatible with phenazone, sodium benzoate, sodium nitrite, and sodium salicylate; caffeine, in half the dose of caffeine citrate ordered, should be used for mixtures containing these incompatible substances. **Store** in airtight containers.

Caffeine citrate has been used similarly to caffeine (p.341) in doses of 120 to 600 mg.

627-m

Acepifylline. Acefylline Piperazine; Piperazine Theophylline Ethanoate. Piperazine bis(theophyllin-7-ylacetate).
$(C_9H_{10}N_4O_4)_2,C_4H_{10}N_2=562.5$.

CAS — 18833-13-1.

A white odourless crystalline powder with a bitter taste. M.p. 260°. Freely **soluble** in water; slightly soluble in alcohol. A 10% solution in water has a pH of about 7.

Adverse Effects, Treatment, and Precautions. As for Aminophylline, p.342. Acepifylline is considered to cause less nausea and gastric irritation than aminophylline and is better tolerated by intramuscular injection.

Uses. Acepifylline is a theophylline derivative which is used similarly to aminophylline (see p.344).

It may be given by mouth in doses of 0.5 to 1 g thrice daily, by rectum as suppositories in doses of 0.5 to 1.5 g daily, or by intramuscular or slow intravenous injection in doses of 500 mg.

A study involving healthy subjects and one patient, indicated that following intravenous administration acepifylline is completely eliminated by the kidneys within 4 hours, and that following administration by mouth absorption is very poor. No theophylline or other xanthine derivatives were detected in serum or urine.— J. Zuidema and F. W. H. M. Merkus (letter), *Lancet*, 1978, *1*, 1318.

Proprietary Preparations

Etophylate *(Delandale, UK)*. Acepifylline, available as 2-ml **Ampoules** of an injection containing 250 mg per ml, for intramuscular or intravenous use; as **Paediatric Suppositories** each containing 100 mg; as **Suppositories** each containing 500 mg; as **Syrup** containing 125 mg in each 5 ml (suggested diluent, syrup); as **Forte Syrup** containing 500 mg in each 5 ml; as **Tablets** of 250 mg; and as scored **Forte Tablets** of 500 mg.

Other Proprietary Names

Dynaphylline *(Canad.)*; Etafillina *(Ital.)*; Etaphylline *(Austral., Fr., Neth., Switz.)*; Etaphylline simple *(Belg.)* Minophylline *(Egypt)*.

A preparation containing acepifylline was also formerly marketed in Great Britain under the proprietary name Heptonal (*Delandale*).

628-b

Aminophylline *(B.P., U.S.P.)*.

Aminophyllinum; Theophylline and Ethylenediamine *(Eur. P.)*; Theophylline Ethylenediamine Compound; Metaphyllin; Theophyllinum et Ethylenediaminum; Theophyllaminum; Euphyllinum; Aminofilina. A mixture of theophylline and ethylenediamine, its composition approximately corresponding to the formula.

$(C_7H_8N_4O_2)_2,C_2H_4(NH_2)_2,2H_2O$=456.5.

CAS — 317-34-0 (anhydrous).

Pharmacopoeias. In *Arg., Aust., Belg., Br., Braz., Chin., Cz., Fr., Ger., Ind., Int., It., Jap., Jug., Mex., Neth., Pol., Port., Roum., Rus., Span., Swiss,* and *Turk. Neth.* also includes anhydrous aminophylline. *U.S.* allows anhydrous or up to 2 molecules of water of crystallisation.

White or slightly yellowish granules or powder with a faintly ammoniacal odour and a bitter taste. It is a stable mixture or combination containing 78 to 84% of anhydrous theophylline and 13 to 14% of ethylenediamine with a variable quantity of water. Aminophylline 1.27 g is approximately equivalent in theophylline content to 1 g of theophylline.

Soluble 1 in 5 of water at 25°, but the addition of ethylenediamine or ammonia solution may be necessary to give complete solution (the solution may become cloudy in the presence of carbon dioxide); practically insoluble in alcohol and ether. A solution in water has a pH of 9.2 to 9.6. Solutions are **sterilised** by autoclaving or by filtration, exposure to carbon dioxide and contact with metal being avoided throughout.

In moist air it gradually loses ethylenediamine and absorbs carbon dioxide with the liberation of theophylline. **Store** in small well-filled airtight containers. Protect from light.

Incompatibility has been reported with acids, chlorpromazine hydrochloride, clindamycin phosphate, corticotrophin, dimenhydrinate, erythromycin gluceptate, hydralazine hydrochloride, hydroxyzine hydrochloride, narcotic analgesics, oxytetracycline hydrochloride, phenytoin sodium, procaine hydrochloride, prochlorperazine salts, promazine hydrochloride, promethazine hydrochloride, sulphafurazole diethanolamine, and vancomycin hydrochloride; with lactose, a yellow or brown colour develops on standing; in the presence of copper, solutions develop a blue colour.

Occasional incompatibility has occurred with cefapirin sodium depending on the strength and composition of the vehicle.

The addition of aminophylline to dextrose injection raised the pH by over 4 units to pH 7.7 to 10.45, so that insulin, which is inactivated above pH 7.5, was incompatible, as was erythromycin gluceptate. Tetracycline hydrochloride lowered the pH to 3.6 to 4 rendering the aminophylline less stable. A mixture of benzylpenicillin and aminophylline in dextrose injection was initially compatible but on standing for 12 hours the pH fell from 8.2 to 6 with the risk of theophylline precipitation.— M. Edward, *Am. J. Hosp. Pharm.*, 1967, *24*, 440.

Other references: R. Misgen, *Am. J. Hosp. Pharm.*, 1965, *22*, 92; J. A. Patel and G. L. Phillips, *ibid.*, 1966, *23*, 409; E. A. Parker (letter), *ibid.*, 1970, *27*, 67; B. B. Riley, *J. Hosp. Pharm.*, 1970, *28*, 228.

Release from suppositories. Blood concentrations of theophylline in 5 persons were measured 2 hours after administration of aminophylline 500 mg or theophylline 400 mg as suppositories or soft gelatin capsules or as a miniature enema. There were large individual variations in blood concentration, but on average there was no significant difference in the theophylline concentration of 4.6 µg per ml attained using glycogelatin, fatty, macrogol, or surfactant bases. A miniature enema containing the equivalent of 500 mg of aminophylline in a 1% methylcellulose '4000' solution gave significantly higher concentrations of about 8.2 µg per ml.— F. Newwald and P. Ackad, *Am. J. Hosp. Pharm.*, 1966, *23*, 347.

There was no appreciable difference, in respect of release of aminophylline, between suppositories of aminophylline in the bases Massa Estarinum B, macrogols, theobroma oil, or Witepsol H15.— H. P. M. Kerckoffs and T. Huizinga, *Pharm. Weekbl. Ned.*, 1967, *102*, 1255, per *Int. pharm. Abstr.*, 1968, *5*, 548.

Aminophylline was more stable in Witepsol H suppository basis than in Lassupol G and was more unstable in theobroma oil.— T. Cieszynski, *Acta Pol. pharm.*, 1971, *28*, 59, per *Pharm. J.*, 1972, *1*, 100.

Further references: J. M. Plaxco *et al.*, *J. pharm. Sci.*, 1967, *56*, 809; J. M. Plaxco and F. Foreman, *ibid.*, 1968, *57*, 698.

Stability in dextrose injection. Aminophylline, about 450 mg per litre, was stable for up to 2 days at 25° in dextrose injection over a pH range of 3.5 to 8.6.— E. A. Parker, *Am. J. Hosp. Pharm.*, 1970, *27*, 67.

Adverse Effects. The side-effects commonly encountered with theophylline and its derivatives are gastro-intestinal irritation and stimulation of the central nervous system.

Aminophylline may cause nausea, vomiting, gastro-intestinal bleeding, visual disorders, insomnia, headache, anxiety, confusion, restlessness, hyperventilation, vertigo, and palpitations; severe overdosage or idiosyncrasy may lead to maniacal behaviour, repeated vomiting with extreme thirst, delirium, hyperthermia, and convulsions. Hypotension may follow intravenous injection, particularly if the injection is too rapid, and sudden deaths have been reported. Aminophylline given by mouth frequently causes gastric irritation with nausea and vomiting. Proctitis may follow repeated administration of suppositories. Intramuscular injections are painful, the pain lasting several hours.

Overdosage in children, particularly with suppositories, can be dangerous, as absorption is unpredictable. It may be characterised by haematemesis, stimulation of the central nervous system, and diuresis.

Plasma concentrations of theophylline greater than 20 µg per ml are considered to be toxic.

The injection over 3 to 5 minutes of aminophylline 200 to 750 mg directly into the right atrium produced a high incidence of cardiac arrest.— S. J. Camarata *et al.*, *Circulation*, 1971, *44*, 688, per *Lancet*, 1972, *1*, 1169.

A review of theophylline poisoning in children.— J. Armand *et al.*, *Lyon méd.*, 1973, *229*, 485.

Case reports of accidental overdosage.— Y. Vaucher *et al.*, *J. Pediat.*, 1977, *90*, 827; D. H. Wells and J. J. Ferlauto, *Pediatrics*, 1979, *64*, 252; P. Gal *et al.*, *Pediatrics*, 1980, *65*, 547; F. E. R. Simons *et al.*, *Am. J. Dis. Child.*, 1980, *134*, 39.

A memorandum circulated to doctors in New Zealand warned of the danger of cerebral ischaemia, convulsions, and cardiotoxicity from overdoses of aminophylline.— *Pharm. J.*, 1974, *1*, 590. Signs of theophylline overdosage in 9 patients included vomiting, impaired consciousness, hyperreflexia, hyperventilation, hypokalaemia, tachycardia, and arrhythmias. Each of 3 patients who died had blood-theophylline concentrations above 65 µg per ml, hypotension, and convulsions. Patients over 50 years appeared to be specially susceptible.— M. Helliwell and D. Berry, *Br. med. J.*, 1979, *2*, 1114.

Excessive release of endogenous catecholamine remained the most logical mechanism of previously unexplained deaths during aminophylline infusion.— N. O. Atuk, *Lancet*, 1974, *1*, 1056.

A premature infant with apnoea and weighing about 1 kg had marked diuresis in response to theophylline 4.3 mg given every 6 hours.— P. A. Nobel and G. S. Light, *J. Pediat.*, 1977, *90*, 825.

Allergy. An allergic reaction to aminophylline in one patient.— D. Wong *et al.*, *J. Allergy & clin. Immunol.*, 1971, *48*, 165. Further reports.— A. E. Fishman, *Ann. Allergy*, 1974, *33*, 161; B. H. Booth *et al.*, *Ann. Allergy*, 1979, *43*, 289.

Depression. Paradoxical depression associated with the use of theophylline in 2 patients.— M. B. Murphy *et al.*, *Br. med. J.*, 1980, *281*, 1322.

Effects on the nervous system. Convulsions. Generalised convulsions occurred in 8 patients, 4 of whom died, whilst receiving aminophylline intravenously in a mean dose of 34 mg per kg body-weight daily. This effect was correlated with a mean serum-theophylline concentration of 53 µg per ml. Four further patients with less serious side-effects had a mean serum-theophylline concentration of 35 µg per ml compared with a mean of 19 µg per ml in 15 patients with no side-effects. Hepatic dysfunction in 11 of the 12 patients with side-effects and high doses contributed to the high serum-theophylline concentrations.— C. W. Zwillich *et al.*, *Ann. intern. Med.*, 1975, *82*, 784. See also M. H. Jacobs and R. M. Senior, *Am. Rev. resp. Dis.*, 1974, *110*, 342.

Generalised and focal motor seizures occurred in 6 patients given aminophylline in dosages ranging from 50 mg per hour intravenously to 500 mg in 30 minutes; one patient was given aminophylline 500 mg as suppositories. Plasma-aminophylline concentrations in 3 patients were 21.5 to 61 µg per ml. One of the patients had a remote history of encephalitis; the seizures were generally resistant to anticonvulsant therapy.— P. R. Yarnell and N. -S. Chu, *Neurology, Minneap.*, 1975, *25*, 819.

The Boston Collaborative Drug Surveillance Program reported that drug-induced convulsions occurred in 2 of 2870 patients given aminophylline.— J. Porter and H. Jick, *Lancet*, 1977, *1*, 587.

Pregnancy and the neonate. Possible aminophylline toxicity in a neonate related to maternal ingestion of aminophylline.— T. F. Yeh and R. S. Pildes (letter), *Lancet*, 1977, *1*, 910.

Urinary retention. Theophylline was associated with urinary retention in 2 middle-aged men with evidence of prostatic enlargement.— G. R. Owens and R. Tannenbaum (letter), *Ann. intern. Med.*, 1981, *94*, 212. See also M. Prakash and J. D. Washburne (letter), *ibid.*, 823.

Treatment of Adverse Effects. Gastric lavage may be used for aminophylline or theophylline overdosage by mouth and enemas for overdosage by rectum. Dialysis and haemoperfusion have been used. Treatment is symptomatic. Fluid and electrolyte balance should be maintained with intravenous fluids and oxygen given as necessary. Convulsions should be controlled by the intravenous administration of diazepam 5 or 10 mg or, if necessary, thiopentone sodium.

The elimination of theophylline in premature infants by exchange transfusion.— B. M. Assael *et al.*, *J. Pediat.*, 1977, *91*, 331.

Inhibition of the absorption of theophylline by activated charcoal.— C. Sintek *et al.*, *J. Pediat.*, 1979, *94*, 314.

Dialysis and haemoperfusion. Haemodialysis effectively removed theophylline from the plasma of one asthmatic anephric patient, and might be of value in the treatment of overdosage.— G. Levy *et al.*, *J. Am. med. Ass.*, 1977, *237*, 1466. See also C. S. Lee *et al.*, *J. clin. Pharmac.*, 1979, *19*, 219; J. N. Miceli *et al.*, *Clin. Toxicol.*, 1979, *14*, 539 (peritoneal dialysis).

Resin haemoperfusion removed theophylline from the plasma of a patient with liver impairment who had seizures which began 2 hours after withdrawal of theophylline when her plasma-theophylline concentration was

46 μg per ml. Although the seizures stopped, coma persisted and the patient subsequently died. The removal of theophylline by resin haemoperfusion was considered to be more rapid, at least for the first 2 hours, than removal by haemodialysis.— C. Lawyer *et al.*, *Ann. intern. Med.*, 1978, *88*, 516.

Charcoal haemoperfusion for 3 hours reduced the theophylline concentration from 146 μg to 31 μg per ml in a 15-year-old girl who had ingested 1.575 g of theophylline as sustained-release tablets about 16 hours earlier. No rebound in drug concentration was seen 8 hours after the end of haemoperfusion.— D. B. Jefferys *et al.*, *Br. med. J.*, 1980, *280*, 1167. Further reports of the successful use of charcoal haemoperfusion: S. M. Ehlers *et al.*, *J. Am. med. Ass.*, 1978, *240*, 474; M. E. Russo, *New Engl. J. Med.*, 1979, *300*, 24.

Precautions. Children are particularly susceptible to the effects of aminophylline or theophylline and they should not be administered more frequently than every 8 hours.

Aminophylline should be administered with caution to elderly patients and those suffering from cardiac disease and liver disease. Intravenous injections must be administered very slowly to prevent dangerous central nervous system and cardiovascular side-effects due to the direct stimulating effect of aminophylline. The bronchodilator and toxic effects of theophylline may be enhanced by sympathomimetics and by administration with other xanthines. Smokers may require increased doses as may patients undergoing routine haemodialysis.

Care should be taken in patients with a history of peptic ulceration.

Treatment with an aminophylline infusion was considered dangerous in conditions such as anaphylactic shock because vasodilatation was increased.— A. G. Cazort (letter), *New Engl. J. Med.*, 1967, *276*, 641.

Aminophylline depressed or completely abolished uterine activity in 60 patients during various stages of the menstrual cycle.— E. M. Coutinho and A. C. V. Lopes, *Am. J. Obstet. Gynec.*, 1971, *110*, 726, per *Int. pharm. Abstr.*, 1972, *9*, 722.

The serum-theophylline concentration immediately after a grand mal convulsion in a man taking aminophylline was 64 μg per ml. Heart failure and fever associated with pneumonia had both decreased theophylline clearance.— R. A. Matthay *et al.*, *Thorax*, 1976, *31*, 470, per *Drugs*, 1977, *14*, 229.

Patients with chronic hepatic cirrhosis had a variable capacity to eliminate theophylline and usual maintenance doses could be hazardous.— K. M. Piafsky *et al.*, *New Engl. J. Med.*, 1977, *296*, 1495. Comments.— C. H. Lawyer *et al.* (letter), *ibid.*, *297*, 1122; A. Mangione *et al.* (letter), *ibid.*, 1123. Reply.— R. I. Ogilvie *et al.* (letter), *ibid.*

In 5 of 6 asthmatic children the plasma half-life of theophylline was strikingly extended during upper respiratory tract infections (influenza A or adenovirus) and one child suffered acute theophylline toxicity; the sixth child (with influenza B infection) had no change in the half-life. The extended half-lives were considered unlikely to be a result of fever since no change was noted in 4 febrile children without evidence of viral infection. Some viral infections might affect theophylline metabolism causing toxic concentrations; alternatively an adequate dose during a viral infection might subsequently be inadequate.— K. C. Chang *et al.*, *Lancet*, 1978, *1*, 1132.

For mention of cross sensitisation to ethylenediamine and to antihistamines, see Ethylenediamine p.44.

Effect of smoking. Young patients who smoked would probably need daily theophylline dosages about twice those of non-smokers and response was likely to be less predictable. Return of theophylline clearance to normal on cessation of smoking was very slow.— S. N. Hunt *et al.*, *Clin. Pharmac. Ther.*, 1976, *19*, 546.

The shorter plasma half-life of theophylline in smokers indicated that they had a more rapid total body clearance.— R. I. Ogilvie, *Ann. intern. Med.*, 1978, *88*, 263.

Interactions, drugs. Evidence that on long-term administration, allopurinol inhibits theophylline metabolism.— R. L. Manfredi and E. S. Vesell, *Clin. Pharmac. Ther.*, 1981, *29*, 224.

Antibiotics. A report of erythromycin enhancing the blood concentrations of theophylline.— L. H. Cummins *et al.* (letter), *Pediatrics*, 1977, *59*, 144. Confirmation of the interaction.— B. J. M. Zarowitz *et al.*, *Clin. Pharmac. Ther.*, 1981, *29*, 601.

Elimination of theophylline was reduced by 50% and serum concentrations were increased in 8 patients with chronic asthma who were also taking triacetyloleandomycin.— M. Weinberger *et al.*, *J. Allergy & clin. Immunol.*, 1977, *59*, 228.

Antineoplastic agents. For reference to a possible interaction between theophylline and lomustine, see Lomustine, p.212.

Barbiturates. Although K.M. Piafsky *et al.* (*Clin. Pharmac. Ther.*, 1977, *22*, 336) reported that phenobarbitone did not affect the disposition of theophylline given intravenously, in a subsequent study (R.A. Landay *et al.*, *J. Allergy & clin. Immunol.*, 1978, *62*, 27) phenobarbitone enhanced the clearance of theophylline from serum.

Beta-adrenoceptor blocking agents. Propranolol reduced theophylline clearance in healthy subjects given aminophylline intravenously. Metoprolol did not reduce clearance in the group as a whole but had a reducing effect in some smokers whose theophylline clearance was initially high.— K. A. Conrad and D. W. Nyman, *Clin. Pharmac. Ther.*, 1980, *28*, 463.

Cimetidine. Evidence that the clearance of theophylline is decreased by cimetidine.— M. A. Campbell *et al.*, *Ann. intern. Med.*, 1981, *95*, 68.

Corticosteroids. In 3 patients with status asthmaticus who were given aminophylline intravenously, serum concentrations of theophylline rose rapidly from the therapeutic range to between 40 and 50 μg per ml when hydrocortisone was given intravenously.— N. Buchanan *et al.*, *S. Afr. med. J.*, 1979, *56*, 1147.

Sympathomimetic agents. Myocardial infarction occurred in a patient with status asthmaticus receiving aminophylline and salbutamol and these agents were considered responsible. Other therapy included antibiotics, hydrocortisone, digoxin, orciprenaline, and adrenaline.— A. Szczeklik *et al.* (letter), *Lancet*, 1977, *1*, 658.

Thiabendazole. An elderly man receiving aminophylline by infusion suffered severe nausea, lethargy, and general malaise, associated with a rise in serum-theophylline concentration from 21 to 46 μg per ml, when he was given thiabendazole.— A. M. Sugar *et al.*, *Am. Rev. resp. Dis.*, 1980, *122*, 501.

Interactions, tests and assays. Theophylline could interfere with the measurement of serum-uric acid concentrations when the reagent used was phosphotungstic acid.— J. Millhouse, *Adverse Drug React. Bull.*, 1974, Dec., 164.

Blood-theophylline concentrations as measured by the spectrophotometric procedure of J.A. Schack and S.H. Waxler (*J. Pharmac. exp. Ther.*, 1949, *97*, 283) could be considerably reduced by the presence of *barbiturates*, *phenytoin*, and *paracetamol*; they could also be reduced by the presence of purine derivatives such as *allopurinol* and *phenylbutazone*. *Hydroxyzine* and large doses of *thiamine* could produce falsely raised values, and *salicylates* totally masked the theophylline spectrum. Elevations due to the presence of *caffeine* were negligible since it was less soluble than theophylline in weak alkali.— A. S. Banner *et al.* (letter), *New Engl. J. Med.*, 1977, *297*, 170.

Concurrent administration of *frusemide*, *sulphathiazole*, *phenylbutazone*, *probenecid*, and *theobromine* could interfere with the Schack and Waxler spectrophotometric assay for plasma-theophylline concentrations to give clinically significant false-positive elevations, whereas *warfarin*, *dicoumarol*, and *salicylic acid* could given significantly lowered results.— L. E. Matheson *et al.*, *Am. J. Hosp. Pharm.*, 1977, *34*, 496.

Sulphamethoxazole in large quantities could interfere with the determination of theophylline concentrations by high-pressure liquid chromatography.— S. A. McKenzie *et al.*, *Archs Dis. Childh.*, 1978, *53*, 167.

Reference to a more specific enzyme immunoassay which can be used to measure theophylline concentrations in serum.— M. Weinberger (letter), *Lancet*, 1978, *2*, 789.

Absorption and Fate. Aminophylline is readily absorbed from the gastro-intestinal tract and from the rectal mucosa. Absorption is rapid from retention enemas but less predictable from suppositories. Theophylline, the active drug, is readily released in the body and effective blood concentrations are rapidly attained after the intravenous injection of aminophylline. Theophylline is less well absorbed from the gastro-intestinal tract than aminophylline.

At least 60% of theophylline may be bound to plasma proteins.

Theophylline is excreted in the urine as metabolites, mainly 1,3-dimethyluric acid and 3-methylxanthine, and about 10% is excreted unchanged.

There are marked variations in theophylline pharmacokinetics. Plasma half-lives for theophylline ranging from 3 to 9 hours and therapeutic plasma concentrations from about 5 to 20 μg per ml have been reported.

Theophylline has also been reported to cross the placenta and to diffuse into breast milk.

Blood concentrations of theophylline were determined in 13 patients after the administration of 500 mg of aminophylline by mouth as uncoated tablets, by retention enema, or by suppository. In 10 patients who received their oral doses after fasting overnight, mean blood concentrations at 1, 2, and 4 hours were 8.7, 8.1, and 6.6 μg per ml respectively; 5.4, 5.4, and 4.3 μg per ml respectively after administration by retention enema; and 3.5, 4.7, and 4.4 μg per ml after administration by suppository. Theophylline concentrations therapeutically effective in asthma or chronic bronchitis were reached, usually within 1 hour, in all patients after oral doses, but were not reached in 5 of 12 patients after rectal administration, nor in 7 of 13 patients after administration in the form of a suppository. Blood concentrations after oral doses in 3 patients who had not fasted were 1.4, 4.5, and 7.7 μg per ml respectively at 1, 2, and 4 hours.— J. P. Lillehei, *J. Am. med. Ass.*, 1968, *205*, 530.

The concentration of theophylline in the saliva was about half the plasma concentration.— V. P. Shah and S. Riegelman, *J. pharm. Sci.*, 1974, *63*, 1283. See also N. N. Khanna *et al.*, *J. Pediat.*, 1980, *96*, 494; S. M. Lena *et al.*, *Postgrad. med. J.*, 1980, *56*, 85.

Prolonged half-life in 8 premature infants.— G. Giacoia *et al.*, *J. Pediat.*, 1976, *89*, 829. See also J. V. Aranda *et al.*, *New Engl. J. Med.*, 1976, *295*, 413. In a study in 54 children aged from 3 months to 6 years, the mean half-life of theophylline of 4.92 hours was longer than previously reported in children and did not appear to be related to age.— G. J. Kadlec *et al.*, *Ann. Allergy*, 1978, *40*, 303.

In a study of 114 adults and 59 children given aminophylline by mouth, apparent theophylline clearance was significantly higher in children than adults. Young children (1 to 9 years) eliminated theophylline more rapidly than older children (10 to 18 years).— D. E. Zaske *et al.*, *J. Am. med. Ass.*, 1977, *237*, 1453. See also P. M. Loughnan *et al.*, *J. Pediat.*, 1976, *88*, 874.

Plasma concentrations and clearance-rates of theophylline in children did not necessarily change proportionately with dose.— M. Weinberger and E. Ginchansky, *J. Pediat.*, 1977, *91*, 820.

The activity of 3-methylxanthine, mainly *in vitro*.— C. G. A. Persson and K. -E. Andersson, *Acta pharmac. tox.*, 1977, *40*, 529.

The metabolism of theophylline in neonates is different from that in adults. In 2 neonates studied, it was metabolised partly to caffeine.— C. Bory *et al.* (letter), *Lancet*, 1978, *2*, 1204. In 24 of 25 premature infants a steady increase in plasma-caffeine concentrations had been noted during administration of theophylline.— M. -J. Boutroy *et al.* (letter), *ibid.*, 830. See also C. Bory *et al.*, *J. Pediat.*, 1979, *94*, 988; M. -J. Boutroy *et al.*, *J. Pediat.*, 1979, *94*, 996; E. Hartemann *et al.*, *Pédiatrie*, 1979, *34*, 273 (18-month-old child); K. -Y. Tserng *et al.*, *Clin. Pharmac. Ther.*, 1981, *29*, 594.

A study of factors affecting theophylline clearances.— W. J. Jusko *et al.*, *J. pharm. Sci.*, 1979, *68*, 1358.

In 18 patients given theophylline 400 mg rectally by enema a mean peak blood concentration of 5.24 μg per ml occurred 2 hours after administration.— M. L. Schilt, *Arzneimittel-Forsch.*, 1978, *28*, 311.

A detailed review of the pharmacokinetics of theophylline.— R. I. Ogilvie, *Clin. Pharmacokinet.*, 1978, *3*, 267.

The methods and rationale for monitoring serum-theophylline concentrations and its practical application.— L. Hendeles *et al.*, *Clin. Pharmacokinet.*, 1978, *3*, 294 and 422.

Further references: M. S. Segal *et al.*, *Ann. Allergy*, 1971, *29*, 135; J. W. Jenne *et al.*, *Clin. Pharmac. Ther.*, 1972, *13*, 349; D. P. Nicholson and T. W. Chick, *Am. Rev. resp. Dis.*, 1973, *108*, 241; R. Koysooko *et al.*, *J. pharm. Sci.*, 1975, *64*, 299; J. H. G. Jonkman *et al.*, *Eur. J. clin. Pharmac.*, 1980, *17*, 379.

Further references to the pharmacokinetics of theophylline in neonates and infants: F. E. R. Simons and K. J. Simons, *J. clin. Pharmac.*, 1978, *18*, 472; P. Bolme *et al., Eur. J. clin. Pharmac.*, 1979, *16*, 133; J. P. Rosen *et al., Pediatrics*, 1979, *64*, 248; J. J. Grygiel and D. J. Birkett, *Clin. Pharmac. Ther.*, 1980, *28*, 456; P. L. Morselli *et al., Clin. Pharmacokinet.*, 1980, *5*, 485; S. M. Somani *et al., J. Pediat.*, 1980, *96*, 1091 (concentrations in serum and CSF).

See also under Dosage in Premature Infants in Uses (below).

Bioavailability. A comparison of the bioavailability of oral theophylline preparations in adults. Absorption was rapid and complete from a solution, uncoated tablets, and chewable tablets and was delayed but still complete from choline theophyllinate tablets with partial enteric-coating. Three of 6 sustained-release theophylline preparations were slowly and completely absorbed but absorption was incomplete and sometimes erratic from the other 3. The authors predicted that serum-theophylline concentrations would fluctuate less between doses with the 3 sustained-release preparations that were reliably absorbed than with uncoated tablets.— M. Weinberger *et al., New Engl. J. Med.*, 1978, *299*, 852.

Further references to bioavailability studies of theophylline and aminophylline preparations: N. E. Bateman *et al., Aust. J. pharm. Sci.*, 1978, *7*, 93; D. D. Shen *et al., J. pharm. Sci.*, 1978, *67*, 916; L. J. Lesko *et al., J. pharm. Sci.*, 1979, *68*, 1392; L. N. Sansom *et al., Eur. J. clin. Pharmac.*, 1979, *16*, 417.

Excretion in breast milk. Irritability occurred in a breast-fed infant when the mother took aminophylline 200 mg every 6 hours. In 5 nursing mothers given aminophylline the ratio of milk concentration of theophylline to serum concentration was about 0.7.— A. M. Yurchak and W. J. Jusko, *Pediatrics*, 1976, *57*, 518. See also G. P. Stec *et al., Clin. Pharmac. Ther.*, 1980, *28*, 404.

Uses. Aminophylline is a soluble derivative of theophylline and is given for its theophylline activity which is considered to be mediated through inhibition of phosphodiesterase with a resulting increase in intracellular cyclic adenosine phosphate (cyclic AMP) concentrations.

Aminophylline or theophylline relaxes smooth muscle and relieves bronchial spasm. It stimulates the myocardium and produces a diminution of venous pressure in congestive heart failure leading to a marked increase in cardiac output. It has a stimulant effect on respiration. In comparison with other xanthines, theophylline has a stronger diuretic effect than caffeine though it has a short duration. It is a more powerful relaxant of smooth muscle than either theobromine or caffeine and it has only a slight stimulant action on the cerebrum.

Aminophylline's main indications are in diseases of the cardiovascular system, asthma, bronchopneumonia, bronchitis, and cardiac, pulmonary, or renal oedema. It has also been employed in the treatment of angina pectoris. Aminophylline is less effective by mouth than by intravenous injection and often causes gastric irritation; administration as enteric-coated tablets or with aluminium hydroxide mixture may reduce irritation but larger doses may be needed. Aminophylline given rectally as suppositories or as a retention enema is of value for preventing attacks of paroxysmal dyspnoea or asthma.

Therapeutic plasma concentrations of theophylline are considered to range from 5 to 20 µg per ml and toxic effects are common above 20 µg per ml.

When a rapid effect is desired, as in Cheyne-Stokes respiration or the acute paroxysms of bronchial asthma, aminophylline is given by slow intravenous injection over a minimum period of 10 to 15 minutes; the dose is 250 to 500 mg in 10 to 20 ml of water. It has also been given by deep intramuscular injection in a dose of 500 mg in 2 ml of water, but such injections are painful. Aminophylline may be given by intravenous infusion in dextrose injection or sodium chloride injection (see also under Dosage, below).

Aminophylline has been given by mouth in doses of 100 to 300 mg three or four times daily, but is more often given rectally as suppositories in a dose of 360 mg once or twice daily. Children have been given aminophylline by suppository in the following doses once or twice daily: up to 1 year, 12.5 to 25 mg; 1 to 5 years, 50 to 100 mg; and 6 to 12 years, 100 to 200 mg.

Reviews on the uses of aminophylline and theophylline: T. G. Tong, *Drug Intell. & clin. Pharm.*, 1973, *7*, 156; J. W. Paterson and G. M. Shenfield, *B.T.T.A. Rev.*, 1974, *4*, 61; *Med. Lett.*, 1975, *17*, 9; J. R. Koup, *Can. J. Hosp. Pharm.*, 1977, *30*, 180; L. Ausburn, *Aust. J. Pharm.*, 1978, *59*, 455; *Curr. med. Res. Opinion*, 1979, *6, Suppl.* 6, 1–176; R. G. Van Dellen, *Mayo Clin. Proc.*, 1979, *54*, 733.

Intravenous injection of aminophylline in man had been shown to cause a 35% increase in cardiac output for about 15 minutes and an increase in glomerular filtration-rate and sodium clearance. The effects on the kidney lasted for 50 to 60 minutes and were not accounted for by the increased cardiac output.— M. F. Lockett and H. L. Gwynne, *J. Pharm. Pharmac.*, 1968, *20*, 688.

Theophylline and other methylxanthines are considered by many workers, including A.N. Corbascio (*Clin. Pharmac. Ther.*, 1971, *12*, 559) and D.C. Webb-Johnson and J.L. Andrews (*New Engl. J. Med.*, 1977, *297*, 476), to exert their action by the inhibition of phosphodiesterase thus increasing the intracellular concentration of cyclic adenosine phosphate (cyclic AMP) and indirectly mimicking some of the physiological actions of adrenaline and isoprenaline. However N.O. Atuk (*Lancet*, 1974, *1*, 1056) reported that J. Vernikos-Danellis and C.G. Harris (*Proc. Soc. exp. Biol. Med.*, 1968, *128*, 1016) had failed to demonstrate any alteration in phosphodiesterase activity in tissues in *rats* after the administration of pharmacologically active doses of theophylline or caffeine. M.S. Manku and D.F. Horrobin (*Lancet*, 1976, *2*, 1115) reported theophylline to be a strong prostaglandin antagonist and weak agonist and D.F. Horrobin *et al.* (*New Engl. J. Med.*, 1977, *297*, 1181) considered that the bronchodilator effects of theophylline were more likely to depend on prostaglandin inhibition since concentrations required to inhibit phosphodiesterase were far higher than could be achieved therapeutically in human plasma. Studies in *rabbits* by S. Moncada and R. Korbut (*Lancet*, 1978, *1*, 1286) suggested that the antithrombotic activity of phosphodiesterase inhibitors such as theophylline depended on the enhancement of prostacyclin which activates adenylcyclase to increase platelet cyclic AMP.

Abnormal glucose tolerance tests and reduced release of insulin were returned to normal in 15 hypocalcaemic non-diabetic patients when their hypocalcaemia was corrected. When 7 similar patients were given theophylline 1 g intravenously over 3 hours insulin release returned to normal despite continued hypocalcaemia. Glucose intolerance was not affected.— O. Gedik and M. S. Zileli, *Diabetes*, 1977, *26*, 813.

Evidence that aminophylline improves diaphragmatic contractility.— M. Aubier *et al., New Engl. J. Med.*, 1981, *305*, 249.

Apnoea. In 10 premature infants apnoeic attacks ceased or became less frequent after the use of 5-mg aminophylline suppositories 6-hourly.— J. A. Kuzemko and J. Paala, *Archs Dis. Childh.*, 1973, *48*, 404.

A review of the use of theophylline, usually by mouth in an alcoholic vehicle, in the treatment of apnoea in the premature infant. Caution was advised until its efficacy had been established by double-blind trials.— H. Mercer and J. M. Gupta, *Med. J. Aust.*, 1977, *2*, 725. See also *J. Am. med. Ass.*, 1976, *235*, 693.

Following resuscitation from an apnoeic episode, administration of theophylline to give a blood concentration of 6.5 µg per ml controlled episodes of periodic breathing associated with bradycardia in a 3-month-old infant. Despite no detected abnormality of breathing the mother noted episodes of pallor at theophylline concentrations of 4.7 µg per ml which resolved when the dosage was increased to give a blood concentration of 9.6 µg per ml.— M. J. Boutroy *et al.* (letter), *Lancet*, 1978, *1*, 1257.

Two premature infants with hyaline membrane disease were successfully weaned from mechanical ventilation within 2 days when given theophylline 1.8 or 2 mg per kg body-weight every 6 hours.— P. A. Barr, *Archs Dis. Childh.*, 1978, *53*, 598. See also N. V. Erkan *et al.* (letter), *ibid.*, 1979, *54*, 81; C. Castalos *et al.* (letter), *ibid.*, 404.

Further references to aminophylline and theophylline in the treatment of apnoea: J. V. Aranda *et al., New Engl. J. Med.*, 1976, *295*, 413; R. Latini *et al., Eur. J. clin. Pharmac.*, 1978, *13*, 203; E. Hadjigeorgiou *et al., Am. J. Obstet. Gynec.*, 1979, *135*, 257 (antepartum administration of aminophylline); T. F. Myers *et al., J. Pediat.*, 1980, *96*, 99.

Asthma and bronchitis. Reviews on aminophylline and theophylline in asthma: A. S. Rebuck, *Drugs*, 1974, *7*, 370; K. M. Piafsky and R. I. Ogilvie, *New Engl. J. Med.*, 1975, *292*, 1218; M. Weinberger and L. Hendeles, *Am. J. Hosp. Pharm.*, 1976, *33*, 1071; P. P. VanArsdel and G. H. Paul, *Ann. intern. Med.*, 1977, *87*, 68; M. Weinberger, *J. Pediat.*, 1978, *92*, 1; *Med. Lett.*, 1978, *20*, 69; C. Green, *Practitioner*, 1979, *223*, 690; *Drug & Ther. Bull.*, 1979, *17*, 91.

It was found that 50 ml of a solution of aminophylline 3 g in 100 ml of alcohol made up to 500 ml with water was quickly absorbed and could abort a moderately severe attack of asthma. In these cases it was often an effective alternative to intravenous therapy and the effects could be seen within 10 to 20 minutes.— H. Herxheimer (letter), *New Engl. J. Med.*, 1974, *291*, 1192.

Theophylline 375 mg given by mouth to 14 asthmatic patients in a double-blind crossover study had a slower onset and longer duration of action than salbutamol 200 µg by aerosol inhalation. There was no significant difference in bronchodilatation produced by salbutamol or theophylline from 1 to 4 hours after administration. The mean peak FEV_1 increases for salbutamol and theophylline were 43.7% at 1 hour and 30.3% at 3 hours respectively. It was considered that simultaneous administration of salbutamol and theophylline could be of use.— B. J. S. Hartnett and G. E. Marlin, *Br. J. clin. Pharmac.*, 1976, *3*, 591. See also J. Barclay *et al., ibid.*, 1981, *11*, 203; G. Lönnerholm *et al., Br. med. J.*, 1981, *282*, 1029.

In a comparative crossover study of bronchodilator effectiveness completed by 18 of 20 patients with chronic bronchitis, aminophylline 225 mg in a sustained release basis (Phyllocontin) given twice daily and increased after 1 week to 450 mg twice daily for the next 3 weeks was considered to have caused a greater improvement in peak expiratory flow-rates with longer lasting relief from attacks of breathlessness than salbutamol 16 mg twice daily for 4 weeks given as salbutamol sulphate in sustained release tablets (Ventolin Spandets). The 2 patients, one in each group of 9, not included in the results withdrew after 3 weeks' treatment because they did not improve.— S. Maneksha, *Curr. med. Res. Opinion*, 1976, *4*, 207. Phyllocontin was also shown to produce a better response than choline theophyllinate.— *idem, Br. J. clin. Pract.*, 1978, *32*, 52.

In a double-blind crossover collaborative study of 28 children with chronic asthma, theophylline in doses ranging from 3.8 to 8.7 mg per kg body-weight four times daily and given generally to produce peak plasma-theophylline concentration of about 10 to 20 µg per ml was more effective than sodium cromoglycate 20 mg four times daily by inhalation. Both agents were also used together when the association produced similar results to theophylline alone but superior results to sodium cromoglycate; 59% of treatment days were symptom-free during cromoglycate therapy compared with 71% during therapy with theophylline or with both compounds. Improvement in pulmonary function was not significantly different with either agent but the association produced a significantly better improvement when compared with sodium cromoglycate. It was considered that a patient inadequately controlled on sodium cromoglycate might gain some benefit from additional therapy with theophylline but that sodium cromoglycate would not benefit those on theophylline. There was no indication for the routine use of both drugs together.— G. Hambleton *et al., Lancet*, 1977, *1*, 381. A report of comparable effects with sodium cromoglycate or a slow-release aminophylline preparation in the prophylaxis of childhood asthma.— A. T. Edmunds *et al., Br. med. J.*, 1980, *281*, 842.

The optimum dose of aminophylline given intravenously for severe asthma resistant to beta-adrenergic stimulants was 375 mg followed by a total daily dose of not more than 1 g. The use of aminophylline in conjunction with beta-adrenergic stimulants in large doses was not recommended because of toxicity.— *Br. med. J.*, 1975, *4*, 65.

Aminophylline in conjunction with adrenaline was no better than adrenaline alone in the initial treatment of acute asthma.— G. W. Josephson *et al., J. Am. med. Ass.*, 1979, *242*, 639. Conflicting evidence.— T. H. Rossing *et al., Am. Rev. resp. Dis.*, 1981, *123*, 190.

Dosage in children. In a double-blind study in 12 children with asthma, aminophylline 6.3 to 10.7 mg per kg body-weight every 6 hours and aminophylline in the same dose plus ephedrine 1.3 to 2.1 mg per kg were significantly more effective than placebo in relieving asthma. Ephedrine did not significantly enhance the effect of aminophylline, but increased the incidence of side-effects. Serum-theophylline concentrations ranged from 8.8 to 25 µg per ml.— M. Weinberger and E. Bronsky, *J. Pediat.*, 1974, *84*, 421.

In a study of 150 asthmatic children aged from about 1 to 19 years, a mean dose of aminophylline 7.5 mg per kg body-weight by mouth resulted in a mean serum-theophylline concentration of about 15 μg per ml. Dose and serum concentrations were not strongly related because of individual differences in rate of metabolism. Those under 10 years needed higher doses than older children.— P. Rangsithienchai and R. W. Newcomb, *J. Pediat.*, 1977, *91*, 325.

From a study involving 156 children and 33 adults recommended maximum oral doses of theophylline in the management of chronic asthma were: 24 mg per kg body-weight daily for children under 9 years, 20 mg per kg daily from 9 to 12 years, 18 mg per kg daily from 12 to 16 years, and 13 mg per kg daily in adults. At these doses about 50% of patients would have serum-theophylline concentrations over 10 μg per ml and 10 to 20% would risk exceeding 20 μg per ml.— R. Wyatt *et al.*, *J. Pediat.*, 1978, *92*, 125. See also M. Weinberger, *ibid.*, 1.

For intravenous doses of aminophylline in children see under Status Asthmaticus and under Dosage (below).

Status asthmaticus. In the treatment of status asthmaticus 500 mg of aminophylline and 200 mg of hydrocortisone sodium succinate should be given intravenously immediately; sympathomimetics by inhalation or injection should be avoided unless oxygen could be administered at the same time. In hospital massive corticosteroid therapy should be continued and if necessary salbutamol aerosol 0.5% should be administered by positive-pressure ventilation in 40% oxygen for 2 to 3 minutes, every 1 to 2 hours; continuous oxygen therapy was essential.— *Br. med. J.*, 1972, *4*, 563.

Aminophylline 4 mg per kg body-weight by slow intravenous injection was recommended together with salbutamol by inhalation and hydrocortisone intravenously in the immediate treatment of status asthmaticus in children.— S. Godfrey, *Br. J. Hosp. Med.*, 1977, *17*, 430. From a study in 50 children it was concluded that aminophylline 6 mg per kg body-weight by intravenous injection over 5 minutes and followed by 1 mg per kg hourly by infusion, in association with hydrocortisone by intravenous bolus injection and then infusion and salbutamol by inhalation, should be given to all children in status asthmaticus with a peak expiratory flow rate of less than 25% of the expected value for height.— S. A. McKenzie *et al.*, *Archs Dis. Childh.*, 1979, *54*, 581.

See also G. Hambleton and M. J. Stone, *Archs Dis. Childh.*, 1979, *54*, 391; K. Selvig *et al.*, *Acta paediat. scand.*, 1979, *68*, 435.

See also under Dosage (below).

Cheyne-Stokes respiration. In 8 patients with Cheyne-Stokes respiration and 6 with emphysema, aminophylline, given over a 5-minute period by intravenous infusion in a dose of 250 mg in 10 ml of saline solution, rapidly abolished periodic breathing, increased ventilation, lowered the arterial pCO_2, and increased the pH of arterial blood in those with Cheyne-Stokes respiration. It was suggested that aminophylline abolished Cheyne-Stokes respiration by lowering the threshold of carbon dioxide tension so that the respiratory response occurred more promptly when the blood carbon dioxide tension rose.— A. R. Dowell *et al.*, *New Engl. J. Med.*, 1965, *273*, 1447.

Dosage. The importance of monitoring serum-theophylline concentrations. The therapeutic index of theophylline is low and individual elimination rates are very variable.— L. Hendeles *et al.*, *Clin. Pharmacokinet.*, 1978, *3*, 294 and 422. It is important to obtain a trough serum-theophylline concentration at the same time on each day.— L. J. Lesko *et al.*, *J. pharm. Sci.*, 1980, *69*, 358. See also L. J. Lesko, *Clin. Pharmacokinet.*, 1979, *4*, 449.

New dosage guidelines for the intravenous administration of aminophylline have been produced by the FDA. All doses should be calculated from lean or ideal body-weight and the safest approach is to individualise dosage according to serum-theophylline concentrations. For patients not already receiving theophylline products a loading dose of 6 mg per kg body-weight of aminophylline is recommended followed by maintenance doses according to the status of the patient, the dose being reduced after 12 hours. Maintenance doses are: for children of 6 months to 9 years, 1.2 mg per kg hourly reduced to 1 mg per kg hourly; children of 9 to 16 years and young adult smokers, 1 mg per kg hourly reduced to 800 μg per kg hourly; nonsmoking adults, 700 μg per kg hourly reduced to 500 μg per kg hourly; older patients and those with cor pulmonale, 600 μg per kg hourly reduced to 300 μg per kg hourly; and patients with congestive heart failure or liver disease, 500 μg per kg hourly reduced to 100 to 200 μg per kg hourly. In patients already receiving theophylline products the loading dose should be adjusted on the basis that each 500 μg per kg of theophylline administered as a loading dose will result in a 1 μg per ml increase in serum-theophylline concentration.— *FDA Drug Bull.*, 1980, *10*, 4. See also *Lancet*, 1980, *1*, 746. Criticism of the interim maintenance dose and a suggestion that it should not be used.— J. E. Murphy and E. S. Ward (letter), *New Engl. J. Med.*, 1980, *303*, 760.

For earlier dosage recommendations for the intravenous administration of aminophylline, see P. A. Mitenko and R. I. Ogilvie, *New Engl. J. Med.*, 1973, *289*, 600; *Lancet*, 1973, *2*, 950; K. M. Piafsky and R. I. Ogilvie, *New Engl. J. Med.*, 1975, *292*, 1218; M. W. Weinberger *et al.*, *J. Am. med. Ass.*, 1976, *235*, 2110; L. Hendeles *et al.*, *Drug Intell. & clin. Pharm.*, 1977, *11*, 12; W. J. Jusko *et al.*, *Ann. intern. Med.*, 1977, *86*, 400; T. R. Kordash *et al.*, *J. Am. med. Ass.*, 1977, *238*, 139.

Dosage in liver failure. Administration in single doses of aminophylline intravenously to 9 patients with chronic alcoholic hepatic cirrhosis (compared with 19 previously studied healthy subjects) indicated that their ability to eliminate theophylline was not easy to predict from the usual laboratory tests of liver function. In 6 of 9 patients the plasma half-life was considerably prolonged and the plasma clearance decreased but the volume of distribution was little affected. For acute therapy, theophylline as aminophylline 6 mg per kg body-weight intravenously over 20 minutes would be safe because of the negligible change in the apparent volume of distribution, but the usually recommended maintenance dose of theophylline could be hazardous in cirrhotic patients. Regular determinations of plasma-theophylline concentrations would help in the calculation of a maintenance dose for cirrhotic patients.— K. M. Piafsky *et al.*, *New Engl. J. Med.*, 1977, *296*, 1495. Comment.— D. G. Shand, *ibid.*, 1527.

Dosage in renal failure. Theophylline can be given in usual doses to patients with renal failure. Concentrations are affected by haemodialysis or peritoneal dialysis.— W. M. Bennett *et al.*, *Ann. intern. Med.*, 1980, *93*, 286.

Obstructive pulmonary disease. The effect of an infusion of 1 g of aminophylline given over 30 minutes was studied in 9 patients with cor pulmonale. Pulmonary vascular resistance fell, and pulmonary artery, brachial artery, and right and left ventricular end-diastolic pressures were significantly reduced. Cardiac output was unchanged.— J. O. Parker *et al.*, *Circulation*, 1966, *33*, 17.

In 10 patients with chronic obstructive pulmonary disease but without cor pulmonale, the infusion, over 30 minutes, of 1 g of aminophylline in 30 ml of Sodium Chloride Injection caused a fall in mean pulmonary artery pressure, right and left ventricular end-diastolic pressure and mean brachial artery pressure, and a rise in heart-rate, respiration-rate, oxygen consumption, and minute ventilation. The calculated total peripheral resistance was reduced.— J. O. Parker *et al.*, *Circulation*, 1967, *35*, 365.

A study of theophylline kinetics in 9 patients with acute pulmonary oedema and 19 healthy subjects. It appeared safe to give a theophylline loading dose of 4.5 mg per kg body-weight (given as aminophylline) intravenously over 20 minutes; this dose was identical to that given for acute asthma. Because of the greater variability of plasma clearance of theophylline in heart failure, plasma concentrations and toxicity could not be predicted after repeated dosage or continuous infusion; benefits of prolonged therapy seemed unlikely to outweigh hazards in such patients.— K. M. Piafsky *et al.*, *Clin. Pharmac. Ther.*, 1977, *21*, 310.

Pregnancy and the neonate. A view that theophylline compounds appear to be the mainstay in the therapy of bronchospasm during pregnancy.— A. M. Weinstein *et al.*, *J. Am. med. Ass.*, 1979, *241*, 1161. Comment on potential problems with the use of theophylline during pregnancy.— J. A. Pollowitz (letter), *ibid.*, 1980, *243*, 651.

Dosage in premature infants. A study of the kinetics of theophylline in 6 premature infants following intravenous infusion (as aminophylline) over periods of 20 minutes; subsequent oral administration was also given to some infants. The apparent volume of distribution of theophylline was only slightly larger than that in children but its half-life of an average of about 30 hours (range about 14 to 58 hours) was 9 times larger, and its relative clearance-rate was decreased almost sevenfold. It was calculated that a loading dose of theophylline 5.5 mg per kg body-weight followed by 1.1 mg per kg every 8 hours would achieve a mean blood concentration of about 8 μg per ml (equivalent to a mean plasma concentration of about 10 μg per ml). Comparative studies with adult plasma indicated reduced theophylline binding by protein of cord plasma from full-term infants (which might be accentuated in premature infants); no significant competition was noted between theophylline and bilirubin.— J. V. Aranda *et al.*, *New Engl. J. Med.*, 1976, *295*, 413. See also G. Giacoia *et al.*, *J. Pediat.*, 1976, *89*, 829.

An effective loading dose of aminophylline in premature infants with apnoea is considered to be 6.2 mg per kg body-weight given intravenously over 20 minutes; this should produce an effective nontoxic serum-theophylline concentration of 12 μg per ml at 1 hour. Serum concentrations are maintained by continuous infusion and 4.4 mg per kg daily is considered to be a safe maximum. The serum half-life in 4 infants ranged from 27 to 45 hours. Choline theophyllinate given by gastric tube is not considered suitable for emergency treatment.— R. A. K. Jones and E. Baillie, *Archs Dis. Childh.*, 1979, *54*, 190. Theophylline 0.5% in alcohol 10% was given by nasogastric tube to 33 similar infants and abolished or alleviated apnoea. A dose of 3 mg per kg given every 8 hours produced mean plasma concentrations of about 14 μg per ml from the 5th day of treatment as measured in 20 of the infants; the half-life was about 30 hours.— J. -L. Brazier *et al.*, *ibid.*, 194. The plasma half-life of theophylline given by nasogastric tube to 6 preterm infants as theophylline sodium glycinate was estimated as 24 to 64 hours. Peak plasma concentrations occurred between 4 and 8 hours.— D. M. King *et al.*, *ibid.*, 238.

Preparations

Enemas

Aminophylline Enema *(U.S.P.)*. An aqueous solution of aminophylline prepared with the aid of ethylenediamine. Potency is expressed in terms of aminophylline dihydrate. pH 9 to 9.5. It contains 172 to 211 mg of ethylenediamine per g of aminophylline dihydrate, but no other substance may be added to adjust the pH.

Injections

Aminophylline Injection *(B.P.)*. Theophylline and Ethylenediamine Injection. A sterile solution in Water for Injections. pH 8.8 to 10.

Aminophylline Injection *(U.S.P.)*. A sterile solution of aminophylline in Water for Injections, or a sterile solution of theophylline in Water for Injections prepared with the aid of ethylenediamine. It contains 23.25 to 26.75 mg of aminophylline dihydrate in each ml. pH 8.6 to 9. It contains 131 to 152 mg of ethylenediamine per g of aminophylline dihydrate, but no other substance may be added to adjust the pH. It must not be used if crystals have separated.

Suppositories

Aminophylline Suppositories *(B.P.)*. Theophylline and Ethylenediamine Suppositories. Suppositories containing aminophylline in a suitable suppository basis. About 1.5 g of aminophylline displaces 1 g of theobroma oil. Store at a temperature not exceeding 30°. *A.P.F.* specifies 400 mg prepared in a 2-g mould for adults and 50 mg prepared in a 1-g mould for children and storage below 25°.

Aminophylline Suppositories *(U.S.P.)*. Suppositories containing aminophylline. Potency is expressed in terms of the dihydrate. Store at a temperature not exceeding 8°.

Tablets

Aminophylline Tablets *(B.P.)*. Theophylline and Ethylenediamine Tablets. Tablets containing aminophylline. Store in airtight containers. Protect from light.

Aminophylline Tablets *(U.S.P.)*. Tablets containing aminophylline. Potency is expressed in terms of the dihydrate. Store in airtight containers.

Proprietary Preparations

Phyllocontin Tablets *(Napp, UK)*. Each contains aminophylline 225 mg in a sustained-release basis. **Phyllocontin Paediatric Tablets**. Each contains aminophylline 100 mg in a sustained-release basis. (Also available as Phyllocontin in *Denm.*, *USA*).

Theodrox *(Riker, UK)*. Tablets each containing aminophylline 195 mg and dried aluminium hydroxide 260 mg.

See also under Ephedrine, p.12.

Other Proprietary Names

Austral.— Androphyllin, Cardophyllin, Carine, Somophyllin; *Canad.*— Aminophyl, Corophyllin, Somophyllin; *Denm.*— Teofylamin; *Fr.*— Inophyline (see also Theophylline Monoethanolamine, p.350); *Ger.*— Euphyllin, Phyllotemp Retard; *Ital.*— Aminomal, Tefamin; *Neth.*— Euphyllin; *S.Afr.*—Euphyllin Retard, Peterphyllin; *Spain*— Eufilina, Godafilin; *Swed.*— Teofyllamin; *Switz.*— Corphyllamin, Escophyllin, Euphyllin, Phyllotemp, Variaphylline L.A.; *USA*— Aminodur, Lixaminol, Mini-lix, Rectalad-Aminophylline, Somophyllin.

Aminophylline was also formerly marketed in Great Britain under the proprietary names Cardophylin (*Fisons*) and Phyldrox Suppositories (*Carlton Laboratories*). A preparation containing aminophylline was also formerly marketed in Great Britain under the proprietary name Riddovydrin (*Riddell*).

629-v

Bamifylline Hydrochloride. AC 3810; CB 8102. 8-Benzyl-7-[2-(*N*-ethyl-*N*-2-hydroxyethylamino)ethyl]theophylline hydrochloride.

$C_{20}H_{27}N_5O_3,HCl=421.9$.

CAS — 2016-63-9 (bamifylline); 20684-06-4 (hydrochloride).

A crystalline solid. M.p. about 185°.

Bamifylline is a theophylline derivative which has been used for the same purposes as aminophylline (see p.344) but has been claimed to cause less gastric irritation. It is readily absorbed from the gastro-intestinal tract and has been reported not to liberate theophylline in the body. Skin reactions have been reported in sensitive persons. It has been given in doses of 600 mg thrice daily, often reduced to 300 mg thrice daily.

The metabolic fate of bamifylline differed markedly from that of theophylline.— L. Dodion *et al.*, *Arzneimittel-Forsch.*, 1969, *19*, 785.

Proprietary Names

Trentadil *(Christiaens, Belg.; Spret-Mauchant, Fr.; Fresenius, Ger.; Padro, Spain; Christiaens, Switz.)*.

Bamifylline hydrochloride was formerly marketed in Great Britain under the proprietary name Trentadil (*Armour*).

630-r

Bufylline. Ambuphylline; Theophylline-aminoisobutanol. 2-Amino-2-methylpropan-1-ol theophyllinate.

$C_{11}H_{19}N_5O_3=269.3$.

CAS — 5634-34-4.

A crystalline solid, slightly **soluble** in water. M.p. about 255°.

Bufylline is a theophylline derivative which is used for the same purposes as aminophylline (see p.344) and has been given in doses of 60 to 120 mg. It has also been given rectally. Bufylline is an ingredient of Nethaprin Dospan and Nethaprin Expectorant, p.13.

Proprietary Names

Buthoid *(Merrell, Canad.)*.

631-f

Choline Theophyllinate *(B.P.)*. Choline Theoph.; Oxtriphylline *(U.S.P.)*; Theophylline Cholinate.

$C_{12}H_{21}N_5O_3=283.3$.

CAS — 4499-40-5.

Pharmacopoeias. In *Br.*, *Chin.*, and *U.S.*

A white crystalline powder, odourless or with a faint amine-like odour and a slightly saline taste. M.p. 185° to 192°. Choline theophyllinate 1.57 g is approximately equivalent in theophylline content to 1 g of theophylline. **Soluble** 1 in less than 1 of water and 1 in 10 of alcohol; very slightly soluble in chloroform and ether. A 1% solution in water has a pH of about 10.3. **Store** at a temperature not exceeding 25° in airtight containers. Protect from light.

Adverse Effects, Treatment, and Precautions. As for Aminophylline, p.342.

A report of a massive overdosage with choline theophyllinate.— T. J. Iberti and R. S. Hammond, *Sth. med. J.*, 1978, *71*, 965.

Absorption and Fate. Choline theophyllinate is readily absorbed from the gastro-intestinal tract.

Serum concentrations of theophylline were higher after the administration of choline theophyllinate by mouth than by rectum, and were higher after administration by either route than after the similar administration of aminophylline.— H. P. M. Kerckhoffs and T. Huizinga, *Pharm. Weekbl. Ned.*, 1967, *102*, 1255, per *Int. pharm. Abstr.*, 1968, *5*, 548.

In 10 asthmatic patients given a 600-mg dose of choline theophyllinate, the mean peak plasma concentration (10.4 µg per ml) was attained after 2 hours; a plasma concentration of 7 µg per ml of theophylline was required for a respiratory effect.— K. B. Bülow *et al.*, *Eur. J. clin. Pharmac.*, 1975, *8*, 115. Plasma-theophylline concentrations and ventilatory function in chronic obstructive pulmonary disease during prolonged treatment with choline theophyllinate by mouth.— *idem*, 119.

Further references.— T. D. Bell *et al.*, *Ann. Allergy*, 1977, *38*, 440; D. S. Sitar *et al.*, *Curr. ther. Res.*, 1977, *21*, 233; T. Bell *et al.*, *Ann. Allergy*, 1980, *44*, 67.

Uses. Choline theophyllinate is a theophylline salt which is used for the same purposes as aminophylline (see p.344). The usual dosage for adults is 100 to 400 mg four times daily, starting with a dose of 200 mg; it should be taken during or after a meal to reduce gastro-intestinal side-effects. The dosage for children aged 1 to 5 years is 50 to 100 mg thrice daily and for children aged 6 to 12 years, 100 to 200 mg thrice daily. Caution is necessary in giving choline theophyllinate to very young children.

In a study of the British Thoracic and Tuberculosis Association, the effects of various combinations of choline theophyllinate 100 mg or 200 mg and salmefamol 0.5 mg or 1 mg on peak expiratory flow rate in 54 patients with reversible airways obstruction were shown to be additive, but enhancement could not be demonstrated. It was considered that the combined use of higher doses of each drug might show an enhanced effect but that the incidence of side-effects would be unacceptable.— A. J. Dyson and I. A. Campbell, *Br. J. clin. Pharmac.*, 1977, *4*, 677.

Dosage in children. Apnoeic attacks in a premature twin were controlled by choline theophyllinate 2 mg per kg body-weight daily by mouth; in the second twin the dose had to be increased to 5 mg per kg, and was associated with 2 episodes of hyperglycaemia and glycosuria.— V. F. Larcher *et al.*, *Archs Dis. Childh.*, 1978, *53*, 757.

In a study to determine a suitable dosage schedule, asthmatic children aged from about 1 to 15 years were given choline theophyllinate either about 8 mg per kg body-weight per dose four times daily or about 10 mg per kg per dose thrice daily. Both schedules produced serum concentrations of theophylline in the therapeutic range, 2 hours after dosing but these were not maintained over an 8-hour dosage interval. The study also showed varying intra-subject blood concentrations of the theophylline.— S. A. McKenzie *et al.*, *Archs Dis. Childh.*, 1978, *53*, 167.

Myasthenia gravis. A 17-year-old girl with refractory fulminating myasthenia gravis responded to the administration of choline theophyllinate with corticotrophin; the maximum response did not occur until after about 10 days' therapy. She was maintained on an oral dose of 800 mg daily.— *J. Am. med. Ass.*, 1971, *216*, 416.

Choline theophyllinate was investigated in 9 patients with myasthenia gravis. The dosage regimen was 300 to 400 mg daily in divided doses increasing to 1.8 to 2.4 g daily within 4 days and then reducing to a maintenance of 1.2 to 1.8 g daily in divided doses. The 5 severely affected patients obtained marked improvement particularly when the drug was used to enhance anticholinesterase or corticotrophin therapy but it had little effect in the patients with mild symptoms and those who responded reasonably well to anticholinesterase medication. Side-effects included tachycardia, anginal pain, and severe nausea.— J. Brumlik *et al.*, *Clin. Pharmac. Ther.*, 1973, *14*, 380.

Preparations

Choline Theophyllinate Tablets *(B.P.)*. Tablets containing choline theophyllinate; they are compression-coated. Store at a temperature not exceeding 25° in airtight containers. Protect from light.

Oxtriphylline Elixir *(U.S.P.)*. An elixir containing choline theophyllinate, with alcohol 18 to 22%. pH 8 to 9. Store in airtight containers. Protect from light.

Oxtriphylline Tablets *(U.S.P.)*. Tablets containing choline theophyllinate; they may be partially enteric-coated. Store in airtight containers.

Proprietary Preparations

Choledyl *(Warner, UK)*. Choline theophyllinate, available as **Syrup** containing 62.5 mg in each 5 ml (dilution not recommended), and as **Tablets** of 100 and 200 mg. (Also available as Choledyl in *Austral.*, *Canad.*, *Denm.*, *Norw.*, *S.Afr.*, *USA*).

Other Proprietary Names

Cholecyl, Teocolina *(Spain)*; Cholegyl, Dilasmyl *(both Neth.)*; Chophyllin *(Denm.)*; Euspirax *(Ger.)*; Sclerofillina, Teofilcolina *(both Ital.)*; Theocoline *(Jap.)*; Theophylline Choline *(Canad.)*.

632-d

Prepared Coffee *(B.P.C. 1968)*. Prep. Coff.; Coffea Praeparata.

Pharmacopoeias. Coffee (Café; Coffeae Semen; Semilla de Café), from *C. arabica*, is included in *Port.* and *Span.*

The kernel of the dried ripe seeds of *Coffea arabica*, *C. liberica*, *C. canephora* (robusta coffee), and other species of *Coffea* (Rubiaceae), roasted until it acquires a deep brown colour and a pleasant characteristic aroma. It contains about 1 to 2% of caffeine. It should be freshly roasted and ground, and used immediately or **stored** in hermetically sealed containers under vacuum or in an inert gas.

Adverse Effects and Precautions. As for Caffeine, p.340.

Comment on the adverse effects associated with coffee drinking.— *Lancet*, 1981, *1*, 256.

A report of 2 deaths associated with the use of coffee enemas.— J. W. Eisele and D. T. Reay, *J. Am. med. Ass.*, 1980, *244*, 1608.

Carcinogenicity. P. Cole (*Lancet*, 1971, *1*, 1335; see also R. Schmauz and P. Cole, *J. natn. Cancer Inst.*, 1974, *52*, 1431) reported a possible association between bladder cancer and coffee drinking but it was not confirmed by R.W. Morgan and M.G. Jain (*Can. med. Ass. J.*, 1974, *111*, 1067). D.H. Shennan (*Br. J. Cancer*, 1973, *28*, 473) concluded that, although there was a strong correlation between coffee consumption and national mortality-rates for renal cancer, other environmental influences were also important. After a retrospective study in 139 patients B. Armstrong *et al.* (*Br. J. Cancer*, 1976, *33*, 127) could find no positive association between coffee consumption and renal cancer.

Coffee, and other foodstuffs containing phenolic substances which were readily oxidised, might significantly increase exposure to carcinogenic *N*-nitrosamines by catalysing their formation in the gastro-intestinal tract.— B. C. Challis and C. D. Bartlett (letter), *Nature*, 1975, *254*, 532.

A report of an unexpected association of pancreatic cancer with coffee consumption in 369 patients with histologically proven cancer of the pancreas when compared with 644 control subjects.— B. MacMahon *et al.*, *New Engl. J. Med.*, 1981, *304*, 630. Data from the Boston Collaborative Drug Surveillance Program which do not support the hypothesis of a positive association between coffee and pancreatic cancer.— H. Jick and B. J. Dinan (letter), *Lancet*, 1981, *2*, 92. Tentative findings of a positive association.— A. Nomura *et al.* (letter), *ibid.*, 415.

Effects on the cardiovascular system. Reports from the Boston Collaborative Drug Surveillance Program (*Lancet*, 1972, *2*, 1278; *New Engl. J. Med.*, 1973, *289*, 63) suggested an association between acute myocardial infarction and coffee consumption which was not confirmed in a controlled study by A.L. Klatsky *et al.* (*J. Am. med. Ass.*, 1973, *226*, 540). More recent studies have also been unable to establish a connection between coffee drinking and the incidence of cardiovascular disease when other risk factors were taken into account (T.R. Dawber *et al.*, *New Engl. J. Med.*, 1974, *291*, 871; C.H. Hennekens *et al.*, *ibid.*, 1976, *294*, 633; K. Yano *et al.*, *ibid.*, 1977, *297*, 405; C.A. Bertrand *et al.*, *New Engl. J. Med.*, 1978, *299*, 315 and 726; S. Heyden *et al.*, *Archs intern. Med.*, 1978, *138*, 1472) and 2 reviews have concluded that a link has not yet been established (*Med. Lett.*, 1977, *19*, 65; *Br. med. J.*, 1977, *2*, 284).

Effects on the gastro-intestinal tract. Heartburn was the major gastro-intestinal symptom associated with drinking coffee in a study of 31 subjects with a history of these symptoms. The heartburn appeared to be associated with lower oesophageal sphincter dysfunction and gastro-oesophageal reflux rather than gastric hypersecretion although symptoms could be modified by a reduction in acid secretion. Intrinsic harmful components in coffee do not appear to be responsible.— S. Cohen, *New Engl. J. Med.*, 1980, *303*, 122.

Interactions. A study on the effects of smoking in association with coffee drinking on blood-cholesterol concentrations.— S. Heyden *et al.*, *Circulation*, 1979, *60*, 22.

Pregnancy and the neonate. There were no dose-related teratological effects in the offspring of female *rats* who had consumed fresh-brewed coffee *ad libitum* as their sole source of liquid for five weeks prior to breeding and throughout gestation.— P. E. Palm, *Toxic. appl. Pharmac.*, 1978, *44*, 1.

Suggestion of ectrodactyly associated with moderately high caffeine intake.— M. F. Jacobson *et al.* (letter), *Lancet*, 1981, *1*, 1415.

No association between coffee consumption and adverse outcomes of pregnancy.— S. Linn *et al.*, *New Engl. J. Med.*, 1982, *306*, 141.

Treatment of Adverse Effects. As for Aminophylline, p.342.

Uses. Coffee has been used in the form of an infusion or decoction as a stimulant and as a flavouring agent in some pharmaceutical preparations.

A decoction is used as a beverage containing up to about 100 mg of caffeine per 100 ml. Preparations of instant coffee may contain up to 40% less caffeine while decaffeinated preparations may contain only about 3 mg per 100 ml.

633-n

Diprophylline (*B.P., Eur. P.*).

Diprophyllinum; Dihydroxypropyltheophyllinum; Dyphylline; Glyphyllinum; Hyphylline. 7-(2,3-Dihydroxypropyl)-1,3-dimethylxanthine; 7-(2,3-Dihydroxypropyl)theophylline.

$C_{10}H_{14}N_4O_4$=254.2.

CAS — 479-18-5.

Pharmacopoeias. In *Aust.*, *Br.*, *Chin.*, *Eur.*, *Fr.*, *Ger.*, *Neth.*, *Nord.*, *Rus.*, and *Swiss.*

A white odourless crystalline powder with a bitter taste. **Soluble** 1 in 3 of water, 1 in 50 of alcohol; slightly soluble in chloroform; practically insoluble in ether. M.p. 160° to 165°. A 1% solution in water is neutral. A 10.87% solution is iso-osmotic with serum. Solutions are **sterilised** by autoclaving or by filtration. **Store** in airtight containers. Protect from light.

An aqueous solution of diprophylline iso-osmotic with serum (10.87%) caused 95% haemolysis of erythrocytes cultured in it for 45 minutes.— E. R. Hammarlund and K. Pedersen-Bjergaard, *J. pharm. Sci.*, 1961, *50*, 24.

Adverse Effects, Treatment, and Precautions. As for Aminophylline, p.342. Diprophylline may cause less nausea and gastric irritation than aminophylline. The intramuscular injection is claimed to be almost painless.

Absorption and Fate. Diprophylline is readily absorbed from the gastro-intestinal tract and from the site of intramuscular injections.

The average half-life of diprophylline was reported to be 2.1 hours.— L. Hendeles and M. Weinberger, *Drug Intell. & clin. Pharm.*, 1977, *11*, 424. See also F. E. R. Simons *et al.*, *J. Allergy & clin. Immunol.*, 1975, *56*, 347, per *Int. pharm. Abstr.* 1976, *13*, 1242.

The bioavailability of a sustained-release preparation of diprophylline.— K. J. Simons *et al.*, *J. clin. Pharmac.*, 1977, *17*, 237.

Diprophylline 600 mg was given by enema to 18 patients; a mean peak blood concentration of 1.56 µg per ml occurred 1 hour after administration.— M. L. Schilt, *Arzneimittel-Forsch.*, 1978, *28*, 311.

In 5 healthy subjects given diprophylline 19 to 28 mg per kg body-weight by mouth a mean peak serum-diprophylline concentration of 24.4 µg per ml (range 19.3 to 36.4 µg per ml) occurred at a mean of 1 hour (range 0.75 to 1.25 hours) after administration. The mean half-life was 1.8 hours (range 1.5 to 2.1 hours). A mean of 83% (range 77 to 88%) of the administered dose was excreted unchanged in the urine after 24 hours. Measurements of faecal excretion in 1 subject accounted for 0.7% of the dose.— K. J. Simons and F. E. R. Simons, *J. pharm. Sci.*, 1979, *68*, 1327.

The extremely rapid clearance of diprophylline was inhibited by probenecid in 5 healthy subjects.— D. C. May and C. H. Jarboe (letter), *New Engl. J. Med.*, 1981, *304*, 791.

Uses. Diprophylline is a theophylline derivative which is used similarly to aminophylline (see p.344), but it is better tolerated by mouth and by intramuscular injection.

The usual dose by mouth is 200 mg thrice daily but up to 400 mg every 6 hours may be necessary for the treatment of acute conditions. It may also be given intramuscularly in a dose of 200 to 500 mg repeated up to thrice daily, by slow intravenous injection to a maximum of 1.5 g in 24 hours, or by rectum in the form of suppositories containing 400 mg. A suggested dose (by mouth or intramuscularly) for children is 5 mg per kg body-weight.

The nicotinate of diprophylline, diniprofylline, has also been used.

Dosage by suppository in children should not exceed 6.6 mg per kg body-weight, repeated every 8 hours if necessary in older children but not more often than 12-hourly in children under 2 years. Early signs of overdosage were vomiting, irritability, and restlessness, followed in more severe cases by haematemesis, maniacal behaviour, delirium, and convulsions; treatment should be symptomatic.— G. Marion (letter), *Can. med. Ass. J.*, 1967, *97*, 1612.

In a double-blind study in 12 patients with severe but partially reversible airway obstruction the bronchodilator effect of 500 mg of aminophylline was greater than that of 500 mg or 1 g of diprophylline. The side-effects of aminophylline were however greater than those of the larger dose of diprophylline and further study with doses of diprophylline higher than those usually recommended was warranted.— L. D. Hudson *et al.*, *Curr. ther. Res.*, 1973, *15*, 367.

Further references: M. Turner-Warwick, *Br. med. J.*, 1957, *2*, 67.

Preparations

Injectabile Glyphyllini (*Nord. P.*). Diprophylline Injection. Diprophylline 10% w/v in Water for Injections. *Dan. Disp.* specifies methyl hydroxybenzoate 0.1% as preservative.

Suppositoria Glyphyllini (*Nord. P.*). Diprophylline Suppositories. Each contains diprophylline 500 mg in adeps solidus (*Nord.P.*).

Tablettae Glyphyllini (*Nord. P.*). Diprophylline Tablets. Each contains diprophylline 250 mg.

Proprietary Preparations

Silbephylline (*Berk Pharmaceuticals, UK*). Diprophylline, available as 2-ml **Ampoules** of an injection containing 250 mg per ml; as **Suppositories** of 400 mg; as **Syrup** containing 100 mg in each 5 ml (suggested diluent, syrup); and as scored **Tablets** of 200 mg. (Also available as Silbephylline in *S.Afr.*).

Other Proprietary Names

Belg.— Neutraphylline; *Canad.*— Aerophylline, Dilin, Protophylline; *Denm.*— Glyfyllin; *Fr.*— Neutraphylline; *Ger.*— Asthmolysin Zäpfchen; *Ital.*— Neutrafillina; *Jap.*— Astmamasitt, Neophyllin M; *Neth.*— Neo-Vasophylline; *Spain*— Difilina; *Switz.*— Dicoryllin, Prophyllen, Synthophylline; *USA*— Airet, Dilin, Dilor, Droxine, Dyflex, Emfabid, Lufyllin, Neothylline.

Diprophylline was also formerly marketed in Great Britain under the proprietary names Lancephylline (*Lancet Pharmaceuticals*, now *Kirby-Warrick*) and Neutraphylline (*Cox-Continental*).

634-h

Etamiphylline Camsylate.

Etamphyllin Camsylate; Diétamiphylline Camphosulfonate. 7-(2-Diethylaminoethyl)-1,3-dimethylxanthine camphor-10-sulphonate; 7-(2-Diethylaminoethyl)theophylline camphor-10-sulphonate.

$C_{23}H_{37}N_5O_6S$=511.6.

CAS — 314-35-2 (etamiphylline); 19326-29-5 (camsylate).

A white crystalline powder. M.p. about 174°. **Soluble** 1 in 2 of water. Solutions in water have a pH of about 7.

Adverse Effects, Treatment, and Precautions. As for Aminophylline, p.342. Etamiphylline camsylate is claimed to cause less gastric irritation than aminophylline and less pain on intramuscular injection.

Uses. Etamiphylline camsylate is a theophylline derivative which is used similarly to aminophylline (see p.344). It has been stated to increase both the rate and depth of respiration to a greater extent than theophylline but its diuretic effects are less.

It is given by mouth in doses of 100 to 300 mg three or four times daily after meals, by intramuscular injection in doses of 700 mg three or four times daily, or by slow intravenous injection, as a 3.5% solution of 350 mg, repeated as required. It is given by rectum once or twice daily as suppositories containing 500 mg. A suggested dose for children is 10 to 100 mg according to age intramuscularly or intravenously or 2.5 mg per kg body-weight and up to 200 mg may be given by mouth or rectally.

Etamiphylline is also used as the hydrochloride and the methiodide.

Proprietary Preparations

Millophylline (*Martindale Pharmaceuticals, UK*). Etamiphylline camsylate, available as 5-ml **Ampoules** of 700 mg for injection; as **Suppositories** (Adult) each containing 500 mg; as **Suppositories** (Child) each containing 200 mg; and as **Tablets** of 100 mg.

Other Proprietary Names

Camphophyline (*Fr.*); Iodaphyline (methiodide) (*Fr.*); Iodafilina (methiodide) (*Spain*); Solufilina simple (hydrochloride) (*Spain*).

635-m

Etofylline (*B.P., Eur. P.*).

Etofyllinum; Aethophyllinum; Hydroxyaethyltheophyllinum; Hydroxyéthylthéophylline; Oxyetophylline. 7-(2-Hydroxyethyl)-1,3-dimethylxanthine; 7-(2-Hydroxyethyl)theophylline.

$C_9H_{12}N_4O_3$=224.2.

CAS — 519-37-9.

Pharmacopoeias. In *Aust.*, *Br.*, *Cz.*, *Eur.*, *Fr.*, *Ger.*, and *Neth.*

A white odourless crystalline powder with a bitter taste. M.p. 161° to 166°.

Soluble in water; slightly soluble in alcohol; sparingly soluble in chloroform; practically insoluble in ether. A 5% solution in water has a pH of 6.5 to 7. Solutions may be **sterilised** by autoclaving or by filtration.

Uses. Etofylline is a theophylline derivative and is used in doses ranging up to 1.5 g daily for the same purposes as aminophylline (see p.344). It is claimed to be well tolerated by mouth and by intramuscular injection and has also been given by slow intravenous injection. It may be given by rectum as suppositories.

Mean regional cerebral blood flow decreased by 16.7% in 10 patients with cerebral ischaemia given etofylline 440 mg intravenously.— H. Herrschaft, *Arzneimittel-Forsch.*, 1976, *26*, 1240.

In 10 healthy subjects given etofylline 300 mg by mouth a mean peak plasma concentration of 7.8 µg per ml occurred 3 hours after administration. Following administration of a tablet containing etofylline 300 mg and fominoben 160 mg the mean peak plasma-etofylline concentration was 10.4 µg per ml after 1.5 hours.— R. Jauch and A. Zimmer, *Arzneimittel-Forsch.*, 1978, *28*, 693.

An improvement of pulmonary haemodynamics was observed in 10 patients with chronic obstructive lung diseases given fominoben 160 mg and etofylline 300 mg thrice daily for 8 to 32 days.— G. Siemon and R. Thoma, *Arzneimittel-Forsch.*, 1978, *28*, 698.

Proprietary Names
Bio-Phyllin *(Bio-Chemical Laboratory, Canad.)*; De-Oxin (nicotinate) *(Berenguer-Beneyto, Spain)*; Dilaphyllin tabletten *(Streuli, Switz.)*; Hesotin (nicotinate) *(Lannacher, Denm.)*; Oxyphylline *(Amido, Fr.)*.

636-b

Heptaminol Acephyllinate. Acéfyllinate d'Heptaminol; Heptaminol Theophylline-7-acetate; Heptaminol Theophylline Ethanoate. The 6-amino-2-methylheptan-2-ol salt of theophyllin-7-ylacetic acid.
$C_8H_{19}NO,C_9H_{10}N_4O_4$=383.4.

CAS — 5152-72-7; 10075-18-0.

Uses. Heptaminol acephyllinate is a theophylline derivative with uses similar to those of aminophylline (see p.344). It has been administered by mouth in doses of 0.5 to 1 g thrice daily, or by intramuscular or intravenous injection.

Proprietary Names
Cariamyl *(Carrion, Fr.; Clin-Midy, Spain; Delalande, Switz.)*; Corophylline *(Gerda, Fr.)*; Funesil*(Sideta, Spain)*; Theo-Heptylon *(Delalande, Ger.)*.

637-v

Kola *(B.P.C. 1949)*. Cola; Cola Seeds; Kola Nuts; Embryo Colae; Semen Colae.

Pharmacopoeias. In *Arg., Aust., Belg., Fr., Pol., Port., Roum., Span.,* and *Swiss.*

The dried cotyledons of *Cola nitida* and *C. acuminata* (Sterculiaceae), containing about 1.5 to 2.5% of caffeine and traces of theobromine. **Store** in a dry place.

Uses. The therapeutic properties of kola derive from its caffeine content (see p.341). It is used in the preparation of cola drinks which may contain up to 20 mg of caffeine per 100 ml.

Preparations

Kola Liquid Extract *(B.P.C. 1949)*. 1 in 1; prepared by percolation with alcohol (60%). *Dose.* 0.6 to 1.2 ml. A similar preparation is included in many pharmacopoeias; several also include a dry extract.

Kola Tincture *(B.P.C. 1934)*. Kola liquid extract 20 ml, alcohol (60%) to 100 ml. *Dose.* 1 to 4 ml. A similar preparation is included in several pharmacopoeias. *Belg. P., Port. P.,* and *Span. P.* also include **Kola Wine** (Vinum Colae).

Labiton *(Laboratories for Applied Biology, UK)*. A mixture containing in each 10 ml dried extract of kola nuts 6.05 mg, caffeine (total) 7 mg, ethyl alcohol 2.8 ml, thiamine hydrochloride 750 µg, aminobenzoic acid 4 mg, syrup 3 g, and glycerophosphoric acid (20%) 0.02 ml. *Dose.* 10 ml twice daily.

Other Proprietary Names
Kobona *(Ger.)*.

638-g

Maté. Paraguay Tea.

The dried leaves of *Ilex paraguensis* (Aquifoliaceae), containing 0.2 to 2% of caffeine.

Uses. Maté is less astringent than tea and is extensively used as a beverage in South America.

Veno-occlusive disease of the liver in a young woman was attributed to the consumption of large quantities of maté tea over a number of years.— J. O'D. McGee *et al., J. clin. Path.,* 1976, *29,* 788.

640-d

Proxyphylline *(B.P., Eur. P.)*. Proxyphyllinum. 7-(2-Hydroxypropyl)-1,3-dimethylxanthine; 7-(2-Hydroxypropyl)theophylline.
$C_{10}H_{14}N_4O_3$=238.2.

CAS — 603-00-9.

Pharmacopoeias. In *Br., Eur., Fr., Ger., Neth.,* and *Nord.*

A white odourless crystalline powder with a bitter taste. Proxyphylline 1.32 g is approximately equivalent in theophylline content to 1 g of theophylline. **Soluble** 1 in 1.5 of water, 1 in 12 of alcohol, 1 in 6 of chloroform, and 1 in 500 of ether; soluble in acetone. M.p. 134° to 136°. A 1% solution is neutral. Solutions may be **sterilised** by autoclaving or by filtration.

Adverse Effects, Treatment, and Precautions. As for Aminophylline, (see p.342). Proxyphylline is reported to cause less gastric irritation than aminophylline.

Absorption and Fate. Proxyphylline is readily absorbed from the gastro-intestinal tract.

Plasma concentrations of theophylline were almost identical for 4 hours following the administration, by mouth or by rectum, of doses of proxyphylline and aminophylline equivalent to 300 mg of theophylline and of intravenous doses equivalent to 200 mg of theophylline.— B. Isakasson and B. Lindholm, *Acta med. scand.,* 1962, *171,* 33.

The biological half-life of proxyphylline was reported to be 4.3 hours.— W. A. Ritschel, *Drug Intell. & clin. Pharm.,* 1970, *4,* 332.

In healthy volunteers a mean peak plasma concentration of about 7 µg per ml was obtained about 30 minutes after a 300 mg dose by mouth. After 400 mg thrice daily for 5 days the mean peak plasma concentration was 18 µg per ml. About 25% of a given dose was excreted unchanged in the urine; the excretion half-life was about 6.5 hours (range 4.8 to 9.2).— C. Graffner *et al., Acta pharm. suec.,* 1973, *10,* 425.

In 18 patients given proxyphylline 600 mg rectally by enema a mean peak blood concentration of 5.3 µg per ml occurred 1 hour after administration.— M. L. Schilt, *Arzneimittel-Forsch.,* 1978, *28,* 311. See also W. A. Ritschel and M. Banarer, *ibid.,* 1973, *23,* 1031.

Uses. Proxyphylline is a theophylline derivative which is used similarly to aminophylline (see p.344), but it is reported to be better tolerated by mouth and by injection. The usual dose by mouth is 300 mg thrice daily but larger doses may be given. It has been given by intramusuclar or slow intravenous injection in doses of 300 to 400 mg and is given rectally as suppositories containing 500 mg.

Proxyphylline 300 mg by mouth was no more effective than a placebo in reducing asthmatic airway obstruction in 12 patients.— K. N. V. Palmer *et al.* (letter), *Br. med. J.,* 1971, *1,* 727.

Proprietary Names
Monophyllin *(AFI, Norw.)*; Neofyllin *(Pharmacia, Denm.)*; Pantafillina *(Ceccarelli, Ital.)*; Purophyllin *(Siegfried, Switz.)*; Spantin *(Pharmacia, Ger.)*; Spasmolysin *(Kade, Ger.)*; Theon *(Draco, Swed.)*.

Proxyphylline was formerly marketed in Great Britain under the proprietary names Brontyl 300 *(Lloyd-Hamol* and Thean *(Astra)*.

641-n

Pyridofylline. Pyridophylline; Pyridoxine *O*-(Theophyllin-7-ylethyl)sulphate. 3-Hydroxy-4,5-bis(hydroxymethyl)-2-methylpyridine 2-(theophyllin-7-yl)ethyl sulphate.
$C_{17}H_{23}N_5O_9S$=473.5.

CAS — 53403-97-7.

Uses. Pyridofylline is a theophylline derivative which is used for purposes similar to those of aminophylline (see p.344). It has been given in doses of 300 to 600 mg daily.

Proprietary Names
Athérophylline *(Merrell Toraude, Fr.)*.

642-h

Tea *(B.P.C. 1949)*. Thea; Chá; Thé; Tee.

Pharmacopoeias. In *Port.* (not less than 1.5% of caffeine) and *Fr.* (not less than 2% of caffeine).

The prepared young leaves and leaf-buds of *Camellia sinensis* (=*C.thea*) (Theaceae). It contains 1 to 4% of caffeine and 7 to 15% of tannin. **Store** in airtight containers. Protect from light.

Tea is used in an infusion as a beverage containing up to about 60 mg of caffeine per 100 ml.

The cardiac effects of tea.— L. Gould *et al., J. clin. Pharmac.,* 1973, *13,* 469.

A review of the nutritional and therapeutic value of tea.— G. V. Stagg and D. J. Millin, *J. Sci. Fd Agric.,* 1975, *26,* 1439.

A woman who had been eating 227 g of tea every 3 to 4 days for about 5 years developed liver dysfunction. Splenomegaly and ascites resolved when she ceased eating tea but liver fibrosis was still present 15 years later. The liver dysfunction could have been due to the tannin content of tea.— K. J. Murphy, *Med. J. Aust.,* 1975, *2,* 428.

Tonic posturing and irritability of the central nervous system occurred in a 7-week-old infant after the ingestion of tea which contained about 75 mg of caffeine.— A. S. Brem *et al., Pediat. Res.,* 1977, *11,* 414.

Chemical basis of quality in tea. I Analysis of freshly plucked shoots, II Analysis of withered leaf and of manufactured tea, and III Correlations of analytical results with tea tasters' reports and valuations.— D. J. Wood *et al., J. Sci. Fd Agric.,* 1964, *15,* 8, 14, and 19.

Effects on iron absorption. Tea produced a 41 to 95% inhibition of iron absorption; the effect was apparently specific for non-haem iron and could be especially useful in the management of patients with thalassaemia intermedia who might absorb large amounts of dietary iron.— P. A. de Alarcon *et al., New Engl. J. Med.,* 1979, *300,* 5.

643-m

Theobromine *(B.P., Eur. P.)*. Theobrominum; Santheose. 3,7-Dihydro-3,7-dimethylpurine-2,6(1*H*)-dione; 3,7-Dimethylxanthine.
$C_7H_8N_4O_2$=180.2.

CAS — 83-67-0.

Pharmacopoeias. In *Arg., Aust., Belg., Br., Braz., Cz., Eur., Fr., Ger., Hung., It., Jug., Mex., Neth., Pol., Port., Roum., Rus., Span.,* and *Swiss.*

A white odourless microcrystalline powder with a bitter taste containing not more than 0.8% caffeine. It sublimes at about 290°. It has weakly acidic properties, combining with bases to form salts by replacement of a hydrogen atom. It also has even weaker basic properties forming, with acids, salts which are decomposed in aqueous solution.

Soluble 1 in 2000 of water, 1 in 150 of boiling water, 1 in 2500 of alcohol, and 1 in 6000 of chloroform; practically insoluble in ether; freely soluble in dilute mineral acids and aqueous solutions of alkali hydroxides; slightly soluble in ammonia. A saturated solution in water has a pH of 5.5 to 7. **Store** in airtight containers. Protect from light.

Solubility. The solubility of theobromine in syrup was 1.4 times that in water.— A. N. Paruta and B. B. Sheth, *J. pharm. Sci.,* 1966, *55,* 896.

Adverse Effects. In large doses, theobromine may cause nausea and anorexia.

Interactions, tests and assays. Theobromine could interfere with the Schack and Waxler spectrophotometric assay for plasma-theophylline concentrations to give significantly false-positive elevations.— L. E. Matheson *et al., Am. J. Hosp. Pharm.,* 1977, *34,* 496.

Pregnancy and the neonate. It was reported that theobromine passed into the breast milk of 6 nursing mothers who had eaten 4 ounces of chocolate containing about 240 mg of theobromine.— B. H. Resman *et al.,* Seventy-eighth Annual Meeting of the American Society for Clinical Pharmacology and Therapeutics,, per *Clin. Pharmac. Ther.,* 1977, *21,* 115. See also *idem, J. Pediat.,* 1977, *91,* 477.

Uses. Theobromine has the general properties of the other xanthines (see p.340). It has a weaker diuretic activity than theophylline and is also a less powerful stimulant of smooth muscle. It has practically no stimulant effect on the central nervous system. Theobromine has been administered as Phenobarbitone and Theobromine Tablets in hypertension but this preparation has no advantage over phenobarbitone alone.

Theobromine has been given in doses of 300 to 600 mg. It is the chief xanthine in the beverage cocoa which may contain more than 200 mg per cup. Theobroma oil may contain up to 2% theobromine.

Studies in healthy subjects on the alterations of theobromine disposition induced by dietary abstention from or exposure to methylxanthines.— D. D. Drouillard *et al.*, *Clin. Pharmac. Ther.*, 1978, *23*, 296.

Proprietary Names

Théosalvose *(Techni-Pharma, Mon.)*.

644-b

Theobromine and Calcium Salicylate. Theobromine Calcium Salicylate; Theosalicin.

CAS — 8065-51-8.

Pharmacopoeias. In *Aust.*, *Nord.*, and *Swiss.*

A double salt or mixture of theobromine calcium [$(C_7H_7N_4O_2)_2Ca$ = 398.4] and calcium salicylate [$(C_7H_5O_3)_2Ca$ = 314.3] in equimolecular proportions.

A white odourless powder with a saline taste containing about 48% of theobromine and 11% of calcium. Slightly **soluble** in water; practically insoluble in alcohol. A saturated solution in water is alkaline to litmus and to phenolphthalein. **Incompatible** with ferric salts and acids. **Store** in airtight containers. Protect from light.

Uses. Theobromine and calcium salicylate has the actions of theobromine, (p.348). It is stated to be less likely to cause gastric irritation than theobromine and sodium acetate or theobromine and sodium salicylate and has been given in doses of 0.5 to 1 g.

Proprietary Preparations

Hypotensive Dellipsoids D 8 *(Pilsworth, UK)*. Coated elliptical tablets each containing theobromine and calcium salicylate 100 mg, glyceryl trinitrate 100 µg, ferrous phosphate 7.5 mg, and chlorophyll 30 mg.

645-v

Theobromine and Sodium Acetate. Theobromine Sodium Acetate; Theobrominum Natricum et Natrii Acetas.

CAS — 8002-88-8.

Pharmacopoeias. In *Int.*, *Mex.*, and *Turk.*

A mixture of theobromine sodium ($C_7H_7N_4NaO_2$ = 202.1) and sodium acetate ($C_2H_3NaO_2$ = 82.0) in approximately equimolecular proportions.

A white, odourless or almost odourless, crystalline, hygroscopic powder with a bitter saline taste, containing about 60% of theobromine.

Soluble 1 in about 1.5 of water, slightly soluble in alcohol, practically insoluble in chloroform and ether. Solutions in water are alkaline to phenolphthalein. **Incompatible** with all acidic substances, alkali carbonates, bicarbonates, borax, sodium phosphate, and ammonium salts. Not to be given with preparations containing sugar or gum. It decomposes in moist air with absorption of carbon dioxide and liberation of theobromine. **Store** in airtight containers. Protect from light.

Uses. Theobromine and sodium acetate has the actions of theobromine (p.348) and has been given in doses of 0.25 to 1 g, up to a maximum of 3 g daily.

646-g

Theobromine and Sodium Salicylate *(B.P. 1953)*. Theobromine Sodium Salicylate; Theobrominum Natricum et Natrii Salicylas; Themisalum; Theobromsal.

CAS — 8048-31-5.

Pharmacopoeias. In *Arg.*, *Aust.*, *Belg.*, *Cz.*, *Hung.*, *Ind.*, *Int.*, *Jug.*, *Pol.*, *Roum.*, *Rus.*, *Span.*, *Swiss*, and *Turk.* The specified minimum percentages of theobromine and of sodium salicylate vary slightly in the various pharmacopoeias.

A mixture of theobromine sodium ($C_7H_7N_4NaO_2$ = 202.1) and sodium salicylate ($C_7H_5NaO_3$ = 160.1) in approximately equimolecular proportions. The dried material contains not less than 46% of theobromine and not less than 41% of sodium salicylate.

A white odourless amorphous powder with a sweetish alkaline taste. **Soluble** 1 in 1 of water; practically insoluble in alcohol, chloroform, and ether. Solutions in water are strongly alkaline to phenolphthalein. **Incompatible** with ammonium and iron salts, sodium bicarbonate, all acid salts, alkaloidal salts, tannins, and free inorganic and organic acids. It decomposes in moist air with absorption of carbon dioxide and liberation of theobromine. **Store** in airtight containers. Protect from light.

Uses. Theobromine and sodium salicylate has the actions of theobromine (p.348) and has been given in doses of 0.6 to 1.2 g.

647-q

Theophylline *(B.P., Eur. P.)*.

Theophyll.; Theophyllinum; Anhydrous Theophylline; Teofilina. 3,7-Dihydro-1,3-dimethylpurine-2,6(1*H*)-dione; 1,3-Dimethylxanthine.

$C_7H_8N_4O_2$=180.2.

CAS — 58-55-9.

Pharmacopoeias. In *Br.*, *Eur.*, *Fr.*, *Ger.*, *Hung.*, *Int.*, *Neth.*, and *Swiss. Ind.*, *It.*, *Pol.*, *Turk.*, and *U.S.* allow anhydrous or monohydrate.

A white odourless crystalline powder with a bitter taste. It is isomeric with theobromine, and forms salts with acids and water-soluble derivatives with alkali metals and amines. M.p. 270° to 274°.

Soluble 1 in 120 of water at 25°, 1 in 80 of alcohol at 25°, and 1 in about 200 of chloroform; very slightly soluble in ether; freely soluble in dilute acids, ammonia, and alkali hydroxide solutions. A saturated solution in water is faintly acid. **Incompatible** with tannins.

Solubility. The solubility of theophylline at 25° increased from 8 mg per ml in water to 8.3 mg per ml in 30% w/w sucrose solution. A further increase in sucrose concentration to that of syrup decreased the solubility to 6.2 mg per ml.— A. N. Paruta and B. B. Sheth, *J. pharm. Sci.*, 1966, *55*, 896.

Sterilisation. Irradiation was not a suitable method of sterilisation for solutions of theophylline.— L. J. Rasero and D. M. Skauen, *J. pharm. Sci.*, 1967, *56*, 724.

648-p

Theophylline Hydrate *(B.P.)*.

Theophylline Monohydrate *(Eur. P.)*; Theophyllinum Monohydricum.

$C_7H_8N_4O_2,H_2O$=198.2.

CAS — 5967-84-0.

Pharmacopoeias. In *Arg.*, *Aust.*, *Belg.*, *Br.*, *Braz.*, *Chin.*, *Cz.*, *Eur.*, *Fr.*, *Ger.*, *Jug.*, *Mex.*, *Neth.*, *Nord.*, *Roum.*, *Rus.*, *Span.*, and *Swiss.* In most pharmacopoeias the title Theophylline is used. *Ind.*, *It.*, *Pol.*, *Turk.*, and *U.S.* allow anhydrous or monohydrate.

Uses. The actions and uses of theophylline are described under Aminophylline, p.342.It is given by mouth in doses of 60 to 200 mg; higher doses are sometimes used. Theophylline is an ingredient of Mersalyl Injection.

Asthma. A view that theophylline by mouth may be used instead of intravenous aminophylline in patients with asthma crises who are already taking oral theophylline. A loading dose of 5 mg per kg body-weight of microfined theophylline (Nuelin) followed by a maintenance regimen of 125 mg every 3 hours in a patient weighing 70 kg is suggested. Theophylline should also be taken regularly by mouth in carefully controlled dosage by nearly all asthmatic patients not responding adequately to treatment with sympathomimetic drugs. Adults taking 125 mg four times daily usually have inadequate blood concentrations of theophylline whereas a dose of 250 mg four times daily leads to nausea, vomiting, headache, or diarrhoea in 25% of adults. To overcome this problem it is suggested that patients start by taking theophylline 125 mg every 6 hours and, with instructions to stop the drug and seek advice if side-effects occur, each dose is then increased by 25 mg every third day to a maximum of 250 mg. Compliance and blood concentrations should be checked at this dose; a trough concentration, measured just before the next dose, of 10 to 20 µg per ml should be achieved. Further increases may be required, involving shorter dosage intervals and very careful monitoring. Children may be given theophylline in doses of 5 mg per kg every 6 hours, increased by 1 mg per kg every third day to a maximum of 7 mg per kg.— H. Guy, *Drugs*, 1980, *19*, 141.

Preparations

Theophylline, Ephedrine Hydrochloride, and Phenobarbital Tablets *(U.S.P.)*. Tablets containing theophylline, ephedrine hydrochloride, and phenobarbitone. The potency of theophylline is expressed in terms of the monohydrate; the *U.S.P.* requires 66% dissolution in 2 minutes. Store in airtight containers.

Theophylline Tablets *(U.S.P.)*. Tablets containing theophylline. Potency is expressed in terms of the monohydrate.

Proprietary Preparations

Labophylline *(Laboratories for Applied Biology, UK)*. Tablets each containing theophylline 100 mg and lysine 74 mg. For chronic bronchitis, asthma, and as an adjunct in diuretic therapy. *Dose.* 1 or 2 tablets 3 or 4 times daily.

Nuelin *(Riker, UK)*. Microcrystalline theophylline, available as tablets of 125 mg. **Nuelin SA.** Theophylline, available as sustained-release tablets of 175 mg. **Nuelin SA-250.** Theophylline, available as sustained-release, scored tablets of 250 mg. (Also available as Nuelin in *Austral.*, *Denm.*, *Norw.*, *S.Afr.*).

In a comparative study involving 8 healthy subjects the bioavailability of Nuelin was not found to be significantly better than that of Theodrox.— J. Apold and O. M. Bakke (letter), *Lancet*, 1979, *1*, 667.

Slo-Phyllin Gyrocaps *(Rona, UK)*. Theophylline, available as sustained-release capsules each containing 60, 125, or 250 mg.

Theocontin *(Napp, UK)*. Theophylline, available as sustained-release tablets of 200 mg.

Theo-Dur *(Fisons, UK)*. Theophylline, available as sustained-release scored tablets of 200 and 300 mg. *Dose.* Initially, 1 tablet 12-hourly; children, half a tablet.

Theograd *(Abbott, UK)*. Theophylline, available as Filmtabs (film-coated tablets) of 350 mg in a porous plastic basis for sustained release. *Dose.* 2 tablets initially, then 1 tablet every 12 hours. (Also available as Theograd in *Neth.*).

Owing to the risk of intestinal obstruction, sustained-release preparations such as Theograd, where the drug is released in transit, but the matrix ghost is often eliminated intact, should not be prescribed in patients with Crohn's disease or other intestinal disease in which strictures may form.— J. L. Shaffer *et al.* (letter), *Lancet*, 1980, *2*, 487.

Theosol Suppositories *(Martindale Pharmaceuticals, UK)*. Each contains theophylline 300 mg.

Uniphyllin Unicontin *(Napp, UK)*. Sustained-release scored tablets each containing theophylline 200 mg. *Dose.* 2 tablets daily for the first week; subsequently, a maximum of 4 tablets once daily.

See also under Ephedrine, p.12..

Other Proprietary Names

Accurbron, Aerolate, Bronkodyl, Elixicon, Elixomin, Labid, Physpan, Slo-phyllin, Somophyllin-T, Sustaire, Theobid, Theocap, Theoclear, Theocot T.D., Theon-300, Theospan, Theovent *(all USA)*; Aminomal, Asmafil *(both Ital.)*; Asperal-T *(Belg.)*; Asthmophylline, Theolixir *(both Canad.)*; Elixophyllin *(Austral., Canad., USA)*; Godafilin, Teolixir Normal *(both Spain)*; Solosin *(Ger.)*; Teofyllin *(Denm.)*; Theo-Dur *(Canad., Denm., Swed., USA)*; Theolair *(Belg., Canad., Neth., Swed., USA)*; Theophyl *(Canad., USA)*.

Preparations containing theophylline were also formerly marketed in Great Britain under the proprietary names Entair (*Duncan, Flockhart*), Rona-Phyllin (*Rona*), Riddospas (*Riddell*), and Theonar (*MCP Pharmaceuticals*).

649-s

Theophylline and Sodium Acetate *(B.P. 1948).* Theophylline Sodium Acetate; Theophyllinum Natricum et Natrii Acetas.

CAS — 8002-89-9.

Pharmacopoeias. In *Aust., Ind.,* and *Int.*

A hydrated mixture of theophylline sodium ($C_7H_7N_4NaO_2$ = 202.1) and sodium acetate ($C_2H_3NaO_2$ = 82.03) in approximately equimolecular proportions, containing not less than 55% of anhydrous theophylline. A white odourless crystalline powder with a bitter salty taste. **Soluble** 1 in 25 of water; practically insoluble in alcohol, chloroform and ether. Solutions in water are alkaline to phenolphthalein. **Incompatible** with acids, ammonium salts, and sodium bicarbonate. It decomposes in moist air with absorption of carbon dioxide and liberation of theophylline. **Store** in airtight containers. Protect from light.

Uses. Theophylline and sodium acetate has the same actions and uses described under Aminophylline, p.342, and has been given in doses of 120 to 300 mg.

650-h

Theophylline Calcium Salicylate

CAS — 37287-41-5.

A hydrated mixture or double salt of theophylline calcium [$(C_7H_7N_4O_2)_2Ca$ = 398.4] and calcium salicylate [$(C_7H_5O_3)_2Ca$ = 314.3] in equimolecular proportions, containing about 48% of anhydrous theophylline.
A white odourless, almost tasteless powder. Slightly **soluble** in water. Aqueous solutions are slightly alkaline.

Uses. Theophylline calcium salicylate has the actions and uses described under Aminophylline, (see p.342).

651-m

Theophylline Monoethanolamine.

Theophylline Olamine *(U.S.P.).* An equimolecular compound of anhydrous theophylline and monoethanolamine.

$C_7H_8N_4O_2,C_2H_7NO$=241.2.

CAS — 573-41-1.

Pharmacopoeias. In *U.S.*

A white or almost white crystalline powder with not more than a slight odour. Theophylline monoethanolamine 1.34 g is approximately equivalent in theophylline content to 1 g of anhydrous theophylline. **Soluble** 1 in 20 of water. **Store** in airtight containers.

Adverse Effects, Treatment, and Precautions. As for Aminophylline, p.342.

Uses. Theophylline monoethanolamine is used for the same purposes as aminophylline (see p.344). In asthma and cardiac disorders the usual dose is 100 to 200 mg three or four times daily. It has also been used as a diuretic in a dose of up to 1 g over a few hours. Theophylline monoethanolamine is also given by rectal instillation of 250 or 500 mg in aqueous solution and as 500-mg suppositories.

Asthma. After the administration of an enema containing theophylline monoethanolamine, serum concentrations of theophylline reached a peak within 60 minutes in about two-thirds of a group of children with intractable asthma. A suitable rectal dose for children was 5 to 6 mg per kg body-weight. Side-effects usually minor and transitory, occurred in 43% of the patients.— J. W. Yunginger *et al., Ann. Allergy,* 1966, *24,* 469.

Preparations

Theophylline Olamine Enema *(U.S.P.).* Theophylline Olamine Solution. A solution of theophylline monoethanolamine. Store at room temperature in airtight containers.

Monotheamin *(Lilly, UK).* Theophylline monoethanolamine, available as capsules of 200 mg.

Other Proprietary Names

Inophyline *(see also Aminophylline, p.345)(Fr.)*; Teoclasma *(Ital.).*

652-b

Theophylline Sodium Glycinate *(U.S.P.).*

Theophylline Sodium Aminoacetate.

CAS — 8000-10-0.

Pharmacopoeias. In *U.S.*

An equilibrium mixture of theophylline sodium ($C_7H_7N_4NaO_2$ = 202.1) and glycine ($C_2H_5NO_2$) = 75.07) in approximately equimolecular proportions, buffered with an additional mole of glycine. The dried substance contains 49 to 52% of theophylline monohydrate. A white crystalline powder with a slight ammoniacal odour and a bitter taste.
Soluble 1 in 6 of water; very slightly soluble in alcohol; practically insoluble in chloroform. A solution in water has a pH of 8.5 to 9.5. A 2.94% solution is iso-osmotic with serum.**Incompatible** with acidic substances. **Store** in airtight containers.

Adverse Effects, Treatment, and Precautions. As for Aminophylline, p.342. Theophylline sodium glycinate is claimed to cause less gastric irritation than aminophylline.

Uses. Theophylline sodium glycinate is used for the same purposes as aminophylline (see p.344). The adult dose by mouth is 300 to 600 mg; for children 1 to 6 years 60 to 120 mg every 6 hours, children 6 to 12 years, 120 to 180 mg every 8 hours.
It has been given by slow intravenous injection, by rectum as suppositories, and was formerly used as an aerosol in the treatment of bronchial asthma.
Theophylline calcium glycinate has also been used.

Preparations

Theophylline Sodium Glycinate Elixir *(U.S.P.).* An elixir containing theophylline sodium glycinate, with alcohol 17 to 23%. pH 8.7 to 9.1.

Theophylline Sodium Glycinate Tablets *(U.S.P.).* Tablets containing theophylline sodium glycinate.

Proprietary Preparations

Nuelin Liquid *(Riker, UK).* Contains theophylline sodium glycinate 120 mg in each 5 ml (suggested diluent, syrup).

Other Proprietary Names

Acet-Am *(calcium and sodium salts)*, Theocyne *(both Canad.)*; Synophylate *(USA)*; Teoglicina *(Ital.).*

Theophylline sodium glycinate was also formerly marketed in Great Britain under the proprietary names Aminomed (*Medo-Chemicals*) and Englate (*Nicholas Laboratories*). A preparation containing theophylline sodium glycinate was formerly marketed under the proprietary name Aminomed Compound (*Medo-Chemicals*).

Camphor and Menthol

262-y

Camphor and its related compounds described in this section are now used mainly for their counter-irritant and rubefacient properties. Menthol has similar uses and in addition is used locally for the relief of respiratory congestive disorders.

263-j

Camphor *(B.P., U.S.P.).* Camph.; Camphora; 2-Camphanone; Camphre du Japon (natural); Camphre Droit (natural); Alcanfor; Cânfora; Kamfer. Bornan-2-one; 1,7,7-Trimethylbicyclo-[2.2.1]heptan-2-one.
$C_{10}H_{16}O$=152.2.

CAS — 76-22-2; 464-49-3 (+); 464-48-2 (−); 21368-68-3 (±).

Pharmacopoeias. In all pharmacopoeias examined except *Eur.* and *Neth.*; some only describe natural camphor and some only synthetic camphor; *Aust.*, *Belg.*, and *Jap.* have separate monographs for natural and synthetic camphor.

Camphor is obtained by distillation from the wood of *Cinnamomum camphora* (Lauraceae) and purified by sublimation, or it may be prepared synthetically. The natural product is dextrorotatory and the synthetic product is optically inactive.

Colourless transparent or white crystals, crystalline masses, blocks, or powdery masses known as 'flowers of camphor', with a penetrating characteristic aromatic odour and a pungent aromatic taste, followed by a sensation of cold. Specific gravity about 0.99. M.p. 174° to 181°.

Soluble 1 in 700 to 800 of water, 1 in 1 of alcohol, 1 in 0.25 of chloroform, 1 in 1 of ether, 1 in 1.5 of turpentine oil, and 1 in 4 of olive oil; practically insoluble in glycerol; freely soluble in carbon disulphide, light petroleum, and fixed and volatile oils. Oily solutions are **sterilised** by maintaining at 150° for 1 hour. **Store** at a temperature not exceeding 25° in airtight containers. A liquid or soft mass is formed when camphor is triturated with betanaphthol, chloral hydrate, menthol, phenol, salol, thymol, and many other crystalline substances. Camphor is readily powdered by triturating with a few drops of alcohol or other volatile organic solvent. It slowly volatilises at ordinary temperatures.

Diffusion through polyethylene. Camphor diffused quickly through polyethylene (Polythene).— O. Weis-Fogh, *Arch. Pharm. Chemi*, 1961, *61*, 736, per *Pharm. J.*, 1961, *2*, 219.

Adverse Effects. Poisoning usually occurs from administration of camphorated oil (camphor liniment) to children in mistake for castor oil. The symptoms include nausea, vomiting, colic, headache, dizziness, a feeling of warmth, delirium, muscle twitching, epileptiform convulsions, depression of the central nervous system, and coma. Breathing is difficult and the breath has a characteristic odour; anuria may occur. Death from respiratory failure is rare though fatalities in children have been recorded from 1 g. There have been reports of instant collapse in infants following the local application of camphor to their nostrils.

Maximum permissible atmospheric concentration 2 ppm.

A man who attempted suicide by the ingestion of 150 ml of camphor liniment suffered peripheral circulatory shock, severe dehydration due to vomiting, and 3 attacks of severe and prolonged grand mal epilepsy. He recovered after gastric lavage, diazepam given intravenously, and intensive supportive treatment. The dose of camphor was believed to be one of the highest to be followed by survival.— R. H. Vasey and S. J. Karayannopoulos (letter), *Br. med. J.*, 1972, *1*, 112.

Of 175 admissions of children (aged 6 months to 5 years) to the Newcastle General Hospital for poisoning, 10 related to the ingestion of camphor liniment.— J. R. Sibert (letter), *Br. med. J.*, 1973, *1*, 803.

Prolonged seizures occurred in a 15-month-old child following skin contact with camphor and 1 year later a brief seizure followed inhalation of a camphor preparation.— R. R. Skoglund *et al.*, *Clin. Pediat.*, 1977, *16*, 901.

Further references: J. H. Trestrail and M. E. Spartz, *Clin. Toxicol.*, 1977, *11*, 151; E. Antman *et al.*, *N.Y. St. J. Med.*, 1978, *78*, 896.

Treatment of Adverse Effects. Empty the stomach by lavage and aspiration. Give a purgative, such as sodium sulphate, 30 g in 250 ml of water. Convulsions may be controlled by the intravenous administration of diazepam 5 to 10 mg or, if necessary, a short-acting barbiturate such as thiopentone sodium.

A 77-year-old man who ingested about 60 ml of camphorated oil developed vomiting and convulsions. Haemodialysis with 8 litres of soya oil for 4½ hours removed 6.56 g of camphor and he recovered.— H. E. Ginn *et al.*, *J. Am. med. Ass.*, 1968, *203*, 230.

Haemoperfusion through amberlite resin was successfully used in the treatment of a 37-year-old man who ingested camphorated oil.— R. Kopelman *et al.*, *J. Am. med. Ass.*, 1979, *241*, 727.

Precautions. It is dangerous to place camphor, e.g. a 20% ointment, into the nostrils of an infant. A small quantity applied in this way may cause immediate collapse.

Absorption and Fate. Camphor is absorbed from all sites. It is hydroxylated in the liver to yield hydroxycamphor metabolites which are then conjugated with glucuronic acid and excreted in the urine. Camphor crosses the placenta.

Uses. Applied externally, camphor acts as a rubefacient and mild analgesic and is employed in liniments as a counter-irritant in fibrositis, neuralgia, and similar conditions. Taken internally it is irritant and carminative and has been used as a mild expectorant and to relieve griping. Use of camphorated oil is discouraged because of its toxicity.

Camphor was formerly administered as a solution in oil by subcutaneous or intramuscular injection as a circulatory and respiratory stimulant, but there is little evidence of its value for this purpose.

A review of the synthesis and properties of camphor.— G. T. Walker, *Mfg Chem.*, 1968, *39* (Feb.), 41.

Preparations

Injections

Camphor Injection *(B.P.C. 1934).* A sterile solution of camphor 10% w/v in olive oil. *Dose.* 0.5 to 2 ml subcutaneously.

In *Port P.* (10% w/v); in *Belg. P.* and *It. P.* (Fiale di Canfora) (10% w/v in a suitable oil); in *Rus. P.* (Solutio Camphorae Oleosa pro Injectionibus) (20% w/v in persic oil).

Linctuses

Camphor Linctus Compound *(A.P.F.).* Camphor spirit compound 1 ml, squill oxymel 1 ml, glycerol 1.5 ml, tolu syrup to 5 ml. *Dose.* 5 to 10ml.

Liniments

Ammoniated Camphor Liniment *(B.P.C. 1968).* Compound Camphor Liniment. Camphor 12.5% w/v, strong ammonia solution 30% v/v, and lavender oil 0.5% v/v, in alcohol. Store in a cool place in airtight containers. *Ind. P.* has a similar preparation.

Camphor Liniment *(B.P. 1973, A.P.F.).* Camph. Lin.; Camphorated Oil. Camphor 20% w/w in arachis oil. Store in a cool place in airtight containers.

In *Port. P.* (10% w/w in olive oil); in *Belg. P.* and *Mex. P.* (10% w/w in any suitable fixed oil).

Spirits

Camphor Spirit *(B.P.C. 1959).* Camphor 10% w/v in alcohol (90%).

Camphor Spirit *(U.S.P.).* Camphor 10 g, alcohol (95.5%) to 100 ml. Store in airtight containers. A similar preparation is included in some other pharmacopoeias.

Camphor Spirit Compound *(A.P.F.).* Camphor 300 mg, benzoic acid 500 mg, anise oil 0.3 ml, alcohol (60%) to 100 ml.

Waters

Camphor Water. Concentrated camphor water 2.5 ml, freshly boiled and cooled water to 100 ml.

Camphor Water *B.P.C. 1968* contained camphor 0.1% and alcohol (90%) 0.2% in water.

Concentrated Camphor Water *(B.P.).* Aq. Camph. Conc. Camphor 4 g, alcohol (90%) 60 ml, water to 100 ml.

Proprietary Preparations

Pernomol *(Laboratories for Applied Biology, UK).* A paint containing camphor 10%, chlorbutol 2%, phenol 0.95%, tannic acid 2.2%, and spirit soap 34%. For chilblains.

A preparation containing camphor was also formerly marketed in Great Britain under the proprietary name Rowalind (*Rowa, Eire*).

Proprietary Preparations Containing Related Substances

Rowachol *(Rowa, Eire: Loveridge, UK).* Liquid contains menthol 32%, menthone ($C_{10}H_{18}O$ = 154.3) 6%, pinene ($C_{10}H_{16}$ = 136.2) 17%, borneol ($C_{10}H_{18}O$ = 154.3) 5%, camphene ($C_{10}H_{16}$ = 136.2) 5%, and cineole 2% in olive oil.

A study of 30 patients with gall-stones and functioning gall-bladder undergoing cholecystectomy indicated that Rowachol reduced the cholesterol-saturation index and may prove to be an effective alternative to chenodeoxycholic acid in the treatment of cholesterol gall-stones.— J. Doran *et al.*, *Gut*, 1977, *18*, A977.

Of 24 patients with gall-stones treated with Rowachol (1 capsule per 10 kg body-weight daily), usually for 6 months, 3 had complete and 4 partial dissolution of gall-stones.— G. D. Bell and J. Doran, *Br. med. J.*, 1979, *1*, 24.

Further references: G. D. Bell *et al.*, *Gut*, 1978, *19*, A972; J. Doran *et al.*, *ibid.*, 1979, *20*, 312.

Rowatinex *(Rowa, Eire: Loveridge, UK).* **Liquid** contains pinene 31%, camphene 15%, borneol 10%, anethole 4%, fenchone 4%, and cineole 3%, in olive oil. **Capsules** each contain 100 mg of Rowatinex Liquid.

264-z

Camphor Monobromide *(B.P.C. 1934).* Monobromated Camphor; Camphora Monobromata; Camphre Bromé; Bromkampfer; Alcanfor Bromuro. 3-Bromocamphor.
$C_{10}H_{15}BrO$=231.1.

CAS — 76-29-9.

Pharmacopoeias. In *Belg.*, *Port.*, *Rus.*, and *Span.*

Colourless prisms with a persistent camphoraceous odour and taste. M.p. 74° to 77°. Practically **insoluble** in water; soluble 1 in 7 of alcohol, 1 in 2 of ether, 1 in 0.5 of chloroform, and 1 in 8 of olive oil; sparingly soluble in glycerol; soluble in sulphuric acid with the formation of a nearly colourless solution. A liquid or soft mass is formed when camphor monobromide is triturated with chloral hydrate, menthol, phenazone, phenol, salol, and thymol.

Incompatible with alkalis. It is stable in air but is decomposed by prolonged exposure to sunlight. **Protect** from light.

Camphor monobromide was formerly administered as tablets or capsules, or as a solution in oil by injection in doses of 120 to 500 mg in the treatment of headache and in certain chronic neurological conditions but it is of doubtful value. Large doses may cause convulsions.

265-c

Rectified Camphor Oil *(B.P.C. 1959).* Essential Camphor Oil; Light Camphor Oil.

CAS — 8008-51-3 (camphor oil).

The lighter fractions, containing not less than 30% w/w of apparent cineole, of the oil obtained as a by-product

in the manufacturing of natural camphor. Its composition varies with the amount of camphor and safrole removed. The heavier fractions of the crude oil, known as 'brown camphor oil' are used as a source of safrole.
A colourless or yellowish liquid with a characteristic camphoraceous odour and taste. Wt per ml 0.870 to 0.918 g. **Soluble** 1 in 3 of alcohol (90%). **Store** in a cool place in well-filled airtight containers. Protect from light.

Rectified camphor oil has been applied externally, undiluted or mixed with an equal quantity of a vegetable oil, as a mild counter-irritant.

266-k

Menthol *(B.P., U.S.P.)*. Mentol. *p*-Menthan-3-ol; 2-Isopropyl-5-methylcyclohexanol.
$C_{10}H_{20}O$=156.3.

CAS — 89-78-1; 1490-04-6; 15356-60-2 (+); 2216-51-5 (−); 15356-70-4 (±).

Pharmacopoeias. In all pharmacopoeias examined except *Eur., Fr., Int.*, and *Neth. Aust., Ger.*, and *Jap.* have separate monographs for laevo-menthol and racemic menthol.

Natural laevo-menthol obtained from the volatile oils of various species of *Mentha* (Labiatae) or synthetic laevo-menthol or racemic menthol.
It occurs as colourless crystals or crystalline powder with a penetrating odour resembling that of peppermint and a warm aromatic taste followed by a local sensation of cold. M.p. of natural or synthetic (−)-menthol 41° to 44°. F.p. of (±)-menthol 27° to 28°, rising on prolonged stirring to 30° to 32°.
Very slightly **soluble** in water and glycerol; soluble 1 in 0.2 of alcohol, 1 in 0.25 of chloroform, 1 in 0.4 of ether, 1 in 4 of olive oil, 1 in 0.7 of light petroleum, and 1 in 6 of liquid paraffin; freely soluble in glacial acetic acid and in fixed and volatile oils. A 5% solution in alcohol is neutral to litmus. **Incompatible** with oxidising agents. **Store** at a temperature not exceeding 25° in airtight containers.
A liquid or soft mass is formed when menthol is triturated with betanaphthol, camphor, chloral hydrate, phenacetin, phenol, resorcinol, thymol, and many other substances.

Measurement of menthol in the vapour above hot water in an open vessel showed that Menthol Inhalation (*B.N.F. 1963*) and Menthol and Eucalyptus Inhalation (*B.P.C. 1963*) were not satisfactory formulations. The menthol from the alcoholic inhalation had vaporised within a minute. Menthol with aromatic oils in a white soft paraffin basis (Vick Vapour-Rub) provided a higher and more prolonged concentration of the aromatic vapours from the open vessel, possibly by retention of the molten basis on the surface of the hot water.— L. E. Coles, *Pharm. J.*, 1968, *2*, 657.

Diffusion through polyethylene. Menthol diffused quickly through polyethylene (Polythene).— O. Weis-Fogh, *Arch. Pharm. Chemi*, 1961, *61*, 736, per *Pharm. J.*, 1961, *2*, 219.

Adverse Effects. Menthol may give rise to hypersensitivity reactions including contact dermatitis. In young children nasal drops containing menthol may cause spasm of the glottis and cases of instant collapse have been reported in infants following local application of menthol. The fatal dose in man has been estimated to be about 2 g.

Hypersensitivity to menthol in a 31-year-old woman was characterised by urticaria, flushing, and headache. A reaction could be induced by a cream containing menthol, peppermint-flavoured toothpaste or candy, menthol cigarettes or even mint jelly.— C. M. Papa and W. B. Shelley, *J. Am. med. Ass.*, 1964, *189*, 546. See also E. M. McGowan, *Archs Derm.*, 1966, *94*, 62.

Of 877 persons with dermatitis or eczema submitted to patch testing with menthol 5% in yellow soft paraffin, 1% gave a positive reaction.— E. Rudzki and D. Kleniewska, *Br. J. Derm.*, 1970, *83*, 543.

Mentholated cigarettes. A woman who smoked 80 mentholated cigarettes daily for 3 months developed insomnia, unsteady gait, thick speech, tremor of the hands, mental confusion, depression, vomiting, and cramp in the legs. Her heart-rate was 44 per minute. The symptoms disappeared when menthol was withheld. Test dosage with 65 mg of menthol thrice daily produced bradycardia and evidence of toxicity after 7 days.— E. Luke (letter), *Lancet*, 1962, *1*, 110. See also B. Highstein and I. Zeligmann, *J. Am. med. Ass.*, 1951, *146*, 816.

Treatment of Adverse Effects. As for Camphor,p.351.

Precautions. It is dangerous to apply an ointment containing menthol to the nostrils of infants; it may cause immediate collapse. Nasal drops may have the same effects.

Absorption and Fate. After absorption, menthol is excreted in the urine and bile as a glucuronide.

Uses. Menthol is chiefly used to relieve symptoms of bronchitis, sinusitis, and similar conditions. For this purpose it may be used as an inhalation, usually with benzoin, as pastilles, often with cineole, or as an ointment with camphor and eucalyptus oil for application to the chest or nostrils (but see Precautions above).
It was formerly used similarly in nasal sprays with light liquid paraffin to relieve catarrh, but the use of oily sprays is undesirable.
Applied to the skin it dilates the vessels, causing a sensation of coldness followed by an analgesic effect.
Menthol relieves itching and is used in creams, lotions, or ointments, often in a strength of 0.25 to 1%, in pruritus and urticaria. Mixtures of equal weights of menthol and chloral hydrate, phenol, or camphor have been applied to carious teeth to relieve pain but they should not be applied repeatedly over short periods.
It has been used for headaches, rheumatic pains, and neuralgia, applied as menthol cones or in a liniment or ointment.
In small doses by mouth menthol has a carminative action.

Estimated acceptable daily intake: up to 200 µg per kg body-weight. Further information was required from toxicity, carcinogenicity, and metabolic studies.— Twentieth Report of the Joint FAO/WHO Expert Committee on Food Additives, *Tech. Rep. Ser. Wld Hlth Org. No. 599*, 1976.

Preparations

Inhalations

Menthol and Benzoin Inhalation *(B.P.)*. Vapor Mentholis et Benzoini. Menthol 2 g, benzoin inhalation to 100 ml. *A.P.F.* (Benzoin and Menthol Inhalation) has menthol 2% in compound benzoin tincture.

Menthol and Eucalyptus Inhalation *(B.P.)*. Vapor Mentholis et Eucalypti. Menthol 2 g, eucalyptus oil 10 ml, light magnesium carbonate 7 g, water to 100 ml.

Menthol and Pine Inhalation *(A.P.F.)*. Menthol 2, pumilio pine oil 5, alcohol (90%) to 100.

Vap. Menthol *(B.N.F. 1963)*. Menthol 1.6% in industrial methylated spirit. *A.P.F.* (Menthol Inhalation) has 2% menthol in alcohol (90%).

Nasal Drops

Menthol and Thymol Nasal Drops *(B.P.C. 1954)*. Narist. Menthol. et Thymol. Menthol 457 mg, thymol 229 mg, cineole 0.208 ml, liquid paraffin to 100 ml.

Ointments

Ceratum Mentholi Compositum *(Dan. Disp.)*. Menthol 1.75 g, thymol 350 mg, camphor 1.5 g, white beeswax 10.5 g, white soft paraffin 85.9 g.

Ung. Menthol. et Eucalyp *(B.N.F. 1963)*. Menthol and Eucalyptus Ointment. Menthol 1 g, eucalyptus oil 4 ml, yellow soft paraffin to 100 g.

Unguentum Mentholi Compositum *(Dan. Disp.)*. Mentolbalsam. Menthol 10, camphor 10, methyl salicylate 25, white beeswax 18, wool fat 37, all by wt.

Pastilles

Menthol and Eucalyptol Pastilles *(B.P.C. 1949)*. Menthol and Eucalyptus Pastilles. Pastilles containing menthol and cineole.

Proprietary Preparations

Karvol Inhalant Capsules *(Crookes Products, UK)*. Contain menthol 35.9 mg, chlorbutol 30 mg, cinnamon oil 12.3 mg, pine oil 85.5 mg, terpineol 67.4 mg, and thymol 3.2 mg. For congestion in the upper respiratory tract. The contents of a capsule should be expressed into a handkerchief, or into 500 ml of hot water, and the vapour inhaled freely.

267-a

Sodium Camsylate. Sodium Camphorsulphonate *(B.P.C. 1949)*. Sodium (+)-camphor-10-sulphonate.
$C_{10}H_{15}NaO_4S$=254.3.

CAS — 21791-94-6.

Pharmacopoeias. In *Belg.* and *Fr.*

Colourless crystals or crystalline hygroscopic powder with a slight odour and a slightly bitter taste. Very **soluble** in water; soluble in alcohol; practically insoluble in ether. Solutions are **sterilised** by heating in an autoclave or by filtration. **Store** in airtight containers.

Sodium camsylate was formerly administered by injection as a 15% aqueous solution as a circulatory and respiratory stimulant. It has been given by injection in a dose of 150 to 300 mg.

Proprietary Names

Camphostyl *(Lacroix, Fr.)*; Cardiocanfene *(Ceccarelli, Ital.)*.

268-t

Validol. A solution of 25 to 30% of menthol in menthyl isovalerate.
$C_{15}H_{28}O_2$=240.4.

CAS — 16409-46-4; 28221-20-7 (both menthyl isovalerate).

Pharmacopoeias. In *Rus.*

A colourless transparent oily liquid with the characteristic odour of menthol. Practically **insoluble** in water; very soluble in alcohol.

Validol has been used in the treatment of certain psychiatric disorders and motion sickness. It has been given in a dose of 120 to 180 mg daily.

Cannabis

841-s

Cannabis *(B.P.C. 1949).* Cannab.; Cannabis Indica; Indian Hemp; Ganja; Guaza; Chanvre; Hanfkraut; Cáñamo Indiano.

CAS — 8063-14-7.

Pharmacopoeias. In *Chin.*, *Ind.*, *Port.*, and *Span.*

The dried flowering or fruiting tops of the pistillate plant of *Cannabis sativa* (Cannabinaceae). In the UK cannabis is defined by law as any part of any plant of the genus *Cannabis*. **Protect** from light.

The active principles of the drug are contained in the resin. The male plant and leaves of the male and female plant are sometimes employed. *Marihuana* usually refers to a mixture of the leaves and flowering tops. *Bhang, dagga, ganja, kif*, and *maconha* are commonly used in various countries to describe similar preparations. *Hashish* and *charas* are names often applied to the resin, although in some countries *hashish* is applied to any cannabis preparation.

A series of cannabinoids has been extracted from the drug, the most important being Δ^9-tetrahydrocannabinol, Δ^8-tetrahydrocannabinol, Δ^9-tetrahydrocannabinolic acid, cannabinol, and cannabidiol. Cannabinol and cannabidiol may be present in large amounts but have little activity. The amount of Δ^9-tetrahydrocannabinol may average 1, 3, and 5% in marihuana, ganja, and hashish respectively.

Synonyms and approximate synonyms for cannabis included: Ait makhlif, Aliamba, Anassa, Anhascha, Assyuni, Bambalacha, Bambia, Bangi-Aku, Bango, Bangue, Bhang, Bhangaku, Canapa, Cangonha, Canhama, Cannacoro, Can-Yac, Caroçuda, Chur ganja, Chutras, Chutsao, Da-boa, Dacha, Dagga, Darakte-Bang, Diamba, Dirijo, Djamba, Djoma, Dokka, Donajuanita, Dormilona, Durijo, Elva, Erva maligna, Erva do norte, Esrar, Fêmea, Fininha, Finote, Fokkra, Fumo brabo, Fumo de caboclo, Gandia, Ganga, Ganja, Ganjila, Gnaoui, Gongo, Gozah, Grahni Sherdool, Greefe, Grifa, Guabza, Guaza, Gunjah, Gunza, Hamp, Haouzi, Hen-Nab, Hursini, Hashish, Igbo, Indische-hennepkruid, Indisk hampa, Intianhamppu, Intsangu, Isangu, Janjah, Jatiphaladya churna, Jea, Juana, Kanab, Karpura rasa, Khanh-Chha, Khanje, Kif, Kif tami, Kinnab, Liamba, Lianda, Maconha, Maconia, Madi, Magiyam, Makhlif, Malva, Maraguango, Marajuana, Marigongo, Marihuana, Mariquita, Maruamba, Matekwane, Mbanje, Meconha, Misari, Mnoana, Momea, Mota, Mulatinha, Mundyadi vatika, Namba, Nsangu, Nwonkaka, Peinka, Penek, Penka, Pito, Pot, Pretinha, Rafe, Rafi, Rafo, Riamba, Rongony, Rora, Rosa Maria, Sabsi, Sadda, Siddhi, Soñadora, Soussi, Subji, Summitates cannabis, Suruma, Tahgalim, Takrouri, Tedrika, Teloeut, Teriaki, Tronadora, Umya, Urumogi, Wee, Wewe, Yamba, Yoruba, Zacate chino, Zerouali, and Ziele konopi indyjskich.

Synonyms and approximate synonyms for cannabis resin included: Bheng, Charas, Charris, Chira, Churrus, Chus, Garaouich, Garawiche, Garoarsch, Gauja, Hachiche, Hascisc, Hashish, Hasis, Hasji's, Hasjisj, Haszysz, Haxixe, Heloua, Kamonga, Malak, Manzul, Momeka, N'rama, and Sighirma.— *Multilingual List of Narcotic Drugs Under International Control*, New York, United Nations, 1968.

842-w

Tetrahydrocannabinol. Δ^1-THC; Δ^9-THC; (−)-Δ^9-*trans*-Tetrahydrocannabinol.
(6a*R*,10a*R*)-6a,7,8,10a-Tetrahydro-6,6,9-trimethyl-3-pentyl-6*H*-dibenzo[*b*,*d*]pyran-1-ol.
$C_{21}H_{30}O_2$=314.5.

CAS — 1972-08-3.

A viscous oil. Practically **insoluble** in water; soluble 1 in 1 of alcohol and acetone and 1 in 3 of glycerol; soluble in fixed oils. **Store** in a cool place in airtight containers.

It accounts for most of the activity of cannabis.

For discussions and studies on the constituents of cannabis, see C. W. Waller, *Pharmac. Rev.*, 1971, *23*, 265; F. K. Klein *et al.* (letter), *Nature*, 1971, *232*, 258; F. W. H. M. Merkus, *ibid.*, 579; P. S. Fetterman *et al.*, *J. pharm. Sci.*, 1971, *60*, 1246; J. L. Neumeyer and R. A. Shagoury, *ibid.*, 1433; R. A. de Zeeuw *et al.*, *J. Pharm. Pharmac.*, 1972, *24*, 1; T. B. Vree *et al.*, *ibid.*, 7; J. W. Fairbairn, *Pharm. J.*, 1972, *2*, 342; C. E. Turner and M. L. Mole (letter), *J. Am. med. Ass.*, 1973, *225*, 639; C. E. Turner *et al.* (letter), *J. pharm. Sci.*, 1973, *62*, 1739; C. E. Turner *et al.*, *ibid.*, 1974, *63*, 1872; M. A. Elsohly and C. E. Turner, *Pharm. Weekbl. Ned.*, 1976, *111*, 1069; M. A. Elsohly *et al.*, *Lloydia*, 1977, *40*, 275; *idem*, *J. pharm. Sci.*, 1978, *67*, 124; D. Bieniek and F. Korte, *Dt. ApothZtg*, 1978, *118*, 1933; B. I. Field and R. R. Arndt, *J. Pharm. Pharmac.*, 1980, *32*, 21.

Stability. Stable emulsions of Δ^9- and Δ^8-tetrahydrocannabinol suitable for parenteral experimental use were prepared using 1 ml of a 10 to 40% solution of cannabinoid in sesame oil with 0.01 to 0.1 ml of polysorbate 80 and 8 to 9 ml of normal saline. Higher concentrations of tetrahydrocannabinol could be incorporated using larger concentrations of polysorbate 80. A 50% solution in alcohol lost about 10% of Δ^9-tetrahydrocannabinol after storage at 5° for 40 days; there was greater deterioration at 22° as measured by the optical density. Dilute solutions of 2% in chloroform were stable for weeks at room temperature and solutions of 10% in sesame oil were stable for up to 60 days.— H. Rosenkrantz *et al.*, *J. pharm. Sci.*, 1972, *61*, 1106.

When cannabis was stored at −18°, 4°, and 22° the content of Δ^9-tetrahydrocannabinol was reduced by 3.8, 5.3, and 6.9% respectively per year. There was greater deterioration at higher temperatures. Cannabis was more stable when protected from light than when stored under nitrogen.— C. E. Turner *et al.*, *J. pharm. Sci.*, 1973, *62*, 1601. Cannabis resin and its preparations were stable for 1 to 2 years if stored in the dark at room temperature. Loss of tetrahydrocannabinol during exposure to light did not lead to increases in cannabinol content, but cannabinol was formed during oxidation in air, in the dark.— J. W. Fairbairn *et al.*, *J. Pharm. Pharmac.*, 1976, *28*, 1.

Δ^9-Tetrahydrocannabinol rapidly diffused into plastics and rubber closures. Binding on to glass could be minimised by silyl pretreatment of the glass. The spectrophotometric pKa′ of Δ^9-THC was 10.6. Solubility in water at 23° was 2.8 mg per litre and in 0.15M NaCl 0.77 mg per litre. Δ^9-THC was readily degraded in acid solutions.— E. R. Garrett and C. A. Hunt, *J. pharm. Sci.*, 1974, *63*, 1056.

Further references: J. M. Parker *et al.*, *J. pharm. Sci.*, 1974, *63*, 970; E. R. Garrett and J. Tsau, *J. pharm. Sci.*, 1974, *63*, 1563.

Dependence. Both the National Commission on Marihuana and Drug Abuse in the USA (*Marihuana: A Signal of Misunderstanding*, First Report of the National Commission on Marihuana and Drug Abuse, Washington, 1972; also known as the Shafer Report) and the LeDain Commission in Canada (*Cannabis*, A Report of the Commission of Inquiry into the Non-medical Use of Drugs, Ottawa, Ministry of National Health and Welfare, 1972) reported that the prolonged heavy use of cannabis could lead to tolerance and psychic dependence but that physical dependence had not been demonstrated. There have been occasional reports of non-specific symptoms such as anorexia, anxiety, insomnia, irritability, restlessness, sweating, headache, and mild gastro-intestinal upsets occurring when cannabis is withdrawn.

There is a positive relationship between the use of cannabis and other drugs of abuse but the role of cannabis, if any, in the progression to these drugs is still not clear.

References: M. M. Glatt, *Br. J. Addict. Alcohol*, 1969, *64*, 109; The Use of Cannabis, *Tech. Rep. Ser. Wld Hlth Org. No. 478*, 1971; *Cannabis: Report by the Advisory Committee on Drug Dependence*, London, HM Stationery Office, 1968; R. Nowlan and S. Cohen, *Clin. Pharmac. Ther.*, 1977, *22*, 550; Twenty-first Report on a WHO Expert Committee on Drug Dependence, *Tech. Rep. Ser. Wld Hlth Org. No. 618*, 1978.

Adverse Effects. Nausea and vomiting may be the first effects of cannabis taken by mouth. The most frequent physical effects of cannabis intoxication are an increase in heart-rate with alterations in blood-pressure, injected conjunctival vessels, and deterioration in motor coordination. The psychological effects include elation, distortion of time and space, irritability, and disturbances of memory and judgement. Anxiety or panic reactions may occur, particularly in inexperienced users. Psychotic episodes of a paranoid or schizophrenic nature, and usually acute, have occurred in subjects taking cannabis, especially in large doses. There is conflicting evidence of atrophic brain changes in heavy smokers of cannabis.

Reports and reviews: A. Lewis, *Cannabis: Report by the Advisory Committee on Drug Dependence*, London, HM Stationery Office, 1968, pp. 40–63; Amphetamines, Barbiturates, LSD and Cannabis, their Use and Misuse, *Reports on Public Health and Medical Subjects No. 124*, London, HM Stationery Office, 1970; The Use of Cannabis, *Tech. Rep. Ser. Wld Hlth Org. No. 478*, 1971. Marihuana and its Surrogates, M. deV. Cotten (Ed.), *Pharmac. Rev.*, 1971, *23*, 262; *Marihuana: A Signal of Misunderstanding*, First Report of the National Commission on Marihuana and Drug Abuse, Washington, 1972; *Cannabis*, A Report of the Commission of Inquiry into the Non-medical Use of Drugs, Ottawa, Ministry of National Health and Welfare, 1972; W. D. M. Paton, *Pharm. J.*, 1972, *2*, 347; G. G. Nahas, *Bull. Narcot.*, 1973, *25*, 9; *Marihuana*, R. Mechoulam (Ed.), New York, Academic Press, 1973; R. Thomas and G. Chesher, *Med. J. Aust.*, 1973, *2*, 229; E. Tylden, *Practitioner*, 1974, *212*, 810; *Marijuana: Effects on Human Behaviour*, L.L. Miller (Ed.), London, Academic Press, 1974; *Pediatrics*, 1975, *56*, 134; *Cannabis and Health*, J.D.P. Graham (Ed.), London, Academic Press, 1976. Interactions of Drugs of Abuse, E. S. Vesell and M. C. Braude (Ed.), *Ann. N.Y. Acad. Sci.*, 1976, *281*, 151–243; *Pharmacology of Marihuana*, M.C. Braude and S. Szara (Ed.), New York, Raven Press, 1976; *Med. Lett.*, 1976, *18*, 69; H. G. Pars *et al.*, *Adv. Drug Res.*, 1977, *11*, 97; D. P. Tashkin *et al.*, *Ann. intern. Med.*, 1978, *89*, 539; G. Milner, *Med. J. Aust.*, 1978, *2*, 420; S. Cohen, *J. Am. med. Ass.*, 1978, *240*, 1761; G. G. Nahas, *ibid.*, 1979, *242*, 2775; *Report of the Expert Group of The Advisory Council on The Misuse of Drugs on The Effects of Cannabis Use*, London, Home Office, 1982; Committee to Study the Health-related Effects of Cannabis and its Derivatives, *Marijuana and Health*, Washington, D.C., National Academy Press, 1982.

Air encephalograms of 10 patients who had smoked cannabis regularly showed evidence of cerebral atrophy.— A. M. G. Campbell *et al.*, *Lancet*, 1971, *2*, 1219. See also *ibid.*, 1240. Similar results in 10 chronic and heavy smokers of cannabis.— M. Evans, *R. Soc. Hlth J.*, 1974, *94*, 15, per *Abstr. Hyg.*, 1974, *49*, 823. There was no evidence of cerebral atrophy in 12 young men, with histories of heavy cannabis smoking, examined by computerised transaxial tomography.— B. T. Co *et al.*, *J. Am. med. Ass.*, 1977, *237*, 1229. A similar report.— J. Kuehnle *et al.*, *ibid.*, 1231.

The cellular pathological effects of cannabis.— *Pharm. J.*, 1974, *1*, 340. See also C. Leuchtenberger *et al.* (letter), *Nature*, 1973, *241*, 137.

The adverse effect of long-term use of cannabis on social characteristics.— B. P. Sharma, *Br. J. Psychiat.*, 1975, *127*, 550; J. Boulougouris *et al.*, *Am. J. Psychiat.*, 1976, *133*, 225, per *Int. pharm. Abstr.*, 1976, *13*, 879.

Cardiovascular effects. A brief review.— *Br. med. J.*, 1978, *1*, 460.

Studies of the cardiovascular effects of tetrahydrocannabinol: R. H. Miller *et al.*, *Am. Heart J.*, 1977, *94*, 740; A. Gash *et al.*, *Ann. intern. Med.*, 1978, *89*, 448; W. J. Crawford and J. C. Merritt, *Int. J. clin. Pharmac. Biopharm.*, 1979, *17*, 191, per *Int. pharm. Abstr.*, 1979, *16*, 1232; C. Kanakis *et al.*, *Ann. intern. Med.*, 1979, *91*, 571; N. L. Benowitz *et al.*, *Clin. Pharmac. Ther.*, 1979, *25*, 440.

A report of pulmonary oedema and acute myocardial infarction in a 25-year-old man who smoked cannabis.— R. Charles *et al.*, *Clin. Toxicol.*, 1979, *14*, 433, per *Int. pharm. Abstr.*, 1980, *17*, 306.

Effect on chromosomes. No significant chromosomal damage was seen in lymphocytes from experienced marihuana smokers.— S. S. Matsuyama *et al.*, *Mutat. Res.*, 1977, *48*, 255.

Effects on the endocrine system. Reduction in plasma-testosterone concentrations, oligospermia, and impotence in male cannabis smokers.— R. C. Kolodny *et al.*, *New Engl. J. Med.*, 1974, *290*, 872. No reduction in plasma-testosterone concentrations.— J. H. Mendelson *et al.*, *ibid.*, *291*, 1051. See also *Br. med. J.*, 1974, *4*, 4.

A report of pubertal arrest in a 16-year-old boy associated with marihuana smoking; he had smoked at least 5 marihuana cigarettes daily since the age of 11 years.— K. C. Copeland *et al.*, *J. Pediat.*, 1980, *96*, 1079.

For a report of rises in chorionic gonadotrophin concentrations in patients smoking marihuana, see under Precautions.

Gynaecomastia. Gynaecomastia occurred in 3 young male patients, intensive smokers of cannabis, one for 6 years and another for 2 years. Tests were performed to rule out other possible causes of gynaecomastia. The chemical similarities of tetrahydrocannabinol and oestradiol were noted.— J. Harmon and M. A. Aliapoulios (letter), *New Engl. J. Med.*, 1972, *287*, 936.

Gynaecomastia in 3 men aged 21 to 30, may have been associated with chronic cannabis smoking. Plasma-prolactin concentrations were raised in all 3, compared with age-matched controls.— S. O. Olusi (letter), *Lancet*, 1980, *1*, 255.

Effect on lymphocytes. Conflicting reports on the effect of marihuana or tetrahydrocannabinol on lymphocytes.— P. Cushman and R. Khurana, *Clin. Pharmac. Ther.*, 1976, *19*, 310; G. S. Rachelefsky and G. Opelz, *Clin. Pharmac. Ther.*, 1977, *21*, 44.

Effect on memory. Tetrahydrocannabinol, even in amounts equivalent to small doses of cannabis, impaired immediate memory in 8 young men.— J. R. Tinklenberg *et al.* (letter), *Nature*, 1970, *226*, 1171. See also L. Miller *et al.* (letter), *ibid.*, 1972, *237*, 172. No effect on academic achievement.— N. Q. Brill and R. L. Christie, *Archs gen. Psychiat.*, 1974, *31*, 713, per *J. Am. med. Ass.*, 1974, *230*, 1213.

Effect on mental and motor performance. Simulated car driving tests were carried out on 8 subjects while under the influence of cannabis, alcohol, or placebo. Both alcohol and cannabis increased the brake time and start time. The effect produced by 70 g of alcohol was equivalent to that produced by the oral ingestion of 300 to 400 mg of cannabis resin containing about 4% of Δ^9-tetrahydrocannabinol.— O. J. Rafaelsen *et al.*, *Science*, 1973, *179*, 920.

In a double-blind trial there was an increase in major errors committed by pilots in flight simulation situations after smoking cannabis (6.3 mg of Δ^9-tetrahydrocannabinol) compared with placebo.— M. P. Meacham *et al.* (letter), *J. Am. med. Ass.*, 1974, *230*, 1258.

A report of a fatal motor accident in which cannabis was at least a contributory factor.— D. Teale and V. Marks, *Lancet*, 1976, *1*, 884.

Herpes simplex. Attacks of herpes simplex (chiefly affecting the shaft of the penis) in a 30-year-old man were closely associated with the smoking of cannabis. Three similar cases had been seen and 2 other cases were known of recurring genital herpes in smokers of cannabis.— B. E. Juel-Jensen (letter), *Br. med. J.*, 1972, *4*, 296.

Pregnancy and the neonate. Conflicting evidence of teratogenicity in *animal* studies.— M. G. Joneja, *Toxic. appl. Pharmac.*, 1976, *36*, 151; P. L. Wright *et al.*, *ibid.*, *38*, 223. See also *Am. Pharm.*, 1978, *NS18* (June), 40.

Psychosis. A review of 79 patients admitted to hospital for treatment of the toxic effects of cannabis showed that the most serious acute syndrome was a toxic confusional psychosis, possibly with disorientation and hallucinations. Lesser symptoms included increasing apprehension, anxiety, tremors, and vomiting.— A. A. Baker and E. G. Lucas, *Lancet*, 1969, *1*, 148.

A discussion of mental disturbances provoked by cannabis.— *Br. med. J.*, 1976, *2*, 1092.

Urinary retention. A report of urinary retention occurring in a 55-year-old man each time after the ingestion of cannabis cigarette butts. He had been smoking cannabis for 5 years without experiencing this effect.— T. A. Burton, *J. Am. med. Ass.*, 1979, *242*, 351.

Treatment of Adverse Effects. Mild panic reactions do not usually require specific therapy; reassurance is generally sufficient. If acute psychotic or paranoid reactions occur, chlorpromazine or possibly diazepam may be given by injection.

Precautions. Cannabis has been reported to affect driving. Although there is little evidence of teratogenicity in man it is considered that cannabis should not be used by pregnant women.

Cannabis and alcohol have additive effects; interactions might be expected between cannabis and a wide range of drugs.

The sedation and respiratory depression caused by oxymorphone was increased by tetrahydrocannabinol, and accompanied by significant tachycardia. Pentobarbitone alone had no significant cardiovascular or respiratory effects, but addition of tetrahydrocannabinol produced severe psychological effects including hallucinations and anxiety in most subjects. These interactions could be significant in anaesthetising regular marihuana users.— R. E. Johnstone *et al.*, *Anesthesiology*, 1975, *42*, 674.

Tetrahydrocannabinol 10 mg by mouth caused severe bronchoconstriction requiring salbutamol therapy in 1 of 6 asthmatic patients; the remaining 5 patients showed variable changes in specific airway conductance. In 6 control subjects, a slight but significant increase in specific airway conductance developed after tetrahydrocannabinol.— R. T. Abboud and H. D. Sanders, *Chest*, 1976, *70*, 480.

Tetrahydrocannabinol and alcohol had an additive effect and significantly decreased perception and cognitive and motor functions in 12 healthy subjects.— G. B. Chesher *et al.*, *Med. J. Aust.*, 1976, *2*, 159. Alcohol possibly interfered with the metabolism of tetrahydrocannabinol.— *idem*, 1977, *1*, 478.

For a brief discussion of the effect of cannabis smoking on drug metabolism, see A. P. Alavares, *Clin. Pharmacokinet.*, 1978, *3*, 462. Evidence that cannabis smoking induces hepatic microsomal enzymes.— R. Uppal *et al.*, *Br. J. clin. Pharmac.*, 1981, *11*, 522.

A spurious rise in chorionic gonadotrophin concentrations was seen in 2 patients with testicular cancer who smoked marihuana. Since raised chorionic gonadotrophin concentrations are used as tumour markers, false-positive results may lead to unnecessary treatment.— M. B. Garnick (letter), *New Engl. J. Med.*, 1980, *303*, 1177.

Absorption and Fate. The active principles of cannabis are absorbed from the gastro-intestinal tract and the lungs. Emulsified preparations of Δ^9-tetrahydrocannabinol have been given by injection.

About 50% of the Δ^9-tetrahydrocannabinol available in cannabis is present in the smoke inhaled from a whole cannabis cigarette. This produces an effect almost immediately, reaches a peak in 20 to 30 minutes, and is dissipated in about 3 to 4 hours. When cannabis or Δ^9-tetrahydrocannabinol is taken by mouth absorption may be slow and irregular. Effects are not seen for 30 minutes to 1 hour and persist for about 8 hours.

Tetrahydrocannabinol is lipophilic and becomes widely distributed in the body. It is extensively metabolised, primarily in the liver, to the active 11-hydroxy derivative; both are extensively bound to plasma proteins. It is excreted in the urine and faeces, sometimes over prolonged periods. Excretion may be more rapid in chronic users.

About 94 to 99% of the 11-hydroxy metabolite of Δ^9-tetrahydrocannabinol was bound to plasma proteins.— M. Widman *et al.*, *J. Pharm. Pharmac.*, 1973, *25*, 453. See also *idem*, 1974, *26*, 914.

Ten minutes after smoking for 5 minutes a cigarette containing 10 mg of Δ^9-tetrahydrocannabinol, plasma concentrations in 3 volunteers were between 19 and 26 ng per ml and had fallen to 5 ng or less within 2 hours.— S. Agurell *et al.*, *J. Pharm. Pharmac.*, 1973, *25*, 554.

Metabolites of Δ^9-tetrahydrocannabinol included 11-hydroxy-Δ^9-tetrahydrocannabinol, 11-nor-9-carboxy-Δ^9-tetrahydrocannabinol, and cannabidiol.— S. J. Gross *et al.* (letter), *Nature*, 1974, *252*, 581.

Studies in *animals* indicated that tetrahydrocannabinol crosses the placenta and is also excreted in breast milk.— *J. Am. med. Ass.*, 1979, *242*, 1299. See also J. T. Wilson *et al.*, *Clin. Pharmacokinet.*, 1980, *5*, 1.

An ester glucuronide of Δ^9-tetrahydrocannabinol-11-oic acid had been identified as a urinary metabolite of tetrahydrocannabinol.— P. L. Williams and A. C. Moffat, *J. Pharm. Pharmac.*, 1980, *32*, 445.

Uses. Cannabis was formerly employed as a sedative or narcotic. It is now rarely used as a therapeutic agent.

In a double-blind crossover study 12 anxious patients undergoing radiotherapy for inoperable bronchial carcinoma received Δ^9-tetrahydrocannabinol 10 mg daily by mouth or a placebo for 7 days. Δ^9-Tetrahydrocannabinol caused drowsiness, improved night sleep, and reduced pain but also increased fatigue and confusion. It was considered to have a beneficial effect on the management of the patients and tolerance did not occur after 7 days.— B. H. Davies *et al.*, *Br. J. clin. Pharmac.*, 1974, *1*, 301.

In a double-blind study on patients suffering continuous pain from malignant neoplasms, 9 of 10 experienced some pain relief after doses of 5, 10, 15, and 20 mg of Δ^9-tetrahydrocannabinol. The higher doses caused considerable drowsiness and sedation; euphoria was very evident in 2 patients.— R. Noyes *et al.*, *J. clin. Pharmac.*, 1975, *15*, 139.

In a 24-year-old epileptic patient regular cannabis smoking in conjunction with therapeutic doses of phenobarbitone and phenytoin controlled seizures while phenobarbitone and phenytoin together did not.— P. F. Consroe *et al.*, *J. Am. med. Ass.*, 1975, *234*, 306. Discussion of cannabis-induced convulsions in *animals*.— P. Martin and P. Consroe, *Science*, 1977, *197*, 1302. Further references: J. M. Cunha *et al.*, *Pharmacology*, 1980, *21*, 175 (cannabidiol; anticonvulsant properties).

In a double-blind, placebo-controlled study, smoking marihuana cigarettes each containing tetrahydrocannabinol 25.2 mg reduced intra-ocular pressure in 16 glaucoma patients who were either normotensive or had systemic hypertension. The greatest reductions in intra-ocular pressure were obtained in the hypertensive patients.— W. J. Crawford and J. C. Merritt, *Int. J. clin. Pharmac. Biopharm.*, 1979, *17*, 191, per *Int. pharm. Abstr.*, 1979, *16*, 1232. Although it had been demonstrated that marihuana could lower intra-ocular pressure in healthy subjects and some glaucoma patients, it is not known whether visual function can be preserved or whether marihuana has any advantage over proved glaucoma medication. Further experimental evidence that it was both safe and effective would be required before it could be used for clinical research in patients with glaucoma.— *J. Am. med. Ass.*, 1979, *242*, 1962. Further references: J. C. Merritt *et al.*, *J. Pharm. Pharmac.*, 1981, *33*, 40.

Spasticity scores in 9 patients with multiple sclerosis were considerably lower after taking capsules containing 5 or 10 mg of tetrahydrocannabinol than after a placebo. Although the greatest effect occurred at 3 hours it persisted for up to 5 hours.— *J. Am. med. Ass.*, 1979, *241*, 2476.

For references covering the pharmacology of cannabis and its principles, see reports and reviews under Adverse Effects.

Anti-emetic effects. Discussions on the use of tetrahydrocannabinol for the control of nausea and vomiting in patients receiving cancer chemotherapy.— M. Rose, *Lancet*, 1980, *1*, 703; *Med. Lett.*, 1980, *22*, 41; D. L. Sweet, *J. Am. med. Ass.*, 1980, *243*, 1265; *Lancet*, 1981, *1*, 255.

Tetrahydrocannabinol has been shown to be effective in controlling severe nausea and vomiting in patients receiving cancer chemotherapy (S.E. Sallan *et al.*, *New Engl. J. Med.*, 1975, *293*, 795). S.E. Sallan *et al.* (*New Engl. J. Med.*, 1980, *302*, 135) and H. Eckert *et al.* (*Med. J. Aust.*, 1979, *2*, 657) subsequently found it to be more effective than prochlorperazine. However, in a study by S. Frytak *et al.* (*Ann. intern. Med.*, 1979, *91*, 825), tetrahydrocannabinol was no more effective than prochlorperazine and patients considered side-effects to be more unpleasant. Similarly, although the anti-emetic effects of tetrahydrocannabinol have been found to be of the same order as those of thiethylperazine and metoclopramide, B.M. Colls (*Lancet*, 1980, *1*, 1187) considered its adverse effects to be a problem and concluded that it could not be recommended as a routine anti-emetic agent in cancer chemotherapy when given by mouth. J.C. Kluin-Nelemans *et al.* (*New Engl. J. Med.*, 1980, *302*, 1364) reported that even though it had a pronounced anti-emetic effect in patients receiving cancer chemotherapy, all patients treated preferred the nausea and the vomiting to therapy with tetrahydrocannabinol. Differences in the effectiveness of tetrahydrocannabinol in various studies may have been due to the age distribution of patients since its adverse effects appear to be more intolerable in older patients (M. Rose, *Lancet*, 1980, *1*, 703; *Med. Lett.*, 1980, *22*, 41). Doses used have ranged from 5 to 15 mg per m^2 body-surface and while 5 mg per m^2 is considered by some authorities (*Med. Lett.*, 1980, *22*, 41) to be the safest starting dose, A.E. Chang *et al.* (*Ann. intern. Med.*, 1979, *91*, 819) considered a dose schedule of 10 mg per m^2 every 3 hours for a total of 5 doses to be associated with substantial therapeutic benefit and minimum toxicity.

Bronchodilation. Tetrahydrocannabinol 50, 100, or 200 µg inhaled from an aerosol produced dose-related bronchodilation in 5 asthmatic subjects. Maximum bronchodilation occurred after 60 minutes and overall bronchodilation lasted for at least 3 hours. The optimum dose appeared to be 100 µg. The patients coughed occasionally after inhalation but no tachycardia was observed.— J. P. R. Hartley *et al.*, *Br. J. clin. Pharmac.*, 1978, *5*, 523.

Further references: L. Vachon *et al.*, *New Engl. J. Med.*, 1973, *288*, 985; D. P. Tashkin *et al.*, *ibid.*, *289*, 336.

For a report of bronchoconstriction in asthmatics, see under Precautions.

Preparations

Tetrahydrocannabinol Injection. Δ^9-Tetrahydrocannabinol 100 mg, alcohol 5 ml, Emulphor EL620 0.6 ml (or polysorbate '80' 1.5 ml), sodium chloride injection to 100 ml. Sterilised by filtration. The solution could be diluted with water without cloudiness.—J.L. Olsen, *et al.* (letter), *J. Pharm. Pharmac.*, 1973, *25*, 344.

The effects of a similar injection containing 5% Emulphor EL620 in *rabbits*.— J. C. Cradock *et al.* (letter), *ibid.*, 345.

843-e

Nabilone. Lilly 109514. (±)-(6a*R*,10a*R*)-3-(1,1-Dimethylheptyl)-6,6a,7,8,10,10a-hexahydro-1-hydroxy-6,6-dimethyl-9*H*-dibenzo[*b,d*]pyran-9-one.
$C_{24}H_{36}O_3$=372.5.

CAS — 51022-71-0.

Nabilone is a synthetic cannabinoid with anti-emetic and anxiolytic properties.

A brief discussion on the effects of nabilone.— *J. Am. med. Ass.*, 1978, *240*, 1469.

In healthy subjects nabilone 1 or 2.5 mg produced relaxation and sedation with mild side-effects including dry mouth, euphoria, tachycardia, and postural hypotension. Side-effects were more pronounced after a 5-mg dose. On repeated dosage tolerance developed to these effects without reducing relaxation.— L. Lemberger and H. Rowe, *Pharmacologist*, 1975, *17*, 210.

Clinical studies involving nabilone were discontinued after neurological toxicity was discovered in *dogs* given high doses continuously over prolonged periods.— *Br. med. J.*, 1979, *2*, 1312. See also M. E. Jarvik, *New Engl. J. Med.*, 1979, *300*, 1330. Further investigation into the toxicity of nabilone in *dogs* has shown that substantial differences exist between the metabolic and kinetic pathways in *dogs* and primates. Accumulation of stereospecific carbinol metabolites does not occur either in *monkeys* or man, and thus further investigation of the compound as an anti-emetic in patients undergoing cancer chemotherapy is proceeding.— R. A. Lucas, *Lilly, Personal Communication,* 1981..

Absorption and fate. Following intravenous administration of radioactively labelled nabilone 500 µg to 5 healthy subjects the half-life of the total radioactivity ranged from 17 to 25 hours (mean 20.6 hours); nabilone was rapidly distributed into tissues and metabolised so that relatively little was detected in plasma after 6 hours, the estimated half-life of the parent compound being only 1.7 hours or about one-twelfth that of the total radioactivity. Following administration of 2 mg by mouth to 2 subjects the estimated half-life of total radioactivity was about 35 hours whereas that of unchanged nabilone was only about 2 hours; the estimated half-life of the carbinol metabolite was about 5 to 10 hours. Following intravenous administration about 67% was eliminated in the faeces and 22% in the urine; similar values were obtained following administration by mouth indicating that most of the oral dose was absorbed. Nabilone and its isomeric carbinol metabolites were noted in faeces but not in urine; at least 6 other metabolites were noted but not identified in urine. The short half-life of nabilone did not correspond to its longer duration of action which suggested that one or more of its metabolites was active.— A. Rubin *et al.*, *Clin. Pharmac. Ther.*, 1977, *22*, 85.

Anti-emetic effect. From the results of 2 double-blind crossover studies, nabilone was shown to be superior to prochlorperazine as an anti-emetic for patients experiencing severe nausea and vomiting during cancer chemotherapy, although side-effects were much more frequent with nabilone. Patients were given nabilone 2 mg or prochlorperazine 10 mg every 6 or 8 hours starting either 30 minutes before or 2 doses before a course of chemotherapy. Of the 113 patients who completed one cycle of chemotherapy with each anti-emetic, 9 (8%) had complete relief of nausea and vomiting with nabilone and none with prochlorperazine; 81 (72%) had a partial response with nabilone but only 36 (32%) with prochlorperazine. Side-effects associated with the use of nabilone were considerable and included: somnolence (85% of patients), dry mouth (84%), dizziness (69%), decreased co-ordination (68%), blurred vision (60%), decreased concentration (50%), depression (20%), euphoria (16%), tachycardia (11%), and anxiety (3%). Side-effects with prochlorperazine were similar but generally much less frequent. Of the 9 patients who stopped anti-emetic treatment because of adverse effects, 5 were taking nabilone and 2 of them experienced serious side-effects after only 2 mg—one had orthostatic hypotension and one, a psychotic reaction with visual hallucinations. Two of the remainder who withdrew had nightmares and one suffered severe lethargy. In spite of these adverse effects 75% of patients chose to receive nabilone during subsequent chemotherapy.— T. S. Herman *et al.*, *New Engl. J. Med.*, 1979, *300*, 1295. Disagreement with the conclusion that nabilone was superior to prochlorperazine.— F. J. Fox (letter), *ibid.*, *301*, 728. Reply.— T. S. Herman (letter), *ibid.*

Further references: T. S. Herman *et al.*, *Biomedicine*, 1977, *27*, 331.

Manufacturers
Lilly, USA.

844-l

Synhexyl. Parahexyl; Pyrahexyl; 5′-Methyl-$\Delta^{6a\text{-}10a}$-tetrahydrocannabinol. 3-Hexyl-7,8,9,10-tetrahydro-6,6,9-trimethyl-6*H*-dibenzo[*b,d*]pyran-1-ol.
$C_{22}H_{32}O_2$=328.5.

CAS — 117-51-1.

Synhexyl is a synthetic analogue of the tetrahydrocannabinols with effects similar to those described above under Tetrahydrocannabinol.

For studies comparing synhexyl and tetrahydrocannabinols, see L. E. Hollister *et al.*, *Clin. Pharmac. Ther.*, 1968, *9*, 783; L. E. Hollister (letter), *Nature*, 1970, *227*, 968; R. T. Pivik *et al.*, *Clin. Pharmac. Ther.*, 1972, *13*, 426.

Carbimazole and other Antithyroid Agents

830-g

The antithyroid agents are used in the treatment of hyperthyroidism, a common form of which is Graves' (Basedow's) disease.

The agents most widely used are thiourea or thiocarbamide derivatives which include the thiouracils and imidazoles (carbimazole and its metabolite methimazole). They act mainly by interfering with the incorporation of iodide into thyroglobulin in the thyroid gland and thus reduce the synthesis of tri-iodothyronine and thyroxine. Any preformed thyroid hormone tends not to be affected by usual doses. Carbimazole is the drug most widely used in Great Britain whereas propylthiouracil and methimazole are used in the United States.

Potassium perchlorate may be used if other antithyroid treatment cannot be tolerated. It acts as an ionic inhibitor and reduces the uptake of iodide by the thyroid as well as causing the release of inorganic iodide already taken up by the gland.

Unlike thyroidectomy or therapy with radioiodine, the antithyroid drugs have a reversible effect on the thyroid. High doses are given initially, usually for 2 to 3 months, until the patient becomes euthyroid. The dose is then reduced to the minimum necessary to maintain this euthyroid state. If treatment is continued for 1 to 2 years about half of the patients have been reported to remain euthyroid for prolonged periods after the drug has been withdrawn but, more recently, lower remission-rates have been attributed to an increased intake of dietary iodine. M.A. Greer *et al.* (*New Engl. J. Med.*, 1977, *297*, 173) have reported good results with short-term therapy (see Propylthiouracil, p.359).

If hyperthyroidism is to be treated by subtotal thyroidectomy, the patient may first be treated with a drug of the thiourea group until euthyroid and then given potassium or sodium iodide or Aqueous Iodine Solution to decrease the vascularity of the gland.

In the treatment of thyrotoxic crisis (thyroid storm) iodine or iodide should be given to prevent further release of thyroid hormone. Propranolol and the antithyroid drugs may also be used.

See Propranolol, p.1329, for its use in the treatment of the symptoms of thyrotoxicosis.

Antithyroid agents were formerly used in animal feeds; this use is banned in a number of countries.

For reviews of hyperthyroidism and its treatment see P. Kendall-Taylor, *Br. med. J.*, 1972, *2*, 337; M. F. Green, *ibid.*, 1974, *1*, 232; C. Laroche *et al.*, *Thérapie*, 1974, *29*, 659; I. M. D. Jackson, *Am. J. Hosp. Pharm.*, 1975, *32*, 933; I. D. Thomas, *Drugs*, 1976, *11*, 119; B. E. W. Brownlie, *ibid.*, 1977, *14*, 376; *Drug & Ther. Bull.*, 1977, *15*, 89; D. W. Slingerland and B. A. Burrows, *J. Am. med. Ass.*, 1979, *242*, 2408; R. Greene, *Prescribers' J.*, 1980, *20*, 73.

Treatment with antithyroid drugs, subtotal thyroidectomy, or radioactive iodine did not influence the underlying cause of thyrotoxicosis. Treatment with antithyroid drugs was usually continued for 1 to 2 years and about half the patients relapsed when treatment ceased. Remissions lasted 10 to 20 years in three-quarters and 6 to 9 years in the remainder of patients. Antithyroid agents were the best initial treatment for young patients and did not permanently damage the thyroid gland but excessive dosage could lead to hypothyroidism. With subtotal thyroidectomy the combined incidence of hypothryoidism and of complications of surgery was relatively high, but surgery was indicated in patients with large goitres, in patients unresponsive to antithyroid drugs for whom treatment with radioactive iodine was contra-indicated, and in patients who were unlikely to take medication regularly. Treatment with radioactive iodine, though convenient, was associated with a delay in response, might need to be repeated, and was associated with a progressive incidence of hypothyroidism; it was usually limited to patients over 40 years of age and was contra-indicated in children and in pregnancy. The treatment of thyroid crisis should include sodium iodide 1 to 2 g by slow intravenous infusion and carbimazole 100 to 200 mg or methylthiouracil 1 to 2 g by mouth.— C. W. H. Havard, *Abstr. Wld Med.*, 1969, *43*, 629.

The role of thyroid-stimulating immunoglobulins in Graves' disease and the effects of surgery, radio-iodine, and carbimazole.— El D. Mukhtar *et al.*, *Lancet*, 1975, *1*, 713.

A survey of the thyroid function of 110 patients in remission from thyrotoxicosis for a mean period of 7.6 years after stopping treatment indicated that long-term follow-up of such patients was desirable if hypothyroidism was to be avoided. A third of the patients who had discontinued antithyroid agents for more than 4 years showed some evidence of thyroid failure.— W. J. Irvine *et al.*, *Lancet*, 1977, *2*, 179.

Investigation of 77 patients with Graves' disease and 300 healthy control subjects showed an association between the thyrotoxicosis and the presence of HLA-B8 antigen and that this association was particularly strong in those who had relapsed after withdrawal of antithyroid therapy. It was considered that thyrotoxic patients positive for HLA-B8 were 1.8 times more likely to relapse after withdrawal of drug treatment than patients negative for this antigen. The absence of the antigen might encourage the use of prolonged antithyroid treatment in the young thyrotoxic patient without gross thyroid enlargement before ablation might be considered.— W. J. Irvine *et al.*, *Lancet*, 1977, *2*, 898. See also A. M. McGregor *et al.*, *ibid.*, 1980, *1*, 1101; P. A. Dahlberg *et al.* (letter), *ibid.*, *2*, 1144.

A discussion on the cause of hyperthyroidism.— *Lancet*, 1979, *2*, 78.

Use in pregnancy. A discussion of the use of antithyroid agents and thyroid concomitantly in hyperthyroidism during pregnancy.— H. A. Selenkow, *Obstet. Gynec.*, 1972, *40*, 117, per *Int. pharm. Abstr.*, 1973, *10*, 218. Arguments against the use of antithyroid agents and thyroid concomitantly in hyperthyroidism during pregnancy.— J. I. Hamburger, *ibid.*, 114, per *Int. pharm. Abstr.*, 1973, *10*, 219.

A review.— G. N. Burrow, *New Engl. J. Med.*, 1978, *298*, 150.

Further references: *Br. med. J.*, 1978, *2*, 977; O. M. Edwards, *Postgrad. med. J.*, 1979, *55*, 340.

831-q

Carbimazole *(B.P.)*. Carbimaz.; Carbimazolum. Ethyl 3-methyl-2-thioxo-4-imidazoline-1-carboxylate.

$C_7H_{10}N_2O_2S$=186.2.

CAS — 22232-54-8.

Pharmacopoeias. In *Br.*, *Chin.*, *Cz.*, *Int.*, and *Turk.*

A white or creamy-white crystalline powder with a characteristic odour; tasteless at first, with a bitter after-taste. M.p. 122° to 125°. **Soluble** 1 in 500 of water, 1 in 50 of alcohol, 1 in 17 of acetone, 1 in 3 of chloroform, and 1 in 330 of ether. **Store** in airtight containers.

Adverse Effects. Side-effects occur most commonly in the first 2 months of treatment and include rashes, nausea, headache, and gastro-intestinal upsets. Occasionally there is drug fever which may also be accompanied by arthralgia. Agranulocytosis is the most serious side-effect, and patients should be instructed to report the development of sore throat, fever, or rashes, as these may sometimes precede abnormal findings in the blood by several days. Alopecia, thrombocytopenia, aplastic anaemia, and hepatitis following carbimazole therapy have also been reported, as occasionally have psychotic reactions.

Cross-sensitivity with other antithyroid agents may sometimes occur.

Antithyroid drugs cross the placenta and may cause foetal or neonatal hypothyroidism and goitre.

Loss of taste occurred in a patient treated with carbimazole.— J. Erikssen *et al.* (letter), *Lancet*, 1975, *1*, 231. See also I. P. Griffith, *Practitioner*, 1976, *217*, 907.

Blood disorders. An analysis of blood dyscrasias reported to the Swedish Adverse Drug Reaction Committee for the 5-year period 1966–70 showed that thrombocytopenia and agranulocytosis attributable to carbimazole had both been reported on 4 occasions. It was estimated that reported figures represented one-third of the true frequency.— L. E. Böttiger and B. Westerholm, *Br. med. J.*, 1973, *3*, 339.

Epidermal necrolysis. Carbimazole might have been responsible for a case of toxic epidermal necrolysis.— A. Lyell, *Br. J. Derm.*, 1967, *79*, 662.

Pregnancy and the neonate. Of 25 children whose mothers had taken carbimazole during pregnancy 5 to 16 years earlier, one had partial adactyly of one foot and the other bilateral congenital cataracts. A third child had a small goitre but was euthyroid, as were all the others.— A. M. McCarroll *et al.*, *Archs Dis. Childh.*, 1976, *51*, 532.

Treatment of Adverse Effects. Antihistamines may be of value in the treatment of mild skin reactions to carbimazole. If blood disorders occur, the drug should be immediately withdrawn and, if necessary, antibiotics, blood transfusions, and corticosteroids should be given.

Precautions. Carbimazole should be given with the utmost caution, or not at all, if there is any degree of tracheal obstruction, as high dosage may produce thyroid enlargement and obstructive symptoms may become marked.

Although there is a risk to the foetal thyroid it is considered that carbimazole may be given during pregnancy but the smallest effective dose should be used and, if possible, treatment should be discontinued 3 or 4 weeks before delivery. Infants should not be breast fed by mothers taking carbimazole.

Patients should be warned to report the development of sore throat, fever, or rashes since these may be indicative of abnormalities in the blood. Also careful consideration should be given to the use of carbimazole in patients with pre-existing blood disorders.

There may be a delayed response in patients who have been treated with iodine and it has been suggested that iodine intake should be reduced during carbimazole therapy.

Absorption and Fate. Carbimazole and the other thioureas are absorbed from the gastro-intestinal tract and are widely distributed throughout the body. They readily cross the placenta and are present in milk during lactation. Carbimazole is metabolised to methimazole which is excreted in the urine, excretion being almost complete in 24 hours.

Methimazole is appreciably bound to plasma proteins and is reported to have an extended plasma half-life in hypothyroid subjects but a reduced half-life in hyperthyroid subjects.

Methimazole was rapidly absorbed in 11 euthyroid subjects with a mean peak plasma concentration of 920 ng per ml achieved one hour after a single dose of 60 mg. The apparent plasma half-life was about 6.4 hours and 11.6% of the dose was excreted in the urine in 24 hours.— J. A. Pittman *et al.*, *J. clin. Endocr. Metab.*, 1971, *33*, 182.

Excretion in breast milk.— L. C. K. Low *et al.* (letter), *Lancet*, 1979, *2*, 1011; L. Tegler and B. Lindstrom (letter), *Lancet*, 1980, *2*, 591.

Uses. Carbimazole, a thiourea derivative, is an antithyroid substance which depresses the formation of thyroid hormone. Its main effect is to reduce the formation of iodotyrosines and hence of tri-iodothyronine and thyroxine.

Carbimazole is used to control Graves' disease and is given by mouth in an initial dosage of 30 to 60 mg daily in divided doses, at 8-hourly intervals, according to the severity of the disorder. This dose is then gradually reduced to the smallest amount that will control the disease. Improvement is usually seen in 1 to 3 weeks and control of symptoms is achieved in 1 to 3 months. Usual maintenance doses are 5 to 20 mg daily. Alternatively, treatment with carbimazole may be continued at the initial dose and thyroxine or liothyronine sodium given to prevent the development of hypothyroidism. A suggested initial dose for children aged 1 year is 7.5 mg daily in divided doses, and for children aged 7 years 15 mg daily.

Marked enlargement of the thyroid is an indication of excessive dosage. Occasionally, eye signs worsen as the condition comes under control. After prolonged administration of carbimazole for many months or years, the disorder may abate spontaneously. It may, however, recur and signs of thyrotoxicosis may reappear within weeks or months of withdrawal of the drug.

Carbimazole is also used in the preparation of patients for subtotal thyroidectomy. The patient is rendered euthyroid with carbimazole and iodine or iodides are given for 10 or 12 days before operation in order to render the gland firmer and less vascular.

Iodine or iodides are normally used in the immediate treatment of thyroid crisis or for the rapid control of a severe fulminating case and propranolol may be given to relieve the cardiovascular symptoms; carbimazole may also be used but only in association with this therapy.

Of 25 thyrotoxic patients who had been treated with carbimazole or methylthiouracil for 1 to 2 years and who were given 200 µg of potassium iodide daily about 56% relapsed, but of another 41 patients who did not receive iodine supplement, only 11 (27%) relapsed. It appeared that the iodine-deficiency state induced by the antithyroid drugs protected the patients from early relapses.— W. D. Alexander *et al.*, *lancet*, 1965, *2*, 866.

In 181 patients with thyrotoxicosis there was no significant difference in response to treatment with iodine-131 between those who had been pretreated with carbimazole and controls.— A. W. G. Goolden and T. R. Fraser, *Br. med. J.*, 1969, *3*, 443.

Thirty patients with hyperthyroidism were treated with carbimazole 10 mg and liothyronine 20 µg every 6 hours. All patients were clinically euthyroid within 2 months. After 3 months the treatment was given as a single daily dose in the morning; there was no evidence of loss of control in follow-up for up to 3 years.— P. H. Wise *et al.*, *Br. med. J.*, 1973, *4*, 143. See also W. D. Alexander *et al.*, *Lancet*, 1966, *2*, 1041; *idem*, 1967, *2*, 681.

In 12 patients with thyrotoxicosis treated with carbimazole, the free thyroxine and tri-iodothyronine indexes fell rapidly, followed by a slightly slower fall in sex-hormone binding globulin (a 'tissue marker' of thyroid action), and generally by a return to normal of the thyrotrophin response to protirelin; the clinical response was more gradual. The dose of carbimazole should be adjusted to maintain biochemical values in the normal range; remaining symptoms should be treated by a beta-blocking agent.— C. H. Mortimer *et al.*, *Br. med. J.*, 1977, *1*, 138.

Further references on the use of carbimazole in thyrotoxic patients: R. G. Twycross and V. Marks, *Br. med. J.*, 1970, *2*, 701; R. C. Lowry *et al.*, *ibid.*, 1971, *2*, 19.

Administration in renal failure. Recommendations for the use of methimazole, to which carbimazole is metabolised, are reported on p.357.

Low-dose therapy. A study of the smallest effective dose of carbimazole indicated that in only one of 4 thyrotoxic patients was there any convincing change in the efficacy of carbimazole in doses above 10 mg daily.— L. C. K. Low *et al.* (letter), *Lancet*, 1979, *1*, 493. See also N. Riccioni *et al.* (letter), *ibid.*, 1087.

Pregnancy and the neonate. Thyroxine 200 to 300µg daily was given with carbimazole in pregnancy; the dose of carbimazole could be reduced by one-third to one-half in the third trimester. In 70 patients so treated there was no foetal goitre or hypothyroidism.— H. A. Selenkow, *Obstet. Gynec.*, 1972, *40*, 117, per *Drugs*, 1973, *6*, 442.

A 29-year-old woman who had had partial thyroidectomy and was on thyroxine maintenance had given birth to an infant with exophthalmos. In a later pregnancy she was given carbimazole and an increased dose of thyroxine. The infant developed signs of thyrotoxicosis one day after birth and was controlled by 3 weeks treatment with carbimazole given in reducing doses starting with 750 µg thrice daily. The child was considered to be completely normal at 2.5 years of age.— I. Ramsay, *Br. med. J.*, 1976, *2*, 1110.

The treatment of foetal thyrotoxicosis should be by giving carbimazole to the mother in doses adjusted to keep the foetal heart-rate between 120 and 160 beats per minute; thyroxine did not readily cross the placenta and could be given to keep the mother euthyroid if necessary.— P. L. Robinson *et al.*, *Br. med. J.*, 1979, *1*, 383.

Short-term therapy. For reference to short-term therapy of hyperthyroidism with carbimazole, see under Propylthiouracil, p.359.

Preparations

Carbimazole Tablets *(B.P.)*. Tablets containing carbimazole. They may be compression-coated.
Store in a cool place in airtight containers.

Neo-Mercazole *(Nicholas, UK)*. Carbimazole, available as scored tablets of 5 mg. (Also available as Neo-Mercazole in *Austral.*, *Canad.*, *Denm.*, *Fr.*, *Norw.*, *S.Afr.*, *Switz.*).

Other Proprietary Names

Basolest *(Neth.)*; Carbazole *(Austral.)*; Carbotiroid *(Ital.)*; Neo-Carbimazole *(Spain)*; Neo-Mercazol *(Belg.)*; Neo-Morphazole, Neo-Thyreostat *(both Ger.)*; Neo-Tireol *(Ital.)*; Neo-Tomizol *(Spain)*.

832-p

Benzylthiouracil. 6-Benzyl-2,3-dihydro-2-thioxopyrimidin-4(1*H*)-one; 6-Benzyl-2-mercaptopyrimidin-4-ol.
$C_{11}H_{10}N_2OS=218.3$.

CAS — 33086-27-0.

Uses. Benzylthiouracil is an antithyroid agent with actions similar to those of Carbimazole, p.356. It has been given in doses of up to 200 mg daily in divided doses with meals.

Proprietary Names
Basdène *(Théraplix, Fr.)*.

833-s

Iodothiouracil Sodium. Iothiouracil Sodium; Athyriodacil Sodique. The dihydrate of the sodium salt of 2,3-dihydro-5-iodo-2-thioxopyrimidin-4(1*H*)-one; the dihydrate of the sodium salt of 5-iodo-2-mercaptopyrimidin-4-ol.
$C_4H_2IN_2NaOS,2H_2O=312.1$.

CAS — 5984-97-4 (iodothiouracil); 3565-15-9 (sodium salt, anhydrous).

Uses. Iodothiouracil sodium, which contains about 40% of iodine, was formerly used in the treatment of hyperthyroidism. It has been given in doses of 150 to 300 mg daily in divided doses.

834-w

Mercaptothiazoline. 3-Thiazoline-2-thiol.
$C_3H_5NS_2=119.2$.

CAS — 96-53-7.

Uses. Mercaptothiazoline has been used in the treatment of hyperthyroidism in doses of 100 mg daily.

835-e

Methimazole *(U.S.P.)*. Mercazolylum; Thiamazole; Tiamazol. 1-Methylimidazole-2-thiol.

$C_4H_6N_2S=114.2$.

CAS — 60-56-0.

Pharmacopoeias. In *Arg.*, *Braz.*, *Chin.*, *Hung.*, *It.*, *Jap.*, *Jug.*, *Nord.*, *Rus.*, and *U.S.*

A white to pale buff crystalline powder with a faint characteristic odour and a slightly bitter taste. M.p. 144° to 147°. **Soluble** 1 in 5 of water, 1 in 5 of alcohol, and 1 in about 5 of chloroform; freely soluble in acetone; slightly soluble in ether. Solutions in water are practically neutral to litmus. **Store** in airtight containers. Protect from light.

Taste. Methimazole, like phenylthiourea and propylthiouracil, had a dualistic taste response and was bitter to nearly 30% of persons tested.— G. H. Hamor and A. Lafdjian, *J. pharm. Sci.*, 1967, *56*, 777.

Adverse Effects, Treatment, and Precautions. As for Carbimazole, p.356.

A 62-year-old woman under treatment with methimazole 10 mg every 8 hours developed swelling of the parotid glands after about 7 weeks of treatment. The swelling disappeared within 3 days when treatment was discontinued, but reappeared in a few hours after a further dose.— R. C. Moehlig (letter), *J. Am. med. Ass.*, 1969, *209*, 1224.

A 13-year-old girl with Graves' disease being treated with methimazole 10 mg daily developed peripheral neuritis after 20 months. The dosage of methimazole was reduced to 2.5 mg daily but toxicity was still evident. On discontinuation of therapy the symptoms disappeared and the patient remained euthyroid.— E. C. Roldan and G. Nigrin, *N.Y. St. J. Med.*, 1972, *72*, 2898.

Loss of taste occurred in a patient treated with methimazole.— J. Erikssen *et al.* (letter), *Lancet*, 1975, *1*, 231.

Loss of libido was reported in a 34-year-old woman taking methimazole.— R. D. Hempel and U. Herter, *Dte GesundhWes.*, 1976, *31*, 2157.

Blood disorders. An analysis of blood dyscrasias reported to the Swedish Adverse Drug Reaction Committee for the 5-year period 1966–70 showed that agranulocytosis attributable to methimazole had been reported on 7 occasions. It was estimated that reported figures represented one-third of the true frequency.— L. E. Böttiger and B. Westerholm, *Br. med. J.*, 1973, *3*, 339.

Liver disease. Jaundice was attributed to methimazole in one patient. Symptoms cleared on substituting propylthiouracil for methimazole.— C. E. Becker *et al.*, *J. Am. med. Ass.*, 1968, *206*, 1787. Another case of jaundice associated with methimazole.— M. G. Fischer *et al.*, *ibid.*, 1973, *223*, 1028.

Pregnancy and the neonate. For reports of the effect of methimazole on the foetus, see Propylthiouracil, p.358.

Absorption and Fate. Methimazole is a metabolite of carbimazole and the absorption and fate of both compounds is described under Carbimazole, p.356.

Uses. Methimazole is an antithyroid agent similar in action to carbimazole (see p.356) and is used for similar purposes. A suitable initial dose is 5 to 20 mg every 8 hours. When the condition is controlled, probably in 1 to 2 months, the dose is reduced to a maintenance dose, usually 5 to 15 mg daily. A suggested initial dose for children is 400 µg per kg bodyweight daily in divided doses; for maintenance this dose may be halved.

Methimazole has been given parenterally in solution in sodium chloride injection.

Methimazole 30 to 40 mg every 8 hours might be given as part of the treatment of hyperthyroid crisis.— S. R. Newmark *et al.*, *J. Am. med. Ass.*, 1974, *230*, 592.

Administration in renal failure. The dose of methimazole should be reduced to 75% of the usual dose in patients with a glomerular filtration-rate of 10 to 50 ml per minute, and to 50% of the usual dose in those with a glomerular filtration-rate of less than 10 ml per minute.— W. M. Bennett *et al.*, *Ann. intern. Med.*, 1980, *93*, 286.

Low-dose therapy. For reference to low-dose therapy of hyperthyroidism, see under Carbimazole, p.357.

Short-term therapy. For reference to short-term therapy of hyperthyroidism with methimazole, see under Propylthiouracil, p.359.

Preparations

Methimazole Tablets *(U.S.P.)*. Tablets containing methimazole. The *U.S.P.* requires 80% dissolution in 30 minutes. Protect from light.

Proprietary Names

Antitiroide GW *(Panthox & Burck, Ital.)*; Danantizol *(Gador, Arg.)*; Favistan *(Asta, Ger.)*; Mercaptol *(Nessa, Spain)*; Metazolo *(Guidi, Ital.)*; Strumazol *(Christiaens,*

Belg.; *Christiaens, Neth.)*; Tapazole *(Lilly, Canad.*; *Lilly, Ital.*; *Lilly, Norw.*; *Lilly, S.Afr.*; *Lilly, Switz.*; *Lilly, USA)*; Thacapzol *(Kabi, Swed.)*; Thycapzol *(GEA, Denm.)*; Tirodril *(Estedi, Spain)*; Tomizol *(Pages Maruny, Spain)*.

836-l

Methylthiouracil *(U.S.P., B.P. 1973)*. Methylthiour.; Methylthiouracilum. 2,3-Dihydro-2-thioxo-6-methylpyrimidin-4(1*H*)-one; 2-Mercapto-6-methylpyrimidin-4-ol.

$C_5H_6N_2OS$=142.2.

CAS — 56-04-2.

Pharmacopoeias. In *Arg., Aust., Braz., Cz., Int., It., Jap., Nord., Pol., Rus., Swiss,* and *U.S.*

A white odourless crystalline powder with a bitter taste. M.p. about 330° with decomposition. **Soluble** 1 in 2000 of water, 1 in 150 of boiling water, and 1 in 800 of alcohol; slightly soluble in acetone, chloroform, and ether; very slightly soluble in dilute mineral acids; freely soluble in solutions of ammonium hydroxide and sodium hydroxide. **Protect** from light.

Uses. Methylthiouracil has an action similar to that of carbimazole (see p.356); it has been given in initial doses of 200 to 400 mg daily, with maintenance doses of 50 to 150 mg daily, but is now little used.

Preparations

Methylthiouracil Tablets *(B.P. 1973)*. Tablets containing methylthiouracil.

Proprietary Names

Atiroid *(Wassermann, Spain)*; Methiocil *(Helvepharm, Switz.)*; Thyreostat *(Herbrand, Ger.)*; Thyrostabil *(Streuli, Switz.)*; Tiouracil *(LEFA, Spain)*.

837-y

Potassium Perchlorate *(B.P.C. 1968)*. Pot. Perchlor.

$KClO_4$=138.5.

CAS — 7778-74-7.

Pharmacopoeias. In *Cz.* and *Hung.*

Odourless colourless crystals or white crystalline powder with a slightly saline taste. It decrepitates on heating and evolves oxygen. Each g represents 7.2 mmol (7.2 mEq) of potassium). **Soluble** 1 in 65 of water and 1 in 15 of boiling water; practically insoluble in alcohol.

WARNING. *The Council of the Pharmaceutical Society of Great Britain advises pharmacists not to supply materials likely to be used for making fireworks, including chlorates, to children under any circumstances. See Pharm. J.,* 1957, *2,* 92; 1970, *1,* 296; 1975, *2,* 459; 1977, *2,* 392.

Adverse Effects. Fatal aplastic anaemia has occurred in a small proportion of patients. Other blood disorders including agranulocytosis, thrombocytopenia, and leucopenia have been reported. Signs of intolerance may precede changes in the blood by several days. The nephrotic syndrome occurs rarely. Nausea and vomiting and hypersensitivity reactions such as maculopapular rashes, fever, and lymphadenopathies may occur, but are infrequent if the daily dosage is kept below 1 g.

For reports of the adverse effects of potassium perchlorate, see Martindale 27th Edn, p. 303.

Treatment of Adverse Effects and Precautions. As for Carbimazole, p.356. Its antithyroid effect can be reversed by iodine.

Absorption and Fate. Potassium perchlorate is absorbed from the gastro-intestinal tract and has a short half-life. It crosses the placenta and is present in milk.

Uses. Potassium perchlorate reduces the uptake of iodide by the thyroid and causes the release of inorganic iodide already taken up by the gland. However, because of toxicity its use is generally limited to patients who cannot tolerate other forms of antithyroid therapy.

Potassium perchlorate may be given in a dose of 200 to 250 mg three or four times a day, reduced after 2 to 4 weeks to 100 to 125 mg three or four times a day. More than 1 g daily should not be given. Treatment has usually to be continued for 12 to 18 months or longer. Thyroid function may remain depressed for some weeks after withdrawal of the drug and signs of hypothyroidism may occur. Potassium perchlorate has been used to prepare patients for partial thyroidectomy when the goitre was small and nodular. Small doses of potassium iodide may be given simultaneously but large doses antagonise the action of the perchlorate.

The effect of potassium perchlorate, given intravenously, in enhancing tumour visibility in brain scanning.— I. Buttfield *et al., J. nucl. Med.,* 1973, *14,* 543, per *Int. pharm. Abstr.,* 1973, *10,* 895.

Potassium perchlorate was routinely given to patients before brain scanning with pertechnetate [^{99m}Tc] to reduce uptake by the choroid plexus and salivary glands. Solutions of potassium perchlorate should not be refrigerated as crystals formed which dissolved only slowly.— C. C. Williams, *Am. J. Hosp. Pharm.,* 1977, *34,* 93.

The use of perchlorate rectally in unconscious patients before brain scintigraphy with pertechnetate (^{99m}Tc).— D. Turner *et al., J. nucl. Med.,* 1977, *18,* 258.

Perchlorate discharge test. Patients were given 10 to 15 µCi of iodine-131 intravenously and 63 minutes later 400 mg of potassium perchlorate by mouth. Counts of the radioactivity of the neck were used to measure the iodine-131 content of the thyroid 60, 90, and 120 minutes after the injection, and studied in relation to the urinary excretion of iodine-131 enabled the discharge of iodine by the thyroid to be calculated. Positive discharge tests implied that the binding of organic iodine by the thyroid was impaired.— R. D. H. Stewart and I. P. C. Murray, *J. clin. Endocr. Metab.,* 1966, *26,* 1050.

Preparations

Potassium Perchlorate Tablets *(B.P.C. 1968)*. Tablets containing potassium perchlorate.

Peroidin *(Larkhall Laboratories, UK)*. Potassium perchlorate, available as tablets of 50 and 200 mg. (Also available as Peroidin in *Austral., Canad.)*.

838-j

Propylthiouracil *(B.P., U.S.P.)*. Propylthiour.; Propylthiouracilum. 2,3-Dihydro-6-propyl-2-thioxopyrimidin-4(1*H*)-one; 2-Mercapto-6-propylpyrimidin-4-ol.

$C_7H_{10}N_2OS$=170.2.

CAS — 51-52-5.

Pharmacopoeias. In *Aust., Br., Braz., Chin., Ger., Ind., Int., It., Jap., Jug., Mex., Nord., Swiss, Turk.,* and *U.S.*

White or pale cream-coloured odourless crystals or crystalline powder with a bitter taste. M.p. 218° to 221°.

Soluble 1 in 700 of water, 1 in about 60 of alcohol, and 1 in 60 of acetone; slightly soluble in chloroform and ether; soluble in solutions of alkali hydroxides. **Protect** from light.

Adverse Effects, Treatment, and Precautions. As for Carbimazole, p.356. Though adverse reactions occur less frequently with propylthiouracil than with methylthiouracil, they are not predictable. A rare complication of therapy with propylthiouracil is a tendency to haemorrhage; it may be controlled by the administration of phytomenadione.

Severe hypoprothrombinaemia developed in a 60-year-old diabetic, hypertensive, hyperthyroid woman after administration of propylthiouracil 300 mg daily for 2 weeks.— G. D'Angelo and L. P. Le Gresley, *Can. med. Ass. J.,* 1959, *81,* 479.

A lupus-like syndrome followed treatment with propylthiouracil.— M. M. Best and C. H. Duncan, *J. Ky St. med. Ass.,* 1964, *62,* 47, per D. Alarcon-Segovia, *Mayo Clin. Proc.,* 1969, *44,* 664.

A 2½-year-old girl with hyperthyroidism became hypothyroid, menstruated, and developed galactorrhoea after treatment with propylthiouracil 25 mg thrice daily; the symptoms disappeared when the dose was halved.— A. Sadeghi-Nejad and B. Senior, *J. Pediat.,* 1971, *79,* 833, per *Int. pharm. Abstr.,* 1972, *9,* 647.

Migratory polyarthritis developed in 2 adolescent girls treated with propylthiouracil.— W. Hung and G. P. August, *J. Pediat.,* 1973, *82,* 852.

In a study of 44 patients with Graves' disease treated with propylthiouracil or methimazole for periods ranging from 7 to 46 months, 6 patients had remission. This low success-rate might have been due to increased daily average dietary intake of iodine.— L. Wartofsky, *J. Am. med. Ass.,* 1973, *226,* 1083.

Reversible tinnitus and loss of hearing occurred in a girl being treated with propylthiouracil.— K. E. Smith and J. S. Spaulding, *Archs Otolar.,* 1972, *96,* 368.

Ingestion of an amount of propylthiouracil considered to be at least 5 g produced no acute effects in a 12-year-old girl.— G. L. Jackson *et al., Ann. intern. Med.,* 1979, *91,* 418.

A report of hypocalcaemia accompanying agranulocytosis in a 28-year-old woman during propylthiouracil therapy.— G. E. Shambaugh *et al., Ann. intern. Med.,* 1979, *91,* 576.

Vasculitis possibly caused by propylthiouracil.— B. D. Houston *et al., Arthritis Rheum.,* 1979, *22,* 925.

Blood disorders. *For reports of blood disorders and haemorrhage associated with propylthiouracil, see Martindale 27th Edn,* p. 304.

Liver disease. A 9-year-old girl developed jaundice and hepatitis 2 months after starting treatment with propylthiouracil 100 mg thrice daily. These effects regressed on withdrawal of the drug.— L. N. Parker (letter), *Ann. intern. Med.,* 1975, *82,* 228.

Hepatic necrosis in a hyperthyroid woman treated with propylthiouracil might have resulted from the sensitisation of her lymphocytes to the drug.— A. A. Mihas *et al., Gastroenterology,* 1976, *70,* 770.

A report of propylthiouracil as the possible cause of a liver disease similar to chronic active hepatitis.— M. S. Fedotin and L. G. Lefer, *Archs intern. Med.,* 1975, *135,* 319. See also M. Weiss *et al., ibid.,* 1980, *140,* 1184.

Pregnancy and the neonate. Goitre in 5 neonates was recorded in infants born to 30 patients given propylthiouracil in 41 pregnancies. The dosage of propylthiouracil appeared to be an important but not the only factor.— G. N. Burrow, *J. clin. Endocr. Metab.,* 1965, *25,* 403.

Exposure to propylthiouracil *in utero* did not appear to have an adverse effect on subsequent growth and development.— G. N. Burrow *et al., Am. J. Dis. Child.,* 1968, *116,* 161.

Transient neonatal goitre occurred in 2 infants, 1 in each of 2 sets of twins, born to mothers who had taken propylthiouracil or methimazole during pregnancy.— S. Refetoff *et al., J. Pediat.,* 1974, *85,* 240.

Propylthiouracil or methimazole was administered to 21 women during 26 pregnancies. Four infants had goitre at birth and of these 3 had neonatal thyrotoxicosis. There were congenital defects in 5 children of 3 mothers.— Q. Mujtaba and G. N. Burrow, *Obstet. Gynec.,* 1975, *46,* 282.

Results emphasising that it is essential to use the smallest possible dose of propylthiouracil in pregnancy and that thyroid function of the neonate should be evaluated carefully.— R. G. Cheron *et al., New Engl. J. Med.,* 1981, *304,* 525.

Absorption and Fate. As for Carbimazole, p.356. Like methimazole, propylthiouracil is reported to have an extended plasma half-life in hypothyroid subjects but a reduced half-life in hyperthyroid subjects.

A study of the metabolism of ^{35}S-labelled antithyroid drugs indicated that propylthiouracil was more rapidly absorbed and excreted and had a shorter biological half-life in the plasma than carbimazole and methimazole. Renal function might have a more important influence on the biological half-life of the drugs than thyroid status.— W. D. Alexander *et al., Br. med. J.,* 1969, *2,* 290.

Studies of the urine-hydroxyproline and urine-calcium concentrations of 30 patients with hyperthyroidism before and after treatment with propylthiouracil suggested that many patients did not achieve a steady metabolic state until about 3 months after starting treatment.— K. Siersbaek *et al.*, *Acta med. scand.*, 1971, *189*, 485, per *Abstr. Wld Med.*, 1971, *45*, 764.

Limited excretion in breast milk.— J. P. Kampmann *et al.*, *Lancet*, 1980, *1*, 736.

Further references: J. Kampmann and L. Skovsted, *Acta pharmac. tox.*, 1975, *37*, 201.

Uses. Propylthiouracil has similar actions to carbimazole (see p.356) but it is thought to inhibit the conversion of thyroxine to tri-iodothyronine as well as depressing the formation of thyroid hormones. In the treatment of hyperthyroidism, the usual dosage is between 200 and 600 mg daily in divided doses, at 8-hourly intervals, until the symptoms have been controlled. The maintenance dose is usually between 50 and 200 mg daily. A suggested initial dose for children aged 6 to 10 years is 50 to 150 mg daily in divided doses, and for children over 10 years 150 to 300 mg daily.

A discussion of the possible use of propylthiouracil in the treatment of alcoholic hepatitis.— *J. Am. med. Ass.*, 1975, *232*, 121.

Propylthiouracil 300 to 400 mg every 8 hours might be given as part of the treatment of hyperthyroid crisis.— S. R. Newmark *et al.*, *J. Am. med. Ass.*, 1974, *230*, 592.

Administration in renal failure. Doses should be reduced to 75% in patients with a glomerular filtration-rate (GFR) of 10 to 50 ml per minute, and to 50% in those with a GFR of less than 10 ml per minute.— W. M. Bennett *et al.*, *Ann. intern. Med.*, 1980, *93*, 286.

Pregnancy and the neonate. Propylthiouracil was probably the drug of choice in the treatment of hyperthyroidism in pregnancy but every effort should be made to avoid maternal hypothyroidism. Since goitres had occurred in only a few infants it was suggested that sufficient maternal thyroid hormone usually crossed the placenta.— G. N. Burrow, *New Engl. J. Med.*, 1978, *298*, 150.

Hyperthyroidism in a 3-month-old boy was treated initially with iodine, then with propylthiouracil 100 mg daily. The child was euthyroid 2.5 months later and the propylthiouracil was gradually reduced and discontinued after 9 months.— H. E. Leszynsky *et al.*, *Pediatrics*, 1971, *47*, 1069.

Thyrotoxicosis in a neonate was treated with propylthiouracil 6 mg at 8-hourly intervals for 2 weeks. Thyrotoxic symptoms reappeared after 2 weeks and were treated with propylthiouracil 6.25 mg twice daily for 8 weeks. The infant then remained euthyroid.— G. J. Robards and J. R. Davis, *Med. J. Aust.*, 1973, *2*, 432. See also S. Samuel *et al.*, *Am. J. Dis. Child.*, 1971, *121*, 440.

Short-term therapy. In a study of 40 patients with thyrotoxicosis (31 previously untreated and 9 previously treated) antithyroid therapy with methimazole or propylthiouracil was discontinued as soon as (or only a few weeks after) the patient became euthyroid. The lasting remission-rates obtained were as good as those in patients who had been treated for a year or more after becoming euthyroid, and avoided the cost and inconvenience of long-term therapy.— M. A. Greer *et al.*, *New Engl. J. Med.*, 1977, *297*, 173. Comment.— L. J. DeGroot, *ibid.*, 212. Disappointing preliminary results with short-term carbimazole therapy, and a recommendation for caution against overenthusiastic adoption of short-term therapy as routine.— W. A. Burr *et al.* (letter), *ibid.*, 1979, *300*, 200. See also H. Tamai *et al.*, *Ann. intern. Med.*, 1980, *92*, 488.

Single daily doses. A single dose of propylthiouracil daily, in most cases 300 mg or less, was sufficient to achieve complete remission in 18 hyperthyroid patients. A dose of 300 mg daily given as a single dose was sufficient to maintain remission in 6 other patients after the condition had been controlled by divided doses of propylthiouracil. In 2 women remission could not be achieved by a single daily dose but was achieved by 300 or 400 mg in divided doses. No remission occurred in 2 patients when treated either with single daily doses or with divided dosage.— M. A. Greer *et al.*, *New Engl. J. Med.*, 1965, *272*, 888.

Of 41 patients with exophthalmic goitre controlled with propylthiouracil or methimazole (2 patients) given at 8-hourly intervals, 28 were still satisfactorily controlled when the total daily dose was given as a single daily dose; 2 further patients were controlled by increasing the dose. A further 9 patients who were treated with single daily doses from the beginning of treatment also gained remissions.— H. Kammer and K. Srinivasan, *J. Am. med. Ass.*, 1969, *209*, 1325.

Further references: G. Gwinup, *J. Am. med. Ass.*, 1978, *239*, 2457.

Preparations

Propylthiouracil Tablets *(B.P.)*. Tablets containing propylthiouracil.

Propylthiouracil Tablets *(U.S.P.)*. Tablets containing propylthiouracil. The *U.S.P.* requires 85% dissolution in 30 minutes.

Proprietary Names

Propycil *(Kali-Chemie, Ger.; Farmades, Ital.)*; Propyl-Thyracil *(Frosst, Canad.)*; Thyreostat II *(Herbrand, Ger.)*; Tiotil *(Pharmacia, Swed.)*.

839-z

Thibenzazoline. 2-Mercaptobenzimidazole-1,3-dimethylol. 1,3-Bis(hydroxymethyl)benzimidazolin-2-thione. $C_9H_{10}N_2O_2S$=210.3.

CAS — 6028-35-9.

M.p. 160° to 162°. **Soluble** in dilute alkalis.

Uses. Thibenzazoline is an antithyroid agent used similarly to carbimazole (see p.356) in the treatment of hyperthyroidism.

Reference: J. A. Ganglberger, *Wien. med. Wschr.*, 1957, *107*, 272, per *J. Am. med. Ass.*, 1957, *164*, 1401.

840-p

Thiouracil *(B.P. 1948)*. 2,3-Dihydro-2-thioxopyrimidin-4(1*H*)-one; 2-Mercaptopyrimidin-4-ol. $C_4H_4N_2OS$=128.1.

CAS — 141-90-2.

Pharmacopoeias. In *Span.*

A white or pale cream-coloured odourless powder with a bitter taste. Slightly **soluble** in water, alcohol, ether, and acids; soluble in solutions of alkali hydroxides.

Uses. Thiouracil has actions similar to those of carbimazole (see p.356) and was formerly used in the treatment of hyperthyroidism. It has been given in doses of 100 to 200 mg.

Thiouracil was suspected of being teratogenic.— M. G. Wilson, *Am. J. Obstet. Gynec.*, 1962, *83*, 818.

Thiouracil had been implicated in the Stevens–Johnson syndrome.— D. B. Coursin, *J. Am. med. Ass.*, 1966, *198*, 113.

An analysis of blood dyscrasias reported to the Swedish Adverse Drug Reaction Committee for the 5-year period 1966–70 showed that agranulocytosis attributable to thiouracil had been reported on 5 occasions. It was estimated that reported figures represented one-third of the true frequency.— L. E. Böttiger and B. Westerholm, *Br. med. J.*, 1973, *3*, 339.

Central and Respiratory Stimulants

1410-k

The central stimulants (sometimes termed analeptics) described in this chapter include the amphetamines and other drugs with less stimulant effect on the central nervous system. Because of abuse for euphoric effect the use of the amphetamines has been discouraged especially as they have a limited sphere of usefulness, chiefly in narcolepsy. The other central stimulants described are generally used for their mild stimulant effect.

Respiratory stimulants increase pulmonary ventilation by their effects on the depth and rate of respiration. They act directly by stimulating the respiratory centre in the medulla or indirectly by their effects on the carotid body. In varying degrees they also stimulate the higher centres of the central nervous system and in doses greater than those employed to stimulate respiration they may cause convulsions. Activity is dependent upon adequate oxygenation and the effects of respiratory stimulants may be diminished in severe hypoxaemia.

Because they generally have a brief duration of action respiratory stimulants have only a limited usefulness in acute respiratory failure. They have been used in respiratory distress after anaesthesia and to hasten arousal after anaesthesia. Respiratory stimulants are generally considered to have no place in the treatment of barbiturate poisoning. In the treatment of respiratory depression due to narcotics such as morphine, specific antagonists should be employed—see the section on Narcotic Antagonists, p.1031.

Apart from the drugs described in this section, other drugs employed to aid respiration include aminophylline (p.344).

Some drugs used as adjuncts in the treatment of obesity have central stimulant effects and are described in the section on Anorectics, (see p.65).

1411-a

Amiphenazole Hydrochloride *(B.P.C. 1959).* Amiphenaz. Hydrochlor.; Amiphenazole Chloride. 5-Phenylthiazole-2,4-diamine hydrochloride.
$C_9H_9N_3S,HCl$=227.7.

CAS — 490-55-1(amiphenazole); 942-31-4 (hydrochloride).

Pharmacopoeias. In *Cz.*

A white or almost white fine crystalline or granular mobile powder; odourless or almost odourless and with a bitter taste. **Soluble** 1 in 16 of water and 1 in 50 of alcohol; slightly soluble in acetone, chloroform, and ether. A 1.5% solution in water has a pH of 4 to 5. Aqueous solutions hydrolyse slowly; injections should be administered immediately after preparation.

Incompatibility. A haze which developed over 3 hours was produced when amiphenazole hydrochloride 600 mg per litre was mixed with methicillin sodium 4 g per litre, methohexitone sodium 2 g per litre, sulphadiazine sodium 4 g per litre, or sulphadimidine sodium 4 g per litre in sodium chloride injection.— B. B. Riley, *J. Hosp. Pharm.*, 1970, *28*, 228.

Sterilisation. Amiphenazole hydrochloride and hydrobromide decomposed on autoclaving when in solution but were stable in the solid state. They were sterilised by dry heat, and the powder was dissolved in Water for Injections using aseptic precautions. The resulting colourless solutions were stable at room temperature for 24 hours.— A. Shulman *et al.*, *Br. med. J.*, 1955, *1*, 1238.

Adverse Effects. Nausea and vomiting, skin rashes, lichenoid, insomnia, and slight twitchings of fingers, shoulders, and neck occasionally occur. Long-term therapy with amiphenazole may lead to bone-marrow depression.

Uses. Amiphenazole is a respiratory stimulant with actions and uses similar to those of nikethamide (see p.367).

It has been given in usual doses of 100 to 150 mg intramuscularly or intravenously. Amiphenazole has been claimed to reduce the respiratory depression and drowsiness caused by morphine and other narcotic analgesics, without significantly reducing their analgesic activity, and has been given in usual doses of 30 mg intramuscularly or intravenously with each dose of narcotic analgesic.

Amiphenazole has also been given by mouth.

Proprietary Names
Daptazile *(Nicholas, Ger.)*; Daptazole *(Nicholas, Neth.; Nicholas, Switz.).*

Amiphenazole hydrochloride was formerly marketed in Great Britain under the proprietary name Daptazole *(Nicholas).*

1412-t

Amphetamine *(B.P. 1958).* Amphet.; Anfetamina; Racemic Desoxynorephedrine. (±)-α-Methylphenethylamine.
$C_9H_{13}N$=135.2.

CAS — 300-62-9.

Pharmacopoeias. In *Arg., Belg., Braz.,* and *Turk.*

A colourless, mobile, slowly volatile liquid with a slight characteristic odour of geranium leaves and an acrid taste. It absorbs carbon dioxide from the air, forming a volatile carbonate. Wt per ml 0.93 to 0.935 g.
Soluble 1 in 50 of water; very soluble in alcohol, chloroform, and ether; readily soluble in acids; soluble in fixed and volatile oils. **Store** in airtight containers. Protect from light.

1413-x

Amphetamine Phosphate. Monobasic Racemic Amphetamine Phosphate; Benzpropaminum Phosphoricum.
$C_9H_{13}N,H_3PO_4$=233.2.

CAS — 139-10-6.

Pharmacopoeias. In *Hung.*

A white odourless crystalline powder with a bitter taste. Amphetamine phosphate 10 mg is approximately equivalent to 8 mg of amphetamine sulphate. Freely **soluble** in water; slightly soluble in alcohol; practically insoluble in chloroform and ether. A 2% solution in water has a pH of 3.5 to 4.5. A 3.47% solution is iso-osmotic with serum.

1414-r

Amphetamine Sulphate *(B.P., Eur. P.).* Amphet. Sulph.; Amphetamine Sulfate *(U.S.P.)*; Amphetamini Sulfas; Phenaminum; Phenopromini Sulphas; Phenylaminopropanum Racemicum Sulfuricum; Psychedrinum.
$(C_9H_{13}N)_2,H_2SO_4$=368.5.

CAS — 60-13-9.

Pharmacopoeias. In *Arg., Aust., Belg., Br., Cz., Eur., Fr., Ger., Ind., Int., It., Jug., Mex., Neth., Nord., Pol., Port., Roum., Rus., Span., Swiss, Turk.,* and *U.S.*

A white odourless crystalline powder with a slightly bitter numbing taste. M.p. about 300° with decomposition. It absorbs insignificant amounts of water at 25° at relative humidities of up to about 90%.
Soluble 1 in 9 of water and 1 in 515 of alcohol; practically insoluble in chloroform and ether. A solution in water has a pH of 5 to 6. A 4.23% solution is iso-osmotic with serum. Solutions are **sterilised** by autoclaving or by filtration. **Incompatible** with alkalis and calcium salts.

Dependence, Adverse Effects, Treatment, and Precautions. As for Dexamphetamine Sulphate, p.361.

Absorption and Fate. Amphetamine is readily absorbed from the gastro-intestinal tract. It is resistant to metabolism by monoamine oxidase and is excreted partly unchanged in the urine with some deaminated and hydroxylated metabolites. Elimination is enhanced in acid urine.

In 4 healthy adults given a single dose of radioactive amphetamine intravenously the half-life was 8 to 10.5 hours when the urine was acidic (pH less than 6) and 16 to 31 hours when the urine was alkaline (pH more than 7.5). Under acidic conditions about 70% of the dose was excreted in 24 hours and 90% during the first 4 days. Under alkaline conditions about 45% was excreted in 24 hours and 70 to 80% during the first 5 days. Under acidic conditions the proportion of unchanged amphetamine was about 4 times greater than that of deaminated metabolites (hippuric and benzoic acids); under alkaline conditions the proportions were about equal. Small amounts of *p*-hydroxynorephedrine and norephedrine were identified.— J. M. Davis *et al.*, *Ann. N.Y. Acad. Sci.*, 1971, *179*, 493. See also L. E. Dring *et al.* (letter), *J. Pharm. Pharmac.*, 1966, *18*, 402; A. H. Beckett *et al.*, *ibid.*, 1969, *21*, 251.

Uses. Amphetamine is an indirectly acting sympathomimetic agent with actions and uses similar to those of dexamphetamine sulphate (see p.362). It is only about one-half as potent as dexamphetamine.

Amphetamine sulphate has been used in the treatment of narcolepsy in doses of 20 to 100 mg daily in divided doses. It has also been advocated for the treatment of hyperkinetic states in children. Amphetamine itself, being volatile, was formerly employed by inhalation from specially constructed inhalers to produce local vasoconstriction. Tolerance develops readily. Amphetamine has also been used as the adipate, aspartate, and phosphate.

Preparations of Amphetamine and its Salts

Amphetamine Sulfate Tablets *(U.S.P.).* Tablets containing amphetamine sulphate.

Amphetamine Sulphate Tablets *(B.P. 1973).* Amphet. Sulph. Tab.; Amphetamine Tablets. Tablets containing amphetamine sulphate.

Proprietary Names
Amfetamin *(sulphate) (DAK, Denm.)*; Benzedrine *(sulphate) (Smith Kline & French, USA)*; Centramina *(sulphate) (Spain)*; Perduretas Anfetamina *(sulphate) (Medea, Spain)*; Simpatina *(sulphate) (LEFA, Spain).*

1415-f

Amphetaminil. *N*-Cyanobenzylamphetamine. α-(α-Methylphenethylamino)-α-phenylacetonitrile.
$C_{17}H_{18}N_2$=250.3.

CAS — 17590-01-1.

Uses. Amphetaminil is a stimulant of the central nervous system which has been given in usual doses of 10 mg daily in fatigue and depressive states.

References.— *Pharmazie*, 1965, *20, Suppl.*, 232; B. Krieg, *Arzneimittel-Forsch.*, 1974, *24*, 133; J. Klosa, *ibid.*, 134; B. Salvesen *et al.*, *ibid.*, 137; H. Honecker and H. Coper, *ibid.*, 1975, *25*, 442.

Proprietary Names
AN 1 *(Voigt, Ger.).*

1416-d

Bemegride *(B.P. 1968).* Bemegridum. 3-Ethyl-3-methylglutarimide; 4-Ethyl-4-methylpiperidine-2,6-dione.
$C_8H_{13}NO_2$=155.2.

CAS — 64-65-3.

Bemegride Sodium ($C_8H_{12}NNaO_2$ = 177.2) was included in the *B. Vet. C. 1965.*

Pharmacopoeias. In *Cz., Ind., Int.,* and *Rus.*

Almost odourless white or almost white flakes or crystalline powder with a bitter taste. M.p. 126° to 128°.
Soluble 1 in 170 of water, 1 in 30 of alcohol, 1 in 12 of acetone, 1 in 4 of chloroform, and 1 in 100 of ether;

soluble in aqueous solutions of alkali hydroxides. A 0.5% solution in water has a pH of 4.5 to 6.5. Solutions are **sterilised** by autoclaving or by filtration. **Store** in airtight containers.

Adverse Effects. Bemegride may sometimes produce retching, vomiting, muscular twitching, and a tendency to hypotension. In excessive dosage it may give rise to convulsions. Confusion and visual hallucinations have been reported after its use in barbiturate poisoning.

Treatment of Adverse Effects. As for Nikethamide, p.367.

Uses. Bemegride is a respiratory stimulant with actions and uses similar to those of nikethamide (see p.367). When given intravenously the effects of bemegride are of brief duration, lasting for only 10 or 20 minutes.

It has been given in usual doses of 25 to 50 mg intravenously.

Preparations

Bemegride Injection *(B.P. 1968).* A sterile 0.5% solution of bemegride, with sodium chloride 0.9% in Water for Injections. Store at room temperature. At lower temperatures, crystals may be deposited; these should be dissolved by warming before use. *Dose.* 10 ml intravenously and repeated as necessary.

The *B.P. 1968* directs that no bactericide should be added to this injection as large volumes may be administered.

Proprietary Names

Bemegrin *(Montedison, Arg.)*; Eukraton *(Nordmark-Werke, Ger.)*; Megimide *(Adcock Ingram, S.Afr.; Inibsa, Spain)*.

Bemegride was formerly marketed in Great Britain under the proprietary name Megimide (*Nicholas*).

1417-n

Camphotamide. Camphétamide. 3-Diethylcarbamoyl-1-methylpyridinium camphor-3-sulphonate. $C_{21}H_{32}N_2O_5S$=424.6.

CAS — 4876-45-3.

Crystals with a slight camphoraceous odour and a bitter taste with a sweet after-taste. M.p. 174° to 175°. **Soluble** in water, alcohol, and ether; practically insoluble in hydrocarbons.

Uses. Camphotamide has been used as a cardiorespiratory stimulant. It is usually given by mouth but has been given by subcutaneous, intramuscular, or intravenous injection.

Proprietary Names

Tonicorine *(Astra, Fr.)*.

1418-h

Dexamphetamine Phosphate.

Dextroamphetamine Phosphate *(U.S.P.)*; Monobasic Dextroamphetamine Phosphate. (+)-α-Methylphenethylamine dihydrogen phosphate.
$C_9H_{13}N,H_3PO_4$=233.2.

CAS — 51-64-9 (dexamphetamine); 7528-00-9 (phosphate).

Pharmacopoeias. In *U.S.*

A white odourless crystalline powder with a bitter taste. Dexamphetamine phosphate 10 mg is approximately equivalent to 8 mg of dexamphetamine sulphate. **Soluble** 1 in 20 of water; slightly soluble in alcohol; practically insoluble in chloroform and ether. A 5% solution in water is dextrorotatory and has a pH of 4 to 5. A 3.62% solution is iso-osmotic with serum.

1419-m

Dexamphetamine Sulphate *(B.P.).*

Dexamphet. Sulph.; Dexamphetamini Sulfas; Dextro Amphetamine Sulphate; Dextroamphetamine Sulfate *(U.S.P.)*.
$(C_9H_{13}N)_2,H_2SO_4$=368.5.

CAS — 51-63-8.

Pharmacopoeias. In *Br., Fr., Ind., Int., Swiss,* and *U.S.*

A white or almost white, odourless, crystalline powder with a slightly bitter saline taste. M.p. 295° to 300°.

Soluble 1 in 9 or 10 of water and 1 in 800 of alcohol; practically insoluble in ether. A 5% solution in water is dextrorotatory and has a pH of 5 to 6. A 4.16% solution is iso-osmotic with serum. **Incompatible** with strong alkalis and calcium salts.

Dependence. Drug dependence of the amphetamine type has been described by the World Health Organization (*Tech. Rep. Ser. Wld Hlth Org. No. 273,* 1964) as a state arising from repeated administration of amphetamine or an agent with amphetamine-like effects, on a periodic or continuous basis. It is characterised by a desire or need to continue taking the drug, by a psychic dependence on the effects of the drug, and by the consumption of increasing doses to obtain greater excitatory and euphoric effects or to combat more effectively depression and fatigue, accompanied by some degree of tolerance. Not all parts of the central nervous system appear to become tolerant at the same rate, so that nervousness and insomnia may persist as the dose is increased.

Persons dependent on amphetamines are prone to accidents, aggressive antisocial behaviour, and, particularly after intravenous injection, to psychotic episodes involving delusions and hallucinations. While dependence of the amphetamine type does not generally include physical dependence, withdrawal is followed by mental and physical depression.

The World Health Organization (*Tech. Rep. Ser. Wld Hlth Org. No. 437,* 1970) has recommended international control of amphetamines (amphetamine, dexamphetamine, and methylamphetamine), methylphenidate, and phenmetrazine because their liability to abuse constitutes a substantial risk to public health and because they have little to moderate therapeutic usefulness.

Reviews and discussions on the dependence, adverse effects, and misuse of amphetamines and amphetamine-like substances.— N. B. Eddy *et al., Bull. Wld Hlth Org.,* 1965, *32,* 721; *J. Am. med. Ass.,* 1966, *197,* 1023 (AMA Committee on Alcoholism and Addiction, and the Council on Mental Health); Amphetamines, Barbiturates, LSD and Cannabis, their Use and Misuse, *Reports on Public Health and Medical Subjects No. 124,* London, HM Stationery Office, 1970.

A review and discussion on the medical and social problems of the amphetamine-dependent mother and her child.— G. Larsson, *Acta paediat. scand.,* 1980, *Suppl.* 278.

For definitions of drug dependence, psychic dependence, physical dependence, and dependence-producing drugs, see *Tech. Rep. Ser. Wld Hlth Org. No. 526,* 1973.

All of 36 addicts had taken amphetamines by mouth before resorting to administration intravenously. Initially, 20 to 40 mg was taken intravenously 3 or 4 times daily and increased to 100 to 300 mg every 2 or 3 hours for 3 to 6 days, or occasionally for 12 days. The patients developed severe tremors and muscle or joint pain, and became exhausted from total lack of sleep, disorganised, tense, and paranoid. Cessation of administration led to prolonged sleep, extreme hunger, and to a semi-comatose state lasting 4 or 5 days. The cycle was usually then repeated. Occasional overdosage resulted in severe chest pain followed by unconsciousness.— J. C. Kramer *et al., J. Am. med. Ass.,* 1967, *201,* 305. See also G. Lloyd, *Br. med. J.,* 1973, *1,* 101.

Adverse Effects. Dexamphetamine is reasonably well tolerated in standard doses, though individuals vary considerably in their reactions. Side-effects which are relatively common include dryness of mouth, metallic taste, anorexia, nausea, constipation or diarrhoea, difficulty in micturition, mydriasis, agitation and restlessness, insomnia, headache, dizziness, and tremor. Changes in libido may also occur and skin rashes have been reported. Particularly with larger doses, the systolic and diastolic blood pressure is increased and tachycardia, anginal pain, or cardiac arrhythmias may occur. Psychotic reactions may develop. Overdosage may give rise to vomiting, abdominal cramps, fever or chilliness, hypotension or hypertension, talkativeness, disorientation, aggressive behaviour, and hallucinations. Central stimulation usually gives way to fatigue and mental depression which may be followed by convulsions, and coma.

Aplastic anaemia and pancytopenia have occasionally been reported after prolonged use.

Amphetamines have dependence-producing properties (see above). Tolerance develops readily.

Carcinogenicity. Of 100 patients with Hodgkin's disease 19 had previously used amphetamines whereas only 3 of 100 controls had used amphetamines.— G. R. Newell *et al., J. natn. Cancer Inst.,* 1973, *51,* 1437. In a study of 315 patients with malignant lymphoma and 38 900 controls there was no association between the occurrence of lymphoma and previous exposure to amphetamines.—A Report from the Boston Collaborative Drug Surveillance Program, *J. Am. med. Ass.,* 1974, *229,* 1462.

Chorea. See under Extrapyramidal Effects (below).

Effects on blood and vascular tissue. *Angiitis.* Angiitis leading to fatal renal failure in a young woman was associated with the intravenous use of amphetamine.— S. I. Rifkin, *Sth. med. J.,* 1977, *70,* 108. See also under Methylamphetamine.

Effects on the gastro-intestinal tract. Abdominal angina in a woman with asymptomatic coeliac-artery compression was considered to be related to the use of dexamphetamine sulphate in combination with a barbiturate.— M. J. R. Ravry (letter), *Ann. intern. Med.,* 1977, *87,* 246.

Effects on growth. Depression of growth in weight and height was noted in 29 hyperactive children who were receiving dexamphetamine 10 to 15 mg daily or methylphenidate 20 to 40 mg daily. Children who had their medication stopped during summer holidays showed a rebound gain in weight. Methylphenidate had less effect on growth than dexamphetamine, particularly at the lower doses.— D. Safer *et al., New Engl. J. Med.,* 1972, *287,* 217. See also *ibid.,* 249.

Further reports of the effect of amphetamines on growth and the secretion of growth hormone.— G. Langer *et al., Archs gen. Psychiat.,* 1976, *33,* 1471; D. Aarskog *et al., J. Pediat.,* 1977, *90,* 136; J. D. Parkes *et al., Br. J. clin. Pharmac.,* 1977, *4,* 343.

Effects on the heart. Cardiomyopathy in a 45-year-old woman with congestive heart failure might have been associated with prolonged intake of high doses of dexamphetamine.— H. J. Smith *et al., Am. Heart J.,* 1976, *91,* 792.

Effects on mental state. A paradoxical response, characterised by increased depression followed by deep sleep, in a hyperkinetic man given dexamphetamine.— J. DeVeaugh-Geiss and A. Joseph, *Psychosomatics,* 1980, *21,* 247.

Reports of psychosis, particularly paranoia, associated with the use of amphetamines.— P. G. Ney, *Can. med. Ass. J.,* 1967, *97,* 1026; *J. Am. med. Ass.,* 1968, *205* (Sept. 9), A39; J. D. Griffith *et al., Archs gen. Psychiat.,* 1972, *26,* 97; M. S. Gold and M. B. Bowers, *Am. J. Psychiat.,* 1978, *135,* 1546.

Extrapyramidal effects. In 3 children and 1 middle-aged woman dyskinesias developed shortly after they were given dexamphetamine sulphate in therapeutic doses (2.5 to 5 mg). In 1 child similar dyskinetic movements were elicited by methylphenidate.— R. M. Mattson and J. R. Calverley, *J. Am. med. Ass.,* 1968, *204,* 400. See also H. H. Eveloff (letter), *ibid.,* 933.

Dexamphetamine worsened existing chorea in some patients and precipitated chorea in a patient with a history of Sydenham's chorea; it had no such effect in healthy persons.— H. L. Klawans and W. J. Weiner, *Neurology, Minneap.,* 1974, *24,* 312.

Gynaecomastia. Gynaecomastia has been clearly associated with the use of amphetamines.— H. E. Carlson, *New Engl. J. Med.,* 1980, *303,* 795.

Overdosage. There was only 1 fatality among 100 patients admitted to hospital after overdosage of amphetamines. Doses ingested were: amphetamine sulphate 25 mg to 2.5 g; dexamphetamine sulphate 10 to 375 mg; and methylamphetamine hydrochloride 10 to 100 mg. Symptoms included tachycardia, hypertension, pyrexia, and unexplained haematological changes. Treatment included gastric lavage, fluids intravenously, and sedation.— *J. Am. med. Ass.,* 1969, *210,* 239.

Reversible renal failure occurred in a 21-year-old subject who ingested about 2 g of amphetamine sulphate.— M. D. Ginsberg *et al., Ann. intern. Med.,* 1970, *73,* 81.

Two patients, aged 18 and 26 years respectively, developed intracranial haemorrhages shortly after taking amphetamines. The first patient had occasionally taken dexamphetamine sulphate, 20 to 30 mg daily, for several months and the day before a brief epileptic seizure he took 50 mg in less than 1 hour. The second patient had injected amphetamine intravenously (dose unknown) about 6 times within 1 month. The hypertensive effect of the drug and a pre-existing vascular lesion were probably the 2 major factors involved in the episodes.— S. J. Goodman and D. P. Becker (letter), *J. Am. med. Ass.*, 1970, *212*, 480.

Pregnancy and the neonate. In 458 mothers who gave birth to infants with congenital malformations, the percentage who had taken compounds of dexamphetamine during pregnancy, including the first 56 days (calculated from the first day of the last menstrual period), was significantly greater than in 911 controls. These results did not prove teratogenicity but suggested that administration should be avoided during pregnancy.— M. M. Nelson and J. O. Forfar, *Br. med. J.*, 1971, *1*, 523. See also O. P. Heinonen *et al.*, *Birth Defects and Drugs in Pregnancy*, Littleton MA, Publishing Sciences Group, 1977, p. 345.

Evaluation of anorectic agents prescribed, during the years 1959–66, to about 2000 pregnant women provided no evidence that the use of amphetamines is associated with the production of severe congenital anomalies. However an excess of oral clefts was observed in the offspring of women who had taken amphetamines during the first 56 days after the last menstrual period. No excess of congenital heart disease was noted in contrast to a previous report (J.J. Nora *et al.*, *Lancet*, 1970, *1*, 1290).— L. Milkovich and B. J. van den Berg, *Am. J. Obstet. Gynec.*, 1977, *129*, 637.

Individual reports of malformations in exposed infants.— M. S. McIntire (letter), *J. Am. med. Ass.*, 1966, *197*, 62 (microcephaly following the use of methylamphetamine hydrochloride in addition to phenobarbitone); R. F. Matera *et al.*, *J. int. Coll. Surg.*, 1968, *50*, 79 (exencephaly); J. N. Levin, *J. Pediat.*, 1971, *79*, 130 (biliary atresia).

Retroperitoneal fibrosis. Mention of drugs incriminated in the development of retroperitoneal fibrosis, including dexamphetamine.— J. R. Curtis, *Br. med. J.*, 1977, *2*, 375.

Treatment of Adverse Effects. In general the management of overdosage with amphetamines involves supportive and symptomatic therapy. In severe overdosage the stomach should be emptied by aspiration and lavage. The use of activated charcoal as an adjunct to gastric lavage has been recommended.

Diazepam may be given to control central nervous system stimulation and convulsions. For marked excitement or hallucinations chlorpromazine may be necessary and, in addition, its alpha-adrenoceptor blocking properties may be useful for the management of hypertension. Severe hypertension may call for the administration of an alpha-adrenoceptor blocking agent, such as phentolamine. Measures should be taken to control increased body temperature.

Active measures to remove the drug from the body, such as forced acid diuresis, have sometimes been advocated for severely poisoned patients who continue to deteriorate despite supportive therapy since amphetamines are basic substances and are excreted to a large extent unchanged in the urine. The hazards of forced acid diuresis generally outweigh any purported benefits but where considered necessary, and provided renal function is adequate, such regimens comprise the administration of sodium chloride injection, dextrose injection, and dextrose injection with added ammonium chloride to maintain the urinary pH below 7. It is essential that serum electrolytes be measured regularly and any adjustments made to the fluid and electrolyte balance as necessary.

Any role of peritoneal dialysis or haemodialysis in the removal of amphetamines from the body is even less well documented.

Adsorption. For comment on the *in vitro* adsorption of dexamphetamine by activated charcoal, see p.79.

Diuresis and dialysis. References.— L. F. Prescott, Limitations of haemodialysis and forced diuresis, in *The Poisoned Patient: the role of the laboratory*, Ciba Foundation Symposium 26, Oxford, Elsevier, 1974, p. 269; J. A. Vale, *Prescribers' J.*, 1978, *18*, 67; J. A. Vale and R. Goulding, *ibid.*, 1979, *19*, 163.

Mental symptoms. In 8 patients amphetamine-induced symptoms were effectively antagonised by haloperidol.— B. Angrist *et al.*, *Am. J. Psychiat.*, 1974, *131*, 817.

For a report of the use of droperidol to control mental symptoms following methylamphetamine overdosage, see under Methylamphetamine, p.366.

Precautions. Dexamphetamine should be given with caution to patients with anorexia, insomnia, or impaired kidney function, and to patients of unstable personality. It should not be given to patients with cardiovascular disease, hypertension, hyperthyroidism, phaeochromocytoma, glaucoma, anxiety, hyperexcitability, or restlessness. Although dexamphetamine itself is not metabolised by monoamine oxidase, as an indirect-acting sympathomimetic it should not be given to patients being treated with a monoamine oxidase inhibitor or within 14 days of stopping such treatment (see Precautions for Phenelzine Sulphate p.128). Dexamphetamine may also diminish the effects of guanethidine and similar antihypertensive agents.

Interactions. Amphetamine was a weak monoamine oxidase inhibitor, but no adverse reactions occurred with this drug because sufficient enzyme remained after inhibition to bring about oxidative deamination of ingested tyramine.— *Br. med. J.*, 1969, *2*, 432. In 5 patients the pressor effect of tyramine was increased by about 2.5 times after the intravenous injection of 10 mg of dexamphetamine but was decreased by about one-third after long-term oral administration of dexamphetamine.— J. H. Cavanaugh *et al.*, *Clin. Pharmac. Ther.*, 1970, *11*, 656.

Cannabis. Studies in healthy subjects revealed no evidence of interaction between marihuana and dexamphetamine; effects of the association were merely additive.— M. A. Evans *et al.*, *Clin. Pharmac. Ther.*, 1976, *20*, 350.

Further references.— J. M. Whyte, *Australas. J. Pharm.*, 1967, *48*, 804.

Diuretics. The rate of urinary excretion of amphetamine and methylamphetamine was markedly retarded in alkaline urine. Care should be exercised when amphetamines were given to patients taking chlorothiazide, acetazolamide or other carbonic anhydrase inhibitors, or to other patients liable to have a high urine pH.— M. Rowland and A. H. Beckett, *Arzneimittel-Forsch.*, 1966, *16*, 1369.

Lithium. Experience with 3 patients suggested that the effects of amphetamine were antagonised by lithium carbonate.— A. Flemenbaum, *Am. J. Psychiat.*, 1974, *131*, 820. See also W. E. Bunney *et al.*, *Ann. intern. Med.*, 1977, *87*, 319.

Monoamine oxidase inhibitors. In 10 patients with essential hypertension, furazolidone produced hypersensitivity to tyramine and amphetamine, inhibition of intestinal monoamine oxidase, and increased urinary excretion of tryptamine. Prolonged administration caused a cumulative inhibition of monoamine oxidase and treatment for more than a few days, in the recommended doses, carried a potential risk of hypertensive crisis.— W. A. Pettinger *et al.*, *Clin. Pharmac. Ther.*, 1968, *9*, 442.

Narcotic analgesics. For reference to the enhancement of morphine-induced analgesia after concurrent administration of dexamphetamine, see Morphine, p.1021.

Interference with diagnostic tests. Dexamphetamine sulphate affected the estimation of urinary 17-oxo-steroids and 17-oxogenic-steroids.— *Adverse Drug React. Bull.*, 1972, June, 104.

Myasthenia. Although amphetamines have not been implicated clinically they do interfere with neuromuscular transmission experimentally and should be used with caution in patients with myasthenia.— Z. Argov and F. L. Mastaglia, *New Engl. J. Med.*, 1979, *301*, 409.

Absorption and Fate. Dexamphetamine is readily absorbed from the gastro-intestinal tract. It is resistant to metabolism by monoamine oxidase and is excreted partly unchanged in the urine with some hydroxylated metabolites. Elimination is enhanced in acid urine. After large doses it may be detected in urine for several days.

In a patient given a single dose of dexamphetamine sulphate, the rate of excretion of amphetamine in the urine depended on the pH. At pH 5 excretion was at a maximum 1 to 2 hours after administration and then fell exponentially. In subjects given dexamphetamine in various formulations the mean half-life was 5 hours.— A. H. Beckett and G. T. Tucker, *J. mond. Pharm.*, 1967, (3), 181.

A review of the literature suggested that tubular reabsorption of dexamphetamine in the kidney did not occur with acid urine. In urine of pH 6 to 7 there was a lower renal clearance of dexamphetamine, suggesting substantial tubular reabsorption.— T. B. Vree *et al.*, *J. Pharm. Pharmac.*, 1969, *21*, 774.

Amphetamine metabolites might be of importance in the development of the paranoid psychosis in chronic abusers.— E. Änggård *et al.*, *Clin. Pharmac. Ther.*, 1973, *14*, 870.

Further studies on the metabolism and excretion of dexamphetamine.— J. L. Rapoport *et al.*, *J. nerv. ment. Dis.*, 1978, *166*, 731; S. H. Wan *et al.*, *Clin. Pharmac. Ther.*, 1978, *23*, 585.

Uses. Dexamphetamine is a sympathomimetic agent with indirect effects on adrenergic receptors. It has alpha- and beta-adrenergic activity. It has a marked stimulant effect on the central nervous system, particularly the cerebral cortex and the respiratory and vasomotor centres. It causes a lessening of fatigue, an increase in mental activity, an elevation of mood, and a general feeling of well-being. However, its indiscriminate use in attempts to increase capacity for work or to overcome fatigue is undesirable. Particularly in high doses, it causes a rise in blood pressure.

Dexamphetamine sulphate is used in the treatment of narcolepsy in doses of 5 to 60 mg daily in divided doses. It has been advocated for the treatment of hyperkinetic states in children. Tolerance develops readily.

Dexamphetamine phosphate has also been used similarly in usual doses of 5 to 10 mg.

Conditions for which dexamphetamine was formerly used include depressive states, enuresis, and postencephalitic parkinsonism. It was also formerly used as an anorectic agent in the treatment of obesity.

Because of their liability to abuse, the use of amphetamines is banned in some countries and limited or discouraged in others including the UK.

Dexamphetamine has also been given as the adipate, saccharate, tannate, and tartrate.

Action. Of 20 normal adults given 10 mg of dexamphetamine, 13 became drowsy with reduced electrical brain activity in the first hour after the drug, whereas the remaining 7 were alert with increased electrical brain activity. Dexamphetamine was not a simple CNS stimulant.— J. J. Tecce and J. O. Cole, *Science*, 1974, *185*, 451.

Diagnostic use. *Prediction of response to antidepressants.* Evidence to suggest an association between the acute activation, euphoria, and antidepressant responses to the administration of a single dose of dexamphetamine and the antidepressant response to imipramine. Further studies are needed to establish the predictive value of dexamphetamine to the successful response to later antidepressant therapy in depressive illnesses.— D. P. van Kammen and D. L. Murphy, *Am. J. Psychiat.*, 1978, *135*, 1179. See also J. Fawcett and V. Siomopoulos, *Archs gen. Psychiat.*, 1971, *25*, 247.

Tardive dyskinesia. In patients with tardive dyskinesia, dexamphetamine intravenously increased dyskinetic movements and it was suggested that it may be of use to diagnose the condition in patients with very minimal or subclinical symptoms or in those where there is some reason to presume the possibility of such a disorder.— R. C. Smith *et al.*, *Am. J. Psychiat.*, 1977, *134*, 763.

Enuresis. Comment on the inefficacy of amphetamines in nocturnal enuresis.— *Drug & Ther. Bull.*, 1977, *15*, 26.

Further references.— R. K. Turner and G. C. Young, *Behaviour Res. Ther.*, 1966, *4*, 225; N. McConaghy, *Med. J. Aust.*, 1969, *2*, 237.

Epilepsy. Experience with dexamphetamine in the management of sleep seizures.— S. Livingston and L. L. Pauli, *J. Am. med. Ass.*, 1975, *233*, 278.

Hyperkinetic states. A review of the use of stimulant drugs (including amphetamines, methylphenidate, and pemoline) for hyperactive children. A medical opinion is often sought for children with behavioural problems.

Typically the child, more often male, is disobedient, quarrelsome, inattentive, and disruptive; he does badly at school, has few, if any, friends, and may be in trouble for stealing or truancy. The parents may complain that the child never settles to play for long and is generally restless. These children, often from disturbed or rejecting homes, respond poorly to psychotherapy or behaviour therapy. In the USA many such children would be diagnosed as 'hyperkinetic' and treated with stimulants but in the UK this diagnosis is much less common and drugs are used much less frequently. Thus the knowledge regarding the efficacy, limitations, and dangers of stimulants in such conditions is mainly in an American context. Stimulant drugs should be considered only for children with poor attention, overactivity, and disruptiveness in school and when clinical and psychometric examination reveals minimal neurological disorders, EEG abnormalities, or deficits in cognitive function. The opinion of a child psychiatrist is also essential. Bad behaviour is not in itself an indication for stimulant therapy.— *Drug & Ther. Bull.*, 1977, *15*, 22. Severe criticism of the use of stimulants for symptoms that are nearly always normal, though annoying, manifestations of children's development.— *Br. med. J.*, 1979, *1*, 1004.

Further reviews and comments on the use of amphetamines and other stimulants in hyperkinetic states.— *Med. Lett.*, 1977, *19*, 53; R. W. Piepho *et al.*, *J. Am. pharm. Ass.*, 1977, *NS17*, 500; W. Ford, *Can. Pharm. J.*, 1978, *111*, 410; C. L. Saccar, *Am. J. Hosp. Pharm.*, 1978, *35*, 544; J. S. Werry, *Drugs*, 1979, *18*, 392.

Reports of the use of amphetamines in hyperkinetic states.— J. G. Millichap and G. W. Fowler, *Pediat. Clins N. Am.*, 1967, *14*, 767 (amphetamine); G. G. Steinberg *et al.*, *Am. J. Psychiat.*, 1971, *128*, 174 (dexamphetamine); L. E. Arnold *et al.*, *Archs gen. Psychiat.*, 1972, *27*, 816 (dexamphetamine and levamphetamine); *idem*, *Am. J. Psychiat.*, 1973, *130*, 165 (dexamphetamine and levamphetamine); *idem*, *Archs gen. Psychiat.*, 1976, *33*, 292 (dexamphetamine and levamphetamine); L. M. Greenberg *et al.*, *Am. J. Psychiat.*, 1972, *129*, 532 (dexamphetamine); M. Buchsbaum and P. Wender, *Archs gen. Psychiat.*, 1973, *29*, 764 (amphetamine); M. L. Wolraieh, *Pediatrics*, 1977, *60*, 512 (dexamphetamine); L. E. Arnold *et al.*, *Archs gen. Psychiat.*, 1978, *35*, 463 (dexamphetamine); W. O. Shekim *et al.*, *J. Pediat.*, 1979, *95*, 389 (dexamphetamine).

Mental disorders. There was no good evidence to date to indicate that central nervous system stimulants or any other agents had any value in the treatment of symptoms associated with senility.— *Med. Lett.*, 1978, *20*, 75.

Raised blood concentrations of phenylacetic acid, the major metabolite of phenylethylamine, which has a close chemical relationship with amphetamine, were found in 10 aggressive psychopaths when compared with 10 control subjects. It was considered that overproduction of phenylethylamine might represent an attempt by the body to compensate for an underlying defect responsible for the aggressive behaviour. Monitoring of such subjects to find those with raised blood concentrations of phenylacetic acid, the major metabolite of phenylethylamine, might identify subjects whose aggressive behaviour might be calmed by administration of amphetamine.— M. Sandler *et al.*, *Lancet*, 1978, *2*, 1269.

In 2 patients long-standing depression was considered to be due to a profound deficiency of brain noradrenaline since it responded only to amphetamine administration. They were therefore given tyrosine 100 mg per kg body-weight daily before breakfast. Within 2 weeks the first patient was able to stop a dose of dexamphetamine of 20 mg daily, and the second was able to reduce a dose of amphetamine 15 mg daily to 5 mg daily.— I. K. Goldberg (letter), *Lancet*, 1980, *2*, 364.

Further references.— A. P. West, *Am. J. Psychiat.*, 1974, *131*, 321 (role in schizophrenia); H. Beckmann and H. Heinemann, *Arzneimittel-Forsch.*, 1976, *26*, 1185 (mania); A. N. G. Clark, *Practitioner*, 1978, *220*, 735; A. N. G. Clark and G. D. Mankikar, *J. Am. Geriat. Soc.*, 1979, *27*, 174 (both senility); A. T. McLellan *et al.*, *New Engl. J. Med.*, 1979, *301*, 1310; H. G. Pope, *ibid.*, 1341 (both role in schizophrenia).

Narcolepsy. The use of dexamphetamine and methylphenidate with clomipramine in narcolepsy and catalepsy.— *Lancet*, 1975, *1*, 845. A view that the alerting effect of amphetamine is unlikely to be the result of the availability of dopamine at receptor centres in the brain.— M. Schachter *et al.* (letter), *Lancet*, 1979, *1*, 831.

Pain. Dexamphetamine 2.5 mg with propranolol 10 mg once to thrice daily relieved pain associated with the spastic colon syndrome in 165 patients. Side-effects included insomnia (46 patients) and supra-umbilical meteorism (27).— F. Lechin *et al.*, *J. clin. Pharmac.*, 1977, *17*, 431.

Preparations of Dexamphetamine and its Salts

Dexamphetamine Tablets *(B.P.)*. Dexamphet. Tab.; Dexamphetamine Sulphate Tablets; Dextroamphetamine Sulphate Tablets. Tablets containing dexamphetamine sulphate.

Dextroamphetamine Phosphate Tablets *(U.S.P.)*. Tablets containing dexamphetamine phosphate.

Dextroamphetamine Sulfate Elixir *(U.S.P.)*. An elixir containing 90 to 110 mg of dexamphetamine sulphate in each 100 ml and from 9 to 11% of alcohol. Store in airtight containers. Protect from light.

Dextroamphetamine Sulfate Tablets *(U.S.P.)*. Tablets containing dexamphetamine sulphate.

Proprietary Preparations of Dexamphetamine and its Salts

Dexedrine *(Smith Kline & French, UK)*. Dexamphetamine sulphate, available as scored tablets of 5 mg. (Also available as Dexedrine in *Belg.*, *Canad.*, *Switz.*, *USA*).

Durophet *(Riker, UK)*. Dexamphetamine 1 part and amphetamine 1 part bonded to an ion-exchange resin, available as capsules of 7.5, 12.5, and 20 mg. For obesity. *Dose.* 1 capsule at breakfast.

Other Proprietary Names of Dexamphetamine and its Salts

Spain— Afatin *(tartrate)*, Dexedrina *(sulphate)*, Maxiton *(tartrate)*, Stil-2 *(sulphate)*, Synatan *(tannate)*; *Switz.*— Amphaetex, Dexamin, Mephadexamin-R *(all sulphate)*; *USA*— Dexampex, Ferndex *(both sulphate)*.

Preparations containing dexamphetamine sulphate were also formerly marketed in Great Britain under the proprietary names Dexamed (*Medo*), Drinamyl, and Steladex (both *Smith Kline & French*). The name Dexamed is also applied to Dexamethasone, see p.467. Preparations containing dexamphetamine and methaqualone, as resin complexes, were formerly marketed under the proprietary name Durophet-M (*Riker*).

1420-t

Dimefline Hydrochloride. DW 62; Rec 7-0267. 8-Dimethylaminomethyl-7-methoxy-3-methyl-2-phenyl-4*H*-chromen-4-one hydrochloride.
$C_{20}H_{21}NO_3,HCl=359.9$.

CAS — 1165-48-6 (dimefline); 2740-04-7 (hydrochloride).

A white crystalline powder with a bitter taste. **Soluble** in water and alcohol; practically insoluble in chloroform and ether.

Uses. Dimefline hydrochloride is a respiratory stimulant which has been given in usual doses of 8 to 16 mg 2 or 3 times daily by mouth, or 8 mg once or twice daily by intramuscular injection.

Proprietary Names

Remeflin *(Recordati, Ital.*; *Jap.*; *Farma-Lepori, Spain*; *Recordati, Switz.)*; Remefline *(Recordati, Belg.)*.

1421-x

Doxapram Hydrochloride *(U.S.P.)*. AHR 619. 1-Ethyl-4-(2-morpholinoethyl)-3,3-diphenylpyrrolidin-2-one hydrochloride monohydrate.

$C_{24}H_{30}N_2O_2,HCl,H_2O=433.0$.

CAS — 309-29-5 (doxapram); 113-07-5 (hydrochloride, anhydrous); 7081-53-0 (hydrochloride, monohydrate).

Pharmacopoeias. In *Braz.* and *U.S.*

A white to off-white, odourless, crystalline powder. M.p. about 220°. **Soluble** 1 in 50 of water; sparingly soluble in alcohol; soluble in chloroform; practically insoluble in ether. A 1% solution in water has a pH of 3.5 to 5. **Incompatible** with alkaline solutions such as aminophylline, frusemide, or thiopentone sodium. **Store** in airtight containers.

Adverse Effects and Treatment. As for Nikethamide, p.367.

Laryngospasm, bronchospasm, dyspnoea, and confusion have also been reported. Thrombophlebitis may follow extravasation during injection.

The margin between the therapeutic dose and the dose producing significant side-effects seems to be greater for doxapram than for many other respiratory stimulants.

Precautions. Doxapram should be given cautiously to patients with heart diseases or obstructive airway disease. It should not be administered to patients with epilepsy or other convulsive disorders, cerebral oedema, cerebrovascular accident, status asthmaticus, severe hypertension, hyperthyroidism, or phaeochromocytoma.

The pressor effects of doxapram may be enhanced by sympathomimetic agents or monoamine oxidase inhibitors.

In 29 patients who received doxapram, 1.5 mg per kg body-weight, during surgery and on awakening from anaesthesia with cyclopropane, ether, halothane, or methoxyflurane, 5 developed arrhythmias related to doxapram. The arrhythmias were not considered to have been hazardous and did not suggest that doxapram was contra-indicated with conventional anaesthetics.— C. R. Stephen and I. Talton, *Anesth. Analg. curr. Res.*, 1966, *45*, 783.

Intravenous injections of doxapram should be given slowly to minimise the haemolysis which had been found to occur *in vitro* when the drug was mixed with blood.— R. J. Trudnowski (letter), *Br. J. Anaesth.*, 1973, *45*, 303.

Absorption and Fate. Doxapram is rapidly metabolised after intravenous injection and metabolites are excreted in the urine.

A rapid fall in plasma-doxapram concentration occurred in 6 healthy subjects following an intravenous bolus injection of doxapram hydrochloride 1.5 mg per kg body-weight and after 1 hour the concentration was less than 2 μg per ml in all subjects. The mean plasma half-life over the period of 4 to 12 hours after administration was 3.4 hours (range 2.4 to 4.1 hours) and 0.4 to 4% of the dose was excreted unchanged in the urine after 24 hours. During infusion of doxapram hydrochloride 3.5 mg per kg per hour for 2 hours to 4 subjects, and for only 1.5 hours to a fifth because of agitation, plasma-doxapram concentration rose steadily to a mean of 4 μg per ml (range 2.7 to 5.2 μg per ml) by the time of termination and thereafter fell rapidly. From 4 to 12 hours the rate of decline appeared to be mono-exponential with a mean half-life of 3.9 hours (range 3.5 to 4.6 hours) and as with the bolus injection the rate of elimination appeared to slow down after 12 hours with a mean half-life of 7.4 hours (range 3.7 to 10.7 hours). A metabolite (AHR 5955) appeared rapidly in plasma, peak concentrations being about 40% of the peak doxapram concentration 2 hours after the termination of the infusion. The mean half-life of this metabolite was 6.5 hours (range 4.0 to 8.5 hours). In 7 subjects given doxapram 300 mg by mouth as an enteric-coated capsule, doxapram was detected in plasma after 1 hour in 1 subject, after 1.5 hours in 4 subjects, and after about 2 hours in the other 2. The mean interval between the first appearance of doxapram and the peak concentration was 2.4 hours (range 0 to 6 hours) and in 2 subjects a second prominent peak was observed 4 hours after the first. A rapid rise also occurred in the plasma concentrations of the metabolite with a mean peak of 680 ng per ml occurring 1 hour after peak doxapram concentrations. The concentrations of doxapram and metabolite were similar with mean plasma half-lives of 7.5 and 9.2 hours respectively over the period of 8 to 24 hours. The systemic availability calculated from comparison of the oral data with the intravenous bolus and infusion data was 60.8 and 59% respectively after correction for dosage. These studies confirmed that renal excretion is a minor route of elimination of doxapram and that oxidation of doxapram (to AHR 5955) is a pathway of metabolism. It is not known whether this metabolite has any pharmacological activity. As the metabolite accumulated more slowly after intravenous administration and as the systemic availability of doxapram by mouth was about 60% it was suggested that significant 'first pass' metabolism of doxapram during absorption of an oral dose may occur. Results from these studies and others have also suggested the possibility of entero-hepatic recirculation and also that biliary excretion may be an important mode of elimination. Doxapram is often administered by constant-rate infusion and although it is generally believed that plasma concentrations fall rapidly when the infusion is discontinued or the rate reduced, these results and those obtained in other patients receiving infusions would indicate that this is not necessarily so after prolonged administration. Also it has been assumed that a plateau concentration of doxapram is rapidly achieved during infusion but only about half of the predicted steady-state concentration was obtained after a 2-hour infusion in the subjects. The pharmacokinetic data would suggest that reasonably steady plasma concentrations could be achieved with a simple oral dosage regimen.— R. H. Robson and L. F. Prescott, *Br. J. clin. Pharmac.*, 1979, *7*, 81. See also R. H. Robson *et al.*, *ibid.*, 1978, *5*, 363P.

See also under Administration in Uses.

Uses. Doxapram hydrochloride is a respiratory stimulant which also has slight vasopressor properties. Its effects are of brief duration apparently lasting for about 5 to 10 minutes following intravenous administration.

It is used in the treatment of respiratory depression following anaesthesia, usually in a dose of 0.5 to 1 mg per kg body-weight intravenously. Further doses may be given at 5-minute intervals to a total dose of 2 mg per kg. It may also be given by intravenous infusion in dextrose injection or sodium chloride injection, initially administered at a rate of 5 mg per minute and then reduced, according to the patient's response, to 1 to 3 mg per minute to a maximum total dosage of 4 mg per kg.

To hasten arousal and return of protective reflexes after anaesthesia, a dose of 1 to 1.5 mg per kg body-weight has been given as a single injection or as 2 injections administered 5 minutes apart.

Administration by mouth has been suggested.

Administration. Following a preliminary report (R.H. Robson and L.F. Prescott, *Br. J. clin. Pharmac.*, 1979, *7*, 81) showing that plasma-doxapram concentrations fall rapidly after intravenous bolus injections and after short-duration infusions and that steady-state concentrations are not achieved for many hours with a constant-rate infusion it was suggested that a variable-rate infusion may overcome these problems. In contrast to some recommendations that the dose be successively increased it is suggested that to achieve an early therapeutic effect the initial infusion-rate should be fast but thereafter reduced to avoid high steady-state concentrations.— J. A. Clements *et al.*, *Eur. J. clin. Pharmac.*, 1979, *16*, 411; *idem*, *J. Pharm. Pharmac.*, 1979, *31*, *Suppl.*, 41P.

See also under Absorption and Fate.

Anaesthesia. Studies on the use of doxapram during or following various anaesthetic procedures.— J. A. H. Davies, *Br. J. Anaesth.*, 1968, *40*, 361 (aid to the passage of a nasal endotracheal tube); P. K. Gupta and J. W. Dundee, *Br. J. Anaesth.*, 1973, *45*, 493 (postoperative arousal agent); P. L. Riddell and G. S. Robertson, *Br. J. Anaesth.*, 1978, *50*, 921 (arousal agent in out-patient general anaesthesia).

See also under Respiratory Depression (below).

Respiratory depression. Studies on the use of doxapram in respiratory depression.— F. E. Noe, *Anesth. Analg. curr. Res.*, 1966, *45*, 479 (postoperative); A. P. Winnie *et al.*, *Anesth. Analg. curr. Res.*, 1971, *50*, 1043 (postoperative); F. S. Arnold *et al.*, *Anesth. Analg. curr. Res.*, 1973, *52*, 643 (reduction of respiratory depression induced by neuroleptanalgesia for bronchoscopy); J. W. Dundee and P. K. Gupta (letter), *Lancet*, 1973, *1*, 1116; P. K. Gupta and J. W. Dundee, *Anaesthesia*, 1974, *29*, 33 and 40 (both references: reduction of respiratory depression induced by narcotics for postoperative analgesia); P. K. Gupta and J. Moore, *J. Obstet. Gynaec. Br. Commonw.*, 1973, *80*, 1002 (in neonates following administration of analgesics or anaesthetics to the mother before childbirth); J. W. Dundee *et al.*, *Anaesthesia*, 1974, *29*, 710 (acute drug overdosage); N. W. Lees *et al.*, *Br. J. Anaesth.*, 1976, *48*, 1197 (postoperative); T. H. Gawley *et al.*, *Br. med. J.*, 1976, *1*, 122 (postoperative with narcotic analgesics); J. E. H. Brice *et al.*, *Archs Dis. Childh.*, 1979, *54*, 981 (in neonates).

Respiratory insufficiency. A comparative study of 5 respiratory stimulants (doxapram, amiphenazole, ethamivan, nikethamide, and prethcamide) in 32 chronic bronchitic patients with acute, moderate to severe, ventilatory failure.— G. Edwards and S. O. Leszczynski, *Lancet*, 1967, *2*, 226. Comment.— H. A. C. Cockburn (letter), *ibid.*, 369.

The use of doxapram in patients with acute respiratory failure associated with chronic obstructive pulmonary disease.— K. M. Moser *et al.*, *New Engl. J. Med.*, 1973, *288*, 427.

Doxapram hydrochloride infused at a rate of 1.25 to 2.5 mg per minute over a period of 19 days was used successfully to manage acute respiratory failure with obesity-hypoventilation syndrome in a 39-year-old woman who weighed about 260 kg.— W. C. Houser and D. P. Schlueter, *J. Am. med. Ass.*, 1978, *239*, 340.

Preparations

Doxapram Hydrochloride Injection *(U.S.P.)*. A sterile solution in Water for Injections. pH 3.5 to 5.

Dopram Infusion *(Robins, UK)*. Contains doxapram hydrochloride 0.2% in dextrose injection. **Dopram Injection.** Contains doxapram hydrochloride 2%, in ampoules of 5 ml. (Also available as Dopram in *Canad., Fr., Ger., Jap., Neth., Norw., NZ, S.Afr., USA*).

Other Proprietary Names

Doxapril *(Ital.)*.

1422-r

Ethamivan *(B.P., U.S.P.)*. Vanillic Acid Diethylamide; Vanillic Diethylamide. *NN*-Diethylvanillamide.

$C_{12}H_{17}NO_3$=223.3.

CAS — 304-84-7.

Pharmacopoeias. In *Br.* and *U.S.*

A white or almost white crystalline powder, odourless or with a faint characteristic odour. M.p. 94° to 99°. **Soluble** 1 in 100 of water, 1 in 2 of alcohol, 1 in 3 of acetone, 1 in 1.5 of chloroform, and 1 in 50 of ether. A 1% solution in water has a pH of 5.5 to 7. **Protect** from light.

Incompatibility. An immediate precipitate occurred when ethamivan 2 g per litre was mixed with chlorpromazine hydrochloride 200 mg per litre, promazine hydrochloride 200 mg per litre, or promethazine hydrochloride 100 mg per litre in dextrose injection and sodium chloride injection. A yellow colour with a precipitate developing over 3 hours occurred when ethamivan was mixed with hydralazine hydrochloride 80 mg per litre in dextrose injection, and an immediate precipitate when mixed with prochlorperazine mesylate 100 mg per litre in sodium chloride injection.— B. B. Riley, *J. Hosp. Pharm.*, 1970, *28*, 228.

Adverse Effects and Treatment. As for Nikethamide, p.367.

Gasping respiration and laryngospasm have also been reported.

Precautions. Ethamivan should not be administered to patients with epilepsy or other convulsive disorders. It has been suggested that it should not be given to patients being treated with a monoamine oxidase inhibitor.

Absorption and Fate. Ethamivan is rapidly metabolised after intravenous injection. It is claimed to be rapidly absorbed from the mucous membranes of the mouth.

Uses. Ethamivan is a respiratory stimulant with actions and uses similar to those of nikethamide (see p.367). Its duration of effect is brief.

It has been given intravenously in usual doses of up to 5 to 10 ml of a 5% solution.

Ethamivan has also been given by mouth.

Preparations

Ethamivan Elixir *(B.P.C. 1973)*. Ethamivan Mixture; Ethamivan Oral Solution. A solution containing ethamivan 5%, alcohol 25%, and glycerol in water. Store in a cool place. The elixir should not be diluted; doses should be measured in a graduated pipette. *Dose.* Premature infants, 0.25 ml; full-term infants, 0.5 ml.

Ethamivan Injection *(U.S.P.)*. A sterile solution in Water for Injections prepared with the aid of sodium hydroxide. pH 9.3 to 9.6. Protect from light.

Clairvan *(Sinclair, UK)*. Ethamivan, available as **Intravenous Injection** containing 5% in ampoules of 2 ml and as **Oral Solution** containing 5% in alcohol (25%).

Other Proprietary Names

Corivanil *(Ital.)*; Romecor *(Ital.)*; Vallimida *(Spain)*; Vandid *(Austral., S.Afr., Switz.)*.

Ethamivan was also formerly marketed in Great Britain under the proprietary name Vandid (*Riker*).

1423-f

Fencamfamin Hydrochloride. H610. *N*-Ethyl-3-phenyl-8,9,10-trinorbornan-2-ylamine hydrochloride; *N*-Ethyl-3-phenylbicyclo[2.2.1]hept-2-ylamine hydrochloride.

$C_{15}H_{21}N,HCl$=251.8.

CAS — 1209-98-9 (fencamfamin); 2240-14-4 (hydrochloride).

Precautions. It is reported that similar precautions should be taken with fencamfamin hydrochloride as with Dexamphetamine Sulphate, p.362.

Uses. Fencamfamin hydrochloride is stated to act as a central stimulant but to have no anorectic activity. It has been given in usual doses of 20 mg at breakfast time and 10 mg at midday in fatigue and depressive states.

Proprietary Preparations

Reactivan *(E. Merck, UK)*. Tablets each containing fencamfamin hydrochloride 10 mg, ascorbic acid 100 mg, cyanocobalamin 10 µg, pyridoxine hydrochloride 20 mg, and thiamine 10 mg. For fatigue. *Dose.* 1 to 2 tablets in the morning and 1 at midday.

1424-d

Flurothyl *(U.S.P.)*. Hexafluorodiethyl Ether; SKF 6539. Bis(2,2,2-trifluoroethyl) ether.

$C_4H_4F_6O$=182.1.

CAS — 333-36-8.

Pharmacopoeias. In *U.S.*

A clear, colourless, volatile, mobile liquid, non-inflammable at room temperature, with a pleasant mild ethereal odour. B.p. about 64°. Specific gravity 1.415 to 1.419. **Soluble** 1 in 500 of water; miscible with alcohol, ether, propylene glycol, and halogenated solvents. **Store** at a temperature not exceeding 40° in single-dose glass ampoules.

Adverse Effects. Loss of memory and confusion may occur and some patients may have prolonged or repeated seizures.

Peripheral circulatory collapse and cardiac arrhythmias may occur, and cardiac infarction has been reported. Headache, nausea, and vomiting have occasionally occurred. Fractures and dislocations are common if muscle relaxants are not administered concurrently. Spontaneous epileptic seizures have followed courses of convulsive therapy.

Intravenous injection may cause thrombosis and extravasation may cause arterial spasm and gangrene.

From experience with its use on more than 2000 occasions, flurothyl was considered to have a good safety record. Methohexitone was preferred to thiopentone because it had less effect on the convulsive threshold. Concomitant treatment with phenothiazines might lead to prolonged or multiple seizures. Delirium had occurred in 2 patients and reversible cardiac arrest in 1. Concomitant use with monoamine oxidase inhibitors was probably contra-indicated; one patient taking phenelzine had persistent hypertension.— B. J. Dolenz, *Am. J. Psychiat.*, 1967, *123*, 1453.

Precautions. Flurothyl should not be given to patients with cardiovascular disease, fever, glaucoma, cerebral oedema, osteoporosis, or respiratory infections. Its use is best avoided during pregnancy.

Concomitant use of tranquillisers, especially phenothiazine derivatives, may increase the tendency to cardiovascular collapse.

For a suggested contra-indication with monoamine oxidase inhibitors, see Adverse Effects, above.

Absorption and Fate. Flurothyl is absorbed through the lungs and about 80% is reported to be excreted through the lungs in 3 minutes.

Uses. Flurothyl stimulates the central nervous system and induces convulsions similar to those produced by electro-convulsive therapy. When inhaled or injected intravenously its action is brief.

Flurothyl has been given by inhalation as an alternative to electro-convulsive therapy in the treatment of severe depression and some schizophrenic conditions. Patients were premedicated with atropine, thiopentone, and suxamethonium; 0.5 to 1 ml of flurothyl was vaporised with oxygen and inhalations taken every 5 seconds until a seizure occurred usually within 40 seconds. It was also given by intravenous injection.

1425-n

Levamphetamine. Laevo-amphetamine. (−)-α-Methylphenethylamine.
$C_9H_{13}N=135.2$.

CAS — 156-34-3.

Uses. Levamphetamine has actions qualitatively similar to those of dexamphetamine (see p.361) but it is less potent.
As the alginate, succinate, or sulphate, it was formerly used as an anorectic agent in the treatment of obesity.

1426-h

Lobelia *(B.P.).* Indian Tobacco; Lobelia Herb.

Pharmacopoeias. In *Aust., Belg., Br., Braz., Chin., Fr., It., Pol., Port.,* and *Span. Br.* also describes Powdered Lobelia.
Ind. specifies the dried aerial parts of Indian lobelia, *Lobelia nicotianifolia*, containing not less than 0.55% of total alkaloids.

The dried aerial parts of *Lobelia inflata* (Lobeliaceae) containing not less than 0.25% of total alkaloids calculated as lobeline.

Adverse Effects. Side-effects include nausea and vomiting, diarrhoea, coughing, headache, tremors, and dizziness. Symptoms of overdosage include profuse diaphoresis, paresis, tachycardia, hypothermia, hypotension, respiratory depression, convulsions, and coma.

A 48-year-old woman with bronchitis and asthma took 2 inhalations of orciprenaline sulphate and inhaled for 5 to 10 minutes the smoke from ignited compound lobelia powder (containing lobelia and stramonium). She collapsed and 5 to 10 minutes later was pale and slightly cyanosed, the skin was moist, and pupils dilated, the bladder was voided, and heart and breath sounds absent. Attempts at cardiac and respiratory resuscitation were unsuccessful. The woman had used the lobelia preparation for 20 years without any ill-effect.— G. McLaren (letter), *Br. med. J.*, 1968, *4*, 456.

Uses. The action of lobelia is due chiefly to lobeline. Tinctures, often in conjunction with iodides, have been used in the treatment of bronchial asthma and chronic bronchitis. Lobelia is contained in a number of 'asthma' powders which are ignited and the fumes inhaled. Their value is limited as they may aggravate chronic bronchitis.

Preparations

Ethereal Lobelia Tincture *(B.P.C. 1973).* Tinctura Lobeliae Aetherea. 1 in 5; prepared by percolation with ether spirit and adjusted to contain 0.05 to 0.075% w/v of alkaloids calculated as lobeline. *Dose.* 0.3 to 1 ml. Store in a cool place in airtight containers.

Simple Lobelia Tincture *(B.P.C. 1949).* Tinctura Lobeliae Simplex; Lobelia Tincture. 1 in 8; prepared by percolation with alcohol (60%). *Dose.* 0.6 to 2 ml.
A similar tincture, usually 1 in 10, is included in several pharmacopoeias.

For preparations of Lobelia and Stramonium, see Stramonium, p.311.

1427-m

Lobeline Hydrochloride *(B.P.C. 1968).* Lobelin. Hydrochlor.; Lobelini Hydrochloridum; Alpha-lobeline Hydrochloride. 2-[6-(β-Hydroxyphenethyl)-1-methyl-2-piperidyl]acetophenone hydrochloride.
$C_{22}H_{27}NO_2,HCl=373.9$.

CAS — 90-69-7 (lobeline); 134-63-4 (hydrochloride).

Pharmacopoeias. In *Aust., Belg., Cz., Ind., Int., It., Pol., Port., Span., Swiss,* and *Turk.*

A white odourless crystalline or granular powder with a bitter taste. M.p. not lower than 180°.
Soluble 1 in 40 of water and 1 in 12 of alcohol; very soluble in chloroform; very slightly soluble in ether. A 1% solution in water has a pH of 4 to 6. Solutions for injection are **sterilised** by filtration and supplied in single-dose containers; no bactericide should be added. **Incompatible** with alkalis, iodides, and tannic acid. **Protect** from light.

1428-b

Lobeline Sulphate.
$(C_{22}H_{27}NO_2)_2,H_2SO_4=773.0$.

CAS — 134-64-5.

Adverse Effects. As for Lobelia.

Uses. Lobeline has a peripheral action very closely resembling that of nicotine.
Lobeline hydrochloride was formerly given intramuscularly in usual doses of 3 to 10 mg as a respiratory stimulant but its effects are transient and uncertain.
Lobeline, by mouth, as the hydrochloride or sulphate, has been claimed to be of value as a smoking deterrent, but results of controlled trials have been disappointing.

Preparations of Lobeline Hydrochloride and Sulphate

Lobeline Injection *(B.P.C. 1968).* Inj. Lobelin.; Lobeline Hydrochloride Injection. A sterile solution of lobeline hydrochloride in Water for Injections. No bactericide should be added. Protect from light.

Some proprietary preparations of lobeline for use as smoking deterrents are listed under Part 3—Formulas of Proprietary Medicines.

Proprietary Names
Habit-X (sulphate) *(Glenden, Switz.)*; Lobatox (sulphate) *(Sobio, Fr.)*; Lobidan (sulphate) *(Berk, S.Afr.; Doetsch, Grether, Switz.)*; Nikoban (sulphate) *(Williams, USA)*; Unilobin (sulphate) *(Badische, Ger.)*.

Lobeline sulphate was also formerly marketed in Great Britain under the proprietary name Lobidan (*Berk Pharmaceuticals*).

1429-v

Meclofenoxate Hydrochloride.

Centrophenoxine Hydrochloride; Clofenoxine Hydrochloride; Clophenoxate Hydrochloride; Deanol 4-Chlorophenoxyacetate Hydrochloride; Meclofenoxane Hydrochloride. 2-Dimethylaminoethyl 4-chlorophenoxyacetate hydrochloride.
$C_{12}H_{16}ClNO_3,HCl=294.2$.

CAS — 51-68-3 (meclofenoxate); 3685-84-5 (hydrochloride).

Pharmacopoeias. In *Roum.*

A white powder. **Soluble**in water. It rapidly hydrolyses in aqueous solution.

Adverse Effects and Precautions. Irritability and lassitude have been reported in patients receiving meclofenoxate. It should not be given to hyperexcitable patients or those with extrapyramidal disorders.

Uses. Meclofenoxate hydrochloride has been claimed to aid cellular metabolism in the presence of diminished oxygen concentrations. It has been given for mental changes in the elderly or following strokes. It has also been given to mentally retarded children. The usual adult dose is 300 mg thrice daily increased, if necessary, to a maximum of 1.5 g daily. A suggested dose for children is 100 mg daily increased, if necessary, by 100 mg daily at intervals of several days to a maximum of 400 mg daily.
Meclofenoxate has also been given intramuscularly and by slow intravenous injection.
To avoid insomnia meclofenoxate should not usually be given later than mid-afternoon.

Proprietary Names
Helfergin *(Promonta, Ger.)*; Lucidril *(Montpellier, Arg.; Lloyd, Austral.; Anphar-Rolland, Fr.; Bracco, Ital.; ICN, Neth.; Adcock Ingram, S.Afr.; Max Ritter, Switz.)*; Luncidril *(Uquifa, Spain)*; Lutiaron, Ropoxyl *(both Jap.)*.

Meclofenoxate hydrochloride was formerly marketed in Great Britain under the proprietary name Lucidril (*Reckitt & Colman*).

1430-r

Methylamphetamine *(B.P.C. 1959).* *d*-Deoxyephedrine; Desoxyephedrine; Methamphetamine. (+)-*N*α-Dimethylphenethylamine.
$C_{10}H_{15}N=149.2$.

CAS — 537-46-2.

A clear, colourless, slowly volatile, mobile liquid with a characteristic odour resembling geranium leaves. Wt per ml 0.921 to 0.922 g.
Slightly **soluble** in water; miscible with alcohol, chloroform, and ether. A saturated solution in water is alkaline to litmus. **Store** in airtight containers.

1431-f

Methylamphetamine Hydrochloride *(B.P. 1973).*

Methylamphet. Hydrochlor.; *d*-Deoxyephedrine Hydrochloride; Desoxyephedrine Hydrochloride; Methamphetamine Hydrochloride; Methamphetamini Hydrochloridum; Methamphetaminium Chloride; Phenylmethylaminopropane Hydrochloride.
$C_{10}H_{15}N,HCl=185.7$.

CAS — 51-57-0.

Pharmacopoeias. In *Aust., Braz., Ger., Ind., Int., Jap., Swiss,* and *Turk.*

White odourless crystals or crystalline powder with a bitter taste. M.p. 172° to 174°. **Soluble** 1 in 2 of water, 1 in 4 of alcohol, and 1 in 5 of chloroform; practically insoluble in acetone and ether. Solutions in water have a pH of about 6. A 2.75% solution is iso-osmotic with serum. Solutions are **sterilised** by autoclaving or by filtration. **Store** in airtight containers. Protect from light.

An aqueous solution of methylamphetamine hydrochloride iso-osmotic with serum (2.75%) caused 97% haemolysis of erythrocytes cultured in it for 45 minutes.— E. R. Hammarlund and K. Pedersen-Bjergaard, *J. pharm. Sci.*, 1961, *50*, 24.

Dependence and Adverse Effects. As for Dexamphetamine Sulphate, p.361.

Marked prostration resembling septic shock, disseminated intravascular coagulation, rhabdomyolysis with myoglobinuria and uraemia appeared to be associated with the intravenous abuse of phenmetrazine or methylamphetamine in 5 patients. From 4 to 11 litres of sodium chloride injection were required in the first 24 hours to maintain blood pressure and urine output suggesting that shock resulted from massive loss of intravascular volume into necrotic muscle.— W. C. Kendrick *et al., Ann. intern. Med.*, 1977, *86*, 381.

Effects on blood and vascular tissue. Angiitis. Abuse of methylamphetamine hydrochloride appeared to be the cause of necrotising angiitis, indistinguishable from periarteritis nodosa, in 14 drug addicts.— B. P. Citron *et al., New Engl. J. Med.*, 1970, *283*, 1003. The suggested causal relationship between drug abuse and necrotising angiitis was not supported by the findings of many thousands of postmortem studies of drug abusers (mainly heroin addicts, though most had used many other drugs) during the past 50 years.— M. M. Baden (letter), *ibid.*, 1971, *284*, 111. Comments.— B. P. Citron and R. L. Peters (letter), *ibid.*, 112.

Effects on mental state. Twelve of 14 patients dependent on amphetamine sulphate developed a typical psychosis after a single large intravenous dose of methylamphetamine hydrochloride.— D. S. Bell, *Archs gen. Psychiat.*, 1973, *29*, 35.

Overdosage. Fatal cerebral haemorrhage in a 25-year-old man associated with the self-administration of methylamphetamine intravenously.— E. R. Olsen, *Angiology*, 1977, *38*, 464.

Pregnancy and the neonate. For reports of malformations following the use of methylamphetamine in pregnancy, see Dexamphetamine Sulphate, p.362.

Treatment of Adverse Effects. As for Dexamphetamine Sulphate, p.362.

Mental symptoms. Droperidol intravenously at a rate of 2.5 mg per minute to a total dose of 13 mg subdued and calmed, within 15 minutes of administration, a patient with agitation, combativeness, and hallucinations following the ingestion of an unknown amount of methylamphetamine.— N. E. Gary and P. Saidi, *Am. J. Med.*, 1978, *64*, 537.

Precautions. As for Dexamphetamine Sulphate, p.362.

Absorption and Fate. Methylamphetamine is readily absorbed from the gastro-intestinal tract and sites of parenteral administration. It is resistant to metabolism by monoamine oxidase and is excreted partly unchanged in the urine. Elimination is enhanced in acid urine.

In 16 hours, 55 to 70% of a dose of methylamphetamine was excreted unchanged in acid urine together with 6 to 7% of amphetamine. Only 0.6 to 2% of methylamphetamine was excreted in alkaline urine.— A. H. Beckett and M. Rowland, *Nature*, 1965, *206*, 1260.

Uses. Methylamphetamine is an indirectly acting sympathomimetic agent with actions and uses similar to those of dexamphetamine sulphate (p.362).

Methylamphetamine hydrochloride has been used as a pressor agent, particularly during anaesthetic procedures, in doses of 15 to 20 mg intramuscularly, or if necessary, 10 to 15 mg intravenously. Methylamphetamine itself, being volatile, was formerly employed by inhalation for the relief of nasal congestion. Tolerance develops readily.

Methylamphetamine was also formerly used as the saccharate.

Hiccup. Methylamphetamine 6 to 12 mg by slow intravenous injection rarely fails to relieve hiccup.— E. N. S. Fry (letter), *Br. med. J.*, 1977, *2*, 704. See also H. C. Voorhoeve, *Ned. Tijdschr. Geneesk.*, 1954, *98*, 3289.

Preparations of Methylamphetamine and its Salts

Methylamphetamine Injection *(B.P. 1973).* Methylamphet. Inj.; Methylamphetamine Hydrochloride Injection. A sterile solution of methylamphetamine hydrochloride in Water for Injections.

Methylamphetamine Tablets *(B.P. 1973).* Methylamphet. Tab.; Methylamphetamine Hydrochloride Tablets. Tablets containing methylamphetamine hydrochloride.

Proprietary Names

Desoxyn *(Abbott, USA)*; Methampex *(Lemmon, USA)*; Pervitin *(Trenker, Belg.*; *Temmler, Ger.*; *Temmler, Switz.)*.

Methylamphetamine hydrochloride was formerly marketed in Great Britain under the proprietary name Methedrine *(Burroughs Wellcome)*.

1432-d

Methylenedioxyamphetamine. MDA; SKF 5. α-Methyl-3,4-methylenedioxyphenethylamine.
$C_{10}H_{13}NO_2$=179.2.

CAS — 4764-17-4.

A white powder. **Soluble** in chloroform and dilute acetic acid.

Methylenedioxyamphetamine is an amphetamine compound with hallucinogenic effects; it has been subject to abuse.

It is chemically related to mescaline and amphetamine and has been widely abused under such names as Mellow Drug of America, Love Drug, Love Pill, or MDA.— K. K. Midha *et al.*, *J. pharm. Sci.*, 1976, *65*, 188.

Further references.— B. Jackson and A. Reed (letter), *J. Am. med. Ass.*, 1970, *211*, 830; K. C. Richards and H. H. Borgstedt, *ibid.*, 1971, *218*, 1826; R. N. Richards, *Can. med. Ass. J.*, 1972, *106*, 256; G. Cimbura, *J. forens. Sci.*, 1972, *17*, 329.

1433-n

Methylphenidate Hydrochloride *(U.S.P.)*.

Methyl Phenidate Hydrochloride. Methyl α-phenyl-α-(2-piperidyl)acetate hydrochloride.
$C_{14}H_{19}NO_2,HCl$=269.8.

CAS — 113-45-1 (methylphenidate); 298-59-9 (hydrochloride).

Pharmacopoeias. In *Braz.*, *Cz.*, *Hung.*, and *U.S.*

Odourless fine white crystalline powder or acicular crystals. Freely **soluble** in water and methyl alcohol; soluble in alcohol; slightly soluble in acetone and chloroform. A 4.07% solution in water is iso-osmotic with serum. Solutions in water are acid to litmus. **Incompatible** with alkalis and with solutions of barbiturates.

Incompatibility. Particulate matter was observed within 2 hours when 1 ml of commercial methylphenidate hydrochloride injection was mixed with 5 ml of sterile water and 1 ml of commercial injection of phenobarbitone sodium or phenytoin sodium.— R. Misgen, *Am. J. Hosp. Pharm.*, 1965, *22*, 92.

Dependence and Adverse Effects. As for Dexamphetamine Sulphate, p.361.

Abuse. Reports of adverse effects following the abuse of methylphenidate by injecting solutions of crushed tablets.— J. Wolf *et al.*, *Ann. intern. Med.*, 1978, *89*, 224 (syndrome of systemic, pulmonary, and musculoskeletal problems); H. Schatz and M. Drake, *J. Am. med. Ass.*, 1979, *241*, 546 (vascular emboli and retinopathy).

Allergy. A 4-year-old girl showed signs of acute conjunctivitis accompanied by an increase in hyperactivity and by skin irritability 30 minutes after taking methylphenidate 5 mg. She had a history of milk allergy but no other known allergies.— C. J. Rothschild and H. Nicol (letter), *Can. med. Ass. J.*, 1972, *106*, 1064. Angioneurotic oedema in one and urticaria in another child occurred during treatment with methylphenidate. Substitution with dexamphetamine produced an urticarial reaction in the first child.— J. Sverd *et al.*, *Pediatrics*, 1977, *59*, 115.

See also under Effects on the Skin (below).

Chorea. See under Extrapyramidal Effects (below).

Effects on growth. In 3 groups of hyperactive children there was no significant difference in long-term efficacy between methylphenidate for 3 to 5 years, chlorpromazine for 18 months to 5 years, or no treatment with drugs. However from the growth curves obtained it was considered possible that some children receiving methylphenidate might fail to grow at the expected rates.— G. Weiss *et al.*, *Can. med. Ass. J.*, 1975, *112*, 159. A report of slowing of growth in an 11-year-old boy who had received methylphenidate 10 mg four times daily from the age of 4 years for hyperkinesis.— M. Barter and H. Kammer (letter), *J. Am. med. Ass.*, 1978, *239*, 1742.

Further reports of the effect of methylphenidate on growth and the secretion of growth hormone.— W. A. Brown, *Archs gen. Psychiat.*, 1977, *34*, 1103; D. Aarskog *et al.*, *J. Pediat.*, 1977, *90*, 136; D. S. Janowsky *et al.*, *Archs gen. Psychiat.*, 1978, *35*, 1384; J. H. Satterfield *et al.*, *ibid.*, 1979, *36*, 212.

See also under Dexamphetamine Sulphate, p.361.

Effects on the heart. Structural alterations in the left ventricular myocardium of a patient were considered to be associated with the administration of methylphenidate for 4½ years.— V. W. Fischer and H. Barner (letter), *J. Am. med. Ass.*, 1977, *238*, 1497.

Further references.— J. E. Ballard *et al.*, *J. Am. med. Ass.*, 1976, *236*, 2870 (increase in heart-rate and blood pressure in children).

Effects on the liver. A 67-year-old woman taking 30 mg of methylphenidate daily developed nausea, vomiting, and dizziness on the first day of treatment; 7 days later serum aspartate aminotransferase (SGOT) and serum alanine aminotransferase (SGPT) values were elevated but returned to normal after methylphenidate was withdrawn. All the symptoms recurred after a challenge with 2.5 mg daily.— C. R. Goodman, *N.Y. St. J. Med.*, 1972, *72*, 2339.

Effects on mental state. Methylphenidate given for the treatment of hyperkinetic states produced a state of catatonic withdrawal in a 6-year-old girl and hallucinations in 2 children aged 10 and 15 years.— A. R. Lucas and M. Weiss, *J. Am. med. Ass.*, 1971, *217*, 1079.

A 36-year-old man who had been using methylphenidate 100 to 200 mg daily intravenously, and his 28-year-old wife who used large amounts intravenously, both developed paranoid psychosis requiring admission to hospital. The husband had withdrawal symptoms of lethargy and sleepiness and the wife symptoms of severe depression when methylphenidate was withdrawn. There were other reports in the literature of methylphenidate-induced psychosis.— J. Spensley and D. A. Rockwell, *New Engl. J. Med.*, 1972, *286*, 880.

Effects on the skin. A rash occurring on 3 occasions in a 73-year-old woman was considered due to methylphenidate; on the third occasion there were numerous large bullae simulating erythema multiforme.— A. J. Weil, *Ann. Allergy*, 1968, *26*, 402.

Extrapyramidal effects. In 1 patient akathisia was associated with methylphenidate hydrochloride and in another akathisia occurring during haloperidol treatment abated when methylphenidate hydrochloride was given.— J. S. Carman (letter), *Lancet*, 1972, *2*, 1093.

Report of tics in 14 children and exacerbations of pre-existing tics in 6 children receiving methylphenidate hydrochloride (10 to 60 mg daily). Following withdrawal of methylphenidate, tics subsided in 13 of the 14 children and symptom intensity returned to previous level in 6.— M. B. Denckla *et al.*, *J. Am. med. Ass.*, 1976, *235*, 1349.

Involuntary movements developed in an 8-year-old boy approximately 2 weeks after increasing the dosage of methylphenidate from 25 to 35 mg daily. Almost 2 years later, when the choreic movements were almost continuous, methylphenidate was discontinued and 2 months later the choreic disorder had disappeared.— W. J. Weiner *et al.*, *Neurology, Minneap.*, 1978, *28*, 1041.

Further references.— I. Extein, *Am. J. Psychiat.*, 1978, *135*, 252 (choreo-athetosis).

Treatment of Adverse Effects. As for Dexamphetamine Sulphate, p.362.

Precautions. Methylphenidate should be given with caution to patients with epilepsy or hypertension or to patients of unstable personality. It should not be given to patients with cardiovascular disease, hyperthyroidism, glaucoma, severe depression, anxiety, hyperexcitability, or restlessness. Methylphenidate should be used with caution in patients being treated with a monoamine oxidase inhibitor or within 14 days of stopping such treatment (see Precautions for Phenelzine Sulphate, p.128). It may also diminish the effects of guanethidine and similar antihypertensive agents.

Gilles de la Tourette's syndrome. Treatment with methylphenidate resulted in exacerbation of symptoms in 2 children with Gilles de la Tourette's disease and in a third with a probable combination of Gilles de la Tourette's disease and minimal brain dysfunction. In one of the two with Gilles de la Tourette's disease imipramine also caused symptoms to become markedly worse.— IFras and J. Karlavage, *Am. J. Psychiat.*, 1977, *134*, 195.

See also under Extrapyramidal Effects in Adverse Effects.

Interactions. *Anticoagulants.* For the effect of methylphenidate on ethyl biscoumacetate, see under Ethyl Biscoumacetate, p.771.

Anticonvulsants. For the effect of methylphenidate on phenytoin and primidone, see under Phenytoin Sodium, p.1240.

Antihypertensives. For the effect of methylphenidate on guanethidine, see under Guanethidine Monosulphate, p.146.

Anti-inflammatory agents. For the effect of methylphenidate on phenylbutazone, see under Phenylbutazone, p.274.

Absorption and Fate. Methylphenidate is readily absorbed from the gastro-intestinal tract. It is rapidly metabolised and excreted in the urine.

Studies on the metabolism and disposition of methylphenidate. Following a single dose of radioactively-labelled methylphenidate by mouth peak radioactivity in plasma, representing mainly metabolites, was observed after about 2 hours with an apparent half-life of 2 to 7 hours. In contrast measurable concentrations of methylphenidate in plasma could be detected after intravenous administration. The pattern of metabolites in urine was similar following both oral and intravenous administration with about 80% of the administered dose excreted as the de-esterified product, ritalinic acid, after 24 hours. Based on this urinary excretion pattern and minimal faecal elimination, absorption after administration by mouth was considered to be essentially complete.— B. A. Faraj *et al.*, *J. Pharmac. exp. Ther.*, 1974, *191*, 535. See also P. G. Dayton *et al.*, *Fedn Proc.*, 1970, *29*, 345.

Further references.— B. L. Hungund *et al.*, *Br. J. clin. Pharmac.*, 1979, *8*, 571.

Uses. Methylphenidate hydrochloride is a sympathomimetic agent with a stimulant effect on the central nervous system. It is used similarly to dexamphetamine sulphate in the treatment of narcolepsy in usual doses of up to 60 mg daily in divided doses; larger doses have been given. It has been advocated for the treatment of hyperkinetic states in children.

Methylphenidate was formerly used in fatigue and depressive states.

Diagnostic use. Reports of the possible diagnostic use of methylphenidate in psychiatry.— D. S. Janowsky and J. M. Davis, *Archs gen. Psychiat.*, 1976, *33*, 304; P. P. Leichner *et al.*, *Can. psychiat. Ass. J.*, 1976, *21*, 489; L. Huey *et al.*, *Psychopharmac. Bull.*, 1977, *13*, 52.

Hyperkinetic states. Reports of the use of methylphenidate in hyperkinetic states.— J. G. Millichap, *J. Am. med. Ass.*, 1968, *206*, 1527; J. L. Rapoport *et al.*, *Archs gen. Psychiat.*, 1974, *30*, 789; J. S. Werry and R. L. Sprague, *Aust. N.Z. J. Psychiat.*, 1974, *8*, 9; J. S. Werry and M. G. Aman, *Archs gen. Psychiat.*, 1975, *32*, 790; R. Gittelman-Klein *et al.*, *ibid.*, 1976, *33*, 1217; R. J. Lever *et al.*, *J. Pediat.*, 1977, *91*, 127; A. D. Nahas and V. Krynicki, *J. nerv. ment. Dis.*, 1977, *164*, 66; R. L. Sprague and E. K. Sleator, *Science*, 1977, *198*, 1274; M. L. Wolraich, *Pediatrics*, 1977, *60*, 512; L. E. Arnold *et al.*, *Archs gen. Psychiat.*, 1978, *35*, 463; R. A. Barkley and C. E. Cunningham, *ibid.*, 1979, *36*, 201; R. T. Brown and E. K. Sleator, *Pediatrics*, 1979, *64*, 408; L. Charles *et al.*, *Develop. Med. Child. Neurology*, 1979, *21*, 758; P. M. Leary *et al.*, *S.Afr. med. J.*, 1979, *55*, 374; R. E. Kauffman *et al.*, *Clin. Pharmac. Ther.*, 1980, *27*, 263.

For comments and criticisms of the use of stimulants in hyperkinetic states, see Dexamphetamine Sulphate, p.362.

Mental disorders. The concomitant use of methylphenidate and tricyclic antidepressants in patients with refractory depression.— R. N. Wharton *et al.*, *Am. J. Psychiat.*, 1971, *127*, 1619, per *Int. pharm. Abstr.*, 1972, *9*, 620.

Further references.— K. Rickels *et al.*, *Clin. Pharmac. Ther.*, 1972, *13*, 595 (depression).

Narcolepsy. The use of dexamphetamine and methylphenidate with clomipramine in narcolepsy and catalepsy.— *Lancet*, 1975, *1*, 845.

Methylphenidate was used in the long-term treatment of 106 patients with narcolepsy and 91% of patients received methylphenidate for more than 2 years. Usual daily doses were in the range 20 to 60 mg and given in 2 doses, after breakfast and after lunch. Marked or moderate improvement of sleep attacks and of psychic tension occurred in 91.5% and 91.4% of patients respectively. Side-effects occurred in 72 patients and included headache, dry mouth, gastro-intestinal disorders, sweating, and micturition disorders. Some side-effects may have been due to antidepressants and hypnotics administered concomitantly. Tolerance and withdrawal syndromes were not observed. Ideas of persecution developed in 8 patients and auditory hallucinations in 1.— Y. Honda *et al.*, *Curr. ther. Res.*, 1979, *25*, 288.

Pain. A study in 60 female patients undergoing abdominal surgery compared the effects of methylphenidate and papaveretum on postoperative pain and peripheral vascular reaction. When the first group recovered consciousness, on complaining of pain, 20 patients were given methylphenidate 40 mg intravenously and 20 papaveretum 20 mg intramuscularly. In the second group, 20 patients were given methylphenidate 40 mg intravenously shortly before the end of the operation. Pain was relieved in all patients but papaveretum had a hypnotic effect whereas all the patients given methylphenidate were alert. Only methylphenidate blocked the peripheral vasoconstrictor reaction to pain.— M. Johnstone, *Br. J. Anaesth.*, 1974, *46*, 778.

Preparations

Methylphenidate Hydrochloride Tablets *(U.S.P.)*. Tablets containing methylphenidate hydrochloride. Store in airtight containers.

Ritalin *(Ciba, UK)*. Methylphenidate hydrochloride, available in **Ampoules** of 20 mg for preparing injections, and as scored **Tablets** of 10 mg. (Also available as Ritalin in *Austral.*, *Canad.*, *Denm.*, *Ger.*, *Ital.*, *Neth.*, *Norw.*, *S.Afr.*, *Switz.*, *USA*).

Other Proprietary Names

Methidate *(Canad.)*; Rilatine *(Belg.)*.

1434-h

Nikethamide *(B.P., Eur. P.)*. Diethylamide Nicotinic Acid; Nikethylamide; Nicethamidum; Nicotinoyldiaethylamidum. *NN*-Diethylnicotinamide; *NN*-Diethylpyridine-3-carboxamide.

$C_{10}H_{14}N_2O = 178.2$.

CAS — 59-26-7.

Pharmacopoeias. In *Aust.*, *Belg.*, *Br.*, *Chin.*, *Cz.*, *Eur.*, *Fr.*, *Ger.*, *Hung.*, *Ind.*, *Int.*, *It.*, *Jug.*, *Mex.*, *Neth.*, *Nord.*, *Pol.*, *Rus.*, *Swiss*, and *Turk*.

A colourless or slightly yellow oily liquid or crystalline solid with a slight characteristic odour and a faintly bitter warming taste. Relative density 1.060 to 1.066. F.p. 23° to 25°. **Miscible** with water, alcohol, acetone, chloroform, and ether. A 25% solution in water has a pH of 6.5 to 7.8. A 5.94% solution is iso-osmotic with serum. Solutions are **sterilised** by autoclaving or by filtration and kept in ampoules. **Incompatible** with alkalis and tannic acid.

An aqueous solution of nikethamide iso-osmotic with serum (5.94%) caused 100% haemolysis of erythrocytes cultured in it for 45 minutes.— E. R. Hammarlund and L. Pedersen-Bjergaard, *J. pharm. Sci.*, 1961, *50*, 24.

Adverse Effects. Side-effects include sweating, nausea and vomiting, sneezing, coughing, flushing of the skin, and pruritus. Anxiety, restlessness, tremor, muscle twitching or rigidity, pyrexia, hypertension, tachycardia, and cardiac arrhythmias have been reported. Large doses may produce epileptiform convulsions and be followed by depression of the central nervous system.

Treatment of Adverse Effects. Convulsions may be controlled by diazepam intravenously or, if necessary, a short-acting barbiturate such as thiopentone sodium.

Uses. Nikethamide is a respiratory stimulant. Its duration of effect is very brief.

It was formerly advocated for the treatment of drug overdosage due to central nervous system depressants but is of no value for such purposes and may be dangerous. It has been suggested that very occasionally nikethamide may be of emergency value as a respiratory stimulant prior to assisted respiration.

Nikethamide has been given in usual doses of 0.5 to 2 g intravenously. It has also been given by mouth and by subcutaneous or intramuscular injection.

Preparations

Cordiaminum *(Rus. P.)*. A sterile 25% solution of nikethamide for oral use or for injection.

Nikethamide Injection *(B.P.)*. A sterile 25% solution in Water for Injections. Sterilised by autoclaving. pH 6 to 8.

Proprietary Names

Cardamin *(Stotzer, Switz.)*; Coracanfor *(Sastre, Spain)*; Coractiv N *(Phyteia, Switz.)*; Coramin *(Ciba, Ger.*; *Ciba, Switz.)*; Coramina *(Ciba, Arg.*; *Ciba, Spain)*; Coramine *(Ciba, Belg.*; *Ciba, Canad.*; *Ciba, Fr.*; *Ciba, Neth.*; *Ciba, USA)*; Cora-Rapide Simple *(Rapide, Spain)*; Corazon *(Grossmann, Switz.)*; Cormed *(Schwarzhaupt, Ger.)*; Juvacor *(Cambridge Laboratories, Austral.)*; Kardonyl *(Casgrain & Charbonneau, Canad.)*; Nicaethacor *(Mepha, Switz.)*; Niketamid *(DAK, Denm.)*; Percoral *(Streuli, Switz.)*.

Nikethamide was also formerly marketed in Great Britain under the proprietary name Coramine (*Ciba*).

1435-m

Oxypinocamphone. 2-Hydroxypinan-3-one.

$C_{10}H_{16}O_2 = 168.2$.

CAS — 10136-65-9.

Uses. Oxypinocamphone is a respiratory stimulant which has been given in usual doses of 120 mg thrice daily.

1436-b

Pemoline. LA 956; Phenilone; 5-Phenylisohydantoin. 2-Imino-5-phenyloxazolidin-4-one.

$C_9H_8N_2O_2 = 176.2$.

CAS — 2152-34-3.

A white crystalline tasteless powder. Practically **insoluble** in water, acetone, and ether; soluble 1 in 100 of propylene glycol.

Adverse Effects. Insomnia, anorexia, nausea, dizziness, headache, drowsiness, and mild depression have been reported. Large doses may cause nervousness and tachycardia and hallucinations may occasionally occur.

Effects on growth. A report of impaired growth in children receiving pemoline.— L. C. Dickinson *et al.*, *J. Pediat.*, 1979, *94*, 538.

Effects on the liver. Of children taking pemoline for hyperkinesis, 2% had elevated concentrations of serum aspartate aminotransferase (SGOT) and serum alanine aminotransferase (SGPT); the effect was stated to be transient and reversible.— *J. Am. med. Ass.*, 1975, *232*, 1204.

Absorption and Fate. Pemoline is absorbed from the gastro-intestinal tract.

Responses achieved in *rats* suggested that magnesium hydroxide might increase the absorption of pemoline.— N. Plotnikoff and P. Meekma, *J. pharm. Sci.*, 1967, *56*, 290.

In healthy subjects given pemoline 40 mg by mouth peak serum concentrations of 1.1 to 1.5 μg per ml occurred 4 to 6 hours after administration with a half-life of 16 to 18 hours. About 35 to 50% of the administered dose was excreted in the urine within 32 hours.— S. Goenechea and G. M. Wagner, *Arzneimittel-Forsch.*, 1977, *27*, 1604.

Further references.— J. -C. Libeer and P. Schepens, *J. pharm. Sci.*, 1978, *67*, 419; N. P. E. Vermeulen *et al.*, *Br. J. clin. Pharmac.*, 1979, *8*, 459.

Uses. Pemoline is a stimulant of the central nervous system which has been given in usual doses of 20 mg after breakfast and lunch for fatigue and depressive states. It has also been advocated for the treatment of hyperkinetic states in children. 'Magnesium pemoline', usually an equimolecular mixture of pemoline and magnesium hydroxide, has been given in a variety of disorders. The magnesium appears to enhance the absorption of pemoline, but the clinical reports have not been convincing.

Hyperkinetic states. Reports of the use of pemoline in hyperkinetic states.— M. Triantafillou (letter), *Br. J. Psychiat.*, 1972, *121*, 577.

For comments and criticisms of the use of stimulants in hyperkinetic states, see Dexamphetamine Sulphate, p.362.

Proprietary Preparations

Ronyl *(Rona, UK)*. Pemoline, available as scored tablets of 20 mg.

Volital *(Laboratories for Applied Biology, UK)*. Pemoline, available as tablets of 20 mg.

Other Proprietary Names

Arg.—Dinergil, Sindromida, Tamilan ('magnesium pemoline'); *Denm.*—Hyton Asa; *Fr.*—Deltamine; *Ger.*—Stimul, Tradon; *Ital.*—Sigmadyn; *S.Afr.*—Dynalert; *Spain*—Tropocer ('magnesium pemoline'); *Switz.*— Stimul; *USA*—Cylert.

Pemoline was also formerly marketed in Great Britain under the proprietary names Cylert (*Abbott*) and Kethamed (*Medo-Chemicals*).

1437-v

Pentetrazol *(B.P., Eur. P.)*. Leptazol; Pentazol; Pentamethazol; Pentylenetetrazol; Pentetrazolum; Corazol; 1,5-Pentamethylenetetrazole. 6,7,8,9-Tetrahydro-5*H*-tetrazoloazepine.

$C_6H_{10}N_4$=138.2.

CAS — 54-95-5.

Pharmacopoeias. In *Arg., Aust., Belg., Br., Cz., Eur., Fr., Ger., Hung., Ind., Int., It., Jug., Mex., Neth., Nord., Pol., Port., Rus., Span., Swiss,* and *Turk.*

Colourless, almost odourless crystals or white crystalline powder with a slightly pungent bitter taste. M.p. 57° to 60°. **Soluble** 1 in less than 1 of water, of alcohol, and of chloroform, and 1 in less than 4 of ether; soluble in carbon tetrachloride. A 10% solution in water has a pH of 5.5 to 7. A 4.91% solution is iso-osmotic with serum. Solutions are **sterilised** by autoclaving or by filtration, avoiding contact with metal. **Protect** from light.

An aqueous solution of pentetrazol iso-osmotic with serum (4.91%) caused 100% haemolysis of erythrocytes cultured in it for 45 minutes.— E. R. Hammarlund and K. Pedersen-Bjergaard, *J. pharm. Sci.*, 1961, *50*, 24.

Pentetrazol in a concentration of 1 to 3% inhibited the growth of *Escherichia coli, Bacillus subtilis, Staphylococcus aureus,* and *Pseudomonas aeruginosa.* This substantiated the statement in the *B.P.* 1958 that no bactericide needed to be added to solutions for injection.— R. J. Gilbert and A. D. Russell, *Pharm. J.*, 1963, *1*, 111.

Adverse Effects. High dosage produces epileptiform convulsions, and overdosage may result in respiratory depression.

Treatment of Adverse Effects. As for Nikethamide, p.367. If pentetrazol has been ingested the stomach should be emptied by aspiration and lavage.

Precautions. Pentetrazol may provoke seizures in patients with epilepsy or other convulsive disorders.

Absorption and Fate. Pentetrazol is readily absorbed after administration by mouth and by injection. It is rapidly metabolised, chiefly in the liver. About 75% of a parenteral dose has been reported to be excreted in the urine.

Peak plasma concentrations of about 2μg per ml were obtained about 2 hours after a dose of 100 mg of pentetrazol by mouth. The drug was excreted in the urine.— W. R. Ebert *et al.*, *J. pharm. Sci.*, 1970, *59*, 1409.

Plasma-pentetrazol concentrations in 3 patients, who were taking the drug regularly, ranged from 1.45 to 3.1 μg per ml when measured 1.25 to 5 hours after a 100-mg dose.— H. W. Jun *et al.*, *J. pharm. Sci.*, 1975, *64*, 1843.

Uses. Pentetrazol is a respiratory stimulant with actions and uses similar to those of nikethamide (see p.367). It has been given in usual doses of 100 mg, administered subcutaneously, intramuscularly, or intravenously. Pentetrazol has been employed in the elderly to alleviate the symptoms of senility. For this purpose it has been given by mouth in a dose of 100 to 200 mg twice or thrice daily, usually in conjunction with nicotinic acid, but its value has not been substantiated in trials.

Pentetrazol has been administered intravenously as an aid to the diagnosis of epilepsy.

Preparations

Leptazol Injection *(B.P.C. 1963).* Inj. Leptazol. A sterile solution of pentetrazol 10% and sodium phosphate 0.25% in Water for Injections, adjusted to pH 7.8 with dilute hydrochloric acid or potassium hydroxide solution. The addition of a bactericide is unnecessary. *Dose.* 0.5 to 1 ml subcutaneously.

Proprietary Names

Cardiazol *(Knoll, Ger.; Medinsa, Spain; Knoll, Switz.)*; Cardiorapide *(Rapide, Spain)*; Metrazol*(Knoll, USA).*

1438-g

Phenatine. *N*-(α-Methylphenethyl)nicotinamide diphosphate; *N*-(α-Methylphenethyl)pyridine-3-carboxamide diphosphate.

$C_{15}H_{16}N_2O,2H_3PO_4$=436.3.

CAS — 139-68-4 (base); 2964-23-0 (diphosphate).

Pharmacopoeias. In *Rus.*

Odourless colourless crystals or white crystalline powder with a bitter saline taste. **Soluble** in water and alcohol; practically insoluble in ether. A 5% solution in water has a pH of 1.8 to 2.4.

Uses. Phenatine is claimed to stimulate the central nervous system in a similar way to dexamphetamine without causing vasoconstriction. It is also claimed that it reduces blood pressure. In the USSR it has been employed similarly to dexamphetamine as a central stimulant; it has also been suggested in the treatment of hypertension.

1439-q

Picrotoxin *(B.P. 1963).* Picrotox.; Picrotoxinum; Cocculin.

$C_{30}H_{34}O_{13}$=602.6.

CAS — 124-87-8.

Pharmacopoeias. In *Arg., Int., It., Mex., Span., Swiss,* and *Turk.*

An active principle from the seeds of *Anamirta cocculus* (=*A. paniculata*) (Menispermaceae).

Odourless, colourless, flexible, shining prismatic crystals or white or nearly white microcrystalline powder, with a very bitter taste. M.p. about 199°.

Soluble 1 in 350 of water, 1 in 35 of boiling water, 1 in 16 of alcohol, and 1 in 3 of boiling alcohol; soluble in glacial acetic acid and solutions of acids and alkali hydroxides; slightly soluble in chloroform and ether. A saturated solution in water is neutral to litmus. Solutions are **sterilised** by autoclaving or by filtration. **Protect** from light.

The potency of picrotoxin solutions diminished as the pH increased above 7.— P. W. Ramwell and J. E. Shaw, *J. Pharm. Pharmac.*, 1962, *14*, 321.

Adverse Effects and Treatment. As for Nikethamide, p.367. As little as 20 mg may cause severe poisoning.

Uses. Picrotoxin is a respiratory stimulant with actions and uses similar to those of nikethamide (p.367). Its duration of effect is brief.

It was formerly given in usual doses of 3 to 6 mg intravenously.

1440-d

Pipradrol Hydrochloride *(B.P.C. 1963).* α-(2-Piperidyl)benzhydrol hydrochloride; αα-Diphenyl-α-(2-piperidyl)methanol hydrochloride.

$C_{18}H_{21}NO,HCl$=303.8.

CAS — 467-60-7 (pipradrol); 71-78-3 (hydrochloride).

Odourless, tasteless, small white crystals or white or almost white crystalline powder. M.p. about 290° with decomposition. **Soluble** 1 in 30 of water, 1 in 35 of alcohol, 1 in 1000 of chloroform, and 1 in 8 of methyl alcohol; practically insoluble in ether. A 1% solution in water has a pH of 5 to 7. **Protect** from light.

Adverse Effects. Pipradrol hydrochloride may cause nausea, anorexia, aggravation of anxiety, hyperexcitability, and insomnia. Epigastric discomfort, skin rash, dizziness, and hallucinations have been reported.

Precautions. Pipradrol hydrochloride is contra-indicated in endogenous depression, in agitated prepsychotic patients, chorea, paranoia, obsessional disorders, and anxiety states, and in patients for whom ECT is indicated.

Uses. Pipradrol hydrochloride is a stimulant of the central nervous system which was formerly given in usual doses of 2 to 6 mg daily in fatigue and some depressive states.

Proprietary Names

Detaril *(ISOM, Ital.)*; Stimolag Fortis *(Lagap, Switz.).*

1441-n

Cropropamide. *NN*-Dimethyl-2-(*N*-propylcrotonamido)butyramide.

$C_{13}H_{24}N_2O_2$=240.3.

CAS — 633-47-6.

1442-h

Crotethamide. 2-(*N*-Ethylcrotonamido)-*NN*-dimethylbutyramide.

$C_{12}H_{22}N_2O_2$=226.3.

CAS — 6168-76-9.

1443-m

Prethcamide. G 5668. A mixture of equal parts by wt of cropropamide and crotethamide.

CAS — 8015-51-8.

Prethcamide is **soluble** in water, alcohol, and ether.

Adverse Effects. Side-effects include headache, paraesthesias, restlessness, muscular twitching, tremors, dyspnoea, and flushing of the skin. Gastro-intestinal disturbances and skin rashes have also been reported.

Precautions. Prethcamide should be given with care to patients with epilepsy.

Uses. Prethcamide is a respiratory stimulant which has been given in usual doses of 400 mg three or four times daily in the treatment of respiratory insufficiency in chronic bronchitis.

It has also been given intramuscularly, by slow intravenous injection, and by intravenous infusion.

Proprietary Preparations

Micoren *(Geigy, UK).* Prethcamide, available as capsules of 400 mg. (Also available as Micoren in *Ger., Ital., Neth., Switz.*).

Other Proprietary Names

Micorene *(Belg.).*

1444-b

Prolintane Hydrochloride. SP 732. 1-(α-Propylphenethyl)pyrrolidine hydrochloride.

$C_{15}H_{23}N,HCl$=253.8.

CAS — 493-92-5 (prolintane); 1211-28-5 (hydrochloride).

A white odourless powder with a bitter taste. M.p. about 133°. **Soluble** in water, alcohol, and chloroform; practically insoluble in ether.

Adverse Effects and Precautions. Dry mouth, nausea, and tachycardia have been reported in patients receiving prolintane. It should be used with care in patients taking monoamine oxidase inhibitors, and should not be given to patients with hyperthyroidism or epilepsy.

Uses. Prolintane hydrochloride is claimed to be a stimulant of the central nervous system. It has been given, in fatigue and to improve appetite usually with vitamin supplements, in a dose of 10 mg twice daily, with the second dose being given not later than mid-afternoon.

Proprietary Preparations

Villescon *(Boehringer Ingelheim, UK).* **Liquid** containing in each 5 ml prolintane hydrochloride 2.5 mg, thiamine hydrochloride 1.67 mg, riboflavine phosphate (sodium salt) 1.36 mg, pyridoxine hydrochloride 500 μg, nicotinamide 5 mg, and alcohol 12.2% w/v (suggested diluent, water) and **Tablets** each containing prolintane hydrochloride 10 mg, thiamine mono-nitrate 5 mg, riboflavine 3 mg, pyridoxine hydrochloride 1.5 mg, nicotinamide 15 mg, and ascorbic acid 50 mg. For the improvement of appetite and mood. *Dose.* 10 ml of liquid or 1 tablet twice daily; children 5 to 12 years, 2.5 to 10 ml.

Other Proprietary Names

Promotil *(Fr.).*

1445-v

Propylhexedrine *(B.P.C. 1973, U.S.P.).*

Propylhexed. (±)-2-Cyclohexyl-*N*,1-dimethylethylamine.

$C_{10}H_{21}N$=155.3.

CAS — 101-40-6; 3595-11-7(±).

Pharmacopoeias. In *Arg.* and *U.S.*

A clear colourless liquid with a characteristic amine-like odour. It slowly volatilises at room temperature and absorbs carbon dioxide from the air. Wt per ml 0.853 to 0.861 g. B.p. about 204°. Very slightly **soluble** in water; miscible with alcohol, chloroform, and ether; soluble in dilute acids. Solutions in water are alkaline to litmus. **Store** in airtight containers.

1446-g

Propylhexedrine Hydrochloride.

$C_{10}H_{21}N,HCl$=191.7.

CAS — 1007-33-6; 6192-95-6(±).

A crystalline solid. M.p. about 127° with decomposition. **Soluble** in water, alcohol, and chloroform; slightly soluble in ether.

Adverse Effects. Excessive inhalation of propylhexedrine may cause stinging, rebound congestion, headache, and temporary enlargement of the nasal turbinates. Chronic rhinitis may follow prolonged use. Ingestion of propylhexedrine hydrochloride may cause mild stimulation of the central nervous system.

Abuse. Results of an examination of 9 deaths following abuse of propylhexedrine by intravenous route using a solution prepared from the cotton pledgets removed from inhalers. In 5 cases a combination of intimal and medial cellular proliferation had produced severe narrowing of pulmonary arterioles; 2 further patients had diffuse pulmonary fibrosis without obvious vascular changes, cardiomegaly being present in both these patients and in 4 of the previous 5. Seven of the 9 subjects had pulmonary foreign-body granulomas containing birefringent material. It was suspected that the mechanism of sudden unexpected death involved cardiac arrhythmias in association with pulmonary hypertension and cor pulmonale. Since the foreign-body granulomas were no different from those found in drug abusers in general they were not considered to be related to the vascular lesions. One death following ingestion of the pledget by mouth was also known.— L. White and V. J. M. DiMaio (letter), *New Engl. J. Med.*, 1977, *297*, 1071. See also R. J. Anderson *et al.*, *Am. J. Med.*, 1979, *67*, 15.

Further references.— P. Marsden and J. Sheldon, *Br. med. J.*, 1972, *1*, 730; J. Johnson *et al.* (letter), *ibid.*, 1972, *3*, 529; D. J. Pallis *et al.*, *Practitioner*, 1972, *209*, 676.

Uses. Propylhexedrine is a volatile sympathomimetic agent which has been used as an inhalant for nasal decongestion. Two inhalations through each nostril have been employed, repeated if necessary every hour.

Propylhexedrine has also been given as the hydrochloride in usual doses of 75 to 100 mg daily in divided doses as an anorectic agent in the treatment of obesity.

Preparations of Propylhexedrine and its Salts

Propylhexedrine Inhalant *(U.S.P.).* Cylindrical rolls of suitable fibrous material impregnated with propylhexedrine, usually with aromatics and contained in an inhaler. Store at a temperature not exceeding 40°.

Proprietary Names

Benzedrex *(Smith Kline & French, Canad.; Smith Kline & French, S.Afr.)*; Eggobesin (hydrochloride) *(Eggochemia, Aust.)*; Eventin (hydrochloride) *(Schering, Austral.; Minden, Ger.; Knoll, S.Afr.; Knoll, Switz.)*; Eventine (hydrochloride) *(Knoll, Belg.).*

Propylhexedrine was also formerly marketed in Great Britain under the proprietary name Benzedrex *(Smith Kline & French).*

1447-q

Tacrine Hydrochloride.

Tetrahydroaminacrine Hydrochloride. 1,2,3,4-Tetrahydroacridin-9-ylamine hydrochloride.

$C_{13}H_{14}N_2,HCl$=234.7.

CAS — 321-64-2 (tacrine); 1684-40-8 (hydrochloride).

A pale yellow crystalline powder with a bitter taste. Readily **soluble** in water. A 1.5% solution has a pH of 4.5 to 6. Solutions are **sterilised** by autoclaving or by filtration.

Adverse Effects. Adverse effects associated with tacrine hydrochloride include nausea and vomiting.

Prolonged respiratory depression followed the use of small doses of suxamethonium given in conjunction with tacrine during an abdominal operation.— P. O. Older *et al.*, *Br. J. Anaesth.*, 1966, *38*, 487.

Uses. Tacrine hydrochloride is an anticholinesterase which was formerly used intravenously in doses of 15 to 60 mg as a respiratory and central nervous system stimulant. It has been used in doses of 30 to 60 mg intravenously as an antagonist to tubocurarine chloride and other non-depolarising muscle relaxants, atropine being required concurrently to control the parasympathomimetic effects. It has also been used in doses of 10 to 15 mg to enhance and prolong the neuromuscular blockade caused by suxamethonium.

References to the use of tacrine.— G. Mendelson (letter), *Med. J. Aust.*, 1975, *1*, 839; *idem*, 1975, *2*, 906 (both orphenadrine overdosage); G. Mendelson (letter), *Med. J. Aust.*, 1976, *2*, 110 (pheniramine overdosage).

Proprietary Names

THA *(Woods, Austral.).*

Tacrine hydrochloride was also formerly marketed in Great Britain under the proprietary name THA *(WB Pharmaceuticals: Boehringer Ingelheim).*

Cetomacrogol and Nonionic Surfactants

430-y

A surfactant is a compound that can reduce the interfacial tension between 2 immiscible phases and this is due to the molecule containing 2 localised regions, one being hydrophilic in nature and the other hydrophobic.

The properties of nonionic surfactants are largely dependent on the proportions of these 2 groups in the molecule. Hydrophilic groups include the oxyethylene group ($-O.CH_2.CH_2-$) and the hydroxyl group ($-OH$). By varying the number of these groups in a hydrophobic molecule, such as a fatty acid, substances are obtained which range from strongly hydrophobic and water-insoluble compounds, such as glyceryl monostearate, to strongly hydrophilic and water-soluble compounds, such as the macrogols (see p.709). These 2 extreme types are not satisfactory as emulsifying agents, though they are useful stabilisers in the presence of efficient emulsifying agents.

Between these extremes are the nonionic emulsifying agents in which the proportions of hydrophilic and hydrophobic groups are more evenly balanced; these include some of the macrogol esters and ethers and sorbitan derivatives.

In addition to their use as emulsifiers some nonionic surfactants may be used in pharmacy as solubilising and wetting agents and nonionic surfactants in general are widely used in various industries.

Since nonionic surfactants do not ionise to any great extent in solution, they are generally compatible with both anionic and cationic substances, but they reduce the antimicrobial action of many preservatives.

In addition to the nonionic surfactants and formulas for emulsion bases given in this section, other nonionic compounds with surface activity such as the higher fatty alcohols and formulas are given in the section on Paraffins and Similar Bases.

Effect on preservatives. A study of the preservation of toilet preparations revealed that nonionic surfactants reduced the antimicrobial action of a number of preservatives; nonionic substances without surface-active properties did not appear to inactivate preservatives. The extent of inactivation varied according to the ratio of surfactant to preservative and appeared to be related to the hydrophilic-lipophilic balance of the surfactant and also to the chemical structure of the preservative. The nonionic surfactants used, each in a concentration of 2%, included Arlacel 83, Nonex 99, polysorbate 80, sucrose monopalmitate, and Texofor D1. Each of these caused complete or partial inactivation of the following preservatives in the concentration in which they were normally employed: Nipastat (0.15%), methyl hydroxybenzoate (0.1%), 2-*p*-chlorophenoxyethanol (0.15%), chlorocresol (0.1%), chlorhexidine acetate (0.01%), benzalkonium chloride (0.1%), phenoctide (0.1%), cetrimide (0.1%), cinnamaldehyde (0.01%), disodium edetate (1%), and potassium hydroxyquinoline sulphate (0.1%). The activity of the following preservatives was not affected by the surfactants in the same concentration (2%) but was reduced when the proportion was increased to 6%: formaldehyde (0.1%), sorbic acid (0.3%), benzoic acid (0.2%), and phenylmercuric nitrate (0.1%).— D. L. Wedderburn, *J. Soc. cosmet. Chem.*, 1958, *9*, 210.

For a critical review of work on the inactivation of preservatives by nonionic surfactants, see D. L. Wedderburn, Preservation of Emulsions against Microbial Attack, *Advances in Pharmaceutical Sciences*, Vol. 1, H.S. Bean *et al.* (Ed.), London, Academic Press, 1964, pp. 195–268.

Fading of dyes. Nonionic surfactants had deleterious effects on the colour stability of indigo carmine, orange G, tartrazine, and other dyes.— M. W. Scott *et al.*, *J. Am. pharm. Ass., scient. Edn*, 1960, *49*, 467.

Hydrophilic-lipophilic balance (HLB). An arbitrary scale of values denoting the relative affinity for oil and water had been devised for the classification of surfactants. Lipophilic materials had low HLB values; e.g. sorbitan sesquioleate had an HLB value of 3.7. Hydrophilic materials had higher values; e.g. polysorbate 80 had an HLB value of 15. Those surfactants having HLB values of about 3 to 6 were used for preparing water-in-oil emulsions; those with HLB values of about 8 to 18 were used for preparing oil-in-water emulsions.— W. C. Griffin, *J. Soc. cosmet. Chem.*, 1949, *1*, 311; *idem*, 1954, *5*, 249.

For HLB values of nonionic and ionic surfactants, see J. T. Davies and E. K. Rideal, *Interfacial Phenomena*, 2nd Edn, London, Academic Press, 1963, pp. 371–83.

The HLB classification as a systematic guide to surfactant selection.— I. A. Morris, *Mfg Chem.*, 1965, *36* (Sept.), 66.

Incompatibility. Tannic acid interacted strongly with polysorbates and macrogol ethers in aqueous solution to give turbid mixtures which were solubilised by the addition of further surfactant. Tannins, which occurred in numerous preparations of natural origin, could give unexpected incompatibilities when such preparations were mixed with surfactants or preparations stabilised with them.— B. N. Kabadi and E. R. Hammarlund, *J. pharm. Sci.*, 1966, *55*, 1069.

Interactions. Nonionic as well as anionic surfactants that contained an ethylene oxide group diminished the activity of clotrimazole against *Candida albicans in vitro*.— K. Iwata and H. Yamaguchi, *Antimicrob. Ag. Chemother.*, 1977, *12*, 206.

Release from suppositories. For a report on the effect of 28 nonionic surfactants on the rate of release of ephedrine from theobroma oil suppositories, see Ephedrine, p.10.

Solubilising properties. For a review of the solubilising properties of surfactants, see B. A. Mulley, Solubility in Systems containing Surface-active Agents, *Advances in Pharmaceutical Sciences*, Vol. 1, H.S. Bean *et al.* (Ed.), London, Academic Press, 1964, pp. 86–194.

Toxicity. A review of toxicity studies on nonionic surfactants, particularly polysorbates.— T. H. Eickholt and W. F. White, *Drug Stand.*, 1960, *28*, 154.

Tests on *rabbit* skin, *in vivo* and *in vitro*, showed that among a range of nonionic surfactants the macrogol ethers caused most irritation, followed by polysorbates and sorbitan esters.— M. Mezei *et al.*, *J. pharm. Sci.*, 1966, *55*, 584.

A short review of the effects of nonionic and other surfactants on the eye. Nonionic surfactants were generally less damaging to the eye than cationic or anionic surfactants.— W. M. Grant, *Toxicology of the Eye*, 2nd Edn, Springfield, Ill, Charles C. Thomas, 1974, pp. 962–7.

The nonionic surfactants used in household detergents were considered to be less toxic than the anionic surfactants. The acute LD_{50} in *animals* ranged from 2 to 10 g or more per kg body-weight. Ingestion might produce gastro-intestinal upset and local contact might produce irritation. Treatment of ingestion included diluting the surfactant with water or milk, the liberal use of demulcents, and, if vomiting had not occurred, emesis or gastric lavage might be required. Appropriate replacement therapy would be necessary if there was excessive vomiting or diarrhoea. Local irritation of the skin or eye could be treated with aqueous washes.— *Bull. Nat. Clearinghouse Poison Control Centers*, Jan.–Feb., 1975.

Patch testing with commonly used synthetic emulsifying agents in over 1200 patients with eczema.— M. Hannuksela *et al.*, *Contact Dermatitis*, 1976, *2*, 201. See also M. Hannuksela, *Int. J. cosmet. Sci.*, 1979, *1*, 257.

Emulsifiers and Stabilisers in Food. In Great Britain, the emulsifiers and stabilisers which may be added to food are controlled by The Emulsifiers and Stabilisers in Food Regulations 1980 (SI 1980: No. 1833) as amended (SI 1982: No. 16) and The Emulsifiers and Stabilisers in Food (Scotland) Regulations 1980 [SI 1980: No. 1888 (S.175)]. The term emulsifier is defined as any substance capable of aiding the formation of the uniform dispersion of 2 or more immiscible substances and a stabiliser is any substance capable of maintaining such a dispersion, but excluding other permitted food additives, caseins and caseinates, proteins and protein hydrolysates, starches, normal straight chain fatty acids derived from food fats, and any natural food substance. The permitted emulsifiers and stabilisers, some of which are limited to specified foods, include: lecithins, ammonium phosphatides, alginic acid, ammonium, calcium, potassium, and sodium alginates, propylene glycol alginate, agar, carrageenan, ceratonia, guar gum, acacia, tragacanth, pectin and amidated pectin, sterculia, xanthan gum, microcrystalline cellulose, methylcellulose, hydroxypropylcellulose, hypromellose, ethylmethylcellulose, carmellose sodium, sodium, potassium, and calcium salts of fatty acids, mono- and di-glycerides of fatty acids and their acetic acid, lactic acid, citric acid, and mono- and di-acetyltartaric acid esters, sucrose esters of fatty acids, sucro-glycerides, polyglycerol esters of fatty acids, of polycondensed fatty acids of castor oil, and of dimerised fatty acids of soya bean oil, oxidatively polymerised soya bean oil, propylene glycol esters of fatty acids, lactylated fatty acid esters of glycerol and propylene glycol, sodium and calcium stearoyl-2-lactylates, stearyl tartrate, polyoxyl 8 and 40 stearates, polysorbates 20, 40, 60, 65, and 80, sorbitan monolaurate, monopalmitate, monostearate, tristearate, and mono-oleate, docusate sodium, and quillaia extract.

Flour may not contain any emulsifier or stabiliser; bread may not contain any emulsifier or stabiliser other than stearyl tartrate, lecithins, mono- and di-glycerides of fatty acids and their lactic acid, citric acid, and mono- or di-acetyltartaric acid esters, or sodium or calcium stearoyl-2-lactylate.

The use of emulsifiers and stabilisers in soft and processed cheeses is limited.

The use of emulsifiers and stabilisers in cocoa and chocolate products is also controlled in Great Britain by The Cocoa and Chocolate Products Regulations 1976 (SI 1976: No. 541) and The Cocoa and Chocolate Products (Scotland) Regulations 1976 [SI 1976: No. 914(S.78)].

Emulsifiers and stabilisers should not be added to drinking milk. The Drinking Milk Regulations 1976 (SI 1976: No. 1883) and The Drinking Milk (Scotland) Regulations 1976 [SI 1976: No. 1888(S.154)] prohibit the alteration of the composition of drinking milk except in relation to the fat content of skimmed milk and semi-skimmed milk.

431-j

Glycol and Glycerol Esters

Hydrophobic properties predominate in the fatty acid esters of glycols and glycerol and these esters are poor emulsifying agents though they are useful stabilisers for both oil-in-water and water-in-oil emulsions. If a small amount of soap, sulphated fatty alcohol, or other surfactant is added to the esters, a 'self-emulsifying' product is formed which is capable of producing satisfactory oil-in-water emulsions. **Acetoglycerides** are mixed glyceryl esters in which the glycerol is esterified partly with a fatty acid and partly with acetic acid.

The chemistry of acetoglycerides and their uses in cosmetics.— H. G. Newman, *J. Soc. cosmet. Chem.*, 1957, *8*, 44.

Variations in the proportion and chain lengths of fatty acids used to esterify glycerol were reflected in the viscosity of cosmetic lotions made to a standard formula (mineral oil 1, glycerol 3, triple-pressed stearic acid 4, macrogol 600 monostearate 3.67, glycerol monoester 1.67, and water to 100, all by wt). The highest viscosities were obtained with glyceryl monomyristate if HLB was disregarded. When formulated to a constant HLB value of 10.6, by varying the macrogol monostearate content, viscosity of the lotions was proportional to chain length of the fatty acid. Mixing the esters reduced the viscosity.— J. Atherton and W. J. Maxcy, *Drug Cosmet. Ind.*, 1967, *100* (Mar.), 50.

For the estimated acceptable daily intakes of fatty and other acid esters of glycerol and polyglycerol esters, see

Seventeenth Report of FAO/WHO Expert Committee on Food Additives, *Tech. Rep. Ser. Wld Hlth Org. No. 539,* 1974.

For background toxicological information on glycerol esters used in food, see *Fd Add. Ser. Wld Hlth Org. No. 5,* 1974.

The Food Additives and Contaminants Committee recommended that mono- and di-glycerides of aliphatic acids of chain length not less than 9 carbon atoms and mono-, di-, and tri-glycerides of oleic acid be permitted as solvents in food.— *Report on the Review of Solvents in Food,* FAC/REP/25, Ministry of Agriculture, Fisheries and Food, London, HM Stationery Office, 1978.

486-g

Diacetylated Monoglycerides *(U.S.N.F.).*

Pharmacopoeias. In *U.S.N.F.*

Consists of glycerol esterified with edible fat-forming acids and acetic acid. A clear liquid. Very **soluble** in alcohol 80%, vegetable oils, and mineral oils; sparingly soluble in alcohol 70%. **Store** in airtight containers. Protect from light.

Diacetylated monoglycerides is an acetoglyceride (see p.370) used as an emulsifying and stabilising agent.

432-z

Diethylene Glycol Monostearate. Diglycol Stearate; Diéthylène Glycol (Stéarate de).

CAS — 106-11-6 (monostearate); 36381-62-1 (monopalmitate).

Pharmacopoeias. In *Fr.*

A white, odourless, tasteless, wax-like solid consisting of a mixture of the palmitic and stearic acid esters of diethylene glycol and containing not less than 40% of monoesters and not more than 7.5% of free glycol. M.p. 44° to 46°. Practically **insoluble** in water; soluble in hot alcohol. It is obtainable in the pure, non-dispersible form, or in the self-emulsifying form containing a small proportion of soap or other primary emulsifying agent.

Diethylene glycol monostearate has the properties of and is used for the same purposes as glyceryl monostearate or self-emulsifying glyceryl monostearate. Diethylene glycol monolaurate and mono-oleate are also available commercially.

433-c

Ethylene Glycol Monostearate. Ethylene Glycol Stearate; Éthylène Glycol (Stéarate d').

CAS — 111-60-4 (monostearate); 4219-49-2 (monopalmitate).

Pharmacopoeias. In *Fr.*

A white, odourless, tasteless, wax-like solid consisting of a mixture of the palmitic and stearic acid esters of ethylene glycol and containing not less than 50% of monoesters and not more than 5% of free ethylene glycol. M.p. 54° to 57°. Slightly **soluble** in water and fixed oils; soluble in hot alcohol and ether. It is obtainable in the pure non-dispersible form or in the self-emulsifying form.

Ethylene glycol monostearate has the properties of and is used for the same purposes as glyceryl monostearate or self-emulsifying glyceryl monostearate. Ethylene glycol monolaurate and mono-oleate are also available commercially.

434-k

Glyceryl Mono-oleate. Monolein.

CAS — 25496-72-4 (mono-oleate).

Pharmacopoeias. In *Aust., Nord.,* and *Swiss. Aust.* specifies not less than 40% of α-monoglycerides calculated as glyceryl mono-oleate with variable amounts of di- and tri-glycerides; *Nord.* specifies not less than 90% of chloroform-soluble glycerides; *Swiss* specifies not more than 5% of free glycerol.

A mixture of the glycerides of oleic acid and other fatty acids, consisting mainly of the mono-oleate.

A yellow to brownish-yellow oily liquid or unctuous mass with a characteristic odour and taste. Practically **insoluble** in water; miscible with alcohol, chloroform, and ether. **Protect** from light. Glyceryl mono-oleate is obtainable in the non-dispersible form or in the self-emulsifying form.

Glyceryl mono-oleate has similar properties to glyceryl monostearate.

435-a

Glyceryl Monostearate *(B.P., Eur. P.).* Glyceroli Monostearas; GMS; Monostearin; Glycérol (Stéarate de).

CAS — 31566-31-1 (monostearate); 26657-96-5 (monopalmitate).

Pharmacopoeias. In *Aust., Br., Eur., Fr., Ger., It., Neth.,* and *Pol.* which all specify not less than about 35% of monoglycerides. Also in *Hung., Jap.,* and *Swiss* without specification. Also in *U.S.N.F.* which specifies not less than 90% of monoglycerides.

A mixture of the monoglycerides of stearic and palmitic acids, together with variable quantities of di- and tri-glycerides. It contains not less than 35% of monoglycerides and not more than 6% of free glycerol. The commercial product is variable in composition.

A white or almost white hard waxy mass, powder, or flakes, greasy to the touch, tasteless and odourless or with a slight fatty taste and odour. M.p. 54° to 60°. Practically **insoluble** in water; it may be dispersed in hot water with the aid of a small amount of soap or other suitable surfactant; soluble 1 in 10 of chloroform, 1 in 100 of ether and methyl alcohol, 1 in 33 of isopropyl alcohol; soluble in hot organic solvents. **Store** in airtight containers. Protect from light.

Stability. Butylated hydroxytoluene and propyl gallate were the most effective antoxidants for glyceryl monostearate and secured its stability during 12 months' storage, irrespective of the container. No oxidation was observed when glyceryl monostearate was stored without any antoxidant for 6 months in aluminium tubes or glass jars.— W. Wisniewski and Z. Golucki, *Acta Pol. pharm.,* 1965, *22,* 293, per *Int. pharm. Abstr.,* 1966, *3,* 382.

Uses. Glyceryl monostearate is a poor water-in-oil emulsifying agent but it is a useful stabiliser of water-in-oil and oil-in-water emulsions in preparations for internal and external use. It has emollient properties. It is usual to add a small amount of soap, sulphated fatty alcohol, or other surfactant, which has the effect of making the product self-emulsifying (see Self-Emulsifying Glyceryl Monostearate) and capable of producing satisfactory oil-in-water emulsions.

Glyceryl monostearate is also used in the food and cosmetic industries.

Preparations

Glyceryl Monostearate Basis. Glyceryl monostearate 12 g, light liquid paraffin 20 g, white soft paraffin 20 g, water 48 g. Melt and mix the ingredients at 70°, stir until emulsified and congealed.—E. Ehrenstein, *Am. prof. Pharm.,* 1950, *16,* 874.

436-t

Self-Emulsifying Glyceryl Monostearate *(B.P.).* Self-emulsifying Monostearin; Self-Emulsifying Mono- and Di-glycerides of Food Fatty Acids; Monostearin Emulsificans; Monostearinum.

Pharmacopoeias. In *Belg.* and *Br.*

A mixture consisting principally of mono-, di- and tri- glycerides of stearic and palmitic acids, and of minor proportions of other fatty acids; it may also contain free fatty acids, glycerol, and soap. It contains not less than 30% of monoglycerides, not more than 7% of free glycerol, and not more than 6% of soap, calculated as sodium oleate, all calculated with reference to the anhydrous substance.

A white to cream-coloured, hard, waxy solid with a faint fatty odour and taste. Practically **insoluble** in water; dispersible in hot water; soluble in hot dehydrated alcohol and hot liquid paraffin; soluble in hot fixed oils, but may give turbid solutions at concentrations below 20%. A 5% dispersion in hot water has a pH of 8 to 10 after cooling.

Because of the presence of soap, it is **incompatible** with acids and high concentrations of ionisable salts, hard water, calcium compounds, zinc oxide, and oxides of heavy metals. Aqueous preparations containing this emulsifying agent should contain an antimicrobial preservative.

The composition, properties, and uses of commercial grades of glyceryl monostearate.— E. S. Lower, *Soap Perfum. Cosm.,* 1960, *33,* 1201 and 1313; *idem,* 1961, *34,* 53.

For a summary of the properties and uses of the various types of self-emulsifying glyceryl monostearate, with formulas, see G. E. Schumacher, *Am. J. Hosp. Pharm.,* 1967, *24,* 290.

Uses. Self-emulsifying glyceryl monostearate is used as an emulsifying agent for oils, fats, solvents, and waxes in the preparation of bases of the non-emulsified, emulsified, and vanishing-cream types.

It is not intended for inclusion in preparations for internal use.

It produces stable fine-grained creams which are reasonably resistant to extremes of temperature but are cracked by acid or calcium ions since the primary emulsifying agent is the added soap. Thin emulsions may be stabilised by the addition of as little as 0.5% of self-emulsifying glyceryl monostearate, provided the viscosity of the product is increased by the use of a thickening agent. For ointments and more viscous creams 5 to 20% may be used.

Aqueous preparations containing self-emulsifying glyceryl monostearate should contain a preservative to prevent fungous or bacterial growth.

487-q

Mono- and Di-glycerides *(U.S.N.F.).*

Pharmacopoeias. In *U.S.N.F.*

Consists of a mixture of glyceryl mono- and di-esters, with small amounts of tri-esters, of fatty acids from edible oils. It may contain suitable stabilisers. Practically **insoluble** in water; soluble in alcohol, chloroform, and ethyl acetate. **Store** in airtight containers. Protect from light.

Mono- and di-glycerides is an emulsifying and stabilising agent.

437-x

Propylene Glycol Monostearate *(U.S.N.F.)*.

Propylene Glycol Stearate; Propylèneglycol (Stéarate de); Prostearin.

CAS — 1323-39-3 (monostearate); 29013-28-3 (monopalmitate).

Pharmacopoeias. In *Fr.* Also in *U.S.N.F.*

U.S.N.F. specifies not less than 90% of monoesters and not more than 1% of free glycerol and propylene glycol; *Fr. P.* specifies not less than 50% of monoesters, not more than 8% of free propylene glycol, and m.p. 33° to 36°.

A variable mixture of the propylene glycol mono- and di-esters of stearic and palmitic acids, consisting mainly of the monoesters.

White wax-like solid, beads, or flakes, with a slight agreeable fatty odour and taste. F.p. not less than 45°. Practically **insoluble** in water but it may be dispersed in hot water with the aid of a small amount of soap or other suitable surfactant; soluble in alcohol, acetone, ether, and in fixed and mineral oils. It is obtainable in the pure, non-dispersible form, or in the self-emulsifying form containing a small proportion of soap or other primary emulsifying agent.

Propylene glycol monostearate is used for the same purposes as glyceryl monostearate or self-emulsifying glyceryl monostearate. Propylene glycol monolaurate and mono-oleate are also available commercially.

Estimated acceptable daily intake of propylene glycol esters of fatty acids; up to 25 mg, as propylene glycol, per kg body-weight.— Seventeenth Report of FAO/WHO Expert Committee on Food Additives, *Tech. Rep. Ser. Wld Hlth Org. No. 539,* 1974.

For background toxicological information, see *Fd Add. Ser. Wld Hlth Org. No. 5,* 1974.

438-r

Proprietary Preparations of Glycol and Glycerol Esters

Included here are a range of proprietary preparations relating to the above monographs.

Abracol GSP *(Bush Boake Allen, UK).* A brand of self-emulsifying glyceryl monostearate, stable in weak acid. It is similar to **Tegacid** *(Goldschmidt, USA).*

Arlacel 165 *(Atlas, UK).* A brand of acid-stable self-emulsifying glyceryl monostearate for use in cosmetic preparations. **Arlacel 186.** A mixture of mono- and di-glycerides of fatty acids. **Arlacels 20** to **85** are sorbitan esters, see p.378.

Cerasynts *(Van Dyk, USA: Black, UK).* A range of glycol and glyceryl esters, including **Cerasynt 945** and **Cerasynt WM** (acid-stable self-emulsifying glyceryl monostearates), **Cerasynt M** (ethylene glycol monostearate), **Cerasynt PA** (propylene glycol monostearate), **Cerasynt Q** (self-emulsifying glyceryl monostearate), and **Cerasynt SD** (glyceryl monostearate).

The name Cerasynt is also applied to a range of macrogol esters, see p.372.

Cithrol *(Croda, UK).* A range of glycol and glycerol esters, including **Cithrol DGMS** (diethylene glycol monostearate), **Cithrol EGMS** (ethylene glycol monostearate), **Cithrol GMO** (glyceryl mono-oleate), **Cithrol GMS** (glyceryl monostearate), and **Cithrol PGMS** (propylene glycol monostearate).

The name Cithrol is also applied to a range of macrogol esters, see p.372.

Dynasan *(Dynamit Nobel, UK).* Single-acid triglycerides of chain length C_{12}, C_{14}, C_{16}, and C_{18}.

Empilan GMS NSE 40 and NSE 90 *(Albright & Wilson, Marchon Division, UK).* Grades of glyceryl monostearate.

Empilan GMS LSE 40, LSE 80, MSE 40, SE 40, and SE 70 *(Albright & Wilson, Marchon Division, UK).* Grades of self-emulsifying glyceryl monostearate.

HA 621 *(Atlas, UK).* A brand of propylene glycol monostearate (HLB 2.5).

Imwitor *(Dynamit Nobel, UK).* A range of glyceryl monostearate emulsifying agents with mono-ester contents of 40 to 90%, including **Imwitor (Emulsfier) 191** and **Imwitor (Emulsifier) 940,** brands which contain respectively 90% and 40% monoglycerides and **Imwitor (Emulsifier) 960,** a brand of a self-emulsifying glyceryl monostearate.

Myvacet *(Eastman, UK).* A range of distilled acetoglycerides prepared from vegetable oils and animal fats.

Myverol *(Eastman, UK).* A range of distilled glycol and glycerol esters containing not less than 90% of mono-esters and based on various vegetable oils and animal fats.

Softigen *(Dynamit Nobel, UK).* **No. 701.** A mixture of partial glycerides of an unsaturated fatty acid containing free hydroxyl groups. **No. 767.** A water-soluble mixture of partial glycerides of natural, saturated, vegetable fatty acids with a chain length of C_8 to C_{12}.

Softisan Ointment Bases *(Dynamit Nobel, UK).* **Nos 100, 133, 134, 138, 142,** and **378** consist of triglycerides of mixtures of naturally-occurring, saturated, even-numbered, straight-chain, vegetable fatty acids of chain length C_8 to C_{18}. **No. 601** is a mixture of triglycerides and partial glycerides of natural vegetable fatty acids with nonionic emulsifying agents, and can be used as a basis with or without water, with which it gives an oil-in-water emulsion.

Witconol *(Witco, UK).* A range of glycol and glycerol esters, including **Witconol F26-46** (polypropylene glycol oleate).

439-f

Macrogol Esters. Polyoxyethylene Esters.

CAS — 9004-99-3.

The hydrophilic properties of the oxyethylene group are weaker than those of the hydroxyl group but by introducing a sufficient number into a fatty acid molecule, substances are produced in which the hydrophilic and hydrophobic properties are sufficiently well balanced for the substances to act as efficient oil-in-water emulsifying agents. They may also be used as wetting and solubilising agents. Since the ester linkage is prone to hydrolysis, these materials are not so resistant to acids and alkalis as the macrogol ethers.

Estimated acceptable total daily intake of polyoxyl 8 stearate and polyoxyl 40 stearate used in combination: up to 25 mg per kg body-weight.— Seventeenth Report of FAO/WHO Expert Committee on Food Additives, *Tech. Rep. Ser. Wld Hlth Org. No. 539,* 1974.

The emulsifying properties and incompatibilities of the macrogol monostearates.— C. A. Johnson and J. A. Thomas, *Pharm. J.,* 1955, *2,* 51.

Of 100 patients with allergic contact dermatitis, 2 gave positive reactions to patch testing with macrogol stearate [molecular weight not specified].— A. A. Fischer *et al., Archs Derm.,* 1971, *104,* 286.

440-z

Polyoxyl 8 Stearate. Macrogol Stearate 400;

Polyoxyethylene 8 Stearate; Polyoxyethylene Glycol 400 Stearate; Polyaethylenglycolum 400 Monostearinicum.

$C_{34}H_{68}O_{10}$ (nominal) = 636.9.

NOTE. Two systems of nomenclature are used for these compounds. The number '8' in the name 'Polyoxyethylene 8 Stearate' refers to the approximate polymer length in oxyethylene units. The number '400' in the name 'Polyoxyethylene Glycol 400 Stearate' refers to the average molecular weight of the polymer chain.

Pharmacopoeias. Substances of similar composition are included in *Aust., Ger.,* and *Swiss. Fr.* includes Stéarate de Polyoxyéthylène-glycol 300, which consists of a mixture of mono- and di-esters of palmitic and stearic acids with macrogol 300. *Fr.* also includes Glycérides Polyoxyéthylénés Glycolysés, which are the products obtained by partial esterification of natural vegetable oils with macrogols of molecular weight between 200 and 400. They consist of glycerides with a certain proportion of macrogol esters.

A mixture of the monostearate and distearate esters of mixed macrogols and the corresponding free glycols, the average polymer length being equivalent to about 8 oxyethylene units.

A cream-coloured, soft, waxy solid with a faint fatty odour and a slightly bitter fatty taste. Congealing range 27° to 29°. **Dispersible** in warm water; soluble in alcohol, acetone, carbon tetrachloride, dioxan, ether, and methyl alcohol; soluble, forming a hazy solution, in light petroleum, liquid paraffin, and fixed oils. **Incompatible** with strong acids and alkalis, phenols, potassium iodide, tannins, and salts of bismuth, mercury, and silver.

For background toxicological information, see *Fd Add. Ser. Wld Hlth Org. No. 5,* 1974.

441-c

Polyoxyl 40 Stearate. Macrogol Stearate

2000; Polyoxyethylene 40 Stearate; Stearethate 40; Polyoxyaethenum Stearinicum; Estearato de Polioxila 40.

$C_{98}H_{196}O_{42}$ (nominal) = 2046.6.

Pharmacopoeias. In *Arg., Braz., Hung., Jap.,* and *Turk.* Also in *U.S.N.F.* Some describe only the monostearate ester.

A mixture of the monostearate and distearate esters of mixed macrogols and the corresponding free glycols, the average polymer length being equivalent to about 40 oxyethylene units.

A waxy solid which is white to light tan in colour and is odourless or has a faint fatty odour. Congealing range 37° to 47°.

Soluble in water, alcohol, acetone, carbon tetrachloride, ether, and methyl alcohol; practically insoluble in liquid paraffin and fixed oils. A 5% solution in water has a pH of 5 to 7. **Store** in airtight containers.

A study of the formation of complexes between polyoxyl 40 stearate and phenol, resorcinol, and other drugs.— D. Chakravarty *et al., Drug Stand.,* 1957, *25,* 137.

For background toxicological information, see *Fd Add. Ser. Wld Hlth Org. No. 5,* 1974.

442-k

Polyoxyl 50 Stearate. Polyoxyethylene 50 Stearate *(U.S.N.F.).*

$C_{118}H_{236}O_{52}$ (nominal) = 2487.1.

Pharmacopoeias. In *U.S.N.F.*

A mixture of the monostearate and distearate esters of mixed macrogols and the corresponding free glycols, the average polymer length being equivalent to about 50 oxyethylene units.

A cream-coloured soft waxy solid with a faint fatty odour. M.p. about 45°. **Soluble** 1 in 0.7 of water, 1 in 13 000 of dehydrated alcohol, 1 in 0.45 of chloroform, and 1 in 14 000 of ether. Soluble in alcohol and isopropyl alcohol. **Store** in airtight containers.

443-a

Proprietary Preparations of Macrogol Esters and Related Compounds

Included here are miscellaneous proprietary preparations of macrogol esters described above and of similar compounds.

Arlatone 285 and 289 *(Atlas, UK).* Oxyethylated esters of fatty acids (HLB 14.4); solubilising agents for cosmetic and pharmaceutical products.

Cerasynt 616, 660, and 840 *(Van Dyk, USA: Black, UK).* Grades of macrogol monostearates.

The name Cerasynt is also applied to a range of glycol and glycerol esters, see p.372.

Cithrol *(Croda, UK).* A range of macrogol mono- and di-esters of lauric, oleic, ricinoleic, and stearic acids.

The name Cithrol is also applied to a range of glycol and glycerol esters, see p.372.

Cremophor EL *(BASF, Ger.: Blagden, UK).* A nonionic emulsifying agent produced by reacting 35 moles of ethylene oxide with 1 mole of castor oil. **Cremophor RH 40** and **Cremophor RH 60.** Nonionic solubilising and emulsifying agents produced by reacting 45 and 60 moles respectively of ethylene oxide with 1 mole of hydrogenated castor oil. **Cremophor S9.** A nonionic emulsifying agent produced by reacting 9 moles of ethylene oxide with 1 mole of stearic acid.

For reports of anaphylactoid reactions, transient haematological and biochemical disturbances, and unusual hyperlipidaemias attributed to the presence of Cremophor EL in the vehicle of various intravenous injections, see A. G. Bagnarello *et al., New Engl. J. Med.,* 1977, *296,* 497; H. B. Niell (letter), *ibid.,* 1479; J. P. Sung and J. G. Grendahl (letter), *ibid., 297,* 786; A. Padfield and J. Watkins (letter), *Br. med. J.,* 1977, *1,* 575; A. R. W. Forrest *et al.* (letter), *ibid., 2,* 1357; C. Lee and E. G. Maderazo, *Antimicrob. Ag. Chemother.,* 1978, *13,* 548; J. Watkins *et al.* (letter), *Lancet,* 1978, *2,* 736; D. Dye and J. Watkins, *Br. med. J.,* 1980, *280,* 1353.

The name Cremophor is also applied to a range of macrogol ethers, see below.

Crodet *(Croda, UK).* A range of macrogol esters of lauric, oleic, and stearic acids, including **Crodet S8** (polyoxyl 8 stearate) and **Crodet S40** (polyoxyl 40 stearate).

Croduret *(Croda, UK).* A range of polyoxyethylated derivatives of hydrogenated castor oil.

Empilan AQ 100 *(Albright & Wilson, Marchon Division, UK).* A brand of macrogol monolaurate with a mean molecular wt of 400.

Empilan BQ 100 *(Albright & Wilson, Marchon Division, UK).* A brand of macrogol mono-oleate with a mean molecular wt of 400.

Emulsynts *(Van Dyk, USA: Black, UK).* A range of nonionic surfactants, including a series of macrogol esters of lauric and oleic acids.

Ethomeens *(Akzo, UK).* A range of polyoxyethylene fatty acid amines, derived from coco, oleic, or tallow acid. **Ethoduomeens** are a range of similar diamines, derived from tallow acid.

Ethomid *(Akzo, UK).* A range of di(polyoxyethylene) fatty acid amides derived from hydrogenated tallow acid or oleic acid.

Etocas *(Croda, UK).* A range of polyoxyethylated derivatives of castor oil.

Gelucire *(Alfa, UK).* A range of semi-solid excipients for encapsulation of liquids into hard gelatin capsules, consisting of the partial glycerides and polyglycides of fatty acids.

Myrj *(Atlas, UK).* A brand name for a range of macrogol stearates, including **Myrj 45** (polyoxyl 8 stearate, HLB 11.1), **Myrj 52** (polyoxyl 40 stearate, HLB 16.9), and **Myrj 53** (polyoxyl 50 stearate, HLB 17.9).

Nonex *(BP Chemicals, UK: Hythe, UK).* A brand name for a range of macrogol esters of fatty acids.

Other Proprietary Names
Labrafil M1944CS *(*polyoxyl 5 oleate; peglicol 5 oleate*) (Fr.).*

444-t

Macrogol Ethers

NOTE. Two systems of nomenclature are used for macrogol ethers. The number '9' in the name 'Nonoxinol 9' refers to the approximate polymer length in oxyethylene units. The number '1000' in the name 'Cetomacrogol 1000' refers to the average molecular weight of the polymer chain.

The macrogol ethers are condensation products prepared by reaction between fatty alcohols or alkyl phenols and ethylene oxide. The ether linkage in these substances confers good stability to acids and alkalis. They are widely used in the preparation of oil-in-water emulsions and as wetting and solubilising agents.

The behaviour of macrogol ethers in emulsions.— *Soap Perfum. Cosm.,* 1968, *41,* 276.

445-x

Cetomacrogol 1000 *(B.P.).* Polyethylene Glycol 1000 Monocetyl Ether.

CAS — 9004-95-9 (m=15).

Pharmacopoeias. In *Br.*

A macrogol ether containing 20 to 24 oxyethylene groups in the polyoxyethylene chain. It is represented by the formula $CH_3.[CH_2]_m.[O.CH_2.CH_2]_n.OH$, where *m* may be 15 or 17 and *n* may be 20 to 24.

An almost odourless cream-coloured waxy unctuous mass which melts, when heated, to a clear brownish-yellow liquid; it has a soapy taste. M.p. not lower than 38°.

Soluble in water, acetone, and alcohol; practically insoluble in light petroleum. Solutions in water are best prepared by sprinkling the powdered wax on hot water, stirring, and allowing to cool. It is **sterilised** by maintaining at 150° for 1 hour. **Incompatible** with phenols and reduces the antibacterial activity of quaternary ammonium compounds. Cetomacrogol may separate from solutions in the presence of a high concentration of electrolytes. **Store** in airtight containers.

Factors affecting autoxidation of aqueous cetomacrogol included temperature, concentration, initial pH, light, metallic impurities, and prior heat treatment or bleaching. Autoxidation could result in an appreciable decrease in solubility.— R. Hamburger *et al., Pharm. Acta Helv.,* 1975, *50,* 10.

Incompatibility. Benzocaine hydrochloride solution (0.25M) was incompatible with 3% cetomacrogol; a yellow colour developed on storage and could be retarded by the addition of antoxidants. Other oxidisable substances were similarly affected in the presence of macrogol groups.— E. Azaz *et al., Pharm. J.,* 1973, *2,* 15.

Pharmaceutical properties. Emulsifying properties and incompatibilities of a series of cetomacrogols.— J. W. Hadgraft, *J. Pharm. Pharmac.,* 1954, *6,* 816.

Uses. Cetomacrogol 1000 is used in the preparation of Cetomacrogol Emulsifying Wax, which can be employed for making oil-in-water emulsions that are unaffected by moderate concentrations of electrolytes and are stable over a wide pH range.

Cetomacrogol 1000 is used to disperse volatile oils in water to form transparent sols; a proportion of 10 parts of cetomacrogol to 1 part of volatile oil is used.

A hydrophilic basis containing cetomacrogol 1000 and a macrogol was used to administer drugs usually given by injection. Insulin was given by rectum or by vagina to diabetic *rats,* and had a hypoglycaemic effect; heparin given similarly had an anticoagulant effect.— E. Touitou *et al., J. Pharm. Pharmac.,* 1978, *30,* 662.

446-r

Lauromacrogols. Macrogol Lauryl Ethers.

CAS — 9002-92-0.

Pharmacopoeias. Jap. includes Lauromacrogol, a macrogol ether prepared by the additive polymerisation of ethylene oxide with lauryl alcohol.

A series of lauryl ethers of macrogols of differing chain lengths.

Lauromacrogols have been used as surfactants and spermicides.

A report of an uncontrolled study in 496 patients with acne of the use of a lauromacrogol in conjunction with calamine and sulphur in skin lotions to promote topical drying and peeling.— S. M. Bluefarb *et al., J. Am. med. Ass.,* 1960, *173,* 40.

447-f

Laureth 4.
$C_{12}H_{25}.[O.CH_2.CH_2]_4.OH$ (nominal)=362.5.

A mixture of monolauryl ethers of macrogols containing an average of 4 oxyethylene groups in the polyoxyethylene chain.

448-d

Laureth 9. Hydroxypolyethoxydodecane; Polidocanol.
$C_{12}H_{25}.[O.CH_2.CH_2]_9.OH$ (nominal)=582.8.

A mixture of monolauryl ethers of macrogols containing an average of 9 oxyethylene groups in the polyoxyethylene chain.

Adverse Effects.
Extensive lichenified and excoriated dermatitis of the perianal and vulval skin in a woman following the use of Anacal Rectal Ointment was attributed, following sensitivity testing, to an ingredient of the ointment, laureth 9.— C. D. Calnan, *Contact Dermatitis,* 1978, *4,* 168.

Uses. Laureth 9 has been used as a local anaesthetic, as a sclerosing agent, and as a spermicide.

The spermicidal activity and toxicity of laureth 9.— D. A. Berberian *et al., Toxic. appl. Pharmac.,* 1965, *7,* 206 and 215.

For a short discussion on the use of laureth 9 as a sclerosing agent, see *Drugs Today,* 1977, *13,* 243.

449-n

Lauromacrogol 400.
$C_{12}H_{25}.[O.CH_2.CH_2]_8.OH$ (nominal)=538.8.

A mixture of monolauryl ethers of macrogols containing an average of 8 oxyethylene groups in the polyoxyethylene chain.

450-k

Nonoxinols. Nonoxynols; Macrogol Nonylphenyl Ethers. α-(4-Nonylphenyl)-ω-hydroxypoly(oxyethylene).

CAS — 26027-38-3.

A series of nonylphenyl ethers of macrogols of differing chain lengths, represented by the formula $C_{15}H_{23}.[O.CH_2.CH_2]_n.OH$. Each nonoxinol name is followed by a number indicating the approximate number of oxyethylene groups in the polyoxyethylene chain.

Nonoxinols are used as surfactants and spermicides.

451-a

Nonoxinol 4. Nonoxynol 4. α-(4-Nonylphenyl)-ω-hydroxytetra(oxyethylene).
$C_{23}H_{40}O_5$ (nominal)=396.6.

CAS — 7311-27-5.

A nonoxinol containing an average of 4 oxyethylene groups in the polyoxyethylene chain.

Nonoxinol 4 is used as a surfactant.

452-t

Nonoxinol 9. Nonoxynol 9. α-(4-Nonylphenyl)-ω-hydroxynona(oxyethylene).
$C_{33}H_{60}O_{10}$ (nominal)=616.8.

A nonoxinol containing an average of 9 oxyethylene groups in the polyoxyethylene chain.

Adverse Effects.
Severe cystitis occurred in a woman who had a contraceptive pessary containing nonoxinol 9 placed inadvertently in her bladder. The bladder was irrigated with copious amounts of saline and she was given ampicillin and antispasmodics. Her acute symptoms slowly resolved over 18 days.— J. E. Gottesman (letter), *New Engl. J. Med.,* 1980, *302,* 633.

Uses. Nonoxinol 9 is employed as a spermicide in several contraceptive preparations.

Encouraging preliminary results with a 5% cream of nonoxinol 9 in the treatment of recurrent genital herpes simplex infection.— H. J. Donsky (letter), *New Engl. J. Med.*, 1979, *300*, 371. Criticism of the use of an uncontrolled study.— G. L. Goodhart and M. E. Guinan (Letter), *ibid.*, 1338. Reply.— H. J. Donsky (letter), *ibid.* Lack of beneficial effect of nonoxinol 9 cream in a double-blind placebo-controlled study in patients with genital herpes simplex.— L. A. Vontrer *et al.*, *Am. J. Obstet. Gynec.*, 1979, *133*, 548.

A discussion on the use of topical spermicides for contraception.— *Med. Lett.*, 1980, *22*, 90.

453-x

Nonoxinol 10. Nonoxynol 10 *(U.S.N.F.)*. α-(4-Nonylphenyl)-ω-hydroxydeca(oxyethylene).
$C_{35}H_{64}O_{11}$ (nominal)=660.9.

Pharmacopoeias. In *U.S.N.F.* which specifies that *n* in the general formula $C_{15}H_{23}.[O.CH_2.CH_2]_n.OH$ varies from 6 to 16.

A colourless to light amber-coloured viscous liquid with an aromatic odour. Specific gravity 1.04 to 1.06. **Soluble** in water and in polar organic solvents. A 1% solution in water has a pH of 6 to 8. **Store** in airtight containers.

Nonoxinol 10 is used as a spermicidal agent. Nonoxinol 11 is similarly used.

454-r

Nonoxinol 15. Nonoxynol 15. α-(4-Nonylphenyl)-ω-hydroxypentadeca(oxyethylene).
$C_{45}H_{84}O_{16}$ (nominal)=881.1.

A nonoxinol containing an average of 15 oxyethylene groups in the polyoxyethylene chain.

Nonoxinol 15 is used as a surfactant.

455-f

Nonoxinol 30. Nonoxynol 30. α-(4-Nonylphenyl)-ω-hydroxytriaconta(oxyethylene).
$C_{75}H_{144}O_{31}$ (nominal)=1541.9.

A nonoxinol containing an average of 30 oxyethylene groups in the polyoxyethylene chain.

Nonoxinol 30 is used as a surfactant.

456-d

Octoxinols.

Octoxynols; Macrogol Tetramethylbutylphenyl Ethers; Octylphenoxy Polyethoxyethanol. α-[4-(1,1,3,3-Tetramethylbutyl)phenyl]-ω-hydroxypoly(oxyethylene).

CAS — 9002-93-1.

A series of tetramethylbutylphenyl ethers of macrogols of differing chain lengths, represented by the formula $C_{14}H_{21}.[O.CH_2.CH_2]_n.OH$. Each octoxinol name is followed by a number indicating the approximate number of oxyethylene groups in the polyoxyethylene chain.

Octoxinols are used as surfactants and spermicides.

457-n

Octoxinol 9.
$C_{32}H_{58}O_{10}$ (nominal)=602.8.

An octoxinol containing an average of 9 oxyethylene groups in the polyoxyethylene chain.

458-h

Octoxynol 9 *(U.S.N.F.)*. Octoxynol 9 is stated to contain an average of 5 to 15 oxyethylene groups in the polyoxyethylene chain.
$C_{34}H_{62}O_{11}$ (nominal number of oxyethylene groups=10)=647.

Pharmacopoeias. In *U.S.N.F.*

It is a clear, pale yellow, viscous liquid with a faint odour and a bitter taste. Specific gravity 1.059 to 1.068. **Miscible** with water, alcohol, and acetone; soluble in toluene; practically insoluble in light petroleum. A 1% w/v solution in water has a pH of 6 to 8. **Store** in airtight containers.

Octoxinol 9 and octoxynol 9 are used as spermicides.

459-m

Polyoxyl 20 Cetostearyl Ether *(U.S.N.F.)*.

Pharmacopoeias. In *U.S.N.F.*

A mixture of the monocetostearyl (mixed hexadecyl and octadecyl) ethers of mixed macrogols, the average polymer length being equivalent to 17.2 to 25 oxyethylene units.
A cream-coloured waxy unctuous mass melting, when heated, to a clear brownish-yellow liquid. **Soluble** in water, alcohol, and acetone; practically insoluble in light petroleum. A 10% solution in water has a pH of 4.5 to 7.5. **Store** in a cool place in airtight containers.

Polyoxyl 20 cetostearyl ether is used as a surfactant.

460-t

Polyoxyl 10 Oleyl Ether *(U.S.N.F.)*. Polyethylene Glycol Mono-oleyl Ether.

CAS — 9004-98-2.

Pharmacopoeias. In *U.S.N.F.*

A mixture of the mono-oleyl ethers of mixed macrogols, the average polymer length being equivalent to 8.6 to 10.4 oxyethylene units. It may contain suitable stabilisers.
A soft white semisolid or pale yellow liquid with a bland odour. **Soluble** in water and alcohol; dispersible in liquid paraffin and propylene glycol with possible separation on standing. **Store** in a cool place in airtight containers.

Polyoxyl 10 oleyl ether is used as a surfactant.

461-x

Tyloxapol *(U.S.P.)*.

CAS — 25301-02-4.

Pharmacopoeias. In *U.S.*

A polymer of 4-(1,1,3,3-tetramethylbutyl)phenol with ethylene oxide and formaldehyde.
A viscous amber liquid, sometimes slightly turbid, with a slight aromatic odour. Slowly but freely **miscible** with water; soluble in chloroform, glacial acetic acid, carbon disulphide, carbon tetrachloride, and toluene. A 5% solution in water has a pH of 4 to 7. Aqueous solutions are **sterilised** by autoclaving; they should not be allowed to come into contact with metals. **Store** in airtight containers.

Adverse Effects.
Effects reported included pharyngitis or pharyngeal burning, bronchospasm, increased congestion in the chest, and a maculopapular rash. Pharyngitis could be avoided by administering the aerosol at a slower rate or by nasal administration. Bronchospasms were reported to have occurred when the aerosol solution was introduced directly into the trachea and occasionally in patients receiving aerosols.— J. B. Miller, *Clin. Med.*, 1967, *74* (Oct.), 37.

Uses. Tyloxapol is a nonionic surfactant of the alkyl aryl polyether alcohol type. Solutions have been used as an aqueous inhalation for hydrating and liquefying tenacious bronchopulmonary secretions. A 0.125% sterile solution is nebulised as a fine dry spray from a suitable device.

462-r

Preparations of Macrogol Ethers

Included below are various official preparations of cetomacrogol.

Cetomacrogol Cream *(B.P.)*. It may be prepared according to the following formulas for use as a diluent where specified: *Formula A,* Cetomacrogol emulsifying ointment 30 g, chlorocresol 100 mg, freshly boiled and cooled water, 69.9 g; *Formula B,* Cetomacrogol emulsifying ointment 30 g, benzyl alcohol 1.5 g, methyl hydroxybenzoate 150 mg, propyl hydroxybenzoate 80 mg, freshly boiled and cooled water 68.27 g. It must be recently prepared unless its microbiological quality is to be assessed. Aluminium tubes should not be used for Formula B creams unless the inner surface of the tubes is coated with a suitable lacquer.

To improve the preservation of the cream (formula A), the incorporation of 10 or 20% propylene glycol and 0.15% chlorocresol was investigated. The partitioning of chlorocresol into the aqueous phase was increased but calculations indicated that binding of cetomacrogol might reduce the effective concentration.— Pharm. Soc. Lab. Rep. P/75/24, 1975.

The physical stability, particularly when stored at refrigerator temperatures, of a cetomacrogol cream (formula A) was slightly reduced by the incorporation of 20% propylene glycol and 0.15% chlorocresol.— Pharm. Soc. Lab. Rep. P/76/16, 1976. Preparations of Betamethasone Valerate Cream *B.P.C. 1973* diluted 1 in 2 or 1 in 10 with this modified cetomacrogol cream exhibited physical stability when stored at 25° for 14 days.— Pharm. Soc. Lab. Rep. P/78/2, 1978..

Cetomacrogol Cream Aqueous *(A.P.F.)*. Non-ionic Cream; Sorbolene Cream. Cetomacrogol emulsifying wax 15 g, liquid paraffin 10 g, white soft paraffin 10 g, chlorocresol 100 mg, propylene glycol 5 ml, freshly boiled and cooled water to 100 g.

Cetomacrogol Emulsifying Ointment *(B.P.)*. Cetomacrogol emulsifying wax 30 g, liquid paraffin 20 g, and white soft paraffin 50 g. Store at a temperature not exceeding 25°.

Cetomacrogol Emulsifying Wax *(B.P.)*. Non-ionic Emulsifying Wax. Cetomacrogol '1000' 20 g, cetostearyl alcohol 80 g.

Pressure Sore Cream *(Guy's Hosp.)*. Cetomacrogol emulsifying wax 10, liquid paraffin 20, Savlon hospital concentrate 1.5, sulphan blue solution 0.1, freshly boiled and cooled water to 100.

Proprietary Preparations of Macrogol Ethers and Related Compounds

Abracol LDS *(Bush Boake Allen, UK)*. An emulsifying agent consisting of a macrogol ether based on a fatty alcohol blended with a macrogol ester; used for oil-in-water emulsions and stable in the presence of electrolytes.

Alevaire *(Winthrop, UK)*. A sterile alkaline solution containing tyloxapol 0.125%, sodium bicarbonate 2%, and glycerol 5%. For the treatment of thickened or excessive bronchopulmonary secretions by inhalation as a fine dry mist. One vol. diluted with 4 vol. of sodium chloride injection may be used as a vehicle for antibiotics for the irrigation of infected bones and joints. (Also available as Alevaire in *Canad., Denm., Swed.*).

Ameroxol OE *(Amerchol, USA: Anstead, UK)*. A range of ethoxylated oleyl alcohols.

Antarox CO *(GAF, UK)*. A range of nonoxinols. Antarox CO is known in *USA* as Igepal CO.

Brij *(Atlas, UK)*. A brand name for a range of macrogol lauryl, cetyl, oleyl, and stearyl ethers.

Cirrasol AEN-XZ *(Atlas, UK)*. An octylphenol/ethylene oxide condensate containing an average of 7.5 oxyethylene groups per molecule.

Collone AC *(ABM Chemicals, UK)*. A macrogol ether emulsifying wax. **Collone NI.** A brand of Cetomacrogol Emulsifying Wax.

Cremophor A6 Solid *(BASF, Ger.: Blagden, UK)*. An ethoxylated saturated fatty alcohol, for use as an oil-in-water or water-in-oil emulsifying agent. **Cremophor**

A25. An ethoxylated saturated fatty alcohol (HLB value 15 to 17), for use as an oil-in-water emulsifying agent.

The name Cremophor is also applied to a range of macrogol esters, see above.

Crodafos *(Croda, UK)*. A brand name for a range of phosphated macrogol ethers based on Volpo products, see below.

For information on the formulation and properties of clear gels prepared from Crodafos, Volpo, and Polychol surfactants, see E. S. Lower and W. H. Harding, *Mfg Chem.*, 1966, *37* (Sept.), 52.

Crodex N *(Croda, UK)*. A brand of Cetomacrogol Emulsifying Wax.

Cyclogol 1000 *(Witco, UK)*. A brand of cetomacrogol 1000.

Cyclogol NI *(Witco, UK)*. A brand of Cetomacrogol Emulsifying Wax.

Empilan KB, KL, KM, and NP Series *(Albright & Wilson, Marchon Division, UK)*. Ranges of macrogol lauryl, cetyl/oleyl, cetyl/stearyl, and nonylphenyl ethers respectively.

Emulsene 1219 *(Bush Boake Allen, UK)*. A nonionic emulsifying agent consisting of a macrogol cetylstearyl ether blended with cetostearyl alcohol. **Emulsene 1220** is similar but produces emulsions of lower viscosity.

Fomescol *(ABM Chemicals, UK)*. A range of macrogol ethers.

Lubrol *(ICI Organics, UK)*. A range of macrogol ethers. **Lubrol N13** is a nonoxinol containing an average of 13 oxyethylene groups per molecule.

Promulgens *(Amerchol, USA: Anstead, UK)*. A range of nonionic emulsifying and gelling agents, stable over a wide pH range, consisting of fatty alcohol/ethylene oxide condensate products.

Surfactant 'T' Series *(BP Chemicals, UK: Hythe, UK)*. A range of nonionic and anionic surfactants.

Synperonics *(ICI Petrochemicals, UK)*. A brand name for a range of macrogol ethers, including nonoxinols and octylphenol/ethylene oxide condensates.

Texofor *(ABM Chemicals, UK)*. A range of macrogol ethers and esters derived from monohydric alcohols (types A and B), saturated (type E) and unsaturated (type M) fatty acids, alkylphenols (type F), and castor oil (type D). **Texofor A1P** is a brand of cetomacrogol 1000.

Volpo CS20 *(Croda, UK)*. A brand of cetomacrogol 1000.

Volpo N *(Croda, UK)*. A brand name for a range of macrogol oleyl ethers; a number following the name indicates the number of oxyethylene groups combined with 1 molecule of oleyl alcohol, and those available include Volpo N 3, 5, 10, 15, and 20.

Other Proprietary Names

Aethoxysklerol *(laureth 9) (Aust., Belg., Ger., Neth., Rus., Swed., Switz.)*; Aetoxisclérol *(laureth 9) (Fr.)*; Lacermuscin *(tyloxapol) (Spain)*; Phlebodestal *(laureth 9) (Ger.)*; Sclerovein *(laureth 9) (Switz.)*; Sotravarix *(laureth 9) (Belg., Switz.)*.

Some Proprietary Contraceptive Preparations of Macrogol Ethers

C-Film *(Potter & Clarke, UK)*. A contraceptive film impregnated with nonoxinol '9' 67 mg, which dissolves to form a gel-like solution.

There were 9 pregnancies in 45 women over a total of 175 months in which C-Film was used as a contraceptive. The Family Planning Association did not recommend the product as a sole contraceptive.— M. Smith *et al.* (letter), *Br. med. J.*, 1974, *4*, 291. See also *Drug & Ther. Bull.*, 1974, *12*, 87; *Pharm. J.*, 1975, *1*, 103.

C-Film was used as the sole contraceptive by 237 women over 1866 months when 14 pregnancies occurred. The use effectiveness rate was calculated as 9 per 100 woman-years. Most of the failures were due to incorrect use of the contraceptive.— N. Raabe and O. Frankman (letter), *Br. med. J.*, 1975, *4*, 286.

Delfen *(Ortho-Cilag, UK)*. A contraceptive available as **Vaginal Cream** (pH 4.5) containing nonoxinol '9' 5% in an oil-in-water emulsion basis, and as **Vaginal Foam** (pH 4.5 to 5) containing nonoxinol '9' 12.5% in an aerosol foam basis. (Also available as Delfen in *Arg., Austral., Belg., Canad., Ger., Neth., Switz., USA*).

Double Check *(Family Planning Sales, UK)*. Contraceptive pessaries containing nonoxinol '9' 6%.

Duragel *(LRC Products, UK)*. A contraceptive gel containing nonoxinol '9' 2%, carbomer 1.4%, glycerol 25%, sodium dinonyl sulphosuccinate 0.1%, and methyl hydroxybenzoate 0.2%. **Duracreme**. A contraceptive cream containing in addition zinc stearate 5%.

Emko Vaginal Foam *(Syntex, UK)*. An aerosol contraceptive containing nonoxinol '9' 8% and benzethonium chloride 0.2%, pH 7.6. (Also available as Emko in *USA*).

Emko Vaginal Foam was used as a contraceptive by 2923 women for 28 322 cycles. The pregnancy rate was 3.98 per 100 woman-years.— G. S. Bernstein, *Contraception*, 1971, *3*, 37, per *Int. pharm. Abstr.*, 1972, *9*, 160.

Genexol *(Rendell, UK)*. Contraceptive pessaries containing nonoxinols '10' and '11' 5% in a basis containing palm kernel oil. (Also available as Genexol in *Switz.*).

Ortho Creme *(Ortho-Cilag, UK)*. A cream (buffered to vaginal pH) containing nonoxinol '9' 2%. For use as a contraceptive with a vaginal diaphragm. (Also available as Ortho-Creme in *Canad., Ger., USA*).

Orthoforms Pessaries *(Ortho-Cilag, UK)*. Contraceptive pessaries containing nonoxinol '9' 5%. (Also available as Ortho-forms in *Belg.*).

Ortho-Gynol *(Ortho-Cilag, UK)*. A vaginal jelly (pH 4.5) containing *p*-di-isobutyl-phenoxypolyethoxyethanol 1%. For use as a contraceptive with a vaginal diaphragm. (Also available as Ortho-Gynol in *Fr., USA*).

Rendell's Pessaries *(Rendell, UK)*. Contraceptive pessaries containing nonoxinols '10' and '11' 5% in a basis containing fractionated palm kernel oil.

Staycept *(Syntex, UK)*. Contraceptive preparations available as **Jelly** containing octoxynol 9 (*U.S.N.F.*) 1% and as **Pessaries** containing nonoxinol '9' 6%.

Two's Company *(Family Planning Sales, UK)*. A composite pack of contraceptive pessaries containing nonoxinols, '10' and '11', 5% and condoms.

Other Proprietary Names

Because Contraceptor, Conceptrol, Encare, Koromex, Koromex II-A *(all nonoxinol 9) (all USA)*; Koromex II *(an octoxinol) (USA)*; Orthodelfen *(nonoxinol 9) (Denm., Fr., Norw.)*; Patenex *(nonoxinol 9) (Ger.)*; Ramses, Semicid, S'Positive *(all nonoxinol 9) (all USA)*.

Contraceptive preparations containing macrogol ethers were also formerly marketed in Great Britain under the proprietary names Antemin (*Napp*) and Preceptin (*Ortho*).

463-f

Poloxamers

CAS — 9003-11-6.

A series of nonionic polyoxyethylene-polyoxypropylene copolymers with the general formula $HO(C_2H_4O)_a(C_3H_6O)_b(C_2H_4O)_cH$, where $a=c$. They are prepared by reacting propylene oxide with propylene glycol to form a polyoxypropylene base chain; as the molecular weight of the chain is increased above 900, it becomes more hydrophobic. By the addition of hydrophilic polyoxyethylene chains to each end of the polyoxypropylene chain, surface-active polymers are obtained. The hydrophilic chains constitute 10 to 80% of the molecule and the molecular weight of the grades varies from about 1000 to over 16 000.

The first 2 digits of the number following the poloxamer name represent, when multiplied by 100, the approximate average molecular weight of the polyoxypropylene portion of the molecule; the third digit represents, when multiplied by 10, the percentage by weight of the polyoxyethylene portion.

The available grades vary from liquids through pastes to solid waxy flakes. Their properties range from hydrophobic liquids practically **insoluble** in water to solids which are very soluble in water and have high HLB values. Some grades are virtually tasteless in the concentrations normally used. Solutions are **sterilised** by autoclaving.

For definitions of individual poloxamers, see *J. Am. med. Ass.*, 1971, *217*, 470; *ibid.*, 1973, *224*, 1294.

Incompatibility. Poloxamers were incompatible with phenol, resorcinol, and betanaphthol in certain concentrations. In formulating preparations containing phenols and poloxamers preliminary experiments should be carried out to find conditions under which precipitation might be avoided.— A. D. Marcus *et al.*, *J. Am. pharm. Ass., pract. Pharm. Edn*, 1956, *17*, 453.

Pluronic L 62 could inactivate quaternary ammoniun compounds.— *J. Am. pharm. Ass., scient. Edn*, 1960, *49*, 430.

Pharmaceutical properties. There were regular trends in all physical properties in the poloxamer series. Water solubility increased with polyoxyethylene content and decreased with polyoxypropylene content, but wetting power showed the reverse effect. The poloxamers were in general soluble in alcohols, aromatic solvents, chlorinated solvents, Carbitols, Cellosolves, higher glycols, and ketones, and insoluble in ethylene glycol, glycerol, kerosene, and mineral oil. The critical micelle concentration was much lower than other nonionic surfactants and conferred high solubilising powers.— L. Raphael, *Mfg Chem.*, 1968, *39* (Jan.), 44.

Adverse Effects. Poloxamers may increase the absorption of liquid paraffin and other fat-soluble substances.

For a survey of the toxicology of the poloxamers in *animals*, see C. W. Leaf, *Soap chem. Spec.*, 1967, *43* (Aug.), 48. See also C. D. Port and P. J. Garvin, *Toxic. appl. Pharmac.*, 1976, *37*, 98; C. D. Port *et al.*, *ibid.*, 1978, *44*, 401.

Uses. Poloxamers are used as emulsifying agents for intravenous fat emulsions, as solubilising agents to maintain clarity in elixirs and syrups, and as wetting agents for antibiotics.

An emulsion of a fluorocarbon with a poloxamer could dissolve oxygen and had been tried in *rats* as a blood substitute. A typical formula was: poloxamer 2.2 g, fluorocarbon FC47 (perfluorotributylamine) 15 to 20 ml, hetastarch 3 g, dextrose 100 mg, potassium chloride 32 mg, magnesium chloride 7 mg, monobasic sodium phosphate 9.6 mg, sodium chloride 54 mg, calcium chloride 18 mg, sodium carbonate to pH 7.44, water to 100 ml. The emulsion was gassed with 95% oxygen and 5% carbon dioxide to adjust pH to 7.44. Streptomycin, penicillin, and phenolsulphonphthalein could be added.— R. P. Geyer, *New Engl. J. Med.*, 1973, *289*, 1077. See also *idem*, *Bull. parent. Drug Ass.*, 1974, *28*, 88; *Lancet*, 1974, *1*, 126.

464-d

Poloxalene. SKF 18,667.
$HO(C_2H_4O)_{12}(C_3H_6O)_{34}(C_2H_4O)_{12}H$ (average)=3000 (approximate).

Uses. Poloxalene is a poloxamer used as a defoaming agent in the treatment of bloat in ruminants.

465-n

Poloxamer 188. Poloxalkol.

$HO(C_2H_4O)_{75}(C_3H_6O)_{30}(C_2H_4O)_{75}H$ (average)=8350 (approximate).

White almost odourless and tasteless waxy flakes. M.p. about 52°. Freely **soluble** in water, alcohol, and chloroform; sparingly soluble in ether; practically insoluble in propylene glycol.

Adverse Effects. As for Poloxamers, above.

Uses. Poloxamer 188 is a nonionic surfactant which is used in medicine for the treatment of constipation. It lowers the surface tension of intestinal fluids, thus softening the faeces, and may be given in conjunction with a laxative such as danthron. The usual dose is 400 to 800 mg daily.

Cardiopulmonary bypass. Pluronic F 68 prevented the accumulation of blood-lipid emboli formed by a pump oxygenator during prolonged cardiopulmonary bypass experiments in *dogs*. It was thereafter used routinely for all operations involving cardiopulmonary bypass. A 10% solution was sterilised by autoclaving and added to heparinised blood at the rate of 600 μg per ml.— J. E. Adams *et al.*, *Surg. Forum*, 1959, *10*, 585.

Intravenous fat emulsions. In a study of the intravenous infusion of fat emulsions, phosphatides, and emulsifying agents, it was found that a solution of Pluronic 'F 68' 0.2% and egg yolk phosphatides 1.2% in 5% dextrose solution gave rise to no reactions when infused on 27 occasions.— O. Schuberth *et al.*, *Acta chir. scand.*, 1961, *Suppl* 278.

466-h

Proprietary Preparations of Poloxamers and Related Compounds

Included here are proprietary preparations of the poloxamers described above and of related copolymers.

Pluronics *(Pechiney, UK).* A range of poloxamers, including **Pluronic F38** (poloxamer 108, a solid grade, HLB 30.5), **Pluronic L62** (poloxamer 182, a liquid grade, HLB 7), and **Pluronic F68** (poloxamer 188, HLB 29).

Supronics *(ABM Chemicals, UK).* A range of polyoxyethylene-polyoxypropylene copolymers, including B and E series.

Tetronics *(Pechiney, UK).* A range of polyoxyethylene-polyoxypropylene copolymers based on ethylenediamine: HLB values range from 2 to 28.

Other Proprietary Names

Alaxin *(poloxamer 188) (USA)*; Alkènide *(a poloxamer) (Fr.)*; Coloxyl *(poloxamer 188) (see also under Docusate Sodium) (Austral.)*; Falkas *(poloxamer 188) (Arg.)*; Idrocol *(poloxamer 188) (Fr.)*; Pliagel *(poloxamer 407) (USA)*.

467-m

Polyvinyl Alcohols

These are complex and variable mixtures obtained by the hydrolysis of polyvinyl acetate.

468-b

Polyvinyl Alcohol *(U.S.P.).*

CAS — 9002-89-5.

Pharmacopoeias. In *U.S.*

A synthetic resin represented by the formula $(-CH_2CHOH-)_n$, where the average value of *n* is 500 to 5000. It is prepared by 87 to 89% hydrolysis of polyvinyl acetate.

White to cream-coloured odourless granules or powder. Freely **soluble** in water; more rapidly soluble at higher temperatures. A 4% solution in water has a pH of 5 to 8.

Uses. Polyvinyl alcohols are strongly hydrophilic and are therefore not very satisfactory as oil-in-water emulsifying agents. About 30% of oil may be emulsified with 1% of polyvinyl alcohol but the emulsion is liable to cream. Solutions in water are viscous mucilages, which resemble those formed by methylcellulose, and they are used in concentrations of 1% to stabilise emulsions which already contain a surfactant such as soap. The viscosity of the mucilages may be greatly increased by incorporating sodium perborate or silicate.

Polyvinyl alcohols may be used to increase the viscosity of ophthalmic preparations thus prolonging contact of the active ingredient with the eye and are present in some ocular lubricants and contact lens wetting solutions. They have also been used in the preparation of jellies which dry rapidly when applied to the skin to form a soluble plastic film; drugs incorporated in the jelly come into intimate contact with the skin and bandaging becomes unnecessary.

A review of methods of manufacture, solubility, reactions, and uses of polyvinyl alcohol.— R. Chudzikowski, *Mfg Chem.*, 1970, *41* (July), 31.

Eye preparations. Polyvinyl alcohol 1.4% in iso-osmotic saline was non-irritant to *rabbits'* eyes when administered subconjunctivally or intra-ocularly.— N. Krishna and B. Mitchell, *Am. J. Ophthal.*, 1965, *59*, 860.

A viscous ophthalmic vehicle containing polyvinyl alcohol 1.4%, sodium chloride 0.9%, and thiomersal 0.001%, and sterilised by autoclaving for 30 minutes at 120°, was found suitable for prolonging the activity in the eye of various alkaloids, antibacterials, steroids, and metallic salts.— I. vonGrósz and G. vonTakácsiNagy, *Arzneimittel-Forsch.*, 1967, *17*, 1213. See also R. Hardberger *et al.*, *Archs Ophthal., N.Y.*, 1975, *93*, 42.

Preparations

For details of jelly preparations containing polyvinyl alcohols, see Martindale 27th Edn, p. 325.

Liquifilm Tears *(Allergan, UK).* Eye-drops containing polyvinyl alcohol 1.4%. For use as artificial tears. (Also available as Liquifilm in *Arg., Austral., Belg., Canad.*).

Polyviol *(Wacker-Chemie, Ger.: Wacker Chemicals, UK).* A range of polyvinyl alcohols. The products are classified on the basis of their viscosity and saponification value.

Other Proprietary Names

Lacril *(Denm.)*; Pre-Sert *(Austral.)*.

469-v

Quillaia *(B.P.).* Quillaia Bark; Quillaiae Cortex; Panama Wood; Soap Bark; Seifenrinde.

CAS — 631-01-6 (quillaic acid).

Pharmacopoeias. In *Arg., Aust., Br., Ind., Nord., Port.,* and *Swiss. Br.* also includes Powdered Quillaia.

The dried inner part of the bark of *Quillaja saponaria* and other species of *Quillaja* (Rosaceae), containing not less than 22% of alcohol (45%)-soluble extractive. Quillaia has an acrid astringent taste. It is odourless but the dust or powder is strongly sternutatory. It contains 2 amorphous saponin glycosides, quillaic acid and quillaiasapotoxin.

Adverse Effects. Quillaia taken by mouth is a violent irritant, producing gastro-enteritis, with nausea, vomiting, epigastric pain, and persistent diarrhoea. In severe poisoning gastro-intestinal lesions may be formed and absorption of quillaia may occur with effects including liver damage, irritation of the bladder, respiratory failure, convulsions, and coma.

Quillaia causes haemolysis of red blood cells *in vitro* and after intravenous administration.

Treatment of Adverse Effects. Empty the stomach by aspiration and lavage and give a demulcent, such as milk, white of egg, or liquid paraffin. The circulation should be maintained with infusions of plasma or suitable electrolyte solutions, and electrolyte and water imbalance should be corrected. If haemolysis is severe, blood transfusions may be necessary. Respiration may require assistance.

Uses. The emulsifying power of the saponins in quillaia is due mainly to their ability to cause a considerable reduction in interfacial tension, and though useful emulsifying agents, they are used mainly as frothing agents. Saponins have little effect on viscosity, and emulsions containing them tend to 'cream' rapidly; for this reason, tragacanth mucilage or another thickening agent is often added. Quillaia causes frothing in water in which it has been macerated.

Quillaia is used, in the form of a liquid extract or tincture, as an emulsifying agent, especially for creosote and tar preparations, for chloroform, and for small quantities of volatile oils. It was formerly given by mouth as a reflex expectorant in bronchitis.

Preparations

Quillaia Liquid Extract *(B.P.).* Quillaia Liq. Ext. 1 in 1; prepared by percolation with alcohol (45%). *Arg. P.* and *Nord. P.* include a similar preparation.

Quillaia Tincture *(B.P.).* Quillaia liquid extract 5 ml, alcohol (45%) to 100 ml. Several other pharmacopoeias include a tincture (usually 1 in 5) prepared by percolation of quillaia with alcohol.

470-r

Saponin *(B.P.C. 1954).* Quillain.

CAS — 8047-15-2.

A mixture containing glycosides, obtained from quillaia. It is a white to light brown, intensely irritating, sternutatory, amorphous powder with a sweetish, afterwards bitter and acrid, burning taste.

Soluble in water and hot alcohol; practically insoluble in most organic solvents. Its solubility in water is increased by the addition of a small amount of alkali. Aqueous solutions froth readily when shaken; the froth is very persistent but is easily dispersed by alcohol or ether.

Saponin has too strong a haemolytic action and is too irritant to the gastro-intestinal tract to be used internally. It has been used to emulsify fixed and volatile oils for external application and as a frothing agent for various technical purposes.

471-f

Sorbitan Derivatives

The elimination of a molecule of water from the hexahydric alcohol sorbitol results in the formation of tetrahydric monocyclic inner ethers or anhydrides called sorbitans; elimination of a second molecule of water yields dihydric dicyclic ethers called sorbides.Esterification of one or more of the hydroxyl groups in the sorbitans with a fatty acid, such as stearic, palmitic, oleic, or lauric acid, produces oil-soluble water-dispersible nonionic *sorbitan esters* with surface-active properties. Derivatives of other polyhydric alcohols, such as mannitol, may be used instead of the sorbitol derivatives. Substances of these types in which the hydrophobic properties just predominate are effective water-in-oil emulsifiers. If the hydrophilic properties of these ether-esters are made more predominant by causing them to react with ethylene oxide so that polyoxyethylene chains are introduced into the molecule, water-soluble nonionic *polysorbates* are produced which are oil-in-water emulsifying agents.

By varying the number of oxyethylene groups introduced into the molecules (in the chemical name this number is often indicated after the word polyoxyethylene) and having different fatty acids in the ether-esters, surfactants with a wide range of properties may be obtained. These nonionic surfactants are pale yellow to reddish-brown oily liquids of varying viscosity, or white, yellowish, or tan, waxy solids or semi-solids with a bitter taste. They are neutral, thermostable, and non-volatile.

Most are **soluble** or dispersible in alcohol, ether, and carbon tetrachloride; some are soluble or dispersible in fixed oils and in mineral oils; the polysorbates are mostly soluble or dispersible in water, but the sorbitan esters are practically insoluble in water. They are miscible with one another. They vary in solubilising power from batch to batch.

Polysorbates are **incompatible** with alkalis, heavy metal salts, phenols, and tannins; they reduce the activity of many preservatives.

The reduction of preservative activity. — J. L. Wailes, *J. pharm. Sci.*, 1962, *51*, 165; N. K. Patel and N. E. Foss, *ibid.*, 1964, *53*, 94; C. K. Bahal and H. B. Kostenbauder, *ibid.*, 1027; M. D. Ray *et al.*, *ibid.*, 1968, *57*, 609.

Polysorbate 80 became bound to cetylpyridinium chloride, crystal violet, chlorpromazine, promethazine, and amethocaine ions in aqueous solutions. This interaction adversely influenced the release and availability for use of these drugs when incorporated in preparations for topical use. No significant interaction was observed with solutions of ephedrine hydrochloride, sulphathiazole sodium, methapyrilene hydrochloride, procaine hydrochloride, and diphenhydramine hydrochloride.— A. R. Hurwitz *et al.*, *J. pharm. Sci.*, 1963, *52*, 893.

Polysorbate 80 in aqueous solutions was salted out by the addition of concentrated solutions of inorganic salts.— Z. Plotkowiak, *Acta Pol. pharm.*, 1971, *28*, 35.

Preservatives for solutions. The following were effective preservatives for solutions of nonionic surfactants: sorbic acid (0.2%), 5-hydroxymethyl-2-furoic acid (0.15%), phenylmercuric borate (0.007%), phenylmercuric nitrate (0.01%), phenylmercuric acetate (0.007%), captan (0.04%), diethylene glycol monomethyl ether (3%), hexylene glycol (3%), and benzalkonium chloride

(0.1%). Complex formation between phenolic and polyoxyethylene groups might account for the failure of various phenolic preservatives.— M. Barr and L. F. Tice, *Pharm. J.*, 1956, *2*, 88.

Solubilising properties. Batches of polysorbate 80 varied in their ability to solubilise vitamin A palmitate in a glycerol and water vehicle.— P. F. G. Boon *et al.*, *J. Pharm. Pharmac.*, 1961, *13*, 200T.

Stability in solution. As aqueous solutions of polysorbates underwent autoxidation on storage it was suggested that stricter standards were needed for the quality control and storage of these materials.— M. Donbrow *et al.*, *J. pharm. Sci.*, 1978, *67*, 1676.

472-d

Polysorbate 20 *(B.P., Eur. P.).* Polysorbatum 20; Sorbimacrogol Laurate 300; Polyoxyethylene 20 Sorbitan Monolaurate; Sorboxaethenum Laurinicum.
$C_{58}H_{114}O_{26}$ (nominal) = 1227.5.

CAS — 9005-64-5.

Pharmacopoeias. In *Br.*, *Eur.*, *Fr.*, *Ger.*, *Hung.*, *It.*, *Neth.*, and *Swiss.* Also in *U.S.N.F.*

A mixture of partial lauric esters of sorbitol and its mono-and di-anhydrides copolymerised with approximately 20 moles of ethylene oxide for each mole of sorbitol and its anhydrides. The lauric acid used for esterification may contain variable amounts of other fatty acids.
A clear yellowish or brownish-yellow oily liquid with a faint characteristic odour and a somewhat bitter taste. Relative density about 1.1; viscosity, at 25°, about 400 cP.
Miscible with water, alcohol, dioxan, ethyl acetate, and methyl alcohol; soluble 1 in 125 of cottonseed oil and 1 in 200 of toluene; practically insoluble in light petroleum, liquid paraffin, and fixed oils. A 5% solution in water has a pH of 5 to 7. **Store** in airtight containers. Protect from light.

427-a

Polysorbate 40. Sorbimacrogol Palmitate 300; Polyoxyethylene 20 Sorbitan Monopalmitate.
$C_{62}H_{122}O_{26}$ (nominal) = 1283.6.

CAS — 9005-66-7.

Pharmacopoeias. In *U.S.N.F.*

A mixture of partial palmitic esters of sorbitol and its mono-and di-anhydrides copolymerised with approximately 20 moles of ethylene oxide for each mole of sorbitol and its anhydrides. A yellow oily liquid with a faint characteristic odour and a somewhat bitter taste. Sp. gr. at 25° about 1.08; viscosity, at 25°, about 600 cP.
Soluble in water, alcohol, acetone, ethyl acetate, methyl alcohol, and cottonseed oil; practically insoluble in liquid paraffin and in fixed oils. **Store** in airtight containers.

474-h

Polysorbate 60 *(B.P., Eur. P.).* Polysorbatum 60; Sorbimacrogol Stearate 300; Polyoxyethylene 20 Sorbitan Mono-stearate; Sorboxaethenum Stearinicum.
$C_{64}H_{126}O_{26}$ (nominal) = 1311.7.

CAS — 9005-67-8.

Pharmacopoeias. In *Br.*, *Eur.*, *Fr.*, *Ger.*, *Hung.*, *It.*, *Neth.*, and *Swiss.* Also in *U.S.N.F.*

A mixture of partial stearic esters of sorbitol and its mono-and di-anhydrides copolymerised with approximately 20 moles of ethylene oxide for each mole of sorbitol and its anhydrides. The stearic acid used for esterification may contain variable amounts of other fatty acids especially palmitic acid.
An opaque lemon-coloured or yellowish-brown semi-gel which becomes a clear liquid at about 24°; it has a faint characteristic odour and a slightly bitter taste. It usually contains a small amount of added water (not more than 3%) to obtain a product liquid at room temperature. Relative density about 1.1; viscosity, at 25°, about 600 cP.
Miscible with water, alcohol, acetone, methyl alcohol, and ethyl acetate; practically insoluble in liquid paraffin and fixed oils. A 5% solution in water has a pH of 5 to 8. **Store** in airtight containers. Protect from light.

475-m

Polysorbate 65. Sorbimacrogol Tristearate 300; Polyoxyethylene 20 Sorbitan Tristearate.
$C_{100}H_{194}O_{28}$ (nominal) = 1844.6.

CAS — 9005-71-4.

A mixture of partial stearic esters, mainly tristearate, of sorbitol and its mono- and di-anhydrides copolymerised with approximately 20 moles of ethylene oxide for each mole of sorbitol and its anhydrides.
A tan-coloured waxy solid with a faint characteristic odour and a waxy somewhat bitter taste. Congealing range 29° to 33°.
Dispersible in water and carbon tetrachloride; soluble in alcohol, acetone, dioxan, ether, light petroleum, liquid paraffin, methyl alcohol, and fixed oils.

476-b

Polysorbate 80 *(B.P., Eur. P.).* Polysorbatum 80; Sorbimacrogol Oleate 300; Polyoxyethylene 20 Sorbitan Mono-oleate; Olethytan 20; Sorethytan 20 Mono-oleate; Polyäthylenglykol-Sorbitan-oleat; Polysorbitanum 80 Oleinatum; Sorboxaethenum Oleinicum.
$C_{64}H_{124}O_{26}$ (nominal) = 1309.7.

CAS — 9005-65-6.

Pharmacopoeias. In *Arg.*, *Aust.*, *Br.*, *Braz.*, *Cz.*, *Eur.*, *Fr.*, *Ger.*, *Hung.*, *It.*, *Jap.*, *Neth.*, *Nord.*, *Port.*, *Roum.*, and *Swiss.* Also in *U.S.N.F.*

A mixture of partial oleic esters of sorbitol and its mono- and di-anhydrides copolymerised with approximately 20 moles of ethylene oxide for each mole of sorbitol and its anhydrides.
A clear yellowish or brownish-yellow oily liquid with a faint characteristic odour and a warm slightly bitter taste. Relative density about 1.08; viscosity, at 25°, about 400 cP.
Miscible with water, alcohol, chloroform, ether, ethyl acetate, and methyl alcohol; soluble 1 in 125 of cottonseed oil; practically insoluble in light petroleum, liquid paraffin, and fixed oils. A 5% w/v solution in water has a pH of 6 to 8. **Store** in airtight containers. Protect from light.

477-v

Polysorbate 85. Sorbimacrogol Trioleate 300; Polyoxyethylene 20 Sorbitan Trioleate.
$C_{100}H_{188}O_{28}$ (nominal) = 1838.6.

CAS — 9005-70-3.

A mixture of partial oleic esters, mainly trioleate, of sorbitol and its mono- and di-anhydrides copolymerised with approximately 20 moles of ethylene oxide for each mole of sorbitol and its anhydrides.
A lemon- to amber-coloured oily liquid with a faint characteristic odour and a somewhat bitter taste. Sp. gr. at 25° about 1.0; viscosity, at 25°, about 300 cP.
Dispersible in water; soluble in alcohol, ethyl acetate, methyl alcohol, and most vegetable oils; soluble in liquid paraffin but produces a hazy solution.

478-g

Sorbitan Monolaurate *(B.P.).* Sorbitan Laurate.
$C_{18}H_{34}O_6$ (nominal) = 346.5.

CAS — 1338-39-2.

Pharmacopoeias. In *Br.* Also in *U.S.N.F.*

A mixture of the partial esters of sorbitol and its mono- and di-anhydrides with lauric acid.
An amber-coloured viscous oily liquid with a characteristic odour. Wt per ml about 1 g; viscosity, at 25°, about 4500 cP.
Practically **insoluble** but dispersible in water and propylene glycol; miscible with alcohol and methyl alcohol; soluble 1 in 100 of cottonseed oil; slightly soluble in ethyl acetate. **Store** in airtight containers.

479-q

Sorbitan Mono-oleate *(B.P.).* Sorbitan Oleate.
$C_{24}H_{44}O_6$ (nominal) = 428.6.

CAS — 1338-43-8.

Pharmacopoeias. In *Br.* Also in *U.S.N.F.*

A mixture of the partial esters of sorbitol and its mono- and di-anhydrides with oleic acid.
An amber-coloured viscous oily liquid with a characteristic fatty odour and a bland taste. Wt per ml about 1 g; viscosity, at 25°, about 1000 cP.
Practically **insoluble** but dispersible in water; miscible with alcohol; soluble in liquid paraffin and fixed oils but produces a hazy solution; slightly soluble in ether; practically insoluble in acetone and propylene glycol. **Store** in airtight containers.

480-d

Sorbitan Monopalmitate. Sorbitan Palmitate.
$C_{22}H_{42}O_6$ (nominal) = 402.6.

CAS — 26266-57-9.

Pharmacopoeias. In *U.S.N.F.*

A mixture of the partial esters of sorbitol and its mono- and di-anhydrides with palmitic acid.
A light cream- to tan-coloured, hard, waxy solid with a characteristic odour and a bland taste. Congealing range 45° to 47°.
Practically **insoluble** in cold water and ethylene glycol; dispersible in warm water; soluble above its melting-point in alcohol, carbon tetrachloride, dioxan, ethyl acetate, methyl alcohol, light petroleum, and toluene; soluble with haze in cottonseed oil and, above 50°, in liquid paraffin.

481-n

Sorbitan Monostearate *(B.P.).* Sorbitan Stearate.
$C_{24}H_{46}O_6$ (nominal) = 430.6.

CAS — 1338-41-6.

Pharmacopoeias. In *Br.* Also in *U.S.N.F.*

A mixture of the partial esters of sorbitol and its mono- and di-anhydrides with stearic acid.
A pale yellow waxy solid with a faint oily odour and a bland taste. F.p. about 50°.
Practically **insoluble** in cold water, acetone, and light petroleum; dispersible in warm water;

soluble 1 in 120 of alcohol; soluble, above 50°, in carbon tetrachloride, methyl alcohol, and toluene; soluble with haze in cottonseed oil and, above 50°, in ethyl acetate and liquid paraffin.

482-h

Sorbitan Sesquioleate.

$C_{33}H_{60}O_{6.5}$ (nominal) = 560.8.

CAS — 8007-43-0.

Pharmacopoeias. In *Jap.* and *Swiss.*

A mixture of the partial mono- and di-esters of sorbitol and its mono- and di-anhydrides with oleic acid.

A pale yellow to light yellowish-brown viscous oily liquid with a faint characteristic odour and a slightly bitter taste. Wt per ml about 1.0 g; viscosity, at 25°, about 1500 cP.

Practically **insoluble** in water and propylene glycol; slightly soluble in alcohol; freely soluble in ether; soluble in liquid paraffin. **Protect** from light.

483-m

Sorbitan Trioleate.

$C_{60}H_{108}O_8$ (nominal) = 957.5.

CAS — 26266-58-0.

A mixture of the partial tri-esters of sorbitol and its mono-and di-anhydrides with oleic acid.

An amber-coloured oily liquid with a characteristic odour and a bland taste. Wt per ml about 0.95 g. Viscosity, at 25°, about 200 cP.

Dispersible in water; soluble in alcohol, acetone, ether, ethyl acetate, fixed oils, and liquid paraffin.

484-b

Sorbitan Tristearate.

$C_{60}H_{114}O_8$ (nominal) = 963.6.

CAS — 26658-19-5.

A mixture of the partial tri-esters of sorbitol and its mono-and di-anhydrides with stearic acid.

A light cream- to tan-coloured, granular, waxy solid with a slight characteristic odour and a bland taste. M.p. about 53°.

Practically **insoluble** in water, alcohol, and methyl alcohol; slightly soluble in carbon tetrachloride, ether, ethyl acetate, and toluene; dispersible in acetone, dioxan, fixed oils, light petroleum, and liquid paraffin.

Adverse Effects. The polysorbates may increase the absorption of liquid paraffin and other fat-soluble substances.

Polysorbate 80 was fed to human subjects in doses of 15 g daily for several months with no evidence of toxicity and the chance of oxalic acid poisoning from the polyoxyethylene component seemed negligible. Increased bowel activity was occasionally observed.— C. N. Jones *et al.*, *Ann. intern. Med.*, 1948, *29*, 1.

Intravenous fat emulsions stabilised by the addition of 0.5% of polysorbate 60 were not toxic to *rats* and *mice*, but were shown to be unsuitable for clinical use as the administration of small quantities caused reactions such as flushing of the face, epigastric or substernal distress, and cough in human patients.— G. F. Lambert *et al.*, *J. Am. pharm. Ass., scient. Edn*, 1956, *45*, 685.

In *rats*, repeated weekly subcutaneous injections of 6% polysorbate 60 induced fibrosarcomas in about 17%.— L. M. Lusky and A. A. Nelson, *Fedn Proc.*, 1957, *16*, Part 1, 318.

Application of polysorbate 60, six times weekly to *mouse* skin (12 g was used on a 25-g animal) produced weak carcinogenic action (2 malignant tumours in 60 mice) but the tumours induced mostly disappeared during the treatment.— P. Shubik (letter), *Soap Perfum. Cosm.*, 1958, *31*, 1166.

Polysorbate 80 was only absorbed to a very small extent. Amounts up to 6 g per day had been given to patients for periods up to 4 years with no serious side-effects.— T. D. Eickholt and W. F. White, *Drug Stand.*, 1960, *28*, 154.

For background toxicological information, see *Fd Add. Ser. Wld Hlth Org. No. 5*, 1974.

A 59-year-old woman who developed contact dermatitis after application of Alphaderm cream to the legs produced a positive patch test to sorbitan monolaurate 5% which was used as an emulsifier in the preparation.— O. A. Finn and A. Forsyth, *Contact Dermatitis*, 1975, *1*, 318.

Of 486 patients with eczema 2 gave positive patch tests to Arlacel '83' 20% and to a combination of Span '60' 5% and Span '80' 5%. In 412 of the patients one gave a positive patch test to a combination of Tween '40' 5% and Tween '80' 5%.— M. Hannuksela *et al.*, *Contact Dermatitis*, 1976, *2*, 105.

Further references: H. Maibach and M. Conant, *Contact Dermatitis*, 1977, *3*, 350 (contact urticaria due to polysorbate 60).

Uses. The sorbitan derivatives, and similar products, produce stable emulsions of fine texture, which are little affected by high concentrations of electrolytes or by changes in pH. The sorbitan esters are active water-in-oil emulsifying agents, while the polysorbates produce oil-in-water emulsions.

In practice, the use of 2 or more of these emulsifying agents has been found to give better results than the use of 1 alone; for example, an oil-in-water emulsion can be prepared using polysorbate 20 as the primary emulsifying agent and sorbitan monolaurate, which is much less hydrophilic, as a stabiliser. By varying the proportions and the types of emulsifying agent used, a complete range of preparations from water-in-oil to oil-in-water emulsions and creams of different texture and consistency may be produced.

These nonionic surfactants are used in pharmacy in the preparation of creams, water-soluble or washable ointments, and suppository bases, and for emulsifying fish-liver oils, vegetable oils, and mineral oils. They are also useful defoaming agents.

The polysorbates, particularly polysorbate 80, are used as solubilising agents for a variety of substances including essential oils, oil-soluble vitamins such as vitamins A and D in multivitamin products, and phenobarbitone. They are also used as wetting agents in the formulation of oral and parenteral suspensions. In medicine they may be used to promote increased absorption of dietary fat in conditions in which steatorrhoea is prominent, such as coeliac disease and sprue.

They are also used as surfactants in insecticide and pesticide sprays, as industrial detergents, in the manufacture of cosmetic creams, and as emulsifiers in the food industry.

The sorbitan esters may be added to paraffin ointment bases to form anhydrous bases capable of absorbing large amounts of water.

Estimated acceptable daily intake of sorbitan monopalmitate, monostearate, and tristearate: up to 25 mg, as total sorbitan esters, per kg body-weight. Estimated acceptable daily intake of polysorbates 20, 40, 60, 65, and 80: up to 25 mg, as total polysorbate esters, per kg body-weight.— Seventeenth Report of FAO/WHO Expert Committee on Food Additives, *Tech. Rep. Ser. Wld Hlth Org. No. 539*, 1974.

Deficiency in fat absorption. A study in 12 patients with steatorrhoea due to bile-salt deficiency suggested that a diet containing polysorbates may result in improved fat absorption.— R. F. G. J. King *et al.*, *Gut*, 1977, *18*, A 426. See also C. N. Jones *et al.*, *Ann. intern. Med.*, 1948, *29*, 1.

Mucoviscidosis. Only 3 of 24 consecutive patients with meconium ileus associated with mucoviscidosis survived for a month or more after surgery for relief of obstruction. Seventeen survived out of the next 23 patients who were given a 1% solution of polysorbate 80 in Tyrode solution in a dose of 5 ml by mouth, 5 to 10 ml by enterostomy, or 10 to 20 ml as an enema, all thrice daily. In 1 of the patients surgery was unnecessary as meconium was passed 36 hours after enemas and oral therapy were started.— A. C. Bowring *et al.*, *J. pediat. Surg.*, 1970, *5*, 338.

Polysorbate 80 oral preparations. The pharmaceutical problems involved in administering polysorbate 80 by mouth in average doses of 8 g daily were considered. When given with a polyhydric alcohol such as glycerol, propylene glycol, or sorbitol, citric acid, a fruit flavour, syrup, or combinations of these agents, the obnoxious taste could be modified to allow ingestion of polysorbate 80 in moderately large volume.— R. Bogash, *Bull. Am. Soc. Hosp. Pharmsts*, 1953, *10*, 365.

Preparation of ointment bases. The rate of release of antibiotic (benzylpenicillin, hamycin, or tetracycline hydrochloride) was increased by the addition to a paraffin basis of 1% of polysorbate 20, 60, or 80.— S. N. Sharma and S. D. Gupta, *Indian J. Pharm.*, 1967, *29*, 309.

Solubilising agent for the preparation of syrups. Polysorbate 20 might be used in the preparation of aromatic syrup of eriodictyon and syrups of tolu and orange. Suitable formulas were: (1) tincture of tolu 2.5, polysorbate '20' 15, glycerol 15, syrup to 50; mix the polysorbate 20 with the tincture, incorporate the glycerol, and add the syrup; (2) orange oil 0.5, polysorbate '20' 3, citric acid monohydrate 0.25, glycerol 5, syrup to 50; mix the orange oil with the polysorbate 20 and add the glycerol; dissolve the citric acid monohydrate in the syrup and add the oil mixture.— W. B. Swafford and W. L. Nobles, *J. Am. pharm. Ass., pract. Pharm. Edn*, 1955, *16*, 223.

Solubilising agent for vaccines. Sorbitan derivatives were used to solubilise aqueous *Clostridium welchii* toxoid in a light mineral oil adjuvant vaccine. The solubilised vaccines gave higher antibody concentrations in *guinea-pigs* than 2 doses of aluminium hydroxide adsorbed vaccine; they were more stable and of lower viscosity than emulsified vaccine.— C. L. J. Coles *et al.*, *J. Pharm. Pharmac.*, 1968, *20*, *Suppl.*, 26S.

Preparations of Sorbitan Derivatives

Emulsifying Wax *(U.S.N.F.)*. A creamy white solid with a characteristic odour, prepared from cetostearyl alcohol containing a polysorbate. M.p. 48° to 52°. It is practically insoluble in water, soluble in alcohol, and freely soluble in chloroform and in ether. A 3% dispersion in water has a pH of 5.5 to 7.0.

For Emulsifying Wax (*B.P.*), see p.1441.

Non-ionic Emulsifying Ointment *(F.N. Belg.)*. Polysorbate'80' 7 g, cetyl alcohol 17 g, sorbitol 15 g, white soft paraffin 25 g, water to 100 g.

Unguentum Emulsificans Non-ionicum *(Hung. P.)*. Nonionic Emulsifying Ointment. Polysorbate '60' 10 g, liquid paraffin 10 g, cetostearyl alcohol 30 g, white soft paraffin 50 g.

Unguentum Hydrophilicum I *(Swiss P.)*. Nonionic Hydrophilic Ointment. Cetyl alcohol 10 g, hydrogenated arachis oil 20 g, polysorbate '60' 5 g, propylene glycol 10 g, methyl hydroxybenzoate 70 mg, propyl hydroxybenzoate 30 mg, water to 100 g.

Unguentum Hydrophilicum Non-ionicum *(Hung. P.)*. Nonionic Hydrophilic Ointment. Nonionic emulsifying ointment 40 g, methyl hydroxybenzoate 140 mg and propyl hydroxybenzoate 60 mg in alcohol 1.8 g, water 58 g.

Proprietary Preparations of Sorbitan Derivatives

Crillets *(Croda, UK)*. A range of polysorbates, including **Crillet 1** (polysorbate 20, HLB 16.7), **Crillet 2** (polysorbate 40, HLB 15.6), **Crillet 3** (polysorbate 60, HLB 14.9), **Crillet 35** (polysorbate 65, HLB 10.5), **Crillet 4** (polysorbate 80, HLB 15), **Crillet 45** (polysorbate 85, HLB 11), and **Crillet 6** (polysorbate 120).

Crills *(Croda, UK)*. A range of sorbitan esters of fatty acids, including **Crill 1** (sorbitan monolaurate, HLB 8.6), **Crill 2** (sorbitan monopalmitate, HLB 6.7), **Crill 3** (sorbitan monostearate, HLB 4.7), **Crill 35** (sorbitan tristearate, HLB 2.1), **Crill 4** (sorbitan mono-oleate, HLB 4.3), **Crill 43** (sorbitan sesquioleate, HLB 3.7), **Crill 45** (sorbitan trioleate, HLB 1.8), and **Crill 6** (sorbitan mono-isostearate).

Polawax *(Croda, UK)*. A pale cream, stable, waxy solid prepared from cetostearyl alcohol and containing a polysorbate. It is an oil-in-water emulsifying and thickening agent, unaffected by heat and by high concentrations of electrolytes. **Polawax A 31** is a modified version for aerosol use.

Sorbanox *(Witco, UK)*. A range of polysorbate emulsifying agents.

Spans *(Atlas, UK)*. A range of sorbitan esters of fatty acids, including **Span 20** (sorbitan monolaurate, HLB 8.6), **Span 40** (sorbitan monopalmitate, HLB 6.7), **Span 60** (sorbitan monostearate, HLB 4.7), **Span 65** (sorbitan tristearate, HLB 2.1), **Span 80** (sorbitan mono-oleate, HLB 4.3), and **Span 85** (sorbitan trioleate, HLB 1.8). **Arlacels 20** to **85** are more highly purified preparations of similar composition. **Arlacel 83** is sorbitan sesquioleate (HLB 3.7).

Tweens *(Atlas, UK)*. A range of polysorbates including **Tween 20** (polysorbate 20, HLB 16.7), **Tween 40** (polysorbate 40, HLB 15.6), **Tween 60** (polysorbate 60, HLB 14.9), **Tween 65** (polysorbate 65, HLB 10.5), **Tween 80**

(polysorbate 80, HLB 15.0), and **Tween 85** (polysorbate 85, HLB 11.0). **Tween 80 TB** is a brand of polysorbate 80 intended specially for use in culture media for *Mycobacterium tuberculosis.*

Other Proprietary Names
Oleosorbate 80 *(*polysorbate 80*) (Fr., Switz.)*; Oleosorbato 80*(*polysorbate 80*) (Spain).*

485-v

Sucrose Esters

Esterification of 1 or more hydroxyl groups in sucrose with a fatty acid such as stearic or palmitic acid produces nonionic compounds which possess surface-active properties.

In the mono-esters of sucrose, esterification takes place in the glucose portion of the sugar. In the di-esters, a second fatty acid group is introduced in the fructose portion of the sugar. Commercial sucrose esters are mixtures of the mono-, di-, and tri-esters of palmitic and stearic acids with sucrose. Varying the proportion of mono-ester from 75 to 29% decreases the HLB value from 14.5 to 6.5.

The sucrose esters are used as dispersing and emulsifying agents in food and cosmetic preparations and have been suggested for use in pharmacy.

Temporary estimated acceptable daily intake of sucrose esters of fatty acids and sucroglycerides: up to 2.5 mg per kg body-weight either individually or as the sum of both. Further metabolic and toxicity studies were required.— Twentieth Report of the Joint FAO/WHO Expert Committee on Food Additives, *Tech. Rep. Ser. Wld Hlth Org. No. 599,* 1976.

For background toxicological information, see *Fd Add. Ser. Wld Hlth Org. No. 5,* 1974.

Further references: L. Osipow *et al., Drug Cosmet. Ind.,* 1957, *80,* 312; L. Osipow *et al., J. Am. Oil Chem. Soc.,* 1958, *35,* 65; H. Hopkins and L. D. Small, *J. Am. pharm. Ass., Scient. Edn,* 1960, *49,* 220; P. Rovesti, *Soap Perfum. Cosm.,* 1962, *35,* 139; R. Colson, *ibid.,* 1962, *35,* 145; S. M. Blaug and D. S. Ebersman, *J. pharm. Sci.,* 1964, *53,* 35; L. Raphael, *Mfg Chem.,* 1965, *36* (Mar.), 63.

Proprietary Preparations
Crodestas *(Croda, UK).* A range of sucrose esters including F-50 (HLB 6.5), F-70 (HLB 7.5), F-110 (HLB 12), F-140 (HLB 13), and F-160 (HLB 14.5).

Chelating Agents and some Drug Antagonists

1030-v

The chelating agents and drug antagonists described in this section are used mainly in the treatment of poisoning by substances such as heavy metals, cyanide, and organophosphorus insecticides, or in the treatment of various physiological disorders, including methaemoglobinaemia, hypercalcaemia, iron storage diseases, and Wilson's disease.

Chelating agents such as desferrioxamine, dimercaprol, penicillamine, and sodium calciumedetate selectively form soluble chelates with metal ions such as lead and mercury and promote the excretion of the metals from the body in a relatively non-toxic form. Chelating agents are also used to lower blood calcium and prevent calcium absorption in hypercalcaemia, and to prevent the formation of stones in cystinuria.

Drug antagonists have more diverse actions and may act by protecting enzyme systems (pralidoxime chloride and sodium nitrite), by reacting chemically with the toxic agent to produce an inactive compound (protamine sulphate and sodium thiosulphate) or by reversing the drug-induced effects (methylene blue).

Drug antagonists described in other sections include narcotic antagonists, sodium phosphate, and folinic acid.

1031-g

Acetylpenicillamine. Acetyl-D-penicillamine; *N*-Acetyl-D-penicillamine. *N*-Acetyl-3,3-dimethyl-D-cysteine. $C_7H_{13}NO_3S$=191.2.

CAS — 15537-71-0.

A white or almost white powder with a characteristic odour.

Uses. Acetylpenicillamine is a derivative of penicillamine. It is a weaker chelating agent than penicillamine, but has been used in the treatment of mercury poisoning. Doses of 250 or 300 mg have been given four times daily.

For some reports of the use of acetylpenicillamine, see Martindale 27th Edn, p. 329.

1032-q

Calcium Trisodium Pentetate. Calcium Trisodium Penthamil; DTPA Ca; NSC-34249. The calcium chelate of the trisodium salt of diethylenetriamine-*NNN'N''N''*-penta-acetic acid.
$C_{14}H_{18}CaN_3Na_3O_{10}$=497.4.

CAS — 12111-24-9.

Adverse Effects. Calcium trisodium pentetate may cause nausea, vomiting, and diarrhoea.

Precautions. Calcium trisodium pentetate should be used with caution in patients with renal disease.

Absorption and Fate. Calcium trisodium pentetate is poorly absorbed from the gastro-intestinal tract. Following parenteral administration it is rapidly excreted in the urine, more than 50% being eliminated within 4 hours and over 90% in 24 hours.

Uses. Calcium trisodium pentetate is a chelating agent that has been employed in the treatment of acute or chronic poisoning by heavy metals such as lead and radioactive metals such as plutonium, and in the treatment of such conditions as haemochromatosis and haemosiderosis.

It was administered by slow intravenous infusion; 1 g was diluted with 200 to 500 ml of dextrose injection or sodium chloride injection. The usual dose was 1 g daily, though doses are reported to have ranged from 0.5 to 7 g daily. It was recommended that at least 2 days without treatment should follow 5 days' treatment. Doses of 25 to 50 mg per kg body-weight have been employed in children.

Calcium trisodium pentetate was also given intramuscularly.

Haemochromatosis. Calcium trisodium pentetate, in doses of approximately 16.7 mg per kg body-weight, was used to measure iron stores in patients with haemochromatosis. The highest amount of the calcium trisodium pentetate-chelatable iron complex in control patients was 1.59 mg, whereas in patients with idiopathic haemochromatosis the range was 15.9 to 29.2 mg. Of 83 patients with chronic liver disease, iron stores in excess of 1.5 g were correctly predicted in 24 using this method.— M. Barry *et al.*, *Gut*, 1970, *11*, 891 and 899.

Haemosiderosis. Calcium trisodium pentetate was used in the treatment of haemosiderosis in 3 patients on haemodialysis, and was shown to be dialysable and capable of binding iron in patients with iron overload. A patient with a serum-iron concentration of 2.56 µg per ml received 36 g of calcium trisodium pentetate in 4-g doses during a 3-week period; an average of 27 mg of iron per dialysis was removed. One patient experienced vomiting when the dose was increased to 4 g. The dosage recommended was 3 g, given during the second hour of dialysis.— C. C. Tisher *et al.*, *Proc. Eur. Dialysis Transplantn Ass.*, 1966, *3*, 43.

Lead poisoning. Nine of 12 workers who had been exposed to lead fumes from 4 weeks to many years had prolonged absorption of lead and 1 had overt signs of lead intoxication. They were given intramuscular injections of 0.5 to 1 g of calcium trisodium pentetate as a 25% solution; 1 patient complained of local discomfort. Calcium trisodium pentetate was as effective as sodium calciumedetate intravenously. A higher mobilisation of lead was produced by the second injection, but in 1 worker no further injections were given because of microhaematuria.— H. G. Brugsch *et al.*, *New Engl. J. Med.*, 1965, *272*, 993.

Calcium trisodium pentetate was formerly marketed in Great Britain under the proprietary name Calcium Chel 330.

Other Proprietary Names

Ditripentat-Heyl *(Ger.).*

Proprietary Preparations of Related Compounds

Chel 330 *(Ciba-Geigy, UK).* A 30% aqueous solution of pentasodium pentetate ($C_{14}H_{18}N_3Na_5O_{10}$=503.3).

1041-p

Cysteamine Hydrochloride. Mercaptamine Hydrochloride; Mercamine Hydrochloride; L-1573 *(cysteamine)*; MEA *(cysteamine)*. 2-Aminoethanethiol hydrochloride.
C_2H_7NS,HCl=113.6.

CAS — 60-23-1 (cysteamine); 156-57-0 (hydrochloride).

White crystals. M.p. about 70°. Cysteamine hydrochloride 147 mg is approximately equivalent to 100 mg of cysteamine **Soluble** in water and alcohol.

Of 6 commercially available preparations (non-pharmaceutical) of cysteamine hydrochloride one contained 40% of cystamine, the oxidation product of cysteamine. A freeze-dried preparation for injection had deteriorated by about 20%. A stable injection could be prepared by dissolving cysteamine hydrochloride in ascorbic acid solution 11.5 mmol per litre, filtering, filling under nitrogen, and sterilising by autoclaving at 115° for 30 minutes.— J. R. B. J. Brouwers and P. Vermeij (letter), *Lancet*, 1976, *2*, 965. There was no need for the ascorbic acid. Freeze-drying need no longer be done since a sterile pyrogen-free injection packed under nitrogen could be prepared using standard manufacturing apparatus and techniques.— F. G. R. Prior (letter), *ibid.*, 1977, *1*, 315.

Adverse Effects. The injection of cysteamine causes nausea, vomiting, and drowsiness; other side-effects reported include malaise, anorexia, and abdominal cramps. Flushing, irritability, meningism, leucopenia, and ventricular tachycardia have been reported.

Precautions. Cysteamine may precipitate hepatic coma in patients with overt hepatic damage.

Uses. Cysteamine has been used in the treatment of severe paracetamol poisoning when it was considered that the patient was at risk of developing severe hepatic damage. It increases the hepatic stores of glutathione, and may prevent the development of toxic metabolites of paracetamol or reduce their toxicity. Other forms of treatment are generally preferred (see Paracetamol, p.269). It is not effective unless given within 10 hours of the overdose of paracetamol. A suggested regimen is to give the equivalent of 2 g of the base by intravenous infusion over 10 minutes, followed by 800 mg in the next 4 hours, and a further 800 mg in the next 16 hours. Appropriate supportive treatment should be given concomitantly.

Cysteamine was considered too toxic for protection against whole body radiation exposure. More effective and safer compounds were being investigated.— T. L. Phillips, *Cancer*, 1977, *39*, 987.

Cystinosis. A 5-year-old child with cystinosis had been treated with cysteamine 60 mg per kg body-weight daily by mouth, with no apparent side-effects and with reduction of leucocyte intracellular cystine content to normal. Three further patients (aged 1, 2, and 4 years) had been started on cysteamine therapy.— L. P. Roy and A. C. Pollard (letter), *Lancet*, 1978, *2*, 729.

A report on the effects of cysteamine therapy in 5 children with nephropathic cystinosis who were treated for up to 30 months. Free cysteamine was given by mouth as a 5% solution in 4 divided doses daily. The initial daily dose of 30 mg per kg body-weight was increased to 60 mg per kg after 4 weeks, to 90 mg per kg after a further 4 weeks, and then maintained at this dose. Cysteamine caused a consistent dose-related decline in concentrations of cystine in leucocytes and extracullular fluid. Glomerular function was stabilised in 2 patients but there was no improvement in renal tubular function or growth velocity. No side-effects were noted. At present cysteamine appears to be the best hope for a specific treatment of this amino acid disorder although more extensive clinical studies are needed to help determine long-term efficacy.— M. Yudkoff *et al.*, *New Engl. J. Med.*, 1981, *304*, 141. Criticism of the study and the view that the suggested effect of cysteamine treatment on the deterioration of glomerular filtration-rate has not been proved.— N. Gretz and F. Manz (letter), *ibid.*, 1171. Mention of a large collaborative study which is in progress to evaluate the effectiveness of cysteamine therapy in nephropathic cystinosis and concern about dose-related toxicity.— J. A. Schneider *et al.* (letter), *ibid.*, 1172. Beneficial results with cysteamine in a child of 16 months.— M. Pococco and G. Tonini (letter), *ibid.* Reply.— M. Yudkoff *et al.* (letter), *ibid.*, 1173.

Further references: E. P. Girardin *et al.*, *J. Pediat.*, 1979, *94*, 838; J. G. Thoene *et al.*, *Pediat. Res.*, 1979, *13*, 374.

Paracetamol poisoning. Reports and discussions on the use of cysteamine hydrochloride in the treatment of paracetamol poisoning: L. F. Prescott *et al.*, *Lancet*, 1974, *1*, 588; L. F. Prescott and H. Matthew (letter), *ibid.*, 998; A. P. Douglas *et al.*, *ibid.*, 1976, *1*, 111; L. F. Prescott *et al.* (letter), *ibid.*, 1976, *1*, 357; R. D. Hughes *et al.* (letter), *ibid.*, 1976, *1*, 536; L. F. Prescott *et al.*, *ibid.*, 1976, *2*, 109; *J. int. med. Res.*, 1976, *4*, *Suppl.* 4;; R. D. Hughes *et al.*, *Br. med. J.*, 1977, *2*, 1395; J. M. Smith *et al.*, *ibid.*, 1978, *1*, 331.

See also under Treatment of Adverse Effects in Paracetamol, p.269.

Preparations

Cysteamine Injection. A stable injection was prepared as follows: cysteamine hydrochloride (of good quality) 600 mg, ascorbic acid 0.0115M solution 30 ml; filter, fill into vials under nitrogen, sterilise by autoclaving at 115° for 30 minutes.—J.R.B.J. Brouwers and P. Vermeij, *Pharm. Weekbl. Ned.*, 1976, *111*, 204.

Proprietary Names

Lambratene *(Bracco, Ital.).*

1034-s

Desferrioxamine Mesylate *(B.P.).* Desferrioxamine Methanesulphonate; Ba-33112; DFOM Mesylate; DFM Mesylate; Deferoxamine Mesylate *(U.S.P.)*; Deferoxamine Mesilate; Desferrioxamine B Mesylate. 30-Amino-3,14,25-trihydroxy-3,9,14,20,25-penta-azatriacontane-2,10,13,21,24-pentaone methanesulphonate. $C_{25}H_{48}N_6O_8,CH_3SO_3H=656.8$.

CAS — 70-51-9 (desferrioxamine); 138-14-7 (mesylate).

Pharmacopoeias. In *Br.* and *U.S.* which also includes Sterile Deferoxamine Mesylate.

A white to cream-coloured odourless or almost odourless powder with a bitter taste. **Soluble** 1 in 5 of water and 1 in 20 of alcohol; practically insoluble in dehydrated alcohol, chloroform, and ether; slightly soluble in methyl alcohol. A 10% solution in water has a pH of 3.5 to 5.5. Solutions in water are stable for not more than a week if stored at room temperature and protected from light. **Store** at a temperature not exceeding 4° in airtight containers. Protect from light.

Adverse Effects. Rapid intravenous injection of desferrioxamine may cause flushing, urticaria, hypotension, and perhaps shock. Local pain may occur with intramuscular injections.

Blurring of vision, abdominal discomfort, diarrhoea, dysuria, fever, pruritus, skin rash, tachycardia, and leg cramps have also been reported. Cataract formation has occurred rarely after prolonged administration.

Pruritus, erythema, and swelling have occurred after prolonged subcutaneous injection.

Allergy. A means of rapid desensitisation for desferrioxamine anaphylactic reaction.— K. B. Miller *et al.* (letter), *Lancet*, 1981, *1*, 1059.

Precautions. Desferrioxamine is contra-indicated in patients with severe renal disease or anuria and should be used with caution in patients with impaired renal function. Skeletal foetal anomalies have occurred in *animals*; its use is therefore best avoided during the first trimester of pregnancy.

Desferrioxamine mesylate could cause a characteristic reddish discoloration of the urine.— R. B. Baran and B. Rowles, *J. Am. pharm. Ass.*, 1973, *NS13*, 139.

Absorption and Fate. Desferrioxamine mesylate is poorly absorbed from the gastro-intestinal tract. The fate of the iron chelate is discussed below.

Uses. Desferrioxamine acts as an iron chelating agent. When given by injection it forms a non-toxic chelate with iron in the tissues and this is rapidly excreted in the urine and in bile. If given by mouth it forms a chelate with iron in the alimentary tract and this is not absorbed.

Desferrioxamine is of value in increasing the urinary excretion of iron in conditions associated with excessive iron storage in the tissues, such as haemochromatosis and haemosiderosis and in iron overload following repeated transfusions as in thalassaemia. For this purpose it is administered intramuscularly, the usual initial dosage being 1 to 1.5 g of the mesylate daily in 1 to 3 injections, followed by a maintenance dose of 0.5 to 1 g daily. Desferrioxamine mesylate 2 g is also given intravenously or preferably by prolonged subcutaneous injection with each unit of blood transfused.

The excretion of iron is greater after intravenous infusion or prolonged subcutaneous injection (which may be provided on an out-patient basis) than after intramuscular administration. Excretion of iron is also generally considered to be increased by ascorbic acid supplements.

Desferrioxamine is also used in the treatment of acute iron poisoning. Theoretically, 100 mg of desferrioxamine mesylate can chelate approximately 8.5 mg of iron. Thus, 5 g can chelate the iron contained in about 10 tablets of ferrous sulphate or ferrous gluconate. In treating acute iron poisoning, speed is essential to block absorption of iron from the alimentary tract. The following procedure has been recommended: inject intramuscularly 2 g of desferrioxamine mesylate dissolved in Water for Injections; wash out the stomach with a 1% solution of sodium bicarbonate; give 5 g of desferrioxamine mesylate in 50 to 100 ml of water by mouth, or by stomach tube, if necessary, to chelate any iron left in the intestine and prevent further absorption; give desferrioxamine mesylate by intravenous infusion at a rate of not more than 15 mg per kg body-weight per hour, with a maximum dosage of 80 mg per kg in 24 hours; if necessary repeat intramuscular injections of 2 g of desferrioxamine mesylate every 12 hours. Solutions for intravenous infusion may be prepared with sodium chloride injection, dextrose injection, or sodium chloride and dextrose injection.

Desferrioxamine has been used as a diagnostic test for iron storage disease by injecting 0.5 to 1 g of the mesylate intramuscularly and estimating the increase in urinary excretion of iron; a 10-fold increase is suggestive of iron overload.

Eye-drops containing 10% have been used for ocular siderosis.

To vials each containing desferrioxamine mesylate 500 mg and ferrioxamine hydrochloride 50 mg was added 6 ml of Water for Injections containing approximately 74 kBq (2 microcuries) of iron-59 as ferric citrate. The resulting solution was injected intravenously in a dose of 0.1 ml per kg body-weight, adjusted to the nearest 0.5 ml. Fluid intake was limited in order to keep the urine volume within 700 ml per 6-hour period. The amount of ferrioxamine hydrochloride formed by chelation with body-iron was determined and expressed in µg per kg body-weight. The method was used to assess total chelatable iron stores.— P. M. Smith *et al.*, *Lancet*, 1967, *1*, 133.

A review of the treatment of iron storage disorders, including chelation with desferrioxamine.— J. W. Halliday and M. L. Bassett, *Drugs*, 1980, *20*, 207.

Administration. In 2 patients with thalassaemia the net iron loss after 750 mg of desferrioxamine given intramuscularly or over 4 hours intravenously was less than 20 mg; the same dose given intravenously over 24 hours led to a loss of over 50 mg of iron R. D. Propper *et al.*, *New Engl. J. Med.*, 1976, *294*, 1421. In 26 patients with disorders associated with iron overload (18 of whom had thalassaemia) constant self-administration of desferrioxamine by the subcutaneous route was 90% as effective on a dose for dose basis as intravenous infusion. There was little immediate toxicity, side-effects being local and reversible pruritus, erythema, and swelling. The method promoted sustained and substantial net iron excretion for at least a year. In 5 patients with appreciably depleted white-cell ascorbic acid concentrations administration of supplementary ascorbic acid markedly increased net desferrioxamine-induced urinary iron excretion; caution was, however, recommended since the potential toxicity of ascorbic acid in patients with iron overload had not been thoroughly investigated.— *idem*, 1977, *297*, 418. Comment.— D. J. Weatherall *et al.*, *ibid.*, 445.

In a study involving 11 patients with β-thalassaemia major and 1 with congenital sideroblastic anaemia receiving routine blood transfusions, desferrioxamine was significantly more effective in increasing iron excretion when given by subcutaneous infusion than by intramuscular injection. The increase in excretion ranged from 62 to 136% (mean 101%) when the infusion was given before transfusion and 19 to 213% (mean 128%) when the infusion was given after transfusion.— M. A. M. Hussain *et al.*, *Lancet*, 1976, *2*, 1278.

Studies in 14 patients with transfusional iron overload suggested that up to 2 g daily of desferrioxamine administered over 12 hours by subcutaneous infusion should be suitable for most patients. Continuous infusion over 24 hours generally offered no advantage over 12-hour administration and might be less acceptable to the patient. Ascorbic acid 1 g twice daily considerably enhanced the iron excretion.— M. A. M. Hussain *et al.*, *Lancet*, 1977, *1*, 977.

A study in young thalassaemic patients indicated that although intramuscular bolus injections of desferrioxamine were inadequate, subcutaneous infusions of desferrioxamine 0.5 to 1 g could promote sufficient iron excretion to achieve iron balance. Adequate iron chelation regimens started early in life might prevent the iron-loading in transfusion-dependent thalassaemic patients. Although older children with a heavier iron load responded to the intramuscular bolus route, their response to subcutaneous infusion was considerably better.— M. J. Pippard *et al.*, *Lancet*, 1978, *1*, 1178.

In 9 patients with iron overload the subcutaneous infusion over 12 hours of 0.5 to 1 g (2 g in 1 patient) of desferrioxamine increased iron excretion by 20 to 125% (mean 62%) compared with the same dose given intramuscularly. Ascorbic-acid saturation was considered to be beneficial.— M. J. Pippard *et al.*, *Clin. Sci. & mol. Med.*, 1978, *54*, 99.

A report of the successful use of desferrioxamine mesylate in 5 patients with excessive iron storage resulting from repeated blood transfusion. Patients received 1 to 4 g per m^2 body-surface daily by continuous intravenous infusion for 12 days, together with ascorbic acid 750 mg daily by mouth. A dose of 2 g per m^2 was nearly as effective as 4 g per m^2.— K. G. Blume *et al.*, *J. Am. med. Ass.*, 1978, *239*, 2149.

Regular subcutaneous infusions of desferrioxamine, 2 to 4 g over 12 hours on 6 nights a week, were given to 34 mainly thalassaemic patients requiring regular blood transfusions and with transfusional iron overload. Ascorbic acid 200 mg daily was given by mouth separately from food. All 34 patients showed a fall in serum-ferritin concentrations, in some almost to normal. Although 2 of the most severely iron-overloaded died during the study, liver function improved as serum-ferritin concentrations fell, and, in all of 17 patients tested, serum-aspartate-aminotransferase (SGOT) concentrations fell; in 5 of 6 patients tested liver-iron concentrations also fell. These early results suggest that this long-term regimen of subcutaneous desferrioxamine infusions might lead to stabilisation of iron stores at normal or near-normal values despite the continued need for transfusions.— A. V. Hoffbrand *et al.*, *Lancet*, 1979, *1*, 947.

A means of administering desferrioxamine entrapped in red cell ghosts to improve chelation.— R. Green *et al.*, *Lancet*, 1980, *2*, 327. Criticism.— G. N. Smith (letter), *ibid.*, 1363. Reply.— R. Green *et al.* (letter), *ibid.* Further comment.— G. N. Smith (letter), *ibid.*, 1981, *1*, 222.

Administration of desferrioxamine 1 or 3 g thrice daily in solution by mouth with meals, to 14 thalassaemic patients aged 3 to 26 years, with varying degrees of iron overload, increased iron excretion above baseline values in every case. Although oral chelation with desferrioxamine was clearly less efficient than the subcutaneous infusion, compliance with subcutaneous infusion is often poor, and oral desferrioxamine may be a useful and acceptable adjunct. The taste can be disguised.— S. T. Callender and D. J. Weatherall (letter), *Lancet*, 1980, *2*, 689. A report of similar findings with desferrioxamine given as the mesylate; the fat-soluble desferrioxamine stearate, however, was found to be relatively ineffective.— A. Jacobs and W. C. Ting (letter), *ibid.*, 794. Doubt as to whether oral desferrioxamine has a place in chelation therapy as an adjunct to subcutaneous infusions in young thalassaemic patients with mild iron overload. In 18 such patients even intravenous administration of desferrioxamine 1 g was not very effective for all (mainly those with lower iron stores).— C. Kattamis *et al.* (letter), *ibid.*, 1981, *1*, 51.

Evidence that low ascorbic acid stores may have reduced the incidence of iron-induced tissue damage in a woman with β-thalassaemia.— A. Cohen *et al.*, *New Engl. J. Med.*, 1981, *304*, 158. Comment on the need for extreme caution when prescribing ascorbic acid for the iron-overloaded patient. More data are awaited from controlled studies, but until results are known the following guidelines are recommended for the physician who chooses to prescribe it: the need for ascorbic acid should be clearly documented by measurements of iron excretion both before and after supplementation, and the oral dose of ascorbic acid should be given an hour or two after the infusion is started, when adequate concentrations of desferrioxamine have been achieved.— A. W. Nienhuis, *ibid.*, 170.

Further references.— B. Cooper *et al.*, *Am. J. Med.*, 1977, *63*, 958; A. Cohen and E. Schwartz, *J. Pediat.*, 1978, *92*, 643; J. H. Graziano *et al.*, *ibid.*, 648; M. Weiner *et al.*, *ibid.*, 653; *Br. med. J.*, 1978, *2*, 782; C. B. Pignatti and P. De Stefano (letter), *ibid.*, 1432.

Dialysis encephalopathy. A 36-year-old man with advanced dialysis encephalopathy obtained a striking improvement following removal of aluminium by means of desferrioxamine. Desferrioxamine 6 g in 500 ml of saline was infused into the arterial line during the first 2 hours of a dialysis, once weekly.— P. Ackrill *et al.* (letter), *Lancet*, 1980, *2*, 692. A report of 5 patients who developed dialysis encephalopathy who are still alive over 2 years after the onset. All have improved considerably from their worst state and 2 are now mentally and neurologically normal. None of them received desferrioxamine or any specific drug therapy apart from anticonvulsants.— M. M. Platts (letter), *ibid.*, 1035. Comment on other factors, including haemofiltration, for the removal of aluminium from patients with dialysis encephalopathy.— J. P. Adhemar *et al.* (letter), *ibid.*, 1311.

Porphyria. Urinary excretion of porphyrin was significantly reduced in 4 patients with delayed cutaneous porphyria who were treated with desferrioxamine.— J. Thivolet *et al.*, *Presse méd.*, 1968, *76*, 367.

Sickle-cell anaemia. In 10 patients with sickle-cell anaemia who had received multiple infusions of red blood cells or repeated partial exchange transfusions the urinary 24-hour excretion of iron following an 18-hour intravenous infusion of desferrioxamine 1.5 g was 5.9 to 28.7 mg (mean 15.1 mg) compared with 0.7 to 2.6 mg in baseline assessments in 5 patients. Excretion of iron in 3 patients given desferrioxamine 750 mg intramuscularly was less than 7 mg. Ascorbic acid given to 3 of the patients (all children) for 3 weeks had no effect on iron excretion. Intensive use of desferrioxamine might retard the accumulation of iron and delay or prevent organ damage.— A. Cohen and E. Schwartz, *J. Pediat.*, 1978, *92*, 659.

Thalassaemia. A detailed account of the total management of thalassaemia major. Long-term therapy with desferrioxamine 0.5 to 1.5 g daily according to weight, by intramuscular injection, is safe and feasible, and can bring patients into iron balance, albeit at high body iron load. The regimen for the management of acute intercurrent illness in the thalassaemic patient includes intravenous infusion of high doses of desferrioxamine to counteract the development of acute iron toxicity due to release from body stores.— B. Modell, *Archs Dis. Childh.*, 1977, *52*, 489.

Major arrhythmias occurred in 7 of 11 patients with thalassaemia, inadequately chelated, and in none of 17 adequately chelated. Chelation appeared to offer some protection against cardiac iron deposition.— S. B. Kaye and M. Owen, *Br. med. J.*, 1978, *1*, 342 and 555.

Further references: B. Modell, *Br. med. Bull.*, 1976, *32*, 270; *Lancet*, 1978, *1*, 479 and 620.

See also above under Administration, p.381.

Tissue stains. In 25 patients with corneal rust stains due to penetration of a foreign body, treatment with 10% desferrioxamine ointment 4 times daily resulted in clearance of rust within 4 days. Rust stains lasted much longer in 15 control patients. There was some conjunctival hyperaemia on the first day of treatment.— A. Valvo, *Am. J. Ophthal.*, 1967, *63*, 98.

Surgical removal of corneal rust rings after injury was more effective than treatment with 5% desferrioxamine ointment.— R. McGuinness and D. Knight-Jones, *Br. J. Ophthal.*, 1968, *52*, 777.

Preparations

Desferrioxamine Eye-drops. Dissolve 500 mg of sterile desferrioxamine mesylate with aseptic precautions in a sterile vehicle containing methylcellulose '4000' 0.5%, benzyl alcohol 1% w/v, Water for Injections to 5 ml. The eye-drops are prepared immediately before use and discarded after 1 week.

Desferrioxamine Injection *(B.P.)*. A sterile solution of desferrioxamine mesylate prepared by dissolving, immediately before use, the sterile contents of a sealed container (Desferrioxamine Mesylate for Injection) in the requisite amount of Water for Injections. Cloudy solutions should be discarded.

Desferrioxamine Ophthalmic Ointment 5%. Desferrioxamine 5% in a basis of cetyl alcohol 0.4%, wool fat 4.6%, white soft paraffin 65%, and liquid paraffin 30%. Apply 4 times daily in ocular siderosis and haematogenous pigmentation of the cornea.—I. Falbe-Hansen, *Acta Ophthal.*, 1966, *44*, 95.

Sterile Deferoxamine Mesylate *(U.S.P.)*. Desferrioxamine mesylate suitable for parenteral use. pH of a 1% solution 4 to 6.

Proprietary Preparations

Desferal *(Ciba, UK)*. Desferrioxamine mesylate, available as powder for preparing injections or for oral use, in vials of 500 mg. (Also available as Desferal in *Austral., Belg., Canad., Denm., Fr., Ger., Ital., Neth., Norw., S.Afr., Swed., Switz., USA*).

Other Proprietary Names

Desferin *(Spain)*.

1035-w

Diacetyl Monoxime. DAM. 3-(Hydroxyimino)butan-2-one.

$C_4H_7NO_2$=101.1.

CAS — 57-71-6.

Soluble in water, chloroform, and light petroleum.

Uses. Diacetyl monoxime has the same actions and uses as pralidoxime chloride (see p.389) but it is less rapidly excreted, and is reported to enter the central nervous system more readily. It has been given intravenously in doses of 1 g at a rate not exceeding 200 mg per minute.

The serum half-life of diacetyl monoxime in man was 7.2 hours after an intravenous dose of 15 mg per kg body-weight.— B. V. Jager *et al.*, *Bull. Johns Hopkins Hosp.*, 1958, *102*, 225. See also *idem*, 203.

1033-p

Dicobalt Edetate. Cobalt Edetate; Cobalt Tetracemate; Cobalt EDTA. Dicobalt ethylenediamine-*NNN'N'*-tetra-acetate.

$C_{10}H_{12}Co_2N_2O_8$=406.1.

CAS — 36499-65-7.

Adverse Effects and Precautions. Dicobalt edetate may cause hypotension, tachycardia, and vomiting; anaphylactic reactions have occurred. Dicobalt edetate should not be injected in conditions other than known cyanide poisoning.

A patient experienced sweating, angina, ventricular ectopic beats, and a red maculopapular rash 36 hours after drug administration; these effects were presumably due to dicobalt edetate.— B. Hillman *et al.*, *Postgrad. med. J.*, 1974, *50*, 171.

Anxiety could mimic the early signs of cyanide poisoning. Several patients had suffered reactions needing intensive care when given dicobalt edetate on suspicion of cyanide poisoning. No adverse effects were seen in 6 patients with confirmed cyanide poisoning. Careful clinical assessment was essential before giving dicobalt edetate.— D. D. Bryson (letter), *Lancet*, 1978, *1*, 92.

In 3 men exposed to cyanide gas and treated with dicobalt edetate side-effects included restlessness, vomiting, profuse diaphoresis, facial and palpebral oedema, retrosternal pain, hypertension, and ventricular tachycardia. The patients survived but it was considered that dicobalt edetate should be reserved for comatose patients not responsive to classical treatment and to patients becoming unconscious despite such treatment.— J. Nagler *et al.*, *J. occup. Med.*, 1978, *20*, 414.

Further references: M. J. McKiernan (letter), *Lancet*, 1980, *2*, 86 (anaphylactic reaction when used as precautionary measure).

Uses. Dicobalt edetate is used in the treatment of severe cyanide poisoning (see p.790). Its use arises from the property of cobalt compounds of forming stable complexes with cyanides; the complexes reduce the potential toxicity of the cobalt itself. Dicobalt edetate has been reported to inactivate about one-eighth of its weight of hydrocyanic acid. A suggested dose is 300 mg administered by intravenous injection, over about 1 minute, as 20 ml of a 1.5% solution. The injection of dicobalt edetate is followed immediately by 50 ml of dextrose injection 50% intravenously through the same needle. The dose may be repeated immediately if necessary and followed by a further injection of dextrose; a further dose of 300 mg of dicobalt edetate may be given 5 minutes later if required.

Oxygen and other resuscitative measures should be used concomitantly.

A 68-year-old man who had ingested sodium cyanide was cyanotic and in respiratory distress when seen by a doctor 15 minutes later; on admission to hospital after a further 40 minutes he was apnoeic, pulseless, and bright pink. The pulse became palpable after the first dose of 300 mg of dicobalt edetate, he developed sinus tachycardia, and the blood pressure rose to 60 mmHg. He was given intensive treatment, gastric lavage, assisted respiration, and a further 14 doses of dicobalt edetate within 36 hours, but died from cardiac arrest 44 hours after admission. It was believed that irreversible brain damage had occurred before treatment was instituted. A blood-cyanide concentration of 5.5 μg per ml on admission (estimated lethal value 2.5 μg per ml) fell during treatment, with a further rise presumably due to further absorption.— B. Hillman *et al.*, *Postgrad. med. J.*, 1974, *50*, 171.

Dicobalt edetate still remained the antidote of choice in cyanide poisoning.— *Lancet*, 1977, *2*, 1167.

Further references: C. L. Evans, *Br. J. Pharmac. Chemother.*, 1964, *23*, 455; G. Paulet, *Urgence méd. chir.*, 1965, *2*, 611; *Br. med. J.*, 1978, *2*, 1141.

Proprietary Preparations

Kelocyanor *(Laroche Navarron, Fr.: Rona, UK)*. Dicobalt edetate, available as a solution containing 300 mg in each 20 ml, in ampoules of 20 ml. (Also available as Kelocyanor in *Fr., S.Afr.*).

1036-e

Dimercaprol *(B.P., B.P. Vet., Eur. P., U.S.P.)*. Dimercap.; Dimercaprolum; BAL; British Anti-Lewisite; Dimercaptopropanol. 2,3-Dimercaptopropan-1-ol.

$C_3H_8OS_2$=124.2.

CAS — 59-52-9.

Pharmacopoeias. In *Aust., Br., Braz., Chin., Cz., Eur., Fr., Ger., Hung., Ind., Int., It., Jap., Jug., Neth., Nord., Pol., Swiss, Turk.*, and *U.S.*

A clear colourless or slightly yellow liquid with an alliaceous odour. The *B.P.* specifies relative density of 1.239 to 1.259; the *U.S.P.* specifies specific gravity of 1.242 to 1.244.

Soluble 1 in 20 of water and 1 in 18 of arachis oil; miscible with alcohol, benzyl benzoate, ether, methyl alcohol, and many other organic solvents. A saturated solution in water has a pH of 5 to 6.5. Solutions in oil are **sterilised** by maintaining at 150° for 1 hour, the air in the containers having been replaced by nitrogen or other suitable gas. **Store** at 2° to 10° in small well-filled airtight containers. Protect from light.

Adverse Effects. The most consistent side-effects produced by dimercaprol are hypertension and tachycardia. Other side-effects include nausea, vomiting, headache, burning sensation of the lips, mouth, throat, and eyes, lachrymation and salivation, tingling of the extremities, a sensation of constriction in the throat and chest, muscle pains and muscle spasm, rhinorrhoea, sweating, restlessness, and abdominal pain. These effects usually reach their maximum in 15 to 20 minutes after the injection and subside in an hour or two. Sterile abscesses may occur. Doses of dimercaprol of 4 to 5 mg per kg body-weight have been reported to produce reactions in about 50% of patients. Large doses may cause convulsions and coma.

Pain may occur at the injection site and infection, leading to pyrexia, has been reported; fever is common in children.

Dimercaprol is irritating to the skin and mucous membranes and imparts a strong odour to the breath.

In a modified 'repeated-insult' patch test, 10% dimercaprol was found to produce extreme sensitisation of the skin.— A. M. Kligman, *J. invest. Derm.*, 1966, *47*, 393.

Studies in *rats* and *mice* indicated that 1,2,3-trimercaptopropane, a common impurity of commercial samples of dimercaprol, was more toxic than dimercaprol and produced more pain on injection.— P. Zvirblis and R. I. Ellin, *Toxic. appl. Pharmac.*, 1976, *36*, 297.

Haemolytic anaemia. Dimercaprol had been reported to cause haemolytic anaemia in certain individuals with a deficiency of glucose-6-phosphate dehydrogenase. The reaction was not considered clinically significant under normal circumstances (e.g. in the absence of infection).— E. Beutler, *Pharmac. Rev.*, 1969, *21*, 73. See also *Chronicle Wld Hlth Org.*, 1974, *28*, 25.

A report of haemolysis during dimercaprol chelation therapy for high blood-lead concentrations in 2 children with a deficiency of glucose-6-phosphate dehydrogenase.— N. Janakiraman *et al.*, *Clin. Pediat.*, 1978, *17*, 485.

Treatment of Adverse Effects. It has been suggested that the administration of an antihistamine might alleviate some of the side-effects of dimercaprol.

Precautions. Dimercaprol should be used with care in patients with hypertension or impaired renal function, or in patients in whom renal insufficiency develops. It should not be used in patients with impaired hepatic function except in the jaundice which may develop in arsenic poisoning. It should not be used in the treatment of poisoning due to cadmium, iron, or selenium.

Absorption and Fate. After intramuscular injection, maximum blood concentrations are attained in about 2 hours; dimercaprol is entirely metabolised or excreted within 6 to 24 hours.

Uses. Dimercaprol combines in the body with arsenic, mercury, and other heavy metals which inhibit the pyruvate-oxidase system by competing for the sulphydryl groups in proteins. It has a greater affinity than the proteins for these metals and the resulting compounds are stable and rapidly excreted by the kidneys.

Dimercaprol is used in the treatment of acute poisoning by arsenic, gold, and mercury; its role in the treatment of poisoning by antimony and bismuth is less well established. It is used in conjunction with sodium calciumedetate (see p.391) in lead poisoning.

In severe arsenical or gold poisoning, 3 to 4 mg per kg body-weight is given intramuscularly at 4-hourly intervals throughout the first 2 days, 4 doses are given on the third day, and 2 for the next 10 days or until recovery is complete. In milder cases 2.5 mg per kg body-weight is given at each injection, 4 injections being given 4 times on each of the first 2 days, 2 injections on the third day, and 1 daily on subsequent days for 10 days or until complete recovery.

Accidental contamination of the eyes with arsenical vesicants has been treated by immediately instilling a 5 to 10% oily solution of dimercaprol into the conjunctival sac. Local applications have also been used in chromium dermatitis.

The recommended dosage for acute mercurial poisoning varies; some authorities suggest a regimen similar to that for severe arsenical or gold poisoning (see above); others suggest an initial injection of 5 mg per kg body-weight followed by 1 or 2 injections of 2.5 mg per kg body-weight daily for 10 days.

In lead poisoning a dose of 3 to 4 mg per kg is given 4-hourly concomitantly with sodium calciumedetate for periods of 2 to 7 days.

The urine should be made alkaline to reduce damage to the kidneys during elimination of the dimercaprol-metal complex.

The use of dimercaprol does not obviate the need for the general treatment of poisoning as outlined under the respective metals.

Gold poisoning. Severe thrombocytopenia in a 56-year-old woman after a course of sodium aurothiomalate was unresponsive to infusions of platelet concentrate or platelet-rich plasma and to corticosteroids. It responded promptly to treatment with dimercaprol 100 mg twice daily intramuscularly for 15 days; the serum-gold concentration of 740 ng per ml (not excessive) fell rapidly to 190 ng per ml and by the end of treatment to less than 100 ng per ml.— J. M. England and D. S. Smith, *Br. med. J.*, 1972, *2*, 748.

Hepatolenticular degeneration. A young woman with hepatolenticular degeneration was treated with dimercaprol continuously for 6 years, during which time she had 2 pregnancies. Clinical improvement was noted during and after each pregnancy and probably resulted from copper mobilisation to meet foetal requirements. There was no biochemical evidence of hepatolenticular degeneration in either child.— F. E. Dreifuss and W. M. McKinney, *J. Am. med. Ass.*, 1966, *195*, 960.

Lead poisoning. There were no deaths in 24 children with acute encephalopathy due to lead poisoning who were treated with sodium calciumedetate and dimercaprol.— J. J. Chisolm, *J. Pediat.*, 1968, *73*, 1.

In lead poisoning with acute encephalopathy or blood-lead concentrations greater than 100 µg per ml dimercaprol and sodium calciumedetate should be used: dimercaprol 4 mg per kg body-weight was given intramuscularly and repeated 4 hours later when sodium calciumedetate 12.5 mg per kg was given intravenously or intramuscularly at a separate site. These doses were repeated every 4 hours for up to 5 days. In patients with less severe poisoning the initial dose of dimercaprol was followed by a dose of 3 mg per kg with sodium calciumedetate 8 mg per kg for 1 to 3 days.— *Med. Lett.*, 1972, *14*, 5.

Mercury poisoning. For reports of the unsuccessful use of dimercaprol in the delayed treatment of 3 cases of poisoning with thiomersal, see J. H. M. Axton, *Postgrad. med. J.*, 1972, *48*, 417.

Rapid and frequent treatment with dimercaprol was necessary in any patient showing symptoms of systemic poisoning after exposure to mercury vapour and should be continued even in the absence of excessive urinary-mercury concentrations.— C. J. Eastmond and S. Holt, *Postgrad. med. J.*, 1975, *51*, 428.

Paracetamol poisoning. Dimercaprol is ineffective in paracetamol poisoning.— L. F. Prescott and N. Wright (letter), *Lancet*, 1974, *2*, 833.

Preparations

Dimercaprol Injection *(B.P.).* BAL Injection. A sterile 5% w/v solution in benzyl benzoate and arachis oil. pH adjusted to 6.8 to 7 with alcoholic ammonia solution. Sterilised, in an atmosphere of nitrogen or other suitable gas, by heating at 150° for one hour. Protect from light.

Dimercaprol Injection *(U.S.P.).* A sterile 9 to 11% w/w solution of dimercaprol in a mixture of benzyl benzoate and vegetable oil.

Injectabile Dimercaproli *(Nord. P.).* Dimercaprol 10 g, benzyl benzoate 20 g, arachis oil to 100 ml.

Proprietary Preparations

Dimercaprol (BAL) Injection *(Boots, UK).* A brand of Dimercaprol Injection *B.P.*, available in ampoules of 2 ml. (Also available as BAL in *Austral., Canad., Fr., Ital., USA*).

Other Proprietary Names

Sulfactin *(Ger.).*

1037-l

Diphenylthiocarbazone. Dithizone. 1,5-Diphenylthiocarbazone.

$C_{13}H_{12}N_4S = 256.3$.

CAS — 60-10-6.

An almost black powder. Practically **insoluble** in water; soluble in carbon tetrachloride, chloroform, and other organic solvents, forming intense green solutions.

Diphenylthiocarbazone is a chelating agent which has been suggested for use in thallium and zinc poisoning. Its value is not established. It has been reported to produce diabetogenic and goitrogenic effects.

References: J. Mathews and A. Anzarut, *Can. med. Ass. J.*, 1968, *99*, 72.

1038-y

Disodium Edetate *(B.P.).*

Edetate Disodium *(U.S.P.)*; Sodium Edetate; Disodium Dihydrogen Edetate; Disodium Edathamil; Disodium Tetracemate; Tetracemindinatrium; Tétracémate Disodique; Titriplex III. Disodium dihydrogen ethylenediamine-*NNN'N'*-tetra-acetate dihydrate.

$C_{10}H_{14}N_2Na_2O_8,2H_2O = 372.2$.

CAS — 139-33-3 (anhydrous); 6381-92-6 (dihydrate).

NOTE. In the USA the title sodium edetate is used to describe the tetrasodium salt.

Pharmacopoeias. In *Br., Fr., Jap., Nord., Turk.*, and *U.S.*

A white odourless crystalline powder with a slightly acid taste. Each g represents approximately 5.4 mmol (5.4 mEq) of sodium. **Soluble** 1 in 11 of water; slightly soluble in alcohol; practically insoluble in chloroform and ether. A 5% solution in water has a pH of 4 to 6. A 4.44% solution is iso-osmotic with serum. Solutions are **sterilised** by autoclaving or by filtration.

Adverse Effects. Nausea, diarrhoea, muscle cramps, and pain at the site of injection often occur during intravenous treatment. Fever, headache, urinary urgency, skin eruptions, and transient hypocoagulability have been reported. Thrombophlebitis has followed the administration of solutions of too high a concentration and a too rapid rate of infusion has resulted in drowsiness, malaise, and vertigo.

Hypocalcaemic tetany can occur if disodium edetate is administered too rapidly or in too concentrated a solution, and convulsions, respiratory arrest, and cardiac arrhythmias can occur.

Albuminuria may follow repeated administration of moderate doses and there may also be tubular necrosis. Oliguria and renal failure have occurred, but generally the damage is not permanent and clears up within a few days after the drug has been withdrawn.

For background toxicological information, see *Fd Add. Ser. Wld Hlth Org. No. 5*, 1974.

Of 23 patients showing sensitivity reactions to ethylenediamine 3 showed a cross-reaction to edetic acid.— K. E. Eriksen (letter), *Archs Derm.*, 1975, *111*, 791.

Treatment of Adverse Effects. Hypocalcaemic tetany can be treated by the administration of an intravenous injection of a calcium salt.

Precautions. Disodium edetate should be used with caution in tuberculosis and is contra-indicated in renal disease.

In 5 patients the excretion of potassium was increased 2- to 6-fold after the infusion of 3 g of disodium edetate in 500 ml of dextrose injection. Disodium edetate should be given with care to patients with potassium deficiency.— T. M. Batchelor *et al.*, *J. Am. med. Ass.*, 1964, *187*, 305.

Absorption and Fate. Disodium edetate is poorly absorbed from the gastro-intestinal tract.

Uses. Disodium edetate is a chelating agent which forms complexes with divalent and trivalent metals. When administered by slow intravenous injection it chelates calcium ions, thereby reducing the serum-calcium concentration, and has the effect of mobilising calcium from the skeleton. The calcium chelate formed is almost completely excreted in the urine within 6 hours.

Disodium edetate has been used in the emergency treatment of hypercalcaemia, it has also been used in digitalis-induced cardiac arrhythmias and vascular disorders. It is also used as a 0.4% solution in the treatment of calcium deposits from lime burns of the eye and in the treatment of calcified corneal opacities, either by topical application after removing the appropriate area of corneal epithelium or by iontophoresis.

Disodium edetate is usually administered as Trisodium Edetate Injection diluted with 500 ml of dextrose injection or sodium chloride injection and is given by slow intravenous infusion over 2 to 4 hours. The usual dose is up to 70 mg per kg body-weight daily for adults, and up to 60 mg per kg for children.

Disodium edetate is used to remove traces of heavy metals from pharmaceutical preparations and so improve their stability (see Antoxidants in the section on Preservatives and Antoxidants p.1281).

Disodium edetate is also used as an anticoagulant for blood taken for haematological investigations.

The uses of edetates as chelating agents in the formulation of liquid pharmaceutical products.— L. Lachman, *Drug Cosmet. Ind.*, 1968, *102* (Feb.), 43.

The presence *in vitro* of disodium edetate, 65 µg per ml, rendered 42 hospital strains of penicillin-resistant *Staphylococcus aureus* organisms susceptible to penicillin.— B. D. Rawal, *Med. J. Aust.*, 1969, *1*, 612.

The reversal *in vitro* of antibiotic resistance in strains of *Pseudomonas aeruginosa* by disodium edetate was shown to be due to a synergistic effect of the disodium edetate-antibiotic combinations.— R. Weiser *et al.*, *Lancet*, 1969, *2*, 619.

Edetic acid enhanced the bactericidal activity *in vitro* of penicillin, streptomycin, and neomycin on *Staph. aureus*. Edetic acid also prevented the development of neomycin-resistant strains.— B. D. Rawal, *Aust. J. Hosp. Pharm.*, 1972, *2*, 20. See also B. G. Charles and B. D. Rawal, *Australas. J. Pharm.*, 1971, *52*, S73.

A review of the uses and efficacy of edetates as synergists to antoxidants.— *Fd Add. Ser. Wld Hlth Org. No. 3*, 1972.

Despite reports that ethylenediaminetetra-acetate (EDTA) abolished rosette formation, EDTA-anti-coagulated blood could be used for rosette testing.— T. R. Fairbanks (letter), *New Engl. J. Med.*, 1976, *294*, 226.

A discussion of the effect of edetic acid on preservative systems used in cosmetics and toiletries.— J. R. Hart, *Cosmet. Toilet.*, 1978, *93* (Dec.), 28.

For references to the enhancement of bactericidal activity by edetates, see Chloroxylenol, p.558.

For a report of the reduction of antibacterial activity of thiomersal by the addition of disodium edetate, see Thiomersal, p.576.

Atherosclerosis. Criticism of the practice of giving disodium edetate chelating therapy for atherosclerosis. There is no acceptable evidence that it is effective and its adverse effects can be lethal.— *Med. Lett.*, 1981, *23*, 51.

Lead poisoning. In patients with lead poisoning, short courses of disodium edetate, 300 to 600 mg daily by intramuscular injection, were well tolerated and satisfactorily increased the urinary excretion of lead. Single intravenous doses of 1 g were useful for diagnostic purposes but not for treatment.— R. Grisler *et al.*, *Medna Lav.*, 1969, *60*, 288.

Multiple sclerosis. Infusions of disodium edetate or sodium bicarbonate improved visual scotoma, nystagmus, and diplopia in 9 patients with multiple sclerosis. Improvement was temporary and was thought to be due to a fall in serum calcium.— F. A. Davis *et al.*, *J. Neurol. Neurosurg. Psychiat.*, 1970, *33*, 723.

Scleromalacia. In a patient with scleromalacia perforans associated with Crohn's disease, disodium edetate 0.5% eye-drops instilled 4 times daily produced beneficial results. It was considered to act as a collagenase inhibitor.— P. J. Evans and P. Eustace, *Br. J. Ophthal.*, 1973, *57*, 330.

Urinary calculus. Irrigation with a warmed alkaline solution of disodium edetate resulted in the complete dissolution of ureteric stones in 3 patients and a reduction in the size of stones in a fourth. The duration of irrigation was 137 to 200 hours in the 3 successes and 723 hours in the fourth patient.— G. J. Heap *et al.*, *Med. J. Aust.*, 1976, *1*, 714.

A discussion of the dissolution of renal calculi.— *Br. med. J.*, 1979, *1*, 1746.

Use in food. Estimated acceptable daily intake: up to 2.5 mg per kg body-weight.— Seventeenth Report of Joint FAO/WHO Expert Committee on Food Additives, *Tech. Rep. Ser. Wld Hlth Org. No. 539*, 1974.

Up to 25 mg of disodium edetate per litre is permitted as an additive to brandy under The Miscellaneous Additives in Food Regulations 1980 (SI 1980: No. 1834) for England and Wales and The Miscellaneous Additives in Food (Scotland) Regulations 1980 [SI 1980: No. 1889 (S. 176)].

Preparations of Disodium and Trisodium Edetate

Disodium Edetate Eye Drops *(A.P.F.)*. Sodium Edetate Eye Drops; EDTA Eye Drops. Disodium edetate 3 g, sodium chloride 300 mg, benzalkonium chloride solution 0.02 ml, Water for Injections to 100 ml. Sterilised by autoclaving.

Disodium Edetate Eye Lotion *(A.P.F.)*. Disodium edetate 400 mg, Water for Injections to 100 ml. Sterilised by autoclaving. For the emergency treatment of burns caused by lime.

Disodium Edetate Eye-drops *(Moorfields Eye Hosp.)*. Disodium edetate 380 mg, sodium acid phosphate 420 mg, sodium phosphate 1.43 g, benzalkonium chloride solution 0.02 ml, Water for Injections to 100 ml. Sterilised by autoclaving. For the inactivation of bacterial collagenase and removal of calcium deposits.

Edetate Disodium Injection *(U.S.P.)*. A sterile solution of disodium edetate in Water for Injections, containing varying amounts of the disodium and trisodium salts as a result of pH adjustment. Potency is expressed in terms of the equivalent amount of anhydrous disodium edetate. pH 6.5 to 7.5.

Trisodium Edetate Injection *(B.P.)*. Trisod. Edetate Inj. A sterile solution containing the equivalent of 20% w/v (limits 18 to 22%) of anhydrous trisodium edetate ($C_{10}H_{13}N_2Na_3O_8$) in Water for Injections made by adding a 10% solution of sodium hydroxide in Water for Injections to 20.8 g of disodium edetate in Water for Injections until a pH of 7.4 is obtained and adding sufficient Water for Injections to produce 100 ml. The solution is distributed into lead-free ampoules and sterilised by autoclaving. pH 7 to 8. The injection should be diluted with sodium chloride injection or dextrose injection before use.

NOTE. 1 g of disodium edetate dihydrate is equivalent to about 962 mg of trisodium edetate.

Proprietary Preparations of Disodium, Trisodium, and Tetrasodium Edetate

Limclair *(Sinclair, UK)*. Trisodium edetate, available as an injection containing 200 mg per ml in ampoules of 5 ml.

Nervanaid B30 *(ABM Chemicals, UK)*. Tetrasodium edetate ($C_{10}H_{12}N_2Na_4O_8$ = 380.2), available as solution.

Nervanaid BA2 *(ABM Chemicals, UK)*. A brand of disodium edetate.

Nervanaid BA3 *(ABM Chemicals, UK)*. A brand of trisodium edetate, technical grade.

Nervanaid BA4 *(ABM Chemicals, UK)*. A brand of tetrasodium edetate. **Nervanaid B conc PDR.** A technical grade of tetrasodium edetate.

Sequestrene NA 2 *(Ciba-Geigy, UK)*. A brand of disodium edetate, technical grade.

Sequestrene NA 3 *(Ciba-Geigy, UK)*. A brand of trisodium edetate, technical grade.

Sequestrene NA4 and Sequestrene 30A *(Ciba-Geigy, UK)*. A brand of tetrasodium edetate, technical grade ($C_{10}H_{12}N_2Na_4O_8$ = 380.2). **Sequestrene 30A** is a 38% solution of tetrasodium edetate.

Other Proprietary Names

Austral.— Sodium Versenate; *USA*— Disotate, Endrate Disodium, Sodium Versenate.

Trisodium edetate was also formerly marketed in Great Britain under the proprietary name Sodium Versenate (*Riker*).

1039-j

Edetic Acid *(U.S.N.F.)*. EDTA; EDTAA; Edathamil; Acide Tetracémique. Ethylenediamine-*NNN′N′*-tetra-acetic acid.

$C_{10}H_{16}N_2O_8$=292.2.

CAS — 60-00-4.

Pharmacopoeias. In *Roum.* Also in *U.S.N.F.*

A white crystalline powder. M.p. above 220° with decomposition. Very slightly **soluble** in water; soluble in solutions of alkali hydroxides.

Edetic acid and its salts have many industrial applications as chelating agents. For their uses in medicine and pharmacy see Disodium Edetate (p.383) and Sodium Calciumedetate (p.391).

Proprietary Preparations

Nervanaid B acid *(ABM Chemicals, UK)*. A brand of edetic acid.

Sequestrene AA *(Ciba-Geigy, UK)*. A brand of edetic acid, technical grade.

1040-q

Magnesium Thiosulphate. Magnesium Hyposulphite.

$MgS_2O_3,6H_2O$=244.5.

CAS — 10124-53-5 (anhydrous).

Pharmacopoeias. In *Fr.*

Colourless or white, odourless, efflorescent crystals. **Soluble** 1 in 2 of water forming slightly alkaline solutions; practically insoluble in alcohol.

Uses. Magnesium thiosulphate has been advocated for the treatment of allergic diseases, administered as tablets of 600 mg or by intramuscular or intravenous injection as a 10% solution. Doses of 0.6 to 2.4 g daily have been given by mouth or 1 to 2 g daily by injection.

Intravenous injections of magnesium thiosulphate were of some value, together with the application of soothing lotions, in treating the pruritus following contact with moths of the genus *Dirphia*.— A. Alvarado (letter), *J. Am. med. Ass.*, 1969, *208*, 867.

Proprietary Names

Emgé Lumière *(Sarbach, Fr.; Sarbach, Switz.)*.

1042-s

Methylene Blue *(U.S.P.)*. Methylthioninii Chloridum; Methylthionine Chloride; Methylenum Caeruleum; Azul de Metileno; Blu di Metilene; Schultz No. 1038; CI Basic Blue 9; Colour Index No. 52015; Tetramethylthionine chloride trihydrate. 3,7-Bis(dimethylamino)phenazathionium chloride trihydrate.

$C_{16}H_{18}ClN_3S,3H_2O$=373.9.

CAS — 61-73-4 (anhydrous); 7220-79-3 (trihydrate).

Pharmacopoeias. In *Arg.*, *Belg.*, *Chin.*, *Cz.*, *Hung.*, *Ind.*, *Int.*, *It.*, *Jap.*, *Mex.*, *Pol.*, *Port.*, *Rus.*, *Span.*, *Swiss*, and *U.S.*; in *Aust.*, *Ger.*, *Jug.*, *Nord.*, and *Roum.* (xH_2O); in *Braz.* (anhydrous or $3H_2O$).
The *B.P. 1973* included the dihydrate.

Dark green, odourless or almost odourless, hygroscopic, crystals or crystalline powder with a bronze-like lustre. It loses 8 to 18% of its weight on drying.

Soluble 1 in 25 of water, 1 in 65 of alcohol, and 1 in 450 of chloroform. A 1% solution in water has a pH of 3 to 4.5. Solutions are **sterilised** by autoclaving or by filtration. **Incompatible** with caustic alkalis, oxidising and reducing substances, and iodides. **Store** in airtight containers.

NOTE. Commercial methylene blue is the double chloride of tetramethylthionine and zinc, and is not suitable for medicinal use.

Preservative for eye-drops. Benzalkonium chloride 0.01% was a suitable preservative for methylene blue eye-drops sterilised by heating at 98° to 100° for 30 minutes.— M. Van Ooteghem, *Pharm. Tijdschr. Belg.*, 1968, *45*, 69.

Adverse Effects. After administration by mouth methylene blue may cause nausea, vomiting, diarrhoea, and dysuria. Nausea, abdominal and chest pain, headache, dizziness, mental confusion, and profuse sweating may occur with large intravenous doses of methylene blue. If injected subcutaneously, it may cause necrotic abscesses. Neural damage has occurred after intrathecal injection of methylene blue.

Radiculomyelopathy developed in a 32-year-old man after the lumbar intrathecal instillation of methylene blue.— P. Schultz and G. A. Schwartz, *Archs Neurol., Chicago*, 1970, *22*, 240.

Necrotic ulcers developed on the feet of a 62-year-old man at the sites of methylene blue injections.— P. M. Perry and E. Meinhard, *Br. J. clin. Pract.*, 1974, *28*, 289.

A 4-year-old boy given methylene blue 1 g intravenously during surgery developed hypotension, tachycardia, and apparent cyanosis. He remained intensely blue for several days.— N. Blass and D. Fung, *Anesthesiology*, 1976, *45*, 458.

Hyperbilirubinaemia secondary to haemolysis, needing 2 exchange transfusions, in a neonate after the intra-amniotic injection of 1 ml of 1% methylene blue, for the diagnosis of suspected premature rupture of membranes.— R. M. Cowett *et al.*, *Obstet. Gynec.*, 1976, *48*, *Suppl.*, 74s. See also F. T. Serota *et al.* (letter), *Lancet*, 1979, *2*, 1142.

In 12 patients undergoing nephrolithotomy the intravenous injection, over 15 seconds, of 20 ml of methylene blue 1% was followed by a mean rise of 35% in arterial blood pressure at 30 seconds, and 29% at 1 minute, with a concomitant fall in renal blood flow. Five patients had transient cardiac arrhythmias associated with the hypertension.— A. A. Birch and W. H. Boyce, *Anesth. Analg. curr. Res.*, 1976, *55*, 674.

Paraparesis progressing to total paraplegia after the lumbar intrathecal injection of methylene blue. Necropsy findings 8 years later are described. The intrathecal use of methylene blue should be abandoned.— M. M. Sharr *et al.*, *J. Neurol. Neurosurg. Psychiat.*, 1978, *41*, 384.

A report of Heinz body haemolytic anaemia in 2 neonates following the use of methylene blue.— I. R. Kirsch and H. J. Cohen, *J. Pediat.*, 1980, *96*, 276. Inadvertent intra-uterine injection of methylene blue in early pregnancy. A normal infant was delivered spontaneously at 40 weeks.— Z. Katz and M. Lancet (letter), *New Engl. J. Med.*, 1981, *304*, 1427.

Precautions. Methylene blue should not be given by subcutaneous or intrathecal injection. It should be used with caution in patients with severe renal impairment.

Methylene blue, 390 mg daily, had been reported to cause haemolytic anaemia in certain individuals with a deficiency of glucose-6-phosphate dehydrogenase. The reaction was not considered clinically significant under normal circumstances (e.g. in the absence of infection).— E. Beutler, *Pharmac. Rev.*, 1969, *21*, 73.

Methylene blue should be diluted to 0.01% prior to use during laparoscopy. Use of undiluted solutions could provoke an acute reaction with signs of pelvic peritonitis lasting for several weeks.— J. C. O'Sullivan (letter), *Br. med. J.*, 1973, *4*, 490 and 564.

Absorption and Fate. Methylene blue is absorbed from the gastro-intestinal tract. It is believed to be reduced in the tissues to the leuco form which is slowly excreted, mainly in the urine, together with some unchanged drug.

Although methylene blue was completely ionised at the pH of the gastro-intestinal tract, it was well absorbed. About 74% of a 10-mg dose was excreted in the urine over 6 days and of this 22% was unchanged and the remainder metabolised to a stabilised form of leucomethylene blue.— A. R. DiSanto and J. G. Wagner, *J. pharm. Sci.*, 1972, *61*, 1086. See also *idem*, 598.

Uses. In high concentrations methylene blue oxidises ferrous iron in haemoglobin to ferric iron, with the production of methaemoglobinaemia. In low concentrations methylene blue is reduced by pyridine nucleotides to leucomethylene blue, which reduces methaemoglobin in the red blood cells to haemoglobin.

Methylene blue is used in the treatment of drug-induced methaemoglobinaemia; it is administered intravenously as a 1% solution in doses of 1 to 4 mg per kg body-weight. It is also of value in the treatment of idiopathic methaemoglobinaemia (not due to abnormal haemoglobin), for which purpose it is given in a daily dose of 300 mg by mouth with large doses of ascorbic acid.

Methylene blue 0.5% solution has been used for the delineation of body structures and fistulas. It was formerly used in a renal-function test, and also in the treatment of urinary-tract infections. Stains on the skin caused by methylene blue may be removed with a hypochlorite solution.

Methylene blue imparts a blue colour to faeces and urine.

Methylene blue was successfully used to stain and identify the parathyroid glands during surgery. In 17 patients examined 41 glands had been identified; as experience with the technique developed identification had become more certain. The dye was given in a dose of 5 mg per kg body-weight as 1% solution diluted with 500 ml of dextrose saline. Maximum staining occurred about 1 hour after infusion and lasted for about 20 minutes. Normal parathyroid gland was stained dusky slate blue and adenomas were stained dark blue to purple. No troublesome side-effects had occurred, though the blue pallor of the patient had to be distinguished from cyanosis.— N. E. Dudley, *Br. med. J.*, 1971, *3*, 680.

In 56 patients with chronic urolithiasis methylene blue 65 mg twice or thrice daily for 18 months or longer seemed to prevent new stone formation in patients with mild metabolic acidosis and renal calculus disease.— M. J. V. Smith, *J. Urol.*, 1972, *107*, 164.

The use of methylene blue in a 36-year-old woman to prevent crystallisation of oxalate after renal transplantation.— J. M. Morgan *et al.*, *Archs Surg., Chicago*, 1974, *109*, 430.

Failure of methylene blue selectively to stain insulinomas in 2 patients.— A. R. Askew (letter), *Br. med. J.*, 1975, *1*, 741.

A discussion of the use of methylene blue for eczema herpeticum.— *J. Am. med. Ass.*, 1975, *233*, 987.

Staining of parotid glands during surgery.— A. D. Cheesman, *Clin. Otolar.*, 1977, *2*, 17.

A technique involving introduction of a 1% solution of methylene blue, 5 ml per kg body-weight, into the fasting stomach, was a safe and effective means of diagnosing gastro-oesophageal reflux in infants and children.— G. Girardi *et al.*, *Lancet*, 1978, *1*, 1236. Methylene blue had also been used in 2 patients with tracheostomies to demonstrate that their respiratory symptoms were due to regurgitation of gastric contents.— D. L. Christie (letter), *ibid.*, *2*, 474.

Preparations

Methylene Blue Injection *(U.S.P.)*. A sterile solution of methylene blue in Water for Injections containing in each ml 9.5 to 10.5 mg of methylene blue trihydrate. pH 3 to 4.5. *Nord. P.* has methylene blue 1 g, sodium sulphate 3.5 g, Water for Injections to 100 ml.

Methylene Blue *(Harvey, USA: Farillon, UK)*. Available as 1% solution, in ampoules of 10 ml.

Other Proprietary Names

Desmoid piller*(Denm.)*; Desmoidpillen *(Ger.)*; Urolene Blue *(USA)*.

Proprietary Preparations of Related Compounds

Panatone *(Paines & Byrne, UK)*. A solution containing leucomethylene blue 5 mg in each 5 ml. For topical application for the delineation of the vagus nerve during vagotomy.

1043-w

Obidoxime Chloride. LüH6. 1,1′-(Oxydimethylene)bis(4-hydroxyiminomethylpyridinium) dichloride.

$C_{14}H_{16}Cl_2N_4O_3$=359.2.

CAS — 7683-36-5 (obidoxime); 114-90-9 (chloride).

Obidoxime chloride has been used to counter poisoning by organophosphorus compounds. Its action, absorption, and elimination are similar to those of pralidoxime chloride (see p.389) but it is reported to exceed pralidoxime in rapidity and degree of cholinesterase reactivation. It has been given in doses of 250 mg by intramuscular or slow intravenous injection.

Obidoxime chloride, commercially available as a stable aqueous solution containing 250 mg per ml, was a more powerful cholinesterase reactivating agent *in vitro* and *in vivo* than pralidoxime, but its toxicity was slightly greater. High doses might penetrate the blood-brain barrier.— Sixteenth Report of WHO Expert Committee on Insecticides, *Tech. Rep. Ser. Wld Hlth Org. No. 356*, 1967.

The predicted time for loss of 10% potency by hydrolysis in a 10% solution of obidoxime chloride in water at pH 3 was about 100 years at 25°.— I. Christenson, *Acta pharm. suec.*, 1968, *5*, 249. See also *idem*, 23.

Obidoxime chloride, 2.5 to 10 mg per kg body-weight, given intramuscularly to 10 healthy men produced dose-related peak plasma concentrations of about 10 to 40 µg per ml after 20 minutes. The average half-life was 82.8 minutes, 84% of the dose being excreted unchanged in the urine in 24 hours. Side-effects included pain at the site of the injection, mild to moderate tachycardia and hypertension, transient paraesthesia and decreased pain sensitivity, and a sensation of warmth in the facial area and taste of menthol.— F. R. Sidell and W. A. Groff, *J. pharm. Sci.*, 1970, *59*, 793. Obidoxime chloride was poorly absorbed from the gastro-intestinal tract and 1-g doses produced peak plasma concentrations of only 1 µg per ml.— *idem*, 1971, *60*, 860.

Obidoxime gave higher plasma concentrations than equal doses of pralidoxime, possibly due to its smaller volume of distribution. It appeared that obidoxime diffused slowly through membranes or into tissues whereas pralidoxime diffused freely. Also obidoxime apparently was reabsorbed by kidney tubules whereas pralidoxime was actively secreted by kidney tubules.— F. R. Sidell *et al.*, *J. pharm. Sci.*, 1972, *61*, 1765.

Proprietary Names

Toxogonin *(E. Merck, Denm.*; *E. Merck, Ger.*; *E. Merck, Neth.*; *Merck, S.Afr.*; *E. Merck, Swed.)*.

1044-e

Penicillamine *(B.P., U.S.P.)*. D-3-Mercaptovaline; D-Penicillamine; (−)-ββ-Dimethylcysteine. 3,3-Dimethyl-D-cysteine.

$C_5H_{11}NO_2S$=149.2.

CAS — 52-67-5.

Pharmacopoeias. In *Br.*, *Cz.*, and *U.S.*

A white or almost white, finely crystalline powder with a slight characteristic odour and a slightly bitter taste. **Soluble** 1 in 9 of water and 1 in 530 of alcohol; practically insoluble in chloroform and ether. A solution in sodium hydroxide solution is laevorotatory. A 1% solution in water has a pH of 4.5 to 5.5. **Store** in airtight containers.

1045-l

Penicillamine Hydrochloride *(B.P. 1973)*. D-Penicillamine Hydrochloride.

$C_5H_{11}NO_2S,HCl$=185.7.

CAS — 2219-30-9.

A white or almost white, hygroscopic, finely crystalline powder with a characteristic odour and an acidic taste. Penicillamine hydrochloride 1.24 g is approximately equivalent to 1 g of penicillamine. **Soluble** 1 in 1 of water, 1 in 1.5 of alcohol, and 1 in 230 of chloroform; practically insoluble in ether. A 1% solution in water has a pH of 1.6 to 2.2. **Store** at a temperature not exceeding 25° in airtight containers.

Penicillamine occurred in 2 crystal forms; this was not clinically important.— J. A. G. Vidler, *Dista*, *J. Pharm. Pharmac.*, 1976, *28*, 663.

Solutions of penicillamine hydrochloride 3% lost 10% of their potency when stored at 20° and pH 6.5 under nitrogen in closed systems for 1.1 years.— J. R. B. J. Brouwers *et al.*, *Pharm. Weekbl. Ned.*, 1977, *112*, 121.

Penicillamine eye-drops were prepared as a 3% solution of the hydrochloride, adjusted to pH 6.5, and sterilised by filtration.— J. R. B. J. Brouwers, *Pharm. Weekbl. Ned.*, 1977, *112*, 155.

Adverse Effects. Anorexia, nausea, and vomiting may occur; reactivation of peptic ulcer has been reported; there may be oral ulceration and stomatitis; impaired taste sensitivity may occur in about 20% of patients. Skin rashes occurring early in treatment are commonly allergic and may be associated with pruritus, urticaria, fever, arthralgia, and lymphadenopathy. Other skin reactions include lupus erythematosus and pemphigoid eruptions. Increased skin fragility, possibly with skin haemorrhage and impaired wound healing, are due to the inhibition of cross-linking of collagen. Leucopenia may occur in up to 2% of patients and thrombocytopenia in up to 4%; other blood disorders include agranulocytosis, aplastic anaemia, eosinophilia, haemolytic anaemia, and thrombocytopenic purpura. Proteinuria may occur; estimates of the incidence range from 6 to 20%; there may be haematuria, and an immune complex membranous glomerulonephritis may progress to a nephrotic syndrome. Other side-effects reported include alopecia, cholestatic jaundice, Goodpasture's syndrome, myasthenia, pancreatitis, and tinnitus.

Patients sensitive to penicillin may react similarly to penicillamine.

Reports and discussions on the adverse effects of penicillamine and their incidence: P. B. Halverson *et al.*, *J. Am. med. Ass.*, 1978, *240*, 1870; W. F. Kean *et al.*, *Arthritis Rheum.*, 1980, *23*, 158; H. B. Stein *et al.*, *Ann. intern. Med.*, 1980, *92*, 24; W. M. O'Brien, *ibid.*, 120.

There were 50 reports of adverse reactions to penicillamine reported to the Committee on Safety of Medicines up to September 1974. These included 22 reports of blood disorders (2 fatal) including thrombocytopenia (9;1 fatal), aplastic anaemia (2;1 fatal), and agranulocytosis (7), and gastro-intestinal effects including haemorrhage.— M. F. Cuthbert, *Curr. med. Res. Opinion*, 1974, *2*, 600.

Very low concentrations of IgA occurred in a 12-year-old girl with Wilson's disease treated with penicillamine. There were reports in the literature of 7 patients with low IgA concentrations among 41 patients with Wilson's disease; most of the 41 had been given penicillamine.— O. Hjalmarson *et al.*, *Br. med. J.*, 1977, *1*, 549. See also W. Proesmans *et al.* (letter), *Lancet*, 1976, *2*, 804; D. R. Stanworth *et al.* (letter), *ibid.*, 1977, *1*, 1001.

Acute polyarthritis in 5 of 32 patients with Wilson's disease appeared to be associated with penicillamine therapy. Joint hypermobility might also be associated with penicillamine therapy although this also appeared to be a feature of the disease itself.— D. N. Golding and J. M. Walshe, *Ann. rheum. Dis.*, 1977, *36*, 99.

In 63 patients with rheumatoid arthritis given 83

courses of penicillamine the following side-effects were encountered: rash (in 15 courses), impaired taste (5), dyspepsia (9), mouth ulcer (6), proteinuria (7), bone-marrow aplasia (1), and nephrotic syndrome (1).— A. S. Weiss, *Am. J. Med.*, 1978, *64*, 114.

Studies in 95 patients with rheumatoid arthritis and in 200 controls suggested that those with the HLA-DR phenotype had an increased risk of developing toxic effects to penicillamine or sodium aurothiomalate.— G. S. Panayi *et al.*, *Br. med. J.*, 1978, *2*, 1326. See also P. H. Wooley *et al.*, *New Engl. J. Med.*, 1980, *303*, 300.

A report of neuromyotonia in a patient taking penicillamine.— J. Reeback *et al.*, *Br. med. J.*, 1979, *1*, 1464.

Acute colitis in a 61-year-old woman was attributed to penicillamine which had been started about 4.5 months earlier; the condition recurred when penicillamine was again given. She was using indomethacin suppositories which were not considered to be involved.— P. Hickling and J. Fuller, *Br. med. J.*, 1979, *2*, 367. See also G. B. Grant (letter), *ibid.*, 555.

Breast enlargement, weight gain, and galactorrhoea occurred in a 25-year-old female taking penicillamine 125 to 250 mg daily for rheumatoid arthritis. Although the galactorrhoea ceased on withdrawal of penicillamine, the weight gain and increase in breast size remained 9 months later.— D. C. N. Thew and I. M. Stewart (letter), *Ann. rheum. Dis.*, 1980, *39*, 200. See also C. Passas and A. Weinstein, *Arthritis Rheum.*, 1978, *21*, 167.

Allergy. A man with a history of penicillin allergy, developed an allergic reaction to the vaginal secretions of his wife who was taking penicillamine for rheumatoid arthritis.— P. C. H. Newbold (letter), *Lancet*, 1979, *1*, 1344.

A report of bronchial spasm and angio-oedema in a woman receiving penicillamine 250 mg thrice daily for rheumatoid arthritis.— K. Tanphaichitr, *Sth. med. J.*, 1980, *73*, 788.

Blood disorders. Haemolytic anaemia and thombocytopenia developed in a woman who had been given penicillamine in mistake for penicillin.— E. E. Harrison and J. W. Hickman, *Sth. med. J.*, 1975, *68*, 113.

Haemolytic anaemia from the use of penicillamine in rheumatoid arthritis was rare. In Wilson's disease haemolytic anaemia might indicate a need to increase, rather than reduce, the dose.— W. H. Lyle, *Dista* (letter), *Lancet*, 1976, *1*, 428.

Haemolytic anaemia, leucopenia, and thrombocytopenia reported in patients with Wilson's disease during treatment with penicillamine might be associated with hepatolenticular degeneration and might not be a toxic effect of the drug.— H. C. Hoagland and N. P. Goldstein, *Mayo Clin. Proc.*, 1978, *53*, 498.

Of 18 deaths ascribed to penicillamine and reported to the Committee on Safety of Medicines between January 1964 and December 1977, fourteen were apparently due to blood disorders, at least 7 of them being marrow aplasias. A further 9 patients with marrow depression, and one suspected case, after taking penicillamine are described.— A. G. L. Kay, *Ann. rheum. Dis.*, 1979, *38*, 232.

Agranulocytosis. In 2 patients.— J. M. Corcos *et al.*, *J. Am. med. Ass.*, 1964, *189*, 265.

Aplastic anaemia. For reports, see E. D. Bird, *Postgrad. med. J.*, 1974, *50*, *Suppl.* 2, 73; A. J. Richards *et al.* (letter), *Lancet*, 1976, *1*, 646; B. Bourke *et al.* (letter), *ibid.*, *2*, 515; W. A. C. McAllister and J. A. Vale (letter), *ibid.*, 631; A. J. Barnett and M. G. Whiteside (letter), *ibid.*, 682; J. L. Gollan *et al.*, *J. clin. Path.*, 1976, *29*, 135; S. Jones *et al.*, *Postgrad. med. J.*, 1978, *54*, 834.

Connective tissue disorders. The effect of penicillamine on collagen.— M. J. O. Francis *et al.* (letter), *Lancet*, 1973, *1*, 773.

A 10.4% mean decrease in skin thickness occurred over a 12-month period in 12 patients with rheumatoid arthritis treated with penicillamine. No significant alteration in skin elasticity was observed over this period.— W. Harvey *et al.*, *Postgrad. med. J.*, 1974, *50*, *Suppl.* 2, 33.

In 5 patients with rheumatoid arthritis given penicillamine the total collagen in skin biopsies tended to decrease and in 4 the proportion of collagen soluble in 5% sodium chloride solution increased. Penicillamine should be used with caution in children as they had a rapid turnover of collagen.— M. J. O. Francis and A. G. Mowat, *Postgrad. med. J.*, 1974, *50*, *Suppl.* 2, 30.

Effect on the eye. Retinal pigment epithelial changes in a patient on long-term penicillamine treatment for Wilson's disease.— J. Dingle and W. H. Havener, *Ann. Ophthal.*, 1978, *10*, 1227.

Effect on the lung. A 48-year-old woman who had taken penicillamine up to 450 mg daily for a year developed dyspnoea, restricted lung function, and an X-ray picture considered to be fibrosing alveolitis. The condition regressed when penicillamine was withdrawn.— C. J. Eastmond, *Br. med. J.*, 1976, *1*, 1506.

There were 15 deaths from non-acute cardiopulmonary disease among 3356 patients treated for more than 6 months with penicillamine; of these 2 were due and 2 possibly due to obliterative bronchiolitis. There was no reason to suppose that penicillamine was involved.— W. H. Lyle, *Dista* (letter), *Br. med. J.*, 1977, *1*, 105. See also D. Brewerton (letter), *ibid.*, 1976, *2*, 1507; G. R. Epler *et al.*, *J. Am. med. Ass.*, 1979, *242*, 528.

Miliary pulmonary infiltrates in a woman treated for 7 weeks with penicillamine.— J. Petersen and I. Møller, *Br. J. Radiol.*, 1978, *51*, 915.

Impairment of taste. During treatment with penicillamine for various conditions, 27 of 173 patients reported decreased taste acuity. The effect generally occurred 4 to 6 weeks after starting treatment and a metallic or salty taste was also noted. Full taste function gradually returned 4 to 8 weeks after treatment was stopped. Dietary supplements of copper or treatment with 5 to 15 mg of copper, as copper sulphate, daily effectively returned taste sensitivity during treatment with penicillamine.— R. I. Henkin *et al.*, *Lancet*, 1967, *2*, 1268. See also H. R. Keiser *et al.*, *J. Am. med. Ass.*, 1968, *203*, 381; A. T. Day and J. R. Golding (letter), *Br. med. J.*, 1973, *3*, 593; W. H. Lyle, *Dista* (letter), *Lancet*, 1974, *2*, 1140.

In 10 patients taking penicillamine, impairment of taste in 6 seemed to coincide with elevated serum concentrations of copper which occurred before copper secretion became maximal.— L. Knudsen and K. Weismann, *Acta med. scand.*, 1978, *204*, 75.

Liver damage. Liver necrosis in one patient was attributed to benorylate and penicillamine that had been given for rheumatoid arthritis.— M. Sacher and H. Thaler (letter), *Lancet*, 1977, *1*, 481.

A 56-year-old man with rheumatoid arthritis developed cholestatic jaundice 4 weeks after penicillamine was added to high-dose aspirin and prednisone therapy; he died in acute renal failure.— D. Barzilai *et al.*, *Ann. rheum. Dis.*, 1978, *37*, 98.

Lupus erythematosus. A 22-year-old woman with hepatolenticular degeneration who received penicillamine, 3 g daily for 1 year, developed a lupus-like syndrome, with aortic regurgitation, fever, pericarditis, pleurisy, and polyarthralgia.— J. P. Harpey *et al.* (letter), *Lancet*, 1971, *1*, 292.

An 18-year-old girl with Wilson's disease developed a syndrome resembling systemic lupus erythematosus with glomerulonephritis after 27 months' therapy with penicillamine. Symptoms subsided on withdrawal of the drug. After 18 months, low-dosage penicillamine therapy was started without producing the lupus-like syndrome.— L. J. Elsas *et al.*, *Ann. intern. Med.*, 1971, *75*, 427.

Report of a lupus-like syndrome occurring in a 47-year-old woman with cystinuria who was treated with penicillamine up to 1.8 g daily.— I. Oliver *et al.* (letter), *J. Am. med. Ass.*, 1972, *220*, 588.

Subacute cutaneous lupus erythematosus developed in a 58-year-old woman treated with penicillamine and benorylate; the condition regressed when penicillamine was withdrawn.— T. Appleboom *et al.* (letter), *Scand. J. Rheumatol.*, 1978, *7*, 64.

Further references: T. M. Harkcom *et al.* (letter), *Ann. intern. Med.*, 1978, *89*, 1012.

Myasthenia gravis. There were 21 cases of myasthenia gravis in the world literature associated with the use of penicillamine in rheumatoid arthritis. The condition was usually reversible when penicillamine was withdrawn though anticholinesterase agents might be required. There were 2 reports involving patients with Wilson's disease.— R. C. Bucknall, *Proc. R. Soc. Med.*, 1977, *70*, *Suppl.* 3, 114.

Nephrotic syndrome. A discussion on penicillamine-induced nephropathy.— *Br. med. J.*, 1981, *282*, 761.

During a 4-year period 31 patients were seen with membranous glomerulonephritis associated with penicillamine. Despite immediate withdrawal of penicillamine at the first sign of proteinuria, 8 patients developed nephrotic syndrome; 11 patients continued treatment for 1 to 7 months before the nephrotic syndrome developed.— G. H. Neild *et al.* (letter), *Lancet*, 1975, *1*, 1201.

Three patients with Wilson's disease who were treated for 2 to 3.5 years with penicillamine 1 to 3.5 g per day developed fatal pulmonary haemorrhages and rapidly progressive glomerulonephritis, characteristic of Goodpasture's syndrome.— I. Sternlieb *et al.*, *Ann. intern. Med.*, 1975, *82*, 673.

Proteinuria in 14 patients taking penicillamine, and nephrotic syndrome in 11.— P. A. Bacon *et al.*, *Q.J. Med.*, 1976, *45*, 661.

Glomerulonephritis in 2 patients taking penicillamine, progressing to fatal renal failure.— H. M. Falck *et al.*, *Acta med. scand.*, 1979, *205*, 133.

Peptic ulcer. Following a report of 2 patients with healed peptic ulcer who developed active peptic ulcers when receiving penicillamine, analysis of at least 1435 patients receiving penicillamine for rheumatoid arthritis showed 8 with reactivation of peptic ulcer.— W. H. Lyle, *Dista* (letter), *Lancet*, 1974, *2*, 285.

Pregnancy and the neonate. O.K. Mjølnerød *et al.* reported (*Lancet*, 1971, *1*, 673) the birth of a child with a generalised connective-tissue defect (lax skin, joint hyperflexibility, vein fragility, varicosities, and impaired wound healing) to a mother who had taken penicillamine 2 g daily for cystinuria throughout pregnancy. L. Solomon *et al.* reported (*New Engl. J. Med.*, 1977, *296*, 54) a similar case with intra-uterine growth retardation, flattened facies, low-set ears, skin laxity, bilateral inguinal hernias, simian creases of the palms, and possible bowel perforation, where the mother had received penicillamine 900 mg daily for rheumatoid arthritis for most of the pregnancy; there was no autopsy evidence of collagen abnormality. They suggested a protective effect in patients with Wilson's disease due to chelation of copper by penicillamine, thus reducing the penicillamine concentration. There have been a number of reports of healthy children born to mothers taking penicillamine, and W.H. Lyle (*Lancet*, 1978, *1*, 606) in a survey of clinicians using penicillamine for cystinuria and rheumatoid arthritis reported on 27 pregnancies in women who had taken penicillamine for part or all of their pregnancies and found no evidence of a teratogenic effect. Penicillamine in high doses is reported to be teratogenic in *rats*.

See also under Precautions.

Skin reactions. A 19-year-old youth developed angular stomatitis and stomatitis of the gums during treatment with penicillamine; the condition was unresponsive to treatment until penicillamine was withdrawn.— R. A. Bennett and E. Harbilas, *Archs intern. Med.*, 1967, *120*, 374.

Skin rash associated with the use of Distamine did not recur when Cuprimine was given.— S. P. Deacon and R. R. Masters (letter), *Br. med. J.*, 1977, *1*, 237.

Severe persistent pemphigus-like stomatitis occurred in a 59-year-old man receiving penicillamine for psoriatic polyarthritis; resolution occurred on cessation of treatment.— P. P. K. Lam, *Br. dent. J.*, 1980, *149*, 180.

Pemphigus. For reports of pemphigus or a pemphigoid eruption associated with the use of penicillamine, see J. Hewitt *et al.* (letter), *Br. med. J.*, 1975, *3*, 371; R. A. Marsden *et al.*, *ibid.*, 1976, *2*, 1423; S. G. Tan and N. R. Rowell, *Br. J. Derm.*, 1976, *95*, 99; M. G. Davies and P. Holt, *Archs Derm.*, 1976, *112*, 1308; O. Scherak *et al.* (letter), *Br. med. J.*, 1977, *1*, 838; J. S. Pegum and A. C. Pembroke (letter), *ibid.*, 1473.

Treatment of Adverse Effects. Many of the adverse effects are reversible when treatment with penicillamine is withdrawn. In patients with Wilson's disease or cystinuria, who need continued treatment, it may be possible to re-introduce treatment, starting with a small dose, but blood disorders, progressive proteinuria, drug fever, or the appearance of a late rash may require complete withdrawal. Corticosteroids or antihistamines may be of value in the treatment of hypersensitivity reactions.

Parakeratitis and alopecia which had developed in an 18-year-old youth with Wilson's disease during treatment for 6 years with penicillamine were found to be due to zinc deficiency, zinc being chelated and excreted during treatment. He responded within 1 month to treatment with zinc acetate 168 mg in the morning followed by penicillamine 250 mg in the evening and at night.— W. G. Klinberg *et al.*, Zinc Deficiency following Penicillamine Therapy, in *Trace Elements in Human Health and Disease*, Vol. 1, A.S. Prasad and D. Oberleas (Ed.), London, Academic Press, 1976, 51.

Penicillamine was successfully re-introduced and administered for at least 13 months in 5 patients with rheumatoid arthritis who had developed proteinuria during the first course of therapy. Proteinuria did not recur. The initial dose was 50 mg, increased by increments of 50 mg to a maintenance dose of 150 mg daily. After 4 months the dose was increased if necessary by increments of 50 mg at intervals of 3 months to 250 mg daily.— H. Hill *et al.*, *Ann. rheum. Dis.*, 1979, *38*, 229.

Nephrotic syndrome. In a pilot study, 13 patients with active rheumatoid arthritis received penicillamine

500 mg daily for 2 weeks then 1 g daily. Azathioprine 50 mg thrice daily was also given in an attempt to prevent proteinuria. Two patients developed proteinuria after 9 or 11 weeks. In a second study azathioprine 50 mg thrice daily was given to 6 patients who had developed nephrotic syndrome during penicillamine therapy. In 3 patients who continued taking penicillamine proteinuria disappeared in 1, was reduced in the second, and disappeared initially but reappeared after 6 months in the third. In the 3 not taking penicillamine, proteinuria was reduced in 1 but not affected in 2.— H. Berry and E. C. Huskisson, *Postgrad. med. J.*, 1974, *50, Suppl.* 2, 61.

Precautions. Penicillamine should not be given with other drugs capable of causing blood disorders. It should be used with care in patients with renal insufficiency. White-cell and platelet counts should be made frequently, the urine should be tested for albumin, and patients closely observed for signs of liver dysfunction, fever, and allergic reactions. Pyridoxine 25 mg daily may be given to patients on long-term therapy since penicillamine increases the requirement for this vitamin. The effects of penicillamine appear to be reduced in patients taking iron supplements simultaneously; at least 2 hours should elapse after a dose of penicillamine before iron is given.

It is recommended that the dose of penicillamine be reduced to 250 mg daily prior to surgery.

There was a significant rise in activity of clotting factors I, II, V, X, and XII in 6 patients with rheumatoid arthritis who were given penicillamine in doses up to 900 mg daily. There was a reduction in partial thromboplastin time but the platelet count remained within normal limits.— H. Zöller *et al., Dt. med. Wschr.*, 1974, *99*, 694.

Lichenoid eruptions occurred in a patient given penicillamine which was found to be an inhibitor of glucose-6-phosphate dehydrogenase. Penicillamine was contra-indicated in patients with glucose-6-phosphate dehydrogenase deficiency.— W. B. J. M. van der Staak and D. W. K. Cotton (letter), *Lancet*, 1975, *1*, 1430.

It was inadvisable to give zinc sulphate and penicillamine together as the latter might be inactivated.— W. H. Lyle, *Dista* (letter), *Lancet*, 1976, *2*, 684.

Effect of gold. Over a period of 5 years, side-effects occurred on 59 occasions in 107 patients during penicillamine therapy. These were classed as renal in 20 patients, haematological in 16, skin in 6, and taste in 16. The frequency of side-effects was related to dose. Of 4 patients with major blood dyscrasias 3 had a history of previous gold therapy.— A. T. Day and J. R. Golding, *Postgrad. med. J.*, 1974, *50, Suppl.* 2, 71.

Of 54 patients who received penicillamine in a controlled trial, 29 had a history of gold therapy. There was no significant difference in the prevalence of rash, thrombocytopenia, and proteinuria between those who had previously had gold therapy and those who had not.— Multicentre Trial Group, *Postgrad. med. J.*, 1974, *50, Suppl.* 2, 77.

Of 114 patients with rheumatoid arthritis treated with penicillamine 75 had previously been treated with gold. While the overall incidence of side-effects was similar in the 2 groups the incidence of bone-marrow depression and skin rash appeared to be increased in those who had previously been treated with gold.— M. Webley and E. N. Coomes, *Br. med. J.*, 1978, *2*, 91. Criticism; absence of statistical evaluation.— D. A. Gough (letter), *ibid.*, 636. The increased incidence of side-effects might be due to underlying Sjögren's syndrome.— L. Fernandes *et al.* (letter), *ibid.*

The incidence of reactions to penicillamine was similar (25 of 59) in patients who had previously received gold therapy and in those who had not (21 of 58). However adverse effects (thrombocytopenia, pemphigus, proteinuria) occurred in 10 of 36 who had shown no reaction to gold and in 15 of 23 who had shown reaction to gold.— H. Hill (letter), *Br. med. J.*, 1978, *2*, 961.

Of 125 patients with rheumatoid arthritis who received only penicillamine 45 developed side-effects whereas of 30 similar patients previously treated with sodium aurothiomalate 27 had a history of gold toxicity and 18 of these 27 patients also reacted adversely to penicillamine. Identical adverse reactions to both penicillamine and gold occurred in 14 patients and the interval between treatments in this group was significantly shorter than in those who developed either differing reactions to both drugs or no reaction to penicillamine after gold therapy. As gold was reported to be stored in tissue for prolonged periods after the end of treatment some adverse reactions to penicillamine may have resulted from the mobilisation of gold in the tissues. It was suggested that in a patient who has reacted adversely to gold, treatment with penicillamine should probably be delayed for at least 6 months, when the risk of further adverse reactions is apparently reduced.— M. J. Dodd *et al., Br. med. J.*, 1980, *280*, 1498. Comments.— A. Calin (letter), *ibid.*, 1980, *281*, 454. Study of 70 patients indicated that there is no increased incidence of adverse reactions to penicillamine in patients who have had an adverse reaction to gold treatment and that there is no increased risk if treatment with penicillamine is started within 6 months of stopping gold therapy.— P. J. Smith and W. R. Swinburn (letter), *ibid.*, 617.

See also Gold Poisoning under Uses.

Porphyria. A study in *rats* indicated that penicillamine would probably not elicit an acute attack in susceptible porphyric individuals.— G. H. Blekkenhorst *et al.* (letter), *Lancet*, 1980, *1*, 1367. Criticisms of extrapolating data obtained from *animal* experiments to the treatment of human disease.— M. J. Brodie (letter), *ibid.*, *2*, 86; A. Gorchein (letter), *ibid.*, 152. Reply.— G. H. Blekkenhorst and L. Eales (letter), *ibid.*, 1250.

See also under Uses.

Pregnancy and the neonate. Since there is no evidence that the elastic and collagen defect induced by penicillamine is in itself lethal and since clinical reversibility seems possible, pregnancy is not contra-indicated in women taking penicillamine. An infant born to a woman taking penicillamine for Wilson's disease had generalised cutis laxa, giving a senescent appearance. By the age of 2 months the infant looked strikingly different, and at the age of 4 months he was normal in external appearance and in physical and neurological development.— A. Linares *et al.* (letter), *Lancet*, 1979, *2*, 43. Comment.— J. M. Walshe (letter), *Lancet*, 1979, *2*, 144.

See also under Adverse Effects.

Wound healing. Failure of normal wound healing occurred in a man who was taking penicillamine. It was suggested that penicillamine be discontinued before elective surgery and that copper supplements might be of benefit in encouraging wound healing.— H. C. Burry, *Postgrad. med. J.*, 1974, *50, Suppl.* 2, 75. In Still's disease and rheumatoid arthritis penicillamine, in moderate dosage for relatively short courses, did not appear seriously to interfere with wound healing.— B. M. Ansell *et al., Proc. R. Soc. Med.*, 1977, *70, Suppl.* 3, 75.

Absorption and Fate. Penicillamine is partially absorbed from the gastro-intestinal tract and reaches peak concentrations in the blood in 1 hour. It is rapidly excreted in the urine, but traces remain in the plasma after 48 hours due to protein binding. About 80% of an intravenous dose is excreted in 24 hours.

In 15 patients with cystinuria receiving a mean dose of 12 200 µmol [1.82 g] of penicillamine daily the mean percentages of the metabolites cysteine-penicillamine disulphide, penicillamine disulphide, and *S*-methyl-D-penicillamine recovered in the urine were 23.6, 12.5, and 3.7% respectively. In 6 patients with Wilson's disease receiving a mean of 9770 µmol [1.458 g] mean recovery was 15.3, 18.2, and 2.2% respectively. In 5 patients with rheumatoid arthritis receiving a mean of 6760 µmol [1.009 g] daily mean recovery was 14.4, 13.2, and 6.1% respectively. Balance studies in 4 patients taking penicillamine showed 26 to 44% of the dose excreted in the urine over 5 to 7 days and 4 to 16% in the faeces. The portion of the dose not accounted for was probably being metabolised in the gut to unidentified metabolites. Radioactive study in 1 patient showed about 35% of a dose in the faeces over 3 days.— D. Perrett, *Proc. R. Soc. Med.*, 1977, *70, Suppl.* 3, 61.

In 6 patients with rheumatoid arthritis receiving chronic penicillamine therapy, plasma-penicillamine concentrations were less than 2 µg per ml 2 hours after being given a 125-mg dose.— J. Mann and P. D. Mitchell, *J. Pharm. Pharmac.*, 1979, *31*, 420.

Uses. Penicillamine is a chelating agent which aids the elimination of certain toxic metal ions. It is therefore used to aid the elimination of copper in the treatment of hepatolenticular degeneration (Wilson's disease).

The suggested initial dose for children or adults is 1 g daily in 4 divided doses before meals, increased as indicated by the urinary copper analyses to 2 g daily if necessary; it is seldom necessary to exceed this dose. A negative copper balance should be attained. Penicillamine should be given in conjunction with a diet low in copper, and a cationic exchange resin may be taken with meals to render dietary copper non-absorbable. Treatment must be continued indefinitely. Penicillamine is also given to patients with asymptomatic disease.

Penicillamine may also be used in the convalescent management of lead poisoning following initial treatment with sodium calciumedetate (see p 391); recommended doses are 20 to 40 mg per kg body-weight daily. It has also been used in poisoning by copper, gold, and mercury.

In cystinuria penicillamine reacts with cystine to form cysteine-penicillamine disulphide which is much more soluble than cystine; penicillamine also reduces the total amount of the amino acid excreted. Renal calculi may therefore be dissolved.

Doses of up to about 2 g daily in divided doses are commonly given, with a range of 0.75 to 4 g daily. It is recommended that treatment be introduced gradually and adjusted according to the individual patient's needs. Children may be given 30 mg per kg body-weight daily in divided doses. Treatment must be continued indefinitely.

Penicillamine has lathyrogenic activity and inhibits the cross-linking of newly synthesised tropocollagen and has therefore been used in the treatment of collagen disorders involving the skin and soft tissues.

Penicillamine is used, as an alternative to sodium aurothiomalate, in the treatment of severe rheumatoid arthritis not responsive to salicylates, other anti-inflammatory agents, physiotherapy, and rest. The initial dose is usually 125 to 250 mg daily, increased by the same amount at intervals of 1 to 3 months. Remission is often achieved with maintenance doses of 500 to 750 mg daily; the daily dose should not normally exceed 1.25 to 1.5 g daily and it is recommended that doses in excess of 500 mg daily be taken in divided doses. If there is no response to treatment for 3 to 4 months with 1 to 1.5 g daily, it should be assumed that there will be no response. After remission has been maintained for 6 months an attempt may be made gradually to reduce the dose at 2- to 3-month intervals. Salicylates, other anti-inflammatory agents, and corticosteroids may be given concomitantly when necessary. A suggested dose of penicillamine for children is: for those under 20 kg, 25 mg twice daily rising to 150 mg thrice daily; for those over 20 kg, 50 mg twice daily rising to 200 mg thrice daily.

A brief review of penicillamine as a chelating agent.— *Br. med. J.*, 1971, *2*, 270.

The chemical basis for the pharmacological and therapeutic effects of penicillamine.— M. Friedman, *Proc. R. Soc. Med.*, 1977, *70, Suppl.* 3, 50.

Two patients with spinal amyotrophy improved when given penicillamine 300 mg thrice daily.— A. Jušić and M. Šoštarko (letter), *Lancet*, 1977, *2*, 1034. No objective beneficial effect was noted in 5 patients with amyotrophic lateral sclerosis.— M. G. Bousser and M. Malier (letter), *ibid.*, 1979, *1*, 168.

Administration in renal failure. Beta-*N*-acetyl glucosaminidase (NAG) excretion, a marker of renal tubular (but not glomerular) damage, was decreased in patients with rheumatoid arthritis given penicillamine 0.5 to 1 g daily, indicating absence of tubular damage.— P. A. Dieppe *et al., Br. med. J.*, 1978, *2*, 664.

Amyloidosis. Partial resolution of primary amyloidosis was obtained in a 59-year-old woman by administration of chemotherapy consisting of penicillamine, melphalan, and prednisone.— J. Corkery *et al.* (letter), *Lancet*, 1978, *2*, 425.

Penicillamine has been used alone in the treatment of primary amyloidosis, but to date without apparent effect on mortality.— *Lancet*, 1978, *2*, 1187.

Ankylosing spondylitis. Two patients with ankylosing spondylitis experienced relief of pain after treatment with penicillamine. One patient with polymyositis had improvement of muscle pain and weakness but a second with muscle weakness but no pain derived no benefit from penicillamine therapy.— D. N. Golding, *Postgrad. med. J.*, 1974, *50, Suppl.* 2, 62.

Arsenic poisoning. Based on experience in treating 4 children (3 of whom survived) the following regimen was proposed for the treatment of arsenic poisoning:

penicillamine 100 mg per kg body-weight daily (up to 1 g daily) in divided doses before food for 5 days. In coma or shock dimercaprol could be given initially, replaced by penicillamine as early as possible.— R. G. Peterson and B. H. Rumack, *J. Pediat.*, 1977, *91*, 661.

Cystinuria. Of 24 patients with cystinuria with calculi treated for at least a year (or until dissolution with penicillamine, in a dose sufficient to reduce the excretion of cystine in the urine to about 200 mg in 24 hours, 10 experienced complete dissolution of calculi, 3 remained free after urolithotomy, 5 had partial dissolution, and 6 no change or growth of calculi.— P. J. Dahlberg *et al.*, *Mayo Clin. Proc.*, 1977, *52*, 533.

Cystinuria in 34 patients had been treated with penicillamine and a high fluid intake; calculi had been dissolved or their formation prevented in most patients. Penicillamine was introduced gradually over 2 to 3 weeks. The usual dose was 500 to 750 mg thrice daily but some patients needed 1 g thrice daily.— A. D. Stephens, *Proc. R. Soc. Med.*, 1977, *70*, *Suppl.* 3, 24.

Experience with 5 patients suggested that penicillamine, not more than 750 mg, taken at 22.00 hours with adequate daily fluid intake, would keep the concentration of cystine in the urine below the saturating concentration, though it did not reduce the 24-hour excretion of cystine. This dose was recommended for the prevention of recurrence of calculi.— P. Purkiss and R. W. E. Watts, *Proc. R. Soc. Med.*, 1977, *70*, *Suppl.* 3, 27.

Further references: R. W. E. Watts, *Postgrad. med. J.*, 1977, *53*, *Suppl.* 2, 7; J. C. Crawhall, *Proc. R. Soc. Med.*, 1977, *70*, *Suppl.* 3, 34.

Eye ulcers. Penicillamine in a constant-delivery device (Ocusert) appeared to benefit a patient with Mooren's ulceration.— P. Wright and B. R. Jones, *Proc. R. Soc. Med.*, 1977, *70*, *Suppl.* 3, 80.

Gold poisoning. In 18 patients who had received gold therapy, urinary and serum concentrations of gold were not significantly affected during treatment with penicillamine, the use of which for the chelation of gold remained speculative.— P. Davis and D. Barraclough, *Arthritis Rheum.*, 1977, *20*, 1413. A similar conclusion.— D. H. Brown and W. E. Smith, *Proc. R. Soc. Med.*, 1977, *70*, *Suppl.* 3, 41.

The occurrence, after 12 days of low-dose penicillamine treatment, of a rash identical to that seen about 10 years previously during gold therapy, and the concomitant resolution of rheumatoid arthritis, suggested that penicillamine had mobilised gold from body tissues.— J. Golding *et al.* (letter), *Br. med. J.*, 1978, *1*, 858.

See also Effect of Gold under Precautions.

Granuloma annulare. A favourable mention of the use of penicillamine in 50 children with granuloma annulare.— E. J. Moynahan, *Proc. R. Soc. Med.*, 1977, *70*, *Suppl.* 3, 73.

Hepatolenticular degeneration. References: J. M. Walshe, *Lancet*, 1968, *1*, 775; *ibid.*, 1021; J. A. Troelstra and H. Holl (letter), *ibid.*, 1094; W. R. Berry *et al.*, *Mayo Clin. Proc.*, 1974, *49*, 405; *Proc. R. Soc. Med.*, 1977, *70*, *Suppl.* 3, 1.

Huntington's chorea. Penicillamine 1 g daily was given to 10 patients with Huntington's chorea. Two patients withdrew from the trial because of skin rashes. Of the 8 remaining patients, 7 improved slightly during the first 3 months, but there was no significant improvement in any patient after 6 months.— E. D. Bird *et al.*, *Postgrad. med. J.*, 1974, *50*, *Suppl.* 2, 24.

Lead poisoning. After treatment for 1 week with penicillamine 0.75 to 1.5 g daily in divided doses, the condition of 14 of 15 workers with lead poisoning was improved. It was suggested that penicillamine, 1.5 g daily, given continuously for 15 to 30 days or until a steady excretion of lead in the urine was obtained, was effective therapy for mild and moderate lead poisoning.— S. Selander *et al.*, *Br. J. ind. Med.*, 1966, *23*, 282.

In 3 patients with poisoning due to tetraethyl lead, penicillamine 900 mg resulted in a mean increase of 85% in lead excreted in the urine.— A. D. Beattie, *Postgrad. med. J.*, 1974, *50*, *Suppl.* 2, 17.

Based on experience in treating 160 children with lead poisoning the following regimen was established for those with erythrocyte protoporphyrin values (EP) at least 10 times normal and blood-lead concentrations of 50 to 60 μg per ml: edetate was given intramuscularly for 5 days, then penicillamine until the EP had decreased to less than 3 to 5 times normal; this usually took 3 months or less. An initial dose of penicillamine 2 g per m^2 body-surface daily for 5 days was followed by 750 mg per m^2 daily in single or divided doses.— J. J. Chisolm, *Pediatrics*, 1974, *53*, 441, per *Abstr. Hyg.*, 1974, *49*, 840.

Further references: A. D. Beattie, *Proc. R. Soc. Med.*, 1977, *70*, *Suppl.* 3, 43.

Liver disease. In a controlled study, penicillamine and prednisone were compared as maintenance therapy in active chronic hepatitis after the disease had been brought under control by corticosteroids. Of 18 patients receiving penicillamine (up to 1.2 g daily), 9 showed little change in liver function tests after 1 year; 9 patients were withdrawn—side-effects (7) and lack of disease control (2). In the 17 patients given prednisone (15 mg daily) 6 were withdrawn—lack of disease control (4), side-effects (1), and carcinomatosis (1). Because of side-effects penicillamine was not the drug of choice for maintenance, but if corticosteroids were contra-indicated penicillamine would be a useful alternative.— R. B. Stern *et al.*, *Gut*, 1977, *18*, 19.

Further references: J. Lange *et al.*, *Dt. med. Wschr.*, 1971, *96*, 139; H. Schnack, *Wien. med. Wschr.*, 1971, *121*, 900; H. Gros *et al.*, *Medsche Klin.*, 1972, *67*, 1277.

Primary biliary cirrhosis. Hepatic and urinary concentrations of copper, and serum concentrations of caeruloplasmin, were elevated in 46 patients with primary biliary cirrhosis. In a double-blind study 19 patients were given penicillamine 250 mg daily increased over 6 weeks to 1 g daily, with a low-copper diet for 1 year while 18 received a placebo. Penicillamine increased the urinary excretion of copper; the median hepatic concentration of copper was significantly reduced by 99 μg per g dry weight compared with an increase of 13 μg per g in those given placebo.— T. B. Deering *et al.*, *Gastroenterology*, 1977, *72*, 1208.

A controlled study of penicillamine in a dose increased to 900 mg daily in 19 patients compared with placebo in 13 controls with primary biliary cirrhosis. There was a significant reduction at 3 months in serum-aspartate-transaminase (SGOT) concentrations in the treated group. At 12 months there was a significant reduction in liver-copper concentrations in the 4 patients assessed in the treated group. Five patients had to withdraw because of severe side-effects. Penicillamine was considered to be of benefit in primary biliary cirrhosis.— S. Jain *et al.* (preliminary communication), *Lancet*, 1977, *1*, 831. In treated patients on a maintenance dose of penicillamine 600 mg daily, circulating immune complexes, all 3 classes of immunoglobulins (IgA, IgG, and IgM), liver-copper concentrations, and aspartate-transaminase (SGOT) concentrations in serum all fell significantly when compared with controls. Bilirubin concentrations increased at a slower rate in treated patients but the significant difference between groups at 12 months was not apparent at 24 months. Alkaline phosphatase concentrations fell in treated patients but not significantly. All these changes were not reflected by a significant change in necrosis and inflammation on liver biopsy but, since an immunological mechanism probably underlay the pathogenesis of primary biliary cirrhosis with accumulation of copper a secondary event, penicillamine might have a beneficial effect on the course of the disease.— O. Epstein *et al.*, *New Engl. J. Med.*, 1979, *300*, 274. Criticisms.— R. D. Soltis and I. D. Wilson (letter), *ibid.*, 1487; R. H. Resnick (letter), *ibid.* Reply.— O. Epstein and H. Thomas (letter), *ibid.* Evidence that penicillamine improves survival in primary biliary cirrhosis.— O. Epstein *et al.*, *Lancet*, 1981, *1*, 1275.

Further references.— D. J. Gottfried (letter), *Lancet*, 1978, *2*, 1158; C. R. Fleming *et al.*, *Mayo Clin. Proc.*, 1978, *53*, 587; M. S. Tanner *et al.*, *Lancet*, 1979, *1*, 1203; J. Evans *et al.*, *Gut*, 1979, *20*, A907; D. R. Triger *et al.*, *Gut*, 1980, *21*, A919.

Mercury poisoning. Penicillamine 1.3 g daily for 12 days then 630 mg daily for 17 days resulted in a marked increase in urinary excretion of mercury accompanied by clinical improvement in a 14-year-old boy suffering from chronic mercury vapour poisoning.— K. F. Swaidman and D. G. Flagler, *Pediatrics*, 1971, *48*, 639, per *Int. pharm. Abstr.*, 1972, *9*, 780.

Penicillamine 250 mg four times daily by mouth for 3 months was of little value in reducing the body burden of mercury in a 31-year-old man who had injected 1 to 2 ml of metallic mercury intravenously but showed no symptoms of mercury poisoning. Although excretion of mercury in the urine increased fivefold when penicillamine therapy was started the estimated excretion of mercury by all routes for the year after the injection was only about 1% of the dose.— J. J. Ambre *et al.*, *Ann. intern. Med.*, 1977, *87*, 451.

Further references: T. Suzuki *et al.*, *Br. J. ind. Med.*, 1976, *33*, 88.

Multiple sclerosis. Improvement in 5 of 9 patients with multiple sclerosis treated with penicillamine 2 to 2.25 g daily, with pyridoxine, zinc, and other vitamin and mineral supplements. A double-blind study was being planned.— M. S. Seelig *et al.*, *J. clin. Psychiat.*, 1978, *39*, 170.

Paracetamol poisoning. The use of penicillamine in the treatment of paracetamol poisoning was abandoned after use in 5 patients; it might enhance the nephrotoxicity of paracetamol overdosage.— L. F. Prescott *et al.*, *Lancet*, 1976, *2*, 109.

Porphyria. For a brief favourable report of 4 patients with porphyria treated with penicillamine, see G. A. Hunter and G. F. Donald (letter), *Br. J. Derm.*, 1970, *83*, 702.

Retinitis pigmentosa. Improvement in 4 patients in the sensorineural deafness associated with retinitis pigmentosa, with concomitant visual improvement during treatment with penicillamine.— D. K. Gahlot *et al.*, *J. Lar. Otol.*, 1977, *91*, 1107.

Rheumatic disorders. Four of 5 patients with palindromic rheumatism had no further attacks for 1 year after being given penicillamine 250 mg daily; the 5th patient had 4 attacks in a year compared with 25 in 6 months before being given penicillamine 750 mg daily.— E. C. Huskisson, *Br. med. J.*, 1976, *2*, 979.

Response of 1 patient, with melting of the cornea associated with rheumatoid arthritis, to penicillamine therapy.— M. I. V. Jayson *et al.*, *Ann. rheum. Dis.*, 1977, *36*, 428.

Rheumatoid arthritis. In a double-blind study of 105 patients with rheumatoid arthritis which was mostly advanced with gross joint destruction and had failed to respond to treatment, 52 were given penicillamine hydrochloride 300 mg increased to 1.8 g daily or penicillamine 250 mg increasing to 1.5 g daily as well as simple analgesics as required, and 53 control patients were given placebo and analgesics. Over one year 22 patients withdrew from treatment with penicillamine, 16 due to adverse reactions which included rash, thrombocytopenia, proteinuria, loss of taste, anorexia, and nausea and vomiting, and 15 patients withdrew from the control group, 9 due to worsening of their condition and 1 because of side-effects. The mean improvement in several symptoms was greater in the patients given penicillamine and no patient in this group had to withdraw from the study because of a deterioration of their arthritis. The administration of copper sulphate in conjunction with penicillamine to 26 patients had no effect on the adverse reactions.— Multicentre Trial Group, *Lancet*, 1973, *1*, 275.

In a multicentre study the effects of penicillamine and gold therapy in rheumatoid arthritis were comparable.— E. C. Huskisson *et al.*, *Ann. rheum. Dis.*, 1974, *33*, 532.

Penicillamine 1 g daily and azathioprine 2.5 mg per kg body-weight daily were equally effective in rheumatoid arthritis.— H. Berry *et al.*, *Br. med. J.*, 1976, *1*, 1052.

Preliminary study in 6 patients with rheumatoid arthritis suggested that a dose of penicillamine 250 mg daily might be adequate though the response to treatment was less rapid.— I. A. Jaffe, *Proc. R. Soc. Med.*, 1977, *70*, *Suppl.* 3, 130.

Of 127 patients with rheumatoid arthritis 109 had responded within a year to small doses of penicillamine—125 mg daily initially, increased if necessary after 3 months to up to 500 mg daily; 18 were not controlled at 500 mg daily. Patients were also subjectively improved.— J. R. Golding *et al.*, *Proc. R. Soc. Med.*, 1977, *70*, *Suppl.* 3, 131.

Further references: K. Miehlke, *Arzneimittel-Forsch.*, 1971, *22*, 1815; *Br. med. J.*, 1973, *3*, 464; D. N. Golding, *Br. J. Hosp. Med.*, 1973, *9*, 805; F. D. Hart, *Pharm. J.*, 1973, *1*, 171; *Drug & Ther. Bull.*, 1973, *11*, 31; M. H. Gordon and G. E. Ehrlich, *J. Am. med. Ass.*, 1974, *229*, 1342; C. G. Barnes, *Prescribers' J.*, 1974, *14*, 73; *Br. med. J.*, 1975, *3*, 120; *Lancet*, 1975, *1*, 1123; *Ann. rheum. Dis.*, 1975, *34*, 273; C. J. Smyth and J. F. Bravo, *Drugs*, 1975, *10*, 394; F. D. Hart, *ibid.*, 1976, *11*, 451; P. Davis and S. S. Bleehen, *Br. J. Derm.*, 1976, *94*, 705; P. Bresloff, *Adv. Drug Res.*, 1977, *11*, 1; O. J. Mellbye and E. Munthe, *Ann. rheum. Dis.*, 1977, *36*, 453; I. K. Tsang *et al.*, *Arthritis Rheum.*, 1977, *20*, 666; J. L. Kalliomäki, *Curr. ther. Res.*, 1977, *21*, 815; A. V. Camp, *Proc. R. Soc. Med.*, 1977, *70*, *Suppl.* 3, 67; *Br. med. J.*, 1978, *1*, 131; *Med. Lett.*, 1978, *20*, 73; P. Makisara *et al.*, *Scand. J. Rheumatol.*, 1978, *7*, 166; H. Berry *et al.*, *Ann. rheum. Dis.*, 1978, *37*, 93; H. F. H. Hill *et al.*, *ibid.*, 1979, *38*, 429; H. A. Capell *et al.*, *ibid.*, 567; E. Munthe *et al.* (letter), *Lancet*, 1979, *2*, 1126; S. Potter, *Med. J. Aust.*, 1979, *1*, *Suppl.*, 19; E. C. Huskisson *et al.*, *Eur. J. Rheumatol. Inflamm.*, 1979, *2*, 294; *J. Rheumatol.*, 1979, *Suppl.* 28, 5–110; H. A. Bird *et al.*, *Ann. rheum. Dis.*, 1980, *39*, 281; O. Börjesson *et al.*, *Acta med. scand.*, 1980, *207*, 93; T. P. Anastassiades, *Can. med. Ass. J.*, 1980, *122*, 405.

Schizophrenia. A favourable report of the use of penicillamine in schizophrenia.— G. A. Nicolson *et al.*, *Lancet*, 1966, *1*, 344. An unfavourable report.— J. W. Affleck *et al.*, *Br. J. Psychiat.*, 1969, *115*, 173.

Scleroderma. Penicillamine was given to 14 children with morphoea in doses from 150 mg to 450 mg daily. Results were good and in all cases clinical improvement was apparent about 2 months after beginning treatment.— E. J. Moynahan, *Postgrad. med. J.*, 1974, *50*, *Suppl.* 2, 39.

In 22 patients with progressive systemic sclerosis 15 had temporary improvement of cutaneous involvement when treated with penicillamine, 125 or 250 mg daily initially increased progressively to obtain a response or to the limit of tolerance, but only 5 had sustained benefit. Seven had initial improvement of joint function but only 3 had sustained benefit. Penicillamine appeared to be of no value for vascular and visceral involvement.— M. I. V. Jayson *et al.*, *Proc. R. Soc. Med.*, 1977, *70*, *Suppl.* 3, 82.

Experience with 6 patients with progressive systemic sclerosis treated with penicillamine in a mean dose of 1.25 g daily for 16 to 48 months showed that such treatment caused skin softening in some patients but did not improve features such as tenosynovitis and Raynaud's syndrome.— P. J. Zilko *et al.*, *Aust. N.Z. J. Med.*, 1977, *7*, 458.

Improvement in clinical status and in capillary circulation in 4 patients with systemic sclerosis (scleroderma) treated with penicillamine 1.2 to 1.8 g daily for 18 to 60 months.— H. Mellstedt *et al.*, *Scand. J. Rheumatol.*, 1977, *6*, 92.

For the use of penicillamine in the treatment of subcutaneous morphoea—a variety of scleroderma, see J. R. Person and W. P. D. Su, *Br. J. Derm.*, 1979, *100*, 371.

Further references.— D. D. Fulghum and R. Katz, *Archs Derm.*, 1968, *98*, 51; C. M. Herbert *et al.*, *Lancet*, 1974, *1*, 187; *Drug & Ther. Bull.*, 1974, *12*, 75.

Preparations

Penicillamine Capsules *(B.P.)*. Capsules containing penicillamine. Store at a temperature not exceeding 30°.

Penicillamine Capsules *(U.S.P.)*. Capsules containing penicillamine 250 mg. Store in airtight containers.

Penicillamine Tablets *(B.P.)*. Tablets containing penicillamine. They are film-coated. Store at a temperature not exceeding 25°.

Proprietary Preparations

Cuprimine *(Merck Sharp & Dohme, UK)*. Penicillamine, available as capsules of 250 mg. (Also available as Cuprimine in *Austral., Canad., Neth., Swed., Switz., USA*).

Distamine *(Dista, UK)*. Penicillamine, available as scored tablets of 50 mg and as tablets of 125 and 250 mg. (Also available as Distamine in *Neth., Switz.*).

Pendramine *(E. Merck, UK)*. Penicillamine, available as scored tablets of 125 and 250 mg.

Other Proprietary Names

Austral.—D-Penamine; *Belg.*—Kelatin; *Denm.*—Dimetylcystein; *Fr.*—Trolovol; *Ger.*—Metalcaptase, Trolovol; *Ital.*—Pemine; *Jap.*—Metalcaptase; *Neth.*—Kelatin; *Pol.*—Cuprenil; *S.Afr.*—Metalcaptase; *Spain*—Cupripen, Sufortanon; *Switz.*—Artamin, Mercaptyl; *USA*—Depen.

Penicillamine was also formerly marketed in Great Britain under the proprietary name Depamine (*Berk Pharmaceuticals*).

1046-y

Pentetic Acid.

DTPA. Diethylenetriamine-*NNN′N″N″*-penta-acetic acid.
$C_{14}H_{23}N_3O_{10}$=393.3.

CAS — 67-43-6.

Pentetic acid is a chelating agent with the general properties of the edetates (see under Disodium Edetate, p.383). The calcium trisodium salt is also used (see p.380).

The use of pentetic acid to increase the stability of ascorbic acid injection solutions.— M. A. Kassem *et al.*, *Pharm. Acta Helv.*, 1972, *47*, 89.

Studies in *mice* and *dogs* showed that pentetic acid with procaine hydrochloride reduced haemorrhage caused by rattlesnake venom.— C. L. Ownby *et al.*, *J. clin. Pharmac.*, 1975, *15*, 419.

1047-j

Pralidoxime Chloride *(U.S.P.)*.

2-PAM Chloride; 2-PAMCl; Pyraloxime Chloride; 2-Pyridine Aldoxime Methochloride. 2-Hydroxyiminomethyl-1-methylpyridinium chloride.
$C_7H_9ClN_2O$=172.6.

CAS — 6735-59-7 (pralidoxime); 51-15-0 (chloride).

Pharmacopoeias. In *U.S.* which also includes Sterile Pralidoxime Chloride.

A white or pale yellow odourless crystalline powder. M.p. 215° to 225° with decomposition. **Soluble** 1 in less than 2 of water and 1 in 100 of alcohol. A 2.87% solution in water is iso-osmotic with serum.

From a review of published data on stability it was concluded that solutions of pralidoxime salts could be stored in a cool place for about 5 years at pH 3, even after sterilisation by heat.— A. W. Boeke, *Pharm. Weekbl. Ned.*, 1978, *113*, 713.

Further references.— R. I. Ellin *et al.*, *J. pharm. Sci.*, 1962, *51*, 141; *ibid.*, 1964, *53*, 1006; *ibid.*, 1143; B. R. Cole and L. Leadbeater, *J. Pharm. Pharmac.*, 1966, *18*, 101.

Adverse Effects. The administration of pralidoxime may be associated with drowsiness, dizziness, disturbances of vision, nausea, tachycardia, headache, hyperventilation, and muscular weakness. Large doses of pralidoxime may cause transient neuromuscular blockade.

When atropine and pralidoxime are given together, the signs of atropinisation may occur earlier than might be expected when atropine is used alone.

Precautions. Pralidoxime should be used cautiously in patients with impaired renal function.

Studies, mostly in *animals*, with various cholinesterase inhibitors given in conjunction with various oximes, including pralidoxime and diacetyl monoxime, suggested that the effects of carbaryl and of diazinon were exaggerated by the concurrent administration of oximes.— R. I. Ellin and J. H. Wills, *J. pharm. Sci.*, 1964, *53*, 1146.

For conflicting reports of the effects of pralidoxime and atropine when the 2 agents were given from the same syringe, see Atropine, p.290.

Absorption and Fate. Pralidoxime chloride is somewhat slowly absorbed from the gastro-intestinal tract. Blood concentrations are more rapidly attained after intramuscular or intravenous injection. It is not bound to plasma proteins, does not readily pass into the central nervous system, and is rapidly excreted in the urine partly unchanged and partly as a metabolite.

The chloride, iodide, dihydrogen phosphate, lactate, and mesylate salts of pralidoxime were administered to human subjects by mouth. Detectable amounts appeared in the blood in 15 minutes and peak concentrations were reached in 2 to 3 hours followed by a decline at first-order rate. Doses of 1.5 and 3.7 g of pralidoxime chloride (equivalent to 8.6 and 21.6 mmol per 70 kg body-weight) gave peak blood concentrations after 2 hours of about 2.6 and 4.3 µg per ml of plasma (equivalent to about 15 and 25 µmol per litre of plasma). A 10-fold increase in dose produced a 3.5-fold increase in peak plasma concentration and the average biological half-life of pralidoxime salts in man was 1.7 hours. About 27% of pralidoxime was recovered from the urine. Iodism occurred in those given the iodide salt but other clinical tests were negative. Probenecid had no effect on pralidoxime excretion.— A. A. Kondritzer *et al.*, *J. pharm. Sci.*, 1968, *57*, 1142. See also A. Sundwall, *Biochem. Pharmac.*, 1960, *5*, 225.

Intramuscular injections of 7.5 or 10 mg per kg body-weight of pralidoxime chloride as a 30% solution gave plasma concentrations exceeding the 4 µg per ml necessary for therapeutic effect. The half-life was 77 minutes, and doses could be repeated hourly.— F. R. Sidell and W. A. Groff, *J. pharm. Sci.*, 1971, *60*, 1224.

The effect of heat and exercise stress on the metabolism and excretion of pralidoxime chloride in 6 healthy adults.— R. D. Schwartz and F. R. Sidell, *Clin. Pharmac. Ther.*, 1973, *14*, 83.

In a study of 6 healthy subjects concomitant intravenous administration of thiamine hydrochloride with pralidoxime chloride prolonged the mean plasma half-life of pralidoxime from 1.1 to 1.55 hours.— J. Josselson and F. R. Sidell, *Clin. Pharmac. Ther.*, 1978, *24*, 95.

Uses. Pralidoxime is used as an adjunct to but *not* as a substitute for atropine in the treatment of poisoning by certain cholinesterase inhibitors. It reactivates the enzyme cholinesterase when the activity of the enzyme is depressed and in this way it indirectly reduces an accumulation of acetylcholine. Atropine, on the other hand, directly counteracts the effects of this accumulation.

Pralidoxime is administered as the chloride, iodide, mesylate, or methylsulphate.

Pralidoxime is not equally antagonistic to all anticholinesterases. It has been reported to be effective in poisoning by some organophosphorus insecticides and miotics including amiton, demeton-methyl, diazinon, dichlorvos, disulfoton, dyflos, fenthion, malathion, mevinphos, parathion, parathion-methyl, phosphamidon, and TEPP, but appears to be relatively ineffective against dimefox, dimethoate, methyl diazinon, mipafox, and schradan, and against carbamate insecticides. It is only slightly effective against overdosage with cholinesterase inhibitors such as neostigmine and pyridostigmine. It is less likely to be effective if given more than 36 hours after exposure.

In the treatment of poisoning by cholinesterase inhibitors, initial measures should include removal of contaminated clothing, washing the skin with soap and water for at least 10 minutes, and irrigation of the eyes, or, if ingested, emptying the stomach by aspiration and lavage, removal of secretions, maintenance of a patent airway, and assisted respiration if necessary. Atropine sulphate should then be given intramuscularly while cyanosis is being corrected, or intravenously. In patients with or without respiratory insufficiency the initial dose is 2 to 4 mg; pralidoxime 1 to 2 g is given concomitantly; further 2-mg doses of atropine may be given every 10 minutes if necessary. In severe poisoning the initial dose of atropine is 4 to 6 mg followed by 2 mg up to every 5 to 10 minutes to maintain full atropinisation; the total required in the first 24 hours will not usually exceed 50 mg; some degree of atropinisation should be maintained for at least 48 hours.

Pralidoxime is administered by intramuscular injection or by slow intravenous injection as a 5% solution in Water for Injections over 5 to 10 minutes. Alternatively the dose may be dissolved in 100 ml of sodium chloride injection and infused over a period of 15 to 30 minutes. Pralidoxime may also be given by subcutaneous injection. A second or even a third dose may be given according to the patient's condition. Treatment should preferably be monitored by the determination of blood-cholinesterase concentrations. A suggested dose for children is 20 to 40 mg per kg body-weight.

If gastro-intestinal symptoms are not severe pralidoxime chloride may be given by mouth; 1 to 3 g may be given 5 times daily.

Pralidoxime iodide could be given to man in doses of 2 g intravenously at a rate of 100 to 300 mg per minute without toxic effects or changes in blood pressure or heart-rate. Repeated intravenous doses totalling over 40 g had been given without side-effects. The chloride could be given intramuscularly and was preferable to the iodide.— Sixteenth Report of the WHO Expert Committee on Insecticides, *Tech. Rep. Ser. Wld Hlth Org. No. 356*, 1967. See also Twentieth Report of the WHO Expert Committee on Insecticides, *Tech. Rep. Ser. Wld Hlth Org. No. 513*, 1973. A similar report.— Third Report of the WHO Expert Committee on Vector Biology and Control, *Tech. Rep. Ser. Wld Hlth Org. No. 634*, 1979.

Ten workers engaged on formulating organophosphorus insecticides were given pralidoxime chloride prophylactically in a dose of 1 g three or four times a week for up to 22 weeks. Concentrations of cholinesterase in red cells fell to below 70% of pre-exposure values in only 1 treated worker but in more than one-half the untreated controls.— G. E. Quinby, *Archs envir. Hlth*, 1968, *16*, 812, per *J. Am. med. Ass.*, 1968, *204* (June 10), A164.

Organophosphorus insecticide poisoning. The use of

11.442 g of atropine over 29 days in a case of unusually severe organophosphorus poisoning.— G. Hopmann and H. Wanke, *Dt. med. Wschr.*, 1974, *99*, 2106.

Pralidoxime chloride in a total of 7 doses each of 1 g daily given by slow intravenous injection over a period of 11 days was effective in the treatment of fenitrothion poisoning in a laboratory technician.— D. J. Ecobichon *et al.*, *Can. med. Ass. J.*, 1977, *116*, 377.

For some further reports of the use of pralidoxime in organophosphorus insecticide poisoning, see Martindale 27th Edn, p. 339.

Preparations

Pralidoxime Chloride Tablets *(U.S.P.)*. Tablets containing pralidoxime chloride.

Sterile Pralidoxime Chloride *(U.S.P.)*. Pralidoxime chloride suitable for parenteral use; it may contain a small amount of sodium hydroxide for the adjustment of the pH. A 5% solution has a pH of 3.5 to 4.5.

Proprietary Names

Protopam Chloride *(Ayerst, Canad.; Ayerst, USA)*.

1048-z

Pralidoxime Iodide.

Pralidoximi Iodidum; Pamium; PAM; P-2-AM; 2-PAMI; 2-PAM Iodide; Pyraloxime Iodide; 2-Pyridine Aldoxime Methiodide. 2-Hydroxyiminomethyl-1-methylpyridinium iodide.

$C_7H_9IN_2O$=264.1.

CAS — 94-63-3.

Pharmacopoeias. In *Chin., Int.,* and *Swiss.*

A yellow, odourless, hygroscopic, crystalline powder with a slight taste. M.p. about 220° with decomposition.

Soluble 1 in 20 of water; practically insoluble in alcohol, chloroform, ether, and light petroleum. Solutions in water have a pH of about 7.5. **Store** in airtight containers. Protect from light.

For reports of the stability of pralidoxime solutions, see p.389.

Adverse Effects and Precautions. As for Pralidoxime Chloride, p.389.

It is contra-indicated in persons hypersensitive to iodine.

Pharyngeal pain. One of the most striking adverse effects of pralidoxime iodide was the production in some men of pharyngeal pain and enlargement of the parotid glands. These effects seemed to be related to the iodide ion and did not occur with pralidoxime chloride or mesylate.— R. I. Ellin and J. H. Wills, *J. pharm. Sci.*, 1964, *53*, 1149.

Absorption and Fate. As for Pralidoxime Chloride, p.389.

Uses. Pralidoxime iodide has uses similar to those of pralidoxime chloride, see p.389.

1049-c

Pralidoxime Mesylate.

Pralidoxime Mesilate; Pralidoxime Methanesulphonate; Pralidoximi Mesylas; 2-PAMM; P2S; RP7676; 2-Pyridine Aldoxime Methyl Mesylate. 2-Hydroxyiminomethyl-1-methylpyridinium methanesulphonate.

$C_8H_{12}N_2O_4S$=232.3.

CAS — 154-97-2.

Pharmacopoeias. In *Nord.* which also includes an injection grade.

A colourless or white, odourless, hygroscopic, crystalline or granular powder with a saline, cooling, slightly bitter taste. **Soluble** 1 in 2 of water and 1 in 12 of alcohol; practically insoluble in chloroform and ether. Solutions are **sterilised** by filtration. **Store** in airtight containers. Protect from light.

For reports on the stability of pralidoxime solutions, see p.389.

Adverse Effects and Precautions. As for Pralidoxime Chloride, p.389.

Absorption and Fate. As for Pralidoxime Chloride, p.389.

Coated tablets containing 400 mg of pralidoxime mesylate were given to 20 volunteers. The therapeutic blood concentration was considered to be 4 µg per ml and this was reached in 20 minutes and maintained for 5 hours in those volunteers who received a dose of 6 to 8 g and in 45 minutes and maintained for 2.5 hours in those who received 4 g. Fasting did not influence blood concentrations. The biological half-life was 1.52 hours and about 32% of a dose was excreted in the urine.— F. R. Sidell *et al.*, *J. pharm. Sci.*, 1972, *61*, 1136.

Uses. Pralidoxime mesylate has uses similar to those of pralidoxime chloride, see p.389.

Pralidoxime mesylate 500 mg intramuscularly gave plasma concentrations of 4 µg per ml within 5 minutes. Higher concentrations were obtained when the injection was given 3 hours after a 4-g dose by mouth. No side-effects were reported but visual disturbances occurred after 3 injections and pain at the injection site was reported after larger doses.— P. Holland *et al.*, *Br. J. Pharmac.*, 1972, *44*, 368P.

1050-s

Pralidoxime Methylsulphate.

Pralidoxime Metilsulfate. 2-Hydroxyiminomethyl-1-methylpyridinium methylsulphate.

$C_8H_{12}N_2O_5S$=248.3.

CAS — 1200-55-1.

Pharmacopoeias. In *It.*

A white odourless or almost odourless crystalline powder. M.p. about 111°. Very **soluble** in water; slightly soluble in chloroform. A 2% solution in water has a pH of 3 to 5. **Incompatible** with acids and alkalis. **Protect** from light.

Uses. Pralidoxime methylsulphate has uses similar to those of pralidoxime chloride (see p.389) and has been given in initial doses of 200 to 400 mg followed by a further dose of 200 mg 30 minutes later.

Proprietary Names

Contrathion *(Rhodia, Arg.; Specia, Fr.; Farmitalia, Ital.)*.

1051-w

Protamine Sulphate.

Protamine Sulfate *(U.S.P.)*; Protamini Sulfas. A purified mixture of simple protein principles obtained from the sperm or the mature testes of fish belonging to the family Clupeidae or Salmonidae.

CAS — 9012-00-4 (protamine); 9009-65-8 (sulphate).

Pharmacopoeias. In *Chin., Jap., Nord.,* and *U.S.*

A white or faintly grey-yellow, odourless, hygroscopic, amorphous or crystalline powder with a slightly acid astringent taste. Sparingly **soluble** in water; very slightly soluble in alcohol; practically insoluble in chloroform and ether. Solutions are **sterilised** by filtration. **Store** at 2° to 8° in airtight containers.

Adverse Effects. Intravenous injections of protamine sulphate, particularly if given rapidly, may cause a sensation of warmth, flushing of the skin, hypotension, bradycardia, and dyspnoea.

The thrombocytopenia that accompanied extracorporeal circulation during cardiac surgery was increased after the injection of protamine sulphate.— J. E. Woods *et al.*, *Mayo Clin. Proc.*, 1967, *42*, 724.

In 15 patients given protamine sulphate 6 mg per kg body-weight after cardiopulmonary bypass there was a transient fall in arterial pressure, a more prolonged increase in pulmonary artery pressure, and a substantial fall in arterial oxygen tension.— J. Jastrzebski *et al.*, *Thorax*, 1974, *29*, 534, per *J. Am. med. Ass.*, 1975, *231*, 100.

Although protamine itself was not thought to be antigenic, hypersensitivity to residual fish antigens remaining after purification could occur in sensitive individuals. During filtration leucophaeresis procedures, 4 of 140 healthy subjects had suffered allergic reactions to protamine sulphate (angioneurotic oedema in 1, urticaria in 2, occipital pain and numbness in 1); 2 of the 4 subjects gave a history of fish allergy.— S. N. Caplan and E. M. Berkman (letter), *New Engl. J. Med.*, 1976, *295*, 172. There was no scientific basis for the routine administration of protamine sulphate 50 mg after a cell-separation procedure. It had not been used in over 700 procedures at the Royal Postgraduate Medical School, London.— N. A. Buskard and J. M. Goldman (letter), *ibid.*, 677.

Evidence that an anaphylactic reaction to protamine was mediated by a complement-dependent IgG skin-sensitising antibody. No adverse reactions occurred in 22 blood component donors given protamine for the first time; of 11 receiving protamine for a second time 4 experienced urticaria with or without bronchospasm or hypotension.— J. D. Lakin *et al.*, *J. Allergy & clin. Immunol.*, 1978, *61*, 102.

Uses. When injected intravenously, protamine sulphate neutralises the anticoagulant action of heparin and is used to check haemorrhage caused by heparin overdosage. Used in excess it has an anticoagulant action.

Each mg of protamine sulphate is stated to neutralise the anticoagulant effect of at least 80 units of heparin (lung) or at least 100 units of heparin (mucous). In some situations, such as dialysis, this variation may be important.

Ideally the dose of protamine sulphate should be titrated against assessments of the coagulability of the patient's blood. Commonly, however, it is given on the basis of 1 mg for each 100 units of heparin which it is desired to neutralise. If protamine sulphate is given 30 minutes after heparin the dose may be reduced to about one-half, to take account of the partial metabolism of the heparin; a similar reduction in dose has been suggested when the heparin is given subcutaneously.

Protamine sulphate is given as a 1% solution, usually at a rate of 0.5 ml per minute. Not more than 50 mg of protamine sulphate should be injected for any one dose; further doses may be required. Some authorities have given up to 50 mg in 1 to 3 minutes with not more than 50 mg in any 10-minute period.

It has also been used to neutralise the effect of heparin given during leucophaeresis procedures.

Because there was little correlation between chemical assays on protamine and heparin and their effects *in vivo*, batches of products could vary and there was no single figure for the amount of protamine required to neutralise an amount of heparin. A dosage such as 1 mg per 100 *U.S.P.* units of heparin given in divided doses until haemostasis was achieved was a useful rule. In addition, the excretion of heparin reduced the amount of protamine required for neutralisation by about 1 mg per minute for an average patient. After extensive and prolonged operations, particularly where the blood had been in contact with foreign surfaces, the neutralisation of heparin with protamine could make the blood incoagulable.— L. B. Jaques, *Can. med. Ass. J.*, 1973, *108*, 1291.

Protamine appears to contain 2 factors: one composed of heparin-neutralising action alone, while the other has some anticoagulant effect. Use of the heparin-neutralising component alone would presumably obviate the present need for precise titration of the amount required.— T. K. Day (letter), *Lancet*, 1979, *2*, 1027.

Preparations

Protamine Sulfate for Injection *(U.S.P.)*. A sterile mixture of protamine sulphate with 1 or more suitable dry diluents. The injection is prepared by the addition of diluent before use. Its solution has a pH of about 6.5 to 7.5.

Protamine Sulfate Injection *(U.S.P.)*. A sterile iso-osmotic solution of protamine sulphate. Store at 2° to 8°.

Protamine Sulphate Injection *(B.P.)*. A sterile solution of protamine sulphate in Water for Injections. Contains not less than 80% of the content of protamine sulphate stated on the label. pH 2.5 to 3.5. Store at 15° to 25°.

Manufacturers

Boots, UK; Weddel, UK.

1052-e

Sodium Calciumedetate *(B.P., B.P. Vet.).*

Sod. Calciumedet.; Natrii Calcii Edetas; Edetate Calcium Disodium; Calcium Disodium Edathamil; Calcium Disodium Edetate; Calcium Disodium Ethylenediamine-tetra-acetate; Calcium EDTA; Edathamil Calcium-disodium; Calcitetracemate Disodique. The dihydrate of the calcium chelate of the disodium salt of ethylenediamine-*NNN'N'*-tetra-acetic acid.

$C_{10}H_{12}CaN_2Na_2O_8,2H_2O$=410.3.

CAS — 62-33-9 (anhydrous).

Pharmacopoeias. In *Br., Fr., Int., It., Jug., Nord., Turk.*, and *U.S. Cz.* includes the anhydrous form. *Fr.* and *U.S.* specify a mixture of the dihydrate and trihydrate but predominantly the dihydrate.

A white or creamy-white, slightly hygroscopic, tasteless crystalline powder or granules, odourless or with a slight odour and a faint saline taste. **Soluble** 1 in 2 of water; very slightly soluble in alcohol; practically insoluble in chloroform and ether. A 20% solution in water has a pH of 6.5 to 8. A 4.5% solution is iso-osmotic with serum. Solutions are **sterilised** by autoclaving or by filtration and kept in containers made from lead-free glass. **Store** in airtight containers.

Incompatibility. A haze developed over 3 hours when sodium calciumedetate 4 g per litre was mixed with amphotericin 200 mg per litre, and a yellow colour when mixed with hydralazine hydrochloride 80 mg per litre in dextrose injection.— B. B. Riley, *J. Hosp. Pharm.*, 1970, *28*, 228.

Adverse Effects. Sodium calciumedetate may cause adverse effects similar to those described under disodium edetate (see p.383), but hypocalcaemic tetany does not occur. Administration by mouth may cause vomiting, diarrhoea, and abdominal cramps. Bone-marrow depression and a histamine-like reaction, with sneezing, nasal congestion, and lachrymation, have been reported.

For background toxicological information, see *Fd Add. Ser. Wld Hlth Org. No. 5*, 1974.

Precautions. The use of sodium calciumedetate is contra-indicated in renal disease.

Absorption and Fate. Sodium calciumedetate is poorly absorbed from the gastro-intestinal tract. After intravenous injection about 50% of a dose is excreted in the urine in 1 hour and over 95% in 24 hours.

Uses. Sodium calciumedetate is used in the treatment of acute or chronic lead poisoning and of lead encephalopathy.Its action is due to its ability to exchange its calcium for lead ions in the blood to form a stable, non-ionisable, water-soluble lead compound which is rapidly excreted unchanged in the urine. This exchange between lead and calcium is selective because other metals such as iron, copper, and cobalt are more strongly bound to tissue proteins. Sodium calciumedetate has also been used in the treatment of porphyria and poisoning by other heavy metals.

Sodium calciumedetate is usually given by intravenous infusion as a 0.5 to 3% solution in dextrose injection or sodium chloride injection. The infusion is usually administered over an hour, to a maximum of 40 mg of anhydrous sodium calciumedetate per kg body-weight, twice daily for 5 days. It may be repeated if necessary after at least 2 days.

In patients with lead encephalopathy and increased intracranial pressure excess fluids must be avoided. Sodium calciumedetate may be given intramuscularly as a 20% solution to which the addition of 1.5% preservative-free procaine hydrochloride has been recommended for local anaesthesia, and the cerebral oedema may be treated by an osmotic diuretic such as mannitol. The daily dose of sodium calciumedetate is divided into 2 to 4 doses and given for 5 days.

Sodium calciumedetate is often used concomitantly with dimercaprol (see p.383).

Sodium calciumedetate has also been given by mouth in the prophylaxis and treatment of lead poisoning, but it has been suggested that absorption of lead may be increased as a result. The usual dose is 4 g of anhydrous sodium calciumedetate daily in divided doses for adults and 60 mg per kg body-weight daily in divided doses for children.

A cream containing sodium calciumedetate 10% has been used in the treatment of chrome ulcers and other contact lesions from heavy metals.

Sodium calciumedetate is also used as a diagnostic test for lead poisoning.

For a brief review of edetates as chelating agents, see *Br. med. J.*, 1971, *2*, 270.

Lead poisoning. A review of the use of chelating agents in workers exposed to lead.— R. Lilis and A. Fischbein, *J. Am. med. Ass.*, 1976, *235*, 2823.

A review of the management of acute lead poisoning in children with chelating agents.— J. J. Chisolm and D. Barlthrop, *Archs Dis. Childh.*, 1979, *54*, 249.

In a study in 16 workers with varying degrees of lead poisoning, sodium calciumedetate had little effect when given by mouth. When given intravenously it increased the excretion of lead and caused significant falls in the urinary excretion of aminolaevulinic acid. Penicillamine, by mouth and intravenously, had a similar effect.— S. Selander, *Br. J. ind. Med.*, 1967, *24*, 272.

The administration of edetate prophylactically for a year to 23 workers in factories for ceramic printing or for producing lead colours was not considered effective in preventing lead poisoning.— R. Reinhold and G. Holzapfel, *Int. Arch. Gewerbepath. Gewerbehyg.*, 1967, *23*, 155.

The intravenous injection of 0.5 or 1 g of sodium calciumedetate in 4 patients with lead intoxication caused an increase in the urinary excretion of lead and in the amount of lead removed by peritoneal dialysis. The use of a small dose of sodium calciumedetate with peritoneal dialysis provided a safe, simple treatment of lead intoxication, with an improvement in the patients' condition which had not been observed when sodium calciumedetate and haemodialysis were used.— H. Mehbod, *J. Am. med. Ass.*, 1967, *201*, 972.

Further references: R. R. G. Warwick and P. F. Gibson, *Br. J. clin. Pract.*, 1973, *27*, 345.

Porphyria. Cutaneous porphyria in 28 patients was treated with sodium calciumedetate; 20 were in continuing remission. Five of 6 patients who failed to benefit from oral treatment gained remission after intravenous therapy. Patients excreting less than 1 mg daily of porphyrins usually benefited from oral treatment with 4 g daily; those excreting up to 2 mg daily usually needed 2 courses of intravenous therapy, each of 5 g daily for 5 days; for those excreting more than 2 mg, repeated intravenous courses might be needed.— G. F. Donald *et al.*, *Br. J. Derm.*, 1970, *82*, 70. See also H. A. Peters (letter), *New Engl. J. Med.*, 1967, *276*, 527.

Use in food. Estimated acceptable daily intake: up to 2.5 mg per kg body-weight.— Seventeenth Report of Joint FAO/WHO Expert Committee on Food Additives, *Tech. Rep. Ser. Wld Hlth Org. No. 539*, 1974.

The use of sodium calciumedetate is permitted in canned fish, canned shellfish, and glacé cherries under The Miscellaneous Additives in Food Regulations 1980 (SI 1980: No. 1834) for England and Wales and The Miscellaneous Additives in Food (Scotland) Regulations 1980 [SI 1980: No. 1889 (S.176)].

Preparations

Disodium Calcium Edetate Eye-drops *(Moorfields Eye Hosp.).* Sodium calciumedetate 4.1 g, chlorhexidine acetate 10 mg, Water for Injections to 100 ml. Sterilised by autoclaving. For the inactivation of epithelial collagenase.

Sodium Calciumedetate Injection *(B.P.).* Sod. Calciumedetate Inj.; Edetate Calcium Disodium Injection *(U.S.P.)* . A sterile solution of sodium calciumedetate in Water for Injections. It contains the equivalent of 18 to 22% of anhydrous sodium calciumedetate. pH 6.5 to 8. It should be diluted with sodium chloride injection or dextrose injection before administration. Store in containers of lead-free glass.

Sodium Calciumedetate Tablets *(B.P. 1973).* Sod. Calciumedetate Tab. Tablets each containing the equivalent of 500 mg of anhydrous sodium calciumedetate.

Proprietary Preparations

Ledclair *(Sinclair, UK).* Sodium calciumedetate, available as 5-ml ampoules of a solution containing the equivalent of 200 mg of anhydrous sodium calciumedetate per ml for intravenous injection after dilution. **Ledclair Cream.** Contains sodium calciumedetate 10%, in a water-miscible basis.

Sequestrene NA2Ca *(Ciba-Geigy, UK).* A brand of sodium calciumedetate, technical grade.

Other Proprietary Names

Calcium Disodium Versenate *(Austral., Canad., USA)*; Calciumedetat *(Ger.)*; Chelante Ipit *(anhydrous) (Ital.)*; Piomburene *(Ital.)*.

1053-l

Sodium Cellulose Phosphate.

The sodium salt of the phosphate ester of cellulose.

CAS — 9038-41-9.

A white to beige-coloured powder. Practically **insoluble** in water. It hydrolyses slowly on storage.

Adverse Effects. Diarrhoea has been reported.

Hypomagnesaemia as a possible side-effect of treatment with cellulose phosphate.— R. A. L. Sutton, *J.R. Coll. Physns*, 1968, *2*, 358.

Precautions. Sodium cellulose phosphate should not be given to patients with renal failure or congestive heart failure.

Uses. Sodium cellulose phosphate has an affinity for calcium ions. When administered by mouth, it binds calcium ions within the intestine and it has been given to diminish absorption of dietary calcium in idiopathic hypercalciuria and calculus formation, osteopetrosis, and hypercalcaemia. The usual dose is 15 g daily in 3 divided doses with meals; children, 10 g daily in 3 divided doses with meals.

Studies on the mechanism of action and effect on calcium metabolism of sodium cellulose phosphate.— C. Y. C. Pak, *J. clin. Pharmac.*, 1973, *13*, 15.

Sodium cellulose phosphate 5 g twice or thrice daily was given to 16 patients with a history of recurrent passage of renal stones and who had probable absorptive hypercalciuria. A low-calcium diet was maintained and magnesium was administered daily by mouth to prevent magnesium depletion. Over a period of 1 to 5 years there was a decrease in urinary excretion of calcium, a decrease in the state of saturation of calcium hydrogen phosphate in the urine and an almost complete cessation of passage of stones or formation of new stones.— C. Y. C. Pak *et al.*, *New Engl. J. Med.*, 1974, *290*, 175. See also *ibid.*, 224.

The mean urinary 24-hour excretion of calcium in 31 patients with hypercalciuria was 430 mg initially and 313 mg after treatment for 6 months with sodium cellulose phosphate 5 g thrice daily.— P. J. Jeffery, *Postgrad. med. J.*, 1976, *52*, 697.

In 19 patients with absorptive hypercalciuria treatment with sodium cellulose phosphate 5 g thrice daily for 6 to 21 months reduced renal stone formation from 1.09 to 0.11 stones per patient per year; a further 8 patients developed hyperoxaluria necessitating withdrawal of treatment.— R. Hautmann *et al.*, *J. Urol.*, 1978, *120*, 712.

Further references: C. E. Dent *et al.*, *Clin. Sci.*, 1964, *27*, 417; A. M. Parfitt *et al.*, *ibid.*, 463; C. E. Dent *et al.*, *Archs Dis. Childh.*, 1965, *40*, 7; C. Y. C. Pak *et al.* (letter), *J. clin. Endocr. Metab.*, 1968, *28*, 1829; J. Marks, *Br. J. Derm.*, 1970, *82*, 1; C. Y. C. Pak, *J. clin. Pharmac.*, 1979, *19*, 451.

Proprietary Preparations

Calcisorb *(Riker, UK).* Sodium cellulose phosphate, available as sachets each containing 4.7 g. Store in a refrigerator if the product is to be kept for more than 1 month. (Also available as Calcisorb in *Belg., Neth., Switz.*).

1054-y

Sodium Diethyldithiocarbamate.
$C_5H_{10}NNaS_2,3H_2O$=225.3.

CAS — 148-18-5 (anhydrous).

White or colourless crystals; **soluble** in water and alcohol.

Uses. Sodium diethyldithiocarbamate has been used in the treatment of nickel carbonyl and thallium poisoning.

An 18-year-old woman with thallium poisoning was treated with sodium diethyldithiocarbamate, 30 mg per kg body-weight daily. Urinary excretion of thallium was increased and there was improvement in the patient's vision, muscular co-ordination, and mental function.— F. W. Sunderman, *Am. J. med. Sci.*, 1967, *253*, 209.

The absorption, elimination, and duration of action of diethyldithiocarbamate in *animals*.— M. R. Craven *et al.*, *J. Pharm. Pharmac.*, 1976, *28, Suppl.*, 38P.

The preparation of enteric-coated capsules of sodium diethyldithiocarbamate. The drug is unstable in gastric acid.— B. K. Evans *et al.*, *J. clin. Hosp. Pharm.*, 1979, *4*, 173.

Cataract. Diethyldithiocarbamate could inhibit the activity of tyrosinase from *Mycobacterium leprae* which was considered to catalyse the oxidation of levodopa or tyrosine to quinones. These quinones might combine with lens proteins to form coloured cataracts.— K. Prabhakaran, *Lepr. Rev.*, 1971, *42*, 11. Quinone formation in the aqueous humour was not considered to be a cause of senile cataract.— A. Pirie and R. van Heyningen (letter), *Lancet*, 1974, *2*, 169.

1055-j

Sodium Nitrite *(B.P.C. 1973, U.S.P.).* Sodii Nitris; Natrii Nitris; Natrium Nitrosum.

$NaNO_2$=69.00.

CAS — 7632-00-0.

Pharmacopoeias. In *Arg., Aust., Belg., Chin., Cz., Ger., Hung., Ind., Mex., Nord., Pol., Roum., Rus., Span., Swiss, Turk.*, and *U.S.*

Colourless or slightly yellow crystals or white or slightly yellow granular powder or white or almost white opaque fused masses or sticks; odourless and deliquescent with a mild saline taste.

Soluble 1 in 1.5 of water and 1 in 160 of alcohol. Solutions in water are alkaline to litmus. A 1.08% solution is iso-osmotic with serum. Solutions are **sterilised** by autoclaving or by filtration. **Incompatible** with oxidising agents, phenazone, acetanilide, caffeine citrate, and morphine. **Store** in airtight containers.

Adverse Effects. Sodium nitrite may cause nausea and vomiting, dizziness, headache, cyanosis, dyspnoea, syncope, hypotension, and cardiovascular collapse. Ionised nitrites readily oxidise haemoglobin to methaemoglobin, causing methaemoglobinaemia.

Sodium nitrite is a precursor for the formation of nitrosamines many of which are carcinogenic in *animals*, but a relationship with human cancer has not been established.

A subject who developed headaches after eating cured meat products also developed headaches after swallowing solutions containing sodium nitrite 10 mg or tyramine hydrochloride 100 mg.— W. R. Henderson and N. H. Raskin, *Lancet*, 1972, *2*, 1162.

Recurrent attacks of muscle pain were reported to occur in 1 subject when he consumed beer containing sodium nitrite as preservative.— B. Williams (letter), *Med. J. Aust.*, 1972, *2*, 390.

For background toxicological information, see *Fd Add. Ser. Wld Hlth Org. No. 5*, 1974.

For a reference to the hazards associated with the use of nitrites as food additives, see *Med. Lett.*, 1974, *16*, 75.

A 36-year-old man who had taken sodium nitrite tablets (1 g daily) for several weeks thinking they were salt tablets became ill after taking 2 g on one hot day. He was obviously cyanosed, perspiring, and quite distressed, but recovered after treatment with oxygen and methylene blue.— L. G. Wilson (letter), *Med. J. Aust.*, 1976, *1*, 505.

Severe cyanosis and dyspnoea developed in a laboratory technician shortly after ingestion of sodium nitrite 30 g in a suicide attempt. Haemodialysis resulted in rapid improvement and after 3 hours the patient was symptom-free.— N. Graben *et al.*, *Dt. med. Wschr.*, 1977, *102*, 865.

Nitrosamines. Nitrosamines as possible environmental carcinogens.— C. L. Walters, *Chem. in Br.*, 1977, *13*, 140.

A review and discussion on naturally occurring toxic substances in foods, including nitrosamines.— R. L. Gross and P. M. Newberne, *Clin. Pharmac. Ther.*, 1977, *22*, 680.

The estimated volatile nitrosamine content of a range of foods in the UK.— T. A. Gough *et al.*, *Nature*, 1978, *272*, 161.

Intake of volatile nitrosamines from consumption of various alcoholic drinks.— E. A. Walker *et al.*, *J. natn. Cancer Inst.*, 1979, *63*, 947, per *Abstr. Hyg.*, 1980, *55*, 398.

For a review of the chemistry of nitrosamine formation, inhibition, and destruction, see M. L. Douglass *et al.*, *J. Soc. cosmet. Chem.*, 1978, *29*, 581.

Discussions on the amount of nitrite in the diet derived from cured meat: R. J. Smith, *Science*, 1978, *201*, 887; P. E. Hartman (letter), *ibid.*, *202*, 260; C. A. Black (letter), *ibid.*, 1979, *203*, 121.

Further references.— *Lancet*, 1968, *1*, 1071; W. Lijinsky and S. S. Epstein, *Nature*, 1970, *225*, 21; W. Lijinsky *et al.* (letter), *ibid.*, 1972, *239*, 165; N. P. Sen *et al.* (letter), *ibid.*, 1973, *241*, 473; *idem*, *245*, 104; *Br. med. J.*, 1973, *4*, 372; A. W. Holmes, *Practitioner*, 1974, *212*, 167; H. Low, *Archs envir. Hlth*, 1974, *29*, 256; P. F. Swann, *J. Sci. Fd Agric.*, 1975, *26*, 1761.

Absorption and Fate. Sodium nitrite is rapidly absorbed after oral administration. About 60% of the absorbed nitrite ion is metabolised in the body, probably partly to ammonia. The remainder is excreted unchanged in the urine.

Uses. Sodium nitrite has an action similar to that of glyceryl trinitrate; it takes effect in about 15 minutes and the action lasts for about an hour.

The principal use of sodium nitrite is in the treatment of cyanide poisoning. It is given intravenously, in conjunction with sodium thiosulphate, as described under Stronger Hydrocyanic Acid (Treatment of Adverse Effects), p.790. The sodium nitrite produces methaemoglobinaemia and the cyanide ions combine with the methaemoglobin to produce cyanmethaemoglobin, thus protecting cytochrome oxidase from the cyanide ions. The cyanmethaemoglobin dissociates, setting free cyanide, which is converted to thiocyanate by the sodium thiosulphate.

Sodium nitrite has been added to aqueous disinfectant solutions to give a concentration of 0.1 to 0.4% in order to prevent rusting of surgical instruments. It is also used as a preservative in foods.

Food preservation. The Preservatives in Food Regulations 1979 (SI 1979: No. 752) as amended (SI 1982: No. 15) and The Preservatives in Food (Scotland) Regulations 1979 [SI 1979: No. 1073 (S.96)] as amended permit as a preservative in certain types of cheese not more than 50 ppm of sodium nitrite and sodium nitrate (both expressed as sodium nitrite) of which not more than 5 ppm may be sodium nitrite. Limits of 150 to 500 ppm of sodium nitrite and sodium nitrate (both expressed as sodium nitrite) are specified for cured meats including cured meat products of which not more than 50 to 200 ppm may be sodium nitrite depending on the type of product.

The Regulations also prohibit the sale of any food specially prepared for babies or young children if it has in it or on it any added sodium nitrite or sodium nitrate.

Estimated acceptable daily intake of nitrites: up to 20 μg per kg body-weight. No change was made from the acceptable daily intake provided in the Seventeenth Report [however, in that report an intake of up to 200 μg per kg was given].— Twenty-third Report of the Joint FAO/WHO Expert Committee on Food Additives, *Tech. Rep. Ser. Wld Hlth Org. No. 648*, 1980.

Preparations

Sodium Nitrite Injection *(B.P.C. 1973).* A sterile solution of sodium nitrite 3% in Water for Injections. It is supplied in single-dose containers. *Dose.* 10 ml by intravenous injection in the treatment of cyanide poisoning.

Sodium Nitrite Injection *(U.S.P.).* A sterile solution of sodium nitrite in Water for Injections. pH 7 to 9.

Proprietary Names

O A R *(Orapharm, Austral.).*

1056-z

Sodium Phytate. Sodium Fytate. The nonasodium salt of *myo*-inositol hexakis(dihydrogen phosphate).
$C_6H_9Na_9O_{24}P_6$=857.9.

CAS — 83-86-3 (phytic acid); 7205-52-9 (nonasodium salt).

Adverse Effects. Nausea, vomiting, diarrhoea, and anorexia may occur during treatment with sodium phytate.

Rickets. The high phytate content of unleavened wheat chapatis was a possible cause of calcium malabsorption and rickets in Asians in Britain.— M. R. Wills and A. Fairney, *Lancet*, 1972, *2*, 406.

Uses. Phytic acid is found in many plants, but particularly in seeds and cereal grains. Sodium phytate reduces the absorption of calcium from the gut. It has been used in the treatment of hypercalcaemia. Doses of up to 9 g daily have been given.

Proprietary Names

Alkalovert (phytic acid) *(Klein, Ger.)*; Iliso *(Made, Spain)*; Phytat D. B. *(Daniel-Brunet, Fr.).*

1057-c

Sodium Thiosulphate *(B.P., B.P. Vet., Eur. P.).* Sodium Thiosulfate *(U.S.P.)*; Sodii Thiosulphas; Sodium Hyposulphite; Natrii Thiosulfas; Natrium Hyposulphurosum; Natrium Thiosulfuricum.

$Na_2S_2O_3,5H_2O$=248.2.

CAS — 7772-98-7 (anhydrous); 10102-17-7 (pentahydrate).

Pharmacopoeias. In all pharmacopoeias examined except *Braz., Int.*, and *Turk.*

Colourless odourless or almost odourless monoclinic prismatic crystals or a coarse crystalline powder with a saline taste; efflorescent in warm dry air; slightly hygroscopic in moist air. It dissolves in its own water of crystallisation at about 49°.

Soluble 1 in 0.5 of water; practically insoluble in alcohol. A 10% solution in water has a pH of 6 to 8.4. A 2.98% solution is iso-osmotic with serum. Solutions are **sterilised** by autoclaving.

Incompatible with salts of heavy metals, oxidising agents, and acids. It is slowly decomposed when boiled in aqueous solution. Aqueous solutions containing carbon dioxide or oxygen are slowly decomposed. If sodium thiosulphate is triturated with chlorates, nitrates, or permanganates, an explosion may occur. **Store** in airtight containers.

Solutions of sodium thiosulphate 50% stored in air developed cloudiness or a deposit after autoclaving. Addition of sodium phosphate 0.5% or 1.2% improved stability but solutions became cloudy or developed a deposit after 12 and 6 weeks respectively at 25°. Solutions containing sodium bicarbonate 0.5% became cloudy or developed a deposit after 12 weeks at 25°. No significant improvement in stability was obtained when the concentration of sodium thiosulphate was reduced to 30% or 15%, or when the injection was sealed under nitrogen.— Pharm. Soc. Lab. Rep., 1975, P/75/3..

Preservative for eye-drops. Phenylmercuric borate 0.005% or benzalkonium chloride 0.01% were suitable preservatives for sodium thiosulphate eye-drops sterilised by filtration.— M. Van Ooteghem, *Pharm. Tijdschr. Belg.*, 1968, *45*, 69.

Adverse Effects. Apart from osmotic disturbances sodium thiosulphate is relatively non-toxic. Large doses by mouth have a cathartic action.

Absorption and Fate. Sodium thiosulphate is poorly absorbed from the gastro-intestinal tract. After intravenous injection it is distributed throughout the extracellular fluid and excreted unchanged in the urine.

The biological half-life of sodium thiosulphate was reported to be 0.65 hours.— W. A. Ritschel, *Drug Intell. & clin. Pharm.*, 1970, *4*, 332.

Uses. The principal medicinal use of sodium thiosulphate is in the treatment of cyanide poisoning. It is given intravenously, in conjunction with sodium nitrite, as described under Stronger Hydrocyanic Acid (Treatment of Adverse Effects), p.790. The sodium nitrite produces methaemoglobinaemia, and the cyanide ions combine with the methaemoglobin to produce cyanmethaemoglobin, thus protecting cytochrome oxidase from the cyanide ions. The cyanmethaemoglobin dissociates, setting free cyanide, which is converted to thiocyanate by the sodium thiosulphate. Sodium thiosulphate is used, as a 20% solution applied once or twice daily, in the treatment of pityriasis versicolor. To prevent relapse, treatment must be continued for weeks or months after infection appears to have been cleared. A 10% solution is used prophylactically against ringworm infection as a foot bath at swimming pools.

Treatment for 3 weeks with sodium thiosulphate solution 10% applied at night virtually eliminated *Pityrosporum orbiculare* infection on the body of a 15-year-old girl. Residual lesions responded to treatment with a selenium sulphide shampoo.— S. O. B. Roberts and J. M. Lachapelle, *Br. J. Derm.*, 1969, *81*, 841.

Pityriasis versicolor might be treated by application of sodium thiosulphate 20% in a 1% cetrimide solution. Treatment should be continued for 6 weeks after an apparent cure to prevent relapse. Areas of depigmentation following infection should be treated with ultraviolet light during the course of treatment.— F. A. Ives, *Br. med. J.*, 1973, *4*, 475.

Estimated acceptable daily intake of sodium thiosulphate as SO_2: up to 700 µg per kg body-weight.— Twenty-second Report of Joint FAO/WHO Expert Committee on Food Additives, *Tech. Rep. Ser. Wld Hlth Org. No. 631*, 1978.

Preparations

Sodium Thiosulphate and Potassium Ferricyanide Eye Lotion *(A.P.F.)*. *Solution A*: sodium thiosulphate 12 g, Water for Injections to 100 ml; sterilised by autoclaving. *Solution B*: potassium ferricyanide 500 mg, Water for Injections to 100 ml; sterilised by autoclaving. *Use:* for silver nitrate burns, equal parts of the 2 solutions are mixed immediately before use.

Sodium Thiosulfate Injection *(U.S.P.)*. A sterile solution of sodium thiosulphate in freshly boiled Water for Injections. pH 8 to 9.5.

Sodium Thiosulphate Injection *(B.P. Vet.)*. A sterile solution of sodium thiosulphate in Water for Injections. Sterilised by autoclaving. *B.P.C. 1973* included a sterile 50% solution in Water for Injections, supplied in single-dose containers in which the air had been replaced by nitrogen or other suitable gas. *Pol. P.* and *Rus. P* have sodium thiosulphate 30% with sodium bicarbonate 2% and *Pol. P.* also has sodium thiosulphate 10% with sodium bicarbonate 0.6%.

Sodium Thiosulphate Lotion *(A.P.F.)*. Sodium thiosulphate 20% in freshly boiled and cooled water. For pityriasis versicolor.

Proprietary Names

Hyposulfène *(Rosa-Phytopharma, Fr.)*; Mikroplex Schwefel *(Herbrand, Ger.)*; S-hydril *(Laves, Ger.)*; Soufre Oligosol *(Labcatal, Fr.)*.

1058-k

Succimer. DIM-SA; DMSA. *meso*-2,3-Dimercaptosuccinic acid.
$C_4H_6O_4S_2$=182.2.

CAS — 304-55-2.

Succimer is chemically related to dimercaprol (see p.382). It is under study for the treatment of arsenic, lead, and mercury poisoning. It is administered by mouth.

Studies in *animals*.— E. Friedheim and C. Corvi (letter), *J. Pharm. Pharmac.*, 1975, *27*, 624; E. Friedheim *et al.*, *ibid.*, 1976, *28*, 711; L. Magos, *Br. J. Pharmac.*, 1976, *56*, 479; L. Magos *et al.*, *Toxic. appl. Pharmac.*, 1978, *45*, 463; J. H. Graziano *et al.*, *J. Pharmac. exp. Ther.*, 1978, *206*, 696; *idem*, *207*, 1051.

Lead poisoning. Encouraging results were obtained following oral administration of succimer to 5 lead-poisoned smelter workers. Although lead excretion was higher in 4 similar subjects who received sodium calciumedetate this might have been because in 2 of these subjects initial lead concentrations were higher. Lead excretion following both of the active therapies was greater than that in 2 untreated control subjects. Succimer was well tolerated; some patients complained of gastric upset when 540 mg (2 capsules) was given on an empty stomach. Succimer had a slight but significant effect on copper excretion, but unlike sodium calciumedetate (which produced an 8-fold rise) had no significant effect on zinc excretion. Succimer was given as 270-mg capsules in an initial dose of 8.4 to 12.7 mg per kg body-weight daily gradually increasing to 28.1 to 42.2 mg per kg daily on the fifth and last day of the course. These initial clinical results are considered quite promising; succimer merited further clinical investigation as an antidote for heavy metal poisoning.— E. Friedheim *et al.*, *Lancet*, 1978, *2*, 1234.

Mercury poisoning. Succimer was given in doses of 500 mg thrice daily for 5 days to 28 workers exposed to mercury. The urinary excretion of mercury was increased, particularly in those with more than 5 years' exposure.— I. E. Okonishnikova and E. E. Rosenberg, *Gig. Truda prof. Zabol.*, 1971, *5*, 29, per *Abstr. Hyg.*, 1972, *47*, 366.

1059-a

Unithiol. Sodium 2,3-dimercaptopropanesulphonate.
$C_3H_7NaO_3S_3$=210.3.

CAS — 4076-02-2.

A fine white crystalline powder. **Soluble** in water.

Uses. Unithiol is a derivative of dimercaprol (see p.382) and has been used in the USSR in the treatment of poisoning by heavy metals. It has been administered subcutaneously or intramuscularly as a 5% solution in Water for Injections or in sodium chloride injection in doses of 5 mg per kg body-weight 3 or 4 times during the first 24 hours, 2 or 3 times on the second day, and once or twice on subsequent days.

Proprietary Names

Dimaval *(Heyl, Ger.)*.

Chloroquine and other Antimalarials

1370-h

Malaria is caused by infection, by the bite of an infected female anopheline mosquito, with sporozoites of the genus *Plasmodium*. Four species are primarily responsible for infection in man: *P. falciparum* causing falciparum (= malignant tertian) malaria which, untreated, may be rapidly fatal; *P. vivax* causing vivax (= benign tertian) malaria; *P. ovale* causing ovale (a mild benign tertian) malaria; and *P. malariae* causing quartan malaria. Patients may sometimes be classified as non-immune if they have not previously or recently been exposed to *Plasmodium* infection and as semi-immune or immune if they have a history of prolonged exposure.

Simply expressed, the *sporozoites* rapidly migrate to the parenchymal cells of the liver (the primary *exoerythrocytic*, or *pre-erythrocytic* phase) where the *schizonts* develop, undergo *schizogony*, rupture the liver cell, and release *merozoites*; some merozoites (not of *P. falciparum*) enter other liver cells (secondary exoerythrocytic phase) and, by repeating the cycle, are responsible for recurrence of malaria; infection within the liver is referred to as the *tissue* phase; other merozoites are released into the blood where they enter red blood cells (*erythrocytic* phase). There development proceeds, through the *trophozoite*, to the mature schizont which, undergoing schizogony, ruptures the cell and releases merozoites; some are destroyed in the plasma while others invade other red blood cells where the process is repeated. Some merozoites give rise within the red blood cells to *gametocytes*; ingestion by and development within the mosquito vector leads to transmission of the disease.

Causal prophylactic drugs would ideally act on the sporozoites; as no effective drug is available the term is applied to drugs acting on pre-erythrocytic forms. The 8-aminoquinolines such as primaquine are active against the primary tissue phase of *P. falciparum* and *P. vivax*; their prophylactic use is limited by their side-effects. Proguanil and pyrimethamine are active against *P. falciparum* and have some action against *P. vivax*.

Tissue schizonticides (anti-relapse drugs) are active against the secondary exoerythrocytic forms of *P. vivax*; the 8-aminoquinolines are effective.

Blood schizonticides act on the asexual erythrocytic forms of all species of *Plasmodium*; active drugs include the 4-aminoquinolines, quinine, and mepacrine; proguanil and pyrimethamine are slowly active against *P. falciparum* and may be effective against *P. vivax*.

Gametocyticidal drugs act on the sexual forms; the 8-aminoquinolines are active; the 4-aminoquinolines, quinine, and mepacrine are active against *P. vivax* and *P. malariae* but have no direct activity against *P. falciparum*.

Sporonticidal drugs, given to humans, inhibit the sporogonic phase in the mosquito; proguanil and pyrimethamine are effective; the action of the 8-aminoquinolines is slower and less prolonged.

The principal antimalarial drugs may be classified into 6 main groups.

1. The *9-aminoacridines*, such as mepacrine (p.399). They have a rapid schizonticidal action and are effective against the gametocytes of *P. vivax* and *P. malariae*, but not against *P. falciparum*; they have largely been replaced by the 4-aminoquinolines and other more recent drugs.
2. The *4-aminoquinolines*, such as amodiaquine (p.397), chloroquine (p.395), and hydroxychloroquine (p.399). They have a rapid schizonticidal action and are effective against the gametocytes of *P. malariae, P. ovale,* and *P. vivax*, but not against *P. falciparum*.
3. The *8-aminoquinolines*, such as primaquine (p.401) and quinocide (p.407). They have a marked effect on gametocytes and are highly active against the primary exoerythrocytic forms of *P. falciparum* and *P. vivax* and the secondary exoerythrocytic form of *P. vivax*.
4. The *biguanides* with dihydrofolate reductase inhibitory activity, such as chlorproguanil (p.398), cycloguanil embonate (p.398), and proguanil (p.401). They have a slow schizonticidal action against all strains of *Plasmodium* and a rapid sporonticidal action against some strains.
5. The *diaminopyrimidines*, such as pyrimethamine (p.402) with actions similar to those of the biguanides; trimethoprim (see p.1484) has been similarly used.
6. The *quinine salts* which have a pronounced schizonticidal action. They are also effective against the gametocytes of *P. malariae* and *P. vivax* (see p.404).

Some other drugs used in the treatment of malaria are dapsone, sulphonamides, and tetracyclines. Vaccination has been attempted and insecticides play a part in mosquito control.

United States Agency for International Development (USAID) and World Health Organization (WHO) workshops on the biology and *in vitro* cultivation of malaria parasites, 7–12 March 1977, New York.— *Bull. Wld Hlth Org.*, 1977, *55*, 121–429.

Programme for combating malaria.— Seventeenth Report of WHO Expert Committee on Malaria, *Tech. Rep. Ser. Wld Hlth Org. No. 640*, 1979.

References to the immunology of malaria.— *Israel J. med. Sci.*, 1978, *14*, May;; *ibid.*, June;; *Bull. Wld Hlth Org.*, 1979, *57*, *Suppl.* 1, 1–290.

Malaria. Reviews of malaria and its prevention and treatment.— W. Peters, *Br. med. Bull.*, 1972, *28*, 28; B. G. Maegraith, *Br. J. Hosp. Med.*, 1972, *8*, 305; R. Drew, *Prescribers' J.*, 1972, *12*, 109; H. A. K. Rowland, *Br. med. J.*, 1972, *2*, 639; *Antimalarial Drugs*, Bulletin No. 2, London, The Ross Institute, 1972; W. Peters, *Postgrad. med. J.*, 1973, *49*, 573; I. F. M. Saint-Yves, *Med. J. Aust.*, 1973, *2*, 1052; Sixteenth Report of WHO Expert Committee on Malaria, *Tech. Rep. Ser. Wld Hlth Org. No. 549*, 1974; C. J. Canfield and R. S. Rozman, *Bull. Wld Hlth Org.*, 1974, *50*, 203; *Br. med. J.*, 1974, *3*, 297; *Drug & Ther. Bull.*, 1974, *12*, 65; E. Barrett-Connor, *Ann. intern. Med.*, 1974, *81*, 219; E. J. Pearlman and A. P. Hall (letter), *ibid.*, 1975, *82*, 590; E. Barrett-Connor (letter), *ibid.*, 591; W. O'Brien, *Practitioner*, 1975, *215*, 487; A. P. Hall, *Br. med. J.*, 1976, *1*, 323; *ibid.*, *2*, 1215; A. M. Geddes, *Adv. Med. Topics Ther.*, 1976, *2*, 1; M. J. Miller, *Prog. Drug Res.*, 1976, *20*, 433; R. H. Black, *Med. J. Aust.*, 1977, *1*, 929; W. Peters, *New Engl. J. Med.*, 1977, *297*, 1261; *Med. Lett.*, 1978, *20*, 17; E. Barrett-Connor, *Ann. intern. Med.*, 1978, *89*, 417; G. M. Trenholme and P. E. Carson, *J. Am. med. Ass.*, 1978, *240*, 2293; D. R. Bell, *Prescribers' J.*, 1978, *18*, 100; *Med. Lett.*, 1979, *21*, 57 and 72; *Med. Lett.*, 1979, *21*, 105; *Guide to the chemotherapy of human malaria*, Scientific Publication No. 373, Washington, Pan American Health Organization, 1979; D. Bell, *J. antimicrob. Chemother.*, 1980, *6*, 7; D. M. Mackay, *Prescribers' J.*, 1980, *20*, 137.

Causal prophylaxis and suppression. Malaria was usually suppressed by a weekly dose of 300 mg of either *chloroquine* or *amodiaquine* base, though in some areas, where the risk of infection was high, a dose of 600 mg of base was given. The treatment was maintained for 4 weeks after leaving the area of infection, and for a much longer period following exposure to *Plasmodium vivax*. Concomitant administration of 45 mg of *primaquine* with chloroquine was of value in areas where *P. vivax* was prevalent but was not always effective against chloroquine-resistant strains of *P. falciparum*. *Proguanil* 100 to 200 mg daily, *chloroproguanil* 20 mg weekly, or *pyrimethamine* 25 or 50 mg weekly had a causal prophylactic effect but resistant parasites had been encountered. *Cycloguanil embonate* in conjunction with acedapsone had been used as a long-acting prophylactic.— Chemotherapy of Malaria, *Tech. Rep. Ser. Wld Hlth Org. No. 375*, 1967.

In areas where indigenous falciparum infections were *resistant* to the 4-aminoquinolines one of the following schedules could be used to provide protection in pregnant women, nursing mothers, infants, and young children (the doses given are for adults): *chloroquine* or *amodiaquine* 300 mg (of base) every 1 or 2 weeks preferably in conjunction with *primaquine* 45 mg (of base) weekly; *quinine* 300 to 600 mg daily; *pyrimethamine* 25 mg weekly; or *proguanil* 100 mg daily. Non-immune subjects spending a limited time in a resistant area should use one of the following schedules for 4 weeks: *proguanil hydrochloride* 100 or 200 mg daily; *pyrimethamine* 25 or 50 mg weekly; *chloroquine* or *amodiaquine* 300 mg weekly or, depending on the risk of infection, *chloroquine* 100 mg daily for 6 days in each week; or *pyrimethamine* 50 mg weekly in conjunction with *sulfadoxine* 1 g or *sulfametopyrazine* 2 g. Suppressive cure of relapsing vivax infection could be achieved in many areas by a course of *chloroquine* 300 mg given with *primaquine* 45 mg once a week for 8 weeks.— Chemotherapy of Malaria and Resistance to Antimalarials, *Tech. Rep. Ser. Wld Hlth Org. No. 529*, 1973.

A WHO warning of the risk to travellers of malaria.— *Chronicle Wld Hlth Org.*, 1978, *32*, 355.

Members of the medical committee of the Hospital for Tropical Diseases made the following recommendations for the prevention of malaria: Africa, Arab States, Pakistan, India (except Eastern India), Pacific Islands—proguanil 200 mg daily (first choice) or chloroquine 300 mg weekly; Eastern India, Bangladesh, South-East Asia, Central and South America, Papua New Guinea—Maloprim one tablet twice weekly or Fansidar one tablet weekly. The doses for children were: under 1 year, one-quarter; 1 to 5 years, one-half; 6 to 12 years, three-quarters of the adult dose.— A. W. Woodruff *et al.* (letter), *Br. med. J.*, 1980, *281*, 1347; *Lancet*, 1980, *2*, 1079. Criticism of the use and dose of Maloprim.— J. Haworth (letter), *Br. med. J.*, 1981, *282*, 70. Reply.— A. W. Woodruff *et al.* (letter), *ibid.*, 989. Report of meetings convened by the Ross Institute on malaria prevention in travellers from the United Kingdom. Fansidar is taken once a week. For the present the prophylactic dose of Maloprim should usually be one tablet a week, but further experience and careful monitoring are required before a final decision can be taken.— *ibid.*, *283*, 214.

Further references: *Br. med. J.*, 1977, *2*, 757; *ibid.*, 1287; L. J. Bruce-Chwatt (letter), *ibid.*, 1978, *1*, 650.

Pregnancy and the neonate. Report of meetings convened by the Ross Institute on malaria prevention in travellers from the United Kingdom, including advice for pregnant women. Although some manufacturers and national authorities recommend that combined antimalarials should not be used by pregnant women and infants, this is not practicable except in the case of neonates. The child of a British parent will not have protective antibodies but, owing to the immaturity of enzyme systems and the practical problems of giving the correct dose, only the least toxic antimalarials should be given prophylactically. Proguanil or chloroquine may be given in areas without resistance; mosquito nets should be used everywhere. Neither of the 2 antimalarial preparations appropriate for chloroquine-resistant areas (Maloprim or Fansidar) is considered by the manufacturers suitable for the first 6 weeks of life; several members of the committee would rely on proguanil and mosquito nets, treating any fever with Fansidar. It was universally thought that no entirely satisfactory strategy was currently available.— *Br. med. J.*, 1980, *283*, 214.

See also under Causal Prophylaxis and Suppression, above.

Treatment. For the treatment of an acute attack of malaria, a 4-aminoquinoline was recommended whenever appropriate. A single 600-mg dose of *chloroquine* base was usually effective for a mild attack of falciparum malaria in partially immune patients but for the non-immune, 900 mg in divided doses was necessary on the first day with smaller doses on the following 2 to 4 days up to a total of 1.5 to 2.4 g. Recrudescence was avoided if small weekly doses of chloroquine were given for 4 to 8 weeks. Attacks of malaria due to *P. malariae*, *P. ovale*, or *P. vivax* were often treated with a course of a 4-aminoquinoline, 1.5 g of base over 3 days, given in conjunction with or followed by *primaquine*, 15 mg of base daily for 14 days. In some countries, *quinocide* was used in place of *primaquine*.— Chemotherapy of Malaria, *Tech. Rep. Ser. Wld Hlth Org. No. 375*, 1967.

Patients in *resistant* areas should be given *quinine* 10 mg per kg body-weight intravenously over at least 10 minutes, repeated if necessary after 6 to 8 hours. When the patient could be treated for more than 2 weeks, *quinine* 2 g daily could be given by mouth for 14 days alone or with *pyrimethamine* 50 mg daily for the first 3 days and *dapsone* 25 mg daily for 30 days, or with *sulphafurazole* or *sulphadiazine* 2 g daily for the first 6 days, or with *sulfametopyrazine* 1 g on the first day repeated if need be on days 5 and 10. Alternatively, *quinine* could be given to children for only 10 days. *Tetracycline* 1 to 2 g, *doxycycline* 200 mg, and *minocycline* 100 to 400 mg daily for 7 days could be effective but were best given with a rapidly acting schizonticide. *Pyrimethamine* 50 mg daily for 3 days with *sulphadiazine* 2 g daily for 5 days and one dose of *pyrimethamine* 50 mg with *dapsone* 100 mg daily for 5 days had been effective. Shorter courses had been used with *trimethoprim* 1.5 g in conjunction with *sulfametopyrazine* 1 g being given daily for 3 days or *pyrimethamine* 50 mg (1 mg per kg) being given once with *sulfadoxine* 1 g (15 mg per kg) or *sulfametopyrazine* 2 g (30 mg per kg) or *dapsone* 200 mg (3 mg per kg).— Chemotherapy of Malaria and Resistance to Antimalarials, *Tech. Rep. Ser. Wld Hlth Org. No. 529*, 1973.

A brief report on a Chinese antimalarial qinghaosu also called artemisinine extracted from *Artemisia annua*. Two synthetic derivatives artemether and artesunate are also being assessed.— L. J. Bruce-Chwatt, *Br. med. J.*, 1982, *284*, 767.

Tropical splenomegaly syndrome. Of 29 patients with the tropical splenomegaly syndrome included in a double-blind trial, 15 received placebo therapy and 14 received malaria prophylaxis. This consisted of primaquine 15 mg daily for 2 weeks (if glucose-6-phosphate dehydrogenase was not deficient) and chloroquine phosphate equivalent to 300 mg of base given weekly. After 15 months, all 14 patients given malaria prophylaxis had significant reduction in splenomegaly; in 11 patients the reduction was in excess of 50% of the original spleen volume. In only 3 control patients was there a significant reduction in splenomegaly; the reduction never exceeded 50%. Younger patients responded significantly better than older ones. Relief of symptoms and improvement in anaemia were more marked in the treatment group.— P. C. Stuiver *et al.*, *Br. med. J.*, 1971, *1*, 426. See also M. N. Lowenthal *et al.*, *ibid.*, 429.

Resistance. Resistance by *Plasmodium* to individual antimalarial compounds has been reported in many parts of the world and often involves cross-resistance to other compounds. It may be partial (decreased sensitivity) or complete (insensitivity). The existence of resistance may require the use of an alternative compound or the use of multiple therapy.

For a review of the geographical distribution of falciparum malaria resistant to 4-aminoquinolines and other antimalarials, see Chemotherapy of Malaria and Resistance to Antimalarials, *Tech. Rep. Ser. Wld Hlth Org. No. 529*, 1973.

The occurrence, control, and surveillance of drug-resistant malaria.— W. H. Wernsdorfer and R. L. Kouznetsov, *Bull. Wld Hlth Org.*, 1980, *58*, 341.

Further references: *Lancet*, 1971, *2*, 855; *Br. med. J.*, 1972, *2*, 604; P. E. Thompson, *Am. J. trop. Med. Hyg.*, 1973, *22*, 139.

1371-m

Chloroquine *(U.S.P.)*. Cloroquina. 7-Chloro-4-(4-diethylamino-1-methylbutylamino)quinoline.

$C_{18}H_{26}ClN_3 = 319.9$.

CAS — 54-05-7.

Pharmacopoeias. In *Braz.* and *U.S.*

A white or slightly yellow odourless crystalline powder with a bitter taste. M.p. 87° to 92°. Very slightly **soluble** in water; soluble in chloroform, ether, and dilute acids.

1372-b

Chloroquine Phosphate *(B.P., U.S.P.)*. Chloroquine Phos.; Chloroquini Diphosphas; Chloroquine Diphosphate; SN 7618; Chlorochinum Diphosphoricum; Chingaminum; Quingamine.

$C_{18}H_{26}ClN_3, 2H_3PO_4 = 515.9$.

CAS — 50-63-5.

Pharmacopoeias. In *Arg.*, *Aust.*, *Br.*, *Braz.*, *Cz.*, *Fr.*, *Hung.*, *Ind.*, *Int.*, *It.*, *Jug.*, *Mex.*, *Nord.*, *Pol.*, *Roum.*, *Rus.*, *Turk.*, and *U.S.*

A white or almost white, odourless or almost odourless powder with a bitter taste. There are 2 forms, one melting at 193° to 195° and the other at 210° to 215°. Chloroquine base 100 mg is approximately equivalent to 161 mg of chloroquine phosphate.

Soluble 1 in 4 of water; very slightly soluble in alcohol; practically insoluble in chloroform and ether. A 10% solution in water has a pH of 3.5 to 4.5. A 7.15% solution in water is iso-osmotic with serum. Solutions are **sterilised** by autoclaving or by filtration. Solutions of pH 4 to 6 are stable when heated but sensitive to light. **Protect** from light.

1373-v

Chloroquine Sulphate *(B.P.)*. Chloroquine Sulph.; Chloroquini Sulfas; RP 3377.

$C_{18}H_{26}ClN_3, H_2SO_4, H_2O = 436.0$.

CAS — 132-73-0 (anhydrous).

Pharmacopoeias. In *Br.*, *Fr.*, and *Int.*

A white or almost white odourless crystalline powder with a bitter taste. M.p. 205° to 210°. Chloroquine base 100 mg is approximately equivalent to 136 mg of chloroquine sulphate.

Soluble 1 in 3 of water; practically insoluble in acetone and alcohol; very sparingly soluble in chloroform and ether; soluble in acetic acid. A 10% solution in water has a pH of 4 to 5. Solutions are **sterilised** by autoclaving or by filtration. **Protect** from light.

Adverse Effects. Chloroquine is generally well tolerated when given in antimalarial doses and adverse effects are rare. The higher doses that may be used over prolonged periods for rheumatoid arthritis are more likely to produce adverse effects.

Side-effects occurring with antimalarial doses are usually reversible on withdrawal of the drug and include headache, gastro-intestinal disturbances such as nausea and vomiting, diarrhoea, and abdominal cramps, pruritus, and macular, urticarial, and purpuric skin eruptions. More severe effects include rare psychotic episodes, convulsions, hypotension and cardiovascular collapse, ECG changes, double vision, and difficulty in focusing the eyes.

Overdosage is especially dangerous in children and after intravenous use. Headache, drowsiness, respiratory and cardiovascular depression, arrhythmias, shock, visual disturbances, and severe gastro-intestinal irritation may be followed by convulsions, respiratory and cardiac arrest, and death.

Prolonged administration of higher doses may lead to corneal and retinal changes. Changes may occur long after the drug has been withdrawn. Pigmented deposits and opacities in the cornea are often reversible if the drug is withdrawn early enough but retinal damage, with macular lesions, defects of colour vision, pigmentation, optic nerve atrophy, scotomas, field defects, and blindness has been reported, and is usually irreversible. The risk of retinopathy is considered to occur when the total cumulative dose ingested exceeds 100 g. Other uncommon adverse effects from prolonged use include loss of hair, bleaching of hair pigment, bluish-black pigmentation of the mucous membranes and skin, photosensitivity, lichen planus-like eruptions, tinnitus, reduced hearing, nerve deafness, neuromyopathy, and myopathy.

Blood disorders have been reported rarely. They include aplastic anaemia, reversible agranulocytosis, thrombocytopenia, and neutropenia.

Bilateral sensorineural deafness after a single dose of chloroquine.— G. S. Dwivedi and Y. N. Mehra, *J. Lar. Otol.*, 1978, *92*, 701.

Peripheral neuropathy and nystagmus occurred in a 49-year-old woman who had been taking chloroquine 250 mg daily for about 5 months.— J. S. Marks, *Postgrad. med. J.*, 1979, *55*, 569.

Blood disorders. Aplastic anaemia was associated with the use of chloroquine in 3 patients. Two patients had received treatment over several months and one of these was later found to have acute myeloblastic leukaemia after receiving chloroquine treatment initially for discoid lupus erythematosus, and later for cerebral malaria. In the third patient aplastic anaemia developed 3 weeks after a short course of chloroquine for malaria.— N. Nagaratnam *et al.*, *Postgrad. med. J.*, 1978, *54*, 108.

Chloroquine-induced haemolysis and acute renal failure in 3 subjects with glucose-6-phosphate dehydrogenase deficiency.— V. P. Choudhry *et al.*, *Trop. geogr. Med.*, 1978, *30*, 331.

Extrapyramidal symptoms. Involuntary movements, often with protrusion of the tongue, occurred in 5 patients after treatment with chloroquine.— E. M. Umez-Eronini and E. A. Eronini, *Br. med. J.*, 1977, *1*, 945. Typical extrapyramidal symptoms occurred in 4 children treated with chloroquine.— S. Singhi *et al.* (letter), *ibid.*, *2*, 520.

Muscle weakness. *For reports of chloroquine-induced myopathy and neuromyopathy, see Martindale 27th Edn.*, p. 345.

Ocular changes. No retinopathy had been detected in thousands of patients taking 500 mg of chloroquine weekly for suppression of malaria, but patients treated with 100 mg daily for other conditions had shown a perceptible rise in the retinal threshold for vision. All the reported cases of retinopathy had concerned patients who had taken 250 mg or more daily for many months, which suggested that doses not exceeding 200 mg daily might be safe for at least 1 year. The disturbing feature of reported cases was the possibility of retinopathy developing several years after chloroquine therapy had been discontinued.— *New Engl. J. Med.*, 1966, *275*, 730. Although most individuals affected with retinopathy had received a total dose of 400 g or more there was probably no safe dose for long-term use.— B. L. Hazleman, *Practitioner*, 1978, *220*, 83.

The diagnosis of a state of premaculopathy, which was reversible.— S. P. B. Percival and I. Meanock, *Br. med. J.*, 1968, *3*, 579. See also S. P. B. Percival and J. Behrman, *Br. J. Ophthal.*, 1969, *53*, 101.

Maculopathy with impaired vision was present in 2% of 95 patients with rheumatoid arthritis who had taken a total of less than 100 g of chloroquine; in about 7% of 93 who had taken 101 to 300 g; in about 10% of 59 who had taken 301 to 600 g; and in 17% of 23 who had taken more than 600 g. Chloroquine retinopathy was present in one woman who had taken about 1000 g. It was considered that a dose of 4 mg per kg body-weight could be taken daily for 10 months a year without risk and that frequent ophthalmological examination was not needed for patients below the age of 50.— A. Elman *et al.*, *Scand. J. Rheumatol.*, 1976, *5*, 161.

Retinal changes developed in 22 of 222 patients receiving long-term chloroquine phosphate treatment in a dose of not more than 250 mg daily. On stopping therapy deterioration of visual acuity occurred in only one and regression of macular changes occurred in 4; there was no progression of retinal changes in the other 17 who showed mild pigmentary disturbance of the macula. The frequency of retinopathy increased with the patients' ages and also with the total dose given (developing in only 10% of those given less than 200 g as against 50% of those receiving more than 600 g). These results indicated that the ocular hazards of long-term chloroquine therapy are low.— J. S. Marks and B. J. Power, *Lancet*, 1979, *1*, 371. A contrary view.— S. Ogawa *et al.* (letter), *ibid.*, 1408.

Overdosage. Suicide of a young man who took the equivalent of 100 mg of chloroquine base per kg body-weight: the accepted toxic limit was usually given as 20 mg per kg. Death from respiratory failure occurred within 2.5 hours.— G. Pille *et al.*, *Med. trop. Marseille*, 1958, *18*, 304, per *Trop. Dis. Bull.*, 1959, *56*, 412.

Chronic poisoning resulting in death occurred in a man who had taken 3 or 4 chloroquine tablets daily to prevent malaria; accidental deaths were also reported in 6 children aged 11 months to 4 years who had each taken up to 5 tablets containing chloroquine.— V. J. M. Di Maio and L. D. Henry, *Sth. med. J.*, 1974, *67*, 1031, per *Abstr. Hyg.*, 1975, *50*, 104.

Non-fatal ingestion of 14.5 g.— P. A. Czajka and P. J. Flynn, *Clin. Toxicol.*, 1978, *13*, 361, per *Int. pharm. Abstr.*, 1980, *17*, 307.

Fatal ingestion of 1.8 g by a 14-month-old child.— L. Allen and W. Plauth, *Morbid. Mortal.*, 1980, *29*, 172, per *Int. pharm. Abstr.*, 1980, *17*, 873.

Pregnancy and the neonate. Chloroquine phosphate was prescribed for a woman during 4 out of 7 pregnancies. Complications in the children included loss of eighth-nerve function, posterior column defects, mental retardation, and neonatal convulsions.— C. W. Hart and R. F. Naunton, *Archs Otolar.*, 1964, *80*, 407, per *J. Am. med.*

Ass., 1964, *190*, 392.

Complete cochlear damage was found in a child whose mother had been treated with chloroquine.— G. J. Matz and R. F. Naunton, *Archs Otolar.*, 1968, *88*, 370, per *J. Am. med. Ass.*, 1968, *206*, 910.

Retinal degeneration in 2 sisters was probably caused by the maternal ingestion of chloroquine daily for 3 years that covered the periods of both pregnancies.— L. Paufique and P. Magnard, *Bull. Socs Ophtal. Fr.*, 1969, *69*, 466.

Skin reactions. In a modified 'repeated-insult' patch test, 25% chloroquine phosphate was found to produce moderate sensitisation of the skin.— A. M. Kligman, *J. invest. Derm.*, 1966, *47*, 393.

Chloroquine and its derivatives have been implicated in erythema multiforme (gravis), the Stevens-Johnson syndrome.— D. B. Coursin, *J. Am. med. Ass.*, 1966, *198*, 113.

Photo-allergic dermatitis appeared in the course of an antimalarial campaign with chloroquinised salt in Guyana but disappeared with the conclusion of the campaign.— G. Giglioli *et al.*, *Trans. R. Soc. trop. Med. Hyg.*, 1967, *61*, 313.

A report of toxic epidermal necrolysis after the ingestion of one tablet of chloroquine.— A. J. Kanwar and O. P. Singh, *Indian J. Derm.*, 1976, *21*, 73.

The problems of chloroquine-induced pruritus in Nigeria.— A. Olatunde, *Afr. J. Med. med. Sci.*, 1977, *6*, 27, per *Trop. Dis. Bull.*, 1977, *74*, 813.

Treatment of Adverse Effects. In gross overdosage prompt treatment is essential. Empty the stomach by inducing emesis or by aspiration and lavage. The use of charcoal has been suggested. Respiration may require assistance and intravenous fluids and vasopressors may be given for hypotension. Ammonium chloride in doses of up to 8 g daily by mouth has been recommended to enhance urinary excretion, but for comments on the hazards of forced diuresis, see under Quinine, p.404. Sodium lactate injection has been given intravenously to counter the depressant effects of chloroquine on the heart. Electrical pacing of the heart may be required. Dialysis procedures appear to offer little benefit.

Precautions. Regular examination for ocular disturbances should be carried out every 3 to 6 months in patients receiving long courses of treatment. Care is necessary in administering chloroquine to patients with impaired liver or renal function or with porphyria or psoriasis. Reactions are more common in alcoholics. Ocular toxicity may render the patient unfit to take charge of vehicles or machinery. Although some adverse foetal effects have been reported with chloroquine, the dangers from malaria, especially the falciparum form, are usually considered to be greater and antimalarial treatment should not be withheld during pregnancy. The concurrent administration of chloroquine with drugs capable of inducing blood disorders, such as gold salts, should be undertaken with caution, if at all.

Systemic administration of chloroquine with triamcinolone was liable to produce exfoliative erythroderma and should be avoided.— C. F. H. Vickers, *Practitioner*, 1969, *202*, 43.

Chloroquine and quinine appeared to be antagonistic when given together for *P. falciparum* malaria.— A. P. Hall (letter), *Trans. R. Soc. trop. Med. Hyg.*, 1973, *67*, 425.

Radiosensitisation by chloroquine.— J. Utley *et al.*, *Radiology*, 1977, *124*, 255.

Resistance. Resistance or reduced sensitivity of *Plasmodium falciparum* to chloroquine or other 4-aminoquinolines has been reported, particularly in South-east Asia and South and Central America, and resistance is spreading. There are also reports of resistance in African countries.

Chloroquine-resistant falciparum malaria in Papua New Guinea.— N. M. Bennett *et al.* (letter), *Med. J. Aust.*, 1979, *1*, 618.

Absorption and Fate. Chloroquine is readily absorbed from the gastro-intestinal tract and about 55% in the circulation is bound to plasma proteins. It accumulates in high concentrations in some tissues, such as the kidneys, liver, lungs, and spleen, and is strongly bound in melanin-containing cells such as those in the eyes and the skin; it is also bound to double-stranded DNA, present in red blood cells containing schizonts. Chloroquine is eliminated very slowly from the body and it may persist in tissues for a prolonged period. Up to 70% of a dose may be excreted unchanged in the urine and up to 25% may be excreted also in the urine as the desethyl metabolite. The rate of urinary excretion of chloroquine is increased at low pH values.

Studies in 4 healthy persons and 5 patients with rheumatoid arthritis who were given 150 mg of chloroquine base daily for 28 days showed that one-third to one-half of the dose was excreted in the urine as chloroquine or its metabolites in the healthy persons and one-half to two-thirds in the patients. About 10% was excreted in the stools. After a single intravenous dose, chloroquine accumulated in ocular and other tissues; concentrations in the iris and choroid were unchanged after 28 days but chloroquine was absent from other tissues after 14 days.— N. J. Zvaifler *et al.*, *Arthritis Rheum.*, 1963, *6*, 799.

Chloroquine could still be detected in the eye of a patient who had taken, 16 years previously, the equivalent of 300 mg of the base weekly for 2 months.— T. Lawwill *et al.*, *Am. J. Ophthal.*, 1968, *65*, 530.

The half-life of chloroquine in healthy people was reported to be about 100 hours.— A. P. Hall, *Trans. R. Soc. trop. Med. Hyg.*, 1977, *71*, 367.

The relationship between plasma concentrations of chloroquine and its side-effects. The pharmacokinetics of chloroquine are dose-dependent.— M. Frisk-Holmberg *et al.*, *Clin. Pharmac. Ther.*, 1979, *25*, 345.

Uses. Chloroquine is used for the suppression and treatment of malaria. It has a rapid schizonticidal effect and appears to affect cell growth by interfering with DNA; its activity also seems to depend on preferential accumulation in the infected erythrocyte. Chloroquine kills the erythrocytic forms of malaria parasites at all stages of development but does not affect the malaria parasite in the human liver cells. It will therefore eliminate malaria caused by *Plasmodium falciparum;* it will not prevent relapse arising from the secondary exo-erythrocytic phase of *P. vivax*, *P. ovale*, or *P. malariae* and additional treatment with an 8-aminoquinoline derivative such as primaquine is required.

For the treatment of an acute attack of malaria a total of 1.5 g of chloroquine base is usually sufficient, the initial dose being 600 mg, followed by 300 mg after 6 to 8 hours and a further 300 mg on each of the 2 following days. In a partially immune person a single dose of 400 to 600 mg usually suffices to terminate an attack. A suggested dosage for treatment in children is 10 mg per kg body-weight (up to 60 kg) followed after 6 hours by 5 mg per kg, then 5 mg per kg daily for 2 days. Alternatively children aged 1 to 4 years may be given 150 mg of base followed 6 hours later by 75 mg, then 75 mg daily for 2 days; children 5 to 8 years, 300 mg followed 6 hours later by 150 mg, then 150 mg daily.

For the treatment of cerebral malaria in an adult, when the patient is unable to swallow, chloroquine in a dose of 200 to 300 mg may be given by intramuscular or intravenous injection as the hydrochloride, phosphate, or sulphate; doses of up to 200 mg may be given at intervals of 6 hours if required, to a total of 800 mg during the first 24 hours. It may be given to a child by intramuscular injection only if absolutely necessary in a dose not exceeding 5 mg per kg; this dose may have to be repeated once 6 hours later. For advice on the problems of parenteral chloroquine therapy in the management of severe falciparum malaria including a reminder of the hazards of intramuscular chloroquine in children and a warning that chloroquine and quinine should not be given simultaneously, see Quinine, p.405.

For the suppression of malaria a dose of 300 mg is given every 7 days during exposure to risk and for 4 to 8 weeks thereafter. A weekly dose of 600 mg may be required for non-immune persons in areas where transmission of infection is intense. When suppressive treatment is prolonged and the total dose of chloroquine exceeds 100 g the use of proguanil or pyrimethamine is recommended. For the suppression of malaria in children, suggested weekly doses are 5 mg of chloroquine per kg body-weight. Alternatively the weekly dose for those aged under 1 year is 37 mg of base, for those aged 1 to 4 years 75 mg, and for those aged 5 to 8 years 150 mg.

Resistance of *Plasmodium falciparum* to chloroquine is common in many areas; in such circumstances proguanil, pyrimethamine, pyrimethamine with sulfadoxine, or chloroquine with primaquine may be used for suppression.

In addition to its antimalarial uses, chloroquine, alone or with emetine hydrochloride or dehydroemetine hydrochloride has also been found to be of value in the treatment of amoebic hepatitis but it has no effect in intestinal amoebiasis—see the section on Metronidazole and some other Antiprotozoal Agents, p.968. For the treatment of amoebic hepatitis and liver abscess, the equivalent of 300 mg of chloroquine base is given by mouth twice daily for 2 days and then once a day for 2 or 3 weeks. Children may be given 6 mg per kg body-weight twice daily for 2 days initially, then 6 mg per kg daily. When intramuscular injections are required for the treatment of amoebiasis, chloroquine may be given in doses of 160 to 200 mg once daily for 10 to 12 days for adults, and 6 mg per kg for children.

Chloroquine has also been found of value in the treatment of skin lesions associated with discoid or subacute lupus erythematosus, but is of less value in the control of systemic symptoms. The usual initial dose is 150 mg of chloroquine base twice or thrice daily, reduced to a maintenance dose of 150 mg or less daily. It has also been used in the management of photoallergic reactions.

Remission of symptoms in rheumatoid arthritis has been effected after 2 or 3 months' treatment with chloroquine; the usual dose is 300 mg daily for 7 to 10 days, then 150 mg daily; but prolonged therapy may give rise to toxic effects (see p.395). Chloroquine has been used in the treatment of giardiasis and of porphyria although it is considered that malarial patients with porphyria should be treated cautiously with chloroquine.

A review of the pharmacological and therapeutic properties of chloroquine. It had been shown to have possible antihistamine properties, to have no effect upon immune mechanisms, and to be without significant clinical sunscreening properties.— W. M. Sams, *Mayo Clin. Proc.*, 1967, *42*, 300.

Chloroquine 3 to 4 mg per kg body-weight was given intravenously or intramuscularly on account of its prostaglandin antagonist properties to 3 infants with patent ductus arteriosus. All 3 improved rapidly and were discharged in a healthy state from the hospital. Surgery which had been considered for ductus closure in all 3 was not required.— G. Collins *et al.* (letter), *Lancet*, 1976, *2*, 810. See also D. R. Lines, *Drugs*, 1977, *13*, 1.

Babesiosis. A report of babesiosis in 1 patient successfully treated with chloroquine phosphate 1.5 g daily for 2 days then 500 mg daily for 2 weeks.— W. B. Scharfman and E. G. Taft, *J. Am. med. Ass.*, 1977, *238*, 1281. A similar report.— M. F. Parry and S. A. Burka, *ibid.*, 1282.

Although chloroquine appeared to be effective for the symptomatic relief of babesiosis in 5 patients there was no correlation between the duration and dosage of chloroquine and the disappearance of parasites from the blood. It was recommended that chloroquine chemotherapy be limited to 2 weeks.— T. K. Ruebush *et al.*, *Ann. intern. Med.*, 1977, *86*, 6.

Clonorchiasis. Chloroquine phosphate, 250 mg thrice daily for 6 weeks, was considered the drug of choice in the treatment of clonorchiasis, and has also been used to combat infection with lung fluke. It did not cure, but produced temporary suppression of ova.— *Med. Lett.*, 1974, *16*, 7.

Malaria. Malaria parasites were found in more than one-third of newly delivered infants born to 50 women in Nigeria. The infants were treated with an intramuscular injection of chloroquine.— N. E. Okeke (letter), *Br. med. J.*, 1970, *3*, 108. Chloroquine was absorbed very rapidly when administered intramuscularly and could cause encephalopathy and convulsions in children. The newborn could be given chloroquine by mouth or subcutaneously.— T. G. Geddes (letter), *ibid.*, 711.

Of 26 children with cerebral malaria treated with chloroquine by intramuscular injection, 15 did not improve and only 10 who were given additional treatment with urea 30% in 10% invert sugar solution to reduce cerebral oedema improved rapidly.— M. E. Kingston, *J. trop. Med. Hyg.*, 1971, *74*, 249, per *Trop. Dis. Bull.*, 1972, *69*, 484.

In malarious areas where the plasmodia were normally sensitive, chloroquine was considered the drug of choice for mass drug administration.— Sixteenth Report of a WHO Expert Committee on Malaria, *Tech. Rep. Ser. Wld Hlth Org. No. 549*, 1974.

In 41 Ethiopian patients with falciparum malaria treated with chloroquine 10 mg per kg body-weight as a single dose, recrudescence of asexual parasitaemia occurred in 11. All recovered after further treatment with chloroquine 25 mg per kg.— D. T. Dennis *et al.*, *Trans. R. Soc. trop. Med. Hyg.*, 1974, *68*, 241.

A recommendation, based on study of serum concentrations, that in non-immune individuals malaria prophylaxis should begin with 600 mg base weekly for 4 weeks and then proceed to 300 mg base weekly.— J. Brohult *et al.* (letter), *Lancet*, 1979, *2*, 522.

Blood transfusion. In malarial zones a single dose of chloroquine 600 mg (calculated as the base) administered to the recipient 24 hours before or on the day of transfusion seemed to protect from induced malaria but it might be prudent to give all non-immune recipients a standard 3-day course of curative antimalarial treatment rather than rely on a single dose of chloroquine.— *Br. med. J.*, 1976, *1*, 542.

Combined therapy. In patients with *P. falciparum* resistant to chloroquine, the addition of dapsone 25 mg daily, to weekly treatment with chloroquine and primaquine was highly effective in preventing patency of infections.— R. B. Eppes *et al.*, *Milit. Med.*, 1967, *132*, 163, per *J. Am. med. Ass.*, 1967, *200* (May 8), A284.

All of 76 patients with falciparum malaria resistant to chloroquine were radically cured by a regimen of chloroquine, pyrimethamine, and sulphafurazole. Reduction of fever was more rapid than in patients given quinine and pyrimethamine. Severe but reversible neutropenia in 15 patients was reduced when the dose of pyrimethamine was reduced to 25 mg thrice daily for 3 days and that of sulphafurazole to 500 mg per dose; but 3% of patients then relapsed.— S. J. Berman, *J. Am. med. Ass.*, 1969, *207*, 128.

Dapsone 25 mg daily was given with the standard prophylactic doses of chloroquine, 300 mg of base weekly, and primaquine, 45 mg of base weekly, to 6 companies of soldiers in Vietnam. Six other companies were given a placebo with the standard prophylactic therapy. Not all the men took the tablets regularly and a total of 263 developed falciparum malaria. Dapsone appeared to have a partial protective effect and prevented the appearance of clinical malaria in a significant proportion.— R. J. T. Joy *et al.*, *Milit. Med.*, 1969, *134*, 493. In a further study, 3 battalions, each of 787 soldiers, took dapsone 25 mg daily for 6 weeks in addition to the standard chloroquine and primaquine. Under combat conditions there were 1.1, 1.3, and 2 malaria cases per 1000 man-days of exposure respectively in the 3 battalions. In 2 control battalions infection-rates were 12.5 and 16.6 per 1000 man-days. There were no side-effects from dapsone. Dapsone was an effective prophylactic, but physical protection from mosquitoes was also important.— R. J. T. Joy *et al.*, *ibid.*, 497.

A mass drug administration campaign covering 80% of the population supplemented spraying with dicophane in an area of vivax malaria in the Ghab district of Syria. The number of patients developing malaria was drastically reduced. The drugs, chloroquine 300 mg and pyrimethamine 25 mg, were administered weekly for 3 months.— E. Onori, *Bull. Wld Hlth Org.*, 1972, *47*, 543.

Six of about 90 students and teachers who had been on a 4-month journey into areas where malaria was endemic developed their first attack (*P. vivax*) 7½ to 10 months after leaving those areas. All had taken chloroquine 500 mg weekly and for 2 weeks after their return. All responded to treatment with chloroquine and primaquine. The latent period might represent an exoerythrocytic resting stage of the parasite.— P. Horstmann, *Br. med. J.*, 1973, *3*, 440.

Chloroquine given by intramuscular injection together with treatment with heparin, dextran, and corticosteroids produced a rapid response and recovery in 32 of 41 patients with cerebral malaria; in an earlier study 4 of 6 patients given chloroquine alone died.— A. D. Mitchell, *S. Afr. med. J.*, 1974, *48*, 1353, per *Trop. Dis. Bull.*, 1974, *71*, 1223.

Medicated cooking salt. For reports and references to the use of cooking salt medicated with chloroquine, see Martindale 27th Edn, p. 347.

Porphyria. Eight patients, all with porphyria cutanea tarda, were treated with chloroquine base 300 mg (given as sulphate) twice weekly for up to 16 weeks. All patients excreted increased amounts of porphyrin in the urine with a peak at 3 to 28 days. Clinical improvement occurred concomitantly. One patient developed an acute reaction with elevation of serum aspartate aminotransferase (SGOT) activity typical of the use of chloroquine in higher doses. The reaction was transient. One patient relapsed over the period of observation of 4 to 12 months. The suggestion that chloroquine acted in porphyria by causing liver damage was questioned.— J. J. F. Taljaard *et al.*, *Br. J. Derm.*, 1972, *87*, 261.

Five patients with porphyria in whom earlier treatment with chloroquine had appeared to correct liver dysfunction showed relapses in 6 months to 3 years after treatment, but responded again to further treatment with chloroquine 500 mg daily for 5 days.— M. J. Kowertz (letter), *J. Am. med. Ass.*, 1975, *233*, 22.

In 10 patients with porphyria cutanea tarda venesection prior to and intermittently during administration of chloroquine phosphate 250 mg daily for 7 days was considered to reduce the incidence of fever, nausea, vomiting, and myalgia, attributed to chloroquine.— G. Swanbeck and G. Wennersten, *Br. J. Derm.*, 1977, *97*, 77.

Chloroquine 125 mg twice weekly for 8 to 18 months had successfully induced remissions lasting 20 months to 4 years in 112 patients with porphyria cutanea tarda; following relapse a further remission could be achieved with the same dose. Another 14 patients had required chloroquine 250 mg twice weekly. Mild and transient serum alanine aminotransferase (SGPT) elevations were noted in 48 patients.— V. Kordac *et al.* (letter), *New Engl. J. Med.*, 1977, *296*, 949.

Further reports.— E. I. Saltzer *et al.*, *Archs Derm.*, 1968, *98*, 496; G. A. Hunter and G. F. Donald (letter), *Br. J. Derm.*, 1970, *83*, 702; M. J. Kowertz, *J. Am. med. Ass.*, 1973, *223*, 515; V. Kordač and M. Semrádová, *Br. J. Derm.*, 1974, *90*, 95; P. Gould, *Br. J. Derm.*, 1978, *98*, 225; G. Goerz and T. Krieg, *Dt. med. Wschr.*, 1978, *103*, 1329; A. Chlumska *et al.*, *Br. J. Derm.*, 1980, *102*, 261.

Rheumatoid arthritis. Treatment with chloroquine gave good results in over 80% of 440 patients with chronic rheumatic disease. Side-effects included gastric intolerance, cholecystopathy, and visual defects in 9% of the patients; treatment was stopped in a few patients because of severe gastritis.— W. Otto and B. Tautenhahn, *Münch. med. Wschr.*, 1966, *108*, 999, per *Int. pharm. Abstr.*, 1966, *3*, 1158.

For an extensive review of rheumatic diseases and their treatment, see *J. Am. med. Ass.*, 1973, *224*, *Suppl.*, 662–805.

Symptoms of palindromic rheumatism were alleviated in most of 18 patients treated with chloroquine phosphate 250 mg daily for 6 to 8 weeks.— D. N. Golding (letter), *Br. med. J.*, 1976, *2*, 1382.

Further references: E. Scull, *Arthritis Rheum.*, 1962, *5*, 30; J. Durant and J. Maitrepierre, *Rhumatologie*, 1964, *16*, 271; C. J. Smyth and J. F. Bravo, *Drugs*, 1975, *10*, 394; I. L. Dwosh *et al.*, *Arthritis Rheum.*, 1977, *20*, 685.

Sarcoidosis. In a double-blind study 52 patients with pulmonary sarcoidosis received chloroquine sulphate, 600 mg daily for 8 weeks and then 400 mg daily for 8 weeks, or a placebo throughout. After 6 months, the chloroquine-treated patients showed significant improvement over the control group, but after 12 months there was no significant difference between them.—A report from the Research Committee of the British Tuberculosis Association, 1967, *Tubercle*, 1967, *47*, 257.

Further references: *Lancet*, 1968, *1*, 736; H. Brodthagen (letter), *ibid.*, 1157; J. G. Scadding, *Prescribers' J.*, 1972, *12*, 125.

Preparations of Chloroquine and its Salts

Injections

Chloroquine Hydrochloride Injection *(U.S.P.)*. A sterile solution of chloroquine in Water for Injections prepared with the aid of hydrochloric acid; it contains in each ml 47.5 to 51.5 mg of $C_{18}H_{26}ClN_3$, 2HCl, equivalent to approximately 38.7 to 42.8 mg of chloroquine base. pH 5.5 to 6.5.

Chloroquine Phosphate Injection *(B.P.)*. Chloroquine Phos. Inj. A sterile solution of chloroquine phosphate in Water for Injections. Sterilised by autoclaving. Potency is expressed in terms of the equivalent amount of chloroquine base. pH 3.5 to 4.5.

Chloroquine Sulphate Injection *(B.P.)*. Chloroquine Sulph. Inj. A sterile solution of chloroquine sulphate in Water for Injections. Sterilised by autoclaving. Potency is expressed in terms of the equivalent amount of chloroquine base. pH 4 to 5.5.

Tablets

Chloroquine Phosphate Tablets *(B.P.)*. Chloroquine Phos. Tab. Tablets containing chloroquine phosphate. They may be film-coated or sugar-coated. The *B.P.* requires 70% dissolution in 45 minutes.

Chloroquine Phosphate Tablets *(U.S.P.)*. Tablets containing chloroquine phosphate.

Chloroquine Sulphate Tablets *(B.P.)*. Chloroquine Sulph. Tab. Tablets containing chloroquine sulphate. The tablets may be sugar-coated or film-coated. The *B.P.* requires 70% dissolution in 45 minutes.

Proprietary Preparations

Aralis *(Winthrop, UK)*. Tablets each containing chloroquine phosphate 75 mg and bismuth glycollylarsanilate 250 mg. For amoebiasis. *Dose.* Adults, 2 tablets thrice daily for 7 days; children under 12 years, ½ to 1 tablet twice daily for 10 to 12 days. (Known in USA as Milibis with Aralen). (Available only in certain countries).

Avloclor *(ICI Pharmaceuticals, UK)*. Chloroquine phosphate, available as scored tablets of 250 mg. (Also available as Avloclor in *Austral.*). (Known in some countries as Klorokin).

Malarivon Syrup *(Wallace Mfg Chem., UK: Farillon, UK)*. Contains chloroquine phosphate 80 mg in 5 ml. **Malarivon Tablets** each contain chloroquine phosphate 250 mg.

Nivaquine *(May & Baker, UK)*. Chloroquine sulphate, available as **Injection** containing the equivalent of 40 mg of chloroquine base per ml, in ampoules of 5 ml; as **Syrup** containing the equivalent of 50 mg of chloroquine base in each 5 ml (suggested diluent, syrup); and as scored **Tablets** of 200 mg. (Also available as Nivaquine in *Arg., Austral., Belg., Fr., Neth., Norw., S.Afr., Spain, Switz.*).

Other Proprietary Names

Aralen *(Austral., Canad., USA)*; Chlorochin *(Switz.)*; Chlorquin *(Austral.)*; Delagil *(Hung.)*; Dichinalex *(Ital.)*; Resochin *(Austral., Denm., Ger., Neth., Norw., Spain, Switz.)*; Resochine *(Belg.)*.

Chloroquine phosphate was also formerly marketed in Great Britain under the proprietary name Resochin *(Bayer)*.

Preparations containing chloroquine phosphate or sulphate were also formerly marketed in Great Britain under the proprietary names Elestol (*Bayer*) and Nivembin (*May & Baker*).

1374-g

Amodiaquine Hydrochloride *(B.P., U.S.P.)*.

Amodiaquini Hydrochloridum; Amodiachin Hydrochloride; SN 10,751. 4-(7-Chloro-4-quinolylamino)-2-(diethylaminomethyl)phenol dihydrochloride dihydrate.

$C_{20}H_{22}ClN_3O,2HCl,2H_2O=464.8$.

CAS — 86-42-0 (amodiaquine); 69-44-3 (hydrochloride, anhydrous); 6398-98-7 (hydrochloride, dihydrate).

Pharmacopoeias. In *Arg., Br., Braz., Fr., Ind., Int.,* and *U.S.*

A yellow, odourless or almost odourless, crystalline powder with a bitter taste. M.p. about 158°. Amodiaquine base 400 mg is approximately equivalent to 522 mg of amodiaquine hydrochloride. **Soluble** 1 in about 22 of water and 1 in about 70 of alcohol; practically insoluble in chloroform and ether. A 2% solution in water has a pH of 3.6 to 4.6. **Store** in airtight containers.

Adverse Effects and Treatment. In therapeutic doses amodiaquine hydrochloride is generally well tolerated but may occasionally give rise to side-effects, including nausea, vomiting, diarrhoea, insomnia, vertigo, and lethargy.

When given for prolonged periods it sometimes causes corneal deposits and a bluish-grey pigmentation of the finger nails, skin, and hard palate. These reactions clear, somewhat slowly, on stopping treatment.

Agranulocytosis and other blood disorders, hepatitis, and peripheral neuropathy have occasionally been reported. Overdosage with amodiaquine would be expected to produce the same effects as overdosage with chloroquine and patients would thus be managed similarly.

Four patients experienced involuntary movements, usually with speech difficulty, after large but not excessive doses of amodiaquine.— M. O. Akindele and A. O. Odejide, *Br. med. J.*, 1976, *2*, 214.

Retinopathy, sometimes reversible, had been reported following treatment with amodiaquine hydrochloride 200 mg daily.— *Med. Lett.*, 1976, *18*, 63.

Precautions. As for Chloroquine, p.396.

Resistance. As for Chloroquine, p.396. Amodiaquine is more effective than chloroquine against some resistant strains of *Plasmodium falciparum*.

Absorption and Fate. Amodiaquine hydrochloride is readily absorbed from the gastro-intestinal tract, and higher concentrations occur in erythrocytes, kidney, liver, lungs, and spleen than in the plasma. Amodiaquine is liberated slowly into the blood and excreted in the urine for at least 7 days after a single dose. Excretion may be hastened in acid urine.

Uses. Amodiaquine hydrochloride is an antimalarial drug which has an action similar to that of chloroquine (see p.396) and is used interchangeably for the same purposes. It is administered by mouth.

For treatment of acute attacks in non-immune subjects a dose equivalent to 600 mg of the base is given followed by 300-mg doses 6, 24, and 48 hours later. A number of variations of this regimen have been used. For partially immune subjects a single dose of 600 mg of the base is often sufficient.

For suppression the usual dose is the equivalent of 300 to 400 mg of base every 7 days. In highly malarious areas 300 mg should be taken twice a week or 200 mg thrice a week. A suggested weekly dose for children is: up to 1 year, 50 mg; 1 to 4 years, 50 to 100 mg; 5 to 8 years, 150 to 200 mg; 9 to 12 years, 200 to 300 mg.

Amodiaquine hydrochloride has been tried in the treatment of giardiasis and hepatic amoebiasis. It has also been tried, with variable success, in the treatment of lepra reactions, lupus erythematosus, rheumatoid arthritis, and urticaria. Amodiaquine has also been used to expel tapeworms.

Giardiasis. Of 42 patients with giardiasis, 34 were apparently cleared of infection following a single-day treatment with amodiaquine, 600 mg for adults and 200 mg for children under 6 years of age. Eight required 2 or 3 further treatments. Re-infection occurred after 2 to 3 weeks in 10% of those cleared.— A. K. Gupta *et al.*, *J. Indian med. Ass.*, 1967, *49*, 117, per *Trop. Dis. Bull.*, 1968, *65*, 427.

Lepra reactions. Of 4 drugs used to relieve 327 episodes of lepra reaction in 62 patients, sodium salicylate proved the most effective. Amodiaquine (200 mg twice daily for 5 days) and stibophen were of similar usefulness and antimony potassium tartrate was least effective. In the more serious cases, amodiaquine was best and in 1 case it desensitised a patient sensitive to sulphones. Most patients preferred amodiaquine.— E. S. Short, *Lepr. India*, 1964, *36*, 24, per *Trop. Dis. Bull.*, 1964, *61*, 679.

Malaria. Amodiaquine 300 mg with primaquine 30 mg once weekly gave slightly better protection against malaria during the 8 months of a field trial with 3000 soldiers in Angola than treatment with cycloguanil embonate and both treatments were better than pyrimethamine. All received initial curative treatment with amodiaquine.— M. T. Leitao, *Revue int. Servs Santé Armées*, 1972, *45*, 877, per *Trop. Dis. Bull.*, 1973, *70*, 834.

In the treatment of 118 children with malaria, amodiaquine 10 to 15 mg per kg body-weight daily in divided doses was considered to be better tolerated than chloroquine since it was less bitter and also more effective in eliminating asexual parasites.— P. O. Fasan *et al.*, *J. trop. Med. Hyg.*, 1974, *77*, 239, per *Trop. Dis. Bull.*, 1975, *72*, 322.

Preparations

Amodiaquine Hydrochloride Tablets *(U.S.P.)*. Tablets containing amodiaquine hydrochloride. Potency is expressed in terms of the equivalent amount of amodiaquine base. The *U.S.P.* requires 75% dissolution in 30 minutes. Store in airtight containers.

Amodiaquine Tablets *(B.P.)*. Tablets containing amodiaquine hydrochloride. Potency is expressed in terms of the equivalent amount of amodiaquine base.

Proprietary Preparations

Basoquin *(Parke, Davis, UK)*. Amodiaquine base, available as **Suspension** containing 150 mg in each 5 ml and as **Tablets** of 150 mg. (Available only in certain countries).

Camoquin *(Parke, Davis, UK)*. Amodiaquine hydrochloride, available as paediatric **Suspension** containing the equivalent of amodiaquine base 50 mg in each 5 ml, and as **Tablets** containing the equivalent of amodiaquine base 200 and 600 mg. (Available only in certain countries).

Other Proprietary Names

Flavoquine *(Fr.)*.

1375-q

Amopyroquine Hydrochloride. PAM 780. 4-(7-Chloro-4-quinolylamino)-2-(pyrrolidin-1-ylmethyl)phenol dihydrochloride.

$C_{20}H_{20}ClN_3O,2HCl = 426.8$.

CAS — 550-81-2 (amopyroquine); 10350-81-9 (dihydrochloride).

A yellow crystalline powder with a very bitter taste.

Uses. Amopyroquine is an analogue of amodiaquine and has similar antimalarial uses. It has been given as a single dose of 150 mg by deep intramuscular injection; children have been given 3 mg per kg body-weight by deep intramuscular injection. It may also be administered by mouth. It has also been used in rheumatoid arthritis.

Amopyroquine hydrochloride was formerly marketed in certain countries under the proprietary name Propoquin *(Parke, Davis)*.

1376-p

Chlorproguanil Hydrochloride *(B.P. 1973)*.

M5943. 1-(3,4-Dichlorophenyl)-5-isopropylbiguanide hydrochloride.

$C_{11}H_{15}Cl_2N_5, HCl = 324.6$.

CAS — 537-21-3 (chlorproguanil).

A white odourless crystalline powder with a bitter taste. **Soluble** 1 in 140 of water and 1 in 50 of alcohol; practically insoluble in chloroform and ether.

Uses. Chlorproguanil is an antimalarial drug with actions and uses similar to those of proguanil (see p.401) but it is more active than proguanil and has a longer duration of action. Resistance has been reported in some areas.

It is given in doses of 20 mg at intervals of 7 days; administration should be continued for 4 weeks after leaving a malarious area.

Malaria. Children aged 6 to 10 years, at 4 schools in Kaduna, Nigeria, were given either 10 mg of chlorproguanil or 12.5 mg of pyrimethamine each week for malaria prophylaxis. After treatment for 3 school terms the incidence of positive blood films was reduced but strains of *P. falciparum* resistant to chlorproguanil were encountered.— J. S. Dodge, *W. Afr. med. J.*, 1967, *16*, 55, per *Trop. Dis. Bull.*, 1967, *64*, 1189.

Preparations

Chlorproguanil Tablets *(B.P. 1973)*. Tablets containing chlorproguanil hydrochloride.

Lapudrine *(ICI Pharmaceuticals, UK)*. Chlorproguanil hydrochloride, available as scored tablets of 20 mg.

1377-s

Cycloguanil Embonate.

Cycloguanil Pamoate; CI 501. Bis[1-(4-chlorophenyl)-1,2-dihydro-2,2-dimethyl-1,3,5-triazine-4,6-diamine] 4,4′-methylenebis(3-hydroxy-2-naphthoate).

$C_{11}H_{14}ClN_5,½(C_{23}H_{16}O_6) = 445.9$.

CAS — 516-21-2 (cycloguanil); 609-78-9 (embonate).

A pale greenish-yellow to yellow odourless crystalline powder. Cycloguanil base 100 mg is approximately equivalent to 177 mg of cycloguanil embonate. Practically **insoluble** in water; sparingly soluble in dimethylformamide.

Adverse Effects. Tenderness, pain, and possibly induration may occur at the site of injection. Allergic-like reactions with urticaria or skin rashes have followed a second injection of cycloguanil. Over a prolonged period, cycloguanil may cause slight depression of haemopoiesis due to interference of the drug in the metabolism of folic acid; the effect may be corrected by an injection of calcium folinate.

Absorption and Fate. Cycloguanil embonate is slowly absorbed into the circulation from a suspension in an oily basis injected intramuscularly. It is mainly excreted in the urine.

Reference: P. G. Contacos *et al.*, *Am. J. trop. Med. Hyg.*, 1966, *15*, 281.

Uses. Cycloguanil is the active metabolite of proguanil (see Proguanil Hydrochloride, p.401) and has similar actions and uses. It is a dihydrofolate reductase inhibitor and has been used for the suppression of malaria, but has gained only limited acceptance. An intramuscular injection of a suspension of fine particles of cycloguanil embonate in an oily basis provides protection for several months against infection. It is of little value in areas where resistance to proguanil or pyrimethamine occurs. For continuous protection in areas with hyperendemic malaria, treatment with cycloguanil and amodiaquine every 4 months has been suggested.

The usual adult dose, by deep intramuscular injection, is the equivalent of 350 mg or 5 to 6 mg per kg body-weight of cycloguanil base every 4 months; children up to 4 years of age may be given 140 mg and children 5 to 10 years of age, 280 mg. The effects of cycloguanil administered by injection have been stated to be prolonged by the concomitant administration by mouth of a single dose of a 4-aminoquinoline such as amodiaquine. Cycloguanil embonate has also been used in the treatment of cutaneous leishmaniasis.

Leishmaniasis. A single injection of cycloguanil embonate in a dose equivalent to 350 mg base was used with no untoward effects in the treatment of a woman, 2 months pregnant, who had cutaneous leishmaniasis. Regression of a large lesion was slow to clear but the pregnancy proceeded normally.— M. Reinhard and H. Wacker, *Dt. med. Wschr.*, 1970, *95*, 2380, per *Trop. Dis. Bull.*, 1971, *68*, 692.

Of 23 patients with cutaneous leishmaniasis who were available for further examination, cycloguanil in a dose equivalent to 210 mg base for children under 7, and 350 mg for adults, caused complete healing in 18 and improvement in 4 patients.— M. Ardehali, *Int. J. Derm.*, 1974, *13*, 26, per *Trop. Dis. Bull.*, 1974, *71*, 800.

Malaria. *For favourable and unfavourable reports of the use of cycloguanil embonate, see Martindale 27th Edn, p. 350.*

Cycloguanil embonate was formerly marketed in certain countries under the proprietary name Camolar (*Parke, Davis*).

1378-w

Cycloquine. Cyclochin; Haloquine. 4-(7-Chloro-4-quinolylamino)-2,6-bis(dihexylaminomethyl)phenol.
$C_{29}H_{41}ClN_4O$=497.1.

CAS — 14594-33-3.

A yellow crystalline powder with a bitter taste. Practically **insoluble** in water; readily soluble in dilute acids; insoluble in dilute alkalis. **Protect** from light.

Uses. Cycloquine resembles chloroquine in its action and has been used in the USSR for the suppression and treatment of malaria. A dose of 300 mg has been given weekly for the suppression of malaria and 300 mg has been given daily for three days in the treatment of acute attacks.

1379-e

Diformyldapsone. DFD; DFDDS; Diformyldiaminodiphenylsulphone. 4,4′-Sulphonylbisformanilide.
$C_{14}H_{12}N_2O_4S$=304.3.

CAS — 6784-25-4.

A crystalline solid. M.p. 267° to 269°. Practically **insoluble** in water; soluble 1 in about 200 of dimethyl sulphoxide. It is most stable at pH 6.

Uses. Diformyldapsone has been used as an antimalarial in doses of 400 to 800 mg weekly, but is given with chloroquine, primaquine, or pyrimethamine, since it has no action on gametocytes.

Diformyldapsone had an approximate half-life of 84 hours.— W. Peters, *Postgrad. med. J.*, 1973, *49*, 573.

Diformyldapsone in doses of 3.2 g twice weekly for 4 weeks damaged the red blood cells in 25 subjects. Smaller doses did not appear to cause haemolysis.— S. A. Cucinell *et al.*, *J. clin. Pharmac.*, 1974, *14*, 51.

Malaria. Diformyldapsone was considered to protect volunteers more effectively against the Vietnam Smith strain of *P. falciparum* than against the Chesson strain of *P. vivax*. There were no reports of methaemoglobinaemia in patients receiving diformyldapsone alone or in conjunction with chloroquine.— Clyde. D.F. *et al.*, *Milit. Med.*, 1971, *136*, 836, per *Trop. Dis. Bull.*, 1972, *69*, 593. See also *idem*, *Milit. Med.*, 1970, *135*, 527.

Diformyldapsone 100 to 800 mg weekly given with chloroquine alone, or with chloroquine and primaquine, suppressed the Smith strain of falciparum malaria in 41 of 45 men and the Brai. strain in 9 men. The combination appeared to be more effective than treatment with chloroquine and primaquine, or than pyrimethamine 25 mg weekly which suppressed the Brai. but not the Smith strain.— D. F. Clyde *et al.*, *Am. J. trop. Med. Hyg.*, 1971, *20*, 1, per *Trop. Dis. Bull.*, 1971, *68*, 1153.

Diformyldapsone given weekly with chloroquine protected 5 of 8 volunteers against falciparum malaria. Better results were noted when volunteers were given dapsone daily with chloroquine or chloroquine and primaquine weekly.— D. Willerson, *Am. J. trop. Med. Hyg.*, 1972, *21*, 138, per *J. Am. med. Ass.*, 1972, *220*, 1382.

Diformyldapsone, 400 to 800 mg with pyrimethamine 25 mg, both given weekly, was considered to provide effective prophylaxis against chloroquine-resistant *P. falciparum* and against *P. vivax*. No toxic side-effects were noted.— D. F. Clyde *et al.*, *Milit. Med.*, 1973, *138*, 418, per *Trop. Dis. Bull.*, 1974, *71*, 15.

1380-b

Hydroxychloroquine Sulphate *(B.P.)*.

Hydroxychloroquine Sulfate *(U.S.P.)*; Oxichlorochin Sulphate; Win 1258-2. 2-{*N*-[4-(7-Chloro-4-quinolylamino)pentyl]-*N*-ethylamino}ethanol sulphate.
$C_{18}H_{26}ClN_3O, H_2SO_4$=433.9.

CAS — 118-42-3 (hydroxychloroquine); 747-36-4 (sulphate).

Pharmacopoeias. In *Br.* and *U.S.*

A white or almost white odourless crystalline powder with a bitter taste. There are 2 forms, one melting at about 198° and the other at about 240°. Hydroxychloroquine sulphate 100 mg is approximately equivalent to 77 mg of hydroxychloroquine base. **Soluble** 1 in 5 of water; practically insoluble in alcohol, chloroform, and ether. A 1% solution in water has a pH of 3.5 to 5.5. **Protect** from light.

Adverse Effects, Treatment, Precautions, and Resistance. As for Chloroquine, p.395.

Hydroxychloroquine was given in an average dose of 800 mg daily for up to 4½ years to 94 patients with lupus erythematosus, rheumatoid arthritis, or scleroderma. The patients had not previously received chloroquine, amodiaquine, mepacrine, or quinine. Corneal deposition occurred in 26 patients; it was reversible in 20, persistent in 3, and 3 were lost to follow-up. There was a rapid rise in incidence after 150 g had been given. One patient who had received 770 g over 26½ months developed retinopathy. A second case of probable retinopathy was subsequently seen in a further patient.— R. V. Shearer and E. L. Dubois, *Am. J. Ophthal.*, 1967, *64*, 245.

Ocular toxicity in 3 of 99 patients after long-term treatment with hydroxychloroquine.— R. I. Rynes *et al.*, *Arthritis Rheum.*, 1979, *22*, 832.

Uses. Hydroxychloroquine sulphate has an antimalarial action similar to that of chloroquine (see p.396) but it is mainly used in the treatment of systemic and discoid lupus erythematosus and rheumatoid arthritis. Treatment is usually started with about 400 to 800 mg daily in divided doses with meals and the dose is reduced to about 200 to 400 mg when a response occurs. In malaria, a suppressive dose of 400 mg every 7 days is used, and in treating an acute attack a dose of 800 mg has been used, followed after 6 to 8 hours by 400 mg and a further 400 mg on each of the 2 following days. Children may be given a weekly suppressive dose equivalent to 5 mg of base per kg body-weight, while for treatment an initial dose of 10 mg per kg may be given, following by 5 mg per kg 6 hours later and again on the second and third days.

In the treatment of giardiasis, the usual dose is 200 mg thrice daily for 5 days.

Hydroxychloroquine sulphate has been used in the treatment of polymorphous light eruptions. The dose is as for rheumatoid arthritis.

Porphyria. Hydroxychloroquine, 400 mg weekly for several months, had been reported to be safe and effective in the treatment of porphyria cutanea tarda.— F. De Matteis, *Br. J. Derm.*, 1972, *87*, 174.

Thrombo-embolic disorders. Of 565 patients who underwent surgery 284 received an injection of hydroxychloroquine sulphate 200 mg with their premedication and then 200 mg eight-hourly by mouth or by injection until discharge from hospital. From postoperative observations and by phlebography it appeared that hydroxychloroquine could be useful in reducing the incidence of deep-vein thrombosis and pulmonary embolism.— A. E. Carter *et al.*, *Br. med. J.*, 1971, *1*, 312.

The incidence of deep-vein thrombosis after surgery was 5% in 107 patients given hydroxychloroquine sulphate compared with 16% in 97 controls. The dose was 1.2 g by mouth in 3 divided doses in the 24 hours before surgery followed by 400 mg every 12 hours after surgery until discharge.— A. E. Carter and R. Eban, *Br. med. J.*, 1974, *3*, 94.

For discussions, see A. S. Gallus and J. Hirsh, *Drugs*, 1976, *12*, 132; A. G. G. Turpie and J. Hirsh, *Br. med. Bull.*, 1978, *34*, 183.

Preparations

Hydroxychloroquine Sulfate Tablets *(U.S.P.)*. Tablets containing hydroxychloroquine sulphate.

Hydroxychloroquine Tablets *(B.P.)*. Tablets containing hydroxychloroquine sulphate. They are sugar-coated.

Plaquenil *(Winthrop, UK)*. Hydroxychloroquine sulphate, available as tablets of 200 mg. (Also available as Plaquenil in *Aust., Austral., Belg., Canad., Denm., Fin., Fr., Iceland, Ital., Neth., Norw., Swed., Switz., USA*).

Other Proprietary Names

Ercoquin *(Denm., Norw., Swed.)*; Quensyl *(Ger.)*.

1381-v

Mefloquine Hydrochloride.

WR 142490. (±)-α-[2,8-Bis(trifluoromethyl)-4-quinolyl]-α-(2-piperidyl)methanol hydrochloride.
$C_{17}H_{16}F_6N_2O, HCl$=414.8.

CAS — 53230-10-7 (mefloquine); 51773-92-3 (hydrochloride).

Adverse Effects. Epigastric discomfort has been reported after doses of 1 g, and nausea and dizziness after doses of 1.75 or 2 g.

Uses. Mefloquine hydrochloride is a 4-quinolinemethanol compound which has schizonticidal activity against malaria parasites. It is active against chloroquine-resistant falciparum malaria.

Malaria. A preliminary study in 17 subjects of the use of mefloquine hydrochloride in single 1-g doses as a prophylactic against drug-resistant malaria.— K. H. Rieckmann *et al.*, *Bull. Wld Hlth Org.*, 1974, *51*, 375.

Thirty-five non-immune volunteers infected with 1 of 3 strains of *Plasmodium falciparum*, 2 of them drug-resistant, were treated with a single oral dose of mefloquine hydrochloride 0.4, 1, or 1.5 g. The infection was cured in 2 of 12 given 0.4 g, 13 of 15 given 1 g, and 8 of 8 given 1.5 g. In 5 partially-immune volunteers infected with *P. vivax* cures were achieved with single doses of 0.4 or 1 g in two, but infection reappeared in the remaining 3 subjects and was subsequently cured with chloroquine and primaquine.— G. M. Trenholme *et al.*, *Science*, 1975, *190*, 792.

None of 21 volunteers bitten by 10 to 15 mosquitoes heavily infected with *P. falciparum* developed malaria when given mefloquine hydrochloride 250 or 500 mg weekly, 500 mg every 2 weeks, or 1 g every 4 weeks. Doses of 250 mg weekly suppressed *P. vivax* infections during drug administration but malaria appeared when treatment ceased.— D. F. Clyde *et al.*, *Antimicrob. Ag. Chemother.*, 1976, *9*, 384.

Of 39 patients with chloroquine-resistant falciparum malaria, 36 (92%) were cleared of infection with no recrudescence after treatment with quinine, sulfadoxine, and pyrimethamine, by the regimen of A.P. Hall (*Br. med. J.*, 1975, *2*, 15; see under Quinine, p.405), while all of 35 were cleared by treatment with quinine followed by a single dose of mefloquine hydrochloride 1.5 g (one patient received only 1 g). Side-effects in 40 patients given mefloquine were: abdominal pain (7), anorexia (6), diarrhoea (6), dizziness (9), nausea (3), vomiting (9), and weakness (3). Side-effects were minimal or absent if at least 12 hours elapsed after the last dose of quinine.— A. P. Hall *et al.*, *Br. med. J.*, 1977, *1*, 1626.

Animal studies of the antimalarial activities of 4-quinolinemethanols including mefloquine and a report of the US Army Malaria Research Program.— L. H. Schmidt *et al.*, *Antimicrob. Ag. Chemother.*, 1978, *13*, 1011.

Of 37 patients with chloroquine-resistant falciparum malaria all were radically cured by a single dose of mefloquine hydrochloride 1.5 g. Side-effects (nausea, vomiting, diarrhoea, dizziness, headache) could probably be reduced by a formulation designed to slow absorption.— E. B. Doberstyn *et al.*, *Bull. Wld Hlth Org.*, 1979, *57*, 275.

Metabolism. Preliminary study in 1 subject given a single dose of mefloquine indicated relatively rapid absorption, extensive distribution, and prolonged elimination phases. Mefloquine was reported to be extensively bound to plasma proteins and to be concentrated in erythrocytes.— J. M. Grindel *et al.*, *J. pharm. Sci.*, 1977, *66*, 834.

The kinetics of mefloquine hydrochloride.— R. E. Desjardins *et al.*, *Clin. Pharmac. Ther.*, 1979, *26*, 372.

1382-g

Mepacrine Hydrochloride *(B.P., Eur. P.)*.

Mepacrini Hydrochloridum; Acrinamine; Quinacrine Hydrochloride *(U.S.P.)*; Quinacrinium Chloride; Acrichinum; Antimalarinae Chlorhydras; Chinacrina. 6-Chloro-9-(4-diethylamino-1-methylbutylamino)-2-methoxyacridine dihydrochloride dihydrate.
$C_{23}H_{30}ClN_3O, 2HCl, 2H_2O$=508.9.

CAS — 83-89-6 (mepacrine); 69-05-6 (dihydrochloride, anhydrous); 6151-30-0 (dihydrochloride, dihydrate).

Pharmacopoeias. In *Arg., Belg., Br., Braz., Eur., Fr., Ger., Hung., Ind., Int., It., Mex., Neth., Nord., Pol., Rus., Span., Swiss, Turk.*, and *U.S.*

A bright yellow odourless crystalline powder with a bitter taste. M.p. about 250° with decomposition. **Soluble** 1 in 35 to 40 of water; soluble in alcohol; slightly soluble in dehydrated alcohol; very slightly soluble in chloroform; practically insoluble in acetone and ether. A 2% solution in water has a pH of 3 to 5. **Incompatible** with alkalis, nitrates, and oxidising agents. **Store** in airtight containers. Protect from light.

Incompatibility. Mepacrine hydrochloride was incompatible with amaranth, benzylpenicillin, sodium alginate, sodium aminosalicylate, sodium carboxymethylcellulose, sodium lauryl sulphate, and thiomersal.— *J. Am. pharm. Ass., pract. Pharm. Edn*, 1952, *13*, 658.

Adverse Effects. Minor effects liable to arise with ordinary doses are dizziness, headache, and mild gastro-intestinal disturbances. Most patients develop a yellow discoloration of the skin. Large doses may give rise to nausea and vomiting and occasionally to transient mental disturbances. A few patients develop chronic dermatoses after prolonged administration of the drug; these may be either lichenoid, eczematoid, or exfoliative in type. Deaths from exfoliative dermatitis and from hepatitis have been reported. The use of mepacrine over prolonged periods may give rise to aplastic anaemia.

Adverse effects of intrapleural instillation include fever and chest pain caused by the inflammatory reaction.

The toxicity arising from prolonged administration has contributed to the decline in the use of mepacrine in malaria.

Two patients had convulsions a few hours after the intrapleural administration of mepacrine hydrochloride 400 mg for malignant effusions. One developed status epilepticus and died; the other was successfully controlled with phenobarbitone intravenously and phenytoin by mouth.— I. Borda and M. Krant, *J. Am. med. Ass.*, 1967, *201*, 1049.

Mepacrine hydrochloride 100 mg daily had been reported to cause haemolytic anaemia in certain individuals with a deficiency of glucose-6-phosphate dehydrogenase. The reaction was not considered clinically significant under normal circumstances (e.g. in the absence of infection).— E. Beutler, *Pharmac. Rev.*, 1969, *21*, 73.

A patient with rheumatoid arthritis treated with mepacrine hydrochloride for about 20 years had developed a blue-black discoloration of the hard palate, the nail beds, and the skin over the shins. The colour disappeared when mepacrine was stopped and reappeared when it was restarted.— M. J. Egorin *et al.*, *J. Am. med. Ass.*, 1976, *236*, 385.

Treatment of Adverse Effects. As for Chloroquine, p.396.

Precautions. Mepacrine enhances the toxicity of the 8-aminoquinoline derivatives such as primaquine by inhibiting their metabolism.

Mepacrine might interfere with fluorimetric estimations of plasma hydrocortisone.— J. Millhouse, *Adverse Drug React. Bull.*, 1974, Dec., 164.

Absorption and Fate. Mepacrine is absorbed from the gastro-intestinal tract and appears in the blood within 2 hours. It becomes concentrated in liver, pancreas, spleen, and lung, and higher concentrations occur in red and white blood cells than in plasma, but it also permeates into all body fluids and crosses the placenta. It has a biological half-life of about 5 days and is excreted only very slowly in the urine and faeces.

Mepacrine hydrochloride was bound to serum proteins *in vitro*.— G. A. Lutty, *Toxic. appl. Pharmac.*, 1978, *44*, 225.

Uses. Mepacrine was formerly widely used for the suppression and treatment of malaria but it has been superseded for these purposes by chloroquine and other more recently introduced antimalarials. Doses ranged from 100 mg daily for suppression and from 900 mg reducing to 300 mg daily for treatment. Mepacrine hydrochloride is used in the treatment of giardiasis; 100 mg thrice daily for 7 days is usually effective, though relapses may occur. A suggested dose for children is 2.7 mg per kg body-weight thrice daily.

It has been used for the expulsion of tapeworms; 100 mg is given at intervals of 5 minutes until a total dose of 1 g is reached.

Instillations of mepacrine hydrochloride or mesylate are used in the symptomatic treatment of neoplastic effusions in the pleura or peritoneum but the treatment is associated with a high frequency of toxic effects.

For the use of mepacrine as an anthelmintic, see A. Davis, *Drug Treatment in Intestinal Helminthiases*, Geneva, World Health Organization, 1973.

Giardiasis. Mepacrine 100 mg thrice daily for 5 to 7 days was usually effective in the treatment of giardiasis, although a second course might be required. The dose for children under 4 years old was one-quarter of the adult dose.— *Br. med. J.*, 1974, *2*, 347.

A 95% cure-rate was obtained in giardiasis after treatment with mepacrine hydrochloride 100 mg thrice daily for 7 days. Dosages in children were: under 1 year, 33 mg thrice daily; 1 to 4 years, 50 mg twice daily; 4 to 8 years, 50 mg thrice daily; over 8 years, 100 mg thrice daily, all for 7 days.— M. S. Wolfe, *J. Am. med. Ass.*, 1975, *233*, 1362.

Further references: G. T. Moore *et al.*, *New Engl. J. Med.*, 1969, *281*, 402; *Med. Lett.*, 1976, *18*, 39; R. E. Raizman, *Am. J. dig. Dis.*, 1976, *21*, 1070.

Malignant effusions. The value of local instillations of mepacrine in controlling effusions in advanced disseminated neoplastic disease was studied in 60 patients. For pleural effusions, an initial dose of 50 to 100 mg was followed by 200 to 400 mg daily for 4 or 5 days; patients with ascites received 100 to 200 mg followed by 400 to 800 mg daily for 3 to 5 days. The mepacrine was dissolved in 10 ml of the effusion fluid which was then re-injected. Of 33 patients clinically evaluated for 2 months or more, objective control of the effusion was maintained in 27 for 2 to 26 months. Fever, often accompanied by leucocytosis and persisting for a few hours to 10 days after completion of treatment, was noted in about half the patients.— J. E. Ultmann *et al.*, *Cancer*, 1963, *16*, 283.

Thirteen patients with neoplastic effusions were treated with mepacrine hydrochloride in doses of 100 to 200 mg daily by local instillations for pleural effusions, and 200 to 400 mg daily for ascites, usually for 3 to 5 days. Clinical benefit with favourable objective changes in all measurable criteria of the disease was seen in 9 patients for periods of up to 27 months. Mild local toxicity was frequent but haematopoietic depression did not occur. No consistent cytolytic changes of tumour cells were observed and response was attributed to the inflammation and fibrosis produced.— M. R. Dollinger *et al.*, *Ann. intern. Med.*, 1967, *66*, 249.

There was a response in 8 of 12 patients with malignant pleural effusions given mepacrine by instillation in small daily doses, and in 19 of 27 given mepacrine as a single dose through a thoracostomy tube. More disturbing and serious toxicity occurred in the second group.— E. R. Borja and R. P. Pugh, *Cancer*, 1973, *31*, 899.

A beneficial effect (less than 500 ml fluid drawn at each pleurocentesis in 3 months) was achieved on 9 of 14 occasions after the instillation of mepacrine (100, 200, and 200 mg respectively on 3 occasions in 1 week), on 4 of 15 occasions after thiotepa (20 mg per instillation), and on 1 of 9 occasions after pleurocentesis alone. Fever and chest pain were limiting factors; mepacrine was suitable if the patient's condition and prognosis was good; otherwise thiotepa or pleurocentesis were preferred.— J. Mejer *et al.*, *Scand. J. resp. Dis.*, 1977, *58*, 319.

Further references: J. A. Hickman and M. C. Jones, *Thorax*, 1970, *25*, 226; M. Lee and D. A. Boyes, *J. Obstet. Gynaec. Br. Commonw.*, 1971, *78*, 843.

Pneumothorax. A patient with cystic fibrosis was treated for pneumothorax on the left side by the instillation of mepacrine hydrochloride 100 mg in 15 ml saline into the intrapleural space on 4 consecutive days. This procedure was repeated 12 months later for pneumothorax on the right. There was no recurrence of pneumothorax on either side before the patient died 11 months after the second treatment after several relapses of chronic pulmonary disease.— J. Kattwinkel *et al.*, *J. Am. med. Ass.*, 1973, *226*, 557. See also R. E. Jones and S. T. Giammona, *Am. J. Dis. Child.*, 1976, *130*, 777.

Tubal occlusion. Two to 4 ml of a 30% aqueous suspension of mepacrine hydrochloride instilled transvaginally once in the immediate postmenstrual phase of 2 consecutive cycles induced tubal occlusion in 93% of 134 women.— Advances in Methods of Fertility Regulation, *Tech. Rep. Ser. Wld Hlth Org. No. 527*, 1973.

Sixty women desiring sterilisation were treated by the application, by cannula within the uterus, of 1 g of mepacrine hydrochloride suspended in 7 ml of sterile water. Of 52 available for examination 4 months later, 22 had bilateral tubal patency and 3 unilateral patency; a further 6 were pregnant. The low success-rate of a single application indicated limited usefulness.— C. Israngkun *et al.*, *Contraception*, 1976, *14*, 75.

Warts. A local injection technique was used in the treatment of warts in children. A 4% solution of mepacrine, in doses of 0.1 to 0.2 ml, was injected into the healthy skin at the base of the wart, 3 to 6 warts being treated at each session. The injections were repeated twice if no response followed the first injection. The treatment was successful in 97 of 112 patients. It sometimes caused slight transient pain.— A. I. Lopatin, *Pediatriya*, 1966, *45*, 71, per *Abstr. Wld Med.*, 1966, *40*, 446.

Preparations

Mepacrine Tablets *(B.P.)*. Tablets containing mepacrine hydrochloride. Protect from light.

Quinacrine Hydrochloride Tablets *(U.S.P.)*. Tablets containing mepacrine hydrochloride. Store in airtight containers.

Proprietary Names

Atabrine *(Winthrop, Canad.)*; Atabrine Hydrochloride *(Winthrop, USA)*.

Mepacrine hydrochloride was formerly marketed in certain countries under the proprietary name Quinacrine *(May & Baker)*.

1383-q

Mepacrine Mesylate. Mepacrine Methanesulphonate *(B.P.C. 1963)*.

$C_{23}H_{30}ClN_3O,2CH_3SO_3H,H_2O=610.2$.

CAS — 316-05-2 (anhydrous).

Bright yellow odourless crystals with a bitter taste. Mepacrine mesylate 120 mg is approximately equivalent to 100 mg of mepacrine hydrochloride. **Soluble** 1 in 3 of water and 1 in 36 of alcohol. A 2% solution in water has a pH of 3 to 5. **Protect** from light. Solutions should not be heated, or stored for any length of time.

Uses. Mepacrine mesylate has actions similar to those of mepacrine hydrochloride, but as it is more soluble than the hydrochloride it has been administered by intramuscular injection in the treatment of severe malaria. A dose of 360 mg has been given in 2 to 4 ml of Water for Injections.

It is given by intrapleural or intraperitoneal instillation in the treatment of neoplastic effusions.

Preparations

Mepacrine Methanesulphonate Injection *(B.P.C. 1963)*. Mepacrine Mesylate Injection. A sterile solution of mepacrine mesylate in Water for Injections, prepared by dissolving, immediately before use, the sterile contents of a sealed container in Water for Injections.

Mepacrine mesylate was formerly marketed in certain countries under the proprietary name Quinacrine Soluble *(May & Baker)*.

1384-p

Pamaquin *(B.P. 1953)*. Gametocidum; Pamachin; Pamaquine Embonate; Plasmoquinum; SN 971. 8-(4-Diethylamino-1-methylbutylamino)-6-methoxyquinoline 4,4′-methylenebis(3-hydroxy-2-naphthoate).

$C_{42}H_{45}N_3O_7=703.8$.

CAS — 491-92-9 (base); 635-05-2 (embonate).

A yellow to orange-yellow odourless powder with a bitter taste. Practically **insoluble** in water; soluble 1 in 20 of alcohol.

Uses. Pamaquin was formerly used in the treatment of malaria but has been superseded by primaquine phosphate.

1385-s

Pentaquine Phosphate. Pentachini Phosphas. 8-(5-Isopropylaminopentylamino)-6-methoxyquinoline phosphate.
$C_{18}H_{27}N_3O,H_3PO_4$=399.4.

CAS — 86-78-2 (pentaquine); 5428-64-8 (phosphate).

Pharmacopoeias. In *Arg.* and *Mex.*

A yellow odourless crystalline powder with a bitter taste. M.p. 188° to 192°. **Soluble** 1 in 25 of water; very slightly soluble in alcohol; practically insoluble in chloroform and ether. **Protect** from light.

Uses. Pentaquine phosphate is an antimalarial with actions and uses similar to those of primaquine phosphate. It has been given in doses of up to 100 mg daily.

1386-w

Plasmocid. Fourneau 710; SN 3115. 8-(3-Diethylaminopropylamino)-6-methoxyquinoline di(methylenebis-salicylate).
$C_{17}H_{25}N_3O,2C_{15}H_{12}O_6$=863.9.

CAS — 551-01-9 (base).

Pharmacopoeias. In *Rus.*

An orange-yellow powder with a slightly bitter taste. Practically **insoluble** in water and in most other organic solvents; slightly soluble in alcohol. **Protect** from light.

Uses. Plasmocid is an antimalarial drug with actions and uses similar to those of primaquine. It was usually administered in conjunction with mepacrine and proguanil. The maximum single dose was 30 mg and the maximum dose in 24 hours was 60 mg. It has been reported to be very toxic to the central nervous system.

1387-e

Primaquine Phosphate *(B.P., U.S.P.)*.

Primaquini Diphosphas; Primachin Phosphate; Primaquinium Phosphate; SN 13,272. 8-(4-Amino-1-methylbutylamino)-6-methoxyquinoline diphosphate.
$C_{15}H_{21}N_3O,2H_3PO_4$=455.3.

CAS — 90-34-6 (primaquine); 63-45-6 (phosphate).

Pharmacopoeias. In *Arg., Br., Braz., Chin., Fr., Jug., Int., Nord., Turk.,* and *U.S.*

An orange-red, odourless or almost odourless, crystalline powder with a bitter taste. M.p. about 200°. Primaquine base 30 mg is approximately equivalent to 53 mg of primaquine phosphate. **Soluble** 1 in about 16 of water; practically insoluble in alcohol, chloroform, and ether. A 1% solution in water has a pH of 2.5 to 3.5. Aqueous solutions should not be heated. **Protect** from light.

Stability. Primaquine was rapidly destroyed in the course of the ordinary preparation of cooked food.— Chemotherapy of Malaria, *Tech. Rep. Ser. Wld Hlth Org. No. 266,* 1961, p. 56.

Adverse Effects. Common symptoms of overdosage are nausea, abdominal pain, and other gastro-intestinal disturbances. Less common side-effects are vomiting and jaundice. Methaemoglobinaemia and bone-marrow depression have also been reported. Haemolytic anaemia may occur in persons with a deficiency of glucose-6-phosphate dehydrogenase.

There were 2 major toxic effects of primaquine therapy: (1) An acute intravascular haemolysis at all doses in those with primaquine-sensitive red blood-cells genetically defective in glucose-6-phosphate dehydrogenase. The haemolysis was usually too slight to be of clinical significance unless the daily adult dose of 15 mg of primaquine base or a once-weekly dose of 60 mg of base was exceeded. The haemolysis was self-limiting since the younger erythrocytes were relatively resistant to the action of the drug. (2) Methaemoglobinaemia, causing dusky cyanosis, abdominal pains, and general weakness, often followed repeated high daily doses, e.g. 30 mg of base; these reactions were usually more severe in persons not susceptible to haemolysis; passage of dark urine was a signal for immediate cessation of treatment.— Chemotherapy of Malaria, *Tech. Rep. Ser. Wld Hlth Org. No. 226,* 1961, pp. 44–7.

Standard prophylactic antimalarial doses of primaquine were given to 1 Negro and 3 Caucasian men with glucose-6-phosphate dehydrogenase deficiency. The haemolytic reaction was mild in the Negro but haemolysis of about 20% of red blood-cells occurred in the Caucasians.— J. N. George *et al., J. Lab. clin. Med.,* 1967, *70,* 80. See also Standardization of Procedures for the Study of Glucose-6-Phosphate Dehydrogenase, *Tech. Rep. Ser. Wld Hlth Org. No. 366,* 1967; G. J. Brewer and C. J. D. Zarafonetis, *Bull. Wld Hlth Org.,* 1967, *36,* 303.

Primaquine had been reported to cause haemolysis in patients with haemoglobin Zürich.— E. Beutler, *Pharmac. Rev.,* 1969, *21,* 73.

Depression and confusion in a patient taking primaquine.— D. Schlossberg (letter), *Ann. intern. Med.,* 1980, *92,* 435.

Treatment of Adverse Effects. As for Chloroquine, p.396.

Precautions. Primaquine should be administered cautiously to persons with any serious systemic disease characterised by a tendency to granulocytopenia. Signs of methaemoglobinuria, indicating haemolysis, should be looked for during treatment. The administration of other bone-marrow depressants or haemolytic agents should be avoided.

The metabolism of primaquine is diminished by mepacrine and its toxicity enhanced.

Resistance. There have been occasional reports of clinical resistance in *P. vivax* infections. Because of the importance of the 8-aminoquinolines in the treatment of relapsing tissue infection, care must be taken to ensure that primaquine resistance does not become a problem through misuse.

In tropical areas where the relapse-rate in vivax malaria was increasing the use of 22.5 or 30 mg of primaquine daily for 14 days after chloroquine was preferred.— P. Charoenlarp and T. Harinasuta, *S.E. Asian J. trop. med. publ. Hlth,* 1973, *4,* 135, per *Trop. Dis. Bull.,* 1974, *71,* 13.

Primaquine 15 mg daily for 21 days was effective treatment for 200 of 209 patients showing malaria relapse after earlier treatment with chloroquine and primaquine in Vietnam. Resistance to primaquine may have been present in 1 patient.— M. H. Kaplan and L. S. Bernstein, *Milit. Med.,* 1974, *141,* 444, per *Abstr. Hyg.,* 1975, *50,* 707.

Further references: R. A. Wiseman (letter), *Br. med. J.,* 1970, *2,* 365; A. P. Hanway, *J.R. Army med. Cps,* 1970, *116,* 108, per *Trop. Dis. Bull.,* 1970, *67,* 1308; D. F. Clyde, *Bull. Wld Hlth Org.,* 1974, *50,* 243.

Absorption and Fate. Primaquine is readily absorbed from the gastro-intestinal tract. Peak plasma concentrations occur about 6 hours after a dose is taken and then rapidly diminish. It is mainly metabolised; little unchanged drug is excreted.

Plasma-primaquine concentrations, and metabolism, in Thai and Caucasian subjects.— J. Greaves *et al., Trans. R. Soc. trop. Med. Hyg.,* 1979, *73,* 328.

Uses. Primaquine is an antimalarial drug which kills the primary exoerythrocytic stages of *Plasmodium falciparum, P. vivax, P. malariae,* and *P. ovale,* and the secondary exoerythrocytic form of all except *P. falciparum.* It also kills gametocytes of all species, or renders them incapable of development in the mosquito, but it has little action on other erythrocytic stages and therefore it should not be used alone in the treatment of a malarial attack. Its mechanism of action is unclear but, appears to involve interference with DNA.

Primaquine is mainly used for the radical cure of *P. vivax* infections. For this purpose, a short intensive course of treatment with a schizonticide such as chloroquine is given to kill any erythrocytic parasites and this is given with or followed by a course of 14 daily doses of primaquine phosphate, each equivalent to 15 mg of the base, to kill the tissue forms. A suggested dose for children is 300 µg per kg body-weight daily for 14 days. The amount of primaquine required varies considerably, depending on the strain of *P. vivax*; infection with the Chesson strain may require daily doses of up to 45 mg. Shorter courses are also less effective.

Primaquine phosphate may be also given every 7 days in a dose equivalent to 45 to 60 mg of the base together with the equivalent of 300 mg of chloroquine or 400 mg of amodiaquine for the suppression of malaria.

Primaquine is also used in conjunction with chloroquine and diformyldapsone or dapsone for the suppression of resistant strains of *P. falciparum.*

Malaria. The activities of racemic primaquine and its (+) and (−) isomers against *Plasmodium cynomolgi* infections in *rhesus monkeys* were identical. However (−)-primaquine was 3 to 5 times as toxic as (+)-primaquine and at least twice as toxic as primaquine. (+)-Primaquine was considered to have a therapeutic index at least twice that of primaquine. (+)-Primaquine could offer advantages over primaquine and a trial in human subjects seemed indicated.— L. H. Schmidt *et al., Antimicrob. Ag. Chemother.,* 1977, *12,* 51.

All except 1 of 137 patients with *P. falciparum* infection were cleared of infection after treatment with chloroquine 600 mg and 5 daily doses of primaquine 15 mg. All of 638 patients were cleared by chloroquine 900 mg in 2 doses and 5 daily doses of primaquine 15 mg.— R. G. Roy *et al., Indian J. med. Res.,* 1975, *63,* 1469, per *Trop. Dis. Bull.,* 1976, *73,* 410.

Some 25% of patients with uncomplicated falciparum malaria given an antimalarial regimen incorporating primaquine 15 mg daily for 5 days (a regimen widely used in South-east Asia) remained potential gametocyte carriers for up to 21 days.— D. Bunnag *et al., Lancet,* 1980, *2,* 91.

Preparations

Primaquine Phosphate Tablets *(U.S.P.).* Tablets containing primaquine phosphate. Protect from light.

Primaquine Tablets *(B.P.).* Tablets containing primaquine phosphate. They are sugar-coated. Potency is expressed in terms of the equivalent amount of primaquine.

Primaquine Phosphate *(ICI Pharmaceuticals, UK).* Available as tablets of 13.2 mg (equivalent to 7.5 mg of the base).

1388-l

Proguanil Hydrochloride *(B.P.)*.

Proguanili Hydrochloridum; Bigumalum; Chloriguane Hydrochloride; Chloroguanide Hydrochloride; Proguanide Hydrochloride; RP 3359; SN 12,837. 1-(4-Chlorophenyl)-5-isopropylbiguanide hydrochloride.
$C_{11}H_{16}ClN_5,HCl$=290.2.

CAS — 500-92-5 (proguanil); 637-32-1 (hydrochloride).

Pharmacopoeias. In *Arg., Br., Ind., Int., It., Rus.,* and *Turk.*

A white odourless crystalline powder with a bitter taste. M.p. about 245°. **Soluble** 1 in 110 of water and 1 in 40 of alcohol; practically insoluble in chloroform and ether. A solution in water has a pH of about 6. **Protect** from light.

Adverse Effects. Proguanil hydrochloride is well tolerated after usual doses; after large doses vomiting, epigastric discomfort, haematuria, and renal irritation may occur.

Blackwater fever was precipitated by proguanil in 2 patients.— I. Singh, *Br. med. J.,* 1953, *1,* 598.

Precautions. Pregnancy is not considered a contra-indication to the prophylactic use of proguanil in malaria.

Resistance. A high degree of resistance appears to develop in all species of *Plasmodium* and in some areas this has limited the usefulness of proguanil. Cross-resistance occurs with other antimalarials.

Reduced susceptibility of human plasmodia to proguanil has been observed since 1948 in Assam, Cambodia, Ghana, Indochina, Indonesia, Kenya, Malaya, New Guinea, Tanganyika, and Thailand. A summary of reported cases of resistance.— Report of a WHO Scientific Group on Resistance of Malaria Parasites to Drugs, *Tech. Rep. Ser. Wld Hlth Org. No. 296,* 1965.

Resistance of *P. falciparum* to proguanil and pyrimethamine could appear after several months and there was world-wide cross-resistance between these drugs.— G. Charmot, Anglo-French Symposium on Control of Tropical Endemic Diseases, May 1969, London,, per *Br. med. J.*, 1969, *2*, 568.

Absorption and Fate. Proguanil is absorbed from the gastro-intestinal tract and peak concentrations in the circulation are attained about 3 hours after the dose is taken; about 75% in the plasma is bound to proteins and high concentrations occur in erythrocytes. The blood concentration rapidly diminishes and about 60% of a dose is excreted unchanged in the urine and about 30% as the active metabolite cycloguanil.

Uses. Proguanil is an antimalarial drug and dihydrofolate reductase inhibitor. It acts like the other antifolate antimalarials by interfering with the folic-folinic acid systems and thus exerts its effect mainly at the time the nucleus is dividing. Since its activity is dependent on its metabolism, proguanil has a slow schizonticidal effect in the blood. It also has some schizonticidal activity in the tissues.

Proguanil is effective against the exoerythrocytic forms of some strains of *Plasmodium falciparum* but it has little or no activity against the exoerythrocytic forms of *P. vivax*. It has a marked sporonticidal effect against some strains of *P. falciparum*; it does not kill the gametocytes, but renders them non-infective for the mosquito while the drug is present in the blood. Malaria parasites in the red blood cells are killed more rapidly by chloroquine or quinine than by proguanil, which is therefore not the best drug to use for the treatment of acute malaria.

When used in the treatment of malaria caused by strains of *P. falciparum*, proguanil kills parasites undergoing schizogony in the red blood cells and also the tissue forms, so that attacks do not recur when treatment is stopped. In the treatment of malaria caused by strains of *P. vivax*, proguanil kills the asexual parasites in the red blood cells but will not always eradicate latent tissue infection, so that attacks of malaria may sometimes recur after treatment is stopped. Because of the development of resistance proguanil should not be used alone for causal prophylaxis or treatment.

For the causal prophylaxis and suppression of symptoms of acute malaria, doses of 100 mg are usually given daily and continued for 4 weeks after leaving the area of infection. In highly malarious areas a daily dose of 200 mg is recommended. A suggested dose for children is: up to 1 year 25 to 50 mg daily, 1 to 4 years 50 mg daily, 5 to 8 years 75 mg daily, and 9 to 12 years 100 mg daily.

Doses of 100 mg of proguanil hydrochloride administered twice a week for 6 months following exposure to infection greatly reduce the chance of relapse in malaria caused by *P. vivax* .

Proguanil has been effective in the suppression of chloroquine-resistant falciparum malaria when given with dapsone 25 mg daily.

Malaria. Dapsone 25 mg daily with proguanil 200 mg was more effective in the prophylaxis of chloroquine-resistant falciparum malaria in soldiers in Vietnam than proguanil alone. No cases of agranulocytosis were reported when dapsone was taken only during the months when *P. falciparum* was epidemic, although several cases were reported when it was taken throughout the year.— R. H. Black, *Med. J. Aust.*, 1973, *1*, 1265.

Tropical splenomegaly syndrome. Proguanil 100 mg daily for 14 months or more, led to a marked improvement in 25 patients with the idiopathic tropical splenomegaly syndrome. Improvement in splenomegaly, hepatomegaly, and a rise in haemoglobin concentrations were first apparent after 3 months, but maximum effect took up to 42 months. A gain in weight was recorded in 16 of 18 patients. Relapse usually followed discontinuance of proguanil, but responded to retreatment.— E. J. Watson-Williams and N. C. Allan, *Br. med. J.*, 1968, *4*, 793.

Proguanil, 100 mg daily for at least 6 months, was given to 43 patients with an initial diagnosis of tropical splenomegaly syndrome. After 6 months' therapy, 32 patients showed a reduction in spleen size while in 11 patients no reduction or an increase in spleen size was noted. In those responding to treatment, serum IgM values were always very high before treatment, falling with the decrease in spleen size due to therapy. Of the other patients, those adequately followed developed identifiable diseases, usually malignant lymphoma or chronic lymphatic leukaemia.— A. -S. Sagoe, *Br. med. J.*, 1970, *3*, 378.

Four patients in whom the symptoms of tropical splenomegaly syndrome were controlled by proguanil relapsed when they defaulted in treatment; symptoms were again controlled when treatment recommenced.— A. S. David-West, *Br. med. J.*, 1974, *3*, 499.

Preparations

Proguanil Tablets *(B.P.)*. Proguanil Hydrochloride Tablets. Tablets containing proguanil hydrochloride.

Paludrine (Known in some countries as Paludrinol) *(ICI Pharmaceuticals, UK)*. Proguanil hydrochloride, available as scored tablets of 100 mg. (Also available as Paludrine in *Austral., Canad., Denm., Neth., Switz.*).

1389-y

Pyrimethamine *(B.P., B.P. Vet., U.S.P.)*.

Pyrimethaminum; BW 50-63; RP 4753; Pirimetamina. 5-(4-Chlorophenyl)-6-ethylpyrimidine-2,4-diamine.

$C_{12}H_{13}ClN_4$=248.7.

CAS — 58-14-0.

Pharmacopoeias. In *Br., Braz., Chin., Fr., Int., Nord.,* and *U.S.*

A white, odourless, tasteless, crystalline powder. M.P. 238° to 242°. Practically **insoluble** in water; soluble 1 in 200 of alcohol and 1 in 125 of chloroform; slightly soluble in acetone; soluble in warm dilute mineral acids. **Store** in airtight containers. Protect from light.

Adverse Effects. Within the usual dose range side-effects are unlikely, but 25 mg given daily over a prolonged period may cause depression of haemopoiesis due to the interference of the drug in the metabolism of folic acid. Skin rashes may also occur.

With larger doses, megaloblastic anaemia, leucopenia, thrombocytopenia, pancytopenia, and atrophic glossitis are more likely. Very large doses cause vomiting, convulsions, and respiratory failure, and deaths have occurred in children.

In a study of 8 children with CNS disease in acute leukaemia given pyrimethamine 75 mg per m² body-surface daily (maximum 100 mg) for 14 days, 2 withdrew because of convulsions or nausea and vomiting. Two of the remaining patients responded but the incidence of side-effects, which included exfoliative dermatitis, dizziness, nausea and vomiting, diarrhoea, and leucopenia, was considered intolerable.— A. H. Ragab (letter), *Lancet*, 1973, *1*, 1061.

Photosensitivity in a 9-year-old boy was attributed to pyrimethamine.— S. A. Craven (letter), *Br. med. J.*, 1974, *2*, 556.

Secondary gout had been reported in 5 to 10% of patients with polycythaemia rubra vera treated with phosphorus-32, busulphan, and pyrimethamine.— *Drug & Ther. Bull.*, 1975, *13*, 73.

Pyrimethamine had been reported to cause aplastic anaemia.— R. H. Girdwood, *Drugs*, 1976, *11*, 394.

Haemolytic anaemia. Pyrimethamine was not considered to cause clinically significant haemolytic anaemia in individuals with glucose-6-phosphate dehydrogenase deficiency under normal circumstances (e.g. in the absence of infection).— E. Beutler, *Pharmac. Rev.*, 1969, *21*, 73.

Pyrimethamine did not cause haemolysis in Chinese patients with glucose-6-phosphate dehydrogenase deficiency.— T. K. Chan *et al.*, *Br. med. J.*, 1976, *2*, 1227.

Overdosage. A 14-month-old child who had ingested 450 mg of pyrimethamine developed vomiting, cyanosis, respiratory distress, unconsciousness, convulsions, tachycardia, and hyperpyrexia, together with blindness, deafness, and ataxia. Treatment included diazepam, oxygen, forced diuresis, and folic acid, and the child recovered. The blindness and deafness slowly regressed but there was residual mental retardation 2 years later. A 4-year-old child who had been given 50 mg of pyrimethamine weekly for 6 months developed severe folic acid-deficient megaloblastic anaemia which responded to blood transfusions and treatment (in the absence of folinic acid) with folic acid.— O. Akinyanju *et al.*, *Br. med. J.*, 1973, *4*, 147.

Pseudolymphoma. A report of fever and cervical, axillary, and inguinal lymphadenopathy in a 9-year-old boy after taking pyrimethamine and sulphadimidine; pyrimethamine was considered responsible. Histologically the neoplasm simulated malignant lymphoma.— J. M. Costello and D. M. O. Becroft, *N.Z. med. J.*, 1977, *86*, 430.

Treatment of Adverse Effects. The stomach should be emptied by aspiration and lavage. Convulsions should be cautiously controlled by the injection of diazepam 5 to 10 mg, and injections of calcium folinate should be given to counter folate deficiency. Respiration may require assistance.

Precautions. When doses high enough to interfere with folic acid metabolism are given, white-cell and platelet counts should be made twice weekly. Subclinical folic acid deficiency may be aggravated by pyrimethamine and the effects of antineoplastic bone-marrow depressants may be enhanced. The administration of folinic acid 10 mg daily has been recommended in order to prevent haematological toxicity due to pyrimethamine.

Pyrimethamine has caused foetal abnormalities in *animals*, but pregnancy is not considered a contra-indication to the prophylactic use of pyrimethamine in malaria. High doses should be avoided during pregnancy unless folinic acid supplements are given. These do not interfere with the antimalarial action.

Pyrimethamine was reported to have delayed haematological recovery in 36 patients with falciparum malaria resistant to chloroquine. Folinic acid should be given.— G. J. Canfield *et al.*, *Milit. Med.*, 1971, *136*, 354, per *Int. pharm. Abstr.*, 1972, *9*, 756.

A soldier under treatment for malaria who developed profound leucopenia and thrombocytopenia was found to have bone-marrow depression and clinically mild tropical sprue. Pyrimethamine could have reduced the already depleted folic acid stores.— J. I. Matthews *et al.*, *Milit. Med.*, 1973, *138*, 280, per *Trop. Dis. Bull.*, 1974, *71*, 13.

Bone-marrow aplasia in a heterozygous beta-thalassaemic youth was attributed to pyrimethamine.— P. Malacarne *et al.* (letter), *Lancet*, 1974, *2*, 904.

For a recommendation that pyrimethamine should not be given to patients between courses of antineoplastic agents because of potential bone-marrow aplasia, see Antineoplastic Agents and Immunosuppressants, p.175.

Interactions. Mild liver toxicity occurred in several patients taking pyrimethamine and lorazepam concomitantly and was confirmed in 2 of 5 women who tolerated each drug without adverse effect when given separately.— M. Briggs and M. Briggs (letter), *Br. med. J.*, 1974, *1*, 40.

Resistance. Resistance or reduced sensitivity of *Plasmodium falciparum* and *P. vivax* to pyrimethamine has been reported. It develops rapidly after the use of pyrimethamine alone in mass treatment or as medicated salt; such use is therefore contra-indicated. There may be cross-resistance to chlorproguanil, cycloguanil, proguanil, and trimethoprim.

For a discussion of resistance to pyrimethamine, see Chemotherapy of Malaria and Resistance to Antimalarials, *Tech. Rep. Ser. Wld Hlth Org. No. 529,* 1973, p. 48.

A report of 4 patients in Papua New Guinea with *Plasmodium falciparum* malaria clinically resistant to pyrimethamine plus sulfadoxine (Fansidar).— B. Darlow *et al.* (letter), *Lancet*, 1980, *2*, 1243. See also G. T. Nurse (letter), *ibid.*, 1981, *1*, 36.

Further references: E. S. Hurwitz *et al.*, *Lancet*, 1981, *1*, 1068 (Fansidar resistance in Thailand); F. Black *et al.*, *Trans R. Soc. trop. Med. Hyg.*, 1981, *75*, 715 (Fansidar resistance in south-east Asia).

Absorption and Fate. Pyrimethamine is absorbed from the gastro-intestinal tract and peak concentrations in the circulation are stated to occur about 2 hours after a dose is taken. It is mainly concentrated in the kidneys, lungs, liver, and spleen. It is only slowly excreted, the average half-life in plasma being about 90 hours; several metabolites appear in the urine. Pyrimethamine is present in the milk of nursing mothers being treated with the drug.

Uses. Pyrimethamine is an antimalarial drug and dihydrofolate reductase inhibitor similar to proguanil hydrochloride, (see p.402).

It has been used alone for the suppression of falciparum and sometimes vivax malaria in doses of 25 to 50 mg every 7 days, treatment being continued for at least 4 weeks after exposure to risk. A suggested dose for children is: up to 1 year, 6.25 mg every 7 days; 1 to 4 years, 6.25 to 12.5 mg; 5 to 8 years 12.5 mg; and 9 to 12 years, 12.5 to 25 mg. More generally pyrimethamine is used in combination with other drugs for both suppression and treatment.

Pyrimethamine interferes with the synthesis of folinic acid by the parasite. Sulphonamides and sulphones act on the same biological pathway at a different point and therefore enhance the action of pyrimethamine. This effect has been utilised in the suppression and treatment of malaria due to most strains of *Plasmodium* including those resistant to chloroquine and pyrimethamine alone. Sulfadoxine is the sulphonamide generally used and for treatment a single dose of 1 to 1.5 g is given with pyrimethamine 50 to 75 mg. The treatment may be given in conjunction with quinine in severe cases (see p.405).

For causal prophylaxis or suppression, sulfadoxine 500 mg with pyrimethamine 25 mg is given every 7 days. Twice or thrice this dose has been given in alternative schedules every 2 or 4 weeks depending on the immunity of the patient. A suggested weekly dose for children is: up to 4 years, one-quarter; 5 to 8 years, one-half; and 9 to 12 years, three-quarters of the adult dose. A similar combined regimen of pyrimethamine and dapsone is used for causal prophylaxis or suppression of malaria, particularly where strains resistant to pyrimethamine or proguanil are present. The usual dose is pyrimethamine 12.5 mg and dapsone 100 mg as a single weekly dose, with half this dose for children aged 5 to 10 years.

Toxoplasmosis may be controlled by the concurrent administration of high doses of pyrimethamine and a sulphonamide such as sulphadiazine. For this purpose pyrimethamine is given in a dose of 50 or 75 mg daily together with sulphadiazine 1 to 4 g daily, reduced according to the patient's response, after 1 to 3 weeks to about half these doses and continued for a further 4 to 5 weeks.

Pyrimethamine was formerly used in the treatment of meningeal leukaemia.

Administration in renal failure. Pyrimethamine could be given in usual doses to patients with renal failure.— W. M. Bennett *et al.*, *Ann. intern. Med.*, 1980, *93*, 62.

Coccidiosis. Coccidiosis due to infection with *Isospora belli* in a poultry farmer was successfully treated with pyrimethamine 75 mg and sulphadiazine 4 g given daily for 21 days, and followed by further treatment with half-doses for 28 days.— J. S. Trier *et al.*, *Gastroenterology*, 1974, *66*, 923, per *Abstr. Hyg.*, 1975, *50*, 708.

A brief discussion of the use of pyrimethamine and a sulphonamide in the treatment of isosporiasis.— R. Knight and S. G. Wright, *Gut*, 1978, *19*, 940.

Leukaemia. Remissions occurred on 2 occasions when pyrimethamine was used to treat episodes of meningeal leukaemia in a patient with adult acute myeloblastic leukaemia. Concentrations in the CSF were 10 to 25% of those in the plasma.— G. F. Geils *et al.*, *Blood*, 1971, *38*, 131, per *Int. pharm. Abstr.*, 1972, *9*, 274.

Experience from treating 12 patients with CNS leukaemia with either pyrimethamine or methotrexate or both indicated that the duration of remission was longer after pyrimethamine and that its haematological side-effects were reversible.— A. C. Boadella and R. P. P. Illa (letter), *Lancet*, 1973, *2*, 1330.

In the treatment of meningeal leukaemia, pyrimethamine should not be used immediately after methotrexate and the dose should not exceed 2 to 3 mg per kg body-weight daily.— J. Armata (letter), *Br. med. J.*, 1973, *4*, 783.

Eight patients in remission from meningeal leukaemia were given pyrimethamine 150 mg daily for 4 days every 3 weeks for a year and 5 sustained a complete remission. Side-effects were common and apart from 1 patient who withdrew because of severe vomiting, usually transitory and tolerable.— J. Hamers *et al.* (letter), *Lancet*, 1974, *1*, 310.

Of 17 adults with previously untreated acute lymphocytic leukaemia 9 achieved complete remissions after induction courses of thioguanine, vincristine, dexamethasone, and pyrimethamine. Seven of the 9 received consolidation and maintenance treatment; 6 of the 17 developed meningeal leukaemia; pyrimethamine provided inadequate prophylaxis for meningeal leukaemia.— A. C. Smyth and P. H. Wiernik, *Clin. Pharmac. Ther.*, 1976, *19*, 240.

Malaria suppression. It had been suggested that young children in areas where falciparum malaria was endemic should be given pyrimethamine 25 mg once a month so that morbidity and mortality might be reduced while not completely suppressing parasitaemia, thus allowing protective antibodies to develop. In 36 Ugandan children this regimen did not prevent all episodes of severe malaria and was associated with low titres of malaria antibodies. It was uncertain whether the predominant cause for these low titres was the pyrimethamine regimen or the frequent courses of chloroquine which were prescribed for all febrile illnesses.— P. S. E. G. Harland *et al.*, *Trans. R. Soc. trop. Med. Hyg.*, 1975, *69*, 261.

Combined use with dapsone. In a double-blind study 280 children living in an area of stable *P. falciparum* malaria were divided into 5 groups and given pyrimethamine 25 mg, pyrimethamine 12.5 mg with dapsone 100 mg, pyrimethamine 12.5 mg with sulfadoxine 125 mg or 250 mg, or placebo tablets, weekly for 52 weeks. Initially, 75% of all the children showed parasitaemia. Pyrimethamine alone caused incomplete suppression of parasitaemia, but after the first dose of the combined drugs there was rapid clearance with almost complete suppression throughout the year. In the control group there was an average crude parasite-rate of 45.2% during the year. At the end of the trial no strains resistant to the combined therapy had emerged.— A. O. Lucas *et al.*, *Trans. R. Soc. trop. Med. Hyg.*, 1969, *63*, 216.

Pyrimethamine and dapsone administered weekly in the malaria transmission season had proved completely active under conditions in which there was partial resistance to pyrimethamine.— G. Charmot, Anglo-French Symposium on Control of Tropical Endemic Diseases, May 1969, London,, per *Br. med. J.*, 1969, *2*, 568.

In 93 workers on a rubber plantation in Malaysia given pyrimethamine 12.5 mg and dapsone 100 mg weekly the parasite infection-rate fell from 35.5% to zero in about 8 weeks, with an occasional breakthrough. In 54 workers given chloroquine 10 mg per kg body-weight weekly the rate fell to about 5% in about 2 weeks; side-effects from chloroquine were troublesome.— J. T. Ponnampalam *et al.*, *J. trop. Med. Hyg.*, 1976, *79*, 220.

Further references: R. M. Harwin, *Cent. Afr. J. Med.*, 1972, *18*, 201, per *Trop. Dis. Bull.*, 1973, *70*, 517; H. E. Segal *et al.*, *J. trop. Med. Hyg.*, 1973, *76*, 285; M. C. Weber *et al.*, *Publ. Hlth, Johannesburg*, 1975, *75*, 355, per *Trop. Dis. Bull.*, 1976, *73*, 485.

For the successful prophylaxis of chloroquine-resistant falciparum malaria with diformyldapsone and pyrimethamine, see Diformyldapsone, p.399.

Combined use with sulfadoxine. The monthly administration of sulfadoxine 1.5 g and pyrimethamine 75 mg was more effective in the prophylaxis of *P. falciparum* malaria than chloroquine or amodiaquine given weekly.— A. Riche and P. Colombo, *Bull. Soc. Path. exot.*, 1971, *64*, 847, per *Trop. Dis. Bull.*, 1973, *70*, 320. A similar report.— D. R. O'Holohan and J. Hugoe-Matthews, *S.E. Asian J. trop. med. publ. Hlth*, 1971, *2*, 164, per *Trop. Dis. Bull.*, 1972, *69*, 182.

Further references: I. Ebisawa *et al.*, *Jap. J. exp. Med.*, 1971, *41*, 209; T. Muto *et al.*, *Jap. J. exp. Med.*, 1971, *41*, 459; A. Z. Shafei, *J. trop. Med. Hyg.*, 1975, *78*, 190.

Malaria treatment. When malaria was caused by a parasite resistant to the recognised antimalarials, the use of sulphones or sulphonamides in conjunction with pyrimethamine could be of value. The long-acting sulphonamide generally used was sulfadoxine. Pyrimethamine 50 mg with sulfadoxine 1 g had produced a high percentage of cures, as had the same regimen followed on the next day by a 500-mg dose of sulfadoxine.— Fourteenth Report of the WHO Expert Committee on Malaria, *Tech. Rep. Ser. Wld Hlth Org. No. 382*, 1968. See also B. Simpson *et al.*, *Trans. R. Soc. trop. Med. Hyg.*, 1972, *66*, 222.

Pyrimethamine 75 mg with sulfametopyrazine 1.5 g as a single dose for adults, or 1 mg per kg body-weight with 25 mg per kg respectively for children, was generally well tolerated in 100 patients with falciparum malaria. Parasitaemia lasted for about 70 hours but up to 7 days in some patients. Two patients died and 1 relapsed during a follow-up of 10 days.— R. Mazaud *et al.*, *Med. trop. Marseille*, 1970, *30*, 759, per *Trop. Dis. Bull.*, 1971, *68*, 925.

In 200 patients given a single dose of pyrimethamine 1.25 mg per kg body-weight together with sulfadoxine 25 mg per kg, *P. falciparum* was suppressed within 39 to 52 hours, compared with 53 to 64 hours among 100 patients given chloroquine 25 to 30 mg per kg over 2 or 3 days. Pyrimethamine 800 µg per kg given with sulfadoxine 16 mg per kg by intramuscular injection to 50 patients who were vomiting but had no cerebral symptoms was not enhanced by quinine. Pyrimethamine 12.5 mg with sulfadoxine 250 mg every 4 weeks was as effective prophylactically in 120 children as pyrimethamine and dapsone in 60 children, or chloroquine in 60. Parasites reappeared after 5 weeks.— H. R. Wolfensberger, *S.E. Asian J. trop. med. publ. Hlth*, 1971, *2*, 39, per *Trop. Dis. Bull.*, 1972, *69*, 593.

Of 25 patients with falciparum malaria resistant to 4-aminoquinolines and treated with sulphadimethoxine or sulfadoxine 1.5 g together with pyrimethamine and primaquine, only 14 were cured and 8 had recrudescences within 28 days.— C. M. Johnson *et al.*, *J. trop. Med. Hyg.*, 1972, *75*, 133, per *Trop. Dis. Bull.*, 1973, *70*, 119.

Recrudescences occurred in 17 of 21 patients with falciparum malaria treated with pyrimethamine 25 mg and dapsone 200 mg compared with 1 of 17 patients treated with sulphadoxine 1 g and pyrimethamine 50 mg. Two other patients in the latter group remained parasitaemic after treatment.— H. E. Segal *et al.*, *Trans. R. Soc. trop. Med. Hyg.*, 1975, *69*, 139. See also J. Verdrager *et al.*, *Bull. Wld Hlth Org.*, 1969, *40*, 319.

In a study in 33 volunteers infected with *Plasmodium falciparum* and treated with pyrimethamine and sulfametopyrazine, acetylator status and plasma concentration of sulphonamide did not correlate with clinical response.— R. L. Williams *et al.*, *Am. J. trop. Med. Hyg.*, 1975, *24*, 734, per *Trop. Dis. Bull.*, 1976, *73*, 739.

Further references: N. A. Tiburskaya *et al.*, *Medskaya Parazit.*, 1971, *40*, 431, per *Trop. Dis. Bull.*, 1971, *68*, 1308; P. Kusnecov *et al.*, *Bull. Wld Hlth Org.*, 1972, *46*, 117; L. Le Pelletier and B. Politur, *Bull. Soc. Path. exot.*, 1973, *66*, 631, per *Trop. Dis. Bull.*, 1974, *71*, 1224; I. Ebisawa *et al.*, *Jap. J. exp. Med.*, 1974, *44*, 151; N. Jaroonvesama *et al.*, *S.E. Asian J. trop. med. publ. Hlth* 1974, *5*, 504; J. J. Picq *et al.*, *Bull. Soc. Path. exot.*, 1975, *68*, 61; A. N. Lewis and J. T. Ponnampalam, *Ann. trop. Med. Parasit.*, 1975, *69*, 1; E. B. Doberstyn *et al.*, *Am. J. trop. Med. Hyg.*, 1976, *25*, 14; E. B. Doberstyn *et al.*, *Bull. Wld Hlth Org.*, 1979, *57*, 275.

For earlier reports of the use of pyrimethamine in the suppression and treatment of malaria, see Martindale, 27th Edn, pp. 355–6.

Mycetoma. Pyrimethamine with sulfadoxine and streptomycin could provide a useful second-line therapy for actinomycetoma.— E. S. Mahgoub, *Bull. Wld Hlth Org.*, 1976, *54*, 303.

Pityriasis. Of 11 patients with pityriasis lichenoides 6 responded strongly to toxoplasmin tests. These 6 were treated with pyrimethamine 50 mg daily for 5 days, repeated after 20 days, with a second course 6 months later; 3 achieved complete cure, 2 a partial remission, and 1 moderate improvement.— N. B. Zlatkov and V. C. Andreev, *Br. J. Derm.*, 1972, *87*, 114.

Pneumonia. Pneumonia due to *Pneumocystis carinii* in 3 patients responded to treatment with pyrimethamine 25 mg once or twice daily and sulphadiazine 1 g four times daily for from 14 to 28 days, but 1 patient died shortly after completion of treatment.— H. B. Kirby *et al.*, *Ann. intern. Med.*, 1971, *75*, 505. See also R. E. Helmer (letter), *ibid.*, 1975, *82*, 124.

A report of effective prophylactic therapy of *Pneumocystis carinii* infection with sulfadoxine and pyrimethamine in infants.— C. Post *et al.*, *Curr. ther. Res.*, 1971, *13*, 273.

Polycythaemia. Five patients with polycythaemia vera were successfully treated with pyrimethamine for periods of 7 months to 2 years in doses of 3 to 75 mg daily. Careful haematological control was necessary.— D. E. Pegg and H. T. Ford, *Br. med. J.*, 1961, *2*, 617. A similar report.— J. S. P. Jones and A. M. Jelliffe, *Clin. Radiol.*, 1963, *14*, 424, per *Abstr. Wld Med.*, 1964, *36*, 41.

Psoriasis. Four of 7 patients with long-standing psoriasis obtained a good response to treatment with pyrimethamine, 750 µg per kg body-weight 12-hourly for 3 doses once a week, increased 4-weekly by 250 µg per kg if tolerated. However, gastro-intestinal effects in 3, haematological effects in 3, suspected hepatotoxicity in 2, and malaise, fatigue, and irritability rendered pyrimethamine no more useful than methotrexate.— N. J. DiBella *et al.*, *Archs Derm.*, 1977, *113*, 172.

Toxoplasmosis. The treatment of choice for toxoplasmosis in infants was pyrimethamine, 2 mg per kg body-weight daily for 3 days and then 1 mg per kg daily, with sulphadiazine 100 mg per kg daily together with calcium folinate 1 mg daily and fresh yeast 100 mg daily to overcome folate antagonism. For adults and children, 50 or 25 mg respectively of pyrimethamine was given daily for 3 days together with conventional doses of sulphadiazine and followed by one-half the dose of pyrimethamine daily thereafter, together with calcium folinate 5 to 15 mg and yeast. Treatment should be maintained for 1 month, provided that improvement occurred within the first 2 weeks. Counts of blood platelets and leucocytes should be performed at least twice weekly to detect early signs of folate antagonism.— H. A. Feldman, *New Engl. J. Med.*, 1968, *279*, 1431.

Comparison of treatment with corticosteroids alone or in conjunction with pyrimethamine and spiramycin in 69 patients with active toxoplasmic retinochoroiditis showed that, while pyrimethamine was the most effective drug, severe side-effects indicated that it should only be used when the lesions might cause permanent damage to the sight. Less severe cases might be treated with spiramycin.— J. Nolan and E. S. Rosen, *Br. J. Ophthal.*, 1968, *52*, 396. See also C. L. Giles, *Am. J. Ophthal.*, 1964, *58*, 611; M. Ghosh *et al.*, *ibid.*, 1965, *59*, 55; M. Alexander and H. U. Stolze, *Advances in Antimicrobial and Antineoplastic Chemotherapy*, Vol. 1, pt 1, Munich, Urban and Schwarzenberg, 1972, p. 493.

Pyrimethamine with sulphonamides were generally considered to be too dangerous for the treatment of toxoplasmosis in pregnant women.— H. Williams, *Postgrad. med. J.*, 1977, *53*, 614.

Preparations

Pyrimethamine Tablets *(B.P.)*. Tablets containing pyrimethamine.

Pyrimethamine Tablets *(U.S.P.)*. Tablets containing pyrimethamine. Store in airtight containers. Protect from light.

Proprietary Preparations

Daraprim *(Wellcome, UK)*. Pyrimethamine, available as scored tablets of 25 mg. (Also available as Daraprim in *Arg., Austral., Belg., Canad., Denm., Ger., Neth., S.Afr., Spain, Swed., Switz., USA*).

Fansidar Injection *(Roche, UK)*. Contains in each ml pyrimethamine 10 mg and sulfadoxine 200 mg, in ampoules of 2.5 ml. Antimalarial. *Dose.* Therapeutic, 5 to 7.5 ml by deep intramuscular injection; children, 1 to 5 ml. (Available only in certain countries).

Fansidar Tablets *(Roche, UK)*. Each scored tablet contains pyrimethamine 25 mg and sulfadoxine 500 mg. Antimalarial. *Dose.* Therapeutic, 2 to 3 tablets as a single dose; children, ½ to 2 tablets. Prophylactic, 1 tablet every 7 days; children, ¼ to ¾ tablet.

Maloprim *(Wellcome, UK)*. Scored tablets each containing pyrimethamine 12.5 mg and dapsone 100 mg. For the prophylaxis of malaria. *Dose.* 1 tablet weekly; children, 5 to 10 years, ½ tablet weekly.

Other Proprietary Names

Erbaprelina *(Ital.)*; Tindurin *(Hung.)*.

1390-g

Quinine *(B.P.C. 1963)*. Quinina; Chininum.

(8*S*,9*R*)-6′-Methoxycinchonan-9-ol trihydrate; (α*R*)-α-(6-Methoxy-4-quinolyl)-α-[(2*S*,4*S*,5*R*)-(5-vinylquinuclidin-2-yl)]methanol trihydrate.

$C_{20}H_{24}N_2O_2,3H_2O$=378.5.

CAS — 130-95-0 (anhydrous).

Pharmacopoeias. In *It.* and *Span. Fr.* has anhydrous.

The chief alkaloid of various species of *Cinchona* (Rubiaceae). It is an optical isomer of quinidine. It is a white, odourless, slightly efflorescent, flaky, granular or microcrystalline powder with a bitter taste. M.p. about 173°.

Very slightly **soluble** in water and glycerol; soluble 1 in 1 of alcohol (90%), 1 in 3 of chloroform, 1 in 4 of ether saturated with water; soluble in carbon disulphide, fixed and volatile oils, dilute acids, and dilute ammonia solution. **Store** in airtight containers. Protect from light.

Adverse Effects. Severe poisoning by quinine or other of the cinchona alkaloids is characterised by headache, fever, vomiting, muscle weakness, excitement, confusion, blindness (possibly permanent), deafness, and loss of consciousness; blood pressure falls, there is a feeble pulse, occasionally renal failure, and death occurs, usually in coma, from respiratory failure. Death may result in a few hours or may be delayed for 1 or 2 days. The average fatal dose is 8 g, though larger doses have been survived, and 4 g usually causes untoward effects.

The repeat administration of quinine in full therapeutic doses may give rise to a train of symptoms known as cinchonism, characterised by tinnitus, headache, nausea, abdominal pain, pruritus, skin rashes, disturbed vision, and temporary blindness.

The administration of quinine to a patient who has previously been suffering from a chronic and inadequately controlled malarial infection may precipitate an attack of blackwater fever. Toxic doses of quinine may cause abortion, but it is unwise on this account to withhold quinine from pregnant women infected with malaria if less toxic antimalarials are not available.

Some patients are hypersensitive to quinine and even small doses may give rise to symptoms of cinchonism, together with angioneurotic oedema, asthma, and other allergic phenomena. Haemolytic anaemia and thrombocytopenia have been reported. As a test for quinine idiosyncrasy a scratch test may be made with a 1 to 10% solution of a quinine salt in physiological saline; redness, oedema, and itching occur within 5 to 15 minutes if the patient is hypersensitive.

Disturbed vision progressing to near blindness within a few hours, numbness of the feet, and mild tinnitus developed in a 51-year-old man after he had ingested quinine sulphate 3 g in 1 day following dosage with 300 mg nightly for several weeks to alleviate leg cramps. Vision improved slowly but was still defective 10 months later.— N. K. Banerji and V. A. Martin, *J. Ir. med. Ass.*, 1974, *67*, 46, per *Pharm. J.*, 1974, *2*, 159. See also G. S. Brinton *et al.*, *Am. J. Ophthal.*, 1980, *90*, 403 (ocular quinine toxicity following overdose).

Mention of acute tubular necrosis as a side-effect of quinine.— J. R. Curtis, *Br. med. J.*, 1977, *2*, 242.

Blood disorders. Positive reactions to the direct Coombs' test occurred in 3 soldiers and was related to the administration of quinine for malaria. They all had haemolysis and 2 also had dermatitis and/or blackwater fever.— M. M. Adver *et al.*, *Ann. intern. Med.*, 1968, *68*, 33, per *J. Am. med. Ass.*, 1968, *203* (Feb. 19), A186.

Quinine 2 g daily was not considered to cause clinically significant haemolytic anaemia in individuals with a deficiency of glucose-6-phosphate dehydrogenase under normal circumstances (e.g. in the absence of infection).— E. Beutler, *Pharmac. Rev.*, 1969, *21*, 73. See also D. J. Weatherall, *Practitioner*, 1978, *221*, 194.

An analysis of blood dyscrasias reported to the Swedish Adverse Drug Reaction Committee for the 5-year period 1966–70 showed that thrombocytopenia attributable to quinine or quinidine had been reported on 26 occasions. It was estimated that reported figures represented one-third of the true frequency.— L. E. Böttiger and B. Westerholm, *Br. med. J.*, 1973, *3*, 339.

Quinine-induced agranulocytosis in a 64-year-old man was confirmed by the inhibition, *in vitro*, of bone-marrow cell cultures by therapeutic concentrations of quinine.— R. Sutherland *et al.*, *Br. med. J.*, 1977, *1*, 605.

Cardiotoxicity. Two Negro men aged 22 and 38 years developed depression of myocardial excitability as a result of injecting themselves with relatively large doses of quinine which was used as an adulterant to diamorphine. In 1 patient, cardiac arrest responded rapidly to external cardiac massage, and atrioventricular block in the second patient gradually lessened as quinine was excreted.— P. Lupovich *et al.* (letter), *J. Am. med. Ass.*, 1970, *212*, 1216.

Erythema multiforme. Quinine had been implicated in erythema multiforme, the Stevens-Johnson syndrome.— D. B. Coursin, *J. Am. med. Ass.*, 1966, *198*, 113.

Fever. Fever due to drug reaction was reported in 26 patients about 8 days after commencement of treatment with quinine which was given to 268 patients experiencing their first attacks of malaria. The fever abated in a mean of 4.6 days after quinine was discontinued.— A. P. Hall, *S.E. Asian J. Trop. med. publ. Hlth*, 1974, *5*, 413, per *Trop. Dis. Bull.*, 1975, *72*, 528.

Pregnancy and the neonate. Jaundice not due to blood group incompatibility developed in a full-term infant with a deficiency of glucose-6-phosphate dehydrogenase born to a woman dependent on multiple daily injections of diamorphine mixed with quinine 30 to 50 mg.— L. Glass *et al.* (letter), *J. Pediat.*, 1973, *82*, 734.

There are a number of reports of congenital malformations, including defects of vision and hearing, in infants born to mothers who had taken quinine, usually in high doses, during pregnancy. The teratogenic risk from therapeutic doses appears to be slight. Brief reviews: T. H. Shepard, *Catalog of Teratogenic Agents*, London, Johns Hopkins, 1973, p. 138; H. Tuchmann-Duplessis, *Monographs on Drugs, Vol. 2, Drug Effects on the Fetus*, G.S. Avery (Ed.), London, Adis, 1975, p. 134; J. L. Schardein, *Drugs as Teratogens*, Cleveland, CRC, 1976, p. 193.

Absence of effect. In 104 children born to mothers monitored by the Collaborative Perinatal Project and found to have been exposed to quinine, and possibly other drugs, at some time during the first 4 months of pregnancy no evidence of a teratogenic effect was found.— O. P. Heinonen *et al.*, *Birth Defects and Drugs in Pregnancy*, Littleton MA, Publishing Sciences Group, 1977, p. 296.

Skin reactions. Five cases of rash attributable to quinine. In 2 men and possibly 3, the rash was caused by the wife's use of a contraceptive pessary containing quinine. In the fourth man, the rash started the day after drinking gin and bitter lemon (3 mg of quinine to 100 ml). In the fifth, the attack was possibly caused by an analgesic tablet containing quinine. All patients gave positive patch tests and negative scratch or intradermal tests.— C. D. Calnan and G. A. Caron, *Br. med. J.*, 1961, *2*, 1750. Similar reports.— R. D. Cundall (letter), *ibid.*, 1964, *1*, 1638; J. A. Savin, *Br. J. Derm.*, 1970, *83*, 546.

Purpura was induced, in a patient previously sensitised to quinine, by drinking bitter lemon.— J. A. Murray *et al.*, *Br. med. J.*, 1979, *2*, 1551.

See also Erythema Multiforme.

Treatment of Adverse Effects. If large doses of quinine or its salts have been recently ingested, the stomach should be emptied by aspiration and lavage and a purgative, such as sodium sulphate 30 g in 250 ml of water, may be given. Elimination of quinine from the body may be assisted by acidification of the urine with ammonium chloride and ensuring an adequate fluid balance, but this has a limited application since quinine is extensively metabolised in the liver with only a small proportion excreted unchanged in the urine (for comments on the hazards of forced diuresis, see under Diuresis, below). Blood pressure should be supported. Signs of haemolytic anaemia may be indicative of a need to treat acute renal failure. Assisted respiration may be necessary to combat respiratory failure. Cardiac rhythm should be monitored.

Vasodilators such as amyl nitrite and nicotinic acid have been given in attempts to reverse visual impairment; beneficial effects have been achieved with stellate ganglion block.

An 18-month-old child who had become unconscious and convulsed after taking an unknown number of quinine sulphate tablets recovered completely after being given an exchange blood transfusion.— A. W. Burrows *et al.*, *Archs Dis. Childh.*, 1972, *47*, 304.

Adsorption. For comment on the *in vitro* adsorption of quinine by activated charcoal, see p.79.

Dialysis. Data indicating that peritoneal dialysis is not a useful method for removal of quinine from the body.— J. V. Donadio *et al.*, *J. Am. med. Ass.*, 1968, *204*, 274.

For a discussion of the limited role of dialysis in the treatment of quinine poisoning, see J. F. Winchester *et al.*, *Trans. Am. Soc. artif. internal Organs*, 1977, *23*, 762.

Diuresis. Forced diuresis has a limited application in the management of drug overdosage to those few drugs that are excreted to a significant extent unchanged in the urine. Forced acid diuresis has been used for poisoning by basic drugs such as quinine but symptomatic treatment is usually adequate and is probably much safer. Forced diuresis should never be undertaken lightly. It is potentially lethal in elderly patients and in those with cardiac and renal disease. Other complications include electrolyte and acid-base disturbances, water intoxication, and cerebral oedema.— L. F. Prescott, Limitations of haemodialysis and forced diuresis, in *The Poisoned Patient: the role of the laboratory*, Ciba Foundation Symposium 26, Oxford, Elsevier, 1974, p. 269.

Stellate ganglion block. After acetylcholine, nicotinic acid, and tolazoline had proved ineffective, stellate ganglion block with 5 ml of 1% lignocaine with adrenaline 1 in 160 000 was repeated 19 times in 7 days and was effective in treating total blindness in a 17-year-old girl after ingestion of a total of 8 g of quinine hydrochloride in 24 hours. Vision was almost normal by the 19th day. Other treatment included dichlorphenamide and potassium chloride.— P. P. Bricknell *et al.*, *Br. med. J.*, 1967, *4*, 400.

A 16-year-old girl who had taken 4.5 g of quinine sulphate with suicidal intent became virtually blind but responded promptly to bilateral stellate ganglion block using bupivacaine. Inhalation of amyl nitrite had produced flushing of the conjunctivae but no subjective visual improvement or fundal changes.— J. L. K. Bankes *et al.*, *Br. med. J.*, 1972, *4*, 85.

A 3-year-old child was completely blind 15 hours after the ingestion of quinine; 28 hours after ingestion he was given bilateral stellate block using bupivacaine, repeated 4½ hours later. After 12 hours central vision was normal but peripheral vision was poor. A month later there were residual pale optic disks and gross attenuation of the retinal vessels.— H. B. Valman and D. C. White, *Br. med. J.*, 1977, *1*, 1065.

Precautions. Quinine is contra-indicated in patients with a history of hypersensitivity and in the presence of haemoglobinuria during malaria or of optic neuritis. It should be used with caution in patients with atrial fibrillation or other serious heart disease. Quinine may cause hypoprothrombinaemia and enhance the effects of anticoagulants. Quinine may cause severe respiratory distress and dysphagia in patients with myasthenia gravis and should be used with care if at all in such patients.

Pregnancy in a patient with malaria is not regarded as a contra-indication to the use of quinine.

Antimalarial agents and especially quinine, when given in inadequate doses, have been implicated in precipitating blackwater fever. However, in some cases deficiency of glucose-6-phosphate dehydrogenase may have been involved.

As quinine has many of the adverse effects and actions of quinidine, see also under Quinidine Sulphate, p.1370.

Chloroquine and quinine appeared to be antagonistic when given together for *P. falciparum* malaria.— A. P. Hall (letter), *Trans. R. Soc. trop. Med. Hyg.*, 1973, *67*, 425.

Interactions. The effect of quinine on the kinetics of digoxin.— M. Wandell *et al.*, *Clin. Pharmac. Ther.*, 1980, *28*, 425.

See also under Digoxin, p.534.

Pregnancy and the neonate. A report of jitteriness in an infant, due to quinine withdrawal. The mother had taken quinine (as tonic water) for the last 17 weeks of pregnancy.— A. N. W. Evans *et al.*, *Practitioner*, 1980, *224*, 315.

Resistance. Resistance of *P. falciparum* has been reported from South American and South-east Asia and cross-resistance has been demonstrated between quinine and the 4-aminoquinolines.

Absorption and Fate. Quinine is almost completely absorbed from the gastro-intestinal tract. Peak concentrations in the circulations are attained about 1 to 3 hours after ingestion and about 70% is bound to proteins in the plasma. Absorption is very slow following subcutaneous or intramuscular injection of quinine salts. Quinine readily diffuses across the placenta. It is degraded in the body, mainly in the liver, and only a small proportion is excreted in the urine unchanged.

In 12 patients with normal renal function who were being treated with quinine for acute falciparum malaria, a dose of 650 mg of quinine sulphate by mouth every 8 hours produced plasma-quinine concentrations of 2.5 to 9.5 µg per ml. Daily urinary excretion of quinine was reported to be usually about 25% of the administered dose.— J. V. Donadio *et al.*, *Lancet*, 1968, *1*, 375.

Further references: C. F. Conway, *Med. J. Aust.*, 1967, *1*, 604; T. Watabe and K. Kayonaga, *J. Pharm. Pharmac.*, 1972, *24*, 625; A. P. Hall *et al.*, *Clin. Pharmac. Ther.*, 1972, *13*, 140.

In 5 volunteers plasma concentrations of quinine were markedly higher during induced *P. falciparum* infection than during control studies. The proportion of unmetabolised quinine in the plasma was increased. The effect was probably due to altered hepatic metabolism during infection. These findings indicated an increased risk of toxicity from conventional doses in patients with severe malarial infection.— G. M. Trenholme *et al.*, *Clin. Pharmac. Ther.*, 1976, *19*, 459.

Excretion in breast milk. The amount of quinine sulphate excreted in the milk of lactating mothers was too small to affect the child.— T. E. O'Brien, *Am. J. Hosp. Pharm.*, 1974, *31*, 844.

Uses. Quinine is a highly active blood schizonticide and suppresses the asexual cycle of development of malaria parasites in the erythrocytes. It is considered to act by interfering with DNA. It has no action on the tissue forms of the malaria parasite and therefore will not prevent relapse of vivax, ovale, or malariae infections; it has no action on *P. falciparum* gametocytes and therefore does not prevent transmission of the infection by the mosquito, but is gametocyticidal against *P. vivax*, *P. ovale*, and *P. malariae*.

Quinine is usually administered as the sulphate, bisulphate, hydrochloride, or dihydrochloride, but other salts have also been used. It is now mainly used in the treatment of *P. falciparum* malaria resistant to other antimalarial drugs.

In the treatment of chloroquine-resistant malaria, 2 g of quinine sulphate or other salt, in divided doses, is given daily for 14 days. Children up to 1 year may be given 100 to 200 mg daily in 2 or 3 divided doses, from 1 to 3 years, 200 to 300 mg, from 4 to 6 years, 300 to 500 mg, from 7 to 11 years, 0.5 to 1 g. These doses are usually given for 10 days. To prevent recrudescence it is often given in conjunction with pyrimethamine, 50 to 75 mg daily for 3 days; sulphonamides such as sulfadoxine or sulphones such as dapsone have also been given with quinine and pyrimethamine. Quinine has also been given with a tetracycline. In severe or complicated disease, a soluble quinine salt, such as the dihydrochloride, may be given in doses of 5 to 10 mg per kg body-weight (usual maximum 500 mg) by intravenous infusion in 500 ml of sodium chloride injection, over a period of 4 hours, at intervals of 12 hours. Therapy should be changed from the intravenous route to the oral route when the disease has been brought under control, and the optimum total number of doses (both oral and intravenous) is 4 to 12. Administration of quinine by intravenous injection is so hazardous that it has been superseded by infusion; nevertheless in the acute emergency of cerebral malaria *slow* intravenous injection of a portion of the dose may be deemed necessary at a suggested rate of 25 mg per minute. For further details, including advice on the problem of parenteral antimalarial therapy in infants, see Malaria (below).

Intramuscular injections of quinine are not generally recommended since they are slower in action than intravenous injections; they are painful and may cause tissue necrosis.

Quinine may be used for the protection of pregnant women, nursing mothers, infants, and young children in areas where *P. falciparum* is resistant to chloroquine. The adult dose is 300 to 600 mg daily. Another use that has been reported is the radical treatment with primaquine of relapsing vivax malaria.

Taken internally in small doses, quinine acts as a bitter; for use as a flavouring agent the dose should not exceed 1 mg per dosage unit. It also has analgesic and antipyretic properties, though the salicylates are more effective; its use for this purpose is not recommended. Night cramps may be relieved by giving 200 to 300 mg of quinine sulphate at night. Quinine has been used to unmask latent myasthenia gravis, but see Precautions.

In Great Britain the content of quinine (calculated as base) in shampoos and hair lotions may not exceed 0.5 and 0.2% respectively.

Malaria. A cure-rate (absence of parasitaemia and no recrudescence within 28 days) of 96% was achieved in 314 patients with chloroquine-resistant *Plasmodium falciparum* malaria after treatment with quinine followed by sulfadoxine and pyrimethamine. Most patients received quinine intravenously—490 mg as the dihydrochloride in 500 ml of sodium chloride injection given over 4 hours. A minimum of 4 doses of quinine, at 8- to 12-hourly intervals, was considered necessary; some patients received 540 mg as the sulphate by mouth every 8 hours. Children were infused with half-strength solution, and in comatose adults the infused dose should not exceed 1 g in 1 to 1.5 litres in 24 hours. With or 8 hours after the last dose of quinine a single dose (for adults) of sulfadoxine 1.5 g plus pyrimethamine 75 mg was given. The cure-rate of 96% exceeded the 85% achieved with quinine alone or sulfadoxine plus pyrimethamine. It was recommended that the combined treatment should be adopted as the standard regimen.— A. P. Hall *et al.*, *Br. med. J.*, 1975, *2*, 15.

A detailed account of the treatment of severe falciparum malaria including guidelines for intravenous antimalarial therapy. Intravenous infusion of an antimalarial drug is the most effective and safest route of administration for severe falciparum malaria because the drug is introduced into the blood stream at a known rate and can be stopped. Oral and intramuscular drugs enter the blood stream at a variable rate and dosage is irrevocable. Quinine is sometimes rapidly fatal by rapid intravenous injection but it is less toxic as an infusion because the peak concentration of the drug is lower. Intramuscular quinine is not very effective and is not recommended; intramuscular chloroquine is often used in Africa but has caused many fatalities.

Quinine is effective against all strains of *P. falciparum* and is definitely more effective than chloroquine against chloroquine-resistant strains. The recommended dosage regimens for chloroquine and quinine are the same: 5 to 10 mg per kg body-weight in 10 ml of fluid per kg body-weight given by intravenous infusion over 4 hours at intervals of 12 hours. However the optimum total number of doses (both oral and intravenous) required is different: about 3 to 6 for chloroquine (half-life about 100 hours in healthy subjects); about 4 to 12 for quinine (half-life about 10 hours in healthy subjects). Therapy should be changed from the intravenous to the oral route when the disease has been brought under control. In falciparum hepatitis the half-life of quinine is prolonged so that the optimum dose of quinine in a patient with hepatic and/or renal failure may be half that of a patient without complications; the metabolism of chloroquine has not yet been determined in relation to the severity of this disease. In cerebral malaria it is essential not to compound the problem with drug neurotoxicity—for example, quinine can cause coma or convulsions; fortunately the coma of cerebral malaria often responds to a small dose of intravenous quinine and one dose may be sufficient to produce awakening.

Much more work is needed on parenteral antimalarial therapy in children. To avoid fluid or drug overload a 100-ml monitoring chamber should be used and if there is delay in starting an intravenous infusion in a seriously ill infant a small dose of antimalarial may be given as an injection—the exact dose would have to be finely judged; for example, 1 mg per kg body-weight of quinine or chloroquine might be injected intravenously then not more than 9 mg per kg infused over 4 hours. A less satisfactory alternative would be to give the balance of the drug intramuscularly—it might be safe to give quinine 9 mg per kg as a single intramuscular injection to a child but intramuscular chloroquine is more dangerous.

Chloroquine alone will cure most cases of chloroquine-sensitive falciparum malaria, but quinine alone will not prevent a recrudescence in chloroquine-resistant cases. At least 2 g of quinine base (4 doses of 500 mg in adults) followed by a single dose of pyrimethamine 75 mg with sulfadoxine 1.5 g (Fansidar) will cure about 95% of patients with the resistant parasite. Chloroquine and quinine should not be used simultaneously since there is evidence of antagonism between them.— A. P. Hall, *Trans. R. Soc. trop. Med. Hyg.*, 1977, *71*, 367.

Emergency infusion of initial 600-mg dose of quinine dihydrochloride over half-an-hour in adult malarial patients with satisfactory cardiovascular status.— L. Wild *et al.* (letter), *Pharm. J.*, 1982, *2*, 128. See above for comment on the hazards of rapid intravenous quinine.

Adult dose of quinine salt 10 mg per kg body-weight, diluted in 250 to 500 ml of dextrose 5% and given every 8 hours by intravenous infusion over 4 hours.— D. A. Warrell *et al.*, *New Engl. J. Med.*, 1982, *306*, 313. Comment on potential toxicity.— A. Hall (letter), *ibid.*, *307*, 317. Clarification; this was a total of 30 mg per kg of quinine salt (equivalent to 25 mg of base) daily and was the amount found needed to achieve therapeutic plasma concentrations in severe falciparum malaria.— D. A. Warrell *et al.* (letter), *ibid.*, 319.

1391-q

Quinine Bisulphate *(B.P.)*. Quinine Acid Sulphate; Neutral Quinine Sulphate; Chininum Bisulfuricum.

$C_{20}H_{24}N_2O_2,H_2SO_4,7H_2O$=548.6.

CAS — 549-56-4 (anhydrous).

Pharmacopoeias. In *Aust.*, *Br.*, *Ind.*, *Port.*, and *Span.*

Odourless colourless crystals or white crystalline powder with a very bitter taste. It effloresces in dry air and becomes yellow when exposed to light. Quinine bisulphate 145 mg is approximately equivalent to 100 mg of quinine.

Soluble 1 in 8 of water, 1 in 1 of boiling water, 1 in 50 of alcohol, 1 in 15 of glycerol, and 1 in 625 of chloroform. A solution in dilute hydrochloric acid is laevorotatory. A 1% solution has a pH of 2.8 to 3.4 and has a blue fluorescence. **Store** in airtight containers. Protect from light.

Uses. Quinine bisulphate has the actions and uses described under quinine (see p.404); it is given in tablet form.

Preparations

Quinine Bisulphate Tablets *(B.P.)*. Quinine Bisulph. Tab.; Quinine Acid Sulphate Tablets. Tablets containing quinine bisulphate. They are film-coated, sugar-coated, or compression-coated. The *B.P.* requires 70% dissolution in 45 minutes and directs that sugar-coated tablets be supplied unless otherwise directed. Tablets which are not sugar-coated should be protected from light.
Store in airtight containers.

Proprietary Names

Biquin *(Adam, Austral.)*; Biquinate *(Knoll, Austral.)*; Dentojel *(Ayerst, Canad.)*; Myoquin *(Fawns & McAllan, Austral.)*; Quinbisan *(Protea, Austral.)*.

1392-p

Quinine Dihydrobromide *(B.P.C. 1934)*. Quinine Acid Hydrobromide; Neutral Quinine Hydrobromide; Chinini Dihydrobromidum; Bibromidrato de Quinina.

$C_{20}H_{24}N_2O_2,2HBr,3H_2O$=540.3.

CAS — 549-47-3 (anhydrous).

Pharmacopoeias. In *Port.*

Yellowish or white crystals or powder. **Soluble** 1 in 7 of water; soluble in alcohol; practically insoluble in ether. Solutions are **sterilised** by autoclaving or by filtration. **Incompatible** with iodides. **Protect** from light.

Uses. Quinine dihydrobromide has been used similarly to quinine dihydrochloride for the preparation of solutions for injection. It has been given in doses of up to 600 mg.

1393-s

Quinine Dihydrochloride *(B.P.)*. Quinine Acid Hydrochloride; Neutral Quinine Hydrochloride; Chinini Bihydrochloridum.

$C_{20}H_{24}N_2O_2,2HCl$=397.3.

CAS — 60-93-5.

Pharmacopoeias. In *Arg.*, *Aust.*, *Belg.*, *Br.*, *Braz.*, *Chin.*, *Ind.*, *Mex.*, *Port.*, *Rus.*, and *Span.*

A white or almost white odourless powder with a very bitter taste. Quinine dihydrochloride 105 mg is approximately equivalent to 100 mg of quinine. **Soluble** 1 in 0.5 of water, 1 in 14 of alcohol, and 1 in 7 of chloroform; practically insoluble in ether. A solution in dilute hydrochloric acid is laevorotatory. A 3% solution in water has a pH of 2 to 3. A 5.07% solution is iso-osmotic with serum. Solutions are **sterilised** by autoclaving or by filtration. **Incompatible** with alkalis, iodides, and tannic acid. **Store** in airtight containers. Protect from light.

Adverse Effects, Treatment, Precautions, and Resistance. As for Quinine, p.404.
The intravenous injection causes a rapid fall in blood pressure and affects the respiratory centre; a careful watch must therefore be kept on the patient's heart and respiration. Care must be taken to ensure that the injection does not infiltrate the walls of the vein or the subcutaneous tissue, or sloughing and fibrosis may result.

Uses. Quinine dihydrochloride has the actions and uses described under quinine (see p.405). It is the most suitable salt of quinine for the preparation of solutions for injection and is usually given by slow intravenous injection as a solution containing not more than 3% in the treatment of malaria in doses of 300 to 600 mg or alternatively in doses of 10 mg per kg body-weight.

Preparations

Quinine Dihydrochloride Injection *(B.P.)*. Quinine Dihydrochlor. Inj. A sterile solution in Water for Injections. Sterilised by autoclaving. pH of 1.5 to 3. For use, as a solution containing not more than 30 mg per ml, by slow intravenous injection. Protect from light.

Quinine Dihydrochloride Tablets *(B.P.C. 1973)*. Quinine Acid Hydrochloride Tablets. Tablets containing quinine dihydrochloride. They may be sugar-coated. Store in airtight containers. Protect from light.

1394-w

Quinine Ethyl Carbonate *(B.P. 1948)*. Euquinina.

$C_{23}H_{28}N_2O_4$=396.5.

CAS — 83-75-0.

Pharmacopoeias. In *Arg.*, *Fr.*, *Ind.*, *Jap.*, *Mex.*, *Port.*, and *Span.*

Odourless, almost tasteless, white masses of silky crystals which darken on exposure to light. M.p. 91° to 95°. Very slightly **soluble** in water; soluble 1 in 2 of alcohol, 1 in 1 of chloroform, and 1 in 10 of ether; readily soluble in dilute acids. A saturated solution in water is slightly alkaline to litmus. **Store** in airtight containers. Protect from light.

Uses. Quinine ethyl carbonate has the actions and uses of quinine (see p.404) and has been given in doses of 300 to 600 mg. As it is almost tasteless it was formerly considered especially useful for the treatment of malaria in children.

1395-e

Quinine Hydrobromide *(B.P.C. 1949)*. Basic Quinine Hydrobromide; Chininum Hydrobromicum; Bromhydrate de Quinine.

$C_{20}H_{24}N_2O_2,HBr,2H_2O$=441.4.

CAS — 549-49-5 (anhydrous).

Pharmacopoeias. In *Arg.* and *Belg.*, which specify $1H_2O$.

Odourless, white, silky, efflorescent crystals with a bitter taste. **Soluble** 1 in about 55 of water, 1 in 1 of boiling water, 1 in 0.7 of alcohol, and 1 in 1 of chloroform, the solution in chloroform being turbid due to separation of water. A 1% solution in water is neutral or slightly alkaline to litmus. **Store** in airtight containers. Protect from light.

Uses. Quinine hydrobromide has the actions and uses of quinine (see p.404).

Proprietary Names

Coqueluśedal Quinine *(Élerté, Fr.)*.

1396-l

Quinine Hydrochloride *(B.P., Eur. P.)*. Chininii Chloridum; Quinini Hydrochloridum; Basic Quinine Hydrochloride; Quininium Chloride; Chininum Hydrochloricum.

$C_{20}H_{24}N_2O_2,HCl,2H_2O$=396.9.

CAS — 130-89-2 (anhydrous); 6119-47-7 (dihydrate).

Pharmacopoeias. In all pharmacopoeias examined except *U.S.*

Colourless, odourless, fine, silky, acicular crystals with a very bitter taste; efflorescent in dry air and becoming gradually yellowish on exposure to light. Quinine hydrochloride 105 mg is approximately equivalent to 100 mg of quinine.

Soluble 1 in 23 of water, 1 in 0.9 of alcohol, 1 in 2 of chloroform to give a turbid solution, and 1 in 7 of glycerol; very slightly soluble in ether; practically insoluble in acetone. A solution in dilute hydrochloric acid is laevorotatory. A 1% solution in water has a pH of 6 to 6.8. Solutions are **sterilised** by autoclaving or by filtration. **Incompatible** with alkalis, iodides, and tannic acid. **Store** in airtight containers. Protect from light.

Masking the taste. Doubling the usual concentration of flavouring agents and increasing the sugar content, adding salt to some flavoured syrups and an excess of citric acid to fruit flavours helped to disguise the taste of quinine hydrochloride. Increasing the viscosity of the solutions and diluting with skimmed or preferably homogenised milk instead of water helped to cover the taste. Cocoa syrup was the best agent for masking the bitter taste.— D. N. Entrekin and C. H. Becker, *J. Am. pharm. Ass., scient. Edn*, 1954, *43*, 693. See also C. J. Eastland, *Pharm. J.*, 1951, *2*, 211; F. G. Drommond and H. G. DeKay, *J. Am. pharm. Ass., pract. Pharm. Edn*, 1954, *15*, 232.

Uses. Quinine hydrochloride has the actions and uses described under quinine (see p.404). It was formerly used in conjunction with urethane as a sclerosing agent in the treatment of varicose veins.

Preparations

Quinine Hydrochloride Tablets *(B.P. 1958)*. Quinine Hydrochlor. Tab. Tablets containing quinine hydrochloride.

Proprietary Names

Kinin *(DAK, Denm.; ACO, Swed.)*.

1397-y

Quinine Salicylate *(B.P.C. 1949)*.

$C_{20}H_{24}N_2O_2,C_7H_6O_3,H_2O$=480.6.

CAS — 750-90-3 (anhydrous).

Pharmacopoeias. In *Span.*

Odourless white silky crystals or a crystalline powder with a bitter taste; it becomes pink on keeping. Very slightly **soluble** in water; soluble 1 in 24 of alcohol and 1 in 25 of chloroform. **Incompatible** with mineral acids—salicylic acid may crystallise out. **Store** in airtight containers. Protect from light.

Uses. Quinine salicylate was formerly employed in the hope of aborting the common cold and influenza and as an analgesic. It has been given in doses of 60 to 300 mg.

1398-j

Quinine Sulphate *(B.P.)*. Quinine Sulfate *(U.S.P.)*; Quinini Sulfas; Basic Quinine Sulphate; Quininium Sulphate; Chinini Sulfas; Chininum Sulfuricum.

$(C_{20}H_{24}N_2O_2)_2,H_2SO_4,2H_2O=782.9$.

CAS — 804-63-7 (anhydrous); 6119-70-6 (dihydrate).

Pharmacopoeias. In all pharmacopoeias examined except *Cz., Eur., Neth.,* and *Nord.*

Colourless odourless acicular crystals or a white or almost white crystalline powder with a very bitter taste, becoming brown on exposure to light. Quinine sulphate 103 mg is approximately equivalent to 100 mg of quinine.

Soluble 1 in about 810 of water, 1 in 35 of boiling water, and 1 in about 95 of alcohol; slightly soluble in chloroform and ether; readily soluble in a mixture of chloroform 2 and dehydrated alcohol 1. A solution in dilute hydrochloric acid is laevorotatory. A 1% suspension in water has a pH of 5.7 to 6.6. **Incompatible** with alkalis and their carbonates, iodides, tannic acid, and mercuric chloride. **Store** in airtight containers. Protect from light.

Quinine sulphate has the actions and uses described under quinine (see p.404). It may be given in tablets, but is not sufficiently soluble for the preparation of injections, the dihydrochloride (see p.406) being generally used. It is also used as a bitter.

Preparations

Capsules

Quinine Sulfate Capsules *(U.S.P.)*. Capsules containing quinine sulphate. Store in airtight containers. Protect from light.

Solutions

Ammoniated Quinine Solution *(B.P.C. 1963)*. Liq. Quinin. Ammon.; Ammoniated Tincture of Quinine. Quinine sulphate 2 g, dilute ammonia solution 10 ml, alcohol (60%) to 100 ml. Store in a cool place. *Dose.* 2 to 4 ml diluted with water.

Suspensions

Quinine Sulfate Oral Suspension *(U.S.P.)*. A suspension containing quinine sulphate 19.8 to 24.2 mg in each ml, with alcohol 3 to 5%; it may contain a suitable antimicrobial agent. Store in airtight containers. Protect from light.

Tablets

Quinine Sulfate Tablets *(U.S.P.)*. Tablets containing quinine sulphate.

Quinine Sulphate Tablets *(B.P.)*. Quinine Sulph. Tab. Tablets containing quinine sulphate. They are film- or sugar-coated. The *B.P.* requires 70% dissolution in 45 minutes and directs that sugar-coated tablets be supplied unless otherwise directed. Tablets which are not sugar-coated should be protected from light.
Store in airtight containers.

Proprietary Names

Adquin *(Adam, Austral.)*; Kinine *(ICN, Canad.)*; Quinate *(Knoll, Austral.)*; Quine *(Rowell, USA)*; Quinoctal *(Fawns & McAllan, Austral.)*; Quinsan *(Prosana, Austral.)*.

1399-z

Quinocide Hydrochloride. Chinocidum; CN 1115; Win 10,448. 8-(4-Aminopentylamino)-6-methoxyquinoline dihydrochloride.

$C_{15}H_{21}N_3O,2HCl=332.3$.

CAS — 525-61-1 (quinocide).

Pharmacopoeias. In *Rus.*

An orange-yellow crystalline powder with a bitter taste. M.p. about 226°. **Soluble** 1 in 2 of water; slightly soluble in alcohol; practically insoluble in acetone and ether.

Uses. Quinocide, a structural isomer of primaquine, has actions and uses similar to those of primaquine phosphate. The dosage may be expressed in terms of the base; 30 mg of quinocide base is approximately equivalent to 38 mg of quinocide hydrochloride. Doses of 30 mg have been given daily.

Experimental evidence suggested that the administration of 30 mg of quinocide could produce significant haemolysis in Negroes with a deficiency of glucose-6-phosphate dehydrogenase.— Standardisation of Procedures for the Study of Glucose-6-Phosphate Dehydrogenase, *Tech. Rep. Ser. Wld Hlth Org. No. 366,* 1967.

Quinocide, in total doses of 234 mg of base, given in conjunction with other schizonticidal drugs during the primary manifestations of induced vivax malaria, greatly reduced the number of relapses, especially long-term relapses.— N. A. Tiburskaia *et al., Bull. Wld Hlth Org.,* 1968, *38,* 447.

1400-z

Totaquine *(B.P. 1953)*. Totaquina.

CAS — 8014-53-7.

Pharmacopoeias. In *Mex.* and *Port.*

A mixture of alkaloids obtained from suitable species of *Cinchona.* A nearly colourless or pale yellowish-grey, or pale brown, odourless powder with a bitter taste, containing not less than 70% of crystallisable cinchona alkaloids of which not less than one-fifth is quinine.

Practically **insoluble** in water; soluble almost completely in warm alcohol and in chloroform; partly soluble in ether and light petroleum. **Store** in airtight containers. Protect from light.

Uses. Totaquine has been used as a substitute for quinine for the treatment of malaria. It has been given in doses of 300 to 600 mg.

Clofibrate and other Lipid Regulating Agents

1340-t

Lipids occur in the blood mainly as cholesterol and triglycerides, with smaller amounts of phospholipids, fatty acids, and fatty acid esters. While free fatty acids are bound to plasma albumin other lipids form complexes with proteins. These lipoproteins differ in composition, size, and density, and may be separated by electrophoresis or ultracentrifugation. They include: *chylomicrons* of density about 0.95 and S_f (flotation unit) value greater than 400 composed largely of exogenous (dietary) triglycerides; *very low-density lipoproteins*, VLDL, pre-β-lipoproteins, of density less than 1.006 and S_f value 20 to 400, composed largely of endogenous triglycerides; *low-density lipoproteins*, LDL, β-lipoproteins, of density 1.006 to 1.063 and S_f value 0 to 20, with a high cholesterol content; *high-density lipoproteins*, HDL, α-lipoproteins, of density 1.063 to 1.21, containing protein about 50%, cholesterol, and phospholipids; and various abnormal lipoproteins. The particle size of the 4 principal lipoproteins decreases progressively from chylomicrons to high-density lipoproteins.

Factors affecting the lipid composition of the blood include the effect of eating, the composition of the diet, posture, age, sex, and genetic and cultural factors.

Lipid disorders of the blood are classified on the basis of the cholesterol and triglyceride concentrations in the blood, and on lipoprotein analysis, all values being determined in fasting samples. Elevations of the cholesterol and triglyceride concentrations, variations in the ratio of their respective concentrations, and the phospholipid concentration provide some guidance, but for full classification lipoprotein analysis is necessary. This may include visual examination, electrophoresis, and ultracentrifugation. Other procedures used include precipitation, nephelometry of samples passed through successive filters of specific pore size, and immunochemical procedures. The results are interpreted in conjunction with the clinical features of the patient, such as the presence of xanthomas or pancreatitis, and with the results of other tests.

The WHO has proposed an international classification of lipoprotein disorders based largely on that suggested by Fredrickson including:

type I, hyperchylomicronaemia, characterised by the presence of chylomicrons and by normal or only slightly increased concentrations of very low-density lipoproteins;

type IIa, hyper-β-lipoproteinaemia, characterised by an elevation in the concentration of low-density lipoproteins and type IIb characterised also by an elevation in the concentration of very low-density lipoproteins;

type III, 'floating β' or 'broad β' pattern, characterised by the presence of very low-density lipoproteins with an abnormal elevated concentration of cholesterol 'floating β' or 'β-VLDL';

type IV, hyperpre-β-lipoproteinaemia, characterised by an elevation in the concentration of very low-density lipoproteins, by no increase in the concentration of low-density lipoproteins, and by the absence of chylomicrons; and

type V, 'hyperpre-β-lipoproteinaemia and chylomicronaemia', characterised by an elevation in the concentration of very low-density lipoproteins and the presence of chylomicrons.

Strisower's classification had no group equivalent to type I; his groups 1 and 2 were equivalent to Fredrickson's type II depending respectively on the presence of tendon xanthomas or the absence of xanthomas; group 3 corresponded; group 4 was equivalent to Fredrickson's type IV and V; group 5 was similar to Fredrickson's type IV but had also an elevation in the concentration of low-density lipoproteins. Strisower's classification is not extensively used.

WHO types II and IV represent the majority of clinical disorders; types III and V are uncommon; type I is rare.

Lipoprotein disorders may be primary, or secondary to a number of underlying diseases.

For details of classifications, see D. S. Fredrickson *et al.*, *New Engl. J. Med.*, 1967, *276*, 34, 94, 148, 215, 273; E. H. Strisower *et al.*, *Am. J. Med.*, 1968, *45*, 488; *Bull. Wld Hlth Org.*, 1970, *43*, 891.

Low-density lipoproteins, very low-density lipoproteins, and chylomicrons could be separated by membrane filtration and nephelometry and were designated S (small), M (medium), and L (large) particles respectively. Abnormal lipoprotein patterns were classified on the basis of abnormalities in the S, M, or L concentrations or in composite abnormalities and on the cholesterol concentration and were partially correlated with WHO and Strisower groups. In 36 healthy subjects correlation with ultracentrifugation was 89% and in 44 patients with abnormal lipoprotein patterns correlation was 75%; discrepancies occurred mainly at borderline values.— M. C. Stone *et al.*, *Clinica chim. Acta*, 1971, *31*, 333.

An analysis of 2 contemporary definitions of type III hyperlipoproteinaemia. Type III hyperlipoproteinaemia might be better defined in terms of the ratio of very low-density lipoprotein cholesterol to plasma-triglycerides.— D. S. Fredrickson *et al.*, *Ann. intern. Med.*, 1975, *82*, 150. Comment.— *ibid.*, 273.

Plasma concentrations of apolipoprotein E exceeding 400 µg per ml (assessed by immunoassay) appeared to be diagnostic of type III hyperlipoproteinaemia.— R. S. Kushwaha *et al.*, *Ann. intern. Med.*, 1977, *87*, 509. See also R. I. Levy and J. Morganroth, *ibid.*, 625.

The diagnosis of familial hypercholesterolaemia in childhood by measuring serum cholesterol.— J. V. Leonard *et al.*, *Br. med. J.*, 1977, *1*, 1566.

Elevated lipid concentrations have long been considered to be associated with atherosclerosis though their precise role remains to be established. Other factors, apart from age, associated with atherosclerosis include hypertension, diabetes, obesity, sedentary occupation, alcohol, and smoking. Many authorities now consider that elevated concentrations of high-density-lipoprotein (HDL) cholesterol have a *protective* effect.

References to the protective effects of HDL cholesterol: *J. Am. med. Ass.*, 1977, *237*, 1066; *Lancet*, 1977, *2*, 808; *ibid.*, 1978, *2*, 1291; A. R. Tall and D. M. Small, *New Engl. J. Med.*, 1978, *299*, 1232; *Med. J. Aust.*, 1978, *2*, 470; *Med. Lett.*, 1979, *21*, 2; P. Williams *et al.*, *Lancet*, 1979, *1*, 72; S. Yaari *et al.*, *Lancet*, 1981, *1*, 1011.

The hypothesis that triglyceride is a cause of coronary heart disease is not proved.— S. B. Hulley *et al.*, *New Engl. J. Med.*, 1980, *302*, 1383.

Treatment depends on appropriate diet, which should be controlled in all patients, the correction of underlying disease, and the effects of different drugs on specific lipoprotein fractions. Type I disorders usually respond to diet alone. Patients with type II may be given cholestyramine or colestipol, possibly with nicotinic acid; dextrothyroxine is also used and, in type IIb disorders, clofibrate. Type III disorders are usually treated with clofibrate or nicotinic acid. Patients with type IV or V disorders may be given clofibrate or nicotinic acid. Patients with Strisower type 5 disorders may be given clofibrate.

Comment on drugs for familial hypercholesterolaemia. Results using colestipol and nicotinic acid are encouraging and seem to indicate the best existing drug treatment for this condition. Combination therapy with a bile-acid-sequestring resin plus nicotinic acid is, however, inconvenient for the patient and continued research into such drugs as probucol is indicated.— *Lancet*, 1981, *1*, 925.

Further reviews and comments: *Med. Lett.*, 1980, *22*, 65; *Br. med. J.*, 1980, *281*, 340; *Drug & Ther. Bull.*, 1980, *18*, 25.

1341-x

Clofibrate

Clofibrate *(B.P., U.S.P.)*. AY-61123; ICI 28,257; NSC-79389; Ethyl Chlorophenoxyisobutyrate; Ethyl Clofibrate. Ethyl 2-(4-chlorophenoxy)-2-methylpropionate.

$C_{12}H_{15}ClO_3$=242.7.

CAS — 637-07-0.

Pharmacopoeias. In *Br., Braz., Chin., Cz., Jap., Neth., Nord., Roum.*, and *U.S.*

A clear colourless to pale yellow liquid with a characteristic faintly acrid odour and a taste acrid at first, becoming sweet. Wt per ml 1.138 to 1.144 g. Practically **insoluble** in water; readily miscible with alcohol, acetone, chloroform, ether, and hexane. **Store** in airtight containers. Protect from light.

Adverse Effects. Side-effects include nausea, gastro-intestinal discomfort, possibly with diarrhoea, drowsiness, headache, and dizziness. Weight gain, pruritus, skin rashes, alopecia, leucopenia, pancreatitis, and cardiac arrhythmias have been reported.

A rise in serum aminotransferase values may occur during therapy; hepatomegaly, apparently not indicative of hepatotoxicity, has occasionally occurred.

A syndrome of muscle pain and weakness, with elevated serum concentrations of creatine kinase, has been reported, occurring particularly in patients with impaired renal function. An increased incidence of gall-stones has been reported in patients taking clofibrate.

Agranulocytosis developed in a 57-year-old woman who was given clofibrate during treatment with anticoagulants and other therapy. Normal granulopoiesis returned after withdrawal of the clofibrate.— B. J. Prout. and E. A. Edwards, *Br. med. J.*, 1963, *2*, 543.

A report of haematological and enzyme changes occurring during treatment with clofibrate in patients with diabetes of juvenile onset.— J. V. Narduzzi *et al.*, *Clin. Pharmac. Ther.*, 1967, *8*, 817. See also K. Dinçol *et al.* (letter), *Lancet*, 1975, *2*, 813.

A 54-year-old man with arteriosclerotic heart disease, treated with clofibrate 2 g daily, developed muscle pain in the legs and premature atrial and ventricular contractions. These symptoms disappeared completely within 4 weeks of discontinuing clofibrate.— J. F. X. McGarvey (letter), *J. Am. med. Ass.*, 1973, *225*, 638.

A woman who had taken clofibrate 2 g daily for 2 years for hypercholesterolaemia developed a lupus-like syndrome with weight loss, anorexia, photophobia, malaise, arthralgias, hepatomegaly, and fever. All symptoms subsided within 2 weeks of discontinuing the drug.— E. J. Howard and S. M. Brown (letter), *J. Am. med. Ass.*, 1973, *226*, 1358.

A report of an increased incidence of angina pectoris, intermittent claudication, pulmonary embolism, and cardiac arrhythmias (other than fibrillation) in patients taking clofibrate.— *J. Am. med. Ass.*, 1975, *231*, 360.

Frequent premature atrial and ventricular contractions and paroxysmal atrial tachycardia occurred in a 63-year-old man with relatively asymptomatic cardiac arrhythmias when he was given clofibrate. Sinus rhythm with no arrhythmias was restored within 2 weeks of stopping clofibrate.— E. K. Chung, *Drug Ther.*, 1975, *5*, 54.

Acute-on-chronic renal failure in 2 patients was precipitated by clofibrate.— S. Dosa *et al.* (letter), *Lancet*, 1976, *1*, 250.

A multicentre study of liver biopsies performed on 40 hyperlipoproteinaemic patients before and after 3 months of clofibrate therapy demonstrated no significant histological changes in fatty infiltration in 13 patients on clofibrate 500 mg daily; of 17 patients with distinct fatty degeneration before therapy with 1.5 g daily, 6 improved, 3 deteriorated, and 8 remained unchanged. No other histological differences were noted between the effects of the 2 dosage regimens and no adverse effects were observed.— P. Schwandt *et al.* (letter), *Lancet*, 1978, *2*, 325.

Granulomatous hepatitis occurred in a 69-year-old woman who had taken clofibrate 2 g daily for 3 months. Liver function had returned to normal on examination 4 weeks after withdrawal of the drug.— E. H. Pierce and D. L. Chesler (letter), *New Engl. J. Med.*, 1978, *299*, 314.

Acute reversible renal failure, due to interstitial nephritis, associated with the use of clofibrate.— A. Cumming, *Br. med. J.*, 1980, *281*, 1529.

Effect on gall-bladder. There were 33 cholecystectomies among 3536 men with high serum-cholesterol concentrations given clofibrate 1.6 g daily compared with 12 in each of 2 groups of 3552 and 3325 men with high and low cholesterol values respectively but not treated with clofibrate. The formation of gall-stones was considered to be associated with clofibrate and not the serum-cholesterol concentration.— J. Cooper *et al.* (letter), *Lancet*, 1975, *1*, 1083.

The cholesterol saturation index of bile was significantly higher in 11 patients treated with clofibrate than in 45 patients with elevated serum-lipid concentrations.— M. C. Bateson *et al.*, *Gut*, 1976, *17*, 814.

Analysis of data obtained during the Coronary Drug Project indicated a significant increase in the development of gall-bladder disease among patients treated with clofibrate (42 cases in 1051 patients) compared with those treated with a placebo (69 cases in 2680 patients).— Coronary Drug Project Research Group, *New Engl. J. Med.*, 1977, *296*, 1185. Comment.— L. R. Krasno and D. C. Harrison (letter), *ibid.*, *297*, 669. A reply.— Coronary Drug Project Research Group (letter), *ibid.*, 1978, *298*, 461.

In 7 patients with hypertriglyceridaemia (2 also had hypercholesterolaemia) given clofibrate 2 g daily for 6 to 18 months the mean concentration of bile acids in the bile fell while that of phospholipids and cholesterol rose; the cholesterol saturation index, considered crucial in the aetiology of gall-stones, rose. These changes were reversed in 5 patients given chenodeoxycholic acid 750 mg daily for a month, and serum concentrations of cholesterol and triglycerides were further significantly reduced. Concomitant treatment with clofibrate and chenodeoxycholic acid might be useful.— M. C. Bateson *et al.*, *Br. med. J.*, 1978, *1*, 1171.

Further references: F. Schaffner, *Gastroenterology*, 1969, *56*, 1111; D. Pertsemlidis *et al.*, *Gastroenterology*, 1974, *66*, 565; *Med. Lett.*, 1977, *19*, 46; *Lancet*, 1977, *2*, 177; M. C. Bateson *et al.*, *Am. J. dig. Dis.*, 1978, *23*, 623.

Effect on taste. Clofibrate could cause taste abnormalities.— I. P. Griffith, *Practitioner*, 1976, *217*, 907.

Impotence. Three men complained of impotence while taking clofibrate; in 2 it resolved when clofibrate was withdrawn; it recurred in one when he was again given clofibrate.— J. Schneider and H. Kaffarnik, *Atherosclerosis*, 1975, *21*, 455.

Of about 5000 patients treated for 4 to 8 years with clofibrate 1.6 g daily 14 ceased treatment because of impotence; a further 58 reported the side-effect significantly more often than in a control group.—Report from the Committee of Principal Investigators, *Br. Heart J.*, 1978, *40*, 1069.

Muscle pain. For reports, see T. Langer and R. I. Levy, *New Engl. J. Med.*, 1968, *279*, 856; J. W. Vester *et al.*, *Clin. Pharmac. Ther.*, 1970, *11*, 689; N. Katsilambros *et al.* (letter), *New Engl. J. Med.*, 1972, *286*, 1110; I. Sekowski and P. Samuel, *Am. J. Cardiol.*, 1972, *30*, 572, per *Int. pharm. Abstr.*, 1973, *10*, 408; M. Denizot *et al.* (letter), *Lancet*, 1973, *1*, 1326; D. Geltner *et al.*, *Postgrad. med. J.*, 1975, *51*, 184; A. M. Pierides *et al.*, *Lancet*, 1975, *2*, 1279; K. W. Rumpf *et al.* (letter), *ibid.*, 1976, *1*, 249; A. G. H. Smals *et al.* (letter), *New Engl. J. Med.*, 1977, *296*, 942.

In patients on dialysis: R. Gabriel and J. M. S. Pearce (letter), *Lancet*, 1976, *2*, 906; Y. Kijima *et al.* (letter), *New Engl. J. Med.*, 1977, *297*, 113.

Overdosage. A 15-year-old boy who attempted suicide by ingesting 49 capsules of clofibrate [strength not stated] complained of headache, pain in the arms, and inability to walk, but no evidence of toxicity was found during the following 5 days.— A. H. Greenhouse, *J. Am. med. Ass.*, 1968, *204*, 402.

Precautions. Clofibrate should not be given to patients with impaired liver or kidney function or with primary biliary cirrhosis. It should not be given in pregnancy.

Clofibrate may enhance the effects of anticoagulant drugs; the dose of anticoagulant should be reduced to about a half when treatment with clofibrate is started, and then increased gradually if necessary. Hypoglycaemia has been reported in patients taking sulphonylurea antidiabetic agents with clofibrate; care should be exercised if the drugs are given concomitantly.

In a 30-year-old woman whose hypercholesterolaemia was controlled with clofibrate, serum-cholesterol concentrations rose on 2 occasions when she took an oral contraceptive.— R. B. W. Smith and I. A. M. Prior (letter), *Lancet*, 1968, *1*, 750.

Muscle pains developed in 5 of 6 patients with the nephrotic syndrome and hyperlipoproteinaemia when they were given clofibrate 1 or 2 g daily. Three of the 5 patients who were also receiving frusemide experienced thirst and polyuria or a marked diuresis, perhaps due to displacement of bound frusemide. Further studies in 4 patients and 4 healthy subjects demonstrated a higher concentration of unbound clofibrate in the serum of 3 of the nephrotic patients, which corresponded to a low serum-albumin concentration, and an increase in urinary unconjugated clofibrate in the nephrotic group. It was recommended that the total daily dose of clofibrate should not exceed 500 mg for each 1 g of albumin per 100 ml of serum.— J. F. Bridgman *et al.*, *Lancet*, 1972, *2*, 506.

Clofibrate could interfere technically with laboratory estimations for vanillylmandelic acid in the urine to produce erroneous lowered results and could interfere biologically with chemical estimations for serum aspartate aminotransferase (SGOT) to produce erroneous raised results.— *Drug & Ther. Bull.*, 1972, *10*, 69.

Clofibrate might give falsely high results in tests for serum protein-bound iodine.— A. J. J. Wood and J. Crooks, *Prescribers' J.*, 1973, *13*, 94.

In 26 patients with type IIa hyperlipoproteinaemia treated with clofibrate 2 g daily mean concentrations of serum-alkaline phosphatase fell from 82.1 to 52.3 units per litre. A similar effect occurred in 5 patients with type IV hyperlipoproteinaemia.— R. W. B. Schade *et al.* (letter), *Lancet*, 1975, *1*, 862.

Interactions. Clofibrate significantly reduced the binding of dantrolene to human serum albumin.— J. J. Vallner *et al.*, *J. pharm. Sci.*, 1976, *65*, 873.

In 19 patients with diabetes taking insulin (3 patients) and/or oral antidiabetic agents, clofibrate 2 g daily had no significant effect on fasting plasma-glucose concentrations.— D. J. Kudzma and S. J. Friedberg, *Diabetes*, 1977, *26*, 291.

Studies in 5 healthy subjects showed that clofibrate did not induce microsomal enzyme activity. When rifampicin, an enzyme inducer, was given concomitantly with clofibrate mean plasma concentrations of clofibric acid were significantly reduced and the half-life shortened, though not significantly.— G. Houin and J. -P. Tillement, *Int. J. clin. Pharmac. Biopharm.*, 1978, *16*, 150.

Absorption and Fate. Clofibrate is readily absorbed from the gastro-intestinal tract. The plasma half-life is about 12 hours. Clofibrate is rapidly hydrolysed in the blood to chlorophenoxyisobutyric acid (clofibric acid) which is extensively bound to plasma proteins. About 85% of a daily dose can be recovered from the urine, 92 to 98% being [illegible] form of a glucuronide conjugate of the acid. Clofibrate appears in breast milk.

Following administration of single doses equivalent to clofibric acid 900 mg to an average of 10 cardiac patients, clofibrate, pyridoxine clofibrate, and clofibride had fairly similar half-lives of 15 to 24 hours with maximum serum concentrations of clofibric acid of about 100 µg per ml. Aluminium clofibrate had a much longer half-life of about 63 hours with a maximum serum concentration of only about 30 µg per ml; this was probably a result of slower release of clofibric acid from its aluminium salt in the intestine. Following twice-daily administration for 12 days clofibrate produced serum concentrations of clofibric acid which were slightly higher than after aluminium clofibrate; the serum concentrations of the latter were, however, considered to be more stable, with less daily variation. The steady-state serum concentrations indicated that the half-life in practice was considerably lower than anticipated from the single-dose studies, probably owing to an increase in the proportion of clofibric acid not bound to plasma proteins.— A. Cailleux *et al.*, *Thérapie*, 1976, *31*, 637. See also C. Harvengt and J. P. Desager, *Int. J. clin. Pharmac. Biopharm.*, 1977, *15*, 1.

Mean blood concentrations of clofibrate in about 5000 patients taking 1.6 g daily were 124 to 171 µg per ml.—Report from the Committee of Principal Investigators, *Br. Heart J.*, 1978, *40*, 1069.

The plasma half-life of total chlorophenoxyisobutyric acid (free and conjugated) was 86.1, 93, and 98.6 hours in 3 patients with renal failure undergoing dialysis 3 times a week and 188.3 and 199.2 hours in 2 patients with renal failure undergoing twice-weekly dialysis. The mean plasma half-life in 5 healthy controls was 17.2 hours.— E. M. Faed and E. G. McQueen, *Br. J. clin. Pharmac.*, 1979, *7*, 407.

Further references: R. Gugler and J. Hartlapp, *Clin. Pharmac. Ther.*, 1978, *24*, 432; R. Gugler, *Clin. Pharmacokinet.*, 1978, *3*, 425.

Uses. Clofibrate reduces elevated plasma concentrations of triglycerides and, to a somewhat smaller extent, elevated plasma concentrations of cholesterol; the effect is particularly evident in a reduction of elevated concentrations of very low-density lipoproteins. In some patients a rise in the concentration of low-density lipoproteins occurs concomitantly.

Clofibrate is the treatment of choice in type III hyperlipoproteinaemia (see p.408) and is also used in type IV and type V hyperlipoproteinaemia; it may be helpful in some patients with type IIb hyperlipoproteinaemia. Xanthomas may regress.

Clofibrate has been used in the long-term treatment and prophylaxis of patients with coronary heart disease; while a reduction in mortality and in the incidence of nonfatal myocardial infarction was reported in some studies, particularly in patients with angina pectoris, a later large WHO study showed a significant increase in total mortality despite a reduced incidence of myocardial infarction. Clofibrate can therefore no longer be recommended for wide-spread use for this purpose.

Clofibrate is given by mouth in a dose of 20 to 30 mg per kg body-weight daily in 2 or 3 divided doses. Treatment must be continuous; if discontinued because of lack of response withdrawal should be gradual.

Clofibrate was formerly used in conjunction with androsterone in the mistaken belief that its action was thereby enhanced.

The findings of a study in 8 patients did not substantiate the suggestion that the action of clofibrate depended upon the displacement of thyroxine.— B. U. Musa *et al.*, *Metabolism*, 1968, *17*, 909, per *J. Am. med. Ass.*, 1968, *206*, 1344.

Clofibrate displaced tryptophan from albumin binding sites. In 8 volunteers treatment for 1 week with clofibrate induced a 50 to 70% fall in the concentration of total tryptophan and a twofold to threefold increase in free tryptophan. The possible antidepressant effect of clofibrate was being studied.— C. R. Sirtori *et al.*, *Clin. Pharmac. Ther.*, 1974, *15*, 219.

Study in 6 patients indicated that one of the mechanisms by which clofibrate reduced raised plasma concentrations of triglycerides was by increasing the activity of lipoprotein lipase in adipose tissue, so increasing plasma-triglyceride clearance.— K. G. Taylor *et al.*, *Lancet*, 1977, *2*, 1106.

Further data on the effects of clofibrate on cholesterol metabolism.— B. J. Kudchodkar *et al.*, *Clin. Pharmac. Ther.*, 1977, *22*, 154.

Mention of the use of clofibrate in familial Mediterranean fever.— R. A. Frayha (letter), *Ann. intern. Med.*, 1977, *87*, 382.

The Committee on Safety of Medicines considered that clofibrate is indicated only in the treatment of exudative diabetic retinopathy, xanthomata, and specific hyperlipoproteinaemias; its use for the prevention of ischaemic heart disease should be discontinued.— *Lancet*, 1980, *2*, 489.

Administration in renal failure. Although clofibrate is not recommended in patients with renal impairment, W.M. Bennett *et al.* (*Ann. intern. Med.*, 1980, *93*, 286) consider that the interval between doses of clofibrate could be extended from 6 hours to 6 to 12 hours in patients with a glomerular filtration-rate (GFR) above 50 ml per minute, to 12 to 18 hours in those with a GFR of 10 to 50 ml per minute, and to 24 to 48 hours in those with a GFR of less than 10 ml per minute. Also A.P. Goldberg *et al.* (*Clin. Pharmac. Ther.*, 1977, *21*, 317) consider that uraemic patients managed by haemodialysis could receive 1 to 1.5 g weekly; this dose had produced the desired decrease in triglyceride concentrations without causing toxicity in 5 such patients.

Cerebrovascular disease. In a double-blind study 20 men with recent cerebral infarction due to occlusive cerebrovascular disease received clofibrate, 500 mg four times daily over a period of 4 years. Eight patients were able to return to work; of the 19 patients receiving a placebo only 3 were able to return. A cooperative trial in another 19 hospitals failed to substantiate the benefit.— S. B. Hirsch *et al.* (letter), *New Engl. J. Med.*, 1972, *287*, 671.

Chyluria. In 10 patients with recurrent chyluria the condition regressed within 12 days during treatment with clofibrate 500 mg thrice daily for 2 to 3 weeks; there was no recurrence in 12 to 18 months.— A. K. R. Choudhury, *J. Indian med. Ass.*, 1976, *66*, 175.

Diabetes insipidus. In 6 patients with vasopressin-responsive diabetes insipidus, clofibrate 2 g daily for 3 to 5 days reduced urine output by a mean of 47%; chlorpropamide 250 mg daily reduced output by a mean of 57%; the mean reductions with clofibrate 2 g plus chlorpropamide 125 mg (5 patients) and clofibrate 2 g plus chlorpropamide 250 mg (4 patients) were 54 and 61% respectively. One patient responded only to combined treatment.— P. Thompson *et al.*, *Metabolism*, 1977, *26*, 749.

Further references.— *Presse méd.*, 1971, *79*, 561; E. Uhlich *et al.*, *Klin. Wschr.*, 1971, *49*, 436; T. Nawar and J. Genest, *Can. med. Ass. J.*, 1972, *107*, 1225; Y. Hamuth and A. M. Gelb (letter), *J. Am. med. Ass.*, 1973, *224*, 1041; E. Suha (letter), *ibid.*, 1974, *228*, 567; L. Perlemuter *et al.*, *Nouv. Presse méd.*, 1975, *4*, 2307.

Diabetes mellitus. In 18 patients with hypertriglyceridaemia and 26 with chemical diabetes, clofibrate 2 g daily for 8 days reduced fasting plasma-glucose concentrations. Glucose tolerance was improved, particularly in those with chemical diabetes. It was considered that clofibrate reduced insulin resistance.— C. Ferrari *et al.*, *Metabolism*, 1977, *26*, 129.

In a double-blind study in 16 patients with coronary heart disease (most had an abnormal response to a glucose-tolerance test, suggesting latent diabetes) treatment for 12 weeks with clofibrate 2 g daily significantly reduced fasting glucose concentrations in spite of a lowered insulin secretion.— S. C. Enger *et al.*, *Acta med. scand.*, 1977, *201*, 563.

In 21 patients, aged about 50 years, with hyperlipidaemia or impaired glucose tolerance, treated in a double-blind crossover study for 4 months with clofibrate 1 g twice daily or a placebo, there was no significant effect of clofibrate on fasting glucose concentrations or on peak serum-insulin concentrations; fasting serum-insulin concentrations fell significantly.— H. Lithell, *Eur. J. clin. Pharmac.*, 1977, *12*, 51.

The hypoglycaemic effect of clofibrate was confirmed in 37 patients by the oral or intravenous glucose-tolerance test. Of 22 diabetic patients given clofibrate 500 mg thrice daily, 11 were insulin-dependent and 6 were taking oral antidiabetic agents. The insulin dose was reduced in 7 and 1 ceased to take the oral antidiabetic agent. Mean fasting blood-glucose concentrations fell from 2.21 to 1.47 mg per ml; glycosuria was reduced; 20 patients were judged to be clinically improved; ketonuria in 3 patients disappeared.— S. I. Csögör and P. Bornemisza, *Clin. Trials J.*, 1977, *14* (1), 15. See also R. D. Miller, *J. Atheroscler. Res.*, 1963, *3*, 694; D. Barnett *et al.*, *Br. J. clin. Pharmac.*, 1977, *4*, 455.

In 11 diabetic patients treated with clofibrate 1 g twice daily for up to 48 weeks there was no significant effect on fasting blood-glucose concentrations. There was no significant effect on cholesterol and the effect on triglycerides was slight.— L. H. Krut *et al.*, *S. Afr. med. J.*, 1977, *51*, 348.

In a study in 22 patients with maturity-onset diabetes, clofibrate 2 g daily was useful in controlling diabetes in 9 patients with poor diabetes control. Plasma-fibrinogen concentrations were significantly reduced in all patients.— J. -C. Daubresse *et al.*, *Br. J. clin. Pharmac.*, 1979, *7*, 599.

Diabetic neuropathy. In a double-blind study 7 of 9 patients with peripheral diabetic neuropathy had relief of pain, paraesthesia, and numbness, and gained an increase in muscle strength and a return of deep tendon reflexes after treatment for a year with clofibrate 2 g daily. Only 1 of 6 patients given a placebo improved.— M. Berenyi *et al.*, *J. Am. Geriat. Soc.*, 1971, *19*, 763.

Diabetic retinopathy. In 23 patients with diabetic exudative retinopathy who were treated with clofibrate 750 mg thrice daily, usually for about 3 years, there was a significant improvement in the extent and severity of the lesions; exudates were cleared completely from both eyes in 6 patients and from 1 eye in 3 patients. Benefit did not occur until treatment had continued for 6 months. In some patients exudates appeared in some areas while disappearing from other areas, and in some patients exudates returned when clofibrate was discontinued. Improvement was not accompanied by increased visual acuity, and was not related to initial serum concentration of cholesterol or triglycerides, or to changes in these values.— L. J. P. Duncan *et al.*, *Diabetes*, 1968, *17*, 458. For similar reports, see J. T. Ireland *et al.*, *J. Atheroscler. Res.*, 1963, *3*, 701; B. P. Harrold *et al.*, *Diabetes*, 1969, *18*, 285; V. R. Kliachko *et al.*, *Sov. Med.*, 1973, *36*, 59.

Effect on fibrinolysis. The effect of clofibrate on fibrinolysis is complex and controversial. S.C. Srivastava *et al.* (*J. Atheroscler. Res.*, 1963, *3*, 640), reported increased fibrinolytic activity in patients treated with clofibrate and androsterone. J.M. Goodhart and H.A. Dewar (*Br. med. J.*, 1966, *1*, 325) and B.M. Rifkind *et al.* (*ibid.*, 678), using clofibrate alone, found no change in fibrinolytic activity. R. Chakrabarti *et al.* (*Lancet*, 1968, *2*, 1007) reported a variable effect on plasma-fibrinogen concentrations and a decrease in fibrinolytic activity in some patients. R.C. Cotton and E.G. Wade, *I.C.I.* (*Lancet*, 1969, *1*, 263) claimed a sustained fibrinolytic effect. Replying, R. Chakrabarti and G.R. Fearnley attributed this discrepancy to differing tests and called for the demonstration of fibrin degradation products, and maintained their view (*Br. med. J.*, 1972, *1*, 247).

A trial specifically designed to repeat the reported effect of clofibrate failed to show any important change in any of 14 measurements of platelet function apart from some prolongation of bleeding time.— J. R. O'Brien (letter), *Br. med. J.*, 1972, *2*, 713.

In 19 patients with type II hyperlipoproteinaemia, intravascular coagulation was demonstrated by increased plasma concentrations of soluble fibrin complexes; there was also activation of the intrinsic coagulation pathway as shown by low concentrations of prekallikrein, kallikrein inhibitors, and factor XII. These effects were reversed after treatment with clofibrate 1.5 to 2 g daily for 6 weeks to 6 months; fibrin degradation products were increased. Though clofibrate did not reduce lipoprotein concentrations in patients with type II hyperlipoproteinaemia, the decrease in intravascular coagulation might help to prevent thrombo-embolic sequelae.— A. C. Carvalho *et al.*, *Circulation*, 1977, *56*, 114.

Clofibrate was reported to decrease antithrombotic activity.— J. R. O'Brien and M. D. Etherington (letter), *Lancet*, 1977, *2*, 1232.

See also below under Intermittent Claudication.

Fat embolism. Lipidaemia was substantially reduced and only 2 instances of fat embolism occurred in 46 patients with bone injury who were treated with clofibrate compared with 79 similar patients who did not receive clofibrate. In the latter group, all had significant lipidaemia, and 27 had some degree of fat embolism. The dosage of clofibrate was 750 mg followed by 500 mg six-hourly for 2 days, then 250 mg six-hourly for 3 days, then 250 mg twice daily for 2 days, then 250 mg daily for 2 days.— M. O'Driscoll and F. J. Powell, *Br. med. J.*, 1967, *4*, 149.

In a double-blind trial involving 119 patients with fractures, there was no evidence to suggest that clofibrate, 1 g twice daily for 6 days, had any significant effect on parameters reflecting fat embolism.— W. G. Cole, *Br. med. J.*, 1971, *4*, 148.

Hyperlipidaemia. In 72 patients with 5 different types of hyperlipidaemia divided on the basis of lipoprotein analysis, clofibrate 2 g daily was beneficial in patients with elevated serum concentrations of low-density lipoproteins without tendinous xanthoma (group 2), in those with elevated concentrations of very low-density lipoproteins and tuberous xanthomas (group 3), and in patients in whom the concentrations of both classes of lipoproteins were raised (group 5), though in the latter group the effect on low-density lipoprotein concentrations was variable. There was little response in patients with tendon xanthomas in addition to elevated serum concentrations of low-density lipoproteins (group 1). In patients with raised concentrations of very low-density lipoproteins and normal concentrations of low-density lipoproteins (group 4) a marked fall in the former occurred usually with a concomitant rise in the latter. When clofibrate caused an increase above normal in low-density lipoprotein concentrations, its use should be discontinued.— E. H. Strisower *et al.*, *Am. J. Med.*, 1968, *45*, 488.

In 2 groups of 10 patients with type II hyperlipoproteinaemia treated with clofibrate 2 g daily for 12 weeks then nicotinic acid 3 g daily for 12 weeks, or vice versa, serum concentrations of cholesterol and phospholipids fell significantly within the first 3 months and continued to fall for the next 3 months. Serum-triglyceride concentrations also fell. Alternating therapy was considered of value.— A. Nordøy and E. Gjone, *Acta med. scand.*, 1970, *188*, 487.

Clofibrate and neomycin were each given in 2-g daily doses to 16 patients mainly with type II hypercholesterolaemia and arteriosclerosis. Serum concentrations of cholesterol were significantly reduced in 15. In some patients the regimen was more effective than either drug alone and could be of value in patients unresponsive to other therapy.— P. Samuel *et al.*, *Circulation*, 1970, *41*, 109.

Clofibrate, 18 to 28 mg per kg body-weight, given in addition to a diet low in fat to 6 children with heterozygous familial (type II) hypercholesterolaemia produced a mean reduction of 33% in the concentration of cholesterol in the serum, in contrast to a mean reduction of 24% with a low-fat diet alone. In another child with homozygous familial hypercholesterolaemia, daily treatment for 2 months with clofibrate, 40 mg per kg body-weight, and cholestyramine 32 g, in conjunction with a restricted diet, reduced the cholesterol concentration by a mean 32%, and all xanthomas decreased in size.— M. M. Segall *et al.*, *Lancet*, 1970, *1*, 641.

In 15 patients with endogenous hypertriglyceridaemia the lipid-lowering effect of clofibrate was enhanced by about 10% by the concomitant use of phenformin.— K. H. Vogelberg, *Dt. med. Wschr.*, 1976, *101*, 1868.

Further references: H. B. Brown *et al.*, *Clin. Pharmac. Ther.*, 1975, *17*, 171; A. P. Goldberg *et al.*, *New Engl. J. Med.*, 1979, *301*, 1073.

For earlier references to the use of clofibrate in hyperlipidaemia, see Martindale 27th Edn, p. 365.

Intermittent claudication. In 62 elderly patients with intermittent claudication treatment for at least 6 months with clofibrate 2 g daily significantly reduced plasma-fibrinogen concentrations and blood viscosity. Stearic-acid and linoleic-acid concentrations in red cells fell and oleic-acid and palmitic-acid concentrations rose. About one-third of the patients improved clinically.— J. A. Dormandy *et al.*, *Br. med. J.*, 1974, *4*, 259. But see also the Coronary Drug Project Research Group, *J. Am. med. Ass.*, 1975, *231*, 360.

Myocardial infarction and ischaemia. Reports of reduced mortality and reduced incidence of non-fatal infarction.—Five-year Study by a Group of Physicians of the Newcastle upon Tyne Region, *Br. med. J.*, 1971, *4*, 767; *Br. med. J.*, 1971, *4*, 775 (Report by a Research Committee of the Scottish Society of Physicians); L. R. Krasno and G. J. Kidera, *J. Am. med. Ass.*, 1972, *219*, 845.

Absence of benefit.— Coronary Drug Project Research Group, *J. Am. med. Ass.*, 1975, *231*, 360. See also Coronary Drug Project Research Group, *New Engl. J. Med.*, 1980, *303*, 1038.

In 40 patients assessed angiographically the effect of clofibrate 2 g daily on the progression of coronary artery disease did not differ significantly from that of a placebo.— K. Cohn *et al.*, *Am. Heart J.*, 1975, *89*, 591.

In a double-blind study in Budapest, Edinburgh, and Prague about 5000 men, aged 30 to 59 at entry, with elevated serum-cholesterol concentrations (group 1) were treated for 4 to 8 (mean 5.3) years with clofibrate 1.6 g daily; about 5000 similar men with high cholesterol concentrations (group 2) and about 5000 with low cholesterol concentrations (group 3) served as controls and received a placebo; about 3500 men in each group completed 5 years of study. Cholesterol concentrations were reduced by 7 to 11%, less than the 15% that had been expected. The incidence of all major episodes of ischaemic heart disease (IHD) was significantly reduced, from 7.4 (per 1000 per year) in group 2 to 5.9 in group 1; the incidence of fatal IHD was not significantly different; the incidence of non-fatal myocardial infarction was significantly reduced from 6.2 to 4.6; the incidence of each of these events was considerably lower in group 3; the incidence of angina pectoris was not significantly different in groups 1 and 2. Subjects most likely to benefit were those in whom cholesterol concentrations were reduced, who had a systolic blood pressure above 135 mmHg, and who smoked. Total deaths within the trial and within 1 year of leaving the trial were significantly higher in group 1 (162) than in group 2 (127); deaths from causes other than IHD were higher—108 compared with 79, possibly due to spuriously low numbers in group 2. An increased mortality from diseases of the liver, gall-bladder, and gastro-intestinal tract might be directly due to clofibrate or indicate that clofibrate promoted excretion of sterols by these tissues. The incidence of cholecystectomies was significantly increased in group 1. Clofibrate could not be recommended as a lipid-lowering agent for wide-spread prevention of ischaemic heart disease.—Report from the Committee of Principal Investigators, *Br. Heart J.*, 1978, *40*, 1069. Discussions.— *Br. med. J.*, 1978, *2*, 1585; *Lancet*, 1978, *2*, 1131; B. Lewis *et al.* (letter), *Lancet*, 1978, *2*, 1302; M. F. Oliver, *New Engl. J. Med.*, 1978, *299*, 1360; R. S. Lees, *New Engl. J. Med.*,

1979, *300*, 491.
Follow-up for more than 4 years after the trial showed a 25% higher mortality in the clofibrate-treated group than in the comparable high-serum-cholesterol group. The implication that there may be a continuing adverse effect on the treated men after leaving the trial is serious. No particular disease accounted for the overall excess in mortality, which was spread over a remarkable range of ordinary everyday causes.— Committee of Principal Investigators, *Lancet*, 1980, *2*, 379 and 490.

Preparations

Clofibrate Capsules *(B.P.)*. Capsules containing clofibrate. Store at a temperature not exceeding 30°.

Clofibrate Capsules *(U.S.P.)*. Capsules containing clofibrate. Protect from light.

Atromid-S (Known in some countries as Amotril, Azionyl) *(ICI Pharmaceuticals, UK)*. Clofibrate, available as capsules of 500 mg. (Also available as Atromid-S in *Arg.*, *Austral.*, *Canad.*, *S.Afr.*, *USA*).

Other Proprietary Names

Arg.—Ateriosan, Atroayerst, Corafen, Elpi, Serotinex; *Austral.*—Arterioflexin, Liprinal, Lostat; *Belg.*—Atromidin, Cartagyl, Liprin; *Canad.*—Claripex, Novofibrate; *Denm.*—Atromidin, Recolip; *Fr.*—Clofibral, Clofirem, Dabical (calcium clofibrate), Lipavlon, Normolipol; *Ger.*—Atheropront, Bioscleran, Regelan, Skleromexe, Sklero-Tablinen, Ticlobran, Xyduril; *Ital.*—Artevil, Atrolen, Atromidin, Citiflus, Cloberat, Clofibral, Clofinit, Fibramid, Geromid, Ipolipid, Lipavil, Lipidicon, Liporan, Nibratol, Normet, Sclerovasal; *Jap.*—Atheromide, Yoclo; *Neth.*—Atromidin, Clofi-ICN; *S.Afr.*—Serolipid; *Spain*—Neo-Atromid; *Swed.*—Aterosol, Atromidin, Recolip; *Switz.*—Apolan, Atheropront, Regelan, Skleromexe.

Clofibrate was also formerly marketed in Great Britain under the proprietary name Liprinal (*Bristol*).

1342-r

Aluminium Clofibrate. Alufibrate. Bis[2-(4-chlorophenoxy)-2-methylpropionato]hydroxyaluminium.
$C_{20}H_{21}AlCl_2O_7$=471.3.

CAS — 24818-79-9.

A white powder. Practically **insoluble** in water, alcohol, and ether.

Uses. Aluminium clofibrate is used similarly to clofibrate in doses of 1.5 to 2 g daily in divided doses in the treatment of hypercholesterolaemia and hypertriglyceridaemia.

For a comparison of the absorption and fate of clofibrate and aluminium clofibrate, see Clofibrate, p.409.

Further references: C. Harvengt and J. P. Desager, *Int. J. clin. Pharmac. Biopharm.*, 1977, *15*, 1.

Proprietary Names
Alofran *(Fedal, Spain)*; Arteriopront *(Hispano Quimica, Spain)*; Aterolip *(Fher, Spain)*; Atherolip *(Parcor, Belg.*; *Millot-Solac, Fr.*; *Vifor, Switz.)*; atherolipin *(Pharma-Schwarz, Ger.)*; Colesnormal *(Miluy, Spain)*; Sepik *(Also, Ital.)*.

1343-f

Aluminium Nicotinate. A complex of aluminium hydroxydinicotinate and nicotinic acid. Each 625 mg represents approximately 450 mg of aluminium hydroxydinicotinate and 155 mg of nicotinic acid, together equivalent to 500 mg of nicotinic acid.

CAS — 1976-28-9.

A white amorphous powder with a slightly acidic taste. Practically **insoluble** in water and alcohol.

Uses. Aluminium nicotinate is used similarly to nicotinic acid (see p.1649) in doses of 1.25 to 2.5 g thrice daily in the treatment of hypercholesterolaemia and hyperlipoproteinaemia.

For the physical and chemical properties of aluminium nicotinate and a summary of clinical reports, see J. P. Mile, *Curr. ther. Res.*, 1965, *7*, 392.

In a study in 60 patients with hypercholesterolaemia, diet alone caused no significant change in serum-cholesterol concentrations but treatment with aluminium nicotinate 500 mg thrice daily, alone or in conjunction with diet, resulted in prompt and sustained reductions in serum cholesterol.— W. B. Parsons, *J. Am. med. Ass.*, 1969, *208*, 1476.

Long-term protection against cardiovascular mortality after daily treatment with aluminium nicotinate 4 g, conjugated oestrogens 1.25 mg, dextrothyroxine 4 mg, or combinations of these, was no better than that achieved with a placebo during a 5-year study of 570 men with an average age of 51 years who had a history of myocardial infarction. Cholesterol concentrations fell during the first 3 months of treatment involving aluminium nicotinate and then rose gradually. Oestrogens had no effect.— Veterans Administration Drug Lipid Co-operative Study Group, *Ann. intern. Med.*, 1972, *76*, 868.

Proprietary Names
Nicalex *(Merrell-National, USA)*; Nicalex Alunitine *(Merrell, Austral.)*.

1344-d

Cholestyramine. MK 135; Cholestyramine Resin *(U.S.P.)*; Colestyramine. The chloride of a strongly basic anion-exchange resin containing quaternary ammonium functional groups which are attached to a styrene-divinylbenzene copolymer (about 2% divinylbenzene).

CAS — 11041-12-6.

Pharmacopoeias. In *U.S.*

A white to buff-coloured, hygroscopic, fine powder, odourless or with a slight amine-like odour. It loses not more than 12% of its weight on drying.
Practically **insoluble** in water, alcohol, chloroform, and ether. A 1% aqueous slurry has a pH of 4 to 6. **Store** in airtight containers.

Effect of structure and added electrolytes on the binding of unconjugated and conjugated bile-salt anions.— W. H. Johns and T. R. Bates, *J. pharm. Sci.*, 1969, *58*, 179. For reports of further studies, see *idem*, 1970, *59*, 329 and 788.

Adverse Effects. The most common side-effect is constipation; diarrhoea, heartburn, and nausea may occur but are usually mild and transient. Faecal impaction may develop and haemorrhoids may be precipitated or exacerbated, with or without bleeding. High dosage may cause steatorrhoea and diminish the absorption of fat-soluble vitamins. There may be a tendency to hyperchloraemic acidosis. Skin rash and pruritus have occasionally occurred. Impairment of calcium absorption may lead to osteoporosis.

Hypoprothrombinaemic haemorrhage developed in a 57-year-old woman during treatment with cholestyramine. It was suggested that fat-soluble vitamins should be given to supplement the diet of patients receiving long-term therapy with cholestyramine.— L. Gross and G. L. Brotman, *Ann. intern. Med.*, 1970, *72*, 95.

Metabolic acidosis developed in a 10-year-old girl with decreased renal function who had been receiving cholestyramine 4 to 8 g daily for 3.5 years.— P. K. Kleinman (letter), *New Engl. J. Med.*, 1974, *290*, 861.

For a brief review of cholestyramine-induced malabsorption, see G. F. Longstreth and A. D. Newcomer, *Mayo Clin. Proc.*, 1975, *50*, 284.

Acidosis and hypernatraemia in infants.— J. V. Hartline (letter), *J. Pediat.*, 1976, *89*, 155; W. A. Primack *et al.*, *ibid.*, 1977, *90*, 1024.

Two infants with intrahepatic cholestasis developed vomiting, constipation, abdominal distension, and partial intestinal obstruction within 12 hours of starting cholestyramine 1 g four times daily. Symptoms subsided when cholestyramine was withdrawn but returned when it was given once more.— J. D. Lloyd-Still, *Pediatrics*, 1977, *59*, 626.

Precautions. Cholestyramine may reduce the absorption of other drugs, particularly acidic drugs such as warfarin, administered concomitantly. Treatment with other drugs should not be given within 1 hour before or about 4 hours after the administration of cholestyramine. Supplements of vitamins A and D should be administered in water-miscible form during prolonged therapy with cholestyramine; supplements of vitamin K may also be necessary.

During treatment with cholestyramine 600 mg per kg body-weight daily for 1 to 2½ years mean serum-folate concentrations decreased from 7.7 to 4.4 ng per ml in 18 children with familial hypercholesterolaemia. Prothrombin times remained normal and although there was a significant decrease in serum concentrations of vitamins A and E, the values remained within the normal range.— R. J. West and J. K. Lloyd, *Gut*, 1975, *16*, 93.

The effect of cholestyramine on the uptake of hydrocortisone from the gastro-intestinal tract.— C. Johansson *et al.*, *Acta med. scand.*, 1978, *204*, 509.

Absorption and Fate. Cholestyramine is not absorbed from the gastro-intestinal tract.

Uses. Cholestyramine exchanges chloride ions for the anions of bile salts which it binds into an insoluble complex that is excreted in the faeces, so preventing the normal reabsorption of bile salts. Each gram of resin exchanges 1.8 to 2.2 g of sodium glycocholate. Bile salts are thus removed from the enterohepatic circulation, leading to increased oxidation of cholesterol to bile acids; there is some increase in the hepatic synthesis of cholesterol but an overall reduction in serum-cholesterol concentrations, particularly in the low-density lipoproteins. Since the uses of cholestyramine are based on the removal of intestinal bile salts it is unlikely that a response will be achieved in patients with complete biliary obstruction.
Cholestyramine is administered by mouth to relieve the pruritus of partial biliary obstruction and the diarrhoea associated with ileal resection, Crohn's disease, vagotomy, and diabetic vagal neuropathy. The usual initial dose is 4 g taken 3 or 4 times daily. When relief occurs a dose of 4 to 8 g daily may be adequate.
Cholestyramine is also used, as an adjunct to diet, in the treatment of type II hyperlipoproteinaemia. The usual dose is 12 to 16 g daily in divided doses. In some cases doses of 36 g daily have been used.
A suggested dose for children over 6 years of age is 80 mg per kg body-weight thrice daily.
Cholestyramine should be administered as a suspension in water or a flavoured vehicle.

Cholestyramine lowered plasma-cholesterol concentrations by binding bile-salt anions in the small intestine, thereby decreasing absorption of exogenous cholesterol as well as increasing the hepatic metabolism of endogenous cholesterol into additional bile salts.— W. H. Johns and T. R. Bates, *J. pharm. Sci.*, 1969, *58*, 179.

Further references: *J. Am. med. Ass.*, 1967, *202* (Oct. 23), A30; *J. Am. med. Ass.*, 1969, *207*, 1959; S. Lindenbaum and T. Higuchi, *J. pharm. Sci.*, 1975, *64*, 1887.

Administration. Cholestyramine given twice daily appeared to be as effective as the same dose given 4 times daily in 7 patients with familial hypercholesterolaemia.— C. B. Blum *et al.*, *Ann. intern. Med.*, 1976, *85*, 287.

Diarrhoea. Intractable diarrhoea in 4 diabetic patients was relieved by the administration of cholestyramine.— J. R. Condon *et al.* (letter), *Br. med. J.*, 1973, *4*, 423.

Diarrhoea, unresponsive to other treatments, ceased in 1 to 3 days in 20 infants given cholestyramine 7.5 to 20 g daily.— M. Berant *et al.* (letter), *J. Pediat.*, 1976, *88*, 153.

The successful use of cholestyramine in 3 patients with chronic diarrhoea due to bile acid malabsorption.— E. H. Thaysen and L. Pedersen, *Gut*, 1976, *17*, 965.

In a double-blind trial, postvagotomy diarrhoea was relieved in 8 of 10 patients given cholestyramine and in 2 of 10 patients given a placebo.— V. M. Duncombe *et al.*, *Gut*, 1977, *18*, 531.

Cholestyramine 4 g thrice daily improved postvagotomy diarrhoea in 12 of 16 patients who had undergone vagotomy, pyloroplasty, and cholecystectomy but in only 6 of 15 who had undergone vagotomy and pyloroplasty.— T. V. Taylor *et al.*, *Lancet*, 1978, *1*, 635.

A favourable response to cholestyramine treatment in a 72-year-old patient with radiation diarrhoea.— J. R. Condon *et al.*, *Postgrad. med. J.*, 1978, *54*, 838.

Further references: J. R. Condon *et al.* (letter), *Br. med. J.*, 1974, *1*, 519; D. Blanckaert and J. P. Farriaux, *Nouv. Presse méd.*, 1976, *5*, 713; J. G. Allan and R. I. Russell, *Br. med. J.*, 1977, *1*, 674; J. R. Brocklehurst and A. C. Walker (letter), *Med. J. Aust.*, 1978, *1*, 504.

Pseudomembranous colitis. Cholestyramine resin was successful in the treatment of diarrhoea and pseudomembranous colitis associated with lincomycin hydrochloride and clindamycin phosphate in 2 patients.— E. J. Burbige and F. D. Milligan, *J. Am. med. Ass.*, 1975, *231*, 1157.

There was a favourable response to cholestyramine in an infant with pseudomembranous colitis.— F. Sinatra *et al.*, *J. Pediat.*, 1976, *88*, 304.

Rapid response of pseudomembranous colitis to cholestyramine in 12 patients.— E. W. Kreutzer and F. D. Milligan, *Johns Hopkins med. J.*, 1978, *143*, 67.

Studies *in vitro* indicated that cholestyramine and colestipol hydrochloride bound the toxin implicated in antibiotic-associated colitis.— T. W. Chang *et al.* (letter), *Lancet*, 1978, *2*, 258. See also R. H. George *et al.* (letter), *ibid.*, 624.

Hyperlipidaemia. Cholestyramine and colestipol were given to 25 patients with familial type II hyperlipoproteinaemia in doses of 20 g daily for 4 months each in a 14-month crossover study, with placebo being given between periods of drug therapy. Plasma-cholesterol and low-density lipoprotein concentrations were equally reduced by both drugs. Colestipol or cholestyramine together with a correct diet were considered effective alternative treatment of familial type II hyperlipoproteinaemia.— C. J. Glueck *et al.*, *J. Am. med. Ass.*, 1972, *222*, 676.

In a controlled study of 47 patients with type II hyperlipoproteinaemia who were also being treated by diet, cholestyramine 4 g four times daily reduced the plasma-cholesterol concentration after 4 weeks by 20.6% and low-density lipoprotein concentration by 27.2% compared with a placebo. When cholestyramine was compared with clofibrate 2 g daily in 10 patients, clofibrate reduced the plasma cholesterol by 11% and the low-density lipoprotein by 4.6% compared with 28% and 38% respectively for cholestyramine.— N. J. Stone, *Ann. intern. Med.*, 1972, *77*, 267.

In 19 children with heterozygous familial hypercholesterolaemia treatment with cholestyramine 8 to 24 g daily in 2 divided doses reduced serum-cholesterol concentrations by a mean of 36%.— R. J. West and J. K. Lloyd, *Archs Dis. Childh.*, 1973, *48*, 370.

An evaluation of the use of cholestyramine in hyperlipoproteinaemia.— *Med. Lett.*, 1974, *16*, 33.

A report on 16 children with familial hypercholesterolaemia managed by diet and cholestyramine 12 or 16 g daily.— C. J. Glueck *et al.*, *Pediatrics*, 1977, *59*, 433.

A study of the dose-effect of cholestyramine in familial hypercholesterolaemia.— J. R. Farah *et al.*, *Lancet*, 1977, *1*, 59. See also R. West and J. K. Lloyd (letter), *ibid.*, 488.

Results of an 8-year follow-up of 35 children with the heterozygous form of familial hypercholesterolaemia indicated that cholestyramine effectively lowers plasma-cholesterol concentrations in this condition, but for long-term use compliance is a problem.— R. J. West *et al.*, *Lancet*, 1980, *2*, 873.

Hyperoxaluria. Cholestyramine 4 g four times daily was given to 4 patients who had developed hyperoxaluria and nephrolithiasis after resection of the lower small intestine. Urinary excretion of calcium oxalate returned to normal and no new kidney stones formed whilst the patients were taking cholestyramine.— L. H. Smith *et al.*, *New Engl. J. Med.*, 1972, *286*, 1371.

Cholestyramine 4 g given four times daily reduced the high urinary oxalate excretion in 6 patients with regional enteritis who had undergone ileal resection to remove an average of 68.7 cm. Results *in vitro* suggested that this might have been due to cholestyramine binding oxalic acid. The severe diarrhoea which was present in 5 patients also improved.— J. Q. Stauffer *et al.*, *Ann. intern. Med.*, 1973, *79*, 383. See also W. F. Caspary (letter), *New Engl. J. Med.*, 1977, *296*, 1357.

Jaundice. Four of 5 children with persistent cholestatic liver disease from early infancy had improvement in liver-function tests after treatment for up to 10 months with cholestyramine 6 to 12 g daily.— R. Nelson *et al.*, *Gut*, 1974, *15*, 825.

Further references: J. L. Asensio and J. P. Crawford (letter), *Lancet*, 1967, *1*, 282; W. A. Arrowsmith *et al.*, *Archs Dis. Childh.*, 1975, *50*, 197; M. Odièvre *et al.*, *Archs Dis. Childh.*, 1978, *53*, 81.

Porphyria. Cholestyramine, 12 g daily in divided doses with meals, produced rapid improvement in 3 patients with porphyria cutanea tarda symptomatica. The formation of photosensitive blisters was decreased and healing hastened. Skin fragility was also decreased.— G. M. Stathers (preliminary communcation), *Lancet*, 1966, *2*, 780.

A child with unusually severe erythropoietic protoporphyria improved when treated with cholestyramine, in doses of 9 to 18 g daily. The treatment was given for periods of 2 and 4 months. Mild hypoprothrombinaemia on 1 occasion was the only side-effect reported.— H. W. Lischner (letter), *Lancet*, 1966, *2*, 1079.

Pruritus. Relief of intractable pruritus in polycythaemia rubra vera with cholestyramine.— I. Chanarin and L. Szur, *Br. J. Haemat.*, 1975, *29*, 669.

A favourable report of the use of cholestyramine 20% ointment to relieve skin irritation around enterostomies.— J. T. Rodriguez *et al.*, *J. Pediat.*, 1976, *88*, 659.

In a double-blind study 4 of 5 patients with uraemic pruritus undergoing haemodialysis were considerably relieved of their pruritus by treatment with cholestyramine 5 g twice daily for 4 weeks; benefit was evident within 4 days. The 5th patient benefited when the dose was doubled. Only 1 of 5 patients given placebo improved. The mechanism of action was not known.— D. S. Silverberg *et al.*, *Br. med. J.*, 1977, *1*, 752. In 5 patients undergoing haemodialysis cholestyramine 5 g twice daily had no effect on pruritus.— R. van Leusen *et al.* (letter), *ibid.*, 1978, *1*, 918.

Preparations

Cholestyramine for Oral Suspension *(U.S.P.)*. A mixture of cholestyramine with suitable excipients, colours, and flavours. The suspension is prepared by the addition of diluent immediately before issue. Store in airtight containers.

Questran *(Bristol-Myers Pharmaceuticals, UK)*. Cholestyramine, available as a powder in sachets of 9 g, each providing 4 g of anhydrous cholestyramine. (Also available as Questran in *Austral., Canad., Denm., Fr., Ital., Neth., Norw., S.Afr., USA*).

Other Proprietary Names

Cuemid *(Austral., Ger., Norw., Swed.)*; Quantalan *(Aust., Ger., Port., Switz.)*.

Cholestyramine was also formerly marketed in Great Britain under the proprietary name Cuemid (*Merck Sharp & Dohme*).

1345-n

Clofibride. MG 46. 3-Dimethylcarbamoylpropyl 2-(4-chlorophenoxy)-2-methylpropionate.
$C_{16}H_{22}ClNO_4$=327.8.

CAS — 26717-47-5.

A pale cream-coloured crystalline powder. Practically **insoluble** in water; soluble in olive oil.

Uses. Clofibride is used similarly to clofibrate in the treatment of hypercholesterolaemia and hypertriglyceridaemia in doses of 1.35 to 2.7 g daily in 2 divided doses.

Clofibride was given in doses of about 1.8 g daily by mouth for 1 to 9 months to 30 patients with various types of hyperlipidaemia. Reductions in total lipids, total cholesterol, and triglycerides were obtained, the best results being in patients with moderate simple hypercholesterolaemia. Results in patients with mixed types of hyperlipidaemia were less good, and poor results were obtained in subjects with dietary-resistant endogenous hypercholesterolaemia. Tolerance was good.— M. Leutenegger *et al.*, *Thérapie*, 1974, *29*, 599.

Metabolism.— C. Harvengt and J. P. Desager, *Int. J. clin. Pharmac. Biopharm.*, 1977, *15*, 1.

Proprietary Names

Lipenan *(Fournier Frères, Belg.; Fournier Frères, Fr.)*.

1346-h

Colestipol Hydrochloride.
U-26 597A. The hydrochloride of a copolymer of diethylenetriamine and 1-chloro-2,3-epoxypropane.

CAS — 26658-42-4; 50925-79-6 (both colestipol); 37296-80-3 (hydrochloride).

Pale yellow odourless tasteless granules. Practically **insoluble** in water.

Adverse Effects and Precautions. As for Cholestyramine, p.411.

The binding of drugs to colestipol hydrochloride *in vitro*.— H. Ko and M. E. Royer, *J. pharm. Sci.*, 1974, *63*, 1914.

A patient developed gall-stones 3 weeks after starting treatment with colestipol.— S. M. Grundy and H. Y. I. Mok, *J. Lab. clin. Med.*, 1977, *89*, 354.

Uses. Colestipol has actions similar to those of cholestyramine (see p.411). Cholesterol concentrations in plasma are reduced while those of triglycerides may be elevated.

It is used in the treatment of type II hyperlipoproteinaemia. The usual dose is 15 to 30 g of the hydrochloride daily in 2 to 4 divided doses. It is taken in water or other suitable flavoured vehicle.

A review of the actions and uses of colestipol.— R. C. Heel *et al.*, *Drugs*, 1980, *19*, 161.

Diarrhoea. *Pseudomembranous colitis. In vitro* studies indicated that cholestyramine and colestipol hydrochloride bound the toxin implicated in antibiotic-associated colitis.— T. W. Chang *et al.* (letter), *Lancet*, 1978, *2*, 258.

Hyperlipidaemia. In a blind crossover study in 26 patients with hypercholesterolaemia, clofibrate 500 mg four times daily for 15 weeks and colestipol 5 g thrice daily before meals had similar effects on serum-cholesterol concentrations but whereas clofibrate also lowered serum-triglyceride concentrations colestipol slightly raised them.— C. A. Dujovne *et al.*, *Clin. Pharmac. Ther.*, 1974, *16*, 291.

Colestipol lowered the serum-cholesterol concentration in diabetic patients controlled with insulin, but not in those receiving oral hypoglycaemic agents.— M. S. Bandisode and B. R. Boshell, *Curr. ther. Res.*, 1975, *18*, 276.

In 25 patients with type II hyperlipoproteinaemia treatment for up to 20 months with colestipol 5 g thrice daily lowered plasma-cholesterol concentrations by a mean of 14% but in only 9 patients was it restored to normal. The response of triglycerides was variable.— A. M. Lees *et al.*, *Atherosclerosis*, 1976, *24*, 129.

Following administration of colestipol 5 g thrice daily before meals, in association with a hypocholesterolaemic dietary regimen, for 3 years to 13 subjects with familial type II hyperlipoproteinaemia an average reduction of 33% was achieved in the serum-cholesterol concentration. No new localisations and sites of xanthoma were noted in patients exhibiting xanthomatosis and in 9 there was improvement of tendon xanthomas after 2 years of treatment.— C. Harvengt and J. -P. Desager, *Clin. Pharmac. Ther.*, 1976, *20*, 310.

A favourable report of the use of colestipol 5 g thrice daily for up to 8 years in patients with hypercholesterolaemia.— J. R. Ryan *et al.*, *Clin. Pharmac. Ther.*, 1977, *21*, 116.

In a single-blind randomised multicentre study in 2278 patients with hypercholesterolaemia, colestipol 5 g thrice daily reduced cholesterol concentrations to a significantly greater extent than a placebo; triglycerides were elevated in both groups. Patients were treated for up to 3 years. Deaths from coronary heart disease were significantly fewer in men receiving colestipol than in those receiving a placebo—9 of 548 compared with 22 of 546. There was no significant difference in mortality in women.— A. E. Dorr *et al.*, *J. chron. Dis.*, 1978, *31*, 5.

Enhanced reduction of low-density-lipoprotein cholesterol in patients with heterozygous familial hypercholesterolaemia by treatment with colestipol with nicotinic acid.— D. R. Illingworth *et al.*, *Lancet*, 1981, *1*, 296. A similar report.— J. P. Kane *et al.*, *New Engl. J. Med.*, 1981, *304*, 251.

Further references: N. E. Miller *et al.*, *Med. J. Aust.*, 1973, *1*, 1223; R. I. Levy and B. M. Rifkind, *Drugs*, 1973, *6*, 12; J. R. Ryan *et al.*, *Clin. Pharmac. Ther.*, 1975, *17*, 83; C. J. Glueck *et al.*, *Pediatrics*, 1976, *57*, 68; M. A. Mishkel and S. M. Crowther, *Curr. ther. Res.*, 1977, *22*, 398.

For a comparison of colestipol and cholestyramine in the treatment of type II hyperlipoproteinaemia, see Cholestyramine, p.412.

Proprietary Preparations

Colestid *(Upjohn, UK)*. Granules containing colestipol hydrochloride, with colloidal silicon dioxide 0.2%, available in 5-g sachets and in bulk. (Also available as Colestid in *Austral., Belg., Ger., NZ, S.Afr., Switz., USA*).

1347-m

Ethanolamine Oxiniacate. Ethanolamine Nicotinate Oxide; Ethanolamine Oxyniacate. 2-Aminoethyl pyridine-1-oxide-3-carboxylate.
$C_8H_{10}N_2O_3$=200.2.

CAS — 36296-31-8.

Uses. Oxiniacic acid reduces elevated triglyceride and cholesterol concentrations in serum and is used as the ethanolamine salt in doses of 1.34 g thrice daily with meals in the treatment of hyperlipidaemia and hypercholesterolaemia.

Proprietary Names
Novacyl *(Astra, Fr.)*.

1348-b

Fenofibrate.
Procetofene; LF-178. Isopropyl 2-[4-(4-chlorobenzoyl)phenoxy]-2-methylpropionate.
$C_{20}H_{21}ClO_4$=360.8.
CAS — 49562-28-9.

A cream-coloured, odourless, tasteless, crystalline powder. Practically **insoluble** in water; soluble in acetone, chloroform, and ether; slightly soluble in alcohol and methyl alcohol.

Adverse Effects. Gastro-intestinal side-effects, muscle pain, and alopecia have been reported. Elevation of serum aminotransferases has occurred.

Precautions. Fenofibrate should not be given to patients with impaired liver or kidney function, and should not be given in pregnancy.

Fenofibrate may enhance the effects of anticoagulant drugs; the dose of anticoagulant should be reduced to about a half when treatment with fenofibrate is started, and then increased gradually if necessary.

Absorption and Fate. Fenofibrate is readily absorbed from the gastro-intestinal tract; the half-life is about 7 hours. The chief metabolite in plasma is the corresponding acid; only about 10% appears unchanged. About 80% of a dose is excreted within 24 hours.

Radioactive fenofibrate 300 mg by mouth was given to 2 healthy subjects. After 4 hours peak plasma concentrations were 28.7 and 18.9 μg per ml respectively and radioactivity declined in the plasma with a half-life of about 7 hours. After 6 days 86.8 and 89.4% of the administered dose respectively had been excreted in the urine with faecal excretion of 8.7 and 1.4% respectively.— R. R. Brodie *et al.*, *Arzneimittel-Forsch.*, 1976, *26*, 896.

Further references: J. P. Desager and C. Harvengt, *Int. J. clin. Pharmac. Biopharm.*, 1978, *16*, 570; P. Drouin *et al.*, *Curr. ther. Res.*, 1979, *26*, 357.

Uses. Fenofibrate has actions and uses similar to those of clofibrate (see p.408). The usual initial dose is 300 mg daily, in 3 divided doses, reduced to a maintenance dose of 200 mg daily, in 2 divided doses, as the lipid concentrations return to normal.

Pharmacology in *animals*.— J. Gurrieri *et al.*, *Arzneimittel-Forsch.*, 1976, *26*, 889.

In 191 patients with various hyperlipoproteinaemias fenofibrate 200 to 400 mg daily lowered cholesterol concentrations by 20 to 36% in types IIa and IIb and triglyceride concentrations by 30 to 50% in types IIb and IV. It appeared that fenofibrate was more potent than clofibrate.— J. Rouffy *et al.*, *Arzneimittel-Forsch.*, 1976, *26*, 901. A similar report.— E. Wülfert *et al.*, *ibid.*, 906.

Preliminary findings in 26 patients with hyperlipoproteinaemia type II or IV given fenofibrate 300 mg daily showed a significant reduction in serum concentrations of cholesterol and triglyceride. There was a significant increase in platelet-count and blood-urea and serum-calcium concentrations and a reduction in phosphate and uric acid concentrations. One patient experienced a transient rise in serum-aminotransferases and another died of pancreatic carcinoma 10 months after receiving fenofibrate for 2 months; there was no *animal* evidence of carcinogenicity.— M. Afschrift *et al.* (letter), *Lancet*, 1977, *2*, 311.

Further references: H. Micheli *et al.*, *Int. J. clin. Pharmac. Biopharm.*, 1979, *17*, 503; P. L. Lauwers, *Curr. ther. Res.*, 1979, *26*, 30; P. Drouin *et al.*, *Curr. ther. Res.*, 1979, *26*, 350.

Uricosuric effect.— J. -P. Desager *et al.*, *J. clin. Pharmac.*, 1980, *20*, 560.

Proprietary Names
Lipanthyl *(Fournier S.A., Fr.; Holphar, Ger.; Falorni, Ital.; Fournier, Switz.)*; Liponat *(Geymonat Sud, Ital.)*; Procetoken *(Bernabó, Arg.)*; Sigurtil *(Sigurtà, Ital.)*.

1349-v

Gemfibrozil.
CI-719. 2,2-Dimethyl-5-(2,5-xylyloxy)valeric acid.
$C_{15}H_{22}O_3$=250.3.
CAS — 25812-30-0.

Adverse Effects. There have been occasional reports of nausea, vomiting, abdominal pain, anorexia, heartburn, and diarrhoea. Drowsiness, allergy, and elevation of serum creatine kinase values have been reported.

Absorption and Fate. Gemfibrozil is readily absorbed from the gastro-intestinal tract; peak concentrations in plasma occur within 2 hours; the half-life is about 1.5 hours; there is evidence of biliary re-absorption. About 50% of a dose is excreted in the urine within 48 hours, chiefly as the conjugate and conjugated metabolites; little is excreted in the faeces.

Uses. Gemfibrozil is used, similarly to clofibrate, in the treatment of hyperlipidaemia. The usual dose is 0.8 to 1.2 g daily in divided doses.

A report of a symposium.— *Proc. R. Soc. Med.*, 1976, *69, Suppl.* 2, 1–120.

In a study in 80 patients, most of whom had type IIa or IIb hyperlipoproteinaemia, the effects of gemfibrozil 0.8 to 1.2 g daily were comparable with those of clofibrate 1.5 g daily.— J. Tuomilehto *et al.*, *Proc. R. Soc. Med.*, 1976, *69, Suppl.* 2, 38.

A favourable report of the use of gemfibrozil 800 mg daily in 5 patients with the nephrotic syndrome.— A. Eisalo *et al.*, *Proc. R. Soc. Med.*, 1976, *69, Suppl.* 2, 47.

Treatment of 14 diabetics; there was no interaction with antidiabetic agents.— I. de Salcedo *et al.*, *Proc. R. Soc. Med.*, 1976, *69, Suppl.* 2, 64.

Effect on platelet function.— V. P. O. Rasi and I. Torsfila, *Proc. R. Soc. Med.*, 1976, *69, Suppl.* 2, 109.

Further references: D. H. Jones *et al.*., *Clin. Trials J.*, 1976, *13* (2), 42; E. R. Nye *et al.*, *N.Z. med. J.*, 1980, *92*, 345.

Manufacturers
Parke, Davis, UK.

1350-r

Halofenate.
MK-185. 2-Acetamidoethyl 4-chloro-α-(3-trifluoromethylphenoxy)phenylacetate.
$C_{19}H_{17}ClF_3NO_4$=415.8.
CAS — 26718-25-2.

Adverse Effects. Nausea and abdominal pain may occasionally occur. Elevations of serum aspartate aminotransferase (SGOT), serum alanine aminotransferase (SGPT), and creatine kinase values have been reported.

Precautions. Halofenate has been reported to diminish the effect of propranolol and to enhance the effect of sulphonylurea antidiabetic agents. It is probable that halofenate enhances the effect of coumarin anticoagulants.

Halofenate reduced the protein binding of phenytoin *in vitro*.— F. E. Karch *et al.* (letter), *Br. J. clin. Pharmac.*, 1977, *4*, 625.

In 5 diabetic patients taking chlorpropamide or tolbutamide, and phenformin, the mean fasting plasma-glucose concentration fell over 6 to 12 weeks when halofenate 0.5 to 1.5 g daily was added to their treatment, and the mean dose of antidiabetic agent was reduced. There was no similar effect in 2 patients taking tolbutamide alone or in 6 taking insulin.— D. J. Kudzma and S. J. Friedberg, *Diabetes*, 1977, *26*, 291.

Abnormal responses to a glucose-tolerance test were present in 6 of 10 patients without overt diabetes. After 24 weeks' treatment with halofenate 0.5 to 1.5 g [daily] abnormal responses were present in 2 of 9, and in none after 48 weeks' treatment.— E. B. Feldman *et al.*, *J. clin. Pharmac.*, 1978, *18*, 241. See also Chlorpropamide, p.853 and Tolbutamide, p.860.

For a report of halofenate reducing the effect of propranolol, see Propranolol Hydrochloride, p.1328.

See also under Absorption and Fate.

Absorption and Fate. Halofenate is absorbed from the gastro-intestinal tract.

Halofenate was metabolised by hydrolysis to the free acid, which was extensively bound to plasma proteins. Testing *in vitro* with the free acid and fresh human blood showed that the drug greatly reduced the binding of salicylic acid and aspirin, whilst it had no effect on the binding of warfarin, dicoumarol, and indomethacin.— H. B. Hucker *et al.*, *J. pharm. Sci.*, 1972, *61*, 1490.

Uses. Halofenate lowers serum-triglyceride but has little effect on serum-cholesterol concentrations. It also reduces serum-uric acid concentrations in patients with hyperuricaemia. The usual dose has been 1 g daily.

The effect on thyroid function.— J. R. Ryan *et al.*, *Clin. Pharmac. Ther.*, 1971, *12*, 464.

Halofenate was a more potent inhibitor of platelet aggregation *in vitro* than clofibrate; it reversed experimentally-induced platelet hypersensitivity.— R. W. Colman *et al.*, *J. Lab. clin. Med.*, 1976, *88*, 282.

Diabetes insipidus. Halofenate 1 g twice daily reduced water intake and urine output in a patient with vasopressin-sensitive diabetes insipidus although not so rapidly as clofibrate 4 g daily.— A. Gattereau *et al.*, *Can. med. Ass. J.*, 1974, *110*, 1275.

Gout. In a double-blind study in 35 patients with gout, halofenate 1 g daily for 48 weeks reduced the mean concentration of uric acid in serum by 27% while probenecid 1 g daily reduced it by 24%. Platelet stickiness was reduced in 6 of 7 patients taking halofenate and in 4 of 11 taking probenecid.— G. B. Bluhm and J. M. Riddle, *Arthritis Rheum.*, 1975, *18*, 388.

Hyperlipidaemia. Serum-triglyceride concentrations and total lipids but not serum-cholesterol concentrations were reduced in 9 patients given halofenate 500 mg twice daily when compared with the response to placebo and there was a fall in serum-uric acid concentrations. It was considered that halofenate displaced thyroxine from thyroid-binding proteins.— J. P. Morgan *et al.*, *Clin. Pharmac. Ther.*, 1971, *12*, 517.

Of 48 patients with raised serum-cholesterol or -triglyceride concentrations included in a double-blind study, 25 received a placebo and 23 received halofenate 1 g once daily. After 48 weeks halofenate had caused a mean reduction in serum-triglyceride concentrations of 49% compared with the placebo while serum-cholesterol concentrations were not significantly affected. There was no significant difference in the incidence of myocardial infarction or mortality-rate between the halofenate and the placebo groups.— W. S. Aronow *et al.*, *Clin. Pharmac. Ther.*, 1973, *14*, 358. There was no difference in the exercise ECG between the 2 sets of patients; this applied equally to patients suffering from angina pectoris and to asymptomatic patients with or without coronary heart disease. Changes in exercise performance or in the ECG did not correlate with serum-cholesterol changes or serum-triglyceride concentrations.— *idem*, 366. Compared with placebo, halofenate caused a mean reduction in serum uric acid of 35%. It was of special value in the treatment of hyperuricaemia and hypertriglyceridaemia.— *idem*, 371. After further treatment of 41 patients for a further 48 weeks there was significant reduction of triglycerides but not of cholesterol.— *idem*, 1974, *15*, 67.

In 6 men with hyperuricaemia and hypertriglyceridaemia halofenate 1 g daily, in conjunction with a purine-free diet, reduced serum-urate concentrations and increased urate excretion. The peak effect occurred 6 to 8 hours after the dose and the effect lasted up to 48 hours.— P. J. Ravenscroft *et al.*, *Clin. Pharmac. Ther.*, 1973, *14*, 547.

In a double-blind, controlled, 48-week study, 9 patients with type IV hyperlipoproteinaemia received halofenate 500 mg twice daily, 9 received clofibrate 1 g twice daily, and 10 received placebo. The mean 48-week plasma triglyceride concentration increased during placebo treatment, decreased significantly during halofenate treatment only on exclusion of a non-compliant patient but decreased significantly during clofibrate therapy regardless of inclusion of a non-compliant patient. The mean 48-week cholesterol concentration was reduced below base-line values by clofibrate only, halofenate had an effect only in the period of 33 to 48 weeks, and only clofibrate reduced very low-density lipoproteins (with concomitant increase in low-density lipoproteins). Halofenate, however, had a more marked hypouricaemic effect. Three patients in the clofibrate group and 5 in the halofenate group with abnormal initial values developed abnormal increases in serum creatine phosphokinase concentrations, and 1 patient in the halofenate group developed general malaise and back pain associated with raised serum aspartate and alanine aminotransferases.— C. A. Dujovne *et al.*, *Clin. Pharmac. Ther.*, 1976, *19*, 352. Study in 12 patients for a further year.— *idem*, *Am. J. med. Sci.*, 1976, *272*, 277.

In a study in 16 patients with type IIb, IV, or V hyperlipoproteinaemia the effect of halofenate (7 patients) on triglycerides was similar to that of clofibrate (9 patients); the effect on cholesterol concentrations was less marked.— E. M. Lorenzo *et al.*, *Curr. ther. Res.*, 1977, *22*, 147.

Further references: A. Jain *et al.*, *Clin. Pharmac. Ther.*, 1970, *11*, 551; W. S. Aronow *et al.*, *Curr. ther. Res.*, 1973, *15*, 902; *idem*, 1974, *16*, 897; *idem*, 1975, *18*, 855; D. R. Bassett *et al.*, *Clin. Pharmac. Ther.*, 1977, *22*, 340; O. Kuntzen *et al.*, *Arzneimittel-Forsch.*, 1978, *28*, 2349.

Manufacturers
Merck Sharp & Dohme, USA.

1351-f

Nafenopin. Nafenoic Acid; Su 13437. 2-Methyl-2-[4-(1,2,3,4-tetrahydro-1-naphthyl)phenoxy]propionic acid.
$C_{20}H_{22}O_3$=310.4.

CAS — 3771-19-5.

Nafenopin has antihyperlipidaemic properties. Study in the USA ceased following a report of liver nodules in *rats*.

References: P. Weiss *et al.*, *Clin. Pharmac. Ther.*, 1970, *11*, 90; J. R. Bianchine *et al.*, *ibid.*, 97; M. Schönbeck *et al.*, *Dt. med. Wschr.*, 1970, *95*, 1761, per *Abstr. Wld Med.*, 1971, *45*, 175; C. A. Dujovne *et al.*, *Clin. Pharmac. Ther.*, 1971, *12*, 117; C. Russo and M. Mendlowitiz, *ibid.*, 676.

1352-d

Nicoclonate. Chlorophenylisobutyl Nicotinate; S 486. 1-(4-Chlorophenyl)-2-methylpropyl pyridine-3-carboxylate.
$C_{16}H_{16}ClNO_2$=289.8.

CAS — 10571-59-2.

A white powder. M.p. about 133°. Slightly **soluble** in water; soluble in alcohol, ether, and acetone.

Uses. Nicoclonate is slowly hydrolysed in the gastro-intestinal tract with the release of nicotinic acid. It is used similarly to nicotinic acid, in doses of 500 mg twice daily with food, in the treatment of hypercholesterolaemia and hyperlipoproteinaemia.

Proprietary Names
Lipidium *(Sedaph, Fr.; Zambeletti, Spain).*

1353-n

Nicofibrate Hydrochloride. Clofenpyride Hydrochloride. 3-Pyridylmethyl 2-(4-chlorophenoxy)-2-methylpropionate hydrochloride.
$C_{16}H_{16}ClNO_3,HCl$=342.2.

CAS — 31980-29-7 (nicofibrate); 17413-51-3 (hydrochloride).

Uses. Nicofibrate is a vasodilator and has hypolipidaemic properties similar to those of clofibrate. It is used in the treatment of hypercholesterolaemia and in arteriosclerotic and diabetic vascular disorders in doses of 400 mg twice or thrice daily.

Proprietary Names
Arterium *(Llorens, Spain)*; Arterium V *(Ist. Chem. Ital., Ital.).*

1354-h

Pentaerythritol Tetra-acetate. Pentaerythrityl Tetra-acetate; Tetra-*O*-acetylpentaerythritol. 2,2-Bis(hydroxymethyl)propane-1,3-diol tetraacetate.
$C_{13}H_{20}O_8$=304.3.

CAS — 597-71-7.

Uses. Pentaerythritol tetra-acetate has been used in the treatment of hypercholesterolaemia and hyperlipidaemia in doses of 4.5 to 6 g daily in divided doses.

1355-m

Polidexide. DEAE-Sephadex; PDX Chloride; Poly[2-(diethylamino)ethyl]polyglycerylene Dextran. Dextran cross-linked with 1-chloro-2,3-epoxypropane (epichlorhydrin) and *O*-substituted with 2-diethylaminoethyl groups, some of them quaternised with diethylaminoethyl chloride.

CAS — 56227-39-5.

Polidexide is an anion-exchange resin which was formerly used similarly to cholestyramine (see p.411) in the treatment of hypercholesterolaemia.

Polidexide was formerly marketed in Great Britain under the proprietary name Secholex (*Pharmacia*).

1356-b

Probucol. DH-581. 4,4′-(Isopropylidenedithio)bis(2,6-di-*tert*-butylphenol).
$C_{31}H_{48}O_2S_2$=516.8.

CAS — 23288-49-5.

Adverse Effects. Diarrhoea occurs in about 10% of patients. Other gastro-intestinal side-effects include flatulence, abdominal pain, nausea, and vomiting. Hyperhidrosis and angioneurotic oedema may occur. There have been reports of increased values for liver-function tests and for blood concentrations of creatine kinase, uric acid, and glucose.

Absorption and Fate. The absorption of probucol from the gastro-intestinal tract is limited and variable, and is stated to be at a maximum if taken with food. Peak concentrations in blood are achieved after 3 or 4 months' treatment. Probucol accumulates in adipose tissue and concentrations fall only slowly, over several months, when treatment is withdrawn. Excretion is considered to be chiefly by the biliary system into the faeces.

Uses. Probucol is used, as an adjunct to diet, to reduce elevated serum-cholesterol concentrations, particularly in type IIa hyperlipoproteinaemia. The effect on triglyceride concentrations is variable and usually slight. The usual dose is 500 mg, with meals, morning and evening.

Probucol reduced serum-cholesterol and serum-phospholipid concentrations in 5 patients and 1 control subject but reduced serum-triglyceride concentrations only in 2 men with mixed lipaemia and diabetes mellitus. Serum-uric acid concentrations increased in 3 patients.— J. W. Drake *et al.*, *Metabolism*, 1969, *18*, 916.

The pharmacology of probucol in man, especially its effects on endocrine function.— T. S. Danowski *et al.*, *Clin. Pharmac. Ther.*, 1971, *12*, 929.

Discussions and reviews: B. F. Murphy, *J. Am. med. Ass.*, 1977, *238*, 2537; *Med. Lett.*, 1977, *19*, 41; R. C. Heel *et al.*, *Drugs*, 1978, *15*, 409.

Hyperlipidaemia. Probucol reduced cholesterol concentrations from 2.96 to 2.53 mg per ml in 2 weeks when given in 500-mg doses twice daily to 40 patients with type II hyperlipoproteinaemia. In a further 15 type IIb patients, cholesterol concentrations were reduced from 3.05 to 2.64 mg per ml and these values remained between 2.46 and 2.63 mg per ml for the 48-week test period. No side-effects occurred.— *J. Am. med. Ass.*, 1973, *223*, 9.

In a controlled crossover study of probucol, 500 mg twice daily compared with a placebo, probucol was slightly more effective than a fat-modified dietary regimen alone in 12 of 19 hyperlipidaemic patients. Of the patients in whom there was an increase or no change in the blood-cholesterol concentration 6 belonged to type IIa and a further patient in this group was excluded from the average because of variation in monthly serum-cholesterol concentrations and in body-weight.— H. B. Brown and V. G. deWolfe, *Clin. Pharmac. Ther.*, 1974, *16*, 44.

In a double-blind placebo-controlled crossover study completed by 30 patients with type II hyperlipidaemia, probucol in association with a modified dietary regimen had a beneficial effect on plasma-cholesterol concentrations; it was equally effective in men and women and in type IIa and IIb hyperlipidaemia; in agreement with previous studies it had no effect on plasma-triglyceride concentrations.— J. LeLorier *et al.*, *Archs intern. Med.*, 1977, *137*, 1429.

Of 62 patients with various hyperlipoproteinaemias given probucol 500 mg twice daily, without dietary restriction, 11 had mean serum-cholesterol concentrations reduced by less than 10% at the end of a year. In 50 treated for a further year cholesterol concentrations were significantly reduced in those with type II and type IIb hyperlipoproteinaemia, with similar reductions in 5 with type IV and one with type V hyperlipoproteinaemia. The effect on triglycerides was variable. Side-effects were minimal.— W. B. Parsons, *Am. Heart J.*, 1978, *96*, 213.

A brief report of a long-term study of probucol in hypercholesterolaemia.— H. L. Taylor *et al.*, *Clin. Pharmac. Ther.*, 1978, *23*, 131.

Comparison of probucol with clofibrate and colestipol in type IIb hyperlipoproteinaemia.— D. B. Hunninghake *et al.*, *Clin. Pharmac. Ther.*, 1980, *27*, 259.

Encouraging results with probucol in familial type II hyperlipoproteinaemia.— J. I. Mann *et al.* (letter), *Lancet*, 1981, *1*, 450.

Further references: D. T. Nash, *J. clin. Pharmac.*, 1974, *14*, 470; T. A. Miettinen and I. Toivonen, *Postgrad. med. J.*, 1975, *51*, *Suppl.* 8, 71; A. F. Salel *et al.*, *Clin. Pharmac. Ther.*, 1976, *20*, 690.

Proprietary Preparations
Lurselle *(Merrell, UK).* Probucol, available as scored tablets of 250 mg. (Also available as Lurselle in *S.Afr.*).

Other Proprietary Names
Lesterol *(Arg.)*; Lorelco *(Canad., USA).*

1357-v

Pyridoxine Clofibrate. 4,5-Bis(hydroxymethyl)-3-hydroxy-2-methylpyridine 2-(4-chlorophenoxy)-2-methylpropionate.
$C_8H_{11}NO_3,C_{10}H_{11}ClO_3$=383.8.

CAS — 29952-87-2.

An equimolecular complex of pyridoxine (see p.1642) and the effective radical of clofibrate (see p.408).

Uses. Pyridoxine clofibrate is used similarly to clofibrate in the treatment of hypercholesterolaemia and hypertriglyceridaemia in doses of 700 mg twice daily.

Proprietary Names
Claresan *(Sarbach, Belg.; Sarbach, Fr.).*

1358-g

Simfibrate. CLY 503. Trimethylene bis[2-(4-chlorophenoxy)-2-methylpropionate].
$C_{23}H_{26}Cl_2O_6$=469.4.

CAS — 14929-11-4.

The simfibrate molecule consists of two clofibrate molecules combined with the loss of a methyl group. Odourless tasteless white or pale yellow crystals or crystalline powder. M.p. about 51°. Very slightly **soluble** in water; very soluble in chloroform.

Uses. Simfibrate is used similarly to clofibrate in the treatment of hypercholesterolaemia and hypertriglyceridaemia in doses of 250 to 500 mg thrice daily.

The absorption of simfibrate.— C. Harvengt and J. -P. Desager, *Curr. ther. Res.*, 1976, *19*, 145.

Simfibrate 1.5 g daily in 3 divided doses for 120 days reduced concentrations of total serum lipids, cholesterol, triglycerides, and lipoproteins in the majority of 26 patients with hyperlipidaemia.— P. Saba *et al.*, *Curr. ther. Res.*, 1977, *22*, 741.

Proprietary Names
Cholesolvin *(Sanders-Probel, Belg.; Cyanamid, Ital.; Jap.)*.

1359-q

Sitosterols

CAS — 12002-39-0; 83-46-5 (β-sitosterol).

A white odourless tasteless powder consisting of a mixture of β-sitosterol ($C_{29}H_{50}O$) and related sterols of plant origin. It contains not less than 95% of total sterols and not less than 85% of unsaturated sterols, calculated as β-sitosterol. Practically **insoluble** in water; slightly soluble in alcohol; freely soluble in carbon disulphide and chloroform.

Adverse Effects. Anorexia, abdominal cramps, and diarrhoea have occurred with large doses.

Uses. Sitosterols appear to reduce absorption of cholesterol and have been used to reduce blood-cholesterol concentrations in patients with type IIa lipoproteinaemia. The usual dose is 3 g thrice daily before meals, increased if necessary up to 30 g daily.

The use of sitosterols in coronary atherosclerosis.— F. P. Riley and A. Steiner, *Circulation*, 1957, *16*, 723.

For a report of an increase in the saturation index of gall-bladder bile in patients given sitosterols, see D. P. Mandgal *et al.*, *Br. med. J.*, 1978, *2*, 851.

Minimal effect on bile saturation.— T. N. Tangedahl *et al.*, *Gastroenterology*, 1979, *76*, 1341.

Preliminary results with sitosterol in 3 patients with familial hypercholesterolaemia.— H. Drexel *et al.* (letter), *Lancet*, 1981, *1*, 1157.

For a report suggesting that β-sitosterol might increase the effect of chenodeoxycholic acid against cholesterol gall-stones, see Chenodeoxycholic Acid, p.646.

Proprietary Names
Cytellin *(Lilly, USA)*; Harzol *(Hoyer, Ger.)*.

1360-d

Tiadenol. LL 1558. 2,2′-(Decamethylenedithio)bisethanol.
$C_{14}H_{30}O_2S_2$=294.5.

CAS — 6964-20-1.

A white powder. Practically **insoluble** in water; soluble in alcohol and chloroform.

Uses. Tiadenol is a hypolipidaemic agent used in the treatment of hypercholesterolaemia and hypertriglyceridaemia in doses of 1.6 to 2.4 g daily in 2 divided doses.

A favourable long-term study of the cholesterol- and triglyceride-lowering effect of tiadenol in 30 patients with type IIa or IIb hyperlipoproteinaemia.— J. Rouffy, *Thérapie*, 1975, *30*, 815.

Favourable results were obtained after administration of tiadenol 2.4 g daily to 7 subjects with moderate type IIa hypercholesterolaemia. Four patients with severe hypercholesterolaemia and xanthomas were more resistant although some beneficial effect was noted.— J. -L. de Gennes *et al.*, *Thérapie*, 1976, *31*, 455.

Further references: P. Saba *et al.*, *Curr. ther. Res.*, 1980, *27*, 677.

Proprietary Names
Braxan *(Bagó, Arg.)*; Eulip *(Robin, Ital.)*; Fonlipol *(Lafon, Fr.; Recordati, Ital.)*; Meralycin *(Disprovent, Arg.)*; Millaterol *(Therapia, Spain)*; Tiaden *(Malesci, Ital.)*; Tiaterol *(Midy, Ital.)*; Tiodenol *(Uquifa, Spain)*.

1361-n

Tibric Acid. CP-18524. 2-Chloro-5-(*cis*-3,5-dimethylpiperidinosulphonyl)benzoic acid.
$C_{14}H_{18}ClNO_4S$=331.8.

CAS — 37087-94-8.

Adverse Effects. Gastro-intestinal disturbances, insomnia, headache, dizziness, and elevation of serum aspartate aminotransferase (SGOT) values have been reported.

Uses. A hypolipidaemic agent used similarly to clofibrate. Doses of 1 to 1.5 g daily have been given.

In 40 patients with type IV hyperlipoproteinaemia mean pretreatment serum-triglyceride concentrations of 2.62 mg per ml fell to 1.7 mg per ml after 1 month's treatment with tibric acid 0.75 to 1 g daily in single or divided doses; the reduction was maintained over 12 months' treatment. Serum-cholesterol concentrations were not affected. Serum creatine kinase values were increased without clinical symptoms.— J. R. Ryan *et al.*, *Clin. Pharmac. Ther.*, 1974, *15*, 218.

In 6 patients with type IV hyperlipoproteinaemia of moderate degree without the presence of chylomicrons, triglyceride concentrations fell significantly after treatment for 24 weeks with tibric acid 0.5 to 1.5 g daily as a single dose. There was no response in 6 similar patients with severe type IV hyperlipoproteinaemia with chylomicrons treated similarly. In 5 patients with severe type IV hyperlipoproteinaemia and chylomicrons, triglyceride and cholesterol concentrations were considerably lowered by the same dose of tibric acid in 3 or 4 divided daily doses for 16 weeks. In 4 patients with moderate type IIa hyperlipoproteinaemia a 20 to 25% reduction in cholesterol concentration was achieved after treatment with divided doses for 16 weeks. Triglyceride and cholesterol concentrations were significantly reduced in 5 patients with type IIb hyperlipoproteinaemia given single daily doses.— G. Noseda and C. R. Sirtori, *Schweiz. med. Wschr.*, 1974, *104*, 1917.

In a double-blind study 50 patients with type IV hyperlipoproteinaemia were treated for 6 weeks with tibric acid 0.5, 0.75, 1, or 1.25 g daily or a placebo. The 2 higher doses of tibric acid were effective in lowering serum-triglyceride concentrations; the effect on cholesterol was less pronounced.— P. Bielmann *et al.*, *Clin. Pharmac. Ther.*, 1975, *17*, 606.

In 20 patients with various primary endogenous hyperlipoproteinaemias given tibric acid 1.5 g daily for 48 weeks plasma-cholesterol concentration was reduced in types II, III, and IV, and plasma triglycerides reduced in types III and IV. No significant effect on plasma lipids was observed in type V patients.— H. -J. Lisch *et al.*, *Arzneimittel-Forsch.*, 1977, *27*, 2017.

In a study in 67 patients with type IV hyperlipoproteinaemia treated under double-blind conditions for 18 weeks with tibric acid 500 mg twice daily, clofibrate 1 g twice daily, or a placebo, tibric acid significantly reduced plasma concentrations of triglycerides in patients with initial high concentrations (more than 3 mg per ml), while clofibrate reduced concentrations in those with low (less than 3 mg per ml) and high concentrations. There was no rebound in triglyceride or cholesterol concentrations when medication ceased.— P. Bielmann *et al.*, *Int. J. clin. Pharmac.*, 1977, *15*, 166.

Manufacturers
Pfizer, USA.

Colchicine Allopurinol and Uricosuric Agents

1000-f

The drugs described in this section are used in the treatment of disorders associated with hyperuricaemia and may be broadly classified as follows: allopurinol, which inhibits the formation of uric acid; the uricosuric agents, benzbromarone, probenecid, and sulphinpyrazone, which increase the excretion of uric acid; and colchicine and colchicum preparations which, while not affecting the formation or excretion of uric acid, have a specific clinical effect in the treatment of acute gout.

Indomethacin (see p.259), naproxen (see p.265), and phenylbutazone (see p.274), and similar agents are also used in the treatment of acute gout.

For reviews of the treatment of gout, see C. G. Barnes, *Practitioner*, 1972, *208*, 101; R. G. Robinson and A. B. Corrigan, *Drugs*, 1972, *3*, 422; *J. Am. med. Ass.*, 1973, *224, Suppl.*, 662–805; L. S. Wallace, *Arthritis Rheum.*, 1975, *18, Suppl.* 6, 847; M. G. Fanelli, *ibid.*, 853; F. D. Hart, *Drugs*, 1976, *11*, 451; *Med. Lett.*, 1976, *18*, 49; J. T. Scott, *Practitioner*, 1977, *219*, 469; F. Sadik *et al.*, *J. Am. pharm. Ass.*, 1977, *NS17*, 36; B. T. Emmerson, *Drugs*, 1978, *16*, 158; M. I. V. Jayson, *Prescribers' J.*, 1978, *18*, 111; D. Morgan, *Aust. J. Pharm.*, 1978, *59*, 507 and 758; P. A. Simkin, *Ann. intern. Med.*, 1979, *90*, 812; R. I. S. Bayliss, *Br. med. J.*, 1979, *1*, 1695; G. R. Boss and J. E. Seegmiller, *New Engl. J. Med.*, 1979, *300*, 1459; J. T. Scott, *Br. med. J.*, 1980, *281*, 1164.

The conservative management of asymptomatic hyperuricaemia.— M. H. Liang and J. F. Fries, *Ann. intern. Med.*, 1978, *88*, 666.

1001-d

Colchicine *(B.P., U.S.P.)*. Colchicinum. (*S*)-*N*-(5,6,7,9-Tetrahydro-1,2,3,10-tetramethoxy-9-oxobenzo[*a*]heptalen-7-yl)acetamide.

$C_{22}H_{25}NO_6$=399.4.

CAS — 64-86-8.

Pharmacopoeias. In *Arg., Aust., Br., Braz., Chin., Cz., Fr., Ger., Ind., Int., It., Jap., Mex., Nord., Port., Span., Swiss, Turk.*, and *U.S.*

Colchicine (*Ind. P.*) is from *Colchicum luteum* and other spp.

An alkaloid obtained from the corm and seeds of the meadow saffron, *Colchicum autumnale* (Liliaceae) and other *Colchicum* spp. It occurs as pale yellow to greenish-yellow, odourless or almost odourless crystals or amorphous scales or powder with a hay-like odour when damped and warmed, and a very bitter taste. It may contain up to 10% of solvent and moisture and not more that 2 to 3% is lost on drying. It darkens on exposure to light. M.p. about 157°.

Soluble 1 in about 20 of water, 1 in 160 of ether; freely soluble in alcohol and chloroform; practically insoluble in light petroleum. Moderately concentrated aqueous solutions may deposit crystals of sesquihydrate, which is less soluble in cold water than the anhydrous alkaloid. A solution in water is laevorotatory. Solutions are **sterilised** by autoclaving or by filtration. **Incompatible** with mineral acids. **Store** in airtight containers. Protect from light.

Stability. No appreciable hydrolysis to colchiceine occurred in neutral and slightly alkaline (pH 8.1) solutions of colchicine during 2 months' storage.— D. R. Wood, *Pharm. J.*, 1957, *1*, 188.

Sterilisation. Colchicine solutions for injection could be sterilised by heating at 115° for 30 minutes, or by heating at 98° to 100° for 30 minutes in the presence of phenylmercuric nitrate 0.002%, or by filtration. Sterilised solutions were stable for at least 6 months if protected from light.— G. Smith *et al.*, *J. Pharm. Pharmac.*, 1963, *15*, 92T. See also *Pharm. J.*, 1963, *2*, 256.

Adverse Effects. Colchicine frequently causes nausea, vomiting, and abdominal pain; these effects may occur even when colchicine is given intravenously. Larger doses may cause profuse diarrhoea, gastro-intestinal haemorrhage, muscle weakness, skin rashes, and renal and hepatic damage, and dehydration and hypotension may follow. Alopecia, peripheral neuritis, and bone marrow depression with agranulocytosis and aplastic anaemia may occur after prolonged treatment.

Extravasation of colchicine given intravenously may cause tissue irritation; thrombophlebitis may occur.

Symptoms of poisoning with colchicine set in only after an interval of 3 to 6 hours, even with large doses. At first there is a feeling of burning and rawness in the mouth and throat and difficulty in swallowing, followed by nausea, abdominal pain, vomiting, profuse blood-stained diarrhoea, colic and tenesmus, spasm of the bladder, and prostration. Anuria, delirium, hypotension, vascular damage, and convulsions may occur, with ascending paralysis. The fatal dose varies; 7 mg of colchicine has caused death, though recovery has occurred after much larger doses.

Fatal agranulocytosis and thrombocytopenia, with bone-marrow hypoplasia, occurred in a patient who had taken colchicine prophylactically in the recommended doses. Obstructive jaundice could have contributed to the toxicity of the drug.— I. B. Boruchow, *Cancer*, 1966, *19*, 541.

Steatorrhoea and a histiocytic lymphoma in the jejunum developed in a 53-year-old man after taking colchicine, 500 µg daily for 3 years, as treatment for gout.— B. J. Boucher and J. T. Wright, *Postgrad. med. J.*, 1973, *49*, 106.

Colchicine stimulated the synthesis of prostaglandins; this might account for the gastro-intestinal side-effects.— A. A. Butt *et al.*, *Gut*, 1974, *15*, 344.

Fatal marrow aplasia in a 70-year-old man given colchicine 10 mg by intravenous injections over 5 days.— Y. K. Liu *et al.*, *Arthritis Rheum.*, 1978, *21*, 731.

Twenty-four hours after instillation of a solution of colchicine 50 mg in sterile water into the urethra for treatment of condyloma acuminata a previously healthy 23-year-old man suffered near-fatal colchicine toxicity. It was recommended that colchicine should only be used with extreme caution, if at all, for the treatment of condyloma acuminata.— R. M. Naidus *et al.*, *Archs intern. Med.*, 1977, *137*, 394.

Epidermal necrolysis. Toxic epidermal necrolysis occurred in a patient who had taken colchicine and alcohol during an acute attack of gout.— A. Lyell, *Br. J. Derm.*, 1967, *79*, 662.

Overdose. Two young women took 28 mg and 39 mg of colchicine respectively in suicide attempts. Nausea, vomiting, colic, and diarrhoea occurred, and later 4 stages of toxic disturbances were observed, marked by cardiovascular, gastro-intestinal, neurological, and dermatological signs. Neither patient became unconscious, and both survived after many months' illness. No specific treatment was possible.— P. Mouren *et al.*, *Presse méd.*, 1969, *77*, 505.

An 18-year-old woman developed the respiratory distress syndrome and died 42 hours after taking about 150 mg of commercial-grade colchicine powder.— R. N. Hill *et al.* (letter), *Ann. intern. Med.*, 1975, *83*, 523.

Death of a 14-year-old girl 13 days after ingesting colchicine 35 mg. Symptoms included paralytic ileus, reversible oliguria, hypotension, Heinz body formation, respiratory distress syndrome, melaena, papilloedema, and grand mal convulsions.— D. Heaney *et al.*, *Am. J. med. Sci.*, 1976, *271*, 233.

Recovery of 3 infants, aged 18 to 26 months, who had ingested colchicine 0.1 to 1 mg per kg body-weight; they received early gastric lavage. A fourth child, aged 23 months, who had ingested 0.4 to 0.8 mg per kg and in whom gastric lavage was not performed until 5 hours after ingestion, died with cardiogenic shock, disseminated intravascular coagulation, haemorrhage, necrotic purpura, and ischaemia of the extremities.— M. Besson-Leaud *et al.*, *Annls Pédiat., Paris*, 1977, *24*, 363.

Survival of a 25-year-old woman given intensive supportive therapy after taking 40 mg of colchicine. Symptoms considered to be consistent with disseminated intravascular coagulation occurred.— A. J. Dodds *et al.*, *Med. J. Aust.*, 1978, *2*, 91.

Pregnancy and the neonate. The incidence of cells with abnormal numbers of chromosomes was increased in 3 patients with gout taking colchicine.— N. R. Ferreira and A. Buoniconti, *Lancet*, 1968, *2*, 1304.

In 7 healthy men maintenance doses of colchicine 1.8 to 2.4 mg daily for 4 to 6 months caused no change in testicular function.— W. J. Bremner and C. A. Paulsen, *New Engl. J. Med.*, 1976, *294*, 1384.

Oligospermia in 11 and amenorrhoea or dysmenorrhoea in 11 of 157 patients with Behçet's disease treated with colchicine.— Y. Mizushima *et al.* (letter), *Lancet*, 1977, *2*, 1037.

For mention that colchicine had no effect on fertility and exhibited no evidence of teratogenicity in patients being treated for familial Mediterranean fever, see under Uses, below.

Treatment of Adverse Effects. In acute poisoning the stomach should be emptied by aspiration and lavage. A purgative, such as sodium sulphate 30 g in 250 ml of water, should be given. Demulcent drinks may be given freely. Respiration may require assistance. The circulation should be maintained and fluid and electrolyte imbalance corrected. Morphine sulphate, 10 mg intramuscularly, may be given to relieve severe abdominal cramps; atropine has also been given.

Precautions. Colchicine should be given with care to old and feeble patients and to those with cardiac, renal, hepatic, or gastro-intestinal disease. Its use is contra-indicated during pregnancy.

It should not be administered by subcutaneous or intramuscular injection.

Significant reduction of the absorption of cyanocobalamin through the ileal mucosa occurred in 19 of 20 persons following the administration of colchicine, 1.9 to 3.6 mg daily. When colchicine was introduced directly into the ileum of 2 persons, less than 5% of the dose of cyanocobalamin was excreted in the urine. The decrease in urinary excretion of cyanocobalamin was accompanied by increased faecal elimination.— D. I. Webb *et al.*, *New Engl. J. Med.*, 1968, *279*, 845.

The administration of colchicine could interfere with measurements of urinary 17-hydroxycorticosteroids.— J. M. Rosenberg and I. S. Kampa, *Drug Intell. & clin. Pharm.*, 1973, *7*, 33.

For a brief review of colchicine-induced malabsorption, see G. F. Longstreth and A. D. Newcomer, *Mayo Clin. Proc.*, 1975, *50*, 284.

Persistent postoperative corneal lesions in 2 children healed only after colchicine, being taken for familial Mediterranean fever, was withdrawn.— B. Z. Biedner *et al.*, *Br. J. Ophthal.*, 1977, *61*, 496.

Absorption and Fate. Colchicine is readily absorbed from the gastro-intestinal tract and is partially deacetylated in the liver; colchicine and its metabolites are excreted in the urine and faeces.

In patients with liver disease, plasma-colchicine concentrations after 2 mg of colchicine were high and disappearance of the drug was rapid, but in patients with gout or severe renal disease plasma concentrations were similar to those of normal patients but rates of disappearance were slower.— S. L. Wallace *et al.*, *Am. J. Med.*, 1970, *48*, 443.

Colchicine achieved a high concentration in the bile and was subject to enterohepatic circulation. This might account for its toxic effects in the gastro-intestinal tract.— *Br. med. J.*, 1974, *1*, 446.

Colchicine was reported to be 50% bound to plasma proteins.— J. J. Vallner, *J. pharm. Sci.*, 1977, *66*, 447.

A peak plasma concentration of 6 ng per ml occurred 2 hours after administration of colchicine 1 mg to a patient. Excretion was prolonged with a long elimination half-life.— J. M. Scherrmann *et al.*, *J. Pharm. Pharmac.*, 1980, *32*, 800.

A study of the kinetics of colchicine in patients with familial Mediterranean fever.— H. Halkin *et al.*, *Clin. Pharmac. Ther.*, 1980, *28*, 82.

Uses. Colchicine is used for the relief of pain in acute gout. It is considered to act against the inflammatory response to the urate crystal. It is not an analgesic and has no effect on blood concentrations of uric acid, nor on uric acid excretion.

The recommended initial dose by mouth is 1 mg followed by 500 µg every 2 or 3 hours until relief is obtained or gastro-intestinal symptoms preclude its further use. The total amount required to relieve the acute attack is usually between 3 and 6 mg, and a total dose of 10 mg should not be exceeded. A course should not be repeated within 3 days. Colchicine may be given by intravenous injection in a dose of 1 or 2 mg in sodium chloride injection, with further doses of 500 µg six-hourly if required to a total of not more than 4 mg in 24 hours. For the prevention of acute episodes, 0.5 to 1 mg is given by mouth, at night or on alternate nights.

Several reports have indicated that colchicine prevents attacks of familial Mediterranean fever.

Colchicine has antimitotic properties; derivatives have been used clinically, particularly in neoplasms of the skin.

The reliability of colchicine as a specific diagnostic agent for acute gout was evaluated in 120 patients, 58 of whom had acute gout; the remainder had various arthritic disorders. Criteria of response were major subsidence of objective joint inflammation within 48 hours of the start of treatment and no recrudescence within 7 days. About 75% of the patients with acute gout responded in this way, but so did 5% of the other patients. A therapeutic trial of colchicine was a useful, but not infallible, diagnostic tool.— S. L. Wallace *et al., J. Am. med. Ass.*, 1967, *199*, 525. The use of colchicine for the diagnosis of acute gout was unreliable and should probably be abandoned.— P. Kinsella (letter), *Br. med. J.*, 1977, *1*, 1086.

Colchicine 500 µg twice daily was effective in the treatment of Mollaret's meningitis.— R. F. Gledhill *et al.* (letter), *Lancet*, 1975, *2*, 415.

A discussion of the antimitotic actions of colchicine in the context of intracellular movements.— F. E. Samson, *A. Rev. Pharmac. Toxic.*, 1976, *16*, 143.

Administration in renal failure. No dose adjustment was required for short-term therapy in renal failure or dialysis.— J. S. Cheigh, *Am. J. Med.*, 1977, *62*, 555.

The interval between doses of colchicine should be extended from 12 hours to 18 hours in patients with a glomerular filtration-rate of less than 10 ml per minute.— W. M. Bennett *et al., Ann. intern. Med.*, 1980, *93*, 286.

Behçet's disease. An analysis on reports of 157 patients with Behçet's disease treated with colchicine showed that 46 patients were much improved, 58 showed some improvement, 42 showed no change, and 11 deteriorated.— Y. Mizushima *et al.* (letter), *Lancet*, 1977, *2*, 1037.

Cirrhosis of the liver. Colchicine 1 to 2 mg daily given for 2 weeks to 7 patients with liver cirrhosis produced a striking clinical improvement. Serum-bilirubin concenrations, which varied from 10 to 55 µg per ml, were lowered in 5 patients to less than 5 µg per ml.— M. Rojkind *et al.* (letter), *Lancet*, 1973, *1*, 38.

Regression of liver fibrosis and clinical improvement in some patients with cirrhosis given colchicine 1 mg daily for 5 days a week.— D. Kershenobich *et al., Gastroenterology*, 1979, *77*, 532.

Malaria. In 22 soldiers with falciparum malaria, colchicine 500 µg was given 2-hourly for 10 doses followed by 500 µg twelve-hourly to a total dose of 6 mg, together with quinine sulphate 650 mg eight-hourly for 14 days. A second group of 38 patients with falciparum malaria received the same dose of quinine sulphate only. With concurrent colchicine-quinine therapy, 77% radical cures were achieved compared with 27% radical cures with quinine alone.— R. C. Reba and T. W. Sheehy, *J. Am. med. Ass.*, 1967, *201*, 553.

Mediterranean fever. In a double-blind crossover study of 13 patients with familial Mediterranean fever, colchicine 500 µg twice daily was effective in reducing the number of attacks. Only one patient experienced more attacks whilst receiving colchicine than a placebo and one had an equal number of attacks.— D. Zemer *et al., New Engl. J. Med.*, 1974, *291*, 932.

In a double-blind crossover trial, 10 patients with familial Mediterranean fever (paroxysmal polyserositis) were given either colchicine 600 µg thrice daily or placebo, in each case for 90 days. The attack-rate was reduced by colchicine, only 5 attacks occurring in 2 patients whereas 59 attacks occurred in 9 patients whilst on placebo.— R. C. Goldstein and A. D. Schwabe, *Ann. intern. Med.*, 1974, *81*, 792.

In a double-blind controlled study of 9 patients with familial Mediterranean fever, a 3-day course of colchicine started at the onset of an attack was effective in aborting attacks in 3 patients and ineffective in 2 patients, whilst the other 4 patients could not be assessed because of an insufficient number of courses. The treatment consisted of colchicine 600 µg every hour for 4 hours then 600 µg every 2 hours for 4 hours on the first day, then 600 µg every 12 hours.— D. G. Wright *et al., Ann. intern. Med.*, 1977, *86*, 162.

Familial Mediterranean fever in 47 patients was treated with colchicine generally in a dose of 500 µg per 25 kg body-weight daily in 1 to 3 doses; 24 had been treated for over a year. Complete remission (marred only by transient failure due to underdosage or lack of compliance) was achieved in 46 patients. Mild diarrhoea and abdominal pain occurred in 3 patients. Five children below the age of 16 years had accelerated growth-rates. Fertility was unaffected (pregnancy in 1 patient and in the wives of 3 others), and no teratogenicity or effect on chromosomal integrity was observed.— M. Levy and M. Eliakim, *Br. med. J.*, 1977, *2*, 808.

Other references: M. Eliakim and A. Licht (letter), *Lancet*, 1973, *2*, 1333; C. A. Dinarello *et al., New Engl. J. Med.*, 1974, *291*, 934; *Br. med. J.*, 1975, *3*, 60; H. A. Reimann, *J. Am. med. Ass.*, 1975, *231*, 64; D. Zemer *et al.* (letter), *New Engl. J. Med.*, 1976, *294*, 170; *Lancet*, 1977, *1*, 1140; R. A. Frayha (letter), *Ann. intern. Med.*, 1977, *87*, 382; M. Ravid *et al., ibid.*, 568; G. Skrinskas *et al., Can. med. Ass. J.*, 1977, *117*, 1416.

Psoriasis. Applications of colchicine 1% facilitated resolution of refractory psoriatic plaques; under occlusive dressings 0.25 and 0.5% concentrations were also effective. It was suggested that its use should at present be limited to small areas in patients resistant to other treatments.— K. H. Kaidbey *et al., Archs Derm.*, 1975, *111*, 33.

Preparations

Colchicine Injection *(U.S.P.)*. A sterile solution of colchicine in Water for Injections prepared with the aid of sodium hydroxide. pH 6 to 7.2. Protect from light.

Colchicine Tablets *(B.P.)*. Tablets containing colchicine. Protect from light.

Colchicine Tablets *(U.S.P.)*. Tablets containing colchicine. The *U.S.P.* requires 75% dissolution in 30 minutes. Protect from light.

Proprietary Names

Colchineos *(Houdé-I.S.H., Fr.)*; Colcin *(Knoll, Austral.)*; Colgout *(Protea, Austral.)*; Coluric *(Adam, Austral.)*.

1002-n

Colchicum Corm *(B.P. 1973)*. Colch. Corm.

The dried corm of the meadow saffron, *Colchicum autumnale* (Liliaceae), containing not less than 0.25% of alkaloids.

Adverse Effects, Treatment, and Precautions. As for Colchicine, above.

Uses. Colchicum corm has been used similarly to colchicine for the relief of pain in acute gout. It has been largely superseded by colchicine.

Preparations

Colchicum and Sodium Salicylate Mixture *(B.P.C. 1973)*. Colchicum tincture 1 ml, sodium salicylate 1 g, potassium bicarbonate 1 g, liquorice liquid extract 0.3 ml, double-strength chloroform water 5 ml, water to 10 ml. It should be recently prepared. *Dose.* 10 to 20 ml.

Colchicum Dry Extract *(B.P. 1948)*. Ext. Colch. Sicc. A dry alcoholic extract of colchicum corm adjusted with lactose to contain 1% of colchicine. *Dose.* 10 to 30 mg.

Colchicum Liquid Extract *(B.P. 1973)*. Colch. Liq. Ext. An alcoholic percolate of colchicum corm adjusted to contain 0.3% of alkaloids.

Colchicum Mixture *(B.P.C. 1954)*. Colchicum tincture 0.94 ml, potassium citrate 2.06 g, chloroform water to 15 ml.

Amended formula. Colchicum tincture 1 ml, potassium citrate 2 g, chloroform water to 10 ml.— *Compendium of Past Formulae 1933 to 1966*, London, The National Pharmaceutical Union, 1969. *Dose.* 15 ml of *B.P.C. 1954* mixture; 10 ml of amended formula.

Colchicum Tincture *(B.P. 1973)*. Colch. Tinct. Colchicum liquid extract 10 ml, alcohol (70%) to 100 ml. It contains 0.03% of alkaloids (600 µg in 2 ml). *Dose.* 0.5 to 2 ml; up to 6 ml daily, in divided doses.

Proprietary Preparations

Rheumatic Dellipsoids D10 *(Pilsworth, UK)*. Tablets each containing colchicum dry extract (*B.P. 1948*) 30 mg, codeine phosphate 7.5 mg, aspirin 250 mg, methyl salicylate 0.003 ml, and aloin 1.5 mg. For gout, rheumatism, lumbago, and sciatica. *Dose.* 1 or 2 tablets thrice daily to a total of not more than 25 tablets; the course may be repeated after an interval of 10 days.

Other Proprietary Names

Colchicum-Dispert *(Ger.)*; Colchysat Bürger *(juice from fresh flowers) (Ger.)*.

1003-h

Colchicum Seed. Colchici Semen; Colchique. The dried ripe seeds of *Colchicum autumnale.*

Pharmacopoeias. In *Arg., Belg., Braz., Fr., Mex., Port., Span.*, and *Turk.*

Braz. and *Port.* specify not less than 0.4% of colchicine; *Arg.* and *Mex.* not less than 0.45%; *Belg., Fr., Span.*, and *Turk.* not less than 0.5%.

Uses. Colchicum seed has actions similar to those of colchicum corm and has been similarly used. A tincture, containing 0.04% to 0.05% of colchicine, is included in some pharmacopoeias.

1004-m

Allopurinol *(B.P., U.S.P.)*. Isopurinol; BW 56-158; HPP. 1*H*-Pyrazolo[3,4-*d*]pyrimidin-4-ol.

$C_5H_4N_4O$=136.1.

CAS — 315-30-0 (allopurinol); 17795-21-0 (sodium salt).

Pharmacopoeias. In *Br., Braz., Cz., Jap.*, and *U.S.*

A white or off-white, odourless or almost odourless, tasteless, microcrystalline powder. Very slightly **soluble** in water and alcohol; practically insoluble in chloroform and ether; soluble in dimethylformamide and dilute solutions of alkali hydroxides.

Allopurinol Sodium. A solution of allopurinol sodium 300 mg in 5 to 10 ml of sodium chloride injection or dextrose injection 5% in water is stated to be stable for 7 days at 4° to 8°, to be incompatible with prednisolone sodium succinate and, in dextrose injection, with mercaptopurine sodium and methotrexate sodium.

The stability of allopurinol in solution.— P. D. Gressel and J. F. Gallelli, *J. pharm. Sci.*, 1968, *57*, 335.

Adverse Effects. The most common side-effect of allopurinol is skin rash which may occur in 3 to 5% of patients and more frequently in patients with renal failure; the rash may be maculopapular, exfoliative, urticarial, or purpuric and its occurrence means that allopurinol should be withdrawn. Further symptoms of hypersensitivity include fever, chills, leucopenia or leucocytosis, eosinophilia, and arthralgia; toxic epidermal necrolysis and the Stevens-Johnson syndrome have been reported. Other side-effects include nausea, vomiting, abdominal pain, diarrhoea, alopecia, headache, drowsiness, and peripheral neuritis. There have been reports of vasculitis and of liver damage.

An acute haemorrhagic lesion of the macula developed in a patient under treatment with allopurinol; the lesion regressed when allopurinol was discontinued.— G. Pinnas, *Archs Ophthal., N.Y.*, 1968, *79*, 786.

A 16-year-old boy with reddish sandy deposits in his urine and repeated haematuria and ureteric colic since infancy was given allopurinol. He developed oxypurine calculi. This complication would be reduced by ensuring a high fluid intake and by producing an alkaline urine.— M. L. Greene *et al., New Engl. J. Med.*, 1969, *280*, 426.

Xanthine stones, 1 to 5 mm in diameter, were found in the kidneys, ureter, and renal pelvis of a 23-year-old man with lymphosarcoma who had received treatment including allopurinol 200 mg four times daily for 6 days.— P. R. Band *et al., New Engl. J. Med.*, 1970, *283*, 354. Comments.— D. C. Blass ('etter), *ibid.*, 1225; D. S. Silverberg (letter), *ibid.*

In 10 patients with gout who had taken allopurinol, 300

to 600 mg daily, for 0.5 to 4 years skeletal muscle biopsy specimens contained crystals of hypoxanthine, xanthine, and oxypurinol; these were not considered significant when compared with the benefits of treatment.— R. W. E. Watts *et al.*, *Q. J. Med.*, 1971, *40*, 1, per *Int. pharm. Abstr.*, 1972, *9*, 231.

Hair loss and ichthyosis had been reported in a woman 6 weeks after a short course of allopurinol.— A. Levantine and J. Almeyda, *Br. J. Derm.*, 1973, *89*, 549.

Anorexia, severe weight loss, general weakness, and malaise, symptoms normally suggestive of malignancy, in a 66-year-old man were considered to be a result of administration of allopurinol for 18 months.— A. Calin (letter), *J. Am. med. Ass.*, 1978, *239*, 497.

Allergy. Allopurinol could cause severe allergic reactions that might be due to a diffuse vasculitis affecting many organs. The illness was prolonged; symptoms included fever, skin rash, eosinophilia, hepatic abnormalities, and acute renal failure. Pre-existing renal disease and the use of thiazide diuretics might be predisposing factors.— J. L. Young *et al.*, *Archs intern. Med.*, 1974, *134*, 553.

Further references: M. W. McKendrick and A. M. Geddes, *Br. med. J.*, 1979, *1*, 988.

See also under Vasculitis, below.

Blood disorders. Allopurinol had been reported to cause aplastic anaemia.— R. H. Girdwood, *Drugs*, 1976, *11*, 394.

Agranulocytosis was associated with allopurinol in a patient with impaired renal function and diabetes mellitus, retinopathy, and neuropathy.— D. G. Wilkinson (letter), *Lancet*, 1977, *2*, 1282.

Neutropenia in 3 obese patients undergoing prolonged total therapeutic starvation, with folate supplements, who also received allopurinol to prevent hyperuricaemia.— I. N. Scobie *et al.*, *Br. med. J.*, 1980, *280*, 1163.

Epidermal necrolysis. A 72-year-old man developed a generalised maculopapular eruption after taking allopurinol 100 mg twice daily for 7 days. This was followed by eosinophilia, toxic epidermal necrolysis, oliguria, uraemia, extensive intracutaneous infections, sepsis, and pneumonia, and he died 21 days after the start of allopurinol.— G. L. Kantor, *J. Am. med. Ass.*, 1970, *212*, 478.

Toxic epidermal necrolysis in 3 patients was attributed to allopurinol.— M. H. Ellman *et al.*, *Archs Derm.*, 1975, *111*, 986.

After 3 weeks' treatment with allopurinol a 54-year-old man developed toxic epidermal necrolysis including pseudomembranous conjunctivitis and ulcerative lesions on the lids and conjunctiva. Punctate corneal ulcers and dry eyes persisted after 14 months; bilateral corneal ulcers developed.— T. O. Bennett *et al.*, *Archs Ophthal., N.Y.*, 1977, *95*, 1362.

Epidermal necrolysis in a 38-year-old man who had been taking allopurinol 200 mg thrice daily for 6 weeks and hydrochlorothiazide 50 mg daily for 2 years.— D. Assaad *et al.*, *Can. med. Ass. J.*, 1978, *118*, 154.

Liver damage. Massive fatal hepatic necrosis developed in a 48-year-old woman who was given allopurinol for hyperuricaemia. Clinical and laboratory findings suggested a hypersensitivity reaction probably due to allopurinol.— R. C. Butler *et al.*, *J. Am. med. Ass.*, 1977, *237*, 473.

Severe cholangitis and pericholangitis with jaundice was attributed to allopurinol in one patient who also developed severe eosinophilia and generalised lymphadenopathy. A skin reaction developed during treatment with allopurinol and amoxycillin.— H. C. Korting and R. Lesch (letter), *Lancet*, 1978, *1*, 275.

Widespread granulomas in the liver of a 47-year-old man appeared to be related to allopurinol which he had taken for 6 years; no granulomas were evident 6 months after allopurinol was discontinued.— A. Medline *et al.*, *Br. med. J.*, 1978, *1*, 1320.

Further references: F. Simmons *et al.*, *Gastroenterology*, 1972, *62*, 101; C. R. Espiritu *et al.*, *Am. J. dig. Dis.*, 1976, *21*, 804; T. D. Boyer *et al.*, *West. J. Med.*, 1977, *126*, 143.

Nephritis. A case of acute interstitial nephritis after 1 month's therapy with allopurinol 300 mg daily. The patient had had normal renal function but had abnormal liver function and hepatomegaly, probably secondary to alcoholic liver disease. It was possible that the nephritis resulted from a cell-mediated hypersensitivity response.— D. R. Gelbart *et al.* (letter), *Ann. intern. Med.*, 1977, *86*, 196.

Vasculitis. Vasculitis with fibrinoid necrosis and an eosinophilic reaction, particularly in the kidney, caused the death of a patient treated with allopurinol.— J. Jarzobski *et al.*, *Am. Heart J.*, 1970, *79*, 116.

Severe arteritis associated with allopurinol in one patient. Prednisone 40 mg daily provided effective treatment.— R. R. Bailey *et al.* (letter), *Lancet*, 1976, *2*, 907.

Precautions. Allopurinol should not be used for the treatment of an acute attack of gout and administration is not advisable immediately after an acute attack. Treatment should be stopped if any skin reactions develop.

Allopurinol should be administered with care to patients with renal or hepatic impairment and doses may need to be reduced. Fluid intake should be such as to maintain a urinary output of not less than 2 litres a day.

It has been suggested that allopurinol should not be given to nursing mothers.

The metabolism of mercaptopurine is inhibited by allopurinol and the dosage of azathioprine or mercaptopurine must be reduced when the drugs are given concomitantly.

In 2 children with a deficiency of hypoxanthineguanine phosphoribosyltransferase, treatment with allopurinol caused up to tenfold increases in the concentration of oxypurine in the plasma, and up to threefold increases in the concentration of oxypurine in CSF. Such treatment might result in exaggeration of CNS dysfunction.— F. M. Rosenbloom *et al.*, *J. Am. med. Ass.*, 1967, *202*, 175.

Allopurinol inhibited the activity of hepatic microsomal drug-metabolising enzymes.— E. S. Vesell *et al.*, *New Engl. J. Med.*, 1970, *283*, 1484.

Allopurinol and oxypurinol could interfere with the spectrophotometric determination of theophylline.— T. F. Woodman *et al.*, *Am. J. Hosp. Pharm.*, 1977, *34*, 984.

Drug interactions. Allopurinol has been reported to increase the incidence of skin rashes in patients taking ampicillin, to increase the half-life of dicoumarol, and to enhance the effect of phenprocoumon. For further details see under the Precautions for each drug.

Possible reduction of the toxicity of fluorouracil by allopurinol.— R. M. Fox *et al.* (letter), *Lancet*, 1979, *1*, 677.

Severe neurotoxicity in 2 patients with chronic lymphocytic leukaemia receiving allopurinol and vidarabine concomitantly.— H. M. Friedman and T. Grasela (letter), *New Engl. J. Med.*, 1981, *304*, 423.

For a report of an increased incidence of bone-marrow toxicity in patients given allopurinol and cyclophosphamide, see Cyclophosphamide, p.200.

Absorption and Fate. Allopurinol is absorbed from the gastro-intestinal tract and is reported to have a plasma half-life of about 1 hour. It is rapidly converted in the body to oxypurinol (alloxanthine) which is also an inhibitor of xanthine oxidase with a reported half-life of 18 to 30 hours. Allopurinol and oxypurinol are not bound to serum proteins and are excreted mainly in urine.

Allopurinol was converted *in vivo* to oxypurinol (alloxanthine). In man, though not in lower animals, this appeared to be reabsorbed by the kidney tubules and was relatively slowly excreted. The slow renal clearance of oxypurinol suggested that part of the therapeutic activity of allopurinol could be due to the maintenance of adequate blood concentrations of its metabolite. This factor could become important when uricosuric agents, which increased oxypurinol excretion, were given with allopurinol.— G. B. Elion, *Ann. rheum. Dis.*, 1966, *25*, 608.

The kinetics of allopurinol.— K. Hande *et al.*, *Clin. Pharmac. Ther.*, 1978, *23*, 598.

Uses. Allopurinol inhibits the action of xanthine oxidase and thus reduces the oxidation of hypoxanthine and xanthine to uric acid. The urinary purine load, normally almost entirely uric acid, is thereby divided between hypoxanthine, xanthine, and uric acid, each with its independent solubility. The reduced concentration of uric acid in plasma facilitates the resolution of tophi and calculi. Hypoxanthine and xanthine may be re-utilised for nucleotide and nucleic acid synthesis, and purine biosynthesis may be reduced.

Allopurinol is administered indefinitely in the treatment of chronic gout; it reduces the concentration of uric acid in plasma with gradual resolution of tophi and reduces the risk of the formation of uric acid calculi. It may be effective in some patients who are unable to tolerate or are unresponsive to uricosuric agents such as probenecid or sulphinpyrazone, particularly in patients with impaired renal function where the impairment prevents the uricosuric agents from inhibiting tubular reabsorption of uric acid.

To reduce the possibility of precipitating acute gout a dose of 100 mg daily may be given initially, increased by 100 mg daily at weekly intervals until the concentration of uric acid in serum is reduced to 60 µg per ml; the average daily dose is 200 to 300 mg for those with mild gout; and 400 to 600 mg for those with moderately severe tophaceous gout. Up to 300 mg may be taken as a single daily dose; larger amounts should be taken in divided doses. Additional therapy with colchicine or an anti-inflammatory agent is sometimes given in the early stages of treatment with allopurinol. Allopurinol is not suitable for the treatment of acute gout.

Allopurinol is also used in the treatment of hyperuricaemia associated with leukaemia or resulting from radiotherapy or the use of antineoplastic agents. A suggested initial dose is 200 mg thrice daily commencing 2 or 3 days before radiotherapy or the commencement of treatment with antineoplastic agents, and adjusted as required to a maintenance dose, usually of 300 to 400 mg daily. For children, the suggested initial dose is 8 mg per kg body-weight daily and this may be increased to 20 mg per kg daily. When given concomitantly with azathioprine or mercaptopurine, the dose of the antineoplastic agent should be reduced to about one-quarter of the usual dose.

Allopurinol is also used for the prophylaxis of uric acid and calcium oxalate calculi, in doses similar to those used for gout, and to prevent hyperuricaemia during treatment with diuretics of the thiazide or similar type.

When changing treatment from a uricosuric agent reduce the dose of the uricosuric agent gradually and increase that of allopurinol gradually over at least 1 to 3 weeks.

Doses should be reduced in patients with impaired renal function; 100 to 200 mg daily should be used if the creatinine clearance is between 10 and 20 ml per minute and not more than 100 mg daily if the creatinine clearance is less. Allopurinol and its metabolite are removed by haemodialysis and doses should be adjusted accordingly or else a single dose of 300 to 400 mg should be given after each dialysis.

Periodic blood counts and tests of kidney and liver function are recommended.

Allopurinol failed to reduce total purine excretion in 7 of 11 patients with excessive uric acid production. These 7 patients each had a marked decrease in hypoxanthine-guanine phosphoribosyltransferase activity. Enzyme activity, however, was normal in 4 additional gouty patients with normal uric acid production in whom a similar failure to depress total purine excretion was observed.— W. N. Kelley *et al.*, *New Engl. J. Med.*, 1968, *278*, 287. See also *Lancet*, 1971, *1*, 73.

Evidence that *in vitro* allopurinol inhibited the synthesis of purines and pyrimidines by a mechanism independent of inhibition of xanthine oxidase.— W. N. Kelley *et al.*, *Ann. N.Y. Acad. Sci.*, 1971, *179*, 588.

Administration. A study in 33 patients who had previously taken allopurinol 400 to 600 mg daily in divided doses indicated that once daily administration was a satisfactory therapeutic regimen.— W. J. C. Currie *et al.*, *Wellcome*, *Br. J. clin. Pharmac.*, 1978, *5*, 90.

Depression. Allopurinol might enhance the activity of tryptophan in depression by blocking appropriate liver enzyme activity. Five of 8 depressed patients treated with both drugs gained remission of symptoms and 2 showed some improvement.— B. Shopsin (letter), *Lancet*, 1976, *1*, 1189.

Gout. The use of allopurinol in the management of drug-induced gout.— *Drug & Ther. Bull.*, 1975, *13*, 73.

A 69-year-old patient with chronic tophaceous gout was treated with allopurinol 100 mg four times daily. Within several months the tophi began to regress but no new bone formation occurred in the areas of pre-existing intraosseous tophi with the result that the digits of the hands and feet became markedly shortened. Although the hands and feet had marked deformities manual dexterity improved as pain and inflammation subsided.— N. L. Gottlieb and R. G. Gray, *J. Am. med. Ass.*, 1977, *238*, 1663.

Hyperuricaemia. Hyperuricaemia was well controlled by allopurinol in a patient with negligible kidney function who was being maintained on long-term, intermittent haemodialysis. He received 400 mg of allopurinol daily. The drug was effectively removed by haemodialysis.— C. P. Hayes *et al.*, *J. Am. med. Ass.*, 1966, *195*, 1089.

An intravenous preparation of sodium allopurinol was used in the treatment of hyperuricaemia secondary to neoplastic disease. The recommended dose was 350 to 700 mg per m^2 body-surface area given as an infusion over 24 hours.— H. E. Kann *et al.*, *Am. J. med. Sci.*, 1968, *256*, 53.

An 8-year-old boy with mild hyperuricaemia, excessive excretion of uric acid, and a seizure disorder unresponsive to anticonvulsants became free of seizures a week after treatment with allopurinol 75 mg daily. He was maintained largely free of seizures and his mental state improved strikingly.— M. Coleman *et al.*, *Archs Neurol., Chicago*, 1974, *31*, 238.

Muscular dystrophy. Of 16 patients with X-linked recessive (Duchenne) muscular dystrophy treated with allopurinol 15 showed initial physical improvement. After 22 months' treatment the 3 who had been barely ambulant were now unable to walk, but of the 12 remaining 6 retained all their initial improvement; 5 had lost some improvement but were still improved; one was a little worse. The original dose of 100 mg daily had been modified for those over 4 years of age: 4 to 6 years, 150 mg; 7 to 9 years, 200 mg; 10 to 12 years, 250 mg; 13 and over, 300 mg.— W. H. S. Thomson and I. Smith (letter), *New Engl. J. Med.*, 1978, *299*, 101.

No evidence of improvement was found in any of 20 adult patients with muscular dystrophy given allopurinol.— P. Bakouche *et al.* (letter), *New Engl. J. Med.*, 1979, *301*, 785.

Administration of allopurinol to 10 children with Duchenne muscular dystrophy was associated with complete recovery of strength in 3 (average age about 3 years), partial recovery in 4 (average age about 9 years), and no change in 3 (average age 10 years).— M. Castro-Gago *et al.* (letter), *Lancet*, 1980, *1*, 1358. Criticism.— D. Gardner-Medwin (letter), *ibid.*, *2*, 92.

Results of an extensive double-blind trial in 25 boys aged 4 to 17 years showed that allopurinol is of no value in the treatment of Duchenne muscular dystrophy.— A. H. Bretag *et al.* (letter), *Lancet*, 1981, *1*, 276.

Psoriasis. Fifty patients with psoriasis, of 8 months' to 32 years' standing, were treated with allopurinol 100 to 400 mg daily. An excellent response (total bleaching of lesions in an average of 30 days, and disappearance of erythema and scaling) was achieved in 25 patients, a good response in 17, and a moderate response in 8. Lesions reappeared when treatment was withdrawn.— P. A. Viglioglia *et al.*, *Dermatologica*, 1970, *141*, 203.

Renal calculi. Allopurinol usually in a dose of 200 mg daily or trichlormethiazide 2 mg twice daily or a combination over periods of about 1 to 7 years reduced the number of calcium oxalate stones formed from a predicted 220 to 22 in a study of 202 patients with idiopathic hypercalciuria or hyperuricosuria or both and a history of recurrent stone formation. In a group of 30 patients without metabolic disorders who received both allopurinol and trichlormethiazide 6 new stones were formed as compared with about 32 predicted. A similar group of 34 untreated patients formed 29 new stones compared with a predicted 33. All patients had some dietary control.— F. L. Coe, *Ann. intern. Med.*, 1977, *87*, 404. See also F. L. Coe and L. Raisen (preliminary communication), *Lancet*, 1973, *1*, 129.

Allopurinol 100 mg daily for 6 months to 5 years appeared to prevent new stone formation in about 60% of 49 patients with a history of calcium oxalate calculi.— M. J. V. Smith, *J. Urol.*, 1977, *117*, 690.

A discussion of the use of allopurinol in the treatment of calcium calculus disease.— *Br. med. J.*, 1977, *2*, 1302.

Reports of the dissolution of renal calculi.— R. Wasko and B. A. Frankenfield (letter), *J. Am. med. Ass.*, 1968, *205*, 801; J. T. Harbaugh, *J. Urol.*, 1968, *100*, 412; A. A. Billings *et al.* (letter), *J. Am. med. Ass.*, 1969, *210*, 2093; J. J. Gertner (letter), *Lancet*, 1973, *1*, 834.

Further references: C. Y. Pak *et al.*, *Am. J. Med.*, 1978, *65*, 593; F. L. Coe, *Archs intern. Med.*, 1978, *138*, 1090; R. Scott *et al.*, *Br. J. Urol.*, 1978, *50*, 455; T. Yü, *Postgrad. Med.*, 1978, *63*, 164; M. Peacock and W. G. Robertson, *Drugs*, 1980, *20*, 225.

Sarcoidosis. The resolution of long-standing sarcoid lesions in 2 patients appeared to be associated with administration of allopurinol.— B. M. Rosof (letter), *New Engl. J. Med.*, 1976, *294*, 447.

Preparations

Allopurinol Tablets *(B.P.)*. Tablets containing allopurinol. They may be film-coated.

Allopurinol Tablets *(U.S.P.)*. Tablets containing allopurinol.

Proprietary Preparations

Caplenal *(Berk Pharmaceuticals, UK)*. Allopurinol, available as scored tablets of 100 and 300 mg.

Zyloric *(Wellcome, UK)*. Allopurinol, available as scored tablets of 100 and 300 mg. (Also available as Zyloric in *Arg., Belg., Denm., Fr., Ger., Ital., Neth., Norw., Spain, Switz.*).

Other Proprietary Names

Arg.— Uroquad; *Austral.*— Capurate, Progout, Zyloprim; *Canad.*— Alloprin, Purinol, Zyloprim; *Denm.*— Apurin; *Ger.*— Bleminol, Cellidrin, Dabrosan, Epidropal, Foligan, Urbol-100, Urobenyl, Urosin, Xanturat; *Hung.*— Milurit; *Ital.*— Allural, Allurit, Uricemil, Uriscel, Urolit, Vedatan; *Jap.*— Adenock, Allozym, Alositol, Anoprolin, Anzief, Aprinol, Ketanrift, Ketobun-A, Masaton, Miniplanor, Monarch, Neufan, Riball, Takanarumin, Uric; *Mex.*— Zyloprim; *Neth.*— Apurin; *Norw.*— Allopur; *NZ*— Zyloprim; *S.Afr.*— Puricos, Zyloprim; *Switz.*— Allopur, Foligan, Lysuron 300; *USA*— Lopurin, Zyloprim.

1005-b

Benzbromarone.
L 2214; MJ 10061. 3,5-Dibromo-4-hydroxyphenyl 2-ethylbenzofuran-3-yl ketone.

$C_{17}H_{12}Br_2O_3$=424.1.

CAS — 3562-84-3.

Adverse Effects. Benzbromarone may cause gastro-intestinal side-effects, especially diarrhoea. Other side-effects occasionally reported include skin rash, allergic conjunctivitis, sandy urine, and renal colic. Joint pains and acute gout have occurred, particularly in patients not given colchicine prophylactically.

Precautions. Benzbromarone should be used with caution in patients with impaired renal function. Salicylates partially antagonise the effect of benzbromarone.

Absorption and Fate. Benzbromarone is absorbed from the gastro-intestinal tract. It is reported to undergo dehalogenation in the liver to form benzarone and bromobenzarone which are partially conjugated with glucuronic acid and excreted in the urine and faeces.

References: J. Brockhuysen *et al.*, *Eur. J. clin. Pharmac.*, 1972, *4*, 125; T. Yu, *J. Rheumatol.*, 1976, *3*, 305.

Uses. Benzbromarone is a uricosuric agent which reduces plasma concentrations of uric acid probably by blocking tubular reabsorption. It is used in the treatment of hyperuricaemia in gout and thiazide-induced hyperuricaemia. The usual dose is 100 mg once daily; up to 300 mg daily has been used. A micronised preparation is also used; 80 mg is stated to be approximately equivalent to 100 mg of the non-micronised material. Colchicine 500 µg may be given 2 or 3 times daily initially to reduce the risk of precipitating acute gout; an adequate fluid intake is recommended.

An extensive review.— R. C. Heel *et al.*, *Drugs*, 1977, *14*, 349.

In 21 men with hyperuricaemia without tophi, micronised benzbromarone 40 or 80 mg daily rapidly reduced plasma concentrations of uric acid; the effect was maintained for one year. Benzbromarone was considered to block tubular reabsorption of uric acid. The effect of benzbromarone was only slightly affected by aspirin.— L. B. Sorensen and D. J. Levinson, *Arthritis Rheum.*, 1976, *19*, 183.

In 12 patients with hyperuricaemia after renal transplantation, treatment with allopurinol 200 mg daily reduced serum concentrations of uric acid by a mean of 19.5%. When these patients and 5 further patients were treated with benzbromarone, usually 50 to 100 mg daily, the mean reduction of uric acid was 35%.— W. Flury *et al.*, *Schweiz. med. Wschr.*, 1977, *107*, 1339.

Further references: N. Zöllner *et al.*, *Klin. Wschr.*, 1968, *46*, 1318, per *J. Am. med. Ass.*, 1968, *206*, 2955; D. P. Mertz, *Münch. med. Wschr.*, 1969, *111*, 491, per *J. Am. med. Ass.*, 1969, *207*, 2495; N. Zöllner *et al.*, *Klin. Wschr.*, 1970, *48*, 426, per *J. Am. med. Ass.*, 1970, *212*, 1091; A. K. Jain *et al.*, *Arthritis Rheum.*, 1974, *17*, 149.

Proprietary Names

Desuric *(Labaz, Belg.; Sigmatau, Ital.; Labaz, Neth.; Labaz, Switz.)*; Désuric *(Labaz, Fr.)*; Max-Uric *(Labinca, Arg.)*; Minuric *(Labaz, S.Afr.)*; Narcaricin *(Heumann, Ger.)*; Normurat *(Grünenthal, Ger.)*; Obason *(Mepha, Switz.)*; Uricovac M *(Labaz, Ger.)*; Urinorm *(Labaz, Spain)*; Urinome *(Jap.)*.

1006-v

Ethebenecid. 4-(Diethylsulphamoyl)benzoic acid.

$C_{11}H_{15}NO_4S$=257.3.

CAS — 1213-06-5.

Adverse Effects. Skin rashes, gastro-intestinal discomfort, and mild sedation have been reported.

Uses. Ethebenecid is a uricosuric agent which has been used similarly to probenecid in the treatment of gout and thiazide-induced hyperuricaemia. The usual daily divided dose was 1 to 3 g.

Ethebenecid was formerly marketed in Great Britain under the proprietary name Urelim *WB Pharmaceuticals.*

1007-g

Oxypurinol. Oxipurinol; Alloxanthine; BW 55-5; NSC-76239. 1*H*-Pyrazolo[3,4-*d*]pyrimidine-4,6-diol.

$C_5H_4N_4O_2$=152.1.

CAS — 2465-59-0.

Oxypurinol is the active metabolite of allopurinol (see p.417).

Sludge and calculus formation in the urinary tract of an 8-year-old boy who had previously received allopurinol was attributed to partial replacement of allopurinol dosage by oxypurinol.— A. R. Landgrebe *et al.*, *New Engl. J. Med.*, 1975, *292*, 626.

A 25-year-old man who was allergic to allopurinol was similarly sensitive to a single dose of oxypurinol 50 mg.— O. Lockard *et al.*, *Ann. intern. Med.*, 1976, *85*, 333.

Manufacturers

Wellcome, USA.

1008-q

Probenecid *(B.P., U.S.P.)*.
Probenecidum. 4-(Dipropylsulphamoyl)benzoic acid.

$C_{13}H_{19}NO_4S$=285.4.

CAS — 57-66-9.

Pharmacopoeias. In *Br., Braz., Chin., Int., Jap., Nord., Swiss, Turk.*, and *U.S.*

A white or almost white, odourless or almost odourless, crystalline powder with a taste at first slightly bitter but becoming unpleasantly bitter. M.p. 198° to 200°.

Practically **insoluble** in water; soluble 1 in 25 of alcohol and 1 in 12 of acetone; soluble in chloroform and in dilute solutions of alkali hydroxides and of sodium bicarbonate; practically insoluble in dilute mineral acids.

Adverse Effects. Probenecid is generally well tolerated, though nausea, vomiting, headache, sore gums, flushing, dizziness, urinary frequency, anaemia, and skin rashes may occasionally occur. On rare occasions an anaphylactic reaction or a hypersensitivity reaction, with fever, dermatitis, and pruritus has occurred and there have been reports of hepatic necrosis, the nephrotic syndrome, and aplastic anaemia. When used in chronic gout, probenecid may precipitate an acute attack, and renal colic or renal calculi, with or without haematuria, may occur. In massive overdosage probenecid causes stimulation of the central nervous system, with convulsions and death from respiratory failure.

A 52-year-old man with gout was given 4 courses of probenecid in doses of about 1 g daily. The first course provoked urticaria. Several months later, and again after 6 years, probenecid brought on nephrosis on 3 occasions. The condition cleared completely when probenecid was withdrawn.— T. F. Ferris *et al.*, *New Engl. J. Med.*, 1961, *265*, 381.

A 49-year-old man took 47.5 g of probenecid in a suicide attempt. He went into a coma and status epilepticus, and his serum urate fell to low levels. No significant changes in calcium or phosphorus metabolism could be demonstrated. The man recovered.— V. J. Rizzuto *et al.*, *Am. J. Med.*, 1965, *38*, 646.

The nephrotic syndrome developed on 2 occasions in a 34-year-old man with gout after he had been treated with probenecid 500 mg twice daily. Symptoms abated when the drug was stopped, and the connection was presumed to be causal.— A. Sokol *et al.*, *J. Am. med. Ass.*, 1967, *199*, 43.

Haemolytic anaemia. Probenecid was not considered to cause clinically significant haemolytic anaemia in individuals with glucose-6-phosphate dehydrogenase deficiency under normal circumstances (e.g. in the absence of infection).— E. Beutler, *Pharmac. Rev.*, 1969, *21*, 73.

Probenecid did not cause haemolysis in Chinese patients with glucose-6-phosphate dehydrogenase deficiency.— T. K. Chan *et al.*, *Br. med. J.*, 1976, *2*, 1227.

Treatment of Adverse Effects. In severe overdosage the stomach should be emptied by aspiration and lavage. Diazepam 5 to 10 mg should be given by intravenous injection to control convulsions. Respiration may need assistance. Anaphylactic reactions may be treated with adrenaline possibly in association with antihistamine and corticosteroid therapy (for details, see Adrenaline, p.4).

Precautions. Salicylates antagonise the action of probenecid and should not be given concomitantly. If probenecid is given concomitantly with methotrexate, the dose of methotrexate should be reduced.

Probenecid should not be given to patients with renal uric acid calculi or blood dyscrasias. It should be used with caution in patients with a history of peptic ulceration.

As well as inhibiting the tubular secretion of some antibiotics probenecid reduces the excretion of aminohippuric acid, some contrast media, dapsone, indomethacin, phenolsulphonphthalein, and sulphobromophthalein sodium. The plasma concentration of conjugated (but not free) sulphonamides may be increased.

A reducing substance has been found in the urine of some patients taking probenecid, and may interfere with Benedict's tests.

Probenecid could interfere with the spectrophotometric assay of theophylline.— L. E. Matheson *et al.*, *Am. J. Hosp. Pharm.*, 1977, *34*, 496.

Drug interactions. Probenecid inhibited the renal excretion of indomethacin in 6 volunteers. Peak blood concentrations 4 hours after administration were about 50% higher after probenecid; after 48 hours they were 6 times the control concentrations and 15% of the peak values.— M. D. Skeith *et al.*, *Clin. Pharmac. Ther.*, 1968, *9*, 89. See also N. Baber *et al.*, *Br. J. clin. Pharmac.*, 1978, *5*, 364P.

The half-life of probenecid was increased after prior treatment with pyrazinamide but protein binding was not affected. The uricosuric effect of probenecid was reduced and prolonged. The excretion of probenecid was increased in alkaline urine.— T. F. Yü *et al.*, *Am. J. Med.*, 1977, *63*, 723.

Enhancement of the effect of frusemide by probenecid.— D. C. Brater, *Clin. Pharmac. Ther.*, 1978, *24*, 548. See also D. E. Smith *et al.*, *J. pharm. Sci.*, 1980, *69*, 571.

Enhancement of the effect of naproxen by probenecid.— R. Runkel *et al.*, *Clin. Pharmac. Ther.*, 1978, *24*, 706.

Prolongation of thiopentone anaesthesia by probenecid.— S. Kaukinen *et al.*, *Br. J. Anaesth.*, 1980, *52*, 603.

For the possible enhancement of the effect of chlorothiazide by probenecid, see Chlorothiazide, p.589.

Absorption and Fate. Probenecid is readily absorbed from the gastro-intestinal tract and is extensively bound to plasma proteins. It is metabolised, and excreted in the urine.

The plasma half-life of probenecid was 4 to 12 hours after doses of 0.5 to 2 g; it was bound to plasma proteins to the extent of 83 to 94%. From 17 to 35.6% of a dose was excreted as the acyl glucuronide and 5.2 to 11% as free probenecid. Four other metabolites had been identified—2 hydroxylated derivatives, a carboxy derivative, and an *N*-depropyl compound.— P. G. Dayton and J. M. Perel, *Ann. N.Y. Acad. Sci.*, 1971, *179*, 399.

From 77 to 88% of a dose of probenecid was found in the urine after administration of 0.5 to 2 g in solution. The major metabolite was probenecid acyl glucuronide which accounted for about 34 to 47% of the dose. Also present in amounts of 8 to 16% were the mono-*N*-propyl, secondary alcohol, and carboxylic acid metabolites mainly in unconjugated forms. The terminal half-lives for excretion of the metabolites, which were about 4 to 6 hours, were not dose-dependent but were limited by their rates of formation. The amount of unchanged probenecid recovered in the urine was about 4 to 13% and appeared to be affected by pH and urine flow-rate. At higher doses the excretion of metabolites was more prolonged and it was suggested that due to its low water solubility probenecid precipitated in the gastro-intestinal tract and its absorption depended on its redissolving.— S. Melethil and W. D. Conway, *J. pharm. Sci.*, 1976, *65*, 861.

Minimal excretion of unchanged probenecid in urine.— R. A. Upton *et al.*, *J. pharm. Sci.*, 1980, *69*, 1254.

Penetration into the CSF.— B. -E. Roos *et al.*, *Eur. J. clin. Pharmac.*, 1980, *17*, 223.

Uses. Probenecid is a uricosuric agent; it promotes excretion of urates by inhibiting tubular reabsorption, which results in a lowering of the elevated concentrations of uric acid in the plasma and in slow depletion of urate tophi in the tissues. It is used in the treatment of gout and to prevent hyperuricaemia during treatment with diuretics of the thiazide or similar type. Probenecid has no analgesic action and is of no value in acute gout, though acute attacks usually diminish some weeks after the beginning of treatment. Acute attacks may be reduced by the concurrent administration of indomethacin (see p.259), naproxen (see p.265), phenylbutazone (see p.274), or colchicine 500 µg twice or thrice daily. Treatment with probenecid should be uninterrupted since any irregularity of dosage leads to reduced output of urates and increased concentrations of uric acid in the plasma.

It is usual to start treatment with doses of 250 mg twice daily increased after a week to 500 mg twice daily and later, if the therapeutic effects are inadequate, by 500-mg increments every 4 weeks, to up to 2 g daily. Probenecid may not be effective in chronic renal insufficiency.

To reduce the risk of urolithiasis, an adequate fluid intake is required and, if necessary, sodium bicarbonate 3 to 7.5 g daily or potassium citrate 7.5 g daily may be given to render the urine alkaline.

When the patient has been free from acute attacks for at least 6 months, and providing the serum concentration of uric acid is within normal limits, the daily dose may be gradually reduced, in stages of 500 mg every 6 months, to the lowest effective maintenance dose.

Probenecid also reduces the tubular excretion of penicillins and may increase the plasma concentrations up to fourfold. It may, therefore, be used as an adjunct to penicillin therapy in conditions where very high or prolonged concentrations of penicillin may be required, such as subacute bacterial endocarditis or the treatment of gonorrhoea. It also similarly enhances the plasma concentrations of some antibiotics of the cephalosporin type. It has no significant effect on the excretion of streptomycin, cephaloridine, chloramphenicol, chlortetracycline, and oxytetracycline.The usual dosage for reducing tubular excretion of penicillins and cephalosporins is 500 mg four times daily, or less in elderly patients with suspected renal impairment. The dosage for children of 2 years and over is 25 mg per kg body-weight initially, followed by 10 mg per kg body-weight every 6 hours. When renal impairment is sufficient to retard the excretion of penicillins, probenecid should not be given concurrently.

Single doses of probenecid 1 g are used in conjunction with penicillins in the single-dose treatment of gonorrhoea.

Probenecid is used in investigational studies to block the transport from the brain into blood of acidic metabolites of monoamine neurotransmitters.

A young woman with calcinosis circumscripta unresponsive to monthly infusions of disodium edetate was given probenecid in gradually increasing doses. Little resolution of the calcinosis occurred until, after 9 months, the dose of probenecid was increased to 2 g daily; resolution had then continued for 3 years. Improvement was probably due to a reduction in the calcium × phosphorus product.— C. E. Dent and T. C. B. Stamp, *Br. med. J.*, 1972, *1*, 216.

A 64-year-old woman with systemic sclerosis and calcification was treated with probenecid 1 g daily for about 4 months. When the patient temporarily discontinued treatment, large bullae containing calcium appeared on the hands and continued to appear for about a week after treatment was reinstituted. The mobility of the hands was improved.— R. MacKie (letter), *Br. med. J.*, 1972, *2*, 768.

In a woman with calcinosis circumscripta and Raynaud's phenomenon calcified deposits decreased in size after treatment with probenecid 2 g daily.— D. Meyers, *Med. J. Aust.*, 1976, *2*, 457.

Probenecid 0.25 to 1 g twice daily was ineffective in 6 patients with chondrocalcinosis articularis.— E. E. Smith and A. St. J. Dixon (letter), *Lancet*, 1976, *2*, 376.

Diagnostic use. The use of probenecid as a biochemical aid in the diagnosis of manic-depressive psychoses.— R. Sjöström, *Eur. J. clin. Pharmac.*, 1973, *6*, 75.

Hypercalciuria. Probenecid, 1 g twice daily, administered to 4 patients with idiopathic hypercalciuria did not affect the urinary excretion of chloride, potassium, and sodium ions, but a sustained increase in the excretion of calcium, citrate, and magnesium, and a temporary increase in the excretion of ammonium occurred. Hydrochlorothiazide, 50 mg twice daily, given with probenecid increased the excretion of calcium, citrate, and magnesium.— D. A. Garcia and E. R. Yendt, *Can. med. Ass. J.*, 1970, *103*, 473.

Preparations

Probenecid Tablets *(B.P.).* Tablets containing probenecid.

Probenecid Tablets *(U.S.P.).* Tablets containing probenecid. The *U.S.P.* requires 80% dissolution in 30 minutes.

Benemid *(Merck Sharp & Dohme, UK).* Probenecid, available as scored tablets of 500 mg. (Also available as Benemid in *Austral., Belg., Canad., Ger., Ital., Neth., S.Afr., Switz., USA*).

Other Proprietary Names

Austral.— Procid; *Belg.*— Probenid; *Canad.*— Benuryl; *Fr.*— Bénémide; *Ital.*— Solpurin, Uroben, Urocid; *Norw.*— Probecid; *S.Afr.*— Panuric, Proben; *Spain*— Probemid; *Swed.*— Probecid.

A preparation containing probenecid was also formerly marketed in Great Britain under the proprietary name ColBenemid (*Merck Sharp & Dohme*).

1009-p

Sulphinpyrazone *(B.P.).* G 28,315; Sulfinpyrazone *(U.S.P.)*; Sulphoxyphenylpyrazolidine.
1,2-Diphenyl-4-(2-phenylsulphinylethyl)pyrazolidine-3,5-dione.
$C_{23}H_{20}N_2O_3S$=404.5.

CAS — 57-96-5.

Pharmacopoeias. In *Br., Braz.,* and *U.S.*

A white, or off-white, odourless powder with a bitter taste. M.p. 130.5° to 135°. Practically

insoluble in water and light petroleum; soluble 1 in 40 of alcohol, 1 in about 10 of acetone, 1 in 2 of chloroform, and 1 in 750 of ether; sparingly soluble in aqueous solutions of alkali hydroxides.

Adverse Effects. Sulphinpyrazone may cause nausea, vomiting, abdominal pain, and skin rash. It may aggravate peptic ulcer and may precipitate acute attacks of gout. Hypersensitivity reactions may occasionally occur. Rare instances of anaemia, agranulocytosis, leucopenia, and thrombocytopenia have been reported. Side-effects similar to those occurring with phenylbutazone (see p.273) and other pyrazoles may possibly occur and blood cell counts should be made at regular intervals. Overdosage may cause ataxia, laboured respiration, convulsions, and coma.

Three of 25 patients with gout who took sulphinpyrazone for 2.8 to 14 years and colchicine intermittently developed fatal acute myelomonocytic leukaemia (2) or multiple myeloma (1). Eight of 22 patients taking sulphinpyrazone for 5 months developed moderate granulocytopenia. Careful haematological control of sulphinpyrazone therapy was essential.— M. W. Witwer *et al.*, *Br. med. J.*, 1976, *2*, 89.

Elevation of creatinine and urea concentrations in a 33-year-old man taking sulphinpyrazone 800 mg daily.— J. Braun, *Archs intern. Med.*, 1976, *136*, 1060.

Oral challenge tests indicating that sulphinypyrazone can induce bronchospasm in patients with aspirin-induced asthma.— A. Szczeklik *et al.* (letter), *New Engl. J. Med.*, 1980, *303*, 702.

Four cases of transient oliguric renal failure associated with the use of sulphinpyrazone.— J. Boelaert *et al.* (letter), *New Engl. J. Med.*, 1980, *303*, 49.

A report of sulphinpyrazone-induced acute renal failure.— D. S. Durham and L. S. Ibels, *Br. med. J.*, 1981, *282*, 609. See also A. L. Linton *et al.*, *Ann. intern. Med.*, 1980, *93*, 735.

Treatment of Adverse Effects. In acute poisoning the stomach should be emptied by aspiration and lavage with sodium bicarbonate solution or other alkaline solution. Respiration may need to be assisted. To control convulsions give diazepam 5 to 10 mg by intravenous injection.

Precautions. Sulphinypyrazone should be given with care to patients with impaired renal function or a history of peptic ulcer. It should not be given to patients with active peptic ulcer.

Because sulphinpyrazone may enhance the effect of coumarin anticoagulants and sulphonylurea hypoglycaemic agents, care should be exercised if they are given concomitantly. The effects of sulphinpyrazone are diminished by salicylates.

Renal-function tests may be invalidated in patients taking sulphinpyrazone.

Sulphinpyrazone prolonged the serum half-life of benzylpenicillin.— J. Kampmann *et al.*, *Clin. Pharmac. Ther.*, 1972, *13*, 516.

The recurrence of myocardial infarction, after withdrawal of warfarin, in 6 of 41 patients who had received sulphinpyrazone plus warfarin, suggested that the combined treatment might predispose to recurrence rather than protect.— J. A. Tulloch and T. C. K. Marr (letter), *Br. med. J.*, 1979, *2*, 133. Apparent interaction with warfarin.— G. G. Nenci *et al.*, *ibid.*, 1981, *282*, 1361.

Absorption and Fate. Sulphinpyrazone is readily absorbed from the gastro-intestinal tract. Over 95% of the sulphinpyrazone in the circulation is bound to plasma proteins. It has been reported to have a biological half-life of about 3 hours after intravenous injection and 25 to 50% of a dose has been reported to be excreted, largely unchanged, in the urine in 24 hours.

In 4 subjects with gout but free from renal or hepatic disease who were given 400 mg of the sodium salt of sulphinpyrazone intravenously, the mean excretion of sulphinpyrazone was reduced from 1.05 mg per minute to 0.25 mg per minute when probenecid was subsequently given. Alkalinisation of the urine did not affect the excretion of sulphinpyrazone. The metabolite of sulphinypyrazone, *p*-hydroxysulphinpyrazone, was similarly affected. The excretion of probenecid was not affected by sulphinpyrazone.— J. M. Perel *et al.*, *Clin. Pharmac. Ther.*, 1969, *10*, 834.

Sulphinpyrazone kinetics after intravenous and oral administration.— J. B. Lecaillon *et al.*, *Clin. Pharmac. Ther.*, 1979, *26*, 611.

Uses. Sulphinpyrazone, an analogue of phenylbutazone, is a uricosuric agent; it promotes excretion of urates by inhibiting tubular reabsorption. It reduces elevated concentrations of uric acid in the blood and causes the slow depletion of urate tophi in the tissues. It is used in the long-term treatment of chronic gout; it has little analgesic action and is of no value in acute gout. The initial dose of sulphinpyrazone is 100 to 200 mg daily, taken with meals or milk. At the beginning of treatment acute episodes of gout may be precipitated. Indomethacin (see p.259), naproxen (see p.265), phenylbutazone (see p.274), or colchicine in a dosage of 500 µg twice or thrice daily may be given concurrently with the aim of reducing the incidence of such attacks. The dosage of sulphinpyrazone is gradually increased over a week until a daily dosage of 600 mg is reached; up to 800 mg daily may be given. After the blood-urate concentration has been controlled, the daily maintenance dose may be reduced to as low as 200 mg.

To reduce the risk of urolithiasis, an adequate fluid intake is required and, if necessary, sodium bicarbonate or potassium citrate may be given to render the urine alkaline.

Sulphinpyrazone has been reported to lengthen platelet survival, to decrease platelet turnover, to inhibit platelet adhesion and aggregation, and to inhibit prostaglandin synthesis by platelets. It has been reported to reduce mortality in patients who have suffered myocardial infarction; the study has, however, been severely criticised.

A review of the pharmacology and therapeutic uses of sulphinpyrazone.— E. H. Margulies *et al.*, *Drugs*, 1980, *20*, 179.

Migraine. Preliminary studies on drugs which affect platelet aggregation suggested that sulphinpyrazone might be effective in reducing the intensity and frequency of headache attacks in patients with migraine.— D. J. Dalessio, *J. Am. med. Ass.*, 1978, *239*, 52.

Paresis. Acute stuttering hemiparesis in a 67-year-old woman was rapidly resolved by treatment with sulphinpyrazone 200 mg thrice daily.— G. Lowe and R. V. Johnston (letter), *Br. med. J.*, 1977, *2*, 125.

Thrombo-embolic and myocardial disorders. Of 52 patients on chronic haemodialysis, 24 received sulphinpyrazone 200 mg thrice daily for 6 months and 28 a placebo. In the sulphinpyrazone group 12 (50%) of the patients had thrombotic episodes in the arteriovenous shunts with 0.18 thrombi per patient-month whereas 24 (86%) of the placebo group had 0.76 thrombi per patient-month. The frequency of arteriovenous shunt revision was also reduced in the sulphinpyrazone group. It was considered that the effectiveness of sulphinpyrazone was due to its suppression of platelet function.— A. Kaegi *et al.*, *New Engl. J. Med.*, 1974, *290*, 304. Similiar results in 16 patients on chronic haemodialysis. The protective effect of sulphinpyrazone in reducing thrombus formation was more apparent in male patients.— D. D. Michie and D. G. Wombolt, *Curr. ther. Res.*, 1977, *22*, 196.

Sulphinpyrazone had been given to 2 patients with thrombotic thrombocytopenic purpura. One patient had had prednisone and a splenectomy with no result and had had no response to aspirin and dipyridamole until sulphinpyrazone was added to the regimen. The other also responded to the simultaneous administration of sulphinpyrazone, aspirin, and dipyridamole.— *Ann. intern. Med.*, 1977, *86*, 102.

In 25 patients with transient cerebral ischaemia suggesting carotid arterial involvement, the platelet survival half-time was significantly reduced (mean 2.5 days) compared with that in 18 healthy subjects (mean 3.7 days). In 19 of the patients treated for 3 to 4 months with sulphinpyrazone, platelet survival was significantly improved from a mean of 2.4 to 2.8 days. Ten patients suffered no more ischaemic attacks and 6 had a reduction in frequency of attacks. Clinical benefit could be predicted from their increased platelet survival.— P. Steele *et al.*, *Stroke*, 1977, *8*, 396.

Discussions.— *Lancet*, 1978, *2*, 245; *Br. med. J.*, 1978, *2*, 454.

For a report of the failure of sulphinpyrazone, used alone, to reduce the incidence of stroke, see Aspirin, p.243.

Effect on platelet function . For discussions of the effect of sulphinpyrazone on platelet function, see J. F. Mustard and M. A. Packham, *Pharmac. Rev.*, 1970, *22*, 97; *idem*, *Drugs*, 1975, *9*, 19; M. Verstraete, *Am. J. Med.*, 1976, *61*, 897; A. S. Gallus and J. Hirsh, *Drugs*, 1976, *12*, 132; J. A. De Muylder and D. Letist, *Acta ther.*, 1977, *3*, 195; D. J. Dalessio, *J. Am. med. Ass.*, 1978, *239*, 228; M. J. Weston (letter), *Lancet*, 1978, *1*, 766; H. J. Weiss, *New Engl. J. Med.*, 1978, *298*, 1344 and 1403; P. Steele *et al.*, *Am. J. Med.*, 1978, *64*, 441; A. S. Gallus, *Drugs*, 1979, *18*, 439.

Myocardial infarction . Results of the Anturane Reinfarction Trial, a randomised, double-blind, multicentre clinical trial involving 1475 eligible patients followed for an average of 8.4 months, comparing sulphinpyrazone 200 mg four times daily (starting 25 to 35 days after infarction) with placebo for the prevention of cardiac death following myocardial infarction, indicated that sulphinpyrazone reduced the incidence of cardiac deaths. Corrected for exposure time, the annual cardiac death-rate was 9.5% in the placebo group and only 4.9% in the sulphinpyrazone group which represented a 48.5% reduction in the overall cardiac mortality in the sulphinpyrazone group; respective figures for sudden cardiac deaths were 6.3% and 2.7% which represented a 57.2% reduction in the sudden cardiac-death rate in the sulphinpyrazone group. Tolerance of sulphinpyrazone was not significantly different from tolerance of placebo.— Anturane Reinfarction Trial Research Group, *New Engl. J. Med.*, 1978, *298*, 289. On completion of the study exposure to therapy was about 16 months for the 1143 patients followed for at least a year. Sulphinpyrazone was of substantial benefit in preventing sudden cardiac death during the high risk period shortly after myocardial infarction. There was no further apparent benefit when treatment was continued beyond the seventh month after infarction. Of 106 deaths in the study group, 105 were cardiac and 59 were sudden. Up to 6 months after infarction there were 17 cardiac deaths in the sulphinpyrazone group, 6 of them sudden, compared with 35 deaths in the placebo group, 24 of these being sudden; in this period the calculated annual sudden death rate in the placebo group was 7% compared with only 1.8% in the sulphinpyrazone group, which represents a 74% reduction in the sudden death rate for those taking sulphinpyrazone. After 6 months the rates of sudden death were comparable and throughout the study the rates of nonsudden death were similar for treated and control groups.— Anturane Reinfarction Trial Research Group, *ibid.*, 1980, *302*, 250.

Comment on uncertainty over the value of sulphinpyrazone in the period after myocardial infarction and the need for further clinical studies.— A. S. Relman, *New Engl. J. Med.*, 1980, *303*, 1476. A report from the FDA on their review of the Anturane Reinfarction Trial, with reasons for the FDA's decision not to approve sulphinpyrazone as effective in reducing mortality in patients with prior myocardial infarction.— R. Temple and G. W. Pledger, *ibid.*, 1488.

Further comments; *Lancet*, 1980, *1*, 295; E. Braunwald, *New Engl. J. Med.*, 1980, *302*, 290; *Lancet*, 1980, *2*, 306; J. C. Forfar *et al.*, *ibid.*, 718; G. P. McNicol, *ibid.*, 736; *Med. Lett.*, 1980, *22*, 25; J. R. A. Mitchell, *Br. med. J.*, 1980, *280*, 1128.

In a double-blind study involving 98 patients with acute myocardial infarction no significant reduction in serious arrhythmias was observed in patients given sulphinpyrazone 200 mg four times daily for up to 10 days compared with those given a placebo. In the sulphinpyrazone-treated group the expected fall in serum-urate concentration was observed but a significant and persistent increase in serum concentrations of urea and creatinine also occurred compared with the placebo group.— R. G. Wilcox *et al.*, *Br. med. J.*, 1980, *281*, 531.

Preparations

Sulfinpyrazone Capsules *(U.S.P.)*. Capsules containing sulphinpyrazone.

Sulfinpyrazone Tablets *(U.S.P.)*. Tablets containing sulphinpyrazone.

Sulphinpyrazone Tablets *(B.P.)*. Tablets containing sulphinpyrazone. The tablets are film-coated.

Proprietary Preparations

Anturan *(Geigy, UK)*. Sulphinpyrazone, available as tablets of 100 or 200 mg. (Also available as Anturan in *Arg.*, *Austral.*, *Belg.*, *Canad.*, *Denm.*, *S.Afr.*, *Spain*, *Switz.*).

Other Proprietary Names

Anturane *(USA)*; Anturano *(Ger.)*; Enturen *(Ital.*, *Neth.)*; Zynol *(Canad.)*.

1010-n

Tisopurine. Thiopurinol; MPP. 1*H*-Pyrazolo[3,4-*d*]-pyrimidine-4-thiol.
$C_5H_4N_4S$=152.2.

CAS — 5334-23-6.

Adverse Effects. Allergic reactions and fever have been reported.

Uses. Tisopurine is claimed to reduce uric acid concentrations by interfering with early stages of its synthesis, thus avoiding increased blood concentrations of hypoxanthine and xanthine. It is used in the treatment of disorders associated with hyperuricaemia, including gout. Doses range from 200 to 400 mg daily.

Comparative enzyme inhibition and protein binding studies of tisopurine with allopurinol, oxypurinol, and mercaptopurine. The mode of action by which tisopurine decreased plasma and urinary uric acid concentrations without increasing hypoxanthine and xanthine excretion was not clear but binding of tisopurine to cellular and serum proteins seemed to play a major role in the body in controlling re-utilisation of the purines and their subsequent excretion as uric acid.— B. M. Dean *et al.*, *Br. J. clin. Pharmac.*, 1974, *1*, 119.

Proprietary Names

Thiopurinol *(Grémy-Longuet, Fr.)*; Uricolyse *(Marxer, Arg.)*.

Colouring Flavouring and Sweetening Agents

2370-w

Medicinal preparations for oral administration are often coloured and flavoured in order to make them acceptable to patients. Highly flavoured media may be required to mask the obnoxious taste of certain drugs, which may be refused or cause nausea and vomiting, particularly on repeated administration. On the other hand, attention has been drawn to the dangers of pleasantly flavoured preparations of potent drugs.

Colouring Agents. Since ancient times, colouring matters from natural sources have been used in foods, medicines, and cosmetics. Natural dyes have now been largely replaced by synthetic ('coal-tar') dyes which provide a much wider range of more stable colours of standard tinctorial power. Synthetic dyes may be broadly classified into 2 groups—acid dyes and basic dyes. Acid dyes form salts with bases, the coloured ion being negatively charged, e.g. amaranth and tartrazine; almost all the permitted dyes used for colouring food and pharmaceutical preparations are sodium salts of sulphonic acids and many of these are azo compounds.

Dyes are also used medicinally as diagnostic agents (see p.515), disinfectants (see p.547), and therapeutic agents.

Lakes, such as the insoluble aluminium or calcium salts of water-soluble dyes, often extended on aluminium hydroxide, are frequently used for colouring uncoated and coated tablets and the shells of gelatin capsules.

A review of colouring agents used in pharmaceutical preparations.— C. J. Swartz and J. Cooper, *J. pharm. Sci.*, 1962, *51*, 89.

A review of colouring agents suitable for food including the anthocyanins, betalaines, carotenoids, and some nonabsorbable polymeric dyes.— *Current Aspects of Food Colorants*, T.E. Furia (Ed.), Cleveland, Ohio, CRC Press, 1977.

The proceedings of the Second European Symposium on dyes in pharmacy.— *Acta pharm. tech.*, 1979, *Suppl.* 8, 7–157. See also *Pharm. J.*, 1978, *2*, 77.

Edible printing inks. A discussion on the factors affecting the printing of information on to tablets and capsules using edible dyes.— D. N. Lykens, *Pharmaceut. Technol.*, 1979, *3*, 57.

COLOUR INDEX NUMBER. The dyes described in the following pages have been given the numbers under which they appear in the Colour Index, published jointly by the Society of Dyers and Colourists and the American Association of Textile Chemists and Colorists.

FADING OF DYES. The colour stability of many dyes is influenced by light, pH, oxidising agents, reducing agents, and surfactants.

Nonionic surfactants had deleterious effects on the colour stability of pharmaceutical dyes.— M. W. Scott *et al.*, *J. Am. pharm. Ass., scient. Edn*, 1960, *49*, 467.

Colour stability of tablets. A series of papers describing methods of assessing stability, influence of light intensity, relative stability of lakes, protective influence of coloured glasses, effect of u.v. absorbers, and dependence of stability on temperature and pH.— T. Urbanyi *et al.*, *J. Am. pharm. Ass., scient. Edn*, 1960, *49*, 163; L. Lachman *et al.*, *ibid.*, 165; L. Lachman *et al.*, *J. pharm. Sci.*, 1961, *50*, 141; C. J. Swartz *et al.*, *ibid.*, 145; L. Lachman *et al.*, *ibid.*, 1962, *51*, 321; C. J. Swartz *et al.*, *ibid.*, 326.

The stability of food colours (USA) in tablets was determined colorimetrically. The results differed from those previously published based on decrease in absorbance. Indigo carmine and tartrazine lakes were the only approved UK food colours tested which were stable under the test conditions.— F. W. Goodhart *et al.*, *J. pharm. Sci.*, 1967, *56*, 63.

Effect of gamma-irradiation. Irradiation with 25 000 Gy had no effect on 10 water-soluble and 9 water-insoluble colouring agents (including 7 lakes).— B. -L. Chang *et al.*, *J. pharm. Sci.*, 1974, *63*, 758.

Fading in the presence of sulphite. Solutions containing about 0.02% of sodium metabisulphite, coloured with various dyes, were liable to fade, especially when the reaction of the solution was alkaline. For bordeaux B, orange G, and trypan blue, the limiting reaction beyond which fading was observed when the solution was made less acid was pH 3, for ponceau 4R it was pH 4, for amaranth pH 5, and for carmoisine and erythrosine pH 6. No fading was observed with red FB, ponceau SX, and tartrazine, from pH 3 to pH 8; with tartrazine, fading was only observed in solutions at pH 4.— *Pharm. J.*, 1956, *1*, 383 (Pharm. Soc. Lab. Rep.).

INCOMPATIBILITY. Since most of the coal-tar colours are sodium salts of organic acids, they may react in solution with cationic drugs such as phenothiazine derivatives and antihistamines to form insoluble compounds.

PERMITTED FOOD, DRUG, AND COSMETIC DYES. The dyes which may be used for colouring foods are subject to some form of legislative control in most countries of the world. The permitted list of food colours in Great Britain consists of (a) the following 'coal-tar' colours: tartrazine, quinoline yellow, *yellow 2G*, sunset yellow FCF or orange yellow S, carmoisine or azorubine, amaranth, ponceau 4R or cochineal red A, erythrosine, *red 2G*, patent blue V, indigo carmine or indigotine, *brilliant blue FCF*, green S or acid brilliant green BS or lissamine green, *brown FK*, *chocolate brown HT*, black PN or brilliant black BN, and (b) the following 'other colours':

1. Beetroot red or betanin, caramel, carbon black or vegetable carbon, chlorophyll, copper complexes of chlorophyll and chlorophyllins, cochineal or carminic acid and its ammonium salts, curcumin, riboflavine or lactoflavine, and *riboflavine-5-phosphate*.
2. The carotenoids: α-carotene, β-carotene, γ-carotene, annatto, bixin, norbixin, capsanthin or capsorubin, lycopene, β-apo-8′-carotenal, and the ethyl ester of β-apo-8′-carotenoic acid.
3. Flavoxanthin, lutein, cryptoxanthin, rubixanthin, violaxanthin, rhodoxanthin, canthaxanthin, and anthocyanins.
4. The following natural substances having a secondary colouring effect: *paprika, turmeric, saffron, sandalwood*, and their *pure colouring principles*.
5. Titanium dioxide and iron oxides and hydroxides.
6. Aluminium, gold, and silver solely for the external colouring of dragées and for the decoration of sugar-coated flour confectionery. Pigment rubine or lithol rubine BK solely for the rind of cheese and *methyl violet* solely for marking raw or unprocessed meat and citrus fruits.
7. The synthetic equivalent identical with the pure colouring principle of the approved natural colouring agents.
8. Except for pigment rubine, the acid forms of the approved colouring agents and the sodium, calcium, potassium, and aluminium salts (lakes).

These colours are also used in the European Economic Community (EEC).

In the USA 3 categories of coal-tar colours were originally allowed under the titles of F D & C Colours (approved for use in food, drugs, and cosmetics), D & C Colours (approved for use in drugs and cosmetics, but not in food) and Ext. D & C Colours (approved for external application but not to lips or mucous membranes) but these titles may no longer correspond to permitted uses.

Colouring agents used in drugs in Great Britain (and the EEC) are those allowed in food with the exception of those in italics, although in Great Britain transitional provisions allowed the use for several years of non-permitted colours that were licensed in Great Britain before 12 December 1977.

The colouring of cosmetics is controlled by legislation and there are special controls on cosmetics intended for application to mucous membranes.

A guide to the legislation affecting the use of colours in cosmetics and toiletries in Great Britain and the EEC. Anomalies between the Cosmetic Products Regulations, 1978 and Directive 76/768/EEC are discussed.— A. Foster, *Int. J. cosmet. Sci.*, 1979, *1*, 221.

CLASSIFICATION OF DYES ACCORDING TO TOXICITY. In 1979 the Food Additives and Contaminants Committee published an Interim Report on the Review of the Colouring Matter in Food Regulations, 1973 (FAC/REP/29). The toxicological evidence available for those colours permitted for use in Great Britain (by the above regulations and subsequent amendments up to and including SI 1978: No. 1787) was reviewed, together with representations relating to 8 other colours. The committee made several recommendations, including: (a) stricter controls should be imposed on the use of permitted colouring matter in food;
(b) as a consequence of suggested definitions of colouring matter, natural food substance, smoking and flavouring substance, future controls on colouring matter should apply only to added colouring matter;
(c) a prohibition should be imposed on the use of colouring matter in foods described either directly or by implication as being specially prepared for infants and young children;
(d) the presence of added citranaxanthin in or on food should not be permitted irrespective of the means by which such addition is effected;
(e) it would be prudent to avoid using methyl violet to mark meat and that it should not be permitted to mark citrus fruit;
(f) new specifications of purity should be included in any future regulations as those in use were unsatisfactory.

About 160 dyes had been classified in accordance with their toxicological evaluation. Only 3 dyes were found to be acceptable for use in food, viz. Amaranth, Sunset Yellow FCF, and Tartrazine. The following 12 colours were harmful and should not be used in food: Auramine, Butter Yellow, Chrysoidine, Guinea Green B, Magenta, Oil Orange SS, Oil Orange XO, Oil Yellow AB, Oil Yellow OB, Ponceau 3R, Ponceau SX, Sudan I.— Eighth Report of FAO/WHO Expert Committee on Food Additives, *Tech. Rep. Ser. Wld Hlth Org. No. 309*, 1965.

A survey of the nature of metallic and organic pigments and dyes used in artists' materials and their toxic hazards to children.— P. Cooper, *Pharm. J.*, 1967, *1*, 233.

An estimated acceptable daily intake of Fast Green FCF of 12.5 mg per kg body-weight had been established after repeated subcutaneous injections to *animals*.— Thirteenth Report of an FAO/WHO Expert Committee on Food Additives, *Tech. Rep. Ser. Wld Hlth Org. No. 445*, 1970.

A temporary estimated acceptable daily intake of up to 1.25 mg per kg body-weight had been established for Annatto (as bixin).— Eighteenth Report of the Joint FAO/WHO Expert Committee on Food Additives, *Tech. Rep. Ser. Wld Hlth Org. No. 557*, 1974.

Background toxicological information on food colours.— *Fd Add. Ser. Wld Hlth Org. No. 6*, 1975.

Benzyl Violet 4B was not to be used in food.— Twenty-first Report of the Joint FAO/WHO Expert Committee on Food Additives, *Tech. Rep. Ser. Wld Hlth Org. No. 617*, 1978.

A discussion on the relative toxicity of various natural and synthetic food dyes.— L. Parente, *Boll. chim.-farm.*, 1978, *117*, 125.

A discussion on intolerance to colouring agents used in foods and drugs.— L. Juhlin, *Acta pharm. tech.*, 1979, *Suppl.* 8, 15.

Preliminary results of a matched case-control study involving 637 matched pairs suggested no excess risk of bladder cancer among dye workers.— R. A. Cartwright *et al.* (letter), *Lancet*, 1979, *2*, 1073.

Hyperkinetic states. A report from the Food and Drug Administration indicated that there was too little evidence to decide whether colours and flavours in food caused hyperactivity in children and suggested that further investigations should be carried out. However, the claimed benefit of the Feingold diet (a diet excluding artificial colours, artificial flavours, selected preservatives, and salicylates) would be difficult to test even if the state of hyperactivity in children were a precise and recognisable entity. The proportion of children who are judged to be hyperkinetic differs greatly throughout the world. Existing evidence suggests that an additive-free diet does alter behaviour in some overactive children but how this happens remains unknown. However, there can be few if any indications for the use of a rigorous additive-free diet in the treatment of hyperactivity. The differences in response to dietary treatment between double-blind studies and those where the participants knew the purpose of the diet indicates a strong placebo effect, suggesting that a psychological approach may be helpful.— *Lancet,* 1979, *2,* 617. See also *Med. Lett.,* 1978, *20,* 55; T. Larkin, *FDA Consumer,* 1977, *11,* (Mar.), 19.

Studies on the use of modified diets in the treatment of hyperactivity in children: P. S. Cook and J. M. Woodhill, *Med. J. Aust.,* 1976, *2,* 85; L. K. Salzman, *ibid.,* 248; J. Breaky, *ibid.,* 508; C. K. Conners *et al., Pediatrics,* 1976, *58,* 154; A. Brenner, *Clin. Pediat.,* 1977, *16,* 652; F. Levy *et al., Med. J. Aust.,* 1978, *1,* 61; J. I. Williams *et al., Pediatrics,* 1978, *61,* 811; J. P. Harley *et al., ibid.,* 818.

Hypersensitivity. For reports of hypersensitivity to colouring agents and cross-sensitivity with aspirin and benzoates, see Tartrazine, p.431.

Toxicity of hair dyes. Chronic administration of dyes and dye intermediates, used in hair colour products in the USA, both topically and by mouth to 3 species of *animals,* gave no indication that hair dyes were toxic to bone marrow as a result of normal use.— C. M. Burnett *et al., Drug chem. Toxicol.,* 1977, *1,* 45, per *Int. pharm. Abstr.,* 1979, *16,* 914.

In a study of chromosomal damage and hair dyes, no excess of chromosomal damage was noted in 60 professional hair tinters compared with 36 control subjects, possibly owing to the protective effect of gloves and poor percutaneous absorption through the hands. A significant excess of chromosomal damage (mainly chromatid breaks) was, however, noted in women with dyed hair compared with matched controls. This latter finding warranted further study in view of the known mutagenicity and carcinogenicity of some hair-dye constituents.— D. J. Kirkland *et al., Lancet,* 1978, *2,* 124.

In a retrospective study of 129 patients with breast cancer and 193 control women the adjusted relative risks for developing breast cancer versus hair dye use were greater than unity but were not generally significant. However, there was a significant relationship between breast cancer and frequency and duration of use of hair dyes. The association was greatest among women over 50 years of age and among those at lower natural risk for breast cancer. Breast cancer was also related to use of hair dyes for 10 or more years before diagnosis. Because of the nature and size of the study further validation of the results is required.— R. E. Shore *et al., J. natn. Cancer Inst.,* 1979, *62,* 277, per *Int. pharm. Abstr.,* 1979, *16,* 912.

See also under Paraphenylenediamine, p.1738.

Flavouring Agents.

The principal flavouring agents used are aromatic oils (p.670) and waters, chloroform (p.746), liquorice (p.691), sweetening agents, such as saccharin (p.429), sorbitol (p.60), and sucrose (p.60), cocoa (p.432), syrups prepared from black currant (p.1657), ginger (p.676), raspberry (p.428), or wild cherry bark (p.432), vanilla (p.432), vanillin (p.432), and imitation flavourings.

In addition to flavouring, some of these agents have other properties; for example, aromatic waters are also carminative and chloroform water is also a preservative. Many flavouring agents, on dilution, form media suitable for the growth of micro-organisms and it is therefore necessary to add suitable preservatives.

CHOICE OF FLAVOUR. The most acceptable flavour for masking an unpleasant taste depends largely on the preference of the individual patient. Colour, odour, viscosity, and local effects on the oral mucosa also influence the acceptability of a preparation to a patient. Children often have flavour preferences quite different from those of adults. Preparations that are to be taken over long periods should not be too highly flavoured; mixed flavours, with no one constituent being readily identifiable, may be preferred for long-term treatments. A flavour which is usually associated with the type of taste to be covered may be useful; for example, orange or gentian is used with bitter alkaloids, and fruit flavours are employed to cover the sour taste of acidic substances.

Substances such as menthol or peppermint oil which produce mild local anaesthesia may help to disguise a variety of tastes. Salty substances are often given in flavoured syrups. The addition of a little sodium chloride may improve the palatability of some preparations. Mucilages and syrups make some tastes less objectionable.

Effervescent tablets, powder, or granules, which release carbon dioxide when added to water, are specially useful for certain unpalatable drugs such as saline substances and aminosalicylates. Ice-cold medicines are sometimes more palatable.

A review of mechanisms of odour and taste with practical considerations of pharmaceutical interest.— K. D. Johnson, *Australas. J. Pharm.,* 1965, *46,* S96.

Improving the palatability of formulated products.— G. E. Schumacher, *Am. J. Hosp. Pharm.,* 1967, *24,* 588 and 713. The choice of sweetening agents.— *idem,* 1968, *25,* 154.

A survey of natural and synthetic sweeteners.— M. K. Cook, *Drug Cosmet. Ind.,* 1975, *117* (Sept.), 44.

Adverse effects. A review of the toxicity of flavouring agents.— C. A. Vodoz, *Perfum. essent. Oil Rec.,* 1966, *57,* 787.

A discussion of possible adverse effects following the usage of sugar substitutes.— A. B. Morrison, *Can. med. Ass. J.,* 1979, *120,* 633.

FLAVOURING AGENTS IN FOODS. In Great Britain recommendations have been made to control flavouring agents in foods. It has been recommended that the following substances be prohibited from such use: coumarin; tonka bean; safrole; sassafras oil; dihydrosafrole; isosafrole; agaric acid; nitrobenzene; dulcamara; pennyroyal oil; oil of tansy; rue oil; birch tar oil; cade oil; volatile bitter almond oil; male fern.

It has also been recommended that flavour modifiers should be controlled in Great Britain by a permitted list which should consist of sodium hydrogen L-glutamate (sodium glutamate), guanosine 5′-disodium phosphate, inosine 5′-disodium phosphate, and sodium 5′-ribonucleotide. It was also recommended that flavour modifiers should not be permitted in foods described directly or by implication as being specially prepared for infants or young children.

In Great Britain, the only artificial sweetener (any chemical compound which is sweet to the taste but does not include any sugar or any polyhydric alcohol) allowed in food in 1982 was saccharin and its sodium and calcium salts. However, the Food Additives and Contaminants Committee (FAC/REP/34) recommended in 1982 that the following bulk sweeteners should be allowed: hydrogenated glucose syrup (a glucose syrup in which all free aldehyde groups have been reduced by hydrogenation), isomalt, mannitol, sorbitol, and xylitol. In addition to saccharin (and its sodium and calcium salts), the intense sweeteners acesulfame potassium and aspartame should be allowed.

A review of flavours and their testing.— *Natural Flavouring Substances, Their Sources, and Added Artificial Flavouring Substances,* Strasbourg, Council of Europe, 1974. See also Seventeenth Report of Joint FAO/WHO Expert Committee on Food Additives, *Tech. Rep. Ser. Wld Hlth Org. No. 539,* 1974, p. 13; FAC/REP/22, London, HM Stationery Office, 1976; FAC/REP/28, London, HM Stationery Office, 1978.

2371-e

Alkanna *(B.P.C. 1949).* Anchusa; Alkanet Root; Dyer's Alkanet; CI Natural Red 20; Colour Index No. 75520 and 75530.

CAS — 517-88-4; 23444-65-7.

The dried root of *Alkanna tinctoria* (Boraginaceae). It contains a red dye, alkannin, $C_{16}H_{16}O_5$, which is **soluble** in oils and fats; alkannin gives a blue colour with alkalis.

Uses. Alkanna is used for colouring toilet preparations of an oily or spirituous nature. It does not appear to have been used in foods. The red colouring matter in alcoholic solution is used in microscopy for the detection of oils and fats.

2372-l

Allura Red AC. CI Food Red 17; Colour Index No. 16035; F D & C No. 40. Disodium 6-hydroxy-5-(6-methoxy-4-sulphonato-*m*-tolylazo)naphthalene-2-sulphonate.

$C_{18}H_{14}N_2Na_2O_8S_2$=496.4.

CAS — 25956-17-6.

A dark red powder. **Soluble** in water.

Effect of gamma-irradiation. Irradiation with 25 000 Gy had no effect on allura red AC.— B. -L. Chang *et al., J. pharm. Sci.,* 1974, *63,* 758.

Uses. Allura red AC is a permitted colouring agent in the USA for use in foods and medicines.

Background toxicological information.— *Fd Add. Ser. Wld Hlth Org. No. 6,* 1975.

In the second interim report of a FDA/National Cancer Institute working group assessing safety data on allura red AC it was reported that the first of 2 studies in *mice* provided no evidence that allura red AC was carcinogenic. The second study still in progress confirms these findings but the working group recommended that a final assessment of allura red AC should be made on completion of this study.— *Ann. intern. Med.,* 1978, *89,* 1.

Estimated acceptable daily intake of allura red: up to 7 mg per kg body-weight; this would be reconsidered.— Twenty-third Report of Joint FAO/WHO Expert Committee on Food Additives, *Tech. Rep. Ser. Wld Hlth Org. No. 643,* 1980.

2373-y

Amaranth *(B.P.C. 1954).* Bordeaux S; CI Food Red 9; CI Acid Red 27; Colour Index No. 16185; F D & C Red No. 2. It consists mainly of trisodium 3-hydroxy-4-(4-sulphonato-1-naphthylazo)naphthalene-2,7-disulphonate.

$C_{20}H_{11}N_2Na_3O_{10}S_3$=604.5.

CAS — 915-67-3.

A reddish-brown, almost odourless powder with a saline taste. **Soluble** 1 in about 15 of water, giving a magenta-red solution; very slightly soluble in alcohol. A 1% solution in water has a pH of about 10.8.

For a report on the fading of amaranth solutions in the presence of sodium metabisulphite, see under Fading in the Presence of Sulphite, p.423.

Effect of gamma-irradiation. Irradiation with 25 000 Gy had no effect on amaranth.— B. -L. Chang *et al., J. pharm. Sci.,* 1974, *63,* 758.

Incompatibility. A report on the mechanism of the incompatibility between amaranth and cetrimide.— B. W. Barry and G. F. J. Russell, *J. pharm. Sci.,* 1972, *61,* 502.

Uses. Amaranth is used as a colouring agent in medicines, foodstuffs, and cosmetics. It is permitted for these uses in Great Britain and by the EEC but is not permitted in the USA.

An account of the reasons why the Food and Drug Administration decided to remove amaranth from the list of colourants permitted for use in food, drugs, and cosmetics in the USA.— *FDA Consumer,* 1976, (Apr.), 18.

Results from 3 studies in *rats* given amaranth 200 mg per kg body-weight yielded no evidence of foetotoxicity.— J. F. Holson *et al., Toxic. appl. Pharmac.,* 1975, *33,* 122. Administration of amaranth dietary regimens containing 300, 900 or 3000 ppm to *dogs* had no teratological or reproductive effects.— K. Mastalski *et al., ibid.*

Temporary estimated accpetable daily intake of amaranth: up to 750 µg per kg body-weight. Long-term feeding studies are required in 2 species, one study to include exposure *in utero* and through lactation.— Twenty-second Report of the FAO/WHO Expert Committee on Food Additives, *Tech. Rep. Ser. Wld Hlth Org. No. 631,* 1978.

Preparations

Amaranth Solution *(B.P.).* Amaranth *food grade of commerce* 1 g, chloroform spirit 20 ml, glycerol 25 ml,

freshly boiled and cooled water to 100 ml.
For colouring medicines, 1% v/v is usually sufficient.

Amaranth Solution *(A.P.F.)*. Red Solution; Liq. Amaranth. A 1% w/v solution of amaranth *food grade of commerce* in chloroform water.

Amaranth Solution Compound *(A.P.F.)*. Amaranth, *food grade of commerce*, 50 mg, tartrazine, *food grade of commerce*, 450 mg, chloroform water to 100 ml. Use 1 to 2% as an orange colouring for an aqueous solution or mixture.

Red Syrup *(A.P.F.)*. Syr. Rubr.; Elixir Rubrum. Amaranth solution 2.5 ml, orange tincture 5 ml, lemon spirit 0.5 ml, concentrated chloroform water 1.5 ml, syrup to 100 ml.

Proprietary Preparations

Evident *(Evident Dental Co., UK: Optrex, UK)*. Dental disclosing solution containing amaranth 5%.

2374-j

Aspartame.

APM; SC 18862. Methyl *N*-L-α-aspartyl-L-phenylalaninate; 3-Amino-*N*-(α-methoxycarbonylphenethyl)succinamic acid.
$C_{14}H_{18}N_2O_5$=294.3.

CAS — 22839-47-0.

An off-white almost odourless crystalline powder with an intensely sweet taste.
Sparingly **soluble** in water at pH 5.2; more soluble in acidic solutions and hot water; slightly soluble in alcohol; very slightly soluble in chloroform; practically insoluble in oils. A 0.8% solution in water has a pH of about 5.3.
In the presence of moisture it hydrolyses to form aspartylphenylalanine and a diketopiperazine derivative, with a resulting loss of sweetness. It is most stable in solution at about pH 4.3. **Store** in airtight containers.

Precautions. Excessive use of aspartame should be avoided by patients with phenylketonuria. Its sweetness is lost during prolonged cooking.

Aspartic acid and sodium glutamate were both neuro-excitatory amino acids which had an additive toxic effect on hypothalamic neurones. As this might be specially damaging to young children, who already receive sodium glutamate in gram quantities in their diet, aspartame should not generally be added to children's food.— J. W. Olney (letter), *New Engl. J. Med.*, 1975, *292*, 1244. See also R. Koch (letter), *ibid.*, 596.

Uses. Aspartame, which has been the subject of protracted investigations, is a sweetening agent about 200 times as sweet as sucrose. Each g provides approximately 17 kJ (4 kcal). It is used to enhance the flavour of uncooked or cold food.

Reviews of sweetening agents including aspartame: G. Chedd, *New Scientist*, 1974, *62*, 299; C. I. Beck, in *Symposium: Sweeteners*, G.E. Inglett (Ed.), Westport, AVI, 1974, p. 164; R. H. Mazur, *ibid.*, p. 159; M. K. Cook, *Drug Cosmet. Ind.*, 1975, *117* (Sept.), 44.

Acceptable daily intake for aspartame: 40 mg per kg body-weight. Aspartame usually contains about 1% of diketopiperazine and may be converted to diketopiperazine in prepared foods; the acceptable daily intake of diketopiperazine is up to 7.5 mg per kg.— Twenty-fourth Report of the Joint FAO/WHO Expert Committee on Food Additives, *Tech. Rep. Ser. Wld Hlth Org. No. 653*, 1980.

Proprietary Names

Canderel *(Searle, Belg.; Searle, Fr.)*; Equal *(Searle, USA)*; Nutrasweet *(Searle, USA)*.

2375-z

Black PN. Brilliant Black BN; CI Food Black 1; Noir Brilliant PN; Colour Index No. 28440. It consists mainly of tetrasodium 4-acetamido-5-hydroxy-6-[7-sulphonato-4-(4-sulphonatophenylazo)-1-naphthylazo]-naphthalene-1,7-disulphonate.
$C_{28}H_{17}N_5Na_4O_{14}S_4$=867.7.

CAS — 2519-30-4.

Pharmacopoeias. In *Fr.*

Black to greyish-black powder or granules. **Soluble** in water and slightly soluble in alcohol.

Uses. Black PN is a permitted colour in Great Britain and the EEC for use in medicines and foods.

Temporary estimated acceptable daily intake of black PN: up to 2.5 mg per kg body-weight. Intestinal cysts were found in *pigs* given black PN in a 90-day feeding study. Further studies are required, preferably including metabolic studies in man.— Twenty-second Report of the Joint FAO/WHO Expert Committee on Food Additives, *Tech. Rep. Ser. Wld Hlth Org. No. 631*, 1978.

Background toxicological information.— *Fd Add. Ser. Wld Hlth Org. No. 6*, 1975.

2376-c

Bordeaux B *(B.P.C. 1949)*. Azorubrum; CI Acid Red 17; Colour Index No. 16180. Consists mainly of disodium 3-hydroxy-4-(1-naphthylazo)naphthalene-2,7-disulphonate.
$C_{20}H_{12}N_2Na_2O_7S_2$=502.4.

CAS — 5858-33-3.

A brown powder. **Soluble** in water, giving a magenta-red solution; moderately soluble in alcohol, giving a purplish-red solution. **Protect** from light.

Uses. Bordeaux B was formerly used as a colouring agent for medicines and foods but has been replaced by other colours as it is not an approved colour for these purposes.

2377-k

Brilliant Blue FCF. Blue EGS; CI Food Blue 2; CI Acid Blue 9; Patent Blue AC; F D & C Blue No. 1; Colour Index No. 42090. Disodium 4′,4″-bis(*N*-ethyl-3-sulphonatobenzylamino)triphenylmethylium-2-sulphonate.
$C_{37}H_{34}N_2Na_2O_9S_3$=792.8.

CAS — 3844-45-9.

Blue powder or granules. **Soluble** 1 in 5 of water, alcohol (75%), and glycerol.

Effect of gamma-irradiation. Irradiation with 25 000 Gy had no effect on brilliant blue FCF.— B. -L. Chang *et al.*, *J. pharm. Sci.*, 1974, *63*, 758.

Uses. Brilliant blue FCF is a permitted colour in Great Britain and the EEC for uses in foodstuffs. In the USA it is also permitted for use in medicines. It has been used to produce green hues in combination with tartrazine.

An estimated acceptable daily intake of 12.5 mg of brilliant blue FCF per kg body-weight had been established after repeated subcutaneous injections to *animals*.— Thirteenth Report of an FAO/WHO Expert Committee on Food Additives, *Tech. Rep. Ser. Wld Hlth Org. No. 445*, 1970.

2378-a

Brown FK. CI Food Brown 1; Chocolate Brown FK. A mixture of 6 azo dyes: sodium 2′,4′-diaminoazobenzene-4-sulphonate; sodium 2′,4′-diamino-5′-methylazobenzene-4-sulphonate; disodium 4,4′-(4,6-diamino-1,3-phenylenebisazo) dibenzenesulphonate; disodium 4,4′-(2,4-diamino-1,3-phenylenebisazo) dibenzenesulphonate; disodium 4,4′-(2,4-diamino-5-methyl-1,3-phenylenebisazo) dibenzenesulphonate; trisodium 4,4′,4″-(2,4-diaminobenzene-1,3,5-triazo)tribenzenesulphonate.

CAS — 8062-14-4.

Red-brown powder or granules. **Soluble** 1 in 5 of water; very slightly soluble in alcohol; practically insoluble in vegetable oils.

Uses. Brown FK is a permitted colour in Great Britain and the EEC for use in foodstuffs.

Results of bacterial mutagenicity studies indicated that 2 of the constituents of brown FK are mutagenic. It was recommended that the use of this colour be restricted pending the results of a further carcinogenicity study in the *rat* and teratology and multigeneration studies.— FAC/REP/29, London, HM Stationery Office, 1979.

2379-t

Calcium Cyclamate *(B.P. 1968)*. Calc. Cyclam.; Calcium Cyclohexanesulfamate; Cyclamate Calcium. Calcium *N*-cyclohexylsulphamate dihydrate.
$C_{12}H_{24}CaN_2O_6S_2,2H_2O$=432.6.

CAS — 139-06-0 (anhydrous); 5897-16-5 (dihydrate).

Pharmacopoeias. In *Nord.*

White odourless or almost odourless crystals or crystalline powder with an intensely sweet taste, even in dilute solution. Hygroscopic in air at relative humidities of more than 70%.
Soluble 1 in 4 of water, 1 in 50 of alcohol, and 1 in 1.5 of propylene glycol; practically insoluble in chloroform and ether. A 10% solution in water has a pH of 5.5 to 7.5. **Incompatible** with nitrites in acid solution; limited compatibility with potassium salts, carbonates, citrates, phosphates, sulphates, and tartrates. Solutions are stable to heat throughout the pH range of 2 to 10. **Store** in airtight containers.

Uses. Calcium cyclamate has similar properties and uses to those of sodium cyclamate (see p.430). When the concentration of calcium cyclamate approaches 0.5% a bitter taste becomes noticeable.
The use of calcium cyclamate as an artificial sweetener in food or soft drinks or as an ingredient in artificial sweetening tablets is no longer permitted in Great Britain—see under Sodium Cyclamate, p.431.
For a temporary estimated acceptable daily intake of cyclamic acid, see Sodium Cyclamate, p.431.

Proprietary Names

Sucaryl Calcium *(Abbott, Canad.)*.

2380-l

Canthaxanthin. CI Food Orange 8; Colour Index No. 40850; E 161 g. β,β-Carotene-4,4′-dione.
$C_{40}H_{52}O_2$=564.9.

CAS — 514-78-3.

Brownish-violet to deep violet crystals. M.p. about 207° to 212° with decomposition. Practically **insoluble** in water and alcohol; very slightly soluble in acetone and vegetable oils; soluble 1 in 10 of chloroform.
When exposed to ultraviolet light or iodine or heated in solution, canthaxanthin forms a mixture of *cis* and *trans* stereoisomers. **Store** under inert gas at low temperature.

Uses. Canthaxanthin is a carotenoid but unlike betacarotene or β-apo-8′-carotenal it possesses no vitamin A activity. It is a permitted colour in Great Britain, the EEC, and the USA for use in medicines and foodstuffs and produces red solutions in oils and orange to red aqueous dispersions. It is used to colour tomato products and may be added to poultry feeds. Canthaxanthin has also been given by mouth to produce an artificial suntan.

The properties and uses of canthaxanthin and other carotenoid pigments.— L. Magid, *Drug Cosmet. Ind.*, 1966, *99* (Nov.), 64.

A review of colouring agents suitable for foodstuffs including canthaxanthin and other carotenoids.— *Current Aspects of Food Colorants*, T.E. Furia (Ed.), Cleveland, Ohio, CRC Press, 1977.

The use of canthaxanthin and other carotenoid pigments for colouring fatty suppositories.— K. Münzel and W. Füller, *Pharm. Acta Helv.*, 1969, *44*, 208.

The estimated acceptable daily intake had been established for the following food colours: canthaxanthin up to 25 mg per kg body-weight; as the sum of the carotenoids β-apo-8′-carotenal, betacarotene, β-apo-8′-carotenoic acid, and its methyl and ethyl esters, up to 5 mg per kg.— Eighteenth Report of the Joint FAO/WHO Expert Committee on Food Additives, *Tech. Rep. Ser. Wld Hlth Org. No. 557*, 1974.

Background toxicological information on canthaxanthin, β-apo-8′-carotenal, betacarotene, and β-apo-8′-carotenoic acid and its ethyl and methyl esters.— *Fd Add. Ser. Wld Hlth Org. No. 6*, 1975.

A discussion on the use of canthaxanthin to colour hard gelatin capsules.— D. Francois *et al.*, *Mfg Chem.*, 1979, *50* (April), 48.

For a report on the use of canthaxanthin in the treatment of photodermatoses, see under Betacarotene, p.1638.

Orobronze, a preparation of canthaxanthin is described on p.1783.

2381-y

Caramel *(B.P.C. 1973).* Burnt Sugar; Saccharum Ustum; Sacch. Ust.

CAS — 8028-89-5.

Pharmacopoeias. In *Ind.* Also in *U.S.N.F.*

A thick, but free-flowing, dark brown liquid, with a slight odour and a bland taste. A 10% w/v solution in water has a wt per ml of 1.023 to 1.025 g.

Miscible with water, dilute alcohol up to about 60%, dilute mineral acids, and sodium hydroxide solution, but precipitated by strong alcohol; immiscible with acetone, chloroform, ether, and light petroleum. A 10% w/v solution in water has a pH of 3 to 5.5.

Caramel (*B.P.C. 1973*) is prepared by heating a suitable water-soluble carbohydrate with a suitable accelerator and adjusting to the required standard with water. Caramel *U.S.N.F.* is prepared from sucrose or dextrose, a small amount of alkali or alkali carbonate or a trace of mineral acid being added while heating; it has a specific gravity of not less than 1.3. In Great Britain caramel permitted for use in food may be a product obtained exclusively by heating sucrose or other edible sugars, or a water-soluble amorphous brown product obtained by heating an edible sugar in the presence of (a) certain organic or mineral acids or sulphur dioxide, or (b) alkali hydroxides or ammonia, or (c) ammonium, sodium, or potassium carbonates, phosphates, sulphates, or sulphites.

Caramel of commerce is made from many raw materials, including sucrose, glucose, liquid glucose, molasses, and invert sugar. It is supplied in various qualities and strengths, with different colour intensities, to suit the various commodities in which it is used.

Uses. Caramel is used as a colouring agent to produce pale yellow to dark brown colours; 2% of a 50% solution in chloroform water is sufficient to colour most liquid preparations. The 50% solution should be recently prepared as it is liable to mould growth.

Some caramels also have flavouring properties. It has no calorific value.

Specifications for various caramels.— *Fd Add. Ser. Wld Hlth Org. No. 2,* 1972; *ibid., No. 7,* 1976.

Background toxicological information.— *Fd Add. Ser. Wld Hlth Org. No. 6,* 1975.

The temporary maximum acceptable daily intake of caramel colours made by the ammonia process was revoked. Temporary estimated acceptable daily intake of caramel colours made by the ammonia-sulphite process: up to 100 mg per kg body-weight when the concentration of 4-methylimidazole should not exceed 200 mg per kg based on the preparation having a colour intensity of 20 000 European Brewery Convention units measured according to BS 3874:1965. Adequate carcinogenicity and teratogenicity studies were required with particular attention to bone and immune competence.— Twenty-first Report of the Joint FAO/WHO Expert Committee on Food Additives, *Tech. Rep. Ser. Wld Hlth Org. No. 617,* 1978. See also Fifteenth Report, *ibid., No. 488,* 1972; Eighteenth Report, *ibid., No. 557,* 1974.

In an Interim Report on the Review of the Colouring Matter in Food Regulations 1973, the Food Additives and Contaminants Committee paid special attention to the safety of caramels used in food. Because of their colouring and flavouring function caramels accounted for about 98% by weight of all colouring matter used in food. There are numerous different caramels in use and not one of these products could be chemically defined. Though some toxicological studies had been carried out on certain caramel products those tested had not been chemically defined and it was therefore impossible to extrapolate from one product to another. The Committee suggested that caramels should be considered as 4 distinct types, categorised according to their method of preparation: (a) burnt sugar (principally used as flavourings); (b) caustic; (c) ammonia; (d) ammonium sulphite. It was also suggested that the permitted number of caramels should be limited and that in the absence of a chemical specification those products permitted should be adequately defined by a full process specification. The British Caramel Manufacturers' Association considered that the needs of the food industry for caramels for colouring could be met by a limited number of caramels and proposed 6 specifications. Since much of the previous toxicological data relates to caramels other than those in the 6 specifications the Committee recommended that the biological properties of the caramels in each specification should be determined.— FAC/REP/29, London, HM Stationery Office, 1979.

Preparations

Caramel Solution *(A.P.F.).* Burnt Sugar Solution *(B.P.C. 1959)*; Liq. Sacch. Ust. Caramel 50% in chloroform water.

2382-j

Carmine *(B.P.C. 1973).* CI Natural Red 4; Colour Index No. 75470. The aluminium lake of the colouring matter of cochineal. It contains about 50% of carminic acid, an anthraquinone glycoside.

CAS — 1390-65-4.

Pharmacopoeias. In *Arg., Belg., Port.,* and *Swiss.* which specify the aluminium-calcium lake.

Light, bright red pieces, readily reducible to powder. It loses 10 to 21% of its weight on drying. Unless precautions are taken during manufacture and transport to prevent contamination, carmine may be infected with salmonella micro-organisms. It must be pasteurised or treated to destroy any viable salmonella organisms.

Insoluble in water and dilute acids; slightly soluble in alcohol; readily soluble in dilute ammonia solution and in other dilute alkaline liquids, giving a dark purplish-red solution. It is **sterilised** by autoclaving; if necessary it should be subsequently dried at 80°. **Store** in airtight containers.

Sterilisation of carmine with alcohol (70%) was effective.— W. F. Garagusi and C. R. Meloni, *Hospitals,* 1968, *42,* 142, per *J. Am. med. Ass.,* 1968, *206,* 431.

Precautions. Carmine should be sterilised before administration by mouth.

Salmonella infection. An epidemic of *Salmonella cubana* enteritis in 21 patients was traced to the contamination of samples of carmine, used as stool markers, with the organism. Prolonged carrier states occurred in several patients. The original source of the infection was believed to be the scale insect from which cochineal was derived. The use of carmine as a food colour represented a potential source of widespread human infection.— D. J. Lang *et al., New Engl. J. Med.,* 1967, *276,* 829.

Salmonella cubana was isolated from the stools of 7 patients who had been given capsules containing carmine as stool markers. The pharmacy stocks of carmine yielded an abundant growth of organisms, including *S. cubana.*— L. E. Komarmy *et al., New Engl. J. Med.,* 1967, *276,* 851.

Uses. Carmine is a permitted colouring agent in Great Britain, the EEC, and USA for use in medicines and foodstuffs. It is also used in cosmetics and toilet preparations, especially tooth powders, dusting-powders, ointments, and mouth-washes. If carmine is used in the solid form, prolonged trituration with a powder is necessary to obtain a good colour and an even distribution; to obtain the maximum colour, carmine should be dissolved in a small quantity of Strong Ammonia Solution before trituration with the powder.

Carmine passes through the gastro-intestinal tract unchanged and is used as a 'marker' in metabolism experiments and when it is desired to check the faeces corresponding to a particular diet or method of treatment; it is given in a dose of 200 to 500 mg in a cachet or gelatin capsule at the commencement of the treatment.

Carmine was given to measure the alimentary transit time in 65 children over the age of 3 suffering from simple chronic constipation. The test was acceptable and had an accuracy of 92%.— S. B. Dimson, *Archs Dis. Childh.,* 1970, *45,* 232, per *J. Am. med. Ass.,* 1970, *212,* 2316.

Preparations

Carmine Solution *(B.P.C. 1949).* Liq. Carmin. Triturate carmine 6 g with dilute ammonia solution 15 ml, add glycerol 35 ml, and heat on a water-bath for 5 minutes or until the carmine is dissolved; cool, add potassium citrate 10 g, and dilute to 100 ml with water; filter if necessary. For colouring neutral or alkaline mouth-washes or mixtures about 1% v/v is used; the colouring matter is precipitated in acid solutions.

2383-z

Carminic Acid. CI Natural Red 4; Colour Index No. 75470. 7-α-D-Glucopyranosyl-3,5,6,8-tetrahydroxy-1-methylanthraquinone-2-carboxylic acid.

$C_{22}H_{20}O_{13}$=492.4.

CAS — 1260-17-9.

Red prismatic crystals. **Soluble** in water and alcohol; slightly soluble in ether; practically insoluble in chloroform.

An anthraquinone glycoside obtained from the dried female insect *Dactylopius coccus* (=*Coccus cacti*) (Coccidae).

Carminic acid is the principal colouring matter of cochineal (p.427). The aluminium or aluminium-calcium lake of carminic acid is carmine (p.426).

Background toxicological information.— *Fd Add. Ser. Wld Hlth Org. No. 6,* 1975.

2384-c

Carmoisine. Azorubine; CI Food Red 3; Colour Index No. 14720. It consists mainly of disodium 4-hydroxy-3-(4-sulphonato-1-naphthylazo)naphthalene-1-sulphonate.

$C_{20}H_{12}N_2Na_2O_7S_2$=502.4.

CAS — 3567-69-9.

Pharmacopoeias. In *Fr.*

A reddish-brown powder. **Soluble** 1 in about 8 of water, forming a magenta-red solution; slightly soluble in alcohol; practically insoluble in vegetable oils. **Incompatible** with acids; stable in the presence of iron salts. **Protect** from light.

For a report on the fading of carmoisine solutions in the presence of sodium metabisulphite, see under Fading in the Presence of Sulphite, p.423.

Temporary estimated acceptable daily intake of carmoisine: up to 1.25 μg per kg body-weight. Further studies are required, including metabolic studies in man.— Twenty-second Report of the Joint FAO/WHO Expert Committee on Food Additives, *Tech. Rep. Ser. Wld Hlth Org. No. 631,* 1978.

Background toxicological information.— *Fd Add. Ser. Wld Hlth Org. No. 6,* 1975.

2385-k

Chlorophyll. CI Natural Green 3; Colour Index No. 75810.

CAS — 479-61-8 (chlorophyll a); 519-62-0 (chlorophyll b).

Chlorophyll is a green colouring matter of plants which is **soluble** in organic solvents and oils but only slightly soluble in water. It is a mixture of 2 closely related substances, chlorophyll a and chlorophyll b. Both constituents are magnesium complexes with a porphyrin structure resembling that of haemoglobin and contain 2 carboxyl groups, one of which is esterified with phytyl alcohol and the other with methyl alcohol. The only difference between the 2 chlorophylls is that a methyl side-chain in chlorophyll a is replaced by a formyl group in chlorophyll b.

Oil-soluble chlorophyll derivatives. Replacement of the magnesium atom by 2 hydrogen atoms using dilute mineral acids produces olive-green water-insoluble phaeophytins. Copper phaeophytins (sometimes called copper chlorophyll complex) can be formed; these are more stable to acids and to light than the chlorophylls.

Water-soluble chlorophyll derivatives. When the chlorophylls are hydrolysed with alkali, phytyl alcohol and methyl alcohol are split off and green water-soluble chlorophyllins are formed. If sodium hydroxide is used, a mixture of sodium magnesium chlorophyllins a and b is the product. Similar water-soluble compounds can be prepared in which the magnesium is replaced by copper to give copper chlorophyllin complex.

Commercial Products. The pure chlorophylls and their derivatives described above are difficult to isolate and are not available commercially. In Great Britain, technical chlorophyll is obtained from lucerne, nettles, or grass, by extraction with alcohol or acetone; after removal of solvent and water-soluble extractives, the product consists of chlorophylls, carotenoids, phosphatides, fatty esters, etc., together with their decomposition products, the nature and amount of which depend on the extraction process.

Uses. Chlorophyll is employed principally as a colouring agent, especially for colouring fats, oils, and soaps. In Great Britain and in the EEC, chlorophyll and the copper complexes of chlorophyll and chlorophyllin are permitted colours for use in food and medicines. In the USA their use for these purposes is restricted so as to permit the use of chlorophyllin in dentifrices only.

Chlorophyll has been used as an external application in the treatment of wounds and ulcers. There is no clear evidence that it does accelerate healing but it has a deodorant action on foul-smelling wounds when kept in constant contact in fairly high concentration and tends to give them a healthy granulating appearance.

Commercial claims for the deodorant effect of chlorophyll tablets or toothpaste on halitosis and other body odours lack scientific proof.

Estimated acceptable daily intake of chlorophyllin copper complex and the sodium or potassium salts: up to 15 mg per kg body-weight.— Twenty-first Report of the Joint FAO/WHO Expert Committee on Food Additives, *Tech. Rep. Ser. Wld Hlth Org. No. 617*, 1978. See also Twenty-second Report of Joint FAO/WHO Expert Committee on Food Additives, *Tech. Rep. Ser. Wld Hlth Org. No. 631*, 1978.

Proprietary Preparations of Chlorophyll and some Derivatives

Amplex C Tablets *(Ashe, UK)*. Each contains 100 mg of chlorophyll derivatives.

Other Proprietary Names

Chloresium, Derifil *(both USA)*; Exodor grün *(Ger.)*; Melodin *(Spain)*; Oligon *(Ger.)*; Sudroma *(Canad.)*; Vulnotox *(Ger.)*.

2386-a

Chocolate Brown HT. CI Food Brown 3; Colour Index No. 20285. Disodium 4,4′-(2,4-dihydroxy-5-hydroxymethyl-1,3-phenylenebisazo)di(naphthalene-1-sulphonate).
$C_{27}H_{18}N_4Na_2O_9S_2$=652.6.

CAS — 4553-89-3.

Brown-black powder or granules. **Soluble** 1 in about 6 of water; practically insoluble in alcohol and isopropyl alcohol; soluble in glycerol.

Uses. Chocolate brown HT is a permitted colour in Great Britain and the EEC for use in foodstuffs.

Temporary estimated acceptable daily intake for Chocolate Brown HT: up to 250 µg per kg body-weight. Multigeneration reproduction/teratology studies and metabolic studies in several species, preferably including man, were required.— Twenty-third Report of the Joint FAO/WHO Expert Committee on Food Additives, *Tech. Rep. Ser. Wld Hlth Org. No. 648*, 1980.

2387-t

Cochineal *(B.P.)*. Coccus; Coccus Cacti; Coccionella; CI Natural Red 4; Colour Index No. 75470.

CAS — 1343-78-8.

Pharmacopoeias. In *Br.*, *Port.*, and *Swiss.*

The dried female insect, *Dactylopius coccus* (=*Coccus cacti*) (Coccidae), containing eggs and larvae. If killed by sulphur or charcoal fumes the insects are a greyish-white colour ('silver-grey') owing to a deposit of wax on the surface. If killed by heat the wax melts and 'black-brilliant' cochineal, which is uniformly purplish-black, is produced. It contains about 10% of carminic acid, an anthraquinone glycoside, and complies with a test for contamination with *Escherichia coli* and Salmonellae. **Store** in a dry place.

Uses. Cochineal is used, in the form of tincture or solution, as a red colouring agent.

An extract of cochineal is a permitted colouring agent in Great Britain, the EEC, and USA for use in food and medicines.

It is also used as a source of carmine.

Background toxicological information.— *Fd Add. Ser. Wld Hlth Org. No. 6*, 1975.

Preparations

Cochineal Solution *(B.P.C. 1949)*. Liq. Cocc.; Liquid Cochineal. Digest cochineal 10 g in a solution of potassium carbonate 1 g in water 60 ml on a water-bath for 2 hours, replacing water lost by evaporation; strain, cool, add alcohol (90%) 20 ml and potassium citrate 10 g, and dilute with water to 100 ml.

Cochineal Tincture *(B.P. 1948)*. Tinct. Cocc. Cochineal 1 in 10 of alcohol (45%) prepared by maceration.

2388-x

Coumarin *(B.P.C. 1934)*. Cumarin; Tonka Bean Camphor; 1,2-Benzopyrone. 2*H*-1-Benzopyran-2-one.
$C_9H_6O_2$=146.1.

CAS — 91-64-5.

Coumarin is the odorous principle of Tonka seed (Tonka or Tonquin bean); it may be prepared synthetically. It occurs as colourless prismatic crystals with a characteristic persistent fragrant odour and a bitter aromatic burning taste. M.p. 68° to 70°.

Soluble 1 in 500 of water and 1 in 50 of boiling water; soluble in most organic solvents and in solutions of alkali hydroxides. **Protect** from light.

Uses. Coumarin is used as a fixative in perfumery. It has been used as a flavouring agent to mask unpleasant odours but this use is now considered undesirable.

It was recommended that coumarin be prohibited for use in foods as a flavouring agent.— *Food Standards Committee Report on Flavouring Agents*, London, HM Stationery Office, 1965.

After coumarin had been taken by mouth, 68 to 92% was excreted as 7-hydroxycoumarin and 1 to 6% as *o*-hydroxyphenylacetic acid during the following 24 hours.— W. H. Shilling *et al.* (letter), *Nature*, 1969, *221*, 664.

Further studies of the pharmacokinetics of coumarin and its metabolites: W. A. Ritschel *et al.*, *Eur. J. clin. Pharmac.*, 1977, *12*, 457; *idem*, *Int. J. clin. Pharmac. Biopharm.*, 1979, *17*, 99, per *Int. pharm. Abstr.*, 1979, *16*, 979.

2389-r

Cyclamic Acid *(B.P. 1968)*. Cyclam. Acid. *N*-Cyclohexylsulphamic acid.
$C_6H_{11}.NH.SO_2.OH$=179.2.

CAS — 100-88-9.

A white, odourless or almost odourless, crystalline powder with a taste which is acid at first and then sweet.

Soluble 1 in 7.5 of water, 1 in 3 of alcohol, 1 in 7 of acetone, 1 in 250 of chloroform, 1 in 12 of glycerol, and 1 in 4 of propylene glycol; practically insoluble in fixed oils. Solutions are strongly acid; a 10% solution in water has a pH of about 1.3. **Incompatible** with nitrites in acid solution; limited compatibility with potassium salts.

Stability. An acidic reaction in cyclamate-sweetened solutions of low dielectric constant should be avoided; the solutions should be buffered to at least 2 pH units above the apparent pK_a of cyclamate in the vehicle.— J. M. Talmage *et al.*, *J. pharm. Sci.*, 1968, *57*, 1073.

Uses. Cyclamic acid has similar properties and uses to those of sodium cyclamate. A 0.2% solution in water has the same tartness as a 0.35% solution of citric acid.

The use of cyclamic acid as an artificial sweetener in food or soft drinks or as an ingredient in artificial sweetening tablets is no longer permitted in Great Britain—see under Sodium Cyclamate, p.431.

For a temporary estimated acceptable daily intake of cyclamic acid, see Sodium Cyclamate, p.431.

2390-j

Dulcin. Phenetolurea. (4-Ethoxyphenyl)urea.
$C_9H_{12}N_2O_2$=180.2.

CAS — 150-69-6.

Pharmacopoeias. In *Span.*

Lustrous colourless crystals or a white crystalline powder with a very sweet taste. **Soluble** 1 in 800 of water, 1 in 50 of boiling water, and 1 in 25 of alcohol.

Uses. Dulcin is a synthetic sweetening agent and has been used in some countries as a substitute for sucrose, being about 250 times as sweet.

Dulcin should not be used as a food additive because of its tumorigenic potentialities.— Eleventh Report of the Joint FAO/WHO Expert Committee on Food Additives, *Tech. Rep. Ser. Wld Hlth Org. No. 383*, 1968.

2391-z

Eosin *(B.P.C. 1963)*. Eosin Y; Éosine Disodique; CI Acid Red 87; Colour Index No. 45380; D & C Red No. 22. The disodium salt of 2′,4′,5′,7′-tetrabromofluorescein.
$C_{20}H_6Br_4Na_2O_5$=691.9.

CAS — 548-26-5; 17372-87-1.

Pharmacopoeias. In *Fr.*

An odourless red crystalline powder. **Soluble** 1 in 3 of water and 1 in 50 of alcohol; practically insoluble in chloroform and ether. **Incompatible** with oxidising agents and acids. A solution in water is yellow to purplish-red with a greenish-yellow fluorescence.

Uses. Eosin has been incorporated in solution-tablets to give a distinctive colour to solutions prepared from them. It is a permitted colour in the USA for use in medicines.

Dermatitis due to lipstick containing eosin was observed in 38 patients. Impurities in the material might have been responsible. Eosin was bound to keratin so that patch testing with cosmetic preparations suspected of being responsible for allergic reactions was not satisfactory. The inclusion of 50% of eosin in a standard lipstick basis or in soft paraffin ensured that an adequate amount was applied for testing purposes.— E. Cronin, *J. Soc. cosmet. Chem.*, 1967, *18*, 681.

The administration or application of eosin could cause photosensitivity.— J. Kalivas, *J. Am. med. Ass.*, 1969, *209*, 1706.

Eosin was bound to serum proteins *in vitro*.— G. A. Lutty, *Toxic. appl. Pharmac.*, 1978, *44*, 225.

2392-c

Erythrosine. Erythrosine BS; Erythrosine Sodium *(U.S.P.)*; CI No. 45430; CI Food Red 14; F D & C Red No. 3. The monohydrate of the disodium salt of 2′,4′,5′,7′-tetraiodofluorescein.
$C_{20}H_6I_4Na_2O_5,H_2O$=897.9.

CAS — 568-63-8; 16423-68-0 (both anhydrous); 49746-10-3 (monohydrate).

Pharmacopoeias. In *Braz.* and *U.S. Fr.* permits disodium or dipotassium salts.

Red or brownish-red odourless hygroscopic powder containing not less than 87% of dye, calculated as $C_{20}H_6I_4Na_2O_5,H_2O$, together with smaller amounts of lower iodinated fluoresceins. **Soluble** in water forming a bluish-red solution that shows no fluorescence in ordinary light; sparingly soluble in alcohol; soluble in glycerol and propylene glycol; practically insoluble in fats and oils. **Store** in airtight containers.

For a report on the fading of erythrosine solutions in the presence of sodium metabisulphite, see under Fading in the Presence of Sulphite, p.423.

For a report of discoloration of tablets containing ethinyloestradiol, norethisterone, and erythrosine, see under Ethinyloestradiol, p.1411.

Effect of gamma-irradiation. Erythrosine was changed from a deep rose colour to a pale pink after irradiation.— *Drug Cosmet. Ind.*, 1973, *113* (Sept.), 136. Irradiation with 25 000 Gy had no effect on erythrosine.— B. -L. Chang *et al.*, *J. pharm. Sci.*, 1974, *63*, 758.

Adverse Effects.

A discussion on the phototoxicity of erythrosine and other colouring agents which have been proposed for use in angiography.— D. P. Valenzeno and J. P. Pooler, *J. Am. med. Ass.*, 1979, *242*, 453.

Precautions.

Erythrosine used to colour capsule shells pink contained sufficient iodine to raise the protein-bound iodine to hyperthyroid values (90 to 110 μg per litre) and depress iodine uptake in a patient taking lithium carbonate. Five subjects who took empty capsule shells for 6 weeks had significantly raised, but not abnormal, protein-bound iodine and iodine uptake was not altered.— S. Haas, *Ann. intern. Med.*, 1970, *72*, 549, per *Int. pharm. Abstr.*, 1970, *7*, 391.

Absorption and Fate.

Erythrosine was bound to serum proteins *in vitro*.— G. A. Lutty, *Toxic. appl. Pharmac.*, 1978, *44*, 225.

Uses. Erythrosine is a permitted colouring agent for medicines and foods in Great Britain, the EEC, and in the USA. It is also used as a disclosing agent for plaque on teeth.

Estimated acceptable daily intake: up to 2.5 mg per kg body-weight.— Eighteenth Report of the Joint FAO/WHO Expert Committee on Food Additives, *Tech. Rep. Ser. Wld Hlth Org. No. 557*, 1974.

Background toxicological information.— *Fd Add. Ser. Wld Hlth Org. No. 6*, 1975.

Preparations

Erythrosine Sodium Topical Solution *(U.S.P.)*. Erythrosine Sodium Solution. A solution of erythrosine in water containing one or more suitable flavours and preservatives. pH 6.8 to 8. Store in airtight containers. Protect from light.

Erythrosine Sodium Soluble Tablets *(U.S.P.)*. Tablets containing erythrosine. Store in airtight containers. Protect from light.

Proprietary Preparations

Ceplac *(Berk Pharmaceuticals, UK)*. Dental disclosing tablets containing erythrosine 6 mg.

En-De-Kay C-Red *(S.S. White, UK)*. Dental disclosing tablets containing erythrosine 2%.

Other Proprietary Names

Disclo *(Austral.)*; Plaquefärbetabletten *(Ger.)*.

2393-k

Ethyl Vanillin *(U.S.N.F.)*. 3-Ethoxy-4-hydroxybenzaldehyde.

$C_9H_{10}O_3$=166.2.

CAS — 121-32-4.

Pharmacopoeias. In *Fr.* Also in *U.S.N.F.*

Fine white or slightly yellowish crystals with a vanilla-like odour and taste. M.p. 76° to 78°. **Soluble** 1 in 100 of water at 50°; soluble 1 in 2 of alcohol; freely soluble in chloroform, ether, and solutions of alkali hydroxides. Solutions in water are acid to litmus. **Store** in airtight containers. Protect from light.

Uses. Ethyl vanillin is used as a flavouring agent and in perfumery to impart the odour and taste of vanilla. It has a finer and more intense odour than vanillin.

Estimated acceptable daily intake: up to 10 mg per kg body-weight.— Eleventh Report of the Joint FAO/WHO Expert Committee on Food Additives, *Tech. Rep. Ser. Wld Hlth Org. No. 383*, 1968.

Proprietary Preparations

Ethavan *(Monsanto, UK)*. A brand of ethyl vanillin.

The proprietary name Vanbeenol has been used in Great Britain by *Bush Boake Allen* for a brand of ethyl vanillin.

2394-a

Green S. Acid Brilliant Green BS; Acid Green S; Lissamine Green; Wool Green B; CI Food Green 4; Colour Index No. 44090. Sodium 1-[4-dimethylamino-α-(4-dimethyliminiocyclohexa-2,5-dienylidene)benzyl]-2-hydroxynaphthalene-3,6-disulphonate.

$C_{27}H_{25}N_2NaO_7S_2$=576.6.

CAS — 3087-16-9.

Soluble 1 in about 12 of water; very slightly soluble in alcohol; slightly soluble in glycerol. It produces bluish-green solutions. It has poor stability to light and alkalis.

Uses. Green S is a permitted colour in Great Britain and the EEC for use in medicines and foodstuffs. It is an ingredient of Green S and Tartrazine Solution (*B.P.*) and Green Solution (*A.P.F.*).

Background toxicological information.— *Fd Add. Ser. Wld Hlth Org. No. 6*, 1975.

Staining of the conjunctiva with Green S was found to be a reasonably specific but inadequately sensitive test for diagnosing early xerophthalmia.— N. Emran and A. Sommer, *Archs Ophthal., N.Y.*, 1979, *97*, 2333.

2395-t

Logwood *(B.P.C. 1949)*. Haematoxylum; CI Natural Black 1; Colour Index No. 75290.

CAS — 8005-33-2.

The unfermented heartwood of *Haematoxylon campechianum* (Leguminosae) containing about 10% of haematoxylin ($C_{16}H_{14}O_6,3H_2O$ = 356.3) with tannin, resin, and a trace of volatile oil. It is dull orange to purplish-red externally and reddish-brown internally. The fermented chips used by dyers are deep red in colour and the haematoxylin is oxidised to haematein ($C_{16}H_{12}O_6$ = 300.3). **Incompatible** with metallic salts, especially those of iron and mercury.

Uses. Logwood is principally used as a dye and extracts are used to colour nylon and silk sutures. Haematein and logwood extracts, in a variety of strengths and degrees of oxidation, are also used for dyeing furs, leather, and textiles, and in histology.

Logwood was formerly used as a mild astringent in diarrhoea.

2396-x

Orange G *(B.P.C. 1954)*. Novaurantia; CI Food Orange 4; Colour Index No. 16230. It consists mainly of disodium 7-hydroxy-8-phenylazonaphthalene-1,3-disulphonate.

$C_{16}H_{10}N_2Na_2O_7S_2$=452.4.

CAS — 1936-15-8.

A yellowish-red, almost odourless powder or crystalline leaflets with a saline taste. **Soluble** 1 in 6 of water, giving an orange-yellow solution; partly soluble in alcohol. A 1% solution in water has a pH of about 8.75. It is unaffected by acids and weak alkalis or, in neutral solution, by light.

Orange G may fade in the presence of some nonionic surfactants.— M. W. Scott *et al.*, *J. Am. pharm. Ass., scient. Edn*, 1960, *49*, 467.

For a report on the fading of Orange G solutions in the presence of sodium metabisulphite, see under Fading in the Presence of Sulphite, p.423.

Adverse Effects.

Allergic dermatitis in workers in a tractor factory was traced to Orange G contained in a rust preventitive oil. Using a colourless oil there were no relapses or new cases.— J. Prout, *Proc. R. Soc. Med.*, 1973, *66*, 261, per *Int. pharm. Abstr.*, 1973, *10*, 841.

Uses. Orange G has been used as a colouring agent for food and medicines but it is not a permitted colour for these uses in Great Britain, the EEC, and the USA.

2397-r

Ponceau 4R. Cochineal Red A; Brilliant Scarlet; Brilliant Ponceau 4RC; Coccine Nouvelle; Rouge Cochenille A; CI Food Red 7; Colour Index No. 16255. Trisodium 7-hydroxy-8-(4-sulphonato-1-naphthylazo)naphthalene-1,3-disulphonate.

$C_{20}H_{11}N_2Na_3O_{10}S_3$=604.4.

CAS — 2611-82-7.

Pharmacopoeias. In *Fr.*

Bright scarlet-red to dark red odourless powder or granules. **Soluble** 1 in about 7 of water; slightly soluble in alcohol; sparingly soluble in glycerol; practically insoluble in vegetable oils.

For a report on the fading of ponceau 4R solutions in the presence of sodium metabisulphite, see under Fading in the Presence of Sulphite, p.423.

Uses. Ponceau 4R is a permitted colour in Great Britain and the EEC for use in medicines and foods.

Temporary estimated acceptable daily intake of ponceau 4R: up to 125 μg per kg body-weight. Metabolic, long-term, and reproduction studies are underway.— Twenty-second Report of the Joint FAO/WHO Expert Committee on Food Additives, *Tech. Rep. Ser. Wld Hlth Org. No. 631*, 1978.

Background toxicological information.— *Fd Add. Ser. Wld Hlth Org. No. 6*, 1975.

Hypersensitivity. For reports of hypersensitivity to ponceau 4R and cross-sensitivity with other azo dyes, aspirin and benzoates, see under Hypersensitivity in Tartrazine, p.431.

2398-f

Quinoline Yellow. Jaune De Quinoléine; Canary Yellow; CI Food Yellow 13; CI Acid Yellow 3; D & C Yellow No. 10; CI No. 47005. The sodium salts of a mixture of the mono- and disulphonic acids (mainly the latter) of quinophthalone or 2-(2-quinolyl)indanedione.

CAS — 8004-92-0.

Pharmacopoeias. In *Fr.*

A dull yellow to greenish-yellow powder or granules. **Soluble** in water. A 0.1% solution is lemon yellow.

Effect of gamma-irradiation. Irradiation with 25 000 Gy had no effect on quinoline yellow.— B. -L. Chang *et al.*, *J. pharm. Sci.*, 1974, *63*, 758.

Uses. Quinoline yellow is a permitted colour in Great Britain and the EEC for use in medicines and foodstuffs. In the USA it is not permitted for use in foodstuffs.

Temporary estimated acceptable daily intake of quinoline yellow: up to 500 μg per kg body-weight. Further studies are required, including metabolic studies in man.— Twenty-second Report of the Joint FAO/WHO Expert Committee on Food Additives, *Tech. Rep. Ser. Wld Hlth Org. No. 631*, 1978.

Background toxicological information.— *Fd Add. Ser. Wld Hlth Org. No. 6*, 1975; *ibid.*, *No. 8*, 1975..

2399-d

Raspberry. Rubus Idaeus; Fructus Rubi Idaei; Framboise; Himbeer. The fresh ripe fruit of *Rubus idaeus* (Rosaceae).

CAS — 8027-46-1.

Pharmacopoeias. In *Arg.*

Uses. Raspberry is used as a colouring and flavouring agent in medicines and foodstuffs.

Preparations

Concentrated Raspberry Juice *(B.P.)*. Prepared from raspberry juice from which the pectin has been removed by the action of pectinase and subsequent clarification, adding to it sufficient sucrose to adjust the wt per ml at 20° to 1.05 to 1.06 g, then concentrating the juice to one-sixth of its original volume and adding sodium metabisulphite or other suitable antimicrobial preservative. Wt per ml 1.30 to 1.36 g. It contains not more than 4700 ppm w/w of SO_2. Store at a temperature not exceeding 25°. Protect from light.

One vol. diluted with 5 vol. of water yields a product equivalent to natural raspberry juice.

Raspberry Syrup *(B.P.)*. Syrupus Rubi Idaei; Syr. Rubi Idaei. Prepared by diluting 1 vol. of Concentrated Raspberry Juice with 11 vol. of syrup. It may contain permitted food-grade colours. It should be freshly prepared, but if it is prepared with precautions which will prevent fermentation, it may be recently prepared when it should be used within 4 weeks of opening the container. Sulphur dioxide content not more than 420 ppm w/w. Wt per ml 1.31 to 1.34 g. Store at a temperature not exceeding 25°. Protect from light. It is intended only for flavouring purposes. If it is used for other purposes it may not comply with food regulations for sulphur dioxide content.

2400-d

Red 2G. Acid Red 1; CI Food Red 10; Ext. D & C Red No. 11; Geranine 2G; Colour Index No. 18050. Disodium 5-acetamido-4-hydroxy-3-phenylazonaphthalene-2,7-disulphonate.
$C_{18}H_{13}N_3Na_2O_8S_2$=509.4.

CAS — 3734-67-6.

Red powder or granules. **Soluble** 1 in about 6 of water; slightly soluble in alcohol; sparingly soluble in glycerol; practically insoluble in isopropyl alcohol and vegetable oils.

Uses. Red 2G is a permitted colour in Great Britain and the EEC for use in foodstuffs.

Temporary estimated acceptable daily intake for Red 2G: up to 6 µg per kg body-weight. Multigeneration reproduction/teratology studies and studies on the bone marrow to elucidate the toxic effects on erythropoiesis were required.— Twenty-third Report of the Joint FAO/WHO Expert Committee on Food Additives, *Tech. Rep. Ser. Wld Hlth Org. No. 648,* 1980.

2401-n

Red Cherry. Cerasus; Griottier; Ginja; Cerise Rouge.

Pharmacopoeias. In *Port.*

The fresh ripe fruit of varieties of the red or sour cherry, *Prunus cerasus* (Rosaceae).

Uses. Red cherry is used as a colouring and flavouring agent.

Preparations

Cherry Juice *(U.S.N.F.).* The juice expressed from the fresh ripe fruit of *P. cerasus,* and containing not less than 1% of malic acid. pH 3 to 4. Store at a temperature not exceeding 40° in airtight containers. Protect from light.

Cherry Syrup *(U.S.N.F.).* Cherry juice 47.5 ml, sucrose 80 g, alcohol 2 ml, water to 100 ml. Store at a temperature not exceeding 40° in airtight containers. Protect from light.

2402-h

Red-Poppy Petal *(B.P.C. 1949).* Rhoeados Petalum; Rhoead. Pet.; Coquelicot; Klatschrose; Petalos de Amapola.

Pharmacopoeias. In *Arg., Belg., Fr., Port.,* and *Span.*

The dried petals of *Papaver rhoeas* (Papaveraceae). **Store** in a cool place, in airtight containers. Protect from light.

Uses. Red-poppy petal has been used in the form of Red-Poppy Syrup as a colouring and sweetening agent for mixtures.

Preparations

Red-Poppy Syrup *(B.P.C. 1949).* Syr. Rhoead. To 40 ml of hot water on a water-bath add gradually red-poppy petal 5.2 g, stirring frequently; remove the vessel from the water-bath and infuse for 12 hours; strain, dissolve sucrose 72.5 g in the infusion using gentle heat, cool, add alcohol (90%) 5 ml, and dilute to 100 ml with water. *Dose.* 2 to 4 ml.

2403-m

Red-Rose Petal *(B.P.C. 1949).* Rosae Petalum; Ros. Pet.; Red Rose Petals; Flos Rosae; Rosae Gallicae Petala; Fleur de Rose; Rosenblüte.

Pharmacopoeias. In *Arg., Fr.,* and *Port. Port.* and *Span.* also include the petals of the cabbage rose, *R. centifolia.*

The petals of the red or Provins rose, *Rosa gallica* (Rosaceae). **Store** in airtight containers in a cool place. Protect from light.

Uses. Red-rose petal has been employed, usually as the acid infusion, for its mild astringent properties and as a colouring agent.

Preparations

Concentrated Acid Infusion of Rose *(B.P.C. 1949).* Inf. Ros. Acid. Conc. Prepared from red-rose petal 20 g, dilute sulphuric acid 10 ml, alcohol (90%) 25 ml, and chloroform water 95 ml. The red-rose petal is macerated with the chloroform water and the resulting liquid is heated to boiling and cooled; the other ingredients are then added and the product is allowed to stand for not less than 14 days before filtering. It is approximately 8 times the strength of the fresh infusion. *Dose.* 2 to 4 ml.

Fresh Acid Infusion of Rose *(B.P.C. 1949).* Inf. Ros. Acid. Rec. Red-rose petal 2.5 g, boiling water 100 g, and dilute sulphuric acid 1.25 ml; infused for 15 minutes and strained. *Dose.* 15 to 30 ml.

2404-b

Saccharin *(B.P., U.S.N.F.).* Benzosulphimide; Gluside; Sacarina; Saccarina; Zaharina. 1,2-Benzisothiazolin-3-one 1,1-dioxide.
$C_7H_5NO_3S$=183.2.

CAS — 81-07-2.

Pharmacopoeias. In *Arg., Br., Fr., Hung., It., Pol., Port., Roum., Span.,* and *Swiss.* Also in *U.S.N.F.*

White odourless or faintly aromatic crystals or crystalline powder with an intensely sweet taste. M.p. 226° to 230°.
Soluble 1 in 290 of water, 1 in 25 of boiling water, 1 in 12 of acetone, 1 in 30 of alcohol, and 1 in 50 of glycerol; slightly soluble in chloroform and ether; readily soluble in dilute ammonia solution and in solutions of alkali hydroxides and, with the evolution of carbon dioxide, in solutions of alkali bicarbonates and carbonates. A saturated solution in water is acid to litmus.

Adverse Effects. Photosensitisation or sensitivity reactions have been attributed to saccharin on rare occasions.

No correlation was shown between the consumption of saccharin during pregnancy and the incidence of spontaneous abortion.— J. Kline *et al., Am. J. Obstet. Gynec.,* 1978, *130,* 708.

Carcinogenic risk. Discussions on the association between the use of artificial sweeteners and bladder cancer: W. L. Pines and N. Glick, *FDA Consumer,* 1977, (May), 10; K. J. Isselbacher and P. Cole, *New Engl. J. Med.,* 1977, *296,* 1348; *Med. Lett.,* 1977, *19,* 75; R. Hoover, *New Engl. J. Med.,* 1980, *302,* 573; *Lancet,* 1980, *1,* 855.

Experiments in *rats* had indicated that tumours of the bladder could be produced by giving 5% of saccharin in the diet over 2 years (equivalent to 175 g daily for life in man). Subsequently in the USA, the Food and Drug Administration (FDA) had recommended that adult intake of saccharin should be limited to 1 g daily (*J. Am. med. Ass.,* 1971, *217,* 412; *ibid.,* 1972, *219,* 990). A study by the FDA using 7.5% of saccharin and a further study by M.O. Tisdel *et al.* (in *Symposium: Sweeteners,* G.E. Inglett (Ed.), Westport, AVI, 1974, p. 145) supported the earlier findings. Further experiments in *rats* (R.M. Hicks *et al., Nature,* 1973, *243,* 347 and 424) suggested that a contaminant of commercial saccharin, *o*-toluene sulphonamide (OTS), might account for co-carcinogenic effects. However, a Canadian study from 1974 to 1977 using pure saccharin and OTS indicated that OTS did not itself produce bladder tumours in the *rat* as bladder tumours were still produced in *rats* fed saccharin free from OTS. The study also raised questions about the safety of using saccharin during pregnancy as *rats* exposed to saccharin *in utero* and during their lifetime developed more malignant tumours (*Science,* 1977, *196,* 276; *ibid.,* 1179; *ibid., 197,* 320). Epidemiological studies by B. Armstrong and R. Doll. (*Br. J. prev. soc. Med.,* 1974, *28,* 233 and *ibid.,* 1975, *29,* 73) and I.I. Kessler (*J. Urol.,* 1976, *115,* 143) had found no evidence in man that saccharin increased the risk of bladder cancer or any other types of cancer (B. Armstrong *et al. Br. J. prev. soc. Med.,* 1976, *30,* 151) but these studies were considered by some (*Med. Lett.,* 1977, *19,* 75; K.J. Isselbacher and P. Cole, *New Engl. J. Med.,* 1977, *296,* 1348) to be too small to detect the degree of increased risk suggested by the *rat* studies. A report from Canada by G.R. Howe *et al.,* (*Lancet,* 1977, *2,* 578) indicated that male users of artificial sweeteners (mainly saccharin) showed a 60% excess of bladder cancer compared to non-users. However the study was considered to have had many shortcomings (*Lancet,* 1977, *2,* 592; A.B. Miller and G.R. Howe (letter), *ibid.,* 1221; *idem,* 1978, *1,* 514). An epidemiological study in the USA by R.N. Hoover and P.H. Strasser (*Lancet,* 1980, *1,* 837) concluded that past artificial sweetener use had had a minimal effect, if any, on rates of bladder cancer. Similar findings had been obtained by A.S. Morrison and J.E. Buring (*New Engl. J. Med.,* 1980, *302,* 537) and by E.L. Wynder and S.D. Stellman (*Science,* 1980, *207,* 1214). It was also concluded that positive associations found in the study by R.N. Hoover and P.H. Strasser, did not by themselves establish a causal link between artificial sweetener use and bladder cancer, but nevertheless, it was noteworthy that the pattern of positive associations was consistent with experimental data suggesting that artificial sweeteners are weakly carcinogenic when given alone, and enhancing when given with other carcinogens.

Animal studies: D. L. Arnold *et al., Toxic. appl. Pharmac.,* 1977, *41,* 164 (*rats*); E. W. McChesney *et al., ibid (monkeys)*; J. M. Taylor *et al., ibid.,* 1980, *54,* 57 (*rats*).

A report by the National Academy of Sciences Committee for a Study on Saccharin and Food Safety Policy concluded that saccharin was a carcinogen, but one of low potency relative to other cancer-producing agents. It was considered to cause bladder cancer in male *rats* and to be most effective in producing cancer when the mother is exposed before pregnancy, the foetus is exposed throughout gestation, and the exposure continues throughout the life of the offspring. It also enhanced the carcinogenic effects of other agents in *rats.*— M. Dolan, *Am. Pharm.,* 1979, *NS19* (Jan.), 54.

Further references: A. Beringer, *Wien. med. Wschr.,* 1973, *123,* 41, per *Int. pharm. Abstr.,* 1974, *11,* 52; S. C. Crocco, *J. Am. med. Ass.,* 1978, *239,* 2035; I. I. Kessler and J. P. Clark, *ibid., 240,* 349; Twenty-first Report of the Joint FAO/WHO Expert Committee on Food Additives, *Tech. Rep. Ser. Wld Hlth Org. No. 617,* 1978; E. K. Yucel (letter), *New Engl. J. Med.,* 1980, *303,* 341; D. Ozonoff (letter), *ibid.;* A. S. Morrison (letter), *ibid.,* 342.

Hypersensitivity. Urticaria occurred in a woman following the ingestion of food containing saccharin.— R. Miller *et al., J. Allergy & clin. Immunol.,* 1974, *53,* 240.

Photosensitivity. Erythema of the face due to photosensitivity caused by saccharin was reported in a patient.— H. J. Kingsley (letter), *Cent. Afr. J. Med.,* 1966, *12,* 243.

Absorption and Fate. Saccharin is readily absorbed from the gastro-intestinal tract. It is almost all excreted unchanged in the urine within 24 to 48 hours.

References: E. W. McChesney and L. Golberg, *Toxic. appl. Pharmac.,* 1973, *25,* 494; W. A. Colburn *et al., Clin. Pharmac. Ther.,* 1981, *30,* 558.

Uses. Saccharin is a synthetic sweetening agent. It is usually considered to have about 550 times the sweetening power of sucrose but this depends to some extent on the strength of solution used, the relative sweetening power being greatest in dilute solution.

Saccharin is used as a substitute for sucrose in diabetes, obesity, and generally where the use of sucrose is undesirable. It has no food value. It is commonly employed in the form of saccharin sodium which is more palatable and comparatively free from the unpleasant after-taste of saccharin; the average amount required is about 1 in 10 000.

In the USA it has been recommended that daily intake should not exceed 1 g.

Under the Soft Drinks Regulations 1964 (SI 1964: No. 760) and the Soft Drinks (Scotland) Regulations 1964 (SI 1964: No. 767) saccharin (including saccharin calcium and saccharin sodium) is a permitted artificial sweetener for soft drinks in Great Britain; it may be used up to a specified maximum proportion together with a specified minimum proportion of added sugar in soft drinks other than those intended for use by diabetics. The Soft Drinks (Amendment) Regulations 1969 (SI 1969: No. 1818) require that any permitted artificial sweetener should be declared on the label.

Under the Artificial Sweeteners in Food Regulations 1969 (SI 1969: No. 1817) saccharin, saccharin calcium, and saccharin sodium are permitted artificial sweeteners in England and Wales for use in the preparation of food, and the composition of tablets containing permitted artificial sweeteners is specified.

The mucociliary function of the Eustachian tube was assessed in 44 patients with dry perforations of the tympanic membrane by placing a saccharin crystal on the mucous membrane of the middle ear and determining the time taken for the patient to taste the saccharin. Although no correlation was found between the results of the saccharin test, an aspiration test, and the Valsalva manoeuvre, the saccharin test was considered to provide adequate information on the mucociliary function and patency of the Eustachian tube.— O. Elbrønd and E. Larsen, *Archs Otolar.*, 1976, *102*, 539.

Temporary estimated acceptable daily intake of saccharin potassium and saccharin sodium: up to 2.5 mg per kg body-weight. Further work required included detailed carcinogenicity and embryotoxicity studies and the initiation of prospective epidemiological studies in high-risk populations.— Twenty-first Report of the Joint FAO/WHO Expert Committee on Food Additives, *Tech. Rep. Ser. Wld Hlth Org. No. 617*, 1978.

The Hornblass saccharin test was found to be more practical and reliable in assessing lachrymal excretory function than the primary Jones fluorescein test, the fluorescein dye disappearance test, and the Schirmer secretory test. In the saccharin test a 2% solution of saccharin was instilled into the inferior conjunctival cul-de-sac and the patient reported when the saccharin could be tasted.— A. Hornblass and T. M. Ingis, *Archs Ophthal., N.Y.*, 1979, *97*, 1654.

For the use of saccharin for the determination of circulation time, see under Saccharin Sodium.

2405-v

Saccharin Calcium *(U.S.P.)*. Calcium Saccharin; Calcium Benzosulphimide. The hydrate of the calcium salt of 1,2-benzisothiazolin-3-one 1,1-dioxide.

$C_{14}H_8CaN_2O_6S_2,3\frac{1}{2}H_2O$=467.5.

CAS — 6485-34-3 (anhydrous); 6381-91-5 (hydrate).

Pharmacopoeias. In *U.S.*

White odourless or faintly aromatic crystals or crystalline powder with an intensely sweet taste. **Soluble** 1 in about 2.5 of water and 1 in about 5 of alcohol.

Saccharin calcium has similar properties and uses to those of saccharin.

Subject to certain conditions, the use of saccharin calcium as an artificial sweetener for soft drinks and for use in the preparation of food is permitted in Great Britain—see under Saccharin.

2406-g

Saccharin Sodium *(B.P., U.S.P.)*. Saccharin Sod.; Sodium Saccharin; Sodium Benzosulphimide; Soluble Gluside; Soluble Saccharin; Saccharinnatrium; Saccharoidum Natricum. The dihydrate of the sodium salt of 1,2-benzisothiazolin-3-one 1,1-dioxide.

$C_7H_4NNaO_3S,2H_2O$=241.2.

CAS — 128-44-9 (anhydrous); 6155-57-3 (dihydrate).

Pharmacopoeias. In *Arg., Aust., Br., Fr., Ger., Hung., Ind., Jap., Jug., Mex., Neth., Nord., Port., Span., Swiss, Turk.,* and *U.S.* Most pharmacopoeias including *U.S.* specify $2H_2O$ usually with a loss on drying of about 12 to 16%. *Br.* specifies a loss of 3 to 15% on drying.

White efflorescent crystals or a white, odourless or faintly aromatic, crystalline powder with an intensely sweet taste. **Soluble** 1 in 1.5 of water and 1 in 50 of alcohol; practically insoluble in chloroform and ether. A 10% solution is neutral or alkaline to litmus but produces no red colour with phenolphthalein. Solutions are **sterilised** by autoclaving. **Store** in airtight containers.

Adverse Effects. As for Saccharin, above.

Uses. Saccharin sodium has similar properties and uses to those of saccharin. It is usually used as tablets or solution. In dilute solution it is about 300 times as sweet as sucrose.

It has also been used to determine the arm-to-tongue circulation time in patients with cardiac disease. A solution of 2.5 g in 5 ml of warm water is rapidly injected into the median basilic vein of the arm held level with the heart, and the time-lapse between the injection and the first perception of a sweet taste in the mouth is noted.

Subject to certain conditions, the use of saccharin sodium as an artificial sweetener for soft drinks and for use in the preparation of food is permitted in Great Britain—see under Saccharin.

Estimated acceptable daily intake: as for Saccharin (above).

The normal circulation time measured using the saccharin method is between 9 and 16 seconds. The circulation time is prolonged in the presence of cardiac failure sometimes up to 45 seconds or more.— F. P. Duras, *Lancet*, 1944, *1*, 303.

Administration of saccharin sodium in a dose of 50 mg in 80 ml of water caused a decrease of 12 to 16% in the blood-sugar concentration of normal persons. Administration of the saccharin in 4 portions during a 40-minute period increased the duration of hypoglycaemia.— H. Kun and I. Horwath, *Proc. Soc. exp. Biol. Med.*, 1947, *66*, 288, per *J. Am. med. Ass.*, 1948, *136*, 502.

Preparations

Saccharin Sodium Oral Solution *(U.S.P.)*. A solution containing saccharin sodium. pH 3 to 5. Store in airtight containers.

Saccharin Sodium Tablets *(U.S.P.)*. Tablets containing saccharin sodium.

Saccharin Solution *(B.P.C. 1954)*. Liq. Saccharin.; Elixir of Saccharin; Elixir Glusidi. Saccharin sodium 7.31 g, alcohol (90%) 12.5 ml, water to 100 ml. The addition of about 1% of this solution is suitable for sweetening most liquid preparations.

Saccharin Tablets *(B.P.C. 1973)*. Prepared from a mixture of saccharin and sodium bicarbonate or from saccharin sodium.

2407-q

Saffron *(Eur. P., B.P.C. 1949)*. Crocus; Croci Stigma; Safran; Estigmas de Azafrán; Azafrán; Açafrão; CI Natural Yellow 6; Colour Index No. 75100.

Pharmacopoeias. In *Arg., Aust., Belg., Eur., Fr., Ger., Jap., Jug., Mex., Neth., Port., Roum., Span.,* and *Swiss.*

The dried stigmas and tops of the styles of *Crocus sativus* (Iridaceae), containing crocines, crocetins, and picrocrocine. **Protect** from light.

Adverse Effects. Early reports indicate that the chief toxic symptoms following poisoning with saffron are flushing of the face, epistaxis, vertigo, vomiting, and bradycardia. Profuse metrorrhagia and menorrhagia may occur. Abortion occurs rarely.

References: P. Fasal and G. Wachner, *Wien. klin. Wschr.*, 1933, *45*, 747.

Uses. Saffron is used as a food dye and flavouring agent. It was once widely used, as a glycerin, syrup, and tincture, for colouring medicines but it has largely been replaced for this purpose by solutions of sunset yellow FCF and tartrazine.

Preparations

Teinture de Safran *(Belg. P., Fr. P.)*. Saffron 1 in 10 of alcohol. Prepared by maceration. *Belg. P.* specifies alcohol 60% and *Fr. P.* specifies alcohol 80%.

2408-p

Sarsaparilla *(B.P.C. 1949)*. Sarsa; Sarsaparilla Root; Salsepareille; Salsaparilha; Smilacis Rhizoma.

Pharmacopoeias. In *Belg., Chin., Jap.,* and *Port. Chin.* and *Jap.* specify *Smilax glabra.*

The dried root of various species of *Smilax* (Liliaceae). It is almost odourless and has a mucilaginous, somewhat sweetish and acrid taste.

Uses. Sarsaparilla, usually in the form of a decoction or extract, has been used as a vehicle and flavouring agent for medicaments.

Leprosy. Sarsaparilla has been traditionally used by Moroccans in treating leprosy, and extracts of *Smilax ornata* have been reported to be effective adjuncts to dapsone therapy.— R. Rollier, *Int. J. Lepr.*, 1959, *27*, 328, per *Lepr. Rev.*, 1960, *31*, 215.

Preparations

Concentrated Compound Sarsaparilla Decoction *(B.P.C. 1949)*. Decoctum Sarsae Compositum Concentratum. Infuse at 70° for one hour sarsaparilla 100 g with water 500 ml at 70°; repeat the infusion twice with similar quantities of water. Exhaust, by boiling with water, guaiacum wood 10 g, and liquorice 10 g. Mix the 3 infusions with the decoction and rapidly evaporate to 75 ml; add sassafras oil 0.05 ml dissolved in alcohol (90%) 22.5 ml, set aside for 14 days, filter, and pour sufficient water over the filter to produce 100 ml.

Sarsaparilla Liquid Extract *(B.P. 1898)*. Extractum Sarsae Liquidum. 1 in 1; prepared by percolation with alcohol (20%), glycerol (10% v/v) being added when adjusting to final volume.

Proprietary Names

Sarsapsor Bürger *(Ysatfabrik, Ger.)*.

2409-s

Sodium Cyclamate *(B.P. 1968)*. Sod. Cyclam.; Sodium Cyclohexanesulphamate; Cyclamate Sodium. Sodium *N*-cyclohexylsulphamate.

$C_6H_{12}NNaO_3S$=201.2.

CAS — 139-05-9.

Pharmacopoeias. In *Neth., Roum.,* and *Swiss.*

White odourless or almost odourless crystals or crystalline powder with an intensely sweet taste, even in dilute solution.

Soluble 1 in 5 of water, 1 in 250 of alcohol, and 1 in 25 of propylene glycol; practically insoluble in chloroform and ether. A 10% solution in water has a pH of 5.5 to 7.5. Solutions are stable to heat throughout the pH range of 2 to 10. **Incompatible** with nitrites in acid solution; limited compatibility with potassium salts.

Adverse Effects and Precautions. In large doses sodium cyclamate causes softness of the stools and an excessive intake may produce diarrhoea. Photosensitisation has been reported. The absorption of lincomycin is reduced by cyclamates.

Chromosome breaks had been induced in human cells, in both white-cell and monolayer cultures, *in vitro*, by sodium and calcium cyclamates in a concentration of 200 µg per ml.— D. Stone *et al.*, *Science*, 1969, *164*, 568.

Studies in 50 women [age not stated] who had ingested artificial sweeteners during pregnancy showed that 29 had given birth to offspring with Down's syndrome. The overall incidence of behavioural problems was 5.4% (10) in the offspring of 185 mothers taking artificial sweeteners and 2% (16) in offspring of 790 mothers who did not take artificial sweeteners. Physical anomalies occurred in 4.4% of offspring of non-users and 9.7% in those of users.— D. Stone *et al.* (letter), *Nature*, 1971, *231*, 53.

Carcinogenic risks. The US Food and Drug Administration had officially acknowledged that the 2 studies which led to the cyclamate ban (J.M. Price *et al.*, *Science*, 1970, *167*, 1131; L. Friedman *et al.*, *J. natn. Cancer Inst.*, 1972, *49*, 751) were unsuitable as studies of carcinogenicity. They had stated that there were too many variables in the first study to permit the incrimination of cyclamates as the cause of tumorogenic response and that the role of cyclamates as carcinogens in the second study was doubtful.— C. E. A. Cook, *Curr. med. Res. Opinion*, 1975, *3*, 218.

A discussion on the possible carcinogenic properties of cyclamates and the FDA ban on cyclamates.— T. H. Jukes, *J. Am. med. Ass.*, 1976, *236*, 1987.

Transitional cell neoplasms and multiple tumours in the bladder were reported in 3 men who had consumed sodium cyclamate 40 mg to 75 mg per kg body-weight daily regularly for from 18 months to 6 years.— M. Barkin *et al.*, *J. Urol.*, 1977, *118*, 258.

For epidemiological studies of the association between the use of artificial sweeteners and the development of bladder cancer, see under Carcinogenic Risks in Saccharin, p.429.

Animal studies. Studies of the carcinogenicity of cyclamates in *animals* with negative results: D. Schmähl, *Arzneimittel-Forsch.*, 1973, *23*, 1466; F. Coulston *et al.*, *Toxic. appl. Pharmac.*, 1977, *41*, 164. See also Eighteenth Report of the FAO/WHO Expert Committee on Food Additives, *Tech. Rep. Ser. Wld Hlth Org. No. 557*, 1974.

Photosensitivity. Reports of photosensitivity due to cyclamates.— T. Kobori and H. Araki, *J. Asthma Res.*, 1966, *3*, 213, per *Br. J. Derm.*, 1968, *80*, 200; S. I. Lamberg, *J. Am. med. Ass.*, 1967, *201*, 747; J. M. Yong and K. V. Sanderson, *Lancet*, 1969, *2*, 1273.

Absorption and Fate. Sodium and calcium cyclamate and cyclamic acid are incompletely absorbed from the gastro-intestinal tract. Some cyclamate is excreted in the urine. Between 10% and 30% of people may metabolise cyclamates to cyclohexylamine which is then in turn excreted in the urine. The amount of cyclohexylamine converted varies greatly between individuals and at different times. This variability may be related to changes in gut flora.

A review of the metabolism of cyclamates.— R. T. Williams, *Ann. N.Y. Acad. Sci.*, 1971, *179*, 141.

Cyclohexylamine was detected in the urine of 1 of 5 healthy subjects given sodium cyclamate in a dose of 3 g on each of 3 consecutive days. The metabolite represented about 0.8% of the dose of cyclamate administered. During the study the total urinary excretion of cyclamate ranged from about 70 to 490 mg daily.— J. S. Leahy *et al.* (letter), *B.I.B.R.A. Inf. Bull.*, 1966, *5*, 669.

Further references: T. R. Davis *et al.*, *Toxic. appl. Pharmac.*, 1969, *15*, 106; M. H. Litchfield and A. A. Swan, *ibid.*, 1971, *18*, 535.

Pregnancy and the neonate. A study of the distribution of cyclamates given during pregnancy.— R. M. Pitkin *et al.*, *Am. J. Obstet. Gynec.*, 1970, *108*, 1043.

The amount of sodium cyclamate excreted in the milk of lactating mothers was too small to affect the child.— T. E. O'Brien, *Am. J. Hosp. Pharm.*, 1974, *31*, 844.

Uses. Sodium cyclamate is a synthetic sweetening agent. In dilute solutions (up to about 0.17%) sodium cyclamate is about 30 times as sweet as sugar but this factor decreases at higher concentrations. When the concentration approaches 0.5%, a bitter taste becomes noticeable.

Sodium cyclamate has been used as a substitute for sucrose by diabetics and others needing to restrict their intake of carbohydrates but its use as an artificial sweetener in food, soft drinks, and artificial sweetening tablets is no longer permitted in Great Britain and in many other countries as little is known of the chronic toxicity of its metabolite cyclohexylamine.

Temporary estimated acceptable daily intake of sodium or calcium cyclamate: up to 4 mg, as cyclamic acid, per kg body-weight. The following studies were required: 1) determination of the no-effect level for cyclohexylamine (CHA) -induced embryotoxicity in the *mouse* 2) determination of the effect of dose on the degree of cyclamate absorption before conversion to CHA; 3) more precise identification of the no-effect level for CHA effects on *rat* testes; and 4) more precise identification in humans of the amount of cyclamate converted to CHA in the gastro-intestinal tract.— Twenty-first Report of the Joint FAO/WHO Expert Committee on Food Additives, *Tech. Rep. Ser. Wld Hlth Org. No. 617*, 1978.

Comparative sweetening power. Sodium cyclamate was compared with saccharin sodium and sucrose as a sweetening agent for pharmaceutical preparations by means of a tasting panel of 30 members. The results suggested that to obtain similar degrees of sweetness in liquid preparations having a pleasantly flavoured basis or consisting of a bitter substance in simple suspension the ratio of concentrations of sucrose, sodium cyclamate, and saccharin sodium was approximately 118:2:1, and for preparations containing a bitter principle in solution 110:1.75:1. The advantages of sodium cyclamate were its 'clean' sweet taste and freedom from the 'off-taste' characteristic of saccharin sodium.— L. G. Brookes, *Pharm. J.*, 1962, *2*, 569.

Proprietary Names

Sucaryl Sodium *(Abbott, Canad.)*; Sucrum 7 *(Lelong, Fr.)*.

2410-h

Sunset Yellow FCF. Jaune Orangé S; Jaune Soleil; CI Food Yellow 3; Orange Yellow S; FD & C Yellow No. 6; Colour Index No. 15985. Disodium 6-hydroxy-5-(4-sulphonatophenylazo)naphthalene-2-sulphonate. $C_{16}H_{10}N_2Na_2O_7S_2$=452.4.

CAS — 2783-94-0.

Pharmacopoeias. In *Fr.*

Orange-red powder or granules. **Soluble** 1 in about 8 of water; slightly soluble in alcohol; sparingly soluble in glycerol; practically insoluble in isopropyl alcohol.

Effect of gamma-irradiation. Irradiation with 25 000 Gy had no effect on sunset yellow FCF.— B. -L. Chang *et al.*, *J. pharm. Sci.*, 1974, *63*, 758.

Uses. Sunset yellow FCF is a permitted colour in Great Britain, the EEC, and the USA for use in foods and medicines. It is an ingredient of Compound Tartrazine Solution (*B.P.*).

Hypersensitivity. For reports of hypersensitivity to sunset yellow FCF and cross-sensitivity with other azo dyes, aspirin, and benzoates, see under Hypersensitivity in Tartrazine, p.431.

2411-m

Tartrazine *(B.P.C. 1954)*. Tartrazin.; Tartrazol Yellow; Jaune Tartrique; CI Food Yellow 4; Colour Index No. 19140; F D & C Yellow No. 5. It consists mainly of trisodium 5-hydroxy-1-(4-sulphonatophenyl)-4-(4-sulphonatophenylazo)pyrazole-3-carboxylate. $C_{16}H_9N_4Na_3O_9S_2$=534.4.

CAS — 1934-21-0.

Pharmacopoeias. In *Fr.*

An orange-yellow powder. **Soluble 1** in 6 of water, giving a golden-yellow solution; slightly soluble in alcohol; practically insoluble in vegetable oils. It is unaffected by acids and weak alkalis or, in neutral solution, by light.

It may fade in the presence of some nonionic surfactants.— M. W. Scott *et al.*, *J. Am. pharm. Ass., scient. Edn*, 1960, *49*, 467.

For a report on the fading of tartrazine solutions in the presence of sodium metabisulphite, see under Fading in the Presence of Sulphite, p.423.

Effect of gamma-irradiation. Irradiation with 25 000 Gy had no effect of tartrazine.— B. -L. Chang *et al.*, *J. pharm. Sci.*, 1974, *63*, 758.

Adverse Effects. Hypersensitivity reactions to tartrazine have been frequently reported. Up to 20% of patients with hypersensitivity to aspirin are also sensitive to tartrazine. Adverse effects following ingestion of preparations containing tartrazine have included acute bronchospasm, urticaria, rhinitis, blurred vision, and angioneurotic oedema. Anaphylactic shock and non-thrombocytopenic purpura have been reported.

Discussions and reviews of adverse reactions to tartrazine: M. S. Cohon, *Drug Intell. & clin. Pharm.*, 1975, *9*, 198; G. A. Settipane, *Compreh. Ther.*, 1977, *3*, 15; *Drug & Ther. Bull.*, 1980, *18*, 53.

Hypersensitivity. Administration of tartrazine 50 mg by mouth to 122 patients with a variety of allergic disorders produced the following reactions: general weakness, flushing, palpitations, blurred vision, rhinorrhoea, feeling of suffocation, pruritus, urticaria and angioneurotic oedema.— I. Neuman *et al.*, *Clin. Allergy*, 1978, *8*, 65.

A report of anaphylactic shock in a patient following treatment with a liquid soap enema containing tartrazine and sunset yellow FCF as colouring agents. Patch testing confirmed hypersensitivity to both tartrazine and sunset yellow FCF. The patient had a past history of a mild seasonal asthma.— J. J. Trautlein and W. J. Mann, *Ann. Allergy*, 1978, *41*, 28.

Further references to hypersensitivity reactions associated with tartrazine: L. J. Smith and R. G. Slavin, *J. Allergy & clin. Immunol.*, 1976, *58*, 456; R. P. Brettle *et al.* (letter), *Lancet*, 1979, *1*, 167.

For a report of severe laryngospasm in a patient after administration of tablets containing tartrazine and propranolol, see under Allergy in Propranolol, p.1325.

Cross-sensitivity. Seven of 8 aspirin-sensitive patients developed asthma, urticaria, or both after 1 to 2 mg of tartrazine.— L. Juhlin *et al.*, *J. Allergy & clin. Immunol.*, 1972, *50*, 92, per *J. Am. med. Ass.*, 1972, *222*, 727. Of 35 patients with aspirin idiosyncrasy only 2 were sensitive to tartrazine.— J. C. Delaney, *Practitioner*, 1976, *217*, 285. Tartrazine could provoke an urticarial reaction in up to 20% of aspirin-sensitive subjects.— G. Settipane *et al.*, *J. Allergy & clin. Immunol.*, 1976, *57*, 541, per A. Taaffe, *Postgrad. med. J.*, 1977, *53*, 732.

Of 39 patients who had reacted with urticaria to provocation with one or more additives used in food and drugs, 19 experienced urticaria after being given tartrazine, and 3 others had signs of hypersensitivity. About 60% of those reacting to tartrazine also reacted to other azo dyes. The dose of tartrazine required to produce a reaction varied from 1 to 18 mg.— G. Michaëlsson and L. Juhlin, *Br. J. Derm.*, 1973, *88*, 525.

Of 100 asthmatic patients undergoing oral provocation tests with low doses of aspirin, benzoic acid, and tartrazine, positive reactions with asthma, rhinitis, or urticaria occurred in 54 tested with tartrazine, 86 with aspirin, and 47 with benzoic acid.— L. Rosenhall and O. Zetterström, *Tubercle*, 1975, *56*, 168.

Of 75 patients with recurrent urticaria and angioneurotic oedema of more than 4 months' duration, 50 were found to be sensitive to the azo dyes tartrazine, sunset yellow FCF, and ponceau 4R, alone or in conjunction with aspirin, or benzoates, or both.— A. -M. Ros *et al.*, *Br. J. Derm.*, 1976, *95*, 19. See also G. Michaëlsson *et al.*, *Archs Derm.*, 1974, *109*, 49.

See also under Allergy, in Aspirin, p.236.

Precautions. A preliminary study indicated that the absorption of tartrazine from the small intestine in *rats* was significantly increased in the presence of docusate sodium. Since tartrazine is not usually well absorbed after administration by mouth, it was considered that this enhancement could be clinically significant.— M. Admans *et al.*, *Aust. J. pharm. Sci.*, 1976, *NS5*, 111.

Uses. Tartrazine is a permitted colouring agent in Great Britain, the EEC, and the USA for use in foods and medicines. With sunset yellow FCF, as in Compound Tartrazine Solution, it forms a substitute for the colouring matter of saffron.

Estimated acceptable daily intake: up to 7.5 mg per kg body-weight. Further toxicological studies in *animals* and man were considered desirable.— Eighth Report of FAO/WHO Expert Committee on Food Additives, *Tech. Rep. Ser. Wld Hlth Org. No. 309*, 1965.

Proposed FDA labelling requirements for preparations containing tartrazine. FDA regulations will require a label declaration of tartrazine as an ingredient when present in foods and in drugs for oral, nasal, vaginal and rectal administration. In addition package inserts for prescription drugs will carry a warning that tartrazine may cause allergic-type reactions (including bronchial asthma) and that sensitivity is frequently seen in patients with aspirin hypersensitivity. The regulations do not apply to externally applied drugs.— *FDA Drug Bull.*, 1979, *9*, 18.

Preparations

Compound Tartrazine Solution *(B.P.)*. Liq. Tartraz. Co.; Liquor Flavus. Tartrazine, food grade of commerce, 750 mg, sunset yellow FCF, food grade of commerce, 100 mg, glycerol 25 ml, chloroform spirit 20 ml, water to 100 ml.

As a colouring agent for medicines 1% v/v of Compound Tartrazine Solution is used.

Green S and Tartrazine Solution *(B.P.)*. Green S, food grade of commerce, 500 mg, tartrazine, food grade of commerce, 500 mg, glycerol 25 ml, chloroform spirit 20 ml, freshly boiled and cooled water to 100 ml.

Green Solution *(A.P.F.)*. Tartrazine, food grade of commerce, 400 mg, green S, food grade of commerce, 50 mg, chloroform water to 100 ml. From 1 to 2% may be used for colouring aqueous solutions and mixtures.

Tartrazine Solution *(A.P.F.)*. Yellow Solution. Tartrazine, food grade of commerce, 0.5% in chloroform water. From 1 to 2% may be used for colouring aqueous solutions or mixtures.

2412-b

Prepared Theobroma *(B.P.C. 1973)*. Prep. Theobrom.; Theobroma Praeparata; Cacao or Cocoa Powder; Non-alkalised Cocoa Powder.

Pharmacopoeias. Nord. includes Cacao which contains 20 to 24% fat. *U.S.N.F.* includes Cocoa (Cacao; Pulvis Theobromae; Pó de Cacau).

The roasted seed of theobroma, *Theobroma cacao* (Sterculiaceae) deprived of most of the shell, pressed to remove a portion of its fat, and finely ground. It should not have undergone any alkalisation. It is often flavoured by the addition of vanillin, ethyl vanillin, or cinnamon. It contains 15 to 30% of fat and 0.5 to 2% of theobromine. *U.S.N.F.* specifies 10 to 22% of non-volatile ether-soluble extractive. A 25% suspension in water has a pH of not more than 6. **Store** in airtight containers.

Adverse Effects.

A review of published reports of allergic reactions and other adverse effects associated with chocolate.— J. H. Fries, *Ann. Allergy*, 1978, *41*, 195.

Uses. Prepared theobroma is used as a basis for tablets and lozenges; the 'chocolate basis' for tablets contains prepared theobroma 15, sucrose 15, and lactose 70. It has also been used for coating tablets and sometimes in the preparation of barium sulphate meal.

Preparations

Cacao Syrup *(F.N. Belg.)*. Cocoa Syrup. Alkalised cocoa powder 18 g, glycerol 10 g, vanilla tincture (1 in 5) 5 g, sucrose 60 g, water to 100 ml.

Cocoa Syrup *(U.S.N.F.)*. Cacao Syrup. Cocoa 18 g, sucrose 60 g, liquid glucose 18 g, glycerol 5 ml, sodium chloride 200 mg, vanillin 20 mg, sodium benzoate 100 mg, water to 100 ml. Boiled for 3 minutes. Store at a temperature not exceeding 40° in airtight containers.

NOTE. Cocoa containing not more than 12% of non-volatile ether-soluble extractive will yield a syrup having a minimum tendency to separate.

Chocolate. Pasta Cacao; Pasta Theobromatis; Theobroma Saccharata. Cocoa nibs finely ground and mixed with powdered sugar and a proportion of cocoa fat, with the addition of a small amount of vanillin or other flavouring. After incorporation of the ingredients, the mixture is subjected to hot milling and then poured into moulds. It contains about 28 to 38% of fat and about 40 to 60% of sugar.

Chocolate powder is sometimes used in the preparation of tablets and lozenges.

2413-v

Theobroma Seed *(B.P.C. 1934)*. Theobromatis Semen; Cacao or Cocoa Seed; Cacau; Cocoa Bean.

Pharmacopoeias. In *Port.*

The fermented and dried seeds of *Theobroma cacao* (Sterculiaceae), containing in the kernel about 1 to 3% of theobromine, a small amount of caffeine, 40 to 60% of solid fat (theobroma oil), and about 2.5% of sugars, mainly sucrose and dextrose. The shell contains about 0.5 to 2% of theobromine.

Heated and deprived of husk and membrane, the theobroma seed yields cocoa nibs. The nibs with most of the oil pressed out produce, when reduced to powder, cocoa for use as a beverage. Before expression of the fat the seeds are often subjected to a process of 'alkalisation' with magnesium carbonate or a solution of sodium, potassium, or ammonium carbonate; the powder is often flavoured with vanillin, ethyl vanillin, or cinnamon.

2414-g

Trypan Blue *(B.P.C. 1954)*. Trypanum Caeruleum; CI Direct Blue 14; Colour Index No. 23850. Tetrasodium 3,3′-[(3,3′-dimethylbiphenyl-4,4′-diyl)bisazo]bis[5-amino-4-hydroxynaphthalene-2,7-disulphonate]. $C_{34}H_{24}N_6Na_4O_{14}S_4$=960.8.

CAS — 72-57-1.

A bluish-grey powder. **Soluble** in water, giving a bluish-violet solution; practically insoluble in alcohol. A 1% solution in water has a pH of about 9.1. Solutions are **sterilised** by autoclaving or by filtration.

For a report on the fading of trypan blue solution in the presence of sodium metabisulphite, see under Fading in the Presence of Sulphite, p.423.

Uses. Trypan blue has been used as a colouring agent in solutions for local application. It has been reported to produce carcinogenic and teratogenic effects in animals after parenteral administration.

Preparations

Trypan Blue Solution *(B.P.C. 1954)*. Liq. Trypan. Caerul. Trypan blue 0.34% w/v in water. As a colouring agent in solutions for local application 1% v/v is used.

Proprietary Names

Parkipan *(Aron, Fr.)*.

2415-q

Turmeric *(B.P.C. 1949)*. Curcuma; Indian Saffron; CI Natural Yellow 3; Colour Index No. 75300. The dried rhizome of *Curcuma longa* (Zingiberaceae).

CAS — 458-37-7.

Pharmacopoeias. In *Chin. Ind.* specifies a volatile oil content of not less than 4%.Témoé-Lawaq (*Fr. P.*) and Javanische Gelbwurz (*Ger. P.*) are the rhizome of *C. zanthorrhiza*, containing not less than 5% (*Fr.*) or 3.5% (*Ger.*) of volatile oil.

Turmeric contains curcumin. 1,7-bis(4-hydroxy-3-methoxyphenyl)hepta-1,6-diene-3,5-dione, $C_{21}H_{20}O_6$ = 368.4] a yellow pigment which dissolves in alcohol to form a deep yellow solution; alkalis change the colour to reddish-brown. It contains also a volatile oil (about 4 to 5%), starch, and resin. **Protect** from light.

Uses. Turmeric is used principally as a constituent of curry powders and other condiments. A tincture is used for the preparation of turmeric paper; it has also been used as a yellow colouring agent, but the colour is fugitive in solution. Turmeric paper is used as an indicator changing from yellow to reddish-brown in alkalis.

Curcumin showed the same amount of inhibition of induced oedema in *rats* as similar doses of cortisone and phenylbutazone, but its action was much reduced in adrenalectomised *rats*. In *mice* larger doses were required of curcumin than of cortisone for the same effect. No fatalities were noted in *mice* receiving a total dose of 2 g curcumin per kg body-weight and it had no antipyretic or analgesic action.— R. C. Srimal and B. N. Dhawan, *J. Pharm. Pharmac.*, 1973, *25*, 447.

Temporary estimated acceptable daily intake of turmeric and curcumin: up to 2.5 mg and 100 µg per kg body-weight respectively. Several studies *in vitro* showed that extracts of tumeric caused chromosome damage. Further studies are in progress.— Twenty-second Report of FAO/WHO Expert Committee on Food Additives, *Tech. Rep. Ser. Wld Hlth Org. No. 631*, 1978.

A preparation containing Rhizoma Curcumae Javanicae was formerly marketed in Great Britain under the proprietary name Rotercholon (*FAIR Laboratories*).

2416-p

Vanilla *(U.S.N.F., B.P.C. 1934)*. Vanilla Beans; Vanilla Pods; Baunilha; Vainilla.

Pharmacopoeias. In *Arg., Mex.,* and *Port.* Also in *U.S.N.F.*

The cured, fully grown, unripe fruit of Madagascar, Mexican, or Bourbon vanilla, *Vanilla planifolia*, or of Tahiti vanilla, *V. tahitensis* (Orchidaceae). It usually contains about 2 to 3% of vanillin. Its odour and flavour are not entirely due to vanillin but depend on the presence of other aromatic substances. Tahiti vanilla contains a lower percentage of vanillin and has an odour slightly different from the other varieties. **Store** at a temperature not exceeding 8° in airtight containers; vanilla which has become brittle should not be used.

Uses. Vanilla is used as a flavouring agent and in perfumery.

Preparations

Vanilla Tincture *(U.S.N.F.)*. 1 in 10; prepared by maceration and percolation with diluted alcohol (about 49%) and containing 20% w/v of sucrose. Store at a temperature not exceeding 40° in airtight containers. Protect from light.

Fr. P. includes a tincture, 1 in 10 in alcohol (80%).

2417-s

Vanillin *(B.P., U.S.N.F.)*. Vanillic Aldehyde; Vainillina. 4-Hydroxy-3-methoxybenzaldehyde. $C_8H_8O_3$=152.1.

CAS — 121-33-5.

Pharmacopoeias. In *Arg., Aust., Belg., Br., Fr., Ger., Hung., Jug., Mex., Nord., Port., Span.,* and *Swiss.* Also in *U.S.N.F.*

White or slightly yellow crystalline needles or powder with an odour and taste of vanilla. It can be extracted from vanilla but it is usually prepared synthetically. M.p. 81° to 83°.

Soluble 1 in 100 of water at 20°, 1 in 20 of water at 80°, 1 in 20 of glycerol; soluble in alcohol, chloroform, and ether, in fixed and volatile oils, and in solutions of alkali hydroxides. A saturated solution in water is acid to litmus. **Incompatible** with oxidising agents and ferric salts. **Store** in airtight containers. Protect from light.

Uses. Vanillin is used as a flavouring agent and in perfumery.

Estimated acceptable daily intake: up to 10 mg per kg body-weight.— Eleventh Report of the Joint FAO/WHO Expert Committee on Food Additives, *Tech. Rep. Ser. Wld Hlth Org. No. 383*, 1968.

Vanillin significantly prolonged the protection time of diethyltoluamide. It was considered that vanillin mixed with some insect repellents could provide protection against mosquito bites for almost 24 hours.— A. A. Khan *et al.*, *Mosquito News*, 1975, *35*, 223, per *Trop. Dis. Bull.*, 1975, *72*, 834.

2418-w

Wild Cherry Bark *(B.P.)*. Prunus Serotina; Virginian Prune; Virginian Prune Bark; Wild Black Cherry Bark; Wild Cherry.

Pharmacopoeias. In *Br.* which also describes Powdered Wild Cherry Bark.

The dried bark of the wild or black cherry, *Prunus serotina* (Rosaceae), known in commerce as Thin Natural Wild Cherry Bark, containing not less than 10% of water-soluble extractive. It has a slight odour and an astringent, aromatic, bitter taste, recalling that of bitter almonds. It contains (+)-mandelonitrile glucoside (prunasin) and an enzyme system, which interact in the presence of water yielding benzaldehyde, hydrocyanic acid, and glucose. Good specimens of the bark yield

0.075 to 0.16% of HCN. **Store** at a temperature not exceeding 25° in a dry place. Powdered bark should be stored at a temperature not exceeding 25° in airtight containers.

Uses. Wild cherry bark, in the form of the syrup, has been used in the treatment of cough but it has little therapeutic value. Its chief use is as a flavouring agent.

Preparations

Wild Cherry Syrup *(B.P.)*. Syr. Prun. Serot.; Syrupus Pruni Serotinae; Virginian Prune Syrup. Prepared from wild cherry bark 15 g, sucrose 80 g, glycerol 5 ml, and water to 100 ml, by percolation with the water and dissolving the sucrose and glycerol in the percolate without the aid of heat. Store at a temperature not exceeding 25°.

Four commercial samples of wild cherry syrup contained no detectable HCN. A sample of syrup freshly prepared in the laboratory (from bark yielding 0.096% of HCN) was found to contain 0.0058% HCN—only 41% of that available in the bark.— *Pharm. J.*, 1961, *2*, 187 (Pharm. Soc. Lab. Rep.).

Wild Cherry Tincture (B.P.C. 1949). Tinct. Prun. Serot.; Tincture of Virginian Prune. Wild cherry bark 20 g, alcohol (90%) 55 ml, water 37.5 ml, and glycerol 10 ml. *Dose.* 2 to 4 ml.

2419-e

Yellow 2G. Acid Light Yellow 2G; Acid Yellow 17; CI Food Yellow 5; Colour Index No. 18965. Disodium 2,5-dichloro-4-[5-hydroxy-3-methyl-4-(4-sulphonatophenylazo)pyrazol-1-yl]benzenesulphonate.
$C_{16}H_{10}Cl_2N_4Na_2O_7S_2$=551.3.

CAS — 6359-98-4.

Light yellow powder or granules. **Soluble** in water; slightly soluble in alcohol; practically insoluble in vegetable oils.

Uses. Yellow 2G is a permitted colour in Great Britain and the EEC for use in foodstuffs and cosmetics

Background toxicological information.— Fd Add. Ser. Wld Hlth Org. No. 6, 1975.

Contrast Media

1550-g

Contrast media (radiopaques) increase the absorption of X-rays as they pass through the body and are used for delineating body structures.

The use of gas (air, oxygen, or carbon dioxide) for visualisation has been described as negative contrast; that of radiopaque agents, positive contrast; when the two are used concomitantly the procedure is called double contrast. Tomography is the procedure whereby a selected plane of the subject is visualised.

Barium sulphate, the principal contrast medium for gastro-intestinal radiography, is described on p.434.

The other contrast media described in this section are iodinated organic compounds whose degree of opacity is directly proportional to their iodine content. They may be divided into 2 main classes depending on whether they are used principally in the examination of urinary and blood systems (urographic and angiographic media) or in the examination of the biliary tract (cholecystographic media).

Urographic and angiographic media, which are salts of moderately strong organic acids, are soluble in water, of comparatively low viscosity in solution, and readily excreted by the kidneys. Those principally used are salts of diatrizoic acid (p.435), iodamide (p.439), iothalamic acid (p.442), ioxitalamic acid (p.443), and metrizoic acid (p.444).

Cholecystographic media are concentrated in the gall-bladder. They are usually given by mouth and include calcium ipodate (p.435), iocetamic acid (p.439), iopanoic acid (p.441), phenobutiodil (p.445), and sodium ipodate (p.445). Salts of iodipamide (p.439), iodoxamic acid (p.441), and of ioglycamic acid (p.441) are given intravenously.

In addition to these 2 main classes, a variety of media are used for the examination of various body cavities.

The adverse effects of water-soluble iodinated contrast media are discussed under Diatrizoic Acid (see p.436).

Intravenous urography was more effective when the patient was in a state of dehydration and urinary osmolality was greater. The meglumine ion had osmotic diuretic properties and the meglumine salts of contrast agents were less effective than sodium salts.— G. T. Benness (letter), *Lancet*, 1968, *2*, 970. See also *idem*, *Australas. Radiol.*, 1968, *12*, 245.

For an account of the visualisation of thrombi in the internal carotid artery using a slow injection of highly concentrated contrast media, see A. E. Hugh, *Br. med. J.*, 1970, *2*, 574.

Reviews. Radiopaques: a review of X-ray contrast media with an extensive bibliography.— N. C. Chenoy, *Pharm. J.*, 1965, *1*, 663.

Reviews and discussions of the nephrotoxicity of X-ray contrast media.— G. E. Schreiner, *J. Am. med. Ass.*, 1966, *196*, 413; *Br. med. J.*, 1971, *3*, 493; R. G. Grainger, *Br. med. Bull.*, 1972, *28*, 191; R. D. Wagoner, *Archs intern. Med.*, 1978, *138*, 353; *Lancet*, 1979, *2*, 835.

A national survey of radiological complications: an interim report.— G. Ansell, *Clin. Radiol.*, 1968, *19*, 175.

Urography: a detailed review.— H. M. Saxton, *Br. J. Radiol.*, 1969, *42*, 321.

The use of lymphangiography in dermatology.— D. D. Munro *et al.*, *Br. J. Derm.*, 1969, *81*, 652.

The use of contrast media to diagnose renal failure.— I. K. Fry and W. R. Cattell, *Br. med. Bull.*, 1971, *27*, 148.

Reviews.— R. G. Grainger, *M & B pharm. Bull.*, 1973, *22*, 38. Urography.— W. Simpson, *ibid.*, 50. Cerebral angiography.— J. V. Occleshaw, *ibid.*, 66. Peripheral arteriography.— J. G. Sowerbutts, *ibid.*, 1974, *23*, 2. Lumbar radiculography.— J. Danziger and S. Bloch, *ibid.*, 14. Angiocardiography and thoracic aortography.— R. G. Grainger, *ibid.*, 26. Radiology of the biliary tract.— L. A. Gillanders, *ibid.*, 38. Lymphography.— J. S. MacDonald, *ibid.*, 50. Gastro-intestinal radiology.— K. Lumsden, *ibid.*, 62. Hysterosalpingography.— J. H. Smitham, *ibid.*, 1975, *24*, 2. Venography.— B. Ross, *ibid.*, 14. Bronchography and laryngography.— *idem*, 26.

A discussion of contrast media.— C. R. Day, *Pharm. J.*, 1977, *1*, 82.

Radiography in the diagnosis of acute cholecystitis.— *Lancet*, 1978, *2*, 457.

Complications of X-ray investigations.— G. Ansell, *Adverse Drug React. Bull.*, 1978, Aug., 252.

A discussion on the use of intravenous urography.— B. Cramer and G. de Lacey, *Br. med. J.*, 1980, *281*, 661.

A brief discussion of the role of mesenteric angiography for the identification of massive bleeding from the large bowel.— *Br. med. J.*, 1980, *280*, 425.

Developments on the use of contrast media in neuroradiology.— B. E. Kendall, *Br. med. Bull.*, 1980, *36*, 273.

1520-d

Acetrizoic Acid *(B.P. 1973)*. Acetriz. Acid; Acidum Acetrizoicum. 3-Acetamido-2,4,6-tri-iodobenzoic acid.

$C_9H_6I_3NO_3$=556.9.

CAS — 85-36-9.

Pharmacopoeias. In *Int.* and *Turk.*

A white or almost white odourless tasteless powder. M.p. about 280° with decomposition. Slightly **soluble** in water, chloroform, and ether; soluble 1 in 20 of alcohol; soluble in solutions of alkali hydroxides. Solutions are **sterilised** by autoclaving or by filtration. **Protect** from light.

1551-q

Sodium Acetrizoate.

$C_9H_5I_3NNaO_3$=578.8.

CAS — 129-63-5.

It contains approximately 65.8% of I. Each g of sodium acetrizoate represents 1.73 mmol (1.73 mEq) of sodium.

Adverse Effects. As for Diatrizoic Acid, p.436.

Pain and spasm may occur during the use of sodium acetrizoate for hysterosalpingography.

Treatment of Adverse Effects. As for Diatrizoic Acid, p.436.

Precautions. As for Diatrizoic Acid, p.437.

It should not be given for hysterosalpingography in the presence of severe cervical or vaginal infection, pelvic infection, cervical erosion, or in pregnancy.

Absorption and Fate. After hysterosalpingography absorption of sodium acetrizoate is complete within about 1 hour. If renal function is not impaired, it is rapidly excreted unchanged in the urine.

Uses. Acetrizoic acid is a contrast medium which, as a 40% solution of sodium acetrizoate, is used for hysterosalpingography.

Sodium acetrizoate has been given parenterally for a variety of diagnostic procedures but has been largely replaced by better tolerated compounds such as the meglumine and sodium salts of diatrizoic or iothalamic acid.

Preparations of Sodium Acetrizoate

Sodium Acetrizoate Injection *(B.P. 1973)*. Sod. Acetrizoate Inj. A sterile solution in Water for Injections of sodium acetrizoate prepared by the interaction of acetrizoic acid and sodium hydroxide; it may contain suitable buffering and stabilising agents. pH 6.5 to 7.5 It is sterilised by autoclaving or by filtration. Protect from light.

Diaginol Viscous *(May & Baker, UK)*. Contains sodium acetrizoate 40% in dextran solution in ampoules of 15 ml. For hysterosalpingography. (Also available as Diaginol Viscous in *Austral.*).

Other Proprietary Names of Sodium Acetrizoate

Densopax *(Arg.)*.

1552-p

Barium Sulphate *(B.P., Eur. P.)*. Barii Sulphas; Barium Sulfate *(U.S.P.)*; Barii Sulfas; Baryum (Sulfate de); Barium Sulfuricum.

$BaSO_4$=233.4.

CAS — 7727-43-7.

Pharmacopoeias. In all pharmacopoeias examined.

A fine, white, odourless, tasteless powder, free from grittiness.

Practically **insoluble** in water and organic solvents; very slightly soluble in acids and alkalis and in solutions of many salts. A 5% suspension in water is neutral to litmus.

CAUTION. *When Barium Sulphate is prescribed the title should always be written out in full to avoid confusion with the poisonous barium sulphide or sulphite.*

Flavouring of suspensions. Barium sulphate suspensions were more acceptable if the chalk-like texture was eliminated with a good suspending agent, such as carmellose sodium, pectin, acacia, or tragacanth, but too viscous a suspension would limit the amount a patient would willingly swallow. The flavour should be tailored to the patients' tastes; children liked sweet tastes while adults did not. Mixtures of flavours in which no single flavour predominated were considered the best. A mild mixture of 3 or 4 flavours such as sweet cherry, wild cherry, raspberry, and orange with some vanilla and then a little of a more sharp flavour such as peppermint, lime, apricot, or citric acid had been found satisfactory. Suspensions were best sweetened.— R. E. Miller, *Am. J. Roentg.*, 1966, *96*, 484.

Adverse Effects. Constipation may occur after barium sulphate enema; impaction, obstruction, and appendicitis have occurred. Intravasation has led to the formation of emboli; deaths have occurred. Perforation of the bowel has led to peritonitis, adhesions, granulomas, and death.

The use of barium sulphate for bronchography, or aspiration into the lungs, has led to phagocytosis of crystalline material into the interstitial tissues or lymph nodes, with granuloma formation. Baritosis, a benign form of pneumoconiosis, occurs in workers exposed to barium sulphate powder.

Cardiac arrhythmias have occurred during the use of barium sulphate enemas.

A healthy 64-year-old man developed fever and pelvic tenderness following a barium enema. This was attributed to the development of sepsis due to increased intracolonic pressure during the enema. Recovery after treatment with antibiotics was uneventful.— E. Larsen (letter), *J. Am. med. Ass.*, 1974, *229*, 639. See also J. L. Hammer, *Sth. med. J.*, 1977, *70*, 1361.

A report of transient bacteraemia in 20 of 175 patients after barium enemas.— J. Le Frock *et al.*, *Archs intern. Med.*, 1975, *135*, 835, per *J. Am. med. Ass.*, 1975, *232*, 1293.

Cardiac arrhythmias. Of 95 patients undergoing barium enema examination, 44 had ECG changes during the procedure; the changes were more frequent in elderly patients and in those with heart disease. In 16 patients the changes were potentially serious.— G. L. Eastwood, *J. Am. med. Ass.*, 1972, *219*, 719.

Significant arrhythmias occurred in 23 of 58 consecutive patients, aged over 60, undergoing barium enema examinations; a further 4 had ST-segment changes. Patients over 60 with a history of cardiac disease, ectopic beats at rest, and significant postural changes of systolic arterial pressure, were considered at risk.— W. R. Roeske *et al.*, *Am. Heart J.*, 1975, *90*, 688, per *Int. pharm. Abstr.*, 1977, *14*, 173.

Further references: C. Z. Berman *et al.*, *J. Am. Geriat. Soc.*, 1965, *13*, 672.

Precautions. The use of barium sulphate enemas may exacerbate ulcerative colitis. Barium sulphate enemas should be used cautiously in elderly patients with pre-existing heart disease.

Uses. Barium sulphate is used as a contrast medium for X-ray examination of the alimentary tract. It is not absorbed and hence does not produce the systemic effects of soluble barium salts. It is given in the form of a suspension, usually with flavouring and suspending agents. The stability of a suspension is improved and the coating of the mucosa facilitated by the use of barium sulphate of very fine particle size.

For X-ray examination of the colon, barium sulphate may be given by enema. Bisacodyl and oxyphenisatin are sometimes employed as adjuvants in preparing the bowel.

A discussion on whether the barium meal is overused.— *Lancet*, 1980, *1*, 1171.

Appendicitis. A barium enema might afford very important information in suspected appendicitis. Preparation of the bowel was unnecessary. The investigation was particularly valuable in young children in the differential diagnosis of acute appendicitis and mesenteric adenitis or gastro-enteritis.— C. S. Soter, *Clin. Radiol.*, 1968, *19*, 410, per *Practitioner*, 1969, *202*, 181.

Bronchography. Bronchography with barium sulphate was carried out in 289 patients. A 50% w/v suspension of barium sulphate in normal saline containing 1.75% of carmellose sodium was used in the earlier stages of the study and in the later stages a similar suspension with hydroxyethylcellulose. It was considered that barium sulphate caused fewer acute reactions than other bronchographic contrast media and, though only slowly eliminated, it did not cause pulmonary fibrosis or other deleterious chronic reactions.— S. W. Nelson *et al.*, *Am. J. Roentg.*, 1964, *92*, 595, per *Abstr. Wld Med.*, 1965, *37*, 144.

Colonic lesions. Massive bleeding from diverticular disease of the colon was stopped by barium enemas in 26 of 28 bleeding episodes in 22 patients. In 5 patients, colonic surgery was carried out.— J. T. Adams, *Archs Surg., Chicago*, 1970, *101*, 457, per *J. Am. med. Ass.*, 1970, *214*, 780.

A discussion on the usefulness of barium enemas.— R. E. Miller and G. Lehman, *J. Am. med. Ass.*, 1976, *235*, 2842.

In a study of 230 patients with intracolonic lesions detected by pre-endoscopic barium contrast studies, 191 (83%) of the results proved to be true-positive and 39 (17%) were false-positive. Results indicated that a 2-day colon preparation, before the initial barium contrast enema would substantially reduce the frequency of false-positive interpretations.— C. O. Knutson *et al.*, *J. Am. med. Ass.*, 1979, *242*, 2206.

Cystic fibrosis. The careful use of a barium sulphate enema was suggested for the reduction of intussusception in patients with cystic fibrosis.— D. S. Holsclaw *et al.*, *Pediatrics*, 1971, *48*, 51, per *Clin. Med.*, 1972, *79* (Dec.), 34.

Dyspepsia. Routine barium-meal examination was of no value in the initial management of uncomplicated dyspepsia; resolution-rates in screened and unscreened patients were comparable.— J. R. W. Lyall and T. E. T. West (letter), *Br. med. J.*, 1977, *2*, 520.

Gastro-intestinal lesions. The detection of intramural haematoma of the gastro-intestinal tract.— C. E. Hughes *et al.*, *Am. J. Surg.*, 1977, *133*, 276.

Oesophagitis. A suspension of barium sulphate, adjusted to pH of 1.7, produced abnormal oesophageal motility in patients with oesophagitis. In 90 of 91 patients, segmented non-peristaltic contractions occurred when the preparation was taken, instead of the progressive peristaltic waves seen in healthy persons.— M. W. Donner *et al.*, *Radiology*, 1966, *87*, 220, per *Abstr. Wld Med.*, 1967, *41*, 239.

Preparations

Barium Sulfate for Suspension *(U.S.P.)*. A dry mixture of not less than 90% of barium sulphate and one or more suitable dispersing and/or suspending agents. It may contain one or more suitable colours, flavours, fluidising agents, and preservatives. pH of a 60% w/w aqueous suspension is 4 to 10. The suspension is prepared by the addition of diluent immediately before issue.

Barium Sulphate for Suspension *(B.P.)*. A dry mixture of not less than 85% of barium sulphate with a suitable dispersing agent and suitable flavouring agents and preservatives. pH of a 75% w/v aqueous suspension 4.5 to 7.

Barium Sulphate Suspension *(B.P.)*. An aqueous suspension containing not less than 75% w/v of barium sulphate with a suitable dispersing agent and suitable flavouring agents and preservatives. pH 4.5 to 7.

Proprietary Preparations

Baritop 100 *(Concept Pharmaceuticals, UK)*. A suspension containing 100% w/v of barium sulphate. For visualisation of the gastro-intestinal tract.

Baritop G Powder *(Concept Pharmaceuticals, UK)*. Contains barium sulphate 97%.

Barosperse *(Mallinckrodt, USA: Camlab, UK)*. A formulation of barium sulphate for the preparation of suspensions for radiography. (Also available as Barosperse in *Canad., Swed., USA*).

Epi-C *(May & Baker, UK)*. Suspension containing barium sulphate 70% w/w. For rectal administration after dilution with an equal volume of water.

Micropaque *(Nicholas, UK)*. **Powder** containing 92% w/w of barium sulphate for preparing suspensions, and **Liquid** containing 100% w/v of barium sulphate. (Also available as Micropaque in *Fr., Ger., Neth., Spain, Switz.*).**Micropaque DC Liquid.** A low viscosity suspension containing 100% w/v of barium sulphate. For radiological examination of the gastro-intestinal tract by the double contrast technique.

Microtrast *(Nicholas, UK)*. A paste containing 70% w/w of barium sulphate for use in the radiographic examination of the oesophagus. (Also available as Microtrast in *Fr., Ger., Neth., Switz.*).

Other Proprietary Names

Arg.—Gastropaque-S; *Austral.*—Baritop, Tixobar; *Belg.*—Neobar, Suspobar; *Canad.*—Gel-Unix, Recto Barium, Unik-Pak; *Denm.*—Barytgen, Danobaryt, Mixobar; *Fr.*—Baryx Colloïdal, Baryxine, Radio-Baryx, Radiopaque, X-Opac; *Ger.*—Unibaryt; *Neth.*—Barium Andreu, Barotrast, Esophotrast, Microbar, Mixobar, Unibaryt; *Norw.*—Mixobar, Topcontral; *Spain*—Microfanox; *Swed.*— Barytgen, Mixobar, Radimix Colon; *Switz.*—Barotrast, Mixobar, Oesobar, Oratrast, Radiobaryt, Radiopaque; *USA*—Esophotrast, E-Z Preparations, Rugar.

Barium sulphate was also formerly marketed in Great Britain under the proprietary name Steripaque (*Nicholas*).

1553-s

Calcium Ipodate.

Calcii Jopodas: Ipodate Calcium *(U.S.P.)*. The calcium salt of 3-(3-dimethylaminomethyleneamino-2,4,6-tri-iodophenyl)propionic acid.

$(C_{12}H_{12}I_3N_2O_2)_2Ca$=1234.0.

CAS — 5587-89-3 (ipodic acid); 1151-11-7 (calcium ipodate).

Pharmacopoeias. In *Nord.* (dihydrate) and *U.S.*

A fine, white or off-white, odourless, crystalline powder, containing approximately 61.7% of I. M.p. about 290°. **Soluble** 1 in 600 of water, 1 in 250 of alcohol, and 1 in 3000 of ether; slightly soluble in chloroform and methyl alcohol. **Store** in airtight containers. Protect from light.

Adverse Effects and Precautions. As for Iopanoic Acid, p.441. Headache has been reported.

Absorption and Fate. Calcium ipodate is absorbed from the gastro-intestinal tract and it appears in the bile within about 30 minutes of a dose. It is reported to be more rapidly absorbed than sodium ipodate. Maximum concentrations are found in the gall-bladder about 10 hours after injection. It is excreted mainly in the urine.

Uses. Calcium ipodate is used as a contrast medium for the examination of the biliary tract. It is given by mouth as an aqueous suspension. For cholecystography, 3 g is given in the evening, about 10 to 12 hours before the examination; a further 3 g may be given early next day 2 to 3 hours before the examination. For cholangiography 3 or 6 g is given and exposures are made every 15 minutes for about 90 minutes commencing 1 hour after the dose is taken. See also under Sodium Ipodate (p.445).

In 73 patients, cholecystography with iopanoic acid 3 g was unsuccessful. Immediately following the X-ray they were given 3 g of calcium ipodate and visualisation of the gall-bladder 5 hours later was adequate in 30 patients and unsuccessful in 30; in 13 patients the gall-bladder was partially opacified.— T. Klepetar *et al.*, *J. Am. med. Ass.*, 1970, *211*, 2154. See also A. W. Robinson, *Br. J. Radiol.*, 1962, *35*, 282.

Preparations

Ipodate Calcium for Oral Suspension *(U.S.P.)*. A dry mixture of calcium ipodate and one or more suitable suspending, dispersing, and flavouring agents. The suspension is prepared by the addition of diluent before issue.

Solu-Biloptin *(Schering, UK)*. Calcium ipodate, available in sachets of 3 g for the preparation of a suspension for oral cholecystangiography. (Also available as Solu-Biloptin in *Austral., Ger., Norw., Swed., Switz.*).

Other Proprietary Names

Oragrafin Calcium *(Canad., USA)*; Solu-Biloptine *(Belg.)*.

1554-w

Diatrizoic Acid

(U.S.P.). Amidotrizoic Acid. 3,5-Diacetamido-2,4,6-tri-iodobenzoic acid.

$C_{11}H_9I_3N_2O_4$=613.9.

CAS — 117-96-4 (anhydrous); 50978-11-5 (dihydrate).

Pharmacopoeias. In *Chin.*, *Fr.*, and *Jap.* (all $2H_2O$); *U.S.* has anhydrous or dihydrate.

An odourless white powder, containing approximately 62% of I, calculated on the anhydrous substance.

Very slightly **soluble** in water and alcohol; practically insoluble in chloroform and ether; sparingly soluble in methyl alcohol; soluble in dimethylformamide and in solutions of alkali hydroxides. **Store** in airtight containers. Protect from light.

1555-e

Meglumine Diatrizoate.

Diatrizoate Meglumine *(U.S.P.)*; Methylglucamine Diatrizoate. *N*-Methylglucamine 3,5-diacetamido-2,4,6-tri-iodobenzoate.

$C_{18}H_{26}I_3N_3O_9$ = 809.1.

CAS — 131-49-7.

Pharmacopoeias. In *Braz.* and *U.S.*

An odourless white powder containing approximately 47.1% of I. Freely **soluble** in water. A solution in water is laevorotatory. Solutions are **sterilised** by autoclaving or by filtration.

1556-l

Sodium Diatrizoate

(B.P.). Sod. Diatrizoate; Diatrizoate Sodium *(U.S.P.)*; Sodium Amidotrizoate. Sodium 3,5-diacetamido-2,4,6-tri-iodobenzoate.

$C_{11}H_8I_3N_2NaO_4$=635.9.

CAS — 737-31-5.

Pharmacopoeias. In *Br. Braz.* and *U.S.* permit up to 10% water. In *Nord.* and *Turk.* as tetrahydrate.

An odourless white powder with a saline taste, containing 4 to 7% of water. It contains approximately 59.9% of I and each g represents 1.57 mmol (1.57 mEq) of sodium, both calculated on the anhydrous substance.

Soluble 1 in 2 of water; slightly soluble in alcohol; practically insoluble in acetone and ether. A 50% solution in water has a pH of 7 to 9. Solutions are **sterilised** by autoclaving or by filtration. **Protect** from light.

Incompatibility. Meglumine diatrizoate was incompatible with promethazine hydrochloride and with diphenhydramine hydrochloride on standing, but compatible with chlorpheniramine and brompheniramine maleates.— C. Riffkin, *Am. J. Hosp. Pharm.*, 1963, *20*, 19.

Precipitation occurred when meglumine and sodium

diatrizoates (as Hypaque 75%) were added to promethazine hydrochloride injection, or when the diatrizoates (as Renovist) were added to brompheniramine maleate or promethazine hydrochloride injections. Meglumine diatrizoate (as Renografin-60) precipitated when added to brompheniramine maleate, diphenhydramine, or promethazine hydrochloride injections.— T. R. Marshall *et al.*, *Radiology*, 1965, *84*, 536.

Adverse Effects. Sodium diatrizoate and other water-soluble iodinated contrast media, given by injection, may cause nausea, a metallic taste, vomiting, sensations of heat, weakress, headache, coughing, sneezing, sweating, retching, lachrymation, pruritus, salivary gland enlargement, pallor, tachycardia, and hypotension. Rarely, convulsions, rigors, ventricular fibrillations, pulmonary oedema, circulatory failure, and cardiac arrest have occurred. Anaphylactic shock and hypersensitivity reactions, with symptoms including dyspnoea, bronchospasm, oedema of the face and glottis, and urticaria, occasionally occur. Fatalities have occurred.

Pain may occur at the injection site and has been followed by extravasation and tissue damage, intramural injection, phlebitis, thrombosis, and embolism.

Paraesthesia, aphasia, hemiplegia, and encephalopathy have occurred after cerebral arteriography. Photophobia, blepharospasm, periorbital and retinal haemorrhage, retinal oedema, and occasionally transient blindness have occurred after carotid angiography.

Injury to the spinal cord has occurred after angiography, and small-bowel injury when the medium has inadvertently been injected into the superior mesenteric artery. Angiocardiography has been followed by haemodynamic changes and ECG changes.

Fibrinolysis and a possible depressant effect on blood coagulation factors has been reported.

Renal failure has occurred after the intravenous use of these media; contributing factors may include renal vasoconstriction, predisposing factors, hypotension, and dehydration. Some authorities consider that large doses of contrast media may be given to patients with renal failure.

Toxic effects after meglumine salts are generally less severe than after equivalent doses of sodium salts. Meglumine salts may have a diuretic effect. Mild diarrhoea may follow the oral or rectal administration of sodium and meglumine diatrizoates for gastro-intestinal examinations. The inhalation of solutions of these salts has caused pulmonary oedema.

An intravenous injection of 1 ml of medium has been given as a test for sensitivity before administration of the main dose but it does not predict hypersensitivity with certainty and severe reactions and fatalities have followed the test dose. An antihistamine or a corticosteroid has been given prior to the administration of contrast medium to reduce the incidence of reactions; antihistamines should not be mixed in the syringe with the contrast medium.

Adequate resuscitative facilities should be available when radiographic procedures are to be employed.

Standard doses of sodium diatrizoate had a uricosuric effect.— A. E. Postlethwaite and W. N. Kelley, *Ann. intern. Med.*, 1971, *74*, 845, per *Abstr. Wld Med.*, 1971, *45*, 799.

In a prospective study of 3509 patients undergoing urography using sodium diatrizoate 25 or 45%, sodium and meglumine diatrizoates, or sodium iothalamate 1287 had no side-effects. Reversible heart failure occurred in 4 patients with pre-existing heart disease given large doses. Allergic reactions usually urticaria, occurred in 52 patients including 13 of 355 with a history of allergy; the incidence of allergic reactions was 3.7% in those with a history of allergy compared with 1.2% in those without. Prophylactic use of an antihistamine did not reduce the incidence or severity of allergic reactions but increased threefold the incidence of flushing. Major reactions occurred in 4 patients—hypotension, bronchospasm, severe vomiting, and dyspnoea with urticaria. Nausea occurred in 286 patients and 90 vomited. Other reactions included warmth (1726), metallic taste (379), visceral sensations, usually an unpleasant feeling in the epigastrium (206), tingling (199), flushing (191), coughing and sneezing (72), and a variety of other symptoms, chiefly sensations in the perineum. Arm pain was usually associated with perivenous injection. Apart from an increased incidence of warmth the speed of injection did not influence side-effects. Up to 600 mg of iodine per kg body-weight should be given rapidly. Special care was needed for small infants, the elderly, patients with renal or hepatic failure, myeloma, heart disease, or a previous major reaction. Full resuscitation facilities should be available.— P. Davies *et al.*, *Br. med. J.*, 1975, *2*, 434.

Of 32 964 patients undergoing excretion urography 6.8% had some side-effects; 1.72% had clinically important side-effects, sometimes severe and life-threatening. Reported estimates of mortality ranged from 1 in 400 000 to 1 in 116 000. Reactions were more common in patients with known hypersensitivity, but the incidence of severe or fatal reactions did not appear to be increased. Of 150 patients who had shown a reaction on previous urography 26 had a clinically important reaction on re-examination. In about 33 000 patients intravenous pretesting failed to identify 559 of 568 who developed significant reactions. Treatment of severe reactions included provision of an adequate airway, oxygen, adrenaline, intravenous fluids, and corticosteroids.— D. M. Witten, *J. Am. med. Ass.*, 1975, *231*, 974.

A brief review of the hazards of radiographic contrast media.— *Drug & Ther. Bull.*, 1975, *13*, 43.

A benign transient eosinophilia developed in 21 of 101 patients who received diatrizoates or meglumine iothalamate. Only 5 of the 21 patients developed any signs of an allergic reaction (urticaria in each patient).— M. E. Vincent *et al.*, *J. Am. med. Ass.*, 1977, *237*, 2629.

A rise in serum-aminotransferase concentrations might occur during treatment with sodium diatrizoate.— F. Clark, *Adverse Drug React. Bull.*, 1977, Oct., 232.

The use of meglumine diatrizoate might have contributed to the death, with bowel necrosis, perforation, and peritonitis, of 2 infants with meconium ileus.— J. C. Leonidas *et al.*, *Radiology*, 1976, *121*, 693. See also T. F. Hogan (letter), *Ann. intern. Med.*, 1977, *87*, 382; S. E. Seltzer and B. Jones, *Am. J. Roentg.*, 1978, *130*, 977.

A report of intravascular haemolysis and renal failure in a 58-year-old man after angiocardiography with diatrizoates (Urografin 370).— J. R. Catterall *et al.*, *Br. med. J.*, 1981, *282*, 779.

Cardiovascular effects. In 18 patients with significant coronary arterial occlusion and 11 normal subjects, 5 to 6 ml of sodium diatrizoate solution 75% introduced into the left or right coronary arteries after a preliminary injection of 2 to 3 ml to verify the position of the cannula produced sinus bradycardia with changes in the ECG suggesting ischaemia, and significant but transitory decrease in both coronary arterial and systemic blood pressures. In a total of 81 cases of selective coronary arteriography, 4 major complications (including ventricular fibrillation in 3 patients) with no deaths had been encountered.— A. Benchimol and E. M. McNally, *New Engl. J. Med.*, 1966, *274*, 1217.

Haemodynamic reactions to injected contrast media were greater with larger doses, more rapid administration, and higher concentrations. Reactions were also determined by the anionic and cationic components of the medium and reactions were reduced by replacing part of the sodium salt with calcium and magnesium salts. The haemodynamic reactions to angiocardiography and aortography were less when the patient was well hydrated and had a normal electrolyte balance.— H. W. Fischer, *Radiology*, 1968, *91*, 66, per *J. Am. med. Ass.*, 1968, *205* (July 29), A141.

Coagulation defects. Abnormalities in the partial prothrombin time, lasting 2 to 3 hours, occurred in 17 of 35 patients given contrast media, and abnormalities of the prothrombin time in 9 of the 35. Studies *in vitro* confirmed the depression of blood coagulation factors.— H. L. Stein and M. W. Hilgartner, *Am. J. Roentg.*, 1968, *104*, 458.

An *in vitro* study showed that diatrizoates increased the prothrombin time, the plasma recalcification time, reduced the fibrinogen content, and increased fibrinolytic activity. In 10 patients the serum-calcium concentration was reduced. In one patient studied there was evidence of a mild anticoagulant effect persisting for 24 hours.— R. Chandra and J. Abraham, *Angiology*, 1973, *24*, 199.

Further references: B. Schulze and H. P. Kaps, *Arzneimittel-Forsch.*, 1977, *27*, 972; B. Schulze *et al.*, *ibid.*, 1978, *28*, 756.

Neurological effects. A 54-year-old woman developed severe muscle spasms following the inadvertent subarachnoid, instead of epidural, administration of a 50% mixture of lignocaine 2% and meglumine diatrizoate 60%. Within 2 hours she began having involuntary spasms in both legs and these lasted throughout the night.— A. Feingold *et al.*, *J. Am. med. Ass.*, 1970, *212*, 879.

Pancreatitis. Direct cholangiography using sodium diatrizoate could cause a transient blockage of the pancreatic duct with a consequent rise in serum-amylase concentration.— D. G. Christian, *Am. J. clin. Path.*, 1970, *54*, 118, per F. Clark, *Adverse Drug React. Bull.*, 1977, Oct., 232.

Acute pancreatitis after translumbar aortography, using sodium iothalamate or meglumine diatrizoate, was probably due to direct damage to the pancreas.— C. W. Imrie *et al.*, *Br. med. J.*, 1977, *2*, 681. The damage might have been due to toxicity of the contrast media.— P. Davies (letter), *ibid.*, 895.

Renal failure. Acute renal failure developed in 12 of 13 diabetic patients with advanced nephropathy who underwent angiocardiography. The patient who did not develop renal failure was not as anaemic as the others and the volume of contrast material needed, 46 ml per m^2 body-surface, was much less than the mean required by the others, 103 ml per m^2.— L. A. Weinrauch *et al.*, *Ann. intern. Med.*, 1977, *86*, 56.

A discussion of the predisposing factors associated with an increased risk of acute renal failure following administration of radiographic contrast media based on a study of 14 patients.— F. A. Krumlovsky *et al.*, *J. Am. med. Ass.*, 1978, *239*, 125.

Acute renal failure precipitated by Urografin in a patient with undiagnosed myoglobulinuria.— C. G. Winearls, *Br. med. J.*, 1980, *281*, 1603.

Further references:. L. A. Bergman *et al.*, *New Engl. J. Med.*, 1968, *279*, 1277; H. A. Feldman *et al.*, *J. Am. med. Ass.*, 1974, *229*, 72; J. A. Diaz-Buxo *et al.*, *Ann. intern. Med.*, 1975, *83*, 155; A. Kamdar *et al.*, *Diabetes*, 1977, *26*, 643.

Skin disorders. Iododerma was reported in 1 patient with renal insufficiency 4 days after he received for urography 120 ml of a diatrizoate preparation (Urografin 76%) corresponding to iodine 45 g; 12 days earlier he had been given metrizoic acid (Isopaque) equivalent to iodine 14 g.— G. Heydenreich and P. O. Larsen, *Br. J. Derm.*, 1977, *97*, 567.

A report of iododerma in a 62-year-old woman following an intravenous pyelogram using diatrizoates (Hypaque) and a lymphangiogram using iodised poppy-seed oil (Lipiodol Ultra-Fluid).— G. P. Sparrow, *J. R. Soc. Med.*, 1979, *72*, 60.

Treatment of Adverse Effects. Urticaria and other mild symptoms of hypersensitivity may be controlled by an intravenous injection of an antihistamine but for the general management of anaphylaxis, see Adrenaline (Allergy and Anaphylaxis), p.4.

Repeated doses of metaraminol tartrate maintained the blood pressure and restored the cerebral circulation in a 55-year-old man who had become hemiplegic after arteriography with meglumine diatrizoate. Dexamethasone, 8 mg initially then 4 mg six-hourly, was also given. In a 50-year-old woman, hemiplegia following arteriography was overcome by an intravenous infusion of noradrenaline tartrate.— G. R. Wise, *New Engl. J. Med.*, 1970, *282*, 610.

Inadvertent injection of water-soluble contrast medium into the subarachnoid space had been treated by irrigating the theca with normal saline and controlling convulsions with curare and artificial ventilation. The same procedure could be used in treating intrathecal overdosage with penicillin.— G. Ansell (letter), *Br. med. J.*, 1970, *3*, 707.

Radiological investigations with sodium diatrizoate, meglumine diatrizoate, and meglumine iodipamide were carried out in 69 patients with a history of adverse reactions to contrast media which included rash reactions in 37, anaphylactoid reactions in 9, and vasomotor reactions in 23. Those patients who had previously developed rash or anaphylactoid reactions were given prednisone 150 mg daily in divided doses starting 18 hours before the procedure and continuing for 12 hours afterwards. The only adverse reactions to the contrast media were 4 mild urticarial responses in patients given prednisone.— B. Zweiman *et al.*, *Ann. intern. Med.*, 1975, *83*, 159. See also R. Patterson and M. Schatz, *ibid.*, 277.

Failure of diphenhydramine and prednisone to prevent a severe anaphylactoid reaction to diatrizoates in a patient with a history of reaction to radiographic contrast media.— J. S. Madowitz and M. J. Schweiger, *J. Am. med. Ass.*, 1979, *241*, 2813.

Precautions. Sodium diatrizoate and other water-soluble contrast media should be used with caution in the presence of severe hepatic and renal impairment, severe hypertension, active tuberculosis, advanced cardiac disease, hyperthyroidism, phaeochromocytoma, or other grave general illness, and in patients with asthma, hay fever, sickle-cell disease, or hypersensitivity to iodine. The administration of iodine-containing contrast media may interfere with thyroid-function tests.

Precipitation of protein in the renal tubules, leading to uraemia, renal failure, and death has occurred in patients with multiple myeloma undergoing urography, possibly due to the additive effect of dehydration; particular care is necessary in such patients.

These media should not be given for hysterosalpingography in the presence of acute inflammatory conditions of the pelvic cavity or in pregnancy. Diatrizoates should not be used for urography in patients with anuria nor should they be injected into the subarachnoid space.

A black coloration developed during the copper-reduction tablet test in 8 of 20 urine samples taken from patients given sodium diatrizoate intravenously for urography. Meglumine diatrizoate, meglumine iothalamate, and meglumine iodipamide behaved similarly *in vitro*.— S. Lee and I. Schoen, *New Engl. J. Med.*, 1966, *275*, 266.

A preparation of sodium and meglumine diatrizoates (Gastrografin) given by mouth interfered with measurements of trypsin activity by spectrophotometric assay.— A. E. Cowen *et al.*, *Gut*, 1972, *13*, 395.

Chromosome damage in 20 infants and children after cardiac catheterisation and angiocardiography with diatrizoates (Renografin-76) was greater than that calculated from the X-ray exposure dose to the patient. Long-term follow-up studies were indicated to determine the long-term hazards of this type of examination.— F. H. Adams *et al.*, *Pediatrics*, 1978, *62*, 312.

Effect on platelet function. There was a 60 to 70% inhibition of platelet function in 2 patients within 20 minutes of an injection of a contrast medium containing meglumine and sodium diatrizoate [Renovist II]. After 3 days there was still a 45% inhibition. *In vitro* studies suggested that the initial effect was due to the chelating agent present in the dye but that the longer term effect was possibly due to the metabolic products of iodinated fatty acids.— L. M. Zir *et al.*, *New Engl. J. Med.*, 1974, *291*, 134.

Platelet aggregation and bleeding time were unaffected in 4 patients who underwent non-cardiac angiography with meglumine and sodium diatrizoates (Renografin 76); plasma concentrations of contrast media were however below those associated with platelet aggregation inhibition *in vitro*. Plasma concentrations in 13 patients who underwent cardiac angiography were higher and 7 had inhibition of platelet aggregation and 3 had prolonged bleeding times. It was not clear if contrast media caused clinically significant bleeding.— G. A. Shapiro *et al.*, *Radiology*, 1977, *124*, 641.

Renal failure in myelomatosis. References suggesting little risk of renal failure in patients with myelomatosus undergoing urography: C. Morgan and W. J. Hammack, *New Engl. J. Med.*, 1966, *275*, 77; E. C. Lasser *et al.*, *J. Am. med. Ass.*, 1966, *198*, 273; M. T. Cwynarski and H. M. Saxton, *Br. med. J.*, 1969, *1*, 486.

Stomal malfunction. Near-fatal haemorrhage in a patient was attributed to precipitation of diatrizoate in an achlorhydric gastric remnant. Diatrizoates should not be used for the investigation of postoperative gastroenterostomy stomal malfunction.— A. L. Gallitano *et al.*, *Radiology*, 1976, *118*, 35.

Absorption and Fate. Diatrizoates in the circulation are not significantly bound to serum proteins. If renal function is not impaired, unchanged sodium diatrizoate is rapidly excreted by glomerular filtration, but traces have been reported to remain in the circulation for 4 days.

Studies with intravenous injections of a 45% solution of sodium diatrizoate showed that plasma concentrations 10 minutes after injection were primarily a function of dose and body size. Excretion in urine was dependent upon glomerular filtration-rate and plasma concentration; the rate of excretion reached a maximum in the first 10 to 20 minutes. Increasing doses up to 1.65 ml per kg body-weight were associated with increasing rates of urine flow and with increasing concentrations of contrast medium in the urine.— W. R. Cattell *et al.*, *Br. J. Radiol.*, 1967, *40*, 561.

During the first month of an infant's life, the excretion of intravenously injected urographic contrast medium was prolonged. Maximum urinary concentrations appeared to be achieved 1 to 3 hours after injection.— M. B. Nogrady and J. S. Dunbar, *Am. J. Roentg.*, 1968, *104*, 289, per *J. Am. med. Ass.*, 1968, *206*, 2161.

A pharmacokinetic study in 10 healthy men showed no significant differences in concentrations in blood and urine between sodium and meglumine diatrizoate.— V. Taenzer *et al.*, *Eur. J. clin. Pharmac.*, 1973, *6*, 137.

Uses. Diatrizoates are used as contrast media in diagnostic radiology, as 25 or 45% solutions of the sodium salt or, when stronger solutions are required, as the meglumine salt of diatrizoic acid or mixtures of the sodium and meglumine salts. The high viscosity of concentrated solutions of the meglumine salt makes them difficult to administer rapidly.

Diatrizoates are given intravenously or by local application for a wide range of diagnostic procedures.

For urography they are given by intravenous injection or infusion, or by retrograde injection into the bladder or via a ureteral catheter.

For examination of the gastro-intestinal tract they may be given by mouth or as an enema. Barium sulphate has been given concomitantly. Tomographic procedures may be used concomitantly to yield additional diagnostic information.

A 22.5 to 45% solution of sodium diatrizoate has been given, with hyaluronidase, intramuscularly; a 22.5% solution has been given, usually with hyaluronidase, subcutaneously. Visualisation is somewhat delayed after these procedures. Diatrizoates are not suitable for myelography.

The lysine salt of diatrizoic acid has also been used.

The visualisation of hepatic amoebic abscess by sodium diatrizoate.— S. Chang *et al.*, *Am. J. trop. Med. Hyg.*, 1974, *23*, 31.

The injection of diatrizoates and azovan blue or indocyanine green was used successfully with xeromammography in 33 of 35 patients for the localisation of breast lesions.— R. W. Wayne and R. E. Darby, *J. Am. med. Ass.*, 1977, *237*, 2219.

Of 30 patients treated for sudden hearing loss with a regimen including vasodilators and meglumine diatrizoate (Hypaque) 9 had a good response, 7 had a moderate response, and 14 had little or no response. Most of the patients who responded were treated within the first month of onset of hearing loss, had no associated vertigo, and had had a hearing loss of less than 90 dB. Of a further 7 patients who complied with these criteria and who were treated using the regimen with vasodilators and meglumine diatrizoate 6 responded to treatment compared with 1 of 8 similar patients who were treated using the regimen without meglumine diatrizoate.— J. J. Shea *et al.*, *Otolaryngology*, 1978, *86*, 667.

A multicentre study of the use of diatrizoates with tomography.— J. S. Morrow, *Curr. ther. Res.*, 1980, *27*, 229.

Cystic fibrosis. A report of the use of sodium diatrizoate in the relief of a residual and late bowel obstruction in 3 infants with cystic fibrosis.— K. F. McPartlin *et al.*, *Br. J. Surg.*, 1973, *60*, 707.

Localisation of placenta. One ml of meglumine diatrizoate 60% was injected into the amniotic sac in 50 women with painless bleeding during the third trimester of pregnancy. This technique permitted correct localisation of the placenta in all but 1 patient, and permitted diagnosis of placenta praevia in 9 patients.— M. L. Blumberg *et al.*, *Am. J. Roentg.*, 1967, *100*, 688, per *Clin. Med.*, 1968, *75* (Apr.), 66.

Malignant effusions. Meglumine diatrizoate, or a mixture of meglumine and sodium diatrizoates, was instilled into the pleural, peritoneal, or tumour cavities of 24 patients with neoplastic disease to delineate tumour masses and to assess the size of the cavities and the freedom of distribution of fluids within the cavities. The dose for peritoneal cavities was 25 to 60 ml and for pleural cavities 25 to 30 ml, given in each case after the removal of most of the fluid.— A. J. Piro *et al.*, *J. Am. med. Ass.*, 1968, *206*, 821.

Urography. After a single intravenous injection of sodium diatrizoate 45%, 2.2 ml per kg body-weight, or an equivalent dose of sodium iothalamate 70%, the kidneys in 20 patients with oliguric renal failure were opacified and the presence or absence of extrarenal obstruction was correctly diagnosed; a nephrogram was not obtained in 1 patient. No adverse reactions or toxic effects occurred. Intravenous urography was not contra-indicated in anuric and oliguric patients and was less hazardous than retrograde pyelography.— C. B. Brown *et al.*, *Lancet*, 1970, *2*, 952.

Adequate diagnostic results were obtained, with no significant side-effects, in 258 urographic studies in 225 patients with reduced renal function; up to 150 ml of Urografin was given undiluted or by infusion.— P. Stage *et al.*, *Acta radiol., Diagnosis*, 1971, *11*, 337, per *Clin. Med.*, 1972, *79* (Oct.), 36.

In 32 patients with acute renal failure, excretion urography using 2.2 ml per kg body-weight of Hypaque 45%, or an equivalent of Conray 420, given intravenously over a period of 3 to 5 minutes permitted delineation of the kidneys in 31 patients and yielded a nephrogram and/or pyelogram of diagnostic value in 27 patients. There were no side-effects.— W. R. Cattell *et al.*, *Br. med. J.*, 1973, *2*, 575.

Venography. Sodium diatrizoate 45% was introduced into a vein on the dorsum of the great toe, from which it flowed directly into the deep veins. The technique, ascending functional cinephlebography, was used to assess the presence or absence of valves and their function.— V. V. Kakkar *et al.*, *Br. med. J.*, 1969, *1*, 810.

Preparations of Diatrizoates

Injections

Diatrizoate Meglumine and Diatrizoate Sodium Injection *(U.S.P.)*. Meglumine Diatrizoate and Sodium Diatrizoate Injection. A sterile solution of meglumine diatrizoate and sodium diatrizoate in Water for Injections, or of diatrizoic acid in Water for Injections prepared with the aid of sodium hydroxide and meglumine. It may contain small amounts of suitable buffers and of sodium calciumedetate or disodium edetate as a stabiliser. pH 6.5 to 7.7. When intended for intravascular use it contains no antimicrobial agents. Protect from light.

Diatrizoate Meglumine Injection *(U.S.P.)*. Meglumine Diatrizoate Injection. A sterile solution of meglumine diatrizoate in Water for Injections or of diatrizoic acid in Water for Injections prepared with the aid of meglumine; it may contain small amounts of suitable buffers and of sodium calciumedetate or disodium edetate as a stabiliser. When intended for intravascular use it contains no antimicrobial agents. pH 6.5 to 7.7. Protect from light.

Diatrizoate Sodium Injection *(U.S.P.)*. Sodium Diatrizoate Injection. A sterile solution of sodium diatrizoate in Water for Injections or a solution of diatrizoic acid in Water for Injections prepared with the aid of sodium hydroxide. It may contain small amounts of suitable buffers and of sodium calciumedetate or disodium edetate as a stabiliser. pH 6.5 to 7.7. When intended for intravascular use it contains no antimicrobial agents. Protect from light.

Meglumine Diatrizoate Injection *(B.P.)*. A sterile solution of meglumine diatrizoate containing a suitable stabilising agent. Sterilised by autoclaving. pH 6 to 7. Protect from light.

Sodium Diatrizoate Injection *(B.P.)*. Sod. Diatrizoate Inj. A sterile solution of sodium diatrizoate in Water for Injections containing suitable buffering and stabilising agents. Sterilised by autoclaving. pH 6 to 7. Protect from light.

Solutions

Diatrizoate Meglumine and Diatrizoate Sodium Solution *(U.S.P.)*. Meglumine Diatrizoate and Sodium Diatrizoate Solution. A solution of diatrizoic acid in water prepared with the aid of meglumine and sodium hydroxide. It may contain small amounts of suitable buffers, disodium edetate, and flavouring agents. pH 6 to 7.6. Not for parenteral use. Store in airtight containers. Protect from light.

Diatrizoate Sodium Solution *(U.S.P.)*. Sodium Diatrizoate Solution. A solution of sodium diatrizoate in water or of diatrizoic acid in water prepared with the aid of sodium hydroxide. It may contain a suitable preservative. pH 4.5 to 7.5. Not for parenteral use. Store in airtight containers. Protect from light.

Proprietary Preparations of Diatrizoates

Gastrografin *(Schering, UK)*. A 76% aqueous solution of sodium and meglumine diatrizoates, in the proportion 1:6.6, with added flavouring agents and a wetting agent. For use, by mouth or rectally, as a contrast medium in the radiological investigation of the gastro-intestinal tract. (Also available as Gastrografin in *Austral., Denm., Norw., Swed., USA*).

A report of the successful use of an iso-osmotic solution of polysorbate 80 and Gastrografin as an enema in the treatment of 5 children with severe bowel obstruction due to meconium or faecal mass.— B. P. Wood and R. W. Katzberg, *Am. J. Roentg.*, 1978, *130*, 747.

Hypaque *(Sterling Research, UK)*. Sodium diatrizoate or a mixture of sodium and meglumine diatrizoates, available as aqueous solutions of the following strengths: **Hypaque 25%** containing sodium diatrizoate 25%, equivalent to 15% of iodine, available in ampoules of 20 ml, and infusion bottles of 250 or 350 ml; **Hypaque 45%** containing sodium diatrizoate 45%, equivalent to 27% of iodine, available in ampoules of 20 and 30 ml; **Hypaque 65%** containing sodium diatrizoate 25.23% and meglumine diatrizoate 50.46%, equivalent to 39% of iodine, available in ampoules of 20 ml; and **Hypaque 85%** containing sodium diatrizoate 28.33% and meglumine diatrizoate 56.67%, equivalent to 44% of iodine, available in ampoules of 20 ml. **Hypaque Sodium**, available as a powder containing sodium diatrizoate, for preparing solutions for oral or rectal use. (Also available as Hypaque in *Austral., Canad., USA*).

Urografin *(Schering, UK)*. Meglumine diatrizoate or a mixture of sodium and meglumine diatrizoates, available as solutions of the following strenths: **Urografin 150 (30%)** containing meglumine diatrizoate 26.1% and sodium diatrizoate 3.9%, equivalent to 14.6% of iodine, available in ampoules of 10 ml and bottles of 250 ml; **Urografin 290 (60%)** containing meglumine diatrizoate 52.1% and sodium diatrizoate 7.9%, equivalent to 29.2% of iodine, available in ampoules of 20 ml and vials of 50 ml; **Urografin 310M** (formerly known as Angiografin) containing meglumine diatrizoate 65%, equivalent to 30.6% of iodine, available in ampoules of 20 ml and vials of 50 ml; **Urografin 325** (formerly known as Urovison) containing meglumine diatrizoate 18% and sodium diatrizoate 40%, equivalent to 32.5% of iodine, available in ampoules of 20 ml and vials of 50 ml; and **Urografin 370 (76%)** containing meglumine diatrizoate 66% and sodium diatrizoate 10%, equivalent to 37% of iodine, available in ampoules of 20 ml and vials of 50, 100, and 200 ml. (Also available as Urografin in *Austral., Denm., Ger., Norw.*).

Other Proprietary Names

Angiografin *(Austral., Ger., Ital., Norw., Swed., Switz.)*; Angiografine *(Belg., Fr.)*; Cardiografin, Cystografin *(both USA)*; Gastrografine *(Fr.)*; Hypaque-Cysto *(USA)*; Peritrast *(Ger.)*; Radiolar-280 *(Spain)*; Radiosélectan *(Fr.)*; Renografin *(USA)*; Reno-M *(Canad., USA)*; Renovist *(USA)*; Triyosom *(Arg.)*; Uropolinum *(Pol.)*; Urovison *(Austral., Denm., Fr., Ger., Norw.)*; Urovist *(Ger., Switz.)*; Urovist S *(Austral.)*.

1521-n

Diodone.

The diethanolamine salt of α-(1,4-dihydro-3,5-di-iodo-4-oxo-1-pyridyl)acetic acid.

$C_{11}H_{16}I_2N_2O_5$=510.1.

CAS — 300-37-8.

Pharmacopoeias. In *Jug. Nord.* and *Swiss* include Diodonum, the acid, $C_7H_5I_2NO_3$ = 404.9.

1557-y

Diodone Injection

(B.P. 1973). Diodone Inj.; Iodopyracet Injection; Cardiotrastum.

Pharmacopoeias. In *Ind.* which specifies 35%, *Rus.* which specifies 35, 50, and 70%, and *Swiss* which specifies 35 and 50%.

A sterile aqueous solution of diodone, prepared in three strengths, viz. diodone injection (35%) containing 17 to 18% w/v of I and having a wt per ml at 20° of 1.18 to 1.2 g, diodone injection (50%) containing 24.2 to 25.8% w/v of I and having a wt per ml at 20° of 1.26 to 1.28 g, and diodone injection (70%) containing 34 to 36% w/v of I and having a wt per ml at 30° of 1.355 to 1.39 g. It may contain a suitable stabilising agent.

A clear almost colourless to straw-coloured liquid with a pH of 7 to 8. A 9.21% solution is iso-osmotic with serum. It should not be allowed to come into contact with metals. It is **sterilised** by autoclaving or by filtration. **Store** at room temperature. Protect from light. Any solid matter which separates on standing should be redissolved by warming before use.

Incompatibility. Precipitation occurred when diodone injection 35% was added to promethazine hydrochloride injection.— T. R. Marshall *et al.*, *Radiology*, 1965, *84*, 536.

Adverse Effects, Treatment, and Precautions. As for Diatrizoic Acid, p.436.

Uses. Diodone has been used as a viscous solution, usually containing 35% of diodone, for ascending urethrography. For hysterosalpingography and salpingography a less viscous 35% solution has been used.

Diodone injection has been given parenterally for a variety of diagnostic procedures.

Proprietary Names

Diodon *(DAK, Denm.)*; Diodrast *(Winthrop, Canad.)*; Joduron *(Bracco, Ital.)*; Perjodal *(Pharmacia, Norw., Pharmacia, Swed.)*; Umbradil *(Astra, Austral.)*.

A preparation containing diodone was formerly marketed in Great Britain under the proprietary name Umbradil (*Astra*).

1558-j

Ethyl Monoiodostearate. A mixture of ethyl 9-iodostearate and ethyl 10-iodostearate (1:1) .

$C_{20}H_{39}IO_2$=438.4.

An oily contrast medium containing approximately 32% w/v of I.

Ethyl monoiodostearate is used for myelography and cerebral ventriculography.

Proprietary Names

Duroliopaque *(Temis, Arg.; Guerbet, Belg.; Guerbet, Fr.; Guerbet, Neth.; Guerbet, Switz.)*.

1559-z

Iobenzamic Acid. *N*-(3-Amino-2,4,6-tri-iodobenzoyl)-*N*-phenyl-β-alanine; 3-(3-Amino-2,4,6-tri-iodo-*N*-phenylbenzamido)propionic acid.

$C_{16}H_{13}I_3N_2O_3$=662.0.

CAS — 3115-05-7.

A white or slightly yellow powder, containing approximately 57.5% of I. Practically **insoluble** in water; slightly soluble in alcohol, acetone, chloroform, and ether; readily soluble in dioxan and dimethylformamide. **Protect** from light.

Iobenzamic acid is a contrast medium which has been given by mouth for the examination of the biliary tract in a dose of 3 g; heavy patients have been given 4.5 g.

Proprietary Names

Bilibyk *(Byk Gulden, Ger.)*; Osbil *(Byk Gulden, Ital.; Österreichische Stickstoffwerke, Switz.)*; Tracebil *(Christiaens, Belg.)*.

Iobenzamic acid was formerly marketed in Great Britain under the proprietary name Osbil (*May & Baker*).

1522-h

Iocarmic Acid.

MP 2032. 5,5′-(Adipoyldiamino)bis(2,4,6-tri-iodo-*N*-methylisophthalamic acid).

$C_{24}H_{20}I_6N_4O_8$=1253.9.

CAS — 10397-75-8.

A white powder. Slightly **soluble** in water; very slightly soluble in alcohol. **Protect** from light.

1560-p

Meglumine Iocarmate.

Iocarmate Meglumine. The di(*N*-methylglucamine) salt of iocarmic acid.

$C_{38}H_{54}I_6N_6O_{18}$=1644.3.

CAS — 54605-45-7.

It contains approximately 46.3% of I.

Adverse Effects. After lumbo-sacral radiculography meglumine iocarmate may cause headache, possibly persistent, nausea and vomiting, pyrexia, back and neck stiffness, lumbar pain, exacerbation of pre-existing pain, epileptiform seizures, syncope, hypotension and sweating, and circulatory collapse. Photophobia, skin rashes, arachnoiditis, and aseptic meningitis have also occurred. Some of these effects may be due to lumbar puncture. Spasm of the lower limbs has led to serious fractures. After cerebral ventriculography, headache, pyrexia, vomiting, and epileptiform seizures may occur. Local swelling and warmth have occurred following knee arthrography.

Bilateral central fracture-dislocation of the hips in a 27-year-old woman after myelography with meglumine iocarmate was attributed to severe clonic spasm. The use of the compound had been abandoned.— J. B. Eastwood *et al.*, *Br. med. J.*, 1978, *1*, 692. See also B. Parker and B. R. Reid (letter), *Br. med. J.*, 1978, *2*, 358.

Mild muscle spasm occurred in 0.5 to 2% of patients investigated by iocarmate myelography; very rarely the spasms were severe. Early intravenous administration of diazepam was important in limiting damage.— R. G. Grainger (letter), *Br. med. J.*, 1978, *1*, 1488.

Treatment of Adverse Effects. Spasm may be treated by the intramuscular or intravenous injection of diazepam 10 mg, repeated if required; larger doses have been given. If hypotension occurs the circulation should be maintained with the infusion of plasma or suitable electrolyte solutions; the intramuscular administration of methoxamine hydrochloride may be of value.

Precautions. The use of meglumine iocarmate should be avoided in patients with a known sensitivity to water-soluble iodinated contrast media, in patients with a history of asthma or epilepsy, in patients with hypotension, and in those taking antihypertensive drugs. It should be used with care in elderly patients and in those with cardiovascular or cerebrovascular disease. Examination should not be repeated within 4 weeks.

Absorption and Fate. After lumbar radiculography meglumine iocarmate disappears from the CSF in 6 to 12 hours; 50 to 60% of a dose is excreted in the urine within 24 hours, and 90% within 3 days; a small amount is excreted in the faeces.

Uses. Iocarmic acid is a contrast medium used, as a 60% solution of meglumine iocarmate, in lumbo-sacral radiculography, in cerebral ventriculography, in knee arthrography, and in hysterosalpingography.

Proprietary Names of Meglumine Iocarmate

Dimer-X *(Temis, Arg.; Guerbet, Belg.; Guerbet, Fr.; Byk Gulden, Ger.; Guerbet, Neth.; Rovi, Spain; Guerbet, Switz.)*; Dirax *(Jap.)*.

Meglumine iocarmate was formerly available in Great Britain under the proprietary name Dimer X (*May & Baker*).

1561-s

Iocetamic Acid *(U.S.P.)*. DRC 1201; MP-620.

N-Acetyl-*N*-(3-amino-2,4,6-tri-iodophenyl)-2-methyl-*β*-alanine; 3-[*N*-(3-Amino-2,4,6-tri-iodophenyl)acetamido]-2-methylpropionic acid.

$C_{12}H_{13}I_3N_2O_3$=614.0.

CAS — 16034-77-8.

A white powder consisting of a mixture of 2 stereoisomers and containing about 62% of I.

Adverse Effects. Iocetamic acid may occasionally cause nausea, abdominal cramp, diarrhoea, and dysuria.

Severe skin reactions occurred in 4 patients within 1 to 10 hours of taking iocetamic acid in doses up to 4.5 g. The rashes disappeared within 2 to 6 days.— M. L. Janower and M. A. Hannon, *Radiology*, 1976, *118*, 301.

Four hours after taking iocetamic acid 4.5 g, a 39-year-old woman developed oedema of the left arm and a macular rash over the rest of the body. Recovery took 4 days and was helped by the intramuscular injection of diphenhydramine.— R. M. Zeit, *Radiology*, 1977, *123*, 590.

Precautions. As for Iopanoic Acid, p.441.

Absorption and Fate. Iocetamic acid is absorbed from the gastro-intestinal tract. It is conjugated in the liver with glucuronic acid and is excreted in the urine; 40% of a dose has been reported to be excreted within 24 hours.

Uses. Iocetamic acid is used as a contrast medium for the examination of the biliary tract. A dose of 3 g is given by mouth 12 to 14 hours before examination. For visualisation of the biliary ducts a further 3 g should be given 3 hours before examination.

In a double-blind study in 85 patients undergoing cholecystography iocetamic acid 3 g produced slightly better visualisation than calcium ipodate 6 g.— M. Muller *et al.*, *Praxis*, 1973, *62*, 1517.

In a study in 51 patients iocetamic acid 4.5 g produced results similar to those produced by sodium tyropanoate 3 g.— D. Wishart and C. Dotter, *Am. J. Roentg.*, 1973, *119*, 429, per *Int. pharm. Abstr.*, 1974, *11*, 185.

In a double-blind study in 726 patients iocetamic acid 4.5 g produced more dense images than iopanoic acid or sodium tyropanoate in patients not given a fatty meal; a fatty meal improved the quality of the image only with iopanoic acid.— R. Stanley *et al.*, *Radiology*, 1974, *112*, 513, per *Int. pharm. Abstr.*, 1975, *12*, 203.

In a study in 800 patients iocetamic acid 3 or 4.5 g, iopanoic acid 3 g, and sodium tyropanoate 3 g produced comparable results. The incidence of cramps was reduced when the dose of iocetamic acid was reduced from 4.5 to 3 g.— R. Parks, *Radiology*, 1974, *112*, 525, per *Int. pharm. Abstr.*, 1975, *12*, 203.

Further references: J. A. Fielding and G. H. Whitehouse, *Clin. Radiol.*, 1979, *30*, 45.

Preparations

Iocetamic Acid Tablets *(U.S.P.)*. Tablets containing iocetamic acid. The *U.S.P.* requires 35% dissolution in 30 minutes and 50% in 60 minutes. Store in airtight containers.

Cholebrin *(Napp, UK)*. Iocetamic acid, available as tablets of 500 mg. (Also available as Cholebrin in *Denm., Norw., Swed.*).

Other Proprietary Names

Cholebrine *(Belg., Canad., Fr., Neth.)*; Colebrin *(Ital.)*; Colebrina *(Arg., Spain)*.

1523-m

Iodamide. Ametriodinic Acid; SH 926. *α*,5-Di(acetamido)-2,4,6-tri-iodo-*m*-toluic acid; 3-Acetamido-5-acetamidomethyl-2,4,6-tri-iodobenzoic acid.

$C_{12}H_{11}I_3N_2O_4$=627.9.

CAS — 440-58-4.

Pharmacopoeias. In *Jap.*

A white odourless crystalline powder. Slightly **soluble** in water and alcohol; practically insoluble in chloroform and ether; sparingly soluble in methyl alcohol; soluble in solutions of sodium hydroxide and sodium carbonate. **Protect** from light.

1524-b

Meglumine Iodamide. Iodamide Meglumine.

The *N*-methylglucamine salt of iodamide.

$C_{19}H_{28}I_3N_3O_9$=823.2.

CAS — 18656-21-8.

It contains approximately 46.3% of I.

1562-w

Sodium Iodamide. Iodamide Sodium.

$C_{12}H_{10}I_3N_2NaO_4$=649.9.

CAS — 10098-82-5.

It contains approximately 58.6% of I. Each g of sodium iodamide represents 1.54 mmol (1.54 mEq) of sodium.

Adverse Effects, Treatment, and Precautions. As for Diatrizoic Acid, p.436.

Uses. Iodamide is used, as its meglumine and sodium salts, as a contrast medium in diagnostic radiology and has properties similar to those of diatrizoic acid (see p.437).

Solutions used contain 65% of meglumine iodamide or mixtures of the meglumine and sodium salts, and are given intravenously or by local application for a wide range of diagnostic procedures.

Comparisons of meglumine iodamide with diatrizoate for intravenous urography: S. Gerzof *et al.*, *Am. J. Roentg.*, 1977, *128*, 211; A. H. Robbins *et al.*, *Am. J. Roentg.*, 1978, *131*, 1043.

Of 22 patients with sensorineural deafness 9 were treated with sodium iothalamate; 2 achieved complete recovery of hearing and 2 partial recovery. Of 13 treated with meglumine and sodium iodamide 7 achieved complete recovery and 1 near-complete recovery. Those responding had some hearing when first seen and had not suffered nausea, vomiting, or vertigo at the onset of sudden deafness. Treatment consisted of the intravenous injection of sodium iothalamate (80%) 1.6 g daily or meglumine and sodium iodamide (80%) 1.6 g daily for at least 4 days and continued for up to 16 days; the dose was increased if needed. The response was greater in those treated promptly.— N. Hirashima, *Ann. Otol. Rhinol. Lar.*, 1978, *87*, 29.

After intravenous administration to 7 healthy subjects, iodamide was eliminated rapidly and almost completely in urine, with negligible formation of metabolites. In 15 patients with renal failure elimination was slower, but still mainly in urine.— L. T. DiFazio *et al.*, *J. clin. Pharmac.*, 1978, *18*, 35. See also A. C. Bollerup *et al.*, *Eur. J. clin. Pharmac.*, 1975, *9*, 63.

Preparations of Iodamides

Meglumine Iodamide Injection *(Jap. P.)*. A sterile aqueous solution prepared from iodamide 24.75 g and meglumine 7.695 g, or iodamide 49.5 g and meglumine 15.39 g, in Water for Injections to 100 ml. pH 6.5 to 7.5. It contains approximately 15 or 30% respectively of I. Protect from light.

Meglumine Sodium Iodamide Injection *(Jap. P.)*. A sterile aqueous solution prepared from iodamide 62.79 g, sodium hydroxide 600 mg, and meglumine 16.59 g, in Water for Injections to 100 ml. pH 6.5 to 7.5. It contains approximately 60% of I. Protect from light.

Uromiro *(E. Merck, UK)*. Meglumine iodamide or a mixture of meglumine and sodium iodamides, available in ampoules of 20 ml and bottles of 50 ml as aqueous solutions of the following strengths: **Uromiro 300** containing meglumine iodamide 65%, equivalent to 30% of iodine; **Uromiro 340** containing meglumine iodamide 18.3% and sodium iodamide 43.4%, equivalent to 34% of iodine; **Uromiro 380** containing meglumine iodamide 70% and sodium iodamide 9.7%, equivalent to 38% of iodine; and **Uromiro 420** containing meglumine iodamide 40.8% and sodium iodamide 39.4%, equivalent to 42% of iodine. (Also available as Uromiro in *Ger., Ital., Neth., Switz.*).

Other Proprietary Names of Iodamides

Isteropac E.R. *(Ital.)*; Jodomiron *(Swed.)*; Opacist E.R. *(Ital.)*; Renovue *(USA)*; Urombrine *(Neth.)*.

1525-v

Iodipamide *(U.S.P.)*. Adipiodone; Bilignostum.

3,3′-Adipoyldiaminobis(2,4,6-tri-iodobenzoic acid).

$C_{20}H_{14}I_6N_2O_6$=1139.8.

CAS — 606-17-7.

Pharmacopoeias. In *Braz., Chin., Cz., Jap., Nord., Rus.,* and *U.S.*

A white, almost odourless, tasteless, crystalline powder. Very slightly **soluble** in water, chloroform, and ether; soluble 1 in 500 of alcohol; freely soluble in dimethylformamide; soluble with the formation of salts in aqueous solutions of alkali carbonates and hydroxides. A saturated solution in water has a pH of 3.5 to 3.9. **Protect** from light.

1526-g

Eglumine Iodipamide. Iodipamide Eglumine.

The di(*N*-ethylglucamine) salt of iodipamide.

$C_{36}H_{52}I_6N_4O_{16}$=1558.3.

It contains approximately 48.9% of I.

1563-e

Meglumine Iodipamide. Iodipamide Meglumine.

The di(*N*-methylglucamine) salt of iodipamide.

$C_{34}H_{48}I_6N_4O_{16}$=1530.2.

CAS — 3521-84-4.

It contains approximately 49.8% of I.

Incompatibility. Meglumine iodipamide was incompatible with chlorpheniramine maleate, diphenhydramine hydrochloride, brompheniramine maleate, or promethazine hydrochloride solutions. Sodium iodipamide was incompatible with diphenhydramine hydrochloride and promethazine hydrochloride.— C. Riffkin, *Am. J. Hosp. Pharm.*, 1963, *20*, 19.

Precipitation occurred when meglumine iodipamide injection (Cholografin) was added to brompheniramine maleate, chlorpheniramine maleate, dimenhydrinate, diphenhydramine hydrochloride, or promethazine hydrochloride injections.— T. R. Marshall *et al.*, *Radiology*, 1965, *84*, 536.

Adverse Effects, Treatment, and Precautions. As for Diatrizoic Acid, p.436.

Iodipamide preparations should not be used in patients with immunoglobulin IgM disorders such as macroglobulinaemia since gelatinous changes may occur in the blood.

Relapse of malaria occurred in 2 patients after the administration of meglumine iodipamide.— D. J. Crosby and A. H. Storm, *Archs intern. Med.*, 1966, *75*, 79, per *J. Am. med. Ass.*, 1966, *197* (July 25), A153.

Standard doses of iodipamide had a uricosuric effect.— A. E. Postlethwaite and W. N. Kelley, *Ann. intern. Med.*, 1971, *74*, 845, per *Abstr. Wld Med.*, 1971, *45*, 799.

Iodipamide was considered to be about 6 times more toxic than other contrast media being used for urography.— G. Ansell, *Adverse Drug React. Bull.*, 1978, Aug., 252.

Hepatotoxicity. A 66-year-old woman suffered a clinically mild but chemically severe hepatotoxic reaction following cholangiography with meglumine iodipamide.— A. E. Stillman, *J. Am. med. Ass.*, 1974, *228*, 1420.

Of 149 patients who received the dose of iodipamide recommended by the manufacturer 13 developed elevated serum aspartate aminotransferase (SGOT) values; of 126 who received twice the dose 23 developed elevated values.— F. J. Scholz *et al.* (letter), *J. Am. med. Ass.*, 1974, *229*, 1724.

Hepatotoxicity occurred in 2 patients following the injection of meglumine iodipamide for cholangiography. Nausea, vomiting, and fever after cholangiography might be indicative of hepatotoxicity.— L. R. Sutherland *et al.*, *Ann. intern. Med.*, 1977, *86*, 437.

A further report; hepatotoxicity occurred on the 4th exposure.— S. Imoto (letter), *Ann. intern. Med.*, 1978, *88*, 129.

Further reports: T. Motoki *et al., Am. J. Gastroent., N.Y.*, 1979, *72*, 71.

Absorption and Fate. Within 10 to 15 minutes of an injection of one of its salts, iodipamide appears in the hepatic duct and the common bile duct, and within 1 hour of the injection it appears in the gall bladder. About 90% of the dose is excreted in the faeces and the remainder in the urine.

Uses. Iodipamide is a contrast medium which is used mainly as its meglumine salt for the examination of the biliary tract when oral procedures are considered unsuitable. It has also been given in conjunction with orally administered cholecystographic media in order to obtain better visualisation in patients with poorly functioning gall-bladders.

It is administered by slow intravenous injection over an average of 10 minutes or by infusion. Doses of 5 to 10 g are employed.

For hysterosalpingography, a viscous 70% solution of meglumine iodipamide has been used.

Preparations of Iodipamides

Iodipamide Meglumine Injection *(B.P.)*. Iodipamide Methylglucamine Injection. A sterile solution of meglumine iodipamide. pH 6.0 to 7.1. It is sterilised by autoclaving.

Iodipamide Meglumine Injection *(U.S.P.)*. Meglumine Iodipamide Injection. A sterile solution of iodipamide in Water for Injections prepared with the aid of meglumine. It may contain small amounts of suitable buffers and of sodium calciumedetate or disodium edetate as a stabiliser. When intended for intravascular use it contains no antimicrobial agents. pH 6.5 to 7.7. Protect from light.

Proprietary Names of Iodipamides

Biligrafin *(Schering, Austral.; Schering, Denm.; Schering, Ger.; Schering, Ital.; Schering, Norw.; Schering, Swed.; Schering, Switz.)*; Biligrafina *(Schering, Arg.)*; Biligrafine *(Schering, Belg.)*; Cholografin *(Squibb, Canad.; Squibb, USA)*; Endocistobil *(Bracco, Ital.)*; Endografin *(Schering, Austral.; Schering, Ger.; Schering, Swed.; Schering, Switz.)*; Intrabilix *(Guerbet, Fr.)*; Transbilix *(Codali, Belg.; Therapex-Unik, Canad.; Guerbet, Denm.; Guerbet, Fr.; Guerbet, Neth.)*.

Meglumine iodipamide was formerly marketed in Great Britain under the proprietary names Biligrafin and Endografin (both *Schering*).

1564-l

Iodised Oil Fluid Injection *(B.P.)*. Ethiodized Oil Injection *(U.S.P.)*; Ethiodized Oil.

CAS — 8001-40-9 (iodised oil).

Pharmacopoeias. In *Br.* and *U.S. Fr.* includes Huile d'Oeillette Iodée.

A sterile iodine addition product of the ethyl esters of the fatty acids obtained from poppy-seed oil. The *B.P.* specifies 37 to 39% w/w of combined iodine. *U.S.P.* specifies 35.2 to 38.9% of combined iodine.

A straw-coloured or amber-coloured, clear, oily liquid which has not more than a slight alliaceous odour, and a bland oily taste. Wt per ml 1.28 to 1.3 g. It decomposes in air and sunlight and develops a dark brown colour.

Practically **insoluble** in water; soluble in acetone, chloroform, ether, and light petroleum. **Store** in an atmosphere of carbon dioxide or nitrogen in previously sterilised single-dose containers sealed by fusion of the glass or by any other method which makes the container gas-tight. Protect from light.

Because of its solvent action on polystyrene, iodised oil injection should not be administered in plastic syringes made with polystyrene.

NOTE. The *B.P.* directs that when Iodised Oil Injection or Iodised Oil is prescribed or demanded, Iodised Oil Fluid Injection be dispensed or supplied.

Adverse Effects and Precautions. The risk of hypersensitivity reactions (see p.436) is greater after the use of iodised oil than after water-soluble iodinated contrast media. Foreign body reactions have occurred. Great care should be taken to avoid vascular structures, because of the danger of oil embolism; it should not therefore be used in areas affected by haemorrhage or local trauma. Iodised oil should be used with care in patients with thyroid dysfunction or a history of allergic reactions. A prior sensitivity test is recommended before its use. The administration of iodine-containing contrast media may interfere with thyroid-function tests.

Conditions associated with the use of iodised vegetable oils for bronchography included lipid granuloma and arteritis obliterans. Pulmonary emboli had also followed injections of iodised oil for lymphangiography or following inadvertent intravenous injection in other examinations such as myelography.— P. D. B. Davies, *Br. J. Dis. Chest*, 1969, *63*, 57.

The use of oily contrast media for hysterosalpingography was dangerous and unnecessary. Oil embolism and pelvic adhesions had occurred, and violent reactions with pelvic abscess in the presence of unsuspected pelvic tuberculosis. Several patients had been seen with bilateral tubal occlusion following an original investigation, using iodised oil, which had shown tubal patency.— F. W. Wright and J. Stallworthy (letter), *Br. med. J.*, 1973, *3*, 632.

In 9 patients given 6 or 7 ml of iodised oil fluid injection into each foot for lymphography there was no fall in forced expiratory volume or vital capacity, though severe breathlessness had been reported by other workers. Gas transfer factor was reduced by a mean of 22%, with the greatest reduction 24 to 48 hours after lymphography. Patients undergoing lymphography should not be submitted to general anaesthesia or irradiation of the mediastinum or lungs until a week had elapsed, and lymphography should not be performed in patients who had had recent radiotherapy.— R. J. White *et al., Br. med. J.*, 1973, *4*, 775.

Consumption coagulopathy and renal impairment in a patient after hepatography with an iodised oil contrast medium.— J. Bernheim *et al., Nouv. Presse méd.*, 1974, *3*, 2635.

Hyperplasia of the thyroid glands observed in several infants who died from Rhesus sensitisation was attributed to the use of iodised oil fluid injection for amniography. It was considered that this contrast medium was contra-indicated in amniography.— D. M. O. Becroft *et al.* (letter), *Lancet*, 1976, *2*, 1191.

Absorption and Fate. Iodised Oil Fluid Injection is relatively rapidly absorbed after hysterosalpingography but may persist for several weeks or months after lymphangiography, and it is only slowly absorbed from most other body sites.

Uses. Iodised Oil Fluid Injection is a contrast medium which is used for lymphangiography and for the visualisation of nasal and other sinuses. It has been used for hysterosalpingography but water-soluble agents are often preferred. The dose is dependent upon the procedure. It is unsuitable for use in bronchography.

The use of iodised oil in treatment of endemic goitre.— I. H. Butfield and B. S. Hetzel, *Bull. Wld Hlth Org.*, 1967, *36*, 243; J. B. Stanbury *et al., Chronicle Wld Hlth Org.*, 1974, *28*, 220.

Over 4 years more than 1000 patients had been submitted to bilateral lymphography, using Iodised Oil Fluid Injection, introduced at a rate of approximately 1 ml in 8 minutes, without clinical evidence of pulmonary complications; the dose was 0.15 ml per kg body-weight divided so that the left side received 0.5 to 1 ml more than the right.— J. W. Davidson (letter), *New Engl. J. Med.*, 1971, *285*, 237.

The use of bilateral pedal lymphography in the assessment of neoplasms of the prostate.— R. M. Paxton *et al., Br. med. J.*, 1975, *1*, 120.

AG 60.99, an emulsion of iodinated poppy-seed oil, given intravenously, showed promise for computerised tomography of the liver and spleen.— R. J. Alfidi and M. Laval-Jeantet, *Radiology*, 1976, *121*, 491.

Proprietary Preparations

Lipiodol Ultra Fluid *(May & Baker, UK)*. Iodised Oil Fluid Injection, available in ampoules of 10 ml. (Also available as Lipiodol Ultra-Fluid in *Canad., Ger., Norw.* and as Lipiodol Ultra-Fluide in *Fr.*).

1565-y

Iodised Oil Viscous Injection *(B.P. 1963)*.

Iodised Oil Visc. Inj.; Iodized Oil Injection; Iodolipolum; Oleum Iodatum; Oleum Iodisatum.

Pharmacopoeias. In *Arg., Ind., Port.* (which has about 20% I), and *Rus.* (about 30% I).

In *Jap.* as Oleum Iodatum Fortius; Oleum Iodatum (*Jap. P.*) is about half this strength (about 20% I).

A sterile iodine addition product of poppy-seed oil. It contains 37 to 40% w/w of combined iodine.

A colourless or yellow, clear, viscous oil which is odourless or has a slightly alliaceous odour and a bland oily taste. Wt per ml 1.34 to 1.37 g. It decomposes in air and sunlight and develops a dark brown colour; it should not be used if it has darkened in colour.

Practically **insoluble** in water; soluble in chloroform, ether, and light petroleum. **Store** in previously sterilised single-dose containers sealed by fusion of the glass or by any other method which makes the containers gas-tight. Protect from light.

Because of its solvent action on polystyrene, iodised oil injection should not be administered in plastic syringes made with polystyrene.

NOTE. The *B.P.* directs that when Iodised Oil Injection or Iodised Oil is prescribed or demanded, Iodised Oil Fluid Injection be dispensed or supplied.

Adverse Effects and Precautions. As for Iodised Oil Fluid Injection.

Iodised Oil Viscous Injection should be used with care in patients with active tuberculosis.

Uses. Iodised oil is a contrast medium which has been used for the examination of the bronchial tract. Postural drainage is recommended after bronchography to minimise the amount of residual material. Any material swallowed should be removed by inducing emesis or by lavage.

Proprietary Preparations

Lipiodol Viscous *(May & Baker, UK)*. Iodised Oil Viscous Injection, available in vials of 20 ml.

Other Proprietary Names

Lipiodol 40% *(Neth.)*.

1566-j

Iodophthalein *(B.P. 1953)*. Iodophthal.; Iodophthalein Sodium; Iodognostum; Soluble Iodophthalein; Tetra-iodophthalein Sodium; Tetrothalein Sodium. Disodium 3′, 3″, 5′, 5″-tetraiodophenolphthalein trihydrate.
$C_{20}H_8I_4Na_2O_4,3H_2O = 919.9$.

CAS — 386-17-4 (tetraiodophenolphthalein); 632-73-5; 2217-44-9 (both disodium salt, anhydrous); 6011-87-6 (disodium salt, trihydrate).

Pharmacopoeias. In *Arg., Ind., Mex., Rus.*, and *Swiss.*

A blue or bluish-violet, odourless, crystalline powder with an astringent saline taste, containing not less than 87% of iodophthalein, calculated on the dried substance. The separated iodophthalein contains 60 to 63% of I.

Soluble 1 in 7 of water; slightly soluble in alcohol. A 9.58% solution in water is iso-osmotic with serum. Solutions are **sterilised** by filtration. **Incompatible** with acidic substances. It slowly absorbs carbon dioxide from the air becoming incompletely soluble due to the formation of tetraiodophenolphthalein. **Store** in airtight containers.

Iodophthalein has been used as a contrast medium for the examination of the biliary tract but toxic reactions frequently followed its use.

1527-q

Iodoxamic Acid. B 10610; SQ 21982. 3,3′-(4,7,10,13-Tetraoxahexadecanedioyldiamino)bis(2,4,6-tri-iodobenzoic acid).
$C_{26}H_{26}I_6N_2O_{10}$=1287.9.

CAS — 31127-82-9.

1567-z

Meglumine Iodoxamate. Iodoxamate Meglumine. The di(*N*-methylglucamine) salt of iodoxamic acid.
$C_{40}H_{60}I_6N_4O_{20}$=1678.4.

CAS — 51764-33-1.

It contains approximately 45.4% of I.

Meglumine iodoxamate is a contrast medium used for cholecystography, by intravenous injection or infusion.

References: E. N. Sargent *et al.*, *Am. J. Roentg.*, 1975, *125*, 251; A. Robbins *et al.*, *Am. J. Roentg.*, 1976, *126*, 70; *idem*, *127*, 257; A. Moss, *Am. J. Roentg.*, 1977, *128*, 931.

Proprietary Preparations of Meglumine Iodoxamate

Endobil *(E. Merck, UK).* Meglumine iodoxamate, available as a solution for intravenous infusion containing 9.91%, equivalent of iodine 45 mg per ml. (Also available as Endobil in *Ital.*).

Other Proprietary Names of Meglumine Iodoxamate

Cholovue *(Neth.)*; Endomirabil *(Ger.)*.

1568-c

Iodoxyl *(B.P. 1958).* Sodium Iodomethamate. Disodium 1,4-dihydro-3,5-di-iodo-1-methyl-4-oxopyridine-2,6-dicarboxylate.
$C_8H_3I_2NNa_2O_5$=492.9.

CAS — 519-26-6.

Pharmacopoeias. In *Arg.*, *Belg.*, *Ind.*, and *It.*

A white odourless powder, containing about 51.5% of I. **Soluble** 1 in 1 of water and 1 in 100 of alcohol; practically insoluble in chloroform and ether. Solutions are **sterilised** by autoclaving or by filtration and must not be allowed to come into contact with metal. **Protect** from light.

Adverse Effects, Treatment, and Precautions. As for Diatrizoic Acid, p.436.

It is more liable to produce local venous reactions than sodium diatrizoate.

Uses. Iodoxyl is a contrast medium which has been used for intravenous urography or retrograde pyelography.

Preparations

Iodoxyl Injection *(B.P. 1958, Ind. P.).* A sterile solution in Water for Injections. Protect from light.

Iodoxyl was formerly marketed in Great Britain under the proprietary name Uropac (*May & Baker*).

1528-p

Ioglycamic Acid. BE419. αα′-Oxybis(3-acetamido-2,4,6-tri-iodobenzoic acid).
$C_{18}H_{10}I_6N_2O_7$=1127.7.

CAS — 2618-25-9.

1529-s

Meglumine Ioglycamate. Ioglycamate Meglumine. The di(*N*-methylglucamine) salt of ioglycamic acid.
$C_{32}H_{44}I_6N_4O_{17}$=1518.1.

CAS — 14317-18-1.

It contains approximately 50.2% of I.

1569-k

Sodium Ioglycamate. Ioglycamate Sodium.
$C_{18}H_8I_6N_2Na_2O_7$=1171.7.

CAS — 3737-71-1.

It contains about 65% of I. Each g of sodium ioglycamate represents 1.71 mmol (1.71 mEq) of sodium.

Adverse Effects, Treatment, and Precautions. As for Diatrizoic Acid, p.436.

Ioglycamates should not be used in patients with immunogobulin IgM disorders such as macroglobulinaemia.

Intravascular precipitation and sudden death occurred in a patient with Waldenström's macroglobulinaemia given an intravenous injection of ioglycamic acid. IgM from this patient produced similar effects in *mice*.— M. Harboe *et al.*, *Lancet*, 1976, *2*, 285.

There were 10 episodes of raised transaminase concentrations with hepatic necrosis in 7 patients given meglumine ioglycamate for infusion cholangiography.— K. Winckler, *Dt. med. Wschr.*, 1978, *103*, 420.

The biliary excretion of ioglycamates was impaired in diabetic patients taking sulphonylureas, and in Scandinavian women taking oral contraceptives.— G. Ansell, *Adverse Drug React. Bull.*, 1978, Aug., 252.

Uses. Ioglycamic acid is a contrast medium which is extensively bound to plasma albumin. It is used, usually as meglumine ioglycamate, for the examination of the biliary tract. Meglumine ioglycamate is given intravenously as a 35% solution over at least 5 minutes or as a 17% solution by infusion over not less than 30 minutes. The bile-ducts are visible 1 to 1½ hours after the start of the examination, and the gall-bladder after about 2 hours. A mixture of the meglumine and sodium salts has also been used. It should not be used within 4 to 7 days of oral cholecystography.

In 50 patients submitted to cholangiography using 30 ml of 35% solution of meglumine ioglycamate and 50 given half the dosage, statistically better results were obtained with the higher dosage. The injection was given over 5 minutes. In 97% of those with intact gall-bladders maximum information was provided by 2 films taken at 60 and 90 minutes respectively. Absence of opacification at 60 minutes was indicative of cystic duct obstruction. In postcholecystectomy patients films at 30 and 60 minutes provided maximum information. Side-effects were nausea (3 patients), a metallic taste (8), and urticaria (2) readily responsive to chlorpheniramine maleate, 10 mg intramuscularly.— G. J. S. Parkin and H. Herlinger, *Gut*, 1974, *15*, 268.

Biliary excretion of meglumine ioglycamate began 20 minutes after the start of its intravenous infusion in 11 patients and was associated with a significant increase in bile flow compared with 10 controls and independently of bile salt secretion which was not significantly affected. Phospholipid and cholesterol secretion were significantly lowered in the treated group. There was a rise in the cholesterol-solubilising capacity of bile during meglumine ioglycamate excretion which suggested the possible development of a drug for dissolving cholesterol gall-stones.— G. D. Bell *et al.*, *Gut*, 1978, *19*, 300.

Plasma binding, renal and biliary excretion studies of meglumine ioglycamate in jaundiced and anicteric patients.— G. D. Bell *et al.*, *Br. J. Radiol.*, 1978, *51*, 251.

Proprietary Preparations of Ioglycamates

Biligram *(Schering, UK).* An aqueous solution of meglumine ioglycamate available as infusion containing 17% in vials of 100 ml, and as injection containing 35% in ampoules of 30 ml. For intravenous cholecystography. (Also available as Biligram in *Belg.*, *Denm.*, *Fr.*, *Ger.*, *Ital.*, *Norw.*, *Swed.*, *Switz.*).

Other Proprietary Names of Ioglycamates

Bilivistan *(Ger., Ital., Norw., Swed.)*; Bilivison *(Ital.)*; Bilograma *(Arg.)*.

1570-w

Iopanoic Acid *(B.P., U.S.P.).* Iopan. Acid; Acidum Iopanoicum; Iodopanoic Acid. 2-(3-Amino-2,4,6-tri-iodobenzyl)butyric acid.
$C_{11}H_{12}I_3NO_2$=570.9.

CAS — 96-83-3.

Pharmacopoeias. In *Arg.*, *Br.*, *Braz.*, *Chin.*, *Cz.*, *Int.*, *Jap.*, *Nord.*, *Roum.*, and *U.S.*

A white to cream-coloured tasteless or almost tasteless powder, odourless or with a faint characteristic odour; it darkens on exposure to light. It contains approximately 66.7% of I. M.p. 152° to 158° with decomposition. Practically **insoluble** in water; soluble 1 in 25 of alcohol; soluble in acetone, chloroform, ether, and aqueous solutions of alkali hydroxides and carbonates. **Store** in airtight containers. Protect from light.

Adverse Effects. Iopanoic acid gives rise occasionally to nausea, vomiting, abdominal cramp, diarrhoea, and, more rarely, dysuria. Pruritus and skin rash have been reported.

Iopanoic acid has a uricosuric effect.

A 50-year-old woman who took iopanoic acid 30 g over 5 hours suffered nausea, vomiting, and diarrhoea, but no other apparent ill effect.— W. D. Hankins, *Radiology*, 1971, *101*, 434.

Hypersensitivity. Submaxillary swelling in 2 patients after administration of sodium ipodate or iopanoic acid could have been hypersensitivity reactions to iodine. Such reactions were rare.— E. C. Lasser, *J. Am. med. Ass.*, 1969, *207*, 2291.

Renal failure. Acute renal insufficiency occurred in 2 patients given iopanoic acid 6 g. Both recovered.— R. M. Rene and S. M. Mellinkoff, *New Engl. J. Med.*, 1959, *261*, 589.

Acute renal failure followed doses of 6 to 15 g of iopanoic acid given to 4 patients for visualisation of the gall-bladder. In one patient an intravenous dose of meglumine iodipamide could have contributed to the reaction. Elderly patients with biliary tract disease might be liable to renal tubular injury from large or repeated doses of iopanoic acid.— C. O. Canales *et al.*, *New Engl. J. Med.*, 1969, *281*, 89.

Thrombocytopenia. All platelets disappeared from the peripheral blood of a woman given two 3-g doses of iopanoic acid. She recovered when treated with prednisone and no subsequent purpura developed though administration of iopanoic acid had previously provoked numerous petechiae on her neck and other skin areas.— G. A. Bishopric, *J. Am. med. Ass.*, 1964, *189*, 771.

Thrombocytopenic purpura occurred after ingestion of iopanoic acid on 3 occasions in a 48-year-old woman.— J. K. Hysell *et al.*, *J. Am. med. Ass.*, 1977, *237*, 361.

Precautions. Iopanoic acid is contra-indicated in severe hepatic or renal disease, and in patients with hypersensitivity to iodine; doses as high as 6 g should not be given to patients with renal impairment. It should not be used in the presence of acute gastro-intestinal disorders since its absorption may be impaired. It should be used with caution in patients with coronary artery disease, severe hyperthyroidism, or cholangitis. Premedication with atropine has been suggested for patients with recent coronary heart disease. The administration of iodine-containing contrast media may interfere with thyroid-function tests.

Small doses of aspirin blocked the uricosuric effect of iopanoic acid.— A. E. Postlethwaite and W. N. Kelley (letter), *J. Am. med. Ass.*, 1972, *219*, 1479.

Absorption and Fate. Iopanoic acid is absorbed from the gastro-intestinal tract and is strongly and extensively bound to plasma protein. It is conjuated in the liver to the glucuronide and about 65% is excreted in the bile and the remainder in the urine. It appears in the gall-bladder about 4 hours after a dose is taken and maximum concentrations occur after about 14 hours. About 50% of a dose is excreted in 24 hours and excretion is complete in about 5 days.

A review of the intestinal absorption, hepatic uptake, biliary excretion, and gall-bladder concentration of iopanoic acid.— R. N. Berk *et al.*, *New Engl. J. Med.*, 1974, *290*, 204.

Excretion in breast milk. The amount of iopanoic acid excreted in the milk of lactating mothers was too small to affect the child.— T. E. O'Brien, *Am. J. Hosp. Pharm.*, 1974, *31*, 844.

Uses. Iopanoic acid is a contrast medium used for the examination of the biliary tract. It is given by mouth with a light fat-free meal about 10 to 15 hours before X-ray examination, the usual dose being 3 g. Adequate fluid intake is desirable. After 2 or 3 exposures have been made, an emulsion or a meal rich in fats is given and as the gall-bladder empties further exposures are made. Adequate visualisation may not occur in patients with substantial gall-bladder disease or advanced liver disease.

An interval of 5 to 7 days should elapse if a repeat examination is to be carried out with double the dose of iopanoic acid. Double doses should not be given to patients with renal disease. Doses of 6 g have often permitted visualisation of the biliary ducts.

For the visualisation of biliary calculi 1 g is given thrice daily after relatively fat-free meals for 4 days and X-ray examination carried out on the morning of the 5th day in the fasting patient.

Sodium iopanoate has been similarly used.

Preparations

Iopanoic Acid Tablets *(B.P., U.S.P.)*. Tablets containing iopanoic acid. Protect from light.

Cistobil *(E. Merck, UK)*. Iopanoic acid, available as tablets of 500 mg. (Also available as Cistobil in *Ital., Spain*).

Telepaque *(Winthrop, UK)*. Iopanoic acid, available as tablets of 500 mg. (Also available as Telepaque in *Arg., Aust., Austral., Belg., Canad., Denm., Fin., Fr., Ger., Ital., Neth., Norw., Spain, Swed., Switz., USA*).

Other Proprietary Names

Bilijodon-Natrium (sodium iopanoate) *(Neth., Swed., Switz.)*; Biliopaco *(Spain)*; Colegraf *(Spain)*; Jopanonsyre *(Denm.)*; Neocontrast, Nigrantil (both *Spain*); Panjopaque (sodium iopanoate) *(Denm.)*; Teletrast *(Swed.)*.

1571-e

Iophendylate Injection *(B.P.)*.

Ethyl Iodophenylundecanoate Injection; Ethyl Iodophenylundecylate Injection. A sterile mixture of stereoisomers of ethyl 10-(4-iodophenyl)undecanoate.

$C_{19}H_{29}IO_2$=416.3.

CAS — 99-79-6 (iophendylate).

Pharmacopoeias. In *Br.*, *Jap.* and *U.S.*, which also includes Iophendylate.

A clear, colourless to pale yellow viscous liquid, odourless or with a faint ethereal odour, darkening on prolonged exposure to air, and containing about 30.5% w/w of I. Wt per ml 1.245 to 1.26 g.

Very slightly **soluble** in water; soluble 1 in 2 of alcohol; miscible with chloroform and ether. It is **sterilised** by filtration. **Store** in previously sterilised single-dose containers sealed by fusion of the glass. Protect from light.

Action on plastics. Polystyrene was soluble in iophendylate and syringes made from polystyrene were rapidly attacked. Syringes made from polypropylene appeared to be unaffected.— J. D. Irving and P. V. Reynolds (letter), *Lancet*, 1966, *1*, 362.

Adverse Effects. Side-effects such as headache, backache, and transient fever are common (10 to 30% of patients are estimated to experience these), and more serious symptoms of allergy and arachnoiditis sometimes occur. Aseptic meningitis has occurred.

Patients with subarachnoid bleeding were considered to be more likely to experience pain after myelography with iophendylate injection.— W. J. Howland *et al.*, *Radiology*, 1966, *87*, 253, per *J. Am. med. Ass.*, 1966, *197* (Aug. 29), A167.

Visual loss occurred in a patient 35 days after myelography with iophendylate; contrast medium was detected along the course of the optic nerve.— K. Tabaddor, *Archs Neurol., Chicago*, 1973, *29*, 435, per *J. Am. med. Ass.*, 1973, *226*, 1374.

Hyperthyroidism, twice previously suspected, was considered to have been precipitated in a 47-year-old man by the injection of 6 ml of Iophendylate Injection.— A. M. Silas and A. G. White (letter), *Br. med. J.*, 1975, *4*, 162.

Chronic urticaria and intermittent anaphylaxis in a man were due to iophendylate used in myelography 17 years previously. After removal of about 8 ml of iophendylate from the spinal canal the patient remained almost totally asymptomatic.— P. Lieberman *et al.*, *J. Am. med. Ass.*, 1976, *236*, 1495.

Focal seizures, which developed in a 30-year-old woman 4 months after a myelogram, were believed to be associated with retained Pantopaque.— M. K. Greenberg and S. C. Vance (letter), *Lancet*, 1980, *1*, 312.

Treatment of Adverse Effects. As for Diatrizoic Acid, p.436.

Precautions. Iophendylate should not be employed when lumbar puncture is contra-indicated, and to avoid subdural and extra-arachnoid extravasation it should not be used within 14 days of a previous lumbar puncture.

Reactions to iophendylate injection used for myelography occurred in 7 of 57 patients; 5 of the 7 patients had definite multiple sclerosis. It was considered that myelography should not be performed if multiple sclerosis was suspected.— P. Kauffmann and W. D. Jeans, *Lancet*, 1976, *2*, 1000.

Absorption and Fate. Iophendylate is very slowly absorbed from the spinal canal; its rate of disappearance has been reported to be about 1 ml per year.

Uses. Iophendylate injection is a contrast medium which is used mainly for myelography. Because of its low viscosity, it is easy to inject; it forms a discrete mass and as much as possible of the material should be removed by aspiration from the spinal column after the examination is complete.

Iophendylate injection has also been used for examination of the third and fourth ventricles, and to visualise the foetus in the amniotic sac prior to intra-uterine blood transfusion.

Iophendylate injection has been used as a basis for the intrathecal injection of phenol in the treatment of severe intractable pain and for the reduction of disabling spasticity (see p.571).

Small tumours of the internal auditory canal could be demonstrated by intraspinal injection of 1 ml of iophendylate and positioning of the patient.— W. E. Hitselberger and W. F. House, *J. Neurosurg.*, 1968, *29*, 214.

During 5 years, iophendylate had been used in 827 patients for examination of the posterior fossa for cerebellopontine angle tumours. There were no serious complications, and the incidence of headache and pain in the back and leg was less than 5%.— B. H. Britton *et al.*, *Archs Otolar.*, 1968, *88*, 608, per *J. Am. med. Ass.*, 1968, *206*, 2764.

Proprietary Preparations

Myodil *(Glaxo, UK)*. Iophendylate Injection, available in ampoules of 3 ml. (Also available as Myodil in *Austral.*).

Other Proprietary Names

Ethiodan *(Canad.)*; Pantopaque *(USA)*.

1572-l

Iophenoxic Acid. Iophenoic Acid. 2-(3-Hydroxy-2,4,6-tri-iodobenzyl)butyric acid.

$C_{11}H_{11}I_3O_3$=571.9.

CAS — 96-84-4.

Iophenoxic acid is a contrast medium which was formerly used for the examination of the biliary tract in a dose of 2 to 6 g.

1573-y

Iopydol. 1-(2,3-Dihydroxypropyl)-3,5-di-iodo-4-pyridone.

$C_8H_9I_2NO_3$=421.0.

CAS — 5579-92-0.

A white crystalline powder containing approximately 60.3% of I. Slightly **soluble** in water.

Iopydol is a contrast medium which is used in conjunction with iopydone for the examination of the bronchial tract. It is administered as an aqueous suspension containing 46% w/v of iopydol and 30.5% w/v of iopydone; the suspension contains approximately 50% w/v of I. Radiological clearing after bronchography is slower than for propyliodone.

For references to the use of iopydol with iopydone, see Martindale 27th Edn, p. 385.

Proprietary Names

Hytrast (iopydol and iopydone) *(Guerbet, Denm.; Guerbet, Fr.)*.

1574-j

Iopydone. 3,5-Di-iodo-4-pyridone.

$C_5H_3I_2NO$=346.9.

CAS — 5579-93-1.

A white crystalline powder containing approximately 73.2% of I. Practically **insoluble** in water.

Iopydone is a contrast medium which is used in conjunction with iopydol for the examination of the bronchial tract.

1530-h

Iothalamic Acid *(B.P., U.S.P.)*.

Iotalamic Acid; Methalamic Acid. 5-Acetamido-2,4,6-tri-iodo-*N*-methylisophthalamic acid.

$C_{11}H_9I_3N_2O_4$=613.9.

CAS — 2276-90-6.

Pharmacopoeias. In *Br.*, *Jap.*, and *U.S.*

A soft, white, odourless, crystalline powder. **Soluble** 1 in 400 of water and 1 in 330 of alcohol; practically insoluble in chloroform and ether; very soluble in solutions of sodium hydroxide and

soluble in other alkali hydroxides. Solutions are **sterilised** by autoclaving. **Protect** from light.
Iothalamic acid is related chemically to acetrizoic acid.

1531-m

Meglumine Iothalamate.

Iothalamate Meglumine. The *N*-methylglucamine salt of iothalamic acid.
$C_{18}H_{26}I_3N_3O_9$=809.1.

CAS — 13087-53-1.

It contains approximately 47.1% of I.

1575-z

Sodium Iothalamate.

Iothalamate Sodium.
$C_{11}H_8I_3N_2NaO_4$=635.9.

CAS — 1225-20-3.

It contains approximately 59.9% of I. Each g of sodium iothalamate represents 1.57 mmol (1.57 mEq) of sodium.

Incompatibility. Precipitation occurred when meglumine iothalamate injection 60% or sodium iothalamate injection 80% was added to promethazine hydrochloride injection.— T. R. Marshall *et al.*, *Radiology*, 1965, *84*, 536.

Adverse Effects, Treatment, and Precautions. As for Diatrizoic Acid, p.436.
Adverse effects with meglumine iothalamate are less severe than with equivalent doses of the sodium salt.

A patient given meglumine iothalamate for lumbar myelography developed temporary paresis of the lower limbs.— B. Steffensen, *Ugeskr. Laeg.*, 1972, *134*, 926.

In 66 patients receiving contrast media there were 10 reactions severe enough to require some treatment; 9 were with meglumine iothalamate and the other with meglumine diatrizoate. Sodium salts should be used in preference to meglumine salts in elderly patients receiving high doses of contrast media.— M. J. G. Smith *et al.*, *Br. J. Radiol.*, 1974, *47*, 566.

In 40 patients undergoing phlebography, usually with about 200 ml of 60% meglumine iothalamate, pain at the injection site and in the calf were common; foot swelling also occurred; skin necrosis occurred as a delayed effect in 1 patient. Retrospective study revealed necrosis of the foot in 3 further patients and gangrene in 2. At the end of examination, in which tourniquets were used above the knee and ankle, the veins were flushed with saline and clearance of the contrast medium encouraged by muscle contraction.— M. L. Thomas and L. M. MacDonald, *Br. med. J.*, 1978, *2*, 317.

Pulmonary oedema associated with contrast media of iothalamates.— A. F. Malins, *Lancet*, 1978, *1*, 413. Comments: P. Davies (letter), *ibid.*, 556; J. Goulton (letter), *ibid.*, 714; D. L. Roback (letter), *ibid.*, 1153.

Acidosis. Routine carotid angiography using meglumine iothalamate under general anaesthesia tended to produce a metabolic acidosis, enhanced by carbon-dioxide retention.— M. Marshall and G. A. Henderson, *Br. J. Radiol.*, 1968, *41*, 190, per *J. Am. med. Ass.*, 1968, *204* (May 6), A271.

Absorption and Fate. Iothalamic acid in the circulation is not significantly bound to serum proteins. If renal function is not impaired, unchanged medium is rapidly excreted, primarily by glomerular filtration. The excretion of the meglumine salt is accompanied by a greater diuresis than accompanies the sodium salt.

Uses. Iothalamic acid is used as its meglumine and sodium salts as a contrast medium in diagnostic radiology and has properties similar to those of diatrizoic acid (see p.437). The meglumine salt of iothalamic acid is generally better tolerated than the sodium salt but the high viscosity of solutions of the meglumine salt makes them difficult to administer rapidly. Solutions used contain up to 80% of the sodium salt, up to 60% of the meglumine salt, or mixtures of the 2 salts.
Iothalamates are given intravenously or by local application for a wide range of diagnostic procedures. For urography they are given by intravenous injection or infusion, or by retrograde injection into the bladder or via a ureteral catheter. For examination of the gastro-intestinal tract they may be given by mouth or as an enema. Barium sulphate may be given concomitantly.
Iothalamates have been given subcutaneously or intramuscularly, sometimes with hyaluronidase. Meglumine iothalamate has been used for ventriculography and lumbar radiculography; it is not suitable for thoracic or cervical myelography.

For some clinical reports of the use of iothalamates, see Martindale 27th Edn, p. 386.

Administration in renal insufficiency. There was no deterioration of renal function in 15 patients, with reduced renal function but free from myelomatosis or diabetes, when they were given large doses of iothalamates for urography or angiography. Avoidance of dehydration and of repeated doses in rapid succession was recommended.— A. Rahimi *et al.*, *Br. med. J.*, 1981, *282*, 1194.

Preparations of Iothalamates

Iothalamate Meglumine and Iothalamate Sodium Injection *(U.S.P.)*. A sterile solution of iothalamic acid in Water for Injections, prepared with the aid of meglumine and sodium hydroxide; it may contain small amounts of suitable buffers and of sodium calciumedetate or disodium edetate as a stabiliser. When intended for intravascular use it contains no antimicrobial agents. pH 6.5 to 7.7. Protect from light.

Iothalamate Meglumine Injection *(U.S.P.)*. A sterile solution of iothalamic acid in Water for Injections, prepared with the aid of meglumine; it may contain small amounts of suitable buffers and of sodium calciumedetate or disodium edetate as a stabiliser. When intended for intravascular use it contains no antimicrobial agents. pH 6.5 to 7.7. Protect from light.

Iothalamate Sodium Injection *(U.S.P.)*. A sterile solution of iothalamic acid in Water for Injections, prepared with the aid of sodium hydroxide; it may contain small amounts of suitable buffers, and of sodium calciumedetate or disodium edetate as a stabiliser. When intended for intravascular use it contains no antimicrobial agents. pH 6.5 to 7.7. Protect from light.

Meglumine Iothalamate Injection *(B.P.)*. A sterile solution of meglumine iothalamate containing suitable stabilising agents. pH 7 to 7.5. The solution is sterilised by autoclaving.Protect from light.

Sodium Iothalamate Injection *(B.P.)*. Sod. Iothalamate Inj. A sterile solution of sodium iothalamate containing suitable stabilising agents. Ph 7 to 7.5. The solution is sterilised by autoclaving. Protect from light.

Proprietary Preparations of Iothalamates

Cardio-Conray *(May & Baker, UK)*. A sterile solution containing meglumine iothalamate 52% and sodium iothalamate 26%, in ampoules of 20 ml and bottles of 50 ml. It contains the equivalent of 400 mg of iodine per ml. For angiocardiography. (Also available as Cardio-Conray in *Austral.*).

Conray 280 *(May & Baker, UK)*. A sterile 60% solution of meglumine iothalamate, in ampoules of 20 ml and bottles of 50 ml. It contains the equivalent of 280 mg of iodine per ml. (Other preparations of iothalamates are available as Conray in *Austral., Canad., Denm., Ger., Ital., Jap., Norw., Swed.*).

Conray 325 *(May & Baker, UK)*. A sterile 54% solution of sodium iothalamate, in ampoules of 20 ml and bottles of 50 ml. It contains the equivalent of 325 mg of iodine per ml.

Conray 420 *(May & Baker, UK)*. A sterile 70% solution of sodium iothalamate, in ampoules of 20 ml and bottles of 50 ml. It contains the equivalent of 420 mg of iodine per ml.

Conray 480 *(May & Baker, UK)*. A sterile 80% solution of sodium iothalamate, available in ampoules of 20 ml. It contains the equivalent of 480 mg of iodine per ml.

Gastro-Conray *(May & Baker, UK)*. A 60% solution of sodium iothalamate, with flavouring and sweetening agents, in bottles of 100 ml. It contains the equivalent of 360 mg of iodine per ml. For visualisation of the gastro-intestinal tract. (Also available as Gastro-Conray in *Austral.*).

Retro-Conray *(May & Baker, UK)*. A sterile 35% solution of meglumine iothalamate, in ampoules of 10 ml. It contains the equivalent of 163 mg of iodine per ml. For retrograde pyelography. (Also available as Retro-Conray in *Austral.*).

Other Proprietary Names of Iothalamates

Angio-Conray *(Canad., Ital.)*; Contrix 28 *(Belg., Fr.)*; Cysto-Conray *(Canad., USA)*; Sombril *(Spain)*; Vascoray *(Denm.)*.

1532-b

Ioxitalamic Acid.

Ioxithalamic Acid; AG 58107. 5-Acetamido-*N*-(2-hydroxyethyl)-2,4,6-tri-iodoisophthalamic acid.
$C_{12}H_{11}I_3N_2O_5$=643.9.

CAS — 28179-44-4.

1533-v

Meglumine Ioxitalamate.

Ioxitalamate Meglumine. The *N*-methylglucamine salt of ioxitalamic acid.
$C_{19}H_{28}I_3N_3O_{10}$=839.2.

CAS — 29288-99-1.

It contains approximately 45.4% of I.

1576-c

Sodium Ioxitalamate.

Ioxitalamate Sodium.
$C_{12}H_{10}I_3N_2NaO_5$=665.9.

CAS — 33954-26-6.

It contains approximately 57.2% of I. Each g of sodium ioxitalamate represents 1.5 mmol (1.5 mEq) of sodium.

Adverse Effects, Treatment, and Precautions. As for Diatrizoic Acid, p.436.

Uses. Salts of ioxitalamic acid (meglumine, sodium, and ethanolamine) are contrast media used for intravenous urography, angiography, and peripheral and selective arteriography; the meglumine salt is also used for hysterosalpingography.

Proprietary Names of Ioxitalamates
Telebrix *(Temis, Arg.*; *Codali, Belg.*; *Guerbet, Denm.*; *Guerbet, Fr.*; *Byk Gulden, Ger.*; *Guerbet, Neth.*; *Guerbet, Switz.)*; Vasobrix *(Guerbet, Denm.*; *Guerbet, Fr.)*.

1577-k

Methiodal Sodium

(U.S.P.). Sodium Methiodal; Sergosin; Urombral. Sodium iodomethanesulphonate.
CH_2INaO_3S=244.0.

CAS — 143-47-5 (methiodal); 126-31-8 (methiodal sodium).

Pharmacopoeias. In *Nord.*, *Rus.*, and *U.S.*

A white odourless crystalline powder with a slight saline taste followed by a sweetish aftertaste, containing approximately 52% of I. On exposure to light it decomposes and becomes yellow.
Soluble 1 in 0.8 of water and 1 in 200 of alcohol; practically insoluble in acetone, chloroform, and ether; very soluble in methyl alcohol. A solution in water has a pH of 5 to 8. Solutions are **sterilised** by autoclaving or by filtration. **Store** in airtight containers. Protect from light.

Adverse Effects, Treatment, and Precautions. As for Diatrizoic Acid, p.436.
After intravenous injection, methiodal sodium has a diuretic effect.

Uses. Methiodal sodium has been used as a contrast medium for the examination of the urinary tract by the intravenous and retrograde routes. For intravenous urography a 40% solution has been given and for retrograde pyelography a 15 to 20% solution is used.

Preparations

Methiodal Sodium Injection *(U.S.P.)*. A sterile solution in Water for Injections. pH 5 to 8.

1578-a

Metrizamide. Win 39103. 2-[3-Acetamido-2,4,6-tri-iodo-5-(*N*-methylacetamido)benzamido]-2-deoxy-D-glucose.
$C_{18}H_{22}I_3N_3O_8$=789.1.

CAS — 31112-62-6.

It contains approximately 48.2% of I. Freely **soluble** in water. **Protect** from light.

Adverse Effects and Treatment. As for Iocarmic Acid, p.438. Metrizamide is claimed to cause fewer side-effects than meglumine iocarmate.

No muscle spasm had been reported in the first 100 000 lumbar myelography examinations using metrizamide.— R. G. Grainger (letter), *Br. med. J.*, 1978, *1*, 1488.

A report of a grand mal seizure after lumbar myelography using metrizamide.— A. R. Wray *et al.* (letter), *Br. med. J.*, 1978, *2*, 1787.

In 100 patients undergoing venography one leg was examined using 50 ml of meglumine iothalamate (280 mg I per ml) and the other leg with metrizamide of comparable iodine content. Immediate pain was experienced by 68 and 15 patients respectively and pain one week later (74 patients) by 37 and 7 patients respectively. Flushing, nausea, vomiting, and foot or calf swelling were also reduced with metrizamide.— M. L. Thomas and H. L. Walters, *Br. med. J.*, 1979, *2*, 1036.

Cervical myelopathy, with arm weakness persisting 6 months later, after lumbar myelography with metrizamide.— M. Bastow and R. B. Godwin-Austen, *Br. med. J.*, 1979, *2*, 1262.

Severe delayed headaches and sometimes distressing nausea and vomiting associated with metrizamide given intrathecally. As these effects were possibly associated with cerebral swelling, iophendylate should be used rather than metrizamide for patients in whom a rise in intracranial pressure due to swelling might be harmful.— L. A. Cala (letter), *Lancet*, 1981, *2*, 922.

For a comparison on the incidence of deep-vein thrombosis following phlebography with metrizamide and Isopaque Cerebral, see under Precautions, Metrizoic Acid, p.444.

Nephrotoxicity. Rapid intravenous injection of metrizamide induced diffuse or focal osmotic nephrosis in 6 of 13 normohydrated patients with various types of kidney disease and various degrees of renal impairment. Renal impairment was mild and transient. Metrizamide nephrotoxicity is comparable to that of ionic contrast media.— J. -F. Moreau *et al.* (letter), *Lancet*, 1978, *1*, 1201.

Precautions. As for Iocarmic Acid, p.438.

Absorption and Fate. Metrizamide is rapidly eliminated from the CSF. It is not significantly bound to plasma albumin.

The pharmacokinetics of metrizamide were investigated after intrathecal injection in the lumbar area of 8 volunteers. There was considerable individual variation. Metrizamide was detected in the blood about 15 minutes after injection with maximum serum concentration in about 2 hours. About half of the dose had disappeared from the CSF in 45 minutes and about 70% of the injected dose was excreted unchanged in the urine within 24 hours.— K. Golman, *J. pharm. Sci.*, 1975, *64*, 405.

Uses. Metrizamide is a non-ionic contrast medium used in lumbar myelography. It is usually given as a freshly prepared 35% solution in a dose of 10 to 15 ml. It may be mixed with CSF if desired.

A review of metrizamide.— *Med. Lett.*, 1980, *22*, 56.

Metrizamide given intrathecally combined with computerised tomography provided a simple, reliable, and safe method for accurately diagnosing a suprasellar mass.— B. P. Drayer and A. E. Rosenbaum (letter), *Lancet*, 1976, *2*, 736.

Computerised tomographic myelography with metrizamide was used in 63 subjects aged 6 days to 21 years. There were no false-positives and one false-negative. Vomiting and headaches occurred in half the children and 10 had fever. Metrizamide was considered better than contrast agents such as iophendylate for the study of the sacral, lumbar, and midthoracic regions.— *J. Am. med. Ass.*, 1977, *237*, 757.

Cerebrospinal-fluid rhinorrhoea in one patient was successfully diagnosed using computerised metrizamide cisternography.— C. Manelfe *et al.* (letter), *Lancet*, 1977, *2*, 1073. See also G. Roberson *et al.*, *Am. J. Roentg.*, 1976, *127*, 965; B. P. Drayer *et al.*, *Radiology*, 1977, *124*, 349.

A double-blind study in 30 patients with heart disease undergoing coronary angiography with either sodium metrizoate or metrizamide indicated that both agents gave good visualisation of the coronary arteries but metrizamide produced less chest pain and heat sensation, a longer coronary transit time, and significantly smaller reductions in diastolic pressure and heart-rate.— I. Enge *et al.*, *Radiology*, 1977, *125*, 317, per *Int. pharm. Abstr.*, 1978, *15*, 822.

Ventriculography using both oxygen and metrizamide proved superior to computerised tomography in revealing the cause of obstructive hydrocephalus. Small tumours and intraventricular cysts, often missed with computerised tomography, were also well demonstrated.— A. Servo and V. Halonen, *J. Neurosurg.*, 1979, *51*, 211, per *J. Am. med. Ass.*, 1979, *242*, 2809.

Further references: *Acta Radiol.*, 1973, *Suppl.*, 1–390; R. G. Grainger *et al.*, *Br. J. Radiol.*, 1976, *49*, 996; J. Sackett *et al.*, *Radiology*, 1977, *123*, 779; W. R. Boyd and G. A. Gardiner, *Am. J. Roentg.*, 1977, *129*, 481; C. Graser *et al.*, *Dt. med. Wschr.*, 1979, *104*, 511; R. D. Strand *et al.*, *Radiology*, 1978, *128*, 405.

Proprietary Preparations

Amipaque *(Nyco, Norw.: Vestric, UK).* Metrizamide, available as vials of 3.75, 6.75, and 13.5 g with 20-ml ampoules of solvent (0.005% sodium bicarbonate solution). (Also available as Amipaque in *Austral., Canad., Denm., Ger., Norw., Swed., Switz., USA*).

1534-g

Metrizoic Acid. 3-Acetamido-2,4,6-tri-iodo-5-(*N*-methylacetamido)benzoic acid.
$C_{12}H_{11}I_3N_2O_4$=627.9.

CAS — 1949-45-7.

Pharmacopoeias. In *Nord.*

A white or almost white, odourless, crystalline powder, tasteless or with a slightly acid taste. On exposure to light it decomposes and becomes yellow.

Soluble 1 in 1200 of water, 1 in 600 of alcohol; practically insoluble in chloroform and ether; soluble in solutions of alkali carbonates and hydroxides. **Protect** from light.

1535-q

Meglumine Metrizoate. Metrizoate Meglumine. The *N*-methylglucamine salt of metrizoic acid.
$C_{19}H_{28}I_3N_3O_9$=823.2.

CAS — 7241-11-4.

It contains approximately 46.2% of I.

1579-t

Sodium Metrizoate. Metrizoate Sodium.
$C_{12}H_{10}I_3N_2NaO_4$=649.9.

CAS — 7225-61-8.

It contains approximately 58.6% of I. Each g of sodium metrizoate represents 1.54 mmol (1.54 mEq) of sodium.

Adverse Effects, Treatment, and Precautions. As for Diatrizoic Acid, p.436.

In 61 patients in whom initial phlebography was normal the fibrinogen uptake test became abnormal after phlebography (60 to 120 ml of meglumine metrizoate; 280 mg I per ml). There was independent evidence of thrombosis in 4 patients. In several patients a uniform clinical picture included pain 5 to 10 hours after phlebography, ascending from the site of injection at the foot to the calf. There was a strong suggestion that thrombosis and embolism could be caused by phlebography.— U. Albrechtsson and C. -G. Olsson, *Lancet*, 1976, *1*, 723.

In a study of the incidence of deep-vein thrombosis following phlebography with Isopaque Cerebral or metrizamide, 90 patients with no signs of thrombosis on first examination were followed up for 6 days. Deep-vein thrombosis was confirmed by a second phlebography in 11 of 42 patients who had received Isopaque Cerebral and in 1 of 48 who had received metrizamide. Further study of whether patients were taking anticoagulants suggested that effective anticoagulant therapy reduced the risk of deep-vein thrombosis after phlebography with hypertonic contrast media. It was recommended that patients not already receiving anticoagulant therapy should be given heparin when phlebography with hypertonic contrast media was performed. It was suggested that 5000 units of heparin should be given intravenously and 5000 to 10 000 units subcutaneously within one hour before phlebography. Additional doses of heparin 5000 units could be given 12 and 24 hours after the procedure to patients confined to bed.— F. Laerum *et al.* (letter), *Lancet*, 1980, *1*, 1141.

Absorption and Fate. Metrizoates are rapidly eliminated after intravenous injection; 86% of a dose has been reported to be recovered in the urine in 6 hours and 95% in 24 hours. Two phases of elimination, with half-lives of about 15 and 105 minutes, have been reported.

Uses. Metrizoic acid is a contrast medium which, as its meglumine and sodium salts, has properties and uses similar to those of the diatrizoates (see p.437). It is used as solutions containing about 53 to 66% of the sodium salt, or about 59 to 66% of the meglumine salt, usually with the addition of small amounts of calcium or calcium and magnesium metrizoates (which are claimed to improve tolerance) for a wide variety of diagnostic procedures. It is not suitable for myelography.

A preparation of meglumine, sodium, and calcium metrizoates (Triosil Meglumine 370) was compared with preparations of meglumine and sodium diatrizoates in patients undergoing coronary arteriography. Electrocardiographic changes were less with the metrizoates than the diatrizoates.— D. Verel *et al.*, *Br. Heart J.*, 1975, *37*, 1049.

Proprietary Preparations of Metrizoates

Isopaque (formerly known as Triosil) *(Nyco, Norw.: Vestric, UK).* Preparations of metrizoates, available as: **Isopaque 350**. A sterile aqueous solution containing in each ml sodium metrizoate 528 mg, calcium metrizoate ($C_{24}H_{20}CaI_6N_4O_8$ = 1294.0) 28 mg, magnesium metrizoate ($C_{24}H_{20}I_6MgN_4O_8$ = 1278.2) 20 mg, and meglumine metrizoate 30 mg, in ampoules of 20 ml and bottles of 50 ml. It contains the equivalent of 350 mg of iodine per ml. For pyelography and angiography. **Isopaque 440**. Contains in each ml sodium metrizoate 660 mg, calcium metrizoate 35 mg, magnesium metrizoate 25 mg, and meglumine metrizoate 38 mg, in ampoules of 20 ml and bottles of 50 ml. It contains the equivalent of 440 mg of iodine per ml. For pyelography and angiography. **Isopaque Cerebral 280**. A sterile aqueous solution containing in each ml meglumine metrizoate 591 mg and calcium metrizoate 11.3 mg, in ampoules of 20 ml and bottles of 50 ml. It contains the equivalent of 280 mg of iodine per ml. For pyelography and angiography. **Isopaque Coronar 370**. Contains in each ml meglumine metrizoate 656.5 mg, sodium metrizoate 101 mg, and calcium metrizoate 11.3 mg, in ampoules of 20 ml and bottles of 50 ml. It contains the equivalent of 370 mg of iodine per ml. For angiography. (Also available as Isopaque in *Canad., Denm., Fr., Swed., USA*). (Known in some countries as Triosil or Ronpacon).

Other Proprietary Names of Metrizoates

Nitigraf *(Spain).*

1580-l

Pheniodol *(B.P. 1958).* Feniodol; Iodoalphionic Acid; Bilitrastum. 3-(4-Hydroxy-3,5-di-iodophenyl)-2-phenylpropionic acid.
$C_{15}H_{12}I_2O_3$=494.1.

CAS — 577-91-3.

Pharmacopoeias. In *Cz.*, *Rus.*, and *Swiss.*

A creamy-white powder with a slight odour and a slight taste followed by local tingling; alkaline solutions have a bitter nauseous taste. It contains about 51% of I. M.p. 158° to 162°.

Practically **insoluble** in water; soluble 1 in 5 of alcohol, 1 in 30 of chloroform, and 1 in 4 of ether; soluble in aqueous alkaline solutions. **Incompatible** with oxidising agents. **Protect** from light.

Pheniodol is a contrast medium which has been used for the examination of the biliary tract in a dose of 3 to 6 g.

1581-y

Phenobutiodil. TH 4114. 2-(2,4,6-Tri-iodophenoxy)butyric acid.
$C_{10}H_9I_3O_3$=557.9.

CAS — 554-24-5.

An almost odourless yellowish-white powder with a slightly bitter taste, containing approximately 68.2% of I. Practically **insoluble** in water; soluble in alcohol, chloroform, dioxan, ether, ethyl acetate, and fixed oils; slightly soluble in light petroleum. Alkaline solutions are unstable and solutions in organic solvents should be **protected** from light.

Adverse Effects and Precautions. As for Iopanoic Acid, p.441.
Frequency of urination may be increased.

Uses. Phenobutiodil is a contrast medium with properties and uses similar to those of iopanoic acid (see p.442). The usual dose is 3 g, increased if necessary for heavy patients to 4.5 g.

Phenobutiodil was formerly marketed in Great Britain under the proprietary name Biliodyl (*May & Baker*).

1582-j

Propyliodone (*B.P., U.S.P.*). Propyliodonum.

Propyl 1,4-dihydro-3,5-di-iodo-4-oxo-1-pyridylacetate.
$C_{10}H_{11}I_2NO_3$=447.0.

CAS — 587-61-1.

Pharmacopoeias. In *Br., Cz., Nord.,* and *U.S.*

A white or almost white, tasteless or almost tasteless, crystalline powder, odourless or with a slight odour, containing approximately 56.8% of I. M.p. 187° to 190°.
Practically **insoluble** in water; soluble 1 in 500 of alcohol, 1 in 150 of chloroform; soluble in acetone and ether. It is **sterilised** by maintaining at 150° for 1 hour; aqueous and oily suspensions for injection are prepared aseptically. **Store** in airtight containers. Protect from light.

Adverse Effects. Propyliodone may give rise to a slight febrile reaction, especially with the aqueous suspension, lasting 24 to 36 hours and sometimes accompanied by coughing. In a few cases, dyspnoea has occurred and, very rarely, transient lobar collapse.

Precautions. Propyliodone should not be used where there is hypersensitivity to iodine. It should be used with care in patients with asthma, bronchiectasis, or pulmonary emphysema. If bilateral examination is necessary in such patients an interval of several days should elapse between the examinations. Use of an excessive volume may result in lobar collapse.
The administration of iodine-containing contrast media may interfere with thyroid-function tests.

Absorption and Fate. After instillation into the lungs some propyliodone may be expectorated and swallowed but the remainder is hydrolysed in the lungs and absorbed. More than 50% of the administered dose is eliminated in the urine within 3 days as di-iodopyridone acetate.

Uses. Propyliodone is a contrast medium used for the examination of the bronchial tract. It may be used in active tuberculosis.
Propyliodone is usually administered in the form of either a 50% aqueous suspension or a 60% oily suspension. Propyliodone gives well-defined bronchograms for at least 30 minutes. Propyliodone has also been used in the investigation of fistulas and sinuses.

Preparations

Propyliodone Oily Suspension *(B.P.).* Sterile Propyliodone Oil Suspension *(U.S.P.)*; Propyliodone Oily Injection. A sterile 60% w/v suspension of propyliodone in arachis oil. It is prepared aseptically. Store below 30°. Protect from light.

Propyliodone Suspension *(B.P.).* Propyliodone Injection. A sterile 50% w/v suspension of propyliodone in Water for Injections containing suitable suspending and dispersing agents; it may contain a suitable buffering agent and antimicrobial preservative. It is prepared aseptically. pH 6 to 7.5. Store between 10° and 30°. Protect from light.

Proprietary Preparations

Dionosil Aqueous *(Glaxo, UK).* A 50% aqueous suspension of propyliodone, in vials of 20 ml. **Dionosil Oily.** A 60% suspension of propyliodone in arachis oil, in vials of 20 ml. (Also available as Dionosil in *Austral., Canad., Ger., Neth., Norw., Swed., Switz.*).

1583-z

Sodium Diprotrizoate. Sodium 2,4,6-tri-iodo-3,5-di(propionamido)benzoate.
$C_{13}H_{12}I_3N_2NaO_4$=664.0.

CAS — 85-16-5 (diprotrizoic acid); 129-57-7 (sodium diprotrizoate).

Sodium diprotrizoate is a contrast medium formerly used for intravenous urography, the usual dose being 20 to 30 ml of a 50% solution.

1584-c

Sodium Iodohippurate. Sodium Ortho-iodohippurate. Sodium α-(2-iodobenzamido)acetate dihydrate.
$C_9H_7INNaO_3,2H_2O$=363.1.

CAS — 147-58-0 (o-iodohippuric acid); 133-17-5 (sodium iodohippurate, anhydrous).

A white crystalline powder with a faint odour and a soapy taste, containing approximately 35% of I. **Soluble** in water yielding a neutral or faintly alkaline solution; soluble in alcohol and dilute solutions of alkali hydroxides. A 5.92% solution is iso-osmotic with serum.

Sodium iodohippurate has been used for intravenous, retrograde, and oral pyelography.

1585-k

Sodium Ipodate. Ipodate Sodium (*U.S.P.*);

Sodium Iopodate. Sodium 3-(3-dimethylaminomethyleneamino-2,4,6-tri-iodophenyl)propionate.
$C_{12}H_{12}I_3N_2NaO_2$=619.9.

CAS — 1221-56-3.

Pharmacopoeias. In *Jap., Nord.,* and *U.S.*

A fine white or off-white, odourless, crystalline powder, containing approximately 61.4% of I. **Soluble** 1 in less than 1 of water, 1 in 2 of alcohol, 1 in 2 of dimethylacetamide, and 1 in 3.5 of dimethylformamide and dimethyl sulphoxide; very slightly soluble in chloroform; freely soluble in methyl alcohol. A 10% solution in water has a pH of 8.9 to 9.9. **Incompatible** with acids and many metallic salts. **Store** in airtight containers. Protect from light.

Adverse Effects and Precautions. As for Iopanoic Acid, p.441.

Hyperthyroidism occurred in 2 patients submitted to cholecystography, using sodium ipodate 3 and 6 g respectively.— B. J. Fairhurst and N. Naqvi, *Br. med. J.*, 1975, *3*, 630. A causal relationship was not established.— R. L. Himsworth *et al.* (letter), *ibid.*, 1975, *4*, 162.

For a report of submaxillary swelling after administration of sodium ipodate, see Iopanoic Acid, p.441.

Absorption and Fate. Sodium ipodate is absorbed from the gastro-intestinal tract and maximum concentrations are found in the gall-bladder about 10 hours after ingestion. It is excreted mainly in the urine.

Uses. Sodium ipodate is a contrast medium used for examination of the biliary tract. It is used similarly to calcium ipodate (see p.435) and in the same doses.

In a study of 4 patients with hyperthyroidism, sodium ipodate 3 g as a single dose by mouth lowered serum concentrations of tri-iodothyronine and thyroxine. It was suggested that sodium ipodate might be useful in the treatment of patients with hyperthyroid Graves' disease.— S. -Y. Wu, *Ann. intern. Med.*, 1978, *88*, 379.

Preparations

Ipodate Sodium Capsules *(U.S.P.).* Capsules containing sodium ipodate. Store in airtight containers.

Biloptin *(Schering, UK).* Sodium ipodate, available as capsules of 500 mg. (Also available as Biloptin in *Arg., Austral., Denm., Ger., Ital., Norw., Swed., Switz.*).

Other Proprietary Names

Biloptine *(Belg., Fr.)*; Oragrafin Sodium *(Canad., USA)*.

1586-a

Sodium Tyropanoate. Tyropanoate Sodium *(U.S.P.)*; Win 8851-2. Sodium 2-(3-butyramido-2,4,6-tri-iodobenzyl)butyrate.
$C_{15}H_{17}I_3NNaO_3$=663.0.

CAS — 27293-82-9 (tyropanoic acid); 7246-21-1 (sodium tyropanoate).

Pharmacopoeias. In *U.S.*

A white odourless hygroscopic powder with a bitter taste. **Soluble** in water, alcohol, and dimethylformamide; very slightly soluble in acetone and ether. **Store** in airtight containers. Protect from light.

Sodium tyropanoate is a contrast medium, containing approximately 57.4% of I, which is used for examination of the biliary tract. It is given by mouth in a dose of 3 g.

References: P. M. Krook and W. H. Bush, *Radiology*, 1978, *127*, 643.

Preparations

Tyropanoate Sodium Capsules *(U.S.P.).* Capsules containing sodium tyropanoate. Store in airtight containers. Protect from light.

Proprietary Names

Bilopaque *(Winthrop, Canad.; Winthrop, Switz.; Winthrop, USA)*; Lumopaque *(Winthrop, Arg.)*.

Corticosteroids

1060-e

The adrenal cortex produces a number of steroids which may be divided into 3 classes; those whose principal pharmacological actions are upon gluconeogenesis, glycogen deposition, and protein and calcium metabolism, together with inhibition of corticotrophin secretion, and anti-inflammatory activity (glucocorticoid actions), namely, cortisone and hydrocortisone; those whose principal actions are upon electrolyte and water metabolism (mineralocorticoid actions), namely, deoxycortone and aldosterone; and the sex corticoids which include mainly androgens.

The naturally occurring corticosteroids in the first 2 classes, except aldosterone which is relatively independent, are secreted under the influence of the anterior pituitary corticotrophic hormone, corticotrophin (see p.486); all 4 have mineralocorticoid actions to a varying degree and they all, with the possible exception of deoxycortone, have some glucocorticoid actions.

In addition to the naturally occurring corticosteroids, many synthetic steroids with similar properties have been introduced. In developing these synthetic analogues the aim has usually been firstly to produce enhanced potency generally and secondly to separate the 2 main pharmacological actions so that, for example, an increase in glucocorticoid actions is not accompanied by a parallel increase in mineralocorticoid effects.

Therapeutically, the mineralocorticoid actions are used in conditions such as Addison's disease and the glucocorticoid actions, which are related to the apparently inseparable anti-inflammatory, anti-allergic, and antirheumatic properties, in conditions such as asthma and rheumatoid arthritis. It appears that a measure of a corticosteroid's potency as a glucocorticoid is the degree of inhibition of corticotrophin secretion it produces.

Publications on corticosteroid therapy: A. B. Myles and J. R. Daly, *Corticosteroid and ACTH Treatment, Principles and Problems*, London, Arnold, 1974.

The chemical structures of the corticosteroids described in this section are all very similar and resemble those of androgens and oestrogens.

The main corticosteroids used systemically are hydroxy compounds (alcohols). They are relatively insoluble in water and the sodium salt of the phosphate or succinate ester is generally used to provide water-soluble forms for injections or solutions. Such esters are readily hydrolysed in the body.

Esterification of corticosteroids at the 17 or 21 positions with fatty acids generally increases the activity on the skin. The formation of cyclic acetonides at the 16 and 17 positions further increases topical anti-inflammatory activity, usually without increasing systemic glucocorticoid activity, and fluorinated corticosteroids also generally have increased topical activity.

Some corticosteroids esterified at the 17 position are much more potent topically than systemically, e.g. beclomethasone dipropionate and betamethasone valerate; they are used by inhalation where their potent anti-inflammatory effect on the lungs has little systemic effect.

In the medical and pharmacological literature the names of unesterified corticosteroids have frequently been used indiscriminately for both the unesterified and esterified forms and it is not always apparent to which form reference is being made. The unesterified form is sometimes qualified by the phrase 'free alcohol'.

Adverse Effects of Corticosteroids. The side-effects associated with the use of corticosteroids in the large doses often necessary to produce a therapeutic response result from excessive action on electrolyte balance, excessive action on other aspects of metabolism including gluconeogenesis, the action on tissue repair and healing, and an inhibitory effect on the secretion of corticotrophin by the anterior lobe of the pituitary gland.

Disturbance of electrolyte balance is manifest in the retention of sodium and water, with oedema and hypertension, and in the increased excretion of potassium with the possibility of hypokalaemic alkalosis. In extreme cases, cardiac failure may be induced. Disturbances of electrolyte balance are common with the naturally occurring corticotrophin, cortisone, deoxycortone, and hydrocortisone, but are less frequent with many synthetic derivatives, such as betamethasone, dexamethasone, methylprednisolone, prednisolone, prednisone, and triamcinolone which have little or no mineralocorticoid activity. Most topically applied corticosteroids may, under certain circumstances, be absorbed in sufficient amounts to produce systemic effects.

Other excessive metabolic effects lead to mobilisation of calcium and phosphorus, with osteoporosis and spontaneous fractures, nitrogen depletion, and hyperglycaemia with accentuation or precipitation of the diabetic state. The insulin requirements of diabetic patients are increased. Increased appetite is often reported.

The effect on tissue repair is manifest in delayed wound healing, and increased liability to infection. There may be peptic ulceration with haemorrhage and perforation but reviews of the literature do not confirm that corticosteroids are associated with an increased incidence of peptic ulceration. The topical application of corticosteroid preparations to the eyes has produced corneal ulcers, raised intra-ocular pressure, and reduced visual function, and systemic administration has caused posterior subcapsular cataract. Increased susceptibility to all kinds of infection, including sepsis, fungous infections, and viral infections, has been reported in patients on corticosteroid therapy; for example, *Candida* infections of the mouth in patients treated with corticosteroids, especially if these are given conjointly with antibiotics, are not uncommon. Application of corticosteroids to the skin has led to loss of skin collagen and subcutaneous atrophy.

The dose of corticosteroid required to diminish corticotrophin secretion with consequent atrophy of the adrenal cortex and the time required for its occurrence vary from patient to patient. Acute adrenal insufficiency may occur during prolonged treatment or on cessation of treatment and may be precipitated by an infection or trauma. Growth retardation in children has been reported and attempts have been made to overcome it by using intermittent dosage (see Uses of Corticosteroids, p.451).

Large doses of corticosteroids, or of corticotrophin, may produce symptoms typical of hyperactivity of the adrenal cortex, with moon-face, sometimes with hirsutism, buffalo hump, flushing, increased bruising, striae, and acne, sometimes leading to a fully developed Cushing's syndrome. If administration is discontinued these symptoms are usually reversed, but sudden cessation is dangerous (see Withdrawal, p.449).

Other adverse effects include amenorrhoea, hyperhidrosis, mental and neurological disturbances, intracranial hypertension, acute pancreatitis, and aseptic necrosis of bone. An increase in the coagulability of the blood may lead to thrombo-embolic complications.

Infections may be masked since corticosteroids have marked anti-inflammatory properties with analgesic and antipyretic effects, and may produce a feeling of well-being.

The administration of corticosteroids may also cause a reduction in the number of circulating lymphocytes.

Muscular weakness is an occasional side-effect of most corticosteroids, particularly when they are taken in large doses, and it is most evident with triamcinolone.

Adverse effects occur, in general, fairly equally with all corticosteroid preparations and their incidence rises steeply if dosage increases much above 7.5 mg daily of prednisolone or its equivalent. Short courses at high dosage for emergencies appear to cause less side-effects than prolonged courses with lower doses.

Adverse reactions were recorded in 121 of 718 patients given prednisone and of these 82 experienced acute reactions which included psychosis in 13, euphoria in 8, gastro-intestinal reactions in 32, and hyperglycaemia in 16. Comparison of these patients with a group of 594 patients given prednisone without any ill effect showed that only the psychiatric reactions were related to dosage.— The Boston Collaborative Drug Surveillance Program, *Clin. Pharmac. Ther.*, 1972, *13*, 694. See also G. P. Lewis *et al.*, *Lancet*, 1971, *2*, 778.

Further reports on the incidence of side-effects associated with corticosteroid therapy: B. L. J. Treadwell *et al.*, *Lancet*, 1964, *1*, 1121; K. Thomsen and H. Schmidt, *Nord. Med.*, 1966, *76*, 1333; Drug Committee of the Research Council of the American Academy of Allergy, *J. Allergy*, 1967, *40*, 87; G. D. Hurrell, *J.R. Coll. gen. Pract.*, 1972, *22*, 387.

Reviews of the adverse effects of corticosteroids: W. S. Bond, *Am. J. Hosp. Pharm.*, 1977, *34*, 479; M. H. Lessof, *Br. J. Hosp. Med.*, 1977, *18*, 360.

Adrenal suppression. A review of inhibition of hypothalamo-pituitary-adrenocortical function associated with corticosteroid administration. Inhibition may persist for 6 to 12 months after treatment is withdrawn and may cause acute adrenal insufficiency with circulatory collapse during stress. In general, suppression of secretion of adrenocorticotrophic hormone and atrophy of the adrenal gland become progressively more definite as doses of corticosteroid exceed physiological amounts, i.e. more than 7.5 mg of prednisolone daily, and as the duration of therapy is prolonged. It is less when the corticosteroid is given as a single dose in the morning, and even less if this morning dose is given on alternate days or less frequently. In patients taking high enough doses of corticosteroids to suppress the adrenals the dose should be increased during any form of stress, and those treated within the last 2 or 3 months should be restarted on therapy. Where the interval since treatment is 3 to 12 months resumption of treatment depends on clinical assessment of signs of adrenal insufficiency. According to the disease and the duration of therapy patients may be weaned from corticosteroids at a rate ranging from 2.5 to 5 mg of prednisolone daily every 2 or 3 days to 2.5 mg every 1 to 3 weeks and possibly less, decrements being made with tablets of 1 mg when the dose has been reduced to 10 mg daily. Suppression may also occur after very short courses of high-dose therapy and since many such patients will be under continuing stress when the drugs are stopped, gradual withdrawal of corticosteroids over 5 to 7 days is preferable.— *Br. med. J.*, 1980, *280*, 813.

The use and interpretation of tests for corticosteroid-impaired hypothalamic-pituitary-adrenocortical function.— J. Landon *et al.*, *Br. J. Derm.*, 1976, *94*, *Suppl.* 12, 61.

For a comparison of the effects of corticosteroids and corticotrophin in depressing hypothalamo-pituitary-adrenal function, see Corticotrophin, p.486.

Controversy surrounding adrenal suppression in patients receiving corticosteroids and cytotoxic therapy: K. S. Wilson *et al.*, *Lancet*, 1976, *1*, 610; A. Naysmith *et al.*, *ibid.*, 715; N. C. Thalassinos *et al.* (letter), *ibid.*, 1238; H. T. Mouridsen and C. Binder (letter), *ibid.*, 1300; R. J. Spiegel *et al.*, *ibid.*, 1979, *1*, 630; M. W. E. Morgan (letter), *ibid.*, 932; K. S. Wilson and A. C. Parker (letter), *ibid.*, 1030; L. Rönnberg and S. Kivinen (letter), *ibid.*, 1345; G. M. Janković (letter), *ibid.*, 1346; H. Olsson *et al.* (letter), *ibid.*

Corticosteroid-induced adrenal suppression has been associated not only with oral, rectal, and parenteral therapy, but has also followed topical application of corticosteroid preparations, particularly those containing potent corticosteroids. Adrenal suppression has also been associated with the use of inhalants, and the topical application of lotions, eye-drops, eye ointments, and nasal preparations.

For reports of adrenal suppression associated with various corticosteroid preparations see under the individual corticosteroid monographs. For further details of the problems associated with adrenal suppression see under Withdrawal, below.

Allergy and anaphylaxis. There have been occasional reports of allergy, and sometimes anaphylaxis, caused by corticosteroids. In some cases the reaction is due to an ingredient used in the manufacture of the corticosteroid preparation.

References: R. J. Coskey and H. G. Bryan (letter), *J. Am. med. Ass.*, 1967, *199*, 136; S. Comaish, *Br. J. Derm.*, 1969, *81*, 919; S. Maddin (letter), *J. Am. med. Ass.*, 1969, *207*, 560; M. D. Alani and S. D. Alani, *Ann. Allergy*, 1972, *30*, 181; S. D. Alani and M. D. Alani, *Contact Dermatitis*, 1976, *2*, 301; N. G. Kounis, *Ann. Allergy*, 1976, *36*, 203; J. A. Romankiewicz and J. E. Franklin (letter), *J. Am. med. Ass.*, 1976, *236*, 1939; T. Menne and K. E. Anderson, *Contact Dermatitis*, 1977, *3*, 337; R. J. Coskey, *Archs Derm.*, 1978, *114*, 115; M. Hayhurst *et al.*, *S. Afr. med. J.*, 1978, *53*, 259; M. R. Partridge and G. J. Gibson, *Br. med. J.*, 1978, *1*, 1521; D. Rubinger *et al.* (letter), *Lancet*, 1978, *2*, 689; K. de Ceulaer and S. N. Papazoglou, *Scott. med. J.*, 1979, *24*, 218; R. F. U. Ashford and A. Bailey, *Postgrad. med. J.*, 1980, *56*, 437.

Carcinogenicity. Studies in *mice* on the potential carcinogenicity of some topical corticosteroids.— M. H. Briggs and M. Briggs, *Br. J. Derm.*, 1973, *88*, 75.

A report of 3 patients who developed Kaposi's sarcoma following prolonged corticosteroid therapy.— R. W. Gange and E. W. Jones, *Clin. exp. Derm.*, 1978, *3*, 135.

For references to the development of various neoplastic disorders after immunosuppressive therapy with azathioprine and a corticosteroid, see under Antineoplastics and Immunosuppressants, p.172.

Diabetogenic effect. A study of factors associated with the development of corticosteroid-induced diabetes, which occurred in 31 (10.8%) of 286 non-diabetic adult renal transplant recipients, observed for a total of 410 patient transplant years. The corticosteroid-induced diabetes had no adverse effects on graft or patient survival.— D. S. David *et al.*, *J. Am. med. Ass.*, 1980, *243*, 532. See also J. E. Woods *et al.*, *J. Am. med. Ass.*, 1975, *231*, 1261.

Effects on the blood and vascular system. Reports of thrombo-embolism in patients receiving corticosteroids: E. Lieberman *et al.*, *J. Pediat.*, 1968, *73*, 320; A. P. Mukherjee *et al.*, *Br. med. J.*, 1970, *4*, 273; B. Wadman and I. Werner (letter), *Lancet*, 1972, *1*, 907; S. A. Uriu and R. D. Reinecke, *Archs Ophthal.*, *N.Y.*, 1973, *90*, 355.

Other reports of corticosteroid effects on blood and vascular tissue: R. Rokseth, *Lancet*, 1960, *1*, 680 (agranulocytosis); M. Floyd *et al.*, *Lancet*, 1969, *1*, 1192 (polymorphonuclear leucocytosis); F. D. Hart, *Br. med. J.*, 1969, *3*, 131 (vasculitis); L. N. Klimova and A. L. Ozerianskaya, *Sov. Med.*, 1972, *72*, 140 (leukemoid reaction); M. G. Britton *et al.*, *Br. med. J.*, 1976, *2*, 73 (leucopenia).

Effects on bones and joints. A description of corticosteroid-induced bone collapse, including critical comments on various descriptive terms for this, which include ischaemic, avascular, or aseptic necrosis of bone.— *Br. med. J.*, 1972, *1*, 581. A review of 95 patients with corticosteroid-induced avascular necrosis, 91 of whom had involvement of the femoral head. The risk of developing this lesion appears to be correlated with the total corticosteroid dose and probably with variations in the dosage regimen. Other related factors are the patients' general health and the disease for which corticosteroids are being given. Many lesions heal with minimal deformity, and symptoms may not be inconsistent with normal living; consequently operation should be deferred and a conservative programme outlined, aimed at minimising deformity.— R. L. Cruess, *J. Bone Jt Surg.*, 1977, *59B*, 308. See also D. E. Fisher and W. H. Brickel, *ibid.*, 1971, *53A*, 859. No evidence of osteonecrosis was observed in 28 children who had been treated with high doses of prednisone for renal disease. It was suggested that previous reports noting a possible association between corticosteroid treatment and avascular necrosis of bone may have been examples of idiopathic avascular necrosis of bone in patients who coincidentally had received or were receiving corticosteroid therapy; most of these patients had conditions which were themselves associated with avascular necrosis of bone or produced a radiographic appearance that might be confused with this condition.— P. J. Gregg *et al.*, *Br. med. J.*, 1980, *281*, 116.

Further references: A. R. Timothy *et al.* (letter), *Lancet*, 1978, *1*, 154 (osteonecrosis in patients receiving combination chemotherapy).

Osteopenia. Studies into the pathogenesis of corticosteroid-induced osteopenia: A. Deding *et al.*, *Acta med. scand.*, 1977, *202*, 253 (mineral and collagen loss); R. G. Klein *et al.*, *J. clin. Invest.*, 1977, *60*, 253 (reduced calcium absorption); R. W. Chesney *et al.*, *Lancet*, 1978, *2*, 1123 (reduced serum concentrations of 1,25-dihydroxycholecalciferol in children); T. J. Hahn *et al.*, *J. clin. Invest.*, 1979, *64*, 655 (altered calcium metabolism).

Rupture of tendon. A report of the rupture of an Achilles tendon in a patient receiving corticosteroid therapy. The rupture was preceded by pain in the heels but the pain disappeared after the rupture; the rupture was not associated with trauma.— S. Pilgaard, *Ugeskr. Laeg.*, 1962, *124*, 1408. Further reports.— G. B. Smaill, *Br. med. J.*, 1961, *1*, 1657; M. A. Cowan and S. Alexander, *ibid.*, 1658; M. L. H. Lee (letter), *ibid.*, 1829; L. T. Ford and J. DeBender, *Sth. med. J.*, 1979, *72*, 827; N. L. Gottlieb and W. G. Riskin, *J. Am. med. Ass.*, 1980, *243*, 1547. See also R. Leach *et al.*, *J. Bone Jt Surg.*, 1978, *60*, 537 (rupture of the plantar fascia).

Effects on the eyes. A comment on eye diseases induced by topically applied corticosteroids, including a warning that the topical use of corticosteroid medications for areas near the eye may result in conjunctival contamination from accumulated amounts of medication.— J. B. Howell, *Archs Derm.*, 1976, *112*, 1529.

Reports and comments on the adverse effects of systemic, topical, or local corticosteroid therapy on the eyes: B. Becker and D. W. Mills, *J. Am. med. Ass.*, 1963, *185*, 884 (glaucoma); G. E. Hewson (letter), *Br. med. J.*, 1964, *1*, 438 (herpes simplex ulceration); H. H. Slansky *et al.*, *Archs Ophthal.*, *N.Y.*, 1967, *77*, 579 (exophthalmos); J. Williamson *et al.*, *Br. J. Ophthal.*, 1969, *53*, 361 (posterior subcapsular cataracts); R. Porter *et al.*, *Br. med. J.*, 1972, *3*, 133; R. Porter and A. L. Crombie (letter), *ibid.*, 1972, *3*, 766; G. H. Hall *et al.* (letter), *ibid.*, 469; C. Leroux-Robert *et al.* (letter), *ibid.*, 586 (posterior subcapsular cataracts); J. S. Berkowitz *et al.*, *Am. J. Med.*, 1973, *55*, 492 (posterior subcapsular cataracts); H. Q. Kirk, *Am. J. Ophthal.*, 1974, *77*, 442 (filtering blebs); J. C. Martins *et al.*, *Am. J. Ophthal.*, 1974, *77*, 433 (uveitis); F. T. Fraunfelder and P. G. Watson, *Br. J. Ophthal.*, 1976, *60*, 227 (perforation); J. Herschler, *Am. J. Ophthal.*, 1976, *82*, 90; Y. Kitazawa, *ibid.*, 492 (glaucoma); R. A. Nozik, *Am. J. Ophthal.*, 1976, *82*, 928 (orbital rim fat atrophy); D. H. Shin *et al.*, *Am. J. Ophthal.*, 1976, *82*, 259 (uveitis); A. R. Foreman *et al.*, *Am. J. Ophthal.*, 1977, *84*, 75 (posterior subcapsular cataracts); H. Shiono *et al.*, *Clin. Pediat.*, 1977, *16*, 726 (posterior subcapsular cataracts); D. Sevel *et al.*, *J. Allergy & clin. Immunol.*, 1977, *60*, 215 (posterior subcapsular cataracts); G. B. Walman *et al.* (letter), *Can. med. Ass. J.*, 1977, *117*, 1257 (posterior subcapsular cataracts).

Inappropriate use. Two women aged 17 and 20 years developed cataracts and glaucoma with permanent visual defects as a result of the indiscriminate prolonged topical application of corticosteroids to relieve ocular irritation associated with contact lenses.— R. M. Burde and B. Becker, *J. Am. med. Ass.*, 1970, *213*, 2075.

Of 6 patients who received accidental intra-ocular injection of depot corticosteroid preparations 2 recovered and 4 became legally blind. The injected material required 6 to 8 weeks to disappear.— T. F. Schlaegel, *Trans. Am. Acad. Ophthal. Oto-lar.*, 1974, *78*, 847. See also R. N. McGrew *et al.*, *Otolaryngology*, 1978, *8*, 147.

Effects on the gastro-intestinal tract. An analysis of 6102 patients in 32 double-blind and 18 non-double-blind studies involving the use of corticosteroids or corticotrophin as treatment failed to show an association between such treatment and an increased prevalence, recurrence, or complications of peptic ulcer.— H. O. Conn and B. L. Blitzer, *New Engl. J. Med.*, 1976, *294*, 473. There was a striking association between corticosteroid therapy and ulcer in some subgroups.— S. B. Green *et al.* (letter), *ibid.*, 1291. Further criticisms.— W. B. Long and Y. -F. Shiau (letter), *ibid.*; J. R. Crass (letter), *ibid.*, 1292; R. A. L. Sturdevant (letter), *ibid.*; A. Lubin (letter), *ibid.*; C. J. McDonald (letter), *ibid.*; A. R. Cooke (letter), *ibid.* Reply.— H. O. Conn and B. L. Blitzer (letter), *ibid.*, 1293; M. Uribe *et al.* (letter), *ibid.*, 1977, *296*, 173. Further comment. It must be concluded that corticosteroids are not associated with peptic ulcer except in the highest dosage regimens.— M. G. Bramble and C. O. Record, *Drugs*, 1978, *15*, 451.

Further references: P. Cushman, *Gut*, 1970, *11*, 534 (no association found in a review of the literature); S. Raptis *et al.*, *Am. J. dig. Dis.*, 1976, *21*, 376 (glucocorticoid-induced hypergastrinaemia); H. Jick and J. Porter, *Lancet*, 1978, *2*, 87 (results of a Boston Collaborative Drug Surveillance Program); S. Seino *et al.*, *Gut*, 1978, *19*, 10 (association with hypergastrinaemia); G. A. Ottonello and A. Primavera, *Stroke*, 1979, *10*, 208 (higher incidence of gastro-intestinal lesions in those dying of cerebral infarction).

Individual reports of adverse gastro-intestinal effects possibly associated with corticosteroid therapy: A. L. Warshaw, *Am. J. Surg.*, 1976, *131*, 442 (colonic perforation).

Effects on growth. Long-term studies of children with asthma, juvenile rheumatoid arthritis, or nephrotic syndrome indicated that treatment with corticosteroids inhibited growth and led to considerable stunting. Corticotrophin when given in adequate dosage to control symptoms led to an increase in the growth-rate.— M. Friedman and L. B. Strang, *Lancet*, 1966, *2*, 568. It had been found that certain children with asthma were predisposed to stunted growth, that some children grew normally while on corticosteroids, and some became stunted on corticotrophin treatment. Small doses such as 5 or 7.5 mg of prednisolone daily usually had no effect on growth.— M. C. S. Kennedy and D. C. Thursby-Pelham (letter), *Lancet*, 1966, *2*, 907. A study of 17 asthmatic children treated with prednisolone or prednisone for at least 6 months indicated that the risk of impairment of growth in height was small with a daily dosage of less than 3 mg per m^2 body-surface but great with dosage exceeding 4 mg per m^2. Skeletal maturation was retarded more than growth in height, but puberty was not delayed.— K. F. Kerrebijn and J. P. M. de Kroon, *Archs Dis. Childh.*, 1968, *43*, 556. In 20 children with Still's disease receiving various treatment regimens, linear growth in those receiving prednisone up to 8 mg daily in 2 divided doses was less than in those receiving prednisone up to 30 mg or corticotrophin up to 20 units as a single morning dose on alternate days. Retardation of growth was not due to an absolute inability to secrete growth hormone.— R. A. Sturge *et al.*, *Br. med. J.*, 1970, *3*, 547. Comments on studies on the effects of corticosteroids on growth in children. The mechanisms are, for the present, obscure, but it appears that the action is peripheral and is reduced by alternate-day regimens.— M. A. Preece, *Postgrad. med. J.*, 1976, *52*, 625.

Further references to the effects of corticosteroids on growth: J. N. Loeb, *New Engl. J. Med.*, 1976, *295*, 547 (physiology); G. G. Shapiro *et al.*, *J. Allergy & clin. Immunol.*, 1976, *57*, 430 (alternate-day methylprednisolone in asthma); R. W. Chesney *et al.*, *Am. J. Dis. Child.*, 1978, *132*, 768 (in childhood glomerular disease).

Effects on the heart. There was a higher incidence of ECG abnormalities in 39 patients with rheumatoid arthritis treated with glucocorticoids than in 33 control patients. The ECG abnormalities were considered to relate to coronary arteriosclerosis.— Y. Ichickawa *et al.* (letter), *Lancet*, 1977, *2*, 828. No confirmation of ECG abnormalities was found when 31 patients receiving a mean daily corticosteroid dose of prednisolone 7 mg were compared with 33 control patients.— I. M. Stewart and J. S. Marks (letter), *ibid.*, 1237.

See also under Effects on Lipid Metabolism.

Individual reports of possible adverse effects of corticosteroids on the heart: A. El-Ghobarey *et al.*, *Br. med. J.*, 1976, *2*, 915 (aortic incompetence).

Effects on immune response. Owing to their immunosuppressant effect administration of corticosteroids in doses greater than those required for physiological replacement therapy is associated with increased susceptibility to infection, aggravation of existing infection, and activation of latent infection. An additional problem is that the anti-inflammatory effect of corticosteroids may mask symptoms until the infection has progressed to an advanced stage; the altered response of the body may also permit the bizarre spread of infections, frequently in aberrant forms, such as disseminated parasitic infections. The risk is greater in patients receiving high doses, or associated therapy with other immunosuppressants such as cytotoxic agents, and in those who are already debilitated. Children receiving high doses of corticosteroids are at special risk from childhood ailments, such as chicken-pox, but vaccination with living organisms is contra-indicated since it too may induce infection, such as disseminated BCG (killed vaccines or toxoids may be given). This increased susceptibility to infection coupled with masking of symptoms may also be caused by topical or local corticosteroid therapy. Thus, topical application to the skin has led to unusual changes such as atypical ringworm infection. Fungal infections, generally restricted to the upper respiratory tract, are associated with corticosteroid inhalations. Severe damage to the eye has followed the ocular use of corticosteroids in herpetic infections, and a similar generalised spread of herpes infection may follow application to the mouth in the presence of herpes infection.

Conversely, the effect of corticosteroids on the symptoms and course of some infections may be life-saving (see Uses). Before embarking on a long-term course of corticosteroid therapy general principles for the reduction of risk of infection include a diligent search for active or quiescent infection and, where appropriate, prevention or eradication of the infection before starting, or concurrent administration of chemoprophylaxis during corticosteroid treatment.

Reviews and studies on corticosteroids and susceptibility to infection: E. C. Rosenow, *Ann. intern. Med.*, 1972, *77,* 977 (review of association with pulmonary infection); D. C. Dale *et al.*, *New Engl. J. Med.*, 1974, *291,* 1154 (reduced susceptibility with alternate-day therapy); A. Engquist *et al.*, *Acta chir. scand.*, 1974, *140,* 343 (increased incidence of postoperative infections); J. J. Rinehart *et al.*, *New Engl. J. Med.*, 1975, *292,* 236 (reduced bactericidal and fungicidal properties of monocytes); D. A. Stevens, *J. Am. med. Ass.*, 1977, *238,* 1668 (comment on the theoretical benefits and hazards of corticosteroids in infectious mononucleosis).

Individual reports of infections associated with systemic or local corticosteroid therapy: T. F. Flynn, *Archs Otolar.*, 1957, *65,* 203 (generalised varicella); G. Slaney and B. N. Brooke, *Lancet*, 1958, *1,* 504 (staphylococcal septicaemia in postoperative patients); W. D. Gingrich, *J. Am. med. Ass.*, 1962, *179,* 602 (mycotic corneal ulcers); G. E. Hewson (letter), *Br. med. J.*, 1964, *1,* 438 (corneal herpes simplex ulceration); T. Cruz *et al.*, *New Engl. J. Med.*, 1966, *275,* 1093 (fatal strongyloidiasis); E. H. Rosenbaum *et al.*, *J. Am. med. Ass.*, 1966, *198,* 737 (generalised vaccinia following smallpox vaccination); G. Roschlau, *Münch. med. Wschr.*, 1967, *109,* 1889 (fatal generalised vaccinia); F. A. Ive and R. Marks, *Br. med. J.*, 1968, *3,* 149 (atypical ringworm); A. Bitoun *et al.*, *Nouv. Presse méd.*, 1972, *1,* 1935 (strongyloidiasis); A. Gershon *et al.*, *J. Pediat.*, 1972, *81,* 1034 (generalised varicella); A. L. Macmillan, *Br. J. Derm.*, 1972, *87,* 496 (atypical scabies and betamethasone valerate ointment); R. Duckworth, *Br. dent. J.*, 1973, *135,* 168 (contra-indication of corticosteroids for herpes infection of the mouth); A. J. A. Ferguson (letter), *Br. med. J.*, 1973, *4,* 485 (atypical Norwegian scabies); R. Clayton and S. Farrow, *Postgrad. med. J.*, 1975, *51,* 657 (atypical Norwegian scabies); D. F. Keren *et al.*, *Johns Hopkins med. J.*, 1975, *136,* 178 (cytomegalovirus colitis); Z. Spirer (letter), *Lancet*, 1975, *1,* 635 (avoidance of progressive varicella by means of gradual withdrawal of corticosteroids and by transfusions of fresh leucocytes and plasma from convalescent adult donors); D. H. Nicholson and E. B. Wolchok, *Archs Ophthal., N.Y.*, 1976, *94,* 248 (ocular toxoplasmosis following systemic therapy); S. A. Sahn and S. Lakshminarayan, *Br. J. Dis. Chest*, 1976, *70,* 195 (activation of tuberculosis); D. V. Coleman *et al.*, *J. clin. Path.*, 1978, *31,* 338 (human polyomavirus infection); W. E. Dismukes *et al.*, *J. Am. med. Ass.*, 1978, *240,* 1495 (disseminated histoplasmosis); M. El-Hennawy and H. Abd-Rabbo, *J. trop. Med. Hyg.*, 1978, *81,* 71 (amoebiasis); J. K. Jain *et al.*, *Am. J. med. Sci.*, 1978, *275,* 209 (localised mucormycosis following intramuscular methylprednisolone); P. C. Stuiver and T. J. L. M. Gould, *Br. med. J.*, 1978, *2,* 394; A. J. Gijsbers *et al.* (letter), *ibid.*, 1372 (amoebiasis); E. Ginzler *et al.*, *N.Y. St J. Med.*, 1979, *79,* 392 (candida arthritis following local injection); B. M. Jenner *et al.*, *Archs Dis. Childh.*, 1979, *54,* 555 (pulmonary candidiasis); S. B. Lucas *et al.* (letter), *Lancet*, 1979, *2,* 1372 (disseminated infection with *Hymenolepis nana*, the dwarf tapeworm, in an immunosuppressed patient); J. W. Millar and N. W. Horne, *Lancet*, 1979, *1,* 1176 (tuberculosis in immunosuppressed patients, especially those receiving more than 10 mg of prednisone daily with other immunosuppressant agents); G. C. Close and I. B. Houston (letter), *Lancet*, 1981, *2,* 480 (fatal haemorrhagic chickenpox).

See also under Carcinogenicity (above).

Effects on the kidneys. Forty-one of 87 patients who were receiving 5 or 10 mg of prednisone daily for asthma reported nocturia. In an investigation on 5 of these patients, there was a decrease in proximal tubular reabsorption at night, leading to a reversal of the normal rhythm of water and electrolyte excretion. This effect was not prevented by giving a single dose of prednisone in the morning and normal rhythm was only regained by stopping corticosteroid therapy.— J. P. Thomas *et al.*, *Clin. Sci.*, 1970, *38,* 415. See also *Br. med. J.*, 1970, *4,* 193.

A patient with polyarteritis nodosa was treated with prednisone 40 mg daily gradually increased to 100 mg daily. When the dose reached 75 mg daily hypercalciuria occurred, the blood-urea concentration rose, and creatinine clearance was reduced. The symptoms gradually remitted when prednisone was progressively withdrawn under azathioprine cover. Corticosteroids might occasionally lead to renal failure in patients with collagen disorders.— J. R. Condon and J. R. Nassim, *Br. med. J.*, 1971, *1,* 327.

Further references: J. R. Curtis, *Br. med. J.*, 1977, *2,* 375; *idem*, *Prescribers' J.*, 1979, *19,* 29 (calcium-containing renal calculi).

Effects on lipid metabolism. In 100 women with asthma who had taken prednisone 5 to 15 mg daily for 4 to 13 years together, in some cases, with corticotrophin or tetracosactrin, the incidence of type IV hyperlipoproteinaemia (endogenous hypertriglyceridaemia) was 21% compared with 4% in 50 healthy women. The incidence of hypercholesterolaemia was not affected significantly. There was no correlation with obesity, diabetes, the dose of prednisone, the duration of treatment, or the previous or present use of corticotrophin or tetracosactrin. The hypertriglyceridaemia could be due to increased hepatic synthesis of very low-density lipoproteins, but the possibility that it might be due to the asthma was not excluded.— A. H. El-Shaboury and T. M. Hayes, *Br. med. J.*, 1973, *2,* 85. See also A. Casaretto *et al.*, *Lancet*, 1974, *1,* 481.

Fatty tumours. Two middle-aged men who received prednisolone, 60 mg daily, for about 2 months and a third who was treated with varying doses of triamcinolone for 4 years developed soft fatty tumours resembling a dewlap in the episternal area.— G. E. Lucena *et al.*, *New Engl. J. Med.*, 1966, *275,* 834.

Effects on mental state. Acute reactions to glucocorticoid therapy with prednisone, among 718 consecutively monitored hospital in-patients, included psychoses in 13 and inappropriate euphoria in 8. The reactions occurred in patients not considered to be emotionally unstable before their onset. Remission followed reduction in dosage, supplemented with brief psychopharmacological drug therapy in the 13 psychotic patients. The latter exhibited hallucinations, delusions or violent behaviour, singly or in combination; 2 patients were profoundly depressed and 6 were maniacal.— The Boston Collaborative Drug Surveillance Program, *Clin. Pharmac. Ther.*, 1972, *13,* 694.

A report of a woman with an intense psychological dependence on prednisone.— H. G. Morgan *et al.*, *Br. med. J.*, 1973, *2,* 93. See also under Withdrawal, p.449.

Further references to studies on the effects of corticosteroids on mental state: R. P. Michael and J. L. Gibbons, *Int. Rev. Neurobiol.*, 1963, *5,* 243 (psychoses); J. C. Gillin *et al.* (letter), *Nature*, 1972, *237,* 398 (effect on sleep); N. Baloch, *Br. J. Psychiat.*, 1974, *124,* 545 (delirium); B. J. Sullivan and J. D. Dickerman, *Pediatrics*, 1979, *63,* 677 (catatonia).

Effects on muscles. Muscle weakness may be caused by potassium loss in patients receiving corticosteroids with a pronounced mineralocorticoid action, such as fludrocortisone. Muscle wasting is caused by the glucocorticoid properties of corticosteroids; it has been particularly noted in patients receiving 9α-fluorinated corticosteroids, such as triamcinolone, but can be caused by any glucocorticoid. For further details see under individual corticosteroid monographs.

Effects on the nervous system. A report of epidural lipomatosis leading to serious neurological complications in a 47-year-old man treated with prolonged high-dose corticosteroid therapy for severe asthma.— D. L. Butcher and S. A. Sahn, *Ann. intern. Med.*, 1979, *90,* 60.

Further references: *J. Am. med. Ass.*, 1970, *212,* 2034 (peripheral neuropathy).

Effects on the pancreas. Up to 30% of patients on moderate doses of corticosteroids might have postmortem evidence of focal pancreatitis, possibly due to vasculitis.— *Adverse Drug React. Bull.*, 1974, Oct., 162.

Of 590 cases of acute pancreatitis seen in a 20-year period, 6 were attributed to corticosteroids; 4 of these were fatal.— J. E. Trapnell and E. H. L. Duncan, *Br. med. J.*, 1975, *2,* 179.

Individual reports of pancreatitis in patients receiving corticosteroids, sometimes in association with other immunosuppressant therapy: T. A. Riemenschneider *et al.*, *Pediatrics*, 1968, *41,* 428; M. Legré *et al.*, *Méd. Chir. dig.*, 1972, *1,* 113; I. Hamed *et al.*, *Am. J. med. Sci.*, 1978, *276,* 211.

Effects on sexual function. A review of drugs and sexual function. Although glucocorticoids have antagonistic effects on androgens in certain respects, replacement doses should cause no problem. Patients requiring supra-physiological doses are often quite seriously ill and this may be the limiting factor.— J. G. B. Millar, *Practitioner*, 1979, *223,* 634.

Effects on the skin. In 12 months, 17 patients who had been taking corticosteroids were admitted to a plastic surgery unit on 21 occasions for extensive skin damage from trivial accidents. All but one had taken corticosteroids for at least 5 years. The length of treatment with corticosteroids was considered more important than daily dosage in contributing to liability to damage; some patients had taken as little as 5 mg of prednisolone daily.— D. J. David, *Br. med. J.*, 1972, *2,* 614.

Individual reports of adverse effects of systemic corticosteroids on the skin: J. T. Cassidy and G. G. Bole, *Ann. intern. Med.*, 1966, *65,* 1008 (cutaneous atrophy following intra-articular injection); E. N. Glick (letter), *Br. med. J.*, 1972, *4,* 300 (depigmentation following subcutaneous injection); H. R. Schumacher, *Ann. rheum. Dis.*, 1977, *36,* 91 (bullous tophi in gout); K. Sedlarik and D. Kirsten, *Dte GesundhWes.*, 1978, *33,* 150 (ulcerating wound); E. J. Feuerman and M. Sandbank, *Acta derm.-vener., Stockh.*, 1979, *59, Suppl.* 85, 59 (superficial porokeratosis); N. L. Gottlieb and N. S. Penneys, *J. Am. med. Ass.*, 1980, *243,* 1260 (spontaneous haemorrhage, tearing, and necrosis associated with prednisone).

Hazards of topical application. A review of the hazards of topical corticosteroid application and a reminder that in addition to adverse effects on the skin, eye disease can be induced by topical corticosteroids and systemic absorption may produce adrenal suppression and collapse.— *Lancet*, 1977, *2,* 487.

After prolonged topical application of fluorinated corticosteroids, mainly betamethasone and fluocinolone, for the treatment of *rosacea*, an aggravation and extension of telangiectasia occurred in 14 patients. In 10 patients, cessation of treatment was followed by severe rebound inflammatory oedema and acute pustular eruption. Telangiectasia improved or cleared within 3 months of cessation of the fluorinated preparations. Treatment with tetracycline 250 mg twice daily for 1 month and then 250 mg daily, and local treatment with hydrocortisone ointment was given when indicated. Fluorinated corticosteroids should not be used in the topical treatment of *rosacea*; hydrocortisone preparations appeared to be harmless.— I. Sneddon, *Br. med. J.*, 1969, *1,* 671.

Of 73 patients (68 women, 5 men) with *perioral dermatitis* seen in 2 years, all but 2 had used fluorinated corticosteroids. Withdrawal of the corticosteroid was usually followed by exacerbation for 8 to 10 days. The condition was then sometimes controlled by hydrocortisone cream 1%, but often required oxytetracycline 250 mg twice daily. Complete recovery usually occurred in patients who ceased using fluorinated corticosteroids. Fluorinated corticosteroids should not be used for trivial inflammation of the face.— I. Sneddon, *Br. J. Derm.*, 1972, *87,* 430. A review of *perioral dermatitis* affecting 259 patients over the 12-year period 1966 to 77 inclusive. The nature of the initial eruption for which the patient sought treatment is not always obvious, but the subsequent course is similar in all cases. Over the subsequent weeks or months erythema, scaling, and grouped micropustules extend around the whole of the perioral area, characteristically sparing a narrow zone close to the vermilion margin of the lips. The cheeks are spared, though some extension may occur outwards from the sides of the nose. A more characteristic extension occurs to the glabella and to the eyelids, though not to the eyebrows. Flushing may be present in some older women but is not a common feature and is not as labile as in the rosaceous patient. The conjunctivae are never suffused. Many aetiological factors were excluded, including the use of fluoridated toothpaste, but all but 9 of the patients gave a clear history of the use of topical corticosteroids, usually strong corticosteroids.— D. S. Wilkinson *et al*, *Br. J. Derm.*, 1979, *101,* 245. Of 43 patients with *perioral dermatitis* most had used potent corticosteroids, but 7 had used hydrocortisone butyrate alone.— J. A. Cotterill, *ibid.*, 259.

Further reviews, comments, and studies on the hazards of topical application of corticosteroids: D. D. Munro, *Br. J. Derm.*, 1976, *94, Suppl.* 12, 67 (adrenal suppression); D. D. Munro, *Topics Ther.*, 1978, *4,* 64 (adrenal suppression); *Br. med. J.*, 1980, *280,* 136 (perioral dermatitis); *Lancet*, 1980, *1,* 75 (perioral dermatitis).

Individual reports of adverse effects following topical application of corticosteroids: J. N. Burry, *Med. J. Aust.*, 1973, *1,* 393 (delayed healing); L. Goldman and W. Kitzmiller, *Archs Derm.*, 1973, *107,* 611 (atrophy of perianal skin); P. E. Romano *et al.*, *Am. J. Ophthal.*, 1977, *84,* 247 (death from Cushing's syndrome following ocular use in a child); H. L. Franco and W. L. Weston, *Pediatrics*, 1979, *64,* 36 (facial eruptions in children); A. W. Nathan and G. L. Rose (letter), *Lancet*, 1979, *1,* 207 (death from Cushing's syndrome).

Effects on the teeth. Only 1 of 43 children who had prolonged treatment with large doses of cortisone was found to have normal teeth. The changes affected the dentine and the enamel.— C. Lanzavecchia *et al.*, *Minerva med., Roma*, 1967, *19,* 13.

Effects on the thyroid. In 2 patients with Hashimoto's thyroiditis, treatment with prednisone apparently precipitated thyrotoxicosis.— W. Singer (letter), *Lancet*, 1966, *1*, 1041.

Effects on zinc concentrations. Serum-zinc concentrations were reduced in 3 patients when treated with corticosteroids; 2 patients had major burns and the third had recently undergone vascular surgery for his low-cardiac-output syndrome.— A. Flynn *et al.*, *Lancet*, 1971, *2*, 1169. Reduced serum-zinc concentrations were found in 10 patients maintained on corticosteroids after bilateral adrenalectomy. In 6 other patients with delayed wound healing who had been given corticosteroids for 6 months to 2 years, serum-zinc concentrations were low. Treatment with zinc sulphate brought about wound healing in 5 of the 6 patients.— *idem*, 1973, *1*, 789. Comment.— G. P. Lewis *et al.* (letter), *ibid.*, 1056. See also R. Ellul-Micallef *et al.*, *Postgrad. med. J.*, 1976, *52*, 148.

Treatment of Adverse Effects of Corticosteroids. The adverse effects of corticosteroids are nearly always due to their use in excess of normal physiological requirements. They should be treated symptomatically, where possible the dosage being reduced or the drug slowly withdrawn.

Acute adrenal insufficiency in corticosteroid-treated patients, whether it be due to accidental abrupt withdrawal of the corticosteroid or the inability of the patient's adrenals to cope with the increased stress of infection or accidental or surgical trauma, must be treated immediately with intravenous injections of hydrocortisone sodium succinate together with infusions of dextrose in 0.9% sodium chloride. Hydrocortisone sodium succinate 100 to 300 mg should be given intravenously immediately, followed by 100 mg intravenously every eight hours. Infusions of dextrose in 0.9% sodium chloride solution should be given in amounts adequate to correct hypoglycaemia, sodium loss, and dehydration; special care must be taken, however, not to overload the circulation. Suitable antibiotic therapy is indicated where the underlying cause is an infection. As the patient recovers, the dose of hydrocortisone sodium succinate may be changed to the intramuscular route before gradually tapering off and re-establishing the patient's original corticosteroid therapy.

Withdrawal of Corticosteroids. The use of pharmacological doses of corticosteroids to treat disease suppresses the endogenous secretion of corticotrophin by the anterior pituitary, with the result that the adrenal cortex becomes atrophied. Sudden withdrawal or reduction in dosage, or an increase in corticosteroid requirements associated with the stress of infection or accidental or surgical trauma, may then precipitate acute adrenal insufficiency. Symptoms of adrenal insufficiency include malaise, muscle weakness, mental changes, muscle and joint pain, desquamation of the skin, dyspnoea, anorexia, nausea, and vomiting, fever, hypoglycaemia, hypotension, and dehydration; deaths have followed the abrupt withdrawal of corticosteroids. For the emergency treatment of acute adrenal insufficiency caused by abrupt withdrawal of corticosteroids, see under Treatment of Adverse Effects (above).

In some instances, withdrawal symptoms may simulate a clinical relapse of the disease for which the patient has been undergoing treatment. Other effects that may occur during withdrawal or change of corticosteroid therapy include benign intracranial hypertension with headache and vomiting and papilloedema caused by cerebral oedema. Latent rhinitis or eczema may be unmasked.

Duration of treatment and dosage appear to be important factors in determining suppression of the pituitary-adrenal response to stress on cessation of corticosteroid treatment, and individual liability to suppression is also important. Administration as a single daily dose in the morning or, where appropriate, on alternate days, reduces the degree of adrenal suppression (for further details see under Uses).

Corticosteroid withdrawal should therefore always be gradual, the rate depending upon the individual patient's response, the dose, and the duration of therapy. Recommendations for initial reduction, stated in terms of prednisolone, vary from as little as steps of 2.5 mg monthly to 2.5 to 5 mg every 3 to 7 days; when the dose has been reduced to the equivalent of prednisolone 10 to 12.5 mg daily, the rate of reduction should be reduced to steps of 1 mg monthly (other sources again suggest intervals of 3 to 7 days). Adrenal function should be monitored throughout withdrawal (see Corticotrophin, p.487 and Tetracosactrin, p.489 for adrenal function tests) and symptoms attributable to over-rapid withdrawal should be countered by resuming a higher dose and continuing the reduction at a slower rate. The administration of corticotrophin does not help to re-establish adrenal responsiveness.

This gradual withdrawal of corticosteroid therapy permits a return of adrenal function adequate for daily needs, but a further one to two years may be required for the return of function necessary to meet the stress of infection, surgical operations, or trauma. On such occasions patients with a history of recent corticosteroid withdrawal should be protected by means of supplementary corticosteroid therapy as described under Precautions, p.449.

Withdrawal. Details of a protocol for the withdrawal of supraphysiological doses of glucocorticoid, involving transfer to hydrocortisone before gradually tapering off.— R. L. Byyny *et al.*, *New Engl. J. Med.*, 1976, *295*, 30.

See also under Adverse Effects (Adrenal Suppression), p.446.

Details of withdrawal symptoms in 5 patients when attempts were made to reduce or discontinue corticosteroids which they had received for many years. Analysis of these 5 patients and of the literature, indicated 4 sub-groups of corticosteroid withdrawal syndrome: type I, symptomatic and biochemical evidence of suppression of hypothalamo-pituitary-adrenal function; type II, recrudescence of the disease for which the corticosteroid was originally prescribed; type III, physical or psychological dependence upon corticosteroids, with normal hypothalamo-pituitary-adrenal function and no recrudescence of underlying disease; and type IV, biochemical evidence of reduced hypothalamo-pituitary-adrenal function without symptoms and without recurrence of underlying disease. Any combination of types I, II, and III may exist.— R. B. Dixon and N. P. Christy, *Am. J. Med.*, 1980, *68*, 224.

Further reviews and studies of corticosteroid withdrawal: T. Livanou *et al.*, *Lancet*, 1967, *2*, 856 (recovery of hypothalamo-pituitary-adrenal function); J. A. Aita, *Postgrad. Med.*, 1974, *55*, 111 (neurological complications); *Br. med. J.*, 1977, *1*, 1117 (dangers of withdrawal of systemic corticosteroids when introducing aerosol therapy).

Individual reports of withdrawal symptoms or exacerbation of the original disease state following withdrawal of corticosteroid therapy: J. Rotstein and R. A. Good, *Archs intern. Med.*, 1957, *99*, 545 (pseudorheumatism); A. E. Walker and J. J. Adamkiewicz, *J. Am. med. Ass.*, 1964, *188*, 779 (raised intracranial pressure); H. Baker and T. J. Ryan, *Br. J. Derm.*, 1968, *80*, 771 (pustular psoriasis); F. E. Hargreave *et al.* (letter), *Br. med. J.*, 1969, *1*, 443 (pseudorheumatism); K. J. Ivey and L. DenBesten, *J. Am. med. Ass.*, 1969, *208*, 1698 (raised intracranial pressure); B. G. R. Neville and J. Wilson, *Br. med. J.*, 1970, *3*, 554 (raised intracranial pressure); R. A. Castelline *et al.*, *Ann. intern. Med.*, 1974, *80*, 593 (heart and lung disorders); W. J. Cunliffe *et al.*, *Br. J. Derm.*, 1975, *93*, 183 (adrenocortical insufficiency on withdrawal of topical therapy); V. P. Gupta and G. E. Ehrlich, *Arthritis Rheum.*, 1976, *19*, 1333 (organic brain syndrome); D. T. Fourie, *S. Afr. med. J.*, 1977, *52*, 301 (raised intracranial pressure following withdrawal of topical betamethasone from an infant); P. M. Trenchard *et al.*, *Postgrad. med. J.*, 1977, *53*, 391 (leuco-erythroblastosis on dexamethasone withdrawal); G. P. Hosking and H. Elliston, *Br. med. J.*, 1978, *1*, 550 (intracranial hypertension, following decreased concentration of hydrocortisone ointment together with reduced absorption due to improvement in eczema).

See also under Adverse Effects (Adrenal Suppression), p.446.

Precautions for Corticosteroids. Unless considered life-saving, systemic administration of corticosteroids is contra-indicated in patients with peptic ulcer, osteoporosis, psychoses, or severe psychoneuroses, and they should be used only with great caution in the presence of congestive heart failure, in patients with diabetes mellitus, infectious diseases, chronic renal failure, and uraemia, and in elderly persons. Patients with active or doubtfully quiescent tuberculosis should not be given corticosteroids except, very rarely, as adjuncts to treatment with antitubercular drugs. Patients with quiescent tuberculosis should be observed closely and should receive chemoprophylaxis if corticosteroid therapy is prolonged. Because of interference with inflammatory and immunological response, corticosteroids are usually contra-indicated (but see p.454) in the presence of acute infections, including herpes zoster and herpes simplex ulceration of the eye. Similarly, patients already receiving corticosteroid therapy are more susceptible to infection, the symptoms of which, moreover, may be masked until an advanced stage has been reached. Vaccination with live vaccine is contra-indicated, but killed vaccines or toxoids may be given (the response may be attenuated in those receiving high corticosteroid doses). Children are at special risk of infection and may require prophylaxis with immunoglobulin.

During long courses of corticosteroid therapy, patients should be seen regularly and, in particular, checked for hypertension, glycosuria, hypokalaemia, gastric discomfort, and mental changes. Sodium intake may need to be reduced and potassium supplements may be necessary. Monitoring of the fluid intake and output, and daily weight records may give early warning of fluid retention; back pain may signify osteoporosis; children are at special risk from raised intracranial pressure; infections should be treated as an emergency. Patients should carry cards (and preferably also wear bracelets) giving full details of their corticosteroid therapy; they and their relatives should be fully conversant with the implications of their therapy and the precautions to be taken.

Measures to compensate for the adrenals' inability to respond to stress (see Withdrawal, p.449) include doubling the dose to cover minor intercurrent illnesses or similar stresses (with intramuscular administration to cover vomiting). Minor surgical procedures may only require intramuscular injection of hydrocortisone sodium succinate 100 mg with the premedication, but major procedures may call for 100 mg intramuscularly every 6 to 8 hours for 3 days. Intravenous infusion of hydrocortisone sodium succinate 100 mg in 0.9% sodium chloride solution may occasionally be required during the procedure if signs of adrenal insufficiency develop (see also below, under Operative Coverage).

Rapid intravenous injection of massive doses of corticosteroids may sometimes cause cardiovascular collapse; the injection should therefore be given over a period of not less than 10 minutes. High doses should not be used for prolonged treatment.

Concurrent administration of barbiturates, phenytoin, or rifampicin may enhance the metabolism and reduce the effects of corticosteroids. Response to anticoagulants may be reduced and, on some occasions, enhanced by corticosteroids. Concurrent administration of corticosteroids or the potassium-depleting diuretics, such as the thiazides or frusemide, may cause excessive potassium loss.

Topical applications of corticosteroids should not be made with an occlusive dressing to large areas of the body because of the increased risk of systemic toxicity and should not, in general, be used in the presence of infection, particularly of the eye. Occasionally they may be used with the addition of a suitable antimicrobial substance in the treatment of infected skin but there is a risk of sensitivity reactions occurring. Corticosteroids should not be applied to ulcers of the leg and long-term topical use is best avoided, especially in children.

Before starting long-term therapy with corticosteroids the following should be undertaken: an evaluation of the patient's pituitary-adrenal status; appropriate tests of carbohydrate metabolism to avoid precipitation of latent diabetes or aggravation of existing diabetes; X-ray films of spine and chest, since osteoporosis was a serious contra-indication and in tuberculosis or other chronic infections corticosteroid therapy could have an unfavourable effect on host-parasite balance; an ECG; and evaluation of blood pressure and renal functions; X-ray films of the upper gastro-intestinal tract in patients with a history of peptic-ulcer diathesis; and evaluation of the patient's psychological predisposition. Severe potassium depletion could occur during the administration of corticosteroids with a diuretic that causes potassium loss. In order to minimise the undesirable side-effects of prolonged corticosteroid therapy, supplementary potassium should be administered and sodium intake restricted, with antacids and a diet containing increased vitamin D and non-irritating foods.— G. W. Thorn, *New Engl. J. Med.*, 1966, *274*, 775.

Abuse and misuse. During a study on percutaneous absorption of topical corticosteroids 18 of 36 infants with dermatitis were found to have been exposed to potent topical fluorinated corticosteroids obtained from relatives, neighbours, or friends. In view of the hazards, patients should be advised to discard any unused potent fluorinated corticosteroids and not pass them on to other individuals.— W. L. Weston *et al.* (letter), *New Engl. J. Med.*, 1977, *297*, 222.

Activation of infection. Although the Center for Disease Control had recommended that chemoprophylaxis which should include isoniazid should be used in patients receiving prolonged corticosteroid therapy and who had positive tuberculin reactivity, experience with 132 treated asthmatics did not indicate that this was necessary especially when considering the toxicity of isoniazid. The patients had received corticosteroids for a mean period of 4.7 years. None had active tuberculosis although only 1 patient had received isoniazid and despite 67 having positive tuberculin responses. Evaluation of tuberculin responses indicated that tuberculin reactivity appeared to be inhibited in patients receiving prednisone in daily doses greater than 19 mg.— M. Schatz *et al.*, *Ann. intern. Med.*, 1976, *84*, 261.

See also under Effects on Immune Response (above).

Interactions. There was an appreciable and consistent increase in plasma corticosteroids after cigarette smoking in man. When corticosteroids were administered the smoking habits of patients might need to be controlled in order to adjust dosage accurately.— A. Kershbaum *et al.*, *J. Am. med. Ass.*, 1968, *203*, 275.

Antacids. Concurrent administration of antacids had no effect on serum concentrations of prednisolone attained.— A. R. Tanner *et al.*, *Br. J. clin. Pharmac.*, 1979, *7*, 397. Magnesium trisilicate and aluminium hydroxide did not affect absorption of prednisolone administered concurrently. Absorption might be reduced if small doses of prednisolone were taken with large doses of antacids.— D. A. H. Lee *et al.* (letter), *Br. J. clin. Pharmac.*, 1979, *8*, 92.

Further references: F. V. Naggar *et al.*, *Pharmazie*, 1977, *32*, 778; V. F. Naggar *et al.*, *J. pharm. Sci.*, 1978, *67*, 1029 (reduced dexamethasone bioavailability with magnesium trisilicate).

A view that weakness and debility attributed to corticosteroids may in fact be due to phosphorus depletion caused by concomitant administration of antacids.— M. Goodman *et al.*, *Am. J. Med.*, 1978, *65*, 868.

Anticoagulants. For the various effects of corticosteroids on anticoagulants see under Heparin and other Anticoagulants, p.762.

Aspirin and other anti-inflammatory analgesics. For the effect of corticosteroids on aspirin, see Aspirin, p.239, and for the effect on phenylbutazone, see Phenylbutazone, p.274.

Barbiturates. The administration of phenobarbitone reduced the plasma half-life of dexamethasone and increased its metabolic clearance-rate in a study in 16 patients with bronchial asthma. In 3 patients dependent on prednisone, there was a marked worsening of symptoms after the administration of phenobarbitone. Improvement occurred when phenobarbitone was discontinued and prednisone requirements could be reduced.— S. M. Brooks *et al.*, *New Engl. J. Med.*, 1972, *286*, 1125. For comments, see C. J. Falliers (letter), *ibid.*, *287*, 201. A reply.— S. M. Brooks and E. E. Werk (letter), *ibid.*

See also Phenytoin and other Anticonvulsants, below.

Cholestyramine. For the effect of cholestyramine on steroids, see Cholestyramine, p.411.

Cytotoxic agents. For the effect of corticosteroids on cyclophosphamide, see Cyclophosphamide, p.200, and on methotrexate, see Methotrexate, p.217.

Insulin. Corticosteroid therapy in 4 diabetic children at first increased their insulin requirements for 1 month and again when corticosteroid dosage was reduced, but insulin dosage returned to normal on stopping the corticosteroid.— J. Guivarch *et al.*, *Annls Pédiat.*, *Paris*, 1967, *43*, 1033, per *J. Am. med. Ass.*, 1967, *200* (June 12), A241. See also P. C. Kansal *et al.*, *Metabolism*, 1976, *25*, 445.

Muscle relaxants. For the effect of corticosteroids on pancuronium, see Pancuronium Bromide, p.994.

Phenytoin and other anticonvulsants. In a woman with temporal lobe astrocytoma control of cerebral oedema with dexamethasone was lost following addition of phenytoin owing to possible acceleration of dexamethasone metabolism; it was re-established by giving the dexamethasone intramuscularly and 2 subsequent relapses again responded to intramuscular administration. The pattern was probably dose-related and much larger doses of dexamethasone by mouth might have maintained a good response. A similar pattern had been noted in 3 other patients; in one it had been possible to reduce the dexamethasone dose on inadvertent omission of phenytoin but return to phenytoin had required it to be increased; in the other two a change in anticonvulsant had permitted reduction in the dexamethasone dose without relapse.— J. McLelland and W. Jack (letter), *Lancet*, 1978, *1*, 1096. Methylprednisolone and its hemisuccinate might be as effective and undergo less metabolic clearance than dexamethasone in patients concurrently receiving phenobarbitone or phenytoin. The switch had been beneficial in 2 patients initially receiving dexamethasone and phenytoin.— F. M. Vincent (letter), *ibid.*, 1360. A report of *primidone*-induced enhancement of corticosteroid metabolism in a woman receiving therapy for congenital adrenal hyperplasia and petit mal.— K. W. Hancock and M. J. Levell (letter), *ibid.*, 1978, *2*, 97.

Further references to interactions between phenytoin and corticosteroids: E. E. Werk *et al.*, *New Engl. J. Med.*, 1969, *281*, 32 (dexamethasone); N. Haque *et al.*, *J. clin. Endocr. Metab.*, 1972, *34*, 44 (dexamethasone); L. B. Petereit and A. W. Meikle, *Clin. Pharmac. Ther.*, 1977, *22*, 912 (prednisolone); L. A. Lawson *et al.*, *Surg. Neurol.*, 1981, *16*, 23 (increased phenytoin concentrations).

Radiopharmaceuticals. For the effect of corticosteroids on gallium uptake, see Gallium-67, p.1389.

Rifampicin. Increased doses of corticosteroids were required by a patient with Addison's disease when given rifampicin. When ethambutol was substituted for rifampicin the corticosteroid dose had to be reduced. Cortisol-production rates increased in 4 patients with pulmonary tuberculosis being given rifampicin and there were signs of hepatic microsomal enzyme induction.— O. M. Edwards *et al.*, *Lancet*, 1974, *2*, 549. See also D. N. Maisey *et al.* (letter), *ibid.*, 896; W. van Marle *et al.* (letter), *Br. med. J.*, 1979, *1*, 1020.

Contrary to expectations, the administration of corticosteroids with rifampicin aggravated neuritis in borderline leprosy and was contra-indicated.— G. J. Steenbergen and R. E. Pfaltzgraff, *Lepr. Rev.*, 1975, *46*, 115. A warning that since rifampicin speeds the metabolism of corticosteroids, leprosy workers may find a poor response to corticosteroid therapy for severe type 2 lepra reaction (ENL reaction), if rifampicin is being given at the same time.— W. H. Jopling and J. H. S. Pettit (letter), *Lepr. Rev.*, 1979, *50*, 331.

Further references to rifampicin diminishing corticosteroid activity: G. A. Buffington *et al.*, *J. Am. med. Ass.*, 1976, *236*, 1958; W. Hendrickse *et al.*, *Br. med. J.*, 1979, *1*, 306.

Sex hormones. Hexoestrol, in doses equivalent to stilboestrol 15 to 100 mg daily, or chlorotrianisene had no effect on various skin disorders in 8 women, but when added to the stable maintenance dose of hydrocortisone or prednisone the skin lesions were controlled and corticosteroid requirements were reduced by about 8 times. Increased concentrations of cortisol binding globulin might have bound and slowed the metabolism of hydrocortisone.— A. S. Spangler *et al.*, *J. clin. Endocr. Metab.*, 1969, *29*, 650.

Sympathomimetics. Studies in 21 asthmatic patients suggested that the plasma half-life of dexamethasone was decreased when it was administered with ephedrine; this did not occur when dexamethasone and theophylline were given together.— S. M. Brooks *et al.*, *J. clin. Pharmac.*, 1977, *17*, 308.

For the effect of hydrocortisone on theophylline metabolism, see Aminophylline, p.343.

Tricyclic antidepressants. For the effect of hydrocortisone on nortriptyline elimination, see Amitriptyline, p.112.

Interference with diagnostic tests. Chlordiazepoxide, chlorpromazine, ethinamate, meprobamate, nalidixic acid, penicillin, phenaglycodol, reserpine, spironolactone, triacetyloleandomycin and other agents could interfere with urinary steroid estimations.— C. L. Cope, *Adrenal Steroids and Disease*, London, Pitman Medical, 1972, p. 125. For further details, see S. Borushek and J. J. Gold, *Clin. Chem.*, 1964, *10*, 41; O. Llerena and O. H. Pearson, *New Engl. J. Med.*, 1968, *279*, 983. Fluorometric estimations for plasma hydrocortisone might be artificially high owing to the presence of fusidic acid, mepacrine, or spironolactone.— J. Millhouse, *Adverse Drug React. Bull.*, 1974, Dec., 164.

Corticosteroids and androgens affected the protein-bound iodine and resin uptake tests of thyroid function by decreasing the quantity of binding protein.— *Adverse Drug React. Bull.*, 1972, June, 104.

Reactions to patch tests were suppressed in 3 of 12 patients by the administration of 40 mg of prednisone daily; in 2 of 15 by 30 mg daily; and in 1 of 16 by 20 mg daily.— E. Feuerman and A. Levy, *Br. J. Derm.*, 1972, *86*, 68. See also R. I. Slott and B. Zweiman, *J. Allergy & clin. Immunol.*, 1974, *54*, 229, per *J. Am. med. Ass.*, 1975, *232*, 211.

The non-specific increase in glomerular filtration-rate due to corticosteroids could be mistakenly interpreted as modification of underlying disease processes.— C. R. P. George (letter), *Lancet*, 1974, *2*, 728.

Evidence that prednisolone does not interfere with tests of hepatic function in healthy subjects.— A. Weiersmüller *et al.*, *Am. J. dig. Dis.*, 1977, *22*, 424.

For the effect of corticosteroids on digoxin radio-immunoassay, see Digoxin, p.534.

Occupational exposure. A report of facial plethora in 12 men engaged in manufacture of a potent glucocorticoid despite adherence to safety regulations; 3 had abnormal responses to tetracosactrin. Such persons should be monitored regularly and should have periods of work not involving corticosteroids.— R. W. Newton *et al.*, *Br. med. J.*, 1978, *1*, 73.

Operative coverage. Recommendations for corticosteroid cover in surgery and general anaesthesia, and criticism of the unnecessarily large cover given to some patients. It is very likely that the shortened cover that should now be recognised will reduce the incidence of wound breakdown. For minor procedures, such as bronchoscopy, where the procedure is short and the patient is expected to be fully conscious shortly after operation and not to require heavy sedation, hydrocortisone sodium succinate 100 mg is given intramuscularly with the premedication. For intermediate operations, such as herniorraphy, where the patient is expected to be awake but may require heavy sedation after operation, hydrocortisone sodium succinate 100 mg is given every 8 hours until the morning after operation, when the usual corticosteroid dose is resumed, by mouth if possible. For major operations, such as colectomy, the cover should be the same as for intermediate operations, but if there is clinical evidence of severe stress or shock, should be continued every 8 hours for the period of stress only, which will usually be for less than 3 days. When severe complications arise the cover will need to be continued, but should be stopped as soon as the period of stress is over. Should a patient who is receiving or has received corticosteroid therapy develop shock unexpectedly, it may be justifiable to give hydrocortisone intravenously, but in most of these patients the collapse will not be due to adrenal failure, but to some complication of the surgery or the disease.— A. B. Myles and J. R. Daly, *Corticosteroid and ACTH Treatment, Principles and Problems*, London, Arnold, 1974, p. 167. See also H. Kehlet and C. Binder, *Br. J. Anaesth.*, 1973, *45*, 1043.

Phaeochromocytoma. A case report of a 69-year-old woman with phaeochromocytoma in whom episodes of hypertension were related to the administration of corticosteroids.— P. Daggett and S. Franks, *Br. med. J.*, 1977, *1*, 84.

Pregnancy and the neonate. *Early pregnancy.* Animal studies by F.C. Fraser *et al.* (*J. cell. comp. Physiol.* 1954, *43*, 237), T. Fainstat (*Endocrinology*, 1954, *55*, 502) and others demonstrated an increase in foetal cleft palate following maternal ingestion of high corticosteroid doses, and cortisone has been used widely as a tool for the investigation of mechanisms responsible for cleft lip and palate. With doses used in clinical practice, however, the risk appears to be low. In an analysis of several hundred cases reported in the literature, A.J.

Popert (*Br. med. J.*, 1962, *1*, 967) concluded that the incidence of cleft palate in exposed children was slightly higher than in a random sample, but that in the small selected group studied, this higher incidence might be fallacious. Although D.W. Warrell and R. Taylor (*Lancet*, 1968, *1*, 117) found an increased incidence of malformations in the children of asthmatic mothers given prednisolone 2.5 to 30 mg daily during pregnancy, J.K. Scott (*Lancet*, 1968, *1*, 208) has suggested that the outcome might have been worse in untreated asthmatic mothers. Moreover, other workers, such as M. Schatz *et al.* (*J. Am. med. Ass.*, 1975, *233*, 804) found no significant increase in the risk of foetal or maternal complications in a study of asthmatic mothers given prednisolone 2.5 to 20 mg daily.

Further studies and surveys on the risks to the foetus of maternal corticosteroid therapy: A. M. Bongiovanni and A. J. McPadden, *Fert. Steril.*, 1960, *11*, 181 (low incidence of cleft palate); D. B. Yackel *et al.*, *Am. J. Obstet. Gynec.*, 1966, *96*, 985 (no association); S. D. Walsh and F. R. Clark, *Scott. med. J.*, 1967, *12*, 302 (no association); H. Serment and H. Ruf, *Bull. Féd. Socs. Gynéc. Obstét. Lang. fr.*, 1968, *20*, 69 (low incidence of cleft palate and other defects); H. O. Nicholson (letter), *Lancet*, 1968, *1*, 117 (no placental insufficiency); A. F. Fleming and N. C. Allan, *Br. med. J.*, 1969, *4*, 461 (no harmful effect); A. S. Goldman *et al.*, *Nature*, 1978, *272*, 464 (*in vitro* studies on human foetal palate cells); J. M. Reinisch *et al.*, *Science*, 1978, *202*, 436 (offspring of women given prednisone throughout pregnancy, significantly lighter).

Late pregnancy. Fears concerning the administration of corticosteroids during late pregnancy relate to their direct adverse effects on the foetus rather than any dysmorphogenic risk. These involve the known side-effects of corticosteroids, such as increased risk of infection and adrenal insufficiency. No such adverse effects were noted by M. Schatz *et al.* (*J. Am. med. Ass.*, 1975, *233*, 804) in the infants of 70 exposed pregnancies, but subclinical adrenal insufficiency has been reported by L.A. Grajwer *et al.* (*J. Am. med. Ass.*, 1977, *238*, 1279) in the infant of a mother given prolonged high-dose dexamethasone therapy for pseudotumor cerebri. Similarly, congenital cytomegalovirus infection was reported by T. J. Evans *et al.* (*Lancet*, 1975, *1*, 1359) in the infant of a woman receiving azathioprine and prednisone for renal transplantation. The potential dangers of maternal diabetogenic effects have been demonstrated by A.S. Gündoğdu *et al.* (*Lancet*, 1979, *2*, 1317) in a study of metabolic changes induced in diabetic women by salbutamol (used in the prevention of premature labour) which could be exacerbated by concomitant administration of dexamethasone (used to promote maturation of the foetal lung) with consequent danger to the foetus. Since the findings of G.G. Liggins and R.N. Howie (*Pediatrics*, 1972, *50*, 515) that administration of a corticosteroid to the mother more than 24 hours before delivery could be used to enhance maturity of the foetal lung and reduce the incidence of respiratory distress syndrome in premature infants (see, particularly, Betamethasone, p.461) investigations have been carried out to evaluate long-term effects on the child. Some adverse long-term effects in exposed *animals* have been demonstrated by M.C. Romano *et al.* (*Pediat. Res.*, 1977, *11*, 1042) and others, suggesting that while such therapy may be suitable for selected infants at risk, it may not be suitable for routine prophylactic administration.

Further references: S. Ohrlander *et al.*, *Obstet. Gynec.*, 1977, *49*, 691 (corticotrophin test to neonates after corticosteroid administration during pregnancy).

For more details concerning the management of the respiratory distress syndrome in infants, see Betamethasone, p.461.

Lactation. For studies demonstrating that corticosteroids are excreted in milk in unimportant amounts, see Prednisolone, p.480.

Absorption and Fate. Corticosteroids, with the exception of deoxycortone, are absorbed from the gastro-intestinal tract. When administered by topical application, particularly under an occlusive dressing or when the skin is broken, or as a pulmonary aerosol inhalation or a rectal enema, sufficient corticosteroid may be absorbed to give systemic effects. Administration by mouth may give a more rapid response than intramuscular injection of an insoluble corticosteroid. Water-soluble forms of corticosteroids giving a rapid response are used for intravenous injection.

Corticosteroids in the circulation are extensively bound to plasma proteins, mainly to globulin and less so to albumin. The corticosteroid-binding globulin has high affinity but low binding capacity, while the albumin has low affinity but large binding capacity. Only unbound corticosteroid has pharmacological effects or is metabolised. The synthetic corticosteroids are less extensively protein bound than hydrocortisone (cortisol). They also tend to have longer half-lives.

Corticosteroids are metabolised mainly in the liver but also in the kidney, and are excreted in the urine. Urinary excretion of 17-hydroxycorticoids is used as an index of adrenal function. The slower metabolism of the synthetic corticosteroids with their lower protein-binding affinity may account for their increased potency compared with the natural corticosteroids.

Uses of Corticosteroids. The corticosteroids are used in physiological doses for replacement therapy in adrenal insufficiency. In primary adrenal insufficiency, such as Addison's disease or after adrenalectomy, both mineralocorticoid and glucocorticoid replacement is needed. In secondary adrenal insufficiency, associated with inadequate corticotrophin secretion, glucocorticoid replacement is usually adequate. Thus, in the treatment of primary adrenal insufficiency hydrocortisone is given by mouth, usually in association with fludrocortisone, to provide supplementary mineralocorticoid replacement, whereas in secondary adrenal insufficiency supplementary mineralocorticoid therapy is not given. The emergency treatment of adrenal insufficiency usually involves intravenous injections of hydrocortisone sodium succinate, together with infusions of sodium chloride and dextrose. Corticotrophin must not be used.

The corticosteroids are used in pharmacological doses for their anti-inflammatory and immunosuppressant glucocorticoid properties, which suppress the clinical manifestations of disease in a wide range of disorders. For these purposes, the synthetic analogues with their considerably reduced mineralocorticoid properties linked with enhanced glucocorticoid properties, are preferred to cortisone and hydrocortisone. Despite the existence of very powerful synthetic glucocorticoids with virtually no mineralocorticoid activity, however, the hazards of inappropriately high glucocorticoid therapy are such that the less powerful prednisolone and prednisone are the glucocorticoids of choice for most conditions, since they allow for a greater margin of safety. There is little to choose between prednisolone and prednisone; prednisolone may be preferred since, like hydrocortisone, it exists in a metabolically active form, whereas prednisone, like cortisone, is inactive and must be converted into its active form by the liver; hence, particularly in some liver disorders, prednisone's bioavailability is less reliable.

Conditions in which glucocorticoid therapy is indicated include allergic disorders, such as bronchial asthma and allergic skin reactions; blood disorders, including auto-immune haemolytic anaemia and idiopathic thrombocytopenic purpura; selected collagen and rheumatic disorders (only rarely rheumatoid arthritis); connective tissue disorders, such as arteritis and systemic lupus erythematosus (but not scleroderma); gastro-intestinal disorders, such as inflammatory bowel disease; some hepatic disorders; neuromuscular disorders, such as myasthenia gravis; some neurological disorders; selected ocular disorders; renal disorders, including the nephrotic syndrome; and severe skin disorders, such as acute exacerbations of eczema, exfoliative dermatitis, and pemphigus.

Some miscellaneous uses for glucocorticoid therapy include raised intracranial pressure, sarcoidosis, the neonatal respiratory distress syndrome, the gastric acid aspiration syndrome, occasionally hypercalcaemia, and acute rheumatic fever with carditis.

The onset of action of glucocorticoids is too slow for the primary treatment of allergic reactions of a life-threatening nature, such as anaphylaxis and laryngeal oedema, but they are used as an adjunct to initial emergency administration of adrenaline, see Adrenaline, p.4.

Glucocorticoids are used in conjunction with antineoplastic agents in regimens for the management of malignant disease as described under Antineoplastic Agents and Immunosuppressants, p.171. They are also given to reduce immune responses after organ transplantations, often in conjunction with azathioprine (p.190).

Although the empirical use of a corticosteroid is appropriate in a life-threatening situation, generally it is advisable not to begin corticosteroid therapy until a definite diagnosis has been made, for otherwise symptoms may be masked to such an extent that a true diagnosis becomes extremely difficult to make.

Doses of corticosteroids higher than those required for physiological replacement will eventually lead to some degree of adrenal suppression, the extent depending on the dose given and its duration of administration. The adrenal glands have a daily output equivalent to approximately 20 mg of hydrocortisone (cortisol), but individual blood-cortisol (hydrocortisone) concentrations may vary widely, and can increase up to tenfold or more during stress. Therefore, during periods of stress, such as during and after surgery and when suffering from intercurrent infections, the corticosteroid dosage of patients must be increased. The effects of different corticosteroids vary qualitatively as well as quantitatively, and it may not be possible to substitute one for another in equal therapeutic amounts without provoking side-effects. Thus, whereas cortisone and hydrocortisone have very appreciable mineralocorticoid (or sodium-retaining) properties relative to their glucocorticoid (or anti-inflammatory) properties, prednisolone and prednisone have considerably less, and others, such as betamethasone and dexamethasone, have none or virtually none. As a rough guide, the approximate equivalent doses of the main corticosteroids in terms of their glucocorticoid (or anti-inflammatory) properties alone, are:

cortisone 25 mg, betamethasone 0.6 mg, dexamethasone 0.75 mg, hydrocortisone 20 mg, methylprednisolone 4 mg, paramethasone 2 mg, prednisolone 5 mg, prednisone 5 mg, triamcinolone 4 mg.

Administration of corticosteroids. Because the therapeutic effects of corticosteroids seem to be of longer duration than the metabolic effects, intermittent treatment with corticosteroids has been used to allow the metabolic rhythm of the body to become re-established while maintaining the therapeutic effects. Regimens of intermittent therapy have usually consisted of short courses of treatment or of the administration of 2 days' doses of corticosteroids as a single dose on alternate days; such alternate-day therapy is only appropriate for corticosteroids with a relatively short duration of action, such as prednisolone.

Corticosteroids are also given in single daily doses at times coinciding with maximum or minimum function of the adrenal cortex in order to enhance or diminish respectively the depressant effects of corticosteroids on the adrenals.

Intra-articular injection of corticosteroids. In the absence of infection and with full aseptic precautions, intra-articular injection is used in the treatment of rheumatoid arthritis, and, sometimes, of osteoarthritis. Cortisone acetate is not suitable for this purpose and hydrocortisone acetate is generally employed. Some of the synthetic analogues such as betamethasone, dexamethasone tebutate, methylprednisolone acetate, prednisolone acetate, prednisolone tebutate, prednisolone pivalate, triamcinolone acetonide, and triamcinolone diacetate may be preferred for some joints because of the small volume of the effective dose. There have been several reports of joint damage after the intra-articular injection of corticosteroids into load-bearing joints—see under Effects on Bones and Joints, p.447.

Topical application of corticosteroids. The topical application of corticosteroids in ointments and lotions often produces dramatic suppression of skin diseases in which inflammation is a prominent feature, e.g. eczema, infantile eczema, atopic dermatitis, dermatitis herpetiformis, contact dermatitis, dermatitis venenata, seborrhoeic dermatitis, neurodermatitis, psoriasis, and intertrigo. However, the disease may return or be exacerbated when corticosteroids are withdrawn if the cause of the condition is not eliminated or treated—see under Withdrawal, p.449.

The resolution of chronic skin lesions such as lichen planus, lichen simplex, keloids, and sarcoidosis of the skin is sometimes hastened by the injection of corticosteroids, sometimes in conjunction with a local anaesthetic, into the lesion.

When applying lotions, creams, or ointments it is possible by means of an occlusive dressing to increase the penetration of the preparation into the skin. The preparation is applied to the affected area and covered by a piece of polyethylene sheet or, for the hands and feet, polyethylene gloves or polyethylene bags. As much as possible of the air between the skin and the polyethylene is expelled and the dressing sealed with adhesive tape. This is left for up to 48 hours and if necessary renewed after the skin has been gently washed and dried. Secondary infection under the occlusive dressing may be a problem but usually clears when treatment is stopped. For comments on adrenal suppression and other hazards associated with the topical application of corticosteroids, see under Adverse Effects, p.446.

Occasionally, corticosteroids may be used with the addition of a suitable antimicrobial substance, such as neomycin, in the treatment of infected skin. For comments on the topical application of preparations containing a corticosteroid and neomycin, see Neomycin Sulphate, p.1189.

Dramatic results have been reported from the topical application of corticosteroids in inflammatory and traumatic diseases of the eye, but the occurrence of herpetic and fungous infections of the cornea and other serious complications militate against their use; eye-drops containing corticosteroids, particularly betamethasone and dexamethasone, should not be used for more than a week except under strict ophthalmic supervision with regular checks of intra-ocular pressure—see under Adverse Effects, p.446, and Precautions, p.449.

Slight stinging or irritation of the skin has been reported after topical application of preparations containing corticosteroids.

Reviews and discussions on the actions and uses of corticosteroids: A. S. Fauci *et al.*, *Ann. intern. Med.*, 1976, *84*, 304; M. W. Greaves, *Postgrad. med. J.*, 1976, *52*, 631; J. C. Melby, *A. Rev. Pharmac. & Toxic.*, 1977, *17*, 511 to 527; C. G. Craddock, *Ann. intern. Med.*, 1978, *88*, 564 (endogenous); S. L. Swartz and R. G. Dluhy, *Drugs*, 1978, *16*, 238; A. M. Dannenberg, *Inflammation*, 1979, *3*, 329.

Studies into the pharmacology of corticosteroids: K. E. Eakins *et al.*, *Br. med. J.*, 1972, *3*, 452 (inhibition of prostaglandin synthesis); G. P. Lewis and P. J. Piper, *Nature*, 1975, *254*, 308 (inhibition of prostaglandin synthesis); W. A. Burr *et al.*, *Lancet*, 1976, *2*, 58 (role in stress with reference to thyroid); M. A. Bray and D. Gordon, *Br. J. Pharmac.*, 1978, *63*, 635 (inhibition of prostaglandin synthesis); A. Danon and G. Assouline, *Nature*, 1978, *273*, 552 (mode of inhibition of prostaglandin synthesis).

Studies on the relative potencies and duration of action of various corticosteroids: A. W. Meikle and F. H. Tyler, *Am. J. Med.*, 1977, *63*, 200 (hydrocortisone, prednisone, and dexamethasone); W. W. Downie *et al.*, *Br. J. clin. Pharmac.*, 1978, *6*, 397 (betamethasone and prednisolone).

For details of the relative potency of topical corticosteroids, see under Skin Disorders, p.458.

Administration. The diurnal rhythm of the adrenal cortex led to about 70% of the daily secretion being made between midnight and 9 am. In the treatment of adrenal cortical hyperplasia a dose of hydrocortisone given at night would be nearly twice as suppressive as the same dose given during the day. However, in treating allergic or collagen disease when suppression of adrenal cortical activity was best avoided a dose of hydrocortisone at about 8 am was indicated. When reducing steroid dosage after treatment, a single dose given at 8 am would be most beneficial and would not inhibit corticotrophin secretion.— C. H. Demos *et al.*, *Clin. Pharmac. Ther.*, 1964, *5*, 721.

The 17-ketogenic steroid excretion resulting when metyrapone was given to block adrenal hydrocortisone production was used to compare the duration of suppression produced by equal anti-inflammatory doses of corticosteroids. Duration of suppression was 3.25 days for betamethasone 6 mg, 2.75 days for dexamethasone 5 mg, 1.25 to 1.5 days for hydrocortisone 250 mg, methylprednisolone 40 mg, prednisolone 50 mg, and prednisone 50 mg, 2 days for paramethasone 20 mg, and 2.25 days for triamcinolone 40 mg. An alternate-day regimen used for prednisone might not be applicable to the longer-acting steroids such as betamethasone and dexamethasone.— J. G. Harter *et al.*, *Arthritis Rheum.*, 1965, *8*, 445. See also J. G. Harter *et al.*, *New Engl. J. Med.*, 1963, *269*, 591; G. L. Ackerman and C. M. Nolan, *ibid.*, 1968, *278*, 405; R. B. Stoughton (letter), *ibid.*, 915; G. L. Ackerman, *ibid.;* R. R. MacGregor *et al.*, *ibid.*, 1969, *280*, 1427.

A study of prednisone administration both with and without potassium supplements in 8 patients with lung disease. Although there were no abnormalities of plasma-potassium concentrations, higher corticosteroid doses were associated with increased potassium excretion. Administration of potassium supplements from the start of treatment might avoid potassium depletion associated with long-term corticosteroid therapy.— G. M. Shenfield *et al.*, *Br. J. Dis. Chest*, 1975, *69*, 171.

Once-daily dosage. Favourable experience with a once-daily dosage regimen of prednisone in doses of up to 15 mg given for periods of 1 to 19 years, in 76 patients suffering from connective tissue or allergic disorders. This method of dosage should be considered in any patient requiring corticosteroid therapy. Prednisone is the corticosteroid of choice since the longer-acting corticosteroids such as betamethasone, dexamethasone, and triamcinolone will eventually cause adrenal suppression, even when given as a single daily dose.— H. F. Klinefelter *et al.*, *J. Am. med. Ass.*, 1979, *241*, 2721.

Alternate-day therapy . A review of alternate-day corticosteroid therapy. Alternate-day therapy with a short-acting corticosteroid such as prednisone or prednisolone is effective and reduces unwanted effects in the long-term treatment of many diseases, especially in children. Even when the drug has to be given daily, as in conditions where pain is prominent, it is worth giving the whole of the patient's daily dose early in the morning.— *Drug & Ther. Bull.*, 1976, *14*, 49.

Studies and comments on alternate-day corticosteroid therapy in both adults and children.— S. D. Walsh and I. W. B. Grant, *Br. med. J.*, 1966, *2*, 796; M. M. Martin *et al.*, *New Engl. J. Med.*, 1968, *279*, 273; D. N. S. Malone *et al.*, *Lancet*, 1970, *2*, 733; H. G. Morris and J. R. Jorgensen, *J. Pediat.*, 1971, *79*, 480; C. J. Falliers *et al.*, *J. Allergy & clin. Immunol.*, 1972, *49*, 156; H. Chai and A. Gilbert, *ibid.*, 1973, *51*, 65; H. G. Morris *et al.*, *J. Allergy & clin. Immunol.*, 1974, *54*, 350; G. G. Shapiro *et al.*, *ibid.*, 1976, *57*, 430 (methylprednisolone); I. Bakran *et al.*, *Int. J. clin. Pharmac. Biopharm.*, 1977, *12*, 57; B. H. Brouhard *et al.*, *J. Pediat.*, 1977, *91*, 343; D. A. Norris, *J. Allergy & clin. Immunol.*, 1978, *61*, 255.

In the elderly . Available evidence to date indicates that basal concentrations of corticotrophin and glucocorticoids are unchanged with age, that the disposal of corticoid is reduced with age, and that the sensitivity of the adrenal gland to corticotrophin is reduced. The importance of these physiological changes for glucocorticoid therapy have not been investigated.— R. E. Vestal, *Drugs*, 1978, *16*, 358.

Administration in hepatic insufficiency. A review of the pharmacokinetics of corticosteroids in patients with liver disease.— M. Uribe and V. L. W. Go, *Clin. Pharmacokinet.*, 1979, *4*, 233.

See also Prednisolone, p.480.

For details of corticosteroid therapy in patients with hepatic insufficiency, see Hepatic Disorders (below).

Administration in renal insufficiency. For details of corticosteroid therapy in patients with impaired renal function see under Organ and Tissue Transplantation and Renal Disorders (below).

Administration in respiratory insufficiency. Comment on the administration of corticosteroids in respiratory insufficiency. The tolerances of these compounds administered acutely suggest that normal pharmacological doses can be given safely.— P. du Sonich *et al.*, *Clin. Pharmacokinet.*, 1978, *3*, 257.

Adrenal hyperplasia. Reviews of the use of corticosteroid therapy in the management of congenital adrenal hyperplasia: G. H. Newns, *Archs Dis. Childh.*, 1974, *49*, 1; G. J. Klingensmith *et al.*, *J. Pediat.*, 1977, *90*, 996.

For details see under Hydrocortisone, p.473.

For the diagnosis of conditions associated with excessive adrenal secretion see under Dexamethasone (Dexamethasone Suppression Tests), p.466.

Adrenal insufficiency or Addison's disease. For the management of acute and chronic primary adrenal insufficiency, see Cortisone, p.464, Hydrocortisone, p.473, and Fludrocortisone, p.470. For the management of adrenal insufficiency secondary to corticosteroid therapy, see Corticosteroids, Treatment of Adverse Effects, p.449.

Allergy and anaphylaxis. For the use of corticosteroids in the management of anaphylactic shock, see Adrenaline, p.4.

Amyloidosis. The use of corticosteroids in the treatment of amyloidosis is controversial but at present there is not sufficient evidence to withhold them when they are indicated in the management of an underlying inflammatory or neoplastic disease.— G. G. Glenner, *New Engl. J. Med.*, 1980, *302*, 1333.

See also under Skin Disorders.

Arteritis. *Polyarteritis nodosa.* Corticosteroid therapy has contributed to an improvement in the course of polyarteritis nodosa.— *Lancet*, 1980, *2*, 407. References: Medical Research Council, *Br. med. J.*, 1960, *1*, 1399; P. P. Frohnert and S. G. Sheps, *Am. J. Med.*, 1967, *43*, 8; M. Sack *et al.*, *J. Rheumatol.*, 1975, *2*, 411.

Further references to corticosteroid therapy in polyarteritis nodosa: D. B. Magilavy *et al.*, *J. Pediat.*, 1977, *91*, 25 (childhood polyarteritis); G. H. Neild and H. A. Lee, *Postgrad. med. J.*, 1977, *53*, 382 (complications of lung granulomata and glomerulonephritis).

Temporal arteritis and polymyalgia rheumatica. An analysis of the course of the disease and the effect of corticosteroid treatment in 53 patients in whom polymyalgia rheumatica or temporal arteritis had been diagnosed between 1967 and 1977. The initial dose of prednisolone was 30 to 40 mg daily for those with evidence of temporal arteritis, and 10 to 20 mg daily for those without; higher starting doses in patients with temporal symptoms were required only for those with ocular complications. Long-term treatment with corticosteroids was found to be safe for most patients, and daily maintenance doses lower than 5 mg in polymyalgia rheumatica and 7.5 to 10 mg in temporal arteritis increased the risk of relapse. Most patients needed treatment for at least 2 to 3 years and therefore withdrawal before the lapse of 1 year is not advisable. Owing to the risk of late relapses, patients taken off corticosteroids should have periodic clinical and laboratory check-ups for at least a year after the end of treatment.— J. von Knorring, *Acta med. scand.*, 1979, *205*, 429. See also *Lancet*, 1979, *2*, 341.

Further references: G. G. Hunder *et al.*, *Ann. intern. Med.*, 1975, *82*, 613 (inadequacy of alternate-day compared with daily or thrice daily prednisone therapy); *Br. med. J.*, 1977, *1*, 1046; Golding J.R. (letter), *ibid.*, 1349; A. G. Freeman and R. W. R. Russell (letter), *ibid.*, 1412 (review and comments, including a strong recommendation that in temporal arteritis a dose of at least 80 mg of prednisolone daily should be given immediately the diagnosis has been made on clinical grounds since patients with giant-cell (temporal) arteritis may occasionally suddenly lose their vision in one or both eyes on an initial dose of only 40 to 50 mg daily); W. Esselinckx *et al.*, *Ann. rheum. Dis.*, 1977, *36*, 219 (difficulty of prednisolone withdrawal in polymyalgia rheumatica); D. G. Model (letter), *Lancet*, 1978, *1*, 340 (reversal in one eye of blindness due to temporal arteritis by means of intravenous methylprednisolone 500 mg).

Aspiration syndrome. In a double-blind study involving 71 children generally with mild to moderate hydrocarbon pneumonitis who received methylprednisolone sodium succinate or placebo together with antibiotic and respiratory care, the results did not support the use of corticosteroids.— M. I. Marks *et al.*, *J. Pediat.*, 1972, *81*, 366.

There is no conclusive clinical or experimental data on which to base the use of corticosteroids in aspiration pneumonia.— J. W. Wynne and J. H. Modell, *Ann. intern. Med.*, 1977, *87*, 466. See also under Pregnancy and the Neonate (Meconium Aspiration Syndrome).

Studies on the effects of corticosteroids in the gastric

aspiration syndrome: J. E. Wolfe *et al.*, *Am. J. Med.*, 1977, *63*, 719 (no significant difference from controls).

Asthma. A review of the general management of asthma including the role of corticosteroid therapy. Just as it is important not to overtreat the mild asthmatic patient, it is equally important to recognise the more severely affected patients and to begin the appropriate treatment at the correct time.— D. W. Empey, *Br. med. J.*, 1978, *2*, 1208.

A discussion on the avoidance of asthma fatalities with emphasis on the importance of the prompt treatment of severe acute asthma. There seems to be little or no danger in giving doses of up to 2 g daily of hydrocortisone intravenously or 100 mg daily of prednisolone by mouth, or both, for short periods in gravely ill patients. Concerning the choice of a bronchodilator drug, there seems to be no place for subcutaneous adrenaline, but intravenous aminophylline remains a useful drug. Intravenous salbutamol, in bolus doses of up to 300 µg or in a dose of 500 µg infused over 60 minutes, appears to be as effective as aminophylline, more rapid in action, and less prone to cause nausea and vomiting, and may eventually replace aminophylline as the standard intravenous preparation for acute asthma. The issue of whether salbutamol is better given intravenously or as an aqueous aerosol, either inhaled spontaneously or delivered from some form of positive-pressure ventilator, has not yet been resolved. If the patient continues to deteriorate despite massive corticosteroid therapy, repeated administration of bronchodilator drugs, and correction of hypoxaemia, dehydration, and metabolic acidosis, then the next urgent indication is tracheal intubation and mechanical ventilation, with heavy sedation to suppress the patient's respiratory drive. Rapid improvement usually follows, and ventilation is seldom required for over 24 hours.— *Br. med. J.*, 1978, *1*, 873. See also *Lancet*, 1979, *2*, 337.

Further reviews on the recognition and general management of asthma: *Drug & Ther. Bull.*, 1976, *14*, 31 (in children); S. Godfrey, *Br. J. Hosp. Med.*, 1977, *17*, 430 (in children); D. C. Webb-Johnson and J. L. Andrews, *New Engl. J. Med.*, 1977, *297*, 758; G. M. Sterling, *Br. med. J.*, 1978, *1*, 1259; H. G. J. Herxheimer (letter), *ibid.*, 1423; C. Green, *Practitioner*, 1979, *223*, 690; A. D. Milner, *Prescribers' J.*, 1980, *20*, 33 (in children).

Long-term corticosteroid therapy, usually with prednisolone or prednisone, was considered a valuable form of treatment in 170 patients with severe bronchial asthma who were followed for up to 13 years. There was no tendency for the efficacy to diminish with prolonged treatment and a temporary increase of steroids was required during exacerbations. Weaning from therapy was associated with a considerable risk of severe attacks of asthma, in which case therapy had to be resumed. Side-effects were related to dosage.— K. Maunsell *et al.*, *Br. med. J.*, 1968, *1*, 661. See also L. Tuft, *Ann. Allergy*, 1979, *42*, 152.

In a study of 90 deaths from asthma outside hospital, only half the patients were taking corticosteroids and then often in inadequate doses.— J. B. Macdonald *et al.*, *Br. med. J.*, 1976, *1*, 1493. See also R. D. Ghannam *et al.*, *Ann. Allergy*, 1968, *26*, 194.

Further studies and comments on the role of corticosteroids in the management of asthma: M. G. Britton *et al.*, *Br. med. J.*, 1976, *2*, 73; J. B. Macdonald (letter), *ibid.*, 300; H. G. J. Herxheimer (letter), *ibid.*, 305 (short-term dosage for severe asthma); H. Harfi *et al.*, *Pediatrics*, 1979, *61*, 829 (high or conventional methylprednisolone dosage for childhood status asthmaticus); S. A. McKenzie *et al.*, *Archs Dis. Childh.*, 1979, *54*, 581 (status asthmaticus in children); C. S. May *et al.*, *Br. J. Dis. Chest*, 1980, *74*, 91 (prednisolone dosage requirements).

See also under Beclomethasone Dipropionate, p.460.

Blood disorders. *Aplastic anaemia.* The value of corticosteroids in aplastic anaemia was not clear and although occasional cases might respond to prednisolone most haematologists believed that it should be avoided although a brief, carefully monitored trial might be justified in chronic cases which had not responded to androgens alone.— C. G. Geary, *Br. med. J.*, 1974, *2*, 432. A detailed review of the treatment of aplastic anaemia.— S. C. Tso *et al.*, *Q.J. Med.*, 1977, *46*, 513. See also Methylprednisolone Sodium Succinate, p.479.

Further references: D. S. Thompson *et al.*, *Postgrad. med. J.*, 1978, *54*, 278 (auto-immune neutropenia in an infant); D. G. Wright *et al.*, *New Engl. J. Med.*, 1978, *298*, 295 (cyclic neutropenia).

Cold-haemagglutinin disease. Despite previously disappointing reports in high-titre cold-haemagglutinin disease, beneficial results were obtained with administration of high doses of corticosteroids to 2 patients with low-titre cold-haemagglutinin disease.— A. D. Schreiber *et al.*, *New Engl. J. Med.*, 1977, *296*, 1490.

Haemangioma. Two infants with giant haemangioma with thrombocytopenia responded satisfactorily to prednisone 20 mg daily, continued in 1 patient for 5 weeks and then tapered off over 2 weeks. Tumours regressed and there was sustained haematological improvement. Prednisone was the treatment of choice for complicated haemangiomas.— J. Evans *et al.*, *Archs Dis. Childh.*, 1975, *50*, 809.

Haemolytic anaemia. Comment on the use of corticosteroid therapy, which is the treatment of choice, for idiopathic warm auto-immune haemolytic anaemia.— T. Flaherty and C. G. Geary, *Br. J. Hosp. Med.*, 1979, *22*, 334.

Hypereosinophilia. In a study of 16 patients with hypereosinophilia and progressive organ-system involvement, prednisone 60 mg daily for 1 week then on alternate days for 3 months gave a good response in 6 of the patients; 5 continued to be controlled on alternate-day therapy. Three of 5 patients who had a partial response and all 5 who had not responded to corticosteroids received hydroxyurea 1 to 2 g daily. Of these patients, some of whom were the most critically ill, 6 had a good response and 2 a partial response. Hydroxyurea was considered to be the drug of choice for corticosteroid-unresponsive patients with the hypereosinophilic syndrome.— J. E. Parrillo *et al.*, *Ann. intern. Med.*, 1978, *89*, 167.

Hypoplastic anaemia. A 24-year-old woman with congenital hypoplastic anaemia (Blackfan-Diamond syndrome) responded favourably to treatment with prednisone.— G. E. Zito and E. C. Lynch, *J. Am. med. Ass.*, 1977, *237*, 991.

Leukaemia. For references on the role of corticosteroids in the treatment of leukaemia, see Antineoplastic Agents and Immunosuppressants, p.178.

Pernicious anaemia. Prednisolone, 20 mg daily by mouth, restored vitamin-B_{12} absorption to near normal values in 7 of 12 women with pernicious anaemia. It had no significant effect on the vitamin-B_{12} absorption or intrinsic factor secretion of 9 healthy normal men or of 5 with chronic superficial gastritis.— R. G. Strickland *et al.*, *Gut*, 1973, *14*, 13.

Sickle-cell anaemia. For comment on the use of dexamethasone in sickle-cell anaemia, see Dexamethasone, p.467.

Thrombocytopenic purpura. Much evidence has accumulated to demonstrate the role of IgG antibody in the genesis of idiopathic thrombocytopenic purpura. Providing the amount of antibody is not too great, prednisone 60 to 100 mg daily usually reduces the amount of antibody on the platelets and raises the platelet count within 2 or 3 weeks. The dose of prednisone can then be rapidly reduced to about 20 mg daily in adults, and subsequently decreased more slowly to the lowest dose that will maintain a normal, or nearly normal, platelet count. This maintenance dose can usually be given on alternate days and, if sufficiently low (no more than 10 to 15 mg daily on alternate days), is probably satisfactory treatment for the patient as long as the auto-immune process may last.— W. F. Rosse, *New Engl. J. Med.*, 1978, *298*, 1139.

Further references: A. I. S. Macpherson and J. Richmond, *Br. med. J.*, 1975, *1*, 64 (postoperative complications in corticosteroid-treated patients undergoing splenectomy); Y. C. Chia and S. J. Machin, *Br. J. clin. Pract.*, 1979, *33*, 55 (failure of prednisolone 60 mg daily for 3 days in tuberculosis-induced thrombocytopenic purpura); M. Karpatkin *et al.*, *New Engl. J. Med.*, 1981, *305*, 936 (maternal administration for an effect on neonatal autoimmune thrombocytopenia).

Bronchitis and emphysema. Corticosteroids usually give no benefit in chronic bronchitis and emphysema, but they are worth a trial in patients with a large response to beta-adrenergic agonists, great variability in their airways obstruction, or sputum eosinophilia.— A. E. Tattersfield, *Br. med. J.*, 1978, *1*, 1123.

Further reviews and studies on the role of corticosteroids in chronic obstructive pulmonary disease: J. A. Evans *et al.*, *Thorax*, 1974, *29*, 401; S. A. Sahn, *Chest*, 1978, *73*, 389; C. Shim *et al.*, *J. Allergy & clin. Immunol.*, 1978, *62*, 363; C. W. Clarke, *Drugs*, 1979, *18*, 226; R. K. Albert *et al.*, *Ann. intern. Med.*, 1980, *92*, 753 (intravenous methylprednisolone).

Cardiac disorders. Although D. Barzilai *et al.* (*Chest*, 1972, *61*, 488) reported a reduction in mortality in patients given hydrocortisone following myocardial infarction, other studies have been unable to demonstrate a beneficial effect. W.M. Vogel and B.R. Lucchesi (*Chest*, 1978, *73*, 444) who advocate further *animal* studies into the problem noted increased severity of arrhythmias in the corticosteroid-treated patients. Similarly, R.W. Peters *et al.*, and J. Heikkila and M.S. Nieminen (*Chest*, 1978, *73*, 483 and 577) could find no significant difference in the size of infarct or in the clinical course of myocardial infarction patients given 2 large doses of methylprednisolone.

Further references to corticosteroids in cardiac disorders: C. P. Aber and E. W. Jones, *Br. Heart J.*, 1965, *27*, 916 (beneficial effect in heart block); Y. Lee, *Curr. ther. Res.*, 1974, *16*, 593 (beneficial effect on arrhythmias); J. V. Z. Maempel, *Israel J. med. Scis*, 1974, *10*, 1126 (enhancement of anti-arrhythmics); L. Gould *et al.*, *J. clin. Pharmac.*, 1975, *15*, 262 (slowed atrioventricular conduction and high-dose methylprednisolone infusion); J. R. Morton *et al.*, *Am. J. Surg.*, 1976, *131*, 419 (no benefit on myocardial preservation in bypass surgery); M. Papadimitriou *et al.* (letter), *Lancet*, 1977, *1*, 1312; D. D. Oakes *et al.* (letter), *ibid.*, 1313; T. J. Buselmeier *et al.* (letter), *ibid.*, *2*, 301 (corticosteroids in uraemic pericarditis); B. Lorell *et al.*, *Am. J. Cardiol.*, 1978, *42*, 143 (cardiac sarcoidosis); H. Kato, *Pediatrics*, 1979, *63*, 175 (Kawasaki disease and coronary involvement).

Convulsions. A review of the treatment of epilepsy in children. Although the long-term follow-up by P.M. Jeavons *et al.* (*Epilepsia*, 1973, *14*, 153) showed no benefit from corticotrophin or corticosteroids in infantile spasms (West's syndrome) there is a suggestion from several workers in this field that those with a short history (less than 4 weeks) may have reasonable hope of benefit from these drugs.— B. Bower, *Br. J. Hosp. Med.*, 1978, *19*, 8. See also R. A. Hrachovy *et al.*, *Epilepsia*, 1979, *20*, 403.

Croup. See under Epiglottitis, Laryngitis, and Croup.

Dental and oral use. Though dressings containing corticosteroids and antibiotics applied to intact or exposed and painful pulps appeared clinically to be miraculous, pathohistological examination of 170 treated teeth showed, without exception, metaplastic changes of pulp tissue, irreversible inhibition of dentine formation, and persistent, chronic inflammation that could lead to slow necrosis. The application of corticosteroids to exposed pulps was contra-indicated if their vitality was to be preserved.— L. J. Baume, *Int. dent. J.*, 1966, *16*, 30. A similar recommendation against this use following *animal* studies.— R. C. Paterson, *Br. dent. J.*, 1976, *140*, 174 and 231.

For the use of corticosteroids in aphthous ulcers, see under Skin Disorders.

Disseminated intravascular coagulation. In patients with disseminated intravascular coagulation, corticosteroids should be used where indicated in the management of the underlying disease, but they should not be used simply because all else has failed.— A. A. Sharp, *Br. med. Bull.*, 1977, *33*, 265.

Drowning. Dramatic improvement in secondary drowning was associated with methylprednisolone 2 g given intravenously. The patient also received frusemide, ampicillin, and oxygen.— E. Oliver *et al.* (letter), *Lancet*, 1978, *1*, 105. It is considered that there is little evidence that corticosteroids are effective in near-drowning and their use could complicate treatment.— P. W. Munt and J. A. Fleetham (letter), *Lancet*, 1978, *1*, 665. See also J. H. Modell *et al.*, *Chest*, 1976, *70*, 231.

Drug overdosage. Measurement of the plasma-11-hydroxycorticosteroid concentrations in 37 patients in various stages of coma due to drug overdosage did not demonstrate any suppression of corticosteroid secretion. The routine administration of corticosteroids to such patients is unnecessary.— J. V. Collins *et al.*, *Lancet*, 1971, *2*, 184.

Epiglottitis, laryngitis, and croup. The use of corticosteroids in acute epiglottitis is logical and widespread although no controlled studies have been carried out.— *Lancet*, 1978, *1*, 1294. Comment on the role of hydrocortisone 100 mg intramuscularly or intravenously in the management of laryngeal obstruction associated with acute laryngitis in infants, which is the commonest cause of croup. No effect is seen for at least 2 hours.— H. B. Valman, *Br. med. J.*, 1980, *280*, 1438.

Conflicting reports on the merits of corticosteroids in croup: A. N. Eden *et al.*, *J. Am. med. Ass.*, 1967, *200*, 403; F. D. Fowler (letter), *ibid.*, 1969, *208*, 1907; J. D. Cherry, *J. Pediat.*, 1979, *94*, 352.

Gastro-intestinal disorders. A discussion on the treatment of inflammatory bowel disease, a generic term which includes both ulcerative colitis and Crohn's disease, but excludes the specific bacterial dysenteries.— T. C. Northfield, *Prescribers' J.*, 1979, *19*, 80. See also *idem*, *Drugs*, 1977, *14*, 198; J. B. Kirsner, *J. Am. med. Ass.*, 1980, *243*, 557.

The following intensive intravenous regimen was used

for 5 days to produce remissions in 36 and improvement in 4 of 49 patients with severe attacks of ulcerative colitis: at least 3 litres of fluid daily comprising sodium chloride injection with dextrose in 0.18% sodium chloride; blood; in some patients nutritional agents with alcohol and laevulose; potassium supplements as required with vitamins B and C; the equivalent of about 44 mg of prednisolone; and tetracycline 1 g daily in divided doses. A hydrocortisone enema was given twice daily. The patients were allowed nothing but sips of water by mouth. After 5 days, patients who showed no improvement should undergo surgery but any deterioration should be treated with immediate surgery. Those in remission resumed normal feeding and were given prednisolone 10 to 15 mg and sulphasalazine 500 mg four times daily by mouth but the 4 who only showed improvement did not respond to oral treatment and had to be treated surgically.— S. C. Truelove and D. P. Jewell, *Lancet*, 1974, *1*, 1067. A report of experience over a period of 5 years with the intensive intravenous regimen incorporating the following minor modifications: a central venous line is usually set up to facilitate intravenous feeding, and instead of adding laevulose and alcohol to the amino-acid infusion, additional calories are supplied as dextrose and Intralipid; if the patient has shown improvement after 5 days but is not symptom-free, addition of azathioprine to the oral regimen is considered. In addition to deterioration in condition, absence of decisive improvement after 5 days is taken as an absolute indication for emergency colectomy before completion of the intravenous regimen. Of 100 courses of the regimen in 87 patients, remission was obtained in 60, improvement in 15, and no change or deterioration occurred in 25.— S. C. Truelove *et al.*, *ibid.*, 1978, *2*, 1086.

Further references to the use of corticosteroids in ulcerative colitis: K. N. Jalan *et al.*, *New Engl. J. Med.*, 1970, *282*, 588 (no increased operative risk in those receiving corticosteroids).

A review of the use of corticosteroids in Crohn's disease with special reference to various aspects of the National Cooperative Crohn's Disease Study in the USA. Impressions gained from 2 large uncontrolled studies that a good initial symptomatic response to prednisone 30 mg daily or its equivalent, is obtained in 75 to 90% of patients, were confirmed in a double-blind controlled trial carried out as part of the National Cooperative Crohn's Disease Study (J.W. Singleton, *Gastroenterology*, 1977, *72*, 1133). Active disease involving the small bowel was especially responsive to corticosteroids, but the extra-intestinal complications and peri-anal disease were as unresponsive to prednisone as to placebo. Previous sulphasalazine therapy seemed to blunt subsequent response to corticosteroids, and the toxicity of corticosteroids at doses high enough to suppress active Crohn's disease was appreciable. The role of prophylactic corticosteroid therapy in both quiescent disease and after complete surgical extirpation of Crohn's disease has been examined in 3 recent controlled studies (L. Bergman and U. Krause, *Scand. J. Gastroenterol.*, 1976, *11*, 651; J.W. Singleton, *Gastroenterology*, 1977, *72*, 1133; R.C. Smith *et al.*, *Gut*, 1978, *19*, 606). Those receiving prophylactic corticosteroid therapy fared no better than those taking placebo or nothing and, in fact, fared noticeably, but not significantly, worse. Thus, prophylactic therapy with corticosteroids is not indicated for Crohn's disease. Although uncontrolled studies indicated a recrudescence of symptoms on withdrawal of corticosteroids, placebo-controlled National Cooperative Crohn's Disease Studies have shown that withdrawal during a quiescent phase is associated with no more relapses than continuation.— J. W. Singleton, *Ann. intern. Med.*, 1979, *90*, 983. See also The National Cooperative Crohn's Disease Study, J. W. Singleton (Ed.), *Gastroenterology*, 1979, *77*, 825-944.

Further references to the use of corticosteroids in Crohn's disease: J. R. Allsop and E. C. G. Lee, *Gut*, 1978, *19*, 729 (no increased operative risk in those receiving corticosteroids); D. J. Atherton *et al.*, *Br. med. J.*, 1978, *1*, 552 (beneficial effect of prednisolone in a boy with genital Crohn's disease).

Further reviews, reports, and studies on the use of corticosteroids in general gastro-intestinal disorders: H. J. Mendelsohn and W. H. Maloney, *Ann. Otol. Rhinol. Lar.*, 1970, *79*, 900 (local therapy for oesophageal stricture); A. J. Wall *et al.*, *Gut*, 1970, *11*, 7 (coeliac disease); L. P. Morandi and P. J. Grob, *Archs intern. Med.*, 1971, *128*, 295 (retroperitoneal fibrosis); J. D. Lloyd-Still *et al.*, *J. Pediat.*, 1972, *81*, 1074 (coeliac crisis); S. Meyers and H. D. Janowitz, *Gastroenterology*, 1978, *75*, 729 (toxic megacolon); J. Powell-Tuck *et al.*, *Scand. J. Gastroenterol.*, 1978, *13*, 833 (once-daily therapy in proctocolitis); M. E. Pickup *et al.*, *Eur. J. Drug Metab. Pharmacokinet.*, 1979, *4*, 87 (prednisolone absorption in coeliac disease).

For further references to the management of inflammatory bowel disease, see Azathioprine, p.191, and Sulphasalazine, p.1482.

Hay fever and allergic rhinitis. See under Rhinitis.

Headache. Results of a double-blind study in 19 patients indicated that a single dose of prednisone 30 mg for acute attacks of cluster headaches gave almost immediate relief, and freedom from symptoms for about 60 days.— J. L. Jamms, *Dis. nerv. Syst.*, 1975, *37*, 375. See also J. R. Couch and D. K. Ziegler, *Headache*, 1978, *18*, 219 (relapse).

For a view on the relative merits of chlorpromazine and prednisone in cluster headache, see Chlorpromazine, p.1515.

Hepatic disorders. A detailed review of the use of corticosteroids in liver disease, possible mechanisms of action, pharmacology, and rational use. Corticosteroids are contra-indicated in uncomplicated viral hepatitis, although they have a limited role in prolonged cholestasis. There has been considerable controversy over the years concerning the place of corticosteroids in the management of fulminant hepatic failure, but the general consensus at present is firmly against the use of corticosteroids. A problem in relation to chronic active hepatitis is that the meaning of the term has evolved since the instigation of some of the major studies, and current criteria are still not universally accepted. There is an established place for corticosteroid therapy in the management of the symptomatic and histologically severe forms, but the use of corticosteroids in hepatitis-B-positive chronic active hepatitis is still controversial. In patients who do benefit from corticosteroid therapy it has been shown that daily administration of prednisone 10 mg in association with azathioprine 50 mg, after an initial month of higher prednisone dose, offers the best chance of disease control, together with the lowest incidence of major corticosteroid side-effects. Assessment of alternate-day therapy has indicated that daily therapy appears to have advantages, but prednisolone has been recommended rather than prednisone, as the serum concentrations are more predictable. There is general agreement that corticosteroid therapy is not indicated in patients with chronic persistent hepatitis, as the condition is virtually asymptomatic, non-progressive, and associated with a good prognosis. If corticosteroids have a role in the management of alcoholic liver disease, it will probably be confined to patients with alcoholic hepatitis who have encephalopathy or a severe coagulation disorder. Corticosteroids often have a dramatic effect on patients with granulomatous hepatitis, but in a large variety of other hepatic disorders, including Wilson's disease, Gilbert's disease, Dubin Johnson syndrome, and hepatic amyloidosis, they have been shown to be of no value. They are of benefit in multi-system diseases that occasionally involve the liver, such as polyarteritis nodosa or systemic lupus erythematosus.— A. R. Tanner and L. W. Powell, *Gut*, 1979, *20*, 1109.

Further reviews on corticosteroid therapy for hepatic disorders: N. A. Auger, *Am. J. Hosp. Pharm.*, 1978, *35*, 1222; *Lancet*, 1978, *2*, 507; *Br. med. J.*, 1980, *281*, 258.

Further comments and studies on the role of corticosteroids alone or with adjunct therapy in hepatic disorders: B. L. Blitzer *et al.*, *Am. J. dig. Dis.*, 1977, *22*, 477 (alcoholic hepatitis); W. C. Maddrey and J. K. Boitnott, *Gastroenterology*, 1977, *72*, 1348 (drug-induced liver disease); *Dt. med. Wschr.*, 1978, *103*, 887 (active chronic hepatitis); H. R. Lesesne *et al.*, *Gastroenterology*, 1978, *74*, 169 (alcoholic hepatitis); W. C. Maddrey *et al.*, *Gastroenterology* 1978, *75*, 193 (alcoholic hepatitis); C. D. R. Pengelly and R. C. Jennings (letter), *Lancet*, 1978, *2*, 632 (cyclophosphamide and corticosteroids in chronic active hepatitis); I. G. Toth (letter), *Lancet*, 1978, *2*, 947 (azathioprine and corticosteroids in chronic active hepatitis); W. Depew *et al.*, *Gastroenterology*, 1980, *78*, 524 (alcoholic hepatitis); A. P. Kirk *et al.*, *Gut*, 1980, *21*, 78 (chronic active hepatitis); E. Sagnelli *et al.*, *Lancet*, 1980, *2*, 395 (risk of hepatitis B virus replication); K. C. Lam *et al.*, *New Engl. J. Med.*, 1981, *304*, 380 (deleterious effect on chronic active hepatitis).

See also under Azathioprine, p.191.

Hypercalcaemia. Despite their unpredictability and the trivial short-term reduction they produce, corticosteroids are still widely used to lower serum-calcium concentrations. Although the hypercalcaemia of sarcoidosis and of vitamin-D intoxication is usually steroid-sensitive and that due to hyperparathyroidism steroid-resistant, this is not invariable. Some authors have considered corticosteroids to be highly effective in the treatment of hypercalcaemia complicating malignant disease whereas others considered them to be ineffective when used alone. Furthermore, the calcium-lowering effect of corticosteroids may take a week to develop, and reductions of less than 0.25 mmol per litre may be all that is achieved.— *Br. med. J.*, 1980, *280*, 204. References: J. Anderson *et al.*, *Lancet*, 1954, *2*, 720 (sarcoidosis with hypercalcaemia); J. V. Verner *et al.*, *Ann. intern. Med.*, 1958, *48*, 765 (vitamin D intoxication); G. Gwinup and B. Sayle, *Ann. intern. Med.*, 1961, *55*, 1001 (hyperparathyroidisim); I. H. Mannheimer, *Cancer*, 1965, *18*, 679 (breast cancer); N. C. Thalassinos and G. F. Joplin, *Lancet*, 1970, *2*, 537 (malignant disease); D. H. Fulmer *et al.*, *Archs intern. Med.*, 1972, *129*, 923.

Hyperpyrexia. A 6-year-old child with suspected malignant hyperpyrexia responded promptly to dexamethasone 4 mg intravenously.— D. G. Raitt and A. J. Merrifield (letter), *Br. med. J.*, 1974, *4*, 656. Dexamethasone 1.5 mg per kg body-weight was successfully used as the sole agent in a patient with malignant hyperpyrexia.— F. R. Ellis *et al.*, *Br. J. Anaesth.*, 1975, *47*, 632. Failure of methylprednisolone in porcine malignant hyperpyrexia.— G. M. Hall *et al.* (letter), *Lancet*, 1977, *2*, 1359.

Infections. Although long-term corticosteroid therapy has an adverse effect on the body's response to infection (see Effects on Immune Response, under Adverse Effects), the judicious use of corticosteroids, usually on a short-term basis, and in conjunction with appropriate chemotherapeutic agents, may have a beneficial effect on the symptoms of selected acute infections, and may on occasions be life-saving.

Individual reports. A comparison of results in patients given corticosteroids with the results in patients not given corticosteroids in *infectious mononucleosis, mumps orchitis*, and *herpes zoster*, suggested that corticosteroid treatment reduced the period of morbidity by about a half. It was considered especially valuable for the management of acute viral infection.— G. E. Breen and P. K. Talukdar, *Lancet*, 1965, *1*, 158.

Two patients with *varicella pneumonia* had a dramatic response to hydrocortisone.— J. P. Anderson (letter), *Lancet*, 1966, *1*, 1097. See also G. E. Breen (letter), *ibid.*, 1268.

Beneficial effects with prednisolone or corticotrophin in a controlled study of patients with severe *infectious mononucleosis*.— C. E. Bender, *J. Am. med. Ass.*, 1967, *199*, 529. See also M. P. Gordon, *Milit. Med.*, 1968, *133*, 303. Over 9 years, prompt symptomatic relief was achieved in 300 students with *infectious mononucleosis* by treatment with dexamethasone. The most satisfactory dosage schedule was 3 tablets of 750 µg taken 4 times the first day, 2 tablets 4 times daily for 2 days, one 4 times daily for 4 days, one 3 times daily for 3 days, one twice daily for 2 days, and one daily for 5 days. Students so treated were only absent from classes for an average of 3 days.— J. B. Riggsbee (letter), *J. Am. med. Ass.*, 1967, *200*, 350. In a double-blind study in 26 students with *infectious mononucleosis* a more rapid response occurred after treatment with prednisone for 12 days (40 mg daily initially, gradually reduced) than after treatment with aspirin.— K. J. Bolden, *J.R. Coll. gen. Pract.*, 1972, *22*, 87.

Prednisone, 10 to 15 mg every 6 hours, was recommended for the treatment of *trichinosis*. Prednisone could be given parenterally if necessary. Treatment should be continued for 5 to 7 days, but if continued for longer the doses should be tapered before withdrawal.— W. E. Herrell, *Clin. Med.*, 1968, *75* (May), 92.

In a patient with *louping-ill virus infection*, treatment with hydrocortisone, 100 mg twice daily by intravenous injection for 5 days and then by gradually reducing intramuscular injections, produced a dramatic effect.— H. E. Webb *et al.*, *Lancet*, 1968, *2*, 255.

Disappearance of nearly all multiple *warts* in 2 children by about the fourth week followed a course of 500 µg of dexamethasone thrice daily for 1 week, 500 µg twice daily for 1 week, then 250 µg thrice daily for 1 week, in conjunction with ascorbic acid 100 mg thrice daily.— T. V. A. Harry, *Practitioner*, 1969, *203*, 356. Similar reports.— K. H. Yeretsian, *ibid.*, 1965, *194*, 824; T. N. Babu, *ibid.*, 1968, *201*, 478.

Corticosteroids were considered to have speeded recovery in 2 children with *laryngeal diphtheria*.— D. A. Roche (letter), *Br. med. J.*, 1969, *1*, 119. See also under Epiglottitis, Laryngitis, and Croup.

An improved survival-rate in patients with *tetanus* given adjunct therapy with betamethasone.— R. K. M. Sanders *et al.*, *Trans. R. Soc. trop. Med. Hyg.*, 1969, *63*, 746; R. K. M. Sanders (letter), *Lancet*, 1970, *2*, 526.

Two patients with *herpes simplex encephalitis* improved after early diagnosis of the disease by EEG and then treatment with dexamethasone.— A. R. M. Upton *et al.* (letter), *Lancet*, 1971, *1*, 290. Comments and criticisms.— M. Longson and T. S. L. Beswick (letter), *ibid.*, 749. Two children with severe encephalitis, probably *herpes simplex encephalitis*, responded dramatically to dexamethasone given parenterally.— A. H. Habel and J. K. Brown (letter), *Lancet*, 1972, *1*, 695.

Prednisolone 15 mg six-hourly for 4 days in *mumps orchitis* often accelerated pain relief and temperature reduction, but corticosteroids did not reduce the risk of testicular atrophy or prevent unilateral orchitis from becoming bilateral.— J. A. Gray, *Br. med. J.*, 1973, *1*, 338.

In *meningococcal disease* corticosteroids are used for their anti-inflammatory action, to combat shock, and as replacement therapy for suspected adrenal involvement. Many paediatricians believe that they have a valuable role in neonatal infection. Routine use in *tuberculous meningitis* has been advocated but others limit their use to proved or threatened spinal block. Corticosteroids have been used widely in meningococcaemia although theoretically they could promote further haemorrhage. In severe and advanced cases of meningitis significant relief from acute cerebral oedema may be obtained with dexamethasone.— J. Stevenson, *Br. med. J.*, 1973, *2*, 411.

Conflicting reports on the merits of the routine use of corticosteroid therapy in the management of *meningitis*, including tuberculous meningitis: J. Bøe *et al.*, *Br. med. J.*, 1965, *1*, 1094; R. A. deLemos and R. J. Haggerty, *Pediatrics*, 1969, *44*, 32; J. A. Escobar *et al.*, *ibid.*, 1975, *56*, 1050; Z. H. Idriss *et al.*, *Am. J. Dis. Child.*, 1976, *130*, 364. See also M. Parsons, *Tuberculous Meningitis: A Handbook for Clinicians*, Oxford, Oxford University Press, 1979.

Routine treatment of *pulmonary tuberculosis* with corticosteroids in addition to tuberculostatics is not advocated; adjunct corticosteroid therapy is indicated in patients who are ill and toxic, and in cases of massive effusions, tuberculous meningitis, or severe drug reactions.— D. K. Stevenson, *Practitioner*, 1974, *212*, 320. Reports of the use of corticosteroids and corticotrophin in conjunction with tuberculostatic agents: Tuberculosis Society of Scotland, *Br. med. J.*, 1957, *2*, 1131; N. W. Horne, *ibid.*, 1960, *2*, 1751; *Tubercle*, 1963, *44*, 484 (report from the Research Committee of the British Tuberculosis Association); *Am. Rev. resp. Dis.*, 1965, *91*, 329 (United States Public Health Service Tuberculosis Therapy Trial); J. R. Johnson *et al.*, *ibid.*, *92*, 376; R. L. Nemir *et al.*, *ibid.*, 1967, *95*, 402; J. R. Johnson *et al.*, *ibid.*, *96*, 62 and 74; S. K. Malik and C. J. Martin, *ibid.*, *100*, 13.

Corticosteroids might be beneficial in the treatment of *whooping cough*.— S. Ware (letter), *Lancet*, 1977, *2*, 872. See also under Epiglottitis, Laryngitis, and Croup.

Although *toxocariasis* is usually benign and self-limiting, the use of corticosteroids may be life-saving in patients with severe respiratory or myocardial involvement. Corticosteroids are also indicated for actively inflamed eyes to prevent further changes leading to retinal detachment.— P. M. Schantz and L. T. Glickman, *New Engl. J. Med.*, 1978, *298*, 436.

A spirited defence of the use of corticosteroids (systemic prenisolone) in *herpes zoster* infection. There is no reliable information suggesting that treatment of zoster with systemic corticosteroids causes dissemination of the disease, except in the immunosuppressed patient.— K. D. Crow and J. P. Ellis (letter), *Br. med. J.*, 1979, *1*, 346. Further references to the use of local or systemic corticosteroid therapy in zoster: E. Epstein (letter), *J. Am. med. Ass.*, 1969, *207*, 2439; W. H. Eaglestein *et al.*, *ibid.*, 1970, *211*, 1681; E. Epstein, *Acta derm.-vener., Stockh.*, 1970, *50*, 69; M. Schreuder and W. T. Fothergill (letter), *Br. med. J.*, 1979, *1*, 818.

For reference to the use of corticosteroids in the management of *cerebral malaria*, see Dexamethasone, p.466.

Infertility. Continuous therapy with prednisone 5 mg thrice daily for 3 to 12 months, or intermittent therapy with methylprednisolone 96 mg daily for 1 to 3 courses of 7 days, improved the fertility of some of 47 men with subfertility caused by antisperm antibodies.— W. F. Hendry *et al.*, *Lancet*, 1979, *2*, 498. See also S. Shulman (letter), *Lancet*, 1976, *2*, 1243. Preliminary findings suggest that administration to the husband of methylprednisolone 96 mg daily for 7 days either for 7 days before the expected commencement of the wife's menstrual cycle or from days 2 to 8 of the cycle may reduce infertility in men whose serum contains antisperm antibodies. Of 7 couples treated, 4 pregnancies have occurred, all 4 when the husband was taking the corticosteroid from days 2 to 8 of his wife's cycle.— M. Katz and R. Newill (letter), *Lancet*, 1980, *1*, 1306.

Further references to corticosteroid therapy in autoimmune infertility: M. De Almeida and J. C. Soufir (letter), *Lancet*, 1977, *2*, 815 (dexamethasone acetate); S. Shulman *et al.*, *Fert. Steril.*, 1978, *29*, 309.

Leucophaeresis. Following administration of dexamethasone 4 mg per m^2 body-surface to 28 healthy leucophaeresis donors no adverse effects were noted on the functional competence of the neutrophils. The practice of administering corticosteroids to produce neutrophilia and increase yields for granulocyte transfusions was therefore not contra-indicated.— L. Glasser *et al.*, *New Engl. J. Med.*, 1977, *297*, 1033. Criticism.— B. A. Mason (letter), *ibid.*, 1978, *298*, 456. Reply.— L. Glasser *et al.* (letter), *ibid.*

Lupus erythematosus. Survival-rates for a group of 209 patients with systemic lupus erythematosus seen before 1968 were compared with another group of 156 patients seen between 1968 and 1975 and showed a marked improvement for the second group. All patients were treated with corticosteroids, but except for 3 patients in the second group none received immunosuppressive therapy. Survival-rates for the first group at 5 and 10 years were 70 and 63% compared to 93 and 84% respectively for the second group. Improvement in survival-rates was largely attributed to better management; in particular, corticosteroid therapy in the second group was adjusted according to both clinical and serological values; it was also attributed to the recent use of newer antibiotics.— J. D. Urman and N. F. Rothfield, *J. Am. med. Ass.*, 1977, *238* 2272. Comments and criticism.— E. L. Dubois *et al.* (letter), *ibid.*, 1978, *239*, 1846.

Comment on the individual variation in corticosteroid prescribing for systemic lupus erythematosus, and on the contribution of corticosteroids to morbidity figures such as the incidence of infection and of osteonecrosis.— G. R. V. Hughes, *Br. med. J.*, 1979, *2*, 1019. Comment on advances in the diagnosis and treatment of collagen disorders including mention that in most patients with systemic lupus erythematosus, corticosteroids are unnecessary.— *ibid.*, 1980, *280*, 170.

See also under Renal Disorders (below).

Mental disorders. Three patients with presenile dementia responded to treatment with hydrocortisone 300 or 400 mg daily by intramuscular injection gradually reduced over a few days followed by maintenance treatment with prednisone, 15 to 30 mg daily by mouth.— R. Chynoweth and J. Foley, *Br. J. Psychiat.*, 1969, *115*, 703.

Muscular disorders. A review of the use of corticosteroids in the treatment of myopathies, particularly polymyositis, dermatomyositis, and myasthenia gravis.— D. Grob, *A. Rev. Pharmac. & Toxic.*, 1976, *16*, 215. See also D. B. Drachman, *New Engl. J. Med.*, 1978, *298*, 186.

Muscular dystrophy. Prednisone was administered in an initial dose of 2 mg per kg body-weight daily to 14 children with Duchenne muscular dystrophy then reduced after 2 to 3 months to an alternate-day schedule of about 60% of the original dose. Improvement occurred in 13 children but 5 deteriorated during treatment. The remaining 8 still showed improvement at 28 months. Prednisone might provide temporary improvement in patients with Duchenne muscular dystrophy.— D. B. Drachman *et al.*, *Lancet*, 1974, *2*, 1409. Criticism.— T. L. Munsat and J. N. Walton (letter), *ibid.*, 1975, *1*, 276.

Further references: J. N. Walton, *Br. med. J.*, 1969, *3*, 639; A. G. Engel and R. G. Siekert, *Archs Neurol., Chicago*, 1972, *27*, 174.

Myasthenia gravis. Of 12 patients with myasthenia gravis given prednisone in gradually increasing doses 7 had good to excellent improvement and 4 moderate. None experienced an increase in weakness. Initially prednisone 25 mg was given on alternate days increasing by 12.5 mg every 3rd dose until a maximum of 100 mg or a lower optimal dose on every alternate day was achieved. Therapy with anticholinesterases was continued at a dosage to give maximum benefit. When the patients' improvement reached a plateau, prednisone was gradually reduced although it could not be withdrawn entirely in any patient.— M. E. Seybold and D. B. Drachman, *New Engl. J. Med.*, 1974, *290*, 81. See also R. B. Jenkins, *Lancet*, 1972, *1*, 765.

A 70-year-old woman with myasthenia gravis was inadequately maintained on pyridostigmine 960 mg daily. There was a dramatic improvement when prednisolone 5 mg thrice daily was added to her treatment, followed by a transient phase of deterioration attributed to cholinergic crisis. The dose of pyridostigmine was gradually reduced and eventually discontinued and the patient was maintained on prednisolone 7.5 mg daily.— P. Dandona *et al.*, *Postgrad. med. J.*, 1977, *53*, 321.

Further references to the role of corticosteroid therapy in myasthenia gravis: J. R. Warmolts *et al.* (letter), *Lancet*, 1970, *2*, 1198; A. Dalby *et al.* (letter), *ibid.*, 1971, *1*, 597; J. R. Warmolts and W. K. Engel, *New Engl. J. Med.*, 1972, *286*, 17; N. G. Brunner *et al.*, *Neurology, Minneap.*, 1972, *22*, 603; M. Seybold and D. B. Drachman, *ibid.*, 1973, *23*, 389; K. C. Fischer and R. J. Schwartzman, *ibid.*, 1974, *24*, 795; J. D. Mann *et al.*, *ibid.*, 1976, *26*, 729.

Correspondence on the use of plasma exchange, either alone or in association with corticosteroid and other immunosuppressant therapy, in the treatment of myasthenia gravis: P. C. Dau *et al.*, *New Engl. J. Med.*, 1977, *297*, 1134; J. Newsom-Davis *et al.* (letter), *ibid.*, 1978, *298*, 456; P. C. Dau *et al.* (letter), *ibid.*, 457; P. O. Behan *et al.*, *Lancet*, 1979, *2*, 438; P. Kornfeld *et al.* (letter), *ibid.*, 629; J. Newsom-Davis and A. Vincent (letter), *ibid.*, 688; P. O. Behan (letter), *ibid.*, 741.

Polymyositis. A recommended therapeutic regimen for severe polymyositis: prednisone 60 mg daily in a single dose; azathioprine 2.5 to 3 mg per kg body-weight daily in divided doses; slow potassium tablets 1.2 g thrice daily; antacids and calcium tablets according to needs. After major improvement or at 6 months, the prednisone should be slowly reduced over 3 months to a maintenance level of 15 to 30 mg on alternate days in a single dose; the other therapy should be continued as before. At 2 years the therapy should be slowly tailed off over 3 months, monitoring for relapse of polymyositis and for adrenocortical failure. Therapy should be re-established if relapse occurs, and every subsequent year attempted withdrawal of therapy should be repeated.— W. G. Bradley, *Br. J. Hosp. Med.*, 1977, *17*, 351. Further reference: R. DeVere and W. G. Bradley, *Brain*, 1975, *98*, 637.

Further references to corticosteroids and other immunosuppressants in muscle-wasting diseases: M. D. Benson and M. A. Aldo, *Archs intern. Med.*, 1973, *132*, 547 (azathioprine in corticosteroid-resistant polymyositis); G. Matell *et al.*, *Ann. N.Y. Acad. Sci.*, 1976, *274*, 659 (myasthenia gravis); P. D. Mohr and T. G. Knowlson, *Postgrad. med. J.*, 1977, *53*, 757 (myositis); T. W. Bunch *et al.*, *Ann. intern. Med.*, 1980, *92*, 365 (alone or with azathioprine in polymyositis).

Neoplastic disorders. In many patients with terminal carcinoma, prednisolone 10 to 15 mg daily would correct hypercalcaemia, reduce fever and weakness, increase appetite, and promote a feeling of well-being.— *Drug & Ther. Bull.*, 1974, *12*, 63. See also B. A. Stoll, *Practitioner*, 1979, *222*, 211.

For reports on the role of corticosteroids in combination chemotherapy for neoplastic disorders, see Antineoplastic Agents and Immunosuppressants, p.177.

Neurological disorders. *Bell's palsy.* Of 186 patients with idiopathic facial paralysis, 94 were treated with corticotrophin and 92 with prednisolone. Complete recovery occurred in 62 and 79 patients respectively, while denervation appeared in significantly more patients given corticotrophin than in those given prednisolone—32 compared with 13. Response was somewhat better in younger than in older patients and if treatment started within 2 days rather than within 4 days of the onset of symptoms. The dose of corticotrophin (depot preparation) was 60 units daily for 5 days, 40 units daily for 2 days, and 20 units daily for 2 days. The dose of prednisolone was 20 mg four times a day for 5 days, thrice daily for 1 day, twice daily for 1 day, daily for 1 day, and 10 mg daily for 1 day. Prednisolone was the treatment of choice for Bell's palsy.— D. Taverner *et al.*, *Br. med. J.*, 1971, *4*, 20. Criticisms.— W. T. Berrill (letter), *ibid.*, 425; M. J. Aminoff, *Postgrad. med. J.*, 1973, *49*, 46.

Prednisone relieved the pain of Bell's palsy and gave fuller recovery to 194 patients compared with 110 untreated patients. There was a more favourable prognosis if the prednisone therapy was started as soon as possible after onset of paralysis. The recommended dose was 60 mg daily for four days tapered off over 10 days to 5 mg daily, starting a second cycle at 60 mg again if there was any recurrence.— K. K. Adour *et al.*, *New Engl. J. Med.*, 1972, *287*, 1268.

A 2-year double-blind study in 51 patients with Bell's palsy showed that corticosteroid treatment was no better than placebo. The regimen used was a total prednisone dose of 410 mg with vitamins or vitamins alone.— M. May *et al.*, *J. Am. med. Ass.*, 1975, *232*, 1203; *ibid.*, *233*, 406.

Further references to the use of corticosteroid therapy in Bell's palsy: S. M. Wolf *et al.*, *Neurology, Minneap.*, 1978, *28*, 158 (favourable).

Guillain-Barré syndrome. In a multicentre study 21 patients with acute polyneuropathy of undetermined aetiology (Guillain-Barré syndrome) received prednisolone 15 mg four times daily for 1 week, 10 mg four times daily for 4 days, and 10 mg thrice daily for 3 days, the dose being subsequently reduced or continued according to clinical judgement; children received doses reduced according to age. Nineteen similar patients did not receive corticosteroids. Analysis of changes in disability grades at one, three, and twelve months indicated that the patients who received prednisolone generally fared worse than the control patients, particularly among patients who entered the trial within a week of the onset of symptoms. These results provided no grounds for the use of corticosteroids in the management of acute inflammatory polyneuropathy.— R. A. C. Hughes *et al.*, *Lancet*, 1978, *2*, 750. Criticism.— R. D. Currier (letter), *ibid.*, 1148. Further criticism.— M. P. McQuillen and H. MSwick (letter), *Lancet*, 1978, *2*, 1209. Reply.— R. A. C. Hughes *et al.* (letter), *ibid.*, 1383.

Further references to the use of corticosteroid therapy in the Guillain-Barré syndrome: R. L. Sullivan and A. G. Reeves (letter), *Lancet*, 1975, *1*, 412; H. M. Swick and M. P. McQuillen, *Neurology, Minneap.*, 1976, *26*, 205.

Correspondence on the use of plasma exchange, either alone or in association with corticosteroid and other immunosuppressant therapy, in the treatment of the Guillain-Barré syndrome: R. P. Brettle *et al.*, *Lancet*, 1978, *2*, 1100; R. L. Levy *et al.* (letter), *ibid.*, 1979, *2*, 741.

Multiple sclerosis. A brief review of studies on the merits of corticosteroid therapy in multiple sclerosis. A current practice is to restrict the use of corticosteroid therapy to the acute demyelinating episode and to prescribe a depot injection of tetracosactrin 0.5 to 1 mg daily for 30 days. Some centres prefer to use an alternate-day dosage of prednisolone (100 mg for 4 to 8 weeks).— L. A. Liversedge, *Br. med. Bull.*, 1977, *33*, 78.

See also under Corticotrophin, p.487.

Intrathecal injection of depot glucocorticoids in patients with multiple sclerosis has been reported to be associated with frequent severe meningeal inflammatory reactions.— J. L. Bernat (letter), *Lancet*, 1977, *1*, 48. See also J. L. Bernat *et al.*, *Neurology, Minneap.*, 1976, *26*, 351.

Further references to the use of corticosteroid therapy in multiple sclerosis: I. Neu *et al.*, *Dt. med. Wschr.*, 1978, *103*, 1368 (intrathecal triamcinolone acetonide); J. Mertin *et al.*, *Lancet*, 1980, *2*, 949; H. Valdimarsson (letter), *ibid.*, 1191; E. H. Jellinek (letter), *ibid.*, 1192; G. S. Plaut (letter), *ibid* (with antilymphocyte immunoglobulin and azathioprine).

Optic neuritis. In a trial in 61 patients with acute demyelinating optic neuritis there was no significant difference in visual acuity, colour vision, and visual fields between those treated with a single retrobulbar injection of triamcinolone 40 mg and controls. Treatment might be justified in those with bilateral disease or poor vision in the second eye, because of a trend to more rapid return of visual acuity.— E. S. Gould *et al.*, *Br. med. J.*, 1977, *1*, 1495.

See also under Corticotrophin, p.487.

Subacute demyelinating polyneuropathy. A report of 10 patients with subacute demyelinating polyneuropathy who obtained a beneficial response to corticosteroid therapy; in one patient the response was initially slight, but became dramatic when azathioprine was added. Prednisone was given in initial single daily doses of 40 to 150 mg, until definite clinical improvement was obtained, and followed by a single-dose alternate-day regimen. After a detailed review of different forms of polyneuropathy, including the Guillain-Barré syndrome, and their response to corticosteroid therapy, it was concluded that subacute demyelination neuropathy appears to be a distinct and clinically identifiable entity in which corticosteroid therapy is indicated.— S. J. Oh, *Archs Neurol., Chicago*, 1978, *35*, 509.

Sudeck's atrophy. A report of a beneficial response to corticosteroid therapy in patients with Sudeck's atrophy (or post-traumatic neurodystrophy) who had failed to improve with other treatment, including intensive physiotherapy. Corticosteroid therapy was usually given as prednisolone 15 to 40 mg daily, gradually reduced after 3 or 4 months; corticotrophin and intramuscular methylprednisolone were also used.— E. N. Glick and B. Helal, *The Hand*, 1976, *8*, 45.

Sydenham's chorea. A retrospective study of 8 young female patients given prednisone 30 to 75 mg daily and/or corticotrophin 30 or 40 units daily usually for periods of not longer than 3 weeks. All 8 patients obtained a favourable and rapid response to corticosteroid therapy suggesting that a controlled study should be carried out.— L. N. Green, *Archs Neurol., Chicago*, 1978, *35*, 53.

Ocular disorders. Ocular disorders and their treatment, including details of those conditions in which topical or systemic corticosteroid therapy is appropriate.— R. A. Thoft, *New Engl. J. Med.*, 1978, *298*, 1239. See also S. I. Davidson, *Prescribers' J.*, 1978, *18*, 139.

Individual reports and studies on the use of corticosteroids in ocular disorders: S. C. Werner, *Lancet*, 1966, *1*, 1004 (high-dose prednisone for exophthalmos); P. G. Watson *et al.*, *Br. J. Ophthal.*, 1968, *52*, 348 (systemic prednisolone for sclero-keratitis); J. R. Cook *et al.*, *Archs Ophthal., N.Y.*, 1972, *88*, 513 (ocular sarcoidosis); S. S. Hayreh, *Br. J. Ophthal.*, 1974, *58*, 981 (anterior ischaemic optic neuropathy); E. M. Eagling *et al.*, *Br. J. Ophthal.*, 1974, *58*, 990 (ischaemic papillopathy); P. G. Watson and S. S. Hayreh, *Br. J. Ophthal.*, 1976, *60*, 163 (scleritis and episcleritis); M. I. V. Jayson and D. L. Easty, *Ann. rheum. Dis.*, 1977, *36*, 428 (ocular rheumatoid arthritis); R. D. Rollinson, *Med. J. Aust.*, 1977, *2*, 50 (optic neuritis); T. A. Makley and A. Azar, *Archs Ophthal., N.Y.*, 1978, *96*, 257 (sympathetic ophthalmica); S. L. Forstot and P. S. Binder, *Am. J. Ophthal.*, 1979, *88*, 186 (therapeutic soft contact lenses for Thygeson's superficial punctate keratopathy).

For the use of subconjunctival or retrobulbar corticosteroid injections to alleviate exophthalmos in patients with thyrotoxicosis, see Methylprednisolone Acetate, p.478.

Organ and tissue transplantation. A general review of transplantation including advances in the control of transplant rejection.— P. S. Russell and A. B. Cosimi, *New Engl. J. Med.* 1979, *301*, 470.

Heart. An account of the management of heart transplants. Immunosuppression starts before operation with loading doses of azathioprine, intravenous methylprednisolone, and antithymocyte immunoglobulin. After operation oral prednisolone is started at 1 mg per kg body-weight [daily], reducing to 500 µg per kg by one month, and 300 µg per kg by 3 months. Azathioprine up to 2.5 mg per kg [daily] is given with the purpose of keeping the white cell count in the region of 5×10^9 per litre. Equine antithymocyte immunoglobulin is given by daily intravenous injection for the first 3 or 4 weeks and is regarded as an important part of the primary immunosuppressive regimen. The dose, which is usually in the range of 10 to 15 mg per kg [daily], is adjusted to suppress the T-cell fraction of the circulating lymphocytes to about 5% of their pre-operative value. If rejection occurs during the period of primary treatment with antithymocyte immunoglobulin, which is uncommon, it is treated with 3 or 4 daily doses of methylprednisolone 1 g. If it occurs later and is mild a short course of antithymocyte immunoglobulin is reinstituted; high-dose pulses of methylprednisolone are added if it is moderate or severe. Mild rejection episodes occurring after the patient has left hospital may be treated by doubling the oral daily dose of prednisolone and then tapering back to maintenance levels over the next 2 weeks. If it is more than mild or if ECG voltages do not recover promptly the patient is admitted for treatment with antithymocyte immunoglobulin and methylprednisolone.— T. A. H. English *et al.*, *Br. med. J.*, 1980, *281*, 699.

Kidney. The standard maintenance regimen for immunosuppression in patients with kidney transplants is azathioprine 3 mg per kg body-weight daily and prednisone 1.5 mg per kg daily. For episodes of acute rejection during the first 3 months after transplanatation up to 3 courses of high-dose corticosteroid can be given intravenously for up to 6 days. The maintenance dose of prednisone is gradually reduced with a maximum dose of 20 to 30 mg daily at 3 months and 10 to 20 mg daily at one year after transplantation. Treatment is usually discontinued if the transplant is not functioning satisfactorily within 3 or 4 months.— N. L. Tilney *et al.*, *New Engl. J. Med.*, 1978, *299*, 1321. Comment on immunosuppression in renal transplantation.— R. D. Guttmann, *ibid.*, 1979, *301*, 1038.

Ten patients with stable renal function at least 2 years after renal transplantation had their sole immunosuppressive therapy of prednisolone 10 mg daily gradually reduced by 1 mg every month. Although 3 patients apparently required only minimal immunosuppression with a daily dose of 5 mg or less, episodes of rejection occurred in 5 patients receiving daily doses below 7 mg. In 2 patients withdrawal of prednisolone was stopped because of the development of symptoms of hypoadrenalism and the deterioration in renal function due to pyelonephritis respectively. It was suggested that although reduction of the prednisolone dose to 7 mg daily in renal transplant recipients more than 2 years after transplantation may be relatively safe, any further reduction should be avoided unless there are extenuating circumstances or the patient is receiving adequate immunosuppressive treatment with azathioprine.— R. B. Naik *et al.*, *Br. med. J.*, 1980, *280*, 1337. See also R. B. Naik *et al.*, *Transplantn Proc.*, 1979, *11*, 39. Comment.— A. J. Robertson *et al.* (letter), *Br. med. J.*, 1980, *280*, 305.

Further studies on the role of corticosteroids as part of the maintenance immunosuppression regimen in patients with kidney transplants: J. L. Anderton *et al.*, *Proc. Eur. Dialysis Transplant Ass.*, 1977, *14*, 342 (minimum corticosteroid requirements); R. L. Burleson, *J. Am. med. Ass.*, 1977, *238*, 201 (alternate-day therapy); H. Kreis *et al.*, *Lancet*, 1978, *2*, 1169; C. Ponticelli *et al.* (letter), *ibid.*, 1979, *1*, 265; A. J. Nicholls *et al.* (letter), *ibid.*, 266; G. Horpacsy (letter), *ibid.*, 321 (controversy surrounding the need for corticosteroids).

There was no significant difference between methylprednisolone given intravenously in 3 doses of 1 g every 12 hours to control 49 episodes of renal allograft rejection and prednisolone given by mouth to control 50 rejection episodes in 3 daily doses of 300, 200, and 100 mg, then reduced by 10 mg daily to a maintenance dose of 10 mg daily. The intravenous schedule reversed 31 rejections and the oral schedule 28 and the only significant difference between the 2 was an increased frequency of fluid retention associated with prednisolone. There was no sign that this schedule of methylprednisolone was nephrotoxic as suggested by J.A. Tremann *et al.* (*Surgery, St. Louis*, 1976, *79*, 370) from *animal* studies.— D. Gray *et al.*, *Lancet*, 1978, *1*, 117. A comparable study but also using antilymphocyte immunoglobulin.— J. L. Touraine and J. Traeger (letter), *ibid.*, 607.

A controlled study in patients with cadaver renal transplants showed that low-dose oral prednisolone with azathioprine provided as effective immunosuppression as azathioprine with high doses of prednisolone and morbidity was less in the low-dose group. There seems little justification for the continued use of high doses of prednisolone in this form of treatment.— P. J. Morris *et al.*, *Lancet*, 1982, *1*, 525.

See also Azathioprine, p.191.

A review of cadaver kidney donor pretreatment using massive doses of corticosteroids and cyclophosphamide.— *Br. med. J.*, 1977, *2*, 1172.

Conflicting views on the benefits of cyclophosphamide and corticosteroid in cadaver kidney pretreatment: R. D. Guttmann *et al.*, *Transplantn Proc.*, 1973, *5*, 663; *idem*, 1975, *7*, 117; H. Zincke and J. E. Woods, *Surgery Gynec. Obstet.*, 1977, *145*, 183; S. N. Chatterjee *et al.*, *ibid.*, 729.

Pancreatitis. A review of the treatment of acute and chronic pancreatitis. The role of corticosteroid therapy in fulminating pancreatitis is not established, but it would appear to be of value in respiratory distress and shock once hypovolaemia has been firmly excluded.— S. Bank *et al.*, *Drugs*, 1977, *13*, 373.

Further references: M. H. Kaplan *et al.*, *Am. J. Surg.*, 1964, *108*, 24 (a 6-year survey with evaluation of corticosteroid therapy).

Polyarteritis nodosa. See under Arteritis.

Polymyalgia rheumatica. See under Arteritis.

Pregnancy and the neonate. For a review of the effects of corticosteroids during pregnancy, see Pregnancy and the Neonate under Precautions.

The mother. Evidence that prednisone, 2.5 mg, given thrice daily for 1 month, markedly reduced the high level of plasma androgens in 5 women with polycystic ovary syndrome.— R. Horton and J. Neisler, *J. clin. Endocr. Metab.*, 1968, *28*, 479.

Evaluation of paramethasone acetate in hypothalamic amenorrhoea.— V. Cortés-Gallegos *et al.*, *Fert. Steril.*, 1978, *29*, 402.

A review of the treatment of herpes gestationis in 41 pregnant women indicated that most patients showed no significant improvement with topical corticosteroid therapy; patients treated systemically usually had a prompt improvement but many required therapy throughout pregnancy.— T. J. Lawley *et al.*, *Archs Derm.*, 1978, *114*, 552.

The infant. Six infants with extensive haemangiomas were treated for about 2 weeks with 20 to 30 mg of prednisone daily by mouth, tapered off over 2 to 4 weeks. In 5 there were remissions, but 3 of them relapsed and were controlled by a second course.— N. C. Fost and N. B. Esterly, *J. Pediat.*, 1968, *72*, 351. See also S. J. Goldberg and E. Fonkalsrud, *J. Am. med. Ass.*, 1969, *208*, 2473.

Results of a placebo-controlled double-blind study of 35 infants with the meconium aspiration syndrome indicated that hydrocortisone is not effective therapy. Indeed, corticosteroid therapy may prolong the duration of oxygen requirement and respiratory distress.— T. F. Yeh *et al.*, *J. Pediat.*, 1977, *90*, 140.

For the prevention of the respiratory distress syndrome, see Betamethasone, p.461.

For a reference to the treatment of neonatal autoimmune thrombocytopenia, see p.453.

Pyrexia. Periodic episodes of fever which had occurred every 21 days for about 8 years in a 66-year-old man and consisted of chills, malaise, anorexia, constipation, muscle stiffness, and fever to 40°, were suppressed by 10 mg of prednisone daily.— D. Thompson (letter), *J. Am. med. Ass.*, 1974, *230*, 208. For the use of corticosteroid therapy in malignant hyperpyrexia, see under Hyperpyrexia, above.

Raised intracranial pressure. For the use of corticosteroid therapy in raised intracranial pressure, see Dexamethasone, p.467.

Renal disorders. A review of the drug therapy of glomerulonephritis, including a discussion on studies attempting to elucidate the role of corticosteroids, with or without other immunosuppressant therapy. Controlled studies carried out to date in *membranous nephropathy* and in *mixed proliferative glomerulonephritis*, employing anti-inflammatory corticosteroids and immunosuppressant drugs have shown no effect other than some short-term benefit from cyclophosphamide (which was not subsequently confirmed) and diminution of proteinuria of membranous patients treated with chlorambucil. Indeed, the mortality of the treated group in the Medical Research Council's trials [D.A.K. Black *et al.*, *Br. med. J.*, 1970, *3*, 421] of corticosteroids alone and with azathioprine was higher than in the control group, which suggests that in some patients the glomerulonephritis was made worse. Few of these trials were ideal and some doubt remains in several directions, so that a further trial of corticosteroids with or without immunosuppressant drugs seems justified.

There also seems to be a case for further trial of indomethacin in *proliferative glomerulonephritis* in doses higher than those of the 100-mg daily dose given by the Medical Research Council to patients with predominantly normal renal function. Reports of successful restoration of declining renal function towards normal have been with higher doses of indomethacin, sometimes accompanied by small doses of cyclophosphamide.

Antithrombin and antiplatelet drugs have usually been given against a background of immunosuppression and this toxic association of drugs should not be given to those whose disease does not satisfy strict criteria for serious disease. Results in patients with *proliferative glomerulonephritis and extensive crescent formation* have been encouraging but it must be remembered that these are obtained in the absence of controlled trials, which will be difficult in these rare, extremely ill patients. In the absence of controlled studies it must be remembered that the prognosis for the patient now includes regular dialysis and transplatation with a reasonable prospect for survival.

Although a considerable improvement has occurred in the prognosis of *lupus nephritis*, several controlled clinical trials, all of them open to criticism, have failed to show any clear advantage of corticosteroid therapy alone, although there are indications that the addition of immunosuppressants, even for a relatively short period, reduces the number of patients subsequently going into renal failure. Our current policy is to use corticosteroids and azathioprine routinely in all patients with severe forms of *lupus nephritis*; some judged to have milder renal disease on histological examination, are managed with corticosteroid therapy alone. The corticosteroid doses are maintained at 10 to 25 mg of prednisone daily, usually at the lower end of this range, in association with azathioprine rather than cyclophosphamide. We have also used anticoagulants and antiplatelet agents and, rarely, pulses of methylprednisolone, in acutely ill patients with *severe crescentic glomerulonephritis*. Plasmaphaeresis has also been tried in acute severe *renal lupus*.

The form of glomerulonephritis described as *minimal-change disease*, which is of unknown aetiology, responds reliably to both corticosteroid and immunosuppressive drugs. Corticosteroids, purine antagonists, and mustard-like drugs considerably accelerate remission of minimal-change disease but, whereas those treated with corticosteroids or purine-antagonists may relapse persistently, cyclophosphamide, at doses of 2.5 to 3 mg per kg body-weight daily for 6 to 8 weeks or longer, induces permanent remission in about a third of these relapsing patients. Administration of corticosteroids at a dose of about 60 mg of prednisone daily will induce remission in over 90% of the patients, and since only half will subsequently relapse, cyclophosphamide or other drugs are not justified as primary treatment except possibly in the elderly where a nephrotic syndrome is more serious and subsequent gonadal function of less importance. Corticosteroids may also be used for subsequent relapses, cyclophosphamide only being introduced when they become unsafe or unsatisfactory. Chlorambucil is reserved for those who relapse after cyclophosphamide therapy, but such patients may respond to lower doses of corticosteroids as if the cyclophosphamide had 'softened' the disease. The impact of diuretics and antibiotics must not be forgotten in this condition which used to carry a mortality of about 50% over 5 years and now has a mortality of less than 5% over 10 years.— J. S. Cameron, *Br. med. J.*, 1977, *1*, 1457 and 1520. In a study of patients with idiopathic nephrotic syndrome, 72 adults with membranous nephropathy and good glomerular function were given either prednisone as a single dose of 100 to 150 mg on alternate days or placebo for at least 8 weeks. This short-term treatment with prednisone appeared to be beneficial and was well-tolerated. During an average follow-up period of 23 months (range 4 to 52 months) only one of 34 patients given prednisone progressed to renal failure compared with 9 of the 38 controls.— *New Engl. J. Med.*, 1979, *301*, 1301 (Report of a Collaborative Study of the Adult Idiopathic Nephrotic Syndrome). Comment.— A. S. Relman, *ibid.*, 1340. Complete remission occurred in 7 patients with nephrotic syndrome accompanied by slight but definite proliferative changes in the glomeruli following treatment with prednisone. A controlled study of the use of corticosteroids in such patients was necessary to verify these results.— H. Rashid *et al.*, *Br. med. J.*, 1980, *281*, 347.

Further reviews and comments: *Lancet*, 1976, *2*, 1121; T. Ehrenreich *et al.* (letter), *ibid.*, 1977, *1*, 100 (immunosuppression in the nephrotic syndrome); *Br. med. J.*, 1977, *2*, 1103 (nephrotic syndrome in children).

Renal transplants. For reference to the use of corticosteroids in the management of renal transplant patients, see Organ and Tissue Transplantation (above).

Further individual reports and comments on the drug treatment of renal disorders: E. S. Cathcart *et al.*, *Lancet*, 1976, *1*, 163; T. Nebout *et al.* (letter), *ibid.*, 1977, *1*, 909; C. Ponticelli *et al.* (letter), *ibid.*, 1063; S. Dosa *et al.*, *Postgrad. med. J.*, 1978, *54*, 628 (high-dose methylprednisolone intravenous pulse therapy for lupus nephritis); T. Ehrenreich *et al.*, *New Engl. J. Med.*, 1976, *295*, 741; C. H. Coggins, *ibid.*, 783; S. Cameron (letter), *ibid.*, 1977, *296*, 49; C. Kleinknecht *et al.* (letter), *ibid.*; L. W. Gold and F. M. Gise (letter), *ibid.*; P. Nussbaum *et al.* (letter), *ibid.*, 50; T. Ehrenreich *et al.* (letter), *ibid.* (controversy surrounding the role of corticosteroids, with or without immunosuppressants, in idiopathic membranous nephropathy); W. E. Grupe *et al.*, *New Engl. J. Med.*, 1976, *295*, 746; C. H. Coggins, *ibid.*, 783; C. Kleinknecht *et al.* (letter), *ibid.*, 1977, *296*, 48; W. E. Grupe *et al.* (letter), *ibid.*; S. Cameron (letter), *ibid.*, 1065 (benefit and risk of chlorambucil in frequently relapsing nephrosis); W. K. Bolton *et al.*, *Am. J. Med.*, 1977, *62*, 60 (alternate-day corticosteroid therapy in idiopathic nephrotic syndrome); R. Counahan *et al.*, *Br. med. J.*, 1977, *2*, 11 (failure of corticosteroid and/or immunosuppressants in Henoch-Schönlein nephritis); B. A. Idelson *et al.*, *Archs intern. Med.*, 1977, *137*, 891 (favourable long-term prognosis in idiopathic nephrotic syndrome associated with early response to corticosteroids); S. Leisti *et al.*, *Lancet*, 1977, *2*, 795; *idem*, *Pediatrics*, 1977, *60*, 334 (role of adrenal suppression in idiopathic nephrotic syndrome relapse); R. J. Levinsky *et al.*, *Lancet*, 1977, *1*, 564 (methylprednisolone pulse therapy in lupus nephritis); C. M. Lockwood *et al.*, *Lancet*, 1977, *1*, 63 (plasma exchange and immunosuppression in fulminating immune-complex crescentic nephritis); J. V. Donadio *et al.*, *New Engl. J. Med.*, 1978, *299*, 1151 (role of cyclophosphamide in addition to corticosteroids for lupus nephritis); C. H. Coggins *et al.*, *New Engl. J. Med.*, 1979, *301*, 1301; L. F. Wright (letter), *ibid.*, 1980, *302*, 921; C. H. Coggins (letter), *ibid.*, 922 (role of corticosteroid in prevention of renal failure secondary to membranous nephropathy); *J. Pediat.*, 1979, *95*, 239 (International Study of Kidney Disease in Children; higher corticosteroid doses in childhood nephrotic syndrome); *Lancet*, 1979, *1*, 401 (report of 'Arbeitsgemeinschaft für Pädiatrische Nephrologie'; comparison of intermittent and alternate-day corticosteroid therapy in children with frequently relapsing minimal-change nephrotic syndrome); M. S. Sabbour and L. M. Osman, *Br. J. Derm.*, 1979, *100*, 113 (advantage of chlorambucil with corticosteroids in lupus nephritis); O. Oredugba *et al.*, *Ann. intern. Med.*, 1980, *92*, 504 (intravenous methylprednisolone in rapidly progressive glomerulonephritis); C. Ponticelli *et al.*, *Br. med. J.*, 1980, *280*, 685 (complete remission in minimal-change nephrotic syndrome using initial high-dose intravenous methylprednisolone); S. A. Williams *et al.*, *New Engl. J. Med.*, 1980, *302*, 929; E. J. Lewis, *ibid.*, 963 (benefit and risk of chlorambucil in addition to corticosteroids in frequently relapsing childhood nephrotic syndrome).

Respiratory disorders. Reports, reviews, and studies on aspects of corticosteroid therapy in various respiratory disorders: *Br. med. J.*, 1972, *4*, 567 (pulmonary aspergillosis); C. C. Smith, *Br. J. clin. Pract.*, 1972, *26*, 151 (pulmonary alveolitis); D. R. Webb and G. D. Currie, *J. Am. med. Ass.*, 1972, *222*, 1146 (pulmonary fibrosis); C. J. Johns *et al.*, *Johns Hopkins med. J.*, 1974, *134*, 271 (pulmonary sarcoidosis); A. Aytac *et al.*, *J. thorac. cardiovasc. Surg.*, 1977, *74*, 145 (foreign body inhalation); C. J. Hewitt *et al.*, *Archs Dis. Childh.*, 1977, *52*, 22 (fibrosing alveolitis); S. K. Teo *et al.*, *Med. J. Aust.*, 1977, *2*, 669 (relapsing polychondritis); P. Y. Holoye *et al.*, *Ann. intern. Med.*, 1978, *88*, 47 (bleomycin pneumonitis); D. J. Pearson and E. C. Rosenow, *Mayo Clin. Proc.*, 1978, *53*, 73; D. E. Dines, *ibid.*, 129 (eosinophilic pneumonia); R. H. Winterbauer *et al.*, *Am. J. Med.*, 1978, *65*, 661 (with azathioprine, for interstitial pneumonitis); B. L. Fanburg, *Am. J. Hosp. Pharm.*, 1979, *36*, 351 (pulmonary sarcoidosis); D. E. Hammerschmidt *et al.*, *Lancet*, 1980, *1*, 947 (adult respiratory distress syndrome).

See also under Aspiration Syndrome, Asthma, Bronchitis and Emphysema, and (for the paediatric respiratory distress syndrome), Betamethasone, p.461.

Rheumatic disorders. Reviews and comments on the use and abuse of corticosteroids in rheumatic disorders.— H. C. Burry, *Drugs*, 1980, *19*, 447; V. Wright and R. Amos, *Br. med. J.*, 1980, *280*, 964; H. F. West (letter), *ibid.*, *281*, 310.

The vogue of systemic corticosteroids in *rheumatoid arthritis* is long over. Even in low dosage their long-term side-effects outweigh their temporary benefit, which long-term trials show to be lost after the first year, following which corticosteroid-treated patients do worse. I do use them for two groups: wage-earners about to lose their job and housewives unable to cope, until gold or pencillamine has taken effect; and in patients in whom all else has failed and whose quality of life is poor. Ideally I try to use them on an alternate-day basis or as a morning daily dose of not more than 5 mg.— J. M. Gumpel, *Br. med. J.*, 1978, *2*, 1068. Systemic corticosteroids should only be used for the complications of *ankylosing spondylitis* such as severe iritis, when doses of up to 10 mg of prednisolone daily suppress the inflammation.— S. M. Doherty and D. A. H. Yates, *Practitioner*, 1980, *224*, 35.

J. G. Schaller, *Arthritis Rheum.*, 1977, *20*, *Suppl.* 2, 537 (juvenile rheumatoid arthritis); P. W. Vanace, *Arthritis Rheum.*, 1977, *20*, *Suppl.* 2, 550 (juvenile rheumatoid arthritis); D. A. H. Yates, *Br. med. J.*, 1977, *1*, 495 (local injections); *Br. med. J.*, 1978, *1*, 600 (local injections); H. A. Bird *et al.*, *Ann. rheum. Dis.*, 1979, *38*, 36 (intra-articular injections); K. De Ceulaer *et al.*, *Ann. rheum. Dis.*, 1979, *38*, 440 (synovial vascular bed).

Frozen shoulder. Comment on the management of frozen shoulder. In patients who present within 3 months of onset, injections of long-acting corticosteroids are often effective in relieving pain and shortening duration of stiffness, but corticosteroid injections and mobilising exercises are usually both painful and ineffective for those who present late. In the small proportion of patients whose symptoms persist beyond 18 months, manipulation under anaesthesia (immediately preceded by corticosteroid injection and followed by active mobilisation for one week) is effective in restoring the range of motion by rupturing the thickened and adherent capsule of the joint.— *Br. med. J.*, 1980, *280*, 1604. See also H. I. Weiser (letter), *Lancet*, 1976, *1*, 589; S. Roy and R. Oldham (letter), *ibid.*, 1322.

Further references to the use of local corticosteroid injections for frozen shoulder: A. W. Fowler (letter), *Lancet*, 1976, *1*, 298 (methylprednisolone acetate).

Palindromic rheumatism. Comment on the management of palindromic rheumatism. Corticosteroids are usually to be avoided but periodic short courses, such as 2 intramuscular injections of methylprednisolone 80 mg in depot form, may be strikingly effective.— *Br. med. J.*, 1979, *2*, 1531.

Tennis elbow. In a study involving 95 patients with tennis elbow local injections of methylprednisolone acetate provided relief in 33 of 36 sites whereas those of lignocaine hydrochloride 1% or sodium chloride 0.9% provided relief in only 7 of 35 and 7 of 29 respectively. It was considered that the beneficial effects of an injection of corticosteroids in tennis elbow were due to their pharmacological effects and not to mechanical distention of the tissues.— B. H. Day *et al.*, *Practitioner*, 1978, *220*, 459.

Further references to the use of local corticosteroid injections for tennis elbow: A. K. Clarke and J. Woodland, *Rheumatol. Rehabil.*, 1975, *14*, 47.

See also under Arteritis, Lupus Erythematosus, and Skin Disorders.

Rheumatic fever. It is hard to find statistical proof that corticosteroids make a difference to the long-term prognosis of acute rheumatic fever but prednisone should be given to those with hyperpyrexia and severe carditis. The usual dose is about 1 mg per kg body-weight daily in 4 divided doses for 7 to 10 days, thereafter reduced by 2.5 mg daily every 5 to 7 days.— E. Davis, *Practitioner*, 1974, *213*, 159.

Studies of corticosteroid therapy in rheumatic fever: S. Friedman *et al.*, *J. Pediat.*, 1962, *60*, 55; Combined Rheumatic Fever Study Group, *New Engl. J. Med.*, 1960, *262*, 895; *idem*, 1965, *272*, 63; *Br. med. J.*, 1965, *2*, 607 (Ten-Year Report by the Rheumatic Fever Working Party of the MRC and the American Council on Rheumatic Fever and Congenital Heart Disease).

Rhinitis. Comment on the ethics of using depot corticosteroids in hay fever. It is generally agreed that they should not be used in patients with mild symptoms, nor in those who respond to antihistamines or sodium cromoglycate. Very severe hay fever is probably better treated with local corticosteroids or, if symptoms are intolerable, by a non-adrenal-suppressive drug such as corticotrophin or tetracosactrin in a zinc complex.— M. K. McAllen, *Practitioner*, 1976, *217*, 492. See also *Drug & Ther. Bull.*, 1979, *17*, 45.

See also under Methylprednisolone Acetate, p.478, and Triamcinolone Acetonide, p.484.

For the intranasal use of corticosteroids in allergic rhinitis, see particularly under Beclomethasone Dipropionate, p.460, and Betamethasone Valerate, p.463.

Sarcoidosis. It should be stressed that in asymptomatic stage I sarcoid, therapy is not required. Corticosteroid treatment is reserved for patients with extensive pulmonary involvement and the attendant dangers of pulmonary fibrosis, or for those with diseases involved with other organ systems sufficient to produce serious or life-threatening illness, such as ocular or myocardial sarcoid or hypercalcaemia. In addition, corticosteroids are useful for control of the fever, weakness, lethargy, and neuropathy sometimes associated with this disorder.— J. E. Kasik, *J. Am. med. Ass.*, 1980, *243*, 1468.

For specific references to corticosteroid therapy in sarcoidosis, see Cardiac Disorders, Ocular Disorders, Respiratory Disorders, and Skin Disorders.

Shock. A discussion on whether corticosteroids should be given in shock. There is insufficient evidence to support the use of corticosteroids in traumatic, haemorrhagic, neurogenic, or cardiogenic shock. Endotoxaemia might respond to very large doses but an adequate prospective study is needed; methylprednisolone and dexamethasone have no therapeutic advantage over hydrocortisone, and the sodium phosphate esters of hydrocortisone have no clinical advantage over the succinate although they are hydrolysed more quickly to the free corticosteroid.— *Drug & Ther. Bull.*, 1976, *14*, 14. See also W. L. Thompson, *Recent Adv. clin. Pharmac.*, 1978, *1*, 123–145.

Conflicting reports on the merits of massive corticosteroid therapy in the treatment of septic shock: R. H. Dietzman *et al.*, *Angiology*, 1969, *20*, 691 (beneficial); H. Seneca and J. P. Grant, *J. Am. Geriat. Soc.*, 1975, *23*, 493 (beneficial); I. M. Ledingham and C. S. McArdle, *Lancet*, 1978, *1*, 1194 (no effect on death-rate).

For the use of corticosteroid therapy in the management of anaphylactic shock, see Adrenaline, p.4.

Shoulder-hand syndrome. Discussion of the conflict on the value of corticosteroids in the reflex sympathetic dystrophy syndrome including the shoulder-hand syndrome.— *Lancet*, 1976, *1*, 1226.

Skin disorders. A detailed review of the clinical pharmacology and therapeutic use of corticosteroids. Guidelines for the correct use of topical corticosteroids are: be prepared to apply an appropriately potent compound to bring the condition under control; continue treatment with a less potent preparation after control is obtained; reduce the frequency of application; if required, continue daily application with the weakest preparation that will control the condition; once healed, tail off treatment; be especially careful in children and in certain anatomical sites, such as the face and flexures. The following is a rough guide to the clinical potencies of topical corticosteroids: *very potent* (*group 1*): beclomethasone dipropionate 0.5%, clobetasol propionate 0.05%, diflucortolone valerate 0.3%, fluocinolone acetonide 0.2%; *potent* (*group 2*): beclomethasone dipropionate 0.025%, betamethasone benzoate 0.025%, betamethasone dipropionate 0.05%, betamethasone valerate 0.1%, desonide 0.05%, desoxymethasone 0.25%, diflorasone diacetate 0.05%, diflucortolone valerate 0.1%, fluclorolone acetonide 0.025%, fluocinolone acetonide 0.025%, fluocinonide 0.05%, fluocortolone 0.5%, fluprednidene acetate 0.1%, flurandrenolone 0.05%, halcinonide 0.1%, hydrocortisone butyrate 0.1%, triamcinolone acetonide 0.1%; *moderately potent* (*group 3*): clobetasone butyrate 0.05%, flumethasone pivalate 0.02%, fluocinolone acetonide 0.01%, fluocortin butylester 0.75%, fluocortolone 0.2%, flurandrenolone 0.0125 to 0.025%, hydrocortisone 1% with urea; *mild* (*group 4*): dexamethasone 0.01%, hydrocortisone or hydrocortisone acetate 0.1 to 1%, methylprednisolone 0.25%. While the borderline between groups 1 and 2 is quite well defined, distinction between those preparations in groups 2 and 3 is not always easy. Some are available in different concentrations, which may be presumed (often erroneously, and seldom on the basis of reliable evidence) to qualify them for inclusion in a different category of clinical potency. There is a several-fold difference in topical absorption of corticosteroids between those absorbed the most and those absorbed the least, and in addition to a large variation in absorption between individuals, there is also a large variation between various anatomical sites which explains the difference in response of different areas to the same corticosteroid formulations. Compared with 1% on the forearm, the scalp absorbs approximately 4%, the forehead 7%, and the scrotum 36%. The groin, axillae and face are also areas of higher penetrability and it is these sites which tend to develop local side-effects more easily.— J. A. Miller and D. D. Munro, *Drugs*, 1980, *19*, 119.

General reviews of topical corticosteroid therapy often with special emphasis on guidelines for safe usage: I. B. Sneddon, *Drugs*, 1976, *11*, 193 (relative potency and hazards of dilution); *Br. med. J.*, 1977, *1*, 1303 (concomitant topical antibiotics); J. J. Leyden and A. M. Kligman, *Br. J. Derm.*, 1977, *96*, 179 (concomitant topical antibiotics); M. J. Busse, *Pharm. J.*, 1978, *1*, 25 (disadvantages of dilution); F. J. Storrs, *J. Am. Acad. Derm.*, 1979, *1*, 95 (regimens for safe systemic usage); L. Hodge, *Drugs*, 1980, *19*, 380 (concomitant topical antibiotics).

Reviews and studies on the relative potency of different corticosteroid topical preparations: B. W. Barry and R. Woodford, *Br. J. Derm.*, 1974, *91*, 323; *idem*, 1975, *93*, 563 (ranking on basis of vasoconstrictor test); J. K. Haleblian, *J. pharm. Sci.*, 1976, *65*, 1417 (review of bioassays for topical corticosteroids); B. S. N. Reddy and G. Singh, *Br. J. Derm.*, 1976, *94*, 191 (ranking on basis of histamine suppressor activity); E. S. Snell, *Br. J. Derm.*, 1976, *94*, *Suppl.* 12, 15 (pharmacological properties and clinical efficacy); L. Wilson, *Br. J. Derm.*, 1976, *94*, *Suppl.* 12, 33 (study of clinical assessment); B. W. Barry and R. Woodford, *J. clin. Pharm.*, 1978, *3*, 43 (modification of the vasoconstrictor assay); C. Delforno *et al.*, *Br. J. Derm.*, 1978, *98*, 619 (correlation with reduction in size of viable cells in the epidermis); G. C. Priestly, *Br. J. Derm.*, 1978, *99*, 253 (effect on collagen synthesis and proliferation *in vitro* of human skin fibroblasts); K. Harnack and H. Meffert, *Derm. Mschr.*, 1979, *165*, 851 (comparison by ultraviolet erythema).

Acne. Resolution of acne cysts could be helped by aspiration followed by the infiltration of triamcinolone acetonide or betamethasone phosphate with betamethasone acetate. This was virtually the only indication for corticosteroids in acne and it had been stated with authority that the only possible indication for the use of topical corticosteroids was to reduce inflammation before an important social event.— R. Carruthers, *Drugs*, 1974, *8*, 217. See also J. Verbov (letter), *Lancet*, 1977, *2*, 925.

Further references to corticosteroids in acne: J. M. Lane *et al.*, *J. Bone Jt Surg.*, 1976, *58A*, 673 (acne arthralgia); M. Gloor *et al.*, *Eur. J. clin. Pharmac.*, 1978, *14*, 53 (potential comedo induction); J. E. Rasmussen, *Pediat. Clins N.Am.*, 1978, *25*, 285 (review); J. L. Burton and E. Saihan, *Br. J. Derm.*, 1979, *101*, *Suppl.* 17, 15 (systemic oestrogen and corticosteroid therapy in women); W. J. Cunliffe, *Br. med. J.*, 1980, *280*, 1394 (review).

Alopecia. Corticosteroids, either injected locally or given systemically usually make the hair regrow. Unfortunately the regrowth is often only temporary and the hazards of long-term treatment with corticosteroids are not justified. Repeated local injections of triamcinolone often induce atrophy of the scalp.— *Br. med. J.*, 1979, *1*, 505.

Further references: F. Pascher *et al.*, *Dermatologica*, 1970, *141*, 193 (topical fluocinolone acetonide); D. Porter and J. L. Burton, *Br. J. Derm.*, 1971, *85*, 272 (local injection of triamcinolone hexacetonide); E. Abell and D. D. Munro, *Br. J. Derm.*, 1973, *88*, 55 (intradermal triamcinolone hexacetonide); W. P. Unger, *Can. med. Ass. J.*, 1973, *108*, 177 (systemic prednisone and topical triamcinolone hexacetonide); J. L. Burton and S. Schuster, *Acta derm.-vener., Stockh.*, 1975, *55*, 493 (single-dose intravenous prednisolone); J. Tofahrn *et al.*, *Z. Haut-u. GeschlKrankh.*, 1976, *51*, 989 (methylprednisolone and dapsone); R. J. Winter *et al.*, *Archs Derm.*, 1976, *112*, 1549 (alternate-day prednisone).

Amyloidosis. Six of 21 patients with lichen amyloidosis improved within 8 weeks after topical application of betamethasone under occlusive dressings, but 2 relapsed when treatment ceased. Three of 5 further patients improved after treatment by intralesional injection of triamcinolone in doses of up to 2 mg twice weekly for 4 weeks. Amyloid substances were still present in the skin during remission.— C. H. Tay and J. L. Dacosta, *Br. J. Derm.*, 1970, *82*, 129. See also under Amyloidosis (above).

Aphthous ulcers. In an investigation in 39 patients, there was no evidence of alteration in incidence or duration of aphthous ulceration following the use for 4 weeks of triamcinolone acetonide (Adcortyl in Orabase) locally, Orabase locally, hydroxyquinoline systemically, carbenoxolone sodium (Biobase) locally, or betamethasone sodium phosphate locally or systemically.— I. T. MacPhee *et al.*, *Br. med. J.*, 1968, *2*, 147.

A double-blind study in 10 patients indicated that topical treatment with betamethasone valerate delivered from an aerosol was more effective than a placebo in the treatment of minor aphthous ulcers, but produced similar results in 2 patients with herpetiform ulcers and 1 patient with Behçet's syndrome.— C. M. Yeoman *et al.*, *Br. dent. J.*, 1978, *144*, 114. See also N. Fisher (letter), *Br. med. J.*, 1979, *1*, 1357.

Further references: R. M. Browne *et al.*, *Lancet*, 1968, *1*, 565 (topical triamcinolone acetonide); W. R. Tyldesley, *Br. dent. J.*, 1973, *135*, 537 (systemic prednisolone).

Atopic dermatitis. An account of the management of atopic dermatitis, including details of the role of corticosteroid therapy. Emphasis is placed on the need to limit the use of high-potency corticosteroid preparations, including the reminder that potent corticosteroids should never be used on the face. The following techniques are recommended for reducing the total amount of high-potency corticosteroid used: maintenance on a low-potency corticosteroid and switch to a high-potency corticosteroid for short periods of time; apply potent corticosteroids only to recalcitrant areas (enhanced by the use of occlusion at night); once daily or alternate day application of a corticosteroid for severe cases, reverting to a low-potency preparation for other applications. Systemic corticosteroids are used infrequently, but in a recalcitrant case, a short course of a systemic corticosteroid will provide time to develop a routine of local management; prednisone in a single morning dose for 7 to 10 days is the drug of choice.— E. M. Moss, *Pediat. Clins N. Am.*, 1978, *25*, 225.

Dermatomyositis. The successful use of moderate doses of prednisone in 8 children with dermatomyositis. Initial treatment was with about 0.7 to 1.5 mg per kg body-weight daily for as short a time as possible, the dose being tapered away after onset of improvement.— V. Dubowitz, *Archs Dis. Childh.*, 1976, *51*, 494. See also K. M. Goel and R. A. Shanks, *ibid.*, 501.

Dermatitis herpetiformis. This is a non-fatal disease but one that causes a great deal of discomfort. Systemic corticosteroid therapy is not particularly effective and is seldom used.— J. A. Savin, *Practitioner*, 1977, *219*, 847.

Eczema and infantile eczema. See under Atopic Dermatitis.

Erythema multiforme. Dramatic symptomatic relief could sometimes be provided in erythema multiforme (the Stevens-Johnson syndrome) by systemic corticosteroids, with an initial dose of 60 mg of prednisone in severe cases.— *Br. med. J.*, 1972, *1*, 63.

From a study of 32 children aged 8 months to 14 years with severe erythema multiforme, recovery among the 17 given prednisone 40 to 80 mg per m^2 body-surface or an equivalent corticosteroid was considered to be less rapid than among the 15 patients given supportive treatment; there was also a significant incidence of medical complications among those given corticosteroids.— J. E. Rasmussen, *Br. J. Derm.*, 1976, *95*, 181.

Keloids. Fluorinated corticosteroids in high concentrations could be applied as creams with occlusive dressings or impregnated in occlusive adhesive tape for the treatment of keloids. Intralesional injections with 0.05 to 0.1 ml of triamcinolone acetonide 1% suspension were commonly used and subcutaneous injection of a local anaesthetic below the keloid would reduce pain associated with the procedure.— D. D. Munro, *Practitioner*, 1974, *212*, 773. See also B. H. Griffith *et al.*, *Plastic reconstr. Surg.*, 1970, *46*, 145.

Lichen planus. Topical corticosteroid therapy is useful in the erosive form of lichen planus of the mouth.— A. D. Macalister, *Drugs*, 1973, *5*, 453.

See also under individual monographs, particularly Betamethasone Valerate, p.463 and Methylprednisolone Acetate, p.478.

Lupus. The use of a cream of triamcinolone acetonide 0.5% was recommended for the treatment of chronic discoid lupus erythematosus. Low-dosage therapy with antimalarial drugs might be justified, under constant supervision, when local corticosteroid therapy was ineffective.— R. K. Winkelmann, *J. Am. med. Ass.*, 1968, *205,* 675. (But see Precautions for Triamcinolone, p.483).

Napkin rashes. Recommendations for the management of *napkin dermatitis.* Topical applications include antibacterial and/or fungicidal agents, usually in association with hydrocortisone. More potent topical corticosteroid applications should not be applied to the skin of infants because of the real danger of dermal atrophy. Treatment of *napkin psoriasis* is with weak tar preparations, or weak corticosteroid preparations alone. Nystatin cream should be used if there is candida infection.— J. Verbov, *Practitioner,* 1978, *220,* 779. Similar recommendation concerning weak corticosteroid therapy in *infantile seborrhoeic dermatitis.*— *idem.*

Panniculitis. A report of relapsing, febrile, nodular, non-suppurative panniculitis (Weber-Christian syndrome) in 2 infants responding to treatment with prednisone.— W. M. Hendricks *et al., Br. J. Derm.*, 1978, *98,* 175.

Polyarteritis nodosa. Most patients with cutaneous polyarteritis nodosa are treated with corticosteroids (up to 20 mg of prednisolone daily) and analgesics. As the conditions become less severe treatment can be discontinued or the dose of prednisolone reduced to 5 to 15 mg daily.— P. Borrie, *Br. J. Derm.*, 1972, *87,* 87.

Pretibial myxoedema. In a prospective study 7 of 9 patients with pretibial myxoedema obtained complete resolution of the plaques after intralesional injections of triamcinolone acetonide. The other 2 obtained partial resolution but did not complete their courses.— P. G. Lang *et al., Archs Derm.*, 1975, *111,* 197.

Pemphigus and pemphigoid. Despite the many problems, systemic corticosteroids remain the first line of treatment of these diseases. The initial dose in pemphigus vulgaris is usually above 100 mg of prednisolone daily (some experts advocate an even higher range) which can be increased within a few days if the blistering does not come under control. Most patients require indefinite maintenance on smaller doses of about 15 mg of prednisolone daily. Pemphigus erythematosus may often be controlled by topical corticosteroid applications alone. Pemphigoid calls for lower doses, often below 50 mg of prednisolone initially, and many patients remit spontaneously within a year or two. Patients with benign mucosal pemphigoid may also require long-term treatment with systemic corticosteroids but these are not always effective and in less severe cases it is probably wise to avoid them.— J. A. Savin, *Practitioner,* 1977, *219,* 847.

In a controlled study in 25 patients with pemphigoid the mean dose of prednisone over 3 years was reduced by 45% in those also given azathioprine 2.5 mg per kg body-weight daily, reduced to half this dosage if the white-cell count fell below 3000 per mm^3. Toxicity and mortality were not increased; the combined regimen should be considered standard.— J. L. Burton *et al., Br. med. J.*, 1978, *2,* 1190. See also A. A. Ahmed *et al., Archs Derm.*, 1977, *113,* 1043.

Further references: J. L. Burton *et al., Br. med. J.*, 1970, *3,* 84 (with azathioprine); H. H. Roenigk and S. Deodhar, *Archs Derm.*, 1973, *107,* 353 (azathioprine alone or with corticosteroids); F. R. Rosenberg *et al., Archs Derm.*, 1976, *112,* 962 (20-year review); M. Skeete and M. W. Greaves, *Br. J. Derm.*, 1976, *95, Suppl.* 14, 23 (massive prednisone dosage); W. F. Lever and G. Schaumburg-Lever, *Archs Derm.*, 1977, *113,* 1236 (immunosuppressants and prednisone; a review of 63 patients); C. I. Harrington and I. B. Sneddon, *Br. J. Derm.*, 1979, *100,* 441 (prednisolone with dapsone).

Psoriasis. A discussion on the treatment of psoriasis and the role of corticosteroid therapy. There is virtually no place for systemic corticosteroids in the treatment of psoriasis. Topical corticosteroids act more quickly, are cleaner, and are therefore more popular than tar or dithranol, but they often fail to achieve complete remission. They tend to fail in the more difficult patient with widespread or inflamed psoriasis; persistence with corticosteroid treatment has almost certainly been responsible for the increase in the past 20 years of the more unpleasant types, such as pustular psoriasis. The relapse-rate after various topical treatments is far less well known and further long-term trials, preferably prospective, are needed. For the moment it must be concluded that the use of topical corticosteroid therapy is no panacea and is not even the best long-term management for most patients with psoriasis. It is useful in localised psoriasis, but not indefinitely, and corticosteroids must not be used in increasing quantities in an attempt to counter clinical deterioration. In long-term treatment the dose of strong corticosteroids should be kept below 25 g weekly and the clinician should watch for early signs of skin atrophy. In more extensive psoriasis the temptation to use topical corticosteroids must be resisted. Some patients may improve a lot when given a strong corticosteroid for up to 6 weeks and not necessarily relapse on gradual withdrawal by replacement with a weaker corticosteroid or a weaker strength of the same one. If they do relapse, an alternative treatment must be sought.— *Br. med. J.*, 1977, *1,* 988. A further review. Topical corticosteroids are most useful when tar and dithranol preparations are poorly tolerated (or, occasionally, ineffective). This often applies to psoriasis of the scalp, flexures, face, palms, and soles. In general the weakest preparation which can clear the psoriasis should be used. It is unwise to persist for more than 3 weeks with continuous treatment with the strongest preparations.— *Drug & Ther. Bull.*, 1978, *16,* 25.

Further reviews and comments on the use of corticosteroids in psoriasis: L. Hodge and J. S. Comaish, *Drugs,* 1977, *13,* 288; J. M. Marks, *Drugs,* 1980, *19,* 429.

For the role of corticosteroid pretreatment in photochemotherapy regimens for psoriasis, see Methoxsalen, p.499.

For a comment on the use of corticosteroids for *napkin psoriasis*, see above.

Pustular psoriasis. Comment on the role of systemic and topical corticosteroid therapy in the precipitation of generalised pustular psoriasis from non-pustular forms of the disease. The value of systemic corticosteroid therapy in the medium- and long-term management of generalised pustular psoriasis is now in doubt, where methotrexate is probably more effective and less toxic.— H. Baker, *Br. J. Derm.*, 1976, *94, Suppl.* 12, 83. See also H. Baker and T. J. Ryan, *Br. J. Derm.*, 1968, *80,* 771; T. J. Ryan and H. Baker, *ibid.*, 1969, *81,* 134; *idem,* 1971, *85,* 407.

Rosacea. Rosacea should not be treated with corticosteroids, even the weakest.— *Br. med. J.*, 1978, *2,* 750.

Sarcoidosis. Prednisone 50 mg given on alternate days was used unsuccessfully to treat a patient with ulcerative sarcoidosis; on gradual reduction of the dose to 35 mg on alternate days no new ulcerations appeared.— M. Meyers and S. Barsky (letter), *Archs Derm.*, 1978, *114,* 447.

Scleroderma. In contrast to their failure in most other types of scleroderma, corticosteroids given by mouth over many months often seem to help in eosinophilic fasciitis.— *Br. med. J.*, 1980, *280,* 506. See also K. Keczkes and J. D. Goode, *Br. J. Derm.*, 1979, *100,* 381.

Further references: J. R. Person and W. P. D. Su, *Br. J. Derm.*, 1979, *100,* 371 (subcutaneous morphoea).

Sun and radiotherapy burns. No proper trials have been done on the use of topical corticosteroids in sunburn, but topical corticosteroids probably do not have a large role.— M. Lane-Brown, *Drugs,* 1977, *13,* 366.

Further references: P. M. Russo and L. J. Schneiderman, *J. fam. Pract.*, 1978, *7,* 1129 (poor results with topical fluocinolone in sunburn); J. P. Glees *et al., Clin. Radiol.*, 1979, *30,* 397 (better results with topical hydrocortisone than topical clobetasone butyrate in radiation burns, but poor results with both).

Urticaria. Corticosteroids are not the treatment of choice for urticaria. Hydrocortisone intravenously or intramuscularly, after adrenaline and an antihistamine, may be life-saving in acute anaphylactic reactions, and corticosteroids are also particularly valuable for severe serum sickness. In the management of other types of acute urticaria and especially chronic urticaria they tend to be disappointing.— R. H. Champion, *Br. med. J.*, 1973, *4,* 730. See also J. Verbov (letter), *Lancet,* 1977, *2,* 925.

Vitiligo. The current treatment of vitiligo is the twice-daily application of 0.1% betamethasone valerate, either in a cream basis or in 50% isopropyl alcohol. If the latest reports of the successful treatment of vitiligo by topical corticosteroid applications are confirmed, methoxsalen would probably not have any place in the treatment of vitiligo.— T. W. Stewart, *Practitioner,* 1976, *217,* 184. See also S. S. Bleehen, *Br. J. Derm.*, 1976, *94, Suppl.* 12, 43.

Further references to the use of corticosteroids in vitiligo: M. Koga, *Br. J. Derm.*, 1977, *197,* 255 (topical application); H. Brostoff and J. Brostoff (letter), *Lancet,* 1978, *2,* 688 (oral, in one patient).

Stroke. Discussions on the role of corticosteroids in stroke: D. C. Anderson and R. E. Cranford, *Stroke,* 1979, *10,* 68; B. G. Parsons-Smith, *Practitioner,* 1979, *223,* 553.

See also Betamethasone, p.461, and Dexamethasone, p.467.

Temporal arteritis. See under Arteritis.

Thyroid disorders. The administration of adrenal glucocorticoids was considered necessary to overcome the abnormal demands on the adrenal cortex during a *thyrotoxic crisis.* During the critical phase of the emergency it was reasonable to give 100 to 300 mg of hydrocortisone daily by intramuscular or intravenous injection, and such doses appeared to have improved the survival-rate.— S. H. Ingbar, *New Engl. J. Med.*, 1966, *274,* 1252.

Hydrocortisone sodium succinate 100 mg daily should be given, initially intravenously and later by intramuscular injection, to patients in *myxoedemic coma* to prevent the onset of adrenocortical shock.— G. A. Smart, *Prescribers' J.*, 1972, *12,* 112.

For the use of subconjunctival or retrobulbar corticosteroid injections to alleviate exophthalmos in patients with *thyrotoxicosis*, see Methylprednisolone Acetate, p.478.

For a comparison of the use of prednisolone, chloroquine, and thyroid in the treatment of *thyroiditis,* see under Thyroid, p.1499.

1061-l

Aldosterone.

Electrocortin. 11β,18-Epoxy-18,21-dihydroxypregn-4-ene-3,20-dione.
$C_{21}H_{28}O_5$=360.4.

CAS — 52-39-1(+).

Adverse Effects. As for Corticosteroids, p.446. Aldosterone has very pronounced mineralocorticoid actions and little effect on carbohydrate metabolism.

Uses. Aldosterone is probably the main mineralocorticoid secreted by the adrenal cortex. It has no anti-inflammatory properties.

Aldosterone has been used in association with a glucocorticoid in the treatment of Addison's disease. It has also been tried in shock when the response to pressor agents is diminished. In acute crisis, 500 µg has been given by slow intravenous injection and repeated several times a day.

Evidence that aldosterone has a half-life of 50 minutes after infusion of 1 mg. About 75% of aldosterone is bound to plasma proteins.— R. E. Peterson, *Ann. N.Y. Acad. Sci.*, 1959, *82,* 846.

Potassium homoeostasis and the roles of insulin and aldosterone.— M. Cox *et al., New Engl. J. Med.*, 1978, *299,* 525.

Adrenal insufficiency. Aldosterone, used instead of deoxycortone, as the mineralocorticoid in the substitution treatment of 4 women with Addison's disease over periods up to 15 months, produced sodium balance in all cases. The cortisone dose remained unchanged. For these patients the daily dose of aldosterone required appeared to be 0.5 to 1 mg subcutaneously, 1 to 2 mg sublingually, and 0.5 to 6 mg by mouth.— H. Warning and J. V. Rosenbeck-Hansen, *Acta med. scand.*, 1963, *174,* 229.

Proprietary Names

Aldocorten *(Ciba, Ger.).*

Aldosterone was formerly marketed in Great Britain under the proprietary name Aldocorten (*Ciba*).

1062-y

Beclomethasone Dipropionate *(B.P., U.S.P.).*

Sch 18020W; Beclometasone Dipropionate; 9α-Chloro-16β-methylprednisolone Dipropionate. 9α-Chloro-11β,17α,21-trihydroxy-16β-methylpregna-1,4-diene-3,20-dione 17,21-dipropionate.
$C_{28}H_{37}ClO_7$=521.0.

CAS — 4419-39-0 (beclomethasone); 5534-09-8 (dipropionate).

Pharmacopoeias. In *Br.* and *U.S.*

A white to creamy-white odourless powder. M.p. about 212° with decomposition. Practically **insol-**

uble in water; soluble 1 in 60 of alcohol and 1 in 8 of chloroform; freely soluble in acetone. A solution in dioxan is dextrorotatory. **Protect** from light.

Adverse Effects, Treatment, Withdrawal, and Precautions. As for Corticosteroids, p.446, p.449. In patients who have been transferred to inhalation therapy, systemic therapy may need to be reinstituted without delay during periods of stress or where airways obstruction or mucus prevents absorption from the inhalation. Candidiasis of the throat and mouth or hoarseness may develop in some patients using aerosol inhalations.

Adrenal suppression. Reports of adrenal insufficiency in patients transferred from systemic corticosteroid therapy to beclomethasone dipropionate aerosol therapy: J. C. Batten *et al.* (letter), *Br. med. J.*, 1973, *1*, 296; R. M. Cayton and P. Howard (letter), *ibid.*, *2*, 547; N. J. Cooke *et al.* (letter), *ibid.*, *4*, 49.

Allergy and asthma. Blood blisters in the mouth of an elderly patient using beclomethasone dipropionate inhalers.— *Med. J. Aust.*, 1979, *1*, 460.

Reports of asthmatic responses to beclomethasone dipropionate inhalations, possibly associated with materials used in their formulation, or with the containers: P. J. Maddern *et al.* (letter), *Med. J. Aust.*, 1978, *1*, 274; J. Godin and J. L. Malo, *Clin. Allergy*, 1979, *9*, 585.

See also under Effects on the Lungs.

Candidiasis. A report on 5½ years of experience with beclomethasone dipropionate aerosol in 600 adults and children with asthma, including comments on the incidence of oropharyngeal candidiasis. Oropharyngeal candidiasis was not a significant problem, but was commoner in patients also taking systemic corticosteroid therapy; it usually responded rapidly to amphotericin lozenges. Our impression is that a drink or a simple gargle after the inhalation of beclomethasone dipropioante aerosol, and improved dental hygiene, has resulted in fewer cases of clinical thrush in recent years.— H. M. Brown *et al.*, *Br. J. clin. Pharmac.*, 1977, *4*, *Suppl.*, 259S. For a view that mouth-washes have no effect on the incidence of candidiasis, see Betamethasone Valerate, p.463.

Differing views on the incidence of oropharyngeal candidiasis in patients using beclomethasone dipropionate by inhalation: L. J. R. Milne and G. K. Crompton, *Br. med. J.*, 1974, *3*, 797; *Lancet*, 1974, *2*, 303 (Preliminary Report of the Brompton Hospital/MRC Collaborative Trial); I. W. B. Grant *et al.* (letter), *ibid.*, 838; M. Turner-Warwick and W. Fox (letter), *ibid.*; H. Kershnar *et al.*, *Pediatrics*, 1978, *62*, 189; F. C. Vogt, *Ann. Allergy*, 1979, *43*, 205.

Effects on the lungs. Pulmonary eosinophilia developed in 3 adults during the gradual withdrawal of systemic corticosteroid therapy following the introduction of beclomethasone dipropionate inhalations.— I. C. Paterson *et al.*, *Br. J. Dis. Chest*, 1975, *69*, 217. Pulmonary eosinophilia in a patient also taking oral corticosteroid therapy.— J. L. Mollura *et al.*, *Ann. Allergy*, 1979, *42*, 326.

Further references to pulmonary eosinophilia in patients inhaling beclomethasone diproprionate: D. W. Hudgel and S. L. Spector, *Chest*, 1977, *72*, 359; L. R. Klotz *et al.*, *Ann. Allergy*, 1977, *39*, 133.

Absorption and Fate. For a brief outline of the absorption and fate of a corticosteroid, see Corticosteroids, p.451.

Beclomethasone dipropionate is readily absorbed after administration by mouth. It has been reported that about 25% of an inhaled dose reaches the lungs.

Beclomethasone dipropionate is considerably more active topically or by inhalation than by mouth.

When applied topically, particularly to large areas, when the skin is broken, or under occlusive dressings, corticosteroids may be absorbed in sufficient amounts to cause systemic effects.

An investigation of the absorption and metabolism of beclomethasone dipropionate administered by mouth to 6 subjects indicated that the selective effect in asthma of inhaled beclomethasone dipropionate did not depend on poor gastro-intestinal absorption. It could, however, depend upon inactivation in the liver.— L. E. Martin *et al.* (letter), *Clin. Pharmac. Ther.*, 1974, *15*, 267.

Uses. Beclomethasone dipropionate is a synthetic glucocorticoid used topically in the treatment of various skin disorders, as described under Corticosteroids (see p.451). It is applied locally as a cream or ointment containing 0.025% or as a 0.5% cream. It may be used under an occlusive dressing to obtain a more intense effect.

Beclomethasone dipropionate exerts a topical effect on the lungs without significant systemic activity at recommended doses and is used by inhalation for the prophylaxis of the symptoms of asthma. It is generally inhaled from a metered aerosol, each metered dose delivering 50 µg.

The adult dosage of the aerosol is 100 µg inhaled 3 or 4 times daily for maintenance treatment; in severe asthma 600 to 800 µg may be inhaled daily initially, subsequently adjusted according to the patient's response; a maximum of 1 mg daily should not be exceeded. In children, 50 or 100 µg may be inhaled 2 to 4 times daily according to the response. An improvement in respiratory function should be obvious within a week.

Changeover from systemic to inhalation therapy should be made very slowly by introducing beclomethasone dipropionate, then after a week reducing the daily systemic corticosteroid dose at the rate of the equivalent of 1 mg of prednisolone at intervals of not less than a week until systemic therapy has been discontinued or until the lowest tolerable dose has been reached.

Although beclomethasone dipropionate is generally inhaled in aerosol form, inhalation capsules are available for patients who experience difficulty in using the aerosol. Owing to differences in the relative bioavailability to the lungs of the 2 preparations a 100-µg dose from an inhalation capsule is approximately equivalent in activity to a 50-µg dose from an aerosol. Recommended maintenance doses of beclomethasone dipropionate from inhalation capsules are therefore 200 µg inhaled 3 or 4 times daily for adults, and 100 µg inhaled 2 to 4 times daily for children. The maximum recommended daily dose remains at 1 mg daily.

Beclomethasone dipropionate is also used as a nasal spray in a dose of 50 µg in each nostril 4 times daily in the prophylaxis and treatment of allergic rhinitis.

Asthma. To define the place of topically active corticosteroid aerosol preparations in asthma, the efficiency of aerosol corticosteroid and alternate-morning single-dose prednisone therapy, given in bioequivalent doses, must be compared directly in patients not previously committed to maintenance corticosteroid therapy. Risk-benefit assessments made during aerosol beclomethasone [dipropionate] treatment of asthmatics, initially taking prednisone daily or on alternate days, support the view that most of the improvement in adrenal function may result from the change from daily to alternate-day (or no) corticosteroids, and that patients already on alternate-day oral prednisone are unlikely to improve their cortisol concentrations significantly after transfer to beclomethasone [dipropionate] aerosol therapy. However, they do not support the notion that improved adrenal function is the only clinical advantage, since in the alternate-day group persistently suppressed (but not worse) adrenal function was coupled with a large improvement in asthma symptoms, which argues for a strong local effect of beclomethasone [dipropionate] aerosol.— J. H. Toogood (letter), *Lancet*, 1979, *2*, 1185; *ibid.*, 1980, *1*, 54. General agreement, and the comment that the physician should select the regimen best suited to the patient's needs. Alternate-day prednisone is less expensive and simpler to administer but sometimes causes excessive weight gain. Inhaled beclomethasone dipropionate is not a viable alternative for infants and toddlers with chronic asthma, causes oral candidiasis in some patients, and is not tolerated by an occasional patient who coughs on inhaling the powder.— M. Weinberger (letter), *ibid.*, 1980, *1*, 316.

Of 40 children treated with beclomethasone dipropionate for 1½ to 6 years, who had had no previous corticosteroid therapy, growth status improved. Assessment of adrenal function in 28 children treated with beclomethasone dipropionate for at least a year, 18 of whom had previously been on prednisolone, showed no evidence of significant adrenal suppression, compared with control children on bronchodilators and sodium cromoglycate, although mean values were slightly lower in children on beclomethasone dipropionate, especially those previously treated with prednisolone. It is unreasonable to restrict the use of beclomethasone dipropionate on the basis of possible adrenal suppression.— G. L. Bhan *et al.* (letter), *Lancet*, 1980, *1*, 96. See also S. Godfrey *et al.*, *J. Allergy & clin. Immunol.*, 1978, *62*, 335.

For further details of the controversy surrounding the merits of beclomethasone dipropionate inhalations compared with alternate-day systemic corticosteroid therapy, see R. Wyatt *et al.*, *New Engl. J. Med.*, 1978, *299*, 1387; S. C. Siegel *et al.* (letter), *ibid.*, 1979, *300*, 986; R. J. Dattwyler and K. J. Bloch (letter), *ibid.*; M. Weinberger and B. Sherman (letter), *ibid.*, 987; *Lancet*, 1979, *1*, 589; H. M. Brown and F. A. Jackson (letter), *ibid.*, 827; H. Herxheimer (letter), *ibid.*; M. Weinberger and B. Sherman (letter), *ibid.*, 871; T. J. H. Clark (letter), *ibid.*, 970; C. J. Falliers (letter), *ibid.*, 932; M. Weinberger (letter), *Lancet*, 1979, *2*, 48; H. M. Brown (letter), *ibid.*, 248.

In a double-blind crossover study of 14 children with severe asthma, beclomethasone dipropionate inhaled as powder from a rotahaler was shown to be as effective as when inhaled as an aerosol. Young children generally preferred to use a rotahaler.— A. T. Edmunds *et al.*, *Archs Dis. Childh.*, 1979, *54*, 233. See also G. Hambleton (letter), *Lancet*, 1978, *2*, 577.

Further studies, reports, and comments on beclomethasone dipropionate therapy in asthma: Brompton Hospital/Medical Research Council, *Br. J. dis. Chest*, 1979, *73*, 121; J. H. Toogood *et al.*, *Bull. int. Un. Tuberc.*, 1979, *54*, 183; P. W. Trembath, *Drugs*, 1980, *20*, 81; H. M. Brown *et al.*, *Practitioner*, 1980, *224*, 847.

Eosinophilic gastro-enteritis. Oral administration of beclomethasone dipropionate 3 mg daily, dissolved in a 0.01% solution of sunflower oil to facilitate contact with the mucosal surface, had a beneficial effect in a woman with intestinal malabsorption due to eosinophilic gastro-enteritis.— K. B. Elkon *et al.*, *S.Afr. med. J.*, 1977, *52*, 838.

Pulmonary fibrosis. A 65-year-old woman with interstitial pulmonary fibrosis needing 30 mg of prednisolone daily responded rapidly to treatment with beclomethasone dipropionate aerosol and prednisolone was reduced to 2.5 mg daily.— J. P. T. Linklater (letter), *Br. med. J.*, 1974, *2*, 672.

Rhinitis. A review of 5 years' experience with the use of beclomethasone dipropionate nasal spray in the treatment of allergic rhinitis. Beclomethasone dipropionate nasal spray was effective in 16 of 23 patients (69%) whose allergic rhinitis was unmasked on withdrawal of systemic corticosteroid therapy for asthma; it was similarly effective in 115 of 169 patients (68%) with perennial allergic rhinitis alone, but a satisfactory response was obtained in only 14 of 31 patients (45%) with nasal polypi. A success-rate of 80% was achieved in 92 patients with seasonal allergic rhinitis. No side-effects were found even when treatment was given daily for up to 5 years. Although nasal biopsies showed no evidence of mucosal damage, further studies are required.— H. M. Brown *et al.*, *Br. J. clin. Pharmac.*, 1977, *4*, *Suppl* 283S.

Skin disorders. For recommendations concerning the correct use of corticosteroids on the skin, and a rough guide to the clinical potencies of topical corticosteroids, see Corticosteroids, p.458.

Preparations

Beclomethasone Cream *(B.P.)*. Beclomethasone dipropionate in very fine powder in a suitable basis. Store at a temperature not exceeding 25° in well-closed containers which minimise evaporation and contamination. Protect from light.

Beclomethasone Ointment *(B.P.)*. A solution of beclomethasone dipropionate in propylene glycol in a paraffin ointment basis. Store at a temperature not exceeding 25°. Protect from light.

Proprietary Preparations

Beconase Nasal Spray *(Allen & Hanburys, UK)*. Beclomethasone dipropionate, available as a pressurised nasal spray delivering 50 µg in each metered dose. For allergic rhinitis. (Also available as Beconase Nasal Spray in *Austral.*, *Belg.*, *Canad.*, *Ger.*, *Neth.*, *S.Afr.*, *Switz.*).

Becotide Inhaler *(Allen & Hanburys, UK)*. Beclomethasone dipropionate, available as a pressurised spray for inhalation delivering 50 µg in each metered dose. For bronchial asthma. **Becotide Rotacaps.** Cartridges each containing beclomethasone dipropionate 100 or 200 µg, in a lactose basis, for administration by inhalation by means of a specially designed inhaler (Rotahaler). (Also available as Becotide in *Austral.*, *Belg.*, *Denm.*, *Fr.*, *Ital.*, *Jap.*, *Neth.*, *Norw.*, *S.Afr.*, *Spain*, *Swed.*, *Switz.*).

NOTE. The availability of beclomethasone dipropionate to the lungs depends upon the formulation used; Becotide

Inhaler and Becotide Rotacaps differ in this respect. See Uses.

Propaderm *(Allen & Hanburys, UK).* Preparations containing beclomethasone dipropionate 0.025%, available as **Cream** [suggested diluent, Cetomacrogol Cream (Formula A)] and **Ointment** (suggested diluent, white soft paraffin). **Propaderm-Forte Cream.** Contains beclomethasone dipropionate 0.5%. (Also available as Propaderm in *Canad., Ital., S.Afr.*).

Propaderm-A Ointment *(Allen & Hanburys, UK).* Contains beclomethasone dipropionate 0.025% and chlortetracycline hydrochloride 3%. **Propaderm-C Cream** and **Ointment** each contain beclomethasone dipropionate 0.025% and clioquinol 3%.

Other Proprietary Names

Aldecin *(Austral., Belg., Denm., Jap., Neth., Swed., Switz.)*; Anceron *(Arg.)*; Beclo-Asma *(Spain)*; Beclovent *(Canad., USA)*; Bronco-turbinal, Clenil, Clenil-A *(all Ital.)*; Dermisone Beclo *(Spain)*; Entyderma, Hibisterin, Korbutone *(all Jap.)*; Propavent *(Arg.)*; Rino-Clenil *(Ital.)*; Sanasthymyl *(Ger.)*; Turbinal *(Ital.)*; Vancenase *(Canad.)*; Vanceril *(Canad., USA)*; Viarox *(Ger., Norw., S.Afr.)*.

A preparation containing beclomethasone dipropionate was also formerly marketed in Great Britain under the proprietary name Propaderm-N *(Allen & Hanburys)*.

1063-j

Betamethasone *(B.P., B.P. Vet., Eur. P., U.S.P.).*

Betameth.; Betamethasonum; Flubenisolonum; 9α-Fluoro-16β-methylprednisolone. 9α-Fluoro-11β,17α,21-trihydroxy-16β-methylpregna-1,4-diene-3,20-dione.

$C_{22}H_{29}FO_5$=392.5.

CAS — 378-44-9.

Pharmacopoeias. In *Br., Braz., Eur., Fr., Ger., It., Jap., Neth., Swiss,* and *U.S.*

A white to creamy-white, odourless, crystalline powder with a bitter taste. M.p. about 240° with decomposition.

Practically **insoluble** in water; soluble 1 in 75 of alcohol, 1 in 15 of warm alcohol, and 1 in 1100 of chloroform; sparingly soluble in acetone, dioxan, and methyl alcohol; very slightly soluble in ether. A solution in dioxan is dextrorotatory. In order to achieve a satisfactory rate of dissolution, betamethasone in ultrafine powder should be used in the preparation of solid dose forms. **Protect** from light.

Adverse Effects and Treatment. As for Corticosteroids, p.446 and p.449.

Its effects on sodium and water retention are less than those of prednisolone or prednisone and approximately equal to those of dexamethasone.

Adrenal suppression. Adrenal suppression following betamethasone enemas: S. G. F. Matts, *Gut,* 1962, *3,* 312.

Withdrawal and Precautions. As for Corticosteroids, p.449.

Absorption and Fate. For a brief outline of the absorption and fate of a corticosteroid, see Corticosteroids, p.451.

Uses. Betamethasone is a synthetic glucocorticoid and has the general properties described under Corticosteroids (see p.451); 600 µg of betamethasone is equivalent in anti-inflammatory activity to about 5 mg of prednisolone. It has been used in the treatment of all conditions for which corticosteroid therapy is indicated, except adrenal-deficiency states for which its lack of sodium-retaining properties makes it less suitable than cortisone or hydrocortisone with supplementary fludrocortisone. It is one of the corticosteroids used for the prevention of the neonatal respiratory distress syndrome, and has also been used to reduce raised intracranial pressure.

Betamethasone has a usual dose range of 0.5 to 9 mg daily in divided doses.

Pregnancy and the neonate. After work showing that the functional maturation of foetal *animal* lungs can be accelerated by stimulation of the foetal adrenal cortex or by administration of glucocorticoids, G.C. Liggins and R.N. Howie, (*Pediatrics,* 1972, *50,* 515) found that intramuscular injection of a preparation containing betamethasone acetate 6 mg and betamethasone phosphate 6 mg, to mothers, more than 24 hours before premature delivery of infants of less than 32 weeks' gestation, was associated with a significant reduction in the incidence of respiratory distress syndrome. In controlled studies using hydrocortisone M. Baden *et al.* (*Pediatrics,* 1972, *50,* 526) and H.W. Taeusch *et al.* (*Pediatrics,* 1973, *52,* 850), found that this benefit did not extend to post-natal administration, and found an increased incidence of ventricular haemorrhage in the treated infants. Other fears concerning prenatal corticosteroid therapy (including possible growth retardation and increased risk of infection) were also expressed, but for the present these adverse effects appear to be outweighed by clinical benefit where corticosteroid therapy is clearly indicated.

This advantage of corticosteroid therapy does not apply to toxaemia of pregnancy where it has been associated with a high incidence of foetal death and is generally contra-indicated. Contrary to other reports, however, in an open study, D.J. Nochimson and R.H. Petrie (*Am. J. Obstet. Gynec.,* 1979, *133,* 449) concluded that pregnancy-related hypertension does not appear to be an absolute contra-indication to glucocorticoid therapy.

In an endeavour to delay the onset of premature labour for long enough to enable corticosteroid therapy to act, beta-receptor stimulants, such as salbutamol, have been given concomitantly; fears, in this case, have been directed at the mutual enhancement of adverse effects.

Further references to corticosteroids and the respiratory distress syndrome: E. Caspi and P. Schreyer (letter), *Lancet,* 1976, *1,* 973 (dexamethasone; need for administration for up to 7 days before delivery); Y. Lefebvre *et al., Am. J. Obstet. Gynec.,* 1976, *125,* 609 (hydrocortisone; intra-amniotic); M. Panter-Brick (letter), *Lancet,* 1976, *2,* 421 (dexamethasone; prophylaxis for an infant with a family history of pulmonary insufficiency); A. B. M. Anderson *et al., Obstet. Gynec.,* 1977, *49,* 471 (betamethasone; placental transfer and metabolism); M. F. Block *et al., Obstet. Gynec.,* 1977, *50,* 186 (betamethasone; time factor not significant; methylprednisolone not beneficial); S. N. Caritis *et al., Am. J. Obstet. Gynec.,* 1977, *127,* 529 (betamethasone; in rhesus-sensitised women); A. Kauppila *et al., Br. J. Obstet. Gynaec.,* 1977, *84,* 124 (dexamethasone; no short-term effect on maternal or infant corticotrophin secretion); A. Lazzarin *et al.* (letter), *Lancet,* 1977, *2,* 1354 (betamethasone; reduced infant polymorphonuclear leucocyte function); R. Osathanondh *et al., J. Pediat.,* 1977, *90,* 617 (dexamethasone; maternal and infant concentrations); W. Siebert *et al., Geburtsch. Frauenheilk.,* 1977, *2,* 149 (betamethasone; similar incidence but reduced mortality); C. Sutton, *Br. med. J.,* 1977, *2,* 1069 (dexamethasone; in diabetic mothers); I. Szabó *et al.* (letter), *Lancet,* 1977, *2,* 243 (prednisolone sodium succinate; advantage of longer interval before delivery); S. Sybulski, *Am. J. Obstet. Gynec.,* 1977, *127,* 871 (betamethasone; rapid recovery of infant adrenal activity); T. F. Yeh *et al., J. Pediat.,* 1977, *90,* 140 (post-natal hydrocortisone; poor results in meconium aspiration syndrome); F. P. Zuspan *et al., Am. J. Obstet. Gynec.,* 1977, *128,* 571 (hydrocortisone; beneficial effect prenatally); D. Bielawski *et al.* (letter), *Lancet,* 1978, *1,* 218 (betamethasone; leukaemoid reaction in infant); J. D. Funkhouser *et al., Pediat. Res.,* 1978, *12,* 1053 (dexamethasone; maternal and infant concentrations); K. D. Gunston and D. A. Davey, *S.Afr. med. J.,* 1978, *54,* 1141 (dexamethasone; with fenoterol); T. R. Johnson and J. Schneider (letter), *New Engl. J. Med.,* 1978, *298,* 56 (betamethasone; chorioamnionitis with foetal and maternal sepsis); A. Kauppila *et al., Obstet. Gynec.,* 1978, *51,* 288 (dexamethasone; with ritodrine); F. Arias *et al., Am. J. Obstet. Gynec.,* 1979, *133,* 894 (betamethasone; lecithin/sphingomyelin ratios); A. M. Butterfill and D. R. Harvey, *Archs Dis. Childh.,* 1979, *54,* 725 (betamethasone; follow-up of treated infants); T. R. Eggers *et al., Med. J. Aust.,* 1979, *1,* 213 (betamethasone; with salbutamol); A. S. Gündoğdu *et al., Lancet,* 1979, *2,* 1317 (hormonal and metabolic effects of salbutamol; possible corticosteroid interaction); A. N. Papageorgiou *et al., Pediatrics,* 1979, *63,* 73 (betamethasone; beneficial effect but increased neonatal hypoglycaemia); H. W. Taeusch *et al., Pediatrics,* 1979, *63,* 64 (dexamethasone; beneficial effect but increased incidence of infection); I. Szabó *et al.* (letters), *Lancet,* 1980, *1,* 320; *idem, 2,* 751 (prednisolone sodium succinate; no benefit below 25 weeks' gestation possibly owing to lack of cortisol receptors in foetal lung).

Induction of labour or abortion. A study indicating, contrary to the findings of previous workers, that a single 20-ml intra-amniotic injection of 18 mg of betamethasone sodium phosphate and betamethasone acetate in physiological saline, had no beneficial effect on the induction of labour, compared with injection of physiological saline 20 ml alone.— Z. Katz *et al., Obstet. Gynec.,* 1979, *54,* 31. Earlier studies suggesting that the technique might be of benefit: J. K. G. Mati *et al., Br. med. J.,* 1973, *2,* 149; U. C. Nwosu *et al., Obstet. Gynec.,* 1976, *47,* 137.

Further references: H. Jensen and P. B. Wright, *Acta obstet. gynec. scand.,* 1977, *56,* 467 (dexamethasone by mouth; induction of labour); R. Baveja *et al., Indian J. med. Res.,* 1979, *69,* 83 (intra-amniotic betamethasone; mid-trimester abortion).

Stroke. Comment on poor results obtained with betamethasone in stroke.— E. G. McQueen (letter), *Br. med. J.,* 1978, *2,* 1230. See also *idem, N.Z. med. J.,* 1978, *87,* 103.

See also under Dexamethasone, p.467.

Preparations

Betamethasone Cream *(U.S.P.).* Betamethasone in a suitable cream basis. Store in airtight containers.

Betamethasone Syrup *(U.S.P.).* A syrup containing betamethasone.

Betamethasone Tablets *(B.P.).* Betameth. Tab. Tablets containing betamethasone. Protect from light.

Betamethasone Tablets *(U.S.P.).* Tablets containing betamethasone.

Proprietary Preparations

Betnelan *(Glaxo, UK).* Betamethasone, available as scored tablets of 500 µg. (Also available as Betnelan in *Belg., Canad., Neth., S.Afr., Spain*).

Other Proprietary Names

Betafluorene (hemisuccinate) *(Ital.)*; Betamamallet *(Jap.)*; Betasona *(Venez.)*; Betnesol (see also under Betamethasone Sodium Phosphate) *(Ger.)*; Celestan (see also under Betamethasone Sodium Phosphate) *(Ger.)*; Célestène (see also under Betamethasone Sodium Phosphate) *(Fr.)*; Celeston (see also under Betamethasone Sodium Phosphate) *(Denm., Norw.)*; Celestona *(Swed.)*; Celestone (see also under Betamethasone Sodium Phosphate and Betamethasone Valerate) *(Austral., Belg., Canad., Ital., Neth., S.Afr., Spain, Switz., USA)*; Corteroid (see also under Betamethasone Sodium Phosphate and Betamethasone Valerate) *(Arg.)*; Cuantin *(Spain)*; Desacort-Beta *(Ital.)*; Hormezon (see also under Betamethasone Valerate) *(Jap.)*; Minisone, No-Reumar, Pertene *(all Ital.)*; Rinderon *(Jap.)*; Sclane (see also under Betamethasone Sodium Phosphate) *(Spain)*.

1064-z

Betamethasone Acetate *(U.S.P.).*

Betamethasone 21-acetate.

$C_{24}H_{31}FO_6$=434.5.

CAS — 987-24-6.

Pharmacopoeias. In *U.S.*

A white to creamy-white odourless powder. M.p. about 165° and, with decomposition, 200° to 220°. Practically **insoluble** in water; soluble 1 in 9 of alcohol and 1 in 16 of chloroform; freely soluble in acetone. A solution in dioxan is dextrorotatory. **Store** in airtight containers.

Betamethasone acetate has the general properties of betamethasone. It is used with betamethasone sodium phosphate as an intramuscular injection in usual daily doses ranging from 0.25 to 4.5 mg of each. It is given by intra-articular injection in usual doses ranging from 0.75 to 6 mg of each, repeated as required.

1065-c

Betamethasone Benzoate *(U.S.P.).*

W 5975. Betamethasone 17α-benzoate.

$C_{29}H_{33}FO_6$=496.6.

CAS — 22298-29-9.

Pharmacopoeias. In *U.S.*

A white or almost white, almost odourless, powder. M.p. about 220° with decomposition.

Practically **insoluble** in water; soluble in alcohol, chloroform, and methyl alcohol. A solution in dioxan is dextrorotatory. **Store** in airtight containers.

Adverse Effects, Treatment, Withdrawal, and Precautions. As for Corticosteroids, p.446, p.449.

Absorption and Fate. For a brief outline of the absorption and fate of corticosteroids, see Corticosteroids, p.451.

When applied topically, particularly to large areas, when the skin is broken, or under occlusive dressings, corticosteroids may be absorbed in sufficient amounts to cause systemic effects.

Uses. Betamethasone benzoate has the general properties of betamethasone and is used by topical application in the treatment of various skin disorders, as described under Corticosteroids (see p.451). It is applied locally as a gel containing 0.025%.

Skin disorders. For recommendations concerning the correct use of corticosteroids on the skin, and a rough guide to the clinical potencies of topical corticosteroids, see Corticosteroids, p.458.

Preparations

Betamethasone Benzoate Gel *(U.S.P.).* A gel containing betamethasone benzoate. Store in airtight containers.

Proprietary Names

Beben *(Parke, Davis, Canad.; Vister, Ital.; Substantia, Neth.)*; Benisone *(Cooper, USA)*; Dermizol *(Roux-Ocefa, Arg.)*; Euvaderm *(Sasse, Ger.)*; Parbetan *(Parke, Davis, Spain)*; Skincort *(Parke, Davis, S.Afr.)*; Uticort *(Parke, Davis, USA)*.

1066-k

Betamethasone Dipropionate *(U.S.P.).*

Sch 11460. Betamethasone 17α,21-dipropionate.

$C_{28}H_{37}FO_7$=504.6.

CAS — 5593-20-4.

Pharmacopoeias. In *U.S.*

A white or creamy-white odourless powder. Practically **insoluble** in water; sparingly soluble in alcohol; freely soluble in acetone and chloroform. A solution in dioxan is dextrorotatory.

Adverse Effects, Treatment, Withdrawal, and Precautions. As for Corticosteroids, p.446, p.449.

Two patients with moderate to severe psoriasis of the scalp developed folliculitis during the second week of treatment with applications of betamethasone dipropionate in alcoholic solution twice daily.— A. Lassus, *Curr. med. Res. Opinion*, 1976, *4*, 365.

Absorption and Fate. For a brief outline of the absorption and fate of corticosteroids, see Corticosteroids, p.451. When applied topically, particularly to large areas, when the skin is broken, or under occlusive dressings, corticosteroids may be absorbed in sufficient amounts to cause systemic effects.

Uses. Betamethasone dipropionate has the general properties of betamethasone (see p.461) and is used by topical application in the treatment of various skin disorders, as described under Corticosteroids (see p.451). It is usually applied as a cream, ointment, or lotion, containing the equivalent of 0.05% of betamethasone. It may also be applied as an aerosol skin spray.

Skin disorders. For recommendations concerning the correct use of corticosteroids on the skin, and a rough guide to the clinical potencies of topical corticosteroids, see Corticosteroids, p.458.

Preparations

Betamethasone Dipropionate Cream *(U.S.P.).* Contains betamethasone dipropionate in a suitable cream basis. Store in airtight containers.

Betamethasone Dipropionate Lotion *(U.S.P.).* Contains betamethasone dipropionate in a suitable lotion basis. Store in airtight containers.

Betamethasone Dipropionate Ointment *(U.S.P.).* Contains betamethasone dipropionate in a suitable ointment basis.

Betamethasone Dipropionate Topical Aerosol *(U.S.P.).* A solution of betamethasone dipropionate in suitable propellents in a pressurised container. Store at a temperature not exceeding 40°.

Proprietary Names

Diproderm *(Schering, Denm.; Essex, Spain; Schering, Swed.)*; Diprosone *(Essex, Arg.; Essex, Austral.; Schering, Belg.; Schering, Canad.; Unilabo, Fr.; Byk Essex, Ger.; Essex, Ital.; Essex, NZ; Scherag, S.Afr.; Schering, Switz.; Schering, USA)*.

1067-a

Betamethasone Sodium Phosphate *(B.P., B.P. Vet., U.S.P.).*

Betameth. Sod. Phos.; Betamethasone Disodium Phosphate. Betamethasone 21-(disodium phosphate).

$C_{22}H_{28}FNa_2O_8P$=516.4.

CAS — 360-63-4 (phosphate); 151-73-5 (sodium phosphate).

Pharmacopoeias. In *Br.* and *U.S.*

A white or almost white, odourless, hygroscopic powder with a bitter taste. The *B.P.* specifies not more than 8% of water; the *U.S.P.* permits up to 10%. Betamethasone sodium phosphate 1.3 mg is approximately equivalent to 1 mg of betamethasone.

Soluble 1 in 2 of water and 1 in 350 of dehydrated alcohol; freely soluble in methyl alcohol; practically insoluble in acetone, chloroform, and ether. A solution in water is dextrorotatory. A 0.5% solution in water has a pH of 7.5 to 9. Solutions are **sterilised** by filtration. Aqueous solutions of pH about 8 are stable if protected from light. Care must be taken to prevent microbial contamination of solutions to avoid hydrolysis by phosphatase. **Store** in airtight containers. Protect from light.

Adverse Effects and Treatment. See Betamethasone, p.461.

There have been reports of joint damage following the intra-articular injection of corticosteroids into load-bearing joints (see under Corticosteroids, p.447).

Prolonged application to the eye of preparations containing corticosteroids has caused increased intra-ocular pressure and reduced visual function.

Effects on the eyes. A 77-year-old man with chronic simple glaucoma became blind after using betamethasone eye-drops 0.1% for 1 year without concomitant miotic drops.— D. O. Crompton (letter), *Med. J. Aust.*, 1966, *2*, 964.

Withdrawal and Precautions. As for Corticosteroids, p.449.

Absorption and Fate. For a brief outline of the absorption and fate of corticosteroids, see Corticosteroids, p.451.

After intradermal injections of 1 ml of Celestone Chronodose (betamethasone sodium phosphate 3 mg, betamethasone acetate 3 mg) plasma-cortisol concentrations in 12 subjects were significantly depressed for 3 days, then returned to normal; after 5-ml doses in 13 subjects there was (paradoxically) less severe depression lasting 4 days and then returning to levels lower than initial levels; after subcutaneous injection of 1 ml and 5 ml (each in 2 subjects) depression lasted 3 and 9 days respectively. After intradermal injection of 5 ml of Kenacort (triamcinolone acetonide 10 mg per ml) in 10 subjects, plasma-cortisol concentrations were only slightly depressed; after subcutaneous injection of 1 ml of Kenacort in 2 subjects there was no appreciable depression and after 5 ml there was transient depression. When intralesional injection of corticosteroids was necessary compounds should be chosen which had a slow effect.— S. T. Zaynoun and I. S. Salti, *Br. J. Derm.*, 1973, *88*, 151.

Uses. Betamethasone sodium phosphate has the general properties of betamethasone (see p.461). It is administered by mouth as tablets and by intramuscular or intravenous injection for intensive therapy or in emergencies. It may also be given as an intravenous infusion and is also injected into joints and soft tissues, usually with a suspension of betamethasone acetate.

Betamethasone sodium phosphate is employed, usually as drops containing 0.1%, in the topical treatment of allergic and inflammatory conditions of eyes, ears, and nose. It was used for the local treatment of aphthous ulcers in the mouth.

Preparations

Betamethasone Eye-drops *(B.P.C. 1973).* Betamethasone Sodium Phosphate Eye-drops; BET. A sterile solution of betamethasone sodium phosphate, with a suitable preservative and stabiliser, in water. The solution is sterilised by filtration. Store in a cool place. Protect from light.

Betamethasone Sodium Phosphate Injection *(B.P.).* Betameth. Sod. Phos. Inj. A sterile solution in Water for Injections containing suitable stabilising agents. Sterilised by filtration. pH 8 to 9. Potency is expressed in terms of the equivalent amount of betamethasone. Store below 30°. Protect from light.

Betamethasone Sodium Phosphate Tablets *(B.P.).* Betameth. Sod. Phos. Tab. Tablets containing betamethasone sodium phosphate. Potency is expressed in terms of the equivalent amount of betamethasone. Protect from light.

Sterile Betamethasone Sodium Phosphate and Betamethasone Acetate Suspension *(U.S.P.).* A sterile preparation containing betamethasone sodium phosphate in solution, and betamethasone acetate in suspension in Water for Injections. pH 6.8 to 7.2. The content of betamethasone sodium phosphate is expressed in terms of the equivalent amount of betamethasone.

Proprietary Preparations

Betnesol *(Glaxo, UK).* Betamethasone sodium phosphate, available as **Drops for Eye, Ear, or Nose** containing 0.1%, with benzalkonium chloride 0.02%; as **Eye Ointment** containing 0.1%; as **Injection** containing the equivalent of 4 mg of betamethasone in each ml, in ampoules of 1 ml; and as scored **Tablets** of 500 µg. (Also available as Betnesol in *Canad., Fr., Ger., Neth., S.Afr., Switz.*).

The name Betnesol is also used as a proprietary name for Betamethasone.

Betnesol-N *(Glaxo, UK).* Preparations containing betamethasone sodium phosphate 0.1% and neomycin sulphate 0.5%, available as **Drops for Eye, Ear, or Nose** with thiomersal 0.005% and as **Eye Ointment**.

Other Proprietary Names

Bentelan *(Ital.)*; Betapred *(Swed.)*; Betallorens *(Spain)*; Betameson *(Ital.)*;Betnasol *(Col., Peru, Port.)*; Bifosona *(Arg.)*; Celestan (see also under Betamethasone) *(Ger.)*; Célestène (see also under Betamethasone) *(Fr.)*; Celeston (see also under Betamethasone) *(Denm., Norw.)*; Celestone (see also under Betamethasone and Betamethasone Valerate) *(Arg., Austral., Belg., Canad., Ital., Neth., S.Afr., Spain, Switz., USA)*; Corteroid (see also under Betamethasone and Betamethasone Valerate) *(Arg.)*; Emilan *(Ital.)*; Linolosal *(Jap.)*; Paucisone *(Ital.)*; Sclane (see also under Betamethasone) *(Spain)*.

Some of these are injections containing betamethasone sodium phosphate with betamethasone acetate.

1068-t

Betamethasone Valerate *(B.P., U.S.P.).*

Betameth. Valerate; Flubenisoloni Valeras; 9α-Fluoro-16β-methylprednisolone 17-Valerate. Betamethasone 17α-valerate.

$C_{27}H_{37}FO_6$=476.6.

CAS — 2152-44-5.

Pharmacopoeias. In *Br.* and *U.S.*

A white to creamy-white, odourless, tasteless powder. M.p. about 190° with decomposition.

Practically **insoluble** in water and light petroleum; soluble 1 in 12 to 16 of alcohol, 1 in 2 of chloroform, and 1 in 50 of isopropyl alcohol; slightly soluble in ether; freely soluble in acetone. A solution in dioxan is dextrorotatory.

Incompatible with alkalis, heavy metals, and metabisulphites. Inactivated by coal tar, salicylic acid, and many other substances. **Store** in airtight containers. Protect from light.

Stability. Preparations of Betamethasone Valerate Cream *B.P.C. 1973* diluted 1 in 2 or 1 in 10 with a modified cetomacrogol cream (formula A) containing

20% propylene glycol and 0.15% chlorocresol exhibited physical stability when stored at 25° for 14 days.— Pharm. Soc. Lab. Rep. P/78/2, 1978.

Studies on the stability of Betnovate Ointment diluted with various semi-solid bases.— Y. W. Yip and A. L. W. Po, *J. Pharm. Pharmac.*, 1979, *31*, 400.

Adverse Effects, Treatment, Withdrawal, and Precautions. As for Corticosteroids, p.446, p.449. In patients who have been transferred to inhalation therapy, systemic therapy may need to be reinstituted without delay during periods of stress or where airways obstruction or mucus prevents absorption from the inhalation. Candidiasis of the throat and mouth or hoarseness may develop in some patients using aerosol inhalations; it has been suggested that the incidence may be reduced by rinsing out the mouth with water after using the inhalation.

Adrenal suppression. In 40 patients who had been treated topically with fluorinated corticosteroids (usually betamethasone valerate) for long periods, mean plasma-corticosteroid concentrations were above 60 ng per ml in 39. Adrenal response as assessed by the insulin test was normal in 37 and was normal or essentially normal in the other 3 when retested 2 to 5 months later after their corticoseroid usage had been reduced by half.— D. D. Munro and D. C. Clift, *Br. J. Derm.*, 1973, *88*, 381. See also L. Wilson *et al.*, *ibid.*, 373.

A 7-month-old boy had 300 g of 0.1% betamethasone valerate ointment applied to the napkin area over 3 months. One week after application ceased he developed signs of raised intracranial pressure comparable with that produced by the sudden withdrawal of systemic corticosteroids.— S. H. Roussounis, *Br. med. J.*, 1976, *2*, 564.

Further references: M. Feiwel *et al.*, *Lancet*, 1969, *1*, 485; A. Kelly *et al.* (letter), *Br. med. J.*, 1972, *4*, 114.

Candidiasis. An assessment of betamethasone valerate aerosol for asthma in which all patients were told to wash out the mouth and throat with water after each inhalation of corticosteroid, hoping to minimise any local adverse effects of the aerosol on the posterior pharyngeal wall which takes the full force of the pressurised spray.— M. K. McAllen *et al.*, *Br. med. J.*, 1974, *1*, 171. A study of the incidence of candidiasis in patients using betamethasone valerate 800 µg daily for the control of asthma. A simple mouthwash procedure did not appear to be of prophylactic value, but oral candidiasis was not, however, clinically important.— J. N. Sahay *et al.*, *Br. J. Dis. Chest*, 1979, *73*, 164.

In 2 women betamethasone valerate, transferred from their husbands during intercourse, was considered to have caused or aggravated vaginal candidal infection.— L. Stankler and P. D. Bewsher, *Br. med. J.*, 1978, *2*, 399.

Absorption and Fate. For a brief outline of the absorption and fate of corticosteroids, see Corticosteroids, p.451.

Betamethasone valerate is absorbed through the skin when applied topically and is absorbed from the gastro-intestinal tract when taken by mouth. Although more potent topically, systemically its effects are comparable with those of betamethasone.

Uses. Betamethasone valerate has the general properties of betamethasone (see p.461) and is used by topical application in the treatment of various skin disorders as described under Corticosteroids (see p.451). Creams, lotions, and ointments contain the equivalent of 0.1% of betamethasone. Rectal ointments containing betamethasone valerate 0.05% and suppositories containing 500 µg are also used. It may be used locally under an occlusive dressing in resistant skin disorders.

Betamethasone valerate is used by inhalation similarly to beclomethasone dipropionate (see p.460) for the prophylaxis of the symptoms of asthma. Each metered dose provides 100 µg of betamethasone valerate. The initial dose for both adults and children is 200 µg inhaled 4 times daily, slowly reduced according to the patient's response to the minimum amount necessary to control the asthma. An improvement in respiratory function should be obvious within a week.

It has been tried by mouth in inflammatory intestinal disorders and has also been given as a retention enema in colitis.

Asthma. For studies aimed at defining the role of corticosteroid inhalations compared with alternate-day prednisolone or prednisone therapy in asthma, see Beclomethasone Dipropionate, p.460.

Rhinitis. Studies of betamethasone valerate in allergic rhinitis: G. J. Archer *et al.*, *Clin. Allergy*, 1975, *5*, 285; D. A. Coffman *et al.*, *Practitioner*, 1975, *215*, 665; J. A. Wilson and S. R. Walker, *J. Lar. Otol.*, 1976, *90*, 201.

Skin disorders. A favourable response was obtained in 17 of 19 patients with oral lichen planus who received betamethasone valerate 400 µg daily either from an aerosol or from pellets allowed to dissolve in the mouth. There was no significant difference between the responses obtained from the use of the aerosol or the pellets. Due to the lower availability of betamethasone from the aerosol it was considered that a dose of 800 µg daily might be needed.— J. S. Greenspan *et al.*, *Br. dent. J.*, 1978, *144*, 83. A confirmation of the effectiveness of betamethasone valerate pellets used over 7 years in oral lichen planus.— K. D. Watts (letter), *Br. dent. J.*, 1978, *144*, 135. See also W. R. Tyldesley and S. M. Harding, *Br. J. Derm.*, 1977, *96*, 659 (using aerosol spray).

For recommendations concerning the correct use of corticosteroids on the skin, and a rough guide to the clinical potencies of topical corticosteroids, see Corticosteroids, p.458.

Preparations

Aerosols

Betamethasone Valerate Topical Aerosol *(U.S.P.)*. Betamethasone Valerate Aerosol. A suspension of betamethasone valerate in suitable propellents in a pressurised container. Potency is expressed in terms of the equivalent amount of betamethasone. Store at a temperature not exceeding 40°.

Applications

Betamethasone Valerate Scalp Application *(B.P.C. 1973)*. Betamethasone Scalp Application; Betamethasone Application; Betamethasone Valerate Application. A solution of betamethasone valerate in aqueous isopropyl alcohol. It may contain a suitable thickening agent. Store in a cool place. Protect from light. This preparation is inflammable; keep away from an open flame. Avoid contact with the eyes. This preparation should not be diluted or mixed with any other preparation.

Creams

Betamethasone Valerate Cream *(B.P.C. 1973)*. Betamethasone Cream. A dispersion of betamethasone valerate in a suitable water-miscible basis containing a buffering agent and chlorocresol as the preservative. Store in a cool place in well-closed containers which prevent evaporation and contamination. When a strength less than that available from the manufacturer is prescribed, the stronger cream may be diluted, taking hygienic precautions, with Cetomacrogol Cream (Formula A). The diluted cream must be freshly prepared and not used more than 1 month after issue.

Betamethasone Valerate Cream *(U.S.P.)*. Contains betamethasone valerate in a suitable cream basis. Potency is expressed in terms of the equivalent amount of betamethasone. Store in airtight containers.

Lotions

Betamethasone Valerate Lotion *(B.P.C. 1973)*. Betamethasone Lotion. A dispersion of betamethasone valerate in a suitable basis. It may contain a preservative. Store at a temperature not exceeding 30° in airtight containers. This preparation should not be diluted or mixed with any other preparation.

Betamethasone Valerate Lotion *(U.S.P.)*. A lotion containing betamethasone valerate. Potency is expressed in terms of the equivalent amount of betamethasone. pH 4 to 6. Store at 15° to 30° in airtight containers. Protect from light.

Ointments

Betamethasone Valerate Ointment *(B.P.C. 1973)*. Betamethasone Ointment. A dispersion of betamethasone valerate in a suitable anhydrous greasy basis. When a strength less than that available from the manufacturer is prescribed, the 0.1% ointment should be diluted with white soft paraffin.

Betamethasone Valerate Ointment *(U.S.P.)*. Contains betamethasone valerate in a suitable ointment basis. Potency is expressed in terms of the equivalent amount of betamethasone. Store at a temperature not exceeding 40° in airtight containers.

Betamethasone Valerate with Chlortetracycline Ointment *(B.P.C. 1973)*. Betamethasone with Chlortetracycline Ointment. Contains betamethasone valerate equivalent to betamethasone 0.1% and chlortetracycline hydrochloride 3% in a suitable anhydrous greasy basis. When a strength less than that available from the manufacturer is prescribed, the ointment should be diluted with white soft paraffin or chlortetracycline ointment, as appropriate.

Proprietary Preparations

Betnovate *(Glaxo, UK)*. Preparations containing betamethasone valerate equivalent to betamethasone 0.1%, available as **Cream, Lotion, Ointment** and as **Scalp Application** in slightly gelled vehicle containing isopropyl alcohol. (Inflammable: keep away from an open flame). Cream and Ointment also available as **Betnovate R.D.**, a ready diluted form containing the equivalent of 0.025% of betamethasone, as well as single-application Flexules. **Betnovate-C**. Preparations containing betamethasone valerate equivalent to betamethasone 0.1% and clioquinol 3%, available as **Cream** and **Ointment** . **Betnovate-N**. Preparations containing betamethasone valerate equivalent to betamethasone 0.1% and neomycin sulphate 0.5%, available as **Cream, Lotion,** and **Ointment**. (Also available as Betnovate in *Austral., Canad., S.Afr., Spain, Switz.*).

Betnovate Compound Suppositories *(Glaxo, UK)*. Each contains betamethasone valerate 500 µg, lignocaine hydrochloride 40 mg, and phenylephrine hydrochloride 2 mg. For haemorrhoids and associated ano-rectal disorders.

Betnovate Rectal Ointment *(Glaxo, UK)*. Contains betamethasone valerate 0.05%, lignocaine hydrochloride 2.5%, and phenylephrine hydrochloride 0.1%. For haemorrhoids and associated ano-rectal disorders.

Bextasol Inhaler *(Glaxo, UK)*. A pressurised spray containing betamethasone valerate, delivering 100 µg in each metered dose.

Other Proprietary Names

Bedermin *(Ital.)*; Beta 21 (valero-acetate) *(Ital.)*; Betacort, Betaderm (both *Canad.)*; Betadival (divalerate) *(Ital.)*; Betnelan-V *(Belg., Lux., Neth.)*; Betnesol-V *(Ger.)*; Betneval *(Fr.)*; Betnevate *(Jap.)*; Betnovat *(Denm., Norw., Swed., Turk.)*; Celestan-V *(Ger.)*; Celestoderm *(Fr., Neth., Norw., Spain)*; Celestoderm-V *(Arg., Belg., Canad., Ital., S.Afr., Switz.)*; Celeston valerat *(Denm.)*; Celestone-M, Celestone-V (both *Austral.)*; Cortico LG *(Ital.)*; Corteroid (see also under Betamethasone and Betamethasone Sodium Phosphate) *(Arg.)*; Dermosol *(Jap.)*; Dermovaleas, Ecoval (both *Ital.)*; Hormezon (see also under Betamethasone), Muhibeta-V, Rinderon V (all *Jap.)*; Rolazote *(Arg.)*; Valisone *(Canad., USA)*.

A preparation containing betamethasone was also formerly marketed in Great Britain under the proprietary name Betnovate-A (*Glaxo*).

1069-x

Clobetasol Propionate.

GR2/925. 21-Chloro-9α-fluoro-11β,17α-dihydroxy-16β-methylpregna-1,4-diene-3,20-dione 17-propionate. $C_{25}H_{32}ClFO_5$=467.0.

CAS — 25122-41-2 (clobetasol); 25122-46-7 (propionate).

A white to creamy-white odourless crystalline powder. M.p. about 195°. Practically **insoluble** in water; soluble 1 in 100 of alcohol and 1 in 1000 of ether; soluble in acetone, dioxan, chloroform, and dimethyl sulphoxide. **Incompatible** with alkalis. **Protect** from light.

Adverse Effects, Treatment, Withdrawal, and Precautions. As for Corticosteroids, p.446, p.449.

Adrenal suppression. In a study to determine the effect of topical application of clobetasol propionate on the hypothalamic-pituitary-adrenal axis, 2 healthy male subjects applied 45 g of clobetasol propionate 0.05% cream weekly to the whole body (excluding head, axillae and genitalia, about 90% of the body-surface), 2 applied 45 g to the limbs (about 50% of the body-surface), 3 applied 90 g to the limbs, 2 applied 90 g to the whole body, and 3 applied 175 g to the whole body. No significant suppression was noted after 45 g weekly whereas all but 1 of those applying 90 g or more showed profound suppression. It was considered that the absence of suppression in 1 subject might explain why a few patients could apply large amounts without developing cushingoid features. Of 13 patients studied, those applying over 50 g weekly all showed signs of suppression and those using over 100 g weekly showed profound suppression with cushingoid symptoms; on withdrawal they had symptoms of adrenocortical insufficiency and developed pustular psoriasis. Patients should not use more than 50 g of cream weekly.— J. A. Carruthers *et al.*, *Br. med. J.*, 1975, *4*, 203. See also C. F. Allenby *et al.*, *ibid.*, 619.

Further references: M. Feiwel and W. F. Kelly (letter), *Lancet*, 1974, *2*, 112; E. Ortega *et al.* (letter), *ibid.*, 1975, *1*, 1200; J. D. Boxley *et al.*, *Br. med. J.*, 1975, *2*, 255; R. C. D. Staughton and P. J. August, *ibid.*, 419.

Effects on the skin. Skin striae developed in 3 psoriatic young women when their previous topical corticosteroid therapy was changed to clobetasol propionate ointment; all were left with some degree of permanent scarring.— R. A. Hardie *et al.*, *Practitioner*, 1977, *219*, 376. Dermal atrophy in patients treated with clobetasol propionate for vitiligo.— R. Clayton, *Br. J. Derm.*, 1977, *96*, 71.

Further references: P. J. Dykes and R. Marks, *Clin. Trials J.*, 1977, *14*, 139.

Absorption and Fate. For a brief outline of the absorption and fate of corticosteroids, see Corticosteroids, p.451.

When applied topically, particularly to large areas, when the skin is broken, or under occlusive dressings, corticosteroids may be absorbed in sufficient amounts to cause systemic effects.

Uses. Clobetasol propionate is a corticosteroid used by topical application in the treatment of various skin disorders, as described under Corticosteroids (see p.451). It is applied as a cream, ointment, or scalp application containing 0.05%.

Skin disorders. For recommendations concerning the correct use of corticosteroids on the skin, and a rough guide to the clinical potencies of topical corticosteroids, see Corticosteroids, p.458.

Proprietary Preparations

Dermovate *(Glaxo, UK).* Preparations containing clobetasol propionate 0.05%, available as **Cream**; as **Ointment**; and as **Scalp Application** in a slightly gelled vehicle containing isopropyl alcohol (Inflammable: keep away from an open flame). Cream and Ointment also available as single-application Flexules. **Dermovate-NN**. Preparations containing clobetasol propionate 0.05%, neomycin sulphate 0.5%, and nystatin 100 000 units per g, available as **Cream** and as **Ointment**. (Also available as Dermovate in *Belg., Canad., Jap., Neth., S.Afr., Switz.*).

Other Proprietary Names

Butavat *(Greece)*; Clobesol *(Ital.)*; Dermadex *(Arg.)*; Dermatovate *(Mex.)*; Dermoval *(Fr.)*; Dermovat *(Denm., Fin., Swed.)*; Dermoxin, Dermoxinale *(both Ger.)*; Psorex *(Niger.)*.

1070-y

Clobetasone Butyrate. GR/1214. 21-Chloro-9α-fluoro-17α-hydroxy-16β-methylpregn-1,4-diene-3,11,20-trione 17-butyrate.

$C_{26}H_{32}ClFO_5$=479.0.

CAS — 54063-32-0 (clobetasone); 25122-57-0 (butyrate).

A white crystalline powder. Practically **insoluble** in water; soluble in many organic solvents.

Adverse Effects, Treatment, Withdrawal, and Precautions. As for Corticosteroids, p.446, p.449.

Effects on the eyes. Studies suggesting that topical clobetasone butyrate may tend to raise intra-ocular pressure less than some other corticosteroids: J. A. Dunne and J. P. Travers, *Br. J. Ophthal.*, 1979, *63*, 762; T. G. Ramsell *et al.*, *ibid.*, 1980, *64*, 43.

Effects on the skin. Studies suggesting that clobetasone butyrate may tend to cause less skin atrophy than some other corticosteroids.— D. V. Stevanovic *et al.*, *Br. J. Derm.*, 1977, *96*, 67; P. J. Dykes and R. Marks, *Clin. Trials J.*, 1977, *14*, 139.

Absorption and Fate. For a brief outline of the absorption and fate of corticosteroids, see Corticosteroids, p.451.

When applied topically, particularly to large areas, when the skin is broken, or under occlusive dressings, corticosteroids may be absorbed in sufficient amounts to cause systemic effects.

Uses. Clobetasone butyrate is a corticosteroid used by topical application in the treatment of various skin disorders, as described under Corticosteroids (see p.451). It is usually employed as a cream or ointment containing 0.05%.

Skin disorders. For recommendations concerning the correct use of corticosteroids on the skin, and a rough guide to the clinical potencies of topical corticosteroids, see Corticosteroids, p.458.

Proprietary Preparations

Eumovate (formerly known as Molivate) *(Glaxo, UK).* Clobetasone butyrate, available as **Cream** containing 0.05%; as **Eye-drops** containing 0.1% and as **Ointment** containing 0.05%. Cream and Ointment also available as single-application Flexules. **Eumovate-N Eye-drops**. Contains clobetasone butyrate 0.1% and neomycin sulphate 0.5%. (Also available as Eumovate in *S.Afr.*).

Trimovate *(Glaxo, UK).* **Cream** containing clobetasone butyrate 0.05%, oxytetracycline calcium equivalent to oxytetracycline 3%, and nystatin 100 000 units per g and **Ointment** containing clobetasone butyrate 0.05%, chlortetracycline hydrochloride 3%, and nystatin 100 000 units per g.

Other Proprietary Names

Emovat *(Denm.)*; Emovate *(Neth.)*.

1071-j

Cloprednol. RS-4691. 6-Chloro-11β,17α,21-trihydroxypregna-1,4,6-triene-3,20-dione.

$C_{21}H_{25}ClO_5$=392.9.

CAS — 5251-34-3.

Adverse Effects, Treatment, Withdrawal, and Precautions. As for Corticosteroids, p.446; p.449.

Absorption and Fate. See Corticosteroids, p.451.

Clopreднol is readily absorbed from the gastro-intestinal tract and has a plasma half-life of only about 100 minutes.

References: E. Ortega *et al.*, *Clin. Pharmac. Ther.*, 1976, *19*, 113 (plasma half-life); E. J. Mroszczak *et al.*, *J. pharm. Sci.*, 1978, *67*, 920 (absorption).

Uses. Clopreднol is a synthetic glucocorticoid with the general properties described under Corticosteroids (p.451). Preliminary studies have suggested that it is about twice as active as prednisolone.

A study of the metabolic effects of clopreднol.— E. Ortega *et al.*, *J. clin. Pharmac.*, 1976, *16*, 122.

Asthma. In a 24-month study involving 20 children with bronchial asthma, treatment with prednisone or prednisolone was substituted by clopreднol administered at half the equivalent daily dose up to a maximum of 12.5 mg daily. Mean pulmonary symptoms score and mean asthma severity score showed no significant change during the study period but 10 of the children were symptomatically improved during clopreднol therapy. Results suggested that clopreднol produced less suppression of hypothalamo-pituitary adrenal function.— U. D. Gavani *et al.*, *J. Am. med. Ass.*, 1979, *242*, 2679.

Further references: G. G. Shapiro *et al.*, *Ann. Allergy*, 1977, *39*, 178A; R. Ellul-Micallef *et al.* (letter), *Br. J. clin. Pharmac.*, 1978, *6*, 91; D. H. Goodman, *Ann. Allergy*, 1978, *40*, 376; G. G. Shapiro *et al.*, *Pediatrics*, 1979, *63*, 747.

Manufacturers

Syntex, USA.

1072-z

Cortisone Acetate *(B.P., Eur. P., U.S.P.).*

Cortisoni Acetas; Compound E Acetate; 11-Dehydro-17-hydroxycorticosterone Acetate. 17α,21-Dihydroxypregn-4-ene-3,11,20-trione 21-acetate.

$C_{23}H_{30}O_6$=402.5.

CAS — 53-06-5 (cortisone); 50-04-4 (acetate).

Pharmacopoeias. In *Arg., Aust., Belg., Br., Braz., Chin., Eur., Fr., Ger., Ind., Int., It., Jap., Jug., Neth., Nord., Pol., Port., Roum., Rus., Swiss, Turk.,* and *U.S.*

A white or almost white, odourless, crystalline powder, tasteless at first, followed by a persistent bitter taste. M.p. about 240° with decomposition. **Soluble** 1 in 5000 of water, 1 in 300 to 350 of alcohol, 1 in 75 of acetone, 1 in 4 of chloroform, and 1 in 30 of dioxan; sparingly soluble in fixed oils; slightly soluble in ether and methyl alcohol. A solution in dioxan is dextrorotatory. **Incompatible** with oxidising agents, particularly in an alkaline medium, mineral acids, and alkalis. **Protect** from light.

It exists in several polymorphic forms. When aqueous suspensions are being prepared all particles should be converted to the most stable of these forms as otherwise crystal growth will occur. Carmellose sodium and polysorbate 80 are suitable suspending and dispersing agents. Benzyl alcohol (1 to 1.5%) and thiomersal (0.01%) are suitable bacteriostatic agents.

In the preparation of sterile suspensions for injections or eye-drops, cortisone acetate may be sterilised by heating at 150° for 1 hour, suspended aseptically in a sterile aqueous vehicle and milled, and then distributed aseptically into suitable sterile containers.

Polymorphism of cortisone acetate. Cortisone acetate may exist in 5 main polymorphic forms. References: R. E. Collard, *Pharm. J.*, 1961, *1*, 113; R. K. Callow and O. Kennard, *J. Pharm. Pharmac.*, 1961, *13*, 723; R. J. Mesley and C. A. Johnson, *ibid.*, 1965, *17*, 329; J. E. Carless *et al.*, *ibid.*, 1966, *18*, *Suppl.*, 190S; *idem*, 1968, *20*, 630 and 639; R. J. Mesley (letter), *ibid.*, 877.

Adverse Effects, Treatment, Withdrawal, and Precautions. As for Corticosteroids, p.446, p.449.

Absorption and Fate. For a brief outline of the absorption and fate of corticosteroids, see Corticosteroids, p.451.

Cortisone acetate is readily absorbed from the gastro-intestinal tract and the cortisone is rapidly converted in the liver to its active metabolite, hydrocortisone (cortisol). The biological half-life of cortisone itself is only about 30 minutes. Absorption of cortisone acetate from intramuscular sites is considerably slower than following oral administration.

The physiological disposition and metabolic fate of cortisone in man.— R. E. Peterson *et al.*, *J. clin. Invest.*, 1957, *36*, 1301.

Uses. Cortisone is a glucocorticoid secreted by the adrenal cortex and has the general properties described under Corticosteroids (p.451).

Cortisone acetate is rapidly effective when given by mouth, and more slowly by intramuscular injection.

Cortisone acetate has appreciable mineralocorticoid properties and it is used mainly for replacement therapy in Addison's disease or chronic adrenocortical insufficiency secondary to hypopituitarism. The normal daily requirement is 25 to 50 mg of cortisone acetate by mouth in divided doses, increased during infection, trauma, or stress. Hydrocortisone (p.473) is now generally preferred since cortisone itself is inactive and must be converted by the liver to hydrocortisone, its active metabolite; hence, in some liver disorders its bioavailability is less reliable.

Additional sodium chloride may be required if there is defective aldosterone secretion, but mineralocorticoid activity is usually supplemented by fludrocortisone acetate by mouth. Acute adrenal insufficiency should be treated with a glucocorticoid such as hydrocortisone given intravenously together with infusions of dextrose in 0.9% sodium chloride solution.

Cortisone acetate has been used in the treatment of many allergic and inflammatory disorders but prednisolone or other synthetic glucocorticoids are generally preferred because of their reduced sodium-retaining properties. It is ineffective when injected into joint capsules or applied to the skin.

Preparations

Cortisone Injection *(B.P.).* Cortisone Acetate Injection. A sterile suspension of cortisone acetate, in very fine particles, in Water for Injections, prepared using aseptic technique, and containing suitable dispersing agents. pH

5 to 7.2. It must not be given intravenously. Store at a temperature not exceeding 25° and avoid freezing. Protect from light.

Cortisone Tablets *(B.P.)*. Cortisone Acetate Tablets. Tablets containing cortisone acetate in fine powder. Protect from light.

Cortisone Acetate Tablets *(U.S.P.)*. Tablets containing cortisone acetate. The *U.S.P.* requires 60% dissolution in 30 minutes.

Sterile Cortisone Acetate Suspension *(U.S.P.)*. A sterile suspension in a suitable aqueous medium. pH 5 to 7.

Proprietary Preparations

Cortelan *(Glaxo, UK)*. Cortisone acetate, available as scored tablets of 25 mg.

Cortisone Acetate *(Merck Sharp & Dohme, UK)*. Available as tablets of 5 mg and scored tablets of 25 mg.

Cortistab *(Boots, UK)*. Cortisone acetate, available as **Injection** containing 25 mg per ml in vials of 10 ml and as scored **Tablets** of 5 and 25 mg.

Cortisyl *(Roussel, UK)*. Cortisone acetate, available as scored tablets of 25 mg.

Other Proprietary Names

Acetisone *(Ital.)*; Adreson *(Belg., Neth.)*; Altesona *(Spain)*; Corlin *(Ind.)*; Cortal *(Swed.)*; Cortate *(Austral.)*; Cortemel *(S.Afr.)*; Cortisol *(Ital.)*; Cortison *(Ger., Norw., Switz.)*; Cortogen *(S.Afr.)*; Cortone *(Austral., Canad., Norw., Swed.)*; Cortone Acetat *(Denm.)*; Cortone Acetate *(USA)*; Cortone Acetato *(Ital.)*; Kortison *(Denm)*; Sterop *(Austral.)*.

NOTE. The name cortisol is also applied to Hydrocortisone.

1073-c

Cortivazol.

H 3625. 11β,17α,21-Trihydroxy-6,16 α-dimethyl-2′-phenyl-2′*H*-pregna-2,4,6-trieno[3,2-*c*]pyrazol-20-one 21-acetate.
$C_{32}H_{38}N_2O_5$=510.7.

CAS — 1110-40-3.

Uses. Cortivazol is a synthetic glucocorticoid with the general properties described under Corticosteroids (see p.446). It has been given by mouth in usual doses of 0.4 to 3.2 mg daily, and by intra-articular injection in doses of 1.25 to 3.75 mg, according to the size of the joint, usually at intervals of one to three weeks.

Proprietary Names

Altim *(Roussel, Fr.)*; Diaster *(Diamant, Fr.)*; Dilaster *(Roussel-Amor Gil, Spain)*; Idaltim (cortivazol acetate) *(Roussel, Arg.)*.

1074-k

Deoxycortone Acetate *(B.P., Eur. P.)*.

Deoxycort. Acet.; Desoxycortone Acetate; Decortone Acetate; Deoxycorticosterone Acetate; Desoxycorticosterone Acetate *(U.S.P.)*; Desoxycortoni Acetas; Cortin. 21-Hydroxypregn-4-ene-3,20-dione 21-acetate.
$C_{23}H_{32}O_4$=372.5.

CAS — 64-85-7 (deoxycortone); 56-47-3 (acetate).

Pharmacopoeias. In *Arg., Aust., Belg., Br., Braz., Cz., Eur., Fr., Ger., Hung., Ind., Int., It., Jug., Mex., Neth., Nord., Pol., Port., Roum., Rus., Swiss, Turk.*, and *U.S.*

Odourless tasteless colourless crystals or white or creamy-white crystalline powder. M.p. 155° to 161°.

Practically **insoluble** in water; soluble 1 in 50 of alcohol, 1 in 30 of acetone, 1 in 1.5 of chloroform, 1 in 170 of ether, 1 in 170 of propylene glycol, 1 in 140 of arachis oil and in other fixed oils, and 1 in 150 of ethyl oleate; sparingly soluble in dioxan. A solution in dehydrated alcohol or dioxan is dextrorotatory. Solutions of deoxycortone acetate in oil are **sterilised** by maintaining at 150° for 1 hour. **Protect** from light.

Effect of gamma-irradiation. Deoxycortone acetate was sterile but slightly decomposed after irradiation with 25 000 Gy.— G. Hortobagyi *et al.*, *Radiosterilization of Medical Products*, Vienna, International Atomic Energy Agency, 1967, p. 25.

Adverse Effects and Precautions. As for Corticosteroids, p.446, and p.449. Overdoses of deoxycortone acetate may produce excessive sodium and water retention, leading to hypertension, oedema, pulmonary congestion, and signs and symptoms of congestive heart failure. Salt restriction is advisable in such cases. Excessive loss of potassium may result in muscular weakness and paralysis.

Effects on bones and joints. Reports of joint pains in patients given deoxycortone acetate alone: K. Kirkeby, *Acta med. scand.*, 1954, *149*, 43.

Hypertension. A 3-week-old child with the adrenogenital syndrome suffered permanent brain damage when hypertensive encephalopathy developed after the subcutaneous implantation of 6 pellets of deoxycortone acetate 125 mg.— J. A. Monteleone, *Pediatrics*, 1969, *43*, 294.

Uses. Deoxycortone is a mineralocorticoid secreted by the adrenal cortex and has the general properties of mineralocorticoids described under Corticosteroids (see p.451).

It has a pronounced effect on sodium retention and potassium excretion but no significant glucocorticoid action. It is destroyed in the gastro-intestinal tract and has only a feeble action when given by mouth.

Deoxycortone acetate has been used in the treatment of Addison's disease and other adrenocortical deficiency states as an adjunct to cortisone or hydrocortisone when these substances alone did not prevent the development of sodium deficiency. For this purpose, however, fludrocortisone given by mouth is now usually preferred.

Deoxycortone acetate is given as an oily intramuscular injection in a usual dose of 1 to 5 mg daily, or as an implant of about 100 to 400 mg every few months according to the patient's response.

Deoxycortone acetate has also been administered sublingually in doses of 2 to 10 mg daily.

Gangrene. For the use of deoxycortone acetate to induce hypertension in the treatment of gangrenous ulcers, see Fludrocortisone Acetate, p.470.

Hypoaldosteronism. A report of a patient with selective hypoaldosteronism whose hyperkalaemia was corrected by deoxycortone acetate 7.5 mg daily.— G. Perez *et al.*, *Ann. intern. Med.*, 1972, *76*, 757.

Preparations

Deoxycortone Acetate Implants *(B.P.)*. Deoxycort. Acet. Implants; Desoxycortone Acetate Pellets. Sterile cylinders prepared by fusion or heavy compression of deoxycortone acetate without the addition of any other substance, distributed singly in sterile containers which are sealed to exclude micro-organisms. Protect from light.

Deoxycortone Acetate Injection *(B.P.)*. Deoxycortone Acet. Inj.; Deoxycortone Injection. A sterile solution in ethyl oleate or other suitable ester, in a suitable fixed oil, or in any mixture of these; it may contain suitable alcohols. Protect from light. On standing, solid matter may separate and should be redissolved by heating before use. For intramuscular injection only.

Similar preparations are included in several pharmacopoeias.

Desoxycorticosterone Acetate Injection *(U.S.P.)*. A sterile solution of deoxycortone acetate in vegetable oil.

Desoxycorticosterone Acetate Pellets *(U.S.P.)*. Sterile implants of compressed deoxycortone acetate without the presence of any binder, diluent, or excipient. Store singly in sterile containers.

Injectabile Desoxicortoni *(Nord. P.)*. Deoxycortone acetate 500 mg, benzyl alcohol 5 g, arachis oil to 100 ml.

Proprietary Names

Cortexon Depot (enanthate) *(Schering, Arg.)*; Corticosterone *(Mitim, Ital.)*; Cortiron *(Schering, Ger.; Schering, Ital.; Schering, Spain)*; Cortiron Depot (enanthate) *(Schering, Ger.; Schering, Ital.)*; Cortisteril *(Ital Suisse, Ital.)*; Cortisteron *(Streuli, Switz.)*; Desoxykorton *(DAK, Denm.)*; Doca *(Organon, Neth.; Organon, Swed.)*; Doca Acetate *(Organon, USA)*; Leocortex *(Leo, Spain)*; Ormossurenol (glucoside) *(Galter, Ital.)*; Percorten *(Ciba, Canad.; Ciba, Spain; Ciba-Geigy, Switz.)*; Percorten Acetate *(Ciba, USA)*; Percorten Hidrosoluble (glucoside) *(Ciba, Spain)*; Percorten wasserlöslich (glucoside) *(Ciba, Ger.; Ciba-Geigy, Switz.)*; Syncorta *(Jap.)*; Syncortyl *(Roussel, Fr.)*.

Deoxycortone acetate was formerly marketed in Great Britain under the proprietary name Deoxycortone Acetate Implants (*Organon*).

1075-a

Deoxycortone Pivalate *(B.P.C. 1973)*.

Deoxycortone Trimethylacetate; Deoxycorticosterone Trimethylacetate; Desoxycorticosterone Trimethylacetate; Desoxycorticosterone Pivalate *(U.S.P.)*; Desoxycortone Pivalate. 21-Hydroxypregn-4-ene-3,20-dione 21-pivalate.
$C_{26}H_{38}O_4$=414.6.

CAS — 808-48-0.

Pharmacopoeias. In *U.S.*

A white or creamy-white, odourless or almost odourless, crystalline powder. M.p. 198° to 206°. Practically **insoluble** in water; soluble 1 in 350 to 500 of alcohol, 1 in 3 of chloroform, 1 in 60 of dioxan, and 1 in 160 of methyl alcohol; sparingly soluble in acetone; slightly soluble in ether and fixed oils. A solution in dioxan is dextrorotatory. **Protect** from light.

Adverse Effects and Precautions. See Deoxycortone Acetate, p.465.

Uses. Deoxycortone pivalate has similar properties and uses to those of deoxycortone acetate. It is administered by intramuscular injection as a suspension of a microcrystalline powder; as it is very slowly absorbed from the site of injection, the therapeutic effect is maintained for about 4 weeks or longer. The usual dose is 25 to 100 mg every 4 weeks.

Adrenal insufficiency. For the use of deoxycortone pivalate as part of a regimen for the management of a woman with Addison's disease who did not take her daily therapy, see Methylprednisolone Acetate, p.478.

Preparations

Deoxycortone Pivalate Injection *(B.P. 1963)*. Deoxycortone Trimethylacetate Injection. A sterile suspension of deoxycortone pivalate, in very fine particles, in Water for Injections containing suitable dispersing, stabilising, and buffering agents, pH 6 to 7. Store at room temperature. Protect from light.

Sterile Desoxycorticosterone Pivalate Suspension *(U.S.P.)*. A sterile suspension of deoxycortone pivalate in an aqueous vehicle. pH 5 to 7. Protect from light.

Percorten M Crystules *(Ciba, UK)*. Deoxycortone pivalate, available for injection as a suspension containing 25 mg per ml, in ampoules of 1 ml. (Also available as Percorten M in *Neth., Spain, Switz.*).

Other Proprietary Names

Percorten Pivalate *(USA)*; Percortene M *(Belg.)*.

1076-t

Desonide.

D2083; Desfluorotriamcinolone Acetonide; 16-Hydroxyprednisolone 16,17-Acetonide. 11β,21-Dihydroxy-16α, 17α-isopropylidenedioxypregna-1,4-diene-3,20-dione.
$C_{24}H_{32}O_6$=416.5.

CAS — 638-94-8.

Adverse Effects, Treatment, Withdrawal, and Precautions. As for Corticosteroids, p.446, p.449.

Absorption and Fate. For a brief outline of the absorption and fate of corticosteroids, see Corticosteroids, p.451.

When applied topically, particularly to large areas, when the skin is broken, or under occlusive dressings, corticosteroids may be absorbed in sufficient amounts to cause systemic effects.

Uses. Desonide is a synthetic corticosteroid used topically in the treatment of various skin disorders as described under Corticosteroids (see p.451). It is applied as a 0.05% cream or ointment.

Skin disorders. For recommendations concerning the correct use of corticosteroids on the skin, and a rough guide to the clinical potencies of topical corticosteroids, see Corticosteroids, p.458.

Proprietary Preparations

Tridesilon *(Dome/Hollister-Stier, UK).* Preparations containing desonide 0.05%, available as **Cream** [suggested diluent, Cetomacrogol Cream (Formula A or B) or Aqueous Cream] and as **Ointment** (suggested diluent, white soft paraffin). (Also available as Tridesilon in *Canad., Ger., USA*).

Other Proprietary Names

Apolar *(Norw., Swed.)*; Locapred *(Fr.)*; PR 100 *(pivalate)*, Prenacid *(sodium phosphate)*, Reticus *(all Ital.)*; Sine-Fluor *(Spain)*; Steroderm *(Ital.)*; Tridésonit *(Fr.)*.

1077-x

Desoxymethasone.

Desoximetasone *(U.S.P.)*; A41-304; Hoe 304; R-2113. 9α-Fluoro-11β,21-dihydroxy-16α-methylpregna-1,4-diene-3,20-dione. $C_{22}H_{29}FO_4$=376.5.

CAS — 382-67-2.

Pharmacopoeias. In *U.S.*

A white or almost white, odourless, crystalline powder. M.p. 208° to 218°. Practically **insoluble** in water; freely soluble in alcohol, acetone, and chloroform. A solution in chloroform is dextrorotatory.

Adverse Effects, Treatment, Withdrawal, and Precautions. As for Corticosteroids, p.446, p.449.

Adrenal suppression. Cushing's syndrome and hirsutism developed in a 45-year-old woman who used a topical corticosteroid cream containing 0.25% of desoxymethasone without occlusive dressings for 5 years to treat psoriasis. At the time of examination she applied about 30 g per day of the cream to extensive lesions. Within 4 months of discontinuation of use of the cream she had normal adrenal function and appearance.— T. Himathongkam *et al., J. Am. med. Ass.*, 1978, *239*, 430.

See also under Corticosteroids, p.446.

Absorption and Fate. For a brief outline of the absorption and fate of corticosteroids, see Corticosteroids, p.451.

When applied topically, particularly to large areas, when the skin is broken, or under occlusive dressings, corticosteroids may be absorbed in sufficient amounts to cause systemic effects.

Uses. Desoxymethasone is a synthetic corticosteroid used in the treatment of various skin disorders as described under Corticosteroids (see p.451). It is applied topically as a 0.05% and a 0.25% cream.

Skin disorders. Reviews of desoxymethasone: *Med. Lett.*, 1977, *19*, 85; R. C. Heel *et al., Drugs*, 1978, *16*, 302.

For recommendations concerning the correct use of corticosteroids on the skin, and a rough guide to the clinical potencies of topical corticosteroids, see Corticosteroids, p.458.

Preparations

Desoximetasone Cream *(U.S.P.).* Contains desoxymethasone in an emollient cream basis. Store at 15° to 30°.

Proprietary Names

Actiderm *(Hoechst, Arg.)*; Flubason *(Albert-Farma, Ital.)*; Ibaril *(Hoechst, Belg.; Hoechst, Denm.; Hoechst, Neth.; Hoechst, Norw.; Hoechst, Swed.)*; Topicorete *(Roussel, Belg.)*; Topicort *(Hoechst, Canad.; Hoechst, USA)*; Topicorte *(Roussel, Fr.; Roussel, Neth.)*; Topiderm *(Roussel-Amor Gil, Spain)*; Topisolon *(Cassella-Riedel, Ger.; Hoechst, S.Afr.; Hoechst, Switz.)*.

1078-r

Dexamethasone

(B.P., B.P. Vet., Eur. P., U.S.P.). Dexameth.; Dexamethasonum; Desamethasone; Dexametasona; 9α-Fluoro-16α-methylprednisolone. 9α-Fluoro-11β,17α,21-trihydroxy-16α-methylpregna-1,4-diene-3,20-dione. $C_{22}H_{29}FO_5$=392.5.

CAS — 50-02-2.

Pharmacopoeias. In *Br., Braz., Cz., Eur., Fr., Ger., Int., It., Jap., Jug., Neth., Roum., Swiss, Turk.*, and *U.S.*

A white or almost white odourless crystalline powder with a slightly bitter taste. M.p. about 250° to 253° with decomposition.

Practically **insoluble** in water; soluble 1 in 42 of alcohol and 1 in 165 of chloroform; sparingly soluble in acetone, dioxan, and methyl alcohol; very slightly soluble in ether. A solution in dioxan is dextrorotatory. **Protect** from light.

When applied topically, the penetration of dexamethasone alcohol through stripped skin was 7 times greater from gelled isopropyl myristate than from soft paraffin.— R. E. Dempski *et al., J. pharm. Sci.*, 1969, *58*, 579.

Stability. Oxidation of the ketol side-chain of dexamethasone was reported to occur in the presence of a base catalyst. Tablets stored at elevated temperatures lost potency, and high relative humidities had very severe effects. Even in the best formulation, containing dexamethasone 500 µg, lactose 88 mg, starch 15 mg, talc 3 mg, magnesium stearate 1.5 mg, and granulated with 20% povidone in alcohol, dexamethasone had a half-life of 542 days at 25° and 60% relative humidity.— S. K. Wahba *et al., J. pharm. Sci.*, 1968, *57*, 1231.

Adverse Effects and Treatment. As for Corticosteroids, p.446 and p.449.

It has little or no effect on sodium and water retention.

There have been reports of joint damage following the intra-articular injection of corticosteroids into load-bearing joints (see under Corticosteroids, p.447).

Prolonged application to the eye of preparations containing corticosteroids has caused increased intra-ocular pressure and reduced visual function.

Adrenal suppression. Reports of adrenal suppression associated with dexamethasone nasal sprays: M. I. Michels *et al., Ann. Allergy*, 1967, *25*, 569; P. K. Champion, *Archs intern. Med.*, 1974, *134*, 750.

See also under Abuse and Misuse (below).

Reports of adrenal suppression associated with dexamethasone eye-drops: P. G. Burch and C. J. Migeon, *Archs Ophthal., N.Y.*, 1968, *79*, 174; K. H. Musson and D. B. Sloan, *J. Pediat. Ophthal.*, 1968, *5*, 33; T. Krupin *et al., Archs Ophthal., N.Y.*, 1976, *94*, 919. For a report of the death of an infant following ocular use of triamcinolone acetonide and dexamethasone sodium phosphate, see Triamcinolone Acetonide, p.484.

Candidiasis. Oropharyngeal candidiasis associated with dexamethasone aerosol inhalation.— M. Dennis and I. H. Itkin, *J. Allergy*, 1964, *35*, 70.

Effects on the eyes. Reports of raised intra-ocular pressure associated with the use of dexamethasone eye-drops: D. O. Crompton, *Med. J. Aust.*, 1966, *1*, 899; G. L. Spaeth, *Archs Ophthal., N.Y.*, 1967, *78*, 714; M. F. Armaly, *Archs Ophthal., N.Y.*, 1967, *78*, 193; J. L. Baum and R. Z. Levene, *Archs Ophthal., N.Y.*, 1968, *79*, 366.

Effects on muscles. Severe myopathy, with bilateral quadriceps wasting, and abdominal bloating, occurred in a man of 58 treated for bronchial asthma with dexamethasone 2.25 mg daily for 11 weeks. The muscle weakness resolved after the substitution of prednisone. In another patient, myopathic changes followed the use of dexamethasone 2 mg daily for 15 months.— D. N. Golding and T. B. Begg, *Br. med. J.*, 1960, *2*, 1129.

Withdrawal and Precautions. As for Corticosteroids, p.449.

Abuse and misuse. Cushing's syndrome developed in a 45-year-old woman who had been using a nasal spray containing dexamethasone (4.5 mg per container) at the rate of one or two containers daily.— L. D. Ortega and R. G. Grande (letter), *Lancet*, 1979, *2*, 96.

Interactions. For references to deterioration of cerebral oedema in patients given phenytoin in addition to dexamethasone, see Corticosteroids, p.450.

Interference with diagnostic tests. 'Decadron' injection included creatinine 8 mg per ml as a solubilising agent and could therefore interfere with serum-creatinine measurements.— M. L. Rogers and C. W. Barrett, *Adverse Drug React. Bull.*, 1974, Aug., 156.

Withdrawal. For references to leuco-erythroblastosis following dexamethasone withdrawal, see Corticosteroids, p.449.

Absorption and Fate. For a brief outline of the absorption and fate of corticosteroids, see Corticosteroids, p.451.

Dexamethasone is readily absorbed from the gastro-intestinal tract. Its biological half-life in plasma is about 190 minutes. Binding of dexamethasone to plasma proteins is less than for most other corticosteroids.

Bioavailability of dexamethasone.— D. E. Duggan *et al., Clin. Pharmac. Ther.*, 1975, *18*, 205. Bioavailability of dexamethasone phosphate.— L. E. Hare *et al., ibid.*, 330.

Further references: J. C. Melby and S. L. Dale, *Clin. Pharmac. Ther.*, 1969, *10*, 344 (dexamethasone phosphate and dexamethasone acetate).

Uses. Dexamethasone is a synthetic glucocorticoid and has the general properties described under Corticosteroids (see p.451); 750 µg of dexamethasone is equivalent in anti-inflammatory activity to about 5 mg of prednisolone.

It has been used in the treatment of all conditions for which corticosteroid therapy is indicated except adrenal-deficiency states for which its lack of sodium-retaining properties make it less suitable than cortisone or hydrocortisone with supplementary fludrocortisone. It is one of the corticosteroids used for the prevention of the neonatal respiratory distress syndrome, and is also used to reduce raised intracranial pressure.

Being a potent pituitary suppressant it is used in the diagnosis of Cushing's syndrome.

Dexamethasone has a usual dose range of 0.5 to 9 mg daily in divided doses.

Cancer chemotherapy. In a study of 17 adults with previously untreated acute lymphocytic leukaemia, use of dexamethasone instead of prednisone in the combination chemotherapy regimen did not reduce the risk of serious infection nor the incidence of meningeal leukaemia.— A. C. Smyth and P. H. Wiernik, *Clin. Pharmac. Ther.*, 1976, *19*, 240.

Croup. For reference to the use of dexamethasone in croup, see under Uses of Corticosteroids (Epiglottis, Laryngitis and Croup), p.453.

Cerebral malaria. Despite some reports of patients with cerebral malaria benefitting from dexamethasone, a double-blind study involving 100 comatose patients with cerebral malaria showed that dexamethasone provided no benefit, prolonged the coma, and increased the incidence of complications.— D. A. Warrell *et al., New Engl. J. Med.*, 1982, *306*, 313. See also R. A. Fishman, *ibid.*, 359.

For references to the use of dexamethasone in other infections associated with raised intracranial pressure, see under Uses of Corticosteroids (Infections), p.454.

Dexamethasone suppression tests. Following a 24-hour collection of urine as a control, dexamethasone 500 µg was given by mouth every 6 hours for 8 doses, then 2 mg every 6 hours for a further 8 doses, and 24-hour urine collections were made. In normal subjects the dexamethasone suppressed corticotrophin secretion by the pituitary with a consequent fall in hydrocortisone production and excretion. In patients with Cushing's syndrome urinary 17-hydroxycorticosteroids were not suppressed by the lower dose. In patients with adrenal cortical hyperplasia but not in those with adrenal tumour, the higher dose suppressed 17-hydroxycorticosteroid excretion.— G. W. Liddle, *J. clin. Endocr. Metab.*, 1960, *20*, 1539. A comparison of the dexamethasone suppression test in 21 patients with Cushing's syndrome, 27 obese patients, and 18 with hirsutism. The most useful criteria for confirming a diagnosis of Cushing's syndrome were a midnight basal 11-hydroxycorticosteroid concentration in excess of 80 ng per ml, a basal 24-hour excretion of 11-hydroxycorticosteroids in excess of 320 µg, and failure of suppression by 2-mg doses of dexamethasone of morning plasma concentrations of 11-hydroxycorticosteroids to less than 60 ng per ml.— D. Mattingly and C. Tyler, *Br. med. J.*, 1972, *3*, 17. The dexamethasone suppression test for the diagnosis of hypercortisolaemic states is considered to be preferable to the assay of urinary free corticosteroid excretion in the presence of abnormal renal function.— J. Gilliland and P. J. Phillips, *J. clin. Path.*, 1978, *31*, 671.

In patients with Cushing's disease a dose of 8 mg of dexamethasone daily usually suppressed the abnormal urinary excretion of 17-hydroxycorticosteroids but in 3 patients with pituitary corticotrophin hypersecretion up to 32 mg daily had been needed for a suppressant effect.— J. E. Linn *et al.*, *New Engl. J. Med.*, 1967, *277*, 403. A 30-year-old woman with Cushing's disease showed no suppression of cortisol secretion with the standard high-dose (up to 8 mg per day) dexamethasone test described by G.W. Liddle (*J. clin. Endocr. Metab.*, 1960, *20*, 1539). Further studies with doses of dexamethasone ranging from 8 to 32 mg daily demonstrated that she metabolised dexamethasone normally but corticotrophin and cortisol secretion were not suppressed. However, exogenous hydrocortisone did have a suppressant effect on corticotrophin secretion and it appears that in this patient the hypothalamic-pituitary-adrenal feedback mechanism failed to recognise dexamethasone as a suppressant corticosteroid.— R. M. Carey, *New Engl. J. Med.*, 1980, *302*, 275. Criticism of the interpretation of these results.— J. Wortsman and J. H. Blank (letter), *ibid.*, *303*, 340; A. W. Meikle *et al.* (letter), *ibid.* Reply.— R. M. Carey (letter), *ibid.*

A dose of dexamethasone, 2 mg by mouth, given between 11.30 pm and midnight, produced a fall of at least 70%, to less than 65 ng per ml, in the plasma-hydrocortisone concentration in normal and obese subjects. In 9 patients with Cushing's syndrome, the plasma hydrocortisone fell to not less than 130 ng per ml.— S. McHardy-Young *et al.*, *Br. med. J.*, 1967, *2*, 740. By a similar method to that used by McHardy-Young it was shown that though normal subjects and most hospital out-patients responded to the test as expected, hospital in-patients did not show a consistent response, possibly due to the disturbance of their diurnal hydrocortisone rhythm by 'hospital stress'.— C. K. Connolly *et al.*, *Br. med. J.*, 1968, *2*, 665.

Dexamethasone failed to produce the expected depression of plasma-hydrocortisone concentration when given to 7 patients who were receiving phenytoin 300 to 400 mg daily. Phenytoin caused less interference with the urinary 17-hydroxycorticosteroid suppression test.— E. E. Werk *et al.*, *New Engl. J. Med.*, 1969, *281*, 32. See also under Precautions for Corticosteroids, p.450.

Dexamethasone 9 mg daily for 2 days was used in 17 patients to suppress plasma-growth hormone concentrations in the differential diagnosis of 2 types of acromegaly. Phentolamine was also used for a suppression test.— K. Nakagawa and K. Mashimo, *J. clin. Endocr. Metab.*, 1973, *37*, 238. See also K. Nakagawa *et al.*, *J. clin. Endocr. Metab.*, 1970, *31*, 502.

Further references: O. Rorstad *et al.*, *Can. med. Ass. J.*, 1976, *115*, 878 (variation according to course of disease); G. F. Oxenkrug (letter), *Lancet*, 1978, *2*, 795 (alcoholism).

Depression. For the potential role of dexamethasone suppression tests in monitoring antidepressant therapy, see Antidepressants, p.110.

Diabetic retinopathy. Dexamethasone-induced corticosteroid glaucoma was used to retard diabetic retinopathy. There was improvement of vision in 38% of the eyes.— J. P. Gills and W. B. Anderson, *Archs intern. Med.*, 1969, *123*, 626. Cataracts in the treated eyes of diabetics given topical dexamethasone for retinopathy. Diabetics were considered to be susceptible to this side-effect.— M. E. Yablonski *et al.*, *Archs Ophthal.*, *N.Y.*, 1978, *96*, 474.

Electroconvulsive therapy. Uncontrolled studies suggesting that intramuscular administration of dexamethasone 4 mg two hours before and two hours after ECT may prevent residual confusion or amnesia. The dexamethasone had no effect on the temporary acute amnesia that is common immediately after ECT.— *J. Am. med. Ass.*, 1979, *241*, 2695.

Hypertension. A father and son with benign hypertension, increased aldosterone secretion, and low plasma-renin activity, not due to adrenocortical tumour or Conn's syndrome, were treated with dexamethasone 2 mg daily. Abnormal symptoms were removed and it was suggested that similar patients be given a trial with dexamethasone before undergoing adrenal surgery.— D. J. A. Sutherland *et al.*, *Can. med. Ass. J.* 1966, *95*, 1109.

A suggestion that in patients with malignant hypertension, dexamethasone should be given before lowering their blood pressure, in an attempt to avoid precipitating blindness.— J. S. Pryor *et al.* (letter), *lancet*, 1979, *2*, 803.

Hirsutism. Unbound testosterone concentrations were consistently elevated in 32 hirsute women. When concentrations were suppressed to normal by dexamethasone 0.5 to 1 mg at night hirsutism was generally improved or ceased to progress after 8 to 10 months of treatment.— J. D. Paulson *et al.*, *Am. J. Obstet. Gynec.*, 1977, *128*, 851.

Further studies on dexamethasone and hirsutism: G. E. Abraham *et al.*, *Obstet. Gynec.*, 1976, *47*, 395; M. H. Kim *et al.*, *Am. J. Obstet. Gynec.*, 1976, *126*, 982; H. L. Judd *et al.*, *ibid.*, 1977, *128*, 408.

Insulin lipoatrophy. A 47-year-old woman had marked lipoatrophy after subcutaneous injections of isophane insulin for 5 months; the addition of dexamethasone to insulin injection resulted in the return of subcutaneous fatty tissue after 8 months.— T. H. Whitley *et al.*, *Curr. ther. Res.*, 1976, *235*, 839. See also D. Kumar *et al.*, *Diabetes*, 1977, *26*, 296.

Postoperative adhesions. For the prevention of postoperative intestinal adhesions, dexamethasone and promethazine were given to 81 patients. The results were very satisfactory.— R. L. Replogle *et al.*, *Ann. Surg.*, 1966, *163*, 580. See also *idem*, *J. Am. med. Ass.*, 1967, *201* (July 3), A32.

Pregnancy and the neonate. For reference to the use of dexamethasone in the respiratory distress syndrome, see Betamethasone, p.461.

Raised intracranial pressure. Asphyxia and cerebral oedema, caused by hanging, in 2 children was successfully treated by the administration of dexamethasone sodium phosphate, 10 mg intravenously then 4 mg intramuscularly every 6 hours, together with oxygen and an infusion of 6% dextran.— J. H. Salmon, *J. Am. med. Ass.*, 1967, *201*, 204. Dexamethasone, 4 mg by intramuscular injection every 6 hours, was successfully used to treat the cerebral oedema which resulted from oxygen deprivation occurring in a man found drowning.— C. Toland, *Br. J. Anaesth.*, 1972, *44*, 616.

Acute irradiation encephalopathy, which developed in a 49-year-old leukaemic man following skull irradiation, resolved within 48 hours of giving dexamethasone 4 mg intravenously four times daily. He was subsequently given dexamethasone 4 mg four times daily for the remainder of the course. Prophylactic administration of dexamethasone might prevent or minimise acute encephalopathy during cranial irradiation.— O. Shalev and R. Silverberg (letter), *Lancet*, 1978, *2*, 574.

Cerebral tumours. Five of 8 patients suffering from metastatic brain tumours treated with dexamethasone 16 mg intramuscularly daily in 4 divided doses (except 1 patient who received 24 mg daily) obtained complete clearing of their neurological defects, and a further 2 were greatly benefited. Improvement was associated with reduction of raised spinal fluid protein and angiographic evidence of resolution of cerebral oedema.— J. D. Weinstein *et al.*, *Neurology, Minneap.*, 1973, *23*, 121. See also B. M. Frier and J. B. McConnell, *Br. med. J.*, 1975, *3*, 208; J. W. Fletcher *et al.*, *J. Am. med. Ass.*, 1975, *232*, 1261; H. J. Ruelen, *Br. J. Anaesth.*, 1976, *48*, 741; A. Lieberman *et al.*, *J. Neurol. Neurosurg. Psychiat.*, 1977, *40*, 678; L. F. Marshall *et al.*, *Ann. Neurol.*, 1977, *1*, 201.

For interactions between dexamethasone and anticonvulsants in patients with cerebral tumours, see under Precautions for Corticosteroids (Interactions), p.450.

Head injuries. Disappointing results with both high- and low-dose dexamethasone in the management of severe head injuries.— P. R. Cooper *et al.*, *J. Neurosurg.*, 1979, *51*, 307. See also S. K. Gudeman *et al.*, *ibid.*, 301 (methylprednisolone).

Further references: H. E. James *et al.*, *Acta Neurochir.*, 1979, *45*, 225 (beneficial results with high-dose dexamethasone).

Rhinitis. Beneficial results with dexamethasone snuff in severe chronic rhinitis.— M. K. McAllen and M. J. S. Langman, *Lancet*, 1969, *1*, 968.

Further references: Drug Committee of the Research Council of the American Academy of Allergy, *J. Allergy*, 1968, *41*, 10.

Sickle-cell anaemia. Administration of dexamethasone 2 mg every 6 hours to 2 siblings with sickle-cell anaemia causes subsidence of symptoms of a crisis within 48 hours. The drug is then tapered off over 3 to 7 days depending on the symptoms. Dexamethasone appears not only to reverse the symptoms but also to decrease the number of crises. Experience with a third sibling, who requires periodic transfusions, has been less good.— B. Robinson (letter), *Lancet*, 1979, *1*, 1088. The use of steroid hormones has been associated with venous thrombosis and may be contra-indicated. Nevertheless, properly controlled studies are indicated.— A. J. Bennett and F. Rosner (letter), *ibid.*, *2*, 474. *In vitro* studies on the blood of 3 patients with homozygous sickle-cell disease indicated that dexamethasone has no effect at the red blood cell level.— I. M. Franklin and D. C. Linch (letter), *ibid.*, 645.

Stroke. In a double-blind study in 118 patients with acute stroke (first episode, treated within 48 hours, not considered due to tumour, injury, or subarachnoid haemorrhage) there was no difference in survival or the grades of disability between those treated with dexamethasone or those treated with a placebo.— G. Mulley *et al.*, *Br. med. J.*, 1978, *2*, 994. Criticism and the view that whether dexamethasone is of value in selected cases of acute cerebral infarction has yet to be determined.— F. C. Rose *et al.* (letter), *ibid.*, 1979, *1*, 55. Further comments and criticisms: A. C. Young (letter), *ibid.*, 1978, *2*, 1230; E. G. McQueen (letter), *ibid.*; J. Freeman *et al.* (letter), *ibid.*, 1500; G. Parsons-Smith (letter), *ibid.*, 1640; R. A. Blattel (letter), *ibid.*, 1641; J. W. Norris (letter), *ibid.*, 1979, *1*, 56.

Further studies on the role of dexamethasone in stroke: L. Candelise and H. Spinnler (letter), *Med. J. Aust.*, 1972, *2*, 335; M. Kaste *et al.*, *Br. med. J.*, 1976, *2*, 1409; J. W. Norris, *Archs Neurol., Chicago*, 1976, *33*, 69.

Test for glaucoma. A description of the use of dexamethasone 0.1% eye-drops to detect open-angle glaucoma.— D. A. Leighton and C. I. Phillips, *Br. J. Ophthal.*, 1970, *54*, 27.

Preparations

Aerosols

Dexamethasone Topical Aerosol *(U.S.P.)*. Dexamethasone Aerosol. Dexamethasone in a suitable lotion basis mixed with suitable propellents in a pressurised container. Store at a temperature not exceeding 40°.

Elixirs

Dexamethasone Elixir *(U.S.P.)*. An elixir containing dexamethasone; it contains 3.8 to 5.7% of alcohol. Store in airtight containers.

Gels

Dexamethasone Gel *(U.S.P.)*. A gel containing dexamethasone. Store at a temperature not exceeding 30° in airtight containers.

Ophthalmic Suspensions

Dexamethasone Ophthalmic Suspension *(U.S.P.)*. A sterile aqueous suspension of dexamethasone containing a suitable antimicrobial preservative; it may contain suitable buffers, stabilising, suspending, and viscosity agents. pH 5 to 6. Store in airtight containers.

Tablets

Dexamethasone Tablets *(B.P.)*. Dexameth. Tab. Tablets containing dexamethasone. Protect from light.

Dexamethasone Tablets *(U.S.P.)*. Tablets containing dexamethasone. The *U.S.P.* requires 70% dissolution in 45 minutes.

Proprietary Preparations

Decadron *(Merck Sharp & Dohme, UK)*. Dexamethasone, available as scored tablets of 500 µg. **Decadron-75**. Dexamethasone, available as scored tablets of 750 µg. (Also available as Decadron in *Arg., Austral., Canad., Denm., Fr., Ger., Ital., Neth., Norw., S.Afr., Swed., Switz., USA*).

Dexacortisyl *(Roussel, UK)*. Dexamethasone, available as scored tablets of 500 µg.

Maxidex *(Alcon, UK: Farillon, UK)*. Eye-drops containing dexamethasone 0.1% and hypromellose 0.5%. (Also available as Maxidex in *Austral., Belg., Canad., Denm., Fr., Neth., S.Afr., Switz.*).

Oradexon-Organon Tablets *(Organon, UK)*. Tablets each containing dexamethasone 500 µg or 2 mg. (Also available as Oradexon in *Austral., Belg., Neth., S.Afr., Spain*).

Other Proprietary Names

Arg.— Dexametosona, Dexa-Scherosana *(also as sodium hydrogen sulphate)*; *Austral.*— Dexmethsone; *Belg.*— Aacidexam *(see also under Dexamethasone Sodium Phosphate)*; *Canad.*— Dexasone, Hexadrol *(see also under Dexamethasone Sodium Phosphate)*; *Ger.*— Cortisumman, Dexalocal, Dexamed *(see also under Dexamethasone Sodium Phosphate and Dexamphetamine Sulphate)*, Dexa-sine, Fortecortin *(see also under Dexamethasone Acetate and Dexamethasone Sodium Phosphate)*, Millicorten, Predni-F, Sokarol; *Ital.*— Decasterolone, Decofluor, Dekacort, Dermadex *(valerate)*, Dermax, Desacort, Desacortone, Desalark *(see also under Dexamethasone Sodium Phosphate)*, Desaval *(valerate)*, Deseronil, Dinormon, Esacortene, Exadion, Firmalone, Fluormone, Fluorocort, Fluorodelta, Fortecortin *(see also under Dexamethasone Acetate and Dexamethasone*

Sodium Phosphate), Luxazone, Methazon-Ion, Topolyn (linoleate), Visumetazone; *Jap.*— Carulon, Corson, Decaderm, Decadrone, Dectan, Dethamedin, Dexamam-allett, Metasolon, Moco, Orgadrone, Sawasone, Sunia Sol-D; *Norw.*— Isopto-Maxidex; *S.Afr.*— Spersadex; *Spain*— Decadeltosona, Decadran (see also under Dexamethasone Sodium Phosphate), Dexa-Aldon, Dexa-Life, Dexa-Scherosona (as sodium hydrogen sulphate), Dexa-Wolner (see also under Dexamethasone Sodium Metasulphobenzoate), Dexafarma, Dexametaluy, Dexamiso, Dexanteric, Dexasan, Falban, Fortecortin (see also under Dexamethasone Acetate and Dexamethasone Sodium Phosphate), Millicorten, Moderix, Solone (see also under Dexamethasone Sodium Phosphate and Prednisolone); *Swed.*— Decacort, Dexacortal, Isopto-Maxidex; *Switz.*— Dexacortin (see also under Dexamethasone Sodium Metasulphobenzoate), Dexalocal, Dexamecortin, Dexa-Rhinosan, Grosodexon, Mephameson, Millicorten; *USA*— Aeroseb-Dex, Decaderm, Decalix, Decaspray, Dexone, Dezone (see also under Dexamethasone Sodium Phosphate), Hexadrol (see also under Dexamethasone Sodium Phosphate), Miral, SK-Dexamethasone.

A preparation containing dexamethasone was also formerly marketed in Great Britain under the proprietary name Decaspray (*Merck Sharp & Dohme*).

1079-f

Dexamethasone Acetate (*B.P. 1963*). Dexameth. Acet.; Dexamethasoni Acetas. Dexamethasone 21-acetate.

$C_{24}H_{31}FO_6$=434.5.

CAS — 1177-87-3 (anhydrous); 55812-90-3 (monohydrate).

Pharmacopoeias. In *Chin.* and *Int. U.S.* includes the monohydrate.

A white or almost white odourless powder. M.p. about 225° with decomposition. Dexamethasone acetate 1.1 mg is approximately equivalent to 1 mg of dexamethasone. Practically **insoluble** in water; soluble 1 in 40 of alcohol, 1 in 25 of dehydrated alcohol, 1 in 33 of chlorform, and 1 in 1000 of ether; freely soluble in acetone, methyl alcohol, and dioxan. A solution in dioxan is dextrorotatory. **Protect** from light.

Uses. Dexamethasone acetate has the same actions and uses as dexamethasone. It is used in ointments containing 0.1 or 0.25% for skin disorders. Capsules containing dexamethasone acetate are used as an insufflation in the palliative treatment of chronic rhinitis; one capsule is used by insufflation daily in 4 divided doses. It has also been given as tablets by mouth, in doses of 0.5 to 10 mg daily in divided doses. The suspension has been given by intramuscular or intralesional injections.

Preparations

Sterile Dexamethasone Acetate Suspension (*U.S.P.*). A sterile suspension of dexamethasone acetate monohydrate in Water for Injections. Potency is expressed in terms of the equivalent amount of dexamethasone. pH 5 to 7.5. Protect from light.

Dexamethasone Acetate Insufflation Capsules (*Paines & Byrne, UK*). Each contains dexamethasone acetate 500 µg in a basis of lactose. For chronic rhinitis. *Dose.* The contents of 1 capsule daily to be inhaled in 4 equal parts.

Other Proprietary Names

Arg.—Decadron AL; *Austral.*— Dexacortisyl; *Fr.*— Acidocort, Dectancyl; *Ger.*— Fortecortin (see also under Dexamethasone and Dexamethasone Sodium Phosphate); *Jap.*— Decadron-A; *Neth.*— Decadron Depot; *Spain*— Decasterolone, Decoderm (see also under Fluprednidene Acetate), Deronil; *USA*— Decadron-LA, Dexacen-La-8.

1080-z

Dexamethasone Isonicotinate. Dexamethasone 21-isonicotinate.

$C_{28}H_{32}FNO_6$=497.6.

CAS — 2265-64-7.

Dexamethasone isonicotinate 1.3 mg is approximately equivalent to 1 mg of dexamethasone.

Uses. Dexamethasone isonicotinate has the actions and uses of dexamethasone. It is used by inhalation similarly to beclomethasone dipropionate (p.460) for the prophylaxis of the symptoms of asthma. It is also used in a nasal spray, and has been given by mouth as tablets and intramuscularly as a long-acting injection.

Results of a crossover study in 8 asthmatic patients indicated that dexamethasone isonicotinate is as effective as beclomethasone dipropionate in the management of asthma. Six patients inhaled dexamethasone isonicotinate 125 µg four times daily and beclomethasone dipropionate 50 µg four times daily, and 2 patients used double these amounts.— Y. Salorinne and L. Klemetti, *IRCS Med. Sci.*, 1979, *7*, 109. See also A. Biedermann, *Wien. med. Wschr.*, 1971, *121*, 331.

Proprietary Preparations

Dexamethasone isonicotinate is an ingredient of Dexa-Rhinaspray, p.33.

Proprietary Names

Auxilosan (*Thomae, Ger.*); Auxison (*Boehringer Sohn, Switz.*); Auxisone (*Boehringer Ingelheim, Belg.*; *Badrial, Fr.*); Azoman (*Boehringer Sohn, Arg.*).

1081-c

Dexamethasone Phenpropionate. Dexamethasone Phenylpropionate. Dexamethasone 21-(3-phenylpropionate).

$C_{31}H_{37}FO_6$=524.6.

CAS — 1879-72-7.

Dexamethasone phenpropionate 1.34 mg is approximately equivalent to 1 mg of dexamethasone.

Uses. Dexamethasone phenpropionate has the general properties of dexamethasone (p.466). It is used in veterinary practice as a long-acting intramuscular injection.

1082-k

Dexamethasone Pivalate. Dexamethasone Trimethylacetate. Dexamethasone 21-pivalate.

$C_{27}H_{37}FO_6$=476.6.

CAS — 1926-94-9.

Dexamethasone pivalate 1.18 mg is approximately equivalent to 1 mg of dexamethasone.

Uses. Dexamethasone pivalate has the general properties of dexamethasone (p.466). It is used in veterinary practice as an intramuscular and an intra-articular injection.

Proprietary Names

Exosterol (*Zyma, Switz.*).

1083-a

Dexamethasone Sodium Metasulphobenzoate. Dexamethasone 21-(sodium *m*-sulphobenzoate).

$C_{29}H_{32}FNaO_9S$=598.6.

CAS — 3936-02-5.

A white crystalline powder. Dexamethasone sodium metasulphobenzoate 1.5 mg is approximately equivalent to 1 mg of dexamethasone. **Soluble** in water; sparingly soluble in acetone and ether.

Dexamethasone sodium metasulphobenzoate has general properties similar to those of dexamethasone (p.466).

Proprietary Preparations

Dexamethasone sodium metasulphobenzoate is an ingredient of Sofradex, p.1166.

Proprietary Names

Dexacortin (see also under Dexamethasone) (*Streuli, Switz.*); Dexa-sol (*Roussel, Belg.*); Dexa-Wolner (see also under Dexamethasone) (*Wolner, Spain*); Hubersona (*Hubber, Spain*); Selftison-F (*Jap.*).

1084-t

Dexamethasone Sodium Phosphate (*B.P., B.P. Vet., U.S.P.*).

Dexamethasonis Natrii Phosphas; Dexamethasone Phosphate Sodium; Fosfato Sódico de Dexametasona; Sodium Dexamethasone Phosphate; Sodium 9α-Fluoro-16α-methylprednisolone 21-Phosphate. Dexamethasone 21-(disodium phosphate).

$C_{22}H_{28}FNa_2O_8P$=516.4.

CAS — 2392-39-4.

Pharmacopoeias. In *Br.*, *Braz.*, *Chin.*, *Jug.*, and *U.S.*

A white or slightly yellow, very hygroscopic, crystalline powder; odourless or with a slight odour of alcohol. It may contain up to 8% of alcohol and up to 16% of alcohol and water. Dexamethasone sodium phosphate 1.3 mg is approximately equivalent to 1 mg of dexamethasone and 1.1 mg of dexamethasone sodium phosphate is approximately equivalent to 1 mg of dexamethasone phosphate.

Soluble 1 in 2 of water, sparingly soluble in dehydrated alcohol; practically insoluble in chloroform and ether; very slightly soluble in dioxan. A 1% solution in water is dextrorotatory and has a pH of 7.5 to 10.5. A 6.75% solution is iso-osmotic with serum. Solutions for injection are **sterilised** by filtration. **Store** in airtight containers. Protect from light.

Contamination. A commercial sample of dexamethasone sodium phosphate solution for injection was found to contain 56% of the labelled concentration and to be extensively contaminated with a white insoluble solid.— E. C. Juenge and J. F. Brower, *J. pharm. Sci.*, 1979, *68*, 551.

Incompatibility. Particulate matter was observed within 2 hours when 1 ml of commercial dexamethasone sodium phosphate injection was mixed with 5 ml of sterile water and 1 ml of commercial injection solution of either prochlorperazine edisylate or vancomycin hydrochloride.— R. Misgen, *Am. J. Hosp. Pharm.*, 1965, *22*, 92. A similar report.— J. A. Patel and G. L. Phillips, *ibid.*, 1966, *23*, 409.

A study on the interaction between dexamethasone sodium phosphate and polymyxin B sulphate in ophthalmic preparations, and the stabilising effect of citrate and phosphate buffers.— M. Aggag and S. A. H. Khahil, *Mfg Chem.*, 1977, *48*, (Dec.), 43.

Adverse Effects and Treatment. See Dexamethasone, p.466. Cardiovascular collapse has been reported following the rapid intravenous injection of large doses of corticosteroids.

A single dose of dexamethasone sodium phosphate 2 mg per kg body-weight given by intravenous infusion at various rates to 30 healthy subjects in a double-blind controlled study produced temporary itching, burning, or tingling, which was most intense in the ano-genital region, in all subjects given the infusion over 2 minutes. This effect was less frequent when the duration of administration was prolonged. Laboratory studies showed no untoward results apart from the expected hyperglycaemic effect.— A. W. Czerwinski *et al.*, *Clin. Pharmac. Ther.*, 1972, *13*, 638.

Effects on the heart. Dexamethasone sodium phosphate 100 mg was administered intravenously to a 43-year-old woman after aortic and mitral valve replacement. Frequent premature ventricular contractions occurred immediately; they were controlled with an intravenous injection of lignocaine. When further doses of dexamethasone were administered severe arrhythmias recurred. These effects might be due to the speed of injection or to the presence of preservatives.— G. B. Schmidt *et al.*, *J. Am. med. Ass.*, 1972, *221*, 1402. Arrhythmias might be caused by hypokalaemia induced by dexamethasone and prophylaxis with potassium chloride in doses of up to 150 mmol (150 mEq) daily could prevent their occurrence.— G. Rao *et al.* (letter), *ibid.*, 1972, *222*, 1185.

Withdrawal and Precautions. As for Corticosteroids, p.449.

Uses. Dexamethasone sodium phosphate has the general properties and uses of dexamethasone (p.466).

It is given by intramuscular or intravenous injection for intensive therapy or in emergencies. Intravenous doses of the equivalent of 2 to 6 mg of dexamethasone phosphate per kg body-weight given slowly over a minimum period of several minutes have been recommended for the treatment of severe Gram-negative septic shock in an attempt to promote rapid vasodilation. These high doses may be repeated within 2 to 6 hours and this treatment should be continued only until the patient's condition is stable and usually for no longer than 48 to 72 hours.

It is used in the treatment of cerebral oedema

caused by anoxia or malignancy. An initial intravenous dose of the equivalent of 10 mg is usually given followed by 4 mg intramuscularly every 6 hours; a response is usually obtained after 12 to 24 hours and dosage may be reduced after 2 to 4 days, and gradually discontinued over 5 to 7 days; those with cerebral malignancy may require maintenance therapy with doses of 2 mg twice or thrice daily. In comatose patients with cerebral oedema due to acute falciparum malaria, dexamethasone sodium phosphate should be given in a dose equivalent to 3 to 10 mg of dexamethasone phosphate every 8 hours.

For intravenous infusion dexamethasone sodium phosphate may be diluted with an appropriate volume of dextrose injection or sodium chloride injection. It is also injected intra-articularly and has been inhaled as an aerosol nasal spray in the treatment of allergic rhinitis. It is used as an ointment or as a solution in the treatment of eye disorders and as a cream in the treatment of skin disorders.

Preparations

Dexamethasone Sodium Phosphate Cream *(U.S.P.)*. A cream containing dexamethasone sodium phosphate. Potency is expressed in terms of the equivalent amount of dexamethasone phosphate. Store in airtight containers.

Dexamethasone Sodium Phosphate Inhalation Aerosol *(U.S.P.)*. A suspension of dexamethasone sodium phosphate in suitable propellents, with alcohol 1.7 to 2.3%, in a pressurised container. Potency is expressed in terms of the equivalent amount of dexamethasone phosphate. Store at a temperature not exceeding 40°.

Dexamethasone Sodium Phosphate Injection *(U.S.P.)*. A sterile solution of dexamethasone sodium phosphate in Water for Injections. pH 7 to 8.5. Potency is expressed in terms of the equivalent amount of dexamethasone phosphate. Protect from light.

Dexamethasone Sodium Phosphate Ophthalmic Ointment *(U.S.P.)*. A sterile eye ointment containing dexamethasone sodium phosphate. Potency is expressed in terms of the equivalent amount of dexamethasone phosphate.

Dexamethasone Sodium Phosphate Ophthalmic Solution *(U.S.P.)*. A sterile solution of dexamethasone sodium phosphate in water. pH 6.6 to 7.8. Potency is expressed in terms of the equivalent amount of dexamethasone phosphate. Protect from light.

Proprietary Preparations

Decadron Injection *(Merck Sharp & Dohme, UK)*. A solution of dexamethasone sodium phosphate containing the equivalent of 4 mg of dexamethasone phosphate in each ml, in vials of 2 ml. **Decadron Shock-Pak.** Dexamethasone sodium phosphate, available as an injection containing the equivalent of 20 mg of dexamethasone per ml, in vials of 5 ml. For slow intravenous injection as an adjunct in the treatment of shock. (Also available as Decadron in *Arg., Austral., Belg., Canad., Neth., Norw., S.Afr., Swed., Switz., USA*).

Oradexon-Organon Injection *(Organon, UK)*. Dexamethasone sodium phosphate, available as an injection containing the equivalent of 4 mg of dexamethasone per ml, in ampoules of 1 ml and vials of 2 ml. (Also available as Oradexon in *Austral., Belg., Neth., Switz.*).

Other Proprietary Names

Austral.— Decasone; *Belg.*— Aacidexam (see also under Dexamethasone); *Canad.*— Hexadrol (see also under Dexamethasone), Novadex; *Denm.*— Decadronfosfat; *Fr.*— Cébédex, Soludécadron; *Ger.*— Decadron-Phosphat, Dexamed (see also under Dexamethasone and Dexamphetamine Sulphate), Fortecortin (see also under Dexamethasone and Dexamethasone Acetate), Totocortin; *Ital.*— Decadron Fosfato, Desalark (see also under Dexamethasone), Eta-Cortilen, Megacort, Soldesam; *Norw.*— Decadron fosfat, Spersadex; *Spain*— Decadran (see also under Dexamethasone), Solone (see also under Dexamethasone and Prednisolone); *Switz.*— Spersadex; *USA*— Dalaron, Dexacen-4, Dexasone, Dezone (see also under Dexamethasone), Hexadrol (see also under Dexamethasone), Savacort-D, Turbinaire Decadron.

1085-x

Dexamethasone Tebutate. Dexamethasone Butylacetate; Dexamethasone Tertiary Butyl Acetate; Dexamethasone TBA. Dexamethasone 21-(3,3-dimethylbutyrate).

$C_{28}H_{39}FO_6$=490.6.

CAS — 24668-75-5.

Dexamethasone tebutate 1.25 mg is approximately equivalent to 1 mg of dexamethasone. Practically **insoluble** in water; soluble in alcohol and acetone.

Uses. Dexamethasone tebutate has the same actions and uses as dexamethasone and is administered by intra-articular injection.

There have been reports of joint damage following the intra-articular injection of corticosteroids into load-bearing joints (see under Corticosteroids, p.447).

Proprietary Names

Decadron TBA *(Merck Sharp & Dohme-Chibret, Fr.; Chibret, Neth.)*; Decadron-TBA *(Merck Sharp & Dohme, Canad.)*.

1086-r

Dexamethasone Trioxa-undecanoate. Dexamethasone Troxundate. Dexamethasone 21-(3,6,9-trioxa)undecanoate.

$C_{30}H_{43}FO_9$=566.7.

CAS — 7743-96-6.

Dexamethasone trioxa-undecanoate 1.44 mg is approximately equivalent to 1 mg of dexamethasone.

Uses. Dexamethasone trioxa-undecanoate has the general properties of dexamethasone (p.466). It is used in veterinary practice as an intramuscular injection (in large animals) or a subcutaneous injection (in small animals) and by intra-articular injection.

1087-f

Diflucortolone Valerate.

6α,9α-Difluoro-11β,21-dihydroxy-16α-methylpregna-1,4-diene-3,20-dione 21-valerate.

$C_{27}H_{36}F_2O_5$=478.6.

CAS — 2607-06-9 (diflucortolone); 59198-70-8 (valerate).

M.p. 200° to 205°. **Soluble** in chloroform; slightly soluble in methyl alcohol; practically insoluble in ether.

Adverse Effects, Treatment, Withdrawal, and Precautions. As for Corticosteroids, p.446, p.449.

Adrenal suppression. From a study of plasma-cortisol concentrations in 20 patients with severe psoriasis diflucortolone valerate ointment 0.3% was reported to cause less adrenal suppression than clobetasol propionate ointment 0.05%.— K. Keczkes *et al.*, *Br. J. Derm.*, 1978, *99*, 417.

Absorption and Fate. For a brief outline of the absorption and fate of corticosteroids, see Corticosteroids, p.451.

When applied topically, particularly to large areas, when the skin is broken, or under occulsive dressings, corticosteroids may be absorbed in sufficient amounts to cause systemic effects.

Uses. Diflucortolone valerate is a synthetic corticosteroid used topically in the treatment of various skin disorders as described under Corticosteroids (see p.451). It is applied as a 0.1% and a 0.3% cream or ointment.

Skin disorders. Diflucortolone valerate as a 0.3% water-in-oil emulsion was equipotent with preparations containing halcinonide, clobetasol propionate, and desoxymethasone, and significantly superior to preparations containing betamethasone dipropionate, betamethasone valerate, and flucinonide in the psoriasis plaque test in 35 patients.— O. Lofferer and R. Reckers, *Arzneimittel-Forsch.*, 1978, *28*, 703.

For recommendations concerning the correct use of corticosteroids on the skin, and a rough guide to the clinical potencies of topical corticosteroids, see Corticosteroids, p.458.

Proprietary Preparations

Nerisone *(Schering, UK)*. Preparations containing diflucortolone valerate 0.1%, available as **Cream** (oil-in-water), **Oily Cream** (water-in-oil), and **Ointment** (anhydrous basis). **Nerisone Forte.** Preparations containing diflucortolone valerate 0.3%, available as **Oily Cream** (water-in-oil) and **Ointment** (anhydrous basis). (Also available as Nerisone in *Fr., NZ, S.Afr.*).

Temetex *(Roche, UK)*. Preparations containing diflucortolone valerate 0.1%, available as **Cream** (oil-in-water), **Ointment** (water-in-oil), and **Fatty Ointment** (anhydrous basis). (Also available as Temetex in *Arg., Ger., S.Afr., Switz.*).

Other Proprietary Names

Nerisona *(Arg., Ger., Ital., Neth., Switz.)*.

1088-d

Fluclorolone Acetonide.

Flucloronide; RS 2252. 9α,11β-Dichloro-6α-fluoro-21-hydroxy-16α,17α-isopropylidenedioxypregna-1,4-diene-3,20-dione.

$C_{24}H_{29}Cl_2FO_5$=487.4.

CAS — 3693-39-8.

A white or almost white odourless, tasteless, crystalline powder. M.p. about 245° with decomposition. Practically **insoluble** in water; soluble 1 in 300 of propylene glycol; soluble in alcohol, chloroform, and methyl alcohol. **Protect** from light.

Adverse Effects, Treatment, Withdrawal, and Precautions. As for Corticosteroids, p.446, p.449.

Absorption and Fate. For a brief outline of the absorption and fate of corticosteroids, see Corticosteroids, p.451.

When applied topically, particularly to large areas, when the skin is broken, or under occlusive dressings, corticosteroids may be absorbed in sufficient amounts to cause systemic effects.

Uses. Fluclorolone acetonide is a synthetic glucocorticoid used topically in the treatment of various skin disorders, as described under Corticosteroids (see p.451). It is usually applied as a 0.025% cream or ointment.

Skin disorders. For recommendations concerning the correct use of corticosteroids on the skin, and a rough guide to the clincal potencies of topical corticosteroids, see Corticosteroids, p.458.

Proprietary Preparations

Topilar *(Syntex, UK)*. Contains fluclorolone acetonide 0.025% in a fatty alcohol-propylene glycol basis.**Topilar Ointment.** Contains fluclorolone acetonide 0.025% in an emollient basis (suggested diluent, white soft paraffin). (Also available as Topilar in *Austral., Denm., Norw.*).

Other Proprietary Names

Cutanit *(Spain)*.

1089-n

Fludrocortisone Acetate *(B.P., U.S.P.)*.

Fludrocort. Acet.; Fludrocortisoni Acetas; 9α-Fluorohydrocortisone 21-Acetate. 9α-Fluoro-11β,17α,21-trihydroxypregn-4-ene-3,20-dione 21-acetate.

$C_{23}H_{31}FO_6$=422.5.

CAS — 127-31-1 (fludrocortisone); 514-36-3 (acetate).

Pharmacopoeias. In *Br., Braz., Chin., Fr., Swiss*, and *U.S.*

A white to pale yellow, odourless or almost odourless, tasteless, hygroscopic, crystalline powder. M.p. of 2 forms about 209° and about 225°

Practically **insoluble** in water; soluble 1 in 50 of alcohol, 1 in 50 of chloroform, and 1 in 250 of ether. A solution in dioxan is dextrorotatory. **Store** in airtight containers. Protect from light.

Adverse Effects. As for Corticosteroids, p.446.

Fludrocortisone acetate has glucocorticoid actions about 15 times as potent as hydrocortisone and mineralocorticoid effects more than 100 times as potent.

Effects on the electrolyte balance. In a 63-year-old man, muscular weakness associated with hypokalaemia and raised serum-creatine phosphokinase concentrations was attributed to fludrocortisone acetate which he had taken for 2½ years in doses of 100 µg three to six times a day for severe postural hypotension. The patient showed no muscular weakness after serum-potassium concentrations were raised by potassium chloride given intravenously and maintained with potassium supplements and a high salt diet.— V. M. Rivera (letter), *J. Am. med. Ass.*, 1973, *225*, 993.

Withdrawal and Precautions. As for Corticosteroids, p.449.

Absorption and Fate. For a brief outline of the absorption and fate of corticosteroids, see Corticosteroids, p.451.

Fludrocortisone is readily absorbed from the gastro-intestinal tract; it is absorbed through the skin when applied topically.

Studies in 5 volunteers showed the absorption of fludrocortisone by mouth to be rapid and complete with maximum blood concentrations after 1.7 hours. After intravenous injection the elimination half-life was 30 minutes.— W. Vogt *et al.*, *Arzneimittel-Forsch.*, 1971, *21*, 1133.

Uses. Fludrocortisone is a synthetic corticosteroid with both mineralocorticoid and glucocorticoid actions as described under Corticosteroids (see p.451).

With a dose that is just sufficient to correct sodium loss in Addison's disease or following total adrenalectomy, the glucocorticoid actions are not sufficient to maintain the patient in normal health; it is therefore given as an adjunct in patients who become sodium deficient on cortisone or hydrocortisone alone. The usual dose of fludrocortisone acetate is 100 or 200 µg daily with a reported range of 100 µg thrice weekly to 300 µg daily.

Fludrocortisone acetate in doses of about 50 to about 200 µg daily may also be given concomitantly with glucocorticoid therapy in the salt-losing form of the adrenogenital syndrome.

Fludrocortisone is also used in the management of severe orthostatic hypotension.

Adrenal insufficiency. A report of 4 patients with Addison's disease who developed hypothyroidism which responded to treatment with cortisone acetate 25 to 30 mg daily or cortisone acetate given in conjunction with fludrocortisone. Since corticosteroid therapy alone might restore normal thyroid function in patients with adrenal insufficiency, it was desirable to delay thyroid treatment until some time after corticosteroid therapy had been started.— H. Gharib *et al.*, *Lancet*, 1972, *2*, 734.

Adrenogenital syndrome. In 4 children with salt-losing congenital adrenal hyperplasia, receiving maintenance doses of hydrocortisone or cortisone acetate, raised plasma concentrations of 17-hydroxyprogesterone and increased plasma renin activity were restored to normal following treatment with fludrocortisone 100 µg daily. It was recommended that these patients should be given mineralocorticoid, in addition to glucocorticoid, therapy at least until adult life.— I. A. Hughes *et al.*, *Archs Dis. Childh.*, 1979, *54*, 350.

Gangrene. Five patients with gangrenous ulcers of the foot due to obliterative arterial disease were treated by a combination of conventional treatment (abstinence from tobacco, bed-positioning, and exercise) and induced hypertension. Fludrocortisone acetate, about 500 µg daily, by mouth or deoxycortone acetate, about 10 mg, sublingually was given together with sodium chloride (as 250-mg tablets) 5 to 15 g daily to provoke a rise in mean arterial blood pressure of about 15 mmHg. Therapy was maintained for several months without troublesome side-effects and blood pressure reverted to normal when treatment ceased. The ulcers, which had been present for 1 to 6 months before treatment, healed.— N. A. Lassen *et al.*, *Lancet*, 1968, *1*, 606. There was little evidence that the observed healing was attributable to the induced hypertension.— I. M. Iedingham and I. G. Schraibman (letter), *ibid.*, 981. The postocclusive blood pressure and the distal blood-flow were increased.— N. A. Lassen *et al.*, *ibid.*

Hypoaldosteronism. The use of fludrocortisone acetate in a patient with hyperkalaemia due to aldosterone deficiency.— J. J. Brown *et al.*, *Br. med. J.*, 1973, *1*, 650. Fludrocortisone in the amelioration of metabolic acidosis in 4 patients with hyporeninaemic hypoaldosteronism.— A. Sebastian *et al.*, *New Engl. J. Med.*, 1977, *297*, 576.

Hypotension. Fourteen diabetic patients with postural hypotension, usually with features of autonomic neuropathy, were treated for 6 to 30 months with fludrocortisone, 100 µg twice daily initially, adjusted as required to a final mean dose of 100 to 400 µg daily. Lying blood pressure was not significantly changed but standing systolic and diastolic pressures rose significantly; 13 patients had symptomatic improvement. Fludrocortisone should be used with care in patients with proteinuria.— I. W. Campbell *et al.*, *Br. med. J.*, 1976, *1*, 872. See also *idem*, *Diabetes*, 1975, *24*, 381, per *J. Am. med. Ass.*, 1975, *233*, 919.

A study of the effects of treatment with fludrocortisone in 7 patients with severe orthostatic hypotension. Doses of 0.3 to 1 mg daily were given for one to 14 years; in some patients the dose was reduced when severe hypertension or hypokalaemia appeared whilst the patient was recumbent. Although blood pressure in the recumbent and standing positions was substantially increased in all patients there was incomplete symptomatic relief; clinical benefit was greatest during the first 6 months of treatment. Increases in blood pressure during the first 10 days of treatment were associated with increases in sodium balance and plasma volume but, in the long term, plasma volume decreased to control values despite further increases in blood pressure. Complications of treatment included recumbent hypertension, cardiomegaly, hypertensive retinopathy, and hypokalaemia; these risks should be borne in mind when long-term treatment with fludrocortisone is considered. In 2 patients, recumbent hypertension after prolonged treatment with fludrocortisone was associated with an increase in total peripheral vascular resistance and not with changes in cardiac output or plasma volumes.— A. V. Chobanian *et al.*, *New Engl. J. Med.*, 1979, *301*, 68. Despite the possible complications of chronic treatment with fludrocortisone it should not be withheld from patients with severe orthostatic hypotension.— R. Walter (letter), *New Engl. J. Med.*, 1979, *301*, 1121. Further comment.— G. Decaux (letter), *ibid.* Reply.— A. V. Chobanian (letter), *ibid.*, 1122.

In the management of orthostatic hypotension fludrocortisone 100 µg daily does not cause fluid retention, but enhances supersensitivity to intravenous noradrenaline and improves standing blood pressure.— R. Bannister, *Lancet*, 1979, *2*, 404.

Further references to fludrocortisone in the management of orthostatic hypotension: L. J. Mahar *et al.*, *Med. J. Aust.*, 1975, *1*, 940 (with tranylcypromine); C. Davidson *et al.*, *Am. J. Med.*, 1976, *61*, 709; B. Davies *et al.*, *Br. J. clin. Pharmac.*, 1979, *8*, 253.

For the use of fludrocortisone in the treatment of severe levodopa-induced postural hypotension, and for the use of fludrocortisone and levodopa in Shy-Drager syndrome, see Levodopa, p.884 and p.887.

Preparations

Fludrocortisone Tablets *(B.P.)*. Fludrocort. Tab. Tablets containing fludrocortisone acetate.

Fludrocortisone Acetate Tablets *(U.S.P.)*. Tablets containing fludrocortisone acetate.

Florinef *(Squibb, UK)*. Fludrocortisone acetate, available as scored tablets of 0.1 and 1 mg. (Also available as Florinef in *Austral.*, *Canad.*, *Denm.*, *Norw.*, *S.Afr.*, *Swed.*).

Other Proprietary Names

Alfa-Fluorone, Alfanonidrone (both *Ital.*); Astonin (base) *(Spain)*; Astonin-H (base) *(Ger.)*; Cortineff *(Pol.)*; Florinef Acetate *(USA)*; Florinef-Acetate *(Switz.)*; Scherofluron *(Ger.)*.

1090-k

Flumethasone. 6α,9α-Difluoro-11β,17α,21-trihydroxy-16α-methylpregna-1,4-diene-3,20-dione. $C_{22}H_{28}F_2O_5$=410.5.

CAS — 2135-17-3.

Uses. Flumethasone is a glucocorticoid with the general properties of the corticosteroids (see p.446); it is used in veterinary practice.

1091-a

Flumethasone Pivalate *(U.S.P.)*.
Flumetasone Pivalate; Flumethasone Trimethylacetate. Flumethasone 21-pivalate. $C_{27}H_{36}F_2O_6$=494.6.

CAS — 2002-29-1.

Pharmacopoeias. In *U.S.*

A white to off-white crystalline powder. Practically **insoluble** in water; soluble 1 in 89 of alcohol, 1 in 350 of chloroform, and 1 in 2800 of ether; slightly soluble in methyl alcohol; very slightly soluble in methylene chloride. A solution in dioxan is dextrorotatory. **Store** in airtight containers. Protect from light.

Adverse Effects, Treatment, Withdrawal, and Precautions. As for Corticosteroids, p.446, p.449.

Adrenal suppression. Adrenocortical suppression associated with extensive topical application of flumethasone pivalate under occlusion.— R. D. Carr and R. G. Wieland, *Archs Derm.*, 1967, *96*, 269.

Effects on the skin. Following a clinical study in 22 patients comparing mild skin atrophy observed in 6 after fluocinolone acetonide and in 1 after flumethasone pivalate, it has been suggested that flumethasone pivalate is more suitable for the long-term treatment of corticosteroid-responsive dermatoses because the associated incidence of skin atrophy is low.— S. Jablonska *et al.*, *Br. J. Derm.*, 1979, *100*, 193.

Absorption and Fate. For a brief outline of the absorption and fate of corticosteroids, see Corticosteroids, p.451.

When applied topically, particularly to large areas, when the skin is broken, or under occlusive dressings, corticosteroids may be absorbed in sufficient amounts to cause systemic effects.

Uses. Flumethasone pivalate is a synthetic glucocorticoid used by topical application in the treatment of various skin disorders as described under Corticosteroids (see p.451). It is usually employed as 0.02% cream, lotion, or ointment.

Preparations

Flumethasone Pivalate Cream *(U.S.P.)*. Contains flumethasone pivalate in a suitable cream basis.

Locorten-Vioform Eardrops *(Ciba, UK)*. Contain flumethasone pivalate 0.02% and clioquinol 1%.

Other Proprietary Names

Locacorten *(Austral., Canad., Denm., Ger., Neth., Norw., Swed., Switz.)*; Locacortene *(Belg.)*; Locorten *(Arg., USA)*; Locorten Simplex *(Ital.)*; Locortene *(Spain)*.

Flumethasone pivalate was also formerly marketed in Great Britain under the proprietary name Locorten *(Ciba)*.

1092-t

Flunisolide.
RS-3999; RS-1320 (acetate). 6α-Fluoro-11β,21-dihydroxy-16α,17α-isopropylidenedioxypregna-1,4-diene-3,20-dione. $C_{24}H_{31}FO_6$=434.5.

CAS — 3385-03-3 (flunisolide); 4533-89-5 (acetate).

Adverse Effects and Treatment. As for Corticosteroids, p.446, and p.449.

A double-blind crossover study in 26 children showed that flunisolide spray 0.025% in aqueous propylene glycol solution, in metered doses providing 25 µg to each nostril thrice daily, was effective in the control of perennial rhinitis. Sixteen children continued to use the spray for 6 months and some could reduce the dose to twice daily or once daily. There was no evidence of adrenal suppression. Four children on long-term treatment experienced transient nasal stinging, and 2 had headache.— J. K. Sarsfield and G. E. Thomson, *Br. med. J.*, 1979, *2*, 95.

Withdrawal and Precautions. As for Corticosteroids, p.449.

Absorption and Fate. For a brief outline of the absorption and fate of corticosteroids, see Corticosteroids, p.451.

A study suggesting that the lack of systemic effect of flunisolide is due to rapid and extensive first-pass metabolism in the liver.— M. D. Chaplin *et al.*, *Clin. Pharmac. Ther.*, 1980, *27*, 402.

Uses. Flunisolide is a synthetic glucocorticoid used as a nasal spray similarly to beclomethasone dipropionate (see p.460) for the prophylaxis and treatment of allergic rhinitis. It is used in a usual initial dose of 50 µg into each nostril twice or thrice daily, subsequently reduced to the lowest dose adequate to control symptoms. Children over 5 years of age may be given 25 µg into each nostril thrice daily.

Rhinitis. A detailed review of studies on intranasal flunisolide in perennial and seasonal rhinitis. In a few well-designed clinical studies flunisolide was as effective as usual doses of intranasal beclomethasone dipropionate in seasonal allergic or perennial (usually allergic) rhinitis. It was usually well tolerated, producing only transient nasal stinging and throat irritation.— G. E. Pakes *et al.*, *Drugs*, 1980, *19*, 397.

Preparations

Syntaris *(Syntex, UK)*. Flunisolide, available as a nasal spray for inhalation delivering about 25 µg in each metered dose. (Also available as Syntaris in *Ger.*).

Other Proprietary Names

Rhinalar *(Canad.)*; Locasyn *(Denm.)*.

1093-x

Fluocinolone Acetonide *(B.P., U.S.P.)*.

6α,9α-Difluoro-16α-hydroxyprednisolone Acetonide. 6α,9α-Difluoro-11β,21-dihydroxy-16α,17α-isopropylidenedioxypregna-1,4-diene-3,20-dione.

$C_{24}H_{30}F_2O_6$=452.5.

CAS — 67-73-2.

Pharmacopoeias. In *Br., Braz., Chin., Jap.,* and *U.S.*

A white or almost white, odourless, tasteless, crystalline powder. M.p. about 270° with decomposition.

Practically **insoluble** in water; soluble 1 in 10 of acetone, 1 in 26 of dehydrated alcohol, 1 in 15 to 25 of chloroform, and 1 in 350 of ether; soluble in methyl alcohol; sparingly soluble in propylene glycol; practically insoluble in light petroleum. A solution in dioxan is dextrorotatory. Strongly alkaline or acidic substances and oxidising agents accelerate the decomposition of fluocinolone acetonide. **Protect** from light.

Studies on the absorption and stability of fluocinolone acetonide in various pharmaceutical preparations: C. W. Barrett *et al.*, *Br. J. Derm.*, 1965, *77*, 576; E. Brode, *Arzneimittel-Forsch.*, 1967, *17*, 103; B. J. Poulsen *et al.*, *J. pharm. Sci.*, 1968, *57*, 928.

Adverse Effects and Treatment. As for Corticosteroids, p.446, and p.449.

Effects on the eyes. Glaucoma in a 22-year-old man who for the past 7 years had applied fluocinolone acetonide ointment 0.01% to the skin of his face, including the eyelids, nightly, for the treatment of eczema.— R. B. Cubey, *Br. J. Derm.*, 1976, *95*, 207.

Withdrawal and Precautions. As for Corticosteroids, p.449.

Absorption and Fate. For a brief outline of the absorption and fate of corticosteroids, see Corticosteroids, p.451.

When applied topically, particularly to large areas, when the skin is broken, or under occlusive dressings, corticosteroids may be absorbed in sufficient amounts to cause systemic effects.

Bioavailability. Variation in the absorption of 2 fluocinolone acetonide formulations.— G. L. Coleman *et al.*, *S. Afr. med. J.*, 1979, *56*, 447.

Uses. Fluocinolone acetonide is a synthetic glucocorticoid and is used by topical application in the treatment of various skin disorders as described under Corticosteroids, (see p.451).

It is applied topically as 0.01%, 0.025%, and 0.2% creams, gels, lotions, or ointments.

Skin disorders. For recommendations concerning the correct use of corticosteroids on the skin, and a rough guide to the clinical potencies of topical corticosteroids, see Corticosteroids p.458.

Preparations

Fluocinolone Acetonide Cream *(U.S.P.)*. A cream containing fluocinolone acetonide. Store in airtight containers.

Fluocinolone Acetonide Ointment *(B.P.)*. Fluocinolone Ointment. An ointment containing fluocinolone acetonide in a suitable basis.

A.P.F. has 0.01% or 0.025% fluocinolone acetonide in 10% w/w liquid paraffin and white soft paraffin to 100%.

Fluocinolone Acetonide Ointment *(U.S.P.)*. An ointment containing fluocinolone acetonide. Store in airtight containers.

Fluocinolone Acetonide Topical Solution *(U.S.P.)*. A solution containing fluocinolone acetonide. Store in airtight containers.

Fluocinolone Cream *(B.P.C. 1973)*. Fluocinolone Acetonide Cream. A dispersion of fluocinolone acetonide in a suitable water-miscible basis containing a preservative mixture of benzyl alcohol and methyl and propyl hydroxybenzoates. Store in a cool place in well-closed containers which prevent evaporation and contamination; aluminium tubes should be internally lacquered. When a strength less than those available from the manufacturer is prescribed, a stronger cream may be diluted, taking hygienic precautions, with Cetomacrogol Cream (Formula B). The diluted cream must be freshly prepared.

Fluocinolone Cream Aqueous *(A.P.F.)*. Fluocinolone Acetonide Cream. Fluocinolone acetonide 10 mg, 25 mg, or 200 mg, cetomacrogol cream aqueous to 100 g.

Proprietary Preparations

Synalar *(ICI Pharmaceuticals, UK)*. Preparations containing fluocinolone acetonide 0.025%, available as **Cream**; as **Gel** in a water-miscible basis; as **Lotion**; and as **Ointment**. **Synalar Forte Cream.** Contains fluocinolone acetonide 0.2%. **Synalar-C. Cream** and **Ointment** each containing fluocinolone acetonide 0.025% and clioquinol 3%. **Synalar-N.** Preparations containing fluocinolone acetonide 0.025% and neomycin sulphate 0.5%, available as **Cream**; **Ointment**; and **Lotion**. (ALso available as Synalar in *Arg., Austral., Belg., Canad., Denm., Fr., Neth., Norw., S.Afr., Spain, Switz., USA*).

Synandone *(ICI Pharmaceuticals, UK)*. **Cream** and **Ointment** each containing fluocinolone acetonide 0.01%.

Other Proprietary Names

Arg.— Flulone; *Canad.*— Dermalar, Fluoderm, Synamol; *Ger.*— Jellin; *Ital.*— Alfabios, Boniderma, Coderma, Cortalar, Cortamide, Cortiderma, Cortiplastol, Dermacort, Dermaisom, Dermaplus, Dermatin, Dermil, Dermofil, Dermolin, Dermomagis, Doricum, Esacinone, Esilon, Fluocinil, Fluocinone, Fluodermol, Fluogisol, Fluomix Same, Fluonide Dermica, Fluordima, Fluoskin, Fluovitef, Isnaderm, Isoderma, Lenar, Leniderm, Localyn, Neoderm, Omniderm, Percutina, Prodermin, Radiocin, Roliderm, Sterolone, Straderm, Topifluor, Ultraderm; *Jap.*— Coriphate, Flucort, Flupollon, Fluvean, Fluzon; *Neth.*— Monoderm; *S.Afr.*— Cortoderm; *Spain*— Alvadermo, Co-Fluocin, Dermisone Fluocinolona, Dermobiomar, Fluocinil, Fluodermo, Gelidina, Intradermo-C, Oxidermiol, Ungovac; *USA*— Fluonid, Synemol.

1094-r

Fluocinonide *(U.S.P.)*.

Fluocinolone Acetonide 21-Acetate. 6α,9α-Difluoro-11β,21-dihydroxy-16α,17α-isopropylidenedioxypregna-1,4-diene-3,20-dione 21-acetate.

$C_{26}H_{32}F_2O_7$=494.5.

CAS — 356-12-7.

Pharmacopoeias. In *U.S.* and *Chin.*

A white to cream-coloured crystalline powder with not more than a slight odour. M.p. about 300° with decomposition.

Practically **insoluble** in water and light petroleum; soluble 1 in 70 of alcohol, 1 in 10 of acetone, and 1 in 10 of chloroform; slightly soluble in methyl alcohol and dioxan; very slightly soluble in ether.

Adverse Effects, Treatment, Withdrawal, and Precautions. As for Corticosteroids, p.446, p.449.

Effects on the skin. Steroid rosacea in children following topical application of fluocinonide.— H. L. Franco and W. L. Weston, *Pediatrics*, 1979, *64*, 36.

Absorption and Fate. For a brief outline of the absorption and fate of corticosteroids, see Corticosteroids, p.451.

When applied topically, particularly to large areas, when the skin is broken, or under occlusive dressings, corticosteroids may be absorbed in sufficient amounts to cause systemic effects.

Uses. Fluocinonide is a synthetic glucocorticoid used by topical application in the treatment of various skin disorders, as described under Corticosteroids (see p.451). It is applied at a concentration of 0.05%.

Skin disorders. For recommendations concerning the correct use of corticosteroids on the skin, and a rough guide to the clinical potencies of topical corticosteroids, see Corticosteroids, p.458.

Preparations

Fluocinonide Cream *(U.S.P.)*. A cream containing fluocinonide. Store in airtight containers.

Fluocinonide Gel *(U.S.P.)*. A gel containing fluocinonide. Store in airtight containers.

Fluocinonide Ointment *(U.S.P.)*. An ointment containing fluocinonide. Store in airtight containers.

Proprietary Preparations

Metosyn *(Stuart, UK)*. Preparations containing fluocinonide 0.05%, available as **FAPG Cream** in a fatty alcohol-propylene glycol basis (the basis is available for use if dilutions are required) and as **Ointment** (suggested diluent, white soft paraffin). (Also available as Metosyn in *Denm., Norw.*).

Other Proprietary Names

Bestasone, Biscosal *(both Jap.)*; Flu 21, Fludex *(both Ital.)*; Lidemol *(Canad.)*; Lidex *(Canad., USA)*; Lidex-E *(USA)*; Topsym *(Ger., Jap., Switz.)*; Topsymin *(Ger., Switz.)*; Topsyn *(Canad., Ital., USA)*; Topsyne *(Belg., Fr., Neth.)*.

1095-f

Fluocortolone.

SH 742; 6α-Fluoro-16α-methyldehydrocorticosterone. 6α-Fluoro-11β,21-dihydroxy-16α-methylpregna-1,4-diene-3,20-dione.

$C_{22}H_{29}FO_4$=376.5.

CAS — 152-97-6.

1096-d

Fluocortolone Hexanoate *(B.P.)*.

Fluocortolone Caproate; SH 770. Fluocortolone 21-hexanoate.

$C_{28}H_{39}FO_5$=474.6.

CAS — 303-40-2.

Pharmacopoeias. In *Br.*

An odourless, white to creamy-white, crystalline powder. M.p. about 244°. Practically **insoluble** in water and ether; very slightly soluble in alcohol and methyl alcohol; soluble 1 in 18 of chloroform; slightly soluble in acetone and dioxan. A solution in dioxan is dextrorotatory. **Protect** from light.

1097-n

Fluocortolone Pivalate *(B.P.)*.

Fluocortolone Trimethylacetate. Fluocortolone 21-pivalate.

$C_{27}H_{37}FO_5$=460.6.

CAS — 29205-06-9.

Pharmacopoeias. In *Br.*

Odourless, white to creamy-white, crystalline powder. M.p. about 187°. Practically **insoluble** in water; soluble 1 in 36 of alcohol and 1 in 3 of chloroform; sparingly soluble in methyl alcohol; freely soluble in dioxan; slightly soluble in ether. A solution in dioxan is dextrorotatory. **Protect** from light.

Adverse Effects, Treatment, Withdrawal, and Precautions. As for Corticosteroids, p.446, p.449.

Absorption and Fate. For a brief outline of the absorption and fate of corticosteroids, see Corticosteroids, p.451.

When applied topically, particularly to large areas, when the skin is broken, or under occlusive dressings, corticosteroids may be absorbed in sufficient amounts to cause systemic effects.

Fluocortolone hexanoate has a longer duration of action than the free alcohol or pivalate ester.

Fluocortolone hexanoate 25 mg per ml as an aqueous crystalline suspension was injected intra-articularly into the knee-joint of 8 patients with chronic rheumatoid arthritis. Synovectomy was performed immediately after or up to 47 days after the injection. Pharmacokinetic studies indicated that the half-life of fluocortolone administered in this manner was 13.5 days and it was recommended that there should be an interval of 2 to 3 weeks between injections.— W. Mützel *et al., Dt. med. Wschr.*, 1979, *104*, 293.

Uses. Fluocortolone is a synthetic glucocorticoid and has the general properties described under Corticosteroids (see p.451).

Fluocortolone is used by topical application in the treatment of various skin disorders, as described under Corticosteroids (see p.451). It is usually employed as ointments containing 0.25% with fluocortolone hexanoate or fluocortolone pivalate 0.1% or 0.25%. Fluocortolone has also been given by mouth.

Clinical and experimental investigations of systemic fluocortolone: H. Breuer *et al., Arzneimittel-Forsch.*, 1965, *15*, 50; K. Winkler, *ibid.*, 53; H. J. Vogt, *ibid.*, 54.

Preparations

Fluocortolone Pivalate and Fluocortolone Hexanoate Ointment *(B.P.)*. An ointment containing fluocortolone pivalate and fluocortolone hexanoate in a suitable basis. Store at a temperature not exceeding 30°.

Proprietary Preparations

Ultradil Plain *(Schering, UK)*. **Cream** and **Ointment** containing fluocortolone hexanoate 0.1% and fluocortolone pivalate 0.1%.

Ultralanum *(Schering, UK)*. An ointment containing fluocortolone 0.25%, fluocortolone hexanoate 0.25%, and clemizole-hexachlorophane 2.5% in a water-in-oil emulsion basis (suggested diluent, Oily Cream). **Ultralanum Plain** available as **Cream** containing fluocortolone hexanoate 0.25% and fluocortolone pivalate 0.25% in an oil-in-water emulsion basis (suggested diluent, Aqueous Cream) and as **Ointment** containing fluocortolone 0.25% and fluocortolone hexanoate 0.25% in a water-in-oil emulsion basis. (Also available as Ultralanum in *Norw., S.Afr.*).

Ultraproct *(Schering, UK)*. **Ointment** containing in each g fluocortolone pivalate 920 µg, fluocortolone hexanoate 950 µg, cinchocaine hydrochloride 5 mg, clemizole undecanoate 10 mg, and hexachlorophane 2.5 mg; and **Suppositories** each containing fluocortolone pivalate 610 µg, fluocortolone hexanoate 630 µg, cinchocaine hydrochloride 1 mg, clemizole undecanoate 5 mg, and hexachlorophane 2.5 mg. For haemorrhoids and similar anorectal disorders.

Other Proprietary Names

Ultralan *(Austral., Ger., Ital., Neth., Spain, Switz.)*.

Preparations containing fluocortolone hexanoate and fluocortolone pivalate were also formerly marketed in Great Britain under the proprietary name Ficoid (*Fisons*).

1098-h

Fluorometholone *(U.S.P.)*. NSC 33001. 9α-Fluoro-11β,17α-dihydroxy-6α-methylpregna-1,4-diene-3,20-dione.

$C_{22}H_{29}FO_4$=376.5.

CAS — 426-13-1.

Pharmacopoeias. In *U.S.*

A white to yellowish-white, odourless, crystalline powder. M.p. about 280° with decomposition. Practically **insoluble** in water; soluble 1 in 200 of alcohol and 1 in 2200 of chloroform; very slightly soluble in ether. A solution in pyridine is dextrorotatory. **Store** in airtight containers. Protect from light.

Adverse Effects, Treatment, Withdrawal, and Precautions. As for Corticosteroids, p.446, p.449.

Effects on the eyes. Evidence that topical application of fluorometholone can significantly raise intra-ocular pressure in a significant number of corticosteroid responders.— R. H. Stewart and R. L. Kimbrough, *Archs Ophthal., N.Y.*, 1979, *97*, 2139.

Absorption and Fate. For a brief outline of the absorption and fate of corticosteroids, see Corticosteroids, p.451.

When applied topically, particularly to large areas, when the skin is broken, or under occlusive dressings, corticosteroids may be absorbed in sufficient amounts to cause systemic effects.

Uses. Fluorometholone is a synthetic glucocorticoid and is used by topical application in the treatment of various skin disorders as described under Corticosteroids (see p.451). It has a local anti-inflammatory action which is approximately 40 times greater than that of hydrocortisone but the effects of the 2 corticosteroids are about equal when they are given by mouth. Fluorometholone is usually employed as a 0.025% cream or ointment.

Skin disorders. For recommendations concerning the correct use of corticosteroids on the skin, and a rough guide to the clinical potencies of topical corticosteroids, see Corticosteroids, p.458.

Preparations

Fluorometholone Cream *(U.S.P.)*. A cream containing fluorometholone.

FML Liquifilm *(Allergan, UK)*. Fluoromethalone, available as a suspension containing 0.1% for ophthalmic use. (Also available as FML in *Canad., Neth., S.Afr.*).

Other Proprietary Names

Cortilet *(Swed.)*; Cortisdin *(Spain)*; Delmeson *(Denm., Switz.)*; Efflumidex Liquifilm *(Ger.)*; Fluaton *(Ital.)*; Flumetholon *(Jap.)*; FML TM *(Belg.)*; Lerna *(Jap.)*; Oxylone *(USA)*; Regresin Sine *(Spain)*; Ursnon *(Jap.)*.

1099-m

Fluperolone Acetate. 9α-Fluoro-21-methylprednisolone Acetate. (21*S*)-9α-Fluoro-11β,17α,21-trihydroxy-21-methylpregna-1,4-diene-3,20-dione 21-acetate.

$C_{24}H_{31}FO_6$=434.5.

CAS — 3841-11-0 (fluperolone); 2119-75-7 (acetate).

A white, odourless, tasteless, crystalline powder. Very slightly **soluble** in water; soluble 1 in 60 of dehydrated alcohol.

Uses. Fluperolone acetate is a synthetic glucocorticoid and has the general properties described under Corticosteroids (see p.446). It has been used topically as a 0.1% cream or ointment.

1100-m

Fluprednidene Acetate. Fluprednideni Acetas; Fluprednylidene 21-Acetate. 9α-Fluoro-11β,17α,21-trihydroxy-16-methylenepregna-1,4-diene-3,20-dione 21-acetate.

$C_{24}H_{29}FO_6$=432.5.

CAS — 2193-87-5 (fluprednidene); 1255-35-2 (acetate).

Pharmacopoeias. In *Nord.*

A white crystalline powder. M.p. about 235°. Practically **insoluble** in water; soluble 1 in 25 of alcohol, 1 in 50 of chloroform, and 1 in 800 of ether; soluble in acetone.

Adverse Effects, Treatment, Withdrawal, and Precautions. As for Corticosteroids, p.446, p.449.

Absorption and Fate. For a brief outline of the absorption and fate of corticosteroids, see Corticosteroids, p.451.

When applied topically, particularly to large areas, when the skin is broken, or under occlusive dressings, corticosteroids may be absorbed in sufficient amounts to cause systemic effects.

Uses. Fluprednidene acetate is a synthetic glucocorticoid and is used by topical application in the treatment of various skin disorders, as described under Corticosteroids (see p.451). It is usually employed as a cream containing 0.1%.

Proprietary Names

Corticoderm *(E. Merck, Denm.; E. Merck, Norw.; E. Merck, Swed.)*; Decoderm *(see also under Dexamethasone Acetate) (Merck, Aust.; Merck, Belg.; E. Merck, Ger.; Bracco, Ital.; E. Merck, Neth.; Merck, S.Afr.; E. Merck, Switz.)*; Décoderme *(Merck-Clévenot, Fr.)*; Emcortina *(Merck, Arg.)*; Etacortin *(Hermal, Ger.)*.

Fluprednidene acetate was formerly marketed in Great Britain under the proprietary name Decoderm (*E. Merck*).

1101-b

Fluprednisolone. 6α-Fluoroprednisolone. 6α-Fluoro-11β,17α,21-trihydroxypregna-1,4-diene-3,20-dione.

$C_{21}H_{27}FO_5$=378.4.

CAS — 53-34-9.

A white to off-white odourless crystalline powder. Practically **insoluble** in water; sparingly soluble in alcohol; slightly soluble in chloroform and ether.

Fluprednisolone could exist in 6 crystalline forms and 1 amorphous form.— J. K. Haleblian *et al., J. pharm. Sci.*, 1971, *60*, 1485.

Uses. Fluprednisolone is a synthetic glucocorticoid with the general properties and uses described under Corticosteroids (see p.446). It has been given in doses of 0.75 to 5.25 mg one to four times daily.

Proprietary Names

Alphadrol *(Upjohn, USA)*; Selectren *(Albert-Farma, Spain)*; Selectren Retard *(acetate) (Albert-Farma, Spain)*; Selectren Soluble *(sodium hemisuccinate) (Albert-Farma, Spain)*; Vladicort *(Spain)*.

1102-v

Flurandrenolone. Fludroxycortide; Flurandrenolide *(U.S.P.)*; 6α-Fluoro-16α-hydroxyhydrocortisone 16,17-Acetonide. 6α-Fluoro-11β,21-dihydroxy-16α,17α-isopropylidenedioxypregn-4-ene-3,20-dione.

$C_{24}H_{33}FO_6$=436.5.

CAS — 1524-88-5.

Pharmacopoeias. In *U.S.*

An odourless, white to off-white, fluffy, crystalline powder. Practically **insoluble** in water and ether; soluble 1 in 72 of alcohol, 1 in 10 of chloroform, and 1 in 25 of methyl alcohol. A solution in chloroform is dextrorotatory. **Store** at a temperature not exceeding 8° in airtight containers. Protect from light.

Adverse Effects and Treatment. As for Corticosteroids, p.446, and p.449.

Effects on the eyes. Glaucoma associated with ocular flurandrenolone application.— R. F. Brubaker and J. A. Halpin, *Mayo Clin. Proc.*, 1975, *50*, 322.

Withdrawal and Precautions. As for Corticosteroids, p.449.

Absorption and Fate. For a brief outline of the absorption and fate of corticosteroids, see Corticosteroids, p.451.

When applied topically, particularly to large areas, when the skin is broken, or under occlusive dressings, corticosteroids may be absorbed in sufficient amounts to cause systemic effects.

Uses. Flurandrenolone is a synthetic glucocorticoid used by topical application in the treatment of various skin disorders as described under Corticosteroids (see p.451). It is usually employed as creams, lotions, or ointments containing 0.0125 to 0.05% or as a polyethylene tape with an adhesive containing 4 µg of flurandrenolone per cm^2 of tape.

Skin disorders. For recommendations concerning the correct use of corticosteroids on the skin, and a rough guide to the clinical potencies of topical corticosteroids, see Corticosteroids, p.458.

Preparations

Flurandrenolide Cream *(U.S.P.)*. A cream containing flurandrenolone. Store in airtight containers. Protect from light.

Flurandrenolide Lotion *(U.S.P.).* A lotion containing flurandrenolone. pH 3.5 to 6. Store in a cool place in airtight containers and avoid freezing. Protect from light.

Flurandrenolide Ointment *(U.S.P.).* An ointment containing flurandrenolone. Store in airtight containers. Protect from light.

Flurandrenolide Tape *(U.S.P.).* Non-porous, pliable, adhesive tape having flurandrenolone impregnated in the adhesive material. Store at 15° to 30°.

Proprietary Preparations

Haelan *(Dista, UK).* **Cream** and **Ointment** each containing flurandrenolone 0.0125%. **Haelan-C. Cream** and **Ointment** each containing flurandrenolone 0.0125% and clioquinol 3%. **Haelan-X. Cream** and **Ointment** each containing flurandrenolone 0.05%. (Also available as Haelan in *Austral.*).

Haelan Tape *(Dista, UK).* Translucent adhesive polyethylene film containing flurandrenolone 4 µg per cm^2.

Other Proprietary Names

Cordran *(USA)*; Drenison *(Canad., Ital.)*; Sermaka *(Ger.)*.

Flurandrenolone was also formerly marketed in Great Britain under the proprietary name Drenison (*Lilly*).

1103-g

Formocortal. 3-(2-Chloroethoxy)-9α-fluoro-11β,21-dihydroxy-16α,17α-isopropylidenedioxy-20-oxopregna-3,5-diene-6-carbaldehyde 21-acetate.
$C_{29}H_{38}ClFO_8$=569.1.

CAS — 2825-60-7.

A white to yellowish, odourless, almost tasteless, fine, crystalline powder. M.p. about 184°.
Practically **insoluble** in water and ether; soluble in alcohol, acetone, ethyl acetate, and methyl alcohol.

Uses. Formocortal is a synthetic glucocorticoid formerly used by topical application in the treatment of various skin disorders as described under Corticosteroids (see p.451). It has been applied as a 0.025% cream, lotion, or ointment.

Proprietary Names
Deflamene *(Montedison, Arg.; Spain)*; Formoftil *(Farmigea, Ital.)*.

Formocortal was formerly marketed in Great Britain under the proprietary name Deflamene (*Montedison now known as Farmitalia Carlo Erba*).

1104-q

Halcinonide.

SQ 18566. 21-Chloro-9α-fluoro-11β-hydroxy-16α,17α-isopropylidenedioxypregn-4-ene-3,20-dione.
$C_{24}H_{32}ClFO_5$=455.0.

CAS — 3093-35-4.

Adverse Effects, Treatment, Withdrawal, and Precautions. As for Corticosteroids, p.446, p.449.

Absorption and Fate. For a brief outline of the absorption and fate of corticosteroids, see Corticosteroids, p.451.
When applied topically, particularly to large areas, when the skin is broken, or under occlusive dressings, corticosteroids may be absorbed in sufficient amounts to cause systemic effects.

Uses. Halcinonide is a synthetic glucocorticoid used by topical application in the treatment of various skin disorders, as described under Corticosteroids (see p.451). It is usually employed as creams or ointments containing 0.025 to 0.1%.

Skin disorders. For recommendations concerning the correct use of corticosteroids on the skin, and a rough guide to the clinical potencies of topical corticosteroids, see Corticosteroids, p.458.

Proprietary Preparations

Halcicomb *(FAIR Laboratories, UK: Squibb, UK).* Preparations containing halcinonide 0.1%, neomycin sulphate 0.25%, and nystatin 100 000 units per g, available as **Cream** and as **Ointment**.

Halciderm Topical *(Squibb, UK).* Halcinonide, available as a cream containing 0.1% (dilution not recommended). (Also available as Halciderm in *Arg., Austral., Belg., Ital., Neth., Switz.*).

Other Proprietary Names

Halcimat *(Ger.)*; Halog *(Canad., Denm., Ger., Norw., S.Afr., Spain, Swed., USA)*.

Halcinonide was also formerly marketed in Great Britain under the proprietary name Halcort (*FAIR Laboratories*).

1105-p

Hydrocortamate Hydrochloride. Ethamicort; Hydrocortisone Diethylaminoacetate Hydrochloride.
11β,17α,21-Trihydroxypregn-4-ene-3,20-dione 21-diethylaminoacetate hydrochloride.
$C_{27}H_{41}NO_6$,HCl=512.1.

CAS — 76-47-1 (hydrocortamate); 125-03-1 (hydrochloride).

Uses. Hydrocortamate hydrochloride is a synthetic glucocorticoid which has been used as an ointment in the treatment of various skin disorders as described under Corticosteroids (see p.451).

1106-s

Hydrocortisone *(B.P., Eur. P., U.S.P.).*

Hydrocort.; Cortisol; Compound F; 17-Hydroxycorticosterone; Hydrocortisonum; Hidrocortisona.
11β,17α,21-Trihydroxypregn-4-ene-3,20-dione.
$C_{21}H_{30}O_5$=362.5.

CAS — 50-23-7.

Pharmacopoeias. In *Arg., Aust., Br., Braz., Chin., Eur., Fr., Ger., Hung., Ind., Int., It., Jap., Jug., Neth., Nord., Pol., Roum., Swiss, Turk.,* and *U.S.*

A white or almost white, odourless, crystalline powder, tasteless at first but followed by a persistent bitter taste. M.p. about 214° with decomposition.
Practically **insoluble** in water and ether; soluble 1 in 40 of alcohol, 1 in 80 of acetone, and 1 in 100 of propylene glycol; slightly soluble in chloroform; very soluble in dioxan. A solution in dioxan is dextrorotatory. Alcoholic solutions, for use in preparing injections, are **sterilised** by filtration. **Protect** from light.

Decomposition occurred at the C-17 side chain and in ring A of hydrocortisone 1% in Polyethylene Glycol Ointment *U.S.P.* The shelf-life based on these studies was 6 months. This could be extended to 9 months with the addition of a 5% excess of hydrocortisone during manufacture.— A. E. Allen and V. D. Gupta, *J. pharm. Sci.*, 1974, *63,* 107.

Hydrocortisone appeared to be unstable at room temperature in water and in Polyethylene Glycol Ointment *U.S.P.* The addition of alcohol and glycerol to water had a stabilising effect.— V. D. Gupta, *J. pharm. Sci.*, 1978, *67,* 299.

Adverse Effects and Treatment. As for Corticosteroids, p.446, and p.449.
There have been reports of joint damage following the intra-articular injection of corticosteroids into load-bearing joints (see under Corticosteroids, p.447).
Prolonged application to the eye of preparations containing corticosteroids has caused increased intra-ocular pressure and reduced visual function.

Withdrawal and Precautions. As for Corticosteroids, p.449.

Absorption and Fate. For a brief account of the absorption and fate of corticosteroids, see Corticosteroids, p.451.
Hydrocortisone is readily absorbed from the gastro-intestinal tract and peak blood concentrations are attained in about an hour. The biological half-life is about 100 minutes. It is more than 90% bound to plasma proteins. It is absorbed more slowly following intramuscular injection and is no longer administered by this route. Hydrocortisone acetate given by mouth is less readily absorbed than hydrocortisone, and it is very poorly absorbed from intramuscular injections; it is also very poorly absorbed from intrasynovial and soft-tissue injections but may be used by these routes to produce a prolonged local effect.
Hydrocortisone is absorbed through the skin, particularly in denuded areas; the acetate is less well absorbed and has a more prolonged action.
Hydrocortisone is metabolised in the liver and most body tissues to hydrogenated and degraded forms such as tetrahydrocortisone and tetrahydrocortisol. These are excreted in the urine, mainly conjugated as glucuronides, together with a very small proportion of unchanged hydrocortisone.

For details of the metabolism of hydrocortisone, see C. L. Cope, *Adrenal Steroids and Disease,* London, Pitman Medical, 1972..

Uses. Hydrocortisone (cortisol) is the main glucocorticoid secreted by the adrenal cortex and has the properties described under Corticosteroids (see p.451). It has properties qualitatively similar to those of cortisone acetate (see p.464) and is used for similar purposes. In fact, hydrocortisone is now preferred to cortisone since it is already pharmacologically active, whereas cortisone must be converted in the liver to hydrocortisone.
Hydrocortisone is administered by mouth for replacement therapy in Addison's disease or chronic adrenocortical insufficiency secondary to hypopituitarism. The normal requirement is 10 to 30 mg daily (usually 20 mg is taken in the morning and 10 mg in the early evening, to mimic the circadian rhythm of the body). Additional sodium chloride may be required if there is defective aldosterone secretion, but mineralocorticoid activity is usually supplemented by fludrocortisone acetate (see p.470) by mouth. Similar doses of hydrocortisone are also given to correct glucocorticoid deficiency in the salt-losing form of adrenal hyperplasia, again in association with fludrocortisone, and together with an adequate sodium intake.
When a rapid effect is required in emergencies such as shock, addisonian or post-adrenalectomy crises, during the acute phase of status asthmaticus, and in allergic emergencies such as laryngeal oedema and drug sensitivity, hydrocortisone may be given by slow intravenous infusion in the form of a water-soluble derivative such as hydrocortisone sodium succinate (p.476) or hydrocortisone sodium phosphate (see p.476).
Hydrocortisone is also used in retention enemas containing about 100 mg and administered once or twice daily.
Hydrocortisone is used by topical application in the treatment of various skin disorders as described under Corticosteroids (see p.451). It is applied as ointments, creams, and lotions containing 0.25 to 2.5%, and has fewer side-effects on the skin and is less liable to induce adrenal suppression than the more potent topical corticosteroids.
Hydrocortisone is given by local injection as the acetate (see p.474). It was formerly given by intramuscular injection as the acetate, but absorption from this site is very poor.
Hydrocortisone palmitate and hydrocortisone valerate are under study.

Adrenal hyperplasia, salt-losing. A study of growth failure in 16 children with the salt-losing form of adrenal hyperplasia. Growth retardation was found to be due to overtreatment related to increased dosage of hydrocortisone at the time of infections often beyond the acute phase of the disease. It is important to establish for each patient the minimal dosage capable of suppressing adrenocortical hyperfunction; this seems to be 30 to 40 mg per m^2 body-surface per 24 hours.— R. Rappaport *et al.*, *J. Pediat.*, 1968, *73,* 760.

Adrenal insufficiency. The inadequate suppression of ACTH by fludrocortisone 100 µg and cortisone acetate 25 to 50 mg or hydrocortisone 30 to 60 mg daily in 12 patients with Addison's disease indicated a secondary pituitary hyperplasia caused by inadequate replacement therapy. This effect might be important in the development of Nelson's syndrome (raised ACTH concentrations, skin pigmentation, and obvious pituitary tumour following bilateral adrenalectomy).— R. Clayton *et al.* (preliminary communication), *Lancet*, 1977, *2*, 954. See also H. K. Kley and H. L. Krüskemper, *Dt. med. Wschr.*, 1978, *103*, 155; S. August *et al.*, *ibid.*, 1979, *104*, 506.

Hyperparathyroidism. As a test to distinguish the hypercalcaemia of hyperparathyroidism from that of other causes, 40 mg of hydrocortisone was given every 8 hours for 10 days and then the dose gradually reduced over the next few days. Calcium concentrations were determined in blood samples taken each morning during the test. In patients with hyperparathyroidism no significant change in hypercalcaemia occurred, but in patients with hypercalcaemia due to other causes plasma-calcium concentrations were consistently and significantly reduced. The test was not used when clinical evidence strongly indicated the cause of hypercalcaemia.— C. E. Dent and L. Watson, *Lancet*, 1968, *2*, 662 and 1198. Experience of the hydrocortisone test and comparison with discriminant analysis indicated that both reach a high level of diagnostic accuracy, and when both point to the same diagnosis the error is less than 1%.— L. Watson *et al.*, *ibid.*, 1980, *1*, 1320. Comment.— *ibid.*, 1339. Criticism of the units used to express the results, and comment on the problem of lack of common methodology.— G. M. Addison (letter), *ibid.*, *2*, 85.

Pregnancy and the neonate. For references to the use of hydrocortisone in the respiratory distress syndrome, see Betamethasone, p.461.

The neonate. Hydrocortisone 10 mg per kg body-weight daily was reported to reverse hypoglycaemia in infants when given intramuscularly in association with a dextrose infusion which was ineffective on its own.— D. Harvey, *Br. J. Hosp. Med.*, 1972, *8*, 65. See also R. D. G. Creery (letter), *Lancet*, 1968, *1*, 594.

Skin disorders. For recommendations concerning the correct use of corticosteroids on the skin, and a rough guide to the clinical potencies of topical corticosteroids, see Corticosteroids, p.458.

Preparations

Creams

Hydrocortisone and Neomycin Cream *(B.P.C. 1973).* Neomycin and Hydrocortisone Cream *(B.P.C. 1963).* Hydrocortisone, of specified particle size, 500 mg, and neomycin cream 99.5 g. A phosphate buffer may be included. Store in a cool place in well-closed containers which prevent evaporation and contamination.

A.P.F. (Aqueous Hydrocortisone and Neomycin Cream) contains hydrocortisone, in ultra-fine powder, 0.5% in aqueous neomycin cream (*A.P.F.*).

Hydrocortisone and Urea Cream *(St. John's Hosp.).* Hydrocortisone 1, urea 10, sodium phosphate 2.5, citric acid monohydrate 0.5, chlorocresol 0.1, emulsifying ointment 30, water to 100.

Hydrocortisone Cream *(B.P.C. 1973).* Hydrocortisone or hydrocortisone acetate, in ultra-fine powder 1 g, chlorocresol 100 mg, cetomacrogol emulsifying ointment 30 g, and freshly boiled and cooled water 68.9 g. A phosphate buffer may be included. Store in a cool place in well-closed containers which prevent evaporation and contamination.

A.P.F. (Hydrocortisone Cream Aqueous) has hydrocortisone or hydrocortisone acetate, in ultra-fine powder, 1% in cetomacrogol cream aqueous.

Hydrocortisone Cream *(U.S.P.).* Cortisol Cream. Hydrocortisone in a suitable cream basis. Store in airtight containers.

Ear-drops

Hydrocortisone and Neomycin Ear Drops *(A.P.F.).* Hydrocortisone 500 mg, neomycin sulphate 500 mg, propylene glycol to 100 ml. Protect from light.

Hydrocortisone Ear Drops *(A.P.F.).* Hydrocortisone 500 mg, propylene glycol to 100 ml. Protect from light.

Enemas

Hydrocortisone Enema *(U.S.P.).* Cortisol Enema. An enema containing hydrocortisone. Store in airtight containers.

Gels

Hydrocortisone Gel *(U.S.P.).* Contains hydrocortisone in a suitable aqueous/alcoholic gel basis. Store in airtight containers.

Injections

Sterile Hydrocortisone Suspension *(U.S.P.).* Sterile Cortisol Suspension. A sterile suspension of hydrocortisone in Water for Injections. pH 5 to 7.

Lotions

Hydrocortisone Lotion *(B.P.C. 1973).* Lot. Hydrocort. Hydrocortisone, of specified particle size, 1 g, chlorocresol 50 mg, self-emulsifying glyceryl monostearate 4 g, glycerol 6.3 g, freshly boiled and cooled water to 100 g. Any other suitable basis may be used. If prepared extemporaneously, the lotion should not be used more than 1 month after preparation.

A.P.F. has a similar preparation but containing glycerol 5 g.

Hydrocortisone Lotion *(U.S.P.).* Cortisol Lotion. Hydrocortisone in a suitable aqueous vehicle. Store in airtight containers.

Ointments

Hydrocortisone and Clioquinol Ointment *(B.P.).* —See p.976.

Hydrocortisone Ointment *(A.P.F.).* Hydrocortisone, in ultra-fine powder, 1 g, liquid paraffin 10 g, wool fat 10 g, and white soft paraffin 79 g.

Hydrocortisone Ointment *(B.P.).* Hydrocort. Oint.; Ung. Hydrocort. Hydrocortisone, in very fine powder, in white soft paraffin or a mixture of white soft paraffin and liquid paraffin, with or without wool fat. Protect from light.

Hydrocortisone Ointment *(U.S.P.).* Cortisol Ointment. Hydrocortisone in a suitable ointment basis.

Unguentum Hydrocortisoni *(Nord. P.).* Hydrocortisone 1 g, propylene glycol 750 mg, cetyl alcohol 5 g, liquid paraffin 19.25 g, soft paraffin 74 g.

Suppositories

Hydrocortisone Suppositories *(B.P.C. 1973, A.P.F.).* Suppositories containing hydrocortisone or hydrocortisone acetate, in ultra-fine powder, in theobroma oil or other suitable fatty basis. About 1.5 g of hydrocortisone or hydrocortisone acetate displaces 1 g of theobroma oil.

Tablets

Hydrocortisone Tablets *(U.S.P.).* Cortisol Tablets. Tablets containing hydrocortisone. The *U.S.P.* requires 70% dissolution in 30 minutes.

NOTE. Many proprietary names used for preparations of hydrocortisone are also applied to preparations of hydrocortisone acetate; see under Hydrocortisone Acetate, p.475.

Cobadex *(Cox Continental, UK).* Cream containing hydrocortisone 0.5 and 1% in a water-repellent silicone basis. **Cobadex-Nystatin.** Ointment containing hydrocortisone 1%, nystatin 100 000 units per g, and benzalkonium chloride 0.2%, in a similar basis.

Cortenema *(Bengué, UK).* Retention enema containing hydrocortisone, partially solubilised, 100 mg in each 60 ml. (Also available as Cortenema in *Canad.*, *USA*).

Cortril *(Pfizer, UK).* Hydrocortisone, available as ointment containing 1 and 2.5% in a water-miscible basis and 1 and 2.5% in a paraffin basis. (Also available as Cortril in *Belg.*, *Canad.*, *USA*).

Cortril Spray *(Pfizer, UK).* An aerosol spray containing hydrocortisone 50 mg per 30 ml. (Also available as Cortril Spray in *S.Afr.*).

Dioderm *(Dermal Laboratories, UK).* Hydrocortisone, available as a cream containing 0.1%. **Dioderm C.** A similar cream containing in addition clioquinol 1%.

Dome-Cort Cream *(Dome/Hollister-Stier, UK).* Contains hydrocortisone 0.125% in a water-miscible emollient basis with a pH of 4 to 5.

Efcortelan *(Glaxo, UK).* Hydrocortisone, available as **Cream** and **Ointment** containing 0.5, 1, and 2.5% and as **Lotion** containing 1%. Cream 1% and Ointment 1% also available as single-application Flexules.

Hydrocortistab *(Boots, UK).* Hydrocortisone, available as **Ointment** containing 1% and as **Tablets** of 20 mg.

Hydrocortisyl *(Roussel, UK).* Hydrocortisone, available as **Skin Cream** and **Skin Ointment** each containing 1%.

Hydrocortone *(Merck Sharp & Dohme, UK).* Hydrocortisone, available as **Ointment** containing 1% and as scored **Tablets** of 10 and 20 mg.

Hydroderm *(Merck Sharp & Dohme, UK).* An ointment containing in each g hydrocortisone 10 mg, neomycin sulphate 5 mg, and bacitracin zinc 1000 units.

Proctosedyl *(Cassenne, UK).* **Ointment** and **Suppositories**: each g of ointment and each suppository contains hydrocortisone 5 mg, cinchocaine hydrochloride 5 mg, framycetin sulphate 10 mg, and esculoside 10 mg. For haemorrhoids.

Uniroid *(Unigreg, UK: Vestric, UK).* **Ointment** containing in each g hydrocortisone 5 mg, neomycin sulphate 5 mg, polymyxin B sulphate 6250 units, and cinchocaine hydrochloride 5 mg. **Suppositories** each containing hydrocortisone 5 mg, neomycin sulphate 10 mg, polymyxin B sulphate 12 500 units, and cinchocaine hydrochloride 5 mg. For haemorrhoids and ano-rectal disorders.

Other Proprietary Names

Arg.—Hidrotisona; *Austral.*—Cort-Dome, Egocort, Hycor, Phiacort, Scheroson F *(hexanoate)*; *Belg.*—Hydro-Adreson SSC; *Canad.*—Cort-Dome, Emo-Cort, Hydro-Cortilean, Manticor, Microcort, Nutracort, Rectocort, Unicort; *Ger.*—Ficortril, Scheroson F *(also as hexanoate)*; *Ind.*—Efcorlin; *Ital.*—Algicortis, Ef-corlin; *Jap.*—Cleiton; *Neth.*—Hydro-Adreson; *S.Afr.*—Hydrocortemel; *Spain*—Bacid, Hidroaltesona, Crema Transcutánea; *Swed.*—Cortiment, Ficortril Hydrocortal, Promecort; *Switz.*—Dermolene, Hydro-Adreson, Hydrocortifor; *USA*—Aeroseb-HC, Barseb HC, Cetacort, Cort-Dome, Cortef, Cortoxide, Cotacort, Dermacort, Eldecort, Hytone, Ivocort, Nutracort, Optef, Proctocort, Rectoid, Tega-cort, Texacort, Ulcort.

A preparation containing hydrocortisone and clemizole-hexachlorophane was formerly marketed in Great Britain under the proprietary name Schericur (*Schering*).

1107-w

Hydrocortisone Acetate *(B.P., Eur. P., U.S.P.).* Hydrocort. Acet.; Cortisol Acetate; Hydrocortisone 21-Acetate; Hydrocortisoni Acetas; Acetato de Hidrocortisona. Hydrocortisone 21-acetate.

$C_{23}H_{32}O_6$=404.5.

CAS — 50-03-3.

Pharmacopoeias. In *Arg.*, *Aust.*, *Belg.*, *Br.*, *Braz.*, *Cz.*, *Eur.*, *Fr.*, *Ger.*, *Hung.*, *Ind.*, *Int.*, *It.*, *Jap.*, *Jug.*, *Neth.*, *Nord.*, *Pol.*, *Port.*, *Roum.*, *Swiss.*, *Turk.*, and *U.S.*

An odourless, white or almost white, crystalline powder, tasteless at first, followed by a persistent bitter taste. M.p. about 220° with decomposition. Hydrocortisone acetate 112 mg is approximately equivalent to 100 mg of hydrocortisone.

Practically **insoluble** in water and ether; soluble 1 in 230 of alcohol, 1 in 150 to 200 of chloroform, and 1 in 1000 of propylene glycol; slightly soluble in dioxan. A solution in dioxan is dextrorotatory. Benzalkonium chloride can be adsorbed and partially inactivated by hydrocortisone acetate; the extent of adsorption of other preservatives is not known. **Protect** from light.

Hydrocortisone acetate particles adsorbed benzalkonium chloride from eye-drops and could leave insufficient residual activity. A commercial eye-drop formulation containing 0.06% benzalkonium chloride had sufficient residual activity to kill *Escherichia coli* despite 66% adsorption.— H. S. Bean and G. Dempsey (letter), *Pharm. J.*, 1972, *2*, 69.

Adverse Effects and Treatment. As for Corticosteroids, p.446, and p.449.

There have been several reports of joint damage following the intra-articular injection of hydrocortisone acetate or other steroids into load-bearing joints (see Corticosteroids, p.447). Prolonged application to the eye of preparations containing corticosteroids has caused increased intra-ocular pressure and reduced visual function.

Withdrawal and Precautions. As for Corticosteroids, p.449.

Absorption and Fate. For a brief outline of the absorption and fate of corticosteroids, see Corticosteroids, p.451. See also Hydrocortisone, p.473.

Hydrocortisone acetate 50 mg was absorbed very quickly following intra-articular injection and was completely absorbed within 1 to 2 days.— L. S. Bain *et al.*, *Ann. phys. Med.*, 1967, *9*, 49.

Uses. Hydrocortisone acetate has the general properties of hydrocortisone (see p.473).

Hydrocortisone acetate is given by intra-articular injection into joints affected by rheumatoid arthritis, osteoarthritis, and other arthritic conditions (see Corticosteroids, p.451). The dose of hydrocortisone acetate for injection into a large joint such as the knee or hip is up to 50 mg; for joints in the hand and wrist 5 to 15 mg may be sufficient. The injections may be repeated at intervals of about 3 weeks.

Hydrocortisone acetate is used by topical application in the treatment of various skin disorders as described under Corticosteroids (see p.451). It is applied as ointments, creams, and lotions containing 0.25 to 2.5%, and has fewer side-effects on the skin and is less liable to cause adrenal suppression than the more potent topical corticosteroids. It is also applied topically as eye-drops and eye ointments containing 0.5 to 2.5%, and used as retention enemas containing about 100 mg.

Skin disorders. For recommendations concerning the correct use of corticosteroids on the skin, and a rough guide to the clinical potencies of topical corticosteroids, see Corticosteroids, p.458.

Preparations

Some official preparations allow the use of hydrocortisone or hydrocortisone acetate; these are described under Hydrocortisone, p.474.

Bandages

Hydrocortisone and Silicone Bandage *(D.T.F.)*. A bandage of white plain-weave cotton cloth impregnated with not less than 175 g per m^2 of a paste of the following composition: hydrocortisone acetate 1 g, silicone fluid 10 g, cetomacrogol '1000' 3 g, cetyl alcohol 4 g, liquid paraffin 5 g, sorbic acid 200 mg, water to 100 g.

Creams

Hydrocortisone Acetate Cream *(U.S.P.)*. Cortisol Acetate Cream. Contains hydrocortisone acetate in a suitable cream basis.

Ear-drops

Hydrocortisone and Neomycin Ear-drops *(B.P.C. 1973)*. A suspension of hydrocortisone acetate, of specified particle size, with appropriate pharmaceutical adjuvants, in a solution of neomycin sulphate in freshly boiled and cooled water. pH 6.5 to 8. Store in a cool place and avoid freezing.

Eye Ointments

Hydrocortisone Acetate Ophthalmic Ointment *(U.S.P.)*. Cortisol Acetate Ophthalmic Ointment. A sterile eye ointment containing hydrocortisone acetate in a suitable basis.

Hydrocortisone and Neomycin Eye Ointment *(B.P.C. 1973)*. A sterile eye ointment containing hydrocortisone acetate and neomycin sulphate, both of specified particle size, in Simple Eye Ointment or any other suitable sterile basis.

Hydrocortisone Eye Ointment *(B.P.C. 1973)*. Hydrocortisone Acetate Eye Ointment. A sterile eye ointment containing hydrocortisone acetate of specified particle size, in Simple Eye Ointment or any other suitable sterile basis.

A.P.F. specifies 2.5% in Eye Ointment basis sterilised at 150° to 160° for not less than 2 hours.

Eye-drops

Hydrocortisone Acetate Ophthalmic Suspension *(U.S.P.)*. Cortisol Acetate Ophthalmic Suspension. A sterile suspension of hydrocortisone acetate in an aqueous medium containing a suitable antimicrobial agent. It may contain suitable buffers and suspending agents. pH 6 to 8. Store in airtight containers.

Hydrocortisone and Neomycin Eye-drops *(B.P.C. 1973)*. A sterile suspension containing up to 1.5% of hydrocortisone acetate, of specified particle size, and 0.5% of neomycin sulphate, with 0.002% of phenylmercuric acetate or nitrate or other suitable preservatives, in water. It may also contain appropriate pharmaceutical adjuvants. pH 6.5 to 8. Store in a cool place and avoid freezing.

Hydrocortisone Eye-drops *(B.P.C. 1973)*. HCOR. A sterile suspension containing up to 1% of hydrocortisone acetate, of specified particle size, with suitable preservatives, in water. It may also contain appropriate pharmaceutical adjuvants. pH 6 to 8. Store in a cool place and avoid freezing.

Injections

Hydrocortisone Acetate Injection *(B.P.)*. Hydrocort. Acet. Inj. A sterile suspension of hydrocortisone acetate in very fine powder, in Water for Injections containing suitable dispersing agents. It is prepared aseptically. It settles on standing but readily disperses on shaking. It is intended for local injection only and is unsuitable for the production of systemic effects. Protect from light.

Hydrocortisone Acetate Subconjunctival Injection *(A.P.F.)*. A sterile suspension of hydrocortisone acetate 2.5%.

Sterile Hydrocortisone Acetate Suspension *(U.S.P.)*. Sterile Cortisol Acetate Suspension. A sterile suspension in a suitable aqueous medium. It may contain suitable buffers and suspending agents. pH 5 to 7.

Lotions

Hydrocortisone Acetate Lotion *(U.S.P.)*. Contains hydrocortisone acetate in a suitable aqueous vehicle. Store in airtight containers.

Ointments

Hydrocortisone Acetate Ointment *(B.P.)*. Hydrocort. Acet. Oint.; Ung. Hydrocort. Acet. Hydrocortisone acetate, in very fine powder, in white soft paraffin or a mixture of white soft paraffin and liquid paraffin, with or without wool fat. Protect from light.

Hydrocortisone Acetate Ointment *(U.S.P.)*. Cortisol Acetate Ointment. Hydrocortisone acetate in a suitable ointment basis.

NOTE. Many proprietary names used for preparations of hydrocortisone acetate are also applied to preparations of hydrocortisone; see under Hydrocortisone, p.474..

Colifoam *(Stafford-Miller, UK)*. Hydrocortisone acetate, available as a foam containing 10%. For ulcerative colitis and proctitis.

Controversy concerning the rectal spreading of Colifoam.— D. J. Hay *et al.*, *Br. med. J.*, 1979, *1*, 1751; M. J. G. Farthing *et al.*, *ibid.*, *2*, 822; D. Hay *et al.* (letter), *ibid.*, 1365; M. J. G. Farthing and M. L. Clark (letter), *ibid.*

Cortacream Bandage *(Smith & Nephew, UK)*. A brand of Hydrocortisone and Silicone Bandage *D.T.F.*

Hydrocortistab *(Boots, UK)*. Hydrocortisone acetate, available as **Cream** containing 1%, as **Eye-drops** containing 1%; as **Eye Ointment** containing 2.5%; and as **Injection** containing 25 mg per ml, in vials of 5 ml.

Hydrocortone Cream *(Merck Sharp & Dohme, UK)*. Contains hydrocortisone acetate 1%. (Also available as Hydrocortone in *Austral.*, *Canad.*, *Neth.*, *Swed.*).

NOTE. Hydrocortone may be applied in different countries to different formulations.

Proctofoam HC *(Stafford-Miller, UK)*. Contains hydrocortisone acetate 1% and pramoxine hydrochloride 1%, in an aerosol with applicator. For haemorrhoids and similar ano-rectal disorders. *Application*: 1 applicator full (approximately 500 mg), per rectum, twice or thrice daily.

Other Proprietary Names

Austral.— Cortef, Cortril, Dermacort, Dermacort 'O', Hydrocortisyl, Hydrosone, Hysone-A, Sigmacort, Siguent Hycor, Squibb-HC; *Belg.*—Cortril, Ophticor H; *Canad.*—Cortamed, Corticreme, Cortiment, Cortril, Hyderm; *Denm.*—Hydrocortisat; *Fr.*—Cortomister; *Ger.*—Ficortril, Litraderm, Scheroson F; *Ital.*—Chemysone, Cortidro, Cortril, Idrocortigamma; *Jap.*—Cortes; *Spain*—Corti-Basileos, Scherosona F, Supralef; *Swed.*—Ficortril, Hydrocortal; *Switz.*—Hydrocortifor; *USA*—Carmol HC, Cortaid, Cortef acetate, Cortifoam, Epifoam, Pramosone.

A preparation containing hydrocortisone acetate was formerly marketed in Great Britain under the proprietary name Pabracort (*Paines & Byrne*).

1108-e

Hydrocortisone Butyrate.

Hydrocortisone 17-Butyrate. Hydrocortisone 17α-butyrate.

$C_{25}H_{36}O_6$=432.6.

CAS — 13609-67-1.

Adverse Effects, Treatment, Withdrawal, and Precautions. As for Corticosteroids, p.446, p.449.

Absorption and Fate. For a brief outline of the absorption and fate of corticosteroids, see Corticosteroids, p.451. See also Hydrocortisone, p.473. When applied topically, particularly to large areas, when the skin is broken, or under occlusive dressings, corticosteroids may be absorbed in sufficient amounts to cause systemic effects.

Uses. Hydrocortisone butyrate is a glucocorticoid used by topical application in the treatment of various skin disorders as described under Corticosteroids (see p.451). It is usually employed as a cream, lotion, or ointment containing 0.1%.

Skin disorders. For recommendations concerning the correct use of corticosteroids on the skin, and a rough guide to the clinical potencies of topical corticosteroids, see Corticosteroids, p.458.

Proprietary Preparations

Locoid *(Brocades, UK)*. Preparations containing hydrocortisone butyrate 0.1% available as **Cream**; as **Scalp Lotion** in an aqueous alcoholic basis (Inflammable: keep away from an open flame); and as **Ointment**. **Locoid C**. Preparations containing hydrocortisone butyrate 0.1% and chlorquinaldol 3%, available as **Cream** and as **Ointment**. (Also available as Locoid in *Austral.*, *Belg.*, *Denm.*, *Neth.*, *Norw.*, *S.Afr.*, *Switz.*).

Other Proprietary Names

Alfason *(Ger.)*; Locoidon *(Ital.)*; Plancol *(Jap.)*.

1109-l

Hydrocortisone Cypionate *(U.S.P.)*. Cortisol Cypionate; Hydrocortisone Cipionate; Hydrocortisone Cyclopentylpropionate. Hydrocortisone 21-(3-cyclopentylpropionate).

$C_{29}H_{42}O_6$=486.6.

CAS — 508-99-6.

Pharmacopoeias. In *U.S.*

A white or almost white, tasteless, crystalline powder, odourless or with a slight odour. Hydrocortisone cypionate 134 mg is approximately equivalent to 100 mg of hydrocortisone. Practically **insoluble** in water; soluble in alcohol, very soluble in chloroform; soluble in glycols and vegetable oils; slightly soluble in ether. A solution in chloroform is dextrorotatory. **Store** at a temperature not exceeding 8° in airtight containers. Protect from light.

Uses. Hydrocortisone cypionate has the general properties of hydrocortisone (see p.473). It is administered by mouth, usually as a flavoured aqueous suspension, and is reported to be more slowly absorbed than hydrocortisone.

Preparations

Hydrocortisone Cypionate Oral Suspension *(U.S.P.)*. Cortisol Cypionate Oral Suspension. A suspension of hydrocortisone cypionate. Potency is expressed in terms of the equivalent amount of hydrocortisone. pH 2.8 to 3.2. Store in airtight containers. Protect from light.

Proprietary Names

Cortef Oral Suspension *(Upjohn, USA)*.

1110-v

Hydrocortisone Hydrogen Succinate.

(B.P.).Hydrocort. Hydrogen Succ.; Cortisol Hemisuccinate; Hémisuccinate d'Hydrocortisone; Hydrocortisone Hemisuccinate *(U.S.P.)*; Hydrocortisonum Hydrogensuccinicum. Hydrocortisone 21-(hydrogen succinate).

$C_{25}H_{34}O_8$=462.5.

CAS — 2203-97-6.

Pharmacopoeias. In *Br.*, *Cz.*, *Fr.*, and *U.S.*

A white or almost white odourless crystalline powder. M.p. 170° to 173° or 210° to 214°. Practically **insoluble** in water; soluble 1 in 40 of alcohol, 1 in 7 of dehydrated alcohol, and 1 in 25 of sodium bicarbonate solution; soluble, with decomposition, in sodium hydroxide solution. A solution in dehydrated alcohol is dextrorotatory. **Store** in airtight containers. Protect from light.

Uses. Hydrocortisone hydrogen succinate has the general properties of hydrocortisone (see p.473) and is used in the preparation of aqueous solutions of hydrocortisone sodium succinate.

Proprietary Names

Oralsone *(Gramon, Arg.; Vinas, Spain)*.

1111-g

Hydrocortisone Sodium Phosphate

(B.P., U.S.P.). Cortisol Sodium Phosphate. Hydrocortisone 21-(disodium phosphate).

$C_{21}H_{29}Na_2O_8P$=486.4.

CAS — 6000-74-4.

Pharmacopoeias. In *Br.* and *U.S.*

A white or light yellow, odourless or almost odourless, hygroscopic powder. The *B.P.* specifies not more than 10% of water; the *U.S.P.* specifies not more than 5% loss on drying. Hydrocortisone sodium phosphate 134 mg is approximately equivalent to 100 mg of hydrocortisone.

Soluble 1 in 4 of water; slightly soluble in alcohol; practically insoluble in dehydrated alcohol, chloroform, dioxan, and ether. A solution in water is dextrorotatory. A 0.5% solution in water has a pH of 7.5 to 9. Solutions are **sterilised** by filtration. **Store** in airtight containers. Protect from light.

No precipitate occurred when hydrocortisone sodium phosphate was added to an injection of heparin.— C. L. J. Coles, *Personal Communication, Glaxo*, 1975.

Incompatibility. For a report of incompatibility between hydrocortisone sodium phosphate and erythromycin lactobionate, see Erythromycin Lactobionate, p.1163.

Hydrocortisone sodium phosphate has the general properties of hydrocortisone (see p.473) and is used by intramuscular or slow intravenous injection. Paraesthesia, especially in the genital region, has been associated with intravenous injections; the phosphate content has been implicated.

Paraesthesia. In a double-blind, placebo-controlled study of 42 healthy subjects, hydrocortisone sodium phosphate in single intravenous doses of 100, 200, or 400 mg (given in a strength of 50 mg per ml over a 2-minute period), was found to have comparable biological effects to those of hydrocortisone sodium succinate 100, 200, or 400 mg (given similarly). Side-effects were, however, more common in the sodium phosphate group with 16 of 18 subjects experiencing ano-rectal itching or burning compared with none of 18 in the sodium succinate group, and 1 of 6 in the placebo group. The effect was observed within 10 seconds to 6 minutes after the start of administration.— E. Novak *et al., Upjohn, USA, Clin. Pharmac. Ther.*, 1976, *20*, 109. Comment on paraesthesia associated with intravenous injection of hydrocortisone sodium phosphate; the phosphate ester should not be used.— *Drug & Ther. Bull.*, 1979, *17*, 71.

Further references to paraesthesia associated with hydrocortisone sodium phosphate.— D. Barltrop and Y. T. Diba (letter), *Lancet*, 1969, *1*, 529; E. S. Snell, *Glaxo* (letter), *Lancet*, 1969, *1*, 530; N. G. Kounis (letter), *Br. med. J.*, 1973, *2*, 663.

Preparations

Hydrocortisone Sodium Phosphate Injection *(B.P.)*. Hydrocort. Sod. Phos. Inj. A sterile solution of hydrocortisone sodium phosphate, with suitable buffering and stabilising agents, in Water for Injections. Sterilised by filtration. Potency is expressed in terms of the equivalent amount of hydrocortisone. pH 7.5 to 8.5. Store at a temperature not exceeding 25° and avoid freezing. Protect from light.

Hydrocortisone Sodium Phosphate Injection *(U.S.P.)*. Cortisol Sodium Phosphate Injection. A sterile buffered solution in Water for Injections. Potency is expressed in terms of the equivalent amount of hydrocortisone. pH 7.5 to 8.5.

Efcortesol Injection *(Glaxo, UK)*. Contains hydrocortisone sodium phosphate equivalent to hydrocortisone 100 mg per ml, in ampoules of 1 and 5 ml.

Other Proprietary Names

Actocortin *(Denm., Ger., Norw., Swed.)*; Actocortina *(Spain)*; Flebocortid-1000 *(Spain)*; Hydrocortone fosfat *(Swed.)*; Idracemi *(Ital.)*; Physiocortison *(Spain)*; Venocortin *(S.Afr.)*.

1112-q

Hydrocortisone Sodium Succinate *(B.P., U.S.P.)*.

Hydrocort. Sod. Succ.; Cortisol Sodium Succinate; Hydrocortisone 21-Sodium Succinate; Succinato Sōdico de Hidrocortisona. Hydrocortisone 21-(sodium succinate).

$C_{25}H_{33}NaO_8$=484.5.

CAS — 125-04-2.

Pharmacopoeias. In *Br., Braz., It.,* and *U.S.*

A white or almost white, odourless, hygroscopic, crystalline powder or amorphous solid. Hydrocortisone sodium succinate 134 mg is approximately equivalent to 100 mg of hydrocortisone.

Soluble 1 in 3 of water, 1 in 34 of alcohol, and 1 in 200 of dehydrated alcohol; very slightly soluble in acetone; practically insoluble in chloroform and ether. A solution in alcohol is dextrorotatory. It is unstable in aqueous solution. Solutions for injection are prepared by dissolving, immediately before use, the sterile contents of a sealed container in Water for Injections. **Store** in airtight containers. Protect from light.

Incompatibility. Hydrocortisone sodium succinate has been reported to be incompatible with amylobarbitone sodium, chloramphenicol sodium succinate, colistin sulphomethate sodium, dimenhydrinate, diphenhydramine hydrochloride, ephedrine sulphate, heparin, hydralazine hydrochloride, kanamycin sulphate, metaraminol tartrate, methicillin sodium, nafcillin sodium, novobiocin sodium, oxytetracycline hydrochloride, pentobarbitone sodium, phenobarbitone sodium, prochlorperazine, promazine hydrochloride, promethazine hydrochloride, quinalbarbitone sodium, tetracycline hydrochloride, and vancomycin hydrochloride; loss of ampicillin potency has been reported. References: R. Misgen, *Am. J. Hosp. Pharm.*, 1965, *22*, 92; J. A. Patel and G. L. Phillips, *ibid.*, 1966, *23*, 409; J. M. Meisler and M. W. Skolaut, *ibid.*, 557; E. A. Parker and H. J. Levin, *ibid.*, 1975, *32*, 943; B. B. Riley, *J. Hosp. Pharm.*, 1970, *28*, 228.

A report of solubility-dependent incompatibility between magnesium sulphate and hydrocortisone sodium succinate which can be circumvented by adding each drug separately to a large-volume parenteral solution with thorough mixing after each addition.— G. L. Fraser (letter), *Am. J. Hosp. Pharm.*, 1978, *35*, 783.

Stability. Hydrocortisone sodium succinate was hydrolysed to hydrocortisone, thus affecting solubility, in intravenous solutions (pH 6.5 to 7.5) containing 250 mg per litre. There was about 3 to 4% loss of potency in 24 hours and about 6 to 8% loss after 48 hours.— E. A. Parker, *Am. J. Hosp. Pharm.*, 1967, *24*, 434. See also R. L. Nedich, *Bull. parent. Drug Ass.*, 1973, *27*, 228.

Hydrocortisone sodium succinate 1 mg per ml was stable for 24 hours at room temperature in Elliott's B Solution, Sodium Chloride Injection, or Lactated Ringer's Injection (*U.S.P.*).— J. C. Cradock *et al.*, *Am. J. Hosp. Pharm.*, 1978, *35*, 402.

Adverse Effects and Treatment. As for Corticosteroids, p.446, and p.449.

Cardiovascular collapse has been reported following the rapid intravenous injection of large doses of corticosteroids.

Muscular weakness and faintness occurred after hydrocortisone 8 mg per kg body-weight intravenously but not after 4 mg per kg. Hypokalaemia in association with the acidaemia and hypoxaemia of acute asthma might precipitate cardiac dysrrhythmias and it was therefore advisable to monitor potassium concentrations after intravenous administration of corticosteroids and to administer potassium supplements sufficient to replace the urinary losses.— J. V. Collins *et al.*, *Lancet*, 1970, *2*, 1047. Severe myopathy in one patient affecting respiratory muscles and those of her limbs was attributed to hydrocortisone sodium succinate given in large doses of up to 3 g in 24 hours for status asthmaticus. Previous therapy had produced no ill effect. Recovery was slow; at 3 weeks the patient could walk unaided and at 2 months there was persistent leg weakness and myopathy. It was recommended that patients with severe asthma should not be given such large doses of hydrocortisone.— I. A. MacFarlane and F. D. Rosenthal (letter), *ibid.*, 1977, *2*, 615. An acute generalised myopathy, considered to be distinct from other forms of corticosteroid myopathy, developed in a patient following treatment with high doses of hydrocortisone intravenously for status asthmaticus.— W. Van Marle and K. L. Woods, *Br. med. J.*, 1980, *281*, 271.

Allergy. Generalised urticaria, together with oedema of the face and lips, occurred in an asthmatic patient within 10 minutes of an intramuscular dose of hydrocortisone sodium succinate 200 mg. The symptoms disappeared within one hour.— R. F. U. Ashford and A. Bailey, *Postgrad. med. J.*, 1980, *56*, 437. See also S. C. Chapman *et al.*, *N.Z. J. Med.*, 1979, *90*, 380.

Effects on the electrolyte balance. Hypernatraemia in 3 patients given high doses of hydrocortisone to treat septic shock.— R. B. Sawyer *et al.*, *Am. J. Surg.*, 1967, *114*, 691.

Withdrawal and Precautions. As for Corticosteroids, p.449.

Absorption and Fate. For a brief outline of the absorption and fate of corticosteroids, see Corticosteroids, p.451. See also Hydrocortisone, p.473.

Uses. Hydrocortisone sodium succinate has the general properties of hydrocortisone (see p.473). It is administered intramuscularly or intravenously for intensive therapy or in emergencies. It is especially useful for intravenous use in acute adrenocortical insufficiency and severe status asthmaticus.

The usual dose is the equivalent of 100 to 500 mg of hydrocortisone, repeated 3 or 4 times in 24 hours, according to the severity of the condition and the patient's response. Children up to 1 year of age may be given 25 mg, 1 to 5 years 50 mg, and 6 to 12 years 100 mg.

In the treatment of severe shock the equivalent of up to 50 mg per kg body-weight in 24 hours has been given by slow intravenous injection over several minutes in divided doses, or by intravenous infusion. In the treatment of severe Gram-negative septic shock single doses of 50 to 150 mg per kg have been given as bolus intravenous injections in an attempt to promote rapid vasodilatation. For intravenous infusion hydrocortisone sodium succinate may be diluted with an appropriate volume of dextrose injection or sodium chloride injection or sodium chloride and dextrose injection.

Patients with adrenal deficiency states require supplements of hydrocortisone during surgical operations and hydrocortisone sodium succinate equivalent to 100 mg of hydrocortisone may be given intramuscularly immediately before surgery in conjunction with intravenous injections if necessary.

In meningitis, daily intrathecal injections of hydrocortisone sodium succinate equivalent to 20 mg of hydrocortisone have been given for a few days, in conjunction with appropriate anti-infective therapy; children may be given 10 to 20 mg.

It is used in the form of lozenges in the treatment of aphthous ulceration in a dose of 2.5 mg four times daily.

A solution of hydrocortisone sodium succinate, usually containing the equivalent of 100 mg of hydrocortisone in 120 ml of physiological saline solution, has been given by slow rectal infusion in the treatment of ulcerative colitis.

A recommendation that hydrocortisone sodium succinate should be used instead of hydrocortisone sodium phosphate since it does not induce paraesthesia on intravenous injection.— *Drug & Ther. Bull.*, 1979, *17*, 71.

Asthma. Hydrocortisone, 4 mg per kg body-weight given intravenously every 140 minutes, produced a plasma-11-hydroxycorticosteroid concentration of 1.5 µg per ml, which was regarded as the minimum necessary in the treatment of acute bronchial asthma.— J. V. Collins *et al.*, *Lancet*, 1970, *2*, 1047.

For details of the emergency management of asthma, see Corticosteroids, p.453.

Operative coverage. For recommendations relating to corticosteroid coverage in surgery and general anaesthesia, see under Precautions for Corticosteroids (Operative Coverage), p.450.

Shock. For comment on the role of high-dose corticosteroid therapy in shock, see under Uses of Corticosteroids (Shock),p.458.

Preparations

Hydrocortisone Lozenges *(B.P.C. 1973)*. Troch. Hydrocort.; Hydrocortisone Sodium Succinate Lozenges. Lozenges containing hydrocortisone sodium succinate. Each lozenge weighs about 100 mg. Store in a cool place in airtight containers.

Hydrocortisone, Penicillin, and Streptokinase Irrigation *(Queen Eliz. Hosp., S. Australia)*. Hydrocortisone (as sodium succinate) 50 mg, benzylpenicillin sodium 600 mg, streptokinase 20 000 units, Water for Injections to 50 ml. Prepare aseptically. Store at 2° to 8°. Used for irrigation of the fallopian tubes.

Hydrocortisone Sodium Succinate for Injection *(U.S.P.)*. Cortisol Sodium Succinate for Injection. A sterile mixture of hydrocortisone sodium succinate and suitable buffers which may be prepared from hydrocortisone sodium succinate or hydrocortisone hydrogen succinate and sodium hydroxide or sodium carbonate. Potency is expressed in terms of the equivalent amount of hydrocortisone. A solution containing the equivalent of 50 mg of hydrocortisone per ml has a pH of 7 to 8.

Hydrocortisone Sodium Succinate Injection *(B.P.)*. Hydrocort. Sod. Succ. Inj. A sterile solution of hydrocortisone sodium succinate in Water for Injections containing suitable buffering agents, prepared by dissolving, immediately before use, the sterile contents of a sealed container (Hydrocortisone Sodium Succinate for Injection) in the requisite amount of Water for Injections. Potency is expressed in terms of the equivalent amount of hydrocortisone. pH of a 6.7% solution, 6.5 to 8.

Proprietary Preparations

Corlan Pellets *(Glaxo, UK)*. Each contains hydrocortisone sodium succinate equivalent to 2.5 mg of hydrocortisone. For aphthous ulceration.
Dose. One pellet 4 times daily; they should not be sucked but kept in the mouth in close proximity to the ulcer. (Also available as Corlan in *Austral., Neth., S.Afr.*).

Efcortelan Soluble *(Glaxo, UK)*. Hydrocortisone sodium succinate, available as powder for preparing injections for intravenous use, in vials each containing the equivalent of hydrocortisone 100 mg, with 2-ml ampoules of Water for Injections. (Also available as Efcortelan Soluble in *Austral., S.Afr.*).

Solu-Cortef *(Upjohn, UK)*. Hydrocortisone sodium succinate, available as powder for preparing injections in vials each containing the equivalent of 100 mg of hydrocortisone, with 2-ml ampoules of Water for Injections. (Also available as Solu-Cortef in *Arg., Austral., Belg., Canad., Denm., Ital., Neth., Norw., S.Afr., Switz., USA*).

Other Proprietary Names

Aacicortisol *(Belg.)*; A-Hydrocort *(USA)*; Buccalsone *(Belg.)*; Efcorlin *(Ind.)*; Emi-Corlin *(Ital.)*; Excerate *(Jap.)*; Flebocortid *(Ital.)*; Hydrocortisyl *(S.Afr.)*; Nordicort *(Austral.)*; S-Cortilean *(Canad.)*; Solu-Cortril *(Arg.)*; Solu-Glyc *(Norw., Swed., Switz.)*; Venocort *(Austral.)*.

1138-k

Hydrocortisone Valerate *(U.S.P.)*. Cortisol 17-Valerate. Hydrocortisone 17-valerate.

$C_{26}H_{38}O_6$=446.6.

CAS — 57524-89-7.

Pharmacopoeias. In *U.S.*

Hydrocortisone valerate is used topically.

Preparations

Hydrocortisone Valerate Cream *(U.S.P.)*. Contains hydrocortisone valerate in a suitable cream basis.

Proprietary Names

Westcort *(Westwood, Canad.; Westwood, USA)*.

1113-p

Medrysone *(U.S.P.)*. 11β-Hydroxy-6α-methylprogesterone; U 8471; Medrisona. 11β-Hydroxy-6α-methylpregn-4-ene-3,20-dione.

$C_{22}H_{32}O_3$=344.5.

CAS — 2668-66-8.

Pharmacopoeias. In *Braz.* and *U.S.*

A white or off-white crystalline powder, odourless or with a slight odour. M.p. about 158° with decomposition. Sparingly **soluble** in water; soluble in chloroform and methylene chloride. A solution in chloroform is dextrorotatory.

Adverse Effects, Treatment, Withdrawal, and Precautions. As for Corticosteroids, p.446, p.449.
Prolonged application to the eye of preparations containing corticosteroids has caused raised intra-ocular pressure and reduced visual function.

A review of medrysone. Medrysone may be less likely than potent glucocorticoids, such as dexamethasone, to cause raised intra-ocular pressure.— *Drugs*, 1971, *2*, 5. Comment.— A. Schwartz and I. H. Leopold, *ibid.*, 1.

Allergy. Delayed hypersensitivity to medrysone.— G. Smolin, *Archs Ophthal., N.Y.*, 1971, *85*, 478.

Absorption and Fate. For a brief outline of the absorption and fate of corticosteroids, see Corticosteroids, p.451.

Uses. Medrysone is a glucocorticoid employed, usually as eye-drops containing 1%, in the topical treatment of allergic and inflammatory conditions of the eye as described under Corticosteroids (see p.451).

Preparations

Medrysone Ophthalmic Suspension *(U.S.P.)*. A sterile suspension of medrysone in a buffered aqueous vehicle containing a suitable antimicrobial agent and preservative. pH 6.2 to 7.5. Store in airtight containers. Protect from light.

Proprietary Names

HMS Liquifilm *(Allergan, Canad.; Allergan, Neth.; Allergan, USA)*; Ipoflogin *(Tubi Lux, Ital.)*; Medrifar *(Farmila, Ital.)*; Ophtocortin *(Winzer, Ger.)*; Sedesterol *(Poen, Arg.)*; Spectramedryn Liquifilm *(Allergan, Ger.)*; Visudrisone *(LOA, Arg.)*.

1114-s

Meprednisone *(U.S.P.)*. 16β-Methylprednisone. 17α,21-Dihydroxy-16β-methylpregna-1,4-diene-3,11,20-trione.

$C_{22}H_{28}O_5$=372.5.

CAS — 1247-42-3.

Pharmacopoeias. In *U.S.*

A white to creamy-white odourless powder. M.p. about 200° with decomposition. **Soluble** 1 in 3300 of water, 1 in 9.6 of chloroform, 1 in 1700 of ether, 1 in 8.7 of methylene chloride, and 1 in 71 of propylene glycol; soluble in alcohol and dioxan. A solution in dioxan is dextrorotatory. **Store** at a temperature not exceeding 40° in airtight containers. Protect from light.

Adverse Effects, Treatment, Withdrawal, and Precautions. As for Corticosteroids, p.446, p.449.

Absorption and Fate. For a brief outline of the absorption and fate of corticosteroids, see Corticosteroids, p.451.

Uses. Meprednisone is a synthetic glucocorticoid with the general properties described under Corticosteroids (see p.451); 4 mg of meprednisone is reported to be equivalent in anti-inflammatory activity to 5 mg of prednisolone.
It may be used in the treatment of all conditions for which corticosteroid therapy is indicated except adrenal-deficiency states, for which its lack of sodium-retaining properties makes it less suitable than cortisone or hydrocortisone with supplementary fludrocortisone. Meprednisone is given in usual doses of 4 to 48 mg daily.

A review of meprednisone.— *Med. Lett.*, 1971, *13*, 106.

Preparations

Meprednisone Tablets *(U.S.P.)*. Tablets containing meprednisone. Store at a temperature not exceeding 40° in airtight containers. Protect from light.

Proprietary Names

Betapar *(Parke, Davis, USA)*; Corti-Bi *(Sidus, Ital.)*.

1115-w

Methylprednisolone *(B.P., U.S.P.)*. Methylprednisolonum; 6α-Methylprednisolone. 11β,17α,21-Trihydroxy-6α-methylpregna-1,4-diene-3,20-dione.

$C_{22}H_{30}O_5$=374.5.

CAS — 83-43-2.

Pharmacopoeias. In *Br., Jap.*, and *U.S.*

A white or almost white odourless crystalline powder, tasteless at first but with a persistent bitter after-taste. M.p. about 240° to 243° with decomposition.
Practically **insoluble** in water; soluble 1 in 100 of dehydrated alcohol, 1 in 530 to 800 of chloroform, and 1 in 800 of ether; sparingly soluble in dioxan and methyl alcohol; slightly soluble in acetone. A solution in dioxan is dextrorotatory. **Store** in airtight containers. Protect from light.

The shelf-life of methylprednisolone in aqueous formulations was dependent upon pH and concentration of polysorbate 80 used. A pH of 4.6 was best. Solubility decreased in the presence of polar additives.— M. I. Amin and J. T. Bryan, *J. pharm. Sci.*, 1973, *62*, 1768.

Photosensitivity. Ultraviolet light and fluorescent lighting caused degradation of methylprednisolone solutions.— W. E. Hamlin *et al.*, *J. Am. pharm. Ass., scient. Edn*, 1960, *49*, 253.

Adverse Effects and Treatment. As for Corticosteroids, p.446, and p.449.
Methylprednisolone may be slightly less likely than prednisone to cause sodium and water retention.

Adrenal suppression. A study of the effect of methylprednisolone on adrenal function.— D. C. Garg *et al.*, *J. clin. Pharmac.*, 1979, *19*, 644.

Withdrawal and Precautions. As for Corticosteroids, p.449.

Absorption and Fate. For a brief outline of the absorption and fate of corticosteroids, see Corticosteroids, p.451.
The half-life of methylprednisolone has been reported to be slightly longer than that of prednisolone.

Uses. Methylprednisolone is a synthetic glucocorticoid with the general properties described under Corticosteroids (see p.451); 4 mg of methylprednisolone is equivalent in anti-inflammatory activity to about 5 mg of prednisolone.
It may be used in the treatment of all conditions for which corticosteroid therapy is indicated except adrenal-deficiency states, for which its lack of sodium-retaining properties makes it less suitable than cortisone or hydrocortisone with supplementary fludrocortisone.
Methylprednisolone has a usual dose range of 4 to 48 mg daily in divided doses, as a single daily dose at 8 a.m., or as a double dose on alternate days.

Preparations

Methylprednisolone Tablets *(B.P.)*. Tablets containing methylprednisolone. Protect from light.

Methylprednisolone Tablets *(U.S.P.)*. Tablets containing methylprednisolone. The *U.S.P.* requires 50% dissolution in 30 minutes.

Medrone *(Upjohn, UK)*. Methylprednisolone, available as scored tablets of 2, 4, and 16 mg.

Other Proprietary Names

Betalona *(Spain)*; Caberdelta-M, Cortalfa, Esametone, Eutisone, Firmacort (all *Ital.*); Horusona *(Spain)*; Medesone *(Ital.)*; Medrate *(Ger.)*; Medrol *(Arg., Austral., Belg., Canad., Denm., Fr., Ital., Norw., S.Afr., Switz., USA)*; Metilbetasone, Metilcort, Metilprednilone, Metilstendiolo (all *Ital.*); Moderin *(Spain)*; Nixolan, Prednilen, Radiosone, Reactenol, Sieropresol, Summicort (all *Ital.*); Suprametil *(Switz.)* Urbason *(Belg., Ger., Ital., Neth., Norw., Spain, Swed., Switz.)*; Urbason-Depot (cypionate) *(Belg., Ger., Switz.)*.

A preparation containing methylprednisolone and aspirin was formerly marketed in Great Britain under the proprietary name Medro-Cordex (*Upjohn*).

1116-e

Methylprednisolone Acetate *(B.P., B.P. Vet., U.S.P.)*. 6α-Methylprednisolone 21-Acetate. Methylprednisolone 21-acetate.

$C_{24}H_{32}O_6$=416.5.

CAS — 53-36-1.

Pharmacopoeias. In *Br.* and *U.S.*

A white or almost white, odourless, crystalline powder. M.p. about 225° with some decomposition. Methylprednisolone acetate 44 mg is approximately equivalent to 40 mg of methylprednisolone. Practically **insoluble** in water; soluble 1 in 250 of chloroform and 1 in 1500 of ether; slightly soluble in alcohol sparingly soluble in acetone and methyl alcohol; soluble in dioxan. A solution in dioxan is dextrorotatory. **Store** in airtight containers. Protect from light.

Adverse Effects and Treatment. As for Corticosteroids, p.446, and p.449.

There have been reports of joint damage following the intra-articular injection of corticosteroids into load-bearing joints (see under Corticosteroids, p.447).

In 8 patients each given 2 intramuscular injections of methylprednisolone acetate 80 mg at 14-day intervals for hay fever, side-effects included exacerbation of peptic ulceration, severe cramps, recurrence of infantile eczema, and anterior uveitis.— M. A. Ganderton and V. H. T. James, *Br. med. J.*, 1970, *1*, 267.

A 30-year-old African woman developed a persistent area of complete depigmentation at the site of an intra-articular injection of methylprednisolone.— E. Bloomfield (letter), *Br. med. J.*, 1972, *3*, 766.

Adrenal suppression. About 18 days after an injection of methylprednisolone the resting plasma cortisol had returned to within the normal range but the response to ACTH remained suppressed for a longer period and the full response was not regained after 60 days.— M. A. Ganderton and V. H. T. James (letter), *Br. med. J.*, 1970, *2*, 362.

Effects on growth. Growth was inhibited in 16 patients with congenital adrenal hyperplasia who were treated with methylprednisolone acetate intramuscularly twice a week in physiological doses. Growth hormone responsiveness returned in 6 selected for study when the shorter-acting cortisone acetate was substituted.— R. S. Stempfel *et al.*, *J. Pediat.*, 1968, *73*, 767.

Withdrawal and Precautions. As for Corticosteroids, p.449.

Activation of infection. Some 15 weeks after a middle-aged man had had 40 mg of methylprednisolone acetate instilled into the lumbar subarachnoid space for sciatica, he developed a severe headache, a temperature of 39.4°, myalgia, and malaise. He was found to have tuberculous meningitis. It was suggested that as methylprednisolone passed very slowly across nervous system membranes, it should be used intrathecally with the greatest caution and the patient examined for latent tuberculous infection.— M. Roberts *et al.*, *J. Am. med. Ass.*, 1967, *200*, 894. Another report of infection following epidural injection of methylprednisolone acetate; the patient had developed a spinal fluid leak.— J. H. Dougherty and R. A. R. Fraser, *J. Neurosurg.*, 1978, *48*, 1023.

Absorption and Fate. For a brief outline of the absorption and fate of corticosteroids, see Corticosteroids, p.451. See also Methylprednisolone, p.477.

Methylprednisolone acetate is absorbed from joints in a few days but is more slowly absorbed following deep intramuscular injection. It is less soluble than methylprednisolone (see p.477).

When applied topically, particularly to large areas, when the skin is broken, or under occlusive dressings, corticosteroids may be absorbed in sufficient amounts to cause systemic effects.

Administration of methylprednisolone acetate 40 mg intramuscularly to 8 men produced measurable plasma concentrations of methylprednisolone for 11 to 17 days. The average peak plasma concentration was 14.8 ng per ml and occurred after 6 to 8 hours.— R. G. Stoll *et al.*, *Clin. Pharmac. Ther.*, 1974, *15*, 220. See also L. S. Bain *et al.*, *Ann. phys. Med.*, 1967, *9*, 49.

An investigation of the systemic absorption of methylprednisolone acetate when given in suspension as a retention enema or by mouth to healthy subjects.— D. C. Garg *et al.*, *Clin. Pharmac. Ther.*, 1979, *26*, 232.

Uses. Methylprednisolone acetate has the general properties of methylprednisolone (see p.477).

An aqueous suspension may be injected directly into joints and soft tissues in the treatment of rheumatoid arthritis, osteoarthritis, bursitis, and similar inflammatory conditions. The dose by intra-articular injection varies from 4 to 80 mg according to the size of the affected joint.

It may also be administered by intramuscular injection for a prolonged systemic effect, the dose varying from 40 mg every 2 weeks to 80 mg weekly; doses of up to 120 mg weekly have been given.

It may be administered by intralesional injection of 20 to 60 mg or by topical application in the treatment of various skin disorders as described under Corticosteroids (see p.451). It is applied as ointments, creams, and lotions containing 0.25% and has fewer side-effects on the skin and is less liable to cause adrenal suppression than the more potent topical corticosteroids. Methylprednisolone acetate may also be used in retention enemas containing 40 to 120 mg.

Adrenal insufficiency. Effective control of Addison's disease and autoimmune hypothyroidism in a woman who did not take her daily therapy correctly, was achieved by giving thyroxine 400 µg weekly, together with methylprednisolone 40 mg intramuscularly weekly, and deoxycortone pivalate 25 mg intramuscularly monthly.— A. R. Fraser and F. Clark (letter), *Lancet*, 1979, *1*, 667.

Anaesthesia and surgery. In a double-blind study of 165 patients undergoing tonsillectomy, local injection of methylprednisolone acetate into each tonsillar fossa reduced postoperative pain compared with normal saline injections, but did not substantially alter other factors such as difficulty in swallowing. The corticosteroid had no effect on the rate of healing.— H. A. Anderson *et al.*, *Archs Otolar.*, 1975, *101*, 86.

Gastro-intestinal disorders. Methylprednisolone given intravenously was effective in controlling severe nausea and vomiting associated with cancer chemotherapy.— B. J. Lee (letter), *New Engl. J. Med.*, 1981, *304*, 486.

Headache. In a double-blind study completed by 40 patients undergoing myelography and 20 undergoing pneumoencephalography, immediate intrathecal instillation after the procedure of methylprednisolone acetate 40 mg in 10 ml of saline solution was effective in preventing headaches compared with a saline placebo. The technique appears to be simple, effective, and safe, although the mode of action of the methylprednisolone acetate suspension was unknown.— J. E. McLennan *et al.*, *Headache*, 1973, *13*, 39. See also S. A. Kulick, *J. Mt Sinai Hosp.*, 1966, *33*, 152.

Nerve root compression. In a double-blind study in 100 patients with lumbar nerve root compression due to lumbar disk degeneration, those treated with an extradural injection of 80 mg of methylprednisolone in 10 ml of normal saline achieved significantly greater relief from pain and more rapid resumption of work than those given a placebo. Injections were given under local anaesthesia and transient sciatic pain was the only side-effect.— T. F. W. Dilke *et al.*, *Br. med. J.*, 1973, *2*, 635.

Ocular disorders. Monthly subconjunctival or retrobulbar injections of a suspension of methylprednisolone acetate, 10 to 15 mg, were found to give encouraging and in some cases dramatic results in treating exophthalmos in patients with thyrotoxicosis. The treatment had been used in 15 patients for 3 years with virtually no side-effects being observed. An addendum reported reversible steroid glaucoma occurring in 1 patient.— M. I. Garber, *Lancet*, 1966, *1*, 958. See also I. D. Thomas and J. K. Hart, *Med. J. Aust.*, 1974, *2*, 484.

A case of chronic toxocaral endophthalmitis in a 13-year-old girl was successfully treated by subconjunctival injections of 50 mg of methylprednisolone acetate (Depo-Medrone) repeated at monthly intervals for 6 months.— J. Nolan, *Br. J. Ophthal.*, 1968, *52*, 276.

Respiratory disorders. Beneficial effect of methylprednisolone in chronic bronchitis and acute respiratory insufficiency.— R. K. Albert *et al.*, *Ann. intern. Med.*, 1980, *92*, 753.

Rhinitis. Three hundred patients with grass pollen hay fever, with or without pollen asthma, were given a course of preseasonal or coseasonal alum-precipitated pyridine extracted grass pollen (Allpyral), or methylprednisolone acetate by injection in a slow-release form (Depo-Medrone) 80 mg at the onset of symptoms, and a second injection not less than 10 days, later just before the expected peak of the pollen cloud. The preseasonal treatment and methylprednisolone were equally effective and were more effective than the coseasonal treatment. Side-effects were more numerous in those receiving the preseasonal treatment, but were mostly local; asthma, urticaria, and rhinitis occurred less frequently. It was considered that the use of a long-acting corticosteroid was not justified in hay fever.— M. A. Ganderton *et al.*, *Br. med. J.*, 1969, *1*, 357. Treatment with prednisolone or prednisolone sodium phosphate in a porous plastic basis, 2.5 or 5 mg daily for four to six weeks, improved 90% of 48 patients with hay fever compared with 68% improvement from an earlier study on methylprednisolone depot injection. Adrenal suppression persisted for a longer time after methylprednisolone than after oral corticosteroid therapy.— M. A. Ganderton and A. W. Frankland (letter), *Lancet*, 1972, *1*, 847. Comment.— W. P. McMillin (letter), *ibid.*, 1025.

For a comment on the ethics of using depot corticosteroids in hay fever, see Corticosteroids, p.458.

Skin disorders. For recommendations concerning the correct use of corticosteroids on the skin, and a rough guide to the clinical potencies of topical corticosteroids, see Corticosteroids, p.458.

Lichen planus, oral . Five patients with lichen planus of the oral mucosa resistant to topical therapy with corticosteroids were given a submucosal injection of methylprednisolone acetate 20 to 40 mg (0.5 to 1 ml of the commercial aqueous suspension). There was a rapid response, lesions healing in 4 patients within 1 week. The fifth patient required another injection of 20 mg before healing occurred.— M. M. Ferguson (letter), *Lancet*, 1977, *2*, 771.

Preparations

Methylprednisolone Acetate Cream *(U.S.P.)*. A cream containing methylprednisolone acetate. Store in airtight containers. Protect from light.

Methylprednisolone Acetate for Enema *(U.S.P.)*. A dry mixture of methylprednisolone acetate with one or more suitable excipients.

Methylprednisolone Acetate Injection *(B.P.)*. A sterile suspension of methylprednisolone acetate, in very fine particles (rarely exceeding 20 µm in diameter), in Water for Injections containing suitable dispersing agents. It is prepared aseptically. pH 3.5 to 7. Not for intravenous use. Store at a temperature not exceeding 30° and avoid freezing. Protect from light. *U.S.P.* (Sterile Methylprednisolone Acetate Suspension) has a similar injection.

Proprietary Preparations

Depo-Medrone *(Upjohn, UK)*. Methylprednisolone acetate, available as an aqueous suspension for injection, containing 40 mg per ml, in vials of 1, 2, and 5 ml, and in disposable syringes of 2 ml. (Also available as Depo-Medrone in *Swed.*). **Depo-Medrone with Lidocaine** contains in addition lignocaine hydrochloride 10 mg per ml and is available in vials of 2 ml.

Medrone Acne Lotion *(Upjohn, UK)*. Contains methylprednisolone acetate 0.25%, aluminium chlorohydroxide complex 10%, and sulphur 5%. For acne vulgaris. To be applied sparingly once or twice daily. **Neo-Medrone Acne Lotion**. Contains, in addition, neomycin sulphate 0.25%.

Medrone Cream *(Upjohn, UK)*. An ointment, with a basis approximating the lipids of human skin, containing methylprednisolone acetate 0.25%. **Neo-Medrone Cream.** Contains, in addition, neomycin sulphate 0.5%. (Also available as Medrone in *Swed.*).

Other Proprietary Names

Betalona *(Spain)*; Depo-Medrol *(Arg., Austral., Belg., Canad., Denm., Fr., Ital., Neth., Norw., S.Afr., Switz., USA)*; Depo-Moderin *(Spain)*; Depot-Medrate *(Ger.)*; D-Med, Dura-Meth *(both USA)*; Emmetipi *(Ital.)*; Medrate *(Ger.)*; Medrol *(Denm.)*; Medrol acetate *(USA)*; Medrol Veriderm *(Ital.)*; Moderin Veriderm *(Spain)*; Mepred, Rep-Pred *(both USA)*; Urbason *(Denm., Ger., Switz.)*; Vériderm Médrol *(Fr.)*.

1117-l

Methylprednisolone Hemisuccinate *(U.S.P.)*. Methylprednisolone Hydrogen Succinate. Methylprednisolone 21-(hydrogen succinate).

$C_{26}H_{34}O_8$=474.5.

CAS — 2921-57-5.

Pharmacopoeias. In *U.S.*

A white or almost white, odourless or almost odourless, hygroscopic solid. Methylprednisolone hemisuccinate 51 mg is approximately equivalent to 40 mg of methylprednisolone. Very slightly **soluble** in water; freely soluble in alcohol; soluble in acetone. A solution in dioxan is dextrorotatory. **Store** in airtight containers.

Methylprednisolone hemisuccinate has the general properties of methylprednisolone (p.477).

1118-y

Methylprednisolone Sodium Succinate

(U.S.P.). Sodium 6α-Methylprednisolone 21-Succinate. Methylprednisolone 21-(sodium succinate).

$C_{26}H_{33}NaO_8$=496.5.

CAS — 2375-03-3.

Pharmacopoeias. In *U.S.*

A white or almost white, odourless, hygroscopic, amorphous powder. Methylprednisolone sodium succinate 53 mg is approximately equivalent to 40 mg of methylprednisolone.

Soluble 1 in 1.5 of water, and 1 in 12 of alcohol; very slightly soluble in acetone; practically insoluble in chloroform and ether. A solution in alcohol is dextrorotatory. **Store** in airtight containers. Protect from light.

Incompatibility. Methylprednisolone sodium succinate is physically incompatible with metaraminol tartrate.— F. E. Turner and J. C. King, *Am. J. Hosp. Pharm.*, 1973, *30*, 128.

Adverse Effects, Treatment, Withdrawal, and Precautions. As for Corticosteroids, p.446, p.449.

Cardiovascular collapse has been reported following the rapid intravenous injection of large doses of corticosteroids.

Methylprednisolone sodium succinate should not be injected into the deltoid muscle since it may cause subcutaneous atrophy.

Comment on the use of large intravenous doses of corticosteroids, with special reference to intravenous methylprednisolone, as much as 1 to 2 g being given at a time. Such massive doses seem to produce few side-effects, provided that the injection is made slowly over 5 to 30 minutes. Some patients have remarked on transient weakness, flushing, or a metallic taste in the mouth, and some have become transiently hypotensive. Since the half-life of the drug is only 2½ hours, plasma concentrations soon fall from their heights. Since prolonged high dosage, as with other corticosteroids, predisposes to septic complications and death, not more than a total of 6 to 8 g is given for kidney-transplant rejection, and if this proves ineffective the kidney is removed.— *Lancet*, 1977, *1*, 633.

Allergy. An account of an anaphylactic reaction to methylprednisolone sodium succinate 40 mg intravenously in a 17-year-old male asthmatic patient.— L. M. Mendelson *et al.*, *J. Allergy & clin. Immunol.*, 1974, *54*, 125. Comment.— *Br. med. J.*, 1974, *4*, 551.

Effects on bones and joints. Severe bilateral knee-pain and tenderness occurred in 4 patients after receiving methylprednisolone 1 g daily for 3 days in the management of kidney-transplant rejections.— K. J. Newmark *et al.* (letter), *Lancet*, 1974, *2*, 229. Similar reports: R. R. Bailey and P. Armour (letter), *ibid.*, 1014; W. M. Bennett and D. Strong (letter), *Lancet*, 1975, *1*, 332.

Absorption and Fate. For a brief outline of the absorption and fate of corticosteroids, see Corticosteroids, p.451. See also Methylprednisolone, p.477.

Uses. Methylprednisolone sodium succinate has the general properties of methylprednisolone (see p.477).

Methylprednisolone sodium succinate may be administered by intramuscular or intravenous injection or by intravenous infusion and it is principally used for short-term emergency treatment. The usual intramuscular or intravenous dose is the equivalent of 10 to 40 mg of methylprednisolone, repeated as required. For slow intravenous infusion methylprednisolone is dissolved in an appropriate volume of dextrose injection or sodium chloride injection or sodium chloride and dextrose injection. The dose in children is determined by the severity of the condition rather than by age, but should generally not be less than 500 µg per kg body-weight daily.

In the treatment of severe shock single doses of the equivalent of up to 30 mg per kg of methylprednisolone have been given as bolus intravenous injections in an attempt to promote rapid vasodilatation. Doses are repeated after 4 hours if necessary. Up to 30 mg per kg intravenously has been given daily for rejection episodes after organ transplantation. Large doses should be given slowly over at least 10 minutes and should generally not be given for prolonged periods.

Retention enemas or rectal irrigations containing the equivalent of 20 to 40 mg of methylprednisolone have been used in the treatment of ulcerative colitis.

Methylprednisolone sodium phosphate is under study.

Blood disorders. Preliminary results suggesting that methylprednisolone by bolus intravenous injection was capable of inducing haematological remissions in some patients with severe aplastic anaemia. Of 6 such patients given methylprednisolone 20 mg per kg body-weight daily by bolus intravenous injection for 3 days, then gradually reduced to 1 mg per kg daily after 3 weeks and continued until the 30th day, 3 achieved a complete remission.— A. Bacigalupo *et al.* (letter), *New Engl. J. Med.*, 1979, *300*, 501.

Raised intracranial pressure. Cerebral tumours . For a suggestion that methylprednisolone may be less liable than dexamethasone to interact with anticonvulsants, see Precautions for Corticosteroids (Interactions), p.450.

Head injuries .For studies on the role of corticosteroid therapy in the management of severe head injuries, see Dexamethasone, p.467.

Preparations

Methylprednisolone Sodium Succinate for Injection *(U.S.P.).* Sterile methylprednisolone sodium succinate with suitable buffers. It may be prepared from methylprednisolone sodium succinate or from methylprednisolone succinate with the aid of sodium carbonate or sodium hydroxide. Potency is expressed in terms of the equivalent amount of methylprednisolone. A solution containing methylprednisolone sodium succinate 50 mg per ml has a pH of 7 to 8.

Solu-Medrone *(Upjohn, UK).* Methylprednisolone sodium succinate, available as powder for preparing injections in two-part vials each containing the equivalent of methylprednisolone 40 mg in 1 ml or 125 mg in 2 ml, with diluent; and also as vials each containing the equivalent of methylprednisolone 0.5, 1, and 2 g, all supplied with diluent.

Other Proprietary Names

A-Methapred *(USA)*; Asmacortone, Mega-star *(both Ital.)*; Medrate Solubile *(Ger.)*; Solu-Medrol *(Austral., Belg., Canad., Denm., Fr., Ital., Neth., Norw., S.Afr., Switz., USA)*; Solu-Moderin *(Spain)*; Urbason Solubile *(Denm., Ger., Ital., Norw., Spain, Swed.)*.

1119-j

Paramethasone Acetate

(U.S.P.). 6α-Fluoro-16α-methylprednisolone 21-Acetate. 6α-Fluoro-11β,17α,21-trihydroxy-16α-methylpregna-1,4-diene-3,20-dione 21-acetate.

$C_{24}H_{31}FO_6$=434.5.

CAS — 53-33-8 (paramethasone); 1597-82-6 (acetate).

Pharmacopoeias. In *U.S.*

A white to creamy-white, fluffy, odourless, crystalline powder. M.p. about 240° with decomposition. Practically **insoluble** in water; soluble 1 in 50 of chloroform, and 1 in 40 of methyl alcohol; soluble in alcohol, acetone, and ether. **Store** in airtight containers.

Adverse Effects, Treatment, Withdrawal, and Precautions. As for Corticosteroids, p.446, p.449.

Absorption and Fate. For a brief outline of the absorption and fate of corticosteroids, see Corticosteroids, p.451.

Uses. Paramethasone acetate is a synthetic glucocorticoid and has the general properties described under Corticosteroids (see p.451); 2 mg of paramethasone is equivalent in anti-inflammatory activity to about 5 mg of prednisolone. It has been suggested for use in the treatment of all conditions in which corticosteroid therapy is indicated except adrenal deficiency states for which its lack of sodium-retaining properties makes it less suitable than cortisone or hydrocortisone with supplementary fludrocortisone.

Preparations

Paramethasone Acetate Tablets *(U.S.P.).* Tablets containing paramethasone acetate.

Proprietary Names

Alfa 6 *(SAM, Ital.)*; Cortidene Depot *(Infal, Spain)*; Cortidene Soluble *(disodium phosphate) (Infal, Spain)*; Depodillar *(Syntex, Belg.; Sarva, Neth.)*; Dilar *(Cassenne, Fr.)*; Dillar *(Syntex, Belg.; Sarva, Neth.)*; Haldrone *(Lilly, USA)*; Metilar *(Syntex, Austral.; Astra-Syntex, Norw.)*; Monocortin *(Grünenthal, Ger.)*; Monocortin Depot *(Grünenthal, Ger.; Grünenthal, Switz.)*; Monocortin S *(disodium phosphate) (Grünenthal, Ger.; Grünenthal, Switz.)*; Paramesone *(Jap.)*; Paramezone *(Recordati, Ital.)*; Soludillar *(disodium phosphate) (Syntex, Belg.)*; Triniol *(Infal, Spain)*.

Paramethasone acetate was formerly marketed in Great Britain under the proprietary names Haldrate (*Lilly*) and Metilar (*Syntex*).

1120-q

Prednisolamate Hydrochloride *(B.P.C. 1963).* Prednisolone 21-Diethylaminoacetate Hydrochloride. 11β,17α,21-Trihydroxypregna-1,4-diene-3,20-dione 21-diethylaminoacetate hydrochloride.

$C_{27}H_{39}NO_6$,HCl=510.1.

CAS — 5626-34-6 (prednisolamate).

A white or almost white odourless crystalline powder. **Soluble** 1 in 7 of water and 1 in 17 of alcohol; very slightly soluble in chloroform; practically insoluble in ether.

Uses. Prednisolamate hydrochloride has been used in some countries as a water-soluble form of prednisolone for intravenous injection.

It was formerly used as an ointment containing 0.25%.

1121-p

Prednisolone

(B.P., B.P. Vet., Eur. P., U.S.P.). Prednisolonum; Deltahydrocortisone; 1,2-Dehydrohydrocortisone; Metacortandralone. 11β,17α,21-Trihydroxypregna-1,4-diene-3,20-dione.

$C_{21}H_{28}O_5$=360.4.

CAS — 50-24-8 (anhydrous); 52438-85-4 (sesquihydrate).

Pharmacopoeias. In *Arg., Br., Braz., Cz., Eur., Fr., Ger., Hung., Ind., Int., It., Jap., Jug., Neth., Nord., Pol., Port., Roum., Rus., Swiss, Turk.,* and *U.S.* (anhydrous or 1½H_2O). *Nord.* also has Prednisolonum Hydratum (1½H_2O).

An odourless, white or almost white, crystalline, hygroscopic powder with a bitter taste. M.p. about 230° to 235° with decomposition.

Soluble 1 in 1300 of water, 1 in 27 of dehydrated alcohol, 1 in 30 of alcohol, 1 in 50 of acetone, and 1 in 180 of chloroform; soluble in dioxan and methyl alcohol. A solution in dioxan is dextrorotatory. **Incompatible** with alkalis. **Store** in airtight containers. Protect from light.

The effect of aqueous suspensions of magnesium trisilicate, magnesium oxide, aluminium hydroxide, calcium carbonate, and magnesium carbonate on prednisolone at 37.5° has been studied. Magnesium trisilicate adsorbed the intact corticosteroid and magnesium oxide produced an alkaline degradation of the side-chain. The other materials were without effect.— T. Chulski and A. A. Forist, *J. Am. pharm. Ass., scient. Edn*, 1958, *47*, 553.

Photosensitivity. Ultraviolet light and fluorescent lighting caused degradation of prednisolone solutions.— W. E. Hamlin *et al.*, *J. Am. pharm. Ass., scient. Edn*, 1960, *49*, 253.

Polymorphism. A study of 3 polymorphs of prednisolone.— P. W. Taylor, *Diss. Abstr.*, 1965, *25*, 5875, per *Int. pharm. Abstr.*, 1966, *3*, 314.

Adverse Effects and Treatment. As for Corticosteroids, p.446, and p.449.

Owing to its less pronounced mineralocorticoid activity prednisolone is less likely than cortisone or hydrocortisone to cause sodium retention, electrolyte imbalance, and oedema.

Prolonged application to the eye of preparations containing corticosteroids has caused increased intra-ocular pressure and reduced visual function.

Withdrawal and Precautions. As for Corticosteroids, p.449.

Absorption and Fate. For a brief outline of the absorption and fate of corticosteroids, see Corticosteroids, p.451.

Prednisolone and prednisone are both readily absorbed from the gastro-intestinal tract, but whereas prednisolone already exists in a metabolically active form, prednisone must be converted in the liver to its active metabolite, prednisolone. In general, this conversion is rapid so that prednisone has a preconversion biological half-life of only about 60 minutes. Hence, although prednisone has been estimated to have only about 80% the bioavailablility of prednisolone, this difference is of little consequence when seen in the light of intersubject variation in the pharmacokinetics of prednisolone itself; bioavailability also depends on the dissolution-rates of the tablet formulations. Nevertheless, prednisolone is the more reliably absorbed of the 2 corticosteroids, particularly in some liver diseases where the conversion of prednisone may be diminished.

Peak plasma concentrations of prednisolone are obtained 1 or 2 hours after administration by mouth, and it has a usual plasma half-life of 2 or 3 hours. Its initial absorption, but not its overall bioavailability, is affected by food.

Prednisolone is extensively bound to plasma proteins, although less so than hydrocortisone (cortisol).

Prednisolone is excreted in the urine as free and conjugated metabolites, together with an appreciable proportion of unchanged prednisolone. Prednisolone crosses the placenta and small amounts are excreted in breast milk.

Prednisolone has a biological half-life lasting several hours, intermediate between those of hydrocortisone (cortisol) and the longer-acting glucocorticoids, such as dexamethasone. It is this intermediate duration of action which makes it suitable for the alternate-day administration regimens which have been found to reduce the risk of adrenocortical insufficiency, yet provide adequate corticosteroid coverage in some disorders such as asthma.

Reviews of the clinical pharmacokinetics of prednisone and prednisolone: M. E. Pickup, *Clin. Pharmacokinet.*, 1979, *4*, 111; J. G. Gambertoglio *et al.*, *J. Pharmacokinet. Biopharm.*, 1980, *8*, 1.

For further details of the metabolism of prednisolone and prednisone, see C. L. Cope, *Adrenal Steroids and Disease*, London, Pitman Medical, 1972.

Recent studies on the pharmacokinetics of prednisolone and prednisone: A. Tanner *et al.*, *Clin. Pharmac. Ther.*, 1979, *25*, 571; F. L. S. Tse and P. G. Welling, *J. Pharm. Pharmac.*, 1979, *31*, 492.

Administration in children. Variability in plasma-prednisolone concentrations was observed from samples taken immediately prior to, and at hourly intervals from 4 to 7 hours, after ingestion of the usual prescribed doses of prednisone by mouth, taken before breakfast, in 29 children with various diseases. In 22 children, the half-life for prednisolone ranged from 84 to 210 minutes; in a further 4 it ranged from 264 to 360 minutes. In most patients, peak concentrations occurred 1 or 2 hours after the dose, but in 5 patients this took 3 to 4 hours, and 3 others had a progressive increase in plasma concentrations during the study period; half-lives could not be calculated for the last 3.— O. C. Green *et al.*, *J. Pediat.*, 1978, *93*, 299.

Administration in hepatic insufficiency. *Comparison of the metabolic effects of prednisolone and prednisone.* Active chronic liver disease or acute viral hepatitis caused lower concentrations and a slower rise to peak concentrations of plasma prednisolone after administration of prednisone than after prednisolone. In patients with inactive chronic liver disease similar concentrations were reached 1 hour after administration of either drug. The amount of prednisolone bound to protein was lower in patients with active liver disease and there was positive correlation between bound prednisolone and serum albumin concentrations; protein binding was not affected by the presence of azathioprine *in vitro*.— L. W. Powell and E. Axelsen, *Gut*, 1972, *13*, 690. Although plasma-prednisolone concentrations were more predictable after administration of prednisolone than after prednisone in 10 healthy subjects, no difference was noted in 25 patients with chronic active hepatitis. In the patients with liver disease, impaired hepatic conversion of prednisone to prednisolone was counteracted by impaired elimination of the prednisolone.— M. Davis *et al.*, *Br. J. clin. Pharmac.*, 1978, *5*, 501. See also S. W. Schalm *et al.*, *Gastroenterology*, 1975, *69*, 863; M. Uribe *et al.*, *Gut*, 1978, *19*, 1131.

Impaired conversion of prednisone to prednisolone in patients with liver cirrhosis.— S. Madsbad *et al.*, *Gut*, 1980, *21*, 52.

Administration in various other clinical states. Studies of the absorption and fate of prednisolone in different clinical states: G. P. Lewis *et al.*, *Ann. N.Y. Acad. Sci.*, 1971, *179*, 729 (increased adverse effects associated with lower plasma albumin concentrations); M. Kozower *et al.*, *J. clin. Endocr. Metab.*, 1974, *38*, 407 (decreased clearance and increased adverse effects); M. E. Pickup *et al.*, *Eur. J. Drug Metab. Pharmacokinet.*, 1979, *4*, 87 (no significant effect on absorption and elimination in coeliac disease); P. R. Elliott *et al.*, *Gut*, 1980, *21*, 49 (different pattern of absorption in acute colitis); C. S. May *et al.*, *Br. J. Dis. Chest*, 1980, *74*, 91 (pharmacokinetics in asthma).

Enteric-coated tablets. Studies and comments on the bioavailabilities of uncoated and enteric-coated tablets of prednisolone. Some studies of enteric-coated tablets have shown poor absorption of prednisolone R. Leclercq and G. Copinschi, *J. Pharmacokinet. Biopharm.*, 1974, *2*, 175; B. Hulme *et al.*, *Br. J. clin. Pharmac.*, 1975, *2*, 317; *Drug & Ther. Bull.*, 1977, *15*, 83; C. G. Wilson *et al.*, *Br. J. clin. Pharmac.*, 1977, *4*, 351; R. G. Henderson *et al.*, *Br. med. J.*, 1979, *1*, 1534; O. N. Fernando and J. Moorhead (letter), *Br. med. J.*, 1979, *1*, 1795; D. A. H. Lee *et al.*, *Br. J. clin. Pharmac.*, 1979, *7*, 523; S. Al-Habet *et al.*, *Br. med. J.*, 1980, *281*, 843; T. G. K. Mant, *Postgrad. med. J.*, 1979, *55*, 421.

Pregnancy and the neonate. The transplacental passage of prednisone and prednisolone in pregnancy near term. In women, the metabolic clearance-rates of prednisolone were significantly lower than those of prednisone and were unaffected by pregnancy or contraceptive medication.— I. Z. Beitins *et al.*, *J. Pediat.*, 1972, *81*, 936.

Lactation. Concentrations of prednisone and prednisolone in human milk 120 minutes after prednisone 10 mg by mouth were 26.7 ng and 1.6 ng per ml.— F. H. Katz and B. E. Duncan (letter), *New Engl. J. Med.*, 1975, *293*, 1154.

Seven lactating women volunteers were given a single 5-mg dose of tritium-labelled prednisolone by mouth. A mean of 0.14% of the radioactivity from the dose was recovered per litre of milk during the following 48 to 61 hours.— S. A. McKenzie *et al.*, *Archs Dis. Childh.*, 1975, *50*, 894.

Rectal absorption. In a study of 8 subjects with proctocolitis receiving a standard 20-mg prednisolone retention enema and 9 healthy volunteers receiving prednisolone 300 µg per kg body-weight by mouth, plasma-prednisolone concentrations indicated that the amount of drug absorbed from rectal administration was about 44% of that absorbed by mouth.— D. A. H. Lee *et al.*, *Gut*, 1979, *20*, 349. See also J. Powell-Tuck *et al.*, *Br. med. J.*, 1976, *1*, 193.

Uses. Prednisolone is a synthetic glucocorticoid with the general properties described under Corticosteroids (see p.451); 5 mg of prednisolone is equivalent in anti-inflammatory activity to about 25 mg of cortisone acetate.

In general, prednisolone is the drug of choice for all conditions in which routine systemic corticosteroid therapy is indicated, except adrenal-deficiency states for which its lack of sodium-retaining properties usually makes it less suitable than cortisone or hydrocortisone (cortisol) with supplementary fludrocortisone. The more potent pituitary-suppressant properties of a glucocorticoid such as dexamethasone (see p.466) may, however, be required for the diagnosis and management of conditions associated with adrenal hyperplasia.

Prednisolone has a usual dose range of 5 to 60 mg daily in divided doses, as a single daily dose at 8 a.m., or as a double dose on alternate days. Alternate-day early-morning dosage regimens produce less suppression of the hypothalamic-pituitary axis and may provide satisfactory control of symptoms in conditions such as allergic or collagen disorders, although they may not provide adequate control where inflammatory symptoms predominate (for further details see under Corticosteroids, Administration, p.452). In long-term therapy dosage should be maintained at not more than about 7 mg daily whenever possible as side-effects inevitably occur with higher dosage.

Prednisolone is applied topically in preparations containing 0.5%.

Adrenal hyperplasia, salt-losing. Data from a study in 6 patients with congenital virilising adrenal hyperplasia. It was concluded that adequate control can be achieved with twice-daily prednisone but not with once daily.— C. A. Huseman *et al.*, *J. Pediat.*, 1977, *90*, 538.

Adrenal insufficiency. In patients undergoing corticotrophin stimulation for suspected Addison's disease prednisolone with deoxycortone acetate or fludrocortisone provided adequate replacement therapy for the hypoadrenalism but did not interfere with the fluorometric method of measuring 11-hydroxycorticosteroids.— P. Sheridan and D. Mattingly, *Lancet*, 1975, *2*, 676.

Diagnosis of pyelonephritis. References to the 'prednisolone provocation test' using intravenous prednisolone in a procedure for the diagnosis of pyelonephritis: Y. J. Katz *et al.*, *Lancet*, 1962, *1*, 1144; P. J. Little and H. E. de Wardener, *ibid.*, 1145; G. Gudowski *et al.*, *Kinderärztl. Prax.*, 1967, *10*, 441.

Marrow-function test. A dose of 40 mg of prednisolone given to 46 normal subjects, 31 patients with bone-marrow depression, and 18 splenectomised patients produced an increase of at least 2000 granulocytes per mm^3 after 5 hours in all but 1 of the normal patients and in the splenectomised patients. In 27 patients with bone-marrow depression the mean increase was 605 granulocytes per mm^3. The normal increase was about 5000 per mm^3 in young persons and less in the elderly.— J. J. Cream, *Br. J. Haemat.*, 1968, *15*, 259, per *Abstr. Wld Med.*, 1969, *43*, 292.

Preparations

Oculentum Prednisoloni *(Nord. P.).* Prednisolone Eye Ointment. Prednisolone 0.5% in a basis of liquid paraffin 1 and yellow soft paraffin 4.

Oculoguttae Prednisoloni *(Nord. P.).* Prednisolone Eye-drops. Prednisolone 10 mg, sodium chloride 750 mg, phenethyl alcohol 500 mg, sterilised water to 100 g. Maintain at 100° for 20 minutes. Protect from light.

Prednisolone Cream *(U.S.P.).* Contains prednisolone in a suitable cream basis. Store in airtight containers.

Prednisolone Tablets *(B.P.).* Tablets containing prednisolone. Protect from light.

Prednisolone Tablets *(U.S.P.).* Tablets containing prednisolone. The *U.S.P.* requires 70% dissolution in 30 minutes.

NOTE. Some proprietary names used for preparations of prednisolone are also applied to preparations of prednisolone acetate; see under Prednisolone Acetate.

Codelcortone *(Merck Sharp & Dohme, UK).* Prednisolone, available as scored tablets of 5 mg.

Delta Phoricol *(Wallace Mfg Chem., UK: Farillon, UK).* Prednisolone, available as tablets of 5 mg.

Deltacortril Enteric *(Pfizer, UK).* Prednisolone, available as enteric-coated tablets of 2.5 and 5 mg. (Also available as Deltacortril in *Belg., Ger., Norw., Spain, Swed.*).

Deltalone *(DDSA Pharmaceuticals, UK).* Prednisolone, available as tablets of 1 mg and scored tablets of 5 mg.

Deltastab *(Boots, UK).* Prednisolone, available as tablets of 1 (scored) and 5 mg.

Hydromycin-D *(Boots, UK).* Preparations containing prednisolone 0.5% and neomycin sulphate 0.5%, available as **Ear/Eye Drops** and as **Ear/Eye Ointment**.

Marsolone *(Marshall's Pharmaceuticals, UK).* Prednisolone, available as tablets of 1 and 5 mg.

Precortisyl *(Roussel, UK).* Prednisolone, available as tablets of 1, 5 (scored), and 25 mg. (Also available as Precortisyl in *Austral.*).

Other Proprietary Names

Austral.— Adnisolone, Delta-Cortef, Deltasolone, Optocort, Panafcortelone, Prelone, Solone (see also under Dexamethasone and Dexamethasone Sodium Phosphate); *Belg.*— Prednicortelone; *Denm.*— Delcortol; *Fr.*— Hydrocortancyl, Predniretard; *Ger.*— Decaprednil, Decortin-H, Dura Prednisolon, Hostacortin H, Precortilon, Predni-Coelin, Predni-H, Scherisolon, Ultracorten-H; *Ital.*— Acepreval, Caberdelta, Cortisolone, Cortomas *(palmitate)*, Deltolio *(palmitate)*, Domucortone, Predartrina; *Jap.*— Derpo PD, Donisolone, Predonine; *Pol.*— Encortolone; *S.Afr.*— Lenisolone, Meticortelone, Predeltilone; *Spain*— Dacortin-H, Delta-Larma, Nisolone *(see also under Prednisolone Succinate)*, Normonsona, Scherisolona; *Switz.*— Dacortin, Meprisolon, Predni-Helvacort; *USA*— Delta-Cortef, Meti-Derm, Prednis, Ropredlone, Sterane, Ulacort.

Preparations containing prednisolone and aspirin were formerly marketed in Great Britain under the proprietary names Cordex and Cordex Forte (*Upjohn*).

1122-s

Prednisolone Acetate *(U.S.P., B.P. 1963)*.

Prednisoloni Acetas. Prednisolone 21-acetate.
$C_{23}H_{30}O_6$=402.5.

CAS — 52-21-1.

Pharmacopoeias. In *Arg., Fr., Ind., Jap., Jug., Pol., Roum., Turk.,* and *U.S.*

An odourless, white or almost white, crystalline powder with a bitter taste. M.p. about 235° with decomposition. Prednisolone acetate 11 mg is approximately equivalent to 10 mg of prednisolone.

Practically **insoluble** in water; soluble 1 in 120 of alcohol, 1 in 170 of dehydrated alcohol, and 1 in 150 of chloroform; slightly soluble in acetone.

A solid dispersion prepared by fusion of prednisolone acetate in macrogol 6000 showed markedly enhanced dissolution in water.— W. L. Chiou and S. Riegelman, *J. pharm. Sci.*, 1971, *60*, 1569.

Adverse Effects, Treatment, Withdrawal, and Precautions. As for Corticosteroids, p.446, p.449.

There have been reports of joint damage following the intra-articular injection of corticosteroids into load-bearing joints (see under Corticosteroids, p.447).

Prolonged application to the eye of preparations containing corticosteroids has caused increased intra-ocular pressure and reduced visual function.

Absorption and Fate. As for Prednisolone, p.480.

It is only slowly absorbed from intramuscular injection sites.

The anti-inflammatory effect of an intra-articular injection of 50 or 100 mg of prednisolone acetate, prednisolone pivalate, or prednisolone tebutate was considered to be related to their solubility and therefore systemic escape from the joint in a study of 46 patients with synovitis affecting at least one knee. At the 50-mg dose prednisolone tebutate had the action of longest duration, the 100-mg dose conferring no advantage; prednisolone acetate had the least effect. A greater action after the 100-mg dose was obtained only with prednisolone acetate.— W. Esselinckx *et al.*, *Br. J. clin. Pharmac.*, 1978, *5*, 447. See also J. S. Reebeck *et al.*, *Ann. rheum. Dis.*, 1980, *39*, 22.

Ocular absorption. Studies on the penetration of prednisolone acetate ophthalmic preparations in the cornea and aqueous humour: A. Kupferman and H. M. Leibowitz, *Archs Ophthal., N.Y.*, 1974, *91*, 377; *idem, Am. J. Ophthal.*, 1976, *82*, 109; H. M. Leibowitz *et al.*, *ibid.*, 1977, *83*, 402; H. M. Leibowitz and A. Kupferman, *Archs Ophthal., N.Y.*, 1979, *97*, 2154.

Uses. Prednisolone acetate has the general properties of prednisolone (see p.480).

It is given by intra-articular injection into joints affected by rheumatoid arthritis, osteoarthritis, and other arthritic conditions; the dosage is approximately the same as with intra-articular injections of hydrocortisone acetate, a single dose of 5 to 50 mg being injected according to the size of the joint.

It is administered by mouth as tablets and may be injected intramuscularly. It has been applied topically in lotions, eye-drops, and ointments, usually containing 0.25 or 0.5%.

Preparations

Sterile Prednisolone Acetate Suspension *(U.S.P.)*. Prednisolone Acetate Suspension, Sterile. A sterile suspension of prednisolone acetate in a suitable aqueous vehicle. pH 5 to 7.5.

NOTE. Some proprietary names used for preparations of prednisolone acetate are also applied to preparations of prednisolone; see under Prednisolone..

Deltastab Injection *(Boots, UK)*. Prednisolone acetate, available as an aqueous suspension containing 25 mg per ml, in vials of 5 ml.

Other Proprietary Names

Austral.— Scherisolon, Ultracortenol; *Belg.*— Ultracortenol; *Canad.*— Meticortelone Aqueous, Pred Forte, Pred Mild; *Denm.*— Ultracortenol; *Fr.*— Hydrocortancyl; *Ger.*— Decortin-H-Kristallsuspension, DuraPrednisolon, Hostacortin H, Inflanefran, Predni-H, Ultracortenol; *Ital.*— Cortipred, Delta-Cortilen, Ibisterolon Pomata, Meticortelone; *Neth.*— Di-Adreson-F, Ultracortenol; *Norw.*— Ultracortenol; *Spain*— Scherisolona; *Switz.*— Pred Forte, Pred Mild, Prednifor, Scherisolon, Ultracortenol; *USA*— Econopred, Meticortelone Acetate, Pred Mild, Savacort.

1123-w

Prednisolone Hexanoate. Prednisolone Caproate. Prednisolone 21-hexanoate.
$C_{27}H_{38}O_6$=458.6.

Freely **soluble** in alcohol, acetone, chloroform, and methyl alcohol. Prednisolone hexanoate 127 mg is approximately equivalent to 100 mg of prednisolone.

Uses. Prednisolone hexanoate has the general properties of prednisolone (see p.479) and has been used as an ointment containing the equivalent of prednisolone 0.15% or as suppositories for the treatment of inflammatory anal conditions.

Proprietary Preparations

Scheriproct *(Schering, UK)*. **Ointment** containing prednisolone hexanoate 0.19%, cinchocaine hydrochloride 0.5%, hexachlorophane 0.5%, and clemizole undecanoate 1% and **Suppositories** each containing prednisolone hexanoate 1.3 mg, cinchocaine hydrochloride 1 mg, hexachlorophane 2.5 mg, and clemizole undecanoate 5 mg. For haemorrhoids, proctitis, pruritus ani, and anal fissures.

1124-e

Prednisolone Pivalate *(B.P.)*.

Prednisolone Trimethylacetate. Prednisolone 21-pivalate.
$C_{26}H_{36}O_6$=444.6.

CAS — 1107-99-9.

Pharmacopoeias. In *Br.*

A white or almost white, odourless, crystalline powder. M.p. about 229°. Practically **insoluble** in water; soluble 1 in 150 of alcohol and 1 in 16 of chloroform. A solution in dioxan is dextrorotatory. Suspensions for injection are prepared aseptically. **Store** in airtight containers. Protect from light.

Adverse Effects, Treatment, Withdrawal, and Precautions. As for Corticosteroids, p.446, p.449.

There have been reports of joint damage following the intra-articular injection of corticosteroids into load-bearing joints (see under Corticosteroids, p.447).

Absorption and Fate. As for Prednisolone, p.480.

It is only slowly absorbed from injection sites.

For a study of the systemic absorption of intra-articular prednisolone pivalate, see Prednisolone Acetate, p.481.

Uses. Prednisolone pivalate has the general properties described under Corticosteroids (see p.451).

It is used for its local anti-inflammatory effect by intra-articular injection in doses of up to 50 mg according to the size of the joint, and by injection into soft tissues. It was formerly applied topically as an ointment, usually containing 0.5%, in the treatment of skin affections.

Rheumatic disorders. Of 46 patients exhibiting mandibular osteoarthrosis who were given a single intra-articular injection of up to 25 mg of prednisolone pivalate, 30 showed complete relief of pain after 6 months, 8 showed long-term improvement, and 8 showed insufficient response or relapsed after 2 or 3 months.— P. A. Toller, *Br. dent. J.*, 1973, *134*, 223.

Preparations

Prednisolone Pivalate Injection *(B.P.)*. Prednisolone Trimethylacetate Injection. A sterile suspension of prednisolone pivalate, in very fine particles (rarely exceeding 20 µm) in Water for Injections containing suitable dispersing, stabilising, and buffering agents. It is prepared aseptically. pH 6 to 7. For local injection only. Store at room temperature. Protect from light.

Ultracortenol *(Ciba, UK)*. Prednisolone pivalate, available as a microcrystalline suspension in an aqueous iso-osmotic buffered solution, containing 50 mg per ml in ampoules of 1 ml. (Also available as Ultracortenol in *Belg., Denm., Ger., Norw., Swed., Switz.*).

NOTE. Ultracortenol may be applied in different countries to different formulations.

Other Proprietary Names

Mecortolon *(Pol.)*.

1125-l

Prednisolone Sodium Metasulphobenzoate.

R 812. Prednisolone 21-(sodium *m*-sulphobenzoate).
$C_{28}H_{31}NaO_9S$=566.6.

CAS — 39175-74-1 (prednisolone metasulphobenzoate).

Prednisolone sodium metasulphobenzoate 157 mg is approximately equivalent to 100 mg of prednisolone. **Soluble** about 1 in 35 of water. Hydrolysed in alkaline solution.

Uses. Prednisolone sodium metasulphobenzoate has the general properties of prednisolone (see p.479). A solution containing the equivalent of 20 mg of prednisolone in 100 ml of water is used as a retention enema.

Evidence that rectally administered prednisolone sodium metasulphobenzoate may have a predominantly local action.— D. A. Lee *et al.*, *Gut*, 1980, *21*, 215.

Proprietary Preparations

Predenema *(Pharmax, UK)*. Contains prednisolone sodium metasulphobenzoate equivalent to prednisolone 20 mg in each 100 ml, in disposable containers of 100 ml.

Other Proprietary Names

Corti-Clyss *(Switz.)*; Désocort, Dulmicort, Solupred *(all Fr.)*.

1126-y

Prednisolone Sodium Phosphate *(B.P., U.S.P.)*.

Prednisolone Sod. Phos. Prednisolone 21-(disodium phosphate).
$C_{21}H_{27}Na_2O_8P$=484.4.

CAS — 125-02-0.

Pharmacopoeias. In *Br., Turk.,* and *U.S.*

A white or slightly yellow hygroscopic powder or granules with a bitter taste, odourless or with a slight odour. The *B.P.* specifies not more than 8% of water; the *U.S.P.* specifies not more than 5% loss on drying. Prednisolone sodium phosphate 27 mg is approximately equivalent to 20 mg of prednisolone.

Soluble 1 in 3 or 4 of water, 1 in 1000 of dehydrated alcohol, and 1 in 13 of methyl alcohol; practically insoluble in chloroform; very slightly soluble in acetone and dioxan. A solution in water is dextrorotatory. A 0.5% solution in water has a pH of 7.5 to 9. Solutions are **sterilised** by filtration or by maintaining at 98° to 100° with a bactericide for 30 minutes. Aqueous solutions having a pH of about 8 are stable if protected from light but particular care must be taken to avoid microbial contamination of the solutions to avoid hydrolysis of the ester by phosphatase. **Store** in airtight containers. Protect from light.

Incompatibility. A reaction in aqueous solution between prednisolone phosphate and sodium metabisulphite, indicated by a rise in pH, suggested the presence of a new soluble compound. Loss of the prednisolone activity was found by biological assay. The extent of the reaction was dependent on the pH, proceeding rapidly at low pH values; the reaction was reversed at a pH of 10 to 12.— P. F. G. Boon and M. J. Busse (letter), *J. Pharm. Pharmac.*, 1961, *13*, 62.

Particulate matter was observed within 2 hours when 1 ml of commercial prednisolone sodium phosphate injection was mixed with 5 ml sterile water and 1 ml of any of the following commercial injection solutions: calcium gluconate, dimenhydrinate, prochlorperazine edisylate, promazine hydrochloride, and promethazine hydrochloride.— R. Misgen, *Am. J. Hosp. Pharm.*, 1965, *22*, 92. See also J. A. Patel and G. L. Phillips, *ibid.*, 1966, *23*, 409.

A haze or precipitate was observed within an hour when an average dose of prednisolone sodium phosphate was mixed in dextrose injection with polymyxin B sulphate.— J. M. Meisler and M. W. Skolaut, *Am. J. Hosp. Pharm.*, 1966, *23*, 557.

The u.v. absorption spectrum of prednisolone sodium phosphate was altered, suggesting incompatibility, when a dilute solution in dextrose injection was mixed with a solution of methotrexate sodium; the spectrum of methotrexate sodium was only slightly affected.— M. P. McRae and J. C. King, *Am. J. Hosp. Pharm.*, 1976, *33*, 1010.

Adverse Effects, Treatment, Withdrawal, and Precautions. As for Corticosteroids, p.446, p.449.

There have been reports of joint damage following the intra-articular injection of corticosteroids into load-bearing joints (see under Corticosteroids, p.447).

Prolonged application to the eye of preparations containing corticosteroids has caused increased intra-ocular pressure and reduced visual function.

Intravenous injections of prednisolone sodium phosphate must be given slowly. No more than 2 ml should be injected intramuscularly into any one site to avoid pain on injection.

Effects on the eyes. After using a proprietary preparation of prednisolone sodium phosphate eye-drops 0.5%, instilled 4 times daily for 3 weeks, 2 (and possibly 5) subjects showed increased intra-ocular pressure in a controlled study with 20 healthy volunteers. Elevated ocular pressures returned to original levels within a week of stopping treatment.— T. G. Ramsell *et al.*, *Br. J. Ophthal.*, 1967, *51*, 398.

Absorption and Fate. As for Prednisolone, p.480.

Prednisolone sodium phosphate is rapidly absorbed after intramuscular injection and it appears in the plasma almost as rapidly as after an intravenous injection. Peak blood concentrations of prednisolone are obtained about an hour after either intravenous or intramuscular administration and the duration of action is about 3 or 4 hours.

Studies covering absorption and fate of oral prednisolone sodium phosphate compared with that of prednisolone: E. Baily *et al.*, *Archs Dis. Childh.*, 1963, *38*, 71; S. G. F. Matts, *Br. J. clin. Pract.*, 1972, *26*, 418.

Ocular absorption. Studies on the penetration of prednisolone sodium phosphate ophthalmic preparations in the cornea and aqueous humour.— A. Kupferman and H. M. Liebowitz, *Archs Ophthal., N.Y.*, 1974, *92*, 331.

Rectal absorption. Urinary excretion of prednisolone was studied in 4 patients with ulcerative colitis. Less than the equivalent of a daily oral dose of 7 mg of prednisolone was absorbed from the rectum after an enema containing 40 mg was given to ulcerative colitis patients. This was unlikely to account for the efficacy of rectal treatment.— W. A. Wood *et al.*, *Br. med. J.*, 1964, *2*, 1045. Studies in 7 patients with ulcerative colitis or Crohn's disease showed that prednisolone 21-phosphate, given as an enema, was absorbed. In 4 patients who retained the enema for at least 2.5 hours plasma-prednisolone concentrations were equal in 1 patient to those achieved after a comparable dose by mouth, higher in 1, and lower in 2.— J. Powell-Tuck *et al.*, *ibid.*, 1976, *1*, 193.

Uses. Prednisolone sodium phosphate has the general properties described under Corticosteroids (see p.451) and it is used for the same purposes as prednisolone (see p.480).

It is administered by intramuscular or intravenous injection, or by intravenous infusion, when oral therapy is not feasible. The usual initial dose is the equivalent of prednisolone phosphate 20 to 100 mg (prednisolone 16 to 80 mg) daily, subsequently adjusted according to the severity of the condition and the patient's response.

It is also used for its local anti-inflammatory effect by injection into joints and soft tissues in doses equivalent to 4 to 16 mg of prednisolone.

It is applied topically as eye-drops or ear-drops containing 0.5%.

It is also administered by retention enema in solutions containing the equivalent of 20 mg of prednisolone and as suppositories containing the equivalent of 5 mg of prednisolone, in the treatment of ulcerative colitis.

Preparations

Prednisolone Enema *(B.P.C. 1973)*. Prednisolone Sodium Phosphate Enema. A solution of prednisolone sodium phosphate in a suitable buffered aqueous vehicle. It may contain stabilising agents and a preservative. pH 5.5 to 7.5. When stored at a temperature not exceeding 25° and protected from light, it may be expected to retain its potency for at least 2 years. *Dose.* The equivalent of 20 mg of prednisolone, once or twice daily as a retention enema.

Prednisolone Eye-drops *(B.P.C. 1973)*. Prednisolone Sodium Phosphate Eye-drops; PRED. Prednisolone sodium phosphate 518 mg, sodium chloride 500 mg, sodium acid phosphate 300 mg, disodium edetate 10 mg, benzalkonium chloride solution 0.02 ml, sodium hydroxide q.s. to pH 8, water to 100 ml. Sterilised by maintaining at 98° to 100° for 30 minutes. Protect from light.

A.P.F. (Prednisolone Sodium Phosphate Eye Drops) has a similar preparation, with 50 mg of disodium edetate in Water for Injections. Sterilised by filtration.

Prednisolone Sodium Phosphate Injection *(B.P.)*. Prednisolone Sod. Phos. Inj. A sterile solution of prednisolone sodium phosphate in Water for Injections. It contains suitable stabilising agents and may contain a suitable buffering agent. Sterilised by filtration. Potency is expressed in terms of the equivalent amount of prednisolone. pH 6 to 9. Store at a temperature not exceeding 15°. Protect from light.

Prednisolone Sodium Phosphate Injection *(U.S.P.)*. A sterile solution of prednisolone sodium phosphate in Water for Injections. Potency is expressed in terms of the equivalent amount of prednisolone phosphate. pH 7 to 8. Protect from light.

Prednisolone Sodium Phosphate Ophthalmic Solution *(U.S.P.)*. A sterile solution of prednisolone sodium phosphate in a buffered aqueous vehicle. Potency is expressed in terms of the equivalent amount of prednisolone phosphate. pH 6.2 to 8.2. Store in airtight containers. Protect from light.

Proprietary Preparations

Codelsol Injection *(Merck Sharp & Dohme, UK)*. A sterile buffered solution containing in each ml prednisolone sodium phosphate equivalent to prednisolone 16 mg, in vials of 2 ml. For intramuscular, intravenous, and intrasynovial injection. (Also available as Codelsol in *Austral., Neth., Swed.*).

NOTE. Codelsol may be applied in different countries to different formulations.

Minims Prednisolone *(Smith & Nephew Pharmaceuticals, UK)*. Sterile eye-drops containing prednisolone sodium phosphate 0.5% in single-use disposable applicators.

Prednesol Tablets *(Glaxo, UK)*. Scored soluble tablets each containing prednisolone sodium phosphate equivalent to prednisolone 5 mg.

Predsol *(Glaxo, UK)*. Prednisolone sodium phosphate, available as **Drops for Eye and Ear** containing 0.5%, with benzalkonium chloride solution 0.04%; as **Retention Enema** containing the equivalent of 20 mg of prednisolone in 100 ml of buffered solution, supplied in a disposable plastic bag with rectal tube; and as **Suppositories** each containing the equivalent of 5 mg of prednisolone. (Also available as Predsol in *Austral., S.Afr.*).

Predsol-N Drops for Eye and Ear *(Glaxo, UK)*. A solution containing prednisolone sodium phosphate 0.5% and neomycin sulphate 0.5%, with thiomersal 0.005%. For inflammatory conditions of the eye or ear.

Other Proprietary Names

Caberdelta *(Ital.)*; Hydeltrasol *(USA)*; Inflamase *(Canad., Ger., USA)*; Metreton *(USA)*; Phortisolone *(Fr.)*; Pred-Clysma *(Denm., Norw.)*; Prednisolona Alonga *(Spain)*; PSP-IV, Savacort-S, Sodasone *(all USA)*; Solucort *(Fr.)*; Ultracorten-H wasserlöslich *(sodium tetrahydrophthalate) (Ger., Switz.)*; Ultracortene-H Hydrosoluble *(sodium tetrahydrophthalate) (Belg.)*.

1127-j

Prednisolone Steaglate.

Prednisolone 21-stearoylglycolate.

$C_{41}H_{64}O_8$=685.0.

CAS — 5060-55-9.

A white powder. M.p. about 105°. Prednisolone steaglate 190 mg is approximately equivalent to 100 mg of prednisolone. **Soluble** in alcohol, acetone, and methyl alcohol.

Adverse Effects, Treatment, Withdrawal, and Precautions. As for Corticosteroids, p.446, p.449.

Absorption and Fate. As for Prednisolone, p.480.

Plasma concentrations are maintained for longer periods than those following equivalent doses of prednisolone.

Blood concentrations after the administration of prednisolone 20 mg and prednisolone steaglate 38 mg (the equivalent of 20 mg of prednisolone) were determined in 10 healthy volunteers. Both the plasma concentration produced by the ester and its plasma half-life were markedly greater than those of prednisolone.— R. Tommasini *et al.*, *Arzneimittel-Forsch.*, 1966, *16*, 172.

Uses. Prednisolone steaglate has the general properties of prednisolone (see p.480); 6.65 mg is claimed to be equivalent in therapeutic activity to 5 mg of prednisolone.

It is used as tablets and as ointments.

Proprietary Preparations

Sintisone *(Farmitalia Carlo Erba, UK)*. Prednisolone steaglate, available as scored tablets of 6.65 mg. (Also available as Sintisone in *Austral., Belg., Ital.*).

Other Proprietary Names

Arg.— Lentosone; *Ital.*— Glitisone, Prenesei, Verisone; *Norw.*— Rolisone; *Spain*— Estilsona.

1128-z

Prednisolone Succinate *(U.S.P.)*.

Prednisolone 21-hydrogen succinate.

$C_{25}H_{32}O_8$=460.5.

CAS — 2920-86-7.

Pharmacopoeias. In *U.S.*

A fine, creamy-white, almost odourless powder with friable lumps. M.p. about 205° with decomposition. Prednisolone succinate 128 mg is approximately equivalent to 100 mg of prednisolone. Very slightly **soluble** in water; soluble 1 in about 6 of alcohol and 1 in about 250 of ether; soluble in acetone; very slightly soluble in chloroform. A solution in dioxan is dextrorotatory. **Store** in airtight containers.

Intravenous solutions diluted to 5 mg per ml in sodium chloride injection or dextrose injection maintained 98% potency for 12 days at 5°, and at a concentration of 25 mg per ml it was stable for 10 days at 25° in the dark.— J. F. Gallelli, *Am. J. Hosp. Pharm.*, 1967, *24*, 425.

Uses. Prednisolone succinate has the general properties and uses of prednisolone (see p.479) and is used by intravenous or intramuscular injection as the sodium salt similarly to prednisolone sodium phosphate.

Preparations

Prednisolone Sodium Succinate for Injection *(U.S.P.)*. Sterile prednisolone sodium succinate, prepared from prednisolone succinate and sodium carbonate, with suitable buffers. Potency is expressed in terms of the equivalent amount of prednisolone. A 2.5% solution in water is clear and has a pH of 6.7 to 7.

Proprietary Names

Alconisolone *(Eliovit, Ital.)*; Di-Adreson-F *(sodium) (Organon, Belg.; Organon, Neth.)*; Endoprenovis *(sodium) (Vister, Ital.)*; Fiasone Parenteral *(Orfi, Spain)*; Hemilagar *(Byk Gulden, Spain)*; Hostacortin H solubile *(sodium) (Hoechst, Ger.)*; Ibisterolon Fiale *(sodium) (Ibi, Ital.)*; Nisolone *(see also under Prednisolone) (Llorente, Spain)*; Precortalon *(sodium) (Organon, Swed.)*; Predonine Water-soluble *(sodium) (Jap.)*; Solu-Dacortin *(sodium) (Merck, Aust.; E. Merck, Austral.; Bracco, Ital.; E. Merck, Switz.)*; Solu-Dacortine *(sodium)*

(Merck, Belg.); Solu-Decortin-H (sodium) *(E. Merck, Ger.)*.

1129-c

Prednisolone Tebutate *(U.S.P.)*. Prednisolone Butylacetate; Prednisolone Tertiary-butylacetate. Prednisolone 21-(3,3-dimethylbutyrate).
$C_{27}H_{38}O_6,H_2O=476.6$.

CAS — 7681-14-3.

Pharmacopoeias. In *U.S.*

A white to slightly yellow hygroscopic powder, odourless or with a characteristic odour. Prednisolone tebutate 132 mg is approximately equivalent to 100 mg of prednisolone. Very slightly **soluble** in water; freely soluble in chloroform and dioxan; soluble in acetone; sparingly soluble in alcohol and methyl alcohol. A solution in chloroform is dextrorotatory. **Store** at a temperature not exceeding 8° in an atmosphere of nitrogen in airtight containers.

Uses. Prednisolone tebutate has the general properties of prednisolone (see p.479) and has been used for its local anti-inflammatory effect by injection into joints or soft tissues. The suggested dose by intra-articular injection was 8 to 30 mg according to the size of the joint.
There have been reports of joint damage following the intra-articular injection of corticosteroids into load-bearing joints (see under Corticosteroids, p.447).

For a study of the systemic absorption of intra-articular prednisolone tebutate, see Prednisolone Acetate, p.481.

Preparations

Sterile Prednisolone Tebutate Suspension *(U.S.P.)*. A sterile suspension of prednisolone tebutate in a suitable aqueous vehicle. pH 6 to 8.

Proprietary Names

Codelcortone TBA *(Merck Sharp & Dohme, Austral.; Chibret, Neth.; Merck Sharp & Dohme, Switz.)*; Hydeltra-TBA *(Merck Sharp & Dohme, USA)*.

Prednisolone tebutate was formerly marketed in Great Britain under the proprietary name Codelcortone-TBA *(Merck Sharp & Dohme)*.

1130-s

Prednisone *(B.P., Eur. P., U.S.P.)*.

Prednisonum; Deltacortisone; Deltadehydrocortisone; 1,2-Dehydrocortisone; Metacortandracin.
17α,21-Dihydroxypregna-1,4-diene-3,11,20-trione.
$C_{21}H_{26}O_5=358.4$.

CAS — 53-03-2.

Pharmacopoeias. In *Arg., Br., Braz., Cz., Eur., Fr., Ger., Ind., Int., It., Jug., Neth., Nord., Pol., Port., Roum., Rus., Swiss, Turk.,* and *U.S.*

A white or almost white, odourless, crystalline powder, with a persistent bitter after-taste. M.p. about 230° with decomposition.
Practically **insoluble** in water; soluble 1 in 150 to 190 of alcohol, 1 in 300 of dehydrated alcohol, and 1 in 200 of chloroform; slightly soluble in dioxan and methyl alcohol. A solution in dioxan is dextrorotatory. **Protect** from light.

Bioavailability. A crossover trial in 22 subjects compared the pharmacokinetics of prednisone tablets having very different dissolution-rates. Peak plasma concentrations of prednisolone were similar after either 1 slowly-dissolving 50-mg prednisone tablet or 10 rapidly-dissolving 5-mg tablets were taken, as were the rate and degree of absorption and plasma half-life (overall mean of 3.25 hours). Dissolution-rate *in vitro* was not a guide to bioavailability.— A. R. DiSanto and K. A. DeSante, *J. pharm. Sci.*, 1975, *64*, 109.

Prednisone is a biologically inert glucocorticoid which is converted to prednisolone in the liver. It has the same chemical relationship to prednisolone as cortisone has to hydrocortisone. The indications and dosage of prednisone for systemic therapy are exactly the same as those for prednisolone but since its bioavailability may, under some circumstances, be less reliable, prednisolone is now the preferred drug. For further details, see Prednisolone, p.480.

Like cortisone, prednisone is not suitable for intra-articular injection or topical application, since its activity depends upon systemic absorption with subsequent conversion into prednisolone.
Studies in healthy subjects indicated that absorption of prednisone was not affected by food.— A. V. Tembo *et al.*, *J. clin. Pharmac.*, 1976, *16*, 620.

Preparations

Prednisone Tablets *(B.P.)*. Tablets containing prednisone. Protect from light.

Prednisone Tablets *(U.S.P.)*. Tablets containing prednisone. The *U.S.P.* requires 80% dissolution in 30 minutes.

Proprietary Preparations

Decortisyl *(Roussel, UK)*. Prednisone, available as tablets of 1 mg and as scored tablets of 5 mg. (Also available as Decortisyl in *Austral.*).

Deltacortone *(Merck Sharp & Dohme, UK)*. Prednisone, available as scored tablets of 5 mg.

Econosone *(DDSA Pharmaceuticals, UK)*. Prednisone, available as tablets of 1 and 5 mg.

Marsone *(Marshall's Pharmaceuticals, UK)*. Prednisone, available as tablets of 1 and 5 mg.

Other Proprietary Names

Arg.— Deltisona, Meticorten; *Aust.*— Parmenison; *Austral.*— Adasone, Deltasone, Panafcort, Presone, Proped, Sone; *Belg.*— Prednicort; *Canad.*— Colisone, Deltasone, Paracort, Winpred; *Denm.*— Delcortin, Predniment; *Fr.*— Cortancyl, Urtilone; *Ger.*— Decortin, Hostacortin, Prednilonga-retard, Predniment, Rectodelt, Ultracorten; *Ital.*— Decorton, Deidrocortisone, Deltacortene, Delta Prenovis, Itacortone (palmitate), Marvidiene; *Norw.*—Deltison Clysma; *Pol.*— Encorton; *S.Afr.*— Deltasone, Meticorten, Panafcort, Predeltin; *Spain*— Cortialer, Dacortin, Delta-Scherosona, Fiasone Oral, Marnisonal, Nisone, Predniartrit, Predni-Wolner, Prednovister, Supopred, Ultracorten; *Swed.*— Deltison; *Switz.*— Meprison, Ultracorten; *USA*— Delta-Dome, Deltasone, Lisacort, Meticorten, Orasone, Prednicen-M, Servisone, SK-Prednisone, Sterapred.

Prednisone was also formerly marketed in Great Britain under the proprietary name Di-Adreson *(Organon)*.

1131-w

Prednisone Acetate *(B.P. 1968)*.

Prednisoni Acetas. Prednisone 21-acetate.
$C_{23}H_{28}O_6=400.5$.

CAS — 125-10-0.

Pharmacopoeias. In *Arg., Chin., Fr., Ind., Int., Jug., Pol., Roum.,* and *Turk.*

A white or almost white, odourless crystalline powder, with a persistent bitter after-taste. M.p. about 240° with decomposition. Prednisone acetate 11 mg is approximately equivalent to 10 mg of prednisone.
Practically **insoluble** in water; soluble 1 in 120 of alcohol, 1 in 160 of dehydrated alcohol, and 1 in 6 of chloroform. **Protect** from light.

Uses. Prednisone acetate has the general properties of prednisone and has been administered by mouth as tablets for the same purposes.

1132-e

Prednylidene. 16-Methylene Prednisolone.
11β,17α,21-Trihydroxy-16-methylenepregna-1,4-diene-3,20-dione.
$C_{22}H_{28}O_5=372.5$.

CAS — 599-33-7.

Uses. Prednylidene has the general properties of prednisolone (p.479) and has been used for similar purposes; 6 mg is equivalent in effect to about 5 mg of prednisolone.

Proprietary Names

Dacorsol (diaminoacetate) *(Igoda, Spain)*; Dacortilen *(Merck, Aust.; Bracco, Ital.; Igoda, Spain; E. Merck, Swed.)*; Decortilen Solubile (diethylaminoacetate hydrochloride) *(E. Merck, Ger.)*; Décortilène *(Merck-Clévenot, Fr.)*.

1133-l

Suprarenal Cortex Injection *(B.P.C. 1959)*. Suprarenal Cort. Inj.; Adrenal Cortex Injection; Suprarenal Cortex Extract.

An aqueous solution of the active principles of suprarenal cortex; it contains a number of steroid compounds the most active of which are corticosterone, dehydrocorticosterone, hydrocortisone, cortisone, and aldosterone. A clear almost colourless liquid, which is odourless, or has a faint garlic-like odour. pH 3.8 to 4. It may be **sterilised** by filtration.

Uses. Suprarenal Cortex Injection was formerly used for the treatment of Addison's disease but it has been superseded by hydrocortisone and other corticosteroids.

Proprietary Names

Biocortone *(SIT, Ital.)*; Cortical *(ION, Ital.)*; Corticopan *(Ist. Chim. Inter., Ital.)*; Cortidin *(Crinos, Ital.)*; Cortigen *(Richter, Ital.)*; Cortine *(Laroche Navarron, Fr.)*; Fluxalgin *(Baer, Ger.)*; Liocortex *(Radiumfarma, Ital.)*; Maxicortex *(Manetti Roberts, Ital.)*; Mencortex *(Menarini, Ital.)*; Novocortex *(Besins-Iscovesco, Fr.)*; Recortex *(Fellows, USA)*; Supracort *(Samil, Ital.)*.

A preparation of suprarenal cortex was formerly marketed in Great Britain under the proprietary name Supracort *(Paines & Byrne)*.

1134-y

Triamcinolone *(B.P.C. 1973, U.S.P.)*.

Fluoxiprednisolonum; 9α-Fluoro-16α-hydroxyprednisolone; Triamcinolonum. 9α-Fluoro-11β,16α,17α,21-tetrahydroxypregna-1,4-diene-3,20-dione.
$C_{21}H_{27}FO_6=394.4$.

CAS — 124-94-7.

Pharmacopoeias. In *Cz., It., Jap., Swiss,* and *U.S.*

A white or almost white, odourless or almost odourless, crystalline powder. M.p. about 262°. **Soluble** 1 in 500 of water and 1 in 240 of alcohol; slightly soluble in methyl alcohol; very slightly soluble in chloroform and ether.

Adverse Effects and Treatment. As for Corticosteroids, p.446, and p.449.
Its effects on sodium and water retention are less than those of prednisolone. Anorexia, weight loss, flushing, depression, and muscle wasting are reported to have been particularly associated with triamcinolone.

Of 47 patients with rheumatoid arthritis treated with triamcinolone in doses of up to 16 mg daily for periods of up to 11 months, 24 experienced serious side-effects. The commonest of these was a typical facial and body flushing which occurred in 17 patients. Mooning of the face occurred in 9 patients, marked hirsuties in 2, dyspepsia in 8, one of whom developed haematemesis and melaena, mental depression in 4, and spontaneous fractures in 2; in 5 patients there was severe weight loss and 4 suffered from rapid symmetrical muscle-wasting of the legs, arms, and shoulders. Of 23 patients receiving less than 6 mg daily, only 3 suffered any discomfort, and it was suggested that this was the highest maintenance dose that could be given over a prolonged period.— P. H. Kendall and M. F. Hart, *Br. med. J.*, 1959, *1*, 682.

Effects on the eyes. Temporary blindness in 1 eye, with diplopia and headaches, followed the injection of triamcinolone suspension into the congested nasal mucous membranes of a woman with allergic rhinitis. Paresis of the left inferior rectus muscle was diagnosed.— R. J. Rowe *et al.* (letter), *J. Am. med. Ass.*, 1967, *201*, 333.

Effects on muscle. Seven patients who had been receiving prolonged high doses of triamcinolone and 3 who had been receiving other fluorinated corticosteroids developed painless muscular atrophy in both thighs and the shoulder girdle so that they were unable to stand up from a sitting position and were scarcely able to walk unaided. In a few of these patients discontinuation of the corticosteroid brought about partial improvement.— H. Kaiser and W. Hochheuser, *Münch. med. Wschr.*, 1972, *114*, 269, per *J. Am. med. Ass.*, 1972, *219*, 1511.

Withdrawal and Precautions. As for Corticosteroids, p.449.

Systemic administration of triamcinolone with chloroquine is liable to produce exfoliative erythroderma and should be avoided.— C. F. H. Vickers, *Practitioner*, 1969, *202*, 43.

Absorption and Fate. For a brief outline of the absorption and fate of corticosteroids, see Corticosteroids, p.451.

Triamcinolone is reported to have a biological half-life in plasma of about 300 minutes. It is bound to plasma albumin to a much smaller extent than hydrocortisone.

References: C. H. Demos *et al.*, *Clin. Pharmac. Ther.*, 1964, *5*, 721.

Triamcinolone is bound to plasma albumin to a smaller extent than hydrocortisone.— J. R. Florini and D. A. Buyske, *J. biol. Chem.*, 1961, *236*, 247.

Uses. Triamcinolone is a synthetic glucocorticoid and has the general properties described under Corticosteroids (see p.451); 4 mg of triamcinolone is equivalent in anti-inflammatory activity to about 5 mg of prednisolone. It has been used in the treatment of all conditions for which corticosteroid therapy is indicated, except adrenal-deficiency states for which its lack of sodium-retaining properties makes it less suitable than cortisone or hydrocortisone with supplementary fludrocortisone.

Triamcinolone has a dose range of 4 to 48 mg daily in divided doses, as a single daily dose at 8 a.m., or as a double dose on alternate mornings.

Preparations

Triamcinolone Tablets *(B.P.C. 1973, U.S.P.)*. Tablets containing triamcinolone.

Adcortyl *(Squibb, UK)*. Triamcinolone, available as scored tablets of 4 mg.

Ledercort *(Lederle, UK)*. Triamcinolone, available as tablets of 2 and 4 mg. (Also available as Ledercort in *Arg.*, *Denm.*, *Ital.*, *Neth.*, *Norw.*, *Spain*, *Switz.*).

Other Proprietary Names

Arg.— Kenacort ; *Austral.*— Kenacort; *Belg.*— Kenacort; *Canad.*— Aristocort, Kenacort; *Fr.*— Kenacort; *Ger.*— Delphicort, Extracort, Triamcet, Triam, Volon; *Ital.*—Albacort, Cinolone, Cortinovus, Delsolone, Flogicort, Ipercortis, Kenacort, Medicort, Sadocort, Triamcort, Trilon, Voncort; *Neth.*— Kenacort; *Spain*— Ditrizin, Trigon; *Switz.*— Kenacort, Triamcort; *USA*— Aristocort, Kenacort, SK-Triamcinolone.

1135-j

Triamcinolone Acetonide *(B.P., B.P. Vet., U.S.P.)*.

9α-Fluoro-11β,21-dihydroxy-16α,17α-isopropylidenedioxypregna-1,4-diene-3,20-dione.

$C_{24}H_{31}FO_6$=434.5.

CAS — 76-25-5.

Pharmacopoeias. In *Br.*, *Braz.*, *Jap.*, *Turk.*, and *U.S.*

A white or cream-coloured, odourless or almost odourless, crystalline powder. Triamcinolone acetonide 11 mg is approximately equivalent to 10 mg of triamcinolone. Very slightly **soluble** in water; soluble 1 in 150 of alcohol, 1 in 11 of acetone, and 1 in 40 of chloroform; very soluble in dehydrated alcohol and methyl alcohol; sparingly soluble in ethyl acetate. A solution in dioxan is dextrorotatory. **Protect** from light.

Adverse Effects, Treatment, Withdrawal, and Precautions. As for Corticosteroids, p.446, p.449. See also Triamcinolone, p.483.

There have been reports of joint damage following the intra-articular injection of corticosteroids into load-bearing joints (see under Corticosteroids, p.447).

Prolonged application to the eye of preparations containing corticosteroids has caused increased intra-ocular pressure and reduced visual function.

Adrenal suppression. Adrenal suppression associated with topical application of triamcinolone cream.— K. S. Taylor *et al.*, *Archs Derm.*, 1965, *92*, 174.

Partial suppression of adrenal function occurred in 1 of 3 healthy persons who applied triamcinolone acetonide 3 mg in Orabase daily to the buccal quadrants of the mouth.— T. Lehner and C. Lyne, *Br. dent. J.*, 1970, *129*, 164.

After 3 peri-ocular injections of triamcinolone acetonide 40 mg monthly, together with 4 times daily topical application of dexamethasone sodium phosphate eye-drops for 4 months, to prevent corneal graft rejection, an 11-month-old girl died from corticosteroid side-effects. It was considered that the toxic effects observed were probably due to the depot triamcinolone.— P. E. Romano *et al.*, *Am. J. Ophthal.*, 1977, *84*, 247.

The incidence of adrenal suppression in asthmatic patients given injections of triamcinolone acetonide.— W. Droszcz *et al.*, *Ann. Allergy*, 1980, *44*, 174.

Candidiasis. Sore throat or hoarseness associated with triamcinolone acetonide inhalations.— W. W. Pingleton *et al.*, *J. Allergy & clin. Immunol.*, 1977, *60*, 254. See also P. Chervinsky and A. J. Petraco, *Ann. Allergy*, 1979, *43*, 80.

Effects on the skin. A report of severe cutaneous atrophy in 2 patients following long-term application of triamcinolone acetonide cream under occlusion.— D. K. Goette, *Sth. med. J.*, 1973, *66*, 542.

Reports of discoloration and atrophy of the skin following local injections of triamcinolone: I. Kikuchi and S. Horikawa, *Archs Derm.*, 1974, *109*, 558; R. A. Nozik, *Am. J. Ophthal.*, 1976, *82*, 928; I. M. Lund *et al.*, *Rheumatol. Rehabil.*, 1979, *18*, 91.

Absorption and Fate. For a brief outline of the absorption and fate of corticosteroids, see Corticosteroids, p.451. See also Triamcinolone, p.484.

When applied topically, particularly to large areas, when the skin is broken, or under occlusive dressings, corticosteroids may be absorbed in sufficient amounts to cause systemic effects. Triamcinolone acetonide is very slowly absorbed when injected intramuscularly.

Uses. Triamcinolone acetonide has the general properties of triamcinolone (see p.484) and is used by topical application in the treatment of various skin disorders as described under Corticosteroids, p.451. It is applied in creams, lotions, and ointments containing 0.1% and also as an aerosol spray.

In the treatment of keloids, lichen planus, lichen simplex, and sarcoidosis of the skin, triamcinolone acetonide may be given by intralesional injection of usually about 0.1 ml of a suspension containing 10 mg per ml. Intralesional injections have also been used in alopecia areata. Triamcinolone acetonide may also be administered intramuscularly as a suspension, usually in a dose of 40 mg, for a prolonged systemic effect; the effects may last for about 3 weeks or longer. Intra-articular injections of 2.5 to 15 mg have been given in the treatment of arthritic joints.

Ainhum. A report of the successful use of local injections of triamcinolone acetonide in ainhum, a disease of dark-skinned people characterised by a groove encircling one or both small toes, resulting usually in spontaneous amputation. Prompt symptomatic relief, followed by partial resolution of the fibrotic band was obtained after monthly intralesional injections of triamcinolone 5 to 7.5 mg.— J. W. Rossiter and P. C. Anderson, *Pharmac. Ther.*, 1976, *15*, 379.

Asthma. Triamcinolone acetonide administered by aerosol inhalation in doses of 0.8 to 2.4 mg daily successfully replaced other corticosteroids in 14 of 18 patients with severe asthma and cortical suppression due to the daily doses equivalent to 5 to 25 mg of prednisone which they had been taking for 3 to 17 years. Adrenal function tests returned to near normal in these 14 patients.— C. J. Falliers (letter), *Lancet*, 1973, *1*, 606. See also M. H. Williams *et al.*, *Am. Rev. resp. Dis.*, 1974, *109*, 538.

Further reports and studies on the role of triamcinolone acetonide aerosol inhalations in respiratory disorders: C. J. Falliers, *J. Allergy & clin. Immunol.*, 1976, *57*, 1; P. Chervinsky, *Ann. Allergy*, 1977, *38*, 192; R. J. Kriz *et al.*, *Chest*, 1977, *72*, 36; W. W. Pingleton *et al.*, *Chest*, 1977, *71*, 782; *idem*, *J. Am. med. Ass.*, 1977, *238*, 2174; M. H. Grieco *et al.*, *Archs intern. Med.*, 1978, *138*, 1337; R. M. Sly *et al.*, *J. Allergy & clin. Immunol.*, 1978, *62*, 76.

Rhinitis. In 42 patients given a single injection of depot methylprednisolone acetate 80 mg at the onset of hay fever symptoms, 42.5% obtained complete relief, 47.5% obtained partial relief, and 10% obtained no relief. Comparable results the next year in 50 patients after a single injection of depot triamcinolone acetonide 80 mg were 63.7, 30.5, and 5.8% respectively. After either injection patients reported relief after 3 days, lasting for 1 to 2 months.— G. Melotte, *Practitioner*, 1973, *210*, 282. See also L. L. Henderson *et al.*, *J. Allergy & clin. Immunol.*, 1973, *52*, 352.

For a comment on the ethics of using depot corticosteroids in hay fever, see Corticosteroids, p.458.

Skin disorders. A review of the use of triamcinolone acetonide and other corticosteroids injected intralesionally for the treatment of a variety of skin disorders.— J. Verbov, *Br. J. Derm.*, 1976, *94*, *Suppl.* 12, 51.

For recommendations concerning the correct use of corticosteroids on the skin, and a rough guide to the clinical potencies of topical corticosteroids, see Corticosteroids, p.458.

Acne. Intralesional injection of minute amounts of triamcinolone acetonide in 2.5% lignocaine caused rapid resolution of acne in 3 to 4 days.— R. M. Adams, *Clin. Med.*, 1972, *79* (Feb.), 26.

For comments on the limited role of corticosteroids in acne, see Corticosteroids, General, p.458.

Psoriasis. In 7 patients with psoriatic dystrophy of finger nails, 21 of 27 nails showed a satisfactory response after deep intradermal injection, by a needleless jet injector, into the matrix area of the nails. The dose was 0.1 ml of 0.5% triamcinolone acetonide solution on 3 occasions at weekly intervals.— E. Abell, *Br. J. Derm.*, 1972, *86*, 79. There was only occasional improvement in oncholysis and relapses were rapid and frequent.— E. Abell and P. D. Samman, *ibid.*, 1973, *89*, 191. See also J. Z. Litt, *Cutis*, 1971, *8*, 569. From a similar trial in 37 patients with psoriatic nail dystrophy it was considered that while deep intradermal injection of triamcinolone acetonide or of triamcinolone hexacetonide might be a useful form of treatment, most of the patients for whom the condition was really troublesome had nail-bed and hyponychial changes in tissues not reached by the injections.— R. D. G. Peachy *et al.*, *Br. J. Derm.*, 1976, *95*, 75. See also T. R. Bedi, *Dermatologica*, 1977, *24*, 155.

Preparations

Triamcinolone Acetonide Cream *(B.P.)*. Triamcinolone Cream. A cream containing triamcinolone acetonide in a suitable basis. Store at a temperature not exceeding 25° in well-closed containers which minimise evaporation and contamination.

When a strength less than those available from the manufacturer is prescribed, the 0.1% cream may be diluted, taking hygienic precautions, with Aqueous Cream. The diluted cream must be freshly prepared and not used more than 14 days after issue.

Triamcinolone Acetonide Cream *(U.S.P.)*. Contains triamcinolone acetonide in a suitable cream basis. Store in airtight containers.

Triamcinolone Acetonide Dental Paste *(B.P.)*. Triamcinolone Dental Paste. Contains triamcinolone acetonide in a suitable basis.

Triamcinolone Acetonide Dental Paste *(U.S.P.)*. Triamcinolone acetonide in a suitable emollient paste. Store in airtight containers.

Triamcinolone Acetonide Ointment *(B.P.)*. Triamcinolone Ointment. An ointment containing triamcinolone acetonide in a suitable basis.

When a strength less than that available from the manufacturer is prescribed, the 0.1% ointment may be diluted with a basis consisting of 1 part wool fat and 9 parts white soft paraffin.

Triamcinolone Acetonide Ointment *(U.S.P.)*. Contains triamcinolone acetonide in a suitable ointment basis.

Sterile Triamcinolone Acetonide Suspension *(U.S.P.)*. A sterile suspension in a suitable aqueous vehicle. pH 5 to 7.5. Protect from light.

Triamcinolone Acetonide Topical Aerosol *(U.S.P.)*. Triamcinolone Acetonide Aerosol. A solution of triamcinolone acetonide in a suitable propellent in a pressurised container. Store at a temperature not exceeding 40°.

Triamcinolone Lotion *(B.P.C. 1973)*. Triamcinolone Acetonide Lotion. A dispersion of triamcinolone acetonide in a suitable lotion basis. When a strength less than that available from the manufacturer is prescribed, the 0.1% lotion may be diluted, taking hygienic precautions, with a 3% solution of carmellose sodium (medium-viscosity grade) in water containing 0.2% methyl hydroxybenzoate and 0.02% propyl hydroxybenzoate. The diluted lotion must be freshly prepared and not used more than 1 month after issue for use.

Proprietary Preparations

Adcortyl *(Squibb, UK)*. Triamcinolone acetonide, available as **Cream** containing 0.1% in a vanishing cream basis [suggested diluent, Cetomacrogol Cream (Formula B)]; as **Ointment** containing 0.1% in Plastibase (a polyethylene and liquid paraffin basis) (suggested diluent, white soft paraffin); and as **Spray** containing 3.3 mg in 50 g.

Adcortyl in Orabase *(Squibb, UK)*. Contains triamcinolone acetonide 0.1% in Orabase, an adhesive basis of gelatin, pectin, and carmellose sodium in Plastibase (a polyethylene and liquid paraffin basis). For the topical treatment of oral lesions.

Adcortyl Intra-articular/Intradermal *(Squibb, UK)*. Triamcinolone acetonide in aqueous suspension containing 10 mg per ml for intra-articular or intracutaneous injection, in ampoules of 1 ml and vials of 5 ml.

Adcortyl with Graneodin (known in USA as Kenalog-S) *(Squibb, UK)*. Preparations containing triamcinolone acetonide 0.1%, neomycin sulphate equivalent to neomycin 0.25%, and gramicidin 0.025%, available as **Cream** in a vanishing basis and as **Ointment**.

Aureocort *(Lederle, UK)*. Preparations containing triamcinolone acetonide 0.1% and chlortetracycline hydrochloride 3%, available as **Cream** in a water-miscible basis and as **Ointment** in a wool fat and white soft paraffin basis.

Aureocort Spray *(Lederle, UK)*. A pressurised spray containing triamcinolone acetonide 0.025% and chlortetracycline hydrochloride 1% in a propellent basis.

Kenalog *(Squibb, UK)*. Triamcinolone acetonide, available as a suspension containing 40 mg per ml, with benzyl alcohol 0.9%, carmellose sodium 0.75%, polysorbate '80' 0.04%, and sodium chloride, in disposable syringes of 1 and 2 ml and vials of 1 ml. (Also available as Kenalog in *Austral., Canad., Denm., USA*).

Ledercort Cream and Ointment *(Lederle, UK)*. Each contains triamcinolone acetonide 0.1%. (Also available as Ledercort in *Arg.,Norw., Spain, Switz.*).

Ledermix *(Lederle, UK)*. **Paste** contains triamcinolone acetonide 1% and demeclocycline calcium equivalent to demeclocycline hydrochloride 3% in a water-soluble cream consisting of triethanolamine, calcium chloride, zinc oxide, sodium sulphite, hard macrogol, and distilled water. For application to exposed tooth pulp under temporary filling. **Cement Powder** contains triamcinolone acetonide 0.6% and demeclocycline 2%, with zinc oxide, Canada balsam, resin, and calcium hydroxide, and is supplied with a hardener consisting of eugenol and turpentine oil; the powder when mixed with hardener sets to a cement. For use as a permanent lining cement for tooth cavities in cases of pulp exposure.

The cream basis of Ledermix Paste was irritant to the pulp of *rat* teeth.— R. C. Paterson, *Br. dent. J.*, 1976, *140,* 174.

Remiderm *(Squibb, UK)*. **Cream** containing triamcinolone acetonide 0.025% and halquinol 0.75% in a vanishing cream basis; **Ointment** containing the same amounts of active ingredients in Plastibase (a polyethylene and liquid paraffin basis); and **Aerosol Spray** containing triamcinolone acetonide 4.95 mg and halquinol 31.2 mg in each container of 75 g.

Remotic Ear Drop Capsules *(Squibb, UK)*. Each contains triamcinolone acetonide 0.025% and halquinol 0.75% in castor oil 0.3 ml.

Silderm *(Lederle, UK)*. Cream containing triamcinolone acetonide 0.1%, neomycin sulphate equivalent to neomycin 0.35%, and undecenoic acid 2.5%.

Tri-Adcortyl Ointment (known in USA as Mycolog Ointment and in some other countries as Kenacomb Ointment) *(Squibb, UK)*. Contains in each g triamcinolone acetonide 1 mg, neomycin sulphate equivalent to neomycin 2.5 mg, gramicidin 250 µg, and nystatin 100 000 units in Plastibase (a polyethylene and liquid paraffin basis). **Tri-Adcortyl Cream** contains the same amounts of active ingredients in a vanishing cream basis. For dermatoses. **Tri-Adcortyl Otic Ointment** contains the same amounts of active ingredients in Plastibase (a polyethylene and liquid paraffin basis). For otitis externa.

Of 159 patients with contact dermatitis 20 were sensitive to ethylenediamine; all had used Tri-Adcortyl cream which contained ethylenediamine.— M. I. White *et al.*, *Br. med. J.*, 1978, *1,* 415.

Tricaderm Solution *(Squibb, UK)*. Contains triamcinolone acetonide 0.2%, salicylic acid 2%, and benzalkonium chloride 0.05%, in an alcoholic basis. For dermatoses of the face and scalp. *Directions.* To be massaged drop by drop into the affected area each night, and on improvement, every 2 or 3 nights for not more than 4 weeks.

Other Proprietary Names

Arg.— Fortcinolona, Trianciterap; *Austral.*— Aristocort, Kenacort-A, Kenalone; *Belg.*— Delphi, Kenacort A, Kenacort A Solubile *(*acetonide dipotassium phosphate*)*; *Canad.*— Triaderm, Trimacort; *Fr.*— Cutinolone Simple, Kenacort-A, Kenacort Retard, Tédarol; *Ger.*— Delphicort, Extracort, Kortikoid, Solodelf, Triam, Volon A, Volon A Solubile *(*acetonide dipotassium phosphate*)*, Volonimat; *Hung.*— Ftorocort; *Ital.*— Eczil, Flogicort, Kenacort-A, Ledercort A; *Jap.*— Rineton, Tricinolon; *Neth.*— Albicort, Kenacort-A, Kenacort A solubile *(*acetonide dipotassium phosphate*)*; *Norw.*— Kenacort-T; *Spain*— Bucalsone, Triaceton, Trigon; *Swed.*— Kenacort-T; *Switz.*— Kenacort-A, Kenacort-A solubile *(*acetonide dipotassium phosphate*)*, Paralen; *USA*— Aristocort, Aristocort A, Aristogel, Cenocort A, Tramacin, Triam-A.

1136-z

Triamcinolone Diacetate *(U.S.P.)*.
Triamcinolone 16α,21-diacetate.

$C_{25}H_{31}FO_8$=478.5.

CAS — 67-78-7.

Pharmacopoeias. In *U.S.*

White to off-white, fine crystalline powder with a slight odour. Loses not more than 6% of its weight on drying. Triamcinolone diacetate 12 mg is approximately equivalent to 10 mg of triamcinolone. Practically **insoluble** in water; soluble 1 in 13 of alcohol, 1 in 80 of chloroform, and 1 in 40 of methyl alcohol; slightly soluble in ether.

Adverse Effects, Treatment, Withdrawal, and Precautions. As for Corticosteroids, p.446, p.449. See also Triamcinolone.

There have been reports of joint damage following the intra-articular injection of corticosteroids into load-bearing joints (see under Corticosteroids, p.447).

Absorption and Fate. For a brief outline of the absorption and fate of corticosteroids, see Corticosteroids, p.451. See also Triamcinolone (above). Triamcinolone diacetate is very slowly absorbed following intramuscular injection.

Uses. Triamcinolone diacetate has the general properties and uses of triamcinolone (see p.484).

It may be administered by intramuscular injection, usually in the form of a suspension containing 40 mg per ml, for a prolonged systemic effect; the usual dose of 40 mg may control symptoms for up to 4 weeks.

Suspensions have been used by intra-articular injection in the local treatment of arthritic joints in usual doses of 5 to 40 mg every 1 to 8 weeks. Intralesional injections may be given for inflammatory skin disorders, ranging from a total of 5 mg in divided doses into small lesions, to a total of 48 mg for large psoriatic plaques; in general, no more than 12.5 mg should be injected into any one injection site.

Triamcinolone diacetate is used by mouth in the form of a syrup containing 2 or 5 mg in 5 ml, in doses similar to those for triamcinolone.

Calcinosis cutis. Triamcinolone diacetate 25 mg injected intralesionally at monthly intervals produced substantial regression of lesions in a 13-year-old patient with calcinosis cutis circumscripta; a total of about 250 mg was given during the first year of treatment.— S. S. Lee *et al.*, *Archs Derm.*, 1978, *114,* 1080.

For a report of calcinosis cutis following intralesional injection of triamcinolone hexacetonide, see p.485.

Preparations

Sterile Triamcinolone Diacetate Suspension *(U.S.P.)*. A sterile suspension in a suitable aqueous vehicle. pH 4.5 to 7.5.

Triamcinolone Diacetate Syrup *(U.S.P.)*. It contains a suitable preservative. Store in airtight containers.

Proprietary Names

Aristocort *(Lederle, USA)*; Cenocort Forte *(Central Pharmacal, USA)*; Cino-40 *(Tutag, USA)*; Delphicort *(Cyanamid-Lederle, Ger.)*; Kenacort *(Squibb, USA)*; Ledercort *(Cyanamid, Spain*; *Lederle, Switz.)*; Ledercort diacetat *(Lederle, Denm.*; *Lederle, Swed.)*; Tédarol *(Specia, Fr.)*; Tracilon *(Savage, USA)*; Tricortale *(Bergamon, Ital.)*.

Triamcinolone diacetate was formerly marketed in Great Britain under the proprietary name Ledercort Depot *(Lederle)*.

1137-c

Triamcinolone Hexacetonide *(U.S.P.)*.
Triamcinolone Acetonide 21-(3,3-Dimethylbutyrate). 9α-Fluoro-11β,21-dihydroxy-16α,17α-isopropylidenedioxypregna-1,4-diene-3,20-dione 21-(3,3-dimethylbutyrate).

$C_{30}H_{41}FO_7$=532.6.

CAS — 5611-51-8.

Pharmacopoeias. In *U.S.*

A white to cream-coloured powder. Practically **insoluble** in water; soluble in chloroform; slightly soluble in methyl alcohol.

Adverse Effects, Treatment, Withdrawal, and Precautions. As for Corticosteroids, p.446, p.449. See also Triamcinolone.

There have been reports of joint damage following the intra-articular injection of corticosteroids into load-bearing joints (see under Corticosteroids, p.447).

Effects on the skin. A report of calcinosis cutis in a patient with nummular eczema following intralesional injection of triamcinolone hexacetonide.— H. P. Baden and L. C. Bonar, *Archs Derm.*, 1967, *96,* 689.

Local cutaneous atrophy associated with injections of triamcinolone hexacetonide.— I. M. Lund *et al.*, *Rheumatol. Rehabil.*, 1979, *18,* 91.

Absorption and Fate. For a brief outline of the absorption and fate of corticosteroids, see Corticosteroids, p.451. See also Triamcinolone (above). Suspensions of triamcinolone hexacetonide are only very slowly released from local injection sites.

Uses. Triamcinolone hexacetonide has the properties and uses of triamcinolone (see p.483).

It is administered by intralesional or sublesional injection in the local treatment of various inflammatory skin lesions usually as a suspension containing 5 mg in 1 ml to give a dosage of up to 80 µg per cm^2 of affected skin. It is also administered intra-articularly in the local treatment of arthritic joints usually as a suspension containing 20 mg in 1 ml in a dose of 2 to 30 mg according to the size of the joint; the effect may last for up to 2 or 3 months. Suspensions of triamcinolone hexacetonide may be diluted with Lignocaine Injection.

Preparations

Sterile Triamcinolone Hexacetonide Suspension *(U.S.P.)*. A sterile suspension in a suitable aqueous vehicle. pH 4 to 8.

Lederspan *(Lederle, UK)*. Triamcinolone hexacetonide, available as an aqueous suspension for injection containing 5 mg per ml in vials of 5 ml (for intralesional injection), and 20 mg per ml in vials of 1 and 5 ml (for intra-articular injection), with polysorbate 80, Sorbitol Solution 50% v/v, and benzyl alcohol 0.9%. (Also available as Lederspan in *Arg., Belg., Denm., Ital., Neth., Norw., Switz.*).

Other Proprietary Names

Aristospan *(Canad., USA)*; Hexatrione *(Fr.)*; Lederlon *(Ger.)*.

Corticotrophin

1461-v

Corticotrophin *(B.P., Eur. P.)*. Corticotropinum; ACTH; Adrenocorticotrophic Hormone; Adrenocorticotropin; Corticotropin.

CAS — 9002-60-2.

Pharmacopoeias. In *Arg., Aust., Br., Braz., Eur., Fr., Ger., Ind., It., Jug., Neth.,* and *Swiss.* Certain pharmacopoeias include only Corticotrophin for Injection.

Corticotrophin is a polypeptide chain comprising 39 amino acids obtained from the anterior lobe of the pituitary gland of the pig and other mammals used by man for food and contains the hormone that increases the rate at which corticoid hormones are secreted by the adrenal gland. It contains not less than 55 units per mg and not more than 5 units of pressor activity per 100 units of corticotrophin activity.

White or almost white hygroscopic flakes or powder. Loses not more than 7% of its weight on drying. Very **soluble** in water. A 1% solution in water has a pH of 3 to 5. Solutions are **sterilised** by filtration. **Store** at a temperature not exceeding 25° in airtight containers. Protect from light. Under such conditions it may be expected to retain its potency for not less than 2 years from the date of manufacture.

Incompatibility. There was loss of clarity when intravenous solutions of corticotrophin were mixed with those of novobiocin sodium or sodium bicarbonate.— J. A. Patel and G. L. Phillips, *Am. J. Hosp. Pharm.*, 1966, *23*, 409. A precipitate formed within 1 hour when aminophylline was mixed with corticotrophin 40 units per litre.— E. A. Parker (letter), *ibid.*, 1970, *27*, 67.

Comment on the stability of corticotrophin *in vitro* in blood.— H. P. J. Bennett and C. McMartin, *Pharmac. Rev.*, 1978, *30*, 247.

Units. 5 units of porcine corticotrophin for bioassay are contained in approximately 50 µg (with lactose 5 mg) in one ampoule of the third International Standard Preparation (1962).

In accordance with the request made in the twenty-sixth report, the National Institute for Biological Standards and Control, London, has obtained a highly purified preparation of human corticotrophin and has studied its activity. There are too few ampoules of this preparation to make it possible to establish it as an international reference material, and a further, larger quantity of similar material is being obtained. The Institute has been requested to arrange an international collaborative study and, in the meantime, to make the material previously studied available to research workers.— Thirtieth Report of WHO Expert Committee on Biological Standardization, *Tech. Rep. Ser. Wld Hlth Org. No. 638*, 1979.

Adverse Effects. Corticotrophin stimulates the adrenals to product cortisol (hydrocortisone) and mineralocorticoids, such as corticosterone; it therefore has the adverse glucocorticoid and the adverse mineralocorticoid properties of corticosteroids (see p.446).

In particular, its mineralocorticoid properties may produce marked sodium and water retention with the risk of hypertension and ultimately heart failure; considerable potassium loss may also occur.

Although corticotrophin has a marked diabetogenic effect, other adverse effects attributable to its glucocorticoid properties are less marked. For example, gastro-intestinal effects and skin atrophy are less evident, it may be less liable to induce osteoporosis, and it appears to cause less growth inhibiton in children.

Corticotrophin also stimulates the adrenals to produce androgens with the result that acne and hirsutism occur more frequently than with corticosteroids.

Whereas corticosteroids replace endogenous cortisol (hydrocortisone) and thereby induce adrenal atrophy, corticotrophin's stimulant effect induces hypertrophy. Withdrawal of corticotrophin is therefore easier than withdrawal of corticosteroids; nevertheless, the ability of the hypothalamic-pituitary-adrenal axis to respond to stress is still reduced, and abrupt withdrawal of corticotrophin may result in symptoms of hypopituitarism (see Withdrawal, below).

Corticotrophin sometimes induces skin pigmentation. It can induce sensitisation and severe allergic reactions may occur.

Thirteen of 19 children, who had been treated with a long-acting preparation of porcine corticotrophin (Acthar Gel) for 5 to 200 weeks, developed circulating antibodies directed mainly against the species-specific part of the molecule. There was no clinical or biochemical evidence that the antibodies impaired the effects of exogenous hormone or blocked endogenous human corticotrophin.— J. Landon *et al.*, *Lancet*, 1967, *1*, 652. For a similar report, see N. Fleischer *et al.*, *J. clin. Invest.*, 1967, *46*, 196.

Corticotrophin is a straight-chain polypeptide consisting of 39 amino acids, only the first 24 of which are biologically active and common to man and cattle, pigs, and sheep. The last 15 amino acids differ between species. The differences could account for the development of antibodies and allergic reactions when animal corticotrophin is injected in man. Amino acids 4 to 11 are identical with the sequence in melanocyte-stimulating hormone and produce the pigmentation of the skin seen in Addison's disease.— *Br. med. J.*, 1969, *2*, 809.

A report of the adverse effects observed in a group of 162 children given corticotrophin for infantile spasms; 60 children suffered pronounced adverse effects and 8 died. The benefits of very high doses of corticotrophin should be reconsidered.— R. Riikonen and M. Donner, *Archs Dis. Childh.*, 1980, *55*, 664.

Adrenal suppression. In 12 patients with rheumatoid arthritis given long-term corticotrophin treatment, the plasma-corticosteroid response in the insulin hypoglycaemia test (IHT) was not significantly different from that in 12 controls, while the response of 12 patients on long-term corticosteroid treatment was significantly depressed. The plasma-corticotrophin response to the IHT was significantly depressed in both the corticosteroid and corticotrophin patients. When, however, the plasma-corticotrophin response was assessed by the area under the concentration/time curve (total secretion) the response in the corticotrophin patients was not significantly different from that in controls. It is possible that treatment with corticotrophin reduces the rate but not the total of corticotrophin secretion. If corticosteroids were given in a single daily dose the suppression of hypothalamo-pituitary-adrenal function might be no greater than that caused by corticotrophin.— J. R. Daly *et al.*, *Br. med. J.*, 1974, *2*, 521. See also J. R. Daly and D. Glass, *Lancet*, 1971, *1*, 476.

Further references: M. E. Carter and V. H. T. James, *Ann. rheum. Dis.*, 1971, *30*, 91.

Allergy. Allergic reactions occurred in 13 patients receiving prednisolone therapy and injections of corticotrophin at 10-day intervals. The reactions usually occurred about half an hour after the sixth injection.— O. Forssman *et al.*, *Acta allerg.*, 1963, *18*, 462.

Effects on bones and joints. Aseptic necrosis of the femur occurred in a 23-year-old man 9 months after receiving 1070 units of corticotrophin over 16 days for retrobulbar neuritis due to multiple sclerosis.— A. E. Good, *J. Am. med. Ass.*, 1974, *228*, 497.

Effects on the electrolyte balance. Severe hyponatraemia occurred in 3 patients following intravenous infusion of corticotrophin in dextrose injection 5% to diagnose adrenocortical insufficiency, despite the administration of about 1 mg of dexamethasone in divided doses. It was recommended that sodium chloride injection should be used as the infusing solution.— L. R. Sheller and O. P. Schumacher, *Ann. intern. Med.*, 1979, *90*, 798. A previous study had shown that natural corticotrophin preparations (Acthar) were contaminated with sufficient amounts of vasopressin to produce water retention even in normal subjects. However the problem of water intoxication could be entirely avoided by using a synthetic corticotrophin preparation (such as Cortrosyn) which had not been found to contain vasopressin and did not produce water retention or hyponatraemia even when infused in salt-free solutions.— G. Baumann (letter), *Ann. intern. Med.*, 1979, *91*, 499. Further speculation on the reason for the hyponatraemia.— M. Geheb *et al.* (letter), *ibid.*, 792. Reply and emphasis that infusion of 5% dextrose seems to cause more problems than infusion of saline.— L. R. Sheeler and O. P. Schumacher (letter), *ibid.*

Effects on the eyes. A 50-year-old women with chronic rheumatoid arthritis who had been treated with corticotrophin, about 20 units intramuscularly daily for 2.5 years, developed posterior subcapsular cataracts and macular lesions in both eyes.— J. Williamson and T. G. Dalakos, *Br. J. Ophthal.*, 1967, *51*, 839.

Effects on the gastro-intestinal tract. A study in patients with multiple sclerosis given corticotrophin provided evidence of increased gastrin secretion in corticosteroid-treated subjects.— S. Raptis *et al.*, *Am. J. dig. Dis.*, 1976, *21*, 376.

Effects on growth. A study in 6 boys, aged 10 to 16 years, who had growth retardation with skeletal and sexual immaturity after being treated for severe asthma for at least 2 years with daily doses of up to 10 mg of prednisone, showed that neither an increase in growth velocity nor any significant change in epiphyseal maturation followed a change to treatment with corticotrophin in doses adequate to suppress symptoms.— A. P. Norman and S. Sanders, *Lancet*, 1969, *1*, 287. Criticisms.— M. Friedman and L. B. Strang (letter), *ibid.*, 527. A reply.— A. P. Norman and S. Sanders (letter), *ibid.*, 626. See also M. Friedman and L. Stimmler, *ibid.*, 1966, *2*, 944.

Further references: P. A. Lee *et al.*, *J. clin. Endocr. Metab.*, 1973, *37*, 389.

Effects on mental state. A report of psychological dependence on corticotrophin.— U. Ehrig and J. G. Rankin (letter), *Ann. intern. Med.*, 1972, *77*, 482.

Effects on the skin. Exudative erythema multiforme developed after one administration of corticotrophin.— E. N. Soloshenko and A. I. Brailovskiĭ, *Klin. Med., Mosk.*, 1975, *53*, 136.

Treatment of Adverse Effects. Adverse effects should be treated symptomatically and the dosage reduced or the drug withdrawn.

Very high doses of ascorbic acid relieved depression associated with prolonged corticotrophin treatment in a 5-year-old girl with chronic active hepatitis.— P. Cocchi *et al.*, *Pediatrics*, 1980, *65*, 862.

Withdrawal. Corticotrophin administration may depress the natural secretion of the hormone sufficiently to cause pituitary hypoplasia. Abrupt withdrawal of corticotrophin may therefore produce symptoms of hypopituitarism and therapy should be stopped gradually. It is easier, however, to withdraw corticotrophin after prolonged administration than to withdraw orally administered corticosteroids. See also Withdrawal under Corticosteroids, p.449.

Precautions. As for Corticosteroids, p.449.

Cushing's syndrome. Occurrence of acute unilateral adrenal haemorrhage in a patient with Cushing's syndrome was associated with repeated doses of corticotrophin and indicated that, as the latter has little diagnostic value in such patients, repeated doses should not be given.— J. F. Redman and F. H. Faas, *Am. J. Med.*, 1976, *61*, 533.

Phaeochromocytoma. Studies in *dogs* demonstrated that corticotrophin causes a prolonged release of catecholamines. This indicates a hazard to the use of corticotrophin in patients with phaeochromocytoma.— J. A. J. H. Critchley *et al.* (letter), *Lancet*, 1974, *2*, 782.

Pregnancy and the neonate. It is probably best not to use corticotrophin during pregnancy since there is some evidence that its use might lead to partial pseudohermaphroditism in the female infant.— I. M. Noble, *Practitioner*, 1974, *212*, 657.

Induction of cleft palate in *hamster* foetuses following administration of high doses of corticotrophin suggested that it was a mild teratogen.— R. M. Shah, *Toxic. appl. Pharmac.*, 1977, *42*, 229. See also under Corticosteroids, p.450.

Absorption and Fate. Corticotrophin is ineffective when given by mouth. It produces rapid effects when administered intravenously but its biological half-life is only about 15 minutes and the effects last only about 2 to 4 hours depending upon the route of injection. Corticotrophin

Gelatin Injection maintains effective concentrations for 12 to 24 hours and Corticotrophin Zinc Hydroxide Injection for up to 48 hours following subcutaneous or intramuscular injection.

A review of studies on the distribution and fate of corticotrophin.— H. P. J. Bennett and C. McMartin, *Pharmac. Rev.*, 1978, *30*, 247.

Uses. Corticotrophin is a naturally occurring hormone of the anterior lobe of the pituitary gland which induces hyperplasia and increase in weight of the adrenal gland. The secretion of adrenocortical hormones, especially hydrocortisone, some mineralocorticoids, such as corticosterone, and, to a lesser extent, of androgens is increased. It has little effect on aldosterone secretion which proceeds independently.

Secretion of corticotrophin by the functioning pituitary gland is controlled by the hypothalamus and is stimulated by a reduction in the concentration of circulating cortisol (hydrocortisone), by an increase in circulating adrenaline, and by conditions of stress. High blood concentrations of hydrocortisone (cortisol) prevent release of corticotrophin and this results in hypofunction of the adrenal gland.

As a therapeutic agent, corticotrophin is used to stimulate the activity of the adrenal cortex and produce a high level of circulating cortisol (hydrocortisone). It is therefore used for conditions for which prednisolone and other corticosteroids are employed systemically (see p.451), with the exception of the adrenal deficiency states and adrenocortical overactivity.

Because of the greater ease with which corticotrophin can be withdrawn it may be preferred to corticosteroids although corticosteroids by mouth are usually preferred because of the ease of administration.

With a view to preventing withdrawal symptoms when corticosteroids are stopped, corticotrophin has been used during the last week of corticosteroid therapy to stimulate an adrenal cortex atrophied by suppression of the anterior pituitary gland. This effect is limited by the inability of the anterior pituitary to respond sufficiently to stimulate the adrenal cortex. In fact, corticotrophin does not help to re-establish adrenal responsiveness and delays recovery by diminishing the ability of the pituitary to respond to low concentrations of endogenous cortisol (hydrocortisone).

Corticotrophin is used as a diagnostic agent to test the secretory activity of the adrenal cortex during and after corticosteroid therapy and in suspected cases of Addison's disease and hypopituitarism. The extent to which the adrenal cortex can respond to corticotrophin may be assessed by measuring the increase in the amount of total 17-hydroxycorticosteroid (usually more correctly termed 17-oxogenic steroid or total ketogenic steroid) or 17-ketosteroid (17-oxosteroid) excreted in the urine after administration of the hormone. Other tests have measured the change in circulating eosinophils and in the excretion of uric acid following the administration of corticotrophin.

Corticotrophin injection is available in two forms: one for intravenous administration and the other for subcutaneous, or intramuscular use. The intravenous injection is usually administered by slow infusion; a dose of 45 to 90 units, according to the age of the patient, over 8 to 24 hours causes maximum adrenal stimulation. The subcutaneous and intramuscular injections may be given in usual doses of 10 to 20 units 4 times daily.

Long-acting preparations of corticotrophin are also used. These include preparations in which the viscosity is increased by the addition of gelatin or in which corticotrophin is combined with zinc hydroxide or sodium carboxymethylcellulose. Dosage depends upon the condition of the patient. Initially, doses of 40 to 80 units daily are usual, though doses of 10 to 120 units have been used. As soon as possible the dosage should be reduced gradually to the minimum necessary to control symptoms. Doses of 20 units twice or thrice weekly may be adequate. These long-acting preparations are administered subcutaneously or intramuscularly and should not be given intravenously; if a rapid therapeutic effect is required, corticotrophin injection should be used although corticosteroids (see p.451) are generally preferred.

Corticotrophin has no effect when applied locally.

Studies and comments on the physiology and pharmacology of corticotrophin: K. H. Falchuk, *New Engl. J. Med.*, 1977, *296*, 1129; J. F. Desforges *et al.*, *ibid.*, 1165 (role in zinc metabolism); J. Volavka *et al.* (letter), *New Engl. J. Med.*, 1979, *300*, 1056 (inhibitory control by endorphins).

Adrenal insufficiency. A 57-year-old man with addisonian crisis of pituitary origin was satisfactorily controlled with hydrocortisone 30 mg daily in divided doses and thyroxine 200 µg each morning, but on discharge from hospital refused to take his tablets. Satisfactory control was therefore obtained by giving corticotrophin 60 units by deep intramuscular injection together with thyroxine 800 µg by mouth twice weekly.— A. W. Nathan *et al.* (letter), *Lancet*, 1979, *1*, 319.

Adrenal-function test. A decrease in circulating eosinophils and a rise in excretion of uric acid consistently followed the administration of 25 mg of corticotrophin intramuscularly to normal subjects and patients with diseases not involving the adrenal cortex. A decrease of 50% or more in the urinary uric acid/creatinine ratio indicated adequate adrenocortical reserve. The test was a measure of the adrenal reserve of hormones regulating the carbohydrate, fat, and protein metabolism and was of value in the diagnosis of adrenal deficiency.— G. W. Thorn *et al.*, *J. Am. med. Ass.*, 1948, *137*, 1005. See also under Tetracosactrin, p.489.

For discussion on hyponatraemia in patients given corticotrophin in dextrose 5% for adrenal-function tests, see under Adverse Effects (Effects on the Electrolyte Balance).

Asthma. Studies on the use of corticotrophin rather than corticosteroids for the management of asthma: I. W. Glick and M. Friedman, *Thorax*, 1969, *24*, 415; D. N. S. Malone *et al.*, *Br. med. J.*, 1972, *3*, 202; A. E. Tribe *et al.*, *Aust. N.Z. J. Med.*, 1973, *3*, 6; J. C. Drever *et al.*, *Br. J. Dis. Chest*, 1975, *69*, 188.

Convulsions. For a comment on the use of corticotrophin in infantile spasms (West's syndrome) see Corticosteroids, p.453.

Infections. Reports of beneficial effects of corticotrophin in infections: R. Barr, *Can. med. Ass. J.*, 1966, *95*, 912 (trichinosis); W. Chin *et al.*, *J. Am. med. Ass.*, 1973, *225*, 740 (cytomegalovirus); J. Richardson (letter), *Br. med. J.*, 1973, *1*, 799; *ibid.*, *2*, 64 (prevention of postherpetic neuralgia).

Lipid disorders. Corticotrophin unexpectedly reduced cholesterol and triglyceride values to normal in an infant with hyperlipoproteinaemia type V.— G. Zamboni and P. Marradi (letter), *Lancet*, 1976, *2*, 264.

Muscular disorders. *Myasthenia gravis.* The short-term massive administration of corticotrophin in 1 or more courses produced gratifying results when tried in 11 severely ill patients with myasthenia gravis (7 of whom had had thymectomies). All the patients were given at least 1 course of corticotrophin, 100 units daily by intramuscular injection for 10 days.— K. E. Osserman and G. Genkins, *J. Am. med. Ass.*, 1966, *198*, 699.

After a total of 38 courses of corticotrophin therapy had been given to 8 patients before and after thymectomy for myasthenia gravis it was concluded that administration of corticotrophin before surgery did not appear to prevent the effectiveness of thymectomy. In 6 patients thymectomy during a remission induced by corticotrophin was also successful. Both therapeutic measures in any order or together were therefore useful for the treatment of myasthenia gravis.— M. S. Shapiro *et al.*, *Archs Neurol., Chicago*, 1971, *24*, 65, per *Abstr. Wld Med.*, 1971, *45*, 773.

Nine patients with myasthenia gravis and ocular symptoms who had not responded adequately to anticholinesterase therapy received corticotrophin 20 to 100 units intramuscularly daily or tetracosactrin 400 to 600 µg daily or on alternate days for 9 days to 8 weeks. Clinical deterioration occurred at first and 4 patients needed assisted respiration. Improvement occurred in all patients in 1 to 2 weeks, usually reaching a maximum after a further week. The clinical condition then usually remained static for several weeks before gradually reverting to its previous level, the total duration of improvement lasting up to 2 years. It was essential to anticipate deterioration during the first 10 days.— F. B. Gibberd *et al.*, *J. Neurol. Neurosurg. Psychiat.*, 1971, *34*, 11, per *Abstr. Wld Med.*, 1971, *45*, 447.

Further references: D. Grob and T. Namba, *J. Am. med. Ass.*, 1966, *198*, 703; T. Namba, *Archs Neurol., Chicago*, 1972, *26*, 144; C. A. Cape and R. A. Utterback, *Neurology, Minneap.*, 1972, *22*, 1160; C. A. Cape, *Archs Ophthal., N.Y.*, 1973, *90*, 292.

See also Corticosteroids, p.455.

Nasal polyp. Corticotrophin 80 units intramuscularly daily for 5 days subsequently reduced by 10 units daily had been used to treat a few patients with nasal polyps. Polyps remaining at the end of the course were very much smaller and were removed. The patients had remained free of symptoms for up to 15 months.— L. R. S. Taylor, *J. Lar. Otol.*, 1973, *87*, 103, per *Drugs*, 1973, *6*, 289.

Neurological disorders. *Bell's palsy.* For the role of corticotrophin in the treatment of idiopathic facial paralysis, see Corticosteroids, p.455.

Delirium tremens. A view that corticotrophin was of value in doses of 25 units every 6 hours, in the treatment of delirium tremens. No more than a total of 150 units should be given.— M. E. Chafetz, *J. Am. med. Ass.*, 1967, *200*, 269.

Guillain-Barré syndrome. A study of corticotrophin has suggested that corticotrophin has little effect on the acute phase of idiopathic polyneuropathy, but seems to promote healing of damaged nerves.— M. P. McQuillen and H. M. Swick (letter), *Lancet*, 1978, *2*, 1209. See also *idem*, *Neurology, Minneap.*, 1976, *26*, 205.

For a discouraging report on the effect of corticosteroids in the Guillain-Barré syndrome, see Corticosteroids, p.455.

Multiple sclerosis. In a multicentre controlled study, 350 patients with multiple sclerosis were treated either with a regimen which included daily injections of corticotrophin or were allocated to a control group given only monthly injections of thiamine 100 mg. In addition to a monthly injection of thiamine, the treated group had a low-salt diet, potassium chloride supplements daily, and a daily intramuscular injection of Corticotrophin Gelatin Injection. The dose of corticotrophin was adjusted to produce just enough 'mooning' of the face to be appreciated by the physician and the dose was not increased during a relapse; it varied between 15 and 25 units daily. Corticotrophin did not appear to prevent deterioration or to reduce the number or severity of relapses. It did not adversely affect the disease process. Side-effects in the treated group included increased blood pressure, depression or psychotic symptoms, gain in weight, glycosuria, hypomania, and osteoporosis. One patient died, probably because corticotrophin was not given when he was admitted to hospital with a severe infection.— J. H. D. Millar *et al.*, *Lancet*, 1967, *2*, 429.

In a continuation of the above study, the withdrawal of corticotrophin over periods of 2 to 9 months from patients with multiple sclerosis did not significantly increase the disability, or frequency or severity of relapses over 1 year.— *idem*, 1970, *1*, 700.

Further references: L. Alexander and L. J. Cass, *Ann. intern. Med.*, 1963, *58*, 454.

See also under Corticosteroids, p.456.

Optic neuritis. In a double-blind trial 50 patients with acute retrobulbar neuritis were treated with either Corticotrophin Gelatin Injection, 40 units daily for 30 days, or with an inert gel of similar composition. Recovery was quicker and more complete in patients who received corticotrophin than in those who received the inert gel.— M. D. Rawson *et al.*, *Lancet*, 1966, *2*, 1044. After 12 months, 24 of the 25 patients treated with corticotrophin and 20 of the 25 patients not treated had regained good visual acuity; the difference in these results was not, however, statistically significant.— M. D. Rawson and L. A. Liversedge (letter), *ibid.*, 1969, *2*, 222. See also under Corticosteroids, p.456.

Sydenham's chorea. For a report on the use of corticotrophin in Sydenham's chorea, see Corticosteroids, p.456.

Pressure-sores. Five out of 42 elderly patients given an intramuscular injection of 80 units of corticotrophin 4 hours before surgery developed pressure-sores compared with 12 of 43 given a placebo. The difference was not significant. However, when only those patients undergoing total-hip replacement were considered, corticotrophin was more effective than the placebo; none of 16 treated patients developed sores compared with 5 of 16 control patients.— A. A. Barton and M. Barton, *Lancet*, 1976, *2*, 443.

Renal disorders. For a review of corticosteroid therapy in the management of renal disorders, see Corticosteroids, p.457.

Diagnostic use. Response to corticotrophin as a sign of adrenal suppression could be used to predict relapse in patients being treated with corticosteroids for the nephrotic syndrome. Of 11 children with subnormal responses to corticotrophin, 10 relapsed within a year; 12 had normal responses and in 6 of these remission from nephrotic syndrome lasted more than 1 year. Adrenal suppression should be avoided in the treatment of the nephrotic syndrome.— S. Leisti *et al.*, *Lancet*, 1977, *2*, 795.

Raised intracranial pressure. A view that high-dose corticotrophin may be superior to dexamethasone in the treatment of cerebral oedema.— I. Lagenstein *et al.* (letter), *Lancet*, 1979, *1*, 1246. Comments.— K. R. Lyen *et al.* (letter), *ibid.*, *2*, 37; T. Deonna and C. Voumard (letter), *ibid.*, 207.

Skin disorders. *Eczema.* In a study lasting for up to 7 years a long-acting corticotrophin preparation (Crookes acth/cmc) had been successfully used, in maintenance doses of from 40 to 80 µg every third day, self-administered by deep subcutaneous injection by 10 patients with eczema. To lessen the risk associated with anaphylactoid reactions the patients are warned to avoid repeated injections if they develop unusual symptoms and to remain in company with another person for an hour after the injection.— D. D. Munro, *Br. J. Derm.*, 1976, *94*, *Suppl.* 12, 135.

Lichen sclerosus et atrophicus. Marked improvement occurred in a patient with generalised bullous and haemorrhagic lichen sclerosus et atrophicus of some years' duration, following treatment with corticotrophin 1 mg on alternate days for 8 doses.— A. di Silverio and F. Serri, *Br. J. Derm.*, 1975, *93*, 215.

Vitiligo. Long-acting corticotrophin 25 to 40 units given twice daily by intramuscular injection for up to 4 courses each of 10 to 12 injections, with intervals of 2 to 4 weeks, caused 80% repigmentation in 16 of 27 patients with vitiligo of from 2 to 16 years duration; a further 6 patients had 50% repigmentation and 4 had 20% or less. There was no response in 1 patient.— B. B. Gokhale and T. B. Gokhale, *Br. J. Derm.*, 1976, *95*, 329.

For further reports of the use of corticotrophin, see under Corticosteroids, p.452.

Preparations

Corticotrophin Injection *(B.P.).* ACTH Inj.; Corticotropini Solutio Iniectabilis *(Eur. P.).* It consists of a sterile solution in Water for Injections, prepared by dissolving, immediately before use, the sterile contents of a sealed container of Corticotrophin for Injection in the requisite amount of Water for Injections. pH 3 to 5. The sealed container may also contain added inert substances. The label on the container must indicate whether the material is intended for intravenous use or for subcutaneous or intramuscular use. Store at a temperature not exceeding 25° in airtight containers sealed to exclude micro-organisms and as far as possible moisture. Protect from light. Under these conditions the contents may be expected to retain their potency for not less than 2 years.

Corticotropin for Injection *(U.S.P.).* A sterile dry mixture which contains corticotrophin and may contain a suitable antimicrobial agent, diluents, and buffers. pH of the reconstituted solution 2.5 to 6.

Corticotropin Injection *(U.S.P.).* A sterile solution in a suitable diluent. It may contain a suitable antimicrobial. pH 3 to 7. Store at a temperature not exceeding 8°. Similar injections are included in several pharmacopoeias.

Proprietary Names

Acethropan *(Hoechst, Ger.)*; Acthar *(Armour, Austral.; Harris, Canad.; Armour, Ital.; Armour, S.Afr.; Armour, USA)*; Acthelea (see also Long-Acting Preparations)*(Elea, Arg.)*; Acortan simplex *(Ferring, Ger.)*; Acton *(Ferring, Swed.)*.

Long-acting Corticotrophin Preparations

CAUTION.*Long-acting corticotrophin preparations should not be administered intravenously. If a rapid therapeutic effect is required, Corticotrophin Injection should be used.*

Corticotrophin Carboxymethylcellulose Injection *(B.P.C. 1973).* A sterile solution of corticotrophin as the carmellose complex in Water for Injections; it is rendered iso-osmotic with serum by the addition of dextrose. Sterilised by filtration. pH 4.5 to 6.5. A clear colourless slightly viscous liquid which does not solidify at 0° to 10°. Store at 2° to 10°. Protect from light. Under these conditions it may be expected to retain its potency for at least 3 years. For subcutaneous use. *Dose.* Determined by the physician according to the patient's needs.

Corticotrophin Gelatin Injection *(B.P.).* ACTH Gel. Inj. A sterile solution of corticotrophin in Water for Injections containing suitably hydrolysed gelatin. Sterilised by filtration. pH 4.5 to 7. It is a pale amber-coloured viscous liquid which may solidify below 25°. Store at 2° to 8°. Protect from light. Under these conditions it may be expected to retain its potency for not less than 18 months. If necessary, the contents should be warmed before use. For subcutaneous or intramuscular use only.

Corticotrophin Zinc Injection *(B.P.).* Corticotrophin Zinc Hydroxide Injection; ACTH Zinc Inj.; Corticotropini Zinci Hydroxidi Suspensio Iniectabilis *(Eur. P.).* A sterile aqueous suspension of corticotrophin with zinc hydroxide made iso-osmotic with blood by the addition of a suitable substance and sodium phosphate is added as a stabiliser. pH 7.5 to 8.5. It is a fine white or almost white suspension. Store at 2° to 8° and avoid freezing. Under these conditions it may be expected to retain its potency for not less than 2 years. The container should be gently shaken before a dose is withdrawn. It is for subcutaneous or intramuscular use only.

Repository Corticotropin Injection *(U.S.P.).* A sterile solution of corticotrophin in partially hydrolysed gelatin. It may contain a suitable antimicrobial agent. It is a colourless or light straw-coloured liquid which may be quite viscid at room temperature. pH 3 to 7.

Sterile Corticotropin Zinc Hydroxide Suspension *(U.S.P.).* A sterile suspension of corticotrophin adsorbed on zinc hydroxide; it contains sodium phosphate. pH 7.5 to 8.5. It is a flocculent white suspension free from large particles after moderate shaking. Store at 15° to 30°.

Proprietary Long-acting Preparations

Acthar Gel *(Armour, UK).* Corticotrophin Gelatin Injection containing 20 units per ml in vials of 5 ml, 40 units per ml in vials of 2 and 5 ml, and 80 units per ml in vials of 5 ml. (Also available as Acthar Gel in *Austral., Canad., Ital., S.Afr., USA*).

ACTH/CMC *(Ferring, UK).* Corticotrophin Carboxymethylcellulose Injection (*B.P.C. 1973*), manufactured from porcine pituitaries, containing 60 units per ml, available in vials of 5 ml. Store at 2° to 10°.

Other Proprietary Names

Arg.— Acthelea (see also above), Actonar; *Austral.*— Cortrophin ZN; *Canad.*— Durackin; *Ger.*— Acortan prolongatum, Depot-Acethropan; *Swed.*— Acton prolongatum, Reacthin; *Switz.*— Cortrophine-Z; *USA*— Cortigel.

Long-acting preparations of corticotrophin were also formerly marketed in Great Britain under the proprietary names Cortico-Gel (*Crookes*), Cortrophin ZN (*Organon*), and Crookes acth/cmc (*Crookes*).

1462-g

Codactide.

α^{1-18} ACTH; Ciba 41795 Ba. [1-D-Serine,17,18-lysine]corticotrophin-(1–18)-octadecapeptide amide; D-Ser-Tyr-Ser-Met-Glu-His-Phe-Arg-Trp-Gly-Lys-Pro-Val-Gly-Lys-Lys-Lys-Lys—NH_2.
$C_{101}H_{158}N_{30}O_{23}S$=2192.6.

CAS — 22572-04-9.

Codactide is a synthetic corticotrophin analogue consisting of the first 18 amino acids of human corticotrophin substituted by D-serine at residue 1 and lysine at residues 17 and 18.

References: J. Keenan *et al.*, *Br. med. J.*, 1971, *3*, 742; W. J. Irvine *et al.*, *Lancet*, 1973, *1*, 1417; P. J. Brombacher *et al.* (letter), *ibid.*, 456; F. Duran *et al.*, *Hormone metab. Res.*, 1975, *7*, 499; G. Geyer and H. Templ, *Dt. med. Wschr.*, 1976, *101*, 1806; J. H. Pratt *et al.*, *Metabolism*, 1976, *25*, 221.

Manufacturers
Ciba, UK.

1463-q

Octacosactrin.

Octacosactid; Tosactide; α^{1-28}-Corticotrophin (human). [25-Aspartic acid, 26-alanine, 27-glycine]corticotrophin-(1–28)-octacosapeptide; Ser-Tyr-Ser-Met-Glu-His-Phe-Arg-Trp-Gly-Lys-Pro-Val-Gly-Lys-Lys-Arg-Arg-Pro-Val-Lys-Val-Tyr-Pro-Asp-Ala-Gly-Glu.
$C_{150}H_{230}N_{44}O_{38}S$=3289.8.

CAS — 47931-80-6.

Octacosactrin is a synthetic polypeptide representing the first 28 amino-acid residues of human corticotrophin.

Given intravenously as the tetra-acetate, 1 mg of octacosactrin is equivalent in activity to about 100 units of corticotrophin. The usual dose is 100 to 250 µg.

Proprietary Names
Actid 1–28 *(Ferring, Ger.)*; Homactid *(Ferring, Swed.)*.

1464-p

Tetracosactrin.

Ciba 30920; Cosyntropin; Tetracosactide; α^{1-24} Corticotrophin; β^{1-24} Corticotrophin. Corticotrophin-(1–24)-tetracosapeptide; Ser-Tyr-Ser-Met-Glu-His-Phe-Arg-Trp-Gly-Lys-Pro-Val-Gly-Lys-Lys-Arg-Arg-Pro-Val-Lys-Val-Tyr-Pro.
$C_{136}H_{210}N_{40}O_{31}S$=2933.5.

CAS — 16960-16-0.

A synthetic polypeptide identical with the first 24 of the 39 amino acids of corticotrophin.

1465-s

Tetracosactrin Acetate *(B.P.).*

Tetracosactrin Hexa-acetate; Tetracosactide Acetate.

CAS — 60189-34-6.

Pharmacopoeias. In *Br.*

A white to yellow amorphous powder containing not less than 76% of peptide, 8 to 13% of acetic acid, and 5 to 16% of water. **Soluble** 1 in 70 of water. A solution in 1% acetic acid is laevorotatory. **Store** in airtight containers.

Tetracosactrin has been reported to be inactivated by enzymes and it has been recommended that it should not be added to infusions of blood or plasma.

Comment on the stability of tetracosactrin *in vitro* in blood.— H. P. J. Bennett and C. McMartin, *Pharmac. Rev.*, 1978, *30*, 247.

Adverse Effects. As for Corticotrophin, p.486. Allergic reactions to tetracosactrin have been reported to be less common than with corticotrophin, but nevertheless serious, and even fatal, reactions have occurred. Tetracosactrin may be used in patients hypersensitive to porcine corticotrophin.

After the use of tetracosactrin (Synacthen Depot), the incidence of pain and lumps at the site of injection was 10% of all injections and occurred at some time in 20% of patients on long-term treatment.— J. A. Weaver (letter), *Br. med. J.*, 1969, *1*, 639. Comment.— J. E. Murphy and J. F. Donald (letter), *ibid.*, *2*, 119.

Adrenal hypertrophy. Most patients with suppression of the hypothalamic-pituitary-adrenal axis due to corticosteroid therapy by mouth recovered adrenal responsiveness within a few weeks of introducing tetracosactrin therapy but normal recovery of the axis could take many months, and defective responses to stress might remain indefinitely in a minority. Overdosage or incautious administration of tetracosactrin might rapidly result in a cushingoid syndrome due to a summation effect of repeated doses at close intervals causing adrenal hypertrophy, and to a depressing effect on corticosteroid-binding globulin resulting in increased concentrations of unbound, and therefore biologically active, cortisol (hydrocortisone). Tetracosactrin therapy should not therefore be given without frequent checks on plasma-cortisol concentrations to adjust the dosage.— M. M. Burns and C. J. Eastman, *Drugs*, 1974, *8*, 241.

Allergy. Experience had shown that the hope that tetracosactrin would cause fewer reactions than natural corticotrophin might not be realised. There had been 2 deaths in patients whose treatment had continued after a mild reaction had occurred with an earlier dose, and serious, even fatal, reactions had occurred at various times during courses of therapy with no mild premonitory symptoms. Although reactions had occurred after the patient had left the doctor's surgery none had occurred more than an hour after injection. The manufacturers had agreed to recommend that patients should remain at the hospital or surgery for a recovery period following an injection, and that self-injection should not normally be recommended.— Committee on Safety of Medicines, *Current Problems Series No. 1*, Sept., 1975.

Individual reports of allergic reactions following injection of tetracosactrin: N. E. Jensen and I. Sneddon (letter), *Br. med. J.*, 1969, *2*, 383; G. Fagg, *Br. J. clin. Pract.*, 1970, *24*, 155; G. Patriarca (letter), *Lancet*, 1971, *1*, 138; P. J. Brombacher *et al.* (letter), *ibid.*, 1975, *1*, 456; P. D. Mohr (letter), *Br. med. J.*, 1975, *4*, 162; J. Porter and H. Jick, *Lancet*, 1977, *1*, 587.

Effects on the blood. In a 27-year-old man with a white-cell count of 9200 to 11 300 per mm^3 (63 to 83% polymorphs), the white-cell count rose after treatment with tetracosactrin—after a total of 4 mg in 5 days it rose to 13 100 per mm^3 (90% polymorphs), and after a further 2 mg in the next 6 days to 23 400 per mm^3 (63% polymorphs). The presence of infection was excluded. The white-cell count fell to its initial value when treatment ceased and stabilised at 16 600 to 17 300 per mm^3 when treatment was recommenced.— A. R. Robinson (letter), *Br. med. J.*, 1972, *4*, 178.

Effects on the eyes. A 45-year-old patient with rheumatoid arthritis developed bilateral macular degeneration following treatment on alternate days with a depot injection containing 1 mg of tetracosactrin. Reduction of the dosage to 250 µg every 72 hours led to an improvement in visual acuity.— J. Williamson and G. Nuki, *Br. J. Ophthal.*, 1970, *54*, 405.

Withdrawal. As for Corticotrophin, p.486.

Precautions. As for Corticosteroids, p.449.

Since reactions may not occur for up to 1 hour after injection sufficient time should be allowed for recovery after administration at the hospital or surgery. Self-administration is not recommended.

Absorption and Fate. Tetracosactrin is inactivated when administered by mouth. Intravenous administration results in a prompt rise in plasma cortisol (hydrocortisone) which can be maintained by a slow infusion. After intramuscular injection, blood-cortisol (hydrocortisone) concentrations reach a peak within an hour and decline to the basal concentration after about 4 hours.

The long-acting depot preparations of tetracosactrin are given by intramuscular injection and produce peak blood-cortisol concentrations in about 8 hours, with raised values for more than 24 hours.

Studies in 4 adults showed that the speed of response in the first 20 to 30 minutes after an intramuscular injection of a long-acting preparation of tetracosactrin was virtually the same as after an intravenous injection of tetracosactrin. Except in cases of extreme collapse, tetracosactrin could be injected intramuscularly.— J. K. Grant (letter), *Lancet*, 1969, *1*, 371. Studies in 6 healthy adults showed that 15 minutes after an intravenous injection of 125 ng of tetracosactrin, plasma-hydrocortisone concentrations were increased by 5 to 189 ng per ml. In 2 patients, 125 ng was as effective as 250 µg.— G. Copinschi *et al.* (letter), *ibid.*, 580.

Estimation of the plasma concentrations of fluorogenic corticosteroids in 6 healthy subjects showed that tetracosactrin powder administered as a nasal insufflation was absorbed efficiently even at low doses.— J. Keenan and M. A. Chamberlain, *Br. med. J.*, 1969, *4*, 407.

Uses. Tetracosactrin is a synthetic polypeptide with general properties and uses similar to those of corticotrophin (see p.487).

Given intravenously as the hexa-acetate, 1 mg of tetracosactrin is equivalent in activity to about 100 units of corticotrophin. It is often used in patients who are allergic or unresponsive to porcine corticotrophin. Tetracosactrin may be given by intravenous, intramuscular, or subcutaneous injection. For diagnostic purposes it is usually given in a single dose of 250 µg intramuscularly. For therapeutic purposes it is usually given by intravenous infusion in a dose of 250 µg in 500 ml of dextrose injection or electrolyte solutions over 6 hours. It may also be given intramuscularly in doses of 250 µg every 3 to 4 hours. Children under 2 years of age may be given 125 µg; children over 2 years of age may be given the adult dose.

Long-acting depot injections of tetracosactrin are intended for intramuscular injection, preferably into the buttock, to provide effects lasting for 1 to 2 days; they are not intended for diagnostic use. By this route tetracosactrin 500 µg on alternate days is approximately equivalent in activity to 1 injection daily of 40 units of corticotrophin gelatin. The usual dose is 0.5 to 1 mg about twice weekly according to the patient's response. In acute conditions, the initial dose may be 1 mg daily for 3 days, subsequently adjusted according to the patient's response. The intial dose for infants is 250 µg daily, for small children, 250 to 500 µg daily, and for children of school age, 0.25 to 1 mg daily; these doses may subsequently be given every 2 to 8 days for maintenance.

Administration. From experiments in normal subjects and in patients previously treated with corticosteroids by mouth or with corticotrophin it was shown that, in terms of mean maximal plasma-hydrocortisone concentrations attained, 1 mg of long-acting tetracosactrin was approximately equivalent to 80 units of Corticotrophin Gelatin Injection. To maintain a continuously elevated hydrocortisone concentration the dose of depot tetracosactrin must be given daily and of corticotrophin twice daily.— G. M. Besser *et al.*, *Br. med. J.*, 1967, *4*, 391. See also T. S. Danowski *et al.*, *J. clin. Endocr. Metab.*, 1968, *28*, 1120; A. H. El-Shaboury, *Br. med. J.*, 1968, *3*, 653; B. L. J. Treadwell and P. M. Dennis, *ibid.*, 1969, *4*, 720.

Adrenal-function test. Providing the patient had not received a glucocorticoid within the previous 12 hours, adrenocortical response was considered to be normal if 2 of the following criteria were fulfilled: the initial plasma-corticosteroid concentration was not less than 60 ng per ml (50 ng per ml in the afternoon and evening); 30 minutes after injection of tetracosactrin 250 µg intramuscularly the increment was not less than 70 ng per ml; 30 minutes after injection the plasma concentration was not less than 180 ng per ml.— W. R. Greig *et al.*, *Postgrad. med. J.*, 1969, *45*, 307. See also J. B. Wood *et al.*, *Lancet*, 1965, *1*, 243; W. R. Greig *et al.*, *J. Endocr.*, 1966, *34*, 411.

Lower and more progressive rises in plasma- and urine-cortisol (hydrocortisone) concentrations occurred in 13 patients with secondary hypoadrenalism than in 10 healthy subjects after an intramuscular injection of a depot preparation of tetracosactrin 1 mg (Synacthen Depot). Plasma measurements carried out at 4 to 6 and 12 to 16 hours could be used to assess adrenal function.— A. Galvão-Teles *et al.*, *Lancet*, 1971, *1*, 557.

Of 48 patients taking glucocorticoids and about to undergo major surgery 17 showed a normal response in plasma concentration of corticosteroids to a single intravenous injection of 250 µg of tetracosactrin, and 13 of these showed a normal hypothalamo-pituitary-adrenal response to surgery, the response in the other 4 being only marginally subnormal. A single injection of tetracosactrin was of value in predicting the hypothalamo-pituitary-adrenal response and the need of added glucocorticoids during stress.— H. Kehlet and C. Binder, *Br. med. J.*, 1973, *2*, 147. Results of a study in 25 patients with various degrees of hypothalamo-pituitary malfunction indicated a high degree of correlation between the increase in plasma-cortisol (hydrocortisone) concentrations during insulin hypoglycaemia and during corticotrophin stimulation, and between peak plasma-cortisol (hydrocortisone) concentrations during the 2 tests. The 30-minute corticotrophin stimulation test employing tetracosactrin therefore appeared to be a reliable means of detecting impaired hypothalamo-pituitary-adrenocortical function.— H. Kehlet *et al.*, *ibid.*, 1976, *1*, 249.

Further references: P. Sheridan and D. Mattingly, *Lancet*, 1975, *2*, 676 (simultaneous investigation and treatment).

Asthma. In children requiring corticosteroid therapy for the management of asthma a lower incidence of growth retardation is associated with the synthetic corticotrophin, tetracosactrin. It may be given in initial doses of 0.5 to 1 mg once or twice weekly, with gradual reduction as a response occurs until the lowest possible dose is reached.— A. B. X. Breslin, *Drugs*, 1979, *18*, 103. For controversy relating to corticotrophin and its effects on growth, see Corticotrophin, p.486.

Individual studies on the use of tetracosactrin in the management of asthma.— S. A. Benos *et al.*, *Acta allerg.*, 1969, *24*, 178; J. E. C. Schook and C. F. Schuller, *Ned. Tijdschr. Geneesk.*, 1971, *115*, 1409.

Neurological disorders. Treatment with tetracosactrin brought about rapid improvement within 6 days in a 12-year-old boy suffering from severe neurological manifestations of rubella.— J. Astruc *et al.*, *Nouv. Presse méd.*, 1973, *2*, 1889.

Multiple sclerosis. For a comment on the use of tetracosactrin in multiple sclerosis, see Corticosteroids, p.456.

Rheumatic disorders. Studies on tetracosactrin therapy in rheumatic disorders: J. E. Murphy and J. F. Donald (letter), *Br. med. J.*, 1969, *1*, 316; F. Prugger, *Wien. med. Wschr.*, 1972, *122*, 259; D. B. P. Tan (letter), *Med. J. Aust.*, 1972, *2*, 52; V. Tsvetkova, *Curr. med. Res. Opinion*, 1977, *4*, 477.

For comments on the limited role of corticosteroid therapy in rheumatic disorders, see Corticosteroids, p.457.

Rhinitis. Beneficial effects in hay fever with twice-weekly depot injections of tetracosactrin 500 µg.— D. F. Harrison and I. M. Stanley, *Practitioner*, 1972, *208*, 680. For a comment on the ethics of using depot corticosteroids in hay fever, see Corticosteroids, p.458.

Skin disorders. *Eczema.* In a study lasting for up to 7 years a long-acting depot injection of tetracosactrin was successfully used with due precautions in maintenance doses of up to 1 mg every third day, self-administered by deep subcutaneous injection by 17 patients with eczema. To lessen the risk associated with anaphylactoid reactions the patients are warned to avoid repeated injections if they develop unusual symptoms and to remain in company with another person for an hour after the injection.— D. D. Munro, *Br. J. Derm.*, 1976, *94*, *Suppl.* 12, 135.

For further reports on the use of corticotrophin and tetracosactrin, see under Corticosteroids, p.451.

Preparations

Tetracosactrin Zinc Injection *(B.P.)*. A sterile aqueous suspension of tetracosactrin acetate with zinc hydroxide and suitable stabilising agents. Potency is expressed in terms of the equivalent amount of peptide. pH 7.8 to 9.2. Store at 2° to 15° and avoid freezing. Under these conditions it may be expected to retain its potency for not less than 3 years.

Synacthen *(Ciba, UK)*. Tetracosactrin acetate, available as an injection containing the equivalent of tetracosactrin 250 µg per ml in buffered aqueous solution, in ampoules of 1 ml. **Synacthen Depot.** Contains in each ml the equivalent of tetracosactrin 1 mg in a zinc phosphate complex for prolonged action, in ampoules of 1 ml and vials of 2 ml. (Also available as Synacthen and/or Synacthen Depot in *Arg.*, *Austral.*, *Belg.*, *Canad.*, *Denm.*, *Ger.*, *Ital.*, *Neth.*, *Norw.*, *S.Afr.*, *Swed.*, *Switz.*).

Other Proprietary Names

Cortrosinta Depot *(Spain)*; Cortrosyn *(Belg., Canad., Ital., Neth.)*; Cortrosyn Depot *(Austral., Belg., Ital., Neth., Norw., S.Afr., Swed., Switz.)*; Nuvacthen, Nuvacthen Depot *(both Spain)*; Synacthène *(Fr.)*.

Tetracosactrin was also formerly marketed in Great Britain under the proprietary name Cortrosyn Depot (*Organon*).

Dermatological Agents

1590-j

The skin is subject to a very wide range of disorders including pruritus, erythema, inflammation, purpura, vesicles and bullae, urticaria, photosensitivity, and disorders of pigmentation and of the scalp.

Some disorders are characteristic of specific diseases and fade as the disease regresses. Some are caused by specific local infections with bacteria and fungi and are best treated by the appropriate antimicrobial agent—see the sections on Penicillins and other Antibiotics, and Griseofulvin and other Antifungal Agents. Many skin disorders are side-effects of therapeutic and other agents, ranging from mild hypersensitivity to the life-threatening Stevens-Johnson syndrome or toxic epidermal necrolysis. There remains a wide range of disorders the aetiology of many of which is poorly understood.

This section describes many of the agents which have been used, often over many years; their pharmacology is often poorly understood.

Agents which have a traditional place in the treatment of skin disorders include dithranol, ichthammol, resorcinol, sulphur, tar, and coal tar. More recent developments include the use of psoralens in psoriasis (see Methoxsalen, p.498) and tretinoin in acne.

Agents with primarily a protective function include calamine, starch, talc, titanium dioxide, and zinc oxide.

Agents used for their antimicrobial activity include chlorquinaldol, hydroxyquinoline sulphate, potassium hydroxyquinoline sulphate, and nitrofurazone.

Agents used to increase pigmentation include dihydroxyacetone, methoxsalen, and trioxsalen.

Agents used to reduce pigmentation include hydroquinone, mequinol, and monobenzone.

Other agents used to protect against sunlight are described under Sunscreen Agents, p.1495.

For the use of corticosteroids in the treatment of skin disorders, see p.451.

For the use of immunosuppressants in the treatment of psoriasis, see p.217.

Cutaneous reactions to drugs.— R. L. Baer and H. Harris, *J. Am. med. Ass.*, 1967, *202*, 710.

Psoriasis and its treatment.— L. Stankler, *Br. med. J.*, 1974, *1*, 27; R. H. Seville, *Practitioner*, 1977, *219*, 833; L. Hodge and J. S. Comaish, *Drugs*, 1977, *13*, 288; R. A. Hardie and J. A. A. Hunter, *Br. J. Hosp. Med.*, 1978, *20*, 13; R. H. Champion, *Br. med. J.*, 1981, *282*, 343.

For the PUVA regimen in the treatment of psoriasis, see Methoxsalen, p.498.

The treatment of dandruff.— *Med. Lett.*, 1977, *19*, 63.

Advances in dermatology.— A. P. Warin, *Br. J. Hosp. Med.*, 1978, *20*, 6.

Acne and its treatment.— W. J. Cunliffe, *Br. J. Hosp. Med.*, 1978, *20*, 24; W. J. Cunliffe, *Br. med. J.*, 1980, *280*, 1394; J. W. Melski and K. A. Arndt, *New Engl. J. Med.*, 1980, *302*, 503; *Med. Lett.*, 1980, *22*, 31.

Contact dermatitis.— C. J. Stevenson, *Br. J. Hosp. Med.*, 1978, *20*, 32.

Cutaneous manifestations of malignancy.— R. C. D. Staughton, *Br. J. Hosp. Med.*, 1978, *20*, 38.

Disorders of cutaneous pigmentation.— R. M. MacKie, *Br. J. Hosp. Med.*, 1978, *20*, 48; A. N. Lerner and J. J. Nordlund, *J. Am. med. Ass.*, 1978, *239*, 1183.

Scabies and its treatment.— M. Orkin and H. I. Maibach, *New Engl. J. Med.*, 1978, *298*, 496.

1591-z

Alcloxa. Aluminium Chlorhydroxyallantoinate; ALCA; RC-173. Chlorotetrahydroxy[(2-hydroxy-5-oxo-2-imidazolin-4-yl)ureato]dialuminium.
$C_4H_9Al_2ClN_4O_7$=314.6.

CAS — 1317-25-5.

Alcloxa is an astringent containing allantoin.

1592-c

Aldioxa. ALDA; RC-172; Aluminium Dihydroxyallantoinate. Dihydroxy[(2-hydroxy-5-oxo-2-imidazolin-4-yl)ureato]aluminium.
$C_4H_7AlN_4O_5$=218.1.

CAS — 5579-81-7.

Aldioxa is an astringent containing allantoin.

Proprietary Preparations

ZeaSorb Powder *(Stiefel, UK).* A dusting-powder containing aldioxa 0.2%, chloroxylenol 0.5%, and pulverised maize core 45%. For moist skin disorders.

Other Proprietary Names

Alanetorin, Alanta-SP, Arlanto, Ascomp *(all Jap.).*

1593-k

Allantoin *(B.P.C. 1934).* Glyoxyldiureide. 5-Ureidohydantoin; 5-Ureidoimidazolidine-2,4-dione.
$C_4H_6N_4O_3$=158.1.

CAS — 97-59-6.

A white, odourless, tasteless, crystalline powder. **Soluble** 1 in 130 of water and 1 in 500 of alcohol; more soluble in hot water and hot alcohol; practically insoluble in ether. A saturated aqueous solution has a pH of about 5.5.

Allantoin is claimed to stimulate tissue formation and hasten wound healing. It appears to have keratin-dispersing activity. It is used in psoriasis and other skin disorders usually in creams and lotions containing 2%.

An evaluation of allantoin.— *Br. med. J.*, 1967, *4*, 535.

Proprietary Preparations

Alphosyl *(Stafford-Miller, UK).* **Cream** and **Lotion** containing allantoin 2% and alcoholic extract of coal tar 5% in a non-greasy basis. For psoriasis. **Alphosyl Application PC.** Contains allantoin 0.2% and alcoholic extract of coal tar 5% in a shampoo basis. For psoriasis of the scalp and other disorders.

Alphosyl HC Cream *(Stafford-Miller, UK).* Contains allantoin 2%, alcoholic extract of coal tar 5%, and hydrocortisone 0.5%. For psoriasis.

1594-a

Azulene. Cyclopentacycloheptene.
$C_{10}H_8$=128.2.

CAS — 275-51-4.

Intensely blue crystals with an odour of naphthalene. M.p. 99°. Practically **insoluble** in water; soluble in organic solvents.

NOTE. The name 'azulene' has also been applied to a series of sesquiterpene derivatives of azulene. Guaiazulene (see p.495) is one such derivative. Another, chamazulene, occurs in chamomile oil (p.673), to which it imparts the blue colour.

Azulene has been reported to have anti-inflammatory properties.

Use in cosmetics and pharmacy: a review.— H. Wirth, *Dragoco Report*, 1968, *15*, 23. Allergic reaction.— E. Cronin, *J. Soc. cosmet. Chem.*, 1967, *18*, 681.

1595-t

Cade Oil *(B.P.C. 1973).* Oleum Cadinum; Juniper Tar *(U.S.P.)*; Juniper Tar Oil; Oleum Juniperi Empyreumaticum; Pix Cadi; Pix Juniperi; Pix Oxycedri; Pyroleum Juniperi; Pyroleum Oxycedri; Goudron de Cade; Kadeöl; Wacholderteer; Alquitrán de Enebro.

Pharmacopoeias. In *Arg., Hung., Mex., Port., Roum., Span., Swiss,* and *U.S.*

Cade oil is obtained by the destructive distillation of the branches and wood of *Juniperus oxycedrus* (Cupressaceae). It is a dark, reddish-brown or nearly black, oily liquid with an empyreumatic odour and an aromatic bitter acrid taste. It contains guaiacol, ethylguaiacol, creosol, and cadinene. Wt per ml 0.97 to 1.01 g. Very slightly **soluble** in water; soluble 1 in 3 of ether; partly soluble in cold alcohol and light petroleum, almost completely soluble in hot alcohol; soluble in amyl alcohol, chloroform, and glacial acetic acid. **Store** at a temperature not exceeding 40°. Protect from light.

Uses. Cade oil has been used as an ointment and shampoo in the treatment of psoriasis and as an ointment in the treatment of eczema. It has been incorporated in medicated soaps and has also been used in seborrhoea.

It was recommended that cade oil be prohibited for use in foods as a flavouring agent.— *Food Standards Committee Report on Flavouring Agents*, London, HM Stationery Office, 1965.

Preparations

Cade Oil Ointment *(B.P.C. 1949).* Ung. Ol. Cadin. Cade oil 25 g, yellow beeswax 12.5 g, and yellow soft paraffin 62.5 g.

Cade Oil Shampoos. (1) Cade oil 2.5 ml, polysorbate '60' 2 g, triethanolamine lauryl sulphate to 100 ml.—W. Swallow, *Pharm. J.*, 1961, *2*, 407.
(2) Cade oil 10% and triethanolamine 10% in soap spirit. For dandruff. Use once weekly, rubbing it in neat and leaving for 2 hours before washing out.—M. Readett, *Practitioner*, 1966, *196*, 630.

Oil of Cade Ointment *(Wycombe Gen. Hosp.).* Cade oil 6 g, precipitated sulphur 3 g, salicylic acid 2 g, emulsifying ointment 89 g.

Proprietary Names

Caditar *(Sarep-Pharmeurop, Fr.).*

1596-x

Cadmium.
Cd=112.41.

CAS — 7440-43-9.

Cadmium is employed in a wide range of manufacturing processes and cadmium poisoning presents a recognised industrial hazard. Maximum permissible atmospheric concentration 50 μg per m^3.

Recommended health-based occupational limits for short-term and long-term exposure to cadmium, and biological limits for cadmium in blood and urine. A short-term exposure level for cadmium oxide fumes and respirable dust of 250 μg Cd/m^3 is recommended for prevention of acute lung reaction provided the time-weighted average is respected. To prevent adverse pulmonary and renal effects in long-term occupational exposure to cadmium the time-weighted average concentration of airborne cadmium fumes or respirable dust should be below 20 $\mu g/m^3$. In the present state of knowledge, a tentative value of 10 $\mu g/m^3$ is recommended. Recommended health-based biological limits for cadmium in blood and urine are 5 μg per litre of whole blood and 5 μg per g creatinine respectively. A revision of these various levels proposed may be required when the results of current epidemiological studies on the carcinogenic properties of cadmium become available.— Report of a WHO Study Group on Recommended Health-Based Limits in Occupational Exposure to Heavy Metals, *Tech. Rep. Ser. Wld Hlth Org. No. 647*, 1980.

Adverse effects. Reviews: *Br. med. J.*, 1967, *2*, 392; *Lan-*

cet, 1968, *1*, 133; G. Kendrey and F. J. C. Roe, *ibid.*, 1969, *1*, 1206; *ibid.*, 1969, *2*, 1346; *ibid.*, 1971, *1*, 382; Report of a WHO Expert Group on Trace Elements in Human Nutrition, *Tech. Rep. Ser. Wld Hlth Org. No. 532*, 1973, 41; L. T. Friberg *et al.*, Cadmium in the Environment, 2nd Edn, Cleveland, Ohio, CRC Press, 1974..

Acute cadmium poisoning could arise from either ingestion or inhalation. The symptoms of poisoning, which occurred within ½ to 3 hours after ingestion, included severe nausea and vomiting, abdominal cramps, occasionally shock, and sometimes haematemesis. Recovery was usually complete within 24 hours and deaths were rare. Acute poisoning from inhalation was relatively rare but was much more dangerous, having a mortality-rate of about 15%. The symptoms were irritation of the eyes, headache, vertigo, cough, constriction of the chest, weakness of the legs, dyspnoea, cyanosis, and bronchopneumonia. Chronic poisoning arose from prolonged exposure (2 or 3 years) to an atmosphere polluted with cadmium fumes or dust. The first obvious symptom of poisoning was a characteristic yellow pigmentation of the teeth, 'the yellow ring of cadmium'; at this stage prophylaxis was possible. Other early symptoms were soreness of the nostrils, 'cadmium sniffles', and loss of smell. Later and more serious symptoms were emphysema and proteinuria; in some cases pain in the back and limbs and bone changes leading to permanent disability had been reported.— F. M. Turner, *Cadmium Poisoning*, AERE Med/M17, UK Atomic Energy Authority Research Group, HM Stationery Office, 1957.

In 6 brands of cigarettes, 70% of the cadmium content of cigarette tobacco passed into smoke.— M. Nandi *et al.*, *Lancet*, 1969, *2*, 1329. Contamination of cigarettes and pipe tobacco by cadmium oxide dust.— M. Piscator *et al.* (letter), *Lancet*, 1976, *2*, 587.

Death after brazing with solder containing 24 to 26% of cadmium.— R. M. Winston (letter), *Br. med. J.*, 1971, *2*, 401. Another death after exposure to cadmium fumes.— J. R. Patwardhan and E. S. Finckh, *Med. J. Aust.*, 1976, *1*, 962. See also P. A. Lucas *et al.* (letter), *Lancet*, 1980, *2*, 205.

Investigation of 27 coppersmiths exposed to cadmium revealed an association between cadmium exposure and renal and some liver impairment, renal stones, and restrictive airways disease when compared with a control group.— R. Scott *et al.*, *Lancet*, 1976, *2*, 396. Experience with 16 cadmium workers, 5 of whom had proteinuria and anaemia 10 years earlier, showed that cadmium-induced proteinuria was reversible.— K. Tsuchiya, *J. occup. Med.*, 1976, *18*, 463, per *Abstr. Hyg.*, 1977, *52*, 135.

Further references: J. S. Anthony *et al.*, *Can. med. Ass. J.*, 1978, *119*, 586; R. Scott (letter), *Lancet*, 1980, *2*, 429; E. King (letter), *ibid.*, 641; E. G. Hughes (letter), *ibid.*; R. M. Winston (letter), *ibid.*, 642.

Cadmium in the environment. Some studies, reviews, and comments on the role of cadmium as an environmental toxin: I. Thornton, *Chem. in Br.*, 1979, *15*, 223; T. C. Harvey *et al.* (letter), *Lancet*, 1979, *1*, 551; E. G. Hughes and M. Stewart (letter), *ibid.*, 727; L. Friberg (letter), *ibid.*, 823; M. Carruthers and B. Smith, *ibid.*, 845; E. G. Hughes and M. Stewart (letter), *ibid.*, 973; C. F. Mills and B. Lawrence (letter), *ibid.*, 1090; M. Carruthers and B. Smith (letter), *ibid.*; L. McDougall (letter), *ibid.*, 1091; D. F. Kraemer *et al.* (letter), *ibid.*, 1241; S. R. Greenberg (letter), *ibid.*, 1242; R. Lauwerys and P. De Wals (letter), *ibid.*, 1981, *1*, 383; R. G. Adams (letter), *ibid.*, 845.

Effect on blood pressure. In 17 untreated hypertensive patients (mean blood pressure 159.8/102.5 mmHg) mean blood-cadmium concentrations were 11.1 ng per ml, compared with 3.4 ng per ml in 10 normotensive subjects.— S. C. Glauser *et al.*, *Lancet*, 1976, *1*, 717.

Autopsy of 76 patients showed no significant correlation between accumulation of cadmium (in liver and kidney) and hypertension or cardiovascular disease.— T. L. M. Syversen *et al.*, *Scand. J. clin. Lab. Invest.*, 1976, *36*, 251, per *Abstr. Hyg.*, 1976, *51*, 934.

No association between blood-cadmium concentration and hypertension was found in a study of 70 hypertensive patients and 70 controls.— D. G. Beevers *et al.*, *Lancet*, 1976, *2*, 1222. See also *ibid.*, 1230; R. Phillip and A. O. Hughes (letter), *Br. med. J.*, 1981, *282*, 2054.

Cadmium in food. Provisional tolerable weekly intake for man: 400 to 500 µg per person or 6.7 to 8.3 µg per kg body-weight.— Sixteenth Report of FAO/WHO Expert Committee on Food Additives, *Tech. Rep. Ser. Wld Hlth Org. No. 505*, 1972. See also *Fd Add. Ser. Wld Hlth Org. No. 4*, 1972.. From analysis of the cadmium content of foodstuffs it was estimated that the average total intake from food and drink in the UK was not more than 250 µg per week.— *Survey of Cadmium in Food*, Minist. Agric. Fish. Fd, London, HM Stationery Office, 1973..

In a review of drinking water standards in April 1972 the WHO recommended that the maximum level of cadmium should be reduced from 0.01 ppm to 0.005 ppm. It also recommended that the intake of cadmium from other sources should be reduced as much as possible.— S. Hernberg, *Chronicle Wld Hlth Org.*, 1973, *27*, 192.

For further details of drinking water standards, see Water p.1669.

The contamination of food by metals, including cadmium.— D. Gloag, *Br. med. J.*, 1981, *282*, 879. See also *J. Am. med. Ass.*, 1979, *242*, 1956.

Metabolism. Study in 21 solderers.— H. Welinder *et al.*, *Br. J. ind. Med.*, 1977, *34*, 221, per *Abstr. Hyg.*, 1977, *52*, 1274.

1597-r

Cadmium Sulphide.
CdS = 144.5.

CAS — 1306-23-6.

A light yellow or orange-coloured powder. Practically **insoluble** in water.

Adverse Effects. See Cadmium (above).

Uses. Cadmium sulphide has been used similarly to selenium sulphide in the control of seborrhoeic dermatitis and dandruff, usually as a shampoo containing 1% of cadmium sulphide suspended in a suitable detergent basis.

Proprietary Names
Biocadmio *(Uriach, Spain)*; Buginol *(GEA, Denm.)*.

1598-f

Calamine *(B.P.)*. Prepared Calamine.

CAS — 8011-96-9.

Pharmacopoeias. In *Br.* and *Chin.*; *Arg.*, *Ind.*, and *U.S.* specify zinc oxide with a small proportion of ferric oxide, yielding on ignition not less than 98% of ZnO.

A basic zinc carbonate coloured with ferric oxide, yielding on ignition 68 to 74% of oxides of zinc and iron. It is an amorphous, impalpable, pink or reddish-brown powder, the colour depending on the variety and amount of ferric oxide present and the process by which it is incorporated. Practically **insoluble** in water; almost completely soluble with effervescence in hydrochloric acid.

Uses. Calamine has a mild astringent action on the skin and is used as a dusting-powder, cream, lotion, or ointment in a variety of skin conditions.

Preparations

Creams and Oily Lotions

Aqueous Calamine Cream *(B.P.)*. Calamine Cream. Calamine 4 g, zinc oxide 3 g, emulsifying wax 6 g, arachis oil 30 g, and freshly boiled and cooled water 57 g. Dissolve the emulsifying wax in the arachis oil with the aid of gentle heat; add 40 g of water at the same temperature and stir until cold; triturate the calamine and zinc oxide with the rest of the water and incorporate in the cream. Store at a temperature not exceeding 25° in well-closed containers which minimise evaporation and contamination.
A.P.F. (Calamine Cream Aqueous) has a similar preparation, but includes cetomacrogol emulsifying wax instead of emulsifying wax. It may be tinted by the addition of up to 1% of caramel solution.

A proposed formula for calamine cream: calamine 4 g, zinc oxide 3 g, cetomacrogol emulsifying wax 5 g, self-emulsifying glyceryl monostearate 5 g, liquid paraffin 20 g, phenoxyethanol 500 mg, water 62.5 g. The cream was stable for 6 months and no difficulties had been encountered in manufacture. Inocula of *Pseudomonas aeruginosa*, *Klebsiella aerogenes*, *Escherichia coli*, *Proteus vulgaris*, and *Staphylococcus aureus* did not survive after 6 hours in the proposed cream.— R. M. Baird, *Pharm. J.*, 1974, *2*, 153.

Further studies on the formulation of calamine cream.— L. S. C. Wan, *Pharm. J.*, 1978, *2*, 533.

Calamine Cream *(St. John's Hosp.)*. Calamine 4, zinc oxide 3, emulsifying wax 2, arachis oil 33.3, water to 100.

Calamine Cream Oily *(A.P.F.)*. Calamine 32 g, oleic acid 0.5 ml, arachis oil 21.5 ml, wool fat 17.5 g, calcium hydroxide solution 30.5 ml. It may be tinted by the addition of up to 1% of caramel solution.

Compound Calamine Application *(B.P.C. 1973)*. Compound Calamine Cream; Compound Calamine Liniment; Linimentum Calaminae Compositum. Calamine 10 g, zinc oxide 5 g, zinc stearate 2.5 g, wool fat 2.5 g, yellow soft paraffin 25 g, and liquid paraffin 55 g.

Oily Calamine Lotion *(B.P.)*. Calamine Liniment; Linimentum Calaminae; Lot. Calam. Oleos. Calamine 5 g, wool fat 1 g, oleic acid 0.5 ml, arachis oil 50 ml, calcium hydroxide solution to 100 ml.
A.P.F. (Calamine Lotion Oily) has a similar preparation and permits the addition of about 0.5% of caramel solution.

Suggested modified formulas for Oily Calamine Lotion. Calamine 5, wool fat 5, zinc stearate 2, oleic acid 1, light liquid paraffin 45, calcium hydroxide solution to 100. This formula would give a satisfactory product when mixed with ichthammol.— J. E. Carless, *Pharm. J.*, 1958, *1*, 419.

The addition of zinc stearate 4% to the formula for Oily Calamine Lotion reduced phase separation; the viscosity increased on storage.— L. S. C. Wan (letter), *Pharm. J.*, 1977, *2*, 457.

Lotions

Calamine Lotion *(B.P., A.P.F.)*. Calam. Lot. Calamine 15 g, zinc oxide 5 g, bentonite 3 g, sodium citrate 500 mg, liquefied phenol 0.5 ml, glycerol 5 ml, freshly boiled and cooled water to 100 ml.
A.P.F. uses sterilised bentonite.

Incorporation of coal tar. To incorporate coal tar 3% in calamine lotion, double the *B.P.* proportion of bentonite should be used. A paste was made of the bentonite with about 20 ml of water, the coal tar added, and mixed thoroughly;the other ingredients were added with trituration (the sodium citrate being dissolved in a little water), water added as necessary, and finally the volume adjusted with water.— *Australas. J. Pharm.*, 1965, *46*, 150.

Incorporation of hydrocortisone. The tendency of hydrocortisone in ultra-fine powder to form aggregates when mixed with calamine lotion or other aqueous vehicle could be overcome by first triturating the hydrocortisone with a viscous liquid such as glycerol (about 5% v/v); the calamine lotion could then be added, in small portions at a time, to produce a satisfactory homogeneous suspension.— G. Smith and A. E. Brooks, *Pharm. J.*, 1964, *2*, 565.

Calamine Lotion *(U.S.P.)*. Calamine *U.S.P.* 8 g, zinc oxide 8 g, glycerol 2 ml, bentonite magma 25 ml, calcium hydroxide topical solution to 100 ml. If a more viscous consistency is desired, the quantity of bentonite magma may be increased to not more than 40 ml. Store in airtight containers.

Modified formula for Calamine Lotion (U.S.P.). Calamine 8 g, zinc oxide 8 g, glycerol 2 ml, microcrystalline cellulose gel (45% w/w Avicel R in water) 2 g, carmellose sodium 2 g, liquefied phenol 1 ml, calcium hydroxide solution to 100 ml. A phenolated lotion with good suspending and spreading properties.— J. E. Haberle, *Am. J. Hosp. Pharm.*, 1968, *25*, 182.

Calamine and Tannic Acid Lotion *(Roy. Marsden Hosp.)*. Calamine 4.4, zinc oxide 4.4, tannic acid 2.2, glycerol 5, water to 100. Should be freshly prepared. Shelf-life 21 days.

Phenolated Calamine Lotion *(U.S.P.)*. Liquefied phenol 1 ml, calamine lotion *U.S.P.* 99 ml. Store in airtight containers.

Ointments

Calamine and Coal Tar Ointment *(B.P.)*. Compound Calamine Ointment; Unguentum Sedativum. Calamine 12.5 g, zinc oxide 12.5 g, strong coal tar solution 2.5 g, hydrous wool fat 25 g, white soft paraffin 47.5 g. Store at a temperature not exceeding 25° in containers which minimise evaporation.

Calamine Ointment *(B.P.)*. Calamine 15 g and white soft paraffin 85 g. Store at a temperature not exceeding 25°.

Proprietary Preparations

Eczederm Cream *(Quinoderm, UK)*. Contains calamine 20.88% and maize starch 2.09% in a cream basis.
Eczederm Cream with Hydrocortisone 0.5%. Contains in addition hydrocortisone 0.5%.

Lacto-Calamine Lotion *(Kirby-Warrick, UK)*. Contains calamine 4%, with hamamelis water 5% and phenol 0.2%.

A preparation containing calamine was also formerly marketed in Great Britain under the proprietary name Calsept (*Norton: Vestric*).

1599-d

Calcium Thioglycollate. Calcium Mercaptoacetate.
Calcium mercaptoacetate trihydrate.
$C_2H_2CaO_2S,3H_2O=184.2$.

A white crystalline powder with a slight sulphidic odour. **Soluble** 1 in 14 of water, more soluble in hot water; very slightly soluble in alcohol and chloroform; practically insoluble in ether. **Store** in airtight containers.

Calcium thioglycollate is used as a depilatory, usually in concentrations of 2 to 7% in creams and lotions made alkaline by the addition of calcium hydroxide. It has been used pre-operatively to avoid shaving.

Review and discussion of epilatory and depilatory methods with particular reference to depilatories containing calcium thioglycollate.— *Lancet*, 1967, *1*, 488.

Pre-operative use.— S. J. A. Powis *et al.*, *Br. med. J.*, 1976, *2*, 1166.

1600-d

Centella. Hydrocotyle; Indian Pennywort.

CAS — 18449-41-7 (madecassic acid); 464-92-6 (asiatic acid); 16830-15-2 (asiaticoside).

The fresh and dried leaves and stems of *Centella asiatica* (=*Hydrocotyle asiatica*) (Umbelliferae). It contains madecassic acid, asiatic acid, and asiaticoside.

Centella has been used in India in skin disease and as a diuretic, and as an adjunct in the treatment of leprosy.

Asiaticoside has been used in the treatment of leprous ulcers (M. Nebout, *Bull. Soc. Path. exot.*, 1974, *67*, 471) and slow-healing wounds (H. Kiesswetter, *Wien. med. Wschr.*, 1964, *114*, 124, per *Int. pharm. Abstr.*, 1964, *1*, 1337).

Proprietary Preparations

Madecassol *(Rona, UK)*. The extract of centella, available as **Ointment** containing 1% and as **Powder** containing 2%. To accelerate cicatrisation and grafting. (Also available as Madecassol in *Belg.*, *Fr.*, *Neth.*).

Other Proprietary Names

Blasteostimulina *(asiaticoside) (Spain)*; Centelase *(Ital.)*; Marticassol *(Fr.)*.

1601-n

Chlorquinaldol. 5,7-Dichloro-2-methylquinolin-8-ol.
$C_{10}H_7Cl_2NO=228.1$.

CAS — 72-80-0.

Pharmacopoeias. In *Roum.*

A green or yellowish-brown crystalline tasteless powder with a pleasant medicinal odour. M.p. about 113°.

Practically **insoluble** in water; soluble in alcohol, acetone, and vegetable oils. **Incompatible** with many metal ions. **Protect** from light and avoid contact with metal.

Chlorquinaldol has the actions and uses of Potassium Hydroxyquinoline Sulphate, p.500. It is applied to the skin as a cream or ointment, usually in a concentration of 3%. It has also been used as a 1% vaginal cream and as 200-mg vaginal tablets.

Following a 200-mg dose of chlorquinaldol, 6 healthy men excreted a mean of 34.9% of the dose in the urine during the following 10 hours.— L. Berggren and O. Hansson, *Clin. Pharmac. Ther.*, 1968, *9*, 67.

Further references: H. Bandmann *et al.*, *Archs Derm.*, 1972, *106*, 335; P. J. Ashurst, *Br. J. clin. Pract.*, 1972, *26*, 263.

Proprietary Preparations

Steroxin *(Geigy, UK)*. Chlorquinaldol, available as an ointment containing 3% in a non-greasy basis. (Also available as Steroxin in *Austral.*).

Steroxin-Hydrocortisone *(Geigy, UK)*. A cream containing chlorquinaldol 3% and hydrocortisone 1%. For inflamed bacterial and fungous skin infections.

Other Proprietary Names

Gyno-Sterosan *(Ger., Neth., Norw.)*; Gynothérax *(Fr., Switz.)*; Siogen *(Neth., Switz.)*; Siogeno *(Ger.)*; Siosteran *(Neth., Switz.)*; Sterosan *(Denm., Ger., Neth., Swed., Switz.)*.

1602-h

Chrysarobin *(B.P.C. 1949)*. Araroba Depurata; commonly but erroneously called Chrysophanic Acid.

Pharmacopoeias. In *Arg.*, *Aust.*, *Ind.*, *Jug.*, *Mex.*, *Nord.*, *Port.*, and *Span.*

A light, odourless, tasteless, yellowish or yellowish-brown, microcrystalline powder, obtained by extraction with benzene from araroba, a substance obtained from cavities in the trunk of *Andira araroba* (Leguminosae). Practically **insoluble** in water; soluble 1 in 400 of alcohol, 1 in 15 of chloroform (usually leaving a small amount of residue), 1 in 160 of ether, in fats, and in alkali hydroxides. **Protect** from light.

Adverse Effects. Chrysarobin is irritating to mucous membranes. Taken internally, it causes diarrhoea, vomiting, and haematuria.

Uses. Chrysarobin has been used as a 1 to 5% ointment in the treatment of parasitic skin infections. It should not be used on the face, genitalia, or scalp, owing to its irritant action, and should not be employed over a large area of skin. The ointment stains the skin and clothing a brownish-violet colour, which may be removed with Dilute Sodium Hypochlorite Solution. Absorption of chrysarobin through the skin causes excretion of a yellow pigment which colours alkaline urine red.

Preparations

Pasta Chrysarobini Composita *(Dan. Disp.)*. Compound Chrysarobin Paste. Chrysarobin 0.1%, pyrogallol 2%, salicylic acid 2%, tar 2%, zinc oxide 34.4%, liquid paraffin 0.8%, soft paraffin to 100%.

Chrysamone *(Andard-Mount, UK)*. Chrysarobin, available as an ointment containing 3 and 5%.

1603-m

Crotamiton *(B.P., U.S.P.)*. Crotam. *N*-Ethyl-*N*-*o*-tolylcrotonamide; *N*-Ethylcrotono-*o*-toluidide.
$C_{13}H_{17}NO=203.3$.

CAS — 483-63-6.

Pharmacopoeias. In *Br.* and *U.S.*

A colourless or pale yellow oily liquid with a faint amine-like odour. Wt per ml 1.004 to 1.009 g. It solidifies partly or completely at low temperatures and it must be completely liquefied by warming before use. The *B.P.* specifies that it is predominantly the (*E*)-isomer, with not more than 15% of the (*Z*)-isomer. *U.S.P.* specifies a mixture of (*E*)- and (*Z*)- isomers.

Soluble 1 in 400 of water; miscible with alcohol, methyl alcohol, and ether. **Store** in small airtight containers. Protect from light.

Adverse Effects and Precautions. Applied topically, crotamiton occasionally causes transient erythema and a sensation of warmth. Crotamiton should not be used in the presence of acute exudative or vesicular dermatitis. It should not be applied near the eyes.

Skin sensitivity to crotamiton, confirmed by patch tests, was seen in 5 patients with eczema during the period 1957/66.— J. K. Morgan, *Br. J. clin. Pract.*, 1968, *22*, 261.

Uses. Crotamiton is an acaricide and in the treatment of scabies a 10% cream or lotion is applied, after first bathing and drying, to the whole of the body surface below the neck particular attention being paid to body folds and creases. A second application is advisable 24 hours later.

A complete change of clothing and bed-linen should be made and a bath should be taken the day after the final application.

Crotamiton is an antipruritic agent and local application gives rapid relief from itching. It is used for the relief of pruritus ani, vulvae, and scroti, senile pruritus, and pruritus associated with various dermatoses. One application is usually effective for 6 to 10 hours.

Preparations

Crotamiton Cream *(U.S.P.)*. A cream containing crotamiton. Store in airtight containers. Protect from light.

Proprietary Preparations

Eurax *(Geigy, UK)*. Crotamiton, available as **Lotion** containing 10% and as **Ointment** containing 10% in a non-greasy basis. (Also available as Eurax in *Austral.*, *Belg.*, *Canad.*, *Fr.*, *Ital.*, *Neth.*, *S.Afr.*, *Swed.*, *Switz.*, *USA*).

Eurax-Hydrocortisone *(Geigy, UK)*. Contains crotamiton 10% and hydrocortisone 0.25% in a vanishing-cream basis. For dermatoses with pruritus.

Other Proprietary Names

Bestloid *(Jap.)*; Crotamitex *(Ger.)*; Euraxil *(Ger., Spain)*.

A preparation containing crotamiton was also formerly marketed in Great Britain under the proprietary name Teevex (*Geigy*).

1604-b

Dextranomer. Dextran cross-linked with epichlorohydrin (1-chloro-2,3-epoxypropane); Dextran 2,3-dihydroxypropyl 2-hydroxypropane-1,3-diyl ether.

CAS — 56087-11-7.

Practically **insoluble** in water.

Precautions. Care should be exercised when dextranomer is used near the eyes.

Spillage may render surfaces very slippery.

Uses. The action of dextranomer depends upon its ability to absorb up to 4 times its weight of fluid, including dissolved and suspended material of molecular weight up to about 5000. The preparation of dextranomer is available in the form of spherical beads which produce a capillary effect.

Dextranomer is used for the cleansing of weeping and infected wounds, including burns and ulcers, and for preparation for skin grafting. The wound is cleansed with water or sodium chloride injection and allowed to remain wet; dextranomer is sprinkled on to a depth of at least 3 mm and covered with a sterile dressing. Occlusive dressings are not recommended as they may lead to maceration around the wound. The dressing is changed once or twice daily, before the layer has become saturated with exudate. The dextranomer layer is washed off with a stream of sodium chloride injection before renewal. All dextranomer must be removed before skin grafting.

Reviews and discussions on the use of dextranomer: *Med. Lett.*, 1978, *20*, 47; *Drug & Ther. Bull.*, 1979, *17*, 9; R. C. Heel *et al.*, *Drugs*, 1979, *18*, 89.

The effect of dextranomer applied once to thrice daily was considered good (decreased secretion, decreased inflammation, and the appearance of granulation tissue) in 36 of 47 patients with leg ulcers and in 23 of 31 patients with miscellaneous wounds; pain was often rapidly relieved; in 15 further patients the time needed to prepare the wound for skin grafting was reduced. In 10 patients studied the prostaglandin content of wound exudate was reduced as inflammation was reduced. In studies *in vitro* in which a suspension of bacteria was drawn into a tube of dextranomer, the greatest concentration of bacteria was found in the highest layer of dextranomer.— S. Jacobsson *et al.*, *Scand. J. plast. reconstr. Surg.*, 1976, *10*, 65.

The degradation of fibrinogen/fibrin combined with continuous removal of wound secretions might explain the favourable clinical effect of dextranomer.— M. Åberg *et al.*, *Scand. J. plast. reconstr. Surg.*, 1976, *10*, 103.

Second- or third-degree burns on 17 hands of 13 patients were successfully treated with dextranomer once to thrice daily, the hands being enclosed in plastic bags. Pain was rapidly relieved; the areas remained soft and pliable; all hands achieved full fucntion. Pain occurring in some patients on the removal of the gel formed by dextranomer and exudate was relieved by immersion in water before removal.— P. Paavolainen and B. Sundell, *Annls Chir. Gynaec. Fenn.*, 1976, *65*, 313.

Dextranomer was effective in the treatment of non-venereal penile ulcers in 25 patients (14 of herpetic origin, 3 caused by dequalinium, and 8 non-specific); ulcers often healed within a week and within 4 weeks in all patients.— A. Lassus *et al.*, *Acta derm.-vener., Stockh.*, 1977, *57*, 361.

Dextranomer was used in the treatment of 130 burnt hands (80 patients); the treated hand was covered with a plastic bag; dextranomer was replaced 3 or 4 times daily for 2 or 3 days, then usually twice daily. Pain was rapidly reduced and no allergic reactions occurred. Good mobility was achieved in 81 of 83 hands not needing grafting and in 38 of 47 grafted hands. The method was considered satisfactory for superficial and deep dermal burns of the hands and as preparation for grafting. For subdermal burns excision was the method of choice.— G. Arturson *et al.*, *Burns*, 1978, *4*, 225.

Further references: S. Jacobsson *et al.*, *Scand. J. plast. reconstr. Surg.*, 1976, *10*, 97; C. -H. Flodén and K. Wikström, *Curr. ther. Res.*, 1978, *24*, 753; A. Flamment, *ibid.*, 1979, *26*, 342; H. L. Brink *et al.*, *ibid.*, 346; E. J. W. McClemont *et al.*, *Br. J. clin. Pract.*, 1979, *33*, 21; N. Thorne, *ibid.*, 263; A. W. Goode *et al.*, *ibid.*, 325.

Proprietary Preparations

Debrisan *(Pharmacia, UK: Farillon, UK)*. Dextranomer, available as beads of diameter 100 to 300 μm. (Also available as Debrisan in *Austral., Denm., Neth., NZ, Norw., S.Afr., Swed., USA*).

Other Proprietary Names

Debrisorb*(Ger.)*.

1605-v

Dihydroxyacetone.

DHA; Ketotriose. 1,3-Dihydroxypropan-2-one.
$C_3H_6O_3$=90.08.

CAS — 96-26-4.

A colourless hygroscopic crystalline solid with a characteristic odour and a sweet cooling taste. The crystals consist of the dimer $(C_3H_6O_3)_2$ which is converted to the monomer on solution or warming.

Slowly **soluble** 1 in 1 of water and 1 in 5 of alcohol; soluble in acetone; slightly soluble in ether. The solubility increases in hot solvents due to the conversion to the monomer. **Incompatible** with amines and their derivatives. **Store** in airtight containers.

Adverse Effects. Skin rashes have occasionally been reported.

Uses. Applied to the skin as a lotion or cream, dihydroxyacetone causes the slow development of a brown coloration similar to that caused by exposure to the sun. The coloration is considered to be due to a reaction with the amino acids of the skin.

A single application may give rise to a patchy appearance; progressive darkening of the skin results from repeated use until a point is reached when no further darkening takes place. If the treatment is stopped the colour starts to fade after about 2 days and disappears completely within 8 to 14 days as the external epidermal cells are lost by normal attrition.

Creams and lotions containing 0.2 to 5% of dihydroxyacetone have been used. The presence of at least 20% of water is recommended; the colour reaction is most rapid in acid media and is facilitated by the addition of a surfactant; no reaction occurs above pH 8. Some preparations have included a sun-screening agent, since dihydroxyacetone gives no protection against sunburn.

The protective effect of a sunscreen filter chemically induced in the skin was evaluated in 18 healthy adults by exposure to direct sunlight. The filter was produced by applying a solution containing dihydroxyacetone 3% and lawsone 0.035%; the solution was applied 6 times before exposure to sunlight. It provided protection for 60 minutes for all the persons, and for 90 minutes for most of them. Increasing the lawsone concentration to 0.13% produced a more effective preparation in some cases. Neither component alone gave significant protection. Washing with soap and water did not remove the filter.— R. M. Fusaro *et al.*, *Archs Derm.*, 1966, *93*, 106.

Dihydroxyacetone 3% and lawsone 0.13% were applied to the skin of 7 patients with erythropoietic protoporphyria 6 to 8 times a day for 48 hours and then thrice daily for 5 days. Patients were then exposed to sunlight and the exposure needed to produce symptoms or lesions observed. Applications were then made 1 to 4 times daily. When contained in a vanishing-cream basis dihydroxyacetone and lawsone protected the patients against sunlight, but did not give adequate protection when freshly mixed in a 50% solution of isopropyl alcohol in water.— R. M. Fusaro and W. J. Runge, *Br. med. J.*, 1970, *1*, 730.

Preservation of blood. For the use of dihydroxyacetone in blood preservation solutions, see Whole Blood, p.322.

Preparations

Artificial Suntan Lotion. Dihydroxyacetone 3 g, Polawax GP '200' 8 g, menthyl salicylate 10 ml, glycerol 2.5 ml, industrial methylated spirit 33 ml, water to 100 ml. Melt the Polawax with part of the water and add the menthyl salicylate; dissolve the dihydroxyacetone in the remaining ingredients and mix the 2 liquids.—W. Swallow, *Pharm. J.*, 1961, *2*, 407.

For other formulas for dihydroxyacetone preparations see *Drug Cosmet. Ind.*, 1960, *87*, 320; E. Futterer, *Cosmet. Perfum.*, 1973, *88*, 31, per *Int. pharm. Abstr.*, 1973, *10*, 900.

1606-g

Dithranol

(B.P.). Anthralin *(U.S.P.)*; Dioxyanthranol. 1,8-Dihydroxy-9-anthrone.
$C_{14}H_{10}O_3$=226.2.

CAS — 1143-38-0.

NOTE. The *B.P.* describes dithranol as a mixture of 1,8-dihydroxy-9-anthrone and its tautomers; the *U.S.P.* describes dithranol as 1,8,9-anthracenetriol.

Pharmacopoeias. In *Belg., Br., Ind., Swiss,* and *U.S.*

A yellow to yellowish-brown, odourless, tasteless, crystalline powder. M.p. 175° to 181°. Practically **insoluble** in water; slightly soluble in alcohol, ether, and glacial acetic acid; soluble in acetone, chloroform, solutions of alkali hydroxides, and fixed oils. The filtrate from a suspension in water is neutral to litmus. **Store** in airtight containers. Protect from light.

CAUTION. *Dithranol is a powerful irritant and should be kept away from the eyes and tender parts of the skin.*

Dithranol pastes stiffened with hard paraffin were stable for at least 18 months, but were less effective after 4 years' storage.— R. H. Seville, *Br. J. Derm.*, 1966, *78*, 269.

The role of the individual ingredients of Dithranol Paste, Full Strength (*Roy. Victoria Infirm., Newcastle*) was studied by selective omission. In pastes containing zinc oxide the presence of salicylic (or benzoic) acid was necessary to prevent the development of pink colour due to interaction between dithranol and zinc oxide; such coloration was indicative of ineffectiveness. Zinc oxide and starch could be omitted without loss of effectiveness provided stiffness was maintained. The effect of dithranol 0.25 or 0.5% in yellow soft paraffin was not affected by the presence or absence of 0.5 or 2% of salicylic acid. If milling facilities were not available, dithranol could be dissolved in chloroform and then dispersed in Lassar's paste.— S. Comaish *et al.*, *Br. J. Derm.*, 1971, *84*, 282. Comment.— F. D. Dean (letter), *ibid.*, *85*, 494. See also T. J. Maloney, *Aust. J. Hosp. Pharm.*, 1977, *7*, 120.

Studies on the discoloration of various dithranol pastes. It was suggested that the application of heat, even indirect, should be avoided in the manufacture of dithranol pastes, and that metal spatulas should not be used.— Pharm. Soc. Lab. Rep. P/79/1, 1979.

Adverse Effects and Precautions. Dithranol may cause a burning sensation when applied to the skin or to lesions, and is irritant to the eyes. Preliminary tests should be carried out before treatment to detect any hypersensitivity. It stains the skin a reddish-brown colour. However, it is considered that the stronger the stain on the psoriasis the greater the improvement. Hair may also be stained.

Initially, dithranol should not be used in a concentration greater than 0.1% nor applied more than once daily. It should not be used in patients with renal disease.

Uses. Dithranol is used in the treatment of psoriasis. Since some patients are hypersensitive to dithranol, a preliminary test for sensitivity should be carried out on a small area of skin. Treatment is commonly started with an ointment or paste containing 0.1%, the strength being gradually increased to 0.5 or 0.6% occasionally to 1%. The preparation is applied to the lesions only; inflammation of surrounding skin may call for temporary withdrawal or the use of a lower strength. Fair patients are more sensitive and an initial strength of 0.05% may be adequate. The face, flexures of skin, and genitalia are particularly sensitive and a strength of 0.01% initially, applied thrice weekly, has been suggested.

Dithranol is a fungicide and has been used in the treatment of ringworm infections and chronic dermatoses.

Psoriasis. The following treatment could be expected to clear the eruptions of psoriasis in 2 to 3 weeks in all but a few patients. The patient soaked for 10 minutes in a warm bath containing coal tar solution 1 in 800. After drying he was exposed to ultraviolet light to produce the slightest erythematous reaction. Each lesion was then obscured with Lassar's paste containing dithranol 0.5%; the paste must be stiff and the melting-point of the paraffin basis should be 46°. The limbs and trunk were covered with stockinette and the patient assumed his clothes and normal routine until the following day when the procedure was repeated. Care must be taken to apply the paste to the psoriasis and not to the normal skin. With widespread eruptions of small pattern, a soft paste, consisting of equal parts of the original dithranol paste and soft paraffin, was applied over the whole affected area and not localised to lesions.— J. T. Ingram, *Br. med. J.*, 1954, *2*, 823. A modified treatment was as effective as the conventional Ingram regimen in 25 patients with psoriasis. It consisted of daily incremental ultraviolet irradiation followed by a hot tar bath and corticosteroid cream application to the lesions every 3 hours. Dithranol 0.1 to 0.4% in a stiff paste was applied overnight. Irritation and staining were minimised and the lesions cleared in an average of 11 days.— E. M. Farber and D. R. Harris, *Archs Derm.*, 1970, *101*, 381, per *Clin. Med.*, 1971, *78* (May), 36.

A theory for the action of dithranol in psoriasis; dithranol combined with deoxyribonucleic acid and other nucleic acids, inhibited the synthesis of nucleic protein, and so diminished cellular proliferation, which was increased in the psoriatic epidermis.— G. Swanbeck and N. Thyresson, *Acta derm.-vener., Stockh.*, 1965, *45*, 344. Using skin biopsies and *in vitro* labelling it was found that there were less DNA-synthesising cells in the lesions of patients with psoriasis after treatment for 1 to 2 weeks with dithranol. There was also an improved development of the granular layer.— S. Lidén and G. M. Lësson, *Br. J. Derm.*, 1974, *91*, 447.

The effects of dithranol in various bases for the treatment of psoriasis.— E. Young, *Br. J. Derm.*, 1970, *82*, 516.

For detailed recommendations on the use of dithranol pastes in psoriasis, see S. Shuster and J. S. Comaish, *Prescribers' J.*, 1973, *13*, 87; L. Stankler, *Br. med. J.*, 1974, *1*, 27; R. H. Seville, *Practitioner*, 1977, *219*, 833.

Reports on 10 patients with psoriasis taking part in a sequential study indicated that remissions were generally longer after the topical use of clobetasol propionate 0.05% than after dithranol 0.25%.— P. J. Marriott and D. D. Munro, *Br. J. Derm.*, 1976, *94*, *Suppl.* 12, 101.

Preparations

Ointments

Anthralin Ointment *(U.S.P.)*. Dithranol Ointment. Dithranol in a soft paraffin or other suitable basis. Protect from light.

Dithranol and Salicylic Acid Ointment (Water-Washable) *(A.P.F.)*. Dithranol 100 mg, salicylic acid 500 mg, liquid paraffin 20 g, emulsifying ointment to 100 g.

Dithranol Ointment *(B.P., A.P.F.)*. Ung. Dithranol. Contains dithranol, in fine powder, in yellow soft paraffin. Store at a temperature not exceeding 25°.

The following formula for a stiffened dithranol ointment appeared to have better patient acceptance than the stiffer pastes: dithranol 0.5%, salicylic acid 0.5%, chloroform 2.5%, equal parts of hard paraffin and white soft paraffin to 100%.— R. H. Seville, *Br. J. Derm.*, 1975, *93*, 205.

Strong Dithranol Ointment *(B.P. 1968)*. Ung. Dithranol. Fort. Dithranol 1% in yellow soft paraffin. Protect from light.

Paints

Dithranol Compound Wart Paint *(Adelaide Child. Hosp.)*. Dithranol 3 g, salicylic acid 25 g, acetone 20 ml, flexible collodion to 100 ml. For warts. It is irritant to normal tissue.

Pastes

Anthralin Pastes *(Rochester Methodist Hosp.)*. Dithranol 0.1 to 0.4, hard paraffin 5, corn starch 46, salicylic acid 1, white soft paraffin to 100. Shelf-life 2 years.

Dithranol and Zinc Paste *(A.P.F.)*. Dithranol 100 mg, zinc and salicylic acid paste to 100 g.

Dithranol Paste *(B.P.)*. Contains dithranol in zinc and salicylic acid paste. Protect from light.

Dithranol Paste, Full Strength *(Roy. Victoria Infirm.)*. Dithranol in Modified Lassar's Paste—Full Strength. Various strengths of dithranol are employed, ranging from 0.025 to 1%. See Lassar's Paste, Modified, Full-Strength *(Roy. Victoria Infirm., Newcastle)*, p.510.

Dithranol Paste, Half Strength *(Roy. Victoria Infirm.)*. A paste containing 0.0125 to 0.6% of dithranol, made with Modified Lassar's Paste—Half Strength. See Lassar's Paste, Modified, Half-Strength *(Roy. Victoria Infirm., Newcastle)*, p.510.

Pomades

Dithranol Pomade *(Bristol Roy. Infirm.)*. Dithranol 300 mg, salicylic acid 300 mg, yellow soft paraffin 4.4 g, emulsifying ointment 95.0 g. Shelf-life 2 years. For psoriasis of the scalp.

Dithranol Pomade *(Leeds Gen. Infirm.)*. Dithranol 0.5 or 1, emulsifying wax 25, and liquid paraffin to 100.

Dithranol Pomade *(Roy. Victoria Infirm.)*. Dithranol q.s., emulsifying wax 25 g, salicylic acid 2 g, liquid paraffin to 100 g.

Dithranol Pomade *(Wycombe Gen. Hosp.)*. Dithranol 400 mg, ascorbic acid 200 mg, liquid paraffin 75.4 g, emulsifying wax 24 g.

Proprietary Preparations

Antraderm *(pHarma-medica, UK: Brocades, UK)*. Dithranol 1% in a solid wax basis. **Antraderm mild.** Contains dithranol 0.5%. **Antraderm forte.** Contains dithranol 2%.

Dithrocream *(Dermal Laboratories, UK)*. Dithranol, available as a cream containing 0.1 and 0.25%.**Dithrocream Forte.** Cream containing dithranol 0.5%.

Dithrolan *(Dermal Laboratories, UK)*. Ointment containing dithranol 0.5% and salicylic acid 0.5%. For psoriasis.

Dithrolan could be diluted with emulsifying ointment if required.— M. Whitefield, *Dermal Laboratories* (letter), *Pharm. J.*, 1978, *1*, 331.

Psoradrate Cream *(Norwich-Eaton, UK)*. Contains dithranol 0.1 or 0.2% in a powder-in-cream basis containing urea. For psoriasis.

Stie-Lasan Ointment *(Stiefel, UK)*. Contains dithranol 0.4% and salicylic acid 0.4% in a basis containing cetyl alcohol, liquid paraffin, white soft paraffin, and sodium lauryl sulphate. For psoriasis.

Other Proprietary Names

Anthra-Derm *(Canad., USA)*; Lasan *(Canad.)*.

1607-q

Dithranol Triacetate.

Dithranol Acetate. 1,8,9-Triacetoxyanthracene.

$C_{20}H_{16}O_6$=352.3.

CAS — 16203-97-7.

Adverse Effects and Treatment. Dithranol triacetate is claimed to be less likely than dithranol to cause burning when applied to the skin. It is irritant to the eyes.

Two patients developed keratitis when a paste containing dithranol triacetate was accidentally introduced into the eye. The first symptoms were blurred or misty vision and were followed by reduced visual acuity and localised oedema. Both patients responded to a few days' treatment with atropine drops daily and prednisolone drops.— M. B. R. Mathalone and D. L. Easty, *Lancet*, 1967, *2*, 195.

Dithranol triacetate was inactive, but on hydrolysis 1,8-diacetoxy-9-anthranol was formed which was active in the unoxidised form. Its activity ceased in alkaline media due to atmospheric oxidation. As the hydrolysis released acetic acid which would be highly irritant to the eye, it was suggested that in cases of accidental eye contamination with dithranol triacetate a mild alkaline irrigation be used.— H. Yarrow, *Dermal Laboratories* (letter), *Lancet*, 1967, *2*, 311.

Uses. Dithranol triacetate is hydrolysed in contact with water to form the active diacetyl compound. It is used in the treatment of psoriasis as a 3% paste applied to the moistened lesions or as a cream or lotion.

Of 41 patients with psoriasis who were treated with a paste containing dithranol triacetate, 25 were cleared of psoriasis or greatly improved. Only 1 patient showed a sensitivity reaction to the paste. Dithranol triacetate had a less intense action than dithranol, and failures among patients using it were attributed to this as well as incorrect use.— F. F. Hellier and M. Whitefield, *Br. J. Derm.*, 1967, *79*, 491.

An evaluation of dithranol triacetate.— *Br. med. J.*, 1967, *1*, 682.

A comparison of dithranol and dithranol triacetate.— C. Hodgson and E. Hell, *Br. J. Derm.*, 1970, *83*, 397.

Proprietary Preparations

Exolan *(Dermal Laboratories, UK)*. Dithranol triacetate, available as cream containing 1%. **Exolan Lotion.** Contains dithranol triacetate 0.1%, coal tar extract 5%, and lecithin 0.4%.

1608-p

Enoxolone. Glycyrrhetinic Acid; Glycyrrhetic Acid. 3β-Hydroxy-11-oxo-olean-12-en-30-oic acid.

$C_{30}H_{46}O_4$=470.7.

CAS — 471-53-4.

A complex triterpene prepared by hydrolysis of glycyrrhizinic acid, a glycoside found in liquorice. The structure of enoxolone bears some resemblance to that of cortisone and there is evidence of the existence of at least 2 isomers.

A white or faintly cream-coloured powder. Very sparingly **soluble** in water; soluble in alcohol, acetone, ether, and methyl alcohol; readily soluble in chloroform.

The active isomers of enoxolone have an anti-inflammatory action and have been used in ointments containing 2% in the treatment of various skin diseases.

Proprietary Names

PO 12 *(Biothérax, Fr.)*.

1609-s

Etretinate.

Ro 10-9359. Ethyl 3-methoxy-15-apo-φ-caroten-15-oate; Ethyl (*all-trans*)-9-(4-methoxy-2,3,6-trimethylphenyl)-3,7-dimethylnona-2,4,6,8-tetraenoate.

$C_{23}H_{30}O_3$=354.5.

CAS — 54350-48-0.

Adverse Effects and Precautions. Side-effects reported following the use of etretinate include dryness of mucous membranes, hair loss, and paronychia.

Etretinate is teratogenic; pregnancy must be avoided during, and for 12 months after cessation of, therapy.

Etretinate is contra-indicated in patients with hepatic or renal impairment; liver-function tests are recommended for patients receiving etretinate therapy.

Patients receiving etretinate should be instructed to avoid dietary supplements of vitamin A.

Cheilitis in 4, dry lips in 2, and paronychia in 2 of 12 patients receiving etretinate.— C. E. Orfanos and U. Runne, *Br. J. Derm.*, 1976, *95*, 101.

Hair loss, paronychia, and elevation of transaminases caused 14% of 196 patients with psoriasis receiving etretinate to stop therapy.— C. E. Orfanos and G. Goerz, *Dt. med. Wschr.*, 1978, *103*, 195.

In a study in over 200 patients with psoriasis given etretinate 76 experienced some hair loss. This usually occurred 5 to 8 weeks after starting therapy after a mean cumulative dose of 1.9 g. Only 4 patients experienced total hair loss. No significant effect on liver function was noted although serum aspartate aminotransferase (SGOT) and serum alanine aminotransferase (SGPT) increased in some individuals. There was no evidence for an increase in light sensitivity after 3 weeks of treatment.— G. Mahrle *et al.*, *Dt. med. Wschr.*, 1979, *104*, 473.

Of 8 patients given etretinate for acne 7 showed mild cheilitis, 5 demonstrated palmar desquamation, and one had diffuse loss of scalp hair which regrew when the drug was stopped. One patient withdrew because of generalised desquamation and erythema.— R. M. MacKie and D. C. Dick (letter), *Lancet*, 1980, *2*, 1300.

Raised plasma lipids associated with etretinate.— G. Michaëlsson *et al.*, *Br. J. Derm.*, 1981, *105*, 201.

Uses. Etretinate is a derivative of tretinoin (p.508). It is given by mouth in the treatment of psoriasis and various other skin disorders.

The recommended initial dosage of etretinate is 0.75 to 1 mg per kg body-weight daily in divided doses (usually 50 to 75 mg daily). If no response has been obtained after 4 weeks this dose may be increased in steps of 10 mg weekly to a maximum total daily dose of 1.5 mg per kg. When a response has been obtained the dosage should be reduced to 0.5 mg per kg daily and taken for a further 6 to 8 weeks.

Comment on the value of etretinate.— *Lancet*, 1981, *1*, 537.

A report of a favourable and rapid response lasting for about 3 months in 1 patient with subcorneal pustular dermatosis to treatment with etretinate in doses of 75 mg daily. The condition did not respond to treatment with corticosteroids, dapsone, levamisole, sulphapyridine or vitamin E. Tretinoin given later caused some reduction in pustules but the patient's condition deteriorated. Side-effects due to etretinate included dry dermatitis of the lips, scaling of unaffected skin and development of haemorrhagic scabs on the lower legs.— E. Folkers and J. Trafelkruyer, *Br. J. Derm.*, 1978, *98*, 681.

Etretinate 1.5 mg per kg body-weight daily in divided doses, reduced gradually after 3 weeks to 300 µg per kg daily caused sequestering of horny skin in 4 patients with epidermolytic hereditary palmaplantar keratoderma, leaving normal-appearing skin with normal surface sensitivity. Side-effects included drowsiness, anorexia and diffuse hair loss, occurring 6 to 8 weeks after treatment. Skin vulnerability experienced by the patients who were manual workers, led to treatment being discontinued.— P. Fritsch *et al.*, *Br. J. Derm.*, 1978, *99*, 561.

A report of the successful use of etretinate in doses of from 25 to 100 mg daily for maintenance treatment of ichthyosis in 5 patients aged 5 to 17 years.— H. Pehamberger *et al.*, *Br. J. Derm.*, 1978, *99*, 319.

Treatment of disseminated superficial actinic porokeratosis with etretinate.— A. -L. Kariniemi *et al.*, *Br. J. Derm.*, 1980, *102*, 213. See also S. Bundino and A. M. Zina, *Dermatologica*, 1980, *160*, 328 (disseminated porokeratosis Mibelli); M. Moriarty *et al.*, *Lancet*, 1982, *1*, 364.

Severe papillomavirus type 5-induced epidermodysplasia verruciformis in a 32-year-old man was treated successfully with etretinate 1 mg per kg body-weight daily by mouth. After 2 months most of his flat wart-like lesions had disappeared, plaques were repigmenting and no longer scaly, and 2 tumours at the inguinal-scrotal margin were much reduced in size. The patient appears to be almost free of causative virus.— M. A. Lutzner and C. Blanchet-Bardon (letter), *New Engl. J. Med.*, 1980, *302*, 1091.

Beneficial results with a synthetic retinoid, etretinate in the treatment of acne. Etretinate was given for 8 weeks at a daily dose of 1 mg per kg body-weight to 8 male patients with severe acne of 2 to 11 years' duration. Of 7 completing the study, 6 showed improvement when assessed photographically, and 5 had fewer acne lesions. Sebum excretion-rate was not measured because it has been reported that the dramatic reduction in sebaceous gland size, observed in patients receiving isotretinoin, is not seen with etretinate.— R. M. MacKie and D. C.

Dick (letter), *Lancet*, 1980, *2*, 1300.

Further references to the use of etretinate in skin disorders: T. Fredriksson and U. Pettersson, *Dermatologica*, 1979, *158*, 60 (pustulosis palmo-plantaris); F. de Mari *et al.* (letter), *Lancet*, 1981, *2*, 936 (bowenoid papulosis of the genitalia); C. Blanchet-Bardon *et al.* (letter), *ibid.*, 1348 (no response in 2 patients with bowenoid papulosis).

Psoriasis. Etretinate given in doses of 75 to 125 mg daily for 2 to 6 weeks and used in conjunction with local treatment with ointment containing salicylic acid 2% in soft paraffin, alone or with added dithranol 0.1%, caused full remission of widespread psoriasis in 5 of 12 male patients aged 21 to 81 years; 4 other patients had 75% flattening of lesions.— C. E. Orfanos and U. Runne, *Br. J. Derm.*, 1976, *95*, 101.

Etretinate up to 100 mg daily by mouth resulted in improvement ranging from satisfactory to excellent in 39 of 55 patients treated for psoriasis and various keratinising dermatoses.— F. Ott, *Schweiz. med. Wschr.*, 1977, *107*, 144.

Of 196 patients with various types of psoriasis given etretinate 1 mg per kg body-weight daily by mouth for 3 to 4 weeks then gradually reduced to 500 µg per kg daily and continued for 6 months 120 had a good response, 45 a moderate response, and 31 no response. In most cases improvement was seen after 2 to 3 weeks of therapy but relapses occurred during long-term treatment. Severe erythrodermic and pustular psoriasis responded particularly well.— C. E. Orfanos and G. Goerz, *Dt. med. Wschr.*, 1978, *103*, 195.

The use of etretinate and ultraviolet-B radiation in the treatment of psoriasis.— C. E. Orfanos *et al.*, *Acta derm.-vener., Stockh.*, 1979, *59*, 241.

Combined treatment of psoriasis with etretinate in low dosage orally and triamcinolone acetonide cream topically.— H. J. Van Der Rhee *et al.*, *Br. J. Derm.*, 1980, *102*, 203.

Further references: B. Dahl *et al.*, *Dermatologica*, 1977, *154*, 261; T. Fredriksson and U. Pettersson, *Dermatologica*, 1978, *157*, 238; A. Lassus, *Br. J. Derm.*, 1980, *102*, 195.

For reports of the use of etretinate with PUVA therapy in psoriasis, see Methoxsalen, p.498.

Proprietary Preparations

Tigason *(Roche, UK)*. Etretinate, available as capsules of 10 and 25 mg.

1610-h

Fuller's Earth *(B.P.C. 1959)*. Terra Fullonica.

CAS — 8031-18-3.

Consists largely of montmorillonite, a native hydrated aluminium silicate, with which very finely divided calcite (calcium carbonate) may be associated.

A fine odourless tasteless powder, varying in colour from almost white to blue-grey or green. Soft and unctuous to the touch. Practically **insoluble** in water and organic solvents; partly soluble in hydrochloric acid. **Sterilised** by maintaining at 150° for 1 hour.

Fuller's earth is an adsorbent which is used chiefly in dusting-powders and toilet powders. Fuller's earth of high adsorptive capacity is used in industry as a clarifying and filtering medium.

It has been used in the treatment of paraquat poisoning.

Preparations

Fuller's Earth Lotion *(Roy. Hallamshire Hosp.)*. Lot. Terr. Silic. Fuller's earth 4.5 g, zinc oxide 4.5 g, glycerol 2 ml, water to 100 ml. Used in dermatitis and eczema. A double-strength lotion, for dilution before use, is sometimes supplied. **Fuller's Earth and Coal Tar Lotion**. Lot. Terr. Silic. et Pic. Coal tar 250 mg, fuller's earth lotion to 100 ml. **Fuller's Earth and Lead Lotion**. Lot. Terr. Silic. et Plumb. Equal quantities of lead lotion and fuller's earth lotion.

Fuller's Earth (Surrey Finest Grade) *(Laporte, UK: ICI Plant Protection, UK)*. Sterilised fuller's earth, suitable for the treatment of paraquat poisoning.

1611-m

Guaiazulene. 1,4-Dimethyl-7-isopropylazulene.
$C_{15}H_{18}$=198.3.

CAS — 489-84-9.

Blue crystals or liquid. Practically **insoluble** in water; poorly soluble in alcohol; soluble in chloroform, ether, fixed and essential oils, and many organic solvents.

Guaiazulene has been reported to have anti-allergic, anti-inflammatory, antipyretic, and antileprotic properties.

Proprietary Names

Azulon *(Homburg, Ger.; Armour, Ital.)*; AZ8 Beris *(Weimer, Ger.)*; Gastrozulen *(Szama, Arg.)*; Szamazulen *(Szama, Arg.)*.

A preparation containing guaiazulene was formerly marketed in Great Britain under the proprietary name Azilex (*Ingasetter*).

1612-b

Hydroquinone *(U.S.P.)*. Quinol; Hydrochinonum. Benzene-1,4-diol.
$C_6H_6O_2$=110.1.

CAS — 123-31-9.

Pharmacopoeias. In *Belg.*, *Braz.*, *Hung.*, and *U.S.*

Fine white crystals or white crystalline powder which darken on exposure to light and air. M.p. 172° to 174°. **Soluble** 1 in 17 of water, 1 in 4 of alcohol, 1 in 51 of chloroform, 1 in 16 of ether, and 1 in 1 of glycerol. **Incompatible** with alkalis, ferric salts, and oxidising agents. **Store** in airtight containers. Protect from light.

Adverse Effects and Treatment. Hydroquinone is irritant and has caused conjunctival changes and depigmentation. Systemic effects are similar to those of phenol (see p.571) and are treated similarly.

Maximum permissible atmospheric concentration 2 mg per m³.

A report of pigmented colloid milium and ochronosis in 35 black women after the use for several years of strong hydroquinone creams in skin areas exposed to sunlight. There was little regresssion after a year or more.— G. H. Findlay *et al.*, *Br. J. Derm.*, 1975, *93*, 613.

In black women hydroquinone 3.5% or 5% creams produced considerably more reactions than lotions of the same strength. Delayed hyperpigmentary reactions and contact-type erythema progressing to hyperpigmentation were the most common reaction. A 3% preparation, regardless of basis, was regarded as the optimum.— B. Bentley-Phillips and M. A. H. Bayles, *S.Afr. med. J.*, 1975, *49*, 1391.

Uses. Hydroquinone is used as a depigmenting agent for the skin in the form of a 2 to 5% ointment. It should be applied only to intact skin. It is also used as an antoxidant for ether and in photographic developers.

The use of hydroquinone in cosmetics and toiletries in Great Britain is controlled under The Cosmetic Products Regulations 1978 (SI 1978: No. 1354).

Reviews of the effects of hydroquinone and other skin lightening agents: B. N. Hemsworth, *J. Soc. cosmet. Chem.*, 1973, *24*, 727; S. S. Bleehen, *ibid.*, 1977, *28*, 407.

Hydroquinone reduced hyperpigmentation in all races by interfering with the tyrosine-tyrosinase-melanin system and had been used as a topical application in 93 patients.— T. B. Fitzpatrick *et al.*, *Archs Derm.*, 1966, *93*, 589, per *J. Am. med. Ass.*, 1966, *196* (May 16), A172.

Twice daily applications for 4 months of an ointment containing 2% of hydroquinone in a hydrophilic basis reduced hyperpigmentation by one-half or more in 8 of 20 patients.— J. Albert and R. I. Goldberg, *Clin. Med.*, 1966, *73* (Mar.), 87.

An ointment containing hydroquinone 5%, tretinoin 0.1%, and dexamethasone 0.1% reduced skin pigmentation in 16 of 19 white women with chloasma associated with oral contraceptives and in 8 of 11 black men with pseudofolliculitis; some improvement was also seen in 25 black patients with acne. The ointment was applied once or twice daily for 2 to 3 months.— O. H. Mills and A. M. Kligman, *J. Soc. cosmet. Chem.*, 1978, *29*, 147.

Preparations

HRH Lotion *(Roy. Hallamshire Hosp.)*. Hydrocortisone 1 g, tretinoin 100 mg, hydroquinone 5 g, butylated hydroxytoluene 50 mg, sodium metabisulphite 100 mg, water 0.4 ml, base solution consisting of equal parts dehydrated alcohol and macrogol 400 to 100 ml. Dissolve the sodium metabisulphite in the water, the rest of the solids in the base solution, then mix. Store in a cool place in airtight containers. Protect from light. Shelf-life up to 6 months. For use as a depigmenting agent.

Hydroquinone Cream *(U.S.P.)*. A cream containing hydroquinone. Protect from light.

Paraffin ointment was found to be a suitable basis, in terms of colour stability, for an ointment containing hydroquinone 2% for skin depigmentation. Hydroquinone 2% in macrogol ointment developed a pink discoloration within 7 days.— Pharm. Soc. Lab. Rep. No. P/68/20, 1968.

Proprietary Names

Eldopaque *(Elder, Canad.; Elder, USA)*; Eldoquin *(Elder, Canad.; Elder, USA)*; Phiaquin *(Robins, Austral.)*.

1613-v

Hydroxyquinoline. Oxine; Oxyquinoline; 8-Quinolinol. Quinolin-8-ol.
C_9H_7NO=145.2.

CAS — 148-24-3.

A white or faintly yellow crystalline powder with a pleasant characteristic odour.

Soluble 1 in 1500 of water; soluble in alcohol, acetone, chloroform, glycerol, fixed oils, liquid paraffin, and mineral acids. **Incompatible** with many metal ions. **Store** in a cool place and avoid contact with metal. Protect from light.

Hydroxyquinoline has properties similar to those of potassium hydroxyquinoline sulphate (see p.500) and has been used for similar purposes. A dusting-powder containing 0.1% has been used as a deodorant.

The use of hydroxyquinoline in cosmetics and toiletries in Great Britain is controlled under The Cosmetic Products Regulations 1978 (SI 1978: No. 1354).

Hydroxyquinoline, and its copper derivative, completely inhibited *in vitro* the growth of the yeast *Malassezia ovalis*, which was associated with dandruff.— J. Brotherton, *Br. J. Derm.*, 1968, *80*, 749.

Hydroxyquinoline and some of its analogues inhibited dental plaque formation *in vitro*.— V. D. Warner *et al.*, *J. pharm. Sci.*, 1975, *64*, 1563.

1614-g

Hydroxyquinoline Sulphate. Chinosolum; Oxine Sulphate; Oxichinolini Sulfas; Oxyquinol; Oxyquinoline Sulphate; 8-Quinolinol Sulphate; Sulfate d'Orthoxyquinoléine. Quinolin-8-ol sulphate.
$(C_9H_7NO)_2,H_2SO_4$=388.4.

CAS — 134-31-6.

Pharmacopoeias. In *Belg.*, *Rus.*, and *Swiss. Fr.* and *Nord.* specify monohydrate.

A light yellow powder with a slight saffron-like odour and a burning taste. M.p. about 178°.

Soluble 1 in 1 of water and 1 in 100 of alcohol; sparingly soluble in glycerol; practically insoluble in chloroform and ether. **Incompatible** with alkalis, iodine, oxidising agents, and many metal ions. **Store** in a cool place and avoid contact with metal. Protect from light.

Hydroxyquinoline sulphate has properties similar to those of potassium hydroxyquinoline sulphate (see p.500) and has been used for similar purposes.

It has been used for preserving syrups in a concentrations of 0.001% and has also been used as an antoxidant synergist since it forms complexes with some heavy metals and thus inhibits catalysis of oxidation by them.

Several iodinated derivatives of hydroxyquinoline are used in the treatment of amoebiasis (see p.968); some of these, notably iodochlorhydroxyquinoline (clioquinol, p.976), are also applied topically in the management of skin infections.

The use of hydroxyquinoline sulphate in cosmetics and toiletries in Great Britain is controlled under The Cosmetic Products Regulations 1978 (SI 1978: No. 1354).

The degree of interaction between hydroxyquinoline sulphate and tuberculin purified protein derivative was small and the preservative activity of hydroxyquinoline sulphate was not reduced.— H. R. Held and S. Landi, *J. pharm. Sci.*, 1974, *63*, 1205.

Proprietary Names

Oxykin *(DAK, Denm.)*; Semori*(Luitpold, Switz.)*; Sérorhinol *(Goupil, Fr.)*; Superol *(Superol, Neth.*; *Superol, S.Afr.)*.

1615-q

Ichthammol *(B.P.)*.

Ammonium Ichthosulphonate; Ammonium Sulpho-Ichthyolate; Ichthyolammonium; Bithyol; Bituminol; Ichthosulphol; Ichthyol; Sulphonated Bitumen; Ammonium Bithiolicum; Ammonium Sulfobituminosum; Ammonium Bituminosulfonicum; Bithiolate Ammonique; Ammonio Sulfoittiolato.

CAS — 8029-68-3.

Pharmacopoeias. In *Arg., Aust., Belg., Br., Chin., Cz., Fr., Ger., Hung., Ind., It., Jap., Jug., Mex., Neth., Nord., Port., Roum., Span., Swiss, Turk.,* and *U.S.*

A reddish-brown to almost black viscous liquid with a strong characteristic empyreumatic odour. It consists mainly of the ammonium salts of the sulphonic acids of an oily substance prepared from the destructive distillation of a bituminous schist or shale, together with ammonium sulphate (about 5 to 7%). It contains not less than 10.5% of organically combined sulphur, calculated on the dried material, of which not more than 25% is in the form of sulphates. It loses not more than 50% of its weight on drying.

Soluble in water; partly soluble in alcohol and ether; soluble in a mixture of equal parts of alcohol and ether; soluble 1 in 9 of glycerol; miscible with soft paraffin, lanolin, and other fats; immiscible with fixed oils and liquid paraffin. **Incompatible** with acids, alkalis, alkaloids, iodides, and salts of iron and lead.

The addition of 2% of a sample of ichthammol to Zinc Cream caused gross separation within 7 days; a second sample of ichthammol gave a stable homogeneous product.—Pharm. Soc. Lab. Rep., *Pharm. J.*, 1961, *2*, 187.

Uses. Ichthammol has only slight bacteriostatic properties; it is slightly irritant to the skin. It has been used in creams and ointments in the treatment of chronic skin diseases. Ichthammol Glycerin is used as ear-drops in inflammatory conditions of the external ear. Tampons of Ichthammol Glycerin or Ichthammol Pessaries are used in cervicitis and vaginitis.

Of 836 persons with dermatitis or eczema submitted to patch testing with ichthammol 5% in yellow soft paraffin, 2.7% gave a positive reaction.— E. Rudzki and D. Kleniewska, *Br. J. Derm.*, 1970, *83*, 543.

Preparations

Creams

Ichthammol and Zinc Cream Oily *(A.P.F.)*. Oily Ichthammol Cream. Ichthammol 5 g, wool fat 15 g, and zinc cream oily 80 g.

Ichthammol Cream. Ichthammol 2 g, calamine 4 g, zinc oxide 3 g, isopropyl myristate 20 g, cetomacrogol emulsifying wax 10 g, white soft paraffin 10 g, chlorocresol 100 mg or phenylmercuric nitrate 5 mg, water to 100 g. Dissolve the chlorocresol (or phenylmercuric nitrate) in 50 ml of hot water and add the ichthammol; stir until homogeneous and disperse the calamine and zinc oxide. Melt together the cetomacrogol emulsifying wax, white soft paraffin, and isopropyl myristate, and add to the aqueous phase at about 60°. Adjust to the final weight with water and stir until cold.—Pharm. Soc. Lab. Rep. No. P/66/27, 1966.

Gelatins

Ichthammol Gelatin *(B.P.C. 1949)*. Ichthammol Jelly; Ammonium Ichthosulphonate Jelly; Ammonium Ichthosulphonate Paste; Ichthammol Paste. Ichthammol 10 g, gelatin 10 g, glycerol 60 g, and water 25 ml. It should be freshly prepared.

Zinc and Ichthammol Gelatin *(B.P.C. 1959)*. Zinc Oxide and Ichthammol Gelatin; Unna's Paste with Ichthammol; Pasta Zinci Oxidi et Ichthammolis. Ichthammol 2 g, zinc oxide 15 g, gelatin 15 g, glycerol 35 g, and water 35 ml. The preparation should be melted by standing the container in hot water, and applied to the skin with a brush, the film produced being covered with a suitable protective.

Glycerins

Ichthammol Glycerin *(B.P.C. 1973)*. Glycerin of Ammonium Ichthosulphonate; Ichthammol Ear Drops *(A.P.F.)*; Ichthammol Paint *(A.P.F.)*. Ichthammol 10% w/w in glycerol.

Lotions

Ichthammol and Calamine Lotion. Ichthammol 2 g, calamine 3 g, linseed oil 28 ml, and lime water 28 ml. Triturate the calamine with the oil until smooth and emulsify with about half of the lime water; disperse the ichthammol in the remainder of the lime water, pour this mixture into the emulsion, and shake vigorously.—Pharm. Soc. Lab. Rep., *Pharm. J.*, 1960, *2*, 454.

Ointments

Ichthammol Ointment *(B.P.)*. Ichthammol 10 g, wool fat 45 g, and yellow soft paraffin 45 g. Store at a temperature not exceeding 25°.

U.S.P. has ichthammol 10, wool fat 10, and yellow soft paraffin 80.

Pessaries

Ichthammol Pessaries *(B.P.C. 1968)*. Pessi Ichthammolis. Prepared by mixing ichthammol with Glycerol Suppositories mass. Unless otherwise specified, pessaries each containing 5% w/w of ichthammol and prepared in 8-g moulds are supplied. They should be recently prepared.

A.P.F. has ichthammol 5% w/w in Glyco-gelatin Gel; each weighs 4 to 5 g.

NOTE. Ichthammol pessaries in a glycerol-gelatin basis must not be overheated or they may become insoluble.

Suppositories

Ichthammol Suppositories *(B.P.C. 1949)*. Supp. Ichtham. Ichthammol 195 mg in Glycerol Suppositories mass sufficient to fill a 1-g mould. They should be freshly prepared.

Suppositories are sometimes made with a basis of theobroma oil; the mixture must be almost set when poured into the mould, otherwise it may separate.

NOTE. Ichthammol suppositories in a glycerol-gelatin basis must not be overheated or they may become insoluble.

Proprietary Names

Adnexol *(Protina, Ger.)*; Bitamon *(Cooper, Switz.)*; Ichthalon *(Ichthyol, Switz.)*; Ichtho-Bad *(Ichthyol, Switz.)*; Ichtho-Cutan *(sodium bituminosulphonate) (Ichthyol, Ger.)*; Ichtholan *(Ichthyol, Ger.)*; Ichthraletten *(Ichthyol, Switz.)*; Ichtopur *(Ichthyol, Ger.)*; Poudre Velours *(Alcon-Couvreur, Belg.)*.

1616-p

Isotretinoin.

Ro 4-3780; 13-*cis*-Retinoic Acid. The 13-*cis*-isomer of retinoic acid (see Tretinoin, p.508).

CAS — 4759-48-2.

Isotretinoin has been used in the treatment of acne and keratinising disorders of the skin, and appears to be less toxic than tretinoin.

Possible use of isotretinoin for the prevention of neoplastic disease in patients at high risk or following resection.— *J. Am. med. Ass.*, 1976, *235*, 1409. See also *J. Am. med. Ass.*, 1978, *240*, 609.

Treatment with isotretinoin, in an initial dose of 1 mg per kg body-weight daily in divided doses increasing at 2 to 3 weekly intervals, was effective in the treatment of some chronic keratinising dermatoses resistant to other treatment. All of 5 patients with lamellar ichthyosis achieved excellent improvement as did 2 of 3 with Darier's disease and one with pityriasis rubra pilaris. Side-effects included cheilitis in 9 of 13 treated and dry nasal mucosa in 2. One patient experienced ocular irritation, blurred vision, arthralgias, and facial dermatitis; all symptoms subsided when treatment was stopped.— G. L. Peck and F. W. Yoder (preliminary communication), *Lancet*, 1976, *2*, 1172. See also *J. Am. med. Ass.*, 1977, *238*, 472.

Treatment for 4 months with isotretinoin was successfully used in 14 patients suffering from severe treatment-resistant acne. An initial dose of 1 mg per kg body-weight daily by mouth was gradually increased to an average of 2 mg per kg daily (range 1 to 3.3 mg per kg) in divided doses. Acne was completely cleared in 13 of the patients; 9 were free of lesions at the end of the 4-month treatment period, 3 during the first 2 months after treatment ended, and one in the tenth month after treatment ended. The remaining patient had a 75% response. In general, facial lesions disappeared rapidly during the first month of treatment whereas those on the trunk, especially in men, took 3 to 4 months to involute. Prolonged remissions averaging 16 months had been noted in all patients and 11 were still completely free of lesions. Treatment was generally well-tolerated but cheilitis and facial dermatitis occurred in all patients and xerosis in 12. Other side-effects included: dry nasal mucosa (9), minor nosebleed (7), conjunctivitis (7), skin fragility (5), and inflamed urethral meatus (2 males). Serum-aminotransferase concentrations were raised transiently in 2 patients. An inhibitory effect on the sebaceous gland was thought to be the probable mode of action of isotretinoin.— G. L. Peck *et al.*, *New Engl. J. Med.*, 1979, *300*, 329. Comments.— P. E. Pochi, *ibid.*, 359; *Lancet*, 1979, *1*, 1222.

In a double-blind dose-response study 8 patients with severe acne unresponsive to conventional therapy received isotretinoin in doses of 100 µg per kg body-weight daily or 0.5 to 1 mg per kg daily. A 75% reduction in sebum excretion-rate was obtained at 4 weeks and all patients had an 80% reduction in their overall acne severity after 16 weeks. Those receiving the high dose of isotretinoin had a greater reduction in sebum-excretion rate, although the clinical response, when expressed as a percentage change, was the same. Clinical side-effects were dose related, the commonest ones being facial dermatitis, xerosis, and cheilitis; one patient developed arthralgia which necessitated dosage reduction from 1 to 0.1 mg per kg daily (the acne continuing to improve on this dose, with no increase in sebum excretion-rate); only one patient had a raised serum-triglyceride concentration, and one with a raised concentration on admission showed no further rise during treatment. Two patients with inflammatory skin diseases (hidradenitis suppurativa and steatocystoma multiplex) who were also treated with isotretinoin, showed no improvement.— H. Jones *et al.*, *Lancet*, 1980, *2*, 1048. Comment.— R. M. MacKie and D. C. Dick (letter), *ibid.*, 1300. See also *Lancet*, 1981, *1*, 537.

Multiple keratoacanthomas in a 43-year-old man responded dramatically to treatment with isotretinoin by mouth. An initial dose of isotretinoin 2 mg per kg body-weight daily was increased weekly until a dose of 6 mg per kg daily was reached in the third week and was continued for the remaining 13 weeks of the study. Adverse effects noted included mild cheilitis, bilateral conjunctivitis, and urethritis. The patient was subsequently given isotretinoin in a maintenance dose of 2 mg per kg daily and has had no new lesions for 18 months; the majority of his remaining lesions were excised surgically without recurrence. The only persistent adverse effect has been a mild cheilitis.— R. P. Haydey *et al.*, *New Engl. J. Med.*, 1980, *303*, 560.

Manufacturers

Roche, UK.

1617-s

Lauroyldiacetylpyridoxine.

L 3763; 3-Lauroyl-4,5-diacetylpyridoxine. 4,5-Bis(acetoxymethyl)-2-methyl-3-pyridyl dodecanoate.

$C_{24}H_{37}NO_6$=435.6.

CAS — 1562-13-6.

Crystals. M.p. 44°. Practically **insoluble** in water; soluble in alcohol, chloroform, ether, and ethylene dichloride.

Lauroyldiacetylpyridoxine is used as a 2% alcoholic solution in the treatment of seborrhoeic dermatitis.

Proprietary Names

Epixine*(Labaz, Belg.*; *Labaz, Fr.)*; Epixyne *(Petersen, S.Afr.)*.

1618-w

Lycopodium *(B.P.C. 1949)*.

Vegetable Sulphur; Bärlappspore.

CAS — 8023-70-9.

Pharmacopoeias. In *Aust., Chin., Cz., Pol., Port.,*

Roum., and *Rus.*

The spores of the clubmoss, *Lycopodium clavatum* (Lycopodiaceae). A pale yellow, very mobile, light powder.

Lycopodium has been used as a dusting-powder for the skin, as a diluent for insufflations for the throat, nose, and ears, and as the basis for medicated snuffs. It was formerly employed as a covering for pills.
Lycopodium is used in quantitative microscopy.
Lycopodium is used in homoeopathic medicine.

1619-e

Mequinol. Hydroquinone Monomethyl Ether. 4-Methoxyphenol.
$C_7H_8O_2$=124.1.

CAS — 150-76-5.

Mequinol is used similarly to monobenzone (see p.499), usually as a 10% cream, in the treatment of hyperpigmentation.

Proprietary Names
Leucobasal *(Biobasal, Switz.)*; Leucodinine B *(Promedica, Fr.)*; Novo-Dermoquinona *(Promesa, Spain)*.

1620-b

Ammoniated Mercury *(U.S.P., B.P. 1973)*.

Hydrargyrum Ammoniatum; Hydrargyri Aminochloridum; Aminomercuric Chloride; Mercuric Ammonium Chloride; Mercury Aminochloride; White Precipitate; Hydrargyrum Amidochloratum; Hydrargyrum Praecipitatum Album.
NH_2HgCl=252.1.

CAS — 10124-48-8.

Pharmacopoeias. In *Aust., Belg., Chin., Cz., Hung., Ind., Int., Jug., Pol., Rus., Turk.*, and *U.S.*
Several pharmacopoeias assign the synonym 'White Precipitate' to Precipitated Mercurous Chloride.

A white odourless powder with an earthy metallic taste. Practically **insoluble** in water, alcohol, and ether; soluble in warm hydrochloric, nitric, and acetic acids, and in solutions of ammonium salts. It is decomposed slowly by warm water and rapidly by boiling water with the formation of a yellow basic compound, NH_2HgCl,HgO. **Incompatible** with alkalis, iodides, and sodium thiosulphate. **Protect** from light.

Adverse Effects and Treatment. As for Mercury, pp.937-8. The topical application of preparations containing ammoniated mercury has resulted in acrodynia and mercury poisoning.

Of 70 patients treated with a 10% ammoniated mercury ointment for psoriasis nearly one-half showed clear evidence of mercury poisoning which included, among other signs, albuminuria, colic, gingivitis, tremors, and erythroderma.— E. Young, *Br. J. Derm.*, 1960, *72*, 449, per *Abstr. Wld Med.*, 1961, *30*, 66.

Acrodynia. Reports of acrodynia.— M. E. R. Stoneman, *Lancet*, 1958, *1*, 938; N. Kesaree (letter), *Br. med. J.*, 1966, *1*, 1111; H. Viani, *Br. J. Derm.*, 1967, *79*, 712.

Hypersensitivity. In a modified 'repeated-insult' patch test, 25% ammoniated mercury was found to produce moderate sensitisation of the skin.— A. M. Kligman, *J. invest. Derm.*, 1966, *47*, 393.

From patch tests carried out in 413 patients with contact dermatoses, 5 were possibly allergic to ammoniated mercury.— E. Epstein, *J. Am. med. Ass.*, 1966, *198*, 517.

Nephrotic syndrome. Of 60 patients (16 men, 44 women) aged 15 to 56 with the nephrotic syndrome, 53% (70% of the women) were using skin-lightening creams containing 5 to 10% of ammoniated mercury or had used such creams. Concentrations of mercury in urine were 90 to 250 ng per ml (mean 150) for those using the creams and 0 to 90 ng per ml (mean 29) for those who had used them. The upper limit for normal was 80 ng per ml. Of 26 patients followed up for 6 months to 2 years, 10 had spontaneous remissions, 2 had remissions after treatment with corticosteroids, and 1 after treatment with cyclophosphamide; 13 did not respond to treatment.— R. D. Barr *et al.*, *Br. med. J.*, 1972, *2*, 131.

Further references: J. L. Turk and H. Baker, *Br. J. Derm.*, 1968, *80*, 623; *Drug Cosmet. Ind.*, 1972, *111* (July), 38; J. W. Kibukamusoke *et al.*, *Br. med. J.*, 1974, *2*, 646.

Neuropathy. A 4-year-old boy was treated with ammoniated mercury ointment for 2 months and developed progressive difficulty in walking. Apart from motor polyneuropathy he developed irritability and eosinophilia. The CSF had a protein content of 1.98 mg per ml and there was also an increase in urinary mercury. He was given dimercaprol to a total dosage of 1.607 g and finally recovered except for absent Achilles reflexes.— A. T. Ross, *J. Am. med. Ass.*, 1964, *188*, 830.

Renal tubular acidosis. Renal tubular acidosis occurred in a 9-month-old girl following the use of 2.5% ammoniated mercury ointment for napkin rash. She recovered after treatment with sodium bicarbonate, dimercaprol, and penicillamine.— P. Husband and W. J. D. McKellar, *Archs Dis. Childh.*, 1970, *45*, 264.

Precautions. Preparations of ammoniated mercury should not be applied to infants and young children as they may cause acrodynia (pink disease). They should not be applied to raw surfaces.

Uses. It is used for external application in ointment form. Ammoniated Mercury Ointment has been applied to the perianal region to destroy threadworms and prevent reinfection; it was formerly used in the treatment of impetigo and other staphylococcal skin infections. The topical application of mercurial preparations is generally considered undesirable.

Psoriasis, particularly of the palms and soles, and of the hyperkeratotic variety, responded better to ammoniated mercury than to steroids. At times it was the only effective treatment.— A. B. Hyman and A. R. Shalita (letter), *New Engl. J. Med.*, 1968, *278*, 337.

Preparations

Adamson's Ointment. Ammoniated mercury 4, salicylic acid 4, coal tar solution 12, paraffin ointment to 100, all by wt.
NOTE. Variations of this formula have been used; some did not contain ammoniated mercury.

Ammoniated Mercury and Coal Tar Ointment *(B.P.C. 1973)*. Unguentum Hydrargyri Ammoniati et Picis Carbonis; Unguentum Picis Carbonis Compositum; Compound Ointment of Coal Tar. Ammoniated mercury 2.5 g, strong coal tar solution 2.5 g, and yellow soft paraffin 95 g. Store in containers which prevent evaporation.

Ammoniated Mercury, Coal Tar, and Salicylic Acid Ointment *(B.P.C. 1973)*. Unguentum Hydrargyri Ammoniati et Picis Carbonis cum Acido Salicylico. Salicylic acid 2 g, ammoniated mercury and coal tar ointment to 100 g. Store in containers which prevent evaporation.

Ammoniated Mercury Ointment *(B.P. 1973)*. Ammon. Mercury Oint.; Ung. Hydrarg. Ammon.; Dilute Ammoniated Mercury Ointment; White Precipitate Ointment; Ung. Hyd. Ammon. Dil. Ammoniated mercury 2.5% in simple ointment.
A similar ointment, usually 5 or 10%, is included in several other pharmacopoeias.

Ammoniated Mercury Ointment *(U.S.P.)*. Contains ammoniated mercury in a suitable oleaginous ointment basis. Protect from light.

Ammoniated Mercury Ophthalmic Ointment *(U.S.P.)*. A sterile eye ointment containing ammoniated mercury in a suitable oleaginous basis.

Ammoniated Mercury, Salicylic Acid and Coal Tar Ointment *(A.P.F.)*. Ammoniated mercury 1 g, salicylic acid 3 g, strong coal tar solution 3 ml, white soft paraffin 50 g, emulsifying ointment to 100 g. The concentration of ammoniated mercury may be increased to 3% for application to limited areas.

Sewell's Oil. Ammoniated mercury ointment 40 g, liquid paraffin to 100 ml. Several other formulas are used.—*Chemist Drugg.*, 1957, *167*, 683.

1621-v

Oleated Mercury *(B.P.C. 1959)*. Hydrargyrum Oleatum; Mercury Oleate.

Pharmacopoeias. In *Ind.*, (as *B.P.C. 1959*); in *Mex.* (25% HgO).

Yellow mercuric oxide 20%, triturated with liquid paraffin 5%, then mixed with oleic acid 75% and heated at 50° until combination is effected. A yellowish unctuous mass. Practically **insoluble** in water; slightly soluble in alcohol and ether; readily soluble in fixed oils. **Protect** from light.

Oleated mercury has been employed in ointment form for uses similar to those of ammoniated mercury.

Preparations

Oleated Mercury Ointment *(B.P. 1953)*. Ung. Hydrarg. Oleat. Oleated mercury 25% in simple ointment; it contains the equivalent of 5% of HgO. Store in a cool place. Protect from light.

Oleated mercury was formerly marketed in Great Britain under the proprietary name Bralium Forte *(Hefa, Ger.)*.

1622-g

Mesulphen *(B.P.C. 1968)*. Mesulfen; Dimethylthianthrene; Dimethyldiphenylene Disulphide. It consists mainly of 2,7-dimethylthianthrene.
$C_{14}H_{12}S_2$=244.4.

CAS — 135-58-0.

Pharmacopoeias. In *Aust.* and *Nord.* Thiantholum (*Jap. P.*) is a mixture of 2,7-dimethylthianthrene and ditolyl disulphide.

A yellow, somewhat viscous, oily liquid with a slight not unpleasant odour, containing about 85 to 90% of dimethylthianthrene and about 25% of organically combined sulphur. Wt per ml 1.195 to 1.215 g. The deposit which frequently forms on standing in the cold should be dissolved by warming and the liquid thoroughly mixed before use. Practically **insoluble** in water; soluble 1 in 18 of alcohol; miscible with acetone, chloroform, ether, and light petroleum.

Mesulphen is a parasiticide and antipruritic agent and has been employed in the treatment of acne, pediculosis pubis, scabies, and seborrhoea. The affected parts are well cleaned and the undiluted mesulphen is applied, with vigorous rubbing, daily for 3 days.

Skin sensitivity to mesulphen, confirmed by patch tests, was seen in 2 patients during the period 1957/66.— J. K. Morgan, *Br. J. clin. Pract.*, 1968, *22*, 261.

Proprietary Names
Mitigal *(Hermal, Ger.*; *Bayropharm, Ital.*; *Bayer, Norw.)*; Soufrol *(Max Ritter, Switz.)*.

1623-q

Methoxsalen *(U.S.P.)*.

Ammoidin; 8-Methoxypsoralen; Metoxaleno; Xanthotoxin. 9-Methoxy-7*H*-furo[3,2-*g*]chromen-7-one.
$C_{12}H_8O_4$=216.2.

CAS — 298-81-7.

Pharmacopoeias. In *Braz.* and *U.S.*

A constituent of the fruits of *Ammi majus*. It occurs as white to cream-coloured, odourless, fluffy crystals. M.p. 143° to 148°.
Practically **insoluble** in water; sparingly soluble in boiling water and ether; freely soluble in chloroform; soluble in boiling alcohol, and in acetone, acetic acid, and propylene glycol. **Protect** from light.

Adverse Effects. Methoxsalen commonly causes nausea and less frequently vomiting, headache, oedema, dizziness, nervousness, insomnia, pruritus, mental excitation, and mental depression. Although methoxsalen is used as a photosensitiser, there may be undesirable skin reactions.
Local application may cause acute vesicular cutaneous photosensitisation. Acute dermatitis may also develop. Exposure to ultraviolet light or sunlight and local treatment should be discontinued if blistering occurs, but oral administration may be continued unless oedema occurs at the same time.

Hypertrichosis, hyperpigmentation, or both occurred in 3 of 100 patients with vitiligo who had been treated with methoxsalen systemically.— G. Singh and S. Lal (letter), *Br. J. Derm.*, 1967, *79*, 501.

Residual oedema of the legs and much cutaneous damage had followed the use of psoralen derivatives for sun-tanning. In a proportion of persons taking psoralens for this purpose, an acute generalised dermatitis with blistering and oedema, and possibly renal complications, could occur. Other side-effects included nausea, vomiting, insomnia, and mental depression. The psoralens might be hepatotoxic.— R. M. B. MacKenna (letter), *Br. med. J.*, 1969, *1*, 254.

Carcinogenicity. Discussion of the cancer risk from PUVA treatment.— *Lancet*, 1978, *1*, 537.

Reports and comments on the possible association between PUVA therapy and carcinogenicity: R. S. Stern *et al.*, *New Engl. J. Med.*, 1979, *300*, 809; J. H. Epstein, *ibid.*, 852; R. W. Morgan (letter), *ibid.*, *301*, 554; R. S. Stern *et al.* (letter), *ibid.*, 555; S. Shuster (letter), *Lancet*, 1979, *1*, 1146; R. G. Jobling and R. B. Coles (letter), *ibid.*

Individual reports of neoplasms in patients treated with PUVA: J. Wagner *et al.*, *Scand. J. Haemat.*, 1978, *21*, 299 (preleukaemia); N. E. Hansen, *ibid.*, 1979, *22*, 57 (acute myeloid leukaemia); C. Hofmann *et al.*, *Br. J. Derm.*, 1979, *101*, 685 (Bowenoid lesions, Bowen's disease, and keratoacanthomas); F. S. Brown *et al.*, *J. Am. Acad. Derm.*, 1980, *2*, 393 (basal cell epitheliomas).

Cytogenetic effects. Extensive chromosome damage was produced in mammalian cells in tissue culture by PUVA treatment [psoralen (P) and high-intensity long-wavelength (u.v.-A) irradiation]. Caution should be exercised in the use of psoralens (such as methoxsalen and trioxsalen) and light therapy since extensive chromosome damage could lead to later malignancy.— M. J. Ashwood-Smith and E. Grant, *Br. med. J.*, 1976, *1*, 342. Possible mechanisms for chromosomal changes.— M. J. Ashwood-Smith and S. Igali (letter), *ibid.*, 1978, *1*, 1138; M. Whitefield *et al.* (letter), *ibid.*, 1418.

See also under Carcinogenicity (above).

Effects on the eyes. Three of 483 patients with psoriasis developed early cataract after a year's treatment with PUVA, and one developed a superficial basal cell carcinoma after 18 months treatment.— W. S. Lynch *et al.*, *Cutis*, 1977, *20*, 477.

Further references: S. Lerman (letter), *New Engl. J. Med.*, 1980, *303*, 941.

Effects on the immune system. Reports and comments on the effect of PUVA on the immune system: G. H. Strauss *et al.*, *Lancet*, 1980, *2*, 556; C. Moss *et al.* (letter), *ibid.*, 922; G. H. Strauss *et al.* (letter), *ibid.*, 1134.

See also under Carcinogenicity (above).

Effects on the liver. Liver injury following administration of methoxsalen during PUVA therapy.— M. Bjellerup *et al.*, *Acta derm.-vener., Stockh.*, 1979, *59*, 371.

Effects on the nails. Onycholysis occurred in a patient treated for mycosis fungoides with methoxsalen and u.v. light.— D. V. Briffa and A. P. Warin (letter), *Br. med. J.*, 1977, *2*, 1150. Two further cases.— L. Zala *et al.*, *Dermatologica*, 1977, *154*, 203. Another report.— R. C. Rau *et al.* (letter), *Archs Derm.*, 1978, *114*, 448.

A report of nail pigmentation in 4 of 14 Indian patients with vitiligo after 2 months' treatment with methoxsalen.— R. P. C. Naik and G. Singh, *Br. J. Derm.*, 1979, *100*, 229.

Effects on the skin. Bullous pemphigoid developed in 2 patients during PUVA treatment; one had a history of bullous pemphigoid, and the other had taken co-trimoxazole which was not considered the precipitating factor.— K. Thomsen and H. Schmidt, *Br. J. Derm.*, 1976, *95*, 568. See also J. K. Robinson *et al.*, *ibid.*, 1978, *99*, 709.

An acneform eruption occurred in a patient with psoriasis treated with methoxsalen and u.v. light.— C. Jones and S. S. Bleehen, *Br. med. J.*, 1977, *2*, 866. See also E. B. Nielsen and J. Thormann, *Acta derm.-vener., Stockh.*, 1978, *58*, 374.

Kaposi's varicelliform eruption developed in a patient with a history of recurrent localised herpes infection 4 days after the start of PUVA therapy.— R. J. Segal and W. Watson, *Archs Derm.*, 1978, *114*, 1067.

Discoid lupus erythematosus possibly associated with PUVA therapy.— H. F. Domke *et al.* (letter), *Archs Derm.*, 1979, *115*, 642.

Contact allergy to methoxsalen, confirmed by patch testing, in 2 patients treated with PUVA.— E. M. Saihan, *Br. med. J.*, 1979, *2*, 20. See also I. Weissmann *et al.*, *Br. J. Derm.*, 1980, *102*, 113.

Reports of severe skin pain after PUVA treatment.— E. Tegner, *Acta derm.-vener., Stockh.*, 1979, *59*, 467; J. Miller and D. D. Munro, *ibid.*, 1980, *60*, 187.

Nevus spilus-like hyperpigmentation in psoriatic lesions during PUVA therapy.— S. Helland and G. Bang, *Acta derm.-vener., Stockh.*, 1980, *60*, 81.

Treatment of Adverse Effects. Overdosage may be treated by emptying the stomach by aspiration and lavage; the patient should be kept in a darkened room for 12 hours.

Precautions. Methoxsalen should not be given concomitantly with any drug known to cause photosensitisation. It should not be given to patients suffering from liver disease, lupus erythematosus, hydroa porphyria, or other disease associated with light sensitivity.

The Committee on Drugs of the American Academy of Pediatrics had recommended that PUVA should not be used for psoriasis in children except under investigational new drug protocols.— S. Segal *et al.*, *Pediatrics*, 1978, *62*, 253.

Absorption and Fate. When taken by mouth methoxsalen is absorbed from the gastro-intestinal tract. Increased photosensitivity is present 1 hour after a dose, reaches a peak at about 2 hours, and disappears after about 8 hours. Up to 80% of a dose is excreted in the urine within 8 hours as the hydroxylated or glucuronide derivatives. Photosensitivity is more persistent after topical application.

In 5 healthy subjects given a single dose of methoxsalen 40 mg mean peak plasma-methoxsalen concentrations were 177 and 324 ng per ml in fasting and non-fasting conditions respectively. No significant differences in time to peak concentrations (about 1.75 hours) or in plasma half-life (about 1 hour) were noted. It was suggested that methoxsalen should be taken in a standardised way in relation to food during ultraviolet light treatment.— H. Ehrsson *et al.*, *Clin. Pharmac. Ther.*, 1979, *25*, 167.

Further references: M. A. Pathak *et al.*, *J. invest. Derm.*, 1974, *62*, 347; N. Fincham *et al.*, *Br. J. Pharmac.*, 1978, *63*, 373P; I. Steiner *et al.*, *Acta derm.-vener., Stockh.*, 1978, *58*, 185; G. Swanbeck *et al.*, *Clin. Pharmac. Ther.*, 1979, *25*, 478; L. Stolk *et al.*, *Br. J. Derm.*, 1981, *104*, 447.

Uses. Methoxsalen increases the formation of melanin pigments in the skin on exposure to ultraviolet light; the stratum corneum is thickened and an inflammatory reaction initiated. It is used to increase tolerance to sunlight and in the treatment of idiopathic vitiligo but has no effect on leucoderma due to infections or trauma.

To increase tolerance to sunlight in light allergy doses usually of 20 mg, may be given daily by mouth with milk or food to minimise side-effects 2 hours before exposure, which should not exceed 30 minutes on the first 3 or 4 days of treatment; treatment should not exceed 2 weeks.

For the treatment of vitiligo a similar dose is used, followed after about 2 hours by exposure to sunlight or ultraviolet light. Treatment is continued for long periods. Liver function tests should be carried out at monthly intervals for the first 3 months of treatment and less frequently thereafter.

Methoxsalen is also applied topically in the treatment of vitiligo. The available 1% solution may need to be diluted 10-fold or 100-fold to avoid excessive reactions. It is applied daily to the affected areas at a rate of 8 to 32 μg per cm^2, followed after 2 hours by exposure to sunlight or ultraviolet light for 30 to 60 seconds, the period of exposure being gradually increased. Treatment should be discontinued if no improvement is noted within 3 months.

Promising results have been reported in psoriasis following the PUVA [psoralen, ultraviolet, A (long-wave, 320-400 nm, black light)] regimen. Excessive DNA synthesis in the lesion is reduced. A psoralen, usually methoxsalen 20 to 50 mg, is given 2 hours before exposure to high-intensity long-wave ultraviolet light. Long-term evaluation continues. Promising results have been reported in mycosis fungoides.

A study in 1500 patients showed that treatment with PUVA gave very good results in patients with psoriasis, acne, bacterial disseminated eczema, herpes zoster, and forms of parapsoriasis and mycosis fungoides. Good results were also reported in patients with herpes simplex and with papular urticaria.— G. Weber, *Br. J. Derm.*, 1976, *95*, *Suppl.* 14, 21.

A report of good to excellent response to PUVA treatment by 6 of 7 patients with lichen planus, treated for an average of 10 weeks.— J. P. Ortonne *et al.*, *Br. J. Derm.*, 1978, *99*, 77.

In a study comparing PUVA and betacarotene in 29 patients with polymorphous light eruption, 9 of 10 treated with PUVA and 6 of 19 treated with betacarotene showed complete remission. All 6 patients treated with both in consecutive years had remissions with betacarotene.— J. A. Parrish *et al.*, *Br. J. Derm.*, 1979, *100*. 187.

The course of psoriatic arthritis in 27 patients receiving PUVA for their psoriasis.— S. G. Perlman *et al.*, *Ann. intern. Med.*, 1979, *91*, 717.

Beneficial results with PUVA in patients with alopecia areata.— A. L. Claudy and D. Gagnaire, *Acta derm.-vener., Stockh.*, 1980, *60*, 171.

Mycosis fungoides. All of 6 patients with mycosis fungoides were clinically improved after PUVA treatment; 5 had complete histological clearance from the epidermis, with a less pronounced effect in the dermis. Methoxsalen 30 to 50 mg was given 2 hours before exposure; treatment was given 3 times a week for 2 to 6 weeks. Side-effects were pruritus and irritation. The treatment might be useful in early and pretumid cases and as an adjunct to electron-beam therapy or radiotherapy in more advanced cases.— L. Hodge *et al.*, *Br. med. J.*, 1977, *2*, 1257.

Seven patients with mycosis fungoides in the plaque stage and one in the erythrodermic stage were cleared of lesions after treatment with methoxsalen, usually 40 mg, followed by irradiation with u.v.-A light thrice weekly followed by maintenance once or twice a week or every 2 weeks. In 4 further patients with plaques and tumours, plaques cleared but tumours were not responsive.— H. H. Roenigk, *Archs Derm.*, 1977, *113*, 1047.

The results obtained in a study of 73 patients with mycosis fungoides at stages 0 to V of the disease confirmed earlier reports that photochemotherapy can produce a complete clinical and histological remission in stages 0 to II. Follow-up data so far indicate that photochemotherapy is able to keep many patients with stage 0 to II disease clear for up to 3 years on maintenance treatment given every one to 4 weeks. Patients at all stages of the disease may relapse when maintenance is withdrawn, and in those with advanced disease fresh lesions may develop despite maintenance treatment. The future role of photochemotherapy in mycosis fungoides will depend upon a comparison of its merits with other proven regimes.— D. V. Briffa *et al.*, *Lancet*, 1980, *2*, 49.

Further references: C. Hofmann *et al.*, *Dt. med. Wschr.*, 1977, *102*, 675.

For reports of the use of PUVA therapy with mustine in mycosis fungoides, see Mustine Hydrochloride, p.223.

Psoriasis. Complete clearing of lesions in 82 of 91 patients with psoriasis after the use of PUVA 3 to 4 times, weekly initially, then weekly to monthly for maintenance. Remissions lasted up to 400 days in some patients.— K. Wolff *et al.*, *Archs Derm.*, 1976, *112*, 943.

Clearance of extensive psoriasis in 88% of 1139 patients after treatment with PUVA 2 or 3 times a week. Remissions were maintained by treatment every 1 to 3 weeks.— J. W. Melski *et al.*, *J. invest. Derm.*, 1977, *68*, 328, per *J. Am. med. Ass.*, 1977, *238*, 2209.

Clearance of psoriasis in 74% of 483 patients after treatment with PUVA.— W. S. Lynch *et al.*, *Cutis*, 1977, *20*, 477.

An excellent response was achieved in 13 of 31 patients with psoriasis and a very good response in a further 11 after treatment with methoxsalen 20 to 60 mg according to body-weight and low-intensity u.v.-A light. Clinical response did not correlate with plasma-methoxsalen concentrations which varied from 2 to 167 ng per ml.— P. Thune and G. Volden, *Acta derm.-vener., Stockh.*, 1977, *57*, 351.

The American Academy of Dermatology warned against the widespread use of PUVA until the following had been fully investigated: the lowest effective irradiation dose, the maintenance irradiation dose, the extent of histopathological change, the measures necessary to prevent ocular and cutaneous injury, and the carcinogenic potential.— *J. Am. med. Ass.*, 1978, *239*, 525. Similar comment by the Psoriasis Association [UK].— *Pharm. J.*, 1977, *1*, 342.

The effect of photochemotherapy in 134 patients with severe plaque-type or palmoplantar psoriasis was enhanced by the prior administration of etretinate compared with photochemotherapy alone in 59 similar patients.— P. Fritsch *et al.*, *Dt. med. Wschr.*, 1978,

103, 1731. See also P. O. Fritsch *et al.*, *J. invest. Derm.*, 1978, *70*, 178; G. Michaëlsson *et al.*, *Br. J. Derm.*, 1978, *99*, 221.

The addition of topical treatment to PUVA treatment could be of value to patients with scalp psoriasis, but fluocinolone acetonide did not interact well with the treatment, dithranol could cause burns, and tar was not effective during a study in 116 patients.— W. L. Morrison *et al.*, *Br. J. Derm.*, 1978, *98*, 125. From a controlled study in 16 patients with psoriasis, pretreatment of lesions with clobetasol propionate 0.05% used twice daily for 1 week prior to treatment with PUVA was considered to have produced a greater and more rapid response than photochemotherapy alone.— P. W. Gould and L. Wilson, *ibid.*, 133. From a study of 90 patients with psoriasis it was reported that combined treatment with PUVA and the topical use of triamcinolone acetonide under occlusion was followed by longer periods of remission than either treatment alone, and PUVA alone was more effective than the corticosteroid used alone.— M. Schmoll *et al.*, *ibid.*, *99*, 693.

Results of the European PUVA study, confirming the dramatic efficacy of PUVA in clearing psoriasis.— T. Henseler *et al.*, *Lancet*, 1981, *1*, 853.

Further references: J. A. Parrish *et al.*, *New Engl. J. Med.*, 1974, *291*, 1207; J. A. Parrish, *Archs Derm.*, 1977, *113*, 1525; J. A. Parrish *et al.*, *ibid.*, 1529; H. H. Roenigk and J. S. Martin, *ibid.*, 1667; L. Fry (letter), *Br. J. Derm.*, 1977, *96*, 327; H. Hönigsmann *et al.*, *ibid.*, 1977, *97*, 119; T. Lakshmipathi *et al.*, *Br. J. Derm.*, 1977, *96*, 587; J. W. Petrozzi and A. M. Kligman, *Archs Derm.*, 1978, *114*, 387; G. A. Wasserman *et al.*, *Can. med. Ass. J.*, 1978, *118*, 1379; S. Rogers *et al.*, *Lancet*, 1979, *1*, 455; D. R. S. Howell (letter), *ibid.*, 772; J. Boer *et al.* (letter), *ibid.*, 773; D. V. Briffa *et al.*, *Br. med. J.*, 1981, *282*, 937.

Discussions.— *Med. Lett.*, 1975, *17*, 39; *Br. med. J.*, 1975, *1*, 474; M. W. Greaves, *Practitioner*, 1976, *217*, 585; K. Wolff *et al.*, *Br. J. Derm.*, 1977, *96*, 1; L. Hodge and J. S. Comaish, *Drugs*, 1977, *13*, 288; *Br. med. J.*, 1978, *2*, 2; *FDA Drug Bull.*, 1978, *8*, 28; E. M. Farber *et al.*, *Br. J. Derm.*, 1978, *99*, 715; *Drug & Ther. Bull.*, 1980, *18*, 1; *J. Am. med. Ass.*, 1980, *243*, 1429.

Topical use. Methoxsalen 0.15% in isopropyl alcohol was applied to the lesions of 74 patients with psoriasis and the whole body was exposed 1 hour later to black light. The lesions were healed in 34 patients after 20 to 34 exposures and greatly improved in 23 patients after 19 to 42 exposures.— G. Weber, *Br. J. Derm.*, 1974, *90*, 317.

Complete clearing of lesions was achieved in 12 of 30 patients with long-standing psoriasis after the application of methoxsalen 1% followed 2 hours later by exposure to u.v.-A light, for 12 to 28 treatments; 9 further patients were markedly improved. Plaque-type and guttate psoriasis responded better than exfoliative dermatitis. Keratotic plaques should be descaled with salicylic acid prior to starting treatment.— J. W. Petrozzi *et al.*, *Archs Derm.*, 1977, *113*, 292.

Further references: I. Willis and D. R. Harris, *Archs Derm.*, 1973, *107*, 358; H. Schaefer *et al.*, *Br. J. Derm.*, 1976, *94*, 363.

Vitiligo. In the treatment of vitiligo, methoxsalen 20 mg and triamcinolone 8 to 12 mg daily followed 2 hours later by exposure to sunshine produced satisfactory responses in 14 of 15 patients.— F. S. Farah *et al.*, *Br. J. Derm.*, 1967, *79*, 89.

If the latest reports of the successful treatment of vitiligo by topical corticosteroids are confirmed, methoxsalen would probably not have any place in the treatment of vitiligo.— T. W. Stewart, *Practitioner*, 1976, *217*, 184. See also S. S. Bleehen, *Br. J. Derm.*, 1976, *94*, *Suppl.* 12, 43.

Preparations

Methoxsalen Topical Solution *(U.S.P.)*. Methoxsalen, 9.2 to 10.8 mg per ml, in a suitable vehicle; it contains 66.5 to 77% of alcohol. Store in airtight containers. Protect from light.

Deltasoralen *(Delta Laboratories, Eire)*. Methoxsalen, available as **Paints** and **Tablets**.

Meladinine *(Delta Laboratories, Eire)*. **Paint** containing methoxsalen and pentosalen and **Tablets** each containing methoxsalen and pentosalen. (Also available as Meladinine in *Fr.*, *Ger.*).

Other Proprietary Names

Geroxalen *(Neth.)*; Meladinin *(Switz.)*; Mopsoralen *(Belg.)*; Oxsoralen *(Austral., Belg., Canad., Ital., Neth., Spain, Switz., USA)*.

1624-p

Monobenzone *(U.S.P.)*. Monobenzyl Ether of Hydroquinone. 4-Benzyloxyphenol.

$C_{13}H_{12}O_2$=200.2.

CAS — 103-16-2.

Pharmacopoeias. In *U.S.*

A white odourless, almost tasteless, crystalline powder. M.p. 117° to 120°. Practically **insoluble** in water; soluble 1 in about 15 of alcohol, 1 in 29 of chloroform, 1 in 14 of ether; soluble in acetone. **Store** at a temperature not exceeding 30° in airtight containers. Protect from light.

Adverse Effects. Monobenzone may cause skin irritation and sensitisation. In some patients, this may only be temporary and need not necessitate complete withdrawal of the drug. In other patients, an eczematous sensitisation may occur. Excessive depigmentation may occur even beyond the areas under treatment and may produce unsightly patches. Some authorities consider that fewer side-effects occur with an ointment containing 10% instead of 20%, though a longer period will then be required to attain depigmentation.

Leucomelanoderma in 347 black patients, with patchy depigmentation and mottled hypermelanosis affecting chiefly the face and neck, appeared to be due to the use of a bleaching cream containing monobenzone 2%.— M. Dogliotti *et al.*, *S. Afr. med. J.*, 1974, *48*, 1555.

Uses. Monobenzone inhibits the action of tyrosinase and thereby prevents the conversion of tyrosine to dihydroxyphenylalanine, a precursor of melanin. It prevents the formation of melanin pigments in the skin without destruction of the melanocytes. It is used locally in the form of an ointment containing up to 20% or a lotion containing 5% as a depigmenting agent in the treatment of excessive pigmentation accompanying such conditions as Addison's disease and pregnancy. It may also be of value in reducing persistent freckles (generalised lentigo). It is applied to the affected parts twice or thrice daily until a satisfactory response had been obtained, and thereafter twice weekly. Excessive exposure to sunlight should be avoided. The results are variable since some patients are resistant to the drug. Depigmentation only becomes apparent when the preformed melanin pigments have been exhausted, and this may take several months. If, however, no improvement is noted after 4 months treatment the use of the drug should be abandoned.

Monobenzone has no effect on melanomas or pigmented naevi.

Preparations

MBEH Ointment *(Roy. Free Hosp.)*. Monobenzone 2.5 to 10 g, industrial methylated spirit 45 ml, propylene glycol 15 ml, macrogol 4000 to 100 g. Shelf-life 1 year. Store in a cool place.

Monobenzone Ointment *(U.S.P.)*. Ointment containing monobenzone. Store at a temperature not exceeding 30° in airtight containers.

Proprietary Names

Aloquin *(Prosana, Austral.)*; Benoquin *(Elder, Canad.; Elder, Switz.; Elder, USA)*; Depigman *(Hermal, Ger.; Hermal, Neth.; Hermal, Switz.)*; Dermochinona *(Chinoin, Ital.)*; Leucodinine *(Covor, Belg.)*.

1625-s

Naphthalan Liquid. Naphthalanum Liquidum.

Pharmacopoeias. In *Hung.*

A complex mixture of hydrocarbons and tars. It is a viscous brownish-black, oil-like liquid with a greenish fluorescence and a characteristic odour. **Immiscible** with water; sparingly soluble in alcohol; soluble in chloroform and light petroleum; miscible with glycerol, oils, fats, and waxes.

Naphthalan liquid has emollient and antiseptic properties and a slight local analgesic action. It has been applied locally as an ointment or cream in the treatment of skin diseases.

1626-w

Nitrofurazone *(B.P., B.P. Vet., U.S.P.)*. Furacilinum; Nitrofural. 5-Nitro-2-furaldehyde semicarbazone.

$C_6H_6N_4O_4$=198.1.

CAS — 59-87-0.

Pharmacopoeias. In *Aust.*, *Br.*, *Braz.*, *Cz.*, *It.*, *Pol.*, *Port.*, *Rus.*, and *U.S.*

A lemon to brownish-yellow odourless or almost odourless, crystalline powder with a bitter taste. M.p. about 236° with decomposition. It slowly darkens on exposure to light and discolours in contact with alkalis.

Soluble 1 in 4200 of water, 1 in 600 of alcohol, and 1 in 350 of propylene glycol; soluble in dimethylformamide; practically insoluble in chloroform and ether; soluble up to 1 in 100 of macrogol mixtures. The filtrate from a 1% suspension in water has a pH of 5 to 7.5. **Store** at a temperature not exceeding 40° in airtight containers. Protect from light.

Adverse Effects. Sensitisation and generalised allergic skin reactions may be produced by continuous applications for 5 days or longer, and intolerance to nitrofurazone, necessitating withdrawal, has been encountered. Cross-sensitisation to other nitrofuran derivatives may occur.

Adverse effects reported following oral administration include polyneuritis, nausea, vomiting, joint pains, and headaches. Nitrofurazone in high doses is carcinogenic in *rats*.

Haemolytic anaemia. Administration of nitrofurazone 1.5 g daily had been reported to produce significant haemolysis in Negroes with a deficiency of glucose-6-phosphate dehydrogenase.— Standardization of Procedures for the Study of Glucose-6-Phosphate Dehydrogenase, *Tech. Rep. Ser. Wld Hlth Org. No. 366*, 1967.

Polyneuritis. A patient given nitrofurazone in the treatment of trypanosomiasis developed a combined sensory and motor peripheral neuropathy which persisted after the drug was withdrawn.— H. C. Spencer *et al.*, *Ann. intern. Med.*, 1975, *82*, 633.

For earlier reports of polyneuritis associated with nitrofurazone, see Martindale 27th Edn, p. 448.

Uses. Nitrofurazone has an antibacterial action against a number of Gram-negative and Gram-positive bacteria. *Pseudomonas* spp. are not generally susceptible. It is used as a local application for superficial wounds, burns, ulcers, and skin infections, and for the preparation of surfaces before skin grafting. It is usually applied in a concentration of 0.2% in a non-greasy ointment basis. A solution of this strength has been used in the treatment of otitis of the middle and external ear. It has also been employed in eye-drops and eye ointments. The solution, diluted 1 in 6, is used for bladder irrigation.

Nitrofurazone has been administered by mouth, either alone or in conjunction with other drugs, in the treatment of trypanosomiasis, mainly in trypanosomal infections that have become refractory to the established trypanocides; a dosage of 1 to 2 g daily, in divided doses, for 5 to 10 days, has been used. In the USSR it has been given by mouth in a dosage of 100 mg four times daily for 5 to 6 days in the treatment of acute bacillary dysentery.

In veterinary medicine, nitrofurazone is used for the treatment of coccidiosis in poultry and farm animals, and necrotic enteritis in pigs.

Studies in 6 healthy men indicated that nitrofurazone was not absorbed from the urethra.— G. Marion-Landais *et al.*, *Eaton, Curr. ther. Res.*, 1976, *19*, 550.

Burns. Nitrofurazone ointment 0.2% was considered to be effective *in vitro* against many of the organisms obtained over an 18-month period from the wounds of burn patients. However, 0.2% nitrofurazone cream was considered to be ineffective.— I. A. Holder *et al.*, *J. antimicrob. Chemother.*, 1979, *5*, 455.

Scabies. Scabies was controlled in most of 30 patients by nitrofurazone as a 0.2% water-soluble ointment.— S. P. R. Chowdhury (letter), *Lancet*, 1977, *1*, 152.

Trypanosomiasis. Nitrofurazone, 22.5 mg per kg body-weight daily in divided doses for 7 days given with supplements of vitamin B group and of ascorbic acid, was generally well tolerated by 5 patients with trypanosomiasis; 1 patient relapsed.— M. N. Lowenthal *et al.* (letter), *Trans. R. Soc. trop. Med. Hyg.*, 1977, *71*, 88. See also T. Ogada, *E. Afr. med. J.*, 1974, *51*, 56, per *Trop. Dis. Bull.*, 1976, *73*, 315.

When melarsoprolol has been unsuccessful in trypanosomiasis nitrofurazone is used as an alternative. Nitrofurazone is given by mouth in an adult dosage of 500 mg three or four times daily for 5 to 7 days. Its use is restricted to hospitals where haematocrit and glucose-6-phosphate dehydrogenase estimations can be done.— Report of a Joint WHO Expert Committee and FAO Expert Consultation on The African Trypanosomiases, *Tech. Rep. Wld Hlth Org. No. 635*, 1979.

Preparations

Creams

Nitrofurazone Cream *(U.S.P.).* Nitrofurazone in a suitable emulsified water-miscible basis. Store at a temperature not exceeding 40° in airtight containers and avoid contact with alkaline materials. Protect from light.

Eye Ointments

Oculentum Nitrofurazoni *(Nord. P.).* Nitrofurazone Eye Ointment. Nitrofurazone 1% in Oculentum Simplex *Nord. P.*, an eye ointment basis containing liquid paraffin 20% and yellow soft paraffin 80%.

Eye-drops

Oculoguttae Nitrofurazoni *(Nord. P.).* Nitrofurazone Eye-drops. Nitrofurazone 15 mg, sodium chloride 900 mg, and Water for Injections 99.09 g. Phenylmercuric nitrate 0.001% is a suitable preservative. Sterilise by autoclaving.

Ointments

Nitrofurazone Ointment *(U.S.P.).* Nitrofurazone Soluble Dressing. Nitrofurazone in a suitable water-miscible basis. Store at a temperature not exceeding 40° in airtight containers and avoid contact with alkaline materials. Protect from light.

Nord. P. has nitrofurazone 200 mg, macrogol '3000' 38 g, macrogol '400' 55.5 g, and water 6.3 g.

Solutions

Nitrofurazone Topical Solution *(U.S.P.).* Nitrofurazone Solution. A solution, miscible with water, containing nitrofurazone. Store at a temperature not exceeding 40° in airtight containers and avoid contact with alkaline materials. Protect from light.

Nord. P. has nitrofurazone 200 mg, macrogol '3000' 25 g, macrogol '400' 40 g, and water 34.8 g.

Tablets

Tabulettae Furacilini *(Rus. P.).* Nitrofurazone Tablets. Tablets each containing nitrofurazone 100 mg.

Proprietary Preparations

Furacin *(Norwich-Eaton, UK).* Nitrofurazone, available as **Soluble Ointment** containing 0.2% in a water-soluble macrogol basis and as **Solution** containing 0.2% in an aqueous macrogol basis (suggested diluent, water). (Also available as Furacin in *Arg., Austral., Canad., Ger., Ital., S.Afr., Spain, Switz., USA*).

Other Proprietary Names

Acutol *(Switz.)*; Furacine *(Belg., Neth.)*; Furesol *(Norw.)*.

1627-e

Pentosalen. Ammidin; Imperatorin; Marmelosin; Isoamylenoxypsoralen. 9-(3-Methylbut-2-enyloxy)-7*H*-furo[3,2-*g*]chromen-7-one.
$C_{16}H_{14}O_4$=270.3.

A constituent of the fruits of *Ammi majus* (Umbelliferae).

Pentosalen has been used with methoxsalen (see p.499) in the treatment of alopecia and vitiligo.

1628-l

Burgundy Pitch *(B.P.C. 1934).* Pix Burgundica; Pix Burgundina; White Pitch; Poix de Bourgogne; Pez de Borgonha.

CAS — 8029-33-2.

Pharmacopoeias. In *Port.* and *Span.*

The purified resinous exudate from the Norway spruce, *Picea abies* (=*P. excelsa*) (Pinaceae).

A hard, brittle, reddish or yellowish-brown substance with an aromatic odour and taste. **Soluble** in alcohol and glacial acetic acid.

Burgundy pitch is a mild counter-irritant and has been used in plasters.

1629-y

Potassium Dichromate *(B.P.C. 1934).* Potassium Bichromate.
$K_2Cr_2O_7$=294.2.

CAS — 7778-50-9.

Pharmacopoeias. In *Swiss.*

Odourless orange-red crystals, granules, or powder with a salty then bitter taste. **Soluble** 1 in 10 of water; practically insoluble in alcohol.

Adverse Effects and Treatment. As for Chromium Trioxide, p.285.

In a modified 'repeated-insult' patch test, 2% potassium dichromate was found to produce extreme sensitisation of the skin.— A. M. Kligman, *J. invest. Derm.*, 1966, *47*, 393.

Of 1205 persons with dermatitis or eczema submitted to patch testing with 0.5% aqueous solution of potassium dichromate, 16.2% gave a positive reaction.— E. Rudzki and D. Kleniewska, *Br. J. Derm.*, 1970, *83*, 543.

Reports of poisoning.— J. Castera *et al.*, *Bull. Méd. lég.*, 1969, *3* (May to June), 134; D. B. Kaufman *et al.*, *Am. J. Dis. Child.*, 1970, *119*, 374, per *J. Am. med. Ass.*, 1970, *212*, 171; B. K. Sharma *et al.*, *Postgrad. med. J.*, 1978, *54*, 414.

Uses. Potassium dichromate is an oxidising agent, rarely used in medicine. It has been applied topically as a 1 to 5% solution to the feet in hyperhidrosis and a 10% solution has been applied as a caustic to warts.

Potassium dichromate (Kalium Bichromicum; Kali. Bich.) is used in homoeopathic medicine.

Preparations

Müller's Fluid. Potassium dichromate 2.5 and sodium sulphate 1 in water 100. It is used for hardening tissues, post mortem, before histological examination.

1630-g

Potassium Hydroxyquinoline Sulphate

(B.P.C. 1973). Potassii Hydroxyquinolini Sulphas; Oxyquinol Potassium; Potassium Oxyquinoline Sulphate. An equimolecular mixture of potassium sulphate and quinolin-8-ol sulphate, containing the equivalent of 50% of quinolin-8-ol.

Pharmacopoeias. In *Aust.*

A pale yellow microcrystalline powder with a slight odour and a bitter taste. It partly liquefies at 172° to 184°. **Soluble** 1 in 2 of water; partly soluble in alcohol; practically insoluble in ether. A 5% solution in water has a pH of about 3. **Incompatible** with many metallic salts. **Store** in a cool place and avoid contact with metal. Protect from light.

Adverse Effects. In some subjects sensitive to potassium hydroxyquinoline sulphate severe irritation and redness may occur.

Uses. Potassium hydroxyquinoline sulphate has antibacterial, antifungal, and deodorant properties and is used, often in conjunction with benzoyl peroxide, in the local treatment of fungous infections, minor bacterial infections, and acne. Potassium hydroxyquinoline sulphate is applied to the skin as creams containing 0.05 to 0.5%. It is also used with hydrocortisone. It has been used as an ingredient of some perspiration deodorants and as a spermicide in a jelly and in pessaries.

A study of the antiviral activity of hydroxyquinolines.— W. Rohde *et al.*, *Antimicrob. Ag. Chemother.*, 1976, *10*, 234.

Proprietary Preparations

Quinoderm *(Quinoderm, UK).* Preparations containing potassium hydroxyquinoline sulphate 0.5% and benzoyl peroxide 10% in an astringent basis, available as **Cream** and **Lotio-Gel**. **Quinoderm Cream with Hydrocortisone** contains in addition hydrocortisone 1%. For acne.

Reference: P. J. Ashurst, *Practitioner*, 1969, *202*, 405.

Quinoped Cream *(Quinoderm, UK).* Contains potassium hydroxyquinoline sulphate 0.5% and benzoyl peroxide 5% in an astringent basis. For athlete's foot.

1631-q

Pumice *(U.S.P.).* Pumice Stone; Lapis Pumicis; Pumex.

CAS — 1332-09-8.

Pharmacopoeias. In *U.S.*

A substance of volcanic origin consisting chiefly of complex silicates of aluminium, potassium, and sodium. Odourless, tasteless, very light, hard, rough, porous greyish masses or gritty, greyish powder. Practically **insoluble** in water and not attacked by acids.

The *U.S.P.* recognises 3 grades of powdered pumice: (1) superfine (=pumice flour)—not less than 97% passes through a No. 200 [US] sieve; (2) fine—not less than 95% passes through a No. 150 sieve and not more than 75% through a No. 200 sieve; (3) coarse—not less than 95% passes through a No. 60 sieve and not more than 5% through a No. 200 sieve.

Powdered pumice is used as a dental and dermal abrasive and as a filtering medium.

Pneumoconiosis caused by pumice dust.— G. Babolini *et al.*, *Bull. int. Un. Tuberc.*, 1979, *54*, 425.

1632-p

Pyrithione Sodium. Sodium Pyridinethione. (1-Hydroxypyridine-2(1*H*)-thionato)sodium.
C_5H_4NNaOS=149.1.

CAS — 1121-30-8 (pyrithione); 15922-78-8 (sodium salt).

An off-white hygroscopic powder with a slight odour. M.p. about 250°. **Soluble** 1 in 2 of water, 1 in 20 of alcohol, and 1 in 5 of dimethyl sulphoxide; freely soluble in glycols; practically insoluble in fixed oils and liquid paraffin. A 2% solution in water has a pH of about 9.1. **Incompatible** with oxidising and reducing agents; with heavy metal ions coloured chelates may be formed. **Store** in airtight containers. Protect from light.

Pyrithione sodium is a bacteriostatic and fungistatic agent active against Gram-positive and Gram-negative organisms. It is used similarly to pyrithione zinc when a water-soluble salt is required.

While less than 1% of pyrithione zinc was absorbed through the skin 13% of pyrithione sodium was absorbed.— C. K. Parekh (letter), *Lancet*, 1978, *1*, 940.

Proprietary Preparations

Sodium Omadine *(Olin, USA: K & K-Greeff, UK).* A brand of pyrithione sodium.

Other Proprietary Names

Fonderma *(Fr., Ital.)*.

1633-s

Pyrithione Zinc.

Zinc Pyridinethione; Zinc 2-Pyridinethiol 1-Oxide. Bis[1-hydroxypyridine-2(1*H*)-thionato]zinc.
$C_{10}H_8N_2O_2S_2Zn$=317.7.

CAS — 13463-41-7.

An off-white powder with a slight odour. Practically **insoluble** in water; very slightly soluble in alcohol; soluble 1 in 20 of dimethyl sulphoxide. **Incompatible** with oxidising and reducing agents, and heavy metal ions. **Protect** from light.

Pyrithione zinc has bacteriostatic and fungistatic properties. It is used similarly to selenium sulphide in the control of seborrhoeic dermatitis and dandruff. It is an ingredient of some proprietary shampoos.

In a double-blind study in 140 persons with dandruff, pyrithione zinc 2% in a shampoo vehicle was as effective as selenium sulphide 2.5% suspension in reducing the dandruff, and both were more effective than a non-medicated shampoo.— N. Orentreich *et al.*, *J. pharm. Sci.*, 1969, *58*, 1279.

A review of antimicrobial agents, including pyrithione zinc and sodium, used in cosmetics.— I. R. Gucklhorn, *Mfg Chem.*, 1970, *41* (Feb.), 30.

In a double-blind study in 170 persons with seborrhoeic dermatitis of the scalp, pyrithione zinc in a shampoo vehicle was more effective than a combination of sulphur, salicylic acid, and hexachlorophane in a shampoo vehicle in reducing the seborrhoeic dermatitis and accompanying itching, though it showed no long-term advantages in the reduction of oiliness. Both were more effective than a non-medicated shampoo.— N. Orentreich, *J. Soc. cosmet. Chem.*, 1972, *23*, 189.

Adsorption on to hair and skin.— T. Okumura *et al.*, *Cosmet. Perfum.*, 1975, *90*, 101.

Adverse effects. Though it had some toxicity on repeated ingestion, little or no pyrithione zinc was absorbed when applied to the intact or abraded skin. It discoloured and was decomposed by u.v. light.— E. W. Brauer *et al.*, *J. invest. Derm.*, 1966, *47*, 174, per *Drug Cosmet. Ind.*, 1967, *100* (Mar.), 155.

Toxicity in *animals*.— M. D. Adams *et al.*, *Toxic. appl. Pharmac.*, 1976, *36*, 523.

Peripheral neuritis with paraesthesia and muscle weakness in one patient was associated with the prolonged use of a shampoo (Head and Shoulders) containing pyrithione zinc 2%. The muscle weakness had disappeared 3 months after stopping the shampoo and 2 years later the paraesthesia had improved by about 75%.— J. E. Beck, *Dome, USA* (letter), *Lancet* 1978, *1*, 444.

Metabolism in *animals*.— C. D. Klaassen, *Toxic. appl. Pharmac.*, 1976, *35*, 581.

Proprietary Preparations

Zinc Omadine *(Olin, USA: K & K-Greeff, UK)*. A brand of pyrithione zinc.

For proprietary preparations of pyrithione zinc for use as shampoos, see Martindale Part 3—Formulas of Proprietary Medicines.

Other Proprietary Names

Danex *(USA)*; Hair Power *(Canad.)*; Sapoderm *(see also under Triclosan) (Austral.)*; Ultrex *(Fr.)*; Zincon *(USA)*.

1634-w

Pyrogallol *(B.P.C. 1949)*. Pyrogallic Acid. Benzene-1,2,3-triol.
$C_6H_6O_3$=126.1.

CAS — 87-66-1.

Pharmacopoeias. In *Aust.*, *Jug.*, *Pol.*, *Port.*, *Span.*, and *Swiss*.

Almost odourless, colourless or grey-yellow feathery crystals or white or yellowish crystalline powder, producing a sensation of coolness on the tongue. M.p. about 133°. It acquires a greyish tint on exposure to air and light.

Soluble 1 in 2 of water, 1 in 1.5 of alcohol, and 1 in 2 of ether. On exposure to air, aqueous solutions acquire a brown colour and an acid reaction. **Incompatible** with alkalis, heavy metal salts, iron salts, and oxidising agents. **Store** in airtight containers. Protect from light.

Adverse Effects. Systemic effects of pyrogallol are similar to those of phenol (see p.571) and in addition include methaemoglobinaemia, haemolysis, and kidney damage; they are treated similarly.

Fatal poisoning followed treatment of psoriasis with an ointment containing pyrogallol. The patient collapsed 5 minutes after covering about two-thirds of the body with ointment. It was estimated that about 10 g of pyrogallol was absorbed.— R. Pewny, *J. Am. med. Ass.*, 1925, *85*, 555.

Uses. Pyrogallol has been used as an ointment (2 to 10% in white soft paraffin) in psoriasis, lupus vulgaris, ringworm, and other parasitic skin diseases, but it is not suitable for application over large areas or denuded surfaces owing to the danger of toxic effects from absorption.

Pyrogallol stains the skin and hair black; skin stains are removed by ammonium persulphate or 10% oxalic acid solution.

Pyrogallol has been used as an ingredient of hairdyes, usually in conjunction with silver nitrate or copper chloride.

The use of pyrogallol in cosmetics and toiletries in Great Britain is controlled under The Cosmetic Product Regulations 1978 (SI 1978: No. 1354).

Preparations

Compound Pyrogallol Ointment. Ung. Pyrogallol. Co. Pyrogallol 2.5 g, salicylic acid 4 g, phenol 2.5 g, white soft paraffin 91 g. Store at 4° to 8°. Protect from light. For a similar preparation, see under Chrysarobin, p.492.

1635-e

Pyrogallol Triacetate. Pyrogalloli Acetas; Lenigallol. 1,2,3-Triacetoxybenzene.
$C_{12}H_{12}O_6$=252.2.

CAS — 525-52-0.

Pharmacopoeias. In *Nord.*

A white, almost odourless, crystalline powder. Practically **insoluble** in water; soluble 1 in 600 of alcohol, 1 in 20 of chloroform, and 1 in 800 of ether. **Incompatible** with alkalis. **Protect** from light.

Pyrogallol triacetate has been used for the same purposes as pyrogallol.

1636-l

Pyroxylin *(B.P., U.S.P.)*. Pyroxylinum; Cellulose Nitrate; Colloxylinum; Soluble Guncotton; Fulmicoton; Kollodiumwolle; Algodão-Polvora.

CAS — 9004-70-0.

Pharmacopoeias. In *Arg.*, *Aust.*, *Belg.*, *Br.*, *Ind.*, *Jap.*, *Mex.*, *Port.*, *Span.*, *Swiss*, and *U.S.*

A nitrated cellulose prepared, under carefully controlled conditions, by treating defatted wood pulp or cotton linters with a mixture of nitric and sulphuric acids and purifying the product. It occurs as white or almost white cuboid granules or fibrous material resembling cotton wool but harsher to the touch and more powdery. It is highly inflammable. The *B.P.* specifies that a solution (10 g in 100 ml) in acetone (95%) has a kinematic viscosity at 20° of 1160 to 2900 centistokes.

Soluble 1 in 25 of a mixture of 1 vol. of alcohol (90%) and 3 vol. of ether, yielding an almost clear and colourless solution; soluble in acetone, amyl acetate, ethyl acetate, methyl alcohol, and glacial acetic acid. **Store** in a cool place loosely packed in airtight containers. Protect from light. It should be kept moistened with not less than 25% of industrial methylated spirit or isopropyl alcohol. When kept in well-closed bottles and exposed to light, it decomposes with the evolution of nitrous vapours, leaving a carbonaceous residue.

Uses. Pyroxylin is used in the preparation of collodions which are applied to the skin for the protection of small cuts and abrasions. Collodions have also been tried as vehicles for the application of drugs when prolonged local action is required but it is possible that the collodion film may inhibit the action of the drug.

Preparations

Collodion *(B.P.)*. A solution of pyroxylin (approximately 10%) in a mixture of alcohol (90%) (or industrial methylated spirit, suitably diluted) 1 volume and solvent ether 3 volumes, diluted with the same mixed solvent to a kinematic viscosity of 405 to 700 cSt.

NOTE. The *B.P.* directs that when Collodion is prescribed or demanded, Flexible Collodion be supplied.

Collodion *(U.S.P.)*. Prepared from pyroxylin 4 g, ether 75 ml, and alcohol 25 ml; it contains not less than 5% w/w of pyroxylin. Store at a temperature not exceeding 30° in airtight containers.

Many other pharmacopieias include a similar collodion, usually with 4 to 5% w/w of pyroxylin.

Flexible Collodion *(B.P.)*. Colophony 2.5 g, castor oil 2.5 g, collodion to 100 ml. Store at a temperature not exceeding 25° in airtight containers

NOTE. This preparation contains much more pyroxylin than the *B.P. 1973* preparation; the flexibility of the film produced is considered to be comparable.

Many other pharmacopoeias include a flexible collodion usually with 4 to 5% w/w of pyroxylin and 3 to 5% w/w of castor oil, but without colophony. *U.S.P.*) has camphor 2 g, castor oil 3 g, and collodion (*U.S.P.*) to 100 g.

Proprietary Preparations

Collodion 33042 *(BDH Chemicals, UK)*. Contains pyroxylin 14% in a basis consisting of equal parts by volume of ether and anhydrous methylated spirit. For preparing permeable membranes.

Necoloidine Solution *(BDH Chemicals, UK)*. Contains pyroxylin 8% in a basis consisting of equal parts by volume of ether and anhydrous methylated spirit. For embedding microscopical sections before cutting.

1637-y

Resorcinol *(B.P., U.S.P.)*. Resorcin; *m*-Dihydroxybenzene; Dioxybenzolum. Benzene-1,3-diol.
$C_6H_6O_2$=110.1.

CAS — 108-46-3.

Pharmacopoeias. In all pharmacopoeias examined except *Eur.*, *Fr.*, *Int.*, *Jap.*, and *Turk.*

Colourless or slightly pinkish-grey, acicular crystals or crystalline powder with a slight characteristic odour and a sweetish pungent taste and a bitter after-taste. M.p. 109° to 112°; it sublimes on further heating. It becomes red on exposure to air and light.

Soluble 1 in less than 1 of water, 1 in 1 of alcohol; freely soluble in ether, and glycerol; soluble in fixed oils; slightly soluble in chloroform; very slightly soluble in carbon disulphide. A 5% solution in water is neutral or acid to litmus but not acid to methyl orange. A 3.3% solution is iso-osmotic with serum.

Incompatible with Nitrous Ether Spirit, ferric salts, and caustic alkalis; it forms a liquid or soft mass when triturated with camphor, menthol, phenol, and certain other substances. **Store** in airtight containers. Protect from light.

Resorcinol formed an insoluble oily liquid with polysorbates but this could be solubilised by increasing the concentration of the polysorbate.— S. S. Ahsan and S. M. Blaug, *Drug Stand.*, 1960, *28*, 95.

Preservative for eye-drops. Benzalkonium chloride 0.01%, phenylmercuric borate 0.005%, or chlorhexidine gluconate 0.02% were suitable preservatives for resorcinol eye-drops sterilised by filtration.— M. Van Ooteghem, *Pharm. Tijdschr. Belg.*, 1968, *45*, 69.

Stabilisation of local preparations. Alpha tocopherol was the best antoxidant for resorcinol preparations containing oil; ascorbic acid and alpha tocopherol were the most effective antoxidants in ointments, and ascorbic acid and sodium metabisulphite were most effective in non-oily liquid preparations.— A. Halpern and H. A. Getz, *J. Am. pharm. Ass., pract. Pharm. Edn*, 1950, *11*, 24.

Adverse Effects and Treatment. Resorcinol is a mild irritant. It may be absorbed through the skin or from ulcerated surfaces and prolonged use may lead to myxoedema due to the anti-thyroid action of the drug. Systemic effects are similar to those of phenol but convulsions may occur more frequently. Resorcinol toxicity is treated as for Phenol, p.571.

Maximum permissible atmospheric concentration 10 ppm.

Of 877 persons with dermatitis or eczema submitted to patch testing with resorcinol 1% in yellow soft paraffin, 2.1% gave a positive reaction.— E. Rudzki and D. Kleniewska, *Br. J. Derm.*, 1970, *83*, 543.

Resorcinol could cause green discoloration of the urine.— J. Karlstrand, *J. Am. pharm. Ass.*, 1977, *NS17*, 735.

Uses. Externally, resorcinol has antipruritic, exfoliative, and keratolytic properties. It is used as a lotion or as an ointment, usually containing 2 to 5%, in the treatment of acne and seborrhoeic skin conditions.

Alcoholic hair lotions containing 2.5% have been employed in the treatment of dandruff but they should not be used on fair hair and before use it is important to free the hair from soap and alkali to avoid discoloration.

The use of resorcinol in cosmetics and toiletries in Great Britain is controlled under The Cosmetic Products Regulations 1978 (SI 1978: No. 1354).

Preparations

Eye-drops

Oculoguttae Resorcinoli *(Nord. P.)*. Resorcinol 1 g, disodium edetate 10 mg, sodium chloride 600 mg, and Water for Injections 98.39 g. Sterilise by autoclaving. Phenethyl alcohol 0.5% is a suitable preservative.

Hair Lotions

Resorcinol Lotion Compound *(A.P.F.)*. Lot. Resorcin. Co. Resorcinol 2.5 g, solvent ether 2.5 ml, castor oil 2.5 ml, spike lavender oil 0.1 ml, alcohol (90%) to 100 ml. Protect from light. This lotion may discolour fair hair.

Lotions

Nomland's Lotion *(Rochester Methodist Hosp.)*. Resorcinol 3 g, glycerol 5 g, borax 1.3 g, starch 6.25 g, calamine 6.25 g, isopropyl alcohol (70%) to 100 ml. Shelf-life 1 year.

Resorcinol and Sulfur Lotion *(U.S.P.)*. Contains resorcinol and sulphur in a suitable hydro-alcoholic vehicle. Store in airtight containers.

Resorcinol and Sulphur Lotion *(A.P.F.)*. Resorcinol 2 g, precipitated sulphur 2 g, calamine 10 g, sterilised talc 10 g, quillaia tincture 0.5 ml, glycerol 10 ml, alcohol (90%) 30 ml, freshly boiled and cooled water to 100 ml. It may be tinted with about 0.5% of caramel solution. Protect from light.

Ointments

Compound Resorcinol Ointment *(B.P.C. 1973)*. Ung. Resorcin. Co. Resorcinol 4 g, bismuth subnitrate 8 g, zinc oxide 4 g, starch 10 g, cade oil 3 g, wool fat 10 g, sodium metabisulphite 200 mg, water 4 g, hard paraffin 2 g, yellow soft paraffin 54.8 g. Store in containers which prevent evaporation.

Compound Resorcinol Ointment *(U.S.P.)*. Resorcinol 6 g, zinc oxide 6 g, bismuth subnitrate 6 g, cade oil 2 g, yellow beeswax 10 g, yellow soft paraffin 29 g, wool fat 28 g, and glycerol 13 g. Store in airtight containers at a temperature not exceeding 30°.

Resorcinol and Salicylic Acid Ointment. Castellani's Ointment. Resorcinol 12 g, salicylic acid 2 g, lanolin and soft paraffin to 100 g. For dhobie itch.

Resorcinol and Sulphur Ointment Compound *(A.P.F.)*. Ung. Resorcin. et Sulphur. Co. Resorcinol 2 g, precipitated sulphur 3 g, salicylic acid 1 g, and simple ointment white 94 g.

Pastes

Resorcinol and Sulphur Paste *(B.P.)*. Resorcinol 5 g, precipitated sulphur 5 g, zinc oxide 40 g, and emulsifying ointment 50 g. Protect from light.

Proprietary Preparations

Acnil *(Fisons, UK)*. A cream containing resorcinol 0.5%, precipitated sulphur 3%, and cetrimide 0.5%. For acne.

Eskamel (known in USA as Acnomel) *(Smith Kline & French, UK)*. Contains resorcinol 2% and sulphur 8% in a greaseless basis. For acne.

Other Proprietary Names

Castel-Minus *(USA)*; Egosol R *(Austral.)*.

1638-j

Resorcinol Monoacetate *(U.S.P.)*. Resorcin Acetate. 3-Acetoxyphenol.

$C_8H_8O_3$=152.1.

CAS — 102-29-4.

Pharmacopoeias. In *U.S.*

A pale yellow or amber viscous liquid with a faint characteristic odour and a burning taste. B.p. about 283° with decomposition. Specific gravity 1.203 to 1.207.

Sparingly **soluble** in water; soluble in alcohol and most organic solvents. A saturated solution in water is acid to litmus. **Store** in airtight containers. Protect from light.

Uses. Resorcinol monoacetate is used for the same purposes as resorcinol; it liberates resorcinol slowly by hydrolysis so that the effects are milder and of longer duration than those of resorcinol. It is less likely than resorcinol to discolour fair hair.

Proprietary Names

Euresol *(Knoll AG, Austral.)*.

A preparation containing resorcinol monoacetate was formerly marketed in Great Britain under the proprietary name Salaphene Gel *(Napp)*.

1639-z

Selenium Sulphide *(B.P.)*. Selenium Sulfide *(U.S.P.)*; Selenium Disulphide.

SeS_2=143.1.

CAS — 7488-56-4.

Pharmacopoeias. In *Br.* and *U.S.*

A bright orange to reddish-brown powder with a faint odour of hydrogen sulphide, and containing 52 to 55.5% of Se. Practically **insoluble** in water; soluble 1 in about 160 of chloroform and 1 in about 1650 of ether; practically insoluble in most other organic solvents.

Adverse Effects. When taken by mouth, selenium sulphide is highly toxic. Symptoms of poisoning include an odour of garlic in the breath, a metallic taste, anorexia, vomiting, anaemia, and fatty degeneration of the liver. Only traces of selenium sulphide are absorbed through the skin.

A 46-year-old woman with an excoriated open eruption on her scalp used a shampoo containing selenium sulphide twice or thrice weekly for 8 months. She developed weakness, anorexia, tremors, sweating, a metallic taste in her mouth, and a smell of garlic in her breath. She completely recovered on ceasing her shampoo, and without specific treatment, in 10 days. During the illness there was an elevation of the urinary porphyrins.— J. W. Ransome *et al.*, *New Engl. J. Med.*, 1961, *264*, 384.

The administration of selenium compounds could cause photosensitivity.— J. Kalivas, *J. Am. med. Ass.*, 1969, *209*, 1706.

The pharmacology and toxicology of selenium.— L. M. Klevay, *Pharmac. Ther.* 1976, *1*, 211.

A review of the toxicity of selenium.— L. Fishbein, in Toxicology of Trace Elements, *Advances in Modern Toxicology*, Vol. 2, R.A. Goyer and M.A. Mehlman (Ed.), London, Wiley, 1977, p. 191. See also L. M. Cummins and E. T. Kimura, *Toxic. appl. Pharmac.*, 1971, *20*, 89; A. W. Kilness and F. H. Hochberg, *J. Am. med. Ass.*, 1977, *237*, 2843; K. Schwarz (letter), *ibid.*, *238*, 2365; L. T. Kurland (letter), *ibid.*; T. K. Daneshmend (letter), *Br. med. J.*, 1978, *2*, 829.

Loss of hair. Repeated use of selenium sulphide shampoo for treatment of seborrhoeic dermatitis in 6 women resulted in loss of hair in varying degrees. When use of the shampoo was discontinued, hair-shedding ceased.— R. W. Grover, *J. Am. med. Ass.*, 1956, *160*, 1397.

In a study of 65 subjects there was no significant increase in the number of damaged hairs after the bi-weekly use of a selenium sulphide shampoo for several months.— N. Orentreich and R. A. Berger, *Archs Derm.*, 1964, *90*, 76, per *Abstr. Wld Med.*, 1965, *37*, 131.

Treatment of Adverse Effects. Empty the stomach by aspiration and lavage and give a purgative, such as sodium sulphate 30 g in 250 ml of water, to promote peristalsis. Urinary excretion may be increased by ascorbic acid given by mouth. Dimercaprol should not be used. Further treatment should be symptomatic.

Ascorbic acid 10 mg per kg body-weight daily might remove the odour of garlic from the breath of workers using selenium and selenium compounds.— *Br. med. J.*, 1973, *4*, 44.

Precautions. Selenium sulphide should not be applied to inflamed or exudative areas, or to extensive areas of the skin. It should not be allowed to enter the eyes.

Uses. Selenium sulphide is used as a shampoo in the treatment of dandruff and seborrhoeic dermatitis of the scalp. The scalp is washed with soap and water, rinsed, and 5 to 10 ml of a suspension containing 2.5% of selenium sulphide is applied together with a small amount of warm water to produce a lather; the hair is rinsed and the application repeated; the suspension should remain in contact with the scalp for a total of 4 to 6 minutes. The hair should be well rinsed after the treatment and all traces of the suspension removed from the hands and nails. Applications are usually made twice weekly for 2 weeks, then once weekly for 2 weeks and then only when necessary. A 1% shampoo is also used.

Selenium sulphide is also used as a 2.5% lotion in the treatment of pityriasis versicolor.

A review of selenium deficiency, metabolism, human requirements and toxicity. Selenium could protect *animals* against the toxic effects of cadmium and of mercury.— Report of a WHO Expert Group on Trace Elements in Human Nutrition, *Tech. Rep. Ser. Wld Hlth Org. No. 532*, 1973.

A committee of the American National Research Council stated that the 150 µg daily of selenium in the average American diet did not need to be supplemented.— *J. Am. med. Ass.*, 1977, *237*, 1068.

Dandruff. In an evaluation of the antidandruff efficacy of 3 shampoos. The shampoo containing selenium sulphide 2.5% was more effective than one containing pyrithione zinc 2% and both were more effective than a non-medicated shampoo.— A. M. Kligman *et al.*, *J. Soc. cosmet. Chem.*, 1974, *25*, 73.

Pityriasis versicolor. Application of 57 to 85 ml of selenium sulphide 2.5% lotion from the neck to the knees (but excluding the genitals) was used to treat pityriasis versicolor in 98 patients; the solution was allowed to dry and was left overnight before washing. Fungi were eliminated by a single treatment in 81 patients, and after a second treatment in 8, but recurrences were common 6 months later. Mild skin irritation occurred in 7 treatments.— A. D. Albright and J. M. Hitch, *Archs Derm.*, 1966, *93*, 460, per *Abstr. Wld Med.*, 1966, *40*, 445.

Preparations

Selenium Sulfide Lotion *(U.S.P.)*. Selenium Sulfide Detergent Suspension. Selenium sulphide in an aqueous stabilised suspension containing a suitable dispersing agent, buffer, and detergent. pH 2 to 6. Store in airtight containers.

Selenium Sulphide Scalp Application *(B.P.)*. Selenium Sulphide Application. A suspension of selenium sulphide in a suitable liquid basis. pH 4 to 5.5. It should not be used within 2 days of the application of hair tints or permanent waving solutions and should not be allowed to come into contact with metals.

Proprietary Preparations

Lenium *(Winthrop, UK)*. A shampoo cream with a non-alkaline basis, containing selenium sulphide 2.5%.

Selsun *(Abbott, UK)*. Selenium sulphide, available as a suspension containing 2.5%, in a detergent basis. (Also available as Selsun in *Austral.*, *Belg.*, *Canad.*, *Denm.*, *Fr.*, *Ger.*, *Ital.*, *Norw.*, *S.Afr.*, *Switz.*, *USA*).

Other Proprietary Names

Austral.—Sebarex; *Canad.*—Exsel, Sebusan; *Denm.*—Selenol; *Ger.*— Selukos; *Norw.*—Selukos; *Spain*—Abbottselsun, Bioselenium, Caspiselenio; *Swed.*—Sebusan, Selukos; *Switz.*—Sebo-Lenium, Selenol, Selukos; *USA*—Exsel, Iosel 250, Selsun Blue, Sul-Blue.

1640-p

Sodium Polymetaphosphate *(B.P.C. 1973)*.

CAS — 50813-16-6.

NOTE. Sodium Hexametaphosphate has been used as a synonym for this substance, but it exists in much higher degrees of polymerisation.

Colourless, translucent, odourless or almost odourless, vitreous deliquescent plates or powder

with a saline and warming taste, containing not less than 85% of $(NaPO_3)_x$ and 8 to 15% of tetrasodium pyrophosphate, $Na_4P_2O_7$.
Slowly **soluble** in water; practically insoluble in alcohol and organic solvents. A 0.25% solution in water has a pH of 7 to 7.5. Aqueous solutions slowly revert to orthophosphate; the rate of hydration is much increased by high temperatures and by the addition of sufficient acid or alkali. **Store** in airtight containers.

Uses. Sodium polymetaphosphate may be used as a 5% dusting-powder in hyperhidrosis and bromidrosis, and as a prophylactic against athlete's foot.
Sodium polymetaphosphate combines with calcium and magnesium ions to form complex soluble compounds. As a water softener, a dilution of 1 in 600 to 1 in 300 is employed for preventing the precipitation of calcium and magnesium compounds when added to water of 20 degrees (English) of hardness. Added to water (1 ppm) in which instruments are boiled, it prevents rusting and deposition of a film if the solution is first made slightly alkaline with sodium carbonate.
In the threshold treatment of boiler-feed waters a concentration of 5 ppm or less is normally used.
It is used in the food industry as a stabiliser.
Similar compounds, of slightly varying composition, and described as Sodium Metaphosphate are used in the food industry as emulsifying agents and chelating agents.

Estimated acceptable daily dietary intake: up to 70 mg as phosphorus per kg body-weight.— Seventh Report of FAO/WHO Expert Committee on Food Additives, *Tech. Rep. Ser. Wld Hlth Org. No. 281*, 1964.

Proprietary Preparations

Calgon *(Albright & Wilson, Medical Division, UK)*. A brand of sodium polymetaphosphate available in several grades. **Calgon S** and **Calgon PT**. Brands of sodium polymetaphosphate (*B.P.C. 1973*).

1641-s

Starch. Amylum; Amidon; Stärke; Almidón; Amido; Amilo.

CAS — 9005-25-8 (starch); 9005-82-7 (α-amylose); 9004-34-6 (β-amylose); 9037-22-3 (amylopectin).

Starches (*B.P., Eur. P.*) may be maize starch (Amylum Maydis), rice starch (Amylum Oryzae), potato starch (Amylum Solani), or wheat starch (Amylum Tritici). Starch (*U.S.N.F.*) is maize starch, wheat starch, or potato starch.

Pharmacopoeias. Some or all of the starches described are included in all pharmacopoeias examined except *Int.*, *Rus.*, and *U.S.*, but in *U.S.N.F.*

Polysaccharide granules obtained from the caryopsis of maize, *Zea mays*, rice, *Oryza sativa*, wheat, *Triticum aestivum* (*T. vulgare*), or from the tubers of potato, *Solanum tuberosum*. Maize starch is also known as corn starch. In tropical or subtropical countries where these starches are not available, the *B.P.* allows the use of tapioca starch—see Cassava Starch, p.504. Starch contains amylose and amylopectin, both polysaccharides based on α-glucose.
A fine, white, odourless, tasteless powder which creaks when pressed between the fingers, or irregular angular masses readily reducible to powder. Maize starch, rice starch, and wheat starch lose not more than 15% of their weight on drying, and potato starch not more than 20% of its weight. At relative humidities between about 25 and 55% at 25°, the equilibrium moisture content is about 10 to 14% for maize, rice, and wheat starches, and 10 to 18% for potato starch. Above about 75% relative humidity, all the starches absorb substantial amounts of moisture.
Practically **insoluble** in cold water and alcohol. When boiled with 50 times their weight of water and cooled, maize, rice and wheat starches give a thin cloudy mucilage, whereas potato starch gives a thicker, more transparent mucilage. A 20% slurry of maize starch or wheat starch has a pH of 4.5 to 7, and of potato starch 5 to 8. **Store** in a cool dry place in airtight containers.

The amylopectin fraction of starch was not very reactive with benzoic acid, *p*-hydroxybenzoic acid, and sorbic acid. The amylose fraction complexed rapidly with these preservatives, probably in a similar manner to the known starch-iodine and starch-alcohol complexes.— Z. Mansour and E. P. Guth, *J. pharm. Sci.*, 1968, *57*, 404.

A review of starch derivatives.— L. Chalmers, *Mfg Chem.*, 1968, *39* (Sept.), 31.

A study of the effect of some binding agents, including maize starch, on the mechanical properties of granules and their compression characteristics.— E. Doelker and E. Shotton, *J. Pharm. Pharmac.*, 1977, *29*, 193.

Disintegrating agents. The long-accepted swelling of starch as a mechanism for tablet disintegration was not demonstrated and could not be related to starch damage during tablet manufacture.— J. T. Ingram and W. Lowenthal, *J. pharm. Sci.*, 1968, *57*, 393.

Rice starch and bentonite were considered the best disintegrants of 6 studied, in that they accelerated disintegration without affecting the mechanical properties of experimental lactose tablets.— A. M. Sakr *et al.*, *Mfg Chem.*, 1973, *44* (Jan.), 37.

A review of starch as a disintegrating agent.— P. Couvreur and M. Roland, *J. Pharm. Belg.*, 1976, *31*, 511, per *Int. pharm. Abstr.*, 1977, *14*, 795.

Further references: R. H. Shangraw, *Drug Cosmet. Ind.*, 1978, *123* (July), 34; J. B. Schwartz and J. A. Zelinskie, *Drug Dev. ind. Pharm.*, 1978, *4*, 463.

Water absorption. The water absorption capacity varied in a predictable way with various combinations and proportions of starch, pregelatinised maize starch, talc, and zinc oxide dispersed in light liquid paraffin, while absorption-rates were unpredictable. Zinc oxide had the best water-absorptive capacity and rate, followed by pregelatinised maize starch. Talc was useless for water absorption in the lipophilic basis. When zinc oxide and pregelatinised maize starch or talc and starch were mixed together, the absorption properties were reduced.— E. D. Sumner *et al.*, *J. pharm. Sci.*, 1969, *58*, 83.

Soluble Starch, which is used as a reagent, is prepared from potato starch or maize starch by a process involving treatment with dilute hydrochloric acid, carefully adjusted so as to destroy the gelatinising power of the starch. Soluble starch shows the microscopical appearance almost unchanged of potato starch or maize starch, but has the property of being readily soluble in hot water to form a transparent mobile liquid.

Banana Starch. As a disintegrating agent in tablets of calcium lactate, calcium carbonate, phenacetin, and phenobarbitone, banana starch compared well with maize starch.— R. P. Patel and G. J. Joshi, *Indian J. Pharm.*, 1959, *21*, 136.

Moriyo Starch. Starch obtained from the polished grain of *Panicum miliare*, commonly used as a diet in India during religious fastings. As a disintegrating agent in tablets of calcium carbonate, calcium gluconate, phenacetin and caffeine, and sulphathiazole, it was superior to maize starch.— R. P. Patel and J. M. Pancholi, *Indian J. Pharm.* 1964, *26*, 313.

Adverse Effects. Granulomatous lesions have been reported following the use of starch glove powders.

The formation of starch gastroliths in some women who ate large quantities of starch during pregnancy.— E. M. Boyd and S. J. Liu, *Can. med. Ass. J.*, 1968, *98*, 492.

The toxicological evaluation of some modified starches.— *Fd Add. Ser. Wld Hlth Org. No. 1*, 1972.

A report of a meningeal reaction to starch glove powder in the CSF after craniectomy.— B. Dunkley and T. T. Lewis, *Br. med. J.*, 1977, *2*, 1391.

Starch granuloma. Some case reports.— J. Neely and J. D. Davies, *Br. med. J.*, 1971, *3*, 625; A. L. Warshaw, *Lancet*, 1972, *2*, 1054; L. Michaels and N. S. Shah (letter), *Br. med. J.*, 1973, *2*, 714; M. Pemberton and M. Johnson (letter), *ibid.*, 1973, *3*, 235; S. P. Pazcoguin *et al.*, *N.Y. St. J. Med.*, 1975, *75*, 1743; J. J. Sternlieb *et al.*, *Archs Surg., Chicago*, 1977, *112*, 458, per *J. Am. med. Ass.*, 1977, *237*, 1878.

Discussions of the hazards of surgical glove dusting-powders.— *Lancet*, 1972, *2*, 74; *Br. med. J.*, 1973, *2*, 502; D. G. Jagelman and H. Ellis, *Br. J. Surg.*, 1973, *60*, 111; H. Ellis, *Postgrad. med. J.*, 1973, *49*, 644; *Br. med. J.*, 1980, *281*, 892.

Uses. Starch is absorbent and is widely used in dusting-powders, either alone or mixed with zinc oxide or other similar substances. Starch is used as a surgical glove powder; because starch granulomas have occurred care should be taken to minimise contamination of the wound.
Ointments containing starch may be used as protective applications in skin diseases. Starch Glycerin and Starch Mucilage have been employed as emollient applications to the skin. The mucilage also forms the basis of some enemas and is used in the treatment of iodine poisoning. Starch has been used as a poultice (10%) and is incorporated in many tablets as a disintegrating agent.

The performance of a starch-tolerance test in addition to a glucose-tolerance test in patients with suspected pancreatic disease would detect an additional 10 to 33% of patients with the disease, compared with those given only a glucose-tolerance test, but at the cost of a 7% increase in false positives.— *Archs intern. Med.*, 1966, *118*, 103, per *J. Am. med. Ass.*, 1966, *197* (Aug. 22), A158.

The use of chemically and enzymically modified starches was only limited by good manufacturing practice.— Seventeenth Report of the FAO/WHO Expert Committee on Food Additives, *Tech. Rep. Ser. Wld Hlth Org. No. 539*, 1974. For background toxicological information on modified starches used in food, see *Fd Add. Ser. Wld Hlth Org. No. 5*, 1974.

Gastro-enteritis. Beneficial results with rice water in treatment of infantile gastro-enteritis.— H. B. Wong (letter), *Lancet*, 1981, *2*, 102.

Preparations

CMTZ Powder *(Rochester Methodist Hosp.)*. Maize starch 50 g, magnesium carbonate 2 g, talc 24 g, zinc oxide 24 g. Shelf-life 2 years.

Starch Calamine Lotion *(Rochester Methodist Hosp.)*. Starch 18.7 g, calamine 6.26 g, phenol 65 mg, glycerol 2 ml, Veegum Regular 1 g, water to 100 ml. Shelf-life 2 years.

Starch Glycerin *(B.P.C. 1963)*. Glycerinum Amyli. A translucent jelly prepared by heating wheat starch 8.5 g with water 17 ml and glycerol 74.5 g. It should be freshly prepared. A similar preparation is included in many pharmacopoeias, sometimes with the title Unguentum Glycerini, the amount of starch varying between 5 and 10%; a suitable preservative, such as methyl hydroxybenzoate, is sometimes included.

Starch Glycerite *(U.S.N.F.)*. Starch 10 g, benzoic acid 200 mg, water 20 ml, glycerol 70 ml, heated at 140° to 144°. It should be freshly prepared. Store in airtight containers.

Starch Mucilage *(B.P.C. 1973)*. Mucilago Amyli. Starch 2.5 g, triturated with water to 20 ml, added to boiling water 80 ml, and again raised to boiling. It should be freshly prepared. *Nord. P.* has soluble starch 8 g and water 92 g.

Sterilisable Maize Starch *(B.P.)*. Absorbable Dusting Powder; Modified Starch Dusting Powder; Starch-derivative Dusting Powder. A white, odourless, free-flowing powder, prepared by treating maize starch by chemical and physical means so that it does not gelatinise on exposure to moisture or steam sterilisation. It contains not more than 2.2% of magnesium oxide and loses not more than 15% of its weight on drying. A 10% suspension in water has a pH of 9.5 to 10.8.
Sterilisable Maize Starch may be sterilised by maintaining the whole of the powder at 150° to 160° for 1 hour, or by spreading in a sufficiently thin layer and exposing to saturated steam at 115° to 118° for 30 minutes.
The *B.P.* requires that when Absorbable Dusting Powder is demanded, Sterilisable Maize Starch must be supplied.
A similar powder (Absorbable Dusting Powder) is described in the *U.S.P.*

Proprietary Preparations

Bio-Sorb *(Surgikos, UK)*. A brand of Sterilisable Maize Starch.

Bio-Sorb Cream *(Surgikos, UK)*. A sterile glove lubricant for application to the hands, consisting of slightly modified Bio-Sorb powder in a rapidly-drying cream basis.

Encapsul *(Laing-National, UK)*. A heat-treated blend of starches for use as an encapsulating agent.

Vulca 90 *(Laing-National, UK)*. A sterilisable maize starch; for use as a dusting-powder basis.

Wheat starch was formerly marketed in Great Britain under the proprietary name Nutregen Wheat Starch (*Energen*).

Preparations of Related Substances

Pregelatinised Maize Starch *(B.P.)*. A white to pale cream-coloured almost odourless powder, dispersible in cold water; prepared by heating an aqueous slurry of maize starch and removing the water from the resulting paste. It contains no added substances and loses not more than 15% of its weight on drying. A 20% dispersion in water has a pH of 5.5 to 8.0.
Store in airtight containers. Tablet excipient.

Pregelatinized Starch *(U.S.N.F.)*. Starch which has been chemically or mechanically processed to rupture all or part of the granules in the presence of water and subsequently dried. Some types are modified to render them compressible and free-flowing. pH of a 10% slurry 4.5 to 7. Tablet excipient.

Proprietary Preparations of Starch Derivatives

Capsul *(Laing-National, UK)*. A brand of heat-treated maize starch ester; for use as an encapsulating agent.

Instant Clearjel *(Laing-National, UK)*. A brand of pregelatinised maize starch which has been esterified; for use as a suspending agent, and binder and tabletting agent.

Jalan *(Laing-National, UK)*. A brand name for a range of starch products, including maize, wheat, potato, farina, and root starch derivatives.

National 1551 *(Laing-National, UK)*. A brand of pregelatinised maize starch; for use as a tablet disintegrant.

1642-w

Cassava Starch. Manihot Starch; Manioc Starch; Amido de Mandioca; Brazilian Arrowroot; Rio Arrowroot; Tapioca Starch.

CAS — 9005-25-8.

Pharmacopoeias. In *Braz.*, *Chin.*, and *Port.*

The starch granules from the rhizomes of bitter cassava, *Manihot utilissima* (=*M. esculenta*) (Euphorbiaceae).
A white odourless tasteless powder. It loses not more than 15% of its weight when dried. Practically **insoluble** in water, alcohol, ether, and most organic solvents. **Store** in a cool dry place.

Cassava starch is used as a substitute for starch and arrowroot. The *B.P.* allows the use of cassava (tapioca) starch in place of starch in tropical and subtropical countries where maize, rice, wheat, or potato starch is not available.

A degenerative neuropathy in Nigeria was possibly due to the high concentration of cyanogenetic material in the outer integument of the tuberous root of cassava contaminating the edible part. Other factors affecting the incidence of degenerative neuropathy could be dietary deficiencies, metabolic abnormalities and infections.— B. O. Osuntokun *et al.*, *Br. med. J.*, 1969, *1*, 547.

A steady diet of cassava inhibited iodine uptake by the thyroid gland. With marginal iodine supply endemic goitre, cretinism, and mental retardation could result.— A. -M. Ermans, *Nature*, 1978, *272*, 121.

Comment on the suspicion that cassava is a pancreatic toxin, and responsible for the development of tropical diabetes.— *Lancet*, 1979, *2*, 341. Comment. The high incidence of diabetes in the Zaire-Zambian border region, a predominantly cassava-eating zone, which has been ascribed to malnutrition, may be due to cassava. In the rest of Zambia where maize is the staple food, diabetes is uncommon.— J. C. Davidson (letter), *ibid.*, 635.

Use as glove powder. Cassava starch produced no granulomas in dogs when a mass of 100 mg was placed on the omentum or subcutaneous tissues. No granulomas or peritonitis attributable to its use had occurred in 15 years of human use.— R. Herrera-Llerandi (letter), *Br. med. J.*, 1973, *3*, 411.

1643-e

Precipitated Sulphur *(B.P.)*. Precipitated Sulfur *(U.S.P.)*; Milk of Sulphur; Lac Sulfuris; Magisterio de Azufre; Soufre Précipité; Gefällter Schwefel; Azufre Precipitado; Enxôfre Precipitado.
S=32.06.

CAS — 7704-34-9.

Pharmacopoeias. In all pharmacopoeias examined except *Chin.*, *Eur.*, *Int.*, and *Neth. Jap.* includes Sulfur but does not specify precipitated or sublimed.

A pale yellow, greyish-yellow, or greenish-yellow, soft, odourless, tasteless, amorphous or microcrystalline powder, free from grittiness. Under a microscope it is seen to consist entirely of grouped amorphous particles free from associated crystals. It melts at about 115° forming a yellow mobile liquid which becomes dark and viscous on heating at about 160°.
Practically **insoluble** in water and alcohol; soluble almost completely in carbon disulphide, the solution depositing the insoluble variety of sulphur on exposure to light; soluble 1 in 60 of chloroform, 1 in 600 of ether, and 1 in 100 of olive oil; soluble in light petroleum and turpentine oil, and in hot aqueous solutions of alkali hydroxides forming polysulphides and thiosulphates. The filtrate from a 20% suspension in water is neutral to litmus.

WARNING. *The Council of the Pharmaceutical Society of Great Britain advises pharmacists not to supply materials likely to be used for making fireworks, including sulphur, to children under any circumstances, and recommends that it should be sold only to persons who are, or appear to be, 18 years of age or over.*

In aqueous lotions containing precipitated sulphur, a few drops of a solution of a surfactant such as docusate sodium was recommended as a 'wetting' agent for the sulphur.— *Pharm. J. N.Z.*, 1957, *19*, No. 8, 21.

Uses. Sulphur is a mild antiseptic and parasiticide and has been widely employed, in the form of lotions or ointments, in the treatment of acne and scabies, though more convenient and effective preparations are available. Lotions of precipitated sulphur with lead acetate have been used to darken grey hair.
When taken by mouth, precipitated sulphur is converted in the small intestine into alkali sulphides which by their irritant action produce a mild laxative effect. It has been employed for this purpose in children as a confection or in lozenges.
Sulphur is used in homoeopathic medicine.

Suspensions of elemental sulphur produced histological evidence of comedone formation when applied to the *rabbit* ear canal. Similar results occurred when 2.5 or 5% suspensions were applied, under occlusive dressings, to the backs of 6 volunteers for 6 weeks. It was considered that, while the application of sulphur suspensions to acne vulgaris reduced the papulo-pustules, it promoted the formation of comedones and so established a vicious circle. The presence of masses of *Corynebacterium acnes* in sulphur-induced comedones cast doubt on the reputed antibacterial activity of sulphur.— O. H. Mills and A. M. Kligman, *Br. J. Derm.*, 1972, *86*, 620. Comment.— R. Carruthers, *Drugs*, 1973, *5*, 337.

Preparations

Baths

Sulfur Bath *(Rochester Methodist Hosp.)*. Precipitated sulphur 12.5 g, dilute sulphuric acid 6.25 ml, sodium thiosulphate 3 g, docusate sodium 1% solution 0.5 ml, water to 100 ml. Add 500 ml to a 190-litre bath. Shelf-life 1 year. Antibacterial and antipruritic.

Sulphur Bath *(B.P.C. 1949)*. Balneum Sulphuris. Sodium acid sulphate 150 g and sodium thiosulphate 150 g in 140 litres of water.

Liniments

Linimentum Sulfuris *(Nord. P.)*. Precipitated sulphur 10 g, carboxymethylcellulose mucilage (*Nord. P.*) 15 g, alcohol 8 g, emulsifying wax 200 mg, water to 100 g.

Lotions

Compound Sulphur Lotion *(B.P.C. 1973)*. Sulphur Compound Lotion. Precipitated sulphur 4 g, alcohol (95%) (or industrial methylated spirit) 6 ml, glycerol 2 ml, quillaia tincture 0.5 ml, calcium hydroxide solution to 100 ml.

Lozenges

Sulphur Lozenges *(B.P.C. 1954)*. Troch. Sulphur. Each contains precipitated sulphur 324 mg and potassium acid tartrate 64.8 mg with sucrose, acacia, and orange tincture.

Ointments

Sulphur and Salicylic Acid Ointment. Sulphur 2% and salicylic acid 1% in HEB Simplex. For the scaling lesions on the scalp in seborrhoeic eczema of infancy.—M. Readett, *Practitioner*, 1966, *196*, 633.

Sulphur Ointment *(B.P.)*. Sulphur Oint.; Ung. Sulphur. Precipitated sulphur 10% in white simple ointment. Store at a temperature not exceeding 25°. *U.S.P.* (Sulfur Ointment) has 10% with liquid paraffin 10% and white ointment 80%.
Scabies has been treated with sulphur ointment after washing with soft soap. Mix equal parts of the ointment and soft paraffin and rub in daily for 3 days. Ointments containing more than 5% or used longer than 3 days may cause dermatitis.

Unguentum Sulfuris *(Roum. P.)*. Precipitated sulphur 10 g, zinc sulphate 10 g, soft soap 15 g, water 5 g, wool fat 6 g, and white soft paraffin 54 g.

Pomades

Pomatum Antipsoricum *(Arg. P.)*. Precipitated sulphur 20%, potassium carbonate 10%, water 10%, wool fat and white soft paraffin of each 30%.

Proprietary Names

Aknaseb *(Prof. Pharm. Corp., Canad.)*; Lotio Alsulfa *(Doak, Canad.)*; Postacne *(Dermik, USA)*; Schwefel-Diasporal *(Protina, Ger.)*; Sufrogel *(Weimer, Ger.)*; Sulfoïdal Robin *(Rosa-Phytopharma, Fr.)*.

1644-l

Sublimed Sulphur *(B.P.C. 1973)*. Sublimed Sulfur *(U.S.P.)*; Flowers of Sulphur; Sulphur Sublimatum; Sulfur Sublimatum Depuratum; Fleur de Soufre; Sublimierter Schwefel; Azufre Sublimado; Enxôfre Sublimado.
S=32.06.

CAS — 7704-34-9.

Pharmacopoeias. In *Arg.*, *Aust.*, *Chin.*, *Ger.*, *Hung.*, *Ind.*, *It.*, *Jug.*, *Port.*, *Span.*, *Swiss*, and *U.S.*
Jap. includes Sulfur but does not specify precipitated or sublimed.

A fine, yellow, tasteless, slightly gritty powder, with a faint and not unpleasant odour and a faint taste. Under a microscope it is seen to consist chiefly of amorphous particles or aggregates, occasionally associated with semi-crystalline masses. It melts at about 115° forming a yellow mobile liquid which becomes dark and viscous on heating at about 160°.
Very slightly **soluble** in water and alcohol; incompletely soluble in carbon disulphide; soluble in chloroform, ether, light petroleum, toluene, and fixed and volatile oils.

Sublimed sulphur has actions and uses similar to those of Precipitated Sulphur, p.504.

Adverse Effects. Metabolic acidosis occurred in a 57-year-old woman who took sublimed sulphur 250 g over a period of 6 days as a folk remedy for malaise and dyspnoea.— J. E. Blum and F. L. Coe, *New Engl. J. Med.*, 1977, *297*, 869.

Preparations

Washed Sulphur. Sulphur Lotum; Sulfur Sublimatum Lotum; Purified Sulphur; Soufre Lavé; Gewaschener Schwefel; Azufre Lavado; Enxôfre Lavado. A fine, odourless, tasteless, yellow, crystalline powder prepared by washing sublimed sulphur with ammoniated water. It is included in many pharmacopoeias.

Dome-Acne *(Dome/Hollister-Stier, UK)*. **Cream** and **Lotion** each containing colloidal sulphur 4% and resorcinol monoacetate 3% in non-greasy bases, and **Medicated Cleanser** containing colloidal sulphur 2% and salicylic acid 2%, with a soya bean emulsion complex. For acne and related conditions.

1645-y

Sulphurated Lime *(B.P.C. 1949)*. Calx Sulphurata; Calcium Sulphide.

CAS — 8028-82-8 (sulphurated lime solution).

A mixture containing calcium sulphate and not less than 50% of calcium sulphide, CaS. It is a greyish-white powder with an odour of hydrogen sulphide and a disagreeable alkaline taste. Sparingly **soluble** in water; soluble in boiling water with decomposition; soluble in solutions of ammonium salts; insoluble in alcohol. **Store** in airtight containers.

Sulphurated lime was formerly given for the treatment of boils, carbuncles, and pustular acne in doses of 15 to 60 mg; it is of doubtful value.

An impure grade of calcium sulphide (Hepar Sulphuris; Hepar Sulph.) is used in homoeopathic medicine.

NOTE. The title Hepar Sulfuris is also applied to Sulphurated Potash—see below.

Preparations

Sulphurated Lime Solution *(B.P.C. 1949).* Sulphurated Lime Lotion; Vleminckx's Solution or Lotion; Calcium Sulfuratum Solutum. Prepared by boiling sublimed sulphur 5 g with calcium hydroxide 2.5 g and water until the sulphur is dissolved and adjusting to 100 ml. It contains polysulphides of calcium equivalent to 4 to 5% of sulphur. Sulphurated Lime Solution has been used, diluted 3 or 4 times, in epidermophytoses and scabies.

Similar solutions are included in several pharmacopoeias. A solution containing calcium polysulphides and known as 'lime-sulphur' is used as a fungicide in horticulture.

Sulfurated Lime Topical Solution *(U.S.P.).* Sulfurated Lime Solution. Prepared by boiling together in water sublimed sulphur 25 g and calcium oxide 16.5 g to produce 100 ml. Store in completely-filled airtight containers.

Dilute 1 in 10 before use.

1646-j

Sulphurated Potash *(B.P.C. 1973).* Sulfurated Potash *(U.S.P.)*; Potassa Sulphurata; Liver of Sulphur; Foie de Soufre; Schwefelleber; Hepar Sulfuris; Kalii Sulfidum.

NOTE. The title Hepar Sulphuris is used in homoeopathic medicine for an impure grade of calcium sulphide—see Sulphurated Lime, above.

Pharmacopoeias. In *Nord., Port., Swiss,* and *U.S.*

A mixture of potassium polysulphides and other potassium compounds, including sulphite and thiosulphate, containing 42 to 45% of sulphur. *U.S.P.* specifies not less than 12.8% of sulphur as sulphide. Greenish-yellow fragments, internally pale liver-brown rapidly changing to greenish-yellow on exposure to air and absorbing moisture and carbon dioxide. It has a bitter acrid alkaline taste and an odour of hydrogen sulphide.

Almost completely **soluble** 1 in 2 of water. Alcohol dissolves only the sulphides. A 10% solution in water is alkaline to litmus. **Incompatible** with acids. **Store** in small airtight containers.

Sulphurated potash is a mild counter-irritant and parasiticide. Applied to the skin it dissolves the epidermis and hair. It is used in skin affections, particularly acne and scabies, in form of a lotion.

Preparations

Sulphurated Lotion *(A.P.F.).* Lot. Sulphurat. Sulphurated potash 5 g, zinc sulphate 5 g, acetone 5 ml, glycerol 5 ml, spike lavender oil 0.2 ml, freshly boiled and cooled water to 100 ml. It should be freshly prepared and used within 7 days.

White Lotion *(U.S.P.).* Lotio Alba. Sulphurated potash 4 g, zinc sulphate 4 g, water to 100 ml. It should be freshly prepared. Store in airtight containers.

When freshly prepared, White Lotion contained zinc monosulphide, zinc polysulphides, zinc hydroxide, and free sulphur suspended in a solution of sulphate, thiosulphate, and potsssium ions. Exposure of the lotion to u.v. light or sunlight resulted in formation of hydrogen peroxide which oxidised sulphides to sulphites and sulphates.— E. P. Guth and Z. Mansour, *J. pharm. Sci.*, 1967, *56,* 376.

Zinc Sulphide Lotion *(B.P.C. 1973).* Sulphurated Potash and Zinc Lotion; Sulphurated Potash Lotion. Sulphurated potash 5 g, zinc sulphate 5 g, concentrated camphor water 2.5 ml, water to 100 ml. It should be freshly prepared.

1647-z

Purified Talc *(B.P.).* Talcum *(Eur. P.)*; Talc *(U.S.P.)*; Powdered Talc; Purified French Chalk; Talcum Purificatum.

CAS — 14807-96-6.

Pharmacopoeias. In all pharmacopoeias examined except *Braz., Chin., Int.,* and *Rus.*

A purified native hydrated magnesium silicate, approximating to the formula $Mg_6(Si_2O_5)_4(OH)_4$; it may contain a small amount of aluminium silicate. A very fine, white, or greyish-white, odourless, tasteless, impalpable, and unctuous powder, which adheres readily to the skin.

Practically **insoluble** in water and in dilute mineral acids and dilute solutions of alkali hydroxides. It is **sterilised** by exposure to ethylene oxide or by heating so that the whole of the material is maintained at 160° for 1 hour.

Talc yielded sufficient nutrient matter when shaken with water to allow the growth of *Pseudomonas aeruginosa.* Peppermint water prepared by shaking with talc was often contaminated.— W. B. Hugo (letter), *Pharm. J.*, 1971, *1,* 194.

Effect of gamma-irradiation. Talc was not affected by gamma-irradiation, except for an increase in the acid-soluble matter.— *The Use of Gamma Radiation Sources for the Sterilisation of Pharmaceutical Products,* London, ABPI, 1960.

Relative adsorptive power of dusting-powders. The adsorptive power of commercial samples of dusting-powders was investigated by J. Rae (*Br. J. Derm.*, 1950, *62,* 319). The results, expressed in terms of the percentage of moisture adsorbed in 24 hours were: precipitated calcium carbonate 2.0; zinc oxide 2.25; lithium stearate 2.75; boric acid 3.5; talc 4.5; 'cosmetic' magnesium carbonate 5.0; titanium dioxide 5.0; aluminium stearate 5.45; calcium stearate 6.5; zinc stearate 6.5; kaolin 6.75; heavy magnesium carbonate 9.0; magnesium stearate 10.25; magnesium trisilicate 13.0; starch 14.25; zinc carbonate 14.75; 'amorphous' silica 15.0.— *Practitioner,* 1950, *165,* 557.

Adverse Effects. Contamination of the tissues with talc is liable to cause granulomas.

Prolonged and intense exposure to talc may produce pneumoconiosis.

Talc is liable to be heavily contaminated with bacteria, including *Clostridium tetani, Cl. welchii,* and *Bacillus anthracis.* When used in dusting-powders, it should be sterilised.

If tablets and capsules were made into crude injections by drug addicts, the talc component might cause pulmonary thromboses. In 2 addicts who injected mixtures of camphorated opium tincture and pyribenzamine tablets, talc in the tablets caused lung lesions.— *J. Am. med. Ass.*, 1966, *195* (Jan. 10), A37.

Pneumoconiosis after the excessive use of cosmetic talcum powder over 20 years.— K. Nam and D. R. Gracey, *J. Am. med. Ass.*, 1972, *221,* 492.

A discussion on the hazards of dust exposure. Purified talc used cosmetically should not provide a health hazard especially in view of improved manufacturing specifications.— *Lancet,* 1977, *1,* 1348. See also G. Y. Hildick-Smith, *Br. J. ind. Med.*, 1976, *33,* 217, per *Abstr. Hyg.*, 1977, *52,* 133.

Abnormal chest X-rays in 15 of 94 workers involved in the processing of talc.— P. Léophonte *et al.*, *Archs Mal. prof. méd. trav.*, 1976, *37,* 513, per *Abstr. Hyg.*, 1976, *51,* 1033.

References to a possible association between ovarian cancer and exposure to cosmetic talc: W. J. Henderson *et al.* (letter), *Lancet,* 1979, *1,* 499; D. L. Longo and R. C. Young, *ibid.*, 1979, *2,* 349; M. L. Newhouse (letter), *ibid.*, 528; F. J. C. Roe (letter), *ibid.*, 744; D. L. Longo and R. C. Young (letter), *ibid.*, 1011; I. M. Phillipson (letter), *ibid.*, 1980, *1,* 48.

Poisoning by aspiration. Case reports of severe respiratory distress, sometimes fatal, in children after the aspiration of talc.— J. J. Molnar *et al.*, *New Engl. J. Med.*, 1962, *266,* 36; W. T. Hughes and T. Kalmer, *Am. J. Dis. Child.*, 1966, *111,* 653, per *Pharm. J.*, 1967, *2,* 533; *Br. med. J.*, 1969, *4,* 5.

Treatment. After aspiration of baby powder by a child, and despite the absence of signs of respiratory depression, intubation was carried out under halothane anaesthesia and intensive bronchial lavage performed. Further treatment consisted of prednisone, ampicillin, humidified air, and acetylcysteine by inhalation. The child suffered no ill effects. This treatment was recommended for children who had aspirated powders especially of talc or zinc oxide. Further symptomatic treatment that might be required included assistance with ventilation and trometamol, not sodium bicarbonate, for respiratory acidosis.— J. Pfenninger and V. D'Apuzzo, *Archs Dis. Childh.*, 1977, *52,* 157. See also *Br. med. J.*, 1969, *4,* 5.

Uses. Purified talc is used in massage and as a dusting-powder to allay irritation and prevent chafing. It is usually mixed with starch and zinc oxide. Talc used in dusting-powders should be sterilised. As purified talc is liable to cause foreign-body granulomas, it is not suitable for dusting surgical gloves. Purified talc is used as a lubricant in making tablets and to clarify liquids.

Talc poudrage has been used to treat recurrent spontaneous pneumothorax and pleural effusions.

Pleural effusion. Favourable reports of the use of talc poudrage in pleural effusions.— G. J. Haupt *et al.*, *J. Am. med. Ass.*, 1960, *172,* 918; R. C. Camishion *et al.*, *Surg. Clins N. Am.*, 1962, *42,* 1521.

The insufflation of iodised talc over the pleural surface eliminated the need for chest aspiration in all but 1 of 21 patients with recurrent malignant pleural effusion.— G. R. Jones, *Thorax,* 1969, *24,* 69, per *J. Am. med. Ass.*, 1969, *207,* 788. See also R. H. Adler and B. W. Rappole, *Surgery, St Louis,* 1967, *62,* 1000, per *J. Am. med. Ass.*, 1968, *203* (Feb. 5), A203.

Preparations

Talc Dusting Powder *(B.P., A.P.F.).* Conspersus Talci; Talc Powder. Purified talc, sterilised, 90 g and starch 10 g.

1648-c

Tar *(B.P.).* Pix Liquida; Pine Tar *(U.S.P.)*; Pix Pini; Pix Abietinarum; Pyroleum Pini; Goudron Végétal; Nadelholzteer; Alquitrán Vegetal; Brea de Pino.

CAS — 8007-45-2.

NOTE. It is known in commerce as Stockholm tar.

Pharmacopoeias. In *Arg., Aust., Belg., Br., Cz., Ind., Mex., Nord., Port., Span., Swiss,* and *U.S.*

Tar is obtained by the destructive distillation of the wood of various trees of the family Pinaceae. It contains hydrocarbons and phenols. It is a dark brown or nearly black viscous bituminous liquid with a characteristic empyreumatic odour and taste; it is heavier than water. Tar has an acid reaction which it imparts to water when shaken with it, and it may thereby be distinguished from coal tar, which has an alkaline reaction.

Very slightly **soluble** in water; soluble 1 in 10 of alcohol (90%) and in acetone, chloroform, ether, glacial acetic acid, and fixed and volatile oils.

When stored for some time tar separates into a layer which is granular in character due to minute crystallisation of catechol, resin acids, etc. and surface layer of a syrupy consistence. **Store** in airtight containers.

Uses. Tar has been used for its antipruritic properties in the treatment of chronic skin diseases, particularly eczema and psoriasis, but it does not relieve pruritus as effectively as coal tar. It has been applied chiefly as ointments.

Internally, tar has been given in the form of a syrup as an expectorant in chronic bronchitis.

Exposure to tars and oils or to ointments containing them could cause acne-like eruptions.— J. M. Hitch, *J. Am. med. Ass.*, 1967, *200,* 879.

Of 4000 patients subjected to patch testing in 5 European clinics 10.3% of males and 9.6% of females showed positive reactions to wood tars 25% in soft paraffin.— H. Bandmann *et al.*, *Archs Derm.*, 1972, *106,* 335.

Proprietary Preparations

Polytar Emollient *(Stiefel, UK).* A bath additive containing tar 7.5%, coal tar topical solution *U.S.P.* 2.5%, arachis oil extract of crude coal tar 7.5%, cade oil 7.5%, and liquid paraffin 35%. For psoriasis, eczema, and pruritic dermatoses.

A report of excessive sweating and weight loss apparently due to daily bathing with Polytar Emollient.— N. B. Simpson and W. J. Cunliffe, *Br. med. J.*, 1979, *1*, 931.

Polytar Liquid *(Stiefel, UK)*. A scalp cleanser containing tar 0.3%, coal tar topical solution *U.S.P.* 0.1%, cade oil 0.3%, arachis oil extract of crude coal tar 0.3%, and oleyl alcohol 1% with triethanolamine lauryl sulphate, lauric diethanolamide, and polysorbate 80, adjusted to pH 5.5. For scalp disorders such as psoriasis, seborrhoea, and pruritus. **Polytar Plus.** Contains in addition hydrolysed animal protein 3%.

Tardrox *(Carlton Laboratories, UK)*. A cream containing tar 1% and halquinol 1.5% in a non-greasy basis. For eczema and psoriasis.

Proprietary Preparations Containing a Tar Distillate

ESTP (Ether-Soluble Tar Paste) *(Martindale Pharmaceuticals, UK)*. A cream containing ether-soluble tar distillate 1.5%, zinc oxide 14%, and starch 12% in an emollient basis. For eczema, psoriasis, and other affections of the skin.

1649-k

Beech Tar. Pix Fagi; Pyroleum Fagi; Oleum Fagi Empyreumaticum.

Pharmacopoeias. In *Aust.* and *Nord.*

A tar obtained by the destructive distillation of the wood of the beech, *Fagus sylvatica* (Fagaceae). It is a dark brown to reddish-brown viscous liquid with a characteristic creosote-like odour and a bitter burning taste; it is heavier than water.

Very slightly **soluble** in water; almost completely soluble in alcohol, chloroform, and ether; slightly soluble in turpentine oil; miscible with soft paraffin, fats, and castor oil; partly soluble in other fixed oils; practically insoluble in glycerol.

Beech tar is used for the same purposes as tar.

Preparations

Spiritus Pyrolei Fagi *(Dan. Disp.)*. Beech Tar Spirit. Beech tar 50 g and alcohol 50 g. Allow to stand for 2 days and filter.

1650-w

Coal Tar *(B.P.)*. Pix Carbonis; Pix Carbon.; Crude Coal Tar; Pix Lithanthracis; Pix Mineralis; Pyroleum Lithanthracis; Oleum Lithanthracis; Goudron de Houille; Steinkohlenteer; Alquitrán de Hulla; Brea de Hulla; Alcatrão Mineral.

CAS — 8007-45-2.

NOTE. Pix Lithanthracis (*Arg. P.*) is Prepared Coal Tar.

Pharmacopoeias. In *Aust., Belg., Br., Cz., Jug., Nord., Port., Roum., Span., Swiss,* and *U.S.*

Coal tar is obtained by the destructive distillation of bituminous coal at about 1000°. The chief constituents are benzene, naphthalene, phenols, and pitch together with small quantities of basic compounds such as pyridine and quinoline.

A thick, nearly black, viscous liquid with a strong characteristic penetrating empyreumatic odour and a sharp burning taste. On exposure to air it gradually becomes more viscous. It burns with a luminous sooty flame. Wt per ml about 1.15 g.

Slightly **soluble** in water; partly soluble in alcohol, acetone, chloroform, ether, carbon disulphide, methyl alcohol, light petroleum, and volatile oils; almost completely soluble in nitrobenzene. A saturated solution in water is alkaline to litmus. **Store** in airtight containers.

Ointments or pastes containing coal tar or an alcoholic solution of coal tar should be made by incorporating the coal tar or coal tar solution in the unheated ointment basis or, if it should be necessary to aid mixing, in the basis which has been slightly warmed.

Variations in composition. Tar of low tar-acid content (14%) and medium naphthalene content (3%) gave relief from pruritus with involution of acute vesicular eruptions. Tar of high tar-acid content (50%) and little or no naphthalene was most effective in psoriasis, lichen simplex, and similar chronic scaly dermatoses.— F. C. Combes, *J. Am. pharm. Ass., pract. Pharm. Edn*, 1954, *15*, 408.

No significant therapeutic differences were noted during a study of 22 patients with stable symmetrical chronic psoriasis when the use of high-temperature tar from coke ovens was compared with low-temperature tar obtained during the manufacture of smokeless fuel.— R. S. Chapman and O. A. Finn, *Br. J. Derm.*, 1976, *94*, 71.

Adverse Effects. Coal tar may cause irritation and acne-like eruptions of the skin. It also has a photosensitising action.

Allergy. From patch tests on 413 patients with contact dermatoses, 4 were found to be allergic to coal tar.— E. Epstein, *J. Am. med. Ass.*, 1966, *198*, 517.

Of 400 patients subjected to patch testing in 5 European clinics 3.4% of males and 3.5% of females showed positive reactions to coal tar 5% in soft paraffin.— H. Bandmann *et al.*, *Archs Derm.*, 1972, *106*, 335.

Further references: E. Rudzki and D. Kleniewska, *Br. J. Derm.*, 1970, *83*, 543.

Carcinogenicity. Findings of an increased risk of skin carcinoma for patients with psoriasis who have had very high exposures to tar and/or ultraviolet radiation. This was not considered to be a contra-indication to use of these agents, but argues for continued careful surveillance for early detection of tumours among patients with psoriasis who receive long-term therapy with tar and ultraviolet radiation. Early detection and treatment results in extremely limited morbidity from skin cancer, which is particularly low when compared to the long-term psychological and physical effects of psoriasis.— R. S. Stern *et al.*, *Lancet*, 1980, *1*, 732. No evidence for an increased risk of skin cancer.— M. R. Pittelkow *et al.*, *Archs Derm.*, 1981, *117*, 465.

Phototoxicity. The phototoxicity of 4 samples of coal tar varied appreciably; the phototoxicity of 2 samples of partially refined tar was lower. It was possible that phototoxicity might provide a measure of therapeutic activity.— K. H. Kaidbey and A. M. Kligman, *Archs Derm.*, 1977, *113*, 592.

Uses. Coal tar is an antipruritic and keratoplastic. It is used in eczema, psoriasis, and other skin affections. Tar acids (see p.575) are used as disinfectants.

The effectiveness of coal tar as a fungicide (against *Trichophyton mentagrophytes*) was increased by its use in water-miscible ointment bases. The use of water-immiscible bases inhibited the antifungal action of the coal tar.— J. C. King and W. R. Lloyd, *J. Am. pharm. Ass., pract. Pharm. Edn*, 1959, *20*, 88.

Eczema. For the use of coal tar preparations in the treatment of eczema, see W. E. De Launey, *Drugs*, 1973, *6*, 400.

Psoriasis. For the effect of topical applications of coal tar on skin mitosis in psoriasis, see L. Fry and R. M. H. McMinn, *Br. J. Derm.*, 1968, *80*, 373.

Applications of coal tar, followed after 24 hours by u.v. irradiations (the Goeckerman regimen), gave good clinical results in psoriasis.— H. O. Perry *et al.*, *Archs Derm.*, 1968, *98*, 178.

There was no evidence that u.v. irradiation increased the effectiveness of treatment in 13 patients with psoriasis treated for at least 14 days with crude coal tar 2 to 6, zinc oxide 30, soft paraffin to 120, or in 10 patients treated with crude coal tar 10% in zinc paste.— E. Young, *Br. J. Derm.*, 1972, *87*, 379.

U.v. light is an important component of the Goeckerman regimen. Treatments with crude coal tar ointment 1% or 6% with u.v. irradiation are superior to treatment with tar ointment alone.— A. R. Marsico *et al.*, *Archs Derm.*, 1976, *112*, 1249.

Further references: L. Stankler, *Br. med. J.*, 1974, *1*, 27; *Drug & Ther. Bull.*, 1978, *16*, 25.

Preparations

Creams

Coal Tar and Zinc Cream Oily *(A.P.F.)*. Coal tar 1 g, castor oil 1 g, and zinc cream oily (*A.P.F.*) 98 g.

Coal Tar Cream. Coal tar 2, cetomacrogol '1000' 5, isopropyl myristate 22, wool fat 15, emulsifying wax 5, water to 100. Dissolve the cetomacrogol in the heated water and disperse the coal tar in the solution. Melt the other ingredients together on a water-bath and mix gradually with the coal tar suspension with constant stirring. This gave a smooth stable cream in which the coal tar was evenly dispersed.—J.W. Hadgraft and R. Wolpert, *Pharm. J.*, 1960, *1*, 509.

Ointments

Coal Tar and Salicylic Acid Ointment *(B.P.)*. Coal tar 2 g, salicylic acid 2 g, emulsifying wax 11.4 g, polysorbate '80' 4 g, liquid paraffin 7.6 g, white soft paraffin 19 g, coconut oil 54 g.

NOTE. Coal Tar and Salicylic Acid Ointment *B.P.C. 1973* was prepared with prepared coal tar.

B.P.C. 1968 had strong coal tar solution [formula as *B.P.C. 1973*] 10 g, salicylic acid 2 g, emulsifying wax 18 g, hard paraffin 10 g, yellow soft paraffin 10 g, and coconut oil 50 g.

Modified formula. Strong coal tar solution *B.P.C. 1973* 10 g, salicylic acid 2 g, Polawax GP '200' 25 g, yellow soft paraffin 23 g, coconut oil 30 g, and castor oil 10 g.—W. Swallow, *J. Hosp. Pharm.*, 1973, *31*, 56.

Coal Tar and Zinc Ointment *(B.P.)*. Strong coal tar solution 10 g, zinc oxide 30 g, and yellow soft paraffin 60 g. Store at a temperature not exceeding 25°.

Coal Tar Ointment *(St. John's Hosp.)*. Coal tar solution 12, hydrous wool fat 10, yellow soft paraffin to 100.

Coal Tar Ointment *(U.S.P.)*. Coal tar 1, polysorbate '80' 0.5, and compound zinc paste 98.5. Store in airtight containers.

Coconut Oil Compound Ointment *(St. John's Hosp.)*. Coal tar solution 12, precipitated sulphur 4, salicylic acid 2, coconut oil 60, yellow soft paraffin 9, and emulsifying wax 13. The coconut oil should not be heated.

Coconut Oil Compound Ointment *(St. Mary's Hosp.)*. Ung. Cocois Co. Coal tar solution 10 g, precipitated sulphur 5 g, salicylic acid 5 g, camphor liniment 10 g, coconut oil 30 g, and emulsifying ointment 40 g.

Zinc and Coal Tar Ointment *(A.P.F.)*. Ung. Zinc. et Pic. Zinc oxide 20 g, coal tar 5 g, castor oil 3 g, and yellow soft paraffin 72 g.

Paints

Coal Tar Paint *(A.P.F.)*. Coal tar 10 g, xylene of commerce 45 ml, acetone to 100 ml. Flammable: keep away from an open flame.

Coal Tar Paint *(B.P.)*. Pigmentum Picis Carbonis. Coal tar 10 g, acetone to 100 ml. Store in airtight containers. Flammable. Keep away from an open flame.

Pastes

Coal Tar and Zinc Paste *(A.P.F.)*. Coal Tar Paste. Coal tar 1 g, castor oil 1 g, and compound zinc paste 98 g.

Coal Tar Paste *(B.P.)*. Pasta Picis Carbonis. Strong coal tar solution 7.5 g and compound zinc paste 92.5 g.

Tar Paste, Mild *(St. John's Hosp.)*. Pasta Picis Mitis; PPM. Coal tar solution 4, zinc oxide 4, boric acid 4, starch 25, emulsifying wax 5, light liquid paraffin 5, yellow soft paraffin to 100.

Zinc and Coal Tar Paste *(B.P.)*. Zinc Oxide and Coal Tar Paste; White's Tar Paste. Coal tar 6 g, zinc oxide 6 g, starch 38 g, emulsifying wax 5 g, and yellow soft paraffin 45 g.

The title White's Tar Paste has also been used for: prepared coal tar 4, zinc oxide 25, soft paraffin to 100.

Pomades

Pomade U.B.H. '69 *(Bristol Roy. Infirm.)*. Coal tar solution 5.95 g, salicylic acid 1.98 g, coconut oil 24.8 g, emulsifying ointment 67.26 g. Shelf-life 2 years.

Tar Pomade *(St. John's Hosp.)*. Coal tar solution 6%, salicylic acid 2%, and emulsifying ointment 92%.

Solutions

Coal Tar Solution *(B.P.)*. Coal tar 20 g, polysorbate '80' 5 g, alcohol (or industrial methylated spirit) to 100 ml. Mix the coal tar with the polysorbate, pour into about 80 ml of alcohol, agitate for one hour, allow to stand for 24 hours, decant, filter, and make up to volume

NOTE. Coal Tar Solution *B.P. 1973* was prepared by maceration from prepared coal tar, see p.507.

Coal Tar Topical Solution *(U.S.P.)*. Coal Tar Solution. Coal tar 20 g, mixed with 50 g of washed sand and macerated for 7 days with 5 g of polysorbate 80 and 70 ml of alcohol, then filtered and adjusted to 100 ml with alcohol.

A similar solution is included in many other pharmacopoeias.

Strong Coal Tar Solution *(B.P.)*. Coal tar 40 g, polysorbate '80' 5 g, alcohol (or industrial methylated spirit) to 100 ml. Mix the coal tar with the polysorbate, pour into about 70 ml of alcohol, agitate for one hour, allow to stand for 24 hours, decant, filter, and make up to volume.

NOTE. Strong Coal Tar Solution *B.P.C. 1973* was prepared by maceration from prepared coal tar, see p.507.

Spirits

Spiritus Pyroleosus Compositus *(Dan. Disp.)*. Compound Tar Spirit. An alcoholic (70%) solution containing resorcinol 2%, salicylic acid 2%, and coal tar spirit (coal tar 25% in a quillaia tincture) 25%.

Proprietary Preparations Containing Coal Tar and Mixtures of Coal Tar Fractions

Carbo-Cort 0.25% *(Dome/Hollister-Stier, UK)*. Cream containing coal tar solution 3% and hydrocortisone 0.25% in a washable non-greasy basis. For inflammatory and pruritic skin conditions.

Carbo-Dome *(Dome/Hollister-Stier, UK)*. Cream containing coal tar solution 10% in a washable non-greasy basis. For psoriasis. (Also available as Carbo-Dome in *Fr.*).

Cor-Tar-Quin *(Dome/Hollister-Stier, UK)*. Cream containing coal tar solution 2%, hydrocortisone 0.5%, and di-iodohydroxyquinoline 1% in a water-miscible non-greasy basis. For bacterial and fungous infections of the skin.

Genisol *(Fisons, UK)*. A liquid containing a mixture of purified coal-tar fractions equivalent to prepared coal tar 2% in a soapless basis. For use as a shampoo in seborrhoea capitis, infantile scurf, and psoriasis of the scalp.

Ionil T *(Alcon, UK: Farillon, UK)*. Shampoo containing coal tar topical solution *U.S.P.* 4.25%, salicylic acid 2%, and benzalkonium chloride 0.2% in an alcoholic basis. For seborrhoeic dermatitis of the scalp.

Meditar Stick *(pHarma-medica, UK: Brocades, UK)*. Coal tar 5% in a solid wax basis.

Psoriderm *(Dermal Laboratories, UK)*. A double-distilled preparation of coal tar available as **Bath Emulsion** containing coal tar 40%; 15 to 30 ml to be added to the bath before use; as **Cream** containing coal tar 6% and lecithin 0.4%; and as **Scalp Lotion** containing coal tar 2.5% and lecithin 0.3% in a foaming basis. For subacute and chronic psoriasis.

Tarcortin *(Stafford-Miller, UK)*. Contains 5% of an alcoholic coal tar extract and hydrocortisone 0.5% in a vanishing cream basis. For eczema and a wide range of dermatoses.

Other Proprietary Names

Balnetar, Estar, Pentrax *(all USA)*; Politar *(Arg.)*; Waxtar *(Denm.)*; Zetar *(USA)*.

Preparations containing coal tar fractions were formerly marketed in Great Britain under the proprietary name Psorox (*Fisons*).

1651-e

Prepared Coal Tar *(B.P. 1973)*.

Prep. Coal Tar; Pix Carbonis Praeparata; Pix Lithanthracis.

NOTE. The name Pix Lithanthracis is also applied to Coal Tar.

Pharmacopoeias. In *Arg.* and *Ind.*

Commercial coal tar heated at 50° for 1 hour. It is a nearly black viscous liquid, brown in very thin layers, with a strongly empyreumatic odour. Practically **insoluble** in water; partly soluble in alcohol (90%) and ether; almost entirely soluble in chloroform.

Ointments or pastes containing prepared coal tar or an alcoholic solution of prepared coal tar should be made by incorporating the prepared coal tar or prepared coal tar solution in the unheated ointment basis or, if it should be necessary to aid mixing, in the basis which has been slightly warmed.

There was considerable variation in the solubility or extractability of coal tar from different sources; four-fold differences were found in the amount of solids dissolved by the same solvent under the same conditions from two samples of prepared coal tar. Greater standardisation was needed in the grades of commercial coal tar selected as starting materials and in the content and, possibly, the nature of the extracted materials.— Pharm. Soc. Lab. Rep P/77/12, 1977.

Prepared coal tar has antipruritic properties and is used in the treatment of eczema, psoriasis, and other skin affections.

Preparations

Emulsions

Coal Tar Emulsion *(Wycombe Gen. Hosp.)*. Tar Wash. Coal tar solution (*B.P. 1973*) 5 ml, emulsifying ointment 5 g, water to 100 ml.

Lotions

Alkaline Coal Tar Lotion *(B.P.C. 1949)*. Lot. Pic. Carbon. Alk. Coal tar solution [formula as *B.P. 1973*] 2.08 ml, sodium bicarbonate 1.25 g, water to 100 ml.

Amended formula. Coal tar solution [formula as *B.P. 1973*] 2 ml, sodium bicarbonate 1.25 g, water to 100 ml.—*Compendium of Past Formulae 1933 to 1966*, London, The National Pharmaceutical Union, 1969.

Ointments

Coal Tar Ointment *(B.P.C. 1934)*. Unguentum Picis Carbonis. Coal tar solution [formula as *B.P. 1973*] 6.25 ml, yellow soft paraffin 93.75 g.

Tar and Salicylic Acid Ointment *(Leeds Gen. Infirm.)*. Coal tar solution (*B.P. 1973*) 6, salicylic acid 2, yellow soft paraffin to 100.

Pastes

Coal Tar Solution Paste *(Leeds Gen. Infirm.)*. Coal tar solution (*B.P. 1973*) 5, zinc oxide 25, soft paraffin to 100.

Pomades

Tar Pomade *(Roy. Victoria Infirm.)*. Coal tar solution (*B.P. 1973*) 6 ml, salicylic acid 2 g, polysorbate '20' 1 g, emulsifying ointment (liquid paraffin 40, emulsifying wax 30, yellow soft paraffin 30) to 100 g.

Solutions

Coal Tar Solution *(B.P.)*. See under Coal Tar (Preparations), p.506.

Coal Tar Solution *(B.P. 1973, A.P.F.)*. Coal Tar Soln.; Liquor Picis Carbonis; Liq. Pic. Carb. A solution made by macerating for 7 days prepared coal tar 20% w/v and quillaia 10% w/v in alcohol (90%) (or industrial methylated spirit, suitably diluted) and filtering. A solution prepared from crude coal tar is included in the *U.S.P.* and many other pharmacopoeias (see above).

Strong Coal Tar Solution *(B.P.)*. See under Coal Tar (Preparations), p.506.

Strong Coal Tar Solution *(B.P.C. 1973)*. Liquor Picis Carbonis Fortis; Coal Tar Solution Strong *(A.P.F.)*. A solution made by macerating for 7 days prepared coal tar 40% w/v and quillaia 10% w/v in alcohol (or industrial methylated spirit) and filtering. This preparation cannot be mixed with alcohol to prepare Coal Tar Solution, as precipitation occurs on dilution.

Proprietary Preparations

See under Coal Tar (above).

1652-l

Birch Tar Oil *(B.P.C. 1949)*.

Oleum Rusci; Oleum Betulae Albae; Oleum Betulae Empyreumaticum; Oleum Betulae Pyroligneum; Pyroleum Betulae; Pix Betulae; Goudron de Bouleau; Birkenteer.

NOTE. Oleum Betulae is Sweet Birch Oil, see p.247.

Pharmacopoeias. In *Nord.* and *Swiss.*

Birch tar oil is obtained by the destructive distillation of the wood and bark of the silver birch, *Betula verrucosa* (=*B. pendula; B. alba*), and the birch, *B. pubescens* (Betulaceae); the distillate is allowed to stand and the oily upper layer separated from the residual tar.

It is a thick brownish-black liquid with an agreeable penetrating odour. Wt per ml 0.915 to 0.95 g. **Soluble** in chloroform, oils, and fats; partly soluble in alcohol.

Birch tar oil has been used in the treatment of eczema, psoriasis, and other chronic skin diseases as a cream or ointment containing up to 8%.

Preparations

Spiritus Pyrolei Betulae *(Dan. Disp.)*. Birch Tar Spirit. Birch tar oil 25 g, ether 37.5 g, and alcohol 37.5 g. Filter if necessary.

1653-y

Tellurium Dioxide.

TeO_2=159.6.

CAS — 7446-07-3.

White crystals. M.p. about 733°. Practically **insoluble** in water.

A 2.5% suspension has been used similarly to selenium sulphide as a shampoo in the treatment of seborrhoeic dermatitis.

The pharmacology and toxicology of tellurium.— L. M. Klevay, *Pharmac. Ther.*, 1976, *1*, 223.

1654-j

Thioxolone.

OL 110. 6-Hydroxy-1,3-benzoxathiol-2-one.

$C_7H_4O_3S$=168.2.

CAS — 4991-65-5.

A white or slightly yellow, odourless, crystalline solid. Practically **insoluble** in water; readily soluble in alcohol, ether, propylene glycol, and isopropyl alcohol. Unstable in the presence of alkalis; stable in acid media.

Thioxolone has been used in the form of a lotion containing 0.2% or an alcoholic solution containing 0.5% in the treatment of acne.

Proprietary Names

Camyna *(Boehringer Ingelheim, Denm.; Boehringer Ingelheim, Norw.; Boehringer Ingelheim, S.Afr.; Boehringer Ingelheim, Swed.)*; Gélacnine *(Furt, Fr.)*; Stepin *(Basotherm, Ger.)*; Vikura Salba *(Jap.)*.

1655-z

Titanium Dioxide *(B.P., U.S.P.)*.

Titanium Oxide; CI Pigment White 6; Colour Index No. 77891.

TiO_2=79.90.

CAS — 13463-67-7.

Pharmacopoeias. In *Aust., Br., Braz., It., Jap., Swiss,* and *U.S.*

A white or almost white, amorphous, infusible, odourless, tasteless powder.

Practically **insoluble** in water, dilute mineral acids, and organic solvents; slowly soluble in hot sulphuric acid; soluble in hydrofluoric acid, and by fusion with alkali hydrogen sulphates and alkali hydroxides or carbonates. A 10% suspension in water is neutral to litmus.

Titanium dioxide has an action on the skin similar to that of zinc oxide and is employed for the relief of pruritus and in certain exudative dermatoses. It absorbs ultraviolet light and is used to prevent sunburn. It is an ingredient of certain face powders and other cosmetics. It is used to pigment and opacify hard gelatin capsules and tablet coatings and as a delustring agent for regenerated cellulose and other man-made fibres. Specially purified grades may be used in food colours.

Preparations

Light-screen Cream. Titanium dioxide 25, magnesium stearate 12.5, butyl stearate 12.5, menthyl salicylate 20, pigment 2, and vanishing cream 28. For protection against sunburn.—R.A. Main, *Practitioner*, 1966, *196*, 654.

Titanium Dioxide Paste *(A.P.F.)*. Titanium Dioxide Magma. Titanium dioxide 20 g, calamine 25 g, light kaolin or light kaolin (natural), sterilised, 10 g, bentonite, sterilised, 1 g, chlorocresol 100 mg, glycerol 15 g, freshly boiled and cooled water to 100 g.

Titanium Dioxide Paste *(B.P.)*. Titanium dioxide 20 g, zinc oxide 25 g, sterilised light kaolin or light kaolin (natural) 10 g, red ferric oxide of commerce 2 g, chlorocresol 100 mg, glycerol 15 g, freshly boiled and cooled water to 100 g. Store in well-closed containers which prevent evaporation. Avoid contact with aluminium.

Proprietary Preparations

Metanium *(Bengué, UK)*. Ointment containing titanium dioxide 20%, titanium peroxide 5%, titanium salicylate

3%, and titanium tannate 0.1%, in a silicone basis. For exudative skin lesions, napkin rash, and bed-sores.

1656-c

Tretinoin *(U.S.P.).* Retinoic Acid; Vitamin A Acid. *all-trans*-Retinoic acid; 15-Apo-β-caroten-15-oic acid; 3,7-Dimethyl-9-(2,6,6-trimethylcyclohex-1-enyl)nona-2,4,6,8-*all-trans*-tetraenoic acid.
$C_{20}H_{28}O_2$=300.4.

CAS — 302-79-4.

Pharmacopoeias. In *U.S.*

A yellow to light-orange crystalline powder. M.p. 179° to 182°.
Practically **insoluble** in water; soluble in ether; slightly soluble in alcohol and chloroform. It is unstable in solution in the presence of strong oxidising agents.

Adverse Effects. The application of tretinoin may cause transitory stinging and a feeling of warmth. Correct application causes erythema similar that of mild sunburn. Sensitivity to u.v. light may be increased. Hypopigmentation and hyperpigmentation have been reported. Allergic dermatitis has occasionally occurred. Excessive application may cause marked redness, discomfort, and peeling without any increase in effect.

The toxicology of tretinoin in *animals*.— R. Kretschmar *et al., Arzneimittel-Forsch.*, 1974, *24*, 1193.

Precautions. Tretinoin should not be applied to the eyes, mouth, or other mucous surfaces, nor to eczematous or abraded skin. It should not be used concomitantly with other topical treatment, especially with keratolytic agents. Excessive exposure to sunlight and the use of u.v. lamps should be avoided.

Exacerbation of atopic eczema occurred in 8 of 9 children with asthma when tretinoin 0.2% in soft paraffin was applied as treatment for keratosis pilaris. Control patients treated with tretinoin noted mild pruritus.— G. G. Krueger *et al., Archs Derm.*, 1972, *105*, 405.

A discussion of the possible increased risk of sun-provoked cancer in patients using tretinoin.— *FDA Drug Bull.*, 1978, *8*, 26. See also H. P. Baden (letter), *New Engl. J. Med.*, 1980, *302*, 1419; J. W. Melski and K. A. Arndt (letter), *ibid.*

Critical comment on the advice (given by Health and Welfare, Canada) that tretinoin was potentially teratogenic and should not be used for the treatment of acne in young women.— F. W. Danby (letter), *Can. med. Ass. J.*, 1978, *119*, 854. Reply upholding the advice.— A. B. Morrison (letter), *ibid.*

Absorption and Fate. Tretinoin appears to be only slightly absorbed from the skin after topical application.

In 4 subjects tretinoin was applied to the skin in a gel and left for 12 hours. About 0.1% of the dose was excreted in the urine within 24 hours.— E. Brode *et al., Arzneimittel-Forsch.*, 1974, *24*, 1188.

Uses. Tretinoin appears to stimulate the epithelium to produce horny cells at a faster rate and to reduce their cohesion, possibly by altering the synthesis or quality of the cement substance which binds horny layer cells into impactions.
Tretinoin is used primarily in the treatment of acne vulgaris in which comedones, papules, and pustules predominate. It is applied as a cream, gel, or alcoholic solution, usually containing 0.025%. The skin should be washed with soap and water to remove excessive oiliness and dried 15 to 20 minutes before applying tretinoin lightly, usually twice daily. There may be apparent exacerbations of the acne during early treatment and a therapeutic response may not be evident for 8 to 12 weeks. When the condition has resolved application for maintenance should be less frequent. Some authorities use a 0.05% or 0.1% preparation once daily. In severe acne antibiotics such as tetracycline may be given concomitantly.
Tretinoin has been used in a number of other skin disorders, including psoriasis where the response has been variable. Derivatives of tretinoin such as etretinate (see p.494) and isotretinoin (see p.496) are given by mouth, and other derivatives are also under study.
For the actions and uses of vitamin A, see p.1635.

A review of the actions and uses of tretinoin.— H. Ashton *et al., Br. J. Derm.*, 1971, *85*, 500.

Tretinoin applied topically, was effective in hypertrophic lichen planus (usually permanently), autosomal dominant ichthyosis, keratoses of the palms or soles, and keratosis pilaris. Tretinoin was too irritating for use in ichthyosis associated with atopic eczema.— S. Gunther, *Cutis*, 1976, *17*, 287.

Topical application of tretinoin 0.05% solution under occlusive tape, had beneficial results in 2 patients with cutaneous metastatic melanoma.— N. Levine and F. L. Meyskens, *Lancet*, 1980, *2*, 224.

Acne. A study in 1056 patients with acne treated with tretinoin. Preparations containing 0.05 or 0.1% were effective. The lower concentration was better tolerated. Good or very good results were achieved in about 70% of patients.— E. Eckstein *et al., Arzneimittel-Forsch.*, 1974, *24*, 1205.

More than 90% reduction in comedones was achieved in 80 men treated with tretinoin 0.05% cream or gel for up to 9 weeks.— R. Engst and P. Linzbach, *Münch. med. Wschr.*, 1976, *118*, 43.

In an 8-week study in 68 patients with acne, tretinoin cream 0.1% was comparable with a benzyl peroxide lotion or acetone gel in respect of comedone reduction and markedly less effective in respect of papule reduction.— L. F. Montes, *Cutis*, 1977, *19*, 681.

Based on experience in treating 387 acne patients with varying schedules of 0.02% and 0.05% tretinoin cream and lotion, it was considered that the best overall benefit was derived from the use of 0.05% cream in the morning and 0.02% lotion at night.— I. Hanojo, *Mod. Med. Asia*, 1977, *13*, 5.

For reviews of the use of tretinoin in the treatment of acne, see *Med. J. Aust.*, 1972, *1*, 204; *Drug & Ther. Bull.*, 1973, *11*, 49; *Med. Lett.*, 1973, *15*, 3; R. C. Heel *et al., Drugs*, 1977, *14*, 401.

Dermatoses. Tretinoin 1% under occlusive dressings was successful in inducing remission which lasted at least 3 months in 3 men with keratosis follicularis. After a period of erythema and scaling, the treated areas converted to normal appearing skin. The treatment had also been used in acne vulgaris, keratosis pilaris, and Kyrle's disease.— J. E. Fulton *et al., Archs Derm.*, 1968, *98*, 396.

Application of tretinoin ointment 0.1 or 0.3% twice daily resulted in the disappearance of lesions in 24 of 51 patients with premalignant keratoses and partial regression in 20. Patients with basal cell carcinoma were treated daily with tretinoin under occlusion; in 5 the lesions regressed completely, in 10 they regressed partially, and there was no response in 1 patient.— W. Bollag and F. Ott, *Schweiz. med. Wschr.*, 1971, *101*, 17, per *Clin. Med.*, 1973, *80* (Feb.), 32.

Two patients with naevus comedonicus were successfully treated by the daily application of 0.1% solution of tretinoin in equal parts of alcohol and propylene glycol for 3 or 4 weeks. Recurrence was prevented by application every 2 or 3 days.— J. W. Decherd *et al., Br. J. Derm.*, 1972, *86*, 528.

It was suggested that to attain a suitable irritation level for the treatment of ichthyosiform dermatoses tretinoin 0.1% or more in a w/o basis should be used whereas for seborrhoeic dermatoses 0.05% or less in an o/w basis was preferred.— D. Schlichting *et al., J. pharm. Sci.*, 1973, *62*, 388.

Four patients with trichostasis spinulosa were successfully treated with daily applications of tretinoin solution 0.05% which expelled the keratin plugs from the hair follicles.— O. H. Mills and A. M. Kligman, *Archs Derm.*, 1973, *108*, 378, per *Int. pharm. Abstr.*, 1974, *11*, 253.

In a double-blind study in patients with ichthyosis or hyperkeratosis tretinoin 0.1% cream applied once or twice daily for 12 weeks was significantly more effective than salicylic acid 2% cream; palmar-plantar keratoses were not responsive.— S. A. Muller *et al., Archs Derm.*, 1977, *113*, 1052.

Pityriasis versicolor. Two to 3 weeks' treatment with twice-daily applications of tretinoin cream 0.05% was effective in 21 of 22 patients with pityriasis versicolor often resistant to other treatment. All of 23 similar patients treated in the same way with tretinoin lotion 0.05% were considered cured. One patient in each group relapsed.— I. Handojo *et al., S.E. Asian J. trop. med. publ. Hlth*, 1977, *8*, 93.

Psoriasis. For variable results in the treatment of psoriasis, see P. Frost and G. D. Weinstein, *J. Am. med. Ass.*, 1969, *207*, 1863; T. Fredriksson, *Dermatologica*, 1971, *142*, 133; A. Macdonald and L. Fry, *Br. J. Derm.*, 1972, *86*, 524; A. Macdonald *et al., ibid.*, *87*, 256; C. E. Organos *et al., ibid.*, 1973, *88*, 167; S. Günther, *ibid.*, *89*, 515; G. L. Peck *et al., Archs Derm.*, 1973, *107*, 245; K. H. Kaidbey *et al., Archs Derm.*, 1975, *111*, 1001.

Solar keratoses. For the use of tretinoin with fluorouracil in the eradication of solar keratoses, especially those on the hands, see Fluorouracil, p.211.

Preparations

Tretinoin Cream *(U.S.P.).* A cream containing tretinoin. Store in airtight containers. Protect from light.

Tretinoin Gel *(U.S.P.).* A gel containing tretinoin. Store in airtight containers. Protect from light.

Tretinoin Topical Solution *(U.S.P.).* Contains tretinoin in a suitable non-aqueous hydrophilic solvent. It contains 50 to 60% of alcohol. Store in airtight containers. Protect from light.

Proprietary Preparations

Retin-A *(Ortho-Cilag, UK).* Preparations containing tretinoin 0.025%, available as **Gel** and alcoholic **Solution**. **Retin A Cream.** Contains tretinoin 0.5%. (Also available as Retin-A in *Austral., Ital., NZ, S.Afr., Switz., USA*).

Other Proprietary Names

Aberel *(Fr., Neth.)*; Aberela *(Norw.)*; A-Acido *(Arg.)*; Acid A Vit *(Belg., Neth.)*; Acnavit *(Denm.)*; Acretin *(Belg.)*; Airol *(Arg., Austral., Denm., Ger., Ital., Norw., S.Afr., Switz.)*; A-vitaminsyre *(Denm.)*; Avitoin *(Norw.)*; Cordes VAS *(Ger.)*; Dermairol *(Swed.)*; Dermojuventus *(Spain)*; Effederm *(Fr.)*; Epi-Aberel *(Ger.)*; Eudyna *(Ger.)*.

1657-k

Trioxsalen *(U.S.P.).* Trioxysalen; 4,5′,8-Trimethylpsoralen. 2,5,9-Trimethyl-7*H*-furo[3,2-*g*]-chromen-7-one.
$C_{14}H_{12}O_3$=228.2.

CAS — 3902-71-4.

Pharmacopoeias. In *U.S.*

A white to off-white or greyish, odourless, crystalline solid. M.p. about 230°. Practically **insoluble** in water; soluble 1 in 1150 of alcohol, 1 in 84 of chloroform, 1 in 43 of methylene chloride, and 1 in 100 of methyl isobutyl ketone. **Protect** from light.

Trioxsalen has the actions and uses of Methoxsalen, p.497. It may be used as an alternative to methoxsalen in the PUVA regimen (see p.498). It has been given in doses of 5 to 10 mg daily 2 to 4 hours before exposure to sunlight or u.v. light up to a maximum of 14 days treatment.

Evaluations of trioxsalen.— *J. Am. med. Ass.*, 1966, *197*, 43; *ibid.*, 1967, *202*, 422.

The urine of subjects given trioxsalen 40 mg was found to contain the fluorescent metabolite 4,8-dimethyl-5′-carboxypsoralen, which was not photosensitising.— B. B. Mandula *et al., Science*, 1976, *193*, 1131.

Psoriasis. Prolonged remissions occurred in 7 patients with chronic psoriasis when treated with oral trioxsalen 10 mg daily for 6 days a week for 3 weeks in conjunction with dithranol therapy.— J. Verbov (letter), *Br. J. Derm.*, 1973, *88*, 518.

A regimen of trioxsalen bathing following by irradiation with u.v. light.— T. Fischer and L. Juhlin (letter), *Archs Derm.*, 1977, *113*, 852. A cautionary note on photosensitisation.— *ibid.*

Further references: MHannuksela and J. Karvonen, *Br. J. Derm.*, 1978, *99*, 703.

Vitiligo. Improvement occurred in 19 of 26 patients with vitiligo treated with methoxsalen or trioxsalen (40 mg for adults, 30 mg for 2 children) 2 hours before exposure to u.v.-A light, twice or thrice weekly for 12 to 14 months. Results with both agents were comparable but trioxsalen caused fewer side-effects.— J. A. Parrish *et al., Archs Derm.*, 1976, *112*, 1531, per *Drugs*, 1977, *14*, 233.

Further references: J. Africk and J. Fulton, *Br. J. Derm.*, 1971, *84*, 151; S. S. Bleehen, *ibid.*, 186; V. N. Sehgal, *ibid.*, *85*, 454; S. S. Bleehen, *ibid.*, 1972, *86*, 54.

Preparations

Trioxsalen Tablets *(U.S.P.)*. Tablets containing trioxsalen. Protect from light.

Proprietary Names

Trisoralen *(Protea, Austral.; Elder, Belg.; Elder, Canad.; Farmochimica Italiana, Ital.; Elder, S.Afr.; Elder, USA).*

Trioxsalen was formerly marketed in Great Britain under the proprietary name Trisoralen *(Elder, USA: Sas).*

1658-a

Xenysalate Hydrochloride. Biphenamine Hydrochloride. 2-Diethylaminoethyl 3-phenylsalicylate hydrochloride; 2-Diethylaminoethyl 2-hydroxy-3-phenylbenzoate hydrochloride.

$C_{19}H_{23}NO_3$, HCl=349.9.

CAS — 3572-52-9(xenysalate); 5560-62-3 (hydrochloride).

Xenysalate hydrochloride has been used similarly to selenium sulphide for the control of seborrhoeic dermatitis of the scalp and dandruff.

Proprietary Names

Sébaklen *(Fumouze, Fr.).*

1659-t

Zinc Carbonate *(B.P.C. 1949)*. Hydrated Zinc Carbonate; Zinci Subcarbonas.

CAS — 3486-35-9 ($ZnCO_3$).

Pharmacopoeias. In *Nord.*

A basic carbonate corresponding approximately, to the formula $ZnCO_3,2ZnO,3H_2O$.

A white, odourless, tasteless, impalpable powder. Practically **insoluble** in water and alcohol; soluble with effervescence in dilute mineral acids and acetic acid; soluble in solutions of ammonia and ammonium carbonate.

Zinc carbonate is mildly astringent and protective to the skin and, in the form of calamine (see p.491), is used in creams, dusting-powders, lotions and ointments.

1660-l

Zinc Oxide *(B.P., Eur. P., U.S.P.)*. Zinci Oxidum; Zinci Oxydum; Zincum Oxydatum; Flores de Zinc; Blanc de Zinc.

ZnO=81.38.

CAS — 1314-13-2.

NOTE. 'Zinc White' is a commercial form of zinc oxide for use as a pigment.

Pharmacopoeias. In all pharmacopoeias examined.

A soft, white or yellowish-white, odourless, tasteless powder, free from grittiness. It gradually absorbs carbon dioxide and moisture when exposed to air. It forms cement-like products when mixed with a strong solution of zinc chloride or with phosphoric acid, owing to the formation of oxy-salts.

Practically **insoluble** in water, alcohol, chloroform, and ether; soluble in dilute mineral acids and in solutions of alkali hydroxides. **Sterilise** by maintaining at 150° for 1 hour. **Store** in airtight containers.

The addition of salicylic acid to ointments and pastes containing zinc oxide was useless since zinc salicylate was rapidly formed; the action of zinc salicylate on the skin was similar to that of zinc oxide.— E. Young and N. Weiffenbach, *Ned. Tijdschr. Geneesk.*, 1959, *103*, 603, per *Am. J. Hosp. Pharm.*, 1959, *16*, 368.

Formation of hydrogen peroxide. When ointments containing zinc oxide and water were melted and exposed to u.v. light, hydrogen peroxide was produced; in the case of fatty ointments containing cholesterol, the amount of hydrogen peroxide was less and the cholesterol was partly oxidised. When kept at temperatures below the melting-point of the ointments, only traces of peroxide could be detected.— H. A. Lozada and E. P. Guth, *Drug Stand.*, 1960, *28*, 73.

Incompatibility. Incompatible with benzylpenicillin.— M. A. Schwartz and F. H. Buckwater, *Australas. J. Pharm.*, 1963, *44*, S86.

Water absorption. For a comparison of the water absorption capacity of zinc oxide and starches in a paraffin basis, see Starch, p.503.

Uses. Zinc oxide is applied externally as a mild astringent for the skin, as a soothing and protective application in eczema, and as a protective to slight excoriations.

When zinc oxide is mixed with a strong solution of zinc chloride, and oxychloride is formed which sets into a hard mass; this forms the basis of some dental cements. A similar product is obtained by mixing zinc oxide with phosphoric acid to form an oxyphosphate. Mixed with clove oil or eugenol, zinc oxide is used as a temporary anodyne dental filling.

For a regimen of treatment of the inhalation of zinc oxide, see Purified Talc, p.505.

Preparations

Bandages

Zinc Paste and Coal Tar Bandage *(B.P.)*. A bandage of a white plain-weave cotton cloth impregnated with not less than 150 g per m^2 of a suitable paste containing zinc oxide and coal tar. The paste contains not less than 6% of zinc oxide. Store at a temperature not exceeding 25°.

Zinc Paste and Ichthammol Bandage *(B.P.C. 1973)*. A bandage of a white open-wove cotton cloth impregnated with not less than 175 g per m^2 of a paste containing zinc oxide and 2% w/w of ichthammol. The paste may have the following composition: zinc oxide 6.25 g, ichthammol 2 g, gelatin 9.4 g, glycerol 37.4 g, sodium propyl hydroxybenzoate 60 mg, water to 100 g.

Zinc Paste Bandage *(B.P.)*. A bandage of a white plain-weave cotton cloth impregnated with not less than 150 g per m^2 of a suitable paste containing zinc oxide. The paste contains not less than 6% of zinc oxide. Store at temperature not exceeding 25°.

Zinc Paste, Calamine and Clioquinol Bandage *(D.T.F.)*. A bandage of a white plain-weave cotton cloth impregnated with not less than 175 g per m^2 of a paste of the following composition: zinc oxide 9.25 g, clioquinol 1 g, calamine 5.75 g, crystal gum 'S' (dextrin) 18.5 g, boric acid 2 g, glycerol 27 g, propyl hydroxybenzoate 62.5 mg, castor oil 1 g, water to 100 g.

Creams

Zinc and Ichthammol Cream *(B.P.)*. Zinc Oxide and Ichthammol Cream. Zinc Cream 82 g, wool fat 10 g, ichthammol 5 g, cetostearyl alcohol 3 g. Store at a temperature not exceeding 25° in well-closed containers which minimise evaporation and contamination.

J. W. Hadgraft and R. Wolpert (*Pharm. J.*, 1960, *1*, 509) have suggested the following formula: zinc oxide 30, ichthammol 5, isopropyl myristate 18, wool fat 9, emulsifying wax 5, cetomacrogol '1000' 5, water to 100.

Zinc Cream *(B.P.)*. Zinc Oxide Cream. Zinc oxide 32 g, oleic acid 0.5 ml, arachis oil 32 ml, wool fat 8 g, calcium hydroxide 45 mg, freshly boiled and cooled water to 100 g. Store at a temperature not exceeding 25° in well-closed containers which minimise evaporation and contamination.

Zinc Cream Oily *(A.P.F.)*. Crem. Zinc. Oleos; Zinc Cream. Zinc oxide 32 g, oleic acid 0.5 ml, arachis oil 21.5 ml, wool fat 17.5 g, and calcium hydroxide solution 30.5 ml.

Zinc Oxide and Diphenhydramine Cream *(B. Vet. C. 1965)*. Zinc oxide 8 g, cetostearyl alcohol 10 g, isopropyl myristate 10 g, cetrimide 1 g, diphenhydramine hydrochloride 1 g, camphor 100 mg, chlorocresol 100 mg, water to 100 g.

Dental Cements

Zinc-Eugenol Cement *(U.S.P.)*. Zinc Compounds and Eugenol Cement. It consists of 2 preparations packed separately: (1) *The Powder.* Zinc oxide 70 g, zinc acetate 500 mg, zinc stearate 1 g, and colophony 28.5 g, (2) *The Liquid.* Eugenol 85 ml and cottonseed oil 15 ml; protect from light. To prepare the cement, mix 10 parts of the powder with 1 part of the liquid to a thick paste immediately before use. The amount of liquid may be varied to give any desired consistency.

Kerr's Sealer. *Powder.* Zinc oxide 41.21 g, precipitated silver 30 g, white resin 16 g, and thymol iodide 12.79 g. *Liquid.* Clove oil 78 g, Canada balsam 22 g. Three parts of powder are mixed with 1 part of liquid. For use as a dental root sealing cement.—A. R. Grieve, *Br. dent. J.*, 1972, *132*, 19.

Dental Pastes

Dental Triozinc Paste *(Jap. P.)*. Past. Triozinc. Dent. (1) *Powder:* zinc oxide 8.2 g, zinc sulphate 900 mg, paraformaldehyde 1 g, thymol 300 mg. The zinc sulphate is heated to 250° until anhydrous, and then mixed with the other ingredients. (2) *Liquid:* cresol 4 g, potash soap 4 g, glycerol 2 g. The powder and liquid are mixed immediately before use.

Dusting-powders

Compound Zinc Dusting-powder *(B.P.C. 1963)*. Compound Zinc Oxide Dusting-powder; Zinc, Starch and Boric Powder; Compound Zinc Oxide and Starch Dusting-powder; Zinc Oxide and Boric Acid Dusting-powder; Pulvis Zinci Compositus. Zinc oxide 25 g, boric acid 5 g, starch 35 g, and sterilised purified talc 35 g. Not to be applied to raw or weeping surfaces.

Conspergens Zinci *(Nord. P.)*. Zinc Dusting-powder. Zinc oxide 10 g, purified talc 90 g.

Zinc and Salicylic Acid Dusting-powder *(B.P.C. 1968)*. Conspersus Zinci et Acidi Salicylici; Zinc Oxide and Salicylic Acid Dusting-powder. Zinc oxide 20 g, salicylic acid 5 g, and starch 75 g.

Zinc, Starch, and Talc Dusting-powder *(B.P.C. 1973)*. Conspersus Zinci, Amyli et Talci; Zinc Oxide and Starch Dusting-powder; Zinc Oxide, Starch, and Talc Dusting-powder; Zinc, Starch and Talc Dusting Powder *(A.P.F.)*. Zinc oxide 1, starch 1, and sterilised purified talc 2.

Gauzes

Zinc Gelatin Impregnated Gauze *(U.S.P.)*. Absorbent gauze impregnated with zinc gelatin that may contain a small amount of ferric oxide. Each 100 g contains 82.5 to 89.5 g of zinc gelatin (*U.S.P.*), equivalent to 6.7 to 9.1% of zinc oxide. Store in airtight containers.

Liniments

Linimentum Phenoli et Zinci Oxydi *(Jap. P.)*. Phenol and Zinc Oxide Liniment. Zinc oxide 10 g, liquefied phenol 2.2 ml, tragacanth 5 g, glycerol 3 ml, water to 100 g.

Linimentum Zinci *(Nord. P.)*. Zinc oxide 12.5 g, talc 12.5 g, alcohol (70%) 12.5 g, glycerol 12.5 g, water 50 g.

Lotions

Lotion F. A lotion with healing and protective properties for use with ileostomy appliances; zinc oxide 25 g, boric acid 666.7 mg, starch 10 g, light kaolin 666.7 mg, diatomite 333.3 mg, magnesium trisilicate 2 g, glycerol 25 ml, bismuth subnitrate 200 mg, aluminium subacetate 1.33 g, water to 100 ml.—*A New Life for Those with a Permanent Ileostomy*, 2nd Edn, London, Ileostomy Association of Great Britain, p. 55.

A similar formula.—J.C. Goligher and M.A. Pollard, *The Care of your Ileostomy*, Leeds, University Dept of Surgery, 1972.

Schamberg's Lotion (Modified) *(Rochester Methodist Hosp.)*. Zinc oxide 8 g, menthol 250 mg, phenol 500 mg, calcium hydroxide solution 46 ml, olive oil to 100 ml. Shelf-life 1 year.

Zinc Talc Lotion *(Rochester Methodist Hosp.)*. Zinc oxide 21 g, talc 21 g, glycerol 12.5 ml, alcohol 12.5 ml, water to 100 ml. Shelf-life 2 years.

Ointments

Hamer's Haemorrhoidal Ointment *(Orsett Hosp.)*. Hammersmith's Cream. Zinc oxide 2 g, camphor liniment 3 g, hydrous wool fat 8 g, and white soft paraffin 4 g. Shelf-life 6 months.

Zinc and Castor Oil Ointment *(B.P., A.P.F.)*. Zinc and Castor Oil Oint.; Zinc and Castor Oil Cream; Zinc Oxide and Castor Oil Ointment; Zinc and Castor Oil. Zinc oxide 7.5 g, castor oil 50 g, cetostearyl alcohol 2 g, white beeswax 10 g, and arachis oil 30.5 g. Store at a temperature not exceeding 25°.

It is used as an emollient and astringent skin application, particularly for infants.

Zinc Ointment *(B.P.)*. Zinc Oint.; Ung. Zinc.; Zinc Oxide Ointment *(A.P.F.)*. Zinc oxide 15% in simple ointment. Store at a temperature not exceeding 25°. This ointment does not mix well with castor oil. Similar ointments are included in many pharmacopoeias most of which specify 10% of zinc oxide.

Zinc Oxide and Ichthammol Ointment *(Jap. P.)*. Ung. Zinc. et Ichtham. Zinc oxide 10 g, ichthammol 9 g, wool fat 9 g, and yellow soft paraffin 72 g.

Zinc Oxide Compound Ointment *(St. Thomas' Hosp.)*. Ignoform Substitute. Zinc oxide 20 g, theobroma oil 2 g, hamamelis water 2 ml, water 16 ml, wool fat 30 g, yellow soft paraffin to 100 g. For X-ray burns.

Zinc Oxide Ointment *(U.S.P.).* Zinc oxide 20 g, liquid paraffin 15 g, white ointment 65 g. Store at a temperature not exceeding 30°.

Zinc Oxide Ointment with Benzoin *(B.P.C. 1949).* Ung. Zinc. Oxid. c. Benzoin. Zinc ointment 70 g and compound benzoin tincture 10 ml.

Pastes

Compound Zinc Paste *(B.P.).* Co. Zinc Paste; Zinc Compound Paste; Zinc Paste; Zinc Paste Compound *(A.P.F.)*; Compound Zinc Oxide Paste; Zinc Oxide Paste *(U.S.P.)*; Lassar's Plain Zinc Paste. Zinc oxide 25, starch 25, and white soft paraffin 50.

Lassar's Paste, Modified, Full-strength *(Roy. Victoria Infirm.).* Lassar's Paste RVI. For use in Dithranol Paste (see p.494). Zinc oxide 24, starch 24, salicylic acid 2, hard paraffin 5 to 10, yellow soft paraffin to 100.

Lassar's Paste, Modified, Half-strength *(Roy. Victoria Infirm.).* Zinc oxide 12, starch 12, salicylic acid 1, hard paraffin 2.5, yellow soft paraffin to 100.

Pasta di Zinco all'Acqua *(It. P.).* Zinc oxide, talc, glycerol, and water, of each equal parts by weight.

Pâte à l'Eau *(Leeds Gen. Infirm.).* Zinc oxide 25 g, purified talc 25 g, glycerol 25 g, calcium hydroxide solution to 100 g. For weeping eczema and other skin conditions.

Pâte à l'Oxyde de Zinc *(F.N. Fr.).* Pâte Zincique de Lassar. Zinc oxide, wheat starch, wool fat, and white soft paraffin, of each equal parts.

Zinc and Coal Tar Paste *(B.P.).* See under Coal Tar, p.506.

Zinc and Salicylic Acid Paste *(B.P.).* Zinc Oxide and Salicylic Acid Paste; Lassar's Paste. Zinc oxide 24 g, salicylic acid 2 g, starch 24 g, and white soft paraffin 50 g.

A.P.F. has salicylic acid 2 g, liquid paraffin 2 g, compound zinc paste 96 g. *Belg. P.* has salicylic acid 1 g, starch 25 g, zinc oxide 25 g, wool fat 24.5 g, white soft paraffin 14.5 g, liquid paraffin 10 g.

Zinc Gelatin *(B.P.C. 1968).* Past. Gelat. Zinc.; Unna's Paste. Zinc oxide 15 g, gelatin 15 g, glycerol 35 g, and water 35 ml.

Zinc gelatin is used as a protective and supportive dressing for varicose ulcers and similar indolent lesions. The leg or foot is thoroughly cleansed and a dusting-powder applied. The paste, previously melted and cooled, is applied with a brush to the affected part and the paste is covered with a gauze bandage. A total of 4 layers of paste is applied, each layer being covered with a gauze bandage. The dressing is left for 3 days to 2 weeks and removed by soaking in warm water.

Zinc Gelatin *(U.S.P.).* Zinc oxide 10 g, gelatin 15 g, glycerol 40 g, and water 35 g. Store in airtight containers. Similar preparations containing 10 to 20% of zinc oxide are included in many pharmacopoeias.

Zinc Oxide and Salicylic Acid Paste *(U.S.P.).* Zinc Oxide Paste with Salicylic Acid; Lassar's Zinc Paste with Salicylic Acid. Salicylic acid 2% in compound zinc paste.

Proprietary Preparations

Calaband *(Seton, UK: Bateman-Jackson, UK).* A bandage of a white plain-weave cotton cloth impregnated with not less than 175 g per m^2 of a paste of the following composition: zinc oxide 9.25 g, calamine 5.75 g, crystal gum 'S' (dextrin) 19.15 g, boric acid 2 g, glycerol 27 g, propyl hydroxybenzoate 200 mg, castor oil 1 g, water to 100 g.

Coltapaste *(Smith & Nephew, UK).* A brand of Zinc Paste and Coal Tar Bandage.

Ichthopaste *(Smith & Nephew, UK).* A brand of Zinc Paste and Ichthammol Bandage.

Icthaband *(Seton, UK: Bateman-Jackson, UK).* A brand of Zinc Paste and Ichthammol Bandage.

Noratex *(Norton, UK: Vestric, UK).* Cream containing zinc oxide 21.8%, talc 7.4%, light kaolin 3.5%, cod-liver oil 2.15%, and wool fat 1.075%.

Pharmakon *(Vine Chemicals, UK).* A pharmaceutical grade of zinc oxide.

Quinaband *(Seton, UK: Bateman-Jackson, UK).* A brand of Zinc Paste, Calamine and Clioquinol Bandage *D.T.F.*

Thrombocytopenia in a 68-year-old woman with myxoedema was attributed to absorption of clioquinol from Quinaband applied to extensive leg ulcers.— A. A. Khaleeli, *Br. med. J.*, 1976, *2*, 562.

Septex Cream No. 1 *(Norton, UK: Vestric, UK).* Contains zinc oxide 7.78%, oleic acid 1%, and cetrimide 0.5%. **Septex Cream No. 2.** Contains zinc oxide 7.4%, boric acid 5.15%, and sulphathiazole 4.94%. For infected skin conditions.

Sudocrem *(Tosara, UK).* Cream containing zinc oxide 15.25%, hydrous wool fat 4%, benzyl benzoate 1.01%, benzyl cinnamate 0.15%, and benzyl alcohol 0.39%.

Tarband *(Seton, UK: Bateman-Jackson, UK).* A brand of Zinc Paste and Coal Tar Bandage.

Thovaline *(Ilon Laboratories, UK).* An ointment containing zinc oxide 19.8%, talc 3.3%, light kaolin 2.5%, cod-liver oil 1.5%, and wool fat 2.5%. For burns, bedsores, and napkin rash. **Thovaline Aerosol** and **Thovaline Impregnated Gauze** contain the same active ingredients as Thovaline.

Viscopaste *(Smith & Nephew, UK).* A brand of Zinc Paste Bandage. (Also available as Viscopaste in *S.Afr.*).

Viscopaste PB7 *(Smith & Nephew, UK).* A cotton bandage impregnated with an oil-in-water cream containing zinc oxide 10%.

Zincaband *(Seton, UK: Bateman-Jackson, UK).* A brand of Zinc Paste Bandage.

Other Proprietary Names

Herisan *(Canad.)*; Oxyplastine *(Fr.)*.

A bandage impregnated with zinc paste with urethane and ichthammol was formerly marketed in Great Britian under the proprietary name Uraband (*Seton Products*).

1661-y

Zinc Salicylate.

$(C_7H_5O_3)_2Zn,3H_2O=393.7$.

CAS — 551-38-2; 16283-36-6 (both anhydrous); 6044-03-7 (trihydrate).

A crystalline powder. **Soluble** in water and alcohol. **Incompatible** with iron salts and mineral acids.

Zinc salicylate is used as an astringent.

Proprietary Preparations

Prehensol *(Dermal Laboratories, UK).* Cream containing zinc salicylate 2% and lecithin 0.5% in a vanishing cream basis. For detergent dermatitis of the hands.

1662-j

Zirconium Dioxide.

Zirconium Oxide; Zirconia; Zirconic Anhydride.

$ZrO_2=123.2$.

CAS — 1314-23-4.

A heavy, white, odourless, tasteless, amorphous powder. Practically **insoluble** in water.

Zirconium dioxide and salts, e.g. zirconium lactate and zirconium oxychloride, have been used in deodorant preparations.

Zirconium dioxide is also used as a contrast medium.

Adverse effects. A Japanese girl developed a non-pruritic papular eruption on the face, forearms and the back of the hands after the use of a lotion containing zirconium dioxide 2% and diphenhydramine hydrochloride 1% for poison oak dermatitis.— W. L. Epstein and J. R. Allen, *J. Am. med. Ass.*, 1964, *190*, 940. A similar report.— G. R. Baler, *Archs Derm.*, 1965, *91*, 145.

Zirconium 10% used in a stick preparation as an antiperspirant might produce granulomas. This was an allergic reaction and was aggravated by the use of soap or hexachlorophane.— P. D. C. Kinmont, *Practitioner*, 1969, *202*, 88. See also W. B. Shelley and H. J. Hurley, *Br. J. Derm.*, 1958, *70*, 75.

Aerosol preparations containing zirconium had been banned by the FDA until extensive safety testing was carried out. Small particles in the air had caused human skin granulomas and toxic effects in the lungs and other organs of experimental *animals*. Non-aerosol antiperspirants containing zirconium were not affected.— *Mfg Chem.*, 1977, *48* (Dec.), 10.

A survey of the adverse effects associated with zirconium used in antiperspirants.— P. Bathe, *Mfg Chem.*, 1978, *49* (July), 72.

1663-z

Some Proprietary Protective Materials

Nobecutane Spray *(Astra, UK).* An aerosol wound dressing consisting of acrylic resin equivalent to total solids 5.7%, ethyl acetate 27.3%, and propellents. When applied to the skin and allowed to evaporate it leaves a tough elastic film impervious to bacteria and other contaminants.

NSB *(Geistlich, UK).* An aerosol spray containing a copolymer of vinylpyrrolidone and vinyl acetate, with solvents and propellents. When sprayed on the skin it provides a flexible, porous, protective film; this may be removed when required with soap and water.

NOTE. This preparation previously also contained noxythiolin.

Op-Site Spray Dressing *(Smith & Nephew, UK).* An aerosol spray containing ethoxyethyl methacrylate and methoxyethyl methacrylate copolymer (Hydron) 3%, in a solvent of ethyl acetate and acetone, with propellents. For the application of a protective film over surgical wounds, dressings, and around stomas.

Other protective materials were also formerly marketed in Great Britain under the proprietary names Aeroplast (*Parke, Davis*) and Hibispray No. 4 Clear Plastic Dressing (*Stuart Pharmaceuticals*).

Dextrans

250-s

Dextrans used therapeutically are polysaccharides (polyanhydroglucoses) produced by the fermentation of sucrose by means of a certain strain of *Leuconostoc mesenteroides* (NCTC No. 10817) and subsequent controlled hydrolysis and fractionation of the high molecular weight dextran thus formed. They may also be produced by other means. The polysaccharides are polymers of glucose in which the linkages between the glucose units are almost entirely of the α-1,6 type, giving predominantly straight chain polymers.

The properties of dextrans administered by injection depend on the molecular structure, the molecular weight distribution, and the average molecular weight of the dextrans used. The term *weight average molecular weight* is used in defining dextrans to indicate that the average molecular weight of dextran preparations is calculated from the proportions by weight of dextrans present and not by taking the numerical average of the molecular weight range.

Dextran injections are given by intravenous infusion to restore or maintain blood volume in the emergency treatment of shock or impending shock due to haemorrhage, burns, surgery, or other trauma. They achieve this effect by maintaining the colloidal osmotic pressure of plasma. As dextran injections have no oxygen-carrying capacity, blood-clotting factors, or plasma proteins, they must not be regarded as substitutes for whole blood or plasma and must be used with caution in order to prevent overhydration or excessive haemodilution. Hetastarch is used for the same purposes as are Polygeline (p.958) and Povidone (p.958).

Dextran 40 Intravenous Infusion has been used to improve capillary blood flow and maintain tissue function in conditions associated with local ischaemia. It has also been used as a priming fluid in extracorporeal circulation procedures.

Both Dextran 70 Intravenous Infusion and Dextran 40 Intravenous Infusion have been suggested for use in the prevention of post-operative thrombosis.

251-w

Dextran 40 Intravenous Infusion *(B.P.)*.

Dextran 40 Injection; Low-Molecular-Weight Dextran. A sterile 9 to 11% w/v solution in dextrose injection or in sodium chloride injection of dextrans of weight average molecular weight about 40 000.

CAS — 9004-54-0 (dextran 40).

Pharmacopoeias. In *Br.* and *Jap. Braz., Jap., Nord.,* and *Roum.* also describe Dextran 40.

It is an almost colourless, slightly viscous solution. **Sterilised** by autoclaving.

It should be **stored** at an even temperature. It should not be used if it is cloudy or if a deposit is present.

Adverse Effects and Treatment. As for Dextran 70 Intravenous Infusion, p.512.

High concentrations of dextran 40 increase urinary viscosity and, in patients with impaired renal function, may cause oliguria; dextran 40 might precipitate renal failure in some patients.

Allergic reaction. References: E. Michelson, *New Engl. J. Med.*, 1968, *278*, 552; E. P. Krenzelok and W. A. Parker, *Minnesota Med.*, 1975, *58*, 454; R. Adar and J. Schneiderman (letter), *J. Am. med. Ass.*, 1977, *237*, 119; J. Ring and K. Messmer, *Lancet*, 1977, *1*, 466.

Renal failure. Infusion of dextran 40 had brought about acute renal failure in 3 patients, apparently through renal ischaemia. Acute failure of an ischaemic kidney was probably related to the increase in urine viscosity.— M. Yudis (letter), *New Engl. J. Med.*, 1967, *276*, 60.

The infusion of dextran 40 in 3 patients with advanced arteriosclerotic vascular disease was followed by acute renal failure. Subsequent experiments on *dogs* suggested that anuria resulted from a reduction of filtration pressure combined with a marked increase in urinary viscosity.— L. Mailloux *et al.*, *New Engl. J. Med.*, 1967, *277*, 1113.

Further references: J. F. Niall and J. C. Doyle (letter), *Lancet*, 1966, *1*, 817; T. O. Morgan *et al.*, *Br. med. J.*, 1966, *2*, 737; N. A. Matheson (letter), *ibid.*, 1198; T. O. Morgan and J. M. Little (letter), *ibid.*, 1967, *1*, 635; N. A. Matheson, *Monogr. surg. Sci.*, 1966, *3*, 303.

For a further report on renal failure associated with administration of dextran injections, see Dextran 70 Intravenous Infusion, p.512.

Precautions. As for Dextran 70 Intravenous Infusion, p.512.

Difficulty in grouping and matching blood occurred in patients who had been given infusions of low-molecular-weight dextrans. The dextrans caused difficulty when proteolytic enzyme techniques were used to match blood.— J. G. Selwyn *et al.* (letter), *Lancet*, 1968, *2*, 1032.

Two patients with multiple fractures who were transfused with blood and low-molecular-weight dextran suffered an onset of haemorrhagic pulmonary oedema. It was suggested that it was dangerous to administer a low-molecular-weight dextran once pulmonary oedema was established.— J. A. O'Garra (letter), *Br. med. J.*, 1970, *4*, 369.

Absorption and Fate. After intravenous infusion of dextran 40, about 60% is excreted in the urine within 6 hours and about 70% within 24 hours. The dextran not excreted is slowly metabolised, mainly in the liver, to carbon dioxide and water. A small amount is excreted into the gastro-intestinal tract and eliminated in the faeces.

Uses. Dextran 40 Intravenous Infusion produces a briefer expansion of plasma volume than dextrans of higher molecular weight. It inhibits the intravascular aggregation of red blood-cells (sludging) and reduces platelet adhesiveness.

It is used to improve blood flow and tissue function in burns and conditions associated with local ischaemia. The dose depends on the condition of the patient. A usual dose is 500 to 1000 ml for 2 days repeated on alternate days for up to 2 weeks, but larger doses may be required, especially in the treatment of burns.

Dextran 40 Intravenous Infusion has also been suggested for use as a prophylactic agent in the prevention of postoperative pulmonary embolism and deep-vein thrombosis. The dose depends on the type of operation and duration of immobilisation. In general 500 ml has been given intravenously immediately prior to, and 500 ml during, the operation and then 500 ml daily for 2 to 3 days and thereafter, according to need, every second or third day for up to 2 weeks.

It has been used as an adjunct to the treatment of shock, 500 ml being given by rapid infusion followed by 500 to 1000 ml given by slow infusion the same day. Further daily doses of 500 ml may be given over the next few days.

It is given before angiography in a dose of 10 to 15 ml per kg body-weight as an infusion over 30 minutes. It has also been given to patients with peripheral vascular disorders in a dose of 500 ml every 12 hours for 4 doses and repeated as required every 3 to 6 months.

Infants may be given 5 ml per kg body-weight and children 10 ml per kg.

It is added to extracorporeal perfusion fluids in doses of up to 20 ml per kg. A 5% solution with electrolytes has been used for the washing and perfusion of organs for transplantation.

A review of the actions and uses of dextran 40.— J. L. Data and A. S. Nies, *Ann. intern. Med.*, 1974, *81*, 500. Comment.— E. F. Schinagl and R. Ali (letter), *ibid.*, 1975, *82*, 722.

In vitro studies indicated that dextran 40 did not reduce blood viscosity; it did however reverse or prevent erythrocyte rouleaux formation and aggregation.— S. Eisenberg, *Am. J. med. Sci.*, 1969, *257*, 336, per *Abstr. Wld Med.*, 1969, *43*, 902.

In 10 patients without haematological or cardiovascular disease the infusion of 500 ml of dextran 40 over 10 to 20 minutes decreased the viscosity of the blood by 14% at the end of the infusion and by a further 4.5% in the next 10 minutes. Calf blood flow increased by 25.2% and a further 4.8% respectively in the same periods. The respective figures after an infusion of 500 ml of compound sodium lactate injection were 10.8% at the end of the infusion with a rise of 3% in the next 10 minutes, and increased blood flow of 21% with a decrease of 10.5% in the next 10 minutes. The greater fall in viscosity after dextran 40 was no greater than would be expected from the greater haemodilution calculated in relation to the packed cell volume. It was concluded that dextran 40 injection had no specific effect on blood viscosity or blood flow.— J. A. Dormandy, *Br. med. J.*, 1971, *4*, 716.

In a study in 54 patients with circulatory disorders, an injection of dextran 40 produced a significant decrease in whole blood viscosity compared with sodium chloride injection.— H. Heidrich and T. Wachta, *Dt. med. Wschr.*, 1978, *103*, 298.

Angiography. Infusions of 500 ml of dextran 40 reduced the incidence of complications in patients undergoing angiography.— P. H. Langsjoen and E. B. Best, *Am. J. Roentg.*, 1969, *106*, 425, per *J. Am. med. Ass.*, 1969, *209*, 805.

Anterior-segment necrosis. Experience gained in treating 5 patients with anterior-segment necrosis of the eye suggested that the acute phase of the condition could be controlled by intravenous infusions of dextran 40.— D. M. O'Day *et al.*, *Lancet*, 1966, *2*, 401.

Caisson disease. Dextran 40 was used in the treatment, without recompression, of a patient with decompression sickness, in order to improve tissue perfusion and normalise platelets.— R. C. Saumarez *et al.*, *Br. med. J.*, 1973, *1*, 151.

Cardiac infarction. An unfavourable report on the use of dextran 40 as an adjunct in the treatment of cardiac infarction.— C. F. Borchgrevink and E. Enger, *Br. med. J.*, 1966, *2*, 1235. A favourable report.— P. H. Langsjoen *et al.*, *Am. Heart J.*, 1968, *76*, 28.

Cardiopulmonary bypass. The use of dextran 40 in oxygenator priming solutions was considered likely to increase the risk of postoperative bleeding, but partial replacement of blood by dextran solutions was considered to reduce the incidence of the sequestration syndrome, which included a reduction in the effective blood volume.— L. P. Rosky and T. Rodman, *New Engl. J. Med.*, 1966, *274*, 833 and 886.

A discussion on the use of dextran 40 during cardiopulmonary bypass.— *Med. Lett.*, 1968, *10*, 3.

Cold injury. In the treatment of the inflammatory and postinflammatory stages of cold injury, the use of dextran 40 had proved beneficial in 2 patients. A suitable adult dosage was 500 ml infused eight-hourly for 48 hours, followed by 500 ml daily for 21 days. Any effects of the treatment would be apparent within 48 hours.— L. Gracey and D. Ingram, *Br. J. Surg.*, 1968, *55*, 302.

Effect on cerebral blood flow. Improved cerebral blood flow occurred in 19 patients after intravenous infusion of 500 ml of dextran 40, and in 16 patients after dextran 70. There was no change in blood flow in 5 patients after 500 ml of sodium chloride injection.— U. Gottstein and K. Held, *Dt. med. Wschr.*, 1969, *94*, 522, per *J. Am. med. Ass.*, 1969, *208*, 187.

A retrospective study in 226 patients with acute cerebral ischaemia treated with vasodilators and 202 patients treated with dextran infusions showed that the death-rate was substantially lower in the dextran-treated patients.— U. Gottstein *et al.*, *Dt. med. Wschr.*, 1976, *101*, 223.

Mean regional cerebral blood flow increased by 9.9% in 12 patients with cerebral ischaemia given 500 ml of low molecular weight dextrans intravenously.— H. Herrschaft, *Arzneimittel-Forsch.*, 1976, *26*, 1240.

In a double-blind study there was no significant benefit, in 20 patients with cerebral infarction, treated with 500 ml of dextran 40 infused over 1 or 2 hours followed by 500 ml every 12 hours for 72 hours, combined with dexamethasone 10 mg intramuscularly followed by 5 mg six-hourly for 7 days, then tapered off. Comparison was with 20 patients treated with placebo.— M. Kaste *et al.*, *Br. med. J.*, 1976, *2*, 1409.

In a controlled trial 100 patients considered to have had stroke due to ischaemic cerebral infarction during the previous 48 hours were treated with either dextran 40 in dextrose injection or with dextrose injection alone. The dose for both was 500 ml initially over 1 hour followed by 500 ml every 12 hours for 3 days. Acute mortality was significantly reduced in patients with severe stroke treated with dextran but survivors were seriously disabled and no significant benefit could be detected 6 months later. No significant benefit was found in patients with less severe stroke treated with dextran 40.— W. B. Matthews *et al.*, *Brain*, 1976, *99*, 193.

Fibrinolytic activity. Dextran 40 in sodium chloride injection was given in doses of 1 to 3 litres, at a rate of 1 litre in 24 hours, by intravenous infusion to 22 patients suffering from peripheral vascular disease. Increased blood fibrinolytic activity occurred in 18 patients 24 to 72 hours after infusion. In a follow up on 10 patients, maximum fibrinolytic activity was seen after 5 to 7 weeks, returning to the original level after 10 to 12 weeks. Considerable variation in the effect was noted. Of the 9 patients in a control group who received sodium chloride injection by intravenous infusion, fibrinolytic activity was increased in 2 and decreased in 5.— W. J. Cunliffe and I. S. Menon, *Br. J. Derm.*, 1969, *81*, 220.

Kidney storage solution. Human kidneys could be stored for 4 to 9 hours without the need for continuous perfusion by flushing them with dextran 40 at 4°, infusing a 10% buffered invert sugar solution, and refrigerating at 4° to 5° until use. Of 60 human kidneys preserved in this way, 45 functioned when transferred to a recipient.— *J. Am. med. Ass.*, 1968, *204* (June 3), A31.

Kidneys were flushed with 100 to 150 ml of dextran 40 in dextrose injection at room temperature. The kidneys were placed in plastic bags, the air expelled, double wrapped, and stored in unsterile ice and water mixture for despatch. Kidneys had survived without a blood supply for nearly 16 hours.— A. D. Barnes *et al.* (letter), *Lancet*, 1972, *1*, 199.

Necrotising enterocolitis. A favourable report on the use of dextran 40 in necrotising enterocolitis and midgut volvulus in infants.— I. H. Krasna *et al.*, *J. pediat. Surg.*, 1973, *8*, 615.

Polycythaemia. Dextran 40 was used simultaneously with venesection as a means of reducing packed cell volume in 8 patients with polycythaemia secondary to hypoxic lung disease.— B. D. W. Harrison *et al.*, *Br. med. J.*, 1971, *4*, 713. See also D. Honeybourne (letter), *Br. med. J.*, 1977, *1*, 52; A. E. Tattersfield, *Br. med. J.*, 1978, *1*, 1123; K. Constantinidis, *Practitioner*, 1979, *222*, 89.

Purpura. Following intravenous administration of dextran 40 in 5% dextrose solution and hydrocortisone over 2½ days, a 17-month-old girl with purpura fulminans complicating chicken-pox showed rapid improvement. Steroids were continued by mouth. Her blood had been virtually uncoagulable, but with this treatment the coagulation time rapidly returned to normal.— H. Smith, *Med. J. Aust.*, 1967, *2*, 685.

Further references: D. L. Cram and R. L. Soley, *Br. J. Derm.*, 1968, *80*, 323.

Scleroderma. A favourable report on the use of dextran 40 in patients with scleroderma.— W. H. Wong *et al.*, *Archs Derm.*, 1974, *110*, 419.

Shock. In 19 of 26 patients with shock, the infusion of dextran 40 gave increase in central venous pressure, cardiac index, plasma volume, and central blood volume, and lesser increases in blood pressure, stroke index, and left ventricular stroke work, as well as decreased mean transit time and total peripheral resistance. Patients with haemorrhage and trauma had increased oxygen consumption. Dextran increased the central venous pressure without improving the cardiac index in 7 patients which suggested limited cardiac function.— P. A. Mohr *et al.*, *Circulation*, 1969, *39*, 379.

Thrombo-embolism. The incidence of postoperative venous thrombo-embolism was significantly less in patients who received 500-ml infusions of dextran solutions during operation than in those who received 5.5% dextrose. The prevention of thrombo-embolism seemed slightly more effective with 10% dextran 40 than with 6% dextran 70.— H. Jansen (letter), *Lancet*, 1970, *1*, 838.

Among patients undergoing total hip replacement, thrombo-embolism occurred in 10% of 113 patients treated prophylactically with dextran 40 for 19 days compared with an incidence of 7.9% among 114 patients treated prophylactically with warfarin for 24 days.— W. H. Harris *et al.*, *J. Am. med. Ass.*, 1972, *220*, 1319.

Further reports of studies in which prophylactic postoperative use of dextran 40 reduced the incidence of thrombosis.— P. H. Langsjoen and R. A. Murray, *J. Am. med. Ass.*, 1971, *218*, 855; C. R. King and J. W. Daly, *Am. J. Obstet. Gynec.*, 1975, *123*, 46; F. van Geloven *et al.*, *Acta med. scand.*, 1977, *202*, 367; U. F. Gruber *et al.*, *Lancet*, 1977, *1*, 207.

Proprietary Preparations

Gentran 40 *(Travenol, UK).* A sterile solution containing 10% of dextran 40 in dextrose injection or sodium chloride injection.

Lomodex 40 *(Fisons, UK).* A sterile solution containing 10% of dextran 40 in dextrose injection or sodium chloride injection. (Also available as Lomodex 40 in *Austral.*).

Perfudex *(Pharmacia, UK: Farillon, UK).* A sterile solution containing 5% of dextrans of weight average molecular weight 40 000 in a balanced salt solution. A wash-through solution for use in organ transplantation. (Also available as Perfudex in *Austral., Belg.*).

Rheomacrodex *(Pharmacia, UK: Farillon, UK).* A sterile solution containing 10% of dextran 40 in dextrose injection or sodium chloride injection. (Also available as Rheomacrodex in *Austral., Belg., Canad., Fr., Ital., Neth., USA*).

Other Proprietary Names

Eudextran *(Ital.)*; Isodex *(Neth.)*; LMD 10% *(Canad., USA)*; Perfadex *(Swed.)*; Plander, Soludex *(both Ital.)*.

252-e

Dextran 70 Intravenous Infusion *(B.P.)*.

Dextran 70 Injection. A sterile 5.5 to 6.5% w/v solution in dextrose injection or in sodium chloride injection of dextrans of weight average molecular weight about 70 000.

CAS — 9004-54-0 (dextran 70).

Pharmacopoeias. In *Br.* and *Jap. Braz., Jap., Nord.*, and *Roum.* also describe Dextran 70.

It is an almost colourless, slightly viscous solution. **Sterilised** by autoclaving. It should be **stored** at an even temperature. It should not be used if it is cloudy or if a deposit is present.

A review of dextrans including their storage and the compatibility of dextran 70 with common additives.— M. C. Smith, *Am. J. Hosp. Pharm.*, 1965, *22*, 273.

Incompatibility. There was loss of clarity when intravenous solutions of dextran were mixed with those of ascorbic acid, chlortetracycline hydrochloride, phytomenadione, or promethazine hydrochloride.— J. A. Patel and G. L. Phillips, *Am. J. Hosp. Pharm.*, 1966, *23*, 409.

Stability. Four dextran solutions were examined in 1954 and again after storage for 5 years at 4°. It was concluded that during the 5-year period there was little, if any, change in the molecular composition of the solutions and none that would be noticeable in clinical use.— W. d'A. Maycock and C. R. Ricketts, *Nature*, 1961, *192*, 174.

When heated at 100°, solutions of dextrans were shown to undergo structural changes. In alkaline solutions, a decrease in reducing power, possibly due to oxidation, occurred. In acid solutions, appreciable hydrolysis and depolymerisation took place resulting in decreased viscosity and increased reducing power.— B. Mondovi *et al.*, *Ital. J. Biochem.*, 1964, *13*, 401.

The stability of a dextran solution (Macrodex) was not affected by prolonged storage, even when subjected to extreme temperature changes including freezing.— O. T. Fure *et al.*, *Pharm. Acta Helv.*, 1975, *50*, 216.

Adverse Effects. Infusions of dextrans may occasionally produce allergic reactions such as urticaria, hypotension, and bronchospasm. Severe anaphylactic reactions may occasionally occur and death may result from cardiac or respiratory arrest. Nausea, vomiting, fever, joint pains, and flushing may occur.

Dextrans might precipitate renal failure in some patients (see also under Dextran 40 Intravenous Infusion).

There were 24 anaphylactic reactions in 34 621 infusions of dextran 60/75 and 4 in 51 261 infusions of dextran 40.— J. Ring and K. Messmer, *Lancet*, 1977, *1*, 466.

From 1968 to 1975 the Swedish Adverse Drug Reaction Committee received 113 reports of anaphylactoid reactions to dextran 70 and 20 reports of anaphylactoid reactions to dextran 40. Five patients died following administration of dextran 70 and 1 patient died after dextran 40. Symptoms were noticed within 10 minutes or before 100 ml had been infused in 96 patients with reactions to dextran 70.— A. -K. Furhoff, *Acta anaesth. scand.*, 1977, *21*, 161.

Reduced incidence of anaphylactoid/anaphylactic reactions following the use of a monovalent hapten dextran preparation with an average molecular weight of 1000 (dextran 1).— K. Messmer *et al.* (letter), *Lancet*, 1980, *1*, 975. Comment.— A. M. Edwards and A. Holland (letter), *ibid.*, 1307.

Reports of anaphylactic reactions to dextran injections.— E. Michelson, *New Engl. J. Med.*, 1968, *278*, 552; R. Brisman *et al.*, *J. Am. med. Ass.*, 1968, *204*, 824; R. Fothergill and G. A. Heaney (letter), *Br. med. J.*, 1976, *2*, 1502; L. H. Fanous *et al.*, *Br. med. J.*, 1977, *2*, 1189; P. D. Wilson and A. D. G. Brown (letter), *Lancet*, 1978, *2*, 899.

Haemorrhage. The use, for 4 months of 1 litre of dextran 70 infused over 12 hours after each major gynaecological operation led to the development of large abdominal haematomas and increased morbidity. Since discontinuing the use of dextran 70, morbidity and the incidence of haematomas were reduced.— A. M. Smith (letter), *Br. med. J.*, 1973, *2*, 777.

A reduction in clotting factor VIII activity occurred on 2 occasions in a 24-year-old woman with thrombotic thrombo-cytopenic purpura when given infusions of dextran 70.— R. J. Raasch, *Am. J. Hosp. Pharm.*, 1979, *36*, 89.

Renal failure. Seven of 8 cases of drug-induced acute renal failure seen in 8 months were due to dextran 40 (6 cases) or dextran 70 (1). Dextran injections had not been withdrawn despite falling urine outputs; 5 patients developed anuria. Dextrans should not be given at a rate faster than 1 litre a day. In addition, they should not be given if urine output was below 1.5 litres a day, or if urine specific gravity rose above 1.045, or if blood urea rose above 600 µg per ml (10 mmol per litre.)— T. G. Feest, *Br. med. J.*, 1976, *2*, 1300.

Treatment of Adverse Effects. Dextran infusions should be discontinued immediately if allergic reactions occur. Administration of adrenaline, corticosteroids, and antihistamines may be necessary, in addition to supportive measures, in the treatment of severe anaphylactic reactions.

Precautions. Dextran infusions are contra-indicated in patients with severe congestive heart failure or cardiac decompensation, thrombocytopenia, renal disease with anuria or severe oliguria, or in those hypersensitive to dextrans. Infusions produce a progressive dilution of oxygen-carrying capacity, coagulation factors, and plasma proteins and may overload the circulation. They should therefore be administered with caution to patients with impaired renal function, clotting defects, haemorrhage, polycythaemia, chronic liver disease, or hypervolaemic disorders, or those at risk of developing pulmonary oedema or congestive heart failure; the haematocrit should not be allowed to fall below 30% and all patients should be observed for early signs of bleeding complications. Patients should be watched closely during the early part of the infusion period, and the infusion stopped immediately if signs of anaphylactic reactions appear.

Dextran injections in dextrose injection without added electrolytes should not be administered through the same transfusion equipment as Whole Blood.

Deficiency of coagulation factors should be corrected and fluid and electrolyte balance maintained. Dehydration should be corrected before or at least during dextran infusions, in order to maintain an adequate urine flow. The effects of anticoagulants may be enhanced by dextran.

Dextrans may interfere with blood grouping and cross matching of blood. Therefore, whenever possible, a sample of blood should be collected before giving the dextran infusion and kept frozen in case such tests become necessary.

The presence of dextran may interfere with the determination of glucose, bilirubin, or protein in blood or urine.

Dextrans might interfere with the measurement of serum-uric acid concentrations when the reagent used was phosphotungstic acid.— J. Millhouse, *Adverse Drug React. Bull.*, 1974, Dec., 164.

See also under Dextran 40 Intravenous Infusion, p.511.

Absorption and Fate. After an intravenous infusion of dextran 70, about 50% has been stated to be excreted unchanged in the urine within 24 hours. Dextran molecules not excreted are metabolised, mainly in the liver, to carbon dioxide and water.

In a study of dextran 70 given to women during and for 6 hours after hysterectomy, half the dose was excreted in about 43 hours and 5 to 10% could be detected in the circulation after 7 days.— J. W. Walkley *et al.*, *J. Pharm. Pharmac.*, 1976, *28*, 29.

Uses. Because the dextran molecules exert a colloidal osmotic pressure similar to that of plasma proteins, dextran 70 is used to produce an expansion of the plasma volume in conditions associated with the loss of plasma proteins. It has also been given to maintain the blood pressure and to prevent surgical shock and deep-vein thrombosis.

After moderate blood loss, 500 ml of dextran 70 may be rapidly infused over 15 minutes, followed by a further 500 ml given over 30 to 45 minutes. For severe haemorrhage, 1 litre may be rapidly infused, and, if necessary, it may be followed by 500 ml administered more slowly, but if there is a great loss of blood, transfusions of whole blood may be necessary. In the treatment of burns it may be necessary to infuse 3 or more litres, with electrolyte replacement solutions, during the first few days. In injury or shock where plasma proteins diffuse into the tissues, 500 ml or more may be required, the rate of infusion being determined by the condition of the patient. In the prevention of postoperative thrombosis, 500 to 1000 ml has been given over 4 to 6 hours initially, followed, if necessary by further doses of 500 ml every other day.

For brief reviews of the use of dextran preparations see C. R. Ricketts, *Prescribers' J.*, 1971, *11*, 138; *Br. J. Anaesth.*, 1973, *45*, 958; A. Doenicke *et al.*, *Br. J. Anaesth.*, 1977, *49*, 681.

Effect on cerebral blood flow. For a comparison of the effect of dextran 40 and dextran 70 on cerebral blood flow, see Dextran 40 Intravenous Infusion, p.511.

Effect on erythrocyte aggregation and platelet adhesiveness. A study *in vitro* to determine the effects on erythrocyte aggregation of solutions of dextrans of average molecular weights ranging from 10 000 to 500 000 showed that solutions of dextrans of weight average molecular weight 40 000 tended to counter aggregation and that at a concentration of 57 mg per ml aggregation was completely reversed in 8 out of 9 samples. Solutions of dextrans of higher and lower average molecular weights were less effective, whilst dextrans of weight average molecular weights of 150 000 and 500 000 invariably resulted in increased aggregation.— J. Engeset *et al.*, *Lancet*, 1966, *1*, 1124.

Studies in 6 healthy men showed that withdrawal of 500 ml of blood and infusion of 500 ml of 6% dextran 70 in sodium chloride injection diminished platelet adhesiveness. Platelet aggregation in response to adenosine diphosphate was also decreased. The changes were most evident 4 hours after the infusion and were maintained for over 24 hours.— P. N. Bennett *et al.*, *Lancet*, 1966, *2*, 1001.

Further references: M. L. Heath *et al.*, *Br. J. Anaesth.*, 1968, *40*, 144; M. L. Heath *et al.*, *Br. J. Anaesth.*, 1969, *41*, 939; H. J. Weiss, *New Engl. J. Med.*, 1978, *298*, 1344 and 1403; J. A. Blakely, *Can. J. Hosp. Pharm.*, 1978, *31*, 11.

Effect on kidney function. Studies in 10 patients during the immediate postoperative period indicated that the effective renal plasma flow increased to a maximum 30% higher than the mean basal level following the intravenous infusion of 500 ml of dextran 40 in dextrose injection. Comparable studies using an infusion of dextran 70 in dextrose injection showed increases of about 50% in the effective renal plasma flow. It was considered that the effects could be due to expansion of plasma volume. Though renal plasma flow had been increased by infusions of dextrans, in the absence of evidence that red blood-cell aggregation was an important factor in the development of acute renal failure, their use prophylactically for that purpose was suggested to be unsound.— N. A. Matheson and J. W. Robertson, *Lancet*, 1966, *2*, 251.

Hyperlipidaemia. Because there might be a risk of platelet aggregation in patients with homozygous hypercholesterolaemia undergoing surgery the following regimen was recommended: 500 ml of dextran 70 given intravenously during the operation and daily for 4 or 5 days thereafter. Aspirin 1 g daily and dipyridamole 50 mg thrice daily should then be given until the plasma-cholesterol concentration stopped falling. Children should receive reduced doses and care should be taken in patients with heart failure.— O. Faergeman *et al.* (letter), *Lancet*, 1976, *2*, 1416.

Malaria. To reduce intravascular 'sludging' of red cells in comatose patients with acute falciparum malaria, 500 ml of dextran 75 should be given every 12 hours.— *Tech. Rep. Ser. Wld Hlth Org. No. 529*, 1973.

Purpura. Purpura fulminans in an 11-year-old boy, which had not responded to antibiotics, corticosteroids, or heparin, was cured by intravenous injections of 6% dextran in saline solution. A dose of 250 ml, corresponding to 500 mg per kg body-weight, was given every third day for about 15 weeks.— J. H. Patterson *et al.*, *New Engl. J. Med.*, 1965, *273*, 734.

Thrombotic thrombocytopenic purpura was treated in 6 patients by immediate splenectomy followed by dextran 70 therapy, 0.5 to 1 litre daily given intravenously for about 2 weeks, and high dosage corticosteroid therapy which was gradually reduced over a period of 6 months. Five patients survived compared with 31 of more than 300 reported in the literature.— J. Cuttner, *J. Am. med. Ass.*, 1974, *227*, 397.

Reports of the use of dextran injection in the treatment of thrombotic thrombocytopenic purpura in 10 patients, unsuccessful in 3. Most patients had previously also received corticosteroids and some had had a splenectomy.— *Ann. intern. Med.*, 1977, *86*, 102.

Shock. For a review of the treatment of cardiac shock and an assessment of the role of dextran injections in the condition, see *Lancet*, 1966, *1*, 645.

Thrombo-embolism. Reviews of the use of dextran in the prevention of postoperative deep vein thrombosis and thrombo-embolism.— *Drug & Ther. Bull.*, 1975, *13*, 41; J. S. Calnan and F. Allenby, *Br. J. Anaesth.*, 1975, *47*, 151; J. F. Mustard and M. A. Packham, *Drugs*, 1975, *9*, 19; A. S. Gallus and J. Hirsh, *Drugs*, 1976, *12*, 132; G. K. Morris and J. R. A. Mitchell, *Br. med. Bull.*, 1978, *34*, 169.

In a double-blind trial 396 patients undergoing elective laparotomy of the gastro-intestinal or biliary tract were given 500 ml of dextran 70 in sodium chloride injection starting at the induction of anaesthesia and a second 500 ml shortly after leaving the theatre; 435 similar patients received sodium chloride injection. Pulmonary embolism occurred in 3 and 13 patients respectively, with deaths in 1 and 7—both significant reductions. The incidence of deep-vein thrombosis, clinically assessed, was not significantly different in 16 and 20 cases respectively. Total deaths within 3 months from thrombo-embolic disease were 4 and 14 respectively. Deaths from other causes were not significantly different. There was close correlation between the clinical assessment of thrombosis and the results of phlebography.— A. Kline *et al.*, *Br. med. J.*, 1975, *2*, 109. Criticism of the comments on the ^{125}I-fibrinogen test.— C. V. Ruckley (letter), *Br. med. J.*, 1975, *2*, 498.

In 50 patients undergoing surgery the incidence of deep-vein thrombosis (34%) was not significantly different, after the prophylactic infusion of 500 ml of dextran 70 (sometimes repeated once or twice) and pneumatic leggings, from that (24%) in 50 controls, but the incidence of pulmonary embolism was significantly reduced from 24 to 8%.— N. L. Browse *et al.*, *Br. med. J.*, 1976, *2*, 1281. See also *Drugs*, 1978, *15*, 325.

In 128 patients undergoing total hip replacement the incidence of calf deep-vein thrombosis (assessed by the fibrinogen uptake test) was similar (above 50%) in 58 treated with warfarin (15 mg 36 hours after surgery, none on the next day, 5 mg next day, then according to the prothrombin time for 3 weeks), in 51 treated with infusions of dextran 70 (1 litre starting with induction of anaesthesia, then 1 litre daily for 3 days, then 500 ml on alternative days for 10 days), and in 19 treated with heparin (5000 units subcutaneously every 12 hours for 3 weeks, commencing the evening before surgery). There was no pulmonary embolism in those given warfarin, a 4% incidence in those given dextran 70, and a 15.8% incidence in those given heparin. The use of warfarin was advocated.— H. M. Barber *et al.*, *Postgrad. med. J.*, 1977, *53*, 130.

In a randomised multicentre study the incidence of deep-vein thrombosis was 22% in 97 patients given 500 ml of dextran 70 in sodium chloride injection before surgery and a further 500 ml postoperatively, significantly less than the 38% incidence in 95 patients treated by intermittent calf compression. In 97 patients treated by both regimens the incidence was 19%. The incidence of pulmonary embolism in the 3 groups was comparable. Median blood loss was not significantly different in the 3 groups but bleeding was more common after dextran.— R. C. Smith *et al.*, *Br. med. J.*, 1978, *1*, 952.

Discussions on dextran versus heparin for the prophylaxis of deep-vein thrombosis.— W. T. Davies (letter), *Lancet*, 1978, *2*, 732; V. V. Kakkar (letter), *ibid.*, 899; G. T. Watts (letter), *ibid.*; P. D. Wilson and A. D. G. Brown (letter), *ibid.*; W. T. Davies (letter), *ibid.*, 1315.

Further references: *J. Am. med. Ass.*, 1968, *206*, 1438; D. London and M. L. Crosfill, *Br. J. clin. Pract.*, 1969, *23*, 158; J. M. Lambie *et al.*, *Br. med. J.*, 1970, *2*, 144; V. V. Kakkar *et al.* (letter), *ibid.*, 540; J. Bonnar and J. Walsh, *Lancet*, 1972, *1*, 614; A. E. Carter and R. Eban, *Br. J. Surg.*, 1973, *60*, 681; U. F. Gruber, *Surg. Clins N. Am.*, 1975, *55*, 679.

Thrombophlebitis. A favourable report on the use of dextran 70 in women with deep thrombophlebitis associated with pregnancy.— R. C. Wallach, *Am. J. Obstet. Gynec.*, 1972, *112*, 613.

Proprietary Preparations of Dextran 70

Gentran 70 *(Travenol, UK)*. A sterile solution containing 6% of dextran 70 in dextrose injection or sodium chloride injection.

Hyskon *(Pharmacia, UK)*. A sterile viscous solution containing 32% of dextrans of weight average molecular weight 70 000 in dextrose injection 10%, in bottles of 100 ml. For hysteroscopy. (Also available as Hyskon in *Swed.*).

Lomodex 70 *(Fisons, UK)*. A sterile solution containing 6% of dextran 70 in dextrose injection or sodium chloride injection.

Macrodex *(Pharmacia, UK: Farillon, UK)*. A sterile solution containing 6% of dextran 70 in dextrose injection or sodium chloride injection. (Also available as Macrodex in *Austral.*, *Belg.*, *Canad.*, *Neth.*, *USA*).

Other Proprietary Names of Dextran 70

Perfudex 70 *(Belg.)*; Soludex *(Ital.)*.

Preparations of Some Other Dextrans

Polyglucinum *(Rus. P.)*. A sterile 6% w/v solution of dextran 60 in 0.9% sodium chloride solution. Sterilised by autoclaving. pH 4.5 to 6.5. Store at −10° to 20°. Used as a plasma substitute.

Experiments to elucidate the physiological action of polyglucin.— V. B. Koziner, *Problemy̆ Gemat. Pereliv. Krovi*, 1965, *10*, 18, per *Abstr. Wld Med.*, 1966, *39*, 345.

253-1

Dextran 110 Intravenous Infusion *(B.P.)*.

Dextran 110 Injection. A sterile 5.5 to 6.5% w/v solution in dextrose injection or in sodium chloride injection of dextrans of weight average molecular weight about 110 000.

CAS — 9004-54-0 (dextran 110).

Pharmacopoeias. In *Br.*

It is an almost colourless, slightly viscous solution. **Sterilised** by autoclaving. It should be **stored** at an even temperature. It should not be used if it is cloudy or if a deposit is present.

Adverse Effects, Treatment, and Precautions. As for Dextran 70 Intravenous Infusion, p.512.

Dextran 110 may cause aggregation of red blood-cells and increase the erythrocyte sedimentation-rate.

Dextrans of high molecular weight (about 110 000) caused rouleaux formation, with the appearance of agglutination, with anti-A and anti-B sera so that blood groups A and B could be mistakenly identified.— M. A. M. Ali, *Prescribers' J.*, 1970, *10*, 60.

Absorption and Fate. After intravenous infusion, dextran 110 is retained in the circulation for 2 or 3 days. The smaller molecules may be excreted unchanged and the larger molecules slowly metabolised to carbon dioxide and water; about 40% has been reported to be excreted in the urine within 24 hours.

Uses. Dextran 110 is used to produce an expansion of the plasma volume in conditions associated with the loss of plasma proteins. It is retained in the circulation long enough for the physiological replacement of plasma proteins. It has also been given to maintain the blood pressure and to prevent surgical shock.

In the treatment of blood loss and burns and in the prevention of shock, it is used similarly to dextran 70 (see p.513). For prophylaxis during surgery associated with blood loss or shock dextran 110 has been infused at an initial rate of 10 to 20 drops per minute immediately after the anaesthetic, and the rate adjusted during the operation to maintain the blood pressure.

Proprietary Preparations

Dextraven 110 *(Fisons, UK)*. A sterile solution containing 6% of dextran 110 in dextrose injection or sodium chloride injection.

254-y

Dextran 150 Intravenous Infusion.

Dextran 150 Injection *(B.P. 1963)*. A sterile 6% w/v solution in dextrose injection or in sodium chloride injection of dextrans of weight average molecular weight about 150 000.

CAS — 9004-54-0 (dextran 150).

It is an almost colourless, slightly viscous solution with a pH of 3.5 to 6.5 for the solution in dextrose injection and a pH of 5 to 7 for the solution in sodium chloride injection. It is **sterilised** by autoclaving or by filtration. It should be **stored** at an even temperature, not exceeding 25°.

Dextran 150 has the actions and uses of Dextran 110 Intravenous Infusion, above. A hyperosmotic 10% injection has also been used.

Allergic reaction. A report of an anaphylactic reaction occurring in a patient given dextran 150 for postoperative hypotension.— J. R. Maltby, *Br. J. Anaesth.*, 1968, *40*, 552.

Proprietary Preparations

Dextraven 150 *(Fisons, UK)*. A sterile solution containing 6% of dextran 150 in dextrose injection or sodium chloride injection. (Also available as Dextraven 150 in *Austral.*).

255-j

Hetastarch.

2-Hydroxyethyl Starch; HES. 2-Hydroxyethyl ether starch.

CAS — 9005-27-0.

A starch that is composed of more than 90% of amylopectin and that has been etherified to the extent that an average of 7 to 8 of the hydroxy groups in each 10 D-glucopyranose units of starch polymer have been converted into hydroxyethyl groups. Mol. wt about 450 000.

Adverse Effects and Precautions. Vomiting, fever, chills, itching, urticaria, and salivary gland enlargement have been reported. The administration of large volumes may interfere with coagulation mechanisms and increase the risk of haemorrhage. It is therefore contra-indicated in patients with severe bleeding disorders.

As hetastarch is excreted relatively slowly, mainly by the kidneys, circulatory overload may occur, especially in patients with impaired renal function, and it is contra-indicated in patients with severe congestive heart failure and renal failure with oliguria or anuria.

There were 14 anaphylactic reactions in 16 405 infusions of hetastarch.— J. Ring and K. Messmer, *Lancet*, 1977, *1*, 466.

There was no adverse effect on renal function in 4 healthy subjects infused with 500 ml of a 6% hetastarch solution in sodium chloride injection on each of 3 consecutive days over 24 to 47 minutes.— J. M. Mishler *et al.*, *Br. J. clin. Pharmac.*, 1977, *4*, 591.

Increases in serum-amylase concentrations occurred in all of 54 patients following infusion of 500 ml of hetastarch 6%. The diagnostic value of serum amylase was limited for 3 to 5 days after infusion.— H. Köhler *et al.*, *Int. J. clin. Pharmac. Biopharm.*, 1977, *15*, 428.

Absorption and Fate. About 40% of a dose of hetastarch is excreted in the urine in 24 hours; the remainder is slowly degraded and excreted over about 2 weeks.

The pharmacokinetics of low molecular weight hetastarch (weight average molecular weight 264 000).— J. M. Mishler *et al.*, *Br. J. clin. Pharmac.*, 1979, *7*, 619.

Changes in the molecular composition of circulating hetastarch following consecutive daily infusions in 4 healthy subjects.— J. M. Mishler *et al.*, *Br. J. clin. Pharmac.*, 1979, *7*, 505. See also *idem*, *J. clin. Path.*, 1980, *33*, 155.

Uses. Hetastarch is used for the same purposes as Dextran 70 Intravenous Infusion (see p.513). The usual dose by infusion of 6% solution in sodium chloride injection is 500 to 1500 ml daily or to a maximum of 20 ml per kg body-weight daily. In acute haemorrhagic shock up to 20 ml per kg per hour has been given.

Hetastarch is also used as an adjunct to leucophaeresis, usually in doses of 250 to 700 ml of the 6% solution; it acts as a sedimenting agent, increasing the yield of granulocytes.

Infusion of 500 ml of 6% hetastarch in 0.9% sodium chloride solution appeared to have no adverse effect on 29 patients. Platelet counts fell 8 hours after infusion but reached pretransfusion levels by 24 hours. Although hetastarch was rapidly excreted in the urine about 60% of the dose remained in the blood after 24 hours. Two patients had unusual bleeding following surgery, which was possibly due to the infusion.— T. F. Solanke, *Br. med. J.*, 1968, *3*, 783. Comments.— R. E. Weston, *McGaw Laboratories* (letter), *ibid.*, 1969, *1*, 125.

A brief review of the actions and uses of hetastarch.— W. L. Thompson, *Recent Adv. clin. Pharmac.*, 1978, *1*, 128. See also W. J. Rudowski, *Br. J. Hosp. Med.*, 1980, *23*, 389; *Med. Lett.*, 1981, *23*, 16.

Further references: W. F. Ballinger *et al.*, *J. surg. Res.*, 1966, *6*, 180; *J. Am. med. Ass.*, 1966, *197* (July 4), A30; S. Gollub *et al.*, *Surgery Gynec. Obstet.*, 1969, *128*, 725; W. L. Thompson *et al.*, *Surgery Gynec. Obstet.*, 1970, *131*, 965; *Lancet*, 1971, *2*, 147.

Proprietary Names

Hespan *(American Critical Care, USA)*; Plasmasteril *(Fresenius, Ger.)*; Volex *(McGaw, USA)*.

Diagnostic Agents

2120-z

In this section are included agents which are administered clinically as an aid to diagnosis or to evaluate body function, as well as a number of proprietary test substances. Also included is the Limulus Test, p.520.
The sections on Contrast Media and Radiopharmaceuticals contain many agents used diagnostically. Many other substances included in other sections may be used for diagnostic purposes although this may not be their main indication.

2121-c

Ametazole Hydrochloride.

Betazole Hydrochloride *(U.S.P.)*; Betazoli Chloridum. 2-(Pyrazol-3-yl)ethylamine dihydrochloride.
$C_5H_9N_3,2HCl = 184.1$.

CAS — 105-20-4 (ametazole); 138-92-1 (hydrochloride).

Pharmacopoeias. In *Nord.* and *U.S.*

A white, almost odourless, hygroscopic, crystalline powder. M.p. not higher than 240°. **Soluble** 1 in 3 of water and 1 in 50 of alcohol; practically insoluble in chloroform; very slightly soluble in ether. A 5% solution in water has a pH of about 3.4. A 1.91% solution is iso-osmotic with serum. **Store** in airtight containers. Protect from light.

Haemolysis. An aqueous solution of ametazole hydrochloride iso-osmotic with serum (1.91%) caused 100% haemolysis of erythrocytes cultured in it for 45 minutes. The solution turned dark brown.— E. R. Hammarland and K. Pedersen-Bjergaard, *J. pharm. Sci.*, 1961, *50*, 24.

Adverse Effects. Ametazole causes side-effects similar to those of histamine acid phosphate (see p.518), but they are usually less severe. Flushing of the skin may occur in about 20% of patients, and headache in about 3%. Urticaria, faintness, and syncope may occur rarely.

During a test for gastric acidity, a 78-year-old woman received ametazole hydrochloride 50 mg subcutaneously. Dyspnoea and nausea developed after 15 minutes, oedema of the lungs after 30 minutes, and death due to irreversible cardiac and respiratory arrest occurred after 40 minutes.— D. Thiede and K. D. Bock, *Medsche Klin.*, 1970, *65*, 29.

Treatment of Adverse Effects and Precautions. As for Histamine Acid Phosphate, p.518.

Uses. Ametazole hydrochloride is an analogue of histamine and is used as a diagnostic agent for testing gastric secretion. It has a less marked effect than histamine on blood pressure and causes only a slight increase in the heart-rate. The effect reaches a peak in about 45 minutes and lasts about 2½ hours. Occasionally it stimulates secretion of hydrochloric acid in patients who do not respond to histamine.
Ametazole hydrochloride may be given in a dose of 500 µg per kg body-weight by subcutaneous or intramuscular injection; this dose produces an effect equivalent to that of about 27.5 µg of anhydrous histamine acid phosphate per kg body-weight. A dose of 50 mg is sometimes given to adults of average weight. Oral doses of 100 mg in 30 ml of water (given by gastric tube) have sometimes been used.

Preparations

Betazole Hydrochloride Injection *(U.S.P.)*. A sterile solution of ametazole hydrochloride in Water for Injections. pH 2.8 to 3.4. Protect from light.

Proprietary Names

Betazol *(Lilly, Ger.)*; Histalog *(Lilly, Canad.*; *Lilly, USA)*; Testazid *(A.L., Norw.)*.

Ametazole hydrochloride was formerly marketed in Great Britain under the proprietary name Histalog *(Lilly)*.

2122-k

Aminohippuric Acid

(U.S.P.). PAHA; *p*-Aminohippuric Acid; Para-aminohippuric Acid; *p*-Aminobenzoylglycine. *N*-4-Aminobenzoylaminoacetic acid.
$C_9H_{10}N_2O_3 = 194.2$.

CAS — 61-78-9 (aminohippuric acid); 94-16-6 (sodium salt).

Pharmacopoeias. In *Cz.*, *Fr.*, and *U.S.*

A white crystalline powder which discolours on exposure to light. M.p. about 195° with decomposition. **Soluble** 1 in 45 of water, 1 in 50 of alcohol, and 1 in 5 of dilute hydrochloric acid; very slightly soluble in carbon tetrachloride, chloroform, and ether; freely soluble, with decomposition, in solutions of alkali hydroxides and carbonates. **Store** in airtight containers. Protect from light.

Stability in solution. Decomposition, through oxidation, of aqueous sodium aminohippurate solutions, especially when exposed to light, could be markedly retarded by the addition of 0.1% of sodium metabisulphite in air-filled ampoules and prevented in nitrogen-filled ampoules for at least 2 weeks in direct sunlight and for 3 years when stored in darkness or diffused light.— T. D. Whittet and A. E. Robinson, *Pharm. J.*, 1964, *2*, 39.

Adverse Effects. Rapid intravenous infusion of sodium aminohippurate may cause nausea and vomiting, vasomotor disturbances, flushing, tingling, cramps, and a feeling of warmth.

Precautions. The estimation of sodium aminohippurate may be affected in patients taking procaine, sulphonamides, or thiazosulphone. Probenecid diminishes the excretion of aminohippuric acid. Clearance is also affected by penicillins and salicylates.

Absorption and Fate. Sodium aminohippurate, administered intravenously to a patient with normal kidney function, is rapidly excreted in the urine.

The biological half-life of aminohippuric acid was reported to be 0.17 hours.— W. A. Ritschel, *Drug Intell. & clin. Pharm.*, 1970, *4*, 332.

Uses. Aminohippuric acid is given by intravenous infusion, as the sodium salt, as a diagnostic agent for the estimation of effective renal plasma flow and, in larger amounts, for the measurement of the renal tubular secretory mechanism.

A dilution method involving sodium aminohippurate had been used to measure the volume of amniotic fluid for the diagnosis of hydramnios.— H. E. Jacoby and D. Charles, *Am. J. Obstet. Gynec.*, 1966, *94*, 910.

For the clearance of aminohippuric acid from amniotic fluid in conditions associated with placental insufficiency, see S. C. Edelberg *et al.*, *Am. J. Obstet. Gynec.*, 1968, *102*, 585.

In 50 normotensive patients without evidence of renal disorder the mean clearance of phenolsulphonphthalein was about 60% of that of aminohippuric acid. From the results of various studies it was suggested that the clearance of phenolsulphonphthalein was a sensitive method in the diagnosis of secretory tubular disorders, whereas clearance of aminohippuric acid was more suitable for assessing renal circulatory disorders.— A. Heidland, *Arch. klin. Med.*, 1968, *214*, 163.

Preparations

Aminohippurate Sodium Injection *(U.S.P.)*. Sodium Aminohippurate Injection. A sterile solution of aminohippuric acid in Water for Injections, prepared with the aid of sodium hydroxide. pH 6.7 to 7.6.

Aminohippurate Sodium 20% Injection *(Merck Sharp & Dohme, UK)*. Contains sodium aminohippurate 20% for intravenous injection, in vials of 10 and 50 ml.

Other Proprietary Names

Nephrotest BAG *(sodium salt) (Ger.)*.

2123-a

Azovan Blue

(B.P. 1958). Azovanum Caeruleum; Evans Blue *(U.S.P.)*; T 1824; CI Direct Blue 53; Colour Index No. 23860. Tetrasodium 6,6′-[3,3′-dimethylbiphenyl-4,4′-diylbis(azo)]bis-[4-amino-5-hydroxynaphthalene-1,3-disulphonate].
$C_{34}H_{24}N_6Na_4O_{14}S_4 = 960.8$.

CAS — 314-13-6.

Pharmacopoeias. In *Arg.*, *Ind.*, *Jap.*, and *U.S.*

A green, bluish-green, or brown, odourless, hygroscopic powder. It loses not more than 15% of its weight on drying. Very **soluble** in water; very slightly soluble in alcohol; practically insoluble in carbon tetrachloride, chloroform, and ether. A 0.5% solution has a pH of 6 to 7. Solutions are **sterilised** by autoclaving or by filtration. **Store** in airtight containers.

Solutions for injection. The following formula gave a stable injection. Azovan blue 500 mg, mannitol 4.65 g, Water for Injections to 100 ml. It was sterilised by autoclaving and filled into ampoules under nitrogen; pH 6 to 6.5.— H. Brunnhofer and K. Steiger, *Pharm. Acta Helv.*, 1959, *34*, 110.

Adverse Effects. Staining of the skin, fading in about 6 weeks, may occur if 3 or more injections are given within 3 days.

Absorption and Fate. After intravenous injection, azovan blue is firmly bound to plasma proteins; it slowly leaves the circulation. It is stated not to penetrate into the CSF, not to cross the placenta, and not to appear in the urine of patients with undamaged kidneys.

Uses. Azovan blue is a dye which has been used for the determination of blood and plasma volumes. The patient should be in the fasting state and have been recumbent for at least 15 minutes. An intravenous injection of up to 5 ml of 0.5% solution of the dye, diluted with about 2 ml of sodium chloride injection, is given into the median antecubital vein of one arm and samples of blood are withdrawn at intervals from the opposite antecubital vein. Mixing with blood is complete in about 9 minutes, or in up to 15 minutes in patients with impaired cardiac function. The concentration of the dye is then determined colorimetrically. The calculated plasma volume is corrected, according to the haematocrit value, to yield the blood volume.

Azovan blue had been used effectively for the localisation of intra-arterial cannulas.— T. Cartmill (letter), *Lancet*, 1962, *2*, 728.

Azovan blue, 5 ml of a 1% solution per 100 ml of dialysing fluid, could be used to assess the effective dialysing area of cellophane filters in dialysing coils.— J. Erben *et al.* (letter), *J. Am. med. Ass.*, 1967, *202*, 72.

The injection of diatrizoates and azovan blue or indocyanine green was used successfully with xeromammography in 33 of 35 patients for the localisation of breast lesions.— R. W. Wayne and R. E. Darby, *J. Am. med. Ass.*, 1977, *237*, 2219.

Preparations

Evans Blue Injection *(U.S.P.)*. A sterile solution of anhydrous azovan blue 4.3 to 4.75 mg per ml in Water for Injections; pH 5.5 to 7.5. *Jap.P.* has a similar preparation.

2124-t

Ceruletide.

Caerulein. 5-oxoPro-Gln-Asp-Tyr(SO_3H)-Thr-Gly-Trp-Met-Asp-Phe—NH_2.
$C_{58}H_{73}N_{13}O_{21}S_2 = 1352.4$.

CAS — 17650-98-5.

NOTE. The name Ceruleinum has been applied to Indigo Carmine, p.519.

Ceruletide is a decapeptide amide isolated from the skin of the Australian frog, *Hyla caerulea*, and other amphibians, or it may be prepared synthetically as a salt, ceruletide diethylamine (FI 6934).

Ceruletide has similar actions to pancreozymin (p.521); when administered by intravenous injection it stimulates gall-bladder contraction and relaxes the sphincter of Oddi.

Ceruletide may be used usually as the diethylamine salt as a diagnostic agent for testing the functional capacity of the pancreas in a dose equivalent to 1 to 2 ng per kg body-weight per minute of ceruletide as an intravenous infusion and has been suggested for the treatment of paralytic ileus. Ceruletide may also be used an an adjunct to cholecystography.

A review of active polypeptides of non-mammalian origin, including ceruletide.— G. Bertaccini, *Pharmac. Rev.*, 1976, *28*, 127.

Bowel movements and normal stool production occurred in 15 patients with paralytic ileus after being given ceruletide 750 ng per kg body-weight intramuscularly every 12 to 24 hours for 1 to 2 days.— A. Agosti *et al.* (letter), *Lancet*, 1971, *1*, 395.

Stimulation of the pancreas with secretin 1 .Clinical unit per kg body-weight together with ceruletide 40 ng per kg followed after 30 minutes by pancreozymin 1 unit per kg led to urine-amylase values far in excess of those normally obtained; under these circumstances the test was of no value in the diagnosis of pancreatitis.— R. Van der Hoeden *et al.*, *Gut*, 1973, *14*, 763.

A single dose of ceruletide 500 ng per kg body-weight intramuscularly had a strong accelerating effect on peristalsis in postoperative patients. Severe pain was often reported at the site of the injection. It was suggested that ceruletide may be of use in the management of postoperative intestinal paralysis.— T. Fumoto and T. Watanuki, *Farmaco, Edn prat.*, 1975, *30*, 579.

Further references.— G. Bertaccini *et al.*, *Br. J. Pharmac.*, 1968, *34*, 291 and 311; G. Bertaccini *et al.*, *Gastroenterology*, 1969, *56*, 862; A. Agosti and G. Bertaccini (letter), *Lancet*, 1969, *1*, 580; A. M. Brooks *et al.*, *New Engl. J. Med.*, 1970, *282*, 535; G. Bertaccini and A. Agosti, *Gastroenterology*, 1971, *60*, 55; E. N. Sargent *et al.*, *Am. J. Roentg.*, 1978, *130*, 1051; S. M. Wetzner *et al.*, *Radiology*, 1979, *131*, 23; J. D. Arnold *et al.*, *Clin. Pharmac. Ther.*, 1980, *27*, 245; V. F. Montero *et al.*, *J. int. med. Res.*, 1980, *8*, 98.

Proprietary Names

Ceosunin (as diethylamine salt) *(Jap.)*; Takus (as diethylamine salt) *(Farmitalia, Ger.)*.

2125-x

Congo Red *(B.P.C. 1973)*.
Rubrum Congoensis; CI Direct Red 28; Colour Index No. 22120. Disodium 3,3′-[biphenyl-4,4′-diylbis(azo)]bis[4-aminonaphthalene-1-sulphonate].
$C_{32}H_{22}N_6Na_2O_6S_2$=696.7.

CAS — 573-58-0.

Pharmacopoeias. In *Hung.*, *Nord.*, and *Span.*

A reddish-brown powder containing not less than 90% of $C_{32}H_{22}N_6Na_2O_6S_2$, calculated on the dried material. It loses not more than 10% of its weight on drying. It usually contains sodium chloride retained from the process of manufacture. **Soluble** 1 in about 25 of water; partly and sparingly soluble in alcohol; practically insoluble in chloroform and ether.

A solution in water has a pH of 8 to 9.5. Solutions are **sterilised** by autoclaving or by filtration. **Store** in airtight containers. Protect from light.

NOTE. The *B.P.C. 1973* standard includes tests for pyrogens and undue toxicity. The grade of congo red that is usually supplied as a microscopical stain is unsuitable for injection.

Solutions could be sterilised by autoclaving at 115° for 30 minutes, or by filtration, and were stable for at least 7 months at room temperature. Storage in a refrigerator was not recommended as crystallisation could occur. Acid solutions were very toxic, and a lower limit of pH 7 should be observed. Solutions should be bright red and clear. The addition of sodium chloride increased the toxicity of the solutions. Solutions containing dextrose could also become dangerous as a result of a fall in pH during autoclaving. A further source of danger was the use of sintered glass filters which had not been completely washed. The use of solutions prepared by dissolving the solid immediately before use was not recommended because there was a danger of incomplete solution of the dye, which was difficult to detect.— G. F. Somers and T. D. Whittet, *J. Pharm. Pharmac.*, 1956, *8*, 1019.

Adverse Effects and Precautions. Congo red may cause staining of the skin if repeated injections are given. Clotting and severe reactions, occasionally fatal, have occurred after large doses or too rapid injection.

It is essential to ensure that the dye is completely dissolved at the time of injection as deaths have been caused by the injection of solutions containing undissolved dye; the solution should be allowed to stand undisturbed for some time and then examined for sediment immediately before use by inverting the container. The solution should be bright red and clear. It may be necessary to warm the solution to about 40° to aid solution. The injection should have a pH of not less than 7. Sodium chloride should not be added as this may precipitate the dye.

Severe substernal pain, cold sweats, visual impairment, and vomiting occurred in 2 women following the intravenous injection of 10 ml of a 1% solution of congo red. One patient died. Previous reports on fatalities were reviewed.— A. M. Abrahamsen, *Nord. Med.*, 1961, *66*, 1473.

Uses. Congo red has been used for the diagnosis of amyloid disease. It is given by slow intravenous injection and the percentage decrease of the dye content of the plasma or serum over a period of 1 hour is estimated colorimetrically. In normal persons, from 10 to 30% of the dye disappears, and in persons with amyloid disease, anything between 30 and 100%. The dose is 1.25 to 3.75 mg per kg body-weight as a 0.5 or 1.5% solution to a maximum of 270 mg; a standard dose of 10 ml of a 1% solution is commonly used.

The biological half-life of congo red was reported to be 2.46 hours.— W. A. Ritschel, *Drug Intell. & clin. Pharm.*, 1970, *4*, 332.

Achlorhydria test. As a screening test for achlorhydria, 500 patients swallowed a capsule containing thread impregnated with congo red, 1 end of the thread being left to protrude to permit recovery. The thread became crimson at pH 7, dark red at pH 5, and purple and then black at lower pH values. There was agreement between the results of the test and gastric analysis in 127 of 136 patients subjected to both procedures.— C. B. Beal and J. E. Brown, *Am. J. dig. Dis.*, 1968, *13*, 113.

Amyloidosis test. Retention of 20% or less of injected congo red in serum was considered to be almost certainly indicative of the presence of amyloid disease; with 21 to 40% retention it was probably present; with 41 to 60% retention the test had no diagnostic value and should be repeated several months later; with 60% or more retention, amyloid disease was excluded. Anaphylactic reactions to the dye were rare.— A. S. Cohen, *New Engl. J. Med.*, 1967, *277*, 628.

An evaluation of the congo red test in the detection of amyloidosis.— *Br. med. J.*, 1968, *4*, 564.

Preparations

Injectabile Congazoni 1% *(Nord. P.)*. Congo red 1 g, sodium acid phosphate 20 mg, sodium phosphate dihydrate 45 mg, mannitol 4.8 g, Water for Injections to 100 ml. pH 6.9 to 7.5. Store in ampoules under an inert gas. Protect from light.

2126-r

Cuprous Thiocyanate.
CuSCN=121.6.

CAS — 1111-67-7.

A white to yellow amorphous powder. Practically **insoluble** in water and alcohol; decomposed by concentrated mineral acids. Soluble in ether and ammonium hydroxide.

Uses. Cuprous thiocyanate has been used, in doses of 500 mg daily, as a marker for faeces and, in doses of 250 mg daily, for the estimation of faecal fat.

Cuprous thiocyanate interfered with radioisotope tests for thyroid function.— A. M. Zalin *et al.* (letter), *Lancet*, 1971, *1*, 1237.

Cuprous thiocyanate used as a continuous marker to assess intestinal calcium absorption in 15 children gave results which were similar to and in good agreement with those obtained with the carmine marker technique.— C. Loirat and H. Mathieu, *Archs Dis. Childh.*, 1977, *52*, 424.

Further references.— M. Dick, *Gut*, 1969, *10*, 408; M. F. Lee *et al.*, *ibid.*, 754.

2127-f

Dichromium Trioxide.
Chromium Oxide; Chromium Sesquioxide; Chromium (III) Oxide.
Cr_2O_3=152.0.

CAS — 1308-38-9.

A light to dark green powder. Practically **insoluble** in water.

Uses. Dichromium trioxide has been used as a marker to enhance the accuracy of estimations of faecal output in metabolic studies. It is not absorbed from the gastro-intestinal tract and is excreted unchanged in the faeces which are generally coloured olive-green. The usual dose is 500 mg thrice daily, or 250 mg six times daily. A suggested dose for children is 250 mg thrice daily.

Radio opaque pellets were superior to dichromium trioxide as markers in studies requiring accurate faecal collections.— W. J. Branch and J. H. Cummings, *Gut*, 1978, *19*, 371.

Further references.— L. G. Whitby and D. Lang, *J. clin. Invest.*, 1960, *39*, 854; G. A. Rose, *Gut*, 1964, *5*, 274.

Dichromium trioxide was formerly marketed in Great Britain under the proprietary name Chromium-Sandoz (*Sandoz*).

2128-d

Direct Blue 1.
Colour Index No. 24410. Tetrasodium 6,6′-[3,3′-dimethoxybiphenyl-4,4′-diylbis(azo)]bis[4-amino-5-hydroxynaphthalene-1,3-disulphonate].
$C_{34}H_{24}N_6Na_4O_{16}S_4$=992.8.

CAS — 2610-05-1.

A blue powder. **Soluble** in water, giving a blue solution; practically insoluble in alcohol.

Uses. Direct blue 1 has an affinity for lymphatic tissue and has been used to delineate lymph nodes during surgery for malignant neoplasms. The skin may be stained blue.

2129-n

Fluorescein *(U.S.P.)*.
3′,6′-Dihydroxyspiro-[isobenzofuran-1(3*H*),9′[9*H*]xanthen]-3-one.
$C_{20}H_{12}O_5$=332.3.

CAS — 2321-07-5.

Pharmacopoeias. In *U.S.*

An odourless yellowish-red to red powder. Practically **insoluble** in water; soluble in dilute solutions of alkali hydroxides. **Store** in airtight containers.

2130-k

Fluorescein Sodium *(B.P., U.S.P.)*.
Fluoresc. Sod.; Fluoresceinum Natricum; Fluorescein Natrium; Obiturin; Sodium Fluorescein; Soluble Fluorescein; Resorcinolphthalein Sodium; Uranin; CI Acid Yellow 73; Colour Index No. 45350; D & C Yellow No. 8. Disodium fluorescein.
$C_{20}H_{10}Na_2O_5$=376.3.

CAS — 518-47-8.

Pharmacopoeias. In *Aust.*, *Br.*, *Braz.*, *Chin.*, *Ind.*, *Int.*, *Jap.*, *Jug.*, *Nord.*, *Swiss*, and *U.S.*

An orange-red, odourless, almost tasteless, hygroscopic powder. The *B.P.* specifies that it loses not more than 10% of its weight when dried; the *U.S.P.* specifies not more than 17% of water. **Soluble** 1 in 1.5 of water, giving a red solution with a strong green fluorescence; a dilute solution is yellowish-green; the fluorescence disappears when the solution is made acid and reappears when it is made alkaline. Soluble 1 in 10 of alcohol; practically insoluble in chloroform and ether. A 0.5% solution has a pH of 8.2 to 8.7. A 3.34% solution in water is iso-osmotic with serum. Solutions are **sterilised** by autoclaving, by filtration, or by maintaining at 98° to 100° for 30 minutes with a bactericide; if sodium bicarbonate is present the container should be sealed before autoclaving and should not be opened until at least 2 hours after the solution has cooled to room temperature. A deposit may form after autoclaving, especially in strong solutions; this deposit may be difficult to detect because of the colour of the solution. **Incompatible** with acids, acid salts, and salts of heavy metals. **Store** in airtight containers. Protect from light.

Fluorescein sodium formed a 1:1 complex with povidone at low fluorescein concentrations.— R. E. Phares, *J. pharm. Sci.*, 1968, *57*, 53.

Sterilisation. Solutions of fluorescein sodium 2% inoculated with *Ps. aeruginosa* were sterile within 3 hours in the presence of phenylmercuric nitrate 0.002% and within 1 hour when phenethyl alcohol 0.4% was also present.— R. M. E. Richards *et al.*, *J. Pharm. Pharmac.*, 1969, *21*, 681.

Adverse Effects. Nausea, vomiting, syncope, and urticaria may occur after intravenous injection of fluorescein sodium. The skin and urine may be transiently coloured.

The application of fluorescein sodium could cause photosensitivity.— J. Kalivas, *J. Am. med. Ass.*, 1969, *209*, 1706.

Of 55 reported adverse reactions following the intravenous injection of fluorescein sodium 37 were of an allergic type and most of these were characterised only by urticaria. Reactions were severe in 16 patients progressing in some instances to shock, respiratory obstruction and arrest, hypotension, cardiac arrest, and myocardial infarction. Reports from various institutions performing fluorescein angiography indicated a mean incidence for all types of reactions of 0.6% and for severe reactions 0.4%.— M. R. Stein and C. W. Parker, *Am. J. Ophthal.*, 1971, *72*, 861.

A 64-year-old man with no previous history of cardiac or pulmonary disease developed acute pulmonary oedema following the intravenous administration of 5 ml of fluorescein sodium 10%. Diuresis, oxygen, positive-pressure respiration and sedation led to recovery.— J. B. Hess and R. I. Pacurariu, *Am. J. Ophthal.*, 1976, *82*, 567.

Reports of and comments on cardiac arrest following fluorescein angiography: E. E. Cunningham and V. Balu, *J. Am. med. Ass.*, 1979, *242*, 2431; J. E. Heffner (letter), *ibid.*, 1980, *243*, 2029; V. Balu (letter), *ibid.*, 2030; P. Lempert (letter), *ibid.*, 1980, *244*, 660; V. Balu (letter), *ibid.*

Uses. A 2% solution of fluorescein sodium is used in ophthalmic practice as a diagnostic agent for detecting corneal lesions and foreign bodies in the eye. When instilled into the eye it does not stain the normal cornea, but ulcers, or parts deprived of epithelium, are stained green and foreign bodies are seen surrounded by a green ring. Since it is applied to abraded corneas, special care should be taken to avoid microbial contamination; eye-drops in single-dose containers are to be preferred.

Fluorescein sodium is used in the fitting of hard contact lenses to ensure a correct fit. The dye is applied to the eye as eye-drops or as sterile fluorescein papers (Kimura papers) and the eye is viewed with a blue light in a darkened room. Any area of contact of the cornea with the contact lens is seen as a dull deep purple patch while all areas of the lens which are clear of the eye surface are coloured with the characteristic yellow-green of fluorescein. Fluorescein sodium should not be used with soft contact lenses as the dye may be absorbed by the lens material.

Fluorescein sodium has been given by rapid intravenous injection, usually in a dose of 500 mg for determination of the circulation time; a suggested dose for children is 15.4 mg per kg body-weight. It has also been given for the examination of the ophthalmic vasculature as a 5 to 25% solution and for the differentiation of malignant and healthy tissue when examined under ultraviolet light.

For visualisation of the gall-bladder and bile ducts 10 ml of a 5% solution may be given intravenously 4 hours before surgery.

In a double-blind crossover study involving 41 healthy subjects and 42 patients with various ophthalmic disorders 3 ml of a 25% solution of fluorescein sodium was significantly superior to 5 ml of a 10% solution in visualisation in healthy subjects and in angiogram quality in patients. No significant difference in the incidence and severity of adverse reactions between the 2 concentrations was observed.— J. Justice *et al.*, *Archs Ophthal., N.Y.*, 1977, *95*, 2015.

Further references.— D. Willerson *et al.*, *Ann. Ophthal.*, 1976, *8*, 833.

Angiography. For the use of fluorescein angiography in patients with various ocular disorders, see M. Best *et al.*, *Br. J. Ophthal.*, 1972, *56*, 6; L. Laatikainen and E. M. Kohner, *ibid.*, 1976, *60*, 411; K. G. Noble *et al.*, *ibid.*, 1977, *61*, 43; L. Laatikainen and R. K. Blach, *ibid.*, 272; N. E. F. Cartlidge *et al.*, *ibid.*, 385.

Carotid artery disease. Ischaemia of the carotid artery could be visualised by fluorescein angiography—3 ml of 20% fluorescein was injected into the antecubital vein and repeat photographs were taken at intervals. An accuracy of 70 to 80% was obtainable.— R. Mapstone and R. McBride, *Br. J. Ophthal.*, 1975, *59*, 664.

A method of assessing internal-carotid-artery disease by giving an intravenous injection of 6 ml of a 10% solution of fluorescein sodium during bilateral compression of the superficial temporal artery.— F. Lund *et al.* (letter), *Lancet*, 1978, *2*, 744. Criticism.— R. R. Lewis and R. G. Gosling (letter), *ibid.*, 839.

Colon viability. The use of fluorescein to evaluate colon viability.— M. B. Myers and G. Cherry, *Surgery Gynec. Obstet.*, 1969, *128*, 97.

Diabetic retinopathy. The retinal vessels were markedly impervious to fluorescein in the blood. In patients with diabetic retinopathy the blood-retinal barrier was reduced permitting escape of fluorescein into the vitreous. The presence of fluorescein, measured by fluorophotometry, in the vitreous of diabetic patients without apparent retinal involvement was an early sign of retinal degeneration.— J. Cunha-Vaz *et al.*, *Br. J. Ophthal.*, 1975, *59*, 649.

Fluorescein leakage could detect diabetic retinopathy before the development of microaneurysms. Angiofluorography should be carried out annually after the onset of diabetes by injecting 10 ml of fluorescein sodium 10% intravenously and taking photographs every second for 10 seconds with a further 2 photographs 15 and 30 minutes after the fluorescein injection.— H. Dorchy and D. Toussaint (letter), *Lancet*, 1978, *1*, 1200.

Retinal fluorography using oral fluorescein.— J. S. Kelley and M. Kincaid, *Archs Ophthal., N.Y.*, 1979, *97*, 2331.

Diagnostic staining. Because fluorescein stained epithelial lesions and rose bengal stained degenerated dead cells, a preparation containing both was recommended for diagnostic staining of the cornea and conjunctiva. The following formula was suggested: fluorescein sodium 50 mg, rose bengal 50 mg, sodium chloride 45 mg, phenylmercuric nitrate 50 µg, and water to 5 ml. Rose bengal also stained normal mucus, which could be differentiated by counterstaining with a solution containing Alcian Blue [8GX, CI 74240] 50 mg and phenylmercuric nitrate 50 µg in 5 ml of water. Mucus cells were stained blue; degenerated cells remained red.— M. S. Norn, *Am. J. Ophthal.*, 1967, *64*, 1078.

Measurement of circulation rate. For details of measurement techniques based on the intravenous injection of fluorescein sodium, see B. M. Gasul *et al.*, *J. Pediat.*, 1949, *34*, 460; A. G. MacGregor and E. J. Wayne, *Br. Heart J.*, 1951, *13*, 80; J. F. Goodwin and S. Kaplan, *Br. med. J.*, 1951, *1*, 1102.

Preparations

Fluorescein Eye Drops *(A.P.F.)*. Gutt. Fluoresc. Fluorescein sodium 250 mg, phenylmercuric nitrate 4 mg, Water for Injections to 100 ml. Sterilised by autoclaving. These eye-drops are dispensed in single-dose containers to avoid contamination by cross-infection.

Fluorescein Eye-drops *(B.P.C. 1973)*. Guttae Fluoresceini; FLN. A sterile solution containing up to 2% of fluorescein sodium in water. The solution is sterilised by autoclaving or by filtration. When sterilised by maintaining at 98° to 100° for 30 minutes it contains 0.002% of phenylmercuric acetate or nitrate. The eye-drops should preferably be supplied in single-dose containers. Eye-drops issued in multidose containers should be discarded after use on a single occasion.

NOTE. Solutions of fluorescein sodium are particularly liable to contamination with *Pseudomonas aeruginosa*.

Fluorescein Sodium Injection *(U.S.P.)*. A sterile solution in Water for Injections. It may contain sodium bicarbonate. pH 8 to 9.8.

Fluorescein Sodium Ophthalmic Strips *(U.S.P.)*. Individual sterile strips of paper; one end of each strip is impregnated with fluorescein sodium.

Injectabile Fluoresceini 20% *(Nord. P.)*. Fluorescein sodium, equivalent to 20 g anhydrous fluorescein sodium, Water for Injections to 100 ml; phenylmercuric nitrate 0.001% is a suitable preservative. Sterilised by autoclaving. To be stored under an inert gas. Protect from light.

Oculoguttae Fluoresceini *(Nord. P.)*. Fluorescein Eye-drops. Fluorescein sodium, equivalent to 1 g of anhydrous fluorescein sodium, phenylmercuric nitrate 1 mg, sodium chloride 600 mg, sterilised water to 100 g. Sterilised by autoclaving. Protect from light.

Proprietary Preparations

Alcon Opulets Fluorescein Sodium 1% *(Alcon, UK: Farillon, UK)*. Sterile eye-drops containing fluorescein sodium 1% in single-use disposable applicators.

Fluor-Amps *(Sas, UK)*. Fluorescein sodium, available as an injection containing 10 or 20%, in ampoules of 5 ml.

Fluorets *(Smith & Nephew Pharmaceuticals, UK)*. Sterile ophthalmic strips, each impregnated at the tip with fluorescein sodium 1 mg. (Also available as Fluorets in *Denm.*).

Fluor-I-Strip *(Ayerst, UK)*. Sterile ophthalmic strips of lint-free paper, each impregnated with fluorescein sodium 9 mg. **Fluor-I-Strip AT.** Similar strips each impregnated with fluorescein sodium 1 mg. (Also available as Fluor-I-Strip and Fluor-I-Strip AT in *Austral.*, *Canad.*).

Minims Fluorescein Sodium *(Smith & Nephew Pharmaceuticals, UK)*. Sterile eye-drops containing fluorescein sodium 1 or 2%, available in single-use disposable applicators. (Also available as Minims Fluorescein Sodium in *Austral.*).

Other Proprietary Names

Fluoresceinnatrium Minims *(Norw.)*; Fluorescite *(Arg., USA)*; Ful-Glo *(Austral., Canad., USA)*; Funduscein *(USA)*; Pancreolauryl-Test *(with fluorescein dilaurate)* *(Ger.)*; Uranina *(Spain)*.

2131-a

Gastrin.

A hormone produced by the gastric mucosa. Chemically, it comprises 2 almost identical peptides, gastrin I and gastrin II.

CAS — 9002-76-0 (gastrin); 9045-90-3 (gastrin I); 39313-26-3 (gastrin II); 18016-68-7 (gastrin II, pig).

In low concentrations, gastrin exerts a powerful stimulating effect on gastric secretion and it has been suggested for use as a test of gastric function. In high concentrations it has an inhibitory effect on gastric secretion.

A review, with references, of the actions of gastrin.— *Lancet*, 1965, *1*, 420. See also G. Bertaccini, *Pharmac. Rev.*, 1976, *28*, 127.

A study in 12 patients showed that the intravenous infusion of gastrin II, 800 ng per kg body-weight per hour, stimulated the motor activity of the antrum of the stomach. It had no detectable effect on the motility of the fundus, right colon, sigmoid, or rectum.— J. J. Misiewicz *et al.*, *Gut*, 1969, *10*, 723.

For a review on the immunological aspects of gastrin, see J. E. McGuigan, *New Engl. J. Med.*, 1970, *283*, 137.

The role of gastrin in gastro-intestinal disorders.— *Br. med. J.*, 1972, *3*, 604. See also R. G. Elmslie, *Med. J. Aust.*, 1974, *1*, 1001; F. P. Brooks, *J. Am. med. Ass.*, 1975, *232*, 357; M. A. Hamboug *et al.*, *Archs Dis. Childh.*, 1979, *54*, 208.

A brief review of the heterogeneity and nomenclature of gastrin.— *Br. med. J.*, 1975, *1*, 112.

A suggestion that gastrin has a role in regulating the

lower oesophageal sphincter.— M. D. Kaye *et al.*, *Gut*, 1976, *17*, 933.

The relationship between renal function and serum concentrations of gastrin.— R. Hällgren *et al.*, *Gut*, 1978, *19*, 207.

Further references.— R. A. Gregory and H. J. Tracy, *J. Physiol.*, 1961, *156*, 523; J. C. Anderson *et al.*, *Nature*, 1964, *204*, 933; G. M. Makhlouf *et al.*, *Lancet*, 1964, *2*, 485; A. G. Wangel and S. T. Callender, *Br. med. J.*, 1965, *1*, 1409; *Lancet*, 1966, *1*, 1022; J. N. Hunt and N. Ramsbottom, *Br. med. J.*, 1967, *4*, 386; A. M. Connell and C. J. H. Logan, *Am. J. dig. Dis.*, 1967, *12*, 277; N. R. Lazarus *et al.*, *Lancet*, 1968, *2*, 248; G. R. Giles *et al.*, *Gut*, 1969, *10*, 730; H. P. Seelig, *Dt. med. Wschr.*, 1972, *97*, 87; *Med. J. Aust.*, 1972, *2*, 459; J. F. Rehfeld *et al.*, *Gut*, 1974, *15*, 102.

2132-t

Histamine.
2-(Imidazol-4-yl)ethylamine.
$C_5H_9N_3$=111.1.

CAS — 51-45-6.

Deliquescent acicular crystals. Freely **soluble** in water, alcohol, and hot chloroform; sparingly soluble in ether.

Histamine is a decarboxylation product of the amino acid histidine. It was first identified in ergot and is widely distributed in the tissues of plants and animals. It is present in a bound and inactive form in the tissues of almost all mammals, the highest concentration being in the lungs; leucocytes also contain appreciable amounts.

The actions and uses of histamine are described below under Histamine Acid Phosphate.

The activity of an aqueous solution of histamine decreased significantly after irradiation. Frozen and dried histamine was unchanged after exposure to irradiation. The effect might explain the radioprotective mechanism of solutions of histamine.— H. C. Sturde and H. J. Heitmann (letter), *Lancet*, 1967, *2*, 1362.

2133-x

Histamine Acid Phosphate *(B.P. 1973).*
Histam. Acid Phos.; Histamine Phosphate *(U.S.P.)*; Histamini Phosphas; Histamine Diphosphate. 2-(Imidazol-4-yl)ethylamine diphosphate.
$C_5H_9N_3,2H_3PO_4$=307.1.

CAS — 51-74-1.

Pharmacopoeias. In *Arg.*, *Aust.*, *Braz.*, *Ind.*, *Int.*, *It.*, *Mex.*, *Span.*, *Turk.*, and *U.S.* Most permit not more than ½H_2O. *B.P. 1973* specified 1 H_2O.

Colourless odourless crystals; stable in air but affected by light. M.p. 130° to 133°. Histamine acid phosphate (anhydrous) 2.76 mg or histamine acid phosphate monohydrate 2.93 mg is approximately equivalent to 1 mg of histamine.

Soluble 1 in 4 of water; slightly soluble in alcohol; practically insoluble in ether. A solution in water has a pH of 3 to 6. A 4.1% solution is iso-osmotic with serum. Solutions are **sterilised** by autoclaving or by filtration and are kept in ampoules. **Store** in airtight containers. Protect from light.

Adverse Effects. Histamine acid phosphate may cause headache, flushing of the skin, general vasodilatation with a fall in blood pressure, tachycardia, bronchial constriction and dyspnoea, visual disturbances, vomiting, and diarrhoea. Reactions may occur at the injection site.

In 60 patients injections of histamine acid phosphate in doses of between about 1 and 3 mg were very much less painful, without loss of the required stimulus to gastric secretion, if used in a strength of about 4 mg per ml with 20 mg of benzyl alcohol added to each ml as a local anaesthetic.— J. E. Lennard-Jones *et al.* (letter), *Br. med. J.*, 1962, *2*, 551.

A report of acute pancreatitis in 2 patients apparently induced by the subcutaneous injection of histamine acid phosphate in doses of about 10 and 40 µg per kg body-weight respectively.— J. J. Schrogie *et al.*, *Gastroenterology*, 1965, *49*, 672.

Signs of erosive gastritis were noted in only 2 of 20 patients prior to the administration of histamine for an augmented histamine test, but after the test severe mucosal hyperaemia was found in 15, acute erosions in 10, diffuse erosion in 1, and overt intraluminal bleeding in 1. Haemorrhage in the fundus neck or lamina propria was common after the administration of histamine.— D. Katz *et al.*, *Am. J. dig. Dis.*, 1969, *14*, 447.

Treatment of Adverse Effects. Severe side-effects or symptoms of overdosage may be treated by the prompt administration of adrenaline.

Histamine shock occurred in 4 patients given the augmented histamine test. Three were given about 40 µg per kg body-weight of histamine acid phosphate by subcutaneous injection preceeded 30 minutes earlier by an intramuscular dose of 50 mg of diphenhydramine. The fourth patient was given 100 mg of ametazole hydrochloride. All patients lost consciousness and the blood pressure and pulse were temporarily unrecordable. One patient was given 0.5 ml of Adrenaline Injection intramuscularly and another was given metaraminol tartrate intravenously. It was considered that the best treatment was to place the patient in the Trendelenburg position and administer adrenaline. The augmented histamine test was contra-indicated in patients with arteriosclerotic disease, cerebral vascular insufficiency, or severe anaemia.— N. I. Blum *et al.*, *J. Am. med. Ass.*, 1965, *191*, 339.

Precautions. Histamine acid phosphate should be given with care to patients with asthma or allergy, and in elderly patients.

Absorption and Fate. Histamine acid phosphate is largely inactive when given by mouth. It exerts a rapid, though transient, effect when given by subcutaneous, intramuscular, or intravenous injection. It is metabolised by methylation and oxidation; the metabolites are excreted in the urine.

The uptake, storage, and release of histamine.— J. P. Green, *Fedn Proc.*, 1967, *26*, 211.

Uses. Histamine given parenterally causes stimulation of smooth muscle, especially of the bronchioles, and lowers blood pressure by dilating the arterioles and capillaries. It also stimulates many of the glands of internal secretion, especially the gastric glands; following administration of histamine, a copious secretion of gastric juice with a high acidity results. This action on the gastric secretion is unaffected by standard antihistamine drugs. Histamine is usually employed in the form of the acid phosphate and has been used, usually by subcutaneous injection, in the treatment of peripheral vascular disease, migraine, and Ménière's disease, but because of the severe systemic effects its value for these purposes is limited.

It is mainly employed as a diagnostic agent to test the secretory action of the stomach as a means of differentiating between the absolute achlorhydria of pernicious anaemia and the relative achlorhydria of carcinoma of the stomach. It has also been used to detect hypersecretion in the Zollinger-Ellison syndrome. It is given as the acid phosphate, in place of a test meal, in a dose of 40 µg per kg body-weight by subcutaneous injection following administration of a large dose of an antihistamine; it is essential to give an antihistamine beforehand.

A solution containing 0.1% of histamine base has been used in the diagnosis of circulatory disturbances such as Raynaud's syndrome. In normal patients, when the solution is pricked into the skin, a red spot followed by a wheal should appear in about 2½ minutes. In Raynaud's syndrome and allied affections this reaction is delayed.

An intracutaneous injection of 0.05 ml of a 1 in 3600 solution of histamine acid phosphate is used to determine histamine sensitivity in patients with Ménière's disease or severe unilateral temporal headache, histamine headache.

A review of histamine.— M. A. Beaven, *New Engl. J. Med.*, 1976, *294*, 30 and 320.

Intravenous use of histamine base in macular degeneration.— D. Macy, *Boswell Hosp. Proc.*, 1975, *1*, 2, per *J. Am. med. Ass.*, 1976, *235*, 1284.

A brief note on the use of histamine acid phosphate in the treatment of dizziness.— J. S. Turner, *Drugs*, 1977, *13*, 382.

Some cardiovascular effects of histamine.— B. A. Callingham, *Pharm. J.*, 1978, *1*, 82.

Augmented histamine test. A modified and augmented histamine test was described as a test of gastric secretion. Thirty minutes after an intramuscular injection of 100 mg of mepyramine maleate, the patient was given a subcutaneous injection of about 40 µg of histamine acid phosphate per kg body-weight as a gastric stimulant. The basal secretion and maximum secretion of hydrochloric acid were measured.— A. W. Kay, *Br. med. J.*, 1953, *2*, 77. Further references: S. J. Konturek and J. Oleksy, *Gastroenterology*, 1967, *53*, 912; K. Jepson *et al.*, *Lancet*, 1968, *2*, 139; H. G. Desai *et al.*, *Postgrad. med. J.*, 1973, *49*, 258; H. G. Desai *et al.*, *Gastroenterology*, 1969, *57*, 636.

Ménière's disease. Histamine could be tried in the treatment of Ménière's disease, but it was probably no more effective than nicotinic acid. A test dose of about 5 µg of histamine acid phosphate should be given intracutaneously and, if no reaction occurred, 1 mg in 250 ml of dextrose injection or of sodium chloride injection was given intravenously over 90 minutes and repeated 2 or 3 times every 48 hours. Vasoconstrictors should be available to deal with severe hypotension. Thereafter, weekly injections of a 0.01% solution were given in doses gradually increasing from 0.3 to 1.5 ml.— *Br. med. J.*, 1970, *1*, 614. See also M. Eszenyi-Halasy, *ibid.*, 1949, *1*, 1121.

Phaeochromocytoma. Histamine was a reliable agent in the diagnosis of phaeochromocytoma. Rapid intravenous injection of 12.5 to 50 µg of the base was invariably followed by a severe flush, headache, and a sharp but fleeting fall in blood pressure. In 5 of 6 patients, with subsequently proved phaeochromocytoma, the patients suddenly blanched and cried in alarm. The blood pressure rose precipitously, greatly in excess of the cold pressor response, and the patients broke out in a profuse sweat, experiencing all the manifestations of a severe spontaneous attack. The test was hazardous in persons with an elevated base-line blood pressure, with weakened vascular systems, or with lowered cardiac reserve.— E. Calkins *et al.*, *J. Am. med. Ass.*, 1951, *145*, 880.

In 28 patients with phaeochromocytoma, a positive response to an intravenous histamine test was noted in 18 out of 24 tested and a positive response to an intravenous phentolamine test in 10 out of 25. Both tests gave positive responses in 11% of tests on patients who did not have a tumour.— S. G. Sheps *et al.*, *Circulation*, 1966, *34*, 473.

Pharmacological tests for phaeochromocytoma have been superseded by chemical assays. Only in exceptional instances are provocative tests, employing glucagon, tyramine, and histamine, justified; they are all dangerous.— P. F. Semple, *Practitioner*, 1979, *223*, 218.

Preparations

Histamine Acid Phosphate Injection *(B.P. 1973).* Histamine Acid Phos. Inj.; Histamine Phosphate Injection; Histamine Injection. A sterile solution of histamine acid phosphate monohydrate in Water for Injections. Protect from light.

Histamine Phosphate Injection *(U.S.P.).* A sterile solution of histamine acid phosphate in Water for Injections. pH 3 to 6. Protect from light.

Akrotherm *(Priory Laboratories, UK).* Ointment containing histamine acid phosphate 0.1%, acetylcholine chloride 0.2%, and oxycholesterol 1%. For chilblains and allied conditions.

2134-r

Histamine Hydrochloride.
Histamine Dihydrochloride. 2-(Imidazol-4-yl)ethylamine dihydrochloride.
$C_5H_9N_3,2HCl$=184.1.

CAS — 56-92-8.

Pharmacopoeias. In *Arg.*, *Cz.*, *Fr.*, *Hung.*, *It.*, *Nord.*, *Pol.*, *Roum.*, and *Swiss.*

Odourless, hygroscopic, colourless crystals or white crystalline powder with an acid saline taste. M.p. about 245° with decomposition. Histamine hydrochloride 1.66 mg is approximately equivalent to 1 mg of histamine. Very **soluble** in water; soluble in alcohol and acetone; practically insoluble in chloroform and ether. A solution in water is acid to litmus. A 2.24% solution is iso-osmotic with serum. Solutions are **sterilised** by autoclaving or by filtration. **Store** in airtight containers. Protect from light.

Histamine hydrochloride is used similarly to histamine acid phosphate.

Haemolysis. An aqueous solution of histamine hydrochloride iso-osmotic with serum (2.24%) caused 79% haemolysis of erythrocytes cultured in it for 45 minutes. The solution and the erythrocytes darkened in colour.— E. R. Hammarlund and K. Pedersen-Bjergaard, *J. pharm. Sci.*, 1961, *50*, 24.

Preparations

Injectabile Histamini *(Nord. P.).* Histamine Injection. A sterile solution of histamine hydrochloride 0.1% and sodium chloride 0.85% in Water for Injections.

Proprietary Names

Alergenol *(LEFA, Spain)*; Histamin *(DAK, Denm.)*.

2135-f

Indigo Carmine *(B.P. 1973).*

Indigotindisulfonate Sodium *(U.S.P.)*; Indicarminum; Sodium Indigotindisulphonate; Ceruleinum; Indigotine; Blue X; CI Food Blue 1; Colour Index No. 73015; FD & C Blue No. 2; Disodium Indigotin-5,5′-disulphonate. Disodium 3,3′-dioxo-2,2′-bi-indolinylidene-5,5′-disulphonate.
$C_{16}H_8N_2Na_2O_8S_2$=466.3.

CAS — 860-22-0.

NOTE. The name Caerulein has been applied to Ceruletide, p.515.

Pharmacopoeias. In *Arg., Belg., Fr., Ind., Jap., Roum.,* and *U.S.*

An almost odourless purplish-blue powder or blue granules with a coppery lustre. The *U.S.P.* specifies not less than 96% calculated on the dried material and a loss on drying of not more than 5%. The *B.P. 1973* specified not less than 90% of $C_{16}H_8N_2Na_2O_8S_2$, calculated on the dried material and a loss of not more than 10% of its weight on drying.

Soluble 1 in 100 of water, being precipitated by sodium chloride; readily soluble in warm water; slightly soluble in alcohol; practically insoluble in most other organic solvents. Solutions are **sterilised** by autoclaving or by filtration. **Store** in airtight containers. Protect from light.

Fading. Indigo carmine might fade in the presence of some nonionic surfactants.— M. W. Scott *et al., J. Am. pharm. Ass., scient. Edn,* 1960, *49*, 467.

Further references: S. A. H. Khalil and S. S. El-Gamal, *Mfg Chem.*, 1978, *49* (May), 52.

Adverse Effects and Precautions. Indigo carmine may cause nausea, vomiting, hypertension, and bradycardia, and occasionally, allergic reactions such as skin rash, pruritus, and bronchoconstriction. A test dose should be given to patients with a history of allergy.

A report of fatal cardiac arrest in 2 patients, aged 73 and 76 years respectively following the administration of indigo carmine 80 mg intravenously. Both had a history of asthmatic bronchitis.— A. M. Voiry *et al., Annls méd. Nancy,* 1976, *15*, 413.

Uses. Indigo carmine has been used to test kidney function. It was usually injected intramuscularly or intravenously in a dose of 10 ml of a 0.4% solution; if the kidneys were functioning normally the urine was coloured blue in about 10 minutes. It was also used to compare the functioning of the 2 kidneys, the appearance of the dye at the ureteric orifices being observed by means of a cystoscope.

It has been used as a blue dye in medicinal preparations but it is relatively unstable. It is used as a food colour (see p.423).

Estimated acceptable daily intake of indigo carmine: up to 2.5 mg per kg body-weight. Information from further studies was desirable.— Thirteenth Report of FAO/WHO Expert Committee on Food Additives, *Tech. Rep. Ser. Wld Hlth Org. No.* 445, 1971.

Preparations

Indigotindisulfonate Sodium Injection *(U.S.P.).* Sodium Indigotindisulfonate Injection. A sterile solution of indigo carmine in Water for Injections. pH 3 to 6.5. Protect from light.

Jap.P. (Indigocarmine Injection) has a similar preparation.

Indigo Carmine *(Hynson, Westcott & Dunning, USA: Farillon, UK).* Indigo carmine, available as a 0.8% solution, in ampoules of 5 ml.

2136-d

Indocyanine Green *(U.S.P.).*

Sodium 2-{7-[1,1-dimethyl-3-(4-sulphobutyl)benz[*e*]indolin-2-ylidene]hepta-1,3,5-trienyl}-1,1-dimethyl-1*H*-benz[*e*]indolio-3-(butyl-4-sulphonate).
$C_{43}H_{47}N_2NaO_6S_2$=775.0.

CAS — 3599-32-4.

Pharmacopoeias. In *U.S.* which also includes Sterile Indocyanine Green.

An olive-brown, dark green, blue-green, dark blue, or black powder, odourless or with a slight odour. It loses not more than 6% of its weight on drying and contains not more than 5% of sodium iodide.

Soluble in water and methyl alcohol; practically insoluble in most other organic solvents. A 0.5% solution in water has a pH of about 6. Aqueous solutions are unstable.

Stability in solution. Solutions of indocyanine green were reported to lose 10% potency in 24 hours at room temperature.— C. J. Latiolais *et al., Am. J. Hosp. Pharm.*, 1967, *24*, 667.

Adverse Effects and Precautions. Care is necessary in administering indocyanine green to patients with severe hepatic impairment as the rate of its elimination may be diminished.

Solutions contain a small amount of sodium iodide and should be used with caution in patients hypersensitive to iodine.

Two patients maintained on haemodialysis experienced headache, diaphoresis, and pruritus when given indocyanine green; a third patient had a severe anaphylactoid reaction.— D. D. Michie *et al., J. Allergy & clin. Immunol.*, 1971, *48*, 235.

A report of allergic-type reactions, one fatal, in 4 patients following the administration of indocyanine green. Two of the patients had no previous history of allergy or asthma.— T. R. Carski *et al.* (letter), *J. Am. med. Ass.*, 1978, *240*, 635.

Absorption and Fate. After intravenous injection indocyanine green is bound to plasma protein. It is rapidly eliminated from the circulation. It is excreted by the liver into the bile.

The mean half-life of indocyanine green, given in doses of 25 mg to 11 patients with normal liver function was 1.3 minutes, compared with 3.9 minutes in 38 patients with liver dysfunction. For 8 patients taking anticonvulsant drugs, 2 on phenylbutazone, 1 on haloperidol, 1 on nitrofurantoin, and 9 addicted to one or more of diamorphine, methadone, morphine, pethidine, or poppy heads the mean half-life was 0.65 minutes. The percentage disappearance-rate per minute from plasma in these 3 groups was 50.6, 24.8, and 115.8 respectively; the highest rates occurred in addicts and were elevated above normal even when liver dysfunction was present.— V. Melikian *et al., Gut,* 1972, *13*, 755.

The mean fractional disappearance-rate of indocyanine green from plasma was significantly faster in 33 healthy women than in 18 healthy men following a single dose of 500 µg per kg body-weight intravenously. No such difference occurred in healthy subjects given 5 mg per kg.— J. F. Martin *et al., Proc. Soc. exp. Biol. Med.*, 1975, *150*, 612.

Uses. Indocyanine green is an indicator dye used for determining cardiac output by the dilution method. It has its peak spectral absorption at about 800 nm, a wavelength at which oxyhaemoglobin and reduced haemoglobin transmit light equally; this permits the continuous recording of dilution curves on whole blood without interference from variations in blood oxygen saturation. The absorption peak is diminished by sodium metabisulphite.

Indocyanine green is given by intravenous injection via a cardiac catheter. The usual dose is 5 mg dissolved in 1 ml of Water for Injections. A suggested dose for children is one-half, and for infants one-quarter, of the adult dose. An average of 5 dilution curves is determined. The total dose should not exceed 2 mg per kg body-weight.

Indocyanine green is also used to test liver function. The usual dose is 500 µg per kg body-weight intravenously.

The use of indocyanine green in dye-dilution studies did not necessitate the measurement of venous and arterial oxygen concentrations. The drug was well tolerated and more than 1000 patients had been studied without untoward effects attributable to the drug. The arbitrary maximum total dose of 2 mg per kg body-weight could be replaced by a dose of 5 mg per kg.— I. J. Fox and E. H. Wood, *Proc. Staff Meet. Mayo Clin.*, 1960, *35*, 732. A report of a symposium on indocyanine green and its clinical use.— *ibid.*, 729–82.

Blood volume estimations with indocyanine green.— E. C. Bradley and J. W. Barr, *Life Sci.*, 1968, *7*, 1001.

The limitations of circulation-time tests.— A. Selzer *et al., Archs intern. Med.*, 1968, *122*, 491.

The use of indocyanine green to detect the source of blood found in pericardial fluid.— J. R. Stone and R. H. Martin, *Ann. intern. Med.*, 1972, *77*, 592.

The injection of diatrizoates and azovan blue or indocyanine green was used successfully with xeromammography in 33 of 35 patients for the localisation of breast lesions.— R. W. Wayne and R. E. Darby, *J. Am. med. Ass.*, 1977, *237*, 2219.

A suggestion that plasma-clearance of indocyanine green, a measure of hepatic blood flow, could be used to predict lignocaine dosage requirements.— R. A. Zito and P. R. Reid, *New Engl. J. Med.*, 1978, *298*, 1160. Criticisms.— N. D. S. Bax *et al.* (letter), *ibid.*, *299*, 662; J. LeLorier (letter), *ibid.* Reply.— P. R. Reid and R. A. Zito (letter), *ibid.*, 663.

Angiography of the choroid. Indocyanine green fluorescence angiography of the choroid gave better visualisation of the choroidal vessels than did fluorescein angiography. Further study was necessary before its clinical usefulness was proved.— A. Craandijk and C. A. Van Beek, *Br. J. Ophthal.*, 1976, *60*, 377.

Further references.— R. W. Flower and B. F. Hochheimer, *Johns Hopkins med. J.*, 1976, *138*, 33.

Liver-function test. Studies on clearance of indocyanine green in which a dichromatic ear densitometer was used showed the usefulness of the dye in detecting mild liver injury. Persons with injury had a normal clearance of 500 µg of the dye per kg body-weight but impairment in removal of 5 mg per kg.— C. M. Leevy *et al., J. Am. med. Ass.*, 1967, *200*, 236.

The advantages of indocyanine green over sulphobromophthalein sodium in liver-function tests were that it was not irritant, it was more completely excreted by the liver without participation of other organs, and there was no enterohepatic circulation.— A. E. Read, *Abstr. Wld Med.*, 1969, *43*, 801.

In 8 patients the mean half-life of indocyanine green (after a 50-mg dose), assessed from ear densitometer recordings, was 3.85 minutes during anaesthesia with nitrous oxide and was increased to 5.61 minutes during anaesthesia with cyclopropane, which was known to reduce liver blood flow. No significant change in half-life occurred in 11 patients during induced hypotension (sodium nitroprusside or lumbar extradural block with lignocaine). The procedure was useful for monitoring of liver function during anaesthesia.— A. R. A. Salam *et al., Br. J. Anaesth.*, 1976, *48*, 231.

Further references.— C. L. Mendenhall and C. M. Leevy, *New Engl. J. Med.*, 1961, *264*, 431; A. R. Cooke *et al., Am. J. dig. Dis.*, 1963, *8*, 244; R. A. Branch *et al., Gut,* 1974, *15*, 837.

Preparations

Sterile Indocyanine Green *(U.S.P.).* Indocyanine green suitable for parenteral use. pH 5.5 to 6.5 in 0.5% solution.

Cardio Green *(Hynson, Westcott & Dunning, USA: Farillon, UK).* Indocyanine green, available in vials of

25 and 50 mg, with solvent, for solution before use. (Also available as Cardio Green in *Canad.*, *USA*).

2137-n

Inulin *(B.P., U.S.P.)*. Alant Starch. Polysaccharide granules obtained from the tubers of *Dahlia variabilis*, *Helianthus tuberosus*, and other genera of the family Compositae.

CAS — 9005-80-5.

Pharmacopoeias. In *Br.*, *Cz.*, and *U.S.*

A white, odourless, tasteless, hygroscopic, amorphous, granular powder. Slightly **soluble** in cold water, freely soluble in hot water; slightly soluble in organic solvents. A 10% solution in hot water is clear and colourless. A 20% solution has a pH of 4.5 to 7. A solution in water is laevorotatory. It is converted into laevulose by hydrolysis with acids. Solutions are **sterilised** by filtration. **Store** in airtight containers.

Absorption and Fate. Inulin is rapidly removed from the circulation following intravenous administration. A trace may be found in the bile, but it is predominantly eliminated in the urine by glomerular filtration. It is not subject to enzymic degradation.

The biological half-life of inulin was variously reported as 0.53 to 1.17 hours.— W. A. Ritschel, *Drug Intell. & clin. Pharm.*, 1970, *4*, 332.

Pregnancy and the neonate. In 5 women who were given intravenous injections of 5 g of inulin during childbirth, the amniotic fluid was found to contain inulin, and inulin was found in cord blood and in foetal urine.— H. Abramovici *et al.*, *Harefuah*, 1969, *77*, 227, per *J. Am. med. Ass.*, 1969, *210*, 752.

Uses. Inulin is used as a diagnostic agent to measure the glomerular filtration-rate. An initial dose of 30 ml of 10% solution is given by slow intravenous injection into a forearm vein and is followed by the intravenous infusion, at a steady rate, of a mixture of 70 ml of a 10% solution and 500 ml of sodium chloride injection into the other forearm. The glomerular filtration-rate is calculated by dividing the amount of inulin excreted per minute in the urine by the concentration in the plasma and correcting for body-surface area.

In a study of various tests of renal function in 73 patients, the best correlation was between the clearance of endogenous creatinine and inulin or sodium thiosulphate; the 24-hour endogenous creatinine clearance test was the most valuable semiquantitative method for the measurement of the glomerular filtration-rate compared with the clearances of inulin and thiosulphate as the standard quantitative methods.— P. Siegenthaler *et al.*, *Schweiz. med. Wschr.*, 1968, *98*, 886.

A method for the measurement of the glomerular filtration-rate by inulin clearance without urine collection; a 10% solution of inulin was given by intravenous injection in a single dose of 30 ml per 70 kg body-weight followed by a sustaining dose given at exactly 0.375 ml per minute for 3 to 4 hours to permit equilibration between the plasma concentration and renal excretion. Clearance was calculated from the rate of infusion, the plasma concentration, and the inulin concentration of the infusion. The assay procedure took account of partial hydrolysis of the infusion to laevulose.— G. A. Rose, *Br. med. J.*, 1969, *2*, 91.

Inulin and endogenous creatinine clearances were closely correlated on 91 occasions in 41 patients. When clearance studies were repeated after an hour in 39 patients, inulin and creatinine clearances varied by as much as 20% from the earlier values. The spontaneous variations of filtration-rate should be recognised. For the inulin clearance determinations a loading dose of 50 mg per kg body-weight was given as 10% solution followed by a constant infusion of 2 ml per minute by infusion pump.— W. M. Bennett and G. A. Porter, *Br. med. J.*, 1971, *4*, 84.

Preparations

Inulin and Sodium Chloride Injection *(U.S.P.)*. A sterile solution, which may be supersaturated, of inulin and sodium chloride in Water for Injections. It contains no antimicrobial agents. pH 5 to 7. Solid matter should be completely redissolved by heating.

Inulin Injection *(B.P.)*. A sterile solution containing inulin 10% and sodium chloride 0.8% in Water for Injections. Sterilised by filtration. pH 5.5 to 6.5. Inulin Injection deposits on storage. Solid matter should be completely redissolved by heating for not more than 15 minutes and cooling before use. The solution should not be reheated.

2138-h

Limulus Test. Limulus Amoebocyte Lysate Test; Limulus Amebocyte Lysate Test; LAL Test.

The limulus test is a test for the presence of bacterial endotoxins and is based on their ability to exhibit a protein coagulation reaction with limulus amoebocyte lysate prepared from the circulating blood cells of the horseshoe crab, *Limulus polyphemus*.

The test may be used for the in-process screening during manufacture of parenteral drugs and solutions and may also be used for the testing of certain pharmaceuticals where the official method for the detection of pyrogens is not applicable. It is not an official alternative to the test for pyrogens.

For the use of the limulus test in the detection of Gram-negative bacterial meningitis, see R. Nachum *et al.*, *New Engl. J. Med.*, 1973, *289*, 931; S. Ross *et al.*, *J. Am. med. Ass.*, 1975, *233*, 1366; N. S. Berman *et al.*, *J. Pediat.*, 1976, *88*, 553.

For an assessment of the limulus test for detecting endotoxaemia, see D. P. Fossard *et al.*, *Br. med. J.*, 1974, *2*, 465.

The limulus test for the detection of endotoxin in blood components or intravenous fluids.— *Pharm. J.*, 1977, *2*, 41. See also D. C. Garratt *et al.*, *ibid.*, 1981, *1*, 112.

Further references.— *Bull. parent. Drug Ass.*, 1977, *31*, 114; C. C. Mascoli and M. E. Weary, *J. parent. Drug Ass.*, 1979, *33*, 81; C. A. de Murphy and T. R. Aneiros, *ibid.*, 1980, *34*, 268; F. C. Pearson and M. Weary, *ibid.*, 103; W. H. Thomas *et al.*, *Pharm. J.*, 1980, *1*, 259.

Proprietary Preparations

E-Toxate *(Sigma, UK)*. A brand of limulus test.

Pyrogent *(Byk-Mallinckrodt, UK)*. A brand of limulus test.

Pyrostat *(Millipore, UK)*. A brand of limulus test.

Pyrotell *(K & K-Greeff, UK)*. A brand of limulus test.

2139-m

Metyrapone *(B.P., U.S.P.)*. SU 4885. 2-Methyl-1,2-di(3-pyridyl)propan-1-one. $C_{14}H_{14}N_2O$=226.3.

CAS — 54-36-4.

Pharmacopoeias. In *Br.* and *U.S.*

A white to light amber, fine, crystalline powder with a characteristic odour. M.p. 50° to 53°. It darkens on exposure to light.

Soluble 1 in 100 of water, 1 in 3 of alcohol and chloroform; soluble in methyl alcohol; soluble in dilute mineral acids forming water-soluble salts. **Store** in a cool place in airtight containers. Protect from light.

Adverse Effects. Metyrapone may give rise to nausea and vomiting thereby causing the test to be abandoned; epigastric pain, headache, sedation, and giddiness have also been reported. Thrombophlebitis has been reported after intravenous injection of the tartrate.

Precautions. Metyrapone should be used with extreme caution in patients with gross hypopituitarism because of the risk of precipitating acute adrenal failure.

Many drugs have been reported to interfere with the estimation of steroids in urine, or decrease the secretion of corticotrophin by the pituitary; these include some analgesics, antibiotics, antihypertensive agents, iodinated contrast media, corticosteroids and sex hormones, diuretics, hypnotics, and tranquillisers; the effect of phenytoin has been reported to persist for 2 weeks. Other medication should therefore be avoided during the metyrapone test.

An abnormal glucose tolerance in a diabetic patient became normal after a metyrapone test and reverted to abnormal a week later.— R. Grinberg and S. Mazar, *N.Y. St. J. Med.*, 1970, *70*, 2341.

Since corticotrophin was associated with a prolonged release of catecholamines in *dogs* there was a hazard to the use of metyrapone in patients with phaeochromocytoma.— J. A. J. H. Critchley *et al.* (letter), *Lancet*, 1974, *2*, 782.

Uses. Metyrapone inhibits the enzyme 11β-hydroxylase responsible for the synthesis of the glucocorticoids cortisone and hydrocortisone (cortisol) from their precursors. The fall in the plasma concentrations of circulating glucocorticoids stimulates the anterior pituitary gland to produce more corticotrophin. This, in turn, stimulates the production of more 11-deoxycortisol and other precursors which are excreted in the urine where they can be measured as a test of glandular function.

Metyrapone is used as a test of hypothalamo-pituitary function. A prior test is performed, using 25 to 50 units of corticotrophin by infusion over 8 hours, to demonstrate the responsiveness of the adrenal cortex. After an interval of 2 days metyrapone is given, usually in a dose of 750 mg every 4 hours for 6 doses. Metyrapone has also been given, as the tartrate, in a dose of 30 mg per kg body-weight in 1 litre of sodium chloride injection or dextrose injection by infusion over 4 hours. A suggested dose by mouth for children is 15 mg per kg body-weight, with a minimum dose of 250 mg every 4 hours for 6 doses.

Assessment is usually based on the 24-hour urinary excretion of 17-hydroxycorticosteroids (usually more correctly termed 17-oxogenic steroids) and 17-ketosteroids (17-oxosteroids). In patients with a normally functioning pituitary gland excretion is increased 2- to 4-fold and about 2-fold respectively. A subnormal response may indicated panhypopituitarism, confirmed by clinical signs, or partial hypopituitarism (limited pituitary reserve). An excessive response is suggestive of Cushing's syndrome. Other investigations may be necessary to identify the specific disorder.

In addition to its inhibitory effect on the synthesis of the glucocorticoids, metyrapone also inhibits, but to a lesser extent, the synthesis of aldosterone. This latter action has been found of value in treating some cases of resistant oedema, but metyrapone should be given in conjunction with a glucocorticoid. This suppresses the normal corticotrophin response to low plasma concentrations of glucocorticoids and thus prevents an increase in the formation of precursors whose effects might counteract the effects of a reduction in aldosterone. The suggested dosage of metyrapone in resistant oedema is 2.5 to 4.5 g daily in divided doses.

The simultaneous evaluation of the secretion of corticotrophin and growth hormone by the metyrapone test.— M. Stahl *et al.*, *Schweiz. med. Wschr.*, 1972, *102*, 1295.

Findings following the use of metyrapone to treat an ectopic carcinoma-induced ACTH syndrome suggested that in addition to inhibiting adrenal 11β-hydroxylation it also blocked earlier steps in cortisol synthesis.— M. Sugawara and G. A. Hagen, *Archs intern. Med.*, 1977, *137*, 102.

Cushing's syndrome. A 16-year-old youth with widespread neoplastic metastases developed Cushing's syndrome while being treated with cyclophosphamide. Treatment with metyrapone 1 to 2 g daily in divided doses reversed the syndrome and permitted a return to normal activity. The patient survived about 20 months.— R. Coll *et al.*, *Archs intern. Med.*, 1968, *121*, 549.

Thirteen patients with Cushing's disease were treated for 2 to 66 months with metyrapone 0.25 g twice daily to 1 g four times daily ; 9 received pituitary irradiation. Clinical features improved rapidly, allowing time for pituitary irradiation to be effective, without worsening in oedema or hypertension or gastro-intestinal symptoms. Lightheadedness occurred in 4 patients for about 20 minutes after each dose; hirsutism was troublesome in some patients.— W. J. Jeffcoate *et al.*, *Br. med. J.*, 1977, *2*, 215. Comment.— D. N. Orth, *Ann. intern. Med.*, 1978, *89*, 128.

Hypercholesterolaemia. Metyrapone could be used for eliminating excess cholesterol from the body. The mechanism of action was unknown.— J. F. Dingman (letter), *New Engl. J. Med.*, 1972, *286*, 1214.

Pituitary-function test. Twenty patients with Cushing's syndrome (11 with adrenocortical hyperplasia and 9 with adrenocortical neoplasms) were given metyrapone 500 mg hourly for 6 hours. In 10 patients with hyperplasia, excretion of 17-hydroxycorticosteroids was doubled and 8 showed a plasma-adrenocorticotrophic hormone response. Most patients with neoplasms showed no significant increased excretion and no plasma-adrenocorticotrophic hormone response.— L. L. Sparks *et al.*, *Metabolism*, 1969, *18*, 175.

A discussion of the relative merits of the metyrapone test and other tests of pituitary function.— *J. Am. med. Ass.*, 1969, *207*, 142.

Metyrapone administered in a single dose of 2 to 3 g at midnight was as effective as the standard metyrapone test (750 mg four-hourly for 6 doses) for assessing pituitary function. Blood for determination of plasma deoxycortisol and adrenocorticotrophic hormone concentrations was obtained from patients at 8 a.m. the following morning, and urine for assay of 11-deoxycorticosteroids was collected from midnight to midnight before and after drug administration.— W. Jubiz *et al.*, *Archs intern. Med.*, 1970, *125*, 472.

Studies in 7 subjects suggested that measurement of the reduction in circulating 11-hydroxycorticosteroids by fluorimetry and of the total plasma-hydroxycorticosteroids by a competitive-protein-binding technique gave a more accurate assessment of pituitary response to metyrapone than did measurement of urinary 17-hydroxycorticosteroids.— M. Nattrass *et al.*, *Lancet*, 1972, *2*, 903.

Evidence to suggest that the metyrapone test was not only useful to screen for adrenal insufficiency but that it could also differentiate between a primary and secondary cause.— L. I. Dolman *et al.*, *J. Am. med. Ass.*, 1979, *241*, 1251.

Further references: A. B. Myles and J. R. Daly, *Corticosteroid and ACTH Treatment*, London, Edward Arnold, 1974, p. 36.

Vitiligo. Metyrapone, given usually by intravenous injection and then by mouth to 10 patients with vitiligo, produced the best results in rapidly progressing cases with a not-too-extensive skin involvement. The largest dose in a patient was 27 g of metyrapone over a period of 3 months.— R. Dolecek (letter), *Br. med. J.*, 1968, *4*, 327.

Preparations

Metyrapone Capsules *(B.P.)*. Capsules containing metyrapone. Store at a temperature not exceeding 30°. Protect from light.

Metyrapone Tablets *(U.S.P.)*. Tablets containing metyrapone. Store at a temperature not exceeding 40° in airtight containers. Protect from light.

Metopirone *(Ciba, UK)*. Metyrapone, available as capsules of 250 mg. (Also available as Metopirone in *Austral., Canad., USA*).

Other Proprietary Names

Metopiron *(Denm., Ger., Ital., Neth., Norw., Swed., Switz.)*.

2140-t

Metyrapone Tartrate.

2-Methyl-1,2-di(3-pyridyl)propan-1-one ditartrate.

$C_{14}H_{14}N_2O,2C_4H_6O_6=526.5$.

CAS — 908-35-0.

Metyrapone tartrate 100 mg is approximately equivalent to 43 mg of metyrapone.

Metyrapone tartrate has been used by intravenous injection in the estimation of pituitary function—see p.520.

Preparations

Metyrapone Tartrate Injection *(U.S.P.)*. A sterile solution in Water for Injections prepared from metyrapone with the aid of tartaric acid. pH 3 to 3.5. Store at a temperature not exceeding 40°. Protect from light.

2141-x

Pancreozymin.

CCK; CCK-PZ. A hormone prepared from the duodenal mucosa of pigs, which stimulates the digestive secretions of the pancreas. It is generally considered that cholecystokinin is identical with pancreozymin; the title cholecystokinin-pancreozymin has also been used.

NOTE. The name Pankreozym has been used for a preparation of pancreatin and diastase.

Soluble in water. **Store** at 2° to 4° in airtight containers.

Units. Various units have been used; in the UK the potency of pancreozymin is expressed as arbitrary Crick-Harper-Raper units based on the amylase content of pancreatic secretion in cats; in Sweden potency is expressed in Ivy dog units based on the increase in gall-bladder pressure after intravenous injection. Correlation between units is complex; the UK manufacturers state that 1 Ivy dog unit is approximately equivalent to 1 Crick-Harper-Raper unit.

Adverse Effects and Precautions. Flushing of the skin may occur, particularly after rapid intravenous injection of pancreozymin. Allergic reactions may occasionally occur, and biliary colic and hypotension have been reported.

See also under Secretin, p.523.

Premedication with diazepam and hyoscine butylbromide prior to endoscopy could delay pancreatic and biliary secretion in response to pancreozymin and secretin.— J. H. B. Saunders *et al.*, *Gut*, 1976, *17*, 351.

Uses. Pancreozymin, administered by intravenous injection, causes an increase in the secretion of pancreatic enzymes, including amylase, lipase, and trypsin, and also stimulates gall-bladder contraction.

Pancreozymin is used as a diagnostic agent in conjunction with secretin for testing the functional capacity of the pancreas and for testing gall-bladder function or bile-duct patency.

A procedure frequently used is to give secretin, 1 to 2 Crick-Harper-Raper units per kg bodyweight, as a freshly prepared solution, by intravenous injection over about 2 minutes, followed after 30 minutes by 1 to 2 units per kg of pancreozymin, as a freshly prepared solution, given by intravenous injection over about 5 minutes. The duodenal secretion is aspirated, measured, and assayed for bicarbonate and enzymes. Gall-bladder function may be assessed by determining the bilirubin content of the aspirate and by visual examination for the presence of bilirubin or cholesterol crystals. Pancreozymin may also be used as an adjunct to cholecystography.

An extensive review.— *Secretin, Cholecystokinin, Pancreozymin and Gastrin*, J.E. Jorpes, and V. Mutt(Eds), Berlin, Springer-Verlag, 1973. See also R. G. Elmslie, *Med. J. Aust.*, 1974, *1*, 1001; G. Bertaccini, *Pharmac. Rev.*, 1976, *28*, 127; P. L. Rayford *et al.*, *New Engl. J. Med.*, 1976, *294*, 1093 and 1157.

In an investigation of 20 patients with the irritable-bowel syndrome given pancreozymin, the 8 patients who usually experienced pain after food showed an increase in intestinal motor activity, associated with pain in 4. Endogenous pancreozymin might be responsible for the functional abdominal pain experienced by patients with this syndrome.— R. F. Harvey and A. E. Read, *Lancet*, 1973, *1*, 1.

In healthy subjects the dose of pancreozymin required to cause gallbladder contraction was 8 times that required to stimulate the secretion of trypsin.— J. R. Malagelada *et al.*, *Gastroenterology*, 1973, *64*, 950.

In 44 controls and 74 patients with possible gall-bladder disease, the gall-bladder, opacified with ipodate sodium, was observed following injection of pancreozymin. There was a high incidence of false positives in the control groups; it was concluded that pancreozymin cholecystography was not helpful in the diagnosis and management of patients with possible acalculous gall-bladder disease.— F. H. Dunn *et al.*, *J. Am. med. Ass.*, 1974, *228*, 997. See also *idem*, *229*, 1283.

Cystic fibrosis. Pancreozymin-secretin tests, performed on 10 children with cystic fibrosis of the pancreas, showed that water and bicarbonate secretion was more severely affected than secretion of enzymes, so that a small volume of pancreatic juice low in bicarbonate and high in enzymes was secreted.— B. Hadorn *et al.*, *Can. med. Ass. J.*, 1968, *98*, 377.

Pancreozymin-secretin test. References to the use of pancreozymin and secretin in the diagnosis of disorders of the pancreas, gall-bladder and biliary tract.— W. Y. Chey *et al.*, *J. Am. med. Ass.*, 1966, *198*, 257; D. C. McGillivray *et al.*, *Can. med. Ass. J.*, 1966, *94*, 1261; K. G. Wormsley, *Scand. J. Gastroenterol.*, 1969, *4*, 623; J. Braganza *et al.*, *Gut*, 1973, *14*, 383; R. Van der Hoeden *et al.*, *Gut*, 1973, *14*, 763; E. A. Eikman *et al.*, *Ann. intern. Med.*, 1975, *82*, 318; J. M. Braganza *et al.*, *Gut*, 1978, *19*, 358; J. M. Braganza and J. J. Rao, *Br. med. J.*, 1978, *2*, 392.

Proprietary Preparations

Cholecystokinin *(Kabi Diagnostica, Swed.)*. Ampoules each containing 40 or 75 Ivy dog units of highly purified pancreozymin with cysteine and cysteine hydrochloride.

Pancreozymin *(Boots, UK)*. Vials each containing approximately 100 Crick-Harper-Raper units of pancreozymin as powder for solution before use.

2142-r

Patent Blue V.

Acid Blue 3; CI Food Blue 5; Colour Index No. 42051. Calcium α-(4-diethylaminophenyl)-α-(4-diethyliminiocyclohexa-2,5-dienylidene)-5-hydroxytoluene-2,4-disulphonate.

$(C_{27}H_{31}N_2O_7S_2)_2Ca=1159.4$.

CAS — 3536-49-0.

NOTE. The name Patent Blue V is also used as a synonym for Sulphan Blue (CI No. 42045)—see p.524.

Pharmacopoeias. In *Fr.*

A dark blue-violet powder. Very **soluble** in water giving a blue solution; slightly soluble in alcohol giving a greenish-blue solution.

Adverse Effects and Precautions. Allergic reactions may occur immediately or after a few minutes and usually consist of erythema, pruritus, and urticaria. More severe reactions, including shock, dyspnoea, and laryngeal spasm, occur rarely. Nausea, hypotension, and tremor have been reported. It should be given with caution to patients with a history of allergy.

Uses. Patent blue V is injected subcutaneously to colour the lymph vessels so that they can be injected with a contrast medium. The usual dose of 0.25 ml of the 2.5% solution diluted with an equal volume of sodium chloride injection or 1% lignocaine hydrochloride injection is injected subcutaneously in each interdigital web space.

Patent blue V is used as a food colour (see p.423).

Proprietary Preparations

Patent Blue V *(May & Baker, UK)*. Patent blue V (CI No. 42051), available as a 2.5% solution in ampoules of 2 ml. For outlining lymph trunks.

2143-f

Penicilloyl-polylysine.

PO-PLL; PPL. A polypeptide compound formed by the interaction of a penicillanic acid and polylysine of an average degree of polymerisation of 20 lysine residues per molecule. The resulting conjugate contains 12 to 15 penicilloyl residues per molecule.

CAS — 53608-77-8.

Soluble in water. Solutions should be **stored** at temperatures not exceeding 4°.

Stability in solution. Solutions of penicilloyl-polylysine in buffered saline at pH 8.2 were stable for 6 months if stored at 4°.— H. E. Voss *et al.*, *J. Am. med. Ass.*, 1966, *196*, 679.

Lyophilised penicilloyl-polylysine lost none of its potency

when stored at 20° or 50° for 84 days; in solution at 20° considerable decomposition occurred in 7 to 14 days.— J. Mikołajczyk *et al.*, *Acta Pol. pharm.*, 1971, *28*, 117.

Adverse Effects and Precautions. Severe allergic reactions have occasionally been reported following administration of penicilloyl-polylysine and further use is contra-indicated in the patients concerned.

Allergic reactions.— E. Ettinger and D. Kaye, *New Engl. J. Med.*, 1964, *271*, 1105; S. S. Resnik and W. B. Shelley, *J. Am. med. Ass.*, 1966, *196*, 740. See also B. B. Levine *et al.* (letter), *ibid.*, *197*, 61.

Uses. Penicilloyl-polylysine is used as a diagnostic agent to detect sensitivity to the penicillins. After a preliminary scratch test it is given in dilute solution by intradermal injection. The development within 15 to 20 minutes of a wheal and of erythema is generally judged a positive reaction.

The possibility of an allergic reaction to treatment with a penicillin is less in patients not reacting to the test, but the test is not unequivocal. The incidence of allergic reactions is stated to be less than 5% in patients showing a negative reaction.

It had been found that 0.005 ml of a 1×10^{-6} molar solution of penicilloyl-polylysine was sufficient to elicit maximum wheal-and-flare reactions; scratch tests with that concentration should always be performed initially to detect hypersensitive subjects.— B. B. Levine *et al* (letter), *J. Am. med. Ass.*, 1966, *197*, 61.

Skin tests with benzylpenicilloyl-polylysine and a 'minor determinant mixture', a mixture of benzylpenicillin and certain of its degradation products, had been carried out in 218 patients who presented with a serious indication for penicillin therapy but also had a history of allergy to penicillin. Of 32 patients with a positive response to both or either test 10 were given gradually increasing doses of penicillin and of these 7 had accelerated allergic reactions. One patient with a positive response whose treatment was initiated with full-dosage penicillin had an immediate urticarial reaction. The 185 patients with a negative response to both tests were given penicillin and one developed a mild accelerated urticarial reaction after 48 hours. One patient found to have dermatographia was not investigated further. Late exanthematic reactions developed in 6 of 185 test-negative and in 3 of 11 test-positive patients given penicillin. It was concluded that the tests, especially a positive reaction to the 'minor determinant mixture', were highly valuable for predicting immediate allergic reactions.— B. B. Levine and D. M. Zolov, *J. Allergy*, 1969, *43*, 231.

Skin tests with benzylpenicillin and benzylpenicilloyl-polylysine in 160 children with suspected allergy to penicillin indicated that these tests were useful to distinguish reactions from other causes than penicillin allergy. Benzylpenicilloyl-polylysine provoked reactions more often than did benzylpenicillin.— C. W. Bierman and P. P. Van Arsdel, *J. Allergy*, 1969, *43*, 267.

It had been shown that if skin tests to penicilloyl-polylysine and to benzylpenicillin were negative, it was very unlikely that immediate or accelerated urticarial reactions would occur with penicillin, even where there was a past history of allergy.— J. S. Comaish, *Br. med. J.*, 1970, *3*, 152.

In an attempt to decrease the frequency of penicillin reactions in a hospital, 2 penicillin antigens, a minor determinant mixture of benzylpenicillin and its derivatives (MDM) and benzylpenicilloyl-polylysine were tested on the skin of each of 218 adults. Fifty of 66 patients with a history of penicillin allergy gave negative results to the tests and 37 of these were subsequently given penicillin without suffering any untoward effects. Ten of 152 patients with no history of penicillin hypersensitivity had positive skin-test reactions and were therefore not given penicillin. The remaining 142 patients had no history of penicillin reactions and a negative result to the skin tests and penicillin was administered without any adverse reactions.— N. F. Adkinson *et al.*, *New Engl. J. Med.*, 1971, *285*, 22.

A survey of 14 000 tests recorded in the literature suggested that the use of penicilloyl-polylysine was safe, more reliable than a history of penicillin allergy, and would reveal sensitivity in patients with no previous history.— W. E. Herrell, *Clin. Med.*, 1972, *79* (Jan.), 12.

Further references.— M. W. Rytel *et al.*, *J. Am. med. Ass.*, 1963, *186*, 894; B. C. Brown *et al.*, *ibid.*, 1964, *189*, 599; *Med. Lett.*, 1978, *20*, 14.

Proprietary Names

Pre-Pen *(Kremers-Urban, USA)*.

2144-d

Pentagastrin *(B.P.)*. AY-6608; ICI 50123.

Boc-βAla-Trp-Met-Asp-Phe—NH_2; *tert*-Butyloxycarbonyl-[β-Ala^{13}]gastrin-(13-17)-pentapeptide amide.

$C_{37}H_{49}N_7O_9S$=767.9.

CAS — 5534-95-2.

Pharmacopoeias. In *Br.* and *Nord.*

A white or almost white odourless powder. M.p. about 229° with decomposition. Practically **insoluble** in water; slightly soluble in alcohol; practically insoluble in chloroform and ether; soluble in dimethyl sulphoxide, dimethylformamide, and dilute ammonia solution. The ammonium salt is soluble 1 in 1000 of water. A solution in dimethylformamide is laevorotatory. **Protect** from light.

Adverse Effects. Pentagastrin may cause nausea, abdominal cramps, flushing of the skin, headache, drowsiness, dizziness, and hypotension.

A 59-year-old man with a gastric ulcer and no history of allergy, hypersensitivity, or drug reactions received pentagastrin 6 µg per kg body-weight subcutaneously. After 7 minutes the patient complained of nausea. After 10 minutes he became dizzy and his heart-rate increased to 100 beats per minute. Later, he complained of cold, desired to defaecate, became sweaty and pallid, and retched; borborygmi were clearly audible; the heart-rate rose to 150 per minute and the blood pressure was 130/70 mmHg. The symptoms disappeared after 1 hour.— M. Aylward and J. B. Bourke (letter), *Lancet*, 1969, *2*, 267.

A 40-year-old man who had received 500 µg of pentagastrin subcutaneously developed extensive rash and pruritus and peri-orbital oedema 17 hours later; the condition responded to treatment with an antihistamine.— C. Wastell and J. MacNaughton (letter), *Br. med. J.*, 1975, *1*, 334.

Atrial fibrillation in a man given pentagastrin and calcium gluconate.— D. Drucker (letter), *New Engl. J. Med.*, 1981, *304*, 1427.

Further references.— J. A. Barrowman *et al.*, *Clin. Pharmac. Ther.*, 1970, *11*, 862; R. F. McCloy and J. H. Baron (letter), *Lancet*, 1977, *1*, 548.

Precautions. Pentagastrin should not be given to patients who have previously shown sensitivity to the drug. It should not be given to patients with acute peptic ulcer and should be given with care to patients with active pancreatic, hepatic, or biliary-tract disease.

The effect of pentagastrin on gastric secretion was significantly reduced by smoking 1 to 2 cigarettes.— A. Wilkinson and D. Johnston, *Gut*, 1969, *10*, 415.

Uses. Pentagastrin is a synthetic polypeptide which when given parenterally has effects similar to those of natural gastrin. It increases gastro-intestinal motility and stimulates the secretion of gastric acid, pepsin, and intrinsic factor. The peak effect occurs over about 10 to 40 minutes. Secretion of pancreatic enzymes is also increased. Pentagastrin is used as a diagnostic agent to test the secretory action of the stomach. The usual dose is 6 µg per kg body-weight by subcutaneous or intramuscular injection; by intravenous infusion the dose is 0.6 µg per kg per hour, in sodium chloride injection, increased if necessary to 6 µg per kg per hour. It has also been used as a snuff. Because the response to pentagastrin is reduced after vagotomy it has been used as a test of the completeness of vagotomy. It has also been suggested as a test for pancreatic function and in the diagnosis of medullary carcinoma of the thyroid.

A brief evaluation.— *Med. Lett.*, 1975, *17*, 60.

The activity of the colon and rectum was increased following intravenous injections of pentagastrin 250 to 500 ng per kg body-weight. Slight increases in ileal activity also occurred. Subcutaneous doses of 1 to 4 µg per kg showed no constant effect.— C. J. H. Logan and A. M. Connell, *Lancet*, 1966, *1*, 996. Pentagastrin, given by intravenous infusion in doses sufficient to raise gastric acid secretion to maximum levels, stimulated motor activity in the gastric antrum; it had no effect on the colon.— J. G. Misiewicz *et al.*, *Gut*, 1967, *8*, 463.

Pentagastrin had been found to produce maximum gastric secretion after doses of 6 µg per kg subcutaneously or during intravenous infusion of 10 ng per kg per minute, indicating that a subcutaneous dose was not fully effective. The half-life of pentagastrin in the circulation was less than 1 minute.— K. N. Wai *et al.*, *J. Pharm. Pharmac.*, 1970, *22*, 923.

The marked increase in lower oesophageal sphincter pressure which occurred when pentagastrin 3 µg per kg body-weight was given subcutaneously to normal fasting subjects was much diminished if the subjects were given a meal prepared from corn oil 15 minutes before the injection of pentagastrin.— O. T. Nebel and D. O. Castell, *Gut*, 1973, *14*, 270.

A study in 4 subjects indicated that pentagastrin might be absorbed intact from the gastro-intestinal tract.— M. T. Morrell and W. M. Keynes (letter), *Lancet*, 1975, *2*, 712.

Further references.— D. T. Caridis *et al.*, *Lancet*, 1968, *1*, 1281; R. S. Gordon (letter), *ibid.*, 1968, *2*, 103; M. H. Pritchard and A. M. Connell, *Gut*, 1969, *10*, 303; V. Eckardt and H. Weigand, *Gut*, 1974, *15*, 706; A. Tarnawski *et al.*, *Gut*, 1978, *19*, 116.

Administration as a snuff. Maximum response of gastric acid to pentagastrin, given in the form of a snuff in lactose in a dose of 1 mg every 10 minutes for 1 hour, was generally not significantly different from the response to pentagastrin given as a continuous intravenous infusion. In 1 patient who had nasal congestion the dose of snuff required to produce comparable effects was greater than that used in the other patients. Pentagastrin was inactive when given sublingually in doses of up to 20 mg.— K. G. Wormsley, *Lancet*, 1968, *1*, 57.

Diagnosis of neoplasms. A preliminary report on the use of pentagastrin in rapid stimulation tests to detect malignant neoplasm of the thyroid.— G. W. Sizemore and V. L. W. Go, *Mayo Clin. Proc.*, 1975, *50*, 53.

Pentagastrin was recommended for the screening of suspected cases of hereditary medullary carcinoma of the thyroid as well as for the early detection of metastases following surgery.— F. M. Ribeiro *et al.* (letter), *Lancet*, 1976, *2*, 1017.

Pentagastrin 5 µg per kg body-weight as an intravenous bolus injection was given to 10 brothers and sisters of 2 patients with proved medullary carcinoma of the thyroid. After pentagastrin the serum-calcitonin concentrations were sufficiently elevated in 4 members for diagnoses of thyroid carcinomas to be made; these were subsequently confirmed histologically.— H. Mulder and C. A. P. F. Su, *Dt. med. Wschr.*, 1977, *102*, 479.

A study in 3 patients with medullary thyroid neoplasms and in 36 asymptomatic relatives of these patients showed that pentagastrin 500 ng per kg body-weight given intravenously over 10 to 15 seconds provided more rapid and effective stimulation of immunoreactive calcitonin release into the blood, within 5 minutes, than did the slow infusion of a calcium salt. The release of calcitonin provided a diagnostic test for the presence of medullary thyroid neoplasm and was positive in 11 persons given pentagastrin and in 3 of them by the use of calcium.— M. Verdy *et al.*, *Can. med. Ass. J.*, 1978, *119*, 29.

Further references.— J. R. Starling *et al.*, *Archs Surg., Chicago*, 1978, *113*, 241.

Effect on gastric secretion. Studies in 204 men showed that after an intramuscular injection of pentagastrin 6 µg per kg body-weight the output of gastric acid was similar to that following an injection of ametazole 2 mg per kg subcutaneously, histamine 40 µg per kg subcutaneously or 40 µg per kg per hour intravenously, or pentagastrin 6 µg per kg subcutaneously or 6 µg per kg per hour intravenously. Samples of gastric secretion were aspirated 10, 20, and 30 minutes after the intramuscular injection of pentagastrin. In 26% of the men given pentagastrin intramuscularly, peak acid output occurred 20 to 40 minutes after the injection so that collection up to 30 minutes after the injection underestimated the peak acid output of these men.—Report of a Multicentre Study, *Lancet*, 1969, *1*, 341.

See also above.

Effect on pancreatic function. In 8 healthy subjects the subcutaneous injection of pentagastrin 6 µg per kg body-weight caused an increase in the volume of duodenal secretion, in the output of lipase and trypsin, and, in 7 of the subjects, in the output of bilirubin. In 3 patients with chronic pancreatitis, there was no increase in the volume of duodenal secretion and no significant increase in the output of lipase and trypsin. In 2 patients who had undergone cholecystectomy the increased output of bilirubin was less than in the controls; in the third patient the output of bilirubin was similar to that in the controls. Pentagastrin was valuable for the study of pancreatic function.— J. E. Valenzuela *et al.*, *Am. J. dig. Dis.*, 1968, *13*, 767.

Preparations

Pentagastrin Injection *(B.P.)*. A sterile solution of pentagastrin in Water for Injections containing ammonium hydroxide. Sterilised by filtration. pH 7 to 8. Store below 20°. Protect from light.
The manufacturer recommends storage below 4°.

Peptavlon *(ICI Pharmaceuticals, UK)*. Pentagastrin, available as an injection containing 250 µg per ml in ampoules of 2 ml. (Also available as Peptavlon in *Austral., Canad., Denm., Norw., Switz., USA*).

Other Proprietary Names

Gastrodiagnost *(Ger.)*.

2145-n

Phenolsulphonphthalein *(B.P.C. 1973)*.

Phenolsulphonphthal.; Phenolsulfonphthalein *(U.S.P.)*; Phenol Red; Fenolsolfonftaleina; PSP.
4,4′-(3*H*-2,1-Benzoxathiol-3-ylidene)diphenol *S,S*-dioxide.
$C_{19}H_{14}O_5S=354.4$.

CAS — 143-74-8.

Pharmacopoeias. In *Chin., Ind., It., Jap., Mex., Nord., Swiss,* and *U.S.*

A bright to dark red, odourless or almost odourless, crystalline powder. **Soluble** 1 in 1500 of water, 1 in 350 of alcohol, and 1 in 500 of acetone; freely soluble in solutions of alkali hydroxides and carbonates, producing a violet-red to deep red colour; practically insoluble in chloroform, ether, and light petroleum. Solutions are **sterilised** by autoclaving or by filtration.

Adverse Effects. Allergic reactions may occasionally occur.

Precautions. Excretion of phenolsulphonphthalein may be affected in patients taking aminohippuric acid, penicillin, probenecid, some sulphonamides, or salicylates.

Absorption and Fate. After intravenous injection, phenolsulphonphthalein is in part bound to plasma proteins, and in a patient with normal kidney function is rapidly excreted, mainly in the urine; some is excreted by the liver. Renal clearance is predominantly by tubular secretion, only a small amount being eliminated by glomerular filtration.

Uses. Phenolsulphonphthalein has been used as a test of renal function by estimating the rate of excretion in the urine after the intravenous injection of 6 mg, with 1.43 mg of sodium bicarbonate, in 1 ml of sodium chloride injection, after a water load of 0.5 to 1 litre. With normal renal function, at least 50% is excreted in the urine in the first hour, or 75% in the first and second hours. The concentration in the urine can be determined colorimetrically after making the urine alkaline with sodium hydroxide solution. Because phenolsulphonphthalein is in part excreted by the liver, abnormally high values may indicate impaired hepatic function. It has also been given intramuscularly.

A review of the phenolsulphonphthalein excretion test of renal function.— G. Dunea and P. Freedman, *J. Am. med. Ass.*, 1968, *204*, 621.

Excretion of only 40% of the dose in 1 hour indicated some kidney impairment, reduction to 20 or 30% was seen in nephritis, and less than 10% showed serious impairment. Drugs which produced a red colour in alkaline urine could falsely elevate readings and indicate normal kidney function. They included danthron and other anthraquinone-containing drugs; formaldehyde-forming drugs also interfered.— F. C. Cross *et al.*, *Am. J. Hosp. Pharm.*, 1966, *23*, 235.

Comparisons were made of tests for renal function using the excretion-rate of phenolsulphonphthalein in urine (PSPU) and the concentration index of phenolsulphonphthalein in plasma (PSPI). PSPU was considered to be satisfactory for co-operative patients with normal urinary systems. Where anatomical and/or functional abnormalities existed, PSPI was preferable.— M. H. Gault *et al.*, *J. Am. med. Ass.*, 1967, *200*, 871.

In 50 normotensive patients without evidence of renal disorder the mean clearance of phenolsulphonphthalein was about 60% of that of aminohippuric acid. From the results of various studies it was suggested that the clearance of phenolsulphonphthalein was a sensitive method in the diagnosis of secretory tubular disorders, whereas clearance of aminohippuric acid was more suitable for assessing renal circulatory disorders.— A. Heidland, *Arch. klin. Med.*, 1968, *214*, 163.

For a report of the use of phenolsulphonphthalein to improve the accuracy of gastric secretion studies, see M. Hobsley and W. Silen, *Gut*, 1969, *10*, 787.

The use of the phenolsulphonphthalein test for the evaluation of the patency of the fallopian tubes.— G. Speck, *Fert. Steril.*, 1970, *21*, 28.

Drug ingestion indicator. The incorporation of phenolsulphonphthalein into a medicament provided a method of checking drug ingestion. The dye was excreted in the urine approximately 2 hours after ingestion. Since the dye was yellow at a pH below 7 the patient was not aware of the presence of the indicator. The addition of sodium bicarbonate to a urine sample caused the indicator to change to a violet colour.— W. L. Ryan *et al.*, *Am. J. Pharm.*, 1962, *134*, 168.

Marker for metabolic studies. The use of phenolsulphonphthalein as a marker compound for the study of intestinal absorption.— A. B. French *et al.*, *Am. J. dig. Dis.*, 1968, *13*, 558.

Residual urine test. A qualitative method of testing for residual urine in the bladder in children: phenolsulphonphthalein, 6 mg in 1 ml, was injected intravenously and urine specimens taken after 3 and 12 hours. The bladder was emptied at least once up to 8 hours after the first specimen. A high concentration of dye in the first specimen and the absence of dye in the second was indicative of normal bladder function.— M. E. MacGregor and C. J. E. W. Williams, *Lancet*, 1966, *1*, 893. See also D. R. Axelrod, *Archs intern. Med.*, 1966, *117*, 74.

Preparations

Phenolsulfonphthalein Injection *(U.S.P.)*. A sterile solution of phenolsulphonphthalein, rendered soluble with sodium bicarbonate or sodium hydroxide, in Water for Injections and made iso-osmotic with sodium chloride. pH 6 to 7.5.

Proprietary Names

Fenolsulfoftalein *(DAK, Denm.)*; PSP-Plasma-Test *(E. Merck, Ger.)*.

2146-h

Rose Bengal Sodium.

Sodium Rose Bengal; Rose Bengal; CI Acid Red 94; Colour Index No. 45440. The disodium salt of 4,5,6,7-tetrachloro-2′,4′,5′,7′-tetraiodofluorescein.
$C_{20}H_2Cl_4I_4Na_2O_5=1017.6$.

CAS — 11121-48-5 (rose bengal); 632-69-9 (disodium salt).

NOTE. Dichlorotetraiodofluorescein (CI Acid Red 93; Ext. D & C Reds Nos. 5 and 6; Colour Index No. 45435) has been used as its disodium or dipotassium salt, for colouring pharmaceutical and cosmetic preparations for external use and as a food colour. The name Rose Bengale has been applied to both CI Acid Red 93 and 94.

A brownish-red solid; **soluble** 1 in 4 of water, giving a clear deep red solution; soluble 1 in 20 of alcohol. Solutions are **sterilised** by autoclaving or by filtration.

Rose bengal was incompatible with phenylmercuric nitrate, benzalkonium chloride, and chlorhexidine, but was compatible with esters of hydroxybenzoic acid.— N. Harb, *J. Hosp. Pharm.*, 1968, *25*, 239.

Uses. Rose bengal sodium is used as the iodine-131-labelled compound, see p.1393, as a diagnostic aid in the determination of hepatobiliary function.

It is also used, as 1% eye-drops, to stain devitalised conjunctival and corneal cells and as an aid in the diagnosis of dry eye. Instillation of this dye may be painful when the conjunctiva is damaged and therefore should only be performed once.

Diagnostic staining. For the use of rose bengal in conjunction with fluorescein sodium for staining the cornea and conjunctiva, see Fluorescein Sodium, p.517.

The use of rose bengal staining for the detection of conjunctival xerosis in nutrition surveys in Indian children.— K. Vijayaraghavan *et al.*, *Am. J. clin. Nutr.*, 1978, *31*, 892.

Preparations

Rose Bengal Eye-drops *(Moorfields Eye Hosp.)*. Rose bengal sodium 1 g, phenylmercuric acetate 2 mg, water to 100 ml.

Minims Rose Bengal *(Smith & Nephew Pharmaceuticals, UK)*. Sterile eye-drops containing rose bengal sodium 1%, in single-use disposable applicators.

NOTE. The *B.P.* allows the synonym ROS to be used for single-dose eye-drops containing rose bengal sodium.

2147-m

Secretin.

A hormone, prepared from the duodenal mucosa of pigs, which stimulates the digestive secretions of the pancreas.

CAS — 17034-35-4.

Soluble in water. **Store** in airtight containers at 2° to 4°.

Secretin solutions in a range of strengths were pumped at a constant rate through a plastic infusion system, including syringe, tubing, and catheter, for 45 minutes. The amount of secretin, measured by radio-immunoassay, decreased on delivery through the system. The reductions in secretin concentrations after 45 minutes were similar in samples of solution from the syringe and catheter tip. The loss of secretin from solution might be due to its binding to plastic; the rate of loss was not related to the original concentration of a solution.— M. Miyata *et al.* (letter), *New Engl. J. Med.*, 1979, *300*, 95.

Units. Various units have been used; in the UK the potency of secretin is expressed as arbitrary Crick-Harper-Raper (CHR) units based on the volume of pancreatic juice secreted in cats; in Sweden potency is expressed as arbitrary Clinical units, the value of which was amended in 1966. Correlation between units is complex; the UK manufacturers state that 1 Clinical unit is approximately equivalent to 4 Crick-Harper-Raper units.

References.— L. V. Gutierrez and J. H. Baron, *Gut*, 1972, *13*, 721.

Adverse Effects. Allergic reactions may occasionally occur. Diarrhoea has occurred in patients given high doses by intravenous infusion.

Changes in the cells of the surface epithelium of the rectal mucosa occurred after an injection of secretin in children.— P. G. Johansen *et al.* (letter), *Nature*, 1968, *217*, 468.

Anaphylactoid local reactions after intradermal injection of secretin occurred in 8 of 8 patients with duodenal ulcer, 2 of 3 with gastric ulcer, 4 of 6 with ulcerative colitis or Crohn's disease, 13 of 23 with other gastro-intestinal diseases, and in possibly 1 of 7 healthy subjects.— H. W. Baenkler *et al.* (letter), *Br. med. J.*, 1975, *2*, 747.

Precautions. The secretin test should be used with caution in patients with acute pancreatitis or with a history of atopic asthma or allergy. An intradermal test for sensitivity has been suggested.

Uses. Secretin, administered by intravenous injection, causes an increase in the secretion by the pancreas of water and bicarbonate into the duodenum. The concentration of insulin in the plasma is also increased in non-diabetic patients. Secretin is usually administered in a dose of 1 to 2 Crick-Harper-Raper units per kg body-weight by slow intravenous injection over about 2 minutes in conjunction with pancreozymin as a diagnostic agent for testing the functional capacity of the pancreas (see p.521). It has also been given by intravenous infusion.

An extensive review.— *Secretin, Cholecystokinin, Pancreozymin and Gastrin*, J.E. Jorpes and V. Mutt (Eds), Berlin, Springer-Verlag, 1973. See also R. G. Elmslie, *Med. J. Aust.*, 1974, *1*, 1001; P. L. Rayford *et al.*, *New Engl. J. Med.*, 1976, *294*, 1093 and 1157.

The use of a simultaneous combined test (secretin, pancreozymin, radioactive selenomethionine, propantheline, X-ray, and cytology) in the evaluation of the pancreas.— S. Nundy *et al.*, *Br. med. J.*, 1974, *1*, 87.

A discussion of gastro-intestinal peptides and the suggestion of the name 'eupeptides'.— D. Wingate, *Lancet*, 1976, *1*, 529.

Hyperparathyroid patients consistently produced very large insulin responses to secretin injection. This large insulin response in hyperparathyroid patients should be investigated as a safe, non-calcium-dependent diagnostic test for primary hyperparathyroidism.— D. J. Sanders *et al.* (letter), *Lancet*, 1980, *2*, 265.

Administration as a snuff. Secretin administered as a snuff in doses of 100 and 75 Clinical units by nasal inhalation was effective in increasing the concentration of bicarbonate in the duodenum. The chloride concentration was decreased.— P. B'hend *et al.*, *Lancet*, 1973, *1*, 509.

In a study of 10 healthy subjects, the pancreatic response to secretin given as a snuff was more than 25 times less than that from secretin given intravenously.— W. Domschke *et al.* (letter), *Lancet*, 1974, *1*, 1348.

Constant infusion test. Secretin, administered by infusion at a rate of 10 CHR units per kg body-weight per hour, caused maximum secretion of bicarbonate into the duodenum in 20 of 24 persons; the response was significantly greater than after intravenous injection over 2 minutes of secretin 2 units per kg. The bicarbonate response of patients with chronic pancreatitis was markedly impaired.— K. G. Wormsley, *Gastroenterology*, 1968, *54*, 197.

Duodenal ulcer. *Diagnosis.* Secretin in a dose of 20 Clinical units given intradermally to 7 patients with duodenal ulcer produced a definite skin reaction due to histamine release in 6. No reactions occurred in 6 control patients. Secretin might be of value in the diagnosis of duodenal ulcer.— H. W. Baenkler *et al.*, *Lancet*, 1977, *1*, 928.

See also under Adverse Effects.

Treatment. Studies in 7 patients with duodenal ulcer indicated that secretin given intravenously suppressed acid secretion in response to a meal or to pentagastrin. Serum-gastrin concentrations were reduced and bicarbonate secretions increased.— S. J. Konturek *et al.*, *Gut*, 1973, *14*, 842.

Experience with 4 patients undergoing haemodialysis for terminal renal failure indicated that infusions of secretin might be useful in reducing the tendency to duodenal ulceration in such patients by inhibiting gastric hypersecretion of acid.— A. M. M. Shepherd *et al.*, *Br. med. J.*, 1974, *1*, 96.

Three patients with a duodenal ulcer received 10 Clinical units per kg body-weight of a long-acting synthetic secretin preparation by subcutaneous injection twice daily for 1 week then once daily for 3 weeks. Improvement in epigastric pain occurred 2 to 8 days after the start of treatment and complete healing of the ulcer occurred after 2 to 3 weeks. Treatment did not result in a fall in basal serum-gastrin concentration nor in a reduced serum-gastrin response to a test meal nor was pancreatic-bicarbonate secretion enhanced.— L. Demling *et al.*, *Scand. J. Gastroenterol.*, 1976, *11*, *Suppl.* 42, 135.

A study involving 14 patients with a duodenal ulcer given a placebo or synthetic porcine secretin 333 µg (approximately equivalent to 18 Clinical units per kg body-weight of natural porcine secretin) by subcutaneous injection every 4 hours was discontinued after 10 days because of transient, asymptomatic, hyperamylasaemia in secretin-treated patients. During the period of study it was considered that secretin was no more effective than a placebo in relieving pain or healing the ulcer.— R. M. Henn *et al.*, *Am. J. dig. Dis.*, 1976, *21*, 921.

Pancreatic arteriography. Radiological visualisation of changes in the pancreatic vessels was improved when secretin was given intra-arterially 1½ minutes prior to the injection of 30 to 50 ml of contrast medium. Of 25 patients examined in this way, 17 showed evidence of pancreatic disease and 1 of neoplastic disease. Visualisation was excellent in 6 of the 7 patients without pancreatic disease, compared with satisfactory visualisation in 10% of the patients examined by arteriography alone.— J. Plessier *et al.*, *Archs Mal. Appar. dig.*, 1968, *57*, 307.

Pancreozymin-secretin test. For references to the use of secretin in conjunction with pancreozymin for testing pancreatic function, see Pancreozymin, p.521.

Zollinger-Ellison syndrome. *Diagnosis.* The infusion over 1 hour of secretin 3 Clinical units per kg body-weight appeared to be of value in the diagnosis of the Zollinger-Ellison syndrome in patients who had not undergone surgery.— S. Bonfils *et al.*, *Gut*, 1974, *15*, 841.

Secretin administered as an intravenous bolus injection was used to diagnose Zollinger-Ellison syndrome in 18 patients with a history of peptic ulcer disease and was preferred to calcium gluconate.— C. W. Deveney *et al.*, *Ann. intern. Med.*, 1977, *87*, 680. A report of a false-positive response of gastrin to a secretin test for diagnosis of the Zollinger-Ellison syndrome in a patient who had achlorhydria and hypergastrinaemia.— R. L. Wollmuth and J. B. Wagonfield (letter), *ibid.*, 1978, *88*, 718.

Further references.— E. L. Bradley and J. T. Galambos (letter), *Lancet*, 1972, *1*, 594.

Proprietary Preparations

Secretin *(Boots, UK).* Vials each containing approximately 100 Crick-Harper-Raper units of secretin as powder for solution before use.

Secretin *(Kabi Diagnostica, Swed.).* Ampoules each containing 75 Clinical units of highly purified secretin with cysteine hydrochloride.

Other Proprietary Names

Secrepan *(Jap.)*.

2148-b

Sincalide. CCK-OP; SQ-19844. Asp-Tyr(SO_3H)-Met-Gly-Trp-Met-Asp-Phe—NH_2; De-1-(5-oxo-L-proline)-de-2-L-glutamine-5-methionine-ceruletide.
$C_{49}H_{62}N_{10}O_{16}S_3$=1143.3.

CAS — 25126-32-3.

A white powder.

Sincalide is the active synthetic C-terminal octapeptide of pancreozymin (p.521) and administered by intravenous injection it stimulates gall-bladder contraction.

Sincalide is used for testing gall-bladder function and is usually given in doses of 20 ng per kg body-weight by intravenous injection over ½ to 1 minute to provide a sample of bile that may be aspirated from the duodenum. It is also used as a diagnostic agent in conjunction with secretin for testing the functional capacity of the pancreas. A suggested procedure is to give secretin by intravenous infusion over 1 hour and 30 minutes after starting this infusion, sincalide 20 ng per kg is infused over a 30-minute period. Sincalide may also be used as an adjunct to cholecystography.

An evaluation of sincalide.— *Med. Lett.*, 1977, *19*, 36.

Maximum gall-bladder contraction occurred in 24 of 40 patients undergoing cholecystography given sincalide 20 ng per kg body-weight by intravenous injection over 1 minute. The remaining 16 patients required a second dose to achieve maximum contraction. Transient mild abdominal pain, cramps, or nausea occurred in 48% of the patients but these were considered to be manifestations of the physiologic actions of sincalide.— E. N. Sargent *et al.*, *Am. J. Roentg.*, 1976, *127*, 267.

Eight patients with chronic pancreatitis became symptom-free during treatment with sincalide given in a dose of 2 drops of a 0.1% solution intranasally thrice daily before meals for 3 weeks. There was also some evidence of improvement in exocrine pancreatic function. Three patients experienced borborygmi and loose stools which stopped when the dose was slightly decreased.— A. Pap and V. Varró (letter), *Lancet*, 1977, *2*, 294.

Proprietary Names

Kinevac *(Squibb, Austral.; Squibb, Canad.; Heyden, Ger.; Squibb, USA).*

2149-v

Sodium Anoxynaphthonate *(B.P. 1963).*

Sod. Anoxynaph.; Sodium Anazolene; CI Acid Blue 92; Colour Index No. 13390. Trisodium 4-[(4-anilino-5-sulpho-1-naphthyl)azo]-5-hydroxynaphthalene-2,7-disulphonate.
$C_{26}H_{16}N_3Na_3O_{10}S_3$=695.6.

CAS — 3861-73-2.

A blue or bluish-black, odourless, hygroscopic powder. It contains 5 to 15% of water. **Soluble** 1 in 30 of water; practically insoluble in alcohol, acetone, and chloroform. Solutions are **sterilised** by autoclaving or by filtration. **Store** in airtight containers.

Adverse Effects. Nausea, vomiting, and rigors have been reported in some patients with single doses of 250 mg or more.

Absorption and Fate. After intravenous injection, sodium anoxynaphthonate is bound to plasma proteins. It is metabolised in the liver and partly excreted in bile; colourless metabolites are excreted in the urine. About 50% of the dye is eliminated from the plasma within 30 minutes.

Uses. Sodium anoxynaphthonate has been used for the determination of blood and plasma volumes, for the measurement of cardiac output, and to define the type and position of intracardiac shunts. It is administered intravenously as a 2% aqueous solution, the usual dose being 5 ml (100 mg). The concentration of the dye in plasma is determined colorimetrically. The dose may be repeated several times up to a total of 500 mg if required.

2150-r

Sulphan Blue *(B.P.C. 1954).*

Sulphanum Caeruleum; Alphazurine 2G; Isosulfan Blue; Blue VRS; Patent Blue V; Acid Blue 1; Colour Index No. 42045. Sodium α-(4-diethylaminophenyl)-α-(4-diethyliminiocyclo-hexa-2,5-dienylidene)toluene-2,5-disulphonate.
$C_{27}H_{31}N_2NaO_6S_2$=566.7.

CAS — 68238-36-8; 129-17-9 (2,4 isomer).

NOTE. The name Patent Blue V is mainly used for CI No. 42051—see p.521. Sulphan blue was formerly described as the 2,4-disulphonate isomer.

A violet powder. **Soluble** in water and partly soluble in alcohol, giving blue solutions. Solutions for injection may be **sterilised** by autoclaving. **Protect** from light.

Adverse Effects and Precautions. Sulphan blue occasionally causes nausea. Allergic reactions and attacks of asthma have occasionally been reported after the intravenous injection of sulphan blue.

Sulphan blue should not be used during surgical shock.

Fatal allergic shock in a burnt patient given 6 ml of a 10% solution of sulphan blue intravenously.— S. Hepps and M. Dollinger, *New Engl. J. Med.*, 1965, *272*, 1281.

Absorption and Fate. Following intravenous injection, sulphan blue is widely distributed in the tissues and may appear in bile, bronchial secretions, faeces, gastro-intestinal secretions, and synovial fluid. It is excreted in the urine, and skin staining disappears in up to 36 hours in children and 48 hours in adults.

Uses. Changes in skin colour occur 1 to 1½ minutes after an intravenous injection of sulphan blue and complete body staining is established in 3 to 5 minutes. This effect is used as a direct visual test of the state of the circulation in healthy and damaged tissues, particularly in assessing tissue viability in burns and soft-tissue trauma. The usual dose is 0.25 to 0.5 ml per kg body-weight of a 6.2% solution by slow intravenous injection. Sulphan blue, suggested dose 1 to 1.5 ml of a 6.2% solution, has been given subcutaneously in lymphangiography to outline lymph trunks.

Sulphan blue has been used as a colouring agent for medicines; it is no longer used for foods.

Lymphangiography. A method for making lymph trunks visible to the naked eye at operation and opaque to X-rays so that radiographs could be made to study their role in disease in man. An 11% solution of sulphan blue was used, about 2 to 2.5 ml being injected subcutaneously between the toes (about 0.5 ml into each web). In this dosage the dye has been found to be without toxic effects. The dye was absorbed into the blood stream and excreted in the urine; the patient became blue in colour but regained a normal complexion in about 24 hours.— J. B. Kinmonth *et al.*, *Br. med. J.*, 1955, *1*, 940. A similar report in which 1 to 1.5 ml of a 6.2% solution was injected into the dorsum of the foot.— G. E. Edwards (letter), *Br. med. J.*, 1962, *1*, 1013.

Marker for intra-arterial injection. To ensure that the catheter bearing the intra-arterial injection of a cytotoxic drug was best placed for the accurate delivery of the drug to the site of the malignant lesion, sulphan blue could be used as a marker. On intra-arterial injection it very rapidly tinted distinctly blue the area served by the artery. This tinting rapidly disappeared but the procedure could be repeated as a check that the therapeutic injection continued to be given into the intended artery. The technique used in 2 patients was that 1 ml of 11% aqueous solution of sulphan blue, which was iso-osmotic with body fluids, was diluted with 4 ml of physiological saline and about 0.5 ml of this diluted solution given by intra-arterial injection into the superior thyroid artery; the injection was repeated, as a check, daily or so during the treatment with intra-arterial methoxtrexate. Delivery of the latter drug to a large malignant lesion near the right ear in the first case and to carcinoma of the tongue in the second was ensured.— A. Engeset *et al.*, *Lancet*, 1962, *1*, 1382.

Preparations

Sulphan Blue Solution *(B.P.C. 1963).* Liq. Sulphan. Caerul. Sulphan blue 60 mg, chloroform water to 100 ml. Protect from light. As a colouring agent for liquids, 1.5 ml per 100 ml is usually sufficient.

Sulphan Blue Solution with Tartrazine *(B.P.C. 1963).* Liq. Sulphan. Caerul. c. Tartraz.; Green Colouring Solution. Sulphan blue 300 mg, tartrazine, food grade of commerce, 300 mg, chloroform water to 100 ml. Protect from light. As a colouring agent for liquids, 1.5 ml per 100 ml is usually sufficient.

Disulphine Blue Intravenous Injection *(ICI Pharmaceuticals, UK).* A sterile solution of sulphan blue 6.2% in ampoules of 10 ml. (Also available as Disulphine Blue in *Ger.*).

2151-f

Sulphobromophthalein Sodium *(B.P.).*

Sulphobromophthal. Sod.; Sodium Sulfobromophthalein; Sulfobromophthalein Sodium *(U.S.P.)*; Bromsulfophthalein Sodium; BSP; SBP. Disodium 4,5,6,7-tetrabromophenolphthalein-3′,3″-disulphonate; Disodium 5,5′-(4,5,6,7-tetrabromophthalidylidene)bis(2-hydroxybenzenesulphonate).

$C_{20}H_8Br_4Na_2O_{10}S_2$=838.0.

CAS — 71-67-0.

Pharmacopoeias. In *Br., Chin., Ind., Jap.,* and *U.S.*

A white, odourless, crystalline, hygroscopic powder with a bitter taste. **Soluble** 1 in 12 of water; practically insoluble in alcohol, acetone, and chloroform. Solutions are **sterilised** by filtration. **Store** in airtight containers. Protect from light.

Purity and stability. Commercial intravenous injections of sulphobromophthalein sodium from 3 manufacturers contained less than 0.1% of impurities such as phenoltetrabromphthalein monosulphonate and trisulphonate. A sample from a fourth manufacturer contained 3.9% of the monosulphonate and 0.2% of other minor derivatives. Chromatography of a solution autoclaved at 120° for 20 minutes showed no breakdown products and solutions were not degraded after storage for up to 4 months.— F. Barbier and G. A. DeWeerdt, *J. pharm. Sci.*, 1968, *57*, 819.

Adverse Effects. Sulphobromophthalein may cause thrombophlebitis when administered intravenously, and inadvertent subcutaneous infiltration may cause irritation and necrosis. Allergic-type reactions, some fatal, have been reported. Urticaria and eczema have also been reported.

An intravenous dose of 5 mg per kg body-weight of sulphobromophthalein sodium was compared with a placebo in 288 volunteers. Venous abnormalities occurred after 24 hours in 10 of 144 subjects given the drug and in 2 of 141 given the placebo. After 72 hours, 21 of 140 subjects given the drug showed venous induration and 4 of 136 given the placebo.— E. M. Schneider, *J. Am. med. Ass.*, 1965, *194*, 339.

In view of the 15 deaths and 27 severe allergic reactions which had been reported in connection with the sulphobromophthalein test, the test was best reserved for cases not readily elucidated by other means.— C. Wierum (letter), *J. Am. med. Ass.*, 1969, *210*, 1102.

After the administration of sulphobromophthalein, severe reactions including cardiac arrest, cyanosis, dyspnoea, and imperceptible pulse, or loss of consciousness, occurred in 3 patients. Storage of sulphobromophthalein at too low a temperature was considered to be the cause of these reactions.— E. Juhl *et al.* (letter), *Lancet*, 1970, *2*, 424. See also T. W. Astin, *Br. med. J.*, 1965, *2*, 408.

Haemolysis associated with the use of sulphobromophthalein.— U. Ballies and K. Leybold, *Dt. med. Wschr.*, 1974, *99*, 1579.

A fixed drug eruption occurred in a patient 8 hours after she was given an injection of sulphobromophthalein; she responded similarly to phenolphthalein given by mouth.— E. L. Smith, *Br. J. Derm.*, 1977, *97*, 106.

Precautions. Sulphobromophthalein should not be given to patients with asthma or allergy, or a history of drug sensitivity.

Because a 5% solution, on standing, may yield a deposit which is not readily visible, ampoules of the solution should, immediately before use, be immersed for 20 minutes in boiling water, well shaken, and cooled to body temperature.

The clearance of sulphobromophthalein may be reduced by drugs which impair hepatic function and has been stated to be reduced by cholagogues, cholecystographic agents, some narcotic analgesics, probenecid, thiazide diuretics, and drugs extensively excreted in bile. The effect of barbiturates is controversial. The colorimetric estimation of sulphobromophthalein has been stated to be affected by other phthalein compounds, heparin, and dyes such as phenazopyridine.

More than 5% of sulphobromophthalein was retained after 45 minutes in 55 of 73 patients with gout and in 12 of 16 with asymptomatic hyperuricaemia, compared with 6 of 30 controls.— R. Grahame *et al.*, *Ann. rheum. Dis.*, 1968, *27*, 19.

Sulphobromophthalein could interfere technically with chemical estimations for total protein in the blood to produce erroneous raised results.— *Drug & Ther. Bull.*, 1972, *10*, 69.

Sulphobromophthalein sodium might give falsely high results in tests for serum protein-bound iodine.— A. J. J. Wood and J. Crooks, *Prescribers' J.*, 1973, *13*, 94.

Absorption and Fate. Sulphobromophthalein sodium, administered intravenously, is bound to plasma proteins. In patients with normal hepatic function it is rapidly excreted in the bile.

In the circulation, sulphobromophthalein was bound to serum albumin. Serum from women who were pregnant or taking oral contraceptives and from blood taken from the umbilical vein could bind more molecules of sulphobromophthalein than serum from control persons. The findings could explain the longer retention of sulphobromophthalein in pregnant women.— J. S. Crawford and H. W. Y. Hooi, *Br. J. Anaesth.*, 1968, *40*, 723.

The biological half-life of sulphobromophthalein was reported to be 5.5 minutes.— W. A. Ritschel, *Drug Intell. & clin. Pharm.*, 1970, *4*, 332.

Uses. Sulphobromophthalein sodium is used as a diagnostic agent for testing the functional capacity of the liver, particularly of its reticuloendothelial cells.

The test is usually performed in the morning after the patient has had a fat-free breakfast; no food must be given during the test. A dose of 5 mg of sulphobromophthalein sodium per kg body-weight is given as a 5% solution by intravenous injection over a period of about 3 minutes. When fluid retention is present, the dose to be given should be calculated from the patient's ideal weight obtained from tables. Forty-five minutes after the injection the amount of dye remaining in the serum is determined colorimetrically. In patients with normal liver function no more than 5 to 7% of the dye is present in the blood 45 minutes after the injection.

A dose of 2 mg per kg has been used but the results are considered less accurate.

In 904 healthy elderly subjects there was no evidence that age affected retention of sulphobromophthalein.— R. S. Koff *et al.*, *Gastroenterology*, 1973, *65*, 300.

Preparations

Sulfobromophthalein Sodium Injection *(U.S.P.).* Sodium Sulfobromophthalein Injection. A sterile solution of sulphobromophthalein sodium 47 to 53 mg per ml in Water for Injections. pH 5 to 6.5. *Jap.P.* has a similar preparation.

Proprietary Names

Bromophthalein *(Abbott, Austral.)*; Bromotaleina *(Igoda, Spain)*; Bromsulphalein *(Hynson, Westcott & Dunning, Canad.)*; Bromthalein *(E. Merck, Ger.; E. Merck, Swed.; E. Merck, Switz.)*; Hepartest *(Biologische Arbeitsgemeinschaft, Ger.)*.

2152-d

Tolonium Chloride. Toluidine Blue O; CI Basic Blue 17; Colour Index No. 52040. 3-Amino-7-dimethylamino-2-methylphenazathionium chloride; 3-Amino-7-dimethylamino-2-methylphenothiazin-5-ium chloride.

$C_{15}H_{16}ClN_3S$=305.8.

CAS — 92-31-9.

NOTE. Distinguish from Toluidine Blue, Colour Index No. 63340.

A green crystalline powder with a bronze lustre. **Soluble** in water giving a blue-violet solution; slightly soluble in alcohol; very slightly soluble in chloroform; practically insoluble in ether.

Uses. Tolonium chloride has been used by intravenous infusion to stain the parathyroid glands. It has also been given by intra-arterial injection. It has also been used for the diagnosis of oral and gastric malignant neoplasms. The urine of patients during treatment assumes a blue-green colour.

Tolonium chloride was formerly used in the treatment of hypermenorrhoea.

Tolonium chloride (toluidine blue O) has been called toluidine blue (see note above). There are numerous reports of the use of toluidine blue for the staining of body tissue, particularly neoplastic tissue; the reports often provide insufficient detail to identify the dye.

In *mice* pretreatment with tolonium chloride or tolonium chloride and methylene blue protected against potentially lethal doses of morphine, codeine, pethidine, levorphanol, methadone, levopropoxyphene, and dextropropoxyphene. Methylene blue alone was not effective.— D. H. Burke and D. E. Mann, *J. pharm. Sci.*, 1974, *63*, 451.

Brief comment on the use of tolonium chloride 2% in the diagnosis of oral cancer.— J. A. Koufman and S. M. Shapshay (letter), *New Engl. J. Med.*, 1977, *297*, 841.

The use of tolonium chloride in the diagnosis of malignant gastric ulcers.— S. Giler *et al.*, *Archs Surg., Chicago*, 1978, *113*, 136.

The problems of using tolonium chloride in the diagnosis of cancer.— *Lancet*, 1982, *1*, 320.

Staining parathyroid glands. In 18 patients tolonium chloride resulted in dark blue coloration of parathyroid glands sufficient to distinguish them from surrounding tissue. Two patients received intra-arterial injections of 5 mg in 4.5 ml of sodium chloride injection; one had transient recurrent laryngeal nerve paralysis. Sixteen received intravenous infusions over 1 hour, usually of 7 mg per kg body-weight; 3 received 10 mg per kg. Eight patients experienced transient hypertension; 10 of the 13 who received 7 mg per kg experienced depression of the T-wave on the ECG and 2 of those who received 10 mg per kg developed multiple premature ventricular and atrial contractions, flattening of the T-waves, and prolongation of the P-Q interval.— R. M. Yeager and E. T. Krementz, *Ann. Surg.*, 1969, *169*, 829.

Tolonium chloride 3.5 to 5 mg per kg body-weight, in 500 ml of sodium chloride injection, was infused intravenously over 30 to 135 minutes in 10 patients. Parathyroid tissue was readily identified in 8 patients by the blue colour. One patient experienced transient S-T depression of the ECG and one, with glucose-6-phosphate dehydrogenase deficiency, experienced a mild haemolytic reaction.— W. Di Giulio and S. M. Lindenauer, *J. Am. med. Ass.*, 1970, *214*, 2302.

Further references.— P. J. Klopper and R. E. Moe, *Surgery, St Louis*, 1966, *59*, 1101; R. J. Hurvitz *et al.*, *Archs Surg., Chicago*, 1967, *95*, 274; A. O. Singleton and J. Allums, *Archs Surg., Chicago*, 1970, *100*, 372.

Proprietary Names
Menodin *(Fabo, Ital.)*.

2153-n

Tyramine Hydrochloride. *p*-Tyramine Hydrochloride; Tyrosamine Hydrochloride. 4-Hydroxyphenethylamine hydrochloride; 4-(2-Aminoethyl)phenol hydrochloride.

$C_8H_{11}NO,HCl=173.6$.

CAS — 51-67-2 (tyramine); 60-19-5 (hydrochloride).

Tyramine hydrochloride 1.27 g is approximately equivalent to 1 g of tyramine.
Soluble in water.

Stability in solution. An aqueous solution of tyramine hydrochloride containing 12.66 mg per ml (equivalent to tyramine 10 mg) with sodium metabisulphite 0.1%, sterilised by filtration, was stable for 1 year when stored in the dark at 4°. Before use it was diluted with sterile iso-osmotic saline.— K. Engelman and A. Sjoerdsma, *J. Am. med. Ass.*, 1964, *189*, 81.

Adverse Effects and Precautions. Palpitations have been reported following the administration of tyramine hydrochloride. For a discussion of the interaction between monoamine oxidase inhibitors and foods rich in tyramine, see Phenelzine Sulphate, p.129.

Uses. Tyramine hydrochloride is a sympathomimetic agent which has indirect effects on adrenergic receptors. It has been used by intravenous injection in the diagnosis of phaeochromocytoma and has been tried by mouth in doses of up to 250 mg daily in the investigation of migraine. It has also been used, as eye-drops, as a mydriatic.

A procedure known as the tyramine pressor test may be used as a measurement of monoamine oxidase inhibitory activity or of amine uptake blocking activity. The ratio of the dose of tyramine by intravenous injection required to produce a given rise in systolic blood pressure, usually of 30 mmHg, during the investigation period to that necessary during a control period is known as the tyramine sensitivity and a value greater than 1 is usually indicative of amine uptake blocking by the test drug and a value less than 1 of monoamine oxidase inhibitory activity. The procedure has also been used to investigate the pressor response in various physiological and diseased states.

After intravenous administration tyramine was rapidly excreted; the equivalent of 70 to 90% of a dose appeared in the urine within 6 hours. It was not concentrated by the formed elements of the blood. About 85% of excreted material consisted of the main metabolite *p*-hydroxyphenylacetic acid and about 6% was free tyramine. Small amounts of 9 other metabolites were detected, 2 of which were probably *N*-acetyltyramine and *p*-hydroxyphenylacetaldehyde.— M. Tacker *et al.* (letter), *J. Pharm. Pharmac.*, 1972, *24*, 247.

Migraine. The relationship of tyramine-induced headache to migraine.— E. Hanington, *Br. med. J.*, 1967, *2*, 550; E. Hanington and A. M. Harper, *Headache*, 1968, *8*, 84, per *J. Am. med. Ass.*, 1968, *206*, 2784.

Orthostatic hypotension. Tyramine on its own or with phenelzine produced severe supine hypertension in 4 patients with orthostatic hypotension but did not influence their hypotensive response to tilting. The addition of phenelzine merely prolonged the induced hypertension but did not affect its pattern. Phenylephrine and ephedrine controlled the postural symptoms but produced recumbent hypertension. Other therapy should be found.— B. Davies *et al.*, *Lancet*, 1978, *1*, 172. Good results were achieved in 3 patients with severe disabling orthostatic hypotension after treatment with tyramine and tranylcypromine. Treatment was continued for 5, 10, and 12 months.— P. M. Trust (letter), *Lancet*, 1978, *1*, 386.

Monoamine oxidase inhibitors and tyramine have been recommended for orthostatic hypotension, but they cause potentially dangerous recumbent hypertension.— R. Bannister, *Lancet*, 1979, *2*, 404.

Further references: R. N. Nanda *et al.*, *Lancet*, 1976, *2*, 1164.

Phaeochromocytoma. Tyramine hydrochloride was proposed for use as a provocative test for diagnosing phaeochromocytoma; in 5 patients with the disease it produced an exaggerated pressor response (an increase of over 20 mmHg in systolic blood pressure) after intravenous injections equivalent to 1 mg or less of tyramine.— K. Engelman and A. Sjoerdsma, *J. Am. med. Ass.*, 1964, *189*, 81.

The tyramine test was evaluated in 46 hypertensive patients and 58 normal controls. In patients with suspected phaeochromocytoma, a first dose of 250 µg was injected and the blood pressure checked every 30 seconds until stable. If there was no response, further injections of 500 µg, 1 mg, and 1.5 mg of tyramine hydrochloride were given. In other patients, only doses of 1 mg and 1.5 mg were used. Positive reactions occurred in 2 patients with phaeochromocytoma and 7 with labile blood pressure. The test was regarded as useful and safe.— R. N. Thurm *et al.*, *J. Am. med. Ass.*, 1966, *196*, 613.

The intravenous tyramine test gave positive results in 19 of 26 patients with phaeochromocytoma and 3 false positive results in 88 patients with hypertension due to other causes. False negative responses to tyramine were commoner among patients with the familial type of phaeochromocytoma associated with medullary carcinoma of the thyroid gland, or among those undergoing treatment with hydrochlorothiazide or phenoxybenzamine. Inhibition of the result by hydrochlorothiazide persisted for up to 4 days, and by phenoxybenzamine for up to 2 weeks after withdrawal. Palpitation was the only side-effect of the test.— K. Engelman *et al.*, *New Engl. J. Med.*, 1968, *278*, 705.

Further references.— S. G. Sheps and F. T. Maher, *J. Am. med. Ass.*, 1966, *195*, 265; W. J. Louis and A. E. Doyle, *Med. J. Aust.*, 1967, *1*, 1023.

Tyramine pressor test. Reports of the use of the tyramine pressor test in various investigations.— W. A. Pettinger *et al.*, *Clin. Pharmac. Ther.*, 1968, *9*, 442 (monoamine oxidase inhibitory activity of furazolidone); K. Ghose *et al.* (preliminary communication), *Lancet*, 1975, *1*, 1317 (pressor response in depression); K. Ghose *et al.* (letter), *Br. J. clin. Pharmac.*, 1976, *3*, 334 (amine uptake blocking activity of desipramine); A. J. Coppen and K. Ghose, *Arzneimittel-Forsch.*, 1976, *26*, 1166 (amine uptake blocking activity of amitriptyline and absence of this effect by mianserin); K. Ghose *et al.*, *Br. med. J.*, 1977, *1*, 1191 (pressor response in migraine and after therapy with indoramin).

Proprietary Names
Mydrial *(Winzer, Ger.)*.

2154-h

Xylose *(B.P., U.S.P.)*. D-Xylose; Wood Sugar. α-D-Xylopyranose.

$C_5H_{10}O_5=150.1$.

CAS — 6763-34-4.

Pharmacopoeias. In *Br.* and *U.S.*

Odourless colourless needles or white crystalline powder with a slightly sweet taste. **Soluble** 1 in less than 1 of water; slightly soluble in alcohol; soluble in hot alcohol. An ammoniacal aqueous solution is dextrorotatory. **Store** at 15° to 30° in airtight containers.

Adverse Effects and Precautions. Xylose may cause diarrhoea, and abdominal discomfort has been reported to last for 24 hours.

After 25-g doses the mean 5-hour urinary excretion of xylose was 5.7 g in 15 healthy subjects compared with 2.1 g in 7 patients with myxoedema and 7.7 g in 6 with thyrotoxicosis.— S. A. Broitman *et al.*, *New Engl. J. Med.*, 1964, *270*, 333.

In the xylose test indomethacin reduced the intestinal absorption of xylose, possibly due to increased intestinal motility. Aspirin reduced the excretion of xylose, possibly by a renal effect.— M. J. Kendall *et al.*, *Br. med. J.*, 1971, *1*, 533.

Absorption and Fate. Xylose is incompletely absorbed from the gastro-intestinal tract. Part of the absorbed xylose is metabolised in the body to carbon dioxide and water and the remainder is excreted unchanged. About 40 to 50% of a dose administered intravenously and about 30% of a dose taken by mouth have been reported to be excreted in the urine within 5 hours.

Studies of the distribution and metabolism of xylose, arabinose, and lyxose.— J. B. Wyngaarden *et al.*, *J. clin. Invest.*, 1957, *36*, 1395.

Uses. Xylose is used for the diagnosis of malabsorption from the gastro-intestinal tract. It is given by mouth, usually in a dose of either 5 or 25 g, with about 500 ml of water. The amount recovered in the urine in 5 hours is estimated; recovery of less than about 16% is generally considered indicative of malabsorption if renal function is not impaired. The amount of xylose recovered decreases with increasing patient age.

In 114 healthy adults the mean amount of xylose excreted in the first 5 hours after a 25-g dose was 5.7 g; in 28 patients who were being treated for sprue the mean amount excreted was 3.5 g, and in 49 patients with untreated sprue 1.4 g. After a 5-g dose the mean amounts for 29, 23, and 25 patients in the same groups were 1.7 g, 1.2 g, and 550 mg respectively. Absorption and excretion of xylose was also reduced, though less consistently, in patients with megaloblastic anaemias or lesions of the small intestine. Cramp and diarrhoea after 25-g doses, though not usually a problem, could be overcome by the use of 5-g doses. In 4 persons given 1 litre of 10% dextrose solution intravenously after the dose of xylose, blood-glucose concentrations exceeded the usual renal threshold while xylose absorption was at its peak, but the urinary excretion of xylose was not affected.— C. E. Butterworth *et al.*, *New Engl. J. Med.*, 1959, *261*, 157. See also R. Santini *et al.*, *Gastroenterology*, 1961, *40*, 772.

In 10 of 13 children with malabsorption probably due to coeliac disease, the 8-hour excretion of xylose was within normal limits (15 to 30%) after a dose of 15 g per m^2 body-surface. The mean excretion of xylose fell to 5.4% when gliadin 5 g per m^2 was given 2 hours before the xylose. The test was considered to be specific for gliadin-dependent coeliac disease.— H. Theile *et al.*, *Z. Kinderheilk.*, 1968, *103*, 247. See also M. J. Kendall *et al.*, *lancet*, 1972, *1*, 667.

The mean 5-hour urinary excretion of xylose after a 5-g dose in 158 healthy Puerto Rican children was 1.44 g; in 17 treated for tropical sprue it was 1.48 g; and in 30 with tropical sprue (untreated) it was 540 mg.— P. J. Santiago-Borrero *et al.*, *Pediatrics*, 1971, *48*, 59.

A retrospective study was made of 152 patients who had undergone the 25-g xylose absorption test; the criteria for abnormal response were a urinary excretion of less than 4 g in 5 hours or a serum concentration of less than 300 µg per ml at 1.5 hours. Of 38 patients with normal jejunal biopsy, 8 gave an abnormal urine response and 3 an abnormal serum response; none gave an abnormal response to both tests. Of 26 patients with normal jejunal biopsy but with definite gastro-intestinal pathology 5 showed an abnormal urine response and 7 an abnormal serum response; 4 gave an abnormal response to both tests. Of 52 patients with Crohn's disease, 19 gave an abnormal urine response and 8 an abnormal serum response; 5 gave an abnormal response to both tests. Of 36 patients with abnormal jejunal biopsy 31 gave an abnormal urine response and 30 an abnormal serum response; none gave a *normal* response to both tests. The concomitant application of urine and serum tests increased the accuracy of the test which had limited usefulness if facilities for jejunal biopsy were available.— G. E. Sladen and P. J. Kumar, *Br. med. J.*, 1973, *3*, 223. While a 25-g xylose test using a 5-hour urinary collection was not a good screening test for coeliac disease, a 5-g test and a 2-hour collection, carefully performed, was a useful guide to small bowel function.— M. J. Kendall (letter), *ibid.*, 405. The 5-g xylose test, with assessment at 2 hours, was helpful in differentiating malabsorption due to enteropathies from other types of malabsorption.— R. Schneider *et al.* (letter), *ibid.*, 540.

Blood-xylose concentrations were measured in 117 children weighing less than 30 kg one hour after they had been given xylose 5 g in 100 to 200 ml of water after a 6-hour fast. Concentrations below 200 µg per ml were detected in 52 of the 53 children with coeliac disease confirmed by biopsy. The 64 children with normal biopsies had concentrations of 200 µg per ml or more as had an additional 40 children with coeliac disease on a gluten-free diet, 22 patients with cystic fibrosis, and 75 control children. It was recommended that for children of less than 30 kg a result of 200 µg per ml or less confirmed by a repeat test should be an indication for small-bowel biopsy.— C. J. Rolles *et al., Lancet,* 1973, *2,* 1043. In an evaluation of the one-hour blood-xylose test in 46 children with untreated coeliac disease there was one false-normal result, six of 102 control subjects gave false-abnormal results; 4 of these were above the 30-kg body-weight limit recommended by Rolles.— U. Schaad *et al., Archs Dis. Childh.,* 1978, *53,* 420.

The xylose tolerance test, as a screening procedure for coeliac disease, was reassessed in 54 children (4 months to 16 years old) with normal renal function. Xylose was given to fasted subjects in a dose of 400 mg per kg body-weight up to a maximum of 7.5 g, as a 3% aqueous solution. The 5- and 24-hour urinary excretion rates of xylose and 3-hour blood-xylose concentrations did not discriminate between subjects with or without coeliac disease. One-hour blood-xylose concentrations were also an unreliable guide.— S. P. Lamabadusuriya *et al., Archs Dis. Childh.,* 1975, *50,* 34. Comment.— C. J. Rolles *et al.* (letter), *ibid.,* 748. A reply.— S. P. Lamabadusuriya *et al.* (letter), *ibid.,* 749.

The one-hour blood-xylose test before and after gluten challenge confirmed the presence of malabsorption of coeliac disease in 15 of 16 infants and children previously diagnosed in early infancy.— C. J. Rolles *et al., Archs Dis. Childh.,* 1975, *50,* 259.

Limitations of the xylose absorption test using 15 g in the diagnosis of coeliac disease.— F. M. Stevens *et al., J. clin. Path.,* 1977, *30,* 76.

A modified one-hour xylose test using a nasoduodenal tube for administration of xylose to neonates.— D. A. Ducker *et al., Archs Dis. Childh.,* 1978, *53,* 690.

The use of the one-hour blood xylose test in the diagnosis of cow's milk protein intolerance in children.— C. L. Morin *et al., Lancet,* 1979, *1,* 1102.

Proprietary Names
Xylo-pfan *(Pfanstiehl, USA).*

2155-m

Glucose Enzymatic Test Strip *(U.S.P.).*

Consists of glucose oxidase, horseradish peroxidase, a suitable substrate for the reaction of hydrogen peroxide catalysed by peroxidase, and other inert ingredients impregnated and dried on filter paper. In human urine of known glucose concentration it reacts in the specified times to produce colours corresponding to the colour chart provided. Store at 15° to 30°.

2156-b

Some Proprietary Test Substances

The preparations listed below include some of the more important tests for the detection of pathological states and for the laboratory control of treatment, and, in general, are limited to those sold under proprietary names from which their use may not be immediately evident. No attempt has been made to cover the very wide range of diagnostic substances and adjuncts used in the laboratory. Also no attempt has been made to cover the radioassays used to determine hormone concentrations or hormone-binding capacities in body fluids.

AccUric *(General Diagnostics, UK).* A colorimetric system for the determination of uric acid.

Acetest *(Ames, UK).* A brand of Diagnostic Nitroprusside Tablets (see under Sodium Nitroprusside, p.168); for detecting the presence of acetone and aceto-acetic acid in urine. Prior administration of phenolsulphonphthalein may cause a false positive reaction. Tests may also be carried out on serum, plasma, or whole blood.

Phenolphthalein and pyrazinamide could cause erroneous results in the Acetest test.— *Drug & Ther. Bull.,* 1972, *10,* 69.

False positive reactions to Acetest tablets had been found during therapy with levodopa.— C. J. Mitchell, *Ames, Chemist Drugg.,* 1978, *209,* 632.

Albustix *(Ames, UK).* Reagent strips for detecting the presence of protein in urine. Strongly alkaline or highly buffered specimens or contamination by quaternary ammonium compounds may cause false positive reactions.

False positive reactions with Albustix had been found during therapy with aminocaproic acid and were most likely to occur in urine containing 25 mg per ml or more of aminocaproic acid.— M. W. Cooksey and M. S. Knapp (letter), *Br. med. J.,* 1968, *1,* 769.

Albym Test *(Boehringer Corp., UK).* Reagent strips for the detection of protein in urine.

AmnicatoR *(Medical Wire, UK).* Reagent strips for determining the pH of the upper vagina to indicate whether or not amniorrhexis, the rupture of the amniotic membranes, has occurred.

Aspergillosis Sero-Diagnostic *(Bencard, UK).* A kit for the detection in serum of antibodies to *Aspergillus fumigatus.*

Atroxin *(Sigma, UK).* A kit for measuring the clotting time of plasma using *Bothrops atrox* venom.

Ausab *(Abbott, UK).* A radio-immunoassay kit for the detection of antibody to hepatitis B surface antigen in serum or plasma.

Auscell *(Abbott, UK).* A haemagglutination test for the detection of hepatitis B surface antigen in serum or recalcified plasma.

Ausria II-125 *(Abbott, UK).* A radio-immunoassay kit for the detection of hepatitis B surface antigen in serum. A confirmatory kit is available.

Auszyme *(Abbott, UK).* An enzyme-immunoassay kit for the detection of hepatitis B surface antigen in serum or plasma.

Azostix *(Ames, UK).* Reagent strips for the detection of urea in blood.

A comparison of Azostix and Urastrat showed Azostix to be more inaccurate and to give results consistently lower than the true values, but because the procedure was simpler and quicker it was preferred to Urastrat for use by general medical practitioners.— J. D. E. Knox, *Practitioner,* 1969, *202,* 280.

In patients with severe acidosis Azostix might give an underestimate of the blood-urea concentration, which might be slightly overestimated in alkalosis.— S. M. Hall and I. W. Preston (letter), *Br. med. J.,* 1971, *3,* 434.

Bili-Labstix *(Ames, UK).* Reagent strips for urine testing, similar to Labstix (see p.528) with the addition of a portion to detect the presence of bilirubin.

An analysis of the 170 (0.35%) false negative tests for urine glucose found in 47 750 consecutive negative urine investigations.— J. S. Mayson *et al.* (letter), *Lancet,* 1973, *1,* 780.

Bilugen Test *(Boehringer Corp., UK).* Reagent strips for urine testing. Colour changes indicate the presence of bilirubin and urobilinogen.

Bilur Test *(Boehringer Corp., UK).* Reagent strips for the detection of bilirubin in serum or urine.

Blue ASO Test *(Fujizoki, Jap.: Diamed, UK).* A kit for the detection of anti-streptolysin-O antibody in serum.

BM-Test 3 *(Boehringer Corp., UK).* Reagent strips for urine testing. Colour changes indicate pH and the presence of protein and glucose. **BM-Test 4.** Indicates nitrite additionally to the tests of BM-Test 3.

BM-Test 5L *(Boehringer Corp., UK).* Reagent strips for urine testing. Colour changes indicate pH and the presence of protein, glucose, ketone, and blood. **BM-Test 6.** Indicates urobilinogen additionally to the tests of BM-Test 5L. **BM-Test 7.** Indicates bilirubin additionally to the tests of BM-Test 6. **BM-Test 8.** Indicates nitrite additionally to the tests of BM-Test 7.

BM-Test Glucose *(Boehringer Corp., UK).* Reagent strips for the detection of glucose in urine.

BM-Test Glycemie 20-800 *(Boehringer Corp., UK).* Reagent strips for the detection of glucose in blood, having two zones with different sensitivities.

References: K. Graham *et al., Br. med. J.,* 1980, *281,* 971; S. Walford *et al.* (letter,), *Lancet,* 1980, *1,* 653; J. E. Earis *et al.* (letter,), *ibid.,* 823; G. D. Podmore and P. R. Beck (letter), *ibid.,* 1981, *1,* 53.

BM-Test Meconium *(Boehringer Corp., UK).* Reagent strips to detect an increased concentration of albumin in the meconium, indicative of cystic fibrosis.

Reference.— I. Antonowicz (letter), *Lancet,* 1976, *1,* 746.

Cephotest *(Nyco, Norw.: BDH Chemicals, UK).* A reagent for determining the activity of the intrinsic clotting system.

Clinistix *(Ames, UK).* Reagent strips for detecting the presence of glucose in urine. The sensitivity of the test may be influenced by inhibiting substances, temperature and pH of the urine, and experience of the user.

Hypochlorites and hydrogen peroxide could cause false positives and levodopa or large doses of ascorbic acid could cause false negatives in the Clinistix test.— *Drug & Ther. Bull.,* 1972, *10,* 69.

Clinitest Reagent Tablets *(Ames, UK).* A brand of Diagnostic Solution-tablets of Copper (see Copper Sulphate, p.931) for indicating the presence and approximate amounts of glucose in urine. A positive reaction is also given by other reducing sugars and other substances, including ascorbic acid and salicylates.

An unusual black-brown colour reaction occurred when Clinitest was used to test the urine of patients who were being treated with cephalothin.— J. Kostis and S. S. Bergen (letter), *J. Am. med. Ass.,* 1966, *196,* 805.

Prior intravenous administration of sodium diatrizoate could cause a greenish-black or black colour.— S. Lee and I. Schoen, *New Engl. J. Med.,* 1966, *275,* 266.

The Clinitest method was accurate in the range 0 to 2% when 5 drops of urine were used; at sugar concentrations over 4% there was reversal of colour which could be confused with lower concentrations. The use of 2 drops of urine eliminated confusion of colour, and the range was extended.— M. M. Belmonte *et al., Diabetes,* 1967, *16,* 557. In a study of 10 juvenile diabetics the Clinitest method using 2 drops of urine could detect up to 5% glycosuria without significant loss of accuracy and was recommended in preference to the 5-drop method.— N. K. Griffin *et al., Archs Dis. Childh.,* 1979, *54,* 371.

Nalidixic acid could cause false positives in the Clinitest test.— *Drug & Ther. Bull.,* 1972, *10,* 69.

An 82-year-old woman developed localised stricture of the oesophagus after swallowing a Clinitest tablet in error for aspirin. Of 16 reports in the literature of ingestion of Clinitest tablets, 13 were followed; strictures developed in 11.— R. J. Payten (letter), *Br. med. J.,* 1972, *4,* 728.

Localised stricture of the oesophagus was reported in 5 children after accidental swallowing of Clinitest tablets. Since the use of lemon juice or vinegar as antidotes to neutralise the sodium hydroxide in the tablets intensified the release of heat and degree of burning, cold milk or tap water were preferred for emergency treatment.— J. D. Burrington, *Ann. thorac. Surg.,* 1975, *20,* 400. See also B. H. Rumack and J. D. Burrington, *Clin. Toxicol.,* 1977, *11,* 27.

A report of the ingestion of Clinitest by 8 patients over 4 years, without serious sequelae. One patient took 47 tablets over 1 month. Earlier reports of Clinitest poisoning were reviewed.— A. Mallory and J. W. Schaefer, *Br. med. J.,* 1977, *2,* 105.

Effervescence during the use of Clinitest and injudicious disposal of residues could lead to the dissemination of pathogens present in the specimen of urine or faeces.— D. Barrie and J. C. Coleman, *Br. med. J.,* 1977, *2,* 368.

Of 100 diabetic patients watched while testing urine with Clinitest tablets only 20 made no mistakes; more time should be spent on initial instruction.— G. M. Shenfield and J. M. Steel, *Practitioner,* 1977, *218,* 147.

If Clinitest tablets are swallowed, large volumes of citric fruit juice or milk with a tablespoon of vegetable oil should be given as soon as possible. Vomiting should not be induced. Contact with the skin or eyes should be treated by copious irrigation with tepid water, for 15 minutes if eyes are affected.— C. J. Mitchell, *Ames, Chemist Drugg.,* 1978, *209,* 632.

Corab *(Abbott, UK).* A radio-immunoassay kit for the detection of antibody to hepatitis B core antigen in serum or plasma.

CRP-Wellcotest *(Wellcome Reagents, UK).* A latex agglutination slide test for the detection of C-reactive protein in serum, in the diagnosis of inflammatory and infectious diseases.

C-Stix *(Ames, UK).* Reagent strips for the estimation of ascorbic acid in urine.

Cytoclair *(Sinclair, UK).* A powder used as a 2% solution to concentrate sputum for the identification of malignant cells.

Cytoclair 2% in sodium chloride solution added to sputum before the preparation of slides or of millipore membrane studies was considered to be of some use in the detection of malignant cells in the sputum of certain patients with primary lung cancer.— J. M. Grainger and O. A. N. Husain, *J. clin. Path.,* 1978, *31,* 585.

Cytur-Test *(Boehringer Corp., UK)*. Reagent strips for the detection of leucocytes in urine.

Dextrostix *(Ames, UK)*. Reagent strips for the approximate estimation of glucose in blood.

Comparison of 267 Dextrostix estimations, with laboratory results showed a general tendency for Dextrostix to underestimate; agreement between the 2 estimations was poorest in the blood-sugar range 90 to 200 mg per 100 ml. There was no tendency to overestimate in the lower ranges.— N. MacKay *et al.*, *Lancet*, 1965, *2*, 269.

Comparison of 516 Dextrostix estimations with laboratory results showed that dextrostix underestimated blood-glucose concentration in all parts of the range by up to 33%.— K. G. M. M. Alberti *et al.*, *Lancet*, 1965, *2*, 319.

The prime cause of discrepant results was differences in the colour discrimination of the technicians who interpreted the results.— J. A. Rock and L. J. Gerende, *J. Am. med. Ass.*, 1966, *198*, 231.

An insulin-dependent diabetic with a venous blood-glucose concentration of 300 µg per ml showed an apparent blood-glucose concentration of 1.75 to 2.5 mg per ml when assessed on capillary blood by Dextrostix. The discrepancy was attributed to a brown discoloration between blood and 70% isopropyl alcohol used for skin swabbing.— S. G. Ball and A. S. B. Hughes (letter), *Br. med. J.*, 1976, *1*, 1279.

The activity of Dextrostix could be validated by dipping a strip into a 2.5 mmol per litre solution of glucose in saturated sodium benzoate; this solution gives a consistent reading of 90 mg per 100 ml.— J. R. Stradling (letter), *Lancet*, 1976, *2*, 690. A better technique and one recommended by the manufacturer was to apply a large drop of the solution to the reagent strip area. The drop should be applied from a nozzle for consistency. This technique gave a consistent reading of 47 mg per 100 ml.— S. J. Iqbal *et al.* (letter), *ibid.*, 1027.

Diafib *(Diamed, UK)*. Bovine fibrinogen for use in coagulation tests.

Diascreen and Diascreen A *(Diamed, UK)*. Reagents for the determination of blood coagulability.

Diastix *(Ames, UK)*. Reagent strips for the estimation of glucose in urine.

A favourable report.— A. D. B. Harrower *et al.*, *Practitioner*, 1974, *213*, 241.

In 3 patients with glycosuria when assessed by Clinistix, no glycosuria was detected by Diastix.— S. E. Browne (letter), *Br. med. J.*, 1977, *2*, 1670.

Dicopac *(Amersham International, UK)*. A radioassay test kit for the determination *in vivo* of vitamin B_{12} absorption.

Dipkit *(Medical Wire, UK)*. Plastic containers with dip spoons containing nutrient media for the detection and quantitative estimation of bacteria in urine.

Discover-2 *(Carter-Wallace, UK)*. A pregnancy test, for use in the home, for the detection of human chorionic gonadotrophin in urine; the result is read at 2 hours. Reagents for a second test are included.

DNA Test *(Fujizoki, Jap.: Diamed, UK)*. A haemagglutination test for the detection of antibodies to double-stranded DNA in systemic lupus erythematosus.

Duo-Spore *(Propper, UK: Horwell, UK)*. Strips prepared from spore suspensions for use as biological monitors for steam, gas, and dry heat sterilisation processes.

DyAmyl-L *(General Diagnostics, UK)*. A colorimetric system for the quantitative determination of amylase in serum and urine.

Fermcozyme 653AM *(Hughes & Hughes, UK)*. A glucose oxidase reagent for use in the determination of blood-glucose concentrations. **Fermcozyme 952DM.** A similar reagent containing in addition peroxidase.

Ferro-Check, Hyland *(Travenol, UK)*. A colorimetric test for the determination of serum iron and serum iron-binding capacity.

Fibrindex *(Ortho Diagnostics, UK)*. Thrombin (human), available as powder for solution before use, for fibrinogen determinations.

Fibros *(Inolex, USA: Horwell, UK)*. Filter papers impregnated with precipitated silver chromate; for the diagnosis of cystic fibrosis of the pancreas by the semi-quantitative determination of excess chlorides in the sweat.

Gammadisk-Digoxin Test Kit *(Wellcome Reagents, UK)*. A radio-immunoassay kit for determination of digoxin in serum or plasma.

Gas-Chex *(Propper, UK: Horwell, UK)*. A sterilisation indicator in which a colour change indicates exposure to and penetration of ethylene oxide.

Gluketur-Test *(Boehringer Corp., UK)*. Reagent strips for urine testing. Colour changes indicate the presence of glucose and ketones.

Gravindex *(Ortho Diagnostics, UK)*. A rapid latex agglutination-inhibition slide test for pregnancy.

The overall accuracy of results obtained with the Gravindex test in 83 specimens of urine was 97.6%.— J. Brodie and H. Mellis, *Practitioner*, 1966, *196*, 821. See also B. M. Hobson, *ibid.*, 1969, *202*, 388.

Protein in the urine might produce false positive reactions.— J. L. Bell, *Lancet*, 1967, *2*, 559.

False positive results to the Gravindex test were obtained when the urine was collected in bottles containing a capsule of boric acid as a preservative. This error was due to the capsule materials and not the boric acid.— R. J. Fallon and B. M. Hobson (letter), *Lancet*, 1973, *1*, 1243.

Haemoccult (formerly known as Hemoccult) *(Norwich-Eaton, UK)*. A test kit comprising of slides impregnated with guaiacum resin and a hydrogen peroxide reagent. For detection of occult blood in faeces.

False-negative results of Hemoccult test in colorectal cancer.— C. D. M. Griffith *et al.*, *Br. med. J.*, 1981, *283*, 472. Correspondence.— K. D. Vellacott *et al.* (letter), *ibid.*, 795; C. D. M. Griffith and J. H. Saunders (letter), *ibid.*; R. Gnauck (letter), *ibid.*

Evidence that cimetidine does not provoke a false-positive reaction in the Hemoccult Test.— P. Herzog and K. H. Holtermüller (letter), *New Engl. J. Med.*, 1981, *305*, 644.

Havab *(Abbott, UK)*. A radio-immunoassay kit for the detection of antibody to hepatitis A virus in serum or plasma.

Limitations of the Havab test for antibody to hepatitis A virus.— J. V. R. Berg *et al.* (letter), *Lancet*, 1979, *1*, 212.

Hema-Combistix *(Ames, UK)*. Reagent strips for urine testing, separately impregnated in 4 portions. Colour changes indicate the pH and the presence of glucose, protein, and blood respectively.

Hemastix *(Ames, UK)*. Reagent strips for detecting the presence of blood in urine. The presence of ascorbic acid in the specimen may reduce the sensitivity of the test.

Hemastix reagent strips could be used to test for occult blood in the stools. Results obtained from 210 specimens were compared with those from a standard test and agreement was found for 87% with 11% false positive and 2% false negative results.— H. Lehmann and E. G. Kitchin (letter), *Lancet*, 1971, *2*, 258.

The iodine in povidone-iodine could cause false positives in tests using orthotolidine reagent used for detecting blood in urine or faeces.— W. N. Hait *et al.* (letter), *New Engl. J. Med.*, 1977, *297*, 1350.

Hemo-Fec *(Med-Kjemi, Norw.: Diamed, UK)*. A test kit for the detection of occult blood in faeces.

Hepanosticon *(Organon Teknika, UK)*. A haemagglutination test for the detection of hepatitis B antigen in serum or plasma.

An evaluation.— E. M. Vandervelde *et al.*, *Lancet*, 1974, *2*, 1066.

Hepanostika *(Organon Teknika, UK)*. An enzyme-immunoassay for the detection of hepatitis B surface antigen in serum.

The Hepanostika test was a suitable alternative to the Ausria II-125 test and was more specific than the Hepanosticon test.— W. Lange *et al.*, *Dt. med. Wschr.*, 1977, *102*, 1581.

Hepatest *(Wellcome Reagents, UK)*. A haemagglutination test for the detection of hepatitis B surface antigen in serum.

Hepanosticon and Hepatest were compared with immunodiffusion and found to be suitable tests for hepatitis B antigen.— A. G. Shattock and A. N. Smith (letter), *Lancet*, 1975, *1*, 227. See also D. Chicot *et al.*, *ibid.*, 345; G. Wolters *et al.* (letter), *ibid.*, 1193.

Hypronosticon *(Organon Teknika, UK)*. A colorimetric kit for the determination of hydroxyproline in urine.

Ictotest *(Ames, UK)*. Reagent tablets for the detection of bilirubin in the urine. Highly pigmented specimens, or specimens containing dyes which give colours in acid media, may mask weak positive reactions.

Six of 45 patients taking mefenamic or flufenamic acid had positive results to tests for excretion of bile in the urine determined by means of Ictotest reagent. It was considered that the positive results probably indicated the presence of drug metabolites rather than bilirubinuria.— R. M. H. Kater, *Med. J. Aust.*, 1968, *1*, 848.

Kernlute *(Ames, UK)*. A test kit for determining the residual binding capacity of serum albumin for bilirubin.

Keto-Diastix *(Ames, UK)*. Reagent strips for the colorimetric estimation of ketone bodies and glucose in urine.

Ketostix *(Ames, UK)*. Reagent strips for detecting the presence of ketones in urine, serum, and plasma. Prior administration of sulphobromophthalein, phenolsulphonphthalein, or phenolphthalein, may cause false positive reactions.

Pyrazinamide could cause erroneous results in the Ketostix test.— *Drug & Ther. Bull.*, 1972, *10*, 69.

Ketostix were used in the diagnosis and management of 50 patients with diabetic coma and precoma. Results were reproducible. Ketostix values of acetoacetate were often lower than those obtained by enzymatic determination. Total ketone values as shown by Ketostix were even less correlated with laboratory values, due to a high 3-hydroxybutyrate to acetate ratio in some patients; 3-hydroxybutyrate was not detected by Ketostix. A negative response to Ketostix in association with a blood pH below 7.2 was an indication for enzymatic determination.— K. G. M. M. Alberti and T. D. R. Hockaday, *Br. med. J.*, 1972, *2*, 565.

Klintex Autoclave Test Papers *(Whitelaw, UK)*. Test papers for placing as indicators in drums and parcels to be autoclaved.

Labstix *(Ames, UK)*. Reagent strips for urine testing, separately impregnated in 5 portions. Colour changes indicate the pH and the presence of protein, glucose, ketones, and blood respectively.

The use of Labstix for assessing protein and glucose concentrations in the CSF.— R. P. Schwartz and J. C. Parke, *J. Pediat.*, 1971, *78*, 677.

Hypochlorites and hydrogen peroxide could cause false positives for glucose and levodopa or large doses of ascorbic acid could cause false negatives in the Labstix tests.— *Drug & Ther. Bull.*, 1972, *10*, 69.

Glycosuria was indicated by Clinistix in 3 patients but not by Labstix.— S. E. Browne (letter), *Br. med. J.*, 1977, *2*, 1670.

Le-Test, Hyland *(Travenol, UK)*. An agglutination slide test for the detection in serum of factors associated with systemic lupus erythematosus.

Luteonosticon *(Organon Teknika, UK)*. A haemagglutination-inhibition test kit for the detection and approximate quantitative estimation of luteinising hormone in urine.

Mecostix *(Ames, UK)*. Reagent strips to detect an increased concentration of albumin in meconium, indicative of cystic fibrosis.

Microsome Test *(Fujizoki, Jap.: Diamed, UK)*. A haemagglutination test for the detection of microsomal antibodies associated with thyroid auto-immune disease.

Microstix-3 *(Ames, UK)*. Reagent strips for the detection of nitrite in urine, indicating bacteriuria, with separate areas for the culture of bacteria.

Comparison with dip slides.— J. M. T. Hamilton-Miller, *Postgrad. med. J.*, 1977, *53*, 248.

An evaluation of the use of Microstix in the examination of 57 urine specimens in general practice showed that nitrite was detected in 53% of 15 specimens found by laboratory culture to have significant bacteriuria, while 2 specimens showed false positive results; in the bacterial incubation test Microstix identified all but 1 specimen with bacteriuria. Growth for total bacterial count was identical for Gram-negative bacteria only. Further studies to evaluate Microstix as a diagnostic agent in general practice were recommended.— R. A. Collacott, *J.R. Coll. gen. Pract.*, 1977, *27*, 104.

Monospot *(Ortho Diagnostics, UK)*. A 1-minute slide test for the diagnosis of infectious mononucleosis.

A short discussion of the tests for infectious mononucleosis. In some individuals the Monospot test may give an anomalous and at present inexplicable false positive result. Nevertheless, these findings are uncommon, and their occasional appearance should not detract from the value of the Monospot test as a rapid and easily available test for mononucleosis due to Epstein-Barr virus.— *Br. med. J.*, 1980, *280*, 1153.

Monosticon *(Organon Teknika, UK)*. A 2-minute slide test for the detection of infectious mononucleosis.

MPS Papers *(Ames, UK)*. A spot test for the detection of increased concentrations of acid mucopolysaccharides in urine, indicative of Hurler's syndrome and related disorders. A low sodium chloride concentration, or the presence of DNA, RNA, or heparin may cause false positive reactions.

Multistix *(Ames, UK)*. Reagent strips for urine testing, separately impregnated in 7 portions. Colour changes indicate the pH and the presence of protein, glucose, ketones, blood, bilirubin, and urobilinogen respectively.

Nephur-Test *(Boehringer Corp., UK)*. Reagent strips for urine testing. Colour changes indicate pH and the presence of blood, glucose, protein, and nitrite.**Nephur-Test + Leucocytes**. Indicates the presence of leucocytes additionally to the tests of Nephur-Test.

Nitur-Test *(Boehringer Corp., UK)*. Reagent strips for the detection of nitrite in urine, indicating bacteriuria. Nitur-Test was formerly marketed in Great Britain under the proprietary name BM-Test Nitrite.

BM-Test Nitrite could not replace the dipslide culture method when only a single random urine sample is available.— J. P. Guignard and A. Torrado (letter), *Lancet*, 1978, *1*, 47.

A study involving 1058 girls aged 5 to 12 years demonstrated that BM-Test Nitrite gave a higher percentage of false negative results than a dipslide culture.— C. A. Sinaniotis *et al.* (letter), *Lancet*, 1978, *1*, 776.

Evaluation of the nitrite dip-strip test in 21 girls with bacteriuria indicated that if this test was used for screening then it would miss 15 to 20% of subjects with Gram-negative bacteriuria and an additional 5% with Gram-positive infections.— C. M. Kunin and J. E. DeGroot, *Pediatrics*, 1977, *60*, 244.

N-Labstix *(Ames, UK)*. Reagent strips for urine testing, separately impregnated in 6 portions. Colour changes indicate the pH and the presence of protein, glucose, ketones, blood, and nitrite respectively.

A study involving 62 patients indicated that although convenient the N-Labstix test was too inaccurate for the diagnosis of urinary infections.— R. A. Collacott, *Practitioner*, 1977, *218*, 123.

N-Multistix *(Ames, UK)*. Reagent strips for urine testing, separately impregnated in 8 portions. Colour changes indicate the pH and the presence of protein, glucose, ketones, bilirubin, blood, nitrite, and urobilinogen respectively.

Normotest *(Nyco, Norw.: BDH Chemicals, UK)*. A reagent containing standardised thromboplastin, factor V, fibrinogen, and calcium. For the estimation of clotting factors II, VII, and X as a test of liver function and as a screening test for deficiences in the extrinsic clotting system.

OK Monitor Strip *(Propper, UK: Horwell, UK)*. A sterilisation indicator in which a colour change indicates exposure to and penetration of steam. **OK Monitor Bags** and **OK Steri-Stik** (self-sealing) bags are also available.

Okokit *(Hughes & Hughes, UK)*. A test kit for the detection of occult blood in faeces. See also under Guaiacum Resin, p.315.

One-A-Day Autoclave Test Sheet *(Propper, UK: Horwell, UK)*. A sterilisation indicator for checking the absence of air in autoclaves.

Ortho Aslo Test *(Ortho Diagnostics, UK)*. A 1-minute latex test for the presence of clinically significant concentrations of anti-streptolysin-O.

Ortho RA Test *(Ortho Diagnostics, UK)*. A 1-minute slide test for the detection of rheumatoid factor in serum.

Oxoid Dip Slide *(Oxoid, UK)*. Sterile plastic containers with slides coated with nutrient media, for the detection and approximate identification and quantitative estimation of bacteria in urine.

In a study in 902 schoolgirls the Oxoid Dip Slide test gave no false negative results with 1.9% of false positives. In a subsequent study in 680 children the incidence of false positives was 4% by the immersion technique and 13.5% by the dipstream technique; the latter figure could be reduced to 1.8%, with a negligible risk of overlooking genuine bacteriuria, by disregarding non-faecal organisms.— B. Edwards *et al.*, *Br. med. J.*, 1975, *2*, 463.

Peroheme 40-c *(BDH Chemicals, UK)*. A reagent system for the detection of occult blood in faeces.

Phenistix *(Ames, UK)*. Reagent strips for the detection of phenylketones (phenylpyruvic acid) and para-aminosalicylic acid in urine.

Phenistix could detect high serum-salicylate concentrations and were of use in the diagnosis of salicylate poisoning.— G. G. Muir and S. Benson, *Br. med. J.*, 1964, *1*, 1686.

The colour change (grey-purple) produced when Phenistix were dipped in urine containing phenothiazines could be distinguished from that produced by urine containing salicylates by placing on the Phenistix a drop of 50% sulphuric acid. The colour due to phenothiazines was enhanced; that due to salicylates was bleached.— *Drug & Ther. Bull.*, 1968, *6*, 103.

Each of 3 tests—paper chromatography test of urine, Guthrie test for phenylalanine in blood, and a modification of the Guthrie test for phenylalanine in urine—was found to be more efficient than the Phenistix test for the detection of phenylketonuria at an early age.—Medical Research Council Working Party on Phenylketonuria, *Br. med. J.*, 1968, *4*, 7. A report on 3 false positive phenylketonuria tests among 35 000 assays.— L. T. Kirby *et al.* (letter), *Lancet*, 1980, *2*, 585.

A deep red-brown coloration occurred when Phenistix was dipped into the urine of infants treated with desferrioxamine for iron poisoning.— H. V. L. Finlay (letter), *Br. med. J.*, 1978, *2*, 356.

Mention of the use of Phenistix in the detection of salicylate abuse.— J. M. Duggan and J. E. Dickeson (letter), *Med. J. Aust.*, 1979, *1*, 340.

Phosphastrate Acid *(General Diagnostics, UK)*. A reagent system for the quantitative colorimetric estimation of acid phosphatase in plasma or serum.

Phosphastrate Alkaline *(General Diagnostics, UK)*. A reagent system for the quantitative colorimetric estimation of alkaline phosphatase in plasma or serum.

Placentex *(Roche, UK)*. An indirect latex agglutination test for pregnancy.

Platelin *(General Diagnostics, UK)*. Standardised freeze-dried platelet factor reagent (partial thromboplastin), containing rabbit-brain cephalin; used in the partial thromboplastin time test and the Hicks-Pitney modification of the thromboplastin generation test. **Platelin Plus Activator** is a platelet factor reagent which also contains a controlled amount of activator.

Predictor *(Chefaro, UK)*. A pregnancy test, for use in the home, for the detection of human chorionic gonadotrophin in urine. The result is read at 2 hours.

Predictor kits were given to 86 women with possible pregnancy for use in their home after a mean of 54 days of amenorrhoea; results in 83 coincided with those obtained with standard tests.— P. R. Grob *et al.* (letter), *Br. med. J.*, 1973, *1*, 112.

Pregnate *(Fisher, USA: Horwell, UK)*. A rapid latex agglutination-inhibition slide test for pregnancy.

Pregnosticon *(Organon Teknika, UK)*. An immunological tube test for pregnancy. The result is read at 2 hours. **Pregnosticon All-In.** A modified version of Pregnosticon with pre-measured reagents. The result is read at 2 hours. Stated to have the same sensitivity as Pregnosticon.

Protein in the urine might produce false positive reactions.— J. L. Bell (letter), *Lancet*, 1967, *2*, 559.

The accuracy of results obtained with the Pregnosticon test in 1103 specimens of urine was 98.9%.— M. B. Hobson, *Practitioner*, 1969, *202*, 388. See also J. Brodie and H. Mellis, *ibid.*, 1966, *196*, 821.

In 19 887 pregnancy tests with Pregnosticon, the accuracy was 99.2%. The sensitivity of the test was such that a positive result was obtained with a urine concentration of chorionic gonadotrophin equivalent to 1 or more units per ml.— B. M. Hobson (letter), *Lancet*, 1969, *2*, 56.

Correct results were obtained in 98.13% of tests of Pregnosticon All-In in 107 patients.— B. Berić and J. Djurdjević, *Arzneimittel-Forsch.*, 1971, *21*, 2030.

The use of Pregnosticon in assessing the prognosis of threatened abortion.— P. R. Grob and F. J. Gibbs, *Practitioner*, 1972, *209*, 79.

Pregnosticon Planotest *(Organon Teknika, UK)*. A 2-minute pregnancy slide test. Stated to be less sensitive than Pregnosticon.

In 300 women tested, Pregnosticon Planotest showed a high degree of reliability for the diagnosis of pregnancy.— P. R. Grob *et al.*, *Practitioner*, 1968, *201*, 811.

The accuracy of results obtained with the Pregnosticon Planotest in 1103 specimens of urine was 98.1%.— B. M. Hobson, *Practitioner*, 1969, *202*, 388.

Pregnostisec *(Organon Teknika, UK)*. A 2-minute slide test for pregnancy with pre-measured reagents. Stated to be less sensitive than Pregnosticon.

Prepurex *(Wellcome Reagents, UK)*. A 2-minute latex agglutination-inhibition slide test for the detection of human chorionic gonadotrophin in urine, particularly in pregnancy.

RAHA Test *(Fujizoki, Jap.: Diamed, UK)*. A haemagglutination test for the detection of rheumatoid factor in serum.

Reflotest-Glucose *(Boehringer Corp., UK)*. Test strips for use with the Reflomat reflectance meter for estimation of glucose in blood and serum.

Rheuma-fac *(Boehringer Corp., UK)*. Latex slide or tube tests for the detection of rheumatoid factors.

Rheuma-Wellcotest *(Wellcome Reagents, UK)*. A 2-minute latex agglutination slide test for the detection of rheumatoid factor in serum.

Sangur-Test *(Boehringer Corp., UK)*. Reagent strips for detecting the presence of blood in urine.

Serameba *(Ames, UK)*. A latex agglutination test to detect antibodies resulting from past or present tissue invasion by *Entamoeba histolytica*.

Serodia-AFP *(Fujizoki, Jap.: Diamed, UK)*. A rapid test for the serological detection and measurement of alpha-fetoprotein in the diagnosis of hepatoma.

Serodia-Anti HBs *(Fujizoki, Jap.: Diamed, UK)*. A haemagglutination test for the detection and titration of antibody to hepatitis B surface antigen.

Serodia-HBs *(Fujizoki, Jap.: Diamed, UK)*. A kit for the serological detection of hepatitis B surface antigen.

Serodia-Myco Test *(Fujizoki, Jap.: Diamed, UK)*. A kit for the rapid serological diagnosis of *Mycoplasma* infections.

Sickledex *(Ortho Diagnostics, UK)*. A kit for the detection of haemoglobin S in blood in conditions such as sickle-cell anaemia.

The presence of haemoglobin S was demonstrated by the Sickledex test in blood from 130 of 619 persons; the results correlated well with those obtained by other testing methods.— M. S. Ballard *et al.*, *J. Pediat.*, 1970, *76*, 117.

Simplastin *(General Diagnostics, UK)*. Standardised, freeze-dried, thromboplastin calcium for use in coagulation tests for prothrombin time.

SPAC Digoxin Kit *(Byk-Mallinckrodt, UK)*. A radioimmunoassay kit for the determination of digoxin in serum.

Strate-Line *(Propper, UK: Horwell, UK)*. A sterilisation indicator in which a colour change indicates exposure to and penetration of steam.

Temp-Plate *(Wahl, USA: Auriema, UK)*. A range of self-adhesive temperature indicators which change colour permanently when a specific temperature (37° to 260°) is reached.

Temptubes *(Propper, UK: Horwell, UK)*. Sealed sterilisation indicator tubes containing pellets which melt and change colour at 121°.**Hi-Speed Temptubes**. Indicator tubes in which the pellets melt and change colour at 133°. **Hi-Dri Temptubes**. Indicator tubes for use in dry heat processes.

Tes-Tape *(Lilly, UK)*. Tape impregnated with enzymes for testing urine for the presence of glucose. Colour changes indicate the presence of 0.1% or more of glucose.

Thrombofax Reagent *(Ortho Diagnostics, UK)*. A coagulation screening test, based upon the partial thromboplastin time test. **Optimised Activated Thrombofax Reagent.** A similar reagent containing, in addition, an activator.

Thrombotest *(Nyco, Norw.: BDH Chemicals, UK)*. A reagent for the determination of blood coagulability, for the control of anticoagulant therapy.

Thrombo-Wellcotest *(Wellcome Reagents, UK)*. A 2-minute latex agglutination slide test for the detection of fibrinogen degradation products in serum or urine.

Thymune-M *(Wellcome Reagents, UK)*. A haemagglutination kit for the detection of thyroid microsomal antibodies in serum. **Thymune-T.** A similar kit for the detection of thyroglobulin antibodies in serum.

Thyroid Test *(Fujizoki, Jap.: Diamed, UK)*. A haemagglutination test for the detection of thyroglobulin autoantibodies associated with thyroid auto-immune disease.

Thyro-Wellcotest *(Wellcome Reagents, UK)*. A 2-minute latex agglutination slide test for the detection of thyroid antibodies in serum.

Timecard *(Propper, UK: Horwell, UK)*. A sterilisation indicator in which colour changes indicate exposure to steam at 121° for 5 to 6, 10 to 13, 17 to 23, or more than 25 minutes. **One-Spot Timecard.** An indicator in which a colour change indicates exposure to steam at 121°. **Hi-Speed Timecard.** An indicator in which a colour change indicates exposure to steam at 133°.

ToxHAtest *(Wellcome Reagents, UK)*. A haemagglutination kit for the detection of antibodies to *Toxoplasma gondii* in serum.

TPHA Kit *(Wellcome Reagents, UK)*. An agglutination kit for the detection of antibodies to *Treponema pallidum* in serum.

TPHA Test Antigen *(Fujizoki, Jap.: Diamed, UK)*. A haemagglutination test for the diagnosis of syphilis.

UCG Slide Test *(Carter-Wallace, UK)*. A kit for pregnancy testing, stated to be suitable for use in retail pharmacies, containing slide tests for the detection of human chorionic gonadotrophin in urine.

Ugen Test *(Boehringer Corp., UK)*. Reagent strips for the detection of urobilinogen in urine.

Urastrat *(General Diagnostics, UK)*. A complete quantitative system for the determination of urea nitrogen in serum.

In 320 blood samples tested, there was a high degree of correlation between urea nitrogen concentrations assessed by the Urastrat test and by standard laboratory methods.— S. Bangerter *et al.*, *Schweiz. med. Wschr.*, 1969, *99*, 110.

Uricase Leo *(Leo, UK)*. A purified uricase preparation for the determination, by u.v. spectrophotometric technique, of uric acid in biological fluids.

Uristix *(Ames, UK)*. Reagent strips having 2 separately impregnated portions for detecting protein and glucose in urine. Strongly alkaline or highly buffered specimens or contamination by quaternary ammonium compounds may give false positive protein reactions.

Urobilistix *(Ames, UK)*. Reagent strips for the detection and estimation of urobilinogen in urine.

Uroscreen *(Pfizer, USA)*. A reagent containing triphenyltetrazolium chloride for the detection of bacteria in urine.

References.— H. G. Jespersen, *Ugeskr. Laeg.*, 1965, *127*, 1548; R. H. Parker *et al.*, *Am. J. med. Sci.*, 1966, *251*, 260; J. Olsen, *Nord. Med.*, 1966, *75*, 270; S. I. Hnatko, *Can. med. Ass. J.*, 1966, *95*, 10; P. J. Constable, *Lancet*, 1966, *2*, 195; B. Resnick *et al.*, *Archs intern. Med.*, 1969, *124*, 165.

Wellcome FDP Kit *(Wellcome Reagents, UK)*. A kit for the measurement, by the haemagglutination-inhibition technique, of fibrinogen in plasma and fibrinogen degradation products in serum and urine.

Digoxin and other Cardiac Glycosides

5800-k

The cardiac glycosides act on the heart by affecting atrioventricular conduction and vagal tone and also have a positive inotropic effect on the failing heart. They are used to slow the heart-rate in atrial arrhythmias, especially atrial fibrillation, and may also be given in congestive heart failure although their role in the long-term treatment of patients with heart failure and sinus rhythm is now questioned.

Therapeutic concentrations are very close to those at which toxicity occurs and since the symptoms of heart disease are similar to the adverse effects of the cardiac glycosides, dosage requires careful control. In emergencies, treatment is started with high initial doses until digitalisation is achieved and then maintained with smaller daily doses equivalent to the daily loss of cardiac glycosides from the body. In situations that are not urgent treatment may be initiated with maintenance doses and a steady state achieved gradually. Special care is necessary in the digitalisation of patients who have recently received cardiac glycosides or prolonged therapy with diuretics. The elderly usually require reduced maintenance doses.

The cardiac glycosides have very similar pharmacological effects but differ considerably in their speed of onset and duration of action. Digitoxin and digitalis are slow to act but their effects persist for 2 or 3 weeks. Ouabain administered intravenously produces its maximum effects within ½ to 2 hours but the effects have disappeared after 1 to 3 days. Medigoxin acts rapidly when given by mouth or intravenously but the duration of action is similar to that of digoxin. Digoxin and lanatoside C are intermediate in speed of onset and duration of action. When rapid digitalisation is necessary, digoxin or ouabain may be given by intravenous injection; medigoxin may also be used.

Digoxin and digitoxin are the cardiac glycosides used most widely and have generally replaced digitalis.

5801-a

Digoxin *(B.P., Eur. P., U.S.P., B.P. Vet.)*.

Digoxinum; Digoxosidum. 3β-[(*O*-2,6-Dideoxy-β-D-*ribo*-hexopyranosyl-(1→4)-*O*-2,6-dideoxy-β-D-*ribo*-hexopyranosyl-(1→4)-2,6-dideoxy-β-D-*ribo*-hexopyranosyl)oxy]-12β,14-dihydroxy-5β,14β-card-20(22)-enolide.

$C_{41}H_{64}O_{14}$=780.9.

CAS — 20830-75-5.

Pharmacopoeias. In *Arg., Br., Braz., Chin., Cz., Eur., Fr., Ger., Hung., Ind., Int., It., Jap., Jug., Neth., Nord., Roum., Swiss, Turk.*, and *U.S.*

A crystalline glycoside obtained from the leaves of *Digitalis lanata*. It occurs as colourless odourless crystals or a white or almost white powder with a bitter taste.

Practically **insoluble** in water, dehydrated alcohol, and ether; soluble 1 in 122 of alcohol (80%) and 1 in 4 of pyridine; slightly soluble in chloroform; freely soluble in a mixture of equal volumes of chloroform and methyl alcohol. A solution in pyridine is dextrorotatory. Alcoholic solutions are **sterilised** by autoclaving. **Incompatible** with acids and alkalis. **Store** in airtight containers. Protect from light.

Effect of gamma-irradiation. Digoxin was slightly discoloured, but no decomposition was apparent after irradiation with 25 000 Gy.— G. Hortobagyi *et al.*, *Radiosterilization of Medical Products*, Vienna, International Atomic Energy Agency, 1967, p. 25.

Stability. A study of the effects of storage upon characteristics *in vitro* and *in vivo* of soft gelatin capsules containing digoxin.— B. F. Johnson *et al.*, *J. Pharm. Pharmac.*, 1977, *29*, 576.

Adverse Effects. Digoxin and the other cardiac glycosides commonly produce side-effects because the margin between the therapeutic and toxic doses is small. There have been many fatalities. Since it is more rapidly excreted, cumulative effects are less likely with digoxin than with digitalis or digitoxin.

Nausea, vomiting, and anorexia may be among the earliest symptoms of digoxin overdosage; diarrhoea, abdominal pain, salivation and sweating may also occur. Certain cerebral effects are also early symptoms of digoxin overdosage and include headache, facial pain, malaise, fatigue, drowsiness, depression, disorientation, mental confusion, aphasia and delirium and hallucinations. Paraesthesia in the extremities and lumbar area, and convulsions have also been reported. Visual disturbances including blurred vision may occur; colour vision may be affected with objects appearing yellow or green, or less frequently red, brown, blue, or white. Allergic and skin reactions are rare; thrombocytopenia has been reported. The cardiac glycosides may have some oestrogenic activity which has been attributed to their structural similarity to the sex hormones. Gynaecomastia occasionally occurs.

The most serious adverse effects are those on the heart and pre-existing congestive heart failure may be aggravated by treatment with digoxin. Frequent ectopic heart beats indicate poisoning of the myocardium. Atrial or ventricular arrhythmias and defects of conduction are common and may be an early indication of overdosage. In general the incidence and severity of arrhythmias is related to the severity of the underlying heart disease. Almost any arrhythmia may ensue, but particular note should be made of multifocal ventricular ectopic beats, bigeminy, ventricular tachycardia, defects of conduction, bradycardia, and paroxysmal atrial tachycardia with heart block.

Hypokalaemia is associated with chronic digoxin toxicity and adverse reactions to digoxin may be precipitated if there is potassium depletion such as may be caused by the prolonged administration of diuretics. Hyperkalaemia occurs in acute overdosage.

The adverse effects of digoxin are similar to the symptoms of cardiac disease and measurement of plasma concentrations is of value in diagnosing overdosage. In general toxicity is likely with plasma concentrations of digoxin above 2 ng per ml but, while mean plasma-digoxin concentrations appear to distinguish between groups of patients who are or are not suffering from digoxin toxicity, there are marked individual variations and concentrations must be interpreted in the light of clinical signs and symptoms. If overdosage is suspected digoxin should be withdrawn.

Of 135 patients who were taking digitalis preparations on admission to hospital, digitalis toxicity was found in 31 (23%) and possible toxicity in 8 (6%). Toxicity was associated with an increased mortality-rate and incidence of advanced heart disease, renal failure, and pulmonary disease; blood concentrations of digitalis were generally higher in patients showing toxicity.— G. A. Beller *et al.*, *New Engl. J. Med.*, 1971, *284*, 989.

The Boston Collaborative Drug Surveillance Program has reported cardiac toxicity in 327 of 3828 hospital in-patients (8.5%) receiving digoxin. The toxicity was life-threatening in 79 patients and fatal in 2. Gastro-intestinal disturbances alone occurred in 119 of the patients (3.1%). Similar adverse effects were reported for digitoxin, digitalis, and ouabain.— D. J. Greenblatt, Digitalis Glycosides, in *Drug Effects in Hospitalized Patients*, R.R. Miller and D.J. Greenblatt (Ed.), London, Wiley, 1976, p. 37. In an assessment of the hazards of intuitive prescribing of digoxin, 437 of 2580 hospital in-patients monitored between 1973 and 1975 were receiving digoxin and 85 (19.5%) developed an adverse reaction. However, side-effects were generally of a relatively benign nature and no deaths were attributed to digoxin. The most striking finding was the high incidence of gastro-intestinal reactions amongst women. There was no clear-cut relationship between side-effects and factors such as previous use of digoxin, low body-weight, renal impairment, and the concomitant use of diuretics, probably because allowance was made for these parameters during prescribing. Doses of digoxin above 700 µg daily were almost invariably associated with side-effects, indicating that the use of loading doses should be abandoned in all but the most urgent cases.— D. A. Henry *et al.*, *Postgrad. med. J.*, 1981, *57*, 358.

An account of an outbreak of digoxin intoxication owing to a change in the tablets affecting bioavailability not announced by the manufacturer.— A. Danon *et al.*, *Clin. Pharmac. Ther.*, 1977, *21*, 643.

Diagnosis of digoxin toxicity. A view that it would be unwise to expect that plasma-digitalis concentrations, red blood cell or salivary electrolytes, or any other available laboratory test will diagnose actual or impending digitalis toxicity reliably enough to serve as a sole basis for clinical decision-making.— T. W. Smith, *New Engl. J. Med.*, 1978, *299*, 545. See also *Lancet*, 1978, *2*, 1188.

Reports of conflicting results when saliva concentrations of calcium and potassium were used to identify digitalis toxicity.— L. Gould *et al.* (letter), *New Engl. J. Med.*, 1972, *286*, 47; M. Swanson *et al.*, *Circulation*, 1973, *47*, 736; R. Avissar *et al.*, *Archs intern. Med.*, 1975, *135*, 1029.

One-fifth of 145 patients admitted to hospital showed clinical signs of digitalis intoxication and had a mean plasma-digoxin concentration of 2.5 ng per ml.— J. Lichey *et al.*, *Dt. med. Wschr.*, 1977, *102*, 1056. First-degree atrioventricular block, atrial ectopic beats, and ventricular ectopic beats were associated with serum-digoxin concentrations between 1.5 and 2.5 ng per ml while higher grade atrioventricular block, atrial tachycardia, and bigeminy were more frequent with concentrations in excess of 3.0 ng per ml.— G. Hennersdorf *et al.*, *Dt. med. Wschr.*, 1977, *102*, 381. In a study of 86 patients receiving digoxin, symptoms of toxicity occurred in 31 patients at serum concentrations which did not differ significantly from concentrations achieved in the remainder. Patients with symptoms of toxicity were distinguished by significantly lower serum-creatinine concentrations and body-weights, but without any variation in creatinine clearance. It is suggested that low muscle mass is only one factor determining individual sensitivity to digoxin.— S. M. Dobbs *et al.*, *Br. J. clin. Pharmac.*, 1977, *4*, 327.

Further references to the correlation of digoxin toxicity with plasma-digoxin concentrations: T. W. Smith and E. Haber, *J. clin. Invest.*, 1970, *49*, 2377, per *Drugs* 1972, *3*, 115; G. A. Beller *et al.*, *New Engl. J. Med.*, 1971, *284*, 989; J. Ingelfinger and P. Goldman, *New Engl. J. Med.*, 1976, *294*, 867; J. Schneider and A. Ruiz-Torres, *Int. J. clin. Pharmac. Biopharm.*, 1977, *15*, 424, per *Int. pharm. Abstr.*, 1978, *15*, 386; J. K. Aronson *et al.*, *Q.J. Med.*, 1978, *NS47*, 111; W. Shapiro, *Am. J. Cardiol.*, 1978, *41*, 852; S. Waldorff and J. Buch, *Clin. Pharmac. Ther.*, 1978, *23*, 19; W. Berman (letter), *Pediatrics*, 1979, *63*, 503; H. Halkin (letter), *ibid.*, 504.

In a controlled study of 46 children receiving digoxin for the treatment of congestive heart failure, digitilisation significantly increased sodium concentrations in the red blood cells whilst potassium concentrations were decreased. Similar, but more marked effects were seen in patients on maintenance therapy, who were diagnosed as suffering from digoxin toxicity, when compared with non-toxic children. The ratio of red cell-sodium to red cell-potassium concentrations was successfully used to identify 32 of 34 patients with digoxin toxicity compared with 30 of 34 who were diagnosed using plasma-digoxin concentrations as a guide to toxicity.— M. W. Loes *et al.*, *New Engl. J. Med.*, 1978, *299*, 501. Comment.— T. W. Smith, *ibid.*, 545. The monitoring of red blood cell electrolytes in adults as a guide to the efficacy and toxicity of digitalis therapy was as effective as the measurement of plasma-digoxin concentrations and saved time and effort.— F. Wessels and H. Losse (letter), *New Engl. J. Med.*, 1979, *300*, 433.

A slow heart-rate in patients taking cardiac glycosides may be indicative of digitalis toxicity although the specificity of this and other cardiac and extracardiac symptoms is low. When toxicity is suspected cardiac glycosides should be withdrawn and serum concentrations measured.— O. Storstein (letter), *Lancet*, 1979, *1*, 445.

Guidelines for the diagnosis of digoxin toxicity in individual patients. Toxicity should be suspected if the plasma-digoxin concentration is greater than 3 ng per ml, or there is hypokalaemia, or there are any two of the following four features: plasma potassium greater than 5 mmol per litre, plasma creatinine greater than 150 μmol per litre, age more than 60 years, or daily maintenance dose at a steady state of more than 6 μg per kg body-weight. Using these guidelines the incidence of overdiagnosis of toxicity in non-toxic patients is 41%.— J. K. Aronson, *Clin. Pharmacokinet.*, 1980, *5*, 137.

See also under Plasma Concentrations in Absorption and Fate (below) and under Administration in Uses (below).

Effects on electrolytes. In 80 patients taking digoxin and in 22 controls, patients showing digoxin toxicity had significantly higher plasma-digoxin concentrations. Plasma-magnesium concentrations were not significantly different in patients or controls; erythrocyte-magnesium concentrations were higher in patients not showing digoxin toxicity. Digitalis-induced ventricular arrhythmias had been reported to be abolished by the use of magnesium chloride.— D. W. Holt and R. Goulding (letter), *Br. med. J.*, 1975, *1*, 627.

In a study of 478 patients, digitalis intoxication was found more frequently in patients with hypomagnesaemia than in those with normal concentrations of magnesium but there was no correlation between serum-magnesium and serum-digitalis concentrations. Nausea, anorexia, extreme fatigue, and flickering of vision were more common in the patients with hypomagnesaemia although nausea and anorexia may have been the cause and not necessarily the symptoms of low serum-magnesium concentrations.— O. Storstein *et al.*, *Acta med. scand.*, 1977, *202*, 445.

Further references to hypomagnesaemia in patients with digitalis toxicity: G. A. Beller *et al.*, *Am. J. Cardiol.*, 1974, *33*, 225; R. B. Singh *et al.*, *Am. Heart J.*, 1976, *92*, 144.

Effects on the eyes. Digitalis might cause green-yellow vision (sometimes red, brown, white), photophobia, haloes around lights, blurred vision, sparks, scintillating scotoma, low intra-ocular pressure, paralysis of extra-ocular muscles, retrobulbar neuritis, cortical blindness, conjunctivitis, and toxic amblyopia.— H. I. Silverman, *Am. J. Optom.*, 1972, *49*, 335.

Further references to the effects of cardiac glycosides on the eyes: D. M. Robertson *et al.*, *Archs Ophthal., N.Y.*, 1966, *76*, 640.

Effects on the gastro-intestinal tract. Marked venous engorgement of the intestine with haemorrhage and oedema of the intestinal wall were found in 10 patients who died after treatment with digitalis, digitoxin, or lanatoside C. Most of the patients had complained of abdominal pain and tenderness during treatment and in some haematemesis or melaena had occurred.— P. C. Gazes *et al.*, *Circulation*, 1961, *23*, 358. See also F. M. Muggia, *Am. J. med. Sci.*, 1967, *253*, 263; H. S. Ko (letter), *J. Am. med. Ass.*, 1974, *227*, 1263; M. Feinroth *et al.*, *Br. med. J.*, 1980, *281*, 838.

Plasma-digoxin concentrations in 104 patients with gastro-intestinal symptoms were significantly higher than in 308 asymptomatic patients. There was wide individual variation and 24% of patients with a concentration of less than 1 ng per ml had symptoms.— D. W. Holt and G. N. Volans (letter), *Br. med. J.*, 1977, *2*, 704.

A report of dysphagia as a symptom of digoxin toxicity.— J. G. Kelton and D. C. Scullin (letter), *J. Am. med. Ass.*, 1978, *239*, 613.

Effects on the heart. Aberrant ventricular complexes in the ECG, particularly if they appear in groups, are considered to be just as serious an index of digitalis toxicity as premature ventricular beats, and require the temporary withdrawal of treatment. It is considered that if digitalis is continued, a transient depression of the atrioventricular pacemaker might produce transient slowing of the ventricular beat followed by acceleration and lead to either ventricular arrest or fibrillation. During 2 years, 8 cases of ventricular arrest with Stokes-Adams seizures followed repeated aberrant ventricular complexes in patients with atrial fibrillation.— L. S. Schwartz and S. P. Schwartz (letter), *New Engl. J. Med.*, 1966, *274*, 804.

In 3 young patients without heart disease ingestion of large amounts of digoxin led to atrioventricular block or sino-atrial exit block; in 2 patients with advanced coronary artery disease multifocal ventricular premature beats, ventricular tachycardia, and ventricular fibrillation developed.— T. W. Smith and J. T. Willerson, *Circulation*, 1971, *44*, 29, per *Clin. Med.*, 1972, *79* (July), 38.

Eleven patients developed double tachycardia in 1 hospital in 1 year. A mortality-rate of 73% was related only to failure to recognise double tachycardia as a symptom of digitalis toxicity. Three of the 4 patients whose digitalis was withdrawn at the onset of double tachycardia survived.— S. H. Wishner *et al.*, *New Engl. J. Med.*, 1972, *287*, 552.

Effects on the mental state. Digitalis is a potent and not rare cause of delirium, which has occurred in 3 to 4% of patients intoxicated with it. Lethargy is not an uncommon manifestation of toxicity, particularly in the bedridden.— H. J. L. Marriott (letter), *J. Am. med. Ass.*, 1968, *203*, 156.

Formed visual hallucinations occurred in 3 elderly patients receiving digoxin. All had high serum-digoxin concentrations. On temporary withdrawal of the drug the concentrations decreased to within the therapeutic range and the hallucinations subsided and never returned.— B. T. Volpe and R. Soave, *Ann. intern. Med.*, 1979, *91*, 865.

Further references to the effects of cardiac glycosides on mental state: D. A. Gorelick *et al.*, *J. nerv. ment. Dis.*, 1978, *166*, 817 (paranoid delusions and auditory hallucinations); M. K. Shear and M. H. Sacks, *Am. J. Psychiat.*, 1978, *135*, 109 (delirium); V. A. Portnoi, *J. clin. Pharmac.*, 1979, *19*, 747 (delirium in the elderly); M. Brezis *et al.* (letter), *Ann. intern. Med.*, 1980, *93*, 639 (nightmares).

Lupus erythematosus. Systemic lupus erythematosus was reported to have occurred following the use of digitalis.— E. C. Rosenow, *Ann. intern. Med.*, 1972, *77*, 977.

Oestrogen-like effects. Mean serum-oestrogen concentrations were increased in 20 postmenopausal women and 18 men who had been taking digoxin for more than 2 years. Mean serum concentrations of luteinising hormone were decreased in both groups and the mean plasma-testosterone concentrations were decreased in the male group.— S. S. Stoffer *et al.*, *J. Am. med. Ass.*, 1973, *225*, 1643.

For reports on the oestrogen-like effects of digitalis, see H. W. Gordon *et al.*, *Am. J. Obstet. Gynec.*, 1966, *94*, 524; D. Burckhardt and J. S. LaDue, *Schweiz. med. Wschr.*, 1968, *98*, 1250; B. Stenkvist *et al.* (letter), *Lancet*, 1979, *1*, 563; E. B. LeWinn (letter), *ibid.*, 1196; D. H. Cove and G. A. Barker (letter), *Lancet*, 1979, *2*, 204.

Overdosage. Within 4 hours of a self-administered intravenous injection of digoxin 200 mg, the serum-digoxin concentration was 52 ng per ml and the plasma-potassium concentration was 11.5 mmol increasing at 4.5 hours to 13.5 mmol per litre. Despite reduction in potassium concentrations by haemodialysis, the cardiac tissue lost all electrical activity.— M. J. Reza *et al.*, *New Engl. J. Med.*, 1974, *291*, 777.

A report of fatal overdosage with digoxin in a 54-year-old woman; the blood-digoxin concentration was 50.4 ng per ml.— D. P. Nicholls, *Postgrad. med. J.*, 1977, *53*, 280.

Further references to overdosage with digoxin: *J. Pediat.*, 1964, *64*, 188; R. Barton and I. Haider, *Practitioner*, 1967, *198*, 538; J. D. Hobson and A. Zettner, *J. Am. med. Ass.*, 1973, *223*, 147; D. L. Citrin *et al.*, *Br. med. J.*, 1973, *2*, 526.

Treatment of Adverse Effects. For the treatment of *chronic poisoning* withdrawal of digoxin or other cardiac glycosides for one or two days may be all that is necessary, with subsequent doses adjusted according to the needs of the patient. Serum electrolytes should be measured and the ECG monitored. If cardiac arrhythmias are severe it may be necessary to give potassium and/or anti-arrhythmic agents as described below.

In the early stages of *acute poisoning* the stomach should be emptied by emesis or aspiration and lavage. Activated charcoal has been given in an attempt to prevent the absorption of cardiac glycosides; cholestyramine is reported to increase the elimination of digitoxin. Attempts to remove cardiac glycosides by dialysis or exchange transfusion have generally been ineffective and the value of haemoperfusion or forced diuresis is controversial. Some authorities consider that a high urinary output should be maintained with agents such as mannitol. There have been varying reports on the effects of frusemide on digoxin excretion; serious electrolyte imbalance may result from the use of such potent diuretics. Cardiac toxicity should be treated under ECG control and serum electrolytes should be monitored. Arrhythmias may be controlled in hypokalaemic patients by giving potassium chloride, by mouth or intravenously, providing that renal function is normal and heart block is not present. Potassium may sometimes be given to normokalaemic patients. Anti-arrhythmic agents given intravenously in the treatment of severe toxicity include phenytoin sodium, lignocaine, and propranolol. Procainamide is generally considered more hazardous but has been used for tachyarrhythmias refractory to other drugs. Phenytoin, propranolol, or procainamide have been given by mouth in the treatment of less severe arrhythmias. Atropine is given intravenously to control bradycardia and in patients with heart block. Pacing may be necessary if atropine is not effective. Cardioversion is used only when other methods fail. Magnesium sulphate has been given intravenously to correct hypomagnesaemia and disodium edetate to correct hypercalcaemia.

In *massive overdosage* progressive hyperkalaemia occurs and is fatal unless reversed. Dextrose infusions and injections of soluble insulin have been given and, if the hyperkalaemia is refractory, dialysis may be tried. Sodium polystyrene sulphonate has been used in less severe hyperkalaemia. Massive overdosage has been treated successfully with Fab fragments of digoxin-specific antibodies.

A review and discussion on the management of acute digoxin poisoning.— B. R. Ekins and A. S. Watanabe, *Am. J. Hosp. Pharm.*, 1978, *35*, 268. Comments.— D. G. Fraser and T. M. Ludden (letter), *ibid.*, 1030; B. R. Ekins and A. S. Watanabe (letter), *ibid.*

All types of arrhythmia may result from the adverse effects of digitalis glycosides, and recognition of the disorder can be difficult. Patients in whom premature ventricular beats, paroxysmal atrial tachycardia with block, nodal tachycardia with or without atrioventricular dissociation, ventricular tachycardia, or atrioventricular nodal block have developed during digitalis therapy should discontinue the drug. In patients with conditions predisposing to tachycardia, such as fever, infection, or hyperthyroidism, attempts to reduce the ventricular beat to 70 to 80 per minute are usually unsuccessful and can result in digitalis overdosage and therefore toxic signs and symptoms. If ectopic tachycardia is present as one of the signs of digitalis toxicity, potassium chloride is the treatment of choice. If the situation is not critical, therapy by mouth is suitable; otherwise an intravenous infusion containing 40 to 60 mmol of potassium per litre might be given, with ECG monitoring for signs of hyperkalaemia. In paroxysmal atrial tachycardia with atrioventricular block there might be paradoxical acceleration of the ventricular-rate, but potassium infusion should then be continued until further slowing of the atrial-rate and termination of the arrhythmia occurs. If digitalis toxicity has caused primary block to the sinoatrial or atrioventricular node, potassium will also depress these tissues and might potentiate the disturbance. In such situations, potassium salts should be avoided unless hypokalaemia is present, and other treatment for primary block employed.— R. M. Stanzler, *New Engl. J. Med.*, 1966, *274*, 1307.

The cellular binding of cardiac glycosides and the effect of potassium: the basis for the use of potassium in the treatment of overdosage with cardiac glycosides.— P. F. Baker and J. S. Willis, *Nature*, 1970, *226*, 521.

Serum-magnesium concentrations in 13 digitalised patients were significantly lower at 0.7 mmol per litre than in 72 controls—0.96 mmol per litre. Four patients with digitalis toxicity had frank hypomagnesaemia. In 19 *dogs* dialysis-induced hypomagnesaemia reduced by 26% the dose of acetylstrophanthidin needed to induce cardiac arrhythmia; sinus rhythm was restored in 13 immediately after the intravenous infusion of 25% magnesium sulphate solution.— R. H. Seller *et al.*, *Am. Heart J.*, 1970, *79*, 57.

Defibrillation and pacing were of more value than drug treatment in 4 patients with massive digoxin overdosage.— J. Asplund *et al.*, *Acta med. scand.*, 1971, *189*, 293, per *Abstr. Wld Med.*, 1971, *45*, 629.

Further references to the treatment of the adverse effects of digoxin: G. L. Ackerman *et al.*, *Ann. intern. Med.*, 1967, *67*, 718 (only a negligible amount of digoxin removed by peritoneal dialysis or haemodialysis); G. Härtel *et al.* (letter), *Lancet*, 1973, *2*, 158 (lower serum-digoxin concentrations in subjects given charcoal); B. H. Rumack *et al.*, *Br. Heart J.*, 1974, *36*, 405 (heart block after 12.5 mg of digoxin reversed by the intravenous injection of phenytoin 25 mg given seven times in 36 hours); W. Shapiro and K. Taubert (letter), *Lancet*, 1975, *2*, 604 (digoxin-induced arrhythmias reversed by the correction of potassium depletion); H. H. Rotmensch *et al.*, *Israel J. med. Sci.*, 1977, *13*, 1109 (phenytoin in the treatment of massive digoxin overdosage).

For the use of phenytoin in the treatment of digitalis-induced arrhythmias, see Phenytoin, p.1243.

For reference to the beneficial effect of canrenoate potassium on digitalis-induced ventricular arrhythmias, see Canrenoate Potassium, p.587.

Digoxin-specific antibodies. Comment on the potential role of digoxin-specific antibodies to detect and treat overdosage with digoxin and digitoxin.— *Lancet*, 1980, *2*, 628.

Results from one patient who had taken 22.5 mg of digoxin showed that digoxin-specific Fab antibody fragments from *sheep* were capable of reversing digoxin toxicity.— T. W. Smith *et al.*, *New Engl. J. Med.*, 1976, *294*, 797.

Digoxin intoxication with severe arrhythmias and generalised heart failure in a 72-year-old man with coronary heart disease and renal failure was successfully treated and sinus rhythm rapidly restored after administration of heterologous digoxin-specific Fab antibody fragments.— T. Hess *et al.*, *Dt. med. Wschr.*, 1979, *104*, 1273.

Forced diuresis. The renal clearance of digoxin was not increased after frusemide infusion in 8 subjects and it would therefore not seem a useful adjunct in the management of digoxin overdosage.— P. Semple *et al.* (letter), *New Engl. J. Med.*, 1975, *293*, 612. Results in 3 patients who attempted suicide with large amounts of digoxin indicate that the prompt administration of frusemide may substantially increase the renal excretion of digoxin.— H. H. Rotmensch *et al.*, *Archs intern. Med.*, 1978, *138*, 1495.

See also under Interactions in Precautions (below).

Haemoperfusion. Reports of the successful use of haemoperfusion in acute digoxin poisoning.— G. H. Gleeson *et al.* (letter), *J. Am. med. Ass.*, 1978, *240*, 2731 (Amberlite column); J. W. Smiley (letter), *ibid.*, 2736 (a macroreticular styrene divinylbenzene copolymer column or a charcoal column). The data presented do not show any beneficial effect and it is considered that haemoperfusion or haemodialysis cannot be effective for a drug like digoxin which has a large volume of distribution.— C. R. Freed *et al.* (letter), *ibid.*, 1979, *241*, 1575.

A report of advanced digoxin toxicity being successfully treated with charcoal haemoperfusion.— T. Marbury *et al.*, *Sth. med. J.*, 1979, *72*, 279.

Further views that charcoal haemoperfusion is of unproven value in the treatment of digoxin overdosage.— S. Pond *et al.*, *Clin. Pharmacokinet.*, 1979, *4*, 329; J. T. Slattery and J. R. Koup, *ibid.*, 395; S. E. Warren and D. D. Fanestil, *J. Am. med. Ass.*, 1979, *242*, 2100; D. A. Rowett (letter), *ibid.*, 1980, *244*, 1558.

For reference to the successful use of charcoal haemoperfusion in digitoxin toxicity, see Digitoxin, p.541.

Ion-exchange resins. Cholestyramine is capable of binding 6.4 ng of digoxin and 14.4 ng of digitoxin per mg of resin *in vitro*; these values are greater than those for colestipol which has been successfully used in treatment; however in the presence of duodenal juice the values were reduced to 2.8 and 4.6 ng per mg respectively. The plasma half-life of digitoxin was reduced from 9.3 to an average of 2.75 days after colestipol administration.— G. Bazzano and G. S. Bazzano, *J. Am. med. Ass.*, 1972, *220*, 828.

A report of cholestyramine having little effect on the absorption and excretion of digoxin.— W. H. Hall *et al.*, *Am. J. Cardiol.*, 1977, *39*, 213.

For the use of cholestyramine in digitoxin toxicity, see Digitoxin, p.541.

Precautions. Digoxin is generally contra-indicated in ventricular arrhythmias and in patients with the Wolff-Parkinson-White syndrome who also have atrial fibrillation. It should be used with caution in heart block; complete heart block may be precipitated if cardiac glycosides are used in partial heart block. It should be used with caution in acute myocarditis such as rheumatic carditis and in patients with advanced heart failure or severe pulmonary disease. The role of digoxin in myocardial infarction is debated. Digoxin should be given with care to patients who have received cardiac glycosides previously. It may enhance the occurrence of arrhythmias in patients undergoing cardiac surgery or cardioversion and should be withdrawn 3 days before such procedures if possible. If cardioversion is essential and digoxin has already been given, low voltage shocks must be used.

Early signs of digoxin toxicity should be watched for and the heart rate should not be allowed to fall below 60 beats per minute. Toxicity may result from administering loading doses too rapidly, from accumulation of maintenance doses, and from the presence of conditions which predispose to toxicity. Digoxin doses should generally be reduced in patients with impaired renal function, in the elderly, and in premature infants; they should be carefully controlled in patients with electrolyte imbalance, or thyroid dysfunction. The effects of digoxin are enhanced by hypokalaemia, hypomagnesaemia, hypercalcaemia, hypoxia, and hypothyroidism and doses may need to be reduced until these conditions are corrected. Hypokalaemia and hypomagnesaemia may follow treatment with the thiazide and similar diuretics. Other potassium-depleting drugs include amphotericin, the corticosteroids, and carbenoxolone. Injections of calcium salts should not be given during digoxin therapy and the drug should be given cautiously to patients receiving parathyroid extract or large doses of vitamin D.

There may be interactions between digoxin and drugs which alter its absorption, interfere with its excretion, or have additive effects on the myocardium.

Reports of gastro-intestinal disturbances interfering with the bioavailability of digoxin: N. Buchanan *et al.*, *J. pharm. Sci.*, 1976, *65*, 914; N. Buchanan, *S. Afr. med. J.*, 1977, *52*, 733 (impaired binding of digoxin *in vitro* in kwashiorkor serum); A. J. Kolibash *et al.*, *Am. Heart J.*, 1977, *94*, 806 (marked decline in serum-digoxin concentration during severe diarrhoea); I. J. McGilveray *et al.* (letter), *Can. med. Ass. J.*, 1979, *121*, 704 (substantial degradation of digoxin in 2 of 3 patients with gastric hyperacidity); C. D. Gerson *et al.*, *Am. J. Med.*, 1980, *69*, 43 (impaired bioavailability of digoxin in patients with a shortened small intestine).

Effects of electrolyte imbalance. Hypokalaemia increased the arrhythmogenic effects of digoxin in *dogs*. Serum-potassium concentrations should be carefully monitored in digitalised patients both as a check against arrhythmias and the possible lessening of the inotropic response to digitalis.— A. Gelbart *et al.* (letter), *Lancet*, 1976, *2*, 850. See also E. Steiness and K. H. Olesen, *Br. Heart J.*, 1976, *38*, 167. Results indicating that the active tubular secretion of digoxin is reduced in hypokalaemic patients.— E. Steiness, *Clin. Pharmac. Ther.*, 1978, *23*, 511.

Insensitivity to digoxin in an 85-year-old man was associated with hypocalcaemia.— D. Chopra *et al.*, *New Engl. J. Med.*, 1977, *296*, 917.

Effects on the heart. First-degree atrioventricular block was not considered a sign of digitalis intoxication and did not in itself contra-indicate its continued administration. Second-degree block should be considered an adverse effect of digitalis, and the dosage should be reduced accordingly.— M. G. Criscitiello, *New Engl. J. Med.*, 1968, *279*, 808. In a retrospective study of 910 hospital patients receiving digoxin therapy and who had plasma-digoxin radioimmunoassays, 64 had been carried out to investigate pulse-rates of below 60. Of 57 of these patients further investigated, only 6 were suffering from digoxin toxicity and no reason for the slow heart-rates could be found in 42. Resting bradycardia with no other sign of toxicity should not be a reason for withholding digitalis.— P. Williams *et al.*, *Lancet*, 1978, *2*, 1340.

A brief report on the occurrence of transient cardiac arrhythmias after single daily maintenance doses of digoxin.— V. Manninen *et al.*, *Clin. Pharmac. Ther.*, 1976, *20*, 266.

For the hazards of the use of cardiac glycosides in heart surgery, see under Heart or Chest Surgery in Uses (below).

Interactions. Reviews of drug interactions occurring with cardiac glycosides.— P. F. Binnion, *Drugs*, 1978, *15*, 369; J. A. Milliken, *Can. med. Ass. J.*, 1979, *121*, 263; D. D. Brown *et al.*, *Drugs*, 1980, *20*, 198.

Anaesthetic agents. A discussion of the effects of anaesthetic agents on digitalis tolerance. Bigeminy has occurred in a digitalised patient after *hexafluorenium* and premature ventricular contractions after *suxamethonium*. Sinus rhythm was restored after the administration of Innovar (fentanyl citrate and droperidol). *Cyclopropane* has been reported to decrease tolerance to digitalis, and *halothane, methoxyflurane, ether, ketamine*, and *Innovar* to increase tolerance. The effect of *diazepam* is controversial.— A. D. Ivankovic, *Anesth. Analg. curr. Res.*, 1972, *51*, 607.

Antacids and other gastro-intestinal agents. In a study involving 10 healthy subjects concurrent administration of *magnesium trisilicate, magnesium hydroxide, aluminium hydroxide*, or *kaolin with pectin* severely reduced the absorption of orally administered digoxin. The mechanism for the interference was not considered to be entirely related to physical adsorption or to changes in gut transit time.— D. D. Brown and R. P. Juhl, *New Engl. J. Med.*, 1976, *295*, 1034.

In 15 healthy subjects given digoxin alone and with a *kaolin-pectin* suspension it was found that the kaolin-pectin suspension reduced both the rate and extent of digoxin absorption. The interaction was virtually eliminated by giving the kaolin-pectin 2 hours after digoxin. The relative extent of absorption of digoxin was reduced by about 20%, although the rate of absorption was not affected, when kaolin-pectin was given 2 hours before digoxin.— K. S. Albert *et al.*, *J. pharm. Sci.*, 1978, *67*, 1582.

Dimethicone did not affect absorption *in vitro* of digoxin; *magnesium trisilicate* reduced absorption by 99.5%.— J. C. McElnay *et al.* (letter), *Br. med. J.*, 1978, *1*, 1554. See also S. A. Khalil, *J. Pharm. Pharmac.*, 1974, *26*, 961.

Study in 4 patients suggested that absorption of digoxin 250 or 500 µg was not affected by concomitant administration of mixtures of *aluminium hydroxide* or *magnesium trisilicate*.— J. Cooke and J. A. Smith (letter), *Br. med. J.*, 1978, *2*, 1166.

Further references to the reduced absorption of digoxin by antacids: P. F. Binnion and M. McDermott (letter), *Lancet*, 1972, *2*, 592 (*kaolin-pectin* and *aluminium and magnesium hydroxides*).

See also under Anticholinergic Agents and Bran (below).

Anti-arrhythmic agents. A review of the interaction between digoxin and *quinidine*. Three groups reported independently that serum-digoxin concentrations were increased when quinidine was given to patients taking digoxin (W. Doering and E. König, *Med. Klin.*, 1978, *73*, 1085; G. Ejvinsson, *Br. med. J.*, 1978, *1*, 279; E.B. Leahey *et al.*, *J. Am. med. Ass.*, 1978, *240*, 533) and it appears that about 90% of patients taking quinidine in association with digoxin will have some increase in serum-digoxin concentrations. The magnitude of the increase is quite variable but, on average, a twofold increase occurs and according to W. Doering (*New Engl. J. Med.*, 1979, *301*, 400) is dependent on the dosage of quinidine. Work by W. Doering (1979) and E.B. Leahey *et al.* (*Archs intern. Med.*, 1979, *139*, 519) suggests that the serum-digoxin concentration starts to rise on the first day of treatment with quinidine and continues to rise until a new steady state is reached at about 5 days; the concentration then remains elevated for as long as quinidine is given. Information on the mechanism of the interaction is sparse. E.B. Leahey *et al.* have suggested that quinidine displaces digoxin from binding sites in tissue. W.D. Hager *et al.* (*New Engl. J. Med.*, 1979, *300*, 1238) have supported this view; they showed that quinidine reduces both the volume of distribution and the renal clearance of digoxin without any change in the elimination half-life. An increase in serum-digoxin concentrations does not necessarily indicate an increase in effect on the heart or other organs but E.B. Leahey *et al.* (1978, 1979) have reported that adverse gastro-intestinal and cardiac effects of digoxin occur when serum digoxin is increased as a result of quinidine administration. In order to prevent the adverse effects of the interaction W. Doering (1979) has suggested that the dose of digoxin should be halved before starting quinidine therapy. However, there is great individual variation in the magnitude of the quinidine-induced increase in serum digoxin and therefore concentrations should be measured 4 or 5 days after starting quinidine to assess whether further adjustment of the digoxin dose is necessary. The patient should also be monitored closely for signs of inadequate or excessive dosage. Studies in small numbers of patients indicate that the anti-arrhythmic agents *lignocaine, disopyramide*, and *procainamide* do not cause an increase in serum-digoxin concentrations.— J. T. Bigger, *New Engl. J. Med.*, 1979, *301*, 779.. A further review. The displacement of digoxin by quinidine from tissue stores may be selective, affecting non-cardiac tissues but not the heart.— *Lancet*, 1980, *2*, 1064. Although the clinical importance of the digoxin-quinidine interaction is still uncertain, digoxin doses should be reduced before starting quinidine and serum-digoxin concentrations should be measured and the dose adjusted accordingly.— E. B. Leahey, *Ann. intern. Med.*, 1980, *93*, 775.

In a study of 6 healthy subjects the positive inotropic effect of digoxin was strongly reduced during concomitant treatment with *quinidine*.— E. Steiness *et al.*, *Clin. Pharmac. Ther.*, 1980, *27*, 791. See also P. D. Hirsh *et al.*, *Am. J. Cardiol.*, 1980, *46*, 863.

Further reports of *quinidine* increasing serum-digoxin concentrations: P. M. Hooymans and F. W. H. M. Merkus (letter), *Br. med. J.*, 1978, *2*, 1022; J. A. Reiffel *et al.*, *Am. J. Cardiol.*, 1978, *41*, 368; D. J. Chapron *et al.*, *Archs intern. Med.*, 1979, *139*, 363; R. Dahlquist *et al.* (letter), *New Engl. J. Med.*, 1979, *301*, 727; D. W. Holt *et al.*, *Br. med. J.*, 1979, *2*, 1401; T. Risler *et al.*, *Dt. med. Wschr.*, 1979, *104*, 1523; T. -S. Chen and H. S. Friedman, *J. Am. med. Ass.*, 1980, *244*, 669; E. B. Leahey *et al.*, *Ann. intern. Med.*, 1980, *92*, 605; T. R. Moench (letter), *New Engl. J. Med.*, 1980, *302*, 864 (reduced serum-digoxin concentrations after withdrawal of quinidine); D. R. Mungall *et al.*, *Ann. intern. Med.*, 1980, *93*, 689; H. J. J. Wellens *et al.*, *Am. Heart J.*, 1980, *100*, 934 (lack of effect on serum digoxin with disopyramide).

Comments on the mechanism of the digoxin-*quinidine* interaction: T. Risler *et al.* (letter), *New Engl. J. Med.*, 1980, *302*, 175; St. G. T. Lee (letter), *ibid.*; K. D. Straub (letter), *ibid.*, 176; K. E. Pedersen and S. Hvidt (letter), *ibid.*; J. R. Powell *et al.* (letter), *ibid.*; W. Doering (letter), *ibid.*, 177; N. H. G. Holford (letter), *ibid.*, 864; J. T. Bigger (letter), *ibid.*

For interactions between digitalis and *verapamil*, see Verapamil, p.1384.

Antibiotics. The absorption of digoxin is impaired by *neomycin*.— J. Lindenbaum *et al.*, *Gastroenterology*, 1976, *71*, 399.

Signs of heart failure and reduced serum-digoxin concentrations were noted when *rifampicin* was given to a woman being treated with digoxin. The patient's cardiac condition could not be controlled by increasing the dose of digoxin, and rifampicin was withdrawn.— C. Novi *et al.* (letter), *J. Am. med. Ass.*, 1980, *244*, 2521.

Antibiotic reversal of digoxin inactivation by gut flora.— J. Lindenbaum *et al.*, *New Engl. J. Med.*, 1981, *305*, 789.

Anticholinergic agents. The mean serum-digoxin concentration of 0.72 ng per ml in 11 patients on maintenance digoxin was reduced to 0.46 ng per ml when given 10 mg of *metoclopramide* thrice daily but returned to normal when metoclopramide was discontinued. *Propantheline* 15 mg thrice daily given in conjunction with digoxin to 13 similar patients caused an increase in mean serum-digoxin concentration in 9 from 1.02 to 1.33 ng per ml. When 8 healthy subjects taking digoxin 500 µg in tablet or liquid form were given propantheline 30 mg, serum-digoxin concentrations increased in those taking digoxin tablets but not in those taking digoxin liquid.— V. Manninen *et al.*, *Lancet*, 1973, *1*, 398. Comment.— W. G. Thompson (letter), *ibid.*, 783; S. Medin and L. Nyberg (letter), *ibid.*, 1393.

Serum-digoxin concentrations were not significantly influenced by *propantheline* in 8 subjects taking Lanoxin. The serum concentrations following the same dose of a slower-dissolving digoxin tablet in the same subjects were lower and were increased by taking the tablet with propantheline.— V. Manninen *et al.* (letter), *Lancet*, 1973, *1*, 1118.

There were no significant variations in concentrations of digoxin excreted in the urine over 8 days despite differences in absorption and rate of absorption measured by means of serum concentrations. It is considered that only tablets with very low dissolution-rates or tablets given to patients with impaired intestinal absorption are affected by drugs altering gastro-intestinal motility.— C. D. Michalopoulos and C. V. Koutoulidis (letter), *Lancet*, 1974, *1*, 167.

The overall mean cumulative urinary excretion of digoxin over 4 days in 10 healthy subjects was significantly lower when they took digoxin 500 µg in tablets containing a large particle size (90 to 106 µm) than after they had received tablets containing standard or micronised digoxin. Prior administration of *propantheline* 15 mg and *metoclopramide* 10 mg respectively reduced and increased the mean cumulative urinary excretion, only when the large particle size preparation was used. It was considered that propantheline and metoclopramide only affected the absorption of digoxin from preparations containing large particle size and having slow dissolution-rates.— B. F. Johnson *et al.*, *Br. J. clin. Pharmac.*, 1978, *5*, 465.

Anticoagulants. A report of *heparin* having a variable but insignificant effect on plasma-digoxin concentrations in patients on haemodialysis.— W. J. F. van der Vijgh and P. L. Oe, *Int. J. clin. Pharmac. Biopharm.*, 1977, *15*, 560.

For reference to digoxin having no effect on plasma-*warfarin* concentrations, see Warfarin Sodium, p.776.

Anticonvulsants. Mention of bradycardia in 3 patients given *carbamazepine* who were also taking digitalis.— J. M. Killian and G. H. Fromm, *Archs Neurol., Chicago*, 1968, *19*, 129.

Administration of digoxin with *phenytoin*, or the treatment of digitalis-induced cardiac arrhythmias with phenytoin could be hazardous. Heart block, which was almost fatal, followed treatment of a 53-year-old man with Down's syndrome with digoxin and phenytoin.— N. M. A. Viukari and K. Aho (letter), *Br. med. J.*, 1970, *2*, 51. In 200 patients the incidence of side-effects was reduced from 22.3% in those given cardiac glycosides to 7% in those given *phenytoin* concomitantly, without adversely affecting the positive inotropic effect.— H. -W. Hansen and H. H. Wagener, *Dt. med. Wschr.*, 1971, *96*, 1866. See also H. Adamska-Dyniewska, *Pol. med. J.*, 1970, *9*, 304, per *Int. pharm. Abstr.*, 1971, *8*, 24.

Administration of *phenytoin* reduced serum-digoxin concentrations in 8 patients receiving maintenance treatment with digoxin. The half-life of digoxin was not affected.— K. Lahiri and N. Ertel, *Clin. Res.*, 1974, *22*, 321A.

Antihypertensive agents. Increased sensitivity to digitalis characterised by frequent ectopic beats and bigeminy has been noted in patients also receiving *reserpine*.— B. Lown *et al.*, *Circulation*, 1961, *24*, 1185, per *Lancet*, 1962, *1*, 843.

Benzodiazepines. Raised plasma-digoxin concentrations were found in 3 patients also taking *diazepam*. Coadministration of diazepam was subsequently found to produce moderate increases of digoxin half-life in plasma, in 5 of 7 healthy subjects, whereas urinary excretion of digoxin was substantially reduced in all 7. Plasma concentrations of digoxin should be carefully monitored in patients also receiving diazepam.— J. R. Castillo-Ferrando *et al.* (letter), *Lancet*, 1980, *2*, 368.

See also under Anaesthetic Agents (above).

Beta-adrenoceptor blocking agents. For interactions between digoxin and *propranolol*, see Propranolol Hydrochloride, p.1328.

Bran. The bioavailability of digoxin was decreased when it was given with a high-fibre diet.— D. D. Brown *et al.*, *Am. J. Cardiol.*, 1977, *39*, 297. There was no significant reduction in the absorption of digoxin when the diet of 12 patients on maintenance therapy was supplemented with bran.— M. N. Woods and J. A. Ingelfinger, *Clin. Pharmac. Ther.*, 1979, *26*, 21.

Diuretics. There are conflicting reports on the effect of *frusemide* on digoxin excretion. R.G. McAllister *et al.* (*J. clin. Pharmac.*, 1976, *16*, 110) found that a single intravenous dose of frusemide 80 mg produced a prompt and brisk diuresis in 3 patients who had been taking digoxin daily for more than 6 months. Urinary excretion of digoxin was increased in direct proportion to the increase in urine volume although no significant changes in serum-digoxin concentrations were found. However, in a study by D.D. Brown *et al.* (*Clin. Pharmac. Ther.*, 1976, *20*, 395) digoxin excretion was not significantly affected by the concurrent administration of frusemide 40 mg daily by mouth for 8 days. Results reported by A.D. Malcolm *et al.* (*Clin. Pharmac. Ther.*, 1977, *21*, 567) and W.J. Tilstone *et al.* (*Clin. Pharmac. Ther.*, 1977, *22*, 389) have also suggested that there is no need to alter loading or maintenance doses of digoxin when frusemide is given concurrently. In an attempt to clarify the effect of frusemide on the serum clearance and renal excretion of digoxin, E. Tsutsumi *et al.* (*J. clin. Pharmac.*, 1979, *19*, 200) gave 6 healthy subjects an oral dose of frusemide 5 hours after an intravenous injection of digoxin. They found that frusemide significantly decreased the serum clearance of digoxin during the diuretic phase and the renal excretion of digoxin after diuresis, although the total amount of urinary digoxin was not affected. Decreased glomerular filtration-rate by volume depletion might have been responsible for the decreased excretion of digoxin although it was considered possible that the tubular secretion of digoxin had been inhibited by frusemide. See also under Forced Diuresis in Treatment of Adverse Effects (above).

There was no evidence that *spironolactone* influenced liver microsomal enzyme activity and digoxin elimination to a significant extent in a study of 8 subjects.— E. E. Ohnhaus and J. P. Masson, *Br. J. clin. Pharmac.*, 1977, *4*, 639P. Following the demonstration by E. Steiness (*Circulation*, 1974, *50*, 103) that *spironolactone* inhibits the tubular secretion of digoxin, the effect of spironolactone on digoxin kinetics has been studied in 4 patients with heart disease and 4 healthy subjects, all of whom were given digoxin intravenously before and after a 5-day course of spironolactone. Plasma concentrations of digoxin were increased by spironolactone and the total clearance of digoxin reduced by 25%. It is suggested that loading and maintenance doses of digoxin may need to be reduced during treatment with spironolactone.— S. Waldorff *et al.*, *Clin. Pharmac. Ther.*, 1978, *24*, 162. See also under Interference with Laboratory Estimations (below).

Ion-exchange resins. Administration of digoxin a few hours before *cholestyramine* avoids interference with the absorption of digoxin.— D. D. Brown *et al.*, *Drugs*, 1980, *20*, 198.

See also Treatment of Adverse Effects (above).

Metoclopramide. For reference to metoclopramide reducing serum concentrations of digoxin, see Anticholinergic Agents (above).

Muscle relaxants. For a report of arrhythmias in digitalised patients after the use of *hexafluorenium* and *suxamethonium*, see Anaesthetic Agents (above).

Quinine. In 6 subjects given quinine sulphate, total body clearance of digoxin after an intravenous dose was decreased by 26%, primarily through a reduction in non-renal clearance. Increased urinary excretion of digoxin was consistent with alterations in the non-renal clearance of digoxin and might be due to changes in the metabolism or biliary secretion of digoxin. Quinine increased the mean elimination half-life of digoxin from 34.2 to 51.8 hours but did not consistently change the volume of distribution. Serum-digoxin concentrations were increased.— M. Wandell *et al.*, *Clin. Pharmac. Ther.*, 1980, *28*, 425.

Sulphonamides. A study in 10 healthy subjects indicated that concurrent administration of *sulphasalazine* with digoxin impaired absorption of digoxin. If concurrent administration of the two drugs was deemed necessary it might be advisable to switch to digitoxin, which, being completely absorbed, is less liable to variations in absorption.— R. P. Juhl *et al.*, *Clin. Pharmac. Ther.*, 1976, *20*, 387.

Sympathomimetic agents. The use of sympathomimetic agents may increase the possibility of cardiac arrhythmias in digitalised patients.— *Med. Lett.*, 1979, *21*, 5.

Vasodilators. In 7 patients stabilised on digoxin, plasma-digoxin concentrations rose progressively by an average of 69% when *amiodarone* 200 mg thrice daily was added to their treatment.— J. O. Moysey *et al.*, *Br. med. J.*, 1981, *282*, 272.

A study in healthy subjects indicated that concomitant administration of *nifedipine* increases plasma-digoxin concentrations.— G. G. Belz *et al.* (letter), *Lancet*, 1981, *1*, 844.

Interference with laboratory estimations. The administration of digoxin could interfere with measurements of urinary 17-hydroxycorticosteroids.— J. M. Rosenberg and I. S. Kampa, *Drug Intell. & clin. Pharm.*, 1973, *7*, 33.

Digoxin might interfere with fluorimetric estimations of urinary catecholamines.— J. Millhouse, *Adverse Drug React. Bull.*, 1974, Dec., 164.

Reports of the presence of various steroid drugs in serum resulting in falsely elevated digoxin concentrations by interfering with the radioimmunoassay for digoxin: J. J. W. Zeegers *et al.*, *Clinica chim. Acta*, 1973, *44*, 109 (prednisone and spironolactone); A. P. Phillips, *Clinica chim. Acta*, 1973, *44*, 333 (canrenone, digitoxin, spironolactone, prednisolone, and prednisone); A. B. T. J. Boink *et al.*, *J. clin. Chem. clin. Biochem.*, 1977, *15*, 261 (cardiac glycosides and spironolactone).

Porphyria. Digoxin probably did not precipitate acute porphyria.— *Drug & Ther. Bull.*, 1976, *14*, 55.

Absorption and Fate. Up to about 70% of a dose of digoxin administered as tablets and 80% of a dose given as elixir is absorbed from the gastro-intestinal tract. Therapeutic plasma concentrations may range from 0.5 to 2.5 ng per ml. Digoxin has a large volume of distribution and is widely distributed in tissues, including the heart, brain, kidneys, liver, and skeletal muscle. The concentration of digoxin in the myocardium is considerably higher than in plasma. From 20 to 30% is bound to plasma protein. Digoxin has been detected in pleural fluid, cerebrospinal fluid, and breast milk; it also crosses the placenta. It has an elimination half-life of 1 to 2 days.

Some metabolism does take place in the liver and limited enterohepatic recycling occurs but digoxin is mainly excreted unchanged in the urine by glomerular filtration; tubular secretion and reabsorption also occurs. After intravenous injection 27% of a dose has been reported to be excreted in the urine within 24 hours, chiefly as digoxin, and 15% excreted in the faeces; 80% of a dose has been recovered in the urine within a week.

Reviews of the pharmacokinetics of cardiac glycosides: H. Lüllmann *et al.*, *Dt. med. Wschr.*, 1971, *96*, 1018; J. E. Doherty *et al.*, *Prog. cardiovasc. Dis.*, 1978, *21*, 141; D. J. Temple *et al.*, *Int. J. Pharmaceut.*, 1979, *2*, 127; A. W. Kelman *et al.*, *Br. J. clin. Pharmac.*, 1980, *10*, 135 (digoxin, medigoxin, and ouabain).

Reviews of the pharmacokinetics of digoxin: J. E. Doherty, *Ann. intern. Med.*, 1973, *79*, 229; H. -J. Gilfrich *et al.*, *Arzneimittel-Forsch.*, 1973, *23*, 1659; E. Iisalo, *Clin. Pharmacokinet.*, 1977, *2*, 1; J. K. Aronson, *Clin. Pharmacokinet.*, 1980, *5*, 137.

Studies on the pharmacokinetics of digoxin: J. R. Koup *et al.*, *J. Pharmacokinet. Biopharm.*, 1975, *3*, 181 (after intravenous bolus and infusion doses); M. Danhof and D. D. Breimer, *Clin. Pharmacokinet.*, 1978, *3*, 39 (saliva-digoxin concentrations); H. R. Ochs *et al.*, *Am. Heart J.*, 1978, *96*, 507 (dose-independent pharmacokinetics); H. R. Ochs *et al.*, *Clin. Pharmac. Ther.*, 1980, *28*, 340 (pharmacokinetics after single and multiple intravenous doses).

Plasma concentrations after the intravenous administration of digoxin were similar in patients with *acute hepatitis* and healthy subjects.— W. Zilly *et al.*, *Clin. Pharmac. Ther.*, 1975, *17*, 302.

A brief discussion on the pharmacokinetics of digoxin in patients with *cardiac failure*.— N. L. Benowitz and W. Meister, *Clin. Pharmacokinet.*, 1976, *1*, 389.

Further references to the pharmacokinetics of digoxin in *cardiovascular disease*: T. Jogestrand (letter), *Lancet*, 1978, *2*, 1104 (an association between higher atrial contraction frequency and greater digoxin binding following cardiac surgery); U. R. Korhonen *et al.*, *Am. J. Cardiol.*, 1979, *44*, 1190 (in acute myocardial infarction); L. R. Tamburrini, *Minerva cardioangiol.*, 1979, *27*, 83 (in hypertension).

The majority of a dose of digoxin is excreted in the urine and *impaired renal function* leads to a decreased rate of elimination and accumulation of digoxin if dosage is not adjusted. Renal clearance of digoxin is very often similar to the creatinine clearance and J.R. Koup *et al.* (*Clin. Pharmac. Ther.*, 1975, *18*, 9) reported a linear relationship between body clearance of digoxin, including renal and nonrenal clearances, and renal clearance of creatinine. The volume of distribution of digoxin is reduced in severe renal impairment.— E. Iisalo, *Clin. Pharmacokinet.*, 1977, *2*, 1. A study on the influence of renal failure on the metabolism and route of excretion of digoxin indicating that it is unlikely that a major change in digoxin metabolism occurs, even in patients with minimal renal function. However, elimination via the biliary tract appears to be much more important in renal failure.— M. H. Gault *et al.*, *Clin. Pharmac. Ther.*, 1979, *25*, 499.

Further references to the pharmacokinetics of digoxin in patients with *renal failure:* J. E. Doherty *et al.*, *Circulation*, 1968, *37*, 865 (renal transplant patients); E. M. Bayliss *et al.*, *Br. med. J.*, 1972, *1*, 338; R. Goulding *et al.* (letter), *ibid.*, 627 (clearance of creatinine and digoxin); F. Grosse-Brockhoff *et al.*, *Dt. med. Wschr.*, 1973, *98*, 1547; M. F. Paulson and P. G. Welling, *J. clin. Pharmac.*, 1976, *16*, 660 (the calculation of serum-digoxin concentrations in patients with normal and impaired renal function); W. J. F. van der Vijgh, *Int. J. clin. Pharmac. Biopharm.*, 1977, *15*, 249 (pharmacokinetics in patients in terminal renal failure, off haemodialysis); *idem*, 255 (patients in terminal renal failure, on haemodialysis); W. J. F. van der Vijgh and P. L. Oe, *ibid.*, 560 (the effect of heparin on digoxin in patients with terminal renal failure); R. D. Okada *et al.*, *Circulation*, 1978, *58*, 1196 (a linear relationship between plasma-digoxin concentrations and dose in patients with normal and impaired renal function).

See also under Protein Binding (below) and under Administration in Renal Failure in Uses.

A brief discussion on the effects of *thyroid dysfunction* on digoxin pharmacokinetics. Plasma-digoxin concentrations have been reported to be lower when patients are thyrotoxic than when they are euthyroid (J.E. Doherty and W.H. Perkins, *Ann. intern. Med.*, 1966, *64*, 489; M.S. Croxson and H.K. Ibbertson, *Br. med. J.*, 1975, *3*, 566; G.M. Shenfield *et al.*, *Eur. J. clin. Pharmac.*, 1977, *12*, 437; J. Bonelli *et al.*, *Int. J. clin. Pharmac. Biopharm.*, 1978, *16*, 302) but J.R. Lawrence *et al.* (*Clin. Pharmac. Ther.*, 1977, *22*, 7) considered that the insensitivity of hyperthyroid patients to digoxin did not have a pharmacokinetic basis. D.H. Huffman *et al.* (*Clin. Pharmac. Ther.*, 1977, *22*, 533) suggested that digoxin absorption might have been impaired and biliary excretion increased in a hyperthyroid patient who required increased digoxin dosage. Some workers have found plasma-digoxin concentrations to be higher in patients when hypothyroid than when euthyroid (J.E. Doherty and W.H. Perkins, *Ann. intern. Med.*, 1966, *64*, 489 and M.S. Croxson and H.K. Ibbertson, *Br. med. J.*, 1975, *3*, 566) although this was not confirmed by G.M. Shenfield *et al.* (*Eur. J. clin. Pharmac.*, 1977, *12*, 437). No reliable interpretation can be placed on the plasma-digoxin concentration in patients with thyroid dysfunction.— J. K. Aronson, *Clin. Pharmacokinet.*, 1980, *5*, 137.

Apart from impairment of digoxin excretion because of impaired renal function, *elderly* patients may have a reduced apparent volume of distribution of digoxin and should therefore be given lower loading doses.— J. K. Aronson, *Clin. Pharmacokinet.*, 1980, *5*, 137.

Further references to the pharmacokinetics of digoxin in *elderly* patients: G. A. Ewy *et al.*, *Circulation*, 1969, *39*, 449 (prolonged half-life); R. Krakauer and E. Steiness, *Clin. Pharmac. Ther.*, 1978, *24*, 454 (digoxin concentrations in choroid plexus, brain, and myocardium); B. Cusack *et al.*, *Clin. Pharmac. Ther.*, 1979, *25*, 772.

A review of the pharmacokinetics of digoxin in *neonates and infants*. In full-term neonates or infants 80 to 90% of a dose of digoxin administered by mouth in liquid form is absorbed, with peak plasma concentrations occurring within 30 to 120 minutes. The rate of absorption may be slower in preterm and low birth-weight infants, with peak concentrations achieved at 90 to 180 minutes, and may be significantly reduced in severe heart failure and in malabsorption syndromes. The intramuscular route should be avoided since the absorption of digoxin is erratic and very slow and tissue necrosis may occur. After the intravenous administration of digoxin there is a rapid distribution phase with an apparent half-life of 20 to 40 minutes followed by a slower exponential decay of plasma concentrations. In full-term neonates digoxin has an apparent volume of distribution of 6 to 10 litres per kg body-weight. Smaller volumes have been noted in premature infants, while in infants the volume may range from 10 to 22 litres per kg which is 1.5 to 2 times reported adult values. The apparent plasma half-life in healthy and sick neonates is generally very long and may range from 20 to 70 hours in full-term neonates or from 40 to 180 hours in preterm neonates. Digoxin is eliminated at a considerably faster rate in infants than in neonates and, in parallel with maturation of kidney function, a marked increase in clearance-rate is usually observed between the second and third month of life. The large apparent volume of distribution, higher clearance values, and greater concentrations of digoxin in the myocardial tissue and red cells of infants might justify the traditional assumption that infants tolerate digoxin better than adults and that higher doses are consequently needed in infants. However, studies have shown that in infants, as in adults, toxic signs become evident at plasma-digoxin concentrations above 3 ng per ml and that the therapeutic range may be 1.5 to 2 ng per ml. It is considered that doses of digoxin used in the past have been too high and that lower doses should be used, especially in premature and full-term neonates.— P. L. Morselli *et al.*, *Clin. Pharmacokinet.*, 1980, *5*, 485. See also G. Wettrell and K. -E. Andersson, *Clin. Pharmacokinet.*, 1977, *2*, 17.

There was no significant difference in serum-digoxin concentrations between 10 mature and 9 premature *infants* given digoxin but the serum half-life was significantly longer in the premature group, median values being 57 and 35 hours for the premature and mature group respectively.— D. Lang and G. von Bernuth, *Pediatrics*, 1977, *59*, 902.

In *neonates* with congestive heart failure the mean half-life of the distribution phase of digoxin was 37 minutes, and 44 hours for the elimination phase; in similar infants the corresponding values were 28 minutes and 19 hours respectively.— G. Wettrell, *Eur. J. clin. Pharmac.*, 1977, *11*, 329.

Studies in 34 *infants* aged 1 week to 2 years given digoxin for congestive heart failure showed that serum concentrations were markedly higher in those aged under 3 months, despite giving weight-adjusted doses.— H. Halkin *et al.*, *Eur. J. clin. Pharmac.*, 1978, *13*, 113. See also H. Halkin *et al.*, *Pediatrics*, 1978, *61*, 184.

Further references to pharmacokinetic studies of digoxin in *infants and children:* W. T. Dungan *et al.*, *Circulation*, 1972, *46*, 983; M. C. Rogers *et al.*, *New Engl. J. Med.*, 1972, *287*, 1010 (serum-digoxin concentrations); R. J. Larese and B. L. Mirkin, *Clin. Pharmac. Ther.*, 1974, *15*, 387 (lack of a relationship between high serum-digoxin concentrations and cardiac arrhythmias in children); R. Gorodischer *et al.*, *Clin. Pharmac. Ther.*, 1976, *19*, 256 (distribution of digoxin in the myocardium, skeletal muscle, erythrocytes, and plasma of infants); M. Kearin *et al.*, *Clin. Pharmac. Ther.*, 1980, *28*, 346 (differences between the binding properties of digoxin in the erythrocytes of neonates and adults).

See also below under Pregnancy and the Neonate.

Absorption. Although steady-state serum digoxin concentrations were obtained in 6 to 7 days in both controls and patients with malabsorption syndromes given digoxin 250 µg daily, the concentrations achieved by the 9 patients were significantly lower than the controls. Absorption was unaffected in 2 patients with pancreatic insufficiency.— W. D. Heizer *et al.*, *New Engl. J. Med.*, 1971, *285*, 257.

In healthy subjects, digoxin given by mouth after fasting or 30 minutes after a meal led to peak plasma concentrations at 30 to 60 minutes, being significantly lower after a meal. There was no significant difference in plasma concentrations in either case after 2 to 8 hours. In a study of 21 patients receiving maintenance digoxin therapy the plasma-digoxin concentration was not significantly altered when digoxin was ingested after food.— R. J. White *et al.*, *Br. med. J.*, 1971, *1*, 380. Studies in 6 healthy subjects demonstrated that ingestion of food decreased the rate but not the extent of absorption of concurrently administered digoxin.— B. F. Johnson *et al.*, *Clin. Pharmac. Ther.*, 1978, *23*, 315.

The absorption of digoxin measured by urinary excretion over a prolonged period was considered to be more accurate than extrapolation of plasma concentrations read up to 6 hours after a dose.— T. Beveridge *et al.* (letter), *Lancet*, 1973, *2*, 499.

Absorption of digoxin was not significantly affected in 7 patients who had undergone jejuno-ileal bypass for massive obesity.— F. I. Marcus *et al.*, *Circulation*, 1977, *55*, 537. Five of 9 patients who had undergone jejuno-ileal bypass showed impaired digoxin absorption.— C. D. Gerson *et al.*, *Am. J. Med.*, 1980, *69*, 43.

Further references to the absorption of digoxin: H. Gault *et al.*, *Clin. Pharmac. Ther.*, 1980, *27*, 16; *idem*, 1981, *29*, 181 (the influence of gastric pH on digoxin biotransformation).

Bioavailability. Variation in the biological availability of digoxin from digoxin preparations has been associated with reports of the content of tablets varying between 28 and 148% of the stated amount, of variability in disintegration, of variability in dissolution ranging from 6 to 92% at 15 minutes, and of up to 7-fold or more differences in serum concentrations. Other factors involved in varying bioavailability include the pharmaceutical formulation and presentation (capsules, solution, or tablets), particle size, and biological factors. The digoxin problem was highlighted in the UK in 1972 by alterations in bioavailability of Lanoxin following changes in manufacturing procedure.

Dissolution-rate is considered to be a better guide to probable bioavailability than a disintegration test. Since digoxin tablets in the UK and USA must now comply with pharmacopoeial standards for dissolution-rates, more uniform absorption from the gastro-intestinal tract should be achieved and there should be fewer problems with variable bioavailability.

Reviews on the bioavailability of digoxin: D. A. Chamberlain, *Adv. Med. Topics Ther.*, 1975, *1*, 49; J. L. Colaizzi *et al.*, *J. Am. pharm. Ass.*, 1977, *NS17*, 635.

Studies in healthy subjects suggested that the bioavailability of digoxin could be increased by administering it as capsules containing 50, 100, or 200 µg of digoxin in solution. The maximum bioavailability from capsules was 88%, compared to 75% with commercially available tablets.— P. F. Binnion, *J. clin. Pharmac.*, 1976, *16*, 461. See also B. F. Johnson *et al.*, *Wellcome*, *Clin. Pharmac. Ther.*, 1976, *19*, 746; B. F. Johnson *et al.*, *Wellcome*, *Br. J. clin. Pharmac.*, 1977, *4*, 209; C. Longhini *et al.*, *Curr. ther. Res.*, 1977, *21*, 909; B. L. Lloyd *et al.*, *Am. J. Cardiol.*, 1978, *42*, 129. In 20 patients given digoxin in their usual dose as tablets for 4 weeks or, in a crossover period, as soft gelatin capsules containing 80% of the tablet dose as a solution in macrogol, mean digoxin concentrations were approximately proportional to the doses given. The introduction of capsules would probably not represent an advance in treatment.— E. M. Rodgers *et al.*, *Br. med. J.*, 1977, *2*, 234.

Further references to the bioavailability of digoxin from capsules.— J. O'Grady *et al.*, *Eur. J. clin. Pharmac.*, 1978, *14*, 357; J. O'Grady *et al.*, *Br. J. clin. Pharmac.*, 1978, *5*, 461; L. Padeletti and A. Brat, *Int. J. clin. Pharmac. Biopharm.*, 1978, *16*, 320; V. Alvisi *et al.*, *Arzneimittel-Forsch.*, 1979, *29*, 1047; E. Astorri *et al.*, *J. pharm. Sci.*, 1979, *68*, 104.

A report of the bioavailability of a digoxin-hydroquinone complex.— F. Bochner *et al.*, *J. pharm. Sci.*, 1977, *66*, 644.

A study of the bioavailability of digoxin from silica matrix formulations.— H. Flasch *et al.*, *Arzneimittel-Forsch.*, 1978, *28*, 326.

Studies *in vitro* indicated that pH influenced the extent of hydrolysis of digoxin and it was suggested that this may account for the variable bioavailability when administered by mouth since gastric pH could modify the composition of digoxin species available for absorption.— L. A. Sternson and R. D. Shaffer, *J. pharm. Sci.*, 1978, *67*, 327. See also S. A. H. Khalil and S. El-Masry, *J. pharm. Sci.*, 1978, *67*, 1358.

Further references to bioavailability studies with various digoxin preparations: C. I. Flasch and N. Heinz, *Arzneimittel-Forsch.*, 1979, *29*, 961; *idem*, 1737; N. Rietbrock *et al.*, *Arzneimittel-Forsch.*, 1979, *29*, 1742; B. Bergdahl *et al.*, *Eur. J. clin. Pharmac.*, 1980, *17*, 443; S. Fletcher and R. S. Summers, *S. Afr. med. J.*, 1980, *57*, 530.

For earlier reports on the bioavailability of oral digoxin preparations, see Martindale 27th Edn, p. 493.

Distribution. Digoxin is widely distributed throughout the body tissues and has a high apparent volume of distribution. Calculated from data given by J.E. Doherty *et al.* (*Ann. intern. Med.*, 1967, *66*, 116) distribution to various tissues is: skeletal muscle, 65%; liver, 13%; heart, 4%, brain, 3%; and kidneys, 1.5%. Numerous studies of the relationship between myocardial tissue concentrations of digoxin and corresponding plasma concentrations have given varying results according to the techniques used and differences in patient populations. Reported ratios between myocardial tissue and plasma concentrations include: figures ranging from 39:1 to 155:1 (J. Coltart *et al.*, *Br. med. J.*, 1972, *2*, 318; *idem*, 1974, *4*, 733), 24:1 (H.-G. Güllner *et al.*, *Clin. Pharmac. Ther.*, 1974, *15*, 208), and 67:1 (G. Härtel *et al.*, *Clin. Pharmac. Ther.*, 1976, *19*, 153). It is suggested that plasma concentrations may be closely related to subcellular concentrations of digoxin which may be of greater therapeutic importance than total myocardial concentrations.— J. K. Aronson, *Clin. Pharmacokinet.*, 1980, *5*, 137.

In a study of 8 patients who had taken digoxin for at least 7 years the ratio between the concentration in myocardial tissue and plasma ranged from 39:1 to 155:1, and between skeletal muscle and plasma from 3:1 to 58:1.— J. Coltart *et al.*, *Br. med. J.*, 1972, *2*, 318.

Further references to myocardial concentrations of digoxin: P. R. Carroll *et al.*, *Aust. N.Z. J. Med.*, 1973, *3*, 400; E. Iisalo and M. Nuutila (letter), *Lancet*, 1973, *1*, 257; S. G. Carruthers *et al.*, *Br. Heart J.*, 1975, *37*, 313.

Digoxin was found to be concentrated in the choroid plexus of infants and adults.— Å. Bertler *et al.* (letter), *Lancet*, 1973, *2*, 1453.

In a patient given digoxin 250 µg every 8 hours for 6 weeks, plasma-digoxin concentrations ranged from 1.5 to 2.1 ng per ml but the CSF concentration was less than 0.2 ng per ml on one occasion and undetectable at all other times.— G. D. Schott and D. Holt (letter), *Lancet*, 1974, *1*, 358. In 10 patients receiving digoxin, and whose plasma-digoxin concentrations were in the therapeutic range, no digoxin was detected in the CSF in 8 and low concentrations in 2.— G. D. Schott *et al.*, *Postgrad. med. J.*, 1976, *52*, 700. In 14 patients maintained on digoxin 125 to 250 µg daily, serum concentrations were 0.43 to 2.15 ng per ml and CSF concentrations 70 to 770 pg per ml. Higher CSF concentrations were found in older patients with a lower body-weight. The results were considered to provide evidence that some effects of digoxin may be mediated via the central nervous system.— J. M. Gayes *et al.*, *J. clin. Pharmac.*, 1978, *18*, 16. See also H. Allonen *et al.*, *Acta pharmac. tox.*, 1977, *41*, 193.

Further references to the distribution of digoxin.— T. Livanou *et al.* (letter), *Lancet*, 1972, *1*, 1027 (in pleural fluid).

Excretion. Studies in 6 patients with biliary fistulas given 0.5 to 1 mg of tritiated digoxin intravenously demonstrated that nearly all the digoxin excreted in the faeces was provided by the bile. About 6.5% of a dose was involved in recycling in the enterohepatic circulation.— J. E. Doherty *et al.*, *Circulation*, 1970, *42*, 867.

The 7-day excretion of digoxin in 20 subjects given digoxin by mouth was 34% in the urine and 15% in the faeces; after intravenous administration in 28 subjects the values were 74 and 11% respectively; and 59 and 1.3% respectively in 6 with biliary fistula, in whom 8.1% was excreted in the bile.— J. E. Doherty *et al.*, *Ann. intern. Med.*, 1972, *76*, 862.

Although hepatic metabolism, biliary excretion, and subsequent intestinal reabsorption of digoxin have been regarded as insignificant, a mean of about 30% of an intravenous dose of tritiated digoxin appeared in the small intestine of 5 healthy subjects in 24 hours.— J. H. Caldwell and C. T. Cline, *Clin. Pharmac. Ther.*, 1976, *19*, 410.

The results of a study on 86 patients suggested that the dietary fat was one of the variables determining the rate of elimination of digoxin.— J. Turner *et al.*, *Br. J. clin. Pharmac.*, 1977, *4*, 489.

Further references to the biliary excretion of digoxin: V. Klotz and K. H. Antonin, *Int. J. clin. Pharmac. Biopharm.*, 1977, *15*, 332, per *Int. pharm. Abstr.*, 1978, *15*, 137.

Metabolism. Although digoxin is reported to be excreted mainly unchanged in the urine there is evidence to suggest that metabolism may sometimes be extensive. Metabolites that have been detected in the urine include digoxigenin, dihydrodigoxigenin, the mono- and bisdigitoxosides of digoxigenin, and dihydrodigoxin. Digoxigenin mono- and bisdigitoxosides are known to be cardioactive whereas dihydrodigoxin is probably much less active than digoxin. The different metabolites cross-react to a different extent with the anti-digoxin antibody used in the radioimmunoassay for digoxin. If digitoxosides are present, plasma-digoxin concentrations will be underestimated whereas digoxigenin results in an overestimate of circulating cardioactivity. In some patients the presence of digitoxosides might account for the occurrence of toxicity at apparently low concentrations of digoxin.— E. Iisalo, *Clin. Pharmacokinet.*, 1977, *2*, 1; J. K. Aronson, *ibid.*, 1980, *5*, 137.

Inactive dihydrodigoxin was present in the urine of 46 of 50 patients given digoxin and represented a mean of 14% of digoxin and metabolites extractable with methylene chloride.— D. R. Clark and S. M. Kalman, *Clin. Pharmac. Ther.*, 1974, *15*, 202. See also U. Peters *et al.*, *Archs intern. Med.*, 1978, *138*, 1074.

Plasma concentrations. Serum and plasma concentrations of digoxin are equivalent.— T. W. Smith and E. Haber, *New Engl. J. Med.*, 1973, *289*, 1063.

The optimum therapeutic serum concentration of digoxin is 0.5 to 2 ng per ml.— E. Iisalo, *Clin. Pharmacokinet.*, 1977, *2*, 1. Plasma (or serum) concentrations of digoxin have not been shown conclusively to be correlated either with the quantity of digoxin in cardiac tissue or with the various measures of its clinical effects. Most workers would prefer to maintain plasma-digoxin concentrations of between 1 and 1.5 ng per ml; it is not clear whether increasing the plasma concentration within the nontoxic range is likely to be of benefit.— J. K. Aronson, *ibid.*, 1980, *5*, 137.

Further discussions on serum-digoxin concentrations: J. E. Doherty, *Ann. intern. Med.*, 1971, *74*, 787; A. Dodek, *Can. med. Ass. J.*, 1977, *117*, 994; M. Weintraub, *Clin. Pharmacokinet.*, 1977, *2*, 205; J. K. Aronson *et al.*, *Q.J. Med.*, 1978, *47*, 111; J. E. Doherty, *J. Am. med. Ass.*, 1978, *239*, 2594; A. Richens and S. Warrington, *Drugs*, 1979, *17*, 488 (therapeutic range, 1 to 2.5 ng per ml).

In 3 patients who were being digitalised, plasma-digoxin concentrations of 0.6 to 1.5 ng per ml were noted, and in 67 patients who were receiving maintenance therapy, concentrations of 0.4 to 5 ng per ml were found. Apart from 3 patients with renal failure with plasma concentrations greater than 4 ng per ml, concentrations were below 3.7 ng per ml. No patient had evidence of digoxin toxicity. Plasma concentrations rose by 0.5 to 1 ng per ml 2 to 4 hours after the administration of digoxin to 4 patients on maintenance therapy, falling to the baseline within 5 to 8 hours.— D. C. Evered *et al.*, *Br. med. J.*, 1970, *3*, 427.

In 116 patients with atrial fibrillation on long-term treatment with digoxin, plasma-digoxin concentrations ranged from less than 0.25 ng per ml to 3.2 ng per ml, mean 1.4 ng per ml, and in 21 of 22 patients with digoxin toxicity from 2 to 5.2 ng per ml, mean 3.1 ng per ml. In 1 patient with digoxin toxicity, the plasma concentration was only 0.7 ng per ml. In patients with good renal function there was a significant correlation between digoxin dosage and plasma concentration. Toxicity was only associated with plasma concentrations of digoxin in excess of 2 ng per ml. The ventricular response to atrial fibrillation correlated poorly with the plasma concentration of digoxin.— D. A. Chamberlain *et al.*, *Br. med. J.*, 1970, *3*, 429.

After administration of digoxin intravenously to 8 digitalised patients with congestive heart failure, initial high blood concentrations were obtained which fell to a plateau after about 4 hours. Following intramuscular injection maximum concentrations developed within 1 to 2 hours; these were higher than the concentrations 2 hours after intravenous injection and were still higher after a further 4 hours. Local tissue damage occurred in *pigs* after intramuscular injections.— E. Steiness *et al.*, *Clin. Pharmac. Ther.*, 1974, *16*, 430.

Further references to the measurement of serum-digoxin concentrations: H. Allonen *et al.*, *Int. J. clin. Pharmac. Biopharm.*, 1978, *16*, 420 (estimations in serum, saliva, and urine); W. G. Kramer *et al.*, *J. Pharmacokinet. Biopharm.*, 1979, *7*, 47, (response intensity and predicted compartmental drug concentrations); L. Balant *et al.*, *J. clin. Hosp. Pharm.*, 1980, *5*, 35 (pharmacokinetic requirements for predicting serum digoxin-concentration during regular therapy). See also Metabolism (above).

Pregnancy and the neonate. Seven pregnant women who received 250 µg of digoxin daily by mouth had a mean plasma-digoxin concentration of 0.6 ng per ml at delivery. Foetal concentrations were within 0.1 ng per ml of the maternal concentration at delivery.— M. C. Rogers *et al.*, *New Engl. J. Med.*, 1972, *287*, 1010.

A study of the milk of 5 women receiving maintenance digoxin therapy for rheumatic heart disease who wished to breast feed their children, indicated that the total daily excretion of digoxin in the milk of mothers with therapeutic serum-digoxin concentrations would not exceed 1 to 2 µg. These amounts were not sufficient to affect the infants.— M. Levy *et al.* (letter), *New Engl. J. Med.*, 1977, *297*, 789. Digoxin could not be detected in the plasma of 2 infants about 10 days after breast feeding had been established. Their mothers had taken digoxin 250 µg daily throughout pregnancy and continued treatment post partum. The estimated daily intake of digoxin in the milk was only 120 ng per kg bodyweight for one infant and 60 ng per kg for the other infant.— P. M. Loughnan, *J. Pediat.*, 1978, *92*, 1019.

Further references to digoxin in pregnancy and the neonate: H. Allonen *et al.*, *Acta pharmac. tox.*, 1976, *39*, 477 (foeto-maternal distribution in early pregnancy); S. Saarikoski, *Br. J. Obstet. Gynaec.*, 1976, *83*, 879 (placental transfer and foetal uptake); V. Chan *et al.*, *Br. J. Obstet. Gynaec.*, 1978, *85*, 605 (placental transfer and excretion into breast milk); J. P. Finley *et al.*, *J. Pediat.*, 1979, *94*, 339 (excretion into breast milk and detection in neonatal serum); L. Padeletti *et al.*, *Int. J. clin. Pharmac. Biopharm.*, 1979, *17*, 82 (placental transfer).

See also above for pharmacokinetic data relating to infants and children.

Protein binding. Reported values for digoxin protein binding have varied from 5 to 60% depending on the methods used, although the figure is usually around 20%. In the present study digoxin was found to be 21.2% bound. Binding was normal in uraemic patients but decreased from 23.5 to 15.4% during haemodialysis.— L. Storstein, *Clin. Pharmac. Ther.*, 1976, *20*, 6. Changes in protein binding during haemodialysis closely resembled those after injection of heparin and it is considered that displacement of digoxin from albumin by free fatty acids is responsible.— L. Storstein and H. Janssen, *ibid.*, 15.

Further references to plasma protein binding of digoxin: D. S. Lukas, *Ann. N.Y. Acad. Sci.*, 1971, *179*, 338 (about 23% bound); L. Storstein, *Clin. Pharmacokinet.*, 1977, *2*, 220 (binding in disease states); N. Verbeke *et al.*, *Eur. J. clin. Pharmac.*, 1979, *16*, 341 (20% measured by ultracentrifugation).

Uses. Digoxin increases the force of myocardial contraction and in heart failure this positive inotropic effect results in an improved cardiac output with a more complete emptying of the ventricle at systole, a reduction in elevated end-diastolic ventricular pressure, and a reduction in the size of the dilated heart. Venous pressure is lowered because the heart is capable of dealing with an increased venous return of blood and not only is the force of systole increased but its length is shortened, giving the heart more time to rest between contractions and more time for the ventricle to fill with venous blood. Improvement in the peripheral circulation secondary to these effects on the heart improves renal function and results in diuresis and the relief of oedema. It will not improve renal function not due to faulty circulation or remove oedema not due to heart failure.

Digoxin also depresses conduction in the heart by a direct effect on the atrioventricular node and bundle of His and indirectly by increasing vagal action and may thus slow the ventricular-rate and produce a relative atrioventricular block. Increased myocardial excitability at high doses may give rise to drug-induced arrhythmias.

Digoxin is used in the treatment of congestive heart failure although the beneficial effect of long-term treatment in patients in sinus rhythm is questioned. Diuretics are often given concomitantly and may be preferred to digoxin as initial treatment in patients with mild congestive heart failure and sinus rhythm. Vasodilators may also be used. There is controversy over the use of digoxin in patients with acute myocardial infarction and over its prophylactic use.

Digoxin is given to slow the ventricular-rate in the management of atrial fibrillation; treatment is usually long term. It has also been given to convert atrial flutter into fibrillation and on subsequent withdrawal of the drug sinus rhythm may be restored. Digoxin should not be used when atrial fibrillation or flutter occurs in patients with the Wolff-Parkinson-White syndrome. It may be given to relieve an attack of paroxysmal atrial or supraventricular tachycardia and has also been given to prevent further attacks. The use of digoxin in paroxysmal ventricular tachycardia is dangerous.

Blood pressure is affected by digoxin only through the action of the drug on the heart and not by any significant effect on the blood vessels or vasomotor centre; low pressures due to decompensation are raised as digoxin improves cardiac function.

When given by mouth, digoxin may take effect in about 1 hour and the maximum effect may be reached in about 6 hours. Its action lasts for up to 6 days.

Higher doses are necessary to provide a chronotropic effect in cardiac arrhythmias than to produce an inotropic effect in congestive heart failure. Dosage should be carefully adjusted to the needs of the individual patient. Factors which may be considered include the patient's age, lean body mass, renal status, thyroid status, electrolyte balance, degree of tissue oxygenation, and the nature of the underlying cardiac or pulmonary disease. Steady-state plasma-digoxin concentrations (in a specimen taken about 6 hours after a dose) of 1 to 2 ng per ml are generally considered acceptable; concentrations in excess of 2 ng per ml may be associated with toxicity. Because of considerable overlap, plasma concentrations are considered inadequate as the sole guide to dosage.

For rapid digitalisation with digoxin, 0.75 to 1.5 mg may be given by mouth followed by 250 µg every 6 hours until the desired therapeutic effect is obtained. Some authorities advocate a total dose of 1 to 1.5 mg given in divided doses every 6 to 8 hours. If there is no great urgency a loading dose is omitted and digitalisation is achieved slowly over a week or more with doses of 125 to 750 µg daily. The usual maintenance dose of digoxin is 250 µg by mouth once or twice daily. In elderly patients therapy should generally be carried out gradually and with smaller doses; maintenance doses of 125 to 250 µg daily are usually adequate.

In urgent cases, provided that the patient has not been treated with cardiac glycosides during the previous 2 weeks, digoxin may be given by slow intravenous injection. The dosage ranges from 0.5 to 1 mg and produces a definite effect on the heart-rate within 10 minutes, reaching a maximum within 1 to 2 hours. A further 500 µg may be given a few hours later if necessary. Alternatively an initial intravenous dose of 250 to 500 µg may be given, followed by 250 µg every 4 to 6 hours to a maximum total dose of 1 mg. Maintenance treatment is then usually given by mouth but intravenous doses of 125 to 500 µg daily have been given if oral administration is not possible. Digoxin has also been given intramuscularly; such injections may be painful.

A suggested dose for infants and children is 10 to 20 µg per kg body-weight by mouth or by injection every 6 hours until the desired therapeutic effect is obtained usually after 2 to 4 doses, then 10 to 20 µg per kg daily, and later adjusted to the optimum maintenance dose. Premature and immature infants are particularly sensitive to digoxin whereas children between one month and 2 years may require relatively larger doses than older children.

Digoxin should not be given subcutaneously as it may give rise to intense local irritation, and when given intravenously it should be administered slowly, care being taken to prevent extravasation.

General reviews on the actions and uses of digoxin and the other cardiac glycosides: D. A. Chamberlain, *Adv. Med. Topics Ther.*, 1975, *1*, 49; J. K. Aronson and D. G. Grahame-Smith, *Br. J. clin. Pharmac.*, 1976, *3*, 639; D. O. Williams, *Prescribers' J.*, 1977, *17*, 66; *Lancet*, 1978, *2*, 1288; *Am. J. Hosp. Pharm.*, 1978, *35*, 1495; M. F. O'Rourke, *Med. J. Aust.*, 1978, *2*, 366; *Drug & Ther. Bull.*, 1979, *17*, 49; A. M. Breckenridge and M. L'E. Orme, *Practitioner*, 1979, *223*, 465; J. F. Bresnahan and R. E. Vlietstra, *Mayo Clin. Proc.*, 1979, *54*, 675; L. H. Opie, *Lancet*, 1980, *1*, 912; A. J. Taggart and D. G. McDevitt, *Drugs*, 1980, *20*, 398.

Action. Discussions on the role of Na^+, K^+-ATPase in the inotropic action of cardiac glycosides.— J. C. Gilbert, *Br. med. J.*, 1976, *2*, 31; T. Akera and T. M. Brody, *Pharmac. Rev.*, 1977, *29*, 187. See also D. B. Morgan *et al.*, *Br. J. clin. Pharmac.*, 1980, *10*, 127 (the sodium and potassium content of erythrocytes in patients treated with digoxin).

Comments on the effects of digoxin on the renin-angiotensin axis.— A. Antonello *et al.* (letter), *Lancet*, 1976, *2*, 850; M. Ferrari *et al.* (letter), *New Engl. J. Med.*, 1979, *301*, 943; R. Lammintausta, *Int. J. clin. Pharmac. Ther. Toxic.*, 1980, *18*, 110.

The role of the nervous system in the cardiovascular effects of digoxin.— R. A. Gillis and J. A. Quest, *Pharmac. Rev.*, 1979, *31*, 19.

Administration. A discussion on pharmacokinetic, pharmacodynamic, and other factors affecting digoxin dosage, with therapeutic guidelines. There is little evidence that prescribing aids such as nomograms or computer programs result in more accurate dosage determination. If patient compliance can be ensured and a preparation of uniform bioavailability is chosen, more accurate initial intuitive prescribing of digoxin should be possible with the help of careful clinical observation, critical use of plasma-digoxin concentrations, and awareness of factors which may modify the individual response such as age, other disease states, and interactions with other drugs.— G. D. Johnston, *Drugs*, 1980, *20*, 494. See also under Adverse Effects (above).

In patients with normal renal function the plasma half-life of digoxin is about 34 hours, and with doses given once or twice daily a steady plasma concentration is reached in 7 to 8 days.— D. A. Chamberlain, *Prescribers' J.*, 1972, *12*, 84.

See also Administration in Renal Failure, below.

Five patients with atrial fibrillation who received a single daily dose of digoxin were monitored for ventricular-rate at rest and during exercise and plasma-digoxin concentrations measured. Plasma-digoxin concentrations ranged from a mean of 3.4 ng per ml 4 hours after a dose to 2 ng per ml 24 hours after a dose but there was no consistent variation in ventricular-rate. On withdrawal of the drug plasma concentrations fell by 30% daily, but the heart-rate increased more slowly; significant chronotropic effect persisted for more than 6 days. Results indicate that a single daily dose of digoxin is sufficient for the control of atrial fibrillation and divided doses are not necessary.— J. C. Zener *et al.*, *J. Am. med. Ass.*, 1973, *224*, 239.

The intravenous injection of loading doses of digoxin could result in high toxic concentrations for prolonged periods. A loading dose of 0.75 to 1 mg was injected into 22 patients at 125 to 750 µg per minute and plasma concentrations remained above the postulated toxic concentration of 2 ng per ml or more for at least 2 hours.— A. Bertler *et al.* (letter), *Lancet*, 1974, *2*, 958. Seven patients were given a total loading dose of digoxin by mouth as a single dose without any adverse effect. They started their maintenance doses 24 hours later.— B. Whiting and D. J. Sumner (letter), *ibid.*, 1393.

A view that digoxin can be given by slow intravenous infusion in 50 ml of dextrose injection over 30 minutes.— C. E. Weber (letter), *Drug Intell. & clin. Pharm.*, 1977, *11*, 306.

Intramuscular injection of digoxin should be discouraged as absorption is about 80% of that from intravenous injection, there is pain and irritation at the site, and creatine phosphokinase concentrations indicate muscle damage from digoxin.— V. E. Muiznicks and D. J. Ricciatti, *Can. J. Hosp. Pharm.*, 1977, *30*, 142. See also D. J. Greenblatt *et al.* (letter), *New Engl. J. Med.*, 1973, *288*, 689; W. S. Lewis and J. E. Doherty (letter), *New Engl. J. Med.*, 1973, *288*, 1077.

Reviews, reports, and comments on the monitoring of plasma-digoxin concentrations.— M. O'Rourke, *Med. J. Aust.*, 1978, *2*, 363; H. G. Washington *et al.*, *Med. J. Aust.*, 1978, *2*, 368; H. Halkin *et al.*, *Israel J. med. Scis*, 1979, *15*, 490; J. N. Cohn, *J. Am. med. Ass.*, 1980, *243*, 1275.

Compliance with prescribed digoxin therapy was estimated by comparing plasma-digoxin concentrations before and after a 10-day period when digoxin consumption was measured. There was non-compliance in 23 of 50 patients studied in general practice.— G. D. Johnston and D. G. McDevitt, *Br. J. clin. Pharmac.*, 1978, *6*, 339. Further references to the problem of non-compliance with digoxin therapy: G. D. Johnston *et al.*, *Br. Heart J.*, 1978, *40*, 1; J. R. Gilbert *et al.*, *Can. med. Ass. J.*, 1980, *123*, 119 (predicting compliance).

Further references to digoxin dosage: R. W. Jelliffe, *Ann. intern. Med.*, 1968, *69*, 703 (dosage schedule); R. W. Jelliffe and G. Brooker, *Chest*, 1970, *58*, 282 (nomogram); R. W. Jelliffe, *J. mond. Pharm.*, 1972, *15*, 53; R. W. Jelliffe *et al.*, *Ann. intern. Med.*, 1972, *77*, 891 (computer-based dosage regimens); C. C. Peck *et al.*, *New Engl. J. Med.*, 1973, *289*, 441 (use of computer); L. B. Sheiner *et al.*, *Ann. intern. Med.*, 1975, *82*, 619 (use of computer); S. M. Dobbs (letter), *Lancet*, 1976, *2*, 694 (dosage schedule); P. Joubert *et al.*, *Clin. Pharmac. Ther.*, 1976, *20*, 676 (ECG assessment); S. M. Dobbs and G. E. Mawer, *Clin. Pharmacokinet*, 1977, *2*, 281 (a discussion on the prediction of dosage requirements); J. Schneider and A. Ruiz-Torres, *Dt. med. Wschr.*, 1977, *102*, 116 (the importance of body-weight); S. M. Dobbs *et al.*, *Br. med. J.*, 1978, *2*, 668 (a 'points' system); P. W. Nicholson *et al.*, *Br. Heart J.*, 1978, *40*, 177 (a method for calculating digoxin dosage).

For further data on plasma concentrations, see under Diagnosis of Digoxin Toxicity in Adverse Effects and under Absorption and Fate (above).

In the elderly. Both loading and maintenance doses of digoxin should be reduced empirically in the small elderly patient with reduced lean body mass and impaired renal function. Plasma-digoxin concentrations correlate with symptoms of toxicity and should be used to achieve optimal maintenance dosage. Patients should be monitored for extra-cardiac symptoms as well as more overt signs of toxicity such as arrhythmias. Not all patients taking digoxin need maintenance therapy and in one study J.L.C. Dall (*Br. med. J.*, 1970, *2*, 705) found that in almost 75% of elderly patients in sinus rhythm, digoxin could be withdrawn safely. B. Whiting *et al.* (*Br. Heart J.*, 1978, *40*, 8) have reported that only about one third of a group of elderly patients were receiving an ideal dose of digoxin and withdrawal of the drug or a revision of dosage was beneficial.— R. E. Vestal, *Drugs*, 1978, *16*, 358. A view that in general digoxin is only necessary when there is rapid atrial fibrillation causing heart failure or signs of incipient failure and in patients with supraventricular paroxysmal tachycardia. Congestive heart failure in elderly patients in sinus rhythm is usually treated with simple diuretic therapy.— J. Williamson, *Practitioner*, 1978, *220*, 749.

Further references to the use of digoxin in elderly patients.— F. I. Caird and R. D. Kennedy, *Age and Ageing*, 1977, *6*, 21; S. Landahl *et al.*, *Acta med. scand.*, 1977, *202*, 437; J. Dimant and W. Merrit, *J. Am. Geriat. Soc.*, 1978, *26*, 378; W. Simonson and D. J. Stennett, *Am. J. Hosp. Pharm.*, 1978, *35*, 943; R. C. Bryan (letter), *J. Am. med. Ass.*, 1980, *243*, 1036; E. K. Chung, *J. Am. med. Ass.*, 1980, *244*, 2561.

See also under Absorption and Fate (above).

In infants and children. In 43 children with cardiac failure of varied aetiology but with normal renal function, digitalisation was established by digoxin (given as Lanoxin paediatric elixir) 50 µg per kg body-weight daily for those under 4 weeks old; 80 µg per kg for those 4 weeks to 2 years; and 50 µg per kg for those over 2 years; these amounts were given in 3 divided doses. Daily maintenance doses were 10, 20, and 10 µg per kg respectively. In 33 patients given the maintenance doses in equal parts every 12 hours, mean plasma-digoxin concentrations were 1.5, 1.6, and 1.3 ng per ml respectively for the 3 age groups. Concentrations in the range 1 to 2 ng per ml were considered satisfactory. In 10 patients given the maintenance dose as a single dose, plasma-digoxin concentrations had fallen to below 1 ng per ml after 24 hours.— J. E. Cree *et al.*, *Br. med. J.*, 1973, *1*, 443.

From a re-evaluation of paediatric dosage schedules it is considered that recommended doses, especially for neonates, are usually unnecessarily high. Doses were calculated using pharmacokinetic principles and maintenance doses aiming to provide average serum-digoxin concentrations of 1.56 ng per ml (2 nmol per litre) during steady-state conditions were 10 µg per kg body-weight daily for neonates, 15 µg per kg daily for 'moderately clearing' infants, and 25 µg per kg daily for 'highly clearing' infants. Calculated loading doses were about

25 μg per kg for neonates and about 35 μg per kg for infants, followed by maintenance therapy 12 hours later. Intravenous loading doses should be about 75% of these oral doses. Preliminary results in 5 full-term neonates with congestive heart failure indicate that the proposed doses in neonates seem rational.— L. Nyberg and G. Wettrell, *Clin. Pharmacokinet.*, 1978, *3*, 453.

An initial dose of digoxin 10 μg per kg body-weight repeated every 4 hours for a total of 4 to 6 doses, intramuscularly, is recommended for infants. Clinical evaluation is necessary before each dose. Maintenance is with doses of 10 μg per kg once or twice daily intramuscularly or by mouth.— D. Pickering, *Br. med. J.*, 1979, *1*, 987. Digoxin can generally be given by mouth to infants but when it has to be given parenterally the intravenous route is preferable although attention should be given to the greater risk of toxicity.— G. Wettrell and K. -E. Andersson, *Clin. Pharmacokinet.*, 1977, *2*, 17.

In a study of digoxin in premature infants a total intravenous loading dose of 30 μg per kg body-weight gave serum concentrations ranging from 1.4 to 7.5 ng per ml (mean 3.5 ng per ml), smaller and more immature infants having higher concentrations. A total dose of 20 μg per kg gave serum concentrations of 1.2 to 3.0 ng per ml (mean 1.73 ng per ml) and there was no difference among various age and weight groups. Half the loading dose was given immediately, followed by a quarter of the dose 8 to 12 hours later and the remaining quarter after a further 8 to 12 hours. Maintenance was continued with one-eighth of the loading dose every 12 hours. Serum concentrations were measured at least 72 hours after digitalisation was begun. Since the two dosage regimens produced the same therapeutic effect a total loading dose of 20 μg per kg of digoxin is recommended for premature infants.— W. W. Pinsky *et al.*, *J. Pediat.*, 1979, *96*, 639.

Ampoules of digoxin for adult use should never be supplied to children's hospital wards; use of the paediatric injection should ensure that a fatal overdose cannot be given.— H. B. Valman, *Br. med. J.*, 1980, *280*, 1588.

Further references to the use of digoxin in infants and children.— H. L. Ellis *et al.* (letter), *Lancet*, 1972, *2*, 325; M. O. Savage *et al.*, *Archs Dis. Childh.*, 1975, *50*, 393; G. Wettrell *et al.*, *Eur. J. clin. Pharmac.*, 1976, *10*, 25 (exchange transfusion removed only small amounts of digoxin from plasma in 2 neonates given digoxin parenterally); J. M. Neutze *et al.*, *N.Z. med. J.*, 1977, *86*, 7; W. Berman *et al.*, *J. Pediat.*, 1978, *93*, 652 (premature infants); N. Buchanan *et al.*, *S. Afr. med. J.*, 1979, *56*, 638; L. F. Soyka, *Hosp. Formul.*, 1979, *14*, 546 (a review including the small dose method of treatment); G. G. S. Sandor *et al.*, *Pediatrics*, 1980, *65*, 541 (neonates).

See also Absorption and Fate (above).

Administration in renal failure. A report of digoxin toxicity in 3 patients being associated with plasma-digoxin concentrations greater than 2 ng per ml at least 6 hours after a dose, due to reduced volumes of distribution. A loading dose of 6 to 10 μg per kg body-weight is recommended for patients in renal failure with the dose being increased incrementally if necessary until a response is achieved. Maintenance doses can be calculated as a percentage of the loading dose using the creatinine clearance as a guide.— J. K. Aronson and D. G. Grahame-Smith, *Br. J. clin. Pharmac.*, 1976, *3*, 1045.

Uraemic patients need lower digoxin doses than patients with normal renal function but should be maintained at the same serum concentrations. Patients on haemodialysis will need still lower doses of digoxin and should be maintained at slightly lower serum concentrations.— L. Storstein and H. Janssen, *Clin. Pharmac. Ther.*, 1976, *20*, 15. See also under Protein Binding in Absorption and Fate (above).

A loading dose of 625 μg of digoxin is suggested as standard, with reduction to 500 μg for those with creatinine clearances of 50 ml per minute and 375 μg for those with clearances of 30 ml per minute.— S. M. Dobbs *et al.*, *Br. med. J.*, 1977, *2*, 168. In most patients with advanced renal failure an appropriate intravenous loading dose of digoxin is 10 μg per kg body-weight.— M. H. Gault *et al.*, *Br. J. clin. Pharmac.*, 1980, *9*, 593.

The normal half-life for digoxin of 36 to 44 hours is increased to 80 to 120 hours in end-stage renal failure. Standard doses should be reduced to 25 to 75% in patients with a glomerular filtration-rate (GFR) of 10 to 50 ml per minute, and to 10 to 25% in those with a GFR of less than 10 ml per minute; the serum concentration 12 hours after a maintenance dose is the best guide to dosage. The loading dose should be reduced in end-stage renal failure. Concentrations of digoxin are not affected by haemodialysis or peritoneal dialysis.— W. M. Bennett *et al.*, *Ann. intern. Med.*, 1980, *93*, 286.

Evidence of cumulation of digoxin metabolites in patients requiring maintenance dialysis for end-stage renal failure. The clinical significance is not known.— T. P. Gibson and H. A. Nelson, *Clin. Pharmac. Ther.*, 1980, *27*, 219.

The use of an equation for calculating maintenance digoxin regimens in 82 patients with renal insufficiency proved unreliable in 57% of patients.— F. Keller *et al.*, *Eur. J. clin. Pharmac.*, 1980, *18*, 433.

Further references to the use of digoxin in renal failure.— L. C. Dettli, *Clin. Pharmac. Ther.*, 1974, *16*, 274; W. J. Jusko *et al.*, *J. clin. Pharmac.*, 1974, *14*, 525; J. G. Wagner, *ibid.*, 329 (theoretical studies on digoxin dosage); E. E. Ohnhaus, *Medsche Klin.*, 1976, *71*, 1867; J. S. Cheigh, *Am. J. Med.*, 1977, *62*, 555 (doses reduced according to creatinine clearance); P. Kramer *et al.*, *J. Dialysis*, 1977, *1*, 689 (elimination through haemofiltration); P. Sharpstone, *Br. med. J.*, 1977, *2*, 36 (dosage intervals increased in renal failure); W. J. F. Van der Vijgh and P. L. Oe, *Int. J. clin. Pharmac. Biopharm.*, 1978, *16*, 540 (use in patients on haemodialysis).

See also under Absorption and Fate (above).

Administration in respiratory insufficiency. A review on the use of digoxin in pulmonary heart disease (cor pulmonale). There has been controversy over the use of digoxin in the treatment of congestive heart failure in patients with cor pulmonale although atrial arrhythmias appear to be legitimate indications for digoxin therapy in such patients. Patients with cor pulmonale may be more susceptible to the adverse effects of cardiac glycosides, especially since they are often elderly, thin, and may have impaired renal function. In general reduced doses are recommended except in the control of atrial fibrillation.— J. E. Doherty *et al.*, *Drugs*, 1977, *13*, 142. The efficacy of digoxin in the treatment of cor pulmonale remains controversial.— L. H. Green and T. W. Smith, *Ann. intern. Med.*, 1977, *87*, 459.

Administration in thyroid dysfunction. Larger doses of cardiac glycosides are required in hyperthyroid patients and lower doses in myxoedemic patients to maintain the same plasma concentrations.— M. Eichelbaum, *Clin. Pharmacokinet.*, 1976, *1*, 339.

A patient with chronic atrial fibrillation with satisfactory ventricular-rate control while receiving digoxin 250 μg daily required increased digoxin dosage after developing hyperthyroidism. After treatment for hyperthyroidism he was again well controlled by digoxin 250 μg daily.— D. H. Huffman *et al.*, *Clin. Pharmac. Ther.*, 1977, *22*, 533.

See also under Absorption and Fate (above).

Cardiac disorders. For the use of digoxin in preventing doxorubicin-induced cardiotoxicity, see Doxorubicin, p.206.

Angina pectoris. A discussion on the use of digoxin and propranolol in the treatment of angina pectoris.— *Lancet*, 1975, *2*, 1136.

Comment on digoxin in the control of atrial arrhythmias associated with angina pectoris.— H. B. Kay, *Drugs*, 1977, *13*, 276.

Arrhythmias. A discussion on paroxysmal supraventricular tachycardia in children; digoxin is considered to be the treatment of choice.— *Br. med. J.*, 1973, *4*, 248. See also L. M. Linde *et al.*, *Pediatrics*, 1972, *50*, 127.

A brief review on the treatment of cardiac arrhythmias including the use of digoxin.— *Med. Lett.*, 1978, *20*, 113.

Elective atrial fibrillation in patients with the pre-excitation syndrome permitted identification of those to whom digitalis might be given; digitalis should be avoided in those in whom the shortest R-R interval during fibrillation was less than 300 msec.— T. D. Sellers *et al.*, *Circulation*, 1977, *56*, 260. See also E. K. Chung, *Am. J. Med.*, 1977, *62*, 252 (a review of the Wolff-Parkinson-White syndrome).

Analysis of 41 patients with multifocal atrial tachycardia underlined the seriousness of this disorder but indicated that it was unlikely to be a manifestation of digitalis toxicity; 15 of 19 patients receiving maintenance digitalis therapy obtained clinical improvement. In 9 further patients digitalised, during an attack, for underlying disorders, digitalis was ineffective in controlling the atrial or ventricular rate.— K. Wang *et al.*, *Archs intern. Med.*, 1977, *137*, 161.

Further references to digoxin in the treatment of arrhythmias.— A. Redfors, *Acta med. scand.*, 1971, *190*, 307 (atrial fibrillation); G. Cargnelli *et al.*, *Int. J. clin. Pharmac. Biopharm.*, 1977, *15*, 384 (with practolol or verapamil in atrial fibrillation).

For reference to the possible beneficial effect of maintenance doses of digitalis glycosides on ventricular tachyarrhythmias, see Acetylstrophanthidin, p.540.

Cardiomyopathy. Digoxin was of little value in the treatment of advanced right-sided endomyocardial fibrosis in patients with sinus rhythm.— *Br. med. J.*, 1974, *4*, 222.

Digoxin 250 μg daily appeared to be suitable treatment for cardiomyopathy in Chagas' disease.— N. Beer *et al.*, *Postgrad. med. J.*, 1977, *53*, 537.

Heart failure. A discussion on the use of digoxin in heart failure. Although digoxin effectively controls the ventricular-rate in patients with supraventricular tachyarrhythmias such as atrial fibrillation, its use as an inotropic agent in patients with heart failure and sinus rhythm is being increasingly questioned. The aim of giving digoxin in heart failure is to increase myocardial contractility but this is only one of the determinants of cardiac performance and diuretics may be used to reduce venous filling pressure or vasodilators to reduce peripheral vascular resistance. There is reasonable evidence that digoxin has an inotropic effect when used in the short term in patients with congestive heart failure and sinus rhythm but in most of these patients it appears to have no long-term stimulant action on the heart and in several studies treatment has been withdrawn without ill effect.— *Br. med. J.*, 1979, *1*, 1103. See also J. Hamer, *ibid.*, 1976, *2*, 220; W. Bleifeld *et al.*, *Am. J. Med.*, 1978, *65*, 203; J. Hamer, *Br. J. clin. Pharmac.*, 1979, *8*, 109; R. Spector, *J. clin. Pharmac.*, 1979, *19*, 692; P. B. Beeson, *New Engl. J. Med.*, 1980, *303*, 1475; J. Hamer, *Recent Adv. clin. Pharmac.*, 1980, *2*, 73.

A discussion on the management of congestive heart failure in infants and children. Except in mild heart failure it is considered that diuretics are required in addition to digoxin.— N. J. Restiaux, *Drugs*, 1977, *13*, 467.

In an attempt to establish the value of maintenance digoxin therapy in heart failure, 46 patients with sinus rhythm or atrial fibrillation who had been stabilised for 3 months on digoxin were allocated in a double-blind manner to placebo or maintenance digoxin and after 6 weeks treatment was crossed over. Sixteen patients deteriorated on placebo, 3 of them developing pulmonary oedema. A reduction in FEV_1 suggested incipient pulmonary oedema in some symptomless patients. Maintenance digoxin was considered to be of value. Experience with these patients suggested that maintenance with diuretics might not be essential.— S. M. Dobbs *et al.*, *Br. med. J.*, 1977, *1*, 749. Criticism.— S. J. Warrington and N. A. J. Hamer (letter), *ibid.*, 1977, *2*, 265. A study in 9 patients indicating that long-term treatment with digoxin improves left ventricular function in congestive heart failure.— S. B. Arnold *et al.*, *New Engl. J. Med.*, 1980, *303*, 1443.

Benefits from digoxin in a controlled study of patients with heart failure but no atrial fibrillation.— D. C. -S. Lee *et al.*, *New Engl. J. Med.*, 1982, *306*, 699.

Digoxin was successfully withdrawn from 33 of 34 patients in sinus rhythm receiving maintenance digoxin therapy whose blood-digoxin concentrations were below 0.8 ng per ml, and from 15 of 22 whose concentrations were between 0.8 and 2 ng per ml. Thus 86% of 56 patients did not appear to have been obtaining any benefit from maintenance digoxin, and concentrations of less than 0.8 ng per ml appeared to be subtherapeutic in most patients. Of the 8 who could not be withdrawn 6 developed atrial fibrillation despite no history of this dysrhythmia in 5. Reintroduction of digoxin rapidly reversed their dysrhythmias, raising the question of whether they had paroxysmal atrial fibrillation or whether digoxin had been exerting an anti-arrhythmic effect.— G. D. Johnston and D. G. McDevitt, *Lancet*, 1979, *1*, 567. Most patients with atrial fibrillation can also be well maintained without digoxin treatment for much of the time.— A. Martin (letter), *ibid.*, 825. Further comment on the need to prescribe digoxin selectively.— R. Lamb (letter), *ibid.* Further comments.— G. S. Crockett (letter), *ibid.*, 920; M. A. K. Ghouri *et al.* (letter), *ibid.*, 1084.

Further reports on the successful withdrawal of digoxin from patients in sinus rhythm.— S. M. Hull and A. Mackintosh, *Lancet*, 1977, *2*, 1054; D. McHaffie and A. Guz (letter), *ibid.*, 1136; H. J. N. Bethell (letter), *ibid.*, 1186; R. Krakauer (letter), *Br. med. J.*, 1978, *2*, 1019.

Heart or chest surgery. There have been conflicting views on the merits of prophylactic digitalisation in patients undergoing heart or chest surgery. A. Selzer *et al.* (*Am. med. Ass.*, 1966, *195*, 549) considered that neither the routine use of digitalis in patients undergoing heart surgery nor its general prophylactic use just after surgery was justified and L.P. Rosky and T. Rodman (*New Engl. J. Med.*, 1966, *274*, 833) reported that large doses of digitalis and the vigorous use of diuretics were inadvisable during the week before heart surgery.

However S.O. Burman (*Ann. thorac. Surg.*, 1972, *14*, 359) found that the incidence of arrhythmias and heart failure and of death was reduced in patients undergoing thoracotomy after digitalisation, usually with digoxin, starting at least 3 days prior to operation, when compared with patients who had not been digitalised pre-operatively. Burman also reported that fewer digitalised patients required digitalis after open-heart surgery than similar patients not given digitalis pre-operatively.

Cardiac surgery appeared to produce an increased sensitivity to digoxin. Of 50 patients undergoing cardiac surgery 37 had postoperative arrhythmias and 17 had arrhythmias compatible with digoxin intoxication although measurements of serum-digoxin concentrations ranged from 0 to 2.8 ng per ml.— M. R. Rose *et al.*, *Am. Heart J.*, 1975, *89*, 288.

Hypertension. Studies on the influence of digoxin on ventricular function and coronary artery haemodynamics in 12 patients with essential hypertension but without heart failure indicated that not only was there no useful therapeutic effect but that a coronary constrictor and ischaemia-inducing effect on the coronary arterial system occurred.— B. E. Strauer, *Dt. med. Wschr.*, 1978, *103*, 1691.

Myocardial infarction. In an assessment of digitalis in acute myocardial infarction, its use was recommended in the presence of supraventricular tachycardia or cardiac failure.— S. H. Rahimtoola and R. M. Gunnar, *Ann. intern. Med.*, 1975, *82*, 234.

The use of digoxin in heart failure immediately after myocardial infarction is controversial but if relief is not obtained by appropriate diuretic therapy and the patient's condition is deteriorating, digoxin should not be withheld.— D. O. Williams, *Prescribers' J.*, 1977, *17*, 66. Verapamil or cardioversion is considered to be the treatment of choice in atrial fibrillation of recent onset in patients with acute myocardial infarction but the combination of heart failure and atrial fibrillation is treated with digoxin. The loading dose of digoxin should be low (500 µg intravenously) to avoid precipitation of arrhythmias.— L. H. Opie, *Lancet*, 1980, *1*, 912.

A view that digoxin 250 µg should be given intravenously for tachycardia in the first-aid treatment of suspected recent myocardial infarction.— *Br. med. J.*, 1979, *2*, 1565. Criticism. Digoxin itself can produce any type of dysrhythmia and its intravenous administration during the acute stage of infarction, when the myocardium is irritable, is dangerous, especially in ventricular tachycardia which may be mistaken for supraventricular arrhythmia.— A. A. Morgan (letter), *ibid.*, 1980, *280*, 251.

Further reports on the effects of digoxin in coronary heart disease.— R. Vogel *et al.*, *Circulation*, 1977, *56*, 355 (improvement of myocardial perfusion in patients with coronary artery disease and left ventricular dysfunction); D. S. Raabe, *Am. J. Cardiol.*, 1979, *43*, 990 (digoxin and vasodilators in congestive heart failure and myocardial infarction); R. A. Goldstein *et al.*, *New Engl. J. Med.*, 1980, *303*, 846 (lack of beneficial effect in heart failure associated with acute myocardial infarction).

Obesity. The use of digoxin or other cardiac glycosides in the treatment of obesity is unwarranted and dangerous.— *FDA Drug Bull.*, 1978, *8*, 21.

Pregnancy and the neonate. In 22 women taking digitalis in their second or later pregnancy, spontaneous onset of labour occurred a week earlier than in 64 comparable women not taking digitalis, and the duration of the first stage of labour was shorter—4.3 hours compared with 8 hours. Apgar scores of the infants at 1 minute were comparable. Digitalis might have a direct effect on the myometrium.— J. B. Weaver and J. F. Pearson, *Br. med. J.*, 1973, *3*, 519.

A study indicating that breast feeding is safe in lactating mothers receiving digoxin therapy.— P. M. Loughnan, *J. Pediat.*, 1978, *92*, 1019.

A view that there are no contra-indications to the use of digoxin in pregnancy.— M. de Swiet, *Prescribers' J.*, 1979, *19*, 59.

Supraventricular tachycardia in a foetus of 29 to 30 weeks' gestation was managed by giving digoxin to the mother.— T. D. Kerenyi *et al.*, *Lancet*, 1980, *2*, 393 and 546.

Foetal congestive heart failure secondary to tachycardia was treated successfully by administration of digoxin to the mother.— J. T. Harrigan *et al.*, *New Engl. J. Med.*, 1981, *304*, 1527.

See also under Absorption and Fate (above).

Raised intracranial pressure. Digoxin reduced the CSF outflow by as much as 78% in 3 patients requiring ventricular drainage. Digitoxin and acetazolamide also reduced the flow but to a lesser extent.— C. R. Neblett *et al.*, *Lancet*, 1972, *2*, 1008.

Respiratory disorders. Digoxin was indicated for the treatment of chronic obstructive airways disease. Dosage should be monitored carefully since digitalis toxicity was an increased risk. Maintenance doses of 125 to 250 µg daily were usually adequate.— J. E. Hodgkin *et al.*, *J. Am. med. Ass.*, 1975, *232*, 1243.

See also Administration in Respiratory Insufficiency (above).

Shock. For reference to the beneficial use of digoxin in septic shock, see Isoprenaline Sulphate, p.17.

Preparations

Digoxin Elixir *(U.S.P.)*. Contains 4.5 to 5.25 mg of digoxin in each 100 ml with alcohol 9 to 11.5%. Store at a temperature not exceeding 40° in airtight containers.

Digoxin Injection *(B.P.)*. Digoxin 25 mg, alcohol (80%) 12.5 ml, propylene glycol 40 ml, citric acid monohydrate 75 mg, sodium phosphate 450 mg, Water for Injections to 100 ml. Sterilised by autoclaving. Contains digoxin 250 µg in 1 ml. pH 6.7 to 7.3. Protect from light.

Digoxin Injection *(U.S.P.)*. A sterile solution in Water for Injections and alcohol (9 to 11%) or other suitable solvents. Store at a temperature not exceeding 40°.

Digoxin Tablets *(B.P.)*. Tablets containing digoxin. The *B.P.* requires 75% dissolution in 45 minutes.

Digoxin Tablets *(U.S.P.)*. Tablets containing digoxin. The *U.S.P.* requires not less than 55% dissolution in 60 minutes for any individual tablet tested and not less than 65% dissolution in 60 minutes for not less than eleven-twelfths of the tablets tested. Store in airtight containers.

Paediatric Digoxin Elixir *(B.P.)*. Digoxin Elixir Paediatric. An elixir containing digoxin 0.005%, alcohol 10%, and sodium phosphate, in a suitable flavoured vehicle which may be coloured. pH 6.8 to 7.2. Contains 50 µg of digoxin in 1 ml. The elixir should not be diluted; the dose should be measured by means of a graduated pipette. Store at a temperature not exceeding 25°. Protect from light.

Paediatric Digoxin Injection *(B.P.)*. Digoxin Paediatric Injection. Digoxin 10 mg, alcohol (80%) 12.5 ml, propylene glycol 40 ml, citric acid monohydrate 75 mg, sodium phosphate 450 mg, Water for Injections to 100 ml. Sterilised by autoclaving. Contains digoxin 100 µg in 1 ml. pH 6.7 to 7.3. Protect from light.

Proprietary Preparations

Digoxin Nativelle *(Wilcox, UK: Lewis, UK)*. Digoxin, available as scored tablets of 250 µg.

Lanoxin *(Wellcome, UK)*. Digoxin, available in 2-ml **Ampoules** of an injection containing 250 µg per ml; as **PG** (paediatric-geriatric) **Elixir** containing 50 µg per ml (dilution not recommended); as **PG Tablets** of 62.5 µg; and as **Tablets** of 125 and 250 µg. (Also available as Lanoxin in *Arg.*, *Austral.*, *Belg.*, *Canad.*, *Ital.*, *Neth.*, *Norw.*, *Switz.*, *USA*).

Other Proprietary Names

Arg.—Cardiogoxin, Lanicor; *Austral.*—Cardiox, Natigoxin, Prodigox; *Belg.*—Cardigox, Digoxine-Sandoz; *Fr.*—Coragoxine, Digoxine Nativelle, Lanoxine; *Ger.*—Allocor (see also under Acetyldigoxin), Digacin, Lanicor, Lenoxin, Novodigal; *Ital.*—Digomal, Dixina, Eudigox, Lanicor, Lanorale; *Neth.*—Lanicor; *S.Afr.*—Purgoxin; *Spain*—Digoxina Nativelle, Lanacordin; *Swed.*—Lanacrist; *Switz.*—Digazolan, Eudigox, Lanicor; *USA*—SK-Digoxin.

5802-t

Acetyldigitoxin. α-Acetyldigitoxin; α-Digitoxin Monoacetate; Digitoxin 3‴-Acetate. 3β-[(*O*-3-*O*-Acetyl-2,6-dideoxy-β-D-*ribo*-hexopyranosyl-(1→4)-*O*-2,6-dideoxy-β-D-*ribo*-hexopyranosyl-(1→4)-2,6-dideoxy-β-D-*ribo*-hexopyranosyl)oxy]-14-hydroxy-5β,14β-card-20(22)-enolide.

$C_{43}H_{66}O_{14}$=807.0.

CAS — 1111-39-3.

Pharmacopoeias. In *Cz.*, *Hung.*, and *Roum.* *Pol.* includes the monohydrate.

The acetyl derivative of digitoxin, in which the acetyl group is attached to the terminal glucose residue of the digitoxose moiety.

A white, odourless, hygroscopic, crystalline powder with a bitter taste. **Soluble** 1 in 6100 of water, 1 in 63 of alcohol, 1 in 12 of chloroform; practically insoluble in ether and light petroleum; soluble in methyl alcohol. **Store** in airtight containers. Protect from light.

Stability. The α-acetyl derivative of digitoxin is preferred to the β-isomer, which is also active, because of its better solubility in water. Under certain conditions deacetylation of α-acetyldigitoxin to digitoxin can occur. In injections and liquid preparations isomerisation can also occur and therefore these preparations should be stored at about 5°. Tablets are considered stable.— L. Szarras *et al.*, *Ann. Pharm. Franç.*, 1965, *23*, 561, per *Pharm. Acta Helv.*, 1966, *41*, 447.

Solutions of α-acetyldigitoxin, as usually prepared, were found to undergo hydrolysis and isomerisation to β-acetyldigitoxin. One sample investigated 19 months after preparation contained only 58% of α-acetyldigitoxin.— A. Ozarowski, *Pharm. J.*, 1965, *2*, 449.

Absorption and Fate.

Acetyldigitoxin has a half-life of between 8.5 and 8.8 days. About 21% of a dose was excreted in the urine in 6 days.— G. Bodem *et al.*, *Arzneimittel-Forsch.*, 1975, *25*, 1448.

Uses. Acetyldigitoxin has the general properties of digoxin (p.531) and has been used similarly in maintenance doses of 100 to 200 µg daily by mouth. It is reported to take effect within 2 to 4 hours of administration and the cardiac action persists for 1 to 3 days.

Proprietary Names

Acetil Digitoxina *(Sandoz, Spain)*; Acylanid *(Sandoz, Arg.*; *Sandoz, Denm.*; *Sandoz, S.Afr.*; *Sandoz, Swed.*; *Sandoz, Switz.)*; Acylanide *(Sandoz-Wander, Belg.*; *Sandoz, Fr.*; *Sandoz, Neth.)*.

5803-x

Acetyldigoxin. α-Acetyldigoxin; Desglucolanatoside C. 3β-[(*O*-3-*O*-Acetyl-2,6-dideoxy-β-D-*ribo*-hexopyranosyl-(1→4)-*O*-2,6-dideoxy-β-D-*ribo*-hexopyranosyl-(1→4)-2,6-dideoxy-β-D-*ribo*-hexopyranosyl)oxy]-12β,14-dihydroxy-5β,14β-card-20(22)-enolide.

$C_{43}H_{66}O_{15}$=823.0.

CAS — 5511-98-8.

Pharmacopoeias. In *Aust.*

A white or almost white odourless powder with a bitter taste. M.p. 210° to 230° with decomposition. Practically **insoluble** in water; slightly soluble in alcohol; very slightly soluble in chloroform; soluble 1 in about 80 of methyl alcohol. Solutions may be **sterilised** by filtration. **Protect** from light.

Uses. Acetyldigoxin has the general properties of digoxin (p.531) and has been used similarly in maintenance doses of 200 to 400 µg daily by mouth. The β isomer is also used.

The pharmacology of acetyldigoxin.— J. Grauwiler *et al.*, *Schweiz. med. Wschr.*, 1966, *96*, 1381, per *Int. pharm. Abstr.*, 1967, *4*, 94. See also P. W. Lücker *et al.*, *Arzneimittel-Forsch.*, 1978, *28*, 1781.

In 122 patients the average digitalising dose of acetyldigoxin was 2.9 mg by mouth and 2 mg intravenously, and the average maintenance dosage was 450 µg by mouth and 275 µg intravenously. The duration of action was 6 to 8 days.— H. Burger and O. Spühler, *Schweiz. med. Wschr.*, 1966, *96*, 1389.

In 150 mainly elderly patients treated with acetyldigoxin the average total digitalisation dose was 2.5 mg by mouth or 1.5 mg intravenously. The latency period following intravenous injection was 0.5 to 2 hours in tachycardia and 2 to 11 hours in atrial fibrillation with tachyarrhythmia. Maintenance dosage was 0.25 to 1 mg by mouth or 200 to 500 µg intravenously. About 65% of a dose given by mouth was absorbed; the effects of a full digitalising dose lasted about 6 days.— M. Bernoulli *et al.*, *Schweiz. med. Wschr.*, 1967, *93*, 83.

The half-life of acetyldigoxin was increased from 24 to 66 hours in patients with impaired renal function.— H. Brass and H. Philipps, *Klin. Wschr.*, 1970, *48*, 972, per *Int. pharm. Abstr.*, 1973, *10*, 641.

Beta isomer. A report of the use of β-acetyldigoxin in 20 patients with heart failure and atrial fibrillation. The dose averaged 2 mg, and the maintenance dose averaged 400 µg. The duration of action of β-acetyldigoxin was on average 6.4 days.— H. Storz, *Dt. med. Wschr.*, 1968, *93*, 523, per *Int. pharm. Abstr.*, 1968, *5*, 1506.

In 4 patients given tritiated β-acetyldigoxin by mouth 90% rapidly passed through the stomach unchanged and was absorbed in the duodenum. Deacetylation to digoxin occurred on passage through the intestinal wall.— H.

Flasch *et al.*, *Arzneimittel-Forsch.*, 1977, *27*, 656.

Therapeutic doses of β-acetyldigoxin given to healthy subjects produced no or only minor ST-segment depression both at rest and during exercise whereas patients with latent coronary insufficiency under similar conditions had significant ST-segment depressions. It was therefore considered that β-acetyldigoxin might be of diagnostic value in the recognition of latent coronary insufficiency.— H. -U. Lehmann *et al.*, *Dt. med. Wschr.*, 1977, *102*, 1335.

Optimal therapeutic serum concentrations of 1.21 to 1.7 ng per ml were produced by β-acetyldigoxin 5 µg per kg body-weight daily by mouth.— J. Schneider and A. Ruiz-Torres, *Dt. med. Wschr.*, 1977, *102*, 116.

Further references to β-acetyldigoxin: J. Bonelli *et al.*, *Int. J. clin. Pharmac. Biopharm.*, 1977, *15*, 288 (the effect of oxyfedrine on absorption); *idem*, 337 (the effect of antacids on absorption).

Proprietary Names

Agolanid *(Sandoz, Spain)*; Allocor *(β-isomer; see also under Digoxin) (Natrapharm, Ger.)*; Cedigocin *(Sandoz, Switz.)*; Cedigocina *(Sandoz, Arg.)*; Cedigocine *(Sandoz-Wander, Belg.)*; Cedigossina *(Sandoz, Ital.)*; Ceverin *(β-isomer) (Pharma-Schwarz, Ger.)*; Decardil *(Trenker, Belg.)*; Digistabil *(Hormonchemie, Ger.)*; Digotab *(β-isomer) (Asta, Ger.)*; Dioxanin *(Boehringer Ingelheim, Ger.)*; Lanadigin *(Promonta, Ger.)*; Novodigal *(Homburg, Belg.)*; Novodigal *(β-isomer) (Beiersdorf, Ger.)*; Sandolanid *(Sandoz, Ger.)*.

5804-r

Acetylstrophanthidin. 3β-Acetoxy-5,14-dihydroxy-19-oxo-5β,14β-card-20(22)-enolide.
$C_{25}H_{34}O_7$=446.5.

CAS — 60-38-8.

A synthetic derivative of strophanthidin, the aglycone of strophanthin.

Acetylstrophanthidin has actions similar to those of digoxin (p.531). It has been stated to have a potency about one-half that of ouabain. Because of its rapid action and rapid elimination it has been used to assess the degree of digitalisation. It has been given, under ECG control, in intravenous doses of 100 to 150 µg at intervals of 5 to 10 minutes, to a maximum of 1.2 mg. The dose given before the appearance of arrhythmias, indicative of toxicity, is a measure of the degree of digitalisation. Deaths have occurred from ventricular fibrillation, and the procedure is considered dangerous by many authorities.

In a study of 142 patients, response to administration of acetylstrophanthidin, 1 mg in 20 ml by slow intravenous injection over a period of 30 minutes, indicated that digitalis glycosides might lessen the frequency of ventricular premature beats. The clinical value of these findings would depend upon whether they also applied to maintenance therapy. Of 29 patients with uncontrollable, life-threatening, ventricular tachyarrhythmias acetylstrophanthidin reduced or abolished ventricular premature beats in 17, and 15 of these obtained a beneficial response to maintenance doses of digitalis glycosides.— B. Lown *et al.*, *New Engl. J. Med.*, 1977, *296*, 301.

Manufacturers

Lilly, UK.

5805-f

Adonis Vernalis. Adonide; Adonis; Adoniskraut; Herba Adonidis.

Pharmacopoeias. In *Aust.*, *Fr.*, *Ger.*, *Pol.*, *Rus.*, and *Span. Rus.* also includes Adonisidum (Adoniside), an aqueous solution of the glycosides of *A. vernalis*. *Ger.* also includes a standardised powder.

The dried aerial parts of *Adonis vernalis* (Ranunculaceae), containing glycosides which resemble digoxin (p.536) in action. **Store** in airtight containers. Protect from light.

Adonis vernalis is inferior to digitalis in its therapeutic effect. It has been administered as an infusion and as a tincture.

5806-d

Convallaria *(B.P.C. 1949)*. Lily of the Valley Flowers; Muguet; Maiblume; Maiglöckchenkraut.

CAS — 3253-62-1 (convallatoxol); 13473-51-3 (convalloside); 13289-19-5 (convallatoxoloside); 508-75-8 (convallatoxin).

Pharmacopoeias. In *Aust.*, *Ger.*, (from *C. majalis* or closely related species); *Pol.*, and *Span. Rus.* specifies aerial parts of *C. majalis* and its varieties and also includes convallatoxin. *Ger.* also includes a standardised powder.

The dried inflorescence of lily of the valley, *Convallaria majalis* (Liliaceae). Several crystalline glycosides have been obtained from the plant including convallatoxol, convalloside, convallatoxoloside, and convallatoxin. **Store** in a cool place.

Convallaria has an action on the heart similar to that of digoxin (p.536).

Solutio Corglyconi 0.06% pro Injectionibus *(Rus. P.)*. Corglycon (total glycosides of convallaria leaves) 60 mg, chlorbutol 400 mg, Water for Injections to 100 ml; in ampoules of 1 ml; 1 ml contains 11 to 16 (frog) units (USSR). Protect from light.

5807-n

Crataegus. Crataegus Oxyacantha; English Hawthorn; Haw; Aubépine; Pirliteiro; Weissdornblätter mit Blüten; Weissdornblüten.

Pharmacopoeias. Belg., *Braz.*, *Fr.*, *Ger.*, *Pol.*, *Port.*, and *Span.* include the dried flowers (used as the extract or tincture). *Ger.* includes the leaves and flowers and also specifies other spp. *Rus.* includes the flowers and dried fruit. *Swiss* includes the dried leaves.

The dried flowers, fruit and leaves of *Crataegus oxyacantha* (=*C. monogyna* and *C. oxyacanthoides*) (Rosaceae) have been used.

Crataegus contains flavonoid glycosides claimed to have cardiotonic properties and has been used similarly to digoxin (p.536) as an extract or tincture.

A review of the active principles of some *Crataegus* spp.— I. Incze *et al.*, *Gyogyszereszet*, 1978, *22*, 167, per *Int. pharm. Abstr.*, 1979, *16*, 76.

Proprietary Names

Cardiplant Schwabe *(Also, Ital.)*; Crasted *(Jap.)*; Crataegol *(Vernin, Fr.)*; Crataegus Gmet *(Oberlin, Fr.)*; Crataegutt *(Schwabe, Neth.)*; Crataegysat Bürger *(Ysatfabrik, Ger.)*; Cratamed *(Redel, Ger.)*; Esbericard *(Schaper & Brümmer, Ger.)*; Oxacant *(Klein, Ger.)*.

5808-h

Cymarin. K-Strophanthin-α. A glycoside extracted from the roots of *Apocynum cannabinum*. 3β-[(2,6-Dideoxy-3-*O*-methyl-β-D-*ribo*-hexopyranosyl)oxy]-5,14-dihydroxy-19-oxo-5β,14β-card-20(22)-enolide.
$C_{30}H_{44}O_9$=548.7.

CAS — 508-77-0.

It is a white to slightly yellowish crystalline powder. Sparingly **soluble** in water; soluble in alcohol and chloroform; sparingly soluble in ether and methyl alcohol. **Protect** from light.

Cymarin has actions similar to those of strophanthin-K (p.545).

A study *in vitro* of the cardiotonic properties of *Apocynum cannabinum* and fractions obtained by chromatography.— J. Desruelles *et al.*, *Thérapie*, 1973, *28*, 103.

Proprietary Names

Alvonal MR *(Gödecke, Ger.)*.

5809-m

Deslanoside *(B.P., U.S.P.)*. Desacetyl-lanatoside C; Deacetyl-lanatoside C. 3β-[(*O*-β-D-Glucopyranosyl-(1→4)-*O*-2,6-dideoxy-β-D-*ribo*-hexopyranosyl-(1→4)-*O*-2,6-dideoxy-β-D-*ribo*-hexopyranosyl-(1→4)-2,6-dideoxy-β-D-*ribo*-hexopyranosyl)-oxy]-12β,14-dihydroxy-5β,14β-card-20(22)-enolide.
$C_{47}H_{74}O_{19}$=943.1.

CAS — 17598-65-1.

Pharmacopoeias. In *Arg.*, *Br.*, *Braz.*, *Chin.*, *Cz.*, *Jap.*, *Nord.*, and *U.S.*

Odourless hygroscopic white crystals or crystalline powder with a bitter taste. The *B.P.* specifies not more than 7% loss of weight on drying; the *U.S.P.* specifies not more than 8%. M.p. about 220°.

Practically **insoluble** in water, chloroform, and ether; soluble 1 in 300 of alcohol and 1 in 200 of methyl alcohol. A solution in pyridine is dextrorotatory. It is more stable in solution than lanatoside C. **Store** in airtight containers. Protect from light.

Adverse Effects, Treatment, and Precautions. As for Digoxin, p.531.

Absorption and Fate. Deslanoside is weakly bound to serum albumin and rapidly passes to other tissues. It has a half-life of about 33 hours. About 20% of the dose administered has been stated to be inactivated daily.

Studies of biliary and urinary excretion of deslanoside given by intravenous injection to 4 patients.— A. Marzo *et al.*, *Farmaco, Edn prat.*, 1980, *35*, 265.

Uses. The actions and uses of deslanoside are similar to those of lanatoside C (p.543). It is usually reserved for the treatment of emergencies although digoxin is generally preferred. Its effects occur 10 to 30 minutes after intravenous administration and the full action on the heart is exerted after about 2 hours; the effects persist for 3 to 6 days.

The suggested rapid digitalising dose of deslanoside is 0.8 to 1.6 mg given by intravenous injection as a single dose or in divided doses over 24 hours. It has also been given by intramuscular injection. For maintenance treatment a cardiac glycoside is then given by mouth; lanatoside C may be used. A suggested digitalising dose for children is 20 to 40 µg per kg body-weight given intravenously as a single dose or in divided doses over 24 hours.

Preparations

Deslanoside Injection *(B.P.)*. A sterile solution of deslanoside 0.02% in Water for Injections containing suitable buffering agents. Sterilised by autoclaving. pH 5.9 to 6.5. Protect from light.

Deslanoside Injection *(U.S.P.)*. A sterile solution in a suitable solvent; it may contain glycerol. pH 5.5 to 7.

Cedilanid Injection *(Sandoz, UK)*. Contains deslanoside 200 µg per ml, in ampoules of 2 ml. (Also available as Cedilanid Injection in *Austral.*, *Canad.*, *Ger.*, *Ital.*, *Norw.*, *S.Afr.*, *Spain*, and *Swed.*).

See also Cedilanid Tablets, p.543.

Other Proprietary Names

Cedilanid-D *(USA)*; Cedilanid Desacetyl *(Denm.)*; Cedilanide *(see also under Lanatoside C) (Belg., Fr., Neth.)*; Desace *(Belg., Fr., Switz.)*; Desaci *(Ital.)*; Verdiana *(Spain)*.

5810-t

Digalen-Neo. A purified aqueous extract of the leaves of *Digitalis ferruginea* (Scrophulariaceae). **Protect** from light.

CAS — 8002-02-6.

Pharmacopoeias. In *Rus.*

Digalen-neo has the general properties of digoxin (p.531) and has been used for similar purposes.

5811-x

Digitalin *(B.P.C. 1954).* Amorphous Digitalin; Digitalinum Purum Germanicum. A standardised mixture of glycosides from the seeds of *Digitalis purpurea*, containing 100 units of activity in 1 g.

A yellowish-white odourless powder with a bitter taste. Very **soluble** in water and alcohol.

Digitalin has actions similar to those of digitoxin (p.541) but is much less potent and is excreted more rapidly. Because of its ready solubility in water it was formerly used for the preparations of solutions for injection.

Digitalin must be distinguished from digitoxin (Digitaline Cristallisée) which is very much more potent.

5812-r

Digitalis Leaf *(B.P., Eur. P.).* Digit. Leaf; Digitalis Folium; Digitalis Purpurea Folium; Digitalis Purpureae Folium; Digitale Pourprée; Digit. Fol.; Digitalis *(U.S.P.)*; Foxglove Leaf; Feuille de Digitale; Fingerhutblatt; Hoja de Digital; Dedaleira.

Pharmacopoeias. In all pharmacopoeias examined, except *Cz.* and *Roum.;* most specify not less than 10 units per g. *Rus.* also allows the leaves of *D. grandiflora* (*D. ambigua*) and specifies 50 to 66 (frog) units (USSR) per g.
Br. also describes Powdered Digitalis Leaf.

The dried leaves of *Digitalis purpurea* (Scrophulariaceae). Digitalis leaf contains a number of glycosides, including digitoxin, gitoxin, and gitaloxin. Several chemical races exist, in some of which a predominance of the glycosides of cardenolide A occurs. The *B.P.* and *Eur. P.* specify not less than 0.3% of total cardenolides, expressed as digitoxin, and calculated with reference to the dried substance. The *U.S.P.* specifies not less than 10 units per g. Aqueous preparations, such as infusions and mixtures, are very unstable. **Store** in airtight containers. Protect from light.

NOTE. When Digitalis, Digitalis Leaf, or Powdered Digitalis Leaf is prescribed, Prepared Digitalis is dispensed.

5813-f

Prepared Digitalis *(B.P.).* Prep. Digit.; Digitalis Praeparata; Powdered Digitalis *(U.S.P.)*; Digitalis Folii Pulvis Standardisatus; Digitalis Pulverata.

Pharmacopoeias. Standardised powders (10 units per g) are included in *Arg., Aust., Belg., Br., Hung., Ind., Int., Jug., Nord., Port., Turk.,* and *U.S. Fr., Ger.,* and *Jap.* (8 to 13 units per g) also describe a powder.

Digitalis leaf reduced to powder, no part being rejected, and biologically assayed, the strength being stated in units per g. For therapeutic purposes it must be adjusted to contain 10 units in 1 g (1 unit in 100 mg). The *B.P.* states that it may be adjusted by admixture with a weaker prepared digitalis or with powdered grass; the *U.S.P.* permits lactose, starch, exhausted marc, or digitalis of higher or lower potency. **Store** in airtight containers. Protect from light.

Units. One unit of digitalis is contained in 76 mg of the third International Standard Preparation (1949) which contains 0.01316 units per mg.

Adverse Effects, Treatment, and Precautions. As for Digoxin, p.531.

A report of poisoning associated with the drinking of herbal tea made from the leaves of *Digitalis purpurea.*— E. S. Dickstein and F. W. Kunkel, *Am. J. Med.,* 1980, *69,* 167. See also A. E. Stillman *et al., Morb. Mortal.,* 1977, *26,* 257.

Absorption and Fate. Digitalis is incompletely absorbed from the gastro-intestinal tract; 20 to 40% of the dose administered has been reported to reach the circulation. It is similarly absorbed from the rectum. Digitalis has a half-life of 4 to 6 days.

Uses. Digitalis has the properties described under digoxin (p.536) and has a similar onset and duration of action to that of digitoxin (p.542). When treatment with a cardiac glycoside is required digoxin or digitoxin is preferred.

Provided that cardiac glycosides have not been given in the previous 10 to 14 days, digitalis as Prepared Digitalis has been used for digitalisation in doses of 1 to 2 g given by mouth over 24 to 48 hours. Alternatively 200 mg has been administered thrice daily for 2 or 3 days followed by half or two-thirds of this dosage for a further 2 or 3 days. Maintenance doses of 60 to 200 mg daily have been given. Elderly patients may require smaller doses.

Preparations

Digitalis Capsules *(U.S.P.).* Capsules containing prepared digitalis. Store in airtight containers.

Digitalis Tablets *(U.S.P.).* Tablets containing prepared digitalis. Store in airtight containers.

Prepared Digitalis Tablets *(B.P.).* Prep. Digit. Tab.; Digitalis Tablets. Tablets containing prepared digitalis. Store in airtight containers.

Proprietary Names

Digifortis *(Parke, Davis, USA)*; Digiglusin *(Lilly, USA)*; Digiplex (an extract of total glycosides from *Digitalis purpurea* leaf) *(Servier, Fr.)*; Digitalysat Bürger *(Ysatfabrik, Ger.)*; Pil-Digis *(Key, USA).*

5814-d

Digitalis Lanata Leaf *(B.P.C. 1973).* Digit. Lanata Leaf; Digitalis Lanatae Folium; Austrian Digitalis; Austrian Foxglove; Woolly Foxglove Leaf.

CAS — 17575-20-1 (lanatoside A).

Pharmacopoeias. In *Arg., Aust., Ger.,* and *Pol. Ger.* also includes a standardised powder.

The dried leaves of the woolly foxglove, *Digitalis lanata* (Scrophulariaceae), containing about 1 to 1.4% of a mixture of cardioactive glycosides, including digoxin, digitoxin, acetyldigoxin, acetyldigitoxin, lanatoside A, and deslanoside. **Store** in airtight containers. Protect from light.

Digitalis lanata leaf is more potent than digitalis leaf and it is used as a source for the manufacture of digoxin and other glycosides.

Preparations

Lantosidum *(Rus. P.).* A purified alcoholic solution of the total glycosides extracted from digitalis lanata leaves. It is a transparent yellow-green to green liquid containing not less than 68% v/v of alcohol and 9 to 12 (frog) units (USSR) per ml. It is administered by mouth.

A preparation containing a complex of glycosides from the leaves of *Digitalis lanata* was formerly marketed in Great Britain under the proprietary name Digilanid *(Sandoz).*

5815-n

Digitoxin *(B.P., Eur. P., U.S.P.).* Digitoxinum; Digitaline Cristallisée; Digitoxoside. 3β-[(O-2,6-Dideoxy-β-D-*ribo*-hexopyranosyl-(1→4)-O-2,6-dideoxy-β-D-*ribo*-hexopyranosyl-(1→4)-2,6-dideoxy-β-D-*ribo*-hexopyranosyl)oxy]-14-hydroxy-5β,14β-card-20(22)-enolide. $C_{41}H_{64}O_{13}$=764.9.

CAS — 71-63-6.

Pharmacopoeias. In all pharmacopoeias examined except *Pol.*

A crystalline glycoside obtained from suitable species of *Digitalis.* The *B.P.* specifies not less than 95% of $C_{41}H_{64}O_{13}$, calculated on the dried substance; the *U.S.P.* specifies not less than 92%. It is a white or pale buff-coloured, odourless, microcrystalline powder with an intensely bitter taste. Practically **insoluble** in water; soluble 1 in 150 of alcohol and 1 in 40 of chloroform; slightly soluble in ether and methyl alcohol; freely soluble in a mixture of equal volumes of chloroform and methyl alcohol. Solutions for injection are **sterilised** by autoclaving. **Incompatible** with acids and alkalis. **Store** in airtight containers. Protect from light.

Stability. Digitoxin lost 15% potency on storage at 100° for 1 month, 24% on heating to 185° for 16 hours, 35% on exposure to u.v. light for 1 month at room temperature, and 54% when suspended in 1M sodium hydroxide solution at 75° for 1½ hours.— L. F. Cullen *et al., J. pharm. Sci.,* 1970, *59,* 697.

Adverse Effects and Treatment. As for Digoxin, p.531.

Digitalis intoxication occurred in 179 patients who took 1 to 3 tablets daily, each containing digitoxin 200 µg and digoxin 50 µg, instead of tablets each containing digoxin 250 µg, for 8 weeks or more, due to a manufacturing error. Fatigue and visual disturbances occurred in 95% of the patients, muscular weakness in 82%, anorexia and nausea in 80%, psychic complaints and abdominal pains in 65%, and dizziness, headache, diarrhoea, and vomiting in about one-half of the patients. Hallucination-like effects occurred in 12 patients. In 48 patients, 105 separate disturbances in rhythm or in atrioventricular conduction occurred. The patients were usually symptom-free from 1 to 4 weeks after withdrawal of the tablets, but 24 patients still had symptoms after 4 weeks. Use of the tablets was believed to have contributed to the death of 6 of 47 patients treated in hospital.— A. H. Lely and C. H. J. van Enter, *Br. med. J.,* 1970, *3,* 737.

In 52 patients taking digitoxin (mean 109 µg daily) and showing no signs of toxicity the mean serum-digitoxin concentration (assessed by radio-immunoassay) was 17 ng per ml compared with 34 ng per ml in 6 further patients taking a similar dose (mean 120 µg daily) but showing ECG signs of toxicity.— T. W. Smith, *J. Pharmac. exp. Ther.,* 1970, *175,* 352.

Further references to the toxicity of digitoxin: J. J. Iacuone, *Am. J. Dis. Child.,* 1976, *130,* 425 (accidental poisoning); O. Storstein *et al., Am. Heart J.,* 1977, *93,* 434 (the incidence of toxicity in patients on maintenance therapy).

Severe digitalis intoxication occurred in a patient considered to have taken about 100 tablets of digitoxin 100 µg. Gastric lavage was performed 3 hours after ingestion. The plasma-digitoxin concentration 21 hours after ingestion was 125 ng per ml (150 ng per ml on admission) when charcoal haemoperfusion was carried out for 8 hours and 1.24 mg of drug was removed. After an interval of one hour a second haemoperfusion was started and removed 870 µg of digitoxin by which time the plasma-digitoxin concentration had fallen to 70 ng per ml and most of the symptoms of intoxication had disappeared. Cholestyramine 4 g was then given thrice daily for 5 days and considered to have increased the elimination of digitoxin.— H. -J. Gilfrich *et al.* (letter), *Lancet,* 1978, *1,* 505. Further references to the removal of digitoxin by charcoal haemoperfusion: H. -J. Gilfrich *et al., Klin. Wschr.,* 1978, *56,* 1179.

Serum-digitoxin concentrations in 2 elderly women with digitoxin toxicity (serum concentrations of 43 and 42 ng per ml respectively) returned to within the therapeutic range (10 to 30 ng per ml) following withdrawal of the drug, correction of hypokalaemia and cardiac arrhythmias where necessary, and 3 doses of cholestyramine 4 g given over 24 hours.— W. J. Cady *et al., Am. J. Hosp. Pharm.,* 1979, *36,* 92.

For reference to the possible danger of using spironolactone in association with cholestyramine in the treatment of digitoxin toxicity, see Precautions (below).

Precautions. As for Digoxin, p.533.

Digitoxin should be used with caution in patients with impaired hepatic function.

Interactions. Digitoxin is bound to plasma protein to the extent of 93%. Binding is not affected by phenylbutazone, sulphadimethoxine, or phenobarbitone, and is slightly reduced by tolbutamide or chlorophenoxyisobutyric acid [compare clofibrate]. It is unlikely that these changes will be clinically significant. In 2 patients receiving digitoxin the plasma concentrations were reduced when phenylbutazone or phenytoin respectively were given concomitantly. This might represent hepatic hydroxylation of digitoxin.— H. M. Solomon *et al., Ann. N.Y. Acad. Sci.,* 1971, *179,* 362.

Antiarrhythmic agents. Quinidine had no statistically significant effect on the distribution or clearance of an intravenous dose of digitoxin in 10 healthy subjects.— H. R. Ochs *et al., New Engl. J. Med.,* 1980, *303,* 672.

Results of a study in 5 healthy subjects indicate that there is a pharmacokinetic interaction between quinidine and digitoxin. Serum-digitoxin concentrations after a single intravenous dose were increased by quinidine, the elimination half-life was prolonged, and both total body and renal clearance of digitoxin were decreased. Unlike studies with digoxin, quinidine did not affect the volume of distribution of digitoxin.— P. E. Fenster *et al.*, *Ann. intern. Med.*, 1980, *93*, 698. See also M. Garty *et al.*, *Ann. intern. Med.*, 1981, *94*, 35.

Antibiotics. Serum-digitoxin concentrations and half-lives were decreased during treatment with *rifampicin* alone or with isoniazid and ethambutol.— U. Peters *et al.*, *Dt. med. Wschr.*, 1974, *99*, 2381.

Barbiturates. In 2 patients with normal renal and hepatic function maintained on digitoxin 100 µg daily the steady-state plasma-digitoxin concentration fell to about half when *phenobarbitone* 60 mg thrice daily was given concomitantly for 12 weeks. In a representative patient the half-life of digitoxin fell from 7.77 to 4.47 days respectively 3 weeks before and 6 weeks after treatment for 8 weeks with phenobarbitone, and the proportions of digoxin and digitoxin in the urine changed from 5.5 and 93% to 13 and 81% respectively.— H. M. Solomon and W. B. Abrams, *Am. Heart J.*, 1972, *83*, 277.

Diuretics. *Spironolactone* altered the pattern of urinary metabolites and decreased the half-life of digitoxin when it was given before an intravenous dose of digitoxin in a study of 8 patients on oral maintenance digitoxin therapy.— K. E. Wirth *et al.*, *Eur. J. clin. Pharmac.*, 1976, *9*, 345. Evidence that concomitant administration of spironolactone increases the half-life of digitoxin. It was also demonstrated that spironolactone given in association with cholestyramine does not enhance the effect of cholestyramine on digitalis elimination and may not be of value in treating digitoxin toxicity. Indeed, the prolongation of digitoxin half-life induced by spironolactone may be harmful in digitoxin-intoxicated patients.— S. G. Carruthers and C. A. Dujovne, *Clin. Pharmac. Ther.*, 1980, *27*, 184.

Sulphonamides. For a report that *sulphasalazine* might be less liable to affect the absorption of digitoxin than that of digoxin, see Digoxin, p.534.

Interference with laboratory estimations. The administration of digitoxin could interfere with measurements of urinary 17-hydroxycorticosteroids.— J. M. Rosenberg and I. S. Kampa, *Drug Intell. & clin. Pharm.*, 1973, *7*, 33.

Absorption and Fate. Digitoxin is readily and completely absorbed from the gastro-intestinal tract. Therapeutic plasma concentrations may range from 10 to 35 ng per ml. Digitoxin has a relatively small volume of distribution when compared with digoxin but it is distributed similarly in the body. It is extensively bound to plasma protein. Digitoxin is very slowly eliminated from the body and is metabolised in the liver, one of the active metabolites being digoxin. Enterohepatic recycling occurs and 60 to 80% of a dose appears in the urine, mainly as metabolites, over 3 weeks. It is also excreted in the faeces. Digitoxin has an elimination half-life of up to 7 days or more.

An account of the clinical pharmacokinetics of digitoxin.— D. Perrier *et al.*, *Clin. Pharmacokinet.*, 1977, *2*, 292.

Digitoxin is bound to plasma protein to the extent of about 97%. In 8 patients given a single dose of 1 mg by mouth, plasma concentrations 30 minutes later were 3.1 to 133.9 ng per ml. Peak concentrations were 19 to 133.9 ng per ml and were reached in ½ to 3 hours. Concentrations fell considerably by 6 hours, fell little over the next 18 hours, and then fell exponentially over about 15 days. At 12 hours the plasma concentration was proportional to the dose in µg per kg body-weight. The plasma half-life was 4.4 to 5.9 days. In 4 patients 22 to 67% of the maximum inotropic effect was evident in 1 hour, with the peak effect in 4 to 6 hours. In patients given maintenance doses plasma concentrations were proportional to the dose. In 4 patients who had been maintained on digitoxin, plasma concentrations at autopsy were 18 to 26 ng per ml, with 30 to 116 ng per g in skeletal muscle, 99 to 205 ng per g in cardiac muscle, 45 to 214 ng per g in the liver, and 117 to 219 ng per g in the kidneys. In 1 patient with a plasma concentration of 134 ng per ml the concentration of digitoxin in the spinal fluid was only 1 ng per ml. Adverse effects were related to plasma concentrations; anorexia, nausea, and vomiting occurred at 40 ng per ml; visual disturbances occurred at concentrations in excess of 50 ng per ml; and cardiac arrhythmias at concentrations in excess of 60 ng per ml. Marked thrombocytopenia occurred in a patient with a concentration of 134 ng per ml. Excretion in the urine and faeces was exponential. Nearly half of a 1-mg dose was recovered, about 60% being in the urine and 40% in the faeces. There was some evidence of tubular reabsorption. Excretion in sweat was negligible.— D. S. Lukas, *Ann. N.Y. Acad. Sci.*, 1971, *179*, 338.

Digitalisation produced higher serum concentrations of digitoxin in children than in adults.— A. C. Giardina *et al.*, *Circulation*, 1975, *51*, 713, per *J. Am. med. Ass.*, 1975, *233*, 832.

Biological half-lives for digitoxin ranging from 2.4 to 16.4 days with a mean half-life of 7.6 days have been reported. This wide variation may be attributed to individual differences in hepatic metabolism of digitoxin and to the use of different assay methods. The shortest mean half-life of 4.8 days was observed with the most specific assay method and the longest mean half-life of 9.8 days with the least specific method.— D. Perrier *et al.*, *Clin. Pharmacokinet.*, 1977, *2*, 292.

Elimination kinetics of digitoxin and its metabolites were not significantly different in 6 patients with severe *renal insufficiency* and in healthy subjects. In 2 of the uraemic patients it was noted that a higher rate of faecal excretion could compensate for the diminished excretion of digitoxin and its metabolites in urine.— H. F. Vöhringer *et al.*, *Clin. Pharmac. Ther.*, 1976, *19*, 387. See also K. Rasmussen *et al.*, *ibid.*, 1972, *13*, 6; D. W. Shoeman and D. L. Azarnoff (letter), *ibid.*, 460 (reduced binding in uraemic patients); L. Storstein, *ibid.*, 1974, *16*, 25; U. Peters *et al.*, *Dt. med. Wschr.*, 1977, *102*, 109.

The pharmacokinetics of digitoxin were changed significantly in 5 patients with the nephrotic syndrome. The apparent volume of distribution of digitoxin was increased and protein binding decreased. Such patients should be maintained at lower serum-digitoxin concentrations than other patients but will need larger doses because of the shortened serum half-life and the increased renal excretion of digitoxin and its cardioactive metabolities.— L. Storstein, *Clin. Pharmac. Ther.*, 1976, *20*, 158.

Absorption. A suggestion that disturbance and delay of gastric emptying accompanied by gastric hypersecretion could enhance acid hydrolysis of digitoxin and contribute to reduced bioavailability.— U. Peters *et al.*, *Arzneimittel-Forsch.*, 1978, *28*, 750.

Bioavailability. A review of the bioavailability of digitoxin.— J. H. Wood *et al.*, *J. Am. pharm. Ass.*, 1976, *NS16*, 467.

In 8 normal males the average plasma half-lives of 2 brands of digitoxin tablets were 8.03 and 9.84 days, with a range of 6.5 to 9.9 days and 5 to 13.7 days respectively.— R. G. Stoll *et al.*, *J. pharm. Sci.*, 1973, *62*, 1615.

Results from studies of digitoxin tablets from 2 manufacturers indicated that there was no correlation between their dissolution-rates *in vitro* and the extent of absorption.— P. M. Hooymans, *Pharm. Weekbl. Ned.*, 1978, *113*, 505.

Further bioavailability studies with digitoxin preparations: L. Nyberg *et al.*, *Can. J. pharm. Sci.*, 1979, *14*, 79.

Distribution. In a study of digitoxin metabolites in the myocardium, the mean ratio of myocardial to serum concentrations of digitoxin and its cardioactive metabolites was found to be 5.4:1. When calculated in terms of free drug the ratio was 200:1 and, since digotoxin is extensively bound to protein, gave a better estimate of affinity to heart tissue.— L. Storstein, *Clin. Pharmac. Ther.*, 1977, *21*, 395.

Excretion. Studies on the excretion of digitoxin and its cardioactive metabolites: J. E. Doherty, *Ann. intern. Med.*, 1973, *79*, 229 (about 27% of a dose is reported to undergo enterohepatic recycling); L. Storstein, *Clin. Pharmac. Ther.*, 1974, *16*, 14 (renal excretion); H. F. Vöhringer and N. Rietbrock, *Clin. Pharmac. Ther.*, 1974, *16*, 796 (metabolism and excretion); L. Stortstein, *Clin. Pharmac. Ther.*, 1975, *17*, 313 (biliary excretion and enterohepatic circulation); R. W. Sattler *et al.*, *Arzneimittel-Forsch.*, 1977, *27*, 1615 (biliary excretion and enterohepatic circulation).

Metabolism. The liver is thought to be the main site of digitoxin metabolism. Hydroxylation transforms digitoxin and its derivatives (digitoxigenin-bis-digitoxoside, digitoxigenin-mono-digitoxoside, and digitoxigenin) to digoxin and its equivalent derivatives. Digitoxin and digoxin metabolites, with successively less sugar, are formed by hydrolysis. All of these metabolites are biologically active and all are inactivated by conjugation with glucuronic or sulphuric acids. A study of digitoxin metabolism in patients on oral maintenance therapy and after a single intravenous dose showed that in both cases digitoxin is the main cardioactive substance in serum and in urine. All known cardioactive metabolites were present but there were differences between the single-dose and steady-state groups. In the steady-state group there was more unchanged digitoxin (89.7% in serum and 87% in urine compared with 80.4% and 56.6% respectively), far less digoxin (less than 1% in the steady-state group compared with 12.5% in serum and 25.5% in urine in the single-dose group), and less hydroxylated metabolites than in the single-dose group.— L. Storstein, *Clin. Pharmac. Ther.*, 1977, *21*, 125. See also L. Storstein and J. Amlie, *ibid.*, 255 (kinetic aspects of digitoxin metabolism); L. Storstein, *ibid.*, 395 (digitoxin metabolites in the myocardium); *idem*, 536 (digitoxin metabolites in patients with renal impairment); L. Storstein and J. Amlie, *ibid.*, 659 (digitoxin metabolism in patients with biliary fistulas).

Plasma concentrations. Serum and plasma concentrations of digitoxin are equivalent.— T. W. Smith and E. Haber, *New Engl. J. Med.*, 1973, *289*, 1063.

Further references to plasma concentrations of digitoxin: W. Shapiro *et al.*, *Archs intern. Med.*, 1972, *130*, 31, per *J. Am. med. Ass.*, 1972, *221*, 523.

Pregnancy and the neonate. Following maternal intravenous injections of digitoxin, the drug was detected in the foetus, with highest concentrations in the heart and kidney. Therapeutic doses were considered harmless to the foetus.— J. B. E. Baker, *Pharmac. Rev.*, 1960, *12*, 37.

Protein binding. Digitoxin has been reported to be 97% bound to serum albumin in healthy subjects. Binding has been slightly reduced in patients with chronic active hepatitis or nephrotic syndrome. Conflicting effects on binding have been noted in uraemic patients; it is reduced in those on haemodialysis and a heparin-induced release of free fatty acids appears to be responsible. Where serum protein binding of digitoxin or digoxin is significantly decreased, total serum concentrations should be maintained below usual therapeutic values.— L. Storstein, *Clin. Pharmacokinet.*, 1977, *2*, 220.

Further references to the protein binding of digitoxin: J. E. Doherty *et al.* (letter), *Lancet*, 1973, *1*, 494 (about 95% bound); A. Brock, *Acta pharmac. tox.*, 1976, *38*, 497; L. Storstein, *Clin. Pharmac. Ther.*, 1976, *20*, 6 and 15; N. Verbeke *et al.*, *Eur. J. clin. Pharmac.*, 1979, *16*, 341 (92% bound; measured by ultracentrifugation).

Uses. Digitoxin has the actions and uses of digoxin (p.536), and is completely and readily absorbed when given by mouth. It is the most potent of the digitalis glycosides and is the most cumulative in action. The onset of its action is slower than that of the other cardiac glycosides; its effects may be evident in about 2 hours and its full effects in about 12 hours after oral administration and somewhat more rapidly after intravenous injection. Its effects persist for about 3 weeks.

As described under digoxin, dosage should be carefully adjusted to the needs of the individual patient. Therapeutic plasma concentrations of digitoxin may range from 10 to 35 ng per ml; higher values may be associated with toxicity. Digoxin may be more suitable for rapid digitalisation but digitoxin can be given to patients who have not received cardiac glycosides during the past 2 weeks. In adults an initial dose of 600 µg may be given, followed by doses of 200 to 400 µg every 6 hours as necessary until a maximum total dose of 1.6 mg has been given over one to two days. For slow digitalisation 200 µg has been given twice daily for 4 days. The maintenance dose varies from 50 to 200 µg daily. Digitoxin may also be given in similar doses by slow intravenous injection when vomiting or other conditions prevent administration by mouth. It has also been given intramuscularly but injections may be painful and absorption is erratic.

Suggested doses of digitoxin for digitalisation in children, to be given in 3 or more divided doses daily by mouth or by injection, are: premature and full-term infants, 22 µg per kg body-weight; 2 weeks to 1 year, 45 µg per kg; 1 to 2 years, 40 µg per kg; and over 2 years, 30 µg per kg. For maintenance one-tenth of the digitalising dose may be given daily.

A brief discussion on pharmacokinetic considerations in the use of digitoxin. A loading dose of digitoxin must be given because of its long half-life; it takes about 5 weeks to reach a steady state of digitalisation. Recommendations vary greatly but in a patient weighing 50 to 70 kg the loading dose should probably be not less than 800 µg and a dose as high as 1.2 mg may be appropriate. A high incidence of toxicity can be expected if the loading dose exceeds 1.8 mg and the daily maintenance dose exceeds 250 µg. It is questionable whether digitoxin is preferable to digoxin. Major advantages of digitoxin are its long duration of action, although this may be a drawback should toxicity occur, and its apparent lack of accumulation in patients with renal failure. However, loading doses must always be given whereas digoxin therapy can often be initiated with maintenance doses. There is great variability in elimination half-lives of digitoxin and in general facilities are lacking for monitoring serum-digitoxin concentrations. Digitoxin is not suitable for the treatment of acute arrhythmias. To change from maintenance treatment with digoxin 250 µg daily to maintenance with digitoxin (assuming that serum-digoxin concentrations are in the therapeutic range) it is suggested that digoxin may be stopped abruptly and digitoxin 400 µg given 24 hours later. This same dose is given on the following day, digitoxin 200 µg on the next day, and thereafter maintenance continued with digitoxin 100 µg daily. To change from maintenance with digitoxin to maintenance with digoxin, digitoxin may be stopped and the anticipated maintenance dose of digoxin started after an interval of 3 treatment-free days.— D. Perrier *et al.*, *Clin. Pharmacokinet.*, 1977, *2*, 292.

Administration in renal insufficiency. From a study of the disposition of digitoxin in 6 subjects with severe renal failure it was concluded that severely reduced renal function did not lead to any substantial change in the disposition of digitoxin and its metabolites.— H. F. Vöhringer *et al.*, *Clin. Pharmac. Ther.*, 1976, *19*, 387. A report of enhanced transformation of digitoxin to dihydrodigitoxin in subjects with renal failure.— G. Bodem and E. V. Unruh, *J. clin. Pharmac.*, 1979, *19*, 195. Doses of digitoxin should be reduced to 50 to 75% in patients with a glomerular filtration-rate of less than 10 ml per minute. Concentrations of digitoxin are not affected by haemodialysis or peritoneal dialysis.— W. M. Bennett *et al.*, *Ann. intern. Med.*, 1980, *93*, 286.

Further references to the administration of digitoxin in renal failure.— J. S. Cheigh, *Am. J. Med.*, 1977, *62*, 555.

See also Absorption and Fate (above).

Preparations

Digitoxin Injection *(U.S.P.)*. A sterile solution in 5 to 50% alcohol; it may contain glycerol or other suitable solubilising agents. Protect from light. *Swiss P.* has 250 µg per ml.

Digitoxin Tablets *(B.P.)*. tablets containing digitoxin.

Digitoxin Tablets *(U.S.P.)*. tablets containing digitoxin. The *U.S.P.* requires not less than 60% dissolution in 30 minutes for each tablet and an average of not less than 85% in 60 minutes. Strongly adsorbent substances such as bentonite should not be used in the manufacture of these tablets.

Guttae Digitoxosidi *(Swiss P.)*. Digitoxin 10 mg, alcohol 10 ml, propylene glycol 40 ml, water to 100 ml.

Proprietary Preparations

Digitaline Nativelle *(Wilcox, UK: Lewis, UK)*. Digitoxin, available as 1-ml **Ampoules** of 200 µg; as a 1 in 1000 **Solution** for oral use; and as **Tablets** of 100 µg. (Also available as Digitaline Nativelle in *Austral., Fr., Neth., Spain, Switz.*).

Other Proprietary Names

Arg.—Digilong, Digimerck, Digitalina Mialhe, Purodigin; *Austral.*—Digitox; *Belg.*—Digitasid, Digitoxine; *Ger.*— Asthenthilo, Digimerck, Ditaven; *Ital.*—Digimerck, Digitalina Nativelle; *Norw.*—Digitrin; *Spain*—Digimerck, Digitalina Bescansa, Digitoxina Simes; *Swed.*—Digitrin; *Switz.*—Digimerck; *USA*—Crystodigin, Purodigin.

5816-h

Erysimin. A glycoside obtained from *Erysimum canescens* (=*E. diffusum*) (Cruciferae). 3β-[(2,6-Dideoxy-β-D-*ribo*-hexopyranosyl)oxy]-5,14-dihydroxy-19-oxo-5β,14β-card-20(22)-enolide dihydrate.
$C_{29}H_{42}O_9,2H_2O=570.7$.

CAS — 630-64-8 (anhydrous).

Pharmacopoeias. In *Rus.*

A white, or slightly greyish or yellowish, crystalline powder, containing 48 to 60.6 (frog) units (USSR) per mg. Slightly **soluble** in water and chloroform; readily soluble in alcohol and methyl alcohol; very slightly soluble in ether; practically insoluble in light petroleum. **Store** in airtight containers. Protect from light.

Erysimin has similar actions to those of strophanthin-K (p.545) and has been given by slow intravenous injection for similar purposes.

5817-m

Gitalin. A mixture of glycosides obtained from *Digitalis purpurea* (Scrophulariaceae), containing 14 to 20% of digitoxin, 13 to 19% of gitaloxin, and 13 to 19% of gitoxin.

CAS — 1405-76-1 (gitalin, amorphous); 3261-53-8 (gitaloxin); 4562-36-1 (gitoxin).

A white or pale buff-coloured amorphous powder. Freely **soluble** in alcohol, acetone, and chloroform; very slightly soluble in ether. **Store** in airtight containers. Protect from light.

Uses. Gitalin has the general properties of digoxin (p.531) and has been used similarly. It has been given by mouth in average maintenance doses of 500 µg daily.

Gitalin was successfully substituted with care for digoxin in 25 patients with stable fibrillation. The average maintenance dose of gitalin was 270 µg daily, compared with 250 µg of digoxin.— A. M. Antlitz and F. L. Barham, *Curr. ther. Res.*, 1967, *9*, 606.

Proprietary Names

Cristaloxine (as gitaloxin) *(Christiaens, Belg.*; *Sedaph, Fr.)*; Formigitil *(Padro, Spain)*; Gitalide *(Padro, Spain)*; Gitaligin *(Schering, USA)*; Verodigeno *(Boehringer Mannheim, Spain)*.

5818-b

Gitoformate. Gitoxin Pentaformate; Pentaformylgitoxin. 3β-[(*O*-2,6-Dideoxy-3,4-di-*O*-formyl-β-D-*ribo*-hexopyranosyl-(1→4)-*O*-2,6-dideoxy-3-*O*-formyl-β-D-*ribo*-hexopyranosyl-(1→4)-2,6-dideoxy-3-*O*-formyl-β-D-*ribo*-hexopyranosyl)oxy]-16β-formyloxy-14-hydroxy-5β,14β-card-20(22)-enolide.
$C_{46}H_{64}O_{19}=921.0$.

CAS — 10176-39-3.

A white powder. Practically **insoluble** in water; slightly soluble in alcohol; very soluble in acetone and chloroform.

Uses. Gitoformate is a synthetic cardiac glycoside with the general properties of digoxin (p.531) and has been used similarly in maintenance doses of 60 to 120 µg daily by mouth.

Proprietary Names

Dynocard *(Madaus, Ger.)*; Formiloxine *(Christiaens, Belg.*; *Menarini, Ital.)*.

5819-v

Lanatoside C *(B.P.)*. Lanatosidum C; Celanide; Celanidum. 3β-[(*O*-β-D-Glucopyranosyl-(1→4)-*O*-3-acetyl-2,6-dideoxy-β-D-*ribo*-hexopyranosyl-(1→4)-*O*-2,6-dideoxy-β-D-*ribo*-hexopyranosyl-(1→4)-2,6-dideoxy-β-D-*ribo*-hexopyranosyl)oxy]-12β,14-dihydroxy-5β,14β-card-20(22)-enolide.
$C_{49}H_{76}O_{20}=985.1$.

CAS — 17575-22-3.

Pharmacopoeias. In *Arg., Aust., Br., Braz., Cz., Hung., Int., Jap., Jug., Mex., Nord., Pol., Roum., Rus., Swiss,* and *Turk.*

Cz. also includes a mixture of lanatosides A, B, and C.

A glycoside obtained from digitalis lanata leaf. It occurs as odourless, colourless or white, hygroscopic crystals or white crystalline powder. It loses not more than 7.5% of its weight on drying. Practically **insoluble** in water, ether, and light petroleum; sparingly soluble in alcohol; soluble 1 in 2000 of chloroform and 1 in 20 of methyl alcohol; soluble in dioxan and pyridine. A solution in methyl alcohol is dextrorotatory. **Store** in airtight containers. Protect from light.

Below pH 3, lanatoside C was largely hydrolysed *in vitro* to digoxin.— S. Aldous *et al.*, *Aust. J. pharm. Sci.*, 1972, *NS1*, 61.

Adverse Effects, Treatment, and Precautions. As for Digoxin, p.531.

Absorption and Fate. Lanatoside C is poorly absorbed from the gastro-intestinal tract. It is weakly bound to serum albumin and rapidly passes to other tissues. About 20% of the dose administered has been stated to be inactivated daily. Its effects disappear after 3 to 6 days. Digoxin is reported to be a metabolite of lanatoside C excreted in the urine.

After administration by mouth, 77% of a dose of lanatoside C was estimated to be absorbed from the gastro-intestinal tract and 23 to 25% was bound to serum albumin. Only 18% of the dose was recovered in the urine as lanatoside C; the remainder was probably digoxin and digoxin metabolites. After intravenous administration 62% of the dose was estimated as recovered in the urine and the half-life for the predominant phase of excretion was 41.3 hours.— H. S. Dengler *et al.*, *Arzneimittel-Forsch.*, 1973, *23*, 64.

The absorption of tritiated lanatoside C was delayed by calcium carbonate and the characteristic double peak of plasma activity was altered, the first peak being reduced and the second increased. Oxyphencyclimine also delayed absorption. These results were consistent with the theory that lanatoside C was converted to digoxin in the gastro-intestinal tract.— R. Thomas and S. Aldous (letter), *Lancet*, 1973, *2*, 1267. Further studies confirmed the belief that lanatoside C is converted into digoxin and its metabolites prior to absorption. Oral administration of lanatoside C might produce lower and more variable concentrations of digoxin in the body.— S. Aldous and R. Thomas, *Clin. Pharmac. Ther.*, 1977, *21*, 647.

Bioavailability. Cedilanid tablets were reformulated in early 1982; they contained the same quantity of lanatoside C, but there was evidence of increased bioavailability and patients would require careful monitoring when being transferred from the old pink tablets to the new white tablets.— *Pharm. J.*, 1982, *1*, 51.

Uses. Lanatoside C is employed for the same purposes as digoxin (p.536). A suggested digitalising dose of lanatoside C is 1.5 to 2 mg daily by mouth in divided doses for 3 to 5 days. The maintenance dose varies from 0.25 to 1.5 mg daily.

Lanatoside A was also formerly used similarly to digoxin. Mixtures of lanatosides A, B, and C have also been used.

Therapeutic serum concentrations of lanatoside C are considered to range from 0.4 to 1 ng per ml compared with 0.8 to 2 ng per ml for digoxin. Of 391 patients taking digoxin or lanatoside C in general practice 159 had serum concentrations lower than 0.8 ng per ml for digoxin or 0.4 ng per ml for lanatoside C; medication was discontinued in 89 patients without clinical deterioration. Dosage was modified in 71 patients.— Liverpool Therapeutics Group, *Br. med. J.* 1978, *2*, 673.

Preparations

Solutio Celanidi 0.02% pro Injectionibus *(Rus. P.)*. Lanatoside C Injection. Lanatoside C 20 mg, alcohol 14.87 ml, glycerol 15 g, Water for Injections to 100 ml; in ampoules of 1 ml. pH 5.5 to 6.5. Sterilised in steam at 100° for 30 minutes. Store in a cool place. Protect from light.

Suppositoria Lanatosidi *(Nord. P.)*. Suppositories each containing 1 mg of lanatoside C in a basis of adeps solidus.

Cedilanid Tablets *(Sandoz, UK)*. Each scored white tablet contains lanatoside C 250 µg. (Also available as Cedilanid Tablets in *Austral., Denm., Ger., Ital., Spain, Swed., Switz., USA*).

See also Cedilanid Injection, p.540.

For the altered bioavailability of Cedilanid, see Absorption and Fate, p.543.

Other Proprietary Names

Austral.—Lanocide; *Belg.*—Cedilanide; *Denm.*—Lanatosid; *Fr.*—Cédilanide; *Ger.*—Celadigal, Lanatosid, Lanimerck, Pandigal (contains lanatosides A, B, and C mixed); *Neth.*— Cedilanide; *Switz.*—Celanat, Dilanat (contains lanatosides A, B, and C mixed), Dilanosid-C.

Cedilanide is also used as a proprietary name for Deslanoside.

5820-r

Medigoxin. β-Methyl Digoxin; β-Methyldigoxin; Metildigoxin. 3β-[(O-2,6-Dideoxy-4-O-methyl-β-D-*ribo*-hexopyranosyl-(1→4)-O-2,6-dideoxy-β-D-*ribo*-hexopyranosyl-(1→4)-2,6-dideoxy-β-D-*ribo*-hexopyranosyl)oxy]-12β,14-dihydroxy-5β,14β-card-20(22)-enolide.
$C_{42}H_{66}O_{14}$=795.0.

CAS — 30685-43-9.

An odourless white crystalline powder. Very slightly **soluble** in water; soluble in alcohol and chloroform.

Adverse Effects, Treatment, and Precautions. As for Digoxin, p.531.

In contrast to digoxin, the rate of decline of radioactivity after intravenous administration of tritiated medigoxin was significantly retarded in patients with acute hepatitis. Delayed demethylation of medigoxin might explain the higher plasma concentrations in patients with liver disease when compared with healthy subjects.— W. Zilly *et al.*, *Clin. Pharmac. Ther.*, 1975, *17*, 302.

Interactions. *Diuretics.* Medigoxin concentrations in serum and urine were not affected in 20 patients given medigoxin 100 or 200 µg daily by the addition of frusemide 80 mg daily to the existing therapy.— R. Baczýnski and F. Kokot, *Dt. med. Wschr.*, 1978, *103*, 662. See also Digoxin, p.534.

Overdosage. A report of a fatal intentional medigoxin overdose.— N. Rietbrock *et al.*, *Dt. med. Wschr.*, 1978, *103*, 1841.

Absorption and Fate. Medigoxin is rapidly and almost completely absorbed from the gastro-intestinal tract and in the steady state a half-life of 54-60 hours has been reported. Demethylation to digoxin occurs. About 60% of an oral or intravenous dose is excreted in the urine as unchanged drug and metabolites over 7 days and 30% appears in the faeces. About 22% of a dose is reported to be lost each day through inactivation or excretion.

Similar mean steady state serum concentrations of about 1.5 ng per ml of medigoxin and digoxin were obtained when 6 healthy subjects took a daily dose of medigoxin 300 µg or digoxin 500 µg respectively. Subjects had a lower medigoxin dose requirement since only 50 to 80% of the digoxin dose was absorbed compared with 70 to 80% of the medigoxin dose. Renal clearances from total serum for digoxin and medigoxin were 126 and 87 ml per minute respectively. Medigoxin was about 22% bound to plasma protein and digoxin about 26%.— G. W. M. Kongola *et al.*, *Br. J. clin. Pharmac.*, 1976, *3*, 954 P. Medigoxin had a half-life of about 2.29 days compared to 1.54 days for digoxin.— F. Keller *et al.*, *Eur. J. clin. Pharmac.*, 1977, *12*, 387. In a crossover study, using a radio-immunoassay technique in 5 healthy subjects, the biological availability of medigoxin significantly exceeded that of digoxin by a factor of 1.6:1. After a single oral dose of medigoxin 800 µg, a mean peak plasma concentration of 10.4 ng per ml was achieved in 15 to 30 minutes compared with a concentration of 5.4 ng per ml in 45 to 75 minutes after digoxin 1 mg. The absorption-distribution phase was 5 to 6 hours for both drugs. About 50% of the medigoxin was excreted in the urine over 96 hours compared with about 47% of the digoxin but it was calculated that under the circumstances of the study the fraction of absorbed medigoxin excreted was about 30% less than the fraction of digoxin eliminated in the urine.— R. P. Hayward *et al.*, *Br. J. clin. Pharmac.*, 1978, *6*, 81.

Further references to the absorption and fate of medigoxin: N. Rietbrock *et al.*, *Eur. J. clin. Pharmac.*, 1975, *9*, 105; D. Boerner *et al.*, *Eur. J. clin. Pharmac.*, 1976, *9*, 307; N. Rietbrock *et al.*, *Eur. J. clin. Pharmac.*, 1976, *9*, 373; B. F. Johnson *et al.*, *Eur. J. clin. Pharmac.*, 1976, *10*, 231 (comparison with digoxin tablets and capsules); P. H. Hinderling *et al.*, *J. pharm. Sci.*, 1977, *66*, 242 (intravenous administration); *idem*, 314 (oral administration); P. H. Hinderling and E. R. Garrett, *ibid.*, 326 (pharmacodynamic correlations); L. Padeletti *et al.*, *Int. J. clin. Pharmac. Biopharm.*, 1979, *17*, 82 (placental transfer).

Uses. Medigoxin has the general properties and uses of digoxin (p.536) but its onset of action is more rapid. When medigoxin is given by mouth or intravenously an effect may appear within 5 to 15 minutes and a maximum effect on the myocardium may be seen in 15 to 30 minutes. The duration of action is similar to or a little longer than that of digoxin; therapeutic serum concentrations are also similar. In stabilised patients 300 µg of medigoxin is as effective as 500 µg of digoxin. Similar doses may be given by mouth or intravenously. For rapid digitalisation medigoxin 200 µg is given thrice daily for 2 to 4 days. Slower digitalisation may be achieved with 200 µg twice daily for 3 to 5 days and maintenance therapy is continued with 200 or 300 µg daily in divided doses. Children have been given 10 µg per kg body-weight every 6 hours, usually for 2 to 4 doses, and then 10 µg per kg daily.

Brief discussions on the actions and uses of medigoxin: *Drug & Ther. Bull.*, 1977, *15*, 79; *Lancet*, 1978, *2*, 1135.

Medigoxin given by mouth or intravenous injection to 9 patients with atrial fibrillation had a maximum effect on slowing the heart-rate within 15 to 20 minutes irrespective of the route of administration.— P. Limbourg *et al.*, *Arzneimittel-Forsch.*, 1973, *23*, 60.

A study of the comparative pharmacodynamics of medigoxin and digoxin in 5 healthy subjects. Although the better gastro-intestinal absorption of medigoxin was reflected in higher blood concentrations of the glycoside this did not result in greater positive inotropic response.— G. Das *et al.*, *Clin. Pharmac. Ther.*, 1977, *22*, 280.

Optimal therapeutic serum concentrations of 1.21 to 1.7 ng per ml were produced by medigoxin 4 µg per kg body-weight daily by mouth.— J. Schneider and A. Ruiz-Torres, *Dt. med. Wschr.*, 1977, *102*, 116.

Comparison of medigoxin and digoxin in the control of atrial fibrillation.— P. Coburn *et al.*, *Br. J. clin. Pharmac.*, 1979, *8*, 53.

Proprietary Preparations

Lanitop *(Roussel, UK).* Medigoxin, available as **Injection** containing 100 µg per ml, in ampoules of 2 ml, and as scored **Tablets** of 100 µg. (Also available as Lanitop in *Arg., Belg., Ger., Neth., Switz.*).

Other Proprietary Names

Lanirapid *(Spain)*; Metidi *(Ital.)*.

5821-f

Meproscillarin. Knoll 570; Ky-18; 4′-O-Methylproscillaridin. 14-Hydroxy-3β-[(4-O-methyl-α-L-rhamnopyranosyl)oxy]-14β-bufa-4,20,22-trienolide.
$C_{31}H_{44}O_8$=544.7.

CAS — 33396-37-1.

NOTE. The name rambufaside was formerly used for meproscillarin.

Colourless crystals. M.p. 213° to 217°. Practically **insoluble** in water; soluble in alcohol and methyl alcohol; slightly soluble in acetone and chloroform.

Stability. Studies on the stability *in vitro* of meproscillarin. Inactivation was greater in more acid solutions.— B. Bergdahl and K. -E. Andersson, *Eur. J. clin. Pharmac.*, 1977, *11*, 267.

Adverse Effects, Treatment, and Precautions. As for Digoxin, p.531.

Absorption and Fate. Meproscillarin is well absorbed from the gastro-intestinal tract and undergoes enterohepatic circulation.

In 5 healthy subjects given 500 µg of tritium-labelled meproscillarin by mouth, peak plasma concentrations of total radioactivity were reached after 1 to 2 hours and in 2 of the subjects a second peak was seen between 6 and 12 hours. The half-life of total radioactivity in plasma was about 51 hours in 4 of the subjects and 19 hours in the fifth; 20% and 56% of the dose was eliminated in the urine and faeces respectively over 7 days. Within 3 hours more than 95% of the radioactivity in plasma and urine consisted of metabolites, the chloroform-insoluble fraction comprising mainly conjugates of meproscillarin. The chloroform-soluble unknown metabolites P_2 and P_3 were anticipated to be cardioactive.— N. Rietbrock and R. Staud, *Eur. J. clin. Pharmac.*, 1975, *8*, 427. The elimination half-life of total plasma radioactivity was about 18 to 30 hours in 4 patients with biliary fistula given tritium-labelled meproscillarin and 29 to 89% of the administered radioactivity was excreted in the bile with 6 to 22% and up to 3% appearing in the urine and faeces respectively.— N. Rietbrock, *Arzneimittel-Forsch.*, 1978, *28*, 540.

In 16 healthy subjects given a single dose of meproscillarin 1.2 mg intravenously or by mouth the mean elimination half-life was about 33 hours. With repeated daily doses a plateau concentration occurred after 3 to 4 days.— G. G. Belz and G. Belz, *Arzneimittel-Forsch.*, 1978, *28*, 535.

No significant difference in plasma concentration was observed between 26 patients with impaired renal function and 7 healthy subjects given meproscillarin 500 µg daily for 2 weeks. It was concluded that, unlike digoxin, dose reduction of meproscillarin in patients with chronic renal failure was unnecessary.— W. D. Twittenhoff *et al.*, *Arzneimittel-Forsch.*, 1978, *28*, 562. Studies involving 9 patients with renal insufficiency associated with cardiac failure given meproscillarin 750 µg daily for 2 weeks indicated that the rapid elimination-rate of meproscillarin was not influenced by renal function.— H. Beckmann *et al.*, *ibid.*, 565. See also G. G. Belz and G. Belz, *ibid.*, 535.

Further references to the absorption and fate of meproscillarin: G. G. Belz *et al.*, *Arzneimittel-Forsch.*, 1976, *26*, 277; J. Weymann *et al.*, *Arzneimittel-Forsch.*, 1978, *28*, 520 (metabolism in *animals*).

Uses. Meproscillarin is the methyl ether of proscillaridin (p.545) and is used similarly to digoxin (p.536). It has been given by mouth in maintenance doses of 500 to 750 µg daily in divided doses and has also been administered intravenously.

In 20 patients with cardiac failure the mean maintenance dose of meproscillarin was 1.71 mg by mouth and 1 mg intravenously daily. Diarrhoea was reported as a side-effect in 9 of the 20 patients.— K. -D. Krämer and H. Hochrein, *Arzneimittel-Forsch.*, 1976, *26*, 579.

Cardiac output and stroke volume in 5 patients with arterial hypertension and left-sided heart failure was increased by up to 25% within 15 minutes of administration of meproscillarin 1 mg by mouth. Heart-rate, arterial blood pressure, and left ventricular filling pressure were unchanged.— W. W. Klein and P. Pavek, *Arzneimittel-Forsch.*, 1978, *28*, 553.

Manifestations of cardiac failure (Friedberg type II and III) were eliminated in 25 patients given meproscillarin 500 to 750 µg daily by mouth for 8 to 10 days during which the cumulative blood concentration had reached 1 to 1.5 mg.— H. Pozenel, *Arzneimittel-Forsch.*, 1978, *28*, 560.

Further studies with meproscillarin: M. Stauch *et al.*, *Arzneimittel-Forsch.*, 1978, *28*, 545; O. Pachinger and P. Probst, *ibid.*, 550; J. Turina and H. P. Krayenbühl, *ibid.*, 555; A. Eckardt *et al.*, *ibid.*, 570.

Proprietary Names

Clift *(Knoll, Ger.)*.

5822-d

Oleandrin. Neriolinum. A glycoside obtained from the oleander, *Nerium oleander* (Apocynaceae). 16β-Acetoxy-3β-[(2,6-dideoxy-3-O-methyl-α-L-*arabino*-hexopyranosyl)oxy]-14-hydroxy-5β,14β-card-20(22)-enolide.
$C_{32}H_{48}O_9$=576.7.

CAS — 465-16-7.

Pharmacopoeias. In *Rus.*

It occurs as colourless odourless acicular crystals with an intensely bitter taste and contains 34 to 40 (frog) units (USSR) per mg. Practically **insoluble** in water and ether; freely soluble in alcohol and chloroform; sparingly soluble in methyl alcohol. **Store** in airtight containers. Protect from light.

Oleandrin has actions similar to those of digoxin (p.531) and has been used for similar purposes.

Preparations

Solutio Neriolini *(Rus. P.).* Oleandrin Solution. Oleandrin 22 mg, alcohol 74 ml, distilled water to 100 ml. It contains 7 to 9 (frog) units (USSR) per ml. Store in a cool place. Protect from light.

Tabulettae Neriolini *(Rus. P.).* Oleandrin Tablets. Each contains oleandrin 100 µg [=3 to 4 (frog) units (USSR)]. Protect from light.

5823-n

Ouabain *(U.S.P., B.P. 1958).* Ouabainum; Strophanthin-G; G-Strophanthin; Strophanthinum; Strophanthoside-G; Uabaina; Ubaína. 3β-(α-L-Rhamnopyranosyloxy)-1β,5,11α,14,19-pentahydroxy-5β,14β-card-20(22)-enolide octahydrate.
$C_{29}H_{44}O_{12},8H_2O$=728.8.

CAS — 630-60-4 (anhydrous); 11018-89-6 (octahydrate).

Pharmacopoeias. In *Arg., Aust., Belg., Cz., Fr., Ger., Ind., Int., It., Jap., Mex., Nord., Pol., Roum., Span., Swiss, Turk.*, and *U.S.* (all $8H_2O$); in *Port.* ($9H_2O$).

A glycoside obtained from the seeds of *Strophanthus gratus* or from the wood of *Acokanthera schimperi* (Apocynaceae) or (*It.* and *Port. P.*) the wood of *A. ouabaio.*

Odourless colourless crystals or white crystalline powder with a bitter taste. M.p. about 190° with decomposition. Slowly **soluble** 1 in 75 of water; soluble 1 in 100 of alcohol and 1 in 30 of methyl alcohol; practically insoluble in chloroform and ether. A solution in water is laevorotatory. Solutions in water are neutral to litmus. Solutions are **sterilised** by autoclaving or by filtration. **Incompatible** with acids, alkalis, and oxidising agents. **Store** in airtight containers. Protect from light.

Adverse Effects, Treatment, and Precautions. As for Digoxin, p.531.

A 57-year-old man with chronic congestive heart failure received ouabain 750 μg intravenously over 3 minutes. About 23 minutes later the patient suddenly became aphasic and left hemiparesis was observed. Blood pressure rose to 255/145 mmHg in about 1 hour and declined over the next 10 hours. The patient died 34 hours after ouabain administration.— R. Kumar *et al.*, *Chest*, 1973, *63*, 105.

Ouabain in small doses could impair short-term memory.— J. T. Archibald and T. D. White (letter), *Nature*, 1974, *252*, 595. See also R. F. Mark and M. E. Watts, *Proc. R. Soc. (Ser. B)*, 1971, *178*, 439.

Absorption and Fate. Absorption of ouabain from the gastro-intestinal tract is unpredictable.

Serum and plasma concentrations of ouabain are equivalent.— T. W. Smith and E. Haber, *New Engl. J. Med.*, 1973, *289*, 1063.

The plasma half-life of ouabain variously reported as 5.5 to 22 hours, was considered to be 19 to 24 hours. In 4 healthy adults given a single intravenous dose a mean of about 26% was excreted in the urine in 18 hours and about 47% in 5 to 6 days. In 3 patients mean faecal excretion in 3 days was 23.4% (range 13.5 to 31.3%) and in 6 days it was 32.9% (range 21.2 to 39.9%). In 4 patients who had undergone cholecystectomy excretion in the bile was 0.7 to 15.8% (mean 5.4%) in 5 to 6 days.— R. Selden *et al.*, *J. Pharmac. exp. Ther.*, 1974, *188*, 615. Following the intravenous administration of 250 μg of ouabain to 6 healthy subjects, the plasma half-life was about 11 hours and 50% of the dose was excreted in the urine in 3 days.— H. -P. Erdle *et al.*, *Dt. med. Wschr.*, 1979, *104*, 976.

The rate of removal of ouabain from plasma by haemodialysis was assessed after a single intravenous injection in 14 dialysis-dependent patients with chronic renal failure. Each patient received ouabain 400 μg (with tritiated ouabain added in 9) at the start of a routine 4-hour haemodialysis. Plasma-ouabain concentrations fell rapidly in the first few hours (from 25.4 to 1.7 ng per ml in the first 4 hours in 1 patient) and then declined exponentially with a mean plasma half-life of 50 hours. Elimination of ouabain from plasma was significantly slower in patients with chronic renal failure than in normal subjects but was more rapid than that of digoxin and digitoxin. Haemodialysis was relatively ineffective for reducing body stores of ouabain and could not be used for treatment of overdosage.— R. Selden and G. Haynie, *Ann. intern. Med.*, 1975, *83*, 15.

Further references to the absorption and fate of ouabain: S. Saarikoski, *Acta pharmac. tox.*, 1980, *46*, 278 (distribution in foetal tissue).

Uses. Ouabain is a cardiac glycoside with actions similar to those of digoxin (p.536). It takes effect in 5 to 10 minutes following intravenous injection and exerts its full action on the heart within ½ to 2 hours, the effect persisting 1 to 3 days. It is used when rapid benefit is required, especially in acute congestive heart failure.

Ouabain is given by slow intravenous injection in a dose of 250 to 500 μg; further injections of 100 μg may be given hourly if needed up to a total dose of 1 mg in 24 hours. Alternatively digitalisation may be continued with digoxin by mouth. Children have been given 5 μg per kg body-weight initially, followed by small doses every 30 minutes until the desired response is obtained or a total dose of 10 μg per kg has been given.

For references to the use of ouabain, see Martindale, 27th Edn, p. 498.

Preparations

Ouabain Injection *(U.S.P.).* A sterile solution of ouabain, 225 to 275 μg per ml, in Water for Injections; it may contain suitable buffers. pH 6 to 7.5. Protect from light. *Jap. P.* also specifies an injection.

Ouabaine Arnaud *(Wilcox, UK: Lewis, UK).* Crystalline ouabain obtained from *S. gratus*, available as 1-ml ampoules of an injection containing 250 μg per ml (for intravenous injection). (Also available as Ouabaine Arnaud in *Austral., Fr., Neth., Spain*).

Other Proprietary Names

g-Strofantin *(Denm., Swed.)*; Ouabaïne Aguettant *(Fr.)*; Purostrophan, Strodival, Strophoperm *(all Ger.)*.

5824-h

Pengitoxin. Pentaacetylgitoxin. 16β-Acetoxy-3β-[(*O*-3,4-di-*O*-acetyl-2,6-dideoxy-β-D-*ribo*-hexopyranosyl-(1→4)-*O*-3-*O*-acetyl-2,6-dideoxy-β-D-*ribo*-hexopyranosyl-(1→4)-3-*O*-acetyl-2,6-dideoxy-β-D-*ribo*-hexopyranosyl)oxy]-14-hydroxy-5β,14β-card-20(22)-enolide.
$C_{51}H_{74}O_{19}$=991.1.

CAS — 7242-04-8.

Pengitoxin is a cardiac glycoside with the general properties of digoxin (p.531) and has been used similarly in maintenance doses of 200 to 400 μg daily by mouth. It has also been given by injection.

Pengitoxin is reported to be metabolised to 16-acetylgitoxin, which is also cardioactive.— K. -O. Haustein, *Eur. J. clin. Pharmac.*, 1978, *13*, 389. Studies of the species-specific deacetylation of pengitoxin showed that the cardioactive glycoside in man is 16-acetylgitoxin.— K. -O. Haustein *et al.*, *ibid.*, *14*, 425.

Proprietary Names

Carnacid-Cor *(TAD, Ger.)*; Cordoval *(Tempelhof, Ger.)*.

5825-m

Periplocin. Glucoperiplocymarin; Periplocoside. A cardiac glycoside isolated from the bark of the silk-vine, *Periploca graeca* (Asclepiadaceae). 3β-[(*O*-β-D-Glucopyranosyl-(1→4)-2,6-dideoxy-3-*O*-methyl-β-D-*ribo*-hexopyranosyl)oxy]-5,14-dihydroxy-5β,14β-card-20(22)-enolide.
$C_{36}H_{56}O_{13}$=696.8.

CAS — 13137-64-9.

White odourless acicular crystals with a very bitter taste. Slightly **soluble** in water; soluble in alcohol and methyl alcohol; very slightly soluble in chloroform and ether; practically insoluble in light petroleum.

Periplocin has actions similar to those of digoxin (p.531) and has been used in the USSR for similar purposes.

5826-b

Proscillaridin. Proscillaridin A; PSC-801. 14-Hydroxy-3β-(α-L-rhamnopyranosyloxy)-14β-bufa-4,20,22-trienolide.
$C_{30}H_{42}O_8$=530.7.

CAS — 466-06-8.

A glycoside obtained from *Scilla maritima* var. *alba* (Liliaceae).

A white crystalline powder. M.p. about 216°. Slightly **soluble** in alcohol; practically insoluble in ether.

Adverse Effects, Treatment, and Precautions. As for Digoxin, p.531.

Absorption and Fate. Proscillaridin is absorbed from the gastro-intestinal tract.

A single dose of proscillaridin 2.5 mg by mouth produced two peak plasma concentrations in 6 healthy subjects. The first appeared between ½ to 1½ hours after the dose (mean 410 pg per ml), and the second at about 10 hours (mean 390 pg per ml). The lowest plasma concentration was at 3 hours (mean 98 pg per ml).— G. G. Belz *et al.*, *Eur. J. clin. Pharmac.*, 1974, *7*, 95. Studies in 6 patients with T-tube drainage of the common bile duct indicated that conjugation was a major route of metabolism of proscillaridin, followed by excretion in bile. It was also suggested that the conjugate could be split in the intestine and reabsorbed, thus accounting for the second peak plasma concentration.— K. -E. Andersson *et al.*, *ibid.*, 1977, *11*, 273.

Studies *in vitro* suggested that if proscillaridin was given before a meal most of the glycoside would be inactivated by acid.— K. -E. Andersson *et al.*, *Eur. J. clin. Pharmac.*, 1975, *8*, 135.

Further references to the absorption and fate of proscillaridin: R. P. Konigstein and A. Lindner, *Wien. med. Wschr.*, 1971, *121*, 53 (pharmacology and use of the 4,5-epoxy derivative); K. -E. Andersson *et al.*, *Eur. J. clin. Pharmac.*, 1977, *11*, 277; K. -E. Andersson *et al.*, *Acta pharmac. tox.*, 1977, *40*, 153; B. Bergdahl, *Arzneimittel-Forsch.*, 1979, *29*, 343.

Uses. Proscillaridin is a cardiac glycoside which is used similarly to digoxin (p.536). It is reported to have a rapid onset and a short duration of action. In patients not previously treated with cardiac glycosides proscillaridin has been given by mouth in initial doses of 1 to 2.5 mg daily, followed by maintenance doses of 0.5 to 2 mg daily.

Digitalisation was achieved in 49 patients with congestive heart failure by giving proscillaridin in doses of 500 μg or 750 μg by mouth every 8 hours. The average maintenance dose was 650 μg daily. After a single intravenous dose of 125 μg of proscillaridin the onset of action occurred at 10 minutes and the maximum effect was noted at 90 minutes.— L. Gould *et al.*, *J. clin. Pharmac.*, 1971, *11*, 135.

Further references to the use of proscillaridin: K. H. Butzengeiger *et al.*, *Dt. med. Wschr.*, 1967, *92*, 2212, per *J. Am. med. Ass.*, 1968, *203* (Jan. 8), A208.

Proprietary Names

Caradrin *(Asta, Ger.; Boehringer Biochemia, Ital.; Boehringer Mannheim, Spain; Laevosan, Switz.)*; Proscillan *(Streuli, Switz.)*; Sandoscill *(Sandoz, Ger.)*; Stellarid *(Zambeletti, Ital.)*; Talucard *(Knoll, Arg.)*; Talusin *(Knoll AG, Austral.; Knoll, Belg.; Biosédra, Fr.; Knoll, Ger.; Knoll, Ital.; Knoll, Neth.; Knoll, Norw.; Knoll, S.Afr.; Knoll, Swed.; Knoll, Switz.)*; Tradenal *(Medinsa, Spain)*; Urgilan *(Sintesa, Belg.; Simes, Ital.)*; Wirnesin *(Inpharzam, Ger.)*; Sucblorin *(Jap.)*.

5827-v

Strophanthin-K *(B.P.C. 1954).* Strophanthin; Kombé Strophanthin; K-Strophanthin; Strophanthoside-K; Estrofantina.

CAS — 11005-63-3.

Pharmacopoeias. In *Arg., Aust., Braz., It., Port., Rus.*, and *Span. Arg.* specifies 40 to 60% of the activity of ouabain. *Rus.* specifies 43 to 58 (frog) units (USSR) per mg.

A mixture of glycosides from strophanthus, adjusted by admixture with a suitable diluent such as lactose so as to possess 40% of the activity of anhydrous ouabain.

A white or yellowish white powder containing microscopic crystals.

Soluble in water and alcohol; very slightly soluble in chloroform; practically insoluble in ether and light petroleum. Solutions for injection, containing a suitable buffering agent such as potassium acid phosphate (2.7%) and adjusted to pH 6.5 by the addition of sodium hydroxide, may be **sterilised** by autoclaving or by filtration. **Incompatible** with acids and alkalis and with tannic acid and lead subacetate. **Store** in airtight containers. Protect from light.

Absorption and Fate.

The half-life of strophanthin-K was increased from 18 to 60 or 70 hours in patients with impaired renal function. Very little glycoside was removed by dialysis.— H. Brass and H. Philipps, *Klin. Wschr.*, 1970, *48*, 972, per *Int. pharm. Abstr.*, 1973, *10*, 641.

In 22 subjects strophanthin-K administered rectally as suppositories containing 0.25, 0.5, and 1 mg reached peak plasma concentrations after 2 hours and peak urine concentrations after 8 hours, with a plasma half-life of 80 hours. About 31% of the drug was absorbed in 24 hours.— P. Ghirardi *et al.*, *Arzneimittel-Forsch.*, 1973, *23*, 1547. See also C. Longhini *et al.*, *Arzneimittel-Forsch.*, 1979, *29*, 827.

Uses. Strophanthin-K has the general properties of digoxin (p.531) and has been used similarly. It is poorly absorbed from the gastro-intestinal tract but acts in 5 to 15 minutes after intravenous injection, the effect lasting about 24 hours. Strophanthin-K has been given intravenously in doses of 125 to 500 μg daily.

Proprietary Names
Estrofosid *(Sandoz, Spain)*; Kombetin *(Boehringer, Arg.; Boehringer Mannheim, Ger.; Boehringer Biochemia, Ital.; Boehringer Mannheim, Spain)*; Myokombin *(Boehringer, Arg.; Boehringer Biochemia, Ital.)*; Strofopan *(Farmasimes, Spain; Simes, Ital.)*; Strophosid *(Sandoz, S.Afr.)*; Trauphantin *(Eifelfango, Ger.)*.

5828-g

Strophanthus *(B.P.C. 1954)*. Strophanthus Seeds.

Pharmacopoeias. In *Belg.*, *Port.*, and *Rus.* (all from *S. kombe*); *Arg.* (from *S. kombe* or *S. hispidus*); *Fr.* (from *S. kombe*, which sometimes includes small amounts of other spp., and *S. gratus;* containing not less than 4% of heterosides expressed as strophanthoside K). *Span.* has separate monographs on Strophanthi Semen (from *S. kombe* and *S. hispidus*) and Strophanthi Grati Semen (from *S. gratus*).

The dried ripe seeds of *Strophanthus kombe* (Apocynaceae), freed from the awns, and containing 7 to 10% of glycosides.

Uses. Strophanthus contains cardiac glycosides and is used principally as a source of strophanthin-K.

The cardiac glycosides of strophanthus are ineffective when administered by mouth.— *Chronicle Wld Hlth Org.*, 1969, *23*, 256.

5829-q

Thevetin. A glycoside obtained from *Thevetia neriifolia* (Apocynaceae).
$C_{42}H_{66}O_{18},3H_2O=913.0$.

CAS — 11018-93-2 (anhydrous).

Thevetin produces typical digitalis actions and is effective 4 to 6 hours after being taken by mouth. It has been used similarly to digoxin (p.536).

Disinfectants and Antiseptics

2200-z

Disinfectants and antiseptics are generally used to destroy or inhibit the growth of pathogenic micro-organisms in the non-sporing or vegetative state.

Considerable confusion exists in the precise definition and usage of the terms disinfectant and antiseptic and further confusion arises because of the difficulties which may occur in distinguishing between them in practice.

According to the British Standard Glossary of Terms Relating to Disinfectants (BS 5283: 1976) the term *disinfectant* is applied to a chemical agent which destroys micro-organisms, but not usually bacterial spores; it does not necessarily kill all micro-organisms, but reduces them to a level which is harmful neither to health nor the quality of perishable goods. The term is applicable to agents used to treat inanimate objects and materials and may also be applied to agents used to treat the skin and other body membranes and cavities. The term *antiseptic* is applied to a chemical agent which destroys or inhibits micro-organisms on living tissues having the effect of limiting or preventing the harmful results of infection.

Sterilisation is the total removal or destruction of all living micro-organisms; a few chemical disinfectants are capable of producing sterility under suitable conditions but, in general, sterility is produced by heat or radiation methods.

Preservatives are used to prevent microbial spoilage of preparations; in pharmacy, preservatives should reduce pathogenic organisms to acceptable numbers or should maintain sterility during use of the preparation. Ideally they should destroy pathogenic organisms.

Some drugs can be used for disinfection and preservation, but those mainly used as preservatives are described in the section on Preservatives and Antoxidants.

Definitions. Besides the terms disinfectant and antiseptic defined above the following were also listed by the British Standards Institution: *bactericide*—a chemical agent which under defined conditions was capable of killing bacteria but not necessarily bacterial spores; *bacteriostat*—a chemical agent which under defined conditions was capable of inhibiting the multiplication of a bacterial population; *fungicide*—a chemical agent which under defined conditions was capable of killing fungi, including their spores.— *Glossary of Terms Relating to Disinfectants*, BS 5283: 1976.

The main types of disinfectants described in this section are aldehydes, cationic surfactants, chlorine and its compounds, dyes, mercurials, phenols and related substances, and some gases and vapours.

The *aldehydes* formaldehyde (p.563) and glutaraldehyde (p.564) are used for disinfection and sterilisation of clean surfaces but are too irritant for use on the skin. Formaldehyde may be used as a vapour.

Cationic surfactants are quaternary ammonium or pyridinium compounds with bactericidal activity against a wide range of Gram-positive and some Gram-negative organisms. They may be used on the skin, where their detergent action is often useful in cleansing dirty wounds. They are also used for cleansing and disinfecting containers and equipment in the food and dairy industries. The quaternary compounds described include benzalkonium chloride (p.549), cetrimide (p.551), cetylpyridinium chloride (p.553), and domiphen bromide (p.561). Their general properties are described under Cetrimide.

Chlorine and chlorine-releasing substances are bactericidal to most Gram-positive and Gram-negative bacteria, some bacterial spores, and some viruses. They also have a deodorant action. Their activity is reduced by organic matter and in alkaline conditions. The main chlorine-releasing compound is sodium hypochlorite solution (p.574); chloramine (p.553), chlorinated lime (p.556), dichlordimethylhydantoin (p.561), halazone (p.565), oxychlorosene (p.570), and sodium dichloroisocyanurate (p.573) also have the general properties described under chlorine (p.557). Hypochlorites have been recommended for disinfecting clean surfaces. Some of the chlorine-releasing substances are used for cleansing foul wounds and ulcers, for disinfecting contaminated water, and since they have low toxicity, for disinfecting utensils in the food industry. Iodine has a similar action.

Two types of *dyes* are used for their antimicrobial action on the skin: the acridine derivatives acriflavine (p.548), aminacrine hydrochloride (p.548), and proflavine hemisulphate (p.572); and the triphenylmethane derivatives brilliant green (p.551), crystal violet (p.560), magenta (p.568), and malachite green (p.568). These dyes are bacteriostatic, particularly against Gram-positive organisms, and have some inhibitory activity against fungi and yeasts.

Gases and *vapours* are used for sterilising objects that cannot be satisfactorily sterilised by heat or chemical means or to sterilise the atmosphere. In general, only surface sterilisation occurs. Gases and vapours are used to sterilise metal or plastic surfaces in some anaesthetic, electrical, and endoscopic equipment, for some plastic components of the heart-lung machine, and for plastic catheters and syringes. Ethylene oxide (p.562) and propiolactone (p.573) are used for these purposes. Formaldehyde may also be used in vapour form.

Mercurials have antibacterial and antifungal activity but are affected by the presence of organic matter. The main mercurial disinfectant is thiomersal (p.576); others used include hydrargaphen (p.567), mercurochrome (p.568), and nitromersol (p.569). Phenylmercuric salts are used as preservatives.

Phenols and chlorinated phenols have a bactericidal action in appropriate concentrations but rapidly lose their effect on dilution or in the presence of organic matter. They are more active in acid conditions and more effective against Gram-positive organisms than against Gram-negative organisms. The more highly substituted phenolic derivatives are more selective in their action than the cruder mixed tar acids and some have antifungal activity. The more selective phenolics are used for skin disinfection and the less-refined products for disinfection of drains and floors and for contaminated bedding and instruments before heat sterilisation. Phenols are also used as preservatives in pharmaceutical preparations. The phenols described in this section include cresol (p.559), phenol (p.570), thymol (p.576), and tar acids and disinfectants (p.574). Chlorinated phenols include bithionol (p.550), chlorocresol (p.558), chloroxylenol (p.558), hexachlorophane (p.566), and triclosan (p.577). Their general properties are described under Phenol.

Other disinfectants described in this section include chlorhexidine salts (p.554) and dibromopropamidine isethionate (p.561). *Chlorhexidine* is a cationic disinfectant, bactericidal against many Gram-positive and Gram-negative organisms but not effective against spores. It is used as a disinfectant for skin and mucous membranes and as a preservative for pharmaceutical preparations.

Substances used as disinfectants or antiseptics and described elsewhere include Alcohol, p.38, Ampholytic Surfactants, p.1443, Hydrogen Peroxide, p.1232, and Iodine, p.863.

Report of the Public Health Laboratory Service Committee on the Testing and Evaluation of Disinfectants, *Br. med. J.*, 1965, *1*, 408.

For reviews of the use of disinfectants, see *Br. med. J.*, 1964, *2*, 1513; J. C. Kelsey and I. M. Maurer, *Mon. Bull. Minist. Hlth*, 1967, *26*, 110; R. B. Kundsin and C. W. Walter, *Practitioner*, 1968, *200*, 15; J. C. Kelsey and I. M. Maurer, *Hlth Trends*, 1971, *3*, 47; J. F. Gardner, *Med. J. Aust.*, 1972, *2*, 1229; *Lancet*, 1978, *2*, 1349; I. M. Maurer, *Hospital Hygiene*, London, Edward Arnold, 1978.

A study of additive and synergistic effects shown by mixtures of some commonly used antibacterial substances *in vitro*.— P. G. Hugbo, *Can. J. pharm. Sci.*, 1976, *11*, 17 and 66.

Disinfectant evaluation. The apparatus and reagents required, the standard techniques and the methods of calculating the various coefficients of disinfectants are fully described in British Standard (BS) Specifications:

The *Rideal-Walker Test*, in BS 541 (*Technique for Determining the Rideal-Walker Coefficient of Disinfectants*), requires distilled-water dilutions of the disinfectant to be tested against broth cultures of the specified micro-organisms.

The *Chick-Martin Test*, in BS 808 (*Modified Technique of the Chick-Martin Test for Disinfectants*), requires the disinfectant to be tested in the presence of a high concentration of organic matter, a yeast suspension being used for this purpose.

The *Crown Agents' Test*, in BS 2462 (*Specification for Black and White Disinfectant Fluids*), is for white fluids only and requires a sterile artifical sea-water dilution of the disinfectant to be tested in the presence of soluble and insoluble organic material.

The *Phenol Coefficient (Staphylococcus) Test*, in BS 2462, is designed to ensure that modified black and modified white fluids are not unduly selective in their bactericidal activity.

A proposed capacity use-dilution test for disinfectants.— J. C. Kelsey and M. M. Beeby, *Mon. Bull. Minist. Hlth*, 1965, *24*, 152. Proposed modification.— A. H. Dodd and J. C. Kelsey, *ibid.*, *25*, 232.

A new test for the assessment of disinfectants.— J. C. Kelsey and G. Sykes, *Pharm. J.*, 1969, *1*, 607.

Two methods of testing stability and long-term effectiveness of disinfectants. Some disinfectants were unstable in that their effectiveness diminished after 7 days' storage; small numbers of organisms which survived in some disinfectants multiplied to more than 10^6 per ml in 5 or 6 days. The concentration of a disinfectant which was effective during the first 24 hours of use was not always effective after being in use for several days.— I. M. Maurer, *Pharm. J.*, 1969, *2*, 529.

Ten disinfectants were evaluated by a capacity use-dilution test. Double the concentration of disinfectant recommended by the manufacturer was usually necessary to pass the test. Only the phenolic compounds were effective tuberculocides.— T. Bergan and A. Lystad, *J. appl. Bact.*, 1971, *34*, 741 and 751.

The sporicidal activity of a number of disinfectants was studied using suspensions of *Bacillus subtilis* spores. Most disinfectants including phenolics, chlorhexidine, a quaternary ammonium disinfectant, formaldehyde solution, and iodophores failed the test. Solutions of hypochlorite 2% in methyl alcohol 50%, and glutaraldehyde 2% in alcoholic suspension were effective in 8 minutes and 3 hours respectively. A suggested method for decontamination of clean heat-sensitive instruments, except those of plated metal, was 15 minutes in a solution of hypochlorite (2000 ppm 'available chlorine'—see p.557) in methyl alcohol 50%.— J. C. Kelsey *et al.*, *J. clin. Path.*, 1974, *27*, 632.

An improved (1974) *Kelsey-Sykes test* for disinfectants.— J. C. Kelsey and I. M. Maurer, *Pharm. J.*, 1974, *2*, 528.

The origin, evolution, and current status of the Kelsey-Sykes test.— D. Coates, *Pharm. J.*, 1977, *2*, 402.

The results of a collaborative assessment of the Kelsey-Sykes test had not been published. Results from 9 commercial laboratories involved showed the test to be suitable for phenolic disinfectants based upon white and clear soluble types. For other types of disinfectant further modification was necessary.— R. A. Cowen, *Pharm. J.*, 1978, *1*, 202.

A discussion on the Kelsey-Sykes test for disinfectants.— W. A. Olsen, *Aust. J. Hosp. Pharm.*, 1980, *9*, 127.

Disinfection of equipment. A brief discussion of the disinfection of ventilators and of the use therein of bacterial filters.— *Br. med. J.*, 1973, *2*, 625.

A discussion of the decontamination of anaesthetic equipment and ventilators.— J. Lumley, *Br. J. Anaesth.*, 1976, *48*, 3.

Recommendations for the use of disinfectants in the disinfection of dental equipment used to treat patients with hepatitis B surface antigen.— *Br. dent. J.*, 1979, *146*, 123.

Disinfection of skin. A review of clinical disinfectants for skin disinfection.— C. L. Odgers, *Aust. J. Hosp. Pharm.*, 1976, *6*, 68.

A 2-minute wash with a liquid soap or detergent antiseptic preparation provided satisfactory pre-operative skin disinfection for surgeons' hands and forearms. Brushing helped to remove dirt and dead epithelial cells, but could cause small excoriations. Brushing for 3 minutes, with careful attention to the finger-nails, before the first operation and washing without the brush prior to each other operation on the list was a reasonable routine for the surgeon.— *Br. med. J.*, 1970, *3*, 418.

The mean reduction in bacterial contamination of operation sites was 79.6 and 74.4% after the application respectively of chlorhexidine 0.5% in alcohol 70% and povidone-iodine (1% available iodine) in alcohol (70%). After 0.1% aqueous benzalkonium chloride and 1% aqueous cetrimide the reductions were 46.2% and 55% respectively. Bacterial counts from hand washings were reduced by 46.7 and 98.2% (after 1 and 6 applications) by Ster-Zac improved liquid soap (containing hexachlorophane 3% and chlorocresol 0.3%) and by 59.9% and 91.4% by Dermofax (containing chlorhexidine gluconate 0.75%, pendecamaine 1.5%, and urea 10%); appreciable reductions were achieved after the use of chlorocresol 0.3%.— H. A. Lilly and E. J. L. Lowbury, *Br. med. J.*, 1971, *3*, 674.

In a study to compare the effect of Hibiscrub (chlorhexidine 4% with detergent), Dermofax (chlorhexidine gluconate 0.75% with detergent), and Disadine (povidone-iodine 7.5% with detergent) the bacterial count of hand washings after a single treatment was reduced by 86.7, 55.5 and 68% respectively; after 6 treatments the reductions were 99.2, 91.8, and 97.7% respectively. To assess their value in the preparation of operation sites, Disadine (povidone-iodine 10%) and chlorhexidine 0.5% aqueous solutions were applied as compresses for 30 minutes and chlorhexidine 0.5% in 70% alcohol and Hibiscrub were rubbed on to the skin with gauze swabs for 2 minutes; mean reductions in bacterial counts were 88.3, 62.7, 80.8, and 71.1% respectively. Repeated washings (on 9 occasions) with Hibiscrub led to a reduction of 98.5% in bacterial count which was further reduced to about one-twentieth of this value by 2 minutes' rubbing with chlorhexidine 0.5% in 70% alcohol. The mean reductions in bacterial count after 2 minutes' washing with chlorocresol 0.3% in soap basis and a preparation containing hexachlorophane 3% with detergent (Disfex) were 29.9 and 51.1% respectively after 1 application and 72.2 and 98.4% after 6 applications. Cetrimide 1% in alcohol 70% reduced the bacterial count by a mean of 69.5% after 2 minutes' swabbing of the hands. Both Hibiscrub and Ster-Zac left considerable antibacterial residue on the skin, effective against *Staphylococcus aureus* and *Escherichia coli*.— E. J. L. Lowbury and H. A. Lilly, *Br. med. J.*, 1973, *1*, 510.

For a review of pre-operative disinfectants for surgeons' and nurses' hands, see *Drug & Ther. Bull.*, 1973, *11*, 99.

The routine bathing of 50 newborn infants in tap water was compared with the bathing of 4 groups of 25 newborn infants with preparations containing lactic acid, hexachlorophane, chlorhexidine gluconate, or phenoxyethanol with hydroxybenzoates. In each case the number of Gram-positive and Gram-negative organisms on the skins of the infants was effectively reduced. Chlorhexidine was less effective than lactic acid or hexachlorophane against pathogens, and hexachlorophane more effective against non-pathogenic organisms, in the concentrations used.— S. I. Hnatko, *Can. med. Ass. J.*, 1977, *117*, 223. See also E. M. Cooperman, *ibid.*, 205.

Use of disinfectants in hospitals. Chemical disinfectants had a narrow antimicrobial spectrum; penetration was often prevented by the presence of soil; they could be inactivated by organic material, soap, some detergents, hard water, and by cork and plastics; and many were unstable. They should be used therefore only when heat sterilisation was not possible. There were 4 main indications for their use in hospitals. For *food hygiene*, hypochlorites or quaternary ammonium compounds were suitable, used after or with a compatible detergent. For *clean surfaces* such as trolley tops, furniture, or walls, hypochlorites, quaternary ammonium compounds, phenolic compounds, or alcohol were suitable. For *contaminated surfaces* or objects, phenolic compounds, a diguanide such as chlorhexidine, or a strong hypochlorite/detergent preparation were suitable. *Skin* and mucous membranes might be disinfected with a phenolic compound or a diguanide. Surgical instruments and catheters should be sterilised though the use of chlorhexidine or glutaraldehyde might be necessary for cystoscopes not capable of withstanding autoclaving. Linen, crockery, and bedpans were best disinfected by heat treatment as part of a routine cleansing procedure. A disinfectant policy needed to be monitored by routine 'in-use' tests which must also detect incorrect dilutions, dilutions kept too long, inadequate preliminary cleaning, inadequate cleaning of containers, and inactivation. Laboratory discard jars, cleaning equipment, and spores, tubercle bacilli, and viruses presented additional problems. The disinfectant policies of 5 hospitals or hospital groups were described.— J. C. Kelsey and I. M. Maurer, The Use of Chemical Disinfectants in Hospitals, *Public Health Laboratory Service Monograph Series No. 2*, London, HM Stationery Office, 1972.

Code of Practice for the Prevention of Infection in Clinical Laboratories and Post-mortem Rooms, London, Department of Health and Social Security, 1978.

Use of disinfectants on farms. For a list of disinfectants and their rate of dilution approved for use in Great Britain in foot-and-mouth disease, swine vesicular disease, fowl pest, and tuberculosis in animals, see The Diseases of Animals (Approved Disinfectants) Order 1978 (SI 1978: No. 32), as amended (SI 1978: No. 934 and SI 1979: No. 37).

Virus disinfection. Fabrics exposed to smallpox virus should be soaked for 2 to 24 hours in one of the following solutions: chlorine preparations in concentrations sufficient to leave 25 ppm of free chlorine, formaldehyde solution at a concentration of 1% or more, or iodophores or quaternary ammonium compounds at a concentration of 1% or more. For disinfection of premises, the disinfectant solution was left in contact for at least 4 hours. When practicable, closed spaces should be disinfected by exposure to formaldehyde vapour for 6 hours.— Second Report of the WHO Expert Committee on Smallpox Eradication, *Tech. Rep. Ser. Wld Hlth Org. No. 493*, 1972. See also *Memorandum on the Control of Outbreaks of Smallpox*, Edinburgh, HM Stationery Office, 1976.

For the disinfection of materials in contact with lassa fever virus, see *Memorandum on Lassa Fever*, Department of Health and Social Security, London, HM Stationery Office, 1976.

Recommendations for precautions in medical care of, and in handling materials from, patients with transmissible virus dementia (Creutzfeldt-Jakob disease).— D. C. Gajdusek *et al.*, *New Engl. J. Med.*, 1977, *297*, 1253.

The virucidal activities of several antimicrobial liquids and foams were determined against rhinoviruses when applied to the hands. Solutions containing iodine 1% in water were most effective and were virucidal when applied immediately after contamination. Foams containing hexachlorophane 0.23% (w/v) with alcohol 58% (v/v) or benzalkonium chloride 0.2% with alcohol 50% (w/w) were less effective and alcohol alone or in a mixture with benzyl alcohol was the least effective preparation.— J. O. Hendley *et al.*, *Antimicrob. Ag. Chemother.*, 1978, *14*, 690.

Recommendations for the use of disinfectants in the disinfection of dental equipment used to treat patients with hepatitis B surface antigen.— *Br. dent. J.*, 1979, *146*, 123.

2201-c

Acriflavine *(B.P.C. 1963).* Acriflavine Hydrochloride. It consists of a mixture of 3,6-diamino-10-methylacridinium chloride hydrochloride and 3,6-diaminoacridine dihydrochloride, the latter being present to the extent of approximately one-third.

CAS — 8063-24-9.

Pharmacopoeias. Similar mixtures to Acriflavine (*B.P.C. 1963*) and Euflavine (*B.P.C. 1949*) are included in several pharmacopoeias but the titles are confused.

An orange-red to red, crystalline, odourless powder with an acid taste. **Soluble** 1 in about 3 of water, 1 in 40 of alcohol, 1 in 4 or less of glycerol, and 1 in 500 of physiological saline; practically insoluble in chloroform, ether, liquid or soft paraffin, and fixed and volatile oils. A precipitate may form in aqueous solutions on dilution or standing. A 1% solution in water has a pH of 1 to 2. Solutions are **sterilised** by autoclaving.
Incompatible with chlorine preparations and with carmellose sodium. Compatible with normal saline if required for immediate use, but deposits after about 24 hours. Concentrations of sodium chloride higher than 5% give a precipitate almost at once.

Acriflavine has properties similar to other acridine derivatives (see p.573)

Photosensitivity. The application of acriflavine could cause photosensitivity.— J. Kalivas, *J. Am. med. Ass.*, 1969, *209*, 1706.

Preparations

Flavazole in Carbowax *(Stoke Mandeville Hosp.).* Acriflavine 54.5 mg, sulphathiazole 46.4 mg, macrogol '4000' 20 g, water to 100 ml. Adjust to pH 6.8 with sodium hydroxide. Autoclave at 115° to 116° for 15 minutes. For bedsores.

Proprietary Names

Diacrid *(Siegfried, Switz.)*; Panflavin *(Chinosolfabrik, Ger.)*.

2202-k

Acrisorcin *(U.S.P.).* Aminacrine 4-Hexylresorcinate. 9-Aminoacridine compound with 4-hexylresorcinol.
$C_{13}H_{10}N_2,C_{12}H_{18}O_2=388.5$.

CAS — 7527-91-5.

Pharmacopoeias. In *U.S.*

A yellow odourless powder. M.p. about 190° with decomposition. **Soluble** 1 in 1000 of water, 1 in 18 of alcohol, 1 in 55 of acetone, 1 in 320 of chloroform, and 1 in 3 of dimethylformamide; very slightly soluble in ether.

Adverse Effects. Skin irritation and photosensitivity may occasionally occur.

Uses. Acrisorcin is an acridine derivative that has been used by topical application of a 0.2% cream in the treatment of tinea versicolor.

Preparations

Acrisorcin Cream *(U.S.P.).* Acrisorcin in a suitable water-miscible basis. Store in airtight containers.

Proprietary Names

Akrinol *(Schering, USA)*.

2203-a

Ambazone. Ambazonum. 4-Amidinohydrazonocyclohexa-2,5-dien-1-one thiosemicarbazone monohydrate.
$C_8H_{11}N_7S,H_2O=255.3$.

CAS — 539-21-9 (anhydrous); 6011-12-7 (monohydrate).

Pharmacopoeias. In *Roum.*

A brown tasteless microcrystalline powder with a faint characteristic odour. Practically **insoluble** in water; very slightly soluble in alcohol; soluble in solutions of acids and of alkali hydroxides.

Ambazone is a bacteriostatic agent which is used in the form of 10-mg lozenges for infections of the mouth and pharynx. It is active against *Streptococcus pyogenes*, *Str. pneumoniae*, and *Streptococcus* spp. *viridans* type.

Proprietary Names

Bridal *(Bayer, Neth.)*; Iversal *(Bayer, Fr.; Bayer, Ger.)*; Primal *(Bayer, Ital.; Bayer, Switz.)*; Primals *(Bayer, Norw.)*.

2204-t

Aminacrine Hydrochloride *(B.P. 1968).*

Aminoacridine Hydrochloride. 9-Aminoacridine hydrochloride monohydrate.
$C_{13}H_{10}N_2,HCl,H_2O=248.7$.

CAS — 90-45-9 (aminacrine); 134-50-9 (hydrochloride, anhydrous).

Pharmacopoeias. In *Arg.*, *Ind.*, and *Nord.*

A yellow odourless crystalline powder with a bitter taste. **Soluble** 1 in 300 of water, 1 in 150 of alcohol, and 1 in 2000 of physiological saline; soluble in glycerol; practically insoluble in chloro-

form and ether. A saturated solution in water is pale yellow with a greenish-blue fluorescence, becoming blue when freely diluted. A 0.2% solution in water has a pH of 5 to 6.5.
Solutions are **sterilised** by autoclaving. The powder is sterilised by maintaining at 150° for 1 hour. **Incompatible** with mineral acids, alkalis, soaps, anionic emulsifying agents, bentonite, methylcellulose, sulphates, and many salts in concentrations greater than 0.5%.

Uses. Aminacrine has properties similar to those of other acridine derivatives (see p.573). It has been used, in a concentration of 0.2%, with other agents in vaginal infections.
It is sometimes preferred to proflavine as it is non-staining.

Preparations

Spiritus Aminoacridini *(Nord. P.).* Aminacrine Spirit. Aminacrine hydrochloride 1 g, alcohol 49.5 g, and water 49.5 g.

Proprietary Names

Aminopt *(Sigma, Austral.).*

2205-x

Amylmetacresol. 6-Pentyl-*m*-cresol; 5-Methyl-2-pentylphenol.
$C_{12}H_{18}O$=178.3.

CAS — 1300-94-3.

A colourless solid with a pleasant odour and taste. M.p. 24°. Practically **insoluble** in water; soluble in alcohol, ether, and oils.

Uses. Amylmetacresol is a disinfectant used chiefly as a mouth-wash or gargle, or as lozenges, in infections of the mouth and throat.

Proprietary Preparations

Strepsils *(Crookes Products, UK).* Lozenges each containing amylmetacresol 600 µg and dichlorobenzyl alcohol 1.2 mg. For minor infections of the mouth and throat. *Dose.* 1 lozenge every 2 or 3 hours. **Strepsils Honey and Lemon.** Contain the same active ingredients in a flavoured basis.

2206-r

Benzalkonium Chloride.

Benzalkonii Chloridum; Benzalkonium Chloratum; Cloreto de Benzalconio. A mixture of alkylbenzyldimethylammonium chlorides of the general formula $[C_6H_5.CH_2.N(CH_3)_2.R]Cl$, in which R represents a mixture of the alkyls from C_8H_{17} to $C_{18}H_{37}$. The *U.S.N.F.* specifies not less than 40% of the $C_{12}H_{25}$ compound, calculated on the dried substance, not less than 20% of the $C_{14}H_{29}$ compound, and not less than 70% of these 2 compounds.

CAS — 8001-54-5.

Pharmacopoeias. In *Arg., Aust., Belg., Braz., Fr., Hung., Int., It., Jap., Jug., Port., Swiss,* and *Turk.* Also in *U.S.N.F.*

A white or yellowish-white amorphous powder, thick gel, or gelatinous pieces with an aromatic odour and a very bitter taste. It contains not more than 15% of water.
Very **soluble** in water, alcohol, and acetone; practically insoluble in ether. A solution in water is usually slightly alkaline and foams strongly when shaken.
Incompatible with soaps and other anionic surfactants, citrates, iodides, nitrates, permanganates, salicylates, silver salts, tartrates, and alkalis. Incompatibilities have been demonstrated with ingredients of some commercial rubber mixes. Incompatibilities have also been reported with other substances including aluminium, fluorescein sodium, hydrogen peroxide, kaolin, hydrous wool fat, and some sulphonamides. Solutions are **sterilised** by autoclaving or by filtration. **Store** in airtight containers. Protect from light.
For precautions to be taken in preparing and storing antiseptic solutions, see under Phenol, p.570.

Total haemolysis occurred when erythrocytes were cultured for 45 minutes in a 0.0027% solution of benzalkonium chl᾿ride in sodium chloride injection. Only slight haemolysis occurred when the strength was reduced to 0.0017%.— H. C. Ansel and D. E. Cadwallader, *J. pharm. Sci.*, 1964, *53,* 169.

Silicone rubber teats, unlike rubber with microcrystalline polyethylene or stearates as a lubricant, did not produce a deposit when benzalkonium chloride was included in eye-drop formulations.— Pharm. Soc. Lab. Rep. P/66/7, 1966.

A dry form of benzalkonium chloride suitable for tableting was produced by complexing with 1.5 to 2 parts of urea.— D. E. Cadwallader and Qamar-Ul-Islam, *J. pharm. Sci.*, 1969, *58,* 238.

The effect of 0.003% benzalkonium chloride against *Pseudomonas aeruginosa* was reduced by 13% in the presence of hypromellose 0.5%.— T. F. J. Tromp *et al.*, *Pharm. Weekbl. Ned.*, 1976, *111,* 561.

A study of the effect of the antibiotic and the preservative on each other's binding to pharmaceutical adjuvants in mixtures containing benzalkonium chloride and ampicillin trihydrate, chloramphenicol, neomycin B sulphate, streptomycin sulphate, or tetracycline hydrochloride.— M. A. El-Nakeeb and M. H. Ali, *Mfg Chem.*, 1976, *47* (Mar.), 37.

It was recommended that the official monographs be amended as benzalkonium solutions obtained from different manufacturers exhibited varying activity which was related to the composition of the benzalkonium chloride. The tetradecyl (C_{14}) homologue had superior antibacterial activity.— R. M. E. Richards and L. M. Mizrahi, *J. pharm. Sci.*, 1978, *67,* 380.

Adsorption. The losses by adsorption of benzalkonium from 30 ml of 0.02% aqueous solution filtered through sintered glass, unglazed porcelain candle, asbestos pad, or membrane filter were 11, 38, 50 to 60, and 14% respectively. In 0.2M acetate buffer (pH 5.9), in 0.33M phosphate buffer (pH 6.9), with disodium edetate 0.1%, or with sodium chloride 0.1% the losses were similar.— N. T. Naido *et al.*, *Aust. J. pharm. Sci.*, 1972, *1,* 16.

Loss in contact with plastics. There was a loss of benzalkonium chloride from its aqueous solution when in contact with polyvinyl chloride, due either to absorption or adsorption or both; the loss was lowest at pH 3, greater in dilute than in stronger solutions, and reduced in the presence of alcohol, glycerol, macrogol 400, and propylene glycol.— W. L. Guess *et al.*, *Am. J. Hosp. Pharm.*, 1962, *19,* 370.

Loss of benzalkonium from solutions stored in polyethylene bottles was caused by interaction between benzalkonium and plasticisers present in the self-adhesive labels, which had been absorbed by the plastic. The solutions became turbid and had blue globules deposited in them.— S. Chrai *et al.*, *Bull. parent. Drug Ass.*, 1977, *31,* 195.

In a series of stability studies loss of benzalkonium chloride from ophthalmic solutions stored in polyethylene bottles was found to be accelerated by the presence of a stearate type mould release agent added to the plastic; solutions showed both hazing and loss of antimicrobial activity presumably due to insoluble complex formation.— B. J. Meakin *et al.*, *J. Pharm. Pharmac.*, 1978, *30, Suppl.*, 15P.

For a report of inactivation of benzalkonium chloride by polyurethane foam, see under Tar Acids, p.575.

Contact lens solutions. The loss of benzalkonium chloride from contact lens solutions by sorption to the polyethylene and polypropylene containers was probably not microbiologically significant.— N. E. Richardson *et al.*, *J. Pharm. Pharmac.*, 1977, *29,* 717.

Benzalkonium chloride was reversibly sorbed into lenses manufactured from polyhydroxyethylmethacrylate.— N. E. Richardson *et al.*, *J. Pharm. Pharmac.*, 1978, *30,* 469.

Loss of activity in presence of cotton. Contamination of cotton pledgets, soaked in a 0.1% aqueous dilution of benzalkonium chloride, with Gram-negative organisms caused infection in 15 patients in a hospital ward. Four patients showed clinical illness and 2 died. Aqueous solutions of quaternary ammonium compounds lost most of their antibacterial properties when brought into contact with cotton, cellulose fibre, or protein.— J. C. Lee and P. J. Fialkow, *J. Am. med. Ass.*, 1961, *177,* 708. See also W. F. Malizia *et al.*, *New Engl. J. Med.*, 1960, *263,* 800.

Cotton fibres in a concentration as low as 4% w/v affected adversely the antibacterial activity (against *Staphylococcus aureus*) of 0.01% and 0.02% solutions of benzalkonium chloride. The adverse effect increased as the amount of cotton fibre was increased.— G. E. Myers and C. Lefebvre, *Can. pharm. J.*, 1961, *94* (July), 55.

Adverse Effects, Treatment, and Precautions. As for Cetrimide, p.552.

Within a few minutes of being inadvertently given an enema of benzalkonium chloride 3%, 2 women experienced sweating and nausea, and died. The viscera were found to be congested and cyanosed. A third woman died soon after using a vaginal douche containing benzalkonium. Death was supposed to have resulted from respiratory paralysis.— G. Gastmeier *et al.*, *Z. ges. gerich. Med.*, 1969, *65,* 96, per *Abstr. Wld Med.*, 1969, *43,* 969.

A report of allergic conjunctivitis occurring in 1 patient after using an ophthalmic solution containing benzalkonium chloride. The patch test reaction to benzalkonium chloride was strongly positive.— A. A. Fisher and M. A. Stillman, *Archs Derm.*, 1972, *106,* 169.

Benzalkonium chloride has been reported to be ototoxic.— J. L. Honigman, *I.C.I. Pharmaceuticals* (letter), *Pharm. J.*, 1975, *2,* 523.

Inflammation of the eye and deterioration of vision 3 days after change of soaking solution, for a soft contact lens, to one containing benzalkonium chloride.— A. R. Gasset, *Am. J. Ophthal.*, 1977, *84,* 169.

A soldier developed toxic contact dermatitis of the ear after wearing an ear-protector which had been disinfected in a solution of benzalkonium chloride.— H. Gall, *Derm. beruf. umwelt,* 1979, *27,* 139.

Uses. Benzalkonium chloride is a quaternary ammonium disinfectant with properties and uses similar to those of the other cationic surfactants as described under Cetrimide, p.552.
A 0.1 to 0.2% solution of benzalkonium chloride has been used for the pre-operative disinfection of unbroken skin, but for application to mucous membranes, denuded skin, wounds, and burns solutions containing up to 0.1% are used. A 0.05 to 0.1% solution has been used in obstetrics. An aqueous solution usually not stronger than 0.005% has been used for irrigation of the bladder and urethra and a 0.0025% solution for retention lavage of the bladder.
Creams containing benzalkonium chloride have been used in the treatment of napkin rash. A 0.0125% solution is used for soaking babies' napkins to prevent napkin rash.
Polyethylene and nylon tubing and catheters have been cleansed by perfusing them with a 0.1% solution to remove air and then immersing them in a solution of the same strength for 24 hours.
Benzalkonium lozenges are used for the treatment of superficial infections of the mouth and throat.
A 0.01% solution of benzalkonium chloride (0.02% v/v of Benzalkonium Chloride Solution) is used as a preservative for some eye-drops of the *B.P.C. 1973* and *U.S.N.F.* It is not suitable for eye-drops containing local anaesthetics. Because some rubbers are incompatible with benzalkonium chloride the *B.P.C. 1973* recommended that, unless the suitability has been established, silicone rubber teats be used on eye-drop containers.
Benzalkonium bromide has been similarly used.

A report of a cluster of *Serratia marcescens* infections complicating cardiopulmonary bypass operations and traced to a contaminated quaternary ammonium disinfectant. Failure of hospital personnel to clean the disinfectant spray bottles before refilling them had enabled the organisms to survive and contaminate the environment. The organisms were subsequently grown in 2 of 4 formulations of quaternary ammonium disinfectant. The danger of using quaternary ammonium compounds as disinfectants rather than cleansers is re-emphasised. Personnel cannot be relied upon to distinguish between disinfectants that can and cannot support bacterial growth, although they should be expected not to top up solutions.— N. J. Ehrenkranz *et al.*, *Lancet,* 1980, *2,* 1289. Criticism.— R. D. Sheets (letter), *ibid.*, 1981, *1,* 727. Reply with correction.— N. J. Ehrenkranz and T. Cleary (letter), *ibid.*, 1154.

The antibacterial effect of benzalkonium chloride (0.003%) was enhanced by 0.175% of benzyl alcohol, phenylpropanol, or phenethyl alcohol. The effect was more than additive, was most pronounced in respect of phenylpropanol, and least pronounced in respect of benzyl alcohol.— R. M. E. Richards and R. J. McBride, *J. pharm. Sci.*, 1973, *62*, 2035.

For the use of phenethyl alcohol with benzalkonium chloride as a preservative for ophthalmic solutions, see Phenethyl Alcohol, p.1288.

Dysentery. For the use of a 0.1% solution of benzalkonium chloride in the control of an outbreak of dysentery, see B. Beer *et al.*, *Mon. Bull. Minist. Hlth*, 1966, *25*, 36.

Ophthalmic solutions. Of a range of substances tested for their bactericidal activity against 13 strains of *Ps. aeruginosa* in ophthalmic solutions, benzalkonium chloride 0.02% had the shortest sterilising time, of 45 minutes; at a concentration of 0.01%, however, it was only effective in 9 hours. The sterilising times of the other substances tested were chlorbutol (0.7%) 9 hours, chlorbutol (0.5%) 12 hours, thiomersal (0.01%) 9 hours, thiomersal (0.02%) 6 hours, methyl hydroxybenzoate (0.2%) with propyl hydroxybenzoate (0.04%) 3 hours, methyl hydroxybenzoate (0.18%) with propyl hydroxybenzoate (0.02%) 6 hours, phenylmercuric nitrate (0.01 and 0.005%) 6 hours, phenethyl alcohol (0.5%) more than 24 hours, polymyxin B sulphate (2000 units per ml) 12 hours, and polymyxin B sulphate (1000 units per ml) 18 hours.— S. R. Kohn *et al.*, *J. pharm. Sci.*, 1963, *52*, 967.

Preparations of Benzalkonium Salts

Lozenges

Benzalkonium Lozenges *(B.P.C. 1973)*. Benzalkonium Chloride Lozenges. Each lozenge weighs about 1 g and contains benzalkonium chloride solution 0.001 ml, menthol 600 µg, thymol 600 µg, eucalyptus oil 0.002 ml, and lemon oil 0.002 ml.

Solutions

Benzalkonium Bromide Solution *(B.P.C. 1968)*. An aqueous solution containing 50% w/v of a mixture of alkylbenzyldimethylammonium bromides. It is a clear colourless or pale yellow syrupy liquid with an aromatic odour and a very bitter taste. A dilution with water is neutral or slightly alkaline to litmus and foams strongly on shaking. Miscible with water, alcohol, and acetone.

Benzalkonium Chloride Solution *(B.P.)*. A solution containing 49 to 51% w/v of benzalkonium chloride. It contains not more than 16% v/v of alcohol or industrial methylated spirit. It is a clear colourless or pale yellow syrupy liquid with an aromatic odour and a very bitter taste. A dilution with water is neutral or slightly alkaline to litmus and foams strongly on shaking. Miscible with water and alcohol.

Benzalkonium Chloride Solution *(U.S.N.F.)*. A solution containing benzalkonium chloride. It may contain a suitable colouring agent and not more than 10% of alcohol. Store in airtight containers and avoid contact with metals. *Int. P.* and *Jap. P.* include a similar solution. *Hung. P.* and *Nord. P.* specify a 10% solution.

Benzalkonium Solution Compound *(A.P.F.)*. Hard Contact Lens Solution. Benzalkonium chloride solution 0.02 ml, disodium edetate 50 mg, sodium chloride 900 mg, Water for Injections to 100 ml. Sterilised by autoclaving.

Proprietary Preparations of Benzalkonium Salts

Capitol *(Dermal Laboratories, UK)*. A gel containing benzalkonium chloride 0.5% in an anionic basis. For dandruff and seborrhoeic dermatitis of the scalp.

Cetanorm *(Norma, UK: Farillon, UK)*. Cream containing benzalkonium chloride 0.1%, aldioxa 0.375%, chlorbutol 0.1%, cetrimide 0.4%, and nonoxinol '9' 2%. For minor wounds and napkin rash.

Drapolene *(Wellcome Consumer Division, UK)*. A cream containing benzalkonium chloride 0.01% and cetrimide 0.2% in a water-miscible basis.

Empigen BAC *(Albright & Wilson, Marchon Division, UK)*. A brand of benzalkonium chloride solution.

Hyamine 3500 *(Rohm & Haas, UK)*. Benzalkonium chloride available as a 50% solution containing 10% of alcohol.

Morpan BC *(ABM Chemicals, UK)*. A brand of benzalkonium chloride solution.

Polycide *(Le-Han, Canad.: Cottrell, UK)*. A solution containing benzalkonium chloride 6.5% and ethylhexadecyldimethylammonium bromide ($C_{20}H_{44}BrN$ = 378.5) 6.5%. For use as a 1% solution for disinfecting surgical and dental instruments.

Roccal *(Winthrop, UK)*. A solution of benzalkonium chloride containing 1%. **Roccal Concentrate** (Roccal 10X) is a solution containing 10%.

Silquat B10 *(Tenneco, UK)*. Benzalkonium chloride, available as a solution containing 10%. **Silquat B50.** A brand of benzalkonium chloride solution.

Stomobar *(Thackray, UK)*. A cream containing benzalkonium chloride 0.5% and chlorhexidine gluconate 0.09%. For use as a barrier cream around stomas.

Stomogel *(Thackray, UK)*. A gel containing benzalkonium chloride 1% and chlorhexidine gluconate 0.1%. For use as an antiseptic and deodorant with ostomy appliances.

Stomosol Concentrate *(Thackray, UK)*. A liquid antiseptic containing benzalkonium chloride 10% and chlorhexidine gluconate 1%. For use as a 1 in 20 solution for general cleansing and skin disinfection.

Toracsol *(Torbet Laboratories, UK)*. A solution containing benzalkonium bromide 2.1%, cetylpyridinium bromide 1%, cetrimide 3.6%, and hexachlorophane 6.7%. For acne.

Vantoc CL *(ICI Organics, UK)*. A brand of benzalkonium chloride solution.

Other Proprietary Names

Austral.—Cetal Conc. A and B, Zephiran; *Canad.*—Benzalchlor-50, Dermo-Sterol, Ice-O-Derm (see also under Other Proprietary Names of Chlorinated Phenols, p.559), Sabol; *Denm.*—Benzalkon, Rodalon; *Fr.*—Ovules Pharmatex; *Ger.*—Laudamonium, Quartamon, Zephirol; *Norw.*—Benzalkon; *Spain*—Armil, Lindemil; *USA*—Zephiran.

Benzalkonium Chloride Solution was also formerly marketed in Great Britain under the proprietary name Cycloton B50 (*Witco*). A range of quaternary ammonium disinfectants was formerly marketed under the proprietary name BTC (*Onyx Chemical Co., USA*). A preparation containing benzalkonium chloride and benzocaine was formerly marketed under the proprietary name Benzets (*Norton*).

Proprietary Preparations of Related Compounds

Rewoquat B 50 (formerly known as Loraquat B 50) *(Rewo, UK)*. A liquid containing benzododecinium chloride (benzyldodecyldimethylammonium chloride) 50%. **Rewoquat QA 100** is an alkylbenzyldimethylammonium saccharinate complex.

Task *(Brentchem, UK)*. A liquid preparation containing didecyldimethylammonium bromide ($C_{22}H_{48}BrN$ = 406.5) with an amphoteric and a nonionic surfactant. For use as a 1% solution for cleansing and disinfecting premises and equipment.

NOTE. The name Task is also applied to a veterinary preparation containing dichlorvos.

Use in dairies. A list of proprietary quaternary ammonium preparations approved for the cleansing and disinfecting of milk containers and appliances is contained in Circular FSH 8/78, Ministry of Agriculture, Fisheries and Food, London HM Stationery Office, 1978.

2207-f

Benzethonium Chloride *(U.S.P.)*.

Benzethonii Chloridum. Benzyldimethyl(2-{2-[4-(1,1,3,3-tetramethylbutyl)phenoxy]ethoxy}ethyl)ammonium chloride.
$C_{27}H_{42}ClNO_2$=448.1.

CAS — 121-54-0.

Pharmacopoeias. In *Arg., Int., Jap., Nord.,* and *U.S.*

White crystals with a mild odour and a very bitter taste. M.p. after drying 158° to 163°.
Soluble 1 in 0.6 of water, 1 in 0.6 of alcohol, and 1 in 1 of chloroform; slightly soluble in ether; practically insoluble in light petroleum. A 1% solution in water is slightly alkaline to litmus and foams strongly when shaken. Solutions are **sterilised** by autoclaving. **Incompatible** with soaps and other anionic surfactants. **Store** in airtight containers. Protect from light.

Total haemolysis occurred when erythrocytes were cultured for 45 minutes in a 0.0022% solution of benzethonium chloride in sodium chloride injection. Only slight haemolysis occurred when the strength was reduced to 0.0015%.— H. C. Ansel and D. E. Cadwallader, *J. pharm. Sci.*, 1964, *53*, 169.

Adverse Effects and Treatment. As for Cetrimide, p.552.

Uses. Benzethonium chloride is a quaternary ammonium disinfectant with properties and uses similar to those of other cationic surfactants as described under Cetrimide, p.552.
It is applied to wounds as an aqueous solution containing about 0.1% and it is used as a 0.2% solution in alcohol and acetone for pre-operative skin disinfection.
Benzethonium chloride is also used for cleansing food utensils and dairy utensils, for the control of algal growth in swimming pools, and as a deodorant and preservative.

Preparations

Benzethonium Chloride Tincture *(U.S.P.)*. Benzethonium chloride 200 mg, alcohol 68.5 ml, acetone 10 ml, and water to 100 ml; it may be coloured. Inflammable. Store in airtight containers. Protect from light.

Benzethonium Chloride Topical Solution *(U.S.P.)*. Benzethonium Chloride Solution. A solution containing benzethonium chloride. Store in airtight containers. Protect from light.

Proprietary Preparations

Hyamine 1622 *(Rohm & Haas, UK)*. A brand of benzethonium chloride.

Other Proprietary Names

Benzalcan, Desamon (both *Switz.*); Phemerol Chloride (*USA*).

2208-d

Benzododecinium Bromide. Benzyldodecyldimethylammonium bromide.
$C_{21}H_{38}BrN$=384.4.

CAS — 10328-35-5 (benzododecinium); 7281-04-1 (bromide).

Pharmacopoeias. In *Cz.*

Benzododecinium bromide is a quaternary ammonium disinfectant present in benzalkonium bromide (see p.550). It is used in a concentration of 0.25% in eye-drops for the treatment of conjunctivitis, keratitis, and blepharitis. Benzododecinium chloride has also been used.

Proprietary Names

Benzo-Davur (benzododecinium chloride); Prorhinel (*Monal, Fr.*) (*Davur, Spain*).

2209-n

Bisdequalinium Diacetate. R 199. 1,1′-Decamethylene-*NN*′-decamethylenebis(4-amino-2-methylquinolinium acetate).
$C_{44}H_{64}N_4O_4$=713.0.

Bisdequalinium diacetate is a bacteriostatic and fungistatic agent applied topically as a cream, gel, or lotion; it is also used in ear-drops in the treatment of otitis media.

Proprietary Names

Alsol (*Also, Ital.*); Salvizol (see also under Dequalinium Chloride, p.561) (*Ravensberg, Belg.*; *Ravensberg, Ger.*; *Grossmann, Switz.*).

2210-k

Bithionol.

Bitionol. 2,2′-Thiobis(4,6-dichlorophenol).
$C_{12}H_6Cl_4O_2S$=356.1.

CAS — 97-18-7.

Pharmacopoeias. In *Arg.*

A white or greyish-white crystalline powder which is odourless or has a slight aromatic or phenolic odour. M.p. 186° to 189°. Practically **insoluble** in water; freely soluble in alcohol, acetone, and ether; soluble in chloroform and in dilute solutions of alkali hydroxides. **Store** in airtight containers. Protect from light.

Adverse Effects. Photosensitivity reactions have occurred in persons using soap containing bithionol. Cross-sensitisation with other halogenated disinfectants has also occurred.

Adverse effects in patients taking bithionol by mouth include anorexia, nausea, vomiting, abdominal discomfort, diarrhoea, salivation, dizziness, headache, and skin rashes.

Reports of photosensitivity.— S. E. O'Quinn *et al.*, *J. Am. med. Ass.*, 1967, *199*, 89; P. D. C. Kinmont, *Practitioner*, 1969, *202*, 88; K. D. Crow *et al.*, *Br. J. Derm.*, 1969, *81*, 180.

Treatment of Adverse Effects. As for Phenol, p.571.

Uses. Bithionol is a bactericide which is effective against Gram-positive cocci. It is no longer applied topically because of photosensitivity reactions.

Bithionol is used in the treatment of paragonimiasis in a dosage of 30 to 50 mg per kg body-weight, given by mouth on alternate days for 10 to 15 doses. In the treatment of clonorchiasis, the same dose has been given. Bithionol has also been used, in a dose of up to 3 g daily on alternate days for 15 doses, in the treatment of fascioliasis. Doses of up to 60 mg per kg body-weight, in 2 divided doses about one hour apart, have been given in tape-worm infection.

Fascioliasis. Bithionol, 3 g daily on alternate days for 28 days, was the treatment of choice in patients infected with the liver fluke, *Fasciola hepatica*. Side-effects included nausea, vomiting, and diarrhoea, and initially the hepatitis might be increased.— A. C. E. Cole, *Practitioner*, 1973, *211*, 528. See also W. L. G. Ashton *et al.*, *Br. med. J.*, 1970, *3*, 500; *Lancet*, 1978, *2*, 196.

Paragonimiasis. Bithionol, 40 mg per kg body-weight on alternate days for 10 or 15 doses, was used for the mass treatment of 1113 patients with infections of *Paragonimus westermani*. One year after treatment sputum samples were free from eggs in 90.8% of those patients and in 73.6% of 53 other patients who received less than 10 doses. Side-effects occurred in 41.2% of 775 patients questioned.— J. S. Kim, *Am. J. trop. Med. Hyg.*, 1970, *19*, 940.

Preliminary results of a study on bithionol in the treatment of an outbreak of paragonimiasis in Nigeria indicated that a dose of 50 mg per kg body-weight on alternate days for 10 doses was effective in over 90% of patients.— C. Nwokolo, *Lancet*, 1972, *1*, 32.

Further reports: S. J. Oh, *Am. J. trop. Med. Hyg.*, 1967, *16*, 585; S. -P. Yang and C. -C. Lin, *Dis. Chest*, 1967, *52*, 220; R. A. Gutman *et al.*, *Am. Rev. resp. Dis.*, 1969, *99*, 255; B. D. Cabrera and P. M. Fevidal, *S.E. Asian J. trop. med. publ. Hlth*, 1974, *5*, 39; G. W. Fischer *et al.*, *J. Am. med. Ass.*, 1980, *243*, 1360.

Proprietary Names

Bitin *(Jap.)*.

2211-a

Brilliant Green *(B.P.)*.
Viride Nitens; CI Basic Green 1; Colour Index No. 42040. 4-(4-Diethylaminobenzhydrylidene)cyclohexa-2,5-dien-1-ylidenediethylammonium hydrogen sulphate.

$C_{27}H_{34}N_2O_4S$=482.6.

CAS — 633-03-4.

Pharmacopoeias. In *Br.*, *Hung.*, and *Ind.*
Viride Nitens (*Rus. P.*) is the oxalate.

Small glistening gold crystals. M.p. about 196°. **Soluble** 1 in 5 of water and 1 in 12 of alcohol. **Incompatible** with anionic, oxidising, and reducing substances.

Incompatible with aqueous suspensions of bentonite.— W. A. Harris, *Australas. J. Pharm.*, 1961, *42*, 583.

The antimicrobial activity of brilliant green was destroyed by prolonged autoclaving at 121°.— W. A. Moats *et al.*, *Appl. Microbiol.*, 1974, *27*, 844.

Adverse Effects. Sensitisation has occasionally occurred.

Sensitisation to brilliant green was observed in 11 patients with eczema. Simultaneous sensitivity to crystal violet and malachite green was found in some patients.— T. Bielicky and M. Novák, *Archs Derm.*, 1969, *100*, 540.

For a report of necrotic skin reaction to brilliant green, see Crystal Violet, p.560.

Uses. Brilliant green is a disinfectant effective against vegetative Gram-positive bacteria but less effective against Gram-negative organisms and ineffective against acid-fast bacteria and bacterial spores. Its activity is greatly reduced in the presence of serum.

It has been applied as a 0.05 to 0.1% solution in water or hyperosmotic saline in the treatment of infected wounds or burns. A solution of brilliant green 0.5% and crystal violet 0.5% has been used for disinfecting the skin.

A paint containing brilliant green 0.5% and mercuric chloride 0.5% in industrial methylated spirit has been used in the treatment of paronychia.

A 0.02% solution in water has been used by aerosol inhalation in the treatment of mycotic infections of the lung.

Preparations

Brilliant Green and Crystal Violet Paint *(B.P.)*. —See under Crystal Violet, p.560.

2212-t

Bromochlorosalicylanilide. 5-Bromo-4′-chlorosalicylanilide; 5-Bromo-*N*-(4-chlorophenyl)-2-hydroxybenzamide.

$C_{13}H_9BrClNO_2$=326.6.

Bromochlorosalicylanilide is an antifungal agent applied topically as a 2% powder and as a solution, cream, or ointment in the prophylaxis and treatment of fungous infections. See also Bromsalans, below.

Proprietary Names

Multifungin *(Knoll, Arg.; Knoll, Ger.; Knoll, Neth.; Knoll, Norw.; Medinsa, Spain)*.

2289-k

Bromsalans.
A series of brominated salicylanilides which possess antimicrobial activity.

CAS — 55830-61-0.

2290-w

Dibromsalan.
NSC 20527. 4′,5-Dibromosalicylanilide; 5-Bromo-*N*-(4-bromophenyl)-2-hydroxybenzamide.

$C_{13}H_9Br_2NO_2$=371.0.

CAS — 87-12-7.

2291-e

Metabromsalan.
NSC 526280. 3,5-Dibromosalicylanilide; 3,5-Dibromo-2-hydroxy-*N*-phenylbenzamide.

$C_{13}H_9Br_2NO_2$=371.0.

CAS — 2577-72-2.

2213-x

Tribromsalan.
ET-394; NSC 20526; TBS. 3,4′,5-Tribromosalicylanilide; 3,5-Dibromo-*N*-(4-bromophenyl)-2-hydroxybenzamide.

$C_{13}H_8Br_3NO_2$=449.9.

CAS — 87-10-5.

An account of the solubilities and industrial applications of bromsalans.— S. J. Hopkins, *Mfg Chem.*, 1965, *36* (Nov.), 63. See also N. H. Molnar, *Soap chem. Spec.*, 1965, *41* (Feb.), 59.

Adverse Effects. There have been many reports of photosensitivity following the use of the various bromsalans as disinfectants in soaps. Cross-sensitisation to other halogenated salicylanilides may occur.

Photosensitisation to bromsalans and related halogenated salicylanilides was considered to result from the conversion of the salicylanilide by light to a more potent contact allergen. Volunteers photosensitised to tribromsalan reacted in irradiated patch tests to dibromsalan and 4′-monobromosalicylanilide, the 2 main photodecomposition products, and the same reaction followed testing with tribromsalan solution irradiated *in vitro*. The final photodecomposition product, monobromosalicylanilide, was a stronger contact allergen than dibromsalan, which was in turn stronger than tribromsalan. The photosensitivity reaction was clinically indistinguishable from contact allergy.— I. Willis and A. M. Kligman, *J. invest. Derm.*, 1968, *51*, 378. See also *idem*, *Archs Derm.*, 1969, *100*, 535; W. M. Sams, *Mayo Clin. Proc.*, 1968, *43*, 783; E. A. Emmett, *J. invest. Derm.*, 1974, *63*, 227; S. Z. Smith and J. H. Epstein, *Archs Derm.*, 1977, *113*, 1372.

Uses. Bromsalans have antibacterial and antifungal activity and were formerly used in medicated soaps. They have also been tried in the treatment of fascioliasis in *sheep*.

In Great Britain the use of bromsalans in cosmetics and toiletries is restricted under the Cosmetic Products Regulations 1978 (SI 1978: No. 1354).

A review of antimicrobial agents, including bromsalans.— I. R. Gucklhorn, *Mfg Chem.*, 1970, *41* (Dec.), 50.

Proprietary Names

Diaphene *(dibromsalan with tribromsalan) (Stecker, USA)*; Temasept I *(dibromsalan with tribromsalan) (Hexcel, USA)*; Temasept IV *(tribromsalan) (Hexcel, USA)*.

2214-r

Cetalkonium Chloride. NSC 32942. Benzylhexadecyldimethylammonium chloride.

$C_{25}H_{46}ClN$=396.1.

CAS — 122-18-9.

A white crystalline powder. Sparingly **soluble** in cold water; soluble in hot water, alcohol, chloroform, ether, and glycerol.

Adverse Effects and Treatment. As for Cetrimide, p.552.

Uses. Cetalkonium chloride is a quaternary ammonium disinfectant with properties and uses similar to those of other cationic surfactants as described under Cetrimide, p.552. It is used, usually in a concentration of 0.01%, in preparations applied to the mouth or throat. It has been used similarly to benzalkonium chloride for hand and instrument disinfection.

Proprietary Names

Baktonium *(Bode, Ger.)*.

A preparation containing cetalkonium chloride was formerly marketed in Great Britain under the proprietary name Throsil Lozenges (*Cox-Continental*).

2215-f

Cethexonium Bromide. Céthéxonium (Bromure de). Hexadecyl(2-hydroxycyclohexyl)dimethylammonium bromide.

$C_{24}H_{50}BrNO$=448.6.

CAS — 6810-42-0 (cethexonium); 1794-74-7 (bromide).

Pharmacopoeias. In *Fr.*

A white or slightly cream-coloured microcrystalline powder with a characteristic odour and a bitter taste. M.p. 75°. Very slightly **soluble** in water; soluble in alcohol; very soluble in chloroform; practically insoluble in light petroleum.

Cethexonium bromide is a quaternary ammonium disinfectant applied topically as a powder, ointment, or mouth-wash; it is also used in nasal drops and eye-drops.

Proprietary Names

Biocidan *(Clin-Comar-Byla, Fr.)*.

2216-d

Cetrimide *(B.P., Eur. P.)*.
Cetrimidum.

Cetrimide consists chiefly of tetradecyltrimethylammonium bromide (= tetradonium bromide) together with smaller amounts of dodecyl- and hexadecyltrimethylammonium bromides. It contains not less than 96% of alkyltrimethylammonium bromides calculated as. $C_{17}H_{38}BrN = 336.4$.

CAS — 8044-71-1.

NOTE. The name cetrimonium bromide was often formerly applied to cetrimide. Cetrimonium bromide (CTAB; cetyltrimethylammonium bromide) is hexadecyltrimethylammonium bromide.

Pharmacopoeias. In *Belg., Br., Braz., Eur., Fr., Ger., Ind., Int., It., Jug., Neth., Swiss,* and *Turk.*

A white to creamy-white, voluminous, free-flowing, hygroscopic powder with a faint characteristic odour and a bitter soapy taste. A solution in water has a low surface tension and foams on shaking. A 2% solution is clear or not more than very slightly opalescent.

Soluble 1 in 2 of water; freely soluble in alcohol. A 1% solution in water has a pH of 5 to 7.5. **Incompatible** with soaps and other anionic surfactants, bentonite, iodine, phenylmercuric nitrate, and alkali hydroxides. Solutions are **sterilised** by autoclaving or by filtration.

Cetrimide is stable in solution. The *B.P.C. 1973* states that solutions containing up to 40% of cetrimide may be stored and subsequently diluted, but in order to guard against contamination with *Pseudomonas* spp., stock solutions should contain at least 7% v/v of alcohol or 4% v/v of isopropyl alcohol. Cork closures should not be used.

Cetrimide is reported to be irritant to nasal mucosa.

For precautions to be taken in preparing and storing antiseptic solutions, see under Phenol, p.570.

Isolates from 63 hospital patients revealed *Pseudomonas maltophilia*, the source being deionised water used for making Savlon solutions. Following a new policy where distilled water and sterilised bottles and caps were used and the solutions replaced weekly no organisms were found in clinical specimens or disinfectant solutions.— M. M. Wishart and T. V. Riley, *Med. J. Aust.*, 1976, *2*, 710.

Compatibility. Quaternary ammonium compounds were inactivated by anionic agents through precipitation or incorporation in micelles, but were compatible with true ampholytic compounds even when the latter were acting as anionic agents. Bactericidal blends of quaternary and anionic surfactants could be formulated using sodium salts of alkylphenyl polyether omega sulphonates [Exonic OP2].— C. D. Moore and D. J. Tennant, *Mfg Chem.*, 1966, *37* (Oct.), 56.

Adverse Effects. When taken by mouth, cetrimide and other quaternary ammonium compounds cause nausea and vomiting; strong solutions may cause oesophageal damage and necrosis. They have depolarising muscle relaxant properties and toxic symptoms include dyspnoea and cyanosis due to paralysis of the respiratory muscles, possibly leading to asphyxia. Depression of the central nervous system (possibly preceded by excitement and with convulsions), hypotension, and coma may also occur. Intra-uterine or intravenous administration may cause haemolysis.

At the concentrations used on the skin, solutions of cetrimide and other quaternary compounds do not generally cause irritation, but some patients become hypersensitive to cetrimide after repeated applications. There have been rare reports of burns with concentrated solutions of cetrimide.

The fatal dose of quaternary ammonium detergents such as benzethonium chloride, benzalkonium chloride, methylbenzethonium chloride, and cetylpyridinium chloride was estimated to be 1 to 3 g. These compounds did not appear to inhibit cholinesterase activity.— J. M. Arena, *J. Am. med. Ass.*, 1964, *190*, 56. See also *Bull. Nat. Clearinghouse Poison Control Centers*, 1975, Jan.–Feb.

Toxic effects from a cetrimide enema.— C. Abrassart, *Rev. méd. Liège*, 1964, *19*, 484.

Cutaneous necrosis of the leg and foot occurred in a 77-year-old woman after the application, under occlusive dressings, of undiluted cetrimide powder to eczema for about 18 days.— P. J. August, *Br. med. J.*, 1975, *1*, 70.

A report of poisoning due to ingesting 30 ml of a solution containing cetrimide 150 mg together with chlorhexidine 15 mg and alcohol. Treatment included the immediate administration of milk and gastric lavage given 1 to 2 hours later; egg white 480 ml was then given. No toxic effects on blood pressure, pulse or respiration were reported.— B. Finlayson and C. Repchinsky, *Can. J. Hosp. Pharm.*, 1978, *31*, 64.

Chemical peritonitis associated with cetrimide washout after hydatid cyst surgery.— D. S. Gilchrist (letter), *Lancet*, 1979, *2*, 1374.

Following liberal irrigation of multiple large hydatid cysts of the liver with cetrimide, a 45-year-old woman developed methaemoglobinaemia with deep cyanosis. This was reversed by intravenous methylene blue 1 mg per kg body-weight. Whenever large amounts of cetrimide are used clinicians should be prepared to reverse the methaemoglobinaemia that may ensue.— A. Baraka *et al.* (letter), *Lancet*, 1980, *2*, 88.

A large burn occurred in a child following the spilling of a shampoo containing cetrimide 12%, on his chest.— J. K. Inman, *Br. med. J.*, 1982, *284*, 385.

Hypersensitivity. Skin sensitivity to cetrimide, confirmed by patch tests, was seen in 46 patients during the period 1957–66.— J. K. Morgan, *Br. J. clin. Pract.*, 1968, *22*, 261.

Treatment of Adverse Effects. Give milk, gelatin solution, or egg white; the use of a mild soap solution has been suggested; avoid alcohol. Assist the respiration and treat shock. Control convulsions by the intravenous injection of diazepam. Emesis and lavage should be avoided if it is believed that a concentrated solution has been ingested.

Precautions. Prolonged and repeated applications of cetrimide to the skin are inadvisable as hypersensitivity may occur.

Quaternary ammonium disinfectants could interfere to produce a blue colour with the Albustix and Labstix qualitative urine tests for protein.— *Drug & Ther. Bull.*, 1972, *10*, 69.

Uses. Cetrimide is a quaternary ammonium disinfectant with properties and uses typical of cationic surfactants. These surfactants dissociate in aqueous solution into a relatively large and complex cation, which is responsible for the surface activity, and a smaller inactive anion. In addition to the emulsifying and detergent properties usually associated with surfactants, the cationic compounds have bactericidal activity against both Gram-positive and Gram-negative organisms but higher concentrations are necessary to kill the latter type; they are, however, relatively ineffective against bacterial spores, acid-fast bacteria, viruses, and fungi.

Cationic surfactants are most effective in neutral or slightly alkaline solution and their bactericidal activity is appreciably reduced in acid media. They are compatible with each other but soaps and other anionic surfactants decrease the activity of cationic surfactants. To effect maximum bactericidal activity it is essential to ensure that any surface to which these agents are applied is freed from soap. Cationic surfactants are also incompatible with the acid dyes.

Quaternary ammonium compounds are bactericidal to Gram-positive organisms but they are relatively ineffective against some Gram-negative organisms; strains of *Pseudomonas aeruginosa* are particularly resistant as are those of *Mycobacterium tuberculosis*. Bacterial spores are likely to survive even prolonged contact with solutions of these compounds. Some cationic surfactants have good activity against *Candida albicans*, but antifungal activity is variable. They combine readily with proteins and the activity of quaternary ammonium compounds is greatly reduced in the presence of blood, cotton, cellulose, and other organic matter.

Quaternary ammonium compounds, particularly cetrimide and benzalkonium chloride, have been employed as aqueous solutions or creams for the pre-operative cleansing of the skin and for cleansing wounds. Aqueous solutions have been used for cleansing contaminated utensils and as preservatives. Quaternary ammonium compounds are not reliable agents for sterilising surgical instruments and heat-labile articles. The sterility of already sterilised surgical instruments, syringes, and similar articles, has been preserved by storing them, completely immersed, in aqueous solutions of these compounds; to retard rusting, 0.4% of sodium nitrite should be added. Before use, the instruments must be thoroughly washed in sterile water or sterile saline solution to remove all traces of the compound.

To suppress the development of ammonia-producing organisms and so prevent napkin rash, babies' napkins may be soaked in a weak solution of a quaternary ammonium compound and allowed to dry without rinsing so that they become impregnated with the compound. Before soaking in the solution, the washed napkins should be freed from soap to avoid soap inhibition of the disinfectant.

For application to the skin, solutions containing 0.1 to 1% of cetrimide have been used. A 0.5% solution in alcohol (70%) was formerly used for pre-operative skin preparation. Solutions containing 1 to 3% of cetrimide are used as shampoos to remove the scales in seborrhoea; care should be taken to prevent the solution from entering the eyes.

A 0.5 to 1% solution may be used for cleansing polyethylene tubing, catheters, and other plastic articles, but the time of immersion should not exceed one hour.

Cetrimide is used in the preparation of Cetrimide Emulsifying Wax, which can be used as an emulsifying agent for producing oil-in-water creams suitable for the incorporation of cationic and nonionic medicaments. For anionic medicaments, Emulsifying Wax and Cetomacrogol Emulsifying Wax are more suitable emulsifying agents.

A review of antimicrobial agents, including cetrimide, used in cosmetics.— I. R. Gucklhorn, *Mfg Chem.*, 1970, *41* (Aug.), 28.

A discussion on the use and misuse of aqueous quaternary ammonium disinfectants.— R. E. Dixon *et al.*, *J. Am. med. Ass.*, 1976, *236*, 2415. For a report re-emphasising the danger of using quaternary ammonium compounds as disinfectants rather than cleansers, and subsequent correspondence, see p.549.

The use of cetrimide as a scolicide in hydatid cyst surgery.— H. Ahrari, *Bull. Soc. Path. exot.*, 1978, *71*, 90, per *Trop. Dis. Bull.*, 1979, *76*, 94.

Antimicrobial activity. Individual components of commercial cetrimide mixture with chains of 12 or 14 carbon atoms had maximum antibacterial activity. The cetyl and stearyl quaternary compounds were less active on their own and formed more stable but virtually inactive emulsions with lauryl to stearyl alcohols. Myristyl alcohol unexpectedly inactivated all the quaternary compounds.— T. L. Welsh *et al.*, *J. pharm. Sci.*, 1967, *56*, 1464.

Effects of surfactants on bactericidal activity. The effect of non-ionic surfactants on the bactericidal activity of cationic surfactants was related to micelle formation and could be minimised by using a ratio of 4:1 or less of a nonionic to cationic and by using a nonionic surfactant with higher critical micelle concentration (CMC) values. The type of nonionic surfactant used was important; poloxamers were less likely than other nonionic surfactants to inactivate cationics because of their micellar characteristics. Other factors such as the addition of urea, or the addition of solvents such as alcohol and glycols which altered CMC values, should be considered, pH could also affect germicidal activity.— I. R. Schmolka, *J. Soc. cosmet. Chem.*, 1973, *24*, 577.

Urinary-tract infections. Application of a cream containing cetrimide 0.5% to the peri-urethral area prior to sexual intercourse might be an effective measure in controlling recurrent urinary-tract infections.— R. R. Bailey, *Drugs*, 1974, *8*, 54.

Preparations

Creams

Cetrimide Cream *(B.P.)*. Contains cetrimide in a suitable basis. It may be prepared to the following formula: cetrimide 500 mg (or a suitable quantity), cetostearyl alcohol 5 g, liquid paraffin 50 g, freshly boiled and cooled water to 100 g. Store at a temperature not exceeding 25° in well-closed containers which minimise evaporation and contamination.

B.P.C. 1973 includes a 0.5% cream to the above formula. *A.P.F.* (Cetrimide Cream Aqueous) has a similar preparation with chlorocresol 0.1%.

Ointments

Cetrimide Emulsifying Ointment *(B.P.)*. Cationic Emulsifying Ointment. Cetrimide 3 g, cetostearyl alcohol 27 g, liquid paraffin 20 g, and white soft paraffin 50 g. Store at a temperature not exceeding 25°.

Paints

Cetrimide and Chlorhexidine Paint *(A.P.F.)*. Cetrimide 500 mg, chlorhexidine gluconate solution 2.5 ml, alcohol 90% 75 ml, freshly boiled and cooled water to 100 ml.

Solutions

Cetrimide Solution *(B.P.C. 1973)*. Strong cetrimide solution 2.5 ml, freshly boiled and cooled water to 100 ml. It contains 1% of cetrimide. It must be freshly prepared, unless it is issued sterile in sealed containers. The solution may be sterilised by autoclaving or by filtration. Unsterilised solution should not be used more than 7 days after issue for use; sterile cetrimide solution should not be used more than 7 days after first opening the container. Avoid contact with cork.

Strong Cetrimide Solution *(B.P.C. 1973)*. A 40% aqueous solution of cetrimide, containing 7.5% v/v of alcohol or industrial methylated spirit and 0.0075% of tartrazine. It may be perfumed. Avoid contact with cork.

Waxes

Cetrimide Emulsifying Wax *(B.P.C. 1973)*. Cationic Emulsifying Wax. Cetrimide 10 g and cetostearyl alcohol 90 g.

Proprietary Preparations

Ceanel Concentrate *(Quinoderm, UK)*. Contains cetrimide 10%, undecenoic acid 1%, phenethyl alcohol 7.5%, in an emollient basis. For cleansing and descaling in seborrhoea capitis, seborrhoeic dermatitis, and psoriasis of the scalp and body.

References: P. J. Ashurst, *Practitioner*, 1967, *198*, 535.

Cetavlex *(ICI Pharmaceuticals, UK)*. Cetrimide, available as cream containing 0.5%. (Also available as Cetavlex in *Austral.*).

Cetavlon *(ICI Pharmaceuticals, UK)*. Cetrimide, available as a solution containing 40%. **Cetavlon PC**. A shampoo solution containing cetrimide 17.5%. For seborrhoea capitis and seborrhoeic dermatitis. (Also available as Cetavlon in *Austral., Denm., Fr., S.Afr., Spain*).

Cetrimide Strong Solution *(ABM Chemicals, UK)*. Cetrimide, available as a 40% aqueous solution.

Crodex C *(Croda, UK)*. A brand of Cetrimide Emulsifying Wax.

Dri-Wash Medical Cleansing Towelette *(Linton, UK)*. Towelettes impregnated with cetrimide 0.5% and chlorhexidine acetate 0.05%. For cleansing the skin prior to blood sampling.

Morpan CHSA *(ABM Chemicals, UK)*. A brand of cetrimide.

Savlodil *(ICI Pharmaceuticals, UK)*. A sterile solution containing cetrimide 0.15% and chlorhexidine gluconate 0.015%. For disinfecting and cleansing skin.

Savlon Hospital Concentrate *(ICI Pharmaceuticals, UK)*. A concentrated antiseptic solution for general purposes, containing cetrimide 15% and chlorhexidine gluconate 1.5%.

Savloclens *(ICI Pharmaceuticals, UK)*. Sachets containing a sterile solution of cetrimide 0.5% and chlorhexidine gluconate 0.05%. For cleansing and disinfecting wounds and burns.

Silquat C100 *(Tenneco, UK)*. A brand of cetrimide.

Travasept 100 *(Travenol, UK)*. A sterile solution containing cetrimide 0.15% and chlorhexidine acetate 0.015%. For cleansing and disinfection of wounds and burns.

Vesagex *(Pharmaceutical Mfg, UK)*. A non-greasy ointment containing cetrimide 1%.

Other Proprietary Names

Arg.—Cetridal, Dermanatal, Solufen; *Austral.*—Savlon D.

Cetrimide was also formerly marketed in Great Britain under the proprietary name Cycloton V (*Witco*). Preparations containing cetrimide were also formerly marketed in Great Britain under the proprietary names Gomaxine Antiseptic Cream (*Riddell* now *Seaford*), Seboderm (*Napp*). Cetrimide Emulsifying Wax was formerly marketed in Great Britain under the proprietary name Cycloton A (*Witco*).

Proprietary Preparations of Some Other Cationic Surfactants

Ambiteric D40 *(ABM Chemicals, UK)*. An aqueous solution (containing about 40%) of an alkyl dimethyl betaine.

The betaines were not true ampholytic agents but behaved as internal salts. Their surface activity was unaffected except by very low pH.— C. D. Moore and A. D. Tennant, *Mfg Chem.*, 1966, *37* (Oct.), 56.

Arquads *(Akzo, UK)*. A range of cationic surfactants derived from quaternary ammonium salts and fatty acids.

Contane *(Diversey, UK)*. A concentrated liquid detergent disinfectant containing a quaternary ammonium compound and nonionic surfactants.

Deogen 3X *(Diversey, UK)*. A concentrated liquid detergent disinfectant containing quaternary ammonium compounds and nonionic detergents. It is stated to be active against staphylococci and Gram-negative bacteria when used in a dilution of 1 in 480 of water.

Dettox ABC *(Reckitt & Colman Pharmaceuticals, UK)*. An antibacterial and cleansing solution containing quaternary ammonium compounds, nonionic surfactants, and a chelating agent, and buffered to pH 8.05. For disinfection of fibre optic instruments, it is diluted 1 in 25; for other purposes, 1 in 50.

Dor *(Simpla, UK)*. A liquid containing a quaternary ammonium compound, alcohol, and perfume. A deodorant for use with ostomies.

Emcol *(Witco, UK)*. A range of cationic surfactants including Emcol CC-9, Emcol CC-36, and Emcol CC-42, diethylmethylpolyoxypropyleneammonium chlorides, Emcol E-607, lapyrium chloride ($C_{21}H_{35}ClN_2O_3$ = 399.0), and Emcol E-607S, an alkoylcolaminoformylmethyl-substituted quaternary ammonium compound.

NOTE. The name Emcol is also applied to a range of anionic surfactants, see under Docusate Sodium, p.1441.

Ethoquads *(Akzo, UK)*. A range of cationic surfactants derived from quaternary ammonium salts and polyoxyethylene fatty acid amines.

Gloquat C *(ABM Chemicals, UK)*. An aqueous solution containing alkylaryltrimethylammonium chloride 50% and isopropyl alcohol 3%. For use as a bactericide. **Gloquat SDE**. Contains 40% of Gloquat C and 40% of a nonionic surfactant.

Use of disinfectants on farms. In Great Britain, Gloquat SD Extra is an approved disinfectant for fowl pest under The Diseases of Animals (Approved Disinfectants) Order 1978 (SI 1978: No. 32), as amended (SI 1978: No. 934).

Hyamine 2389 *(Rohm & Haas, UK)*. An aqueous solution of quaternary ammonium compounds stated to contain methyldodecylbenzyltrimethylammonium chloride 40% and methyldodecylxylylenebistrimethylammonium chloride 10%. For use in formulating disinfectant solutions.

Rewoquat B 41 *(Rewo, UK)*. A liquid containing 50% of an alkyltriethanolammonium chloride complex.

Morpan CHA *(ABM Chemicals, UK)*. A bactericidal powder containing hexadecyltrimethylammonium bromide not less than 95%.

Resistone QD *(ABM Chemicals, UK)*. An aqueous solution containing alkylaryltrialkylammonium chloride 50%.

Tricidal *(Wingfield, UK)*. A concentrated liquid disinfectant containing tetradecyltrimethylammonium bromide and other surfactants. For use in formulating disinfectant solutions.

Vantropol FHC *(ICI Organics, UK)*. A concentrated liquid detergent disinfectant based on cationic surfactants and a nonionic detergent. For general cleaning and disinfection it is used as a 0.3% solution.

2217-n

Cetylpyridinium Chloride *(B.P., U.S.P.)*.

Cetylpyridinii Chloridum. 1-Hexadecylpyridinium chloride monohydrate.

$C_{21}H_{38}ClN, H_2O$=358.0.

CAS — 7773-52-6 (cetylpyridinium); 123-03-5 (chloride, anhydrous); 6004-24-6 (chloride, monohydrate).

Pharmacopoeias. In *Br., Fr., Hung., Int., Nord.,* and *U.S.*

A white powder with a slight characteristic odour and a bitter taste. The *B.P.* specifies not less than 98% of the monohydrate. The *U.S.P.* specifies not less than 99% calculated on the anhydrous basis. M.p. 79° to 84°.

Soluble 1 in 20 of water; very soluble in alcohol and chloroform; slightly soluble in ether. A 1% solution in water has a pH of 5 to 5.4 and foams strongly when shaken. **Incompatible** with soaps and other anionic surfactants. **Store** in airtight containers.

For precautions to be taken in preparing and storing antiseptic solutions, see under Phenol, p.570.

Adverse Effects and Treatment. As for Cetrimide, p.552.

Uses. Cetylpyridinium chloride is a cationic disinfectant with properties and uses similar to those of other cationic surfactants as described under Cetrimide, p.552.

A 0.1% to 1% aqueous solution is applied to intact skin, a 0.1% solution is used for minor wounds. For mucous membranes or large areas of exposed tissue a 0.01 to 0.05% solution is employed.

Lozenges and mouth-washes containing cetylpyridinium chloride are used for the treatment of superficial infections of the mouth and throat.

In a double-blind crossover study in 100 subjects, use of a mouth-wash containing cetylpyridinium chloride 0.05% after meals reduced plaque accumulation in all subjects.— J. D. Holbeche *et al.*, *Aust. dent. J.*, 1975, *20*, 397. See also J. Llewelyn, *Br. dent. J.*, 1980, *148*, 103.

Gargling with a cetylpyridinium chloride solution reduced the bacterial count in children with tonsillitis and pharyngitis.— C. A. L. Vermooten, *Curr. ther. Res.*, 1977, *21*, 893.

A study of the use of a solution of cetylpyridinium bromide 1% for decontamination of sputum samples from patients with tuberculosis.— Z. Mokhtari, *Bull. int. Un. Tuberc.*, 1980, *55*, 51.

Preparations

Cetylpyridinium Chloride Lozenges *(U.S.P.)*. Lozenges containing cetylpyridinium chloride.

Cetylpyridinium Chloride Topical Solution *(U.S.P.)*. Cetylpyridinium Chloride Solution. A solution containing cetylpyridinium chloride. Store in airtight containers.

Proprietary Preparations

Merocet *(Merrell, UK)*. A solution containing cetylpyridinium chloride 0.05% and alcohol 14%. To be used full strength or with an equal volume of water as a gargle or mouth-wash.

Merocets *(Merrell, UK)*. Lozenges each containing cetylpyridinium chloride 0.066%. *Dose.* 1 lozenge to be dissolved slowly in the mouth as required.

Other Proprietary Names

Cepacol *(Austral., USA)*; Dobendan *(Ger.)*; Hiozon *(Denm.)*; Nedermin *(cetylpyridinium bromide) (Spain)*; Pyrisept *(Norw.)*; Zepacole *(Spain)*.

2218-h

Chloramine *(B.P., Eur. P.)*.

Chloraminum; Chloramidum; Chloramine T; Mianin; Natrium Sulfaminochloratum; Tosylchloramidum Natricum; Cloramina. Sodium *N*-chlorotoluene-*p*-sulphonimidate trihydrate.

$C_7H_7ClNNa\ O_2S, 3H_2O$=281.7.

CAS — 127-65-1 (anhydrous).

NOTE. The name Chloramin is applied to a preparation of chlorpheniramine maleate.

Pharmacopoeias. In *Aust., Belg., Br., Cz., Eur., Fr., Ger., Hung., It., Jug., Mex., Neth., Nord., Port., Span.,* and *Swiss.*

White or slightly yellow crystalline powder with a faint odour of chlorine and an unpleasant bitter taste. It contains about 25% w/w of 'available chlorine' (see p.557). It effloresces in air, losing chlorine and becoming yellow in colour and less soluble in water.

Soluble 1 in 7 of water, 1 in 2 of boiling water, and 1 in 7 of glycerol; soluble 1 in 12 of alcohol with slow decomposition; practically insoluble in chloroform, ether, and liquid paraffin. A 5% solution in water has a pH of 8 to 10. A 4.1% solution is iso-osmotic with serum. **Incompatible**

with alcohol, hydrogen peroxide, and many other substances. The stability of solutions may be improved by buffering at pH 9. **Store** in a cool place in airtight containers. Protect from light.

Adverse Effects. Vomiting, cyanosis, circulatory collapse, frothing at the mouth, and respiratory failure can occur within a few minutes of chloramine ingestion. Fatalities have occurred.

Chloramine in tap water has caused haemolysis in patients undergoing dialysis.

A report of allergic asthma in 7 workers occupationally exposed to chloramine. All showed a positive response to a prick test, and symptoms did not recur when exposure to chloramine ceased.— M. S. Bourne *et al.*, *Br. med. J.*, 1979, *2*, 10. Bronchospasm due to exposure to chloramine in a 43-year-old man was delayed for several hours after exposure.— T. J. Charles (letter), *Br. med. J.*, 1979, *2*, 334.

Haemodialysis. Chloramine, if added to public water supplies, was a hazard to patients undergoing dialysis. It readily passed through dialysis membranes and oxidised haemoglobin to methaemoglobin while inhibiting the hexose-monophosphate shunt to enhance the oxidative changes. Red-cell survival could be reduced, haemolytic intravascular disease occur, and the patient become highly sensitive to drugs such as sulphonamides which induced methaemoglobinaemia. Chloramine could be removed from tap water by filtration through activated charcoal, boiling, or vacuum extraction. Treatment with ascorbic acid could reverse the haemolytic process.— C. M. Kjellstrand *et al.*, *Nephron*, 1974, *13*, 427.

Chloramines were present in tap water used in 2 dialysis centres. Heinz bodies were present in the red blood cells from 10 of 12 patients. *In vitro* methaemoglobin rose from a mean of 2.31% in cells incubated with purified water to a mean of 5.27% in cells incubated in tap water. Four months after the routine use of ascorbic acid 2 g in each 120 litres of dialysate, Heinz bodies were present in only 2 patients.— J. Botella *et al.*, *Proc. Eur. Dialysis Transplant Ass.*, 1977, *14*, 192.

A severe Heinz-body haemolytic anaemia which developed in approximately half of 20 patients undergoing haemodialysis coincided with the reintroduction of chloramine as a disinfectant to the Brisbane tap water. After the introduction of a carbon filter to the system the mean haemoglobin concentrations rose to pre-chloramine values.— D. J. Birrell *et al.*, *Med. J. Aust.*, 1978, *2*, 288.

Further references: Y. Yawata *et al.*, *Ann. intern. Med.*, 1973, *79*, 362; J. W. Eaton *et al.*, *Science*, 1973, *181*, 463.

Treatment of Adverse Effects. Empty the stomach by aspiration or lavage. Assist respiration if necessary. Sodium nitrite and sodium thiosulphate can be given as directed for cyanide poisoning (see p.790).

Uses. Chloramine is an organic derivative of chlorine with the bactericidal actions and uses of chlorine (see p.557).

It is stable at an alkaline pH but is much more active in acid media. It releases hypochlorous acid more slowly and is less active than hypochlorite solutions.

Chloramine has been employed as a wound disinfectant and general surgical antiseptic. It is non-irritant. A 2% solution may be used for the irrigation of wounds. More dilute solutions have been used as a mouth-wash and for application to mucous membranes. The solutions should be freshly prepared.

For the treatment of drinking water containing little organic matter, 5 mg of chloramine may be added to each litre—see Chlorine Treatment of Water, p.557.

Chloramine has been used as a spermicide.

Adenovirus type 8 virus on applanation tonometers or gonioscopes was inactivated by immersion for 15 minutes in 0.6% chloramine solution. The use of a 5% solution for 10 minutes was suggested.— D. L. Barnard *et al.*, *Br. med. J.*, 1973, *2*, 165.

Preparations

Vaselinum Chloramini *(Dan. Disp.)*. Chloramine 1% in yellow soft paraffin.

Proprietary Names

Clonazone *(Daufresne, Switz.)*; Clorina Heyden *(Químicos, Spain)*; Dercusan *(Spain)*; Gineclorina *(Químicos, Spain)*; Hydroclonazone *(Grimault, Fr.; Promedica, Switz.)*; Klortee *(Protea, Austral.)*.

Preparations containing chloramine were formerly marketed in Great Britain under the proprietary names Gynomin (*Napp*), Rendell Foam (*Rendell*), Santronex (*Rendell*).

2219-m

Chloramine B. Chlorogenium. Sodium *N*-chlorobenzenesulphonimidate sesquihydrate.
$C_6H_5ClNNaO_2S,1\frac{1}{2}H_2O=240.6$.

CAS — 127-52-6 (anhydrous).

Pharmacopoeias. In *Hung.* and *Roum.*

White or yellowish-white crystals or crystalline powder with a faint odour of chlorine and an unpleasant bitter taste. It contains about 29% w/w of 'available chlorine' (see p.557).

Soluble in water and alcohol; practically insoluble in chloroform and ether. Solutions in water are alkaline to litmus and to phenolphthalein. **Store** in a cool place in airtight containers. Protect from light.

Chloramine B is used for the same purposes as chloramine.

2220-t

Chlorhexidine Acetate *(B.P.)*.

Chlorhexidine Diacetate. 1,1′-Hexamethylenebis[5-(4-chlorophenyl)biguanide] diacetate.
$C_{22}H_{30}Cl_2N_{10},2C_2H_4O_2=625.6$.

CAS — 55-56-1 (chlorhexidine); 56-95-1 (acetate).

Pharmacopoeias. In *Br.* and *Chin.*

A white to pale cream, odourless or almost odourless microcrystalline powder with a bitter taste. **Soluble** 1 in 55 of water and 1 in 15 of alcohol; very slightly soluble in glycerol and propylene glycol.

Solutions are **sterilised** by autoclaving at 115° for 30 minutes; solutions should not be alkaline.

It is stable at ordinary temperatures but when heated it decomposes with the production of trace amounts of 4-chloroaniline. Aqueous solutions slowly decompose with the formation of trace amounts of 4-chloroaniline. **Store** in a cool place in airtight containers. Protect from light.

For precautions to be taken in preparing and storing antiseptic solutions, see under Phenol, p.570.

As a precaution against contamination with *Pseudomonas* spp., stock solutions should contain at least 7% v/v of alcohol or 4% v/v of isopropyl alcohol.

2221-x

Chlorhexidine Gluconate Solution *(B.P.)*.

Chlorhex. Glucon. Soln. An aqueous solution containing 19 to 21% of chlorhexidine gluconate. 1,1′-Hexamethylenebis[5-(4-chlorophenyl)biguanide] digluconate.
$C_{22}H_{30}Cl_2N_{10},2C_6H_{12}O_7=897.8$.

CAS — 18472-51-0 (chlorhexidine gluconate).

Pharmacopoeias. In *Br.*

It is an almost colourless to pale straw-coloured, clear or slightly opalescent, odourless or almost odourless liquid with a bitter taste. Wt per ml 1.06 to 1.07 g.

Miscible with water, with up to 5 parts of alcohol, and with up to 3 parts of acetone. A 5% v/v dilution in water has a pH of 5.5 to 7. **Sterilise** by autoclaving at 115° for 30 minutes or by filtration. The solutions should not be alkaline.

Store at a temperature not exceeding 25° in airtight containers. Protect from light.

For precautions to be taken in preparing and storing antiseptic solutions, see under Phenol, p.570.

As a precaution against contamination with *Pseudomonas* spp., stock solutions should contain at least 7% v/v of alcohol or 4% v/v of isopropyl alcohol.

NOTE. Commercial 5% concentrate contains a nonionic surfactant to prevent precipitation on dilution with hard water and is not suitable for use on mucous membranes; dilutions of the 20% concentrate should be used for this purpose.

2222-r

Chlorhexidine Hydrochloride *(B.P.)*.

Chlorhexidine Dihydrochloride; AY 5312. 1,1′-Hexamethylenebis[5-(4-chlorophenyl)biguanide] dihydrochloride.
$C_{22}H_{30}Cl_2N_{10},2HCl=578.4$.

CAS — 3697-42-5.

Pharmacopoeias. In *Br.* and *Jap.*

A white or almost white, odourless, crystalline powder with a bitter taste. M.p. 255° with decomposition.

Soluble 1 in 1700 of water, 1 in 450 of alcohol, and 1 in 50 of propylene glycol; slightly soluble in methyl alcohol; practically insoluble in glacial acetic acid. **Sterilise** by maintaining at 150° for 1 hour.

It is stable at ordinary temperatures but when heated it decomposes with the formation of trace amounts of 4-chloroaniline. It is less readily decomposed than chlorhexidine acetate and may be heated at 150° for 1 hour without appreciable production of 4-chloroaniline. It absorbs insignificant amounts of moisture at temperatures up to 37° and relative humidities up to about 80%. **Store** in a cool place in airtight containers. Protect from light.

For precautions to be taken in preparing and storing antiseptic solutions, see under Phenol, p.570.

As a precaution against contamination with *Pseudomonas* spp., stock solutions should contain at least 7% v/v of alcohol or 4% v/v of isopropyl alcohol.

Chlorhexidine Incompatibilities. Chlorhexidine is incompatible with soaps and other anionic materials. Chlorhexidine acetate is incompatible with potassium iodide. At a concentration of 0.05%, chlorhexidine is incompatible with borates, bicarbonates, carbonates, chlorides, citrates, phosphates, and sulphates, forming salts of low solubility which may precipitate from solution only after standing for 24 hours. At dilutions of 0.01% or more, these salts are generally soluble.

Cork closures and cork liners should not be used for containers of chlorhexidine solutions as chlorhexidine is inactivated by cork.

Fabrics which have been in contact with chlorhexidine solution may develop a brown stain if bleached with a hypochlorite. A perborate bleach may be used instead.

The losses by adsorption of chlorhexidine acetate from 30 ml of a 0.01% aqueous solution filtered through sintered glass, unglazed porcelain candle, asbestos pad, or membrane filter were 21, 47 to 68, 97 and 2% respectively. In 0.2 M acetate buffer the respective losses were 1, 40 to 77, 47, and 5%.— N. T. Naido *et al.*, *Aust. J. pharm. Sci.*, 1972, *1*, 16.

Contact lens solutions. Chlorhexidine was sorbed on to polyhydroxymethylmethacrylate contact lenses; desorption occurred in sodium chloride solution.— N. E. Richardson *et al.*, *J. Pharm. Pharmac.*, 1978, *30*, 469.

Sorption of chlorhexidine by hard contact lenses.— D. L. MacKeen and K. Green, *J. Pharm. Pharmac.*, 1979, *31*, 714.

Concentrations of chlorhexidine gluconate in a soft contact lens solution were reduced to a greater extent when stored in the dark for 6 months in amber or clear glass bottles than when similarly stored in polypropylene or polyethylene containers. Although concentrations of thiomersal in the solution were similarly affected when the solution was stored in the plastic containers they were unchanged when stored in the glass containers.— C. M. McTaggart *et al.*, *J. Pharm. Pharmac.*, 1979, *31*,

Suppl., 60P.

Haemolysis. In common with some other preservatives, chlorhexidine caused trace haemolysis *in vitro* at a concentration of 20 µg per ml and total haemolysis at 110 µg per ml. The mode of action and effective concentration of chlorhexidine against micro-organisms and erythrocytes were similar. Haemolytic activity was reduced by the addition of higher molecular weight macrogols or dimethyl sulphoxide 15%.— H. C. Ansel, *J. pharm. Sci.*, 1967, *56*, 616.

Inactivation. Solutions of chlorhexidine gluconate could solubilise the less soluble diacetate. Chlorhexidine was partly inactivated by polysorbate 80.— D. D. Heard and R. W. Ashworth, *J. Pharm. Pharmac.*, 1968, *20*, 505.

After storage for 72 hours, a decrease of more than 90% in the concentration of chlorhexidine acetate 0.05% occurred in aqueous suspensions containing insoluble magnesium compounds or starch; smaller losses occurred in the presence of insoluble zinc and calcium compounds.— T. J. McCarthy, *J. mond. Pharm.*, 1969, *12*, 321.

Nonionic and quaternary surfactants used to prevent the precipitation of inorganic chlorhexidine salts on dilution of concentrates with hard water could reduce the availability of chlorhexidine. In a 0.1% chlorhexidine gluconate solution the loss of availability due to 0.1% of a macrogol ether was 30% while with 1% it was over 90%. A nonoxynol and polysorbate 80 also decreased the availability of chlorhexidine. Alcohol reduced the interaction of chlorhexidine with the surfactant and a 10% solution of alcohol increased the activity of chlorhexidine acetate in a 0.04% solution with 1% polysorbate 80 by 50%.— N. Senior, *J. Soc. cosmet. Chem.*, 1973, *24*, 259.

Binding of chlorhexidine to tragacanth reduced the antibacterial activity of chlorhexidine.— T. J. McCarthy and J. A. Myburgh, *Pharm. Weekbl. Ned.*, 1974, *109*, 265, per *Pharm. J.*, 1974, *2*, 16.

Stability. Production of 4-chloroaniline was in excess of the *B.P.* limit when 0.01% solutions of chlorhexidine acetate were autoclaved at 115° for 30 minutes but not when they were heated at 100° for 30 minutes.— D. A. Norton, *J. Hosp. Pharm.*, 1967, *24*, 328.

Since A.I. Scott and E. Eccleston (*Proc. Eur. Soc. Stud. Drug Toxicity*, 1966, *8*, 195) concluded from animal experiments that the daily absorption of 500 mg of 4-chloroaniline would allow a wide margin of safety against methaemoglobinaemia, the risk of toxicity from this source was very slight, as autoclaved 0.01% solutions of chlorhexidine acetate or gluconate would only contain 300 µg per litre of 4-chloroaniline.— R. R. Goodall *et al.*, *I.C.I.*, *Pharm. J.*, 1968, *1*, 33.

The degradation of chlorhexidine gluconate to 4-chloroaniline during autoclaving of 0.02% solutions increased with increase of pH and was negligible up to about pH 7. Even above this pH there was an insignificant effect on the bactericidal activity of chlorhexidine.— F. Jaminet *et al.*, *Pharm. Acta Helv.*, 1970, *45*, 60.

Temperatures greater than 110° greatly increased the decomposition of chlorhexidine acetate during autoclaving. Decomposition was least at pH 5 to 6. Chlorhexidine gluconate was more liable to decomposition than the acetate. Autoclaved solutions darkened on exposure to direct sunlight when stored in polypropylene or polyethylene bottles but not when stored in glass bottles.— J. Dolby *et al.*, *Pharm. Acta Helv.*, 1972, *47*, 615.

Adverse Effects and Treatment. Skin sensitivity to chlorhexidine has occasionally been reported. Strong solutions may cause irritation of the conjunctiva and other sensitive tissues. Ototoxicity has been reported. Inadvertent bladder irrigation with concentrated solutions may cause haematuria.

Chlorhexidine is poorly absorbed from the gastro-intestinal tract. Up to 2 g daily by mouth has been taken in metabolic experiments.

Toxic effects due to ingestion of chlorhexidine should be treated by gastric lavage.

Toothpastes or mouth-washes containing chlorhexidine softened the oral epithelium and could cause aphthous ulcers.— G. Y. Caldwell, *Practitioner*, 1970, *204*, 581.

The side-effects of chlorhexidine gluconate and chlorhexidine acetate mouth-washes (0.1 and 0.2%) were evaluated in 50 subjects over a period of 4 months. Lesions of the oral mucosa occurred in 11 persons, including 1 control, and were severe in 3. Discoloration occurred in 12% of front tooth surfaces within the first 4 weeks, and 62% of silicate cement fillings in these areas were discoloured. In 12 subjects the tongue became discoloured.— L. Flötra *et al.*, *Scand. J. dent. Res.*, 1971, *79*, 119.

Hydrophilic contact lenses stored overnight in soaking solutions containing chlorhexidine acetate 0.005% produced mild irritation in the eyes of *rabbits* fitted with the lenses. After 21 days' use corneal opacities had developed in 2 out of 3 *rabbits*.— M. Davies, *J. Pharm. Pharmac.*, 1973, *25*, *Suppl.*, 134P. A similar report.— D. L. MacKeen and K. Green, *J. Pharm. Pharmac.*, 1978, *30*, 678.

Precautions. Chlorhexidine should not be used on the brain, meninges, or perforated ear-drum. Syringes and needles that have been immersed in chlorhexidine solutions should be thoroughly rinsed with Water for Injections before use for spinal injection.

Chlorhexidine could interfere to produce a blue colour with the Albustix and Labstix qualitative urine tests for protein.— *Drug & Ther. Bull.*, 1972, *10*, 69.

Chlorhexidine was detected in low concentrations in the venous blood of 5 of 24 infants after bathing with a preparation containing chlorhexidine gluconate 4% (Hibiscrub). No adverse effects due to percutaneous absorption of chlorhexidine were reported.— J. Cowen *et al.*, *Archs Dis. Childh.*, 1979, *54*, 379. Low or undetectable concentrations after the use of powder containing chlorhexidine 1%.— V. G. Alder *et al.*, *Archs Dis. Childh.*, 1980, *55*, 277.

Chlorhexidine used as a skin disinfectant before blood sampling may interfere with microbiological assays of antibiotics and should not be used before such a procedure.— P. Larsson and M. Rylander (letter), *J. antimicrob. Chemother.*, 1980, *6*, 682.

Uses. Chlorhexidine is a disinfectant which is effective against a wide range of vegetative Gram-positive and Gram-negative bacteria; it is ineffective against acid-fast bacteria, bacterial spores, fungi, and viruses. It is more effective against Gram-positive than Gram-negative bacteria, some species of *Pseudomonas* and *Proteus* being relatively less susceptible. Chlorhexidine is most active at a neutral or slightly alkaline pH, but its activity is reduced by blood and other organic matter.

Chlorhexidine gluconate is used in disinfectant solutions, creams, and gels. A 0.5% solution in alcohol (70%) is used for the pre-operative disinfection of the skin, and a 0.05% aqueous solution is used as a wound disinfectant. A 0.05% solution in glycerol is used for urethral disinfection and catheter lubrication, and a 0.02% solution for bladder irrigation. A 1% cream is used in obstetrics. A 0.02% solution containing sodium nitrite 0.1% is used for the storage of sterile instruments.

Chlorhexidine acetate is used for skin disinfection and, in a concentration of 0.01%, as a preservative for eye-drops.

Chlorhexidine hydrochloride has been used in creams and dusting powders; a cream containing 0.1% of chlorhexidine hydrochloride and 0.5% of neomycin sulphate is used in the prophylaxis and treatment of nasal carriers of staphylococci.

For general disinfectant purposes a mixture of chlorhexidine gluconate and cetrimide is often used.

For a review of the action and uses of chlorhexidine, with formulas of disinfectant solutions, see J. Dolby *et al.*, *J. Hosp. Pharm.*, 1972, *30*, 223 and 244.

For an extensive review of the properties of chlorhexidine salts, their formulation, toxicity, and uses in medicine and cosmetics, see N. Senior, *J. Soc. cosmet. Chem.*, 1973, *24*, 259. See also D. G. Higgins, *Chemist Drugg.*, 1974, *201*, 518.

Chlorhexidine acetate, 250 mg per 500-ml bottle, was used for the preservation of urine specimens awaiting estimation of glucose.— G. E. Lovatt and B. Coates (letter), *Br. med. J.*, 1973, *4*, 296.

An 0.02% aqueous solution of chlorhexidine inhibited the growth of pathogens in the water of flower vases.— K. S. Johansen *et al.* (letter), *Lancet*, 1974, *1*, 359.

Acne. In an uncontrolled study of 48 patients with acne, the twice-daily application of chlorhexidine was associated with a clearance of the acne in 9 and improvement in 8. Forty of the patients were considered to have made some progress during treatment.— S. A. Khan (letter), *Br. med. J.*, 1975, *4*, 346.

Antimicrobial activity. A 1 in 5000 dilution of a 20% solution of chlorhexidine gluconate (0.004%) killed 100% of type 1 strains of *Neisseria gonorrhoeae* and 80 to 99% of type 4 strains. Chlorhexidine might be tried as a genital disinfectant for the prophylaxis of gonorrhoea.— S. A. Waitkins and I. Geary, *Br. J. vener. Dis.*, 1975, *51*, 267, per *Abstr. Hyg.*, 1975, *50*, 1238.

Diminished activity. The antibacterial activity of chlorhexidine acetate 0.005% against *Staphylococcus aureus* was reduced by between 70 and 100% by 1% of kaolin, magnesium trisilicate, aluminium magnesium silicate, or bentonite.— R. T. Yousef *et al.*, *Can. J. pharm. Sci.*, 1973, *8*, 54.

Enhanced activity. The antibacterial effect of chlorhexidine acetate 0.002% was enhanced by benzyl alcohol, phenylpropanol, and phenethyl alcohol, all 0.175%.— R. M. E. Richards and R. J. McBride, *J. pharm. Sci.*, 1973, *62*, 2035.

Aphthous ulcers. In a double-blind study in 12 patients with aphthous ulcers a mouth-wash containing 0.1% of chlorhexidine gluconate used thrice daily and retained in the mouth for 1 minute reduced the incidence, discomfort, and duration of the ulcers. An astringent mouth-wash containing zinc chloride and zinc sulphate was without effect.— M. Addy *et al.*, *Br. dent. J.*, 1974, *136*, 452.

In a double-blind crossover study of 20 patients chlorhexidine gluconate as a 1% gel reduced the duration and severity of aphthous ulcers but did not affect the incidence of ulceration. The gel appeared to be less effective than the mouth-wash.— M. Addy *et al.*, *Br. dent. J.*, 1976, *141*, 118.

Burns. The addition of chlorhexidine hydrochloride or gluconate 0.2% w/v to silver sulphadiazine cream used in the treatment of burns reduced the isolation-rate of *Staphylococcus aureus* in 51 patients to 9.2% compared with 34% in 91 patients treated with silver sulphadiazine alone. Gram-negative organisms were isolated in 11.1% compared with 18.6% and the number of uninfected patients rose from 52% to 81%.— A. M. Clarke *et al.* (letter), *Lancet*, 1971, *2*, 661. See also *idem*, *Med. J. Aust.*, 1975, *1*, 413; M. Pannier *et al.*, *Nouv. Presse méd.*, 1976, *5*, 207.

Dental use. A 66% reduction in plaque formation and a 24% reduction in gingival inflammation compared with controls was observed in 40 patients, aged 19 to 39 years, when they each used 10 ml of chlorhexidine acetate or gluconate 0.1 or 0.2% solution as a mouth-wash twice daily for 8 weeks. In the 2 months after the teeth were scaled and polished, the plaque reduction was 84% and the gingival index was reduced by 43%. There was no significant difference between the 0.2% and the 0.1% solution.— L. Flötra *et al.*, *Scand. J. dent. Res.*, 1972, *80*, 10.

Toothbrush application of 1% chlorhexidine gluconate gel reduced both plaque formation and gingival inflammation.— M. A. Bassiouny and A. A. Grant, *Br. dent. J.*, 1975, *139*, 323.

A mouth-wash of chlorhexidine gluconate 0.2% used in doses of 10 ml twice daily produced improvement in gingival inflammation in a controlled study of 55 patients. Improvement was increased when scaling had also been carried out. Mild side-effects included soreness of the tongue or mucosa and changes in taste.— T. C. A. O'Neil, *Br. dent. J.*, 1976, *141*, 276.

Chlorhexidine gel 1% brushed on to the teeth twice daily for a month caused a small reduction in dental plaque and gingivitis, and stained the teeth brown.— *Drug & Ther. Bull.*, 1976, *14*, 47.

In a double-blind study of 56 children with gingivitis, the use of a chlorhexidine gluconate gel (1%) as a toothpaste every night for 4 weeks was not more effective than placebo in improving the gingivitis. At the end of the 4-week period the gel produced a slightly greater reduction in plaque formation than placebo but 4 weeks later there was no difference. Tooth staining occurred in 75% of children given the gel, compared with 25% on placebo, and 4 weeks after stopping treatment 45% were still stained.— D. F. Hajos *et al.*, *Br. dent. J.*, 1977, *142*, 366.

Chlorhexidine as a 0.2% mouth-wash alleviated the pain of aphthous ulceration but was of little or no value in the treatment of chronic gingivitis and periodontitis.— *Drug & Ther. Bull.*, 1978, *16*, 23.

Use of a mouth-wash solution containing chlorhexidine 0.2% before operation was effective in reducing microbial contamination from debris produced by the use of ultrasonic scalers.— K. F. Muir *et al.*, *Br. dent. J.*, 1978, *145*, 76.

Mouth-washes containing chlorhexidine gluconate 0.2% were not particularly useful in eradicating *Klebsiella* spp. from the mouths of patients with denture stomatitis.— W. P. Holbrook and C. Russell (letter), *Br. dent. J.*, 1979, *146*, 3.

Disinfection of skin. Estimation, by 3 different techniques, of the bacterial population of abdominal skin before and after disinfection indicated that virtually all non-sporing bacteria could be eliminated by swabbing for 30 seconds with 0.5% chlorhexidine in 70% alcohol.— S. Selwyn and H. Ellis, *Br. med. J.*, 1972, *1*, 136.

A comparison was made of the value of chlorhexidine 4% (Hibiscrub), povidone-iodine (Disadine), and hexachlorophane emulsion 3% as surgical scrubs in 228, 222, and 416 operations respectively, assessment being made on the number of colonies grown from hands which had been gloved throughout the operation. Hibiscrub was marginally more effective than hexachlorophane emulsion and, because the surgical team expressed preference (on non-bacteriological grounds) for it, had replaced hexachlorophane emulsion for routine use. Disadine was much less effective than either of the other 2 preparations.— H. G. Smylie *et al.*, *Br. med. J.*, 1973, *4*, 586.

Viable bacterial counts on the hands were reduced by a mean of 97.9% by the application to the hands of 0.5% chlorhexidine gluconate in 95% alcohol rubbed in until dry, by 65.1% by the application for 2 minutes of 0.5% chlorhexidine gluconate in water, by 86.7% by the application for 2 minutes of a 4% chlorhexidine gluconate detergent solution, and by 91.8% by a 0.1% solution of tetrabromo-*o*-cresol in 95.3% alcohol, rubbed in till dry. After 6 successive applications in 2 days the respective reductions were 99.7%, 91.8%, 99.2%, and 99.5%.— E. J. L. Lowbury *et al.*, *Br. med. J.*, 1974, *4*, 369.

Klebsiella spp. were transmitted to nurses' hands on 17 of 47 occasions after nursing procedures involving patients infected with klebsiella in an intensive care ward. Washing the hands with chlorhexidine 4% skin cleanser reduced infection on the hand by 98% on 19 of 23 occasions and reduced infection completely on 14 of 23 occasions. The incidence of klebsiella infection in patients fell from 22 and 22.6% (for each of 2 years) to 15.5% when chlorhexidine hand washing became routine before passing from one patient to the next.— M. Casewell and I. Phillips, *Br. med. J.*, 1977, *2*, 1315.

In a study comparing the efficacy of bar soaps with that of established agents in hand disinfection in hospitals, alcoholic chlorhexidine 0.5% was found to be superior to povidone-iodine soap, povidone-iodine surgical scrub, povidone-iodine alcoholic solution 0.1% and chlorhexidine surgical scrub.— J. D. Jarvis *et al.*, *J. clin. Path.*, 1979, *32*, 732.

Powders containing chlorhexidine 1% or hexachlorophane 0.33% were equally effective in preventing colonisation and infection of the skin of newborn infants by *Staphylococcus aureus* but the skin became profusely colonised by coagulase-negative staphylococci, irrespective of the powder used.— V. G. Alder *et al.*, *Archs Dis. Childh.*, 1980, *55*, 277.

Prophylaxis during immunosuppression. A regimen suggested by the Royal Marsden Hospital leukaemia unit to give practical decontamination for patients with acute non-lymphoblastic leukaemia. Neomycin sulphate, colistin sulphate, nystatin, and amphotericin are given in association with application of chlorhexidine obstetric cream 1% to vagina and vulva twice daily; chlorhexidine mouth-washes (0.02% aqueous) are used only if necessary.— J. G. Watson and B. Jameson (letter), *Lancet*, 1979, *1*, 1183.

Trachoma. In a study of 49 patients with trachoma, eye-drops containing chlorhexidine 50 µg per ml were considered to be as effective as topical treatment with oxytetracycline hydrochloride and polymyxin B or co-trimoxazole given by mouth. Since chlorhexidine is unable to penetrate mammalian cells, any effect it exerted may have been due to inactivation of free elementary bodies of *Chlamydia trachomatis* in the eye.— I. T. Nisbet *et al.*, *Antimicrob. Ag. Chemother.*, 1979, *16*, 855.

Urethral syndrome. Symptoms of frequency and dysuria in women, without evidence of urinary-tract infection, generally responded to urethral dilatation and instillation of chlorhexidine. Some women who had not reached the menopause improved when treated with quinestradol.— R. M. Jameson (letter), *Lancet*, 1969, *1*, 256.

Preparations

Creams

Chlorhexidine Cream *(B.P.)*. Contains chlorhexidine gluconate solution in a suitable basis. It may be prepared to the following formula: chlorhexidine gluconate solution, a suitable quantity, liquid paraffin 10 g, cetomacrogol emulsifying wax 25 g, freshly boiled and cooled water to 100 g. Store at a temperature not exceeding 25° in well-closed containers which minimise evaporation and contamination. *A.P.F.* (Chlorhexidine Cream Aqueous) specifies 1%.

Dusting-powders

Chlorhexidine Dusting Powder *(B.P.)*. Chlorhexidine hydrochloride 0.5% in sterilisable maize starch. Sterilised in quantities of not more than 30 g in suitable containers by maintaining the whole powder for 1 hour at 150° to 155°.

Ear-drops

Chlorhexidine Ear Drops *(A.P.F.)*. Chlorhexidine acetate 50 mg, freshly boiled and cooled water to 100 ml.

Gels

Chlorhexidine Gel *(A.P.F.)*. Chlorhexidine gluconate solution 2.5 ml, tragacanth 2.5 g, glycerol 25 g, freshly boiled and cooled water to 100 g. Protect from light.

Irrigations

Chlorhexidine Irrigation *(A.P.F.)*. Chlorhexidine gluconate solution 0.1 ml, Water for Injections to 100 ml. Sterilised by autoclaving.

Mouth-washes

Chlorhexidine Mouth-wash *(D.P.F.)*. Chlorhexidine gluconate solution 1 ml, alcohol (95 per cent) 7 ml, freshly boiled and cooled water to 100 ml. It may contain suitable colouring and flavouring agents. To be used undiluted.

Solutions

Dilute Chlorhexidine Solution *(B.P.C. 1973)*. Alcoholic Chlorhexidine Solution. Chlorhexidine gluconate solution 2.5 ml, carmoisine, food grade of commerce, 50 mg, alcohol (or industrial methylated spirit or isopropyl alcohol) 70 ml, freshly boiled and cooled water to 100 ml. Shelf life 1 year; 3 years if prepared with isopropyl alcohol.

F.N. Belg. includes a similar preparation.

Proprietary Preparations of Chlorhexidine and its Salts

Bactigras *(Smith & Nephew, UK)*. A sterile tulle dressing impregnated with chlorhexidine acetate 0.5%. (Also available as Bactigras in *Austral., Canad., S.Afr.*).

Chlorhexidine Acetate Irrigations *(Travenol, UK)*. Chlorhexidine acetate, available as sterile solutions containing 0.02 and 0.05%.

Corsodyl Dental Gel (known in some countries as Hibitane Dental Gel) *(ICI Pharmaceuticals, UK)*. Contains chlorhexidine gluconate 1%. For gingivitis. **Corsodyl Mouthwash.** Contains chlorhexidine gluconate 0.2%.

Cyteal *(Concept Pharmaceuticals, UK)*. A solution containing chlorhexidine gluconate solution 0.5%, chlorocresol 0.3%, and hexamidine di-isethionate 0.1%. For skin cleansing and disinfection.

Dispray 1 Quick Prep *(Stuart, UK)*. A liquid aerosol spray containing industrial methylated spirit (acetone-free) 70% and chlorhexidine gluconate 0.5% with a propellent. For disinfecting skin prior to injection.

Dispray 2 Hard Surface Disinfectant *(Stuart, UK)*. A liquid aerosol spray containing chlorhexidine gluconate 0.02% in industrial methylated spirit (acetone-free) 70%. For disinfection of trolleys, gas cylinders, and similar equipment.

A possible toxic and explosive hazard from the use of Dispray 2 Hard Surface Disinfectant.— A. T. Chamberlain (letter), *Pharm. J.*, 1977, *1*, 366. The quantities considered were quite excessive.— D. Ganderton, *ICI Pharmaceuticals* (letter), *ibid.*, 442.

Eludril Mouthwash *(Concept Pharmaceuticals, UK)*. Contains chlorhexidine gluconate 0.1%, chloroform 0.5%, and chlorbutol 0.1%. **Eludril Spray**. A pressurised spray containing chlorhexidine gluconate 0.05% and amethocaine hydrochloride 0.015%. For mouth and throat infections.

Hibidil *(ICI Pharmaceuticals, UK)*. Sachets containing a sterile aqueous solution of chlorhexidine gluconate 0.05%.

Hibiscrub *(ICI Pharmaceuticals, UK)*. Contains chlorhexidine gluconate 4%. For hand cleansing prior to surgery and other procedures. (Also available as Hibiscrub in *Belg., Denm., Fr., Norw., S.Afr., Switz.*).

Hibisol Hand Rub *(ICI Pharmaceuticals, UK)*. Contains chlorhexidine gluconate solution 2.5%, isopropyl alcohol 70%, and emollients. For skin disinfection.

Hibitane *(ICI Pharmaceuticals, UK)*. A brand of chlorhexidine, available as acetate and as hydrochloride in powder form, and as gluconate in 20% solution (Chlorhexidine Gluconate Solution *B.P.*). (Also available as Hibitane in *Austral., Denm., Fr., Neth., Norw., S.Afr., Spain, Switz., USA*).

Hibitane Antiseptic Cream *(ICI Pharmaceuticals, UK)*. Contains chlorhexidine gluconate 1%. **Hibitane Antiseptic Lozenges**. Each contains chlorhexidine hydrochloride 5 mg and benzocaine 2 mg. For infections of the mouth and throat. *Dose*. 1 lozenge every 2 hours.

Hibitane 5% Concentrate contains chlorhexidine gluconate 5% with a surfactant in a red-coloured aqueous solution. **Hibitane Obstetric Cream** contains chlorhexidine gluconate 1% in a pourable water-miscible basis.

Naseptin *(ICI Pharmaceuticals, UK)*. A cream containing chlorhexidine hydrochloride 0.1% and neomycin sulphate 0.5%. For nasal application to nasal carriers of staphylococci.

References: P. M. Rountree *et al.*, *Med. J. Aust.*, 1962, *2*, 367.

pHiso-MED *(Winthrop, UK)*. Contains chlorhexidine gluconate 4%.

NOTE. pHiso-MED previously contained hexachlorophane 3%.

Rotersept Spray *(Roterpharma, UK)*. An aerosol spray containing chlorhexidine gluconate 0.2%. For the prevention of puerperal mastitis and the treatment of chapped nipples. (Also available as Rotersept Spray in *Belg., Neth.*).

Sterets H *(Schering-Prebbles, UK)*. Swabs saturated with 70% isopropyl alcohol solution containing chlorhexidine acetate 0.5%. For skin cleansing prior to injection.

Other Proprietary Names of Chlorhexidine and its Salts

Austral.—Cetal, Chlorohex, Hexol, Hexophene, Hibiclens, Savlon Medicated Powder; *Belg.*—Hibident, Hibigel, Sterilon; *Canad.*—Hibicare; *Denm.*—Rødhex; *Fr.*—Vitacontact; *Ger.*—anti Plaque, Chlorhexamed, Hibiclens; *Jap.*—Maskin; *Neth.*—Sterilon; *Norw.*—Hexidin; *Switz.*—Elgydium, Plak-out; *USA*—Hibiclens.

Preparations containing chlorhexidine or its salts were also formerly marketed in Great Britain under the proprietary names Dermofax (*Hough, Hoseason*), Medi-Prep, Medi-Sache, Medi-Swabs (H) (all *Pharmax*).

2223-f

Chlorinated Lime *(B.P.)*. Calx Chlorinata; Bleaching Powder; Chloride of Lime; Calcaria Chlorata; Calcii Hypochloris; Calcium Hypochlorosum; Calx Chlorata; Chlorure de Chaux; Chlorkalk; Cloruro de Cal; Cal Clorada.

CAS — 7778-54-3.

Pharmacopoeias. In *Arg., Belg., Br., Chin., Fr., Ind., Jap., Nord., Pol., Span.*, and *Swiss*.

A dull white powder with a characteristic odour, containing not less than 30% w/w of 'available chlorine' (see p.557). It becomes moist and gradually decomposes in air, carbon dioxide being absorbed and chlorine evolved.

Partly **soluble** in water and alcohol. Aqueous solutions are strongly alkaline. **Incompatible** with acids, ammonium salts, sulphur, and many organic compounds. It is decomposed by hydrochloric acid with the evolution of chlorine. **Store** in a cool place in airtight containers. Protect from light.

Adverse Effects, Treatment, and Precautions. As for Strong Sodium Hypochlorite Solution, p.574.

Uses. Chlorinated lime has the bactericidal actions and uses of chlorine (see below).

Its action is rapid but brief, the 'available chlorine' being soon exhausted by combination with organic material. It is used to disinfect faeces, urine, and other organic material, and as a cleansing agent for water-closets, drains, and effluents.

Chlorinated lime is a powerful bleaching agent and will decolorise most dyes.

Chlorinated lime is used in the preparation of Surgical Chlorinated Soda Solution which has been employed as a wound disinfectant, by continuous or frequent irrigation. Infected wounds are rapidly cleansed and disinfected, but the solution must be renewed at least every 2 hours, and the irrigation may give rise to localised oedema and delayed healing. The surrounding skin must be protected by smearing with soft paraffin to prevent irritation.

Chlorinated Lime and Boric Acid Solution has been used as a disinfectant lotion and wet dressing, but it is not used for wound irrigation since it may prove irritant to the tissues.

Dakin's solution and liquid paraffin. As an alternative to eusol and liquid paraffin, a satisfactory preparation might be prepared with equal volumes of double-strength Dakin's solution and liquid paraffin and 5% of Unemul. It provided an adequate dispersion which separated a little on standing but was easily redispersed on shaking. There was little loss of 'available chlorine' after storage at 18° for 23 days. Similar preparations made with cetomacrogol 1000, wool fat, cetostearyl alcohol, or oleic acid in place of Unemul lost their 'available chlorine' much more rapidly.— P. A. Grigg, *Pharm. J.*, 1962, *1*, 101.

Eusol. Eusol had an initial pH of 8.35 and an 'available chlorine' content of 0.39% w/v. After 4 weeks' storage at room temperature, the residual chlorine content was still in excess of *B.P.C.* limits. However at 37°, losses in excess of this limit occurred in just over one week. Strong Sodium Hypochlorite Solution 3 ml diluted to 100 ml in water had an initial pH of 11.55 and an 'available chlorine' content of 0.37%. Losses of 'available chlorine' on storage were slight. Addition of 1.25% of boric acid to this solution lowered the pH to 7.5 and resulted in rapid losses of 'available chlorine'. Dakin's solution had an initial pH of 12.2 and an 'available chlorine' content of 0.521%. Strong Sodium Hypochlorite Solution 4.5 ml in water to 100 ml had an initial pH of 11.7 and 'available chlorine' content of 0.515%. After 4 weeks' storage at room temperature and at 37°, losses of 'available chlorine' were slight. The amount of 0.1 M hydrochloric acid required to reduce 10 ml of solution to pH 7 was 4.95 ml for Eusol, 18.6 ml for Dakin's solution, and 4.8 and 1.9 ml for sodium hypochlorite solutions diluted to 0.37 and 0.52% 'available chlorine' respectively.— Pharm. Soc. Lab. Rep. P/71/22, 1971.

Eusol and liquid paraffin. Equal parts of eusol and liquid paraffin could be satisfactorily emulsified with either Unemul 5% or white beeswax 1%. Loss of potency over 23 days was ½% and 7% respectively.— F. H. Summers and C. R. McLaughlin (letter), *Lancet*, 1968, *2*, 1299.

Preparations

Calcium Hypochlorite Solution *(A.P.F.)*. Eusol. Chlorinated lime 1.25 g, boric acid 1.25 g, calcium hydroxide 1.25 g, water to 100 ml. Contains approximately 0.3% w/v (3000 ppm) of 'available chlorine'.

Chlorinated Lime and Boric Acid Solution *(B.P.)*. Eusol. Chlorinated lime 1.25 g, boric acid 1.25 g, water to 100 ml. It contains not less than 0.25% w/v (2500 ppm) of 'available chlorine'. Store at a temperature not exceeding 20° in well-filled airtight containers. Protect from light. It deteriorates on storage and should be used within 2 weeks.

Diluendum Calcis Chloratae *(Nord. P.)*. A solution containing 2.5% w/w calcium hypochlorite; Aqua Calcis Chloratae (*Nord. P.*) contains 0.5% calcium hypochlorite and is freshly prepared by diluting the Diluendum with water.

Surgical Chlorinated Soda Solution *(B.P.C. 1973)*. Liq. Sod. Chlorinat. Chir.; Dakin's Solution. Prepared from chlorinated lime, sodium carbonate, boric acid, and freshly boiled and cooled water, the proportions varying with the amount of 'available chlorine' in the chlorinated lime. It contains 0.5 to 0.55% w/v (5000 to 5500 ppm) of 'available chlorine'. It should be recently prepared. Store in a cool place in well-filled airtight containers. Protect from light.

'Tropical' Bleaching Powder. Consists of chlorinated lime with an excess of unslaked lime. It is stable even in hot climates.

2224-d

Chlorine.

Cl=35.453.

CAS — 7782-50-5 (Cl_2).

Chlorine has a potent bactericidal action. It is used as liquid chlorine for the chlorination treatment of water, but for most other purposes it is used in the form of hypochlorites, organic chloramines, chlorinated hydantoins, chlorinated isocyanurates, and similar oxidising compounds capable of releasing chlorine.

In the presence of water these compounds produce hypochlorous acid and hypochlorite ion and it is generally considered that the lethal action on organisms is due to chlorination of cell protein or enzyme systems by nonionised hypochlorous acid. The activity of most of the compounds decreases with increase of pH, the activity of solutions of pH 4 to 7 being greater than those of higher pH values. However, stability is usually greater at an alkaline pH.

Chlorine is capable of killing bacteria, and some fungi, yeasts, algae, viruses, and protozoa when used in sufficient concentration. It is reported to be almost ineffective against acid-fast bacteria and relatively ineffective against spores. Its activity is readily reduced by the presence of organic matter, particularly proteins or large numbers of micro-organisms.

Conventionally and confusingly the potency of chlorine disinfectants is expressed in terms of 'available chlorine'. This is based on the concept of chlorine gas (Cl_2) as the reference substance. Two atoms of chlorine (2 × Cl) yield in water one molecule of hypochlorous acid (on which activity is based), while hypochlorites and chloramines yield one molecule of hypochlorous acid for each atom of chlorine. Thus the assayed chlorine in such compounds has to be multiplied by 2 to produce 'available chlorine'. The term 'active chlorine' has been used confusingly for either 'available chlorine' (Cl_2) or combined chlorine (Cl).

Because they have relatively low residual toxicity, chlorine compounds are useful for the disinfection of relatively clean impervious surfaces, such as babies' feeding bottles, baths, wash-basins, trolleys, and food and dairy equipment. A concentration of 200 to 250 ppm of 'available chlorine' is used, though lower concentrations may be adequate if a detergent is added to ensure wetting of the surface. For food and dairy equipment where there is likely to be organic contamination, 250 to 300 ppm is used. For disinfecting equipment and surfaces contaminated by blood and to minimise the risk of transmission of hepatitis, solutions containing 10 000 ppm of 'available chlorine' are used.

The hypochlorites were once extensively used for disinfecting and deodorising wounds and body cavities.

Bromine (see p.338) and iodine (see p.863) are also used as disinfectants.

Adverse Effects. Chlorine gas is an irritant producing inflammation of the conjunctiva and when inhaled causing pain and spasm of the larynx and bronchi. There is a feeling of burning and suffocation. Coughing occurs, and if high concentrations are inhaled syncope and almost immediate death may follow. The irritant effect of chlorine may produce extensive pulmonary oedema with cyanosis, venous engorgement, and rapid respiration. There may be vomiting and excitement; acidosis may develop. Death may follow within 24 hours from either circulatory failure or pulmonary oedema.

Maximum permissible atmospheric concentration 1 ppm.

In 7 chemical workers exposed to chlorine gas for 3 to 45 minutes, side-effects included chest pains, a choking sensation, conjunctivitis, crepitations, cyanosis, dyspnoea, headache, and muscle pains. Cough and sputum, which varied from mucoid to mucopurulent, developed in 5. The effects lasted from 3 to 9 days. Respiratory failure in 3 patients and hypoxaemia in 4 were treated with oxygen therapy; hypoxaemia persisted for 4 days in 1 patient with severe symptoms.— F. X. M. Beach *et al.*, *Br. J. ind. Med.*, 1969, *26*, 231.

Damage to the respiratory tract by chlorine was attributed to its oxidising activity and this might be enhanced if intensive oxygen therapy was carried out.— L. Adelson and J. Kaufman, *Am. J. clin. Path.*, 1971, *56*, 430.

Pulmonary oedema occurred in an 83-year-old woman as a result of inhaling chlorine released from a mixture of sodium hypochlorite and sodium bisulphate contained in 2 household cleaners.— F. L. Jones (letter), *J. Am. med. Ass.*, 1972, *222*, 1312.

A report of reversible airways obstruction in 3 children after bathing in a chlorine-sterilised swimming pool. The children had no history of asthma but had an atopic background. Other children had had to leave the pool after developing coughs and sore throats. The pool had been treated with chlorine dioxide, generated by the addition of hydrochloric acid to sodium hypochlorite in a mixing chamber; an excessive concentration of chlorine or chlorine compound may have been used.— C. P. Mustchin and C. A. C. Pickering, *Thorax*, 1979, *34*, 682. Comment.— *Lancet*, 1979, *2*, 1342.

Repeated deliberate inhalation of chlorine in 1 patient.— P. Rafferty, *Br. med. J.*, 1980, *281*, 1178. A report of 2 further incidents of voluntary chlorine inhalation suggests that some individuals may be unusually insensitive to chlorine-induced irritation. Workers should be warned that concentrations of chlorine which can be tolerated for short periods without undue discomfort can still cause serious injury which may not be immediately apparent.— F. Dewhurst (letter), *Br. med. J.*, 1981, *282*, 565.

Further references: R. H. Wheater, *J. Am. med. Ass.*, 1974, *230*, 1064.

Precautions. Rice cooked in chlorinated water had been shown to have had a greatly reduced concentration of thiamine.— C. S. Farkas (letter), *Can. med. Ass. J.*, 1980, *122*, 1356.

Treatment of Adverse Effects. Conjunctivitis may require frequent irrigations of Sodium Chloride Eye Lotion. Respiratory distress should be treated with inhalations of oxygen, and antibiotics should be given to prevent bronchopneumonia. Corticosteroids may be required to minimise pulmonary damage. Acidosis may require the intravenous use of sodium bicarbonate or other suitable alkalising agent. Intravenous fluids may be given cautiously to correct electrolyte imbalance.

Chlorine Treatment of Water. On a large scale, chlorine gas is used to disinfect public water supplies. On a smaller scale, the use of chlorine compounds is more convenient and sodium hypochlorite, chloramine, and halazone are used. After satisfying the chlorine demand (the amount of chlorine needed to react with organic matter and other substances), a residual content of 0.2 to 0.4 ppm 'available chlorine' (see p.557) should be maintained for at least 15 minutes, though more is required for alkaline waters with a pH of 9 or more. For the disinfection of potentially contaminated water a concentration of 0.5 to 1 ppm for at least 30 minutes is recommended. The unpleasant taste of residual chlorine may be removed by adding a little citric acid or sodium thiosulphate.

For use in small swimming pools, sodium hypochlorite may be added daily to maintain a residual 'available chlorine' concentration of 0.25 to 1 ppm. Chloramine and the isocyanurates (see Sodium Dichloroisocyanurate, p.573) may also be used. To minimise irritation of the eyes, a pH of 7.5 to 8 should be maintained.

Disinfection of water. For the chlorination of public water supplies to control waterborne viruses, see S. L. Chang, *Bull. Wld Hlth Org.*, 1968, *38*, 401. See also *J. Am. med. Ass.*, 1975, *233*, 1316.

For a comparison of the use of chlorine and iodine for the disinfection of water in swimming pools, see A. P. Black *et al.*, *Am. J. publ. Hlth*, 1970, *60*, 535.

Under ideal conditions, 4 ppm of free chlorine would kill amoebic cysts in water in 30 minutes; in field conditions up to 200 ppm could be required.— W. P. Stamm, *Lancet*, 1970, *2*, 1355.

The Purification of the Water of Swimming Pools, Department of the Environment, London, HM Stationery Office, 1975.

A review of the disinfection of water in public swimming pools.— W. H. Humphrey, *R. Soc. Hlth J.*, 1978, *98*, 22, per *Abstr. Hyg.*, 1978, *53*, 421.

Use in dairies. A list of proprietary preparations based on available chlorine approved for the cleansing and disinfection of milk containers and appliances is contained in Circular FSH 8/78, Ministry of Agriculture, Fisheries and Food, London, HM Stationery Office, 1978.

2225-n

Chloroazodin (*U.S.P., B.P.C. 1949*). Chlorazodin. α,α′-Azobis(N^2-chloroformamidine).
$C_2H_4Cl_2N_6$=183.0.

CAS — 502-98-7.

Pharmacopoeias. In *Arg.* and *U.S.*

Bright yellow needles or flakes with a faint odour of chlorine and a slightly burning taste, containing about 77% w/w of 'available chlorine' (see p.557). It explodes without melting at about 155°. Very slightly **soluble** in water and chloroform; slightly soluble in glycerol and triacetin; sparingly soluble in alcohol. Solutions in glycerol and alcohol decompose rapidly on warming and all its solutions decompose on exposure to light. **Store** in airtight containers. Protect from light. Its decomposition is accelerated by contact with metals.

Chloroazodin aqueous solution liberates chlorine very slowly, giving a prolonged action. It has been used as a wet dressing and for irrigating infected wounds.

Preparations

Chloroazodin Topical Solution (*U.S.P.*). Contains chloroazodin 0.26% in triacetin. Store in airtight containers. Protect from light. Avoid contact with metals.

2226-h

Chlorocresol (*[illegible]*). Chlorocresolum; Chlorkresolum; PCMC; Parachlorometacresol. *p*-Chloro-*m*-cresol; 4-Chloro-3-methylphenol.
C_7H_7ClO=142.6.

CAS — 59-50-7.

Pharmacopoeias. In *Aust., Belg., Br., Fr., Ind., Int., It., Jug., Nord., Swiss,* and *Turk.*

Colourless or almost colourless crystals or crystalline powder with a characteristic, not tarry, phenolic odour; it is volatile in steam. M.p. 64° to 66°.
Soluble 1 in 260 of water, 1 in 50 of boiling water, and 1 in 0.4 of alcohol; soluble in acetone, chloroform, ether, fixed oils, glycerol, terpenes, and solutions of soap and alkali hydroxides. Solutions in water may be **sterilised** by autoclaving and solutions in oil or glycerol by maintaining at 160° for 1 hour. Solutions in water acquire a yellowish colour on exposure to light and air. **Protect** from light.
For precautions to be taken in preparing and storing antiseptic solutions, see under Phenol, p.570.

Total haemolysis occurred when erythrocytes were cultured for 45 minutes in a 0.06% solution of chlorocresol in sodium chloride injection. Only slight haemolysis occurred when the strength was reduced to 0.052%.— H. C. Ansel and D. E. Cadwallader, *J. pharm. Sci.*, 1964, *53*, 169.

A study of the effect of the antibiotic and preservative on each other's binding to pharmaceutical adjuvants in mixtures containing chlorocresol and ampicillin trihydrate, chloramphenicol, neomycin B sulphate, streptomycin sulphate, or tetracycline hydrochloride.— M. A. El-Nakeeb and M. H. Ali, *Mfg Chem.*, 1976, *47* (Mar.), 37.

Incompatibilities. Solutions of the following substances were incompatible with chlorocresol: hydrated calcium chloride, carbachol, codeine phosphate, diamorphine hydrochloride, digitalin, ergometrine, homatropine hydrobromide, papaveretum, physostigmine salicylate (unless sodium metabisulphite was added), quinine hydrochloride, sodium cacodylate, sodium chloride, sodium glycerophosphate, sodium morrhuate, thiamine hydrochloride, and strychnine hydrochloride.— J. S. McEwan and G. H. Macmorran, *Pharm. J.*, 1947, *1*, 260.

Incompatible with methylcellulose.— W. E. Harris, *Australas. J. Pharm.*, 1961, *42*, 583.

At a concentration up to 0.1%, chlorocresol was compatible with Cetomacrogol Cream *B.P.C.* Concentrations greater than this impaired stability and increased the tendency to form a granular preparation.— Pharm. Soc. Lab. Rep. P/70/15, 1970.

In the presence of polysorbate '80' 1% chlorocresol 0.1% had almost no antibacterial activity against *Staphylococcus aureus*.— R. T. Yousef *et al.*, *Can. J. pharm. Sci.*, 1973, *8*, 54.

Adverse Effects and Treatment. As for Phenol, p.571.
Chlorocresol is much less toxic than phenol. Sensitisation reactions may follow the application of strong solutions to the skin.

Hydrophilic contact lenses which were stored overnight in soaking solutions containing chlorocresol 0.1% caused severe irritation within a few days in the eyes of *rabbits* fitted with the lenses.— M. Davies, *J. Pharm. Pharmac.*, 1973, *25, Suppl.*, 134P.

Hypersensitivity occurred in a patient given heparin preserved with chlorocresol. Chlorocresol was considered to be responsible.— E. J. Ainley *et al.* (letter), *Lancet*, 1977, *1*, 705.

Uses. Chlorocresol is a potent disinfectant with low toxicity; it is more active in acid than in alkaline solution.
It may be used in a concentration of 0.2% in the process of sterilisation by heating with a bactericide and, in a concentration of 0.1%, in aqueous injections issued in multidose containers to maintain sterility during the withdrawal of successive doses. It should not be employed for these purposes in solutions for use by intrathecal, intracisternal, or peridural injection, or in solutions for intravenous injections where the dose exceeds 15 ml.
In a concentration of 0.05% it was formerly used as a preservative for eye-drops.
It is also used as a preservative in creams and other preparations for external use which contain water but its effectiveness is reduced if oils, fats, or nonionic surfactants are present.

Heating at 100° for 30 minutes with chlorocresol 0.1% was much less effective than autoclaving in killing the spores of *Bacillus stearothermophilus*. The use of 0.2% of chlorocresol was more effective but was irritant to eyes.— R. A. Anderson, *J. Hosp. Pharm.*, 1969, *26*, 48.

Microbial contamination of label dampers in a hospital pharmacy department was eliminated when saturated chlorocresol solution was used as the damping liquid.— R. M. Baird, *J. Hosp. Pharm.*, 1972, *30*, 105.

Pain. Of 66 patients with cancer treated by injections of chlorocresol in glycerol, 48 were relieved of pain. The usual strength of solution used was 2% chlorocresol in glycerol. The usual dose was 0.75 ml injected into the subarachnoid space and repeated after 3 weeks. The injection could be repeated once or twice without causing dysfunction. Though there was a slight delay in relief from pain when compared with phenol injections, there was diffusion of 43% into the cerebrospinal fluid in 1 hour. In 13 patients previously untreated, 10 were relieved by injections of 3.3 or 5% chlorocresol, but the risk of complications was greater. Of 38 patients previously untreated, 30 were relieved of pain by 2% chlorocresol without the development of complications. It was considered that chlorocresol was better than phenol in relieving pain in cancer and was more reliable though the effect was not instantaneous.— R. M. Maher, *Lancet*, 1963, *1*, 965 and 1157. The sterilisation and stability of chlorocresol 2% in glycerol. The solution was satisfactorily sterilised by maintaining it at 160° for 1 hour. No decomposition occurred, though 1 batch turned slightly pink on heating. Further examination showed that this discoloration occurred with certain batches of chlorocresol and was usually attributed to the presence of traces of heavy metals. After 3 months' storage no decomposition could be detected.—Pharm. Soc. Lab. Rep., *Pharm. J.*, 1963, *1*, 378.

Proprietary Preparations

See Proprietary Preparations of Chlorinated Phenols, p.559.

2227-m

Chlorothymol. Monochlorothymol. 6-Chlorothymol; 4-Chloro-2-isopropyl-5-methylphenol.
$C_{10}H_{13}ClO$=184.7.

CAS — 89-68-9.

White crystals or a crystalline granular powder with a characteristic odour and a very pungent aromatic taste. M.p. 59° to 61°. It darkens with age, becoming yellowish or brownish, and is affected by light. Slightly **soluble** in water; soluble 1 in 0.5 of alcohol, 1 in 2 of chloroform, 1 in 1.5 of ether, and 1 in 10 of light petroleum; soluble in dilute solutions of sodium hydroxide. **Store** at room temperature and avoid prolonged excessive heat. Protect from light.

Chlorothymol is a potent bactericide but is intensely irritating to mucous membranes. Its activity is markedly reduced by organic matter.

2228-b

Chloroxylenol (*B.P., B.P. Vet.*). PCMX; Parachlorometaxylenol. 4-Chloro-3,5-xylenol; 4-Chloro-3,5-dimethylphenol.
C_8H_9ClO=156.6.

CAS — 88-04-0.

Pharmacopoeias. In *Arg.* and *Br.*

White or cream-coloured crystals or crystalline powder with a characteristic odour; volatile in steam. M.p. 114° to 116°. **Soluble** 1 in 3000 of water, 1 in 200 of boiling water, 1 in 1 of alcohol; soluble in ether, terpenes, fixed oils, and solutions of alkali hydroxides.
For precautions to be taken in preparing and storing antiseptic solutions, see under Phenol, p.570.

The activity of chloroxylenol in solution was reduced by cetomacrogol 1000.— A. G. Mitchell, *J. Pharm. Pharmac.*, 1964, *16*, 533.

The microbiological activity of chloroxylenol against *Bacillus subtilis, Pseudomonas aeruginosa,* and *Aspergillus niger* was reduced by interaction with polysorbate 80 and activity against the *Bacillus* and *Pseudomonas* was also reduced by interaction with methylcellulose and macrogol 6000.— M. D. Ray *et al.*, *J. pharm. Sci.*, 1968, *57*, 609.

Adverse Effects. As for Phenol, p.571.
It is less toxic than phenol. In the recommended dilutions it is generally non-irritant but eczematous reactions have followed its use.

Skin sensitivity to Dettol (containing chloroxylenol), confirmed by patch tests, was seen in 4 patients during the period 1957–66.— J. K. Morgan, *Br. J. clin. Pract.*, 1968, *22*, 261.

Contact dermatitis due to chloroxylenol in 7 individuals.— F. Storrs, *Contact Dermatitis*, 1975, *1*, 211.

Precautions. Solutions should not be applied repeatedly to the skin and wet dressings should not be left in contact as skin sensitivity may occur.

Absorption and Fate. About one-third of ingested chloroxylenol is excreted in the urine conjugated with glucuronic acid and sulphuric acid.

Uses. Chloroxylenol is a disinfectant of low toxicity, which is active against streptococci but less active against staphylococci and almost inactive against certain Gram-negative organisms, including *Pseudomonas aeruginosa* and *Proteus vulgaris*. It is inactive against bacterial spores. Its activity is reduced in the presence of blood or serum.
It is used chiefly in the form of Chloroxylenol Solution. Dilutions are: for wounds, 5%; for external use in obstetrics, 2.5%; for vaginal douching, 0.5%; for the disinfection of instruments, 5% in 70% alcohol. A tincture containing chloroxylenol 1.44% is used undiluted for pre-operative skin disinfection.

A review of antimicrobial agents, including chloroxylenol, used in cosmetics.— I. R. Gucklhorn, *Mfg Chem.*, 1970, *41* (Oct.), 49.

Enhanced activity. Dettol diluted with freshly made 0.5% sodium polyphosphate or 0.1% edetic acid solutions had increased bactericidal activity.— J. A. Myers, *Chemist Drugg.*, 1968, *189*, 220.

Enhancement of the effect of chloroxylenol, against *Pseudomonas aeruginosa*, by edetic acid.— J. Dankert and I. K. Schut, *J. Hyg., Camb.*, 1976, *76*, 11; A. D. Russell and J. R. Furr, *J. appl. Bact.*, 1977, *43*, 253. See also R. Lyth, *Reckitt & Sons* (letter), *Chemist Drugg.*, 1968, *189*, 259.

Preparations

Chloroxylenol Solution *(B.P., A.P.F.)*. Roxenol. Chloroxylenol 5 g, terpineol 10 ml, alcohol (or industrial methylated spirit) 20 ml, castor oil 6.3 g, potassium hydroxide 1.36 g, oleic acid 0.75 ml, freshly boiled and cooled water to 100 ml. Dissolve the potassium hydroxide in 1.5 ml of water, add a solution of the castor oil in 6.3 ml of alcohol, mix, allow to stand for 1 hour or until a small portion remains clear when diluted with 19 times its vol. of water, and add the oleic acid; mix the terpineol with a solution of the chloroxylenol in the remainder of the alcohol, pour into the soap solution and adjust to 100 ml with water.

See also below, under Proprietary Preparations of Chlorinated Phenols.

2229-v

Proprietary Preparations of Chlorinated Phenols

Bristol Pine Disinfectant (known in some countries as Prinsyl) *(Tenneco, UK)*. A germicide solution containing chlorinated phenols 2% with terpenes in a solution of a vegetable-oil soap; RW coefficient 5 to 6. For use as a 2.5 to 12.5% solution for general disinfection.

CX 140 *(BTP Cocker Chemicals, UK)*. A mixture of chlorinated xylenols, mainly dichloroxylenol, solubilised with isopropyl alcohol, for use in formulating disinfectants.

CX 41 *(BTP Cocker Chemicals, UK)*. A mixture of chlorinated xylenols for use in formulating disinfectants.

Dettol *(Reckitt & Colman Pharmaceuticals, UK)*. A liquid germicide containing chloroxylenol 4.8%. For use as a 5% solution for wounds, and as a 5% solution in alcohol (70%) for disinfection of instruments. (Also available as Dettol in *Neth.*). **Surgical Dettol.** A tincture containing chloroxylenol 1.44% and terpineol 1.8% for pre-operative skin disinfection. **Instrument Dettol.** A liquid containing chloroxylenol 6.25%, for the disinfection of surgical instruments; it forms a clear solution with soft or distilled water and with alcohol. **Dettol Lotion.** Contains chloroxylenol 1.3% and edetic acid 0.2%; for surgical, medical, and obstetric use. **Dettol Cream.** A water-miscible cream containing chloroxylenol 0.3%, triclosan 0.3%, and edetic acid 0.2%. For minor wounds. **Dettol Mouthwash.** A concentrated mouth-wash and gargle containing chloroxylenol 1.02% with menthol, peppermint oil, anise oil, and other ingredients.

A 66-year-old woman who had ingested an estimated 300 ml of Dettol was unconscious 90 minutes later with a blood pressure of 90/0 mmHg. Consciousness returned 6½ hours after ingestion and blood pressure rose transiently to 130/60 mmHg; 21 hours after ingestion the patient was confused and there were signs of pulmonary oedema. Oliguria was treated by peritoneal dialysis but the patient died. Treatment should include the administration of liquid paraffin, forced alkaline diuresis, exchange transfusion, early dialysis, and assisted respiration.— D. Meek *et al.*, *Postgrad. med. J.*, 1977, *53*, 229.

A 70-year-old woman who ingested 350 ml of Dettol with suicidal intent experienced coma, arreflexia, miosis, impaired respiration, hypotension, hypothermia, and ECG evidence of ischaemia. After treatment with gastric lavage, oxygen, and dopamine she began to recover consciousness in 6 to 8 hours and was fully conscious in 24 hours.— P. Joubert *et al.*, *Br. med. J.*, 1978, *1*, 890.

A report of 10-year addiction to Dettol, by ingestion and the use of Dettol-soaked pessaries.— J. S. Khan *et al.*, *Br. med. J.*, 1979, *1*, 791.

Stridor requiring prolonged intubation and tracheostomy in a 22-month-old child who had ingested up to 125 ml of Dettol.— L. N. J. Archer, *Br. med. J.*, 1979, *2*, 19.

Gomaxide *(Seaford, UK)*. A liquid germicide containing chlorinated xylenols, chlorophyll, and terpineol in a detergent basis. For use as a 25% solution for disinfection of instruments.

Halocide 10 *(BTP Cocker Chemicals, UK)*. Chlorinated benzyl phenol with some benzyl phenol. A liquid preparation with bactericidal and fungicidal properties for use in the formulation of disinfectants.

HEB 'A' (Anerythene) *(Waterhouse, UK)*. A non-greasy cream containing chlorocresol 0.2%, with glycerol and olive oil. For roughness and dryness of the skin and for napkin rash.

Hycolin (known in *Austral.* as Medol) *(Pearson, UK)*. A disinfectant fluid containing 16% of a mixture of chloroxylenol, chlorocresol, chlorophene, sodium *o*-phenylphenate, and sodium pentachlorophenate in a basis of anionic emulsifier and alcohol; RW coefficient 9 to 10. For use as a 0.5 to 2% solution for general disinfection.

Hycolin Antibacterial Cream *(Pearson, UK)*. Contains Hycolin 2.5% and triclosan 0.25%, in a vanishing-cream basis. For use as a hand cream by nursing and medical staff.

Hycolin Liquid Soap *(Pearson, UK)*. Contains Hycolin 5% and triclosan 0.5%. For use in washing and disinfecting the hands.

Ibcol *(Jeyes, UK)*. A liquid non-staining germicide containing chlorinated phenols and aromatic substances; RW coefficient 3 to 5. For use as a general disinfectant. **Ibcol Extra.** A similar germicide containing chlorinated phenols and aromatic substances; RW coefficient 5 to 7. For use as a 1 in 160 solution for general disinfection.

Izal Antiseptic *(Sterling Industrial, UK)*. A concentrated disinfectant containing dichloroxylenol 1.25%, *o*-benzyl-*p*-chlorophenol 1.25%, and terpenes 4.5%, in an alcohol/soap/water basis; RW coefficient 7 to 11.

Jeypine *(Jeyes, UK)*. A liquid non-staining germicide containing chlorinated phenolic compounds and aromatic oils.

Multiguard *(Spearhead, UK)*. A disinfectant based on dichloroxylenol; RW coefficient 3 to 4.

Novasapa *(Pharmaceutical Mfg, UK)*. A bactericidal solution containing a halogenated cresol, a tertiary amine, and sodium citrate. For use undiluted for the rapid disinfection of instruments in the cold.

Pynol *(Wellcome, UK)*. A non-staining disinfectant containing chloroxylenols and pine oil.

Sterillium *(Pearson, UK)*. A disinfectant fluid containing 12% of the mixture of phenolic substances contained in Hycolin; RW coefficient 6 to 7. A 1.5% dilution is used for general disinfection; a dilution of 0.2 to 2% is used for laundry or linen disinfection.

Wright's Vaporizing Fluid *(LRC Products, UK)*. A liquid containing chlorocresol 10%. For use in Wright's Vaporizer for congestion in whooping cough, the common cold, and catarrh.

A survey of poisoning by Wright's Vaporizing Fluid.— H. M. Wiseman *et al.*, *Postgrad. med. J.*, 1980, *56*, 166.

Zal *(Sterling Health)*. A disinfectant fluid containing chlorinated and benzylated phenols and pine oil in a saponaceous basis; RW coefficient 3.5. For use as a 1 in 70 solution for general disinfection.

Other Proprietary Names of Chlorinated Phenols

Espadol Quirúrgico *(Arg.)*; Ice-O-Derm (see also under Benzalkonium Chloride, p.550) *(Canad.)*; Metasep *(USA)* (all containing chloroxylenol).

A preparation containing chloroxylenols was also formerly marketed in Great Britain under the proprietary name Zant *(Evans Medical)*.

2230-r

Clorophene. Clorfene; Septiphene. 2-Benzyl-4-chlorophenol.

$C_{13}H_{11}ClO$=218.7.

CAS — 120-32-1.

White or pink irregular flakes with a slight phenolic odour. M.p. about 49°. Practically **insoluble** in water; soluble in most organic solvents and in solutions of alkalis. **Protect** from light.

Clorophene is stated to have a high phenol coefficient against a wide range of bacteria and fungi. It is used in disinfectant solutions and soaps.

Proprietary Preparations

Santophen 1 *(Monsanto, UK)*. Clorophene, available as flakes or as a 75% w/w solution in isopropyl alcohol.

Other Proprietary Names

Manusept Emulsion *(Switz.)*.

2231-f

Cresol *(B.P.)*. Cresolum; Cresolum Crudum; Cresylic Acid; Kresolum Venale; Tricresol; Tricresolum; Trikresolum.

CAS — 1319-77-3; 95-48-7 (o-cresol); 108-39-4 (m-cresol); 106-44-5 (p-cresol).

Pharmacopoeias. In *Arg., Aust., Belg., Br., Chin., Hung., Ind., Int., It., Jap., Jug., Mex., Nord., Pol., Port., Roum., Span., Swiss,* and *Turk.* Also in *U.S.N.F.*

NOTE. Some grades of mixed cresols may be equivalent to Tar Acids, see p.574.

An almost colourless to pale brownish-yellow liquid, becoming darker with age or on exposure to light, with a characteristic odour resembling phenol, but more tarry, and consisting of a mixture of cresols and other phenols obtained from coal tar. An aqueous solution has a pungent taste. *B.P.* specifies that at least 80% distils between 195° and 205° and not more than 2% distils below 188°. Wt per ml 1.029 to 1.044 g. *U.S.N.F.* specifies a mixture of isomeric cresols from coal tar or petroleum; at least 90% distils between 195° and 205°; specific gravity 1.030 to 1.038.

o-Cresol ($CH_3.C_6H_4.OH$ = 108.1) is a colourless deliquescent solid, becoming yellow on keeping; m.p. about 30°, b.p. about 191°. *m*-Cresol is a colourless or yellowish liquid; m.p. about 10°, b.p. about 202°; slightly soluble in water; readily soluble in organic solvents. *p*-Cresol is a crystalline solid; m.p. about 36°, b.p. about 201°; slightly soluble in water; readily soluble in alcohol and ether.

Almost completely **soluble** 1 in 50 of water; miscible with alcohol, chloroform, ether, and glycerol; freely soluble in fixed and volatile oils; soluble in solutions of alkali hydroxides. A 2% solution in water is neutral to bromocresol purple. **Store** in airtight containers. Protect from light.

For precautions to be taken in preparing and storing antiseptic solutions, see under Phenol, p.570.

Total haemolysis occurred when erythrocytes were cultured for 45 minutes in a 0.25% solution of cresol in sodium chloride injection. Only slight haemolysis occurred when the strength was reduced to 0.225%. For *m*-cresol the same effect occurred at strengths of 0.3% and 0.26% respectively.— H. C. Ansel and D. E. Cadwallader, *J. pharm. Sci.*, 1964, *53*, 169.

Adverse Effects and Treatment. As for Phenol, p.571.

Maximum permissible atmospheric concentration 5 ppm.

A 62-year-old woman who had swallowed 150 ml of a solution of cresol and soap (Lysol) underwent peritoneal dialysis for 23 hours with the removal of 130 mmol of potassium. She then received 500 ml of a 5% solution of sodium bicarbonate and standard doses of hydrocortisone and ampicillin. Potassium supplements were also given for 4 days after dialysis. The patient slowly recovered. Peritoneal dialysis might have been useful in preventing a precipitate rise in serum potassium, which was possibly an important factor in early deaths due to cresol poisoning.— B. B. Thomas (letter), *Br. med. J.*, 1969, *3*, 720.

Methaemoglobinaemia developed in 2 patients following poisoning by Lysol. One also developed massive intravascular haemolysis 3 days later. These effects were considered to be due to a direct oxidant action on the red cells.— T. K. Chan *et al.*, *Blood*, 1971, *38*, 739.

Absorption and Fate. Cresols are absorbed and metabolised in the same way as phenol (see p.571).

Uses. Cresol has a similar action to phenol. The majority of common pathogens are killed in about 10 minutes by solutions containing 0.3 to 0.6% of cresol but spores require higher concentrations for a much longer time.

It is used as Cresol and Soap Solution as a general disinfectant for hospital and domestic use but it has been largely superseded by less irritant phenolic disinfectants. The bactericidal activity of Cresol and Soap Solution varies with the soap used. Linseed and castor oil soaps given the highest values, oleic acid the lowest. In any concentration in which it is an effective germicide it is caustic to the skin and unsuitable for skin and wound disinfection.

Cresol has sometimes been used in place of phenol in lotions and ointments, and has been used in a concentration of 0.3%, as a preservative for solutions for injections.

The cresols are widely used in commercial disinfectants, see p.575.

The addition of electrolytes such as sodium chloride, sodium benzoate, and sodium salicylate and non-electrolytes such as alcohol and glycerol to Cresol and Soap Solution *B.P. 1968* formulations resulted in increased bactericidal activity.— M. A. F. Gadalla *et al.*, *Arzneimittel-Forsch.*, 1974, *24*, 901.

For the use of cresol with formaldehyde (formocresol) in the sterilisation of dental cones, see Formaldehyde Solution, p.564.

Preparations

Cresol and Soap Solution *(B.P. 1968)*. Liq. Cresol. Sap.; Saponated Cresol Solution; Lysol. Cresol 50% v/v in a saponaceous solvent; the solvent is prepared by the interaction of suitable fixed oils, or their fatty acids, and potassium and/or sodium hydroxide, together with water. Miscible up to 10% v/v with water and in all proportions with alcohol. A 5% v/v solution in water is clear and shows no opalescence after standing for 3 hours.

A similar preparation is included in many pharmacopoeias.

NOTE. The use of the name Lysol is limited; in some countries it is a trade-mark and may be applied to a product of different composition.

Use of disinfectants on farms. For the rate of dilution of preparations containing Cresol and Soap Solution *B.P. 1968* approved for use as a disinfectant in Great Britain for specified diseases in animals, see The Diseases of Animals (Approved Disinfectants) Order 1978 (SI 1978: No. 32), as amended (SI 1978: No. 934 and SI 1979: No. 37).

See also Proprietary Preparations containing Cresols, Tar Acids, or other Phenols, p.575.

2232-d

Crystal Violet *(B.P.)*. Viola Crystallina; Medicinal Gentian Violet; Methylrosaniline Chloride; Pyoctaninum Caeruleum; CI Basic Violet 3; Colour Index No. 42555; Hexamethylpararosaniline Hydrochloride. 4-[4,4′Bis(dimethylamino)benzhydrylidene]cyclohexa-2,5-dien-1-ylidenedimethylammonium chloride.

$C_{25}H_{30}ClN_3$=408.0.

CAS — 548-62-9.

Pharmacopoeias. In *Br., Chin., Fr., Ind.*, and *Nord. Arg., Braz., Hung., Jap., Jug.*, and *Swiss* include mixtures of hexamethylpararosaniline hydrochloride with the tetramethyl- and pentamethyl-compounds.

Gentian violet *U.S.P.* is hexamethylpararosaniline hydrochloride usually admixed with penta- and tetra-methylpararosaniline hydrochloride.

The name methyl violet—CI Basic Violet 1; Colour Index No. 42535—has been used as a synonym for crystal violet, but is applied to a mixture of the hydrochlorides of the higher methylated pararosanilines consisting principally of the tetramethyl-, pentamethyl-, and hexamethyl compounds.

Greenish-bronze odourless or almost odourless crystals or powder. It loses not more than 9% of its weight on drying. **Soluble** 1 in 200 of water and 1 in 30 of glycerol; very soluble in alcohol; soluble in chloroform; practically insoluble in ether. Solutions are **sterilised** by autoclaving.

NOTE. The original material supplied in Great Britain contained certain homologues of hexamethylpararosaniline hydrochloride and was appreciably more soluble in water than crystal violet. It was often prescribed as a 1 or 2% solution in water, and much of the early published work refers to this more soluble but less pure material. Pharmacists are sometimes called upon to prepare 1 or 2% solutions of crystal violet in water though the pure dye is soluble only 1 in 200. Solutions of greater strength than 0.5% can be prepared by the addition of alcohol, but are not suitable for use on mucous membranes.

Effect of pH. Crystal violet was more effective against *Escherichia coli, Staphylococcus aureus, Streptococcus faecalis*, and *Bacillus subtilis* at pH 8 than pH 6. *E. coli* was most resistant. It was considered that crystal violet formed a non-ionised complex with the bacteria.— E. Adams, *J. Pharm. Pharmac.*, 1967, *19*, 821.

Incompatibility with zinc cream. Zinc cream with crystal violet lost its colour within 24 hours. The preparation remained satisfactory for a longer period (11 days in the case of the *B.P.* cream) when additional oleic acid was added before the dye was incorporated.— G. S. Riley, *Pharm. J.*, 1954, *2*, 106.

Inhibitory effect of bentonite. The antibacterial activity of crystal violet was inhibited in suspension of bentonite with which it formed a stable complex.— W. A. Harris, *Australas. J. Pharm.*, 1961, *42*, 583.

Preparation of 1% and 2% solutions. For the preparation of a 1% solution of crystal violet in water the addition of 15 to 20% of alcohol was required; for a 2% solution 25 to 30% of alcohol was required. Dilute solutions of glycerol were found to be poor solvents for crystal violet.—Pharm. Soc. Lab. Rep., *Pharm. J.*, 1957, *1*, 205.

Removal of stains. *From carpets.* A little soapless detergent was brushed on and rubbed several times with a moist sponge until all the detergent was removed.—Pharm. Soc. Lab. Rep., *Pharm. J.*, 1956, *1*, 383.

From the skin. Dilute hydrochloric acid was applied and rinsed immediately under running water; a second application and rinse might be necessary.—Pharm. Soc. Lab. Rep., *Pharm. J.*, 1961, *2*, 187.

Adverse Effects. Crystal violet is usually well tolerated but may cause nausea, vomiting, diarrhoea, griping, headache, dizziness, lassitude, and ulceration of mucous membranes. Cationic dyes should not be applied to the eyes.

In vitro, crystal violet was capable of interacting with DNA of living cells (indicating possible carcinogenicity); this suggested a need to re-evaluate its use clinically.— H. S. Rosenkranz and H. S. Carr (letter), *Br. med. J.*, 1971, *3*, 702.

A report of 3 patients who developed necrotic skin reactions after the topical application of a 1% aqueous solution of crystal violet. Other cases had been observed. The areas involved included the submammary folds, the genitalia, the gluteal fold, and the toe-webs. A similar reaction was produced in 2 subjects by the application of 1% crystal violet or brilliant green to stripped skin.— A. Björnberg and H. Mobacken, *Acta derm.-vener., Stockh.*, 1972, *52*, 55.

All of 6 neonates treated with aqueous gentian violet 0.5 or 1% for oral candidiasis developed oral ulceration not attributable to the candidiasis.— P. Horsfield *et al.* (letter), *Br. med. J.*, 1976, *2*, 529. A further report.— R. W. John, *ibid.*, 1968, *1*, 157.

Epistaxis. Nosebleeds in apple packers were caused by dust from the packing trays dyed blue with crystal violet.— G. E. Quinby, *Archs environ. Hlth*, 1968, *16*, 485.

Uses. Crystal violet is a disinfectant effective against some vegetative Gram-positive bacteria, particularly *Staphylococcus* spp., and some pathogenic yeasts such as *Candida* spp. It is much less active against Gram-negative bacteria and ineffective against acid-fast bacteria and bacterial spores. Its activity is greatly reduced in the presence of serum.

A 0.5% aqueous solution is applied topically in the treatment of candidal infections of the mouth, boils, chronic ulcers, and mycotic skin affections and a solution containing 0.5% of crystal violet and 0.5% of brilliant green has been used for pre-operative skin disinfection. It has been used as cream and pessaries for vaginal infections.

Crystal violet was formerly used in the treatment of strongyloid and threadworm infection.

A form of crystal violet is used for marking raw and unprocessed meat and citrus fruits.

A 1% aqueous solution of crystal violet was successfully used in the conservative treatment of 3 infants with giant exomphalos and avoided the risk of mercury intoxication associated with the use of mercurochrome solutions.— M. C. K. Chan (letter), *Archs Dis. Childh.*, 1980, *55*, 167. Comment.— D. C. S. Gough, *ibid.*

Neonatal infections. The effectiveness of a compound crystal violet paint (triple dye), hexachlorophane, and liquid soap in reducing staphylococcal colonisation in newborn infants was evaluated in a study of 1117 infants. Staphylococcal cord colonisation-rates were 10.5% using the paint, 41.1% using hexachlorophane, and 71.5% using the soap. The nasal colonisation-rates were 12.4, 15.8, and 48.3% respectively. The paint was applied to the cords of a further 1147 infants. The cord colonisation-rate was 1.8% and the nasal colonisation-rate was 5.2%. Triple dye was considered to be an effective agent for maintaining low staphylococcal colonisation-rates in nurseries for the newborn.— R. S. Pildes *et al.*, *J. Pediat.*, 1973, *82*, 987.

Umbilical care using a triple dye reduced the incidence of streptococcal infection in a neonatal nursery, compared with hexachlorophane or a control group.— E. R. Wald *et al.*, *Am. J. Dis. Child.*, 1977, *131*, 178.

In a study in 284 neonates treatment of the umbilical cord stump with triple dye reduced colonisation with *Staphylococcus aureus* compared with treatment with silver sulphadiazine, but colonisation with streptococci and Gram-negative bacilli was increased.— W. T. Speck *et al.*, *Am. J. Dis. Child.*, 1977, *131*, 1005.

Skin marking ink. Skin could be marked for surgical purposes by applying Compound Crystal Violet Paint (*B.P.C. 1954*) and when dry painting over with Weak Iodine Solution. The marks produced withstood rigorous pre-operative skin preparation and could be used on patients who were not hypersensitive to iodine.— A. W. Asscher *et al.* (letter), *Lancet*, 1968, *2*, 638.

Thrush. Mucosal use of crystal violet solution should be limited to twice daily for a maximum of 4 days.— J. Verbov (letter), *Br. med. J.*, 1976, *2*, 639.

Preparations

Creams

Gentian Violet Cream *(U.S.P.)*. It contains gentian violet *U.S.P.* 1.2 to 1.6%, calculated as anhydrous hexamethylpararosaniline hydrochloride, in a suitable cream basis. Store at a temperature not exceeding 40° in airtight containers.

Ointments

Unguentum Violae Cristallisatae Forte *(F.N. Belg.)*. Strong Ointment of Crystal Violet; Pommade au Cristal Violet Forte. Crystal violet 1, zinc oxide 20, starch 20, wool fat 20, soft paraffin 20, and calcium hydroxide solution 19, all by wt.

Unguentum Violae Cristallisatae Mite *(F.N. Belg.)*. Weak Ointment of Crystal Violet; Pommade au Cristal Violet Faible. Crystal violet 0.5, zinc oxide 20, starch 20, wool fat 20, soft paraffin 20, and calcium hydroxide solution 19.5, all by wt.

Paints

Brilliant Green and Crystal Violet Paint *(B.P.)*. Liquor Tinctorium; Pigmentum Tinctorium; Pigmentum Caeruleum; Brilliant Green and Crystal Violet Solution; Crystal Violet Paint Alcoholic; Blue Paint; Bonney and Browning's Blue Paint. Brilliant green and crystal violet of each 500 mg, alcohol (90%) (or industrial methylated spirit, suitably diluted) 50 ml, and water to 100 ml. Store in airtight containers.

Compound Crystal Violet Paint *(B.P.C. 1954)*. Pig. Violae Crys. Co.; Triple Dye; Pigmentum Triplex. Crystal violet 229 mg, brilliant green 229 mg, proflavine hemisulphate 114 mg, water to 100 ml.

Crystal Violet Paint *(B.P.)*. Gentian Violet Paint. Crystal violet 500 mg, freshly boiled and cooled water to 100 ml. Store at a temperature not exceeding 25° in airtight containers.

Pessaries

Crystal Violet Pessaries *(B.P.)*. Pess. Violae Crys. Pessaries containing crystal violet in Glycerol Suppositories mass. Store at a temperature not exceeding 25°. *A.P.F.* has 0.5% in Glyco-gelatin Gel.

Solutions

Gentian Violet Topical Solution *(U.S.P.)*. Gentian Violet Solution. Contains gentian violet (*U.S.P.*) equivalent to hexamethylpararosaniline hydrochloride 0.95 to 1.05% with alcohol 8 to 10%. Store in airtight containers. *F.N. Belg.* includes a similar preparation.

Proprietary Names

Genapax *(Key, USA)*.

2233-n

Dequalinium Acetate *(B.P. 1973)*. Decalinium Acetate. 1,1′-Decamethylenebis(4-amino-2-methylquinolinium acetate).

$C_{34}H_{46}N_4O_4$=574.8.

CAS — 6707-58-0 (dequalinium); 4028-98-2 (acetate).

A white or pinkish-buff, odourless, slightly hygroscopic powder with a bitter taste. M.p. about

280° with decomposition.
Soluble 1 in 2 of water and 1 in 12 of alcohol. A 5% solution in water has a pH of 6 to 8. **Store** in airtight containers. Protect from light.

2234-h

Dequalinium Chloride *(B.P.)*.
Decalinium Chloride; Decaminum. 1,1′-Decamethylenebis(4-amino-2-methylquinolinium chloride).
$C_{30}H_{40}Cl_2N_4$=527.6.

CAS — 522-51-0.

Pharmacopoeias. In *Br.* and *Rus.*

A creamy-white odourless powder with a bitter taste. M.p. about 315° with decomposition. Slightly **soluble** in water; soluble 1 in 30 of boiling water and 1 in 200 of propylene glycol. **Incompatible** with soaps and other anionic surfactants, with phenol, and with chlorocresol. **Store** in airtight containers.

Adverse Effects and Precautions. Ulceration and necrosis has occasionally followed application of dequalinium to occluded skin. It should not be applied to skin in the ano-genital area.

Pure and impure preparations of dequalinium chloride produced positive skin reactions in 309 of 6000 patients routinely given patch tests. Reactions were more common in patients with leg ulceration or varicose eczema.— O. P. Salo *et al.*, *Acta allerg.*, 1968, *23*, 490.

Necrosis. Evidence has been found connecting dequalinium preparations, especially when used in the treatment of balanitis, with the occasional development of necrosis. It was recommended that dequalinium preparations should not be used in the treatment of this condition or in circumstances where the skin was occluded.— R. B. Coles *et al.* (letter), *Lancet*, 1964, *2*, 531; *idem*, *Br. med. J.*, 1964, *2*, 688.

Uses. Dequalinium is an antibacterial and antifungal agent, active against many Gram-positive and Gram-negative bacteria and against *Borrelia vincenti, Candida albicans,* and some species of *Trichophyton.* The action is little affected by the presence of serum. It is used in the form of lozenges in the treatment of infections of the mouth and throat.

Proprietary Preparations of Dequalinium Salts

Dequadin *(Farley, UK).* Dequalinium chloride, available as lozenges of 250 µg. (Also available as Dequadin in *Austral., Canad., Denm., Ital., S.Afr., Spain, Switz.*).

Labosept Pastilles *(Laboratories for Applied Biology, UK).* Each contains dequalinium chloride 250 µg.

Other Proprietary Names of Dequalinium Salts

Belg.—Angils; *Denm.*—Danical; *Ger.*—Dequafungan, Dequavagyn, Eriosept, Evazol, Optipect Halstabletten, Phylletten, Soor-Gel *(salicylate)*, Sorot; *Ital.*—Decabis, Osangin; *Jap.*—SP; *Neth.*—Gargilon; *Norw.*—Dekadin, Salvizol *(see also under Bisdequalinium Diacetate, p.550)*; *Switz.*—Grocreme.

Dequalinium chloride was also formerly marketed in Great Britain under the proprietary name Hexilin (*Farley*).

2235-m

Diacetylaminoazotoluene. Diacetazotol; Pellidol. 4-Diacetylamino-2′,3-dimethylazobenzene.
$C_{18}H_{19}N_3O_2$=309.4.

CAS — 83-63-6.

Pharmacopoeias. In *Aust., Span.,* and *Swiss.*

A yellowish-red crystalline powder with a slight odour. M.p. about 74°. Practically **insoluble** in water; soluble 1 in 20 of alcohol (90%); soluble in chloroform, ether, fats, oils, and soft paraffin. **Protect** from light.

Diacetylaminoazotoluene is chemically related to scarlet red (see p.573) and has been used medicinally for similar purposes, as a 2% ointment in soft paraffin and as a 5% dusting-powder.

Of 612 persons with dermatitis or eczema submitted to patch testing with diacetylaminoazotoluene 2% in yellow soft paraffin, 2.1% gave a positive reaction.— E. Rudzki and D. Kleniewska, *Br. J. Derm.*, 1970, *83*, 543.

2236-b

Dibromopropamidine Isethionate *(B.P.)*.
Dibromopropamidine Isetionate. 4,4′-Trimethylenedioxybis(3-bromobenzamidine) bis(2-hydroxyethanesulphonate).
$C_{17}H_{18}Br_2N_4O_2,2C_2H_6O_4S$=722.4.

CAS — 496-00-4 (dibromopropamidine); 614-87-9 (isethionate).

Pharmacopoeias. In *Br.*

A white or almost white, odourless, crystalline powder with a bitter taste.
Soluble 1 in 2 of water, 1 in 60 of alcohol, and 1 in 20 of glycerol; practically insoluble in chloroform, ether, fixed oils, and liquid paraffin. A 5% solution in water has a pH of 5 to 7. Aqueous solutions are **sterilised** by filtration. **Store** in airtight containers.

Uses. Dibromopropamidine isethionate has antibacterial and antifungal properties. It is active against pyogenic cocci and *Staphylococcus aureus,* and against certain Gram-negative bacteria including *Escherichia coli, Proteus vulgaris,* and some strains of *Pseudomonas aeruginosa.* Its antibacterial action is not considered to be inhibited by pus or blood.
It is used as a 0.15% cream for the treatment of surface infections and as a first-aid dressing for minor burns and other injuries. It may also be used in impetigo, sycosis barbae, ringworm, and otitis externa, and in skin grafting. An eye ointment containing 0.15% of dibromopropamidine isethionate is used in the treatment of blepharitis, acute and chronic conjunctivitis, and other infections of the eye.
The embonate has been used in lozenges.

Proprietary Preparations

Brolene Eye Ointment *(May & Baker, UK).* Contains dibromopropamidine isethionate 0.15%. (Also available as Brolene Eye Ointment in *Austral., S.Afr.*).

Brulidine *(May & Baker, UK).* Dibromopropamidine isethionate, available as a cream containing 0.15% in a water-miscible basis. (Also available as Brulidine in *Austral., S.Afr.*).

A preparation containing dibromopropamidine isethionate was also formerly marketed in Great Britain under the proprietary name Otamidyl (*May & Baker*).

2237-v

Dichlordimethylhydantoin. 1,3-Dichloro-5,5-dimethylhydantoin; 1,3-Dichloro-5,5-dimethylimidazolidine-2,4-dione.
$C_5H_6Cl_2N_2O_2$=197.0.

A white or faintly cream-coloured powder containing about 72% w/w of 'available chlorine' (see p.557). M.p. 132°. Slightly **soluble** in water; freely soluble in chloroform. An aqueous solution has a pH of about 4.4.

Adverse Effects and Treatment. As for Strong Sodium Hypochlorite Solution, p.574.
Maximum permissible atmospheric concentration 200 µg per m^3.

Uses. Dichlordimethylhydantoin is used as a source of chlorine, for sterilising babies' feeding bottles, and as a bleach.

Proprietary Preparations

Hydan *(ABM Chemicals, UK).* A brand of dichlordimethylhydantoin.

2238-g

Dichlorobenzyl Alcohol. Dybenal. 2,4-Dichlorobenzyl alcohol.
$C_7H_6Cl_2O$=177.0.

CAS — 1777-82-8.

Dichlorobenzyl alcohol is an antiseptic, it is an ingredient of Strepsils lozenges (see p.549).

Proprietary Preparations

Myacide SP *(Boots, UK).* A brand of dichlorobenzyl alcohol.

2239-q

Dichloroxylenol *(B.P.C. 1959).* Dichlorometaxylenol. 2,4-Dichloro-3,5-xylenol; 2,4-Dichloro-3,5-dimethylphenol.
$C_8H_8Cl_2O$=191.1.

CAS — 133-53-9.

White or creamy-white crystals or crystalline powder with a characteristic odour. M.p. 93.5° to 95°. Volatile in steam. **Soluble** 1 in 5000 of water, in alcohol, ether, terpenes, fixed oils, and solutions of alkali hydroxides.

Dichloroxylenol is a bactericide with actions similar to those of chloroxylenol (p.558) and may be used for the same purposes.

2240-d

Dodecarbonium Chloride. Benzyl(dodecylcarbamoylmethyl)dimethylammonium chloride.
$C_{23}H_{41}ClN_2O$=397.0.

CAS — 100-95-8.

Crystals with a bitter taste. M.p. 147° to 148°. **Soluble** in water and alcohol; practically insoluble in acetone and ether.

Dodecarbonium chloride is a quaternary ammonium disinfectant with properties and uses similar to those of other cationic surfactants as described under Cetrimide, p.551.

Proprietary Names

Straminol *(Bracco, Ital.).*

2241-n

Dofamium Chloride. Phenamylium Chloride; G 25,268. Dimethyl[2-(*N*-methyldodecanamido)ethyl]-[(phenylcarbamoyl)methyl]ammonium chloride.
$C_{25}H_{44}ClN_3O_2$=454.1.

CAS — 54063-35-3.

Dofamium chloride is a quaternary ammonium disinfectant which has been used in the treatment of superficial infections of the mouth and throat.

Dofamium chloride was formerly marketed in Great Britain under the proprietary name Desogen Lozenges (*Geigy*).
The name Desogen has also been applied to preparations of toloconium methylsulphate.

2242-h

Domiphen Bromide *(B.P.)*.
Phenododecinium Bromide; NSC 39415. It consists chiefly of dodecyldimethyl(2-phenoxyethyl)ammonium bromide.
$C_{22}H_{40}BrNO$=414.5.

CAS — 13900-14-6 (domiphen); 538-71-6 (bromide).

Pharmacopoeias. In *Br.* and *Chin.*

Colourless or faintly yellow crystalline flakes with a bitter soapy taste. M.p. 106° to 116°. **Soluble** 1 in less than 2 of water, 1 in less than 2 of alcohol, and 1 in 30 of acetone. A 10% solution in water is almost colourless and not more than slightly opalescent; it foams on shaking. A 1% solution in water has a pH of 6.4 to 7.6. **Incompatible** with soaps and other anionic surfactants, alkali hydroxides, proflavine, physostigmine, and fluorescein. **Store** in a cool place in

airtight containers. Protect from light.
For precautions to be taken in preparing and storing antiseptic solutions, see under Phenol, p.570.

Adverse Effects and Treatment. As for Cetrimide, p.552.

Uses. Domiphen bromide is a quaternary ammonium disinfectant with properties and uses similar to those of other cationic surfactants as described under Cetrimide, p.552. It also has some antifungal activity.
Lozenges each containing 500 µg of domiphen bromide have been used in the prophylaxis and treatment of infections of the mouth and throat. Solutions containing 0.01 to 0.5% were formerly used for a variety of applications.

A review of antimicrobial agents, including domiphen bromide, used in cosmetics.— I. R. Gucklhorn, *Mfg Chem.*, 1970, *41* (Sept.), 82.

Proprietary Preparations

Bradosol Lozenges *(Ciba, UK)*. Each contains domiphen bromide 500 µg. (Also available as Bradosol in *Canad.*, *Denm.*).

Other Proprietary Names

Neo-Bradoral *(Switz.)*.

2243-m

Ethacridine Lactate. Acrinol; Acrinol Lactate; Lactoacridine; Aethacridinium Lacticum. 6,9-Diamino-2-ethoxyacridine lactate.
$C_{15}H_{15}N_3O,C_3H_6O_3$=343.4.

CAS — 442-16-0 (ethacridine); 1837-57-6 (lactate).

Pharmacopoeias. In *Cz.*, *Jug.*, *Pol.*, and *Rus.*; in *Aust.*, *Ger.*, *Jap.*, *Port.*, *Roum.*, and *Swiss* as monohydrate.

A yellow odourless crystalline powder with an astringent bitter taste. M.p. about 245° with decomposition. Slowly **soluble** 1 in 15 of water, 1 in 9 of boiling water, and 1 in about 150 of alcohol. It forms yellow fluorescent solutions which are stable to boiling. A 2% solution in water has a pH of 5.5 to 7. **Store** in airtight containers. Protect from light.

Ethacridine was incompatible with several macrogol derivatives.— S. Gecgil, *Eczac. Bült.*, 1971, *13*, 40, per *Int. pharm. Abstr.*, 1972, *9*, 658.

Adverse Effects. Hypersensitivity reactions have been reported.
Of 316 persons with dermatitis or eczema submitted to patch testing with ethacridine lactate 1% in yellow soft paraffin, 2.9% gave a positive reaction.— E. Rudzki and D. Kleniewska, *Br. J. Derm.*, 1970, *83*, 543.

Uses. Ethacridine lactate has properties similar to other acridine derivatives (see p.573). It has been used as a surgical disinfectant as a 0.025 to 1% solution. Ointments (1%), dusting-powders (2.5%), and gauze (0.2%) have been used on the skin. It has been taken by mouth in doses of 25 to 100 mg.

Ethacridine lactate was used in Japan to induce abortions. No fatalities had been reported.— Y. Manabe (letter), *J. Am. med. Ass.*, 1969, *210*, 1091. Further references to the use of ethacridine lactate for induction of abortion; K. Edström, *Bull. Wld Hlth Org.*, 1979, *57*, 481.

In patients with nonparasitic diarrhoea 18 of 21 treated with ethacridine lactate 600 mg daily for 5 days were cured in 3 days or less, compared with 11 of 15 treated with a combination of phanquone 60 mg, clioquinol 600 mg, and oxyphenonium bromide 6 mg daily for 5 days, and 10 of 21 given a placebo.— N. Madanagopalan *et al.*, *Curr. ther. Res.*, 1975, *18*, 546.

After tritiated ethacridine lactate 200 mg was given by mouth in an aqueous solution to 3 healthy volunteers faecal elimination was complete after 4 days and accounted for 99% of the dose.— T. J. Rising *et al.*, *Arzneimittel-Forsch.*, 1977, *27*, 872.

Proprietary Names

Antidiar 200 (see also under Dried Aluminium Hydroxide) *(Hoechst, Arg.)*; Hectalin *(Jap.)*; Metifex *(Cassella-med, Ger.)*; Rimaon *(Jap.)*; Rivanol *(Chinosolfabrik, Ger.)*.

2244-b

Ethylene Oxide. Oxirane.

C_2H_4O=44.05.

CAS — 75-21-8.

A colourless mobile liquid below its b.p. of 10.7°. A colourless gas with a not unpleasant odour, reminiscent of bruised apples, at ordinary temperature. Flash-point less than −29°. Concentrations of 3.3 to 80% v/v in air are explosive but the range can be narrowed by the addition of carbon dioxide and mixtures containing 43% v/v or more of carbon dioxide cease to be explosive. **Soluble** in water, alcohol, and ether.

CAUTION. *Mixtures of ethylene oxide with oxygen or air are explosive. Ethylene oxide should not be used in the presence of an open flame or of any electrical apparatus liable to produce a spark.*

Absorption and desorption of ethylene oxide.— D. A. Gunther, *Am. J. Hosp. Pharm.*, 1969, *26*, 45.

Solubility of ethylene oxide in selected plasticisers.— W. L. Guess and A. B. Jones, *Am. J. Hosp. Pharm.*, 1969, *26*, 180.

Adverse Effects. Ethylene oxide vapour irritates the nose and eyes and may also cause nausea and vomiting, diarrhoea, headache, vertigo, central nervous system depression, dyspnoea, and pulmonary oedema. Liver and kidney damage may occur. Fatalities have occurred. Symptoms may be delayed half an hour after exposure and may persist for a few days. Excessive exposure of the skin to liquid or solution causes burns and blistering.
Maximum permissible atmospheric concentration 50 ppm.

Plastics used in medical and pharmaceutical devices were often sterilised by ethylene oxide, but the residual ethylene oxide could produce haemolysis of red blood cells and could kill cell cultures.— R. K. O'Leary and W. L. Guess, *J. pharm. Sci.*, 1968, *57*, 12.

Ethylene chlorohydrin, formed from ethylene oxide in the presence of chloride ions in the material being sterilised, was toxic in *animals* when injected intradermally, and also cytotoxic in cell cultures.— W. H. Lawrence *et al.*, *J. pharm. Sci.*, 1971, *60*, 568. The haemolytic activity of ethylene chlorohydrin was less than 15% of the haemolytic activity of ethylene oxide.— D. A. Gunther, *Am. J. Hosp. Pharm.*, 1974, *31*, 684.

A sudden increase in the frequency of tracheal stenosis after tracheotomy and prolonged artificial respiration was due to insufficient removal of ethylene oxide after sterilisation of the tracheotomy cannulas; the cannulas had been kept for 48 hours before use. It was suggested that at least 8 days should elapse after sterilisation with ethylene oxide before the instruments are used.— J. M. Mantz *et al.*, *Sem. Hôp. Paris*, 1972, *48*, 3367.

Polyvinyl chloride materials previously sterilised by gamma irradiation produced toxic ethylene chlorohydrin when resterilised by ethylene oxide.— R. M. G. Boucher, *Am. J. Hosp. Pharm.*, 1972, *29*, 661.

For toxicological data, see 1971 Evaluations of some Pesticide Residues in Food, *Pestic. Residue Ser. Wld Hlth Org. No. 1*, 1972.

A report of 1st to 3rd degree burns occurring postoperatively or postpartum in 19 women. The gowns and sheets used were found to contain 16 to 50 times the safe residual concentration of ethylene oxide.— L. Biro *et al.*, *Archs Derm.*, 1974, *110*, 924.

A patient on chronic haemodialysis developed systemic allergic reactions associated with the use of a plastic and rubber connecting tube, in an arteriovenous shunt, which had been sterilised by ethylene oxide.— J. Poothullil *et al.*, *Ann. intern. Med.*, 1975, *82*, 58.

A report of neurotoxicity in 4 workers exposed to ethylene oxide.— J. A. Gross *et al.*, *Neurology, Minneap.*, 1979, *29*, 978.

Workers who had been employed for more than one year by a company producing ethylene oxide had been studied from 1960 to 1961. No significant differences had been found between workers permanently working in the ethylene oxide manufacturing area, those who had previously worked in this area, those working there intermittently and a further group who had never worked in ethylene oxide production. However a subgroup of individuals with high exposure had decreased haemoglobin concentrations and significant lymphocytosis. When workers were followed up from 1961 to 1977, those who had been exposed full-time to ethylene oxide production (first 2 groups above) showed a considerable excess mortality, this being mainly due to an increased incidence of leukaemia, stomach cancer, and diseases of the circulatory system. Although malignancies could not be linked to any particular chemical associated with ethylene oxide production it was considered that ethylene oxide and ethylene dichloride, possibly together with ethylene chlorohydrin or ethylene, were the causative agents.— C. Hogstedt *et al.*, *Br. J. ind. Med.*, 1979, *36*, 276. See also C. Hogstedt *et al.*, *J. Am. med. Ass.*, 1979, *241*, 1132.

Uses. Ethylene oxide is lethal to insects and is a bactericide and fungicide which is effective against most micro-organisms, including viruses. It is used as a fumigant for foodstuffs and textiles and as an agent for the gaseous sterilisation of pharmaceutical and surgical materials.
The principal disadvantage of ethylene oxide is that it forms explosive mixtures with air, but this may be overcome by using mixtures containing 10% ethylene oxide in carbon dioxide or halogenated hydrocarbons, or by removing at least 95% of the air from the apparatus before admitting either ethylene oxide or a mixture of 90% ethylene oxide in carbon dioxide.
Certain fluorinated hydrocarbons form non-inflammable mixtures with ethylene oxide; mixtures of dichlorodifluoromethane and trichlorofluoromethane with 9 to 12% w/w of ethylene oxide are most commonly employed. The advantages of these mixtures over the carbon dioxide mixture are that they permit a higher partial pressure of ethylene oxide in the exposure chamber at the same total pressure and that the liquefied mixture can be stored in containers of a much lighter weight (e.g. small disposable cans) than the steel cylinders required for the carbon dioxide mixture.
Effective sterilisation by ethylene oxide depends on exposure time, temperature, humidity, the amount and type of microbial contamination, and the partial pressure of the ethylene oxide in the exposure chamber. The material being sterilised must be permeable to ethylene oxide if occluded micro-organisms are present. The bactericidal action is accelerated by increase of temperature; a temperature of about 55° can be used for most thermolabile materials. Concentrations of between 500 and 1000 mg of ethylene oxide per litre are used. The exposure time may vary from 2 hours at elevated temperatures to 16 to 36 hours at lower temperatures.
Moisture is essential for sterilisation by ethylene oxide and the gas is most effective at a relative humidity of about 35%. However, in practice, dry micro-organisms need to be rehydrated before ethylene oxide can be effective, so a conditioning period in a suitable atmosphere should be used before sterilisation. Relative humidities of 40 to 60% are used. Control of physical factors does not assure sterility, and the process should be monitored.
Many materials, particularly plastics, rubber, and leather, absorb ethylene oxide freely during the exposure period and because of its toxic nature, all traces of the gas must be removed before the sterilised materials can be used; this may be achieved by ventilation or drawing sterile air through the load.

The sterilising properties of ethylene oxide, its applications, and equipment for ethylene oxide sterilisation.— *Recent Developments in the Sterilisation of Surgical Materials*, London, The Pharmaceutical Press, 1961, pp. 59–106.

A small-scale method of sterilisation of plastic articles by ethylene oxide.— M. Florentine and L. P. Schiff, *Am. J. Hosp. Pharm.*, 1967, *24*, 367.

Ethylene oxide was not a reliable sterilisation method for disposable syringes; spores could be trapped between the plunger seal and the barrel.— S. D. Rubbo and J. F. Gardner, *J. appl. Bact.*, 1968, *31*, 164.

A method for sterilising small items with 84% ethylene oxide.— R. M. Smith and J. A. Young, *Br. J. Anaesth.*, 1968, *40*, 909.

For information on fumigation with ethylene oxide and precautions against fire and explosion, see *Fumigation with Ethylene Oxide*, London, HM Stationery Office, 1969.

For an extensive review of the use of ethylene oxide in sterilisation, see J. J. Roxon, *Aust. J. pharm. Sci.*, 1973, *NS2*, 65. See also *Med. J. Aust.*, 1974, *1*, 686.

Residues of not more than 1000 ppm of ethylene oxide for implanted materials and not more than 150 ppm for parenteral solutions were suggested as safe concentrations.— S. R. Andersen, *Bull. parent. Drug Ass.*, 1973, *27*, 49.

The recommended maximum concentration of ethylene oxide residues in biological materials which come in contact with sensitive biological tissues was 100 ppm.— T. O. McDonald *et al.*, *Bull. parent. Drug Ass.*, 1973, *27*, 153.

A discussion of sterilisation by means of ethylene oxide.— R. R. Ernst, *Acta pharm. suec.*, 1975, *12*, *Suppl.*, 44.

A discussion of the permeability of packaging materials to ethylene oxide.— D. A. Gunther, *Bull. parent. Drug Ass.*, 1976, *30*, 152.

A discussion on the use of ethylene oxide for sterilisation of cosmetics.— R. H. Gilmour, *Soap Perfum. Cosm.*, 1978, *51*, 498, per *Int. pharm. Abstr.*, 1979, *16*, 351.

Aeration time. After sterilisation with ethylene oxide, a plastic cardiac catheter required at least 48 hours' aeration, while a rubber Foley catheter needed a minimum of 72 hours' aeration before clinical use.— T. Matsumoto *et al.*, *Archs Surg., Chicago*, 1968, *96*, 464.

After aeration at room temperature for 24 hours following sterilisation of polyethylene and polypropylene with ethylene oxide gas, the concentration of gas decreased from as much as 3.2 mg per g of plastic to about 200 µg per g and no significant toxicity was observed in the systems used for testing.— R. K. O'Leary *et al.*, *J. pharm. Sci.*, 1969, *58*, 1007.

Minimum aeration time was required for non-reinforced medical-grade silicone sheeting sterilised by ethylene oxide; however, dacron-reinforced silicone sheeting released the gas at a much slower rate and a mininum aeration time of 24 hours was recommended.— J. D. White and T. J. Bradley, *J. pharm. Sci.*, 1973, *62*, 1634.

Residues from materials sterilised with ethylene oxide and aerated at 50° for 8 hours caused less haemolysis of red blood cells than residues from materials aerated at room temperature for 24 hours.— D. A. Gunther, *Am. J. Hosp. Pharm.*, 1974, *31*, 558.

Further references: J. B. Stetson *et al.*, *Anethesiology*, 1976, *44*, 174.

Proprietary Preparations

Etox *(Rentokil, UK)*. A mixture of ethylene oxide 90% and carbon dioxide 10%.

Sterethox *(ICI Mond, UK)*. A mixture of ethylene oxide 12% w/w and dichlorodifluoromethane 88% w/w. For the sterilisation of medical and surgical equipment.

A mixture of ethylene oxide 10% and carbon dioxide 90% was formerly marketed in Great Britain under the proprietary name Cartox (*Rentokil*).

2245-v

Euflavine *(B.P.C. 1949)*. Neutral Acriflavine; Neutroflavin.

Pharmacopoeias. See under Acriflavine, p.548.

An orange-red or brownish-red powder with a faint odour and a very bitter taste. It consists of a mixture of 3,6-diamino-10-methylacridinium chloride and 3,6-diaminoacridine monohydrochloride. The latter is usually present to the extent of between 30 and 40%. Slightly **soluble** in water and alcohol; soluble 1 in 4 of warm water; practically insoluble in chloroform, ether, fixed oils, and liquid paraffin.

Euflavine has properties similar to other acridine derivatives (see p.573).

Vasectomy. The slow injection of 2.5 ml of 0.1% euflavine solution into the distal end of each vas deferens during vasectomy was considered sufficiently spermicidal to eliminate the need for examination of semen for non-motility or azoospermia.— D. Urquhart-Hay, *Br. med. J.*, 1973, *3*, 378. None of the 110 specimens reported on was completely aspermic. The need for 2 consecutive counts was emphasised.— L. N. Jackson (letter), *ibid.*, 589.

Spermatozoa were killed within 20 minutes in 0.1% euflavine at 30° *in vitro*. The injection of 2.5 ml of solution into the vas should be accompanied by the instruction not to urinate for 2½ to 3 hours. Sperm examinations should still be performed.— J. Slome (letter), *Br. med. J.*, 1973, *4*, 233.

In 200 vasectomies where 0.1% euflavine solution was used as spermicide, 2 definite and 2 probable failures occurred.— I. S. Edwards, *Med. J. Aust.*, 1977, *1*, 847.

Preparations

Euflavine Lint *(B.P.C. 1973)*. Absorbent lint impregnated with 0.08 to 0.2% of euflavine.

2246-g

Formaldehyde Solution *(B.P.)*. Formaldehydi Solutio; Formalin; Formol.

CAS — 50-00-0.

NOTE. The use of the name Formalin is limited; in some countries it is a trade-mark.

Pharmacopoeias. In all pharmacopoeias examined except *Braz.*, *Chin.*, *Eur.*, *Fr.*, and *Neth.* The specified content of formaldehyde varies slightly but is usually about the same as the *B.P.*

Formaldehyde Solution is an aqueous solution containing 34 to 38% w/w of CH_2O (= 30.03) with methyl alcohol as a stabilising agent to delay polymerisation of the formaldehyde to solid paraformaldehyde. The *U.S.P.* specifies not less than 36.5% of CH_2O. It is a colourless liquid with a characteristic, pungent, irritating odour and a burning taste. Wt per ml about 1.08 g. **Miscible** with water and alcohol; immiscible with chloroform and ether. **Incompatible** with ammonia, gelatin, phenols, and oxidising agents. **Store** in a moderately warm place (above 15°) in airtight containers. A slight white deposit may form on keeping and develops more rapidly if the solution is kept in a cold place. Protect from light.

NOTE. When a 1% solution of formaldehyde is prescribed 1 vol. of Formaldehyde Solution diluted to 100 vol. with water should be dispensed.

Solutions of formaldehyde 10% in propylene glycol or ethylene glycol were odourless. When diluted with water the solutions remained odourless; bactericidal and sporicidal activities of aqueous solutions were satisfactory.— R. Trujillo and K. F. Lindell, *Appl. Microbiol.*, 1973, *26*, 106.

Adverse Effects. Formaldehyde vapour is irritant to the eyes, nose, and respiratory tract, and may cause coughing, dysphagia, spasm of the larnyx, bronchitis, and pneumonia. Asthma has been reported after repeated exposure.

Concentrated solutions applied to the skin cause whitening and hardening. Contact dermatitis and sensitivity reactions have occured after the use of conventional concentrations and after contact with residual formaldehyde in resins.

Ingestion of formaldehyde solution causes intense pain, with inflammation, ulceration, and necrosis of mucous membranes. There may be vomiting, haematemesis, blood-stained diarrhoea, haematuria, and anuria; acidosis, vertigo, convulsions, and circulatory failure may occur. Death has occurred after the ingestion of about 30 ml. If the patient survives 48 hours, recovery is probable.

Maximum permissible atmospheric concentration 2 ppm.

A brief discussion on formaldehyde toxicity with special reference to industrial exposure.— *Lancet*, 1979, *2*, 620. General hazards of formaldehyde, including mention of Urea-formaldehyde foam insulation.— *Lancet*, 1981, *1*, 926. Correspondence.— D. D. Bryson (letter), *ibid.*, 1263; J. M. Berger and S. H. Lamm (letter), *ibid.*, 1264.

Irreversible ureteric obstruction occurred in a 73-year-old man with carcinoma of the bladder after treatment with formaldehyde solution to control bladder haemorrhage. Irrigation with formaldehyde solution (3.7% formaldehyde) had been successfully carried out 2 months previously.— P. G. Fishbein *et al.*, *J. Am. med. Ass.*, 1974, *228*, 872.

Haemolysis during chronic haemodialysis was due to formaldehyde eluted from filters.— E. P. Orringer and W. D. Mattern, *New Engl. J. Med.*, 1976, *294*, 1416.

Low concentrations of formaldehyde solution induced an antigenic change in human red blood cells which caused them to react with the anti-N sera found in certain patients undergoing haemodialysis. The use of formaldehyde for the sterilisation of home dialysis equipment might be implicated in changes in the patient's immune system and might be a possible cause of the failure of future renal grafts.— D. W. Gorst *et al.*, *J. clin. Path.*, 1977, *30*, 956.

Hypersensitivity. In a modified 'repeated-insult' patch test, 5% formaldehyde solution was found to produce strong sensitisation of the skin.— A. M. Kligman, *J. invest. Derm.*, 1966, *47*, 393.

Of 1205 persons with dermatitis or eczema submitted to patch testing with 2% aqueous solution of formaldehyde, 6.3% gave a positive reaction.— E. Rudzki and D. Kleniewska, *Br. J. Derm.*, 1970, *83*, 543.

Of 4000 patients subjected to patch testing in 5 European clinics 3.1% of males and 3.8% of females showed positive reactions to formaldehyde.— H. Bandmann *et al.*, *Archs Derm.*, 1972, *106*, 335.

For reports of formaldehyde-induced asthma, see D. J. Hendrick and D. J. Lane, *Br. med. J.*, 1975, *1*, 607; A. Sakula (letter), *Lancet*, 1975, *2*, 816; D. J. Hendrick and D. J. Lane, *Br. J. ind. Med.*, 1977, *34*, 11. See also *Lancet*, 1977, *1*, 790.

Further references: S. E. O'Quinn and C. B. Kennedy, *J. Am. med. Ass.*, 1965, *194*, 593; J. L. Danto, *Can. med. Ass. J.*, 1968, *98*, 652; F. N. Marzulli and H. I. Maibach, *J. Soc. cosmet. Chem.*, 1973, *24*, 399; Y. G. Al-Nashi and A. A. Al-Rubayi, *Br. dent. J.*, 1977, *142*, 52.

Carcinogenicity. Some evidence of nasal cancers in *rats* (but not in *mice*) exposed to formaldehyde vapours.— O. M. Jensen (letter), *Lancet*, 1980, *2*, 480. See also P. F. Infante *et al.* (letter), *ibid.*, 1981, *2*, 980; W. K. C. Morgan (letter), *ibid.*, 981.

Treatment of Adverse Effects. Contaminated skin should be washed with soap and water. After ingestion give water, milk, charcoal, and/or demulcents. Alleviate shock; acidosis may require the intravenous administration of sodium bicarbonate or sodium lactate. Dilute solutions of ammonia may be given to convert the formaldehyde to hexamine. The use of haemodialysis has been suggested.

Gastric lavage and emesis should be avoided if concentrated solutions have been ingested.

Absorption and Fate. Formaldehyde is rapidly metabolised to formic acid in the body tissues, especially in the liver and erythrocytes; the formic acid may then be excreted as carbon dioxide and water, excreted in the urine as formate, or metabolised to labile methyl groups.

Uses. Formaldehyde Solution is a disinfectant effective against vegetative bacteria, fungi, and many viruses, but it is only slowly effective against bacterial spores and acid-fast bacteria. Formaldehyde reacts with proteins, which may reduce its activity against micro-organisms. Its sporicidal effect is greatly increased by increase in temperature. It has little penetrating power and readily polymerises and condenses on surfaces.

The effectiveness of formaldehyde gas depends on dissolving in a film of moisture before acting on micro-organisms, and in practice a relative humidity of 75% is necessary.

When applied to the unbroken skin, formaldehyde hardens the epidermis, renders it tough and whitish, and produces a local anaesthetic effect.A solution containing Formaldehyde Solution 3% has been used for the treatment of warts on the palms of the hands and soles of the feet. Sweating of the feet may be treated by the application of 1 part of Formaldehyde Solution in 3 parts of glycerol or 5 to 10 parts of alcohol but such applications are liable to produce sensitisation reactions.

After surgical removal of hydatid cysts, diluted Formaldehyde Solution, 0.5 to 2% in water, may be used for irrigating the cavities to destroy scolices. It is generally too irritant for use on mucous membranes but it has been used in mouthwashes as an antiseptic and hardening agent for the gums. In dentistry it has been used as a paste with thymol, cresol, glycerol, and zinc oxide as a mummifying agent for residual pulp tissue, and with equal parts of cresol or creosote as a dressing for septic root canals.

Formaldehyde gas is used for the disinfection of rooms; a spray has also been used. When vaporisation is effected by heat, 500 ml of Formaldehyde Solution added to 1 litre of water is boiled in a stainless steel vessel over an electric hot-plate; this volume is sufficient for 30 m^3 of air space. Alternatively, 170 g of potassium permanganate added to 500 ml of Formaldehyde Solution will cause violent boiling within 10 seconds and the production of sufficient moist formaldehyde gas to disinfect the same cubic capacity. During fumigation, the room must be effectively sealed and maintained at a temperature above 18°; contact with the vapour must continue for more than 6 hours and preferably overnight.

Formaldehyde Solution does not damage metals or fabrics but it should not be used for their disinfection when other more reliable methods are possible. In the disinfection of blankets and bedding, it has been used as a vapour; the amount of Formaldehyde Solution used must allow for absorption by the materials. It has also been used as a solution for presoaking before laundering, and as part of a dry-cleaning process. Formaldehyde Solution is also used for the disinfection of the membranes in dialysis equipment.

Formaldehyde Solution 10% in saline is used as a preservative for pathological specimens. It is not suitable for preserving urine for subsequent examination.

In applications where a solid form is required, paraformaldehyde is used (see p.570).

The use of formaldehyde in cosmetics and toiletries is restricted in Great Britain under The Cosmetics Products Regulations 1978 (SI 1978: No. 1354).

The bactericidal activity of formaldehyde adsorbed on various surfaces was greatest at 83% relative humidity. Cotton had a greater affinity for formaldehyde than either glass or stainless steel. Formaldehyde 15 to 27 µg per ml was bacteriostatic in nutrient broth and concentrations greater than 27 µg per ml were bactericidal.— J. R. Braswell *et al.*, *Appl. Microbiol.*, 1970, *20*, 765.

Studies on formaldehyde-steam sterilisation: V. Handlos, *Arch. Pharm. Chemi, scient. Edn*, 1979, *7*, 1 and 12.

Disinfection of blankets and bedding. Formaldehyde disinfection was most effective when applied at a high formaldehyde concentration, high temperature, and a relative humidity of 80 to 90%. Mycobacteria were rather more resistant to formaldehyde than micrococci, and *Bacillus subtilis* spores were 2 or 3 times more resistant than micrococci. Smallpox crusts were not sterilised even after exposure to formaldehyde vapour for 24 hours. Formaldehyde gas could not be recommended for the disinfection of fabrics contaminated with smallpox virus or anthrax spores or for the disinfection of articles contaminated with tubercle bacilli. Materials should be arranged to allow the best possible access of the gas to all surfaces. Fabrics absorbed much formaldehyde, though this effect was lessened with temperatures reaching 100°.—Committee on Formaldehyde Disinfection of the Public Health Laboratory Service, *J. Hyg., Camb.*, 1958, *56*, 488.

For further references to the use of Formaldehyde Solution in the disinfection of blankets and bedding, see *Chemical disinfection of hospital woollen blankets in laundering*, Joint Report by British Launderers' Research Association and the International Wool Secretariat, April 1962; J. C. Dickinson and R. E. Wagg, *J. appl. Bact.*, 1967, *30*, 340; V. G. Alder *et al.*, *J. appl. Bact.*, 1971, *34*, 757.

Disinfection of dental cones. A cold technique using a solution of formaldehyde 48.5%, cresol 48.5%, and glycerol 3% (formocresol) was considered effective for the sterilisation of gutta percha dental cones. Exposure of contaminated cones to the vapour from this solution in a closed atmosphere rendered *Staphylococcus aureus, Corynebacterium striatum, Bacillus subtilis, Escherichia coli*, and *Streptococcus faecalis* nonviable in 16 hours.— E. S. Senia *et al.*, *J. Am. dent. Ass.*, 1977, *94*, 887.

Disinfection of equipment. Formaldehyde in low-temperature steam was an efficient sterilising agent comparable with ethylene oxide. Penetration into narrow tubes was poor. Most fabrics, plastics, and instruments were unharmed. The exposures routinely used were 2 hours at 80° for deep penetration, and 2 hours at 70° for shallow penetration. Five ml of 38% formaldehyde solution was used for each ft^3 of autoclave space and the air was evacuated.— V. G. Alder *et al.*, *J. clin. Path.*, 1966, *19*, 83.

The 400-litre tanks of a haemodialysis machine were sterilised with Formaldehyde Solution 1% in hot water. The formalin was removed with 3 rinses, each of 100 litres, of softened tap water. The rinsing process was adjudged satisfactory when the washings failed to reduce a Clinitest tablet.— E. Bowers (letter), *Lancet*, 1967, *1*, 44.

Surfaces of ampoules and some equipment used to maintain a newborn infant free from micro-organisms were sterilised with a solution containing Formaldehyde Solution 10% and Tego 1% followed by a solution of peracetic acid 2%.— R. D. Barnes *et al.*, *Lancet*, 1969, *1*, 168.

For a favourable report of the use of formaldehyde and steam at 80° for the disinfection of endoscopes, see V. G. Alder *et al.*, *Br. med. J.*, 1971, *3*, 677.

Disinfection of rooms. For a discussion of the practical aspects of the disinfection of rooms with formaldehyde, see *Mon. Bull. Minist. Hlth*, 1958, *17*, 270.

In a test, 750 ml of Formaldehyde Solution with 225 g of potassium permangante for vaporisation was used to disinfect a 1500-ft^3 room. Though an adequate formaldehyde concentration (1 mg per litre) was produced the relative humidity remained too low. It was recommended that the official method should be modified by doubling the quantity of formaldehyde solution; each 500 ml of solution required 170 g of potassium permanganate, but if possible part of the formaldehyde should be vapourised by heat.— M. M. Beeby *et al.*, *J. Hyg., Camb.*, 1967, *65*, 115.

Disinfection of rooms contaminated by smallpox virus could be achieved by exposure to formaldehyde vapour—by boiling 500 ml of commercial formalin solution with 1 litre of water for each 30 m^3 or by adding permanganate 170 to 200 g to a similar solution.— Second Report of the WHO Expert Committee on Smallpox Eradication, *Tech. Rep. Ser. Wld Hlth Org. No. 493*, 1972. Advice on virus disinfection including the use of formaldehyde.— Department of Health and Social Security and the Welsh Office, *Memorandum on the Control of Outbreaks of Smallpox*, London, HM Stationery Office, 1975. See also *Memorandum on the Control of Outbreaks of Smallpox*, Edinburgh, HM Stationery Office, 1976.

For the limited effectiveness of formaldehyde fumigation against virus-infected cockroaches, see C. A. Bartzokas *et al.*, *J. Hyg., Camb.*, 1978, *80*, 125.

Neoplasm of the bladder. Intravesical instillation of 10% formalin under general anaesthesia proved a satisfactory method of dealing with bleeding and strangury of inoperable carcinoma of the bladder. No permanent side-effects or complications had been observed. Repeated courses of treatment had been used for symptomatic relapses.— R. B. Brown, *Med. J. Aust.*, 1969, *1*, 23. A further reference.— C. Servadio and I. Nissenkorn, *Cancer*, 1976, *37*, 900.

See also under Adverse Effects.

Storage of allografts. For the storage of bone and cartilage allografts in formaldehyde solutions, see N. A. Preobrazhensky and V. D. Melanin, *Archs Otolar.*, 1977, *103*, 567.

Use of disinfectants on farms. In Great Britain, Formaldehyde Solution diluted 1 in 10 with water is an approved disinfectant for foot-and-mouth disease and swine vesicular disease under the Diseases of Animals (Approved Disinfectants) Order 1978 (SI 1978: No. 32), as amended (SI 1978: No. 934).

Warts. Results of a retrospective survey of 446 children and a prospective survey of 200 children indicated that the advantages of formalin therapy for plantar warts are considerable, but it must be remembered that technique is all-important. In the initial stages of treatment 3% formalin solution was used. The patient was instructed to remove scale and dead tissue from the top of the wart by scraping with a nail-file or the side of the blade of a pair of scissors. The wart-bearing portion of the sole was then soaked in the 3% formalin solution for 15 to 20 minutes (stressing that the wart must not be placed in contact with the bottom of the receptacle). The whole process was repeated each night. To avoid the development of interdigital cracks due to hardening of the skin, if the warts were near toe clefts the patients were instructed to place a little soft paraffin between the toes before starting treatment. If there was little hardening of the skin after 3 weeks of treatment, the concentration of formalin was increased to 5%, 7% or even 10%. As a result of the survey in all 646 children, it was shown that formalin foot-soaks used each night for 6 to 8 weeks will cure 80% of all plantar warts up to 1 cm in diameter. Larger warts should be curetted after 3 weeks of treatment with formalin. By these means the recurrence and reinfection rates are reduced to extremely low levels; in addition the method is simple and painless.— C. F. H. Vickers, *Br. med. J.*, 1961, *2*, 743. Comment.— *ibid.*, 1972, *2*, 586 (5%). See also M. H. Bunney, *Drugs*, 1977, *13*, 445 (solution, gel, or ointment in strengths varying from 3 to 20%).

Preparations

Dowling's Wart Paint *(Bristol Roy. Infirm.)*. Formaldehyde solution 5 ml, salicylic acid 12 g, acetone 12 ml, flexible collodion to 100 ml.

Formaldehyde and Salicylic Acid Paint *(A.P.F.)*. Formaldehyde solution 10 ml, salicylic acid 10 g, acetone 40 ml, alcohol (90%) to 100 ml. For warts.

Formaldehyde Lotion *(A.P.F.)*. Formalin Lotion. Formaldehyde solution 3 ml, water to 100 ml. It must be freshly prepared.

Formaldehyde Mouth-wash *(B.P.C. 1959)*. Collut. Formaldehyd. Formaldehyde solution 3.13 ml, peppermint water to 100 ml. To be diluted with 10 times its vol. of warm water before use.

Amended formula. Formaldehyde solution 3 ml, peppermint water to 100 ml.—*Compendium of Past Formulae 1933 to 1966*, London, The National Pharmaceutical Union, 1969.

Formaldehyde Solution with Soap *(B.P.C. 1934)*. Liq. Formaldehyd. Sap. Formaldehyde solution 20 ml, soft soap 40 g, alcohol (90%) (or industrial methylated spirit, suitably diluted) 30 ml, water to 100 ml. A disinfectant and deodorant solution.

Similar solutions, sometimes perfumed with lavender, are included in several pharmacopoeias.

Formalin Water *(Jap. P.)*. Aqua Formalinata. A 1% w/v solution of formaldehyde (CH_2O) in water.

Pict's Solution *(Aberdeen Roy. Infirm.)*. Formaldehyde solution 250 ml, sodium chloride 4 g, sodium bicarbonate 8 g, sodium sulphate 20 g, water to 2250 ml. Shelf-life 1 year. For preservation of tissue specimens.

Proprietary Preparations

Emoform *(Pharmaceutical Mfg, UK)*. A toothpaste containing formaldehyde solution 1.3%. For hypersensitive teeth. **Emoform Mouth Bath.** Contains formaldehyde solution 1.626%, sodium chloride 8%, potassium sulphate 0.652%, sodium phosphate 0.325%, sodium sulphate 0.28%, sodium fluoride 0.05%, and chlorbutol 0.04%.

Veracur Gel *(Typharm, UK)*. Contains formaldehyde solution 1.5% in a water-miscible basis. For warts. *Directions.* Apply twice daily and cover with plaster; protect surrounding skin with soft paraffin.

Other Proprietary Names

Formitrol *(Ital., Spain, Switz.)*; Lysoform *(Ger., Neth.)*.

2247-q

Acid Fuchsine. Acid Magenta; Acid Roseine; Acid Rubine; CI Acid Violet 19; Colour Index No. 42685.

The disodium or diammonium salt of the trisulphonic acid of magenta.

Glistening green granules or a dark red powder. **Soluble** in water; practically insoluble in alcohol. A 1% solution in water has a pH of about 5.

Acid fuchsine is used as a microscopic stain. It was formerly used in the treatment of vaginal infections.

Preparations containing acid fuchsine were formerly marketed in Great Britain under the proprietary name Pruvagol (*Norgine*).

2248-p

Glutaraldehyde.

Glutaral; Glutaric Dialdehyde. Pentane-1,5-dial.

$C_5H_8O_2$=100.1.

CAS — 111-30-8.

A liquid. **Soluble** in water and alcohol. Solutions

in water are slightly acid and are stable for long periods when stored in a cool place. Alkaline solutions rapidly lose activity; when buffered at pH 7.5 to 8.5 they are stable for about 2 weeks.

Adverse Effects. As for Formaldehyde Solution, p.563.

Glutaraldehyde is less irritant to skin and mucous membranes than formaldehyde but it may cause dermatitis and sensitisation.

Maximum permissible atmospheric concentration 0.2 ppm.

Hypersensitivity. A report of 5 patients with contact dermatitis due to glutaraldehyde. Three were dental assistants using glutaraldehyde for sterilisation and 2 were using it dermatologically. All patients also had positive patch tests to glutaraldehyde-tanned leather although it had been thought that the glutaraldehyde was irreversibly bound to leather collagen.— W. P. Jordan *et al.*, *Archs Derm.*, 1972, *105*, 94. A similar report.— K. V. Sanderson and E. Cronin (letter), *Br. med. J.*, 1968, *3*, 802.

Of 9 subjects sensitised to glutaraldehyde 6 showed an allergic response when challenged by patch test a year later. Each of these 6 tolerated the application of 25% glutaraldehyde to the sole of the foot for 7 days, while each of 5 tested developed severe dermatitis within 48 hours when 2.5% glutaraldehyde was applied to the antecubital fossa.— H. I. Maibach and S. D. Prystowsky, *Archs Derm.*, 1977, *113*, 170.

Uses. Glutaraldehyde is a disinfectant which is rapidly effective against vegetative forms of Gram-positive and Gram-negative bacteria. It is also effective against acid-fast bacteria, bacterial spores, some fungi, and viruses. Aqueous solutions show optimum activity between pH 7.5 and 8.5, though solutions at acid pH values are more stable. The activity of glutaraldehyde is reported to be unaffected by up to 20% of serum.

A 2% aqueous solution buffered to pH 7.5 to 8.5 is used for the sterilisation of endoscopic instruments, thermometers, rubber or plastic equipment, and for other equipment which cannot be sterilised by heat. Complete immersion in the solution for 15 to 20 minutes is sufficient for rapid disinfection of thoroughly cleansed instruments but exposure for 10 hours is necessary for sterilisation.

A 5 or 10% solution is used for the treatment of warts; it should not be used for facial or anogenital warts.

Glutaraldehyde was used as a tanning agent for leather.— W. P. Jordan *et al.*, *Archs Derm.*, 1972, *105*, 94.

In 2 patients with localised epidermolysis bullosa topical application of glutaraldehyde 10% was beneficial but irritation and skin sensitisation limited its use.— J. P. DesGroseilliers and P. Brisson, *Archs Derm.*, 1974, *109*, 70.

Antimicrobial activity. Sterility was attained in 20 minutes when catheters and cystoscopes, previously immersed in water containing 'mixed organisms', were immersed in a 2% solution of glutaraldehyde (Cidex) but when 50% blood was added to the water containing contaminating organisms, some organisms survived.— P. W. Ross, *J. clin. Path.*, 1966, *19*, 318.

An aqueous 2% solution of glutaraldehyde adjusted to pH 8 with 0.3% sodium bicarbonate was rapidly bactericidal against spores of *Bacillus anthracis* and *Clostridium tetani* and a 1% solution acted more quickly than a 4% solution of formaldehyde. A 0.05% alkaline solution rapidly killed Gram-negative and Gram-positive bacteria; 1 and 2% solutions were not appreciably affected by 10% serum or 2.5% yeast. Glutaraldehyde in 2% alkaline solution was slowly bactericidal to *Myobacterium tuberculosis* but was less effective than formaldehyde, iodine, alcohol, or Sudol; 3 hours or more should be allowed for sterilisation. It was also effective against *Trichophyton interdigitale* but less effective against *Aspergillus niger*. Glutaraldehyde was much more effective at pH 8 than at pH 4 and potency increased with temperature. After storage for a month, a 2% alkaline solution lost half its activity against *B. anthracis* spores. Alkaline glutaraldehyde was as active in 70% v/v isopropyl alcohol as in water, but less active in 70% v/v alcohol.— S. D. Rubbo *et al.*, *J. appl. Bact.*, 1967, *30*, 78.

A 1% solution of glutaraldehyde was fungicidal to 17 species of fungi including 3 yeasts known to cause nail infections.— N. Dabrowa *et al.*, *Archs Derm.*, 1972, *105*, 555.

The increased activity of glutaraldehyde at alkaline pH was not due to any change in the free aldehyde equilibrium with pH but was considered to result from an effect of alkali on the bacterial surface.— J. A. King *et al.*, *J. pharm. Sci.*, 1974, *63*, 804.

Glutaraldehyde solution 2% effectively disinfected stainless steel cylinders, neoprene O rings, and polyvinyl tubing infected with *Bacillus subtilis, Escherichia coli, Pseudomonas aeruginosa, Staphylococcus aureus, Clostridium sporogenes,* and *Mycobacterium smegmatis*.— W. -D. Leers *et al.*, *Can. J. Hosp. Pharm.*, 1974, *27*, 17.

At pH 7.9 glutaraldehyde solution 0.5% reduced by 99.99% the viable counts of 4 species of filamentous fungi and the yeast *Saccharomyces cerevisiae*, after contact for 90 minutes.— S. P. Gorman and E. M. Scott, *J. appl. Bact.*, 1977, *43*, 83.

A study of the surface disinfectant effect of glutaraldehyde in the gas-aerosol phase at different humidities and temperatures. At a temperature of 22 to 27° and a relative humidity of 80%, glutaraldehyde in a gas-aerosol concentration of 15 to 20 mg per m^3 reduced the viable count of *Escherichia coli, Pseudomonas aeruginosa, Micrococcus luteus, Serratia marcescens, Staphylococcus aureus,* and *Streptococcus faecium* by 90% within 5 minutes and similarly reduced the spore count of *Bacillus subtilis* subsp. *niger, B. cereus,* and *B. megaterium* in 45 minutes. In spite of its low volatility glutaraldehyde was more effective than formaldehyde.— Å. Bovallius and P. Ånäs, *Appl. & environ. Microbiol.*, 1977, *34*, 129.

Further reference: J. S. Kuipers and T. F. J. Tromp, *Pharm. Weekbl. Ned.*, 1973, *108*, 169.

Dental use. Glutaraldehyde in conjunction with calcium hydroxide as an effective pulp dressing after pulpotomy.— D. R. Hannah, *Br. dent. J.*, 1972, *132*, 227.

Disinfection of equipment. Glutaraldehyde solution after 10 hours left an aldehyde residue which created problems on delicate plastic instruments.— R. M. G. Boucher, *Am. J. Hosp. Pharm.*, 1972, *29*, 661.

A 2.5% buffered solution of glutaraldehyde eradicated *Pseudomonas aeruginosa* from endoscopes in all of 5 tests following disinfection for 15 minutes whereas alcohol 70% was not considered satisfactory.— A. T. R. Axon *et al.*, *Lancet*, 1974, *1*, 656.

Glutaraldehyde 0.025 and 0.125% prevented germination of *Bacillus subtilis* and *B. pumilus* spores, while concentrations of 2% were sporicidal.— S. Thomas and A. D. Russell, *J. appl. Bact.*, 1974, *37*, 83.

Complete disinfection of anaesthetic apparatus using buffered glutaraldehyde (Cidex) was only possible when the apparatus was dismantled and air totally eliminated.— R. H. George, *Br. J. Anaesth.*, 1975, *47*, 719.

Description of a rapid and simple method for the disinfection of endoscopic equipment between successive examinations by immersion for 2 minutes in an activated 2% aqueous solution of glutaraldehyde (Cidex). Cleaning with tap water or an aqueous solution of 1% cetrimide and 0.1% chlorhexidine was inadequate.— D. L. Carr-Locke and P. Clayton, *Gut*, 1978, *19*, 916. Serious problems with staff sensitivity.— A. T. R. Axon *et al.*, *Lancet*, 1981, *1*, 1093.

A study of the absorption of glutaraldehyde by various types of plastic and rubber tubing after exposure to a 2% alkaline buffered solution. Absorption was generally greater for rubber tubing than plastic tubing, being highest in silicone rubber, latex rubber, and polyvinyl chloride. There was no accumulation of glutaraldehyde in polyvinyl chloride or silicone rubber tubing after repeat exposures to the solution but residual amounts did increase in latex rubber. A single 10-minute rinse in water appeared to reduce the amount of residual glutaraldehyde in most materials tested to a concentration which gave a sufficient level on safety for acute toxicity on blood cells but immersion in water for 2 hours or more was required to reduce concentrations in polyvinyl chloride, latex rubber, and silicone rubber to any significant extent. Careful washing and extended soaking procedures to remove glutaraldehyde prior to repeated treatment was recommended for materials like latex rubber that accumulated glutaraldehyde.— B. Osterberg, *Arch. Pharm. Chemi, scient. Edn*, 1978, *6*, 241.

Discussions on the useful life of acid and alkaline solutions of glutaraldehyde and their corrosive effects on equipment: G. Ayliffe *et al.* (letter), *Br. med. J.*, 1979, *1*, 1019; T. D. Duffy and E. G. P. Powell (letter), *ibid.*, 1426; R. M. G. Boucher (letter), *ibid.*, *2*, 444; A. C. Mair (letter), *ibid.*, 673; J. A. King (letter), *ibid.*, 797; R. M. G. Boucher (letter), *ibid.*, 1440; A. C. Mair, *ibid.*, 1980, *280*, 403.

For the use of glutaraldehyde in renal dialysis units, see Strong Sodium Hypochlorite Solution, p.574.

Hyperhidrosis. Glutaraldehyde 10% solution, applied on alternate evenings, was moderately effective for hyperhidrosis of the feet but it stained the skin yellow and occasionally caused allergic hypersensitivity.— *Br. med. J.*, 1978, *2*, 1479.

Earlier references: L. Juhlin and H. Hansson, *Archs Derm.*, 1968, *97*, 327; W. Frain-Bell, *Practitioner*, 1969, *202*, 79; K. Sato and R. L. Dobson, *Archs Derm.*, 1969, *100*, 564.

Onychomycosis. A 10% aqueous solution of glutaraldehyde was applied to 21 toe-nails on 4 patients with onychomycosis. Superficial infection was eliminated after 4 to 6 weeks' treatment. Whole-thickness infection of the nail required 4 months' treatment.— D. W. R. Suringa, *Archs Derm.*, 1970, *102*, 163.

Warts. An unbuffered solution of glutaraldehyde 25% was successful in the treatment of warts.— I. D. London (letter), *Archs Derm.*, 1971, *104*, 440. Glutaraldehyde 10% buffered with sodium bicarbonate to pH 7.5 could be applied daily to plantar warts. This treatment was painless but lengthy.— *Br. med. J.*, 1972, *3*, 170.

Glutaraldehyde 10% in an aqueous alcoholic solution was an effective and convenient treatment for warts.— C. F. Allenby, *Br. J. clin. Pract.*, 1977, *31*, 12.

Further references: *Drug & Ther. Bull.*, 1977, *15*, 97.

Preparations

Glutaral Concentrate *(U.S.P.)*. A solution of glutaraldehyde 50% w/w in water. pH 3.7 to 4.5. Store at a temperature not exceeding 40° in airtight containers. Protect from light.

Glutaral Disinfectant Solution *(U.S.N.F.)*. A solution containing glutaraldehyde. pH 2.7 to 3.7. Store at a temperature not exceeding 40° in airtight containers. Protect from light.

Proprietary Preparations

ASEP *(Galen, UK)*. A 2% solution of glutaraldehyde to which an activating liquid is added before use to make a buffered solution, which is stable for 14 days; a corrosion inhibitor is included.

Cidex *(Surgikos, UK)*. A 2% solution of glutaraldehyde to which an activating powder is added before use to make a buffered alkaline solution, which is stable for 14 days; the activator also acts as a corrosion inhibitor. **Cidex Long-Life.** A similar solution for use up to 28 days.

Glutarol *(Dermal Laboratories, UK)*. Glutaraldehyde, available as a 10% solution. For warts.

Pantasept *(Adroka, Switz.: Martindale Samoore, UK)*. A concentrated liquid containing glutaraldehyde 30%. For disinfection of ophthalmic instruments.

Totacide 28 *(Tenneco, UK)*. A 2% solution of glutaraldehyde to which an activating liquid is added before use to make a buffered alkaline solution, which is stable for 28 days; the activator also acts as a corrosion inhibitor.

Verucasep *(Galen, UK)*. Glutaraldehyde, available as a 10% water-miscible gel. For warts.

Other Proprietary Names

Sonacide *(USA)*; Sterihyde *(Jap.)*.

2249-s

Halazone *(U.S.P., B.P.C. 1954)*. Halazonum; Pantocide. 4-(Dichlorosulphamoyl)benzoic acid. $C_7H_5Cl_2NO_4S$=270.1.

CAS — 80-13-7.

Pharmacopoeias. In *Nord., Rus.*, and *U.S.*

A white crystalline powder with a strong odour of chlorine, containing about 52% of 'available chlorine' (see p.557). M.p. about 194° with decomposition.

Very slightly **soluble** in water, chloroform, and ether; soluble 1 in 140 of alcohol; soluble in glacial acetic acid and aqueous solutions of alkali hydroxides and carbonates. Solutions are unstable and rapidly lose chlorine. **Store** in airtight containers. Protect from light.

Uses. Halazone has the properties of chlorine (see p.557) in aqueous solution and is used for the disinfection of drinking water. One tablet containing 4 mg of halazone, with sodium carbonate and sodium chloride, is sufficient to treat about a litre of water (500 ml for heavily contaminated water), in about 30 minutes to 1 hour. The taste of residual chlorine may be removed by adding sodium thiosulphate.

The addition of halazone to river water in concentrations ranging from 1 to 50 mg per litre reduced the bacterial counts on average by 73 to 99% after 48 hours' incubation. At concentrations of less than 1 mg per litre the bacterial counts usually increased.— H. W. Hackenberg, *Bull. Hyg., Lond.*, 1964, *39*, 1062.

Preparations

Halazone Tablets for Solution *(U.S.P.)*. Solution-tablets containing halazone. One 4-mg tablet in 200 ml of water has a pH of not less than 7. Protect from light.

Tabulettae Pantocidi *(Rus. P.)*. Pantocide Tablets. Each contains halazone 8.2 mg, anhydrous sodium carbonate 3.6 mg, and sodium chloride 108.2 mg.

2250-h

Hexachlorophane *(B.P., B.P. Vet.)*. Hexachlorophene *(U.S.P.)*; G 11. 2,2′-Methylenebis(3,4,6-trichlorophenol).

$C_{13}H_6Cl_6O_2$=406.9.

CAS — 70-30-4.

Pharmacopoeias. In *Arg., Aust., Br., Braz., Hung., Ind., Jug., Nord., Swiss,* and *U.S.*

A white or pale buff tasteless crystalline powder which is odourless or has a slight phenolic odour. M.p. 161° to 167°.

Practically **insoluble** in water; soluble 1 in 3.5 of alcohol, 1 in less than 1 of acetone, and 1 in less than 1 of ether; soluble, possibly with turbidity, in chloroform; soluble in dilute solutions of alkali hydroxides; soluble, with the aid of heat, in vegetable oils. **Sterilise** by dry heat (but see m.p.). **Store** in airtight containers. Protect from light.

For precautions to be taken in preparing and storing antiseptic solutions, see under Phenol, p.570.

Activity and inactivation in solution. The antibacterial activity of hexachlorophane was reduced in the presence of polysorbate 80.— S. H. Hopper and K. M. Wood, *J. Am. pharm. Ass., scient. Edn*, 1958, *47*, 317.

Hexachlorophane was incompatible with benzalkonium chloride. The maximum loss of activity occurred at an approximate equimolar concentration of each component.— G. Walter and W. Gump, *J. pharm. Sci.*, 1962, *51*, 770.

The antibacterial activity of hexachlorophane was reduced in alkaline media. Products including hexachlorophane should have a pH between 5 and 6. Reduction in pH from 8 to 6 caused a fourfold increase in antibacterial activity. In addition, preparations should not contain large amounts of nonionic surfactants, which depressed or inactivated hexachlorophane completely.— G. Walter and W. Gump, *Soap chem. Spec.*, 1963, *39* (July), 55.

Phenylmercuric acetate and nitromersal enhanced the effect of hexachlorophane against *Candida albicans, Staphylococcus aureus, Escherichia coli, Bacillus subtilis,* and *Streptococcus faecalis, in vitro.* A vanishing cream containing hexachlorophane 0.5% and phenylmercuric acetate 0.05% was more effective than a similar cream containing only hexachlorophane 0.5% when tested *in vivo* against *Microsporum canis* and *Trichophyton mentagrophytes*.— F. S. Barr *et al.*, *J. pharm. Sci.*, 1970, *59*, 262.

Discoloration of detergent solutions. Hexachlorophane was extremely sensitive to iron, and to avoid discoloration due to traces of this metal in the detergent, it was advisable to incorporate a sequestrant such as disodium edetate (0.1 to 0.5%).— M. Bell, *Specialities*, 1965, *1*, 16.

Adverse Effects. Following ingestion, anorexia, nausea, vomiting, diarrhoea, abdominal pain, dehydration, shock, confusion, cyanosis, and anuria may occur. Convulsions and coma may follow. Central nervous stimulation and convulsions have occurred after absorption of hexachlorophane from burns and damaged skin.

Photosensitivity and skin sensitisation have occurred occasionally after repeated use of hexachlorophane.

There have been reports showing that hexachlorophane can be absorbed through the skin of infants in amounts sufficient to produce spongy lesions of the brain, sometimes fatal; the reports are not unanimous. In some countries, preparations containing more than a specified percentage of hexachlorophane are available only on medical prescription. Also in some countries the concentration of hexachlorophane in cosmetics is limited to 0.1% as a preservative, and such preparations may not be used for babies or for personal hygiene.

Reviews of the toxicity of hexachlorophane.— R. D. Kimbrough, *Archs envir. Hlth*, 1971, *23*, 119; *Br. med. J.*, 1972, *1*, 705; *Can. med. Ass. J.*, 1973, *108*, 1475; V. D. Plueckhahn, *Drugs*, 1973, *5*, 97; E. G. McQueen, *ibid.*, 154; *Adverse Drug React. Bull.*, 1974, Feb., 144.

A woman who had accidentally ingested 200 ml of a detergent emulsion containing hexachlorophane 3% prior to an abdominal hysterectomy vomited once during the operation and once afterwards. The following day she became febrile and later lethargic and confused and died despite antibiotic and corticosteroid therapy. The concentration of hexachlorophane in the blood was 35 µg per ml.— L. D. Henry and V. J. DiMaio, *Milit. Med.*, 1974, *139*, 41.

A 10-year-old boy died from hexachlorophane toxicity following extensive topical treatment with hexachlorophane for a 25% burn. Late symptoms included hyperthermia, weakness of the lower extremities, and cerebral oedema.— R. Chilcote *et al.*, *Pediatrics*, 1977, *59*, 457.

Eighteen children, aged 3 months to 3 years, were admitted to hospital [in 1972] after application to the napkin area several times daily of a dusting-powder containing, in error, hexachlorophane 6%. Symptoms included severe erythema of the napkin area, anorexia, vomiting, fever, agitation, drowsiness, coma, tremor, abnormal movements, ocular involvement, intracranial hypertension, acute transverse myelitis, leg paralysis, paraplegia, and abnormalities of the EEG. Four children died within 3 to 5 days; in 2 subjected to necropsy brain weight was increased, the spinal cord was swollen, and there was massive cystic spongiosis. Of the survivors 2 had spastic paraplegia, one had bilateral pyramidal signs, and 11 apparently recovered completely.— F. Goutières and J. Aicardi, *Br. med. J.*, 1977, *2*, 663.

An 8-day-old child was accidentally fed 10 to 15 ml of a 3% solution of hexachlorophane (pHisohex). The child immediately spit up milky fluid and later had diarrhoea and began vomiting. Treatment with gastric lavage and aspiration was given and activated charcoal was left in the stomach. Six hours after ingestion the child was lethargic and poorly responsive to painful stimulation. Two hours later the child had facial twitching. Jitteriness and excitability increased over the first 12 to 18 hours but had notably diminished by day 3 and had disappeared entirely at the time of discharge at 14 days. There were no sequelae at follow-up at 2½ years of age.— J. Herskowitz and N. P. Rosman, *J. Pediat.*, 1979, *94*, 495.

A 31-year-old woman developed severe bilateral optic atrophy without any other systemic evidence of neurotoxicity after taking 10 to 15 ml of hexachlorophane emulsion (pHisohex) daily for 10 to 11 months. She had also applied large amounts to her face every day.— T. L. Slamovits *et al.*, *Am. J. Ophthal.*, 1980, *89*, 676.

Aphthous ulcers. Toothpastes or mouth-washes containing hexachlorophane softened the oral epithelium and could cause aphthous ulcers.— G. Y. Caldwell, *Practitioner*, 1970, *204*, 581.

Brain damage. R.D. Kimbrough and T.B. Gaines (*Archs environ. Hlth*, 1971, *23*, 114) reported cystic vacuolation in the white matter of the brains of *rats* fed hexachlorophane 25 mg per kg body-weight daily, and E.R. Hart *et al.* (*Toxic. appl. Pharmac.*, 1974, *29*, 117) reported similar effects in *monkeys*. There have been a number of reports of vacuolation of the brain in newborn infants washed with hexachlorophane, though the condition has also been seen in infants apparently not exposed to hexachlorophane. V.D. Plueckhahn and R.D. Collins (*Med. J. Aust.*, 1976, *1*, 815) reported that infants at risk of vacuolation were premature infants weighing 2 kg or less at birth who received 3 or more washings with hexachlorophane. However, they followed more than 800 premature infants, most of whom underwent total body washing with hexachlorophane 3% on 4 or more occasions (and who were therefore considered at risk of developing CNS vacuolation), and considered that the children's progress had not been adversely affected. There have been reports of increased neonatal staphylococcal infection since the use of hexachlorophane has been restricted. Opinion remains divided.

References: G. A. Hall and I. M. Reid (letter), *Lancet*, 1972, *2*, 1251; H. Powell *et al.*, *J. Pediat.*, 1973, *82*, 976; R. M. Shuman *et al.*, *Morb. Mortal.*, 1973, *22*, 93; *idem*, *Pediatrics*, 1974, *54*, 689; *idem*, *Archs Neurol., Chicago*, 1975, *32*, 320; V. D. Plueckhahn, *Med. J. Aust.*, 1973, *1*, 93; *idem*, *Pediatrics*, 1973, *51*, 368; V. D. Plueckhahn and R. B. Collins, *Med. J. Aust.*, 1976, *1*, 815; J. M. Gowdy and A. G. Ulsamer, *Am. J. Dis. Child.*, 1976, *130*, 247.

The toxicity and effectiveness of hexachlorophane in the prevention of sepsis in neonatal units.— J. G. Kensit, *J. Antimicrob. Chemother.*, 1975, *1*, 263; V. D. Plueckhahn *et al.*, *Med. J. Aust.*, 1978, *2*, 555; V. D. Plueckhahn, *Aust. J. Hosp. Pharm.*, 1979, *9*, 84.

A review of the possible toxicity of hexachlorophane in neonates.— *Br. med. J.*, 1977, *1*, 337. Comments.— B. D. Corner *et al.* (letter), *ibid.*, 636; E. G. McQueen and D. G. Ferry (letter), *ibid.*, 637; M. D. Young and G. Treadway, *Winthrop* (letter), *ibid.*, 904; J. M. Gowdy (letter), *ibid.*, 1977, *2*, 1353.

Dermatitis. Scrotal dermatitis in 6 patients attributed to particles of hexachlorophane precipitated in bath water.— H. Baker and M. J. Lloyd (letter), *Br. J. Derm.*, 1967, *79*, 727. A similar report in 10 patients.— H. Baker *et al.*, *Archs Derm.*, 1969, *99*, 693.

Hexachlorophane caused primary irritation in open and closed patch tests when a concentration of 0.5% was incorporated in paraffin, propylene glycol, or olive oil.— *Drug Cosmet. Ind.*, 1972, *111* (July), 38.

Hexachlorophane 0.1% in propylene glycol caused primary irritation in 17 of 72 subjects when closed patch test methods were used, but concentrations of 10% in olive oil, isopropyl myristate, paraffin, and macrogol did not cause irritation (propylene glycol alone caused irritation by closed patch test). In *animals* hexachlorophane had a more potent primary irritancy than any other halogenated compound studied.— F. Morikawa *et al.*, *J. Soc. cosmet. Chem.*, 1974, *25*, 113.

Further references: D. S. Wilkinson, *Contact Dermatitis*, 1978, *4*, 172 (scrotal dermatitis).

Pregnancy and the neonate. According to H. Halling, in 6 hospitals in Sweden there were 25 severe foetal malformations and 46 minor deformities among 460 births to nurses who washed their hands 10 to 60 times a day with hexachlorophane 0.5% liquid soap or pHisohex (3%). The incidence (15%) was much higher than that (3%) in the general Swedish population, and than that (3.4%) in 233 nurses who did not use hexachlorophane.— *J. Am. med. Ass.*, 1978, *240*, 513. The cases quoted were composed of 'clusters' of malformation and were not selected because of exposure to hexachlorophane; in other hospitals the outcome of pregnancy was comparable with that in the general population. The malformation-rate (3%) in the general population referred to serious malformations.— B. Källén (letter), *ibid.*, 1585. A study conducted by the Swedish National Board of Health and Welfare in 30 048 infants born during 1973-75 to women employed in hospitals also found a 'cluster' of seriously malformed infants similar to those found by H. Halling *et al.* but failed to identify any likely teratogenic factor. Perinatal death rates and malformation rates did not differ between 3007 infants born to women who had worked in 31 hospitals with extensive use of hexachlorophane and 1653 infants born to women who had worked in 18 hospitals where hexachlorophane was not used or only used sporadically.— B. Baltzar *et al.* (letter), *New Engl. J. Med.*, 1979, *300*, 627.

Further references: D. T. Janerich, *J. Am. med. Ass.*, 1979, *241*, 830.

Treatment of Adverse Effects. Empty the stomach by aspiration and lavage.

The administration of 60 ml of olive oil, or other vegetable oil, to delay absorption, has been suggested. Symptoms should be treated symptomatically.

Peritoneal dialysis was of minimal benefit in the treatment of a 7-year-old boy who had ingested about 1 g of pHisohex.— R. M. Boehm and P. A. Czajka, *Clin. Toxicol.*, 1979, *14*, 257, per *Int. pharm. Abstr.*, 1980, *17*, 407.

Precautions. Hexachlorophane should not be applied to mucous membranes, large areas of skin, or to burnt or damaged skin and should not be applied under occlusive dressings. It should be used with caution on infants, especially premature and low birth-weight infants, and preferably only for the control of outbreaks of staphylococcal infection in nurseries.

Absorption and Fate. Hexachlorophane is absorbed from the gastro-intestinal tract and through intact and denuded skin. Percutaneous absorption may be significant in premature infants and through damaged skin. Hexachlorophane crosses the placenta.

Fifty infants were washed daily in hospital for periods of 1 to 11 days with a mean of 3.5 g of a 3% solution of hexachlorophane added to 50 to 100 ml of water. The concentration of hexachlorophane (derived from maternal vaginal use or use during delivery) in cord-blood samples taken at birth ranged from 3 to 182 ng per ml (mean 22 ng per ml) and concentrations in venous blood at the time of discharge ranged from 9 to 646 ng per ml (mean 109 ng per ml).— A. Curley *et al.* (preliminary communication), *Lancet*, 1971, *2*, 296.

Plasma-hexachlorophane concentrations of 50 to 140 ng per ml occurred in infants, prior to discharge from a maternity unit, who had been washed with 2 ml of a 3% hexachlorophane emulsion which was allowed to dry on the skin. Washing was repeated on alternate days until discharge after up to 6 weeks.— V. D. Plueckhahn and J. Banks (letter), *Med. J. Aust.*, 1972, *1*, 1327.

The mean concentration of hexachlorophane immediately after birth in the cord-blood of 14 infants who were subsequently dusted with a powder containing hexachlorophane 0.33% in quantities of no more than 5 mg of hexachlorophane daily was 44 ng per ml (range 10 to 120 ng). One other infant had 1.88 µg per ml which suggested contamination at the time of sampling. After 8 days of dusting the mean concentration in a sample of blood taken from the heels of all 15 infants was 180 ng per ml (range 40 to 500 ng). These concentrations were not harmful.— V. G. Alder *et al.* (letter), *Lancet*, 1972, *2*, 384. See also W. A. Gillespie *et al.*, *J. Hyg., Camb.*, 1974, *73*, 311.

In 5 low birth-weight infants bathed daily for 21 to 56 days with 3 to 4 ml of hexachlorophane 3% emulsion diluted with water, blood concentrations ranged from 0.21 to 1.1 µg per ml with a mean of 0.482 µg per ml. None of the infants had abnormal neurological signs.— A. E. Kopelman, *J. Pediat.*, 1973, *82*, 972, per *Int. pharm. Abstr.*, 1974, *11*, 33. Hexachlorophane 650 ng per g was found in stored cerebral tissue from a 6-day-old premature infant with spongiform myelinopathy to whom a 3% detergent hexachlorophane solution had been applied daily on the face, napkin area, and umbilicus.— J. M. Anderson *et al.*, *Br. med. J.*, 1975, *2*, 175.

The mean blood concentration of hexachlorophane in operating room personnel who regularly scrubbed with hexachlorophane emulsion 3% was 220 ng per ml compared with 30 ng per ml in randomly chosen patients.— H. R. Butcher *et al.*, *Archs Surg.*, 1973, *107*, 70. See also B. Calesnick *et al.*, *Toxic. appl. Pharmac.*, 1974, *29*, 108.

Plasma concentrations of hexachlorophane in adults after the application of a corticosteroid ointment, which also contained hexachlorophane 1.4%, to the skin were comparable with those in infants after whole-body hexachlorophane washings.— P. G. T. Bye *et al.*, *Br. J. Derm.*, 1975, *93*, 209.

During 2 staphylococcal epidemics hexachlorophane 3% was used in a neonatal intensive care unit. In 27 infants the blood concentration of hexachlorophane after the 9th bath was 0.148 to 2.775 µg per ml, being highest in infants of low birth weight, and in those with abraded or erythematous skin. In the second group of 27 infants concentrations were 0.15 to 4.35 µg per ml; all of 8 infants weighing less than 1.1 kg had concentrations above 1 µg per ml. The infant with the highest concentration had impaired liver function and developed symptoms consistent with hexachlorophane toxicity. In 6 infants the hexachlorophane half-life was 6.1 to 44.2 hours.— E. E. Tyrala *et al.*, *J. Pediat.*, 1977, *91*, 481.

Uses. Hexachlorophane is a disinfectant with bactericidal activity against Gram-positive organisms, but it is much less active for Gram-negative organisms. It has bacteriostatic activity against *Staphylococcus aureus* in high dilutions. Like most phenols it is most active at a slightly acid pH but some activity is retained in the presence of soap solutions. The activity of hexachlorophane is reduced in the presence of blood. Preparations of hexachlorophane are liable to contamination with Gram-negative organisms such as species of *Pseudomonas* and *Salmonella*, which are resistant to its action.

Hexachlorophane is mainly used in soaps and creams in a concentration of 0.25 to 3%. After repeated use of these preparations for several days there is a marked diminution of the bacterial flora due to accumulation of hexachlorophane in the skin.

A preparation containing 3% is used for the disinfection of the hands of surgeons and others and, when other measures are not effective, for the control of staphylococcal infection in the newborn. Thorough rinsing is recommended before drying.

A 0.3% dusting powder has been applied to the cord stumps of the newborn.

The use of hexachlorophane in cosmetics and toiletries is restricted in Great Britain under The Cosmetic Products Regulations 1978 (SI 1978: No. 1354).

A discussion of the absorption, toxicity, and usage of hexachlorophane.— *Drug & Ther. Bull.*, 1972, *10*, 53. See also *Med. Lett.*, 1973, *15*, 1.

Following an outbreak of cervical abscesses due to *Staphylococcus aureus* in infants at 2 maternity hospitals, hexachlorophane powder 0.3% was applied to the axillae, groin, and umbilicus of all infants when napkins were changed, a hexachlorophane detergent preparation was used by the staff for hand washing, and the nasal carriers among the staff were treated with a cream containing chlorhexidine and neomycin. Babies were always changed in their cots and bathed only before discharge from the hospital. No further outbreaks occurred.— G. A. J. Ayliffe *et al.* (letter), *Lancet*, 1972, *2*, 479.

Powders containing chlorhexidine 1% or hexachlorophane 0.33% were equally effective in preventing colonisation and infection of the skin of newborn infants by *Staphylococcus aureus* but the skin became profusely colonised by coagulase-negative staphylococci, irrespective of the powder used.— V. G. Alder *et al.*, *Archs Dis. Childh.*, 1980, *55*, 277.

For other reports of the use of hexachlorophane, see Martindale 27th Edn, p. 524.

Preparations

Hexachlorophane Drench *(B. Vet. C. 1965).* Hexachlorophane 5 g, liquid paraffin 15 ml, arachis oil, or other suitable vegetable oil of commerce, to 100 ml. It is used in fascioliasis in ruminants.

Dusting-powders

Hexachlorophane Dusting-powder *(B.P.C. 1973).* Hexachlorophane 300 mg, zinc oxide 3 g, sterilisable maize starch 96.7 g. Distribute, in quantities of not more than 30 g, into suitable glass containers with perforated reclosable lids or into other suitable containers, and sterilise by heating the whole for 1 hour at 150° to 155°.

Emulsions

Hexachlorophene Cleansing Emulsion *(U.S.P.).* Hexachlorophene Detergent Lotion. Hexachlorophane in a suitable aqueous vehicle. It contains no colouring agents. pH of a 2:1 dilution in water, 5 to 6. Store in airtight non-metallic containers. Protect from light.

Ointments

Unguentum Hexachloropheni 1% *(Hung. P.).* Hexachlorophane 1 g, oleyl oleate 10 g, cetostearyl alcohol 10.8 g, sodium lauryl sulphate 1.2 g, sorbitol 5 g, Solutio Conservans (*Hung. P.*) 1 g, water to 100 g.

Soaps

Hexachlorophene Liquid Soap *(U.S.P.).* A 0.225 to 0.26% w/w solution of hexachlorophane in a 10 to 13% solution of a potassium soap. It may contain suitable water-hardness controls. The inclusion of nonionic detergents in amounts greater than 8% w/w may decrease the bacteriostatic activity of this preparation. Store in airtight containers. Protect from light.

Solutions

Concentrated Hexachlorophane Solution *(B.P.C. 1973).* Hexachlorophane 10 g, sodium hydroxide 1 g, alcohol (or industrial methylated spirit) 40 ml, freshly boiled and cooled water to 100 ml. Protect from light. Avoid contact with cork. *Directions.* Add 30 ml to a bath of water (100 to 150 litres). If necessary, a suitable water softener should be added to the water before adding the solution.

Proprietary Preparations

Ster-Zac Antibacterial Soap *(Hough, Hoseason, UK).* Contains hexachlorophane 2%. **Ster-Zac Antibacterial Shaving Foam.** Contains hexachlorophane 1% and triclosan 0.1%.

Ster-Zac DC Skin Cleanser *(Hough, Hoseason, UK).* A cream containing hexachlorphane 3% and an alkylphenoxy polyether sulphonate. For pre-operative hand cleansing.

Ster-Zac Powder *(Hough, Hoseason, UK).* A dusting-powder containing hexachlorophane 0.33% and zinc oxide 3% in a basis of sterilised talc. For the prophylaxis of skin and cord stump infections.

Other Proprietary Names

Fisohex *(Arg.)*; Gamophen Surgical Soap *(Switz.)*; Germibon *(Spain)*; Hexaphenyl *(Canad.)*; Phaisohex *(Denm., Iceland, Norw.)*; Phisoscrub *(USA)*; Sumasept *(Norw.)*.

The name Gamophen is also applied to a preparation containing triclosan.

Preparations containing hexachlorophane were also formerly marketed in Great Britain under the proprietary names Steridermis Washing Cream, Zalpon Antibacterial Washing Cream (both *Sterling Industrial*).

2251-m

Hexamidine Isethionate.

Hexamidine Isetionate. 4,4′-(Hexamethylenedioxy)dibenzamidine bis(2-hydroxyethanesulphonate).

$C_{20}H_{26}N_4O_2,2C_2H_6O_4S = 606.7$.

CAS — 3811-75-4 (hexamidine); 659-40-5 (isethionate).

NOTE. The name Hexamidinum is a synonym for primidone.

Hexamidine isethionate has bactericidal, bacteriostatic, and fungistatic properties and is used as a 0.1% solution for infections of the ears and eyes, as a mouth-wash, and for wounds and infections of the skin.

Proprietary Names

Désomédine *(Chauvin-Blache, Fr.; Chauvin-Blache, Switz.)*; Hexomedine *(Theraplix, Belg.; Théraplix, Fr.; Théraplix, Neth.; Rhodia, Spain; Théraplix, Switz.)*; Opthamedine *(de Bournonville, Belg.)*; Ophtamedine *(Bournonville, Neth.)*.

2252-b

Hydrargaphen.

Hydraphen; Hygraphen. µ-[3,3′-Methylenebis(naphthalene-2-sulphonato)]-bis(phenylmercury).

$C_{33}H_{24}Hg_2O_6S_2 = 981.8$.

CAS — 14235-86-0.

An amorphous powder. Practically **insoluble** in water. **Incompatible** with metals, halides, and sulphides. Metal or PVC containers should not be used.

Adverse Effects and Treatment. As for Mercury, pp.937-8.

Uses. Hydrargaphen is a disinfectant with antibacterial and antifungal properties. Its activity is not inhibited by pus or blood. It is used in the treatment of vaginitis, and was formerly used as a solution or tincture in the treatment of wounds, burns, and infections of the skin.

For a comparison of hydrargaphen and povidone-iodine in the treatment of cervical erosions, see Povidone-Iodine, p.867.

Proprietary Preparations

Conotrane *(WB Pharmaceuticals, UK: Boehringer Ingelheim, UK).* A cream containing hydrargaphen 0.05% and dimethicone '350' 20%. For bedsores.

Penotrane *(WB Pharmaceuticals, UK: Boehringer Ingelheim, UK).* Hydrargaphen, available as pessaries of 1.5 and 5 mg.

Other Proprietary Names

Versotrane *(Austral.)*.

2253-v

Laurolinium Acetate. 4-Amino-1-dodecyl-2-methylquinolinium acetate.
$C_{24}H_{38}N_2O_2$=386.6.

CAS — 6803-62-9 (laurolinium); 146-37-2 (acetate).

A faintly pink microcrystalline powder. M.p. about 168°. **Soluble** 1 in 5 of water, 1 in 3 of alcohol, and 1 in 2 of chloroform.

Laurolinium acetate is a cationic surfactant which has been used for skin disinfection.

2254-g

Magenta *(B.P.C. 1973).* Fuchsine; Basic Fuchsine; Basic Fuchsin *(U.S.P.)*; Basic Magenta; Fuchsinum; Rosaniline Hydrochloride; Aniline Red; CI Basic Violet 14; Colour Index No. 42510.

CAS — 569-61-9 (pararosaniline hydrochloride); 632-99-5 (rosaniline hydrochloride).

Pharmacopoeias. In *Hung.* and *U.S.*

A mixture of the hydrochlorides of pararosaniline {4-[(4-aminophenyl)(4-iminocyclohexa-2,5-dien-1-ylidene)methyl]aniline} and rosaniline {4-[(4-aminophenyl)(4-iminocyclohexa-2,5-dien-1-ylidene)methyl]-2-methylaniline}. The dried material contains not less than 85% of dyestuff, calculated as rosaniline hydrochloride ($C_{20}H_{20}ClN_3$ = 337.9).
Odourless, iridescent green crystals, or a dark green, lustrous, crystalline powder. **Soluble** in water, alcohol, and amyl alcohol forming deep red solutions; practically insoluble in ether. It loses not more than 10% of its weight on drying. **Incompatible** with oxidising and reducing agents.
In Great Britain, the manufacture of magenta and auramine, and any process in the course of which these substances are formed, are controlled by the Carcinogenic Substances Regulations 1967 (SI 1967: No. 879).

Uses. Magenta is a disinfectant effective against Gram-positive bacteria and some fungi. Magenta Paint (Castellani's paint) has been used in the treatment of superficial dermatophytoses, especially when moist eczematous dermatitis is present.

Magenta was considered unsafe for use in food.— Eighth Report of the Joint FAO/WHO Expert Committee on Food Additives, *Tech. Rep. Ser. Wld Hlth Org. No. 309,* 1965.

Magenta was a controlled substance under the Carcinogenic Substances Regulations 1967, the provisions of which required that those engaged in the manufacture of magenta should undergo 6-monthly medical examinations; this was good reason for considering its disuse in the treatment of fungous skin lesions.— G. Whitwell (letter), *Lancet,* 1968, *2,* 110. A protest against the suggestion that the clinical use of magenta should be discontinued.— A. Castellani (letter), *ibid.,* 287.

Preparations

Carbol-Fuchsin Topical Solution *(U.S.P.).* Magenta 300 mg, phenol 4.5 g, resorcinol 10 g, acetone 5 ml, alcohol 10 ml, water to 100 ml. Store in airtight containers. Protect from light.

Magenta Paint *(B.P.C. 1973, A.P.F.).* Castellani's Paint; Fuchsine Paint. Magenta 400 mg, boric acid 800 mg, phenol 4 g, resorcinol 8 g, acetone 4 ml, alcohol (90%) (or industrial methylated spirit, suitably diluted) 8.5 ml, water to 100 ml. Store in a cool place in airtight containers. Protect from light.
A.P.F. has freshly boiled and cooled water.
F.N. Belg. includes a similar preparation.

Methaemoglobinaemia in a 6-week-old child following topical use of a solution containing magenta, boric acid, phenol, and resorcinol.— E. Lundell and R. Nordman, *Ann. clin. Res.* 1973, *5,* 404.

Phenol was found in the urine of 4 of 16 infants with seborrhoeic eczema treated with Magenta Paint applied twice daily for 48 hours.— S. C. F. Rogers *et al., Br. J. Derm.,* 1978, *98,* 559.

2255-q

Malachite Green. Viride Malachitum; CI Basic Green 4; Colour Index No. 42000. [4-(4-Dimethylaminobenzhydriylidene)cyclohexa-2,5-dienylidene]dimethylammonium chloride.

NOTE. *B.P.C. 1949* defined malachite green as an acid oxalate of anhydrobis (4-dimethylamino)triphenylmethanol.

Green plates with a metallic sheen. **Soluble** 1 in 15 of water and 1 in 15 of alcohol. A 1% solution in water has a pH of about 1.4. **Store** in airtight containers.

Malachite green is a disinfectant with actions and uses similar to those of brilliant green (see p.551).

In vitro, malachite green was capable of interacting with the DNA of living cells (indicating possible carcinogenicity); this suggested a need to re-evaluate its use clinically.— H. S. Rosenkranz and H. S. Carr (letter), *Br. med. J.,* 1971, *3,* 702.

2256-p

Mercurochrome *(B.P.C. 1954).* Merbromin; Mercurodibromofluorescein; Mercurescéine Sodique; Disodium 2,7-dibromo-4-hydroxymercurifluorescein. The disodium salt of [2,7-dibromo-9-(2-carboxyphenyl)-6-hydroxy-3-oxo-3*H*-xanthen-5-yl]hydroxymercury.
$C_{20}H_8Br_2HgNa_2O_6$=750.7.

CAS — 129-16-8.

NOTE. The use of the name Mercurochrome is limited; in some countries it is a trade-mark.

Pharmacopoeias. In *Braz., Fr., Jap., Port., Span.,* and *Swiss.*

Odourless greenish iridescent scales or granules, containing 24 to 27% of Hg, calculated on the dried substance.
Soluble 1 in 1 of water, giving a dark red solution which shows green fluorescence on dilution; practically insoluble in alcohol, acetone, chloroform, and ether. **Incompatible** with acids, most alkaloidal salts, and many local anaesthetics. *Solutions should not be boiled or autoclaved.* Solutions may be **sterilised** by filtration. **Store** in airtight containers.
For precautions to be taken in preparing and storing antiseptic solutions, see under Phenol, p.570.
For a note on the incompatibility of mercurials with aluminium and steel, see under Mercuric Chloride, p.939.

Alcoholic and aqueous solutions of mercurochrome 2% were relatively stable when stored for 5 months in hermetically sealed bottles at a temperature below 40°. The presence of a precipitate indicates a strong alkalinity that could induce toxicity.— M. Balin *et al., Annls pharm. fr.,* 1979, *37,* 71.

Adverse Effects and Treatment. As for Mercury, pp.937-8.

A report of contact dermatitis attributed to mercurochrome.— G. Camarasa, *Contact Dermatitis,* 1976, *2,* 120.

Mercurochrome used in topical antiseptic preparations was toxic to epidermal cells.— *Med. Lett.,* 1977, *19,* 83.

A report of fatal mercury poisoning from mercurochrome treatment of infected omphalocele. The high tissue concentrations of mercury might have contributed to cardiac arrest.— T. -F. Yeh *et al.* (letter), *Lancet,* 1978, *1,* 210. See also *idem, Clin. Toxicol.,* 1978, *13,* 463.

A 59-year-old woman had a 2% aqueous solution of mercurochrome applied to her surgical wounds and decubitus areas after surgery for an oesophageal stricture. By day 22 her blood contained 700 ng per ml of mercury and on day 23 she died in therapy-resistant shock. Aplastic anaemia, confirmed at autopsy, was tentatively ascribed to mercurochrome treatment.— P. H. T. J. Slee *et al., Acta med. scand.,* 1979, *205,* 463.

Uses. Mercurochrome is a weak disinfectant; in the presence of organic material its effect is greatly reduced. A 2% solution in a mixture of alcohol, acetone, and water has been used for skin infection and a 1% solution was formerly used for bladder and urethral irrigation.
Stains on the skin caused by mercurochrome may be removed with chlorinated soda solution.

Proprietary Names

Cinfacromin *(Cinfa, Spain)*; Cromo Utin *(Deiters, Spain)*; Curichrome *(Goupil, Fr.)*; Mercromina *(Lainco, Spain)*; Mercrotona *(Orravan, Spain)*; Mercurasept *(Sauter, Switz.)*; Mercuro Clinico *(Llano, Spain)*; Mercurocromo *(Perez Jimenez, Spain)*; Super Cromer Orto *(Normon, Spain)*.

2257-s

Methyl Bromide. Bromomethane; Monobromomethane.
CH_3Br=94.94.

CAS — 74-83-9.

A colourless non-inflammable gas with a burning taste; odourless in low concentrations or with a chloroform-like odour at high concentrations. B.p. 4.5°. Sparingly **soluble** in water; freely soluble in alcohol, chloroform, and ether.

Adverse Effects. Methyl bromide is a vesicant. Toxic effects after inhalation or percutaneous absorption include dizziness, headache, anorexia, nausea, vomiting, abdominal pain, blurred vision, weakness, ataxia, confusion, hyperactivity, convulsions, pulmonary oedema, and coma. Renal failure may occur and death may be due to circulatory collapse or respiratory failure. Onset of symptoms may be preceded by a latent period. Concentrations of 1% or more are irritant to the eyes.
Rubber absorbs and retains methyl bromide and should not therefore be used in protective clothing.
Maximum permissible atmospheric concentration 15 ppm.

A review of 10 cases of methyl bromide poisoning.— C. H. Hine, *J. occup. Med.,* 1969, *11,* 1.

For toxicological data, see 1971 Evaluations of some Pesticide Residues in Food, *Pestic. Residue Ser. Wld Hlth Org. No. 1,* 1972.

Further references: *J. Am. med. Ass.,* 1976, *236,* 1510.

Treatment of Adverse Effects. Remove the patient to fresh air, remove contaminated clothing, and wash the skin with water. Dimercaprol (see p.383) may be of value if given during the latent period. Toxic effects should be treated symptomatically. The patient should be kept at rest for at least 48 hours.

Uses. Methyl bromide is used as a gaseous disinfectant in concentrations of 3.5 g per litre at relative humidities between 30 and 60%; it has low antimicrobial activity but good penetrating power.
Methyl bromide is used as an insecticidal fumigant for soil and stored dried foodstuffs, and for the disinfection of fresh fruit and vegetables in plant quarantine procedures.
When supplied in small cans for fumigation of enclosed spaces, it contains not less than 2% w/w of chloropicrin as a lachrymatory warning agent.
Methyl bromide has been used with carbon tetrachloride in some fire extinguishers. It is also used as a refrigerant, and for the disinfection of spacecraft.

Residues in diet. The maximum acceptable concentration of methyl bromide in cereals after fumigation: 50 ppm in raw cereals, 10 ppm in milled cereals, and 0.5 ppm in bread and other cooked cereal products.— Report of the 1971 Joint FAO/WHO Meeting on Pesticide Residues in Food, *Tech. Rep. Ser. Wld Hlth Org. No. 502,* 1972.

Maximum acceptable daily intake of inorganic bromide, derived from bromine-containing fumigants and other sources: 1 mg per kg body-weight.— Report of the 1972 Joint FAO/WHO Meeting on Pesticide Residues in Food, *Tech. Rep. Ser. Wld Hlth Org. No. 525,* 1973.

2258-w

Methylbenzethonium Chloride *(U.S.P.)*.

Benzyldimethyl(2-{2-[2(*or* 3)-methyl-4-(1,1,3,3-tetramethylbutyl)phenoxy]ethoxy}ethyl)ammonium chloride monohydrate.

$C_{28}H_{44}ClNO_2,H_2O=480.1$.

CAS — 25155-18-4 (anhydrous); 1320-44-1 (monohydrate).

Pharmacopoeias. In *U.S.*

White hygroscopic crystals with a mild odour and a very bitter taste. M.p. after drying 159° to 163°. **Soluble** 1 in less than 1 of water, alcohol, and ether; practically insoluble in chloroform. Solutions in water are neutral or slightly alkaline to litmus. **Store** in airtight containers.

Adverse Effects and Treatment. As for Cetrimide, p.552.

Uses. Methylbenzethonium chloride is a quaternary ammonium disinfectant with properties and uses similar to those of other cationic surfactants, as described under Cetrimide, p.552.

It has been used principally to prevent ammoniacal dermatitis and skin irritation due to contact with urine, faeces, or perspiration; a 0.004 to 0.005% solution is used for rinsing babies' napkins and the undergarments and bedlinen of incontinent children and adults, or a cream, ointment, or dusting-powder (0.055 to 0.1%) may be applied locally.

Preparations

Methylbenzethonium Chloride Lotion *(U.S.P.)*. An emulsion containing methylbenzethonium chloride. pH 5.2 to 6. Store in airtight containers.

Methylbenzethonium Chloride Ointment *(U.S.P.)*. An ointment containing methylbenzethonium chloride. pH of a 1 in 100 dispersion, 5 to 7. Store in airtight containers.

Methylbenzethonium Chloride Powder *(U.S.P.)*. Methylbenzethonium chloride in a suitable fine powder basis free from grittiness. pH of a 1 in 100 dispersion, 9 to 10.5.

Proprietary Preparations

Hyamine 10-X *(Rohm & Haas, UK)*. A brand of methylbenzethonium chloride.

Other Proprietary Names

Diaparene *(USA)*; Vi-Medin *(Canad.)*.

2259-e

Miristalkonium Chloride.

Myristylbenzalkonium Chloride. Benzyldimethyltetradecylammonium chloride.

$C_{23}H_{42}ClN=368.0$.

CAS — 139-08-2.

Miristalkonium chloride is used with other antimicrobial agents in lozenges for the treatment of throat infections.

2260-b

Myristyl-gamma-picolinium Chloride.

4-Methyl-1-tetradecylpyridinium chloride.

$C_{20}H_{36}ClN=326.0$.

CAS — 7631-49-4 (myristyl-gamma-picolinium); 2748-88-1 (chloride).

A fine white, or almost white, crystalline powder. **Soluble** in water and alcohol. A 0.1% solution in water has a pH of 4.5 to 6.

Myristyl-gamma-picolinium chloride is a cationic surfactant which is used as an antimicrobial preservative in some pharmaceutical products.

2261-v

Nitromersol *(U.S.P.)*.

5-Methyl-2-nitro-7-oxa-8-mercurabicyclo[4.2.0]octa-1,3,5-triene.

$C_7H_5HgNO_3=351.7$.

CAS — 133-58-4.

Pharmacopoeias. In *U.S.*

A brownish-yellow to yellow odourless tasteless powder or granules. Very slightly **soluble** in water, alcohol, acetone, chloroform, and ether; soluble in alkalis and in ammonia with the formation of salts. **Store** in airtight containers. Protect from light.

For a note on the incompatibility of mercurials with aluminium and steel, see under Mercuric Chloride, p.939.

Adverse Effects and Treatment. As for Mercury, pp.937-8.

Nitromersol occasionally gives rise to hypersensitivity reactions.

Nitromersol had been reported to be ototoxic.— J. L. Honigman, *I.C.I. Pharmaceuticals* (letter), *Pharm. J.*, 1975, *2*, 523.

Nitromersol used in topical antiseptic preparations was toxic to epidermal cells.— *Med. Lett.*, 1977, *19*, 83.

Uses. Nitromersol is a disinfectant effective against some of the commoner pathogenic organisms including *Staphylococcus aureus, Escherichia coli,* and *Streptococcus pyogenes.* It is not effective against spores and acid-fast bacteria and its activity is greatly reduced in the presence of blood and organic matter. It is used as the sodium salt.

Nitromersol is used for disinfection of the skin prior to surgical treatment as a 0.5% alcohol-acetone-aqueous solution. A 0.2% solution is applied to the skin for the treatment of minor cuts.

A 0.04% solution has been used for the disinfection of surgical instruments but does not sterilise; it should not be used for those made of aluminium.

Preparations

Nitromersol Tincture *(U.S.P.)*. Nitromersol 500 mg, sodium hydroxide 100 mg, acetone 10 ml, alcohol 52.5 ml, water to 100 ml; it may be coloured. Store in airtight containers. Protect from light.

Nitromersol Topical Solution *(U.S.P.)*. Nitromersol Solution. Nitromersol 200 mg, sodium hydroxide 40 mg, sodium carbonate monohydrate 425 mg, water to 100 ml. Store in airtight containers. Protect from light. Dilutions of this solution should be freshly prepared as they tend to precipitate on standing.

2262-g

Noxythiolin.

Noxytiolin. 1-Hydroxymethyl-3-methyl-2-thiourea.

$C_3H_8N_2OS=120.2$.

CAS — 15599-39-0.

A white crystalline powder which decomposes between 88° and 90°. **Soluble** 1 in 10 of water. Solutions for irrigation should be freshly prepared. **Store** in a cool place.

There was a considerable increase in the toxicity of noxythiolin solutions with age and after autoclaving, probably due to formation of formaldehyde.— B. P. Block, *Clin. Trials J.*, 1967, *4*, 629.

Adverse Effects.

Widespread filmy plastic-type adhesions developed in 2 boys who had had peritoneal lavage with noxythiolin during surgery; a causal relationship was suspected.— M. A. Morris (letter), *Br. med. J.*, 1977, *1*, 1355. Clinical experience and a number of published papers did not support the suggestion that noxythiolin caused adhesions.— R. D. Rosin (letter), *ibid.*, 1664.

Uses. Noxythiolin has wide antibacterial and antifungal actions. It probably acts by slowly releasing formaldehyde in solution. It has been used, usually as a 1 to 2.5% solution in water, for the irrigation of body cavities and fistulas. In the treatment of bladder infections the intense burning sensation frequently experienced may be relieved by the addition of a local anaesthetic such as amethocaine hydrochloride. It has also been applied topically in gels and sprays.

Noxythiolin released formaldehyde when stored at 37° for 18 hours. In aqueous buffer solutions of pH 4, 7, and 10, containing noxythiolin 1%, most of the theoretical content of formaldehyde was released but in urine at pH 5.5 only 15% of the maximum was slowly released. The inhibitory action of noxythiolin on *Escherichia coli, Pseudomonas aeruginosa,* and *Staphylococcus aureus* could be accounted for by the amount of formaldehyde released.— D. Kingston, *J. clin. Path.*, 1965, *18*, 666.

A gel containing noxythiolin inserted into the vagina the night before radiotherapy successfully eliminated the odour of necrotic tumour tissue and micro-organisms normally released on removing gynaecological radium applicators and gauze.— I. J. Kerby (letter), *Lancet*, 1973, *2*, 1340.

Antimicrobial activity. Noxythiolin was bactericidal *in vitro* to Gram-negative bacteria which were resistant to the commonly used antibacterial agents, and was stated to be active in the presence of serum. *Proteus* organisms were less susceptible than most, and MICs for some strains of *Proteus* were 5 mg per ml. Such concentrations could be obtained by topical application, but were only bactericidal after 24 hours' contact with the bacteria, so that several applications of the preparation would be necessary each day.— D. Horsfield, *Clin. Trials J.*, 1967, *4*, 625.

Twelve strains of *Ps. aeruginosa,* 3 of *Klebsiella aerogenes,* and 2 of *E. coli* were resistant to noxythiolin. Some antibiotic-resistant pseudomonads were resistant to noxythiolin. Sensitivity of the infecting organism should be established before noxythiolin was used.— B. Chattopadhyay, *Br. med. J.*, 1977, *2*, 1121.

Of 51 isolates of *Bacteroides fragilis* 18 had an MIC of noxythiolin of 125 µg per ml, 28 had an MIC of 250 µg per ml, and 5 had an MIC of 500 µg per ml. One strain with a minimum bactericidal concentration of 2 mg per ml, determined by plating, required 2 hours exposure at 10 mg per ml for killing. Routine tests were of limited value.— R. H. George and D. E. Healing (letter), *Br. med. J.*, 1977, *2*, 1478.

Dental use. A paste of noxythiolin 50% in a macrogol basis was considered to prevent periapical infection when incorporated into the root treatment of pulpless anterior teeth.— G. D. C. Kennedy *et al.*, *Br. dent. J.*, 1977, *143*, 77.

Osteomyelitis. Four patients with osteomyelitis of the tibia were treated with noxythiolin instillation, 2.5% in water, after irrigations with penicillin, streptomycin, tetracycline, and then chloramphenicol had failed. Treatment with noxythiolin was carried out twice daily for 5 days. Complete resolution of infection was confirmed on the fifth day; there was progressive healing with closure of the wounds.— A. T. Williams, *Clin. Trials J.*, 1967, *4*, 634.

Peritonitis. Of 23 patients with faecal peritonitis who were treated with noxythiolin, 2.5 to 5 g in 100 ml of water intraperitoneally, 20 recovered and 3 died (2 from pulmonary embolism and 1 from multiple residual abscesses).— M. K. Browne and J. L. Stoller, *Br. J. Surg.*, 1970, *57*, 525.

Of 9 patients with severe peritonitis given up to 1.5 litres of a 1% solution of noxythiolin in sodium chloride injection intraperitoneally at the time of operation, followed by a continuous intraperitoneal infusion of 1 litre daily for up to 72 hours postoperatively, only 2 cases showed significant evidence of wound infection.— R. G. Pickard, *Br. J. Surg.*, 1972, *59*, 642.

Urinary-tract infections. Noxythiolin was instilled after intermittent catheterisation of the bladder in 42 patients as a 1 or 2.5% solution and chlorhexidine 0.02% solution in a further 40 patients. Three noxythiolin-treated patients and 9 chlorhexidine-treated patients developed urinary infections.— I. R. McFadyen, *Clin. Trials J.*, 1967, *4*, 654.

Wound infections. The postoperative application of noxythiolin to wounds was less effective than a placebo in preventing infection, and its use had been abandoned.— K. C. Calman *et al.* (letter), *Br. med. J.*, 1971, *4*, 232.

Proprietary Preparations

Noxyflex *(Geistlich, UK)*. Noxythiolin in vials of 2.5 g with amethocaine hydrochloride 10 mg, foı preparing solutions for the irrigation of body cavities and fistulas. **Noxyflex 'S'** is similar but without amethocaine. (Also available as Noxyflex in *Fr.*).

A preparation containing noxythiolin was also formerly marketed in Great Britain under the proprietary name Gynaflex (*Geistlich*).

2263-q

Octaphonium Chloride *(B.P.)*. Octafonium Chloride; Phenoctide. Benzyldiethyl{2-[4-(1,1,3,3-tetramethylbutyl)phenoxy]ethyl}ammonium chloride monohydrate.
$C_{27}H_{42}ClNO,H_2O$=450.1.

CAS — 15687-40-8 (anhydrous).

Pharmacopoeias. In *Br.*

A white, odourless or almost odourless, crystalline powder. **Soluble** 1 in 5 of water; soluble in alcohol and chloroform. A 1% solution in water has a pH of 5 to 6.

Uses. Octaphonium chloride is a quaternary ammonium disinfectant with properties and uses similar to those of other cationic surfactants as described under Cetrimide, p.551. It also has antifungal properties.

2264-p

Oxychlorosene. Monoxychlorosene. The hypochlorous acid complex of a mixture of the phenyl sulphonate derivatives of aliphatic hydrocarbons.
$C_{20}H_{34}O_3S,HOCl$=407.0.

CAS — 8031-14-9.

A fine white powder with an odour of chlorine. Slowly **soluble** in water, followed by rapid hydrolysis; it decomposes in organic solvents. A 0.5% solution has a pH of about 5.5.

Uses. Oxychlorosene is a chlorine disinfectant with the actions and uses described under Chlorine, p.557.
A 0.1 to 0.4% solution of the sodium salt of oxychlorosene is used for cleansing wounds.

Proprietary Preparations

Clorpactin XCB *(Guardian, USA: Farillon, UK)*. Oxychlorosene, available in containers of 5 g. A 0.5% solution (or more concentrated in certain cases) in sodium chloride injection is used to irrigate the wound during surgery for cancer; contact for not less than 5 minutes is necessary. (Also available as Clorpactin XCB in *USA*)
Clorpactin WCS-90 is sodium oxychlorosene; it is used in aqueous solution (0.1 to 0.4%) as a topical antiseptic for local infections, to remove necrotic debris in massive infections, and to counteract offensive discharges. (Also available as Clorpactin WCS-90 in *Canad., USA*).

2265-s

Parachlorophenol *(U.S.P.)*. 4-Chlorophenol.
C_6H_5ClO=128.6.

CAS — 106-48-9.

Pharmacopoeias. In *Aust., Braz., Nord., Pol., Swiss,* and *U.S.*

White or pink crystals with a characteristic phenolic odour. M.p. about 42°.
Soluble 1 in 60 of water; very soluble in alcohol, chloroform, ether, glycerol, solutions of alkali hydroxides, and fixed and volatile oils; soluble in liquid paraffin and melted soft paraffin. A 1% solution in water is acid to litmus. **Store** in airtight containers. Protect from light.

Total haemolysis occurred when erythrocytes were cultured for 45 minutes in a 0.15% solution of parachlorophenol in sodium chloride injection. Only slight haemolysis occurred when the strength was reduced to 0.11%.— H. C. Ansel and D. E. Cadwallader, *J. pharm. Sci.*, 1964, *53*, 169.

Adverse Effects and Treatment. As for Phenol, p.571.

Uses. Parachlorophenol is a disinfectant effective against many Gram-negative organisms. It was formerly used as a 0.25% solution in physiological saline for the irrigation of sinus tracts.

Preparations

Camphorated Parachlorophenol *(U.S.P.)*. Parachlorophenol 35 g and camphor 65 g, triturated until the mixture liquefies. Store in airtight containers. Protect from light. It is employed in dentistry in the treatment of infected root canals. A 5 to 20% solution in glycerol has been used for the treatment of infection of the buccal mucosa. A 1 to 2% ointment has been used in keratitis.

Camphorated parachlorophenol was the least irritant of the antiseptics based on phenol and was effective against most of the organisms likely to be found in root canals.— I. Curson, *Br. dent. J.*, 1966, *121*, 381.

2266-w

Paraformaldehyde *(B.P.C. 1973)*. Paraform; Paraformic Aldehyde; Polymerised Formaldehyde; Paraformaldehydum; Trioxyméthylène.
$(CH_2O)_n$.

CAS — 30525-89-4.

Pharmacopoeias. In *Aust., Belg., Jap., Jug., Nord., Pol., Port.,* and *Span.*

A solid polymer of formaldehyde containing not less than 95% of CH_2O. It is a white amorphous powder or friable mass, with a pungent odour. It volatilises at 100° and is readily converted into formaldehyde when heated to this temperature in the presence of water.
Practically **insoluble** in cold water, alcohol, and ether; soluble in boiling water with depolymerisation, and in solutions of alkali hydroxides. A 5% suspension in water is neutral to litmus. **Store** in airtight containers.

Adverse Effects and Treatment. As for Formaldehyde Solution, p.563.

Uses. Paraformaldehyde has the properties and uses of formaldehyde (see p.563) and is used as a source of formaldehyde. For disinfecting rooms it has been vapourised by heating but as it produces a dry gas it is less satisfactory for this purpose than Formaldehyde Solution. Tablets prepared for disinfecting rooms by vaporisation should be coloured by the addition of a suitable blue dye.
Paraformaldehyde is also used in lozenges. In dentistry, it has been used as an obtundent for sensitive dentine and as an antiseptic in mummifying pastes and for root canals.

Mummifying pastes. For details of the use of paraformaldehyde, often with cresols, in pastes for mummification of dental pulp, see I. Curson, *Br. dent. J.*, 1966, *121*, 519.

Preparations

Conspergens Paraformaldehydi *(Nord. P.)*. Paraformaldehyde Dusting-powder. Paraformaldehyde 5 g, lavender oil 200 mg, potato starch 20 g, purified talc 74.8 g.

Dental Paraformaldehyde Paste *(Jap. P.)*. Past. Paraform. Dent. Paraformaldehyde 35 g, procaine hydrochloride 35 g, hydrous wool fat 30 g.

Formaldehyde Lozenges *(B.P.C. 1973)*. Formalin Throat Tablets; Formamint Tablets. Each lozenge weighs about 1 g, and contains paraformaldehyde 10 mg, menthol 2.5 mg, citric acid monohydrate 20 mg, and lemon oil 0.0006 ml. Store in a cool place in airtight containers. These lozenges are liable to deteriorate on storage.
NOTE. The use of the names Formalin and Formamint is limited; in some countries they are trade-marks.

Pulp Devitalising Paste for Teeth. Paraformaldehyde 1 g, lignocaine 60 mg, propylene glycol 0.5 ml, macrogol '1500' 1.3 g, carmine 10 mg.—P. Hobson, *Br. dent. J.*, 1970, *128*, 275.

2267-e

Phenol *(B.P., U.S.P.)*. Phenolum; Carbolic Acid; Phenyl Hydrate; Fenol. Hydroxybenzene.
$C_6H_5.OH$=94.11.

CAS — 108-95-2.

Pharmacopoeias. In all pharmacopoeias examined except *Eur., Roum.,* and *Rus.*

Colourless or faintly pink deliquescent crystals or crystalline masses, becoming pink on keeping, with a characteristic, not tarry, odour and, in dilute solution, a sweetish pungent taste. *U.S.P.* permits the addition of a suitable stabilising agent. F.p. 40° to 41°; b.p. about 181°.
Soluble 1 in 12 to 15 of water, 6 in 1 of alcohol, 2 in 1 of chloroform, 5 in 1 of ether, 3 in 1 of glycerol, 1 in 100 of liquid paraffin, 1 in about 10 of castor oil, and in fixed and volatile oils; readily soluble in caustic alkalis, forming phenoxides (phenates, phenolates). At 20°, 100 parts are liquefied by 10 of water and will dissolve about a further 30 parts of water; on further addition of water the liquid separates into 2 layers, one a solution of phenol in water, the other a solution of water in phenol, until about 1200 parts of water have been added, when a solution of phenol in water is formed. A saturated solution in water at 20° is clear and is alkaline to methyl orange. A 2.8% solution in water is iso-osmotic with serum.
Solutions in oil and glycerol are **sterilised** by maintaining the whole of the material, in hermetically sealed containers, at 150° for 1 hour; aqueous solutions are sterilised by autoclaving.
Incompatible with alkaline salts, acetanilide, phenazone, piperazine, quinine salts, phenacetin, and iron salts. It coagulates albumin and gelatinises collodion. It forms a liquid or semi-solid mass with camphor, chloral hydrate, menthol, resorcinol, thymol, and certain other substances. **Store** in a cool place in airtight containers. Protect from light.
NOTE. Unless otherwise specified, aqueous solutions of phenol should be coloured with amaranth or other suitable red dye.
Preparation and Storage of Antiseptic Solutions. As aqueous solutions of phenol and other antiseptics are liable to contamination with resistant organisms, the *B.P.C. 1973* recommended that solutions be prepared with freshly distilled or freshly boiled water and transferred to thoroughly cleansed, preferably sterile, containers, that cork closures or cork liners be not used, and that the contents be not used later than 1 week after first opening a container. Solutions for application to broken skin or to eyes or for introduction into body cavities such as the bladder must be sterile.

CAUTION. *Phenol is caustic to the skin.*

2268-l

Liquefied Phenol *(B.P.)*. Liq. Phenol.; Liquefied Carbolic Acid; Phénol Aqueux; Verflüssigtes Phenol. A solution of water in phenol; it contains 80% w/w of phenol.

Pharmacopoeias. In *Br., Ind.,* and *Turk.* (77 to 81.5% w/w); in *Swiss* (82 to 85.5% w/w); in *It.* (82 to 86.5% w/w); in *Jap.* and *Pol.* (both not less than 88% w/w); in *U.S.* (not less than 89% w/w); in *Aust., Belg., Hung., Nord.,* and *Port.* (all about 90% w/w).

A colourless or faintly coloured caustic liquid with a characteristic and not tarry odour. It forms a clear solution on the addition of 11 parts of water; **Miscible** with alcohol, ether, and glycerol; a mixture with an equal volume of glycerol is miscible with water. Wt per ml 1.055 to 1.06 g. **Store** in airtight containers. Protect from light. It may congeal or deposit crystals if stored below 4°; it should be completely melted before use.

NOTE. When phenol is to be mixed with collodion, fixed oils, or paraffins, melted phenol crystals should be used and not Liquefied Phenol.

CAUTION. *Liquefied Phenol is caustic to the skin.*

Total haemolysis occurred when erythrocytes were cultured for 45 minutes in a 0.54% solution of phenol in sodium chloride injection. Only slight haemolysis occurred when the strength was reduced to 0.49%.— H. C. Ansel and D. E. Cadwallader, *J. pharm. Sci.*, 1964, *53*, 169.

Inactivation by nonionic surfactants. To maintain the same activity in a 5% solution of polyoxyl stearates the concentrations of phenol, cresol, chlorocresol, thymol, chloroxylenol, and hexachlorophane should be increased by factors of 2, 4, 8, 30, and 800 respectively. Macrogols had little effect on the antibacterial activity of phenols.— K. Thoma *et al.*, *Archs. Pharm., Weinheim*, 1970, *303*, 289.

Incompatibility with lignocaine. The following injection solution produced a precipitate: liquefied phenol 12 ml, lignocaine hydrochloride 1 g, zinc sulphate 8 g, glycerol 24 ml, Water for Injections to 100 ml. It was found that the lignocaine hydrochloride and the zinc sulphate caused the phenol to come out of solution. A clear solution was obtained either by increasing the concentration of glycerol to 50% of the final volume or by replacing the glycerol with propylene glycol in the original concentration. The latter procedure was preferred as the solution was less viscous.—Pharm. Soc. Lab. Rep., *Pharm. J.*, 1959, *1*, 9.

Incompatibility with polymers. Weak solutions of polysorbates reacted with phenol to give an insoluble oily liquid; this could be solubilised by increasing the concentration of the polysorbate.— S. S. Ahsan and S. M. Blaug, *Drug Stand.*, 1960, *28*, 95.

Aqueous solutions containing phenol with macrogol 4000 or poloxamer 188 were turbid if the ratio of polymer to phenol was low but cleared on adding more macrogol or poloxamer 188.— J. Jacobs *et al.* (letter), *J. Pharm. Pharmac.*, 1972, *24*, 586.

Adverse Effects. When taken by mouth, phenol causes extensive local corrosion, with pain, nausea, vomiting, sweating, and diarrhoea. Initially fleeting excitation may occur but it is quickly followed by unconsciousness. There is depression of the central nervous system, with circulatory and respiratory failure. Pulmonary oedema may develop, and damage to the liver and kidneys may lead to organ failure. Death usually occurs from respiratory failure; fatalities have been reported after 1 to 15 g by mouth.

Severe or fatal poisoning may occur from the absorption of phenol from unbroken skin or wounds. Applied to skin, phenol causes blanching and corrosion. Aqueous solutions as dilute as 10% may be corrosive.

Maximum permissible atmospheric concentration 5 ppm.

Cresols and other phenolic substances have similar, but often milder, effects.

A 38-year-old woman who had regularly not worn protective gloves while cleaning sputum jars with phenol complained of a lime green coloration of her urine. The urine was found to contain a phenol derivative calculated as phenol 10 µg per ml.— J. Balassa (letter), *Br. med. J.*, 1970, *2*, 589.

Of 621 persons with dermatitis or eczema submitted to patch testing with a 1% aqueous solution of phenol 0.3% gave a positive reaction.— E. Rudzki and D. Kleniewska, *Br. J. Derm.*, 1970, *83*, 543.

Skin depigmentation occurred in 12 hospital workers exposed to phenolic disinfectants, particularly *p*-t-butylphenol and *p*-t-amylphenol, and from subsequent studies in these patients and in a further 6 volunteers it was concluded that many phenolic compounds were capable of causing depigmentation if appied to the skin under occlusion in an irritating concentration.— G. Kahn, *Archs Derm.*, 1970, *102*, 177.

A 44-year-old laboratory technician who had been exposed to phenols over a period of 13 years developed phenol marasmus. His health deteriorated and he suffered loss of appetite, weight loss, dark urine, and pains in the limbs. After cessation of all exposure to phenol and cresol the patient slowly recovered but dark urine persisted for several months.— R. R. Merliss, *J. occup. Med.*, 1972, *14*, 55.

Treatment of Adverse Effects. If phenol has been swallowed, empty the stomach by aspiration and lavage, taking care to avoid perforation. Castor oil may be added to the water to dissolve phenol and delay absorption; 50 ml of castor oil may be left in the stomach. Remove contaminated clothing and wash the skin with glycerol, vegetable oil, alcohol, or soap and water. Keep the patient warm and treat pulmonary oedema, systemic acidosis, respiratory failure, and circulatory failure symptomatically. Respiration may have to be assisted.

Adsorption. For comment on the *in vitro* adsorption of phenol by activated charcoal, see p.79.

Removal from skin. Phenol splashes should be treated by removing all contaminated clothing and rubbing the contaminated skin for at least 10 minutes with swabs soaked in glycerol, a liquid macrogol, or a mixture containing a liquid macrogol 70 parts and methylated spirit 30 parts. If these solvents were not immediately available, swabs soaked in water should be used initially.— CIA Medical Committee, London, British Chemical Industry Safety Council, 1970. See also T. G. Pullin *et al.*, *Toxic. appl. Pharmac.*, 1978, *43*, 199.

Precautions. Solutions should not be applied to large wounds since sufficient phenol may be absorbed to give rise to toxic symptoms. Wet dressings containing phenol should not be applied to the fingers or toes.

A report of paraplegia following coeliac plexus block with a 6% aqueous phenol solution.— E. J. Galizia and S. K. Lahiri, *Br. J. Anaesth.*, 1974, *46*, 539.

Anaesthesia and paresis of the legs, improving only to a very limited extent before death 32 days later from bronchopneumonia, appeared to be due to inadvertent entry into the subarachnoid space of phenol used for chemical sympathectomy.— R. C. Smith *et al.*, *Br. med. J.*, 1978, *1*, 552.

For a report that phenol was found in the urine of infants with seborrhoeic eczema following treatment with applications of Magenta Paint, see under Magenta, p.568.

Absorption and Fate. Phenol is absorbed from the gastro-intestinal tract and through skin and mucous membranes. It is metabolised to phenylglucuronide and phenyl sulphate, and small amounts are oxidised to catechol and quinol which are mainly conjugated. The metabolites are excreted in the urine; on oxidation to quinones they may tint the urine green.

Subjects exposed to phenol vapour (without skin contact) in concentrations of 5 to 25 mg per m^3 for a total of 7 hours daily retained 60 to 88% of the inhaled quantity. Retention ranged from 17.8 to 62.8 mg and an average of 99% of this dose was excreted in the urine in 24 hours. Subjects exposed for less then 6 hours to similar concentrations but with a separate air supply retained 8.6 to 47.7 mg from absorption through the skin.— J. K. Piotrowski, *Br. J. ind. Med.*, 1971, *28*, 172.

Uses. Phenol is a disinfectant effective against vegetative Gram-positive and Gram-negative bacteria, but only very slowly effective against spores and acid-fast bacteria. It is also active against certain viruses. Phenol is more active in acid solution; its activity is affected by blood and organic matter.

Aqueous solutions of 0.2 to 1% are bacteriostatic while stronger solutions are bactericidal; this action varies with the organism, strength of solution, and temperature.

When strong solutions of phenol are applied to the skin or mucous membranes, the surface becomes white and opaque owing to precipitation of proteins and a slough is formed; after preliminary slight irritation, the area becomes numb due to paralysis of the sensory nerve endings.

Weaker solutions (up to 2%) have been used as dressings for small wounds. A 0.5 to 1% solution has been used for its local anaesthetic effect to relieve itching. A 0.2 to 0.5% solution with glycerol may be used as a mouth-wash or gargle and dilute solutions of alkaline phenates are used similarly but they are unlikely to have a significant antimicrobial effect.

In dentistry, Liquefied Phenol has been used as an obtundent or analgesic for sensitive dentine. A 5% solution of phenol may be used to devitalise the pulp in deciduous teeth.

The antibacterial and caustic properties of phenol are greatly reduced if it is dissolved in alcohol, glycerol, or fixed oils.

Phenol Glycerin diluted with glycerol is employed as a paint in inflammatory conditions of the mouth and throat and in infections of the middle and external ear. Oily Phenol Injection is injected into the tissues around internal haemorrhoids as an analgesic thrombotic agent.

Phenol 30 to 125 mg is administered intrathecally as a 5% w/w solution in glycerol (Phenol and Glycerol Injection 0.5 to 2 ml) for the alleviation of spasticity and severe intractable pain in malignant neoplasm and solutions of 5 to 20% in Iophendylate Injection or glycerol have been used intrathecally for the reduction of disabling spasticity. Aqueous solutions of phenol 6% have also been used for chemical sympathectomy. Solutions containing 5% phenol have been used as disinfectants for excreta.

The use of phenol in cosmetics and toiletries is restricted in Great Britain under the Cosmetic Products Regulations 1978 (SI 1978: No. 1354).

Molluscum contagiosum could be treated by pricking liquefied phenol into each lesion with a sharpened stick.— F. A. Ive, *Br. med. J.*, 1973, *4*, 475.

A mixture of phenol, water, liquid soap, and croton oil containing approximately 50% of phenol was used for chemical face peeling in the treatment of facial wrinkling. The liquid was applied to the face after thorough cleansing and left for 24 hours under an occlusive dressing. In a group of about 1575 patients there was no evidence of systemic toxicity. Hypertrophic scarring occasionally occurred.— *J. Am. med. Ass.*, 1974, *228*, 898. See also R. P. Ariagno and D. R. Briggs, *Trans. Am. Acad. Ophthal. Oto.-lar.*, 1975, *80*, 536.

Liquefied phenol applied to the nail-bed, nail-fold, and sulci was highly successful for destroying the matrix after removal of ingrowing nails.— A. Shepherdson, *Practitioner*, 1977, *219*, 725. A favourable report of cauterisation for 3 minutes with phenol 88% for onychogryphosis or ingrowing toenail.— T. Andrew and W. A. Wallace, *Br. med. J.*, 1979, *1*, 1539. Further references: P. F. Cameron, *ibid.*, 1981, *283*, 821; P. J. Read (letter), *ibid.*, 1125; W. R. Murray and J. E. Robb (letter), *ibid.*; P. A. G. Helmn (letter), *ibid.*

Enlarged prostate. Fifty patients with benign enlargement of the prostate received an average of 3.2 intraprostatic injections each of 2 to 3 ml of a solution containing: phenol 0.6 ml, glacial acetic acid 0.6 ml, glycerol 1.2 ml, water to 28 ml. Of 29 available for follow-up, 13 had a normal urine stream for 3 years or more and 12 for 1 to 3 years. Histologically there was evidence of haemorrhage or gross necrosis and scarring, but no evidence of inflammation. The procedure was valuable for selected patients with acute retention.— J. J. Shipman *et al.*, *Br. med. J.*, 1974, *3*, 734.

Haemorrhoids. In a controlled study in 60 patients with internal haemorrhoids, the overall results were satisfactory after 6 months in about one-half the patients treated by injections of 3 to 5 ml of 5% phenol in almond oil or by injection of oil alone, and excellent in three-quarters of patients treated by rubber ring ligation. Phenol injections were very effective in controlling bleeding.— C. G. Clark *et al.*, *Br. med. J.*, 1967, *2*, 12. The amount of Oily Phenol Injection required varied from 2 to 6 ml per haemorrhoid; in small haemorrhoids 3 injections of 3 ml might be used.— A. B. G. Carden, *Drugs*, 1972, *4*, 75. Up to 10 ml of phenol 5% in almond or arachis oil could be used for each haemorrhoid; a total of not more than 10 ml should be given at one time.— R. E. B. Tagart, *Practitioner*, 1974, *213*, 141.

Hydrocele. A solution containing phenol 2.5%, dextrose 25%, and glycerol 25% was used for the treatment of hydrocele and epididymal cysts—5 ml was injected for cysts of up to 15 ml, and up to 20 ml for those of 400 to 600 ml; repeated injections might be needed.— G. E. Moloney, *Br. med. J.*, 1975, *3*, 478. Based on experience in 19 patients similarly treated treatment might be successful in hydroceles of moderate size if the volume injected was not less than 1 volume for every 50 volumes aspirated; it was probably inadvisable for hydroceles of larger size and was considered unsuccessful for epididymal cysts. Similar results were obtained with sodium tetradecyl sulphate.— H. Thomson and M. Odell, *ibid.*, 1979, *2*, 704. Assessment 1 or 2 years after treatment of 56 patients showed 95% cure for hydroceles and 100% for epididymal cysts. Side-effects and complications were minimal. Treatment for hydroceles of more than 500 ml was not recommended unless surgery was precluded.— J. R. Nash (letter), *ibid.*, 1980, *280*, 182.

Pain. For reports and discussions of the use of phenol in the relief of pain, see M. Swerdlow, *Anaesthesia*, 1967, *22*, 568; J. W. Warrick (letter), *Br. med. J.*, 1969, *1*, 122; *J. Am. med. Ass.*, 1969, *207*, 855; M. D. Churcher, *Practitioner*, 1973, *210*, 243; S. Lifshitz *et al.*, *Obstet. Gynec.*, 1976, *48*, 316; A. Rubin and B. Master (letter), *Br. med. J.*, 1978, *1*, 790; J. W. Lloyd, *ibid.*, 1980, *281*, 432; *ibid.*, 549.

Pilonidal sinus. Injection of liquefied phenol was used to treat pilonidal sinus in 20 patients. None complained of pain or discomfort, but there was an inflammatory reaction in 2 patients probably due to inadvertent injection into the tissues around the sinus.— F. O. Stephens and D. R. Sloane, *Med. J. Aust.*, 1968, *1*, 395.

Further references: B. A. Maurice and R. K. Greenwood, *Br. J. Surg.*, 1964, *51*, 510.

Spasticity. In 68 patients with spasticity due to cerebrovascular accidents, spinal cord injuries, and cerebral palsy, 126 peripheral nerves were blocked with aqueous phenol solution. The period of effectiveness ranged from 2 to 743 days, with an average of 308 days. Seven nerve blocks were repeated. Gain and loss of voluntary movement following the blocks were observed. Ten patients developed paraesthesias. Muscle atrophy and osteoporosis could be prevented by this simple method.— A. A. Khalali and H. B. Betts, *J. Am. med. Ass.*, 1967, *200*, 1155. A similar report.— D. Halpern and F. E. Meelhuysen, *ibid.*, 1152.

Further references: A. N. Győry, *Drugs*, 1980, *20*, 309.

Preparations

Dental Preparations

Dental Phenol with Camphor *(Jap. P.).* Phenol c. Camph. Dent. Phenol 35 g, camphor 65 g.

Ear-drops

Phenol Ear-drops *(B.P.C. 1973).* Phenol glycerin 40 ml, glycerol to 100 ml. They contain about 6.4% w/w of phenol.

CAUTION. *Dilution with water renders the ear-drops caustic; glycerol may be used as a diluent.*

Gargles and Mouth-washes

Alkaline Phenol Mouth-wash *(D.P.F.).* Collut. Phenol. Alk.; Phenol and Alkali Mouth-wash. Liquefied phenol 3 ml, potassium hydroxide solution 3 ml, amaranth solution 1 ml, water to 100 ml. To be diluted with 10 times its vol. of warm water before use.

Phenol Gargle *(B.P.C. 1973).* Garg. Phenol.; Carbolic Acid Gargle. Phenol glycerin 5 ml, amaranth solution 1 ml, water to 100 ml; it contains about 1% w/v of phenol. It should be diluted with an equal vol. of warm water before use.

Glycerins

Phenol Glycerin *(B.P., Ind. P.).* Phenol 16% w/w in glycerol. Store in airtight containers.

CAUTION. *Dilution with water renders this preparation caustic; glycerol may be used as a diluent.*

Phenol Glycerin is too strong to use undiluted. It may be diluted with an equal volume of glycerol for use as an antiseptic and analgesic paint in the treatment of mouth ulcers and tonsillitis. It is used in the preparation of Phenol Ear-drops..

Injections

Hackett's Sclerosing Solution. Zinc sulphate-phenol stock 4 ml, amethocaine hydrochloride solution (0.15%) 42 ml, sodium chloride injection 42 ml. The formula for zinc sulphate-phenol stock is zinc sulphate 8 g, liquefied phenol 12 ml, glycerol 24 ml, distilled water to 100 ml.—*Br. med. J.*, 1961, *1*, 522.

Oily Phenol Injection *(B.P.).* Inj. Phenol. Oleos.; 5% Phenol in Oil Injection. A sterile 5% w/v solution of phenol in almond oil. Sterilised by heating at 150° for one hour. For the treatment of haemorrhoids.

Comparison of the subsequent histological changes showed that in the treatment of piles the effect of injection of almond oil and of injection of almond oil containing 5% phenol was similar. It was concluded that the symptomatic improvement was due to almond oil rather than to phenol.— C. W. Graham-Stewart, *Br. med. J.*, 1962, *1*, 213.

Phenol and Glycerol Injection *(B.P.).* Phenol and Glycerin Injection. Phenol 5 g, glycerol, previously dried at 120° for one hour, to 100 g. The solution is distributed in dry ampoules, sealed, and sterilised by heating at 150° for 1 hour. Protect from light. *Dose.* By intrathecal injection for the relief of pain and spasticity, 0.5 to 2 ml.

Phenol and Silver Nitrate in Glycerol. Dissolve, aseptically, phenol 1 g in sterile glycerol 24 ml in a dry sterile bottle; add 0.3 ml of a sterile 5% solution of silver nitrate in Water for Injections and adjust to 25 ml with Water for Injections. The final injection contains 600 µg of silver nitrate in a 4% solution of phenol in glycerol. —R.M. Maher, *Lancet*, 1960, *1*, 895. For lumbosacral injection for pain.

Phenol in Iophendylate Injection. Dissolve, aseptically, the requisite amount of phenol in the sterile Iophendylate Injection.—V.H. Mark *et al.*, *New Engl. J. Med.*, 1962, *267*, 589.

Lotions

Phenol Lotion *(B.P.C. 1954).* Carbolic Acid Lotion. Liquefied phenol 2.6 ml, amaranth solution 0.104 ml, water to 100 ml. To be diluted with an equal vol. of warm water before use.

Amended formula. Liquefied phenol 2.6 ml, amaranth solution 0.1 ml, water to 100 ml.—*Compendium of Past Formulae 1933 to 1966*, London, The National Pharmaceutical Union, 1969.

Ointments

Salicylated Phenol Ointment *(Jap. P.).* Phenol 3 g, salicylic acid 5 g, white soft paraffin or other suitable ointment basis to 100 g, with aromatics.

Paints

Phenol with Camphor *(B.P.C. 1949).* Carbolic Camphor; Paint of Phenol with Camphor. Phenol 25 g triturated with camphor 75 g, until liquefied. It is immiscible with water and glycerol.

Phenol with Camphor may be used to relieve toothache due to exposed pulp; it has also been used to treat athlete's foot. It is not intended for use over extensive areas and should not be applied to the face.

Proprietary Preparations

Chloraseptic *(Norwich-Eaton, UK).* Liquid containing phenol and sodium phenolate equivalent to total phenol 1.4%, with sodium borate, menthol, thymol, and glycerol. For use as a spray or gargle in mouth and throat infections. (Also available as Chloraseptic in *USA*).

See also under Some Proprietary Preparations containing Cresols, Tar Acids, or other Phenols, p.575.

Other Proprietary Names

Fenicado *(Spain)*; Paoscle *(Jap.)*.

2269-y

Picloxydine. 1,1′-[Piperazine-1,4-diylbis(formimidoyl)]bis[3-(4-chlorophenyl)guanidine]. $C_{20}H_{24}Cl_2N_{10}$=475.4.

CAS — 5636-92-0.

Picloxydine is a disinfectant with actions similar to those of chlorhexidine gluconate (see p.554).

It has been used, as digluconate, with benzalkonium chloride, in a detergent basis for the cleansing and disinfection of surfaces.

References: A. M. Gordon, *J. clin. Path.*, 1969, *22*, 496; J. M. H. Boyce and H. M. Meddick (letter), *Br. med. J.*, 1974, *1*, 38; S. Morris *et al.* (letter), *Med. J. Aust.*, 1976, *2*, 110; M. Guinness and J. Levey (letter), *ibid.*, 392; T. W. Ostrowski and A. K. Sutherland (letter), *ibid.*, 1977, *1*, 78; I. M. Maurer (letter), *ibid.*, 308.

A preparation containing picloxydine digluconate was formerly marketed in Great Britain under the proprietary name Resiguard (*Nicholas*).

2270-g

Polynoxylin. Poly{-[bis(hydroxymethyl)ureylene]methylene}, a condensation product of formaldehyde and urea with the formula.
$(C_4H_8N_2O_3)_n$.

CAS — 9011-05-6.

An amorphous, white, odourless, tasteless powder. Decomposes at 200° without melting. Slightly **soluble** in water.

Uses. Polynoxylin has wide antibacterial and antifungal actions. It may act by the release of formaldehyde. It has been used as a cream, aerosol, or powder, usually containing 10%, for the treatment of infections of the skin. It has also been used in lozenges for infections of the mouth.

Polynoxylin and noxythiolin evolved formaldehyde when stored at 37° for 18 hours.— D. Kingston, *J. clin. Path.*, 1965, *18*, 666.

Antimicrobial activity. Polynoxylin inhibited 169 of 170 strains of *Proteus vulgaris*, *Pr. morganii*, *Salmonella typhi*, *Klebsiella pneumoniae*, *Pseudomonas aeruginosa*, *Streptococcus faecalis*, *Str. pyogenes*, *Staphylococcus aureus*, *Escherichia coli*, *Kleb. aerogenes*, and *Enterobacter cloacae* grown on solid media. The only resistant organism was a strain of *Enterobacter cloacae*. Strains of *Staph. aureus* which were resistant to the usual antibiotics were less susceptible than antibiotic-sensitive strains to the action of polynoxylin.— G. Wernsdorfer and W. H. Wernsdorfer, *Arzneimittel-Forsch.*, 1967, *17*, 1204.

Mouth infections. Polynoxylin lozenges, used thrice daily or up to 8 a day, were tested against a placebo over a period of 14 days in 2 double-blind trials in 30 patients with denture stomatitis due to infection by *Candida albicans*. Only 2 patients showed improvement: 1 on placebo and 1 on polynoxylin.— H. I. B. Phillips, *Br. dent. J.*, 1970, *128*, 78.

Polynoxylin in concentrations recommended by the manufacturer had no effect on the numbers of *Candida albicans* in the mouths of patients; tests *in vitro* confirmed the drug's inactivity.— J. JWilliamson (letter), *Br. dent. J.*, 1970, *129*, 102.

Proprietary Preparations

Anaflex *(Geistlich, UK).* Polynoxylin, available as **Aerosol** containing 2%; as **Cream** containing 10%; as **Paste** containing 10%; as **Powder** containing 10%; and as **Lozenges** each containing 30 mg. (Also available as Anaflex in *Austral.*, *Denm.*, *Neth.*, *Switz.*).

Ponoxylan Gel *(Berk Pharmaceuticals, UK).* Contains polynoxylin 10% in a macrogol basis. (Also available as Ponoxylan in *Austral.*, *S.Afr.*).

Other Proprietary Names

Larex *(Switz.)*.

2271-q

Proflavine Hemisulphate *(B.P.C. 1973).* Neutral Proflavine Sulphate; Proflavine. 3,6-Diaminoacridine sulphate dihydrate.
$(C_{13}H_{11}N_3)_2,H_2SO_4,2H_2O$=552.6.

CAS — 92-62-6 (proflavine).

Pharmacopoeias. In *Belg.* and *Ind.* as monohydrate.

An orange to red, odourless or almost odourless, hygroscopic, crystalline powder with a bitter taste. **Soluble** 1 in 300 of water, 1 in 1 of boiling water, and 1 in 35 of glycerol; very slightly soluble in alcohol; practically insoluble in chloroform and ether. A saturated solution in water has a pH of 6 to 8, is deep orange in colour, and gives a green fluorescence when freely diluted. A 0.1% solution in physiological saline is clear or almost clear and does not visibly deteriorate when stored for 24 hours in the dark. **Store** in airtight containers. Protect from light.

A solution prepared by dissolving proflavine hemisulphate 0.4% and tannic acid 4% in hot water became cloudy and developed a gummy deposit on cooling. Inclusion of 40% or more of glycerol resulted in a clear solution.— Pharm. Soc. Lab. Rep. P/71/26, 1971.

Removal of stains. A flavine stain is easily removed from the skin by scrubbing immediately with a household detergent (or soap) and hot water. For old stains immerse the skin in hot water and then rub with a piece of lemon, or wash with a dilute solution of sulphurous or hydrochloric acid.

Adverse Effects. Hypersensitivity reactions to proflavine have been reported occasionally.

Skin sensitivity to proflavine hemisulphate, confirmed by patch tests, was seen in 3 patients during the period 1957–66.— J. K. Morgan, *Br. J. clin. Pract.*, 1968, *22*, 261.

Discussions of a possible risk of carcinogenicity after the use of photoactive dyes such as neutral red or proflavine, followed by exposure to fluorescent light, in herpes simplex infections.— *Med. Lett.*, 1974, *16*, 111; R. S.

Berger and C. M. Papa, *J. Am. med. Ass.*, 1977, *238*, 133.

Uses. The acridine derivatives, proflavine, acriflavine, aminacrine, ethacridine, and euflavine, are slow-acting disinfectants. They are bacteriostatic against many Gram-positive bacteria but less effective against Gram-negative organisms; in the concentrations usually employed they are not effective against *Proteus vulgaris, Pseudomonas aeruginosa,* some strains of *Escherichia coli,* and acid-fast bacteria. They have little antifungal activity and solutions are liable to grow moulds. Their activity is increased in alkaline solutions and is not reduced by tissue fluids. The acridines are absorbed on to dressings.

The acridine derivatives have been used for the treatment of infected wounds or burns and for skin disinfection. Prolonged treatment may delay healing. They have also been used for the treatment of local infections of the ear, mouth, and throat.

Herpes. In a preliminary study with 28 women suffering from recurrent herpes with antibodies to herpes virus, proflavine 0.1% was painted on the patients' ulcers and exposed to incandescent or fluorescent light at a distance of 15 to 20 cm for at least 10 minutes. The dye was applied and exposed to light a second time. Fifteen of these women experienced immediate relief compared with 8 of 20 with primary disease.— *J. Am. med. Ass.*, 1973, *226*, 528. See also R. H. Kaufman *et al.*, *Am. J. Obstet. Gynec.*, 1973, *117*, 1144; *J. Am. med. Ass.*, 1975, *231*, 79.

In a study in 36 male patients with genital herpes simplex infection the area of the lesions after proflavine photo-inactivation remained larger for longer than after the use of idoxuridine or placebo, the healing time was slower, and virus could be isolated for longer.— P. K. Taylor and N. R. Doherty, *Br. J. vener. Dis.*, 1975, *51*, 125.

Proflavine hemisulphate was no more effective than placebo when used with photo-inactivation in the treatment of 157 women with genital herpes simplex infection.— R. H. Kaufman *et al.*, *Am. J. Obstet. Gynec.*, 1978, *132*, 861, per *Int. pharm. Abstr.*, 1980, *17*, 320.

See also under Adverse Effects.

Preparations

Proflavine Cream *(B.P.C. 1973).* Flavine Cream; Proflavine Emulsion. Proflavine hemisulphate 100 mg, chlorocresol 100 mg, yellow beeswax 2.5 g, wool fat 5 g, freshly boiled and cooled water 25 g, and liquid paraffin 67.3 g. Store in a cool place in containers which prevent evaporation and contamination.

Proflavine Cream (*B.P.C.*) had little or no antibacterial activity when tested *in vitro* against 6 pathogenic organisms, as the proflavine hemisulphate was in the aqueous phase of a water-in-oil emulsion and was not released. Other salts of proflavine with a series of acids were tried in the same basis, and a water-in-oil cream containing 0.8% w/w of proflavine *n*-valerate, soluble in both oil and water, was found to be the most active. However, the hemisulphate was readily released from an oil-in-water cream and exhibited antibacterial activity. A suggested formula: proflavine hemisulphate 100 mg, cetomacrogol emulsifying wax 15 g, liquid paraffin 20 g, water to 100 g.— A. H. Fenton and M. Warren, *Pharm. J.*, 1962, *1*, 5.

2272-p

Propamidine Isethionate *(B.P.C. 1949, B. Vet. C. 1965).* Propamidin. Isethion.; Propamidine Isetionate. 4,4′-Trimethylenedioxydibenzamidine bis(2-hydroxyethanesulphonate).

$C_{17}H_{20}N_4O_2,2C_2H_6O_4S$=564.6.

CAS — 104-32-5 (propamidine); 140-63-6 (isethionate).

A white or nearly white, odourless, granular, hygroscopic powder with a bitter taste. **Soluble** 1 in 5 of water, 1 in 33 of alcohol, and in glycerol; practically insoluble in organic solvents. **Store** in airtight containers.

Uses. Propamidine isethionate has antibacterial and antifungal properties. It is active against *Staphylococcus aureus, Streptococcus pyogenes,* and certain other streptococci and clostridia, but not against *Pseudomonas aeruginosa, Proteus vulgaris,* or *Escherichia coli.* Its action is not reduced by tissue fluids, serum, or pus.

Propamidine isethionate is used similarly to dibromopropamidine isethionate (see p.561) as a 0.15% cream for the treatment of minor burns and wounds. Treatment for more than 10 days may cause a superficial necrosis of the granulations and lead to reinfection.

An ophthalmic solution containing 0.1% of propamidine isethionate is used for the treatment of conjunctivitis. Treatment should not be prolonged for more than a week.

Proprietary Preparations

Brolene Eye Drops *(May & Baker, UK).* Contain propamidine isethionate 0.1%. (Also available as Brolene Eye Drops in *Austral.*).

M & B Antiseptic Cream *(May & Baker, UK).* Contains propamidine isethionate 0.15% in a water-miscible basis. (Also available as M & B Antiseptic Cream in *Austral., S.Afr.*).

2273-s

Propiolactone.

β-Propiolactone; BPL. Propiono-3-lactone.

$C_3H_4O_2$=72.06.

CAS — 57-57-8.

A colourless liquid with a pungent odour. Its vapour is not explosive or inflammable. B.p. about 162°, with rapid decomposition. **Soluble** 1 in 3 of water; miscible with acetone, chloroform, and ether. **Incompatible** with alcohol. It hydrolyses to hydracrylic acid, slowly in the absence of added moisture, but rapidly and completely in aqueous solutions. It is stable when **stored** in airtight glass containers at 5° to 10°.

In aqueous solution, the half-life of propiolactone was 18 hours at 10°, 3½ hours at 25°, and 20 minutes at 50°.— S. H. Hopper, *Am. J. Hosp. Pharm.*, 1961, *18*, 388.

Adverse Effects. Propiolactone vapour is a caustic vesicant, extremely irritating to the skin, eyes, and mucous membranes. Inhalation of the vapour causes headache, sweating, epigastric pain, and tachycardia. The liquid has shown carcinogenic activity in *animals*.

The biological and chemical aspects of propiolactone as a carcinogen.— F. Dickens, *Br. med. Bull.*, 1964, *20*, 96.

Uses. Propiolactone vapour is a highly effective disinfectant which is active against vegetative Gram-positive and Gram-negative bacteria, acid-fast bacteria, fungi, and viruses. It is rather less effective against bacterial spores.

Propiolactone vapour has been used for the gaseous sterilisation of pharmaceutical and surgical materials and for disinfecting large enclosed areas. It has low penetrating power and for effective sterilisation a propiolactone concentration of 2 to 5 mg per litre of air and a relative humidity of about 80% for 2 hours at 24° are required. These concentrations are obtained by heating or atomising propiolactone in an enclosed space.

Propiolactone has been used as a 0.2 to 1% aqueous solution for the sterilisation of tissues for grafting. It is used for the sterilisation of rabies vaccine. It is not suitable for sterilising nylon, polystyrene, or polyvinyl chloride.

Suitable apparatus for promoting vaporisation of propiolactone by heating the liquid in an air-stream, by atomisation, or by drawing a vacuum.— H. F. Allen and J. T. Murphy, *J. Am. med. Ass.*, 1960, *172*, 1759.

A method for disinfecting large enclosures with propiolactone.— D. R. Spiner and R. K. Hoffman, *Appl. Microbiol.*, 1960, *8*, 152.

The chemical and physical properties of propiolactone and tests of its reliability as a gaseous bactericide.— S. H. Hopper, *Am. J. Hosp. Pharm.*, 1961, *18*, 388.

The use of propiolactone for the disinfection of enclosed areas.— C. W. Bruch, *Am. J. Hyg.*, 1961, *73*, 1.

Propiolactone, 1% in water or pH 6.8 phosphate buffer, killed *Escherichia coli, Bacillus subtilis* spores, and *Aspergillus niger* spores within 40 minutes.— W. Hazeu and H. J. Hueck, *Antonie van Leeuwenhoek*, 1965, *31*, 295.

The moisture content and location of water in the bacterial cell was an important factor in disinfection by propiolactone vapour. Higher atmospheric humidities were required to kill desiccated spores exposed to propiolactone than those required for non-desiccated spores.— R. K. Hoffman, *Appl. Microbiol.*, 1968, *16*, 641.

The use of propiolactone to sterilise pig heart valves.— J. A. Myers, *Chemist Drugg.*, 1969, *192*, 232.

The effect of combined propiolactone and ultraviolet irradiation treatment on hepatitis B virus.— A. M. Prince and W. Stephan (letter), *Lancet*, 1980, *2*, 917.

Proprietary Names

Betaprone *(Fellows, USA).*

2274-w

Scarlet Red *(B.P.C. 1959).* Rubrum Scarlatinum; Biebrich Scarlet R Medicinal; Sudan IV; Scharlachrot; CI Solvent Red 24; Colour Index No. 26105. 1-[4-(*o*-Tolylazo)-*o*-tolylazo]naphth-2-ol.

$C_{24}H_{20}N_4O$=380.4.

CAS — 85-83-6.

Pharmacopoeias. In *Aust.*

A dark reddish-brown, odourless powder. Practically **insoluble** in water; soluble 1 in 15 of chloroform; slightly soluble in alcohol; soluble in oils, fats, and warm soft paraffin. **Protect** from light.

Adverse Effects. Ointments containing more than 5% of scarlet red are irritant and may cause systemic effects.

Uses. Scarlet red has been used, usually as a 5% ointment, to promote the growth of epithelium in the treatment of wounds, burns, and ulcers.

Preparations

Scarlet Red Ointment *(B.P.C. 1954).* Ung. Rub. Scarlat.; Unguentum Rubrum. Scarlet red 5% in yellow simple ointment.

2275-e

Sodium Bithionolate. Sodium Bitionolate. Disodium 2,2′-thiobis(4,6-dichlorophenolate).

$C_{12}H_4Cl_4Na_2O_2S$=400.0.

CAS — 6385-58-6.

Sodium bithionolate is a bactericide with actions and uses similar to those of bithionol, p.550.

2276-l

Sodium Dichloroisocyanurate.

Sodium Troclosene; Sodium Dichloro-*s*-triazinetrione. The sodium salt of 1,3-dichloro-1,3,5-triazine-2,4,6(1*H*,3*H*,5*H*)-trione.

$C_3Cl_2N_3NaO_3$=219.9.

CAS — 2893-78-9.

A white crystalline or granular powder containing about 64% of 'available chlorine' (see p.557). **Soluble** 1 in 4 of water. A 1% solution has a pH of about 6.

Adverse Effects and Treatment. As for Strong Sodium Hypochlorite Solution, below.

Uses. Sodium dichloroisocyanurate has the actions and uses of chlorine (see p.557) but its activity is only slightly affected by pH over the range 6 to 10. It is used for disinfecting babies' feeding bottles and napkins, and in various commercial bleach detergents and scouring powders as a relatively stable source of chlorine.

Dichloroisocyanuric acid ($C_3HCl_2N_3O_3$ = 198.0), potassium dichloroisocyanurate (potassium troclosene, troclosene potassium, $C_3Cl_2KN_3O_3$ = 236.1), and trichloroisocyanuric acid (symclosene, $C_3Cl_3N_3O_3$ = 232.4) are similarly used.

The addition of half of a tablet containing sodium dichloroisocyanurate 500 mg in an effervescent basis (Simpla Tablets) to 1.1 litres of water produced a solution containing from 156 to 206 ppm of 'available chlorine'. The neutral solution made with these tablets retained a potency well above 125 ppm for 7 days. A daily output of about 400 infants' feeding bottles had been sterilised by standing for several days in a solution of sodium dichloroisocyanurate. The solution was prepared from 400 tablets in 200 gallons of water in a stainless steel tank and was replaced twice weekly; urine collecting bottles could be sterilised similarly. A diluted sodium hypochlorite solution (Milton) had a lower initial strength but lost less potency on keeping.— W. T. Wing, *J. Hosp. Pharm.*, 1970, *28*, 47. A similar report.— *idem*, 1972, *30*, 157.

Solutions prepared from sodium dichloroisocyanurate effervescent tablets had a significantly higher bactericidal capacity than stabilised solutions of sodium hypochlorite against *Escherichia coli* and retained satisfactory levels of activity in the presence of 2% milk. The hypochlorite solution was inactivated by milk.— S. F. Bloomfield, *Lab. Pract.*, 1973, *22*, 672, per *Abstr. Hyg.*, 1974, *49*, 3. Sodium dichloroisocyanurate was also more active than sodium hypochlorite against *Salmonella typhi*, *Pseudomonas aeruginosa*, *Staphylococcus aureus* , and *Klebsiella aerogenes* and of similar activity against *Candida albicans*. Differences in activity between sodium dichloroisocyanurate and sodium hypochlorite were not entirely due to pH effects.— S. F. Bloomfield and G. A. Miles, *J. appl. Bact.*, 1979, *46*, 65.

A review of the toxicity and chemical and bacteriological properties of cyanuric acid and chlorinated isocyanurates and their application to swimming pool disinfection.— E. Canelli, *Am. J. publ. Hlth*, 1974, *64*, 155.

See also The Purification of the Water of Swimming Pools, Department of the Environment, London, HM Stationery Office, 1975.

Proprietary Preparations of Chlorinated Isocyanurates

ACL 56 *(Monsanto, UK)*. A brand of sodium dichloroisocyanurate dihydrate. **ACL 59**. A brand of potassium dichloroisocyanurate. **ACL 60**. A brand of sodium dichloroisocyanurate. **ACL 66**. A complex of trichloroisocyanuric acid and potassium dichloroisocyanurate in the ratio 1:4. **ACL 85**. A brand of trichloroisocyanuric acid.

Babysafe Tablets *(Kirby-Warrick, UK)*. Each effervescent tablet contains sodium dichloroisocyanurate 500 mg. **Babysafe-5 Tablets**. Each contains sodium dichloroisocyanurate 5 g.

Fi-Clor 91 *(Chlor-Chem, UK)*. A brand of trichloroisocyanuric acid; also available as tablets (Fi-Tab S/D and Fi-Clor Tablets, Maxi and Mini).

Fi-Clor Clearon *(Chlor-Chem, UK)*. A brand of sodium dichloroisocyanurate dihydrate; also available **Granules** and as **Tablets** (Fi-Tab R/D).

Kirbychlor Tablets *(Kirby-Warrick, UK)*. Each effervescent tablet contains sodium dichloroisocyanurate 2.5 g.

Multichlor *(Spearhead, UK)*. Tablets containing dichloroisocyanuric acid and sodium bicarbonate, with a detergent and a trace of sodium chlorate. One tablet dissolved in 1 gallon of water provides a solution containing 200 ppm of 'available chlorine'. For the disinfection of medical equipment.

Puritabs *(Kirby-Warrick, UK)*. Each effervescent tablet contains sodium dichloroisocyanurate 17 mg. **Puritabs-Maxi.** Each effervescent tablet contains sodium dichloroisocyanurate 425 mg. For treating drinking water. One Puritabs tablet dissolved in 1 litre of water, or 1 Puritabs-Maxi tablet dissolved in 25 litres, provides a solution containing 10 ppm of 'available chlorine'. (Also available as Puritabs and Puritabs-Maxi in *Austral.*).

Reddichlor Tablets *(Reddish Detergents, UK)*. Contain dichloroisocyanuric acid and sodium bicarbonate, with a detergent and a trace of sodium chlorate. One tablet dissolved in 1 gallon of water provides a solution containing 200 ppm of 'available chlorine'. For the disinfection of dairy and medical equipment.

Simpla Tablets *(Ashe, UK)*. Each contains sodium dichloroisocyanurate 500 mg.

Tricidechlor *(Wingfield, UK)*. A brand of sodium dichloroisocyanurate dihydrate.

2277-y

Strong Sodium Hypochlorite Solution
(B.P.).

Pharmacopoeias. In *Br.*

An aqueous solution containing not less than 8% w/w (80 000 ppm) of 'available chlorine' (see p.557), prepared by absorption of chlorine in sodium hydroxide solution. It decreases in strength fairly rapidly and should be used as soon as possible after preparation. It may contain suitable stabilising agents. **Store** at a temperature not exceeding 20° away from acids in well-filled airtight bottles, closed with a glass stopper or suitable plastic cap. Protect from light. It should not be stored for longer than a few months. The solution is alkaline and must be diluted before use.

Adverse Effects. Hypochlorite solutions release hypochlorous acid upon contact with gastric juice and acids, and ingestion causes irritation and corrosion of mucous membranes with pain and vomiting. A fall in blood pressure, delirium, and coma may occur. Inhalation of hypochlorous fumes causes coughing and choking and may cause severe respiratory tract irritation and pulmonary oedema.

An 18-year-old attendant developed onycholysis of all her fingernails after adding 16% sodium hypochlorite solution to swimming-pool water daily for several weeks. The nails grew normally when she ceased using the preparation. Onycholysis developed the following year when she again used the hypochlorite solution.— R. J. Coskey (letter), *Archs Derm.*, 1974, *109*, 96.

A young girl had suffered episodes of vomiting, abdominal pain, and bronchopneumonia over a period of years, which were finally traced to her habit of sucking socks bleached with sodium hypochlorite.— F. X. Loeb and T. L. King, *Am. J. Dis. Child.*, 1974, *128*, 256.

Treatment of Adverse Effects. If sodium hypochlorite solution is ingested, give water, milk, or other demulcents; antacids and sodium thiosulphate 1% solution may be of value.

Precautions. Topically applied hypochlorites may dissolve blood clots and cause bleeding.

Sodium hypochlorite could interfere with the Clinistix and Labstix qualitative urine tests for glucose to produce false positive results.— *Drug & Ther. Bull.*, 1972, *10*, 69.

Traces of sodium hypochlorite solution adhering to utensils for preparing feeds of pooled human milk for premature infants increased dietary sodium intake by 50% in a series of 9 paired estimations.— A. Lucas (letter), *Lancet*, 1977, *2*, 144.

Uses. Sodium hypochlorite solutions have the actions and uses of chlorine (see p.557). They are commonly used for the rapid disinfection of hard surfaces, food and dairy equipment, and babies' feeding bottles, but their alkalinity and rapid inactivation by organic matter are disadvantages. Only diluted solutions containing up to 0.5% of 'available chlorine' are suitable for use on the skin and in wounds.

As with other chlorine-containing solutions, an alkaline pH is required for stability, though hypochlorites are more active at a slightly acid pH.

A solution of sodium hypochlorite containing 200 ppm of 'available chlorine' was effective in destroying Sabin type 2 poliomyelitis virus on babies' napkins soiled by infants excreting the virus.— W. E. Jordan *et al.*, *Am. J. Dis. Child.*, 1969, *117*, 313, per *J. Am. med. Ass.*, 1969, *207*, 2119.

To reduce the risk of transmission of hepatitis in renal dialysis units, haemodialysis equipment and surfaces contaminated with blood or other body fluid should be disinfected with a strong hypochlorite solution containing 10 000 ppm of 'available chlorine'. A weak solution containing 1000 ppm was suitable for objects not known to be soiled. These solutions should be freshly diluted each day in carefully cleansed containers. Glutaraldehyde as a 2% solution should be used for surgical instruments and metal parts liable to corrosion. After soaking in disinfectant to remove blood, contaminated equipment should whenever possible be autoclaved.— *Hepatitis and the Treatment of Chronic Renal Failure*, Report of the Advisory Group 1970–2, London, DHSS, 1973.

A short discussion on the use of sodium hypochlorite solutions for the inactivation of hepatitis A and B viruses.— J. A. Bryan (letter), *J. Am. med. Ass.*, 1974, *230*, 961.

Human breast milk expressed hygienically into sterilised glass containers which had been rinsed in 1% sodium hypochlorite solution had a lower bacterial count (within 4 hours) than samples expressed into sterile glass containers.— C. L. Jones *et al.*, *Br. med. J.*, 1979, *2*, 1320.

Disinfection of equipment. Haemodialysis tanks were sterile after circulation for 20 minutes of 290 ml of 5.25% sodium hypochlorite solution in 25 litres of tap water at 50° and pH 8.6. After 6 to 8 hours of dialysis, total bacterial counts were about 40 000 per ml.— P. M. Tierno, *Appl. Microbiol.*, 1968, *16*, 1259.

A mixture of methyl alcohol 50% and sodium hypochlorite solution which gave a solution of 2000 ppm of 'available chlorine' was highly sporicidal against spores of *Bacillus subtilis* and was effective within 10 minutes and up to 8 hours after preparation; it might be of use for the disinfection of instruments sensitive to heat.— D. Coates and J. E. Death, *J. clin. Path.*, 1978, *31*, 148. By buffering sodium hypochlorite solution or alcohol and sodium hypochlorite mixtures in the pH range 7.6 to 8.1, high sporicidal activity could be obtained with low concentrations of alcohol and sodium hypochlorite.— J. E. Death and D. Coates, *ibid.*, 1979, *32*, 148.

Disinfection of water. Sodium hypochlorite solution in tap water, containing 5 ppm 'available chlorine', inactivated cercarias of *Schistosoma mansoni* in 1 to 2.5 minutes at pH 5, in 3 minutes at pH 7.5, and in about 30 minutes at pH 10 at 20°. The latter time was reduced to about one-fifth at 40° but increasing the 'available chlorine' to about 15 ppm only reduced the times slightly. Cercarias were inactivated in 30 minutes by 0.3 ppm at pH 5, 0.6 ppm at pH 7.5, and 5 ppm at pH 10.— L. P. Frick and G. V. Hillyer, *Milit. Med.*, 1966, *131*, 372. Sodium hypochlorite 10 ppm killed all cercarias of *Schistosoma mansoni* and *S. haematobium* in drinking water within 10 minutes. Halazone tablets were only slowly soluble and left a taste but had an immediate cercaricidal effect.— P. J. Fripp *et al.*, *S. Afr. med. J.*, 1972, *46*, 1819.

For the use of sodium hypochlorite for the bacteriological control of a hydrotherapy pool, see A. F. Barnard, *Community Med.*, 1972, *129*, 87.

Sterilisation of feeding bottles. A freshly prepared hypochlorite solution containing 100 to 200 ppm of 'available chlorine' might be used for sterilising infants' feeding bottles. The cleaned bottles and teats should be totally submerged in the solution for 3 hours; it was preferable for the individual bottle and teat of each child to be soaked in a separate bowl of hypochlorite solution and for the bowls to be kept on shelves in a covered-in cupboard. A warm solution was preferable to a cold solution. Bottles and teats should be handled as little as possible after removal from the hypochlorite solution in preparation for the feed.—Report of a MRC Working Party, *Mon. Bull. Minist. Hlth*, 1953, *12*, 209 and 214. See also *Br. med. J.*, 1963, *1*, 970.

Infant feeds produced by a hospital milk kitchen were found to be contaminated by Gram-negative bacteria. Mixing containers, dispensers, and bottles had been cleansed and then sterilised with a 1% hypochlorite solution, diluted 1 in 80, but taps which could not be cleansed before disinfection were the source of contamination. Terminal heat sterilisation, with aseptically prepared feeds and disposable bottles or sterile feeds 'ready to use' was recommended as a replacement for chemical disinfection.— G. A. J. Ayliffe *et al.*, *Lancet*, 1970, *1*, 559.

In 758 households, 48% of the mothers disinfected feeding bottles and teats with sodium hypochlorite solution, 30% boiled the bottles and teats, and 11% used both processes. Assuming 5 or fewer colonies of bacteria per bottle or teat to be acceptable, 78% of the bottles and 70% of teats disinfected with hypochlorite were satisfactory compared with 46% and 34% respectively following boiling.— J. A. D. Anderson and A. Gatherer, *Br. med. J.*, 1970, *2*, 20.

Preparations

Antiforminum Dentale *(Jap. P.)*. Dental Sodium Hypochlorite Solution. A solution containing not less than 3% of sodium hypochlorite prepared from chlorinated lime 12 g, anhydrous sodium carbonate 8.5 g, and water to 100 ml.

Dilute Sodium Hypochlorite Solution *(B.P.)*. An aqueous solution containing 0.9 to 1.1% w/w of 'available chlorine'. It may contain stabilising agents and sodium chloride. Store at a temperature not exceeding 20° away from acids in well-filled airtight bottles. Protect from light.

Similar solutions are included in some other pharmacopoeias.

Eau de Javelle. A title which has been applied to preparations of potassium hypochlorite, prepared from chlorinated lime and potassium carbonate.

Labarraque's Solution. The *U.S.N.F. XIV (1975)* directed that when this solution was ordered Sodium Hypochlorite Solution [now *U.S.P.*] diluted with an equal volume of water be dispensed.

Sodium Hypochlorite Solution *(U.S.P.)*. A solution containing 4 to 6% w/w of NaOCl. Store in airtight containers at a temperature not exceeding 25°. Protect from light. It is not suitable for application to wounds. Similar solutions are included in some other pharmacopoeias.

For other preparations containing hypochlorites, see under Chlorinated Lime, p.557.

Proprietary Preparations

Chloros *(ICI Mond, UK)*. A relatively stable sodium hypochlorite solution available as a general disinfectant, and as a special grade (Agricultural) for sterilising dairy equipment. The former contains not less than 10% and the latter 11% ± 0.5% by weight of 'available chlorine' when dispatched from the works.

Deosan Green Label Steriliser *(Diversey, UK)*. A solution of low alkalinity containing 10% of 'available chlorine'. For use as a general antiseptic and for disinfection of kitchen utensils and crockery.

Diversol BX *(Diversey, UK)*. A crystalline powder containing a sodium hypochlorite-sodium phosphate complex and a bromine salt, which react to produce sodium hypobromite; contains 3% of 'available halogen'. For use as a general disinfectant and for disinfection of equipment and utensils.

Hospital Milton *(Richardson-Vicks, UK)*. A stabilised 1% sodium hypochlorite solution with standardised salt and free alkali content. **Milton 2**. A similar solution containing sodium hypochlorite 2%. For use as general antiseptics.

Hyposan and Voxsan *(Voxsan, UK)*. Sodium hypochlorite solutions containing 12.5% of 'available chlorine'. The former is used mainly in dairying for sterilising milk bottles, etc., and the latter in water purification.

Milton Crystals *(Richardson-Vicks, UK)*. Crystals containing potassium monopersulphate (K_2SO_5=190.3) and sodium chloride, yielding sodium hypochlorite in aqueous solution. For treatment of infant feeding utensils.

Parozone *(Jeyes, UK)*. Solutions of sodium hypochlorite containing 5 or 10% of 'available chlorine'. For use as a general disinfectant. Parozone Plus. Contains in addition a detergent.

Other Proprietary Names

Bactot *(Arg.)*; Hygeol *(Canad.)*.

Use in dairies. A list of proprietary sodium hypochlorite solutions approved for the cleansing and disinfecting of milk containers and appliances is contained in Circular FSH 8/78, Ministry of Agriculture, Fisheries and Food, London, HM Stationery Office, 1978.

2278-j

Succinchlorimide. *N*-Chlorosuccinimide; 1-Chloropyrrolidine-2,5-dione.
$C_4H_4ClNO_2$=133.5.

CAS — 128-09-6.

A white crystalline powder with an odour and taste of chlorine, containing about 53% of 'available chlorine' (see p.557). **Soluble** 1 in 70 of water. **Protect** from light.

Succinchlorimide has been used for water disinfection.

2279-z

Tar Acids

Tar acids are phenolic substances derived from the distillation of coal tar or, more recently, petroleum fractions. The lowest boiling fraction of coal tar, distilling at 188° to 205°, consists of mixed cresol isomers forming cresol *B.P.* The middle fraction, known as 'cresylic acids', distils at 205° to 230° and consists of cresols and xylenols. The 'high-boiling tar acids', distilling at 230° to 290°, consist mainly of alkyl homologues of phenol, with naphthalenes and other hydrocarbons.

Adverse Effects. As for Phenol, p.571.

Tar acids are generally very irritant and corrosive to the skin, even when diluted to concentrations used for disinfection.

Uses. Tar acids are used in the preparation of a range of disinfectant fluids used for household and general disinfection purposes.

The low-boiling range cresols produce fluids with low Rideal-Walker coefficients but their activity is not greatly reduced in the presence of organic matter. The cresylic acid fraction produces fluids with RW coefficients of 8 to 10 and the high-boiling fraction produces fluids with RW coefficients of 20 or more.

This higher activity is greatly reduced by organic matter and is reflected in very much lower Chick-Martin coefficients. The higher boiling fractions are also more selective in action and less uniformly effective against Gram-positive organisms than the low-boiling range cresols.

The addition of chlorinated phenols to tar acids increases the RW coefficient but such mixtures are more selective and affected to a greater degree by organic matter. Hydrocarbons are often used to enhance the activity of the tar acids in disinfectant fluids; they also help to reduce crystallisation of phenols in cold weather.

Fluids based on tar acids are used similarly, but they must be used in adequate concentration as activity is markedly reduced by dilution.

Specifications for **disinfectants containing tar acids** are given in a British Standard Specification (BS 2462: 1961) and described as follows.

Black Fluids. Homogeneous solutions of coal-tar acids, or similar acids derived from petroleum, or any mixture of these, with or without hydrocarbons and with a suitable emulsifying agent. Black Fluids are miscible, yielding stable emulsions, with artificial hard water in all proportions from 1 to 5%. They are preferred when the undiluted fluid is required to be stable for long periods near freezing point.

White Fluids. Finely dispersed emulsions of coal-tar acids, or similar acids derived from petroleum, or any mixture of these, with or without hydrocarbons. White Fluids are miscible, yielding stable emulsions, with artificial sea water in all proportions from 1 to 5%, and may be required to produce no visible loss of whiteness in bleached cotton fabric. White Fluids can be used with all kinds of water; they mix readily with abnormally hard or saline waters and are, therefore, especially suitable for use with them. They are more stable after dilution than black fluids.

Modified Black Fluids and **Modified White Fluids** may contain, as an addition, any other active ingredients, but if these are used, the type and amount must be disclosed, if required, to the prospective buyer.

Black Fluids and White Fluids are classified in groups according to their germicidal value and the method of testing employed: the groups are designated by group letters which indicate the type of fluid (i.e. black or white), and the germicidal value according to the method of test. There are 6 designations of black fluids: group BA (Rideal-Walker coefficient not less than 4); group BB (RW coefficient not less than 10); group BC (RW coefficient not less than 18); group BE (Chick-Martin coefficient not less than 1); group BF (CM coefficient not less than 3); and group BG (CM coefficient not less than 4.4). There are 7 designations of white fluids; 6 of these, groups WA, WB, WC, WE, WF, and WG, have the same minimum RW or CM coefficients as the corresponding black fluids; the seventh white fluid, group WD, has a minimum Crown Agents' coefficient of 10 and a minimum RW coefficient of 18.

For Modified Black and Modified White Fluids, the Phenol Coefficient (Staphylococcus), determined by a specified method, must be stated by the manufacturer in addition to the RW coefficient.

The fluids are required to be free from objectionable smell, to be packed in containers not liable to deleterious interaction with them, and to be labelled with certain particulars including directions for dilution.

Inactivation by plastics. Incompatibilities between polyurethane foam and disinfectant solutions of Hycolin, Sudol, and benzalkonium were detected by bacteriological examination.— D. A. Leigh and C. Whittaker (letter), *Br. med. J.*, 1967, *3*, 435.

Sudol and Hycolin disappeared partially from solutions in which plastic sponges of polyvinyl acetate were immersed, probably due to adsorption.— L. Steingold *et al.* (letter), *Br. med. J.*, 1967, *3*, 620.

In an investigation of the effect of polyvinyl acetate, polyurethane, and cellulose sponges on the germicidal activity of phenolic disinfectants, cellulose sponge appeared to be the plastic of choice to avoid loss of phenolic germicide from solution.— J. W. Gibson *et al.*, *Izal* (letter), *Br. med. J.*, 1967, *4*, 804.

Recommended dilutions. For use as general disinfectants in hospitals, black and white fluids (BS 2462) and clear soluble fluids of the lysol type (but not chlorinated phenols) with a Chick-Martin coefficient of at least 1.5 should be used at dilutions of not more than 50 times the CM coefficient in clean situations. Where there was heavy organic contamination, a dilution of not more than 20 times the CM coefficient should be used.—Report by the Public Health Laboratory Service Committee on the Testing and Evaluation of Disinfectants, *Br. med. J.*, 1965, *1*, 408.

Virus disinfection. Advice on virus disinfection including the use of white fluid.— Department of Health and Social Security and the Welsh Office, *Memorandum on the Control of Outbreaks of Smallpox*, London, HM Stationery Office, 1975.

See also Scottish Home and Health Department, *Memorandum on the Control of Outbreaks of Smallpox*, Edinburgh, HM Stationery Office, 1976.

2280-p

Some Proprietary Preparations containing Cresols, Tar Acids, or other Phenols

Clearsol *(Tenneco, UK)*. A disinfectant containing 40% of xylenols and ethyl phenols with a detergent system consisting of sulphated alcohols. For general hospital disinfection dilute 1 in 100 to 1 in 200.

Disinfection of urinals. Clearsol 1% used similarly to Hycolin (see p.559) was considered a suitable alternative to Hycolin for disinfecting urinals.— A. M. Emmerson and V. E. Franks (letter), *Lancet*, 1975, *2*, 232.

Use of disinfectants on farms. In Great Britain, Clearsol is an approved disinfectant for tuberculosis in *animals* under The Diseases of Animals (Approved Disinfectants) Order 1978 (SI 1978: No. 32), as amended (SI 1978: No. 934).

Creolin *(Pearson, UK)*. A disinfectant of the black fluid type prepared from refined coal-tar oils, containing 20 to 22% of the less toxic, higher-boiling homologues of phenol; RW coefficient 5 to 7. For use as a general disinfectant dilute 1 in 200.

Cresolox *(Tenneco, UK)*. A range of disinfectants of the black and white fluid types.

Desderman *(Sterling Industrial, UK)*. A solution for hand disinfection containing alcohol, 3,4,5,6-tetrabromo-*o*-cresol ($C_7H_4Br_4O$=423.7), and surfactants.

Izal Germicide *(Sterling Industrial, UK)*. A disinfectant of the white fluid type containing 35 to 40% of a high-boiling phenolic fraction. It is miscible with water, saline, alcohol, and glycerol; RW coefficient at least 18. For general purposes dilute 1 in 600.

Use of disinfectants on farms. In Great Britain Izal Germicide is an approved disinfectant for fowl pest and tuberculosis in *animals* under The Diseases of Animals (Approved Disinfectants) Order 1978 (SI 1978: No. 32), as amended (SI 1978: No. 934).

Jeyes' Fluid *(Jeyes, UK)*. A solution of the black fluid type, made from coal tar products; RW coefficient 26 to 28. For household purposes and general disinfection.

Lyseptol *(Philip Harris, UK)*. A solution for preserving and sterilising surgical instruments, containing cresol and soap solution 1.5%, solvent ether 25%, and alcohol to 100%.

Printol Hospital Disinfectant *(Tenneco, UK)*. A disinfectant containing 15% of the higher-boiling homologues of phenol. It is stated to have a higher germicidal potency than cresol and soap solution, to be free from corrosive action, and to retain its potency in the presence of organic contamination. RW coefficient 6.5. For use, it is diluted 1 in 50 to 1 in 100.

Stericol Hospital Disinfectant *(Sterling Industrial, UK)*. A solution containing xylenols in an alcoholic anionic detergent basis, stated to be active against Gram-negative and Gram-positive organisms. For use as a 1% or 2% solution.

Sterilite *(Tenneco, UK).* A range of disinfectants of the white fluid type. **Sterilite 18/20** contains 30 to 35% of phenols; RW coefficient 18 to 20.

Sudol *(Tenneco, UK).* A disinfectant containing 50% v/v of a closely-cut fraction of phenolic homologues consisting chiefly of xylenols and ethyl phenols; RW coefficient 7. For use as a 0.5 to 0.75% solution.

Use of disinfectants on farms. In Great Britain, Sudol is an approved disinfectant for fowl pest and tuberculosis in *animals* under The Diseases of Animals (Approved Disinfectants) Order 1978 (SI 1978: No. 32), as amended (SI 1978: No. 934).

2281-s

Thiomersal *(B.P.).* Thiomersalate; Thimerosal *(U.S.P.)*; Mercurothiolate; Sodium Ethyl Mercurithiosalicylate; Mercurothiolate Sodique.

The sodium salt of (2-carboxyphenylthio)ethylmercury.

$C_9H_9HgNaO_2S$=404.8.

CAS — 54-64-8.

Pharmacopoeias. In *Arg., Br., Braz., Hung., It., Pol., Swiss,* and *U.S.*

A light cream-coloured crystalline powder with a slight characteristic odour containing about 50% of Hg.

Soluble 1 in 1 of water and 1 in 8 of alcohol; soluble in methyl alcohol; practically insoluble in ether. A 1% solution in water has a pH of 6 to 8. Solutions are **sterilised** by autoclaving or by filtration. **Incompatible** with acids, iodine, heavy metal salts, and many alkaloids. **Store** in airtight containers. Protect from light.

The rate of oxidation of thiomersal in solution is greatly increased by traces of copper ions. In slightly acid solution thiomersal may be precipitated as the corresponding acid which undergoes slow decomposition with the formation of insoluble products.

For precautions to be taken in preparing and storing antiseptic solutions, see under Phenol, p.570.

For a note on the incompatibility of mercurials with aluminium and steel, see under Mercuric Chloride, p.939.

Total haemolysis occurred when erythrocytes were cultured for 45 minutes in a 2% solution of thiomersal in sodium chloride injection. Only slight haemolysis occurred when the strength was reduced to 1.5%.— H. C. Ansel and D. E. Cadwallader, *J. pharm. Sci.*, 1964, *53*, 169.

Thiomersal could be sorbed by polyethylene and polypropylene leading to almost complete loss of preservative from contact lens solutions.— N. E. Richardson *et al.*, *J. Pharm. Pharmac.*, 1977, *29*, 717.

Inactivation. The inactivation of thiomersal by rubber.— S. Wiener, *J. Pharm. Pharmac.*, 1955, *7*, 118; J. Birner and J. R. Garnet, *J. pharm. Sci.*, 1964, *53*, 1426.

Stability of solutions. Dilute aqueous solutions of thiomersal were fairly stable to heat but labile to light, less stable to heat when acid than when alkaline, most stable to light at pH 5 to 7, and unstable to heat but not to light in the presence of Cu, Fe, or Zn ions, but not Ca or Mg ions; thiomersal was adsorbed by rubber caps even at 0°. It was concluded that eye-drops containing thiomersal should be stored in light-resistant containers with no direct contact with rubber caps and that they should be buffered at pH 6 to 7.— K. Tsuji *et al.*, *Arch. pract. Pharm.*, 1964, *24*, 110.

Adverse Effects and Treatment. As for Mercury, pp.937-8. Hypersensitivity reactions, usually with erythema and papular or vesicular eruptions, occasionally occur. Allergic conjunctivitis has been reported.

A patient suffered a burn 5 cm in diameter at the site of contact with an aluminium foil diathermy electrode after pre-operative preparation with thiomersal 0.1% in 50% alcohol. Subsequent investigation showed that considerable heat was generated when such a solution came into contact with aluminium.— H. T. Jones, *Br. med. J.*, *1972* 2, 504.

For a report of 6 cases of poisoning, 5 of them fatal, resulting from the presence of 1000 times the normal quantity of thiomersal in a preparation of chloramphenicol for intramuscular injection, see J. H. M. Axton, *Postgrad. med. J.*, 1972, *48*, 417.

Thiomersal had been reported to be ototoxic.— J. L. Honigman, *ICI Pharmaceuticals* (letter), *Pharm. J.*, 1975, *2*, 523.

Of 13 children with exomphalos (umbilical hernia) treated with a tincture of thiomersal, 10 had died. Tissue concentrations of mercury were above the minimum toxic concentrations in 6 examined. Neurological examination of 1 survivor showed no evidence of minimum mercury damage. It was recommended that organic mercurial disinfectants should be heavily restricted or withdrawn from hospital use as absorption occurred readily through intact membranes.— D. G. Fagan *et al.*, *Archs Dis. Childh.*, 1977, *52*, 962.

Thiomersal used in topical antiseptic preparations was toxic to epidermal cells.— *Med. Lett.*, 1977, *19*, 83.

A study into the penetration of mercury (in thiomersal) from ophthalmic preservatives into the human eye. The study indicated that significant amounts of mercury may be found in the cornea and aqueous shortly after brief exposure of abnormal corneas to organic mercurials such as may occur in the course of normal ophthalmological procedures.— A. F. Winder *et al.*, *Lancet*, 1980, *2*, 237.

Hypersensitivity. Of 100 patients with allergic contact dermatitis, 2 gave positive reactions to patch testing with thiomersal.— A. A. Fisher *et al.*, *Archs Derm.*, 1971, *104*, 286. See also H. Möller, *Acta derm.-vener., Stockh.*, 1977, *57*, 509.

False positive reactions to old tuberculin were attributed to the presence of thiomersal. In 63 subjects with positive thiomersal reactions, nearly all had positive reactions to old tuberculin but 23 had negative reactions to PPD, which contained no thiomersal.— H. Hansson and H. Möller, *Scand. J. infect. Dis.*, 1971, *3*, 169.

Delayed hypersensitivity reactions to intradermal injections of thiomersal 1 in 10 000 were noted in 9 of 44 patients. The reactions took the form of erythema and induration.— H. Mizutari (letter), *New Engl. J. Med.*, 1973, *289*, 1424.

A report of laryngeal obstruction attributed to sensitivity to thiomersal.— H. Maibach, *Contact Dermatitis*, 1975, *1*, 221.

Pregnancy and the neonate. An increased rate of malformation was found in 56 children born to mothers monitored by the Collaborative Perinatal Project and found to have been exposed to thiomersal, and possibly other drugs, at some time during the first 4 months of the pregnancy.— O. P. Heinonen *et al.*, *Birth Defects and Drugs in Pregnancy*, Littleton MA, Publishing Sciences Group, 1977, p. 296.

Uses. Thiomersal is bacteriostatic and fungistatic. Its activity is not significantly reduced by serum, but is reduced by whole blood. It is less effective and less toxic than mercuric chloride. A 0.1% tincture has been used for pre-operative skin disinfection and a 0.1% aqueous solution has been employed for application to wounds and raw surfaces.

For ophthalmic purposes and for urethral irrigation or application to nasal mucous membranes, aqueous solutions of 0.02% have been used. A cream or tincture containing thiomersal 0.1% has been employed to treat mycotic skin infections.

Thiomersal, 0.01 to 0.02%, is used as a preservative in biological products.

The use of thiomersal in cosmetics and toiletries is restricted in Great Britain under the Cosmetic Products Regulations 1978 (SI 1978: No. 1354).

The antibacterial activity of thiomersal solutions was reduced by the addition of disodium edetate and also by the addition of sodium thiosulphate.— R. M. E. Richards and J. M. E. Reary, *J. Pharm. Pharmac.*, 1972, *24, Suppl.*, 84P.

Thiomersal and alcohol 50% were equally effective as preservatives in urinary cytology but thiomersal was preferred since it did not increase the volume of the specimen, nor did it affect cytopreparation and it permitted a higher cell yield.— M. E. Beyer-Boon *et al.*, *J. clin. Path.*, 1979, *32*, 168.

Preparations

Thimerosal Tincture *(U.S.P.).* Thiomersal 100 mg, alcohol 52.5 ml, acetone 10 ml, ethylenediamine 20 mg, ethanolamine 100 mg, water to 100 ml. It may be coloured. It should be made and stored in glass or suitably resistant metal containers. Inflammable. Store at a temperature not exceeding 40° in airtight containers. Protect from light.

Thimerosal Topical Aerosol *(U.S.P.).* Thiomersal Aerosol. An alcoholic solution of thiomersal mixed with suitable propellents in a pressurised container. Thiomersal 100 mg, ethanolamine 29.2 mg, edetic acid 2.11 mg, water 0.61 ml, acetone 10 ml, alcohol to 100 ml. Sufficient propellent is added during filling. It should be made and stored in glass or suitably resistant metal containers. It may be coloured. Inflammable. Store at a temperature not exceeding 40°. Protect from light.

Thimerosal Topical Solution *(U.S.P.).* Thiomersal Solution. Thiomersal 100 mg, ethylenediamine 20 mg, ethanolamine 100 mg, sodium chloride 800 mg, borax 140 mg, water to 100 ml. pH 9.6 to 10.2. It may be coloured. It should be made and stored in glass or suitably resistant metal containers. Store at a temperature not exceeding 40° in airtight containers. Protect from light.

Proprietary Preparations

Merthiolate *(Lilly, UK).* Thiomersal, available as a coloured tincture containing 0.1% in alcohol 50%, with acetone. (Also available as Merthiolate in *Austral., Canad., S.Afr., USA*).

Other Proprietary Names

Colluspray *(Belg.)*; Merseptyl *(Fr.)*; Nutramersal *(S.Afr.)*; Vitaseptol *(Fr.)*.

2282-w

Thymol *(B.P.).* Thymolum; Timol; Isopropylmetacresol; Acido Timico. 2-Isopropyl-5-methylphenol.

$C_{10}H_{14}O$=150.2.

CAS — 89-83-8.

Pharmacopoeias. In *Arg., Aust., Belg., Br., Ger., Hung., Ind., Int., It., Jap., Mex., Pol., Port., Roum., Rus., Span., Swiss,* and *Turk.* Also in *U.S.N.F.*

Colourless crystals or white crystalline powder with a characteristic pungent aromatic odour and taste. M.p. 48° to 51°; when melted it remains liquid at a considerably lower temperature.

Soluble 1 in 1000 of water, 1 in 0.3 of alcohol, 1 in 0.6 of chloroform, 1 in 0.7 of ether, 1 in 200 of glycerol, and 1 in 2 of olive oil; soluble in glacial acetic acid, caustic alkalis, fixed and volatile oils, and fats. A 4% solution in alcohol (50%) is neutral to litmus. **Incompatible** with iodine, alkalis, and oxidising agents. It liquefies with camphor, chloral hydrate, menthol, phenol, and certain other substances. **Store** in airtight containers. Protect from light.

For precautions to be taken in preparing and storing antiseptic solutions, see under Phenol, p.570.

Adverse Effects and Treatment. As for Phenol, p.571.

When taken by mouth, thymol is less toxic than phenol. It is irritant to the gastric mucosa. Rashes may occur. Fats and alcohol increase absorption and aggravate the toxic symptoms.

Thymol and other phenols could cause green or dark discoloration of the urine which could become black on standing.— R. B. Baran and B. Rowles, *J. Am. pharm. Ass.*, 1973, *NS13*, 139.

Absorption and Fate. Thymol is completely absorbed from the intestine. About 50% is excreted in the urine as the sulphate and glucuronide together with some thymolquinone.

Uses. Thymol is a more powerful disinfectant than phenol but its use is limited by its low solubility in water. It has the disadvantages that it is irritant to tissues and its bactericidal properties are greatly reduced in the presence of proteins.

Thymol is used chiefly as a deodorant in mouth-washes and gargles. Mixed with phenol and camphor it is used in dentistry to prepare cavities before filling, and mixed with zinc oxide it forms a protective cap for the dentine. Externally, thymol has fungicidal properties and has been used in dusting-powders for the treatment of fungous skin infections.

Thymol (0.01%) is added as an antoxidant to halothane, trichloroethylene, and tetrachloroethylene. Thymol, 10% in isopropyl alcohol, has been used to preserve urine.

Thymol had only a low solubility in water and was a poor bactericide. Its use as a disinfectant even for clinical thermometers was not recommended.—Report by the Public Health Laboratory Service Committee on the Testing and Evaluation of Disinfectants, *Br. med. J.*, 1965, *1*, 408.

Herpes. Fifteen patients with herpes of the genitalia were treated topically with thymol (as Listerine) twice daily. Symptomatic relief was obtained in 14 days with gradual healing of the lesions. There had been one recurrence in 8 months.— H. M. Radman, *Md St. med. J.*, 1978, *27*, 49. See also V. Knight and M. W. Noall (letter), *New Engl. J. Med.*, 1976, *294*, 337.

Use in food. The Food Additives and Contaminants Committee recommended that, on the grounds of safety, thymol could continue to be used as a stabiliser for solvents used in food.— *Report on the Review of Solvents in Food*, FAC/REP/25, Ministry of Agriculture, Fisheries and Food, London, HM Stationery Office, 1978.

Preparations

Compound Thymol Glycerin *(B.P.)*. Glycerinum Thymolis Compositum. Thymol 50 mg, sodium bicarbonate 1 g, borax 2 g, sodium benzoate 800 mg, sodium salicylate 520 mg, menthol 30 mg, cineole 0.13 ml, pumilio pine oil 0.05 ml, methyl salicylate 0.03 ml, alcohol (90%) (or industrial methylated spirit, suitably diluted) 2.5 ml, glycerol 10 ml, sodium metabisulphite 35 mg, carmine, food grade of commerce, 30 mg, dilute ammonia solution 0.075 ml, water to 100 ml. pH 7.1 to 7.6. To be diluted with about 3 times its vol. of warm water before use; diluted solutions should be prepared immediately before use.

Modified formula. Fading and discoloration of Compound Thymol Glycerin during storage could be minimised by increasing the sodium metabisulphite to 50 mg per 100 ml and by protecting from light.—Pharm. Soc. Lab. Rep. No. P/69/33, 1969.

Reports of contamination of Compound Thymol Glycerin.— M. H. Hughes (letter), *Lancet*, 1972, *1*, 210; T. A. Rees (letter), *ibid.*, 532.

A study suggesting that phenol might be worth investigating as a potential preservative of Compound Thymol Glycerin.— Pharm. Soc. Lab. Rep. P/78/9, 1978. Confirmation that phenol 0.5% was physically compatible with Compound Thymol Glycerin. Initial studies also suggested that cinnamon oil and citral appeared worthy of further investigation as preservatives.— Pharm. Soc. Lab. Rep. P/80/3, 1980.

Compound Thymol Mouth-wash *(B.P.C. 1949)*. Collut. Thymol. Co. Thymol 30 mg, liquefied phenol 0.52 ml, potassium hydroxide solution 0.52 ml, methyl salicylate 0.01 ml, peppermint oil 0.01 ml, bordeaux B solution 1.04 ml, water to 100 ml. To be diluted with 3 times its vol. of warm water before use.

Amended formula. Thymol 30 mg, liquefied phenol 0.52 ml, potassium hydroxide solution 0.52 ml, methyl salicylate 0.01 ml, peppermint oil 0.01 ml, amaranth solution 1 ml, water to 100 ml.—*Compendium of Past Formulae 1933 to 1966*, London, The National Pharmaceutical Union, 1969.

Compound Thymol Solution-tablets *(B.P.C. 1963)*. Solv. Thymol. Co. Each contains thymol 3.24 mg, sodium bicarbonate 324 mg, borax 324 mg, phenol 32.4 mg, and amaranth 650 µg. One solution-tablet to be dissolved in 60 ml of warm water.

Thymol Mouth-wash Compound *(A.P.F.)*. Collut. Thymol. Alb.; Liq. Thymol. Co. Thymol 150 mg, menthol 10 mg, benzoic acid 800 mg, methyl salicylate 0.05 ml, cineole 0.05 ml, glycerol 2 ml, alcohol (90%) 20 ml, water to 100 ml. Dilute with 7 vol. of water for use as a gargle or mouth-wash.

2292-l

Dithymol Di-iodide. 4,4′-Bis(iodo-oxy)-5,5′-di-isopropyl-2,2′-dimethyl-1,1′-biphenyl.
$C_{20}H_{24}I_2O_2$=550.2.

CAS — 552-22-7.

2283-e

Thymol Iodide *(B.P.C. 1949)*. Dithymol Diiodide; Iodothymol; Timol Ioduro. A mixture of iodine derivatives of thymol, chiefly dithymol di-iodide, containing not less than 43% of iodine.

NOTE. The name iodothymol is also applied to an anthelmintic compound (see p.94).

Pharmacopoeias. In *Port.* and *Swiss.*

A reddish-brown or buff-coloured, almost tasteless, bulky, amorphous powder with a slight aromatic odour. Practically **insoluble** in water, glycerol, and sodium hydroxide solution; slightly soluble in alcohol; soluble in chloroform, ether, soft paraffin, and fixed and volatile oils, usually leaving a slight residue. **Incompatible** with alkalis, mercuric chloride, and metallic oxides. **Protect** from light.

Thymol iodide is insoluble and has little or no antiseptic action but acts as an absorbent and protective.
It has been used in dusting-powders and ointments, and in dental root filling preparations.

2284-l

Tribromometacresol. 2,4,6-Tribromo-*m*-cresol; 2,4,6-Tribromo-3-methylphenol.
$C_7H_5Br_3O$=344.8.

CAS — 4619-74-3.

Tribromometacresol is an antifungal agent used in the treatment of dermatomycoses. It is applied topically as an aerosol spray containing 2%. It should be applied with caution to suppurating mycoses; it should not be applied near the eyes or mucous membranes.

Proprietary Names

Triphysan *(Dumex, Denm.)*; Tri-Physol *(Sigma, Austral.)*.

2285-y

Triclobisonium Chloride. Hexamethylenebis{dimethyl[1-methyl-3-(2,2,6-trimethylcyclohexyl)propyl]ammonium chloride}.
$C_{36}H_{74}Cl_2N_2$=605.9.

CAS — 7187-64-6 (triclobisonium); 79-90-3 (chloride).

A white or nearly white, almost odourless, crystalline powder. M.p. about 243°. Freely **soluble** in water, alcohol, and chloroform; practically insoluble in ether. **Protect** from light.

Triclobisonium chloride is a quaternary ammonium compound with properties and uses similar to those of other cationic surfactants as described under Cetrimide, p.551. It has been reported to have activity against *Candida albicans* and *Trichomonas vaginalis*. It has been applied topically as a 0.1% ointment or cream in the treatment of skin infections and as a 0.1% cream or pessaries in the treatment of vaginitis.

2286-j

Triclocarban.

3,4,4′-Trichlorocarbanilide. 1-(4-Chlorophenyl)-3-(3,4-dichlorophenyl)urea.
$C_{13}H_9Cl_3N_2O$=315.6.

CAS — 101-20-2.

A fine white odourless powder. M.p. 250° to 256°. Practically **insoluble** in water: soluble 1 in 25 of acetone, 1 in 100 of propylene glycol, and 1 in 100 of dimethyl phthalate; soluble 1 in 10 to 1 in 4 of macrogols.

Macrogol 400 monolaurate increased the solubility of triclocarban, resulting in increased bactericidal activity.— A. E. Elkhouly and R. C. S. Woodroffe, *J. appl. Bact.*, 1973, *36*, 387.

Adverse Effects and Precautions. When subjected to prolonged high temperatures triclocarban can decompose to form toxic chloroanilines, which can be absorbed through the skin.

Mild photosensitivity has been seen in patch testing.

An outbreak of methaemoglobinaemia in 18 infants (12 premature) in a nursery in a 5-week period ceased when the laundry process applied to clothing and napkins was revised. The process had involved washing in detergent, blueing, a chemical rinse containing triclocarban 2%, neutralising, drying and autoclaving. — R. O. Fisch *et al.*, *J. Am. med. Ass.*, 1963, *185*, 760.

Eight patients developed methaemoglobinaemia after receiving an enema prepared from soap containing about 2% of triclocarban. Three days prior to the incident the procedure for preparing the soap gel had been changed to include heating near to boiling-point for several hours. Laboratory tests showed that boiling reduced the triclocarban content of the soap gel (pH 9.5) and led to the formation of primary amines.— R. R. Johnson *et al.*, *Pediatrics*, 1963, *31*, 222.

Cutaneous and mucosal lesions.— H. Barrière, *Therapeutique*, 1973, *49*, 685.

Uses. Triclocarban is a non-phenolic disinfectant. It is bacteriostatic against Gram-positive organisms in high dilutions but is less effective against Gram-negative organisms and some fungi. It is used in soaps, usually in a concentration of 2%, for similar purposes to hexachlorophane, and has been applied in solutions, powders, and ointments for the control of skin infections.

A review of antimicrobial agents, including triclocarban, used in cosmetics.— I. R. Gucklhorn, *Mfg Chem.*, 1970, *41* (Feb.), 30.

Proprietary Preparations

Cutisan *(Martindale Pharmaceuticals, UK: Farillon, UK)*. Triclocarban, available as **Ointment** containing 2%; as **Powder** containing 1%; and as **Solution** containing 1%. For infected skin conditions, leg ulcers, and burns. (Also available as Cutisan in *Fr.*).

TCC *(Monsanto, UK)*. A brand of triclocarban.

Other Proprietary Names

Arg.—Ungel; *Belg.*—Solubacter; *Fr.*—Nobacter, Septi-von-Lavril, Solubacter.

A preparation containing triclocarban was also formerly marketed in Great Britain under the proprietary name Crinagen (*Pharmax*).

2287-z

Triclosan.

Cloxifenol; CH 3565. 5-Chloro-2-(2,4-dichlorophenoxy)phenol.
$C_{12}H_7Cl_3O_2$=289.5.

CAS — 3380-34-5.

A white to off-white crystalline powder or soft agglomerates with a slightly aromatic odour. M.p. 55° to 57°.Practically **insoluble** in water; very soluble in most organic solvents; soluble 1 in 3 of 4% sodium hydroxide solution. **Protect** from light.

Adverse Effects. Contact dermatitis has occasionally been reported.

From studies on the percutaneous absorption of triclosan in *rats*, it was calculated that the absorbed dose from a shampoo preparation (0.05% triclosan) in a woman would be about 4.8 µg per kg body-weight and from an aerosol (0.1% triclosan) 24.9 µg per kg. These doses were considered to have no effect in humans.— J. G. Black and D. Howes, *J. Soc. cosmet. Chem.*, 1975, *26*, 205.

Uses. Triclosan is bacteriostatic against Gram-positive and most Gram-negative organisms. It has little activity against *Pseudomonas* spp., yeasts, or fungi. It is used in surgical scrubs, soaps, and deodorants in concentrations of 0.05 to 2%.

Review of properties and microbiological activity.— T. E. Furia and A. G. Schenkel, *Soap chem. Spec.*, 1968, *44* (Jan.), 47.

Handwashing for 2 minutes with soap containing triclosan 0.75% was less effective in removing skin bacteria than washing with soap containing hexachlorophane 2%.

After 6 applications over 2 days of a cream containing triclosan 2%, skin bacteria were reduced as effectively as by 4% chlorhexidine gluconate detergent solution and slightly more effectively than by 3% hexachlorophane detergent cream.— H. A. Lilly and E. J. L. Lowbury, *Br. med. J.*, 1974, *4*, 372.

Proprietary Preparations

Gamophen Antiseptic Soap *(Surgikos, UK)*. Contains triclosan 1.5%.
The name Gamophen is also applied to a preparation containing hexachlorophane.

Irgasan DP300 *(Ciba-Geigy, UK)*. A brand of triclosan, available as a powder.

Ster-Zac Bath Concentrate *(Hough, Hoseason, UK)*. Contains triclosan 2%. For the prevention of cross-infection and secondary infection via bathing. *Directions*. 30 ml to be added to the bath or 1 ml to 5 litres.

Zalclense Bactericidal Washing Cream *(Sterling Industrial, UK)*. A gel containing triclosan 2% in an emollient saponaceous basis.

Other Proprietary Names

Adasept *(Canad.)*; Lipo-Sol *(Switz.)*; Sapoderm *(*see also under Pyrithione Zinc*) (Austral.)*; Tersaseptic *(Canad.)*.

2288-c

Trinitrophenol *(B.P.C. 1959)*. Carbazotic Acid; Picric Acid; Picrinic Acid. 2,4,6-Trinitrophenol.

$C_6H_3N_3O_7$=229.1.

CAS — 88-89-1.

Pharmacopoeias. In *Arg., Port., Span.,* and *Swiss.*

Bright yellow odourless crystals with a very bitter taste. **Soluble** 1 in 90 of water, 1 in 10 of alcohol (90%), 1 in 50 of chloroform, and 1 in 50 of ether. A 1% solution in water has a pH of about 1.35. **Incompatible** with alkaloids, aromatic hydrocarbons, and phenols. It should be stored mixed with an equal weight of water; it must not be stored in glass-stoppered bottles.
Trinitrophenol burns readily and explodes when heated rapidly or when subjected to percussion. For safety in handling it is usually supplied mixed with not less than half its weight of water. It combines with metals to form salts, some of which are very explosive.

Adverse Effects. Dermatitis, skin eruptions, and severe itching may occur. Absorption through abraded skin or by ingestion has caused vomiting, pain, and diarrhoea, progressing to haemolysis, hepatitis, anuria, and convulsions. The metabolic-rate is increased, causing pyrexia.
Maximum permissible atmospheric concentration 100 µg per m^3.

Uses. Trinitrophenol has disinfectant properties and was formerly used, mainly as a 1% aqueous solution, in the treatment of burns. Because of its toxic effects it is now rarely used in medicine.
The use of trinitrophenol in cosmetics and toiletries is restricted under the Cosmetic Products Regulations 1978 (SI 1978: No. 1354).

2293-y

Some Proprietary Ostomy Deodorants

Atmocol *(Thackray, UK)*. A deodorant spray for use with colostomies and ileostomies.

Chironair Odour Control Liquid *(Downs, UK)*. A deodorant for use with colostomies and ileostomies.

Nilodor *(Loxley, UK)*. A deodorant liquid for use with colostomies and ileostomies.

No-Roma *(Salt, UK)*. A deodorant liquid for use with colostomies and ileostomies.

Ostobon *(Coloplast, UK)*. A deodorant powder for use with ostomies.

Translet Plus One (formerly known as Ostomy Plus One) *(Franklin Medical, UK)*. A deodorant liquid for use with colostomies and ileostomies.

Translet Plus Two (formerly known as Ostomy Plus Two) *(Franklin Medical, UK)*. A deodorant liquid for use with colostomies and ileostomies.

Disulfiram and Citrated Calcium Carbimide

2731-t

Disulfiram *(B.P., U.S.P.).* Disulfiramum; Éthyldithiourame; TTD. Tetraethylthiuram disulphide. $C_{10}H_{20}N_2S_4$=296.5.

CAS — 97-77-8.

Pharmacopoeias. In *Aust., Br., Cz., Hung., Jug., Roum., Swiss,* and *U.S.*

A white or almost white, odourless or almost odourless powder with a slightly bitter taste. M.p. 69° to 73°. Practically **insoluble** in water; soluble 1 in 65 of alcohol, 1 in 2 of chloroform, 1 in 20 of ether; soluble in acetone and carbon disulphide; slightly soluble in light petroleum. The pH of a solution obtained by shaking 1 g with 30 ml of water is 6 to 8. **Store** in airtight containers. Protect from light.

Adverse Effects. Disulfiram when taken alone may give rise to a number of side-effects including an unpleasant taste, gastro-intestinal upsets, body odour, bad breath, drowsiness, headache, impotence, and occasionally allergic dermatitis. Peripheral and optic neuritis and psychotic reactions may also occur. Hepatitis has been reported.

The effects of the disulfiram-alcohol interaction are described under Uses. However, severe reactions may follow the ingestion of even small quantities of alcohol; these include marked respiratory depression, cardiovascular collapse, cardiac arrhythmias, acute congestive heart failure, unconsciousness, convulsions, and sudden death.

Maximum permissible atmospheric concentration 2 mg per m^3.

Unpleasant colostomy odours occurred in a patient when taking disulfiram in doses of 125, 250, and 500 mg daily.— S. I. Miller (letter), *J. Am. med. Ass.*, 1977, *237,* 2602.

A study of the role of disulfiram metabolites in its toxicity. Carbon disulphide was considered to be responsible for the behavioural and neurological effects of disulfiram. A dose of 125 mg of disulfiram daily might increase the risk of arteriosclerotic cardiovascular disease by a factor of 3 or 4.— J. M. Rainey, *Am. J. Psychiat.*, 1977, *134,* 371, per *Int. pharm. Abstr.*, 1977, *14,* 1079.

Cardiovascular effects. See under Citrated Calcium Carbimide, p.580.

Central effects. A report of an acute organic brain syndrome developing in 5 patients treated with disulfiram. No patient had taken alcohol. Symptoms resolved 2 to 21 days after disulfiram was withdrawn.— S. T. Knee and J. Razani, *Am. J. Psychiat.*, 1974, *131,* 1281, per *Int. pharm. Abstr.*, 1975, *12,* 1120.

Grand mal seizures occurred in a patient who had been taking disulfiram for 6 months.— T. R. P. Price and P. M. Silberfarb (letter), *Am. J. Psychiat.*, 1976, *133,* 235, per *Int. pharm. Abstr.*, 1976, *13,* 927.

Acute paranoid psychosis, considered to be a toxic encephalopathy, occurred in a man who had taken disulfiram 250 mg daily for 16 months for the treatment of alcoholism; a second patient became disorientated and lethargic and then had a generalised tonic-clonic seizure 3 weeks after commencing treatment with disulfiram 500 mg daily, and further neurological symptoms followed. In both patients recovery followed withdrawal of disulfiram.— J. R. Hotson and J. W. Langston, *Archs Neurol., Chicago,* 1976, *33,* 141.

Depression. A brief discussion of the role of disulfiram in causing depression.— F. A. Whitlock and L. E. J. Evans, *Drugs,* 1978, *15,* 53.

Effects on the liver. A 44-year-old man developed hypersensitivity hepatitis on 2 separate occasions following ingestion of disulfiram.— E. B. Keeffe and F. W. Smith, *J. Am. med. Ass.*, 1974, *230,* 435.

A 49-year-old Negro developed jaundice after taking disulfiram on 2 occasions.— H. J. Eisen and A. L. Ginsberg (letter), *Ann. intern. Med.*, 1975, *83,* 673.

Six patients developed signs of liver damage 3 to 25 weeks after starting to take disulfiram. All developed coma and 5 died. A causal relationship was suspected.— L. Ranek and P. B. Andreasen, *Br. med. J.*, 1977, *2,* 94.

Further references to disulfiram and hepatitis.— S. J. Morris *et al.*, *Gastroenterology,* 1978, *75,* 100.

For reference to a characteristic hepatic lesion in some patients taking disulfiram, see Citrated Calcium Carbimide, p.580.

Effect on serum-cholesterol concentration. In patients being treated for habitual alcohol consumption disulfiram 500 mg daily for 3 weeks was associated with an increase in serum-cholesterol concentration. This was in contrast to other patients who received disulfiram 250 mg, disulfiram and pyridoxine 50 mg daily or pyridoxine alone and who experienced a fall in serum cholesterol. A further group of alcoholic patients who received no medication had an expected fall in serum cholesterol during a 3-week period of abstinence thus indicating that a decrease in serum cholesterol was apparently not due to pyridoxine. Chronic disulfiram therapy thus might increase the incidence of arteriosclerotic cardiovascular disease.— L. F. Major and P. F. Goyer, *Ann. intern. Med.*, 1978, *88,* 53.

Peripheral neuropathy. A discussion of peripheral neuropathy and disulfiram.— *Lancet,* 1971, *2,* 649.

Reports of neuropathies developing in patients taking disulfiram.— W. G. Bradley and R. L. Hewer, *Br. med. J.*, 1966, *2,* 449; G. Moddel *et al.*, *Archs Neurol., Chicago,* 1978, *35,* 658; C. P. Watson *et al.*, *Can. med. Ass. J.*, 1980, *123,* 123; *idem,* 270.

Pregnancy and the neonate. A report of 2 infants with severe limb-reduction anomalies whose mothers had taken disulfiram during pregnancy. Only 2 similar cases had previously been reported.— A. H. Nora *et al.* (letter), *Lancet,* 1977, *2,* 664.

A view that the foetal-alcohol syndrome is induced by acetaldehyde. In a woman taking disulfiram even a few drops of alcohol could result in an acetaldehyde concentration high enough to injure the foetus.— P. V. Véghelyi and M. Osztovics (letter), *Lancet,* 1979, *2,* 35.

Treatment of Adverse Effects. The stomach should be emptied by aspiration and lavage if tablets have been taken recently. Gastro-intestinal or neurological disturbances should be treated symptomatically and the patient should abstain from alcohol for at least a week and probably longer as reactions have occurred as long as 14 days after stopping disulfiram.

When severe reactions follow the administration of alcohol with disulfiram assisted respiration or oxygen may be needed. Treatment with 0.5 to 1 g of sodium ascorbate, administered by slow intravenous infusion, has been suggested. The circulation should be maintained with infusions of plasma or suitable electrolyte solutions. An antihistamine may be of value.

Precautions. Disulfiram is contra-indicated in the presence of cardiovascular disease, overt psychosis, and drug dependence. Disulfiram should not be given to patients known to be hypersensitive to it or to thiuram compounds. It should be used with caution in the presence of diabetes mellitus, epilepsy, impaired hepatic or renal function, respiratory disorders, cerebral damage, or hypothyrodism. It is probably best avoided in pregnancy.

Disulfiram should not be given to patients who have recently taken alcohol. Patients should be fully aware of the disulfiram-alcohol interaction. Alcohol-based medicines should be avoided, and alcohol-based preparations should not be applied topically.

Disulfiram inhibits enzyme induction and may thus interfere with the metabolism of drugs taken at the same time. It enhances the effects of the coumarin anticoagulants and phenytoin. The toxicity of isoniazid may be increased. Acute psychoses or confusional states have been reported when disulfiram and metronidazole are given concomitantly. Paraldehyde should not be administered to patients receiving disulfiram.

Chlorpromazine, diazepam, or an antihistamine may inhibit the alcohol reaction in patients taking disulfiram.

For a recommendation that careful cardiovascular assessment is required before treatment with disulfiram, see Citrated Calcium Carbimide, p.580.

Interactions. Disulfiram given to *mice* and *dogs* also given paraldehyde produced slight increases in blood concentrations of paraldehyde and delayed blood clearance leading to a prolonged hypnotic effect. Blood concentrations of acetaldehyde were somewhat higher and more prolonged in animals given both compounds but were far short of those achieved following the administration of alcohol to disulfiram-treated animals.— M. L. Keplinger and J. A. Wells, *Fedn Proc. Fedn Am. Socs exp. Biol.*, 1956, *15,* 445.

Seven alcoholic patients with tuberculosis who were receiving isoniazid showed changes in behaviour and coordination when treatment with disulfiram was started. It was possible that isoniazid and disulfiram together blocked 2 of the 3 metabolic pathways of dopamine. The resulting increase in methylated products of dopamine might be responsible for the mental changes seen in the patients.— H. C. Whittington and L. Grey, *Am. J. Psychiat.*, 1969, *125,* 1725.

Amitriptyline appeared to enhance the reaction occurring with disulfiram or citrated calcium carbimide and alcohol.— W. A. G. MacCallum (letter), *Lancet,* 1969, *1,* 313. Animal studies employing disulfiram confirmed these findings.— J. Hendtlass (letter), *Med. J. Aust.*, 1977, *1,* 758.

Disulfiram was found to prolong the plasma-phenazone half-life in healthy subjects and to reduce the excretion of 4-hydroxy-3-methoxymandelic acid in the urine indicating altered dopamine metabolism.— E. S. Vesell *et al.*, *Clin. Pharmac. Ther.*, 1971, *12,* 785.

Administration of either isomer of tranylcypromine to *rats* pretreated with disulfiram caused a toxic reaction; following administration of the (−)-isomer the reaction occurred sooner and was more pronounced.— D. F. Smith and M. Shimizu (letter), *J. Pharm. Pharmac.*, 1976, *28,* 858.

A study in *rats* showed an increased incidence of morbidity and mortality in animals exposed to a combination of ethylene dibromide and disulfiram. The clinical significance was not known but the advisability of continued occupational exposure to ethylene dibromide by patients receiving disulfiram was uncertain.— H. B. Plotnick (letter), *J. Am. med. Ass.*, 1978, *239,* 1609. See also R. E. Yodaiken, *ibid.*, 2783.

A report of hypersensitivity to disulfiram occurring in a patient with rubber contact sensitivity.— P. K. Webb *et al.*, *J. Am. med. Ass.*, 1979, *241,* 2061.

For the effect of disulfiram on the disposition of benzodiazepines, see Diazepam, p.1522.

Absorption and Fate. Disulfiram is absorbed from the gastro-intestinal tract. The maximum effect usually occurs 12 hours after ingestion. Disulfiram is slowly eliminated from the body. About 20% of a dose is excreted unchanged in the faeces and the remainder is excreted as metabolites in the urine. Carbon disulphide is reported to be a final metabolite.

Uses. Disulfiram is used in the treatment of chronic alcoholism. It is not a cure and the treatment is likely to be of little value unless it is undertaken with the willing cooperation of the patient and is employed in conjunction with psychotherapy.

Taking alcohol, even small quantities, after the administration of disulfiram evokes an extremely unpleasant syndrome of systemic reactions. This effect is due to the inhibition of the oxidation of acetaldehyde, the primary metabolite of alcohol, causing an increase of acetaldehyde in the blood. The effects of disulfiram therapy arise within 10 minutes after the ingestion of alcohol. They commence with flushing of the face and injection of the conjunctiva, followed by a sensation of heat, throbbing headache, tachycardia, irritation of the throat, and a feeling of giddiness. There may be, in addition, nausea, vomiting, sweating, accelerated and deepened respiration, chest pain, blurred vision, confusion, and a marked fall in blood pressure. The effects last for ½ to 1 hour in mild cases and for several hours in severe cases.

The intensity and duration of symptoms vary greatly with different individuals and even quite small doses of alcohol may sometimes be followed by alarming reactions. Because of this, it is advisable to carry out the initial treatment in hospital where the patient can be kept under close supervision. Treatment with disulfiram is started with a high dose for a few days and is then continued with a small maintenance dose. Some physicians give a test dose of 10 to 15 ml of alcohol on the fifth day of treatment to study the patient's reactions, especially blood pressure and heart-rate; a second dose may be given after 15 minutes if the reaction is not marked. However, such a test dose should not be given to patients over 50 years of age.

A suggested dose is 800 mg of disulfiram on the first day of treatment, reduced by 200 mg daily to a daily dose of 200 mg and then to the lowest effective maintenance dose, usually 100 to 200 mg daily, which is preferably taken in the morning.

Disulfiram controlled hypertension and hyperkinesia induced by levodopa, possibly by inhibiting the conversion of dopamine to noradrenaline. When disulfiram was withdrawn the side-effects returned.— E. Birket-Smith and J. V. Andersen (letter), *Lancet*, 1973, *1*, 431.

Reactions to the administration of disulfiram were used as an index of susceptibility to carbon disulphide.— D. Djuric *et al.*, *Archs envir. Hlth*, 1973, *26*, 287, per *J. Am. med. Ass.*, 1973, *224*, 1442.

Disulfiram blocked the formation of the eggshell in female schistosomes and had a beneficial effect in *mice* infected with *Schistosoma mansoni*. However, its usefulness might be limited by its rapid reversibility.— J. L. Seed *et al.*, *Am. J. trop. Med. Hyg.*, 1979, *28*, 508, per *Trop. Dis. Bull.*, 1980, *77*, 59.

Antimalarial activity of disulfiram *in vitro*.— L. W. Scheibel *et al.*, *Proceedings of the National Academy of Sciences of the USA*, 1979, *76*, 5303, per *Trop. Dis. Bull.*, 1980, *77*, 361.

Alcoholism. A review of the proposed mechanism of the disulfiram-alcohol interaction and its management.— R. M. Elenbaas, *Am. J. Hosp. Pharm.*, 1977, *34*, 827.

A review of disulfiram and its use in the treatment of alcoholism.— *Med. Lett.*, 1980, *22*, 1. See also E. M. Sellers *et al.*, *New Engl. J. Med.*, 1981, *305*, 1255.

The reaction occurring when a patient taking either disulfiram or citrated calcium carbimide consumed alcohol was not always sufficiently unpleasant to be a deterrent, but the effect could be enhanced by concomitantly taking amitriptyline, 25 mg thrice daily. No untoward side-effects occurred.— W. A. G. MacCallum (letter), *Lancet*, 1969, *1*, 313.

In a study of 128 alcoholic patients treated for 1 year with disulfiram 250 mg daily, disulfiram 1 mg daily (a pharmacologically ineffective dose) or placebo, there were no statistically significant differences in total abstinence, percentage of drinking days, days worked, or percentage of appointments kept. Disulfiram is probably of limited value in the treatment of alcoholism, and fear of a disulfiram-alcohol reaction occurring might be as important as the reaction itself.— R. K. Fuller and H. P. Roth, *Ann. intern. Med.*, 1979, *90*, 901.

A double-blind, placebo-controlled study in non-alcoholic subjects supporting the claim by alcoholics that by taking several small alcoholic drinks over a few hours they can diminish the effects of disulfiram and eventually drink with impunity. The diminution was more pronounced for calcium carbimide than for disulfiram.— J. E. Peachey *et al.* (letter), *Lancet*, 1981, *1*, 943. The effect of disulfiram might have worn off.— M. Phillips (letter), *ibid.*, *2*, 210.

Use of implants. Ten 100-mg implant tablets of disulfiram were inserted into the abdominal musculature of 47 alcoholic patients on 70 occasions. The period of alcohol abstinence which followed was significantly longer than that after previous treatment which, in 39 patients, had included disulfiram given by mouth.— M. T. Malcolm and J. S. Madden, *Br. J. Psychiat.*, 1973, *123*, 41.

In a controlled study of 45 alcoholics, 22 who had 1 g of disulfiram implanted achieved an average period of abstinence after discharge of 5.4 months compared with only 1.9 months in the controls.— C. R. Whyte and P. M. J. O'Brien, *Br. J. Psychiat.*, 1974, *124*, 42.

Of 62 patients who had received disulfiram implants, only 3 had symptoms which could have been a reaction when they later drank alcohol. Blood-disulfiram concentrations were above 1 µg per ml (considered a therapeutic concentration) on only 8 of 31 occasions in the first week and even in these patients concentrations were less than 1 µg per ml within about 7 weeks.— M. T. Malcolm *et al.*, *Br. J. Psychiat.*, 1974, *125*, 485.

From a study of 62 alcoholic patients seen monthly for the first 6 months after they had received disulfiram implants it was considered that the predominant benefits were psychological, and the pharmacological action was minimal.— S. A. Kline and E. Kingstone, *Can. med. Ass. J.*, 1977, *116*, 1382. Comment, emphasising the importance of the pharmacological action of disulfiram as a deterrent for the alcoholic patient.— A. Wilson (letter), *ibid.*, *117*, 722. Reply.— S. A. Kline and E. Kingstone (letter), *ibid.*, 727.

Preparations

Disulfiram Tablets *(B.P.)*. Tablets containing disulfiram. Protect from light.

Disulfiram Tablets *(U.S.P.)*. Tablets containing disulfiram. Store in airtight containers. Protect from light.

Antabuse 200 *(Weddel, UK)*. Disulfiram, available as scored tablets of 200 mg. (Also available as Antabuse in *Austral., Belg., Canad., Ital., S.Afr., USA*).

Other Proprietary Names

Abstensyl *(Arg.)*; Abstinyl *(Switz.)*; Antabus *(Denm., Ger., Neth., Norw., Spain, Swed., Switz.)*; Antietil *(Ital.)*; Antivitium *(Spain)*; Aversan *(Norw.)*; Espéral *(Fr.)*; Refusal *(Neth.)*; Ro-Sulfiram-500 *(USA)*.

2732-x

Citrated Calcium Carbimide.

A mixture of 1 part by weight of highly purified calcium carbimide (calcium cyanamide) with 2 parts by weight of citric acid.

CAS — 8013-88-5.

Adverse Effects. Drowsiness, fatigue, tinnitus, impotence, frequent micturition, and skin rash have been reported. Hypothyroidism may rarely develop after prolonged administration. Mild or transitory leucocytosis has been reported in patients taking citrated calcium carbimide.

Cardiovascular effects. In the course of treatment for alcoholism abnormal ECGs developed during drinking trials in 4 of 19 patients who received calcium carbimide 50 mg daily, and in 3 of 7 patients who received disulfiram 500 mg daily. Four of the 19 patients on citrated calcium carbimide and 6 of 11 patients on disulfiram also had hypotension at these times.— M. S. Levy *et al.*, *Am. J. Psychiat.*, 1967, *123*, 1018.

Potentially dangerous cardiovascular changes occurred in 3 alcoholic subjects participating in studies of the citrated calcium carbimide/alcohol interaction. Hypotension with bradycardia can occur during the citrated calcium carbimide or disulfiram interaction due to enhanced vagal tone, as a result of retching or vomiting. Careful cardiovascular assessment is required before treatment with either compound.— J. E. Peachey *et al.*, *Clin. Pharmac. Ther.*, 1981, *29*, 40.

Effects on the liver. Evidence of an unusual liver cell alteration in alcoholics taking cyanamide to discourage alcohol consumption. The lesion has now been seen in 4 patients taking cyanamide alone, one taking cyanamide and disulfiram, one who had been taking disulfiram alone for a very long time, and one who had been taking disulfiram in addition to many other drugs. The characteristic hepatic alteration has been seen in every patient taking cyanamide and may be a predictable lesion in alcoholics taking this drug.— J. J. Vázquez and S. Cervera (letter), *Lancet*, 1980, *1*, 361.

Peripheral neuropathy. Peripheral neuropathy attributed to calcium carbimide in a patient also taking haloperidol.— T. M. Reilly, *Lancet*, 1976, *1*, 911.

Treatment of Adverse Effects. As for Disulfiram, p.579.

Precautions. Citrated calcium carbimide should be used with caution in patients with coronary artery disease or myocardial disease. It should not be given to patients who have recently taken alcohol.

It is reported that paraldehyde may precipitate a citrated calcium carbimide/alcohol reaction while metronidazole may exacerbate such a reaction. See also under Disulfiram, p.579.

Calcium carbimide had no effect on serum concentrations of phenytoin or on the excretion of its metabolite in 4 subjects given both compounds. Disulfiram increased the serum concentration of phenytoin and reduced excretion of the metabolite in 2 subjects. Calcium carbimide had no effect on serum concentrations of phenobarbitone.— O. V. Olesen, *Archs Neurol., Chicago*, 1967, *16*, 642.

For a recommendation of cardiovascular assessment before treatment with citrated calcium carbimide, see under Adverse Effects.

Uses. Citrated calcium carbimide acts similarly to disulfiram (see p.579). The usual dose is 50 mg once or twice daily.

As with disulfiram, successful results can only be achieved if the treatment is undertaken with the willing cooperation of the patient and in conjunction with psychotherapy.

Alcoholism. A brief discussion of citrated calcium carbimide in the reduction of alcohol consumption.— E. M. Sellers *et al.*, *New Engl. J. Med.*, 1981, *305*, 1255.

Possible intra-individual variability in the calcium carbimide/alcohol interaction.— J. F. Brien *et al.*, *Clin. Pharmac. Ther.*, 1980, *27*, 426. For a study indicating that the effects of disulfiram and calcium carbimide can be reduced by taking several small alcoholic drinks over a few hours, see Disulfiram, p.580.

Proprietary Preparations

Abstem *(Lederle, UK)*. Citrated calcium carbimide, available as tablets of 50 mg.

Other Proprietary Names

Dipsan *(Austral., Denm., Neth., S.Afr., Swed., Switz.)*; Temposil *(Canad.)*.

Diuretics

2300-t

Diuretics promote the excretion of water and electrolytes by the kidneys. They are used in the treatment of patients with conditions such as congestive heart failure or hepatic, renal, or pulmonary disease when salt and water retention has resulted in oedema or ascites. The disease process in these conditions is not generally affected by the diuretic treatment.

Diuretics are also used, either alone, or in association with other antihypertensive agents, in the treatment of raised blood pressure.

Diuretics have also been used for oedema and hypertension in pregnancy but the value of such therapy has now been questioned. Similarly, they have been used for tension and weight gain associated with the premenstrual syndrome, but such use has little rationale and carries the risk of exacerbating the problem of fluid retention.

The principal groups of diuretics described in this section are:

1. Thiazides (benzothiadiazines), typified by chlorothiazide (p.587), and certain other compounds, often with structural similarities to the thiazides including: bendrofluazide, p.584, benzthiazide, p.585, chlorthalidone, p.591, clopamide, p.592, clorexolone, p.593, cyclopenthiazide, p.593, cyclothiazide, p.593, hydrochlorothiazide, p.600, hydroflumethiazide, p.602, mefruside, p.605, methyclothiazide, p.607, metolazone, p.607, polythiazide, p.609, quinethazone, p.609, trichlormethiazide, p.615.
They inhibit sodium and chloride reabsorption in the kidney tubules. They also promote potassium excretion.
2. Bumetanide (p.585), ethacrynic acid (p.594), and frusemide (p.596), which are carboxylic acids, produce an intense diuresis of relatively short duration. They are sometimes termed 'loop' or 'high-ceiling' diuretics.
3. Aldosterone inhibitors, such as spironolactone (p.609) and canrenone (p.587). They also diminish the excretion of potassium.
4. Mercurial diuretics, typified by mersalyl (described under Mersalyl Acid, p.606), including: chlormerodrin, p.587, meralluride, p.606, mercaptomerin, p.606.
They inhibit sodium reabsorption at sites probably lower than the proximal kidney tubule; they also promote potassium excretion. Their action is enhanced by acidification of the urine.
5. Carbonic anhydrase inhibitors, including: acetazolamide, p.581, dichlorphenamide, p.593, ethoxzolamide, p.595, methazolamide, p.607.
They are also used to reduce intra-ocular pressure in glaucoma.
6. Osmotic diuretics, such as mannitol (p.603) and urea (p.616), which reduce the water content of the body by physical means.They are used to reduce or prevent cerebral oedema and to promote the excretion of drugs such as aspirin and some barbiturates.
7. Other diuretics, such as amiloride (p.583) and triamterene (p.614) which diminish the excretion of potassium and may be used in conjunction with other diuretics to counter their potassium-depleting effects.

The xanthines, which are described in the section on Caffeine and other Xanthines (p.340), are also used as diuretics and laevulose (p.54) is used as an osmotic diuretic.

The pharmacology and use of diuretics.— T. O. Morgan, *Drugs*, 1978, *15*, 151.

Further general reviews and comments on diuretics: P. D. Lief, *Am. Heart J.*, 1978, *96*, 824; G. J. Green and A. M. Breckenridge, *Pharm. J.*, 1979, *1*, 384.

Hypertension. A discussion of the treatment of mild hypertension.— G. E. Bauer and S. N. Hunyor, *Drugs*, 1978, *15*, 80.

Further reviews and comments on the use of diuretics in hypertension: F. J. Goodwin, *Topics Ther.*, 1978, *4*, 167; D. Robertson and A. S. Nies, *Recent Adv. clin. Pharmac.*, 1978, *1*, 55; M. Joy, *Practitioner*, 1979, *223*, 178; D. G. McDevitt, *ibid.*, 228; L. T. Bannan *et al.*, *Br. med. J.*, 1980, *281*, 982; *idem*, 1053.

Oedema. A review of the use of diuretics and relief of oedema.— A. Lant, *Topics Ther.*, 1978, *4*, 150.

Further reviews and comments on the use of diuretics in oedema: W. Bleifeld *et al.*, *Am. J. Med.*, 1978, *65*, 203; *Br. med. J.*, 1979, *1*, 148; *Lancet*, 1979, *1*, 253; G. A. Porter, *J. Am. med. Ass.*, 1980, *244*, 1614.

Premenstrual syndrome. A review of drugs for the treatment of premenstrual tension, including criticism of claims made on behalf of diuretics. There is no basis for the belief that fluid retention is a cause of premenstrual tension.— *Br. J. Psychiat.*, 1979, *135*, 576.

Further references: P. E. Preece *et al.*, *Br. med. J.*, 1975, *4*, 498 (lack of benefit in mastalgia).

Toxaemia of pregnancy. A brief review of drug therapy for severe pre-eclampsia and eclampsia. Diuretic therapy may be indicated if there is gross fluid retention, evidence of impending renal necrosis or, in the longer term, to enhance the action of antihypertensive agents, such as hydralazine. Hypovolaemia is a feature of severe pre-eclampsia, however, even though oedema may be gross, and diuretics should be used with caution.— B. M. Hibbard, *Practitioner*, 1978, *221*, 847.

Diuretics should not be used routinely for the medical management of moderate hypertension in pregnancy, because controlled trials have shown that they are not beneficial.— *Br. med. J.*, 1980, *280*, 1483.

2301-x

Acetazolamide *(B.P., U.S.P.)*.
Acetazolam; Acetazolamidum. 5-Acetamido-1,3,4-thiadiazole-2-sulphonamide; *N*-(5-Sulphamoyl-1,3,4-thiadiazol-2-yl)acetamide.
$C_4H_6N_4O_3S_2$=222.2.

CAS — 59-66-5.

Pharmacopoeias. In *Br.*, *Braz.*, *Chin.*, *Cz.*, *Fr.*, *Hung.*, *Ind.*, *It.*, *Jap.*, *Jug.*, *Nord.*, *Roum.*, *Swiss*, *Turk.*, and *U.S.*

A fine, white to yellowish-white, odourless, tasteless, crystalline powder. M.p. about 260° with decomposition.

Soluble 1 in 1400 of water, 1 in 400 of alcohol, and 1 in 100 of acetone; practically insoluble in carbon tetrachloride, chloroform, and ether; soluble in solutions of alkali hydroxides

2302-r

Acetazolamide Sodium.
Sodium Acetazolamide.
$C_4H_5N_4NaO_3S_2$=244.2.

CAS — 1424-27-7.

Acetazolamide sodium 275 mg is approximately equivalent to 250 mg of acetazolamide. A freshly prepared 10% solution in water has a pH of 9 to 10. A 3.85% solution is iso-osmotic with serum.

Adverse Effects. Side-effects of acetazolamide therapy occur fairly frequently and consist mainly of drowsiness and numbness and tingling of the face and extremities. Fatigue, excitement, thirst, headache, dizziness, ataxia, hyperpnoea, tinnitus, hearing loss, and gastro-intestinal disturbances occasionally occur. Transient myopia has also been reported. In patients with hepatic cirrhosis, it may cause disorientation. Fever and skin reactions of an allergic type have been reported. Isolated cases, some fatal, of agranulocytosis, aplastic anaemia, thrombocytopenia, crystalluria, kidney stones, and renal lesions have occurred.

Appreciable losses of potassium and sodium during prolonged therapy with acetazolamide may result in a tendency towards hypokalaemic acidosis.

Intramuscular injections are painful owing to the alkalinity of the solution.

Allergy. A 54-year-old man with glaucoma who was treated with acetazolamide 500 mg daily for 26 days developed a generalised erythematous rash and became delirious, dehydrated, markedly jaundiced, with peripheral circulatory failure, and died from hepatic coma and anuria. Drug-induced hypersensitivity and hepatitis due to acetazolamide was suspected.— A. Kristinsson, *Br. J. Ophthal.*, 1967, *51*, 348.

Diabetogenic effect. Acetazolamide could exacerbate diabetes mellitus.— *Drug & Ther. Bull.*, 1973, *11*, 5.

Effects on the blood. *Agranulocytosis or aplastic anaemia.* Fatal bone-marrow depression, with anaemia, leucopenia, and thrombocytopenia, developed in a 66-year-old man after treatment with acetazolamide 500 mg twice daily for 3½ months.— G. W. Englund (letter), *J. Am. Med. Ass.*, 1969, *210*, 2282.

Mention of 2 cases of fatal aplastic anaemia or agranulocytosis in one year probably due to acetazolamide.— W. H. W. Inman, *Br. med. J.*, 1977, *1*, 1500.

Further references: F. G. Hoffman *et al.*, *New Engl. J. Med.*, 1960, *262*, 242.

Thrombocytopenic purpura. Fatal thrombocytopenic purpura in a patient was associated with acetazolamide.— J. T. Corbett (letter), *Br. med. J.*, 1958, *1*, 1122.

Effects on endocrine function. Hirsutism occurred in a 2½-year-old girl after treatment for 16 months with acetazolamide for congenital glaucoma. There was no evidence of virilisation.— I. S. Weiss, *Am. J. Ophthal.*, 1974, *78*, 327.

Effects on the eyes. Examination of 100 drainage operations (Scheie's) showed that acetazolamide had an adverse effect on the outcome of the operation.— W. H. G. Douglas and T. G. Ramsell, *Br. J. Ophthal.*, 1969, *53*, 472.

Effects on the kidneys. *Crystalluria.* Anuria preceded by backache and haematuria developed in 2 patients following short courses of acetazolamide. A high fluid intake was recommended for patients taking acetazolamide to reduce the risk of crystalluria.— T. Higenbottam *et al.*, *Postgrad. med. J.*, 1978, *54*, 127.

Further references: R. T. Orchard *et al.* (letter), *Br. med. J.*, 1972, *3*, 646; S. A. Howlett, *Sth. med. J.*, 1975, *68*, 504.

Renal stones. A 21-year-old man with chronic glaucoma treated with acetazolamide 250 mg five times daily developed a calcium stone in the left ureter.— M. B. Pepys (letter), *Lancet*, 1970, *1*, 837.

Further references: M. A. Rubenstein and J. G. Bucy, *J. Urol.*, 1975, *114*, 610; N. G. Kingsley, *Aust. J. Hosp. Pharm.*, 1977, *7*, 95.

Effects on the liver. For a report of liver damage associated with acetazolamide administration, see Allergy (above).

Effects on mental state. Apparent exacerbation of his chronic paranoid schizophrenia developed in a 69-year-old man given acetazolamide 250 mg thrice daily for glaucoma. He returned to his previously adequate level of social behaviour on reduction of the dosage.— T. O. Rowe (letter), *Am. J. Psychiat.*, 1977, *134*, 587.

Effects on sexual function. A complex of malaise, fatigue, weight loss, anorexia, depression, and loss of libido occurred in 44 of 92 patients with chronic glaucoma during therapy with acetazolamide or methazolamide. These patients were found to be significantly more acidotic than those who did not experience such side-effects.— D. L. Epstein and W. M. Grant, *Archs Ophthal., N.Y.*, 1977, *95*, 1378.

Lupus erythematosus. Lupus erythematosus has been implicated as a side-effect of treatment with acetazolamide.— P. Cohen and F. H. Gardner, *J. Am. med. Ass.*, 1966, *197*, 817.

Treatment of Adverse Effects. As for Chlorothiazide, p.589. It has been reported that acidosis associated with overdosage with carbonic anhydrase inhibitors may respond to bicarbonate administration.

Precautions. Acetazolamide is contra-indicated in the presence of sodium or potassium depletion, in idiopathic renal hyperchloraemic acidosis, in conditions such as Addison's disease and adrenal failure, and in marked hepatic or renal failure. It should not be used in chronic noncongested closed-angle glaucoma since it may mask deterioration of the condition. Its use is best avoided in the first trimester of pregnancy. It should be given with care to patients likely to develop acidosis or with diabetes mellitus.

By rendering the urine alkaline acetazolamide enhances the effects of amphetamines and reduces the effects of hexamine and its compounds; it may increase the plasma concentration of quinidine. The diuretic effect of acetazolamide is diminished if ammonium chloride is taken concomitantly. Acetazolamide may enhance anticonvulsant-induced osteomalacia. Concurrent administration of acetazolamide and aspirin may result in severe acidosis.

For a contra-indication to the use of acetazolamide in the long-term management of chloridorrhoea, see Gastro-intestinal disorders under Uses.

Interactions. Antacids. The use of concurrent sodium bicarbonate therapy enhances the risk of calculus formation in patients taking acetazolamide.— M. A. Rubenstein and J. G. Bucy, *J. Urol.*, 1975, *114*, 610.

Aspirin. The acidosis caused by carbonic anhydrase inhibitors may increase the likelihood and severity of salicylate toxicity in patients taking salicylates, and conversely the acidosis caused by salicylates may increase the likelihood and severity of the acidotic syndrome complex in patients taking carbonic anhydrase inhibitors.— C. J. Anderson *et al.*, *Am. J. Ophthal.*, 1978, *86*, 516.

Diuretics. For competition between acetazolamide and chlorthalidone for binding sites in blood cells, see Chlorthalidone, p.591.

Lignocaine and other local anaesthetics. For the effect of acetazolamide on procaine, see Procaine Hydrochloride, p.921.

Phenytoin and other anticonvulsants. For severe osteomalacia in patients taking acetazolamide with phenytoin and other anticonvulsants, see Phenytoin, p.1240.

For a suggestion that concurrent administration of acetazolamide impairs the absorption of primidone, see Primidone, p.1254.

Interference with diagnostic tests. The administration of acetazolamide could interfere with measurements of urinary 17-hydroxycorticosteroids.— J. M. Rosenberg and I. S. Kampa, *Drug Intell. & clin. Pharm.*, 1973, *7*, 33.

Pregnancy and the neonate. Acetazolamide is mostly unavailable for transfer into the foetal compartment following administration in pregnancy because it is firmly bound to carbonic anhydrase within the red blood cell.— K. Adamsons and I. Joelsson, *Am. J. Obstet. Gynec.*, 1966, *96*, 437.

A recommendation, based on results in *animals*, that carbonic anhydrase inhibitors should not be used in early pregnancy.— T. H. Maren, *Archs Ophthal., N.Y.*, 1971, *85*, 1.

An infant with a large sacrococcygeal teratoma was born prematurely to a woman who had taken acetazolamide for glaucoma until the nineteenth week of pregnancy. A cause and effect relationship is not proposed.— F. Worsham *et al.*, *J. Am. med. Ass.*, 1978, *240*, 251.

Absorption and Fate. Acetazolamide is fairly rapidly absorbed from the gastro-intestinal tract with peak plasma concentrations occurring about 2 hours after administration by mouth. It has been estimated to have a plasma half-life of about 4 hours. It is tightly bound to carbonic anhydrase and accumulates in tissues containing this enzyme, particularly red blood cells and the renal cortex; it is bound to plasma proteins. It is excreted unchanged in the urine, renal clearance being enhanced in alkaline urine.

The pharmacokinetics of acetazolamide in relation to its use in the treatment of glaucoma and its effects as an inhibitor of carbonic anhydrase.— B. Lehmann *et al.*, *Adv. Biosci.*, 1969, *5*, 197.

Further references: T. H. Maren *et al.*, *Bull. Johns Hopkins Hosp.*, 1954, *95*, 199; T. H. Maren and B. Robinson, *ibid.*, 1960, *106*, 1; W. F. Bayne *et al.*, *J. pharm. Sci.*, 1975, *64*, 402.

Bioavailability. In 20 healthy subjects given acetazolamide 250 mg the mean peak plasma-acetazolamide concentration for 5 separate batches of tablets from a single manufacturer was 6.90, 8.55, 8.60, 11.28, and 11.44 µg per ml respectively. It was suggested that these results demonstrated bio-inequivalence.— G. J. Yakatan *et al.*, *J. pharm. Sci.*, 1978, *67*, 252.

Further references: F. Theeuwes *et al.*, *Archs Ophthal., N.Y.*, 1978, *96*, 2219.

Red cell binding. Following administration of a single dose of acetazolamide 250 mg to 5 healthy subjects the range of peak plasma concentrations was 10 to 18 µg per ml over a period of 1 to 3 hours after dosage; this was about half those reported after a 500-mg dose. Red blood cell concentrations were higher and declined slowly; at 24 to 31 hours after dosage the ratio of red blood cell to plasma concentrations was greater than 4:1. Saliva concentrations were constant for each individual and were about 1% of those of plasma.— S. M. Wallace *et al.*, *J. pharm. Sci.*, 1977, *66*, 527.

Uses. Acetazolamide is an inhibitor of carbonic anhydrase. By inhibiting the reaction catalysed by carbonic anhydrase in the renal tubules, acetazolamide increases the excretion of bicarbonate and of cations, chiefly sodium and potassium, and so promotes an alkaline diuresis.

Continuous administration of acetazolamide is associated with metabolic acidosis and associated loss of diuretic activity. Therefore, although acetazolamide has been used as a diuretic, its effectiveness diminishes with continuous use, and it has largely been superseded by agents such as the thiazides or frusemide. For diuresis the usual dose is 250 to 375 mg daily or on alternate days. A suggested dose for children is 5 mg per kg body-weight daily.

By inhibiting carbonic anhydrase in the eye acetazolamide decreases intra-ocular pressure and is used in the pre-operative management of closed-angle glaucoma, or as an adjunct in the treatment of open-angle glaucoma. In the treatment of glaucoma the usual dose is 0.25 to 1 g daily, in divided doses for amounts over 250 mg daily.

Acetazolamide is also used, either alone or in association with other anticonvulsants, for the treatment of various forms of epilepsy, in doses of 0.25 to 1 g daily. A suggested dose for children for glaucoma or epilepsy is 8 to 30 mg per kg daily.

When oral administration is impracticable, similar doses of acetazolamide sodium may be given by intramuscular or preferably by intravenous injection.

When treatment is prolonged, or in susceptible patients, loss of potassium may be sufficient to produce hypokalaemia; potassium supplements should then be given as for Chlorothiazide (see p.589).

Action. A detailed account of the chemistry, physiology, and inhibition of carbonic anhydrase.— T. H. Maren, *Physiol. Rev.*, 1967, *47*, 595–781.

Administration in renal failure. The interval between doses of acetazolamide should be extended from 6 hours to 12 hours in patients with a glomerular filtration-rate (GFR) of 10 to 50 ml per minute; it should be avoided in patients with a GFR of less than 10 ml per minute.— W. M. Bennett *et al.*, *Ann. intern. Med.*, 1980, *93*, 286.

Cardiac disorders. *Angina pectoris.* A brief discussion of experimental studies of the effect of acetazolamide in patients with angina pectoris.— M. A. Nevins, *J. Am. med. Ass.*, 1974, *229*, 804.

Open-heart surgery. In 6 patients with alkalosis after open-heart surgery pH was rapidly corrected and respiratory and cardiac distress reduced in 5 by treatment with acetazolamide 250 mg six-hourly.— P. B. Sabawala and A. S. Keats, *Clin. Pharmac. Ther.*, 1974, *15*, 218.

Epilepsy. Acetazolamide was first used as an anticonvulsant in petit mal absences. It has been used in catamenial (menstrual) epilepsy because of its diuretic action. However, it is a poor diuretic but in practice may help to control a number of types of generalised epilepsy, especially myoclonic astatic epilepsy. It is essentially an adjuvant anticonvulsant.— P. M. Jeavons, *Practitioner*, 1977, *219*, 542.

Further references: J. Holowach and D. L. Thurston, *J. Pediat.*, 1958, *53*, 160; I. P. Ross, *Lancet*, 1958, *2*, 1308; H. Kutt and S. Louis, *Drugs*, 1972, *4*, 227.

For a further comment on the role of acetazolamide in epilepsy, see Sulthiame, p.1255.

Gastro-intestinal disorders. *Chloridorrhoea.* Administration of acetazolamide 125 mg every 8 hours to a 5-year-old child with congenital chloridorrhoea and metabolic alkalosis. Serum-bicarbonate concentrations were decreased but the underlying problem of chloride loss was exacerbated. Acetazolamide is therefore contra-indicated for the long-term management of this condition.— E. B. Clark and J. A. Vanderhoof, *J. Pediat.*, 1977, *91*, 148.

Pancreatitis. In 26 patients with acute pancreatitis, acetazolamide was effective in reducing the volume of pancreatic secretion.— M. C. Anderson and M. K. Copass, *Am. J. dig. Dis.*, 1966, *11*, 367.

Further references: K. H. Grözinger, *Surgery, St Louis*, 1966, *59*, 319; W. P. Dyck *et al.*, *Gastroenterology*, 1972, *62*, 547.

Ménière's disease. Acetazolamide was used to treat 60 patients with Ménière's disease, during an 8-year period. The best results were seen in patients younger than 45 years who had suffered from the disease for less than 5 years. After a low-salt diet and restricted fluids for 3 days, acetazolamide, 500 mg followed by 3 evenly spaced doses of 250 mg, was given on the fourth day, 4 doses of 250 mg on the fifth day, and 250 mg thrice daily for the next 10 days.— G. Varga *et al.*, *J. Lar. Otol.*, 1966, *80*, 250.

Mountain sickness. Acetazolamide 250 mg twice daily for 4 days given to 71 unacclimatised hikers when they reached a height of 3340 m in the Himalayas significantly reduced the incidence of acute mountain sickness in those who had flown to a starting point for their hike at 2800 m. The severity of the condition also appeared to be reduced.— P. H. Hackett *et al.*, *Lancet*, 1976, *2*, 1149. Doubts on the value of acetazolamide.— L. E. Ramsay (letter), *ibid.*, 1977, *1*, 540.

A plea that sedatives should not be given at high altitude and the view that acetazolamide improves sleep at high altitude.— J. R. Sutton *et al.* (letter), *Lancet*, 1979, *1*, 165.

In studies on 9 hypoxaemic mountaineers, acetazolamide reduced periodic breathing and improved arterial oxygenation during sleep at high altitude. In a study of 32 healthy men at sea level, acetazolamide increased ventilation at any percentage of oxygenation. It seems likely that acetazolamide diminishes sleep hypoxaemia by increasing ventilation; by improving oxygenation at high altitude it might ameliorate the symptoms of acute mountain sickness.— J. R. Sutton *et al.*, *New Engl. J. Med.*, 1979, *301*, 1329. Comments.— J. W. Bauman and J. Boyle (letter), *ibid.*, 1980, *302*, 813; N. H. Edelman and T. V. Santiago (letter), *ibid.* Reply.— A. C. P. Powles *et al.* (letter), *ibid.*, 814.

The subjective view of 4 experienced climbers was that acetazolamide 500 mg daily (as a sustained-release preparation) facilitated acclimatisation. It is not, however, a panacea for acclimatisation and does not obviate the need for slowness in exposure to great heights; a climber treated for severe cerebral oedema at 6000 metres and his companion with early pulmonary oedema had taken 10 days to acclimatise to this height and were taking acetazolamide daily at the same time. Side-effects of acetazolamide included diuresis of up to 1 to 2 litres extra daily, increased wakefulness at night, and painful peripheral paraesthesia.— A. Pines (letter), *Lancet*, 1980, *2*, 807.

In a double-blind placebo-controlled study 10 men taking slow-release capsules of acetazolamide 500 mg daily had fewer symptoms of acute mountain sickness at 5000 metres than 10 control men.— Birmingham Medical Research Expeditionary Society Mountain Sickness Study Group, *Lancet*, 1981, *1*, 180. Comment.— J. R. Sutton *et al.* (letter), *ibid.*, 552. Reply.— A. R. Bradwell *et al.* (letter), *ibid.*, 730.

A similar study.— M. K. Greene *et al.*, *Br. med. J.*, 1981, *283*, 811.

Further references: S. M. Cain and J. E. Dunn, *J. appl. Physiol.*, 1966, *21*, 1195; S. A. Forwand *et al.*, *New Engl. J. Med.*, 1968, *279*, 839.

Muscular and rheumatic disorders. The disappearance of a ganglion on the left wrist while a patient was being treated with acetazolamide for glaucoma suggested that synovial fluid tension was reduced as well as aqueous humour tension.— J. B. Cleland (letter), *Br. med. J.*, 1969, *3*, 361.

Hypokalaemic periodic paralysis. Acetazolamide 375 to 500 mg daily was an effective prophylactic agent in 2 patients with severe hypokalaemic periodic paralysis, and was well tolerated. Preliminary observations in 5 other patients given acetazolamide showed a striking improvement in 3.— J. S. Resnick *et al.*, *New Engl. J. Med.*, 1968, *278*, 582. In treating a further 12 patients, doses of 125 mg of acetazolamide were given thrice daily to children and 250 mg two to six times daily to adults. There was dramatic improvement in 10 of the 12 and this lasted for up to 43 months. Chronic weakness between attacks in 10 patients was improved in 8.— R. C. Griggs *et al.*, *Ann. intern. Med.*, 1970, *73*, 39.

Further references: R. J. Viskoper *et al.*, *Am. J. med. Sci.*, 1973, *266*, 119; B. Hoskins *et al.*, *Archs Neurol., Chicago*, 1974, *31*, 187; F. Q. Vroom *et al.*, *ibid.*, 1975, *32*, 385.

Paramyotonia congenita. Acetazolamide was tested on a patient with paramyotonia congenita, a condition marked by myotonia exacerbated by cold and exercise, and episodic weakness. Although acetazolamide had been used in the treatment of periodic paralysis, in this patient each administration of acetazolamide resulted in marked quadriparesis, although the myotonia was improved.— J. E. Riggs *et al.*, *Ann. intern. Med.*, 1977, *86*, 169.

Ocular disorders. *Cataract extraction.* The use of acetazolamide in cataract extraction.— L. M. Fine, *Archs Ophthal., N.Y.*, 1965, *73*, 19, per *J. Hosp. Pharm.*, 1965, *22*, 113.

Further references: B. Beidner *et al.*, *Am. J. Ophthal.*, 1977, *83*, 565.

Glaucoma. Acetazolamide 250 mg with a potassium salt 1 g six-hourly is used to reduce aqueous flow in simple glaucoma. For long-term therapy, carbonic-anhydrase inhibitors are disappointing because of tiresome side-effects and a tendency to lose effectiveness.— J. Winstanley, *Practitioner*, 1969, *202*, 751. A further brief comment.— S. I. Davidson, *Prescribers' J.*, 1978, *18*, 139.

In patients taking acetazolamide for the control of glaucoma, a further diuretic such as chlorothiazide could be given concomitantly for its saliuretic effect.— *J. Am. med. Ass.*, 1974, *227*, 1175.

In a short-term dose-response study completed by 9 patients with ocular hypertension, acetazolamide was given in single doses of 63, 125, 250, and 500 mg. Although plasma concentrations increased progressively with higher doses, the maximum fall in intra-ocular pressure exhibited a plateau effect with no difference between doses of 63 and 125 mg and very little average additional effect from 250 or 500 mg. A minor increase in the duration of response was observed with the 250-mg dose compared to lower doses, but 500 mg showed no further effect. A long-term study was now necessary.— B. R. Friedland *et al.*, *Archs Ophthal., N.Y.*, 1977, *95*, 1809. Comment.— T. J. Zimmerman, *Ann. Ophthal.*, 1978, *10*, 509.

Further references: G. L. Spaeth, *Archs Ophthal., N.Y.*, 1967, *78*, 578; P. R. Lichter *et al.*, *Am. J. Ophthal.*, 1978, *85*, 495; F. G. Berson *et al.*, *Archs Ophthal., N.Y.*, 1980, *98*, 1051; P. Jaeger *et al.* (letter), *New Engl. J. Med.*, 1980, *303*, 702.

Raised intracranial pressure. For the use of acetazolamide in hydrocephalus, see J. Mealy and D. T. Barker, *J. Pediat.*, 1968, *72*, 257; R. J. Schain, *Am. J. Dis. Child.*, 1969, *117*, 621; P. Visudhiphan and S. Chiemchanya, *J. Pediat.*, 1979, *95*, 657.

For a report of acetazolamide reducing CSF production, see Digoxin, p.539.

Renal disorders. *Renal calculi.* Criticism of the suggested use of acetazolamide as a supplement to sodium bicarbonate for alkalinisation of the urine in patients with a tendency to form uric acid and cystine calculi.— R. H. Davis (letter), *J. Am. med. Ass.*, 1975, *233*, 138; D. F. McDonald (letter), *ibid.* A reply.— L. B. Berman (letter), *ibid.*

Respiratory disorders. Studies in 8 patients with chronic obstructive lung disease who had chronic respiratory acidosis with superimposed metabolic alkalosis showed that correction of the alkalosis by the administration of acetazolamide, in 7 instances, or of ammonium chloride, in 3 instances, was followed by substantial improvement in clinical symptoms and in arterial oxygen pressures.— R. Bear *et al.*, *Can. med. Ass. J.*, 1977, *117*, 900.

Acetazolamide 500 mg by mouth induced bicarbonaturia and resulted in improved oxygenation in 2 patients with chronic obstructive pulmonary disease and congestive heart failure who had developed alkalosis following intravenous administration of frusemide 40 mg.— P. D. Miller and A. S. Berns, *J. Am. med. Ass.*, 1977, *238*, 2400.

Preparations

Acetazolamide Tablets *(B.P.)*. Tablets containing acetazolamide.

Acetazolamide Tablets *(U.S.P.)*. Tablets containing acetazolamide. The *U.S.P.* requires 70% dissolution in 45 minutes.

Sterile Acetazolamide Sodium *(U.S.P.)*. A sterile powder suitable for parenteral use prepared from acetazolamide with the aid of sodium hydroxide. Potency is expressed in terms of the equivalent amount of acetazolamide. pH of a 10% solution 9 to 10.

Proprietary Preparations

Diamox *(Lederle, UK)*. Acetazolamide, availabe as **Tablets** of 250 mg and as **Sustets** (sustained-release capsules) of 500 mg. (Also available as Diamox in *Austral., Belg., Canad., Denm., Fr., Ger., Ital., Neth., Norw., S.Afr., Spain, Swed., Switz., USA*).

Diamox Sodium *(Lederle, UK)*. Acetazolamide sodium, available as powder for preparing injections in vials each containing the equivalent of 500 mg of acetazolamide.

Other Proprietary Names

Acetamide *(Spain)*; Atenezol *(Jap.)*; Défiltran *(Fr.)*; Didoc *(Jap.)*, Diuramid *(Pol.)*; Diuriwas *(Ital.)*; Edemox *(Spain)*; Glaucomide *(Austral.)*; Glauconox *(Spain)*; Glaupax *(Denm., Ger., Norw., Swed., Switz.)*; Inidrase *(Ital.)*; Oratrol *(Arg.)*.

2303-f

Ambuside. EX 4810. 5-Allylsulphamoyl-2-chloro-4-(3-hydroxybut-2-enylideneamino)benzenesulphonamide; N^1-Allyl-4-chloro-6-(3-hydroxybut-2-enylideneamino)benzene-1,3-disulphonamide.
$C_{13}H_{16}ClN_3O_5S_2=393.9$.

CAS — 3754-19-6.

Adverse Effects, Treatment, and Precautions. As for Chlorothiazide, p.588.

Uses. Ambuside is a diuretic which has certain structural similarities to the thiazides and has actions and uses similar to those of chlorothiazide (see p.589).

In the treatment of oedema the usual initial dose is 20 to 30 mg daily, reduced to a dose of 10 to 20 mg thrice weekly for maintenance. In the treatment of hypertension the usual dose is 5 to 10 mg daily or 10 mg on alternate days.

When treatment is prolonged, or in susceptible patients, loss of potassium may be sufficient to produce hypokalaemia; potassium supplements should then be given as for chlorothiazide.

Proprietary Names

Hydrion *(Robert et Carrière, Fr.)*.

2304-d

Amiloride Hydrochloride *(B.P.)*.

Amipramizide; MK 870. *N*-Amidino-3,5-diamino-6-chloropyrazine-2-carboxamide hydrochloride dihydrate.
$C_6H_8ClN_7O,HCl,2H_2O=302.1$.

CAS — 2609-46-3 (amiloride); 2016-88-8 (hydrochloride, anhydrous).

Pharmacopoeias. In *Br.*

An odourless or almost odourless pale yellow to greenish-yellow powder. **Soluble** 1 in 200 of water and 1 in 350 of alcohol; practically insoluble in chloroform and ether. **Protect** from light.

Adverse Effects. Amiloride hydrochloride may cause nausea, vomiting, abdominal pain, diarrhoea or constipation, paraesthesia, thirst, dizziness, skin rash, pruritus, weakness, muscle cramps, and minor psychiatric or visual changes. Orthostatic hypotension and rises in blood-urea-nitrogen concentrations have been reported. Its potassium-sparing effect may lead to hyperkalaemia. Occasional abnormalities in liver-function tests have been reported.

Effects on the blood. Striking eosinophilia in a patient taking amiloride. It was not possible to determine whether this was related to the drug.— B. N. Singh *et al.*, *Br. med. J.*, 1967, *1*, 143.

Effects on the electrolyte balance. Studies in 9 patients with hypertension and 14 with cardiac failure, who had been taking daily one or two tablets containing amiloride hydrochloride 5 mg and hydrochlorothiazide 50 mg for at least 6 months for diuresis, showed that there were no significant changes in their plasma concentrations of potassium, sodium, bicarbonate, or urea during treatment.— P. S. Burge and E. Montuschi, *Curr. med. Res. Opinion*, 1976, *4*, 260.

Calcium. In 6 healthy persons, treatment with amiloride for 7 days produced significant hypercalciuria, not consistently related to the excretion of magnesium or potassium. Three patients with marked hypercalciuria showed no correlation between urinary excretion of calcium and sodium, while 1 with marked and 2 with moderate or no hypercalciuria showed a correlation.— K. V. Johny *et al.*, *Australas. Ann. Med.*, 1969, *18*, 267.

Potassium. Plasma-potassium concentrations rose above 5 mmol (5 mEq) per litre in 3 of 6 patients treated with amiloride. The plasma-potassium concentrations rose from 4.1 to 6.7 mmol (4.1 to 6.7 mEq) per litre after 3 days' treatment in a patient who received amiloride 40 mg daily, and a rise from 3.8 to 5.3 mmol (3.8 to 5.3 mEq) per litre followed 2 days' treatment with amiloride 10 mg daily in another patient. Treatment with amiloride increased the urinary sodium/potassium ratio.— I. Surveyor and R. A. Saunders (letter), *Lancet*, 1968, *2*, 516.

Further references: A. F. Lant *et al.*, *Clin. Pharmac. Ther.*, 1969, *10*, 50.

Effects on the kidneys. In a study involving 24 patients small rises in blood-urea concentrations were common with amiloride.— C. Davidson and I. M. Gillebrand, *Br. Heart J.*, 1973, *35*, 456.

Further references: B. Senewiratne and S. Sherlock, *Lancet*, 1968, *1*, 120; P. Vesin *et al.*, *Schweiz. med. Wschr.*, 1969, *99*, 21.

Effects on the liver. A report of raised serum aspartate aminotransferase (SGOT) values in a patient receiving amiloride. There was no evidence of myocardial infarction.— A. G. A. Heffernan (letter), *Lancet*, 1968, *1*, 361.

Effects on taste perception. Amiloride was not tolerated in 3 of 24 patients because of nausea or alteration in taste.— C. Davidson and I. M. Gillebrand, *Br. Heart J.*, 1973, *35*, 456.

Further references: *Br. med. J.*, 1979, *1*, 398.

Treatment of Adverse Effects. As for Spironolactone, p.610.

Precautions. Amiloride should not be given to patients with hyperkalaemia or progressive renal failure, and should not be given with other potassium-sparing diuretics. Potassium supplements should not be given with amiloride. In patients with impaired renal function it may result in the rapid development of hyperkalaemia. It should be given with care to patients likely to develop acidosis, to patients with diabetes mellitus, and to those with impaired hepatic or renal function. Amiloride should be discontinued before glucose-tolerance tests are given to patients with diabetes mellitus. Serum electrolytes and blood-urea-nitrogen should be estimated periodically.

Absorption and Fate. Amiloride is incompletely absorbed from the gastro-intestinal tract; peak serum concentrations are achieved about 3 or 4 hours after administration by mouth. It is excreted unchanged in the urine and *animal* studies have shown little evidence of any biliary excretion. Amiloride has been estimated to have a serum half-life of about 6 hours.

In 5 fasting subjects who were given 20 mg of amiloride hydrochloride by mouth, the peak serum concentration occurred after 3 hours. The serum half-life was 6 hours. About one-half the dose appeared in the urine, the rate of excretion being highest in the first 24 hours, and about 40% was found in the faeces. There was no evidence of metabolites.— P. Weiss *et al.*, *Clin. Pharmac. Ther.*, 1969, *10*, 401.

Further references: E. Schmid and G. Fricke, *Pharmacol. Clin.*, 1969, *1*, 110; A. J. Smith and R. N. Smith, *Br. J. Pharmac.*, 1973, *48*, 646.

Enterohepatic recycling. Less than 2% of a dose of amiloride was excreted in the bile of a *dog* following intravenous administration of amiloride.— J. E. Baer *et al.*, *J. Pharmac. exp. Ther.*, 1967, *157*, 472.

Uses. Amiloride is a mild diuretic which appears to act mainly on the distal renal tubules. It takes effect about 2 hours after administration by mouth and its diuretic action has been reported to persist for about 24 hours. The full effect may be delayed until after several days of treatment. Like spironolactone, it increases the excretion of sodium and chloride and reduces the excretion of potassium. Unlike spironolactone, however, it does not appear to act by inhibiting aldosterone. Amiloride does not inhibit carbonic anhydrase.

Amiloride adds to the natriuretic but diminishes the kaliuretic effects of other diuretics, and is mainly used as an adjunct to the thiazides, frusemide, and similar diuretics, to conserve potassium, in the treatment of refractory oedema associated with hepatic cirrhosis and congestive heart failure. It has little effect in the treatment of hypertension. Amiloride hydrochloride is usually given in a dose of 10 mg daily (or 5 mg twice daily) which may be increased, if necessary, to a maximum of 20 mg daily.

Potassium supplements should not be given.

Reviews and comments on amiloride: *Drug & Ther. Bull.*, 1971, *9*, 47; *ibid.*, 1972, *10*, 30; M. E. Kosman, *J. Am. med. Ass.*, 1974, *230*, 743.

Action. Studies in *animals* and in healthy subjects suggested that amiloride has a primary direct effect on the distal renal tubule. Although chemically distinct, amiloride has some structural similarities to triamterene and at many points behaves in a similar manner.— W. I. Baba *et al.*, *Clin. Pharmac. Ther.*, 1968, *9*, 318. *Animal* studies suggesting some disparities between the mode of action of amiloride and triamterene.— J. T. Gatzy, *J. Pharmac. exp. Ther.*, 1971, *176*, 580.

Further references: J. E. Baer *et al.*, *J. Pharmac. exp. Ther.*, 1967, *157*, 472; F. P. Brunner, *Schweiz. med. Wschr.*, 1967, *97*, 1542; M. B. Bull and J. H. Laragh, *Circulation*, 1968, *37*, 45; G. Hitzenberger *et al.*, *Clin. Pharmac. Ther.*, 1968, *9*, 71.

Administration. A study indicating that absorption from the gastro-intestinal tract was significantly higher when a dose was followed by a 4-hour fast.— E. Schmid and G. Fricke, *Pharmacol. Clin.*, 1969, *1*, 110.

Administration in renal failure. Hyperkalaemia occurred following amiloride administration to some cirrhotic patients with impaired renal function.— S. Yamada and T. B. Reynolds, *Gastroenterology*, 1970, *59*, 833.

In patients with impaired renal function serum-amiloride concentrations can be expected to be increased.— P. Weiss *et al.*, *Clin. Pharmac. Ther.*, 1969, *10*, 401.

Further references: C. F. George (letter), *Br. J. clin. Pharmac.*, 1980, *9*, 94.

Cardiac disorders. In 24 patients, most of whom had valvular heart disease, receiving at least 80 mg of frusemide daily, potassium supplements were replaced by amiloride 20 mg daily; serum-potassium concentrations rose slightly within a week; total exchangeable potassium rose within the first 3 months but was not significantly different at 6 months. Amiloride may be more effective than potassium supplements in maintaining plasma-potassium concentrations.— C. Davidson and I. M. Gillebrand, *Br. Heart J.*, 1973, *35*, 456.

Further references: C. F. George *et al.*, *Lancet*, 1973, *2*, 1288.

Hepatic disorders. Discussions, reviews, and comments on amiloride and other potassium-sparing diuretics in cirrhosis of the liver: P. Vesin, *Postgrad. med. J.*, 1975, *51*, 545; *Br. med. J.*, 1978, *1*, 66.

Amiloride 10 mg twice daily, given with either frusemide or ethacrynic acid, was successful in relieving fluid retention in 23 of 24 patients with ascites due to hepatic cirrhosis. Doses of frusemide and ethacrynic acid were adjusted to keep the urinary excretion of sodium at 2 to 3 times the daily intake; the dose of frusemide required ranged from 40 to 300 mg daily and the dose of ethacrynic acid from 50 to 100 mg daily. The effect of the treatment was unpredictable. On occasions it produced a moderate or massive diuresis. Potassium depletion occurred in 5 of the patients and the safety of the treatment relied upon a dietary intake of 70 mmol (70 mEq) of potassium daily.— B. Senewiratne and S. Sherlock, *Lancet*, 1968, *1*, 120.

When used alone in 72 patients with cirrhosis and ascites, amiloride in a dose of 15 to 30 mg daily produced a satisfactory natriuresis in 80%. There was no hypokalaemia or alkalosis but acidosis and hyperkalaemia occurred in some patients, mainly with impaired renal function.— S. Yamada and T. B. Reynolds, *Gastroenterology*, 1970, *59*, 833.

Further references: V. H. Sethy *et al.*, *J. clin. Pharmac.*, 1968, *8*, 309; P. Vesin *et al.*, *Schweiz. med. Wschr.*, 1969, *99*, 21.

Hypertension. The blood pressure of 10 hypertensive patients was reduced by the administration of amiloride 10 mg twice daily but the effect was less than that of hydrochlorothiazide 50 mg twice daily.— E. A. Gombos *et al.*, *New Engl. J. Med.*, 1966, *275*, 1215.

Amiloride, alone or in conjunction with hydrochlorothiazide, had little effect on blood pressure in 17 patients with hypertension. Combined administration produced more natriuresis than either drug alone and amiloride appeared to cause withdrawal of sodium from compartments not usually affected by thiazide diuretics. A substantial part of the sodium lost might represent an exchange of sodium for cellular potassium.— H. Kampffmeyer and J. Conway, *Clin. Pharmac. Ther.*, 1968, *9*, 350.

Further references: A. Schwartz *et al.*, *J. clin. Pharmac.*, 1969, *9*, 217; A. C. Antcliff *et al.*, *Br. J. clin. Pract.*, 1972, *26*, 413; P. S. Burge and E. Montuschi, *Curr. med. Res. Opinion*, 1976, *4*, 260; V. R. Pearce *et al.*, *Postgrad. med. J.*, 1978, *54*, 533.

Associated with aldosteronism. A 70-year-old woman with hyperaldosteronism, intolerant of spironolactone, was treated with amiloride 40 mg daily for 6 weeks. Systolic and diastolic blood pressure fell, serum concentrations of sodium and bicarbonate fell, and serum concentrations of potassium, chloride, and urea rose. She was maintained on 20 mg daily.— D. Kremer *et al.*, *Br. med. J.*, 1973, *2*, 216.

Further references: C. N. Braren *et al.*, *Am. J. Med.*, 1968, *45*, 480; J. B. Ferriss *et al.*, *Am. Heart J.*, 1978, *96*, 97.

Preparations

Amiloride Hydrochloride Tablets *(B.P.)*. Amiloride Hydrochlor. Tab.; Amiloride Tablets. Tablets containing amiloride hydrochloride.

Midamor *(Morson, UK)*. Amiloride hydrochloride, available as tablets of 5 mg. (Also available as Midamor in *Austral., Neth., Norw., S.Afr., Swed., Switz.*).

Moduretic *(Merck Sharp & Dohme, UK)*. Tablets each containing amiloride hydrochloride 5 mg and hydrochlorothiazide 50 mg. Diuretic. *Dose.* 1 or 2 tablets daily, increased if necessary up to 4 tablets daily.

Other Proprietary Names

Arumil *(Ger.)*; Modamide *(Fr.)*; Nirulid *(Denm.)*; Pandiuren *(Arg.)*.

2305-n

Aminometradine *(B.P.C. 1959)*. Aminometramide. 1-Allyl-6-amino-3-ethylpyrimidine-2,4(1*H*,3*H*)-dione. $C_9H_{13}N_3O_2$=195.2.

CAS — 642-44-4.

Aminometradine is a relatively weak diuretic which has been used to control oedema in patients with mild congestive heart failure. Its adverse effects include headache, nausea, diarrhoea, and vomiting. It has been given in doses of 200 to 800 mg daily in divided doses on 3 days a week, or on alternate days.

2306-h

Bendrofluazide *(B.P., B.P. Vet.)*.

Bendrofluaz.; Bendroflumethiazide *(U.S.P.)*; Bendroflumethiazidum; Benzydroflumethiazide; FT 81. 3-Benzyl-3,4-dihydro-6-trifluoromethyl-2*H*-1,2,4-benzothiadiazine-7-sulphonamide 1,1-dioxide. $C_{15}H_{14}F_3N_3O_4S_2$=421.4.

CAS — 73-48-3.

Pharmacopoeias. In *Br., Braz., Chin., Fr., Int., It.*, and *U.S.*

A white or cream-coloured, odourless or almost odourless, tasteless, crystalline powder. M.p. about 220° with decomposition.

Practically **insoluble** in water; soluble 1 in 17 of alcohol, 1 in 1.5 of acetone, and 1 in 500 of ether; practically insoluble in chloroform. **Store** in airtight containers.

Adverse Effects, Treatment, and Precautions. As for Chlorothiazide, p.588.

Adverse reactions to bendrofluazide and propranolol for the treatment of mild hypertension.— Report of Medical Research Council Working Party on Mild to Moderate Hypertension, *Lancet*, 1981, *2*, 539.

Effects on the electrolyte balance. *Phosphate.* In 7 of 14 patients with hypercalciuria, prolonged use of bendrofluazide induced hypophosphataemia which was irreversible in 2 patients after withdrawal of treatment. Renal tubular reabsorption of phosphate was reduced in these 2 patients. Renal tubular damage could have been caused by prolonged intracellular potassium deficiency and resulted in a failure to reabsorb phosphate. The absence of bone disease in these patients was attributed to their normal intestinal phosphate absorption.— J. R. Condon and R. Nassim (letter), *Br. med. J.*, 1970, *1*, 110.

Effects on the eyes. A study indicating that usual therapeutic doses of bendrofluazide interfere with colour vision.— J. Laroche and C. Laroche, *Annls pharm. fr.*, 1972, *30*, 433.

Interactions. *Lithium.* For the effect of bendrofluazide in reducing renal clearance of lithium, see Lithium Carbonate, p.1539.

Oedema. For reference to the possible role of diuretics including bendrofluazide in exacerbating and perpetuating idiopathic oedema, see Oedema, under Adverse Effects of Chlorothiazide, p.588.

Absorption and Fate. Unlike chlorothiazide, bendrofluazide has been reported to be completely absorbed from the gastro-intestinal tract, and there are indications that it is fairly extensively metabolised; about 30% is excreted unchanged in the urine. It is estimated to have a plasma half-life of about 3 or 4 hours, its biological half-life being much longer.

Following a dose of bendrofluazide 10 mg by mouth to 4 healthy subjects peak plasma concentrations ranged from 56 to 107 ng per ml at 2 to 2.5 hours after administration. The plasma half-life averaged 2.7 hours.— B. Beermann *et al.*, *Eur. J. clin. Pharmac.*, 1976, *10*, 293. A chronic placebo-controlled study in 8 hypertensive subjects. The plasma half-life averaged about 4 hours.— *idem*, 1978, *13*, 119.

Following administration of bendrofluazide 10 mg to 9 healthy subjects a mean peak plasma-bendrofluazide concentration of about 86 ng per ml (range 56 to 107 ng per ml) was obtained after about 2 hours (range 90 to 150 minutes); this declined with a mean half-life of 3 hours which agreed well with previous findings of 150 minutes in *dogs* (J.J. Piala, *et al.*, *J. Pharmac. exp. Ther.*, 1961, *134*, 273). About 30% of the dose was recovered in the urine within 48 hours, over 90% of this in the first 12 hours, but most of the drug was eliminated through non-renal mechanisms. Since bendrofluazide has been reported by H.R. Brettell *et al.* (*Archs intern. med.*, 1964, *113*, 373) to be completely absorbed, this indicates that it is approximately 70% metabolised.— B. Beermann *et al.*, *Clin. Pharmac. Ther.*, 1977, *22*, 385.

Protein binding. Bendrofluazide is 94% bound to human serum albumin *in vitro*.— A. Ågren and T. Bäck, *Acta pharm. suec.*, 1973, *10*, 223.

Uses. Bendrofluazide is a thiazide diuretic with actions and uses similar to those of chlorothiazide (see p.589). Diuresis is initiated in about 2 hours and lasts for 12 to 18 hours or longer. Its inhibitory action on carbonic anhydrase is weak.

In the treatment of oedema the usual initial dose is 5 mg daily, reduced to a dose of 2.5 mg daily or 5 mg on alternate days; in some cases initial doses of 10 to 20 mg may be necessary. A suggested initial dose for children is up to 400 µg per kg body-weight daily, reduced to 50 to 100 µg per kg for maintenance.

In the treatment of hypertension the usual dose is 2.5 to 10 mg daily, either alone, or in conjunction with other antihypertensive agents; some sources have recommended initial doses of up to 20 mg daily.

When treatment is prolonged, or in susceptible patients, loss of potassium may be sufficient to produce hypokalaemia; potassium supplements should then be given as for chlorothiazide.

Hyperkalaemia, familial. Successful treatment of familial hyperkalaemia in a 9-year-old girl with bendrofluazide 2.5 mg twice daily. It is considered probable that she would eventually have developed significant hypertension and it is hoped to prevent this with long-term bendrofluazide therapy.— M. R. Lee and D. B. Morgan (letter), *Lancet*, 1980, *1*, 879. See also M. R. Lee *et al.*, *Q.J. Med.*, 1979, *48*, 245.

Hypertension. In a study of 19 patients with severe hypertension not properly controlled by beta-blocking agents, the addition of bendrofluazide 5 or 10 mg daily without potassium supplements produced a further fall in mean pressure of about 12%. There was no difference between the effect of either dose. Plasma-potassium concentrations were significantly reduced and although in half the patients given bendrofluazide the concentration fell below 3.6 mmol per litre within 1 month they came to no apparent harm. Prazosin 2 or 5 mg thrice daily reduced the blood pressure by about 15% and this reduction was dose-dependent. Giving both bendrofluazide and prazosin was considered to produce an additive effect. When the beta-blocker was withdrawn from patients taking either bendrofluazide or prazosin the systolic pressure rose. It was considered that patients with high initial blood pressures would be likely to require an agent additional to a beta-blocker and that a single daily dose of a thiazide diuretic would usually produce a further useful fall in blood pressure with few side-effects. The effectiveness of this dual therapy could be assessed in 2 weeks. If a third agent was required then prazosin could be added to the regimen, although side-effects such as dizziness might then be produced.— A. J. Marshall *et al.*, *Lancet*, 1977, *1*, 271.

Results of a 6-year follow-up of 53 previously untreated middle-aged men with mild to moderately severe essential hypertension treated with bendrofluazide 2.5 to 5 mg daily with potassium chloride 0.57 to 1.14 g daily compared with 53 similar men given propranolol 80 to 160 mg daily. If the blood pressure was not controlled by the higher doses hydralazine 25 to 50 mg thrice daily was added. After 6 years 34 patients in the bendrofluazide group and 27 in the propranolol group had their originally allocated drug alone for the entire follow-up. The blood-pressure reduction was the same in both groups. Since both drugs can be given once daily and the incidence of side-effects (which decreased significantly over the first year of treatment and then stabilised) was similar, and since diuretics are cheaper, they should at present be the drug of choice for this type of hypertension in patients for whom they are not contra-indicated.— G. Berglund and O. Andersson, *Lancet*, 1981, *1*, 744. Comment.— *ibid.*, 763.

Further references to the use of bendrofluazide in hypertension, either alone, or in conjunction with other anti-hypertensive agents: T. Q. Spitzer and B. A. Harris, *Curr. ther. Res.*, 1975, *17*, 75; O. Andersson *et al.*, *Läkartidningen*, 1976, *73*, 1824; W. A. I. Rushford *et al.*, *Acta ther.*, 1977, *3*, 117; M. Spira, *Curr. med. Res. Opinion*, 1977, *5*, 252; R. G. Wilcox and J. R. A. Mitchell, *Br. med. J.*, 1977, *2*, 547; R. L. Agrawal *et al.*, *J.R. Coll. gen. Pract.*, 1979, *29*, 602; J. S. Horvath *et al.*, *Med. J. Aust.*, 1979, *1*, 626; N. B. Karatzas *et al.*, *J. int. med. Res.*, 1979, *7*, 215; A. J. Marshall *et al.*, *Br. J. clin. Pharmac.*, 1980, *10*, 217; L. R. Solomon and P. M. Dawes, *J. int. med. Res.*, 1980, *8*, 34.

For a report of the MRC Working Party on Mild to Moderate Hypertension, which uses bendrofluazide in one of the basic treatment regimens, see Antihypertensives, p.135.

Oedema. In a double-blind trial in 90 women with varicose veins, the administration of bendrofluazide, 5 mg each morning during the premenstrual week, resulted in significantly more relief of pain when compared with aspirin or a placebo.— W. G. Fegan and M. Henry, *Practitioner*, 1968, *201*, 784.

For reference to the possible role of diuretics in exacerbating and perpetuating idiopathic oedema, see Oedema, under Adverse Effects of Chlorothiazide, p.588.

Osteoporosis. The use of bendrofluazide in regimens using ergocalciferol and dihydrotachysterol to treat osteoporosis.— J. R. Condon *et al.*, *Postgrad. med. J.*, 1978, *54*, 249.

Pregnancy and the neonate. *Suppression of lactation.* In 40 patients bendrofluazide 5 mg twice daily for 5 days was as effective as a synthetic oestrogen in the suppression of lactation.— M. Healy (letter), *Lancet*, 1961, *1*, 1353.

Renal disorders. Bendrofluazide 10 mg daily given to 9 patients with hypercalciuria for 3 or 4 periods of 6 days, decreased the urinary excretion of calcium to about one-half the original concentration.— A. R. Harrison and G. A. Rose, *Clin. Sci.*, 1968, *34*, 343.

Bendrofluazide 5 to 10 mg daily has proved a cheap and effective treatment in many cases of renal stones associated with hypercalciuria.— G. A. Rose, *Practitioner*, 1977, *218*, 74.

Preparations

Bendrofluazide Tablets *(B.P.)*. Tablets containing bendrofluazide.

Bendroflumethiazide Tablets *(U.S.P.)*. Tablets containing bendrofluazide. Store in airtight containers.

Proprietary Preparations

Aprinox *(Boots, UK)*. Bendrofluazide, available as tablets of 2.5 and 5 mg. (Also available as Aprinox in *Austral.*).

Berkozide *(Berk Pharmaceuticals, UK)*. Bendrofluazide, available as tablets of 2.5 mg and scored tablets of 5 mg.

Centyl *(Burgess, UK)*. Bendrofluazide, available as tablets of 2.5 mg and scored tablets of 5 mg. (Also available as Centyl in *Denm.*, *Norw.*).

Centyl K *(Burgess, UK)*. Tablets each containing bendrofluazide 2.5 mg in an outer layer and potassium chloride 573 mg (potassium 7.7 mmol; 7.7 mEq) in a slow-release core.

Neo-NaClex *(Duncan, Flockhart, UK)*. Bendrofluazide, available as scored tablets of 5 mg. (Also available as Neo-NaClex in *Austral.*). **Neo-NaClex-K**. Tablets each containing bendrofluazide 2.5 mg and, in a separate slow-release layer, potassium chloride 630 mg (potassium 8.4 mmol; 8.4 mEq).

Owing to the risk of intestinal obstruction, sustained-release preparations such as Centyl K and Neo-NaClex-K, where the drug is released in transit, but the matrix ghost is often eliminated intact, should not be prescribed in patients with Crohn's disease or other intestinal disease in which strictures may form.— J. L. Shaffer *et al.* (letter), *Lancet*, 1980, *2*, 487.

Urizide *(DDSA Pharmaceuticals, UK)*. Bendrofluazide, available as tablets of 5 mg.

Other Proprietary Names

Arg.—Tesical, Urinagen; *Austral.*—Aprinox-M, Pluryl; *Belg.*—Pluryl Forte; *Canad.*—Naturetin; *Fr.*—Naturine; *Ger.*—Sinesalin; *Ital.*—Notens, Polidiuril, Salural, Sodiuretic; *Neth.*—Pluryl; *Swed.*—Salures; *Switz.*—Sinesalin; *USA*—Naturetin.

2307-m

Benzthiazide *(U.S.P., B.P.C. 1963)*. P 1393.

3-Benzylthiomethyl-6-chloro-2*H*-1,2,4-benzothiadiazine-7-sulphonamide 1,1-dioxide.
$C_{15}H_{14}ClN_3O_4S_3=431.9$.

CAS — 91-33-8.

Pharmacopoeias. In *U.S.*

A white crystalline powder with a characteristic odour and a bitter taste. M.p. about 240°. Practically **insoluble** in water, chloroform, and ether; soluble 1 in 100 of acetone; slightly soluble in alcohol; freely soluble in dimethylformamide and in solutions of alkalis. A suspension in water has a pH of about 5. **Store** in airtight containers.

Adverse Effects, Treatment, and Precautions. As for Chlorothiazide, p.588.

Diabetogenic effect. Twenty-five patients with well-controlled mild diabetes were given courses of benzthiazide. Hyperglycaemia promptly occurred in 13 of 15 patients given 50 mg thrice daily but, generally, this disturbance was not seen in 5 patients receiving 50 mg daily or in 5 who received 50 mg thrice daily together with 4.8 g of aspirin daily. Other effects were elevation of the serum concentrations of uric acid in each of the 3 groups, by 13%, 12%, and 9% respectively. The blood urea rose when 50 mg of benzthiazide was given thrice daily but not when it was given once daily. The aspirin prevented a worsening of the diabetes (perhaps by simply reducing appetite) but it did not materially affect the tendency of the concentration of uric acid to rise and it did not hinder the rise in blood urea which occurred with large doses of benzthiazide.— J. W. Runyan, *New Engl. J. Med.*, 1962, *267*, 541.

Uses. Benzthiazide is a thiazide diuretic with actions and uses similar to those of chlorothiazide (see p.589). Diuresis is initiated in about 2 hours and lasts for about 12 hours.

The initial dose in the treatment of oedema is 50 to 200 mg daily, followed by a maintenance dose of 50 to 150 mg daily. A suggested initial dose in children is 1 to 4 mg per kg body-weight daily in divided doses. In the treatment of hypertension, the usual dose is 25 to 50 mg twice daily, either alone or in conjunction with other anti-hypertensive agents.

When treatment is prolonged, or in susceptible patients, loss of potassium may be sufficient to produce hypokalaemia; potassium supplements should then be given as for chlorothiazide.

Preparations

Benzthiazide Tablets *(U.S.P.)*. Tablets containing benzthiazide. Store in airtight containers.

Proprietary Names

Aquatag *(Tutag, USA)*; Exna *(Robins, Canad.*; *Robins, USA)*; Fovane *(Pfizer, Belg.)*; Hydrex *(Trimen, USA)*.

2308-b

Benzylhydrochlorothiazide. Su 6227. 3-Benzyl-6-chloro-3,4-dihydro-2*H*-1,2,4-benzothiadiazine-7-sulphonamide 1,1-dioxide.
$C_{14}H_{14}ClN_3O_4S_2=387.9$.

CAS — 1824-50-6.

White odourless crystals or crystalline powder. M.p. about 269°. Practically **insoluble** in water; soluble in acids.

Benzylhydrochlorothiazide is a thiazide diuretic with actions and uses similar to those of chlorothiazide (see p.587). It has been given in initial doses of 4 to 8 mg twice daily, reduced to twice or thrice weekly for maintenance.

Proprietary Names

Behyd *(Jap.)*; 3 BT *(Jap.)*.

2309-v

Boldo *(B.P.C. 1934)*. Boldo Leaves.

CAS — 8022-81-9 (boldo leaf oil); 476-70-0 (boldine); 1398-22-7 (boldoglucin).

Pharmacopoeias. In *Arg.*, *Belg.*, *Cz.*, *Fr.*, *It.*, *Port.*, *Roum.*, *Span.*, and *Swiss.*

The dried leaves of *Peumus boldus* (Monimiaceae). It contains the alkaloid boldine (about 0.1%), the glycoside boldin or boldoglucin, and about 2% of volatile oil.

Boldo has been employed as a diuretic in the form of a tincture (1 in 10; in doses of 0.5 to 2 ml). The alkaloid boldine was formerly used in the treatment of hepatic congestion.

2310-r

Bumetanide. Ro 10-6338. 3-Butylamino-4-phenoxy-5-sulphamoylbenzoic acid.

$C_{17}H_{20}N_2O_5S=364.4$.

CAS — 28395-03-1.

A white odourless crystalline powder with a slightly bitter taste. M.p. about 230°. **Protect** from light.

Incompatibility. Bumetanide should not be added to infusion fluids with an acid reaction because of the risk of sedimentation.— R. N. Brogden *et al.*, *Drugs*, 1975, *9*, 4.

Adverse Effects. Probably the most common side-effect to be associated with bumetanide therapy is fluid and electrolyte imbalance after either single large doses or prolonged administration.

Other side-effects reported include nausea and dizziness, vomiting, abdominal discomfort, skin rashes, muscle cramps (which are sometimes severe, especially with high-dose therapy), gynaecomastia, leucopenia, and thrombocytopenia. Raised blood concentrations of glucose and uric acid may occur.

The 17 reports of adverse reactions to bumetanide received by the Committee on Safety of Medicines were: skin and muscle reactions (10), including 6 reports of muscular pain, thrombocytopenia (3), granulocytopenia or leucopenia (2), nausea and dizziness (1), and gynaecomastia (1). Two reactions proved fatal.— M. F. Cuthbert, *Committee on Safety of Medicines*, *Postgrad. med. J.*, 1975, *51*, *Suppl.* 6, 51.

Diabetogenic effect. In a long-term study in 29 patients with cardiac failure bumetanide did not precipitate glycosuria and was considered relatively safe to use in patients with diabetes mellitus.— M. M. Kubik and E. Bowers (letter), *Lancet*, 1975, *2*, 991. See also M. M. Kubik *et al.*, *Br. J. clin. Pract.*, 1976, *30*, 11.

Effects on the ears. Three patients with hearing loss associated with frusemide were able to tolerate bumetanide.— E. Bourke (letter), *Lancet*, 1976, *1*, 917.

Effects on the liver. Minor abnormalities in liver function noted in patients receiving bumetanide.— L. E. Murchison *et al.*, *Br. J. clin. Pharmac.*, 1975, *2*, 87.

Effects on the muscles. Mention of curious muscle stiffness, with tenderness to compression and pain on movement, in association with bumetanide therapy. The calf muscles were the first to be affected; shoulder girdle and thigh muscle tenderness also occurred in 2 patients, and one patient also had neck stiffness. The side-effect appeared to be dose-related for the individual patients.— J. E. Barclay and H. A. Lee, *Postgrad. med. J.*, 1975, *51*, *Suppl.* 6, 43.

Effects on the pancreas. Increased serum-α-amylase values were observed in 4 of 11 patients with renal impairment and receiving bumetanide. In 3 of the patients the effect was dose-related. The cause was unknown; one possibility was a subclinical pancreatitis with some extrahepatic cholestasis.— F. Lynggaard and N. Bjørndal (letter), *Lancet*, 1977, *2*, 1355.

Effects on the skin. *Erythema multiforme.* A skin reaction of the Stevens-Johnson type occurred in a patient with cirrhosis of the liver given bumetanide for 212 days.— H. Ring-Larsen, *Acta med. scand.*, 1974, *195*, 411, per *Drugs*, 1975, *9*, 4.

Treatment of Adverse Effects. As for Chlorothiazide, p.589.

Precautions. As for Chlorothiazide, p.589.
Bumetanide should be used with care in patients with prostatic hypertrophy or impairment of micturition.

A report indicating that indomethacin may decrease the effect of bumetanide.— D. C. Brater and P. Chennavasin, *Clin. Pharmac. Ther.*, 1980, *27*, 421.

Absorption and Fate. Bumetanide is completely and fairly rapidly absorbed from the gastro-intestinal tract. It has a plasma elimination half-life of about 1½ hours. It is extensively bound to plasma proteins, and is mainly excreted in the urine, partly unchanged and partly in the form of metabolites; variable amounts are also excreted in the faeces.

Bumetanide was rapidly and virtually completely absorbed following administration of 2 mg by mouth to 3 healthy subjects and 1 subject with diabetes mellitus and a biliary T-tube. Peak plasma concentrations were reached in about 30 minutes and the half-lives ranged from 1.2 to 1.8 hours (average 1.5 hours). From 77 to 85% of the dose was excreted in the urine and in the 3 healthy subjects 11 to 19% in the faeces; in the subject with the biliary T-tube 14.4% was excreted into the bile (with a further 4.6% found in the faeces being presumed to have been lost from the bile during sampling intervals). After 48 hours about 80% of the dose had been excreted, about half as unchanged bumetanide (a higher proportion of the unchanged drug being excreted in the early stages). Metabolites of bumetanide mainly included conjugates and side-chain oxidative metabolites.— S. C. Halladay *et al.*, *Clin. Pharmac. Ther.*, 1977, *22*, 179.

The fate of bumetanide labelled with carbon-14 was studied in 4 healthy subjects given 500 µg by mouth or intravenous injection. It was completely and rapidly absorbed from the gastro-intestinal tract, bound extensively to plasma proteins, partly metabolised, and excreted rapidly, mainly in the urine. Peak plasma radioactivity occurred 1.5 hours after oral administration. The total radioactive urinary excretion amounted to 80% over about 18 hours following both routes of administration; faecal excretion amounted to 9 and 16% following the intravenous and oral doses respectively. The elimination half-life was 1.5 hours. Four metabolites were detected in the urine and during the first 6 hours these represented 16 and 19% of the intravenous and oral doses respectively. Maximum diuresis occurred in the first 30 minutes following intravenous administration and between 30 and 60 minutes following oral administration; diuresis lasted for 3 to 4 hours.— P. J. Pentikäinen *et al.*, *Br. J. clin. Pharmac.*, 1977, *4*, 39.

Further references: P. W. Feit *et al.*, *J. pharm. Sci.*, 1973, *62*, 375; D. L. Davies *et al.*, *Clin. Pharmac. Ther.*, 1974, *15*, 141; W. R. Dixon *et al.*, *J. pharm. Sci.*, 1976, *65*, 701; U. Busch *et al.*, *Arzneimittel-Forsch.*, 1979, *29*, 315; P. J. Pentikäinen *et al.*, *Clin. Pharmac. Ther.*, 1980, *27*, 278.

Protein binding. In a study involving 4 healthy subjects over 90% of an intravenous dose of bumetanide was bound to plasma proteins at 30 minutes. No bumetanide was detected in the red blood cells.— P. J. Pentikäinen *et al.*, *Br. J. clin. Pharmac.*, 1977, *4*, 39.

Uses. Although chemically unrelated, bumetanide is a diuretic with actions and uses similar to those of frusemide (see p.598). Diuresis is initiated within about 30 minutes to an hour after a dose by mouth, and lasts for about 4 hours; after intravenous injection its effects are evident within a few minutes and last for about 2 hours.
In the treatment of oedema, the usual dose is 1 mg by mouth in the morning; a second dose may be given 6 to 8 hours later if necessary. In some cases higher doses may be needed; severe cases have required gradual titration of the bumetanide dosage up to 20 mg or more daily. In emergency or when oral therapy cannot be given 1 mg may be administered by intramuscular or intravenous injection, subsequently adjusted according to the patient's response. A recommended dose for pulmonary oedema is 1 to 2 mg by intravenous injection, repeated 20 minutes later if necessary. Alternatively, 2 to 5 mg may be given over 30 to 60 minutes in 500 ml of infusion fluid consisting of dextrose 5%, sodium chloride 0.9%, or sodium chloride 0.18% with dextrose 4% (but see above under Incompatibility).
When treatment is prolonged, or in susceptible patients, loss of potassium may be sufficient to produce hypokalaemia; potassium supplements should then be given as for chlorothiazide (see p.589). When very high doses are used careful laboratory control is essential as described under the uses for frusemide (p.598; high-dose therapy).

Reviews and symposium reports on the actions, uses, and pharmacokinetics of bumetanide: *Drug & Ther. Bull.*, 1974, *12*, 49; R. N. Brogden *et al.*, *Drugs*, 1975, *9*, 4; *Lancet*, 1975, *2*, 860; *Postgrad. med. J.*, 1975, *51*, *Suppl.* 6,.

Action. In 4 healthy subjects bumetanide caused an increasing natriuresis when given in increasing doses from 0.5 to 3 mg. Onset of action occurred within 30 minutes, and peak effect at 90 minutes, with a return to base-line values by 270 minutes. In 18 oedematous patients given (on 21 occasions) bumetanide, frusemide, or placebo, the effect of bumetanide 1 or 2 mg was comparable with that of frusemide 40 or 80 mg. In 11 patients given bumetanide 1 mg daily for 8 days the mean sodium excretion increased by 100% and that of potassium by 30%. Some patients unresponsive to frusemide 80 mg responded to bumetanide 2 mg.— M. J. Asbury *et al.*, *Br. med. J.*, 1972, *1*, 211.

Intergroup difference due to different dietary intake was noted in a comparative study of frusemide and bumetanide in English and German subjects but results in both groups indicated that the bumetanide:frusemide dosage equivalence was 1:60 and not 1:40 as had been reported elsewhere.— R. A. Branch *et al.*, *Clin. Pharmac. Ther.*, 1976, *19*, 538. A double-blind placebo-controlled study in 9 healthy subjects comparing bumetanide with frusemide supported previous findings that on a weight basis bumetanide was 40 times as potent as frusemide. Results also confirmed that it belongs to the same pharmacological class as frusemide and ethacrynic acid. Bumetanide had a less rapid onset of effect than frusemide, changes in the different parameters appearing 40 to 60 minutes after its administration whereas frusemide produced changes in 20 to 40 minutes.— S. Carrière and R. Dandavino, *Clin. Pharmac. Ther.*, 1976, *20*, 424.

Further references: E. Bourke *et al.*, *Eur. J. Pharmac.*, 1973, *23*, 283; S. -G. Karlander *et al.*, *Eur. J. clin. Pharmac.*, 1973, *6*, 220; A. Bellerup *et al.*, *Acta pharmac. tox.*, 1974, *34*, 305; H. C. Seth *et al.*, *Br. J. clin. Pract.*, 1975, *29*, 7; M. M. Kubik *et al.*, *Br. J. clin. Pract.*, 1976, *30*, 11; K. J. Berg *et al.*, *Eur. J. clin. Pharmac.*, 1976, *9*, 265; P. H. Mackie *et al.*, *Br. J. clin. Pharmac.*, 1976, *3*, 613; L. E. Ramsay *et al.*, *Br. J. clin. Pharmac.*, 1978, *5*, 243.

Administration. In 10 patients there was significantly increased diuresis and sodium excretion, but not potassium excretion, when their stabilised doses were taken in 2 divided doses at 8 am and 6 pm compared with a single stabilised dose taken in the morning.— K. R. Hunter and P. N. Underwood, *Postgrad. med. J.*, 1975, *51*, *Suppl.* 6, 91.

Studies have indicated that the rate of diuresis due to bumetanide is reduced and its onset delayed if given after food.— M. Homeida *et al.*, *Br. J. clin. Pharmac.*, 1976, *3*, 969P.

Administration in renal failure. Bumetanide could be given in usual doses to patients with renal failure.— W. M. Bennett *et al.*, *Ann. intern. Med.*, 1980, *93*, 286.
See also under Renal Disorders (below).

Cardiac disorders. *Heart failure.* In studies in 106 patients with congestive heart failure bumetanide 1, 2, 3, and 4 mg was comparable in effect to frusemide 40, 80, 120, and 160 mg respectively. There was a trend to the development of hypokalaemia and hypochloraemia. After treatment of 21 patients for 3 months pre-existing hyperuricaemia was significantly increased; there was no evidence of a diabetogenic effect. Bumetanide could be given concomitantly with thiazides, mercaptomerin, triamterene, or spironolactone.— K. H. Olesen *et al.*, *Acta med. scand.*, 1973, *193*, 119.

In 12 infants with heart failure a single oral dose of bumetanide 15 µg per kg body-weight produced significant diuresis and sodium excretion. In a long-term study in 13 similar infants, bumetanide, which was given with a potassium supplement, was considered to be an effective diuretic; doses ranged from 15 µg per kg on alternate days to 100 µg per kg daily. No significant side-effects occurred.— O. C. Ward and L. K. T. Lam, *Archs Dis. Childh.*, 1977, *52*, 877.

Further references: A. Pines *et al.*, *Br. J. clin. Pract.*, 1974, *28*, 311; W. R. Murdoch and W. H. R. Auld, *Postgrad. med. J.*, 1975, *51*, 10; C. Kourouklis *et al.*, *Curr. med. Res. Opinion*, 1976, *4*, 422; M. M. Kubik *et al.*, *Br. J. clin. Pract.*, 1976, *30*, 11; B. B. Singh and D. A. L. Watt, *Curr. med. Res. Opinion*, 1976, *4*, 117; B. Sigurd and K. H. Olesen, *Am. Heart J.*, 1977, *94*, 168; M. Varricchio *et al.*, *Farmaco, Edn prat.*, 1980, *35*, 349.

Mitral stenosis. Bumetanide 2 mg was injected into the right heart catheter of 12 patients with mitral stenosis undergoing cardiac catheterisation. Results confirmed that bumetanide is a very potent diuretic that changes haemodynamic parameters towards normal in patients with mitral stenosis.— A. M. Abrahamsen, *Acta med. scand.*, 1977, *201*, 481.

Hepatic disorders. Bumetanide 0.5 to 4 mg daily appeared to be a satisfactory diuretic in the treatment of ascites in 15 of 17 patients with chronic liver disease.— P. J. A. Moult, *Gut*, 1974, *15*, 988.

Further references: R. F. Maronde and M. Quinn, *Clin. Pharmac. Ther.*, 1977, *21*, 110; G. Nicholson, *Curr. med. Res. Opinion*, 1977, *4*, 675.

Hypertension. No evidence of hypokalaemia was found in 12 mildly hypertensive patients given bumetanide 500 µg twice daily for a 6-month period, 6 of whom also received potassium supplements. Bumetanide did not have a sustained antihypertensive effect, it caused hyperuricaemia, and minor abnormalities of liver function were noted.— L. E. Murchison *et al.*, *Br. J. clin. Pharmac.*, 1975, *2*, 87.

Renal disorders. Brief details of 12 patients with oedema and varying degrees of renal impairment treated with bumetanide in doses of 1.5 to 25 mg daily.— J. A. Barclay and H. A. Lee, *Postgrad. med. J.*, 1975, *51 Suppl.* 6, 43. In 7 patients with chronic renal failure bumetanide 5 or 10 mg daily produced diuresis and sodium excretion comparable with that of frusemide 100 mg in 6 patients and less than that produced by frusemide 200 to 400 mg in 5 patients.— M. E. M. Allison *et al.*, *ibid.*, 47.

Further references: T. E. G. Jones and G. Kurien (letter), *Br. med. J.*, 1977, *2*, 1419 (acute renal failure).

Urology. Bumetanide 250 to 500 µg intravenously was given to 42 patients to induce forced diuresis following urological surgery. This avoided the external flushing by nephrostomy or use of a bladder catheter in such patients.— E. Lindstedt *et al.*, *Läkartidningen*, 1976, *73*, 508.

Proprietary Preparations

Burinex *(Leo, UK).* Bumetanide, available as an **Injection** containing 500 µg per ml in ampoules of 2, 4, and 10 ml, and as scored **Tablets** of 1 and 5 mg. (Also available as Burinex in *Belg., Denm., Ital., Neth., Norw., S.Afr., Swed., Switz.*) **Burinex K**. Tablets containing bumetanide 500 µg in an outer layer and potassium chloride 573 mg (potassium 7.7 mmol; 7.7 mEq) in a slow-release wax core.

Owing to the risk of intestinal obstruction, sustained-release preparations such as Burinex K, where the drug is released in transit, but the matrix ghost is often eliminated intact, should not be prescribed in patients with Crohn's disease or other intestinal disease in which strictures may form.— J. L. Shaffer *et al.* (letter), *Lancet*, 1980, *2*, 487.

Other Proprietary Names

Aquazone *(Spain)*; Bonures *(Swed.)*; Butinat *(Arg.)*;

Cambiex *(Arg.)*; Diurama *(Ital.)*; Fontego *(Ital.)*; Fordiuran *(Ger., Spain)*; Lunetoron *(Jap.)*; Segurex *(Arg.)*.

2311-f

Buthiazide. Butizide; Thiabutazide. 6-Chloro-3,4-dihydro-3-isobutyl-2*H*-1,2,4-benzothiadiazine-7-sulphonamide 1,1-dioxide.
$C_{11}H_{16}ClN_3O_4S_2$=353.8.

CAS — 2043-38-1.

Pharmacopoeias. In *Roum.*

An odourless white crystalline powder. Slightly **soluble** in water. Soluble in alcohol and in solutions of alkali hydroxides.

Adverse Effects, Treatment, and Precautions. As for Chlorothiazide, p.588.

Uses. Buthiazide is a thiazide diuretic with actions and uses similar to those of chlorothiazide (see p.589). It has been given in doses of 5 to 15 mg daily on 2 or 3 days weekly for the treatment of oedema. It has also been given in doses of 2.5 to 10 mg daily for hypertension.

Proprietary Names
Eunéphran *(Servier, Fr.)*; Saltucin *(Boehringer Mannheim, Ger.)*.

2312-d

Canrenone.
Aldadiene; RP 11614; SC 9376. 3-Oxo-17α-pregna-4,6-diene-21,17β-carbolactone.
$C_{22}H_{28}O_3$=340.5.

CAS — 976-71-6.

Stability. For a study of the stability of canrenone and factors affecting its conversion to canrenoate potassium, see E. R. Garrett and C. M. Won, *J. pharm. Sci.*, 1971, *60*, 1801.

2313-n

Canrenoate Potassium.
Potassium Canrenoate; Aldadiene Potassium; MF 465a; SC-14266. Potassium 17β-hydroxy-3-oxo-17α-pregna-4,6-diene-21-carboxylate.
$C_{22}H_{29}KO_4$=396.6.

CAS — 4138-96-9 (canrenoic acid); 2181-04-6 (canrenoate potassium).

Soluble in water at pH 8.5 or above. At a lower pH canrenone is formed.

The formulation of an injection of canrenoate potassium using alcohol.— E. R. Garrett and T. W. Hermann, *J. pharm. Sci.*, 1972, *61*, 717.

Adverse Effects, Treatment, and Precautions. As for Spironolactone, p.610.

Discomfort is reported to occur at the site of injections of canrenoate potassium.

Effects on the heart. A report of a cardiac arrhythmia apparently associated with intravenous canrenoate potassium administration in one patient.— W. J. Mroczek *et al.*, *Clin. Pharmac. Ther.*, 1974, *16*, 336.

Interactions. *Fludrocortisone.* In 12 healthy subjects who were receiving fludrocortisone, single doses of canrenoate potassium 100, 150, or 200 mg caused a paradoxical dose-related increase in urinary potassium excretion 12 to 16 hours after administration; this was possibly related to increased urine volume. Similar results were obtained with spironolactone, but the dose-effect relationship was not clear.— L. E. Ramsay *et al.*, *Eur. J. clin. Pharmac.*, 1977, *11*, 101.

Absorption and Fate. As for Spironolactone, p.610.

Micronisation increases the absorption of canrenone.

Canrenoate potassium is suitable for intravenous administration.

Canrenoate potassium is excreted mainly in the urine in the form of canrenone and the glucuronide of the hydroxy acid.— A. Karim *et al.*, *J. pharm. Sci.*, 1971, *60*, 708.

For studies on the pharmacokinetics of canrenone and canrenoate potassium, see Spironolactone, p.610.

Uses. Canrenone has actions and uses similar to those of spironolactone (see p.611) of which it is a metabolite. It has been given in doses of 50 to 200 mg daily or on alternate days, in one to three divided doses; up to 300 mg daily has been given.

Canrenoate potassium is a soluble form of canrenone suitable for parenteral administration. It may be given in doses of 200 mg twice or thrice daily by slow intravenous injection (over a period of not less than 3 minutes). It has been recommended that single doses of 400 mg and daily doses of 800 mg should not be exceeded. It is also given by intravenous infusion in a 5% solution of dextrose or a 0.9% solution of sodium chloride.

Action. Canrenoate potassium 200 mg dissolved in 10 ml of saline was administered intravenously over a period of 2 minutes twice daily for 7 days to 3 healthy subjects. An anti-mineralocorticoid effect was noted which appeared to be similar in magnitude and action to spironolactone; a cardiac arrhythmia apparently related to canrenoate was noted in 1 subject. The only advantage of canrenoate potassium over spironolactone appeared to be that it could be administered parenterally.— W. J. Mroczek *et al.*, *Clin. Pharmac. Ther.*, 1974, *16*, 336. In 3 healthy subjects given canrenoate potassium 200 mg intravenously there was no consistent natriuresis for the following 6 hours, and no change in glomerular filtration-rate or renal plasma flow. It has minimal diuretic activity in the absence of hyperaldosteronism.— L. M. Hofmann *et al.*, *ibid.*, 1975, *18*, 748.

Anabolism. A study indicating improved nitrogen balance in patients receiving canrenoate potassium 600 to 800 mg daily in addition to total parenteral nutrition during the first 5 post-operative days following abdominal surgery. The effect was particularly marked in elderly subjects.— P. Guinot and Y. Metivier, *Clin. Ther.*, 1977, *1*, 56. See also Y. Metivier *et al.*, *Agressologie*, 1976, *17*, 313.

Cardiac disorders. *Digitalis-induced arrhythmias.* Intravenous administration of canrenoate potassium 400 to 700 mg had an anti-arrhythmic effect in 8 of 12 patients believed to be suffering from digitalis-induced ventricular arrhythmias. The anti-arrhythmic effect lasted from a few minutes to several hours.— B. K. Yeh *et al.*, *Am. Heart J.*, 1976, *92*, 308.

Hepatic disorders. In 12 patients with liver cirrhosis canrenoate potassium 200 mg intravenously significantly reduced the excretion of magnesium for up to 48 hours after the dose.— P. Lim and E. Jacob, *Br. med. J.*, 1978, *1*, 755.

Further references: P. Boivin and R. Fauvert, *Revue int. Hépat.*, 1969, *19*, 241 (canrenone).

Proprietary Preparations

Spiroctan-M *(MCP Pharmaceuticals, UK)*. Canrenoate potassium, available as solution for injection containing 10 mg per ml, in ampoules of 20 ml.

Other Proprietary Names of Canrenone and Canrenoate Potassium

Aldactone *(Ger.)*; Osiren (see also under Spironolactone) *(Switz.)*; Osirenol *(Denm., Norw.)*; Osyrol (see also Spironolactone) *(Ger.)*; Phanurane *(Fr.)*; Sincomen pro injectione *(Ger.)*; Soldactone *(Belg., Ital., Neth., S.Afr., Switz.)*; Venactone *(Ital.)*.

2314-h

Chlorazanil Hydrochloride. ASA-226. *N*-(4-Chlorophenyl)-1,3,5-triazine-2,4-diamine hydrochloride.
$C_9H_8ClN_5,HCl$=258.1.

CAS — 500-42-5 (chlorazanil); 2019-25-2 (hydrochloride).

Chlorazanil hydrochloride is a diuretic that has been given in usual doses of 150 mg twice or thrice weekly. It is contra-indicated in patients with hepatic coma, hypokalaemia, or renal insufficiency with anuria.

Proprietary Names
Orpidan *(Heumann, Ger.)*.

2315-m

Chlormerodrin *(B.P.C. 1959)*. Promeranum; Chlormeroprin; Mercurylurée. (3-Chloromercuri-2-methoxypropyl)urea; Chloro(2-methoxy-3-ureidopropyl)mercury.
$C_5H_{11}ClHgN_2O_2$=367.2.

CAS — 62-37-3.

Pharmacopoeias. In *Rus.*

A white odourless powder with a bitter metallic taste. M.p. about 150°.

Soluble 1 in 150 of water, 1 in 300 of alcohol, and 1 in 100 of methyl alcohol; very slightly soluble in chloroform; practically insoluble in acetone and ether; soluble in solutions of alkali hydroxides. A 0.5% solution in water has a pH of 4.3 to 5.

Uses. Chlormerodrin is a mercurial diuretic with actions and uses similar to those of mersalyl acid (see p.606), but which is suitable for oral administration. It has been given by mouth in doses of 18.3 to 73.2 mg daily, equivalent to 10 to 40 mg of mercury daily.

Proprietary Names
Orimercur *(Reder, Spain)*.

2316-b

Chlorothiazide *(B.P., U.S.P.)*.
Chlorothiaz.; Chlorothiazidum; Clorotiazida. 6-Chloro-2*H*-1,2,4-benzothiadiazine-7-sulphonamide 1,1-dioxide.
$C_7H_6ClN_3O_4S_2$=295.7.

CAS — 58-94-6.

Pharmacopoeias. In *Arg., Br., Braz., Fr., Int., It., Nord., Port., Turk.,* and *U.S.*

A white or almost white, odourless, crystalline powder with a slightly bitter taste. M.p. about 340° with decomposition.

Practically **insoluble** in water; soluble 1 in 650 of alcohol and 1 in 100 of acetone; practically insoluble in chloroform and ether; slightly soluble in methyl alcohol; freely soluble in dimethylformamide and dimethyl sulphoxide; soluble in solutions of alkali hydroxides. Alkaline solutions undergo decomposition, due to hydrolysis, upon standing. **Store** in airtight containers.

2317-v

Chlorothiazide Sodium.
Sodium Chlorothiazide.
$C_7H_5ClN_3NaO_4S_2$=317.7.

CAS — 7085-44-1.

A crystalline solid. **Soluble** in water.

Chlorothiazide sodium 537 mg is approximately equivalent to 500 mg of chlorothiazide.

Incompatibility. There was loss of clarity when intravenous solutions of chlorothiazide sodium were mixed with those of insulin, narcotic analgesics, noradrenaline acid tartrate, procaine hydrochloride, prochlorperazine maleate, promazine hydrochloride, promethazine hydrochloride, streptomycin sulphate, tetracycline hydrochloride, or vancomycin hydrochloride.— J. A. Patel and G. L. Phillips, *Am. J. Hosp. Pharm.*, 1966, *23*, 409.

An immediate precipitate occurred when chlorothiazide 2 g per litre was mixed with chlorpromazine hydrochloride 200 mg per litre, promazine hydrochloride 200 mg per litre, or promethazine hydrochloride 100 mg per litre, and a yellow colour with a precipitate developed over 3 hours when chlorothiazide was mixed with hydralazine hydrochloride 80 mg per litre in dextrose injection or sodium chloride injection. A yellow colour was produced when chlorothiazide was mixed with polymyxin B sulphate 2 mega units per litre in dextrose injection. A haze developed over 3 hours when the drug was mixed with prochlorperazine mesylate 100 mg per litre in sodium chloride injection, but an immediate precipitate was formed when they were mixed in dextrose injection.— B. B. Riley, *J. Hosp. Pharm.*, 1970, *28*, 228.

Chlorothiazide sodium was incompatible with amikacin sulphate.— B. C. Nunning and A. P. Granatek, *Curr. ther. Res.*, 1976, *20*, 417.

Stability. Chlorothiazide was slowly hydrolysed in alkaline solution. The solid sodium salt was stable and could be dissolved in Water for Injections, sodium chloride injection, or dextrose injection, for intravenous use. Solutions were found to be incompatible (formation of precipitate) with hydralazine and reserpine but compatible with protoveratrines A and B, pentolinium tartrate, cryptenamine acetate, alkavervir, and mecamylamine hydrochloride. Chlorothiazide (free acid) was stable in aqueous suspension at pH 6.5 and under. Suspensions prepared with tragacanth in a syrup vehicle were satisfactory; the particle size averaged 5 µm and there was no evidence of caking even after storage at higher temperatures. The addition of citrus flavours helped to mask the slightly bitter taste.— W. F. Charnicki *et al.*, *J. Am. pharm. Ass., scient. Edn*, 1959, *48*, 656.

Adverse Effects. Side-effects which occur occasionally with chlorothiazide include allergies, skin rashes, thirst, epigastric pain, anorexia, gastric irritation, nausea, vomiting, diarrhoea, constipation, photosensitivity, dizziness, headache, muscle spasm, weakness, inflammation of the salivary gland, loss of libido, and paraesthesias. Acute pancreatitis has been reported. Adverse effects such as pneumonitis, jaundice, and blood disorders including agranulocytosis, aplastic anaemia, thrombocytopenia, and leucopenia have occasionally occurred. Postural hypotension which may be accentuated by alcohol, antihypertensives, barbiturates, or narcotics has occurred. Hyperparathyroidism has been associated with thiazide diuretic therapy, and changes in serum lipids have been noted.

Thiazide diuretics may provoke hyperglycaemia and glycosuria in diabetic and other susceptible patients. They may cause hyperuricaemia and precipitate attacks of gout in some patients. Administration of thiazide diuretics may be associated with electrolyte imbalances including hypochloraemic alkalosis, hyponatraemia, and hypokalaemia. Hypokalaemia intensifies the effect of digitalis on cardiac muscle and administration of digitalis or its glycosides may have to be temporarily suspended. Hyponatraemia may occur in patients with severe congestive heart failure who are very oedematous, particularly with large doses in conjunction with restricted salt in the diet. The urinary excretion of calcium is reduced. Hypomagnesaemia has also occurred.

Intestinal ulceration has occurred following the administration of tablets containing thiazides with an enteric-coated core of potassium chloride (see also under Potassium Chloride, p.629).

Allergy. See Vasculitis under Effects on the Skin.

Diabetogenic effect. Deterioration of glucose tolerance occurred in all of 90 patients (70 with initial hyperglycaemia) treated for 6 to 10 months with chlorothiazide and other antihypertensives.— F. Khan and G. Spergel (letter), *Lancet*, 1976, *1*, 808. See also P. J. Lewis *et al.*, *ibid.*, 564.

No significant difference in glucose-tolerance tests was noted in 10 asymptomatic diabetic patients given frusemide 40 mg daily, dihydrochlorothiazide 50 mg daily, or ethacrynic acid 50 mg daily, each for a week. The diabetogenic effect of thiazides does not constitute a contra-indication to the use of the compounds in asymptomatic diabetes.— A. Káldor *et al.*, *Int. J. clin. Pharmac. Biopharm.*, 1975, *11*, 232.

Effects on the blood. *Agranulocytosis.* Agranulocytosis in an 84-year-old man who took 1 g of chlorothiazide thrice weekly, or so, for 21 months was attributed to chlorothiazide.— W. E. Ince, *Practitioner*, 1962, *189*, 74.

Haemolysis. The possibility that neonatal damage might result from the use of thiazide derivatives in obstetric practice was raised by the reports of Heinz-body haemolysis in 2 newborn infants of mothers who received thiazide derivatives in pregnancy.— J. D. Harley *et al.* (letter), *Br. med. J.*, 1964, *1*, 696.

Thrombocytopenia. Thrombocytopenia and other haematological abnormalities occurred in 7 newborn babies whose mothers had received thiazide drugs antepartum. One baby died. The thiazides given were chlorothiazide, hydrochlorothiazide, and methyclothiazide, and the period of treatment varied from 3 days to 3 months. Other drugs were also given in 6 of the pregnancies.— S. U. Rodriguez *et al.*, *New Engl. J. Med.*, 1964, *270*, 881. See also Precautions (Pregnancy and the Neonate).

Thrombocytopenic purpura occurred in a 37-year-old woman who had received 500 mg of chlorothiazide twice daily for 9 months. There was a depression both of thrombocyte production and of the leucocytes but they returned to normal within 10 days of stopping the drug.— R. McMurdo, *Practitioner*, 1964, *192*, 403.

Effects on the brain. Transient cerebral ischaemic attacks occurred in 3 elderly patients following treatment with thiazide diuretics.— A. B. Carter (letter), *Lancet*, 1965, *2*, 1127.

Transient cerebral ischaemia (pallor, drowsiness, confusion, coma, slow-wave EEG) occurred in 6 children, 3 of whom inadvertently swallowed large quantities of chlorothiazide but the remainder of whom received normal therapeutic doses.— N. J. O'Doherty (letter), *Lancet*, 1965, *2*, 1297.

Further references: H. Weisberg *et al.*, *Gastroenterologia, Basel*, 1966, *105*, 321.

Effects on the electrolyte balance. *Calcium.* Thiazide diuretics reduced the urinary excretion of calcium by about 40% in patients with intact parathyroid glands but not in patients with hypoparathyroidism.— S. Middler *et al.*, *Metabolism*, 1973, *22*, 139.

See also under Effects on the Parathyroid Glands, below.

Magnesium. Of 135 patients who had received long-term diuretic therapy 14 were found to have hypomagnesaemia; this was attributed to complicating diseases in 10 of the patients which included malignancies, chronic alcoholism, diabetes mellitus, epilepsy, and renal failure. It was considered that hypomagnesaemia might be an infrequent adverse reaction to diuretic treatment and routine determinations of serum-magnesium concentrations could be confined to patients with disorders predisposing them to hypomagnesaemia.— K. Laake *et al.*, *Curr. ther. Res.*, 1978, *23*, 730.

Further references: P. Lim and E. Jacob, *Br. med. J.*, 1972, *3*, 620.

Potassium. For studies and reviews on the need for potassium supplements in patients taking diuretics, see under Uses.

Sodium. Symptoms of hyponatraemia with sodium deficit occurred in 4 patients without cardiac failure taking diuretics. Symptoms were lethargy, weakness, slowing of cerebration, anorexia, and nausea, possibly progressing to coma and convulsions; there was no peripheral oedema. The condition, which could easily be missed if plasma-electrolyte concentrations were not measured, responded to the administration of sodium and potassium and the withdrawal of diuretics.— C. J. C. Roberts *et al.*, *Br. med. J.*, 1977, *1*, 210. Of 44 patients with hyponatraemia (plasma-sodium concentration below 125 mmol per litre) 13 were taking diuretics; 5 were taking frusemide and 8 thiazides.— P. G. E. Kennedy *et al.*, *Br. med. J.*, 1978, *2*, 1251.

Further references: M. P. Fichman *et al.*, *Ann. intern. Med.*, 1971, *75*, 853.

Zinc. For a report suggesting that long-term thiazide therapy may carry with it the risk of zinc deficiency, see Adverse Effects of Hydrochlorothiazide, p.601.

Effects on the eyes. A study indicating that usual therapeutic doses of chlorothiazide interfere with colour vision.— J. Laroche and C. Laroche, *Annls pharm. fr.*, 1972, *30*, 433.

Effects on the gall-bladder. Findings from a case-controlled drug surveillance programme of an association between the incidence of acute cholecystitis and the use of thiazide-containing drugs.— L. Rosenberg *et al.*, *New Engl. J. Med.*, 1980, *303*, 546.

Effects on the kidneys. Thiazide diuretics can produce acute renal failure by over-enthusiastic use producing saline depletion and hypovolaemia and also, occasionally, by a hypersensitivity reaction. They can occasionally cause the formation of non-opaque urate calculi.— J. R. Curtis, *Br. med. J.*, 1977, *2*, 242 and 375.

For a report of a possible hypersensitivity reaction to thiazide diuretics or frusemide, resulting in reversible renal failure, see Frusemide, p.596.

Effects on lipid metabolism. A report of increased plasma-triglyceride concentrations occurring in patients given thiazide diuretics.— B. F. Johnson *et al.* (letter), *Lancet*, 1976, *1*, 1019. See also R. P. Ames and P. Hill, *Am. J. Med.*, 1976, *61*, 748.

A 9-month study in 18 men receiving thiazide therapy for mild essential hypertension indicated that although serum uric acid and blood glucose concentrations increased, the effect on serum lipid concentration was negligible.— S. G. Chrysant *et al.*, *Angiology*, 1976, *27*, 707.

The pathological significance of the modest serum lipid changes, first noted with chlorthalidone therapy, is still unclear. If the patient requires and responds well to a diuretic, withdrawal does not seem warranted at the present time.— E. D. Freis, *J. Am. med. Ass.*, 1978, *240*, 1997. A similar view.— R. W. Gifford, *ibid.*

Comment on serum-cholesterol concentrations and thiazides.— A. Amery *et al.* (letter), *Lancet*, 1980, *2*, 473.

Further references: A. Helgeland *et al.*, *Am. J. Med.*, 1978, *64*, 34.

Effects on the muscles. Drugs which cause hypokalaemia might make myasthenia worse.— *Drug & Ther. Bull.*, 1977, *15*, 29.

Effects on the pancreas. Evaluation by the Medicines Evaluation and Monitoring Group of drugs taken before hospital admission by 100 patients with acute pancreatitis compared with 100 control patients indicated a greater preponderance of diuretics in the pancreatitis group. Further analysis was required before any conclusions could be drawn.— D. C. Moir (letter), *Lancet*, 1978, *2*, 369.

Further references: D. H. Johnston and A. L. Cornish, *J. Am. med. Ass.*, 1959, *170*, 2054; J. B. Bourke *et al.*, *Lancet*, 1978, *1*, 706.

Effects on the parathyroid glands. Six patients who had been treated with chlorothiazide (3 patients), hydrochlorothiazide (2), or polythiazide (1), for 2 to 8 years for hypertension, developed hyperparathyroidism. In *animals*, hypercalcaemia, hypophosphataemia, and hypertrophy of the parathyroid glands had been associated with the administration of thiazides. Calcium and phosphate concentrations in serum should be monitored in patients receiving thiazides.— E. Paloyan *et al.*, *J. Am. med. Ass.*, 1969, *210*, 1243. See also A. M. Parfitt, *New Engl. J. Med.*, 1969, *281*, 55.

Effects on the skin. Thiazides could cause photosensitisation, purpuric eruptions, eruptions resembling erythema multiforme, and eruptions resembling lichen planus.— R. L. Baer and H. Harris, *J. Am. med. Ass.*, 1967, *202*, 710. See also J. L. Verbov, *Br. J. clin. Pract.*, 1968, *22*, 229.

The most common cutaneous reaction to chlorothiazide was a lichenoid eruption but petechial and erythematous ones were also seen.— N. Thorne, *Practitioner*, 1973, *211*, 606.

Eczema. Thiazide diuretics, which are sulphonamide derivatives, may produce eczematous eruptions if given to patients sensitised by topical use of sulphonamides.— J. Verbov, *Practitioner*, 1979, *222*, 400.

Purpura. Purpura caused by thiazide diuretics, and the structurally similar drug, frusemide, may be either thrombocytopenic or non-thrombocytopenic.— J. Verbov, *Practitioner*, 1979, *222*, 400.

Vasculitis. In a series of 25 elderly patients with necrotising vasculitis in the skin, 11 were on thiazides and 3 on chlorthalidone; 13 of the 25 had haematuria during the course of their vasculitis. In the 1 patient in whom provocative tests were tried there were reactions to hydrochlorothiazide and chlorthalidone.— A. Björnberg and H. Gisslén, *Lancet*, 1965, *2*, 982. See also H. Kjellbo *et al.*, *ibid.*, *1*, 1034.

Lupus erythematosus. Systemic lupus erythematosus is reported to have occurred following the use of thiazide diuretics.— E. C. Rosenow, *Ann. intern. Med.*, 1972, *77*, 977.

Oedema. The commonest cause of so-called idiopathic oedema is the taking of diuretics, the effect of which may, in some patients, take at least a year to wear off.— G. A. MacGregor and H. E. de Wardener (letter), *Lancet*, 1979, *2*, 355. See also G. A. MacGregor *et al.*, *ibid.*, *1*, 397. Criticisms of this view: D. H. P. Streeten (letter), *ibid.*, 775; M. G. Dunnigan and J. R. Lawrence (letter), *ibid.*, 776. Further discussion on whether idiopathic oedema is a result of diuretic abuse.— O. M. Edwards and R. G. Dent (letter), *ibid.*, 1188; G. Lagrue *et al.* (letter), *ibid.* See also *ibid.*, 1980, *1*, 1066.

Further references: G. A. MacGregor *et al.*, *Lancet*, 1975, *1*, 489.

Pregnancy and the neonate. A patient who became comatose during the fourth month of pregnancy had taken chlorothiazide in an estimated total of 80 g over 3 weeks. She had extremely low serum-sodium and serum-potassium concentrations, and hypochloraemic alkalosis. She died probably as a result of pneumonia leading to cerebral hypoxia, superimposed on the effects of severe salt depletion.— B. S. Schifrin *et al.*, *Obstet. Gynec.*, 1969, *34*, 215.

An association between thiazide diuretics and neonatal hypoglycaemia. Analysis of 32 hypoglycaemic infants showed that 15 mothers had taken thiazides during pregnancy. Of the 14 infants with no obvious predisposing factor for their hypoglycaemia, 8 of the mothers had taken thiazide diuretics.— B. Senior *et al.* (letter), *Lancet*, 1976, *2*, 377.

See also under Effects on the Blood, above.

Treatment of Adverse Effects. Hypokalaemia in patients treated with thiazide diuretics may be avoided or treated by the administration of foods with a high potassium content, or by concurrent administration of potassium (but see the discussion on potassium supplements, under Uses) or a potassium-sparing diuretic. With the exception of patients with conditions such as liver failure or kidney disease, chloride deficiency is usually mild and does not require specific treatment. Apart from the rare occasions when it is life-threatening, dilutional hyponatraemia is best treated with water restriction rather than salt therapy; in true hyponatraemia, appropriate replacement is the treatment of choice.

In massive overdosage, treatment should be symptomatic and directed at fluid and electrolyte replacement. In the case of recent ingestion gastric lavage should be carried out. Phenylbutazone has been recommended to treat acute attacks of gout.

Precautions. Chlorothiazide and other thiazide diuretics should be used with caution in patients with impaired hepatic or renal function, or with diabetes mellitus or adrenal disease. They may precipitate attacks of gout in susceptible patients. All patients should be carefully observed for signs of fluid and electrolyte imbalance, especially in the presence of vomiting or during parenteral fluid therapy.

Chlorothiazide and other thiazide diuretics may enhance the toxicity of digitalis glycosides by depleting serum-potassium concentrations. They may enhance the neuromuscular blocking action of non-depolarising muscle relaxants, such as tubocurarine. They may enhance the effect of antihypertensive agents such as guanethidine, methyldopa, and rauwolfia alkaloids, while postural hypotension associated with thiazide diuretic therapy may be enhanced by concomitant ingestion of alcohol, barbiturates, or narcotics. The potassium-depleting effect of thiazide diuretics may be enhanced by corticosteroids, corticotrophin, or carbenoxolone. They may diminish the response to pressor amines, such as noradrenaline. Concomitant administration of thiazide diuretics and lithium is not generally recommended since the association may lead to toxic blood concentrations of lithium. Blood-glucose concentrations should be monitored in patients taking antidiabetic agents, since requirements may change.

Thiazide diuretics may interfere with a number of diagnostic tests, including tests for parathyroid function; serum concentrations of protein-bound iodine may increase without signs of thyroid disturbance.

Interactions. A discussion of interactions, including desirable interactions, between diuretics and other drugs.— J. E. Crook and A. S. Nies, *Drugs*, 1978, *15*, 72.

Aspirin and other anti-inflammatory analgesics. Since phenylbutazone promotes sodium and water retention it might diminish the activity of diuretics.— R. M. Pearson and C. W. H. Havard, *Br. J. Hosp. Med.*, 1974, *12*, 812.

For references to the reversal or blunting of the antihypertensive effect of diuretics and propranolol by indomethacin, see Propranolol, p.1328.

Ion-exchange resins. Gastro-intestinal absorption of chlorothiazide in 10 patients was reduced by colestipol both when the drugs were ingested simultaneously (4 patients) and when chlorothiazide was ingested 1 hour prior to colestipol (6 patients).— R. E. Kauffman and D. L. Azarnoff, *Clin. Pharmac. Ther.*, 1973, *14*, 886.

Lithium. For the effect of concomitant administration of a thiazide diuretic on serum-lithium concentrations, see Lithium Carbonate, p.1539.

Phenytoin. Because phenytoin had been reported to enhance hyperglycaemia care was necessary if it was given concomitantly with diabetogenic drugs such as corticosteroids or thiazide diuretics.— I. H. Stockley, *Pharm. J.*, 1972, *2*, 105.

Probenecid. Pretreatment with probenecid in 5 healthy subjects caused a significant increase in sodium excretion and urinary volume excretion after the intravenous administration of chlorothiazide 500 mg compared to values in the same subjects after only chlorothiazide. This increase was associated with a prolonged diuresis of chlorothiazide rather than an increase in intensity. No significant increase occurred when a dose of 1 g of chlorothiazide was employed.— D. C. Brater, *Clin. Pharmac. Ther.*, 1978, *23*, 259.

Vitamin D. Hypercalcaemia occurred in 5 of 12 patients with hypoparathyroidism treated with vitamin D when they were also treated with thiazide diuretics.— A. M. Parfitt, *Ann. intern. Med.*, 1972, *77*, 557.

Further references: A. M. Parfitt, *J. clin. Invest.*, 1972, *51*, 1879.

See also under Uses.

Interference with diagnostic tests. Thiazide diuretics could interfere biologically with chemical estimations for calcium and glucose in the blood to produce erroneous raised results.— *Drug & Ther. Bull.*, 1972, *10*, 69.

The administration of chlorothiazide could interfere with measurements of urinary 17-hydroxycorticosteroids.— J. N. Rosenberg and I. S. Kampa, *Drug Intell. & clin. Pharm.*, 1973, *7*, 33.

For a report that thiazide diuretics interfere with protein-bound iodine determinations, see Hydrochlorothiazide, p.601.

Pregnancy and the neonate. Uric acid and creatinine concentrations in amniotic fluid were markedly raised in 10 pregnant women with pre-eclampsia receiving thiazide diuretics. Because of the potential harmful effects of increased concentrations of these substances on the foetus, routine prolonged therapy with thiazide diuretics is not recommended in women with pre-eclampsia.— C. J. McAllister *et al.*, *Am. J. Obstet. Gynec.*, 1973, *115*, 560.

Evidence of reduced placental perfusion associated with hydrochlorothiazide administration supported the conclusion that thiazide diuretics represent a potential hazard to the foetus.— N. F. Gant *et al.*, *Am. J. Obstet. Gynec.*, 1975, *123*, 159.

Of 50 282 children born to mothers monitored by the Collaborative Perinatal Project 280 were found to have been exposed to diuretics, and possibly other drugs, at some time during the first 4 months of the pregnancy. In general exposure to diuretics was not associated with the production of malformations but a slight association with respiratory malformations was suggested.— O. P. Heinonen *et al.*, *Birth Defects and Drugs in Pregnancy*, Littleton MA, Publishing Sciences Group, 1977, p. 371.

The risk of thrombocytopenia in the foetus in association with thiazide diuretic therapy during pregnancy has been exaggerated and it should not be thought of as a contra-indication to the therapy of heart failure during pregnancy.— M. de Swiet, *Prescribers' J.*, 1979, *19*, 59.

For a warning that chlorothiazide is an inappropriate diuretic for jaundiced infants, see Precautions for Frusemide, p.597.

Absorption and Fate. Chlorothiazide is poorly but fairly rapidly absorbed from the gastro-intestinal tract. It has been estimated to have a plasma half-life of about 1 or 2 hours, and a biological half-life of up to about 12 hours. It is distributed throughout the extracellular tissues but is reported to accumulate in the kidneys; it is excreted unchanged in the urine. Chlorothiazide crosses the placental barrier and small amounts are reported to be excreted in breast milk.

Measured by a high-pressure liquid chromatographic method the mean percentage of a dose of chlorothiazide excreted in the urine by 4 healthy subjects within 48 hours of administration was 25% after a 250-mg dose and 14% after a 500-mg dose; a significant amount was excreted between 24 and 48 hours. The plasma half-life for chlorothiazide ranged from 1 to 1.8 hours and the biological half-life from 8 to 12 hours.— V. P. Shah *et al.*, *Curr. ther. Res.*, 1978, *24*, 366.

Interference by urinary constituents could cause appreciable errors in chlorothiazide bioavailability estimates based on colorimetric procedures. High-pressure liquid chromatography should be the analytical method of choice for urinary excretion-based bioavailability studies on chlorothiazide and, perhaps, other thiazide diuretics.— D. E. Resetarits and T. R. Bates, *J. pharm. Sci.*, 1979, *68*, 126. A study on the bioavailability of chlorothiazide tablets. It appeared that in general chlorothiazide was not well absorbed from the gastro-intestinal tract after administration by mouth.— A. B. Straughn *et al.*, *ibid.*, 1099.

Problems of bioavailability had been reported with 500-mg tablets of chlorothiazide.— *Pharm. J.*, 1981, *2*, 265.

Further references to absorption studies on chlorothiazide: R. E. Kauffman and D. L. Azarnoff, *Clin. Pharmac. Ther.*, 1973, *14*, 886; M. C. Meyer and A. B. Straughn, *Curr. ther. Res.*, 1977, *22*, 573; O. I. Corrigan and K. M. O'Driscoll, *J. Pharm. Pharmac.*, 1980, *32*, 547.

Pregnancy and the neonate. In 11 nursing mothers given chlorothiazide 500 mg the concentration in breast milk was less than an estimated 1 mg per litre. The risk to the infant was therefore remote.— M. W. Werthmann and S. V. Krees, *J. Pediat.*, 1972, *81*, 781.

Protein binding. *In vitro* studies show that chlorothiazide is fairly strongly bound to plasma proteins. The nature of the bond seems to be non-ionic.— A. Breckenridge and A. Rosen, *Biochim. biophys. Acta*, 1971, *229*, 610.

Uses. Chlorothiazide and the other thiazides (which are chemically related to the sulphonamides) are diuretics which reduce the reabsorption of electrolytes from the renal tubules, thereby increasing the excretion of sodium and chloride ions, and consequently of water. Potassium ions are excreted to a lesser extent. They also reduce carbonic-anhydrase activity so that bicarbonate excretion is increased, but this effect is generally small compared with the effect on chloride excretion and does not appreciably alter the acid-base balance or the pH of the urine.

The thiazides also have a slight lowering effect on the blood pressure and enhance the effects of other antihypertensive agents. Paradoxically, they have an antidiuretic effect in patients with diabetes insipidus.

Chlorothiazide, like the other thiazide diuretics, is used in the treatment of oedema associated with congestive heart failure, and renal and hepatic disorders. It is also used in hypertension, either alone, or as an adjunct to other antihypertensive agents.

Chlorothiazide and the other thiazide diuretics are also used in oedema associated with corticosteroid therapy; they may enhance the potassium-depleting action of corticosteroids (see under Precautions).

Chlorothiazide and the other thiazide diuretics are no longer recommended for the routine treatment of toxaemia of pregnancy, although their cautious use is still advocated for some aspects of the management of pre-eclampsia, for example when there is cardiac failure (see under Pregnancy and the Neonate).

The use of diuretic therapy has been advocated for the oedema accompanying premenstrual tension in otherwise healthy subjects although such use has little rationale. It has been suggested that this use of diuretic therapy may, however, exacerbate the conditions for which it was originally prescribed. Less common uses of chlorothiazide and other thiazide diuretics include the treatment of diabetes insipidus and hypercalciuria.

Following oral administration of chlorothiazide a response is usually obtained in about 2 hours and the diuresis is maintained for up to about 12 hours. The usual dose of chlorothiazide for diuresis is 0.5 to 1 g once or twice daily; therapy on alternate days or on 3 to 5 days weekly may be adequate.

In the treatment of hypertension chlorothiazide may be given in an initial dose of 0.5 to 1 g daily, given as a single or divided dose; up to 2 g daily may be given in divided doses.

Concurrent administration of potassium supplements or foods rich in potassium (such as citrus fruits, bananas, dried fruits, and fresh tomatoes) has usually been recommended to prevent the development of hypokalaemia associated with thiazide diuretic therapy. Recent studies however have cast doubt on the need for potassium supplements in many patients taking thiazide diuretics, particularly in hypertension, and have conversely emphasised the hazards of hyperkalaemia following inappropriate potassium supplementation, particularly in the elderly. Plasma-potassium concentrations should be monitored in patients taking thiazide diuretics; potassium supplements or potassium-sparing diuretics should be added only when appropriate. Hypokalaemia is a particular hazard in patients with cirrhosis or in those receiving digitalis therapy.

A suggested dose of chlorothiazide in children is 25 mg per kg body-weight daily in two divided doses. Infants up to the age of 6 months may require up to 35 mg per kg daily in two divided doses.

Chlorothiazide has also been given intravenously as the sodium salt, in doses of 0.5 to 1 g once or twice daily; it is not suitable for subcutaneous or intramuscular injection.

Action. A study on the mechanism of action of thiazide diuretics in hypertension. First, volume depletion may blunt environmental pressor stimuli while at the same time enhancing depressor influences. Second, volume depletion may lower blood pressure by the baroreceptor reflexes. Third, and most likely, the haemodynamic changes may involve feedback autoregulatory responses as originally suggested by L. Tobian (*Archs intern. Med.*, 1974, *133*, 959 and *Fedn Proc.*, 1974, *33*, 138), inducing 'reverse autoregulation' which leads to a decrease in total peripheral resistance.— S. Shah *et al.*, *Am. Heart J.*, 1978, *95*, 611.

In a double-blind placebo-controlled crossover study completed by 9 women with hypertension due to severe renal failure, chlorothiazide 500 mg twice daily for 6 weeks caused a significant reduction in standing and supine blood pressure, without postural hypotension, and without any natriuretic effect, stable sodium balance being reflected in stable body-weight and urinary sodium excretion. These data indicate that thiazides have an antihypertensive effect independent of their diuretic action, and favour a direct vasodilator action, rather than 'reverse autoregulation' secondary to extracellular-fluid-volume depletion.— B. Jones and R. S. Nanra, *Lancet*, 1979, *2*, 1258. Criticism. Although the report is of interest it does not prove that diuretics have an independent antihypertensive effect.— W. M. Bennett (letter), *ibid.*, 1980, *1*, 256. See also H. G. Langford (letter), *ibid.*, 203.

Further references: R. FBing *et al.*, *Lancet*, 1979, *2*, 121.

Administration. *In the elderly.* A discussion of the proper role of diuretics in the elderly.— *Br. med. J.*, 1978, *1*, 1092.

Further reviews: R. H. Briant, *Drugs*, 1977, *13*, 225; R. E. Vestal, *ibid.*, 1978, *16*, 358.

A double-blind placebo-controlled study was carried out on the effects of withdrawal of diuretic therapy from 54 elderly patients in whom its use was not deemed mandatory. These patients were given placebo tablets while 52 similar patients continued to take diuretics. During the following 12 weeks resumption of diuretic therapy was required in only 8. These results indicated that many patients receive diuretics who do not need them. It was concluded that elderly people receiving long-term diuretic therapy without obvious current indication should have them withdrawn under careful supervision so that those who needed them can be identified.— M. L. Burr *et al.*, *Age and Ageing*, 1977, *6*, 38. See also *idem* (letter), *Br. med. J.*, 1977, *1*, 976.

A study of the prevalence of diuretic therapy and associated hypokalaemia in 128 male and 361 female geriatric out-patients, receiving mainly thiazide or loop diuretics. Hypokalaemia had developed in 1 of 44 men and 25 of 134 women receiving diuretic therapy but no difference in serum-potassium concentration relating to the prescription of potassium supplements could be demonstrated for either sex. It was concluded that moderate and severe degrees of hypokalaemia can follow even small doses of diuretics in the elderly, this occurring more frequently in women than men, and that small amounts of potassium chloride cannot be relied upon to prevent this. Periodic control of serum-potassium concentration is necessary if severe diuretic-associated hypokalaemia is to be avoided.— R. Krakauer and M. Lauritzen, *Dan. med. Bull.*, 1978, *25*, 126.

Further references: G. Jackson *et al.*, *Lancet*, 1976, *2*, 1317.

Administration and potassium. A detailed account of diuretic therapy and potassium metabolism, and a reassessment of the need, effectiveness, and safety of potassium therapy.— J. P. Kassirer and J. T. Harrington, *Kidney Int.*, 1977, *11*, 505.

Further reviews and recommendations: L. E. Ramsay and M. H. Ramsay, *Practitioner*, 1977, *219*, 529; H. J. Dargie, *Prescribers' J.*, 1978, *18*, 83; *Drug & Ther. Bull.*, 1978, *16*, 73; L. B. Jellett, *Drugs*, 1978, *16*, 88; T. O. Morgan, *ibid.*, 1979, *18*, 218.

A study of the potassium status of 151 patients with chronic heart disease with particular reference to the long-term effects of diuretics plus potassium supplementation in 83. Among the 83 the total body-potassium deficit appeared in those taking frusemide to be no more than 3.6% for men and 5.5% for women; also 12 had low plasma-potassium concentrations (less than 3.5 mmol per litre) but without any clinical symptoms or ECG changes. It was considered that when patients with heart failure are given diuretics then potassium supplements should be given so as to maintain an acceptable plasma-potassium concentration rather than given on the basis of an assumed cellular potassium depletion.— C. Davidson *et al.*, *Lancet*, 1976, *2*, 1044. See also *idem*, *Postgrad. med. J.*, 1978, *54*, 405.

A study suggesting that cellular uptake of potassium from potassium supplements is dependent upon the correction of magnesium deficiency.— T. Dyckner and P. O. Wester, *Br. med. J.*, 1978, *1*, 822.

Potassium supplements or potassium-retaining diuretics are given with potent diuretics because potassium depletion in patients with heart failure has been attributed to their actions. A review of the literature, however, suggests that the reported decrease in body potassium compared with results in healthy subjects, is not due to diuretics, and that there is no evidence that severe cellular depletion of potassium was ever common in patients with heart failure. The apparent deficiences of potassium which have been repeatedly observed could be due to failure to match patients and controls, and to muscle wasting.— D. B. Morgan *et al.*, *Postgrad. med. J.*, 1978, *54*, 72.

An analysis of the literature suggested that the risk of appreciable hypokalaemia (less than 3 mmol per litre) was small in patients with heart failure or hypertension given diuretics. In patients with severe heart failure or renal or liver disease the use of a potassium-sparing diuretic was preferable.— D. B. Morgan and C. Davidson, *Br. med. J.*, 1980, *280*, 905. Comments.— J. L. C. Dall (letter), *ibid.*, 1123; R. C. Hamdy *et al.* (letter), *ibid.*, 1187.

A study of the computerised records of analysis of electrolyte concentrations of 58 000 patients in hospital indicated that diuretics were an infrequent source of severe hypokalaemia.— *Lancet*, 1980, *1*, 520. Comment.— K. A. Manley (letter), *ibid.*, 880.

Further references: C. J. Edmonds and B. Jasani, *Lancet*, 1972, *2*, 8; R. J. Manner *et al.*, *Clin. Med.*, 1972, *79* (Nov.), 15; R. P. S. Edmondson *et al.*, *Lancet*, 1974, *1*, 12; P. R. Wilkinson *et al.*, *ibid.*, 1975, *1*, 759; R. W. Pain and P. J. Phillips (letter), *ibid.*, 1975, *2*, 77; S. Carney *et al.*, *Med. J. Aust.*, 1975, *1*, 803; D. H. Lawson *et al.*, *Q. J. Med.*, 1976, *45*, 469; W. D. Alexander *et al.*, *Postgrad. med. J.*, 1977, *53*, 117; A. Kohvakka *et al.*, *Acta med. scand.*, 1979, *205*, 319.

Enteric-coated potassium formulations. Deprecation of the fact that cases of small-bowel ulceration continue to be reported in patients given thiazide preparations containing enteric-coated potassium. Such preparations have no apparent advantages over less dangerous formulations containing potassium chloride (such as embedding the drug in a wax core) and should be removed from the market.— *Drug & Ther. Bull.*, 1977, *15*, 67.

References to bowel ulceration following the use of diuretic preparations containing enteric-coated potassium, including HydroSaluric-K and Salupres: *Br. med. J.*, 1972, *1*, 797; J. M. Jefferson and P. Aukland (letter), *Br. med. J.*, 1974, *1*, 456; B. L. D. Phillips, *Br. J. clin. Pract.*, 1974, *28*, 143; J. R. Ball (letter), *Lancet*, 1976, *1*, 495; D. A. Makey (letter), *Lancet*, 1977, *1*, 704; J. Tresadern *et al.*, *Br. med. J.*, 1977, *2*, 1124.

Administration in hepatic failure. See under Hepatic Disorders.

Administration in renal failure. Thiazide diuretics are generally ineffective in patients with a glomerular filtration-rate below 30 ml per minute.— W. M. Bennett *et al.*, *Ann. intern. Med.*, 1980, *93*, 286. See also *idem*, *Clin. Pharmac. Ther.*, 1977, *22*, 499.

See also under Renal Disorders.

Cardiac disorders. The use of diuretics in the treatment of congestive heart failure in children.— N. J. Restiaux, *Drugs*, 1977, *13*, 467.

Diabetes insipidus. The antidiuretic effect of chlorothiazide and hydrochlorothiazide in 12 infants and children and 1 adult with diabetes insipidus.— N. J. O'Doherty, *Can. med. Ass. J.*, 1962, *86*, 559. See also M. G. Schotland *et al.*, *Pediatrics*, 1963, *31*, 741.

Treatment with thiazide diuretics usually reduces urine output by 25 to 50% in patients with diabetes insipidus.— R. Utiger, *J. Am. med. Ass.*, 1969, *207*, 1699.

Diagnostic use. *Aldosteronism.* Intravenous infusion of chlorothiazide lacks specificity and sensitivity as a screening test for primary hyperaldosteronism.— W. L. McGuffin and J. C. Gunnells, *Archs intern. Med.*, 1969, *123*, 124, per *J. Am. med. Ass.*, 1969, *207*, 1364.

Hyperparathyroidism. For provocative tests of parathyroid activity, chlorothiazide together with phosphate deprivation was used to investigate the incidence of primary hyperparathyroidism in patients with idiopathic hypercalciuria.— P. Adams *et al.*, *Br. med. J.*, 1970, *4*, 582.

Glaucoma. For the concomitant use of acetazolamide and chlorothiazide, see Acetazolamide (Ocular Disorders), p.583.

Hepatic disorders. Results of a controlled study indicated that diuresis, aiming at a modest rate of diuresis, can be accomplished in patients with decompensated alcoholic liver disease and ascites of recent onset, without serious complications that can be attributed to diuretic therapy.— P. B. Gregory *et al.*, *Gastroenterology*, 1977, *73*, 534.

See also under Spironolactone, p.611.

In children. Comment on the use of diuretic therapy for ascites and oedema associated with hepatic diseases in children. Hypokalaemia and dehydration are particular risks with frusemide and the thiazide diuretics. Spironolactone is the logical diuretic to use; it may be adequate used alone, or the addition of a small dose of frusemide or a thiazide diuretic may yield the desired diuresis.— D. M. Danks (letter), *J. Pediat.*, 1976, *88*, 695.

Hypertension. A review of the use of thiazide diuretics in the treatment of hypertension.— *Drug & Ther. Bull.*, 1975, *13*, 101.

A reduction in blood pressure following treatment chiefly with thiazides, usually chlorothiazide 250 mg daily 5 days a week, in 100 geriatric patients with hypertension, led to a near-halving of the death-rate, when compared with a control group of 83 untreated patients of comparable age, blood pressure, and associated diseases.— W. W. Priddle *et al.*, *J. Am. Geriat. Soc.*, 1968, *16*, 887.

Further references: W. M. Smith *et al.*, *Ann. intern. Med.*, 1964, *61*, 829.

For a study comparing long-term thiazide diuretic therapy with propranolol in mild to moderately severe essential hypertension, see Bendrofluazide, p.585.

Effect on plasma renin. Studies in 8 patients with essential hypertension, treated with thiazide diuretics for 6 to 24 months, indicated that during the reduction in blood pressure there was persistent plasma-volume contraction but increased peripheral renin activity.— R. C. Tarazi *et al.*, *Circulation*, 1970, *41*, 709.

Support for the view that stimulation of the renin-angiotensin system limits the hypotensive effect of diuretics.— C. I. Johnston *et al.*, *Lancet*, 1979, *2*, 493.

Further references: E. D. Vaughan *et al.*, *Circulation Res.*, 1978, *42*, 376.

Hypoglycaemia. For the use of diazoxide with chlorothiazide in hypoglycaemia, see Diazoxide, p.144.

Hypoparathyroidism. The thiazide diuretics may help to maintain more normal serum-calcium concentrations in hypoparathyroid patients.— J. Lemann *et al.*, *New Engl. J. Med.*, 1979, *301*, 535.

For details of the controversy surrounding the use of thiazide diuretics in hypoparathyroid patients, see under Chlorthalidone, p.592.

See also under Precautions.

Lithium therapy. A study in 13 patients indicated that concurrent administration of thiazide diuretics induced clinically significant elevations in serum-lithium concentrations with an enhanced response in refractory manic-depressive patients.— J. M. Himmelhoch *et al.*, *Am. J. Psychiat.*, 1977, *134*, 149.

Further references: J. Forrest *et al.*, *J. clin. Invest.*, 1974, *53*, 1115.

See also under Precautions.

Oedema. A review of the management of idiopathic oedema. In most patients the condition is no more than an inconvenience and should be dealt with by reassurance and possibly support tights or elastic stockings. In a minority where the oedema causes severe discomfort and even dyspnoea the patient may respond to a dietary regimen containing no added salt. Only if this fails should a diuretic be given.— *Drug & Ther. Bull.*, 1976, *14*, 101. See also under Adverse Effects.

Associating a thiazide diuretic with a loop diuretic is

very useful in refractory oedema. Loop diuretics supply ample sodium at the distal sites of the nephron, inducing accelerated reabsorption at these sites, which is effectively depressed by a thiazide.— P. Franzén (letter), *Br. med. J.*, 1979, *1*, 823.

Paget's disease of bone. Beneficial effects were obtained in 8 of 9 patients with Paget's disease, using a regimen designed to raise plasma-calcium concentrations and thus stimulate endogenous calcitonin production. A low phosphorus dietary regimen was given, together with aluminium hydroxide to bind phosphorus in the gut. Oral calcium was given between meals and a thiazide diuretic (methyclothiazide) was given to raise plasma-calcium concentrations.— R. A. Evans, *Aust. N.Z. J. Med.*, 1977, *7*, 259.

Pregnancy and the neonate. Hypertension of pregnancy. A review of drug therapy for severe pre-eclampsia and eclampsia. Diuretic therapy may be indicated if there is gross fluid retention, evidence of impending acute renal necrosis, or in the longer term to enhance the action of antihypertensive drugs, such as hydralazine. Hypovolaemia is a feature of severe pre-eclampsia, however, even though oedema may be gross, and diuretics should be used with caution. With some diuretics there are also added risks of producing excessive sodium depletion, pancreatitis, and thrombocytopenia, and they should probably only be used when blood pressure control is difficult or when there is cardiac failure.— B. M. Hibbard, *Practitioner*, 1978, *221*, 847.

Further reviews and comments: B. M. Hibbard and M. Rosen, *Br. J. Anaesth.*, 1977, *49*, 3; M. de Swiet, *Prescribers' J.*, 1979, *19*, 59.

In a study involving 3083 pregnant women, aged 17 or under, the use of thiazide diuretics protected the mother against toxaemia and significantly reduced perinatal mortality and prematurity. Chlorothiazide 500 mg daily was given to 936 patients and 404 received chlorthalidone in a dose of 50 mg daily. A similar control group of 1743 pregnant patients also aged 17 or under received no thiazides. A 10% or more increase in arterial pressure and albuminuria (not caused by infection) developed in 5% of the treated patients and in 15% of those untreated. In the treated group, perinatal mortality was 0.7% and the prematurity-rate was 5%; the corresponding figures for the untreated group were 5% and 12% respectively— F. A. Finnerty and F. J. Bepko, *J. Am. med. Ass.*, 1966, *195*, 429.

In a controlled study of 153 pregnant women who had shown high weight gain between the 20th and 30th week of gestation, there was no significant reduction in the incidence of pre-eclampsia in those treated by diet or thiazide diuretic compared with controls. This result was in spite of body fat being reduced by dieting and total body water by the diuretic, cyclopenthiazide 500 µg daily with potassium.— D. M. Campbell and I. MacGillivray, *Br. J. Obstet. Gynaec.*, 1975, *82*, 572.

See also under Adverse Effects and Precautions.

Premenstrual syndrome. A review of drugs for the treatment of premenstrual tension, including criticism of claims made on behalf of diuretics. There is no basis for the belief that fluid retention is a cause of premenstrual tension.— *Br. J. Psychiat.*, 1979, *135*, 576.

Further references: E. C. Jungck *et al.*, *J. Am. med. Ass.*, 1959, *169*, 112; B. P. Appleby, *Br. med. J.*, 1960, *1*, 391.

For reference to the possible role of diuretics in exacerbating and perpetuating idiopathic oedema, see Oedema, under Adverse Effects (above).

Renal disorders. *Renal calculus.* Chlorothiazide 500 mg twice daily was being widely used to prevent the recurrence of renal calculi.— T. Mathew, *Drugs*, 1974, *8*, 62.

A suggestion that the increased urinary excretion of zinc might contribute to the beneficial effect of thiazide diuretics in preventing renal stones.— M. Cohanim and E. R. Yendt, *Johns Hopkins med. J.*, 1975, *136*, 137.

The use of thiazide diuretics in the treatment of calcium nephrolithiasis.— D. V. Weber *et al.*, *Ann. intern. Med.*, 1979, *90*, 180.

The rate of stone formation was reduced to a similar extent by thiazide and by placebo in a controlled study of 62 patients.— P. Brocks *et al.*, *Lancet*, 1981, *2*, 124. Comment and criticism: J. C. Birkenhäger *et al.* (letter), *ibid.*, 578; G. Graziani *et al.* (letter), *ibid.*; D. J. Sherrard (letter), *ibid.*, 644.

Further references: C. Y. C. Pak and K. Holt, *Metabolism*, 1976, *25*, 665; C. Y. C. Pak *et al.*, *J. Lab. clin. Med.*, 1977, *89*, 891.

Trauma. The use of diuretics in acute renal failure following trauma.— H. A. Lee, *Br. J. Anaesth.*, 1977, *49*, 697.

Vertigo. For a brief note on the use of some diuretics in the treatment of dizziness, see J. S. Turner, *Drugs*, 1977, *13*, 382.

Preparations

Chlorothiazide Oral Suspension *(U.S.P.)*. A suspension containing chlorothiazide. pH 3.5 to 4. Store in airtight containers.

Chlorothiazide Sodium for Injection *(U.S.P.)*. A sterile mixture of chlorothiazide sodium, prepared from chlorothiazide with the aid of sodium hydroxide, and mannitol. Potency is expressed in terms of the equivalent amount of chlorothiazide. The solution has a pH of 9.2 to 10.

Chlorothiazide Tablets *(B.P., U.S.P.)*. Tablets containing chlorothiazide.

Proprietary Preparations

Saluric *(Merck Sharp & Dohme, UK)*. Chlorothiazide, available as scored tablets of 500 mg.

Other Proprietary Names

Austral.— Azide, Chlotride, Diubram, Diuret, Diurone; *Denm.*— Chlotride; *Fr.*— Diurilix; *Ital.*— Clotride; *Neth.*— Chlotride; *Norw.*— Chlotride; *S.Afr.*— Chlotride; *Spain*— Saluretil; *Swed.*— Chlotride; *USA*— Diuril, SK-Chlorothiazide.

2318-g

Chlorthalidone *(B.P., U.S.P.)*. Chlortalidone; G33182. 2-Chloro-5-(1-hydroxy-3-oxoisoindolin-1-yl)benzenesulphonamide.

$C_{14}H_{11}ClN_2O_4S = 338.8$.

CAS — 77-36-1.

Pharmacopoeias. In *Br.*, *Braz.*, *Cz.*, *It.*, *Jug.*, and *U.S.*

A white or yellowish-white, odourless or almost odourless, tasteless, crystalline powder. M.p. about 220° with decomposition.

Practically **insoluble** in water; soluble 1 in 150 of alcohol, 1 in 650 of chloroform, and 1 in 25 of methyl alcohol; slightly soluble in ether; soluble in solutions of alkali hydroxides.

Adverse Effects, Treatment, and Precautions. As for Chlorothiazide, p.588.

Epidermal necrolysis has been reported with chlorthalidone.

Abuse. Hypokalaemia occurred in 3 women who had abused frusemide and chlorthalidone.— F. H. Katz *et al.*, *Ann. intern. Med.*, 1972, *76*, 85.

Diabetogenic effect. Of 16 patients given chlorthalidone (average total dose 14.9 g over an average of 114 days) the glucose tolerance was unchanged in 10 and slightly reduced in 3. One patient developed diabetes mellitus and 2 others had a considerably reduced carbohydrate tolerance, which was irreversible in 1 patient.— O. O. Andersen and I. Persson, *Br. med. J.*, 1968, *2*, 798.

A 43-year-old man with diabetes mellitus developed hyperosmolar, hyperglycaemic, nonketotic coma after treatment with chlorthalidone for hypertension. The coma occurred 5 days after he received the last dose of chlorthalidone. This reaction was delayed because the drug was poorly absorbed from the gastro-intestinal tract.— J. Curtis *et al.*, *J. Am. med. Ass.*, 1972, *220*, 1592.

Effects on the blood. *Agranulocytosis.* A 54-year-old woman developed agranulocytosis attributable to chlorthalidone after a total dosage of 1.5 g over 5 weeks. Prompt withdrawal of the drug was followed by complete recovery.— M. Klein, *J. Am. med. Ass.*, 1963, *184*, 310.

Further references: M. A. Neaverson (letter), *Lancet*, 1964, *2*, 208; R. J. Plumridge, *Aust. J. Pharm.*, 1973, *54*, 486.

Effects on the electrolyte balance. *Calcium.* A woman treated with chlorthalidone for mild hypertension developed mild hypercalcaemia which was responsive to changes in chlorthalidone dosage.— F. J. Palmer (letter), *J. Am. med. Ass.*, 1974, *229*, 267. Chlorthalidone had caused permanent hypercalcaemia in patients with hyperparathyroidism.— A. Weinberger *et al.* (letter), *ibid.*, 1975, *231*, 134.

Potassium. In 23 hypertensive patients receiving chlorthalidone, 100 mg on alternate days, potassium depletion was treated by 1 of 3 drugs. Triamterene 50 mg twice daily was apparently ineffective. Spironolactone 25 mg twice daily markedly reduced potassium loss, while a preparation of potassium chloride completely reversed previous deficits in total exchangeable potassium.— T. J. McKenna *et al.*, *Br. med. J.*, 1971, *2*, 739.

Effects on the eyes. A study indicating that usual therapeutic doses of chlorthalidone interfere with colour vision.— J. Laroche and C. Laroche, *Annls pharm. fr.*, 1972, *30*, 433.

Effects on the kidneys. A report of reversible acute renal failure considered to be associated with the use of chlorthalidone given to a 58-year-old man with hypertension who had had a transient cerebral ischaemic attack.— S. T. Peskoe *et al.*, *J. med. Ass. Ga*, 1978, *67*, 17.

Inappropriate secretion of antidiuretic hormone. Chlorthalidone 100 mg daily induced inappropriate secretion of antidiuretic hormone in a 60-year-old woman with mild hypertension and nephrolithiasis.— R. Luboshitzky *et al.*, *J. clin. Pharmac.*, 1978, *18*, 336.

Effects on lipid metabolism. Mean serum-cholesterol concentrations rose by 5.2% and serum-triglyceride concentrations by 25.7% in 32 hypertensive patients treated by diet and chlorthalidone 50 mg twice weekly to 100 mg daily for about 6 months. Only 15 of the 32 were significantly affected and the mean increases in these 15 were 13.9 and 51.9% respectively. In 31 similar patients with lower initial blood pressure treated by diet mean serum-cholesterol concentrations fell by 4.7% and triglyceride concentrations did not change.— R. P. Ames and P. Hill, *Lancet*, 1976, *1*, 721. Analysis of data from the Framingham Heart Study did not reveal any rise in serum-cholesterol concentration in patients taking diuretics; neither was there a rise in blood-glucose concentration.— W. B. Kannel *et al.* (letter), *ibid.*, 1977, *1*, 1362. There was a significant increase in plasma-cholesterol and plasma-triglyceride concentrations in patients receiving chlorthalidone during a study of the treatment of mild hypertension.— H. Schnaper *et al.* (letter), *ibid.*, *2*, 295.

Further references: A. I. Goldman *et al.*, *J. Am. med. Ass.*, 1980, *244*, 1691; C. Joos *et al.*, *Eur. J. clin. Pharmac.*, 1980, *17*, 251.

Effect on the muscles. Probably the first reported case of hypokalaemic vacuolar myopathy associated with chlorthalidone occurred in a 56-year-old woman. Severe hypokalaemia was induced by chlorthalidone in therapeutic doses of 50 mg daily for 5 days a week and abuse of laxatives ('magnesium laxative'). Treatment initially with prednisolone, given because of an incorrect tentative diagnosis, had an adverse effect but subsequent potassium chloride 40 mmol (40 mEq) twice daily increased to 140 mmol (140 mEq) daily resulted in complete recovery.— S. J. Oh *et al.*, *J. Am. med. Ass.*, 1971, *216*, 1858.

Effects on the pancreas. Massive acute haemorrhagic pancreatitis in an elderly woman was considered to be associated with chlorthalidone administration.— T. Prigogine *et al.* (letter), *Acta clin. belg.*, 1978, *33*, 272.

Effects on sexual function. Chlorthalidone has been reported to have some adverse effects on sexual function.— *Med. Lett.*, 1977, *19*, 81.

Sexual dysfunction, characterised by impotence or decreased libido, was associated with the administration of chlorthalidone in 5 men. In all patients sexual function improved on stopping, or reducing the dose of chlorthalidone.— J. Stessman and D. Ben-Ishay, *Br. med. J.*, 1980, *281*, 714.

Interactions. *Acetazolamide.* A study in 2 healthy subjects indicated that chlorthalidone and acetazolamide competed for the same binding sites in the blood cells. These showed greater affinity for acetazolamide which was able to inhibit the uptake of chlorthalidone into the red cells and also to displace chlorthalidone already attached to the binding sites.— B. Beermann *et al.*, *Clin. Pharmac. Ther.*, 1975, *17*, 424.

Oedema. For reference to the possible role of diuretics in exacerbating and perpetuating idiopathic oedema, see Oedema, under Adverse Effects of Chlorothiazide, p.588.

Pregnancy and the neonate. In the infants born to 9 women given chlorthalidone for toxaemia of pregnancy concentrations of 0.43 to 1.60 µg per ml were measured in cord blood of 8 at delivery. Treatment of the mothers was continued for 3 days after delivery, and concentrations of 90 to 860 ng per ml were found in milk on the third day. It was recommended that mothers receiving chlorthalidone should not breast-feed, as the infants might be less able than adults to eliminate it.— B. A. Mulley *et al.*, *Eur. J. clin. Pharmac.*, 1978, *13*, 129.

Absorption and Fate. Chlorthalidone is incompletely absorbed from the gastro-intestinal tract to give peak plasma concentrations about 2 to 4 hours after a dose. Its prolonged terminal half-life of several days has been reported to be due to its strong binding to red blood cells. It is mainly excreted unchanged in the urine, but there is also evidence for an additional, presumably metabolic, route of elimination. It crosses the placental barrier and is excreted in breast milk.

A report of studies on the absolute bioavailability of chlorthalidone in healthy subjects and hospital in-patients. The long half-life appears to be mainly due to its strong binding to red blood cells. Data following intravenous as well as oral administration provided evidence for an important route of elimination of chlorthalidone in addition to the renal route. It was presumed to be metabolic; no evidence of significant biliary excretion was noted.— H. L. J. Fleuren *et al.*, *Eur. J. clin. Pharmac.*, 1979, *15*, 35.

Further references: M. G. Tweeddale and R. I. Ogilvie, *J. pharm. Sci.*, 1974, *63*, 1065; H. L. Fleuren and J. M. van Rossum, *J. Pharmacokinet. Biopharm.*, 1977, *5*, 359; H. L. J. Fleuren *et al.*, *Clin. Pharmac. Ther.*, 1979, *25*, 806; B. A. Mulley *et al.*, *Eur. J. clin. Pharmac.*, 1980, *17*, 203.

Red cell binding. An *in vitro* study of the binding of chlorthalidone to human blood components. In the absence of red blood cells about 75% was bound to plasma proteins (mainly albumin) at a concentration range of 0.02 to 7.7 μg per ml. In whole blood, however, at concentrations of about 15 to 20 μg per ml, at least 98% was preferentially contained in the red blood cell fraction. Above this concentration the percentage of drug in the red blood cells decreased, and that in the plasma increased, indicating the presence of a saturable receptor in the red blood cells, which was identified as carbonic anhydrase. Chlorthalidone is much less strongly bound to albumin than carbonic anhydrase.— W. Dieterle *et al.*, *Eur. J. clin. Pharmac.*, 1976, *10*, 37.

Further references: P. Collste *et al.*, *Eur. J. clin. Pharmac.*, 1976, *9*, 319; W. Riess *et al.*, *ibid.*, 1977, *12*, 375; G. D. Parr *et al.*, *J. Pharm. Pharmac.*, 1979, *31*, *Suppl.*, 42P.

Uses. Chlorthalidone is a diuretic which has certain structural similarities to the thiazides and has actions and uses similar to those of chlorothiazide (see p.589).

Diuresis is initiated in about 2 hours and lasts for 48 hours or longer. Its inhibitory action on carbonic anhydrase is only weak.

In the treatment of oedema the usual dose is 100 to 200 mg on alternate days; single initial doses of up to 400 mg have been given. A suggested initial dose in children is 2 mg per kg body-weight 3 times a week.

The usual dose in the treatment of hypertension is 50 mg daily, either alone, or in conjunction with other antihypertensive agents; in some cases initial doses of 100 mg may be necessary.

In diabetes insipidus an initial dose of 100 mg twice daily has been recommended reduced to a maintenance dose of 50 mg daily.

When treatment is prolonged, or in susceptible patients, loss of potassium may be sufficient to produce hypokalaemia; potassium supplements should then be given as for chlorothiazide.

Administration in renal failure. The interval between doses of chlorthalidone should be extended from 24 hours to 48 hours in patients with a glomerular filtration-rate of less than 10 ml per minute.— W. M. Bennett *et al.*, *Ann. intern. Med.*, 1980, *93*, 286.

Cardiac disorders. *Angina pectoris.* A double-blind crossover trial in 9 patients suffering from angina pectoris compared the effects of chlorthalidone 50 mg daily and a placebo over 4-week treatment periods. In 7 patients chlorthalidone was associated with improvement.— C. B. Floyd and J. G. Domenet, *Practitioner*, 1973, *210*, 559.

Hypertension. Dose-dependent antihypertensive effects were not observed in 37 patients with mild to moderate essential hypertension given chlorthalidone. In 25 patients the greatest reduction in mean diastolic blood pressure occurred with chlorthalidone 25 or 50 mg daily while the remaining 12 patients required a dose of 100 or 200 mg daily.— M. G. Tweeddale *et al.*, *Clin. Pharmac. Ther.*, 1977, *22*, 519. See also B. J. Materson *et al.*, *ibid.*, 1978, *24*, 192.

In a crossover study in 33 hypertensive patients there was no significant difference between the antihypertensive effect of chlorthalidone 50 to 100 mg daily and frusemide 40 to 80 mg daily. Concomitant antihypertensive therapy remained the same throughout the study. Potassium supplements were required by 17 patients during the chlorthalidone period alone and by 2 patients during both drug periods.— M. E. Davidov *et al.*, *Curr. ther. Res.*, 1979, *25*, 1.

Further references to the use of chlorthalidone in hypertension, either alone, or in conjunction with other antihypertensive agents: J. M. Bryant *et al.*, *J. Am. med. Ass.*, 1965, *193*, 1021; *Practitioner*, 1965, *194*, 270 (Report No. 68 of the General Practitioner Research Group); D. W. Richardson *et al.*, *Circulation*, 1968, *37*, 534; J. J. Healy *et al.*, *Br. med. J.*, 1970, *1*, 716; D. B. Toubles *et al.*, *Am. Heart J.*, 1971, *82*, 312; W. J. Louis *et al.*, *Med. J. Aust.*, 1973, *2*, 23; C. Bengtsson *et al.*, *Br. med. J.*, 1975, *1*, 197; S. Carney *et al.*, *Med. J. Aust.*, 1976, *2*, 692; T. J. J. M. Bloem and J. M. Kerkhof, *Clin. Ther.*, 1977, *1*, 228; A. H. Griep, *Curr. ther. Res.*, 1978, *24*, 1; M. H. R. Sheriff *et al.*, *Acta ther.*, 1978, *4*, 51; R. Buoninconti *et al.*, *J. int. med. Res.*, 1979, *7*, 519; M. Kubik *et al.*, *Clin. Pharmac. Ther.*, 1979, *25*, 25; M. Bergström *et al.*, *Curr. ther. Res.*, 1980, *27*, 805; R. J. Noveck *et al.*, *Clin. Pharmac. Ther.*, 1980, *28*, 581; Y. K. Seedat, *Br. med. J.*, 1980, *281*, 1241.

Effect on plasma renin. In a study of 50 patients with essential hypertension 10 of 13 patients with low-renin activity, 13 of 28 with normal-renin activity and 2 of 9 with high-renin activity responded to treatment with chlorthalidone 100 mg daily for 6 weeks. Increases in plasma-renin activity and particularly in the excretion-rate of aldosterone were higher in nonresponders than in responders. Factors governing the sensitivity of the aldosterone response to renin stimulation might determine the effectiveness of antihypertensive diuretics.— M. A. Weber *et al.*, *Ann. intern. Med.*, 1977, *87*, 558.

Further references: D. K. Falch *et al.*, *Curr. ther. Res.*, 1979, *26*, 372.

Hypoparathyroidism. Administration of chlorthalidone 50 mg daily in association with a salt-restricted dietary regimen, given to 7 hypoparathyroid patients for periods of up to 25 months, effectively controlled the symptoms of hypoparathyroidism without incurring the hypercalcaemia or hypercalciuria associated with vitamin-D therapy. Neither the diuretic therapy nor the salt-restricted dietary regimen were as effective alone.— R. H. Porter *et al.*, *New Engl. J. Med.*, 1978, *298*, 577. Chlorothiazide 500 mg daily added to the regimen of a 14-year-old boy with hypoparathyroidism had no noticeable effect on plasma or urinary concentrations of calcium.— J. M. Gertner and M. Genel (letter), *ibid.*, 1478. Metabolic alkalosis was a common complication of treatment with thiazides and there was potential danger if they were used in hypoparathyroid patients with endogenous metabolic alkalosis.— U. S. Barzel (letter), *ibid.* Reply.— W. N. Suki (letter), *ibid.*, 1479. Further criticism.— D. A. McCarron (letter), *ibid.*, *299*, 900. Reply.— W. N. Suki (letter), *ibid.* Further comment.— C. N. de Deuxchaisnes *et al.* (letter), *ibid.*, 1979, *300*, 140.

Premenstrual syndrome. A double-blind study indicating that chlorthalidone is no more effective than placebo in relieving the premenstrual syndrome.— B. Mattsson and B. V. Schoultz, *Acta psychiat. scand.*, 1974, *255*, *Suppl.*, 75.

Further references: H. Kramer, *S.Afr. med. J.*, 1962, *36*, 4.

For reference to the possible role of diuretics in exacerbating and perpetuating idiopathic oedema, see Oedema, under Adverse Effects of Chlorothiazide, p.588.

Preparations

Chlorthalidone Tablets *(B.P.)*. Tablets containing chlorthalidone.

Chlorthalidone Tablets *(U.S.P.)*. Tablets containing chlorthalidone.

Hygroton *(Geigy, UK)*. Chlorthalidone, available as scored tablets of 50 and 100 mg. (Also available as Hygroton in *Arg., Austral., Belg., Canad., Denm., Fr., Ger., Neth., Norw., S.Afr., Swed., Switz., USA)*. **Hygroton-K.** Sustained-release tablets each containing chlorthalidone 25 mg and potassium chloride 500 mg (potassium 6.7 mmol; 6.7 mEq).

Owing to the risk of intestinal obstruction, sustained-release preparations such as Hygroton-K, where the drug is released in transit, but the matrix ghost is often eliminated intact, should not be prescribed in patients with Crohn's disease or other intestinal disease in which strictures may form.— J. L. Shaffer *et al.* (letter), *Lancet* 1980, *2*, 487.

Other Proprietary Names

Higrotona *(Spain)*; Hydro-long *(Ger.)*; Igrolina, Igroton *(both Ital.)*; Novothalidone *(Canad.)*; Renon *(Ital.)*; Urid *(Austral.)*; Uridon *(Canad.)*; Urolin, Zambesil *(both Ital.)*.

2319-q

Clofenamide. Monochlorphenamide. 4-Chlorobenzene-1,3-disulphonamide.
$C_6H_7ClN_2O_4S_2$=270.7.

CAS — 671-95-4.

Clofenamide is a diuretic with general properties similar to those described under dichlorphenamide (see p.593). It has been given in doses of 200 to 400 mg daily on 2 or 3 days a week.

Effects on the eyes. A study indicating that usual therapeutic doses of clofenamide interfere with colour vision.— J. Laroche and C. Laroche, *Annls pharm. fr.*, 1972, *30*, 433.

2320-d

Clopamide. DT 327. 4-Chloro-*N*-(2,6-dimethylpiperidino)-3-sulphamoylbenzamide.
$C_{14}H_{20}ClN_3O_3S$=345.8.

CAS — 636-54-4.

A white or almost white, almost odourless crystalline powder. M.p. about 246°. **Soluble** 1 in about 250 of water, 1 in about 100 of dehydrated alcohol, and 1 in about 250 of chloroform.

Adverse Effects, Treatment, and Precautions. As for Chlorothiazide, p.588.

Diabetogenic effect. In 15 diabetic patients not receiving insulin, clopamide 30 mg daily caused a significant elevation in the blood-glucose concentration.— B. H. Hicks *et al.*, *Metabolism*, 1973, *22*, 101.

Effects on the eyes. A study indicating that usual therapeutic doses of clopamide interfere with colour vision.— J. Laroche and C. Laroche, *Annls pharm. fr.*, 1972, *30*, 433.

Interactions. *Antibiotics.* For the effect of clopamide on the urinary elimination of chloramphenicol, see Chloramphenicol, p.1138.

Uses. Clopamide is a diuretic which has certain structural similarities to the thiazides and has actions and uses similar to those of chlorothiazide (see p.589). Diuresis is initiated in about 2 hours and lasts for up to 24 hours. In the treatment of oedema the usual initial dose is 40 to 60 mg daily, reduced to a maintenance dose of 20 to 40 mg daily or intermittently. The usual dose in the treatment of hypertension is 20 to 40 mg daily, either alone, or in conjunction with other antihypertensive agents.

When treatment is prolonged, or in susceptible patients, loss of potassium may be sufficient to produce hypokalaemia; potassium supplements should then be given as for chlorothiazide.

Action. A study in subjects without apparent cardiac or renal impairment showed that clopamide was an effective natriuretic agent with a rapid onset of action. The optimum dose was 60 mg, the effects of which lasted for 16 hours.— F. J. Radcliff *et al.*, *Curr. ther. Res.*, 1968, *10*, 103.

Further references: J. P. Radó *et al.*, *J. clin. Pharmac.*, 1969, *9*, 99.

Cardiac disorders. *Heart failure.* Beneficial results on oedema in patients with congestive heart failure following administration of clopamide.— G. L. Donnelly *et al.*, *Curr. ther. Res.*, 1969, *11*, 137.

Further references: T. Winsor and W. J. Wells, *J. new Drugs*, 1966, *6*, 155; B. W. Johansson, *Svenska Läkartidn.*, 1967, *64*, 4945; P. H. J. Theobald, *Med. J. Aust.*, 1967, *2*, 15.

Hepatic disorders. Clopamide seemed more suitable than hydrochlorothiazide in the treatment of patients with hyperammonaemia.— I. Szám *et al.* (letter), *Lancet*, 1969, *2*, 602.

Hypertension. After 3 days free from antihypertensive agents, clopamide 25 mg twice daily gave as good a control of hypertension as 50 mg twice daily in 14 hypertensive patients on a constant daily diet containing potassium 50 to 60 mmol (50 to 60 mEq) and sodium 80 to 100 mmol (80 to 100 mEq). Exchangeable potassium and serum-potassium concentrations fell slightly while urinary potassium loss, beginning after the peak sodium diuresis, was equal to dietary intake. Clopamide

50 and 100 mg produced identical water and chloride diuresis, while sodium diuresis increased after 100 mg.— F. K. Bauer, *J. clin. Pharmac.*, 1969, *9*, 16.

Further references to the use of clopamide in hypertension, either alone, or in conjunction with other antihypertensive agents: R. P. Faupel and R. Gotzen, *Dt. med. Wschr.*, 1978, *103*, 1602; D. Crowder and E. G. M. Cameron, *Curr. med. Res. Opinion*, 1979, *6*, 342; E. Török *et al.*, *ibid.*, 193; W. Reiterer, *ibid.*, 1980, *6*, 552.

Proprietary Preparations

Brinaldix *(Sandoz, UK)*. Clopamide, available as scored tablets of 20 mg. (Also available as Brinaldix in *Austral., Belg., Denm., Fr., Ger., Ital., Neth., Norw., Spain, Swed., Switz.*) **Brinaldix K.** Effervescent tablets each containing clopamide 20 mg, potassium bicarbonate 400 mg, and potassium chloride 600 mg providing potassium 12 mmol (12 mEq), with anhydrous citric acid 800 mg.

Other Proprietary Names

Adurix *(Denm.)*.

2321-n

Clorexolone. M&B 8430; RP 12833. 6-Chloro-2-cyclohexyl-3-oxoisoindoline-5-sulphonamide.
$C_{14}H_{17}ClN_2O_3S$=328.8.

CAS — 2127-01-7.

A white crystalline powder. M.p. about 266°. Very slightly **soluble** in water; soluble in solutions of alkali hydroxides.

Adverse Effects, Treatment, and Precautions. As for Chlorothiazide, p.588.

Diabetogenic effect. In 15 diabetic patients not receiving insulin, clorexolone 25 mg daily caused a significant elevation in the blood-glucose concentration.— B. H. Hicks *et al.*, *Metabolism*, 1973, *22*, 101.

Further references: J. L. Verbov *et al.*, *Br. J. clin. Pract.*, 1966, *20*, 351.

Effects on the eyes. A study indicating that usual therapeutic doses of clorexolone interfere with colour vision.— J. Laroche and C. Laroche, *Annls pharm. fr.*, 1972, *30*, 433.

Uses. Clorexolone is a diuretic which has certain structural similarities to the thiazides and has actions and uses similar to those of chlorothiazide (see p.589). It has a diuretic action lasting 24 to 48 hours.

In the treatment of oedema, 25 to 100 mg may be given daily or on alternate days. In the treatment of hypertension, the usual dose is 10 to 25 mg daily, either alone, or in conjunction with other antihypertensive agents. For diabetes insipidus a dose of 10 to 20 mg daily has been suggested.

When treatment is prolonged, or in susceptible patients, loss of potassium may be sufficient to produce hypokalaemia; potassium supplements should then be given as for chlorothiazide.

Action. Clorexolone given by mouth did not affect glomerular filtration-rate, and its action appeared to be primarily on the kidney tubules, inhibition of carbonic anhydrase playing no significant part. Natriuresis was independent of aldosterone antagonism and was at least in part due to selective inhibition of sodium reabsorption in the distal tubules.— W. I. Baba *et al.*, *Clin. Pharmac. Ther.*, 1966, *7*, 212.

No significant differences were found in the metabolic and antihypertensive effects of clorexolone and hydrochlorothiazide.— R. P. Russell *et al.*, *Clin. Pharmac. Ther.*, 1969, *10*, 265.

Further references: A. F. Lant *et al.*, *Clin. Pharmac. Ther.*, 1966, *7*, 196.

Hypertension. Clorexolone was given for up to 12 months to 23 out-patients with mild to moderate hypertension. Five of them were already taking a sympatholytic drug but this was stopped in 2. The usual dose of clorexolone was 10 mg twice daily but doses of 10 mg daily and 10 mg thrice weekly were also tried. In 3 patients who were unresponsive to 20 mg daily, the dose was increased to 25 mg twice daily with little further effect.— F. O. Simpson, *Curr. ther. Res.*, 1964, *6*, 21.

Proprietary Preparations

Nefrolan *(May & Baker, UK)*. Clorexolone, available as scored tablets of 10 mg. (Also available as Nefrolan in *Austral., S.Afr.*).

2322-h

Couch-grass *(B.P.C. 1934)*. Agropyrum; Twitch; Graminis Rhizoma; Chiendent.

Pharmacopoeias. In *Pol.* and *Swiss.*

The rhizome of *Agropyron repens*(=*Triticum repens*) (Gramineae). It contains glucose, mannitol, inositol, and triticin (a carbohydrate resembling inulin).

Couch-grass is a mild diuretic which has been used in the treatment of infections of the urinary tract. It has usually been employed as a decoction (1 in 20; in doses of 15 to 60 ml) or as a liquid extract (1 in 1) in doses of 4 to 8 ml.

2323-m

Cyclopenthiazide *(B.P.)*.

Cyclopenthiaz.; Su 8341. 6-Chloro-3-cyclopentylmethyl-3,4-dihydro-2*H*-1,2,4-benzothiadiazine-7-sulphonamide 1,1-dioxide.
$C_{13}H_{18}ClN_3O_4S_2$=379.9.

CAS — 742-20-1.

Pharmacopoeias. In *Br.*

A white, odourless, almost tasteless powder. Practically **insoluble** in water; soluble 1 in 12 of alcohol and 1 in 600 of chloroform; soluble in acetone and in ether.

Adverse Effects, Treatment, and Precautions. As for Chlorothiazide, p.588.

Oedema. For reference to the possible role of diuretics in exacerbating and perpetuating idiopathic oedema, see Oedema, under Adverse Effects of Chlorothiazide, p.588.

Uses. Cyclopenthiazide is a thiazide diuretic with actions and uses similar to those of chlorothiazide (see p.589). Diuresis is induced in 1 to 2 hours and lasts up to about 12 hours.

In the treatment of oedema the usual initial dose is 0.5 to 1 mg daily, reduced to a dose of 250 to 500 µg daily or 500 µg on alternate days. In the treatment of hypertension the usual dose is 250 to 500 µg daily either alone, or in conjunction with other antihypertensive agents. The maximum effective daily dose of cyclopenthiazide is reported to be 1.5 mg, and to be rarely required.

When treatment is prolonged, or in susceptible patients, loss of potassium may be sufficient to produce hypokalaemia; potassium supplements should then be given as for chlorothiazide.

References to the use of cyclopenthiazide: J. V. Hodge *et al.*, *N.Z. med. J.*, 1962, *61*, 258 (hypertension). Report No. 24 of the General Practitioner Research Group, *Practitioner*, 1962, *188*, 679 (heart failure or varicose veins); W. A. Forrest, *Br. J. clin. Pract.*, 1978, *32*, 326 (hypertension).

Pregnancy and the neonate. *Hypertension of pregnancy.* A study indicating that administration of cyclopenthiazide produced no significant reduction in the incidence of pre-eclampsia in high-weight-gain primigravidas, compared with similar control women.— D. M. Campbell and I. MacGillivray, *Br. J. Obstet. Gynaec.*, 1975, *82*, 572.

See also under Precautions for Chlorothiazide, p.589.

Preparations

Cyclopenthiazide Tablets *(B.P.)*. Tablets containing cyclopenthiazide.

Navidrex *(Ciba, UK)*. Cyclopenthiazide, available as scored tablets of 500 µg. (Also available as Navidrex in *Austral., Belg., Denm., Ger., Neth., S.Afr., Switz.*).

Navidrex-K *(Ciba, UK)*. Tablets each containing cyclopenthiazide 250 µg in an outer coating and potassium chloride 600 mg (potassium 8.1 mmol; 8.1 mEq) in a slow-release wax core.

Owing to the risk of intestinal obstruction, sustained-release preparations such as Navidrex-K, where the drug is released in transit, but the matrix ghost is often eliminated intact, should not be prescribed in patients with Crohn's disease or other intestinal disease in which strictures may form.— J. L. Shaffer *et al.* (letter), *Lancet*, 1980, *2*, 487.

2324-b

Cyclothiazide *(U.S.P.)*.

MDi 193. 6-Chloro-3,4-dihydro-3-(norborn-5-en-2-yl)-2*H*-1,2,4-benzothiadiazine-7-sulphonamide 1,1-dioxide.
$C_{14}H_{16}ClN_3O_4S_2$=389.9.

CAS — 2259-96-3.

Pharmacopoeias. In *U.S.*

A white or almost white, almost odourless powder. M.p. 217° to 225° with a range not exceeding 4°. Practically **insoluble** in water and chloroform; soluble 1 in 70 of alcohol and 1 in 30 of methyl alcohol; freely soluble in acetone.

Adverse Effects, Treatment, and Precautions. As for Chlorothiazide, p.588.

Inappropriate secretion of antidiuretic hormone. Cyclothiazide, 5 mg daily for 5 days then 10 mg daily for 2 days, increased the secretion of antidiuretic hormone in a 63-year-old woman, causing an impairment in the excretion of a water load, and an inability to dilute urine. Hyponatraemia with clouding of consciousness and incoherence also occurred. These symptoms disappeared after discontinuation of the drug.— J. Horowitz *et al.*, *J. clin. Pharmac.*, 1972, *12*, 337.

Uses. Cyclothiazide is a thiazide diuretic with actions and uses similar to those of chlorothiazide (see p.589). Diuresis is initiated in about 2 hours and lasts for 18 to 24 hours.

In the treatment of oedema the usual initial dose is 1 to 2 mg daily, reduced to a dose of 1 or 2 mg on alternate days or twice or thrice weekly. A suggested initial dose for children is 20 to 40 µg per kg body-weight daily.

In the treatment of hypertension the usual dose is 2 mg daily, either alone, or in conjunction with other antihypertensive agents; in some cases doses of 2 mg up to thrice daily may be required.

When treatment is prolonged, or in susceptible patients, loss of potassium may be sufficient to produce hypokalaemia; potassium supplements should then be given as for Chlorothiazide.

Preparations

Cyclothiazide Tablets *(U.S.P.)*. Tablets containing cyclothiazide.

Proprietary Names

Anhydron *(Lilly, USA)*; Doburil *(Boehringer Ingelheim, Austral.; Pharmacia, Denm.; Boehringer Sohn, Spain)*.

2325-v

Dichlorphenamide *(B.P., U.S.P.)*. Diclofenamide; Diclofenamidum. 4,5-Dichlorobenzene-1,3-disulphonamide.
$C_6H_6Cl_2N_2O_4S_2$=305.2.

CAS — 120-97-8.

Pharmacopoeias. In *Br., Chin.,* and *U.S.*

A white or almost white crystalline powder with a slight characteristic odour and taste followed by a bitter after-taste. M.p. about 240°.

Practically **insoluble** in water and chloroform; soluble 1 in 30 of alcohol; slightly soluble in ether; freely soluble in pyridine; soluble in solutions of alkali hydroxides and carbonates.

Adverse Effects. As for Acetazolamide, p.581. Blood disorders do not appear to have been reported.

Effects on the kidneys. Four of 7 patients given 50 mg of dichlorphenamide 4 times daily developed a rise in blood urea to between 550 and 700 mg per litre. It rapidly returned to normal after therapy ceased.— E. Wahl and C. F. McCarthy (letter), *Lancet*, 1961, *1*, 620.

Precautions. As for Acetazolamide, p.581.

Dichlorphenamide should be employed with caution in the presence of pulmonary disorders when there is a severe loss of pulmonary ventilation.

Uses. Dichlorphenamide is an inhibitor of carbonic anhydrase which has actions similar to those of acetazolamide (see p.582); unlike acetazolamide it has also been reported to cause an increase in the excretion of chlorides. When given by mouth, its effect begins within 1 hour and lasts for up to 12 hours.

Dichlorphenamide is used to reduce intra-ocular pressure

in glaucoma. The usual initial adult dose is 100 to 200 mg, then 100 mg every 12 hours, followed by a maintenance dose of 25 to 50 mg once to thrice daily. When treatment is prolonged, or in susceptible patients, loss of potassium may be sufficient to produce hypokalaemia; potassium supplements should then be given as for Chlorothiazide.

Respiratory disorders. A report of some improvement in the blood gases of bronchial patients able to tolerate long-term dichlorphenamide therapy. There was no symptomatic improvement.— W. M. Nelson and W. F. M. Wallace, *Br. med. J.*, 1965, *1*, 759.

Further references: B. Mann, *Dis. Chest*, 1963, *43*, 285; A. Naimark and R. M. Cherniack, *Can. med. Ass. J.*, 1966, *94*, 164.

Preparations

Dichlorphenamide Tablets *(B.P., U.S.P.)*. Tablets containing dichlorphenamide.

Daranide *(Merck Sharp & Dohme, UK)*. Dichlorphenamide, available as scored tablets of 50 mg. (Also available as Daranide in *Austral., Belg., Canad., Neth., Swed.*).

Oratrol *(Alcon, UK: Farillon, UK)*. Dichlorphenamide, available as scored tablets of 50 mg. (Also available as Oratrol in *Austral., Belg., Fr., Neth., Spain, Switz.*).

Other Proprietary Names

Antidrasi *(also as sodium salt) (Arg., Ital.)*; Fenamide *(Ital.)*; Glauconide *(Spain)*; Glaumid *(Ital.)*; Hipotensor Oftalmico *(Spain)*; Oralcon *(Denm., Swed.)*; Tensodilen *(Spain)*.

2326-g

Disulphamide *(B.P.C. 1968)*. 5-Chlorotoluene-2,4-disulphonamide.

$C_7H_9ClN_2O_4S_2$=284.7.

CAS — 671-88-5.

A white or creamy-white, odourless, tasteless, crystalline powder. **Soluble** 1 in 500 of water, 1 in 50 of alcohol, and 1 in 1000 of ether; slightly soluble in chloroform.

Disulphamide is a diuretic which has certain structural similarities to the thiazides and has actions and uses similar to those of chlorothiazide (see p.587) but which also inhibits the action of carbonic anhydrase, thereby increasing the excretion of bicarbonate ions, as described under acetazolamide (see p.582). Potassium supplements should be given, where deemed necessary, as for chlorothiazide (see p.589).

In the treatment of oedema the usual initial dose was 200 mg daily for 5 days a week or on alternate days, reduced to 100 mg daily.

Preparations

Disulphamide Tablets *(B.P.C. 1968)*. Tablets containing disulphamide.

Proprietary Names

Diluen *(Libra, Ital.)*; Toluidrin *(Radiumfarma, Ital.)*.

2327-q

Epithiazide. Epitizide. 6-Chloro-3,4-dihydro-3-(2,2,2-trifluoroethylthiomethyl)-2*H*-1,2,4-benzothiadiazine-7-sulphonamide 1,1-dioxide.

$C_{10}H_{11}ClF_3N_3O_4S_3$=425.8.

CAS — 1764-85-8.

A white crystalline powder with a faint characteristic odour. Practically **insoluble** in water; soluble in alkaline solutions.

Epithiazide is a thiazide diuretic with actions and uses similar to those of chlorothiazide (see p.587). It is given in doses of 4 mg twice or thrice daily as an ingredient of Thiaver (see p.136).

2363-e

Ethacrynate Sodium. Etacrynate Sodium; Sodium Etacrynate; Sodium Ethacrynate.

$C_{13}H_{11}Cl_2NaO_4$=325.1.

CAS — 6500-81-8.

Pharmacopoeias. In *Chin. U.S.* includes Ethacrynate Sodium for Injection.

2328-p

Ethacrynic Acid *(B.P., U.S.P.)*. Acidum Etacrynicum; Etacrynic Acid *(Eur. P.)*; Etacrynsäure; MK 595. [2,3-Dichloro-4-(2-ethylacryloyl)phenoxy]acetic acid.

$C_{13}H_{12}Cl_2O_4$=303.1.

CAS — 58-54-8.

Pharmacopoeias. In *Br., Chin., Eur., Fr., Ger., Neth., Nord.*, and *U.S.*

A white or almost white, odourless or almost odourless, crystalline powder. M.p. about 123°. Very slightly **soluble** in water; soluble 1 in 1.6 of alcohol, 1 in 6 of chloroform, and 1 in 3.5 of ether. Solutions of the sodium salt are stable at pH 7 and room temperatures for short periods and less stable at higher pH values and temperatures. **Incompatible** with solutions with a pH below 5. It forms water-soluble compounds with hydroxides, alkali carbonates, and ammonia. **Store** in airtight containers.

CAUTION. *Ethacrynic acid, especially in the form of dust, is irritating to the skin, eyes, and mucous membranes.*

Incompatibility. There were changes in the u.v. spectra indicating chemical change and possible incompatibility when ethacrynate sodium was added to sodium chloride injection containing hydralazine hydrochloride, procainamide hydrochloride, or tolazoline hydrochloride. A precipitate occurred with reserpine injection (Serpasil). Ethacrynate sodium appeared to be compatible with chlorpromazine hydrochloride, prochlorperazine edisylate, and promazine hydrochloride.— P. N. Catania and J. C. King, *Am. J. Hosp. Pharm.*, 1972, *29*, 141.

It has been recommended that ethacrynic acid may be dissolved in a 5% solution of dextrose for infusion or slow injection, but if this has a pH below 5 the resulting solution may be cloudy and should not be used. In addition, ethacrynic acid should not be mixed with whole blood or blood derivatives; if it is desired to give ethacrynic acid at the same time as a blood transfusion it should be given independently.

Adverse Effects. The most common side-effect associated with ethacrynic acid therapy is fluid and electrolyte imbalance after either single large doses or prolonged administration.

Anorexia, dysphagia, nausea and vomiting, and diarrhoea may also occur; profuse watery diarrhoea is an indication for stopping ethacrynic acid therapy. Gastro-intestinal bleeding has been associated with ethacrynic acid; vertigo, tinnitus and deafness, which may not be reversible, may rarely occur particularly following high-dose parenteral therapy. Liver damage and paraesthesia have also been reported.

Other side-effects reported are allergy, skin rashes, purpura, headache, blurred vision, confusion, fatigue, fever, muscle spasm, hypotension, gynaecomastia, pancreatitis, and blood disorders, including agranulocytosis, neutropenia, and thrombocytopenia.

Ethacrynic acid may provoke hyperglycaemia and glycosuria, but probably to a lesser extent than the thiazide diuretics; hypoglycaemia has also been reported following large doses in 2 uraemic patients. It may cause hyperuricaemia and precipitate attacks of gout in some patients. Unlike the thiazide diuretics it increases the urinary excretion of calcium.

Local irritation and pain may follow accidental extravasation of the intravenous injection.

An account of the toxic effects of ethacrynic acid.— F. D. Schwartz *et al.*, *Am. Heart J.*, 1970, *79*, 427, per *Drugs*, 1971, *1*, 492.

Abuse. Abuse of mefruside and ethacrynic acid by a 46-year-old nurse led to hypokalaemia, polyuria, and raised plasma-renin concentrations without hyperaldosteronism.— C. Fuchs *et al.*, *Dt. med. Wschr.*, 1977, *102*, 1319.

Diabetogenic effect and hypoglycaemia. High doses of ethacrynic acid induced symptomatic hypoglycaemia with convulsions in 2 patients with uraemia.— J. F. Maher and G. E. Schreiner, *Ann. intern. Med.*, 1965, *62*, 15.

Ethacrynic acid 200 mg daily and hydrochlorothiazide 200 mg daily each reduced glucose tolerance when tested in 24 patients with essential hypertension. The effect was more pronounced with hydrochlorothiazide than with ethacrynic acid; the latter showed its most pronounced effect in diabetic subjects.— R. P. Russell *et al.*, *J. Am. med. Ass.*, 1968, *205*, 11.

One patient with heart failure developed hyperosmolar hyperglycaemic coma after 3 months' treatment with ethacrynic acid 200 to 400 mg daily in divided doses. Patients should be monitored for the development of hyperglycaemia.— A. J. Cowley and R. S. Elkeles (letter), *Lancet*, 1978, *1*, 154.

Further references: O. O. Andersen and I. Persson, *Br. med. J.*, 1968, *2*, 798.

Effects on the blood. *Agranulocytosis.* A report of fatal agranulocytosis in association with ethacrynic acid.— J. G. Walker, *Ann. intern. Med.*, 1966, *64*, 1303.

Haemolysis. The addition of ethacrynic acid in concentrations greater than 2 mmol per litre caused immediate damage to red cells in whole blood. Frusemide did not have this effect.— J. Lieberman and W. Kaneshiro (letter), *Lancet*, 1971, *1*, 911.

Haemolytic anaemia. Suspected haemolytic anaemia in a patient receiving ethacrynic acid therapy.— M. Hanna, *Med. J. Aust.*, 1966, *1*, 534.

Effects on the ears. The Boston Collaborative Drug Surveillance Program monitored consecutively 32 812 medical inpatients. Drug-induced deafness occurred in 2 of 184 patients given ethacrynic acid.— J. Porter and H. Jick, *Lancet*, 1977, *1*, 587. See also Boston Collaborative Drug Surveillance Program, *J. Am. med. Ass.*, 1973, *224*, 515.

Deafness accompanied by nystagmus occurred in a patient following the slow intravenous infusion of 100 mg of ethacrynic acid; the side-effects resolved within 1 hour.— I. H. Gomolin and E. Garshick (letter), *New Engl. J. Med.*, 1980, *303*, 702.

Further references: G. J. Matz *et al.* (letter), *J. Am. med. Ass.*, 1968, *206*, 2119; V. K. G. Pillay *et al.*, *Lancet*, 1969, *1*, 77; R. H. Mathog and W. J. Klein, *New Engl. J. Med.*, 1969, *280*, 1223; W. D. Meriwether *et al.*, *J. Am. med. Ass.*, 1971, *216*, 795.

Effects on the electrolyte balance. *Calcium and magnesium.* In 3 healthy adults ethacrynic acid, 50 mg intravenously, increased the excretion of calcium and magnesium in the urine. A similar effect was observed in 3 patients given 200 to 400 mg daily in divided doses by mouth.— F. E. Demartini *et al.*, *Proc. Soc. exp. Biol. Med.*, 1967, *124*, 320.

Potassium. Ethacrynic acid caused little loss of potassium at low levels of sodium excretion.— J. B. Puschett and A. Rastegal, *Clin. Pharmac. Ther.*, 1974, *15*, 397.

Effects on the gastro-intestinal tract. Symptoms of gastro-intestinal intolerance, consisting of indigestion, nausea, vomiting, or occasional diarrhoea, occurred in 7 of 40 out-patients given ethacrynic acid therapy.— A. C. Newell, *Med. J. Aust.*, 1970, *1*, 320.

Of 26 294 hospital in-patients monitored by the Boston Collaborative Drug Surveillance Program, major gastro-intestinal bleeding occurred in only 57. Of these 57 patients, 37 had been receiving ethacrynic acid, heparin, warfarin, corticosteroids, or aspirin-containing drugs either alone or in different associations. The highest percentage of bleeds relative to patients exposed occurred in those receiving ethacrynic acid intravenously alone (4.5%) or by mouth in association with heparin or corticosteroids (6.3%).— Jick H. and J. Porter, *lancet*, 1978, *2*, 87.

Further references: D. Slone *et al.*, *J. Am. med. Ass.*, 1969, *209*, 1668; W. H. Wilkinson *et al.* (letter), *ibid.*, *210*, 347; D. Slone *et al.* (letter), *ibid.*

Effects on the kidneys. Transient bilateral abdominal pain, radiating to the genitalia, occurred in a patient a few minutes after taking ethacrynic acid.— N. G. Kounis (letter), *Br. med. J.*, 1973, *3*, 641.

Effects on the liver. A 25-year-old man developed hepatocellular damage on 3 occasions probably due to ethacrynic acid which he had taken in dosages varying from 50 to 200 mg daily for periods of 1 to 7 weeks. On 2 occasions the jaundice regressed when ethacrynic acid was discontinued, but on the third occasion the jaundice persisted and he died in congestive cardiac failure.— K. K. Datey *et al.*, *Br. med. J.*, 1967, *3*, 152.

Effects on the skin. Purpura. A report of a patient in whom extensive purpuric and ecchymotic rashes might have been associated with ethacrynic acid administration. The patient subsequently died and among other post-mortem findings, there was extensive gastro-duodenal ulceration.— A. K. Pain (letter), *Br. med. J.*, 1967, *1*, 634.

Oedema. For reference to the possible role of diuretics in exacerbating and perpetuating idiopathic oedema, see Oedema, under Adverse Effects of Chlorothiazide, p.588.

Treatment of Adverse Effects. As for Chlorothiazide, p.589.

Precautions. As for Chlorothiazide, p.589.

Ethacrynic acid should be used with care in patients with prostatic hypertrophy or impairment of micturition.

Ethacrynic acid may enhance the nephrotoxicity of the aminoglycoside antibiotics such as gentamicin, kanamycin, neomycin, and streptomycin. The risks of gastro-intestinal bleeding associated with ethacrynic acid administration may be enhanced by concurrent administration of anticoagulants.

Interactions. *Antibiotics.* For the effect of ethacrynic acid on the urinary elimination of chloramphenicol, see Chloramphenicol, p.1138.

Anticoagulants. A study of haemolytic reactions and drug interactions in 500 warfarin-treated patients. Among interactions not previously noted clinically was one with ethacrynic acid.— J. Koch-Weser, *Clin. Pharmac. Ther.*, 1973, *14*, 139.

Further references: J. Koch-Weser, *Am. Heart J.*, 1975, *90*, 93.

For reference to gastro-intestinal bleeding associated with concurrent administration of heparin and ethacrynic acid, see Heparin, p.765.

Absorption and Fate. Ethacrynic acid is fairly rapidly absorbed from the gastro-intestinal tract. *Animal* studies have indicated that it has a short half-life and is excreted both in the bile and the urine, partly unchanged and partly in the form of metabolites. It is bound to plasma proteins.

Animal studies on the absorption and fate of ethacrynic acid.— K. H. Beyer *et al.*, *J. Pharmac. exp. Ther.*, 1965, *147*, 1.

Uses. Although chemically unrelated, ethacrynic acid is a diuretic with actions and uses similar to those of frusemide (see p.598). Diuresis is initiated within about 30 minutes after a dose by mouth, and lasts for about 6 hours; after intravenous injection of its sodium salt, the effects are evident within a few minutes and last for about 2 hours.

In the treatment of oedema, the usual initial dose is 50 mg in the morning, taken with or immediately after food; in some cases higher doses may be necessary, and severe cases have required gradual titration of the ethacrynic acid dosage up to a maximum of 400 mg daily, but the effective dose range is usually between 50 and 150 mg daily. Dosage of 100 mg or more daily should be given in divided doses, and it is preferable for all doses to be taken with food. Maintenance doses may be taken daily or intermittently and are usually less than the initial doses.

In emergency, such as acute pulmonary oedema, or when oral therapy cannot be given, ethacrynic acid may be given by slow intravenous injection or intravenous infusion as its salt, ethacrynate sodium, in a dose equivalent to 50 mg of ethacrynic acid dissolved in 50 ml of dextrose 5%(but see above under Incompatibility) or sodium chloride 0.9% solution; should a subsequent injection be required the site should be changed to avoid thrombophlebitis. Single doses of 100 mg have been given intravenously in critical situations. It is not suitable for subcutaneous or intramuscular injection.

For children a suggested initial dose of ethacrynic acid is 25 mg daily by mouth, cautiously increased as necessary by 25 mg daily.

When treatment is prolonged, or in susceptible patients, loss of potassium may be sufficient to produce hypokalaemia; potassium supplements should then be given as for chlorothiazide (see p.589). If very high doses are used careful laboratory control is essential as described under the uses for frusemide (p.598; high-dose therapy).

Action. A review of short-acting diuretics. The mode of action of ethacrynic acid is similar to that of frusemide. It is unsuitable for parenteral use because of its low solubility and the pain injection causes.— *Drug & Ther. Bull.*, 1979, *17*, 48.

A report of detailed *animal* studies into the mode of action of ethacrynic acid.— K. H. Beyer *et al.*, *J. Pharmac. exp. Ther.*, 1965, *147*, 1.

Administration. *In children.* In infants under 1 year of age with cardiac failure the dose of ethacrynic acid is 1 mg per kg body-weight intravenously repeated after 12 hours if necessary, or 3 mg per kg daily by mouth.— D. Goldring *et al.*, *Pediatrics*, 1971, *47*, 1056.

Further references: A. W. Sparrow *et al.*, *Pediatrics*, 1968, *42*, 291.

Administration in renal failure. Ethacrynic acid should be avoided in patients with a glomerular filtration-rate of less than 10 ml per minute.— W. M. Bennett *et al.*, *Ann. intern. Med.*, 1980, *93*, 286.

See also under Renal Disorders (below).

Cardiac disorders. Heart failure. Reports of beneficial results with ethacrynic acid in patients with right or left heart failure: P. M. Buckfield and M. Hamilton, *J. Ther.*, 1966, *1* (2), 5; H. Oelert and F. Sebening, *Dt. med. Wschr.*, 1968, *93*, 1550; A. Ramirez and W. H. Abelmann, *Archs intern. Med.*, 1968, *121*, 320; M. Scheinman *et al.*, *Am. J. Med.*, 1971, *50*, 291.

Diabetes insipidus. Three boys with nephrogenic diabetes insipidus were given ethacrynic acid intravenously, and in 2 the urinary output was decreased. The 2 who responded were then treated with ethacrynic acid by mouth, 150 mg initially and then up to 100 and 200 mg daily. Sodium intake was controlled. Both required supplements of potassium chloride, 75 to 120 mmol (75 to 120 mEq) daily, and both developed hyperuricaemia.— D. M. Brown *et al.*, *Pediatrics*, 1966, *37*, 447.

A study of the mechanism of the antidiuretic effect of saliuretic drugs, including ethacrynic acid, in diabetes insipidus.— G. Ramos *et al.*, *Clin. Pharmac. Ther.*, 1967, *8*, 557.

Hepatic disorders. Reports on the use of ethacrynic acid alone or with other diuretics in cirrhosis of the liver, emphasising the hazards of powerful diuretics in hepatic disorders: F. L. Lieberman and T. B. Reynolds, *Gastroenterology*, 1965, *49*, 531; Sherlock S. *et al.*, *Lancet*, 1966, *1*, 1049.

For later reports on powerful diuretic therapy in hepatic disorders, see Hepatic Disorders under Uses of Frusemide, p.599.

Hypertension. Oedema associated with cardiac failure was satisfactorily controlled in 57 ambulant patients given ethacrynic acid 50 to 250 mg every other day; blood pressure was reduced in hypertensive patients.— D. G. Wombolt *et al.*, *Clin. Med.*, 1971, *78* (Mar.), 24.

Pulmonary oedema. Results of a comparative study involving ethacrynic acid in pulmonary oedema indicated that clinical improvement did not depend upon rapidity of diuresis but was secondary to the underlying cardiac disorder.— M. Lesch *et al.*, *New Engl. J. Med.*, 1968, *279*, 115.

Further references: S. L. Fine and R. I. Levy, *New Engl. J. Med.*, 1965, *273*, 583.

For further studies on the role of rapid-acting diuretics in pulmonary oedema, see under Frusemide, Action, p.598, and Mountain Sickness and Pulmonary Oedema, p.599.

Renal disorders. Of 22 patients with oedema and severe chronic renal failure who received on average 150 mg of ethacrynic acid daily for 9 days, in only 3 did diuresis not occur.— K. D. G. Edwards *et al.*, *Med. J. Aust.*, 1967, *1*, 375.

Two patients with oliguric acute renal failure, unresponsive to mannitol, were successfully treated with mannitol and ethacrynic acid.— R. G. Auger *et al.*, *J. Am. med. Ass.*, 1968, *206*, 891.

Further references: M. Kaye *et al.* (letter), *Lancet*, 1968, *1*, 1255.

For conflicting views on the merits of diuretic therapy in renal failure, see Frusemide (Renal Disorders), p.600.

Renal tubular acidosis. A patient with renal tubular acidosis, early renal insufficiency, and osteomalacia responded to treatment with ethacrynic acid 50 mg daily for 2 years. Urinary pH decreased and systemic acidosis disappeared. Osteomalacia receded and despite the hypercalciuric effect of ethacrynic acid, nephrocalcinosis did not get worse.— E. Heidbreder *et al.* (letter), *Lancet*, 1973, *1*, 52.

Preparations

Ethacrynate Sodium for Injection *(U.S.P.)*. A sterile, freeze-dried powder, prepared by the neutralisation of ethacrynic acid with the aid of sodium hydroxide. Potency is expressed in terms of the equivalent amount of ethacrynic acid. A solution, equivalent to 0.1% of ethacrynic acid, has a pH of 6.3 to 7.7.

Ethacrynic Acid Tablets *(B.P., U.S.P.)*. Tablets containing ethacrynic acid.

Proprietary Preparations

Edecrin *(Merck Sharp & Dohme, UK)*. Ethacrynic acid, available as scored tablets of 50 mg. (Also available as Edecrin in *Belg.*, *Canad.*, *Denm.*, *Ital.*, *Neth.*, *NZ*, *Norw.*, *Spain*, *Switz.*, *USA*).

Edecrin Injection *(Merck Sharp & Dohme, UK)*. Vials each containing ethacrynate sodium equivalent to 50 mg of ethacrynic acid, as powder for preparing intravenous injection.

Other Proprietary Names

Crinuryl *(Israel)*; Edecril *(Austral., Jap.)*; Edecrina *(Swed.)*; Édécrine *(Fr.)*; Hydromedin *(Ger.)*; Reomax *(Ital.)*; Taladren *(Ital.)*; Uregyt *(Hung.)*.

2329-s

Ethiazide. 6-Chloro-3-ethyl-3,4-dihydro-2*H*-1,2,4-benzothiadiazine-7-sulphonamide 1,1-dioxide.

$C_9H_{12}ClN_3O_4S_2$=325.8.

CAS — 1824-58-4.

Adverse Effects, Treatment, and Precautions. As for Chlorothiazide, p.588.

Uses. Ethiazide is a thiazide diuretic which has actions and uses similar to those of chlorothiazide (see p.589).

In the treatment of oedema the usual dose is 2.5 to 5 mg twice daily; it may be given on alternate days or intermittently according to the patient's response. In the treatment of hypertension the usual dose is 2.5 to 5 mg twice daily, either alone, or in conjunction with other antihypertensive agents. Higher doses have also been cited.

When treatment is prolonged, or in susceptible patients, loss of potassium may be sufficient to produce hypokalaemia; potassium supplements should then be given as for Chlorothiazide.

2330-h

Ethoxzolamide *(U.S.P.)*. Ethoxyzolamide. 6-Ethoxybenzothiazole-2-sulphonamide.

$C_9H_{10}N_2O_3S_2$=258.3.

CAS — 452-35-7.

Pharmacopoeias. In *U.S.*

A white or slightly yellow, odourless, crystalline powder. M.p. 189° to 195°. Practically **insoluble** in water; slightly soluble in alcohol, chloroform, and ether.

Adverse Effects and Precautions. As for Acetazolamide, p.581.

Uses. Ethoxzolamide is an inhibitor of carbonic anhydrase with actions and uses similar to those of acetazolamide (see p.582). Its effects last for about 10 hours.

In the treatment of glaucoma it is given in doses of 125 mg four times daily subsequently reduced to 62.5 mg four times daily if possible; an initial dose of 250 mg may be given.

Preparations

Ethoxzolamide Tablets *(U.S.P.)*. Tablets containing ethoxzolamide.

Proprietary Names

Cardrase *(Upjohn, Austral.*; *Upjohn, USA)*; Ethamide *(Allergan, USA)*; Glaucotensil *(Farmila, Ital.)*; Poenglausil *(Poen, Arg.)*; Redupresin *(Thilo, Ger.)*.

2331-m

Frusemide *(B.P., B.P. Vet.)*. Furosemide *(U.S.P.)*; Furosemidum; LB 502. 4-Chloro-*N*-furfuryl-5-sulphamoylanthranilic acid; 4-Chloro-2-furfurylamino-5-sulphamoylbenzoic acid. $C_{12}H_{11}ClN_2O_5S = 330.7$.

CAS — 54-31-9.

Pharmacopoeias. In *Br., Braz., Chin., Cz., Eur., Fr., Ger., Jap., Jug., Neth., Nord., Turk.,* and *U.S.*

A white or slightly yellow, odourless, almost tasteless, crystalline powder. M.p. about 206° with decomposition.

Practically **insoluble** in water and chloroform; soluble 1 in 75 of alcohol, 1 in 850 of ether, and 1 in 15 of acetone; freely soluble in dimethylformamide and solutions of alkali hydroxides; soluble in methyl alcohol. **Protect** from light.

Solutions for injection are prepared with the aid of sodium hydroxide, giving solutions with a pH of about 9 which can be **sterilised** by autoclaving or filtration. Such solutions should not be mixed or diluted with dextrose injection or other acidic solutions.

Stability. Stability studies of frusemide in aqueous solutions.— A. G. Ghanekar *et al., J. pharm. Sci.,* 1978, *67,* 808. See also K. A. Shah *et al., ibid.,* 1980, *69,* 594.

Adverse Effects. The most common side-effect associated with frusemide therapy is fluid and electrolyte imbalance after either single large doses or prolonged administration.

Other side-effects are relatively uncommon, and include allergy, nausea, diarrhoea, blurred vision, dizziness, headache, pancreatitis, photosensitivity, skin rashes, muscle spasm, and hypotension. Agranulocytosis, aplastic anaemia, thrombocytopenia, and leucopenia have been reported. Liver damage and paraesthesia have also been reported. Tinnitus and deafness may rarely occur. In particular, during high-dose parenteral frusemide therapy, transient deafness may occur if the infusion-rate exceeds 4 mg per minute.

Frusemide may provoke hyperglycaemia and glycosuria, but probably to a lesser extent than the thiazide diuretics. It may cause hyperuricaemia and precipitate attacks of gout in some patients. Unlike the thiazide diuretics, it increases the urinary excretion of calcium.

A brief review of the clinical hazards of the powerful diuretics, frusemide and ethacrynic acid. By far the most frequently encountered problem is excessive depletion of blood volume, which can lead to profound shock, frequently complicated by hypokalaemia, and ending in death. Metabolic abnormalities comprise the second group of adverse effects from injudicious use of frusemide and ethacrynic acid; these include hypokalaemia, hyponatraemia, and metabolic or 'contraction' alkalosis. Less commonly, frusemide worsens carbohydrate tolerance; hyperuricaemia is frequent.— V. J. Plumb and T. N. James, *Mod. Concepts cardiovasc. Dis.,* 1978, *47,* 91.

Of 553 hospital in-patients receiving frusemide 220 experienced 480 adverse reactions. Considering only the most serious reactions, electrolyte disturbances occurred in 130 patients, extracellular volume depletion in 50, hepatic coma in 20, and other toxic effects in 20. Adverse reactions were more common in patients with cirrhosis of the liver.— C. A. Naranjo *et al., Am. J. Hosp. Pharm.,* 1978, *35,* 794. See also *idem, Clin. Pharmac. Ther.,* 1979, *25,* 154 (in cirrhosis).

The incidence of adverse effects attributed to frusemide in 585 hospital patients was: volume depletion (in 85), hyperuricaemia (54), hypokalaemia (21, equally in those with or without potassium supplements), hyponatraemia (6), gastro-intestinal effects (6), confusion (2), rash (1), thrombocytopenia (1), and glycosuria (1). Adverse effects were not related to renal function; in only 3 patients were adverse effects considered life-threatening (hypokalaemia in 2). Adverse effects were dose-related.— J. Lowe *et al., Br. med. J.,* 1979, *2,* 360.

Further references: D. J. Greenblatt *et al., Am. Heart J.,* 1977, *94,* 6; M. Spino *et al., Can. med. Ass. J.,* 1978, *118,* 1513.

Abuse. Hypokalaemia occurred in 3 women who had abused frusemide and chlorthalidone.— F. H. Katz *et al., Ann. intern. Med.,* 1972, *76,* 85.

Deprecation of the use by jockeys of diuretics—usually frusemide 80 to 120 mg.— D. Price (letter), *Br. med. J.,* 1973, *1,* 804.

A woman had regularly taken frusemide 1.2 to 1.6 g daily for periods up to several weeks in an effort to lose weight. She had no evidence of renal dysfunction or other symptoms except malaise or fatigue and occasionally disturbances in potassium and chloride levels.— E. J. Howard (letter), *J. Am. med. Ass.,* 1976, *235,* 146.

Allergy or collapse. Death occurred in 2 elderly men almost immediately after they were given an injection of frusemide. Both patients had heart disease and mild diabetes.— I. Machtey (letter), *Lancet,* 1968, *2,* 1301. Thirty seconds after an injection of frusemide a 7-year-old boy with the nephrotic syndrome collapsed with cardiac and circulatory arrest, and subsequently died. Although he had previously received frusemide both orally and intravenously, it was concluded that he had a cardiac arrest caused by hypersensitivity to frusemide.— C. P. Rance (letter), *ibid.,* 1969, *1,* 1265.

A report of cross allergy between glisoxepide, glibenclamide, frusemide, and probenecid in a 55-year-old diabetic man.— B. Ummenhofer and D. Djawari, *Dt. med. Wschr.,* 1979, *104,* 514.

See also under Effects on the Skin (below).

Diabetogenic effect. Frusemide 80 mg once or twice daily was associated with the worsening of diabetes mellitus in one patient with heart failure and the precipitation of diabetes in another. Patients should be monitored for the development of hyperglycaemia.— A. J. Cowley and R. S. Elkeles (letter), *Lancet,* 1978, *1,* 154.

Further references: S. Toivonen and O. Mustala (letter), *Br. med. J.,* 1966, *1,* 920; P. R. W. Tasker and P. F. Mitchell-Heggs, *ibid.,* 1976, *1,* 626; A. A. Khaleeli and A. L. Wyman, *Postgrad. med. J.,* 1978, *54,* 43.

Effects on the blood. In a study of 204 patients, biochemical changes in the blood occurred in 117. These changes were certainly or probably induced by frusemide and were accompanied by clinical effects in 13 of these patients. It was considered that all patients receiving frusemide should be carefully monitored.— M. Spino *et al., Can. med. Ass. J.,* 1978, *118,* 1513.

Agranulocytosis or aplastic anaemia. Mention of 2 cases of fatal aplastic anaemia or agranulocytosis in one year probably due to frusemide.— W. H. W. Inman, *Br. med. J.,* 1977, *1,* 1500.

Leucopenia. Leucopenia associated with the ingestion of frusemide 1 g daily occurred in a 49-year-old male renal transplant patient. The white-cell counts returned to normal within 10 days of stopping frusemide.— J. P. Wauters, *Br. med. J.,* 1975, *4,* 624.

Effects on the circulation. A report of leg ischaemia or superficial gangrene in 5 patients taking frusemide (plus amiloride in 3 patients). Dramatic improvement occurred on withdrawal of diuretics and rehydration.— D. A. O'Rourke and J. E. Hede, *Br. med. J.,* 1978, *1,* 1114.

Effects on the ears. Reversible hearing loss in the medium- and high-frequency range occurred in 9 of 15 uraemic patients who were given intravenous infusions of 1 g of frusemide at the rate of 25 mg per minute. Very slight reversible impairment of hearing occurred in 4 of 10 patients given 600 mg at the rate of 15 mg per minute. There were no ototoxic effects in 10 patients who were given high doses of frusemide by slow infusion or by mouth for a prolonged period. Loss of hearing was considered to be a function of speed of infusion of frusemide.— A. Heidland and M. E. Wigand, *Klin. Wschr.,* 1970, *48,* 1052.

A report of permanent deafness in 6 patients following administration of frusemide during periods of impaired renal function. The onset of deafness was insidious and gradually progressive for up to 6 months after frusemide therapy.— C. A. Quick and W. Hoppe, *Ann. Otol. Rhinol. Lar.,* 1975, *84,* 94.

Further references: G. H. Schwartz *et al., New Engl. J. Med.,* 1970, *282,* 1413; S. I. Rifkin *et al., Sth. med. J.,* 1978, *71,* 86; K. L. Gallagher and J. K. Jones, *Ann. intern. Med.,* 1979, *91,* 744.

Effects on the electrolyte balance. In 2 healthy subjects and 5 patients frusemide 80 mg caused no significant change in sodium, calcium, or magnesium concentrations in plasma; potassium and chloride fell; packed cell volume, protein, inorganic phosphorus, and urate rose; creatinine and urea rose after an initial fall. Frusemide causes acute changes in the concentrations of several plasma components and should be considered in any assessment of electrolyte disturbances.— T. O. Haug, *Br. med. J.,* 1976, *2,* 622.

Calcium. Following administration of frusemide 80 mg by mouth to 14 healthy subjects, a marked diuresis was accompanied by a highly significant increase in calcium excretion during the subsequent 8 hours. This effect could not be accounted for by any change in glomerular filtration-rate, but might have been due to decreased tubular reabsorption.— J. A. Tambyah and M. K. L. Lim, *Br. med. J.,* 1969, *1,* 751. Following administration of frusemide by intravenous injection and by mouth, there was a marked hypercalciuria in the subsequent 4 hours, which was then followed by hypocalciuria, so that the overall 24-hour calcium excretion might be little changed.— M. S. Knapp and D. A. Heath (letter), *ibid.,* *2,* 248.

Despite the traditional view that frusemide administration lowers serum-calcium concentrations, they were raised in 11 of 13 male subjects by administration of 40 mg daily, for 3 weeks. It is suggested that low doses by mouth increase serum-calcium concentrations but that doses above 60 mg daily may depress them owing to urinary losses.— P. T. Chandler and S. A. Chandler, *Sth. med. J.,* 1977, *70,* 571.

Frusemide therapy in hypoparathyroid patients could result in hypocalcaemic tetany. In 6 hypoparathyroid patients the administration of frusemide 40 mg every 12 hours for 4 days produced a significant decrease in serum concentrations of ionised calcium. In 5 patients there was also an increase in urinary calcium excretion.— P. A. Gabow *et al., Ann. intern. Med.,* 1977, *86,* 579.

Effects on the eyes. Mention of blurring of vision in association with frusemide therapy.— *J. Am. med. Ass.,* 1967, *200,* 979.

A study indicating that usual therapeutic doses of frusemide interfere with colour vision.— J. Laroche and C. Laroche, *Annls pharm. fr.,* 1972, *30,* 433.

Effects on the gastro-intestinal tract. Although results of a Boston Collaborative Drug Surveillance Program involving 26 294 hospital in-patients supported the hypothesis that ethacrynic acid could cause gastro-intestinal bleeding, it did not implicate frusemide.— H. Jick and J. Porter, *Lancet,* 1978, *2,* 87.

Effects on the kidneys. Dose-related bilateral loin pain developed in a patient taking frusemide and was considered to be due to calyceal dilatation.— B. P. Harrold (letter), *Lancet,* 1973, *1,* 888. See also N. G. Kounis (letter), *Br. med. J.,* 1973, *3,* 641.

Reversible renal failure associated with intestitial nephritis occurred in 4 patients with glomerulonephritis. It was considered that a hypersensitivity reaction to frusemide, taken by all 4, or a thiazide, taken by 3 could have been the cause, as renal function improved on cessation of the diuretics and administration of prednisone.— H. Lyons *et al., New Engl. J. Med.,* 1973, *288,* 124. See also T. J. Fuller *et al., J. Am. med. Ass.,* 1976, *235,* 1998.

Effects on lipid metabolism. A study of the effects of frusemide on plasma lipoproteins in healthy subjects.— C. Joos *et al., Eur. J. clin. Pharmac.,* 1980, *17,* 251.

Effects on the liver. Two reports of hepatic dysfunction in association with frusemide therapy.— *Japan med. Gaz.,* 1979, *16* (Apr. 20), 12.

Further references: J. R. Mitchell *et al.* (letter), *Nature,* 1974, *251,* 508.

Effects on the muscles. Mention of periodic muscle cramps associated with frusemide therapy.— D. E. Hutcheon and G. Leonard, *J. clin. Pharmac.,* 1967, *7,* 26.

Effects on the nervous system. Mention of paraesthesias in the finger tips and toes associated with frusemide therapy.— D. E. Hutcheon and G. Leonard, *J. clin. Pharmac.,* 1967, *7,* 26.

A report of severe generalised paraesthesia on 2 occasions in a cirrhotic patient following intravenous administration of frusemide. The mechanism was not understood and there were no clinical findings of anaphylaxis.— B. J. Materson, *J. Florida med. Ass.,* 1971, *58,* 34.

Effects on the pancreas. Brief case reports of 3 patients who developed pancreatitis after receiving frusemide intravenously. The incidence was considered to be small.— N. Buchanan and R. D. Cane (letter), *Br. med. J.,* 1977, *2,* 1417.

Further references: A. E. Wilson *et al.* (letter), *Lancet,* 1967, *1,* 105; D. M. Davies (letter), *ibid.,* 1386; P. E. Jones and M. H. Oelbaum, *Br. med. J.,* 1975, *1,* 133; P. Strunge (letter), *ibid.,* *3,* 434; T. Call *et al., Am. J. dig. Dis.,* 1977, *22,* 835; F. B. Thomas *et al., Gastroenterology,* 1977, *73,* 221; B. Ø. Kristensen *et al., Br. med. J.,* 1980, *281,* 978.

Effects on the skin. Skin reactions to frusemide are rare.— N. Thorne, *Practitioner,* 1973, *211,* 606.

Erythema multiforme. A 65-year-old man developed erythema multiforme after treatment with a total dosage of 280 mg of frusemide by mouth. The rash and bullae resolved within 31 days.— T. P. Gibson and P. Blue (letter), *J. Am. med. Ass.*, 1970, *212*, 1709.

Further references: C. Zugarman and E. J. La Voo (letter), *Archs Derm.*, 1980, *116*, 518.

Photosensitivity. Epidermolysis bullosa in 7 patients was attributed to frusemide which had been taken in doses of 0.5 to 2 g daily for 2 months to 3 years. The lesions persisted for 3 to 9 weeks and then regressed even when frusemide was continued.— A. C. Kennedy and A. Lyell, *Br. med. J.*, 1976, *1*, 1509.

Bullae and blistering of exposed areas of the skin occurred soon after the dose of frusemide was increased or high doses given in 4 patients with chronic renal failure. The reaction was considered to be phototoxic. There was no blistering following intermittent high intravenous doses of frusemide in 2 of these patients after the daily doses were discontinued and replaced by doses of ethacrynic acid, or in 1 patient when the high intermittent doses were given following a kidney transplant.— J. N. Burry and J. R. Lawrence, *Br. J. Derm.*, 1976, *94*, 495.

Frusemide had relatively high activity, similar to the phenothiazines, in an *in vitro* test for photosensitivity, and this might be the basis of reported skin reactions associated with its use.— D. E. Moore, *J. pharm. Sci.*, 1977, *66*, 1282.

Further references: K. Keczkes and M. J. Farr (letter), *Br. med. J.*, 1976, *2*, 236; G. Heydenreich *et al.*, *Acta med. scand.*, 1977, *202*, 61.

Purpura. Purpura caused by thiazide diuretics, and the structurally similar drug, frusemide, may be either thrombocytopenic or non-thrombocytopenic.— J. Verbov, *Practitioner*, 1979, *222*, 400.

Vasculitis. Cutaneous necrotising vasculitis in a 72-year-old man was presumably caused by an allergic reaction to frusemide.— W. H. Hendricks and R. S. Ader (letter), *Archs Derm.*, 1977, *113*, 375.

Gout. Gout occurred in 2 elderly men who had received frusemide, each for about 3 months, in daily doses of 80 mg by mouth.— J. McSherry, *Practitioner*, 1968, *201*, 809.

Further references: D. M. Humphreys, *Br. med. J.*, 1966, *1*, 1024.

Oedema. For reference to the possible role of diuretics in exacerbating and perpetuating idiopathic oedema, see Oedema, under Adverse Effects of Chlorothiazide, p.588.

Treatment of Adverse Effects. As for Chlorothiazide, p.589.

Precautions. As for Chlorothiazide, p.589.

Frusemide is probably best avoided in the first trimester of pregnancy. It should be used with care in patients with prostatic hypertrophy or impairment of micturition. Frusemide may enhance the nephrotoxicity of cephaloridine and the aminoglycoside antibiotics, such as gentamicin, kanamycin, neomycin, and streptomycin.

Interactions. *Anaesthetics.* For the effect of frusemide during halothane anaesthesia, see Halothane, p.742.

Antibiotics. Studies in *animals* demonstrating enhancement of ear and kidney damage resulting from concurrent administration of frusemide and aminoglycoside antibiotics.— I. Ohtani *et al.*, *Chemotherapy, Tokyo*, 1977, *25*, 2348.

For the effect of frusemide on cephaloridine and gentamicin, see Cephaloridine,p.1126, and Gentamicin Sulphate, p.1168. For the effect of frusemide on chloramphenicol, see Chloramphenicol, p.1138.

Anticonvulsants. In 14 epileptic patients taking phenytoin and phenobarbitone (and in some cases other anticonvulsants) the mean diuretic effect of frusemide 20 mg was 68% of that in 10 healthy subjects and the peak effect was delayed from about 2 hours to about 4 hours. The diuretic effect of frusemide 40 mg in 17 epileptic patients was 51% of that in 10 healthy controls. The diuretic effect of frusemide 20 mg given intravenously to 12 epileptic patients was 50% of that in 5 healthy controls.— S. Ahmad, *Br. med. J.*, 1974, *3*, 657. In 5 healthy men absorption of frusemide and the maximum concentration in blood were reduced by about 50% when phenytoin 100 mg thrice daily was taken for 10 days. Serum and renal clearance of frusemide were not changed. The mechanism was not clear but was not due to stimulation of microsomal enzymes.— A. Fine *et al.*, *ibid.*, 1977, *2*, 1061.

For the effect of frusemide on phenobarbitone, see Phenobarbitone, p.814.

Aspirin and other anti-inflammatory analgesics. Reports indicating that *aspirin* and other nonsteroidal anti-inflammatory agents can diminish the diuretic effect of frusemide: K. J. Berg, *Eur. J. clin. Pharmac.*, 1977, *11*, 111; *idem*, 117; H. Valette and E. Apoil (letter), *Br. J. clin. Pharmac.*, 1979, *8*, 592; E. Bartoli *et al.*, *J. clin. Pharmac.*, 1980, *20*, 452; A. C. Yeung Laiwah and R. A. Mactier, *Br. med. J.*, 1981, *283*, 714.

Results of a study suggesting that frusemide therapy may be ineffective in infants receiving *indomethacin* for patent ductus arteriosus.— Z. Friedman *et al.*, *J. Pediat.*, 1978, *93*, 512.

A pharmacokinetic evaluation of the attenuation of the diuretic effect of frusemide by indomethacin.— D. E. Smith *et al.*, *J. Pharmacokinet. Biopharm.*, 1979, *7*, 265.

Absence of effect of diflunisal on the diuretic action of frusemide.— J. A. Tobert *et al.*, *Clin. Pharmac. Ther.*, 1980, *27*, 289.

For the effect of frusemide on indomethacin, see Indomethacin, p.258.

Chloral hydrate. Administration of frusemide to a patient who had been given chloral hydrate 8 and 12 hours previously on 2 occasions resulted in a sensation of heat, flushes, tachycardia, elevation of blood pressure to 160/90 mmHg, and severe diaphoresis. The reaction lasted 15 minutes. No adverse effects occurred after administration of frusemide alone.— M. Malach and N. Berman, *J. Am. med. Ass.*, 1975, *232*, 638. A retrospective study among 43 patients who had received both chloral hydrate and frusemide showed that 1 patient given frusemide 80 mg intravenously 8 hours after chloral hydrate had suffered a similar reaction; of 2 further patients who had possibly been affected, 1 had subsequently taken both drugs without side-effects.— M. P. Pevonka *et al.*, *Drug Intell. & clin. Pharm.*, 1977, *11*, 332.

Digoxin. For the effect of frusemide on serum-digoxin concentrations, see Digoxin, p.534.

Diuretics. Studies were made in 10 patients of possible interaction between frusemide and hydrochlorothiazide given in maximum therapeutic dosage intravenously. It was concluded that frusemide and hydrochlorothiazide were not synergistic.— A. O. Robson *et al.*, *Lancet*, 1964, *2*, 1085.

During a study in 6 healthy subjects no evidence was found of any interaction between frusemide and spironolactone, other than the desired conservation of potassium on pretreatment with spironolactone.— M. Homeida *et al.*, *Clin. Pharmac. Ther.*, 1977, *22*, 402.

For reference to severe electrolyte disturbances occurring in patients given metolazone concurrently with frusemide, see Metolazone, p.607.

Lithium. For a report on the absence of effect of frusemide on serum-lithium concentrations, see Lithium Carbonate, p.1539.

Muscle relaxants. For reference to the enhancement of tubocurarine-induced neuromuscular blockade by frusemide, see Tubocurarine Chloride, p.999.

Probenecid. Reduction in the renal clearance of frusemide by concurrent administration of probenecid.— J. Honari *et al.*, *Clin. Pharmac. Ther.*, 1977, *22*, 395.

Further references: B. Odlind and B. Beermann, *Clin. Pharmac. Ther.*, 1980, *27*, 784; D. E. Smith *et al.*, *J. pharm. Sci.*, 1980, *69*, 571.

Interference with diagnostic tests. Frusemide, 20 mg intravenously, given to promote diuresis in tests for the localisation of urinary-tract infections, reduced the bacterial count in ureteric and bladder urine by a factor of 100 in a third of the patients. Thus it was impossible to distinguish renal from bladder infections.— K. F. Fairley (letter), *Lancet*, 1969, *1*, 1212.

Frusemide could interfere with the Schack and Waxler spectrophotometric assay for plasma-theophylline concentrations to give significantly false-positive elevations.— L. E. Matheson *et al.*, *Am. J. Hosp. Pharm.*, 1977, *34*, 496.

Porphyria. A study in *rats* indicated that frusemide should be regarded as potentially hazardous for patients with a hereditary hepatic porphyria.— G. H. Blekkenhorst *et al.* (letter), *Lancet*, 1980, *1*, 1367. Criticisms of extrapolating data obtained from *animal* experiments to the treatment of human disease.— M. J. Brodie (letter), *ibid.*, *2*, 86; A. Gorchein (letter), *ibid.*, 152.

Pregnancy and the neonate. A study indicating that frusemide is a potent displacer of bilirubin and should be used with caution in jaundiced infants.— S. Shankaran *et al.*, *J. Pediat.*, 1977, *90*, 642. A study indicating that on a molar basis, chlorothiazide, frusemide, and ethacrynic acid are at least as potent as sulphafurazole in displacing bilirubin from albumin. Frusemide and ethacrynic acid, when used in the recommended doses of 1 mg per kg body-weight, would probably not produce a significant increase in free bilirubin in most infants, but the weaker diuretic, chlorothiazide, in its recommended dose of 15 to 20 mg per kg, would result in substantially higher plasma concentrations, and hence would be an inappropriate alternative to frusemide for diuretic therapy in jaundiced infants.— R. P. Wennberg *et al.*, *ibid.*, 647. Confirmation that a single dose of frusemide 1 mg per kg body-weight does not displace bilirubin from the albumin binding site. Doses greater than 1.5 mg per kg or repeated doses could potentially do so.— J. V. Aranda *et al.*, *ibid.*, 1978, *93*, 507.

The use of frusemide in late pregnancy should be avoided if the adequacy of placental perfusion was suspect.— D. C. Dukes, *Practitioner*, 1978, *220*, 285.

Absorption and Fate. Frusemide is incompletely but fairly rapidly absorbed from the gastro-intestinal tract. It has a biphasic half-life in the plasma with a terminal elimination phase that has been estimated to range up to about 1½ hours. It is up to 99% bound to plasma proteins, and is mainly excreted in the urine, largely unchanged, but also in the form of the glucuronide and free amine metabolites. Variable amounts are also excreted in the bile, non-renal elimination being considerably increased in renal failure. Frusemide crosses the placental barrier and is excreted in milk.

A detailed review of the clinical pharmacokinetics of frusemide.— R. E. Cutler and A. D. Blair, *Clin. Pharmacokinet.*, 1979, *4*, 279.

Further reviews: J. Prandota and M. Witkowska, *Eur. J. Drug Metab. Pharmacokinet.*, 1976, *1*, 177; L. Z. Benet, *J. Pharmacokinet. Biopharm.*, 1979, *7*, 1.

In subjects without cardiac or renal disease, frusemide produced peak plasma concentrations 30 and 60 minutes after intramuscular and oral administration respectively. About 80% of the dose appeared in urine within 24 hours after an intramuscular or intravenous injection. In 2 subjects given frusemide by mouth, 26 and 54% respectively was excreted in urine and 2.1% in faeces. Most of the drug excreted in the urine was passed during the first 4 hours, irrespective of the route of administration.— B. Calesnick *et al.*, *Proc. Soc. exp. Biol. Med.*, 1966, *123*, 17.

In 8 healthy subjects frusemide was detected in the serum within 10 minutes after an 80-mg dose in the fasting state, reached a mean peak of 2.2 μg per ml at 60 to 70 minutes and was scarcely detectable 3 or 4 hours after a dose. When the dose was taken after food concentrations were delayed, lower (mean 1 μg per ml), and more persistent. It was calculated that 40 to 60% of a dose was absorbed in the fasting state and 30 to 50% of a dose was excreted in the urine in 24 hours.— M. R. Kelly *et al.*, *Clin. Pharmac. Ther.*, 1974, *15*, 178.

In 4 healthy males given frusemide 20 to 120 mg intravenously, the apparent volume of distribution averaged 11.4% of body-weight and was unaffected by dosage. Marked diuresis occurred in all subjects with a peak flow-rate 20 to 60 minutes after injection and a duration of action of 6 hours, both independent of dosage. Frusemide was 95% bound to plasma proteins and had an average plasma half-life of 29.5 minutes with a clearance of 162 ml per minute. Renal excretion accounted for 92% of the administered dose, 8% being eliminated by other mechanisms. In 5 functionally anephric patients who received 2 separate doses of frusemide 120 mg intravenously, 1 dose during dialysis, average distribution volume was 17.8% of body-weight, average plasma half-life 80.7 minutes, and average plasma clearance 105 ml per minute; these data suggested a greater rate of non-renal elimination than in healthy subjects. Frusemide was not measurably cleared across the dialyser.— R. E. Cutler *et al.*, *Clin. Pharmac. Ther.*, 1974, *15*, 588. See also under Uses (Administration in Renal Failure).

Confirmation in 6 healthy subjects that despite reduced bioavailability of frusemide given by mouth the total diuretic response is the same as after intravenous administration.— R. A. Branch *et al.*, *Br. J. Pharmac.*, 1976, *57*, 442P. The response to frusemide was determined by the concentration of drug in the tissue compartment rather than in plasma.— *idem*, *Br. J. clin. Pharmac.*, 1977, *4*, 121.

Evidence of reduced bioavailability of frusemide in oedema and suggestion that the intravenous route be tried before a diagnosis of diuretic resistance is made.— B. G. Odlind and B. Beermann, *Br. med. J.*, 1980, *280*, 1577.

Further references: A. Greither *et al.*, *Am. J. Cardiol.*, 1976, *37*, 139 (absorption in heart failure); F. Andreasen *et al.*, *Eur. J. clin. Pharmac.*, 1978, *14*, 237 (reduced serum clearance in severe hypertension); B. Beermann *et al.* (letter), *Br. J. clin. Pharmac.*, 1978, *6*, 537 (bioavailability of different brands); J. E. Cruz *et al.*, *Int. J. Pharmaceut.*, 1979, *2*, 275 (*in vitro*study on bioavailability).

Metabolism. Studies suggesting that frusemide induces its own metabolism, probably forming a glucuronide.— F. Andreasen and E. Mikkelsen, *Eur. J. clin. Pharmac.*, 1977, *12*, 15.

Animal studies on frusemide metabolites: G. J. Yakatan *et al.*, *J. pharm. Sci.*, 1976, *65*, 1456.

Pregnancy and the neonate. Study in 12 patients suggested that the pharmacokinetics of frusemide were not modified by gestosis of pregnancy. In one woman delivered 3.5 hours after receiving frusemide the concentration in the mother and in umbilical artery blood were comparable; in a second woman delivered of twins 7.5 hours after frusemide the concentration in the umbilical artery was about one-third.— E. Riva *et al.*, *Eur. J. clin. Pharmac.*, 1978, *14*, 361.

A study of the pharmacokinetic disposition and protein binding of frusemide in 8 newborn infants. Plasma clearance was remarkably slow, with an 8-fold prolongation of the plasma half-life.— J. V. Aranda *et al.*, *J. Pediat.*, 1978, *93*, 507. Mean peak diuresis and electrolyte excretion occurred within 1 hour and the effects were discernible for about 5 hours in 9 neonates with fluid overload after the intravenous or intramuscular administration of frusemide 1 mg per kg body-weight. Of 4 infants who had relatively poor responses 3 were asphyxiated compared to none of 5 with good responses and it was suggested that perinatal asphyxia may decrease the response to frusemide.— W. -C. R. Woo *et al.*, *Clin. Pharmac. Ther.*, 1978, *23*, 266.

Further references: R. A. Vota *et al.*, *Am. J. Obstet. Gynec.*, 1975, *123*, 621 (amniotic fluid); J. W. Wladimiroff, *Br. J. Obstet. Gynaec.*, 1975, *82*, 221 (foetal urine); B. S. Ross *et al.*, *J. Pediat.*, 1978, *92*, 149 (pharmacology in neonates).

See also under Precautions and Uses.

Protein binding. Frusemide was 95% bound to plasma proteins.— R. E. Cutler *et al.*, *Clin. Pharmac. Ther.*, 1974, *15*, 588.

Further references: J. Prandota and A. W. Puritt, *Clin. Pharmac. Ther.*, 1975, *17*, 159 (in nephrotic children); R. Zini *et al.*, *Eur. J. clin. Pharmac.*, 1976, *10*, 139 (*in vitro* binding).

Uses. Frusemide is a potent diuretic with a rapid action. Its effects are evident within 1 hour after a dose by mouth and last for about 4 to 6 hours; after intravenous injection its effects are evident in about 5 minutes and last for about 2 hours. It has been reported to exert inhibiting effects on electrolyte reabsorption in the proximal and distal renal tubules and in the ascending loop of Henle. Excretion of sodium, potassium, and chloride ions is increased and water excretion enhanced. It has no effect on carbonic anhydrase. Frusemide is used similarly to chlorothiazide (see p.589) and may be effective in patients unresponsive to thiazide diuretics. It is also used in the treatment of renal insufficiency and, where appropriate, in forced diuresis regimens for the management of poisoning with some drugs, such as the barbiturates (see Phenobarbitone, p.812).

Unlike the thiazide diuretics where, owing to their flat dose-response curve, very little is gained by increasing the dose, frusemide has a steep dose-response curve, which gives it a wide therapeutic range.

In the treatment of oedema, the usual initial dose is 40 mg once daily, reduced to 20 mg daily or 40 mg on alternate days; in some patients doses of 80 mg or more daily may be required (given as a single dose or in 2 divided doses). Severe cases may require gradual titration of the frusemide dosage up to 600 mg daily. In emergency or when oral therapy cannot be given, 20 to 40 mg may be administered by intramuscular or slow intravenous (over 1 to 2 minutes) injection; a second dose can be given not less than 2 hours later, according to the patient's response. A recommended dose for pulmonary oedema is 40 or 50 mg by slow intravenous injection (over 1 to 2 minutes), followed by a second dose one to one-and-a-half hours later according to the patient's response. Sources in the *USA* have recommended that if an initial slow intravenous injection of 40 mg (over 1 to 2 minutes) does not produce a satisfactory response within one hour, the dose may be increased to 80 mg given slowly intravenously.

For children, the usual dose by mouth is 1 to 3 mg per kg body-weight daily or on alternate days; suggested doses by injection are 0.5 to 1.5 mg per kg.

In the treatment of hypertension, frusemide is given in doses of 40 to 80 mg daily, either alone, or in conjunction with other antihypertensive agents. Doses of 40 to 80 mg have also been given by slow intravenous injection for hypertensive crises.

When treatment is prolonged, or in susceptible patients, loss of potassium may be sufficient to produce hypokalaemia; potassium supplements should then be given as for chlorothiazide (p.589).

High-dose therapy. In the treatment of acute or chronic renal failure an ampoule of frusemide 250 mg (in a 25-ml ampoule) may be added to about 225 ml of sodium chloride injection or compound sodium chloride infusion and infused over one hour. If urine output is insufficient within the next hour, this dose may be followed by 500 mg (in 2 ampoules of 25 ml) added to an appropriate infusion fluid, the total volume of which must be governed by the patient's state of hydration, and infused over 2 hours. If a satisfactory urine output has still not been achieved within one hour of the end of the second infusion then a third dose of 1 g may be infused over 4 hours. The rate of infusion should never exceed 4 mg per minute. In oliguric or anuric patients with significant fluid overload, the injection may be given without dilution directly into the vein, using a constant-rate infusion pump with a micrometer screw-gauge adjustment; the rate of administration should still never exceed 4 mg per minute. If the response to either method of administration is satisfactory, the effective dose (of up to 1 g) may then be given daily. Dosage adjustments should subsequently be made according to the patient's response. Alternatively, treatment may be maintained by mouth; 500 mg should be given by mouth for each 250 mg required by injection.

In the treatment of chronic renal insufficiency, an initial dose of 250 mg may be given by mouth, increased, if necessary in steps of 250 mg every 4 to 6 hours to a maximum of 2 g; the effective dose may be given daily (as a single dose); dosage adjustments should subsequently be made according to the patient's response.

During treatment with these high-dose forms of frusemide therapy, careful laboratory control is essential. Fluid balance and electrolytes should be carefully controlled and, in particular, in patients with shock, measures should be taken to correct the blood pressure and circulating blood volume, before commencing this type of treatment. High-dose frusemide therapy is contra-indicated in renal failure caused by nephrotoxic or hepatotoxic agents, and in renal failure associated with hepatic coma.

A review of the efficacy of frusemide and bumetanide in the treatment of thiazide-resistant salt and water retention.— *Drug & Ther. Bull.*, 1979, *17*, 47.

Action. A study suggesting that frusemide is eliminated predominantly by proximal tubular secretion, and that tubular, rather than plasma, concentration is the main determinant of its diuretic effect. The renal tubular site of action of frusemide is still debated, but most of the evidence points to the thick ascending limb of Henle's loop as the primary area of frusemide action, with somewhat conflicting results regarding its proximal tubular effect.— J. Honari *et al.*, *Clin. Pharmac. Ther.*, 1977, *22*, 395. See also M. Homeida *et al.*, *ibid.*, 402.

An investigation into the action of frusemide in pulmonary oedema, and the recommendation that continuous high-dosage oxygen therapy should be used concurrently.— H. W. Iff and D. C. Flenley, *Lancet*, 1971, *1*, 616. Comment and the view that the main value of rapidly acting diuretics is to reduce left-ventricular end-diastolic pressure, and thus reduce the risk of acute left-ventricular failure. Their action is likely to remove lung water and improve gas exchange in the lung, but this effect is relatively slow and is likely to be of long-term rather than immediate benefit.— A. E. Tattersfield and M. W. McNicol (letter), *ibid.*, 911. For an earlier view that frusemide causes fluid to be removed from the pulmonary circulation before its produces diuresis, see under Mountain Sickness and Pulmonary Oedema (below).

Further references to studies on the mode and site of action of frusemide: P. A. F. Morrin, *Can. J. Physiol. Pharmac.*, 1966, *44*, 129; H. Weinstein and V. Solis-Gil, *Curr. ther. Res.*, 1966, *8*, 435; K. K. Gupta *et al.* (letter), *Lancet*, 1967, *1*, 1386; C. E. Leme *et al.*, *Metabolism*, 1967, *16*, 871; P. G. F. Nixon, *Lancet*, 1968, *2*, 146; J. P. Radó and L. Borbély (letter), *Lancet*, 1968, *1*, 1434; J. Stribrná and O. Schück, *Medsche Klin.*, 1968, *63*, 103; U. Veltkamp *et al.*, *Arzneimittel-Forsch.*, 1968, *18*, 1207; I. M. Baird and N. Longhurst, *Curr. med. Res. Opinion*, 1972, *1*, 134; R. E. Cutler *et al.*, *Clin. Pharmac. Ther.*, 1974, *15*, 588; T. W. Wilson *et al.*, *Clin. Pharmac. Ther.*, 1975, *18*, 165; J. D. Lazar and P. Z. Kissner (letter), *ibid.*, 1976, *19*, 598; T. W. Wilson (letter), *ibid.*, 599; L. E. Ramsay *et al.* (letter), *Br. J. clin. Pharmac.*, 1975, *2*, 361; P. H. Mackie *et al.*, *Br. J. clin. Pharmac.*, 1976, *3*, 613; S. B. Stallings *et al.*, *Am. J. Hosp. Pharm.*, 1979, *36*, 68.

Administration. *In children.* A study of the safety and efficacy of frusemide, in the treatment of salt and water retention in infants and children with cardiac and renal disorders. A total of 106 paediatric in-patients received 137 courses of frusemide therapy, which was found to be safe and effective in the doses given. The following dosage regimens are recommended: frusemide 1 mg per kg body-weight intravenously, increasing by increments of 1 mg per kg for each dose, until satisfactory diuresis is obtained; for continuing therapy 2 mg per kg is given by mouth in the morning, increased by increments of 1 mg per kg until diuresis is achieved; no more than one or two doses are given daily unless the situation is critical, and it is usually not necessary to use a single dose greater than 4 mg per kg; potassium supplements are given if the diuretic is needed for more than a few days.— M. A. Engle *et al.*, *Pediatrics*, 1978, *62*, 811.

Further references: H. A. Repetto *et al.*, *J. Pediat.*, 1972, *80*, 660 (glomerulonephritis); J. Prandota and A. W. Pruitt, *Pharmacologist*, 1974, *16*, 220 (nephrotic children); A. W. Pruitt and A. Boles, *J. Pediat.*, 1976, *89*, 306 (glomerulonephritis).

In the elderly. Comment on the use of antihypertensive and diuretic drugs in the elderly. The use of powerful diuretics, such as frusemide, can cause painful distention of the bladder in men with prostatic hypertrophy.— *Med. Lett.*, 1979, *21*, 43.

Further references: *Prescribers' J.*, 1970, *10*, 46.

For reference to the risk of hypokalaemia in elderly patients receiving diuretic therapy, see Chlorothiazide, p.590.

Administration and potassium. The influence of sodium and potassium supplements, given for 10 days, on the diuretic response to a single dose of frusemide 80 mg was investigated in a crossover study in 12 healthy subjects. On the addition of potassium chloride 96 mmol daily to the normal diet, excretion of potassium after frusemide was higher and the Na/K ratio lower than when the subjects had received no supplement. On the addition of sodium chloride 100 mmol daily, potassium excretion after frusemide was lower and the Na/K ratio higher than when no supplement was given. There was no significant change in sodium excretion after frusemide with either sodium or potassium supplements. These differences in response to frusemide were smaller than those anticipated after an earlier study (R.A. Branch *et al.*, *Clin. Pharmac. Ther.*, 1976, *19*, 538).— R. A. Branch *et al.*, *Br. J. Pharmac.*, 1978, *64*, 285.

Further references: H. J. Dargie *et al.*, *Br. med. J.*, 1974, *4*, 316; C. J. Edmonds (letter), *ibid.*, 1975, *1*, 36.

For comments, discussions, and studies on the role of potassium supplementation in diuretic therapy, see Chlorothiazide, p.590.

Administration in renal failure. Investigations in 12 patients in advanced renal failure who received frusemide 1 g in 100 ml dextrose injection, infused intravenously over a period of 30 minutes, and frusemide 1 g by mouth, on separate occasions, indicated that in uraemic patients without concurrent liver disease non-renal frusemide clearance should be adequate to prevent drug cumulation even after a dose of 1 g daily. The average elimination half-life was about 10 hours. The intravenous route appeared to be preferable for the treatment of patients with end-stage kidney disease as absorption was erratic after administration by mouth and the diuretic response was generally reduced.— C. M. Huang *et al.*, *Clin. Pharmac. Ther.*, 1974, *16*, 659. Studies in 'diuretic-resistant' patients indicated that frusemide 240 mg produced the same diuresis whether given intravenously or by mouth.— M. R. Kelly *et al.*, *Curr. ther. Res.*, 1977, *21*, 1.

In a comparative study of 5 healthy subjects and 17 patients with various degrees of renal impairment the half-life of frusemide in the healthy subjects ranged from 0.49 to 1.20 hours (average 0.86 hours) which was longer than that found by R.E. Cutler *et al.* (*Clin. Pharmac. Ther.*, 1974, *15*, 588). In those with renal failure the half-life ranged from 1.15 to 24.58 hours which agreed with C.M. Huang *et al.*(*Clin. Pharmac. Ther.*, 1974, *16*, 659). No correlation was found between half-life and creatinine clearance, but plasma clearance of frusemide correlated with creatinine clearance despite large interindividual variations. In 1 patient who received radioactively labelled frusemide the main route of elimination was noted to be the faeces and although the half-life was only 1.55 hours the rate of elimination of metabolites was decreased. It was noted that high doses of frusemide often used in renal failure might not always be necessary and could lead to toxic concentrations in the blood since the patient with a half-life of 24.58 hours obtained a good diuretic response to frusemide 160 mg daily.— B. Beermann *et al.*, *Clin. Pharmac. Ther.*, 1977, *22*, 70.

Further references: L. F. Gregory *et al.*, *Archs intern. Med.*, 1970, *125*, 69; A. Lucas *et al.*, *Biomedicine*, 1976, *24*, 45; H. J. Rose *et al.*, *Clin. Pharmac. Ther.*, 1977, *21*, 141; S. Harding and A. J. Munro (letter), *Br. med. J.*, 1978, *2*, 1431; J. Petersen *et al.* (letter), *ibid.*, 1790; W. J. Tilstone and A. Fine, *Clin. Pharmac. Ther.*, 1978, *23*, 644; A. Rane *et al.*, *ibid.*, *24*, 199.

See also under Absorption and Fate.

Cardiac disorders. Heart failure. Indications that frusemide may have a beneficial haemodynamic effect on the heart, independent of its diuretic effect: K. Dikshit *et al.*, *New Engl. J. Med.*, 1973, *288*, 1087; S. Piepenbrock *et al.*, *Dt. med. Wschr.*, 1977, *102*, 1661.

The successful use of frusemide by infusion (4 to 16 mg per hour) in 10 patients with congestive heart failure unresponsive to single doses of 120 mg by mouth.— D. H. Lawson *et al.*, *Br. med. J.*, 1978, *2*, 476. See also J. M. B. Gray *et al.*, *Br. J. clin. Pharmac.*, 1978, *6*, 461P.

Further references: M. Davidov *et al.*, *J. Am. med. Ass.*, 1967, *200*, 824; B. Levy, *J. clin. Pharmac.*, 1977, *17*, 420; D. C. Brater *et al.*, *Clin. Pharmac. Ther.*, 1980, *28*, 182; D. Hutcheon *et al.*, *J. clin. Pharmac.*, 1980, *20*, 59.

Myocardial infarction. Frusemide 40 mg was administered routinely by intravenous infusion to 50 patients with recent myocardial infarction. Left heart failure was effectively controlled in 80% of patients, without the use of digitalis. No adverse effects occurred.— E. Stock, *Med. J. Aust.*, 1970, *1*, 480.

Further references: J. Kiely *et al.*, *Circulation*, 1973, *48*, 581.

Diabetes insipidus and inappropriate secretion of antidiuretic hormone. In a patient with diabetes insipidus an intravenous injection of 40 mg of frusemide had an antidiuretic effect lasting for about 30 hours and a dose of 120 mg lasted for 42 hours. An intravenous dose of hydrochlorothiazide, 300 mg, produced an antidiuresis lasting for at least 72 hours.— J. P. Radó *et al.* (letter), *Lancet*, 1967, *2*, 568.

While patients with hyponatraemia due to inappropriate secretion of antidiuretic hormone could be treated by restricting fluid intake such treatment could be too slow, and infusions of hypertonic saline were only transiently effective because of rapid excretion. A 27-year-old woman was therefore given frusemide 1 mg per kg body-weight intravenously, repeated as required, and electrolyte losses were replaced with 3% sodium chloride infusions with potassium supplements, and her confusion and convulsions were relieved. Four other patients had been similarly treated. Mean plasma-sodium concentrations rose from 120 to 133 mmol (120 to 133 mEq) per litre within 10 hours.— D. Hantman *et al.*, *Ann. intern. Med.*, 1973, *78*, 870.

Further references: J. Torretti and I. Zanzi, *Metabolism*, 1967, *16*, 529 (diabetes insipidus); G. Decaux *et al.*, *New Engl. J. Med.*, 1981, *304*, 329 (inappropriate secretion of antidiuretic hormone).

Diagnostic use. *Renography.* In 3 patients, partial ureteric obstruction was diagnosed with the aid of renograms made during diuresis induced by frusemide. Frusemide was given in a dose of 40 mg by intravenous injection and in 1 patient was preceded by an intravenous infusion of 1 litre of a 2.5% solution of sodium chloride.— J. P. Radó *et al.* (letter), *Lancet*, 1967, *2*, 1419.

Enuresis. In 3 children aged 8 to 12 years, treatment with frusemide 20 mg in the evening effectively prevented nocturnal enuresis.— W. Dobson, *Practitioner*, 1968, *200*, 568.

Epilepsy. Concurrent administration of frusemide 40 mg thrice daily for 4 weeks reduced the frequency of focal fits in 9 of 11 epileptic patients whose fits had been poorly controlled by conventional long-term therapy. Five of 14 patients experienced drowsiness (severe enough to require withdrawal of 3), possibly due to raised serum-phenobarbitone concentrations.— S. Ahmad *et al.*, *Br. J. clin. Pharmac.*, 1976, *3*, 621.

Hepatic disorders. Ascitic fluid was withdrawn from 6 of 8 men with liver cirrhosis and massive ascites, and re-infused intravenously. Frusemide 40 mg was infused intravenously after 3 ascitic fluid transfusions, and repeated to maintain a high urinary output. The other 2 men received frusemide 40 mg alone, followed by 20 mg per hour by constant infusion until three 30-minute collections of urine had been made, whereupon they received ascitic fluid intravenously. In the first group, ascitic fluid infusion alone did not alter the urinary volume or sodium excretion. The combined infusion raised the glomerular filtration-rate and the renal plasma flow-rate. Urinary volume and sodium and potassium excretion increased. Frusemide alone given to patients in the second group increased urinary volume and sodium and potassium excretion but did not alter the glomerular filtration-rate or the renal plasma flow-rate, both of which increased when ascitic fluid was added to the treatment.— G. Eknoyan *et al.*, *New Engl. J. Med.*, 1970, *282*, 713.

Results of a controlled study (using spironolactone and/or frusemide in the active drug group) indicated that diuresis aiming at a modest rate of diuresis can be accomplished in patients with decompensated alcoholic liver disease and ascites of recent onset, without serious complications that can be attributed to diuretic therapy.— P. B. Gregory *et al.*, *Gastroenterology*, 1977, *73*, 534.

Further references: A. Z. Shafei *et al.*, *J. trop. Med. Hyg.*, 1967, *70*, 286; A. El-Badry *et al.*, *J. Egypt. med. Ass.*, 1964, *47*, 594 (schistosomal ascites); F. Sadikali, *Br. J. clin. Pract.*, 1973, *27*, 222 (with spironolactone); R. K. Fuller *et al.*, *J. Am. med. Ass.*, 1977, *237*, 972 (with spironolactone); E. J. Thompson *et al.*, *Clin. Pharmac. Ther.*, 1977, *21*, 392 (with triamterene); C. A. Naranjo *et al.*, *Clin. Pharmac. Ther.*, 1979, *25*, 154.

In children. Comment on the use of diuretic therapy for ascites and oedema associated with hepatic diseases in children. Hypokalaemia and dehydration are particular risks with frusemide and the thiazide diuretics. Spironolactone is the logical diuretic to use; it may be adequate used alone, or the addition of a small dose of frusemide or a thiazide diuretic may yield the desired diuresis.— D. M. Danks (letter), *J. Pediat.*, 1976, *88*, 695.

Hypercalcaemia. Diuresis, resulting in a fall in serum-calcium concentrations of 23 to 38 µg per ml, occurred after a dose of frusemide of 80 to 100 mg intravenously in 8 patients with serum-calcium concentrations of 123 to 184 µg per ml due to various causes. Urinary losses of magnesium, potassium, sodium, and water were measured and replaced.— W. N. Suki *et al.*, *New Engl. J. Med.*, 1970, *283*, 836.

Frusemide has little place in the treatment of hypercalcaemia; it is not uniformly successful, it requires very large volumes of intravenous fluids requiring careful monitoring of electrolytes, and its effectiveness diminishes after a few days.— C. R. Paterson, *Postgrad. med. J.*, 1974, *50*, 158.

Further references: S. S. Najjar *et al.*, *J. Pediat.*, 1972, *81*, 1171 (in infants); J. P. Fillastre *et al.*, *Curr. ther. Res.*, 1973, *15*, 641 (in neoplastic diseases).

See also under Adverse Effects, Effects on the Electrolyte Balance.

Hypertension. Single intravenous injections of frusemide, 40 to 300 mg, reduced the blood pressure by 15% or more in 21 of 62 patients with mild to moderate hypertension who received less than 100 mg, and in 20 of 22 given more than 120 mg. The greatest effect occurred 2 to 2.5 hours after injection, and lasted 10 to 12 hours. Repeated weekly injections showed no development of tolerance during 8 weeks. In 16 similar patients given frusemide by mouth doses exceeding 120 mg consistently reduced the blood pressure.— M. Davidov *et al.*, *Circulation*, 1967, *36*, 125, per *Abstr. Wld Med.*, 1968, *42*, 95.

In 27 hypertensive patients whose blood pressure was not controlled by 3 or more drugs including a thiazide diuretic, a change in therapy, either by substituting frusemide for the thiazide or by adding spironolactone, resulted in a significant fall in blood pressure and loss of weight.— L. E. Ramsay *et al.*, *Br. med. J.*, 1980, *281*, 1101.

Further references: L. Wertheimer *et al.*, *Archs intern. Med.*, 1971, *127*, 934; W. J. Mroczek *et al.*, *Am. J. Cardiol.*, 1974, *33*, 546; R. J. Young *et al.*, *Br. med. J.*, 1980, *280*, 1579.

Comparative studies with other antihypertensive agents: J. Anderson *et al.*, *Q. J. Med.*, 1971, *40*, 541 (hydrochlorothiazide); J. Anderson and J. G. Nievel, *Clin. Trials J.*, 1977, *14*, 119 (hydrochlorthiazide); W. J. Mroczek *et al.*, *Curr. ther. Res.*, 1978, *24*, 824 (hydrochlorothiazide); M. E. Davidov *et al.*, *Curr. ther. Res.*, 1979, *25*, 1 (chlorthalidone); O. D. Holland *et al.*, *Archs intern. Med.*, 1979, *139*, 1015 (hydrochlorothiazide).

Once-daily administration. There was no significant difference between the mean arterial blood pressure obtained in 38 patients with hypertension when they took frusemide 80 mg as a once-daily dose for a mean of 191 days and in 2 divided doses for a mean of 173 days. Other antihypertensive therapy remained unchanged. Of 13 patients who had complained of nocturia during the twice-daily regimen, none reported this during the once-daily administration.— M. E. Davidov and W. J. Mroczek, *Curr. ther. Res.*, 1978, *23*, 300.

High-dose therapy. In 10 patients with severe hypertension (7 with essential arterial hypertension) frusemide in doses of 0.12 to 4 g daily produced a significantly greater reduction in blood pressure than previous conventional antihypertensive medication; maintenance doses were 40 mg to 2 g daily. Patients received dietary and/or supplementary sodium up to 680 mmol (680 mEq) daily and all received potassium 60 to 150 mmol (60 to 150 mEq) daily.— F. Cantarovich *et al.*, *Nephron*, 1974, *12*, 133.

Renin categorisation. A simple screening test for hypertension in outpatients was assessed in 40 hypertensive patients. Frusemide 60 mg was taken by mouth and plasma-renin activity measured 5 hours later. The results fell into 4 groups: exteme hyporeninaemia (primary aldosteronoma), suppressed renin (confirmed suppressed-renin hypertension), normal renin (essential hypertension), and elevated renin (renovascular hypertension). Identification of patients requiring further evaluation for remediable secondary causes was possible. All medication should be withheld for at least 1 week before testing because many drugs affected plasma-renin activity.— L. Wallach *et al.*, *Ann. intern. Med.*, 1975, *82*, 27. See also N. M. Kaplan *et al.*, *Ann. intern. Med.*, 1976, *84*, 639.

Mountain sickness and pulmonary oedema. A study in 7 patients recovering from high altitude pulmonary oedema, given frusemide 40 mg by intracardiac injection, showed a distinct reduction in pulmonary volume before general diuresis occurred. This supports the suggestion of R.W. Biagi and B.N. Bapat (*Lancet*, 1967, *1*, 849) that frusemide moves fluid from the pulmonary circulation before it produces a diuresis.— M. L. Bhatia *et al.*, *Br. med. J.*, 1969, *2*, 551.

See also under Acetazolamide Sodium, p.582.

Prostatectomy. A litre of sodium chloride infusion was given to 110 patients 1 hour prior to prostatectomy, and frusemide 80 mg was given intravenously after bladder closure to ensure rapid diuresis, minimising blood-clot formation and postoperative oozing. A further 5 litres of saline and dextrose-saline were given over 24 hours. The average 24-hour urinary output was 4.5 litres, 40% being passed in the first 3 hours. Eight patients received further intramuscular injections of frusemide 40 mg as the urine was blood-stained. Bladder washouts were not necessary, the postoperative urinary infection-rate was 8% at 1 week after operation, and clot retention was not a problem.— C. R. Williams, *Br. J. Surg.*, 1972, *59*, 190. See also D. M. Essenhigh and B. R. Eustace, *Br. J. Urol.*, 1969, *41*, 579.

Pregnancy and the neonate. *Antenatal diagnosis of renal agenesis.* Negative scanning for a foetal bladder following administration of frusemide to the mother to increase foetal urine production, strongly supports a diagnosis of renal agenesis (Potter syndrome).— R. P. Balfour and K. M. Laurence (letter), *Lancet*, 1980, *1*, 317. See also M. J. N. Keirse and R. H. Meerman, *Obstet. Gynec.*, 1978, *52*, 64.

Hypertension of pregnancy. Frusemide, 160 to 320 mg, administered in conjunction with thiazides and diazoxide, where necessary, to 37 pregnant women with severe toxaemia produced complete clearance of oedema, a fall in arterial pressure, and a decrease in albuminuria in all of them. Mild oedema in a further 16 pregnant out-patients was cleared by the addition of frusemide, 40 mg every second or third day, to thiazide therapy. Following its sole use in a further 35 out-patients, excessive diuresis occurred in 4; this unpredictability precludes its routine use as a sole diuretic in out-patients.— F. A. Finnerty, *Am. J. Obstet. Gynec.*, 1969, *105*, 1022.

Three patients with toxaemia of pregnancy were controlled by frusemide 40 to 80 mg and methyldopa 1.25 to 2 g daily with appropriate sedatives and tranquillisers and fluid intake of 1.5 to 2 litres daily. Delivery by caesarean section was successful in each patient although all 3 infants suffered from meconium ileus attributed to methyldopa and which was fatal in 1 infant.— A. D. Clark *et al.* (letter), *Lancet*, 1972, *1*, 35. Comment.— I. MacGillivray (letter), *ibid.*, 198.

Lactation. Frusemide 40 mg each morning for 3 to 6 days was effective for the suppression of lactation.— R. G. H. Wade (letter), *Br. med. J.*, 1977, *1*, 442. See also *ibid.*, 1973, *2*, 711.

The neonate. Frusemide was given by intravenous injection in 3 doses each of 1.5 mg per kg body-weight to 7 premature babies with severe respiratory distress syndrome (RDS) during the first 24 hours of life. When compared with an untreated group of 13 infants with less severe RDS, frusemide produced a 4-fold increase in urine volume and a 10-fold increase in urine-sodium and -calcium excretion. Frusemide was not recommended for routine management of infants with RDS because there was no improvement in blood-gas tensions in the 5 infants in which they were measured and because of the possibility of severe dehydration.— M. O. Savage *et al.*, *Archs Dis. Childh.*, 1975, *50*, 709.

Further references: K. H. Marks *et al.*, *Pediatrics*, 1978, *62*, 785.

See also under Precautions for Frusemide (Pregnancy and the Neonate) and Adverse Effects, Precautions, and Uses for Chlorothiazide (Pregnancy and the Neonate).

Raised intracranial pressure. Twenty patients scheduled for craniotomy were given mannitol 1 g per kg body-weight or frusemide 1 mg per kg, intravenously. Results indicated that intracranial pressure increased significantly at the onset of diuresis after mannitol and decreased significantly on completion of diuresis, and postoperatively. After frusemide the intracranial pressure decreased at peak diuresis, on completion of diuresis and postoperatively. Moreover, changes in serum-electrolyte values and osmolality were less with frusemide. Accordingly frusemide should replace mannitol in neurosurgery, especially when the patient already has increased intracranial pressure, an altered blood-brain barrier, or increased pulmonary water content, or in those with pre-existing cardiac and electrolyte abnormalities.— J. E. Cottrell *et al.*, *Anesthesiology*, 1977, *47*, 28.

Further references: S. G. F. Matts, *Br. J. clin. Pract.*, 1972, *26*, 361; J. Thilmann and H. Zeumer, *Dt. med. Wschr.*, 1974, *99*, 932.

Renal disorders. Advocation by F. Cantarovich *et al.* (*Br. med. J.*,1973, *4*, 449) and others, of the routine use of high-dose frusemide therapy in renal failure, has been criticised by G. Ganeval *et al.* (*Br. med. J.*, 1974, *1*, 244) and others.

References to conflicting views on the role of high-dose frusemide therapy in renal failure: *Frusemide in Renal Failure*, Proceedings of a Conference, Stockholm, 1969, *Postgrad. med. J.*, 1971, *47* (Apr.), *Suppl.*; Y. K. Seedat, *S. Afr. med. J.*, 1972, *46*, 1371; *Lancet*, 1973, *2*, 134; S. A. J. Naqvi (letter), *Br. med. J.*, 1974, *2*, 278; S. Karayannopoulos (letter), *Br. med. J.*, 1974, *2*, 278; P. J. C. Vereerstraeten *et al.*, *Nephron*, 1974, *14*, 333; J. Rodés *et al.*, *Postgrad. med. J.*, 1975, *51*, 492; A. N. Minuth *et al.*, *Am. J. med. Sci.*, 1976, *271*, 317; V. Borirakchanyavat *et al.*, *Postgrad. med. J.*, 1978, *54*, 30; A. L. Linton (letter), *Practitioner*, 1979, *222*, 159; D. B. Evans, *ibid.*

Nephrotic syndrome. Five patients with the nephrotic syndrome with gross oedema and hypoalbuminaemia received frusemide in maximum doses of 320 mg to 1 g daily for up to 50 days. Albumin infusions were necessary to initiate a diuresis in 2 patients. As oedema disappeared renal function improved in 4 patients.— P. D. Snashall, *Br. med. J.*, 1971, *1*, 319.

Transplants. Renal allograft recipients rapidly became dependent on diuretics. Potent diuretics such as frusemide should be used sparingly and not discontinued abruptly.— M. K. Chan *et al.*, *Br. med. J.*, 1979, *1*, 1604. Criticism; the factors which led to the initial oedema had not been altered.— L. E. Ramsay (letter), *ibid.*, *2*, 131. Reply.— M. K. Chan *et al.* (letter), *ibid.*, 132.

Trauma. A study in 54 critically ill surgical patients indicated that frusemide does not protect against renal failure, and may cause it by producing hypovolaemia.— C. E. Lucas *et al.*, *Surgery, St Louis*, 1977, *82*, 314.

Respiratory disorders. The addition of oral diuretics to the regimen used in the treatment of respiratory failure resulted in striking improvements in the respiratory function of 4 patients. They were given frusemide 40 mg, either once or twice daily, and in addition some were given spironolactone 25 mg four times daily.— M. I. M. Noble *et al.*, *Lancet*, 1966, *2*, 257.

See under Pregnancy and the Neonate, for reference to the use of frusemide in respiratory distress syndrome in neonates.

Preparations

Frusemide Injection *(B.P.)*. A sterile solution of frusemide sodium, prepared from frusemide and sodium hydroxide, in Water for Injections. Potency is expressed in terms of the equivalent amount of frusemide. pH 8.7 to 9.3. Sterilise by autoclaving. Protect from light.

Frusemide Tablets *(B.P.)*. Tablets containing frusemide.

Furosemide Injection *(U.S.P.)*. A sterile solution of frusemide in Water for Injections, prepared with the aid of sodium hydroxide. Potency is expressed in terms of frusemide. pH 8.5 to 9.3. Protect from light.

Furosemide Tablets *(U.S.P.)*. Tablets containing frusemide. Store in airtight containers. Protect from light.

Proprietary Preparations

Diumide-K *(Napp, UK)*. Tablets each containing frusemide 40 mg and potassium chloride 600 mg (potassium 8 mmol; 8 mEq) in a separate layer for sustained release.

Dryptal *(Berk Pharmaceuticals, UK)*. Frusemide, available as **Injection** containing 10 mg per ml, in ampoules of 2, 5, and 25 ml, and as scored **Tablets** of 40 and 500 mg.

Frusetic *(Unimed, UK)*. Frusemide, available as scored tablets of 40 mg.

Frusid *(DDSA Pharmaceuticals, UK)*. Frusemide, available as tablets of 40 mg. (Also available as Frusid in *Austral.*).

Fur-O-Ims *(IMS, UK)*. Frusemide, available as tablets of 20, 40, 80, 100, 250, and 500 mg.

Lasikal *(Hoechst, UK)*. Tablets each containing frusemide 20 mg and, in a separate slow-release layer, potassium chloride 750 mg (potassium 10 mmol; 10 mEq).

Owing to the risk of intestinal obstruction, sustained-release preparations such as Lasikal, where the drug is released in transit, but the matrix ghost is often eliminated intact, should not be prescribed in patients with Crohn's disease or other intestinal disease in which strictures may form.— J. L. Shaffer *et al.* (letter), *Lancet*, 1980, *2*, 487.

Lasilactone *(Hoechst, UK)*. Capsules each containing frusemide 20 mg and spironolactone 50 mg. For resistant oedema and hypertension. *Dose.* 1 to 4 capsules daily.

Lasix *(Hoechst, UK)*. Frusemide, available as Injection containing 10 mg per ml, in ampoules of 2, 5, and 25 ml; as **Paediatric Liquid** (supplied as granules for preparation with water before use) containing 5 mg in each 5 ml; and as scored **Tablets** of 20, 40, and 500 mg. (Also available as Lasix in *Austral.*, *Belg.*, *Canad.*, *Denm.*, *Ger.*, *Ital.*, *Neth.*, *Norw.*, *S.Afr.*, *Switz.*, *USA*).

Lasix + K *(Hoechst, UK)*. A composite pack designed for the daily administration of one scored 40-mg tablet of frusemide and two 750-mg sustained-release tablets of potassium chloride, each containing 10 mmol (10 mEq) of potassium.

Min-I-Jet Frusemide Injection *(IMS, UK)*. A cartridge assembly containing a solution of frusemide 10 mg per ml, in vials of 2, 4, 8, 10, 12, 25, and 50 ml.

Other Proprietary Names

Alg.— Lasilix; *Arg.*—Errolon; *Austral.*— Aquamide, Uremide, Urex, Urex-M; *Canad.*— Furoside, Neo-Renal, Novosemide, Uritol; *Chile*— Laxur; *Denm.*— Diural, Furix, Impugan, Nicorol; *Fr.*— Lasilix; *Ger.*— Fusid, Hydro-rapid, Sigasalur; *Jap.*— Arasemide, Franyl, Moilarorin, Promedes; *Mor.*— Lasilix; *Neth.*— Lasiletten; *Norw.*— Diural, Impugan; *S.Afr.*— Aquasin; *Spain*— Diurolasa, Seguril; *Swed.*— Impugan; *Switz.*— Impugan; *Tun.*— Lasilix.

2332-b

Hydrobentizide. Dihydrobenzthiazide. 3-Benzylthiomethyl-6-chloro-3,4-dihydro-2*H*-1,2,4-benzothiadiazine-7-sulphonamide 1,1-dioxide.
$C_{15}H_{16}ClN_3O_4S_3$=433.9.

CAS — 13957-38-5.

Adverse Effects, Treatment, and Precautions. As for Chlorothiazide, p.588.

Uses. Hydrobentizide is a thiazide diuretic which has actions and uses similar to those of chlorothiazide (see p.589). In the treatment of hypertension the usual dose is 20 to 30 mg daily, in conjunction with other antihypertensive agents.

2333-v

Hydrochlorothiazide *(B.P., B.P. Vet., U.S.P.)*.

Hydrochlorothiaz.; Hydrochlorothiazidum; Hidroclorotiazida. 6-Chloro-3,4-dihydro-2*H*-1,2,4-benzothiadiazine-7-sulphonamide 1,1-dioxide.
$C_7H_8ClN_3O_4S_2$=297.7.

CAS — 58-93-5.

Pharmacopoeias. In *Br.*, *Braz.*, *Chin.*, *Cz.*, *Hung.*, *Int.*, *It.*, *Jap.*, *Jug.*, *Nord.*, *Pol.*, *Roum.*, *Turk.*, and *U.S.*

A white or almost white odourless or almost odourless crystalline powder with a slightly bitter taste. M.p. about 268° with decomposition. Practically **insoluble** in water, chloroform, ether, and dilute mineral acids; soluble 1 in 200 of alcohol and 1 in 20 of acetone; sparingly soluble in methyl alcohol; freely soluble in dimethylformamide, *n*-butylamine, and solutions of alkali hydroxides. **Store** in airtight containers.

Adverse Effects and Treatment. As for Chlorothiazide, p.588.

Erythema multiforme (the Stevens-Johnson syndrome) has been reported.

Allergy. Two women developed pulmonary oedema after they had each taken 50 mg of hydrochlorothiazide, as an aid to dieting in 1 case and for mild hypertension in the other. Both reactions were considered to be idiosyncratic.— A. D. Steinberg, *J. Am. med. Ass.*, 1968, *204*, 825. See also R. T. Bell and M. Lippmann, *Archs intern. Med.*, 1979, *139*, 817.

Acute severe allergic pneumonitis occurred in a patient on 2 occasions within 1 hour of taking hydrochlorothiazide. Challenge with hydrochlorothiazide provoked a third reaction.— C. Beaudry and L. Laplante, *Ann. intern. Med.*, 1973, *78*, 251.

Diabetogenic effect. Hyperglycaemia which occurred in 11 of 24 patients treated with hydrochlorothiazide 50 mg twice daily for 6 to 10 weeks was only partly corrected by administration of potassium supplements. There was no correlation between the changes in blood sugar and serum-potassium concentrations; the mechanism of the effect was not understood.— K. F. McFarland and A. A. Carr, *J. clin. Pharmac.*, 1977, *17*, 13.

Results of a double-blind controlled study by the European Working Party on Hypertension in the Elderly in which 119 elderly hypertensive subjects were followed-up for 1 year and 48 for 2 years, indicated that those who received hydrochlorothiazide and triamterene (together with methyldopa if necessary) had impaired glucose tolerance compared with those who received placebo. The impairment was noted within 2 years although studies by P.J. Lewis *et al.*, (*Lancet*, 1976, *1*, 564) have shown that in younger patients this might take over 5 years to develop. The theoretical risk of a small increase in blood-sugar concentration was expected to be offset by the decreased risk associated with blood pressure reduction and this information should be provided by the overall results of the trial.— A. Amery *et al.*, *Lancet*, 1978, *1*, 681.

Further references: A. Breckenridge *et al.*, *Lancet*, 1967, *1*, 61; V. Zamrazil *et al.*, *Metabolism*, 1967, *16*, 445; B. H. Hicks *et al.*, *ibid.*, 1973, *22*, 101.

Effects on the blood. *Agranulocytosis.* A 76-year-old woman who had taken 50 mg of hydrochlorothiazide daily for 6 months developed agranulocytosis and uraemia which were probably attributable to the drug.— M. B. Chrein and I. L. Rubin, *J. Am. med. Ass.*, 1962, *181*, 54.

Haemolytic anaemia. A report of haemolytic anaemia

induced by hydrochlorothiazide.— J. M. Vila *et al.*, *J. Am. med. Ass.*, 1976, *236*, 1723.

Thrombocytopenia. Thrombocytopenic purpura occurred in a 55-year-old woman with congestive heart failure treated with hydrochlorothiazide.— M. H. Gesink and H. A. Bradford, *J. Am. med. Ass.*, 1960, *172*, 556.

Effects on the electrolyte balance. *Calcium.* Hypercalcaemia occurred in a patient given hydrochlorothiazide 50 mg twice daily for mild hypertension.— C. G. Duarte *et al.*, *New Engl. J. Med.*, 1971, *284*, 828.

Total calcium and ionised calcium serum concentrations were increased in 9 healthy subjects given hydrochlorothiazide 50 mg twice daily for 25 days. There was no significant alteration in serum concentrations of immunoreactive parathyroid hormone.— R. M. Stote *et al.*, *Ann. intern. Med.*, 1972, *77*, 587.

Further references: R. Makin *et al.*, *Can. med. Ass. J.*, 1979, *121*, 591.

Potassium. A 48-year-old woman developed hypokalaemia after taking hydrochlorothiazide 50 mg daily for about a month and 100 mg daily for about a week.— P. D. Redleaf and I. J. Lerner, *J. Am. med. Ass.*, 1968, *206*, 1302.

For a report of hypokalaemia during treatment with hydrochlorothiazide and salcatonin, unresponsive to supplementary potassium by mouth, see Calcitonin, p.1074.

Sodium. A 46-year-old man with untreated hypothyroidism, who was given hydrochlorothiazide 50 mg daily and a low-salt diet for the treatment of congestive heart failure, developed hyponatraemia and water intoxication. Hyponatraemia occurred on a subsequent occasion when hydrochlorothiazide was given. The absence of hypokalaemia suggested that the hyponatraemia was not simply diuretic-induced.— A. Q. Mataverde *et al.*, *J. Am. med. Ass.*, 1974, *230*, 1014.

Hyponatraemia occurred on 3 occasions in a patient with psychogenic polydipsia while taking hydrochlorothiazide.— V. V. Gossain *et al.*, *Postgrad. med. J.*, 1976, *52*, 720. A similar report: H. R. Beresford, *J. Am. med. Ass.*, 1970, *214*, 879.

A report of hyponatraemia in 4 elderly patients taking hydrochlorothiazide.— C. A. Pinnock (letter), *Br. med. J.*, 1978, *1*, 48. See also A. I. Polanska and D. N. Baron (letter), *ibid.*, 175.

Further references: G. J. Gilbert (letter), *New Engl. J. Med.*, 1966, *274*, 1153; M. P. Fichman *et al.*, *Ann. intern. Med.*, 1971, *75*, 853.

Zinc. Occasional findings of subnormal serum-zinc concentrations in patients receiving thiazide therapy suggested that long-term thiazide therapy carries with it the risk of zinc deficiency.— M. Cohanim and E. R. Yendt, *Johns Hopkins med. J.*, 1975, *136*, 137.

Effects on the eyes. A study indicating that usual therapeutic doses of hydrochlorothiazide interfere with colour vision.— J. Laroche and C. Laroche, *Annls pharm. fr.*, 1972, *30*, 433.

Effects on the kidneys. A 43-year-old woman, who took hydrochlorothiazide 25 mg and triamterene 50 mg every second day for 10 days before menstruation for premenstrual oedema, suffered from renal colic following each dose of diuretic. Surgical investigation revealed a partial urinary-tract obstruction.— A. F. Delevett and M. Recalde (letter), *J. Am. med. Ass.*, 1973, *225*, 992.

Acute interstitial nephritis in 1 patient associated with the administration of hydrochlorothiazide.— A. L. Linton *et al.*, *Ann. intern. Med.*, 1980, *93*, 735.

Effects on lipid metabolism. A study confirming a possible adverse effect of hydrochlorothiazide on plasma-lipid concentrations.— P. van Brummelen *et al.*, *Curr. med. Res. Opinion*, 1979, *6*, 24.

Further references: A. Helgeland *et al.*, *Am. J. Med.*, 1978, *64*, 34; C. Joos *et al.*, *Eur. J. clin. Pharmac.*, 1980, *17*, 251.

Effects on the parathyroid glands. A 55-year-old man developed 3 parathyroid adenomas 11 years after the removal of 3 similar adenomas. It was suggested that hydrochlorothiazide, 30 mg daily, taken for 9 of the 11 intervening years, might have induced the recurrence of the adenomas.— L. Balizet, *J. Am. med. Ass.*, 1973, *225*, 1238.

Further references: T. Christensson *et al.*, *Archs intern. Med.*, 1977, *137*, 1138.

Effects on sexual function. A 33-year-old man reported difficulty in sustaining erection after he had commenced antihypertensive treatment with hydrochlorothiazide, up to 50 mg daily; the difficulty was enhanced when hydralazine in gradually increasing doses was also taken, but rapid improvement occurred when all medication was discontinued.— H. Keidan (letter), *Can. med. Ass. J.*, 1976, *114*, 874.

Effects on the skin. *Photosensitivity.* A report of photosensitivity in 2 patients probably due to hydrochlorothiazide.— *Japan med. Gaz.*, 1976, *13* (Sept. 20), 9.

Precautions. As for Chlorothiazide, p.589.

Interactions. *Antibiotics.* For the effect of hydrochlorothiazide on the urinary elimination of chloramphenicol, see Chloramphenicol, p.1138.

Probenecid. The urinary excretion of calcium, magnesium, and citrate was greater when hydrochlorothiazide and probenecid were given concomitantly than when hydrochlorothiazide was given alone. Probenecid prevented or abolished thiazide-induced increases in serum concentrations of uric acid but did not affect thiazide-induced excretion of monovalent ions.— D. A. Garcia and E. R. Yendt, *Can. med. Ass. J.* 1970, *103*, 473, per *Int. pharm. Abstr.*, 1971, *8*, 704.

Interference with diagnostic tests. A report that hydrochlorothiazide interferes with protein-bound iodine determinations for thyroid function.— H. Mehbod *et al.*, *Archs intern. Med.*, 1967, *119*, 283.

Absorption and Fate. Hydrochlorothiazide is incompletely but fairly rapidly absorbed from the gastro-intestinal tract. It has been estimated to have a plasma half-life of about 3 or 4 hours with a subsequent longer terminal phase; its biological half-life is up to about 12 hours. It appears to be preferentially bound to red blood cells. It is excreted unchanged in the urine. Hydrochlorothiazide crosses the placental barrier and is excreted in breast milk.

A review of the pharmacokinetics of hydrochlorothiazide.— B. Beermann and M. Groschinsky-Grind, *Eur. J. clin. Pharmac.*, 1977, *12*, 297.

Further reviews: M. C. Meyer *et al.*, *J. Am. pharm. Ass.*, 1976, *NS16*, 47 (bioavailability); A. Melander, *Clin. Pharmacokinet.*, 1978, *3*, 337 (bioavailability).

Following administration of hydrochlorothiazide 5 mg to 4 healthy subjects most was absorbed from the upper small intestine and a little from the stomach; maximum blood concentrations were reached after 60 to 120 minutes; up to 10 hours the plasma half-life was a mean of 3.8 hours with a possible second phase thereafter; peak concentrations about 3.5 times those in plasma occurred in red blood cells after 3 to 4 hours. Four hours after receiving 75 mg by mouth 1 healthy subject had a maximum plasma concentration of 428 ng per ml which declined in 2 phases with half-lives of 1.73 and 13.1 hours respectively. Following intravenous administration to 2 healthy subjects the half-life was 3.2 hours in one and 4.3 hours in the second, and maximum concentrations in the red blood cells about 3 times as high as in plasma were reached after 50 to 120 minutes. Urinary excretion of hydrochlorothiazide closely followed the fall in plasma concentration and after oral administration 70% of the dose was recovered from the urine within 4 days, generally about half in the first 12 hours; 11.4% to 24.5% of the oral dose was found in the faeces whereas after intravenous administration over 90% was recovered in the urine with only 1% to 4.3% in the faeces. Biliary excretion was thus negligible and gastro-intestinal absorption about 60% to 80%. Absorption and excretion after chronic administration of therapeutic doses by mouth to 3 hypertensive patients followed a similar pattern with peak plasma concentrations after 3 to 4 hours and peak red blood cell concentrations after 4 to 5 hours; the range of maximum plasma concentration was 260 to 616 ng per ml with red blood cell concentrations about 3 times as high; plasma half-lives during the first 12 hours varied from 3 to 6.3 hours and in the blood cells 3.2 to 7 hours; urinary recovery was of the same magnitude as in the healthy subjects but delayed excretion in 1 may have been due to decreased renal function.— B. Beermann *et al.*, *Clin. Pharmac. Ther.*, 1976, *19*, 531.

The gastro-intestinal absorption of hydrochlorothiazide was enhanced when it was given with food; this was probably due to delayed passage through the small intestine.— B. Beermann and M. Groschinsky-Grind, *Eur. J. clin. Pharmac.*, 1978, *13*, 125. A report of reduced absorption of hydrochlorothiazide in 5 patients who had previously undergone intestinal shunt surgery. The uptake of hydrochlorothiazide may depend on transit time through the small intestine.— L. Backman *et al.*, *Clin. Pharmacokinet.*, 1979, *4*, 63.

No correlation was shown between the plasma concentration of hydrochlorothiazide and reduction in blood pressure among 9 previously untreated hypertensive patients given doses of 12.5 to 75 mg daily.— B. Beermann and M. Groschinsky-Grind, *Eur. J. clin. Pharmac.*, 1978, *13*, 195.

Further references: W. J. A. Vandenheuvel *et al.*, *J. pharm. Sci.*, 1975, *64*, 1309.

Red cell binding. In 2 healthy subjects given hydrochlorothiazide 50 mg by mouth, peak plasma concentrations of 428 and 450 ng per ml occurred 2.5 and 2 hours respectively after administration. Whole blood concentrations occurring after 3 hours were about 2.5 times the value of plasma concentrations.— E. Redalieu *et al.*, *J. pharm. Sci.*, 1978, *67*, 726.

Uses. Hydrochlorothiazide is a thiazide diuretic with actions and uses similar to those of chlorothiazide (see p.589). Diuresis is initiated in about 2 hours and lasts for up to 12 hours.

In the treatment of oedema the usual initial dose is 50 to 100 mg daily, reduced to a dose of 25 to 50 mg daily or on alternate days; in some cases initial doses of up to 200 mg daily may be necessary. A suggested initial dose for children is 2 mg per kg body-weight daily in 2 divided doses.

In the treatment of hypertension the usual dose is 25 to 100 mg daily, either alone, or in conjunction with other antihypertensive agents.

When treatment is prolonged or in susceptible patients, loss of potassium may be sufficient to produce hypokalaemia; potassium supplements should then be given as for chlorothiazide.

Action. A study in 14 hypertensive patients was considered to provide additional evidence that the antihypertensive effect of prolonged hydrochlorothiazide therapy results mainly from reduced total peripheral resistance associated with a mild, but persistent, contraction in plasma volume.— J. G. R. de Carvalho *et al.*, *Clin. Pharmac. Ther.*, 1977, *22*, 875.

Administration. *Enteric-coated potassium formulations.* For references to bowel ulceration following the use of diuretic preparations containing enteric-coated potassium, including HydroSaluric-K and Salupres, see Chlorothiazide, Administration and Potassium, p.590.

Administration in renal failure. The pharmacokinetics of hydrochlorothiazide were altered in congestive heart failure and in 3 patients gastro-intestinal absorption was reduced to about 50% of that seen in healthy controls. The plasma half-life correlated with the endogenous creatinine clearance.— B. Beermann and M. Groschinsky-Grind, *Br. J. clin. Pharmac.*, 1979, *7*, 579.

Cardiac disorders. *Heart failure.* Hydrochlorothiazide and polythiazide were given to 30 patients with chronic congestive heart failure. The dose of polythiazide was 1, 2, or 4 mg daily and of hydrochlorothiazide 50, 100, or 200 mg daily. Each drug was given for 7 days with a week of placebo treatment in between. After hydrochlorothiazide 100 mg maximum excretion of sodium occurred within the first 12 hours and continued for 48 hours; after polythiazide 4 mg maximum excretion occurred within 12 to 36 hours and continued for 72 hours. Both drugs caused the same loss of potassium. The trial showed that there was no significant difference in the efficiency of the drugs after repeated administration.— D. E. Hutcheon and G. B. Leonard, *J. Am. med. Ass.*, 1963, *185*, 640.

See also Administration in Renal Failure, above.

Diabetes insipidus. Four patients with diabetes insipidus associated with deficiency of antidiuretic hormone responded well to treatment with hydrochlorothiazide. A further 4 members of the same family responded to chlorpropamide 500 mg daily.— A. A. Driedger and A. L. Linton, *Can. med. Ass. J.*, 1973, *109*, 594.

Hypernatraemia. Long-term therapy with hydrochlorothiazide 50 mg four times daily benefited a woman who suffered from chronic hypernatraemia and mental confusion without polyuria or polydipsia. The patient's urine-concentrating capacity was improved by chlorpropamide, 250 to 500 mg daily for 5 days, and by tolbutamide, 2 g daily for 3 days.— J. H. Mahoney and A. D. Goodman, *New Engl. J. Med.*, 1968, *279*, 1191.

Hypertension. In a double-blind 6-month crossover study in 30 patients with hypertension both hydrochlorothiazide 50 mg twice daily and frusemide 40 mg twice daily significantly reduced blood pressure but the fall was consistently greater with hydrochlorothiazide especially with respect to systolic pressure.— M. A. Araoye *et al.*, *J. Am. med. Ass.*, 1978, *240*, 1863. Criticism.— H. R. Dettelbach and D. A. Bennett (letter), *ibid.*, 1979, *242*, 712. A reply.— M. A. Araoye *et al.* (letter), *ibid.*

Further references to studies involving hydrochlorothiazide in the treatment of hypertension: Veterans Administration Cooperative Study Group on Antihypertensive Agents, *J. Am. med. Ass.*, 1967, *202*, 1028; J. Anderson *et al.*, *Q. J. Med.*, 1971, *40*, 541; D. M. Burley, *Ciba* (letter), *Lancet*, 1972, *1*, 597; G. Berglund and O. Andersson, *Eur. J. clin. Pharmac.*, 1976, *10*, 177; J. P. Chalmers *et al.*, *Med. J. Aust.*, 1976, *1*, 650; T. B. Cocke *et al.*, *J. clin. Pharmac.*, 1977, *17*, 334; Veterans Administration Cooperative Study Group on Antihypertensive Agents, *J. Am. med. Ass.*, 1977, *237*, 2303; R. H. Barnes and L. G. Eichner, *Curr. ther. Res.*, 1978, *24*, 786; J. W. Hollifield and P. E. Slaton, *Curr. ther. Res.*, 1978, *24*, 818; N. M. A. Walter *et al.*, *Med. J. Aust.*, 1978, *1*, 509; *Br. med. J.*, 1979, *2*, 1456; C. Bengtsson, *Curr. ther. Res.*, 1979, *26*, 394; M. Danielson and J. Kjellberg, *ibid.*, 383; R. M. Goodfellow, *Curr. med. Res. Opinion*, 1979, *6*, 371; O. B. Holland *et al.*, *Archs intern. Med.*, 1979, *139*, 1015; G. Schrijver and M. H. Weinberger, *Clin. Pharmac. Ther.*, 1979, *25*, 33; G. Berglund and O. Andersson, *Curr. ther. Res.*, 1980, *27*, 360; A. Lutterodt *et al.*, *Clin. Pharmac. Ther.*, 1980, *27*, 324; P. van Brummelen *et al.*, *ibid.*, 328.

Migraine. Hydrochlorothiazide, 25 mg thrice daily for 3 days, twice daily for 10 days, and once daily for 1 week, was given to 12 women with migraine. In 5 patients pain was stopped, and no relapse occurred during observation for 1½ years. Three patients experienced satisfactory improvement, 2 could not tolerate the drug, and 2 made no response.— L. Loubal, *Farmakoter. Zpr.*, 1967, *13*, 59, per *Int. pharm. Abstr.*, 1967, *4*, 1353.

Pregnancy and the neonate. Hypertension of pregnancy. No clear benefit from the continuous prophylactic use of hydrochlorothiazide from early in pregnancy was demonstrated by a random, double-blind assessment in 1030 women. Of these, 28% were teenagers and 39% were nulliparas. The dose of hydrochlorothiazide was 50 mg daily, and the patients who received it became more hypokalaemic and hyperuricaemic, though none showed clinical symptoms. The use of hydrochlorothiazide was not found significantly to affect the incidence of pre-eclampsia, hypertension, premature delivery, congenital abnormalities, or perinatal mortality. However, only 7.7% of the drug-treated patients made excessive gains in weight compared with 13.9% of the placebo group.— G. W. Kraus *et al.*, *J. Am. med. Ass.*, 1966, *198*, 1150.

See also under Precautions for Chlorothiazide, p.589.

Renal disorders. Hydrochlorothiazide 50 mg twice daily appeared to be effective in preventing the formation of calcium stones in the urinary tract of 67 patients with idiopathic hypercalciuria, urinary infection, or renal calculi with no apparent cause.— E. R. Yendt, *Can. med. Ass. J.*, 1970, *102*, 497. See also *idem*, 614.

Further references: E. R. Yendt *et al.*, *Am. J. med. Sci.*, 1966, *251*, 449; C. Y. C. Pak, *Clin. Pharmac. Ther.*, 1973, *14*, 209; M. Cohanim and E. R. Yendt, *Johns Hopkins med. J.*, 1975, *136*, 137.

Vertigo. Results with hydrochlorothiazide in Ménière's disease are largely inconclusive.— *Drug & Ther. Bull.*, 1971, *9*, 42.

Further references: I. Norell *et al.*, *Acta Oto-lar.*, 1962, *54*, 447; I. Klockhoff and U. Lindblom, *ibid.*, 1967, *63*, 347.

Preparations

Hydrochlorothiazide Tablets *(B.P.)*. Tablets containing hydrochlorothiazide.

Hydrochlorothiazide Tablets *(U.S.P.)*. Tablets containing hydrochlorothiazide. The *U.S.P.* requires 60% dissolution in 30 minutes.

Proprietary Preparations

Direma *(Dista, UK)*. Hydrochlorothiazide, available as tablets of 25 and 50 mg.

Esidrex *(Ciba, UK)*. Hydrochlorothiazide, available as scored tablets of 25 and 50 mg. **Esidrex-K.** Tablets each containing hydrochlorothiazide 12.5 mg in an outer layer and potassium chloride 600 mg (potassium 8.1 mmol; 8.1 mEq) in a slow-release wax core. (Also available as Esidrex in *Austral.*, *Belg.*, *Canad.*, *Denm.*, *Fr.*, *Ital.*, *Neth.*, *Norw.*, *Spain*, *Swed.*, *Switz.*).

Owing to the risk of intestinal obstruction, sustained-release preparations such as Esidrex-K, where the drug is released in transit, but the matrix ghost is often eliminated intact, should not be prescribed in patients with Crohn's disease or other intestinal disease in which strictures may form.— J. L. Shaffer *et al.* (letter), *Lancet*, 1980, *2*, 487.

HydroSaluric *(Merck Sharp & Dohme, UK)*. Hydrochlorothiazide, available as scored tablets of 25 and 50 mg.

Other Proprietary Names

Arg.—Diurex, Hidrenox, Tandiur; *Austral.*—Dichlotride, Neo-Flumen; *Belg.*—Dichlotride; *Canad.*—Diuchlor H, Hydro-Aquil, HydroDIURIL, Natrimax, Neo-Codema, Novohydrazide, Urozide; *Ger.*—Di-Chlotride, Esidrix; *Ital.*—Atenadon, Diclotride, Didral, Diidrotiazide, Dixidrasi, Idrodiuvis, Idrofluin, Idrolisin, Neo Minzil; *Jap.*—Chlothia, Maschitt, Newtolide, Pantemon; *Neth.*—Dichlotride; *Norw.*—Dichlotride; *S. Afr.*—Dichlotride, Urirex; *Spain*—Catiazida, Diursana-H, Hidrosaluretil, Neoflumen; *Swed.*—Dichlotride; *USA*—Chlorzide, Delco-Retic, Diucen-H, Esidrix, Hydro-Z, HydroDIURIL, Hydrozide, Jen-Diril, Lexor, Loqua, Mictrin, Oretic, Ro-Hydrazide, SK-Hydrochlorothiazide, Thiuretic.

Preparations containing hydrochlorothiazide were also formerly marketed in Great Britain under the proprietary names HydroSaluric-K and Salupres (*Merck Sharp & Dohme*).

2334-g

Hydroflumethiazide *(B.P., U.S.P.)*.

Hydroflumethiaz.; Hydroflumethiazidum; Trifluoromethylhydrothiazide. 3,4-Dihydro-6-trifluoromethyl-2*H*-1,2,4-benzothiadiazine-7-sulphonamide 1,1-dioxide.

$C_8H_8F_3N_3O_4S_2$=331.3.

CAS — 135-09-1.

Pharmacopoeias. In *Br.*, *Int.*, *Nord.*, and *U.S.*

White or cream-coloured, odourless or almost odourless, tasteless, glistening crystals or crystalline powder. M.p. 270° to 275°. **Soluble** 1 in 3000 of water and 1 in about 50 of alcohol; soluble 1 in 4 of acetone; practically insoluble in chloroform and ether. A 1% suspension in water has a pH of 4.5 to 7.5. **Store** in airtight containers.

Adverse Effects, Treatment, and Precautions. As for Chlorothiazide, p.588.

Interactions. *Lithium.* For the effect of hydroflumethiazide in reducing the renal clearance of Lithium, see under Lithium Carbonate, p.1539.

Absorption and Fate. Hydroflumethiazide is incompletely but fairly rapidly absorbed from the gastro-intestinal tract. It appears to have a biphasic biological half-life with an estimated alpha-phase of about 2 hours and an estimated beta-phase of about 17 hours; it has a metabolite with a longer half-life, which is extensively bound to the red blood cells. Hydroflumethiazide is excreted in the urine; its metabolite has also been detected in the urine.

In 5 healthy subjects and 9 patients with heart failure given hydroflumethiazide about 6 µmol per kg body-weight peak concentrations in plasma and peak excretion-rates occurred within the first 4 hours. The mean half-lives (α-phase) were 1.91 and 2.12 hours in healthy subjects and patients respectively, and (β-phase) 16.6 and 9.6 hours. About 47% of the dose was recovered from the urine in healthy subjects and patients; a small amount was recovered as 2,4-disulphamoyl-5-trifluoromethylaniline.— O. Brørs *et al.*, *Eur. J. clin. Pharmac.*, 1978, *14*, 29.

After a dose of hydroflumethiazide of 100 to 150 mg by mouth, only 0.051% was excreted in bile compared with 34.9% in urine during the first 6 hours after administration.— O. Brørs *et al.*, *Eur. J. clin. Pharmac.*, 1979, *15*, 287.

Further references: P. J. McNamara *et al.*, *J. clin. Pharmac.*, 1978, *18*, 190; G. J. Yakatan *et al.*, *J. clin. Pharmac.*, 1977, *17*, 37; O. Brørs and S. Jacobsen, *Eur. J. clin. Pharmac.*, 1979, *16*, 125.

Protein and red cell binding. Hydroflumethiazide is 74% bound to human serum albumin *in vitro*.— A. Agren and T. Bäck, *Acta pharm. suec.*, 1973, *10*, 223.

Evidence of extensive binding of 2,4-disulphamoyl-5-trifluoromethylaniline, a metabolite of hydroflumethiazide, to red blood cells.— O. Brørs and S. Jacobsen, *Eur. J. clin. Pharmac.*, 1979, *15*, 281.

Uses. Hydroflumethiazide is a thiazide diuretic with actions and uses similar to those of chlorothiazide (see p.589). Diuresis is initiated in about 2 hours and lasts for about 12 to 18 hours.

In the treatment of oedema the usual initial dose is 50 to 200 mg daily, in one or two divided doses, reduced to a dose of 25 to 50 mg on alternate days or intermittently. A suggested initial dose for children is 1 mg per kg body-weight daily, reduced for maintenance.

In the treatment of hypertension the usual dose is 50 to 100 mg daily in one or two divided doses, either alone, or in conjunction with other antihypertensive agents.

When treatment is prolonged, or in susceptible patients, loss of potassium may be sufficient to produce hypokalaemia; potassium supplements should then be given as for chlorothiazide.

Action. Hydroflumethiazide did not significantly inhibit carbonic anhydrase.— J. H. Jones and J. V. Jones, *Br. med. J.*, 1959, *2*, 928.

Hypertension. A recommendation for the combined use of hydroflumethiazide, 200 mg daily, with potassium supplement, methyldopa, up to 1.5 g daily in divided doses, and bethanidine sulphate, in order to maintain the standing diastolic pressure below 100 mmHg.— M. Hamilton, *Prescribers' J.*, 1972, *12*, 38.

Preprations

Hydroflumethiazide Tablets *(B.P.)*. Tablets containing hydroflumethiazide.

Hydroflumethiazide Tablets *(U.S.P.)*. Tablets containing hydroflumethiazide. Store in airtight containers.

Hydrenox *(Boots, UK)*. Hydroflumethiazide, available as tablets of 50 mg. (Also available as Hydrenox in *Austral.*).

Other Proprietary Names

Di-Ademil *(Austral.)*; Diucardin *(Canad., USA)*; Enjit *(Jap.)*; Leodrine *(Fr.)*; Rivosil *(Ital.)*; Robezon *(Jap.)*; Rontyl *(Denm., Neth., Norw.)*; Saluron *(USA)*; Salurona *(Spain)*.

Hydroflumethiazide was also formerly marketed in Great Britain under the proprietary name NaClex (*Glaxo*).

NOTE. In the USA, NaClex (*Robins*) was formerly used as a proprietary name for benzthiazide.

2335-q

Indapamide.

SE 1520. 4-Chloro-*N*-(2-methylindolin-1-yl)-3-sulphamoylbenzamide hemihydrate.

$C_{16}H_{16}ClN_3O_3S,\frac{1}{2}H_2O$=374.8.

CAS — 26807-65-8 (anhydrous).

Adverse Effects, Treatment, and Precautions. As for Chlorothiazide, p.588.

Diabetogenic effect. Following administration of a single dose of indapamide 40 mg to 6 healthy subjects no increases in blood-sugar concentrations occurred.— D. B. Campbell and E. M. Phillips, *Eur. J. clin. Pharmac.*, 1974, *7*, 407.

Effects on the electrolyte balance. A study indicating that indapamide does not significantly modify the exchangeable potassium and sodium pools after treatment.— R. Isaac *et al.*, *Curr. med. Res. Opinion*, 1977, *5*, *Suppl.* 1, 64. See also G. Onesti *et al.*, *ibid.*, 83.

A report of very severe hypokalaemia in an elderly man given indapamide for hypertension.— O. Rodat and J.-P. Hamelin, *Nouv. Presse méd.*, 1978, *7*, 3054.

Further references: A. Richard *et al.*, *Nouv. Presse méd.*, 1977, *6*, 1409.

Effects on lipid metabolism. Mention of increases in the serum cholesterol concentrations of 12 patients undergoing long-term indapamide therapy.— J. C. Demanet *et al.*, *Curr. med. Res. Opinion*, 1977, *5*, *Suppl.* 1, 129.

Interactions. *Disopyramide.* Cardiac arrhythmias in a 64-year-old hypertensive man with suspected latent coronary insufficiency were considered to have been cause by the hypokalaemic action of indapamide together with the effect of concomitant disopyramide administration.— C. Cosma *et al.*, *Nouv. Presse méd.*, 1978, *7*, 3455.

Absorption and Fate. Indapamide is rapidly absorbed from the gastro-intestinal tract. It has a biphasic plasma half-life with an initial alpha-phase of about 1.5 to 2 hours and a terminal beta-phase of up to about 20 hours. It is extensively metabolised, the metabolites being slowly excreted in the urine and faeces over about a week; only about 5% is excreted in the urine unchanged. Indapamide is about 80% bound to plasma proteins but is preferentially taken up in the red blood cells.

A review of the pharmacokinetics and metabolism of indapamide.— D. B. Campbell *et al.*, *Curr. med. Res. Opinion*, 1977, *5, Suppl.* 1, 13.

Following oral administration of radioactively labelled indapamide 10 mg to 4 healthy subjects it was rapidly absorbed with peak plasma concentrations occurring after 30 minutes. Decay followed a bi-exponential curve with mean half-lives of 1.7 and 17.8 hours. Indapamide was extensively metabolised with less than 5% of the dose excreted in the urine unchanged. Radioactivity was slowly eliminated into urine (60%) and faeces (20%) over a period of 8 days.— D. B. Campbell *et al.*, *Br. J. clin. Pharmac.*, 1976, *3*, 971P.

Further references: D. B. Campbell and E. M. Phillips, *Eur. J. clin. Pharmac.*, 1974, *7*, 407.

Metabolism. A study of the metabolism of indapamide in *mice* and *rats*.— B. L. Furman, *Curr. med. Res. Opinion*, 1977, *5, Suppl.* 1, 33.

Protein and red cell binding. Binding of indapamide to human plasma protein was 79% but concentrations 4 times higher were found in the red blood cells. About one hour after oral administration about 30% of the total dose was located in red blood cells, and was found to be reversibly bound to the carbonic anhydrase fraction.— D. B. Campbell *et al.*, *Br. J. clin. Pharmac.*, 1976, *3*, 971P.

Uses. Indapamide is a diuretic which has certain structural similarities to frusemide as well as the thiazides and has actions and uses similar to those of chlorothiazide (see p.589). Diuresis is initiated within about 1 to 2 hours and has been reported to last for up to 36 hours. Its inhibitory action on carbonic anhydrase is only weak. In the treatment of oedema it has been given in doses of 2.5 to 5 mg daily; higher doses were used in initial studies. In the treatment of hypertension the usual dose is 2.5 mg daily, either alone, or in conjunction with other antihypertensive agents; higher doses are not recommended since the diuretic effect may become apparent without appreciable additional antihypertensive effect.

When treatment is prolonged, or in susceptible patients, loss of potassium may be sufficient to produce hypokalaemia; potassium supplements should then be given as for chlorothiazide.

Action. Reviews, reports, and discussions on the mode of action and uses of indapamide: *Curr. med. Res. Opinion*, 1977, *5, Suppl.* 1, 1-174; *Clin. Trials J.*, 1978, *15* (3), 103; *Postgrad. med. J.*, 1981, *57, Suppl.* 2, 1–73.

Animal studies suggesting that the antihypertensive activities of indapamide are dissociated from its diuretic activity.— L. G. Beregi, *Curr. med. Res. Opinion*, 1977, *5, Suppl.* 1, 3.

Studies in *rats* suggested that indapamide has a direct action on the vascular bed, and mode of action different from that of hydrochlorothiazide.— L. Finch *et al.*, *J. Pharm. Pharmac.*, 1977, *29*, 739.

A study in 6 healthy subjects, given indapamide 10 mg, indicated that its primary site of action in man is the proximal end of the distal tubule.— J. Pitone *et al.*, *Clin. Pharmac. Ther.*, 1978, *23*, 125.

Further references: G. Onesti *et al.*, *Curr. med. Res. Opinion*, 1977, *5, Suppl.* 1, 83; M. Laubie and H. Schmitt, *ibid.*, 89; F. Lenzi and T. Di Perri, *ibid.*, 145; G. Onesti *et al.*, *Clin. Pharmac. Ther.*, 1977, *21*, 113.

Hypertension. Results of a small preliminary study indicated that indapamide 2.5 to 5 mg daily is an effective antihypertensive agent in some patients with mild to moderate hypertension, and is free of significant short-term side-effects. Further studies, however, are needed in a larger patient population to delineate its place in therapy. The study was a placebo-controlled 12-week single-blind trial involving 14 hypertensive patients and completed by 10, of whom 2 also took propranolol. Associated with the change in blood pressure, a gradual decrease in supine pulse-rate occurred during indapamide administration, with a mean fall of 10%. Side-effects possibly associated with drug therapy were: nocturia (1), nocturia and constipation (1), and giddiness and migraine (1; a known migraine sufferer).— P. Turner *et al.*, *Curr. med. Res. Opinion*, 1977, *5, Suppl.* 1, 124.

Evidence that indapamide has an antihypertensive effect in doses of 0.5 to 1 mg daily. It is unlikely, however, that these doses will be useful in the clinical treatment of hypertension.— M. Fernandes *et al.*, *ibid.*, 60.

Further references: S. Witchitz *et al.*, *Thérapie*, 1974, *29*, 109; S. Hamilton and D. Kelly, *J. Ir. med. Ass.*, 1977, *70*, 462; E. Uhlich *et al.*, *Curr. med. Res. Opinion*, 1977, *5, Suppl.* 1, 71; J. C. Canicave and F. X. Lesbre, *ibid.*, 79; J. G. Hashida, *ibid.*, 116; J. C. Demanet *et al.*, *ibid.*, 129; D. A. Kelly and S. Hamilton, *ibid.*, 137; F. P. Casar, *ibid.*, 157; P. Schlesinger *et al.*, *ibid.*, 159; E. W. Andries *et al.*, *ibid.*, 165; C. B. Coutinho *et al.*, *Clin. Pharmac. Ther.*, 1980, *27*, 296.

Proprietary Preparations

Natrilix *(Servier, UK)*. Indapamide, available as tablets of 2.5 mg. (Also available as Natrilix in *Ger.*, *Ital.*, *S.Afr.*).

Other Proprietary Names

Fludex *(Fr., Neth., Switz.)*; Ipamix *(Ital.)*.

2336-p

Isosorbide. AT-101. 1,4:3,6-Dianhydro-D-glucitol.
$C_6H_{10}O_4$=146.1.

CAS — 652-67-5.

A crystalline solid. M.p. about 62°.

Adverse Effects and Precautions. These may be anticipated to be as for Urea, p.616, but isosorbide has been reported to be less irritant; it is, nevertheless, unpalatable, and gastro-intestinal irritation is common.

Adverse effects reported following administration of isosorbide include vomiting, diarrhoea, loss of weight, irritability, and elevated blood-urea-nitrogen values. Creatinine clearance has been reported to be significantly increased.

Adverse effects noted during isosorbide administration for hydrocephalus included persistent vomiting, marked irritability, doughy skin, failure to gain weight, and elevated blood-urea-nitrogen values.— D. B. Shurtleff and P. W. Hayden, *J. clin. Pharmac.*, 1972, *12*, 108.

Effects on the kidneys. Surprisingly, creatinine clearance was significantly increased during isosorbide diuresis (possibly as a result of decreased tubular reabsorption).— J. H. Nodine *et al.*, *Clin. Pharmac. Ther.*, 1973, *14*, 196.

Interactions. *Diuretics.* Findings of synergy between isosorbide and hydrochlorothiazide.— J. H. Nodine *et al.*, *Clin. Pharmac. Ther.*, 1973, *14*, 196.

Absorption and Fate. Isosorbide is fairly rapidly absorbed from the gastro-intestinal tract. It is excreted unchanged in the urine with a plasma half-life of about 8 hours.

A study of the pharmacodynamics and pharmacokinetics of isosorbide. In 6 healthy subjects isosorbide was found to be rapidly absorbed from the gastro-intestinal tract with a mean absorption half-life of 0.35 hour (range 0.22 to 0.53 hour). In 4 healthy subjects it was found to be excreted unchanged in the urine with a mean serum disappearance half-life of 7.13 hours (range 4.9 to 9.49 hours) after a single dose of 100 g and 8.25 hours (range 5.43 to 10.60 hours) after repeated doses of 100 g daily for 2 weeks. This difference was neither clinically nor statistically different. Abdominal discomfort was the only side-effect reported.— J. H. Nodine *et al.*, *Clin. Pharmac. Ther.*, 1973, *14*, 196.

Uses. Isosorbide is an osmotic diuretic which, unlike mannitol, (p.604) is readily absorbed from the gastro-intestinal tract and, unlike urea (p.616), is not too irritant for administration by mouth.

It is given in doses of about 2 g per kg body-weight four times daily for the treatment of hydrocephalus. It has also been used in raised intra-ocular pressure and in oedema associated with cirrhosis of the liver.

Action. A study of the diuretic effect of isosorbide in healthy subjects.— F. J. Troncale *et al.*, *Am. J. med. Sci.*, 1966, *251*, 188.

Further references: J. H. Nodrine *et al.*, *Clin. Pharmac. Ther.*, 1973, *14*, 196.

Administration in hepatic failure. A suggestion of some reduced absorption of isosorbide in patients with cirrhosis of the liver.— O. Gagnon *et al.*, *Am. J. med. Sci.*, 1967, *254*, 284.

See also under Hepatic Disorders (below).

Glaucoma. Isosorbide 1.5 g per kg body-weight reduced intra-ocular pressure in 40 glaucomatous eyes and 18 normal eyes. The side-effects were minimal.— O. P. Kulshrestha and R. N. Mittal, *Br. J. Ophthal.*, 1972, *56*, 439.

Further references: B. Becker *et al.*, *Archs Ophthal.*, *N.Y.*, 1967, *78*, 147; K. S. Mehra and R. Singh, *ibid.*, 1971, *86*, 623; *Med. Lett.*, 1974, *16*, 83.

Hepatic disorders. Isosorbide, usually in a dose of 1 g per kg body-weight, given as a cooled 50% solution before or after the morning meal to 21 patients with liver cirrhosis or fluid retention, was nearly as effective in producing diuresis as mannitol given intravenously. Higher daily doses were given in 2 or 3 divided doses to avoid nausea. Since isosorbide produced less increase of plasma volume, it might be safer than mannitol for patients with oesophageal varices, raised central venous pressure, or impending congestive heart failure.— O. Gagnon *et al.*, *Am. J. med. Sci.*, 1967, *254*, 284.

Raised intracranial pressure. *Hydrocephalus.* Isosorbide 2 g per kg body-weight every 6 hours was given to 34 selected patients, 2 days to 11 months old (1 of 15 years on shunt removal), with infantile hydrocephalus. If effective the dose was reduced to 1 to 1.5 g per kg every 6 hours after 3 weeks. If ineffective, 2 g per kg was given every 4 hours for a limited period. Treatment was given from periods of a few days to 11 months and was successful, shunt therapy not being needed, in 10 of 15 patients; operation was delayed in 9 of 19 more severely affected patients. Reversible toxic effects included hypernatraemia, diarrhoea, vomiting, and loss of weight. Isosorbide was of value in infants with uncomplicated infantile hydrocephalus with a cerebral mantle of 20 mm or more and in those with spina bifida and a cerebral mantle of at least 15 to 25 mm. Surgery was successfully delayed in infants with posthaemorrhagic and postmeningitic hydrocephalus.— J. Lorber, *Archs Dis. Childh.*, 1975, *50*, 431.

Further references: P. W. Hayden *et al.*, *Pediatrics*, 1968, *41*, 955; D. B. Shurtleff and P. W. Hayden, *J. clin. Pharmac.*, 1972, *12*, 108; D. B. Shurtleff *et al.*, *J. Pediat.*, 1973, *83*, 651; J. Lorber, *Clin. Pediat.*, 1975, *14*, 916; I. Blumenthal *et al.* (letter), *Lancet*, 1976, *1*, 756; J. Lorber, *Med. Problems Paediat.*, 1977, *18*, 178.

2337-s

Lithium Benzoate *(B.P.C. 1934)*.
$C_7H_5LiO_2$=128.1.

CAS — 553-54-8.

Pharmacopoeias. In *Fr.* and *Port.*

An odourless light white powder or small crystalline scales with a sweetish saline taste. Each g represents 7.8 mmol (7.8 mEq) of lithium. **Soluble** 1 in 3 of water and 1 in 15 of alcohol; **incompatible** with acids and alkali carbonates.

Lithium benzoate has been used as a diuretic and urinary disinfectant. Its use cannot be recommended because of the pharmacological effect of the lithium ion (see Lithium Carbonate, p.1535).

2338-w

Mannitol *(B.P., U.S.P.)*. Manna Sugar; Mannite; Manita. D-Mannitol.

$C_6H_{14}O_6$=182.2.

CAS — 69-65-8.

Pharmacopoeias. In *Aust.*, *Belg.*, *Br.*, *Braz.*, *Chin.*, *Cz.*, *Fr.*, *It.*, *Jap.*, *Nord.*, *Port.*, *Roum.*, *Span.*, *Swiss*, *Turk.*, and *U.S.*

A hexahydric alcohol related to mannose ($C_6H_{12}O_6$ = 180.2). It is isomeric with sorbitol. A white odourless crystalline powder or granules with a sweetish taste. M.p. 165° to 169°.

Soluble 1 in 6 of water and 1 in 18 of glycerol; slightly soluble in alcohol and pyridine; practically insoluble in chloroform and ether; soluble in solutions of alkali carbonates and hydroxides. A 5.07% solution in water is iso-osmotic with serum. Solutions are **sterilised** by autoclaving or by filtration.

Incompatibility. Mannitol solutions, 20% or stronger, could be salted out by potassium or sodium chloride.— J. Jacobs, *J. Hosp. Pharm.*, 1969, *27*, 341.

Flocculent precipitation occurred when a 25% solution of mannitol was allowed to contact plastic.— E. Epperson (letter), *Am. J. Hosp. Pharm.*, 1978, *35*, 1337. Plastic surfaces may act as nuclei for crystallisation to occur at a rapid rate, thereby providing atypically small crystals when supersaturated mannitol injections are used. Resolubilisation with the aid of heat is of no benefit since rapid recrystallisation may occur. Where volume intake is not a major concern this problem may be overcome by diluting the supersaturated injection to 18% or less with water before contact with the plastic container or administration device. In all cases, however, a filtration device should be used during the administration of the fluid.— R. L. Nedich, *Travenol* (letter), *ibid.*

Mannitol should never be added to whole blood for transfusion or given through the same set by which blood is being infused. For details of the adverse effects of mannitol on red blood cells, see Effects on the Blood under Adverse Effects.

Stability. There was no physical or chemical change in a mannitol injection nor any change in potency after 5 autoclavings. Mannitol injections could therefore be heated or autoclaved repeatedly if crystals appeared as a result of storage.— B. S. R. Murty and J. N. Kapoor, *Am. J. Hosp. Pharm.*, 1975, *32*, 826.

Tablet excipient. For the use of mannitol as a tablet excipient, see Kee-Neng Wai *et al.*, *J. pharm. Sci.*, 1962, *51*, 1076; R. G. Daoust and M. J. Lynch, *Drug Cosmet. Ind.*, 1963, *93*, 26; J. L. Kanig, *J. pharm. Sci.*, 1964, *53*, 188; E. J. Mendell, *Mfg Chem.*, 1972, *43* (May), 43.

Adverse Effects. The most common side-effect associated with mannitol therapy is fluid and electrolyte imbalance; in patients with diminished cardiac reserve expansion of the extracellular fluid volume is a special hazard. Other side-effects reported may be associated with hypersensitivity reactions.

When given by mouth, mannitol causes diarrhoea; nausea and vomiting may also occur. Intravenous infusion of mannitol has been associated with nausea, vomiting, thirst, headache, dizziness, chills, fever, tachycardia, chest pain, hyponatraemia, urinary retention, dehydration, blurred vision, convulsions, urticaria, pulmonary oedema, and hypotension or hypertension. Extravasation of the solution may cause oedema and skin necrosis; thrombophlebitis may occur.

Allergy. Within 3 to 6 minutes of the commencement of an infusion of 20% mannitol solution, a 65-year-old woman, with a history of allergy to penicillin, procaine, and other agents, showed an allergic reaction including sneezing, rhinorrhoea, swollen tongue, dyspnoea, wheals on the chest, cyanosis, and loss of consciousness. Later, skin testing showed a positive reaction to mannitol solution. Her hypersensitivity could have originated from desensitisation injections containing fungous products with a mannitol content, which had been given 40 years earlier.— G. L. Spaeth *et al.*, *Archs Ophthal., N.Y.*, 1967, *78*, 583.

Further references: J. D. Lamb and J. A. M. Keogh, *Can. Anaesth. Soc. J.*, 1979, *26*, 435.

Effects on the blood. Agglutination and irreversible crenation of erythrocytes occurred when blood was mixed with varying proportions of a 10% mannitol solution. It was suggested that intravenous infusions should be carefully controlled and administered at a slow rate.— B. E. Roberts and P. H. Smith, *Lancet*, 1966, *2*, 421. The significance of the results in relation to adverse effects in sickle-cell disease.— F. I. D. Konotey-Ahulu (letter), *ibid.*, 591; B. E. Roberts and P. H. Smith (letter), *ibid.* A further comment.— J. H. Samson (letter), *ibid.*, 1191.

Effects on the electrolyte balance. Sodium. Severe hyponatraemia in a 69-year-old man who required 30 to 40 litres of mannitol 3% for bladder irrigation during transurethral prostatic resection.— M. A. Kirschenbaum, *J. Urol.*, 1979, *121*, 687.

Further references: A. Aviram *et al.*, *Am. J. Med.*, 1967, *42*, 648.

Effects on the gastro-intestinal tract. For a report of potentially explosive intracolonic hydrogen concentrations in patients receiving mannitol, see under Bowel Preparation in Uses.

Effects on the heart. Mannitol, given to *dogs* after coronary occlusion, hindered the development of collateral circulation.— H. O. Hirzel and E. S. Kirk, *Circulation*, 1977, *56*, 1006.

Effects on the kidneys. Focal osmotic nephrosis occurred in a patient after the administration of mannitol 20% intravenously.— W. E. Goodwin and H. Latta, *J. Urol.*, 1970, *103*, 11.

Treatment of Adverse Effects. Treatment of overdosage with mannitol should be symptomatic and, in particular, directed at correction of fluid and electrolyte imbalance.

Precautions. Mannitol is contra-indicated in patients with pulmonary congestion or pulmonary oedema, intracranial bleeding (except during craniotomy), congestive heart failure (in patients with diminished cardiac reserve expansion of the extracellular fluid may lead to fulminating congestive heart failure), and in patients with renal failure unless a test dose has produced a diuretic response (if renal flow is inadequate, expansion of the extracellular fluid may lead to acute water intoxication).

All patients given mannitol should be carefully observed for signs of fluid and electrolyte imbalance.

Interactions. Muscle relaxants. For reference to a suggestion that mannitol may enhance tubocurarine-induced neuromuscular blockade, see Tubocurarine Chloride, p.999.

Interference with diagnostic tests. Evidence that mannitol causes false-positive estimations of ethylene glycol.— I. J. Gilmour *et al.* (letter), *New Engl. J. Med.*, 1974, *291*, 51.

Absorption and Fate. Only small amounts of mannitol are absorbed from the gastro-intestinal tract, but any that is absorbed passes thence to the liver to be metabolised ultimately to carbon dioxide. Following intravenous injection mannitol is excreted rapidly by the kidneys before any very significant metabolism can take place in the liver.

Absorption and distribution. Studies on the duodenum and ileum of *dogs* indicated that although mannitol is absorbed at a slow, but appreciable, rate from both, in the duodenum hyperosmotic mannitol solution causes a profuse secretion of water and sodium into the lumen to produce an iso-osmotic solution, whereas in the ileum there is merely a continued slow absorption of both water and mannitol.— W. Hindle and C. F. Code, *Am. J. Physiol.*, 1962, *203*, 215.

Mannitol, given to patients undergoing cardiopulmonary bypass, required over 3 hours for distribution in the extracellular fluid. In the next 24 hours, 83% was recovered in the urine. Approximately 20% of mannitol filtered by the glomeruli was reabsorbed by the tubules.— G. A. Porter *et al.*, *J. Surg. Res.*, 1967, *7*, 447.

Further references: R. Dominguez *et al.*, *J. Lab. clin. Med.*, 1947, *32*, 1192; J. R. Elkinton, *J. clin. Invest.*, 1947, *26*, 1088.

Metabolism. A study indicating that mannitol is partially absorbed from the gastro-intestinal tract, and that some of the absorbed mannitol is excreted unchanged in the urine and some is metabolised, presumably in the liver, to carbon dioxide. No difference was noted between the metabolism of mannitol in cirrhotic subjects and those with healthy liver function. As the dose increased, inducing diarrhoea, the proportion of mannitol in the faeces increased. Very little metabolism was noted after intravenous administration of 10 g.— S. M. Nasrallah and F. L. Iber, *Am. J. med. Sci.*, 1969, *258*, 80.

Further references: J. K. Clark and H. G. Barker, *Proc. Soc. exp. Biol. Med.*, 1948, *69*, 152; A. N. Wick *et al.*, *ibid.*, 1954, *85*, 188.

Uses. Mannitol, an isomer of sorbitol, has little significant energy value, since it is largely eliminated from the body before any metabolism can take place. Mannitol is generally administered by intravenous infusion as an osmotic diuretic but it has also been given by mouth to remove fluid by inducing purgation. Careful monitoring of fluid balance, electrolytes, and vital signs is necessary during infusion to prevent fluid and electrolyte imbalance, including circulatory overload. The more concentrated solutions of mannitol are supersaturated; crystals may be redissolved by warming before use; the administration set should include a filter. Mannitol is not suitable for subcutaneous or intramuscular injection.

The adult dose of mannitol ranges from 50 to 200 g by intravenous infusion in a 24-hour period, but an adequate response is generally achieved with a dosage of 100 g in 24 hours. The rate of administration is usually adjusted to maintain a urine flow of at least 30 to 50 ml per hour. The total dosage, the concentration, and the rate of administration depend on the fluid requirement, the urinary output, and the nature and severity of the condition being treated.

Mannitol may be used to treat patients with renal failure (oliguria) or those suspected of inadequate renal function, provided a test dose of about 200 mg per kg body-weight (about 50 ml of a 25% solution or 100 ml of a 15% solution) given by intravenous infusion over 3 to 5 minutes produces a diuresis of at least 30 to 50 ml per hour during the next 2 to 3 hours; a second test dose is permitted if the response to the first is inadequate. The usual dose to treat oliguria is 50 to 100 g of a 15 to 25% solution, and 50 to 100 g may be given as a 5 to 25% solution to prevent acute renal failure during cardiovascular and other types of surgery, or following trauma.

To reduce raised intracranial pressure or raised intra-ocular pressure in neurosurgery or ophthalmology, mannitol is given by rapid infusion as a 15 to 25% solution in a dose of 1.5 to 2 g per kg body-weight over 30 to 60 minutes.

Where appropriate, a 5% solution of mannitol is used in diuresis regimens for the management of poisoning (see under Phenobarbitone, p.812).

Mannitol has been used for the determination of the glomerular filtration-rate; mannitol is given intravenously and its concentration in plasma and urine is measured at specified time intervals, permitting calculation of the volume of plasma in ml per minute which must have been filtered at the glomeruli to provide the amount found in the urine.

A 2.5% solution of mannitol has been used for irrigating the bladder during the transurethral resection of the prostate.

Mannitol has also been used as a diluent and excipient in pharmaceutical preparations.

Temporary estimated acceptable daily intake of mannitol: up to 50 mg per kg body-weight.— Twentieth Report of the Joint FAO/WHO Expert Committee on Food Additives, *Tech. Rep. Ser. Wld Hlth Org. No. 599*, 1976.

Administration in renal failure. Administration of hyperosmotic solutions of mannitol could cause considerable expansion of the extracellular fluid even when urine flow exceeded 5 ml per minute. Severe oliguria could follow and the patient might need dialysis for the relief of pulmonary oedema.— A. Polak and A. G. Morgan (letter), *Lancet*, 1968, *1*, 1310.

A study in 40 patients with glomerular filtration rates ranging from 2 to 100 ml per minute indicated that mannitol can be used successfully as an osmotic diuretic even in patients with low glomerular filtration rates.— P. Metaxas *et al.*, *Am. J. med. Sci.*, 1970, *259*, 175. See also R. G. Luke *et al.*, *ibid.*, 168.

Mannitol is ineffective and hazardous in primary acute or chronic renal failure.— J. S. Cheigh, *Am. J. Med.*, 1977, *62*, 555.

Further references: A. Aviram *et al.*, *Am. J. Med.*, 1967, *42*, 648; E. Pitakenen *et al.*, *Ann. clin. Res.*, 1976, *8*, 368.

See also under Renal Disorders (below).

Bowel preparation. Mannitol was effective for preparing the bowel for barium enema. One litre of 10% solution was consumed within 30 minutes early on the day of (afternoon) examination. Bowel clearance was better than that achieved with a 3-day low-residue diet, followed by magnesium sulphate, castor oil, and bisacodyl rectally.— K. R. Palmer and A. N. Khan, *Br. med. J.*, 1979, *2*, 1038. See also G. L. Newstead and B. P. Morgan, *Med. J. Aust.*, 1979, *2*, 582.

A study demonstrating potentially explosive intracolonic hydrogen concentrations in patients given mannitol for bowel preparation.— S. J. La Brooy *et al.*, *Lancet*, 1981, *1*, 634. Data indicating that mannitol is a safe preparation for colonoscopy even when diathermy is to be used.— I. Trotman and R. Walt (letter), *ibid.*, 848.

Cardiac disorders. Heart failure. Nine patients with chronic heart failure, which had not responded to diuretic therapy, benefited from the administration of 1 litre of mannitol 20% solution by mouth over a period of 2 hours. Diarrhoea began 30 minutes after the first glass of mannitol solution and continued for about 6 hours. Three of the patients (all with cardiac oedema) subsequently responded to diuretic therapy that had previously been ineffective. Six patients with oedema associated with renal failure and one with oedema associated with cirrhosis of the liver also benefited.— J. W. James and R. A. Evans, *Br. med. J.*, 1970, *1*, 463.

Drug overdosage. Of 23 patients with aspirin or barbiturate poisoning given mannitol to induce diuresis, haemodialysis was necessary in 1 due to oliguria and pulmonary oedema. Retention of mannitol occurred in all the patients, ranging from 27 to 314 g. Great caution is necessary during this treatment as retention of mannitol can lead to movement of water into the extracellular fluid.— A. G. Morgan *et al.*, *Q. J. Med.*, 1968, *37*, 589.

Catharsis, preferably using an orally administered saturated solution of mannitol, presents far too many hazards in the treatment of drug poisoning, despite its value in paraquat poisoning. The frequently associated loss of gut mobility presents an ideal situation for increased absorption of the now further diluted poison. Catharsis by other agents is likely to add the toxic effect of the cathartic to that of the poison for which it is being given.— S. Locket, *Br. J. Hosp. Med.*, 1978, *19*, 200.

Glaucoma. Comments on the use of mannitol in raised intra-ocular pressure.— D. P. Durkee and B. G. Bryant, *Am. J. Hosp. Pharm.*, 1978, *35*, 682.

A report of the prevention of glaucoma by the use of mannitol and acetazolamide in a 29-year-old man undergoing haemodialysis.— P. Jaeger *et al.* (letter), *New Engl. J. Med.*, 1980, *303*, 702.

Hepatic disorders. Massive diarrhoea was produced by the administration by mouth of 2 litres of 10% mannitol over about 4 hours to 11 patients with cirrhosis and ascites and to 3 normal controls. The average stool volume in 24 hours was just over 4 litres. Significant amounts of sodium—mean 155 mmol (155 mEq)—and potassium—mean 75 mmol (75 mEq)—and about 2 litres of fluid were thus removed from the body within 24 hours.— P. M. Gertman *et al.*, *J. Am. med. Ass.*, 1966, *197*, 257.

Further references: J. W. James and R. A. Evans, *Br. med. J.*, 1970, *1*, 463.

Pregnancy and the neonate. *Termination of pregnancy.* Mannitol, 200 ml of a 25% solution instilled into the amniotic cavity, induced abortion in 6 of 12 women.— I. L. Craft and B. D. Musa (letter), *Br. med. J.*, 1971, *2*, 49.

Pulmonary oedema. A report on experience with mannitol in pulmonary oedema.— C. H. Carter (letter), *J. Am. med. Ass.*, 1967, *201*, 275.

Raised intracranial pressure. A brief account of the role of mannitol in the control of cerebral oedema. For the best effects, mannitol should be given rapidly and in an adequate dosage to maximise the osmotic gradient. A typical dose is 1 g per kg body-weight given over approximately 10 minutes, unless the intracranial pressure is being monitored in which case smaller doses may be tried. If mannitol is required more often than every 3 to 4 hours the serum osmolality must be followed closely; if this rises above 320 mosmol per litre and the intracranial pressure remains elevated, administration of more mannitol is likely to lead to renal failure, metabolic acidosis, and death.— J. D. Miller, *Br. J. Hosp. Med.*, 1979, *21*, 152.

Further references: J. A. Pierce, *Anesth. Analg. curr. Res.*, 1966, *45*, 407; E. Young and R. F. Bradley, *New Engl. J. Med.*, 1967, *276*, 665; E. Ramos *et al.*, *J. Am. med. Ass.*, 1968, *205*, 590.

For a recommendation that frusemide be used instead of mannitol when diuresis is required in patients with pre-existing raised intracranial pressure, and in those who have pre-existing cardiac and electrolyte abnormalities, see Frusemide, p.600.

Reye's syndrome. Mannitol was considered to be the single most effective drug for rapidly reducing intracranial pressure in children with Reye's syndrome. A dose of 1 g per kg body-weight intravenously produced an effect within 5 minutes and the intracranial pressure remained low for 90 to 150 minutes thereafter.— B. A. Shaywitz *et al.*, *Pediatrics*, 1977, *59*, 595. Reye's syndrome was successfully treated in 18 children using a specific protocol which included the intravenous infusion of mannitol 2 g per kg body-weight every four hours or more frequently if intraventricular pressure was high. Only 2 patients had neurological sequelae 2 weeks after discharge.— S. L. Newman *et al.* (letter), *New Engl. J. Med.*, 1978, *299*, 1079. A warning of the dangers of mannitol in the treatment of Reye's syndrome. An 11-year-old girl with the syndrome, given mannitol 1 g per kg body-weight every 4 hours and additional doses of up to 0.5 g per kg hourly for rises in intracranial pressure, developed severe hyperosmolarity by the third day which may have contributed to her death.— J. Schmidley *et al.* (letter), *ibid.*, 1979, *301*, 106. Further comment.— S. L. Newman (letter), *ibid.*, 945.

Further references: G. W. Kindt *et al.*, *J. Am. med. Ass.*, 1975, *231*, 822.

Renal disorders. Mannitol had been used to restore renal tubular function and urinary output in shock. When urinary flow diminished or the presence of tubular pigment or debris was suspected, 1 to 2 litres of 10% mannitol was infused, after a test dose, at a rate of 50 to 60 ml per hour.— J. J. Byrne, *New Engl. J. Med.*, 1966, *275*, 659.

In patients who had had a rising blood-urea concentration and were oliguric after shock, mannitol should not be given until deficits of water, electrolytes, plasma, or blood had been made good.— R. G. Luke and A. C. Kennedy (letter), *Lancet*, 1968, *1*, 1310.

Prophylaxis. Twenty-two men, aged 54 to 73 years, undergoing resection of an aneurysm of the abdominal aorta, were given, as a prophylactic against the renal failure thought to accompany the aortic clamping, either standard pre-operative management (intravenous dextrose-saline solution begun an hour before operation and replaced by blood as required) or 500 ml of 5% mannitol during the 90 minutes before induction, and a further 200 ml of 20% mannitol after the operation had started. No patient in either group developed acute renal failure but 3 who received no mannitol became severely oliguric; there were no comparable cases in the group receiving mannitol.— R. J. Luck and W. T. Irvine, *Lancet*, 1965, *2*, 409.

In a small controlled study, the occurrence of postoperative renal failure in jaundiced patients was reduced by mannitol-induced diuresis. Beginning 1 to 2 hours before operation, 500 ml of a 10% solution was infused, and for 48 hours after operation renal flow was maintained at more than 1 ml per minute with infusions of 5% mannitol.— J. L. Dawson, *Ann. R. Coll. Surg.*, 1968, *42*, 163. See also *idem*, *Br. med. J.*, 1965, *1*, 82.

A review of the diagnosis and management of septic shock, including details of 3 case histories. Mannitol infusion may save patients with poor renal function from developing acute renal failure.— G. C. Hanson, *Postgrad. med. J.*, 1974, *50*, 288.

Indication that mannitol infusion prevents radiocontrast-induced acute renal failure.— C. W. Old and L. M. Lehrner (letter), *Lancet*, 1980, *1*, 885. Criticism.— J. A. Becker (letter), *ibid.*, 1147.

Further references: K. G. Barry *et al.*, *New Engl. J. Med.*, 1961, *264*, 967; L. P. Rosky and T. Rodman, *ibid.*, 1966, *274*, 886; R. I. Mazze and K. G. Barry, *Anesth. Analg. curr. Res.*, 1967, *46*, 61.

For conflicting reports on the benefit of mannitol in reducing the nephrotoxicity of amphotericin, see p.717.

Preparations

Mannitol and Sodium Chloride Injection *(U.S.P.)*. A sterile solution of mannitol and sodium chloride in Water for Injections; it contains no antimicrobial agents. pH 4.5 to 7.

Mannitol Injection *(U.S.P.)*. A sterile solution of mannitol in Water for Injections; it contains no antimicrobial agents. pH 4.5 to 7.

Mannitol Intravenous Infusion *(B.P.)*. Mannitol Injection. A sterile solution in Water for Injections. Sterilised by autoclaving. pH 4.5 to 7. Store at 20° to 30°; crystals depositing at lower temperatures should be dissolved by warming before use.

Proprietary Preparations

Mannitol 25% Injection *(Merck Sharp & Dohme, UK)*. Mannitol, available as a 25% solution for intravenous injection, in ampoules of 50 ml.

Mannitol Injections *(Boots, UK)*. Mannitol, available as 10 and 20% solutions, for intravenous infusion.

Mannitol Solutions *(Egic, Fr.: Servier, UK)*. Mannitol, available as 10 and 20% solutions, for intravenous infusion.

Osmitrol *(Travenol, UK)*. Mannitol, available as aqueous solutions, for intravenous injection, containing 10, 15 and 20%. (Also available as Osmitrol in *Austral.*, *Canad.*).

Other Proprietary Names

Isotol *(Ital.)*; Manicol *(Fr.)*; Mannistol *(Ital.)*; Mannit TM *(Jap.)*; Osmofundin *(Switz.)*; Osmosal *(Spain)*; Osmosol *(Austral.)*; Resectisol *(USA)*.

2339-e

Mebutizide. 6-Chloro-3-(1,2-dimethylbutyl)-3,4-dihydro-2*H*-1,2,4-benzothiadiazine-7-sulphonamide 1,1-dioxide.

$C_{13}H_{20}ClN_3O_4S_2$=381.9.

CAS — 3568-00-1.

Mebutizide is a thiazide diuretic with actions and uses similar to those of chlorothiazide (see p.587). It has been given in doses of 7.5 to 30 mg daily.

Proprietary Names

Neoniagar *(Sintesa, Belg.)*.

2340-b

Mefruside. Bay 1500; FBA 1500. 4-Chloro-N^1-methyl-N^1-(tetrahydro-2-methylfurfuryl)benzene-1,3-disulphonamide.

$C_{13}H_{19}ClN_2O_5S_2$=382.9.

CAS — 7195-27-9.

A white odourless powder. M.p. 148° to 149°. Practically **insoluble** in water; soluble in dilute solutions of sodium hydroxide.

Adverse Effects, Treatment, and Precautions. As for Chlorothiazide, p.588.

Abuse. Abuse of mefruside and ethacrynic acid by a 46-year-old nurse led to hypokalaemia, polyuria, and hyperreninism without hyperaldosteronism.— C. Fuchs *et al.*, *Dt. med. Wschr.*, 1977, *102*, 1319.

Absorption and Fate. Mefruside is absorbed from the gastro-intestinal tract and has been reported to be metabolised, and excreted in the bile and urine.

A study of the metabolism and kinetics of mefruside in *rats*. Mefruside was rapidly and almost completely absorbed from the gastro-intestinal tract and was extensively metabolised. The constitution of the metabolites was elucidated and its main metabolite was shown to be pharmacologically active. About two-thirds of a dose was excreted in the urine; about one-third was excreted in the faeces, after both oral and intravenous administration, establishing the existence of biliary excretion. A single study in man has demonstrated that there are similarities between man and *rats* in the metabolism and kinetics of mefruside.— B. Duhm *et al.*, *Arzneimittel-Forsch.*, 1967, *17*, 672.

Pharmacokinetics of mefruside and two active metabolites in healthy subjects.— H. L. J. Fleuren *et al.*, *Eur. J. clin. Pharmac.*, 1980, *17*, 59.

Uses. Mefruside is a diuretic which has certain structural similarities to frusemide as well as the thiazides and has actions and uses similar to those of chlorothiazide (see p.589). Diuresis is initiated in about 2 hours and lasts for about 20 to 24 hours. Its inhibitory action on carbonic anhydrase is only weak.

In the treatment of oedema the usual dose is 25 to 50 mg daily, reduced to a dose of 25 mg daily or on alternate days; in some cases initial doses of 75 to 100 mg daily may be necessary.

In the treatment of hypertension the usual dose is 25 mg daily, either alone, or in conjunction with other antihypertensive agents; initial doses of 25 to 50 mg daily have been recommended; alternate-day maintenance dosage has also been advocated.

When treatment is prolonged, or in susceptible patients, loss of potassium may be sufficient to produce hypokalaemia; potassium supplements should then be given as for chlorothiazide.

Action. A review. Mefruside is an oral diuretic agent whose efficacy and mechanism of action resemble those of the thiazide diuretics. The choice of the name mefruside is unfortunately liable to cause confusion with frusemide.— *Drug & Ther. Bull.*, 1972, *10*, 19 and 28.

Further reviews: R. N. Brogden *et al.*, *Drugs*, 1974, *7*, 419.

A study of the acute effects of mefruside in man. It was concluded that mefruside is a long-acting oral diuretic with an efficacy and mechanism of action similar to the thiazide diuretics. The similarities extend to include a weak inhibitory action on carbonic anhydrase.— C. B. Wilson and W. M. Kirkendall, *J. Pharmac. exp. Ther.*, 1970, *171*, 288. Similar findings in *dogs* suggesting that mefruside has a mechanism of action similar to the thiazide diuretics without any unique features.— *idem*, *173*, 422.

Further references to the action of mefruside: KMeng and G. Kroneberg, *Arzneimittel-Forsch.*, 1967, *17*, 659; W. H. R. Auld and W. R. Murdoch, *Br. med. J.*, 1971, *4*, 786; D. Kerr (letter), *ibid.*, 1972, *1*, 176.

References to the use of mefruside: G. Dean *et al.*, *S. Afr. med. J.*, 1971, *45*, 323 (hypertension); S. J. Jachuck (letter), *Br. med. J.*, 1972, *3*, 590 (hypertension); H. B. Allen and D. A. Lee, *Curr. med. Res. Opinion*, 1973, *1*, 547 (oedema and hypertension); T. J. J. M. Bloem and J. M. Kerkhof, *Clin. Ther.*, 1977, *1*, 228 (hypertension).

Proprietary Preparations

Baycaron *(Bayer, UK)*. Mefruside, available as scored tablets of 25 mg. (Also available as Baycaron in *Arg., Austral., Belg., Denm., Ger., Jap., Neth., Norw., Swed.*).

Other Proprietary Names

Mefrusal *(Ital.)*.

2341-v

Meralluride *(B.P.C. 1959)*.

CAS — 113-50-8 (meralluride); 129-99-7; 8069-64-5 (both sodium salt).

Pharmacopoeias. In *Cz.*

A white to slightly yellow powder, consisting of a mixture of {3-[3-(3-carboxypropionyl)ureido]-2-methoxypropyl}hydroxymercury ($C_9H_{16}HgN_2O_6$=448.8) and theophylline in approximately equimolecular proportions.

Slightly **soluble** in water; soluble in hot water, glacial acetic acid, and solutions of alkali hydroxides; practically insoluble in alcohol, chloroform, and ether. A saturated solution is acid to litmus. **Store** in airtight containers. Protect from light.

Uses. Meralluride is a mercurial diuretic with actions and uses similar to those of mersalyl acid (see below). It has been reported to cause little pain on intramuscular injection, and has even been given subcutaneously although this may cause a painful local reaction.

Meralluride is administered as a solution of the sodium compound containing the equivalent of 39 mg of mercury and 43.6 mg of theophylline in each ml, the usual dose being 1 to 2 ml intramuscularly once or twice weekly. It is advisable to give an initial dose of 0.5 ml or less to test the tolerance of the patient to the drug. The diuretic action of meralluride is enhanced by previous administration of ammonium chloride.

2342-g

Mercaptomerin Sodium *(U.S.P.)*.

Sodium Mercaptomerin. The disodium salt of carboxymethylthio[3-(3-carboxy-2,2,3-trimethylcyclopentanecarboxamido)-2-methoxypropyl]mercury.

$C_{16}H_{25}HgNNa_2O_6S$=606.0.

CAS — 20223-84-1 (mercaptomerin); 21259-76-7 (mercaptomerin sodium).

Pharmacopoeias. In *Arg., Ind., Jap., Nord.,* and *U.S.*

A white hygroscopic powder or amorphous solid having a characteristic honeycomb structure. M.p. about 175°.

Freely **soluble** in water; soluble in alcohol; slightly soluble in chloroform and ether. A 2% solution in water is neutral or slightly alkaline to litmus. Injection solutions should be stored at 2° to 8° and should not be used if they develop a colour or precipitate. **Store** in airtight containers.

Adverse Effects and Precautions. As for Mersalyl Acid, below. It appears to produce fewer local reactions than other mercurial diuretics.

Uses. Mercaptomerin sodium is a mercurial diuretic with actions and uses similar to those of mersalyl acid (see below).

It may be given by subcutaneous injection, though local reactions may occasionally be encountered. Care must be taken to give the injection beneath the subcutaneous fat, to make the injections at different sites, and to avoid oedematous areas.

Mercaptomerin sodium is administered intramuscularly or subcutaneously as a 12.5% solution, the usual dose being 125 mg (1 ml, equivalent to about 40 mg of mercury) daily if required and the dosage range 25 to 250 mg. It is advisable to give a low initial dose of 0.5 ml or less to test the tolerance of the patient to the drug. The diuretic action of mercaptomerin sodium is enhanced by preliminary acidification of the urine with ammonium chloride. Suggested intramuscular doses for children are: up to 3 kg body-weight, 16 mg; 3 to 7 kg, 31 mg; 8 to 15 kg, 63 mg; 16 to 25 kg, 94 mg; over 25 kg, 125 mg; from once weekly to once daily.

Medical nephrectomy. Daily intramuscular injections of mercaptomerin sodium were used in 2 patients to obtain medical nephrectomy to control massive proteinuria in the nephrotic syndrome complicating irreversible renal failure. Treatment lasted 5 to 10 days, one patient receiving a total of 800 mg of mercury and the second 1280 mg.— M. M. Avram and H. I. Lipner (letter), *New Engl. J. Med.*, 1976, *295*, 1080.

Preparations

Mercaptomerin Sodium Injection *(U.S.P.)*. Sodium Mercaptomerin Injection. A sterile solution in Water for Injections, containing 118 to 132 mg in 1 ml. pH 8 to 9.5. Store at 2° to 8°. Protect from light.

Nord. P. (Injectabile Mercaptomerini) is similar.

Proprietary Names

Thiomerin *(Wyeth, Canad.; Wyeth, USA)*.

2343-q

Mercurophylline Sodium. Mercurophylline; Mercurofilina.

CAS — 8012-34-8.

Pharmacopoeias. In *Ind. Aust.* and *Hung.* include Mercamphoramidum, (Mercamphamidum) ($C_{14}H_{25}HgNO_5$=487.9).

A white or slightly yellow, odourless, moderately hygroscopic powder, consisting of a mixture of the sodium salt of [3-(3-carboxy-2,2,3-trimethylcyclopentanecarboxamido)-2-methoxypropyl]-hydroxymercury ($C_{14}H_{24}HgNNaO_5$=509.9) and theophylline in approximately equimolecular proportions.

Soluble 1 in 5 of water; soluble in alcohol; practically insoluble in ether and mineral oils. Solutions in water are alkaline to litmus. **Store** in airtight containers. Protect from light.

Mercurophylline sodium is a mercurial diuretic with actions and uses similar to those of mersalyl acid (see below). It has been given in doses of 200 mg daily by mouth, and 135 mg once or twice weekly by intramuscular injection. It has also been given intravenously.

Proprietary Names

Novurit *(Llorens, Spain)*.

2344-p

Merethoxylline Procaine. A mixture of the procaine salt of anhydro-*o*-{*N*-[3-hydroxymercuri-2-(2-methoxyethoxy)propyl]carbamoyl}phenoxyacetic acid ($C_{28}H_{39}HgN_3O_8$=746.2) and theophylline in the molecular proportion 1:1.4; available as a solution.

CAS — 8063-37-4.

Uses. Merethoxylline procaine has actions and uses similar to those of mersalyl acid (see below) but causes less local irritation. Merethoxylline procaine is administered by deep subcutaneous or intramuscular injection. It is used as a solution providing in each ml merethoxylline ($C_{15}H_{19}HgNO_6$=509.9) 100 mg (equivalent to 39.3 mg of Hg), procaine 45 mg, and theophylline 50 mg. A preliminary dose of 0.5 ml of the solution should be injected as a test for sensitivity. The average subsequent dose of the solution is 2 ml daily and alternative injection sites should be used to reduce the possibility of local reactions. It should not be administered to patients hypersensitive to procaine.

Proprietary Names

Dicurin Procaine *(Lilly, USA)*.

2345-s

Mersalyl Acid *(B.P. 1973)*.

Mersal. Acid; Acidum Mersalylicum; Mersalylum Acidum. A mixture of {3-[2-(carboxymethoxy)benzamido]-2-methoxypropyl}hydroxymercury and its anhydrides.

$C_{13}H_{17}HgNO_6$=483.9.

CAS — 486-67-9 ($C_{13}H_{17}HgNO_6$).

Pharmacopoeias. In *Ind., Int.,* and *Swiss*; in *Nord.* which describes the anhydride, $C_{13}H_{15}HgNO_5$.

A white, odourless, slightly hygroscopic powder. Sparingly **soluble** in water and dilute mineral acids; readily soluble in solutions of alkali hydroxides. **Store** in airtight containers.

Effect of gamma irradiation. At 25 000 Gy, mersalyl acid became grey and at 250 000 Gy greyish-brown; an odour of charring was noted; the total mercury content was not significantly affected but mercuric salts, absent in the original material, were present after irradiation. Mersalyl Injection *B.P.* at 25 000 Gy became yellow and opalescent with a black precipitate which increased significantly at 250 000 Gy; there was a marked decrease in pH; mercuric salts were present and the content of organic mercury was halved at 250 000 Gy.— *The Use of Gamma Radiation Sources for the Sterilisation of Pharmaceutical Products*, London, ABPI, 1960.

2346-w

Mersalyl Sodium *(B.P.C. 1959)*.

Mersalyl. The sodium salt of mersalyl acid.

$C_{13}H_{16}HgNNaO_6$=505.9.

CAS — 492-18-2.

Pharmacopoeias. In *Arg., Aust., Jug., Mex.,* and *Turk.*

A white, odourless, deliquescent powder with a bitter taste.

Soluble 1 in 1 of water, 1 in 3 of alcohol, and 1 in 2 of methyl alcohol; practically insoluble in chloroform and ether. Solutions in water are alkaline to litmus. A 9.06% solution is iso-osmotic with serum.

Incompatible with acids, metals, and reducing agents. Aqueous solutions containing sodium chloride or other salts decompose with the formation of toxic compounds except in the presence of some substance, such as theophylline, which inhibits decomposition. **Store** in airtight containers. Protect from light.

Adverse Effects. The most frequently occurring adverse effects following the administration of mersalyl are stomatitis, gastric disturbance, vertigo, febrile reactions, and skin eruptions and irritation. Diarrhoea and hypersensitivity reactions may occur. It has been reported that some patients may be sensitive to mersalyl, but tolerant to other mercurial compounds. Thrombocytopenia, neutropenia, and agranulocytosis have followed the use of mercurial diuretics. Overdosage may cause severe dehydration and uraemia.

Prolonged administration of mersalyl may cause depletion of electrolytes and water in the body and consequent weakness and hypotension. Hypochloraemic alkalosis is a common feature.

Intravenous injection may cause severe hypotension and cardiac arrhythmias and has been followed by sudden death.

For specific details of adverse effects associated with the administration of mercurials, see under the adverse effects of mercury (p.937).

Effects on the kidneys. In a review of the association between heart disease and the nephrotic syndrome, it was found that mercurial diuretics had been given in 23 of 24 cases and could well have been implicated.— P. J. Hilton *et al.*, *Br. med. J.*, 1968, *3*, 584. See also *idem* (letter), 1969, *2*, 115.

Further references: M. Riddle *et al.*, *Br. med. J.*, 1958, *1*, 1274; J. Burston *et al.*, *ibid.*, 1277.

Precautions. Mersalyl should be used with great care in patients having frequent extrasystoles, those who have suffered recent myocardial infarction, those with severe colitis, and those receiving digitalis therapy. Mersalyl should not be given to patients with impaired renal function or acute nephritis. Repeated injections are contra-indicated when there is no resulting diuresis.

Interference with diagnostic tests. Mercurial diuretics could interfere technically with chemical estimations for protein-bound iodine to produce erroneous lowered results.— *Drug & Ther. Bull.*, 1972, *10*, 69.

Absorption and Fate. Mersalyl acid is incompletely and slowly absorbed from the gastro-intestinal tract and is completely and rapidly absorbed from intramuscular injection sites. Most of an injected dose is rapidly excreted in urine in the form of a mersalyl-cysteine complex; excretion is virtually complete within 24 hours.

Uses. Mersalyl acid, in the form of its salts, is a powerful diuretic which acts on the renal tubules, increasing the excretion of sodium and chloride, in approximately equal amounts, and of water. Diuresis occurs in 1 to 2 hours and lasts for about 12 hours. The diuresis may diminish after a few injections, even though the oedema persists, due to the development of hypochloraemic alkalosis.

It has been used in the treatment of oedema and ascites in cardiac failure and in ascites due to cirrhosis of the liver, in nephrotic oedema, and in carefully selected patients with subacute and chronic nephritis provided that there is no serious impairment of renal function. It has largely been superseded by oral diuretics such as the thiazides and frusemide.

Mersalyl acid is usually given as the sodium salt (mersalyl) in conjunction with theophylline in the form of Mersalyl Injection, as this lessens the local irritant reaction and increases stability. It is given by deep intramuscular injection. Its diuretic action may be increased by producing a mild acidosis before administering the injection by giving 3 doses, each of 2 g, of ammonium chloride on the previous day, or a single 2-g dose of ammonium chloride 2 hours before the mersalyl injection.

The patient's tolerance to Mersalyl Injection may be tested by giving a preliminary intramuscular injection of 0.5 ml. In the absence of signs of intolerance, such as haematuria, diarrhoea, or irritation of the skin, a larger dose, of 1 to 2 ml, may be given the next morning.

The intervals between injections depend on the therapeutic response. Usually, the dose is repeated every third or fourth day and reduced to weekly administration when the condition of the patient improves.

Administration in renal failure. Mercurials are ineffective and nephrotoxic in patients with advanced renal disease and should be avoided.— W. M. Bennett, *Drugs*, 1979, *17*, 111. Mercurial diuretics should not be given to patients with a glomerular filtration-rate less than 50 ml per minute.— W. M. Bennett *et al.*, *Ann. intern. Med.*, 1980, *93*, 286.

Diabetes insipidus. A study of the mechanism of the antidiuretic effect of saliuretic drugs, including mercurials, in diabetes insipidus.— G. Ramos *et al.*, *Clin. Pharmac. Ther.*, 1967, *8*, 557.

Preparations

Mersalyl Injection *(B.P. 1973)*. Mersalyl and Theophylline Injection. A sterile solution containing 10% w/v of mersalyl sodium and 5% w/v of theophylline, prepared by dissolving mersalyl acid and theophylline in a solution of sodium hydroxide and sterilised by heating with a bactericide (phenylmercuric nitrate) or by filtration. pH 7.6 to 8.2. Protect from light in glass ampoules. Avoid contact with metal. *Dose.* 0.5 to 2 ml intramuscularly, on alternate days.

2347-e

Methazolamide *(U.S.P.)*. *N*-(4-Methyl-2-sulphamoyl-Δ^2-1,3,4-thiadiazolin-5-ylidene)acetamide.
$C_5H_8N_4O_3S_2$=236.3.

CAS — 554-57-4.

Pharmacopoeias. In *U.S.*

A white or faintly yellow crystalline powder with a slight odour. M.p. about 213°. Very slightly **soluble** in water and alcohol; slightly soluble in acetone; soluble in dimethylformamide. **Protect** from light.

Adverse Effects and Precautions. As for Acetazolamide, p.581.

Effects on the blood. *Aplastic anaemia.* Non-fatal aplastic anaemia in an 83-year-old man was probably associated with methazolamide administration.— J. L. Gangitano *et al.*, *Am. J. Ophthal.*, 1978, *86*, 138.

Reports of aplastic anaemia in 2 patients and agranulocytosis in 1 patient given methazolamide for the treatment of glaucoma.— T. P. Werblin *et al.*, *J. Am. med. Ass.*, 1979, *241*, 2817.

Further references: N. Wisch *et al.*, *Am. J. Ophthal.*, 1973, *75*, 130.

Uses. Methazolamide is an inhibitor of carbonic anhydrase with actions and uses similar to those of acetazolamide (see p.582). Its action is less prompt but of longer duration than that of acetazolamide, lasting for 10 to 18 hours. In the treatment of glaucoma, it is given in doses of 50 to 100 mg twice or thrice daily.

The diuretic activity of methazolamide is less pronounced than that of acetazolamide.

Ocular disorders. A study in patients with open-angle glaucoma suggesting that a dose of 100 mg of methazolamide twice daily may represent for most patients a reasonable balance between desired and undesired effects. There were indications that methazolamide may enhance its own metabolism, presumably by enzyme induction.— K. Dahlen *et al.*, *Archs Ophthal., N.Y.*, 1978, *96*, 2214.

Further references: R. A. Stone *et al.*, *Am. J. Ophthal.*, 1977, *83*, 674.

Preparations

Methazolamide Tablets *(U.S.P.)*. Tablets containing methazolamide.

Proprietary Names

Neptazane *(Lederle, Canad.*; *Théraplix, Fr.*; *Lederle, USA)*.

2348-l

Methyclothiazide *(U.S.P.)*. 6-Chloro-3-chloromethyl-3,4-dihydro-2-methyl-2*H*-1,2,4-benzothiadiazine-7-sulphonamide 1,1-dioxide.
$C_9H_{11}Cl_2N_3O_4S_2$=360.2.

CAS — 135-07-9.

Pharmacopoeias. In *U.S.*

A white or almost white, odourless or almost odourless, crystalline powder.

Very slightly **soluble** in water and chloroform; soluble 1 in about 90 of alcohol; sparingly soluble in methyl alcohol; soluble in solutions of alkali hydroxides and carbonates; freely soluble in acetone and pyridine.

Adverse Effects, Treatment, and Precautions. As for Chlorothiazide, p.588.

Uses. Methyclothiazide is a thiazide diuretic with actions and uses similar to those of chlorothiazide (see p.589). Diuresis is initiated in about 2 hours, and lasts for about 24 hours.

In the treatment of oedema the usual initial dose is 2.5 to 10 mg daily, reduced to a dose of 2.5 to 5 mg daily. A suggested dose for children is 50 to 200 µg per kg body-weight daily. In the treatment of hypertension the usual dose is 2.5 to 5 mg daily, either alone, or in conjunction with other antihypertensive agents; in some cases doses of 10 mg may be necessary.

When treatment is prolonged, or in susceptible patients, loss of potassium may be sufficient to produce hypokalaemia; potassium supplements should then be given as for chlorothiazide.

Hypertension. Tablets containing methyclothiazide 5 mg and deserpidine 250 or 500 µg (Enduronyl) produced a clinically significant blood pressure response in 25 of 26 hypertensive patients. In most cases 1 tablet daily was adequate and treatment was continued for 5 to 8 months.— H. W. Kimmerling, *Curr. ther. Res.*, 1967, *9*, 75.

Methyclothiazide 5 mg daily failed to lower the blood pressure in 9 hypertensive young adults, despite a 10% reduction in plasma volume. In a further 9 young adults with normal blood pressure methyclothiazide 5 or 10 mg daily produced a similar reduction in plasma volume but had no effect on blood pressure. It was suggested that young adults tend to have an efficient homoeostatic mechanism, which limits the efficacy of diuretics in hypertension.— R. D. Gordon *et al.*, *Eur. J. clin. Pharmac.*, 1977, *12*, 403.

In a study of 117 hypertensive patients given methyclothiazide 5 mg daily, it was found that some responded to therapy within 4 weeks, whereas others had a modest reduction in blood pressure in the first 4 weeks followed by a plateau lasting about 2 weeks, then a further reduction during the following 6 weeks. Increasing the dose to 10 mg did not enhance the final response, suggesting that late responses are not due to increasing the dose. Thiazide therapy should be tried in hypertensive patients for at least 8 to 12 weeks before adding another drug.— K. Soghikian and D. E. Bartenbach, *Sth. med. J.*, 1977, *70*, 1397.

Further references: F. H. Stern, *J. Am. Geriat. Soc.*, 1962, *10*, 256; A. S. Leon *et al.*, *Dis. Chest*, 1962, *42*, 626; R. J. Carpenter *et al.*, *Clin. Med.*, 1967, *74* (May), 65; *Practitioner*, 1978, *220*, 969 (Report No. 198 of the General Practitioner Research Group).

Preparations

Methyclothiazide Tablets *(U.S.P.)*. Tablets containing methyclothiazide.

Proprietary Preparations

Enduron *(Abbott, UK)*. Methyclothiazide, available as scored tablets of 5 mg. (Also available as Enduron in *Austral., Belg., Spain, USA*).

Enduronyl *(Abbott, UK)*. Scored tablets each containing methyclothiazide 5 mg and deserpidine 250 µg. **Enduronyl Forte**. Scored tablets each containing methyclothiazide 5 mg and deserpidine 500 µg. For hypertension. *Dose.* Initial, 1 Enduronyl tablet daily; maintenance, according to response, ½ an Enduronyl tablet to 2 Enduronyl Forte tablets daily.

Other Proprietary Names

Aquatensen *(USA)*; Duretic *(Canad.)*; Endurona *(Swed.)*; Enduron-M *(Austral.)*; Thiazidil *(Fr.)*.

2349-y

Metolazone. SR 720-22. 7-Chloro-1,2,3,4-tetrahydro-2-methyl-4-oxo-3-*o*-tolylquinazoline-6-sulphonamide.
$C_{16}H_{16}ClN_3O_3S$=365.8.

CAS — 17560-51-9.

Colourless crystals. It is polymorphic; m.p. of one crystalline form about 227°, and of the other about 270°. Sparingly **soluble** in water; more soluble in alkalis and organic solvents. **Protect** from light.

Adverse Effects and Treatment. As for Chlorothiazide, p.588.

Convulsions. Two patients experienced acute muscle cramps with impairment of consciousness and epileptiform movements after taking metolazone 5 mg (single dose) or 2.5 mg daily for 3 days.— M. X. Fitzgerald and N. J. Brennan, *Br. med. J.*, 1976, *1*, 1381. Doubt as to the association with metolazone.— G. H. Gunson, *Penwalt* (letter), *ibid.*, 1976, *2*, 476.

Effects on the electrolyte balance. Studies and comments on the effects of metolazone on the electrolyte balance: S. Fotiu *et al.*, *Clin. Pharmac. Ther.*, 1974, *16*, 318; J. B. Puschett and A. Rastegar, *Clin. Pharmac. Ther.*, 1974, *15*, 397; W. M. Bennett and G. A. Porter, *Curr. ther. Res.*, 1977, *22*, 326.

See also under Precautions (Interaction with Frusemide).

Effects on the muscles. Muscle cramps associated with metolazone therapy.— J. L. Cangiano *et al.*, *Curr. ther. Res.*, 1974, *16*, 778.

Precautions. As for Chlorothiazide, p.589.

Interactions. *Frusemide.* Addition of metolazone to a regimen which included frusemide improved diuresis and augmented blood pressure control in 2 patients with severe hypertension and moderately severe renal failure. In 5 patients with refractory heart failure, however, the response was less satisfactory, and severe abnormalities in electrolytes developed. This association of diuretics should be used with caution.— W. D. Black *et al.*, *Sth. med. J.*, 1978, *71*, 380.

Further references: R. F. Gunstone *et al.*, *Postgrad. med. J.*, 1971, *47*, 789.

Absorption and Fate. Metolazone is incompletely but fairly rapidly absorbed from the gastro-intestinal tract. It is extensively bound to plasma proteins and to red blood cells. It has been estimated to have a plasma half-life of about 8 hours, its biological half-life being much longer. It is mainly excreted in the urine, largely unchanged but partly as inactive metabolites; there is also some biliary excretion. Metolazone crosses the placental barrier and is excreted in breast milk.

Following administration of metolazone intravenously to healthy subjects the plasma concentration fell bi-exponentially and almost 90% was excreted in the urine as metolazone or its metabolites over a period of 6 days. After administration by mouth to healthy subjects about 64% was considered to be absorbed but this was reduced to about 40% in some cardiac patients. In patients with renal failure plasma clearance was 20 ml per minute compared with 110 ml in the healthy subjects.— W. J. Tilstone *et al.*, *Clin. Pharmac. Ther.*, 1974, *16*, 322.

Protein and red cell binding. A study in 8 healthy subjects indicated that metolazone is rapidly absorbed following oral administration, and rapidly distributed into the red blood cells and bound to plasma protein, so that only a small amount remains in the plasma free fraction.— K. N. Modi *et al.*, *Fedn Proc.*, 1970, *29*, 276.

Uses. Metolazone is a diuretic which has certain structural similarities to the thiazides and has actions and uses similar to those of chlorothiazide (see p.589). It has no effect on carbonic anhydrase. Diuresis is initiated in about 1 hour and the effect lasts for 12 to 24 hours.

In the treatment of oedema the usual dose is 5 to 10 mg daily; in some cases doses of 20 mg or more may be required. It has been recommended that not more than 80 mg should be given in any 24-hour period, but there does not appear to be any recently published evidence of a daily dose of up to 80 mg being used.

In the treatment of hypertension the usual dose is 2.5 to 5 mg daily, either alone, or in conjunction with other antihypertensive agents.

When treatment is prolonged, or in susceptible patients, loss of potassium may be sufficient to produce hypokalaemia; potassium supplements should then be given as for chlorothiazide.

Action. A review of the uses and adverse effects of metolazone. As an antihypertensive metolazone appeared to have similar clinical efficacy and toxicity to the thiazide diuretics. Its prolonged plasma half-life did not appear to be an advantage in the treatment of hypertension.— *Drug & Ther. Bull.*, 1978, *16*, 87.

Further references: *Med. Lett.*, 1979, *21*, 40.

In a modified double-blind crossover study in 21 patients with hypertension there were no significant differences in antihypertensive effect, excretion of sodium, potassium, and chloride, and concentrations of blood-urea-nitrogen, uric acid, or glucose after a 100-g load, between 3 treatments: hydrochlorothiazide 50 mg daily, metolazone 2.5 mg daily, and metolazone 5 mg daily.— R. M. Pilewski *et al.*, *Clin. Pharmac. Ther.*, 1971, *12*, 843.

Further references: J. W. Smiley *et al.*, *Clin. Pharmac. Ther.*, 1972, *13*, 336; B. J. Materson *et al.*, *Curr. ther. Res.*, 1972, *14*, 545.

Administration in renal failure. Metolazone has some efficacy in far-advanced renal failure but it is ineffective with glomerular filtration-rates less than 10 ml per minute.— W. M. Bennett, *Drugs*, 1979, *17*, 111. Metolazone can be given in usual doses to patients in renal failure. Concentrations of metolazone are not affected by haemodialysis.— W. M. Bennett *et al.*, *Ann. intern. Med.*, 1980, *93*, 286.

See also Renal Disorders, below.

Cardiac disorders. *Congestive heart failure.* In 30 patients with congestive heart failure, the administration of metolazone resulted in weight loss, reduction of systolic and diastolic blood pressure in normotensive and hypertensive patients, hypokalaemia, decreased serum chloride, and increased serum uric acid and creatinine levels. The dose of metolazone was 5, 10, or 15 mg daily for 3 weeks, then 2.5, 5, or 10 mg daily for 12 weeks.— B. A. Levey and R. F. Palmer, *Curr. ther. Res.*, 1975, *18*, 641.

Hepatic disorders. In 20 patients with chronic liver disease and ascites, the ascites was greatly reduced by treatment with metolazone in 8 patients, and a further 10 patients responded when also given amiloride or spironolactone. Some very high doses of metolazone were given but results indicated that 5 mg is a suitable starting dose. The incidence of electrolyte disturbances was high—hypokalaemia in 16, hypochloraemia in 7, and encephalopathy in 7. Azotaemia occurred in only 1 patient and the drug might be useful if renal function was greatly impaired.— P. Hillenbrand and S. Sherlock, *Br. med. J.*, 1971, *4*, 266.

Further references: D. T. Lowenthal and L. Shear, *Archs intern. Med.*, 1973, *132*, 38; G. R. Lang *et al.*, *Clin. Pharmac. Ther.*, 1977, *21*, 234; M. Epstein *et al.*, *Curr. ther. Res.*, 1977, *21*, 656.

Hypertension. Metolazone was given to 22 patients with hypertension, 11 of whom were taking other antihypertensive agents; the dose was 1 to 10 (mean 5.5) mg daily. An excellent response (reduction of more than 20 mmHg in mean arterial blood pressure) occurred in about 13 patients, with a good response (reduction of 10 to 20 mmHg) in a further 7. Hypokalaemia occurred in 6 patients, hyperglycaemia in 2, and hyperuricaemia in 2. Other persistent side-effects were dizziness (4), weakness (2), muscle cramps (2), headache (2), and nocturia (5). Transient side-effects were more common and included also nausea, diarrhoea, and insomnia.— J. L. Cangiano *et al.*, *Curr. ther. Res.*, 1974, *16*, 778.

A study in 57 non-oedematous hypertensive patients indicated that metolazone in doses of 1, 2.5, and 5 mg daily appeared to be equally effective in antihypertensive effect, and much the same as chlorthalidone 100 mg daily. There were no differences in the incidences of hypokalaemia.— S. Fotiu *et al.*, *Clin. Pharmac. Ther.*, 1974, *16*, 318.

Metolazone gave good control of blood pressure in 8 hypertensive patients treated for 30 to 42 months; doses ranged from 4 to 40 mg daily. All patients required potassium supplements. No serious side-effects were noted, though 2 patients had raised serum-uric acid concentrations and one had raised serum aspartate aminotransferase (SGOT).— L. Dornfeld and R. E. Kane, *Curr. ther. Res.*, 1977, *21*, 265.

There was a striking clinical improvement and reduction in oedema in 8 patients with chronic essential hypertension whose fluid retention had not been controlled by large doses of ethacrynic acid or frusemide alone, when metolazone 5 mg daily was added to the regimen.— C. Venkata *et al.*, *Curr. ther. Res.*, 1977, *22*, 686.

Further references: B. J. Materson *et al.*, *Curr. ther. Res.*, 1974, *16*, 890; L. Dornfeld and R. E. Kane, *ibid.*, 1975, *18*, 527; M. P. Sambhi *et al.*, *J. clin. Pharmac.*, 1977, *17*, 214; H. Masters, *Curr. ther. Res.*, 1978, *23*, 584; R. H. Timpson, *ibid.*, 709; J. F. Winchester *et al.*, *Clin. Pharmac. Ther.*, 1980, *28*, 611.

Oedema. In 3 patients (one with heart failure and 2 with cirrhosis of the liver) with oedema resistant to frusemide 320 mg daily, the addition of metolazone 5 to 20 mg daily produced a marked diuresis. All patients required potassium supplements.— M. Epstein *et al.*, *Curr. ther. Res.*, 1977, *21*, 656.

See also Precautions (Interaction with Frusemide).

Premenstrual tension. A report of the treatment of premenstrual symptoms with metolazone.— A. Werch and R. E. Kane, *Curr. ther. Res.*, 1976, *19*, 565.

For reference to the possible role of diuretics in exacerbating and perpetuating idiopathic oedema, see Oedema, under Adverse Effects of Chlorothiazide, p.588.

Renal disorders. In a study in 10 patients with chronic renal failure and 10 patients with the nephrotic syndrome previous diuretic therapy was replaced with metolazone 2.5 to 20 mg once daily; treatment with antihypertensives and corticosteroids was continued. Fluid retention, oedema, and blood pressure were controlled in most patients. One patient with oedema resistant to frusemide alone and to metolazone 40 mg daily responded to frusemide 160 mg daily with metolazone 30 mg. Three patients required potassium supplements.— R. R. Paton and R. E. Kane, *J. clin. Pharmac.*, 1977, *17*, 243.

See also Precautions (Interaction with Frusemide).

Further references: H. J. Dargie *et al.*, *Br. med. J.*, 1972, *4*, 196; W. M. Bennett and G. A. Porter, *J. clin. Pharmac.*, 1973, *13*, 357.

Proprietary Preparations

Metenix 5 *(Hoechst, UK).* Metolazone, available as tablets of 5 mg.

Other Proprietary Names

Diulo *(Austral., USA)*; Zaroxolyn *(Canad., Ger., S.Afr., Switz., USA)*.

Metolazone was also formerly marketed in Great Britain under the proprietary name Zaroxolyn (*Pennwalt Pharmaceuticals: Farillon*).

2350-g

Muzolimine.

Bay g 2821. 3-Amino-1-[1-(3,4-dichlorophenyl)ethyl]-2-pyrazolin-5-one.

$C_{11}H_{11}Cl_2N_3O = 272.1$.

CAS — 55294-15-0.

Adverse Effects. Probably the most common side-effect to be associated with muzolimine therapy would be fluid and electrolyte imbalance after either single large doses or prolonged administration.

A report of toxicological studies on muzolimine in *mice, rats, rabbits,* and *dogs*. The only presenting symptom was excessive diuresis and, apart from the kidney, no other organs were damaged. Renal impairment was considered to be a result of the excessive diuresis. Studies in pregnant *rabbits* and *rats* revealed no embryotoxic or teratogenic effects.— D. Lorke and P. Mürmann, *Curr. med. Res. Opinion*, 1977, *4*, 716.

Treatment of Adverse Effects. As for Chlorothiazide, p.589.

Precautions. As for Chlorothiazide, p.589. Muzolimine should be used with care in patients with prostatic hypertrophy or impairment of micturition.

Absorption and Fate. Muzolimine is fairly rapidly absorbed from the gastro-intestinal tract. It has a biphasic half-life in the plasma with an initial distribution phase of about 3 or 4 hours and a terminal elimination phase of up to about 17 hours. It has been suggested that muzolimine is metabolised, and excreted primarily in the bile.

A study of the pharmacokinetics of muzolimine in *dogs*, healthy subjects, and patients with renal failure. Peak plasma concentrations were obtained within an hour of administration of 40 mg by mouth to 3 healthy subjects, and disappearance from the plasma was biphasic with an initial half-life of about 3 hours and a terminal elimination half-life of 13 to 17 hours. Similar results were obtained in patients with renal failure. It was assumed that in man muzolimine is excreted in the bile, possibly after biotransformation, with urinary elimination a minor pathway.— W. Ritter, *Curr. med. Res. Opinion*, 1977, *4*, 564. See also D. Loew *et al.*, *Eur. J. clin. Pharmac.*, 1977, *12*, 341 (initial plasma half-life of 3 to 4.5 hours and terminal half-life of 6 to 14 hours).

In a study comparing the effects of single doses of muzolimine 40 mg in 2 healthy subjects and 7 cardiac patients, the pharmacokinetics did not appear to be significantly affected by cardiac disorders. Peak plasma concentrations were obtained 1 to 3 hours after administration and declined biphasically. In 5 of the patients the half-life of the alpha (distribution) phase ranged from 2.3 to 4.7 hours (in the other 2 it could not be determined), and in the healthy subjects it was 2.3 and 2.9 hours. The beta phase was 7.4 to 22.4 hours in the patients and 12.4 to 14.6 hours in the healthy subjects.— O. Brørs *et al.*, *Eur. J. clin. Pharmac.*, 1979, *15*, 105.

Uses. Although chemically unrelated, muzolimine is a diuretic which has been reported to have actions and uses similar to those of frusemide (see p.598); its duration of action is reported to be more prolonged. Diuresis is initiated within about 30 minutes to an hour after a dose by mouth, and lasts for about 6 to 7 hours; some significant diuresis is still detectable for about 10 hours. In the treatment of oedema doses of 40 to 80 mg have been given daily; higher doses have also been used.

Action. A study involving 10 patients with heart failure, 5 with severe renal insufficiency, and 2 healthy subjects indicated that muzolimine has a site of action in the thick ascending limb of Henle's loop, that it may also exert an additional effect on the proximal tubule, and that it has a log-linear dose-response curve for doses of 20 to 160 mg. It was concluded that muzolimine appeared to be a high-ceiling diuretic similar to frusemide but with a longer duration of action.— K. J. Berg *et al.*, *Pharmatherapeutica*, 1976, *1*, 319.

In a double-blind study in 12 healthy subjects muzolimine 30 mg was shown to have a similar saliuretic effect to frusemide 40 mg.— D. Loew *et al.*, *Eur. J. clin. Pharmac.*, 1977, *12*, 341.

Further reports of clinical pharmacological studies into the mode of action of muzolimine: D. Loew, *Curr. med. Res. Opinion*, 1977, *4*, 455; M. Mussche and N. Lameire, *ibid.*, 462; E. Schnurr *et al.*, *Pharmatherapeutica*, 1977, *1*, 415.

Cardiac disorders. Heart failure. Single doses of muzolimine 40 mg and frusemide 40 mg were given to 12 patients with heart failure and associated oedema in a double-blind crossover study. In terms of total excretion muzolimine was slightly more effective than frusemide but the difference did not reach statistical significance. The duration of action was prolonged compared to frusemide.— P. Fauchald and E. Lind, *Pharmatherapeutica*, 1977, *1*, 409.

Further references: K. J. Berg *et al.*, *Pharmatherapeutica*, 1976, *1*, 319; W. Klein *et al.*, *Arzneimittel-Forsch.*, 1977, *27*, 2377; O. Brørs *et al.*, *Curr. med. Res. Opinion*, 1980, *6*, 431.

Hepatic disorders. In a 7-day double-blind study completed by 22 patients with hepatogenic ascites, muzolimine 80 mg daily with spironolactone 100 mg thrice daily was superior to frusemide 80 mg daily with a similar dose of spironolactone, or to a similar dose of spironolactone with placebo.— F. Heinrich *et al.*, *Curr. med. Res. Opinion*, 1977, *4*, 706.

Raised intracranial pressure. Beneficial results using muzolimine for the control of CSF pressure in patients with supra-tentorial tumours. It was not suitable for use alone, but might be of value in association with other agents.— A. Hartmann *et al.*, *Arch. Psychiat. NervKrankh.*, 1977, *224*, 351.

Renal disorders. A study of the efficacy of muzolimine in 18 non-oedematous patients with advanced renal failure. In patients with a glomerular filtration-rate of 5 to 10 ml per minute the efficacy of muzolimine was similar to that of frusemide and ethacrynic acid; below 3 ml per minute muzolimine lost its effect. As with frusemide, sodium clearance became more pronounced after high doses (360 mg by mouth), so that there is a risk of hyponataemia after high doses.— A. Röckel, *Curr. med. Res. Opinion*, 1977, *4*, 574. In a double-blind crossover study involving 11 patients with advanced renal failure both frusemide and muzolimine had an excellent saliuretic effect. Whereas that of frusemide generally wears off after 12 hours, the effect of muzolimine lasted for a much longer period of time. Muzolimine had a more pronounced effect on potassium excretion in all groups and in all time periods.— P. Schmidt *et al.*, *Eur. J. clin. Pharmac.*, 1978, *14*, 399.

Further references: A. D. Canton *et al.*, *Br. med. J.*, 1981, *282*, 595.

Manufacturers
Bayer, Ger.

2351-q

Paraflutizide. LD 3612; Parafluthiazide. 6-Chloro-3-(4-fluorobenzyl)-3,4-dihydro-2*H*-1,2,4-benzothiadiazine-7-sulphonamide 1,1-dioxide.
$C_{14}H_{13}ClFN_3O_4S_2$=405.8.

CAS — 1580-83-2.

Paraflutizide is a thiazide diuretic with actions and uses similar to those of chlorothiazide (see p.587). It has been given in doses of 5 to 15 mg daily for 5 days each week.

2352-p

Polythiazide *(B.P., U.S.P.)*. P 2525. 6-Chloro-3,4-dihydro-2-methyl-3-(2,2,2-trifluoroethylthiomethyl)-2*H*-1,2,4-benzothiadiazine-7-sulphonamide 1,1-dioxide.
$C_{11}H_{13}ClF_3N_3O_4S_3$=439.9.

CAS — 346-18-9.

Pharmacopoeias. In *Br.* and *U.S.*

A white or almost white crystalline powder with an alliaceous odour. M.p. 207° to 217° with decomposition. Practically **insoluble** in water and chloroform; soluble 1 in 40 in alcohol; soluble in methyl alcohol and acetone. **Store** in airtight containers. Protect from light.

Adverse Effects, Treatment, and Precautions. As for Chlorothiazide, p.588.

Absorption and Fate. Polythiazide is fairly readily absorbed from the gastro-intestinal tract, and *animal* studies have indicated that it is fairly extensively metabolised; about 25% is reported to be excreted unchanged in the urine. It has been estimated to have a plasma elimination half-life of about 26 hours.

In 18 healthy subjects given polythiazide 1 mg a mean plasma concentration of 3.22 ng per ml occurred 5 hours after administration, with mean plasma half-lives for absorption and elimination of 1.2 and 25.7 hours respectively. Within 48 hours a mean of 20.34% of the administered dose had been excreted unchanged in the urine of 13 subjects. It can be concluded that about 25% of the dose is cleared intact by the kidney, the remainder presumably cleared after metabolic changes as well as by elimination in the faeces. Studies *in vitro* indicated that about 83.5% of polythiazide is bound to plasma proteins.— D. C. Hobbs and T. M. Twomey, *Clin. Pharmac. Ther.*, 1978, *23*, 241.

Uses. Polythiazide is a thiazide diuretic with actions and uses similar to those of chlorothiazide (see p.589). Diuresis is initiated within about 2 hours after administration, and lasts for 24 to 48 hours.

In the treatment of oedema the usual initial dose is 2 mg daily, reduced to a dose of 1 to 2 mg daily or less; in some cases initial and maintenance doses of 4 mg daily may be necessary.

In the treatment of hypertension the usual initial dose is 2 mg daily, either alone, or in conjunction with other antihypertensive agents; the maintenance dose is 1 to 4 mg daily.

When treatment is prolonged, or in susceptible patients, loss of potassium may be sufficient to produce hypokalaemia; potassium supplements should then be given as for chlorothiazide.

References to the use of polythiazide: D. E. Hutcheon and G. B. Leonard, *J. Am. med. Ass.*, 1963, *185*, 640 (heart failure); W. E. Samson, *Am. J. med. Sci.*, 1965, *249*, 571 (hypertension); E. M. Newton, *J. Ther.*, 1966, *1* (1), 28 (hypertension); R. D. Mann and D. Jackson, *Practitioner*, 1966, *196*, 293 (hypertension); J. F. Sanders, *Clin. Med.*, 1968, *75* (June), 59 (hypertension); J. Guevara *et al.*, *Clin. Pharmac. Ther.*, 1977, *21*, 105 (hypertension); T. Pitkäjärvi *et al.*, *Curr. ther. Res.*, 1977, *21*, 169 (hypertension).

Preparations

Polythiazide Tablets *(B.P.)*. Tablets containing polythiazide. Protect from light.

Polythiazide Tablets *(U.S.P.)*. Tablets containing polythiazide. Store in airtight containers. Protect from light.

Nephril *(Pfizer, UK)*. Polythiazide, available as scored tablets of 1 mg. (Also available as Nephril in *Austral.*).

Other Proprietary Names
Drenusil *(Ger., S.Afr.)*; Renese *(Belg., Canad., Denm., Fr., Neth., Norw., Spain, Swed., Switz., USA)*.

2353-s

Prorenoate Potassium. Potassium Prorenoate; SC-23992. Potassium 6α,7α-dihydro-17β-hydroxy-3-oxo-3′*H*-cyclopropa[6,7]-17α-pregna-4,6-diene-21-carboxylate.
$C_{23}H_{31}KO_4$=410.6.

CAS — 49848-01-3 (prorenoic acid); 49847-97-4 (potassium salt).

Adverse Effects, Treatment, and Precautions. As for Spironolactone, p.610.

Uses. Prorenoate potassium has actions and uses similar to those of spironolactone (see p.611). It has been given in doses of about 40 mg daily.

Action. In a double-blind study involving 6 healthy subjects aged 18 to 35 years, the responses to prorenoate potassium 40 mg were similar to those to spironolactone 100 mg. Spironolactone had a slightly higher activity as regards sodium excretion whereas potassium retention was greater after prorenoate potassium but the differences were not significant. Prorenoate potassium was, however, significantly more active than spironolactone when the amount of potassium spared was expressed per unit of sodium excreted, thus demonstrating a qualitative difference. Both drugs showed significant activity between 2 to 16 hours after administration.— L. E. Ramsay *et al.*, *Br. J. clin. Pharmac.*, 1976, *3*, 475.

Further references: L. M. Hofmann *et al.*, *J. Pharmac. exp. Ther.*, 1975, *194*, 450; L. E. Ramsay *et al.*, *Br. J. clin. Pharmac.*, 1975, *2*, 271; *idem*, *Clin. Pharmac. Ther.*, 1975, *18*, 391.

Manufacturers
Searle, UK.

2354-w

Quinethazone *(U.S.P.)*. Chinethazonum. 7-Chloro-2-ethyl-1,2,3,4-tetrahydro-4-oxoquinazoline-6-sulphonamide.
$C_{10}H_{12}ClN_3O_3S$=289.7.

CAS — 73-49-4.

Pharmacopoeias. In *U.S.*

A white to yellowish-white crystalline powder. Very slightly **soluble** in water; slightly soluble in alcohol; sparingly soluble in pyridine; freely soluble in solutions of alkali hydroxides and carbonates.

Adverse Effects, Treatment, and Precautions. As for Chlorothiazide, p.588.

Effects on the skin. Photosensitivity. A patient who developed photosensitivity when given quinethazone had had similar reactions to chlorothiazide and hydrochlorothiazide.— R. C. Miller and V. S. Beltrani, *Archs Derm.*, 1966, *93*, 346.

Absorption and Fate. Quinethazone is fairly rapidly absorbed from the gastro-intestinal tract and has a fairly prolonged duration of action. It crosses the placental barrier and is excreted in milk.

Uses. Quinethazone is a diuretic which has certain structural similarities to the thiazides and has actions and uses similar to those of chlorothiazide (see p.589). Diuresis is initiated within about 2 hours after administration and lasts for 18 to 24 hours.

In the treatment of oedema the usual dose is 50 to 100 mg daily; in some cases doses of 200 mg daily may be necessary.

In the treatment of hypertension the usual dose is 50 to 100 mg daily, either alone, or in conjunction with other antihypertensive agents.

When treatment is prolonged, or in susceptible patients, loss of potassium may be sufficient to produce hypokalaemia; potassium supplements should then be given as for chlorothiazide.

References: R. H. Seller *et al.*, *Clin. Pharmac. Ther.*, 1962, *3*, 180 (clinical pharmacology); G. Sandler, *Br. med. J.*, 1964, *2*, 288 (heart failure); B. J. Fairhurst, *J. Ther.*, 1966, *1* (3), 5 (hypertension); W. E. Parkes *et al.*, *Practitioner*, 1969, *203*, 194 (hypertension).

Preparations

Quinethazone Tablets *(U.S.P.)*. Tablets containing quinethazone. Store in airtight containers.

Aquamox *(Lederle, UK)*. Quinethazone, available as tablets of 50 mg. (Also available as Aquamox in *Austral., Belg., Canad., Denm., Ger., Ital., Neth., Norw., Swed., Switz.*).

Other Proprietary Names
Hydromox *(USA)*.

2355-e

Spironolactone *(B.P., U.S.P.)*. Espironolactona; Spirolactone; SC 9420. 7α-Acetylthio-3-oxo-17α-pregn-4-ene-21,17β-carbolactone acid γ-lactone.
$C_{24}H_{32}O_4S$=416.6.

CAS — 52-01-7.

Pharmacopoeias. In *Br., Braz., Chin., Cz., It., Jap., Nord.,* and *U.S.*

A white to light tan powder with a slightly bitter taste; it is odourless or has a slight odour of thio-acetic acid. M.p. 198° to 207°. Practically

insoluble in water; soluble 1 in 80 of alcohol, 1 in 3 of chloroform, and 1 in 100 of ether; soluble in ethyl acetate; slightly soluble in methyl alcohol and fixed oils. A solution in chloroform is laevorotatory. **Protect** from light.

Adverse Effects. Spironolactone may give rise to headache and drowsiness, and gastro-intestinal disturbances, including cramp and diarrhoea. Ataxia, mental confusion, hirsutism, deepening of the voice, menstrual irregularities, impotence, and skin rashes have been reported as side-effects. Gynaecomastia is not uncommon and in rare cases breast enlargement may persist. Transient increases in blood-urea-nitrogen concentrations may occur, and mild acidosis has been reported. Spironolactone has been demonstrated to cause tumours in *rats*.

Spironolactone may cause hyponatraemia and hyperkalaemia.

A survey indicated that of 788 patients who received spironolactone 164 developed side-effects. These included hyperkalaemia in 8.6%, dehydration in 3.4%, hyponatraemia in 2.4%, gastro-intestinal disorders in 2.3%, neurological disorders in 2% and rash, gynaecomastia, and unspecified effects.— Boston Collaborative Drug Surveillance Program Research Group, *J. Am. med. Ass.*, 1973, *255,* 40.

Carcinogenicity. A report of breast cancer in 5 patients who had taken spironolactone with hydrochlorothiazide for prolonged periods.— S. D. Loube and R. A. Quirk (letter), *Lancet,* 1975, *1,* 1428. Evidence against a substantial association between spironolactone and breast cancer.— H. Jick and B. Armstrong (letter), *ibid.*, *2,* 368.

Long-term studies in *rats* have shown that spironolactone can cause tumours.— *FDA Drug Bull.*, 1976, *6,* 33.

Effects on the electrolyte balance. *Calcium.* Spironolactone appears to act directly on tubular transport to increase calcium excretion.— M. R. Wills *et al.*, *Clin. Sci.*, 1969, *37,* 621. Hypercalciuria in 10 volunteers taking spironolactone 400 mg daily and in 4 taking a placebo was attributed to the calcium content of the tablets.— R. C. Prati *et al.*, *J. Lab. clin. Med.*, 1972, *80,* 224.

Chloride. During treatment with spironolactone 6 patients with advanced alcoholic cirrhosis developed hyperchloraemic acidosis.— P. A. Gabow *et al.*, *Ann. intern. Med.*, 1979, *90,* 338. Comment.— D. W. Nierenberg (letter), *ibid.*, *91,* 321. Reply.— P. A. Gabow *et al.* (letter), *ibid.*, 322.

Magnesium. Reduced clearance of magnesium by spironolactone.— T. Mountokalakis *et al.*, *Klin. Wschr.*, 1975, *53,* 633. Slight increase in magnesium loss in several cirrhotic patients receiving spironolactone.— J. L. Campra and T. B. Reynolds, *Am. J. dig. Dis.*, 1978, *23,* 1025.

Further references: P. G. Wheeler *et al.*, *Gut,* 1977, *18,* 683.

Potassium. A report of a 69-year-old man with near-fatal cardiac arrhythmia caused by spironolactone-induced hyperkalaemia. He had a high dietary potassium intake. Survival followed intravenous therapy with sodium bicarbonate.— C. Pongpaew *et al.*, *Chest,* 1973, *63,* 1023.

Hyperkalaemic muscular paralysis, responsive to insulin, in a patient taking spironolactone.— E. O. Udezue and B. P. Harrold, *Postgrad. med. J.*, 1980, *56,* 254.

Further references: E. Herman and J. P. Radó, *Archs Neurol., Chicago,* 1966, *15,* 74; J. P. Radó *et al.*, *J. Am. Geriat. Soc.*, 1968, *16,* 874.

Effects on endocrine function. A discussion on, and details of, investigations into the oestrogenic effects of spironolactone, which include decreased libido, impotence, and gynaecomastia in men, and menstrual irregularity and painful breast enlargement in women. Spironolactone interferes with testosterone biosynthesis but studies imply that this is inadequate to explain the oestrogen-like side-effects of spironolactone therapy; its anti-androgen action at receptor sites may offer a more convincing explanation. On the other hand, the menstrual irregularity may be explained by its reduction of 17-hydroxylase activity.— D. L. Loriaux *et al.*, *Ann. intern. Med.*, 1976, *85,* 630.

Further references: J. I. Levitt, *J. Am. med. Ass.*, 1970, *211,* 2014; P. Corvol *et al.*, *Nouv. Presse méd.*, 1976, *5,* 691; R. Caminos-Torres *et al.*, *J. clin. Endocr. Metab.*, 1977, *45,* 255; L. I. Rose *et al.*, *Ann. intern. Med.*, 1977, *87,* 398.

Effects on the gastro-intestinal tract. Haematemesis secondary to gastric ulceration occurred in a patient being treatment with spironolactone.— A. Mackay and R. D. Stevenson (letter), *Lancet,* 1977, *1,* 481.

Further references: J. J. Brown *et al.* (letter), *Br. med. J.*, 1969, *4,* 688; D. Kremer *et al.*, *ibid.*, 1973, *2,* 216.

Effects on sexual function. Details of gynaecomastia and impotence complications of spironolactone therapy.— D. J. Greenblatt and J. Koch Weser, *J. Am. med. Ass.*, 1973, *223,* 82.

See also under Effects on Endocrine Function (above).

Effects on the skin. *Lichen planus.* A report of lichen-planus-like skin eruptions which developed in a 62-year-old woman who was taking digoxin, propranolol, diazepam, spironolactone, and iron tablets. Flares of the lichen-planus-like eruption seemed to be associated with administration of spironolactone and there was evidence of resolution when spironolactone was withdrawn.— T. F. Downham (letter), *J. Am. med. Ass.*, 1978, *240,* 1138.

Gout. A comment that spironolactone has not been implicated as a cause of hyperuricaemia.— G. R. Boss and J. E. Seegmiller, *New Engl. J. Med.*, 1979, *300,* 1459.

Lupus erythematosus. A patient experienced a cutaneous reaction to spironolactone resembling lupus erythematosus.— M. S. Uddin *et al.*, *Cutis,* 1979, *24,* 198.

Oedema. For reference to the possible role of diuretics in exacerbating and perpetuating idiopathic oedema, see Oedema, under Adverse Effects of Chlorothiazide, p.588.

Treatment of Adverse Effects. Hyperkalaemia may be treated by giving a diuretic which causes the excretion of potassium, by the injection of dextrose with insulin, or by the use of an appropriate ion-exchange resin. For further details see under the treatment of adverse effects of potassium (p.628).

Precautions. Spironolactone should not be given to patients with hyperkalaemia or progressive renal failure, and should not be given with other potassium-sparing diuretics. Potassium supplements should not be given with spironolactone. It should be given with care to patients with impaired hepatic or renal function. Although spironolactone has not been shown to have any effect on carbohydrate metabolism, it should be given with care to patients with diabetes mellitus, who may be predisposed to hyperkalaemia. It should also be given with care to patients likely to develop acidosis. Serum electrolytes and blood-urea-nitrogen should be estimated periodically.

Spironolactone enhances the effects of other antihypertensive agents and may diminish vascular responses to noradrenaline. Spironolactone is not suitable for nursing mothers.

Interactions. It is suggested that spironolactone is a weak enzyme inducer in some individuals.— S. A. Taylor *et al.* (letter), *J. Pharm. Pharmac.*, 1972, *24,* 598. No evidence in a study of 8 subjects that spironolactone induces liver microsomal enzyme activity.— E. E. Ohnhaus and J. P. Masson, *Br. J. clin. Pharmac.*, 1977, *4,* 639P.

Further references: D. H. Huffman *et al.*, *Pharmacology,* 1973, *10,* 338 (evidence of enzyme induction).

Ammonium chloride. A 58-year-old woman receiving spironolactone 25 mg four times a day and potassium chloride about 50 mmol (50 mEq) daily developed acidosis about 20 days after starting ammonium chloride 4 g daily; renal function was adequate. Three factors might have contributed; increased acid load due to ammonium chloride, decreased ability of the kidney to excrete hydrogen ions due to the aldosterone-antagonist effect of spironolactone, and increased acid load due to hyperkalaemia.— M. L. Mashford and M. B. Robertson (letter), *Br. med. J.*, 1972, *4,* 298.

Aspirin and other anti-inflammatory analgesics. The urinary sodium excretion induced by spironolactone was reduced by 30% in 7 volunteers after a single dose of aspirin 600 mg.— M. G. Tweeddale and R. I. Ogilvie, *New Engl. J. Med.*, 1973, *289,* 198. Aspirin did not appear to alter the effect of spironolactone on blood pressure, serum electrolytes, urea nitrogen, or plasma renin activity in 5 patients with low-renin essential hypertension and 2 with hypertension associated with primary aldosteronism.— J. W. Hollifield, *Sth. med. J.*, 1976, *69,* 1034. In a double-blind study in 6 healthy subjects the administration of aspirin 600 mg with spironolactone 50 mg significantly reduced the urinary excretion and the fractional excretion of its active metabolite, canrenone, 4 to 6 hours later.— L. E. Ramsay *et al.*, *Eur. J. clin. Pharmac.*, 1976, *10,* 43.

Digoxin and other cardiac glycosides. For conflicting reports on the effects of concomitant administration of spironolactone on digoxin pharmacokinetics, see Digoxin, p.534.

For the effect of spironolactone on digitoxin, see Digitoxin, p.542.

Fludrocortisone. For reference to a paradoxical increase in urinary-potassium excretion on concomitant administration of spironolactone and fludrocortisone, see Canrenoate Potassium, p.587.

Mitotane. For a report of the inhibition of the action of mitotane by concomitant administration of spironolactone, see Mitotane, p.222.

Narcotic analgesics. An allergic pruritic reaction to a preparation of dextropropoxyphene, aspirin, caffeine, and phenacetin was considered to trigger spironolactone-induced gynaecomastia in one patient. The pruritus and breast swelling resolved when both the preparation and spironolactone were withdrawn. The reintroduction of spironolactone produced no ill effect but the effects returned when the dextropropoxyphene preparation was reinstituted.— A. A. Licata and F. C. Bartter (letter), *Lancet,* 1976, *2,* 905.

Interference with diagnostic tests. Reports and studies on the interference of spironolactone with diagnostic tests: *Drug & Ther. Bull.*, 1972, *10,* 69 (blood-cortisol concentrations); S. C. Lowder and G. W. Liddle, *New Engl. J. Med.*, 1974, *291,* 1243 (diagnosis of low plasma-renin activity); E. V. Young Lai *et al.*, *Hormone metab. Res.*, 1975, *7,* 364 (progesterone and oestrogen radioassay); Y. S. Tan *et al.*, *J. clin. Endocr. Metab.*, 1975, *41,* 791 (deoxycortone radio-assay); J. Lichey *et al.*, *Dt. med. Wschr.*, 1977, *102,* 1056; *idem*, *Int. J. clin. Pharmac. Biopharm.*, 1977, *15,* 557 (digoxin radio-immunoassay); J. W. Taylor (letter), *J. Am. med. Ass.*, 1978, *240,* 2248 (digoxin radio-immunoassay).

Pregnancy and the neonate. In a study of a nursing mother taking spironolactone 25 mg four times daily the estimated maximum quantity of canrenone (the principle metabolite) ingested by the infant in the breast milk was 0.2% of the daily dose.— D. L. Phelps and A. Karim, *J. pharm. Sci.*, 1977, *66,* 1203.

Absorption and Fate. Spironolactone is incompletely, but fairly rapidly, absorbed from the gastro-intestinal tract, the extent of absorption depending on particle size and formulation. Canrenone, which is an active metabolite, has a biphasic plasma half-life of about 4 and 17 hours. Spironolactone is excreted in the urine and in the faeces, in the form of metabolites. It is extensively bound to plasma proteins. Spironolactone or its metabolites may cross the placental barrier, and canrenone is excreted in breast milk.

A review of the disposition, metabolism, pharmacodynamics, and bioavailability of spironolactone.— A. Karim, *Drug Metab. Rev.*, 1978, *8,* 151.

A detailed study of the absorption, excretion, and metabolism of spironolactone in 5 healthy men. About 3 hours after single doses of spironolactone 200 mg in alcoholic solution by mouth mean peak serum concentrations of the dethioacetylated metabolite, canrenone (415 ± 145 ng per ml), were obtained and subsequently declined in 2 phases with a half-life of 4.42 hours from 2.5 to 12 hours and about 17 hours from 12 to 72 hours. Spironolactone was excreted as its metabolites both in urine and faeces.— A. Karim *et al.*, *Clin. Pharmac. Ther.*, 1976, *19,* 158. In a study of 23 healthy men who received spironolactone 200 mg once daily or 50 mg four times daily for 15 days steady-state blood concentrations of canrenone were obtained 3 to 4 days after either regimen. With the once-daily regimen maximum and minimum concentrations were about 500 and 100 ng per ml whereas the minimum concentration with the multiple-dose regimen was about 200 ng per ml, but the post steady-state half-life of the active metabolite, canrenone, was longer following the single-dose regimen suggesting that the optimum spironolactone dosage should be twice or even once daily.— *idem*, 177.

Further references: J. Hettiarachchi and L. E. Ramsay, *Br. J. clin. Pharmac.*, 1979, *7,* 426P; U. Abshagen *et al.*, *Eur. J. clin. Pharmac.*, 1979, *16,* 255.

Bioavailability. Studies in healthy subjects indicated that administration of spironolactone with food increased the amount of canrenone, its active metabolite, which entered the general circulation.— A. Melander *et al.*, *Clin. Pharmac. Ther.*, 1977, *22*, 100.

A single-blind, randomised, crossover study involving 6 healthy subjects showed no differences in bioavailability between 2 commercial preparations of spironolactone. Following administration of spironolactone 100 mg twice daily for 6 days a mean peak serum-canrenone concentration of about 500 ng per ml occurred about 3 hours after a dose.— H. Rameis *et al.*, *Dt. med. Wschr.*, 1979, *104*, 881.

Further references: M. J. Tidd *et al.*, *Int. J. clin. Pharmac. Biopharm.*, 1977, *15*, 205; G. Raptis *et al.*, *Drug Dev. ind. Pharm.*, 1978, *4*, 389.

Metabolism. A study in 12 healthy subjects suggested that canrenone was not the only active metabolite of both spironolactone and canrenoate potassium.— L. E. Ramsay *et al.*, *Br. J. clin. Pharmac.*, 1976, *3*, 607. A study in healthy subjects comparing single doses of spironolactone and canrenoate potassium indicated that, on a weight or molar basis, canrenoate potassium was only about a third as potent although its effects were qualitatively similar. It thus appeared that canrenone is not the principal pharmacological metabolite of spironolactone; the major part of the diuretic activity might be associated with minor, sulphur-containing metabolites.— *idem*, *Clin. Pharmac. Ther.*, 1976, *20*, 167. See also *idem*, 1977, *21*, 602.

Following administration of spironolactone 200 mg to healthy subjects at home and to cirrhotic and non-cirrhotic patients in hospital about 3% of the administered dose appeared in the urine as canrenone after 3 days in all groups of patients, with healthy subjects showing the most rapid elimination of the metabolite. The elimination of canrenone appeared to be dose-related as spironolactone 50 mg gave a considerably lower percentage of the metabolite in the urine.— A. Váradi *et al.*, *Arzneimittel-Forsch.*, 1977, *27*, 1618.

Further references: E. Gerhards and R. Engelhardt, *Arzneimittel-Forsch.*, 1963, *13*, 972; G. T. McInnes *et al.*, *Br. J. clin. Pharmac.*, 1980, *9*, 295P; *idem*, *Clin. Pharmac. Ther.*, 1980, *27*, 363.

Protein binding. Protein binding of spironolactone and canrenone exceeded 89% at plasma concentrations of 550 and 710 ng per ml respectively.— A. Karim *et al.*, *Clin. Pharmac. Ther.*, 1976, *19*, 158.

Further references: A. S. Ng *et al.*, *J. pharm. Sci.*, 1980, *69*, 30.

Uses. Spironolactone, a steroid with a structure resembling that of the natural adrenocortical hormone, aldosterone, acts on the distal portion of the renal tubule as a competitive inhibitor of aldosterone. It thus increases sodium and water excretion and reduces potassium excretion. It acts both as a diuretic and as an antihypertensive agent.

Spironolactone is reported to have a relatively slow onset of action, requiring 2 or 3 days for maximum effect, and a similarly slow diminishment of action over 2 or 3 days on discontinuation.

Spironolactone is used in the treatment of refractory oedema associated with congestive heart failure, cirrhosis of the liver, or the nephrotic syndrome. For these purposes it is frequently given with the thiazides, frusemide, and similar diuretics, where it adds to their natriuretic but diminishes their kaliuretic effects, hence conserving potassium. In hepatic disorders, in view of its slower onset of action, it has been recommended that it be given a few days before concomitant therapy with potassium-losing diuretics in order to prevent induction of exacerbation of hypokalaemia with the associated risk of coma. Spironolactone has also been used as an antihypertensive agent, particularly in the diagnosis and treatment of primary hyperaldosteronism.

Spironolactone is usually given in an initial dose of 100 mg daily in divided doses, subsequently increased as necessary; some patients may require doses of up to 400 mg daily. It is given in doses of 400 mg daily for the diagnosis of hyperaldosteronism; in doses of 100 to 400 mg daily for the pre-operative management of hyperaldosteronism; and in the lowest effective dosage for long-term maintenance therapy in the absence of surgery. A suggested initial dose of spironolactone for children is 3 mg per kg body-weight daily, in divided doses.

Potassium supplements should not be given with spironolactone.

A detailed review of the chemistry, pharmacokinetics, mechanisms of action, uses, and unwanted effects of spironolactone.— H. R. Ochs *et al.*, *Am. Heart J.*, 1978, *96*, 389.

Further reviews and discussions on spironolactone: *Drug & Ther. Bull.*, 1972, *10*, 30; M. E. Kosman, *J. Am. med. Ass.*, 1974, *230*, 743; *Med. Lett.*, 1975, *17*, 86.

Action. *Animal* studies on the aldosterone-antagonist action of spironolactone: R. M. Salassa *et al.*, *J. clin. Endocr. Metab.*, 1958, *18*, 787; C. M. Kagawa *et al.*, *J. Pharmac. exp. Ther.*, 1959, *126*, 123; T. Uete and E. H. Venning, *Proc. Soc. exp. Biol. Med.*, 1962, *109*, 760; J. Crabbe, *Acta endocr., Copenh.*, 1964, *47*, 419.

A study in patients with primary hyperaldosteronism, indicating that the antihypertensive effect is nonspecific and largely dependent on salt and water balance.— E. L. Bravo *et al.*, *Clin. Pharmac. Ther.*, 1974, *15*, 201. See also *idem*, *Circulation*, 1973, *48*, 491.

A study suggesting that mineralocorticoid excess is rarely responsible for essential hypertension, and that the beneficial role of spironolactone cannot be fully explained by mineralocorticoid antagonism.— B. I. Hoffbrand *et al.*, *Br. med. J.*, 1976, *1*, 682.

Absence of correlation between the antihypertensive effect of spironolactone and changes in body-weight or plasma-renin activity.— R. I. Ogilvie *et al.*, *Clin. Pharmac. Ther.*, 1977, *21*, 113.

Further references: B. E. Karlberg *et al.*, *Am. J. Cardiol.*, 1976, *37*, 642.

Administration. For reference to the enhanced bioavailability of spironolactone when given with food, see under Absorption and Fate.

Administration in hepatic failure. A study suggesting that the metabolism of spironolactone is unaltered in patients with liver disease.— U. Abshagen *et al.*, *Eur. J. clin. Pharmac.*, 1977, *11*, 169.

In 5 patients with chronic liver disease the mean elimination half-life of canrenone, a major metabolite of spironolactone, was about 59 hours, and in 7 patients with congestive heart failure about 37 hours, compared to 20.5 hours in healthy subjects. However, there was no evidence of accumulation of canrenone in plasma.— L. Jackson *et al.*, *Eur. J. clin. Pharmac.*, 1977, *11*, 177.

Further references: W. Sadée *et al.*, *Eur. J. clin. Pharmac.*, 1974, *7*, 195.

See also under Hepatic Disorders (below).

Administration in renal failure. Potassium-sparing diuretics are best avoided in patients with impaired renal function because of the risk of hyperkalaemia and because decline in renal function has been observed with spironolactone, triamterene, and amiloride.— R. R. Bailey (letter), *Br. med. J.*, 1978, *1*, 1618.

Further references: J. S. Cheigh, *Am. J. Med.*, 1977, *62*, 555; W. M. Bennett *et al.*, *Ann. intern. Med.*, 1980, *93*, 286.

Aldosteronism. For the use of spironolactone in hypertension associated with hyperaldosteronism, see under Hypertension.

Carcinoma. Suppression of plasma androgens by spironolactone in castrated men with carcinoma of the prostate.— P. C. Walsh and P. K. Siiteri, *J. Urol.*, 1975, *114*, 254.

Cardiac disorders. *Cor pulmonale.* A study of the effects of canrenoate potassium intravenously and spironolactone by mouth in cor pulmonale.— U. Hüttemann and K. P. Schüren, *Klin. Wschr.*, 1972, *50*, 953.

Heart failure. Beneficial effect of spironolactone on cardiac arrhythmias associated with severe heart failure.— A. Tourniaire *et al.*, *Sem. Hôp. Paris*, 1969, *45*, 1388.

Diabetes insipidus. In 3 children with diabetes insipidus, spironolactone, in doses of 100 to 400 mg six-hourly, reduced urinary output. In 1 child, the addition of chlorothiazide 250 mg to spironolactone 200 mg every 6 hours reduced urine flow, which was further reduced by a low-sodium diet.— A. Kowarski *et al.*, *Bull. Johns Hopkins Hosp.*, 1966, *119*, 413, per *Abstr. Wld Med.*, 1967, *41*, 587.

Endocrine disorders. A 19-year-old girl with amenorrhoea, hirsutism, and hypertension was treated with spironolactone and hydrochlorothiazide. Satisfactory control of blood pressure was accompanied by a decrease in serum-testosterone concentrations, with a softening of facial hair. Spironolactone might be an alternative treatment to oral contraceptives or corticosteroids in some women with excessive androgen production.— K. P. Ober and J. F. Hennessy, *Ann. intern. Med.*, 1978, *89*, 643.

Further references: D. L. Loriaux *et al.*, *Ann. intern. Med.*, 1976, *85*, 630; A. Boiselle and R. R. Tremblay, *Fert. Steril.*, 1979, *32*, 276; G. Shapiro and S. Evron, *J. clin. Endocr. Metab.*, 1980, *51*, 429.

For the use of spironolactone in hypertension associated with hyperaldosteronism, see under Hypertension.

Hepatic disorders. A review of the management of hepatic ascites, with special reference to the value of spironolactone, and emphasis on the merits of slow increase in dosage. Potassium depletion is common in patients with cirrhosis and may itself precipitate hepatic encephalopathy, therefore oral potassium supplements should be prescribed at the start of treatment. However, spironolactone prevents the later development of hypokalaemia and potassium supplements are best withdrawn after a few days.— *Br. med. J.*, 1978, *1*, 66.

Further reviews and comments: P. Vesin, *Postgrad. med. J.*, 1975, *51*, 545.

Fourteen patients with cirrhosis of the liver, due to chronic alcoholism, and with persistent ascites received spironolactone in a daily dose of 100 or 150 mg where the initial urinary sodium/potassium ratio exceeded 1. Up to 1 g daily was given to patients where the urinary sodium/potassium ratio was initially less than 1. Ethacrynic acid or frusemide was given, in addition, to 3 patients in whom diuresis did not occur within 3 or 4 days of reversal of the ratio. In all patients a sustained uncomplicated diuresis was achieved without the occurrence of hypokalaemia and hepatic encephalopathy. Mild hyperkalaemia, which occurred in 2 patients after complete diuresis, responded to discontinuance of therapy or a reduced dosage of spironolactone.— R. C. Eggert, *Br. med. J.*, 1970, *4*, 401.

In 10 patients with cirrhosis of the liver and ascites, spironolactone in doses of 200 mg daily together with frusemide produced more effective diuresis than spironolactone in doses of 100 mg daily. The addition of prednisolone to therapy produced increased diuresis.— N. Papadoyanakis *et al.*, *Br. J. clin. Pract.*, 1972, *26*, 27.

Spironolactone 150 mg daily or triamterene 300 mg daily (distal diuretics) together with a low-sodium diet was recommended for the treatment of ascites in patients with cirrhosis of the liver who had low sodium excretion but high free water clearance. Frusemide 40 to 80 mg daily was added if satisfactory diuresis was not obtained.— V. Arroyo and J. Rodés, *Postgrad. med. J.*, 1975, *51*, 558.

Spironolactone 200 mg daily for 4 to 14 days reduced plasma concentrations of bile acids in 15 patients with liver cirrhosis or bile-duct obstruction. It had no effect on the bile of 8 healthy controls.— T. Feher *et al.* (letter), *Lancet*, 1976, *2*, 51. Spironolactone did not lower serum-bile-salt concentrations in 12 patients with cirrhosis but elevated the concentrations.— A. A. Mihas *et al.* (letter), *Lancet*, 1977, *1*, 914.

A report of excellent results in 9 of 10 patients with hepatic cirrhosis given spironolactone 300 mg daily, increased every sixth day if necessary by 100 mg, to a maximum of 600 mg daily. Spironolactone was well tolerated and no serious electrolyte disturbance was noted other than hyperkalaemia (in 3 patients). Because of the risk of hyperkalaemia this treatment regimen is not suitable for patients with renal dysfunction or those taking potassium supplements. A small fall in serum-magnesium concentrations occurred in several patients.— J. L. Campra and T. B. Reynolds, *Am. J. dig. Dis.*, 1978, *23*, 1025.

Further references: H. Gold *et al.*, *J. clin. Pharmac.*, 1971, *11*, 125; *idem*, 1972, *12*, 35; G. R. Lang *et al.*, *Clin. Pharmac. Ther.*, 1977, *21*, 234.

For further reports on the use of spironolactone in the treatment of hepatic cirrhosis and cardiac oedema, see Frusemide, p.599.

In children. A favourable report on experience with spironolactone in over 60 children with liver disease. In at least 75% of these patients spironolactone alone produced a satisfactory diuresis within 24 to 36 hours of a first administration. An initial dose of 25 mg twice daily was used for infants under 12 months of age and an initial dose of 25 mg thrice daily for those aged 12 months to 2 years of age. In the 25% of infants where diuresis did not occur, it was always obtained by addition of a small dose of frusemide or a thiazide. Providing these drugs are given after satisfactory saturation with spironolactone, serious potassium depletion is rarely seen.— D. M. Danks (letter), *J. Pediat.*, 1976, *88*, 695.

Hypertension. In a double-blind crossover study of 24 hypertensive patients, 13 of whom had normal and 11 of whom had low renin activity, administration of spironolactone had no advantage over hydrochlorothiazide in either group. Side-effects were significantly higher following spironolactone administration and included skin eruption, lassitude, gastro-intestinal complaints, and breast swelling and tenderness in men.— R. K. Ferguson *et al.*, *Clin. Pharmac. Ther.*, 1977, *21*, 62.

Further references: L. C. Johnston and H. G. Grieble, *Archs intern. Med.*, 1967, *119*, 225; B. M. Winer *et al.*, *J. Am. med. Ass.*, 1968, *204*, 775; *Practitioner*, 1971, *206*, 412 (Report No. 158 of the General Practitioner Research Group); A. Froment and H. Milon, *Presse méd.*, 1971, *79*, 577; J. G. Douglas *et al.*, *J. Am. med. Ass.*, 1974, *227*, 518; N. M. A. Walter *et al.*, *Med. J. Aust.*, 1978, *1*, 509; F. Alhenc-Gelas *et al.*, *Am. J. Med.*, 1978, *64*, 1005; D. H. Hull *et al.*, *Aviat. Space & Environ. Med.*, 1978, *49*, 503; W. P. Leary *et al.*, *J. int. med. Res.*, 1979, *7*, 29; D. Levitt, *Curr. med. Res. Opinion*, 1979, *6*, 136; G. Berglund and O. Andersson, *Curr. ther. Res.*, 1980, *27*, 360; J. G. R. DeCarvalho *et al.*, *Clin. Pharmac. Ther.*, 1980, *27*, 53; K. R. Madwar, *Curr. ther. Res.*, 1980, *27*, 190; E. N. Mngola, *J. int. med. Res.*, 1980, *8*, 199.

Associated with aldosteronism. In 67 patients with hypertension, raised plasma concentrations of aldosterone, and low plasma concentrations of renin, there was an inverse correlation between aldosterone and renin concentrations. After treatment with spironolactone 50 to 400 mg daily for at least 4 weeks, blood pressure was reduced from a mean of 201/122 to 159/101 mmHg 3 to 5 weeks after starting treatment. The response was comparable in those with or without adrenocortical adenoma and was greater in those with lower initial blood-urea concentrations. In 32 patients subjected to surgery, usually for adrenocortical adenoma, there was good correlation between postoperative hypotensive response and prior response to spironolactone.— J. J. Brown *et al.*, *Br. med. J.*, 1972, *2*, 729. Hypertension due to hyperaldosteronism; its physiology and treatment.— *idem*, 391.

A detailed account of the surgical and medical management of patients with low-renin (primary) hyperaldosteronism. In patients with a good response to pre-operative spironolactone, surgical removal of the tumour-bearing gland is usually the treatment of choice. Long-term spironolactone therapy is, however, an acceptable alternative, and if it is not tolerated, amiloride may be substituted.— J. B. Ferriss *et al.*, *Am. Heart J.*, 1978, *96*, 97. See also *idem*, *Br. med. J.*, 1975, *1*, 135.

Further reports and comments: D. G. Beevers *et al.*, *Am. Heart J.*, 1973, *86*, 404; B. E. Karlberg *et al.*, *Br. med. J.*, 1976, *1*, 251; P. F. Semple, *Practitioner*, 1979, *223*, 218; *Lancet*, 1979, *2*, 1221.

Mental disorders. Six manic-depressive patients who were well maintained on lithium therapy but who found its side-effects unacceptable were changed to spironolactone 25 mg four times daily. Over a follow-up period of 12 to 18 months 5 of the 6 were maintained satisfactorily. Spironolactone might act by stabilising a presynaptic membrane in the hypothalamus against fluctuations of aldosterone seen in manic disease.— N. H. Hendler, *J. nerv. ment. Dis.*, 1978, *166*, 517.

Migraine. A patient with a long history of recurrent migraine twice a month was free from symptoms for 9 months while receiving 225 mg of spironolactone daily.— E. Stanford (letter), *Lancet*, 1968, *1*, 1038.

Mountain sickness. Two of 6 unacclimatised climbers taking spironolactone 25 mg thrice daily starting 48 hours before reaching 3000 m developed acute mountain sickness compared with 5 of 6 similar climbers taking a placebo. A larger study was needed to confirm the value of spironolactone.— G. V. Brown *et al.* (letter), *Lancet*, 1977, *1*, 855.

Further references: T. T. Currie *et al.*, *Med. J. Aust.*, 1976, *2*, 168; A. C. McFarlane (letter), *ibid.*, 923; T. T. Currie (letter), *ibid.*, 1977, *1*, 419; J. A. Snell and E. P. Cordner, *ibid.*, 828; A. C. McFarlane (letter), *ibid.*, *2*, 616; G. Turnbull (letter), *Br. med. J.*, 1980, *280*, 1453; D. H. Meyers (letter), *ibid.*, *281*, 1569; L. D. Rutter (letter), *ibid.*, 618.

See also under Acetazolamide Sodium, p.582.

Premenstrual syndrome. A report of a double-blind crossover study, involving 18 women with premenstrual tension and 10 control women, during 4 menstrual cycles, comparing spironolactone 25 mg four times daily from the 18th to the 26th day of the cycle, with placebo. Spironolactone had a beneficial effect on weight gain and mood in most of those with premenstrual syndrome. There was no evidence to support the hypothesis that aldosterone concentrations were higher in the symptomatic group and it is probable that spironolactone acted purely through its diuretic effect.— P. M. S. O'Brien *et al.*, *Br. J. Obstet. Gynaec.*, 1979, *86*, 142.

For reference to the possible role of diuretics in exacerbating and perpetuating idiopathic oedema, see Oedema, under Adverse Effects of Chlorothiazide, p.588.

Urology. In a double-blind controlled trial in patients with prostatic hypertrophy, treatment with spironolactone 50 mg twice daily resulted in an overall improvement compared with placebo after 3 months but this had disappeared when assessed again at 6 months.— J. E. Castro *et al.*, *Br. J. Surg.*, 1971, *58*, 485, per *Proc. R. Soc. Med.*, 1972, *65*, 126.

Preparations

Spironolactone Tablets *(B.P.)*. Tablets containing spironolactone. They may be flavoured. Protect from light.

Spironolactone Tablets *(U.S.P.)*. Tablets containing spironolactone. Store in airtight containers. Protect from light.

Proprietary Preparations

Aldactide 25 *(Searle, UK)*. Scored tablets each containing spironolactone 25 mg and hydroflumethiazide 25 mg. *Dose.* Oedematous conditions, 4 tablets daily initially, then 1 to 8 tablets daily; essential hypertension, 1 to 4 tablets daily.

Aldactide 50 *(Searle, UK)*. Scored tablets each containing spironolactone 50 mg and hydroflumethiazide 50 mg. *Dose.* Oedematous conditions, 2 tablets daily initially, then 1 to 4 tablets daily; essential hypertension, 1 to 2 tablets daily.

Aldactone *(Searle, UK)*. Spironolactone, available as scored tablets of 25 mg and tablets of 100 mg. (Also available as Aldactone in *Austral.*, *Canad.*, *Denm.*, *Fr.*, *Ger.*, *Ital.*, *Neth.*, *Norw.*, *S.Afr.*, *Swed.*, *Switz.*, *USA*). The name Aldactone is also used in some countries as a proprietary name for canrenoate potassium.

Diatensec *(Searle, UK)*. Spironolactone, available as tablets of 50 mg.

Spiroctan *(MCP Pharmaceuticals, UK)*. Spironolactone, available as **Capsules** of 100 mg and **Tablets** of 25 and 50 mg. (Also available as Spiroctan in *Neth.*).

Other Proprietary Names

Arg.—Aldactone-A; *Austral.*—Spirotone; *Denm.*—Osiren *(see also under Canrenoate Potassium)*, Spirix, Spiron; *Ger.*—Aldopur, Osyrol *(see also under Canrenoate Potassium)*, Sincomen, Spiro; *Hung.*—Verospirone; *Ital.*—Idrolattone, Sincomen, Spirolang, Uractone; *Jap.*—Aldactone-A, Alexan, Almatol, Alpamed, Aporasnon, Dira, Hokuraton, Lacalmin, Lacdene, Nefurofan, Noidouble, Osyrol *(see also under Canrenoate Potassium)*, Pirolacton, Suracton, Urusonin; *Neth.*—Aldactone-A; *Norw.*—Osiren *(see also under Canrenoate Potassium)*; *S.Afr.*—Sincomen; *Spain*—Aldactone-A; *Switz.*—Osiren *(see also under Canrenoate Potassium)*; *USA*—Altex.

2356-l

Teclothiazide Potassium. Tetrachlormethiazide. The potassium salt of 6-chloro-3,4-dihydro-3-trichloromethyl-2*H*-1,2,4-benzothiadiazine-7-sulphonamide 1,1-dioxide.

$C_8H_6Cl_4KN_3O_4S_2$=453.2.

CAS — 4267-05-4 (teclothiazide); 5306-80-9 (potassium salt).

A white crystalline powder. **Soluble** in water and solutions of alkalis; practically insoluble in most organic solvents.

Teclothiazide potassium is a thiazide diuretic with actions and uses similar to those of chlorothiazide (see p.587). It has been given in doses of 110 to 220 mg daily for 3 or 4 days each week.

Teclothiazide potassium was formerly marketed in Great Britain under the proprietary name Deplet (*Marshall's Pharmaceuticals*).

2357-y

Tienilic Acid. SKF 62698; Ticrynafen. [2,3-Dichloro-4-(2-thenoyl)phenoxy]acetic acid.

$C_{13}H_8Cl_2O_4S$=331.2.

CAS — 40180-04-9.

Adverse Effects. Severe liver damage has been associated with tienilic acid therapy which has resulted in a number of deaths; for this reason tienilic acid has been withdrawn in some countries.

Like chlorothiazide, administration of tienilic acid may be associated with electrolyte imbalances, notably hypokalaemia; it has also been associated with reduced glucose tolerance and increased plasma-triglyceride concentrations. Unlike chlorothiazide, tienilic acid has a uricosuric action and reduces, rather than raises, plasma concentrations of uric acid; its prolonged administration has not therefore been associated with the development of gout. During initial therapy its uric acid mobilising action has precipitated acute attacks of gout and renal failure in hyperuricaemic subjects.

Other side-effects occasionally reported include: gastro-intestinal symptoms (including dyspepsia, nausea, abdominal pain, stomach cramps, and constipation), headache, drowsiness, vertigo, dry mouth, leg muscle cramps and weakness, joint pain, back pain, nervousness, allergy, skin rashes or urticaria, palpitations, chest pain, orthostatic hypotension, and urinary frequency.

Reversible changes in blood-urea-nitrogen and creatinine concentrations have been noted.

Allergy. Tienilic acid has been given safely to patients allergic to the thiazides.— *Med. Lett.*, 1979, *21*, 61.

A serum sickness type of reaction with rash and arthralgias occurred in a woman receiving both tienilic acid and quinidine. It was not known which agent was responsible.— K. T. Weber and A. P. Fishman, *Postgrad. med. J.*, 1979, *55*, *Suppl.* 3, 58.

Diabetogenic effect. No significant difference was noted between the deterioration in glucose tolerance in patients with mild maturity-onset diabetes given hydrochlorothiazide or tienilic acid.— F. G. McMahon *et al.*, *Postgrad. med. J.*, 1979, *55*, *Suppl.* 3, 75. See also E. D. Frohlich *et al.*, *ibid.*, 98.

Effects on the electrolyte balance. During a comparative study both hydrochlorothiazide and tienilic acid significantly reduced serum concentrations of potassium and chloride and increased serum bicarbonate content. Four patients developed hypokalaemia; in 2 it was severe enough to require potassium supplements during tienilic acid therapy.— E. D. Frohlich *et al.*, *Postgrad. med. J.*, 1979, *55*, *Suppl.* 3, 98.

Calcium. Tienilic acid had a definite hypocalciuric effect in healthy subjects although this was less marked than with hydrochlorothiazide.— G. Lemieux *et al.*, *Nephron*, 1978, *20*, 54.

Effects on endocrine function. A man had to start shaving twice daily three days after starting tienilic acid therapy; he had not done this for 15 years. A woman with previous thining of hair felt that regrowth of fine hair at the hairline slowed when she started tienilic acid.— H. J. Waal-Manning *et al.*, *Postgrad. med. J.*, 1979, *55*, *Suppl.* 3, 85.

Effects on the gastro-intestinal tract. Dyspepsia associated with tienilic acid therapy.— H. J. Waal-Manning *et al.*, *Postgrad. med. J.*, 1979, *55*, *Suppl.* 3, 85.

Effects on the heart. A patient complained of chest pain on several occasions after receiving tienilic acid.— M. Nemati *et al.*, *J. Am. med. Ass.*, 1977, *237*, 652.

Premature ventricular and atrial contractions in 2 patients taking tienilic acid were relieved by supplemental potassium therapy to restore normokalaemia.— E. D. Frohlich *et al.*, *Postgrad. med. J.*, 1979, *55*, *Suppl.* 3, 98.

Effects on the kidneys. A 45-year-old woman developed oliguric renal failure 5 days after starting treatment with tienilic acid; acute uric acid nephropathy was probably the cause. Dehydrated patients and those who have been taking thiazides must have a washout period and be rehydrated before tienilic acid is given.— W. M. Bennett *et al.* (letter), *New Engl. J. Med.*, 1979, *301*, 1179. Acute renal failure occurred in 2 patients within hours of a single dose of tienilic acid.— L. H. Cohen *et al.* (letter), *ibid.*, 1180. An untoward reaction to tienilic acid has been reported in about 0.05% of patients; it has usually been limited to hypertensive patients with raised uric-acid concentrations whose treatment has been changed to tienilic acid without a diuretic-free period or adequate hydration. The reaction is characterised by flank or abdominal pain, noted within hours of the first dose, followed by nausea, vomiting, uraemia, transient oliguria, and rarely, anuria. Treatment of the reaction has included hydration and administration of allopurinol with or without loop diuretics although, in general, disturbances have cleared within 7 to 10 days of discontinuing tienilic acid regardless of the measures used. It appears that the reaction may be avoided if patients are adequately hydrated before starting treatment with tienilic acid and other diuretics discontinued 3 days beforehand.— T. Selby, *Smith Kline & French, USA* (letter), *ibid.* See also M. Nemati *et al.*, *J. Am. med. Ass.*, 1977, *237*, 652; G. Lelievre *et al.*, *Nouv. Presse méd.*, 1978, *7*, 2654.

Increases in serum creatinine and blood-urea-nitrogen concentrations noted during a 24-month study of tienilic acid were considered disquieting.— R. Okun and M. A. Beg, *Postgrad. med. J.*, 1979, *55*, *Suppl.* 3, 103. The transitory rise in serum creatinine concentrations associated with tienilic acid therapy is a feature common to all diuretics, especially in high dosage, and reflects a reduction in glomerular filtration rate.— A. Lant, *ibid.*, 133.

Effects on lipid metabolism. Significant increases in plasma triglyceride concentrations during tienilic acid therapy.— E. D. Frohlich *et al.*, *Postgrad. med. J.*, 1979, *55*, *Suppl.* 3, 98.

Further references: M. A. Nadal *et al.*, *Curr. ther. Res.*, 1978, *23*, 286 (reduction); A. Morgan *et al.*, *Postgrad. med. J.*, 1979, *55*, *Suppl.* 3, 63 (increase).

Effects on the liver. Some findings of abnormal liver function tests, mainly rises in serum aspartate aminotransferase (SGOT) in patients receiving tienilic acid. More information is needed concerning possible hepatic toxicity.— H. J. Waal-Manning *et al.*, *Postgrad. med. J.*, 1979, *55*, *Suppl.* 3, 85. No evidence of hepatotoxicity in 11 patients given tienilic acid.— E. D. Freis, *ibid.*, 92.

Tienilic acid had been withdrawn from the U.S. market because of strong suspicion of hepatic damage; 56 cases had been reported. Damage was predominantly hepatocellular, with fever, malaise, and abdominal pain; jaundice occurred in about 60% of cases. Toxicity usually occurred 1 to 3 months after starting treatment, and was generally reversible.— *FDA Drug Bull.*, 1980, *10*, 3. Regret for the ban on tienilic acid. Although a recent report gives the number of deaths as 24 and the number of cases of liver damage as 363, the relation between these events and tienilic acid is not proven.— F. O. Simpson and H. J. Waal-Manning (letter), *Lancet*, 1980, *1*, 978. Further regret for the withdrawal of tienilic acid. Symptomless hepatotoxicity was noted in 2 of 8 patients studied, but both admitted to very high alcohol consumption.— D. G. Beevers and J. M. Walker (letter), *ibid.*, 1417.

Further comments on the withdrawal of tienilic acid.— *Lancet*, 1980, *2*, 681.

Effects on the skin. *Dermatitis.* Generalised dermatitis in a patient taking tienilic acid.— Veterans Administration Cooperative Study Group on Antihypertensive Agents, *New Engl. J. Med.*, 1979, *301*, 293.

Gout. Changing from a thiazide diuretic to tienilic acid appeared to precipitate acute attacks of gout in 2 patients with hyperuricaemia. By increasing excretion and mobilisation of urate, tienilic acid might precipitate acute attacks of gout in a similar manner to uricosuric agents. Perhaps hyperuricaemic, hypertensive patients should receive a concomitant course of indomethacin or colchicine for several weeks to prevent acute gout.— R. S. King; B. A. Wichman (letter), *New Engl. J. Med.*, 1979, *301*, 1065; *idem*, 1980, *302*, 242.

Further references: M. A. Nadal *et al.*, *Curr. ther. Res.*, 1978, *23*, 286.

Treatment of Adverse Effects. As for Chlorothiazide, p.589.
It has been recommended that acute gout, caused by the urate-mobilising action of initial tienilic acid therapy, should be treated with agents such as indomethacin or colchicine.
Acute renal failure associated with initial tienilic acid therapy, which is probably due to urate precipitation in the kidneys, has been managed with hydration and administration of allopurinol, with or without loop diuretics (such as frusemide).

Acute renal failure associated with initial tienilic acid therapy was treated with sodium bicarbonate and allopurinol.— W. M. Bennett *et al.* (letter), *New Engl. J. Med.*, 1979, *301*, 1179. General supportive measures, including hydration and administration of allopurinol, with or without loop diuretics, have been used to treat this reaction.— T. Selby, *Smith Kline & French, USA* (letter), *ibid.*, 1180.

Precautions. As for Chlorothiazide, p.589.
Severe liver damage has been associated with tienilic acid therapy which has resulted in a number of deaths; for this reason tienilic acid has been withdrawn in some countries.
Despite its uricosuric properties, tienilic acid is not suitable for the treatment of gout, because it is a diuretic. It has been recommended that tienilic acid therapy should not be initiated in patients being treated with other diuretics or within 3 days of stopping such treatment, and should only be initiated in adequately hydrated patients.
The effect of warfarin may be enhanced by concurrent administration of tienilic acid, and the uricosuric action of tienilic acid may be diminished by concurrent administration of aspirin (the plasma concentrations of which may, in turn, be raised by tienilic acid).

Interactions. Comments that no evidence of inhibition of microsomal oxidation or induction of enzymes has been found in association with tienilic acid, but that tienilic acid may participate in some drug interactions because of its high level of protein binding.— *Postgrad. med. J.*, 1979, *55*, *Suppl.* 3, 67.

Aspirin and other anti-inflammatory analgesics. Concurrent administration of aspirin 650 mg significantly diminished the uricosuric effect of tienilic acid, probably by inhibiting uric acid secretion. Tienilic acid tended to inhibit salicylate excretion.— J. W. Dubb *et al.*, *Postgrad. med. J.*, 1979, *55*, *Suppl.* 3, 47.

Diuretics. Acute renal insufficiency occurred in a woman given tienilic acid in addition to amiloride.— D. Hillion *et al.*, *Nouv. Presse méd.*, 1979, *27*, 2284.

Phenytoin and other anticonvulsants. A woman receiving phenytoin 300 mg daily developed dizziness, slurred speech, confusion, and ataxia on addition of tienilic acid. She gradually recovered on withdrawal of tienilic acid.— K. T. Weber and A. P. Fishman, *Postgrad. med. J.*, 1979, *55*, *Suppl.* 3, 58.

Pyrazinamide. Blunting of the uricosuric effect of tienilic acid by pyrazinamide.— G. Lemieux *et al.*, *Nephron*, 1978, *20*, 54.

Warfarin. For enhancement of the effect of warfarin by tienilic acid, see Warfarin Sodium, p.780.

Absorption and Fate. Tienilic acid is rapidly absorbed from the gastro-intestinal tract with peak plasma concentrations obtained about 3 or 4 hours after administration. It has been reported to have a plasma half-life of about 3 hours and is excreted in the urine partly unchanged and partly in the form of metabolites. *Animal* studies have also demonstrated biliary excretion. It is very extensively bound to plasma proteins.

A total mean peak plasma concentration of tienilic acid and its metabolites of about 11 µg per ml occurred 3 hours after administration of tienilic acid 250 mg by mouth to 8 healthy subjects. Excretion in the urine after 24 hours accounted for about 40% of the administered dose.— B. Hwang *et al.*, *J. pharm. Sci.*, 1978, *67*, 1095.

A study of the kinetics and acute effects of tienilic acid in 4 healthy subjects. In 3 of the 4 subjects peak plasma concentrations occurred within 1 to 2 hours of oral ingestion; the fourth subject absorbed the drug more slowly and achieved peak plasma concentrations at 6 hours. The decline in plasma concentrations of tienilic acid was approximately mono-exponential with a half-life ranging from 2 to 3.3 hours.— A. J. Wood *et al.*, *Clin. Pharmac. Ther.*, 1978, *23*, 697.

Studies in healthy subjects demonstrated that tienilic acid is well absorbed, giving peak concentrations 3 or 4 hours after oral administration. It is rapidly excreted in the urine, both unchanged and after undergoing extensive metabolic transformation by reduction and oxidation. About 60% of the doses given were not accounted for in the urine, suggesting either that other metabolites exist, or that biliary excretion may be an additional factor; another factor might be incomplete absorption.— J. W. Dubb *et al.*, *Postgrad. med. J.*, 1979, *55*, *Suppl.* 3, 47.

Protein binding. *In vitro* studies demonstrating that tienilic acid is approximately 99.5% bound to serum protein at therapeutic concentrations.— A. J. Wood *et al.*, *Clin. Pharmac. Ther.*, 1978, *23*, 697.

Uses. Although chemically related to ethacrynic acid, tienilic acid is a diuretic with uses similar to those of chlorothiazide (see p.589). Unlike chlorothiazide it also has a uricosuric action, which, it has been considered, might be of benefit to hypertensive patients who are also hyperuricaemic. Diuresis lasts for up to about 12 hours.
Severe liver damage has been associated with tienilic acid therapy which has resulted in a number of deaths; for this reason tienilic acid has been withdrawn in some countries.
In the treatment of hypertension tienilic acid has been given in usual doses of 250 mg daily initially gradually increased to a maximum of 1 g daily, either alone, or in conjunction with other antihypertensive agents. Patients must be adequately hydrated and not receiving other diuretic therapy before starting tienilic acid treatment.
When treatment is prolonged, or in susceptible patients, loss of potassium may be sufficient to produce hypokalaemia; potassium supplements should then be given as for chlorothiazide.

Reviews, comments and symposia on tienilic acid: *Med. Lett.*, 1979, *21*, 61; *Nephron*, 1979, *23*, *Suppl.* 1;; *Postgrad. med. J.*, 1979, *55*, *Suppl.* 3;; E. D. Frohlich, *New Engl. J. Med.*, 1979, *301*, 1378; M. E. Kosman, *J. Am. med. Ass.*, 1979, *242*, 2876.

Action. On the basis of its dichlorophenoxyacetic acid structure, tienilic acid appears to be related to ethacrynic acid, but it differs chemically in being non-reactive with cysteine *in vitro*, with which ethacrynic acid reacts avidly. Studies in *dogs* subsequently suggested that tienilic acid was thiazide-like, presumably because of the similar site of action in the cortical diluting segment of the distal tubule. Thus, the pattern of electrolyte response, the maximum natriuresis obtained, the comparable chloruresis, the modest kaliuresis, the prolonged duration of activity and natriuresis in alkalotic and acidotic *dogs*, all support the conclusion of a thiazide-like response, with the exception of uricosuria.— A. R. Maass and I. B. Snow, *Postgrad. med. J.*, 1979, *55*, *Suppl.* 3, 37.

In a double-blind crossover study in 13 patients with hypertension tienilic acid 250 mg in the morning produced a fall in blood pressure similar to that produced by spironolactone 100 mg or bendrofluazide 5 mg. Tienilic acid caused a fall in potassium concentration similar to that caused by bendrofluazide, but decreased the plasma-urate concentration and increased urate clearance.— C. J. C. Roberts *et al.*, *Br. med. J.*, 1979, *1*, 224.

Further references: G. Lemieux *et al.*, *Nephron*, 1978, *20*, 54; R. M. Stote *et al.*, *Clin. Pharmac. Ther.*, 1978, *23*, 456.

Administration. To avoid possible renal impairment associated with the uricosuric activity of tienilic acid, therapy should be started with low doses and after neutralisation of the urine.— G. Lohmöller *et al.*, *Postgrad. med. J.*, 1979, *55*, *Suppl.* 3, 68.

Cardiac disorders. *Heart failure.* Results of 2 double-blind studies demonstrated that tienilic acid is as effective as hydrochlorothiazide in patients with heart failure.— K. T. Weber and A. P. Fishman, *Postgrad. med. J.*, 1979, *55*, *Suppl.* 3, 58.

Hypertension. In a crossover study 17 hyperuricaemic, hypertensive patients whose blood pressure was well controlled by cyclopenthiazide, sometimes in association with a beta-blocker, took tienilic acid instead of the cyclopenthiazide for 3 months, followed by cyclopenthiazide for a further 3 months, while 19 similar patients took their established cyclopenthiazide regimen for the first 3 months, followed by tienilic acid. The antihypertensive effect of a mean dose of 210 mg of tienilic acid was similar to that of a mean dose of 410 µg of cyclopenthiazide, and at these doses there was no significant difference between the 2 drugs on pulse-rate or body-weight. The mean serum-uric acid concentration after tienilic acid therapy, however, was only 290 µmol per litre compared with 500 µmol per litre for cyclopenthiazide. Side-effects in the tienilic acid group included indigestion in 3 patients and abnormal liver-function tests in 3 patients (not definitely associated with tienilic acid); there was no ototoxicity.— P. Bolli *et al.*, *Lancet*, 1978, *2*, 595.

In a placebo-controlled double-blind four-way crossover study of 16 hypertensive subjects tienilic acid 250 mg daily and propranolol 80 mg twice daily for 6 weeks, effectively reduced blood pressure, and had an additive effect in association, compared with the same doses of tienilic acid and propranolol given alone. There was no evidence of antagonism or enhancement of effect between the two drugs. Tienilic acid had the advantage over thiazide diuretics that it reduced serum-urate concentrations; in addition, the hypokalaemic effect of tienilic acid was corrected by propranolol. Tienilic acid reduced the circulating basophil count, although it was considered that such an effect of a drug might be commoner than suspected; it also caused a small fall in haemoglobin.— R. M. Pearson *et al.*, *Lancet*, 1979, *1*, 697.

In a double-blind randomised study, 240 men with mild to moderate hypertension took either tienilic acid, 250 or 500 mg, or hydrochlorothiazide, 50 or 100 mg, once daily for 6 weeks. All 4 regimens were associated with significant reductions in systolic and diastolic blood pressure although tienilic acid 250 mg daily appeared to be less effective. Serum concentrations of uric acid were significantly reduced by both doses of tienilic acid but rose in patients taking hydrochlorothiazide. Mean serum-potassium concentrations were reduced in all 4 groups. Mean serum-creatinine concentrations rose significantly more in patients on tienilic acid although the absolute increase was not great. Of these patients 189 continued treatment for a total of 6 months, doses being individually titrated up to a maximum of tienilic acid 1 g daily or hydrochlorothiazide 200 mg daily. At the end of 6 months blood pressure had been similarly reduced by both drugs. Treatment was generally well tolerated although there was more postural dizziness in patients taking tienilic acid.— Veterans Administration Cooperative Study Group on Antihypertensive Agents,

New Engl. J. Med., 1979, *301*, 293.

Further references: J. Furrer *et al.*, *Schweiz. med. Wschr.*, 1978, *108*, 1983; G. Lemieux *et al.*, *Can. med. Ass. J.*, 1978, *118*, 1074; A. H. B. Gillies and T. O. Morgan, *Br. J. clin. Pharmac.*, 1978, *6*, 357; O. Andersson *et al.*, *Postgrad. med. J.*, 1979, *55*, *Suppl.* 3, 110; E. D. Freis, *ibid.*, 92; E. D. Frohlich *et al.*, *ibid.*, 98; R. E. Noble and M. A. Beg, *ibid.*, 120; R. Okun and M. A. Beg, *ibid.*, 103; R. M. Pearson *et al.*, *ibid.*, 115; F. Zacharias, *ibid.*, 81.

Effects on plasma renin. Raised plasma renin activity and raised urinary aldosterone associated with tienilic acid therapy.— *Postgrad. med. J.*, 1979, *55*, *Suppl.* 3, 91.

Proprietary Names

Diflurex *(Anphar-Rolland, Fr.; Max Ritter, Switz.)*; Selcryn *(RIT, Belg.)*.

2358-j

Triamterene *(B.P., U.S.P.).* Triamterenum; SKF8542. 6-Phenylpteridine-2,4,7-triamine.

$C_{12}H_{11}N_7$=253.3.

CAS — 396-01-0.

Pharmacopoeias. In *Br.*, *Braz.*, *Chin.*, *It.*, *Jap.*, and *U.S.*

A yellow odourless crystalline powder, almost tasteless at first and with a slightly bitter aftertaste.

Soluble 1 in 1000 of water, 1 in 3000 of alcohol, 1 in 4000 of chloroform, 1 in 30 of formic acid, and 1 in 85 of 2-methoxyethanol; very slightly soluble in acetic acid and dilute mineral acids; practically insoluble in ether and dilute solutions of alkali hydroxides. Acidified solutions give a blue fluorescence. **Store** in airtight containers. Protect from light.

Adverse Effects. Nausea and vomiting, diarrhoea, hypotension, headache, dryness of the mouth, and skin rash have been reported. Rises in blood-urea-nitrogen concentrations have been reported. Its potassium-sparing effect may lead to hyperkalaemia. Hyperuricaemia may also occur. Other disturbances in electrolyte metabolism and acidosis have been reported. Allergic reactions and photosensitivity have occasionally occurred and there have been rare reports of megaloblastic anaemia and thrombocytopenic purpura.

Allergy. Fever and rigor were associated with the use of triamterene in a 53-year-old woman.— M. A. Safdi (letter), *New Engl. J. Med.*, 1980, *303*, 701.

Effects on the blood. *Megaloblastic anaemia.* A patient with cirrhosis of the liver developed megaloblastosis after 2 weeks' treatment with triamterene. The dihydrofolate reductase activity of bone marrow was inhibited and it was considered that triamterene should be used with caution in patients, such as pregnant women and alcoholics, with reduced stores of folate.— J. Corcino *et al.*, *Ann. intern. Med.*, 1970, *73*, 419.

Further references: F. L. Lieberman and J. R. Bateman, *Ann. intern. Med.*, 1968, *68*, 168; M. Renoux *et al.*, *Nouv. Presse méd.*, 1976, *5*, 641; B. Pillegand *et al.*, *ibid.*, 1977, *6*, 3004; K. Wilms *et al.*, *Dt. med. Wschr.*, 1979, *104*, 814.

Effects on the electrolyte balance. *Calcium and magnesium.* A study indicating that magnesium depletion could be a possible complication of triamterene therapy. It is unlikely that it would produce significant elevation of serum-calcium concentrations in non-azotaemic patients.— B. R. Walker *et al.*, *Clin. Pharmac. Ther.*, 1972, *13*, 245.

Further references: S. Hänze and H. Seyberth, *Klin. Wschr.*, 1967, *45*, 313.

Potassium. In 6 patients given chlorthalidone 100 mg daily for 7 days mean serum-potassium concentration fell from 4.38 to 3.3 mmol per litre and whole body potassium decreased by about 10% but continuation of treatment with chlorthalidone 50 mg daily and triamterene 150 mg daily led to correction of the potassium concentrations after 1 to 2 weeks. In a further 9 patients given hydrochlorothiazide 50 mg daily with triamterene 100 mg daily for 6 months no significant change in potassium concentrations occurred.— G. E. Schäfer *et al.*, *Dt. med. Wschr.*, 1977, *102*, 1838.

Further references: K. B. Hansen and A. D. Bender, *Clin. Pharmac. Ther.*, 1967, *8*, 392.

Effects on the eyes. A study indicating that usual therapeutic doses of triamterene slightly interfere with colour vision.— J. Laroche and C. Laroche, *Annls pharm. fr.*, 1972, *30*, 433.

Effects on the kidneys. Capsules of a triamterene-hydrochlorothiazide mixture (50 or 75 mg/25 mg) given to 23 patients with congestive heart failure produced in 15 a rise in the blood-urea-nitrogen concentrations. The rise was attributed to a reduction in glomerular filtration-rate and this reduced the clinical value of the mixture.— H. Sevelius and J. P. Colmore, *J. new Drugs*, 1965, *5*, 43.

Kidney stones, apparently formed from triamterene, were passed by a woman who had been taking 300 to 350 mg daily for 2½ years.— B. Ettinger *et al.*, *Ann. intern. Med.*, 1979, *91*, 745. See also E. L. Socolow (letter), *ibid.*, 1980, *92*, 437.

For a report of renal colic induced by triamterene and hydrochlorothiazide, see Hydrochlorothiazide, p.601.

Gout. A study suggesting that triamterene is unlikely to produce significant elevation of serum concentrations of uric acid in non-azotaemic patients, although uric acid retention has been shown with the chronic use of the drug.— B. R. Walker *et al.*, *Clin. Pharmac. Ther.*, 1972, *13*, 245.

Further references: R. J. Sperber and A. C. DeGraff, *Am. Heart J.*, 1965, *69*, 134; W. I. Cranston *et al.*, *ibid.*, *70*, 455.

Treatment of Adverse Effects. As for Spironolactone, p.610.

Parenteral folate therapy has been used to reverse megaloblastic anaemia.

Use of blood transfusions and folinic acid for megaloblastosis in a cirrhotic woman receiving triamterene.— B. Pillegand *et al.*, *Nouv. Presse méd.*, 1977, *6*, 3004.

Precautions. Triamterene should not be given to patients with hyperkalaemia or progressive renal failure, and should not be given with other potassium-sparing diuretics. Potassium supplements should not be given with triamterene. It should be given with care to patients likely to develop acidosis, to patients with diabetes mellitus, or those with impaired hepatic or renal function, or with a history of gout. Serum electrolytes and blood-urea-nitrogen should be estimated periodically.

Triamterene may interfere with the fluorescent measurement of quinidine; it may slightly colour the urine blue.

It has been suggested that triamterene therapy should be withdrawn gradually in order to prevent a theoretical rebound loss of potassium.

Absorption and Fate. Triamterene is incompletely but fairly rapidly absorbed from the gastro-intestinal tract. It has been estimated to have a plasma half-life of about 2 hours. It is extensively metabolised and is mainly excreted in the urine in the form of metabolites with some unchanged triamterene; variable amounts are also excreted in the bile. *Animal* studies have indicated that triamterene crosses the placental barrier and is excreted in milk.

Following administration of triamterene 100 or 200 mg by mouth to 7 healthy subjects and intravenous administration to 2, rapid and extensive metabolism occurred, the metabolite 2,4,7-triamino-6-*p*-hydroxyphenylpteridine being found in the plasma as soon as 30 minutes after a dose and at a concentration of up to 12 times that of the parent drug, and in the urine at 1.5 hours (again at a much higher concentration than the parent drug). Excretion also occurred in the bile after either oral or intravenous administration, with faecal excretion being the primary route in 1 subject. Absorption was prolonged in another subject, who was hyperlipidaemic, with both triamterene and metabolite persisting in the plasma. Bioavailability of triamterene was low, following administration by mouth, being estimated at 30 to 70%; peak plasma concentrations were also low with wide intersubject variation (92 to 280 ng per ml, following administration of 200 mg to 3 of the subjects, reached 2 to 4 hours after the dose). The overall plasma half-life of triamterene was about 1½ to 2½ hours. Both oral and intravenous studies in 1 subject indicated that metabolism was the same by either route.— A. W. Pruitt *et al.*, *Clin. Pharmac. Ther.*, 1977, *21*, 610.

Further references: U. Gundert-Remy *et al.*, *Eur. J. clin. Pharmac.*, 1979, *16*, 39.

Bioavailability. Studies with experimental tablets and capsules containing triamterene and hydrochlorothiazide, in a 2:1 ratio mixture, showed that the tablets led to approximately twice as much excretion of hydrochlorothiazide and 3 times as much triamterene as the capsules.— P. J. Tannenbaum *et al.*, *Clin. Pharmac. Ther.*, 1968, *9*, 598.

Metabolites. Determination of the metabolites of triamterene.— B. Grebian *et al.*, *Arzneimittel-Forsch.*, 1976, *26*, 2125.

Protein binding. In 7 of 8 healthy subjects, the binding of triamterene to plasma ranged from 43% to 53%. In one hyperlipidaemic subject it was 72%; *in vitro* studies indicated that this was probably due to the solubility in the lipid-protein phase.— A. W. Pruitt *et al.*, *Clin. Pharmac. Ther.*, 1977, *21*, 610.

Further references: J. B. Lassen and O. E. Nielsen, *Acta pharmac. tox.*, 1963, *20*, 309; M. M. Reidenberg and J. Affrime, *Ann. N.Y. Acad. Sci.*, 1973, *226*, 115.

Uses. Triamterene is a mild diuretic which appears to act mainly on the distal renal tubules. It produces a diuresis in about 2 to 4 hours, reaching a maximum effect in about 6 hours. The full effect may be delayed until after several days of treatment. Like spironolactone, it increases the excretion of sodium and chloride and reduces the excretion of potassium. Unlike spironolactone, however, it does not appear to act by inhibiting aldosterone. It slightly increases the excretion of bicarbonate though it does not appear to inhibit carbonic anhydrase activity.

Triamterene adds to the natriuretic but diminishes the kaliuretic effects of other diuretics, and is mainly used as an adjunct to the thiazides, frusemide, and similar diuretics, to conserve potassium, in the treatment of refractory oedema associated with hepatic cirrhosis, congestive heart failure, and the nephrotic syndrome. It has little effect in the treatment of hypertension.

When given alone, the suggested range of dosage is 150 to 250 mg daily; 100 mg twice daily, after breakfast and lunch, is considered to be the optimum dose, preferably on alternate days for maintenance therapy. More than 300 mg daily should not be given. Smaller doses are suggested initially when other diuretics are being given.

In children, when given alone, a suggested initial dose is 1 to 2 mg per kg body-weight twice daily. Potassium supplements should not be given.

Reviews and comments on triamterene: *Drug & Ther. Bull.*, 1972, *10*, 30; M. E. Kosman, *J. Am. med. Ass.*, 1974, *230*, 743.

Action. Results of a study in *rats* and in healthy subjects indicated that the action of triamterene is not due to aldosterone antagonism, but is probably a direct effect on the renal tubules.— W. I. Baba *et al.*, *Br. med. J.*, 1962, *2*, 756.

Further references: B. R. Walker *et al.*, *Clin. Pharmac. Ther.*, 1972, *13*, 245.

References to *animal* studies: V. D. Wiebelhaus *et al.*, *Fedn Proc.*, 1961, *20*, 409; A. P. Crosley *et al.*, *Ann. intern. Med.*, 1962, *56*, 241.

Administration. *In the elderly.* Use of triamterene in association with hydrochlorothiazide in 549 elderly patients. Of 189 who had normal serum-potassium concentrations before treatment, 5% developed hypokalaemia and 12% developed hyperkalaemia.— A. D. Bender *et al.*, *J. Am. Geriat. Soc.*, 1967, *15*, 166.

Administration in hepatic failure. For the possible use of triamterene in the diagnosis of hepatic failure, see under Hepatic Disorders (below).

Administration in renal failure. Triamterene could be given in usual doses in mild or moderate renal failure. It should be avoided in patients with a glomerular filtration-rate of less than 10 ml per minute.— W. M. Bennett *et al.*, *Ann. intern. Med.*, 1980, *93*, 286.

Further references: J. B. Lassen and O. E. Nielsen, *Acta pharmac. tox.*, 1963, *20*, 309; J. S. Cheigh, *Am. J. Med.*, 1977, *62*, 555.

Cardiac disorders. *Cardiac arrhythmias.* In 20 patients with valvular heart disease taking digoxin and either thiazides or frusemide the mean leucocyte-potassium concentration (in mmol per litre of cell water) was 109, compared with 146 in 10 patients receiving neither digoxin nor diuretics. The value rose to 130 in 10 patients when triamterene 200 mg daily was added to their diuretic regimen. Triamterene might be of value in digitalis-induced arrhythmias and open-heart surgery where depletion of cellular potassium jeopardised myocardial function.— E. K. Donaldson *et al.*, *Br. med. J.*, 1976, *1*, 1254.

Heart failure. Administration of triamterene in association with hydrochlorothiazide in 23 patients with congestive heart failure provided effective diuresis with little potassium loss, but there was an unacceptably high incidence of uraemia.— H. Sevelius and J. P. Colmore, *J. new Drugs*, 1965, *5*, 43.

Hepatic disorders. A discussion of the use of the potassium-sparing diuretics, including triamterene, in cirrhosis of the liver.— P. Vesin, *Postgrad. med. J.*, 1975, *51*, 545.

Further references to triamterene in hepatic cirrhosis: E. J. Thompson *et al.*, *Clin. Pharmac. Ther.*, 1977, *21*, 392 (with frusemide).

For the use of triamterene in the treatment of ascites in patients with cirrhosis of the liver, see Spironolactone, p.611.

Diagnosis. Reduced metabolism of triamterene could be used as a test of liver function.— P. G. Dayton *et al.*, *Pharmacologist*, 1976, *18*, 153.

Hypertension. In a double-blind trial spironolactone 400 mg daily was effective in controlling hypertension in all of 17 patients with low-renin essential hypertension. A combination of hydrochlorothiazide 100 mg and triamterene 200 mg daily was effective in 14 of these patients.— J. G. Douglas *et al.*, *J. Am. med. Ass.*, 1974, *227*, 518.

Further references: E. C. Clark *et al.*, *Sth. med. J.*, 1979, *72*, 798; J. G. R. DeCarvalho *et al.*, *Clin. Pharmac. Ther.*, 1980, *27*, 53.

Preparations

Triamterene Capsules *(B.P.)*. Capsules containing triamterene. Store at a temperature not exceeding 30°.

Triamterene Capsules *(U.S.P.)*. Capsules containing triamterene. Store in airtight containers. Protect from light.

Proprietary Preparations

Dyazide (known in some countries as Dytenzide) *(Smith Kline & French, UK)*. Scored tablets each containing triamterene 50 mg and hydrochlorothiazide 25 mg. For oedema and mild to moderate hypertension. *Dose.* 1 or 2 tablets daily, after meals, increased if necessary up to 4 tablets daily.

Dytac *(Smith Kline & French, UK)*. Triamterene, available as capsules of 50 mg. (Also available as Dytac in *Austral., Belg., Neth., S.Afr.*).

Dytide *(Smith Kline & French, UK)*. Capsules each containing triamterene 50 mg and benzthiazide 25 mg. For oedema. *Dose.* 1 to 3 capsules daily after meals.

Other Proprietary Names

Diesse *(hydrochloride) (Ital.)*; Diucelpin *(Jap.)*; Dyrenium *(Canad., Switz., USA)*; Jatropur *(Ger.)*; Natrium *(hydrochloride)(Ital.)*; Tériam *(Fr.)*; Triamteril *(Ital.)*; Urocaudal *(Spain)*.

2359-z

Trichlormethiazide *(U.S.P.)*. Trichlormethiazidum.

6-Chloro-3-dichloromethyl-3,4-dihydro-2*H*-1,2,4-benzothiadiazine-7-sulphonamide 1,1-dioxide.

$C_8H_8Cl_3N_3O_4S_2$=380.6.

CAS — 133-67-5.

Pharmacopoeias. In *Jap.* and *U.S.*

A white or almost white, odourless or almost odourless, crystalline powder. M.p. about 274° with decomposition. Very slightly **soluble** in water, chloroform, and ether; soluble 1 in 48 of alcohol, 1 in about 9 of dioxan, and 1 in about 5 of dimethylformamide; freely soluble in acetone; soluble in methyl alcohol.

Adverse Effects, Treatment, and Precautions. As for Chlorothiazide, p.588.

A 51-year-old woman took 2 mg of trichlormethiazide twice daily. After about 4 months' therapy she developed non-thrombocytopenic purpura due apparently to capillary fragility with a prolonged bleeding time.— L. R. Loftus and H. O. Loyd, *J. Am. med. Ass.*, 1962, *180*, 410.

Uses. Trichlormethiazide is a thiazide diuretic with actions and uses similar to those of chlorothiazide (see p.589). Diuresis is initiated in about 2 hours, and lasts about 24 hours.

In the treatment of oedema the usual dose is 2 to 4 mg daily; initial doses of 2 to 4 mg twice daily may be given.

In the treatment of hypertension the usual dose is 2 to 4 mg daily, either alone, or in conjunction with other antihypertensive agents; in some patients initial doses of 2 to 4 mg twice daily may be necessary.

When treatment is prolonged, or in susceptible patients, loss of potassium may be sufficient to produce hypokalaemia; potassium supplements should then be given as for chlorothiazide.

References: D. D. Gellman, *Can. med. Ass. J.*, 1963, *89*, 66 (hypertension); E. E. Reisman, *Angiology*, 1963, *14*, 59 (heart failure); S. S. Fajans *et al.*, *J. clin. Invest.*, 1966, *45*, 481 (hypoglycaemia); F. L. Coe, *Ann. intern. Med.*, 1977, *87*, 404; *idem*, *Archs intern. Med.*, 1978, *138*, 1090 (renal stones).

Preparations

Trichlormethiazide Tablets *(U.S.P.)*. Tablets containing trichlormethiazide. Store in airtight containers.

Proprietary Names

Achletin, Anatran, Anistadin, Aponorin, Carvacron, Chlopolidine, Cretonin, Intromene, Kubacron, Sanamiron, Schebitran, Tachionin, Tolcasone *(all Jap.)*; Diu-Fortan *(Lazar, Arg.)*; Esmarin *(E. Merck, Ger.)*; Fluitran *(Schering, Denm.*; *Essex, Ital.*; *Schering, NZ*; *Schering, Norw.)*; Flutra *(Schering, Swed.)*; Hidroalogen *(Bicsa, Spain)*; Metahydrin *(Merrell-National, USA)*; Naqua *(Schering, USA)*; Triflumen *(Ausonia, Spain)*.

2360-p

Trometamol. Tromethamine *(U.S.P.)*;

THAM; TRIS; Trihydroxymethylaminomethane; Tris(hydroxymethyl)aminomethane. 2-Amino-2-(hydroxymethyl)propane-1,3-diol.

$C_4H_{11}NO_3$=121.1.

CAS — 77-86-1.

Pharmacopoeias. In *Chin.*, *Nord.*, and *U.S.*

A white crystalline powder with a slight characteristic odour and a saline taste. M.p. 168° to 172°.

Soluble 1 in 1.25 of water and 1 in about 45 of alcohol; slightly soluble in acetone and ether; practically insoluble in carbon tetrachloride and chloroform. A 5% solution in water has a pH of 10 to 11.5. A 3.6% (0.3M) solution is iso-osmotic with serum. **Store** in airtight containers.

Injections are prepared by dissolving the requisite quantity of trometamol in Water for Injections immediately before use.

The alkalinity of trometamol solutions precluded their sterilisation by heat in glass because of silicate formation.— G. G. Nahas, *Clin. Pharmac. Ther.*, 1963, *4*, 784. Solutions could be sterilised by autoclaving.— C. Rauch *et al.*, *Pharm. Ztg, Berl.*, 1964, *109*, 693.

Stability in solution. A 0.3M solution of trometamol for intravenous use was stable for a 'few hours' after reconstitution.— C. J. Latiolais *et al.*, *Am. J. Hosp. Pharm.*, 1967, *24*, 667.

Dextran solution 10% administered intravenously in conjunction with trometamol prolonged its action and reduced the rate of alkalisation.— G. Kienle *et al.*, *Medsche Welt, Stuttg.*, 1969, *20*, 1389, per *J. Am. med. Ass.*, 1969, *209*, 817.

Adverse Effects and Precautions. Great care must be taken to avoid extravasation at the injection site as solutions may cause tissue damage. Local inflammation may follow administration and venospasm and phlebitis have occurred.

Respiratory depression and hypoglycaemia may occur and the respiration may require assistance. Trometamol is contra-indicated in anuria and should be administered cautiously in patients with impaired renal function. Hyperkalaemia has been reported in patients with renal impairment.

Blood concentrations of carbon dioxide, bicarbonate, glucose, and electrolytes, and blood pH should be monitored during infusion of trometamol.

Pregnancy and the neonate. *Necrosis.* Haemorrhagic liver necrosis was found at post mortem in 22 of 67 infants who had received trometamol (3 to 90 ml of a 1.2M solution) and bicarbonate—2 to 34 mmol (2 to 34 mEq)—in the treatment of the respiratory distress syndrome. The injections were made into the umbilical vein. Those who had injections via the umbilical artery, or who had received bicarbonate only, were not affected.— V. E. Goldenberg *et al.*, *J. Am. med. Ass.*, 1968, *205*, 81. The 1.2M solution had a pH of 10.2. Concentrated alkaline solutions should not be administered in the central or peripheral veins of infants whose circulation might be impaired. Many workers used 0.3M solutions, administered at the rate of 6 ml per hour, or slowly in doses of 3 to 5 ml.— G. G. Nahas (letter), *ibid.*, *206*, 1793.

Accidental intra-arterial injection of trometamol produced severe haemorrhagic necrosis in 2 newborn girls and was fatal in 1.— H. Rehder and E. Heiming, *Archs Dis. Childh.*, 1974, *49*, 76.

Bladder necrosis developed in an infant given trometamol in a 10% dextrose solution by umbilical artery catheter.— M. J. Mihatsch *et al.*, *J. Urol.*, 1974, *111*, 835.

Absorption and Fate. Trometamol is rapidly excreted unchanged in the urine. About 75% of the dose is excreted within 8 hours and the remainder within 3 days.

Uses. Trometamol is an organic amine base which combines not only with cations of fixed or metabolic acids but also with hydrogen ions from carbonic acid to form bicarbonate and a cationic buffer. When infused intravenously it causes an osmotic diuresis. It is capable of penetrating into intracellular compartments. It has been used in the treatment of metabolic, respiratory, diabetic, and postoperative acidosis, in acidosis associated with cardiopulmonary bypass and cardiac arrest, and for the correction of acidosis due to the use of citrated blood.

The dose used should be the minimum required to increase the pH of the blood to within normal limits. The usual dose is 300 mg per kg body-weight administered intravenously as a 0.3M solution over a period of not less than 1 hour. Severe acidosis may require higher doses but the dose should not exceed 500 mg per kg body-weight.

Trometamol has also been added to citrated blood to correct the acidity before infusion.

Acidosis. In burned patients. The use of trometamol in the treatment of acidosis following severe burns.— J. R. Hinshaw and L. M. Cramer, *Clin. Med.*, 1968, *75* (Jan.), 49.

Further references: H. Ewerbeck *et al.*, *Dt. med. Wschr.*, 1966, *91*, 1333.

In neonates. In 65 babies with the respiratory distress syndrome, there were 11 episodes of apnoea after the administration of trometamol solution 3.6 or 7%; there was a greater incidence of intraventricular haemorrhage among babies given the 7% solution than among those given the 3.6% solution. Because sodium bicarbonate solution 8.4% did not cause respiratory depression in a further 32 babies (23 of whom had the respiratory distress syndrome), it was favoured in the treatment of acidaemia in the newborn baby with respiratory distress syndrome.— N. R. C. Roberton, *Archs Dis. Childh.*, 1970, *45*, 206.

Further references: T. K. Oliver (letter), *New Engl. J. Med.*, 1966, *275*, 1203; G. G. Nahas (letter), *ibid.*; J. H. P. Jonxis, *Pädiat. Pädol.*, 1967, *3*, 231; P. K. J. van Vliet and J. M. Gupta, *Archs Dis. Childh.*, 1973, *48*, 249.

In shock. In shock, acidosis which had led to diminished vascular and cardiac tone could be corrected by administering sodium bicarbonate or trometamol 0.3M solution. Trometamol conferred no sodium ions but influenced intracellular acidosis by undergoing 30% ionisation. Hazards associated wtih its use included respiratory depression, hypokalaemia, and hypoglycaemia and frequent monitoring was necessary of arterial and venous pH, venous carbon-dioxide tension, and glucose and electrolyte concentrations in blood. The guiding formula for the dose of trometamol was: mmol trometamol = 0.3 × body-weight (kg) × mmol deficiency of bicarbonate ion.— J. J. Byrne, *New Engl. J. Med.*, 1966, *275*, 659.

In status asthmaticus. With the possible exception of status asthmaticus, where both trometamol and sodium bicarbonate might relieve bronchospasm, few if any clinical circumstances were considered to exist where the transient effect of trometamol on pCO_2 had been of significant value.— H. L. Bleich and W. B. Schwartz (letter), *New Engl. J. Med.*, 1966, *275*, 1204.

Further references: M. H. Holmdahl *et al.*, *Presse méd.*, 1967, *75*, 957.

Cardiopulmonary bypass. Stored blood adjusted to approximately normal pH with trometamol, then recalcified and heparinised, was suitable for priming the pump oxygenator and replacing blood losses during open-heart surgery. Its viscosity was less than that of fresh blood, and the osmotic diuresis due to the trometamol would improve renal function.— L. P. Rosky and T. Rodman, *New Engl. J. Med.*, 1966, *274*, 883 and 886.

Further references: K. Taguchi *et al.*, *Surgery, St Louis*, 1968, *63*, 252.

Pregnancy and the neonate. *Infant foods.* The suggested use of trometamol to increase the pH of reconstituted cows' milk for infant feeding.— V. C. Harrison and G. Peat, *Br. med. J.*, 1972, *4*, 515.

For references to the use of trometamol for acidosis in neonates see Acidosis (above).

Preparations

Tromethamine for Injection *(U.S.P.)*. A sterile lyophilised mixture of trometamol with potassium chloride and sodium chloride. Its solution has a pH of 10 to 11.5.

Proprietary Names

Addex-THAM *(Pharmacia, Swed.)*; Alcaphor *(Bellon, Fr.)*; Basionic *(RIT, Belg.)*; Thamesol *(Baxter, Ital.)*; Trisaminol *(Bellon, Fr.)*.

Trometamol was formerly marketed in Great Britain under the proprietary name Tham-E (*Abbott*).

2361-s

Urea *(B.P., U.S.P.)*. Carbamide; Ureum.

$NH_2.CO.NH_2$=60.06.

CAS — 57-13-6.

Pharmacopoeias. In *Aust.*, *Br.*, *Cz.*, *Hung.*, *Ind.*, *Jap.*, *Jug.*, *Mex.*, *Neth.*, *Nord.*, *Pol.*, *Port.*, *Swiss*, *Turk.*, and *U.S.*

Colourless, slightly hygroscopic, odourless or almost odourless, prismatic crystals or pellets, or white crystalline powder, with a cooling saline taste. M.p. 132° to 135°.

Soluble 1 in 1 to 1.5 of water, 1 in 10 to 12 of alcohol, and 1 in 1.5 of boiling alcohol; practically insoluble in chloroform and ether.

Solutions in water are neutral to litmus. A 1.63% solution is iso-osmotic with serum. Solutions are **sterilised** by filtration. **Incompatible** with nitric acid, nitrites, alkalis, and formaldehyde. Solutions in water hydrolyse during storage, liberating ammonia and carbon dioxide. **Store** in airtight containers.

An aqueous solution of urea iso-osmotic with serum (1.63%) caused 100% haemolysis of erythrocytes cultured in it for 45 minutes.— E. R. Hammarlund and K. Pedersen-Bjergaard, *J. pharm. Sci.*, 1961, *50*, 24.

Incompatibility. Urea should never be added to whole blood for transfusion or given through the same set by which blood is being infused. For details of the adverse effects of urea on red blood cells, see above and see also under Effects on the Blood, under Adverse Effects.

Stability. Urea in solution or when moist slowly hydrolysed to carbon dioxide and ammonia, whilst heat, acids, and alkalis increased the rate of hydrolysis. However, little decomposition was evident in solutions stored at either 16° or 4° for 1 month.— R. H. Sutaria and F. H. Williams, *Publ. Pharm.*, 1960, *17*, 168, 225, and 281.

The degree of degradation of 2M, 4M, 6M and 8M solutions of urea at 25°, 35°, and 45° was extremely small.— H. L. Welles *et al.*, *J. pharm. Sci.*, 1971, *60*, 1212.

Sterilisation. Dry sterile urea suitable for intravenous use could be prepared by first sterilising a concentrated solution by filtration and subsequently drying under vacuum at temperatures not exceeding 100°. Irradiation with ultraviolet light and washing with ether were unreliable methods.— R. H. Sutaria and F. H. Williams, *Publ. Pharm.*, 1960, *17*, 168, 225, and 281.

Adverse Effects. Urea may cause gastric irritation with nausea and vomiting when given by mouth. Intravenous administration may cause headache, nausea, vomiting, confusion, and a fall in blood pressure. Continued administration of urea may lead to excessive loss of sodium and potassium.

The intravenous administration of hyperosmotic solutions of urea may cause venous thrombosis or phlebitis at the site of injection and only large veins should be used for infusion. Extravasation may cause sloughing or necrosis.

Topical applications may be irritant to inflamed skin or exudative lesions.

Effects on the blood and vascular system. Fatal intracranial haemorrhage was provoked in a 54-year-old hypertensive man, suffering from cerebrovascular disease, who was given 90 g of urea in 1 litre of normal saline by slow intravenous infusion as a test of kidney function.— S. Marshall and F. Hinman, *J. Am. med. Ass.*, 1962, *182*, 813.

In healthy subjects the infusion of a 6M solution of urea in 10% invert sugar solution caused intravascular haemolysis similar to that in patients with sickle-cell anaemia.— T. A. Bensinger *et al.*, *Blood*, 1973, *41*, 461.

For reports of disseminated intravascular coagulation in women given urea for termination of pregnancy, see under Pregnancy and the Neonate, below.

Pregnancy and the neonate. Disseminated intravascular coagulation, attributed to urea, occurred in a 24-year-old woman given urea and oxytocin for termination of pregnancy.— M. F. B. Grundy and E. R. Craven, *Br. med. J.*, 1976, *2*, 677.

A report of haemorrhage due to coagulopathy in 2 women undergoing mid-trimester termination of pregnancy using hyperosmotic urea solution.— R. T. Burkman *et al.*, *Am. J. Obstet. Gynec.*, 1977, *127*, 533.

Precautions. Urea should not be used in patients with marked impairment of hepatic or renal function or with dehydration; it should not be used in the presence of active intracranial bleeding other than as a preliminary to prompt surgical operation.

Extreme care is essential to prevent accidental extravasation of urea infusions; to avoid phlebitis and thrombosis urea should not be infused in the veins of the lower limbs of elderly subjects.

Infusions of urea must be given slowly.

Absorption and Fate. Urea is fairly rapidly absorbed from the gastro-intestinal tract but causes gastro-intestinal irritation. It is excreted unchanged in the urine.

A discussion of the excretion of urea.— J. R. Robinson, *Med. J. Aust.*, 1967, *2*, 277. A study of plasma urea kinetics during urea infusion.— P. R. Yarnell *et al.*, *Clin. Pharmac. Ther.*, 1972, *13*, 558.

Uses. Urea is an osmotic diuretic with a low renal threshold. The ability to excrete urea is markedly impaired when renal damage has occurred and it has therefore been employed in a test for renal efficiency, 15 g being administered in 100 ml of water.

Urea has been used intravenously in the treatment of acute increases in intracranial pressure due to cerebral oedema. It has also been given to maintain the output of urine during surgical procedures. Urea has been largely superseded by mannitol for these purposes. It has also been used to decrease intra-ocular pressure in acute glaucoma.

In cerebral oedema, decompression may be produced by the intravenous infusion of 40 to 80 g of urea, but not exceeding 1.5 g per kg body-weight daily, as a 30% solution in 5 or 10% dextrose or 10% invert sugar solution, at a rate not exceeding 4 ml per minute. A similar dose as a 4% solution has been used to combat oliguria during surgery.

The range of dosage for children is 0.1 to 1.5 g per kg body-weight in 24 hours.

Urea, by mouth, in doses of up to 20 g from 2 to 5 times daily, as a 40% solution in water or carbonated beverages, has been given as maintenance therapy following intensive intravenous use for the relief of cerebral oedema.

Hyperosmotic solutions of urea have also been given by intra-amniotic injection for the termination of pregnancy. Oxytocin, by intravenous injection, is often given concomitantly. Urea is also given prior to the intra-amniotic injection of dinoprostone.

Urea is used as a 10% cream for the treatment of ichthyosis and hyperkeratotic skin disorders. Anaesthetic, bactericidal, and keratolytic properties have been claimed for urea, but the effect in skin disorders is probably dependent upon increased hydration.

Diabetes insipidus and inappropriate secretion of antidiuretic hormone. Urea given by mouth for inappropriate secretion of antidiuretic hormone in a patient with tuberculous meningitis.— G. Decaux *et al.*, *J. Am. med. Ass.*, 1980, *244*, 589. See also *idem*, *Am. J. Med.*, 1980, *69*, 99.

Urea in doses of 30 g or 60 g daily by mouth produced improvement in 7 patients with inappropriate secretion of antidiuretic hormone.— G. Decaux and F. Genette, *Br. med. J.*, 1981, *283*, 1081.

Glaucoma. Comments on the use of urea in raised intra-ocular pressure.— D. P. Durkee and B. G. Bryant, *Am. J. Hosp. Pharm.*, 1978, *35*, 682.

Migraine. The use of urea in migraine: B. Southwell (letter), *Br. med. J.*, 1962, *2*, 550; J. C. A. Norman and B. J. Mead (letter), *ibid.*, 924; B. J. Mead, *Practitioner*, 1964, *193*, 796.

Neoplasms. Over a period of 3 years 112 patients with basal or squamous cell skin carcinoma were treated with urea injected around the lesions and later by debridement and the topical application of urea powder. Complete remission occurred in 65 and considerable improvement in 27 of the patients.— E. D. Danopoulos and I. E. Danopoulou, *Lancet*, 1974, *1*, 115. Beneficial results were also obtained in patients with tumours of the liver given 2 to 2.5 g four to six times daily.— *idem* (letter), 132.

Tumours in 8 patients with epibulbar malignancies of the eyes were successfully treated with urea as a sterilised powder applied to the surface of the eye, a 10% subconjunctival injection, and a 10% instillation.— E. D. Danopoulos *et al.*, *Br. J. Ophthal.*, 1975, *59*, 282.

Otitis media. In children suffering from secretory otitis media, 'glue ear', the viscous mucus filling the middle ear was liquefied by slowly injecting through the antero-inferior quadrant of the tympanic membrane 1½ to 2 ml of 8M (approx. 50%) urea solution. About 5 minutes later the liquefied mucus oozed through the puncture in the tympanic membrane into the auditory canal.— F. Bauer, *J. Lar. Otol.*, 1968, *82*, 717.

Pregnancy and the neonate. *Termination of pregnancy.* Mid-trimester abortion occurred in a mean of 22.3 hours in 257 of 295 patients after the intra-amniotic injection of 200 ml of freshly prepared 45% urea solution, followed by infusion of oxytocin. In 38 in whom abortion had not occurred within 50 hours the foetus was macerated allowing easy evacuation by suction curettage.— W. G. Smith *et al.*, *Am. J. Obstet. Gynec.*, 1977, *127*, 228.

Further references: J. O. Greenhalf and P. L. C. Diggory, *Br. med. J.*, 1971, *1*, 28; M. Pugh *et al.* (letter), *ibid.*, 345; I. Craft and B. Musa, *Lancet*, 1971, *2*, 1058; J. O. Greenhalf, *Br. J. clin. Pract.*, 1972, *26*, 24; R. J. Smith and J. Newton, *J. Obstet. Gynaec. Br. Commonw.*, 1973, *80*, 135; P. C. Weinberg and M. K. Shepard, *Obstet. Gynec.*, 1973, *41*, 451; J. M. Paine *et al.*, *ibid.*, 1974, *43*, 295; S. O. Anteby *et al.*, *ibid.*, 765; S. Segal *et al.*, *Br. J. Obstet. Gynaec.*, 1976, *83*, 156.

For the use of dinoprost and dinoprostone with urea to induce abortion, see Dinoprost Trometamol, p.1356, and Dinoprostone, p.1358.

Raised intracranial pressure. *Malaria.* All of 10 children with cerebral malaria and continuous convulsions improved rapidly after the intravenous infusion over about 2 hours of urea 1 g per kg body-weight, given as 30% solution in 10% invert sugar solution.— M. E. Kingston, *J. trop. Med. Hyg.*, 1971, *74*, 249.

Renal disorders. *Diagnosis of renal hypertension.* To test for hypertension due to unilateral renovascular disease, contrast medium for a standard intravenous pyelogram was injected, then 15 to 18 minutes later an infusion of 40 g of urea in 500 ml of normal saline was given over 15 minutes. Radiographs were taken at 3-minute intervals from the start of this infusion until both pyelograms showed dilution or there was a clear difference between the 2 kidneys. A positive test was indicated when the collecting system of 1 kidney retained the contrast medium in dense concentration for at least 6 minutes longer than the other.— A. R. Remmers *et al.*, *Am. J. Roentg.*, 1969, *107*, 750.

Further references: R. L. Fein *et al.*, *J. Urol.*, 1969, *101*, 12.

Respiratory disorders. For conflicting reports of the

merits of urea as a mucolytic agent, see D. Waldron-Edward and S. C. Skoryna, *Can. med. Ass. J.*, 1966, *94*, 1249; J. Lieberman, *J. Am. med. Ass.*, 1967, *202*, 694; M. C. F. Pain and M. A. Denborough, *Med. J. Aust.*, 1967, *2*, 68.

Sickle-cell disease. Comment on the use of urea in the treatment of sickle-cell anaemia. Although the results of the cooperative studies dampened almost all enthusiasm in the United States for any form of urea therapy, work continues in Africa on the possible effectiveness of long-term oral administration for the prevention of crises.— J. Dean and A. N. Schechter, *New Engl. J. Med.*, 1978, *299*, 804.

Further reviews and comments: *Lancet*, 1974, *2*, 762.

Favourable reports on the use of urea in the management of sickle-cell anaemia: R. M. Nalbandian *et al.*, *Am. J. med. Sci.*, 1971, *261*, 309; *idem*, *Am. J. Path.*, 1971, *64*, 405.

Unfavourable reports on the use of urea in the management of sickle-cell anaemia: E. Opio and P. M. Barnes, *Lancet*, 1972, *2*, 160; J. I. Brody (letter), *New Engl. J. Med.*, 1972, *287*, 616; E. C. Lipp *et al.*, *Ann. intern. Med.*, 1972, *76*, 765; B. H. Lubin and F. A. Oski, *J. Pediat.*, 1973, *82*, 311; Cooperative Urea Trials Group, *J. Am. med. Ass.*, 1974, *228*, 1120 and 1125. Multiple criticism of the Cooperative Urea Trials Group.— R. M. Nalbandian; R. L. Henry (letter), *J. Am. med. Ass.*, 1974, *229*, 1285. A reply.— P. R. McCurdy (letter), *ibid.*, *230*, 1386.

Further references to the use of urea in sickle-cell disease: R. M. Nalbandian *et al.*, *Am. J. med. Sci.*, 1971, *261*, 325 (oral use for prophylaxis).

Skin disorders. Reviews and discussions on the use of urea cream.— *Drug & Ther. Bull.*, 1971, *9*, 29; H. Ashton *et al.*, *Br. J. Derm.*, 1971, *84*, 194; *Med. Lett.*, 1973, *15*, 104.

Epidermal thinning, associated with a decreased number of DNA-synthesising cells, provoked by application of a 10% solution of urea for 8 weeks, suggested that additional or preliminary treatment with urea may enhance the effectiveness of topical drugs.— W. Wohlrab, *Dermatologica*, 1977, *155*, 97.

Eczema. In a double-blind comparison in 50 patients a cream containing urea 10% and hydrocortisone 1% (Calmurid HC) was as effective as betamethasone valerate cream 0.1% in the treatment of atopic eczema. Six patients who had excoriated skin reported initial smarting when urea and hydrocortisone cream was applied.— J. Almeyda and L. Fry, *Br. J. Derm.*, 1973, *88*, 493.

Further references: T. C. Hindson, *Archs Derm.*, 1971, *104*, 284; S. A. Khan, *Practitioner*, 1978, *221*, 265; R. S. Chapman, *ibid.*, 1979, *223*, 713.

Ichthyosis and hyperkeratosis. Excellent results were achieved in all of 17 patients with ichthyosis treated with 10% urea cream and in 10 of 11 patients with hyperkeratosis of the hands and feet. Fewer patients with atopic dermatitis, disseminated neurodermatitis, and hand dermatitis responded, and there was no response in those with psoriasis, solar keratitis, or perioral dermatitis.— M. Rosten, *Aust. J. Derm.*, 1970, *11*, 142.

In a double-blind trial in 55 patients, a cream containing 10% urea (Calmurid) was no more effective than aqueous cream in the treatment of hyperkeratoses.—Report No. 179 of the General Practitioner Research Group, *Practitioner*, 1973, *210*, 294.

In 14 patients with ichthyosis, treatment for 3 weeks with 10% urea cream caused an increase of about 100% in the ability of skin scales to retain water. The effect of urea in ichthyosis was probably due to its hygroscopic effect.— K. Grice *et al.*, *Acta derm.-vener., Stockh.*, 1973, *53*, 114.

Further references: F. M. Pope *et al.*, *Br. J. Derm.*, 1972, *86*, 291 (ichthyosis); C. Blair, *Br. J. Derm.*, 1976, *94*, 145 (ichthyosis).

Neoplasms. For the use of urea in the treatment of neoplasms, see above.

Psoriasis. Absence of beneficial effect of urea cream in psoriasis.— M. Rosten, *Aust. J. Derm.*, 1970, *11*, 142.

Results of a preliminary double-blind study completed by 8 patients with psoriasis indicated that dithranol 0.1% in a basis containing urea 17% applied to one half of the body, was twice as effective as the basis alone, applied to the other half. The basis alone did have some beneficial effect.— D. B. Buckley, *Curr. med. Res. Opinion*, 1978, *5*, 489.

Preparations

Sterile Urea *(U.S.P.)*. Urea suitable for parenteral use.

Urea Injection *(B.P. 1973)*. A sterile solution of urea in dextrose injection 5% or 10%, prepared by dissolving, immediately before use, the sterile contents of a sealed container in the requisite amount of dextrose injection. The sealed container also contains a small proportion of citric acid. Urea Injection deteriorates on storage. For the treatment of raised intracranial pressure.

Proprietary Preparations

Alphaderm *(Norwich-Eaton, UK)*. Cream containing urea 10%, adsorbed on a polysaccharide matrix and dispersed in a slightly oily basis, with hydrocortisone 1%.

Aquadrate *(Norwich-Eaton, UK)*. Urea, available as a cream containing 10%, adsorbed on a polysaccharide matrix and dispersed in a slightly oily basis. (Also available as Aquadrate in *Austral.*).

Calmurid *(Pharmacia, UK: Farillon, UK)*. Cream containing urea 10% in a stabilising emulsified basis. **Calmurid HC.** Contains in addition hydrocortisone 1%. (Also available as Calmurid in *Arg., Belg., Canad.*).

Nutraplus *(Alcon, UK: Farillon, UK)*. **Cream** and **Lotion** each containing urea 10% in an unperfumed emulsion basis. (Also available as Nutraplus in *Austral., USA*).

Ureaphil *(Abbott, UK)*. Urea, available as powder in bottles of 40 g for preparing intravenous injections. (Also available as Ureaphil in *USA*).

Other Proprietary Names

Austral.—Aquacare-HP, Nutraplus; *Canad.*—Carmol; *Denm.*—Carbaderm; *Jap.*—Keratinamin, Pastaron, Urepearl; *Norw.*—Calmuril; *Swed.*—Calmuril; *USA*—Aquacare, Carmol, Gormel, Nutraplus, Ultra-Mide.

Urea was also formerly marketed in Great Britain under the proprietary name Urevert (*Travenol*).

2362-w

Xipamide.

BE 1293. 4-Chloro-5-sulphamoylsalicylo-2′,6′-xylidide; 4-Chloro-2-hydroxy-2′,6′-dimethyl-5-sulphamoylbenzanilide.
$C_{15}H_{15}ClN_2O_4S = 354.8$.

CAS — 14293-44-8.

A white crystalline substance with a bitter taste and a faint odour. Practically **insoluble** in water; soluble in alcohol; very soluble in acetone; slightly soluble in chloroform and ether. M.p. about 260° (with decomposition).

Adverse Effects, Treatment, and Precautions. As for Chlorothiazide, p.588.

Absorption and Fate. Unlike chlorothiazide, xipamide has been reported to be completely absorbed from the gastro-intestinal tract. Absorption is fairly rapid with peak plasma concentrations occurring within 1 or 2 hours of oral administration. It is 99% bound to plasma proteins, and is excreted in the urine, partly unchanged and partly in the form of the glucuronide and free amine metabolites. It is reported to have a plasma half-life of about 5 to 8 hours, its biological half-life being much longer. Only traces of xipamide are normally excreted in the bile but extensive biliary excretion has been noted in subjects with renal failure.

The clinical pharmacokinetics of xipamide.— F. W. Hempelmann and P. Dieker, *Arzneimittel-Forsch.*, 1977, *27*, 2143.

Uses. Xipamide is a diuretic which has certain structural similarities to frusemide as well as the thiazides and has actions and uses similar to those of chlorothiazide (see p.589). Diuresis is initiated in about 1 or 2 hours and lasts for about 12 hours.

In the treatment of oedema the usual initial dose is 40 mg daily, subsequently reduced to 20 mg daily, according to the patient's response; in resistant cases doses of 80 mg daily may be required. In the treatment of hypertension the usual dose is 20 mg daily, as a single morning dose, either alone, or in conjunction with other antihypertensive agents; this may be increased to 40 mg daily, as a single morning dose, if necessary.

When treatment is prolonged, or in susceptible patients, loss of potassium may be sufficient to produce hypokalaemia; potassium supplements should then be given as for chlorothiazide.

Action. A review of the actions and uses of xipamide.— *Drug & Ther. Bull.*, 1979, *17*, 74.

A study in 26 healthy subjects indicated that the diuretic, saliuretic and kaliuretic effects of xipamide 20, 40 and 60 mg were similar and generally resembled those of hydrochlorothiazide 50 or 100 mg or frusemide 40 mg; frusemide had a relatively shorter duration of action.— W. P. Leary and A. C. Asmal, *Curr. ther. Res.*, 1978, *24*, 662. See also *idem*, 656; W. P. Leary *et al.*, *ibid.*, 1980, *27*, 16.

Further references: K. H. G. Piyasena *et al.*, *Curr. med. Res. Opinion*, 1975, *3*, 121; C. H. Gold and M. Viljoen, *Clin. Pharmac. Ther.*, 1979, *25*, 522.

Administration in renal failure. The plasma elimination half-life of xipamide was markedly prolonged in 2 subjects with renal failure. The amount eliminated in the faeces was increased and the proportion excreted in the urine as the glucuronide was also increased. The glucuronide was also detected in the plasma of one patient. Although xipamide is highly bound to plasma proteins, some was removed from plasma by haemodialysis.— F. W. Hempelmann and P. Dieker, *Arzneimittel-Forsch.*, 1977, *27*, 2143.

Hypertension. In a double-blind crossover study on 46 patients with mild to moderate hypertension, xipamide 20 or 40 mg once daily was significantly more effective than a placebo in reducing blood pressure. There was no significant difference between the effects of the two doses. Xipamide acted for at least 22 hours. Reported side-effects were dizziness and tiredness.— J. C. P. Weber *et al.*, *Br. J. clin. Pharmac.*, 1977, *4*, 283.

Further references: R. D. Harding *et al.*, *Clin. Trials J.*, 1974, *11*, 45; P. S. Davies and B. N. C. Prichard, *J. int. med. Res.*, 1975, *3*, 389; V. H. Heimsoth, *Int. J. clin. Pharmac. Biopharm.*, 1977, *15*, 260; W. P. Leary *et al.*, *Curr. ther. Res.*, 1978, *24*, 884; M. Castro, *Curr. med. Res. Opinion*, 1980, *6*, 416; S. Lentini *et al.*, *J. int. med. Res.*, 1980, *8*, 38.

Renal disorders. *Nephrotic syndrome.* Beneficial results with xipamide in patients with the nephrotic syndrome. Side-effects included hypokalaemia, hyperglycaemia, and hyperuricaemia.— C. H. Gold and M. Viljoen, *S. Afr. med. J.*, 1978, *54*, 569.

Proprietary Preparations

Diurexan *(E. Merck, UK)*. Xipamide, available as scored tablets of 20 mg.

Other Proprietary Names

Aquafor *(Ital.)*; Aquaphor *(Ger.)*.

NOTE. The name Aquaphor has also been applied to a water-soluble ointment basis.

Electrolytes

1150-y

The maintenance of normal body function is dependent upon the interplay of many systems including neurological, cardiorespiratory, and renal. However, central to all is the fluid and electrolyte medium in which all cells are bathed and which constitutes the body's transport system. Homoeostasis is the term applied to systems regulation as a whole in the body and has particular relevance to body fluids.

The body water is conveniently divided into extra- and intracellular compartments separated by the cell membrane which is freely permeable to water. With some exceptions, osmotic equilibrium is maintained across this membrane. Electroneutrality between anions and cations is present in the water outside cells (extracellular) and that inside cells (intracellular) but there may be an electrochemical gradient across membranes.

In the extracellular space the principal cations in plasma are sodium, potassium, calcium, and magnesium. The principal anions are chloride, bicarbonate, phosphate, sulphate, derivatives of organic acids (lactate, citrate), and protein. Measurements of extracellular (plasma) concentration are sometimes limited to sodium (or sodium and potassium), chloride, and bicarbonate. Assuming measurement only of sodium, bicarbonate, and chloride, the sum of the concentrations of sodium plus unmeasured cations (calcium, magnesium, potassium) equals the sum of the concentrations of bicarbonate and chloride plus unmeasured anions (phosphate, protein, sulphate, derivatives of organic acids). The difference between the concentrations of unmeasured anions and unmeasured cations is sometimes called the *anion gap*; variations in the anion gap are said to have value in the diagnosis of some disorders.

The expressions of concentrations of electrolytes in terms of mass concentration (e.g. mg per litre) is of little clinical value. This led initially to the expression of concentrations in terms of milliequivalents (mEq), a milliequivalent of an ion being one thousandth of the gram equivalent weight of the substance. More recently and in the interests of expressing both the law of mass action and the osmotic importance of ions, the mole has assumed some prominence. The mole is the SI unit for 'amount of substance'. The millimole (mmol) is recommended for the expression of ionic concentration. For monovalent ions the concentration in mEq and in mmol is numerically identical; for divalent ions the concentration in mEq is numerically twice that of the concentration in mmol.

The mechanisms involved in homoeostasis are complex and often inter-related. The principal factors, as far as electrolytes and fluids are concerned, are: maintenance of blood volume and osmolality, acid-base balance, and the role of specific ions.

The osmotic effects of solutions are expressed in terms of osmolality (molar concentration per 1000 g of solvent) or osmolarity (molar concentration per 1000 g of solution); the unit usually used is the milliosmole (mosmol)—the effect of an mmol of an undissociated substance or of an mmol of each of the separate ions of a dissociated substance. At a given temperature, the osmotic effect of an ideal solution (a dilute solution in which those molecules capable of dissociation are fully dissociated) depends upon the number of particles (molecules and ions) present in the solution. As the concentration increases the actual situation deviates from this 'ideal' situation and a correction factor known as the osmotic coefficient must be applied. Deviation from the 'ideal' situation is slight in solutions within the physiological range. Osmolality may be determined by measuring the depression of the freezing point or of vapour pressure. Because the difference between osmolality and osmolarity is slight at physiological values, the osmotic concentration of electrolyte solutions is often expressed as mosmol per litre. Knowledge of the osmotic concentration indicates whether a solution is hypo-, iso-, or hypertonic. Useful information may be obtained by such measurements in blood and urine.

Maintenance of Blood Volume Osmolality.. Water comprises approximately 60% of body weight; the volume of the intracellular compartment is almost twice that in the extracellular compartment. While the concentrations of specific ions in these compartments vary widely, there is a dynamic equilibrium between the compartments and their osmotic pressures are equal. Intake of water comes from food, drink, and the product of metabolism; loss takes place in urine, faeces, through the skin (as insensible transudative loss and as sensible perspiration), and in expired air.

Maintenance of body fluid volume (including that of the blood) is by the interaction of two main systems: the hypothalamic-posterior pituitary-renal axis which responds to changes in extracellular osmolality, and the renin-angiotensin-aldosterone (kidney-adrenal) system which is activated by changes in volume. Increase or decrease in water content causes decrease or increase of osmolality which adjusts the response of the hypothalamic 'osmostat' so controlling the rate of release of antidiuretic hormone. Increase or decrease of volume alters pressure relations in the juxtaglomerular apparatus of the kidney, resulting in the release of more or less renin which sets the conversion of angiotensinogen in blood into angiotensin I. The lung converts this substance to angiotensin II which has an effect on the peripheral vasculature and alters aldosterone release from the adrenal cortex. Aldosterone regulates sodium concentration by the kidney and thus adjusts extracellular volume.

Classification of disorders of blood volume and osmolality is complex and the nomenclature is varied and often confusing. While certain 'pure' depletions or excesses can be considered theoretically, they seldom occur as such in practice; e.g. dehydration theoretically means water loss; in practice loss of sodium and other ions usually occurs concomitantly though to a lesser degree and clinicians use the term to mean extracellular fluid volume depletion. Nomenclature also tends to vary depending on the starting point of analysis be this volume depletion, sodium depletion in extracellular fluid, or total sodium depletion in the body.

Disorders of blood volume and osmolality may arise from various causes including excessive loss of fluids and electrolytes in vomiting, diarrhoea, fistulas, haemorrhage, burns, and excessive perspiration; from excessive or inappropriate (in terms of electrolyte content) replacement of losses; from adrenal, renal, or cardiac disorders; and from inappropriate secretion of antidiuretic hormone.

Diagnosis depends upon a careful study of the history, probable fluid and electrolyte intake, probable fluid and electrolyte loss based upon weight loss and the known composition of body fluids, blood pressure, pulse, colour and temperature of the skin, elasticity of the skin, moisture of mucous membranes, size and appearance of tongue, state of consciousness and characteristics of respiration. Judicious use of laboratory data is sometimes also of value.

Eight categories are noted below: they should not be considered to be mutually exclusive and alternative titles should not be considered to be synonymous.

(a) Volume depletion with proportionate loss of water and sodium; iso-osmotic contraction; acute extracellular fluid volume deficit; real (distinct from apparent) sodium depletion; sodium dehydration; salt depletion; saline depletion. Treatment consists of restoration of volume with sodium chloride injection or a multiple electrolyte fluid, often with the addition of dextrose.

(b) Volume depletion where the loss of water exceeds the loss of sodium; hyperosmotic contraction; hyperosmotic dehydration; water dehydration; true dehydration; water depletion; apparent sodium excess (see hypernatraemia). Treatment consists of restoration of volume of water; water by mouth, 5% dextrose injection, and multiple electrolyte solutions have been used.

(c) Volume depletion where the loss of sodium exceeds the loss of water; hypo-osmotic contraction; hypo-osmotic dehydration; salt-depleted hyponatraemia (see hyponatraemia). This is rare but may occur if water and sodium losses are replaced with water only. Treatment consists of restoration of volume with the supply of adequate sodium.

(d) Volume excess with proportionate retention of water and sodium (as in cardiac failure); iso-osmotic expansion; extracellular fluid volume excess; oedema. Treatment consists of reduction of sodium intake and the use of diuretics; ion-exchange resins have also been used.

(e) Volume excess where the retention of water exceeds that of sodium; hypo-osmotic expansion; apparent sodium depletion; sodium dilution; dilutional hyponatraemia; water intoxication (see hyponatraemia). Treatment consists of water restriction and the use of osmotic diuretics or sodium chloride.

(f) Volume excess where the retention of sodium exceeds that of water; hyperosmotic expansion; real (distinct from apparent) sodium excess. A suitable diuretic will promote loss of water and sodium.

(g) Elevated concentration of sodium in plasma without volume change; sodium excess of extracellular fluid; hypernatraemia. The term hypernatraemia is also applied to elevated concentrations of sodium in plasma irrespective of volume (see hypernatraemia). Dextrose injection, sodium chloride injection 0.45%, and balanced electrolyte solutions with a low sodium content have been used in treatment. Too rapid replacement is to be avoided because of the risk of causing cerebral oedema and convulsions.

(h) Reduced concentrations of sodium in plasma without volume change; sodium deficit of extracellular fluid; hyponatraemia. The term hyponatraemia is also applied to reduced concentrations of sodium in plasma irrespective of volume (see hyponatraemia). Sodium chloride injection 0.9% may be given or, cautiously, sodium chloride injection 3% or 5%. However, hyponatraemia is most often the consequence of severe illness for which the mechanism remains obscure. Hyperosmotic infusions are rarely of value in such circumstances and the cause must be corrected if the plasma concentration is to rise.

Acid-base Balance.. The pH of plasma is normally maintained at about 7.38, chiefly by means of buffer mechanisms (haemoglobin, protein, phosphate, the bicarbonate-carbonic acid system) and by respiratory and renal mechanisms. The principal disorders of acid-base balance are:

Respiratory acidosis: retention of carbon dioxide in the body due to reduced ventilation as a result of mechanical or muscular impairment, diseases of the lungs, or CNS depression because of narcotic analgesics, barbiturates, and other

depressants. Renal mechanisms will tend partially to correct the imbalance. Treatment is directed primarily to removal or correction of the basic defect. Sodium bicarbonate has been given by infusion but is contra-indicated because it affects respiratory stimulation.
Respiratory alkalosis: excessive excretion of carbon dioxide from the body due to hyperventilation as a result of emotional factors, fever, hypoxia, the early stages of salicylate poisoning, and CNS lesions. Renal mechanisms tend to correct the imbalance. Treatment consists of re-breathing of expired air or the administration of carbon dioxide 5%. Compound sodium chloride injection has also been given, the high chloride content reducing the bicarbonate load. The condition is usually self-correcting.
Metabolic acidosis: the loss of proton acceptors (base) or the accession of an acid load. Loss of proton acceptors is exemplified by the loss of bicarbonate in excessive diarrhoea or intestinal intubation; accession of acid load occurs in many conditions—excessive acid production as in diabetic acidosis, lactic acidosis, exercise, inadequate or inappropriate food intake, lack of oxygen such as occurs in cardiac arrest or when large volumes of tissue are underperfused (e.g. a mesenteric or peripheral arterial embolus); excessive acid retention as in renal insufficiency; and excessive administration of acidifying salts such as ammonium chloride. Respiratory and renal mechanisms will tend to correct the imbalance. Treatment is directed primarily to removal or correction of the underlying defect. Sodium bicarbonate is often given by infusion; multiple electrolyte solutions containing lactate have also been used.
Metabolic alkalosis: the retention of excess bicarbonate in the body. Causes include, excessive use of bicarbonate, loss of hydrogen ion by vomiting or the result of potassium depletion induced by Cushing's syndrome, the use of corticosteroids or diuretics, and dietary deficiency. Respiratory and renal mechanisms will tend to correct the imbalance. Treatment consists of the supply of adequate chloride ions to replace bicarbonate and the administration of potassium supplements, for example, as potassium chloride and sodium chloride injection. Infusions of ammonium chloride have been used but are not generally recommended.

Role of Specific Ions.. For information on the role of the cations, calcium, magnesium, potassium, and sodium, see p.619, p.625, p.628, and p.633 respectively.
Chloride. Chloride is the principal anion of plasma, being present in a concentration of about 103 mmol per litre. It is readily exchangeable for other anions, particularly bicarbonate. An adequate supply of chloride is therefore essential in treating alkalosis.
Bicarbonate. Bicarbonate is the second most plentiful anion in plasma, being present in a concentration of about 26 mmol per litre. It is the principal anion involved in acid-base balance (see above).
Phosphate. Phosphate is present in plasma in a concentration of about 2 mEq per litre. There is an inverse relationship between the concentration of phosphate and that of calcium. Phosphate is involved in the metabolism of carbohydrates and lipids, in the storage and transfer of energy, as a buffer, and in the renal excretion of hydrogen ions. For further information, see under Sodium Phosphate, p.641.
Sulphate. Sulphate is present in plasma in a concentration of about 1 mEq per litre. It is involved in the formation of cartilage and in the detoxification of phenols.
Anions of organic acids. The principal acids involved are citric and lactic acids. The concentration of these anions in plasma is about 5 mEq per litre. In the presence of adequate hepatic function, lactate is metabolised to bicarbonate; therefore lactate is often present in electrolyte solutions for its alkalinising effect. For further information, see under Sodium Lactate, p.640.
Protein. Protein is present in plasma in a concentration of about 16 mEq per litre. It does not readily cross capillary membranes and therefore has a role in the maintenance of osmotic pressure inside the vascular compartment. It also acts as a buffer. Deficit of protein in plasma may be treated with appropriate blood fractions.

Fluid, electrolyte, and acid-base balance.— H. T. Randall, *Surg. Clins N. Am.*, 1976, *56*, 1019.

The hypertonic state.— P. U. Feig and D. K. McCurdy, *New Engl. J. Med.*, 1977, *297*, 1444.

Intravenous fluid therapy.— D. H. Lawson and D. A. Henry, *Am. J. Hosp. Pharm.*, 1977, *34*, 1332.

Fluid therapy during surgery.— D. R. Bevan, *Br. J. Hosp. Med.*, 1978, *19*, 445.

The assessment of acid-base balance.— J. Norman, *Br. J. Anaesth.*, 1978, *50*, 45.

Electrolyte studies: potassium, chloride, and acid-base M. D. Burke, *Postgrad. Med.*, 1978, *64*, 205.

Electrolyte and metabolic changes in patients with myocardial infarction.— C. T. G. Flear and P. Hilton, *Br. med. J.*, 1979, *1*, 1242.

Metabolic alkalosis in 2 patients was corrected by aggressive fluid replacement. Plasma-protein equivalency should be considered whenever plasma-anion-gap values are interpreted. Since almost all moderate to severe metabolic alkalosis is associated with a substantial amount of extracellular volume contraction, special attention should be given to this effect of plasma proteins; metabolic acidosis is not the only cause of an elevated anion gap.— N. E. Madias *et al.*, *New Engl. J. Med.*, 1979, *300*, 1421.

The diagnostic importance of an increased serum anion gap.— P. A. Gabow *et al.*, *New Engl. J. Med.*, 1980, *303*, 854.

Further references: H. J. Carroll and M. S. Oh, *Water, Electrolyte, and Acid-Base Metabolism*, Philadelphia, Lippincott, 1978.

1151-j

Calcium Salts.

Ca=40.08.

Calcium is an essential body electrolyte. It is involved in the maintenance of normal muscle and nerve function, is essential for normal cardiac function, and is essential to the clotting of blood.
The concentration of calcium in plasma is, in health, maintained very close to 2.5 mmol per litre; 50 to 60% is present in ionised form; up to about 10% is present as diffusible complexes with organic acids; the remainder is present as non-diffusible complexes with proteins. Variations in the concentration of ionised calcium are responsible for the symptoms of hypercalcaemia and hypocalcaemia.
There is a dynamic equilibrium between the calcium in blood and that in the skeleton. Homoeostasis is mainly regulated by the parathyroid hormone, by calcifonin, and by vitamin D. Excess of parathyroid hormone mobilises calcium from the bones and increases the concentration of calcium in blood and other extracellular fluid, including the proportion of ionic compared with bound calcium; parathyroid hormone increases the tubular reabsorption of calcium, but calcium excretion may be increased in hyperparathyroidism. Calcitonin exerts a rather rapid but only brief effect in increasing the uptake of calcium by bone and so lowers the concentration of calcium in extracellular fluid. Calcium is also mobilised from the bones by 1,25-dihydroxycholecalciferol, the active metabolite of vitamin D. These effects are largely interdependent. There is an inverse relationship between the concentration of calcium and phosphate in blood.
The total body content of calcium is about 1 kg, of which about 99% is present in bone. Symptoms of hypercalcaemia are described below under Adverse Effects while those of hypocalcaemia are described under the Uses section.
The soluble calcium salts described in this section are used in the treatment of calcium deficiency; they may be given by mouth or by injection. Less soluble salts are used as antacids or as dietary supplements.
Other calcium salts, described elsewhere, include calcium carbonate and calcium glycerophosphate.
Other drugs affecting calcium metabolism include the diphosphonates, fluorides, and mithramycin.

NOTE. Each g of calcium represents approximately 25 mmol (49.9 mEq).

Adverse Effects. When given by mouth calcium salts may cause constipation (see under Calcium Carbonate, p.76). Intravenous injection of calcium salts may cause nausea, vomiting, a chalk-like taste, tingling of the skin, peripheral vasodilatation, sweating, and hypotension.
The principal causes of hypercalcaemia are hyperparathyroidism and excessive intake of vitamin D. It may also occur as idiopathic infantile hypercalcaemia, in neoplastic disease either because of bone destruction or more rarely because a tumour secretes parathyroid-like hormone, after prolonged immobilisation, in sarcoidosis, hyperthyroidism, and the milk-alkali syndrome, and, because of increased ionisation of calcium, in acidosis.
Symptoms of hypercalcaemia may include anorexia, nausea, vomiting, constipation, abdominal pain, muscle weakness, thirst, polyuria, drowsiness, confusion, bone pain due to demineralisation, nephrocalcinosis, loss of renal concentrating capacity, renal calculi, and, in severe cases, cardiac arrhythmias, coma, and cardiac arrest.

Hard tap-water was inadvertently used in place of softened water in the haemodialysis of 10 patients. The mean plasma-calcium concentrations rose from 2.31 to 3.75 mmol and the mean magnesium concentration from 1.25 to 1.95 mmol per litre. Vomiting, which had been infrequent, occurred in 17 of 23 dialyses. Patients complained of extreme weakness and lethargy and a sensation of skin warmth was reported on 9 occasions. The lack of any severe complications was attributed to the antagonism between calcium and magnesium, both of which were increased in concentration.— R. M. Freeman *et al.*, *New Engl. J. Med.*, 1967, *276*, 1113. See also H. K. Schulten *et al.*, *Dt. med. Wschr.*, 1968, *93*, 387.

In a study of myocardial concentrations of magnesium and calcium in heart muscle taken at necropsy, after allowance had been made for a number of factors, samples from patients who died from ischaemic heart disease contained a mean magnesium concentration 23 µg per g lower and a mean calcium concentration 4 µg per g higher than the mean for samples obtained from patients who died from other causes. There was no evidence of any association between concentrations of magnesium and calcium in tissue samples and in the domestic tap water of the various areas.— P. C. Elwood *et al.*, *Lancet*, 1980, *2*, 720.

Hypertension. Reversible hypertension occurred on 4 occasions in a woman during episodes of hypercalcaemia caused by hyperparathyroidism, vitamin D toxicity (2 occasions), and calcium infusion respectively. It was suggested that hypertension might be directly related to hypercalcaemia in some patients.— M. Blum *et al.*, *J. Am. med. Ass.*, 1977, *237*, 262.

Pregnancy and the neonate. Of 50 282 children born to mothers monitored by the Collaborative Perinatal Project, 1007 had been exposed to calcium-containing compounds, and possibly other drugs, at some time during the first 4 months of the pregnancy. Although no relationship between malformations in general and calcium exposure was noted, an association with central nervous system malformations was detected which required independent confirmation.— O. P. Heinonen *et al.*, *Birth Defects and Drugs in Pregnancy*, Littleton MA, Publishing Sciences Group, 1977, p. 401.

Treatment of Adverse Effects. Calcium intake should be reduced to a minimum and large amounts of fluid given to combat dehydration and reduce renal deposition of calcium. In mild to moderate hypercalcaemia sodium phosphates may be given by mouth (see Neutral Phosphates, p.642). In more severe cases, reduction of serum-calcium concentrations has been achieved by the intravenous infusion of sodium phosphate, sodium sulphate, sodium chloride, or sodium citrate. Sodium chloride and sodium sulphate promote a calciuresis which may be increased by concomitant administration of frusemide or ethacrynic acid; thiazide diuretics are not effective. All these treatments should be used with caution in patients with impaired renal or cardiac function. Disodium edetate has also been used but renal damage may occur with large doses.

Calcitonin and corticosteroids are effective in reducing serum-calcium concentrations in a variety of hypercalcaemic states. In neoplastic diseases mithramycin has been used.

A discussion on the treatment of severe hypercalcaemia including details of the emergency treatment, and the role of corticosteroids, calcitonin, and inorganic phosphate.— *Br. med. J.*, 1980, *280*, 204.

The use of peritoneal dialysis with a calcium-free dialysate was successful for the treatment of severe hypercalcaemia in one patient.— P. J. Heyburn *et al.*, *Br. med. J.*, 1980, *280*, 525.

Further references: *Lancet*, 1967, *2*, 501; C. E. Dent (letter), *ibid.*, 613; B. Nielsen (letter), *ibid.*, 1090.

Precautions. Solutions of calcium salts, particularly calcium chloride, are irritant, and care should be taken to prevent extravasation during intravenous injection. Intravenous injections should be given slowly as high blood concentrations may cause vasodilatation and depress cardiac function leading to hypotension and syncope. Calcium salts should be given cautiously to patients with impaired renal function or a history of renal stone formation.

Calcium enhances the effects of digitalis on the heart and may precipitate digitalis intoxication; parenteral calcium therapy is contra-indicated in patients receiving cardiac glycosides. Calcium salts reduce the absorption of tetracyclines.

Intravenous injections of calcium salts, usually the gluconate, in doses of up to 9 mg of elemental calcium per kg body-weight given within an hour produced an increase in gastric secretion of acid and pepsin. Marked bradycardia with sinus arrhythmia followed the administration of calcium and the change in heart-rate was inversely related to the rise and fall in gastric secretion. Bradycardia and the secretory response was abolished by atropine.— R. A. Smallwood, *Gut*, 1967, *8*, 592.

Calcium administration could increase secretion of gastrin and could increase gastric acid secretion enormously in patients with Zollinger-Ellison syndrome.— J. E. McGuigan, *Mayo Clin. Proc.*, 1973, *48*, 634.

Atrial fibrillation after injection of calcium gluconate and pentagastrin for the early detection of medullary thyroid carcinoma.— D. Drucker (letter), *New Engl. J. Med.*, 1981, *304*, 1427.

Administration in renal failure. In 15 patients with chronic renal failure 23 episodes of hypercalcaemia occurred associated with the use of calcium-containing products. In most cases the dose of calcium was within the normal therapeutic range. Calcium concentrations should be monitored during calcium therapy in patients with renal failure.— N. Graben *et al.*, *Dt. med. Wschr.*, 1977, *102*, 1903. See also under Absorption and Fate, below.

Absorption and Fate. Calcium is absorbed from the small intestine; about one-third of ingested calcium is absorbed; absorption decreases with age and may be more efficient when the body is deficient in calcium or from diets deficient in calcium. Absorption of calcium is increased by 1,25-dihydroxycholecalciferol, the active metabolite of vitamin D.

Calcium is excreted in sweat, bile, pancreatic juice, saliva, urine, faeces, and milk. Up to 400 mg may be excreted in the urine daily; the amount is directly related to the excretion of sodium ions and is also increased by increased dietary magnesium. Urinary excretion of calcium decreases when increased amounts of phosphorus are ingested and increases when the phosphorus intake is reduced.

The nature of circulating calcium is discussed above.

In 30 patients with advanced renal failure, intestinal calcium absorption in the first 2 hours was delayed compared with 31 healthy subjects; between 2 and 6 hours there was little difference; absorption continued between 6 and 25 hours to a greater degree in the patients with renal failure. This alteration in calcium absorption might have been due to a defect in the renal production of 1,25-dihydroxycholecalciferol.— A. S. Brickman *et al.*, *J. Lab. clin. Med.*, 1974, *84*, 791.

The dissociation of the absorption of calcium and phosphate after cadaveric renal transplantation.— K. Farrington *et al.*, *Br. med. J.*, 1979, *1*, 712.

The measurement of serum-calcium concentrations.— *Lancet*, 1979, *1*, 858. Comments: R. B. Payne and B. E. Walker (letter), *ibid.*, 1248; P. J. Phillips *et al.* (letter), *ibid.*, *2*, 156. See also S. C. Conceicao *et al.*, *Br. med. J.*, 1978, *1*, 1103.

A discussion on the urinary excretion of calcium.— J. Lemann *et al.*, *New Engl. J. Med.*, 1979, *301*, 535.

Human Requirements. The average adult requires about 12.5 mmol (500 mg) of calcium per day. Adequate amounts of calcium are present in the average diet and supplements are seldom necessary except for growing children and pregnant and lactating women, whose requirements are greater, and those on parenteral nutrition.

A critical review of recommendations for human requirements of calcium.— C. R. Paterson, *Postgrad. med. J.*, 1978, *54*, 244.

Recommended daily intake of calcium: infants up to 1 year, 600 mg; boys and girls, 1 to 8 years, 600 mg; 9 to 14 years, 700 mg; 15 to 17 years, 600 mg; adults, 500 mg; during pregnancy, 3rd trimester, 1.2 g; during lactation, 1.2 g.— Report by the Committee on Medical Aspects of Food Policy, *Reports on Health and Social Subjects, No. 15*, London, HM Stationery Office, 1979.

The US National Research Council recommended the following daily dietary allowances of calcium: infants up to 6 months, 360 mg; 6 to 12 months, 540 mg; children aged 1 to 10 years, 800 mg; males and females 11 to 18 years, 1.2 g; over 19 years, 800 mg; during pregnancy and lactation, 1.2 g.— *Recommended Dietary Allowances*, 9th Edn, Washington, The National Research Council, 1980.

Uses. Calcium salts are used mainly in the treatment of calcium deficiency and hypocalcaemia.

Signs of hypocalcaemia may occur when the serum-calcium concentration falls below 2.25 mmol per litre. The principal causes of hypocalcaemia are hypoparathyroidism and deficiency of vitamin D. Hypocalcaemia may occur in malnutrition or dietary deficiency, in steatorrhoea, acute pancreatitis, or renal insufficiency, after excessive intake of fluoride or transfusion of citrated blood, and, because of decreased ionisation, in alkalosis.

Symptoms may include paraesthesia, laryngospasm, muscle cramps, increased muscle excitability leading to tetany, convulsions, mental changes, alterations in the skin, fungous infections, and prolongation of the Q-T interval on the ECG.

In simple deficiency states calcium salts may be given by mouth in doses to provide up to 50 mmol (100 mEq) of calcium daily, with adequate vitamin D to aid absorption.

In acute hypocalcaemia parenteral administration is necessary; typical doses are 2.25 to 4.5 mmol (4.5 to 9 mEq) of calcium, usually as 10% calcium gluconate or glubionate, by slow intravenous injection, repeated as required. In neonatal tetany 2.7 mmol (5.4 mEq) has been given 4-hourly by mouth; intravenous therapy may be necessary to control convulsions.

Calcium is used as an adjunct in the treatment of severe hyperkalaemia; a typical dose is 2.25 to 4.5 mmol (4.5 to 9 mEq), usually as 10% calcium gluconate, by slow intravenous injection, repeated as required under ECG control.

Calcium has been used in the treatment of hypermagnesaemia; a typical dose is 2.25 to 4.5 mmol (4.5 to 9 mEq) intravenously.

Calcium salts are given for their inotropic effect in cardiac resuscitation. Doses of 1.7 to 3.4 mmol (3.4 to 6.8 mEq) have been given intravenously as 2.5 to 5 ml of 10% calcium chloride, and repeated after 10 minutes; intracardiac injections are very occasionally necessary; calcium gluconate is used similarly. Calcium salts are also used for the prevention of hypocalcaemia in exchange transfusions.

Intravenous injections of calcium have been used for the acute colic of lead poisoning, and in the treatment of fluoride poisoning.

Calcium therapy may arrest or slow down the rate of bone demineralisation in osteoporosis.

Calcium has been given as an infusion of the gluconate in sodium chloride injection as a test for osteomalacia or osteoporosis and parathyroid function. Normal results are fairly clear but abnormal results cannot always be interpreted.

Calcium carbonate is used as an antacid (see p.76).

The phosphates of calcium are slightly soluble in water and soluble in acid and have been used as antacids and as sources of calcium but they are generally regarded as inert and suitable for use as excipients.

Bone pain. All of 14 patients with bone pain associated with primary biliary cirrhosis obtained relief from pain in 3 to 12 days from the commencement of a 12-day course of 4-hour daily infusions of calcium (as gluconate) 1.5 or 15 mg per kg body-weight. Pain relief was achieved more rapidly after the higher dose but remissions lasted 2 to 3 months after low or high doses and were again induced by a repeated course in 5 patients.— A. B. Ajdukiewicz *et al.*, *Gut*, 1974, *15*, 788.

See also under Osteoporosis, below.

Calcium-infusion test. After 3 days on a low calcium diet, 15 mg per kg body-weight of calcium, as gluconate, in sodium chloride injection was infused over 4 hours. Urinary and plasma calcium was measured. Of 98 patients tested, the 21 'normal' patients excreted 33 to 53% of the calcium in 12 hours and 12 with osteomalacia and steatorrhoea excreted 1.5 to 26.8%. Excretion of calcium was normal or raised in osteoporosis.— B. E. C. Nordin and R. Fraser, *Lancet*, 1956, *1*, 823. Further tests for osteoporosis.— J. M. Finlay *et al.*, *ibid.*, 826.

The only possible value of a calcium-infusion test (calcium gluconate in 5% dextrose) was that a normal result might exclude osteomalacia; however, an abnormal result could not be interpreted.— J. V. Lever *et al.*, *Br. med. J.*, 1967, *3*, 281.

In a modification of the classical calcium-infusion test phosphorus excretion during the last 12 hours of the infusion day was compared with that during the same period of the preceding day. In 15 normal subjects phosphorus excretion was depressed by a mean of 51.5%; in 13 patients with hyperparathyroidism (due to adenoma or hyperplasia) phosphorus excretion was less affected and the range was outside that of normal subjects; values returned to normal in 13 patients after parathyroidectomy.— C. Y. C. Pak, *Ann. N.Y. Acad. Sci.*, 1971, *179*, 450. See also C. Y. C. Pak *et al.*, *Archs intern. Med.*, 1972, *129*, 48, per *Lancet*, 1972, *1*, 578.

A calcium-infusion test was evaluated as a diagnostic aid for carcinoid and related tumours.— E. L. Kaplan *et al.*, *Am. J. Surg.*, 1972, *123*, 173, per *Int. pharm. Abstr.*, 1973, *10*, 945.

Failure of calcium infusion as a provocation test for insulinoma.— J. L. Miller *et al.* (letter), *New Engl. J. Med.*, 1981, *304*, 1430.

Calcium-loading test. Administration by mouth of a large dose of calcium citrate suspension (100 mg of calcium per kg body-weight) produced a significantly greater rise in serum and urine calcium in 9 hypercalciuric patients with renal stone disease than in 9 healthy controls. Hypercalciuria was generally due to hyperabsorption, and oral calcium loading might give a better diagnostic test of this condition than a 24-hour urine collection on a free diet.— M. Peacock *et al.*, *Br. med. J.*, 1968, *2*, 729.

A test feed containing calcium lactate, 385 mg per kg body-weight (50 mg of calcium per kg), dissolved in dextrose solution 5% (30 ml per g of calcium lactate) was given after a 4- to 5-hour fast in children aged 2 months to 2.5 years. Fifteen children with various disorders all showed normal fasting serum-calcium concentrations. Twelve children with idiopathic hypercalcaemia showed exaggerated response to the calcium-loading test. In 2 patients, full recovery from the disease was associated with the reversion of the test to normal.— D. G. D. Barr and J. O. Forfar, *Br. med. J.*, 1969, *1*, 477.

Cardiac resuscitation. Recommendations concerning calcium chloride, at the National Conference on Standards for Cardiopulmonary Resuscitation and Emergency Cardiac Care held in May 1973. Calcium chloride increases myocardial contractility, prolongs systole, and enhances ventricular excitability. Sinus impulse formation can be suppressed, and sudden death has been described following a rapid intravenous injection of calcium chloride, particularly in fully digitalised patients. Calcium chloride is useful in profound cardiovascular collapse (electromechanical dissociation). It may be useful in restoring an electrical rhythm in instances of asystole and may enhance electrical defibrillation. The absolute dose of calcium required in cardiac arrest emergencies is difficult to determine and may vary widely. The usual recommended dose of calcium chloride is 2.5 to 5 ml of a 10% solution (1.7 to 3.4 mmol of calcium; 3.4 to 6.8 mEq). Where required, this amount should be injected intravenously as a bolus at intervals of 10 minutes. Calcium gluconate provides less ionisable calcium per unit volume; if it is used, the dose should be 10 ml of a 10% solution. Calcium can also be administered as calcium gluceptate.—American Heart Association and the National Academy of Sciences-National Research Council, *J. Am. med. Ass.*, 1974, *227, Suppl.*, 833–868. See also Adrenaline, p.5.

Calcium and the myocardium, cardiac pacemakers, and vascular smooth muscle.— A. Fleckenstein, *A. Rev. Pharmac. Toxic.*, 1977, *17*, 149–166.

Dialysis. From acute and long-term observations, the optimum calcium concentration of dialysis fluid for maintenance haemodialysis was considered to be 60 ± mg per litre [1.5 ± 0.05 mmol per litre].— A. J. Wing, *Br. med. J.*, 1968, *4*, 145.

The metacarpal index was reduced in most of 11 patients dialysed with a solution containing calcium 5 mg per 100 ml, indicating a loss of cortical bone. This was not seen in patients using a solution containing calcium 7 mg per 100 ml.— J. M. Bone *et al.*, *Lancet*, 1972, *1*, 1047.

In a study in 11 patients undergoing dialysis the use of a dialysate containing calcium 1.6 mmol per litre raised ionised calcium concentrations appropriately and prevented hyperparathyroidism.— S. Conceicao *et al.*, *Proc. Eur. Dialysis Transplant Ass.*, 1977, *14*, 229.

Effect on gastric secretion. In 15 healthy subjects, intragastric instillation of calcium gluconate 2 g increased gastric acid secretion in 11, and increased serum-gastrin concentration in 12.— M. J. Brodie *et al.*, *Gut*, 1977, *18*, 111.

Calcium gluconate by intravenous infusion was used to diagnose Zollinger-Ellison syndrome in 20 patients with a history of peptic ulcer disease. However, secretin was preferred.— C. W. Deveney *et al.*, *Ann. intern. Med.*, 1977, *87*, 680.

See also under Precautions, above.

Hyperkalaemia. For the use of calcium salts in the management of hyperkalaemia, see under Potassium Salts, Treatment of Adverse Effects, p.628.

Hypocalcaemia. Small doses of calcium gluconate (up to 9 ml of 10% solution intravenously in 24 hours, or by mouth) relieved neonatal hypocalcaemia in 35 infants.— N. R. C. Roberton and M. A. Smith, *Archs Dis. Childh.*, 1975, *50*, 604. See also O. Troughton and S. P. Singh, *Br. med. J.*, 1972, *4*, 76; D. R. Brown *et al.*, *J. Pediat.*, 1976, *89*, 973; M. Moya and E. Doménech, *Archs Dis. Childh.*, 1978, *53*, 784; L. Sann *et al.*, *Archs Dis. Childh.*, 1980, *55*, 611.

Hypotension. Hypotension which was successfully treated with calcium chloride 2 g intravenously was considered to have been caused by hypocalcaemia in an 11-year-old uraemic girl.— C. Chaimovitz *et al.* (letter), *J. Am. med. Ass.*, 1972, *222*, 86.

Muscle cramps. Intravenous injections of calcium gluconate should not be given for muscle cramps in athletes.— *J. Am. med. Ass.*, 1975, *232*, 1169.

Osteitis deformans. Relief from pain and increased mobility occurred in 8 of 9 patients with Paget's disease of bone given 15 mg of calcium, as calcium gluconate, per kg body-weight by intravenous infusion in 1 litre of sodium chloride injection daily over 4 hours for 10 days. Serum-alkaline phosphatase concentrations, which were raised in 8 patients, were reduced by 30% during and after the infusion.— R. Sekel (letter), *Lancet*, 1973, *1*, 372. The biochemical benefits of calcium infusions might be temporary.— A. Rapoport *et al.* (letter), *ibid.*, 1128.

In 8 of 9 patients with Paget's disease of bone, bone pain was relieved after 20 to 70 days' treatment with calcium 0.5 to 1 g thrice daily, with aluminium hydroxide, methyclothiazide, and a low-phosphorus diet. At 120 days the mean alkaline phosphatase value was reduced to 58% of the original value; this effect was maintained after 200 days of treatment.— R. A. Evans, *Aust. N.Z. J. Med.*, 1977, *7*, 259.

Osteoporosis. In 59 premenopausal and 36 postmenopausal women the overnight ratio of calcium : creatinine clearance was greater in the postmenopausal women, suggesting that calcium metabolism increased with age. The ratio was not significantly different when two Sandocal tablets were given before retiring at night. In postmenopausal osteoporosis, calcium supplements should be given as a single large dose immediately before retiring at night.— P. E. Belchetz *et al.*, *Br. med. J.*, 1973, *2*, 510.

Calcium gluconate relieved the symptoms of spinal osteoporosis in 16 of 19 patients when given as a course of 6 to 12 infusions containing 8.75 g. Concurrent corticosteroid therapy in 5 patients did not affect the response.— J. Shafar, *Br. J. clin. Pract.*, 1973, *27*, 405.

Alternating calcium and phosphorus infusions were given to 5 patients with severe osteoporosis, daily for 6 to 8 weeks, then 2 or 3 times a week for 10 to 12 months. There was rapid relief from bone pain, a cessation of spontaneous fractures, and some evidence of increased bone formation.— M. M. Popovtzer *et al.*, *Am. J. Med.*, 1976, *61*, 478.

From a study of 95 postmenopausal women with osteoporosis of the spine, assessment of cortical bone loss, compression fracture-rate, and calcium balance suggested that useful treatments might be calcium (1.2 g Ca daily), hormones (ethinyloestradiol 25 µg daily for 3 weeks in 4, or norethisterone 5 mg daily), or alfacalcidol (1 or 2 µg daily) with hormones. Treatment with vitamin D (10 000 to 50 000 units daily) or alfacalcidol alone was not effective and might be harmful; the usefulness of calcium with vitamin D was equivocal.— B. E. C. Nordin *et al.*, *Br. med. J.*, 1980, *280*, 451.

Discussions on the use of calcium in the treatment of postmenopausal osteoporosis: B. E. C. Nordin, *Drugs*, 1979, *18*, 484; *Med. Lett.*, 1980, *22*, 45.

Rickets. Severe rickets developed in a 10-month-old child owing to calcium deficiency alone. Vitamin-D intake had been adequate.— S. W. Kooh *et al.*, *New Engl. J. Med.*, 1977, *297*, 1264.

1152-z

Calcium Acetate *(B.P.)*. Dried Calcium Acetate.

$C_4H_6CaO_4$=158.2.

CAS — 62-54-4.

Pharmacopoeias. In *Br.*

A white, odourless or almost odourless, hygroscopic powder with a bitter taste. It may contain up to 7% of water. Each g (anhydrous) represents approximately 6.3 mmol (12.6 mEq) of calcium and the equivalent of bicarbonate. Calcium acetate 3.95 g is approximately equivalent to 1 g of calcium.

Soluble 1 in 3 of water and 1 in 500 of alcohol (90%); practically insoluble in chloroform and ether. A 5% solution in water has a pH of 7.2 to 8.2. **Incompatible** with soluble carbonates, phosphates, sulphates, and salts of weak acids. **Store** in airtight containers.

Adverse Effects, Treatment, and Precautions. As for Calcium Salts, p.619.

Uses. Calcium acetate is used as a convenient stable source of calcium in haemodialysis solutions. It is also used as a food preservative.

1153-c

Calcium Chloride *(B.P., Eur. P., U.S.P.)*.

Calc. Chlor.; Calcium Chloride Dihydrate; Calcii Chloridum; Calcii Chloridum Siccatum; Calcium Chloratum; Cloruro de Calcio; Cloruro de Calcio Cristalizado; Cloreto de Cálcio.

$CaCl_2,2H_2O$=147.0.

CAS — 10035-04-8.

Pharmacopoeias. In *Arg., Br., Braz., Chin., Eur., Fr., Ger., It., Jap., Mex., Neth., Nord., Swiss,* and *U.S.*

White, hygroscopic, odourless, crystalline powder or granules with a bitter warming saline taste. At relative humidities up to 10 to 30% it is hygroscopic, and deliquescent under damper conditions. It contains about 76% of $CaCl_2$. Each g represents approximately 6.8 mmol (13.6 mEq) of calcium and 13.6 mmol (13.6 mEq) of chloride. Calcium chloride (dihydrate) 3.67 g is approximately equivalent to 1 g of calcium.

Soluble 1 in 1.2 of water, 1 in 0.7 of boiling water, 1 in about 4 of alcohol, and 1 in 2 of boiling alcohol. A 5% solution in water has a pH of 4.5 to 9.2. A 1.7% solution in water is iso-osmotic with serum. A suitable preservative in eye-drops is phenylmercuric acetate 0.002%. Solutions are **sterilised** by autoclaving or by filtration. **Incompatible** with soluble carbonates, phosphates, sulphates, and tartrates; with amphotericin, cephalothin sodium, chlorpheniramine maleate, chlortetracycline hydrochloride, oxytetracycline hydrochloride, and tetracycline hydrochloride. Occasional incompatibilities, depending on concentration, have occurred with sodium bicarbonate. **Store** in airtight containers.

Preservative for eye-drops. Benzalkonium chloride 0.01% was a suitable preservative for calcium chloride eye-drops sterilised by heating at 98° to 100° for 30 minutes or by filtration, and chlorhexidine gluconate 0.02% when sterilised by filtration.— M. Van Ooteghem, *Pharm. Tijdschr. Belg.*, 1968, *45*, 69.

1154-k

Calcium Chloride Hexahydrate. Calcii Chloridum Crystallisatum; Hydrated Calcium Chloride; Calcium Chloratum Crystallisatum; Chlorure de Calcium Cristallisé; Cloruro Cálcico; Cloreto de Cálcio Cristalizado. Calcium chloride hexahydrate.

$CaCl_2,6H_2O$=219.1.

CAS — 7774-34-7.

In the *B.P. 1953*, and earlier editions, the name Calcium Chloride was applied to the anhydrous salt, $CaCl_2$ = 111.0, and the hexahydrated salt had the title Hydrated Calcium Chloride. In the *B.P. 1958*, and later editions, the name Calcium Chloride was applied to the hexahydrate but by the *B.P. 1973* this title is applied to the dihydrate..

Pharmacopoeias. In *Aust., Braz., Hung., Ind., Int., Jug., Nord., Pol., Port., Roum., Rus., Span.,* and *Turk.*
Belg. specifies the tetrahydrate, $CaCl_2,4H_2O$ = 183.0.

Colourless, odourless, very deliquescent crystals with a slightly bitter taste, containing about 50% of $CaCl_2$. At relative humidities below 20% it is efflorescent and above 30% deliquescent. Each g represents approximately 4.6 mmol (9.1 mEq) of calcium and 9.1 mmol (9.1 mEq) of chloride. Calcium chloride hexahydrate 5.47 g is approximately equivalent to 1 g of calcium.

Soluble 1 in 0.2 of water and 1 in 0.5 of alcohol. An aqueous solution has an almost neutral reaction. A 20% solution in water is clear and colourless. A 2.5% solution in water is iso-osmotic with serum. **Sterilisation** and **incompatibilities** as for Calcium Chloride. **Store** at a temperature not exceeding 25° in airtight containers.

Other forms occurring in commerce are anhydrous calcium chloride and 'fused' calcium chloride; the latter contains variable amounts of water.

Details of some calcium chloride injections and comment on the considerable confusion between the labelling of the dihydrate and the hexahydrate.— B. Hughes (letter), *Pharm. J.*, 1977, *1*, 182. Correction.— *ibid.*, 230.

Adverse Effects, Treatment, and Precautions. As for Calcium Salts, p.619.

Solutions of calcium chloride are irritant and cause necrosis if injected intramuscularly. Intravenous injections must be given very slowly to reduce the risk of cardiovascular collapse. Calcium chloride is irritant to the stomach and must be given well diluted with water.

Metabolic acidosis. If treatment with calcium chloride by mouth was continued for longer than 2 days in neonates, metabolic acidosis was liable to occur.— A. Mizrahi *et al.*, *New Engl. J. Med.*, 1968, *278*, 1163.

Absorption and Fate. As for Calcium Salts, p.620.
Calcium chloride is poorly absorbed by mouth. After intravenous administration the chloride ions may produce acidosis and a mild diuretic effect.

Uses. Calcium chloride has the actions of calcium salts (see p.620) and is administered by slow intravenous injection as a 5 to 10% solution of the dihydrate in doses of up to 1 g (6.8 mmol). Calcium chloride is reported to provide a more reliable increase in extracellular ionised calcium concentration but, since it is highly irritant to the tissues and produces sloughing in the event of leakage outside the veins, calcium gluconate is often preferred.
When administered by mouth calcium chloride produces more gastric irritation than other soluble calcium salts. It is unpalatable in mixtures, the taste being very difficult to mask. Doses of 1 to 2 g of the dihydrate (6.8 to 13.6 mmol) have been used.

Reasons why calcium chloride rather than calcium gluconate should be the calcium salt of choice for parenteral indications: first, the body's retention of calcium chloride is greater and more predictable than its retention of calcium gluconate; second, the increase in extracellular ionised calcium concentration is unpredictable for the gluconate; finally, the positive inotropic effect of calcium chloride is greater than that of calcium gluconate.— L. I. G. Worthley and P. J. Phillips (letter), *Lancet*, 1980, *2*, 149.

Cardiac resuscitation. For the role of calcium salts in cardiac resuscitation, see p.621.

Preparations

Calcium Chloratum Solutum *(Cz. P., Hung. P.)*. Diluendum Calcii Chloridi 50% *(Nord. P.)*. A solution containing 50% w/w of calcium chloride hexahydrate in water. *Rus. P.* also includes a 10% w/v solution for injection.

Calcium Chloride Injection *(U.S.P.)*. A sterile solution of calcium chloride in Water for Injections. pH 5.5 to 7.5.

Min-I-Jet Calcium Chloride Injection *(IMS, UK)*. A cartridge assembly containing a solution of calcium chloride 100 mg per ml, in vials of 10 ml.

Other Proprietary Names

Chloro-Calcion *(Fr.)*.

1155-a

Anhydrous Calcium Chloride. Cloruro de Calcio.
$CaCl_2$=111.0.

CAS — 10043-52-4.

Pharmacopoeias. In *Arg.*

Dry, white, very deliquescent masses or granules, with a warm bitter taste, containing not more than 10% of water. Each g represents approximately 9 mmol (18 mEq) of calcium and 18 mmol (18 mEq) of chloride. **Soluble** 1 in 1.5 of water and 1 in 3 of alcohol. A 1.3% solution in water is iso-osmotic with serum. **Store** in airtight containers.
Anhydrous Calcium Chloride was included in the *B.P. 1953*, and earlier editions, with the title Calcium Chloride; in the *B.P. 1958*, and later editions, this title was applied to the hexahydrate but by the *B.P. 1973* it was applied to the dihydrate.

Anhydrous calcium chloride is used as a drying agent in desiccators and for package testing. It must not be administered by injection.

1156-t

Calcium Glubionate.

Calcium Gluconate Lactobionate Monohydrate; Calcium Gluconogalactogluconate Monohydrate. Calcium D-gluconate lactobionate monohydrate.
$(C_{12}H_{21}O_{12},C_6H_{11}O_7)Ca,H_2O$=610.5.

CAS — 31959-85-0 (anhydrous); 12569-38-9 (monohydrate).

Soluble in water. Each g represents approximately 1.6 mmol (3.3 mEq) of calcium. Calcium glubionate monohydrate 15.2 g is approximately equivalent to 1 g of calcium.

Adverse Effects, Treatment, and Precautions. As for Calcium Salts, p.619.

Uses. Calcium glubionate has the actions and uses of calcium salts, p.620. It is used similarly to calcium gluconate as an injection or syrup.
Up to about 20 g (32.8 mmol; 65.5 mEq of calcium) has been given daily. When intravenous therapy is needed 5 to 10 ml of solution providing 1.2 to 2.3 mmol (2.3 to 4.6 mEq) is used; it may also be given intramuscularly, except to children.

Proprietary Preparations

Calcium-Sandoz *(Sandoz, UK)*. **Ampoules** each containing 10 ml of a solution of calcium glubionate equivalent to calcium gluconate 10% (10 ml≡93 mg Ca; 2.3 mmol), and **Syrup** containing calcium glubionate 21% and calcium lactobionate 14% (15 ml≡calcium gluconate 3.5 g; 325 mg Ca; 8.1 mmol). (Also available as Calcium-Sandoz in *Austral., Canad., Denm., Fr., Norw., Switz.*).

Other Proprietary Names

Neo-Calglucon *(USA)*.

1157-x

Calcium Gluceptate.

Calcium glucoheptonate.
$C_{14}H_{26}CaO_{16}$=490.4.

CAS — 17140-60-2; 29039-00-7.

Pharmacopoeias. In *U.S.* which allows anhydrous or with varying amounts of water of crystallisation (equivalent to $2H_2O$ or $3\frac{1}{2}H_2O$).

A white or faintly yellow amorphous powder with an acrid taste. The hydrated forms may lose part of their water of crystallisation on standing. Each g represents approximately 2 mmol (4 mEq) of calcium. Calcium gluceptate (anhydrous) 12.2 g is approximately equivalent to 1 g of calcium.
Freely **soluble** in water; practically insoluble in alcohol and many other organic solvents. A 10% solution in water has a pH of 6 to 8.
Incompatible with cephalothin sodium and magnesium sulphate; incompatibilities have occurred with novobiocin sodium, prednisolone sodium phosphate, prochlorperazine, and, depending on concentration, with phosphates.

The chemical and physicochemical characteristics of a monoclinic crystalline form of the hydrated calcium gluceptate containing $3\frac{1}{2}$ H_2O. This crystalline form, which is slightly soluble in water, is responsible for crystallisation of calcium gluceptate in pharmaceutical syrup preparations. Heating calcium gluceptate to between 115° and 120°, or the preparation to above 80°, destroyed this form of calcium gluceptate.— R. Muller *et al.*, *Annls pharm. fr.*, 1979, *37*, 301.

Adverse Effects, Treatment, and Precautions. As for Calcium Salts, p.619.
Mild local reactions may occur after intramuscular injection.

Severe superficial tissue necrosis followed perivenous infiltration in 6 patients receiving infusions of calcium salts. Three of the patients were receiving calcium gluceptate.— *Lancet*, 1976, *1*, 291.

Uses. Calcium gluceptate has the actions of calcium salts (see p.620). It is given intramuscularly or by slow intravenous injection as a solution containing the equivalent of 18 mg of calcium per ml. Intramuscular injection should be avoided in children if possible.

Cardiac resuscitation. For the role of calcium salts in cardiac resuscitation, see p.621.

Preparations

Calcium Gluceptate Injection *(U.S.P.)*. A sterile solution of calcium gluceptate in Water for Injections. It contains the equivalent of 17 to 19 mg of Ca in each ml. pH 5.6 to 7.

1158-r

Calcium Gluconate *(B.P., B.P. Vet., Eur. P.)*.

Calc. Glucon.; Calcii Gluconas; Calcium Glyconate; Calcium Gluconicum. Calcium D-gluconate monohydrate.
$C_{12}H_{22}CaO_{14},H_2O$=448.4.

CAS — 299-28-5 (anhydrous).

Pharmacopoeias. In all pharmacopoeias examined except *U.S.* which has anhydrous.

A white, odourless, tasteless, crystalline or granular powder containing about 9% of calcium. Each g represents approximately 2.2 mmol (4.5 mEq) of calcium. Calcium gluconate 11.2 g is approximately equivalent to 1 g of calcium.
Slowly **soluble** 1 in 30 of water; soluble 1 in 5 of boiling water; practically insoluble in alcohol, chloroform, and ether. Solutions in water are neutral to litmus. Solutions are **sterilised** by autoclaving. **Incompatible** with oxidising agents, citrates, and soluble carbonates, phosphates, and sulphates; with amphotericin, cephalothin sodium, cephazolin sodium, clindamycin phosphate, magnesium sulphate, novobiocin sodium, and prednisolone sodium phosphate; incompatibilities have occurred with oxytetracycline hydrochloride, prochlorperazine, sodium bicarbonate, streptomycin sulphate, and tetracycline hydrochloride.
Calcium gluconate readily forms supersaturated solutions which are relatively stable when free from suspended particles of solid matter; the stability of the solutions may be increased by the addition of a suitable stabiliser such as calcium saccharate.

Incompatibility. The solubility of calcium gluconate rose initially from 1 in 30 to 1 in 20 in the presence of an equal weight of *sodium citrate* but precipitation of calcium citrate occurred after 2 days. In 10% supersaturated solutions the addition of sodium citrate caused immediate precipitation of calcium citrate.— *Pharm. J.*, 1961, *2*, 187 (Pharm. Soc. Lab. Rep.).

Adverse Effects, Treatment, and Precautions. As for Calcium Salts, p.619.

Soft-tissue calcification occurred in 3 infants due to extravasation of calcium gluconate infusions.— P. Berger *et al.*, *Am. J. Roentg.*, 1974, *121*, 109.

Nine neonates were given calcium gluconate intravenously, with care to avoid extravasation. Three to 20 days later 5 developed subcutaneous nodules, with induration and brown discoloration, and 4 developed lesions resembling abscesses or cellulitis; all had X-ray evidence of calcification.— R. S. Ramamurthy *et al.*, *Pediatrics*, 1975, *55*, 802.

Five infants given calcium gluconate 10% (5% in one) via an umbilical artery catheter located in the lower abdominal aorta developed blanching or erythema of the buttocks or thighs progressing in some instances to necrosis. Three infants had occult blood in the stools.— L. S. Book *et al.*, *J. Pediat.*, 1978, *92*, 793.

Absorption and Fate. As for Calcium Salts, p.620.

Uses. Calcium gluconate has the actions of calcium salts (see p.620). Being tasteless and nonirritant to the stomach, it is a more acceptable salt for administration by mouth than the chloride or lactate but it contains less calcium and is less soluble (unless stabilised) than these salts.
Calcium gluconate is usually administered by mouth as tablets; the usual dose is 1 to 5 g, repeated as required. A suggested dose for children is 100 or 125 mg per kg body-weight, given up to 4 times daily. For a more rapid effect it may be given intravenously usually as 10 to 20 ml of a 10% solution. The same dose may also be given intramuscularly. Intramuscular injections are not recommended for children.

For a view that calcium chloride rather than calcium gluconate is the calcium salt of choice for parenteral preparations, see Calcium Chloride, p.622.

Cardiac resuscitation. For the role of calcium salts in cardiac resuscitation, see p.621.

Preparations

Calcium Gluconate Injection *(B.P.)*. Calc. Glucon. Inj. A

sterile solution of calcium gluconate in Water for Injections; not more than 5% of the calcium gluconate may be replaced with calcium saccharate, or other suitable harmless calcium salt, as a stabiliser. Solutions are supersaturated and must be completely free from solid particles.
Many pharmacopoeias contain a similar injection.

Calcium Gluconate Injection *(U.S.P.)*. A sterile solution of anhydrous calcium gluconate in Water for Injections. It may contain small amounts of calcium saccharate or other suitable calcium salts as stabilisers; sodium hydroxide may be added to adjust the pH to 6 to 8.2.

Calcium Gluconate Tablets *(B.P.)*. Tablets containing calcium gluconate. If they are intended to be chewed before being swallowed they are prepared in a chocolate-flavoured basis.

Calcium Gluconate Tablets *(U.S.P.)*. Tablets containing anhydrous calcium gluconate.

Effervescent Calcium Gluconate Tablets *(B.P.)*. Tablets containing calcium gluconate; they should be dissolved in water immediately before use. Store at a temperature not exceeding 25° in airtight containers.

Proprietary Preparations

Calcium Gluconate Gel *(Industrial Pharmaceutical, UK)*. For the treatment of hydrofluoric acid burns.

Other Proprietary Names

Vical *(Ital.)*; Weifa-Kalk *(Norw.)*.

Proprietary Preparations of Related Salts

Sandocal *(Sandoz, UK)*. Effervescent tablets each containing calcium lactate gluconate 3.08 g (equivalent to calcium gluconate 4.5 g) providing 400 mg Ca (10 mmol), 137 mg Na (6 mmol), and 176 mg K (4.5 mmol), with anhydrous citric acid 1.1 g. *Dose*. 1 to 5 tablets daily.

1159-f

Calcium Hydrogen Phosphate *(B.P., B.P. Vet., Eur. P.)*.

Calcii Hydrogenophosphas; Calcii et Hydrogenii Phosphas; Calcium Hydrophosphoricum; Calcium Monohydrogen Phosphate; Dibasic Calcium Phosphate *(U.S.P.)*; Dicalcium Orthophosphate; Dicalcium Phosphate; Phosphate Mono-acide de Calcium; Phosphate Secondaire de Calcium; Fosfato Bicalcio; Fosfato Monocálcico. Calcium hydrogen orthophosphate dihydrate.
$CaHPO_4,2H_2O=172.1$.

CAS — 7757-93-9 (anhydrous); 7789-77-7 (dihydrate).

Pharmacopoeias. In *Arg., Aust., Belg., Br., Eur., Fr., Ger., Hung., Ind., It., Jap., Jug., Mex., Neth., Nord., Pol., Port., Rus., Span.,* and *Swiss.* Also in *U.S.* which also permits anhydrous calcium hydrogen phosphate. The title Calcium Phosphoricum is used in *Hung.* The *Nord.* title is Calcii Phosphas.

A white, odourless, tasteless, crystalline powder with a slightly acid reaction; it may effloresce on exposure to air. It contains about 23% of calcium and about 18% of phosphorus. Calcium hydrogen phosphate 4.29 g is approximately equivalent to 1 g of calcium.
Practically **insoluble** in water and alcohol; sparingly soluble in dilute acetic acid; soluble in dilute hydrochloric or nitric acid. On heating with water it is partially decomposed. It may lose water on exposure to air.

The term brushite has been used to describe crystals of $CaHPO_4$, $2H_2O$ found in the urine.— G. Pylypchuk *et al., Can. med. Ass. J.*, 1979, *120*, 658. See also C. Y. Pak, *J. clin. Invest.*, 1969, *48*, 1914.

Adverse Effects, Precautions, and Absorption and Fate. As for Calcium Salts, p.619. As there is little absorption, there is little danger of systemic adverse effects.

Uses. Calcium hydrogen phosphate is used as a calcium supplement. It has been given in doses of up to 2 g. It is of no value in the treatment of acute manifestations of calcium deficiency.
It is used in fine powder as an abrasive in toothpastes.

For the use of dicalcium phosphate dihydrate in tablet manufacture by direct compression, see E. J. Mendell, *Mfg Chem.*, 1972, *43* (May), 43.

Dental caries. For a review of the use of calcium hydrogen phosphate and other phosphates in preventing dental caries, see *Lancet*, 1968, *1*, 1187.
The addition of 3% of dicalcium phosphate dihydrate to sweets reduced the incidence of dental caries in permanent teeth compared with the consumption of sweets containing 3% of flour but not compared with sweets similar to those commercially available. In deciduous teeth the incidence of dental caries was reduced compared with either control group.— F. P. Ashley *et al., Br. dent. J.*, 1974, *136*, 361 and 418.

Preparations

Dibasic Calcium Phosphate Tablets *(U.S.P.)*. Tablets containing calcium hydrogen phosphate. Potency is expressed in terms of the dihydrate.

Emcompress *(Mendell, USA: K & K-Greeff, UK)*. A brand of calcium hydrogen phosphate, suitable for use as a direct compression agent in tablet manufacture.

Other Proprietary Names

DCP 340 *(Austral., Canad.)*.

1160-z

Calcium Lactate *(B.P., B.P. Vet., Eur. P., U.S.P.)*.

Calcii Lactas; Calc. Lact.
$C_6H_{10}CaO_6,xH_2O=218.2$.

CAS — 814-80-2 (anhydrous); 41372-22-9 (hydrate); 5743-47-5; 63690-56-2 (both pentahydrate).

Pharmacopoeias. In all pharmacopoeias examined except *Cz.* and *Jug.*

A white or almost white efflorescent crystalline or granular powder, odourless or with a slight not unpleasant odour and a slight taste. The *B.P.* specifies 24 to 30% loss on drying; the *U.S.P.* specifies 22 to 27% (pentahydrate), 15 to 20% (trihydrate), 5 to 8% (monohydrate), or not more than 3% (dried form). Each g (pentahydrate) represents approximately 3.2 mmol (6.5 mEq) of calcium. Calcium lactate (pentahydrate) 7.69 g is approximately equivalent to 1 g of calcium.
Soluble 1 in 20 of water at 25°; freely soluble in boiling water; soluble 1 in 1500 of alcohol; practically insoluble in chloroform and ether. A 4.5% solution in water is iso-osmotic with serum. **Incompatible** with soluble carbonates, phosphates, and sulphates, and with oxidising agents. The pentahydrate effloresces on exposure to air and becomes anhydrous when heated at 120°. **Store** in airtight containers.

Adverse Effects, Treatment, Precautions, and Absorption and Fate. As for Calcium Salts, p.619.

Uses. Calcium lactate has the actions of calcium salts (see p.620). It is much less irritant that the chloride and may be administered by mouth as tablets or in solution in doses of 1 to 5 g.

Preparations

Calcium Lactate Tablets *(B.P.)*. Tablets containing calcium lactate.

Calcium Lactate Tablets *(U.S.P.)*. Tablets containing calcium lactate. Potency is expressed in terms of the pentahydrate. Store in airtight containers.

1161-c

Calcium Laevulinate.

Calcium Levulinate *(U.S.P.)*; Calcii Levulinas; Calcium Laevulate; Lévulinate Calcique. Calcium 4-oxovalerate dihydrate.
$C_{10}H_{14}CaO_6,2H_2O=306.3$.

CAS — 591-64-0 (anhydrous); 5743-49-7 (dihydrate).

Pharmacopoeias. In *Aust., Belg., Braz., Chin., Nord., Span., Swiss,* and *U.S.*

A white crystalline or amorphous powder with an odour suggestive of burnt sugar and a bitter salty taste. M.p. 119° to 125°. Each g represents approximately 3.3 mmol (6.5 mEq) of calcium. Calcium laevulinate 7.64 g is approximately equivalent to 1 g of calcium.
Soluble 1 in 2.5 of water and 1 in 800 of alcohol; practically insoluble in acetone, chloroform, and ether. Solutions are **sterilised** by autoclaving or by filtration. A 10% solution in water has a pH of 7 to 8.5. A 3.6% solution is iso-osmotic with serum. **Incompatible** with alkalis, soluble carbonates, phosphates, and sulphates. **Store** in airtight containers.

Sterilisation. During autoclaving of 10% solutions of calcium laevulinate a slight turbidity was produced, due to calcium carbonate which apparently was formed by oxidation of laevulinate. The addition of 0.01% of ascorbic acid before sterilisation prevented the formation of the turbidity.— F. Ernerfeldt and E. Sandell, *Pharm. Acta Helv.*, 1952, *27*, 48.

Adverse Effects, Treatment, Precautions, and Absorption and Fate. As for Calcium Salts, p.619.

Uses. Calcium laevulinate is given by injection in the same manner as calcium gluconate, over which it has the advantage of a higher calcium content. It is given intramuscularly or intravenously as a 10% solution in doses of 1 g (3.3 mmol).

Preparations

Calcium Levulinate Injection *(U.S.P.)*. A sterile solution of calcium laevulinate in Water for Injections. pH 6 to 8.

Proprietary Names

Levucal *(Eddé, Canad.)*.

1162-k

Calcium Phosphate *(B.P.)*.

Precipitated Calcium Phosphate; Neutral Calcium Phosphate; Tribasic Calcium Phosphate *(U.S.N.F.)*; Tricalcium Phosphate; Calcium Orthophosphate; Phosphate Tertiaire de Calcium; Fosfato Tricalcico. It consists mainly of tricalcium diorthophosphate, $Ca_3(PO_4)_2$, together with calcium phosphates of a more acidic or basic character.

CAS — 7758-87-4 [$Ca_3(PO_4)_2$].

Pharmacopoeias. In *Arg., Br., Hung., Ind., Mex., Port., Roum., Span.,* and *Swiss.* Also in *U.S.N.F.*

A white, odourless or almost odourless, tasteless, amorphous powder, containing not less than 90% of calcium phosphates calculated as $Ca_3(PO_4)_2$, i.e. about 34.9% of calcium and about 18% of phosphorus. *U.S.N.F.* specifies 34 to 40% of calcium. At relative humidities between about 15 and 65%, the equilibrium moisture content at 25° is about 2%, but at relative humidities above about 75% it absorbs small additional amounts of moisture.
Practically **insoluble** in water and alcohol; soluble in dilute mineral acids.

Effect of low- and high-humidity ageing on the hardness, disintegration time, and dissolution-rate of calcium phosphate-based tablets.— Z. T. Chowhan and A. A. Amaro, *Drug Dev. ind. Pharm.*, 1979, *5*, 545.

Adverse Effects and Precautions. As for Calcium Salts, p.619. As little calcium phosphate is absorbed, there is little danger of systemic adverse effects.

Absorption and Fate. Calcium phosphate is soluble in gastric acid but is largely insoluble in the intestine and is poorly absorbed.

Uses. Calcium phosphate has been used as a dietary supplement when both calcium and phosphorus are required but is of little use as a therapeutic source of calcium and phosphorus. It has been used as an antacid in doses of about 4 g.
Calcium phosphate is a useful non-hygroscopic diluent for powders and vegetable extracts but it should not be used as a diluent in calciferol pre-

parations because it may considerably modify the absorption of high doses of the vitamin. It is used as a tablet excipient particularly in compression-coated tablets, and in fine powder as an abrasive in toothpastes.

Calcium phosphate Calcarea Phosphorica; Calc. Phos. is used in homoeopathic medicine.

Estimated acceptable total daily dietary phosphorus load: up to 70 mg per kg body-weight, attention being given to the reverse relationship with calcium intake.— Seventeenth Report of the FAO/WHO Expert Committee on Food Additives, *Tech. Rep. Ser. Wld Hlth Org. No. 539,* 1974.

Proprietary Names

Calcevidol *(Farmochimica Italiana, Ital.)*; Kafoma *(Ferring, Swed.)*; Trikalkol *(Laves, Ger.)*.

1163-a

Calcium Saccharate. Calcii Saccharas; Calcium D-Saccharate. Calcium D-glucarate tetrahydrate.
$C_6H_8CaO_8,4H_2O$=320.3.

CAS — 5793-88-4 (anhydrous); 5793-89-5 (tetrahydrate).

Pharmacopoeias. In *Int., Nord.,* and *Turk.*

A white, odourless, tasteless, crystalline powder. Each g represents approximately 3.1 mmol (6.2 mEq) of calcium. Calcium saccharate 8 g is approximately equivalent to 1 g of calcium. **Soluble** 1 in 3000 of water; slightly soluble in boiling water; practically insoluble in alcohol, chloroform, and ether. A saturated solution in water is neutral to litmus. **Store** in airtight containers.

Calcium saccharate is employed as a stabilising agent in solutions of calcium gluconate for injection.

1164-t

Calcium Sodium Lactate *(B.P., B.P. Vet.).*

Calc. Sod. Lact.
$2C_3H_5NaO_3,(C_3H_5O_3)_2Ca,4H_2O$=514.4.

Pharmacopoeias. In *Br.*

A white deliquescent powder or granules with a slight characteristic odour and a slightly acid, bitter taste. Each g represents approximately 1.9 mmol (3.9 mEq) of calcium and 3.9 mmol (3.9 mEq) of sodium. Calcium sodium lactate 12.83 g is approximately equivalent to 1 g of calcium. It melts when heated above 100° and loses water of crystallisation on further heating.

Soluble 1 in 14 of water and 1 in 25 of boiling alcohol; practically insoluble in ether. **Store** in airtight containers.

Adverse Effects, Precautions, and Absorption and Fate. As for Calcium Salts, p.619.

Uses. Calcium sodium lactate has the actions of calcium salts (see p.620). It is given in doses of 0.3 to 2 g (0.6 to 3.9 mmol of calcium).

Preparations

Calcium Sodium Lactate Tablets *(B.P.C. 1973).* Tablets containing calcium sodium lactate. Store in airtight containers.

1165-x

Calcium Sulphate. Calcium Sulfate *(U.S.N.F.)*; Gypsum *(dihydrate)*; Gypsum Fibrosum *(dihydrate)*.
$CaSO_4$=136.1.

CAS — 7778-18-9 (anhydrous); 10101-41-4 (dihydrate).

Pharmacopoeias. In *U.S.N.F.* which specifies the dihydrate or the anhydrous material. *Jap. P.* specifies the dihydrate.

A white to yellowish-white odourless fine powder. Slightly **soluble** in water; soluble in dilute hydrochloric acid.

Calcium sulphate is used as an inert excipient for the preparation of tablets by direct compression. Dried calcium sulphate (see below) known as plaster of Paris, is the hemihydrate.

References: L. A. Bergman and F. J. Bandelin, *J. pharm. Sci.,* 1965, *54,* 445; C. J. Swartz and W. L. Suydam, *ibid.,* 1050.

1166-r

Dried Calcium Sulphate *(B.P.).*

Exsiccated Calcium Sulphate; Calcined Gypsum; Gypsum Siccatum; Plaster of Paris; Sulphate of Lime; Calcii Sulfas Hemihydricus; Calcium Sulphuricum Ustum; Plâtre Cuit; Gebrannter Gips; Yeso Blanco; Gêsso.
$CaSO_4,\frac{1}{2}H_2O$=145.1.

CAS — 7778-18-9 (anhydrous); 10034-76-1; 26499-65-0 (both hemihydrate).

Pharmacopoeias. In *Arg., Aust., Br., Cz., Ger., Hung., Ind., Jap., Jug., Mex., Pol., Port., Span.,* and *Swiss.*

A white or almost white, odourless or almost odourless, tasteless hygroscopic powder. The *B.P.* permits the presence of suitable setting accelerators or decelerators. Slightly **soluble** in water; more soluble in dilute mineral acids; practically insoluble in alcohol. A 20% suspension in water has a pH of 6 to 7.6.

When mixed with a little water it forms a smooth paste which rapidly sets to a hard mass, but if completely dehydrated or heated above 200°, or if much atmospheric moisture has been absorbed, it loses this property. Deterioration is indicated either by too rapid setting or by very slow setting, the set mass being more or less weakened and friable according to the degree of deterioration. The setting-time is retarded by adding a colloid such as dextrin, acacia, methylcellulose, or glue, or any substance which will decrease the solubility, such as alcohol or citrates, and is accelerated by gypsum, sodium chloride, alum, or potassium sulphate. **Store** in airtight containers.

Uses. Dried calcium sulphate is used for the preparation of Plaster of Paris Bandage which is used for the immobilisation of limbs and fractures. Extemporaneously the dried calcium sulphate may be spread thickly on check muslin or book muslin before rolling; after rolling, the bandage is thoroughly moistened and wound round the limb. The bulk of the mass increases slightly as the plaster sets. Alternatively, dried calcium sulphate is mixed to a thin cream, in the proportion of 1 part to 1.5 or 2 parts of water, and the bandaging material passed through the cream immediately before applying to the limb; a 5% solution of dextrin may be used in place of water. The plaster should be set within 15 minutes.

Dried calcium sulphate is also employed for making dental casts.

A review of new materials for the immobilisation of fractures.— D. M. Hunt, *Br. J. Hosp. Med.,* 1980, *24,* 273.

An account of an outbreak of plaster-associated pseudomonas infection. Since the outbreak, plaster casts have been made up with sterile water in an autoclaved stainless-steel bowl, and no further plaster-related wound infections had been observed.— E. T. Houang *et al.* (letter), *Lancet,* 1981, *1,* 728. See also E. G. Dowsett (letter), *ibid.,* 954.

Preparations

Plaster of Paris Bandage *(B.P.).* P.O.P. Bandage; Plaster of Paris Dressing. Bleached cotton gauze impregnated with dried calcium sulphate (not less than 85%) and suitable adhesives and setting-time modifiers. Store at a temperature not exceeding 25°.

Proprietary Preparations

Cellona *(Lohmann, Ger.: Athrodax, UK).* A brand of Plaster of Paris Bandage.

Gypsona Plaster of Paris Bandages *(Smith & Nephew, UK).* A brand of Plaster of Paris Bandage of low plaster loss containing about 90% w/w of plaster.

Plastic support materials are described under Plastics in Part 2.

Substitutes for Plaster of Paris Bandage

Cellamin *(Lohmann, Ger.: Athrodax, UK).* A cotton bandage impregnated with dried calcium sulphate and a synthetic resin. A light-weight alternative to Plaster of Paris Bandage.

Orthoflex *(Johnson & Johnson Orthopaedic, UK).* An elasticated cotton gauze impregnated with dried calcium sulphate. For the initial, closely-conforming layer of a cast, followed by another reinforcing material.

Zoroc *(Johnson & Johnson Orthopaedic, UK).* A cotton bandage impregnated with dried calcium sulphate and a melamine-formaldehyde resin. A light-weight alternative to Plaster of Paris Bandage.

1167-f

Calcium Tetrahydrogen Phosphate. Acid Calcium Phosphate; Monobasic Calcium Phosphate; Monocalcium Phosphate; Phosphate Monocalcique; Phosphate Diacide de Calcium; Phosphate Primaire de Calcium; Fosfato Monocalcico. Calcium tetrahydrogen diorthophosphate monohydrate.
$CaH_4(PO_4)_2,H_2O$=252.1.

CAS — 7758-23-8 (anhydrous).

Pharmacopoeias. In *Arg., Belg., Jap., Span.,* and *Swiss.* In *Port.* with $2H_2O$.

White odourless deliquescent crystals, granules, or powder, with a strong acid taste and reaction. It contains about 16% of calcium and about 24.6% of phosphorus. Calcium tetrahydrogen phosphate 6.29 g is approximately equivalent to 1 g of calcium.

Partly **soluble** in water, with decomposition; practically insoluble in alcohol; soluble in dilute hydrochloric and nitric acids. **Store** in airtight containers.

Calcium tetrahydrogen phosphate is chiefly used in the flour-milling trade and in baking.

1168-d

Hydroxyapatite. A natural mineral with composition similar to that of the mineral in bone. Decacalcium dihydroxide hexakis (orthophosphate).
$3Ca_3(PO_4)_2,Ca(OH)_2$=1004.6.

CAS — 1306-06-5.

Hydroxyapatite is used as a source of calcium and phosphorus in deficiency states.

Proprietary Preparations

Ossopan *(Robapharm, Switz.: Welbeck, UK).* Preparations containing hydroxyapatite in a proteinaceous basis, available as **Powder** providing in each g calcium 176 mg and phosphorus 82 mg and as **Tablets** each providing calcium 43 mg and phosphorus 20 mg. Calcium supplement. *Dose.* One or two 5-ml spoonfuls before food, or up to 16 tablets daily. (Also available as Ossopan in *Fr.*).

A study of Ossopan and its mineral content in the treatment of osteoporosis.— R. A. Durance *et al., Clin. Trials J.,* 1973, *10* (3), 67.

A favourable report of the use of Ossopan for prophylaxis of osteoporosis in corticosteroid-treated rheumatoid arthritis.— K. H. Nilsen *et al., Br. med. J.,* 1978, *2,* 1124.

1169-n

Preparations of Calcium with Vitamin D

Calcium with Vitamin D Tablets *(B.P.C. 1973).* Each contains calcium sodium lactate 450 mg (or calcium lactate 300 mg, or an appropriate quantity of a mixture of calcium sodium lactate and calcium lactate), calcium phosphate 150 mg, and ergocalciferol 12.5 µg (equivalent to 500 units of vitamin D activity). Each tablet contains not less than 79 mg of Ca. Store in a cool place in airtight containers. *Dose.* 1 tablet, to be crushed before administration.

Bee stings. A view that Calcium with Vitamin D Tablets were effective in controlling the swelling that follows bee stings. A dose of 2 tablets three times a day had been used.— D. A. Long (letter), *Prescribers' J.*, 1980, *20*, 52.

Proprietary Preparations

Chocovite *(Medo Chemicals, UK)*. Tablets each containing calcium gluconate 500 mg and ergocalciferol 15 µg (600 units) in a chocolate-flavoured basis. *Dose.* 1 to 3 tablets thrice daily.

Preparations of calcium with vitamin D were also formerly marketed in Great Britain under the proprietary names Calcinate (*LRC Products*) and Caldecium (*Kerfoot*).

1170-k

Magnesium Salts.

Mg=24.305.

Magnesium is an essential body electrolyte. It is the second most important cation in intracellular fluid, is a cofactor in numerous enzyme systems, is involved in phosphate transfer, muscle contractility, and neuronal transmission, and is believed to be essential for the structural stabilisation of nucleic acids. Its activity is often competitive with that of calcium.

The concentration of magnesium in intracellular fluid and plasma is about 15 and 0.75 to 1.1 mmol per litre respectively. About one-third of the magnesium in plasma is bound to plasma protein; most of the remainder is ionised. The total body content of magnesium is about 1000 mmol, of which about 50% occurs in bone. Symptoms of hypermagnesaemia are described below under Adverse Effects while those of hypomagnesaemia are described under the Uses section.

NOTE. Each g of magnesium represents approximately 41.1 mmol (82.3 mEq).

Adverse Effects. Hypermagnesaemia has occurred after dialysis when the dialysate contained excess magnesium, after the intravenous use of magnesium sulphate in toxaemia of pregnancy, after the prolonged use of magnesium sulphate as a purgative, after the excessive use of magnesium-containing antacids, and especially in renal insufficiency. Symptoms of hypermagnesaemia, which may begin to appear when the plasma-magnesium concentration exceeds 2 mmol per litre, include flushing of the skin, thirst, hypotension due to vasodilatation, drowsiness, loss of tendon reflexes due to neuromuscular blockade, weakness, respiratory depression, cardiac arrhythmias, coma, and cardiac arrest.

An extensive review of hypermagnesaemia and its effects.— J. P. Mordes and W. E. C. Wacker, *Pharmac. Rev.*, 1977, *29*, 273.

Severe, life-threatening respiratory depression due to hypermagnesaemia occurred in a 35-year-old man 14 days after irrigation of the renal pelvis with a urologic solution containing magnesium oxide (0.38%), citric acid (3.24%), and calcium carbonate (0.43%).— D. B. Jenny *et al.*, *J. Am. med. Ass.*, 1978, *240*, 1378.

Treatment of Adverse Effects. Hypermagnesaemia may be corrected by the intravenous injection of 10 to 20 ml of 10% Calcium Gluconate Injection. Dialysis and correction of fluid deficit may be of value.

Human Requirements. The average diet contains 10 to 20 mmol of magnesium daily, adequate for normal requirements. Much of the intake is excreted in the urine and the excess in the faeces. Excretion in the urine is reduced in magnesium deficiency.

The US National Research Council recommended the following daily dietary allowances for magnesium: infants up to 6 months, 50 mg; 6 to 12 months, 70 mg; children aged 1 to 3 years, 150 mg; 4 to 6 years, 200 mg; 7 to 10 years, 250 mg; males 11 to 14 years, 350 mg; 15 to 18 years, 400 mg; over 19 years, 350 mg; females over 11 years, 300 mg; during pregnancy and lactation, 450 mg.— *Recommended Dietary Allowances*, 9th Edn, Washington, National Research Council, 1980.

Uses. Plasma concentrations of magnesium are not a complete measure of deficiency but are generally considered the most useful guide available. Deficiency is usually associated with deficiency of calcium and potassium, but the relationship is not clearly defined. Deficiency may occur due to reduced intake, malabsorption, and excessive loss due to vomiting, diarrhoea, and drainage from fistulas; it is commonly associated with alcoholism, pancreatitis, aldosteronism, and may occur in renal tubular necrosis, after the use of diuretics, after the infusion of magnesium-free fluids, especially in diabetic acidosis.

Symptoms, which may occur if the plasma-magnesium concentration falls below 0.5 mmol per litre, include muscle tremor and weakness, tetany due to increased muscle excitability, ataxia, hyperreflexia, tachycardia, mental disturbances of a hyperactive kind, convulsions, cardiac arrhythmias, and cardiac arrest.

Magnesium salts are poorly absorbed from the gastro-intestinal tract and are used as saline purgatives. However, sufficient magnesium is absorbed from the gastro-intestinal tract to replace many deficiency states if magnesium is given by mouth as magnesium hydroxide mixture; magnesium is also absorbed from preparations of magnesium carbonate or oxide. In severe deficiency states, magnesium sulphate may be given intramuscularly or magnesium chloride or sulphate may be administered intravenously. Magnesium acetate and chloride are used as sources of magnesium ions in dialysis solutions.

For a review of magnesium deficiency, metabolism, human requirements, and toxicity, see Report of a WHO Expert Group on Trace Elements in Human Nutrition, *Tech. Rep. Ser. Wld Hlth Org. No. 532*, 1973, 32. See also W. E. C. Wacker and A. F. Parisi, *New Engl. J. Med.*, 1968, *278*, 658, 712, and 772; A. S. Prasad, *Trace Elements and Iron in Human Metabolism*, Chichester, John Wiley, 1978.

A discussion of factors controlling the urinary excretion of magnesium and of hypocalcaemia due to magnesium deficiency.— S. G. Massry, *A. Rev. Pharmac. & Toxic.*, 1977, *17*, 67.

Cardiac disorders. Analysis of the hearts of 64 Canadian males who had died as a result of accidents demonstrated that those who had lived in soft water areas had a mean magnesium heart concentration of 206.7 µg per g while those from hard water areas had a mean concentration of 22.3 µg per g.— T. W. Anderson *et al.* (letter), *Lancet*, 1973, *2*, 1390.

The regional differences in mortality from cardiovascular disease in Finland could be due to differences in the magnesium content of the soil; the high death-rates were associated with low magnesium concentrations.— H. Karppanen and P. J. Neuvonen (letter), *Lancet*, 1973, *2*, 1390. See also M. Bloch, *Br. J. Hosp. Med.*, 1973, *9*, 91; M. S. Seelig (letter), *Br. med. J.*, 1975, *3*, 647.

Forty-two patients with acute myocardial infarction and 9 with acute coronary insufficiency had reduced serum-magnesium concentrations compared with 80 healthy control subjects and 14 patients with chest pains not of cardiac origin.— A. S. Abraham *et al.*, *New Engl. J. Med.*, 1977, *296*, 862. Comments.— J. Zonszein and R. P. Sotolongo (letter), *ibid.*, *297*, 170. Reply.— A. S. Abraham *et al.* (letter), *ibid.*

In a study of myocardial concentrations of magnesium and calcium in heart muscle taken at necropsy, after allowance had been made for a number of factors, samples from patients who died from ischaemic heart disease contained a mean magnesium concentration 23 µg per g lower and a mean calcium concentration 4 µg per g higher than the mean for samples obtained from patients who died from other causes. There was no evidence of any association between concentrations of magnesium and calcium in tissue samples and in the domestic tap water of the various areas.— P. C. Elwood *et al.*, *Lancet*, 1980, *2*, 720.

Further references.— J. S. Bradshaw and G. Dean, *Practitioner*, 1976, *216*, 673.

Diabetic retinopathy. The mean serum-magnesium concentration in 71 insulin-dependent diabetics who had had diabetes for 10 to 20 years was significantly lower than in 194 controls. The magnesium concentration was significantly lower in those with more severe retinopathy than in those with less severe retinopathy.— P. McNair *et al.*, *Diabetes*, 1978, *27*, 1075.

Comment on the possible association between hypomagnesaemia and diabetic retinopathy.— *Lancet*, 1979, *1*, 762.

The mean plasma-magnesium concentration in 582 diabetics was 0.74 mmol per litre compared with 0.81 mmol per litre in 140 controls but there was no evidence thus far of soft-tissue magnesium depletion. A causal relationship between hypomagnesaemia and the vascular complications of diabetes was not yet established.— H. M. Mather and G. E. Levin (letter), *Lancet*, 1979, *1*, 924.

Hypomagnesaemia. A review of the physical and psychiatric symptoms of hypomagnesaemia, including a case report.— R. C. W. Hall and J. R. Joffe, *J. Am. med. Ass.*, 1973, *224*, 1749. A discussion of disorders of magnesium metabolism in infancy.— *Br. med. J.*, 1973, *4*, 373.

A discussion of the association of magnesium deficiency and diuretic therapy.— *Br. med. J.*, 1975, *1*, 170. See also P. Lim and E. Jacob, *ibid.*, 1972, *3*, 620.

A discussion of magnesium deficiency.— *Lancet*, 1976, *1*, 523.

Renal calculi. A brief discussion of the possible role of magnesium in the prevention of renal calculi.— A. Hodgkinson, *Postgrad. med. J.*, 1977, *53*, Suppl. 2, 25.

1171-a

Magnesium Acetate *(B.P.)*.

$C_4H_6MgO_4,4H_2O$=214.5.

CAS — 142-72-3 (anhydrous); 16674-78-5 (tetrahydrate).

Pharmacopoeias. In *Br.*

Odourless or almost odourless colourless crystals or a white crystalline powder. M.p. about 80°. Each g represents approximately 4.7 mmol (9.3 mEq) of magnesium and the equivalent of bicarbonate.

Soluble 1 in 1.5 of water and 1 in 4 of alcohol. A 5% solution in water has a pH of 7.5 to 8.5.

Adverse Effects and Treatment. As for Magnesium Salts, p.625.

Uses. Magnesium acetate is used as a source of magnesium ions in haemodialysis solutions.

1172-t

Magnesium Chloride *(B.P., B.P. Vet., Eur. P., U.S.P.)*.

Mag. Chlor.; Magnesii Chloridum; Magnesium Chloratum; Chlorure de Magnésium Cristallisé; Cloreto de Magnésio.

$MgCl_2,6H_2O$=203.3.

CAS — 7786-30-3 (anhydrous); 7791-18-6 (hexahydrate).

Pharmacopoeias. In *Arg.*, *Br.*, *Cz.*, *Eur.*, *Fr.*, *Ger.*, *It.*, *Jug.*, *Neth.*, *Nord.*, *Port.*, and *U.S.* The *B.P.* also describes Magnesium Chloride for Dialysis.

Colourless odourless hygroscopic crystals with a bitter taste. When heated at 100° it loses 2 molecules of water of crystallisation and at 110° it begins to lose hydrogen chloride, forming basic salts. Each g represents approximately 4.9 mmol (9.8 mEq) of magnesium and 9.8 mmol (9.8 mEq) of chloride.

Soluble 1 in 1 of water and 1 in 2 of alcohol. Solutions are **sterilised** by autoclaving or by filtration. A 5% solution in water has a pH of 4.5 to 7. A 2.02% solution is iso-osmotic with serum. **Store** in airtight containers.

Adverse Effects. As for Magnesium Salts, p.625.

Uraemic pruritus, unresponsive to conventional treatments, in a patient undergoing chronic haemodialysis was promptly relieved when the magnesium concentration of the dialysate was lowered to produce a predialysis serum-magnesium concentration of 0.57 mmol per litre.— H. Graf *et al.*, *Br. med. J.*, 1979, *2*, 1478.

Hypermagnesaemia. Six patients were accidentally dialysed with a solution containing an excessive amount of magnesium—7.5 mmol per litre instead of the usual

0.75 mmol per litre. After about 3 hours of dialysis symptoms of hypermagnesaemia occurred, including blurring of vision, flushing of the face, weakness, and inability to stand. These effects were rapidly reversed after a further dialysis with a known normal dialysate fluid.— J. R. Govan *et al.*, *Br. med. J.*, 1968, *2*, 278.

Treatment of Adverse Effects. As for Magnesium Salts, p.625.

Uses. Magnesium chloride is used primarily as a source of magnesium ions in haemodialysis and peritoneal dialysis solutions. It has been used in the treatment of hypomagnesaemia.

Two children with vitamin D-resistant rickets responded to treatment with magnesium chloride.— V. Reddy and B. Sivakumar, *Lancet*, 1974, *1*, 963.

Hypocalcaemia in a patient with diarrhoea and tetany responded only to treatment with magnesium.— P. Vesin *et al.* (letter), *Lancet* 1974, *2*, 110.

Encouraging results were obtained in 120 patients suffering from stasis ulcers (44), varicose eczema (36), varicose eczema with superimposed contact eczema (20), severe intertrigo (13), cutaneous angiitis (4), Darier's disease (1), widespread capillary haemangioma with ulceration (1), and benign familial chronic pemphigus (1), and treated with a hypertonic cream or lotion containing magnesium chloride, camphor, and other ingredients (Miol). All lesions were initially infected and 96 patients obtained substantial clinical improvement which was maintained for at least a month.— P. W. M. Copeman and S. Selwyn, *Br. med. J.*, 1975, *4*, 264. Criticism.— K. Haeger (letter), *ibid.*, 1976, *1*, 155. A reply.— S. Selwyn and P. Copeman (letter), *ibid.*, 399.

The use of potassium and magnesium solutions to produce elective cardiac arrest (cardioplegia) for open-heart surgery.— *Lancet*, 1981, *1*, 24.

Hypomagnesaemia. Significant falls in serum-magnesium concentrations occurred in 8 of 20 patients with burns; 5 had symptoms of magnesium deficiency. Treatment with magnesium chloride, 4 g daily by mouth or an intravenous infusion of 25 mmol in 500 ml of 0.85% sodium chloride injection, generally produced marked improvement. It was suggested that magnesium deficiency might cause or aggravate psychiatric symptoms in burnt patients.— A. Broughton *et al.*, *Lancet*, 1968, *2*, 1156.

A report of the use of magnesium chloride in a 4-month-old infant with primary hypomagnesaemia; treatment was continued for 4 years.— P. J. Milla *et al.*, *Gut*, 1979, *20*, 1028.

Hypoparathyroidism. A 13-year-old girl with hypoparathyroidism failed to show any improvement in her hypocalcaemia when treated with ergocalciferol or with dihydrotachysterol and calcium salts. Treatment with ergocalciferol and 12.5 mmol of magnesium given as magnesium chloride and citrate brought about prompt improvement.— A. Rösler and D. Rabinowitz, *Lancet*, 1973, *1*, 803. A similar report of magnesium depletion in hypoparathyroidism.— M. E. Scott (letter), *ibid.*, 1005.

Preparations

Delbet's Isotonic Solution. Solutio Isotonica Delbet. A 2% solution of magnesium chloride in water. Used as a wound dressing.

Magnesium Chloride Mixture *(Bristol Roy. Infirm.)*. Magnesium chloride 5 g, lemon syrup 3 ml, raspberry syrup 3 ml, chloroform water to 10 ml. It should be freshly prepared. Each 10 ml provides 25 mmol of Mg. Used in magnesium deficiency from hepatic cirrhosis due to chronic alcoholism.

Another formula. Magnesium chloride 10 g, water freshly boiled and cooled 8 ml, liquorice liquid extract 5 ml, syrup to 20 ml. Each 20 ml provides 50 mmol of Mg. Sodium benzoate 0.1% or potassium sorbate 0.134% were suitable preservatives.—Pharm. Soc. Lab. Rep. P/78/1, 1978.

Miol *(Comprehensive Pharmaceuticals, UK)*. **Cream** containing magnesium chloride 1.5%, sodium chloride 2.1%, calcium chloride 0.2%, alcloxa 1%, chlorphenesin 0.1%, and camphor 4% and **Lotion** containing magnesium chloride 1.42%, sodium chloride 1.98%, calcium chloride 0.17%, alcloxa 1%, and camphor 1%. For pruritic, inflammatory, and ulcerative conditions of the skin and mucosa.

Other Proprietary Names

Slow Mag *(S.Afr.)*.

1173-x

Magnesium Citrate.

$C_{12}H_{10}Mg_3O_{14}$=451.1.

CAS — 3344-18-1.

Uses. Magnesium citrate is used as a mild purgative preferably on an empty stomach with a substantial fluid intake. The usual dose of Magnesium Citrate Oral Solution *U.S.P.* is 200 ml as a single dose.

After chronic abuse of magnesium citrate a 62-year-old woman with adequate renal function became lethargic and developed severe refractory hypotension. She was found to have extreme hypermagnesaemia [6.25 mmol per litre] and a perforated duodenal ulcer. There was a transient rise in blood pressure after a bolus dose of calcium chloride. Peritoneal dialysis reduced the serum-magnesium concentration and reversed the hypotension but the patient subsequently died.— J. P. Mordes *et al.*, *Ann. intern. Med.*, 1975, *83*, 657.

Preparations

Magnesium Citrate Oral Solution *(U.S.P.)*. Magnesium Citrate Solution; Magnesia Lemonade; Limonata Aerata Laxans; Limonade Citro-Magnésienne; Limonada Purgante. A colourless or slightly yellow, clear, effervescent liquid with a sweet acidulous taste, prepared by dissolving magnesium carbonate 15 g in a solution of anhydrous citric acid 27.4 g (or the equivalent amount of citric acid monohydrate) in water, adding syrup 60 ml, heating to boiling-point, adding lemon oil 0.1 ml previously triturated with talc 5 g, and filtering while hot. The mixture is cooled, diluted to 350 ml, and potassium bicarbonate 2.5 g or if citric acid monohydrate is used sodium bicarbonate 2.1 g added. The container is immediately stoppered and shaken; the solution may be further carbonated by the use of carbon dioxide under pressure. The solution is sterilised or pasteurised. Store at 8° to 30°.

A similar preparation is included in several pharmacopoeias.

Proprietary Names

Citro-Mag *(Rougier, Canad.)*; National Laxative *(Therapex-Unik, Canad.)*.

1203-w

Magnesium Gluconate *(U.S.P.)*. Magnesium D-gluconate (1:2) dihydrate.

$C_{12}H_{22}MgO_{14},2H_2O$=450.6.

CAS — 3632-91-5 (anhydrous); 59625-89-7 (dihydrate).

Pharmacopoeias. In *U.S.*

Colourless odourless tasteless crystals or a white powder or granules. Each g represents approximately 2.2 mmol (4.4 mEq) of magnesium. Freely **soluble** in water; very slightly soluble in alcohol; practically insoluble in ether. A 5% solution in water has a pH of 6 to 7.8.

Magnesium gluconate is used as a source of magnesium.

Preparations

Magnesium Gluconate Tablets *(U.S.P.)*. Tablets containing magnesium gluconate. Potency is expressed in terms of the equivalent amount of anhydrous magnesium gluconate.

Proprietary Names

Erimag *(ICN, Canad.)*; GYN *(Amfre-Grant, USA)*; Mikroplex Magnesium *(Herbrand, Ger.)*; Ultra Mg *(Sopar, Belg.)*.

1174-r

Magnesium Sulphate *(B.P., B.P. Vet., Eur. P.)*. Mag. Sulph.; Magnesium Sulfate *(U.S.P.)*; Magnesii Sulfas; Magnesium Sulfuricum Heptahydricum; Epsom Salts; Sal Amarum; Sel Anglais, Sel de Sedlitz.

$MgSO_4,7H_2O$=246.5.

CAS — 10034-99-8.

Pharmacopoeias. In all pharmacopoeias examined except *Int.*

Odourless, brilliant, colourless crystals or a white crystalline powder with a cool saline bitter taste. It effloresces in warm dry air and is converted to the monohydrate when heated at 150° to 160°. The last molecule of water of crystallisation is expelled at about 280°. Each g represents approximately 4.1 mmol (8.1 mEq) of magnesium and of sulphate.

Soluble 1 in 1.5 of water and 1 in 0.5 of boiling water; practically insoluble in alcohol; slowly soluble 1 in 1 of glycerol. A 5% solution in water has a pH of 5 to 9.2. A 6.3% solution is iso-osmotic with serum. Solutions are **sterilised** by autoclaving or by filtration.

Incompatible with polymyxin B sulphate, with sodium and potassium tartrates, with soluble phosphates and arsenates, and with alkali carbonates and bicarbonates unless in dilute solution; with potassium or ammonium bromide, concentrated solutions give a precipitate of the double sulphate. **Store** in a cool place in airtight containers.

Incompatibility. There was loss of clarity when intravenous solutions of magnesium sulphate were mixed with those of calcium gluconate, novobiocin sodium, procaine hydrochloride, or sodium bicarbonate.— J. A. Patel and G. L. Phillips, *Am. J. Hosp. Pharm.*, 1966, *23*, 409.

Magnesium sulphate was reported to be incompatible with concentrated solutions of sodium iodide.— K. P. Van Der Linde and R. K. Campbell, *Drug Intell. & clin. Pharm.*, 1977, *11*, 30.

Adverse Effects. As for Magnesium Salts, p.625. Though magnesium is poorly absorbed following oral administration, there may be sufficient accumulation to produce toxic effects if given to a patient with impaired renal function.

Death could occur within 2 hours of oral or rectal administration of magnesium sulphate in children with intestinal worms, or in other patients whose gut had become unusually permeable to magnesium sulphate. Extreme thirst and a feeling of heat were signs of poisoning. Calcium gluconate 1 g should be injected intravenously as soon as possible.— D. W. Fawcett and J. P. Gens, *J. Am. med. Ass.*, 1943, *123*, 1028.

A woman with a reduced gastric volume and a gastric stoma developed profound prostration with respiratory depression after taking an estimated 70 g of magnesium sulphate for bowel preparation. Her clinical condition improved dramatically within minutes of receiving an intravenous injection of calcium gluconate.— A. K. Aucamp *et al.* (letter), *Lancet*, 1981, *2*, 1057.

In 14 women who had received magnesium sulphate intravenously for eclampsia or pre-eclampsia the concentration of magnesium in the maternal blood at delivery was 1.5 to more than 7 mmol per litre, and the concentration in cord blood was 1.55 to 5.75 mmol per litre. The mean comparable values for healthy individuals were 0.88 and 0.93 mmol respectively. Several of the infants had reduced muscle tone, a weak cry, cyanosis, and respiratory depression; the symptoms could not be correlated with magnesium concentrations. While hypoxia might be responsible for some of the symptoms, they were consistent with hypermagnesaemia. The infants usually improved within 24 to 48 hours.— P. J. Lipsitz and I. C. English, *Pediatrics*, 1967, *40*, 856.

The mothers of 2 infants born with hypermagnesaemia and striking abdominal distension had received magnesium sulphate 25 to 39 g on the day before delivery.— M. M. Sokal *et al.*, *New Engl. J. Med.*, 1972, *286*, 823. Comment.— J. A. Pritchard (letter), *ibid.*, *287*, 48. Reply.— M. R. Koenisberger, *ibid.*

When 22 healthy persons were given 20.55 mmol of magnesium as magnesium sulphate by intravenous infusion, there was a decrease in serum-calcium concentration, an increase in the urinary excretion of calcium, an initial decrease in serum phosphate values, and a decrease in the urinary excretion of phosphate. The last 2 factors were considered to be indicative of a role of magnesium in parathyroid function.— T. H. Mountokalakis *et al.* (letter), *J. Am. med. Ass.*, 1972, *221*, 195.

Treatment of a newborn infant having suspected hyaline membrane disease with a magnesium sulphate enema produced fatal systemic magnesium intoxication.— E. W. Outerbridge *et al.*, *J. Am. med. Ass.*, 1973, *224*, 1392. Comment.— D. Stowens (letter), *ibid.*, *225*, 751.

Bolus intravenous injections of magnesium sulphate frequently produced slowing of maternal respirations and hypotension in women with toxaemia in labour; there was occasional transient apnoea.— B. K. Young and H. M. Weinstein, *Obstet. Gynec.*, 1977, *49*, 681.

A report of acute pulmonary oedema in 2 patients given magnesium sulphate and betamethasone to prevent premature labour.— J. P. Elliott *et al.*, *Am. J. Obstet. Gynec.*, 1979, *134*, 717.

Cardiopulmonary arrest in a pregnant woman given a probable overdose of magnesium sulphate.— J. H. McCubbin *et al.* (letter), *Lancet*, 1981, *1*, 1058.

Treatment of Adverse Effects. As for Magnesium Salts, p.625.

Precautions. The use of magnesium sulphate is inadvisable in patients with impaired renal function and in children with intestinal parasitic diseases.

Magnesium therapy was dangerous in patients with renal failure. Both antacids and enemas containing magnesium salts were contra-indicated in such patients. Magnesium sulphate should not be given by injection for nephritic convulsions unless hypomagnesaemia had been confirmed and the serum concentration of magnesium was monitored. The intravenous route for administering magnesium sulphate was potentially the most hazardous and should be employed only for the immediate control of convulsions threatening life. Severe respiratory depression usually accompanied serum-magnesium concentrations of 7.5 mmol per litre, and the disappearance of the knee-jerk reflex was an indicator of incipient toxicity.— W. E. C. Wacker and A. F. Parisi, *New Engl. J. Med.*, 1968, *278*, 772.

Parenteral administration of magnesium sulphate and either tubocurarine or suxamethonium to 2 women with pre-eclampsia demonstrated the possible hazards of this treatment due to the enhancement of the action of muscle relaxants by magnesium.— M. M. Ghoneim and J. P. Long, *Anesthesiology*, 1970, *32*, 23. See also A. J. C. de Silva, *Br. J. Anaesth.*, 1973, *45*, 1228.

Absorption and Fate.

Plasma-magnesium concentrations of 36.8 μg per ml were measured at birth in 16 premature infants and 5 full-term infants, whose mothers had received magnesium therapy. The maternal plasma concentration was 42 μg per ml and this was the plasma concentration measured in the infants when 2 hours old. The neonatal half-life was 43 hours and plasma concentrations in the infants did not fall to a normal value for about a week.— B. C. Dangman and T. S. Rosen, *Pediat. Res.*, 1977, *11*, 415.

Uses. Magnesium sulphate is a saline purgative. Such purgatives act because they are not readily absorbed from the intestine. When taken by mouth in dilute solution they reduce the normal absorption of water from the intestine with the result that the bulky fluid contents distend the bowel, active reflex peristalsis is excited, and evacuation of the contents of the intestine follows. With higher concentrations water is withdrawn from the tissues. Magnesium may also cause purgation by the release of cholecystokinin. The usual dose as a saline purgative is 5 to 15 g, and the best results are obtained by taking the dose in about 250 ml of water, preferably before breakfast. A suggested dose for children is 100 to 250 mg per kg body-weight. Magnesium sulphate has been used like sodium sulphate to hasten the excretion of drugs in overdosage and of other toxic substances. Doses of up to 30 g in 250 ml of water have been used.

A 50% solution of magnesium sulphate in water, in a dose of 60 to 180 ml, has been given as an enema.

When introduced into the circulation, magnesium sulphate acts as a depressant to the central nervous system and has been used to lower intracranial pressure and to control the convulsions in acute uraemia and eclampsia. The usual intramuscular dose is 1 to 5 g, as a 25 or 50% solution, repeated up to 6 times daily if necessary. Intravenously 1 to 4 g may be given as a 10 or 20% solution at a rate not exceeding 150 mg per minute. It may also be given by infusion. The blood pressure should be monitored during each injection.

Because of its osmotic action it has been employed locally in various inflammatory conditions.

Magnesium sulphate is a common ingredient of aperient mineral waters.

There were reports in the literature of surgery being performed under anaesthesia induced by magnesium sulphate, but in 2 persons the administration of magnesium sulphate by slow intravenous infusion, until the serum concentration of magnesium was about 10 times the initial value of 0.7 mmol per litre, failed to induce anaesthesia. The patients remained aware of their surroundings, were conscious to pain, and vision and hearing were not affected.— G. Somjen *et al.*, *J. Pharmac. exp. Ther.*, 1966, *154*, 652.

Arterial disease. Magnesium sulphate in angina pectoris and other cardiovascular disorders.— S. E. Browne, *Practitioner*, 1969, *202*, 562. See also *idem*, 1964, *192*, 781. Ineffectiveness in angina pectoris.— Z. Voslářová, *Čas. Lék. česk.*, 1965, *104*, 292.

Cardiac arrhythmia. Intravenously administered magnesium sulphate, 100 mg per kg body-weight, had an anti-arrhythmic effect in 18 of 27 patients with ventricular fibrillation due to hypothermia. Defibrillation was noted within 3 to 9 minutes after administration of magnesium sulphate.— B. Büky, *Br. J. Anaesth.*, 1970, *42*, 886. A similar report.— K. D. Chadda *et al.*, *Am. J. Cardiol.*, 1973, *31*, 98, per *Int. pharm. Abstr.*, 1973, *10*, 413. See also P. I. Parkinson and D. S. P. Dickson (letter), *Br. med. J.*, 1969, *3*, 175. See also under Hypokalaemia.

Eclampsia. In the treatment of eclampsia, the following dosage of magnesium sulphate was recommended: initially 4 g by intravenous injection, subsequent doses by intramuscular injection according to body-weight. Signs of magnesium toxicity might appear at serum concentrations above 2 mmol per litre.— *Med. Lett.*, 1969, *11*, 38.

An account of the standardised treatment of 154 consecutive cases of eclampsia, treated over a period of 20 years, using magnesium sulphate, in association with hydralazine if necessary to control diastolic pressures exceeding 110 mmHg, and intravenous fluid therapy. The magnesium sulphate dosage regimen was: intravenous injection of magnesium sulphate 4 g as 20 ml of a 20% solution, given over at least 3 minutes, followed immediately by intramuscular injection of magnesium sulphate 10 g as 20 ml of a 50% solution (5 g being injected into the upper outer quadrant of each buttock); every 4 hours thereafter magnesium sulphate 5 g as 10 ml of a 50% solution was injected intramuscularly into alternate buttocks after ascertaining that the knee jerk (patellar reflex) was present, urine flow had been 100 ml or more in the previous 4 hours, and respirations were not depressed.— J. A. Pritchard and S. A. Pritchard, *Am. J. Obstet. Gynec.*, 1975, *123*, 543. Mention of the use of an initial infusion, rather than intravenous injection, to avoid the risk of respiratory depression.— C. E. Flowers, *ibid.*, 549.

Mention of the use of magnesium sulphate, by infusion, to maintain a serum-magnesium concentration of 3 to 4 mmol per litre, in 169 patients with eclampsia or pre-eclampsia.— W. A. Andersen and G. M. Harbert, *Am. J. Obstet. Gynec.*, 1977, *129*, 260.

A brief discussion of the use of magnesium sulphate in pre-eclampsia and eclampsia; the aim was to achieve a magnesium concentration of 3 to 4 mmol per litre.— B. M. Hibbard and M. Rosen, *Br. J. Anaesth.*, 1977, *49*, 3.

Further references: L. Speroff, *Am. J. Cardiol.*, 1973, *32*, 582.

Effect on gastro-intestinal tract. In 20 patients with the irritable bowel syndrome the administration of magnesium sulphate 100 mg per kg body-weight in 150 ml of water caused a prompt increase in colon motility, particularly in those in whom eating produced pain. The effect was considered due to magnesium sulphate-induced release of cholecystokinin.— R. F. Harvey and A. E. Read, *Gut*, 1973, *14*, 983.

From studies in 18 patients undergoing routine pancreatic investigations it was concluded that magnesium sulphate was a satisfactory purgative for speeding the intestinal transit of pancreatic enzymes and did not stimulate the mean output of bicarbonate or trypsin in response to exogenous secretin and cholecystokinin-pancreozymin.— J. H. B. Saunders *et al.*, *Gut*, 1976, *17*, 435.

Further references.— J. Malagelada *et al.*, *Am. J. dig. Dis.*, 1978, *23*, 481.

Hypocalcaemia, neonatal. Magnesium sulphate in neonatal hypocalcaemia.— T. L. Turner *et al.*, *Lancet*, 1977, *1*, 283.

Hypokalaemia. In 34 patients with suspected magnesium deficiency generally due to diuretic therapy, infusions of potassium chloride did not affect the potassium concentration in muscle; when magnesium sulphate was first given the potassium concentration was then increased, and there was a significant decrease in the incidence of ventricular ectopic beats.— T. Dyckner and P. O. Wester, *Am. Heart J.*, 1979, *97*, 12.

Hypomagnesaemia. For a review of reports of hypomagnesaemia in children and a discussion of its significance and treatment, see *Lancet*, 1967, *1*, 712.

A sequential trial involving 52 malnourished Nigerian children showed that children given intramuscular injections of magnesium sulphate solution 50% rapidly acquired a good appetite; subnormal temperature and hypotension were corrected within 24 hours. Inactive and fretful children became more alert and mobile. The dose was usually 1 ml for children weighing less than 9 kg or 1 to 1.5 ml for heavier children, given every 12 hours for 1 to 3 days, then once daily. In some hypotensive children premature withdrawal of magnesium therapy led to death, but persistence sometimes produced a dramatic improvement.— J. L. Caddell, *New Engl. J. Med.*, 1967, *276*, 535. See also J. L. Caddell and D. R. Goddard, *ibid.*, 533.

Of 40 young children in hospital with convulsions, tremors, or muscular twitchings, 13 were found to have hypomagnesaemia without hypocalcaemia. Recovery occurred either spontaneously or after daily doses of 0.5 to 2 ml of an injection containing 50% of magnesium sulphate, usually given in divided doses of 0.5 ml one to four times daily.— H. B. Wong and Y. F. Teh, *Lancet* 1968, *2*, 18.

Hyponatraemia. Eight patients with severe congestive heart failure, oedema, hyponatraemia, and an increasing resistance to diuretic treatment had high concentrations of sodium and chloride and low concentrations of potassium and magnesium in skeletal muscle. Administration of 30 mmol of magnesium sulphate in 5.5% dextrose produced an increase in concentrations of sodium in serum, while concentrations of sodium and chloride in skeletal muscle fell and concentrations of potassium in skeletal muscle rose.— T. Dyckner and P. O. Wester, *Lancet*, 1981, *1*, 585.

Premature labour. Magnesium sulphate given intravenously for prevention of premature labour (abolition of contractions for at least 24 hours).— C. M. Steer and R. H. Petrie, *Am. J. Obstet. Gynec.*, 1977, *129*, 1.

Preparations

Magnesium Sulfate Injection *(U.S.P.)*. A sterile solution of magnesium sulphate in Water for Injections. pH of a 5% solution 5.5 to 7. *Nord. P.* specifies 20%.

Magnesium Sulphate Bath *(B.P.C. 1949)*. Balneum Magnesii Sulphatis. Magnesium sulphate 480 g in 140 litres of water.

Magnesium Sulphate Enema *(B.P.C. 1959)*. Magnesium sulphate 50% in water. *Rectal dose.* 60 to 180 ml.

Magnesium Sulphate Mixture *(B.P.)*. Mist. Mag. Sulph.; Mistura Alba. Magnesium sulphate 4 g, light magnesium carbonate 500 mg, concentrated peppermint emulsion 0.25 ml, double-strength chloroform water 3 ml, water to 10 ml. It should be recently prepared.
Dose. 10 to 20 ml.

Proprietary Preparations

Fletchers' Disposable Magnesium Sulphate Retention Enema *(Pharmax, UK)*. A 50% solution of magnesium sulphate in a plastic bag, containing 130 ml, fitted with a rectal tube.

Other Proprietary Names

Addex-Magnesium *(Swed.)*; Sulmetin Simple Endovenoso *(Spain)*.

Proprietary Names of some other Magnesium Compounds

Mg-Plus (magnesium-protein complex)*(USA)*.

1175-f

Dried Magnesium Sulphate *(B.P.)*. Dried Mag. Sulph.; Exsiccated Magnesium Sulphate; Mag. Sulph. Exsic.; Dried Epsom Salts.

CAS — 7487-88-9.

Pharmacopoeias. In *Arg., Aust., Belg., Br., Cz., Hung., Ind., Jug., Nord., Pol., Rus.,* and *Swiss.*

A white odourless powder with a bitter saline taste, prepared by heating magnesium sulphate at 100° until it has lost about 25% of its weight; it contains 62 to 70% of $MgSO_4$.

Soluble 1 in 2 of water; more rapidly soluble in hot water; practically insoluble in alcohol. A

37.5% solution in water may be slightly turbid at first but becomes clear in a few minutes. A 7.5% solution in water is neutral to phenol red. **Store** in airtight containers.

Uses. Dried magnesium sulphate is employed when the use of the hydrated salt would be disadvantageous. As Magnesium Sulphate Paste it is used as an application to boils and carbuncles but prolonged or repeated use may damage the surrounding skin.

Preparations

Magnesium Sulphate Paste *(B.P.).* Past. Mag. Sulph.; Morison's Paste. Dried magnesium sulphate, after heating at 150° or 130°, 45 g, glycerol, heated at 120° for 1 hour and cooled, 55 g, and phenol 500 mg. Heat about 70 g of dried magnesium sulphate for 1½ hours at 150° or for 4 hours at 130° or longer if necessary, to ensure that the dried powder contains at least 85% of $MgSO_4$ and allow to cool in a desiccator; mix 45 g of this powder in a warm mortar with the phenol dissolved in the glycerol. It should be stirred before use.
Collapsible tubes are not considered suitable containers for this preparation.

1176-d

Potassium Salts.

K=39.098.

Potassium is an essential body ion. It is the principle cation of intracellular fluid and is intimately involved in cell function and metabolism. It is essential for carbohydrate metabolism and glycogen storage and for protein synthesis. It is intimately involved in transmembrane potential and has profound effects on muscle, including heart muscle.
The concentration of potassium in intracellular fluid and plasma is about 160 and 3.5 to 5 mmol respectively per litre.
The total body content of potassium is about 3500 mmol depending on the size of the non-fat mass. The concentration of potassium in plasma is not a reliable indication of total body stores.
Potassium turnover is to a certain extent the consequence of that of sodium. The conservation of sodium by the kidney is by exchange for either potassium or hydrogen ion, preferably the former. In consequence, when low intake of both sodium and potassium pertains, then sodium is conserved while potassium loss continues. Symptoms of hyperkalaemia are described below under Adverse Effects while those of hypokalaemia are described under the Uses section.
The uses of the potassium salts described in this section are dependent largely on the extent to which they are absorbed when taken by mouth. Those which are readily absorbed are used mainly in the prevention and treatment of potassium deficiency or as mild diuretics and those less well absorbed have been used as saline purgatives.

NOTE. Each g of potassium represents approximately 25.6 mmol (25.6 mEq).

Adverse Effects. The toxicity of potassium salts by mouth in healthy individuals is slight, since potassium is rapidly excreted in the urine. With some salts, such as potassium chloride, nausea, vomiting, diarrhoea, and abdominal cramps may occur. Also the administration of potassium salts, particularly in enteric-coated tablets, may cause intestinal ulceration; see under Potassium Chloride and Potassium Gluconate.
Hyperkalaemia may occur after excessive intake (including the excessive transfusion of stored blood), after the use of potassium-sparing diuretics, in adrenal cortical insufficiency, renal failure, and acidosis, and after tissue trauma. Symptoms include paraesthesia of the extremities, listlessness, mental confusion, weakness, paralysis, hypotension, cardiac arrhythmias, heart block, and cardiac arrest. Adverse effects may occur from the intravenous injection of even small doses of potassium salts when excretion is delayed, as in the presence of renal insufficiency.

An 84-year-old woman died about 90 minutes after drinking with suicidal intent a liquid preparation containing at least 540 mmol of potassium. About 1 hour after ingestion the patient had a grand mal convulsion followed by coma; her blood pressure was unrecordable. Intravenous administration of metaraminol and 20 ml of 10% calcium gluconate was without effect. No vomiting or diarrhoea occurred.— M. Kaplan, *Ann. intern. Med.*, 1969, *71*, 363.

Hyperkalaemia occurred in acute renal failure, severe acidosis, trauma associated with muscle necrosis, adrenal insufficiency, after the use of potassium-sparing diuretics, and after excessive oral or parenteral administration of potassium. It had been considered minimal if serum concentrations did not exceed 6.5 mmol per litre, moderate between 6.5 and 8 mmol per litre, and severe above 8 mmol per litre. Cardiac arrhythmias appeared above 5.5 mmol per litre and clinical signs above 6.5 mmol per litre. Cardiac arrhythmias or a concentration above 6.5 mmol per litre generally called for immediate treatment.— S. R. Newmark and R. G. Dluhy, *J. Am. med. Ass.*, 1975, *231*, 631.

Treatment of Adverse Effects. Potassium-containing foods must be eliminated from the diet and potassium-retaining diuretics withdrawn. Severe cardiac toxicity, which requires immediate attention, may be treated by the intravenous injection, over 1 to 5 minutes, of 10 to 20 ml of Calcium Gluconate Injection 10%, with ECG monitoring. Serum concentrations of potassium may be reduced by infusions of dextrose, 300 to 500 ml per hour of 10 or 25% solution, containing up to 10 units of insulin for each 20 g of dextrose, or by the infusion of sodium bicarbonate solution.
Mild hyperkalaemia may be treated with sodium polystyrene sulphonate (see p.870), administered by mouth or as an enema. In severe hyperkalaemia, treatment with haemodialysis or peritoneal dialysis may become necessary.
Hyperkalaemia associated with hyponatraemia may respond to treatment with infusions of sodium salts.

The first requirement of treatment was to reverse the ECG changes; for this purpose 10 to 20 ml of 10% calcium gluconate or 10% calcium chloride was given by slow intravenous injection over 5 to 10 minutes; the effect was transitory and the injection would need to be repeated, under ECG control. Hyperkalaemia could be reduced by the rapid intravenous injection of 44 mmol of sodium bicarbonate which transferred potassium from extracellular to intracellular sites; for each 0.1 unit rise in pH the serum-potassium concentration would fall by 0.5 to 1 mmol per litre. Further infusions would be required. Dextrose reduced the serum-potassium concentration by increasing glycogen and potassium storage and by facilitating intracellular potassium transport; 500 to 1000 ml of 10% dextrose was given over 1 hour with 10 to 15 units of insulin. Sodium polystyrene sulphonate, given as an enema, removed 1 mmol of potassium for each g of resin; 30 g in 100 to 200 ml was retained for 4 hours and repeated 2 or 3 times daily; it could also be given by mouth in sorbitol solution. The method was too slow for the treatment of acute hyperkalaemia. Peritoneal dialysis and haemodialysis were effective but slow.— S. R. Newmark and R. G. Dluhy, *J. Am. med. Ass.*, 1975, *231*, 631. See also N. G. Levinsky, *New Engl. J. Med.*, 1966, *274*, 1076.

Precautions. Potassium salts should be administered by mouth in well-diluted solutions. Intravenous injections should be given slowly as high blood concentrations may affect cardiac function. Potassium salts should be given cautiously to patients with renal or adrenal insufficiency, acute dehydration, or heat cramp. Care should be exercised if potassium salts are given concomitantly with potassium-sparing diuretics.

Administration of dextrose with potassium to potassium-depleted patients could cause a decrease in serum-potassium concentration associated with the metabolism of glucose. The decrease in serum potassium could precipitate dangerous ventricular arrhythmias in patients with severe potassium depletion and in those receiving digitalis. When such patients required intravenous potassium therapy it was recommended that the concentration of potassium in dextrose be relatively high to minimise the danger.— A. S. Kunin *et al.*, *New Engl. J. Med.*, 1962, *266*, 228.

Studies in 5 healthy subjects indicated a circadian variation in response to potassium infusion. It was suggested that additional care should be taken when administering potassium infusions at night.— M. C. Moore-Ede *et al.*, *Clin. Pharmac. Ther.*, 1978, *23*, 218.

Absorption and Fate. Potassium salts other than the phosphate, sulphate, and tartrate are generally readily absorbed from the gastro-intestinal tract. Potassium is excreted mainly by the distal tubules of the kidney; 5 to 10 mmol a day may be excreted in the faeces, and some in perspiration. The urinary excretion of potassium continues even when intake is low, and faecal losses may be large in the presence of diarrhoea.

Human Requirements. It has been suggested that the average adult requires about 20.5 to 33.3 mmol of potassium daily. The normal diet provides 60 to 100 mmol of potassium daily.
Foods reported to be rich in potassium include apricots, avocados, bananas, cherries, dried fruits, tomatoes, beans (butter and haricot), and potatoes.

For the potassium content of certain foods, see *Manual of Nutrition*, Ministry of Agriculture, Fisheries and Food, London, HM Stationery Office, 1970; F. J. Salter and R. E. Pearson (letter), *J. Am. med. Ass.*, 1970, *212*, 1526; A. A. Paul and D. A. T. Southgate, *The Composition of Foods*, London, HM Stationery Office, 1978.

Uses. Hypokalaemia may occur due to decreased intake (malnutrition, alcoholism, starvation) or due to increased loss (vomiting, diarrhoea, fistulas) and commonly occurs in acid base disturbances characterised by alkalosis, aldosterone excess, Cushing's syndrome, during recovery from diabetic acidosis, periodic familial paralysis, and renal tubular dysfunction. Losses are increased after burns, stress, trauma, surgery, and during the use of thiazide diuretics and related substances. The excessive use of corticosteroids is said to increase renal losses but the data is conflicting.
Deficiency of potassium ions may cause vomiting, abdominal distension, paralytic ileus, acute muscular weakness, reduced or absent reflexes, paralysis, paraesthesia, mental clouding, dyspnoea, respiratory failure, polydipsia and an inability to concentrate urine, hypotension, cardiac dilatation, cardiac arrhythmias and coma. Hypokalaemia increases the potential toxicity of digitalis and other cardiac glycosides.
There is no uniform correlation between plasma concentrations of potassium and total body stores. Up to 300–400 mmol of potassium may be lost in an adult without change in plasma concentrations. Clinical signs of deficiency may occur whenever the plasma-potassium concentration falls below 3.5 mmol per litre. The need for potassium and the dosage should therefore be based on the patient's history and clinical condition, only supplemented by plasma-potassium estimation. Treatment should preferably be given by mouth but in acute potassium deficiency a solution of potassium chloride or acetate may be administered intravenously.
For administration by mouth doses of up to 40 mmol 3 or 4 times daily may be required with frequent measurement of concentration in plasma. For intravenous use up to 80 to 120 mmol may be needed daily; it should be given under ECG control in a solution containing not more than 40 mmol per litre at a rate not exceeding 30 mmol per hour, preferably after the infusion of one litre of potassium-free solution, to demonstrate adequate renal function. It may also be given with sodium chloride to replace simultaneously sodium and chloride losses due to excess loss as in vomiting and diarrhoea. Prophylactically solutions are given containing electrolytes, including potassium, in amounts broadly similar to those in plasma, to replace electrolytes and fluids lost in vomiting, diarrhoea, and after injury.
There are differences in judgement concerning

the need for potassium supplements in patients taking diuretics (see p.581). When potassium supplements are given, they should preferably be given on the days other than those on which the diuretic is administered. The usual daily dose is up to 40 to 80 mmol of potassium.

Potassium salts may be given in the treatment of cumulative digitalis poisoning —see p.532.

Potassium salts have a low renal threshold and excretion promotes diuresis. The phosphate, sulphate, and tartrate salts of potassium may be given by mouth to reduce the normal absorption of water from the intestine and, by promoting peristalsis, to cause evacuation of the intestine. They act promptly when administered as a dilute solution but rather more slowly if given as a concentrated solution.

Potassium salts by mouth are more irritant than the corresponding sodium salts and should be taken after meals. Unless enteric coated, potassium chloride tablets should be crushed and dissolved in water before administration. As potassium deficiency is often associated with hypochloraemic alkalosis, adequate amounts of chloride ions should be administered concomitantly.

Some potassium salts are used as sodium-free condiments when sodium intake must be restricted.

A study of total body potassium in non-dialysed and dialysed patients with chronic renal failure.— K. Boddy *et al.*, *Br. med. J.*, 1972, *1*, 771.

Equations for the prediction of exchangeable body potassium according to weight, height, age, and sex.— F. Skrabal *et al.*, *Br. med. J.*, 1973, *2*, 37.

Discussions of the use of potassium supplements.— *Drug & Ther. Bull.*, 1972, *10*, 47; T. O. Morgan, *Drugs*, 1973, *6*, 222; *Lancet*, 1974, *2*, 1123; *Br. med. J.*, 1974, *4*, 307; M. E. Kosman, *J. Am. med. Ass.*, 1974, *230*, 743; L. Beeley, *Adverse Drug React. Bull.*, 1980, Oct., 304; *idem*, *J. R. Coll. Physns*, 1980, *14*, 58.

A discussion of the treatment of hyperkalaemia and hypokalaemia.— S. R. Newmark and R. G. Dluhy, *J. Am. med. Ass.*, 1975, *231*, 631.

A discussion of potassium metabolism and diuretics in cirrhosis of the liver.— P. Vesin, *Postgrad. med. J.*, 1975, *51*, 545.

The indications for potassium therapy and the hazards associated with its use.— D. H. Lawson, *Br. J. Hosp. Med.*, 1976, *16*, 392.

Potassium-containing salt substitutes as a source of potassium.— J. A. Sopko and R. M. Freeman, *J. Am. med. Ass.*, 1977, *238*, 608.

Potassium homoeostasis and the roles of insulin and aldosterone.— M. Cox *et al.*, *New Engl. J. Med.*, 1978, *299*, 525.

Electrolyte studies: potassium, chloride, and acid-base.— M. D. Burke, *Postgrad. Med.*, 1978, *64*, 205.

A discussion on hypokalaemia and potassium depletion and their management with potassium supplements or potassium-sparing diuretics.— T. O. Morgan, *Drugs*, 1979, *18*, 218.

A discussion on the active transport of sodium and potassium ions.— K. J. Sweadner and S. M. Goldin, *New Engl. J. Med.*, 1980, *302*, 777.

Cardiac disorders. For studies on regimens of potassium, dextrose, and insulin in myocardial infarction, see p.630.

Diabetes. References to the use of potassium supplements in patients with diabetic acidosis or diabetic coma are provided under insulin, see p.847.

Paralysis. Comment on the management of familial hypokalaemic periodic paralysis. The mainstay of prophylaxis and treatment continues to be potassium.— *Lancet*, 1981, *1*, 1140. Further references: T. Johnsen, *Dan. med. Bull.*, 1981, *28*, 1.

1177-n

Potassium Acetate *(B.P., U.S.P.)*.

Potassii Acetas; Kalii Acetas.

$CH_3.CO_2K = 98.14$.

CAS — 127-08-2.

Pharmacopoeias. In *Br., Braz., Ind., Pol., Port., Rus., Span.*, and *U.S.*

A solution of potassium acetate is included in *Aust., Jug.*, and *Pol.* (all about 33%). *Jap.* has 38%.

Colourless crystals or a white crystalline powder; odourless or with a faint acetous odour and a saline, slightly alkaline taste. It is deliquescent in moist air. Each g represents approximately 10.2 mmol (10.2 mEq) of potassium.

Soluble 1 in 0.5 of water and 1 in about 3 of alcohol. A 5% solution in water has a pH of 7.5 to 9.5. A 1.53% solution is iso-osmotic with serum. **Incompatible** with acids and with silver, mercury, and iron salts. **Store** in airtight containers.

Adverse Effects, Treatment, and Precautions. As for Potassium Salts, p.628.

Uses. Potassium acetate may be used similarly to potassium chloride for the prevention and treatment of potassium deficiency.

Potassium acetate is also used as a source of potassium in solutions for haemodialysis and peritoneal dialysis.

Potassium acetate has been used as a diuretic.

It is added to solutions for hardening and preserving tissues in order to preserve their natural colour (e.g. Kaiserling's solutions) and it is also used as a food preservative.

Preparations

Potassium Acetate Injection *(U.S.P.)*. A sterile solution of potassium acetate in Water for Injections. pH (of a 1% solution) 5.5. to 8. To be diluted before use.

Trikates Oral Solution *(U.S.P.)*. A solution of potassium acetate, potassium bicarbonate, and potassium citrate in water. Store in airtight containers. Protect from light.

1178-h

Potassium Bicarbonate *(B.P.C. 1973, U.S.P.)*.

Pot. Bicarb.; Potassium Hydrogen Carbonate; Kalium Bicarbonicum; Potassii Bicarbonas; Carbonato Monopotássico.

$KHCO_3 = 100.1$.

CAS — 298-14-6.

Pharmacopoeias. In *Arg., Braz., Ger., Ind., Mex., Nord., Pol., Port., Span., Swiss*, and *U.S.*

Colourless, odourless or almost odourless, transparent prisms or white granular powder with a saline, feebly alkaline taste. Each g represents approximately 10 mmol (10 mEq) of potassium.

Soluble 1 in 3 of water; practically insoluble in alcohol. A 1% solution in water has a pH of not more than 8.6.

Adverse Effects, Treatment, and Precautions. As for Potassium Salts, p.628.

Uses. Potassium bicarbonate has been used for the prevention and treatment of potassium deficiency. It is an alkalinising agent and has been used as a diuretic.

It has been used similarly to sodium bicarbonate as an antacid, but it is unsuitable for intravenous use in the treatment of metabolic acidosis because of the pharmacological effect of the potassium ion.

Preparations

Effervescent Potassium Tablets *(B.P.C. 1968)*. Tab. Pot. Efferv. Each contains potassium bicarbonate 500 mg, potassium acid tartrate 300 mg, anhydrous citric acid 200 mg, sucrose 200 mg, and saccharin sodium 5 mg (representing 6.6 mmol of potassium). Store in a cool place in well-filled airtight containers. The tablets should be dissolved in water before administration.

1179-m

Potassium Chloride *(B.P., Eur. P., U.S.P.)*.

Pot. Chloride; Potassii Chloridum; Kalii Chloridum; Kalium Chloratum; Cloreto de Potássio.

$KCl = 74.55$.

CAS — 7447-40-7.

Pharmacopoeias. In all pharmacopoeias examined.

Odourless, colourless, cubical, elongated, or prismatic crystals or white crystalline powder with a saline taste. It is anhydrous and decrepitates when heated. Each g represents approximately 13.4 mmol (13.4 mEq) of potassium.

Soluble 1 in 3 of water, 1 in 400 of alcohol (90%), and 1 in 16 of glycerol; practically insoluble in dehydrated alcohol and ether. A solution in water is neutral to litmus. A 1.19% solution in water is iso-osmotic with serum. Solutions are **sterilised** by autoclaving or by filtration. **Incompatible** with silver, lead, and mercury salts.

Addition to intravenous fluids. Transient unconsciousness in 2 patients was attributed to hyperkalaemia due to inadequate mixing of concentrated potassium chloride solution added to intravenous fluids in flexible plastic containers.— R. H. P. Williams, *Br. med. J.*, 1973, *1*, 714. See also E. E. A. Watkins and H. L. Daniels (letter), *Pharm. J.*, 1973, *1*, 71; W. Woodside *et al.*, *J. Hosp. Pharm.*, 1973, *31*, 192.

Incompatibility. A haze developed over 3 hours when potassium chloride 4 g per litre was mixed with amphotericin 200 mg per litre in dextrose injection.— B. B. Riley, *J. Hosp. Pharm.*, 1970, *28*, 228.

Mixtures. Potassium chloride mixtures made with lemon syrup, with or without concentrated chloroform water, and with benzoic acid or the hydroxybenzoates remained clear after 4 weeks' storage at room temperature in white flint glass bottles. These solutions all had a pH of 2 to 2.3; without lemon syrup the mixtures had a pH of about 5 and became cloudy.— Pharm. Soc. Lab. Rep. No. P/69/2, 1969.

Release and absorption from tablets. For reports, see C. G. Barlow (letter), *J. Pharm. Pharmac.*, 1965, *17*, 822; M. Payne, *Pharm. J.*, 1966, *1*, 657; C. Graffner and J. Sjögren, *Acta pharm. suec.*, 1971, *8*, 13; U. Otto and G. Rooth, *ibid.*, 1973, *10*, 337; D. Ben-Ishay and K. Engelman, *Clin. Pharmac. Ther.*, 1973, *14*, 250; D. L. Levene (letter), *Can. med. Ass. J.*, 1973, *108*, 1480; J. A. Rider *et al.*, *J. Am. med. Ass.*, 1975, *231*, 836.

Adverse Effects, Treatment, and Precautions. As for Potassium Salts, p.628.

There have been numerous reports of intestinal ulceration, sometimes with haemorrhage and perforation or with the late formation of strictures, after the use of enteric-coated tablets of potassium chloride. Gastric ulceration has also been reported. Ulceration has also occurred after the use of sustained-release tablets.

Comments on the dangers of slow-release potassium tablets.— *Med. Lett.*, 1975, *17*, 73.

Of 60 patients on potassium chloride therapy 18 had impaired absorption of vitamin B_{12}.— I. P. Palva *et al.*, *Acta med. scand.*, 1972, *191*, 355.

A comment on the possible hazards of nausea, retching, and vomiting brought on by the unpleasant taste of potassium chloride in solution. Three patients suffered life-threatening cardiovascular complications immediately after or during ingestion of potassium chloride solution; 2 subsequently died. Nausea with eructation or vomiting preceded the complications. When fluctuations in cardiac output and arterial pressure are undesirable, potassium replacement should be given intravenously, especially if the patient complains of nausea.— F. H. Messerli and N. D. Pappas (letter), *Lancet*, 1980, *2*, 919. Intravenous potassium administration is not without hazard. Oral supplements might safely be given as the potassium gluconate solution (Katorin).— J. Smith (letter), *ibid.*, 1135. Emphasis that potassium must be given as the chloride.— R. G. Benians (letter), *ibid.*, 1300.

Hyperkalaemia. Hyperkalaemia occurred in 179 (3.6%) of 4921 patients given potassium supplements, with a mean peak concentration of 6 mmol per litre; 13 had concentrations greater than 7.5 mmol per litre. Adverse effects of potassium were considered to have contributed to the death of 7 patients, to have threatened the lives of 21 more, with hyperkalaemia as the principal factor, and to have produced considerable morbidity in a further 29. Other side-effects included gastro-intestinal effects (60), phlebitis (4), and arrhythmias (3). Potassium supplements should be given with caution particularly to the elderly and to those with impaired renal function.—Boston Collaborative Drug Surveillance Programme, *Q.J. Med.*, 1974, *43*, 433.

Excessive use of potassium-containing salt substitutes resulted in hyperkalaemia with cardiac arrhythmia in 2 patients who had an impaired ability to excrete potassium due to congestive heart failure, uraemia, and administration of spironolactone.— V. Yap *et al.*, *J. Am. med. Ass.*, 1976, *236*, 2775.

Although a 25-year-old woman with sickle-cell haemoglobinopathy had a normal response to acute potassium loading she developed life-threatening hyperkalaemia after receiving only modest amounts of potassium chloride over 3 days. It was recommended that potassium should be administered with caution to patients with sickle-cell haemoglobinopathy.— P. Mitnick *et al.* (letter), *Ann. intern. Med.*, 1979, *91*, 319.

Rapid development of life-threatening hyperkalaemia following overdose with slow-release potassium tablets.— R. N. Illingworth and A. T. Proudfoot, *Br. med. J.*, 1980, *281*, 485.

Uses. Potassium chloride is mainly used in the prevention and treatment of potassium deficiency—see under Potassium Salts, p.628. As it contains chloride ions it is employed in the treatment of hypokalaemia associated with hypochloraemic alkalosis. It may be administered by mouth in a dilute solution or as slow-release tablets in which it is contained in a wax matrix.

In acute potassium deficiency, a solution of potassium chloride may be administered intravenously; administration should be slow and under ECG control.

Potassium chloride is used in the treatment of cumulative digitalis poisoning—see p.532. It may be administered intravenously if the patient is unable to tolerate treatment by mouth.

There should be careful mixing when adding concentrated potassium chloride solutions to infusion fluids (see p.629).

Cardiac disorders. The role of potassium in cardiac failure.— *Br. med. J.*, 1977, *1*, 469.

Myocardial infarction. A regimen which included insulin, potassium, and dextrose, with other supportive treatment, reduced the mortality-rate in patients with myocardial infarction from 28.2 to 11.7%.— B. Mittra, *Lancet*, 1965, *2*, 607; *idem*, 1966, *2*, 1438.

In a controlled study in 840 patients with recent myocardial infarction, a regimen of potassium, dextrose, and insulin did not significantly affect the chances of survival.—Report by the MRC Working-Party on the Treatment of Myocardial Infarction, *Lancet*, 1968, *2*, 1355. A similar conclusion following the treatment of 200 patients.— B. L. Pentecost *et al.*, *ibid.*, 1968, *1*, 946. A study in 15 patients undergoing cardiac catheterisation showed that there was no consistent increased uptake of potassium by the myocardium when they were given potassium, dextrose, and insulin. The findings confirmed the conclusions of the MRC Working-Party.— H. Ikram and J. S. Pryor (letter), *ibid.*, 1969, *1*, 104.

Discrepancies in the results of the polarising treatment of myocardial infarction with potassium, dextrose, and insulin were due to different methods of treatment.— D. Sodi-Pallares *et al.* (letter), *Lancet*, 1969, *1*, 1315.

A discussion of the role of potassium, dextrose, and insulin in the treatment of myocardial infarction.— *Lancet*, 1972, *2*, 1295.

In 70 patients with proven acute myocardial infarction free fatty acid concentrations were significantly reduced after the infusion into the right atrium for 48 hours, at a rate of 0.5 to 2 ml per kg body-weight per hour, of a solution containing in each litre dextrose 300 g, insulin 50 units, and potassium chloride 80 mmol. The mortality-rate was 11 of 70 compared with 19 of 64 similar patients not so treated.— W. J. Rogers *et al.*, *Am. Heart J.*, 1976, *92*, 441.

A favourable report on the use of a concentrated glucose-insulin-potassium mixture as an infusion after acute myocardial infarction.— *J. Am. med. Ass.*, 1977, *237*, 1070.

Preparations

Elixirs

Potassium Chloride Elixir *(U.S.P.)*. An elixir containing potassium chloride and alcohol about 18%. pH 5.7 to 6.7. Store in airtight containers.

Injections

Cardioplegia Injection *(St. Thomas' Hosp.)*. Potassium chloride 5.965 g, magnesium chloride 16.265 g, procaine hydrochloride 1.364 g, Water for Injections to 100 ml. Pack into 20 ml ampoules and seal under nitrogen. Sterilise by autoclaving. Add 20 ml to 1 litre of Ringer's Injection (*U.S.P.*) or Compound Sodium Chloride Injection (*B.P.C. 1959*) and administer by local infusion to the coronary arteries during cardiopulmonary bypass. Contains in each 20 ml potassium 16 mmol, magnesium 16 mmol, and procaine 1 mmol. A similar preparation is used at *Gt Ormond St Child. Hosp.* and at *Bristol Roy. Infirm.*

Potassium Chloride and Dextrose Intravenous Infusion *(B.P.)*. Potassium Chloride and Dextrose Injection; Pot. Chlor. and Dextrose Inj. A sterile solution of potassium chloride and anhydrous dextrose or dextrose monohydrate for parenteral use in Water for Injections. It is sterilised, immediately after preparation, by autoclaving. pH 3.5 to 5.5. Rapid infusion may be harmful. Store at a temperature not exceeding 25°.

Potassium Chloride and Sodium Chloride Intravenous Infusion *(B.P.)*. Potassium Chloride and Sodium Chloride Injection; Pot. Chlor. and Sod. Chlor. Inj. A sterile solution of potassium chloride and sodium chloride in Water for Injections. Sterilised by autoclaving. Rapid infusion may be harmful.

Potassium Chloride Injection *(U.S.P.)*. A sterile solution in Water for Injections. pH 4 to 8. To be diluted before use.

Potassium Chloride, Sodium Chloride and Dextrose Intravenous Infusion *(B.P.)*. Potassium Chloride, Sodium Chloride and Dextrose Injection; Pot. Chlor., Sod. Chlor. and Dextrose Inj. A sterile solution of potassium chloride, sodium chloride 0.17 to 0.19%, and anhydrous dextrose 3.8 to 4.2% (or the equivalent of dextrose monohydrate for parenteral use) in Water for Injections. Sterilise immediately by autoclaving. pH 3.5 to 5.5. Store at a temperature not exceeding 25°. It may cause the separation of solid particles from glass containers; solutions containing such particles must not be used. Rapid infusion may be harmful.

Strong Potassium Chloride Solution *(B.P. 1973)*. Sterile Potassium Chloride Solution *(B.P. 1968)*. A sterile 15% solution of potassium chloride in Water for Injections. pH 5 to 7. It contains approximately 20 mmol (20 mEq) of potassium and of chloride in 10 ml and must be diluted before use with not less than 50 times its vol. of sodium chloride injection or other suitable diluent.

Mixtures

Mixtura Kalii Chloridi *(Dan. Disp.)*. Potassium chloride 3.3 g, sweet orange-peel tincture 5 g, syrup 20 g, and water 71.7 g. Each 15 ml contains about 500 mg of potassium chloride [providing 6.7 mmol of potassium and of chloride].

Potassium Chloride Mixture *(A.P.F.)*. Potassium chloride 1 g, lemon syrup 2 ml, concentrated chloroform water 0.25 ml, water to 10 ml.

Each 10 ml contains 13.4 mmol of potassium and of chloride.

Solutions

Bretschneider's Solution No. 3. Sodium chloride 70 mg, potassium chloride 75 mg, magnesium chloride 20 mg, procaine hydrochloride 200 mg, mannitol 4.35 g, water for injections to 100 ml. For cardioplegia in aortic valve surgery.—T. Søndergaard *et al.*, *J. cardiovasc. Surg.*, 1975, *16*, 288,.

The use of potassium and magnesium solutions to produce elective cardiac arrest (cardioplegia) for open-heart surgery.— *Lancet*, 1981, *1*, 24.

Kidney Preservation Solution. Solution C_4. Potassium chloride 112 mg (1.5 mmol; 1.5 mEq), potassium acid phosphate 205 mg (potassium 1.5 mmol), potassium phosphate trihydrate 970 mg (potassium 8.5 mmol), sodium bicarbonate 84 mg (1 mmol), procaine hydrochloride 10 mg, heparin 500 units, phenoxybenzamine 2.5 mg, dextrose 2.5 g, magnesium sulphate 738 mg (3 mmol), Water for Injections to 100 ml. pH 7. The first 6 ingredients were dissolved in the Water for Injections and sterilised by autoclaving. A faint turbidity occurred when phenoxybenzamine was added in the preparation of solution C_4 but cleared within 24 hours. Dextrose and magnesium sulphate were each added as 50% solutions immediately before use. The solution was used for cold (0° to 4°) perfusion of *dogs'* kidneys before transplantation and increased the storage life to 30 hours by replacing losses of intracellular potassium and magnesium. Solution C_3 contained no phenoxybenzamine.—G.M. Collins *et al.*, *Lancet*, 1969, *2*, 1219.

Collins' preservation solution (C_4) had proved superior to other solutions such as balanced salt solution for the preservation of human kidneys. It had been used regularly for this purpose without any stability problems.— H. Collste *et al.* (letter), *Lancet*, 1970, *2*, 780.

Of 29 human kidneys perfused with Collins' C_3 preservative solution before storage on ice for up to 12 hours, 24 functioned immediately when transplanted.— L. C. J. Hartley *et al.*, *New Engl. J. Med.*, 1971, *285*, 1049.

The effect of ischaemic injury on kidneys preserved in Collins' C_4 solution.— R. W. G. Johnson, *Br. J. Surg.*, 1972, *59*, 765.

A modification of Collins' C_4 solution: potassium chloride 112 mg, potassium acid phosphate 205 mg, potassium phosphate trihydrate 740 mg, sodium bicarbonate 84 mg, procaine hydrochloride 10 mg, phenoxybenzamine 2.5 mg, heparin 500 units, chlorpromazine 1.6 mg, dextran '40' 5 g, dextrose 2.5 g, Water for Injections to 100 ml. The electrolytes were dissolved in 50 ml of Water for Injections and sterilised by autoclaving.

A few hours before use, heparin, chlorpromazine, and phenoxybenzamine were added and the solution filtered. Finally 50 ml of 10% Rheomacrodex in 5% dextrose was added and the osmolality adjusted with dextrose. This solution and hyperbaric oxygen were used in the preservation of *dog* kidneys which had been subjected to periods of warm ischaemia.— M. E. Snell *et al.*, *Br. J. Surg.*, 1972, *59*, 886.

A comparison of 146 first-graft transplants with kidneys preserved in Collins' solution and 401 preserved on the Belzer machine.— E. A. Clark *et al.*, *Lancet*, 1973, *1*, 361. Favourable results with the Belzer technique.— H. C. Miller *et al.* (letter), *ibid.*, 880.

Kidneys should not be stored for periods as long as 24 hours in Collins' preservative solution because of potential damage.— R. M. R. Taylor *et al.* (letter), *Lancet*, 1973, *1*, 551.

Two preservation solutions were used successfully to preserve *canine* kidneys for up to 72 hours and to protect ischaemic kidneys subjected to normothermia for up to 3 hours. The first was a modified Collins' solution which contained in each 100 ml potassium chloride 112 mg, potassium acid phosphate 205 mg, potassium phosphate trihydrate 970 mg, sodium bicarbonate 84 mg made hyperosmolar (410 mosmol per litre) with mannitol 5 g, and provided the following electrolytes: potassium 11.5 mmol, sodium 1 mmol, chloride 1.5 mmol, and bicarbonate 1 mmol. The second solution contained in each 100 ml, potassium acid phosphate 476 mg, potassium phosphate trihydrate 970 mg, potassium bicarbonate 230 mg, sodium bicarbonate 126 mg, mannitol 3.75 g to give an osmolarity of 430 mosmol per litre, and magnesium chloride. This provided the following electrolytes: potassium 12.6 mmol, sodium 1.4 mmol, chloride 1.6 mmol, bicarbonate 2 mmol, and magnesium 0.8 mmol.— S. A. Sacks *et al.*, *Lancet*, 1973, *1*, 1024. A modified formula.— J. Y. Masude *et al.*, *Am. J. Hosp. Pharm.*, 1975, *32*, 397.

The high concentration of magnesium was the cause of the precipitation that was sometimes seen in Collins' C_4 solution.— L. T. Welch and W. J. Flanigan (letter), *Lancet*, 1973, *2*, 1444.

Phenoxybenzamine produced a turbidity that lasted for 24 to 48 hours in Collins' C_4 solution; kidneys perfused with this turbid solution did not recover function.— Z. F. Braf and H. Boichis (letter), *Lancet*, 1974, *1*, 563.

A modified method of preparing Collins' C_3 solution, including disodium edetate.— V. Fenton-May and C. Jones (letter), *Pharm. J.*, 1975, *1*, 448.

Phenoxybenzamine, heparin, and procaine hydrochloride had been eliminated without ill effect.— G. M. Collins and N. A. Halasz (letter), *Lancet*, 1975, *1*, 220.

Cardiac arrest occurred during renal transplantation when the vascular clamps were removed from a kidney that had been preserved in Collins' solution. Study in 8 further cases showed transient increases of up to 5.3 mmol in the potassium concentration in the right atrium following the removal of clamps. Changes were minimal when the clamps were slowly released.— J. P. Soulillon *et al.*, *Nephron*, 1977, *19*, 301.

Potassium Chloride for Oral Solution *(U.S.P.)*. A dry mixture of potassium chloride and one or more suitable diluents, colouring, and flavouring agents. Store in airtight containers.

Potassium Chloride Oral Solution *(U.S.P.)*. A solution containing potassium chloride. It may contain up to 7.5% of alcohol. Store in airtight containers.

Tablets

Potassium Chloride Tablets *(B.P. 1973)*. Pot. Chloride Tab. Tablets containing potassium chloride. The tablets should be dissolved in water before administration.

Store in airtight containers.

Proprietary Preparations

Cellular Repair Solution (Nabarro's Solution) *(Boots, UK)*. A solution for intravenous infusion containing potassium chloride 0.149%, potassium phosphate 0.087%, sodium chloride 0.117%, magnesium chloride 0.024%, and anhydrous dextrose 5%, providing in each litre potassium 30 mmol, sodium 20 mmol, magnesium 1 mmol, and chloride 42 mmol.

Kay-Cee-L *(Geistlich, UK)*. Potassium chloride, available as a sugar-free syrup containing 5 mmol in each 5 ml.

K-Contin *(Napp, UK).* Potassium chloride, available as tablets of 600 mg (8 mmol of potassium and of chloride), in a slow-release basis.

Kloref *(Cox Continental, UK).* Effervescent tablets each containing betaine hydrochloride 740 mg, potassium bicarbonate 455 mg, potassium chloride 140 mg, and potassium benzoate 50 mg; providing, on solution, potassium chloride 500 mg (6.7 mmol of potassium and of chloride). **Kloref-S.** Effervescent granules in sachets each containing potassium chloride 500 mg, potassium bicarbonate 1.35 g, and betaine hydrochloride 2.07 g providing, on solution, potassium chloride 1.5 g (20 mmol of potassium and of chloride).

Leo K *(Leo, UK).* Potassium chloride, available as tablets of 600 mg (8 mmol of potassium and of chloride), in a slow-release wax basis. (Also available as Leo-K in *S.Afr.*).

Owing to the risk of intestinal obstruction, sustained-release preparations such as Leo K, where the drug is released in transit, but the matrix ghost is often eliminated intact, should not be prescribed in patients with Crohn's disease or other intestinal disease in which strictures may form.— J. L. Shaffer *et al.* (letter), *Lancet*, 1980, *2*, 487.

Nu-K *(Consolidated Chemicals, UK).* Potassium chloride, available as sustained-released Capsules of 600 mg.

Paediatric Electrolyte Solution *(Boots, UK).* A solution for intravenous infusion containing potassium chloride 0.149%, potassium phosphate 0.13%, sodium lactate molar solution 1.825%, sodium chloride 0.117%, hydrochloric acid 0.042%, and anhydrous dextrose 5%, providing in each litre potassium 35 mmol, sodium 38 mmol, chloride 45 mmol, and bicarbonate (as lactate) 18 mmol.

Sando-K *(Sandoz, UK).* Effervescent tablets each containing potassium chloride 600 mg and potassium bicarbonate 400 mg, providing potassium 12 mmol and chloride 8 mmol, with anhydrous citric acid 800 mg.

Slow-K *(Ciba, UK).* Tablets each containing potassium chloride 600 mg (8 mmol of potassium and of chloride), in a slow-release wax core. (Also available as Slow-K in *Austral., Canad., Jap., S.Afr., USA*).

A 15-month-old child died after ingesting 8 Slow-K tablets. He had vomited and been unconscious for several hours before admission to hospital when his serum-potassium concentration was 9.9 mmol per litre; he died 75 minutes later with a serum-potassium concentration of 14 mmol per litre.— C. Bacon (letter), *Br. med. J.*, 1974, *1*, 389.

Reports of oesophageal, gastric, or intestinal stricture or ulceration after the use of Slow-K.— A. D. Howie and R. W. Strachan, *Br. med. J.*, 1975, *2*, 176; S. J. Heffernan and J. J. Murphy (letter), *ibid.*, 746; M. A. Farquharson-Roberts *et al.*, *ibid.*, *3*, 206; F. Sandor, *J. R. Coll. gen. Pract.*, 1976, *26*, 595; F. G. McMahon and K. Akdamar (letter), *New Engl. J. Med.*, 1976, *295*, 733; S. M. Weiss *et al.* (letter), *ibid.*, 1977, *296*, 111.

Owing to the risk of intestinal obstruction, sustained-release preparations such as Slow-K, where the drug is released in transit, but the matrix ghost is often eliminated intact, should not be prescribed in patients with Crohn's disease or other intestinal disease in which strictures may form.— J. L. Shaffer *et al.* (letter), *Lancet*, 1980, *2*, 487.

Other Proprietary Names

Arg.—Celeka, Durules-K; *Austral.*— Chlorvescent, K-San, Kay Ciel, Span-K; *Belg.*— Chloropotassuril, Kalium Durettes, Steropotassium, Ultra-K-Chlor; *Canad.*— Kaochlor, Kay Ciel, K-Lyte/Cl, K-10 Solution, Roychlor; *Denm.*— Kaleorid, Kalinorm; *Fr.*—Kaleorid, Potassion (see also under Potassium Gluconate); *Ger.*— Kalinor, Kalium-Duriles, Rekawan; *Ital.*—Kadalex, Lento-Kalium; *Neth.*—Kalium Durettes; *Norw.*— Kaleorid, Kalilente, Kalium Duretter, Kali-Retard; *S.Afr.*—Peter-Kal, Lento-K; *Spain*—Miopotasio, Potasion (see also under Potassium Gluconate); *Swed.*—Kaleorid, Kalilente, Kalipor, Kalitabs, Kalium Duretter; *Switz.*—Kaliglutol; *USA*— Kaochlor, Kaochlor S-F, Kaon-Cl, Kato, Kay Ciel, Klor, Klor-Con, K-Lor, Klorfen, Klorvess 10% Liquid, Klotrix, K-Lyte/Cl, Pan-Kloride, PfiKlor, Rum-K.

Potassium chloride was also formerly marketed in Great Britain under the proprietary name Kalium Durules (*Astra*).

Some Proprietary Sodium-free Condiments

Ruthmol *(Cantassium Co., UK: Dendron, UK).* A sodium-free salt substitute containing potassium chloride 50%, lactose and potato starch.

Selora (known in some countries as Neocursal and Neocurtasal) *(Winthrop, UK).* A sodium-free salt substitute containing potassium chloride 92.05%, hydrated calcium silicate 1%, glutamic acid 1.15%, and potassium glutamate 5.79%.

1180-t

Potassium Citrate *(B.P., Eur. P., U.S.P.).*

Pot. Cit.; Kalii Citras; Kalium Citricum; Tripotassium Citrate.

$C_6H_5K_3O_7,H_2O=324.4$.

CAS — 866-84-2 (anhydrous); 6100-05-6 (monohydrate).

Pharmacopoeias. In *Br., Chin., Eur., Fr., Ger., Hung., Ind., Neth., Nord., Port.,* and *U.S.*

Transparent, odourless, hygroscopic crystals or a white granular powder with a fresh saline taste. Each g represents approximately 9.25 mmol (9.25 mEq) of potassium.

Soluble 1 in 1 of water and 1 in 2.5 of glycerol; practically insoluble in alcohol, chloroform, and ether. A solution in water has a pH of 7.5 to 9. **Incompatible** with calcium and strontium salts. Aqueous solutions, owing to their slight alkalinity, may react with acidic substances. **Store** in airtight containers.

Adverse Effects, Treatment, and Precautions. As for Potassium Salts, p.628.

Hyperkalaemia caused by potassium citrate mixture.— J. J. Browning and K. S. Channer, *Br. med. J.*, 1981, *283*, 1366.

Uses. Potassium citrate, after absorption, is metabolised and acts similarly to sodium bicarbonate in rendering the urine less acid. It has a less marked purgative action than potassium tartrate. Its use is followed by a mild diuresis. Potassium citrate is employed in the treatment of inflammatory conditions of the bladder and to prevent crystalluria during treatment with sulphonamides. It may also be used as a potassium supplement (see under Potassium, p.628). Potassium citrate is given in a dose of up to 10 g daily in divided doses; it is usually administered in mixtures.

Cholera. Potassium loss during cholera could be replaced by mouth. Green coconut water contained 70 mmol per litre; 170 g for each litre of stool would prevent significant depletion. Potassium citrate 10% solution could be given in 15-ml doses (diluted) 3 or 4 times daily.— Second Report of WHO Expert Committee on Cholera, *Tech. Rep. Ser. Wld Hlth Org. No. 352*, 1967.

Urinary-tract infections. The use of Potassium Citrate Mixture alone was to be condemned in the treatment of urinary-tract infection; it might allay symptoms but did not eradicate bacteriuria.— R. R. Bailey, *Drugs*, 1974, *8*, 54.

Preparations

Mixtura Kalii Citratis *(Nord. P.).* Potassium citrate 8 g, citric acid monohydrate 500 mg, water 41.5 g, methyl hydroxybenzoate 100 mg, black currant syrup 50 g. Store in a cool place. Each 10 ml contains about 8.6 mmol of potassium.

Potassium Citrate and Citric Acid Oral Solution *(U.S.P.).* Contains, in each 100 ml, potassium citrate 20.9 to 23.1 g and citric acid monohydrate 6.34 to 7.02 g in a suitable aqueous vehicle, providing approximately 2 mmol of potassium per ml. pH 4.9 to 5.4. Store in airtight containers.

Potassium Citrate and Hyoscyamus Mixture *(A.P.F.).* Mist. Pot. Cit. et Hyoscy. Potassium citrate 2 g, citric acid monohydrate 400 mg, hyoscyamus liquid extract 0.2 ml, quillaia tincture 0.1 ml, lemon syrup 1 ml, concentrated chloroform water 0.2 ml, water to 10 ml. *Dose.* 10 to 20 ml well diluted with water. Each 10 ml contains about 18.5 mmol of potassium.

Potassium Citrate and Hyoscyamus Mixture *(B.P.C. 1973).* Mist. Pot. Cit. et Hyoscy. Potassium citrate 3 g, citric acid monohydrate 500 mg, hyoscyamus tincture 2 ml, syrup 2.5 ml, quillaia tincture 0.1 ml, lemon spirit 0.05 ml, double-strength chloroform water 2 ml, water to 10 ml. *Dose.* 10 ml well diluted with water. It should be recently prepared. Each 10 ml contains about 27.8 mmol of potassium.

Hyoscyamine was stabilised by the high electrolyte concentration produced by potassium citrate and citric acid, which tended to prolong the shelf-life of the mixture.— S. A. H. Khalil and S. El-Masry, *J. Pharm. Pharmac.*, 1978, *30*, 664.

Potassium Citrate and Sodium Bicarbonate Mixture *(A.P.F.).* Potassium citrate 1 g, sodium bicarbonate 750 mg, orange syrup 1 ml, concentrated chloroform water 0.2 ml, water to 10 ml. *Dose.* 10 to 20 ml, well diluted with water. Each 10 ml contains about 9 mmol of potassium and about 8.9 mmol of sodium.

Potassium Citrate Mixture *(A.P.F.).* Mist. Pot. Cit. Potassium citrate 2 g, citric acid monohydrate 400 mg, lemon syrup 1 ml, concentrated chloroform water 0.2 ml, water to 10 ml. *Dose.* 10 to 20 ml, well diluted with water. Each 10 ml contains about 18.5 mmol of potassium.

Potassium Citrate Mixture *(B.P.).* Mist. Pot. Cit. Potassium citrate 3 g, citric acid monohydrate 500 mg, syrup 2.5 ml, quillaia tincture 0.1 ml, lemon spirit 0.05 ml, double-strength chloroform water 3 ml, water to 10 ml. *Dose.* 10 ml, well diluted with water. Children: up to 1 year, 2.5 ml; 1 to 5 years, 5 ml; 6 to 12 years, 10 ml. It should be recently prepared and well diluted with water before use. When a dose less than or not a multiple of 5 ml is prescribed, the mixture should be diluted to 5 ml, or a multiple, with syrup. Such dilutions must be freshly prepared and not used more than 2 weeks after issue. Each 10 ml contains about 27.8 mmol of potassium.

For a report of incompatibility when Potassium Citrate Mixture was prepared with or diluted with syrup preserved with hydroxybenzoates, see under Sucrose, p.61.

Potassium Citrate Mixture CF *(A.P.F.).* Potassium Citrate Mixture for Children. Potassium citrate 1 g, citric acid monohydrate 200 mg, lemon syrup 1 ml, concentrated chloroform water 0.1 ml, water to 5 ml. *Dose.* 5 ml, diluted with water. Each 5 ml contains about 9.25 mmol of potassium.

Potassium Citrate Mixture for Infants *(B.P.C. 1959).* Mist. Pot. Cit. pro Inf. Potassium citrate 731.2 mg, citric acid monohydrate 146.4 mg, benzoic acid solution 0.083 ml, amaranth solution 0.033 ml, syrup 1.33 ml, chloroform water to 4 ml. *Dose.* 4 to 8 ml, well diluted with water. ***Amended formula.*** Dispense Potassium Citrate Mixture.—*Compendium of Past Formulae 1933 to 1966*, London, The National Pharmaceutical Union, 1969.

Tricitrates Oral Solution *(U.S.P.).* Contains, in each 100 ml, potassium citrate 10.45 to 11.55 g, sodium citrate dihydrate 9.5 to 10.5 g, and citric acid monohydrate 6.34 to 7.02 g in a suitable aqueous vehicle, providing approximately 1 mmol of potassium and 1 mmol of sodium per ml. pH 4.9 to 5.4. Store in airtight containers.

Proprietary Preparations

Effercitrate Tablets *(Typharm, UK).* Each contains the equivalent of 1.5 g of potassium citrate and 250 mg of citric acid in an effervescent basis; each contains 13.9 mmol (13.9 mEq) of potassium.

Other Proprietary Names

Efferkal *(Switz.)*; Kacitrin *(Switz.)*; Kajos *(Norw., Swed.)*; Kation *(Ital.)*.

1181-x

Potassium Gluconate *(B.P.C. 1973, U.S.P.).*

Potassium D-gluconate.

$CH_2OH.[CH(OH)]_4.CO_2K=234.2$.

CAS — 299-27-4.

Pharmacopoeias. In *U.S.* which permits anhydrous or the monohydrate.

A white or yellowish-white, odourless or almost odourless, crystalline powder or granules with a slightly bitter taste. Each g represents approximately 4.3 mmol (4.3 mEq) of potassium.

Soluble 1 in 3 of water; very slightly soluble in alcohol; practically insoluble in dehydrated alcohol, chloroform, and ether. A solution in water has a pH of about 7 and is colourless and stable. Solutions are **sterilised** by autoclaving or by filtration. **Store** in airtight containers.

Adverse Effects, Treatment, and Precautions. As for Potassium Salts, p.628.

Intestinal ulceration. An obese alcoholic woman who had been taking hydrochlorothiazide and a preparation of potassium gluconate in aqueous solution (Kaon Elixir) developed an acute, obstructive, jejunal ulcer.

The possibility that such a preparation could, like enteric-coated potassium chloride, cause small-bowel ulceration should be kept in mind.— O. S. Warr and J. P. Nash, *J. Am. med. Ass.*, 1967, *199*, 217.

Uses. Potassium gluconate is almost tasteless and is convenient for oral administration for the prevention and treatment of potassium deficiency—see under Potassium Salts, p.628.

For discussions on whether potassium should be given as the gluconate or the chloride for potassium replacement therapy in patients receiving diuretics, see under Potassium Chloride, p.629.

Preparations

Potassium Gluconate Elixir *(U.S.P.)*. Contains potassium gluconate and alcohol 4.5 to 5.5%. Potency is expressed in terms of anhydrous potassium gluconate. Store in airtight containers. Protect from light.

Potassium Gluconate Mixture. Potassium gluconate 5 g, citric acid monohydrate 3 g, benzoic acid solution 0.2 ml, orange syrup 4 ml, chloroform water to 20 ml. Each 20 ml contains about 21.4 mmol of potassium.—Pharm. Soc. Lab. Rep. No. 883, 1962.

Potassium Gluconate Tablets *(U.S.P.)*. Tablets containing potassium gluconate. Potency is expressed in terms of anhydrous potassium gluconate. Store in airtight containers.

Proprietary Names

Gluconsan *(Jap.)*; Kalium Beta *(Beta, Arg.)*; Kalium-Hausmann *(Asta, Ger.)*; Kaon *(Montpellier, Arg.; Adria, Canad.; Adria, USA)*; Kaoplus *(Fulton, Ital.)*; Potasion *(gluceptate)(see also under Potassium Chloride)(Delagrange, Spain)*; Potasoral *(Galepharma, Spain)*; Potassion *(gluceptate)(see also under Potassium Chloride)(Delagrange, Fr.)*; Potassium Égic*(Egic, Fr.)*; Potassium-Rougier *(Rougier, Canad.)*; Potassuril *(Cochard, Belg.)*; Royonate *(Roy, Canad.)*; Sirokal *(Egic, Belg.)*; Ultra K *(Sopar, Belg.)*.

Potassium gluconate was formerly marketed in Great Britain under the proprietary name Katorin (*Boots*).

1182-r

Potassium Metaphosphate *(U.S.N.F.)*. Potassium Polymetaphosphate; Potassium Kurrol's Salt.
$(KPO_3)_x$.

CAS — 7790-53-6.

Pharmacopoeias. In *U.S.N.F.*

A straight-chain polyphosphate, having a high degree of polymerisation, containing the equivalent of about 59 to 61% of P_2O_5.
It is a white odourless powder. Practically **insoluble** in water; soluble in dilute solutions of sodium salts, forming viscous solutions.

Potassium metaphosphate is used as a buffering agent, and as a fat emulsifier and moisture-retaining agent in foods.

1184-d

Dibasic Potassium Phosphate *(U.S.P.)*. Dipotassium Monophosphate; Dipotassium Phosphate; Potassium Phosphate. Dipotassium hydrogen orthophosphate.
K_2HPO_4=174.2.

CAS — 7758-11-4.

Pharmacopoeias. In *U.S.*

A colourless or white, deliquescent, tasteless, granular powder. Each g represents approximately 11.5 mmol (11.5 mEq) of potassium. **Soluble** 1 in 3 of water; very slightly soluble in alcohol. A 5% solution in water has a pH of 8.5 to 9.6.

Commercial potassium phosphate injections containing monobasic potassium phosphate and potassium phosphate varied considerably in composition and in their phosphorus content; the valence of phosphate was dependent on pH; phosphate content should be expressed in mmol.— S. J. Turco and W. A. Burke, *Hosp. Pharm.*, 1975, *10*, 320.

Adverse Effects, Treatment, and Precautions. As for Potassium Salts, p.628.

A 9-year-old boy with severe diabetic ketoacidosis responded to intravenous fluids, bicarbonate, insulin, and potassium phosphate (given to replace depleted stores of 2,3-diphosphoglycerate). However, 28 hours after the start of treatment he had hypocalcaemia, hypomagnesaemia and hyperphosphataemia due to phosphate overload. It was suggested that in the treatment of diabetic ketoacidosis a combination of potassium phosphate and potassium chloride might be preferable to the use of potassium phosphate alone.— R. J. Winter *et al.*, *Am. J. Med.*, 1979, *67*, 897.

Uses. Dibasic potassium phosphate has been used as a saline purgative (see under Potassium Salts, p.628) in doses of 0.6 to 2 g. It has also been used similarly to sodium phosphate (see p.642) in the treatment of calcium and phosphate metabolic disorders.
A potassium phosphate (Kalium Phosphoricum, Kali Phos.) is used in homoeopathic medicine.

Estimated acceptable total daily dietary phosphorus load: up to 70 mg per kg body-weight, attention being given to the reverse relationship with calcium intake.— Seventeenth Report of the FAO/WHO Expert Committee on Food Additives, *Tech. Rep. Ser. Wld Hlth Org. No. 539*, 1974.

1183-f

Monobasic Potassium Phosphate *(U.S.N.F.)*. Potassium Acid Phosphate; Potassium Biphosphate; Monopotassium Phosphate. Potassium dihydrogen orthophosphate.
KH_2PO_4=136.1.

CAS — 7778-77-0.

Pharmacopoeias. In *U.S.N.F.*

Colourless crystals or a white odourless granular or crystalline powder with a saline taste. Each g represents approximately 7.3 mmol (7.3 mEq) of potassium. **Soluble** 1 in 4.5 of water; practically insoluble in alcohol. A 1% solution in water has a pH of about 4.5. A 2.1% solution is iso-osmotic with serum. **Store** in airtight containers.

The haemolytic effect of phosphate buffer solutions.— J. R. Phillips and D. E. Cadwallader, *J. pharm. Sci.*, 1971, *60*, 1033.

Adverse Effects, Treatment, and Precautions. As for Potassium Salts, p.628.

Uses. Monobasic potassium phosphate has been used, in doses of 1 to 4 g, as a saline purgative (see under Potassium Salts, p.628). It may also be used similarly to sodium phosphate (see p.642) in the treatment of calcium and phosphate metabolic disorders, and as a buffering agent.

Preparations

Amphoteric Lotion *(Moorfields Eye Hosp.)*. Universal Buffer. Monobasic potassium phosphate (KH_2PO_4) 7 g, sodium phosphate ($Na_2HPO_4,12H_2O$) 18 g, and Water for Injections 85 ml. pH about 7. Sterilised by filtration. For the first aid treatment of chemical splashes in the eye.

See also Sodium Phosphate Irrigation, p.642.

Potassium Phosphates Injection *(U.S.P.)*. A sterile solution of monobasic potassium phosphate and dibasic potassium phosphate in Water for Injections. It contains no bacteriostatic agent or other preservative. pH 6.2 to 6.8. To be diluted before use.

Sørensen's Phosphate Buffer Solutions, pH 5 to 8. *Solution A:* a 0.907% w/v (0.067 M) solution of monobasic potassium phosphate (KH_2PO_4) in water. *Solution B:* a 2.39% w/v (0.067 M) solution of sodium phosphate ($Na_2HPO_4,12H_2O$) in water.
To prepare buffer solutions at the following pH values, take the corresponding stated volume of *solution A* and make up to 100 ml with *solution B:* pH 5.0: 99.2 ml; pH 5.4: 97.3 ml; pH 5.6: 95.5 ml; pH 6.0: 88.9 ml; pH 6.4: 75.4 ml; pH 6.6: 65.3 ml; pH 7.0: 41.3 ml; pH 7.4: 19.7 ml; pH 7.6: 12.8 ml; pH 8.0: 3.7 ml.

Proprietary Preparations

Travenol Electrolyte Solution B with 20% Dextrose *(Travenol, UK)*. A sterile solution for intravenous infusion containing monobasic potassium phosphate, anhydrous dextrose, and sodium metabisulphite, and providing in each litre potassium 60 mmol and phosphate 60 mmol.

Other Proprietary Names

K-Phos Original *(USA)*.

1185-n

Potassium Sulphate *(B.P.C. 1949)*. Potassii Sulphas; Kalium Sulfuricum; Tartarus Vitriolatus.
K_2SO_4=174.3.

CAS — 7778-80-5.

Pharmacopoeias. In *Arg., Aust., Belg., Fr., Hung., Jap., Nord., Pol., Port., Span.,* and *Swiss.*

Colourless odourless crystals or white powder with a saline, slightly bitter taste. Each g represents approximately 11.5 mmol (11.5 mEq) of potassium. **Soluble** 1 in 10 of water and 1 in 4 of boiling water; practically insoluble in alcohol and ether; slightly soluble in glycerol. A 5% solution in water is neutral to litmus. A 2.11% solution in water is iso-osmotic with serum. Solutions are **sterilised** by autoclaving or by filtration.

Adverse Effects, Treatment, and Precautions. As for Potassium Salts, p.628.

Uses. Potassium sulphate has been used, in doses of 1 to 3 g, in dilute solution as a saline purgative (see under Potassium Salts, p.628).

1186-h

Potassium Acid Tartrate *(B.P.C. 1973)*.

Pot. Acid. Tart.; Potassium Hydrogen Tartrate; Purified Cream of Tartar; Potassium Bitartrate; Kalium Hydrotartaricum; Tartarus Depuratus; Weinstein.
$C_4H_5KO_6$=188.2.

CAS — 868-14-4.

Pharmacopoeias. In *Arg., Aust., Belg., Ind., It., Neth., Pol., Port., Roum.,* and *Span.*

Odourless or almost odourless colourless crystals or white crystalline powder with a pleasant acid taste. It absorbs insignificant amounts of moisture at 25° at relative humidities up to about 90%. Each g represents approximately 5.3 mmol (5.3 mEq) of potassium.
Soluble 1 in 190 of water and 1 in 16 of boiling water; practically insoluble in alcohol, chloroform, and ether; readily soluble in dilute mineral acids and in solutions of alkalis or borax. A 0.5% solution in water has a pH of 3.5 to 4. Solutions are **sterilised** by autoclaving or by filtration.

Adverse Effects, Treatment, and Precautions. As for Potassium Salts, p.628.

Uses. Potassium acid tartrate is used as a saline purgative in doses of up to 4 g (see under Potassium Salts, p.628). It has also a mild diuretic action and was used for this action as Imperial Drink. Potassium acid tartrate has been used as a dusting-powder for surgical rubber gloves.

1187-m

Potassium Tartrate *(B.P.C. 1949)*. Pot. Tart.; Normal, or Neutral, Potassium Tartrate.
$(C_4H_4K_2O_6)_2,H_2O$=470.6.

CAS — 921-53-9 (anhydrous).

Pharmacopoeias. In *Port.*

Odourless, colourless, deliquescent crystals, or white crystalline powder, with a cooling saline taste. Each g represents approximately 8.5 mmol (8.5 mEq) of potassium. **Soluble** 1 in 0.5 of water; practically insoluble in alcohol. A solution in water has a pH of 7 to 8.

Adverse Effects, Treatment, and Precautions. As for Potassium Salts, p.628.

For background toxicological information, see *Fd Add. Ser. Wld Hlth Org. No. 5*, 1974.

Uses. Potassium tartrate has been used, in doses of 2 to 16 g, in dilute solution as a saline purgative (see under Potassium Salts, p.628).

Estimated acceptable daily intake: up to 30 mg, as tartaric acid, per kg body-weight.— Seventeenth Report of the FAO/WHO Expert Committee on Food Additives, *Tech. Rep. Ser. Wld Hlth Org. No. 539*, 1974.

Proprietary Names
K-Med *(ICN, Canad.)*; Nati-K *(Sabex, Canad.; Synlab, Fr.; Nativelle, Switz.)*; Wel-K *(Welcker-Lyster, Canad.)*.

1188-b

Sodium Salts.
Na=22.98977.

Sodium is the principal cation in the extracellular space where it is mainly complemented by the anion chloride. The sodium ion is the main osmotic component of the extracellular space—the blood plasma and the fluids in the tissues around the cells (normal concentration 140 mmol per litre).

Because the extracellular water is about 15 litres in a healthy adult and the normal sodium concentration 140 mmol per litre, 2000 to 2100 mmol of sodium are found in the extracellular space. Intracellular sodium is only 10 mmol per litre, thus with 25 litres of intracellular water there is a further 250 mmol of sodium in the cells. Finally, there is some sodium in bone (about 450 mmol) which is less freely exchangeable. The body therefore contains about 40 mmol (40 mEq) of sodium per kg bodyweight.

About 100 to 200 mmol of sodium is ingested daily in the typical diet and a similar amount is excreted, chiefly in the urine; primitive diets are relatively low in sodium. The body can adapt to a wide range of intakes by adjustment of renal excretion. Thus if intake falls to zero renal output will not normally exceed 5 mmol daily. Similarly up to 300 mmol daily can normally be tolerated without ill effects, though the volume of extracellular fluid will be increased by about 10%.

Symptoms of hypernatraemia are described below under Adverse Effects while those of hyponatraemia are described under the Uses section.

NOTE. Each g of sodium represents approximately 43.5 mmol (43.5 mEq).

Equations for the prediction of exchangeable body sodium according to weight, height, age, and sex.— F. Skrabal *et al., Br. med. J.*, 1973, *2*, 37.

Adverse Effects. Sodium excess may be caused by inadequate fluids, excessive fluid losses (hot weather, fever, diarrhoea), excessive administration of sodium including the overfeeding or inappropriate feeding of infants, overloading with dextrose during parenteral feeding, brain injury, impaired renal function, and aldosteronism.

Sodium 'excess' may take two forms. The first form is a rise in extracellular concentration (hypernatraemia, a plasma-sodium concentration of more than 147 mmol per litre) which may be the consequence of too little available water or over-provision of sodium against a low excretion-rate. The second form is too much sodium and water in the body without change in extracellular concentration.

Hypernatraemia is characteristic of excessive administration including the overfeeding or inappropriate feeding of infants, in brain injury and acute water lack. It is also sometimes seen in patients who are overloaded with dextrose during parenteral feeding.

Symptoms of hypernatraemia may include restlessness, weakness, thirst, reduced salivation and lachrymation, swollen tongue, flushing of the skin, pyrexia, dizziness, headache, oliguria, hypotension, tachycardia, delirium, hyperpnoea, and respiratory arrest.

Retention of sodium and water—isotonic retention or iso-osmotic expansion because the plasma concentration is unchanged—leads to the accumulation of extracellular fluid (oedema). This may affect the cerebral, pulmonary, or peripheral circulations. It is the consequence of heart failure, renal failure, increased adrenocortical activity, the administration of corticosteroids, or excessive administration of sodium after operation or injury (when there is a renal restriction on sodium excretion).

Hypernatraemia.— E. J. Ross and S. B. M. Christie, *Medicine, Baltimore*, 1969, *48*, 441.

Hypernatraemia and elevated urinary osmolality in babies nursed under radiant heaters.— R. W. A. Jones *et al., Br. med. J.*, 1976, *2*, 1347.

Discussions of a possible association between cot deaths and hypernatraemia.— J. S. Robertson and V. Parker, *Lancet*, 1978, *2*, 1012. H. C. Milligan (letter), *ibid.*, 1979, *1*, 42.

Hypernatraemia was uncommon in adults; of 16 224 patients 20 had plasma-sodium concentrations in excess of 154 mmol per litre: 8 had diabetes mellitus, 8 a primary intracranial disorder, and 4 dehydration with no other common factor.— P. Daggett *et al., Br. med. J.*, 1979, *1*, 1177.

The incidence of hypernatraemia in infant deaths in Sheffield had fallen from 1.6 per 1000 live births in 1973 to 0.7 in 1974, 0.2 in 1975 and 1976, and zero in 1977 and 1978. This might reflect the removal of high-sodium foods, increased breast-feeding, and education on child care.— R. Sunderland and J. L. Emery, *Br. med. J.*, 1979, *2*, 575.

Adverse effects following dialysis. Hypertension, cerebral oedema, and deterioration in general health in 4 patients immediately after peritoneal dialysis was due to the high sodium content (146 to 148 mmol per litre) of solutions labelled as containing 'approximately 141 mmol per litre'.— P. G. Bisson and K. M. Bailey, *Br. med. J.*, 1979, *1*, 1322.

Treatment of Adverse Effects. Hypernatraemia requires the use of sodium-free fluids and the cessation of excessive sodium intake. Very occasionally dialysis has been needed in severe hypernatraemia.

Iso-osmotic overload is managed by sodium and water restriction plus measures to increase renal sodium and water loss such as 'loop diuretics' (e.g., frusemide) or, in specific circumstances, antimineralocorticoid agents.

Treatment of hypernatraemic dehydration in infancy.— A. Banister *et al., Archs Dis. Childh.*, 1975, *50*, 179.

A regimen for the treatment of hypernatraemia in children.— R. A. Cockington *et al., Med. J. Aust.*, 1977, *1*, 957.

Precautions. Sodium salts should be used cautiously in patients with cardiac failure, hypertension, impaired renal function, peripheral and pulmonary oedema, and in toxaemia of pregnancy.

Uses. Alkaline sodium salts, such as sodium bicarbonate, are used as antacids to neutralise excess hydrochloric acid in the gastric secretion. Sodium bicarbonate is also administered, usually by intravenous injection, in the treatment of metabolic acidosis; sodium lactate and sodium acetate are used similarly. Sodium chloride is used, by mouth and by injection, to replace excessive losses of sodium or chloride ions. The phosphate, sulphate, and tartrate salts, which are poorly absorbed from the gastro-intestinal tract, retain water in the lumen of the bowel by an osmotic effect and have purgative actions. When administered in dilute solution evacuation of the contents of the intestine follows. With higher concentrations water is drawn into the bowel from the tissues to restore osmotic equilibrium. Purgative action is sometimes slower because the increased intraluminal volume develops only gradually.

Sodium 'deficit' may take two forms. The first form is associated with an inappropriate ratio of sodium to water in the extracellular space (hyponatraemia), and is usually the result of an excessive amount of water in the body, in turn caused by failure of renal excretion often accompanied by the over-administration of hypo-osmotic fluids. Low plasma sodium concentrations are also found in seriously ill patients from whatever cause. Symptoms of hyponatraemia (water intoxication) may include anorexia, fatigue, muscle weakness, diarrhoea, abdominal cramps, confusion, hypotension, tachycardia, weakened pulse, cyanosis, hypothermia, pitting oedema, oliguria, and convulsions.

The second form of sodium deficit is when sodium and water are both lost, usually at the concentration found in extracellular fluids. Because of the jealous conservation of sodium by the normal kidney, such loss is nearly always by an extrarenal route such as loss of intestinal secretions by vomiting, diarrhoea, fistula, or gastro-intestinal suction. Excessive sweating with water replacement only is a further cause. In Addison's disease the kidney cannot conserve sodium and the losses take place by this route. A similar state may be found in chronic renal disease.

Features of iso-osmotic fluid loss include thirst, dizziness, postural hypotension, low urine output, and ultimately shock because of fall in the plasma volume. Hyponatraemia, because it is the consequence of water overload, usually responds to water restriction. In ill patients provision of carbohydrate energy (dextrose), potassium, and insulin may correct the extracellular/intracellular distribution of water and so raise plasma-sodium concentrations.

Extrarenal isotonic sodium and water deficiency is mainly treated by the use of 0.9% sodium chloride injection, Ringer-lactate solution, 0.18% sodium chloride in 4% dextrose injection, or balanced electrolyte solutions.

Too rapid replacement with a solution low in sodium content is to be avoided because of the risk of causing cerebral oedema and convulsions.

Electrolyte changes after burn injury and effect of treatment.— P. Hinton *et al., Lancet*, 1973, *2*, 218.

For a discussion on heat stroke, heat exhaustion, and heat cramps, see K. S. Cho and S. H. Lee, *Bull. Wld Hlth Org.*, 1978, *56*, 205.

Electrolyte studies: sodium and water.— M. D. Burke, *Postgrad. Med.*, 1978, *64*, 147.

Water balance and hyponatraemia.— D. B. Morgan and T. H. Thomas, *Clin. Sci.*, 1979, *56*, 517.

A discussion on the active transport of sodium and potassium ions.— K. J. Sweadner and S. M. Goldin, *New Engl. J. Med.*, 1980, *302*, 777.

Serum-sodium concentration after surgical operation.— S. Chan *et al., Br. J. Surg.*, 1980, *67*, 711.

Abnormalities of cell volume regulation and their functional consequences.— A. S. Pollock and A. I. Arieff, *Am. J. Physiol.*, 1980, *239*, F195.

The mechanisms and management of hyponatraemia.— C. T. G. Flear *et al., Lancet*, 1981, *2*, 26.

Hyponatraemia of the newborn due to maternal fluid overload.— W. O. Tarnow-Mordi *et al., Br. med. J.*, 1981, *283*, 639.

1189-v

Sodium Acetate *(B.P., Eur. P., U.S.P.)*.
Sod. Acet.; Natrii Acetas; Sodii Acetas; Natrium Aceticum.

$CH_3.CO_2Na,3H_2O$=136.1.

CAS — 127-09-3 (anhydrous); 6131-90-4 (trihydrate).

Pharmacopoeias. In *Br., Braz., Eur., Fr., Ger., Hung., Jap., Neth., Nord. Pol.,* and *U.S.* which also allows the anhydrous form. The material described in *Eur. P.* is not necessarily suitable for dialysis.

Colourless crystals or a white crystalline powder or flakes, odourless or with a slight odour of acetic acid, and a slightly bitter saline taste. It effloresces in warm dry air. Each g represents approximately 7.3 mmol (7.3 mEq) of sodium and of acetate.

Soluble 1 in 0.8 of water and 1 in 19 of alcohol; practically insoluble in chloroform and ether. A 5% solution in water has a pH of 7.5 to 9.2. **Sterilise** by autoclaving or by filtration. **Store** in airtight containers.

Adverse Effects, Treatment, and Precautions. As for Sodium Salts, p.633.

Uses. Sodium acetate is used as a source of sodium ions in solutions for haemodialysis and peritoneal dialysis (see under Sodium Chloride, p.636); it is preferred to sodium bicarbonate because of its greater solubility and because the sterilisation process is less complicated.

It is also occasionally used, usually in conjunction with other electrolytes, by intravenous infusion for the correction of acidosis and to replace electrolyte losses. It has been given by mouth, in doses of 1.5 g, to render the urine less acid and to promote a mild diuresis.

In a study *in vitro* sodium acetate added to protein hydrolysate solutions inhibited the growth of *Escherichia coli* and *Staphylococcus aureus* but did not inhibit *Candida albicans*. Inhibition of *Pseudomonas aeruginosa* could not be attributed solely to sodium acetate and may have been related to the pH of the solution.— G. Frech *et al.*, *Am. J. Hosp. Pharm.*, 1979, *36*, 1672.

Acidosis. Acetate solutions in the treatment of metabolic acidosis: R. A. Cash *et al.*, *Lancet*, 1969, *2*, 302; H. E. Eliahou *et al.*, *Br. med. J.*, 1970, *4*, 399.

Dehydration. In 18 adults, the dehydration and acidosis of cholera were treated with 1 of 3 solutions given intravenously; initially administered rapidly to correct dehydration and then at a rate to replace losses in stools and urine. After 24 hours of treatment, the most rapid correction of acidosis was attained with a compound sodium bicarbonate solution which contained 133 mmol per litre of sodium, 99 mmol per litre of chloride, 14 mmol per litre of potassium, and 48 mmol per litre of bicarbonate. Adequate restoration of the acid-base balance was obtained in patients with acidosis of moderate severity with either of 2 solutions which were cheaper and could be stored for long periods in hot climates, namely a cholera replacement solution (NAMRU-2), which contained per litre 120 mmol of sodium, 100 mmol of chloride, 10 mmol of potassium, and 30 mmol of acetate, or a lactated Ringer's solution which contained per litre 130 mmol of sodium, 109 mmol of chloride, 4 mmol of potassium, and 28 mmol of lactate.— R. H. Watten *et al.*, *Lancet*, 1969, *2*, 512.

Dialysis. Acetate was converted quantitatively by the body to bicarbonate and could be used to replace bicarbonate in haemodialysis solutions. This obviated the difficulty of mixing a concentrated solution of bicarbonate with magnesium and calcium solutions before dilution with water in a proportioning pump. Because the clearance-rate of acetate was lower than bicarbonate, acetate concentrations of 35 to 40 mmol per litre should be used to maintain serum bicarbonate at 25 mmol per litre.— C. M. Mion *et al.*, *Trans. Am. Soc. artif. internal Organs*, 1964, *10*, 110.

Sodium acetate reduced the bacterial count in 44 of 45 inoculates and eliminated bacteria in 11 of 15 inoculates of *Staphylococcus aureus* and 2 of 15 of *Escherichia coli*, but no complete killing occurred in sodium lactate dialysates. Substitution of sodium lactate by sodium acetate 43 mmol per litre in peritoneal dialysis solutions was recommended to reduce the risk of peritonitis.— J. A. Richardson and K. A. Borchardt, *Br. med. J.*, 1969, *3*, 749.

Preparations

Sodium Acetate Injection *(U.S.P.)*. A sterile solution of anhydrous sodium acetate in Water for Injections. pH 6 to 7. To be diluted before use.

1190-r

Sodium Bicarbonate *(B.P., B.P. Vet., Eur. P., U.S.P.)*.

Sod. Bicarb.; Baking Soda; Natrii Hydrogenocarbonas; Sodium Acid Carbonate; Sodium Hydrogen Carbonate; Sodium Hydrocarbonate; Natrii Bicarbonas; Natrium Bicarbonicum; Carbonate Monosodique; Sal de Vichy.
$NaHCO_3$=84.01.

CAS — 144-55-8.

Pharmacopoeias. In all pharmacopoeias examined except *Int.*

A white odourless crystalline powder with a saline slightly alkaline taste. Each g represents approximately 11.9 mmol (11.9 mEq) of sodium. When heated it decomposes, and is converted to anhydrous sodium carbonate at 250° to 300°. At relative humidities up to about 80%, the equilibrium moisture content is less than 1%, but at relative humidities above 85%, it rapidly absorbs excessive amounts of moisture and this may be associated with decomposition by loss of carbon dioxide. When intended for oral use only (Sodium Bicarbonate Oral Powder) the *U.S.P.* permits suitable added substances.

Soluble 1 in 11 of water with slow decomposition; practically insoluble in alcohol and ether. A 5% solution in water has a pH of not more than 8.6. A 1.39% solution in water is iso-osmotic with serum. Sodium bicarbonate, 20 parts, is neutralised by approximately 16.7 parts of citric acid monohydrate or approximately 17.9 parts of tartaric acid. Solutions in water slowly decompose at ordinary temperatures with partial conversion into the normal carbonate; the decomposition is accelerated by agitation or warming. Solutions are **sterilised** by autoclaving or by filtration. For sterilisation by autoclaving, the solution is placed in the final container and carbon dioxide is passed into it for 1 minute before sealing; the container is sealed so as to be gas-tight and then autoclaved, and is not opened until at least 2 hours after it has cooled to room temperature. The *B.P.* specifies that such solutions may contain not more than 0.01% of disodium edetate (see below).

Incompatible with acids, acidic salts, dopamine hydrochloride, pentazocine lactate, many alkaloidal salts, aspirin, and with bismuth salicylate. The darkening of salicylates is intensified by sodium bicarbonate. **Store** in airtight containers.

Incompatibility. There was loss of clarity when intravenous solutions of sodium bicarbonate were mixed with those of corticotrophin, hydromorphone hydrochloride, insulin, magnesium sulphate, methicillin sodium, narcotic salts, noradrenaline acid tartrate, pentobarbitone sodium, procaine hydrochloride, promazine hydrochloride (in dextrose injection), streptomycin sulphate, tetracycline hydrochloride, thiopentone sodium, vancomycin hydrochloride, lactated Ringer's injection, sodium lactate injection, or Ringer's Injection (*U.S.P.*).— J. A. Patel and G. L. Phillips, *Am. J. Hosp. Pharm.*, 1966, *23*, 409.

A haze or precipitate was observed within an hour when an average dose of sodium bicarbonate was mixed in dextrose injection with oxytetracycline hydrochloride. Calcium chloride and gluconate were also precipitated at certain concentrations.— J. M. Meisler and M. W. Skolaut, *Am. J. Hosp. Pharm.*, 1966, *23*, 557.

Solubility in glycerol. The solubility of sodium bicarbonate in aqueous glycerol solutions was least in a solution of 75% glycerol and increased rapidly with increased concentrations of glycerol.— S. D. Fitzgerald, *Australas. J. Pharm.*, 1966, *47*, S82.

Solutions for injection. Disodium edetate is incorporated in solutions for injection to prevent any cloudiness or sediment due mainly to calcium carbonate and traces of magnesium and other metals. The *B.P.* allows not more than 0.01% of disodium edetate and specifies, as does the *U.S.P.*, that solutions containing visible particles should not be used. J.W. Hadgraft who reported with B.D. Hewer (*Pharm. J.* 1964, *1*, 544 and 648) that a concentration of 0.01% would prevent the formation of a deposit subsequently found it desirable (*Lancet*, 1966, *1*, 603) to increase the concentration of disodium edetate to 0.02%.

Alternatively, the difficulty may be overcome by preparing a solution according to the method described under 'Sterilisation' (see above) then removing the deposit by filtering through a bacteria-proof filter, using positive pressure, and re-autoclaving. Solutions so prepared have remained clear after storage for several months.

For discussions of the problems of preparation of injections of sodium bicarbonate, see H. L. Daniels, *Lancet*, 1966, *1*, 548; G. Smith, *ibid.*, 658; Y. Marzouk, *J. Hosp. Pharm.*, 1967, *24*, 64.

Stability. A sterile 7.5% solution of sodium bicarbonate remained stable in polypropylene syringes for up to 100 days at 12° to 14° or up to 45 days at 23°. Care was necessary to prevent loss of carbon dioxide and to maintain the pH below 8.— C. I. Hicks *et al.*, *Am. J. Hosp. Pharm.*, 1972, *29*, 210. See also P. P. DeLuca and R. J. Kowalsky, *ibid.*, 217.

Eye lotions of sodium bicarbonate 2% preserved with chlorocresol and/or phenethyl alcohol were sterilised by filtration or by autoclaving. Filtered solutions had a higher initial pH (8.25 to 8.9) than autoclaved solutions (7.4 to 8), but the pH of filtered solutions decreased during storage at room temperature. As deposition or discoloration occurred in some solutions after 2 to 3 months, a shelf-life of less than 2 months was suggested.— Pharm. Soc. Lab. Rep. P/74/6, 1974.

Sterilisation. Sodium bicarbonate eye lotion 3.5% contaminated with *Pseudomonas aeruginosa* was sterilised within 1 hour by phenylmercuric nitrate 0.002% with phenethyl alcohol 0.4%, chlorocresol 0.05%, chlorocresol 0.05% with phenethyl alcohol 0.4%, or chlorocresol 0.05% with edetic acid 0.05%.— R. M. E. Richards and R. J. McBride, *Br. J. Ophthal.*, 1971, *55*, 734.

Adverse Effects, Treatment, and Precautions. As for Sodium Salts, p.633.

Rapid reversal of acidosis in infants by infusion of hyperosmotic solutions of sodium bicarbonate could lead to hyperosmolality.— L. Finberg, *Pediatrics*, 1967, *40*, 1031. For a similar comment, see E. de H. Lobo (letter,), *Br. med. J.*, 1966, *1*, 1360.

Cerebral oedema occurred in 4 patients (3 died) with ketoacidosis treated with 200 to 300 mmol of sodium bicarbonate given as 8.4% solution in less than an hour.— J. Moore (letter,), *Br. med. J.*, 1975, *3*, 540.

Studies in 10 healthy subjects indicated that metabolic alkalosis, induced by the injection of sodium bicarbonate, might have a depressant effect on respiration.— T. Nishino *et al.*, *Br. J. Anaesth.*, 1977, *49*, 331.

A report on tissue necrosis following commonly used intravenous infusions, including 8 cases after infusion of sodium bicarbonate.— N. R. Gaze, *Lancet*, 1978, *2*, 417. A further case.— I. T. Jackson and D. W. Robinson, *Scott. med. J.*, 1976, *21*, 200.

A study of the incidence of intraventricular haemorrhage in 100 infants indicated that there was no relationship between intraventricular haemorrhage and the amount of sodium bicarbonate administered intravenously or the concentration of sodium obtained. However, rapid infusion of hyperosmolar solutions of sodium bicarbonate was associated with a significant increase in the incidence of intraventricular haemorrhage and it was recommended that in the treatment of persistent metabolic acidosis in the neonate sodium bicarbonate should be given slowly as a dilute (M/4) solution.— L. Papile *et al.*, *J. Pediat.*, 1978, *93*, 834. See also J. S. Wigglesworth *et al.*, *Archs Dis. Childh.*, 1976, *51*, 755.

Uses. Sodium bicarbonate neutralises the acid secretion in the stomach with the liberation of carbon dioxide. After absorption it is retained by the kidney to meet any deficit of bicarbonate in the plasma, e.g. in metabolic acidosis. In the absence (in health) of such a deficit it is excreted by the kidney; the urine is rendered less acid, with accompanying diuresis.

Sodium bicarbonate is given by mouth in the treatment of simple hyperchlorhydric dyspepsia to relieve pain; it is given with bitters, such as gentian, 30 minutes before meals to neutralise excessive secretion in the stomach. It is also used in the treatment of vomiting in children; care should be taken to avoid excessive amounts in infants. For the treatment of renal acidosis without glomerular failure, sodium bicarbonate may be given; an initial dose of 120 mmol (120 mEq) daily reduced later to 60 mmol daily has been suggested.

Solutions containing up to 4.2% (0.5 mmol per ml) of sodium bicarbonate are administered intravenously for the rapid correction of acidosis and solutions containing up to 8.4% (1 mmol per ml) are used for the initial treatment of metabolic acidosis caused by cardiac arrest. Solutions containing 1.26% are used in regimens for forced alkaline diuresis as described under Phenobarbitone, p.812.

For its action in rendering mucus less viscous, sodium bicarbonate is added to spray solutions and washes for the throat and nose and it is taken as an expectorant.

A 3.5% solution in warm water is used as an eye lotion and a 5% solution as ear-drops to soften and remove wax. A 1 to 2% solution is used as a rinsing solution for contact lenses.

Solutions containing 1 to 4% of sodium bicarbonate are used as vaginal douches.

The use of ear-drops which contained sodium bicarbonate 1 g, glycerol 12 g, water to 28 ml in patients with wax in the ears, followed 20 to 30 minutes later by syringing with a warm aqueous solution of sodium bicarbonate 4 g to 570 ml, had always been effective in removing wax.— H. G. Morris-Jones (letter), *Br. med. J.*, 1968, *4*, 835.

Sodium bicarbonate 20% in talc was an effective deodorant since it combined with the fatty acids formed by decomposition of apocrine sweat and epithelial debris and rendered them inoffensive.— P. D. C. Kinmont, *Practitioner*, 1969, *202*, 88.

Extravasation following the inadvertent administration of doxorubicin hydrochloride subcutaneously was treated by immediate infiltration into the same area of 5 ml of an 8.4% solution of sodium bicarbonate followed by dexamethasone 4 mg.— J. I. Zweig and B. Kabakow (letter), *J. Am. med. Ass.*, 1978, *239*, 2116.

Correspondence on whether bicarbonate values are better expressed as actual or standard bicarbonate: A. Lawrie and B. P. Golda (letter), *Lancet*, 1979, *2*, 201; P. J. Horsey (letter), *ibid.*, 311; A. W. Grogono (letter), *ibid.*, 631; T. A. Hyde (letter), *ibid.*, 796; P. J. N. Howorth (letter), *ibid.*, 849; E. B. Love (letter), *ibid.*, 1015; L. Tibi *et al.* (letter), *ibid.*, 1139.

Acidosis. Severity of metabolic acidosis as a determinant of bicarbonate requirements.— S. Garella *et al.*, *New Engl. J. Med.*, 1973, *289*, 121.

The incidence of hypernatraemia in neonates was reduced from 8.8 to 0.6% when sodium bicarbonate, given usually for the correction of acidosis associated with respiratory distress, was given by slow infusion, diluted so that the daily sodium intake was less than 8 mmol per kg body-weight. The corresponding decrease in frequency of intracranial haemorrhage was possibly due to this less vigorous use of sodium bicarbonate.— M. A. Simmons *et al.*, *New Engl. J. Med.*, 1974, *291*, 6.

A controlled study in 62 premature infants with acidosis showed that the use of sodium bicarbonate, in addition to dextrose infusions and other supportive measures, was not more effective than the use of dextrose and other supportive measures alone.— A. J. Corbet *et al.*, *J. Pediat.*, 1977, *91*, 771.

Controlled treatment with sodium bicarbonate, 4.8 to 14.1 mmol per kg body-weight daily, reversed the impaired growth associated with renal tubular acidosis in 8 children and prevented growth retardation in 2 infants.— E. McSherry and R. C. Morris, *J. clin. Invest.*, 1978, *61*, 509, per *J. Am. med. Ass.*, 1978, *239*, 1849.

See also under Cardiac Resuscitation, below.

Asthma. Bronchial lavage with a 1% solution of sodium bicarbonate was considered to be a valuable addition to the intensive treatment of severe status asthmaticus.— N. E. Williams and J. W. Crooke, *Lancet*, 1968, *1*, 1081.

Although sodium bicarbonate was given almost routinely to patients with severe asthma and respiratory acidosis this treatment was still unproved. Its use could sometimes be deleterious and could delay institution of other important measures. Apart from in emergency situations when severe metabolic acidosis accompanies respiratory acidosis, such as may occur in respiratory arrest, respiratory acidosis should be corrected by improving alveolar ventilation R. P. McCombs *et al.*, *J. Am. med. Ass.*, 1979, *242*, 1521.

Cardiac resuscitation. Cardiac arrest was rapidly followed by metabolic acidosis. A concentration of 8.4% sodium bicarbonate was recommended with a reasonable dose being 100 mmol when resuscitation began and while ventilation was maintained. Larger or repeated doses demanded caution.— *Lancet*, 1976, *1*, 946. See also R. Rackwitz *et al.* (letter), *ibid.*, 474; L. I. G. Worthley (letter), *ibid.*,.

Of 22 infants with neonatal cardiac arrest unresponsive to cardiac massage for 4 minutes or longer 14 responded and achieved a heart-rate of 120 beats per minute within 90 seconds of the intracardiac injection of sodium bicarbonate 2 to 4 mmol, with continued massage.— E. Hey, *Br. J. Anaesth.*, 1977, *49*, 25.

Porphyria cutanea tarda. Treatment of porphyria cutanea tarda in 4 patients with sodium bicarbonate for 10 weeks to 9 months. Blistering and ulceration after exposure to sunlight were reduced or completely alleviated.— S. E. Wiegand *et al.*, *Archs Derm.*, 1969, *100*, 544.

Renal calculi. For the use of sodium bicarbonate 5 to 15 g daily in the treatment of uric acid renal calculi, see T. Mathew, *Drugs*, 1974, *8*, 62.

Respiratory distress. A study in 225 infants with the respiratory distress syndrome indicated that treatment with sodium bicarbonate in 10% dextrose given intragastrically was of limited value and could be harmful. Intermittent positive-pressure respiration remained the treatment of choice.— M. E. R. Stoneman and R. M. Owens, *Archs Dis. Childh.*, 1968, *43*, 155.

Intravenous infusion of sodium bicarbonate and dextrose solutions appeared to benefit neonates with hyaline membrane disease.— P. G. Savignoni *et al.*, *Acta paediat. scand.*, 1969, *58*, 1.

Rapid infusion of 0.9 M sodium bicarbonate in 18 neonates with metabolic acidosis and respiratory distress.— S. R. Siegel *et al.*, *Pediatrics*, 1973, *51*, 651.

Sickle-cell disease. In a crossover study in 18 children sodium bicarbonate daily, to maintain in general a neutral or alkaline urine, did not significantly reduce the incidence of sickle-cell crisis.— J. R. Mann and J. Stuart, *Pediatrics*, 1974, *53*, 414.

In a study in 84 patients with sickle-cell crises (116 crises) there was no significant difference between treatment with the sodium bicarbonate in invert sugar solution, urea in invert sugar solution, and invert sugar solution alone. The dose of sodium bicarbonate used was 1 mmol per kg body-weight per hour for 3 hours, then 0.36 mmol per kg per hour for 45 hours.— Cooperative Urea Trials Group, *J. Am. med. Ass.*, 1974, *228*, 1120.

Preparations

Baths

Effervescent Bath *(B.P.C. 1949).* Balneum Effervescens. Sodium bicarbonate 480 g and sodium hydrogen sulphate 240 g in 140 litres.

Effervescent Bath with Chlorides *(B.P.C. 1949).* Balneum Effervescens cum Chloridis. Effervescent Bath with the addition of sodium chloride 1.44 kg and anhydrous calcium chloride 240 g in 140 litres.

Ear-drops

Sodium Bicarbonate Ear Drops *(B.P., A.P.F.).* Auristillae Sodii Bicarbonatis. Sodium bicarbonate 5 g, glycerol 30 ml, freshly boiled and cooled water to 100 ml. The ear-drops should be recently prepared.

Eye Lotions

Sodium Bicarbonate Eye Lotion *(A.P.F.).* Collyr. Sod. Bicarb.; Alkaline Eye Lotion. Sodium bicarbonate 3.5% in Water for Injections. Prepared and sterilised similarly to Sodium Bicarbonate Eye Lotion *(B.P.C. 1968).*

Sodium Bicarbonate Eye Lotion *(B.P.C. 1968).* Collyrium Sodii Bicarbonatis. A 3.5% solution of sodium bicarbonate in water. The solution is filtered, transferred to the final containers, a stream of carbon dioxide is passed through the solution for 1 minute, and the containers are closed to exclude micro-organisms and sterilised by autoclaving. The containers should not be opened until at least 2 hours after the solution has cooled to room temperature. Alternatively, the solution may be sterilised by filtration and transferred to the final sterile containers which are then closed. The lotion is used undiluted. It should be discarded 24 hours after first opening the container.

Sodium Bicarbonate Eye Lotion has been known as Factory Eye Drops No. 2. Current regulations require that factory first-aid boxes contain an 'approved eye ointment'–sulphacetamide eye ointment 6 or 10%.

Injections

Sodium Bicarbonate Intravenous Infusion *(B.P.).* Sodium Bicarbonate Injection; Sod. Bicarb. Inj. A sterile solution in Water for Injections; it may contain not more than 0.01% of disodium edetate. A 1.4% solution provides 167 mmol of sodium and of bicarbonate per litre.

Sodium Bicarbonate Injection *(U.S.P.).* A sterile solution in Water for Injections, the pH of which may be adjusted by the addition of carbon dioxide. pH 7 to 8.5.

Mixtures

Paediatric Sodium Bicarbonate Mixture *(B.P.C. 1973).* Mistura Carminativa pro Infantibus. Sodium bicarbonate 50 mg, ginger syrup 0.2 ml, concentrated dill water 0.1 ml, syrup 1.85 ml, double-strength chloroform water 2.5 ml, water to 5 ml. It should be recently prepared. *Dose.* Children, up to 1 year, 5 ml; 1 to 5 years, 10 ml.

Powders

Pulvis Alcalina Bourget *(F.N. Belg.).* Bourget's Alkaline Powder. Sodium bicarbonate 8 g, sodium phosphate ($2H_2O$) 4 g, anhydrous sodium sulphate 2 g.

Pulvis Alcalinus *(Roum. P.).* Powder for Bourget's Solution. Sodium bicarbonate 600 mg, sodium phosphate ($2H_2O$) 400 mg, anhydrous sodium sulphate 200 mg. Dissolve in water to make 100 ml of Bourget's Solution. *Port.P.* (Pó de Sais de Sódio) specifies anhydrous sodium phosphate.

Tablets

Compound Sodium Bicarbonate Tablets *(B.P.).* Co. Sod. Bicarb. Tab.; Soda Mint Tablets. Each contains sodium bicarbonate 300 mg and peppermint oil 0.003 ml. They should be allowed to dissolve slowly in the mouth. Store at a temperature not exceeding 25°.

Sodium Bicarbonate Tablets *(U.S.P.).* Tablets containing sodium bicarbonate.

Proprietary Preparations

Baritop Effervescent Tablets *(Concept Pharmaceuticals, UK).* Tablets each containing sodium bicarbonate 35 mg, tartaric acid 35 mg, calcium carbonate 5 mg, and dimethicone 3 mg. For production of gas in radiography of the gastro-intestinal tract. *Dose.* 20 to 30 tablets.

Beogex *(Pharmax, UK).* **Adult suppositories** each containing sodium bicarbonate 1.08 g and anhydrous sodium acid phosphate 1.32 g in an inert basis and **paediatric suppositories** each containing sodium bicarbonate 700 mg and anhydrous sodium acid phosphate 700 mg; when inserted into the rectum, contact with the moist mucous lining causes the release of a predetermined amount of carbon dioxide which distends the lower bowel, inducing peristalsis. For constipation.

Carbex *(Ferring, UK: Henleys, UK).* Granules available in sachets each containing sodium bicarbonate 1.25 g and activated dimethicone 42 mg, supplied with solution containing anhydrous citric acid 10%. For production of gas in radiography of the gastro-intestinal tract. *Dose.* The contents of 1 sachet to be placed on the back of the tongue, and swallowed with 10 ml of solution.

Liquid Gaviscon *(Reckitt & Colman Pharmaceuticals, UK).* Suspension containing in each 10 ml sodium bicarbonate 267 mg and sodium alginate 500 mg (sodium 6.3 mmol), with saccharin. For conditions associated with gastric reflux. *Dose.* 10 to 20 ml after meals and at bedtime.

See also Gaviscon, p.73.

Other Proprietary Names

Neut *(USA)*; Segmentan *(Ger.)*; Sodibic *(Austral.)*.

1191-f

Sodium Chloride *(B.P., Eur. P., U.S.P.).* Sod. Chlor.; Sodii Chloridum; Natrii Chloridum; Natrii Chloretum; Natrium Chloratum; Salt; Chlorure de Sodium; Cloreto de Sódio.

$NaCl = 58.44$.

CAS — 7647-14-5.

Pharmacopoeias. In all pharmacopoeias examined.

Odourless colourless crystals or white crystalline powder with a saline taste. It contains no added substances. Each g represents approximately 17.1 mmol (17.1 mEq) of sodium and of chloride. **Soluble** 1 in 3 of water, 1 in 250 of alcohol, and 1 in 10 of glycerol. A 0.9% solution in water is iso-osmotic with serum.

Solutions are **sterilised** by autoclaving or by filtration. Solutions, when stored, may cause separation of solid particles from glass containers and solutions containing such particles must not be used. **Incompatible** with silver, lead, and mercury salts. **Store** in airtight containers.

NOTE. Domestic or table salt may contain sodium iodide, and magnesium carbonate as an anticaking agent.

Effect of gamma-irradiation. A 0.9% sodium chloride solution for irrigation of the anterior chamber of the eye was packed in 10-ml polystyrene syringes, each enclosed in 2 heat-sealed polyethylene envelopes, and sterilised by irradiation to 25 000 Gy. No toxic effects were observed in 200 eyes.— A. J. Ogg, *Radiosterilization of Medical Products*, Vienna, International Atomic Energy Agency, 1967, p.49.

Adverse Effects and Treatment. As for Sodium Salts, p.633. Hyperosmotic solutions are irritant to the gastro-intestinal mucosa and may cause nausea, vomiting, and diarrhoea. The use of hyperosmotic solutions of sodium chloride to induce abortions has led to cardiovascular shock, central nervous system disorders, haemolysis, renal necrosis, and death. Death has also followed the use of sodium chloride to induce emesis.

Sodium chloride poisoning due to the substitution of sugar by salt was described in 14 infants, 6 of whom died. Poisoning was characterised by convulsions, muscular twitchings, vomiting, thirst, fever, and respiratory distress. Postmortem examination showed haemorrhagic encephalopathy. Peritoneal dialysis with dextrose injection was used in 4 babies; 1 died. The greatest fall in concentration of serum sodium was from 274 to 154 mmol per litre after 6 dialyses. It was considered that the use of potassium in the dialysing solution was contra-indicated and that a solution containing 7% or 8% of dextrose would have been preferable.— L. Finberg *et al.*, *J. Am. med. Ass.*, 1963, *184*, 187.

Of 71 infants in a maternity ward, 18 became seriously ill after being given feeds prepared with sugar which had become mixed with salt. In 17 cases dyspnoea occurred and 1 infant had convulsions. Rapid respiration and slight fever occurred in most instances and enlarged liver in 6 with pitting oedema in 1. Profuse vomiting in 6 infants, 2 of whom vomited blood, was reported. Cerebral irritation was noted in 4.— *Clinica pediat.*, 1964, *3*, 1. Further similar reports: A. L. Picchioni, *Am. J. Hosp. Pharm.*, 1961, *18*, 617; M. E. Calvin *et al.*, *New Engl. J. Med.*, 1964, *270*, 625.

Intravascular haemolysis in a woman with non-ketotic hyperglycaemic diabetic coma was possibly caused by the infusion of large volumes of 0.18% sodium chloride injection.— S. W. Blackwell and C. J. Burns-Cox, *Postgrad. med. J.*, 1973, *49*, 656.

Hypertension. For comments on the possible role of sodium chloride restriction in hypertension, see Antihypertensives, p.135.

Toxicity following intra-amniotic injection. The use of hyperosmotic saline solutions to induce abortion had been associated with severe complications including cardiovascular shock, CNS disorders, haemolysis, and renal necrosis. More than 60 fatalities occurred in Japan in the years 1949–53.— Y. Manabe (letter), *J. Am. med. Ass.*, 1969, *210*, 2091.

Febrile reactions occurred in 18.5% of 302 patients undergoing saline abortion studied retrospectively, and in 25.6% of 43 studied prospectively. Only a small proportion of the reactions could be attributed to bacterial infection.— C. R. Steinberg *et al.*, *Obstet. Gynec.*, 1972, *39*, 673.

Of 13 946 healthy women undergoing saline-induced abortion, 1964 experienced haemorrhage, 237 pelvic infection, 426 haemorrhage and infection, 467 fever, and 109 miscellaneous side-effects. Additionally 61 had saline-specific complications, including severe disturbance of blood coagulation (8), hyponatraemia (5), hypernatraemia (2), hyperpyrexia (3), and convulsions (1); 42 had less severe symptoms of saline leakage, such as pain at instillation.— C. Tietze and S. Lewit, *Stud. Fam. Plann.*, 1973, *4*, 133.

It was reported that intra-amniotic injection of dinoprost for mid-trimester abortion caused more complications than hyperosmotic saline similarly administered and that both methods caused more complications than curettage or evacuation. These findings were questioned and were not considered to reflect clinical experience in mid-trimester abortion.— *Med. Lett.*, 1977, *19*, 25.

Other reports and references.—Acute renal failure.— G. M. Eisner and J. S. Piver, *New Engl. J. Med.*, 1968, *279*, 360. Endometritis in 2 women.— P. B. Thurstone, *J. Am. med. Ass.*, 1969, *209*, 229. Extensive myometrial necrosis.— A. C. Wentz and T. M. King, *Obstet. Gynec.*, 1972, *40*, 315; D. R. Gupta and N. H. Cohen, *J. Am. med. Ass.*, 1972, *220*, 681; R. S. Galen *et al.*, *Am. J. Obstec. Gynec.*, 1974, *120*, 347, per *Int. pharm. Abstr.*, 1975, *12*, 356.

Coagulation changes. Changes in coagulation factors consistent with disseminated intravascular coagulation occurred in patients in whom pregnancy was terminated during the second trimester by the intra-amniotic injection of hyperosmotic saline.— R. W. Stander *et al.*, *Obstet. Gynec.*, 1971, *37*, 660, per *Br. med. J.*, 1973, *1*, 19.

Studies in 40 patients undergoing abortion by intra-amniotic injection of hyperosmotic saline suggested activation of the coagulation mechanism with a mild secondary activation of the fibrinolytic system, but only 1 clinical problem associated with thrombosis or haemorrhage occurred in 1500 infusions.— F. D. Brown *et al.*, *Obstet. Gynec.*, 1972, *39*, 538.

After the intra-amniotic injection of sodium chloride solution 20% to induce abortion in 12 women, there was a decrease in blood fibrinogen, and an increase in fibrinogen-fibrin breakdown products. Observation of 6 normal deliveries showed only a slight increase in fibrinogen-fibrin breakdown products.— J. L. Spivak *et al.*, *New Engl. J. Med.*, 1972, *287*, 321.

A report of haemorrhage due to coagulopathy in 6 women undergoing mid-trimester abortion using hyperosmotic sodium chloride solution.— R. T. Burkman *et al.*, *Am. J. Obstet. Gynec.*, 1977, *127*, 533.

Toxicity following intrathecal injection. Alarming but transient ECG changes occurred in patients treated with hyperosmotic saline solution for intractable pain. In patients who received a lumbar intrathecal injection, there was a striking increase in heart-rate and ventricular ectopic beats occurred in 3 patients. Other symptoms included peripheral cyanosis, sweating, and muscular fasciculation. A cisternal injection was followed by reduced heart-rate, amounting in 2 cases to sinus bradycardia, and other symptoms included vertigo, nystagmus, and vomiting. The side-effects were not considered contra-indications to the use of the technique.— M. C. McKean and E. Hitchcock (letter), *Lancet*, 1968, *2*, 1083.

Toxicity following use as emetic. Saline emetics should either never be used, or advice on their use should be carefully stated and widely circulated.— *Br. med. J.*, 1977, *2*, 977. Sodium chloride should not be used as an emetic.— W. O. Robertson (letter), *Br. med. J.*, 1977, *2*, 1022. A similar view.— W. K. Schwartz and H. B. Finke (letter), *J. Am. med. Ass.*, 1978, *240*, 1338; *Fedl Register*, 1978, *43*, 33701, per *Int. pharm. Abstr.*, 1979, *16*, 725.

For reports of toxicity and fatalities following the use of sodium chloride as an emetic, see Martindale 27th Edn, p. 1447.

Precautions. As for Sodium Salts, p.633.

Sodium chloride injection should be administered cautiously by intravenous injection to young children and the elderly. More dilute solutions, made iso-osmotic by the addition of dextrose, are generally preferred.

In geriatric patients, sodium chloride should be administered cautiously. An injection of 0.18% sodium chloride in dextrose injection 4% was suitable or dextrose injection 5% could be given. The central venous pressure should not exceed 10 cm of saline.— R. Simpson (letter), *Br. med. J.*, 1970, *1*, 110.

Hyperkalaemia and hypernatraemia in 7 well-nourished infants given an oral solution similar to the one recommended by UNICEF for rehydration. It is felt that for well-nourished children, under one year of age, treatment with UNICEF-type solutions should not last more than 24 hours.— A. Kahn and D. Blum (letter), *Lancet*, 1980, *1*, 1082. Criticisms and comments: M. L. Clements *et al.* (letter), *ibid.*, *2*, 34; W. A. M. Cutting (letter), *ibid*; M. Santosham *et al.* (letter), *ibid.*, 583; J. H. Tripp and J. T. Harries (letter), *ibid.*, 793; M. L. Clements *et al.* (letter), *ibid.*, 854; W. A. M. Cutting (letter), *ibid.*

Comment on the hazards of administering sodium chloride to patients, for example those with uncontrolled diabetes mellitus, whose plasma-sodium concentration is only spuriously low, owing to large amounts of solid matter in the plasma, chiefly lipids and protein.— *Lancet*, 1980, *2*, 1121. Comments.— R. Swaminathan and D. B. Morgan (letter), *ibid.*, 1981, *1*, 96; P. E. R. Madsen (letter), *ibid.*

Absorption and Fate. Sodium chloride is readily absorbed from the gastro-intestinal tract. It is present in all body fluids but is mainly found in the extracellular fluid. The amount of sodium chloride normally lost in the sweat is small and the osmotic equilibrium is maintained by the excretion of surplus amounts in the urine.

Jejunal absorption of sodium ions from a solution of sodium chloride was slow but the rate was markedly increased by the concomitant administration of bicarbonate ions and dextrose.— G. E. Sladen and A. M. Dawson (letter), *Nature*, 1968, *218*, 267.

Discussions of electrolyte metabolism in hepatic failure.— *Postgrad. med. J.*, 1975, *51*, 523–57.

Uses. Sodium chloride is the principal salt involved in maintaining the osmotic tension of the blood and tissues; changes in osmotic tension influence the movement of fluids and diffusion of salts in cellular tissues.

Excess of sodium chloride acts as a saline diuretic in patients who are not dehydrated; in a dosage of 10 to 12 g a day, by aiding excretion, sodium chloride is of value in the treatment of poisoning by bromides or iodides.

Severe sweating, such as occurs when heavy work is done in a hot atmosphere, may cause a marked loss of sodium chloride, producing muscle cramps and involuntary tremors. This can be prevented or relieved by taking sufficient saline drink (a 0.5% salt solution is suitable) to compensate for the loss of sodium chloride in the sweat.

In Addison's disease, the patient loses large quantities of sodium chloride in the urine, owing to deficiency of cortical hormones. Additional salt is necessary to maintain the electrolyte balance, and as much as 10 to 15 g of sodium chloride by mouth daily in enteric-coated capsules or tablets, or a mixture of sodium citrate, chloride, and bicarbonate may be given. During replacement therapy with mineralocorticoids care must be taken to ensure that abnormal retention of sodium chloride, with resultant oedema, does not occur.

In cardiac and kidney diseases a salt-free or salt-poor diet is sometimes employed.

Solutions containing sodium chloride are extensively used for the prevention or correction of fluid and electrolyte deficits or imbalance in a wide range of clinical situations (see below and p.633). Oral administration may be effective but usually such solutions must be given intravenously.

During prolonged courses of treatment the inclusion of lactate reduces the risk of the development of acidosis; 1 volume of sodium lactate injection with 2 volumes of sodium chloride injection 0.9% has been used.

All of these solutions should be adjusted to the needs of the individual patient, particularly for infants and young children, and for patients undergoing surgery.

Sodium chloride injections have been administered subcutaneously, including to infants, by hypodermoclysis, in conjunction with hyaluronidase, which facilitates the absorption of the fluid.

For rectal administration, half-strength saline is usually employed as it is more readily absorbed than physiological saline. Saline irrigations are also used to wash out the colon and antigrade bowel lavage with up to 12 litres of saline is now common.

Sterile hyperosmotic solutions of sodium chloride are given by extra-amniotic and intra-amniotic injection to induce abortion (but see under Adverse Effects).

Sodium chloride, with other electrolytes and dextrose, formulated to simulate an ideal extracellular fluid, is used as a dialysis solution in the treatment of renal failure or to assist in the elimination of toxic substances from the body. In haemodialysis, the exchange of ions between the solution and the patient's blood is made across a synthetic semipermeable membrane. In intraperitoneal dialysis, the exchange is made across the membranes of the peritoneal cavity. Solutions for intraperitoneal dialysis must be sterile.

The osmolality of the solutions may be increased by the addition of increased amounts of dextrose so as to aid the removal of water from the body, and by decreasing the concentration of specific electrolytes in the solutions it is possible to increase selectively the removal of electrolytes from the blood.

Dextrose facilitates the absorption of sodium from the intestinal tract. Solutions of sodium chloride and dextrose, often with added sodium bicarbonate and potassium chloride, are therefore used for oral rehydration in acute diarrhoea and cholera. A number of variant formulas are in use.

Sodium chloride has been used as an emetic, but is not without danger—see under Adverse Effects.

Sodium chloride (Natrium muriaticum; Nat. Mur.) is used in homoeopathic medicine.

A discussion on crystalloids versus colloids for plasma replacement.— *Lancet*, 1979, *1*, 1385. Comment.— J. A. R. Smith (letter), *ibid.*, *2*, 156.

Asthma diagnosis. Inhalation of different concentrations of ultrasonically nebulised saline to detect non-immunologically mediated bronchial hyperreactivity.— R. E. Schoeffel *et al.*, *Br. med. J.*, 1981, *283*, 1285.

Corneal erosion. Recurrent corneal erosion in 60 patients was treated initially with chloramphenicol ointment or eye-drops, with debridement if necessary. Prophylaxis with 5% sodium chloride ointment at night kept 32 patients symptom-free, with improvement in a further 16. Deteroration was common when treatment was stopped. It was not clear whether the lubricant or desiccant effect of the ointment was the more important.— N. Brown and A. Bron, *Br. J. Ophthal.*, 1976, *60*, 84.

Dehydration. A review of oral therapy for acute diarrhoea.— *Lancet*, 1981, *2*, 615.

In patients with cholera, replacement of fluid and electrolytes was based on restoration of a full pulse and filling of neck veins and, in adults, upon plasma specific gravity. For adults 2 units of sodium chloride injection followed by 1 unit of 1.39% sodium bicarbonate were suitable, or 3 units of sodium chloride injection followed by one of 2% sodium bicarbonate. Iso-osmotic sodium lactate could be used instead of sodium bicarbonate. After replacement of the initial loss, sodium chloride injection was administered at the rate at which fluid was lost in the stool. Potassium losses could be replaced by mouth; with green-coconut water–70 mmol potassium per litre–170 g for each litre of stool, or with potassium citrate solution 10% in 15-ml doses (diluted) 3 or 4 times daily. In children under 10 years of age, a solution with a bicarbonate or sodium lactate content of 48 mmol per litre reduced the fatality-rate to 0.6% in over 300 cases. The use of a solution (5-4-1 solution) containing sodium chloride 0.5%, sodium bicarbonate 0.4%, and potassium chloride 0.1%, obviated the need for potassium replacement by mouth.— WHO Expert Committee on Cholera, Second Report, *Tech. Rep. Ser. Wld Hlth Org. No. 352*, 1967.

A brief discussion of salt supplements in the tropics.— *Br. med. J.*, 1974, *2*, 497.

A comparison was made between 3 intravenous regimens for the treatment of hypernatraemic dehydration in 28 infants up to 15 weeks old. Group A (10 infants) were given sodium chloride 0.45% in dextrose 5% at 100 ml per kg estimated rehydrated body-weight per 24 hours. Group B (9 infants) received the same infusion at 150 ml per kg body-weight per 24 hours, and Group C (9 infants) received sodium chloride 0.18% in dextrose 4.3% at 100 ml per kg body-weight per 24 hours. In all groups potassium chloride, 26 mmol per litre, was added to the infusion once urine was passed, unless plasma-potassium concentration was still high. Rehydration was achieved within 48 hours in groups B and C but much more slowly in group A. Group B showed a comparatively high incidence of convulsions during treatment. Rehydration could be achieved most safely by the regimen used in group C, with the early addition of potassium.— A. Banister *et al.*, *Archs Dis. Childh.*, 1975, *50*, 179.

Diarrhoea was common in infants in developing countries and was probably the major cause of deaths. It was caused by bacterial or viral infection and led to dehydration. Early replacement of water and electrolyte losses and maintenance of adequate nutrition were essential. Oral rehydration facilitated prompt treatment. Absorption of dextrose from the small bowel remained intact even in severe diarrhoea; sodium was absorbed concomitantly in approximately equimolar amounts. Sucrose could be used if dextrose was not available. Oral replacement was adequate for patients with mild or moderate dehydration (up to 7% loss of body-weight). Thirst was a useful guide to the volume required; puffy eyelids indicated excess. Maintenance volumes showed equal stool losses. Vomiting might occur during initial treatment but small volumes given frequently were usually acceptable. Normal intake of food should continue. Antibiotics should not be given routinely. Adequate renal function was essential. Dextrose malabsorption occurred in about 3% of patients with acute diarrhoea; oral replacement was not recommended for such patients or for premature infants or infants aged less than 1 month.— N. F. Pierce and N. Hirschhorn, *Chronicle Wld Hlth Org.*, 1977, *31*, 87.

A rehydrating solution containing sodium 50 mmol per litre, rather than 90 mmol per litre, was considered to be preferable for use in infants because of its lower sodium concentration, and because it eliminated the need for administration of additional water.— A. Chatterjee *et al.*, *Archs Dis. Childh.*, 1978, *53*, 284.

A 'diarrhoea treatment solution', similar in composition to Dacca solution but containing only 118 mmol of sodium per litre, and with the addition of 44 mmol per litre of dextrose, was suitable for the intravenous treatment of diarrhoea and cholera. Patients treated with Dacca solution might, if renal function was compromised, suffer salt intoxication in the absence of oral intake of water.— M. M. Rahaman *et al.*, *Bull. Wld Hlth Org.*, 1979, *57*, 977.

Discussions and further references.— D. R. Nalin *et al.*, *Lancet*, 1968, *2*, 370; R. A. Cash *et al.*, *ibid.*, 1970, *2*, 549; *Br. med. J.*, 1970, *4*, 2; P. L. de V. Hart (letter), *ibid.*, 1971, *1*, 49; A. G. Ironside, *ibid.*, 1973, *1*, 284; *Lancet*, 1975, *1*, 79; *Br. med. J.*, 1975, *4*, 539; D. R. Bell, *ibid.*, 1976, *2*, 1240; D. R. Nalin and R. A. Cash (letter), *Lancet*, 1976, *2*, 957; C. R. Pullan *et al.*, *Br. med. J.*, 1977, *1*, 619; *ibid.*, *2*, 119; M. D. Holdaway, *Drugs*, 1977, *14*, 383; *Chronicle Wld Hlth Org.*, 1977, *31*, 421; *Bull. Wld Hlth Org.*, 1977, *55*, 87 (report of a Field Trial by an International Study Group); *Drug & Ther. Bull.*, 1978, *16*, 1; C. McCord (letter), *Lancet*, 1978, *1*, 1207; Nalin D.R. *et al.*, *ibid.*, 1978, *2*, 277; D. A. Sack *et al.*, *ibid.*, 280; *ibid.*, 300; L. Rees and C. G. D. Brook, *Lancet*, 1979, *1*, 770; *Drug & Ther. Bull.*, 1979, *17*, 51; M. M. Rahaman *et al.*, *Lancet*, 1979, *2*, 809; D. Pizarro *et al.*, *Bull. Wld Hlth Org.*, 1979, *57*, 983; P. Hutchins *et al.*, *J. Hyg.*, *Camb.*, 1979, *82*, 15, per *Abstr. Hyg.*, 1979, *54*, 444; D. R. Nalin *et al.*, *Trans. R. Soc. trop. Med. Hyg.*, 1979, *73*, 10; W. A. M. Cutting and A. D. Langmuir, *ibid.*, 1980, *74*, 30.

A formula for Oral Rehydration Salts (Unicef) is given below under Preparations.

Dialysis. Some general references: R. A. Branch *et al.*, *Br. med. J.*, 1971, *1*, 249; *Lancet*, 1972, *2*, 582; E. G. Lowrie *et al.*, *New Engl. J. Med.*, 1973, *288*, 863; V. Parsons *et al.*, *Postgrad. med. J.*, 1975, *51*, 515; D. B. Evans, *Br. med. J.*, 1977, *1*, 1585; J. A. P. Trafford *et al.*, *ibid.*, 1979, *1*, 518; L. Sellars *et al.*, *ibid.*, 520.

A discussion on the use of dialysis for the treatment of irreversible uraemia.— T. Manis and E. A. Friedman, *New Engl. J. Med.*, 1979, *301*, 1260 and 1321. Comments.— C. F. Bolton (letter), *ibid.*, 1980, *302*, 755; D. G. Oreopoulos (letter), *ibid.* Reply.— T. Manis and E. A. Friedman (letter), *ibid.*

Data indicating that patient morbidity is affected by the dialysis regimen.— E. G. Lowrie *et al.*, *New Engl. J. Med.*, 1981, *305*, 1176.

Haemodialysis. Cramps occurred during haemodialysis in 195 of 397 (49%) dialyses carried out using a solution containing sodium 132.5 mmol per litre compared with 131 episodes in 563 (23%) dialyses using 145 mmol of sodium per litre.— W. K. Stewart *et al.*, *Lancet*, 1972, *1*, 1049.

In a double-blind crossover study in 17 patients undergoing maintenance haemodialysis with a solution containing sodium 134 mmol per litre, 2 experienced no cramp. In the 15 experiencing cramp the frequency was reduced by 26% and the severity by 30% by the use of 14 Slow Sodium tablets during each period of dialysis. Blood pressure and body-weight were not affected.— G. R. D. Catto *et al.*, *Br. med. J.*, 1973, *3*, 389.

Experience with 19 patients with hypertension indicated that haemodialysis with isonatric dialysate containing 145 mmol per litre instead of the conventional 132.5 mmol per litre was consistent with the maintenance of good control of blood pressure, with the advantage of relative freedom from cramp.— W. K. Stewart and L. W. Fleming, *Postgrad. med. J.*, 1974, *50*, 260.

Formulas for haemodialysis solutions are given below, under Preparations.

Peritoneal dialysis. A study of the heat loss induced in a patient by peritoneal dialysis with cold dialysate and a suggestion of its use in malignant hyperpyrexia.— J. Gjessing *et al.*, *Br. J. Anaesth.*, 1976, *48*, 469.

Peritoneal dialysis in chronic renal failure.— *Lancet*, 1978, *2*, 303.

Discussions of chronic ambulatory peritoneal dialysis in the treatment of chronic renal failure: *Br. med. J.*, 1979, *2*, 229; *Med. Lett.*, 1979, *21*, 69.

Formulas for peritoneal dialysis solutions are given below, under Preparations.

Hydatid cyst. An account of the management of hydatid disease and mention of preference for hypertonic saline 10% as a scolicidal agent after aspiration of the cyst.— D. L. Morris, *Br. J. Hosp. Med.*, 1981, *25*, 586.

Lavage. Since the absorption of some drugs could be enhanced by the presence of water in the gastro-intestinal tract it was suggested that in the emergency treatment of overdoses of lipid-insoluble drugs, gastric lavage with physiological saline would be preferable to lavage with water.— G. Williams and J. L. Maddocks (letter), *Br. J. clin. Pharmac.*, 1975, *2*, 543.

A whole-gut perfusion technique using an iso-osmotic electrolyte solution for thorough cleansing of the bowel.— P. Woo *et al.*, *Br. med. J.*, 1976, *1*, 433.

Bronchial lavage. Bronchial lavage with 800 to 1500 ml of a solution of sodium chloride greatly improved the condition of 56 of 92 patients with obstructive lung disease. The procedure was performed under anaesthesia.— H. T. Thompson *et al.*, *Thorax*, 1966, *21*, 557.

Pain. Permanent pain relief was produced in a period up to approximately 6 months in 44% of patients with intractable pain due to benign conditions and in 15% of patients with malignant disease by the intrathecal administration of 20 ml of a 10 to 15% solution of sodium chloride. Sphincter disturbances occurred in 8% and muscle weakness in 3% of patients.— E. Hitchcock and M. N. Prandini, *Lancet*, 1973, *1*, 310.

Local infiltration of lignocaine 1.5% or physiological saline into pericranial tender spots were both found to have a beneficial effect on attacks of common migraine.— P. Tfelt-Hansen *et al.* (letter), *Lancet*, 1980, *1*, 1140.

For a report indicating that local injection of physiological saline provides better relief of myofascial pain than local injection of mepivacaine 0.5%, see p.902.

For reports of the use of solutions of sodium chloride with benzyl alcohol for local anaesthesia, see Benzyl Alcohol, p.40.

Pancreatitis. Peritoneal lavage, using sodium chloride injection, for the assessment of severity of acute pancreatitis.— I. R. Pickford *et al.*, *Br. med. J.*, 1977, *2*, 1377.

Shock. Following injections of hyperosmotic (7.5%) sodium chloride solution 100 to 400 ml, reversal of refractory hypovolaemic shock was promptly achieved in 11 of 12 patients in terminal hypovolaemic shock. The injections were given in portions of 50 ml over 3 to 5 minutes, and repeated at intervals of 10 to 15 minutes. Nine of these patients were ultimately discharged from hospital.— J. de Felippe *et al.*, *Lancet*, 1980, *2*, 1002. Agreement that hypertonic solutions are efficacious.— D. K. Brooks (letter), *ibid.*, 1256. Further comment.— P. J. Horsey (letter), *ibid.*

Tattoo removal. The use of sodium chloride in the abrasive removal of tattoos.— W. A. Koerber and N. M. Price, *Archs Derm.*, 1978, *114*, 884; A. M. M. Strong and I. T. Jackson, *Br. J. Derm.*, 1979, *101*, 693; *Lancet*, 1980, *1*, 577; M. D. Catterall (letter), *ibid.*, 981.

Termination of pregnancy. From 1955 to 1976, mid-trimester abortions and inductions of labour were performed in 213 women by instillation of a 30% sodium chloride solution into the amniotic sac. Up to 250 ml of amniotic fluid was replaced over 10 to 15 minutes with a quantity of solution 10 to 15 ml more than the volume withdrawn. Oxytocin and antibiotics were not injected into the amniotic cavity. Curettage was performed where the foetus was less than 600 g or the abortion appeared incomplete. The mean time from instillation to abortion was 25.4 hours; 11 patients required a second instillation a week later. From a follow-up of 103 patients 2 to 22 years after abortion it was concluded that the use of 30% sodium chloride solution was safe and rapid and rarely resulted in late sequelae. Early complications had included fever in 8 patients and haemorrhage in 2. Hypermenorrhoea developed in 8 patients and oligomenorrhoea in one. Following gynaecological examination it was considered that hydrosalpinx, cervical incompetence, or intrauterine adhesions in 3 patients were possibly attributable to the use of saline for abortion.— R. Borenstein *et al.*, *Int. J. Fert.*, 1980, *25*, 88.

Wounds. The aims of treatment were: to reduce infection; to remove necrotic, purulent, or foreign material; and to facilitate wound repair. The second and third objectives were achieved by salt baths which however had little place in the treatment of small clean wounds.— *Br. med. J.*, 1974, *3*, 622.

Preparations

Baths

Sodium Chloride Bath *(B.P.C. 1949)*. Balneum Sodii Chloridi. Sodium chloride 3.36 kg in 140 litres.

Dialysis Solutions

Haemodialysis Solutions. Haemodialysis Fluids; Dialysing Solutions for Artificial Kidney

Concentrated Haemodialysis Solution (35×) *(B.P.C. 1973)*. Sodium chloride 194.5 g, sodium acetate 166.6 g, dextrose monohydrate 70 g, potassium chloride 2.6 g, freshly boiled and cooled water to 1 litre. One litre of concentrate is diluted with 34 litres of the appropriate type of water for each 35 litres required in the artificial kidney.

After dilution with purified water 1 litre of solution contains about 130 mmol of sodium, 1 mmol of potassium, 35 mmol of bicarbonate (as acetate), and 96 mmol of chloride.

Purified water, potable water softened by base exchange, or potable water may be used for diluting the concentrated solution. The quantity of sodium may need to be adjusted to take into account the sodium content of the water, and calcium and magnesium (as acetate or chloride) may need to be added to give concentrations, in the diluted solutions, of 1.5 to 2 mmol of calcium and 0.45 to 0.75 mmol of magnesium. Concentrated haemodialysis solutions are supplied in suitable glass or plastic containers which do not release ions or harmful substances into the solution. Though the solutions are not required to be sterile, hygienic precautions should be taken to prevent heavy bacterial contamination.

Concentrated Haemodialysis Solution (40×) *(B.P.C. 1973).* Sodium chloride 222.4 g, sodium acetate 190.4 g, dextrose monohydrate 80 g, potassium chloride 4 g, lactic acid 4 ml, freshly boiled and cooled water to 1 litre. The solution should be stored in a warm place as it is liable to deposit crystals on keeping. One litre of concentrate is diluted with 39 litres of the appropriate type of water (see above) for each 40 litres required in the artificial kidney.

After dilution with purified water 1 litre of solution contains about 130 mmol of sodium, 1.3 mmol of potassium, 36 mmol of bicarbonate (as acetate), and 96 mmol of chloride.

Intraperitoneal Dialysis Solutions. Intraperitoneal Dialysis Fluids; Peritoneal Dialysis Solutions

Intraperitoneal Dialysis Solution (Acetate) *(B.P.C. 1973).* Sodium chloride 5.56 g, sodium acetate 4.76 g, calcium chloride dihydrate 220 mg, magnesium chloride 152 mg, sodium metabisulphite 150 mg, anhydrous dextrose 17 g, Water for Injections to 1 litre. Dissolve, filter, and sterilise by autoclaving; a rapid-cooling autoclave should be used to minimise caramelisation of the dextrose.

The solution contains in each litre about 130 mmol of sodium, 1.5 mmol of calcium, 0.75 mmol of magnesium, 100 mmol of chloride, and 35 mmol of bicarbonate (as acetate).

The solutions are slightly hyperosmotic; when a more rapid removal of excess water is required, the osmolarity may be increased by using up to 7% of dextrose. Potassium chloride is usually administered separately in accordance with the needs of the patient. Intraperitoneal dialysis solutions are supplied in suitable glass or plastic containers which do not release ions or harmful substances into the solution. The solutions are not suitable for intravenous injection. Any portion remaining after the contents are first used should be discarded.

Intraperitoneal Dialysis Solution (Lactate) *(B.P.C. 1973).* Sodium chloride 5.6 g, lactic acid and sodium hydroxide equivalent to sodium lactate 5 g, calcium chloride dihydrate 260 mg, magnesium chloride 150 mg, sodium metabisulphite 50 mg, anhydrous dextrose 13.6 g, Water for Injections to 1 litre. The sodium lactate may be obtained from lactic acid 3.8 ml and sodium hydroxide 1.8 g using the *B.P.* method for the preparation of Sodium Lactate Intravenous Infusion; a correction to the formula must be made for the sodium chloride produced by neutralisation of the excess sodium hydroxide by hydrochloric acid. Dissolve the other ingredients in a portion of the water, mix with the sodium lactate solution, filter, and sterilise by autoclaving; A rapid-cooling autoclave should be used to minimise caramelisation of the dextrose.

The solution contains in each litre about 140 mmol of sodium, 1.8 mmol of calcium, 0.75 mmol of magnesium, 100 mmol of chloride, and 45 mmol of bicarbonate (as lactate).

Eye Preparations

Sodium Chloride Eye Lotion *(B.P.).* Sodium chloride 900 mg, water to 100 ml. The solution is filtered, transferred to the final containers, which are then closed to exclude micro-organisms, and sterilised by autoclaving.

The lotion is used undiluted. It should be discarded 24 hours after first opening the container.

NOTE. The *B.P.* permits the title SALINE for single-dose eye-drops containing sodium chloride 0.9%.

Sodium Chloride Ophthalmic Solution *(U.S.P.).* A sterile iso-osmotic solution of sodium chloride; it contains a buffer and may contain suitable antimicrobial and stabilising agents. pH 7 to 7.2. Store in airtight containers.

Inhalations

Sodium Chloride Inhalation *(U.S.P.).* A sterile solution of sodium chloride in water containing no antimicrobial agents or other added substances. pH 4.5 to 7.

Injections

Bacteriostatic Sodium Chloride Injection *(U.S.P.).* A sterile solution of sodium chloride 0.9% in Water for Injections, containing one or more suitable antimicrobial agents.

Compound Sodium Chloride Injection *(B.P.C. 1959).* Ringer's Injection; Ringer's Solution for Injection. Sodium chloride 860 mg, potassium chloride 30 mg, calcium chloride hexahydrate 48 mg, Water for Injections to 100 ml. Sterilised immediately by autoclaving or by filtration.

A similar injection, with slight variations of formula, is included in many pharmacopoeias. The *U.S.P.* formula is given below (Ringer's Injection).

Dacca Solution. 5-4-1 Solution. Sodium chloride 0.5%, sodium bicarbonate 0.4%, potassium chloride 0.1%. For electrolyte replacement treatment in cholera.

Dextrose and Sodium Chloride Injection *(U.S.P.).* A sterile solution of anhydrous dextrose or dextrose monohydrate and sodium chloride in Water for Injections containing no antimicrobial agents. pH 3.5 to 6.5.

Ringer's Injection *(U.S.P.).* Ringer's Solution *(Jap. P.).* A sterile solution containing sodium chloride 860 mg, potassium chloride 30 mg, calcium chloride (dihydrate) 33 mg, and Water for Injections to 100 ml. It contains no antimicrobial agents. pH 5 to 7.5.

Each litre contains approximately 147.5 mmol of sodium, 156 mmol of chloride, 4 mmol of potassium, and 2.25 mmol of calcium.

Sodium Chloride and Dextrose Intravenous Infusion *(B.P.).* Sodium Chloride and Dextrose Injection; Sod. Chlor. and Dextrose Inj. A sterile solution of sodium chloride and anhydrous dextrose or dextrose monohydrate for parenteral use in Water for Injections. The solution is sterilised immediately after preparation by autoclaving. pH 3.5 to 5.5. Store at a temperature not exceeding 25°.

Sodium Chloride Injection *(U.S.P.).* A sterile solution of sodium chloride in Water for Injections containing no antimicrobial agents. pH 4.5 to 7.

Sodium Chloride Intravenous Infusion *(B.P.).* Sodium Chloride Injection; Sod. Chlor. Inj.; Physiological Saline Solution for Injection; Normal Saline Solution for Injection; Physiological Sodium Chloride Solution for Injection. A sterile solution of sodium chloride in Water for Injections. Sterilised by autoclaving. Store at a temperature not exceeding 25°.

A 0.9% solution is iso-osmotic with human blood plasma and also with the lachrymal secretion. It contains 154 mmol (154 mEq) of sodium and of chloride per litre. The *B.P.* requires that the concentration be stated as 150 mmol per litre. In *Martindale* this injection is intended when no strength is specified for sodium chloride injection.

This injection is included in many other pharmacopoeias.

NOTE. When Normal Saline Solution for Injection is prescribed, a 0.9% injection is supplied.

CAUTION. Physiologically normal solutions (0.9%) of sodium chloride should not be confused with chemically normal (molar; 5.85%) solutions of sodium chloride.

Mixtures

Compound Sodium Chloride Mixture *(B.P.C. 1973).* Sodium chloride 200 mg, sodium bicarbonate 500 mg, double-strength chloroform water 5 ml, water to 10 ml. It should be recently prepared. *Dose.* 10 to 20 ml in a tumblerful of hot water, sipped slowly.

Mouth-washes

Compound Sodium Chloride Mouthwash *(B.P.).* Sodium Chloride Compound Mouthwash; Collut. Sod. Chlor. Co. Sodium chloride 1.5 g, sodium bicarbonate 1 g, concentrated peppermint emulsion 2.5 ml, double-strength chloroform water 50 ml, water to 100 ml. To be diluted with an equal volume of warm water before use.

Powders

Compound Sodium Chloride and Dextrose Oral Powder *(B.P.).* Compound Sodium Chloride and Dextrose Powder; Sodium Chloride and Dextrose Compound Powder; Electrolyte Powder. Each powder contains sodium chloride 500 mg, dextrose [monohydrate] 20 g, potassium chloride 750 mg, and sodium bicarbonate 750 mg; it may contain suitable flavouring agents. One powder dissolved in sufficient recently boiled and cooled water to make 500 ml of solution provides sodium 17.5 mmol, potassium 10 mmol, chloride 18.5 mmol, bicarbonate 9 mmol, and dextrose 100 mmol. The solution should not be used more than 24 hours after preparation. For infantile diarrhoea. A powder containing two-fifths of the above quantities to make 200 ml of solution is also available.

Oral Rehydration Salts *(Unicef).* Sodium chloride 3.5 g, potassium chloride 1.5 g, sodium bicarbonate 2.5 g, [anhydrous] dextrose 20 g. For solution in 1 litre of water. *Dose.* infants, 1 litre in 24 hours; children, 1 litre in 8 to 24 hours. Each litre of solution provides approximately 90 mmol of sodium, 20 mmol of potassium, 80 mmol of chloride, and 30 mmol of bicarbonate.

Solutions

Cholera Replacement Solution. Sodium bicarbonate 400 mg, sodium chloride 400 mg, potassium chloride 150 mg, dextrose 2 g, water to 100 ml. Each 100 ml provided the following mmol: sodium 11.6; potassium 2.1; chloride 8.9; bicarbonate 4.8; and dextrose 11. For oral replacement of faecal fluid losses in cholera. Potassium citrate 270 mg or anhydrous potassium acetate 250 mg could be used instead of potassium chloride, but sodium chloride should then be increased to 550 mg and sodium bicarbonate reduced to 200 mg.—R.W. Goodgame and W.B. Greenough, *Ann. intern. Med.*, 1975, *82*, 101.

Elliott's B Solution. Artificial Spinal Fluid. Sodium chloride 730 mg, potassium chloride 30 mg, calcium chloride (dihydrate) 20 mg, magnesium sulphate 30 mg, sodium phosphate heptahydrate 20 mg, dextrose 80 mg, sodium bicarbonate 190 mg, phenol red 10 μg, Water for Injections to 100 ml.—M.J. Duttera *et al.* (letter), *Lancet*, 1972, *1*, 540.

Gastro-intestinal Replacement Solution. From a study of the electrolyte concentration of gastro-intestinal aspirations from a number of patients, a formula for a gastro-intestinal replacement solution was recommended. It contained in 1 litre sodium 100 mmol, potassium 12 mmol, ammonium 10 mmol, chloride 122 mmol. Laevulose 100 g or anhydrous dextrose 50 g could also be added. Each 100 ml of solution contained sodium chloride 590 mg, potassium chloride 90 mg, ammonium chloride 53 mg, and anhydrous dextrose 5 g or laevulose 10 g. Gastro-intestinal aspirations could be replaced by this solution volume for volume every 6 hours. In 1 hour 500 ml could be given.—E.A. Badoe, *Br. med. J.*, 1970, *3*, 622.

Hanks's Balanced Salt Solution. *Stock solution:* sodium chloride 8 g, potassium chloride 400 mg, magnesium sulphate 200 mg, calcium chloride (dihydrate) 140 mg (dissolved separately), sodium phosphate (dihydrate) 60 mg (=120 mg of dodecahydrate), monobasic potassium phosphate 60 mg, anhydrous dextrose 1 g, water to 100 ml; add 10 ml of 0.2% phenol red solution (see under Skin Bank Fluid, p.638) and 0.4 ml of chloroform, and store at room temperature. The final solution used for tissue preservation was made by diluting the stock solution 1:10 and autoclaving 20-ml quantities in screw-capped Pyrex bottles; to each bottle was added 0.5 ml of autoclaved 1.4% sodium bicarbonate solution; the solution was stored in a refrigerator for equilibration of the CO_2 to pH 7.6 before finally tightening the caps.—J.H. Hanks and R.E.Wallace, *Proc. Soc. exp. Biol. Med.*, 1949, *71*, 196.

This solution is very similar to Balanced Salt Solution, described under Skin Bank Fluid, below.

Ringer's Irrigation *(U.S.P.).* Ringer's Solution. A sterile solution containing sodium chloride 860 mg, potassium chloride 30 mg, calcium chloride (dihydrate) 33 mg, and Water for Injections to 100 ml. pH 5 to 7.5. It should not be used for injection or for irrigations that might result in absorption into the blood.

Ringer-Locke Solution *(B.P.C. 1934).* Sodium chloride 900 mg, potassium chloride 42 mg, anhydrous calcium chloride 24 mg, anhydrous dextrose 100 mg, sodium bicarbonate 50 mg, water to 100 ml.

Similar solutions have also been used and have also been called Locke's Solution.

Ringer-Tyrode Solution *(B.P.C. 1934).* Sodium chloride 800 mg, potassium chloride 20 mg, anhydrous calcium chloride 20 mg, magnesium chloride 1 mg, anhydrous dextrose 100 mg, sodium acid phosphate 5 mg, sodium bicarbonate 100 mg, water to 100 ml.

Skin Bank Fluid. SBF. Balanced salt solution (10×) 8 ml, Water for Injections 67 ml, plasma AB^+ (or A^+) 20 ml. Mix; sterilise by filtration. Add sterile solution of neomycin sulphate 50 mg in Water for Injections 5 ml.

Balanced Salt Solution 10×. BSS. Sodium chloride 8 g, calcium chloride (dihydrate) 140 mg, anhydrous dextrose 910 mg, potassium chloride 400 mg, magnesium sulphate 200 mg, monobasic potassium phosphate 60 mg, sodium phosphate (heptahydrate) 90 mg (=120 mg of dodecahydrate), phenol red solution 0.2% 10 ml (see below), Water for Injections to 100 ml.

Phenol Red Solution 0.2%. Phenol red (phenolsulphonphthalein) 240 mg, 0.05N sodium hydroxide solution 13 ml (or sufficient to give pH 6.8), Water for Injections to 120 ml.—O.M. Netzer, *Am. J. Hosp. Pharm.*, 1960, *17*, 28.

Sodium Chloride Irrigation *(U.S.P.).* A sterile solution of sodium chloride in Water for Injections. It contains no antimicrobial agents; it should not be used for injection or for irrigations that might result in absorption into the blood.

Sodium Chloride Solution *(B.P.).* Liq. Sod. Chlor.; Normal Saline. Sodium chloride 0.9% in freshly boiled and cooled water. It should not be used for injection.

Tyrode's Solution. Sodium chloride 800 mg, potassium chloride 20 mg, anhydrous calcium chloride 20 mg, magnesium chloride 10 mg, sodium acid phosphate 5 mg, sodium bicarbonate 100 mg, anhydrous dextrose 100 mg, water to 100 ml.—M.V. Tyrode, *Archs Pharmacodyn.*, 1910, *20*, 205.

Solution-tablets

Sodium Chloride Solution-tablets *(B.P.C. 1954).* Solvellae Sodii Chloridi. One solution-tablet containing 2.25 g dissolved in 250 ml of water forms a 0.9% solution of sodium chloride.

Sodium Chloride Tablets for Solution *(U.S.P.).* Tablets containing sodium chloride with no added substance.

Tablets

Sodium Chloride and Dextrose Tablets *(U.S.P.).* Tablets containing sodium chloride and dextrose monohydrate.

Sodium Chloride Tablets *(B.P.).* Sod. Chlor. Tab. Tablets containing sodium chloride. They should be dissolved in water before administration.

Sodium Chloride Tablets *(U.S.P.).* Tablets containing sodium chloride.

Proprietary Preparations

Alcon Opulets Sodium Chloride *(Alcon, UK: Farillon, UK).* Sterile eye-drops containing sodium chloride 0.9%, in single-use disposable applicators.

Balanced Salt Solution Alcon, BSS *(Alcon, UK: Farillon, UK).* A sterile iso-osmotic solution containing sodium chloride 0.49%, potassium chloride 0.075%, calcium chloride 0.048%, magnesium chloride 0.03%, sodium acetate 0.39%, and sodium citrate 0.17%. For ophthalmic irrigation.

Dextrolyte *(Cow & Gate, UK).* A solution containing sodium chloride, sodium lactate, and potassium chloride, with dextrose monohydrate 3.6%; providing approximately these ions in each 100 ml; sodium 3.5 mmol, potassium 1.34 mmol, and chloride 3.05 mmol. For oral electrolyte replacement.

Dialaflex 61 *(Boots, UK).* A solution for peritoneal dialysis in plastic containers of 1 litre, containing sodium chloride 0.56%, sodium lactate 0.5%, calcium chloride 0.026%, magnesium chloride 0.015%, dextrose monohydrate 1.36%, and sodium metabisulphite 0.005%, providing in each litre sodium 141 mmol, calcium 1.8 mmol, magnesium 0.75 mmol, chloride 100.8 mmol, and lactate 44.6 mmol, with dextrose monohydrate 13.6 g. **Dialaflex 62** is a similar solution containing the same constituents in the same proportion except that the dextrose monohydrate is 6.36% and sodium metabisulphite 0.012%; the sodium content is 141 mmol per litre and dextrose monohydrate content 63.6 g per litre. **Dialaflex 63** differs from Dialaflex 61 only in that it contains sodium chloride 0.5%, providing sodium 130 mmol and chloride 90.5 mmol per litre.

Dianeal with 1.36% Dextrose *(Travenol, UK).* A solution for peritoneal dialysis containing sodium chloride 0.56%, anhydrous dextrose 1.36%, sodium lactate 0.5%, calcium chloride dihydrate 0.026%, and magnesium chloride 0.015%, in Water for Injections, and providing the following ions per litre—sodium 141 mmol, chloride 101 mmol, calcium 1.75 mmol, magnesium 0.75 mmol, and lactate 45 mmol. **Dianeal with 3.86% Dextrose.** A similar solution containing anhydrous dextrose 3.86%. **Dianeal 130 with 1.36% Dextrose.** A similar solution containing sodium chloride 0.5% providing 130 mmol of sodium per litre. **Dianeal 130 with 1.36% Dextrose and Potassium.** A similar solution providing in addition 2.5 mmol of potassium per litre.

Dianeal 137 with 1.36% Dextrose *(Travenol, UK).* A solution for peritoneal dialysis containing sodium chloride 0.57%, anhydrous dextrose 1.36%, sodium lactate o.39%, calcium chloride dihydrate 0.0257%, and magnesium chloride 0.0152%, providing in each litre sodium 132 mmol, calcium 1.75 mmol, magnesium 0.75 mmol, chloride 102 mmol, and lactate 35 mmol. **Dianeal 137 with 3.86% Dextrose.** A similar solution containing anhydrous dextrose 3.86%. **Dianeal K 139 with 1.36% Dextrose.** A similar solution to Dianeal 137 with 1.36% Dextrose, providing in addition potassium 2 mmol per litre. **Dianeal K 139 with 3.86% Dextrose.** A similar solution to Dianeal 137 with 3.86% Dextrose, providing in addition potassium 2 mmol per litre.

Dioralyte *(Armour, UK).* Sachets each containing sodium chloride 200 mg, potassium chloride 300 mg, sodium bicarbonate 300 mg, and dextrose monohydrate 8 g, providing (after reconstitution to 200 ml with water) sodium 7 mmol, potassium 4 mmol, chloride 7.5 ml, and bicarbonate 3.5 mmol approximately. For oral electrolyte replacement.

An evaluation of Dioralyte.— *Drug & Ther. Bull.*, 1979, *17*, 51.

Effervescent Saline Tablets *(Southon-Horton, UK).* Each contains sodium chloride 300 mg, sodium acid phosphate 30 mg, and potassium citrate 30 mg, providing sodium 5.3 mmol and chloride 5.1 mmol.

Electrosol *(Macarthys, UK).* Tablets each containing sodium chloride 200 mg, potassium chloride 160 mg, and sodium bicarbonate 200 mg in an effervescent basis. Eight tablets dissolved in 1 litre of water provide a solution containing 46.5 mmol sodium, 17 mmol potassium, 44.5 mmol chloride, and 19 mmol bicarbonate. For oral electrolyte replacement. *Dose.* Adults and children, 1 to 3 litres over 24 hours; infants, 150 to 200 ml per kg body-weight to a maximum of 1.5 litres over 24 hours. NOTE. The name Electrosol is also applied to a veterinary preparation of different composition.

Iodised Sodium Chloride Tablets *(Southon-Horton, UK).* Enteric-coated tablets each containing sodium chloride 800 mg (13.7 mmol of sodium and of chloride), with potassium iodide 1 in 100 000.

Minims Saline *(Smith & Nephew Pharmaceuticals, UK).* Sterile eye-drops of sodium chloride 0.9% available in single-use disposable applicators. (Also available as Minims Saline in *Austral.*).

Plasma-Lyte *(Travenol, UK).* A range of electrolyte solutions for intravenous use. For replacing severe losses: **Plasma-Lyte 148 in Water,** providing in each litre the following ions—sodium 140 mmol, potassium 5 mmol, magnesium 1.5 mmol, chloride 98 mmol, bicarbonate (as acetate) 27 mmol, and 23 mmol of gluconate; **Plasma-Lyte 148 in 5% Dextrose,** containing also anhydrous dextrose 5% (880 kJ per litre); and **Plasma-Lyte with 10% Travert,** providing in each litre the following ions—sodium 140 mmol, potassium 10 mmol, calcium 2.5 mmol, magnesium 1.5 mmol, chloride 103 mmol, acetate 47 mmol, and lactate 8 mmol with invert sugar 10% (1600 kJ per litre). For maintenance: **Plasma-Lyte M in 5% Dextrose,** providing in each litre the following ions—sodium 40 mmol, potassium 16 mmol, calcium 2.5 mmol, magnesium 1.5 mmol, chloride 40 mmol, acetate 12 mmol, and lactate 12 mmol, with anhydrous dextrose 5% (800 kJ per litre).

Renalyte *(Macarthys, UK).* A range of concentrates for the preparation of solutions for haemodialysis.

Slow Sodium *(Ciba, UK).* Sodium chloride, available as sustained-release tablets of 600 mg. Each represents approximately 10.3 mmol of sodium and of chloride. (Also available as Slow Sodium in *S.Afr.*).

Evaluations of Slow Sodium.— *Drug & Ther. Bull.*, 1971, *9*, 98; E. M. Clarkson *et al.*, *Br. med. J.*, 1971, *3*, 604.

Owing to the risk of intestinal obstruction, sustained-release preparations such as Slow Sodium, where the drug is released in transit, but the matrix ghost is often eliminated intact, should not be prescribed in patients with Crohn's disease or other intestinal disease in which strictures may form.— J. L. Shaffer *et al.* (letter), *Lancet*, 1980, *2*, 487.

Sterets Normasol *(Schering-Prebbles, UK).* A sterile topical irrigation solution containing sodium chloride 0.9%, in sachets of 25 ml.

Other Proprietary Names

Addex-Natriumklorid *(Swed.)*; Adsorbonac *(Canad.)*; Fyskosal *(Norw., Swed.)*; Humist, Hypersal *(both USA)*; Koksalt *(Swed.)*; Natrilentin *(Norw., Swed.)*; Ocean Mist *(USA)*; Øyebadevann *(Norw.)*; Vésirig *(Fr.)*.

1192-d

Sodium Acid Citrate *(B.P.).* Sod. Acid Cit.; Sodii Citras Acidus; Natrium Citricum Acidum; Natrii Hydrocitras pro Injectionibus; Disodium Hydrogen Citrate.

$C_6H_6Na_2O_7,1\frac{1}{2}H_2O=263.1$.

CAS — 144-33-2 (anhydrous).

Pharmacopoeias. In *Br., Hung.*, and *Rus.*

A white odourless powder with a saline taste. Each g represents approximately 7.6 mmol (7.6 mEq) of sodium.

Soluble 1 in less than 2 of water; practically insoluble in alcohol. A 3% solution in water has a pH of 4.9 to 5.2. Solutions are **sterilised** by autoclaving or by filtration.

Adverse Effects, Treatment, and Precautions. As for Sodium Salts, p.633.

Uses. Sodium acid citrate is used as an anticoagulant, generally in solution with dextrose, to prevent the clotting of blood intended for transfusion.

When very large transfusions are needed, the dose of sodium acid citrate may affect the patient's coagulation; in these circumstances heparinised blood should be used.

It has also been used to render the urine less acid and to promote a mild diuresis.

Preparations

Acid Citrate Dextrose Solution (ACD) *(B.P.).* See under Sodium Citrate.

Proprietary Names

Citralka *(Parke, Davis, Austral.; Parke, Davis, Belg.; Parke, Davis, Canad.)*.

1193-n

Sodium Citrate *(B.P., Eur. P., U.S.P.).* Sod. Cit.; Trisodium Citrate; Natrii Citras; Natrium Citricum; Natrii Citras pro Injectionibus; Tribasic Sodium Citrate.

$C_6H_5Na_3O_7,2H_2O=294.1$.

CAS — 68-04-2 (anhydrous); 6132-04-3 (dihydrate).

Pharmacopoeias. In all pharmacopoeias examined, but the following have $5\frac{1}{2}H_2O$: *Aust., Rus.*, and *Span. Braz.* and *U.S.* specify anhydrous or dihydrate.

White odourless granular crystals or crystalline powder with a saline taste; slightly deliquescent in moist air and efflorescent in warm dry air. Each g represents approximately 10.2 mmol (10.2 mEq) of sodium.

Soluble 1 in less than 2 of water; practically insoluble in alcohol and ether. A 5% solution in water has a pH of 8 to 10. A 3.02% solution is iso-osmotic with serum. Solutions are **sterilised** by autoclaving or by filtration. Solutions when stored may cause separation of particles from glass containers and solutions containing such particles must not be used. **Store** in airtight containers.

Adverse Effects, Treatment, and Precautions. As for Sodium Salts, p.633.

The indiscriminate addition of sodium citrate tablets to infants' feeds was to be discouraged; it added to the sodium content of the faeces (possibly already high because of use of excessive amounts of milk powder) and might contribute to the risk of hypernatraemia.— R. S. Shannon and R. P. C. Barclay (letter), *Br. med. J.*, 1974, *2*, 503.

Uses. Sodium citrate, after absorption, is metabolised and has actions similar to those of sodium bicarbonate (see p.634). It has a less marked purgative action than sodium tartrate or sodium potassium tartrate.

It is employed in the treatment of inflammatory conditions of the bladder and to prevent crystalluria during treatment with sulphonamides. It is usually administered in mixtures in doses of 3 to 6 g.

It is added to milk in the feeding of infants and invalids to prevent the formation of large curds. For invalids, from 60 to 180 mg of sodium citrate is added to each 40 ml of milk, for infant feeding, a solution containing 125 mg in 5 ml of water is added to each feed (but see under Adverse Effects).

Sodium citrate prevents the clotting of blood *in vitro;* a 3% solution has been used for washing out syringes and apparatus before collection of blood. It is used as an anticoagulant for Whole Blood. When very large transfusions are needed the dose of sodium citrate may affect the patient's coagulation; in these circumstances heparinised blood should be used.

A sterile 3 or 4% solution has been used postoperatively for bladder irrigation.

The use of citric acid and its calcium, potassium, and sodium salts in food was limited only by good manufacturing practice.— Seventeenth Report of the Joint FAO/WHO Expert Committee on Food Additives, *Tech. Rep. Ser. Wld Hlth Org. No. 539*, 1974.

For background toxicological information, see *Fd Add. Ser. Wld Hlth Org. No. 5*, 1974.

Acid aspiration syndrome. A single dose of 15 ml of 0.3M sodium citrate had been given as an antacid on 1396 occasions before the induction of general anaesthesia for obstetric procedures; no case of aspiration had occurred. To increase palatability the dose was presented in 20% syrup; such a preparation was stable (as judged by pH) at 4° or room temperature for at least 8 weeks.— E. Abouleish and I. A. Schenle (letter), *Br. J. Anaesth.*, 1977, *49*, 394. Based on *in vitro* studies sodium citrate 0.3M was less effective than magnesium trisilicate mixture for preventing the acid aspiration syndrome during anaesthesia.— J. B. Hester and M. L. Heath, *Br. J. Anaesth.*, 1977, *49*, 595. See also S. K. Lahiri *et al.*, *Br. J. Anaesth.*, 1973, *45*, 1143.

Sickle-cell anaemia. In 10 patients with sickle-cell disease the duration of pain was significantly less in patients treated with codeine and sodium citrate by mouth, or with sodium lactate intravenously, than in 8 patients given codeine without an alkali. Sodium citrate was given in doses of 60 ml of a 10% solution diluted with water to a volume of 400 ml every 2 hours for 24 hours with tapering doses thereafter.— L. Barreras and L. W. Diggs, *J. Am. med. Ass.*, 1971, *215*, 762.

Preparations

Effervescent Granules

Sodium Citro-tartrate Effervescent Granules *(B.P.C. 1959)*. Gran. Sod. Citro-tart. Efferv. Prepared from sodium bicarbonate 51 g, citric acid monohydrate 18 g, tartaric acid 27 g, and sucrose 15 g. *Dose.* 4 to 8 g.

Irrigations

Sterile Sodium Citrate Solution for Bladder Irrigation *(B.P.C. 1973)*. Sodium citrate 3 g, dilute hydrochloric acid 0.2 ml, freshly boiled and cooled water to 100 ml. Sterilise by autoclaving or by filtration. Store in containers sealed to exclude micro-organisms. Not suitable for injection.

A.P.F. (Sodium Citrate Irrigation) has 4% in Water for Injections.

Mixtures

Sodium Citrate Mixture *(B.P.C. 1973)*. Sodium citrate 3 g, citric acid monohydrate 500 mg, syrup 2.5 ml, lemon spirit 0.05 ml, quillaia tincture 0.1 ml, double-strength chloroform water 3 ml, water to 10 ml. It should be recently prepared. When a dose less than 5 ml is prescribed, the mixture should be diluted to 5 ml with syrup. Such dilutions must be freshly prepared and not used more than 2 weeks after issue. *Dose.* Well diluted with water, adults, 10 to 20 ml; children, up to 1 year, 2.5 ml; 1 to 5 years, 5 ml; 6 to 12 years, 10 ml.

For a report of incompatibility when Sodium Citrate Mixture was prepared with or diluted with syrup preserved with hydroxybenzoates, see under Sucrose, p.61.

Sodium Citrate Mixture *(A.P.F.)*. Mist. Sod. Cit. Sodium citrate 2 g, citric acid monohydrate 400 mg, lemon syrup 1 ml, concentrated chloroform water 0.2 ml, water to 10 ml. *Dose.* 10 to 20 ml well diluted with water.

Sodium Citrate Mixture CF *(A.P.F.)*. Sodium Citrate Mixture for Children. Sodium citrate 1 g, citric acid monohydrate 200 mg, lemon syrup 1 ml, concentrated chloroform water 0.1 ml, water to 5 ml. *Dose.* 5 ml diluted with water.

Solutions

Acid Citrate Dextrose Solution (ACD) *(B.P.)*. A sterile solution of sodium citrate and citric acid (or sodium acid citrate) with dextrose monohydrate for parenteral use (or anhydrous dextrose) in Water for Injections. Sterilise by autoclaving. pH 4.5 to 5.5. Store in containers sealed to exclude micro-organisms. Protect from light. Four formulas are given. *Formula A:* sodium citrate 2.2 g, citric acid monohydrate 800 mg (or anhydrous citric acid 730 mg), dextrose monohydrate for parenteral use 2.45 g (or anhydrous dextrose 2.24 g), and Water for Injections to 100 ml. *Formula B*: 1.32 g, 480 mg (or 440 mg), 1.47 g (or 1.34 g) respectively, and Water for Injections to 100 ml. *Formula C*: sodium acid citrate 2.9 to 4 g, dextrose monohydrate for parenteral use 2.5 g (or anhydrous dextrose 2.29 g), and Water for Injections to 100 ml. *Formula D*: 2 to 2.5 g, 3 g (or 2.74 g) respectively, and Water for Injections to 100 ml. For the anticoagulation and preservation of blood 15 ml, 25 ml, 15 ml, and 28.6 ml respectively are added to 100 ml of blood.

U.S.P. (Anticoagulant Citrate Dextrose Solution) has Solution A and Solution B with the same formulas as Formula A and Formula B respectively.

Anticoagulant Sodium Citrate Solution *(U.S.P.)*. A sterile solution in Water for Injections containing 3.8 to 4.2% of sodium citrate dihydrate or an equivalent amount of anhydrous sodium citrate. pH 6.4 to 7.5. It contains no antimicrobial agents.

Citrate Phosphate Dextrose Solution *(B.P.)*. Sodium citrate 2.63 g, citric acid monohydrate 327 mg, dextrose monohydrate for parenteral use 2.55 g (or anhydrous dextrose 2.32 g), sodium acid phosphate (dihydrate) 251 mg, and Water for Injections to 100 ml. Sterilise by autoclaving. pH 5 to 6. Store in containers sealed to exclude micro-organisms. Protect from light. For the anticoagulation and preservation of blood 14 ml is added to 100 ml of blood.

U.S.P. (Anticoagulant Citrate Phosphate Dextrose Solution) varies only in the degree of hydration of the ingredients permitted; the final product is identical.

Sodium Citrate and Citric Acid Oral Solution *(U.S.P.)*. Sodium Citrate and Citric Acid Solution. A solution of sodium citrate dihydrate 10% and citric acid monohydrate 6.34 to 7.02% in a suitable aqueous vehicle. pH 4 to 4.4. Store in airtight containers.

Tablets

Sodium Citrate Tablets *(B.P.)*. Sod. Cit. Tab. Tablets containing sodium citrate. Starch, in a proportion of not more than 10%, may be used as a disintegrating agent and magnesium stearate, in a proportion of not more than 0.5%, may be used as a lubricant; other materials may not be present. Store in airtight containers.

These tablets are intended for use in infant feeding; they should be dissolved in water and the solution added to the feed.

Proprietary Preparations

Micralax *(Smith Kline & French, UK)*. A micro-enema stated to contain sodium citrate 450 mg, sodium alkylsulphoacetate 45 mg, sorbic acid 5 mg, and glycerol, sorbitol, and water to 5 ml; supplied in a plastic tube fitted with rectal nozzle. An evacuant enema. *Dose.* 5 ml.

Microlet *(Ayerst, UK)*. A micro-enema stated to contain sodium citrate 450 mg, sodium lauryl sulphoacetate 45 mg, and glycerol 625 mg, with potassium sorbate, sorbitol, citric acid, and water to 5 ml; supplied in a plastic tube fitted with a rectal nozzle. An evacuant enema. *Dose.* 5 ml.

Relaxit *(Pharmacia, UK: Farillon, UK)*. A micro-enema containing sodium citrate 450 mg, sodium lauryl sulphate 75 mg, sorbic acid 5 mg, and glycerol and sorbitol solution to 5 ml. An evacuant enema. *Dose.* 5 ml.

Sodium Citrate 3% for Irrigation *(Travenol, UK)*. A sterile irrigation solution containing sodium citrate 3%. For bladder irrigation.

Other Proprietary Names

Citrosodina *(Ital.)*; Citrosodine Longuet *(Belg.)*.

Proprietary Names of Sodium Citrotartrates

Citravescent *(Protea, Austral.)*; Urade *(Warner, Austral.)*.

1194-h

Sodium Lactate.

$C_3H_5NaO_3$=112.1.

CAS — 72-17-3.

Pharmacopoeias. In *Aust.*, *Chin.*, *Ger.*, *Nord.*, and *Roum.* with differing percentages of $C_3H_5NaO_3$.

A colourless or slightly yellow moist crystalline mass or viscous hygroscopic liquid; odourless, or with a slight odour, and a slightly saline, warm taste. It usually contains 70 to 80% $C_3H_5NaO_3$. 1 g of $C_3H_5NaO_3$ represents approximately 8.9 mmol (8.9 mEq) of sodium and of lactate.

Soluble in water, alcohol, and glycerol; practically insoluble in chloroform, ether, and fixed oils. A 1.72% w/v solution of sodium lactate in water is iso-osmotic with serum. Solutions are **sterilised** by autoclaving or by filtration.

Incompatibility has been reported with novobiocin sodium, oxytetracycline hydrochloride, sodium bicarbonate, sodium calciumedetate, and sulphadiazine sodium.

NOTE. Sodium lactate for medicinal purposes is usually prepared in solution by neutralising dilute lactic acid with sodium hydroxide. Solutions of sodium lactate, on keeping, may cause separation of small solid particles from glass containers; solutions containing such particles must not be used.

Adverse Effects, Treatment, and Precautions. As for Sodium Salts, p.633.

Its use is contra-indicated in patients with severe liver damage who would be unable to convert lactate to bicarbonate.

In 2 patients with essential hypertension blood pressure rose by about 20 mmHg within half an hour of ingesting 5 g of sodium lactate; in a third patient with thyrotoxicosis and hypertension there was a fall in blood pressure of about 20 mmHg.— R. V. Sellwood (letter), *Med. J. Aust.*, 1974, *1*, 22.

Weakness, decreased vital capacity, and decreased grip strength occurred in 6 of 7 patients with myasthenia gravis given infusions of sodium lactate.— B. M. Patten *et al.*, *Neurology, Minneap.*, 1974, *24*, 986.

In 5 diabetic patients given Compound Sodium Lactate Intravenous Infusion during surgery the rise in plasma-glucose concentration was significantly higher than in diabetics not given this solution; it was recommended that it be not given to diabetics.— D. J. B. Thomas and K. G. M. M. Alberti, *Br. J. Anaesth.*, 1978, *50*, 185.

Uses. Sodium lactate, after absorption, is metabolised in 1 to 2 hours to bicarbonate; it then has similar actions to those of sodium bicarbonate (see p.634). It is usually administered intravenously as a solution containing 1.85% of sodium lactate, which represents about 165 mmol of sodium per litre. The rate of injection should not exceed 300 ml per hour.

Sodium lactate is also given by injection with sodium chloride, potassium chloride, and calcium chloride, the concentration of electrolytes in the injection being similar to those in human blood.

Sodium lactate has various industrial uses; it is used as a humectant and as a substitue for glycerol.

The use of Compound Lactate Intravenous Infusion, given for 24 hours by epidural infusion, alleviated or prevented headache in 16 women in whom the dura had been accidentally punctured during the initiation of epidural block for obstetric analgesia.— J. S. Crawford, *Br. J. Anaesth.*, 1972, *44*, 598.

In a study of the utilisation of sodium L(+) lactate and racemic sodium lactate solutions when given intravenously to 5 healthy subjects, D(−) lactate was metabolised more slowly and excreted more readily than L(+) lactate. The presence of D(−) lactate altered the rate of metabolism and the renal excretion of L(+) lactate. It was considered that the use of the L(+) isomer would be preferable to the racemic mixture.— H. Connor *et al.*, *Clin. Sci. & mol. Med.*, 1978, *55* (Sept.), 10p.

Cholera. Lactated Ringer's Injection was suitable as the sole intravenous solution for use in children with cholera or severe diarrhoea provided that 5% dextrose solution, potassium hydrogen citrate, and tetracycline could be given by mouth.— D. Mahalanabis *et al.*, *Bull. Wld Hlth Org.*, 1972, *46*, 311.

Shock. In the treatment of shock, lactated Ringer's solution was preferable to saline as it avoided metabolic acidosis when large volumes were required or when renal function was impaired.— T. Shires, *J. Am. med. Ass.*, 1973, *225*, 1131. See also J. A. Barnett and J. P. Sanford, *ibid.*, 1969, *209*, 1514.

Sickle-cell anaemia. In a double-blind study, in which 21 patients were treated on 43 occasions for sickle-cell vaso-occlusive crises, intravenous infusion of 0.1667M sodium lactate was no more effective than dextrose-saline infusion.— Cooperative Urea Trials Group, *J. Am. med. Ass.*, 1974, *228*, 1129.

Use in surgery. In a comparative study of 18 patients undergoing surgery of the rectum or colon the 9 who were given 750 ml of Compound Sodium Lactate Intravenous Infusion per hour during the operation and 1 litre on the 2nd, 3rd, and 4th days postoperatively in addition to the normal fluids had no reduction in plasma volume or central venous pressure compared with the 9 control patients. In addition these 9 patients showed no reduction of urine, urinary sodium excretion, and the urinary sodium/potassium ratio.— T. T. Irvin *et al.*, *Lancet*, 1972, *2*, 1159.

Preparations

Compound Sodium Lactate Intravenous Infusion *(B.P.)*. Compound Sodium Lactate Injection; Co. Sod. Lact. Inj.; Hartmann's Solution for Injection; Ringer-Lactate Solution for Injection. A sterile solution containing 0.37 to 0.42% of total Cl, 0.025 to 0.029% of $CaCl_2,2H_2O$, and 0.23 to 0.28% w/v of $C_3H_6O_3$, prepared by dissolving 115 mg of sodium hydroxide in 20 ml of Water for Injections, adding 0.24 ml of lactic acid, autoclaving the solution at 115° to 116° for 1 hour, cooling, cautiously adding dilute hydrochloric acid (about 0.1 ml) until 0.15 ml of the solution give a full orange colour with 0.05 ml of phenol red solution, mixing this solution with a solution of sodium chloride 600 mg, potassium chloride 40 mg, and calcium chloride 27 mg in 70 ml of Water for Injections, then adjusting with Water for Injections to 100 ml, filtering, and immediately sterilising by autoclaving. pH 5 to 7. The injection contains approximately 131 mmol of sodium, 5 mmol of potassium, 2 mmol of calcium, 29 mmol of bicarbonate (as lactate), and 111 mmol of chloride per litre. Store at a temperature not exceeding 25°.

Darrow's Solution. Sodium lactate 0.59%, potassium chloride 0.26%, sodium chloride 0.4%. Each litre provides sodium 121 mmol, potassium 35 mmol, chloride 103 mmol, and bicarbonate (as lactate) 53 mmol.
NOTE *U.S.N.F. XIII* (1970) included this preparation under the title Lactated Potassic Saline Injection.

Lactated Ringer's Injection *(U.S.P.).* A sterile solution of calcium chloride, potassium chloride, sodium chloride, and sodium lactate in Water for Injections. It contains 285 to 315 mg of sodium, 14.1 to 17.3 mg of potassium, 4.9 to 6 mg of calcium, 368 to 408 mg of chloride, and 231 to 261 mg of lactate in each 100 ml, providing in each litre sodium approximately 124 to 137 mmol, potassium 3.6 to 4.4 mmol, calcium 1.22 to 1.5 mmol, chloride 104 to 115 mmol, and lactate 26 to 29 mmol. It contains no antimicrobial agents. pH 6 to 7.5.

Sodium Lactate Intravenous Infusion *(B.P.).* Sodium Lactate Injection; Sod. Lact. Inj. A sterile 1.75 to 1.95% w/v solution of sodium lactate in Water for Injections, prepared by dissolving 670 mg of sodium hydroxide in 40 ml of Water for Injections, adding 1.4 ml of lactic acid, autoclaving the solution at 115° to 116° for 1 hour, cooling, cautiously adding Dilute Hydrochloric Acid (about 0.2 ml) until 0.15 ml of the solution give a full orange colour with 0.05 ml of phenol red solution, adding Water for Injections to 100 ml, filtering, and immediately sterilising by autoclaving. pH 5 to 7. The injection is approximately one-sixth molar and contains approximately 167 mmol of sodium and of bicarbonate (as lactate) per litre. Store at a temperature not exceeding 25°.
A similar injection is included in some pharmacopoeias.

Sodium Lactate Injection *(U.S.P.).* Sterile Sodium Lactate Solution (*U.S.P.*) in Water for Injections, or a sterile solution of lactic acid in Water for Injections prepared with the aid of sodium hydroxide. pH 6.0 to 7.3.

Sodium Lactate Solution *(U.S.P.).* An aqueous solution containing not less than 50% w/w of sodium lactate. pH 5 to 9. Store in airtight containers.

1195-m

Sodium Acid Phosphate *(B.P., B.P. Vet.).*

Sod. Acid Phos.; Sodii Phosphas Acidus; Sodium Dihydrogen Phosphate; Sodium Biphosphate (monohydrate) *(U.S.P.)*; Monosodium Orthophosphate; Mononatrii Phosphas; Natrii Biphosphas; Natrium Phosphoricum Monobasicum.
Sodium dihydrogen orthophosphate dihydrate.
$NaH_2PO_4,2H_2O=156.0$.

CAS — 7558-80-7 (anhydrous); 10049-21-5 (monohydrate); 13472-35-0 (dihydrate).

Pharmacopoeias. In *Arg., Aust., Belg., Br., Ger., Hung., Ind., Int., Jug., Nord.,* and *Swiss* (all with $2H_2O$); in *Braz., Chin., Mex., Pol.,* and *U.S.* (all with $1H_2O$).

Odourless colourless crystals or white crystalline powder with an acid saline taste. Each g represents approximately 6.4 mmol (6.4 mEq) of sodium and 6.4 mmol (6.4 mEq) of phosphate and contains approximately 198.5 mg of phosphorus. When heated it loses its water of crystallisation at 100°, melts with decomposition at 205° forming sodium hydrogen pyrophosphate, $Na_2H_2P_2O_7$, and at 250° leaves a final residue of sodium metaphosphate, $NaPO_3$.
Soluble 1 in 1 of water; practically insoluble in alcohol, chloroform, and ether. A 5% solution in water has a pH of 4.2 to 4.6 and effervesces with sodium carbonate. A 2.77% solution of the dihydrate, a 2.45% solution of the monohydrate, and a 2.10% solution of the anhydrous salt are iso-osmotic with serum. Solutions are **sterilised** by autoclaving or by filtration.

Adverse Effects, Treatment, and Precautions. As for Sodium Salts, p.633. See also under Sodium Phosphate, below.

Hypernatraemic dehydration occurred in a 4-year-old child with congenital megacolon who had been given 4 hyperosmotic sodium enemas in a week. The concentration of sodium in the serum rose to 166 mmol per litre and returned to normal within 48 hours after electrolyte therapy. Similar changes were reproduced experimentally in *dogs*.— E. W. Fonkalsrud and J. Keen, *J. Am. med. Ass.*, 1967, *199*, 584.

Tetany occurred in a 3-month-old infant receiving an unknown quantity of a laxative preparation (Sal Hepatica) containing sodium acid phosphate, sodium bicarbonate, and citric acid monohydrate.— M. Levitt *et al., J. Pediat.*, 1973, *82*, 479.

A report of tetany on 2 occasions after the use of a hyperosmotic phosphate enema in an 11-year-old girl with chronic pyelonephritis and dehydration.— R. W. Chesney and P. B. Haughton, *Am. J. Dis. Child.*, 1974, *127*, 584.

Rectal damage in 3 patients receiving hyperosmotic phosphate enemas led to necrosis of the anal area in 2. Methylprednisolone was given intravenously to the other patient with good results.— J. B. Pietsch *et al., Can. med. Ass. J.*, 1977, *116*, 1169.

Uses. Sodium acid phosphate is poorly absorbed from the gastro-intestinal tract and retains water in the lumen of the intestine. When taken by mouth in dilute solution it acts as a saline purgative and produces a watery evacuation of the bowel. It is also administered rectally as an enema.
Sodium acid phosphate is given by mouth to render the urine more acid. It is given with sodium phosphate (see below) in the treatment of hypercalcaemia.

Dental caries. Preliminary results of a study in 500 children indicated that the addition of 1% of sodium acid phosphate to a presweetened breakfast cereal significantly reduced the incidence of dental caries.— G. K. Stookey *et al., J. Am. dent. Ass.*, 1967, *74*, 752.

Effect on urine pH. Sodium acid phosphate 1 g four-hourly was less effective than ammonium chloride 1 g six-hourly in rendering acid the urine of gynaecological patients.— J. M. Beazley, *Br. J. clin. Pract.*, 1968, *22*, 101.

Preparations

Phosphates Enema *(B.P.).* Sodium Phosphates Enema. *Formula A.* Sodium acid phosphate 16 g, sodium phosphate 6 g, freshly boiled and cooled water to 100 ml. *Formula B.* Sodium acid phosphate 10 g, sodium phosphate 8 g, freshly boiled and cooled water to 100 ml. Both formulas may include a suitable preservative.

Sodium Phosphates Enema *(U.S.P.).* Sodium Phosphate and Biphosphate Enema. A solution of sodium acid phosphate (monohydrate) 15.2 to 16.8% and sodium phosphate (heptahydrate) 5.7 to 6.3% in water. It may be prepared from sodium phosphate with the aid of phosphoric acid. pH 5 to 5.8.

Sodium Phosphates Injection *(U.S.P.).* A sterile solution of sodium acid phosphate and sodium phosphate in Water for Injections. It contains no bacteriostatic agent or other preservative. pH 5.5 to 6. To be diluted before use.

Sodium Phosphates Oral Solution *(U.S.P.).* Sodium Phosphate and Biphosphate Oral Solution. A solution of sodium acid phosphate (monohydrate) 45.6 to 50.4% and sodium phosphate (heptahydrate) 17.1 to 18.9% in water. It may be prepared from sodium phosphate with the aid of phosphoric acid. pH 4.4 to 5.2. Store in airtight containers.

Proprietary Preparations

Fletchers' Disposable Phosphate Enema *(Pharmax, UK).* An aqueous solution of sodium acid phosphate 12.8 g and sodium phosphate 10.24 g in a plastic bag containing 128 ml and fitted with a rectal tube.

Phosphate-Sandoz *(Sandoz, UK).* Effervescent tablets each containing anhydrous sodium acid phosphate 1.936 g, sodium bicarbonate 350 mg, potassium bicarbonate 315 mg, and anhydrous citric acid 800 mg, providing phosphorus 500 mg, sodium 20.4 mmol, and potassium 3.1 mmol. For hypercalcaemia. *Dose.* Up to 6 tablets, dissolved in water, daily. (Also available as Phosphate-Sandoz in *Austral.*).

1196-b

Sodium Phosphate *(B.P., Eur. P.).*

Sod. Phos.; Sodii Phosphas; Disodium Hydrogen Phosphate; Dibasic Sodium Phosphate; Disodium Phosphate; Natrii Phosphas; Natrium Phosphoricum; Phosphate Disodique. Disodium hydrogen orthophosphate dodecahydrate.
$Na_2HPO_4,12H_2O=358.1$.

CAS — 7782-85-6 (heptahydrate); 10039-32-4 (dodecahydrate).

Pharmacopoeias. In *Arg., Br., Cz., Eur., Fr., Ger., Hung., Ind., It., Jap., Neth., Pol., Port., Roum., Span.,* and *Swiss. Aust., Belg., Jug.,* and *Nord.* specify $2H_2O$, and *Mex.* and *U.S.* specify $7H_2O$.

Colourless, odourless, efflorescent, transparent crystals with a salty slightly alkaline taste. Each g represents approximately 5.6 mmol (5.6 mEq) of sodium and 2.8 mmol of phosphate and contains approximately 86.5 mg of phosphorus. When heated at 40° it fuses; at 100° it loses its water of crystallisation; at a dull-red heat it is converted to the pyrophosphate $Na_4P_2O_7$.
Soluble 1 in 5 of water; practically insoluble in alcohol. A 2% solution in water has a pH of 9 to 9.2. A 4.45% solution of the dodecahydrate, a 3.33% solution of the heptahydrate, and a 2.23% solution of the dihydrate are iso-osmotic with serum. Solutions are **sterilised** by autoclaving or by filtration. **Incompatible** with alkaloidal salts, particularly those of strychnine, and with chloral hydrate, lead acetate, phenazone, and resorcinol. **Store** in airtight containers.

The haemolytic effect of phosphate buffer solution.— J. R. Phillips and D. E. Cadwallader, *J. pharm. Sci.*, 1971, *60*, 1033.

Adverse Effects, Treatment, and Precautions. As for Sodium Salts, p.633.
Long-term administration by mouth or the intravenous injection as a neutral solution may lead to extraskeletal calcification. Hypotension has occurred after intravenous injection. Hyperphosphataemia and hypocalcaemia has occurred in children after the use of phosphate enemas.

Two patients with hypercalcaemia relapsed into coma and died after phosphate therapy. One received an intravenous infusion of 1 litre of a phosphate buffer which contained 100 mmol of phosphate, 162 mmol of sodium, and 19 mmol of potassium; the other was treated initially with 25 mmol of phosphate 6-hourly by mouth, followed by 50 mmol of phosphate as a buffer solution by intravenous infusion over 1 hour. It was suggested that intravenous infusions of buffer solutions of phosphates should be given cautiously and that the initial dose should not exceed 50 mmol. It was necessary to take frequent readings of the blood pressure during the infusion and for 24 hours afterwards.— S. Shackney and J. Hasson, *Ann. intern. Med.*, 1967, *66*, 906.

A 40-year-old man with disseminated squamous cell carcinoma became hypercalcaemic 7 weeks before death, and was treated with repeated doses of inorganic phosphate. Extensive extraskeletal calcification was found after death. It was recommended that phosphate therapy be postponed until other hypercalcaemia therapy had been tried. Extreme caution was necessary in patients with renal insufficiency and chronic hyperphosphataemia.— R. W. Carey *et al., Archs intern. Med.*, 1968, *122*, 150.

Extraskeletal calcification developed in 7 of 9 patients (5 hypercalcaemic and 4 normocalcaemic) who were treated for 9 to 87 months with a solution of phosphates with a neutral reaction. The solution was given in daily doses containing 10 to 20 g of sodium phosphate and sodium acid phosphate in 4: 1 proportions.— F. J. Dudley and C. R. B. Blackburn, *Lancet*, 1970, *2*, 628. Comments and replies.— D. S. Bernstein and P. Pletka (letter), *ibid.*, 1032; F. J. Dudley (letter), *ibid.*; A. G. Schoch (letter), *ibid.*, 1363.

Coma developed in a 6-week-old infant given an overdose of a hyperosmotic preparation of sodium phosphate and sodium acid phosphate by mouth.— M. S. Smith *et al., J. Pediat.*, 1973, *82*, 481.

A 64-year-old man with primary hyperparathyroidism was given elemental phosphorus 2.2 to 3.2 g daily, as sodium phosphate and sodium acid phosphate in solution, by mouth. Acute hyperphosphataemia and acute persistent renal insufficiency developed after 8 days' treatment. On the last 2 days large doses of 4.5 and

6.7 g had been given inadvertently.— G. Ayala *et al.* (letter), *Ann. intern. Med.*, 1975, *83*, 520.

There was experimental and circumstantial evidence that hyperphosphataemia might damage renal function in the uraemic state.— *Lancet*, 1978, *1*, 753.

Uses. Sodium phosphate is poorly absorbed from the gastro-intestinal tract and retains water in the lumen of the intestine. When taken by mouth in dilute solution it acts as a saline purgative and produces a watery evacuation of the bowel. It also has a mild diuretic action and renders the urine less acid. Doses are reported to range from 2 to 16 g.

Sodium phosphate, usually in conjunction with other phosphates to give solutions with an approximately neutral reaction, is administered by mouth and by intravenous infusion in the treatment of calcium and phosphorus metabolic disorders. The incautious use of phosphate infusions has been associated with dangerous hypocalcaemia, particularly in initially hypercalcaemic patients.

The absorption, metabolism, and excretion of phosphorus.— J. T. Irving, *Calcium and Phosphorus Metabolism*, London, Academic Press, 1973.

Estimated acceptable total daily dietary phosphorus load: up to 70 mg per kg body-weight, attention being given to the reverse relationship with calcium intake.— Seventeenth Report of the FAO/WHO Expert Committee on Food Additives, *Tech. Rep. Ser. Wld Hlth Org. No. 539*, 1974.

For background toxicological information, see *Fd Add. Ser. Wld Hlth Org. No. 5*, 1974.

Dental caries. For reviews of the role of phosphates in the prevention of dental caries, see J. Beveridge *et al.*, *Med. J. Aust.*, 1967, *2*, 54; *Lancet*, 1968, *1*, 1187; J. Beveridge *et al.*, *Med. J. Aust.*, 1968, *1*, 120 (particular reference to the use of sugar phosphates); B. M. Smythe, *Australas. J. Pharm.*, 1971, *52*, 248.

Effect on urine pH. Sodium phosphate 1 g four-hourly was less effective than potassium citrate 2 g four- to six-hourly in rendering alkaline the urine of gynaecological patients and took longer to promote a change of pH.— J. M. Beazley, *Br. J. clin. Pract.*, 1968, *22*, 101.

Hypercalcaemia. In 20 patients with hypercalcaemia due to multiple myeloma, lymphoma, carcinoma, hyperparathyroidism, and vitamin-D overdosage, inorganic phosphate was administered either by mouth as the disodium or dipotassium salt or by intravenous infusion over 6 to 8 hours of 1 litre of a solution containing anhydrous sodium phosphate 1.15% (0.081M) and potassium acid phosphate 0.259% (0.019M) at a pH of 7.4. In 16 patients, phosphate invariably induced a prompt reduction in the serum calcium to normal or near normal.— R. S. Goldsmith and S. H. Ingbar, *New Engl. J. Med.*, 1966, *274*, 1. Only one-half the intravenous dose previously recommended should be given initially; the remainder should not be given until the blood-calcium response had been determined. The alteration was made following the occurrence of hypocalcaemia in 2 patients.— R. S. Goldsmith and S. H. Ingbar (letter), *ibid.*, 284.

Of 13 patients with hypercalcaemia due to carcinoma who were given phosphate therapy, 7 rapidly reached normal serum-calcium concentrations and the rest showed decreases of 16 to 33%. A striking clinical improvement was evident in most patients and the blood urea was usually unchanged or fell while the serum phosphate altered variably. An oral preparation of anhydrous sodium phosphate 3.66 g, sodium acid phosphate 1 g, orange syrup 16 ml, and water to 60 ml was used when the clinical condition permitted; the normal daily dose was 180 ml (equivalent to about 3 g of elemental phosphorus). For patients who were vomiting, an intravenous infusion of a solution of anhydrous sodium phosphate 0.081M and potassium acid phosphate 0.019M per litre was given in a dose of 330 ml (equivalent to about 1 g of elemental phosphorus) over 6 to 8 hours.— N. Thalassinos and G. F. Joplin, *Br. med. J.*, 1968, *4*, 14.

A study in 32 patients and 12 controls given, on a total of 59 occasions, an infusion of 0.1M sodium phosphate buffered to pH 7.4 indicated that patients with hypercalcaemia were more sensitive than controls to the effect of phosphate, as were patients with rickets or osteomalacia, osteoporosis, chronic renal failure, and Paget's disease. Phosphate treatment appeared useful in many cases of hypercalcaemia and possibly useful in osteoporosis or osteomalacia. Other forms of treatment were preferable for most cases of hypercalcaemia.— T. C. B. Stamp, *Clin. Sci.*, 1971, *40*, 55.

Comment on the management of severe hypercalcaemia, including the role of phosphates. The risks of treatment with phosphates are less when they are given by mouth rather than intravenously, but there may be little choice in the desperately ill patient who is vomiting or in coma. In these circumstances 50 mmol of a neutral solution should be infused over 6 to 8 hours, and only one dose should be given in any 24 hours. The serum-calcium concentration may begin to fall within minutes, but the reduction continues for several hours after the end of the infusion.— *Br. med. J.*, 1980, *280*, 204.

Hypophosphataemia. The pathophysiology and clinical characteristics of severe hypophosphataemia.— J. P. Knochel, *Archs intern. Med.*, 1977, *137*, 203.

A discussion of renal hypophosphataemia.— *Lancet*, 1978, *2*, 878.

The treatment of severe hypophosphataemia.— R. D. Lentz *et al.*, *Ann. intern. Med.*, 1978, *89*, 941. See also *Lancet*, 1981, *2*, 734.

For the use of sodium phosphate in the assessment of the response to treatment with ergocalciferol in patients with hypophosphataemia, see p.1659.

Osteoporosis. Experience in 5 patients suggested that long-term infusion treatment with phosphate and calcium alternately might produce lasting relief in osteoporosis.— M. M. Popovtzer *et al.*, *Am. J. Med.*, 1976, *61*, 478.

In 14 patients with dialysis-induced osteomalacia without hypophosphataemia the use of phosphate-enriched dialysis fluid for 6 months, with alfacalcidol, did not reduce the osteomalacia.— T. G. Feest *et al.*, *Br. med. J.*, 1978, *1*, 18.

Renal calculi. A solution of phosphates with a neutral reaction (Neutra-Phos) was recommended, in a dosage providing 1.5 to 2 g of elemental phosphorus daily in 4 divided doses, for the treatment of renal lithiasis. Diarrhoea often occurred in the first 2 weeks of therapy. A stone could be passed during the first few months, probably as a result of loosening or dissolution of the stone.— L. H. Smith, *J. Am. med. Ass.*, 1966, *195*, 708.

Further references.— G. A. Rose, *Practitioner*, 1977, *218*, 74; R. W. E. Watts, *Postgrad. med. J.*, 1977, *53*, *Suppl.* 2, 7; A. Hodgkinson, *ibid.*, 25; M. Peacock and W. G. Robertson, *Drugs*, 1980, *20*, 225.

Rickets. Results in 11 children indicating that a regimen of calcitriol and phosphate is beneficial in the treatment of vitamin D-resistant rickets. Long-term administration of phosphate, as Joulie's solution, alone or in association with ergocalciferol induced mineralisation of the epiphyseal plate but not of the endosteal bone surface, whereas phosphate in association with calcitriol 0.25 to 1 μg daily greatly improved the mineralisation of trabecular bone.— F. H. Glorieux *et al.*, *New Engl. J. Med.*, 1980, *303*, 1023.

'Neutral Phosphates'. Solutions of various phosphate salts in proportions to give an approximately neutral reaction, usually pH 7.4, have been given in the treatment of hypercalcaemia associated with conditions such as vitamin-D toxicity, malignant neoplasm, and hyperparathyroidism and also in disorders of calcium or phosphorus metabolism. The usual dose is the equivalent of 1 g of elemental phosphorus daily increasing, if necessary, to 3 g or more daily in divided doses. Similar solutions have also been employed intravenously in the treatment of severe hypercalcaemia but should be replaced by oral treatment as soon as possible. For comments on the hazards of intravenous phosphates see under Sodium Phosphate (above).

Preparations

Buffer Solutions. For formulas of phosphate buffers from pH 4.5 to 8.5, see G.E. Schumacher, *Am. J. Hosp. Pharm.*, 1966, *23*, 628.

Phosphate Mixture. Joulie's Solution. Sodium phosphate 13.6 g, 85% phosphoric acid 5.88 g, water to 100 ml. The solution has a pH of 4.9, contains 1725 millios-moles per litre, and provides 30.4 mg of inorganic phosphorus per ml. *Dose.* 15 ml every 4 hours, 5 times daily. —F.H. Glorieux *et al.*, *New Engl. J. Med.*, 1972, *287*, 481.

Sodium Phosphate Irrigation. Buffered Phosphate Irrigation (Ophthalmic). Sodium phosphate 18 g, monobasic potassium phosphate 7 g, and water 85 ml. An antidote to both acids and alkalis in the treatment of splashes of corrosive liquids in the eye.—L.G. Morgan, *Br. med. J.*, 1961, *2*, 466. The solution could be sterilised by autoclaving.—Pharm. Soc. Lab. Rep., *Pharm. J.*, 1961, *2*, 187.

See also Amphoteric Lotion, p.632.

For some other preparations containing sodium phosphate, see under Sodium Acid Phosphate.

Proprietary Preparations

Phosphates Solution *(Boots, UK)*. A solution for intravenous infusion containing sodium phosphate 2.9% and potassium acid phosphate 0.259%, providing in each litre 162 mmol of sodium, 19 mmol of potassium, and 100 mmol of phosphate.

Other Proprietary Names

Mikroplex Phosphor *(Ger.)*.

1197-v

Anhydrous Sodium Phosphate *(B.P.C. 1959)*.

Exsiccated Sodium Phosphate; Dried Sodium Phosphate. Disodium hydrogen orthophosphate.

Na_2HPO_4=142.0.

CAS — 7558-79-4 (anhydrous).

Pharmacopoeias. In *Arg.*, *Ind.*, *Span.*, and *Swiss. U.S.* includes Dried Sodium Phosphate, Na_2HPO_4,xH_2O (loss on drying not more than 5%).

A white odourless hygroscopic powder with a saline taste. **Soluble** 1 in 12 of water; practically insoluble in alcohol. A 2% solution in water has a pH of 9 to 9.2. A 1.75% solution in water is iso-osmotic with serum. Each g represents approximately 14.1 mmol (14.1 mEq) of sodium, and 7 mmol (about 14 mEq) of phosphate and contains 218.1 mg of phosphorus. **Store** in airtight containers.

Anhydrous sodium phosphate has the actions and uses of sodium phosphate and has been given in doses of 2 to 4 g. It is used for preparing effervescent granules and powders.

Preparations

Effervescent Sodium Phosphate *(U.S.P.)*. Granules from dried sodium phosphate 20% with sodium bicarbonate, tartaric acid, and citric acid monohydrate. Store in airtight containers.

1198-g

Sodium Potassium Tartrate *(B.P.C. 1973)*.

Sod. Pot. Tart.; Sodii et Potassii Tartras; Potassium Sodium Tartrate *(U.S.P.)*; Rochelle Salt; Seignette Salt; Kalium-natrium Tartaricum; Tartarus Natronatus.

$C_4H_4KNaO_6,4H_2O$=282.2.

CAS — 304-59-6 (anhydrous); 6381-59-5 (tetrahydrate).

Pharmacopoeias. In *Aust.*, *Belg.*, *Cz.*, *Fr.*, *Hung.*, *Ind.*, *It.*, *Mex.*, *Neth.*, *Port.*, *Roum.*, *Span.*, *Swiss*, and *U.S.*

Odourless or almost odourless colourless crystals or white crystalline powder, with a cooling saline taste. It effloresces in warm dry air. Each g represents approximately 3.5 mmol (3.5 mEq) of potassium and of sodium. Solutions in water have a pH of 7 to 8.

Soluble 1 in 1 of water; very slightly soluble in chloroform and ether; practically insoluble in alcohol. **Incompatible** with acids, calcium and lead salts, magnesium sulphate, and silver nitrate. **Store** in airtight containers.

Adverse Effects, Treatment, and Precautions. As for Sodium Salts, p.633.

Uses. Sodium potassium tartrate is poorly absorbed from the gastro-intestinal tract and retains water in the lumen of the intestine. When taken by mouth in dilute solution it acts as a saline purgative and produces a watery evacuation of the bowel. It is the main constituent of Seidlitz powder (Compound Effervescent Powder) which provides 7.5 g or 15 g of sodium potassium tartrate per dose.

The tartrates of the alkali metals are less readily absorbed than the citrates. Their purgative action is therefore greater while their diuretic action and effect in reducing the acidity of the urine is less pronounced.

Sodium potassium tartrate is used in the food industry in some countries as a stabiliser in cheese and meat products.

Estimated acceptable daily intake: up to 6 mg, calculated as tartaric acid, per kg body-weight.— Seventh Report of FAO/WHO Expert Committee on Food Additives, *Tech. Rep. Ser. Wld Hlth Org. No. 281*, 1964.

Preparations

Compound Effervescent Powder *(B.P.C. 1973)*. Pulv. Efferv. Co.; Seidlitz Powder. Sodium potassium tartrate, in powder, 7.5 g, sodium bicarbonate, in powder, 2.5 g, in blue paper. Tartaric acid, in powder, 2.5 g, in white paper. *Dose*. Dissolve the contents of the blue paper in a tumblerful of cold or warm water, then add the contents of the white paper and drink the liquid while it is effervescing.

Double-strength Compound Effervescent Powder *(B.P.C. 1973)*. Pulv. Efferv. Co. Dup.; Double-strength Seidlitz Powder. Formula as for Compound Effervescent Powder but with double the amount (15 g) of sodium potassium tartrate.

Strong Compound Effervescent Powder *(B.P.C. 1959)*. Pulv. Efferv. Co. Fort.; Extra-strong Seidlitz Powder. Formula as for Compound Effervescent Powder but with 50% more (11.25 g) of sodium potassium tartrate.

1199-q

Sodium Sulphate *(B.P., B.P. Vet., Eur. P.)*.

Sod. Sulph.; Sodium Sulfate *(U.S.P.)*; Sodii Sulphas; Glauber's Salt; Natrii Sulphas; Natrii Sulfas Decahydricus; Natrium Sulfuricum Crystallisatum.

$Na_2SO_4,10H_2O=322.2$.

CAS — 7727-73-3.

Pharmacopoeias. In all pharmacopoeias examined except *Int.* and *Jap.*

Colourless odourless crystals or white crystalline powder with a bitter saline taste; efflorescent in dry air. Each g represents approximately 6.2 mmol (6.2 mEq) of sodium. The crystals liquefy at 33°. The anhydrous salt fuses at red heat without decomposition.

Soluble 1 in 2.5 of water at 20° and 1 in 0.5 at 100°; it partially dissolves in its own water of crystallisation at about 33°; practically insoluble in alcohol, chloroform, and ether; soluble 1 in 30 of glycerol. It readily forms a supersaturated solution in water when a saturated solution, prepared at a temperature above 33°, is cooled. Solutions in water are neutral to litmus. A 3.95% solution is iso-osmotic with serum. Solutions are **sterilised** by autoclaving or by filtration.

Incompatible with barium, calcium, lead, mercury, silver, and strontium, with which it forms insoluble salts. **Store** in airtight containers.

Adverse Effects, Treatment, and Precautions. As for Sodium Salts, p.633.

In 3 young children, infantile diarrhoea was caused by drinking well water which contained over 2 mg per ml of dissolved solids, mainly sodium, sulphate (over 600 µg per ml), chloride, and bicarbonate. The sulphate was considered to have been the laxative agent and it was suggested that waters with a sulphate content of more than 400 µg per ml were unsuitable for infant feeding. Older children and adults tolerated the well water.— L. Chien *et al.*, *Can. med. Ass. J.*, 1968, *99*, 102.

Uses. Sodium sulphate is poorly absorbed from the gastro-intestinal tract and retains water in the lumen of the intestine. When taken by mouth in dilute solution it acts as a saline purgative and produces a prompt watery evacuation of the bowel.

In the treatment of severe hypercalcaemia, 1 to 4 litres of a 3.89% solution of sodium sulphate has been administered intravenously over 9 to 15 hours.

A 12 to 25% lotion has been used for its osmotic effect in infected wounds.

Sodium sulphate has sometimes been used to hasten the excretion of drugs in overdosage and other toxic substances; when so used the dose is usually about 30 g in 250 ml of water.

Preparations

Lot. Sod. Sulph *(N.F. 1955)*. Sodium Sulphate Lotion. Sodium sulphate 21.9 g, chlorocresol 87.5 mg, water to 100 ml. It may crystallise in cold weather; the crystals should be redissolved by warming before use.

Amended formula. Sodium sulphate 22 g, chlorocresol 88 mg, water to 100 ml.—*Compendium of Past Formulae 1933 to 1966*, London, The National Pharmaceutical Union, 1969.

Sodium Sulfate Injection *(U.S.P.)*. A sterile concentrated solution of sodium sulphate in Water for Injections, which upon dilution is suitable for parenteral use. pH 5 to 6.5. It should be diluted to 3.89% before use.

Further preparations of sodium sulphate are described under Anhydrous Sodium Sulphate (below).

Proprietary Names

Liquisulf *(Cophar, Switz.)*.

1200-q

Anhydrous Sodium Sulphate *(B.P., Eur. P.)*.

Anhyd. Sod. Sulph.; Natrii Sulfas Anhydricus; Exsiccated Sodium Sulphate; Dried Sodium Sulphate; Exsiccated Glauber's Salt; Dried Glauber's Salt; Natrium Sulfuricum Siccatum.

$Na_2SO_4=142.0$.

CAS — 7757-82-6.

Pharmacopoeias. In *Arg., Aust., Belg., Br., Chin., Cz., Eur., Fr., Ger., Hung., Ind., It., Jap., Jug., Neth., Nord., Pol., Port., Span.*, and *Swiss*.

A white odourless hygroscopic powder with a bitter saline taste. Each g represents approximately 14.1 mmol (14.1 mEq) of sodium.

Soluble 1 in 5 of water; practically insoluble in alcohol. A 1.61% solution in water is iso-osmotic with serum. **Store** in airtight containers.

Anhydrous sodium sulphate has the actions and uses of sodium sulphate. It is also used for preparing effervescent granules and powders and in other preparations for which the powdered crystals of sodium sulphate are not suitable.

Preparations

Artificial Carlsbad Salt *(B.P.C. 1949)*. Sal Carolinum Factitium. Prepared from sodium sulphate 55, potassium sulphate 1, sodium chloride 10, and sodium carbonate 35. *Dose*. 2 to 6 g.

Artificial Hunyadi Janos Salt. Anhydrous sodium sulphate 450, magnesium sulphate 950 dried to 500, sodium chloride 50. *Dose*. 1.3 to 4 g.

Effervescent Artificial Carslbad Salt *(B.P.C. 1949)*. Sal Carolinum Factitium Effervescens. Prepared from anhydrous sodium sulphate 9, sodium potassium tartrate 38, sodium chloride 3, sodium bicarbonate 33, saccharin 0.05, and tartaric acid 16.95. *Dose*. 4 to 8 g.

Effervescent Sodium Sulphate Granules *(B.P.C. 1949)*. Gran. Sod. Sulph. Efferv. Granules prepared from crystalline sodium sulphate 50 g (dried until it has lost about 55% of its weight), citric acid monohydrate 21 g, tartaric acid 24 g, and sodium bicarbonate 50 g. *Dose*. 4 to 16 g.

Sal Carolinum Factitium *(Jap. P., Nord. P., Pol. P.)*. Sal Carlsbadense Factitium; Pulvis Caroli; Alkaline Laxative Salt. Contains anhydrous sodium sulphate 44, potassium sulphate 2, sodium chloride 18, sodium bicarbonate 36. *Dose*. 5 g; 6 g in 1 litre of water is approximately equivalent to the natural water. *Marienbad Salt* is similar.

Sal Emsanum Facticium. Artificial Ems Salt. Anhydrous sodium sulphate 10, potassium sulphate 10, sodium chloride 265, and sodium bicarbonate 715.

Sal Vichy Artificiale *(Pol. P.)*. Artificial Vichy Salt. Anhydrous sodium sulphate 40, anhydrous sodium phosphate 20, potassium bicarbonate 35, sodium chloride 75, sodium bicarbonate 830.

1201-p

Sodium Tartrate.

$C_2H_4O_2(CO_2Na)_2,2H_2O=230.1$.

CAS — 868-18-8 (anhydrous); 6106-24-7 (dihydrate).

White almost tasteless crystals or granules. **Soluble** 1 in 3 of water; practically insoluble in alcohol.

Sodium tartrate has been used as a purgative in doses of 10 to 20 g. It is used in the food industry in some countries as a sequestrant and stabiliser in meat products.

Estimated acceptable daily intake: up to 30 mg, as L(+)-tartaric acid, per kg body-weight.— Twenty-first Report of the Joint FAO/WHO Expert Committee on Food Additives, *Tech. Rep. Ser. Wld Hlth Org. No. 617*, 1978.

For background toxicological information, see *Fd Add. Ser. Wld Hlth Org. No. 5*, 1974.

Proprietary Names

Limonade Asepta *(Rodeca, Canad.)*.

1202-s

Proprietary Preparations of Some Other Electrolyte Solutions

Addamel *(KabiVitrum, UK)*. A solution containing calcium chloride, copper chloride, ferric chloride, magnesium chloride, manganese chloride, potassium iodide, sodium fluoride, zinc chloride, and sorbitol, providing in each 10-ml ampoule the following ions: calcium 5 mmol, magnesium 1.5 mmol, and chloride 13.3 mmol, with trace amounts of copper, iron, manganese, zinc, fluoride, and iodide. For use as a supplement during parenteral nutrition.

Difusor *(Boots, UK)*. A range of sterile pyrogen-free solutions for peritoneal dialysis.

Flowfusor *(Boots, UK)*. A range of sterile irrigation solutions.

Ped-El *(KabiVitrum, UK)*. A solution containing calcium chloride, copper chloride, ferric chloride, magnesium chloride, manganese chloride, phosphoric acid, potassium iodide, sodium fluoride, zinc chloride, and sorbitol, providing in each 20-ml vial the following ions: calcium 3 mmol, phosphorus 1.5 mmol, and chloride 7 mmol, with trace amounts of copper, iron, magnesium, manganese, zinc, fluoride, and iodide. For use as a supplement during parenteral nutrition in infants.

Polyfusor *(Boots, UK)*. A range of sterile solutions for intravenous infusion, in disposable plastic containers.

Steriflex *(Boots, UK)*. A range of sterile solutions for intravenous infusion in disposable plastic containers.

Travenol Electrolyte Solution A with 20% Dextrose *(Travenol, UK)*. A sterile solution for intravenous infusion containing magnesium chloride, calcium chloride dihydrate, zinc acetate, manganese chloride, and anhydrous dextrose, and providing in each litre the following ions—magnesium 28 mmol, calcium 26 mmol, zinc 0.08 mmol, manganese 0.04 mmol, chloride 108 mmol, and acetate 0.16 mmol.

Uromatic *(Travenol, UK)*. A range of sterile bladder irrigation solutions in plastic containers.

Viaflex *(Travenol, UK)*. A range of sterile solutions for intravenous infusions, in disposable plastic containers.

Enzymes Choleretics and other Digestive Agents

3700-x

This section describes some enzymes of mammalian, bacterial, and plant origin which are used therapeutically, bile salts and some choleretic compounds.

3701-r

Acetylcysteine *(U.S.P.)*. *N*-Acetylcysteine.

N-Acetyl-L-cysteine.

$C_5H_9NO_3S$=163.2.

CAS — 616-91-1.

Pharmacopoeias. In *Braz., Chin.,* and *U.S.*

A white crystalline deliquescent powder with a slight acetic odour. M.p. 104° to 110°.

Soluble 1 in 5 of water and 1 in 4 of alcohol; practically insoluble in chloroform and ether. A solution is dextrorotatory. A 1% solution in water has a pH of 2 to 2.8. A 4.58% solution in water is iso-osmotic with serum.

Incompatible with most metals, with rubber, with oxygen and oxidising substances, and with erythromycin lactobionate, oleandomycin phosphate, oxytetracycline hydrochloride, and tetracycline hydrochloride. Some antibiotics may be inactivated if nebulised with acetylcysteine. **Store** in airtight containers.

The activity of 6 penicillins, of cephaloridine, and of tetracycline was reduced *in vitro* in the presence of 5% acetylcysteine. Erythromycin and fusidic acid were unaffected. Acetylcysteine by inhalation had no measurable effect upon the blood concentrations of cloxacillin in 1 patient.— D. Lawson and B. A. Saggers (letter), *Br. med. J.*, 1965, *1,* 317.

An aqueous solution of acetylcysteine iso-osmotic with serum (4.58%) caused 100% haemolysis of erythrocytes cultured in it for 45 minutes. The solution turned dark green-brown.— C. Sapp *et al., J. pharm. Sci.,* 1975, *64,* 1884.

Adverse Effects. Side-effects reported include bronchospasm, nausea, vomiting, stomatitis, and rhinorrhoea. Chills and fever have occurred occasionally. Haemoptysis has been reported in a few patients.

Thirty minutes after the start of an acetylcysteine infusion for paracetamol overdosage, a 20-year-old woman developed an anaphylactoid reaction, with a generalised erythematous rash, itching, nausea, vomiting, dizziness, and severe breathlessness; there was bronchospasm with tachycardia. The infusion was immediately withdrawn and she was given chlorpheniramine 10 mg and intravenous hydrocortisone 100 mg. Her symptoms settled over the next 30 minutes and the signs of bronchospasm resolved. Her initial serum-paracetamol concentration was then reported to be low, indicating no further need for specific therapy.— N. G. Walton *et al.* (letter), *Lancet,* 1979, *2,* 1298.

Treatment of Adverse Effects. Bronchospasm may usually be quickly relieved by the administration of a sympathomimetic agent in aerosol form.

Precautions. Acetylcysteine should be used with caution in elderly patients with severe respiratory insufficiency or in asthmatic patients.

Acetylcysteine inhibited 12 of 13 strains of *Pseudomonas aeruginosa* at concentrations of 2 to 20 μg per ml. Only 1 of 8 strains of *Staphylococcus aureus* was inhibited at 20 μg per ml while none of 10 strains of *Klebsiella* and *Enterobacter* species was affected. An additive effect was demonstrated against *Ps. aeruginosa* with combinations of acetylcysteine with carbenicillin or ticarcillin. Antagonism against this organism was demonstrated with combinations of acetylcysteine and gentamicin or tobramycin; antagonism against *Kl. pneumoniae* was also demonstrated with acetylcysteine and gentamicin. It was suggested that, although acetylcysteine and aminoglycoside antibiotics were chemically compatible, they should not be administered at the same time by aerosol in patients with cystic fibrosis because of the possibility of local inactivation of the antibiotic.— M. F. Parry and H. C. Neu, *J. clin. Microbiol.,* 1977, *5,* 58.

Absorption and Fate. Acetylcysteine is absorbed from the gastro-intestinal tract.

A single 100 mg labelled dose of acetylcysteine given to 10 patients with various respiratory or cardiac diseases was found to be rapidly absorbed with peak plasma concentrations in 2 to 3 hours and concentrations remaining high after 24 hours. Lung tissue concentrations measured in 5 patients were high and comparable with those in plasma 5 hours after administration. Acetylcysteine was also found in the bronchial mucus.— D. Rodenstein *et al., Clin. Pharmacokinet.,* 1978, *3,* 247.

Uses. Acetylcysteine is a mucolytic agent which is used as the sodium salt, as an adjunct to other therapy, to reduce the viscosity of pulmonary secretions in cystic fibrosis of the pancreas and other conditions where mucolytic therapy is required. Acetylcysteine is most active in concentrations of 10 to 20% at a pH of 7 to 9. It is administered by direct instillation of 1 to 2 ml of a 10 to 20% solution every 1 to 4 hours or by nebulisation of 2 to 5 ml of a 20% solution or 4 to 10 ml of a 10% solution through a face mask or mouthpiece 3 or 4 times daily. It may be administered by nebulisation every 2 to 6 hours if necessary. Mechanical suction of the liquefied secretions may be necessary. Nebulisers containing metal or rubber components should not be used.

Acetylcysteine is also used in the treatment of paracetamol poisoning. An initial dose of 150 mg of acetylcysteine per kg body-weight as a 20% solution may be given intravenously over 15 minutes, followed by an intravenous infusion of 50 mg per kg in 500 ml of dextrose injection over the next 4 hours and then 100 mg per kg in one litre of dextrose injection over the next 16 hours. Acetylcysteine is reported to be very effective when administered within 8 hours of paracetamol overdosage with the protective effect diminishing after this time and being ineffective when administered later than 15 hours after ingestion. Acetylcysteine has also been given by mouth in the treatment of paracetamol poisoning.

Bronchitis and pulmonary disease. Large quantities of proteinaceous material were removed from the lungs of 3 patients with alveolar proteinosis by lavage with sodium chloride solution with acetylcysteine.— J. Ramirez-R, *Archs intern. Med.,* 1967, *119,* 147.

A 10% solution of acetylcysteine was as effective as a 20% solution when nebulised, and more effective than sodium chloride solution in thinning sputum and in increasing its volume in 70 patients with chronic obstructive pulmonary disease. Neither acetylcysteine nor sodium chloride caused spirometric changes in most patients, but the 10% solution of acetylcysteine was less frequently associated with bronchial obstruction than the 20% solution.— S. R. Hirsch and R. C. Kory, *J. Allergy,* 1967, *39,* 265.

Acetylcysteine was administered in doses of 500 to 600 mg by intramuscular or intravenous injection, or by mouth, to 27 patients with chronic bronchitis or bronchiectasis. The drug was effective by all routes in reducing sputum viscosity but had a more rapid action when administered intravenously. Acetylcysteine administered systemically seemed an effective alternative to its topical use.— C. Grassi *et al., Curr. ther. Res.,* 1973, *15,* 165.

In a double-blind study in 30 patients with asthma, the inhalation by aerosol twice daily of 6 ml of acetylcysteine and isoprenaline solution was superior, in terms of pulmonary function and reduced sputum viscosity, to saline and isoprenaline solution.— W. C. Grater and A. Cato, *Curr. ther. Res.,* 1973, *15,* 660.

Two patients with status asthmaticus who had not responded to other treatments and one patient with mucous impaction of the left main-stem bronchus were successfully treated by instillation of acetylcysteine followed by aspiration. Five to 10 ml of a 10% solution was administered to the first 2 patients but because of the viscosity of this strength the 3rd patient received a 5% solution (30 ml). None of the patients had additional bronchospasm.— J. C. Donaldson *et al., Ann. intern. Med.,* 1978, *88,* 656.

Further references: P. N. Paez *et al., Can. med. Ass. J.,* 1966, *95,* 522; K. M. Moser and P. G. Rhodes, *Dis. Chest,* 1966, *49,* 370; R. C. Kory *et al., Dis. Chest,* 1968, *54,* 504; C. Grassi and G. C. Morandini, *Eur. J. clin. Pharmac.,* 1976, *9,* 393; A. Cato and I. Goldstein, *J. int. med. Res.,* 1977, *5,* 175; N. Lemy-Debois *et al., Acta ther.,* 1978, *4,* 125.

Candidiasis. A 24-year-old diabetic, who had achlorhydria and a gastric infection of *Candida albicans* unresponsive to nystatin and amphotericin, was treated with acetylcysteine. After gastric lavage, 30 ml of a 20% solution of acetylcysteine was given by mouth, and gastric lavage repeated after about 3 hours with good results. The dose was repeated before retiring. The treatment was given for 2 days and resulted in moderate diarrhoea. X-ray examination showed a normal ventricle. A further 2 patients with massive gastric mycosis had been effectively treated.— E. Ståhl *et al.* (letter), *Lancet,* 1969, *1,* 1022.

Cystic fibrosis. The use of a 10% solution of acetylcysteine for bronchial lavage was compared with that of sodium chloride solution in 14 patients with cystic fibrosis. Acetylcysteine lavage produced a significant increase in the carbon-dioxide tension of arterial blood and a decrease in arterial-oxygen tension immediately after the procedure. The converse effects were observed after lavage with sodium chloride solution. Pulmonary function was impaired with both agents from 48 to 72 hours after lavage and 3 patients developed pneumonia within 3 days. The use of acetylcysteine significantly increased the dangers of bronchial lavage and sodium chloride solution was preferable for this purpose.— G. Cezeaux *et al., J. Am. med. Ass.,* 1967, *199,* 15.

Pulmonary secretions in patients with cystic fibrosis were effectively dispersed *in vitro* by 20% acetylcysteine and less effectively by 10% acetylcysteine. A daily dose of 10 ml of 20% acetylcysteine solution was given in 3 or 4 divided treatments by aerosol to 9 patients with cystic fibrosis and 1 patient with bronchiectasis. Each treatment was followed by inhalation of 1 ml of 10% propylene glycol. All 10 patients showed clearing of the upper respiratory tract but the treatment did not affect the condition of the lower respiratory tract.— R. Denton *et al., Am. Rev. resp. Dis.,* 1967, *95,* 643.

In 5 children with cystic fibrosis, abdominal pain was relieved after 1 week during treatment with acetylcysteine 10% given in 5-ml doses 4 times daily in a flavoured drink for 1 to 2 weeks, followed by thrice daily for 1 to 2 weeks, then twice daily for 1 to 2 weeks, and then once daily or less frequently.— M. Gracey *et al., Archs Dis. Childh.,* 1969, *44,* 404.

Further references: H. W. Reas, *J. Pediat.,* 1964, *65,* 542; S. J. Stamm and J. Docter, *Dis. Chest,* 1965, *47,* 414.

Cystinuria. A favourable report of the use of acetylcysteine in the treatment of 6 cystinuric stone-forming patients.— W. P. Mulvaney *et al., J. Urol.,* 1975, *114,* 107.

Further references: A. D. Smith *et al., Urology,* 1979, *13,* 422.

Gold poisoning. For the use of acetylcysteine in the treatment of gold poisoning, see Sodium Aurothiomalate, p.933.

Ileus. A report of the successful use of solutions of acetylcysteine 10% adminstered rectally and by mouth in the treatment of meconium ileus in a 2-day-old girl.— T. E. Simpson *et al., Mayo Clin. Proc.,* 1968, *43,* 725.

Acetylcysteine 4% solution had no adverse effect on the colon or intestine of *rats.* A suspension of barium sulphate with acetylcysteine 4% was suggested for use rectally in anatomically uncomplicated meconium ileus.— M. Schiller *et al., Am. J. Surg.,* 1971, *122,* 22.

Kerato-conjunctivitis sicca. Three patients with non-sicca filamentary keratitis were successfully treated with eye-drops of acetylcysteine sodium 20%, applied 4 times daily for 2 or 3 weeks. Fifteen patients with filamentary keratitis sicca were similarly treated with relief of symptoms, especially photophobia, in all but 2.— R. B. Jones and H. V. Coop, *Trans. ophthal. Soc. U.K.,* 1965, *85,* 379.

In a double-blind crossover study on 30 patients with kerato-conjunctivitis sicca, acetylcysteine produced significantly better objective results than treatment with artificial tears.— M. J. Absolon and C. A. Brown, *Br. J. Ophthal.,* 1968, *52,* 310.

A 5 or 10% solution of acetylcysteine in hypromellose was less irritant to the eye than a 20% solution.— *Drug & Ther. Bull.,* 1974, *12,* 81.

Twenty patients with kerato-conjunctivitis of Sjögren's syndrome which had failed to respond to other treatment and displayed mucous shreds and corneal filaments were treated with acetylcysteine for 1 year. A 5% solution, adjusted to pH 8.4 with sodium bicarbonate, was instilled at least 4 times daily. After 1 year, 6 patients (30%) showed objective and subjective improvement.— J. Williamson *et al.*, *Br. J. Ophthal.*, 1974, *58*, 798.

Further references: P. Wright, *Practitioner*, 1975, *214*, 631.

Paracetamol poisoning. Reviews discussing the use of acetylcysteine in paracetamol overdosage: L. F. Prescott, *Hlth Bull., Dep. Hlth Scotl.*, 1978, *36*, 204; H. E. Bye, *Duncan, Flockhart, Pharm. J.*, 1979, *2*, 407; *Med. Lett.*, 1979, *21*, 98; *Drug & Ther. Bull.*, 1980, *18*, 81; T. J. Meredith and G. N. Volans, *Recent Adv. clin. Pharmac.*, 1980, *2*, 129.

Acetylcysteine improved survival in *mice* given toxic doses of paracetamol without affecting the hepatic covalent binding of paracetamol. The protective effect was different from that of cysteamine.— J. G. Gerber *et al.* (letter), *Lancet*, 1977, *1*, 657.

Of 100 cases of paracetamol poisoning 60 were considered at high risk of developing liver damage—plasma-paracetamol concentration above a line joining 300 μg per ml at 4 hours and 45 μg per ml at 15 hours on a semilogarithmic graph. None of 19 given acetylcysteine intravenously within 8 hours of ingestion developed severe liver damage; 1 of 14 developed liver damage when given acetylcysteine after 8 to 10 hours; 3 of 7 treated after 10 to 12 hours; 5 of 9 treated after 12 to 15 hours; and 9 of 11 treated after 15 to 24 hours. There was no renal impairment in those treated within 10 hours. Treatment consisted of 150 mg per kg body-weight in 200 ml of dextrose injection given over 15 minutes, followed by 50 mg per kg in 500 ml of dextrose over 4 hours and 100 mg per kg in 1 litre of dextrose over the next 16 hours. There were no obvious side-effects. Acetylcysteine was the treatment of choice. Treatment should include gastric lavage within 4 hours and in unconscious patients; acetylcysteine in those with paracetamol concentrations above a treatment line of 200 μg per ml at 4 hours and 30 μg per ml at 15 hours, and in those who had taken more than 7.5 g more than 8 hours previously and in whom plasma concentrations were not yet available. A case could be made for lowering the treatment line to 150 μg per ml at 4 hours and 25 μg per ml at 15 hours. Although acetylcysteine by mouth has been used for paracetamol poisoning in the USA most severely poisoned patients develop early nausea and vomiting making oral treatment impracticable. There seems to be no place for oral treatment of severe paracetamol poisoning when effective intravenous treatment is available.— L. F. Prescott *et al.*, *Br. med. J.*, 1979, *2*, 1097. Criticism. It was suggested that methionine by mouth was just as effective as acetylcysteine intravenously in the treatment of acute paracetamol poisoning.— J. A. Vale *et al.* (letter), *ibid.*, 1435. A reply. Acetylcysteine intravenously must remain the treatment of choice.— L. F. Prescott *et al.* (letter), *ibid.*, 1980, *1*, 46.

Further references to the use of acetylcysteine in paracetamol poisoning: L. Lyons *et al.* (letter), *New Engl. J. Med.*, 1977, *296*, 174 (oral administration); R. G. Peterson and B. H. Rumack, *J. Am. med. Ass.*, 1977, *237*, 2406 (oral administration); R. D. Scalley and C. S. Conner, *Am. J. Hosp. Pharm.*, 1978, *35*, 964 and 1349 (oral administration); W. G. Maurer and J. Zeisler (letter), *ibid.*, 1025 (oral and intravenous administration); H. Carloss *et al.*, *Sth. med. J.*, 1978, *71*, 906 (oral administration).

Patency of endotracheal tubes. To prevent obstruction of endotracheal tubes during mechanical ventilation in infants, 0.1 or 0.2 ml of a solution of acetylcysteine was introduced into the tube hourly and half an hour later the secretions were aspirated. The mucolytic solution apparently had no harmful effect on the trachea or bronchi. It was ineffective in removing obstructions caused by blood.— R. King (letter), *Lancet*, 1967, *1*, 900.

Preparations

Acetylcysteine Eye-drops *(Moorfields Eye Hosp.)*. Eye-drops containing acetylcysteine 5 or 10% prepared by dilution of a 20% solution with Hypromellose Eye-drops. Adjusted to pH 9 with sodium hydroxide 4% solution. Prepared aseptically.

Acetylcysteine Solution *(U.S.P.)*. A sterile solution in water prepared with the aid of sodium hydroxide. pH 6.5 to 7.5. Store in airtight containers. Store in a refrigerator after opening. A change in colour to light purple does not indicate impairment of safety or efficacy.

Proprietary Preparations

Airbron *(Duncan, Flockhart, UK)*. A sterile neutral aqueous solution containing the equivalent of 20% of acetylcysteine, available in ampoules of 2 ml and vials of 10 ml. If only a portion of a vial is used, the remainder should be stored in a refrigerator and used within 96 hours. (Also available as Airbron in *Canad.*).

Parvolex *(Duncan, Flockhart, UK)*. Acetylcysteine, available as an injection containing 200 mg per ml, in ampoules of 10 ml.

Other Proprietary Names

Fluimucil *(Ger., Ital., Neth., Spain, Switz.)*; Inspir *(Swed.)*; Lysomucil *(Belg.)*; Mucofilin Sol *(Jap.)*; Mucolyticum *(Ger.)*; Mucomist *(Ital.)*; Mucomyst *(Arg., Austral., Belg., Canad., Denm., Fr., Neth., Norw., Swed., Switz., USA)*; Nac *(Canad.)*.

3702-f

Amylase.

An enzyme catalysing the hydrolysis of α-1,4-glucosidic linkages of polysaccharides such as starch, glycogen, or their degradation products.

CAS — 9000-92-4.

Amylases may be classified according to the manner in which the glucosidic bond is attacked. Endoamylases attack the α-1,4-glucosidic linkage at random.Alpha-amylases are the only types of endoamylases known and yield dextrins, oligosaccharides, and monosaccharides. The more common alpha-amylases include those isolated from human saliva, mammalian pancreas, *Bacillus subtilis*, *Aspergillus oryzae*, and barley malt. Exoamylases attack the α-1,4-glucosidic linkage only from the non-reducing outer polysaccharide chain ends. They include beta-amylases and glucoamylases (amyloglucosidases) and are of vegetable or microbial origin. Beta-amylases yield beta-limit dextrins and maltose and glucoamylases yield glucose.

Adverse Effects. Hypersensitivity reactions have been reported.

A report of allergic responses in workers exposed to fungal α-amylase derived from *Aspergillus oryzae*. These responses were not obtained with α-amylase derived from *Bacillus subtilis*. These findings have implications for workers in the flour milling and bakery industries.— M. L. H. Flindt (letter), *Lancet*, 1979, *1*, 1407.

Uses. Amylase is used in the production of predigested starchy foods and for the conversion of starch to fermentable sugars in the brewing and fermentation industries.

Amylase from various sources has also been used as a digestant. An alpha-amylase obtained from a non-pathogenic variant of *Bacillus subtilis* has also been suggested for use as an adjunct to standard therapy in the treatment of inflammation and oedema but is of unproven value.

Preparations

Compound Diastase and Sodium Bicarbonate Powder *(Jap. P.)*. Diastase 20 g, sodium bicarbonate 60 g, magnesium oxide 15 g, powdered gentian 5 g. *Usual dose.* 6 g daily.

Diastase *(B.P.C. 1934)*. Amylase; Maltin. A mixture of amylolytic enzymes obtained by precipitation with alcohol from an infusion of malt. *Dose.* 60 to 300 mg. A similar preparation is included in *Jap. P.* and *Port. P.*.

Diastase and Sodium Bicarbonate Powder *(Jap. P.)*. Diastase 20 g, sodium bicarbonate 30 g, calcium carbonate 40 g, magnesium oxide 10 g. *Usual dose.* 6 g daily.

Proprietary Names of Amylases

Buccalase *(Winthrop, Austral.)*; Maxilase *(Millot-Solac, Fr.; Perrier, Switz.)*; Oramyl *(Sandoz, Fr.)*; Taka-Diastasa *(Parke, Davis, Spain)*.

An amylase preparation was formerly marketed in Great Britain under the proprietary name Taka-Diastase *(Parke, Davis)*.

3703-d

Anethole Trithione. SKF 1717; Trithioparamethoxyphenylpropene. 5-(4-Methoxyphenyl)-3*H*-1,2-dithiole-3-thione.
$C_{10}H_8OS_3$=240.4.

CAS — 104-46-1 (anethole); 532-11-6 (trithione).

Orange-coloured crystals with a very bitter taste. M.p. 111°. Practically **insoluble** in water; soluble in chloroform and carbon disulphide; slightly soluble in acetone, ether, and acetic acid.

Anethole trithione is used as a choleretic. The usual dose is 50 mg daily in divided doses, before meals; children, 12.5 to 25 mg. It is also used in salivary insufficiency in doses of 25 mg thrice daily. Anethole trithione may cause discoloration of the urine.

Proprietary Names

Felviten *(Grünenthal, Ger.)*; Mucinol *(Kali-Chemie, Ger.)*; Sialor *(Charton, Canad.)*; Sulfarlem *(Latema, Belg.; Latéma, Fr.; Farmades, Ital.; Noristan, S.Afr.; Latéma, Switz.)*.

3704-n

Brinolase. Astra 1652; Brinase; CA-7; Protease I. A fibrinolytic enzyme from *Aspergillus oryzae*.

CAS — 9000-99-1.

Adverse Effects. Pyrexia, paraesthesia, nausea, diarrhoea, drowsiness, skin rash, tachycardia, chest pain, vascular spasm and pain, thrombosis at the injection site, oedema after extravasation, haematoma, transient acute renal insufficiency, and anaphylaxis have been reported.

Allergic symptoms had been noted in employees of a pharmaceutical company working with the proteolytic enzyme brinolase.— M. Forsbeck and L. Ekenvall (letter), *Lancet*, 1978, *2*, 524.

Uses. Brinolase has fibrinolytic and proteolytic activity and lowers the plasmin-inhibitory activity of the serum. Its thrombolytic effect is inversely proportional to the concentration of inhibitors in the blood (protease resistance).

It has been used for clearing blocked haemodialysis cannulas. Because cellular immune mechanisms appear to be related to the fibrinolytic system it has also been tried in leukaemia and neoplastic disease.

Action. A review of the development and uses of brinolase.— *Can. med. Ass. J.*, 1968, *98*, 789.

Brinolase has a direct effect not only on fibrin but also on other substrates such as fibrinogen, prothrombin, and factors V and VII. It has been claimed to be effective in lysing intravascular fibrin without undue bleeding.— V. V. Kakkar and M. F. Scully, *Br. med. Bull.*, 1978, *34*, 191.

Intermittent claudication. All of 14 patients with intermittent claudication had their walking ability increased after treatment with brinolase. Initially 100 mg was given intravenously each week in 200 ml of sodium chloride injection, but in the absence of side-effects was then given daily.— *Med. News, Lond.*, 1973, *5* (May 7), 1.

Neoplasms. Reports of the use of brinolase in neoplastic diseases.— R. D. Thornes *et al.*, *Cancer Res.*, 1972, *32*, 280; E. T. O'Brien *et al.*, *Lancet*, 1968, *1*, 173; R. D. Thornes, *ibid.*, 1968, *2*, 1220; R. D. Thornes *et al.* (letter), *ibid.*, 1973, *1*, 1386; R. D. Thornes, *ibid.*, 1974, *2*, 382.

Patency of cannulas. Use in clearing blocked haemodialysis cannulas.— W. H. E. Roschlau, *Can. med. Ass. J.*, 1968, *98*, 757; A. W. Perry, *ibid.*, 762; G. Pedroni *et al.*, *Farmaco, Edn prat.*, 1972, *27*, 60.

Thrombo-embolic disorders. Local treatment with brinolase resulted in recanalisation of occlusions in 2 of 7 patients with thrombotic and 2 patients with embolic arterial occlusions.— D. Nyman *et al.*, *Schweiz. med. Wschr.*, 1974, *104*, 1865, per *J. Am. med. Ass.*, 1975, *232*, 97.

Further references: F. Lund *et al.*, *Angiology*, 1975, *26*, 534.

Proprietary Names

Brinastrase *(Astra, Norw.; Astra, Swed.)*.

3705-h

Bromelains. Bromelins; Plant Protease Concentrate.

CAS — 9001-00-7.

A concentrate of proteolytic enzymes derived from the pineapple plant, *Ananas comosus* (=*A. sativus*) (Bromeliaceae). A buff-coloured powder. Slightly **soluble** in water; practically insoluble in alcohol, chloroform, and ether.

The properties and assay methods of bromelains.— Bromelain, in *Pharmaceutical Enzymes*, R. Ruyssen and A. Lauwers (Ed.), Gent, E. Story-Scientia, 1978, p. 107.

Units. One Rorer unit of protease activity is defined as that amount of enzyme which hydrolyses a standardised casein substrate at pH 7 and 25° so as to cause an increase in absorbance of 0.00001 per minute at 280 nm.

One FIP unit of bromelain activity is contained in that amount of a standard preparation, which hydrolyses a suitable preparation of casein (FIP controlled) under the standard conditions at an initial rate such that there is liberated per minute an amount of peptides, not precipitated by a specified protein precipitation reagent which gives the same absorbance as 1 µmol of tyrosine at 275 nm.

Adverse Effects. Bromelains may cause nausea, vomiting, and diarrhoea. Menorrhagia has occasionally occurred. Hypersensitivity reactions have been reported and have included skin reactions and asthma.

A report of bronchial asthma experienced by 2 patients after exposure to bromelains.— F. Galleguillos and J. C. Rodriguez, *Clin. Allergy*, 1978, *8*, 21.

Of 6 workers sensitised to papain 5 showed positive skin tests to bromelains and 2 of them also showed immediate asthmatic reactions after bronchial challenge with bromelains. It was considered that this provided evidence for immunological cross-reaction between bromelains and papain.— X. Baur and G. Fruhmann, *Clin. Allergy*, 1979, *9*, 443.

Precautions. Bromelains should be given with care to patients with abnormal blood-clotting mechanisms or severely impaired hepatic or renal function and to patients taking anticoagulants.

Uses. Bromelains is used as an adjunct in the treatment of soft tissue inflammation and oedema associated with trauma and surgery.

The suggested initial dose is 100 000 Rorer units 4 times daily, followed by a maintenance dose of 50 000 units 4 times daily or 100 000 units twice daily.

Action. A review— W. M. Cooreman *et al.*, *Pharm. Acta Helv.*, 1976, *51*, 73.

Claims made for the immediate proteolytic and mucolytic effects of bromelains were not substantiated. A spasmolytic effect was suggested; it might be of use in the treatment of dysmenorrhoea.— S. L. B. Duncan *et al.*, *Lancet*, 1960, *2*, 1420.

The protease activity of bromelains was inhibited by the addition of human serum. Given in a gelatin capsule to volunteers it produced no detectable proteolytic activity in blood and no inactivation of fibrinolysis.— H. Lang *et al.*, *Arzneimittel-Forsch.*, 1969, *19*, 939.

Inflammation. The use of bromelains in acute sinusitis.— R. E. Ryan, *Headache*, 1967, *7*, 13.

In a trial of bromelains in 74 boxers with bruises of the face and haematomas of the orbits, lips, ears, chest, and arms, 2 tablets [each 50 000 units] were given 4 times daily for 4 days, or until all signs of bruising had disappeared; within 4 days bruising was cleared in 58 of those given bromelains but in only 10 of 72 controls.— G. L. Blonstein, *Practitioner*, 1969, *203*, 206.

Thrombo-embolic disorders. Bromelains had been used successfully in the treatment of central retinal vein thrombosis.— L. F. Gray, *Sth. med. J.*, 1969, *62*, 11.

Proprietary Preparations

Ananase Forte *(Rorer, UK)*. Bromelains, available as enteric-coated tablets of 100 000 Rorer units.

Other Proprietary Names

Ananase *(Austral., Ital., USA)*; Extranase *(Belg., Fr.)*; Proteolis *(Ital.)*; Resolvit *(Switz.)*; Rogorin *(Ital.)*; Traumanase *(Ger., Switz.)*.

3706-m

Chenodeoxycholic Acid. Chenodiol; Chenic Acid; CDCA. 3α,7α-Dihydroxy-5β-cholan-24-oic acid.

$C_{24}H_{40}O_4$=392.6.

CAS — 474-25-9.

Adverse Effects. Chenodeoxycholic acid may cause diarrhoea and pruritus. A transient rise in liver-function test values has been reported.

Diarrhoea. Dosage reduction owing to diarrhoea was required by one of 16 patients given chenodeoxycholic acid 500 mg daily, 5 of 64 given 750 mg daily, and 9 of 40 given 1 g daily with a further one of the 40 requiring discontinuation. Additional side-effects included skin itching in 2 patients which resolved without dosage reduction; one patient stopped therapy owing to a non-specific symptomatic digestive disturbance. There were no other signs of increased toxicity with the 1-g dose except the diarrhoea.— M. C. Bateson *et al.*, *Lancet*, 1978, *1*, 1111.

Results of a placebo-controlled double-blind crossover study of chenodeoxycholic acid 15 mg per kg body-weight daily in 7 patients with radiolucent gall-stones indicated that although loose stools and/or increased bowel frequency might occur in the first few days of chenodeoxycholic acid therapy this was of short duration and did not call for dosage reduction or discontinuation of therapy.— E. Corazziari *et al.* (letter), *Lancet*, 1978, *2*, 266.

Effects on the liver. In healthy persons and patients with gall-stones given chenodeoxycholic acid about 20% of lithocholate (the main bacterial metabolite and probably responsible for the reported liver damage in *animals*) was absorbed from the colon and then conjugated and sulphated to substances rapidly excreted in the faeces. A defective sulphation of lithocholate in the *rhesus monkey* had recently been reported. This difference in metabolism provided a simple explanation for the consistent toxicity of chenodeoxycholic acid in the *monkey* and its apparent safety in man.— R. N. Allan *et al.*, *Gut*, 1976, *17*, 405 and 413. A factor reducing the toxic potential of chenodeoxycholic acid was the epimerisation to ursodeoxycholic acid, which was not a preferred precursor for lithocholic acid.— *Lancet*, 1978, *1*, 805. See also G. Salen *et al.*, *J. clin. Invest.*, 1974, *53*, 612; T. Fedorowski *et al.*, *Gastroenterology*, 1977, *73*, 1131; A. Stiehl *et al.*, *ibid.*, 1978, *75*, 1016.

Hepatic sinusoidal dilatation was associated with chenodeoxycholic acid.— V. G. Levy *et al.* (letter), *Lancet*, 1978, *1*, 206.

Pregnancy and the neonate. The offspring of *monkeys* given chenodeoxycholic acid during pregnancy had congenital hepatic, renal, and adrenal abnormalities.— R. Heywood *et al.* (letter), *Lancet*, 1973, *2*, 1021. A report of species difference between *monkey* and man in the metabolism of chenodeoxycholic acid.— R. N. Allan *et al.*, *Gut*, 1976, *17*, 405 and 413.

Opinions differed on the wisdom of giving chenodeoxycholic acid to women of childbearing age and to women taking oral contraceptives.— *Lancet*, 1978, *1*, 805.

Precautions. Chenodeoxycholic acid should not be administered to patients with chronic liver disease or inflammatory diseases of the small intestine and colon.

Pregancy and the neonate. See above under Adverse Effects.

Absorption and Fate. Chenodeoxycholic acid is absorbed from the gastro-intestinal tract and some is conjugated in the liver before being excreted into the bile. Under the influence of intestinal bacteria the free and conjugated forms undergo 7α-dehydroxylation to lithocholic acid some of which is excreted directly in the faeces and the rest absorbed mainly to be conjugated and sulphated by the liver. The sulphated compounds being water-soluble are then excreted in the faeces. Chenodeoxycholic acid also undergoes epimerisation to ursodeoxycholic acid.

For reports on the metabolism of chenodeoxycholic acid, see G. Salen *et al.*, *J. clin. Invest.*, 1974, *53*, 612; G. P. van Berge-Henegouwen and A. F. Hofmann, *Gastroenterology*, 1977, *73*, 300; T. Fedorowski *et al.*, *ibid.*, 1131; A. Stiehl *et al.*, *ibid.*, 1978, *74*, 572; *idem*, *75*, 1016.

Uses. Chenodeoxycholic acid is a naturally occurring bile acid. When given by mouth it reduces the ratio of cholesterol to bile salts plus phospholipids in bile and so causes desaturation of cholesterol-saturated bile associated with gall-stones.

Chenodeoxycholic acid is used for the dissolution of cholesterol-rich gall-stones in patients with a functioning gall-bladder. It is considered to be ineffective against calcified or pigment-containing stones or in those patients with a non-functioning gall-bladder. The usual dose is 10 to 15 mg per kg body-weight daily in divided doses. The duration of treatment appears to be correlated with the size of the stone. It has been recommended that treatment continues for 3 months after dissolution.

Chenodeoxycholic acid has also been used in hyperlipidaemia.

Arthritis. Sixteen patients with rheumatoid arthritis had been treated with chenodeoxycholic acid 0.75 to 1 g daily for 3 to 11 weeks. Initially there was deterioration of joint pain and general condition, sometimes with fever; this was followed, usually after about 6 weeks of treatment, by obvious remission of the disease and a reduction in ESR.— A. Bruusgaard and R. B. Andersen (letter), *Lancet*, 1976, *1*, 700.

Gall-stones. Reviews and discussions on the use of chenodeoxycholic acid in the dissolution of gall-stones.— I. A. D. Bouchier, *Br. med. J.*, 1976, *2*, 870; *ibid.*, 1977, *1*, 1119; R. G. Batey, *Drugs*, 1977, *14*, 116; *Lancet*, 1978, *1*, 805; *Br. med. J.*, 1978, *2*, 309; *ibid.*, 847; *Drug & Ther. Bull.*, 1978, *16*, 69; G. D. Bell, *Prescribers' J.*, 1979, *19*, 87; P. Carruthers-Czyzewski, *Can. J. Hosp. Pharm.*, 1979, *32*, 113; J. A. Summerfield, *Br. J. Hosp. Med.*, 1979, *21*, 482; J. H. Iser and A. Sali, *Drugs*, 1981, *21* 90.

The effect of chenodeoxycholic acid in desaturating bile with cholesterol was due to a reduction in the output of cholesterol and not to increased output of bile salts or phospholipids.— T. C. Northfield *et al.*, *Gut*, 1973, *14*, 826. Fasting gall-bladder bile in 6 patients with gall-stones became less saturated with cholesterol during treatment with chenodeoxycholic acid 1 to 2.25 g daily. There was an increase in the size of the bile-acid pool of chenodeoxycholic acid.— T. C. Northfield *et al.*, *Gut*, 1975, *16*, 12.

In 4 of 11 patients, gall-stones were dissolved or markedly reduced in size after treatment for 3 to 18 months with chenodeoxycholic acid. Two further patients with recurrent cholangitis had a marked reduction in the number of attacks. The overall ratio of cholesterol to bile salts plus phospholipids was not markedly changed but there were wide individual changes.— O. James *et al.*, *Gut*, 1973, *14*, 827.

An analysis of chenodeoxycholic acid in the treatment of various gall-stones in 70 patients. Radiolucent gall-stones in functioning gall-bladders in 25 patients dissolved completely in 10 patients and partially in 6 after more than 6 months' treatment with chenodeoxycholic acid. An effective dose was 14 to 15 mg per kg body-weight daily. Small stones reappeared in 2 of the 10 patients 8 and 10 months after treatment had been discontinued. A fasting bile unsaturated with cholesterol after 1 to 3 months' treatment was an indication that the treatment should be successful.— J. H. Iser *et al.*, *New Engl. J. Med.*, 1975, *293*, 378.

A controlled study of 29 patients with gall-stones indicated that β-sitosterol might enhance the effect of chenodeoxycholic acid against cholesterol gall-stones.— A. Gerolami and H. Sarles (letter), *Lancet*, 1975, *2*, 721. Study in 15 patients showed that the effect of chenodeoxycholic acid on the saturation index of gall-bladder bile was enhanced by a low-cholesterol diet. Surprisingly there was a rise in the saturation index when patients were given sitosterols.— D. P. Maudgal *et al.*, *Br. med. J.*, 1978, *2*, 851. The reduction in the saturation index of bile was small and probably not of biological significance.— J. M. Watts *et al.* (letter), *ibid.*, 1979, *1*, 200.

Intrahepatic cholesterol stones in 2 men aged 34 and 46 years were dissolved within 8 and 2 months respectively by retrograde instillation of chenodeoxycholic acid via a T-drain. Both patients then received chenodeoxycholic acid 750 mg daily by mouth to prevent recurrence of the stones.— P. Czygan *et al.*, *Dt. med. Wschr.*, 1977, *102*, 518.

A syndrome of resistance to chenodeoxycholic acid therapy.— P. N. Maton *et al.*, *Gut*, 1977, *18*, A976.

Given in doses effective to desaturate bile, chenodeoxycholic acid seemed to decrease the absorption of dietary cholesterol.— M. P. de Leon *et al.*, *Gut*, 1978, *19*, A972.

Calcification of gall-stones in 2 patients during treatment with chenodeoxycholic acid.— M. J. Whiting *et al.*, *Gut*, 1980, *21*, 1077.

Two doses of chenodeoxycholic acid, 750 mg daily and 375 mg daily and a placebo were compared in The National Cooperative Gallstone Study. Treatment was for 2 years and covered 916 patients with radiolucent gall-stones. The 750-mg dose provided complete dissolution in 13.5% of patients compared with 5.2% for the 375-mg dose and 0.8% for placebo. Thin patients or those with small gall-stones or serum-cholesterol concentrations of 2.27 mg or more per ml appeared to respond best. However, biliary symptoms and the need for surgery were not diminished, diarrhoea was frequent, hepatic dysfunction occurred, causing 3% of patients to withdraw, and there was an increase in serum concentrations of total and low-density lipoprotein cholesterol.— L. J. Schoenfield *et al.*, *Ann. intern. Med.*, 1981, *95*, 257. Comment.— K. J. Isselbacher, *ibid.*, 377. Further comment including concern at the adverse effects and criticism of the doses being low and fixed. An optimum dose was considered to be 15 mg per kg body-weight; higher doses may be required by the very obese patient.— *Lancet*, 1981, *2*, 905.

Further references: R. G. Danzinger *et al.*, *New Engl. J. Med.*, 1972, *286*, 1; J. L. Thistle and A. F. Hofmann, *ibid.*, 1973, *289*, 655; D. Bainton *et al.* (letter), *Lancet*, 1974, *1*, 562; H. Y. I. Mok *et al.*, *ibid.*, *2*, 253; M. J. Coyne *et al.*, *New Engl. J. Med.*, 1975, *292*, 604; *Br. med. J.*, 1977, *1*, 1119; U. Leuschner and M. Leuschner, *Dt. med. Wschr.*, 1979, *104*, 629.

Administration. In patients commencing treatment with chenodeoxycholic acid, there was an interval of up to 4 weeks before bile became undersaturated with cholesterol. After stopping therapy, bile returned to its supersaturated state in less than 3 weeks. It was concluded that intermittent therapy would prolong the time required for dissolution of gall-stones.— J. H. Iser *et al.*, *Gut*, 1977, *18*, 7.

Studies had shown that administration of chenodeoxycholic acid for 4-day periods followed by 3-day breaks was effective. Studies on a larger scale seemed justified since intermittent treatment was safer and cheaper.— V. Ferrari (letter), *Lancet*, 1978, *1*, 1314.

Results of a comparative dosage study of chenodeoxycholic acid 0.5, 0.75, or 1 g daily administered for up to 4 years to 96 patients with radiolucent gall-stones, indicated that treatment for radiolucent gall-stone dissolution should be started with 1 g daily where tolerated; it seemed reasonable to continue this dosage indefinitely since recurrence could occur on reduction of dosage, but more work was needed on this aspect of therapy. A success-rate of 50% could be expected and although the place of dissolution therapy remained to be established, it seemed suitable for patients unfit or unwilling to undergo surgery.— M. C. Bateson *et al.*, *Lancet*, 1978, *1*, 1111. Criticism of the use of a fixed dose of chenodeoxycholic acid.— R. H. Dowling and P. N. Maton (letter), *ibid.*, 1978, *2*, 378. Reply.— M. C. Bateson *et al.* (letter), *ibid.*, 379.

In 8 obese patients (more than 125% ideal body-weight) with gall-stones the mean biliary cholesterol saturation index was higher than in 8 non-obese patients (not more than 2% above ideal body-weight). After treatment with chenodeoxycholic acid 13 to 15 mg per kg body-weight daily for at least a month bile remained supersaturated in the obese patients but became unsaturated in the non-obese patients. Partial or complete dissolution of gall-stones occurred in 5 of the 8 non-obese patients after 6 to 18 months treatment and in none of the obese patients. When the dose of chenodeoxycholic acid was increased to a mean of 18.6 mg per kg in the obese patients the bile became unsaturated and 4 of the group eventually showed partial gall-stone dissolution.— J. H. Iser *et al.*, *Br. med. J.*, 1978, *1*, 1509.

In 16 patients with gall-stones the mean saturation index of bile before treatment was 1.28; this was reduced to 0.78 after treatment for one month with chenodeoxycholic acid 14 to 16 mg per kg body-weight daily given at bedtime, compared with 0.92 when the dose was given in the morning or as 3 divided doses with meals. There was no increase in bowel frequency.— D. P. Maudgal *et al.*, *Br. med. J.*, 1979, *1*, 922.

Hyperlipidaemia. In a double-blind crossover study of 9 patients receiving dietary treatment for hypertriglyceridaemia, chenodeoxycholic acid 250 mg thrice daily for 3 months reduced fasting hypertriglyceridaemia by a mean of 22% compared with placebo, and without reciprocally raising high-density lipoprotein (HDL) concentrations. This absence of effect on HDL concentrations was confirmed in 19 men with gall-stones given chenodeoxycholic acid 250 mg three or four times daily. Chenodeoxycholic acid might be a useful alternative to clofibrate without the hazard of inducing gall-stones but neither agent is likely to have any significant effect on HDL-cholesterol.— M. C. Bateson and J. Iqbal (letter), *Lancet*, 1979, *1*, 930. See also M. C. Bateson *et al.*, *Br. J. clin. Pharmac.*, 1978, *5*, 249.

Further references: G. D. Bell *et al.*, *Br. med. J.*, 1973, *3*, 520; N. E. Miller and P. J. Nestel (preliminary communication), *Lancet*, 1974, *2*, 929; B. Angelin *et al.*, *Clin. Sci & mol. Med.*, 1978, *54*, 451; E. Camarri *et al.*, *Int. J. clin. Pharmac. Biopharm.*, 1978, *16*, 527.

For the effect of chenodeoxycholic acid in reducing the clofibrate-induced raised cholesterol saturation index of bile, and in enhancing the effect of clofibrate, see Clofibrate, p.409.

Migraine. In a preliminary double-blind study, 17 patients with migrainous headaches who received chenodeoxycholic acid 250 mg thrice daily suffered fewer attacks than 18 similar patients who received a placebo, but the findings required confirmation.— V. G. Lévy *et al.* (letter), *New Engl. J. Med.*, 1978, *298*, 630.

Proprietary Preparations

Chendol *(Weddel, UK).* Chenodeoxycholic acid, available as capsules of 125 mg. (Also available as Chendol in *Austral., Port., Spain*).

Chenofalk *(Armour, UK).* Chenodeoxycholic acid, available as capsules of 250 mg. (Also available as Chenofalk in *Arg., Aust., Belg., Chile, Ger., Hong Kong, Ital., Kuwait, Mex., Neth., Peru, Phillipp., Switz., Taiwan, Thai.*).

Other Proprietary Names

Belg.—Chenolith, Kebilis; *Chile*—Hepanem; *Denm.*—Chendal; *Fr.*—Chénodex; *Ger.*—Cholanorm, Hekbilin; *Ital.*—Chenocol, Chenossil, Fluibil; *Neth.*—Cheno-Caps; *Spain*—Carbilcolina, Chelobil, Chemicolina, Chenodecil, Chenomas, Quenobilan; *Switz.*—Ulmenid.

3707-b

Cholic Acid.

Cholalic Acid. 3α,7α,12α-Trihydroxy-5β-cholan-24-oic acid.
$C_{24}H_{40}O_5$=408.6.

CAS — 81-25-4.

Pharmacopoeias. In *Aust.*

A white crystalline powder with a bitter taste. Slightly **soluble** in water, chloroform, and ether; soluble in alcohol.

Uses. Cholic acid is a naturally occurring bile acid. It has been used as the acid or sodium salt for the dissolution of gall-stones.

Absorption.— P. Samuel *et al.*, *J. clin. Invest.*, 1968, *47*, 2070.

Cholic acid 250 mg thrice daily improved faecal frequency and consistency in 4 of 5 patients with long-standing constipation.— G. W. Hepner and A. J. Hofmann, *Mayo Clin. Proc.*, 1973, *48*, 356.

Estimated acceptable daily intake of cholic and deoxycholic acid and their salts: up to 1.25 mg per kg body-weight.— Seventeenth Report of FAO/WHO Expert Committee on Food Additives, *Tech. Rep. Ser. Wld Hlth Org. No. 539*, 1974. For background toxicological information, see *Fd Add. Ser. Wld Hlth Org. No. 5*, 1974.

Gall-stones. A favourable report of the use of sodium cholate solution by perfusion to assist in the removal of retained stones in the common bile duct after cholecystectomy.— C. Lansford *et al.*, *Gut*, 1974, *15*, 48.

Cholic acid 250 mg and soya-bean lecithin 750 mg were given thrice daily by mouth for 6 months to 11 patients with radiolucent gall-stones; the stones disappeared in 2 patients.— J. Toouli *et al.* (preliminary communication), *Lancet*, 1975, *2*, 1124.

Further references: A. M. Molokhia *et al.* (letter), *J. pharm. Sci.*, 1975, *64*, 2029; M. C. Bateson and I. A. D. Bouchier, *Gut*, 1977, *18*, A977.

3708-v

Chymopapain.

Bax 1526. A proteolytic enzyme isolated from the latex of papaya (*Carica papaya*), differing from papain in electrophoretic mobility, solubility, and substrate specificity. Molecular weight approximately 27 000.

CAS — 9001-09-6.

Units. One nanokatal is defined as the amount of chymopapain which produces 1 nanomole of *p*-nitroaniline per second from *N*-α-benzoyl-DL-arginine -*p*-nitroanilide substrate at pH 6.4 and 37°. One CTE unit is defined as the amount of chymopapain which produces from acid-denatured haemoglobin at pH 4 in 1 minute a hydrolysate with an optical density at 275 nm equal to that of a solution containing tyrosine 1 μg per ml.

Adverse Effects. Chymopapain injection may cause allergic reactions including urticaria, angio-oedema, erythema, pruritus, shock, cardiac arrest, laryngeal oedema, and bronchospasm. Severe muscle spasm and an increase in back pain are common reactions. Paraplegia, arachnoiditis, subarachnoid haemorrhage, and pulmonary embolism have occurred. Other reported reactions include headache, nausea and vomiting, pyrexia, ileus, urinary retention, thrombophlebitis, pancreatitis, paraesthesias, foot-drop, meningismus, and toxic psychosis.

Between 0.3 and 1% of patients were allergic to chymopapain and some had suffered severe anaphylactic reactions.— *J. Am. med. Ass.*, 1974, *229*, 747.

Of 1200 patients given chymopapain anaphylactic reactions occurred in 9, rash in 15, and urticaria in 11. Foot-drop occurred in 3 patients, 2 of whom recovered completely. Concomitant administration of an antihistamine and a corticosteroid reduced the incidence of anaphylactic reactions to 2 in 600.— L. L. Wiltse *et al.*, *J. Am. med. Ass.*, 1975, *231*, 474. Comment.— B. J. Sussman (letter), *ibid.*, *234*, 271. Reply.— L. L. Wiltse (letter), *ibid.*, 272.

Further references: C. E. Graham (letter), *Med. J. Aust.*, 1973, *2*, 406; R. Rajagopalan *et al.*, *Anesth. Analg. curr. Res.*, 1974, *53*, 191; B. J. Sussman, *J. Neurosurg.*, 1975, *42*, 389; J. C. Maroon *et al.*, *J. Neurol. Neurosurg. Psychiat.*, 1976, *39*, 508; C. Watts *et al.*, *Anesthesiology*, 1976, *44*, 437.

Treatment of Adverse Effects. Anaphylactic reactions should be treated with adrenaline, possibly in association with antihistamine and corticosteroid therapy. For detailed recommendations concerning the management of anaphylaxis, see Adrenaline, p.4.

Precautions. Chymopapain should not be used in those patients with a known sensitivity to papaya proteins or in patients with active infectious disease.

Drugs and equipment for the emergency management of anaphylactic reactions should always be to hand when giving patients chymopapain; the risk of allergic reactions associated with chymopapain is so high that no patient should ever receive it more than once.

Uses. Chymopapain is used as an injection into the intervertebral disk in the treatment of sciatic pain secondary to herniation of intervertebral disks of the lumbar spine. The aim of this treatment, termed chemonucleolysis, is to dissolve the disk.

Chymopapain injection should be administered under local anaesthesia; if general anaesthesia is used endotracheal intubation is essential. A recommended dose for a single intervertebral disk is 8 mg (5 nanokatals) with a maximum dose per disk of 10 mg (6.25 nanokatals); the maximum permissible total dose to the patient is 20 mg (12.5 nanokatals).

In a series of 1200 patients with recurrent low-back pain or sciatica, chemonucleolysis with 6 to 8 mg of chymopapain per disk space was carried out. Of 455 patients followed up for 1 year, results were excellent to good in 285, fair in 58, and poor in 112.— L. L. Wiltse *et al.*, *J. Am. med. Ass.*, 1975, *231*, 474. Comment.— A. S. Russell (letter), *ibid.*, *233*, 1164. Reply.— L. L.

Wiltse, *ibid.* Criticism.— B. J. Sussman (letter), *ibid.*, *234*, 271. Reply.— L. L. Wiltse (letter), *ibid.*, 272.

Injection of chymopapain was of doubtful value in the treatment of back pain due to disk degeneration without nerve-root irritation.— *J. Am. med. Ass.*, 1975, *231*, 554.

In a double-blind study involving 66 patients with herniated lumbar disks not responsive to conservative treatment there was no statistically significant difference in incidence or quality of improvement between those given an intradiskal injection of chymopapain and those given a placebo.— P. R. Schwetschenau *et al.*, *J. Neurosurg.*, 1976, *45*, 622.

A prospective study involving 480 patients who underwent enzymatic dissolution of the nucleus pulposus with chymopapain. A favourable response to chemonucleolysis was obtained in 158 of the 225 patients with the clinical criteria for a disk herniation. Those patients who had undergone a previous operation, had spinal stenosis, or had psychogenic components to the disability had very poor results.— J. A. McCulloch, *J. Bone Jt Surg.*, 1977, *59B*, 45.

A discussion of the use of chymopapain in intervertebral disk disorders.— *Br. med. J.*, 1977, *2*, 1107. See also *ibid.*, 1974, *2*, 625; *Lancet*, 1975, *1*, 1022.

Further references: L. Smith, *J. Am. med. Ass.*, 1964, *187*, 137; L. Smith and J. E. Brown, *J. Bone Jt Surg.*, 1967, *49B*, 502; D. S. Weiner and I. Macnab, *Can. med. Ass. J.*, 1970, *102*, 1252; C. E. Graham, *Med. J. Aust.*, 1974, *1*, 5; M. J. Javid, *J. Am. med. Ass.*, 1980, *243*, 2043.

Preparations

Discase *(Travenol, UK)*. Chymopapain, available as injection in vials containing 20 mg (12.5 nanokatals) with cysteine hydrochloride monohydrate 3.5 mg and disodium edetate 0.37 mg. After reconstitution the injection may be stored at room temperature for up to 30 minutes or at 2° to 8° for up to 4 hours.

3709-g

Chymotrypsin *(B.P., Eur. P.)*. Chymotrypsinum; α-Chymotrypsin.

CAS — 9004-07-3.

Pharmacopoeias. In *Br., Cz., Eur., Fr., Ger., It., Neth.*, and *U.S.*

A proteolytic enzyme obtained by the activation of chymotrypsinogen extracted from bovine pancreas.

Chymotrypsin (*B.P., Eur. P.*) contains not less than 4 microkatals in each mg, and not less than 5 microkatals in each mg if intended for ophthalmic use. Chymotrypsin (*U.S.P.*) contains not less than 1000 *U.S.P.* units in each mg, calculated on the dry basis. Despite the different unit systems, American and European material appear to have approximately the same potency on a weight basis. See below under Units.

A white to yellowish-white odourless crystalline or amorphous powder; the amorphous form is hygroscopic. Sparingly **soluble** in water. A 1% solution has a pH of 3 to 5. **Incompatible** with adrenaline and hydrogen peroxide. Stable in the dry state but solutions deteriorate rapidly. Solutions have a maximum stability at pH 3 and a maximum activity at about pH 8. **Store** at 2° to 8° in sealed containers. Protect from light.

The properties and assay methods of chymotrypsin.— Chymotrypsin, in *Pharmaceutical Enzymes*, R. Ruyssen and A. Lauwers (Ed.), Gent, E. Story-Scientia, 1978, p. 41.

Stability. The stability of chymotrypsin was increased by the addition of calcium ions. It was inactivated by heavy metals, organophosphorus compounds, and chloramphenicol.— International Commission for the Standardisation of Pharmaceutical Enzymes, *J. mond. Pharm.*, 1965, *8*, 5.

Units. Chymotrypsin is assayed for potency on the basis of its proteolytic activity and the potency of commercial products has been expressed in various units based on different methods of assay.

There are 2 principal methods of assay. One method is based on the use of a denatured haemoglobin substrate; the other is based on the hydrolysis of *N*-acetyl-L-tyrosine ethyl ester by chymotrypsin at the ester linkage.

Chymotrypsin (*B.P., Eur. P.*) is assayed for potency, by comparison with a reference standard, in terms of its ability to digest *N*-acetyl-L-tyrosine ethyl ester at 25° and the hydrolysis is followed potentiometrically. One microkatal is the enzymic activity producing the hydrolysis of 1 μmol of substrate per second under the conditions specified in the assay.

Chymotrypsin (*U.S.P.*) is assayed for potency, by comparison with a reference standard, in terms of its ability to digest *N*-acetyl-L-tyrosine ethyl ester at 25°. The hydrolysis is followed spectrophotometrically by measurement of the light absorption at 237 nm and the potency is determined by the average change in absorption per minute. One *U.S.P.* Chymotrypsin Unit is the activity causing a change in absorption of 0.0075 per minute under the conditions specified in the assay. An approximate correlation that has been given is 1 microkatal equals 275 *U.S.P.* units.

One FIP unit of chymotrypsin hydrolyses 1 μmol of *N*-acetyl-L-tyrosine ethyl ester per minute.

One Armour unit and 2½ Denver (or Wallace or Wampole) units are equivalent to 1 *U.S.P.* unit. One microkatal is equivalent to 60 FIP units.

Adverse Effects. Chymotrypsin may cause nausea, vomiting, diarrhoea, and skin rash. Local irritation has occurred occasionally after buccal administration and pain, swelling, and erythema have been noted at the site of injection after intramuscular administration.

Chymotrypsin is antigenic and severe allergic reactions have occasionally followed its intramuscular injection; it has been suggested that, where allergy is suspected, a sensitivity test should be made before injection.

Increased intra-ocular pressure, loss of vitreous humour, corneal oedema, striation, and uveitis have occurred following its use in ophthalmology.

Chymotrypsin, in a dose 200 times the recommended amount, was tolerated without postoperative complications in a patient who received 5000 Armour units in 1 ml instead of 25 units in 0.25 ml. It was suggested that in some cases the routine concentration might safely be exceeded without undue risk.— P. K. Ray, *Br. J. Ophthal.*, 1964, *48*, 230, per *J. Hosp. Pharm.*, 1964, *21*, 238.

After uncomplicated intracapsular cataract extraction on 343 eyes, with and without chymotrypsin, severe glaucoma occurred in 72.5% when chymotrypsin was used and mild glaucoma in 27.6% without it. The glaucoma was self-limiting, required no treatment, and did not appear to cause damage.— R. E. Kirsch *et al.*, *Archs Ophthal., N.Y.*, 1964, *72*, 612, per *Int. pharm. Abstr.*, 1965, *2*, 1000.

Precautions. Chymotrypsin should be used with caution in patients with abnormal blood-clotting mechanisms, or with severe hepatic disease. It is inadvisable to use chymotrypsin in ocular surgery for patients under 20 years of age or for patients with congenital cataracts with high vitreous pressure and a gaping incisional wound.

Intracapsular extraction of the lens in cataract surgery by injection of chymotrypsin should not be attempted in children under 10 years of age since serious complications, unrelated to the enzyme, might ensue due to special conditions existing in the eyes of young patients.— J. Barraquer and J. Rutllan, *Postgrad. Med.*, 1964, *35*, 57, per *Int. pharm. Abstr.*, 1964, *1*, 239.

Benzylpenicillin inhibited the zonulolytic properties of chymotrypsin and should not be used until zonulolysis was complete.— M. P. Coke, *Am. J. Ophthal.*, 1967, *63*, 1706, per *J. Hosp. Pharm.*, 1967, *24*, 375.

Uses. Chymotrypsin is used in ophthalmology for the dissection of the zonule of the lens, thus facilitating intracapsular cataract extraction with less trauma to the eye. For this purpose a 1 in 5000 or 1 in 10 000 solution of chymotrypsin in a sterile diluent such as sodium chloride injection is usually employed.

Chymotrypsin is given with the intention of reducing soft tissue inflammation and oedema from abscesses and ulcers, or associated with traumatic injuries, and to promote liquefaction of secretions of the upper respiratory tract in patients suffering from asthma, bronchitis, pulmonary diseases, and sinusitis.

Chymotrypsin may be administered by mouth, usually in doses of 20 000 to 40 000 *U.S.P.* units 4 times daily, by intramuscular injection of 5000 *U.S.P.* units once to thrice daily, or topically as an ointment. Chymotrypsin is also administered by mouth in conjunction with trypsin.

Blood clots in the eye. Chymotrypsin given 2 to 3 days after massive vitreous haemorrhage in a patient with sickle-cell anaemia produced rapid clearing of vision.— F. I. D. Konotey-Ahulu (letter), *Lancet*, 1972, *2*, 714.

Dental surgery. Chymar, given intramuscularly the night before operation and daily for 3 days following the removal of impacted wisdom teeth, did not aid in reducing the swelling.— J. H. Sowray, *Br. dent. J.*, 1961, *110*, 130.

Treatment with 1 or 2 tablets, each containing approximately 20 mg of crystalline chymotrypsin, given 4 times daily, reduced the swelling after dental surgery or maxillofacial injuries in 56 patients. Swelling after 24 hours was about one-third of that expected.— F. Wigand and E. Messer, *Clin. Med.*, 1967, *74* (July), 29.

Detection of cancer cells. For the parenteral administration of chymotrypsin to aid the early detection of cancer cells in sputum, see M. Takahashi *et al.*, *Acta cytol.*, 1967, *11*, 61.

The use of chymotrypsin in gastric exfoliative cytology.— L. L. Brandborg *et al.*, *Gastroenterology*, 1969, *57*, 500.

Trauma. A report of the use of chymotrypsin following episiotomy.— H. D. Bumgardner and G. I. Zatuchni, *Am. J. Obstet. Gynec.*, 1965, *92*, 514.

Whipworm infections. Injections of chymotrypsin, 10 to 40 mg daily in 2 to 4 doses, given in conjunction with enemas of sodium bicarbonate for 20 days, resulted in the cure of 6 of 18 children with massive whipworm (*Trichuris*) infections and improvement in 4.— R. Alonso Fiel, *Revta cub. Med. trop.*, 1967, *19*, 45, per *Trop. Dis. Bull.*, 1968, *65*, 917.

Preparations

Chymotrypsin for Ophthalmic Solution *(U.S.P.)*. Sterile chymotrypsin suitable for ophthalmic use. pH 4.3 to 8.7 after reconstitution.

Proprietary Preparations

Chymar *(Armour, UK)*. Chymotrypsin, available in vials of 5000 *U.S.P.* units, for solution in sodium chloride injection, for intramuscular use. (Also available as Chymar in *Austral., S.Afr., Switz.*).

Chymar-Zon *(Armour, UK)*. Chymotrypsin, for use in cataract surgery, in vials of 750 *U.S.P.* units supplied with 10-ml vials of sodium chloride injection. (Also available as Chymar-Zon in *Austral.*).

Deanase DC Tablets *(Consolidated Chemicals, UK)*. Each enteric-coated tablet contains 10 mg of delta-chymotrypsin (a proteolytic enzyme related to α-chymotrypsin). For inflammation. *Dose.* 2 tablets twice daily for 3 days, then 1 twice daily.

Zonulysin *(Henleys, UK)*. Chymotrypsin, available as powder in ampoules containing 1.5 microkatals (300 *U.S.P.* units), with 1-ml ampoules of sodium chloride injection. For use in cataract surgery. (Also available as Zonulysin in *S.Afr.*).

Other Proprietary Names

Arg.—Zonulasi; *Austral.*—Catarase, Kimopsin, Zolyse; *Canad.*—Alpha Chymolean, Catarase, Quimotrase, Zolyse, Zonulyn; *Fr.*—Alphacutanée, Aphlozyme; *Ger.*—Catarase; *Ind.*—Alfapsin; *Ital.*—Alfa-Chimo, Zonulasi; *Jap.*—Kimopsin; *Switz.*—Chymoser, Quimotrase, Zolyse; *USA*—Alpha Chymar, Avazyme.

Chymotrypsin was also formerly marketed in Great Britain under the proprietary name Chymar Aqueous (*Armour*).

3710-f

Cicrotoic Acid. Acidum Cicrotoicum; AD 106. 3-Cyclohexyl-3-methylacrylic acid.
$C_{10}H_{16}O_2$=168.2.

CAS — 25229-42-9.

Cicrotoic acid is a choleretic. It has been given in doses of 500 mg thrice daily initially, followed by 500 mg twice daily.

Proprietary Names
Accroibile *(Théraplix, Fr.).*

3711-d

Cinametic Acid. 4-(2-Hydroxyethoxy)-3-methoxycinnamic acid.
$C_{12}H_{14}O_5$=238.2.

CAS — 35703-32-3.

Cinametic acid is a choleretic. It has been given in doses of 500 to 750 mg daily.

Proprietary Names
Transoddi *(Millet, Arg.; Anphar-Rolland, Fr.).*

3712-n

Cyclobutyrol Sodium. Sodium 2-(1-hydroxycyclohexyl)butyrate.
$C_{10}H_{17}NaO_3$=208.2.

CAS — 512-16-3 (cyclobutyrol); 1130-23-0 (sodium salt).

Cyclobutyrol sodium is a choleretic. It has been given in doses of 0.5 to 1 g daily, by mouth, in divided doses with meals and in doses of 500 mg intramuscularly or intravenously daily or on alternate days to a total dose of 3 g in 12 days.

Proprietary Names
Bis-bil *(Isola-Ibi, Ital.)*; Cytinium (cyclobutyrol betaine) *(Roques, Fr.)*; Epa-Bon *(Sierochimica, Ital.)*; Hebucol *(Logeais, Belg.; Logeais, Fr.; Logeais, Switz.)*; Lipotrin (acid) *(Jap.)*; Secrobil *(Medital, Ital.)*; Tri-bil *(Biologici Italia, Ital.)*; Tribilina *(Farge, Ital.).*

3713-h

Cyclovalone. Divanillidenecyclohexanone. 2,6-Divanillylidenecyclohexanone.
$C_{22}H_{22}O_5$=366.4.

CAS — 579-23-7.

Crystals. M.p. 178° to 179°. **Soluble** in water and alcohol.

Cyclovalone is a choleretic. It has been given in doses of 300 to 900 mg daily in divided doses.

Proprietary Names
Vanidene *(Belgana, Belg.)*; Vanilon *(Uquifa, Spain)*; Vanilone *(Nicholas, Fr.).*

3714-m

Cynara. Artichoke Leaf; Artichaut; Alcachôfra.

Pharmacopoeias. In *Braz.* and *Roum.*

The leaves of the globe artichoke, *Cynara scolymus* (Compositae).

NOTE. The Jerusalem artichoke is *Helianthus tuberosus* (Compositae).

Cynara is reputed to have diuretic and choleretic properties.

Proprietary Names
Chophytol *(Rosa-Phytopharma, Fr.; CT, Ital.).*

3715-b

Cynarine. Cynarin; 1,5-Dicaffeoylquinic Acid. 1-Carboxy-4,5-dihydroxy-1,3-cyclohexylene bis(3,4-dihydroxycinnamate).
$C_{25}H_{24}O_{12}$=516.5.

CAS — 1182-34-9.

Cynarine is an active ingredient of cynara (see above). It is used as a choleretic in doses of 200 to 250 mg thrice daily. It is also used for the treatment of hyperlipidaemia and has been given in doses of 500 mg twice daily initially followed by 250 mg twice daily for maintenance therapy.

Cynarine 500 mg daily induced a significant reduction of the hypercholesterolaemia, the concentration of pre-β-lipoproteins, the β/α-lipoprotein ratio, and the patients' body-weight, when compared with a placebo in a controlled trial in 60 patients.— M. Montini *et al.*, *Arzneimittel-Forsch.*, 1975, *25*, 1311. See also W. H. Hammerl *et al.*, *Wien. med. Wschr.*, 1973, *123*, 601.

Proprietary Names
Cinarcaf *(Sierochimica, Ital.)*; Listrocol *(Farmitalia, Ger.).*

3716-v

Dehydrocholic Acid *(U.S.P.).* Chologon; Triketocholanic Acid; Acido Dehidrocolico. 3,7,12-Trioxo-5β-cholan-24-oic acid.
$C_{24}H_{34}O_5$=402.5.

CAS — 81-23-2.

Pharmacopoeias. In *Aust., Cz., Hung., It., Jap., Jug., Mex., Pol., Rus.*, and *U.S.*

A white fluffy odourless powder with a bitter taste. M.p. 231° to 242° with a range of not more than 3°. Practically **insoluble** in water; soluble 1 in 100 of alcohol, 1 in 35 of chloroform, 1 in 130 of acetone, 1 in 135 of acetic acid and ethyl acetate, and 1 in 2200 of ether at 15°; solutions in alcohol and chloroform are usually slightly turbid; soluble in glacial acetic acid and in solutions of alkali hydroxides and carbonates. A 2% solution in dioxan is dextrorotatory.

Precautions. Dehydrocholic acid is contra-indicated in complete mechanical biliary obstruction and in severe hepatitis.

Uses. Dehydrocholic acid increases the volume of the bile without increasing its total content of bile salts and pigments. It is given after surgery of the biliary tract to flush the common duct and drainage tube, and may be useful to wash away small calculi obstructing the flow through the common bile duct. It has been used to outline the bile ducts at operation, and to accelerate the appearance of the gall-bladder shadow and hasten removal of residual dye from the biliary tract in cholecystography.

It has also been used for the temporary relief of constipation.

Dehydrocholic acid has been given as a choleretic in usual doses of 250 to 750 mg thrice daily.

Preparations

Dehydrocholic Acid Tablets *(U.S.P.).* Tablets containing dehydrocholic acid.

Dehydrocholic Acid Tablets *(Evans Medical, UK).* Each contains dehydrocholic acid 250 mg.

The proprietary name Dehydrocholin was formerly used in Great Britain for dehydrocholic acid.

Other Proprietary Names
Bio-Cholin *(Canad.)*; Biochol *(Jap.)*; Chetocolina *(Ital.)*; Cholan-DH *(USA)*; Choleubil (see also under Sodium Dehydrocholate) *(Switz.)*; Cholypyl *(Canad.)*; Decholin (see also under Sodium Dehydrocholate) *(Canad., Ger., Ital., Switz., USA)*; Dehidrocolin *(Spain)*; Deidrocolico, Deidrocolit, Deidrosan (ethyl dehydrocholate), Dicolan (see also under Sodium Dehydrocholate), Didrocolo (all *Ital.*); Dycholium (see also under Sodium Dehydrocholate) *(Canad., Fr.)*; Hepahydrin *(USA)*; Idrocrine *(Canad.)*; Neocholan *(USA).*

3717-g

Deoxyribonuclease. Pancreatic Dornase; Desoxyribonuclease.

CAS — 9003-98-9.

An enzyme obtained by fractional precipitation from aqueous acid extracts of beef pancreas, followed by dialysis, sterilisation by filtration, and lyophilisation.

A white powder. **Soluble** in water.

Deoxyribonuclease requires magnesium ions for its activation and is inhibited by anions which remove them. Stable in the dry state for approximately 2 years at 4°. Solutions have a maximum activity at pH 6 to 7.

Units. The unit of activity is based on the rate of decrease in viscosity of a solution of thymus deoxyribonucleic acid when digested by deoxyribonuclease. One dornase viscosity unit of activity is defined as that amount of enzyme which causes a drop of 1 viscosity unit in the viscosity of thymus deoxyribonucleic acid in 10 minutes at 30°, where the flow-time of water is taken as 1 viscosity unit. One mg of purified deoxyribonuclease has been reported as having an activity of approximately 90 000 units.

Adverse Effects. Irritation of the respiratory tract and bronchospasm have been reported. Allergic reactions may occur after prolonged use.

A 12-month-old Indian boy with *Haemophilus influenzae* meningitis was treated with antibiotics and sulphadiazine sodium. He was also given an intrathecal injection of 134 000 units of deoxyribonuclease on the 2nd, 4th, 6th, 9th, and 12th hospital day. His condition improved but fever and nuchal rigidity persisted until the 14th hospital day. Another intrathecal injection of deoxyribonuclease on the 23rd hospital day provoked fever and nuchal rigidity and a temporary increase in the concentrations of protein in the CSF, thus demonstrating that the prolongation of symptoms was due to the deoxyribonuclease and not to the persistence of meningitis.— R. H. Parker *et al.*, *J. Am. med. Ass.*, 1965, *192*, 169.

Uses. Deoxyribonuclease acts directly upon deoxyribonucleoprotein and deoxyribonucleic acid, causing rapid depolymerisation with a resulting decrease in viscosity of purulent material. It acts only on extracellular matter and disintegrating cells.

Inhalation therapy with aerosols of 50 000 to 500 000 units of deoxyribonuclease daily has been employed to reduce the viscosity of pulmonary secretions and to facilitate the expectoration of sputum in bronchopulmonary infections. It may also be used by irrigation.

Deoxyribonuclease has been used locally in abscesses and haematomas in concentrations of 1 million units in 2 to 3 ml of sodium chloride injection and as a solution containing 1 million units in 50 ml of sterile water for bladder irrigation. It has also been given intramuscularly or intravenously in a dose of 1 million units every other day.

The use of an intrathecal injection of up to 1 million units of deoxyribonuclease in 5 ml of sodium chloride injection has been suggested in the treatment of meningitis.

Proprietary Preparations

Deanase *(Consolidated Chemicals, UK).* Deoxyribonuclease, available as powder (stated to be synergised with magnesium ions) in vials of 250 000 and 1 million units for preparing injections or solutions for inhalation. (Also available as Deanase in *Spain*).

Other Proprietary Names
Dinase *(Ital.).*

3718-q

Dextranase

CAS — 9025-70-1.

An enzyme which breaks down the dextran-binding dental plaque.

For a review of dextranase and dental caries, see S. A. Leach, *Br. dent. J.*, 1969, *127*, 325.

For a discussion of the use of dextranase and proteolytic enzymes in the removal of dental plaque, and some formulas, see P. Alexander, *Mfg Chem.*, 1972, *43* (June), 45.

3719-p

Di-isopromine Hydrochloride. *NN*-Di-isopropyl-3,3-diphenylpropylamine hydrochloride.
$C_{21}H_{29}N,HCl=331.9$.

CAS — 5966-41-6 (di-isopromine); 24358-65-4 (hydrochloride).

Crystals. M.p. 175° to 176°. **Soluble** in water, alcohol, chloroform, and methyl alcohol; practically insoluble in ether and aqueous alkaline solutions.

Di-isopromine hydrochloride is an antispasmodic used with sorbitol in visceral disorders. It has been given in doses of 2 to 4 mg thrice daily before meals.

Proprietary Names of Di-isopromine Hydrochloride with Sorbitol
Agofell *(Janssen, Ger.*; *Janssen, S.Afr.)*; Bilagol *(Leo, Swed.)*; Do-Bil *(Dompè, Ital.)*; Galbil *(Janssen, Denm.)*; Mégabyl *(Janssen-Le Brun, Fr.)*.

3720-n

Dimecrotic Acid. 2,4-Dimethoxy-*β*-methylcinnamic acid.
$C_{12}H_{14}O_4=222.2$.

CAS — 7706-67-4.

Dimecrotic acid is a choleretic used as the magnesium salt ($C_{24}H_{26}MgO_8=466.8$). It has been given in doses of 50 mg three or four times daily with meals.

Proprietary Names
Hépadial *(Biocodex, Fr.)*.

3721-h

Dimethylphenylacetic Acid. 2-Methyl-2-phenylpropionic acid.
$C_{10}H_{12}O_2=164.2$.

CAS — 826-55-1.

Dimethylphenylacetic acid has been given by mouth as a choleretic and intravenously as an adjunct to cholecystographic contrast media. It has been given in doses of 250 to 500 mg by mouth thrice daily after meals and in doses of 0.5 to 1 g intravenously.

3722-m

Fenipentol. 1-Phenylpentan-1-ol; *α*-Butylbenzyl alcohol.
$C_{11}H_{16}O=164.2$.

CAS — 583-03-9.

A colourless or pale yellow liquid with a bitter pungent taste. Practically **insoluble** in water; miscible with acetone, alcohol, chloroform, and methyl alcohol. **Store** in airtight containers. Protect from light.

Fenipentol is a choleretic. It has been given in doses of 100 to 200 mg thrice daily after meals.

Proprietary Names
Kol *(Mitim, Ital.)*; Pancoral *(Jap.)*; Pentabil *(OFF, Ital.)*; Sapem *(Craveri, Arg.)*.

3723-b

Florantyrone. 4-(Fluoranthen-8-yl)-4-oxobutyric acid.
$C_{20}H_{14}O_3=302.3$.

CAS — 519-95-9.

A yellow crystalline powder. Practically **insoluble** in water; moderately soluble in alcohol and solutions of alkali hydroxides and carbonates.

Florantyrone has actions and uses similar to those of dehydrocholic acid (see p.649). Doses of 0.75 to 1 g daily have been given.

References: J. R. Kirkpatrick *et al.*, *Gut*, 1974, *15*, 830.

Proprietary Names
Bilyn *(Janus, Ital.)*; Cistoplex *(Borromeo, Ital.)*; Idroepar *(Nagel, Ital.)*; Zanchol *(Searle, Arg.*; *Searle, Belg.)*.

3724-v

Hyaluronidase *(B.P.)*. Hyaluronidase for Injection.

CAS — 9001-54-1.

Pharmacopoeias. In *Arg., Br., Braz., Chin., Cz., Ind.*, and *It. U.S.* includes Hyaluronidase for Injection.

An enzyme which depolymerises the mucopolysaccharide hyaluronic acid. It is prepared from the testes and semen of mammals and purified by fractional precipitation of an aqueous extract, followed by dialysis, sterilisation by filtration, and freeze-drying of the resulting solution; hydrolysed gelatin or a suitable non-protein stabilising agent may be added to the purified preparation.

A sterile, white or yellowish-white, odourless powder, or an almost colourless glass-like solid, containing not less than 300 International units per mg and not less than 10 000 units per mg of tyrosine present. *U.S.P.* specifies not more than 0.25 µg of tyrosine for each unit of hyaluronidase, i.e. not less than 4000 units of hyaluronidase for each mg of tyrosine.

Very **soluble** in water; practically insoluble in alcohol, acetone, and ether. A 0.3% solution in water has a pH of 4.5 to 7.5. A 1% solution in water is clear and not more than faintly yellow.

Hyaluronidase is destroyed by heating at 100° for 30 minutes. Aqueous solutions prepared by dissolving the freeze-dried material in Water for Injections are unstable. Solutions for injection are prepared by dissolving, immediately before use, the sterile contents of a sealed container in Water for Injections; a stabilised solution is available in some countries.

Store in a cool dry place in single-dose containers sealed to exclude micro-organisms.

The properties and assay methods of hyaluronidase.— Hyaluronidase, in *Pharmaceutical Enzymes*, R. Ruyssen and A. Lauwers (Ed.), Gent, E. Story-Scientia, 1978, p. 217.

Effect of gamma-irradiation. Gamma-irradiation of hyaluronidase caused a marked loss of potency; at 25 000 Gy the loss was about 30% and at 250 000 Gy over 90%.— *The Use of Gamma Radiation Sources for the Sterilisation of Pharmaceutical Products*, London, ABPI, 1960.

Incompatibility. There was loss of clarity when solutions of hyaluronidase were mixed with those of adrenaline hydrochloride or heparin.— J. A. Patel and G. L. Phillips, *Am. J. Hosp. Pharm.*, 1966, *23*, 409.

Units. Approximately 2000 units of hyaluronidase, bovine are contained in one ampoule of the first International Standard Preparation (1955). One ampoule contains 10 tablets, each containing approximately 20 mg of dried material.

The International and *U.S.P.* units are equivalent.

The *U.S.P.* unit is equivalent to the earlier *U.S.N.F.* unit.

One International unit of hyaluronidase was approximately equivalent to 1 Turbidity Reducing unit and to 3.3 Viscosity Reducing Units.— International Commission for the Standardisation of Pharmaceutical Enzymes, *J. mond. Pharm.*, 1965, *8*, 5.

Adverse Effects and Precautions. Sensitivity to hyaluronidase occasionally occurs. Hyaluronidase should be administered with caution to patients with infections; because of the danger of spreading infection, the enzyme generally should not be injected into or around an infected area. It has been suggested that the presence of malignancy may similarly be a contra-indication to the use of hyaluronidase. The administration of salicylates is reported to inhibit the spreading action of hyaluronidase. It should not be administered by intravenous injection.

Hyaluronidase, injected subconjunctivally into 24 eyes, increased refraction by up to 3 dioptres. The effect began 5 to 6 days after injection, reached a peak after about 10 days, and persisted for several weeks.— G. Treister *et al.*, *Archs Ophthal., N.Y.*, 1969, *81*, 645, per *J. Am. med. Ass.*, 1969, *208*, 1204.

Uses. Hyaluronidase is an enzyme which has a specific action on the mucopolysaccharide, hyaluronic acid, a component of the mucoprotein ground substance or tissue cement of the tissue spaces, thereby reducing its viscosity and rendering the tissues more readily permeable to injected fluids.

Therapeutically, hyaluronidase is employed to increase the speed of absorption and to diminish discomfort due to subcutaneous or intramuscular injection of fluids, to promote resorption of excess fluids and extravasated blood in the tissues, and to increase the effectiveness of local anaesthesia.

In hypodermoclysis, hyaluronidase is used to aid the subcutaneous administration of relatively large volumes of fluids, especially in infants and young children, where intravenous injection is difficult. The addition of up to 1500 International units to 500 to 1000 ml of fluids will enable the injection to be given subcutaneously at the rate of 10 ml per minute. Hyaluronidase may be added to the injection fluid or may be injected into the site before the fluid is administered. Dextrose should always be administered as a hypo-osmotic solution, and, if there is dehydration, electrolytes should only be given to infants and children as a hypo-osmotic solution. Care should be taken in the treatment of children to control the speed and total volume administered and to avoid over-hydration.

The diffusion of local anaesthetics is accelerated by the addition of 1000 to 1500 units of hyaluronidase to each 20 ml of the anaesthetic solution. This is of value in the reduction of fractures and in pudendal block in midwifery. When hyaluronidase is added to a local anaesthetic, the duration of anaesthesia may be shortened. The addition of adrenaline to the hyaluronidase anaesthetic mixture prolongs the anaesthesia without affecting the spread.

Resorption of accumulations of blood and fluid, as in traumatic or postoperative oedema or haematoma, may be hastened by the infiltration of hyaluronidase dissolved in sodium chloride injection. Inflammatory reactions following the accidental leakage of irritant substances from intravenous infusions may be minimised by infiltration of this solution.

Substances used in radiography, such as diodone, are rapidly absorbed from the site of intramuscular injection with the aid of hyaluronidase, thus providing an alternative to the commoner intravenous technique in pyelography. Maximum opacity in the kidney is found 15 to 45 minutes after the injection of diodone in conjunction with hyaluronidase.

Hyaluronidase has been used subcutaneously in fibrositis and muscular rheumatism. It has also been used in ophthalmology.

Results of a pilot study in 6 patients suggested that intra-arterial injection of a highly purified preparation of hyaluronidase (GL-Enzyme, *Biorex*) may be of benefit in severe peripheral arterial disease.— J. B. Elder *et al.* (letter), *Lancet*, 1980, *1*, 648.

Ankylosing spondylitis. Most of 20 patients with Bechterew's disease benefited after intravenous injection every 2 to 3 days of 1500 to 9000 units of hyaluronidase; benefit was noted, after an initial aggravation of pain, after 3 to 12 injections. Patients received 10 to 53 injections with a total dose of 27 000 to 240 000 units.— H. Bellman *et al., Dte GesundhWes.*, 1972, *27*, 2391, per *Int. pharm. Abstr.*, 1973, *10*, 665.

Asthma. Thirty-four patients with asthma or allergic rhinitis were treated with hyaluronidase by a method of 'transepidermal hyposensitisation' in which a mixture of enzyme and allergen, contained in a small cup of 1-ml capacity, was maintained in contact with a scarification on the patient's forearm for 24 hours. Successful results were obtained in 33 patients, presumably due to induction of tolerance to the allergens. There were no side-effects. From the results with 200 other patients it appeared that the method might be effective in severe corticosteroid-dependent asthma and other allergic conditions provided the multiple allergens responsible could be identified. β-Glucuronidase and *N*-acetyl-β-glucosaminidase, contaminants of commercial testicular hyaluronidase, might be essential for its desensitising action.— L. M. McEwen *et al.* (letter), *Br. med. J.*, 1967, *2*, 507.

Myocardial infarction. Intravenous administration of hyaluronidase 500 units per kg body-weight every 6 hours for 48 hours to 46 patients starting within 8 hours of the clinical onset of acute myocardial infarction appeared to reduce the extent of myocardial necrosis compared with 45 similar control patients.— P. R. Maroko *et al., New Engl. J. Med.*, 1977, *296*, 898. Comment.— H. L. Rutenberg (letter), *ibid.*, *297*, 224. Reply.— E. Braunwald (letter), *ibid.*

Further references: P. R. Maroko *et al., Ann. intern. Med.*, 1975, *82*, 516.

Parenteral fluid administration. For details of the treatment of dehydration in elderly subjects by adding hyaluronidase to parenteral fluids to facilitate their administration by subcutaneous route, see R. G. Simpson, *Practitioner*, 1977, *219*, 361.

Preparations

Hyaluronidase for Injection *(U.S.P.)*. Sterile hyaluronidase suitable for parenteral use. Store at 15° to 30°.

Hyaluronidase Injection *(B.P.C. 1973)*. A sterile solution of hyaluronidase, prepared by dissolving, immediately before use, the sterile contents of a sealed container in Water for Injections. The sealed container should be stored in a cool place. The injection decomposes on storage and should be used immediately after preparation. Not for intravascular injection.

Hyaluronidase Injection *(U.S.P.)*. A sterile solution in Water for Injections. pH 6.4 to 7.4. It may contain suitable stabilisers. Store at 2° to 8°.

Proprietary Preparations

Hyalase *(Fisons, UK)*. Hyaluronidase for injection, available in ampoules of 1500 International units for solution before use. (Also available as Hyalase in *Austral.*, *S.Afr.*).

Lasonil *(Bayer, UK)*. An ointment containing in each 100 g hyaluronidase 15 000 International units and a heparinoid (obtained by sulphation of polysaccharides from the cell walls of certain *Penicillium* strains) equivalent to 5000 units of heparin. For superficial thrombosis, bruising, and varicose conditions.

A report of oleogranuloma in a 57-year-old man following the rectal administration of Lasonil.— M. G. Greaney and P. R. Jackson, *Br. med. J.*, 1977, *2*, 997.

Other Proprietary Names

Aust.—Permease; *Belg.*—Hyason; *Canad.*—Wydase; *Denm.*—Penetrase; *Ger.*—Kinetin; *Ital.*—Jalovis, Jaluran; *Neth.*—Hyason; *Norw.*—Penetrase; *Spain*—Kinaden; *Swed.*—Hyalas; *Switz.*—Hyason, Permease; *USA*—Wydase.

3725-g

Hymecromone.
Imecromone; LM-94. 7-Hydroxy-4-methylcoumarin.

$C_{10}H_8O_3$=176.2.

CAS — 90-33-5.

Hymecromone is a choleretic and biliary antispasmodic. Diarrhoea may occasionally occur. It has been given in doses of 400 mg thrice daily before meals.

Proprietary Names

Bicolic *(Unifa, Arg.)*; Bilicanta *(Boehringer Mannheim, Spain)*; Cantabilin *(Formenti, Ital.)*; Cantabiline *(Lipha, Belg.*; *Médicia, Fr.)*; Cholspasmin forte *(Lipha, Ger.)*; Eurogale *(Spain)*; Cumarote-C, Himecol *(both Jap.)*; Medilla *(Omega, Arg.)*.

3726-q

Mesna.
Mesnum; UCB 3983. Sodium 2-mercaptoethanesulphonate.

$C_2H_5NaO_3S_2$=164.2.

CAS — 19767-45-4.

Mesna is a mucolytic agent used in bronchitic disorders. Cough and bronchospasm may occur. The usual dose is 0.6 to 1.2 g administered by a nebuliser.

Mention of the uroprotective action of mesna against cyclophosphamide in *animals*.— N. Brock *et al., Arzneimittel-Forsch.*, 1979, *29*, 659. Results of a single-blind crossover study involving 8 patients with advanced bronchial carcinoma given ifosfamide 2 g per m^2 body-surface by intravenous bolus demonstrated a uroprotective effect of mesna against the antineoplastic agent. Mesna was given in a dose of 400 mg per m^2 by intravenous bolus injection 0, 4, and 8 hours after ifosfamide. Pharmacokinetic studies demonstrated that, although it appears to inactivate acrolein, the metabolite of ifosfamide responsible for bladder toxicity, mesna does not appear to interfere with the metabolism of ifosfamide itself, or its active metabolite, isofosforamide mustard. There is every reason to assume that mesna will also protect against cyclophosphamide-induced urothelial damage, since the mechanism of toxicity is identical.— B. M. Bryant *et al., Lancet*, 1980, *2*, 657. Two months after receiving high-dose cyclophosphamide therapy before total-body irradiation for bone-marrow transplantation, a 37-year-old man with acute myeloid leukaemia developed delayed-type cyclophosphamide cystitis although he had received mesna, forced diuresis, and urine alkalinisation as adjunct therapy. Mesna may only prevent early haemorrhagic cystitis or alternatively, the ratio of mesna to cyclophosphamide may need increasing when unusually high doses of cyclophosphamide are given.— B. Löwenberg *et al.* (letter), *ibid.*, 1195. A hope that mesna may have a role in preventing cyclophosphamide-induced irreversible bladder fibrosis.— J. A. Murray (letter), *ibid.*

Respiratory disorders. In a double-blind crossover study in 31 subjects with chronic bronchitis who inhaled daily 6 ml of a 20% solution of mesna changes in pulmonary function were clinically insignificant but subjective clinical improvement was noted by most subjects. In 18 subjects substantially more sputum was produced than after sodium chloride solution.— S. N. Steen *et al., Clin. Pharmac. Ther.*, 1974, *16*, 58.

Further references: S. R. Hirsch *et al., Thorax*, 1970, *25*, 737; V. Kyncl *et al., J. int. med. Res.*, 1979, *7*, 423.

Proprietary Names

Mistabron *(UCB, Belg.*; *UCB, Neth.*; *UCB, S.Afr.*; *UCB, Switz.)*; Mistabronco *(UCB, Ger.)*; Mucofluid *(UCB, Belg.*; *UCB, Fr.*; *UCB, Ger.)*.

3727-p

Methochalcone.
Trimethoxychalcone; CB1314. 2′,4,4′-Trimethoxychalcone.

$C_{18}H_{18}O_4$=298.3.

CAS — 18493-30-6.

Methochalcone is a choleretic. It has been given in doses of 1 to 1.5 g daily in divided doses with meals.

Proprietary Names

Agobilex *(Farmaroma, Ital.)*; Auxibilina *(Granata, Ital.)*; Chemicol *(Beta, Ital.)*; Cholesteril *(Tosi-Novara, Ital.)*; Choligen *(Ital Suisse, Ital.)*; Colazid *(Nagel, Ital.)*; Colerex *(Tiber, Ital.)*; Megalip *(Biotrading, Ital.)*; Solvocolo *(Farmacologico Milanese, Ital.)*; Spechol *(Molteni, Ital.)*; Trimecolo *(AMSA, Ital.)*; Vésidryl *(Clin-Comar-Byla, Fr.)*.

3728-s

Muramidase.
Lysozyme; Globulin G_1.

CAS — 9001-63-2.

A crystalline polypeptide mucolytic enzyme, widely distributed in nature. It is present in tears, egg-white, nasal mucus, lungs, serum, leucocytes, and many other tissues and secretions of animals, and in certain plants. Its chemical properties vary according to the method used for its extraction. It is fairly stable in acid solution and is unaffected by heat up to about 55°.

The properties and assay methods of muramidase.— Lysosyme, in *Pharmaceutical Enzymes*, R. Ruyssen and A. Lauwers (Ed.), Gent, E. Story-Scientia, 1978, p. 167.

Adverse Effects. Hypersensitivity reactions have been reported.

Two fatalities occurred after the first intramuscular injection of 25 mg of muramidase to 2 infants, 1 aged 10 months and the other 20 months. Both had constitutional eczema and the deaths were ascribed to typical allergy. The therapeutic use of a protein substance, such as muramidase, was certainly not free from danger, especially in patients under 3 years of age.— R. Luvoni, *Minerva medicoleg.*, 1963, *83*, 130, per *Abstr. Wld Med.*, 1964, *36*, 139.

Uses. Muramidase is a mucopolysaccharidase which is active against Gram-positive bacteria, possibly by transforming the insoluble polysaccharides of the cell wall to soluble mucopeptides. It is also active against some viruses and some Gram-negative bacteria.

Muramidase has been used in the treatment of bacterial and viral infections in widely varying doses of up to 100 to 600 mg daily. Doses of up to 2 g daily appear to have been used. Doses of 125 and 250 mg have been given intravenously or intramuscularly. A 2% solution has been used as eye-drops in the treatment of keratitis. Muramidase has been claimed to enhance the activity of some antimicrobial preparations when given concomitantly.

A report of a symposium on muramidase.— P. Rentchnick, *Méd. Hyg., Genève*, 1964, *22*, 377.

In 24 patients with herpes zoster treated with muramidase, 1 g daily by mouth, very good control was achieved in 7, good control in 10, and moderate control in 4.— G. F. Strani, *Minerva derm.*, 1968, *43*, 288, per *Abstr. Hyg.*, 1969, *44*, 722.

When muramidase was given with penicillin, chloramphenicol, or nitrofurantoin, the growth of staphylococci was more effectively inhibited than by the antibiotics alone. The growth of *Escherichia coli* was unaffected by muramidase and was inhibited only by the chloramphenicol or nitrofurantoin part of the preparations.— W. Ritzerfeld, *Arzneimittel-Forsch.*, 1969, *19*, 674.

Proprietary Names

Antalzyme *(Vifor, Switz.)*; Buco-Lysozima *(Poen, Arg.)*; Fisiozima *(Neopharmed, Ital.)*; Lisobase Lacrimale *(Tubi Lux, Ital.)*; Lisozimina *(Volpino, Arg.)*; Aibel D, Eggtose, Leftose, Lysorzym, Neuzym, Toyolyzom-DS *(all Jap.)*.

Many of these preparations are of muramidase chloride.

3729-w

Osalmid.
Oxaphenamide; L 1718. 4′-Hydroxysalicylanilide.

$C_{13}H_{11}NO_3$=229.2.

CAS — 526-18-1.

Pharmacopoeias. In *Rus.*

A white or purplish-grey odourless powder. M.p. about 176°. Practically **insoluble** in water; readily soluble in alcohol and alkalis; sparingly soluble in ether. **Protect** from light.

Osalmid is a choleretic. It has been given in doses of 250 to 750 mg twice daily.

Proprietary Names

Driol *(Labaz, Belg.*; *Labaz, Switz.)*; Bichol, Bilecoll, Cholatin, Coypanon, Galerite, Gallocol, Isechol, Loibnal, Marionchol, Neodekoll, Sawacol, Shikichol, Taichol, Tanjuron, Yoshichol *(all Jap.)*.

3730-m

Ox Bile Extract *(B.P. 1948)*. Extractum Fellis Bovini; Ext. Fell. Bov.

CAS — 8008-63-7.

Pharmacopoeias. Fresh Ox Bile is included in *Arg., Mex., Port.,* and *Span.*

Fresh ox bile 1000 ml is evaporated to 250 ml and the product shaken with alcohol (90%) 500 ml; the mixture is set aside until the solid matter has subsided, the supernatant solution heated to remove most of the alcohol, and the residue evaporated to the consistence of a firm extract.

A dark yellowish-green plastic mass with a disagreeable bitter taste, containing sodium glycocholate, $C_{26}H_{42}NNaO_6$=487.6, and sodium taurocholate, $C_{26}H_{44}NNaO_7S$=537.7.

Soluble 2 in 1 of water; soluble in alcohol; practically insoluble in ether. **Store** in a cool place in airtight containers, preferably not in glass-stoppered bottles.

Uses. Ox bile extract has been given in the treatment of some conditions in which there is a deficiency of bile in the intestinal tract; doses of 0.3 to 1 g have been employed. It is usually given in enteric-coated capsules or tablets. It may also be used to stimulate intestinal peristalsis in chronic constipation.

The mean half-life of sodium taurocholate was 1.65 days in 10 healthy individuals and 1.16 days in 7 patients with gall-stones.— E. W. Pomare and K. W. Heaton, *Gut*, 1973, *14*, 885.

Proprietary Preparations of Bile Salts

Opobyl *(Bailly, Fr.: Bengué, UK).* Pills each containing desiccated liver 50 mg, sodium tauroglycocholate 50 mg, boldo extract 10 mg, podophyllin 2 mg, euonymus extract 2 mg, and aloes 20 mg. For biliary insufficiency and constipation. *Dose.* 1 or 2 pills before or after meals.

Veracolate *(Warner, UK).* Tablets each containing bile salts 70 mg, cascara dry extract 65 mg, phenolphthalein 32 mg, and capsicum oleoresin 3 mg. For biliary insufficiency, constipation, and similar conditions. *Dose.* 1 tablet with water thrice daily after meals, or 2 tablets with water at bedtime.

Other Proprietary Names

Desicol *(Austral.)*; Felkreon *(Ger.)*.

A preparation containing bile salts was also formerly marketed in Great Britain under the proprietary name Taxol(*Cox-Continental*).

3731-b

Pancreatin *(B.P., B.P. Vet.)*. Pancreat.; Pancreatinum.

CAS — 8049-47-6.

Pharmacopoeias. Pancreatin is included in most pharmacopoeias. The potency varies.

NOTE. Based on miminum potencies Pancreatin *B.P. 1980* has about 1.4 times the protease activity, 1.3 times the lipase activity, and twice the amylase activity of the *B.P. 1973* material, which had about 2.5 times the activity of the *B.P. 1968* material.

Based also on minimum potencies Pancreatin *B.P. 1980* has about 3.5 times the protease activity, 10 times the lipase activity, and 4 times the amylase activity of the *U.S.P.* material.

A preparation of mammalian pancreas containing enzymes having protease, lipase, and amylase activity; it may contain sodium chloride.

It is a white or buff-coloured amorphous powder free from unpleasant odour. Each g of pancreatin contains not less than 1400 units of free protease activity, not less than 20 000 units of lipase activity, and not less than 24 000 units of amylase activity.

Soluble or partly soluble in water forming a slightly turbid solution; practically insoluble in alcohol and ether. **Incompatible** with acids, strong alcohol, caustic alkalis, heavy metal ions, and tannins. Its greatest activity is exhibited in neutral or faintly alkaline media. Its proteolytic activity is rapidly destroyed in the presence of more than traces of acids, by strong alkalis, by excess of alkali carbonate, or by boiling in aqueous solution. Solutions in water are precipitated by heat, acids, strong alcohol, metallic salts, and tannic acid. **Store** at a temperature not exceeding 15° in airtight containers.

The *U.S.P.* includes Pancreatin, a cream-coloured amorphous powder with a faint characteristic not unpleasant odour, containing in each g not less than 25 000 *U.S.P.* units of protease activity, not less than 2000 *U.S.P.* units of lipase activity, and not less than 25 000 *U.S.P.* units of amylase activity. It may be labelled as a whole-number multiple of the 3 minimum activities, or may be diluted with lactose, sucrose containing up to 3.25% of starch, or pancreatin of lower digestive power. Store at a temperature not exceeding 30° in airtight containers.

Units. The *B.P.* and *U.S.P.* units of protease activity depend upon the rate of hydrolysis of casein, those of lipase activity depend upon the rate of hydrolysis of olive oil, and those of amylase activity depend upon the rate of hydrolysis of starch. One *B.P.* unit of protease activity is approximately equivalent to 62.50 *U.S.P.* units, 1 *B.P.* unit of lipase activity is approximately equivalent to 1 *U.S.P.* unit, and 1 *B.P.* unit of amylase activity is approximately equivalent to 4.15 *U.S.P.* units. *U.S.P.* units are equivalent to the former *U.S.N.F.* units.

FIP units of protease, lipase, and amylase activity are approximately equivalent to *B.P.* units.

A comparative assessment *in vitro* of pancreatic extract preparations.— A. M. Howell *et al.*, *J. Hosp. Pharm.*, 1975, *33*, 143.

Assay *in vitro* of 16 different commercial pancreatic preparations for lipase, trypsin, chymotrypsin, proteolytic activity, and amylase demonstrated wide variation between preparations, in particular the lipase content varied from 10 to 3600 units per product unit. *In vivo* studies demonstrated correlation with the *in vitro* results and indicated that, despite theoretical advantages, enteric coating could reduce the clinical effectiveness of pancreatic extracts. Most commercial preparations contained inadequate amounts of lipase and required a lipase supplement.— D. Y. Graham, *New Engl. J. Med.*, 1977, *296*, 1314. Comments.— J. H. Meyer, *ibid.*, 1347; T. L. Yeh and M. L. Rubin (letter), *ibid.*, *297*, 615; R. Kirshen (letter), *ibid.*, 616. From an *in vitro* study simulating the conditions in which orally administered pancreatin is exposed in the human stomach it was concluded that administration of uncoated pancreatin in powder form may result in substantial loss of enzymic activity.— D. T. Graham *et al.*, *Med. J. Aust.*, 1979, *1*, 45. Criticisms of the extrapolation of *in vitro* results to *in vivo* situations.— G. L. Barnes and P. D. Phelan (letter), *ibid.*, 282; B. Allen and G. Giles (letter), *ibid.*

The properties and assay methods of pancreatin.— Pancreatin, in *Pharmaceutical Enzymes*, R. Ruyssen and A. Lauwers (Ed.), Gent, E. Story-Scientia, 1978, p. 57.

Adverse Effects. Pancreatin may cause buccal and perianal soreness, particularly in infants. Hypersensitivity reactions have been reported; these may be sneezing, lachrymation, or skin rashes.

In 3 children taking preparations of pancreatic extracts (Pancrex V powder, Pancrex V Forte), severe mouth ulceration and angular stomatitis, causing dysphagia, loss of weight, and pyrexia, were attributed to digestion of the mucous membrane due to retention of the preparations in the mouth before swallowing.— C. W. Darby (letter), *Br. med. J.*, 1970, *2*, 299.

Hypersensitivity. A report of bronchospasm in 4 men exposed to pancreatin powder in which a high proportion of particles had a diameter less than 10 microns—none had shown hypersensitivity reactions to pancreatin previously despite contact for several years.— B. J. Ferry (letter), *Med. J. Aust.*, 1975, *2*, 809.

Attacks of bronchial asthma were induced in a patient by handling pancreatin.— A. Sakula (letter), *Lancet*, 1977, *2*, 193.

Hypersensitivity to pancreatic extracts in parents of patients with cystic fibrosis.— F. J. Twarog *et al.*, *J. Allergy & clin. Immunol.*, 1977, *59*, 35.

Hyperuricosuria. Hyperuricosuria was reported in 3 children who had been given pancreatic extracts in daily doses in excess of the prescribed dose for the treatment of cystic fibrosis.— F. B. Stapleton *et al.*, *New Engl. J. Med.*, 1976, *295*, 246. See also S. Nousia-Arvanitakis *et al.*, *J. Pediat.*, 1977, *90*, 302.

Confirmation that ribonuclease activity in the pancreatic supplements also contributes by producing the purine bases that are uric-acid precursors.— W. A. Gahl *et al.* (letter), *New Engl. J. Med.*, 1977, *297*, 1349.

Salmonellal infections. *Salmonella agona* infection in 2 infants in hospital was traced to the use of contaminated pancreatin. *S. agona, S. brandenberg,* and *S. infantis* were identified in the offending batch.— E. J. G. Glencross, *Br. med. J.*, 1972, *2*, 376.

Microbial contamination was reduced in preparations of pancreatin treated with isopropyl alcohol 88.2 or 90% for 20 hours; the enzymatic properties of pancreatin were not affected.— B. Lüssi-Schlatter and P. Speiser, *Pharm. Acta Helv.*, 1974, *49*, 41.

Salmonellosis due to very slight contamination of porcine pancreatin with *S. schwarzengrund* was reported in an infant being treated for cystic fibrosis.— A. Lipson (letter), *Lancet*, 1976, *1*, 969.

A report of salmonellal contamination of preparations of pancreatin producing infection in children with cystic fibrosis. In one child the infecting dose was considered to be less than 44 organisms. Stringent control on salmonellal contamination was required.— A. Lipson and A. Meikle, *Archs Dis. Childh.*, 1977, *52*, 569.

Uses. Pancreatin hydrolyses fats to glycerol and fatty acids, changes protein into proteoses and derived substances, and converts starch into dextrins and sugars. It is given by mouth in conditions of pancreatic deficiency such as pancreatitis and fibrocystic disease of the pancreas. It is available in the form of powder, capsules which are intended to be opened before use and the contents sprinkled on the food, tablets which are enteric-coated, or granules which may contain suitable enteroprotective substances. If pancreatin is mixed with liquids or feeds the resulting mixture should not be allowed to stand for more than 1 hour prior to use.

A suggested dose is up to 8 g daily in divided doses. Pancreatin has sometimes been given together with large doses of sodium bicarbonate, but the possibility of alkalosis should be borne in mind. Other antacids and histamine H_2-receptor antagonists, such as cimetidine, have also been given in conjunction with pancreatin in an attempt to lessen destruction of pancreatin by the gastric acids.

Pancreatin is also used for the preparation of predigested or peptonised foods, such as milk, gruel, arrowroot, and other farinaceous foods. The preparation is maintained at 38° for 15 minutes (or longer if complete peptonisation is desired) and then heated to boiling point to destroy the enzymes.

For 4 weeks, in a double-blind study, 28 elderly patients with impaired digestive ability received a polyvalent digestive enzyme product (Combizym) and 16 a placebo—2 tablets thrice daily with each meal. The enzyme product was significantly superior in its effects on dyspepsia and gastro-intestinal symptoms, in reducing abdominal circumference, and in gain in weight. No untoward effects were observed.— M. S. Kataria and D. Bhaskarrao, *Br. J. clin. Pract.*, 1969, *23*, 15. See also S. Karani *et al.*, *ibid.*, 1971, *25*, 375.

Pancreatic extracts were useful in the treatment of cystic fibrosis, pancreatic insufficiency in adults, and after partial gastrectomy. There was no scientific basis for the widespread administration of pancreatic extracts for indigestion or hypothetical pancreatic disease.— *Br. med. J.*, 1970, *2*, 161.

Cystic fibrosis. A discussion of the use of pancreatin in the treatment of children with cystic fibrosis.— C. M. Anderson, *Prescribers' J.*, 1972, *12*, 45.

A study of the biliary bile-salt composition of 26 children with cystic fibrosis (14 of whom were temporarily off enzyme therapy), 7 children with cholelithiasis, and 13 control children. The lipid composition of fasting bile from the untreated children with cystic fibrosis was found to be abnormal and comparable to that of the children with gall-stones. Enzyme supplements in cystic fibrosis thus had the additional role of preventing gall-stones in cystic fibrosis as well as controlling diarrhoea, reducing overt steatorrhoea, and maintaining nutrition. Further work was needed on the early and optimum treatment of pancreatic insufficiency to prevent the development of eventual hepatic complications.— C. C. Roy *et al.*, *New Engl. J. Med.*, 1977, *297*, 1301.

In children with cystic fibrosis the greatest reduction in steatorrhoea and loss of faecal bile acid was achieved by giving a diet in which some long-chain triglycerides were replaced by medium-chain triglycerides, with pancreatic enzymes. A lesser reduction was obtained by giving a normal diet with pancreatic enzymes, or by replacing some long-chain with medium-chain triglycerides.— C. A. Smalley *et al.*, *Archs Dis. Childh.*, 1978, *53*, 477.

Further references: M. C. Goodchild *et al.*, *Br. med. J.*, 1974, *3*, 712.

Pancreatic insufficiency. *Reviews.* For reviews and discussions on the use of pancreatic extracts in the treatment of pancreatic insufficiency, see *Lancet*, 1977, *2*, 73; S. Banks *et al.*, *Drugs*, 1977, *13*, 373; W. I. Austad, *ibid.*, 1979, *17*, 480.

In a patient with pancreatic insufficiency, steatorrhoea, and malabsorption of cyanocobalamin, the absorption of cyanocobalamin was increased after treatment with pancreatic extracts and further increased after the addition of sodium bicarbonate.— E. LeBauer *et al.*, *Archs intern. Med.*, 1968, *122*, 423.

The administration of pancreatic extracts with antacids, during treatment with an H_2-antagonist, permitted satisfactory normalisation of digestion in patients with pancreatic exocrine insufficiency.— J. H. B. Saunders *et al.*, *Br. med. J.*, 1977, *1*, 418.

In a comparative study involving 6 healthy subjects and 6 patients with pancreatic insufficiency, ingestion of pancreatin ('Viokase') 8 tablets four times daily (given before, during, and after food) was no less effective than 2 tablets hourly from 7 a.m. to 10 p.m. and appeared to correct azotorrhoea more often. With either regimen steatorrhoea was persistently less well controlled than azotorrhoea possibly because less lipase activity reached the ligament of Treitz; this emphasised the need for adjunct therapy (such as the use of H_2-receptor antagonists) to inhibit gastric acid secretion and thus prevent acid denaturation of the enzymes.— E. P. DiMagno *et al.*, *New Engl. J. Med.*, 1977, *296*, 1318. Comment.— J. H. Meyer, *ibid.*, 1347.

In a study of 6 patients with advanced pancreatic insufficiency steatorrhoea was significantly reduced by administration of pancreatin, but concurrent administration of supplementary antacids was no more effective than pancreatin alone, nor was administration of an enteric-coated pancreatic preparation although, in this case, steatorrhoea was abolished in 2 patients. Concurrent administration of cimetidine with pancreatin, however, further reduced steatorrhoea in all the patients, abolishing it in 4. Adjunct cimetidine administration might benefit patients who failed to respond to pancreatic enzyme replacement alone. In contrast, faecal nitrogen excretion was corrected in nearly all the patients by all the treatment regimens.— P. T. Regan *et al.*, *New Engl. J. Med.*, 1977, *297*, 854. See also P. T. Regan *et al.*, *Mayo Clin. Proc.*, 1978, *53*, 79.

Further references: R. P. Knill-Jones *et al.*, *Br. med. J.*, 1970, *4*, 21; F. P. Diggins, *Paines & Byrne* (letter), *ibid.*, 1971, *1*, 115.

Preparations

Pancreatic Extract *(B.P.)*. A preparation of mammalian pancreas containing enzymes having protease, lipase, and amylase activity; it may contain a suitable diluent. The minimum potency is half that of Pancreatin *B.P.* Store at a temperature not exceeding 15°.

Pancreatin Capsules *(U.S.P.)*. Capsules containing pancreatin *U.S.P.* Store in airtight containers.

Pancreatin Granules *(B.P.)*. Granules containing pancreatin; they may contain enteroprotective substances. Store at a temperature not exceeding 15°.

Pancreatin Tablets *(B.P.)*. Tablets containing pancreatin. They are enteric-coated and either film-coated or sugar-coated. Store at a temperature not exceeding 15°.

Pancreatin Tablets *(U.S.P.)*. Tablets containing pancreatin *U.S.P.* Store in airtight containers.

Proprietary Preparations Containing Pancreatin and Pancreatic Enzymes

Combizym *(Luitpold-Werk, UK: Farillon, UK)*. Tablets each containing, in an inner core, 220 mg of pancreatin (amylase activity as *U.S.P.*, protease activity 4 times *U.S.P.* and lipase activity 17 times *U.S.P.*) and, in an outer layer, 120 mg of a mixture of proteases, amylase, cellulase, and hemicellulases. **Combizym Compositum.** Tablets containing, in an outer layer, 120 mg of a mixture of proteases, amylase, cellulase, and hemicellulase, and, in an inner core, 400 mg of pancreatin (as above) and 60 mg of ox bile extract. For disorders of the gastro-intestinal system. *Dose.* Combizym: 1 or 2 tablets during meals; Combizym Compositum: 1 tablet during or after each meal.

Cotazym *(Organon, UK)*. An extract of hog pancreas in capsules each containing lipase not less than 14 000 FIP units, amylase not less than 10 000 FIP units, and protease not less than 500 FIP units. For pancreatic insufficiency. (Also available as Cotazym in *Ital.*). **Cotazym B.** Tablets each containing pancreas having lipase not less than 5400 FIP units, cellulase, and ox bile extract equivalent to cholic acid 30 mg. For digestive disorders. *Dose.* Cotazym: the contents of 6 capsules daily, sprinkled on food; Cotazym B: 2 tablets thrice daily with meals.

NOTE. In *Austral.* and *USA* Cotazym is defined as pancrelipase.

Depropanex *(Merck Sharp & Dohme, UK)*. A physiologically standardised deproteinated extract of pancreas in vials of 10 ml. Vasodilator and antispasmodic. *Dose.* Intramuscularly; 1 to 5 ml. (Also available as Depropanex in *Arg.*).

Enzypan *(Norgine, UK)*. Tablets each containing, in an outer layer, pepsin 12 mg and, in an enteric-coated core, pancreatin equivalent to 180 mg of pancreatin *B.P. 1968* and dried ox bile 60 mg. For digestive enzyme deficiencies.

Fermentogran *(Keimdiät, Ger.: Thomson & Joseph, UK)*. A product, prepared by growing specific moulds on bran, containing amylase, protease, lipase, and other enzymes. For use as an additive in pharmaceutical, dietary, and cosmetic preparations.

Nutrizym *(E. Merck, UK)*. Tablets each containing, in an enteric-coated core, pancreatin 400 mg (lipase 9000 *B.P.* units, protease 400 *B.P.* units, and amylase 9000 *B.P.* units) and ox bile extract 30 mg, and, in an outer layer, bromelains 50 mg. For pancreatic insufficiency. *Dose.* 1 to 2 tablets with each meal.

Pancrex Granules *(Paines & Byrne, UK)*. Pancreatin, available as enteric-coated granules containing in each g not less than 300 *B.P.* units of protease activity, not less than 5000 *B.P.* units of lipase activity, and not less than 4000 *B.P.* units of amylase activity. (Also available as Pancrex in *Austral.*).

Pancrex V Powder *(Paines & Byrne, UK)*. Pancreatin, containing in each g not less than 1400 *B.P.* units of protease activity, not less than 25 000 *B.P.* units of lipase activity, and not less than 30 000 *B.P.* units of amylase activity. **Pancrex V Capsules** each containing not less than 430 *B.P.* units of protease activity, not less than 8000 *B.P.* units of lipase activity, and not less than 9000 *B.P.* units of amylase activity. **Pancrex V Tablets** and **Pancrex V Forte Tablets** are enteric-coated and contain respectively not less than 110 and 330 *B.P.* units of protease activity, not less than 1900 and 5600 *B.P.* units of lipase activity, and not less than 1700 and 5000 *B.P.* units of amylase activity. (Also available as Pancrex V in *Austral.*, *Ital.*).

Other Proprietary Names

Pancreon *(Ital.)*; Pankreon *(Swed.)*; Panteric *(Canad.)*; Viokase *(Austral., USA)*.

The empty capsules used for Viokase dissolved rapidly in pooled gastric or duodenal juice indicating potential destruction of pancreatin in this preparation.— T. A. Robb *et al.* (letter), *Lancet*, 1980, *2*, 544.

Pancreatin was also formerly marketed in Great Britain under the proprietary name Protopan (*Pharmaceutical Mfg*). Preparations containing pancreatic enzymes were also formerly marketed in Great Britain under the proprietary names Panar and Zypanar (both *Armour*).

3732-v

Pancrelipase *(U.S.P.)*.

CAS — 53608-75-6.

Pharmacopoeias. In *U.S.*

A preparation obtained from the pancreas of the hog. It is a cream amorphous powder with a faint characteristic, not offensive odour, containing enzymes, principally lipase, with protease and amylase; it contains in each g not less than 100 000 *U.S.P.* units of protease activity, not less than 24 000 *U.S.P.* units of lipase activity, and not less than 100 000 *U.S.P.* units of amylase activity. Its greatest activity is exhibited in neutral or faintly alkaline media. It is inactivated by more than traces of acids, by large amounts of alkali, or by excess of alkali carbonate. **Store** in airtight containers.

NOTE. Based on minimum potencies, pancrelipase has about 4 times the protease activity, 12 times the lipase activity, and 4 times the amylase activity of pancreatin *U.S.P.* and about 1.14 times the protease activity, 1.20 times the lipase activity, and equal amylase activity of pancreatin *B.P.*

Units. See Pancreatin, p.652.

Uses. Pancrelipase has the actions and uses of pancreatin (see p.652). The dose is the equivalent of 8000 to 24 000 *U.S.P.* units of lipase activity before each meal or snack, or according to the patient's needs.

Enteric-coated microspheres of pancrelipase (Pancrease) produced a significant improvement in 12 patients with alcohol-induced chronic pancreatitis and deficiency of pancreatic enzymes. In 2 patients who also had a severe deficiency of duodenal bicarbonate, 325 mg of sodium bicarbonate was given with each meal.— G. Salen and A. Prakash, *Curr. ther. Res.*, 1979, *25*, 650.

Preparations

Pancrelipase Capsules *(U.S.P.)*. Capsules containing not less than 30 000 *U.S.P.* units of protease activity, not less than 8000 *U.S.P.* units of lipase activity, and not less than 30 000 *U.S.P.* units of amylase activity. Store at a temperature not exceeding 25° in airtight containers.

Pancrelipase Tablets *(U.S.P.)*. Tablets containing not less than 30 000 *U.S.P.* units of protease activity, not less than 8000 *U.S.P.* units of lipase activity, and not less than 30 000 *U.S.P.* units of amylase activity. Store at a temperature not exceeding 25° in airtight containers.

Proprietary Names

Cotazym *(Organon, Austral.; Organon, USA)*; Ilozyme *(Adria, USA)*; Ku-Zyme HP *(Kremers-Urban, USA)*; Pancrease *(Johnson & Johnson, USA)*.

NOTE. In the UK Cotazym is not defined as pancrelipase.

The empty capsules used for Cotazym, the Australian preparation of pancrelipase, dissolved rapidly in pooled gastric or duodenal juice indicating potential destruction of pancrelipase in this preparation.— T. A. Robb *et al.* (letter), *Lancet*, 1980, *2*, 544.

3733-g

Papain *(U.S.P., B.P.C. 1954)*.

CAS — 9001-73-4.

Pharmacopoeias. In *Arg.*, *Ind.*, *It.*, and *U.S.*

A proteolytic enzyme or mixture of enzymes prepared from the juice of the unripe fruit of *Carica papaya* (Caricaceae). The *U.S.P.* specifies not less than 6000 *U.S.P.* units per mg.

An amorphous or slightly granular, white to light brown powder with a characteristic odour and faint pepsin-like taste.

Partly **soluble** in water; practically insoluble in alcohol, chloroform, and ether; soluble in glycerol. A 2% solution in water has a pH of 4.8 to 6.2. The maximum proteolytic activity occurs at pH 5 to 8. Papain is very liable to deterioration. **Store** in a cool place in airtight containers. Protect from light.

Proteolytic activity was considerably impaired by oxidation.— R. R. Thomson, *Q.J. Pharm. Pharmac.*, 1938, *11*, 125.

Papain had a wider range of activity and was more difficult to destroy than either trypsin or pepsin. It was active in acid or alkaline medium; the optimum pH was 5. Its optimum temperature zone was above that favourable to bacteria and it could therefore be used for long periods of digestion without bacterial contamination.— A. F. Watson *et al.*, *Q.J. Pharm. Pharmac.*, 1938, *11*, 391.

The structure of papain.— J. Drenth *et al.*, *Nature*, 1968, *218*, 929.

The properties and assay methods of papain.— Papain,

in *Pharmaceutical Enzymes*, R. Ruyssen and A. Lauwers (Ed.), Gent, E. Story-Scientia, 1978, p. 95.

Units. One *U.S.P.* unit of papain activity is the activity that releases the equivalent of 1 μg of tyrosine from a specified casein substrate under the conditions of the assay, using the enzyme concentration that liberates 40 μg of tyrosine per ml of test solution.
One FIP unit of papain is defined as the enzyme activity which under specified conditions hydrolyses 1 μmol of *N*-benzoyl-L-arginine ethyl ester per minute.

Adverse Effects. Allergic reactions have followed repeated inhalations of papain powder.

Extensive destruction of the oesophageal wall, with perforation, resulted from the use of a papain suspension given to treat an obstruction caused by impacted meat. The patient had been given 1.2 g of papain over a 12-hour period. Ten days after a thoracotomy, the descending thoracic aorta ruptured, and she died from haemorrhage.— J. W. Holsinger *et al.*, *J. Am. med. Ass.*, 1968, *204*, 734.

Of 120 workers in contact with papain who were examined over a 3-year period, 15 had evidence of allergic reactions, such as bronchial asthma, urticaria, or both. A further 3 workers gave positive reactions to patch tests and intradermal tests but had no discomfort.— C. Nava, *Medna Lav.*, 1969, *60*, 732, per *Abstr. Hyg.*, 1970, *45*, 740.

Papain solution caused pruritus in blister-base tests in all of 20 subjects.— J. Kirby *et al.*, *Br. med. J.*, 1974, *4*, 693.

Allergic asthma following exposure to papain in a factory worker.— M. L. H. Flindt, *Lancet*, 1978, *1*, 430.

Of 6 workers sensitised to papain 5 showed positive skin tests to bromelains and 2 of them also showed immediate asthmatic reactions after bronchial challenge with bromelains. It was considered that this provided evidence for immunological cross-reaction between bromelains and papain.— X. Baur and G. Fruhmann, *Clin. Allergy*, 1979, *9*, 443.

Uses. Papain consists chiefly of a mixture of papain and chymopapain, proteolytic enzymes which hydrolyse polypeptides, amides, and esters, especially at bonds involving basic amino acids, or leucine or glycine, yielding peptides of lower molecular weight. It is widely used as a meat tenderiser and in the clarification of beverages.

A brief discussion of the properties of papain.— J. L. Breeling, *J. Am. med. Ass.*, 1969, *210*, 2100.

The use of papain in scarring disorders of the eye.— G. L. Starkow and W. I. Sawinych, *Klin. Mbl. Augenheilk.*, 1971, *159*, 755, per *Int. pharm. Abstr.*, 1973, *10*, 668.

Jellyfish stings could be treated by sprinkling papain (or papain-containing meat tenderisers) on to the wetted affected area and allowing it to remain until stinging abated.— J. S. Loder (letter), *J. Am. med. Ass.*, 1973, *226*, 1228.

Papain given as enteric-coated tablets in a dose of 1.98 g with every meal reversed a malabsorption syndrome incompletely controlled by a gluten-free diet and considered to be due to a transient gluten intolerance.— M. Messer and P. E. Baume (letter), *Lancet*, 1976, *2*, 1022.

Papain-tenderised meat. The Minister of Agriculture, Fisheries and Food had been advised by the Food Standards Committee that they could see no hazard to human health from the consumption of meat tenderised by the pre-slaughter injection of papain. The process consisted in injecting a concentrated preparation of papain into the animal's blood system via the jugular vein about half an hour before the animal was slaughtered. The blood distributed the papain throughout the body tissues so that all the meat contained small quantities of papain which tenderised the tissues when the meat was cooked.— *Pharm. J.*, 1964, *1*, 166.

Preparations

Papain Tablets for Topical Solution *(U.S.P.)*. Tablets containing papain. pH of a solution of one tablet in 10 ml of water 6.9 to 8. Store in airtight containers. Protect from light.

Proteolytic Enzymes from *Carica papaya*. A mixture of proteolytic enzymes from *Carica papaya*. It is assayed for potency by means of a milk-clotting method and the potency is expressed in units, 1 unit (Warner-Chilcott) being defined as that quantity which will clot 2.64 microlitres of milk substrate in 2 minutes at 40°.

These enzymes have been proposed in doses of 10 000 to 20 000 units for oral and buccal use in treating oedema and inflammation in episiotomy but their value has not been established. Urticaria, pruritus, dizziness, nausea, vomiting, and diarrhoea have been observed following their administration and it is possible that sensitisation may occur. They should not be used simultaneously with anticoagulants or in patients with generalised or systemic infections or with disorders of blood coagulation. They are supplied as tablets each containing 10 000 units.

Clinical reports.— C. P. Vallis and M. H. Lund, *Curr. ther. Res.*, 1969, *11*, 356; H. T. Holt, *ibid.*, 621; M. H. Lund and R. R. Royer, *Archs Surg., Chicago*, 1969, *98*, 180; F. Caci and G. M. Gluck, *J. Am. dent. Ass.*, 1976, *93*, 325.

Proprietary Names of Proteolytic Enzymes from *Carica papaya*

Benase *(Ferndale, USA)*; Papase *(Parke, Davis, USA)*; Tromasin *(Warner, Arg.*; *Warner, Austral.*; *Warner, S.Afr.)*; Vermizym *(Schwab, Ger.)*.

3734-q

Pectinase. PG; Pectolase; Pectin-polygalacturonase.

CAS — 9032-75-1.

Pharmacopoeias. In *Aust.* and *Nord.*

Pectinase is an enzyme produced by most thallophytes. It hydrolyses pectin and pectic acids (polygalacturonic acids) and is used in wine making and in the manufacture of fruit juices to reduce their viscosity.

3735-p

Penicillinase.

An enzyme produced by many strains of bacteria. The commercial product is obtained by fermentation from cultures of a strain of *Bacillus cereus* or *Bacillus subtilis*.

CAS — 9001-74-5.

A white powder. **Soluble** in water. Stable at room temperature when dry but it deteriorates in solution. Solutions are stable at 2° to 8° for 1 week.

Units. One Levy unit is defined as that amount which inactivates 59.3 units of benzylpenicillin (sodium or potassium salt) per hour *in vitro* at 25° and pH 7 in the presence of an excess of penicillin.

Adverse Effects. An intramuscular injection may be followed by local soreness, erythema, and oedema. Fever, chills, skin rash, dyspnoea, and weakness occasionally occur. Hypersensitivity reactions have been reported.

Uses. Penicillinase catalyses the hydrolysis of penicillin to produce penicilloic acid which is biologically inactive and relatively non-antigenic.
Penicillinase has been given intramuscularly in the treatment of allergic reactions to penicillin; it acts within about 1 hour to destroy penicillin in the body fluids and remains active for at least 4 days. The injection of 800 000 Levy units should be made when the allergic symptoms, such as urticaria, oedema, and fever, first appear. This dose may be repeated within 3 to 7 days if necessary; it is advisable not to give more than 3 injections in each course of treatment.
The action of penicillinase intramuscularly is too slow to be effective in immediate allergic reactions; for this purpose it has been given intravenously in conjunction with adrenaline, antihistamines, and other supportive measures. Penicillinase is not effective against allergic reactions caused by penicillinase-resistant penicillins such as methicillin and cloxacillin. Penicillinase is also used, prior to culture, to inactivate any penicillin in clinical specimens.

Proprietary Names

Compenase *(Commonwealth Serum Laboratories, Austral.)*.

Penicillinase was formerly marketed in Great Britain under the proprietary name Neutrapen *(Riker)*.

3736-s

Pepsin *(B.P.C. 1959)*. Saccharated Pepsin.

CAS — 9001-75-6.

Pharmacopoeias. In *Arg., Aust., Chin., Cz., Ger., Hung., Ind., It., Jug., Neth., Pol., Port., Roum., Span.*, and *Swiss*. In *Jap.* as Saccharated Pepsin.

A substance containing a proteolytic enzyme present in the gastric juice of animals and obtained from the mucous membrane of the stomach of certain animals commonly used for food.
A white or light buff-coloured amorphous powder or translucent scales with a faintly meaty odour and a slightly acid or saline taste. It is active in acid media only; maximum activity occurs at pH 1.8. It dissolves not less than 2500 times its weight of coagulated egg albumen, and may be diluted to this strength with lactose or sucrose; varieties which dissolve up to 10 000 times their weight of coagulated egg albumen are available in commerce.
Soluble in water giving an opalescent solution; practically insoluble in alcohol, chloroform, and ether. A 2% solution in water is acid to litmus. **Incompatible** with alcohol, alkalis, tannins, and salts of heavy metals. Its proteolytic activity is destroyed by boiling its solution, by heating in the presence of alkali, and by pancreatic enzymes in neutral solution. Pepsin solutions are reduced in proteolytic activity by agitation and storage, particularly at or above normal room temperatures. It is active in the presence of dilute acid but its activity is destroyed by more than about 0.5% of HCl.
It absorbs moisture on exposure to air, particularly in powder form. Pure dry pepsin is, however, stable up to 100°. **Store** in a cool place in airtight containers.

A review of the properties and assay methods of pepsin. The activity required for pharmaceutical pepsin should fall between 0.5 and 0.7 FIP units per mg.— Pepsin, in *Pharmaceutical Enzymes*, R. Ruyssen and A. Lauwers (Ed.), Gent, E. Story-Scientia, 1978, p. 85.

Units. One FIP unit of pepsin activity is contained in that amount of the standard preparation, which upon incubation at 25° for 1 minute with a suitable preparation of pure haemoglobin will cause the decomposition of the haemoglobin to such an extent that the amount of hydroxyaryl substances liberated will, upon reaction with Folin-Ciocalteu reagent, result in the formation of a coloured solution of equal intensity to that resulting from the reaction of 1 μmol of tyrosine with the reagent.

Uses. Pepsin is a proteolytic enzyme which is secreted by the stomach and controls the degradation of proteins into proteoses and peptones. It hydrolyses polypeptides including those with bonds adjacent to aromatic or dicarboxylic L-amino-acid residues.
Pepsin has been given in doses of up to 1 g with dilute hydrochloric acid to increase the digestive power of the gastric juice when there is a deficiency of pepsin secretion, but is not considered to be of value. In acid media, pepsin destroys pancreatin and in neutral or alkaline media it is destroyed by pancreatin.

Pepsinogens and pepsins: a review.— M. D. Turner, *Gut*, 1968, *9*, 134.

For a review of the uselessness of pepsin in achlorhydria, see S. Buchs, *Dt. med. Wschr.*, 1971, *96*, 1925, per *Germ. Med.*, 1972, *2*, 64.

Preparations

Glycerin of Pepsin *(B.P.C. 1934)*. Glycer. Pepsin. Pepsin 10 g, hydrochloric acid 1.15 ml, glycerol 60 ml, water to 100 ml. *Dose.* 4 to 8 ml.

Glycerin of Pepsin *(B.P.C. 1949)*. Glycer. Pepsin.; Stronger Glycerin of Pepsin *(B.P.C. 1934)*. Pepsin 15 g, dilute hydrochloric acid 5 ml, glycerol 50 ml, simple elixir 5 ml, water to 100 ml. *Dose.* 2 to 4 ml.

Pepsin Lemonade *(Jap. P.).* Saccharated pepsin 1 g, dilute hydrochloric acid 0.5 ml, syrup 10 ml, water to 100 ml.

3737-w

Phenylpropanol. SH 261; Ethyl Phenyl Carbinol; α-Hydroxypropylbenzene. 1-Phenylpropan-1-ol; α-Ethylbenzyl alcohol.
$C_9H_{12}O=136.2$.

CAS — 93-54-9.

An oily liquid with a weak ester-like odour and a sweetish slightly irritating taste. **Miscible** with alcohol, ether, methyl alcohol, toluene, and olive oil.

Phenylpropanol is a choleretic. The usual dose is 100 to 200 mg thrice daily with meals.

Proprietary Names
Bilergon *(Limas, Ital.)*; Ejibil *(Sopar, Belg.)*; Eufepar *(Arnaldi, Ital.)*; Felicur *(Schering, Austral.*; *Schering, Arg.*; *Asche, Ger.).*

3738-e

Piprozolin. Gö 919; W 3699. Ethyl (3-ethyl-4-oxo-5-piperidinothiazolidin-2-ylidene)acetate.
$C_{14}H_{22}N_2O_3S=298.4$.

CAS — 17243-64-0.

Colourless crystals. M.p. about 86°. Practically **insoluble** in water.

Piprozolin is a choleretic. It has been given in doses of 100 to 200 mg thrice daily. Piprozolin may cause discoloration of the urine.

Studies on the absorption and fate of piprozolin.— K. -O. Vollmer *et al., Arzneimittel-Forsch.*, 1977, *27*, 502; V. Gladigau and I. Ehret, *ibid.*, 512.

In open and controlled studies in 1545 patients piprozolin was significantly better than a placebo in the treatment of patients with gall-bladder diseases and intestinal disorders. No significant side-effects occurred with piprozolin therapy.— E. Schleicher, *Arzneimittel-Forsch.*, 1977, *27*, 520.

Proprietary names
Probilin *(Gödecke, Ger.*; *Substancia, Spain).*

3739-l

Plasmin. Plasmin (Human); Fibrinolysin (Human). A proteolytic enzyme derived from the activation of human plasminogen by highly purified streptokinase.

CAS — 9004-09-5 (human).

A white powder. **Soluble** in water. Solutions for injection should be freshly prepared. **Store** at 2° to 8.°

The properties and assay methods of plasmin.— Plasmin, in *Pharmaceutical Enzymes*, R. Ruyssen and A. Lauwers (Ed.), Gent, E. Story-Scientia, 1978, p. 123.

Incompatibility. Plasmin 200 mg was 'physically incompatible' with oxytocin 0.5 units, thiopentone sodium 250 mg, or promazine 100 mg in 100 ml of dextrose injection.— R. D. Dunworth and F. R. Kenna, *Am. J. Hosp. Pharm.*, 1965, *22*, 190.

Units. 8 units of plasmin are contained in approximately 1 ml of a solution of partially purified plasmin in glycerol 50% in one ampoule of the first International Reference Preparation (1976).

One FIP unit of plasmin is defined as the enzyme activity which under the specified standard conditions in the course of 1 minute gives rise to the formation of peptides soluble in perchloric acid with an absorbance at 275 nm equal to that of 1 μmol of tyrosine.

One MSD unit is defined as the amount that will lyse a standard fibrin clot in 10 minutes under the conditions specified in the assay.

Adverse Effects. A transitory febrile response may occur 3 to 10 hours after administration of plasmin. Haemorrhage may occur. Side-effects may also include reactions such as chills, nausea, vomiting, tachycardia, hypotension, dizziness, headache, and muscle pain; some authorities consider that allergic reactions are caused by the streptokinase component of plasmin. Jaundice has been reported following treatment with plasmin.

A severe systemic reaction occurred in a 39-year-old man after an intravenous injection of purified human plasmin. Immunological studies suggested that both streptokinase and plasmin antibodies were responsible for the reaction.— P. W. Boyles, *J. Am. med. Ass.*, 1959, *170*, 1045.

Further references: J. L. Ambrus *et al., Am. J. Cardiol.*, 1960, *6*, 462, per *Lancet*, 1961, *1*, 754.

Precautions. Plasmin should be used with caution in patients with cardiac arrhythmias, or immediately after anaesthesia or surgery. Care is necessary in patients with abnormal blood-clotting mechanisms or severe hepatic dysfunction and in conditions associated with haemorrhage. Blood coagulability should be checked frequently.

Uses. Plasmin has fibrinolytic properties and also contains a plasminogen-activator. It has been used for the treatment of thrombotic disorders and has been given as an adjunct to anti-coagulant therapy. Dosage will depend on clinical response. A suggested dose was 50 000 to 100 000 MSD units per hour by intravenous infusion for 1 to 6 hours daily for 3 or 4 days if necessary. Bovine plasmin has been used in conjunction with deoxyribonuclease for the debridement of wounds.

3740-v

Prozapine Hydrochloride. Hexadiphane Hydrochloride. 1-(3,3-Diphenylpropyl)perhydroazepine hydrochloride.
$C_{21}H_{27}N,HCl=329.9$.

CAS — 3426-08-2 (prozapine); 13657-24-4 (hydrochloride).

Prozapine hydrochloride is an antispasmodic used with sorbitol in visceral disorders. It has been given in doses of 2 to 6 mg daily taken in water before meals.

Proprietary Names
Norbiline *(Fournier Frères, Fr.*; *Semar, Spain).*

3741-g

Rennet *(B.P.C. 1934).* Rennin; Chymosin; Seriparium. The partially purified, milk-curdling, proteolytic enzyme from the glandular layer of the fourth or true digesting stomach of the calf.

CAS — 9042-08-4.

It occurs as greyish- or yellow-white slightly hygroscopic scales or powder with a peculiar but not unpleasant odour and a characteristic slightly saline taste. Slowly **soluble** in water and dilute alcohol, the solutions being more or less opalescent. **Store** in a cool place.

Rennet hydrolyses polypeptides to peptides of lower molecular weight and is used for the preparation of junkets and in making cheese.

Commercial preparations of microbial rennet could be produced by the controlled fermentation of *Bacillus cereus*, nonpathogenic species of *Endothia parasitica*, or *Mucor miehei* or *M. pusillus.— Fd. Add. Ser. Wld Hlth Org. No. 2*, 1972.

For background toxicological information on microbial rennets, see *Fd Add. Ser. Wld Hlth Org. No. 6*, 1975.

3742-q

Sodium Dehydrocholate. Sodium Triketocholanate; Deidrocolato de Sódio. Sodium 3,7,12-trioxo-5β-cholan-24-oate.
$C_{24}H_{33}NaO_5=424.5$.

CAS — 145-41-5.

Pharmacopoeias. In *Braz.* and *Swiss.*

A colourless crystalline powder with a bitter taste. **Soluble** in water and alcohol. A solution in water is alkaline to litmus. **Store** in airtight containers.

Sodium dehydrocholate was incompatible with protein hydrolysate, invert sugar, and laevulose; a haze or precipitate occurred within 24 hours with dextrose 5, 10, or 20%, within 6 hours with dextrose 50%, and within 1 hour with dextrose 5% in Lactated Ringer's Solution.— W. D. Kirkland *et al., Am. J. Hosp. Pharm.*, 1961, *18*, 694.

Adverse Effects. When administered by intravenous injection, sodium dehydrocholate may cause nausea, vomiting, diarrhoea, bradycardia, muscular hyperactivity, headache, hypotension and tachycardia, dyspnoea, fever, skin rashes, and allergic reactions. Fatalities have followed rapid intravenous injections. Extravasation may lead to local reactions.

Precautions. As for Dehydrocholic Acid, p.649. It should be injected with care.

Uses. Sodium dehydrocholate has the actions and uses of dehydrocholic acid (see p.649).

It is usually given by slow intravenous injection of a 20% solution, a dose of 3 to 5 ml (0.6 to 1 g) being given on each of 3 successive days.Daily doses of up to 3 g have sometimes been used.

It has also been used as a diagnostic aid in the determination of the arm-to-tongue circulation time, from 3 to 5 ml of a 20% solution being injected into a cubital vein, with the patient in the supine position. The time is recorded from the beginning of the injection to the perception of a bitter taste. The normal range is from 8 to 16 seconds. The routine use of sodium dehydrocholate for the determination of the circulation time is not generally recommended because of the severe side-effects.

Preparations

Dehydrocholate Sodium Injection *(U.S.P.).* Sodium Dehydrocholate Injection. A sterile solution of sodium dehydrocholate in Water for Injections, usually prepared by neutralising dehydrocholic acid, pH 8.5 to 9.5. Protect from light. *Jap. P.* includes a similar injection. *Aust. P.* and *Swiss P.* include a 20% injection.

Proprietary Names
Choleubil *(see also under Dehydrocholic Acid) (Ibsa, Switz.)*; Decholin *(see also under Dehydrocholic Acid) (Cassella-Riedel, Ger.)*; Deidroepar *(Bucaneve, Ital.)*; Dicolan *(see also under Dehydrocholic Acid) (Biologici Italia, Ital.)*; Dycholium *(see also under Dehydrocholic Acid) (Théraplix, Fr.).*

3743-p

Sodium Deoxycholate. Sodium Desoxycholate. Sodium 3α,12α-dihydroxy-5β-cholan-24-oate.
$C_{24}H_{39}NaO_4=414.6$.

CAS — 302-95-4.

A white powder. **Soluble** in water. A 10% solution has a pH of 8 to 10.

Sodium deoxycholate is used as a solubilising agent and in the manufacture of vaccines.

Estimated acceptable daily intake of cholic and deoxycholic acid and their salts: up to 1.25 mg per kg body-weight.— Seventeenth Report of FAO/WHO Expert Committee on Food Additives, *Tech. Rep. Ser. Wld Hlth Org. No. 539*, 1974. For background toxicological information, see *Fd Add. Ser. Wld Hlth Org. No. 5*, 1974..

In 16 healthy adults given deoxycholic acid, 100 to 150 mg daily in divided doses for a mean of 2 weeks, the cholesterol content of the bile rose in 10. Since deoxycholic acid was formed in the colon excessive absorption might predispose to gall-stones.— T. S. Low-Beer and E. W. Pomare, *Br. med. J.*, 1975, *1*, 438.

3744-s

Sodium Tauroglycocholate *(B.P.C. 1954).* Bile Salts.

CAS — 11006-55-6.

A yellowish-brown hygroscopic powder with an odour resembling that of fresh bile, a sweet taste, and a bitter after-taste; it contains not less than 65% of bile acids. **Soluble** 2 in 1 of water; soluble in alcohol; practically insoluble in ether. **Store** in a cool place in airtight containers, preferably not in glass-stoppered bottles.

Sodium tauroglycocholate has been given in doses of 120 to 400 mg to assist emulsification of fats and the absorption of oil-soluble vitamins where there is a deficiency of biliary secretion. It is best administered in capsules.

3745-w

Streptodornase. Streptococcal Deoxyribonuclease. A deoxyribonuclease, or a specific series of such enzymes, produced by the growth of haemolytic streptococci.

CAS — 37340-82-2.

Units. 2400 units of streptodornase are contained in approximately 1 mg of extract which also contains streptokinase, with lactose 5 mg, in one ampoule of the first International Standard Preparation (1964). The U.S. unit has been defined as that amount of the enzyme which causes a change in the relative viscosity of a 0.15% solution of deoxyribonucleic acid from 5 to 4 in 10 minutes at 30°.

Uses. Streptodornase, in the presence of magnesium ions, depolymerises deoxyribonucleic acid and deoxyribonucleoprotein which are constituents of purulent exudates and account for much of their viscosity. It is used only in conjunction with streptokinase.

Preparations

See under Streptokinase-Streptodornase, p.658.

3746-e

Streptokinase *(B.P.).* A protein obtained from culture filtrates of certain strains of haemolytic streptococcus group C, which has the property of activating human plasminogen to form plasmin, and has been purified to contain not less than 600 International units of streptokinase activity per microgram of bacterial protein nitrogen. After purification it is mixed with a stabiliser and buffering agents.

CAS — 9002-01-1.

Pharmacopoeias. In *Br.*

A sterile white powder or friable solid. Freely **soluble** in water and normal saline. A solution in freshly boiled and cooled water containing 5000 units per ml has a pH of 6.8 to 7.5. It is unstable in dilute solutions; solutions of the purified material containing more than 10 000 units per ml are reasonably stable for about 6 hours at 4°. Solutions have a maximum activity in neutral media and are inactivated below pH 5 or above pH 9. **Store** in airtight containers at 2° to 8° and protect from light; under these conditions the powder may be expected to retain its potency for 2 years.

Units. 3100 units of streptokinase are contained in approximately 1 mg of extract which also contains streptodornase, with lactose 5 mg, in one ampoule of the first International Standard Preparation (1964). The Christensen or U.S. unit is the quantity of streptokinase that will lyse a standard blood clot completely in 10 minutes. The Christensen unit is equivalent to the International unit.

Adverse Effects. Streptokinase may cause fever and haemorrhage. Cerebral, peripheral, and pulmonary embolisms have occurred. Streptokinase is antigenic and allergic reactions may occur. A transient rise in serum-transaminase concentrations has occasionally been reported.

Effects on the blood. In 5 patients massive blood plasmocytosis occurred 7 to 9 days after beginning therapy with streptokinase. One patient also had clinical signs of serum sickness.— P. W. Straub *et al.*, *Schweiz. med. Wschr.*, 1974, *104*, 1891.

Effects on the kidney. A 50-year-old man developed temporary and reversible changes in renal function 10 days after starting therapy with streptokinase.— L. Spangen *et al.*, *Acta med. scand.*, 1976, *199*, 335.

A report of acute renal failure in a 65-year-old man due to diffuse cholesterol crystal embolisation during streptokinase treatment.— F. W. Rieben *et al.*, *Dt. med. Wschr.*, 1979, *104*, 1447.

Effects on the liver. Severe intra-abdominal bleeding with spontaneous rupture of the liver and spleen occurred in 3 and 1 patients respectively during treatment with streptokinase for deep vein thrombosis. Liver disease was not found in any of the patients.— B. Eklöf *et al.*, *Vasa*, 1977, *6*, 369. The same study.— L. Norgren *et al.*, *Läkartidningen*, 1978, *75*, 777.

Effects on the nerves. Femoral neuropathy developed in a 52-year-old woman 12 hours after the end of streptokinase therapy for ergotism. It was suggested the neuropathy resulted from bleeding into the iliac and psoas muscle sheaths.— A. Ganel *et al.*, *Angiology*, 1979, *30*, 192.

Treatment of Adverse Effects. Fever may be reduced by the concomitant administration of corticosteroids. Haemorrhage may be treated by the administration of fresh blood, fibrinogen, tranexamic acid, or aminocaproic acid, or aprotinin in pregnant patients.

Precautions. Streptokinase should not be given to patients with severe hypertension, coagulation defects, cerebral metastases, or with haemorrhagic diathesis such as peptic ulcer, or to patients following recent surgery or trauma. It should not be given for occlusion of the carotid or vertebral arteries. Its use should also be avoided during the first 16 to 18 weeks of pregnancy because of the risk of placental separation. It is also contra-indicated in patients with streptococcal infections or sub-acute bacterial endocarditis, and in patients who have been treated with streptokinase within the preceding 3 months. It has been suggested that streptokinase should not be used during menstruation. It should be used with care in the elderly, in patients with atrial fibrillation, severe hepatic or renal insufficiency, in patients convalescing from streptococcal infections, after parturition, or in conjunction with drugs, such as aspirin or dipyridamole, affecting platelet function. It has also been suggested that heparin and oral anticoagulants should not be administered during treatment with streptokinase. It has been recommended that during streptokinase therapy invasive procedures, including intramuscular injections, should be avoided.

Uses. Streptokinase rapidly activates plasminogen, indirectly by means of a streptokinase-plasminogen complex, to plasmin (see p.655), a proteolytic enzyme which has fibrinolytic effects and can be used to dissolve intravascular blood clots. Streptokinase is given by intravenous infusion in the treatment of thrombo-embolic disorders such as pulmonary embolism and arterial and venous occlusions. It is most likely to be effective if given as soon as possible after the occurrence of the embolism. It has also been tried in myocardial infarction. High antibody titres to streptokinase develop after 7 to 10 days' treatment or after streptococcal infections and may persist for 4 to 6 months. In such patients and in children a streptokinase resistance test may be performed and the dose necessary to neutralise circulating antibodies calculated (titrated initial dose). This dose is given by intravenous infusion in dextrose injection or sodium chloride injection over 30 to 60 minutes, followed by maintenance doses usually of 100 000 International units per hour for up to 5 days. The maintenance dose for children can be calculated on the basis of 20 units per ml of blood volume per hour. Since most patients have a low antibody titre, some authorities use a standard initial dose, usually of 250 000 to 600 000 units. Most authorities recommend the use of the equivalent of 100 mg of hydrocortisone with the initial dose to reduce the risk of allergic reactions. Because thrombolytic activity rapidly fades when treatment ceases, anticoagulant therapy with heparin by intravenous infusion and then with oral anticoagulants must follow. Streptokinase has also been administered by intrapleural instillation in doses of 250 000 units in 100 ml of sodium chloride injection. Streptokinase is also used topically in conjunction with streptodornase (see Streptokinase-Streptodornase, p.658).

Action. For detailed reviews and comments on the action and uses of streptokinase, see *Postgrad. med. J.*, 1973, *49* (Aug.), *Suppl.* 5; R. N. Brogden *et al.*, *Drugs*, 1973, *5*, 357–445; M. Verstraete, *ibid.*, 353; A. S. Gallus and J. Hirsch, *ibid.*, 1976, *12*, 132; *Br. med. J.*, 1977, *1*, 927; V. V. Kakkar and M. F. Scully, *Br. med. Bull.*, 1978, *34*, 191; W. R. Bell and A. G. Meek, *New Engl. J. Med.*, 1979, *301*, 1266. Summary of an NIH Consensus Conference, *Br. med. J.*, 1980, *280*, 1585.

Further references relating to the action and uses of streptokinase.— D. Ogston and A. S. Douglas, *Drugs*, 1971, *1*, 228; J. C. Fratantoni and T. L. Simon, *New Engl. J. Med.*, 1975, *293*, 1073; P. T. Flute, *Br. J. Hosp. Med.*, 1976, *16*, 135; J. M. Porter and S. H. Goodnight, *Am. J. Surg.*, 1977, *134*, 217; V. J. Marder, *Ann. intern. Med.*, 1979, *90*, 802.

Administration. A study of the biochemical changes noted during intermittent administration of streptokinase to 9 patients with chronic obliterative arterial disease and 8 patients with venous occlusion. An initial dose of 600 000 units was given intravenously over 30 minutes followed by 250 000 units every 24 hours for 3 days given intravenously over about 5 minutes. It was concluded that controlled clinical trials were necessary to compare the relative therapeutic effect of intermittent infusions with continuous administration of streptokinase.— M. Verstraete *et al.*, *Thromb. Haemostasis*, 1978, *39*, 61.

A favourable report of the use of an equimolar preparation of streptokinase-human plasminogen complex in 26 patients with chronic arterial occlusion and stenosis of the lower-limb arteries or thrombosis of the subclavian veins.— M. Martin *et al.*, *Dt. med. Wschr.*, 1978, *103*, 1953.

Behçet's disease. Thrombophlebitis associated with Behçet's disease in 2 patients responded to treatment with streptokinase.— T. Chajek and M. Fainaru, *Br. med. J.*, 1973, *1*, 782. See also D. A. Tibbutt *et al.* (letter), *ibid.*, *3*, 236.

Ergotism. For a report of the use of streptokinase in the treatment of arterial insufficiency due to ergotism, see Ergotamine Tartrate, p.665.

Haemolytic disorders. Disseminated intravascular coagulation and peripheral necrosis, unresponsive to heparin therapy, resulting from malaria infection in a 9-year-old boy was successfully treated with streptokinase and blood preparations. The initial dose of streptokinase was 200 000 units followed by 50 000 units hourly for 30 hours.— I. R. Edwards, *Br. med. J.*, 1980, *280*, 1252.

Haemolytic-uraemic syndrome. A brief report of streptokinase followed by heparin being used in 36 children with the haemolytic-uraemic syndrome.— L. Monnens *et al.* (letter), *Lancet*, 1972, *1*, 692. See also J. M. Bergstein *et al.* (letter), *ibid.*, 448; M. H. Winterborn *et al.* (letter), *ibid.*, 1071.

The use of streptokinase in 5 children with the haemolytic-uraemic syndrome and a discussion of the problems involved.— J. Stuart *et al.*, *Br. med. J.*, 1974, *3*, 217.

Further references: H. R. Powell and H. Ekert, *J. Pediat.*, 1974, *84*, 345.

Purpura fulminans. The successful use of streptokinase in a patient with purpura fulminans.— F. E. Preston and I. R. Edwards, *Br. med. J.*, 1973, *3*, 329.

Myocardial infarction. For reviews on streptokinase in myocardial infarction, see T. L. Simon *et al.*, *Ann. intern. Med.*, 1973, *79*, 712; J. M. Sullivan, *New Engl. J. Med.*, 1979, *301*, 836; *Br. med. J.*, 1979, *2*, 1017.

There was a mortality-rate of 19% in 357 patients with myocardial infarction who received streptokinase within 24 hours compared with 27.4% in 339 comparable patients treated with heparin. Re-infarction was less common in patients given streptokinase.—Report of a European Working Party, *Br. med. J.*, 1971, *3*, 325. Criticism.— R. Heikinheimo (letter), *ibid.*, *4*, 361.

In a multicentre study 302 patients with acute myocardial infarction were treated with streptokinase and their progress compared with 293 controls. There was no significant difference in mortality up to 6 weeks and 6 months after infarction; the incidence of cardiac failure and re-infarction was comparable; major arrhythmias were reduced in the streptokinase group, as were venous thrombosis and pulmonary and systemic embolism. There was no case for the routine use of streptokinase in myocardial infarction.— C. P. Aber *et al.*, *Br. med. J.*, 1976, *2*, 1100.

In a multicentre study, streptokinase reduced mortality at 6 months in selected medium- and high-risk patients with acute myocardial infarction who were admitted to a coronary care unit within 12 hours of the onset of symptoms. Criteria for entry into the study were very stringent and of 2338 patients originally assessed only 8 high-risk and 307 medium-risk patients were admitted. Patients were given either streptokinase 250 000 units infused in dextrose injection over 20 minutes, followed by 100 000 units hourly for 24 hours, or dextrose infusions only. All patients also received anticoagulant therapy. Within 6 months, 24 of 155 (15.6%) evaluable patients given streptokinase had died compared with 48 of 157 (30.6%) control patients.—Report of a European Cooperative Study Group, *New Engl. J. Med.*, 1979, *301*, 797. Comment.— J. M. Sullivan, *ibid.*, 836.

Further references: R. Schmutzler *et al.*, *Dt. med. Wschr.*, 1966, *91*, 581; V. Hiemeyer *et al.*, *Klin. Wschr.*, 1969, *47*, 371; L. Benda *et al.*, *Dt. med. Wschr.*, 1971, *96*, 771; N. Dioguardi *et al.*, *Lancet*, 1971, *2*, 891; J. H. N. Bett *et al.*, *ibid.*, 1973, *1*, 57; J. H. N. Bett *et al.*, *Med. J. Aust.*, 1977, *1*, 553; J. E. Markis *et al.*, *New Engl. J. Med.*, 1981, *305*, 777.

Neoplasms. Streptokinase and brinolase, separately or together, were given to 18 anergic patients with various neoplasms to induce proteolysis and convert the anergic state to one where the patient reacted to skin tests. Eleven patients converted from the anergic state. Seven patients eventually relapsed with tumour recurrence but 4 remained converted at 14 to 26 weeks.— R. D. Thornes (preliminary communication), *Lancet*, 1974, *2*, 382.

Patency of cannulas. Between 100 000 and 250 000 units of streptokinase dissolved in 5 ml of sodium chloride injection had been used to remove clots in Scribner shunts. The solution was introduced into the thrombosed segment of the shunt, left for 2 hours, and then removed by aspiration with a syringe.— J. Vermylen *et al.* (letter), *Lancet*, 1967, *2*, 1368.

In 22 patients maintained on regular dialysis, streptokinase was used on 73 occasions for blocked arterial or venous cannulas; 50 000 to 100 000 units in 2 to 4 ml of solvent was injected, the cannula was clamped for an hour, and then aspirated. Patency lasting longer than a month was achieved on 36 occasions.— L. Arisz *et al.*, *Postgrad. med. J.*, 1973, *49* (Aug.), *Suppl.* 5, 99.

On 2 occasions streptokinase 10 000 units in 5 ml of sodium chloride solution was successfully used to clear partially blocked central venous catheters.— J. E. Gilligan *et al.* (letter), *Lancet*, 1979, *2*, 1189.

Pregnancy and the neonate. A 29-year-old woman in the 32nd week of pregnancy developed acute massive pulmonary embolism after surgery. She was successfully treated with streptokinase and subsequently a healthy child was delivered with no evidence of adverse effect. Extensive postpartum haemorrhage was controlled by discontinuing streptokinase, the administration of aminocaproic acid, and fundal massage. In retrospect it was suggested that streptokinase be discontinued 4 to 6 hours before anticipated delivery and that aprotinin be used instead of aminocaproic acid.— R. J. C. Hall *et al.*, *Br. med. J.*, 1972, *4*, 647.

Streptokinase had been used in moderately high dosage (250 000 to 750 000 units initially, then 200 000 units per hour for 8 hours, then 100 000 units per hour) in 24 pregnant patients without adverse effect on the foetus. Streptokinase did not appear to cross the placenta, but streptokinase antibodies did.— H. Ludwig, *Postgrad. med. J.*, 1973, *49* (Aug.), *Suppl.* 5, 65.

Further references.— C. Walther and H. Koestering, *Dt. med. Wschr.*, 1969, *94*, 32; T. Skiftis, *Geburtsch. Frauenheilk.*, 1971, *31*, 568; A. G. Amias (letter), *Br. med. J.*, 1977, *1*, 1414.

Thrombo-embolic disorders. A review of the use and side-effects of streptokinase in the treatment of pulmonary embolism and deep-vein thrombosis.— *Med. Lett.*, 1978, *20*, 37.

Thrombolytic therapy in treatment.—Summary of an NIH Consensus Conference, *Br. med. J.*, 1980, *280*, 1585.

Of 30 patients with deep-vein thrombosis of the leg of less than 4 days' duration, 10 patients received heparin 10 000 units in 5 minutes, then 10 000 to 15 000 units every 6 hours; 10 received streptokinase, 500 000 units in 30 minutes and then 900 000 units every 6 hours; and 10 received ancrod, 80 units in 6 hours followed by 80 units in 15 minutes and 40 to 80 units every 6 hours. Treatment was given by continuous intravenous infusions usually for 5 days and was followed with anticoagulants by mouth. Thrombolysis was more effective with streptokinase than with either heparin or ancrod, and side-effects, mainly bleeding, occurred least in those treated with ancrod.— V. V. Kakkar *et al.*, *Br. med. J.*, 1969, *1*, 806. See also *idem*, 810.

Streptokinase was infused continuously for 3 days in 170 patients with chronic vascular occlusions and stenoses in the lower half of the body. Results were very promising in the treatment of stenoses of the iliac arteries (42 successes in 73 limbs), and 3 of 4 cases of narrowing of the aorta also responded. Long-standing vascular occlusions of the large arteries (abdominal aorta and common iliac artery) were also resolved with streptokinase. Peripheral occlusions were not responsive. Because of the danger of thrombosis, anticoagulants were administered both during and after lysis.— M. Martin *et al.*, *J. Am. med. Ass.*, 1970, *211*, 1169. See also M. Verstraete *et al.*, *Ann. intern. Med.*, 1971, *74*, 377.

In patients with recent thrombo-embolic occlusions of limb arteries who were treated with at least 1 million units of streptokinase, the frequency of clearing of iliac, femoral, and popliteal artery occlusions increased when treatment was started within 72 hours of occlusion. A significantly higher clearing-rate and a significantly lower mortality-rate occurred when the initial dose given in the first 30 minutes of treatment was less than 500 000 units, as compared with patients receiving larger initial doses of streptokinase. An initial dose in excess of 500 000 units appeared to be dangerous. Maintenance therapy was given at a dose of 100 000 units per hour for 72 hours unless clearing occurred. Bleeding complications occurred in 16 of 85 patients, and were not related to streptokinase dosage. Other side-effects included psychological disturbances in 14 patients, shock in 3, and renal insufficiency in 4. During streptokinase therapy 5 patients had an acute cerebrovascular accident and 8 developed thrombo-embolic complications.— A. Amery *et al.*, *Br. med. J.*, 1970, *4*, 639.

Streptokinase 600 000 units infused over 30 minutes and preceded by either 90 mg or 120 mg of plasminogen in sodium chloride injection infused over 4 to 6 hours was given daily for 5 days to 12 patients with subacute deep-vein thrombosis confirmed by phlebography. This treatment was considered to be clinically successful in 11 of the patients whereas in 5 patients given streptokinase only, 3 still had symptoms after 5 days. Phlebography showed that 8 of the 12 given both drugs had complete clearing of involved veins compared with no change in thrombi of the 5 given streptokinase alone.— V. V. Kakkar *et al.*, *Lancet*, 1975, *2*, 674.

Further references: A. V. Persson *et al.*, *Archs Surg., Chicago*, 1973, *107*, 779; G. E. Mavor *et al.*, *Br. J. Surg.*, 1973, *60*, 468; D. A. Tibbutt *et al.*, *Br. J. Haemat.*, 1974, *27*, 407; F. Duckert *et al.*, *Br. med. J.*, 1975, *1*, 479; J. Rösch *et al.*, *Am. J. Roentg.*, 1976, *127*, 553; H. Arnesen *et al.*, *Acta med. scand.*, 1978, *203*, 457; H. -G. Jester, *Dt. med. Wschr.*, 1978, *103*, 1922; *Lancet*, 1981, *1*, 1035.

Cerebral occlusions. The use of streptokinase in cerebral artery occlusion.— W. Dahlman *et al.*, *Nervenarzt*, 1972, *43*, 272.

Pelvic occlusions. A significant improvement occurred in the degree of stenosis in 10 patients with 13 stenoses in the pelvic area treated with streptokinase 30 000 units per hour for 72 hours. Heparin and oral anticoagulants were also used.— J. Bopp *et al.*, *Dt. med. Wschr.*, 1977, *102*, 198.

Pulmonary occlusions. A discussion of the use of streptokinase in the treatment of pulmonary embolism.— D. A. Tibbutt and C. N. Chesterman, *Drugs*, 1976, *11*, 161. See also *Drug & Ther. Bull.*, 1980, *18*, 45.

Of 23 patients with massive pulmonary embolism, 15 received streptokinase 600 000 units in the first half hour followed by 100 000 units per hour, usually for a total of 72 hours, and 8 received heparin in a dose adequate to prolong the whole-blood clotting time by a factor of 2 to 3, the dosage ranging from 40 000 to 60 000 units in 24 hours. The drugs were infused through a pulmonary artery catheter. There was significantly greater resolution of pulmonary embolism at 72 hours after streptokinase than after heparin therapy.— G. A. H. Miller *et al.*, *Br. med. J.*, 1971, *2*, 681.

Thirty patients with life-threatening pulmonary embolism were treated with heparin or streptokinase. In 23 who completed 72 hours' treatment, streptokinase was significantly more effective in improving the angiographic score (assessing the thrombus and peripheral perfusion) and in reducing pulmonary arterial systolic and mean pressures. The 7 patients who failed to complete the treatment had high initial angiographic scores and most underwent surgery, which was probably indicated for high scores and systemic arterial systolic pressures of less than 100 mmHg. The respective doses were 600 000 units of streptokinase or 5000 units of heparin in 100 ml of sodium chloride injection or dextrose injection, each with hydrocortisone 100 mg, infused into the pulmonary artery, followed by hourly infusions of 100 000 units of streptokinase or 2500 units of heparin. Dosage was controlled by daily monitoring of coagulation tests. Side-effects of streptokinase (peripheral vasodilatation in 1 patient, a widespread pruritic erythematous rash in 1 patient, and fever frequently) were not considered more severe than the side-effects of heparin.— D. A. Tibbutt *et al.*, *Br. med. J.*, 1974, *1*, 343.

A study in 40 patients with pulmonary embolism indicated that the thrombolytic agents, streptokinase and urokinase, allow more complete resolution of thromboemboli than do heparin and oral anticoagulants. It is suggested that the sequence of therapy in venous thrombo-embolism should be lysis of thrombo-emboli, followed by preventative treatment with anticoagulants.— G. V. R. K. Sharma *et al.*, *New Engl. J. Med.*, 1980, *303*, 842. Comments on the frequency of bleeding complications.— D. Goodenberger (letter), *ibid.*, 1981, *304*, 360; G. V. R. K. Sharma and A. A. Sasahara (letter), *ibid.*, 361.

Further references: J. Hirsh *et al.*, *Br. med. J.* 1968, *4*, 729; *idem*, *Lancet*, 1967, *2*, 593; G. A. H. Miller *et al.*, *Br. med. J.*, 1969, *1*, 812; M. J. Goldberg, *Br. J. clin. Pract.*, 1970, *24*, 523; R. Gibson, *Practitioner*, 1970, *204*, 262; G. A. H. Miller *et al.*, *Am. Heart J.*, 1977, *93*, 568; B. Ly *et al.*, *Acta med. scand.*, 1978, *203*, 465.

For a comparative study of streptokinase and urokinase in pulmonary embolism, see Urokinase, p.660.

See also under Adverse Effects (above).

Renal occlusions. The use of streptokinase in renal occlusion.— E. Streicher *et al.*, *Dt. med. Wschr.*, 1971, *96*, 1086; E. Böttger *et al.*, *Fortschr. Geb. RöntgStrahl. NuklMed.*, 1971, *115*, 742.

Retinal occlusions. In a random controlled study 20 patients with central retinal vein occlusion received a course of streptokinase followed by anticoagulant therapy and 20 received no specific therapy. Although the beneficial effect was small, vision after 12 months (6 months in 2 patients) was significantly better in the streptokinase group and only 1 treated patient developed thrombotic glaucoma compared with 4 in the control group. Vitreous haemorrhage with permanent loss of vision occurred in 3 patients probably as a result of streptokinase therapy and accordingly streptokinase only appeared to have a limited role in the treatment of central retinal occlusion.— E. M. Kohner *et al.*, *Br. med. J.*, 1976, *1*, 550.

Further references: H. Rossmann, *Postgrad. med. J.*, 1973, *49* (Aug.), *Suppl.* 5, 105.

Preparations

Streptokinase Injection *(B.P.)*. A sterile solution of streptokinase prepared immediately before use by dissolving the contents of a sealed container (Streptokinase for Injection) in the requisite amount of Water for Injections.

Kabikinase *(KabiVitrum, UK)*. Streptokinase, available as powder for solution before use, in vials of 100 000, 250 000, and 600 000 units for intravascular therapy. (Also available as Kabikinase in *Austral., Belg., Ger., Neth., S.Afr., Switz.*).

Streptase *(Hoechst, UK)*. Streptokinase, available in vials of 100 000, 250 000, and 750 000 units for preparing solutions for intravascular use and in ampoules of 5000 units for diagnostic use. (Also available as Streptase in *Austral., Belg., Denm., Fr., Ger., Ital., Neth., Norw., S.Afr., USA*).

Other Proprietary Names

Kabikinas *(Denm., Norw., Swed.)*.

3747-l

Streptokinase-Streptodornase. A mixture of streptokinase and streptodornase.

CAS — 8048-16-6.

Solutions deteriorate rapidly in potency at room temperature but are stable at 2° to 10° for 7 days. Solutions have a maximum activity in neutral media. **Store** at a temperature not exceeding 4° when the powder may be expected to retain its potency for 18 months.

After storage for 2 years in excess of the manufacturer's expiry date, and after irradiation with 12 Gy, no change in the fibrinolytic activity of streptokinase-streptodornase (Varidase) was detected.— E. Szirmai *et al.*, *Arzneimittel-Forsch.*, 1967, *17*, 50.

Units. 3100 units of streptokinase and 2400 units of streptodornase are contained in approximately 1 mg of extract, with lactose 5 mg, in one ampoule of the first International Standard Preparation (1964). The Christensen or U.S. unit is also used for streptokinase; it is equivalent to the International unit.

Adverse Effects. A pyogenic reaction may occur after instillation of streptokinase-streptodornase into closed body cavities but this may be minimised by frequent drainage. Other reactions include malaise, nausea, leucocytosis, and gastro-intestinal discomfort. Allergic reactions may occasionally occur.

In 22 patients treated buccally or rectally for 8 days with a preparation containing streptokinase-streptodornase, the incidence of antibodies to streptokinase was higher (17 of 22) 3 or 4 weeks after treatment than initially (8 of 22), and antibody titres were significantly increased. No significant changes in antibody titre occurred during 6 months in 13 controls. Antigenic material from streptokinase appeared to be absorbed from the oral and rectal mucosa and possibly from other parts of the gastro-intestinal tract.— F. Bachmann, *J. Lab. clin. Med.*, 1968, *72*, 228, per *J. Am. med. Ass.*, 1968, *206* (Sept. 30), A174.

Treatment of Adverse Effects. Fever may be treated with corticosteroids.

Precautions. Streptokinase-streptodornase should not be employed in the presence of active haemorrhage or acute cellulitis without suppuration, as it may interfere with clotting or encourage the spread of infections. Where bronchopleural fistulas have previously existed, there is a danger of reopening, especially in active tuberculosis. Injection of the enzymes into the peritoneal cavity after operations to prevent adhesions may result in leakage from sutured wounds or in secondary haemorrhage. Streptokinase-streptodornase is antigenic and high anti-enzyme titres may occur; in such cases doses may need to be increased. Streptokinase-streptodornase must not be given intravenously.

Uses. Streptokinase-streptodornase combines the fibrinolytic effects of streptokinase and the effect of streptodornase in lysing pus and is used topically or by instillation into closed body cavities to remove clotted blood or fibrinous or purulent accumulations. It is used as an adjunct in the treatment of haemothorax, haematoma, empyema, and suppurative lesions. It has been proposed for oral use as an adjunct in the treatment of oedema and trauma. Streptokinase-streptodornase is used topically in solutions containing 5000 International units of streptokinase and 1250 U.S. units of streptodornase per ml applied as wet dressings or by other suitable means. For instillation into closed cavities, a solution containing 200 000 units of streptokinase and 50 000 units of streptodornase has been suggested for large spaces, and 10 000 to 15 000 units of streptokinase and 2500 to 3750 units of streptodornase for small spaces such as in the treatment of maxillary sinus empyema. Provision must be made for adequate drainage. The suggested oral dose is 10 000 units of streptokinase and 2500 units of streptodornase 4 times daily. Streptokinase-streptodornase has also been given by intramuscular injection. It has also been administered by aerosol for thinning purulent, tenacious, bronchial secretion.

Streptokinase-streptodornase given by mouth in a single dose containing 1 million units of streptokinase caused no fibrinolytic activity in the plasma; streptokinase was not absorbed when given by mouth.— W. Fischbacher, *Schweiz. med. Wschr.*, 1967, *97*, 211, per *Int. pharm. Abstr.*, 1967, *4*, 574.

Periarthritis. Of 50 patients with humero-scapular periarthritis who took 4 Varidase tablets daily for 7 days, there was full restoration of function in 11 and only in 18 was there slight residual restriction of movement.— A. Hopf and H. W. Schmitt, *Dt. med. Wschr.*, 1964, *89*, 1691, per *Abstr. Wld Med.*, 1965, *37*, 124.

Skin testing. A preparation of streptokinase-streptodornase 5 units (streptokinase 4 units and streptodornase 1 unit) per 0.1 ml given intradermally is used as a skin test for delayed hypersensitivity. The erroneous use of a 1000 unit per 0.1 ml solution resulted in an accentuated delayed hypersensitivity reaction in 3 patients with fever and a markedly indurated, erythematous, and painful area at the injection site.— H. K. Steinman and P. G. Tuteur (letter), *New Engl. J. Med.*, 1979, *300*, 46.

Swelling and bruising. In a controlled study in 120 patients with superficial injuries, those treated with streptokinase 10 000 units and streptodornase 2500 units (Varidase tablets), 4 times daily for 5 days, showed greater improvement after 1 week than an untreated group. Disappearance of pain and swelling from the injury site was more rapid and an earlier return to normal function was evident.— M. Matta and G. L. Mouzas, *Practitioner*, 1972, *209*, 343. See also Report No. 27 of the General Practitioner Research Group, *Practitioner*, 1962, *189*, 89.

Wound healing. Streptokinase-streptodornase was not of value for debridement of deep bedsores, but was useful in the treatment of inflamed tissue beneath skin flaps after surgery.— M. RSather *et al.*, *Drug Intell. & clin. Pharm.*, 1977, *11*, 160.

Proctocolectomy was performed in 3 patients with Crohn's disease and 4 with ulcerative colitis. Varidase solution (1 vial dissolved in 20 ml of sodium chloride 0.9%) was instilled into the perineal wound daily in the first postoperative week. Wound healing occurred in 5 patients within 12 weeks. Treatment with Varidase solution in 6 patients with chronic suppurating perineal sinuses following proctocolectomy diminished suppuration and inflammation but wound healing did not occur.— S. Fasth *et al.*, *Curr. ther. Res.*, 1978, *24*, 813.

Proprietary Preparations

Varidase *(Lederle, UK)*. Vials each containing streptokinase 100 000 International units and streptodornase 25 000 U.S. units as powder for preparing solutions for topical use. **Varidase Oral Tablets** each contain streptokinase 10 000 International units and streptodornase 2500 U.S. units. (Also available as Varidase in *Austral.*, *Ger.*).

3748-y

Sutilains *(U.S.P.)*. BAX 1515.

CAS — 12211-28-8.

Pharmacopoeias. In *U.S.*

A cream-coloured powder containing proteolytic enzymes derived from *Bacillus subtilis*. It contains not less than 2 500 000 *U.S.P.* Casein units of proteolytic activity per g. A 1% solution has a pH of 6.1 to 7.1. **Store** at 2° to 8° in airtight containers.

Units. One *U.S.P.* Casein unit of proteolytic activity is contained in the amount of sutilains which when incubated at 37° with 35 mg of denatured casein, produces in 1 minute a hydrolysate whose absorbance at 275 nm is equal to that of a tyrosine solution containing 1.5 µg of *U.S.P.* Tyrosine Reference Standard per ml. The *U.S.P.* unit is equivalent to the earlier *U.S.N.F.* unit.

Adverse Effects. Pain, paraesthesia, bleeding, and transient dermatitis may occur.

Precautions. Contact with the eyes should be avoided. It should not be used in major body cavities, wounds containing exposed nerves or nervous tissues, or in fungating neoplastic lesions.

Uses. Sutilains is a proteolytic agent used for wound debridement. The wound should be moist, and cleansed of antiseptics such as benzalkonium chloride, hexachlorophane, iodine, nitrofurazone, silver nitrate, or those containing heavy metals which may reduce activity.

Preparations

Sutilains Ointment *(U.S.P.)*. A sterile ointment containing sutilains in a suitable ointment basis. Store at 2° to 8° in airtight containers.

Proprietary Names

Travase *(Flint, USA)*.

3749-j

Timonacic. ATC; Thioproline; NSC-25855. Thiazolidine-4-carboxylic acid.

$C_4H_7NO_2S$=133.2.

CAS — 444-27-9.

NOTE. The name ATC has also been used for a combination of paracetamol and trichloroethanol (4-acetamidophenyl 2,2,2-trichloroethyl carbonate).

Crystals. M.p. about 195°. Sparingly **soluble** in cold water; readily soluble in hot water, acids, and alkalis; practically insoluble in alcohol.

Timonacic is used as a choleretic. It has also been used as an adjuvant to the treatment of psoriasis and acne. It has been given in doses of 200 mg twice daily initially, followed by 100 mg twice daily for maintenance treatment.

A report of beneficial results, with no side-effects, following administration of the sodium salt of timonacic to patients with advanced cancer. A mild antitumour effect was noted with a dose of timonacic, 5 mg per kg body-weight daily intravenously or by mouth; definite activity was noted with 20 mg per kg intravenously for 5 days every 3 weeks, with complete remission in 2 patients when this was increased to 40 mg per kg. A regimen of 40 mg per kg intravenously daily appeared to be the most effective, with complete clinical remission 1 month after therapy began in all of 4 patients, which had so far lasted for 1 to over 2.5 months, no patient having discontinued therapy.— A. Brugarolas and M. Gosalvez, *Lancet*, 1980, *1*, 68. A warning concerning the toxicity of timonacic. Overdosage induces status epilepticus and coma within 15 minutes to an hour of ingestion. The toxic dose is especially low in young children whose blood-brain barrier is less effective, and seizures may occur with doses of 30 mg per kg body-weight and are always reported with more than 50 mg per kg; in adults seizures have been recorded with 60 mg per kg. These neurological disturbances are associated with initial transient hypoglycaemia followed by longer-lasting hyperglycaemia, and sometimes with hyperthermia. Seizures are readily controlled with diazepam, but EEG disturbances may persist for several weeks or even months. There have also been a number of cases of auditory sequelae (deafness or hypacusia).— R. Garnier *et al.* (letter), *ibid.*, 365. Toxicological studies on the sodium salt have indicated that the oral form of timonacic is more toxic than the intravenous form. Possibly it is hydrolysed in the stomach to yield cysteine and formaldehyde. Following intravenous injection it is rapidly eliminated unchanged in the urine which is why it is proposed to administer it to cancer patients at a dosage of 40 mg per kg body-weight daily by injection (in divided doses every six hours).— M. Gosálvez (letter), *ibid.*, 597. Further comment on the possible antitumour action of timonacic.— T. F. Slater (letter), *ibid.*. In a study of 5 patients timonacic had no beneficial effect on the tumours, and all patients showed progressive disease while on treatment. Three patients had somnolence and mild confusion one week after starting treatment, and one of these subsequently had frank psychosis with paranoid delusions.— A. P. Sappino and I. E. Smith (letter), *ibid.*, 1980, *2*, 417. Further evidence that timonacic is toxic to the CNS and a report that it also disturbs renal function. Lack of therapeutic effect was noted.— S. Nasca *et al.* (letter), *ibid.*, 1981, *1*, 778.

Proprietary Names

Detoxepa *(Ayerst, Ital.)*; Hepalidine *(Riker, Arg.*; *Riker, Fr.)*; Heparegen *(Gramon, Arg.)*; Héparégène *(Syntex, Switz.)*; Tiazolidin *(UCM-Difme, Ital.)*.

3750-q

Tocamphyl. The diethanolamine salt of 1-*p*-tolylethyl hydrogen (+)-camphorate.

$C_{19}H_{26}O_4,C_4H_{11}NO_2$=423.5.

CAS — 5634-42-4.

Tocamphyl is a choleretic agent obtained from turmeric (see p.432). It has been given in doses of 200 mg thrice daily.

Proprietary Names

Hépatoxane *(Élerté, Fr.).*

3751-p

Trypsin. Crystalline Trypsin; Trypsin Crystallized.

CAS — 9002-07-7.

Pharmacopoeias. In *Cz., Fr., It., Roum., Rus.,* and *U.S.* Crystallized Trypsin *U.S.P.* is crystallised from an extract of bovine pancreas. It contains not less than 2500 *U.S.P.* units in each mg, calculated on the dry basis.

A proteolytic enzyme (protease) obtained from mammalian pancreas by aqueous acid or alcoholic extraction of its precursor trypsinogen and subsequent conversion to trypsin.

A white to yellowish-white, odourless, crystalline or amorphous powder. **Soluble** in water; practically insoluble in alcohol, chloroform, ether, and glycerol. A solution in water has a pH of about 3 to 5. Stable in the dry state. Solutions retain about 80% of their activity for 24 hours at room temperature at pH 3; they should be freshly prepared; the stability in solution increases in the presence of calcium ions. Trypsin is most active at pH 7.6 to 8. **Store** in a cool place in airtight containers.

The properties and assay methods of trypsin.— Trypsin, in *Pharmaceutical Enzymes,* R. Ruyssen and A. Lauwers (Ed.), Gent, E. Story-Scientia, 1978, p. 33.

Activity. Trypsin purified electrophoretically had a specific activity of just over 8000 *N.F.* units per mg.— R. C. Peterson, *J. pharm. Sci.,* 1966, *55,* 49.

Stability. The addition of calcium chloride to ointments of trypsin in a macrogol basis prevented excessive loss of proteolytic activity. Trypsin ointment containing 600 mg of calcium chloride (dihydrate) in 100 g lost 20% of its activity in 6 months at room temperature and at 37°; without the calcium chloride the loss was 68%.— J. A. Bush, *J. pharm. Sci.,* 1962, *51,* 697.

Units. Trypsin is assayed for potency on the basis of its proteolytic activity and the potency of commercial products has been expressed in various units based on different methods of assay.

There are 2 principal methods of assay. One is based on the use of a denatured haemoglobin substrate; the other is based on the hydrolysis of *N*-benzoyl-L-arginine ethyl ester by trypsin at the ester linkage. Crystallized Trypsin *U.S.P.* is assayed for potency, by comparison with a reference standard, in terms of its ability to digest *N*-benzoyl-L-arginine ethyl ester hydrochloride at 25°. The hydrolysis is followed spectrophotometrically by measurement of the light absorption at 253 nm and the unit is determined by the average change in absorption per minute. One *U.S.P.* Trypsin unit is the activity causing a change in absorption of 0.003 per minute under the conditions specified in the assay. The *U.S.P.* unit is equivalent to the earlier *U.S.N.F.* unit.

One FIP unit of trypsin activity is contained in that amount of the standard preparation which, under specified conditions, hydrolyses 1 μmol of *N*-benzoyl-L-arginine ethyl ester as the hydrochloride per minute. The hydrolysis is followed potentiometrically.

One Armour unit is equivalent to 1 *U.S.P.* unit. One Anson unit is equivalent to 160 000 *U.S.P.* units.

Adverse Effects. Allergic reactions with symptoms of fever, skin rash, and, occasionally, angioneurotic oedema and urticaria may follow intramuscular injections or instillation of solutions into closed cavities. Reactions may be diminished by prior administration of an antihistamine. It has been suggested that where allergy is suspected, a sensitivity test should be made before injection. Application of the dry powder to surface lesions may cause a severe burning sensation. Intramuscular injections may be followed by pain and induration at the site of injection. A leucocytosis may also occur.

A 43-year-old man who had developed a cough and vasomotor rhinitis while working for 7 years in a factory processing trypsin, and then had daily asthma attacks, was shown by skin testing to have become sensitive to trypsin. Aerosol preparations containing trypsin should be used with care in patients with asthma.— B. Zweiman *et al., J. Allergy,* 1967, *39,* 11, per *Abstr. Wld Med.,* 1967, *41,* 512.

Precautions. Trypsin should not be employed in patients with severe hepatic insufficiency and should be given cautiously to patients with renal damage or irregularities of the blood-clotting mechanism. It should not be given intravenously or applied topically to bleeding areas or ulcerated carcinomas. Topical application should be used with caution in tuberculous empyema and in bronchopleural fistula caused by tuberculosis. It should not be used for a week after pulmonary haemorrhage.

Uses. Trypsin is a proteolytic enzyme which catalyses the hydrolysis of proteins, polypeptides, amides, and esters at bonds involving the carboxyl group of L-arginine and L-lysine. It is therefore used for the removal of coagulated blood, exudate, and necrotic tissue as an adjunct in the treatment of necrotic wounds and ulcers, abscesses, empyemas, haematomas, sinuses, and fistulas, and to separate eschar in second-degree burns. It has no effect on viable tissue because of the presence of inhibitors. It may be applied as a dry powder, the lesion being moistened if necessary with sodium chloride injection, as wet compresses of a solution containing about 10 000 *U.S.P.* units per ml, or by instillation of a similar solution. Powder dressings may be applied every 15 to 30 minutes for small lesions and every 3 hours for large areas; wet dressings or irrigations may be repeated 3-hourly. For intrapleural use 25 ml of a solution containing 10 000 *U.S.P* units per ml is instilled once or twice daily after prior aspiration of the intrapleural space and irrigation with sodium chloride injection. An antihistamine is given concomitantly to prevent reactions due to the absorption of products of hydrolysis.

Trypsin is also used as an aerosol solution containing up to 125 000 *U.S.P.* units in 3 ml of sodium chloride injection for the liquefaction of viscous sputum; such solutions may be irritant. Trypsin has been given intramuscularly in doses of 12 500 to 25 000 *U.S.P.* units daily. Trypsin is also given by mouth in conjunction with chymotrypsin.

Back pain. Tablets containing trypsin and chymotrypsin (Chymoral) were given to 28 patients with back pain sufficiently severe to necessitate bed rest. The dose was 2 tablets 4 times daily for 2 days, then one 4 times daily for 8 days. Straight-leg raising appeared to be improved, but pain, tenderness, and mobility were not different in treated patients and patients receiving a placebo.— K. Hingorani, *Br. J. clin. Pract.,* 1968, *22,* 209.

Cystic fibrosis. There were no significant changes in ventilatory function or in the clinical findings in 11 children with varying degrees of ventilatory deficiency due to cystic fibrosis who were given 1 Chymoral tablet, containing trypsin and chymotrypsin, 6-hourly for 3 months.— J. P. Stanfield, *Br. med. J.,* 1963, *1,* 727.

Trauma. Treatment of football injuries with tablets containing trypsin and chymotrypsin (Chymoral) resulted in more rapid healing of muscular and other soft-tissue injuries than ligamentous injuries and overall the results were better than with previous treatments.— P. S. Boyne and H. Medhurst, *Practitioner,* 1967, *198,* 543.

A trypsin-chymotrypsin mixture effectively reduced inflammation and associated oedema in minor injuries sustained by 111 patients.— J. E. Buck and N. Phillips, *Br. J. clin. Pract.,* 1970, *24,* 375.

Further references to the use of trypsin with chymotrypsin in traumatic conditions.— S. D. Soule *et al., Am. J Obstet. Gynec.,* 1966, *95,* 820 (episiotomy); J. L. Blonstein, *Practitioner,* 1967, *198,* 547 (boxing injuries); W. F. Rathgeber, *S. Afr. med. J.,* 1971, *45,* 181 (sporting injuries); A. De N'Yeurt, *J.R. Coll. gen. Pract.,* 1972, *22,* 633 (vasectomy); T. Winsor, *J. clin. Pharmac.,* 1972, *12,* 325 (first-degree burns); W. F. Rathgeber, *Clin. Med.,* 1973, *80* (Aug.), 39 (tenosynovitis of the forearm).

Tuberculosis. Eight children in Mexico with tuberculous meningo-encephalitis were given intrathecal injections of trypsin and chymotrypsin (usually 2 mg of each in 5 ml every third day, increased in severe cases to 3 mg of each in 3 ml daily) together with chemotherapeutic agents, but not corticosteroids. Recovery of motor function was complete in 5 patients and partial in 3. Intracranial hypertension developed in 3 patients and hydrocephalus in 1. Compared with the general death-rate of 50%, the treatment appeared to reduce intracranial complications. One child had fever and skin rash after an injection made with a solvent containing hydrolysed gelatin, but not after aqueous injections.— O. H. D. Marquez and F. G. Segur, *Médicina, Mex.,* 1968, *48,* 61, per *Abstr. Wld Med.,* 1968, *42,* 800.

Ulcers and bedsores. In the treatment of post-thrombotic leg ulcers, use of an ointment containing proteolytic enzymes (Chymacort ointment) promoted more rapid healing than the ointment basis without enzymes.— B. Gordon, *Br. J. clin. Pract.,* 1975, *29,* 143.

Bedsores in a group of patients treated with a spray containing trypsin, peru balsam, and castor oil were reported to have healed twice as rapidly as controls treated without medication.— M. R. Sather *et al., Drug Intell. & clin. Pharm.,* 1977, *11,* 163.

Preparations

Crystallized Trypsin for Inhalation Aerosol *(U.S.P.).* Trypsin Crystallized for Aerosol. Prepared by freeze-drying. Store at a temperature not exceeding 40°.

Proprietary Preparations

Chymacort Ointment *(Armour, UK).* Contains in each g proteolytic activity (provided by a concentrate of chymotrypsin and trypsin) 10 000 Armour units and hydrocortisone acetate 10 mg.

Chymoral *(Armour, UK).* Enteric-coated tablets of trypsin and chymotrypsin, each tablet providing total enzyme activity of 50 000 Armour units. For inflammatory oedema due to trauma or surgery, and the reduction of the viscosity of bronchial exudates. *Dose.* 2 tablets 4 times daily, half an hour before meals; children, 1 tablet 4 times daily. **Chymoral Forte.** Tablets of twice the above strength.

Trypure Novo *(Novo, UK: Farillon, UK).* Pure crystalline trypsin stabilised with a small amount of an inert calcium salt and stated to contain about 4000 *U.S.P.* units per mg, available as **Powder** for preparing solutions in vials of 50 mg together with vials of 15 ml of diluent containing sodium chloride 0.9% and hydroxybenzoates; as **Dispersible Powder** containing 1% in sprinkler-bottles of 5 g together with 45 ml of wetting solution containing lignocaine hydrochloride 2%, cetrimide 0.1%, and sodium chloride 0.47%; and as **Spray** containing 1% in an aerosol together with 45 ml of wetting solution. (Also available as Trypure Novo in *Denm., Ger., Ital., Neth., Norw., Switz.*).

Other Proprietary Names

Tryptar *(Austral.).*

Trypsin was also formerly marketed in Great Britain under the proprietary name Tryptar (*Armour*).

3752-s

Urokinase. An enzyme obtained from human urine, or from tissue cultures of human kidney cells.

CAS — 9039-53-6.

A colourless freeze-dried powder. **Soluble** in water. Stable at 4° when dry. Aqueous solutions are stable for about 3 days at 4°. **Store** at 4°.

The properties and assay methods of urokinase. It was generally admitted that preparations of urokinase obtained from the extraction of human urine must be able to activate plasminogen to plasmin for an activity of 24 FIP units per mg of protein.— Urokinase, in

Pharmaceutical Enzymes, R. Ruyssen and A. Lauwers (Ed.), Gent, E. Story-Scientia, 1978, p. 133.

An investigation of some commercially available urokinase preparations for contamination by biologically active substances.— M. Nobuhara *et al., J. clin. Hosp. Pharm.,* 1979, *4,* 179.

Units. 4800 units of urokinase are contained in approximately 1.8 mg of urokinase, with lactose 5 mg, in one ampoule of the first International Reference Preparation (1968). See also abstracts below.

In Great Britain potency is also expressed in arbitrary units known as Ploug units. One Ploug unit is approximately equivalent to 1.5 International units.

In the USA, potency has been expressed in CTA Units (National Heart Institute Committee on Thrombolytic Agents). One CTA unit is approximately equivalent to 1 International unit.

One FIP unit of urokinase hydrolyses 1 μmol of *N*-α-acetyl-glycyl-L-lysine methyl ester acetate per minute. One FIP unit is equivalent to 546 Ploug units and approximately to 780 CTA units.

Since the definition of the international unit, urokinase preparations have been shown to have 2 forms of different molecular weight (33 000 and 55 000). It is not yet known whether these 2 forms have different pharmacological properties or half-lives however, they may be partly responsible for variations in assay results.— *Tech. Rep. Ser. Wld Hlth Org. No. 610,* 1977.

The isolation, from commercial preparations, of a third urinary urokinase with a molecular weight of 22 000 had been reported.— Urokinase, in *Pharmaceutical Enzymes,* R. Ruyssen and A. Lauwers (Ed.), Gent, E. Story-Scientia, 1978, p. 133.

Adverse Effects, Treatment, and Precautions. As for Streptokinase, p.656. Serious allergic reactions may be less likely to occur with urokinase than with streptokinase.

Sickle-cell disease was a contra-indication to the use of urokinase.— F. I. D. Konotey-Ahulu (letter), *Lancet,* 1972, *2,* 714.

The conversion of plasminogen to plasmin by urokinase can be inhibited by aminocaproic acid and tranexamic acid but this conversion is not inhibited by aprotinin.— Urokinase, in *Pharmaceutical Enzymes,* R. Ruyssen and A. Lauwers (Ed.), Gent, E. Story-Scientia, 1978, p. 133.

Uses. Urokinase directly converts plasminogen to plasmin (see p.655) a proteolytic enzyme which has fibrinolytic effects.

Urokinase is used to lyse fibrin or blood clots in the eye. For hyphaemia, doses of 5000 to 7500 International units dissolved in 2 ml of sodium chloride injection are used. Doses of up to 37 500 units have sometimes been employed. For vitreous haemorrhage, solutions of 7500 to 37 500 units dissolved in 0.5 to 1.5 ml of Water for Injections may be used.

It is also used to lyse clots in arterio-venous shunts in doses of 5000 to 37 500 units. In the treatment of pulmonary embolism urokinase is given by intravenous infusion in initial doses of 4400 units per kg body-weight over 10 minutes, followed by 4400 units per kg per hour for 12 hours.

Action. For detailed reviews and comments on the action and uses of urokinase, see A. S. Gallus and J. Hirsh, *Drugs,* 1976, *12,* 132; V. V. Kakkar and M. F. Scully, *Br. med. Bull.,* 1978, *34,* 191; W. R. Bell and A. G. Meek, *New Engl. J. Med.,* 1979, *301,* 1266; P. Wolf (letter), *ibid.,* 1980, *302,* 812; M. S. Hansen and I. Clemmensen (letter), *ibid.,* 813; W. R. Bell and A. G. Meek (letter), *ibid.* Summary of an NIH Consensus Conference, *Br. med. J.,* 1980, *280,* 1585.

Further references relating to the action and uses of urokinase: P. T. Flute, *Br. J. Hosp. Med.,* 1976, *16,* 135; J. M. Porter and S. H. Goodnight, *Am. J. Surg.,* 1977, *134,* 217; V. J. Marder, *Ann. intern. Med.,* 1979, *90,* 802.

Leucocytes and the leucocyte-plasma interaction are both important in the fibrinolytic action of urokinase.— L. A. Moroz *et al., New Engl. J. Med.,* 1979, *301,* 1100.

Administration. Urokinase, obtained from urine or from tissue culture, was given to 30 patients with pulmonary embolism in doses of 2000 CTA units per lb body-weight initially over 10 minutes followed by 2000 CTA units per lb hourly for 12 hours. The results demonstrated biochemical equivalence and equal safety for the two types of urokinase when administered at this dose, and it seemed reasonable to expect that they are equally effective in altering haemodynamic and clinical parameters of patients with pulmonary embolism.— V. J. Marder *et al., J. Lab. clin. Med.,* 1978, *92,* 721.

See also under Thrombo-embolic Disorders, below.

Blood clots in the eye. Reviews and comments on the use of urokinase in the treatment of vitreous haemorrhage.— *Br. J. Ophthal.,* 1977, *61,* 499; *Br. med. J.,* 1978, *1,* 940.

Treatment of 27 patients with unresolved vitreous haemorrhage with urokinase, at a usual dose of 25 000 Ploug units by intravitreal injection gave the following results; 10 eyes showed marked improvement; 9 eyes improved subjectively, 10 remained unchanged and 3 became worse. Hypopyon, which resolved within 5 to 6 days occurred in 22 eyes and transient glaucoma was noted in some patients.— J. S. Chapman-Smith and G. W. Crock, *Br. J. Ophthal.,* 1977, *61,* 500. Criticism.— G. A. Peyman *et al., ibid.,* 1978, *62,* 70. A reply.— J. S. Chapman-Smith and G. W. Crock, *ibid.,* 71.

Further references: D. Pierse and H. LeGrice (preliminary communication), *Lancet,* 1963, *2,* 1143; J. Williamson and J. V. Forrester (letter), *ibid.,* 1972, *2,* 488; W. N. Dugmore and M. Raichand (letter), *ibid.,* 660; J. Williamson and J. V. Forrester (letter), *ibid.,* 1973, *1,* 888; J. Williamson (letter), *Br. med. J.,* 1973, *2,* 666; J. Forrester and J. Williamson, *Lancet,* 1973, *2,* 179; P. Sternberg *et al.* (letter), *New Engl. J. Med.,* 1980, *302,* 812.

Haemolytic disorders. In the treatment of acute microangiopathic disease, urokinase might be indicated when other measures failed.— S. M. Rosen *et al.* (letter), *Br. med. J.,* 1970, *3,* 465.

Postpartum renal failure. In a 26-year-old woman with acute renal failure postpartum urokinase, given by the catheter used for renal arteriography, increased the blood flow but did not restore renal function.— M. Cochran *et al., Br. med. J.,* 1977, *1,* 1257.

Renal cortical necrosis. A report of the local infusion of urokinase and heparin into the renal arteries of 4 patients with impending renal cortical necrosis.— F. E. Jones *et al., Br. med. J.,* 1975, *4,* 547.

Myocardial infarction. Of 17 patients with acute myocardial infarction, treated within 14 hours with urokinase 3630 CTA units per kg body-weight initially, then 3630 CTA units per kg per hour for 8 hours, 14 survived. The study was considered to demonstrate the feasibility of the use of urokinase.— G. I. Litman *et al., Am. J. Cardiol.,* 1971, *27,* 636. A contrary view.— T. L. Simon *et al., Ann. intern. Med.,* 1973, *79,* 712.

In a controlled study of 341 patients with acute cardiac infarction urokinase produced a fibrinolytic state but did not influence the mortalityrate compared with placebo during a 1-year follow-up.—A European Collaborative Study, *Lancet,* 1975, *2,* 624.

Further references: *J. Am. med. Ass.,* 1974, *228,* 1629; R. D. Sautter *et al.* (letter), *ibid., 230,* 34; M. S. Mazel *et al., J. Am. Geriat. Soc.,* 1975, *23,* 419; P. Babeau and P. Pras, *Annls Med. intern. Paris,* 1977, *128,* 219.

Thrombo-embolic disorders. A review of the use and side-effects of urokinase in the treatment of pulmonary embolism and deep-vein thrombosis.— *Med. Lett.,* 1978, *20,* 37.

Thrombolytic therapy in treatment.—Summary of an NIH Consensus Conference, *Br. med. J.,* 1980, *280,* 1585.

Urokinase given intra-arterially was successful in clearing occlusions of the radial and ulnar arteries in a 47-year-old man.— B. J. Boucher *et al., Postgrad. med. J.,* 1973, *49,* 365.

A report of the use of urokinase and heparin in 32 patients 1 to 6 weeks after deep-vein thrombosis.— G. Trübestein *et al., Dt. med. Wschr.,* 1979, *104,* 1241.

Further references.— D. Silver, *Archs Surg., Chicago,* 1968, *97,* 910; G. Patron *et al., Thérapie,* 1975, *30,* 695.

Cerebral occlusions. A pilot study of urokinase therapy in cerebral infarction.— A. P. Fletcher *et al., Stroke,* 1976, *7,* 135.

Further references: A. Larcan *et al., Thérapie,* 1977, *32,* 259.

Pulmonary occlusions. A discussion of the use of urokinase in the treatment of pulmonary embolism.— D. A. Tibbutt and C. N. Chesterman, *Drugs,* 1976, *11,* 161. See also *Drug & Ther. Bull.,* 1980, *18,* 45.

Urokinase 200 000 to 300 000 Ploug units infused into the pulmonary artery over 2 hours in 8 patients with major pulmonary embolism produced rapid improvement in 7 patients. Two died of recurrent emboli, 1 of whom had improved with urokinase.— I. R. Edwards *et al., Lancet,* 1973, *2,* 409.

In a controlled multicentre study of 160 patients with proven recent pulmonary embolisms, 82 were treated with urokinase 2000 CTA units per lb body-weight infused intravenously over 10 minutes followed by 2000 CTA units per lb each hour for 12 hours and 78 were given heparin 75 units per lb intravenously followed by 10 units per lb each hour for 12 hours. All patients were then given heparin intravenously for 5 days and treatment was continued for 14 days with either heparin or warfarin. Assessments showed that patients given urokinase had a quicker resolution of their emboli, 31% showing considerable improvement at 24 hours, and that patients with massive emboli appeared to benefit most. Bleeding complications occurred in 45% of patients during the first 24 hours of urokinase treatment and during the first 2 weeks in 27% of patients given heparin.—A National Cooperative Study of the American Heart Association, *Circulation,* 1973, *47, Suppl.* II 1. Comments.— *Lancet,* 1973, *1,* 1427; *J. Am. med. Ass.,* 1974, *227,* 1168.

In a comparative trial 167 patients with pulmonary embolism received either urokinase for 12 or 24 hours or streptokinase. A loading dose of 4400 CTA units of urokinase per kg body-weight was followed by 4400 CTA units per kg body-weight per hour by constant infusion for either 12 or 24 hours. A loading dose of 250 000 units of streptokinase given over 20 to 30 minutes was followed by 100 000 units per hour by constant infusion for 24 hours. Heparin was administered as necessary to control prothrombin time. In clot resolution, urokinase therapy for 24 hours was no more effective than urokinase therapy for 12 hours, but slightly more effective than streptokinase therapy for 24 hours. There was no significant difference in mortality or bleeding complications between groups. Allergic reactions occurred in 3 patients treated with streptokinase.—A Cooperative Study, *J. Am. med. Ass.,* 1974, *229,* 1606.

Further references: M. Brochier *et al., Sem. Hôp. Paris,* 1973, *49,* 1825; K. J. Dickie *et al., Am. Rev. resp. Dis.,* 1974, *109,* 48.

Proprietary Preparations

Abbokinase *(Abbott, UK).* Urokinase, obtained from tissue cultures of human kidney cells, available as powder for preparing injections, in vials of 250 000 International units with mannitol 25 mg and sodium chloride 25 mg. (Also available as Abbokinase in *USA.*

Ukidan *(Serono, UK).* Urokinase, obtained from human male urine, available as powder for preparing solutions, in vials each containing 5000 or 25 000 International units. (Also available as Ukidan in *Ital.*).

Urokinase *(Leo, UK).* Urokinase, obtained from human male urine, available as powder for preparing solutions, in ampoules each containing 5000, 25 000, or 100 000 Ploug units equivalent to 7500, 37 500, or 150 000 International units.

Other Proprietary Names

Breokinase *(USA)*; Wakamoto 6000 *(Jap.).*

3753-w

Ursodeoxycholic Acid. Ursodesoxycholic Acid; UDCA. 3α,7β-Dihydroxy-5β-cholan-24-oic acid.

$C_{24}H_{40}O_4$=392.6.

CAS — 128-13-2.

Pharmacopoeias. In *Jap.*

A white odourless crystalline powder with a bitter taste. M.p. about 199°. Practically **insoluble** in water; freely soluble in alcohol and glacial acetic acid; slightly soluble in chloroform; very slightly soluble in ether.

Adverse Effects and Precautions. As for Chenodeoxycholic Acid, p.646.

Absorption and Fate. Ursodeoxycholic acid is absorbed from the gastro-intestinal tract and undergoes enterohepatic circulation. In comparison with chenodeoxycholic acid (see p.646), less ursodeoxycholic acid undergoes bacterial degradation to lithocholic acid.

References: T. Fedorowski *et al., Gastroenterology,* 1977, *73,* 1131; A. Stiehl *et al., ibid.,* 1978, *75,* 1016.

Uses. Ursodeoxycholic acid is the 7β-epimer of chenodeoxycholic acid (seep.646) and is used similarly for the dissolution of gall-stones. The usual dose is 450 to 600 mg daily in 2 divided doses after meals; the second dose should be taken after the evening meal. Ursodeoxycholic acid has also been used by mouth in the treatment of hepatic disorders or as the sodium salt by intravenous injection.

For reports on the actions of ursodeoxycholic acid, see T. Fedorowski *et al.*, *Gastroenterology*, 1977, *73*, 1131; N. Carulli *et al.*, *Gut*, 1978, *19*, A994; A. Stiehl *et al.*, *Gastroenterology*, 1978, *75*, 1016; E. Roda *et al.*, *Dig. Dis. Sci.*, 1979, *24*, 123.

Gall-stones. For reviews and discussions on the dissolution of gall-stones, including mention of the use of ursodeoxycholic acid, see *Br. med. J.*, 1978, *2*, 309; *ibid.*, 847.

There was complete or partial dissolution of gall-stones in 8 of 31 patients given ursodeoxycholic acid 150 or 600 mg daily in divided doses for at least 6 months. There was no change in 13 patients given placebo. It was considered that the minimum effective dose was 2.8 mg per kg body-weight daily. Gall-stones greater than 10 mm in diameter did not respond. The only side-effect appeared to be a 21% reduction in serum-triglyceride concentrations.— S. Nakagawa *et al.*, *Lancet*, 1977, *2*, 367.

Ursodeoxycholic acid 150 mg thrice daily was given to 68 patients with gall-stones and a functioning gall-bladder for at least 6 months. Stones disappeared or were reduced in size or number in 24 of 46 patients with no calcification of the stones and in 6 of 22 with some calcification.— M. Okumura *et al.*, *Gastroenterol. Jap.*, 1977, *12*, 469.

Ursodeoxycholic acid initially in doses of about 5, 10, and 15 mg per kg body-weight daily then adjusted individually was evaluated in 9 patients with radiolucent gall-stones. Two additional patients withdrew in the first month to undergo surgery for severe biliary colic or transient obstructive jaundice. The fate of the gall-stones was assessed in 3 of the 9 patients at 6 months; there was complete dissolution in 1 with partial dissolution in the other 2. Dissolution with ursodeoxycholic acid as with chenodeoxycholic acid might be mediated by a reduction in hepatic cholesterol synthesis. Biliary cholesterol saturation was reduced. Ursodeoxycholic acid had advantages over chenodeoxycholic acid in being effective at about a half to two-thirds the dose, in not causing diarrhoea, and in not affecting liver-transaminase values. A recommended dose was 10 mg per kg daily.— P. N. Maton *et al.*, *Lancet*, 1977, *2*, 1297. See also P. N. Maton *et al.*, *Clin. Sci. & mol. Med.*, 1978, *54*, 32p.

Treatment of 12 patients, suffering from gall-stones, with ursodeoxycholic acid 250 mg or 500 mg daily for one month in a crossover study reduced biliary-cholesterol concentration to normal but cholesterol saturation indices did not fall consistently. Most patients reported improved abdominal symptoms.— M. C. Bateson *et al.*, *Gut*, 1978, *19*, A972.

It was concluded from studies in 120 patients with radiolucent gall-stones who were treated with chenodeoxycholic acid (CDCA) and 22 similar patients given ursodeoxycholic acid (UDCA) that UDCA had comparable efficacy to CDCA at two-thirds of the dose, did not cause diarrhoea, and might replace CDCA.— G. Williams *et al.*, *Gut*, 1978, *19*, A94.

Calcification of radiolucent gall-stones during treatment with ursodeoxycholic acid.— M. C. Bateson *et al.*, *Br. med. J.*, 1981, *283*, 645.

Further references: K. Kutz and A. Schulte (letter), *Gastroenterology*, 1977, *73*, 632; G. Salvioli *et al.*, *Curr. ther. Res.*, 1979, *26*, 995; M. C. Bateson *et al.*, *Gut*, 1980, *21*, 305.

Hyperlipidaemia. In a double-blind crossover study 12 patients with primary endogenous hypertriglyceridaemia were given ursodeoxycholic acid 250 mg thrice daily for one month or chenodeoxycholic acid 250 mg thrice daily for one month. Despite their close chemical relationship and similar effects on biliary cholesterol, results indicated that, unlike chenodeoxycholic acid, ursodeoxycholic acid does not lower increased serum-triglyceride concentrations.— M. C. Bateson and J. Iqbal (letter), *Lancet*, 1979, *2*, 151.

Steatorrhoea. In a preliminary study of 6 patients with steatorrhoea after ileal resections, ursodeoxycholic acid 250 mg was given before meals for 4 days. Replacement of bile acid with ursodeoxycholic acid reduced steatorrhoea and diarrhoea and daily faecal fat fell by a mean of 15%. In a further patient given ursodeoxycholic acid 4 g daily there was a 50% reduction in faecal fat.— T. M. Cox *et al.*, *Gut*, 1978, *19*, A970.

Proprietary Preparations

Destolit *(Merrell, UK)*. Ursodeoxycholic acid, available as tablets of 150 mg.

Other Proprietary Names

Deursil, Ursacol *(both Ital.)*; Urso *(Jap.)*; Ursochol *(Neth.)*.

3754-e

Vanitiolide. Vanitiolidum. 4-(Thiovanilloyl)morpholine; 4-(4-Hydroxy-3-methoxythiobenzoyl)morpholine.
$C_{12}H_{15}NO_3S$=253.3.

CAS — 17692-71-6.

Vanitiolide is a choleretic. It has been given in doses of 500 mg thrice daily, before meals, for up to 10 days.

Proprietary Names

Bildux *(Millot-Solac, Fr.)*.

3755-l

Proprietary Preparations of Other Mixed Enzymes

Vasolastine *(Enzypharm, UK: Rona, UK)*. A solution for intramuscular injection in ampoules of 2 ml each containing enzymes of lipid metabolism 8000 Enzypharm units, amine oxidase 4000 Enzypharm units, and tyrosinase 4000 Enzypharm units. For atheroscleosis and associated symptoms. *Dose.* Initially, 2 ml daily, reducing to 2 ml thrice weekly; maintenance, 2 ml once to twice weekly.

Atherosclerosis. In a double-blind study in 38 patients with atherosclerosis, Vasolastine was given intramuscularly, 2 ml daily for 6 days per week for 2 weeks, then thrice weekly for 4 weeks, and was compared with a placebo. Vasolastine appeared to be capable of favourably affecting both hypercholesterolaemia and defective metabolism which might cause excess deposition of cholesterol and other lipids in the arterial wall.— J. P. Saunders, *Br. J. clin. pract.*, 1967, *21*, 341.

Coma. Of 37 patients with coma due to various causes, but not to damage caused by haemorrhage, 25 responded to treatment with Vasolastine and Coliacron, together with conventional treatment, and were conscious within 3 to 6 hours of commencement of treatment. The dose was 4 ml each of Vasolastine and of Coliacron initially, by intramuscular injection, followed by 2 ml every hour until there was a response and then every 2 or 4 hours. There were no side-effects.— P. E. van Coller, *Med. Proc.*, 1968, *14*, 102.

Injectable preparations containing mixed enzymes were formerly marketed in Great Britain under the proprietary names Coliacron, Interacton, and Rheumajecta (all *Enzypharm*).

Ergot and Ergot Derivatives

1500-t

Seven isomeric pairs of alkaloids have been isolated from ergot: ergocristine and ergocristinine (ergotinine), ergotamine and ergotaminine, ergocryptine and ergocryptinine, ergocornine and ergocorninine (ψ-ergotinine), ergosine and ergosinine, ergostine and ergostinine, ergometrine (ergonovine, ergobasine, ergostetrine, ergotocine) and ergometrinine. Ergotoxine, the first active substance to be isolated from ergot was later found to be a mixture of ergocristine, ergocornine, and ergocryptine.

The first 12 of these alkaloids are derivatives of lysergic or isolysergic acid combined with polypeptide groups. In ergometrine and ergometrinine, however, the polypeptide group is replaced by propanolamine, which accounts for their greater solubility in water. Ergomonamine, which unlike all the other alkaloids is not an indole derivative, has also been isolated. The first named of each of the isomeric pairs is laevorotatory and physiologically active while the second is dextrorotatory and has little physiological activity. The active alkaloids show a general tendency to form additive compounds; they crystallise with solvent of crystallisation and they form crystalline equimolecular compounds such as sensibamine (ergotamine and ergotaminine) and ergoclavine (ergosine and ergosinine). The nature and quantity of the alkaloids present in ergot vary with the geographical source.

Semi-synthetic derivatives of ergot alkaloids have been prepared. Hydrogenation of one of the double bonds of lysergic acid produces stable dihydrogenated alkaloids such as dihydroergotamine. The addition of an amine to lysergic acid and *N*-methyllysergic acid has led to the production of methylergometrine and methysergide respectively.

The ergot alkaloids were the first alpha-adrenoceptor blocking agents discovered but in general side-effects prevent the administration of doses that could produce more than minimal blockade in man. Different alkaloids and their derivatives have varying degrees of blocking activity; dihydrogenated alkaloids are potent blocking agents while compounds such as ergometrine and methylergometrine, which lack a polypeptide side-chain in their structure, possess little or none of this activity. The stimulation of smooth muscle, especially that of the blood vessels and the uterus, has been attributed to a direct action but it has also been suggested to be due, in part at least, to an alpha-adrenoceptor agonist action. Thus the alkaloids may be considered to be a series of partial agonists. Ergot alkaloids also produce complex excitation and depression of the central nervous system. The overall vasodilatation produced by co-dergocrine is believed to be predominantly due to a central action. There is also evidence that ergot derivatives interact with many other systems, including serotonin and dopamine receptors. The alkaloids of ergot and their derivatives have many clinical applications. Ergometrine and methylergometrine are used in obstetrics and ergotamine, dihydroergotamine, and lysuride are used mainly for the relief of migraine. Co-dergocrine and nicergoline are employed for their vasodilator properties and metergoline is used similarly to bromocriptine (see p.894). Also included in this section is methysergide which is also used mainly for the relief of migraine.

The chemistry and pharmacology of the alkaloids of ergot.— A. Stoll, *Pharm. J.*, 1965, *1*, 605.

Some aspects of receptor pharmacology of ergotamine.— H. O. Schild, *Postgrad. med. J.*, 1976, *52, Suppl.* 1, 9. See also W. H. Aellig, *Postgrad. med. J.*, 1976, *52, Suppl.* 1, 21.

An historical view on ergot alkaloids.— A. Hofmann, *Pharmacology*, 1978, *16, Suppl.* 1, 1.

General pharmacology of ergot alkaloids.— J. R. Boissier, *Pharmacology*, 1978, *16, Suppl.* 1, 12.

Preparations of Mixed Ergot Alkaloids

Ergotal *(Rus. P.)*. A mixture of phosphates of ergot alkaloids. A grey powder with a slight characteristic odour; very sparingly soluble in water.

Solutio Ergotali 0.05% pro Injectionibus *(Rus. P.)*. Ergotal 50 mg, tartaric acid 1 g, sodium metabisulphite 8 mg, chlorbutol 50 mg, Water for Injections to 100 ml; in ampoules of 1 ml.

Tabulettae Ergotali *(Rus. P.)*. Tablets each containing ergotal 1 mg, with excipient q.s. to 100 mg.

1501-x

Ergot *(B.P.C. 1968)*. Secale Cornutum; Rye Ergot; Ergot de Seigle; Grano Speronato; Mutterkorn; Cornezuelo de Centeno; Esporão de Centeio; Cravagem de Centeio.

Pharmacopoeias. In *Arg., Aust., Fr., Ind., Int., Port., Roum., Rus., Span.*, and *Turk.*

The sclerotium of the fungus *Claviceps purpurea* (Hypocreaceae) developed in the ovary of the rye, *Secale cereale* (Gramineae), containing not less than 0.15% of total alkaloids, calculated as ergotoxine, and not less than 0.01% of water-soluble alkaloids, calculated as ergometrine. Ergot should be thoroughly dried, kept entire, and stored in a cool place. If powdered and stored without the immediate removal of the fat the alkaloidal content decreases.

NOTE. When Ergot or Powdered Ergot is prescribed, Prepared Ergot is dispensed.

1502-r

Prepared Ergot *(B.P.C. 1968)*. Prep. Ergot.; Ergota Praeparata; Secalis Cornuti Pulvis Standardisatus.

Pharmacopoeias. In *Arg., Aust., Ind., Int.*, and *Turk.* which all specify about 0.2% of total alkaloids.

Powdered and defatted ergot adjusted to contain 0.15% of total alkaloids, calculated as ergotoxine. A purplish-brown powder with an unpleasant odour and taste. **Store** in a cool place in airtight containers. Protect from light.

A comparison of alkaloid contents of Argentine and European ergot.— G. E. Ferraro *et al.* (letter), *J. Pharm. Pharmac.*, 1976, *28*, 729.

Adverse Effects. Symptoms of acute poisoning are nausea, vomiting, diarrhoea, thirst, coldness of the skin, pruritus, weak pulse, numbness and tingling of the extremities, confusion, and unconsciousness.

Chronic ergotism may result from therapeutic overdosage, especially following administration to patients with severe infection, such as puerperal fever, and to patients with liver disease or hyperthyroidism. Circulatory disturbances due to vasoconstriction and thrombi formation are usually the first symptoms to appear, including coldness of the skin, severe muscle pains, and vascular stasis resulting in dry peripheral gangrene. Anginal pain, tachycardia or bradycardia, and hypotension or hypertension may occur. Other symptoms are headache, nausea, vomiting, diarrhoea, dizziness, and weakness of the legs; miosis has been reported. Nervous symptoms are confusion, drowsiness, hemiplegia, and convulsions.

Epidemic ergot poisoning, arising from the ingestion of ergotised rye bread, is now seldom seen. Two forms of epidemic toxicity, which rarely occur together, have been described, a gangrenous form characterised by agonising pain of the extremities of the body followed by dry gangrene of the peripheral parts, and a rarer nervous type giving rise to paroxysmal epileptiform convulsions.

A report of an outbreak of ergotism, attributed to the ingestion of infected wild oats (*Avena abyssinica*), in Wollo, Ethiopia.— B. King (letter), *Lancet*, 1979, *1*, 1411.

Treatment of Adverse Effects. Treatment of acute poisoning is symptomatic. The stomach should be emptied by aspiration and lavage. Amyl nitrite inhalations may be given.

In cases of chronic poisoning, treatment consists of complete withdrawal of the drug and attempts to prevent gangrene by maintaining an adequate circulation in the affected parts. Vasodilators may be tried, together with mechanical procedures to restore the circulation.

Nausea and vomiting may be controlled by the intramuscular injection of 25 to 50 mg of chlorpromazine or of a comparable dose of a related phenothiazine.

Precautions. Ergot is contra-indicated in patients with severe hypertension, severe or persistent sepsis, vascular disease, or impaired hepatic or renal function. It is also contra-indicated in pregnancy, for the induction of labour, or during the first stage of labour. If used during the second stage of labour it should be done so under obstetric supervision and not until after delivery of the anterior shoulder of the infant. Numbness or tingling of the extremities indicate the need to discontinue ergot alkaloids.

The vasoconstrictor effects of ergot are enhanced by sympathomimetic agents such as adrenaline. The effects of ergot on the parturient uterus are diminished by halothane.

Pregnancy and the neonate. Ergot alkaloids in the milk of nursing mothers gave infants symptoms of ergotism, such as vomiting, diarrhoea, weak pulse and unstable blood pressure. Care should be taken when giving nursing mothers preparations containing ergot alkaloids for the treatment of migraine.— J. A. Knowles, *J. Pediat.*, 1965, *66*, 1068.

Ergot alkaloids impaired lactation by inhibition of maternal pituitary prolactin secretion.— *J. Am. med. Ass.*, 1974, *227*, 676.

The amount of methylergometrine excreted in breast milk was unlikely to affect the suckling infant.— R. Erkkola *et al.*, *Int. J. clin. Pharmac. Biopharm.*, 1978, *16*, 579.

Absorption and Fate. Ergot alkaloids are incompletely absorbed from the gastro-intestinal tract. Different alkaloids are absorbed to varying degrees. They are probably metabolised in the liver. The alkaloids are excreted mainly in the bile with only small amounts appearing in the urine.

For various studies on the pharmacokinetics of ergot derivatives see P. Loddo *et al.*, *Boll. chim.-farm.*, 1976, *115*, 570 (co-dergocrine); W. H. Aellig and E. Nüesch, *Int. J. clin. Pharmac. Biopharm.*, 1977, *15*, 106 (co-dergocrine, dihydroergotamine, and ergotamine); R. Mäntylä *et al.*, *Int. J. clin. Pharmac. Biopharm.*, 1978, *16*, 254 (methylergometrine); H. Allonen *et al.*, *Int. J. clin. Pharmac. Biopharm.*, 1978, *16*, 340 (methylergometrine); V. Ala-Hurula *et al.*, *Eur. J. clin. Pharmac.*, 1979, *15*, 51 (ergotamine); V. Ala-Hurula *et al.*, *Eur. J. clin. Pharmac.*, 1979, *16*, 355 (ergotamine).

Uses. Ergot stimulates smooth muscle, especially of the blood vessels and uterus.

The action of ergot depends on its alkaloidal content, especially of ergotamine, ergotoxine, and ergometrine. Of these, ergometrine is the only one which produces a rapid oxytocic effect by mouth and the use of this alkaloid is usually preferred to preparations of the whole drug because of the more exact dosage which can be given, the specific action on the uterine muscle, and the fact that it has much less tendency to give rise to gangrene.

Ergot has been given as capsules or tablets of prepared ergot in usual doses of 150 to 500 mg.

The liquid extract loses its activity very rapidly, especially when diluted in mixtures.

Preparations

Ergot Liquid Extract *(B.P.C. 1954).* Prepared by macerating and percolating defatted ergot with alcohol (50%) acidified with tartaric acid. It contains, when fresh, 0.06% w/v of alkaloids, and, after storage, not less than 0.04%. It loses activity on keeping, the rate being rapid at ordinary temperatures but slower at refrigerator temperatures. Store in a cool place in completely filled containers. *Dose.* 0.6 to 1.2 ml. A similar liquid extract is included in some pharmacopoeias.

Ergot Tablets *(B.P.C. 1968).* Prepared Ergot Tablets. Tablets containing prepared ergot. Store in a cool place in airtight containers.

1503-f

Co-dergocrine Mesylate.

Co-dergocrine Methanesulphonate; Dihydroergotoxine Mesylate; Dihydroergotoxine Methanesulphonate; Dihydrogenated Ergot Alkaloids; Hydrogenated Ergot Alkaloids; DEA; DHAE. A mixture in equal proportions of dihydroergocornine mesylate ($C_{31}H_{41}N_5O_5,CH_4O_3S$ = 659.8), dihydroergocristine mesylate ($C_{35}H_{41}N_5O_5,CH_4O_3S$ = 707.8), and α- and β-dihydroergocryptine mesylates ($C_{32}H_{43}N_5O_5,CH_4O_3S$ = 673.8) in the ratio 2:1.

CAS — 11032-41-0 (co-dergocrine); 8067-24-1 (mesylate).

NOTE. Ergoloid mesylates is a similar substance: the only difference in the definition is that the ratio of α- and β-dihydroergocryptine mesylates is quoted as 1.5 to 2.5:1.

M.p. 196° to 206° with decomposition.

Caffeine increased the aqueous solubility of co-dergocrine in 0.1 N hydrochloric acid and pH 6.65 phosphate buffer. This might assist absorption of co-dergocrine *in vivo* thus increasing its effectiveness.— M. A. Zoglio and H. V. Maulding, *J. pharm. Sci.*, 1970, *59*, 215. For a similar report on the increased solubility of dihydroergocristine mesylate, a component of co-dergocrine, with caffeine, proxyphylline, and theophylline, see H. V. Maulding and M. A. Zoglio, *J. pharm. Sci.*, 1970, *59*, 384.

Adverse Effects. Side-effects of co-dergocrine mesylate include nausea, vomiting, headache, blurred vision, skin rashes, nasal stuffiness, flushing of the skin, and orthostatic hypotension.

Local irritation has been reported following sublingual administration.

A study indicating that usual therapeutic doses of co-dergocrine mesylate interfere with colour vision.— J. Laroche and C. Laroche, *Annls pharm. fr.*, 1972, *30*, 433.

Of 8 patients given co-dergocrine mesylate 1.5 mg thrice daily for the treatment of dementia, 3 developed severe sinus bradycardia associated with general deterioration in their condition, necessitating withdrawal of the treatment.— A. C. D. Cayley *et al.*, *Br. med. J.*, 1975, *4*, 384. No sinus bradycardia had been observed in 40 elderly patients in whom the dose was built up to 1.5 mg thrice daily over 3 weeks.— C. Cohen (letter), *ibid.*, 581.

Absorption and Fate. See Ergot, p.662.

Uses. Co-dergocrine mesylate produces a generalised peripheral vasodilatation and a fall in arterial pressure.

It is used with the intention of treating symptoms of mild to moderate impairment of mental function in the elderly in doses of up to 4.5 mg daily by mouth. It is also given sublingually in doses of 0.75 to 3 mg daily. It has been given in a dose of 300 to 600 µg daily by intramuscular, intra-arterial, subcutaneous, or slow intravenous injection.

Cerebrovascular disease. In a double-blind study over 12 weeks of 57 patients with cerebrovascular insufficiency associated with cerebral arteriosclerosis, co-dergocrine mesylate was more effective than a placebo in improving physical, social, and psychological functions.— D. B. Rao and J. R. Norris, *Johns Hopkins med. J.*, 1972, *130*, 317.

In a double-blind study in 10 patients (mean age 66.1 years) with clinical symptoms of cerebrovascular insufficiency and slowing of the EEG frequency, treated for 12 weeks with co-dergocrine mesylate 1.5 mg thrice daily, there was significant improvement in headache, vertigo, fatigue, sleep disturbances, and depression compared with 10 similar patients (mean age 70.5 years) treated with placebo. Clinical improvement correlated with improvement in the EEG pattern.— A. Arrigo *et al.*, *Curr. ther. Res.*, 1973, *15*, 417.

In a double-blind study in 47 elderly patients with organic brain syndrome treatment with co-dergocrine mesylate 1 mg thrice daily for 12 weeks led to improvement in 16 of 18 parameters compared with 11 of 18 parameters in those given placebo. After 24 weeks improvement was present in 15 of 18 parameters in patients given co-dergocrine mesylate and in 2 of 18 in those given placebo.— C. M. Gaitz *et al.*, *Archs gen. Psychiat.*, 1977, *34*, 839.

There was no convincing evidence that co-dergocrine mesylate was effective for the treatment of any condition associated with impairment of mental function in the elderly.— *Med. Lett.*, 1977, *19*, 61. See also *ibid.*, 1974, *16*, 21; *ibid.*, 1976, *18*, 39.

A favourable report of the use of co-dergocrine mesylate in elderly patients with cerebrovascular insufficiency.— J. Kugler *et al.*, *Dt. med. Wschr.*, 1978, *103*, 456.

Dyskinesia. Of 6 patients with tardive dyskinesia following long-term therapy with phenothiazines 1 lost all symptoms of the dyskinesia and the others showed some improvement after treatment with co-dergocrine mesylate 4.5 mg daily for 6 weeks.— J. Hajioff (letter), *Br. med. J.*, 1978, *2*, 834.

Proprietary Preparations

Hydergine *(Sandoz, UK).* Co-dergocrine mesylate, available as scored tablets of 1.5 mg and tablets of 4.5 mg. (Also available as Hydergine in *Belg., Canad., Fr., S.Afr.*).

Other Proprietary Names

Circanol, Deapril-ST *(both USA)*; Hydergin *(Denm., Ger., Swed.)*; Hydergina *(Arg., Ital., Spain)*; Progeril *(Ital.)*.

Other Proprietary Names of Similar Compounds

Circanol, Dacoren, DCCK, DH-Ergotoxin-forte, Ergoplus *(all Ger.)*; Ischelium *(Ital.)*; Optamine *(Fr.)* *(all similar to co-dergocrine mesylate, but ratio of α- and β-dihydroergocryptine mesylates not specified)*; Decme, Enirant, Nehydrin *(all Ger.)*; Diertina *(Ital., Switz.)*; Diertine *(Spain)*; Insibrin *(Arg.)* *(all dihydroergocristine mesylate)*; Redergam *(Hung.)*; Ségolan *(Fr.)* *(both co-dergocrine esylate)*.

1504-d

Dihydroergotamine Mesylate *(U.S.P.)*.

Dihydroergotamine Methanesulphonate; Dihydroergotaminium Methansulfonicum. 9,10-Dihydro-12′-hydroxy-2′-methyl-5′α-benzyl-ergotaman-3′,6′,18-trione methanesulphonate. $C_{33}H_{37}N_5O_5,CH_3SO_3H$=679.8.

CAS — 511-12-6 (dihydroergotamine); 6190-39-2 (mesylate).

Pharmacopoeias. In *Cz., Jug., Swiss,* and *U.S.*

A white to slightly yellowish or an off-white to slightly red microcrystalline powder with a slight odour. **Soluble** 1 in 125 of water, 1 in 90 of alcohol, 1 in 175 of chloroform, and 1 in 2600 of ether; soluble in acetone. A 2.5% solution in a mixture of alcohol, chloroform, and ammonia is laevorotatory. Solutions are **sterilised** by filtration. A 0.1% solution in water has a pH of 4.4 to 5.4. **Store** in a cool place in an atmosphere of nitrogen in hermetically sealed containers. Protect from light.

Adverse Effects and Treatment. As for Ergot, p.662. There is a reduced risk of gangrene.

Mention of retroperitoneal fibrosis as a side-effect of dihydroergotamine.— J. R. Curtis, *Br. med. J.*, 1977, *2*, 375.

A 42-year-old woman who had taken dihydroergotamine 10 mg daily for 2 weeks and then 20 mg in a day had symptoms suggestive of chronic renal failure, later considered to be acute renal failure in diuretic phase.— C. D. Pusey and D. J. Rainford, *Br. med. J.*, 1977, *2*, 935.

A report of ergotism following treatment with dihydroergotamine mesylate and triacetyloleandomycin.— A. Franco *et al.* (letter), *Nouv. Presse méd.*, 1978, *7*, 205.

Precautions. As for Ergot, p.662.

In the presence of coronary disease, dihydroergotamine mesylate should be given by mouth only.

Absorption and Fate. See Ergot, p.662.

Uses. Dihydroergotamine has diminished oxytocic and vasoconstrictor effects compared with ergotamine.

Dihydroergotamine mesylate is used mainly for the treatment of migraine and may give relief in some cases of headache of vascular origin. In the treatment of migraine it is most effective when given subcutaneously or intramuscularly in doses of 1 to 2 mg, the patient usually responding within 15 to 30 minutes. The dose may be repeated if necessary. It has been given intravenously in doses of up to 2 mg. In mild attacks, 1 to 3 mg may be given by mouth and repeated every half hour if necessary to a total dose of 10 mg. A dose of 1 or 2 mg has been given thrice daily to reduce the frequency and severity of attacks. It has also been administered with caffeine.

Dihydroergotamine mesylate is also used in conjunction with a low-dose heparin regimen in the prophylaxis of postoperative deep-vein thrombosis. A suggested dose is 500 µg subcutaneously every 8 to 12 hours, starting 2 hours before surgery and continued for at least 7 to 10 days postoperatively.

When given in single intramuscular doses or in repeated doses by mouth, dihydroergotamine was found to diminish the intensity and duration of the psychotomimesis induced by lysergide.— K. A. Flügel and R. Stoerger, *Arzneimittel-Forsch.*, 1966, *16*, 235.

Diarrhoea. In 121 of 123 patients with diarrhoea due to various causes, dihydroergotamine 1 or 2 mg by mouth before meals or 1 mg by intramuscular injection rapidly reduced the frequency of bowel movements. The remaining 2 patients were successfully treated with diphenoxylate.— F. Lechin *et al.*, *J. clin. Pharmac.*, 1977, *17*, 339.

Hypotension. Haemodynamic studies indicated that dihydroergotamine may have beneficial effects in circulatory disturbances that are characterised by impaired venomotor regulation, such as orthostatic hypotension.— S. Mellander and I. Nordenfelt, *Postgrad. med. J.*, 1976, *52*, *Suppl.* 1, 17.

In 10 patients given dihydroergotamine mesylate 1 mg intramuscularly peak plasma concentration occurred after about 30 minutes. It was suggested that dihydroergotamine given intramuscularly 15 to 30 minutes before spinal anaesthesia may prevent the hypotension caused by spinal or epidural anaesthetics.— H. Hilke *et al.*, *Int. J. clin. Pharmac. Biopharm.*, 1978, *16*, 277.

In 6 patients with autonomic insufficiency and orthostatic hypotension blood pressure was increased after dihydroergotamine given intravenously. Of 4 patients given the drug by mouth one was controlled on 10 mg daily and 3 on 30 mg daily.— G. Jennings *et al.*, *Br. med. J.*, 1979, *2*, 307. The apparent failure of 2 patients with postural hypotension to respond to dihydroergotamine by mouth was attributed to low bioavailability of the drug as both patients greatly improved following dihydroergotamine intravenously.— I. N. Olver *et al.*, *ibid.*, 1980, *281*, 275.

Dihydroergotamine 1 mg daily intramuscularly relieved the hypotension which resulted from poisoning with a nitrophenylurea rodenticide.— N. L. Benowitz *et al.*, *Ann. intern. Med.*, 1980, *92*, 387.

Retinal hypotension. Good results followed treatment with dihydroergotamine in 21 of 24 patients with postural retinal hypotension.— P. G. Moreau and P. Pichon, *Annls Oculist.*, 1968, *201*, 801.

Use in surgery. In 150 patients given heparin 5000 units and dihydroergotamine 500 µg daily the incidence of postoperative deep-vein thrombosis and pulmonary embolism was 8.7 and 2.7% respectively compared with 19.8 and 5.5% in 162 patients receiving heparin 5000 units twice daily. In 50 patients not receiving prophylactic therapy the incidence was 30 and 14% respectively.— K. Koppenhagen *et al.*, *Dt. med. Wschr.*, 1977, *102*, 1374.

In a randomised study the incidence of deep-vein thrombosis in 50 patients undergoing abdominal surgery and given heparin calcium, 5000 units subcutaneously 2 hours before surgery and then 4-hourly for 7 days or longer, was 4% compared with 20% in 50 given dihydroergotamine mesylate 500 μg subcutaneously before surgery and then 12-hourly; the difference was significant. The incidence was 4% in 48 further patients given heparin calcium 5000 units, compared with 6% in 49 given heparin 2500 units per dose plus dihydroergotamine; the difference was not significant. The incidence was 52% in 50 patients undergoing hip surgery and given heparin in 5000-unit doses for 10 to 14 days compared with 20% in 50 given heparin in 5000-unit doses plus dihydroergotamine; the difference was significant and such continued treatment was considered of value.— V. V. Kakkar *et al.*, *J. Am. med. Ass.*, 1979, *241*, 39.

Preparations

Dihydroergotamine Mesylate Injection *(U.S.P.)*. A sterile solution in Water for Injections. pH 3.2 to 4. Protect from light.

Dihydergot *(Sandoz, UK)*. Dihydroergotamine mesylate, available as **Injection** containing 1 mg per ml, in ampoules of 1 ml; as **Oral Solution** containing 2 mg per ml; and as scored **Tablets** of 1 mg. (Also available as Dihydergot in *Arg., Austral., Belg., Denm., Ger., Jap., Neth., Norw., S.Afr., Spain, Switz.*).

Other Proprietary Names

Fr.—Ikaran, Séglor; *Ger.*— DET MS, DH-Ergotamin-retard, Tonopres; *Ital.*—Diidergot; *Swed.*—Orstanorm; *Switz.*— Ergotonin; *USA*—D.H.E. 45.

1505-n

Dihydroergotamine Tartrate *(B.P.)*.
$(C_{33}H_{37}N_5O_5)_2,C_4H_6O_6$=1317.5.

CAS — 5989-77-5.

Pharmacopoeias. In *Br.*

Odourless colourless crystals or a white or almost white crystalline powder. M.p. about 203° with decomposition. Very slightly **soluble** in water; sparingly soluble in alcohol; soluble in pyridine. A 1% solution in pyridine is laevorotatory. A 0.25% suspension in water has a pH of 4 to 5.5. **Protect** from light.

There is little evidence of use of dihydroergotamine tartrate.

1506-h

Ergometrine Maleate *(B.P., Eur. P.)*.

Ergometr. Mal.; Ergometrinii Maleas; Ergometrini Maleas; Ergonovine Maleate *(U.S.P.)* Ergonovine Bimaleate; Ergometrinhydrogenmaleat; Maleato de Ergonovina. *N*-[(*S*)-2-Hydroxy-1-methylethyl]-D-lysergamide hydrogen maleate; 9,10-Didehydro-*N*-[(*S*)-2-hydroxy-1-methylethyl]-6-methylergoline-8β-carboxamide hydrogen maleate.

$C_{19}H_{23}N_3O_2,C_4H_4O_4$=441.5.

CAS — 60-79-7 (ergometrine); 129-51-1 (maleate).

Pharmacopoeias. In all pharmacopoeias examined except *Port.* and *Rus.*

A white or yellowish, odourless, slightly hygroscopic, microcrystalline powder. It darkens with age and on exposure to light. M.p. about 185° with decomposition. **Soluble** 1 in 40 of water at 25° and 1 in 100 of alcohol at 25°; practically insoluble in chloroform and ether. Solutions in water and alcohol give a blue fluorescence. A 1% solution in water is dextrorotatory and has a pH of 3 to 5. Solutions are **sterilised** by autoclaving and kept in ampoules, the air in the containers having been replaced by nitrogen or other suitable gas.

Store at a temperature not exceeding 8° in an atmosphere of nitrogen or other suitable gas in hermetically sealed containers. Protect from light.

Effect of gamma-irradiation. At 25 000 Gy a 2% aqueous solution of ergometrine maleate developed a yellow opalescence and at 250 000 Gy it became greenish-brown with a flocculent deposit. Ergometrine maleate injection was more affected; it became pale brown and opalescent at 25 000 Gy and buff-coloured with a dark brown precipitate at 250 000 Gy. The pH increased from 3.1 to 4.7 at 25 000 Gy and to 5.58 at 250 000 Gy.— *The Use of Gamma Radiation Sources for the Sterilisation of Pharmaceutical Products*, London, ABPI, 1960.

Adverse Effects. Adverse effects do not appear to occur as frequently with ergometrine maleate as with other ergot alkaloids. Those that have been observed include headache, vertigo, tinnitus, abdominal pain, nausea, vomiting, hypertension, chest pain, palpitation, dyspnoea, and bradycardia. Ergometrine shows less tendency to produce gangrene than ergotamine.

A 20-year-old woman suffering from metrorrhagia after her delivery 8 days previously was given 200 μg of ergometrine maleate by mouth thrice daily to a total of 3.6 mg. Both feet became cold and numb and later, purple. Ergometrine maleate was discontinued.— W. Bross *et al.*, *Lancet*, 1963, *1*, 85.

Ergometrine might cause blurred vision, optic oedema, and concentric constriction of visual fields.— H. I. Silverman, *Am. J. Optom.*, 1972, *49*, 335.

Symmetrical gangrene of the extremities associated with the use of dopamine subsequent to ergometrine administration.— N. Buchanan *et al.*, *Intensive Care Med.*, 1977, *3*, 55.

Chromosomal aberrations. Chromosomal aberrations in cultured leucocytes were noted after 4 hours' exposure to dilute solution of ergometrine maleate.— L. F. Jarvik and T. Kato (letter), *Lancet*, 1968, *1*, 250.

Pregnancy and the neonate. The Poland anomaly (a congenital defect) was possibly related to the use of ergometrine for attempted abortion.— T. J. David, *New Engl. J. Med.*, 1972, *287*, 487. See also B. MacMahon, *New Engl. J. Med.*, 1972, *287*, 514.

Convulsions, ventilatory failure, and water intoxication in a neonate following the accidental administration of ergometrine 500 μg with synthetic oxytocin 5 units (Syntometrine) intramuscularly. Following therapy with anticonvulsants and assisted respiration the infant made an uneventful recovery.— M. F. Whitfield and S. A. W. Salfield, *Archs Dis. Childh.*, 1980, *55*, 68.

Hypertension. A 17-year-old girl in labour was given 500 μg of ergometrine maleate intramuscularly as the head crowned and after 12 minutes her blood pressure rose sharply. It fell again 30 minutes after papaveretum 20 mg had been given, and then 25 minutes later she developed severe frontal headache, a further increase in blood pressure, and typical generalised eclamptic convulsions. Morphine and paraldehyde controlled the fits which could only be attributed to ergometrine. In reports by H.G. Hamilton (*Am. J. Obstet. Gynec.*, 1953, *65*, 503) and I.R. McFadyen (*Lancet*, 1960, *2*, 1009), ergometrine was also considered the causative factor in cases of postpartum eclampsia in previously normotensive patients.— A. M. Hassim (letter), *Br. med. J.*, 1964, *2*, 1327.

Postpartum administration of ergometrine in 4 patients resulted in hypertension in 3 (with eclampsia in 1) and cardiac arrest in the fourth. Blood pressure rose to 180/130 mmHg, 190/165 mmHg, and 180/120 mmHg respectively and responded to hydralazine in 2 patients and spontaneously in the third. Cardiac arrest responded to cardiac massage. It was suggested that ergometrine should not be used routinely in obstetrics.— D. J. Browning, *Med. J. Aust.*, 1974, *1*, 957.

Further references.— G. N. Cassady *et al.*, *J. Am. med. Ass.*, 1960, *172*, 1011; C. A. D. Ringrose, *Can. med. Ass. J.*, 1962, *87*, 712.

Precautions. As for Ergot, p.662. Ergometrine maleate should be given with caution to patients with toxaemia.

Pregnancy and the neonate. Ergometrine maleate was given in a dose of 500 μg intravenously as an oxytocic following delivery of the child to 266 pregnant patients requiring general anaesthesia for caesarean section or instrumental delivery. A marked rise in both systolic and diastolic pressures, exceeding in many cases 20 mmHg, was noted in patients suffering from hypertensive toxaemia. No significant pressor response occurred in normotensive patients and there was little or no response in patients with chronic hypertension.— T. W. Baillie, *Br. med. J.*, 1963, *1*, 585.

The period after delivery of a child was a dangerous time for women with heart disease and the administration of ergometrine 250 μg was considered to be less hazardous than the risk of a third-stage haemorrhage.— D. D. Moir (letter), *Br. med. J.*, 1970, *1*, 563.

Vasoconstrictive effects made the use of ergometrine undesirable for obstetric patients who had cardiovascular, respiratory, or renal diseases, chronic anaemia, or toxaemia of pregnancy; oxytocin was preferable in such cases, its hypotensive effect being less if it was given to patients in the lithotomy position.— M. Johnstone, *Br. J. Anaesth.*, 1972, *44*, 826.

In a study in 148 patients who had received oxytocin infusions during the first and second stages of labour and who had received epidural analgesia blood loss was similar in those given ergometrine 500 μg intravenously or oxytocin 5 units intravenously after delivery of the anterior shoulder of the infant; the incidence of nausea, retching, and vomiting was 46% in those receiving ergometrine and nil in those receiving oxytocin. Oxytocin was preferable to ergometrine during epidural analgesia, particularly in patients with heart disease, pre-eclampsia, hypertension, phaeochromocytoma, thyrotoxicosis, and coronary insufficiency.— J. E. Moodie and D. D. Moir, *Br. J. Anaesth.*, 1976, *48*, 571.

A woman given ergometrine 500 μg intravenously following caesarean section had absent peripheral pulses, without cyanosis, for about 2 hours after the injection; she had had symptoms of Raynaud's syndrome before her pregnancy and had developed pre-eclamptic toxaemia at 34 weeks of gestation.— B. H. Valentine *et al.*, *Br. J. Anaesth.*, 1977, *49*, 81.

Absorption and Fate. See Ergot, p.662.

Uses. Ergometrine has a much more powerful action on the uterus than most of the other alkaloids of ergot, the difference being more marked on the puerperal uterus than on the normal non-pregnant uterus. Its main action is the production of contractions and its action is more prolonged than that of oxytocin. Uterine stimulation occurs about 8 minutes after administration by mouth of therapeutic doses in solution and contractions become less frequent after about an hour. Injection of ergometrine causes uterine contractions to begin more rapidly, in about 5 minutes if given intramuscularly or about 1 minute if given intravenously. Following intramuscular injection of ergometrine with oxytocin contractions are reported to occur within 2 or 3 minutes.

The most extensive use of ergometrine maleate is in the active management of the third stage of labour and in the treatment of postpartum haemorrhage.

In the active management of the third stage of labour of normal confinements, ergometrine maleate is frequently administered under obstetric supervision, usually as a combined injection containing ergometrine maleate 500 μg with synthetic oxytocin 5 units intramuscularly, following the delivery of the anterior shoulder of the infant during the second stage of labour. Delivery of the placenta is assisted while the uterus is firmly contracted. It is generally considered that this active management reduces the risk of primary postpartum haemorrhage. Ergometrine maleate alone in doses of 200 μg is used in the USA in the above manner. Doses of 200 to 500 μg are given intramuscularly in the treatment of primary postpartum haemorrhage, usually on completion of the third stage of labour. In emergences 200 μg may be given intravenously.

For the treatment of mild secondary postpartum haemorrhage, ergometrine maleate, by mouth, in doses of 200 μg two to four times daily or 500 μg thrice daily may be used.

Ergometrine maleate was also used in the treatment of migraine but was generally less effective than ergotamine tartrate.

The venoconstrictor effects of ergometrine maleate.— O. G. Brooke and B. F. Robinson, *Br. med. J.*, 1970, *1*, 139.

Studies suggested that ergometrine administered immediately after coitus significantly reduced the conception rate.— E. M. Coutinho *et al.*, *Am. J. Obstet. Gynec.*, 1976, *126*, 48.

Detection of coronary heart disease. The effects of ergometrine maleate in 60 patients with and without coronary heart disease. All of 5 patients with variant angina (cyclic rest pain with transient ST-segment elevation) were identified but the procedure was less useful than the exercise test in detecting myocardial ischaemia. Patients with clinical variant angina or hypertension received 50 μg intravenously, repeated over 5 minutes to a maximum of 200 µg; other patients received 200 µg. Prolonged chest pain unresponsive to glyceryl trinitrate, or myocardial infarction, did not occur, but because of the risk the procedure should not be used outside specialised units.— R. C. Curry *et al.*, *Circulation*, 1977, *56*, 803.

Further references.— J. S. Schroeder *et al.*, *Am. J. Cardiol.*, 1977, *40*, 487; F. A. Heupler *et al.*, *ibid.*, 1978, *41*, 631; J. L. Gerry *et al.*, *J. Am. med. Ass.*, 1979, *242*, 2858.

Pregnancy and the neonate. A short discussion on the traditional uses of ergot compounds in obstetrics.— A. C. Turnbull, *Postgrad. med. J.*, 1976, *52*, *Suppl.* 1, 15.

In a double-blind trial, 250 µg was as effective as 500 µg of ergometrine maleate given intravenously after completion of the second stage of labour for achieving haemostasis in the third stage of labour and in preventing primary postpartum haemorrhage. Postpartum haemorrhage was related to genital tract trauma rather than to the dose of ergometrine administered.— J. D. Paull and G. J. Ratten, *Med. J. Aust.*, 1977, *1*, 178.

Further references.— C. Wilson (letter), *Med. J. Aust.*, 1974, *2*, 715.

Ergometrine with oxytocin. In a clinical study, the intramuscular injection of ergometrine with oxytocin (Syntometrine), given with the birth of the anterior shoulder in the active management of the third stage of labour and the prophylaxis of postpartum haemorrhage, resulted in a significant reduction in the incidence of postpartum haemorrhage compared with the intramuscular injection of ergometrine; in both primigravidas and multigravidas the frequency of postpartum haemorrhage was approximately halved. There was no increase in the incidence of retention of the placenta.— M. P. Embrey *et al.*, *Br. med. J.*, 1963, *1*, 1387.

Ergometrine maleate 500 µg, with oxytocin 5 units (Syntometrine), administered intramuscularly, was more effective in controlling blood loss in the third stage of labour that when ergometrine maleate 500 µg was given alone, though there was less marked advantage when compared with ergometrine maleate 1 mg intramuscularly. There was a suspicion that the risk of retention of the placenta was greater in cases treated with Syntometrine than in those treated with ergometrine 500 µg, though this was significant only at the 20% level. Compared with cases treated with 1 mg of ergometrine there was little difference in the incidence of this complication.— W. O. Chukudebelu *et al.*, *Br. med. J.*, 1963, *1*, 1390.

A retrospective study of 1392 deliveries indicated that the incidence of post-partum haemorrhage and heavy loss was reduced when ergometrine maleate 500 µg and oxytocin 5 units (Syntometrine 1 ml) was given intramuscularly after delivery of the anterior shoulder, compared to ergometrine 500 µg only.— O. Djahanbakhch *et al.*, *Br. J. clin. Pract.*, 1978, *32*, 137.

Further references.— J. McGrath and A. D. H. Browne, *Br. med. J.*, 1962, *2*, 524; J. Kemp, *ibid.*, 1963, *1*, 1391; S. K. Basu and H. G. I. Shanks, *Practitioner*, 1964, *192*, 784; R. J. Beard *et al.*, *Br. J. clin. Pract.*, 1973, *27*, 13.

Preparations

Injections

Ergometrine and Oxytocin Injection *(B.P.)*. A sterile solution of ergometrine maleate and synthetic oxytocin in Water for Injections; the acidity is adjusted to pH 3.3 by the addition of maleic acid (limits: pH 2.9 to 3.5); it may contain suitable stabilisers. Sterilise by filtration. Store at a temperature not exceeding 25° in ampoules in which the air has been replaced by nitrogen or other suitable gas. It should be protected from light both during and after preparation. Under these circumstances it may be expected to retain its potency for not less than 2 years.

Ergometrine Injection *(B.P.)*. Ergonovine Maleate Injection. A sterile solution of ergometrine maleate in Water for Injections free from dissolved air, adjusted to pH 3 with maleic acid (limits: pH 2.7 to 3.5). It may contain suitable stabilisers. Sterilised by autoclaving in an atmosphere of nitrogen or other suitable gas. It should be protected from light both during and after preparation. *Nord. P.* includes an injection (Injectible Ergometrini) with sodium chloride and hydrochloric acid.

Ergonovine Maleate Injection *(U.S.P.)*. A sterile solution of ergometrine maleate in Water for Injections. pH 2.7 to 3.5. Store at a temperature not exceeding 8°. Protect from light.

Tablets

Ergometrine Tablets *(B.P.)*. Ergonovine Maleate Tablets. Tablets containing ergometrine maleate. Protect from light.

Ergonovine Maleate Tablets *(U.S.P.)*. Tablets containing ergometrine maleate.

Proprietary Preparations

Syntometrine *(Sandoz, UK)*. An injection containing ergometrine maleate 500 µg and oxytocin 5 units in each ml, in ampoules of 1 ml. For the prevention and treatment of postpartum haemorrhage. *Dose.* 1 ml by intramuscular injection.

Other Proprietary Names

Ergomine *(Austral.)*; Ergotrate *(Arg., Austral., Canad., S. Afr., USA)*; Ermalate *(Austral.)*; Ermetrine *(Belg., Neth.)*.

1507-m

Ergometrine Tartrate. Ergonovinum Tartaricum; Ergometrini Tartras.
$(C_{19}H_{23}N_3O_2)_2,C_4H_6O_6=800.9$.

CAS — 129-50-0.

White or slightly reddish-yellow, odourless, very light, matted masses of acicular crystals with a bitter taste. It may contain 2 molecules of methanol of crystallisation. **Soluble** in water and alcohol; slightly soluble in chloroform and ether. **Store** in airtight containers. Protect from light.

Ergometrine tartrate has similar actions to the maleate.

A preparation containing ergometrine tartrate was formerly marketed in Great Britain under the proprietary name Neo-Femergin (*Sandoz*).

1508-b

Ergotamine Tartrate *(B.P., Eur. P.)*.

Ergotam. Tart.; Ergotaminii Tartras; Ergotamini Tartras. 12′-Hydroxy-2′-methyl-5′α-benzyl-ergotaman-3′,6′,18-trione tartrate.
$(C_{33}H_{35}N_5O_5)_2,C_4H_6O_6=1313.4$.

CAS — 113-15-5 (ergotamine); 379-79-3 (tartrate).

Pharmacopoeias. In all pharmacopoeias examined except *Arg., Chin., Rus.*, and *Span.*

The tartrate of ergotamine, an alkaloid obtained from certain species of ergot; it may contain 2 molecules of methanol of crystallisation. It occurs as colourless odourless crystals or as a white or yellowish-white crystalline powder. M.p. about 180° with decomposition.

Soluble 1 in about 500 of water, addition of tartaric acid often being necessary to maintain a clear solution; soluble 1 in 500 of alcohol; practically insoluble in chloroform and ether. A solution of ergotamine in chloroform is laevorotatory. A 0.25% suspension in water has a pH of 4 to 6. Solutions are **sterilised** by filtration and distributed into ampoules, the air in which is replaced with nitrogen or other suitable gas, and the ampoules are immediately sealed. **Store** at a temperature not exceeding 8° in an atmosphere of nitrogen in hermetically sealed containers. Protect from light.

Caffeine increased the solubility of ergotamine tartrate at gastric and intestinal pH *in vitro* so that ergotamine was not precipitated. This might assist absorption of ergotamine and explain the greater effect claimed for a mixture of caffeine and ergotamine in migraine.— M. A. Zoglio *et al.*, *J. pharm. Sci.*, 1969, *58*, 222.

Stability in solution. The stability and degradation of ergotamine tartrate in aqueous solution.— B. Kreilgard and J. Kisbye, *Arch. Pharm. Chemi, scient. Edn*, 1974, *2*, 1 and 38.

Adverse Effects. As for Ergot, p.662.

In large repeated doses, ergotamine can produce all the symptoms of ergot poisoning and fatalities have been reported from its use. In some cases it may increase nausea and vomiting in migraine attacks before giving relief.

A report of ergotamine abuse in 5 patients, 1 of whom later abused methysergide.— R. N. Lucas and W. Falkowski, *Br. J. Psychiat.*, 1973, *122*, 199.

A 38-year-old woman developed venous thrombosis of the leg after an intramuscular injection of 500 µg of ergotamine tartrate.— U. Mintz *et al.*, *Postgrad. med. J.*, 1974, *50*, 244.

Two cases of ergotamine toxicity in which ischaemia of all extremities and bilateral foot-drop occurred in one patient and unilateral leg ischaemia and transient monocular blindness in the other.— G. C. Merhoff and J. M. Porter, *Ann. Surg.*, 1974, *180*, 773.

Subclinical ergotism was detected in a group of 29 patients who had been taking ergotamine regularly for at least one year. One additional patient had evidence of arterial insufficiency in the foot but the other 29 had reduced foot-systolic blood pressure indicating a risk of arterial insufficiency. There was a significant rise in blood pressure in all 13 patients who succeeded in stopping ergotamine treatment.— H. Dige-Petersen *et al.*, *Lancet*, 1977, *2*, 65.

Mention of retroperitoneal fibrosis as a side-effect of ergotamine.— J. R. Curtis, *Br. med. J.*, 1977, *2*, 375.

Acute myocardial ischaemia occurred in 2 patients after doses of 2 and 10 mg of ergotamine. The patients had previously been taking up to 2 and 40 mg respectively of ergotamine weekly.— N. J. C. Snell *et al.*, *Postgrad. med. J.*, 1978, *54*, 37.

A suggestion of association between angina pectoris and sudden death in the absence of atherosclerosis and the ingestion of ergotamine tartrate 8.75 mg over the preceding 9 days by a middle-aged woman.— C. R. Benedict and D. Robertson, *Am. J. Med.*, 1979, *67*, 177.

Acute ergotism in 2 patients receiving ergotamine tartrate and triacetyloleandomycin.— N. T. Matthews and J. H. Havill, *N.Z. med. J.*, 1979, *89*, 476.

Autonomic dysaesthesia due to ergot toxicity, confused with progression of chronic back pain.— P. J. D. Evans *et al.*, *Br. med. J.*, 1980, *281*, 1621.

Arterial aneurysm associated with ergotamine tartrate in one patient.— M. Pajewski *et al.* (letter), *Lancet*, 1981, *2*, 934.

Further references.— E. Hokkanen *et al.*, *Headache*, 1978, *18*, 95; M. Zicot *et al.*, *Angiology*, 1978, *29*, 495.

Treatment of Adverse Effects. As for Ergot, p.662.

A 30-year-old nurse with severe headache was given ergotamine tartrate 2 mg at once and then 4 times daily to a total of 40 mg. Spasm of veins and arteries developed and gangrene was threatened. Heparin and tolazoline produced limited recovery.— J. J. Cranley *et al.*, *New Engl. J. Med.*, 1963, *269*, 727.

A woman who had used 18 rectal suppositories containing ergotamine tartrate 2 mg and caffeine 100 mg in 18 hours developed lower extremity cyanosis which was not relieved by hydralazine hydrochloride. An intravenous infusion of sodium nitroprusside was started at a rate of 50 µg per minute. The infusion was stopped after 20 hours but restarted 3 hours later at a rate of 123 µg per minute because of coldness of the feet and continued for 15 hours. The patient recovered fully.— N. H. Carliner *et al.*, *J. Am. med. Ass.*, 1974, *227*, 308. Intra-arterial infusion of sodium nitroprusside 16 µg per minute slowly increased to 300 µg per minute over the next 45 minutes alleviated signs of peripheral ergotism in a 33-year-old patient. The infusion was continued for 9 hours and gradually decreased to 32 µg per minute and then given at this rate intravenously for a further 96 hours.— C. W. O'Dell *et al.*, *Radiology*, 1977, *124*, 73.

Streptokinase was used effectively for the treatment of arterial insufficiency in the leg of a woman who had for 3 years been using suppositories containing ergotamine tartrate for treatment of headaches.— B. Brismar *et al.*, *Acta chir. scand.*, 1977, *143*, 319.

A 37-year-old woman had vasoconstriction affecting the legs after a high intake of ergotamine tartrate for migraine. Treatment consisted of anticoagulants, tolazoline, nerve blocks, phentolamine, sodium nitroprusside, methylprednisolone, and injection of dextran 40. Blood pressure fell, and after initial frusemide-induced diuresis acute renal failure developed necessitating dialysis. While injection of dextran 40 had been known to cause acute renal failure ergotamine was possibly responsible.— J. Webb (letter), *Br. med. J.*, 1977, *2*, 1355.

A report of the successful treatment of vasospasm owing to ergotism in 2 women by means of intravenous infusion of sodium nitroprusside 25 µg per minute increased by 25 µg per minute at intervals of 5 to 15 minutes to maximum infusion rates of 100 and 150 µg per minute. Total doses of 80 and 100 mg were given over about 32 and 16 hours respectively. Epidural block with bupivacaine had been unsuccessful.— P. K. Andersen *et al.*, *New Engl. J. Med.*, 1977, *296*, 1271.

Ergotamine-induced severe peripheral vascular ischaemia in a 30-year-old woman was successfully treated with intravenous phentolamine 10 mg every 8 hours and intravenous heparin 3000 units every 4 hours for 4 days. Pethidine hydrochloride was used to relieve pain.— C. A. Attah, *N.Y. St. J. Med.*, 1977, *77*, 2257.

In a 39-year-old woman who had been taking ergotamine tartrate 4.5 mg daily for 4 days, intravenous infusion of sodium nitroprusside 1 µg per kg body-weight per minute rapidly alleviated ischaemic signs in her upper limbs; increase of the rate to 2 µg per kg per minute alleviated those in her lower limbs. Her feet again became ischaemic on reducing the rate to 1 µg so the rate of 2 µg was maintained for 36 hours; on discontinuation of therapy there were no signs of vasconstriction.— B. Eurin *et al.* (letter), *New Engl. J. Med.*, 1978, *298*, 632.

Infusion of glyceryl trinitrate successfully alleviated the symptoms of ergotism in a 41-year-old woman admitted with a 12-hour history of pain, coldness, discoloration, and numbness in her right foot. She had been using half a suppository of Gynergen Comp (each suppository containing ergotamine tartrate 2 mg and caffeine 100 mg) up to 5 times weekly for the preceding 10 years and daily for the preceding 5 months; 5 weeks before admission she had also started treatment with propranolol 120 mg daily. She was treated with a continuous intravenous infusion from a glass bottle containing glyceryl trinitrate 50 mg (10 ml of glyceryl trinitrate 0.5% in alcohol) in 500 ml of dextrose solution 5.5%. The infusion was discontinued after 11 hours, and the maximum infusion rate was 3.2 µg per kg body-weight per minute. During the infusion the patient had a brief headache of her usual migraine type; no other untoward effects were noted.— B. Husum *et al.* (letter), *Lancet*, 1979, *2*, 794.

Ergotamine-induced peripheral ischaemia in a patient successfully treated with prazosin hydrochloride 1 mg thrice daily by mouth.— D. S. Cobaugh, *J. Am. med. Ass.*, 1980, *244*, 1360.

In 2 patients with imminent gangrene of the extremities caused by ergot-induced arteriospasm after taking ergotamine tartrate, arterial dilatation by a balloon-tipped catheter produced an immediate and sustained reversal of the arteriospasm, together with a dramatic relief of symptoms and signs. The patients had not responded to standard therapy including heparin, vasodilators, and sympathetic blockade.— E. Shifrin *et al.*, *Lancet*, 1980, *2*, 1278.

Further references.— T. L. Whitsett *et al.* (letter), *Am. Heart J.*, 1978, *96*, 700; G. A. Skowronski *et al.*, *Med. J. Aust.*, 1979, *2*, 8.

Dialysis. A 13-month-old girl swallowed about 15 mg of ergotamine tartrate and 1 g of phenobarbitone in Bellergal tablets and was unconscious 5 hours later. The stomach was washed out immediately but the respiration-rate continued to fall and peritoneal dialysis was started. The intravenous injection of 2 doses, each of 20 ml of 10% mannitol solution, provided forced diuresis. Nine hours later the child was fully conscious and continued to recover.— E. M. Jones and B. Williams, *Br. med. J.*, 1966, *1*, 466.

Peritoneal dialysis was effective in the treatment of ergotamine tartrate overdosage.— E. M. Jones (letter), *Br. med. J.*, 1970, *3*, 222.

Pain relief. Peripheral arterial insufficiency with paraesthesia in the toes and soles of both feet occurred in a 28-year-old woman following ingestion of large doses of ergotamine tartrate for migraine. She received 500-ml intravenous infusions of dextran 40, containing heparin 5000 units, 8-hourly, until she had received 2 litres. Large doses of analgesics were required to alleviate the severe burning pain in her legs as they became warmer. The patient recovered completely after withdrawal of the drug.— S. T. Yao *et al.*, *Br. med. J.*, 1970, *3*, 86.

A 43-year-old woman developed bilateral thigh and calf claudication after taking 4 mg ergotamine tartrate daily for 2 to 3 weeks. Severe leg pain in a 22-year-old woman was caused by 6 to 8 mg ergotamine tartrate daily for 1 week. Pain in both patients was relieved by lumbar blocks with phenol.— C. W. Imrie, *Br. J. clin. Pract.*, 1973, *27*, 457.

Precautions. As for Ergot, p.662. Ergotamine tartrate should not be administered prophylactically, as prolonged use may give rise to gangrene.

A 68-year-old woman with headache developed cyanosis of the tongue 3 hours after the administration of ergotamine tartrate 500 µg intramuscularly and again 6 days later after two 1-mg tablets given with an interval of 6 hours. Partial necrosis of the tongue resulted. Temporal arteritis was later diagnosed and it was suggested that ergotamine should be used with caution in elderly patients with headache until temporal arteritis was ruled out.— J. R. Wolpaw *et al.*, *J. Am. med. Ass.*, 1973, *225*, 514.

Interactions. A 61-year-old man who was regularly using Cafergot suppositories twice daily for migraine was given propranolol 30 mg daily as additional prophylaxis; the patient's feet became progressively more purple and painful.— J. F. Baumrucker (letter), *New Engl. J. Med.*, 1973, *288*, 916. There were no adverse reactions in 50 patients with migraine who received simultaneous doses of ergotamine and propranolol. It was noted that the above patient received 4 mg of ergotamine daily, which was much higher than the accepted limit and it was suggested that the patient had ergotism rather than an interaction with propranolol.— S. Diamond (letter), *ibid.*, *289*, 159.

Liver disease. Ergotamine tartrate caused prolonged arteriospasm when given to a 23-year-old woman with viral hepatitis. A cumulative effect was considered to have been caused by the impairment of detoxification mechanisms in the diseased liver.— A. I. Katz and S. G. Massry, *Archs intern. Med.*, 1966, *118*, 62.

Cramps and signs of peripheral vasoconstriction on exposure to cold which had been experienced by a 39-year-old woman with migraine who had been taking preparations containing ergotamine for 5 years, became progressively worse and she developed nausea, lassitude, and jaundice. Despite treatment she died from acute hepatic necrosis, presumably of viral origin. It was suggested that ergotamine poisoning followed defective hepatic detoxication. The use of ergotamine preparations should be avoided, so far as possible, in the presence of liver disease.— M. J. Whelton *et al.*, *Gut*, 1968, *9*, 287.

Migraine. The symptoms of migraine were similar to those of ergotamine overdosage and included malaise, nausea, and vomiting. The use of further ergotamine to relieve the symptoms could lead to patients taking more than 12 mg weekly. One patient took up to 60 mg in a week. Using simple analgesics while ergotamine was withdrawn, most patients were improved within 2 weeks.— M. Wilkinson, *Pharm. J.*, 1973, *1*, 276.

Of 1000 patients with migraine taking ergotamine seen in 11 months 43 had intractable headache; 20 took 10 to 20 mg weekly, 14 took 20 to 30 mg weekly, and 9 took 30 to 70 mg weekly. Headache was often accentuated at first when ergotamine was withdrawn, reducing in frequency and severity in 1 to 14 days.— G. Wainscott *et al.* (letter), *Br. med. J.*, 1974, *2*, 724.

A number of patients seen in 2 migraine clinics appeared to be suffering from ergotamine tartrate overdosage. It was considered that ergotamine-induced headache could occur with doses as low as 1 mg daily by mouth or 250 µg daily intramuscularly.— F. C. Rose and M. Wilkinson, *Br. med. J.*, 1976, *1*, 525.

Absorption and Fate. See Ergot, p.662.

Uses. Ergotamine tartrate has marked vasconstrictor effects and a powerful action on the uterus, comparable to that of ergometrine. Following intramuscular injection uterine contractions begin after about 20 minutes and the effect is prolonged. Its action is also delayed following intravenous administration. It is used mainly for the relief of migraine. The smallest dose should be given and the patient should lie down in a quiet darkened room for 2 hours afterwards. The earlier in the attack that it is given the smaller the dose needed and the more effective the treatment. The usual dose is 1 to 2 mg administered by mouth, preferably sublingually, and the dose may be repeated, if necessary, 0.5 to 1 hour later. Not more than 6 mg should be administered in a day and not more than 10 mg in a week. Absorption from oral doses is variable. It is often given with caffeine.

Subcutaneous or intramuscular administration is preferable for more certain and more rapid action. A dose of 250 to 500 µg is given by subcutaneous or intramuscular injection and repeated if necessary. Not more than 1 mg should be administered in a week. Ergotamine tartrate may be administered by oral inhalation. One dose containing 360 µg may be inhaled at the onset of the attack, and repeated, if necessary, after 5 minutes. Up to 3 inhalations may be required. No more than 6 should be taken in a day and not more than 15 in a week.

Ergotamine may also be administered rectally in the form of suppositories. These usually contain caffeine in addition, which is claimed to enhance their action. The rate of absorption by this route is fairly constant and it provides an effective method of treatment, particularly in refractory cases of migraine. The dose is 2 mg repeated once or twice at hourly intervals. Not more than 3 suppositories should be used in a day and not more than 5 in a week.

For a report of the venoconstrictor effects of ergotamine tartrate, see O. G. Brooke and B. F. Robinson, *Br. med. J.*, 1970, *1*, 139.

Migraine. In a semi-blind study in 59 patients who suffered from migraine, a preparation containing ergotamine tartrate, cyclizine, and caffeine (Migril) was found to be as effective in relieving symptoms as a preparation containing buclizine, paracetamol, and codeine (Migraleve). As treatment with Migraleve could be given continuously, it should be tried before Migril.—Report No. 184 of the General Practitioner Research Group, *Practitioner*, 1973, *211*, 357.

Studies of the cerebral blood flow of an 18-year-old woman during a migraine attack indicated that cerebral perfusion was not involved in the effect of ergotamine.— J. W. Norris *et al.*, *Br. med. J.*, 1975, *3*, 676.

A short discussion on the traditional uses of ergot compounds in the treatment of migraine.— J. B. Foster, *Postgrad. med. J.*, 1976, *52*, *Suppl.* 1, 12.

Further references to the use of ergotamine, in various dosage forms, in the treatment of migraine.— T. Dalsgaard-Nielsen, *Nord. Med.*, 1968, *80*, 942; W. E. Waters, *Br. med. J.*, 1970, *2*, 325; J. C. Moir (letter), *ibid.*, 599; D. S. Freestone (letter), *ibid;* W. E. Waters (letter), *ibid.*, *3*, 164; G. N. Volans, *Adv. Med. Topics Ther.*, 1976, *2*, 156; J. M. Bradfield, *Drugs*, 1976, *12*, 449; D. Thrush, *Br. med. J.*, 1978, *2*, 1004; W. E. Waters (letter), *ibid.*, 1228.

Preparations

Inhalations

Ergotamine Aerosol Inhalation *(B.P.C. 1973).* An aerosol spray in a pressurised canister, containing a fine suspension of ergotamine tartrate in a suitable mixture of aerosol propellents. Usual strength: provides 360 µg in each metered dose. It may contain a surfactant, stabilising agents, and other adjuvants. Store in a cool place. *Dose.* 1 dose at the onset of symptoms, repeated at intervals of 5 minutes, if necessary, to a maximum of 6 doses daily. Fifteen doses weekly should not be exceeded.

Injections

Ergotamine Injection *(B.P.).* A sterile solution prepared by dissolving ergotamine tartrate in Water for Injections; it contains alcohol, glycerol, and sufficient tartaric acid to adjust the pH to 3.3 (limits 2.8 to 3.8). Of the total alkaloidal content not less than 50% and not more than 70% is present as ergotamine tartrate. Sterilise by filtration and store in ampoules in which the air has been replaced by nitrogen or other suitable gas. Protect from light.

Ergotamine Tartrate Injection *(U.S.P.).* A sterile solution of ergotamine tartrate and the tartrates of its epimer, ergotaminine, and of other related alkaloids, in Water for Injections to which tartaric acid or suitable stabilisers have been added, containing in each ml 450 to 550 µg of total alkaloids. The content of ergotamine tartrate is 52 to 74% of the total alkaloidal content, and the content of ergotaminine tartrate is not more than 45% of the total alkaloidal content. pH 3.5 to 4. Protect from light.

Suppositories

Ergotamine Tartrate and Caffeine Suppositories *(U.S.P.).* Suppositories containing ergotamine tartrate and caffeine. Store at a temperature not exceeding 25° in airtight containers. Protect unwrapped suppositories from light.

Tablets

Ergotamine Tablets *(B.P.).* Compressi Ergotamini Tartratis. Tablets containing ergotamine tartrate. The tablets are sugar-coated.

Ergotamine Tartrate and Caffeine Tablets *(U.S.P.).* Tablets containing ergotamine tartrate and caffeine. The *U.S.P.* requires 70% dissolution of ergotamine tartrate and 75% dissolution of caffeine in 30 minutes. Protect from light.

Ergotamine Tartrate Tablets *(U.S.P.).* Tablets containing ergotamine tartrate. Protect from light.

Proprietary Preparations

Cafergot Tablets *(Wander, UK).* Each contains ergotamine tartrate 1 mg and caffeine 100 mg. For migraine. *Dose.* 2 tablets at the onset of symptoms, followed if necessary by 1 tablet every half-hour up to a maximum of 6 tablets in 1 day or 10 in any 1 week. When the total effective dose is known, this may be taken as a single initial dose.

Cafergot Suppositories *(Wander, UK).* Each contains ergotamine tartrate 2 mg and caffeine 100 mg. For migraine. *Dose.* 1 to be administered at the onset of symptoms, repeated if necessary up to a maximum of 3 suppositories in 1 day or 5 in any 1 week. When the total effective dose is known, this may be administered as a single initial dose.

Effergot *(Wander, UK).* Scored effervescent tablets each containing ergotamine tartrate 2 mg and caffeine 50 mg. For migraine. *Dose.* 1 tablet, dissolved in water, at the onset of symptoms, followed if necessary by ½ tablet every half-hour up to a maximum of 3 tablets in 1 day or 5 in any 1 week.

Lingraine *(Winthrop, UK).* Sublingual tablets each containing ergotamine tartrate 2 mg. (Also available as Lingraine in *Austral.*).

Medihaler Ergotamine *(Riker, UK).* An aerosol spray containing ergotamine tartrate 9 mg per ml and delivering 360 µg in each metered dose. For migraine. *Dose.* 1 inhalation at the onset of symptoms, repeated if necessary at intervals of 5 minutes up to a maximum of 6 inhalations in 24 hours or 15 in 1 week. (Also available as Medihaler Ergotamine in *Austral., Belg., Canad.*).

Migril *(Wellcome, UK).* Scored tablets each containing ergotamine tartrate 2 mg, caffeine hydrate 100 mg, and cyclizine hydrochloride 50 mg. For migraine. *Dose.* 1 or 2 tablets at the onset of symptoms, followed if necessary by ½ to 1 tablet at half-hourly intervals up to a maximum of 4 tablets for any single attack, or 6 in any 1 week.

Other Proprietary Names

Arg.—Gynergeno; *Austral.*—Gynergen; *Belg.*—Gynergene; *Canad.*—Ergomar, Gynergen; *Denm.*—Ergotamin-Medihaler, Gynergen; *Fin.*—Eximigrex; *Fr.*—Gynergène; *Ger.*—Ergotamin Medihaler; *Ital.*—Ergotan, Gynergen; *Jap.*—Migretamine; *Neth.*—Exmigra, Gynergeen; *Norw.*—Lingrene; *S.Afr.*—Ergate; *Spain*—Gynergeno; *Swed.*—Lingrän; *Switz.*—Gynergen; *USA*—Ergomar, Ergostat, Gynergen.

Preparations containing ergotamine tartrate were also formerly marketed in Great Britain under the proprietary names Ergodryl *(Parke, Davis)*, Femergin *(Wander)*, and Orgraine *(Organon)*.

1509-v

Ergotoxine Esylate. Ergotoxine Ethanesulphonate. Ergotoxine is a mixture of the 3 isomorphous alkaloids ergocornine, ergocristine, and ergocryptine.
$C_{31}H_{39}N_5O_5,C_2H_5SO_3H = 671.8$.

CAS — 8006-25-5 (ergotoxine); 8047-28-7 (esylate).

Colourless crystals. Sparingly **soluble** in water; more soluble in alcohol. **Store** in a cool place in an atmosphere of nitrogen in hermetically sealed containers. Protect from light.

Adverse Effects, Treatment, and Precautions. As for Ergot, p.662.

Uses. Ergotoxine esylate was formerly used as an oxytocic and in the treatment of migraine in doses of 0.5 to 1 mg, subcutaneously or intramuscularly.

1510-r

Lysuride Maleate.

Lisuride Maleate; Methylergol Carbamide Maleate. 3-(9,10-Didehydro-6-methylergolin-8α-yl)-1,1-diethylurea hydrogen maleate.
$C_{20}H_{26}N_4O,C_4H_4O_4 = 454.5$.

CAS — 18016-80-3 (lysuride); 19875-60-6 (maleate).

Adverse Effects. Nausea, vomiting, headache, drowsiness, dizziness, vertigo, mental effects, muscle aches and pains, coldness of the limbs, tachycardia, and hypotension have been reported.

Uses. Lysuride maleate is an ergot derivative and has been called an ergoline. It is a serotonin antagonist. It is also reported to be a dopamine agonist.

Lysuride maleate is given for the prophylaxis of migraine. The usual dose is 25 µg thrice daily.

Acromegaly. A single dose of lysuride 300 µg significantly reduced plasma concentrations of growth hormone and prolactin in 12 acromegalic patients. Plasma concentrations of growth hormone and prolactin were consistently suppressed in 2 of these patients given lysuride in a gradually increasing dose over 10 days to 300 µg four times daily and continued at this dose for 2 weeks.— A. Liuzzi *et al.*, *J. clin. Endocr. Metab.*, 1978, *46*, 196.

Inhibition of lactation. Lysuride in a dose of up to 600 µg daily inhibited lactation.— L. De Cecco *et al.*, *Br. J. Obstet. Gynaec.*, 1979, *86*, 905.

Migraine. Five serotonin antagonists were assessed in 290 patients who suffered from headaches with features of migraine. Lysuride maleate 25 to 50 µg thrice daily was found to be no more effective than placebo in the prevention of migraine.— J. W. Lance *et al.*, *Br. med. J.*, 1970, *2*, 327.

In a 3-month double-blind study involving 253 patients, lysuride maleate 25 µg thrice daily was as effective as methysergide maleate 2 mg thrice daily for the prophylaxis of migraine. Of those treated with lysuride 53% noted a 50% or more reduction in number of attacks and of those treated with methysergide 51% noted a comparable reduction in frequency. Side-effects caused 17 and 39% of patients receiving lysuride and methysergide respectively to withdraw from the study.— W. M. Herrmann *et al.*, *Headache*, 1977, *17*, 54.

Lysuride maleate 25 µg thrice daily was significantly superior to a placebo for the prophylaxis of migraine in a 3-month double-blind study involving 132 patients. Side-effects caused 12 and 5 patients receiving lysuride and placebo respectively to withdraw from the study.— B. W. Somerville and W. M. Herrmann, *Headache*, 1978, *18*, 75. See also W. M. Herrmann *et al.*, *J. int. med. Res.*, 1978, *6*, 476.

Parkinsonism. Studies in *rats* suggested that lysuride may be useful in the treatment of Parkinson's disease.— D. Loos *et al.*, *Naunyn-Schmiedebergs Arch. Pharmac.*, 1977, *300*, 195.

A report of the gradual replacement of bromocriptine by lysuride in 11 patients with moderate to severe Parkinson's disease, taking bromocriptine alone or with levodopa; domperidone was given to relieve nausea. Five patients were withdrawn owing to increase in akinesia and tremor (3), persistent nausea (1), and visual hallucinations and disorientation (1). The remaining 6 are taking lysuride 2.4 to 4.8 mg daily 2 months after starting the drug, the dosage of levodopa remaining unchanged. Improvement was noted in one patient and no change in 5; the efficacy of lysuride did not diminish over the 8 weeks. It was concluded that lysuride has definite antiparkinsonian action, with 1 mg having approximately the same antiparkinsonian potency as 12 to 15 mg of bromocriptine.— M. Schachter *et al.* (letter), *Lancet*, 1979, *2*, 1129. See also A. N. Lieberman *et al.* (letter), *ibid.*

Lysuride was given in a dose of 0.2 to 6 mg daily in three divided doses to 12 parkinsonian patients with levodopa-induced oscillations. Oscillations improved in one patient. Four patients reported an improvement in mobility during 'on' periods. Adverse effects were frequent and dose-limiting; they included gastro-intestinal upsets in 6 patients, an increase in peak-dose choreoathetosis in 2, and toxic confusional states with visual hallucinations in 2.— A. J. Lees and G. M. Stern (letter), *Lancet*, 1981, *2*, 577.

Further references: A. N. Lieberman *et al.*, *Clin. Pharmac. Ther.*, 1980, *27*, 266; *idem*, 1981, *29*, 261.

Pituitary tumours. Serial computed tomographic evidence for the almost complete disappearance of a large prolactinoma in a patient treated for 2 years with lysuride.— G. Verde *et al.* (letter), *Lancet*, 1979, *2*, 582.

Proprietary Names

Cuvalit *(Schering, Ger.)*; Lysenyl *(Cz.)*.

1511-f

Metergoline.

Methergoline; MCE; FI6337. Benzyl *N*-(1,6-dimethylergolin-8β-ylmethyl)carbamate.
$C_{25}H_{29}N_3O_2 = 403.5$.

CAS — 17692-51-2.

Uses. Metergoline is an ergot derivative and has been called an ergoline. It is a serotonin antagonist. It is also reported to be a dopamine agonist.

Metergoline is used for the inhibition of lactation. The usual dose is 12 mg daily, in divided doses, for about 7 days. It has also been given in doses of 1 to 2 mg intramuscularly. Metergoline has also been tried in the prophylaxis of migraine.

A short review on the mechanism of action of some ergot alkaloids, including metergoline.— E. E. Müller *et al.*, *Pharmacology*, 1978, *16*, *Suppl.* 1, 63.

Acromegaly. A single dose of metergoline 4 mg depressed plasma concentrations of growth hormone and prolactin in 6 patients with acromegaly. The responses resembled those observed after administration of levodopa and bromocriptine. Plasma concentrations of the 2 hormones remained suppressed during treatment in 3 of the patients given metergoline 2 mg four times daily for 6 days.— G. Delitala *et al.*, *J. clin. Endocr. Metab.*, 1976, *43*, 1382.

Galactorrhoea-amenorrhoea syndrome. A 33-year-old woman with amenorrhoea and galactorrhoea of 10 years' duration complaining of infertility received metergoline 4 mg twice daily. During treatment galactorrhoea decreased, but did not cease, and after 2 months when plasma-prolactin concentration was reduced to about 50 ng per ml (normal less than 25 ng per ml) ovulation and conception occurred. Metergoline was discontinued and a healthy infant was delivered after an uneventful pregnancy.— P. G. Crosignani *et al.*, *Br. J. Obstet. Gynaec.*, 1977, *84*, 386.

A 39-year-old woman with amenorrhoea, galactorrhoea, and hyperprolactinaemia due to a prolactin-secreting pituitary microadenoma received metergoline 8 to 12 mg daily for 8 months. Galactorrhoea promptly decreased, but did not cease, and after 3 months of therapy regular menstrual periods occurred which persisted for 2 months after withdrawal of therapy. Presumptive evidence of ovulation was obtained in some instances by determination of progesterone and gonadotrophin in serum. Serum-prolactin concentration was reduced during therapy; a rebound above pretreatment value followed withdrawal of metergoline.— C. Ferrari *et al.*, *Fert. Steril.*, 1978, *30*, 237.

Inhibition of lactation. Metergoline reduced the elevated plasma-prolactin concentrations in 78 lactating women. Lactation was suppressed within 5 days in 59 of 69 women given 4 mg twice daily for 5 days when started within 24 hours of delivery. In 9 women given metergoline from the 4th day congestion and discomfort were rapidly relieved. There were no side-effects.— G. Delitala *et al.*, *Br. med. J.*, 1977, *1*, 744.

Metergoline 4 mg thrice daily for 5 days inhibited lactation in 20 women when administered within 24 hours of delivery and suppressed lactation in a further 10 when administered within 48 to 72 hours of delivery. After stopping therapy only 3 women showed a mild rebound of lactation, breast engorgement, or pain, which was relieved by a few additional days of treatment. Plasma-prolactin concentrations were significantly reduced.— P. G. Crosignani *et al.*, *Obstet. Gynec.*, 1978, *51*, 113.

Proprietary Names

Liserdol *(Farmitalia, Ital.)*.

1512-d

Methylergometrine Maleate *(B.P. 1973).*

Methylergometrine Mal.; Methylergonovine Maleate *(U.S.P.)*; Methylergonovinium Bimaleate; Methylergobasine Maleate. *N*-[(*S*)-1-(Hydroxymethyl)propyl]-D-lysergamide hydrogen maleate; 9,10-Didehydro-*N*-[(*S*)-1-(hydroxymethyl)propyl]-6-methylergoline-8β-carboxamide hydrogen maleate.
$C_{20}H_{25}N_3O_2,C_4H_4O_4 = 455.5$.

CAS — 113-42-8 (methylergometrine); 57432-61-8 (maleate).

Pharmacopoeias. In *Braz.*, *Jap.*, *Jug.*, *Nord.*, *Turk.*, and *U.S.*

A white or pinkish-tan, odourless, crystalline powder with a bitter taste. It darkens on exposure to light. M.p. 185° to 195° with decomposition.

Soluble 1 in 200 of water and 1 in 140 of alcohol giving a blue fluorescence; practically insoluble in chloroform and ether. A 0.02% solution in water has a pH of 4.4 to 5.2. Solutions are **sterilised** by autoclaving or by filtration; before autoclaving or after filtration, the solution is distributed into ampoules, the air in which is replaced by nitrogen or other suitable gas. **Store** at a temperature not exceeding 8° in an atmosphere of nitrogen in hermetically sealed containers. Protect from light.

Adverse Effects. As for Ergometrine Maleate, p.664.

Pregnancy and the neonate. Hypertension. Mean venous pressure in the umbilical cord was 430 mm blood in 23 women given methylergometrine maleate 200 µg when the foetal head crowned compared with a mean pressure of 269 mm blood in 51 women who did not receive an oxytocic. An abrupt increase in venous pressure might be harmful to infants with cardiovascular disorders.— A. T. LeDonne and L. McGowan, *Obstet. Gynec.*, 1967, *30*, 103.

Precautions. As for Ergot, p.662.

It should be given with caution to patients with toxaemia.

Absorption and Fate. See Ergot, p.662.

Uses. Methylergometrine maleate has an action on the uterus similar to that of ergometrine maleate (see p.664). Uterine contractions occur within 5 to 10 minutes of administration by mouth, 2 to 5 minutes after intramuscular injection, and ½ to 1 minute after intravenous injection.

Methylergometrine maleate may be used similarly to ergometrine maleate in the management of the third stage of labour of normal confinements. It is given in doses of 200 µg intramuscularly, under obstetric supervision, following the delivery of the anterior shoulder of the infant during the second stage of labour and delivery of the placenta is then usually assisted while the uterus is firmly contracted.

In the treatment of postpartum haemorrhage doses of 200 µg intramuscularly are also used, usually on completion of the third stage of labour. It may also be given by slow intravenous injection over at least 60 seconds in a dose of 100 to 200 µg. If uterine inertia or haemorrhage persists, the dose may be repeated at intervals of 2 to 4 hours.

For the treatment of subinvolution or during postpartum convalescence, 125 to 250 µg may be given by mouth 3 or 4 times a day for up to 7 days.

Preparations

Methylergometrine Injection *(B.P. 1973).* Methylergometrine Maleate Injection. A sterile solution of methylergometrine maleate in Water for Injections free from dissolved air. The acidity is adjusted to pH 3.2 (limits: pH 2.9 to 3.5) with maleic acid. Protect from light.

Methylergometrine Tablets *(B.P. 1973).* Methylergometrine Maleate Tablets. Tablets containing methylergometrine maleate. The tablets are sugar-coated.

Methylergonovine Maleate Injection *(U.S.P.).* A sterile solution of methylergometrine maleate in Water for Injections. pH 2.7 to 3.5. Protect from light.

Methylergonovine Maleate Tablets *(U.S.P.).* Tablets containing methylergometrine maleate. The *U.S.P.* requires 70% dissolution in 30 minutes. Store in airtight containers. Protect from light.

Proprietary Names

Basofortina *(Sandoz, Arg.)*; Levospan *(Jap.)*; Methergin *(Sandoz, Austral.*; *Sandoz-Wander, Belg.*; *Sandoz, Denm.*; *Sandoz, Fr.*; *Sandoz, Ger.*; *Sandoz, Ital.*; *Sandoz, Neth.*; *Sandoz, Norw.*; *Sandoz, S.Afr.*; *Sandoz, Spain*; *Sandoz, Swed.*; *Sandoz, Switz.)*; Methergine *(Sandoz, USA)*.

1513-n

Methysergide Maleate *(B.P., U.S.P.).* 1-Methyl-D-lysergic Acid Butanolamide Maleate.

N-[1-(Hydroxymethyl)propyl]-1-methyl-D-lysergamide hydrogen maleate; 9,10-Didehydro-*N*-[1-(hydroxymethyl)propyl]-1,6-dimethylergoline-8β-carboxamide hydrogen maleate.

$C_{21}H_{27}N_3O_2,C_4H_4O_4$=469.5.

CAS — 361-37-5 (methysergide); 129-49-7 (maleate).

Pharmacopoeias. In *Br.* and *U.S.*

A white to yellowish-white or reddish-white, odourless or almost odourless, crystalline powder. It loses not more than 7% of its weight on drying. Methysergide 1 mg is approximately equivalent to 1.33 mg of methysergide maleate.

Soluble 1 in 500 of water, 1 in 125 of methyl alcohol, 1 in 165 of alcohol, and 1 in 10 000 of chloroform; practically insoluble in ether. A solution is dextrorotatory. A 0.2% solution in water has a pH of 3.7 to 4.7. **Store** at 2° to 8° in airtight containers. Protect from light.

The addition of caffeine increased the aqueous solubility of methysergide maleate independently of pH.— M. A. Zoglio and H. V. Maulding, *J. pharm. Sci.*, 1970, *59*, 1836.

Adverse Effects. Adverse effects, which resemble those of ergot (see p.662), may be frequent, and may necessitate withdrawal of methysergide in some patients; rebound headaches may occur if it is withdrawn suddenly.

Common reactions are nausea, vomiting, epigastric pain, dizziness, and drowsiness. Other effects include diarrhoea, constipation, restlessness, weakness, ataxia, vertigo, increase in weight, leg cramps, peripheral oedema, arterial spasm, paraesthesias of the extremities, confusion, insomnia, psychic effects, dermatitis, loss of hair, pain in joints and muscles, increased anginal pain, tachycardia, and orthostatic hypotension. Neutropenia and eosinophilia have also been reported.

Retroperitoneal fibrosis with obstruction of abdominal vessels, pleural fibrosis, and fibrotic changes in heart valves have occurred in some patients after taking methysergide for prolonged periods. Most changes are reversible when the drug is discontinued.

In 850 patients with migraine, methysergide 1 to 8 mg daily, benefited 45% without side-effects and 12% were not benefited at all. Side-effects in the remaining 43% included weight gain (30%), severe oedema (4%), severe depression (2%), pain in the calves (26%), disturbed vision (1%), and loss of hair (1%); 3% were completely intolerant of the drug.— N. Leyton (letter), *Lancet*, 1964, *1*, 830.

For a report of methysergide abuse, see R. N. Lucas and W. Falkowski, *Br. J. Psychiat.*, 1973, *122*, 199.

Effects on mental state. In 57 patients treated with methysergide, treatment was discontinued in 4 because of hallucinations, in 3 because of nightmares, and in 2 because of psychosis possibly precipitated by methysergide.— A. R. Hale and A. F. Reed, *Am. J. med. Sci.*, 1962, *243*, 92.

Further references.— I. Persyko, *J. nerv. ment. Dis.*, 1972, *154*, 299.

Fibrosis. *Cardiac.* Endocardial fibrosis indicated by cardiac murmurs developed in 48 patients receiving methysergide. The murmurs gradually regressed in 27 of the patients when methysergide was discontinued. Retroperitoneal fibrosis was present in 9 patients and pleuropulmonary fibrosis in 2. Methysergide should be used with great caution in patients with existing cardiac disease.— D. S. Bana *et al.*, *Am. Heart J.*, 1974, *88*, 640.

A 48-year-old man who had taken methysergide, 4 mg daily for 4 years, and who died from a pulmonary infection was found on necropsy to have thickening of the chordae and heart valve cusps by a layer of avascular fibrous tissue.— K. A. Misch, *Br. med. J.*, 1974, *2*, 365.

A 52-year-old woman who had taken methysergide intermittently for 3 years (average dose 5 mg daily, with abstinence for 3 to 4 weeks every 6 months) developed tricuspid, aortic, and mitral valve insufficiency, and myocardial fibrosis.— J. W. Mason *et al.*, *Circulation*, 1977, *56*, 889.

Pleuropulmonary. A 50-year-old man and a 37-year-old woman receiving methysergide, 3 mg and 3 to 6 mg daily respectively, developed extensive pleural fibrosis. Bilateral pleural effusions also occurred in the man. These abnormalities rapidly improved following withdrawal of methysergide therapy.— W. Hindle *et al.*, *Br. med. J.*, 1970, *1*, 605.

A 77-year-old woman who had taken methysergide daily for 10 years for migraine headache and who, 5 years previously had been evaluated for pleural fibrosis, subsequently developed constrictive pericarditis.— R. C. Orlando *et al.*, *Ann. intern. Med.*, 1978, *88*, 213.

Further references.— O. Lindeneg and A. Kok-Jensen, *Nord. Med.*, 1968, *79*, 681.

Retroperitoneal. Six months after the removal of a kidney, a 59-year-old man was found to have retroperitoneal fibrosis involving a ureter. He had taken methysergide daily for about 3 years for migraine but had discontinued treatment a few weeks prior to the first operation. Because the fibrosis did not regress when the drug was withdrawn it was suggested that in some predisposed individuals methysergide might initiate a process which became self-perpetuating.— F. D. Schwartz and G. Dunea, *Lancet*, 1966, *1*, 955.

Methysergide daily, taken for headaches for periods of 9 to 54 months, was considered to be responsible for the development of retroperitoneal fibrosis in 27 patients; cardiac murmurs developed in 6 of them. Fibrotic changes, affecting the aorta, heart valves, and pulmonary tissues, also occurred in a few of the patients and it was suggested that methysergide should be contra-indicated in patients with valvular heart disease, rheumatic arthritis, chronic pulmonary disease and collagen diseases. The need for regular examination of patients receiving methysergide was stressed.— J. R. Graham *et al.*, *New Engl. J. Med.*, 1966, *274*, 359.

A report of the successful treatment of methysergide-induced retroperitoneal fibrosis by means of corticosteroid therapy.— J. Paccalin *et al.*, *Thérapie*, 1976, *31*, 231.

For other reports of retroperitoneal fibrosis, see D. C. Utz *et al.*, *J. Am. med. Ass.*, 1965, *191*, 983; J. E. Conley *et al.*, *ibid.*, 1966, *198*, 808; N. C. Kerbel, *Can. med. Ass. J.*, 1967, *96*, 1420; R. Seymour, *Med. J. Aust.*, 1968, *1*, 59; A. H. Elkind *et al.*, *J. Am. med. Ass.*, 1968, *206*, 1041; W. J. Farrell *et al.*, *ibid.*, 1969, *207*, 1909; L. V. Wagenknecht, *Münch. med. Wschr.*, 1972, *114*, 585.

Haemolytic anaemia. A report of reversible haemolytic anaemia in a middle-aged woman who took methysergide daily for about 5 years.— P. H. Slugg and R. S. Kunkel, *J. Am. med. Ass.*, 1970, *213*, 297.

Lupus erythematosus. Methysergide had been suspected of inducing a syndrome resembling systemic lupus erythematosus.— *Adverse Drug React. Bull.*, 1973, Dec., 140.

Vascular disorders. Thrombophlebitis occurred in a 9-year-old girl, 2 weeks after starting treatment with methysergide for migraine. Complete recovery followed anti-coagulant therapy and withdrawal of methysergide maleate but phlebitis recurred when methysergide was restarted.— G. M. Fenichel and S. Battiata, *J. Pediat.*, 1966, *68*, 632.

A 39-year-old woman developed classical intestinal ischaemia following treatment with methysergide maleate 4 to 8 mg daily for 9 months. When methysergide was withdrawn, abdominal angina was immediately relieved, there was a gain in weight, and the abdominal murmur disappeared. Narrowing of the mesenteric artery branches, which was demonstrated by an arteriogram, disappeared 11 weeks after withdrawal of methysergide.— R. E. Buenger and J. A. Hunter, *J. Am. med. Ass.*, 1966, *198*, 558. A similar report.— J. Katz and R. M. Vogel, *J. Am. med. Ass.*, 1967, *199*, 124.

During long-term treatment with methysergide for migraine, 3 middle-aged patients suffered cardiac infarction (1 died), and 1 patient had acute coronary insufficiency. An ECG after exertion was recommended in all patients over the age of 40 in whom the use of methysergide was contemplated.— P. Hudgson *et al.* (letter), *Lancet*, 1967, *1*, 444.

Following the ingestion of methysergide maleate 8 mg daily for about 22 months, a 43-year-old woman developed vasculitis involving the iliac vessels with secondary ureteral obstruction, bilateral hydronephrosis and diminution of renal function. The symptoms slowly disappeared when methysergide maleate was withdrawn.— H. B. Miles and W. M. Tappan (letter), *J. Am. med. Ass.*, 1968, *203*, 431.

Acute arterial spasm of the lower extremities, characterised by pain in the calves when walking and tingling in the feet, occurred in a patient after treatment with methysergide 1 mg daily for 5 days. Improvement occurred after withdrawal of therapy.— K. Raw and H. Gaylis, *S. Afr. med. J.*, 1976, *50*, 1999.

Occlusion of the left brachial artery occurred in a patient after 2 months' therapy with methysergide maleate 4 to 6 mg daily. The patient was asymptomatic 4 days after withdrawal of methysergide.— F. M. Ameli *et al.*, *Can. J. Surg.*, 1977, *20*, 158.

Precautions. Methysergide maleate should not be given to pregnant patients or to patients with peripheral vascular disturbances, severe hypertension, coronary artery disease, heart valve disease, thrombophlebitis, pulmonary or collagen diseases, impaired hepatic or renal function, sepsis, or malnutrition. It should be used with caution in patients with oedema or peptic ulcer.

In order to diminish the side-effects of methysergide maleate taken for the prophylactic treatment of severe migraine, a rise in the sedimentation-rate in the absence of infection or other obvious cause might act as a warning for discontinuance of the drug.— M. T. Sweetnam (letter), *Br. med. J.*, 1970, *2*, 599.

For the enhancement of tolbutamide activity by methysergide maleate, see Tolbutamide, p.860.

Uses. Methysergide maleate is a potent serotonin antagonist. It has only slight oxytocic and vasoconstrictor effects. It is used as a prophylactic agent in the management of severe recurrent migraine, but the mode of action by which it prevents migraine is unknown. It is ineffective in the treatment of acute attacks of migraine or in the treatment of muscle tension headaches.

Methysergide maleate is usually given in a dosage equivalent to 2 to 6 mg of methysergide base daily in divided doses with meals, with the initial dose preferably given at bedtime. Careful and regular observation of the patient is essential because of the high incidence of side-effects. After 6 months' treatment the dosage of methysergide should be gradually reduced over 2 or 3 weeks and then discontinued for at least a month for reassessment. In patients receiving methysergide maleate, the dose of ergotamine required to control acute attacks of migraine may need to be reduced.

Methysergide is also used to control the diarrhoea associated with carcinoid disease and has been used in the treatment of mania.

Reviews.— J. R. Graham, *Practitioner*, 1967, *198*, 302.

Erythromelalgia. Methysergide 2 mg thrice daily relieved erythromelalgia in a 13-year-old girl previously treated without success with chlorpheniramine maleate or atropine. After 3 months of therapy, a maintenance dose of only 4 mg daily was necessary.— B. N. Catchpole, *Lancet*, 1964, *1*, 909. See also H. Pepper, *J. Am. med. Ass.*, 1968, *203*, 1066.

Headache. A comparative study of the use of methysergide, ergometrine and ergotamine in the relief of chronic recurrent headache in 105 patients.— M. A. Barrie *et al.*, *Q. J. Med.*, 1968, *37*, 319.

Patients with cluster headache who did not respond to ergotamine might be relieved by methysergide 3 to 6 mg daily or by pizotifen 1.5 to 3 mg daily for the duration of the bout.— *Br. med. J.*, 1975, *4*, 425.

Mania. In a controlled study, 8 of 10 patients who had suffered from typical manic attacks for 3 to 12 weeks benefited from treatment with methysergide. Methysergide, in gradually increasing doses, was given by injection for the first 2 days, by injection and mouth during the following 2 days, and subsequently by mouth only. Methysergide inhibited excessive psychomotor activity and drive, and sleeping habits became normal. Seven patients assumed transient depression but no serious side-effects were noticed.— L. Haškovec and K. Souček (letter), *Nature*, 1968, *219*, 507.

In a double-blind controlled trial there was no evidence that methysergide 6 mg daily was better than placebo in the treatment of 10 patients with mania. For talk and behavioural disturbance, methysergide was significantly less effective than placebo.— A. J. Coppen *et al.*, *Lancet*, 1969, *2*, 338. See also W. G. Dewhurst (letter), *ibid.*, 490; A. J. Coppen (letter), *ibid;* L. Haškovec (letter), *ibid.*, 902.

Further references.— W. G. Dewhurst (letter), *Lancet*, 1969, *1*, 624; J. H. Court and F. M. M. Mai, *Med. J. Aust.*, 1970, *2*, 526.

Migraine. In a double-blind crossover study, 50 patients with migraine were given methysergide 4 mg daily for 3 months and a placebo for a similar period. There was a significant reduction in duration of severe headache and a small reduction in frequency of attacks with methysergide. Patients in whom oedema and subsequent diuresis were a feature appeared to benefit most.— J. Whewell, *Br. med. J.*, 1966, *2*, 394.

Methysergide, given prophylactically in a dosage of 3 mg daily for 3 months to 67 patients with migraine, was effective in preventing or diminishing attacks in 26.9% compared with a response in 9% when a placebo was given. Patients with premenstrual migraine seemed much less likely to respond.— O. de S. Pinto and R. Greene, *Practitioner*, 1967, *198*, 129.

Five serotonin antagonists were assessed in 290 patients who suffered from headaches with features of migraine. Methysergide 1 to 2 mg thrice daily was more effective in the prevention of migraine than pizotifen in a dose of 1.5 to 3 mg thrice daily, and both were more effective than a placebo. Improvement after treatment with cyproheptadine 4 to 8 mg thrice daily or methdilazine 8 to 16 mg morning and night was better than placebo treatment, but the improvement-rates did not reach statistical significance. Lysuride maleate 25 to 50 µg thrice daily was found to be no more effective than placebo in the prevention of migraine. Side-effects after methysergide and lysuride maleate included muscle pains and cramps, coldness of the limbs, epigastric discomfort, and nausea. Drowsiness was the most common side-effect of the other drugs.— J. W. Lance *et al.*, *Br. med. J.*, 1970, *2*, 327.

Myoclonus. A report of the successful use of methysergide in the treatment of long-standing myoclonus.— P. Bedard and R. Bouchard (letter), *Lancet*, 1974, *1*, 738. Methysergide produced only slight improvement in 1 out of 3 patients with postanoxic myoclonus.— M. H. Van Woert and V. H. Sethy (letter), *ibid.*, 1285. Methysergide failed to have any benefit in a similar patient who deteriorated. Clonazepam produced some improvement.— F. Romero *et al.* (letter), *ibid.*, 1975, *1*, 395.

Narcolepsy. Methysergide gave as good a control of sleep attacks as dexamphetamine in 5 patients with narcolepsy, but the cataplexy, present in 4, was less well controlled. Two patients developed severe calf claudication during treatment.— A. R. Wyler *et al.*, *Archs Neurol., Chicago*, 1975, *32*, 265.

Preparations

Methysergide Maleate Tablets *(U.S.P.)*. Tablets containing methysergide maleate. The *U.S.P.* requires 70% dissolution in 30 minutes. Store in airtight containers.

Methysergide Tablets *(B.P.)*. Tablets containing methysergide maleate; they are sugar-coated. Protect from light.

Deseril *(Wander, UK)*. Methysergide maleate, available as tablets each containing the equivalent of 1 mg of methysergide base. (Also available as Deseril in *Austral., Belg., Denm., Neth., Norw., S.Afr.*).

Other Proprietary Names

Deseril retard *(Ger., Norw., Switz.)*; Désernil *(Fr.)*; Deserril *(Ital.)*; Sansert *(Canad., Swed., USA)*.

1514-h

Nicergoline.

FI 6714. 10α-Methoxy-1,6-dimethylergolin-8β-ylmethyl 5-bromonicotinate. $C_{24}H_{26}BrN_3O_3$=484.4.

CAS — 27848-84-6.

A yellowish-white crystalline powder. Practically **insoluble** in water; soluble in alcohol, acetone, chloroform, and dilute acetic acid; slightly soluble in ether. M.p. 136° to 138°.

Adverse Effects. Gastro-intestinal side-effects, flushing of the skin, drowsiness, vertigo, and insomnia may occur. Hypotension, particularly following parenteral administration, has been reported and the effects of antihypertensive agents may be enhanced.

Of 359 patients with cerebrovascular insufficiency treated with nicergoline intramuscularly for 5 days and then 15 mg daily by mouth for 1 month side-effects occurred in 25, necessitating withdrawal of therapy in 11. The reactions included hot flushes (6), general malaise (8), agitation (2), hyperacidity (3), nausea (1), diarrhoea (3), and dizziness and somnolence (2).— J. Dauverchain, *Arzneimittel-Forsch.*, 1979, *29*, 1308.

Uses. Nicergoline is an ergot derivative (an ergoline). It is used as a vasodilator in the treatment of acute or chronic cerebral or peripheral circulatory insufficiency. The usual dose is 5 mg thrice daily; 2 mg may be given intramuscularly twice daily; 2 to 8 mg has been given by slow intravenous infusion.

Metabolism.— F. Arcamone *et al.*, *Biochem. Pharmac.*, 1972, *21*, 2205.

A favourable report on the effect of nicergoline 30 mg daily by mouth for 30 days on the reduced hearing of old age in 30 patients.— G. Aliprandi and V. Tantalo, *Arzneimittel-Forsch.*, 1979, *29*, 1287. See also A. Pech and P. Gitenet, *Annls Otolaryngol. Chir. cervicofac.*, 1975, *92*, 625.

The use of nicergoline in fluorescence retinographic studies in ophthalmology.— M. Borgioli *et al.*, *Arzneimittel-Forsch.*, 1979, *29*, 1311.

Cerebrovascular disease. In an uncontrolled study in 25 patients with chronic cerebral insufficiency, nicergoline in a daily dosage increased over 9 days to 4 mg parenterally and 10 mg by mouth improved the symptoms in a high proportion of patients. Cerebral perfusion seen by serial angiography was also improved.— F. P. Bernini *et al.*, *Farmaco, Edn prat.*, 1977, *32*, 32.

Further references.— L. D. Iliff *et al.*, *J. Neurol. Neurosurg. Psychiat.*, 1977, *40*, 746; J. Dauverchain, *Arzneimittel-Forsch.*, 1979, *29*, 1308.

Peripheral vascular disease. In 10 healthy subjects and 24 with atherosclerosis the infusion of nicergoline 5 mg increased perfusion of the lower limbs, particularly in the affected limbs. The effect was not produced by phentolamine and could not be attributed to a central effect nor to alpha-adrenergic blockade.— F. Boismare *et al.*, *Thérapie*, 1974, *29*, 925.

In 36 patients with arteritis of the lower limbs an infusion of nicergoline 5 mg increased the circulation. After treatment for 1 month with 15 mg daily by mouth 22 patients were clinically improved. The failure of a second infusion to increase circulation was considered due to vasodilatation produced by oral therapy.— J. C. Schrub *et al.*, *Thérapie*, 1975, *30*, 407.

Proprietary Names

Sermion *(Montedison, Arg.; Specia, Fr.; Farmitalia, Ger.; Farmitalia, Ital.; Spain; Carlo Erba & Deutsche Farmitalia, Switz.)*; Varson *(Almirall, Spain)*.

Essential Oils and Aromatic Carminatives

4600-n

Essential oils are volatile odorous principles which are soluble in alcohol but only to a very limited extent in water. Chemically they are mixtures of esters, aldehydes, alcohols, ketones, and terpenes. In many pharmacopoeias volatile oils are described as ethereal oils (aetherolea). Other names used include ätherische öle, esencias, essences, essências, essentiae, and olea aetherea.

Taken internally, the volatile oils, as a group, exert a mild irritant action on the mucous membranes of the mouth and the digestive tract, which induces a feeling of warmth and increases salivation. Their excretion takes place through the lungs, skin, and kidneys. Taken after meals they are carminative and are employed for the relief of gastric discomfort and of flatulent colic and also to counteract the griping action of purgatives. They have also been inhaled for the relief of congestive respiratory disorders.

When applied to the intact skin essential oils have an irritant and rubefacient action, causing first a sensation of warmth and smarting, which is followed by a mild local anaesthesia. For this reason they are used as counter-irritants and cutaneous stimulants in the treatment of chronic inflammatory conditions, and to relieve neuralgia and rheumatic pains. They may also cause sensitisation. Care should be taken to avoid blistering.

The use of essential oils for flavouring medicines is described in the section on Colouring, Flavouring, and Sweetening Agents, p.424.

Information on essential oils and their preparations not included in the following section is given under the drugs from which they are manufactured.

Storage. Essential oils should be stored in a cool place in small, well-filled, airtight containers, protected from light.

The solubilisation in water of essential oils, flavours, and perfumes using nonionic surfactants.— B. Angla, *Soap Perfum. Cosm.*, 1966, *39*, 375. See also K. Thoma and G. Pfaff, *J. Soc. cosmet. Chem.*, 1976, *27*, 221.

An *in vitro* study of antifoaming and carminative actions of volatile oils.— N. Harries *et al.*, *J. clin. Pharm.*, 1978, *2*, 171.

The use of a preparation of *d*-limonene for dissolving gallstones.— H. Igimi *et al.*, *Am. J. dig. Dis.*, 1976, *21*, 926.

The structurally related terpinoids citral, citronellol, geranyl acetate, linalol, and linalyl acetate which are present in a number of essential oils are rapidly absorbed in the body. Citronellol, geraniol, and citral follow the same metabolic pathway, undergoing oxidation to carboxylic acids. Some is then decarboxylated and the remaining portion is oxidised to yield 2,6-dimethyl-2,6-octadienedioic acid from citral and geraniol or the dihydro form of the acid from citronellol. Some of the acid from citral or geraniol may be further reduced to the dihydro acid. At low doses, decarboxylation is the major metabolic route; at high doses, some terpinoids may be excreted unchanged. Excretion is rapid with little enterohepatic circulation. Linalol is readily conjugated to its glucuronide. An estimated acceptable daily intake of up to 500 µg per kg body-weight was established for citral, geranyl acetate, citronellol, linalol, and linalyl acetate, expressed as citral. Temporary estimated acceptable daily intakes were also established for *trans*-anethole (up to 2.5 mg per kg), (+)-carvone and (−)-carvone (up to 1 mg per kg), cinnamaldehyde (up to 700 µg per kg), and eugenol (up to 2.5 mg per kg). Estimated acceptable daily intakes are given for methyl anthranilate (up to 1.5 mg per kg), and methyl *N*-methylanthranilate (up to 200 µg per kg).— Twenty-third Report of Joint FAO/WHO Expert Committee on Food Additives, *Tech. Rep. Ser. Wld Hlth Org. No. 648*, 1980.

Antimicrobial activity. For reports of the antimicrobial activity of essential oils and their vapours, see J. C. Maruzzella and L. Liguori, *J. Am. pharm. Ass., scient. Edn*, 1958, *47*, 250; J. C. Maruzzella and P. A. Henry, *ibid.*, 294; *idem*, 471; J. C. Maruzzella, *Soap Perfum. Cosm.*, 1960, *33*, 835; J. C. Maruzzella and N. A. Sicurella, *J. Am. pharm. Ass., scient. Edn*, 1960, *49*, 692; J. C. Maruzzella *et al.*, *J. pharm. Sci.*, 1961, *50*, 665; J. C. Maruzzella, *ibid.*, 1963, *52*, 601.

Antoxidants for essential oils. See under Alkyl Gallates, p.1282.

Standard for essential oils. In addition to those standards noted under the oils included in *Martindale*, the British Standards Institution publishes British Standard Specifications for Cananga Oil (BS 2991/1:1965), Patchouli Oils (BS 2991/10/11:1965), Vetiver Oil (BS 2999/15:1965), Paraguay Petitgrain Oil (BS 2999/27:1972), Grapefruit Oil (BS 2999/44:1972), Lime Oils (BS 2999/45/46:1972), Mandarin Oil (BS 2999/47:1972), Wild Marjoram Oil (BS 2999/48:1972), Rosewood Oil (BS 2999/51:1972), and Litsea Cubeba Oil (BS 2999/55:1975).

Adverse Effects and Treatment. Excessive doses of essential oils are irritant to the gastro-intestinal tract and may cause nausea, vomiting, and diarrhoea. There may be occasional irritation of the urinary tract and aggravation of pre-existing inflammatory conditions. There may be initial excitement. Convulsions may occur. Severe poisoning leads to respiratory failure. The CNS may be depressed leading to stupor and respiratory failure, or stimulated leading to excitement and convulsions.

In acute poisoning the stomach should be emptied by aspiration and lavage. Give a saline purgative, such as sodium sulphate 30 g in 250 ml of water, unless catharsis is already present. Demulcent drinks may be given. Large volumes of fluid should be given provided renal function is adequate.

In studies in *mice* of the toxicity of the vapours of certain essential oils, it was found that with oils of aniseed, pine, dill, and juniper, the concentration causing the death of 50% of the mice in 12 hours ranged from 0.8 to 1.5 mg per litre and the highest concentration at which all animals survived for 21 days was from 120 to 200 µg per litre. In 2 investigations of 49 and 45 persons respectively who had worked in contact with essential oils for 3 to 12 years, somnolence, headache, pain in the region of the liver, cough, enlargement of the liver, increased urobilinogen in the urine, and albuminuria were noted in a considerable proportion of the workers. The concentration of essential oils in the air in the working environment was from 5 to 378 µg per litre. The maximum permissible level was considered to be 10 µg per litre.— Z. Kowalski *et al.*, *Medycyna Pr.*, 1962, *13*, 69, per *Bull. Hyg., Lond.*, 1962, *37*, 1030.

For a report of photodermatitis after the use of a preparation containing various perfume oils, see (Starke, J.C.), *Archs Derm.*, 1967, *96*, 62, per *J. Am. med. Ass.*, 1967, *201*, (July 24), A143.

4601-h

Achillea. Milfoil; Yarrow; Millefolii Herba; Millefeuille; Schafgarbe.

Pharmacopoeias. In *Aust.*, *Hung.*, *Pol.*, and *Swiss*. *Roum.* includes the oil (Aetheroleum Millefolii).

The dried flowering tops of yarrow, *Achillea millefolium* (Compositae). It contains a volatile oil (about 0.25%), aconitic acid (=achilleic acid), an alkaloid (achilleine), a bitter principle (ivain), and tannin.

Achillea has been used for a great variety of medicinal purposes. It is stated to have diaphoretic, stimulant, and haemostatic properties.

4602-m

Ajowan. Trachyspermum; Ptychotis.

The dried ripe fruits of *Trachyspermum ammi* (=*Carum copticum*) (Umbelliferae), containing about 4 to 6% of volatile oil.

4603-b

Ajowan Oil *(B.P.C. 1934)*. Ptychotis Oil.

CAS — 8001-99-8.

Pharmacopoeias. In *Ind.*

The oil distilled from the fruits of *Trachyspermum ammi*. It contains not less than 40% of thymol.

Ajowan has been used as a carminative and antispasmodic. The oil has been used similarly. It is a commercial source of thymol.

An aqueous extract from roasted seeds of *Trachyspermum ammi* was found to have cholinomimetic effects.— G. Devasankaraiah *et al.*, *Br. J. Pharmac.*, 1974, *52*, 613.

4604-v

Amber Oil *(B.P.C. 1949)*. Oleum Succini; Rectified Amber Oil.

CAS — 8002-67-3.

A pale yellow or brownish-yellow liquid with a penetrating odour and a burning acrid taste, obtained by the destructive distillation of certain resins or by distilling resin oil. Wt per ml 0.845 to 0.9 g.

Soluble in alcohol, chloroform, ether, and fixed oils. **Store** in a cool place in airtight containers. Protect from light.

Amber oil has properties similar to those of turpentine oil and is used in liniments.

4605-g

Amomum. The seed mass of *Amomum xanthioides* (Zingiberaceae).

Pharmacopoeias. In *Jap.*, which also specifies Powdered Amomum.

Ind.P.C. includes the dried ripe or nearly ripe seeds of *Amomum aromaticum* (Bengal Cardamom) or *A. subulatum* (Nepal or Greater Cardamom) (Zingiberaceae).

Amomum has been used as a substitute for cardamom.

4606-q

Anethole *(U.S.N.F.)*. Anethol; Anetol; *p*-Propenylanisole. (*E*)-1-Methoxy-4-(prop-1-enyl)benzene.

$C_{10}H_{12}O$ = 148.2.

CAS — 104-46-1; 4180-23-8 (E).

Pharmacopoeias. In *Braz.* Also in *U.S.N.F.*

A white or faintly yellow crystalline mass, melting at or above 23° to a colourless or faintly yellow liquid with a sweet taste and the characteristic odour of aniseed. It is obtained from anise oil or other sources or prepared synthetically. The *U.S.N.F.* specifies specific gravity of 0.983 to 0.988.

Very slightly **soluble** in water; soluble 1 in 2 of alcohol; soluble in chloroform and ether. A solution in alcohol is neutral to litmus. **Store** in airtight containers. Protect from light.

Uses. Anethole is used for the same purposes as anise oil.

Temporary estimated acceptable daily intake of *trans*-anethole: up to 2.5 mg per kg body-weight. Anethole is rapidly metabolised. Long-term studies in *mice* and *rats* though not totally satisfactory indicate that *trans*-anethole is probably not a carcinogen. Adequate long-term feeding studies are required.— Twenty-third Report of the Joint FAO/WHO Expert Committee on Food Additives, *Tech. Rep. Ser. Wld Hlth Org.* No. 648, 1980.

Proprietary Names
Monasirup *(Arznei Müller-Rorer, Ger.).*

4607-p

Aniseed *(B.P., Eur. P.).* Anise; Anise Fruit; Anisi Fructus; Fructus Anisi Vulgaris; Anis Vert; Anice; Anis Verde.

Pharmacopoeias. In *Arg., Aust., Belg., Br., Cz., Eur., Ger., Hung., It., Neth., Pol., Port., Roum., Rus., Span.,* and *Swiss.*

The dried ripe fruit of *Pimpinella anisum* (Umbelliferae), containing not less than 2% v/w of volatile oil. **Powdered Aniseed** is greenish yellow or brownish green. **Store** in a cool dry place. Protect from light.

4608-s

Star Anise *(B.P.C. 1934).* Anisum Stellatum; Star Anise Fruit; Anisum Badium; Badiana; Anis Étoilé; Badiane de Chine; Sternanis; Anís Estrellado.

Pharmacopoeias. In *Arg., Aust., Braz., Chin., Fr.,* and *Port.*

The dried ripe fruit of *Illicium verum* (Magnoliaceae), containing about 5% of volatile oil. **Store** in a cool dry place.
Japanese Star Anise, *Illicium anisatum* (=*I. religiosum*), is smaller and less regular in appearance, and contains a poisonous principle sikimin. The volatile oil contains safrole.

4609-w

Anise Oil *(B.P., U.S.N.F.).* Aniseed Oil; Oleum Anisi; Essence d'Anis; Esencia de Anís.

CAS — 8007-70-3.

Pharmacopoeias. In *Arg., Aust., Belg., Br., Cz., Ger., Hung., Ind., Jug., Mex., Neth., Nord., Pol., Port., Roum., Span., Swiss,* and *Turk.* Also in *U.S.N.F.*

A colourless or pale yellow oil obtained by distillation from aniseed or star anise. It has a characteristic odour and a sweet aromatic taste. It contains about 80 to 90% of anethole. Wt per ml 0.978 to 0.992 g. F.p. not below 15°.
Soluble 1 in 3 of alcohol (90%), sometimes with a slight opalescence. It can be cooled considerably below 15° without becoming solid provided it is undisturbed. If the oil has crystallised it should be melted completely and mixed before use. Exposure to air causes polymerisation and some oxidation with the formation of *p*-methoxybenzaldehyde (anisaldehyde) and anisic acid. **Store** at a temperature not exceeding 25° in well-filled airtight containers. Protect from light.

The Pharmaceutical Society's Department of Pharmaceutical Sciences found that PVC bottles softened and distorted fairly rapidly in the presence of anise oil, which should not be stored or dispensed in such bottles.— *Pharm. J.,* 1973, *1,* 100.

The solubility of anise oil in macrogol esters.— K. Thoma and G. Pfaff, *J. Soc. cosmet. Chem.,* 1976, *27,* 221.

Uses. Aniseed or anise is carminative and mildly expectorant; it is used mainly as anise oil or as preparations of the oil which is a common ingredient of cough mixtures and lozenges. The oil is also a flavouring agent. *Dose:* 0.05 to 0.2 ml.

For the antimicrobial activity of *Illicium verum,* see R. N. Patel, *Indian J. Pharm.,* 1968, *30,* 43.

Preparations

Anise Emulsion *(B.P.C. 1954).* Emuls. Anis. Anise oil 2 ml, quillaia liquid extract 0.25 ml, water to 100 ml. Store in a warm place. *Dose.* 0.3 to 2 ml.

Anise Spirit *(B.P.C. 1949).* Sp. Anis. Anise oil 10 ml, alcohol (90%) to 100 ml. *Dose.* 0.3 to 1.2 ml.

Anise Water. Concentrated anise water 2.5 ml, freshly boiled and cooled water to 100 ml.

Concentrated Anise Water *(B.P.).* Anise Water Concentrated *(A.P.F.)*; Aqua Anisi Concentrata. Anise oil 2 ml, alcohol (90%) 70 ml, water to 100 ml; shaken with 5 g of sterilised talc and filtered.

Aqua Anisi *(Arg. P.).* Agua de Badiana. Star anise 10 g and water 200 ml; distil 100 ml.

Syrupus Anisi *(Arg. P.).* Jarabe de Anise. Sucrose 85 g, aqua anisi to 100 ml.

4610-m

Apiol *(B.P.C. 1934).*

CAS — 523-80-8.

Pharmacopoeias. In *Port.* and *Span.*

A green oil with a peculiar odour and a disagreeable taste, obtained by alcoholic extraction from the dried ripe fruits of parsley, *Petroselinum crispum* (=*Carum petroselinum*) (Umbelliferae). Wt per ml about 1.1 g. Practically **insoluble** in water; soluble in alcohol and ether.

Apiol has been used as an emmenagogue but is of doubtful therapeutic value.

Acute haemolytic anaemia, thrombocytopenic purpura, nephrosis, and hepatic dysfunction resulted from taking 36 capsules of a proprietary compound, each capsule containing 300 mg of apiol.— L. Lowenstein and D. H. Ballew, *Can. med. Ass. J.,* 1958, *78,* 195.

4611-b

Bay Oil *(B.P.C. 1949).* Oleum Myrciae; Myrcia Oil.

CAS — 8006-78-8.

NOTE. Laurel Leaf Oil (Bay Leaf Oil) is obtained from the leaves of *Laurus nobilis* (Lauraceae).

A yellow oil, darkening rapidly on exposure to air, with a pleasant odour and spicy taste, obtained by distillation from the leaves of *Pimenta acris* (=*P. racemosa*) (Myrtaceae) and probably other allied species. It contains 50 to 65% v/v of phenols. Wt per ml 0.94 to 0.985 g. **Soluble** when freshly distilled, 1 in 1 of alcohol; soluble in glacial acetic acid.

Standard for bay oil. A British Standard Specification for Bay Oil (BS 2999/16: 1972) is published by the British Standards Institution.

The principal use of bay oil is in the preparation of bay rum, which is used as a hair lotion and as an astringent application to the face after shaving.

Preparations

Compound Bay Spirit *(B.P.C. 1949).* Sp. Myrc. Co.; Compound Myrcia Spirit; Compound Pimento Spirit. Bay oil 0.875 ml, orange oil 0.062 ml, pimento oil 0.062 ml, quassia dry extract 86 mg, saponin 31 mg, alcohol (90%) 64 ml, water to 100 ml. Dissolve the oils, the extract, and the saponin in the alcohol and adjust to volume with water; set aside for 8 days, add a little talc, and filter.
Similar preparations, coloured brown, are sold as Bay Rum.

4612-v

Benzaldehyde *(B.P., U.S.N.F.).* Artificial Essential Oil of Almond.

$C_6H_5.CHO = 106.1$.

CAS — 100-52-7.

Pharmacopoeias. In *Belg., Br., Braz., Hung., Mex.,* and *Port.* Also in *U.S.N.F.*

A clear colourless strongly refractive liquid with a characteristic odour of bitter almonds and a burning aromatic taste. Wt per ml 1.043 to 1.049 g.
Soluble 1 in 350 of water; miscible with alcohol, ether, and fixed and volatile oils. B.p. about 178°. It becomes yellowish on keeping and oxidises in air to benzoic acid. **Store** in a cool place in well-filled airtight containers. Protect from light.

Solubility in water. A gravimetric method of determining the solubility of benzaldehyde in water was described and the result obtained compared with that given by gas chromatography. The solubilities given by the 2 methods at 25° were 1 in 153 and 1 in 152 respectively which was in marked contrast with the International Critical Table 1928, which gave 3 g per litre (1 in 333) at room temperature, and the Merck Index 1960, which gave 1 in 350 of water.— A. G. Mitchell *et al., J. Pharm. Pharmac.,* 1964, *16,* 632. A third method of determination of the solubility of benzaldehyde in water was described, based on refractive index measurements. The resulting solubility figures given by this method were 1 in 143 to 1 in 145 at 25°.— J. E. Carless and J. Swarbrick, *J. Pharm. Pharmac.,* 1964, *16,* 633.

Uses. Benzaldehyde is used as a flavouring agent in the place of volatile bitter almond oil. A syrup containing 0.2% of Benzaldehyde Spirit may be used as an alternative to Wild Cherry Syrup.

Estimated acceptable daily intake: up to 5 mg per kg body-weight as total benzoic acid from all food additive sources.— Eleventh Report of the Joint FAO/WHO Expert Committee on Food Additives, *Tech. Rep. Ser. Wld Hlth Org. No. 383,* 1968.

Preparations

Benzaldehyde Spirit *(B.P.).* Benzaldehyde 1 ml, alcohol (90%) 80 ml, water to 100 ml.
Store in a cool place in well-filled airtight containers. Protect from light.

Compound Benzaldehyde Elixir *(U.S.N.F.).* Benzaldehyde 0.05 ml, vanillin 100 mg, orange-flower water 15 ml, alcohol 5 ml, syrup 40 ml, water to 100 ml. Store in airtight containers. Protect from light.

4613-g

Bergamot Oil *(B.P.C. 1949).* Oleum Bergamottae; Bergamot Essence.

CAS — 8007-75-8.

Pharmacopoeias. In *Arg., Fr., Port.,* and *Span.*

A greenish or brownish-yellow oil with a characteristic fragrant odour and a bitter aromatic taste, obtained by expression from the fresh peel of fruit of *Citrus bergamia* (Rutaceae). It contains about 40% w/w of esters calculated as linalyl acetate ($C_{12}H_{20}O_2$). Wt per ml 0.876 to 0.881 g.
Soluble 1 in 2 of alcohol; soluble in glacial acetic acid and in most fixed oils; practically insoluble in glycerol and propylene glycol.

Standard for bergamot oil. A British Standard Specification for Bergamot Oil (BS 2999/32: 1971) is published by the British Standards Institution.

Bergamot oil is chiefly employed in perfumery, especially in preparations for the hair, and in suntanning preparations.

An estimated acceptable daily intake of up to 500 µg per kg body-weight was established for citral, geranyl acetate, citronellol, linalol, and linalyl acetate, expressed as citral.— Twenty-third Report of Joint FAO/WHO Expert Committee on Food Additives, *Tech. Rep. Ser. Wld Hlth Org. No. 648,* 1980 (see also p.670 for the absorption of these terpinoids).

5-Methoxypsoralen, a constituent of bergamot oil, known also as bergapten, caused phototoxic reactions of the skin in the presence of long wavelength ultraviolet light and was considered to be only slightly less active than methoxsalen.— S. T. Zaynoun *et al., Br. J. Derm.,* 1977, *96,* 475. See also S. T. Zaynoun, *J. Soc. cosmet. Chem.,* 1978, *29,* 247.

Brief discussions on the possible cancer hazard associated with 5-methoxypsoralen in suntan preparations: M. J. Ashwood-Smith (letter), *Br. med. J.,* 1979, *2,* 1144; P. Forlot (letter), *ibid.,* 1980, *280,* 648; P. Kersey (letter), *ibid.,* 940; I. Hook (letter), *ibid.,* 1537.

For further information on adverse effects associated with the use of methoxypsoralens, see under Methoxsalen, p.497.

Preparations

Cologne Spirit. Spiritus Coloniensis *(B.P.C. 1949)*; Aqua Coloniensis. A form of Eau de Cologne prepared from bergamot oil 1.25 ml, lemon oil 0.5 ml, neroli oil 0.2 ml, rosemary oil 0.15 ml, thyme oil 0.05 ml, concentrated orange-flower water 0.3 ml, water 4.17 ml, and alcohol (90%) to 100 ml.

Proprietary Names
Bergolio *(Pierrel, Ital.)*.

4614-q

Betel *(B.P.C. 1934).* Betel Leaf; Betel Pepper.

The dried leaves of *Piper betle* (Piperaceae). It contains a volatile oil, tannins, and diastase.

Betel is reputed to have stimulant and carminative properties.
It is used in India as a masticatory; in Malaysia, the leaves are usually mixed with lime and scrapings of areca nut.

4615-p

Volatile Bitter Almond Oil *(B.P.C. 1959).* Oleum Amygdalae Volatile Purificatum; Purified Volatile Bitter Almond Oil; Bitter Almond Oil FFPA; Oleum Amygdalae Amarae sine Acido Prussico; Oleum Amygdalae Amarae (s.AP); Oleum Amygdalae Amarae sine Acido Hydrocyanico.

CAS — 8013-76-1 (bitter almond oil).

Pharmacopoeias. In *Arg.*

Obtained, by distillation with water, from the cake left after pressing out the fixed oil from bitter almonds or peach or apricot kernels. The crude distilled oil is freed from hydrogen cyanide by treatment with calcium hydroxide and ferrous sulphate, followed by redistillation. It contains not less than 95% w/w of benzaldehyde.
A colourless or pale yellow liquid with an odour and taste of bitter almond. Wt per ml about 1.044 g. **Soluble** 1 in 300 of water, 1 in 2 of alcohol (70%), in ether, and fixed and volatile oils; slightly soluble in mineral oils; practically insoluble in glycerol. On exposure to air it is rapidly oxidised and benzoic acid is deposited as a crystalline mass. **Store** in a cool place in small well-filled airtight containers. Protect from light.

Uses. Volatile bitter almond oil has been employed as a flavouring agent for emulsions and for culinary purposes.

It was recommended that volatile bitter almond oil be prohibited for use in foods as a flavouring agent.— *Food Standards Committee Report on Flavouring Agents*, London, HM Stationery Office, 1965.

4616-s

Cajuput Oil *(B.P.C. 1973).* Oleum Cajuputi; Cajuput Essence.

CAS — 8008-98-8.

The title Niaouli Essence has been applied to Cajuput Oil.

Pharmacopoeias. In *Arg., Port.,* and *Span.*

A colourless, yellow, or green oil with an agreeable camphoraceous odour and a bitter, aromatic, camphoraceous taste, obtained by distillation from the fresh leaves and twigs of certain species of *Melaleuca* such as *M. cajuputi* and *M. leucadendron* (Myrtaceae). It contains 50 to 65% w/w of cineole. Wt per ml 0.910 to 0.923 g.
Soluble 1 in 2 of alcohol (80%), becoming less soluble with age; miscible with alcohol (90%). **Store** in a cool place in well-filled airtight containers. Protect from light.

Cajuput oil obtained from the leaves of *Melaleuca cajuputi* contained about 10% of a crystalline phenolic compound 3,5-dimethyl-4,6-di-*O*-methylphloroacetophenone. This would explain its reputed antiseptic properties and the green colour due to chelation of copper distillation vessels.— J. B. Lowry (letter), *Nature*, 1973, *241*, 61.

Uses. Cajuput oil is employed externally as a stimulant and mild rubefacient in rheumatism. It is an ingredient of some ointments and liniments. It has been given internally as a carminative.

4617-w

Capsicum *(B.P.C. 1973).* Capsic.; Chillies; Capsici Fructus; Piment Rouge; Spanischer Pfeffer; Pimentão.

CAS — 404-86-4 (capsaicin).

NOTES. Ground cayenne pepper of commerce is normally a blend of varieties. Paprika is from *Capsicum annuum* var. *longum*; it is milder than capsicum.

Pharmacopoeias. Belg., Hung., Jap., Pol., and *Port.* all specify *C. annuum. Ind.* specifies *C. annuum* or *C. frutescens. Aust.* and *Span.* specify *C. annuum* var. *longum. It.* specifies *C. annuum, C. fastigiatum,* or *C. frutescens. Ger.* and *Swiss* specify *C. frutescens.*

The dried ripe fruits of *Capsicum annuum* var. *minimum* and small-fruited varieties of *C. frutescens* (Solanaceae). It contains not less than 0.5% of the pungent principle capsaicin ((*E*)-8-methyl-*N*-vanillylnon-6-enamide, $C_{18}H_{27}NO_3$ = 305.4). **Store** in a cool dry place. Protect from light.

Uses. Capsicum has a carminative action but it is mainly used externally as a counter-irritant in lumbago, neuralgia, and rheumatism.

The properties, reactions, and uses of capsaicin.— G. T. Walker, *Mfg Chem.*, 1968, *39* (June), 35.

Capsaicin, the active principle of capsicum, caused erythema and burning, but not vesication, when applied to the skin.— J. G. Smith *et al., J. invest. Derm.*, 1970, *54*, 170, per *J. Am. med. Ass.*, 1970, *211*, 1726.

Intragastric infusion of powdered red chillies (0.8 or 1.6 g per hour) caused a rapid and marked increase in the DNA content of gastric aspirate, indicating exfoliation of epithelial cells from the gastric mucosa.— H. G. Desai *et al., Gut*, 1973, *14*, 974.

4618-e

Capsicum Oleoresin *(B.P.C. 1973).* Oleores. Capsic.; Capsicin; Capsicum Extract.

CAS — 8023-77-6.

Pharmacopoeias. In *Belg.* and *Ind.*

It is made by extracting capsicum with hot acetone or alcohol (90%) and evaporating the solvent, extracting the residue with cold alcohol (90%), and removing the alcohol by evaporation. It is a thick dark reddish-brown liquid with an intensely pungent taste containing not less than 8% of capsaicin.
Soluble in alcohol, acetone, ether, chloroform, volatile oils, and fats; soluble with opalescence in fixed oils. **Store** in airtight containers. If separation occurs it should be warmed and mixed before use.

CAUTION. *Capsicum oleoresin is a powerful irritant and even a minute quantity produces an intense burning sensation in contact with the eyes and tender parts of the skin. The use of a dilute solution of potassium permanganate on the skin, and of Cocaine Eye-drops for the eyes, may allay the irritation.*

Uses. Capsicum oleoresin is used for the same purposes as capsicum. *Dose:* 0.6 to 2 mg.

Preparations

Dressings

Capsicum Cotton Wool *(B.P.C. 1973).* Capsicum Cotton. Absorbent cotton wool impregnated with capsicum oleoresin (equivalent to about 0.05% of capsaicin), methyl salicylate (about 1%), and an orange-brown dye.

Capsicum Self-adhesive Plaster *(B.P.C. 1963).* Capsicum Plaster. Cotton or rayon or cotton and rayon cloth of plain weave spread evenly with a self-adhesive plaster mass containing about 1% of capsicum oleoresin. The cloth may be perforated, and the adhesive surface is covered by a protective layer of muslin or other suitable material.

Gauze and Capsicum Cotton Tissue *(B.P.C. 1973).* Capsicum Tissue. Capsicum cotton wool enclosed in tubular absorbent gauze which is tinted orange-brown.

Ointments

Capsicum Ointment *(B.P.C. 1973).* Unguentum Capsici. Capsicum oleoresin 1.5 g, emulsifying wax 5 g, and simple ointment 93.5 g. *Belg. P.* has 20% in an emulsified basis.

Compound Capsicum Ointment *(B.P.C. 1949).* Ung. Capsic. Co.; Chillie Paste. Capsicum oleoresin 2 g, menthol 10 g, chloral hydrate 10 g, camphor 10 g, and yellow soft paraffin 68 g.

Tinctures

Capsicum Tincture *(B.P.C. 1973).* Prepared by macerating capsicum oleoresin 320 mg with alcohol (90%) 100 ml. *Dose.* 0.3 to 1 ml. A tincture prepared from capsicum, usually 1 in 10, is included in some pharmacopoeias.

An ointment containing capsicum oleoresin 1.2%, camphor 5.25%, terpentine oil 9.75%, and eucalyptus oil 2.5%, was formerly marketed in Great Britain under the proprietary name Capsolin (*Parke, Davis*).

4619-l

Caraway *(B.P., U.S.N.F.).* Carum; Caraway Fruit; Caraway Seed; Fructus Carvi; Cumin des Prés; Kümmel; Alcaravia.

Pharmacopoeias. In *Aust., Br., Ger., Hung., Ind., Pol., Port., Roum.,* and *Swiss.* Also in *U.S.N.F.*

The dried ripe fruits of *Carum carvi* (Umbelliferae). The *B.P.* specifies not less than 3.5% v/w of volatile oil. **Powdered Caraway** (*B.P.*) (Cari Pulvis) contains not less than 2.5% v/w of volatile oil. **Store** at a temperature not exceeding 25° in a dry place; the powdered drug should be kept in airtight containers. Protect from light.

4620-v

Caraway Oil *(B.P.).* Oleum Cari; Oleum Carui; Oleum Carvi; Kümmelöl.

CAS — 8000-42-8.

Pharmacopoeias. In *Aust., Br., Cz., Ger., Hung., Ind., Jug.,* and *Roum.* Also in *U.S.N.F.*

A colourless or pale yellow oil with a characteristic odour and taste, obtained by distillation from freshly crushed caraway. The *B.P.* specifies that it contains 53 to 63% w/w of ketones calculated as carvone, $C_{10}H_{14}O$; the *U.S.N.F.* specifies not less than 50% v/v of *d*-carvone. Wt per ml 0.902 to 0.912 g.
Soluble 1 in 7 or 8 of alcohol (80%); soluble in chloroform and ether. **Store** at a temperature not exceeding 25° in well-filled airtight containers. Protect from light.

Uses. Caraway is an aromatic carminative and is employed as caraway water for the flatulent colic of infants. Caraway water is a vehicle for children's mixtures. *Dose:* 0.05 to 0.2 ml (oil).

Temporary estimated acceptable daily intake of (+)-carvone and (−)-carvone: up to 1 mg per kg bodyweight. Further biochemical and metabolic studies are required.— Twenty-third Report of Joint FAO/WHO Expert Committee on Food Additives, *Tech. Rep. Ser. Wld Hlth Org. No. 648*, 1980.

Preparations

Caraway Water. Concentrated caraway water 2.5 ml, freshly boiled and cooled water to 100 ml.

Concentrated Caraway Water *(B.P.C. 1973).* Aq. Cari Conc. Caraway oil 2 ml, alcohol (90%) 60 ml, water to 100 ml; shaken with 5 g of sterilised talc and filtered. *Dose.* 0.3 to 1 ml.

4621-g

Cardamom Fruit *(B.P.).* Cardam. Fruit; Cardamomi Fructus.

Pharmacopoeias. In *Br., Ind., Jap.,* and *Port.*
Arg. and *U.S.N.F.* specify Cardamom Seed recently removed from the fruit.

The dried, nearly ripe fruit of *Elettaria cardamomum* var. *minuscula* (Zingiberaceae). Only the seeds are used in making preparations of cardamom; they are removed from the fruit when required for use; they have a strongly aromatic odour and an aromatic slightly bitter taste and contain not less than 4% v/w of volatile oil. The fruit should be **stored** in a cool dry place; the seeds should not be stored after removal from the fruit.

4622-q

Cardamom Oil *(B.P.)*. Ol. Cardamom.

CAS — 8000-66-6.

Pharmacopoeias. In *Br.* Cardamom Oil (*U.S.N.F.*) is distilled from the seeds.

A colourless or pale yellow oil with an aromatic pungent odour and taste, distilled from crushed cardamom fruit. It contains cineole, limonene, and terpineol. Wt per ml 0.917 to 0.94 g. **Soluble** 1 in 6 of alcohol (70%). **Store** at a temperature not exceeding 25° in well-filled airtight containers. Protect from light.

Uses. Preparations of cardamom fruit and oil are used as carminatives and as flavouring agents. *Dose:* 0.03 to 0.2 ml (oil).

Preparations

Aromatic Cardamom Tincture *(B.P.)*. Arom. Cardam. Tinct.; Tinctura Carminativa. Cardamom oil 0.3 ml, caraway oil 1 ml, cinnamon oil 1 ml, clove oil 1 ml, strong ginger tincture 6 ml, alcohol (90%) to 100 ml.

Compound Cardamom Tincture *(B.P.)*. Co. Cardam. Tinct. Cardamom oil 0.045 ml, caraway oil 0.04 ml, cinnamon oil 0.0225 ml, glycerol 5 ml, with cochineal, in alcohol (60%) to 100 ml.

Compound Cardamom Tincture *(U.S.N.F.)*. Prepared by macerating cardamom seed 2 g, cinnamon *U.S.N.F.* 2.5 g, and caraway 1.2 g with glycerol 5 ml and diluted alcohol to 100 ml. The tincture may be coloured. Store at a temperature not exceeding 40° in airtight containers. Protect from light.

4623-p

Cassia Bark *(B.P.C. 1949)*. Cassiae Cortex; Cassia Cinnamon; Chinese Cinnamon; Cinnamon Bark; Cinnamomum; Canela-da-China.

Pharmacopoeias. In *Chin., Hung., Ind., Jap.,* and *Roum.*

The dried bark of *Cinnamomum cassia* (Lauraceae) containing not less than 1% v/w of volatile oil. **Powdered Cassia** (*B.P.C. 1949*) contains not less than 0.7% v/w of oil. **Store** in a cool dry place; the powdered drug should be kept in airtight containers.

4624-s

Cassia Oil *(B.P.C. 1949)*. Oleum Cassiae; Cinnamon Oil *(U.S.N.F.)*; Chinese Cinnamon Oil; Oleum Cinnamomi; Oleum Cinnamomi Cassiae.

CAS — 8007-80-5.

Pharmacopoeias. In *Chin., Hung., Ind.,* and *Jap.* Also in *U.S.N.F.*

A mobile yellowish or brownish oil with a fragrant pungent odour and a sweetish, spicy, burning taste, obtained by steam distillation from the leaves and twigs of *Cinnamomum cassia*, and rectified by distillation. It darkens with age or exposure to light, and becomes more viscous. The *U.S.N.F.* specifies not less than 80% v/v of aldehydes, and a specific gravity of 1.045 to 1.063. **Soluble** 1 in 2 of alcohol (70%), 1 in 1 of alcohol, and 1 in 1 of glacial acetic acid. **Store** at a temperature not exceeding 40° in well-filled airtight containers. Protect from light.

Standard for cassia oil. A British Standard Specification for Cassia Oil (BS 2999/17: 1972) is published by the British Standards Institution.

Uses. Cassia Oil has properties resembling those of cinnamon oil but the odour is less fragrant and more pungent and the taste is harsher. It is used as a flavouring agent. Cassia bark also has properties similar to those of cinnamon.

Temporary estimated acceptable daily intake of cinnamaldehyde: up to 700 µg per kg body-weight. Further studies are required.— Twenty-third Report of Joint FAO/WHO Expert Committee on Food Additives, *Tech. Rep. Ser. Wld Hlth Org. No. 648*, 1980.

4625-w

Cedar Wood Oil *(B.P.C. 1949)*. Oleum Cedri; Red Cedar Oil.

CAS — 8000-27-9.

An almost colourless or slightly yellow somewhat viscous oil with a mild, persistent, characteristic odour, obtained by distillation from the wood of *Juniperus virginiana* (Cupressaceae) and other species of red cedar. It consists almost entirely of cedrene, ($C_{15}H_{24}$), a liquid sesquiterpene. Wt per ml 0.936 to 0.97 g. **Soluble** 1 in 20 to 1 in 10 of alcohol (90%).

Standard for Virginian cedarwood oil. A British Standard Specification for Virginian Cedarwood Oil (BS 2999/57: 1975) is published by the British Standards Institution.

Cedar wood oil is used in perfumery and as a clearing agent in microscopy. A thickened form, with the addition of resins, is used in microscopy as an immersion oil.

4626-e

Celery *(B.P.C. 1949)*. Apium; Celery Fruit; Celery Seed.

CAS — 8015-90-5 (celery oil).

The dried ripe fruits of cultivated plants of celery, *Apium graveolens* (Umbelliferae), containing not less than 1.5% v/w of volatile oil.

Standard for celery oil. A British Standard Specification for Celery Oil (BS 2999/2: 1965) is published by the British Standards Institution.

Celery has been used as a domestic remedy for rheumatism. The oil from the fruits has been used as an antispasmodic.

4627-l

Chamomile Flowers *(B.P.)*. Anthemis; Chamomile; Roman Chamomile; Roman Chamomile Flowers; Anthemidis Flores; Anthemidis Flos; Flos Chamomillae Romanae; Camomille Romaine; Manzanilla Romana.

Pharmacopoeias. In *Arg., Aust., Belg., Br., Eur., Fr., Ger., It., Jug., Neth.,* and *Span.*

The dried flowerheads of the cultivated double variety of *Anthemis nobilis* (Compositae), containing not less than 0.7% v/w of volatile oil. **Store** in well-closed containers. Protect from light.

4628-y

Chamomile Oil *(B.P.C. 1949)*. Oleum Anthemidis; English Chamomile Oil; Roman Chamomile Oil.

CAS — 8015-92-7.

Pharmacopoeias. In *Swiss.*

The oil obtained by distillation from the recently dried flowerheads of *A. nobilis*. It is blue when fresh (due to the presence of chamazulene) but becomes greenish and then brownish-yellow. It has a strong, pleasant, aromatic odour and a burning taste. It contains esters of angelic and tiglic acids. Wt per ml 0.897 to 0.91 g. **Soluble** 1 in 6 of alcohol (70%) and 1 in less than 1 of alcohol (90%); soluble in propylene glycol; practically insoluble in glycerol.

Adverse Effects.

Anaphylactic shock had been reported with chamomile tea. Allergic rhinitis may occur in atopic subjects known to be sensitive to ragweed pollen.— W. H. Lewis (letter), *J. Am. med. Ass.*, 1978, *240*, 109. See also C. L. Casterline (letter), *ibid.*, 1980, *244*, 330.

Uses. Chamomile flowers have been used as an aromatic bitter; large doses are emetic. An infusion, 'chamomile tea' is a domestic remedy for indigestion. A poultice of the flowers is sometimes applied externally in the early stages of inflammation. Chamomile is an ingredient of some hair preparations. Chamomile oil has been used as an aromatic carminative; *dose:* 0.03 to 0.2 ml.

Proprietary Preparations

Kamillosan *(Norgine, UK)*. Ointment containing chamomile flowers extract 10%, chamomile oil 0.5%, and hexylresorcinol 0.4%. For cracked nipples and nappy rash.

4629-j

Cineole *(B.P.C. 1973)*. Eucalyptol; Cajuputol.

1,8-Epoxy-*p*-menthane; 1,3,3-Trimethyl-2-oxabicyclo[2.2.2]octane.

$C_{10}H_{18}O = 154.3$.

CAS — 470-82-6.

Pharmacopoeias. In *Arg., It., Mex., Port., Span.,* and *Swiss.*

A colourless liquid with an aromatic camphoraceous odour and a pungent cooling taste, obtained from eucalyptus oil, cajuput oil, and other oils. Wt per ml 0.922 to 0.924 g. F.p. not lower than 0°. B.p. about 175°.

Practically **insoluble** in water; soluble 1 in 2 of alcohol (70%); miscible with alcohol, glacial acetic acid, light liquid paraffin, and fixed and volatile oils. **Store** in a cool place in airtight containers. Protect from light.

Adverse Effects and Treatment. As for Eucalyptus Oil, p.675.

Uses. Cineole has the action and uses of eucalyptus oil but is less irritating to mucous membranes. It is used with other counter-irritants in some compound ointments. It has antimicrobial properties and is used in dentifrices (0.25%). It has also been used as a softening agent to adapt gutta percha fillings and cones to cavities and root canals of teeth. It has been used in many proprietary nasal preparations, but oily solutions inhibit ciliary movement and may cause lipoid pneumonia. Cineole has been reported to induce liver enzymes.

Inhalant capsules containing cineole and other essential oils were formerly marketed in Great Britain under the proprietary name Calyptol (*Smith & Nephew Pharmaceuticals*).

4630-q

Cinnamon *(B.P., U.S.N.F.)*. Cinnam.; Cinnamomi Cortex; Cinnamon Bark; Ceylon Cinnamon; Ceylonzimt; Cannelle Dite de Ceylan; Canela; Canela do Ceilão; Zimt.

Pharmacopoeias. In *Aust., Belg., Br., Braz., Fr., Ind., Mex., Neth., Port., Roum., Span.,* and *Swiss.* Also in *U.S.N.F. Mex.* specifies not less than 2.5% v/w of volatile oil, *Aust.* and *Braz.* not less than 1.5%, *Swiss* not less than 1.4%, *Arg.* not less than 1.3%, *Neth.* not less than 1.2%, and *Belg.* not less than 0.7%. *U.S.N.F.* specifies *C. loureirii* and not less than 2.5% of volatile oil.

The *B.P.* specifies dried inner bark of the shoots of coppiced trees of Ceylon cinnamon, *Cinnamomum zeylanicum* (Lauraceae) containing not less than 1.2% v/w of volatile oil. The *U.S.N.F.* specifies the dried bark of *Cinnamomum loureirii* containing not less than 2.5% v/w of volatile oil. **Powdered Cinnamon** (*B.P.*) contains not less than 1% v/w of volatile oil. **Store** in a cool dry place; the powdered drug should be kept in airtight containers. Protect from light.

4631-p

Cinnamon Oil *(B.P.)*. Cinnam. Oil; Oleum Cinnamomi; Ceylon Cinnamon Bark Oil; Aetheroleum Cinnamomi Zeylanici; Essence de Cannelle de Ceylan; Zimtöl; Esencia de Canela.

CAS — 8007-80-5.

Pharmacopoeias. In *Arg., Aust., Belg., Br., Cz., Fr., Ind., Mex., Roum., Span.,* and *Swiss. Arg.* and *Mex.* have not less than 80% v/v aldehydes; *Aust., Cz.,* and *Swiss* have 65 to 76% w/w; *Belg.* has 55 to 74% w/w; *Span.* has 65 to 75% v/v; *Fr.* has 65 to 75% w/w; *Ind.* has 55 to 70% w/w; and *Roum.* 66 to 76% v/v.

Cinnamon Oil in *Chin. P., Jap. P.,* and *U.S.N.F.* is Cassia Oil.

A yellow oil with the characteristic odour and taste of cinnamon, obtained by distillation from cinnamon. It becomes reddish-brown with age. It contains 60 to 80% w/w of aldehydes, calculated as cinnamaldehyde (C_9H_8O), with eugenol, phellandrene, and other terpenes. Wt per ml 1.000 to 1.040 g.

Soluble 1 in 3 of alcohol (70%), with slight opalescence, and 1 in 0.3 of alcohol (90%); soluble in propylene glycol and in most fixed oils; practically insoluble in glycerol and mineral oils. **Store** in well-filled airtight containers, at a temperature not exceeding 25°. Protect from light.

Adverse Effects.

Three patients developed acute contact sensitivity of the mouth after changing to a new brand (Close-Up) of toothpaste containing cinnamon oil. Symptoms subsided within 1 week when the use of the toothpaste ceased. Each patient responded positively to a patch test of cinnamon oil 0.5% in soft paraffin.— L. G. Millard (letter), *Br. med. J.,* 1973, *1,* 676.

Further reports of sensitivity to cinnamon: V. Kirton and D. S. Wilkinson (letter), *Br. med. J.,* 1973, *2,* 115; T. E. Drake and H. I. Maibach, *Archs Derm.,* 1976, *112,* 202; M. J. Roberts (letter), *Br. med. J.,* 1976, *2,* 47; C. G. T. Mathias *et al., Archs Derm.,* 1980, *116,* 74.

Uses. Cinnamon and cinnamon oil are carminative and are largely used as flavouring agents. The oil is occasionally used as an inhalation and as a spray, but oily solutions are not recommended because they inhibit ciliary movement and may cause lipoid pneumonia. Cinnamon oil has sometimes been used as a preservative. *Doses:* 0.3 to 1.2 g (cinnamon); 0.05 to 0.2 ml (oil).

Temporary estimated acceptable daily intake of cinnamaldehyde: up to 700 µg per kg body-weight. Further studies are required.— Twenty-third Report of Joint FAO/WHO Expert Committee on Food Additives, *Tech. Rep. Ser. Wld Hlth Org. No. 648,* 1980.

Preparations of Cinnamon and Cinnamon Oil

Spirits

Cinnamon Spirit *(B.P.C. 1949).* Sp. Cinnam. Cinnamon oil 1 in 10 of alcohol (90%). *Dose.* 0.3 to 1.2 ml.

Syrups

Syrupus Cinnamoni *(Arg. P.).* Jarabe de Canela; Cinnamon Syrup. Sucrose 85 g in distilled cinnamon water to 100 ml.

Tinctures

Cinnamon Tincture *(B.P.C. 1949).* Tinct. Cinnam. Prepared by percolating cinnamon 1 with 5 of alcohol (70%). *Dose.* 2 to 4 ml.

Waters

Cinnamon Water. Concentrated cinnamon water 2.5 ml, freshly boiled and cooled water to 100 ml.

Concentrated Cinnamon Water *(B.P.).* Aq. Cinnam. Conc. Cinnamon oil 2 ml, alcohol (90%) 60 ml, water to 100 ml; shaken with 5 g of sterilised talc and filtered.

Distilled Cinnamon Water *(B.P.C. 1949).* Aq. Cinnam. Dest. Cinnamon 10 g and water 200 ml; distil 100 ml. *Dose.* 15 to 30 ml.

4632-s

Cinnamon Leaf Oil. Ol. Cinnam. Fol.

CAS — 8015-96-1.

Pharmacopoeias. In *Ind.*

Distilled from the leaves of *Cinnamomum cassia* and other species of *Cinnamomum.* It is a dark brown limpid liquid with a penetrating fragrant odour, resembling that of cinnamon and of clove, and a very pungent taste. It contains 70 to 90% of eugenol. Wt per ml about 1.05 g.

Soluble 1 in 3 of alcohol (70%). **Store** in a cool place in airtight containers. Protect from light.

Standard for cinnamon leaf oil. A British Standard Specification for Cinnamon Leaf Oil (BS 2999/3: 1965) is published by the British Standards Institution.

Cinnamon leaf oil is used in India as a substitute for clove oil.

For the temporary estimated acceptable daily intake of eugenol, see p.676.

4633-w

Citronella Oil *(B.P.C. 1973).* Oleum Citronellae.

CAS — 8000-29-1.

Pharmacopoeias. In *Aust., Belg., Cz., Roum.,* and *Swiss. Aust.* and *Roum.* give Oleum Melissae Indicum as a synonym for citronella oil.

A pale to deep yellow oil with a pleasant characteristic odour, obtained by distillation from *Cymbopogon nardus* or *C. winterianus* (Gramineae) or varietal or hybrid forms of these species. The chief constituents are geraniol ($C_{10}H_{18}O$) and citronellal ($C_{10}H_{18}O$).

There are 2 main types of citronella oil in commerce, differing in odour and composition and known as Ceylon oil and Java oil. Ceylon oil has a wt per ml of 0.895 to 0.905 g and contains about 10% of citronellal and about 18% of geraniol; Java oil has a wt per ml of 0.88 to 0.895 g and contains about 35% of citronellal and about 21% of geraniol. **Soluble** 1 in 4 of alcohol (80%) forming a clear or slightly opalescent solution. **Store** in a cool place in well-filled airtight containers. Protect from light.

Standard for citronella oils. British Standard Specifications for Ceylon Citronella Oil (BS 2999/18: 1972) and Java Citronella Oil (BS 2999/19: 1972) are published by the British Standards Institution.

Uses. Citronella oil was used as an insect repellent. It is chiefly used as a perfume, particularly for soaps and brilliantines. Hypersensitivity has been reported.

Preparations

Aqua Citronellae *(Belg. P.).* Eau de Citronelle; Citronella Water. Citronella spirit *(Belg. P.)* 3 g, water 97 g. Must be freshly prepared.

Spiritus Citronellae *(Belg. P.).* Esprit de Citronelle; Citronella Spirit. Citronella oil 1 g, alcohol (80%) 99 g.

4634-e

Clove *(B.P.).* Caryophyllum; Caryoph.; Cloves; Clou de Girofle; Giroflier; Gewürznelke; Cravinho; Cravo-da-India.

Pharmacopoeias. In *Aust., Br., Fr., Hung., Ind., Jap., Neth., Port.,* and *Swiss.*

The dried flower-buds of *Syzygium aromaticum* (=*Eugenia caryophyllus; Caryophyllus aromaticus; E. aromatica; Jambosa caryophyllus*) (Myrtaceae), containing not less than 15% v/w of volatile oil, of which about 85 to 92% consists of eugenol. **Powdered Clove** (*B.P.*) contains not less than 12% v/w of volatile oil. Clove has a strong, characteristic, aromatic, spicy odour and an aromatic pungent taste. **Store** in a cool dry place; the powdered drug should be kept in airtight containers. Protect from light.

4635-l

Clove Oil *(B.P., U.S.N.F.).* Oleum Caryophylli; Ol. Caryoph.; Essence de Girofle; Nelkenöl; Esencia de Clavo.

CAS — 8000-34-8.

Pharmacopoeias. In *Arg., Aust., Br., Fr., Ger., Hung., Ind., It., Jap., Jug., Mex., Neth., Port., Roum., Span.,* and *Swiss.* Also in *U.S.N.F.*

A colourless or pale yellow oil with the characteristic odour and taste of clove, obtained by distillation from clove. It darkens and thickens with age and on exposure to air; it should not be allowed to come into contact with iron or zinc. It contains 85 to 90% v/v of eugenol. Wt per ml 1.041 to 1.054 g.

Soluble 1 in 2 of alcohol (70%); miscible with alcohol (90%), ether, and with glacial acetic acid. **Store** at a temperature not exceeding 25° in well-filled airtight containers. Protect from light.

The Pharmaceutical Society's Department of Pharmaceutical Sciences found that PVC bottles softened and distorted fairly rapidly in the presence of clove oil, which should not be stored or dispensed in such bottles.— *Pharm. J.,* 1973, *1,* 100.

The solubility of clove oil in macrogol esters.— K. Thoma and G. Pfaff, *J. Soc. cosmet. Chem.,* 1976, *27,* 221.

Standard for clove oils. British Standard Specifications for oils of clove bud, leaf, and stem (BS 2999/20/21/22: 1972) and Indonesian Clove Leaf Oil (BS 2999/54: 1975) are published by the British Standards Institution.

Uses. Clove oil is an antispasmodic and carminative and is sometimes used in the treatment of flatulent colic. *Doses:* clove, 120 to 300 mg; clove oil, 0.05 to 0.2 ml. Applied externally clove oil is irritant, rubefacient, and slightly analgesic. It has been used in liniments with olive oil. Clove oil is used as a domestic remedy for toothache, a plug of cotton wool soaked in the oil being inserted in the cavity of the carious tooth; repeated application may damage the gingival tissues. Mixed with zinc oxide, it is used as a temporary anodyne dental filling, though eugenol (see p.676) is often preferred.

It is also used in dentifrices (1 to 3%) as a flavouring agent. It has useful preservative properties.

For the temporary estimated acceptable daily intake of eugenol, see p.676.

When a mixture of zinc oxide and clove oil was inserted into the tooth sockets of *dogs* at the time of extraction healing was delayed, clot formation inhibited, and severe inflammation produced. Pain relief following the paste being packed into dry sockets might result from the secondary destruction of local nerve endings associated with the increased inflammation. Such a method of achieving analgesia was questionable.— L. Summers and L. R. Matz, *Br. dent. J.,* 1976, *141,* 377.

Preparations

Clove Water. Concentrated clove water 2.5 ml, freshly boiled and cooled water to 100 ml.

Concentrated Clove Infusion *(B.P.C. 1954).* Inf. Caryoph. Conc. Clove 1 in about 5; prepared by maceration with alcohol (25%). *Dose.* 2 to 4 ml. Clove Infusion is prepared by diluting 1 vol. of this concentrated infusion to 8 vol. with water.

Concentrated Clove Water *(B.P.C. 1934).* Aq. Caryoph. Conc. Clove oil 2 ml, alcohol (90%) 60 ml, water to 100 ml; shaken with talc and filtered. *Dose.* 0.3 to 1 ml.

Toothache Drops. Odontalgicum. Chlorbutol 25 g, clove oil to 100 ml.

4636-y

Copaiba *(B.P.C. 1949).* Balsam of Copaiba; Balsamum Copaivae; Terebinthina Copaiferae.

CAS — 8001-61-4.

Pharmacopoeias. In *Port.* and *Span.*

The oleoresin obtained from the trunk of *Copaifera lansdorfii* and other species of *Copaifera* (Leguminosae). The most important varieties are known as Pará, Maranham, Maracaibo, and Savanilla copaiba. It is a yellow to golden-brown viscous liquid with a characteristic odour and a slightly bitter, acrid, persistent taste. Wt per ml 0.958 to 0.993 g.

Miscible with dehydrated alcohol, carbon disulphide, ether, and fixed and volatile oils; soluble in an equal volume of light petroleum (b.p. 50° to 60°) but precipitates on adding more solvent.

Copaiba is carminative. It has been used as a urinary antiseptic in chronic cystitis and gonorrhoeal urethritis, but it has an irritant action on the mucous membrane of the gastro-intestinal tract and may give rise to digestive disturbances and to a morbilliform rash.
Copaiba oil has been used similarly.

4637-j

Coriander *(B.P.)*. Coriand.; Coriander Fruit; Coriander Seed; Fruto de Cilantro; Coentro.

Pharmacopoeias. In *Aust., Belg., Br., Fr., Hung., Ind., Pol., Port.,* and *Span.*

The dried ripe fruits of *Coriandrum sativum* (Umbelliferae), containing not less than 0.3% v/w of volatile oil.
Powdered Coriander (*B.P.*) (Coriandri Pulvis) contains not less than 0.2% v/w of volatile oil.
Store at a temperature not exceeding 25° in a dry place; the powdered drug should be kept in airtight containers.

4638-z

Coriander Oil *(B.P.)*. Oleum Coriandri; Ol. Coriand.

CAS — 8008-52-4.

Pharmacopoeias. In *Arg., Br., Cz.,* and *Ind.* Also in *U.S.N.F.*

A colourless or pale yellow oil with the characteristic odour and taste of coriander, obtained by distillation from coriander. The flavour becomes less pleasant with age. It contains about 65 to 80% of alcohols, chiefly (+)-linalol (coriandrol), together with terpenes. Wt per ml 0.863 to 0.87 g.
Soluble 1 in less than 1 of alcohol (90%), 1 in 3 of alcohol (70%), in chloroform, and ether. **Store** at a temperature not exceeding 25° in well-filled airtight containers. Protect from light.

Standard for coriander oil. A British Standard Specification for Coriander Oil (BS 2999/33: 1971) is published by the British Standards Institution.

Uses. Coriander oil is aromatic, stimulant, and carminative. *Dose:* 0.05 to 0.2 ml.

An estimated acceptable daily intake of up to 500 µg per kg body-weight was established for citral, geranyl acetate, citronellol, linalol, and linalyl acetate, expressed as citral.— Twenty-third Report of the Joint FAO/WHO Expert Committee on Food Additives, *Tech. Rep. Ser. Wld Hlth Org. No. 648*, 1980 (See also p.670 for the absorption of these terpinoids).

4639-c

Cubeb *(B.P.C. 1954)*. Cubeba; Cubeb Berries; Cubeb Fruit; Tailed Pepper.

Pharmacopoeias. In *Span.*

The dried, unripe, fully grown fruit of *Piper cubeba* (Piperaceae), containing not less than 15% v/w of volatile oil. **Store** in a cool dry place.

4640-s

Cubeb Oil *(B.P.C. 1949)*. An oil obtained by distillation from cubeb.

CAS — 8007-87-2.

It is a colourless, pale yellow, or bluish-green liquid with a warm characteristic odour and a camphoraceous taste. Wt per ml 0.905 to 0.925 g. **Soluble** 1 in 18 of alcohol (90%); miscible with dehydrated alcohol. **Store** in a cool place in airtight containers. Protect from light.

Standard for cubeb oil. A British Standard Specification for cubeb oil (BS 2999/5: 1965) is published by the British Standards Institution.

Cubeb oil was formerly employed, usually as an emulsion or in capsules, as a urinary antiseptic. It is used as a flavouring agent.

4641-w

Dill *(B.P.C. 1954)*. Anethum; Dill Fruit.

NOTE. Indian Dill is the dried ripe fruits of *Anethum sowa.*

Pharmacopoeias. In *Ind.*

The dried ripe fruit of *Anethum graveolens* (Umbelliferae), containing not less than 2.5% v/w of volatile oil. **Powdered Dill** (*B.P.C. 1954*) contains not less than 2% v/w of volatile oil. **Store** in a cool dry place; the powdered drug should be kept in airtight containers.

4642-e

Dill Oil *(B.P.)*. Oleum Anethi; European Dill Seed Oil.

CAS — 8016-06-6.

NOTE. Indian Dill Seed Oil (East Indian Dill Seed Oil) is obtained from *Anethum sowa.* American Dillweed Oil (Dill Herb Oil) is obtained from the stalks, leaves, and seeds of *A. graveolens..*

Pharmacopoeias. In *Br.* and *Ind.*

A colourless or pale yellow oil obtained by distillation from dill. It darkens with age and has a characteristic odour, resembling that of caraway, and a sweet aromatic and subsequently pungent taste. It contains 43 to 63% of carvone ($C_{10}H_{14}O$). Wt per ml 0.895 to 0.91 g.
Soluble 1 in 1 of alcohol (90%) and 1 in 10 of alcohol (80%); soluble in propylene glycol; practically insoluble in glycerol. **Store** at a temperature not exceeding 25° in well-filled airtight containers. Protect from light.

Uses. Dill oil, usually in the form of dill water, is used as an aromatic carminative, especially in the treatment of flatulence in infants. The adult dose of dill oil is 0.05 to 0.2 ml.

Temporary estimated acceptable daily intake of (+)-carvone and (−)-carvone: up to 1 mg per kg body-weight. Further biochemical and metabolic studies are required.— Twenty-third Report of Joint FAO/WHO Expert Committee on Food Additives, *Tech. Rep. Ser. Wld Hlth Org. No. 648*, 1980.

Preparations

Concentrated Dill Water *(B.P.C. 1973)*. Aqua Anethi Concentrata. Dill oil 2 ml, alcohol (90%) 60 ml, water to 100 ml; shaken with 5 g of sterilised talc and filtered. *Dose.* 0.3 to 1 ml.

Dill Water. Concentrated dill water 2.5 ml, freshly boiled and cooled water to 100 ml.

4643-l

Elemi *(B.P.C. 1934)*. Manila Elemi.

CAS — 9000-75-3.

Pharmacopoeias. In *Port.* and *Span.*

An oleoresin exuded through the bark of *Canarium luzonicum* (Burseraceae). Firm yellow granular masses with a fragrant balsamic odour and a bitter spicy taste.

The properties of elemi are similar to those of turpentine and it has been employed in the form of an ointment (20% in simple ointment) as a local stimulant.
The name elemi is applied commercially to a large number of resins other than Manila elemi.

4644-y

Eucalyptus Oil *(B.P., Eur. P., U.S.N.F.)*. Oleum Eucalypti; Eucalypti Aetheroleum; Essence d'Eucalyptus Rectifiée; Esencia de Eucalipto.

CAS — 8000-48-4.

Pharmacopoeias. In *Arg., Aust., Belg., Br., Chin., Cz., Eur., Fr., Ger., Hung., Ind., It., Jap., Jug., Neth., Pol., Port., Roum., Rus., Span.,* and *Swiss.* Also in *U.S.N.F. Arg., Belg., Fr., Port., Roum.,* and *Span.* include Eucalyptus Leaves from *E. globulus* and *Rus.* the leaves from *E. cinerea* and *E. globulus.*

A colourless or pale yellow oil with a characteristic aromatic camphoraceous odour and a pungent camphoraceous cooling taste, obtained by rectifying the oil distilled from the fresh leaves and terminal branches of various species of *Eucalyptus* (Myrtaceae) (*E. globulus, E. fruticetorum = E. polybractea,* and *E. smithii* are used) which yield oils containing a large proportion of cineole (eucalyptol) but little phellandrene. It contains not less than 70% w/w of cineole; it also contains (+)-α-pinene and other terpenes and may contain small quantities of phellandrene. Wt per ml 0.906 to 0.925 g.
Very slightly **soluble** in water; soluble 1 in 5 of alcohol (70%); miscible with alcohol (90%), dehydrated alcohol, oils, fats, and paraffins. **Store** at a temperature not exceeding 25° in well-filled containers. Protect from light.
'Lemon-scented' Eucalyptus Oil is obtained from *E. citriodora* and contains about 70% of citronellal.

Standard for eucalyptus oils. British Standard Specifications for Eucalyptus Oil obtained from *E. citriodora* (BS 2999/23: 1972) and Eucalyptus Oil from *E. globulus* (BS 2999/53: 1975) are published by the British Standards Institution.

Adverse Effects and Treatment. See under Essential Oils, p.670. The symptoms of poisoning are epigastric burning, nausea and vomiting, dizziness and muscular weakness, miosis, tachycardia, and a feeling of suffocation. Cyanosis, delirium and convulsions may occur. Deaths have been recorded from doses varying from 3.5 to 21 ml.

For a report of the successful use of mannitol and dialysis in the treatment of poisoning by eucalyptus oil, see F. W. Gurr and J. G. Scroggie, *Australas. Ann. Med.*, 1965, *14*, 238, per *Int. pharm. Abstr.*, 1966, *3*, 589.

Uses. Eucalyptus oil has the general properties of essential oils (see p.670).
Eucalyptus oil has been taken by mouth for catarrh. To relieve cough in chronic bronchitis and asthma it is inhaled with steam, sometimes with the addition of menthol, pine oil, and Compound Benzoin Tincture. Mixed with menthol, camphor, or pine oil, it is used in 'dry' inhalers. Oily spray solutions containing eucalyptus oil and other volatile oils have also been used for the relief of catarrh but oily solutions are not recommended because they inhibit ciliary movement and may cause lipoid pneumonia. A 1% ointment has been used in rhinitis and a 25% liniment as a rubefacient. *Dose:* 0.05 to 0.2 ml.

Eucalyptus oils—a review of their constituents, properties, and uses in medicine, perfumery, and industry.— A. S. Ramaswamy, *Pharmaceutist*, 1965, *11*, 11.

4645-j

Eugenol *(B.P., U.S.P.)*. Eugen.; Eugenic Acid; 4-Allylguaiacol. 4-Allyl-2-methoxyphenol. $C_{10}H_{12}O_2$=164.2.

CAS — 97-53-0.

Pharmacopoeias. In *Belg., Br., Jug., Nord., Pol., Swiss,* and *U.S.*

A colourless or pale yellow liquid with an odour of clove and a spicy pungent taste; it may be obtained from clove oil. Wt per ml 1.064 to 1.068 g. B.p. about 254°.
Practically **insoluble** in water; soluble 1 in 2 of alcohol (70%); miscible with alcohol, chloroform, ether, fixed oils, and glacial acetic acid; soluble in aqueous sodium hydroxide. The filtrate from a 10% suspension in water has a pH of 4 to 7.

Eugenol darkens in colour with age or on exposure to air. Avoid contact with iron and zinc. **Store** at a temperature not exceeding 25° in well-filled airtight containers. Protect from light.

Adverse Effects.

Eugenol was a primary irritant and sensitiser and had caused contact dermatitis in dental surgeons.— I. B. Sneddon and R. C. Glew, *Practitioner*, 1973, *211*, 321.

Uses. Eugenol has similar properties to clove oil (see p.674). It is employed in dentistry as a flavouring agent and mild rubefacient in dentifrices, as an obtundent for hypersensitive dentine, caries, or exposed pulp, and mixed with zinc oxide, as a temporary anodyne dental filling.

Isoeugenol, used in perfumery for its carnation-clove odour, for the manufacture of vanillin, and as a flavouring agent, is obtained by heating eugenol with potassium hydroxide.

Temporary estimated acceptable daily intake of eugenol: up to 2.5 mg per kg body-weight. Carcinogenicity studies are continuing.— Twenty-third Report of the Joint FAO/WHO Expert Committee on Food Additives, *Tech. Rep. Ser. Wld Hlth Org. No. 648*, 1980.

4646-z

Fennel *(B.P.C. 1973).* Foeniculum; Fennel Fruit; Fennel Seed; Fenouil; Fenouil Doux; Fenchel; Fruto de Hinojo; Funcho.

Pharmacopoeias. In *Aust., Belg., Chin., Cz., Fr., Ger., Hung., Ind., Jap., Neth., Pol., Port., Roum., Rus., Span.,* and *Swiss.* Specifications for volatile content range from 1.4 to 4%.

The dried fruits of cultivated plants of *Foeniculum vulgare* var. *vulgare* (= *F. capillaceum; F. dulce*) (Umbelliferae), containing not less than 1.2% v/w of volatile oil. **Powdered Fennel** (*B.P.C. 1973*) contains not less than 1% v/w of volatile oil. **Store** in a cool dry place; the powdered drug should be stored in airtight containers. Protect from light.

4647-c

Fennel Oil *(B.P.C. 1949).* Oleum Foeniculi; Aetheroleum Foeniculi; Esencia de Hinojo; Essência de Funcho.

CAS — 8006-84-6.

Pharmacopoeias. In *Arg., Aust., Cz., Ger., Hung., Ind., Jap., Jug., Neth., Nord., Pol., Roum.,* and *Swiss.* Also in *U.S.N.F.*

A colourless or pale yellow oil with a characteristic aromatic odour and a bitter camphoraceous taste, obtained by distillation from fennel. It contains anethole and about 20% of fenchone ($C_{10}H_{16}O$ = 152.2). Wt per ml 0.95 to 0.98 g. **Soluble** 1 in 1 of alcohol (90%). If solid matter separates it should be melted and mixed before use. **Store** in a cool place in airtight containers. Protect from light.

Uses. Fennel oil is an aromatic carminative. It is given to infants in the form of fennel water for the treatment of flatulence. The adult dose of fennel oil is 0.03 to 0.2 ml.

Preparations

Concentrated Fennel Water *(B.P.C. 1934).* Aq. Foenic. Conc. Fennel oil 2 ml, alcohol (90%) 60 ml, water to 100 ml; shaken with talc and filtered. *Dose.* 0.3 to 1 ml. *Hung. P.* has a similar preparation with 2% of polysorbate 20.

Fennel Water. Concentrated fennel water 2.5 ml, freshly boiled and cooled water to 100 ml.

4650-e

Galanga *(B.P.C. 1934).* China Root; Chinese Ginger; East Indian Root; Galangal; Lesser Galangal; Rasna.

Pharmacopoeias. In *Ind.* and *Swiss.*

The dried rhizome of the lesser galangal, *Alpinia officinarum* (Zingiberaceae), containing about 0.5 to 1.5% v/w of volatile oil.

Galanga is aromatic and carminative and similar in its effects to ginger.

4651-l

Galanga Major. Greater Galangal; Java Galangal.

The dried rhizome of the greater galangal, *Alpinia galanga* (Zingiberaceae).

Galanga major has been used in India as an aromatic carminative and in rheumatism and catarrhal affections.

Essential oil obtained from the rhizomes of *Alpinia galanga* had antibacterial activity against a variety of Gram-negative and Gram-positive organisms.— A. K. Bhargava and C. S. Chauhan, *Indian J. Pharm.*, 1968, *30*, 150.

4652-y

Geranium Oil *(B.P.C. 1959).* Oleum Geranii; Aetheroleum Pelargonii; Pelargonium Oil; Rose Geranium Oil.

CAS — 8000-46-2.

Pharmacopoeias. In *Cz.* and *Nord.*

A colourless, greenish, or brownish oil with a pleasant rose-like odour, obtained by distillation from the aerial parts of various species and hybrid forms of *Pelargonium* (Geraniaceae). It contains citronellol ($C_{10}H_{20}O$) and geraniol ($C_{10}H_{18}O$), free and as tiglates, together with some linalol. French and African oils contain not less than 20% w/w and Bourbon oil not less than 25% w/w of esters, calculated as geranyl tiglate, $C_{15}H_{24}O_2$. Wt per ml 0.889 to 0.9 g (French and African) or 0.883 to 0.892 g (Bourbon).

Algerian Geranium Oil, obtained from *Pelargonium graveolens*, contains 13 to 29.5% w/w of esters, calculated as geranyl tiglate.

Soluble 1 in 3 of alcohol (70%) with not more than a slight opalescence. **Store** in a cool place in well-filled airtight containers. Protect from light.

Standard for geranium oils. British Standard Specifications for Kenya, North Africa, and Réunion geranium oils (BS 2999/24/25/26: 1972) are published by the British Standards Institution.

Uses. Geranium oil is used for perfuming toothpowders, ointments, talcum powders, and various cosmetics.

An estimated acceptable daily intake of up to 500 µg per kg body-weight was established for citral, geranyl acetate, citronellol, linalol, and linalyl acetate, expressed as citral.— Twenty-third Report of Joint FAO/WHO Expert Committee on Food Additives, *Tech. Rep. Ser. Wld Hlth Org. No. 648*, 1980 (See also p.670 for the absorption of these terpinoids).

4653-j

Ginger *(B.P.).* Zingiber; Zingib.; Gingembre; Ingwer; Gengibre.

Pharmacopoeias. In *Aust., Belg., Br., Chin., Ind., Jap., Mex., Port.,* and *Swiss.*

The *B.P.* specifies scraped or unscraped rhizome of *Zingiber officinale* (Zingiberaceae), known in commerce as unbleached Jamaica ginger, and containing zingiberene, gingerol, and terpene derivatives. It contains not less than 4.5% of alcohol (90%)-soluble extractive and not less than 10% of water-soluble extractive. **Powdered Ginger** (*B.P.*) is light yellow or yellowish-brown. **Store** in a cool dry place; the powdered drug should be kept in airtight containers.

The chemistry of the pungent principles of ginger.— N. Pravatoroff, *Mfg Chem.*, 1967, *38* (Mar.), 40.

Uses. Ginger has carminative properties and has sometimes been added to purgatives in the belief that it prevents griping. Ginger is also used as a flavouring agent. *Dose:* 0.25 to 1 g.

The reduction of motion sickness by ginger.— D. B. Mowrey and D. E. Clayson, *Lancet*, 1982, *1*, 655.

Preparations

Ginger Oleoresin *(B.P.C. 1968).* Oleores. Zingib.; Gingerin. The acetone-soluble matter of ginger. Store in airtight containers. *Dose.* 15 to 60 mg.

Ginger Syrup *(B.P.C. 1973, A.P.F., Ind. P.).* Syrupus Zingiberis. Strong ginger tincture 5 ml, syrup to 100 ml. *Dose.* 2.5 to 5 ml.

Strong Ginger Tincture *(B.P.).* Strong Ginger Tinct.; Tinct. Zingib. Fort.; Ginger Essence; Essence of Ginger. Prepared by percolating ginger 50 g with alcohol (90%) to 100 ml.

Ind. P. has a similar tincture; *Belg. P.* and *Mex. P.* specify 1 in 5.

Weak Ginger Tincture *(B.P.).* Weak Ginger Tinct.; Tinct. Zingib. Mit.; Ginger Tincture. Strong ginger tincture 20 ml, alcohol (90%) to 100 ml.

4654-z

Juniper *(B.P.C. 1934).* Juniper Berry; Juniper Fruit; Baccae Juniperi; Juniperi Fructus; Genièvre; Wacholderbeeren; Zimbro.

Pharmacopoeias. In *Aust., Belg., Cz., Ger., Hung., Port., Roum., Rus.,* and *Swiss.*

The dried ripe fruits of *Juniperus communis* (Cupressaceae). It contains 0.5 to 2% of volatile oil and about 10% of resin.

4655-c

Juniper Oil *(B.P.C. 1949).* Oleum Juniperi; Juniper Berry Oil; Essence de Genièvre; Wacholderöl.

CAS — 8012-91-7.

Pharmacopoeias. In *Aust., Fr., Hung., Jug., Roum.,* and *Swiss.*

The oil distilled from the dried ripe fruits of *J. communis.* It is a colourless or pale greenish-yellow limpid liquid with a characteristic odour and a somewhat bitter burning taste. Wt per ml 0.859 to 0.89 g.

Soluble 1 in 4 of alcohol, becoming less soluble and more viscid with age; miscible with most organic solvents; practically insoluble in glycerol and propylene glycol. **Store** in a cool place in airtight containers. Protect from light.

Juniper oil is carminative and has been used in flatulence and colic. It has been used as a diuretic but it should not be employed during pregnancy or in the presence of renal disease. *Dose:* 0.03 to 0.2 ml.

Preparations

Juniper Spirit *(B.P.C. 1949).* Sp. Junip. Juniper oil 10 ml, alcohol (90%) to 100 ml. *Dose.* 0.3 to 1.2 ml.

Oleum Juniperi Ligni. Juniper Wood Oil. A trade name for a fictitious juniper oil supposed to be made from juniper wood but usually a mixture of juniper berry oil and turpentine oil.

4656-k

Laurel Berries. Bay-laurel Berries; Sweet Bay Berries; Lauri Fructus; Baie de Laurier; Lorbeerfrucht.

Pharmacopoeias. In *Swiss. Arg., Aust.,* and *Port.* specify the expressed oil (Oleum Lauri).

The dried ripe berries of *Laurus nobilis* (Lauraceae), containing about 1% of an aromatic volatile oil and about 25% of fixed oil.

Laurel berries were reputed to have carminative, emmenagogue, and diuretic properties. The oil is sometimes used in stimulating liniments.

Laurel Leaf Oil, obtained by distillation, is used as a flavouring agent.

4658-t

Lavender Flower. Flos Lavandulae.

Pharmacopoeias. In *Hung.*, *Port.*, and *Span.*

The dried flowers or flowering tops of *Lavandula officinalis* (= *L. spica* L.; *L. vera*) (Labiatae).

4659-x

Lavender Oil *(B.P., U.S.N.F.).* Oleum Lavandulae; Lavender Flower Oil; Essência de Alfazema; Esencia de Alhucema; Esencia de Espliego.

CAS — 8000-28-0.

Pharmacopoeias. The title of lavender oil is used in many pharmacopoeias usually to describe oil obtained from *L. officinalis* (=*L. spica* L. =*L. vera*). Lavender Oil *B.P.* is from *L. intermedia* or *L. angustifolia.* Lavender Oil *U.S.N.F.* is from *L. angustifolia*, or produced synthetically. It contains not less than 35% of total esters calculated as linalyl acetate.

A colourless or pale yellow or yellowish-green oil with a characteristic fragrant odour reminiscent of the flowers and a slightly bitter pungent taste, obtained by distillation from the fresh flowering tops of *Lavandula intermedia* (English oil) or of *L. angustifolia* (= *L. officinalis*) (foreign oil) (Labiatae). Lavender Oil *U.S.N.F.* may also be produced synthetically.
English oil has a wt per ml of 0.875 to 0.895 g, and is **soluble** 1 in 3 of alcohol (80%). Foreign oil has a wt per ml of 0.878 to 0.892 g, and is soluble 1 in 4 of alcohol (70%). Solutions in alcohol may be slightly opalescent. The oils become less soluble with age. English oil contains chiefly free linalol and some cineole but little linalyl acetate. French oil contains chiefly linalol, the total amount being about the same as that in the English oil, and linalyl acetate but only traces of cineole. English oil is usually considered to have the finer odour but the fresh floral note of the French oil is enhanced in those oils having higher contents of linalyl acetate. **Store** at a temperature not exceeding 25° in well-filled airtight containers. Protect from light.

Standard for lavender oil. A British Standard Specification for French Lavender Oil (BS 2999/34: 1971) is published by the British Standards Institution.

The solubility of lavender oil in macrogol esters.— K. Thoma and G. Pfaff, *J. Soc. cosmet. Chem.*, 1976, *27*, 221.

Uses. Lavender oil has been used as a carminative and as a colouring and flavouring agent. It is sometimes applied externally as an insect repellent. Its chief use is in perfumery and it is occasionally used in ointments and other pharmaceutical preparations to cover disagreeable odours. It is a preservative. *Dose:* 0.05 to 0.2 ml.

An estimated acceptable daily intake of up to 500 µg per kg body-weight was established for citral, geranyl acetate, citronellol, linalol, and linalyl acetate, expressed as citral.— Twenty-third Report of Joint FAO/WHO Expert Committee on Food Additives, *Tech. Rep. Ser. Wld Hlth Org. No. 648*, 1980 (See also p.670 for the absorption of these terpinoids).

Preparations

Compound Lavender Tincture *(B.P.C. 1949).* Tinct. Lavand. Co. Prepared from lavender oil 0.5 ml, rosemary oil 0.05 ml, cinnamon 1 g, nutmeg 1 g, and red sanders wood 2 g, by macerating with 90 ml of alcohol (90%) for 7 days, filtering, and adjusting with more alcohol (90%) to 100 ml. *Dose.* 2 to 4 ml.

Coronation Solution *(Bristol Roy. Infirm.).* Thymol 712.5 mg, lavender oil 0.9375 ml, glacial acetic acid 0.9375 ml, citronella oil 0.1 ml, Tween '80' 0.05 ml, industrial methylated spirit '66OP' to 100 ml. Dilute one part with two parts of industrial methylated spirit '66OP', and one part of water. Allow to evaporate in an open vessel or apply to absorbent material. Shelf-life 1 year. Used to mask odours.

Lavender Spirit *(B.P.C. 1934).* Sp. Lavand. Lavender oil 10 ml, alcohol (90%) to 100 ml. *Dose.* 0.3 to 1.2 ml. *Nord. P.* has lavender oil 2 g and alcohol 98 g. *Swiss P.* has lavender oil 300 mg and alcohol (63%) 99.7 g.

4660-y

Spike Lavender Oil *(B.P.C. 1968).* Oleum Lavandulae Spicatae; Ol. Lavand. Spic.; Spike Oil.

CAS — 8016-78-2.

The oil from *Lavandula latifolia* (= *L. spica* DC.) (Labiatae). It contains linalol, cineole (up to about 20%), and camphor.
A colourless or pale yellow liquid with an odour of lavender and cineole. Wt per ml 0.894 to 0.915 g.
Soluble 1 in 4 of alcohol (65%) sometimes with a faint opalescence on further dilution with alcohol (65%); soluble in propylene glycol and in most fixed oils; slightly soluble in glycerol and mineral oil. **Store** in a cool place in well-filled airtight containers. Protect from light.

Standard for spike lavender oil. A British Standard Specification for Spike Lavender Oil (BS 2999/42: 1971) is published by the British Standards Institution.

Spike lavender oil resembles lavender oil in its properties and is mainly used in perfumery.

An estimated acceptable daily intake of up to 500 µg per kg body-weight was established for citral, geranyl acetate, citronellol, linalol, and linalyl acetate, expressed as citral.— Twenty-third Report of Joint FAO/WHO Expert Committee on Food Additives, *Tech. Rep. Ser. Wld Hlth Org. No. 648*, 1980 (See also p.670 for the absorption of these terpinoids).

Proprietary Names

Tavipec-Montavit *(Sagitta, Ger.).*

4657-a

Lavandin Oil

CAS — 8022-15-9.

The oil from hybrids of *Lavandula latifolia* × *L. officinalis* (Labiatae) containing 20 to 28% of esters calculated as linalyl acetate; it has characteristics of both lavender and spike lavender oils.
A greenish-yellow liquid with an odour similar to lavender but slightly camphoraceous. Wt per ml about 0.89 g. **Soluble** 1 in 4 of alcohol (70%).

Standard for lavandin oil. A British Standard Specification for Lavandin Oil (BS 2999/6: 1965) is published by the British Standards Institution.

Lavandin oil is a substitute for lavender oil and is more fragrant than spike lavender oil; it is used largely in the soap industry and as a source of linalol and linalyl acetate.

An estimated acceptable daily intake of up to 500 µg per kg body-weight was established for citral, geranyl acetate, citronellol, linalol, and linalyl acetate, expressed as citral.— Twenty-third Report of Joint FAO/WHO Expert Committee on Food Additives, *Tech. Rep. Ser. Wld Hlth Org. No. 648*, 1980 (See also p.670 for the absorption of these terpinoids).

4661-j

Lemon Grass Oil *(B.P.C. 1954).* Oleum Graminis Citrati; Indian Melissa Oil; Indian Verbena Oil; Lemongrass Oil; Essência de Capim-Limão.

CAS — 8007-02-1.

NOTE. The synonym Indian Melissa Oil is sometimes applied to Citronella Oil.

Pharmacopoeias. In *Ind.* (from *C. flexuosus* only).

The oil is obtained by distillation from *Cymbopogon flexuosus* and *C. citratus* (Gramineae). Indian or 'Cochin' lemon grass oil, the principal lemon grass oil of commerce, is from *C. flexuosus* which is indigenous to India, and the so-called 'West Indian' oil is from *C. citratus* which is widely cultivated in India, Guatemala, Haiti, East and West Africa, and other tropical countries. The Indian oil is a reddish-yellow or brownish-red mobile liquid with a very strong verbena-like odour, while the 'West Indian' oil is pale yellow to yellowish-brown and has an odour similar to but somewhat lighter in character than that of the Indian oil.
The oils contain not less than 70% w/w of aldehydes, calculated as citral, $C_{10}H_{16}O$. Wt per ml 0.893 to 0.906 g (Indian) and 0.87 to 0.895 g ('West Indian'). **Soluble** 1 in 3 (Indian) or incompletely soluble ('West Indian') in alcohol (70%); soluble in mineral oils; freely soluble in propylene glycol; practically insoluble in glycerol. **Store** in a cool place in well-filled airtight containers. Protect from light.

Standard for lemon grass oils. British Standard Specifications for East Indian and West Indian Lemon Grass Oils (BS 2999/35/36: 1971) are published by the British Standards Institution.

Uses. Lemon grass oil was formerly given as a carminative but is now employed mainly in perfumery and as a source of citral. It is used as a flavouring agent.

An estimated acceptable daily intake of up to 500 µg per kg body-weight was established for citral, geranyl acetate, citronellol, linalol, and linalyl acetate, expressed as citral.— Twenty-third Report of Joint FAO/WHO Expert Committee on Food Additives, *Tech. Rep. Ser. Wld Hlth Org. No. 648*, 1980 (See also p.670 for the absorption of these terpinoids).

Lemon grass oil had considerably less activity than dicophane, dieldrin, and malathion as a contact insecticide against flies and mosquitoes. Flies and mosquitoes exposed to a saturated vapour of the oil were killed in 60 minutes and 20 minutes respectively. As a repellent, lemon grass oil had 10 to 15% of the activity of dimethyl phthalate.— B. K. Tiwari *et al.*, *Indian J. exp. Biol.*, 1966, *4*, 128, per *Trop. Dis. Bull.*, 1967, *64*, 571.

4662-z

Lemon Oil *(B.P., U.S.N.F.).* Oleum Limonis; Ol. Limon.; Aetheroleum Citri; Oleum Citri; Essence de Citron; Citronenöl; Esencia de Cidra; Essência de Limão.

CAS — 8008-56-8.

Pharmacopoeias. In *Arg.*, *Aust.*, *Belg.*, *Br.*, *Cz.*, *Ger.*, *Hung.*, *Ind.*, *It.*, *Jug.*, *Mex.*, *Pol.*, *Port.*, *Roum.*, *Span.*, and *Swiss.* Also in *U.S.N.F.*

A pale yellow or greenish-yellow oil with a characteristic odour and a warm, aromatic, slightly bitter taste, obtained by expression from fresh lemon peel, and consisting chiefly of (+)-limonene ($C_{10}H_{16}$) which, together with small quantities of other terpenes, constitutes about 90% of the oil. The *B.P.* specifies not less than 3.5% w/w of aldehydes calculated as citral. $C_{10}H_{16}O$. The quality of the oil is not determined solely by its citral content. Wt per ml 0.85 to 0.856 g. The *U.S.N.F.* specifies 2.2 to 3.8% of aldehydes, calculated as citral, for California-type Lemon Oil and 3 to 5.5% for Italian-type Lemon Oil.
Soluble 1 in 12 of alcohol (90%), the solution having a slight opalescence; miscible with dehydrated alcohol, glacial acetic acid, and carbon disulphide. **Store** at a temperature not exceeding 25° in well-filled airtight containers. Protect from light.

Uses. Lemon oil is carminative but it is chiefly used as a flavouring agent.

An estimated acceptable daily intake of up to 500 µg per kg body-weight was established for citral, geranyl acetate, citronellol, linalol, and linalyl acetate, expressed as citral.— Twenty-third Report of Joint FAO/WHO Expert Committee on Food Additives, *Tech. Rep. Ser. Wld Hlth Org. No. 648*, 1980 (See also p.670 for the absorption of these terpinoids).

The use of a preparation of *d*-limonene for dissolving gallstones.— H. Igimi *et al.*, *Am. J. dig. Dis.*, 1976, *21*, 926.

4663-c

Terpeneless Lemon Oil *(B.P.)*. Oleum Limonis Deterpenatum.

Pharmacopoeias. In *Br.*

A colourless or pale yellow oil with the characteristic odour and taste of lemon, prepared by concentrating lemon oil *in vacuo* until most of the terpenes have been removed, or by solvent partition. It consists chiefly of citral ($C_{10}H_{16}O$) with considerable quantities of esters, chiefly geranyl acetate ($C_{12}H_{20}O_2$) and linalyl acetate ($C_{12}H_{20}O_2$). It contains not less than 40% w/w of aldehydes calculated as citral. Wt per ml 0.88 to 0.895 g.

Soluble 1 in 1 of alcohol (80%). **Store** at a temperature not exceeding 25° in well-filled airtight containers. Protect from light.

Uses. Terpeneless lemon oil is used almost exclusively as a flavouring agent. It has the advantages of being stronger in flavour and odour and more readily soluble than the natural oil. One volume of the terpeneless oil is equivalent in flavour to about 20 volumes of lemon oil. A 1% v/v solution in alcohol (70%) is generally used for culinary purposes.

An estimated acceptable daily intake of up to 500 µg per kg body-weight was established for citral, geranyl acetate, citronellol, linalol, and linalyl acetate, expressed as citral.— Twenty-third Report of Joint FAO/WHO Expert Committee on Food Additives, *Tech. Rep. Ser. Wld Hlth Org. No. 648*, 1980 (See also p.670 for the absorption of these terpinoids).

Preparations

Lemon Spirit *(B.P., A.P.F.)*. Sp. Limon. Terpeneless lemon oil 10% v/v in alcohol (96%).

Lemon Syrup *(B.P.)*. Syrupus Limonis; Syr. Limon. Lemon spirit 0.5 ml, citric acid monohydrate 2.5 g, invert syrup 10 ml, syrup to 100 ml. Store at a temperature not exceeding 25°.

A.P.F. has a similar preparation without invert syrup and containing concentrated chloroform water 1.5 ml.

Lemon Syrup Neutral *(A.P.F.)*. Lemon spirit 0.5 ml, concentrated chloroform water 1.5 ml, syrup to 100 ml.

4664-k

Dried Lemon Peel *(B.P.)*. Limonis Cortex Siccatus.

Pharmacopoeias. In *Br.*

The dried outer part of the pericarp of the ripe or nearly ripe fruit of *Citrus limon* (Rutaceae). The dried peel contains not less than 2.5% v/w of volatile oil. **Store** in airtight containers.

4665-a

Fresh Lemon Peel *(B.P. 1958)*. Limonis Cortex Recens; Citri Cortex; Pericarpium Citri; Epicarpo de Limão.

Pharmacopoeias. In *Fr., Ind., Port.,* and *Swiss.*

The outer part of the fresh pericarp of the ripe or nearly ripe fruit of *Citrus limon* (Rutaceae).

Uses. Lemon peel is used principally as a flavouring agent.

Preparations

Lemon Tincture *(B.P. 1958)*. Tinct. Limon. Prepared by macerating fresh lemon peel 1 in 2 of alcohol (60%). Store in a cool place. Protect from light. *Dose.* 1 to 2 ml. *Fr. P.* has a similar preparation.

4666-t

Mace. Macis.

NOTE. The name mace is also applied to a solution of chloroacetophenone (a tear-gas) in organic solvents.

Pharmacopoeias. In *Port.*

The arillode of the seed of *Myristica fragrans* (Myristicaceae). It contains 7 to 14% of a volatile oil which closely resembles nutmeg oil.

4667-x

Mace Oil

CAS — 8007-12-3.

A volatile oil obtained by distillation from mace. It is very similar to nutmeg oil (p.679).

As with nutmeg, large doses of mace may cause epileptiform convulsions; a teaspoonful of powdered mace has caused severe toxic symptoms.

A youth in a hospital for juvenile narcotic addicts drank a suspension made with powdered mace. After 4 to 5 hours he became hot, weak, and dizzy. He received routine treatment for toxic shock and afterwards complained only of heaviness in the abdomen. Recovery was rapid and complete.— *N.Y. St. J. Med.*, 1965, *65*, 2270, per *Pharmacy Dig.*, 1966, *30*, 103.

4668-r

Matricaria Flowers *(B.P., Eur. P.)*. German Chamomile; Matricaria; Chamomilla; Flos Chamomillae; Flos Chamomillae Vulgaris; Matricariae Flos; Camomile Allemande; Kamillenblüten; Manzanilla Ordinaria; Camomilla.

CAS — 8002-66-2 (Matricaria oil).

Pharmacopoeias. In *Arg., Aust., Br., Cz., Eur., Fr., Ger., Hung., It., Jug., Neth., Pol., Port., Roum., Rus., Span.,* and *Swiss. Aust., Hung.,* and *Swiss* also include Matricaria Oil which is inferior in odour to chamomile oil.

The dried flowerheads of *Matricaria chamomilla* (Compositae), containing not less than 0.4% v/w of volatile oil. **Powdered Matricaria** *(B.P.C. 1949)* contains not less than 0.2% v/w of volatile oil. **Store** in a cool place in airtight containers. Protect from light.

Uses. Matricaria is used for the same purposes as chamomile (see p.673).

α-Bisabolol was isolated from the oil of *Matricaria chamomilla*, and anti-inflammatory activity was demonstrated in the *rat*. α-Bisabolol was much less toxic than guaiazulene.— V. Jakovlev and A. Von Schlichtegroll, *Arzneimittel-Forsch.*, 1969, *19*, 615.

Ventricular catheterisation studies in 12 patients with heart disease showed that chamomile tea prepared from matricaria had no significant cardiac effects. A marked hypnotic effect was observed; approximately 10 minutes after drinking the tea, 10 patients fell into a deep sleep lasting about 90 minutes.— L. Gould *et al.*, *J. clin. Pharmac.*, 1973, *13*, 475. See also N. R. Farnsworth and B. M. Morgan (letter), *J. Am. med. Ass.*, 1972, *221*, 410.

Antifungal activity of constituents of matricaria.— M. Szalontai *et al.*, *Acta pharm. hung.*, 1976, *46*, 232, per *Int. pharm. Abstr.*, 1977, *14*, 800.

4669-f

Melaleuca Oil *(B.P.C. 1949)*. Oleum Melaleucae; Tea Tree Oil; Ti-tree Oil.

CAS — 8022-72-8.

NOTE. Though the synonym Ti-tree Oil has been used for melaleuca oil (e.g. in *B.P.C. 1949*), the name Ti-tree is also applied to species of *Cordyline* (Liliaceae) indigenous to New Zealand.

A colourless or pale yellow oil with a pleasant characteristic odour and a terebinthinate taste, obtained by distillation from the leaves of the Australian tea tree, *Melaleuca alternifolia* (Myrtaceae).

It contains about 50 to 60% w/w of terpenes, cineole (up to 10%), and terpineol to which the odour is largely due. Wt per ml 0.89 to 0.9 g. **Soluble** 1 in 3 of alcohol (90%). **Store** in a cool place in airtight containers. Protect from light.

Melaleuca oil has been added to many disinfectant preparations.

4670-z

Melissa. Balm; Melissenblatt.

Pharmacopoeias. In *Aust., Belg., Fr., Ger., Roum., Span.,* and *Swiss.*

The leaves or leaves and tops of *Melissa officinalis* (Labiatae) a fragrant lemon-scented herb, containing a small amount (about 0.1%) of volatile oil. **Protect** from light.

4671-c

Melissa Oil. Balm Oil; Lemon Balm Oil; Esencia de Melisa.

CAS — 8014-71-9.

Pharmacopoeias. In *Arg.*

A yellow oil with an odour and taste resembling lemon, obtained by distillation from *Melissa officinalis*. It contains citral. Wt per ml about 0.91 g.

Melissa has carminative and diaphoretic properties. It is an ingredient of a number of aromatic spirits and aromatic waters. A compound aromatic spirit (Karmelitergeist; Agua Carmelitana), prepared from a mixture of fresh melissa herb, lemon peel, cinnamon, nutmeg, coriander, and other aromatics, has been used as a digestive stimulant and as a fragrant stimulating application to the skin.

An estimated acceptable daily intake of up to 500 µg per kg body-weight was established for citral, geranyl acetate, citronellol, linalol, and linalyl acetate, expressed as citral.— Twenty-third Report of Joint FAO/WHO Expert Committee on Food Additives, *Tech. Rep. Ser. Wld Hlth Org. No. 648*, 1980 (See also p.670 for the absorption of these terpinoids).

The essential oils from melissa had antibacterial and sedative actions. A polyphenolic fraction showed antiviral activity.— I. Morelli, *Boll. chim.-farm.*, 1977, *116*, 334, per *Int. pharm. Abstr.*, 1978, *15*, 388.

4672-k

Black Mustard *(B.P.C. 1949)*. Sinapis Nigra; Graine de Moutarde Noire; Moutarde Jonciforme; Schwarzer Senfsame; Semilla de Mostaza; Mostarda Preta.

Pharmacopoeias. In *Aust., Belg., Fr., Mex., Port., Roum., Span.,* and *Swiss. Fr.* specifies the seeds of *B. juncea. Swiss* allows *B. nigra, B. juncea,* and other species.

The dried ripe seeds of *Brassica nigra* (= *B. sinapioides*) (Cruciferae). It contains the glycoside sinigrin (potassium myronate) and the enzyme myrosin, which interact in the presence of water to yield allyl isothiocyanate (0.8 to 2%). **Store** in a dry place.

4673-a

White Mustard *(B.P.C. 1949)*. Sinapis Alba.

The dried ripe seeds of *Brassica alba* (Cruciferae). It contains the glycoside sinalbin and the enzyme myrosin. **Store** in a dry place.

Bath Mustard is a mixture of black and white mustard in coarse powder. *Mustard Bran* consists chiefly of the powdered seed coats of black mustard. *Mustard Flour* consists of powdered black and white seeds from which the seed coats have been largely removed.

Uses. Mustard flour is used mainly as a condiment. It has been used as an emetic. It causes redness and a feeling of warmth when applied to the skin or mucous membranes and acts as a counter-irritant when applied as a poultice (2% in linseed poultice). It may blister tender skins.

Added to hot water is has been used as a foot-bath.

Preparations

Mustard Bath *(B.P.C. 1949)*. Balneum Sinapis. Bath mustard, of commerce, 360 g in about 140 litres.

4674-t

Expressed Mustard Oil *(B.P.C. 1954)*. Ol. Sinap. Express.; Black Mustard Oil.

CAS — 8007-40-7.

Pharmacopoeias. Ind. P. specifies the oil from *B. juncea.*

A brownish-yellow or greenish-brown oil with a slight odour and a mild, not unpleasant taste; expressed from black mustard seeds (*Brassica nigra*), which contain about 27% of fixed oil.

Slightly **soluble** in alcohol; miscible with ether, chloroform, and light petroleum. Wt per ml about 0.917 g. **Store** in a cool place in airtight containers. Protect from light.

Expressed mustard oil has been used as a mild rubefacient.

4675-x

Volatile Mustard Oil *(B.P.C. 1949)*.
Oleum Sinapis Volatile; Allyl Isothiocyanate; Essence of Mustard; Allylsenföl.

CAS — 57-06-7.

Pharmacopoeias. In *Aust., Belg., Hung., Pol., Port.,* and *Roum.*

It is prepared synthetically or distilled from black mustard seeds after expression of the fixed oil and maceration in tepid water to allow interaction between the glycoside sinigrin and the enzyme myrosin.

It is a colourless or pale yellow mobile liquid with an intensely pungent irritating odour and an acrid taste, containing not less than 92% w/w of allyl isothiocyanate, (C_3H_5CNS = 99.15). Wt per ml 1.007 to 1.02 g.

Soluble 1 in 150 of water and 1 in 10 of alcohol (70%); miscible with organic solvents. **Store** in a cool place in airtight containers. Protect from light.

CAUTION. *Volatile Mustard Oil is a powerful vesicant and irritant and should not be inhaled or tasted undiluted.*

Uses. Volatile mustard oil is an extremely powerful irritant and when applied undiluted it causes rapid blistering of the skin. Diluted with alcohol (1 in 50) or as Mustard Liniment it is used as a counter-irritant and rubefacient.

Preparations

Mustard Liniment *(B.P.C. 1949)*. Lin. Sinap. Volatile mustard oil 3.5 ml, camphor 5.5 g, castor oil 12.5 ml, alcohol (90%) to 100 ml.

Spiritus Sinapis *(Aust. P.)*. Mustard Spirit; Senfspiritus. Volatile mustard oil 2 g and alcohol 98 g.

Similar preparations are included in several pharmacopoeias.

4676-r

Neroli Oil *(B.P.C. 1949)*.
Oleum Neroli; Orange Flower Oil *(U.S.N.F.)*; Orange-flower Oil; Esencia de Azahar; Essência de Flor de Laranjeira.

CAS — 8016-38-4.

Pharmacopoeias. In *Arg., Aust., Belg., Mex., Port.,* and *Swiss.* Also in *U.S.N.F.*

A pale yellow, slightly fluorescent oil, becoming reddish-brown on exposure to air and light, with an intense characteristic odour and a sweet aromatic taste with a bitter after-taste, obtained by distillation from the flowers of the bitter-orange tree, *Citrus aurantium* (Rutaceae). It contains the methyl ester of anthranilic acid, methyl anthranilate ($C_8H_9NO_2$), to which the odour is stated to be due. It may become turbid or solid at low temperatures. It is neutral to litmus. Wt per ml 0.865 to 0.88 g.

Soluble 1 in 2 of alcohol (80%), the solution becoming turbid on the addition of more of the alcohol. **Store** in a cool place in airtight containers. Protect from light.

Standard for neroli oil. A British Standard Specification for Neroli Oil (BS 2999/8: 1965) is published by the British Standards Institution.

Uses. Neroli oil is used as a flavouring agent and in perfumery.

Estimated acceptable daily intake of methyl anthranilate: up to 1.5 mg per kg body-weight and of methyl *N*-methylanthranilate: up to 200 µg per kg.— Twenty-third Report of Joint FAO/WHO Expert Committee on Food Additives, *Tech. Rep. Ser. Wld Hlth Org. No. 648,* 1980.

Preparations

Concentrated Orange-flower Water *(B.P.C. 1949)*. Aq. Aurant. Flor. Conc. Neroli oil 0.62 ml, alcohol (90%) 60 ml, water to 100 ml ; shaken with talc and filtered. **Triple orange-flower water** (Aq. Aurant. Flor. Trip.) and **Orange-flower water** may be prepared by diluting the concentrated water with 12 times and 39 times its volume of water respectively.

Elixir Aromaticum *(Swiss P.)*. Elixir Gari. Saffron 100 mg, clove 150 mg, nutmeg 150 mg, cinnamon 200 mg, alcohol 20 g, brandy 10 g, syrup 56 g, and orange-flower water *(Swiss P.)* 15 g. Prepared by maceration in the alcohol, adding the other liquids, and filtering.

Orange Flower Water *(U.S.N.F.)*. A saturated solution prepared by distilling the fresh flowers of *C. aurantium* with water and removing the excess volatile oil from the clear aqueous portion of the distillate. Neutral or only slightly acid to litmus. Store in airtight containers.

Arg. P., Turk. P., and *Swiss P.* include a similar preparation.

4677-f

Niaouli Oil. Essence de Niaouli.

CAS — 8014-68-4.

NOTE. The title Niaouli Essence has been applied to Cajuput Oil.

Pharmacopoeias. In *Arg., Belg., Neth., Port., Roum., Span.,* and *Swiss. Neth. P.* specifies *Melaleuca quinquenervia.*

A colourless or yellowish oil with a characterstic cineole-like odour and a bitter aromatic taste, obtained by distillation from the fresh leaves of *Melaleuca viridiflora* (Myrtaceae). It contains about 60% v/v of cineole. **Soluble** 1 in 4 of alcohol (70%) and 1 in 1 of alcohol (80%).

Niaouli oil has been given in rhinitis, laryngitis, and various respiratory diseases. *Dose:* 0.05 to 0.3 ml.

Preparations

Syrupus Olei Aetheri Niaouli *(Arg. P.)*. Jarabe de Esencia de Niaouli. Niaouli oil 0.2 ml, alcohol (95%) 5 ml, sucrose 85 g, water 100 ml.

Proprietary Names

Gomenol *(Gomenol, Fr.)*; Gomenoléo *(Gomenol, Fr.)*; Vaseline Gomenolée *(Gomenol, Fr.)*.

Niaouli oil was formerly marketed in Great Britain under the proprietary names Gomenol and Gomenoleo (*Napp*).

4679-n

Nutmeg *(B.P.C. 1973)*.
Myristica; Nux Moschata; Muscade; Nuez Moscada; Noz Moscada.

Pharmacopoeias. In *Ind., Port., Span.,* and *Swiss.*

The dried kernels of the seeds of *Myristica fragrans* (Myristicaceae), containing not less than 5% v/w of volatile oil. It contains about 35% of solid fat, the chief fatty acid constituents of which are myristic acid (about 60%) and smaller amounts of palmitic, oleic, linoleic, and lauric acids. **Powdered Nutmeg** (*B.P.C. 1973*) contains not less than 4% v/w of volatile oil. **Store** in a cool place in airtight containers.

4678-d

Nutmeg Oil *(B.P., U.S.N.F.)*.
Oleum Myristicae; Myristica Oil; Essence de Muscade; Ätherisches Muskatöl; Essência de Moscada; Esencia de Nuez Moscada.

CAS — 8008-45-5.

Pharmacopoeias. In *Arg., Aust., Br., Ind.,* and *Swiss.* Also in *U.S.N.F.*

A volatile oil obtained by distillation from nutmeg. It is a colourless, pale yellow or pale green liquid with an odour and taste of nutmeg. It consists chiefly of terpenes, including α-pinene and β-pinene, and a small proportion of myristicin. It is scarcely distinguishable from volatile oil of mace and frequently no commercial distinction is made between the two. Wt per ml 0.86 to 0.88 g (West Indian oil) and 0.885 to 0.915 g (East Indian oil). West Indian oil is **soluble** 1 in 4 of alcohol (90%), East Indian 1 in 3. **Store** at a temperature not exceeding 25° in well-filled airtight containers. Protect from light.

Standard for nutmeg oils. British Standard Specifications for East Indian and West Indian Nutmeg Oil (BS 2999/37/38: 1971) are published by the British Standards Institution.

Adverse Effects and Treatment. As for Essential Oils, p.670.

Nutmeg, taken in large doses may cause nausea and vomiting, flushing or sometimes shivering, dry mouth, tachycardia, disorientation, stupor or stimulation of the central nervous system possibly with epileptiform convulsions, miosis sometimes followed by mydriasis, and euphoria and hallucinations.

A review of the toxic effects and uses of nutmeg.— A. T. Weil, *Bull. Narcot.,* 1966, *18* (4), 15.

Within 4 hours of taking 28 g of nutmeg in water and orange juice, a 19-year-old woman felt cold and shivery. This was followed after 6 to 8 hours by severe vomiting accompanied by hallucinations. For a week she had poor concentration and was disorientated. The hallucinogen in nutmeg was believed to be myristicin.— D. J. Panayotopoulos and D. D. Chisholm (letter), *Br. med. J.,* 1970, *1,* 754. A similar report.— R. A. Faguet and K. F. Rowland, *Am. J. Psychiat.,* 1978, *135,* 860.

Within 3 days of receiving ground nutmeg 9 teaspoonfuls daily to control the diarrhoea associated with medullary carcinoma of the thyroid, a patient complained of dry eyes and mouth, blurred vision, dizziness, tingling, and feelings of depersonalisation and remoteness. The symptoms gradually subsided as the dose was reduced.— G. S. Venables *et al.* (letter), *Br. med. J.,* 1976, *1,* 96.

Ingestion of freshly ground nutmeg 1.5 to 4 g three to four times daily for 2 days by 2 subjects produced constipation, but no aspirin-like effect on biphasic platelet aggregation was noted. Both subjects also felt lightheaded, slightly disorientated, occasionally nauseated, flushed, and had nasal congestion and very dry mouths; pupil size was unaffected.— W. H. Dietz and M. J. Stuart (letter), *New Engl. J. Med.,* 1976, *294,* 503.

Uses. Nutmeg is aromatic and carminative. It is the source of Nutmeg Oil, and a solid fat, Expressed Nutmeg Oil (see p.697). Nutmeg oil is mildly rubefacient. Nutmeg appears to inhibit prostaglandin synthesis.

In a 41-year-old woman with medullary carcinoma of the thyroid and diarrhoea probably due to elevated plasma-prostaglandin concentrations, persistent diarrhoea following thyroidectomy responded to treatment with powdered nutmeg, a prostaglandin inhibitor, one teaspoonful 9 times daily.— J. A. Barrowman *et al., Br. med. J.,* 1975, *3,* 11. See also *idem* (letter), 160. See also above under Adverse Effects.

A 27-year-old man with intractable diarrhoea due to Crohn's disease unresponsive to conventional therapy obtained marked improvement within 24 hours of taking nutmeg [powdered] one teaspoonful 4 times daily. Correlating well with his clinical response, serum-prostaglandin E_1 concentrations fell, suggesting that the secretory watery diarrhoea seen in Crohn's disease might be prostaglandin-mediated.— I. Shafran *et al.* (letter), *New Engl. J. Med.*, 1977, *296*, 694.

4680-k

Orange Oil *(B.P.)*. Oleum Aurantii; Sweet Orange Oil; Essence of Orange; Essence of Portugal; Arancia Dolce Essenza; Essência de Laranja.

CAS — 8008-57-9.

Pharmacopoeias. In *Br.*, *It.*, and *Jap.* Also in *U.S.N.F.* Bitter orange oil is included in *Belg.*, *Port.*, and *Span.*

It is obtained by mechanical means from the fresh peel of the sweet orange *Citrus sinensis* (Rutaceae) and contains at least 90% of (+)-limonene ($C_{10}H_{16}$). The *B.P.* specifies not less than 1% w/w of aldehydes calculated as decanal ($C_{10}H_{20}O$). The *U.S.N.F.* describes California-type Orange Oil and Florida-type Orange Oil and specifies 1.2 to 2.5% of aldehydes calculated as decanal.

Distilled orange oil is inferior, the effects of heat and steaming being detrimental to the oxygenated compounds.

The *B.P.C. 1954* and earlier editions allowed also bitter orange oil, from *C. aurantium*. This oil is chemically almost identical with sweet orange oil but it can be distinguished by its odour and bitter taste.

A yellow, orange, or yellowish-brown liquid with an odour characteristic of orange and a mild and aromatic taste. Wt per ml 0.842 to 0.848 g.

Soluble 1 in 7 of alcohol (90%) but rarely with the formation of bright solutions on account of the presence of waxy non-volatile substances; miscible with dehydrated alcohol and carbon disulphide; soluble 1 in 1 of glacial acetic acid. The oil deteriorates on keeping, acquiring a disagreeable terebinthinate taste. **Store** at a temperature not exceeding 25° in well-filled airtight containers. Protect from light.

Standard for orange oil. A British Standard Specification for Sweet Orange Oil (BS 2999/43: 1971) is published by the British Standards Institution.

Uses. Orange oil is used as a flavouring agent and in perfumery.

Preparations

Aromatic Elixir *(U.S.N.F.)*. Orange oil *U.S.N.F.* 0.24 ml, lemon oil *U.S.N.F.* 0.06 ml, coriander oil 0.024 ml, anise oil 0.006 ml, syrup 37.5 ml, alcohol about 25 ml, and water to 100 ml; shaken with talc (3 g) and filtered.

Compound Orange Spirit *(U.S.N.F.)*. Orange oil *U.S.N.F.* 20 ml, lemon oil *U.S.N.F.* 5 ml, coriander oil 2 ml, anise oil 0.5 ml, alcohol to 100 ml. Store at a temperature not exceeding 8° in airtight containers. Protect from light.

4681-a

Terpeneless Orange Oil *(B.P.)*. Oleum Aurantii Deterpenatum.

Pharmacopoeias. In *Br.*

A yellow or orange-yellow oil with the characteristic odour and taste of orange, prepared by concentrating orange oil *in vacuo* until most of the terpenes have been removed, or by solvent partition. It consists chiefly of the free alcohols (+)-linalol and (+)-terpineol, with considerable quantities of aldehydes, chiefly decanal, and small amounts of esters. It contains not less than 18% w/w of aldehydes calculated as decanal, $C_{10}H_{20}O$. Wt per ml 0.855 to 0.88 g.

Soluble 1 in 1 of alcohol (90%). **Store** at a temperature not exceeding 25° in well-filled airtight containers. Protect from light.

Uses. Terpeneless orange oil is used as a flavouring agent. It has the advantages of being stronger in flavour and odour and more readily soluble than the natural oil.

An estimated acceptable daily intake of up to 500 µg per kg body-weight was established for citral, geranyl acetate, citronellol, linalol, and linalyl acetate, expressed as citral.— Twenty-third Report of Joint FAO/WHO Expert Committee on Food Additives, *Tech. Rep. Ser. Wld Hlth Org. No. 648*, 1980 (See also p.670 for the absorption of these terpinoids).

Preparations

Compound Orange Spirit *(B.P.)*. Spiritus Aurantii Compositus; Sp. Aurant. Co. Terpeneless orange oil 0.25 ml, terpeneless lemon oil 0.13 ml, coriander oil 0.625 ml, anise oil 0.425 ml, alcohol (90%) to 100 ml.

4682-t

Dried Bitter-Orange Peel *(B.P.)*. Aurantii Amari Cortex; Aurantii Cortex Siccatus; Pericarpium Aurantii; Corteza de Naranja Amarga; Flavedo Aurantii Amara; Pomeranzenschale.

Pharmacopoeias. Most pharmacopoeias include the dried or fresh peel from either bitter orange or sweet orange (*C. sinensis*).

Fr. includes the peel, flower, and leaf of the bitter orange (Bigaradier; Oranger à Fruit Amer) and the fresh peel of the sweet orange (Oranger à Fruit Doux). *Jap. P.* includes the immature fruit of *C. aurantium* spp. or their allied plants

The dried outer part of the pericarp of the ripe or nearly ripe fruit of the bitter orange, *Citrus aurantium* (Rutaceae). The dried peel contains not less than 2.5% v/w of volatile oil. Preparations of orange peel darken in colour with salts of iron. The dried peel should be **stored** in airtight containers. Protect from light.

Uses. Dried bitter-orange peel is used as a flavouring agent and for its bitter and carminative properties. The fresh peel has been used in preparing orange tinctures and syrups.

Preparations

Elixirs

Simple Elixir *(B.P.C. 1949)*. Elix. Simp. Orange tincture [fresh bitter-orange peel 1 in 4 in alcohol (90%)]7.5 ml, syrup 40 ml, chloroform water to 100 ml. Add 2.5 g of purified talc, allow to stand for a few hours with occasional shaking, and filter. *Dose.* 4 to 8 ml.

Extracts

Orange Liquid Extract *(B.P.C. 1949)*. Ext. Aurant. Liq. Dried bitter-orange peel (about 1 in 1); prepared by maceration in alcohol (70%). *Dose.* 0.6 to 1.2 ml. A similar extract is included in some pharmacopoeias.

Infusions

Concentrated Compound Orange Peel Infusion *(B.P.C. 1954)*. Inf. Aurant. Co. Conc. Macerate dried bitter-orange peel 20 g, dried lemon peel 8 g, and bruised clove 2.5 g in alcohol (25%) 100 ml for 48 hours and press out the liquid; macerate the marc with alcohol (25%) 35 ml for 24 hours and press out the liquid; mix the expressed liquids, allow to stand 14 days, and filter. *Dose.* 2 to 4 ml. Compound Orange Peel Infusion is prepared by diluting 1 vol. of this concentrated infusion to 8 vol. with water.

Concentrated Orange Peel Infusion *(B.P.)*. Conc. Orange Peel Inf.; Infusum Aurantii Concentratum. Dried bitter-orange peel (1 in 2.7), prepared by maceration in alcohol (25%).

Orange Peel Infusion is prepared by diluting 1 vol. of this concentrated infusion to 10 vol. with water.

Syrups

Aromatic Syrup *(A.P.F.)*. Syr. Aromat. Orange tincture 5 ml, lemon spirit 0.5 ml, concentrated chloroform water 1.5 ml, syrup to 100 ml.

Aromatic Syrup *(B.P.C. 1949)*. Syr. Aromat. Orange liquid extract 6.25 ml, cinnamon water 25 ml, syrup to 100 ml. Mix the liquid extract and the cinnamon water with a little purified talc or light kaolin, filter, and add the syrup. *Dose.* 2 to 4 ml.

Orange Syrup *(B.P.)*. Syrupus Aurantii.
Orange tincture 6 ml, syrup to 100 ml.
A.P.F. has a similar formula with concentrated chloroform water.
A similar syrup is included in many pharmacopoeias.

Orange Syrup *(U.S.N.F.)*. Sweet orange peel tincture 5 ml, anhydrous citric acid 500 mg, and talc 1.5 g, mixed with water 40 ml, and filtered until clear with enough water to make a filtrate of 45 ml. Dissolve sucrose 82 g in the filtrate without the use of heat, and dilute to 100 ml with water. Store at a temperature not exceeding 8° in airtight containers.

Tinctures

Bitter Tincture *(Jap. P.)*. Dried bitter-orange peel 5 g, swertia 500 mg, zanthoxylum fruit 500 mg, alcohol (70%) to 100 ml. Prepare by maceration or percolation.

Orange Tincture *(B.P.)*. Tincture Aurantii. Dried bitter-orange peel 11 in 100; prepared by percolation with alcohol (70%). Orange Tincture *B.P.C. 1968* was prepared by macerating fresh bitter-orange peel 1 in 2 of alcohol (90%).
Many pharmacopoeias include an orange tincture.

Sweet Orange Peel Tincture *(U.S.N.F.)*. Prepared by macerating fresh sweet-orange peel 1 in 2 of alcohol. Store at a temperature not exceeding 40° in airtight containers. Protect from light.

4683-x

Origanum

CAS — 8007-11-2 (origanum oil).

NOTE. The name Origanum has been applied to several other labiate plants which have been used medicinally or for culinary purposes. Confusion exists also over the name Origanum Oil—see under Thyme Oil, p.684.

Pharmacopoeias. In *Cz.*

The fresh or dried flowering tops of marjoram, *Origanum vulgare* (Labiatae), containing a volatile oil.

Origanum has been used as an aromatic carminative and in cough syrups. It has also been employed externally in healing lotions for wounds, usually in conjunction with other herbs.

4684-r

Orris *(B.P.C. 1949)*. Iridis Rhizoma; Orris Rhizome; Orris Root.

Pharmacopoeias. In *Port.*

The peeled and dried rhizome of *Iris germanica*, *I. pallida*, and *I. florentina* (Iridaceae). It has a fragrant violet-like odour and a slightly aromatic and bitter somewhat irritating taste. It contains 0.1 to 0.2% of volatile substance, known as Concrete Oil of Orris or Butter of Orris, which is pale yellow and solid at ordinary temperatures (m.p. about 40°) and composed of about 85% of myristic acid, the remainder being a mixture of irone ($C_{14}H_{22}O$), oleic acid, methyl myristate, and other esters. The rhizome also contains starch, sugar, and a little resin.

Powdered orris is yellowish-white to pale yellow in colour.

Orris has been used as an ingredient of toilet powders but it may cause allergic reactions in hypersensitive persons. It has also been used in toothpowders and toothpastes and the oil has been used as a flavouring agent. A formerly popular dusting-powder, known as Violet Powder, contained 12.5% of orris with bergamot and neroli oils and starch; Syrup of Violets, originally made from violet petals, was later prepared from a tincture of orris and coloured with a violet dye. Volatile oil of orris is used as a basis for violet perfumes.

4685-f

Palmarosa Oil. East Indian Geranium Oil; Turkish Geranium Oil; Essência de Palma-rosa.

CAS — 8014-19-5.

A colourless or slightly yellow oil with a characteristic fragrant rose-like odour, obtained by distillation from the leaves of *Cymbopogon martini* var. *motia* (Gramineae). It contains 75 to 95% of geraniol ($C_{10}H_{18}O$) together with geranyl acetate ($C_{12}H_{20}O_2$).

Soluble 1 in 3 of alcohol and 1 in 5 of alcohol (60%); soluble with opalescence in mineral oil; practically insoluble in glycerol.

Standard for palmarosa oil. A British Standard Specification for Palmarosa Oil (BS 2999/49: 1972) is published by the British Standards Institution.

Palmarosa oil is used in cosmetics, particularly as a perfume for soaps. It is a source of a high grade of geraniol.

An estimated acceptable daily intake of up to 500 µg per kg body-weight was established for citral, geranyl acetate, citronellol, linalol, and linalyl acetate, expressed as citral.— Twenty-third Report of Joint FAO/WHO Expert Committee on Food Additives, *Tech. Rep. Ser. Wld Hlth Org. No. 648,* 1980 (See also p.670 for the absorption of these terpinoids).

4686-d

Parsley. Petroselinum; Persil. *Petroselinum crispum* (=*P. sativum; Apium petroselinum; Carum petroselinum*) (Umbelliferae).

Pharmacopoeias. Cz. specifies the root. *Port.* specifies the fruit and the root.

4687-n

Parsley Oil *(B.P.C. 1934).* Oleum Petroselini; Parsley Seed Oil; Parsley Fruit Oil.

CAS — 8000-68-8.

A thick colourless or yellowish oil distilled from parsley fruit. Wt per ml about 1.05 g. **Soluble** 1 in 8 of alcohol (80%). **Store** in airtight containers. Protect from light. It contains apiole ($C_{12}H_{14}O_4$) which separates in crystals at low temperatures.

Standard for parsley oil. A British Standard Specification for Parsley Oil (BS 2999/9: 1965) is published by the British Standards Institution.

Both the fruit and the roots of parsley have been used medicinally as diuretics and emmenagogues.

The oil has similar properties to apiol (see p.671). It is also used as a flavouring agent.

4688-h

Black Pepper *(B.P.C. 1949).* Piper Nigrum; Pepper; Piper; Pimenta.

CAS — 8006-82-4 (black pepper oil).

Pharmacopoeias. In *Aust.* and *Port.*

The dried unripe fruits of *Piper nigrum* (Piperaceae), containing a pungent resin, chavicine, with piperine, piperidine, and 1 to 2.5% of volatile oil. **Store** in a cool dry place.

Standard for pepper oil. A British Standard Specification for Pepper Oil (BS 2999/12: 1965) is published by the British Standards Institution.

Black pepper stimulates the taste-buds, producing a reflex increase in gastric secretion. It has diaphoretic and diuretic properties. The distilled oil (Black Pepper Oil) is used as a flavouring agent.

4689-m

White Pepper *(B.P.C. 1949).* Piper Album.

The ripe fruits of *Piper nigrum* (Piperaceae) deprived of the outer part of the pericarp. It contains less volatile oil than black pepper. **Store** in a cool dry place.

White pepper is used for the same purposes as black pepper but is less aromatic.

4690-t

Peppermint Leaf *(B.P., Eur. P.).* Peppermint *(U.S.N.F.)*; Mentha Piperita; Menthae Piperitae Folium; Menth. Pip.; Menthe Poivrée; Pfefferminzblätter; Hoja de Menta; Hortelã-Pimenta.

Pharmacopoeias. In *Arg., Aust., Belg., Br., Cz., Eur., Fr., Ger., Hung., It., Jug., Neth., Pol., Port., Roum., Rus., Span.,* and *Swiss.* Also in *U.S.N.F.*

Chin. P. specifies *M. haplocalyx. Jap. P.* specifies *M. arvensis* var. *piperascens.*

The dried leaves of *Mentha* × *piperita* (Labiatae), containing not less than 1.2% v/w of volatile oil. There are 2 varieties known as black peppermint and white peppermint. **Store** in a cool dry place in well-closed containers which prevent loss of volatile oil. Protect from light.

4691-x

Peppermint Oil *(B.P., Eur. P., U.S.N.F.).* Menthae Piperitae Aetheroleum; Oleum Menthae Piperitae; Ol. Menth. Pip.; Essence de Menthe Poivrée; Pfefferminzöl; Essência de Hortelã-Pimenta.

CAS — 8006-90-4.

Pharmacopoeias. In *Arg., Aust., Belg., Br., Cz., Eur., Ger., Hung., Ind., It., Jug., Mex., Neth., Nord., Pol., Port., Roum., Rus., Span.,* and *Swiss.* Also in *U.S.N.F.* Mentha Oil (*Jap. P.*) is from *M. arvensis* var. *piperascens. Ger. P.* also has a similar oil. Mentha Oil (*Ind.P.*) is from various species of *Mentha. Belg.* specifies *M. piperita* or *M. arvensis* var. *piperascens.* Oleum Menthae (*Chin. P.*) is from *M. haplocalyx.*

The oil obtained by distillation from the fresh flowering tops of *Mentha* × *piperita* (Labiatae) and rectified if necessary.

It is a colourless, pale yellow, or greenish-yellow liquid with the characteristic odour of peppermint and a pungent aromatic cooling taste. It contains menthol, menthone, menthyl acetate, and terpenes; unrectified oil contains dimethyl sulphide. The *B.P.* specifies 4.5 to 10% w/w of esters, calculated as menthyl acetate, $C_{12}H_{22}O_2$, not less than 44% w/w of free alcohols calculated as menthol, and 15 to 32% of ketones calculated as menthone, $C_{10}H_{18}O$. The *U.S.N.F.* specifies not less than 5% of esters calculated as menthyl acetate and not less than 50% of total menthol, free and as esters. Menthol separates on cooling to a low temperature, especially when seeded with menthol crystals. Wt per ml 0.9 to 0.912 g.

Soluble 1 in 4 of alcohol (70%) with slight opalescence and 1 in 0.5 of alcohol (90%), the solution sometimes becoming turbid on adding more alcohol (90%); miscible with dehydrated alcohol. It darkens in colour and becomes viscous on keeping. **Store** at a temperature not exceeding 25° in well-filled airtight containers. Protect from light.

The Pharmaceutical Society's Department of Pharmaceutical Sciences found that PVC bottles softened and distorted fairly rapidly in the presence of peppermint oil, which should not be stored or dispensed in such bottles.— *Pharm. J.,* 1973, *1,* 100.

The solubility of peppermint oil in macrogol esters.— K. Thoma and G. Pfaff, *J. Soc. cosmet. Chem.,* 1976, *27,* 221.

Standard for peppermint oils. British Standard Specifications for Peppermint Oil (BS 2999/39: 1971) and Dementholized Mentha Arvensis Oil (BS 2999/56: 1975) are published by the British Standards Institution.

Adverse Effects. Peppermint oil may cause allergic reactions.

Idiopathic auricular fibrillation in 2 patients addicted to 'peppermints'. Normal rhythm was restored when peppermint-sucking ceased.— J. G. Thomas (letter), *Lancet,* 1962, *1,* 222.

An acute allergic reaction in the mouth, neck, and throat was traced to peppermint oil contained in a toothpaste.— I. L. F. Smith, *Br. dent. J.,* 1968, *125,* 304.

Recurrent attacks of muscle pain were reported in 2 patients when they consumed large quantities of confectionery flavoured with peppermint oil.— B. Williams (letter), *Med. J. Aust.,* 1972, *2,* 390.

Uses. Peppermint oil is an aromatic carminative; it relieves gastric and intestinal flatulence and colic and is employed with purgatives to prevent griping. It is given in doses of 0.05 to 0.2 ml. It is also used to flavour dental preparations. Peppermint Water is used as a basis for mixtures.

The effect of peppermint on the gastro-oesophageal sphincter was studied in 24 healthy fasting subjects by the administration by catheter of 15 drops of peppermint spirit in 30 ml of water, 5 minutes after the introduction of 400 to 1500 ml of air. In 22 subjects sphincter pressure fell and reflux occurred within 1 to 7 minutes. In 2 subjects relaxation of the sphincter did not occur. In 3 subjects given peppermint without air, the sphincter pressure fell but there was less marked reflux. Saline given to 7 controls had no effect.— C. J. Sigmund and E. F. McNally, *Gastroenterology,* 1969, *56,* 13, per *Abstr. Wld Med.,* 1969, *43,* 653.

In a double-blind crossover study in 16 patients peppermint oil 0.2 ml in enteric-coated capsules, 1 or 2 thrice daily, was more effective than placebo in relieving the symptoms of the irritable bowel syndrome.— W. D. W. Rees *et al., Br. med. J.,* 1979, *2,* 835. It is essential that the peppermint capsules are enteric-coated; the use of uncoated capsules may lead to gastric irritation.— D. Slagel, *Tillotts* (letter), *Pharm. J.,* 1979, *2,* 557.

Preparations

Emulsions

Concentrated Peppermint Emulsion *(B.P.).* Peppermint oil 2 ml, polysorbate '20' 0.1 ml, double-strength chloroform water 50 ml, freshly boiled and cooled water to 100 ml. When diluted to 40 times its volume with freshly boiled and cooled water it yields a preparation equivalent in strength to Peppermint Water.

Concentrated Peppermint Emulsion *B.P.C. 1973* was prepared from peppermint oil 2 ml, quillaia liquid extract 0.1 ml, double-strength chloroform water 50 ml, freshly boiled and cooled water to 100 ml.

In studies on peppermint-flavoured mixtures of the *B.P.C.,* growth of a large *Pseudomonas* inoculum was halted in those mixtures flavoured with a 1 in 40 dilution of a peppermint emulsion containing 0.25% chloroform but not in preparations containing dilutions of Concentrated Peppermint Water.— J. McKenny, *J. Hosp. Pharm.,* 1972, *30,* 188.

Spirits

Peppermint Spirit *(B.P.).* Spiritus Menthae Piperitae; Sp. Menth. Pip.; Peppermint Essence; Essence of Peppermint. Peppermint oil 10 ml, alcohol (90%) to 100 ml. Clarify if necessary by shaking with sterilised talc and filtering.

A.P.F. uses alcohol (95%).

Peppermint Spirit *(U.S.P.).* Essence of Peppermint. Peppermint oil 10% v/v in alcohol in which 1% w/v of coarsely powdered peppermint leaves (previously macerated in water for 1 hour and then expressed) has been macerated for 6 hours. Store in airtight containers. Protect from light.

Waters and Solutions

Concentrated Peppermint Water *(B.P. 1973).* Conc. Peppermint Water; Peppermint Water Concentrated *(A.P.F.)*; Aq. Menth. Pip. Conc. Peppermint oil 2 ml, alcohol (90%) 60 ml, water to 100 ml; shaken with talc and filtered. It is 40 times as strong as peppermint water. *Dose.* 0.25 to 1 ml.

Diluendum Menthae *(Hung. P.).* Concentrated Peppermint Oil Solution. Peppermint oil 200 mg, polysorbate '20' 2 g, alcohol (95%) 20 g, water 77.8 g.

Mentha Water *(Jap. P.).* Mentha oil 0.2 ml, water to 100 ml.

Peppermint Water *(B.P. 1973).* Aq. Menth. Pip. Concentrated peppermint water 2.5 ml, freshly boiled and cooled water to 100 ml.

Peppermint Water *(U.S.N.F.).* A saturated solution of peppermint oil in water. Store in airtight containers.

Proprietary Preparations

Colpermin *(Tillotts, UK).* Peppermint oil, available as enteric-coated capsules of 0.2 ml.

4692-r

Pimento *(B.P.C. 1934).* Pimenta; Allspice; Jamaica Pepper.

The dried full-grown unripe fruits of *Pimenta officinalis* (Myrtaceae), containing 3 to 4.5% v/w of volatile oil.

4693-f

Pimento Oil *(B.P.C. 1949).* Ol. Piment.; Pimenta Oil; Allspice Oil.

CAS — 8006-77-7.

A yellow or yellowish-red oil, which darkens with age, with a characteristic odour and a spicy pungent taste, obtained by distillation from pimento. It contains not less than 60% v/v of eugenol. Wt per ml 1.03 to 1.045 g.
Miscible with alcohol (90%); soluble 1 in 3 of alcohol (70%). **Store** in a cool place in airtight containers. Protect from light.

Standard for pimento oils. British Standard Specifications for Oils of Pimento Fruit and Leaf (BS 2999/28/29: 1972) are published by the British Standards Institution.

Pimento oil has been used as a carminative and as a flavouring agent.

For the temporary estimated acceptable daily intake of eugenol, see p.676.

4694-d

Pimpinella. Pimpinella Root; Racine de Boucage; Bibernellwurzel.

Pharmacopoeias. In *Swiss.*

The dried rhizome and roots of the burnet saxifrage, *Pimpinella saxifraga*, and the greater burnet saxifrage, *P. major* (= *P. magna*) (Umbelliferae).

Pimpinella is an aromatic carminative.

4695-n

Pine Oil. Aromatic Pine Oil *(B.P.C. 1949).*

CAS — 8002-09-3.

A colourless to pale yellow oil with a characteristic pinaceous odour and a bitter taste, obtained by extraction and fractionation or by steam distillation from the wood of *Pinus palustris* and other species of *Pinus* (Pinaceae).
It consists mainly of tertiary and secondary terpene alcohols the main constituent being α-terpineol. Wt per ml about 0.94 g. **Miscible** with alcohol.

There is a British Standard Specification for light-duty aromatic disinfectant fluids of low mammalian toxicity containing substituted phenols (which include pine oil) (BS 5197: 1976). This does not apply to disinfectants for use in hospitals, or in other situations where there is a high risk from infectious disease.

Pine oil is extensively used in so-called pine disinfectants which are employed for general disinfecting and deodorising purposes.

A 31-year-old woman induced an abortion by instilling into her uterus about 75 to 150 ml of a 1 in 3 mixture of pine oil and soap (Hexol) in water. She developed acute renal failure within 24 hours, with vomiting and widely distributed pain. The uraemia slowly cleared, and an episode of acute pyelonephritis was successfully treated with cephalothin sodium. Anaemia, present when the patient was admitted to hospital, persisted for nearly 6 months, and a peripheral neuropathy which occurred 4 weeks after abortion gradually subsided. Renal biopsy about 6 weeks after admission to hospital indicated focal fibrosis and tubular atrophy.— D. L. Gornel and R. Goldman, *J. Am. med. Ass.*, 1968, *203*, 146.

Preparations

Pine Oil Inhalation *(Roy. Nat. T. N. and E. Hosp.).* Pine oil 8, light magnesium carbonate 5, water to 100.

4696-h

Pulegium Oil *(B.P.C. 1934).* Pennyroyal Oil.

CAS — 8007-44-1.

A yellow or greenish-yellow oil distilled from fresh pennyroyal herb, *Mentha pulegium* (Labiatae), containing not less than 85% of the ketone, pulegone ($C_{10}H_{16}O$). It has a strong aromatic mint-like odour and an aromatic taste. Wt per ml about 0.94 g.
Soluble 1 in 3 of alcohol (70%). **Store** in airtight containers. Protect from light.

Standard for pulegium oil. A British Standard Specification for Pulegium Oil (BS 2999/50: 1972) is published by the British Standards Institution.

Pulegium oil was formerly used as an emmenagogue. Severe toxic effects have followed its use as an abortifacient with convulsions and death.

It was recommended that pulegium oil be prohibited for use in foods as a flavouring agent.— *Food Standards Committee Report on Flavouring Agents,* London, HM Stationery Office, 1965.

4697-m

Pumilio Pine Oil *(B.P.).*

Oleum Pini Pumilionis; Pine Needle Oil *(U.S.N.F.)*; Dwarf Pine Needle Oil; Essence de Pin de Montagne; Latschenöl.

CAS — 8000-26-8.

Pharmacopoeias. In *Aust., Br., Cz., Hung., It., Roum.,* and *Swiss.* Also in *U.S.N.F.*

A colourless or faintly yellow oil with a pleasant aromatic odour and a bitter pungent taste, obtained by distillation from the fresh leaves of *Pinus mugo* var. *pumilio* (Pinaceae), a variety of mountain pine. The *B.P.* specifies that it contains 4 to 10% w/w of esters, calculated as bornyl acetate, $C_{12}H_{20}O_2$. The *U.S.N.F.* specifies 3 to 10% of esters. Wt per ml 0.858 to 0.87 g.
Soluble 1 in 10 of alcohol, with opalescence. **Store** at a temperature not exceeding 25° in well-filled airtight containers. Protect from light.

Uses. Pumilio pine oil is inhaled with steam, sometimes with the addition of menthol, eucalyptus oil, and Compound Benzoin Tincture to relieve cough and nasal congestion. It has been applied externally as a rubefacient in the treatment of sprains and fibrositis.

Proprietary Names
Macoel *(Mack, Reichenhall, Ger.).*

4698-b

Oleum Pini Sylvestris. Fir-wool Oil; Scotch Pine Needle Oil.

Pharmacopoeias. In *Hung.*

A colourless or yellowish oil with an aromatic turpentine-like odour distilled from the fresh leaves of the Scotch pine, *Pinus sylvestris*, containing 1.5 to 5% of esters, calculated as bornyl acetate. The oil now sold under this name is often a distillate from the leaves and twigs of various conifers.

4699-v

Rose Oil *(U.S.N.F., B.P.C. 1949).*

Oleum Rosae; Otto or Attar of Rose; Esencia de Rosa.

CAS — 8007-01-0.

Pharmacopoeias. In *Arg., Port., Span.,* and *Swiss.* Also in *U.S.N.F.*
Swiss allows the oil of *R. damascena* and *R. gallica; Arg.* allows the use of *R. damascena, R. centifolia,* and other species; *Span.* and *U.S.N.F.* allow the oil of *R. damascena, R. alba, R. centifolia, R. gallica,* and varieties of these species.

An oil obtained by distillation from the fresh flowers of the damask rose, *Rosa damascena* (Rosaceae) and other species. It is a pale yellow semi-solid crystalline mass at ordinary temperatures with a strong characteristic fragrant odour and a slightly sweet mild taste. The principal constituents are geraniol ($C_{10}H_{18}O$) and citronellol ($C_{10}H_{20}O$). Wt per ml, at 30°, 0.852 to 0.862 g. It yields turbid solutions with alcohol. **Store** in a cool place in airtight containers. Protect from light.

Uses. Rose oil is largely employed in perfumery and toilet preparations and has been used in lozenges, dentifrices, and ointments.

An estimated acceptable daily intake of up to 500 μg per kg body-weight was established for citral, geranyl acetate, citronellol, linalol, and linalyl acetate, expressed as citral.— Twenty-third Report of Joint FAO/WHO Expert Committee on Food Additives, *Tech. Rep. Ser. Wld Hlth Org. No. 648,* 1980 (See also p.670 for the absorption of these terpinoids).

Preparations

Concentrated Rose Water *(B.P.C. 1949).* Aq. Ros. Conc. Rose oil 1 ml, alcohol (90%) 50 ml, water to 100 ml; shaken with talc and filtered. It is about 40 times as strong as rose water. **Rose Water** may be prepared by diluting, immediately before use, 1 vol. of triple rose water with 2 vol. of water, 1 vol. of concentrated rose water with 39 vol. of water, or 1 vol. of stronger rose water with 1 vol. of water.

Rose Water Ointment *(B.P.C. 1949).* Cold Cream; Galen's Cerate. Rose water 20 ml, white beeswax 18 g, borax 1 g, almond oil 61 g, and rose oil 0.1 ml. Protect from light.

Rose Water Ointment *(U.S.P.).* Cetyl esters wax 12.5 g, white beeswax 12 g, almond oil 56 g, borax 500 mg, stronger rose water 2.5 ml, water 16.5 ml, and rose oil 0.02 ml (to make about 100 g). It must be free from rancidity. Store in airtight containers. Protect from light.

Stronger Rose Water *(U.S.N.F.).* A saturated solution of the odoriferous principles of the flowers of *R. centifolia,* prepared by distilling the fresh flowers with water and separating the excess volatile oil from the clear aqueous portion of the distillate. It should be stored in containers which allow a limited access of fresh air.
The *U.S.N.F.* states that Stronger Rose Water diluted with an equal volume of water may be supplied when Rose Water is required.

Triple Rose Water *(B.P.C. 1934).* The undiluted rose water of commerce, prepared by distillation from the fresh flowers of *R. damascena;* it is a saturated aqeuous solution of the volatile oil.

4700-v

Rosemary Oil *(B.P.C. 1973).*

Oleum Rosmarini; Oleum Roris Marini; Essence de Romarin; Rosmarinöl; Esencia de Romero; Essência de Alecrim.

CAS — 8000-25-7.

Pharmacopoeias. In *Arg., Aust., Belg., Cz., Ger., Mex., Port., Span.,* and *Swiss.*

An oil obtained by distillation from the flowering tops or leafy twigs of rosemary, *Rosmarinus officinalis* (Labiatae). It contains 2 to 5% of esters, notably bornyl acetate ($C_{12}H_{20}O_2$) and 10 to 18% of free alcohols including borneol ($C_{10}H_{18}O$) and linalol ($C_{10}H_{18}O$). It is a colourless or pale yellow oil with a characteristic odour and a warm bitter camphoraceous taste. Wt per ml 0.893 to 0.91 g.
Soluble 1 in 10 of alcohol (80%), with slight turbidity, and 1 in 1 of alcohol (90%) with not more than slight opalescence. **Store** in a cool place in well-filled airtight containers. Protect from light.

Standard for rosemary oil. A British Standard Specification for Rosemary Oil (BS 2999/40: 1971) is published by the British Standards Institution.

Uses. Rosemary oil is carminative and mildly irritant. It is chiefly used as Rosemary Spirit in hair lotions. It is an ingredient of Soap Liniment *B.P.C. 1973.*

An estimated acceptable daily intake of up to 500 µg per kg body-weight was established for citral, geranyl acetate, citronellol, linalol, and linalyl acetate, expressed as citral.— Twenty-third Report of Joint FAO/WHO Expert Committee on Food Additives, *Tech. Rep. Ser. Wld Hlth Org. No. 648*, 1980 (See also p.670 for the absorption of these terpinoids).

Preparations

Rosemary Spirit *(B.P.C. 1949)*. Sp. Rosmarin. Rosemary oil 10 ml, alcohol (90%) to 100 ml. *Dose.* 0.3 to 1.2 ml.

4701-g

Rue *(B.P.C. 1934)*. Ruta; Herb of Grace; Herbygrass; Rutae Herba.

The dried herb *Ruta graveolens* (Rutaceae), containing a small amount of volatile oil (about 0.1%).

4702-q

Rue Oil *(B.P.C. 1934)*. Oleum Rutae.

CAS — 8014-29-7.

A pale yellow oil with a characteristic sharp unpleasant odour and an acrid taste, obtained by distillation from rue. It contains about 90% of methyl nonyl ketone ($C_{11}H_{22}O$) with small amounts of other ketones, esters, and phenols. Wt per ml about 0.84 g. **Soluble** 1 in 3 of alcohol (70%); soluble in mineral oil and in most fixed oils.

Rue oil and infusions of rue were formerly used as antispasmodics and emmenagogues. Rue oil is a powerful local irritant.

Rue (Ruta grav.) is used in homoeopathic medicine.

It was recommended that rue oil be prohibited for use in foods as a flavouring agent.— *Food Standards Committee Report on Flavouring Agents*, London, HM Stationery Office, 1965.

Identification of rue oil ingredients.— D. H. E. Tattje *et al., Pharm. Weekbl. Ned.*, 1974, *109*, 881, per *Int. pharm. Abstr.*, 1978, *15*, 437.

4703-p

Safrole *(B.P.C. 1949)*. Safrol; Synthetic Sassafras Oil.
4-Allyl-1,2-methylenedioxybenzene.
$C_{10}H_{10}O_2$=162.2.

CAS — 94-59-7.

A colourless or yellowish oil with an odour of sassafras and a sharp taste. Wt per ml 1.096 to 1.1 g. M.p. not below 11°. F.p. not below 10°. **Soluble** 1 in 3 of alcohol (90%) and 1 in 10 of alcohol (80%); practically insoluble in water. **Store** in airtight containers.

Safrole has similar properties to sassafras oil; it is too toxic for internal use. It is the chief constituent of sassafras oil but it is mostly obtained from rectified camphor oil. It is provisionally allowed in cosmetic products in EEC countries in concentrations up to 0.01%.

It is recommended that safrole be prohibited for use in foods as a flavouring agent.— *Food Standards Committee Report on Flavouring Agents*, London, HM Stationery Office, 1965.

The absorption, metabolism, and excretion of safrole.— M. S. Benedetti *et al., Toxicology*, 1977, *7*, 69.

4704-s

Sage *(B.P.C. 1934)*. Salvia; Feuilles de Sauge; Salbeiblätter.

CAS — 8022-56-8 (sage oil).

Pharmacopoeias. In *Aust., Ger., Hung., Jug., Pol., Port., Roum., Rus.*, and *Swiss. Cz.* includes sage herb. *Ger.* also specifies *Salvia triloba*.

The dried leaves of the red or garden sage, *Salvia officinalis* (Labiatae), containing 1 to 2.5% of volatile oil. Protect from light. **Dalmatian Sage Oil** contains not less than 50% of ketones, calculated as thujone.

Spanish Sage Oil is obtained from *S. lavandulae* or *S. hispanorium* and has a different odour.

Standard for oil of spanish sage. A British Standard Specification (BS 2999/13: 1965) for Oil of Spanish Sage, from *S. lavandulae*, is published by the British Standards Institution.

Sage has carminative properties and is used as a flavouring agent for meat.

4705-w

Sandalwood Oil *(B.P.C. 1949)*. Oleum Santali; Oil of Santal Wood; East Indian Sandalwood Oil; Sandal Wood Oil.

CAS — 8006-87-9.

NOTE. West Indian Sandalwood Oil is obtained from *Amyris balsamifera* (Rutaceae).

Pharmacopoeias. In *Port.* and *Span.*

An oil obtained by distillation from the heartwood of *Santalum album* (Santalaceae).

It is a pale yellow or nearly colourless, viscid oil with a peculiar, faint, persistent odour and unpleasant, nauseous taste, containing not less than 2% w/w of esters and not less than 90% w/w of free alcohols. Wt per ml 0.968 to 0.983 g.

Soluble 1 in less than 1 of alcohol (90%), 1 in 5 of alcohol (70%), in chloroform and ether. **Store** in a cool place in airtight containers. Protect from light.

Standard for sandalwood oils. British Standard Specifications for East Indian Sandalwood Oil and Amyris Oil (BS 2999/30/52: 1972) are published by the British Standards Institution.

Sandalwood oil was formerly employed, often in conjunction with cubeb, as a urinary antiseptic. Oils of sandalwood are also used in perfumery.

Proprietary Names

Gelosantal *(Pohl, Ger.)*.

4706-e

Australian Sandalwood Oil *(B.P.C. 1949)*.

An oil obtained by distillation from *Eucarya spicata* (= *Santalum spicatum*) (Santalaceae).

It is a colourless or pale yellow oily liquid with a characterstic odour and unpleasant taste, containing not less than 90% w/w of free alcohols. Wt per ml 0.964 to 0.974 g.

Soluble 1 in 3 to 6 of alcohol (70%). **Store** in a cool place in airtight containers. Protect from light.

Standard for Australian sandalwood oil. A British Standard Specification for Australian Sandalwood Oil (BS 2999/31: 1972) is published by the British Standards Institution.

Australian sandalwood oil has been used for similar purposes to sandalwood oil.

4707-l

Sassafras *(B.P.C. 1949)*. Sassafras Bark.

The dried inner bark of the root of *Sassafras albidum* (= *S. officinale; S. variifolium*) (Lauraceae) containing not less than 3% v/w of volatile oil. **Store** in a cool dry place.

4708-y

Sassafras Oil *(B.P.C. 1954)*. Oleum Sassafras.

CAS — 8006-80-2.

Pharmacopoeias. In *Port.* and *Span.*

An oil distilled from the root or root bark of *Sassafras albidum* (Lauraceae) (American oil), or from the wood of certain species of *Ocotea* (Lauraceae) (Brazilian oil). It is a pale yellow, greenish-yellow, or reddish oil with a characteristic odour and an aromatic taste, containing 80 to 90% of safrole (American oil) or 85 to 95% of safrole (Brazilian oil). Wt per ml 1.064 to 1.078 g (American), 1.08 to 1.094 g (Brazilian).

Soluble 1 in 3 of alcohol (90%) (American) or 1 in 4 of alcohol (90%) (Brazilian). **Store** in a cool place in well-filled airtight containers. Protect from light.

Standard for sassafras oil. A British Standard Specification for Brazilian Sassafras Oil (BS 2999/41: 1971) is published by the British Standards Institution.

Neither sassafras nor the oil should be taken internally; the use of herb teas of sassafras may lead to a large dose of safrole. Large doses of sassafras oil cause fatty changes in the liver and kidneys. It has rubefacient properties. It has been used to destroy pediculi but more effective agents are available.

It was recommended that sassafras oil be prohibited for use in foods as a flavouring agent.— *Food Standards Committee Report on Flavouring Agents*, London, HM Stationery Office, 1965.

4709-j

Savin *(B.P.C. 1934)*. Sabina; Savin Tops; Sabinae Cacumina.

The fresh or dried young shoots of *Juniperus sabina* (Cupressaceae) containing 1 to 4% of volatile oil together with tannin and resin.

4710-q

Savin Oil *(B.P.C. 1934)*. Oleum Sabinae.

CAS — 8024-00-8.

A colourless or yellowish liquid with a characteristic odour and a bitter pungent camphoraceous taste. **Soluble** 1 in 2 of alcohol (90%).

Savin oil was formerly used as an emmenagogue but in addition to pelvic congestion it may cause haematuria and violent gastro-intestinal irritation. Serious and fatal cases of poisoning have resulted from its use as a supposed abortifacient. It is a violent irritant both externally and internally.

4711-p

Siberian Fir Oil *(B.P.C. 1949)*. Oleum Abietis; Fir Oil; Pine Oil *(B.P. 1932* and *B.P.C. 1949* synonym*)*; Siberian Fir Needle Oil.

CAS — 8002-09-3.

A colourless or pale yellow oil with an agreeable pinaceous odour and a pungent taste, obtained by distillation from the fresh leaves of *Abies sibirica* (Pinaceae). It contains 33 to 45% w/w of esters, calculated as bornyl acetate, $C_{12}H_{20}O_2$. Wt per ml 0.9 to 0.92 g.

Soluble 1 in 1 of alcohol (90%). **Store** in a cool place in airtight containers. Protect from light.

Siberian fir oil has similar properties to pumilio pine oil but the latter has a more pleasant odour. It is also used as a flavouring agent.

4712-s

Spearmint *(U.S.N.F.)*. Mentha Viridis; Mint.

Pharmacopoeias. In *Hung.* which specifies varieties of *M. spicata* and *M. aquatica*. Also in *U.S.N.F.* which specifies *M. spicata* (Common Spearmint) and *M. cardiaca* (Scotch Spearmint).

The dried leaves and flowering tops of spearmint, *Mentha spicata* (= *M. viridis*) or of *M. cardiaca* (Labiatae).

4713-w

Spearmint Oil *(B.P., U.S.N.F.)*. Oleum Menthae Viridis; Oleum Menthae Crispae.

CAS — 8008-79-5.

Pharmacopoeias. In *Br.* Also in *U.S.N.F.*

A colourless, pale yellow or greenish-yellow oil with the characteristic odour of spearmint and a warm and slightly bitter taste, obtained by distillation from fresh flowering spearmint, *Mentha spicata* (= *M. viridis*), or Scotch Spearmint, *M. cardiaca* or *M.* × *cardiaca* (= *M. arvensis* × *M. spicata*) (Labiatae). It becomes darker and viscous on keeping. It contains not less than 55% w/w of carvone ($C_{10}H_{14}O$). Wt per ml 0.917 to 0.934 g.

Soluble 1 in 1 of alcohol (80%); the solution may

become opalescent on the addition of more alcohol (80%). **Store** at a temperature not exceeding 25° in well-filled airtight containers. Protect from light.

Standard for spearmint oil. A British Standard Specification for Spearmint Oil (BS 2999/14: 1965) is published by the British Standards Institution.

Uses. Spearmint oil has similar properties to peppermint oil. It is used as a carminative and as a flavouring agent. *Dose:* 0.05 to 0.2 ml.

Temporary estimated acceptable daily intake of (+)-carvone and (−)-carvone: up to 1 mg per kg body-weight. Further biochemical and metabolic studies are required.— Twenty-third Report of Joint FAO/WHO Expert Committee on Food Additives, *Tech. Rep. Ser. Wld Hlth Org. No. 648,* 1980.

Preparations

Concentrated Spearmint Water *(B.P.C. 1959).* Aq. Menth. Vir. Conc. Spearmint oil 2 ml, alcohol (90%) 60 ml, water to 100 ml; shaken with talc and filtered. *Dose.* 0.3 to 1 ml.

Spearmint Water. Concentrated spearmint water 2.5 ml, freshly boiled and cooled water to 100 ml.

4714-e

Terebene *(B.P.C. 1959).* Terebenum.

CAS — 1335-76-8.

A mixture of dipentene [(±)-limonene] and other hydrocarbons obtained by shaking turpentine oil with sulphuric acid, added in successive small quantities, and distilling the separated product in a current of steam.

It is a colourless or very pale yellow liquid with an agreeable odour resembling fresh-sawn pine-wood, and a terebinthinate taste. Wt per ml 0.857 to 0.865 g.

Very slightly **soluble** in water; soluble 1 in 6 of alcohol (90%); miscible with dehydrated alcohol, chloroform, and ether. **Store** in a cool place in well-filled airtight containers. Protect from light.

Adverse Effects and Treatment. See under Essential Oils, p.670.

Uses. Terebene closely resembles turpentine oil in its properties but its odour is more agreeable. It is an aromatic ingredient of some pastilles.

About 0.4 ml may be added to 500 ml of hot water and the vapour inhaled to relieve nasal congestion and cough.

Preparations

Terebene Inhalation *(B.P.C. 1949).* Terebene 8.33 ml, light magnesium carbonate 6.8 g, water to 100 ml.

AMENDED FORMULA. Terebene 8.3 ml, light magnesium carbonate 6.8 g, water to 100 ml.—*Compendium of Past Formulae 1933 to 1966,* London, The National Pharmaceutical Union, 1969.

4715-l

Terpineol *(B.P., B.P. Vet.).*

$C_{10}H_{18}O$=154.3.

CAS — 8000-41-7; 98-55-5 (α); 2438-12-2 [(±)-α].

Pharmacopoeias. In *Arg.* and *Br.*

A mixture of isomers in which (±)-α-terpineol [*p*-menth-1-en-8-ol] largely predominates.

It is a colourless, slightly viscous, optically inactive liquid which may deposit crystals; it has a pleasant lilac-like odour and a bitter slightly pungent taste. Wt per ml 0.931 to 0.935 g.

Very slightly **soluble** in water; soluble 1 in 2 of alcohol (70%); soluble in chloroform, ether, and fixed oils; slightly soluble in glycerol.

Uses. Terpineol has disinfectant and solvent properties and is used in Chloroxylenol Solution (see p.559) and similar preparations. It is also used as a flavouring agent.

4716-y

Thyme *(B.P.C. 1949).* Thymi Herba; Rubbed Thyme; Common Thyme; Garden Thyme; Timo.

Pharmacopoeias. In *Arg., Aust., Cz., Ger., Hung., It., Neth., Nord., Pol.,* and *Roum. Jug.* and *Swiss* include the leaves only. *Ger.* also specifies *Thymus zygis.*

The dried leaves and flowering tops of the 'garden thyme', *Thymus vulgaris* (Labiatae), containing not less than 1% of volatile oil. It has an agreeable odour and an aromatic warming taste. **Store** in a cool place in airtight containers. Protect from light.

4717-j

Thyme Oil *(B.P.C. 1949).* Oleum Thymi; Ol. Thym.; Esencia de Tomillo; Essência de Tomilho.

CAS — 8007-46-3.

NOTE. In the *B.P.C. 1949,* Oil of Origanum was given as a synonym for Thyme Oil, but true oil of origanum is derived from *T. capitatus* and *Origanum* spp.; it may contain up to 75% of phenols..

Pharmacopoeias. In *Arg., Aust., Fr., Mex., Pol., Roum., Span.,* and *Swiss* (all from *T. vulgaris* only).

A yellow or dark reddish-brown liquid with a strong pleasant odour and a biting, persistent, cooling taste, obtained by distillation from the leaves and flowering tops of *Thymus vulgaris* and other species of *Thymus* and of species of *Origanum* (Labiatae). It contains not less than 40% v/v of phenols (thymol and carvacrol, $C_{10}H_{14}O$). Wt per ml 0.9 to 0.955 g. **Soluble** 1 in 2 of alcohol (80%). **Store** in a cool place in airtight containers. Protect from light.

Uses. Thyme has carminative properties due to its content of volatile oil. The liquid extract has been used as an ingredient of cough linctuses. It is used as a flavouring agent.

Thyme oil has antimicrobial, antispasmodic, and carminative properties. Externally, it has been employed in conjunction with olive and other oils as a rubefacient and counter-irritant.

A success-rate of 85% was achieved in 6 weeks in 17 children aged 3 to 18 with enuresis by the administration of a small wineglassful of distilled thyme tea at bedtime.— D. R. Somerset, *Practitioner,* 1972, *208,* 577.

Preparations

Thyme Liquid Extract *(B.P.C. 1949).* Ext. Thym. Liq. Thyme 100 g is exhausted by percolation first with a mixture of glycerol 10 ml, alcohol (90%) 25 ml, and water 65 ml, and then with a mixture of alcohol (90%) 1 vol. and water 3 vol.; the first 85 ml of percolate is reserved; the remainder of the percolate is evaporated to a soft extract, dissolved in the reserved portion, and diluted to 100 ml with the second menstruum. *Dose.* 0.6 to 4 ml. A similar preparation is included in some pharmacopoeias.

4718-z

Wild Thyme. Herba Serpylli; Mother of Thyme; Serpolet; Quendel.

Pharmacopoeias. In *Fr., Hung., Roum.,* and *Swiss.*

The dried leaves and flowering tops of *Thymus serpyllum* (Labiatae), containing up to 0.6% of volatile oil.

Wild thyme has similar properties to thyme.

4719-c

Turpentine. Terebinthina; Terebinthina Communis; Trementina de Burdeos.

NOTE. The name Turpentine is sometimes applied in commerce to unrectified turpentine oil.

Bordeaux Turpentine is a variety of turpentine obtained chiefly from the cluster pine, *Pinus pinaster* (= *P. maritima*) (Pinaceae), in SW France.

The oleoresin obtained as an exudate from various species of *Pinus* (Pinaceae). It occurs as yellowish-orange to yellow opaque masses with a characteristic odour and taste. **Soluble** in alcohol, chloroform, ether, and glacial acetic acid.

4720-s

Turpentine Oil *(B.P., B.P. Vet.).* Oleum Terebinthinae; Rectified Turpentine Oil; Spirits of Turpentine; Aetheroleum Terebinthinae; Oleum Terebinthinae Depuratum; Essence de Térébenthine; Esencia de Trementina.

CAS — 8006-64-2.

Pharmacopoeias. In *Arg., Aust., Belg., Br., Chin., Cz., Ger., Hung., Ind., Jap., Mex., Nord., Pol., Port., Roum., Rus., Span.,* and *Swiss* (as crude or rectified oil, or both).

The oil obtained by distillation and rectification from turpentine, an oleoresin obtained from various species of *Pinus* (Pinaceae). It consists principally of pinenes with smaller amounts of other terpenes.

It is a clear bright colourless liquid with a characteristic odour and a pungent, somewhat bitter taste, both of which become stronger and less pleasant on storage and on exposure to air. Wt per ml 0.855 to 0.868 g.

Soluble 1 in 7 of alcohol (90%) and 1 in 3 of alcohol (96%); miscible with dehydrated alcohol, carbon disulphide, chloroform, ether, glacial acetic acid, fixed oils, and light petroleum. **Incompatible** with oxidising agents. On exposure to air, it undergoes rapid change especially in the presence of moisture; it becomes viscous and yellow and acquires an acid reaction, the wt per ml increases, the b.p. rises, and the solubility in alcohol increases. **Store** at a temperature not exceeding 25° in well-filled airtight containers. Protect from light.

Adverse Effects and Treatment. See under Essential Oils, p.670.

In poisoning with turpentine oil there may be haematuria, albuminuria, and coma; the urine may have an odour of violets. A dose of 140 ml (15 ml in children) may be fatal.

The application to the skin of liniments containing turpentine oil may cause vesicular eruption, urticaria, and vomiting in susceptible persons.

Maximum permissible atmospheric concentration 100 ppm.

Severe chemical peritonitis and pulmonary oedema occurred in a woman following the self-administration of an intra-uterine injection of turpentine oil with the object of inducing abortion.— M. F. Quander and J. E. Mosely, *Obstet. Gynec.,* 1964, *24,* 572.

Symptoms of toxicity occurred among workers in a factory producing shoe-cream containing dyes and turpentine, and included giddiness, burning and reddening of the face and throat, burning and itching of the anus, painful defaecation, and painful and frequent micturition. Three workers had bladder ulcers, 2 had rectal inflammation, 1 had leucocytosis, and 1 had renal inflammation. The symptoms were considered due to inhalation and absorption through the skin of turpentine, together with the use of alpha-pinene in high concentration.— F. Nürnberger, *Zentbl. ArbMed. ArbSchutz,* 1967, *17,* 301, per *Abstr. Hyg.,* 1968, *43,* 895.

A 9-year-old boy who drank an indeterminate volume of turpentine and a 15-year-old boy whose home had had the floors cleaned with turpentine, developed profuse petechiae on the body-surface and in the mouth. The thrombocyte count was considerably lowered and the bleeding time prolonged. The bone marrow became normoblastic and there was abundant erythropoiesis. After prednisolone 15 mg daily the thrombocyte count and bleeding time became normal within 10 days, and the bone-marrow changes subsided within 14 days.— P. Wahlberg and D. Nyman (letter), *Lancet,* 1969, *2,* 215.

Of 1205 persons with dermatitis or eczema submitted to patch testing with turpentine 10% in arachis oil, 4.3% gave a positive reaction.— E. Rudzki and D. Kleniewska, *Br. J. Derm.,* 1970, *83,* 543. Of 4000 patients subjected to patch testing in 5 European clinics 5.2% of males and 6.4% of females showed positive reactions to turpentine oil.— H. Bandmann *et al., Archs Derm.,* 1972, *106,* 335.

A study of pulmonary function abnormalities in children

following hydrocarbon pneumonitis due to ingestion and aspiration of turpentine.— D. Gurwitz *et al.*, *Pediatrics*, 1978, *62*, 789, per *Int. pharm. Abstr.*, 1979, *16*, 456.

Uses. Turpentine oil has the therapeutic action characteristic of many of the essential oils (see p.670), but it is rarely given internally. It is excreted by the kidneys, lungs, and skin. Externally, turpentine oil is a rubefacient and is employed in liniments for rheumatic pains and stiffness. Turpentine has also been employed as a rubefacient, but the oil is preferred.

Myiasis in 14 patients caused by maggots in the ear was treated by turpentine oil, given as ear-drops, and douching. The parasite was removed in 6 patients; pain and severe inflammation occurred in 3 patients. Ether ear-drops were effective in the remaining 8 patients and caused no pain.— R. Sharan and D. K. Isser, *J. Lar. Otol.*, 1978, *92*, 705.

Preparations

Dutch Drops. Haarlem Drops. A limpid brownish-red liquid containing turpentine oil 15, sulphur 1, and linseed oil 4, by wt. It has been given in doses of 0.3 to 2 ml for lumbago and rheumatism.

The liquid has been prepared in Denmark and Holland as follows: heat, in an iron vessel large enough to allow frothing, 4 parts linseed oil and 1 part sulphur to 165° stirring until mixture drops off stirrer with a glossy appearance. Remove from heat. Add 15 parts (by wt) turpentine oil, agitate until solution is complete or nearly so, and filter.

Turpentine Liniment *(B.P.)*. Turpent. Lin.; Lin. Terebinth. Turpentine oil 65 ml, camphor 5 g, soft soap 7.5 g, and freshly boiled and cooled water 22.5 ml.

An improved method of manufacture.—L.S.C. Wan (letter), *Pharm. J.*, 1976, *1*, 206. Confirmation.—B. Jones (letter), *ibid.*, 371.

White Liniment *(B.P.)*. Linimentum Album; Lin. Alb.; White Embrocation; Linimentum Commune. Turpentine oil 25 ml, oleic acid 8.5 ml, dilute ammonia solution 4.5 ml, ammonium chloride 1.25 g, and water 62.5 ml.

4721-w

Venice Turpentine.

Terebinthina Laricina; Larch Turpentine; Térébenthine de Venise; Terebintina de Veneza; Trementina de Alerce; Trementina de Venecia.

CAS — 8007-41-8.

Pharmacopoeias. In *Port.*, *Span.*, and *Swiss.*

The oleoresin from the larch, *Larix decidua* (=*L. europaea*) (Pinaceae). Commercial Venice turpentine is usually a factitious substance made from colophony, linseed oil, and turpentine oil.

A viscous amber-coloured fluid with a characteristic agreeable odour and a pungent bitter taste. It contains about 15 to 20% of volatile oil. When a thin layer is exposed to air it very slowly hardens; when mixed with magnesium oxide it does not solidify. Alcoholic solutions are slightly acid to litmus.

Soluble 1 in 5 of alcohol; soluble in acetone, chloroform, ether, ethyl acetate, glacial acetic acid, and toluene; miscible with fixed and volatile oils; partly soluble in petroleum spirit and carbon disulphide. **Protect** from light.

Venice turpentine has been used as an ingredient of ointments and plasters.

4722-e

Zedoary

Pharmacopoeias. In *Jap. Chin.* also allows *Curcuma aromatica* and *C. kwangsiensis.*

The rhizome of *Curcuma zedoaria* (Zingiberaceae), resembling ginger in odour and taste.

Zedoary has been used as an aromatic stimulant and carminative.

Expectorants

2000-q

Small doses of drugs such as ipecacuanha and squill, ammonium salts, some volatile oils, and potassium iodide have been administered in the belief that they act reflexly, irritating the gastric mucosa and so stimulating respiratory-tract secretions, but there is little evidence to show that expectorants are effective.

Clearance of sputum may be aided by humidifying the respiratory tract with hot drinks or by inhalation of water or sodium chloride aerosols. The inhalation of a surfactant such as Tyloxapol (p.374) may be of assistance. Bromhexine and other mucolytic agents such as Acetylcysteine (p.644), Chymotrypsin (p.648), and Trypsin (p.659) are reported to aid the removal of sputum by altering its structure.

2001-p

Adhatoda *(B.P.C. 1949).* Arusha; Vasaka.

CAS — 6159-55-3 (vasicine).

Pharmacopoeias. In *Ind.*

The fresh or dried leaves of *Adhatoda vasica* (Acanthaceae). Adhatoda contains a bitter crystalline alkaloid, vasicine (peganine), and adhatodic acid.

Adhatoda has been given as an expectorant in doses of 1 to 2 g. Large doses are irritant and cause vomiting and diarrhoea.

Preparations

Vasaka Liquid Extract *(Ind. P.).* Adhatoda Liquid Extract. 1 in 1; prepared by percolation with alcohol (40%). *Dose.* 1 to 2 ml.

Vasaka Syrup *(Ind. P.).* Adhatoda Syrup. Vasaka liquid extract 50 ml, glycerol 10 ml, syrup to 100 ml. *Dose.* 2 to 4 ml.

2002-s

Ambroxol. NA 872. *trans*-4-(2-Amino-3,5-dibromobenzylamino)cyclohexanol.
$C_{13}H_{18}Br_2N_2O$=378.1.

CAS — 18683-91-5.

Ambroxol is a metabolite of bromhexine (see p.687) and has similar actions and uses. It has been given in doses of 45 to 60 mg daily by mouth as the hydrochloride. The hydrochloride has also been administered by inhalation and injection.

Pharmacology in animals.— P. C. Curti, *Arzneimittel-Forsch.*, 1974, *24*, 847; J. Iravani and G. N. Melville, *ibid.*, 849; S. Püschmann and R. Engelhorn, *ibid.*, 1978, *28*, 889.

In 5 healthy subjects given approximately 250 µg per kg body-weight of radio-labelled ambroxol a mean peak blood concentration equivalent to about 140 ng of ambroxol per ml occurred 1 hour after administration with an elimination half-life of about 22 hours. About 80% and 8% respectively of the radioactivity was subsequently found in the urine and faeces.— R. Hammer *et al.*, *Arzneimittel-Forsch.*, 1978, *28*, 899.

Metabolism of ambroxol in 8 healthy subjects was similar when given by mouth or intravenously. The two major metabolites were identified as 6,8-dibromo-3-(*trans*-4-hydroxycyclohexyl)-1,2,3,4,-tetrahydroquinazoline and 3,5-dibromoanthranilic acid. Ambroxol and its metabolites were also converted to conjugates, mainly glucuronides.— R. Jauch *et al.*, *Arzneimittel-Forsch.*, 1978, *28*, 904.

Bronchitis. In a 4-week double-blind study in 30 patients with chronic obstructive bronchitis, ambroxol 45 mg daily was more effective than bromhexine 36 mg daily.— K. J. Wiessmann and K. Niemeyer, *Arzneimittel-Forsch.*, 1978, *28*, 918.

In an open study involving 52 patients with acute bronchitis and 46 with chronic bronchitis, ambroxol 45 to 90 mg daily by mouth produced a marked reduction in coughing and dyspnoea as well as an improvement in expectoration. No side-effects were observed.— P. Göbel and H. Rensch, *Arzneimittel-Forsch.*, 1978, *28*, 929.

Similar results in 165 patients with respiratory disorders receiving ambroxol 15 mg daily by inhalation.— H. Hoffmann, *ibid.*, 931.

Studies involving 40 patients indicated that ambroxol may be useful in the therapy of postoperative bronchitis. The recommended daily dose was 30 mg intravenously for 5 to 7 days with 15 mg once or twice daily by inhalation.— R. Kranicke, *Arzneimittel-Forsch.*, 1978, *28*, 934.

Silicosis. Ambroxol was considered to be more effective in patients with silicosis than in patients with chronic obstructive bronchitis. It was suggested that the twofold action of ambroxol as a secretolytic and surfactant stimulant would account for the increased activity in the silicosis patients.— P. C. Curti and H. D. Renovanz, *Arzneimittel-Forsch.*, 1978, *28*, 922.

Proprietary Names

Mucosolvan *(hydrochloride) (Thomae, Ger.).*

2003-w

Strong Ammonium Acetate Solution.

(B.P.). Ammonium Acetate Solution Strong; Liq. Ammon. Acet. Fort.

CAS — 631-61-8 (ammonium acetate); 8013-61-4 (ammonium acetate solution).

Pharmacopoeias. In *Br.* and *Ind.*

Solutions of ammonium acetate are included in *Arg.P.* (14.5 to 15.5% w/v), *Belg.P.* (15 to 15.5% w/w), *Mex.P.* 19.5 to 22.5% w/v), *Roum.P.* (15.5% w/w), and *Span.P.* (20% w/w).

A thin syrupy liquid with an odour of ammonia and acetic acid. It is prepared by neutralising glacial acetic acid with ammonium bicarbonate and a sufficient quantity of Strong Ammonia Solution, and diluting the product with freshly boiled and cooled water. It contains 55 to 60% w/v of ammonium acetate ($CH_3CO_2NH_4$ = 77.08) and a 10% solution in water has a pH of 7 to 8. Wt per ml 1.085 to 1.095 g. **Store** in bottles of lead-free glass.

NOTE. The *B.P.* and *A.P.F.* direct that when Ammonium Acetate Solution or Dilute Ammonium Acetate Solution is prescribed or demanded, Strong Ammonium Acetate Solution diluted to 8 times its volume with freshly boiled and cooled water be supplied.

Adverse Effects. Large doses of ammonium salts irritate the gastric mucosa and may produce nausea and vomiting. Toxic effects of the ammonium ion arising from infusion of ammonium acetate are similar to those of terminal liver failure. However, ingestion is unlikely to produce these effects.

Absorption and Fate. Ammonium acetate is reported to be completely metabolised, producing urea and free acetate.

Uses. Ammonium acetate has a mild expectorant, diaphoretic, and diuretic action. It is given as the strong solution in doses of 1 to 5 ml or as the dilute solution in doses of 8 to 30 ml.

Preparations

Dilute Ammonium Acetate Solution *(B.P. 1953).* Liq. Ammon. Acet. Dil.; Spirit of Mindererus. Strong ammonium acetate solution 1, water to 8, by vol. Store in bottles of lead-free glass. *Dose.* 8 to 30 ml.

Saline Mixture *(B.P.C. 1968).* Mist. Salin.; Diaphoretic Mixture. Sodium citrate 500 mg, sodium nitrite 30 mg, strong ammonium acetate solution 0.5 ml, concentrated camphor water 0.25 ml, water to 10 ml. It must be freshly prepared. *Dose.* 10 to 20 ml.

2004-e

Ammonium Bicarbonate

(B.P.). Ammon. Bicarb.
NH_4HCO_3=79.06.

CAS — 1066-33-7.

Pharmacopoeias. In *Br.* and *Ind.*

A fine, white, slightly hygroscopic, crystalline powder, white crystals, or glassy colourless solid, with a slightly ammoniacal odour and a pungent taste. It volatilises rapidly at 60° with dissociation into ammonia, carbon dioxide, and water; volatilisation takes place slowly at ordinary temperatures if slightly moist.

Soluble 1 in 5 of water; practically insoluble in alcohol. **Incompatible** with acids, iron salts, and salts of alkaline earths. **Store** in a cool place in airtight containers.

NOTE. The *B.P.* directs that when Ammonium Carbonate is prescribed or demanded Ammonium Bicarbonate be supplied.

Adverse Effects. Large doses of ammonium bicarbonate can produce nausea and vomiting.

Uses. Ammonium bicarbonate is irritant to mucous membranes and is used in doses of 200 to 600 mg as a reflex expectorant. It also has a carminative action.

Preparations

Ammonia and Ipecacuanha Mixture *(B.P.).* Mist. Ammon. et Ipecac.; Mistura Expectorans; Mist. Expect. Ammonium bicarbonate 200 mg, liquorice liquid extract 0.5 ml, ipecacuanha tincture 0.3 ml, concentrated camphor water 0.1 ml, concentrated anise water 0.05 ml, double-strength chloroform water 5 ml, water to 10 ml. The mixture should be recently prepared. *Dose.* 10 ml.

Senega and Ammonia Mixture *(A.P.F.).* Mist. Seneg. et Ammon. Ammonium bicarbonate 250 mg, compound camphor spirit 1 ml, liquorice liquid extract 0.5 ml, concentrated senega infusion 0.5 ml, concentrated chloroform water 0.25 ml, water to 10 ml. *Dose.* 10 to 20 ml.

2005-l

Ammonium Carbonate *(U.S.N.F.).* Ammon. Carb.; Carbonato de Amonio.

CAS — 8000-73-5.

Pharmacopoeias. In *Arg.*, *Fr.*, *It.*, *Mex.*, *Port.*, and *Span.* Also in *U.S.N.F.*

A white powder or hard white or translucent masses with an ammoniacal odour and a sharp ammoniacal taste, consisting of a variable mixture of ammonium bicarbonate and ammonium carbamate, $NH_2.CO_2.NH_4$. It yields 30 to 34% of NH_3. On exposure to air it loses ammonia and carbon dioxide. Slowly **soluble** 1 in 4 of water, and 1 in 5 of glycerol; partly soluble in alcohol. It is decomposed by hot water. A solution in water is alkaline to litmus. **Store** at a temperature not exceeding 30° in airtight containers. Protect from light.

NOTE. The *B.P.* directs that Ammonium Bicarbonate be supplied when Ammonium Carbonate is prescribed or demanded.

Ammonium carbonate has been used as an expectorant in doses of 300 to 600 mg.

2006-y

Ammonium Chloride

(B.P., Eur. P., U.S.P.). Ammon. Chlor.; Ammonii Chloridum; Ammonium Chloratum; Muriate of Ammonia; Sal Ammoniac; Cloruro de Amonio.
NH_4Cl=53.49.

CAS — 12125-02-9.

Pharmacopoeias. In all pharmacopoeias examined except *Cz.*, *Jap.*, *Int.*, *Rus.*, and *Turk.*

Odourless, somewhat hygroscopic, white crystalline powder or colourless crystals with a cooling saline taste. Each g represents 18.69 mmol (18.69 mEq) of chloride.

Soluble 1 in 2.7 of water, 1 in 1.4 of boiling water, 1 in 100 of alcohol, and 1 in 8 of glycerol. A 5% solution in water has a pH of 4.6 to 6. A 0.8% solution is iso-osmotic with serum. Solutions are **sterilised** by autoclaving or by filtration.

Incompatible with alkalis, carbonates of alkaline earths, and lead and silver salts. **Store** in airtight containers.

An aqueous solution of ammonium chloride iso-osmotic with serum (0.8%) caused 93% haemolysis of red blood cells cultured in it for 45 minutes. Sodium chloride 0.65% or dextrose 4% prevented haemolysis when added to ammonium chloride 0.8% solution. Haemolysis was only about 20% in ammonium chloride solution 4%, and the degree of haemolysis increased with concentrations up to 7%.— E. R. Hammarlund and K. Pedersen-Bjergaard, *J. pharm. Sci.*, 1961, *50*, 24.

Incompatibility. Ammonium chloride was incompatible with chlortetracycline hydrochloride, nitrofurantoin sodium, novobiocin sodium, sulphadiazine sodium, and warfarin sodium. There was loss of clarity when intravenous solutions of ammonium chloride were mixed with dimenhydrinate, narcotic analgesics, or sulphafurazole diethanolamine.— J. A. Patel and G. L. Phillips, *Am. J. Hosp. Pharm.*, 1966, *23*, 409.

Adverse Effects. Large doses of ammonium chloride may cause nausea, vomiting, thirst, headache, hyperventilation, and progressive drowsiness, and lead to profound acidosis and hypokalaemia.

Maximum permissible atmospheric concentration of ammonium chloride fumes, 10 mg per m^3.

Treatment of Adverse Effects. Acidosis and electrolyte loss may be corrected by the intravenous administration of sodium bicarbonate or sodium lactate and hypokalaemia treated by the administration of a suitable potassium salt by mouth.

Precautions. Ammonium chloride is contra-indicated in the presence of impaired hepatic or renal function.

Ammonium chloride and other drugs producing acidosis might cause anoxia and acidosis in patients with sickle-cell anaemia, with resulting haemolysis or thrombosis.— T. M. French, *J. Hosp. Pharm.*, 1970, *28*, 19.

Absorption and Fate. Ammonium chloride is effectively absorbed from the gastro-intestinal tract. The ammonium ion is converted into urea in the liver; the anion thus liberated into the blood stream and extracellular fluid causes a metabolic acidosis and decreases the pH of the urine; this is followed by transient diuresis.

Absorption. In healthy persons, absorption of ammonium chloride given by mouth was practically complete. Only 1 to 3% of the dose was recovered in the faeces.— P. Richards *et al.*, *Lancet*, 1967, *2*, 845.

Uses. A mild acidosis is produced by the administration of ammonium chloride by mouth in a dose of 2 g, and this is used in the treatment of urinary-tract infections when a low urinary pH is required, and to aid the excretion of basic drugs, such as amphetamine in cases of overdosage. Ammonium chloride has been given to increase the diuretic effect of mercurial diuretics (see Mersalyl Acid, p.607). It has also been used to hasten the elimination of lead in the treatment of lead poisoning but more effective treatments are now available.

It is given by mouth or injection to replace chloride lost during vomiting or severe sweating. The usual dose by intravenous infusion is up to 500 ml of a 2% solution over 3 hours.

Ammonium chloride, in doses of 300 mg to 1 g, is used as an ingredient of expectorant cough mixtures but it is doubtful whether its irritant action on the gastric mucous membrane contributes to any expectorant action.

Large doses of ammonium chloride should be given in enteric-coated tablets. Liquorice liquid extract is commonly used to disguise its taste in liquid medicines.

Ammonium chloride, 6 g per m^2 body-surface daily in 4 divided doses for 3 days, produced significantly smaller falls in urinary pH in rachitic infants than in non-rachitic infants. Vitamin D given to the infants with rickets corrected the abnormality.— C. F. Whitten, *J. Pediat.*, 1966, *69*, 80.

Preparations

Injections

Ammonium Chloride Injection *(U.S.P.).* A sterile solution of ammonium chloride in Water for Injections. Hydrochloric acid may be added to adjust the pH (of a 10% solution) to 4 to 6.

Mixtures

Ammonium Chloride and Morphine Mixture *(B.P.).* Mist. Ammon. Chlorid. Co.; Mist. Ammon. Chlor. Sed.; Mistura Tussi Sedativa. Ammonium chloride 300 mg, ammonium bicarbonate 200 mg, chloroform and morphine tincture 0.3 ml, liquorice liquid extract 0.5 ml, water to 10 ml. It should be recently prepared. Contains about 500 µg of anhydrous morphine in 10 ml. *Dose.* 10 ml.

Ammonium Chloride Mixture *(A.P.F.).* Mist. Ammon. Chlorid.; Expectorant Mixture; Mist. Expect. Ammonium chloride 1 g; ipecacuanha tincture 0.25 ml, aromatic ammonia spirit 0.5 ml, liquorice liquid extract 0.5 ml, concentrated chloroform water 0.25 ml, water to 10 ml. *Dose.* 10 to 20 ml.

Ammonium Chloride Mixture *(B.P.).* Mist. Ammon. Chlor. Ammonium chloride 1 g, aromatic ammonia solution 0.5 ml, liquorice liquid extract 1 ml, water to 10 ml. It should be recently prepared. *Dose.* 10 ml.

Tablets

Ammonium Chloride Tablets *(B.P.C. 1973).* Tablets containing ammonium chloride. They may be enteric-coated and the coating may be coloured.

Ammonium Chloride Tablets *(U.S.P.).* Enteric-coated tablets containing ammonium chloride. Store in airtight containers.

Proprietary Names

Chlorammonic *(Promedica, Fr.)*; Expigen *(Pharmacia, Denm.)*; Gen-Diur *(Leo, Spain)*.

Ammonium chloride was formerly marketed in Great Britain under the proprietary name Nuseals Ammonium Chloride (*Lilly*).

2007-j

Angelica. Angelicae Radix; Archangelica.

Pharmacopoeias. In *Aust.*, *Fr.*, and *Port. Jap.* specifies *Angelica acutiloba* and *Angelica dahurica.Chin.* specifies *Angelica dahurica*, *Angelica dahurica* var. *taiwaniana*, *Angelica pubescens*, and *Angelica sinensis*.

The dried rhizome and roots of *Angelica archangelica* (Umbelliferae). The fruits (Angelicae Fructus) have also been used. The rhizome and roots contain about 0.3 to 1% and the fruits about 1% of volatile oil.

Angelica has diaphoretic and expectorant properties; it was administered as a powder in doses of 0.6 to 2 g, or as an infusion (1 in 20).

2008-z

Bromhexine Hydrochloride *(B.P.).* NA 274.

2-Amino-3,5-dibromo-*N*-cyclohexyl-*N*-methylbenzylamine hydrochloride.

$C_{14}H_{20}Br_2N_2,HCl=412.6$.

CAS — 3572-43-8 (bromhexine); 611-75-6 (hydrochloride).

Pharmacopoeias. In *Br.* and *Chin.*

A synthetic derivative of vasicine, the active principle of *Adhatoda vasica* (see p.686). A white or almost white, odourless or almost odourless, crystalline powder. M.p. about 237°. Practically **insoluble** in water and acetone; soluble 1 in 100 of alcohol, 1 in 300 of chloroform, and 1 in 50 of methyl alcohol. **Protect** from light.

Adverse Effects. Gastro-intestinal side-effects may occur occasionally and a transient rise in serum aminotransferase values has been reported.

Precautions. Bromhexine should be given cautiously to patients with gastric ulceration.

Absorption and Fate. Bromhexine hydrochloride is absorbed from the gastro-intestinal tract and peak plasma concentrations have occurred after 1 hour. Most of a dose is excreted in the urine mainly as metabolites; only a small amount is excreted in the faeces. Ambroxol (p.686) is a metabolite of bromhexine.

References: Z. Kopitar *et al.*, *Eur. J. Pharmac.*, 1973, *21*, 6; R. Jauch *et al.*, *Arzneimittel-Forsch.*, 1975, *25*, 1954.

Uses. Bromhexine hydrochloride has been reported to change the structure of bronchial secretions and to increase the volume and reduce the viscosity of sputum.

It is administered in bronchitis and other respiratory conditions as an aid to expectoration, with variable results. The usual adult dose is 8 to 16 mg three or four times daily. Suggested dosage for children under 5 years is 4 mg twice daily, and for children aged 5 to 10 years, 4 mg four times daily.

It is also given by deep intramuscular or slow intravenous injection in doses of 8 to 24 mg daily; up to 20 mg in 500 ml of dextrose injection or up to 40 mg in 500 ml of sodium chloride injection, may be given by slow intravenous infusion.

When bromhexine was given in a dose of 8 mg thrice daily to 5 subjects, the viscosity of uninfected bronchial mucus was reduced, usually within 5 days, and the microscopical appearance of the acid mucopolysaccharide of the mucus changed from unbroken thick continuous fibres to complete fragmentation within 10 days. When treatment ceased the viscosity rose and there was a tendency to the re-establishment of a complete fibre system.— R. A. Bruce and V. Kumar, *Br. J. clin. Pract.*, 1968, *22*, 289.

Effects on the eye. Oral mucolytic agents such as bromhexine did not control the symptoms or signs of excess conjunctival mucus in patients with keratoconjunctivitis sicca.— P. Wright, *Trans. ophthal. Soc. U.K.*, 1971, *91*, 119.

Improvement in tear secretion occurred in 65 of 81 patients with keratoconjunctivitis sicca given bromhexine 0.2% eye-drops. Symptoms returned when the drops were discontinued but improvement recurred when the drops were reinstated.— H. Rossmann, *Dt. med. Wschr.*, 1974, *99*, 408.

A study involving 29 patients suggested that bromhexine 16 mg thrice daily was of value in relieving dry eye associated with Sjögren's syndrome; there was no effect on salivary-gland function.— K. Frost-Larsen *et al.*, *Br. med. J.*, 1978, *1*, 1579. Comment. Only 3 of the 29 satisfied the definition of Sjögren's syndrome.— I. Mackie and D. V. Seal (letter), *ibid.*, *2*, 638. A study involving 14 patients with Sjögren's syndrome, including 5 with sicca syndrome, and 11 healthy subjects indicated that bromhexine 16 mg four times daily for 2 weeks was no more effective than a placebo in this syndrome.— L. M. Tapper-Jones *et al.*, *ibid.*, 1980, *280*, 1356. Criticism.— R. Manthorpe *et al.* (letter), *ibid.*, *281*, 1216. Reply.— L. M. Tapper-Jones *et al.*, *ibid.*

Further references: R. L. Blandford *et al.*, *Br. med. J.*, 1979, *1*, 1323.

Otitis media. Bromhexine hydrochloride 8 mg twice daily was ineffective in the treatment of chronic secretory otitis media in 79 children.— H. W. Elcock and I. J. Lord, *Br. J. clin. Pract.*, 1972, *26*, 276.

Respiratory disease. In a double-blind multicentre study in 42 patients with chronic bronchitis and non-purulent sputum treated for four 3-week periods with bromhexine 16 mg thrice daily or a placebo and assessed subjectively and by evaluation of their clinical status, there was a trend in favour of bromhexine in some parameters but not of statistical significance. Bromhexine could not be recommended for the routine treatment of bronchitis.—A report to the Research Committee of the British Thoracic and Tuberculosis Association, *Br. J. Dis. Chest*, 1973, *67*, 49. For similar reports in patients with chronic bronchitis or other respiratory disease, see M. Gent *et al.*, *Lancet*, 1969, *2*, 1094; J. H. M. Langlands, *ibid.*, 1970, *1*, 448.

Bromhexine hydrochloride was effective in the treatment of 11 patients with sinusitis in an uncontrolled trial.— D. R. Oliver (letter), *Med. J. Aust.*, 1974, *2*, 794.

Bromhexine was no better than placebo in preventing

postoperative bronchopneumonia following upper abdominal surgery in a study of 70 patients. However, patients considered to be at high risk gained some protection from bromhexine.— S. A. Hargrave *et al.*, *Br. J. Dis. Chest*, 1975, *69*, 195.

In a 10-week double-blind crossover trial completed by 10 patients with chronic bronchitis, treatment with bromhexine 72 mg daily resulted in significantly increased sputum volume, a significantly Higher peak expiratory flow-rate, and an improvement in auscultatory findings, compared with placebo. Side-effects were headache and nausea in 1 (withdrew from trial) and dizziness and dry mouth in 1 who reduced dosage to 8 mg thrice daily.— M. L. Armstrong, *Med. J. Aust.*, 1976, *1*, 612. See also W. F. D. Hamilton *et al.*, *Br. med. J.*, 1970, *3*, 260.

Use with oxytetracycline. The average mean daily content of tetracycline in the sputum of 10 patients treated for acute exacerbations of chronic bronchitis with oxytetracycline and 24 mg of bromhexine was greater than in 10 patients treated only with oxytetracycline in the same dosage.— H. Burgi *et al.* (letter), *Lancet*, 1968, *2*, 406.

Further references to bromhexine increasing oxytetracycline concentrations in sputum and in nasal mucus: T. D. Brogan *et al.*, *Br. J. clin. Pract.*, 1972, *26*, 555; J. Offermeier *et al.*, *S. Afr. med. J.*, 1972, *46*, 1509; P. H. Bach and W. P. Leary, *ibid.*, 1512.

Preparations

Bromhexine Hydrochloride Tablets *(B.P.)*. Bromhexine Hydrochlor. Tab. Tablets containing bromhexine hydrochloride.

Bisolvomycin *(Boehringer Ingelheim, UK)*. Capsules each containing bromhexine hydrochloride 8 mg and oxytetracycline hydrochloride 250 mg. For respiratory infections associated with viscous sputum. *Dose.* 1 capsule 4 times daily.

Bisolvon *(Boehringer Ingelheim, UK)*. Bromhexine hydrochloride, available as 2-ml **Ampoules** of an injection containing 2 mg per ml; as **Elixir** containing 4 mg in each 5 ml, with chloroform 17.5 mg (suggested diluent, water or Sorbitol Solution); and as **Tablets** of 8 mg.(Also available in *Austral., Belg., Denm., Ger., Ital., Jap., Lux., Neth., Norw., S.Afr., Spain, Swed., Switz.*).

Other Proprietary Names

Aletor *(Spain)*; Bromcilate (bromhexine camsylate) *(Spain)*; Broncokin *(Ital.)*; Dakroy Biciron, Ophtosol (both *Ger.*).

2009-c

Cocillana *(B.P.)*. Grape Bark; Guapi Bark; Huapi Bark.

CAS — 1398-77-2.

Pharmacopoeias. In *Br.* which also describes Powdered Cocillana.

The dried bark of *Guarea rusbyi* and closely related species (Meliaceae) containing not less than 3.5% of alcohol (60%)-soluble extractive.

Uses. Cocillana is used as an expectorant and, in large doses, as an emetic. It has been used as an alternative to ipecacuanha in the treatment of coughs. It is administered as the liquid extract, usually in conjunction with other expectorants.

Preparations

Cocillana Liquid Extract *(B.P.C. 1973)*. 1 in 1; prepared by percolation with alcohol (60%). *Dose.* 0.5 to 1 ml.

2010-s

Creosote *(B.P.C. 1959)*. Creasote; Wood Creosote; Kreosotum.

CAS — 8021-39-4.

Pharmacopoeias. In *Belg., Ind., It., Jap., Pol., Port., Span.*, and *Swiss.*

A colourless or pale yellow highly refractive liquid with a penetrating smoky odour and burning taste, consisting of a mixture of guaiacol, creosol, and other phenols obtained by fractional distillation from wood tar. B.p. 200° to 225°. Wt per ml 1.08 to 1.10 g. **Soluble** 1 in 150 of water; miscible with most organic solvents. It is neutral or slightly acid to litmus. **Incompatible** with strong oxidising agents and ferric and silver salts. **Store** in airtight containers. Protect from light.

Commercial creosote used for timber preservation is obtained by distillation from coal tar.

Adverse Effects, Treatment, and Precautions. As for Phenol, p.571.

Creosote could cause dark green discoloration of the urine.— R. B. Baran and B. Rowles, *J. Am. pharm. Ass.*, 1973, *NS13*, 139.

Absorption and Fate. Creosote is absorbed from the gastro-intestinal tract and conjugates, with glucuronic and sulphuric acids, appear in the urine. When administered by mouth it is not excreted by the lungs.

Uses. Creosote possesses disinfectant and expectorant properties and has been used in bronchitis and bronchiectasis. It has been given in doses of 0.12 to 0.6 ml. Because of its local analgesic effect it was formerly applied to tooth cavities.

Preparations

Creosote and Potassium Iodide Mixture *(B.P.C. 1949)*. Creosote 0.125 ml, potassium iodide 343.5 mg, quillaia tincture 0.16 ml, liquorice liquid extract 1.25 ml, tolu syrup 1.88 ml, anise water to 15 ml. *Dose.* 15 to 30 ml. ***Amended formula.*** Creosote 0.1 ml, potassium iodide 300 mg, quillaia tincture 0.15 ml, liquorice liquid extract 1 ml, tolu syrup, 1.5 ml, anise water to 10 ml.—*Compendium of Past Formulae 1933 to 1966*, London, The National Pharmaceutical Union, 1969.

Mist. Creosot *(N.F. 1939)*. Creosote 0.06 ml, juniper spirit 0.06 ml, syrup 1.8 ml, water to 15 ml. *Dose.* 15 ml. ***Amended formula.*** Creosote 0.05 ml, juniper spirit 0.05 ml, syrup 1.5 ml, water to 10 ml.—*Compendium of Past Formulae 1933 to 1966*, London, The National Pharmaceutical Union, 1969.

2011-w

Creosote Carbonate *(B.P.C. 1934)*. Creosotal; Kreosoti Carbonas.

CAS — 8001-59-0.

Pharmacopoeias. In *Belg.* and *Port.*

A mixture of the carbonates of the various constituents of creosote. It is a colourless or amber-coloured syrupy liquid, odourless and tasteless or with a faint creosote-like odour and taste. Wt per ml about 1.16 g. Practically **insoluble** in water and glycerol; soluble in alcohol, chloroform, ether, and fixed and volatile oils. **Protect** from light.

As creosote carbonate is comparatively tasteless and is non-irritant to the stomach it has been employed in place of creosote, but is of doubtful therapeutic value. It may be given in capsules or in milk in doses of 0.3 to 1.2 ml.

2012-e

Eriodictyon *(U.S.N.F., B.P.C. 1934)*. Mountain Balm; Yerba Santa.

CAS — 8013-08-9.

Pharmacopoeias. In *U.S.N.F.*

The dried leaves of *Eriodictyon californicum* (= *E. glutinosum*) (Hydrophyllaceae). It has an aromatic odour and a balsamic bitter taste which becomes sweetish and slightly acrid. **Store** in airtight containers. Protect from light.

Uses. Eriodictyon has been used as a bitter and as an expectorant. It has the property of masking the taste of quinine and many other bitter drugs and it is mainly used for this purpose, usually in the form of an aromatic syrup. It has been given in doses of 1 to 4 g.

Preparations

Aromatic Eriodictyon Syrup *(U.S.N.F.)*. Aromatic Yerba Santa Syrup; Syrupus Corrigens. Prepared from eriodictyon fluidextract 3.2 ml, potassium hydroxide solution (1 in 20) 2.5 ml, compound cardamom tincture *U.S.P.* 6.5 ml, lemon oil 0.05 ml, clove oil 0.1 ml, alcohol 3.2 ml, sucrose 80 g, magnesium carbonate 500 mg, water to 100 ml. Store at a temperature not exceeding 40° in airtight containers. Protect from light.

Eriodictyon Fluidextract *(U.S.N.F.)*. Yerba Santa Fluidextract. 1 in 1; prepared by percolation with a mixture of alcohol 4 vol. and water 1 vol. Store at a temperature not exceeding 40° in airtight containers. Protect from light.

2013-l

Euphorbia *(B.P.C. 1954)*. Euphorbia Herb; Euphorbia Pilulifera; Snake Weed.

Pharmacopoeias. In *Chin.*

The dried entire plant of *Euphorbia hirta* (= *E. pilulifera*) (Euphorbiaceae) containing not less than 16% of alcohol (45%)-soluble extractive.

Euphorbia has been used in the form of a liquid extract or tincture in the treatment of coughs and asthma.

2030-y

Euphorbium *(B.P.C. 1934)*.

Pharmacopoeias. In *Nord., Port., Span.*, and *Swiss.*

The dried latex from the stem of *Euphorbia resinifera.*

Euphorbium is emetic and powerfully purgative but it is not used internally on account of its violent action and its tendency to cause acute nephritis. The powder is violently sternutatory. Externally, it acts as a vesicant and was used for this purpose in veterinary medicine.

2014-y

Garlic *(B.P.C. 1949)*. Allium; Ajo.

Pharmacopoeias. In *Chin., Span.*, and *Swiss.*

The fresh bulb of *Allium sativum* (Lilaceae). It has a very strong and disagreeable odour and a strongly pungent and persistent taste. It yields 0.1 to 0.3% of a volatile oil containing allyl propyl disulphide and diallyl disulphide. **Stored** in a cool dry place with free access of air it may be kept for about 6 months after harvesting.

Garlic has expectorant, diaphoretic, disinfectant, and diuretic properties and has been used in doses of 2 to 8 g. The juice was formerly used alone, or in a syrup, in the treatment of pulmonary conditions. Administration of preparations of garlic to children is dangerous and fatalities have been recorded.

The larvicidal principles of garlic active against the *Culex* mosquito were found to be diallyl di- and trisulphides. Natural and synthetic samples proved larvicidal at 5 ppm.— S. V. Amonkar and A. Banerji, *Science*, 1971, *174*, 1343.

A report of allergic contact dermatitis to garlic.— E. Bleumink *et al.*, *Br. J. Derm.*, 1972, *87*, 6.

Garlic juice and the extracted essential oil prevented the hyperlipaemia and blood coagulation changes following fat ingestion in 5 healthy subjects.— A. Bordia and H. C. Bansal (letter), *Lancet*, 1973, *2*, 1491. See also G. S. Sainani *et al.* (letter), *Lancet*, 1976, *2*, 575.

An extract of garlic called allicin possessed antifungal activity against *Candida, Cryptococcus, Trichophyton, Epidermophyton,* and *Microsporum* spp. *in vitro.*— Y. Yamada and K. Azuma, *Antimicrob. Ag. Chemother.*, 1977, *11*, 743.

For a discussion of the antibacterial properties of garlic, see V. D. Sharma *et al.*, *Indian J. expl. Biol.*, 1977, *15*, 466.

Application of thin slices of garlic bulb was reported to aid healing during repair of perforations of the eardrum in 17 of 18 patients at a Chinese hospital.— *Br. med. J.*, 1977, *2*, 324.

Analysis of the relationship of garlic and onion consumption to mortality from ischaemic heart disease in 27 countries did not demonstrate any protective effect of garlic.— C. Buck *et al.* (letter), *Lancet*, 1979, *2*, 104.

Evidence of a platelet aggregation inhibitor in garlic.— T. Ariga *et al.* (letter), *Lancet*, 1981, *1*, 150. See also D. J. Boullin (letter), *ibid.*, 776.

Hypertension. In 5 consecutive cases of hypertension, garlic reduced the blood pressure to satisfactory levels.— V. Srinivasan (letter), *Lancet*, 1969, *2*, 800.

Preparations

Garlic Juice *(B.P.C. 1949).* Succus Allii. Bruise garlic 80 g and express the juice; mix the marc with water 20 ml and again express the juice; repeat the operation until the volume of the mixed juice and washings amounts to 80 ml, and add alcohol (90%) 20 ml; allow to stand for 14 days, and decant or filter. *Dose.* 2 to 4 ml.

Garlic Syrup *(B.P.C. 1949).* Syr. Allii. Garlic juice 20 ml, sucrose 80 g, acetic acid (6 per cent) 20 ml, water 20 ml. *Dose.* 2 to 8 ml.

2015-j

Grindelia *(B.P.C. 1949).* Gum Plant; Gumweed; Tar Weed.

Pharmacopoeias. In *Belg.* and *Fr.* which also allow *G. humilis, G. robusta,* and *G. squarrosa. Span.* and *Port.* specify *G. robusta; Port.* also allows *G. squarrosa.*

The dried leaves and flowering tops of *Grindelia camporum* (Compositae) containing not less than 20% of alcohol (90%)-soluble extractive. **Store** in a cool dry place.

Grindelia has expectorant properties and has been stated to exert a spasmolytic effect. It has been used as a liquid extract or a tincture in the treatment of asthma and bronchitis. Large doses sometimes cause renal disturbances. Its nauseous taste may be masked with chloroform or glycerol.

Preparations

Grindelia Liquid Extract *(B.P.C. 1949).* Ext. Grindel. Liq. Grindelia 100 g is exhausted by percolation with alcohol (90%), the alcohol is removed by distillation, and the residue is dissolved in water 50 ml to which 10 g of sodium bicarbonate has previously been added; after effervescence has ceased, the solution is adjusted to 100 ml with alcohol (90%) and filtered. *Dose.* 0.6 to 1.2 ml.

2016-z

Guaiacol *(B.P.C. 1949).* Gaïacol; Methyl Catechol.

CAS — 90-05-1 (2-methoxyphenol).

Pharmacopoeias. In *Arg., Fr., It., Mex., Port., Roum., Span.,* and *Swiss.*

A colourless or almost colourless oily liquid or crystals with a penetrating aromatic odour and a caustic taste, obtained as a liquid by fractional distillation of wood-tar creosote or, usually as crystals, by synthesis.

The main constituent is 2-methoxyphenol, $CH_3O.C_6H_4.OH$ = 124.1. Wt per ml (liquid) about 1.12 g; m.p. (crystals) about 28°. It tends to become yellowish on exposure to light.

Soluble 1 in 80 of water; miscible with alcohol, chloroform, ether, glacial acetic acid, and fixed and volatile oils; soluble 1 in 1 of glycerol but separates out on the addition of water. **Incompatible** with ferric salts, camphor, menthol, and chloral hydrate. **Protect** from light.

Guaiacol has disinfectant properties similar to those of creosote. It has been used as an expectorant in doses of 0.3 to 0.6 ml. Adverse effects are similar to those of Phenol, p.571.

2017-c

Guaiacol Carbonate *(B.P.C. 1949).* Duotal. Bis(2-methoxyphenyl) carbonate.

$(CH_3O.C_6H_4.O)_2.CO$ = 274.3.

CAS — 553-17-3.

Pharmacopoeias. In *Port.* and *Span.*

Guaiacol carbonate is the carbonic ester of guaiacol. It is a white, almost odourless, tasteless, crystalline powder. M.p. 83° to 88°. Practically **insoluble** in water; soluble 1 in 70 of alcohol and 1 in 20 of ether; readily soluble in chloroform; slightly soluble in glycerol and fixed oils. It is decomposed by alcoholic potassium hydroxide solution and guaiacol separates from the solution on the addition of excess acid.

Guaiacol carbonate has the actions of guaiacol but is less irritant. It has been used in doses of 0.3 to 1 g. It liberates guaiacol slowly and incompletely in the intestines, the larger part passing through the alimentary tract unchanged.

2018-k

Guaiphenesin *(B.P.).* Guaiacyl Glyceryl Ether; Guaiacol Glycerol Ether; Guaifenesin *(U.S.P.)*; Glyceryl Guaiacolate; Glycerylguayacolum; Guajacolum Glycerolatum. 3-(2-Methoxyphenoxy)propane-1,2-diol.

$C_{10}H_{14}O_4$ = 198.2.

CAS — 93-14-1.

Pharmacopoeias. In *Aust., Br., Cz., Roum.,* and *U.S.*

White or slightly grey crystals or crystalline aggregates, odourless or with a slight characteristic odour and with a bitter taste. M.p. 78° to 82° with a range of not more than 3°.

Soluble 1 in 33 of water at 20°, 1 in 11 of alcohol and of chloroform, and 1 in 100 of ether; soluble 1 in 15 of glycerol with warming, 1 in 15 of propylene glycol, and 1 in 80 of sorbitol syrup. A 2% solution in water has a pH of 5 to 7. Aqueous solutions are stable and may be **sterilised** by autoclaving. **Store** in airtight containers.

Adverse Effects and Precautions. Gastro-intestinal discomfort and drowsiness have been reported. Very large doses cause nausea and vomiting.

A metabolite of guaiphenesin was found to produce an apparent increase in urinary 5-hydroxyindoleacetic acid, and guaiphenesin could thus interfere with the diagnosis of the carcinoid syndrome. Patients being evaluated for the carcinoid syndrome should therefore discontinue any preparation containing guaiphenesin for 24 hours before the collection of urine specimens for the determination of 5-hydroxy indolcactic acid. Acctanilidc, mcphcncsin, and methocarbamol had been reported to cause similar false positive reactions, and hexamine mandelate and some phenothiazine derivatives to cause false negative reactions.— A. T. Pedersen *et al., J. Am. med. Ass.,* 1970, *211,* 1184. See also P. D. Reeme, *Hosp. Formul. Mgmt,* 1970, *5,* 15, per *Int. pharm. Abstr.,* 1973, *10,* 26.

Hypouricaemia (serum-urate concentrations of less than 20 µg per ml) in 6 patients could have been due to guaiphenesin. Therapeutic doses for 3 days reduced serum urate by up to 30 µg per ml in 4 patients.— C. M. Ramsdell and W. N. Kelley, *Ann. intern. Med.,* 1973, *78,* 239.

Absorption and Fate. Guaiphenesin is readily absorbed from the gastro-intestinal tract. It is rapidly metabolised and excreted in the urine.

Guaiphenesin was rapidly absorbed from the gastro-intestinal tract, blood concentrations of 1.4 µg per ml occurring 15 minutes after a dose of 600 mg in 3 healthy fasting men. It was rapidly eliminated from the circulation, having a half-life of 1 hour, and was not detectable in the blood after 8 hours.— W. R. Maynard and R. B. Bruce, *J. pharm. Sci.,* 1970, *59,* 1346.

The major urinary metabolite of guaiphenesin was indentified as β-(2-methoxyphenoxy)lactic acid.— W. J. A. VandenHeuvel *et al., J. pharm. Sci.,* 1972, *61,* 1997.

Uses. Guaiphenesin is reported to reduce the viscosity of tenacious sputum and is used as an expectorant. It has been given in doses of 100 to 200 mg every 2 to 4 hours.

When given by mouth or by injection in large doses, guaiphenesin has a relaxant effect on skeletal muscle similar to that of mephenesin which it closely resembles structurally, but this effect is not produced by the doses normally employed in the treatment of cough.

Guaiphenesin was no better than water in lowering the viscosity of 27 sputum specimens obtained from chronic bronchitics. Doses of 0.8 to 1.6 g daily had no effect on sputum or respiratory function when compared with placebo in 11 patients with chronic bronchitis.— S. R. Hirsch *et al., Chest,* 1973, *63,* 9.

From a study in 239 patients it was reported that guaiphenesin reduced cough frequency and intensity in patients with dry or productive cough, and helped to thin sputum, when compared to placebo.— R. E. Robinson *et al., Robins, Curr. ther. Res.,* 1977, *22,* 284.

A report of a double-blind crossover study in 19 patients with chronic bronchitis showed that guaiphenesin was not significantly better that a placebo in aiding clearance of secretion from the lungs.— D. B. Yeates *et al., Am. Rev. resp. Dis.,* 1977, *115, Suppl.* 4, 182.

Effects on blood. A dose of 200 mg of guaiphenesin was found to prolong the activated-plasma clotting time in 22 healthy volunteers. The same dose, given to 12 healthy volunteers, was found to reduce platelet adhesiveness significantly.— R. D. Eastham and E. P. Griffiths, *Lancet,* 1966, *1,* 795.

Guaiphenesin 200 mg given as a single dose to 5 healthy subjects was associated with transient abnormality in platelet aggregation patterns determined 1 hour after ingestion, showing some inhibition of secondary aggregation but less marked than that observed in other subjects given chlorpromazine or aspirin. Mean bleeding times as determined by a modified Ivy technique were prolonged by single doses of aspirin but were not affected by guaiphenesin; thrice-daily doses of indometacin given for 3 days caused some prolongation.— G. R. Buchanan *et al., Am. J. clin. Path.,* 1977, *68,* 355.

Preparations

Guaifenesin Capsules *(U.S.P.).* Capsules containing guaiphenesin. Store in airtight containers.

Guaifenesin Syrup *(U.S.P.).* A syrup containing guaiphenesin and alcohol 3 to 4%. pH 2.3 to 3. Store in airtight containers.

Guaifenesin Tablets *(U.S.P.).* Tablets containing guaiphenesin. Store in airtight containers.

Guaiphenesin Linctuses. (1) *Lemon-flavoured.* Guaiphenesin 2 g, glycerol 10 ml, chloroform spirit 10 ml, menthol 10 mg, compound tartrazine solution 0.2 ml, water 10 ml, modified lemon syrup to 100 ml.

(2) *Tolu-flavoured.* Guaiphenesin 2 g, glycerol 10 ml, chloroform spirit 10 ml, menthol 10 mg, amaranth solution 1 ml, tolu solution 10 ml, invert syrup 20 ml, syrup to 100 ml.

Modified lemon syrup contains lemon spirit 0.5 ml, citric acid monohydrate 2.5 g, invert syrup 20 ml, syrup to 100 ml.

Both lemon-flavoured and tolu-flavoured guaiphenesin linctuses remained stable for 6 months when stored at temperatures from −5° to 37°.— Pharm. Soc. Lab. Rep. No. P/65/21, 1965. See also G. Smith, *Pharm. J.,* 1966, *1,* 165.

Proprietary Preparations

Dimotane Expectorant *(Robins, UK).* Contains in each 5 ml guaiphenesin 100 mg, brompheniramine maleate 2 mg, phenylephrine hydrochloride 5 mg, and phenylpropanolamine hydrochloride 5 mg (suggested diluent, syrup). **Dimotane Expectorant DC** contains in addition hydrocodone tartrate 1.8 mg in each 5 ml. *Dose.* 5 to 10 ml four times daily; children, 1 to 3 years, 1 to 2.5 ml; 3 to 6 years, 2.5 to 5 ml; 6 to 12 years, 5 ml.

Dimotane with Codeine *(Robins, UK).* Contains in each 5 ml guaiphenesin 100 mg, codeine phosphate 10 mg, brompheniramine maleate 2 mg, phenylephrine hydrochloride 5 mg, and phenylpropanolamine hydrochloride 5 mg (suggested diluent, syrup). For cough. *Dose.* 5 to 10 ml four times daily.

Dimotane with Codeine Paediatric *(Robins, UK).* Contains in each 5 ml guaiphenesin 50 mg, codeine phosphate 3 mg, brompheniramine maleate 1 mg, phenylephrine hydrochloride 2.5 mg, and phenylpropanolamine hydrochloride 2.5 mg (suggested diluent, syrup). *Dose.* 3 to 6 years, 5 ml four times daily; 6 to 12 years, 5 to 10 ml.

Exyphen *(Norton, UK: Vestric, UK).* An elixir containing in each 5 ml guaiphenesin 80 mg, brompheniramine maleate 2 mg, phenylephrine hydrochloride 4.75 mg, and phenylpropanolamine hydrochloride 5 mg. For cough. *Dose.* 5 to 10 ml four times daily; children, 2.5 to 5 ml three or four times daily.

Noradran Bronchial Syrup *(Norma, UK: Farillon, UK).* Contains in each 5 ml guaiphenesin 25 mg, diphenhydramine hydrochloride 5 mg, diprophylline 50 mg, and ephedrine hydrochloride 7.5 mg. *Dose.* 10 ml every 4 hours; children over 5 years, 5 ml.

Pholcomed Expectorant (formerly known as Pulmodrine Expectorant) *(Medo Chemicals, UK).* Contains in each 5 ml guaiphenesin 62.5 mg and methylephedrine hydrochloride 625 µg. *Dose.* 10 to 20 ml thrice daily; children, 2.5 to 5 ml.

Robitussin *(Robins, UK).* An expectorant mixture containing in each 5 ml guaiphenesin 100 mg (suggested diluent, syrup). (Also available as Robitussin in *Austral., Canad., Ital.*).

Robitussin AC *(Robins, UK).* Contains in each 5 ml guaiphenesin 100 mg, codeine phosphate 10 mg, and pheniramine maleate 7.5 mg (suggested diluent, syrup). For coughs. *Dose.* 5 to 10 ml four times daily; children, 6 to 12 years, 5 ml.

Other Proprietary Names
Belg.—Resyl; *Canad.*—Balminil Expectorant, Broncho-Grippex, Corutol Expectorant, Demo-Cineol Expectorant Syrup, Gaiapect, Motussin, Resyl, Sedatuss Expectorant, Tussanca; *Ger.*—Myoscain 'E', Reorganin; *Ital.*—Broncovanil; *Spain*—Resyl; *Swed.*—Resyl; *Switz.*—Guajasyl, Resyl; *USA*—2/G Expectorant, Glycotuss, Glytuss, Guiatuss, Hytuss, Hytuss-2X, S-T Expect.

A preparation containing guaiphenesin was also formerly marketed in Great Britain under the proprietary name Riddovydrin Elixir (*Riddell*now *Seaford*).

2019-a

Ipecacuanha *(B.P., Eur. P.)*. Ipecacuanhae Radix; Ipecac; Ipecacuanha Root; Brechwurzel.

CAS — 8012-96-2.

Pharmacopoeias. In all pharmacopoeias examined except *Chin.* and *Rus. Br.* also describes Powdered Ipecacuanha.

The dried root, or rhizome and roots, of *Cephaëlis ipecacuanha* (= *Uragoga ipecacuanha*) (Rubiaceae), known in commerce as Matto Grosso (Rio) or Minas (Brazilian) ipecacuanha or of *C. acuminata*, known in commerce as Cartagena (Colombia), Nicaragua, Panama, or Costa Rica ipecacuanha, or of a mixture of both species. It contains not less than 2% of total alkaloids, calculated as emetine. *U.S.P.* specifies not less than 2% of ether-soluble alkaloids of which not less than 90% is emetine and cephaëline; the content of cephaëline is equal to, to not more than twice, that of emetine. Matto Grosso ipecacuanha contains 2 to 2.4% of alkaloids, of which 60 to 75% is emetine and about 26% cephaëline; Colombian ipecacuanha contains 2.1 to 2.45% of alkaloids, Nicaraguan 2.65 to 3%, and Costa Rican 2.9 to 3.5%, of which emetine constitutes 30 to 50% in these 3 varieties.

Ipecacuanha has a slight odour and a bitter, nauseous and acrid taste. **Store** in airtight containers. Protect from light.

NOTE. The *B.P.* directs that when Ipecacuanha, Ipecacuanha Root, or Powdered Ipecacuanha is prescribed, Prepared Ipecacuanha must be dispensed.

2020-e

Prepared Ipecacuanha *(B.P., Eur. P.)*. Ipecacuanhae Pulvis Normatus; Prep. Ipecac.; Ipecacuanhae Radicis Pulvis Standardisatus; Ipecacuanha Praeparata; Radix Ipecacuanhae Titrata; Powdered Ipecac *(U.S.P.)*.

Pharmacopoeias. In *Aust., Br., Eur., Fr., Ger., Ind., Int., It., Jap., Mex., Neth., Turk.,* and *U.S.*

Finely powdered ipecacuanha adjusted with powdered ipecacuanha of lower alkaloidal strength or powdered lactose to contain 1.9 to 2.1% of total alkaloids, calculated as emetine. **Store** in a cool place in airtight containers. Protect from light.

Adverse Effects. Ipecacuanha has an irritant effect on the gastro-intestinal tract and large doses may give rise to persistent vomiting and bloody diarrhoea; mucosal erosions of the entire gastro-intestinal tract have been reported. Albuminuria may also occur. Effects on the heart may vary from mild depression or inversion of T-waves to bradycardia or myocardial infarction and may be due to the specific cardiotoxicity of emetine. This combined with dehydration due to vomiting may cause vasomotor collapse followed by death in some patients. Emetine is also known to accumulate in muscle and may interfere with muscle fibre contractility of heart muscle.

There have been several reports of ipecacuanha poisoning due to the unwitting substitution of ipecac fluidextract (*U.S.P. XVI*) for ipecac syrup (*U.S.P.*); the fluidextract is about 14 times the strength of the syrup.

A review of the toxicology of ipecacuanha.— B. R. Manno and J. E. Manno, *Clin. Toxicol.*, 1977, *10,* 221.

Treatment of Adverse Effects. Prolonged vomiting should be controlled by the intramuscular injection of 25 to 50 mg of chlorpromazine or of a comparable dose of a related phenothiazine. Fluid and electrolyte imbalance should be corrected.

Precautions. Ipecacuanha should not be used as an emetic in patients in a state of coma or shock or in patients who have ingested corrosive substances when the dangers from aspiration are greater than those from ingestion; neither should it be given with milk or after charcoal. Ipecacuanha is therefore unsuitable as an emetic for patients who have taken overdoses of antiemetic drugs such as phenothiazines, or other depressants, when the dose may be ineffective or vomit may be inhaled.

A 23-month-old girl who swallowed 10 to 12 pipamazine tablets (5 mg) was given about 90 ml of ipecacuanha syrup. She became drowsy with tachycardia, low blood pressure, and constricted pupils. She was treated by gastric lavage and intravenous 5% dextrose solution, and the tachycardia and ECG abnormalities were controlled with a cardiac pacemaker. She recovered after about 6 hours. The ipecacuanha probably failed to cause emesis because of the depressant action of pipamazine on the vomiting centre. It was considered that poisoning by anti-emetics and phenothiazine derivatives should be treated by prompt gastric lavage rather than by an emetic.— J. MacLeod, *New Engl. J. Med.*, 1963, *268,* 146.

Results of a controlled crossover study of 9 subjects indicated that concurrent administration with milk delayed the speed of action of Ipecac Syrup [*U.S.P.*]. When possible Ipecac Syrup should be given with water.— R. J. Varipapa and G. M. Oderda (letter), *New Engl. J. Med.*, 1977, *296,* 112.

Studies *in vitro* indicated that activated charcoal adsorbed substantial quantities of emetine. These results substantiated previous suggestions that charcoal and ipecacuanha syrup should not be given together for the treatment of poisoning.— D. O. Cooney, *J. pharm. Sci.*, 1978, *67,* 426.

Uses. Ipecacuanha is used as an expectorant in doses of 25 to 100 mg (approximately 0.5 to 2 mg of total alkaloid) and is also used in larger doses as an emetic for selected patients. Vomiting usually occurs within 30 minutes of administration by mouth of an emetic dose due to the irritant effect on the gastro-intestinal tract. There is evidence that ipecacuanha also has a central action.

Ipecacuanha with opium, as in Dover's powder, has traditionally been given as a diaphoretic in the early stages of febrile affections, often in conjunction with aspirin.

For an emetic action, ipecacuanha is given followed by a copious drink of water or fruit juice. Adults may be given doses of 21 to 42 mg of total alkaloids represented by 15 to 30 ml of Paediatric Ipecacuanha Emetic Mixture *(B.P.)* or of Ipecac Syrup *(U.S.P.)*. Children aged 6 to 18 months may be given 14 mg of total alkaloids, represented by 10 ml of Paediatric Ipecacuanha Emetic Mixture *(B.P.)* or of Ipecac Syrup *(U.S.P.)*; older children may be given 21 mg, represented by 15 ml of Paediatric Ipecacuanha Emetic Mixture *(B.P.)* or of Ipecac Syrup *(U.S.P.)*. Doses may be repeated after 20 minutes if emesis has not occurred.

Ipecacuanha is used in homoeopathic medicine.

The routine addition of ipecacuanha to drugs subject to abuse, as had been suggested, could not be recommended at present due to conflicting evidence. There was no evidence that ipecacuanha prevented the abuse of preparations in which it was an ingredient, and *animal* experiments had shown that it might enhance the action of barbiturates. The production of nausea and vomiting by some drugs did not prevent their abuse.— J. M. Gowdy (letter), *New Engl. J. Med.*, 1970, *283,* 936.

Emesis in acute poisoning. Ipecac Syrup (*U.S.P.*) was used to produce emesis in 250 children suffering from accidental poisoning. Vomiting occurred in 98% and the average time of action was less than 20 minutes. The initial dose was 15 ml followed by 200 ml of water or clear fluid. A further dose of 15 ml of Ipecac Syrup was repeated once if no vomiting occurred within 20 to 25 minutes. Emesis with Ipecac Syrup was contra-indicated in poisoning with corrosive or petroleum products; gastric lavage was preferable in unconscious patients.— D. H. S. Reid (letter), *Lancet*, 1969, *1,* 261. A similar report.— J. J. Alpert (letter), *ibid.*, 728. See also S. B. Malcolm and J. A. Kuzemko, *Practitioner*, 1969, *202,* 666.

Although vomiting could be readily induced by Ipecac Syrup (*U.S.P.*) all the ingested poison might not be effectively removed. If there was any doubt then gastric aspiration and lavage should be instituted, using a wide-bore stomach tube.— H. Matthew, *Br. med. J.*, 1971, *1,* 519.

In a survey of 82 children given Ipecacuanha Syrup (*A.P.F.*) on admission to hospital in the treatment of poisoning, 75 vomited after 1 dose. Five were given a second dose and 4 of these vomited. Emesis was induced by other means in children who did not vomit. The average delay before treatment was about 50 minutes and the average delay between administration of ipecacuanha syrup and vomiting was about 15 minutes. Recommended doses were: under 1 year, 10 ml; 1 to 2 years, 15 ml; 2 to 4 years, 20 ml; over 4 years, 25 ml. The dose was followed by 200 ml of fluid to facilitate emesis.— O. Jonas and N. Smyth, *Aust. J. Pharm.*, 1975, *56,* 607.

A comparison of Ipecac Syrup (*U.S.P.*) 15 ml and Ipecacuanha Syrup (*A.P.F.*) 15 or 30 ml in 105 adults with accidental or intentional poisoning showed no significant differences in emetic response either between the different formulations or between different dosages. It was suggested that the dose of Ipecacuanha Syrup (*A.P.F.*) could be reduced from 50 ml to 30 ml.— K. F. Ilett *et al.*, *Med. J. Aust.*, 1977, *2,* 91.

Of 232 patients with drug overdose given Ipecac Syrup (*U.S.P.*) vomiting was induced after a single dose in 188 and after two doses in 34; 7 patients were classified as ipecac failures and 3 became lethargic or convulsed as a result of the overdose before vomiting began. Results in patients who had ingested anti-emetics were similar. Doses used were: 12 months to 5 years, 15 ml followed by 240 ml of water; children over 5 years and adults, 30 ml followed by 360 ml of water.— A. S. Manoguerra and E. P. Krenzelok, *Am. J. Hosp. Pharm.*, 1978, *35,* 1360.

Further references: J. A. Hurst and A. M. Dozzi, *Med. J. Aust.*, 1975, *2,* 432; *Br. med. J.*, 1975, *4,* 483; *ibid.*, 1977, *2,* 977; R. Goulding and G. N. Volans, *Proc. R. Soc. Med.*, 1977, *70,* 766; *Med. Lett.*, 1979, *21,* 70.

Preparations

Extracts

Ipecacuanha Liquid Extract *(B.P.)*. Ipecac. Liq. Ext. Prepared by percolation with alcohol (80%) and adjusted to contain 1.9 to 2.1% w/v of total alkaloids calculated as emetine; about 2 mg in 0.1 ml. *Dose:* 0.025 to 0.1 ml (expectorant).

Several pharmacopoeias include similar liquid or dry extracts or compound extracts, some containing considerably higher concentrations of total alkaloids.

Linctuses

Paediatric Ipecacuanha and Squill Linctus *(B.P.C. 1973)*. Ipecacuanha and Squill Linctus Paediatric; Mist. Tuss. Rubra pro Inf. Ipecacuanha tincture 0.1 ml, squill tincture 0.15 ml, compound orange spirit 0.0075 ml, black currant syrup 2.5 ml, syrup to 5 ml. Store in a cool place. *Dose.* Children, 5 ml.

Mixtures

Alkaline Ipecacuanha Mixture *(B.P.C. 1963)*. Ipecacuanha and Alkali Mixture; Mist. Ipecac. Alk.; Mist. Expect. Alk. Ipecacuanha tincture 0.625 ml, sodium bicarbonate 685.5 mg, ammonium bicarbonate 205.5 mg, chloroform water to 15 ml. *Dose.* 15 to 30 ml.

Amended formula. Ipecacuanha tincture 0.5 ml, sodium bicarbonate 500 mg, ammonium bicarbonate 200 mg, chloroform water to 10 ml.—*Compendium of Past Formulae 1933 to 1966*, London, The National Pharmaceutical Union, 1969.

Ipecacuanha and Morphine Mixture *(B.P.)*. Mistura Tussi Nigra. Ipecacuanha tincture 0.2 ml, chloroform and morphine tincture 0.4 ml, liquorice liquid extract 1 ml, water to 10 ml. It should be recently prepared. 10 ml contains 700 µg of anhydrous morphine. *Dose.* 10 ml.

Ipecacuanha and Squill Mixture *(A.P.F.)*. Cough Mixture. Ipecacuanha tincture 0.25 ml, compound camphor spirit 1 ml, tolu syrup 1 ml, squill oxymel 1 ml, concentrated chloroform water 0.15 ml, concentrated anise water 0.15 ml, water to 10 ml. *Dose.* 10 ml.

Ipecacuanha and Squill Mixture CF *(A.P.F.).* Expectorant Mixture for Children. Ipecacuanha tincture 0.1 ml, compound camphor spirit 0.25 ml, squill oxymel 1 ml, water to 5 ml. *Dose.* 5 ml.

Paediatric Ipecacuanha and Ammonia Mixture *(B.P.C. 1973).* Ipecacuanha tincture 0.1 ml, ammonium bicarbonate 30 mg, sodium bicarbonate 100 mg, tolu syrup 0.5 ml, double-strength chloroform water 2.5 ml, water to 5 ml. It should be recently prepared. *Dose.* Children, up to 1 year, 5 ml; 1 to 5 years, 10 ml.

Paediatric Ipecacuanha Emetic Mixture *(B.P.).* Paediatric Ipecacuanha Emetic Draught; Paediatric Ipecacuanha Emetic; Ipecacuanha Paediatric Emetic Draught. Ipecacuanha liquid extract 0.7 ml, hydrochloric acid 0.025 ml, glycerol 1 ml, syrup to 10 ml. *Dose.* Children 6 months to 18 months, 10 ml; 18 months to 5 years, 15 ml.

Paediatric Ipecacuanha Mixture *(B.P.C. 1973).* Ipecacuanha tincture 0.1 ml, sodium bicarbonate 100 mg, tolu syrup 1 ml, double-strength chloroform water 2.5 ml, water to 5 ml. It should be recently prepared. *Dose.* Children up to 1 year, 5 ml; 1 to 5 years, 10 ml.

A similar preparation containing liquorice liquid extract and anise water was supplied as Mist. Tuss. pro Inf.

For a report of incompatibility when Paediatric Ipecacuanha Mixture was prepared with or diluted with syrup preserved with hydroxybenzoates, see under Sucrose, p.61.

Paediatric Opiate Ipecacuanha Mixture *(B.P.C. 1973).* Ipecacuanha tincture 0.1 ml, camphorated opium tincture 0.15 ml, sodium bicarbonate 100 mg, tolu syrup 1 ml, double-strength chloroform water 2.5 ml, water to 5 ml. It should be recently prepared. *Dose.* Children, up to 1 year, 5 ml; 1 to 5 years, 10 ml.

For a report of incompatibility when Paediatric Opiate Ipecacuanha Mixture was prepared with or diluted with syrup preserved with hydroxybenzoates, see under Sucrose, p.61.

Powders

Ipecacuanha and Opium Powder *(B.P.C. 1973).* Pulvis Ipecacuanhae Compositus; Ipecac and Opium Powder; Dover's Powder; Compound Ipecacuanha Powder. Prepared ipecacuanha 10 g, powdered opium 10 g, lactose 80 g. It contains 1% of anhydrous morphine; 6 mg in 600 mg. Store and supply in airtight containers. *Dose.* 300 to 600 mg.

Many pharmacopoeias include a similar powder, sometimes with potassium sulphate or with equal parts of potassium nitrate and potassium sulphate or with starch or mannitol in place of lactose.

Syrups

Ipecac Syrup *(U.S.P.).* Prepared by percolation from powdered ipecac *U.S.P.* 7 g, glycerol 10 ml, syrup to 100 ml. It contains 123 to 157 mg of ether-soluble alkaloids in each 100 ml. Store in airtight containers.

Ipecacuanha Syrup (Emetic) *(A.P.F.).* Ipecacuanha liquid extract 6 ml, dilute acetic acid 2.5 ml, glycerol 10 ml, syrup to 100 ml. *Dose.* 30 ml; children under 2 years, 15 ml; 2 to 3 years, 20 ml; 3 to 4 years, 25 ml.

Tablets

Ipecacuanha and Opium Tablets *(B.P.C. 1973, Ind. P.).* Tab. Ipecac. et Opii; Dover's Powder Tablets. Tablets containing ipecacuanha and opium powder. Store in a cool place in airtight containers. *Dose.* 300 to 600 mg.

Tinctures and Wines

Ipecacuanha Tincture *(B.P.).* Ipecac. Tinct. Ipecacuanha liquid extract 10 ml, dilute acetic acid 1.65 ml, alcohol (90%) 21 ml, glycerol 20 ml, water to 100 ml. Set aside for not less than 24 hours and filter. It contains 0.19 to 0.21% w/v of total alkaloids, calculated as emetine; about 2 mg in 1 ml. *Dose:* 0.25 to 1 ml (expectorant).

A similar tincture is included in many pharmacopoeias. The *B.P.* directs that Ipecacuanha Tincture be dispensed when Ipecacuanha Wine is prescribed.

NOTE. Ipecacuanha tincture of the *B.P. 1953* and earlier editions was half the strength of the above tincture in terms of ipecacuanha liquid extract (5 ml in 100 ml) and contained 0.1% w/v of total alkaloids.

Proprietary Preparations

Linituss *(Ayrton, Saunders, UK).* Contains in each 5 ml ipecacuanha liquid extract 0.02 ml, chloroform and morphine tincture 0.4 ml, squill vinegar 0.4 ml, camphorated opium tincture 0.2 ml, liquorice liquid extract 0.35 ml, capsicum tincture 0.02 ml, tolu syrup 0.125 ml, and linseed (as infusion) 40 mg. For cough. *Dose.* 5 ml in water every 4 hours.

Tussifans *(Norton, UK: Vestric, UK).* A children's cough mixture containing in each 5 ml ipecacuanha liquid extract 0.013 ml, belladonna liquid extract 0.007 ml, potassium citrate 250 mg, anise oil 0.0015 ml, tolu syrup 0.4 ml, and squill syrup 0.3 ml. *Dose.* 2.5 to 10 ml.

A preparation containing ipecacuanha was also formerly marketed in Great Britain under the proprietary name Pectomed (*Medo-Chemicals*).

2021-l

Liquorice *(B.P.).* Liquorice Root *(Eur. P.)*; Glycyrrhiza; Liquiritiae Radix; Glycyrrhizae Radix; Licorice Root; Réglisse; Süssholzwurzel; Raiz de Regaliz; Alcaçuz; Orozuz.

Pharmacopoeias. In all pharmacopoeias examined except *Int.*, *Mex.*, *Turk.*, and *U.S.* Many allow peeled or unpeeled liquorice. Most pharmacopoeias specify not less than 20 to 30% of water-soluble extractive. Also in *U.S.N.F. Br.* also describes Powdered Liquorice.

Liquorice consists of the dried unpeeled root and stolons of *Glycyrrhiza glabra* (Leguminosae) containing not less than 25% of water-soluble extractive, including about 7% of glycyrrhizin consisting of the potassium and calcium salts of glycyrrhizinic acid (a glucoside of glycyrrhetinic acid). Glycyrrhiza *U.S.N.F.* is the dried rhizome and roots of *Glycyrrhiza glabra*, known in commerce as Spanish Licorice, *G. glabra* var. *glandulifera*, known in commerce as Russian Licorice, or of other varieties.

It has a characteristic odour and a slightly aromatic sweet taste. **Store** in airtight containers. Protect from light.

Adverse Effects. Liquorice may cause reversible sodium retention and potassium loss leading to hypertension, water retention, and electrolyte imbalance.

A 53-year-old man, who was previously healthy, developed fulminant congestive heart failure after eating 700 g of liquorice candy over a period of about 1 week. He had hypertension, hypokalaemic alkalosis, suppressed aldosterone and renin levels, oedema, headache, and weakness. He improved following treatment with a 2-g sodium diet and then spironolactone, 25 mg thrice daily for 1 week.— T. J. Chamberlain (letter), *J. Am. med. Ass.*, 1970, *213*, 1343.

A 51-year-old man was admitted to hospital with hypokalaemia and hypertension. A diagnosis of pseudoaldosteronism was made when it was discovered that 2 months before admission he had begun eating 70 g of liquorice sticks daily. His condition returned to normal within one month of stopping the liquorice.— L. K. Wash and J. D. Bernard, *Am. J. Hosp. Pharm.*, 1975, *32*, 73.

In 14 volunteers who ingested confectionery liquorice 100 or 200 g daily (equivalent to glycyrrhizinic acid 0.7 to 1.4 g) for up to 4 weeks there were significant falls in mean plasma-renin activity, plasma concentrations of angiotensin II, and plasma and urine concentrations of aldosterone. Plasma-potassium concentrations fell by up to 1.5 mmol per litre. Liquorice should be avoided by patients with hypertension or circulatory disorders.— M. T. Epstein *et al.*, *Br. med. J.*, 1977, *1*, 488. See also *idem*, 209.

A report of hypokalaemia, hypomagnesaemia, myopathy, and cardiac arrest in a 58-year-old woman who had been ingesting 1.8 kg of liquorice sweets per week; she recovered after potassium and magnesium supplementation.— B. Bannister, *Br. med. J.*, 1977, *2*, 738. Hypomagnesaemia and metabolic alkalosis might have been responsible.— J. Montoliu (letter), *ibid.*, 1352. A reply.— B. A. Bannister *et al.* (letter), *ibid.*

In addition to hypokalaemia, hyporeninaemia, and low aldosterone excretion, a young woman also developed hyperprolactinaemia with amenorrhoea, after eating excessive amounts of liquorice for several years. When the liquorice was stopped the blood pressure returned to normal within 2 weeks, menstruation returned after 6 months when the hormone concentrations had returned to normal, and severe headaches which she had been suffering did not recur.— S. Werner *et al.* (letter), *Lancet*, 1979, *1*, 319.

A report of severe hypokalaemia, complete flaccid paralysis of all limbs, and myoglobinuria in a 70-year-old woman who had ingested intermittently for 2 to 3 years small amounts of a liquorice-containing mixture as a laxative.— A. M. M. Cumming *et al.*, *Postgrad. med. J.*, 1980, *56*, 526.

Profound muscular weakness, with hypokalaemia, hypertension, renal potassium wasting, metabolic alkalosis, sodium retention, and depressed renin, in an 85-year-old man was associated with the chewing of large quantities of tobacco. The tobacco contained about 8.3% of liquorice paste with a glycyrrhizinic acid content of 0.15%.— J. D. Blachley and J. P. Knochel, *New Engl. J. Med.*, 1980, *302*, 784. See also A. Synhaivsky (letter), *ibid.*, *303*, 463; J. D. Blachley and J. P. Knochel (letter), *ibid.*

Further references: E. G. Gross *et al.*, *New Engl. J. Med.*, 1966, *274*, 602 (hypokalaemic myopathy with myoglobinuria); F. Lai *et al.* (letter), *ibid.*, 1980, *303*, 463 (hypokalaemic myopathy).

Uses. Liquorice is demulcent and expectorant. The liquid extract is used in cough mixtures and as a flavouring agent in mixtures containing nauseous medicines such as ammonium chloride, the alkali iodides, quinine, creosote, and cascara liquid extract, but it should only be prescribed in alkaline or neutral solution. Powdered liquorice was used as an absorbent pill excipient. A decoction with linseed has been used as a domestic treatment for cough and bronchitis. Liquorice has also been used as a sweetener.

Liquorice has mild anti-inflammatory and mineralocorticoid properties associated with the presence of glycyrrhizin and has occasionally been used in place of the corticosteroids. Deglycyrrhizinised liquorice has a reduced mineralocorticoid activity and is used in the treatment of peptic ulcer.

A review of glycyrrhizin as a sweetener.— M. K. Cook and B. H. Gominger, in *Symposium, Sweeteners*, G.E. Inglett (Ed.), Westport, AVI, 1974, p. 211. See also J. E. Hodge and G. E. Inglett, *ibid.*, p. 216.

For a report of the use of deglycyrrhizinised liquorice to reduce the toxicity of nitrofurantoin, see Nitrofurantoin, p.1048.

Mineralocorticoid action. A woman with auto-immune Addison's disease escaped the consequences of adrenal failure for a long period due to the sodium-retaining properties of liquorice, which she ingested in large quantities as a sweet.— E. J. Ross (letter), *Br. med. J.*, 1970, *2*, 733. For a similar report, see J. A. Cotterill and W. J. Cunliffe, *Lancet*, 1973, *1*, 294.

Peptic ulcers. Thirty-three patients with gastric ulcer were treated for 4 weeks with either capsules of deglycyrrhizinised liquorice, 760 mg thrice daily after food, or inactive but identical capsules. In 7 of 16 patients who received the active treatment, ulcers appeared to be healed when viewed radiologically compared with 1 of 17 patients in the control group. The average reduction in ulcer size was 78% in patients treated with deglycyrrhizinised liquorice and 34% in the others. No patients developed oedema; average increases in weight were 1.1 and 0.87 kg for patients receiving treatment and control respectively. Serum electrolytes were not determined routinely.— A. G. G. Turpie *et al.*, *Gut*, 1969, *10*, 299. See also S. N. Tewari and F. C. Trembalowicz, *Gut*, 1968, *9*, 48.

Carbenoxolone and deglycyrrhizinised liquorice were shown to be equally effective in the treatment of gastric ulcer in 37 patients.— J. A. C. Wilson, *Br. J. clin. Pract.*, 1972, *26*, 563.

An increase in the dose of deglycyrrhizinised liquorice (Caved-S) from 8 tablets daily for 8 weeks in 20 patients to 12 tablets daily for 16 weeks in another 20 patients increased the proportion of patients wich duodenal ulcer who were free from relapse during follow-up for 1 year.— S. N. Tewari and A. K. Wilson, *Practitioner*, 1973, *210*, 820.

An evaluation of the pharmacological properties of a deglycyrrhizinised liquorice preparation (Caved-S) and its use in the treatment of gastric and duodenal ulcers.— R. N. Brogden *et al.*, *Drugs*, 1974, *8*, 330. See also M. J. S. Langman, *ibid.*, 1977, *14*, 105.

In an uncontrolled study of 32 patients with duodenal ulcer complete or partial healing occurred in all cases after administration of deglycyrrhizinised liquorice (Caved-S) tablets in a dose of 2 tablets 5 times daily. For optimal results it appeared to be important that the tablets should be chewed thoroughly and swallowed on an empty stomach while standing.— W. Larkworthy and P. F. L. Holgate, *Practitioner*, 1975, *215*, 787.

In a study in 34 patients with duodenal ulcer, half of whom were treated with deglycyrrhizinised liquorice 900 mg five times daily or placebo for 8 weeks, as capsules or in a chewing-gum basis, there was no endoscopic evidence of any greater beneficial effect of the active medication over the placebo.— W. Larkworthy *et al.*, *Br. med. J.*, 1977, *2*, 1123. For a similar conclusion from a study of 96 patients with gastric ulcer treated for 4 weeks see K. D. Bardhan *et al.*, *Gut*, 1978, *19*, 779.

In a 2-year double-blind trial the effect of deglycyrrhizinised liquorice in a dose of five 450-mg capsules daily was compared with that of placebo in the prevention of recurrence of healed gastric ulcer. The incidence of recurrence, 5 of 11 (45%) and 13 of 22 (59%) respectively, was not significantly different.— D. Hollanders *et al.*, *Br. med. J.*, 1978, *1*, 148. For similar conclusions from earlier studies, see H. Feldman and T. Gilat, *Gut*, 1971, *12*, 449. A Multicentre Trial, *Br. med. J.*, 1971, *3*, 501; A. Engqvist *et al.*, *Gut*, 1973, *14*, 711.

Preparations

Elixirs

Elixir Pectorale *(Swiss P.)*. Liquorice liquid extract 40, dilute ammonia solution 4, anise oil 0.1, alcohol 16, and fennel water 40. A similar preparation is included in *Pol. P.* (Elixir Glycyrrhizae).

Liquor Pectoralis *(Dan. Disp.)*. Elixir Pectorale; King of Denmark's Chest Mixture. A liquorice liquid extract 40, water 44.5, ammonia solution (5M) 4, fennel oil 0.03, anise oil 0.17, and alcohol 11.3, all by wt.

Extracts

Crude Glycyrrhiza Extract *(Neth. P.)*. A dried aqueous extract in blocks or sticks.

Glycyrrhiza Fluidextract *(U.S.N.F.)*. A 1 in 1 extract; prepared by maceration and percolation with boiling water, followed by evaporation after the addition of dilute ammonia solution and finally adding one-third of its volume of alcohol. Store at a temperature not exceeding 40° in airtight containers. Protect from light.

Liquorice Extract *(B.P.C. 1973)*. Extractum Glycyrrhizae. A soft extract prepared by percolating liquorice with chloroform water and evaporating the percolate. Store in a cool place. *Dose*. 0.6 to 2 g. *It. P.* and *Jap. P.* include a similar extract.

Liquorice Liquid Extract *(B.P.)*. Liquorice Liq. Ext.; Ext. Glycyrrh. Liq.; Glycyrrhiza Liquid Extract. A water percolate of liquorice, evaporated to a wt per ml of 1.198 g and mixed with a quarter of its volume of alcohol (90%). Allow to stand for at least 4 weeks and filter.

Pure Glycyrrhiza Extract *(U.S.N.F.)*. Prepared by percolating liquorice with boiling water, adding dilute solution of ammonia to the percolate, boiling, filtering and evaporating to a pilular consistence.

Solazzi. A liquorice extract in stick form.

Lozenges

Liquorice Lozenges *(B.P.C. 1973)*. Trochisci Glycyrrhizae; Brompton Cough Lozenges. Each lozenge contains liquorice extract 200 mg, anise oil 0.03 ml, and simple basis for lozenges q.s.

Powders

Compound Liquorice Powder *(B.P.C. 1973)*. Pulvis Glycyrrhizae Compositus; Pulv. Glycyrrh. Co. Peeled liquorice 16 g, senna leaf 16 g, fennel 8 g, sublimed sulphur 8 g, and sucrose 52 g. *Dose*. 5 to 10 g. A similar powder is included in several pharmacopoeias.

Proprietary Preparations

Ammoniated Glycyrrhizin *(MacAndrews & Forbes, UK)*. The ammonium salt of a triterpenoid derived from liquorice. It is claimed to be about 50 times sweeter than sucrose and 100 times sweeter in the presence of sucrose; it is used with sucrose as a sweetening agent.

Caved-S *(Cedona, Neth.: Tillotts, UK)*. Tablets each containing deglycyrrhizinised liquorice (not more than 3% glycyrrhizinic acid) 380 mg, dried aluminium hydroxide 100 mg, light magnesium carbonate 200 mg, and sodium bicarbonate 100 mg. For gastric and duodenal ulcers. *Dose*. Gastric ulcer; 2 tablets thrice daily; in duodenal ulcer this dose may be increased if necessary to a maximum of 2 tablets 6 times daily; to be chewed, then swallowed with a drink of water.

Magnasweet *(MacAndrews & Forbes, UK)*. A range of ammoniated glycyrrhizins derived from liquorice. For use as sweetening agents.

Rabro *(Sinclair, UK)*. Tablets each containing deglycyrrhizinised liquorice (not more than 3% glycyrrhizinic acid) 400 mg, magnesium oxide 100 mg, calcium carbonate 500 mg, and frangula bark 25 mg. For peptic ulcer. *Dose*. 1 or 2 tablets thrice daily after meals; to be chewed, then swallowed with a drink of water.

Other Proprietary Names

Rucedal *(Neth.)*.

Deglycyrrhizinised liquorice was also formerly marketed in Great Britain under the proprietary name Ulcedal (*Boehringer Ingelheim*).

2022-y

Potassium Guaiacolsulfonate *(U.S.P.)*. Potassium Guaiacolsulphonate; Kalium Guajacolsulfonicum; Kalii Sulfoguaiacolas; Sulfagaïacol. Potassium hydroxymethoxybenzenesulphonate hemihydrate.
$C_7H_7KO_5S,½H_2O=251.3$.

CAS — 1321-14-81 (anhydrous); 78247-49-1 (hemihydrate).

Pharmacopoeias. In *U.S.* Also in *Aust.*, *Belg.*, *Fr.*, *It.*, *Neth.*, *Pol.*, *Port.*, *Roum.*, and *Span.* none of which specify hemihydrate.

A white odourless or slightly aromatic powder with a bitter-sweet taste. **Soluble** 1 in 8 of water; practically insoluble in alcohol, acetone, ether, and oils. A solution in water is neutral or alkaline to litmus. **Incompatible** with ferric salts. **Store** in airtight containers. Protect from light.

Potassium guaiacolsulfonate has been used as an expectorant in bronchitis and as an intestinal antiseptic in doses of 0.5 to 1 g.

Proprietary Names

Broncovanil *(Scharper, Ital.)*; Silborina *(Bucaneve, Ital.)*.

2023-j

Primula Rhizome. Primelwurzel; Racine de Primevére; Schlüsselblumenwurzel.

Pharmacopoeias. In *Aust.*, *Cz.*, *Ger.*, *Jug.*, *Pol.*, and *Roum.* which specify *P. veris* and *P. elatior*. *Hung.* specifies *P. veris* and *P. vulgaris*.

The dried rhizome and roots of the cowslip, *Primula veris* (= *P. officinalis*), the oxlip, *P. elatior*, and the primrose, *P. vulgaris* (Primulaceae) containing saponins.

Primula rhizome has been used similarly to senega root as an expectorant.

2024-z

Saponaria. Soapwort; Bouncing Bet; Fuller's Herb.

Pharmacopoeias. In *Pol.*, *Port.*, *Roum.*, and *Span.* Saponariae Albae Radix (*Hung. P.*) is from *Gypsophila paniculata* (Caryophyllaceae) (Maiden's Breath) and is used as a tincture. Saponaria (*Roum. P.*) is from *S. officinalis* or *G. paniculata*.

The dried root of *Saponaria officinalis* (Caryophyllaceae).

The action of saponaria is attributed to its saponin constituents. It has been used as an expectorant and diuretic, usually as a decoction or infusion. *Pol. P.* includes a tincture.

2025-c

Senega Root *(B.P.)*. Senega; Seneca Snakeroot; Rattlesnake Root; Polygala.

CAS — 1260-04-4 (polygalic acid).

Pharmacopoeias. In *Arg.*, *Aust.*, *Belg.*, *Br.*, *It.*, *Jap.*, *Mex.*, *Nord.*, *Port.*, *Span.*, and *Swiss*. *Br.* also describes Powdered Senega Root.

Polygala (*Jap. P.*) is the dried root of *Polygala tenuifolia* (= *P. sibirica*) and Chinensis, Chinensis Root or Indian Senega, is the dried root of *P. chinensis*; they are used for the same purposes as senega.

The dried root and root crown of *Polygala senega* or certain closely related species of *Polygala* or a mixture of these. It contains not less than 29% of alcohol (60%)-soluble extractive. **Protect** from light.

Uses. Senega root contains 2 glycosidal saponins, senegin and polygalic acid, which are not absorbed but are reported to irritate the gastric mucosa and give rise to the reflex secretion of mucus in the bronchioles. It is employed, usually with other expectorants, in the treatment of chronic bronchitis. It has been used in doses of 2.5 to 5 ml of the concentrated infusion, or 0.3 to 1 ml of the liquid extract.

Preparations

Concentrated Senega Infusion *(B.P.)*. Conc. Senega Inf. 1 in 2; prepared by percolation with alcohol (25%) and made faintly alkaline by the addition of dilute ammonia solution.

Senega Infusion is prepared by diluting 1 vol. of this concentrated infusion to 10 vol. with water.

Infusum Polygalae

Senega root, bruised, 2 g, boiling water to 100 ml. Infuse for 20 minutes, filter, and adjust to volume.

Senega and Ammonia Mixture *(A.P.F.)*. See p.686.

Senega Liquid Extract *(B.P.)*. Senega Liq. Ext. 1 in 1; prepared by percolation with alcohol (60%) and made faintly alkaline with dilute ammonia solution.

A similar preparation is included in several pharmacopoeias.

Senega Syrup *(Jap. P.)*. Senega root 4 g, alcohol (10%) to 50 ml, sucrose 78 g, water to 100 ml. Prepared by macerating the senega in the dilute alcohol, filtering, and dissolving the sucrose in the filtrate. *Dose*. 1.5 to 3 ml.

Senega Tincture *(B.P.C. 1973)*. Senega liquid extract 20 ml, alcohol (60%) to 100 ml. *Dose*. 2.5 to 5 ml.

Sirupus Polygalae *(Belg. P.)*. Liquid extract of senega 5 g, syrup 95 g.

2026-k

Squill *(B.P.)*. Scilla; White Squill; Scillae Bulbus; Cebolla Albarrana; Scille; Meerzwiebel; Bulbo de Escila; Cila.

Pharmacopoeias. In *Arg.*, *Br.*, *Ger.*, *Port.*, *Span.*, and *Swiss*. *Br.* also describes Powdered Squill.

The dried sliced bulb of the white or Mediterranean squill *Drimia maritima* (=*Urginea maritima, U. scilla*) (Liliaceae), with the membranous outer scales removed, and containing not less than 68% of alcohol (60%)-soluble extractive. It contains scillarin A and scillarin B, both of which are active; the former is a pure crystalline glycoside, the latter a mixture of glycosides.

Store at a temperature not exceeding 25° in a dry place. Powdered squill is very hygroscopic and should be stored in a desiccated atmosphere.

Adverse Effects. These include nausea and vomiting. Violent purging has been reported. It has a digitalis-like action on the heart. When given intravenously 800 µg of squill total glycosides is claimed to be equivalent in potency to digitoxin 900 µg.

Treatment of Adverse Effects. Empty the stomach if necessary by aspiration and lavage. Cardiac irregularities should be treated as described under Digoxin, p.532.

Precautions. Squill should not be given to patients with impaired renal function. Its use is inadvisable in patients with cardiac disorders.

Uses. Squill has an irritant effect on the gastric mucosa and is used for its reflex expectorant action. It has been given in doses of 60 to 200 mg, as the oxymel, elixir, tincture, or vinegar.

It was recommended by the Food Additives and Contaminants Committee that squill be prohibited for use in foods as a flavouring agent.— *Report on the Review of Flavourings in Food*, FAC/REP/22, Minist. Agric. Fish. Fd, London, HM Stationery Office, 1976.

Rat poison. During a campaign in Alexandria to poison rats in order to eradicate plague-carrying fleas, the most effective preparation was the following tallow bait: white squill 60 g, flour 180 g, tallow 60 g, common salt 500 mg. The ingredients were well mixed with sufficient water and provided enough for 300 baits.— A. G. Hussein, *Bull. Wld Hlth Org.*, 1955, *13*, 27.

Preparations

Squill Elixir *(B.P.)*. Squill Syrup; Syr. Scill. Squill vinegar 45 ml, sucrose 80 g, water to 100 ml.

Squill Liquid Extract *(B.P.)*. Squill Liq. Ext.; Ext. Scill. Liq. 1 in 1; prepared by percolation with alcohol (70%).

Squill Oxymel *(B.P.)*. Oxymel Scill.; Oxymel of Squill. Contains the equivalent of about 5% of squill or Indian squill in acetic acid, purified honey, and water.

Squill Tincture *(B.P.)*. Tinct. Scill. 1 in 10; prepared by maceration with alcohol (60%).

A similar tincture is included in several pharmacopoeias.

Squill Vinegar *(B.P.)*. Vinegar of Squill; Acetum Scillae. 1 in 10; prepared by maceration of squill or Indian squill with (6 per cent) acetic acid.

A preparation containing squill syrup was formerly marketed in Great Britain under the proprietary name Sedatussin (*Lilly*).

2027-a

Indian Squill *(B.P.)*. Urginea.

Pharmacopoeias. In *Br.* and *Ind.*

The bulb of *Drimia indica* (=*Urginea indica*) (Liliaceae), with the outer membranous scales removed, usually sliced and dried, and containing about 20 to 50% of alcohol (60%)-soluble extractive. It contains cardiac glycosides similar to those in squill and about 35 to 40% of mucilage. **Store** at a temperature not exceeding 25° in a dry place. The powdered form is hygroscopic and should be stored in a desiccated atmosphere. The *B.P.* permits the use of Indian squill in place of squill for the preparation of Squill Oxymel and Squill Vinegar.

Indian squill has the actions and uses of Squill (see p.692).

From a comparison of the potencies in *guinea pigs* of tinctures prepared from European and from Indian squill there was considered to be little possibility of overdosage with cardiac glycosides from the normal use of Indian squill.— F. S. Hakim *et al.* (letter), *J. Pharm. Pharmac.*, 1976, *28*, 81.

2028-t

Red Squill

CAS — 507-60-8 (scilliroside).

A red variety of *Urginea maritima*, which contains, in addition to cardiac glycosides, an active principle, scilliroside.

Red squill is very toxic to rats and is incorporated in rat pastes; it acts on the central nervous system. Its use as a poison is prohibited in the UK by the Animals (Cruel Poisons) Regulations 1963 (SI 1963: No. 1278).

Red squill was not considered acceptable to animals other than rodents, but poisoning was reported to have occurred in *cattle, sheep, chickens,* and *dogs.* Since it was extremely irritating to the skin it should be handled with rubber gloves. The Committee endorsed its use from the standpoint of safety.— Safe Use of Pesticides, Twentieth Report of the WHO Expert Committee on Insecticides, *Tech. Rep. Ser. Wld Hlth Org. No. 513*, 1973.

2029-x

Terpin Hydrate *(U.S.P., B.P.C. 1968)*.

Terpene Hydrate; Terpine; Terpinol. *p*-Menthane-1,8-diol monohydrate; 4-Hydroxy-α,α,4-trimethylcyclohexanemethanol monohydrate.

$C_{10}H_{20}O_2,H_2O=190.3$.

CAS — 80-53-5 (anhydrous); 2451-01-6 (monohydrate).

Pharmacopoeias. In *Arg., Belg., Hung., Ind., It., Mex., Port., Roum., Rus., Span., Swiss,* and *U.S.*

Colourless glistening crystals or white powder with a slightly aromatic but not terebinthinate odour and a somewhat bitter taste. M.p. after drying about 103°. It effloresces in dry air. **Soluble** 1 in 200 of water, 1 in 35 of boiling water, 1 in 13 of alcohol, 1 in 3 of boiling alcohol, 1 in 140 of chloroform, and 1 in 140 of ether; soluble in glycerol and volatile oils. A 1% solution in hot water is neutral to litmus. **Store** in airtight containers.

Adverse Effects. Epigastric pain may follow the ingestion of terpin hydrate on an empty stomach.

Terpin hydrate given with codeine was considered to have caused liver damage.— D. Faierman and S. Jacobs, *Mt Sinai J. Med.*, 1973, *40*, 56.

Uses. Terpin hydrate has been stated to increase bronchial secretion directly and to assist expectoration. It is given in doses of 125 to 300 mg every 6 hours but doses of up to 600 mg have been used.

For a review of terpin hydrate including an evaluation of its toxicity and of its status as an expectorant, together with some suggested formulas for elixirs, see E. D. Sumner, *J. Am. pharm. Ass.*, 1968, *8*, 250.

Preparations

Terpin Hydrate and Codeine Elixir *(U.S.P.)*. Codeine 10 mg, terpin hydrate elixir to 5 ml. Store in airtight containers.

Terpin Hydrate and Dextromethorphan Hydrobromide Elixir *(U.S.P.)*. Dextromethorphan hydrobromide 10 mg, terpin hydrate elixir to 5 ml. Store in airtight containers.

Terpin Hydrate Elixir *(U.S.P.)*. Terpin hydrate 85 mg, glycerol 2 ml, syrup 0.5 ml, alcohol 2.15 ml, benzaldehyde 0.00025 ml, sweet orange peel tincture 0.1 ml (or orange oil 0.005 ml dissolved in alcohol 0.075 ml), water to 5 ml. Store in airtight containers.

Proprietary Preparations

Coterpin *(Ayrton, Saunders, UK)*. An elixir containing in each 5 ml terpin hydrate 30 mg, codeine phosphate 15 mg, menthol 8 mg, pumilio pine oil 0.0025 ml, cineole 0.004 ml, and glycerol 1.7 ml. For cough. *Dose.* 5 to 10 ml with water.

Tercoda *(Sinclair, UK)*. An elixir containing in each 5 ml terpin hydrate 8 mg, codeine phosphate 8 mg, cineole 0.02 ml, and menthol 4 mg. *Dose.* 5 to 10 ml in a little water.

Terpalin *(Norton, UK: Vestric, UK)*. An antitussive elixir containing in each 5 ml terpin hydrate 6.5 mg, codeine phosphate 13 mg, cineole 0.002 ml, and menthol 1.5 mg. *Dose.* 5 to 10 ml thrice daily; children, 2.5 to 5 ml.

Terpoin *(Hough, Hoseason, UK)*. Contains in each 5 ml terpin hydrate 9.15 mg, guaiphenesin 50 mg, cineole 4.15 mg, codeine phosphate 18.3 mg, and menthol 18.3 mg. *Dose.* 5 to 10 ml every 3 hours if necessary.

Fixed Oils

7350-d

Fats and fixed oils of vegetable origin consist mainly of triglycerides (fatty acid esters of glycerol), which may be simple triglycerides, in which the 3 hydroxyl groups of glycerol are esterified with the same acid, or mixed triglycerides, in which 2 or 3 different acids may be present. The term fixed is used to describe the nonvolatile nature of these oils. The triglycerides of fats are mainly solids at ordinary temperatures and are chiefly composed of saturated fatty acid esters. The triglycerides of fixed oils are mainly liquids at ordinary temperatures and are chiefly composed of unsaturated fatty acid esters.

When taken in the diet fixed oils provide 38 kJ (9 kcal) per g. For further information on the use of oils as a source of energy, see the section on Amino Acids and Nutritional Agents, p.47.

Medium-chain Triglycerides are described under Fractionated Coconut Oil, p.696.

Fixed oils are liable to become rancid, a change which may arise as a result of several different types of chemical reaction, including hydrolysis of the glycerides, oxidation of saturated fatty acids to ketones, and oxidation at double bonds of unsaturated fatty acids. Antoxidants are described on p.1281.

Several pharmacopoeias include a vegetable oil for injection. In some the oil is specified and is frequently arachis oil; castor oil and sesame oil are also used. Fixed oils not included in this section are described under the compounds from which they are manufactured.

Coronary heart disease. A critical appraisal of evidence for the role of diet in coronary heart disease.— G. V. Mann, *New Engl. J. Med.*, 1977, *297*, 644. Criticisms.— W. J. Walker (letter), *ibid.*, 1978, *298*, 106; T. M. Vogt (letter), *ibid.*, 107; M. W. Hinds (letter), *ibid.*; N. J. Stone (letter), *ibid.* Reply.— G. V. Mann (letter), *ibid.*, 108. Further criticisms.— P. Leren (letter), *ibid.*; C. S. Vil *et al.* (letter), *ibid.*, 109.

Intravenous emulsions. Intravenous emulsions are discussed under Cottonseed Oil (p.696), Soya Oil (p.698), and Amino Acids and Nutritional Agents (p.48).

Malabsorption of fats. For the use of medium-chain triglycerides in the treatment of conditions associated with malabsorption of fat, see Fractionated Coconut Oil, p.696.

Unsaturated Fatty Acids

Unsaturated fatty acids occur in large amounts in the oils and fats of certain seeds, such as linseed and maize, and in some animal fats. The name *Vitamin F* has been applied to a mixture of unsaturated fatty acids, including linoleic, linolenic, and arachidonic acids, which have been found essential for the growth of *rats*, and may be essential for man.

Unsaturated fatty acids and oils containing a high proportion of them have been given to lower blood-cholesterol and lipid concentrations in patients with hypercholesterolaemia. The relationship between hypercholesterolaemia and atherosclerosis and the value of treatment in atherosclerosis or coronary heart disease is the subject of much investigation. The relationship between unsaturated fatty acids, particularly linoleic acid, and multiple sclerosis is also under investigation.

For further information on the treatment of hyperlipidaemia, see under Clofibrate and other Lipid Regulating Agents, p.408.

Unsaturated fatty acids are sometimes given by mouth or applied externally in eczema and other skin diseases.

Serum-cholesterol concentrations were reduced in 5 of 6 healthy subjects, plasma-triglyceride concentrations reduced in 3, and faecal excretion of sterols reduced in all 6 when they received a diet containing fats enriched with linoleic acid from animals fed on unsaturated seed oils compared with a control diet of unsaturated fats.— P. J. Nestel *et al.*, *New Engl. J. Med.*, 1973, *288*, 379.

Replacement of the normal saturated fatty acids in the diet of 19 men with polyunsaturated fatty acids (mainly linoleic acid) altered platelet-function tests suggesting reduced platelet activation when compared with 20 control men.— J. R. O'Brien *et al.*, *Lancet*, 1976, *2*, 995.

As a preparation of linoleic and linolenic acids (Naudicelle) had an immunosuppressive effect on lymphocytes *in vitro* it was tried in patients with rheumatoid arthritis. Preliminary results of a pilot study showed that the preparation in a dose of 2.1 g daily might be beneficial, although any benefit was not obvious until after 3 months' treatment.— J. N. McCormick *et al.* (letter), *Lancet*, 1977, *2*, 508.

Coronary heart disease. For a review of dietary fat content in relation to coronary heart disease, see R. W. D. Turner, *Practitioner*, 1979, *222*, 601.

Changing the diet in a long-stay institution in Helsinki so that for 6 years dairy fat was replaced by vegetable fat (mainly soya oil) was not associated with any significant difference for intra-hospital comparison in the number of coronary deaths. However, the incidence of major ECG changes was lower than in patients on normal diets.— I. Turpeinin *et al.*, *Int. J. Epidemiol.*, 1979, *8*, 99, per *Lancet*, 1979, *2*, 919.

A study on diet and death-rates in 7 countries did not prove that saturated fatty acids in the diet caused increased mortality, but findings were consistent with the hypothesis that risk of early death is increased by diet saturates in populations in which coronary disease is a major death cause.— A. Keys *et al.*, *Lancet*, 1981, *2*, 58.

Multiple sclerosis. The possible benefit of γ-linolenate given as Naudicelle in multiple sclerosis.— H. J. Meyer-Rienecker *et al.* (letter), *Lancet*, 1976, *2*, 966.

A discussion on the relevance of fatty acids in multiple sclerosis.— J. Mertin and C. J. Meade, *Br. med. Bull.*, 1977, *33*, 67. An account of the treatment and management of multiple sclerosis with reference to dietary fats.— L. A. Liversedge, *ibid.*, 78.

In a double-blind study in 152 patients with chronic progressive multiple sclerosis there was no evidence that linoleic acid or linoleic acid with linolenic acid (Naudicelle) provided any greater benefit than control treatment with oleic acid.— D. Bates *et al.*, *Br. med. J.*, 1977, *2*, 932. Criticism of statements regarding the biochemistry.— H. Sinclair (letter), *ibid.*, 1217.

γ-Linolenate (in Naudicelle) could be used to treat active cases of multiple sclerosis with recurrent episodes and patients with a first sign or symptom of multiple sclerosis. It might be of value if given prophylactically to children born into families showing a susceptibility to multiple sclerosis.— E. J. Field (letter), *Lancet*, 1978, *1*, 780.

In a double-blind study the 'attack score' (measuring severity and intensity of attacks) in 29 patients with acute remitting multiple sclerosis, given linoleic acid 23 g daily for 2 years as a spread, was significantly lower than in 29 controls. There was no reduction in the frequency of attacks in 29 further patients given linoleic acid 2.92 g and γ-linolenic acid 340 mg daily (as 8 capsules of Naudicelle); the number of patients who deteriorated was significantly higher than in a control group.— D. Bates *et al.*, *Br. med. J.*, 1978, *2*, 1390. Comments.— E. J. Field (letter), *ibid.*, 1979, *1*, 411; A. G. Hassam and M. A. Crawford (letter), *ibid.* Reply.— D. Bates *et al.* (letter), *ibid.*, 683.

Failure of linoleic acid to show therapeutic benefit in multiple sclerosis.— D. W. Paty *et al.*, *Acta neurol. scand.*, 1978, *58*, 53.

Naudicelle capsules contained tartrazine which blocked the conversion of polyunsaturated fatty acids to prostaglandins. Preliminary study had shown some good results in patients treated with evening primrose oil without tartrazine, especially when given with colchicine.— D. F. Horrobin *et al.* (letter), *Br. med. J.*, 1979, *1*, 199. Naudicelle capsules no longer contained tartrazine.— *ibid.*, 417.

Further references: *Lancet*, 1979, *2*, 131; R. H. Dworkin (letter), *ibid.*, 1981, *1*, 1153.

Proprietary Preparations of Unsaturated Fatty Acids

Efamol *(Agricultural Holdings, UK: Britannia Health, UK).* Capsules each stated to contain 500 mg of evening primrose oil (from *Oenothera biennis* or other spp.) and stated to include γ-linolenic acid 45 mg with vitamin E 10 mg or capsules each stated to contain 250 mg of evening primrose oil, safflower oil 200 mg, linseed oil 50 mg, and vitamin E 10 mg.

A modest but significant improvement in patients with atopic eczema given Efamol, 4 capsules twice daily; children were given half the adult dose.— C. R. Lovell *et al.* (letter), *Lancet*, 1981, *1*, 278.

Esoban Barrier Cream *(Southon-Horton, UK).* Contains unsaturated fatty acids of the linoleic-linolenic group and hexachlorophane 0.25%. For protection of the skin against acids, alkalis, suds, formaldehyde, and phenolic and urea resins.

Evening Primrose Oil Capsules *(Evening Primrose Oil Co., UK).* Capsules each containing 250 or 500 mg of evening primrose oil (from *Oenothera biennis* or other spp.), stated to contain γ-linolenic acid 8.3%.

Naudicelle (known in some countries as Preglandin) *(Bio-Oil Research, UK).* Capsules of evening primrose oil 0.6 ml each containing triglyceride esters of linoleic acid 70% and γ-linolenic acid 7%.

Syngran *(Keimdiät, Ger.: Thomson & Joseph, UK).* Consists of the ethyl esters of linoleic and other unsaturated fatty acids. For use in dermatological and cosmetic preparations. **Syngran-W** is a similar water-soluble preparation.

A preparation containing unsaturated fatty acids derived from cod-liver oil was formerly marketed in Great Britain under the proprietary name Rowaskleron (*Rowa, Eire*).

7352-h

Almond Oil *(B.P., U.S.N.F.).* Oleum Amygdalae; Ol. Amygdal.; Expressed Almond Oil; Sweet Almond Oil; Huile d'Amande; Mandelöl; Aceite de Almendra.

CAS — 8007-69-0.

Pharmacopoeias. In *Arg., Belg., Br., Port., Rus., Span.*, and *Swiss* which specify *Prunus dulcis* var. *dulcis* or var. *amara. Fr., It.*, and *Mex.* specify oil from *Prunus dulcis* var. *dulcis. Aust.* specifies oil from *Prunus dulcis* var. *amara* or var. *communis* (=var. *sativa*). *U.S.N.F.* specifies oil from varieties of *Prunus dulcis*.
Fr. also specifies Huile de Noyaux, an oil obtained from various species of *Prunus*.

A pale yellow oil with a slight characteristic odour and a bland nutty taste, consisting of glycerides chiefly of oleic acid, with smaller amounts of linoleic, myristic, and palmitic acids. It is expressed, without the application of heat, from the seeds of the bitter or the sweet almond, *Prunus dulcis (Prunus amygdalis; Amygdalis communis)* var. *amara* or var. *dulcis* (Rosaceae). Almond oil remains clear at −10° for 3 hours; f.p. about −18°.

Practically **insoluble** in alcohol; miscible with chloroform, ether, and light petroleum. Wt per ml 0.912 to 0.916 g. It is **sterilised** by maintaining at 150° for 1 hour. **Store** in a cool place in well-filled airtight containers. Protect from light.

Uses. Almond oil is nutritive and demulcent and may be administered in the form of an emulsion. The usual dose is 15 to 30 ml. Externally, it is applied as an emollient for chapped hands. It is sometimes used in the preparation of cold creams, brilliantines, hair lotions, and other toilet articles. It is also employed as a solvent in Oily Phenol Injection, used in the treatment of haemorrhoids.

Preparations

Emulsio Oleoso-Saccharata *(Swiss P.).* Emulsion d'Huile d'Amande Sucrée. Almond oil 10 g, acacia 10 g, orange-flower water 10 g, syrup 15 g, water 55 g.

7353-m

Arachis Oil *(B.P.).* Oleum Arachidis; Oleum Arachis; Ol. Arach.; Ground-nut Oil; Nut Oil; Peanut Oil *(U.S.N.F.)*; Earth-nut Oil; Huile d'Arachide; Erdnussöl; Óleo de Amendoim.

CAS — 8002-03-7.

Pharmacopoeias. In *Arg., Aust., Belg., Br., Cz., Fr., Ger., Ind., Int., It., Jap., Mex., Nord., Pol., Port.,* and *Swiss.* Also in *U.S.N.F.* (Peanut Oil) which specifies oil from the seed kernels of one or more of the cultivated varieties of *A. hypogaea.*
Fr. and *Pol.* also have arachis oil for injection.

The refined fixed oil obtained from the seeds of *Arachis hypogaea* (Leguminosae). It is a pale yellow oil with a faint nutty odour and a bland nutty taste consisting of glycerides, chiefly of oleic and linoleic acids, with smaller amounts of other acids. Wt per ml 0.909 to 0.916 g. It becomes cloudy at about 3° and partly solidifies at lower temperatures.
The unrefined oil may sometimes contain toxic substances.
Practically **insoluble** in alcohol; miscible with carbon disulphide, chloroform, ether, and light petroleum. It is **sterilised** by maintaining at 150° for 1 hour. On exposure to air it thickens very slowly and may become rancid. **Store** at a temperature not exceeding 40° in well-filled airtight containers. Protect from light. If it has solidified, it should be completely melted and mixed before use.

Aflatoxin was not detected in samples of refined arachis oil tested, but 5 out of 16 samples of crude ground-nut oil contained aflatoxin B1; aflatoxin G1 was also found.— Y. H. Chong and C. G. Beng, *Med. J. Malaya,* 1965, *20,* 49, per *Bull. Hyg., Lond.,* 1966, *41,* 631.

Sterilisation. Owing to the comparative resistance to heat of *Bacillus cereus, B. licheniformis,* and *B. subtilis* in arachis oil, maize oil, and sesame oil, a time and temperature study was made. Results showed that heating at 170° for 2 hours was realistic for sterilisation of injections using arachis, maize, or sesame oils, whereas heating at 150° for 1 hour was inadequate. There was also evidence that oils which contained fatty acid chains of low molecular weight required less heat for sterilisation.— D. Pasquale *et al., Bull. parent. Drug Ass.,* 1964, *18,* 1.

Uses. Arachis oil has properties similar to those of olive oil (see p.697) and is used for the same purposes. Emulsions containing arachis oil and dextrose have been administered by continuous intragastric infusion as part of a nitrogen-free diet. It has been used in drops for softening ear wax.

The seed membrane of *Arachis hypogaea* was reputed to contain a haemostatic principle; controlled trials failed to show any subjective or objective effect in patients with haemophilia.— M. Verstraete, *Haemostatic Drugs,* The Hague, Martinus Nijhoff, 1977, p. 145.

Proprietary Preparations

Fletchers' Arachis Oil Retention Enema *(Pharmax, UK).* Arachis oil 130 ml in a plastic bag fitted with a rectal tube.

Cerumol (known in Switz., and formerly also marketed in Great Britain, as Cerumenol) *(Laboratories for Applied Biology, UK).* Ear-drops containing turpentine oil 10%, paradichlorobenzene 2%, and chlorbutol 5%, in arachis oil. For the removal of wax from the ear.

Cerumol, Dioctyl Ear Capsules, olive oil, Waxsol, and Xerumenex were compared with Sodium Bicarbonate Ear-drops in 124 geriatric patients with bilateral impacted hard wax. Ears in which Cerumol, olive oil, or Waxsol had been used were easier to syringe than those in which Sodium Bicarbonate Ear-drops had been used, but syringing was more difficult when Dioctyl Ear Capsules or Xerumenex had been used. Cerumol was significantly more effective than Sodium Bicarbonate Ear-drops but a significant difference between Cerumol and olive oil or Waxsol could not be demonstrated.— J. G. Fraser, *J. Lar. Otol.,* 1970, *84,* 1055.

For a comparison of Cerumol and Waxsol for softening wax in the ear, see under Docusate Sodium, p.1441.

Oilatum Cream *(Stiefel, UK).* Contains arachis oil 21% and povidone 1% in an oil-in-water emulsion basis. An emollient for dry skin.

Oilatum Soap *(Stiefel, UK).* A skin cleanser containing unsaponified arachis oil 7.5% and salts of higher molecular weight fatty acids. For use in place of ordinary soaps in dry skin disorders.

Prosparol *(Duncan, Flockhart, UK).* An emulsion containing arachis oil 50%, glyceryl monostearate 3%, polysorbate '60' 1%, sodium benzoate 0.1%, and butylated hydroxyanisole 0.01%. A food of high energy value (providing 19MJ per litre) for administration by mouth or by nasogastric tube and for use as a fatty meal during cholecystography.

X-Vac *(Forrest, Austral.: Schering, UK).* Arachis oil, available as emulsion containing 0.25%. For inducing contraction of the gall-bladder during cholangiography.

7354-b

Hydrogenated Arachis Oil.

Oleum Arachidis Hydrogenatum; Gehärtetes Erdnussöl.

Pharmacopoeias. In *Aust.* and *Swiss.*

An almost white soft fat which is transparent in layers of 1 cm when melted. M.p. 37° to 42°. Five parts take up 1 part of water.
Slightly **soluble** in dehydrated alcohol; readily soluble in chloroform, ether, and light petroleum. **Store** in airtight containers. Protect from light.

Hydrogenated arachis oil is used in the preparation of fatty ointments.

7355-v

Castor Oil *(B.P., Eur. P., B.P. Vet., U.S.P.).*

Oleum Ricini; Ricini Oleum; Ol. Ricin.; Huile de Ricin; Rizinusöl; Aceite de Ricino.

CAS — 8001-79-4.

Pharmacopoeias. In all pharmacopoeias examined except *Braz. Fr.* also describes the seed.

The fixed oil expressed, without the application of heat, from the seeds of *Ricinus communis* (Euphorbiaceae), containing about 80% of the triglyceride of ricinoleic acid. It is a nearly colourless or slightly yellow transparent viscid oil with a slight odour and taste which is bland at first, but afterwards slightly acrid. Relative density 0.952 to 0.965. On cooling to 0° it remains clear, but congeals to a yellowish mass at −18°.
Soluble 1 in 2.5 of alcohol; miscible with dehydrated alcohol, chloroform, ether, carbon disulphide, and glacial acetic acid; miscible with one-half its vol. of light petroleum but only partially soluble in 2 vol. It is **sterilised** by maintaining at 150° for 1 hour. **Store** at a temperature not exceeding 40° in well-filled airtight containers. Protect from light.
When castor oil is intended for parenteral administration it must contain no added antoxidant. When, for other purposes, such addition is authorised, the name and quantity of the added antoxidant is stated on the label.

Basis for steroid hormones. The solubilities of hydroxyprogesterone hexanoate, oestradiol valerate, testosterone, and progesterone were higher in castor oil than in sesame or arachis oil. A series of injection formulas which contained hydroxyprogesterone hexanoate and oestradiol valerate were tested in *animal* and human subjects. Results showed that the most acceptable oil solvent was castor oil with a mixture of benzyl alcohol and benzyl benzoate. This gave prolonged action and was well tolerated.— C. Riffkin *et al., J. pharm. Sci.,* 1964, *53,* 891.

Adverse Effects. The administration of castor oil by mouth, particularly in large doses, may produce nausea, vomiting, colic, and severe purgation.
The seeds of *Ricinus communis* contain a toxic protein, ricin (see p.1751).

Hypersensitivity to castor oil seeds. A woman who had worn a necklace which included the seeds of *Ricinus communis* experienced a severe allergic reaction when a seed was broken. Two earlier mild episodes, and pruritus of the neck, were believed to have been caused by the necklace.— S. D. Lockey and L. Dunkelberger (letter), *J. Am. med. Ass.,* 1968, *206,* 2900. See also R. Wolfromm *et al., Presse méd.,* 1967, *75,* 2157.

Precautions. Castor oil should be used with caution during pregnancy or menstruation. It should not be used when abdominal pain, intestinal obstruction, nausea, or vomiting is present.
Castor oil given in doses that exert a laxative effect may inhibit the absorption of fat-soluble vitamins.

Castor oil in doses that exert a laxative effect is reported to inhibit the absorption of fat-soluble vitamins, notably vitamin A and vitamin D. Doses of up to 4 g do not appear to affect absorption in adults and the Committee considered this to be the no-effect value.— Twenty-third Report of Joint FAO/WHO Expert Committee on Food Additives, *Tech. Rep. Ser. Wld Hlth Org. No. 648,* 1980.

Uses. Castor oil is a purgative acting on the small intestine. It takes effect in 2 to 8 hours. It is best administered in milk or fruit juice, in capsules, or as an emulsion.
It is given in doses of about 15 ml to empty the bowel and remove flatus before X-ray examination but other purgatives are often preferred.
Castor oil is a soothing application to the conjunctiva and allays irritation due to foreign bodies in the eye, and it has been employed for making solutions of alkaloidal bases for ophthalmic purposes.
Castor oil is used externally for its emollient effect and is employed in such preparations as Zinc and Castor Oil Ointment. Castor oil may be employed as the solvent in some injections and is often used as an ingredient of spirituous hair lotions.

Use in food. The Food Additives and Contaminants Committee recommended that castor oil be permitted for use as a solvent in food and recommended a maximum concentration of ricin in food as consumed of 1 ppm.— *Report on the Review of Solvents in Food,* FAC/REP/25, Ministry of Agriculture, Fisheries and Food, London, HM Stationery Office, 1978.

Estimated acceptable daily intake of castor oil: up to 700 µg per kg body-weight.— Twenty-third Report of Joint FAO/WHO Expert Committee on Food Additives, *Tech. Rep. Ser. Wld Hlth Org. No. 648,* 1980.

Preparations

Aromatic Castor Oil *(U.S.P.).* Cinnamon oil *(U.S.N.F.)* 0.3 ml, clove oil 0.1 ml, saccharin 50 mg, vanillin 100 mg, alcohol 3 ml, castor oil to 100 ml. Store in airtight containers.

Castor Oil Capsules *(U.S.P.).* Capsules containing castor oil. Store at 15° to 30° in airtight containers.

Castor Oil Emulsion. Castor oil 36 g, vanillin 20 mg, saccharin calcium 130 mg, sodium metabisulphite 100 mg, sodium benzoate 100 mg, citric acid monohydrate 50 mg, methylcellulose '4000' 750 mg, methyl salicylate 0.13 ml, water to 100 ml. The methylcellulose and methyl salicylate were mixed in the castor oil; the remaining ingredients were dissolved in water and added slowly to the oils, then homogenised.—G.E. Schumacher, *Am. J. Hosp. Pharm.,* 1967, *24,* 143.

Proprietary Preparations

Minims Castor Oil *(Smith & Nephew Pharmaceuticals, UK).* Sterile eye-drops containing castor oil in single-dose disposable applicators.
NOTE. The code CAS OIL is permitted in Great Britain for single-dose eye-drops of castor oil.

Other Proprietary Names

Laxopol *(Ger.)*; Neoloid *(USA)*; Ricifruit, Unisoil *(both Canad.)*; Wonderolie *(Neth.).*

7356-g

Hydrogenated Castor Oil *(U.S.N.F.).*

CAS — 8001-78-3.

Pharmacopoeias. In *U.S.N.F.*

Refined, bleached, hydrogenated, and deodorised castor oil consisting mainly of the triglyceride of hydroxystearic acid. It is a white crystalline wax. M.p. 85° to 88°. Practically **insoluble** in water and most common organic solvents. **Store** at a temperature not exceeding 40° in airtight containers.

Hydrogenated castor oil is used as a stiffening agent.

7357-q

Fractionated Coconut Oil *(B.P.).* Thin Vegetable Oil.

Pharmacopoeias. In *Br. Ger.* has a similar preparation (Triglycerida mediocatenalia) obtained from vegetable oils.

It is prepared from the fixed oil obtained from the dried solid part of the endosperm of the coconut, the fruit of *Cocos nucifera* (Palmae), by hydrolysis, fractionation of the liberated fatty acids and re-esterification. It consists of a mixture of triglycerides containing only short- and medium-chain saturated fatty acids, mainly octanoic and decanoic acids.

It is a clear pale yellow odourless or almost odourless liquid with a characteristic taste. It solidifies at about 0°, and has a low viscosity even at temperatures near its solidification point. Wt per ml 0.94 to 0.95 g.

Practically **insoluble** in water; miscible with alcohol, chloroform, and ether. It is **sterilised** by maintaining at 150° for 1 hour. **Store** at a temperature not exceeding 25° in well-filled airtight containers. Protect from light.

NOTE. Coconut oil is described in the section on Paraffins and Similar Bases, p.1066.

Adverse Effects and Precautions. Abdominal pain and diarrhoea have been reported in patients taking diets based on medium-chain triglycerides.

Patients with cirrhosis of the liver have impaired hepatic clearance of fatty acids and administration of large quantities of medium-chain triglycerides may lead to increased blood and spinal fluid concentrations of fatty acids and to hepatic coma.

In 21 patients with cirrhosis of the liver given coconut oil 60 ml as a single dose or 30 ml twice daily for from 1 week to 6 months, there was no evidence of significant changes in the EEG nor of clinical deterioration.— M. H. Morgan *et al.*, *Gut*, 1974, *15*, 180.

Uses. Fractionated coconut oil has been used as a basis for the preparation of oral suspensions of drugs unstable in aqueous media.

Fractionated coconut oil is used as a source of medium-chain triglycerides. Diets based on medium-chain triglycerides are used in conditions associated with malabsorption of fat, such as cystic fibrosis, enteritis, and steatorrhoea, and following intestinal resection. Medium-chain triglycerides are more readily hydrolysed than long-chain triglycerides and are not dependent upon biliary or pancreatic secretions for absorption from the gastro-intestinal tract. They provide 35 kJ (8.3 kcal) per g.

A discussion of the clinical uses of medium-chain triglycerides.— D. C. Ruppin and W. R. J. Middleton, *Drugs*, 1980, *20*, 216.

In 11 infants with cystic fibrosis, the frequency, bulk, and offensiveness of stools was reduced during treatment with a diet based on medium-chain triglycerides.— M. Gracey *et al.*, *Archs Dis. Childh.*, 1969, *44*, 401.

Medium-chain triglycerides were ineffective in 14 patients with decompensated extrahepatic biliary atresia with irreversible growth failure.— C. C. Roy and A. Weber (letter), *J. Pediat.*, 1972, *80*, 528.

Replacement of part of the dietary fat by medium-chain triglycerides (Portagen) and addition of cholestyramine, 4 g thrice daily, caused a marked reduction in the number of stools in 10 of 11 patients and in the amount of fat excreted daily in 4 of these who had developed diarrhoea and steatorrhoea after abdominal surgery. Substitution of long-chain by medium-chain triglycerides caused a similar reduction in steatorrhoea in 4 patients restudied after 4 to 11 months.— C. N. Williams and R. C. Dickson, *Can. med. Ass. J.*, 1972, *107*, 626.

Six children with intestinal lymphangiectasia were treated with a low-fat diet supplemented with medium-chain triglycerides for 3 to 8 years. Marked symptomatic relief was maintained as long as the diet was continued.— W. L. Tift and J. K. Lloyd, *Archs Dis. Childh.*, 1975, *50*, 269.

A study in 34 premature infants showed that there was a positive correlation between the absorption of fat and that of calcium and of magnesium and that the absorption of all 3 was improved when medium-chain triglycerides were present in the feeds. The correlation was stronger for calcium than for magnesium, and for both absorption was increased when the dietary content of the triglycerides was increased from 40% to 80%.— P. Tantibhedhyangkul and S. A. Hashim, *Pediatrics*, 1978, *61*, 537.

Further references to the use of medium-chain triglycerides: P. R. Holt, *Gastroenterology*, 1967, *53*, 961; N. J. Greenberger *et al.*, *Ann. intern. Med.*, 1967, *66*, 727; A. Feres *et al.*, *Am. J. dig. Dis.*, 1967, *12*, 65; B. J. Smits *et al.*, *Gut*, 1968, *9*, 28; F. X. Pi-Sunyer *et al.*, *Diabetes*, 1969, *18*, 96; M. Gracey *et al.*, *Archs Dis. Childh.*, 1970, *45*, 445; G. G. Graham *et al.*, *Am. J. Dis. Child.*, 1973, *126*, 330.

Proprietary Preparations of Fractionated Coconut Oil or Triglycerides from Medium-chain Fatty Acids

Alembicol D *(Alembic Products, UK).* A brand of Fractionated Coconut Oil.

Liquigen *(Scientific Hospital Supplies, UK).* An emulsion containing 52% of triglycerides from medium-chain fatty acids, mainly C_8 and C_{10} fatty acids. For use in fat malabsorption syndromes.

MCT Oil *(Bristol-Myers Pharmaceuticals, UK).* A mixture of triglycerides from medium-chain fatty acids, mainly C_8 and C_{10} fatty acids. For use in fat malabsorption syndromes. (Also available as MCT Oil in *Austral., USA*).

MCT Oil *(Scientific Hospital Supplies, UK).* A mixture of triglycerides from medium-chain fatty acids, mainly C_8 and C_{10} fatty acids. For use in fat malabsorption syndromes.

Medium Chain Triglyceride (MCT) Oil *(Cow & Gate, UK).* A mixture of triglycerides from straight-chain fatty acids, mainly C_8 and C_{10} fatty acids. For use in fat malabsorption syndromes.

Miglyols *(Dynamit Nobel, UK).* Triglycerides of medium-chain saturated fatty acids including linolenic acid. **Miglyol Gel** is Miglyol 812 gelled with an organically substituted montmorillonite. Solvents, stabilisers, and bases for pharmaceutical products.

Neobee *(PVO International, USA: Alfa, UK).* A range of emollient oils derived from triglycerides and propylene glycol diesters.

Wecobee *(PVO International, USA: Alfa, UK).* A range of triglycerides derived from edible vegetable oils, and claimed to have similar properties to theobroma oil.

7358-p

Cottonseed Oil *(U.S.N.F., B.P. 1968).* Oleum Gossypii Seminis; Ol. Gossyp. Sem.; Cotton Oil; Aceite de Algodon; Oléo de Algodoeiro.

CAS — 8001-29-4.

Pharmacopoeias. In *Arg.* and *Mex.* Also in *U.S.N.F.*

The refined fixed oil obtained by expression or solvent extraction from the seeds of the cotton plant, *Gossypium hirsutum*, and other cultivated species of *Gossypium* (Malvaceae).

It is a pale yellow or yellow, odourless or nearly odourless oil with a bland taste. Specific gravity 0.915 to 0.921.

Slightly **soluble** in alcohol; miscible with carbon disulphide, chloroform, ether, and light petroleum. It is **sterilised** by maintaining at 150° for 1 hour. **Store** at a temperature not exceeding 40° in well-filled airtight containers. Protect from light. At temperatures below 10° particles of solid fat may separate from the oil and at temperatures between 0° and −5° it congeals; the oil should be remelted and thoroughly mixed before any of it is used.

Adverse Effects. Reactions characterised by dyspnoea, cyanosis, myalgia, nausea, vomiting, headache, lumbar pains, flushing, and hypotension have been reported during the intravenous infusion of cottonseed oil emulsions.

Patients receiving fat emulsions over prolonged periods may exhibit the 'overload syndrome', manifested by bone-marrow depression, anaemia, thrombocytopenia, thrombotic episodes, jaundice, and persistent hyperlipidaemia. The effects are reversible on discontinuing the infusion.

A report of reversible fat embolism after repeated infusions of fat emulsions.— M. Goulon *et al.*, *Nouv. Presse méd.*, 1974, *3*, 13, per *Thérapie*, 1975, *30*, 381.

Uses. Cottonseed oil has properties similar to those of olive oil and is used for the same purposes. Emulsions containing 40% w/v of cottonseed oil are used in single doses of 60 ml as a high fat meal during cholecystography.

Emulsions containing 10 and 15% w/v of cottonseed oil have been given by slow intravenous infusion as a source of energy or when a nitrogen-free diet was required. Because of its high content of unsaturated fatty acids cottonseed oil has been used in the dietary control of hypercholesterolaemia.

An extract of cottonseed oil, gossypol (p.1714), is used as an antifertility agent in males.

Intravenous nutrition. *For details of the use and precautions of cottonseed oil in intravenous nutrition, see Martindale, 27th Edn,* p. 1032.

Proprietary Names

Neo-Cholex *(Horner, Canad.).*

Preparations containing cottonseed oil were formerly marketed in Great Britain under the proprietary name Lipiphysan (*Égic, Fr.: Servier*).

7359-s

Ethyl Oleate *(B.P.).* Ethylis Oleas; Aethylis Oleas. $C_{20}H_{38}O_2$=310.5.

CAS — 111-62-6.

Pharmacopoeias. In *Br., Fr., Ind., Int., It.,* and *Swiss.* Also in *U.S.N.F.*

An almost colourless or pale yellow oily mobile liquid with a slight but not rancid odour and with a taste somewhat resembling that of olive oil. It consists of the ethyl esters of oleic acid and related high molecular weight fatty acids. It may contain a suitable antoxidant. Practically **insoluble** in water; miscible with alcohol, chloroform, ether, fixed oils, liquid paraffin, and most other organic solvents. Wt per ml 0.869 to 0.874 g. It is **sterilised** by heating at 150° for 1 hour. Ethyl oleate dissolves some types of rubber and causes others to swell. It oxidises on exposure to air; the air in partially filled containers should be replaced by nitrogen or other suitable inert gas. **Store** in a cool place in small well-filled airtight containers or in an atmosphere of nitrogen. Protect from light.

Uses. Ethyl oleate has properties similar to those of almond and arachis oil but is less viscous and more rapidly absorbed by the tissues. It is used as a vehicle in oily injections and liniments.

7360-h

Linseed Oil *(B.P. 1963, B.P. Vet.).* Oleum Lini; Flaxseed Oil; Huile de Lin; Leinöl; Aceite de Linaza.

CAS — 8001-26-1.

Pharmacopoeias. In *Arg., Aust., Cz., Hung., Ind., Jug., Nord., Pol., Port., Roum., Span.,* and *Swiss. Arg.* also allows other species of Linaceae.

The fixed oil expressed from the ripe seeds of linseed, *Linum usitatissimum*(Linaceae), and subsequently clarified. It is a clear yellowish-brown oil with a faint characteristic odour and a bland unpleasant taste, gradually thickening on exposure to air and forming, when spread in a thin film, a hard transparent varnish. Wt per ml 0.925 to 0.93 g. Much commercial oil has a marked odour and an acrid taste.

Soluble 1 in 40 of dehydrated alcohol; slightly soluble in alcohol; miscible with chloroform, ether, carbon disulphide, light petroleum, and turpentine oil. **Store** in a cool place in well-filled airtight containers.

Uses. Linseed oil is used in veterinary medicine as a purgative for horses and cattle. It is no longer used as a purgative in man.

Boiled linseed oil ('boiled oil') is linseed oil heated with litharge, manganese resinate, or other driers, to a temperature of about 150° so that metallic salts of the fatty acids are formed and cause the oil to dry more rapidly. It must not be used for medicinal purposes.

Hydrolysed linseed oil as well as linolenic acid, which is present in linseed oil, inhibited methicillin-resistant *Sta-*

phylococcus aureus in vitro.— M. I. McDonald *et al.* (letter), *Lancet*, 1981, *2*, 1056.

7361-m

Maize Oil *(B.P.)*. Oleum Maydis; Ol. Mayd.; Huile de Maïs; Corn Oil *(U.S.N.F.)*.

CAS — 8001-30-7.

Pharmacopoeias. In *Br.*, *Fr.*, and *Jap.* Also in *U.S.N.F.*

The refined fixed oil obtained from the embryos of maize, *Zea mays* (Gramineae). It is a clear light to golden yellow oil with a faint characteristic odour and taste. It consists mainly of the glycerides of oleic acids and linoleic acids and smaller proportions of palmitic and stearic acids. Wt per ml 0.915 to 0.923 g.

Practically **insoluble** in alcohol; miscible with chloroform, ether, and lirht petroleum. It is **sterilised** by maintaining at 150° for 1 hour. **Store** at a temperature not exceeding 25° in well-filled airtight containers. Protect from light.

Sterilisation. For a report on the sterilisation of oils used for the preparation of injections, see Arachis Oil, p.695.

Uses. Maize oil has properties similar to those of olive oil. Because of its high content of unsaturated acids, maize oil has been given instead of oils and fats with high concentrations of saturated acids in patients with hypercholesterolaemia, particularly following myocardial infarction, but the value of such treatment has not been established in atherosclerosis or coronary heart disease.

Cholecystography. A preparation based on maize oil emulsion (GB Prep Emulsion) was used before cholecystography in 33 patients. There was a good contraction of the gall bladder in 79%.— N. Delelis and P. Lachance, *Can. med. Ass. J.*, 1967, *96*, 1417.

Proprietary Preparations

Biocorno *(Keimdiät, Ger.: Thomson & Joseph, UK)*. An oil prepared from the embryos of maize and of wheat, with added vitamin A and cholecalciferol. For use, in place of other vegetable oils, in pharmaceutical and cosmetic preparations.

Esoban Ointment *(Southon-Horton, UK)*. Contains maize oil 37.5%, zinc oxide 9.6%, wool fat 7.5%, linseed oil fatty acids 7%, and urea 0.56%. For dermatitis and allergic skin conditions.

Other Proprietary Names

Huile Diétex *(Fr.)*.

7362-b

Expressed Nutmeg Oil. Mace Butter; Adeps Myristicae; Oleum Nucistae; Beurre de Muscade; Muskatnussöl.

CAS — 8007-12-3.

A bright orange solid fat obtained from nutmeg or mace by hot expression. **Soluble** in alcohol, chloroform, and ether.

Expressed nutmeg oil is a mild counter-irritant and has been incorporated in plasters and hair lotions.

7363-v

Olive Oil *(U.S.N.F., B.P. 1973)*. Oleum Olivae; Azeite.

CAS — 8001-25-0.

Pharmacopoeias. In *Arg.*, *Aust.*, *Belg.*, *Cz.*, *Fr.*, *Ger.*, *It.*, *Jap.*, *Jug.*, *Mex.*, *Port.*, *Span.*, *Swiss*, and *Turk.* Also in *U.S.N.F.*

The fixed oil expressed from the ripe fruits of *Olea europaea* (Oleaceae). The oil may be refined. It consists of glycerides, mainly with oleic acid, with smaller amounts of palmitic, linoleic, stearic, and myristic acids. It is a pale yellow or light greenish-yellow oil with a slight characteristic odour and taste and a faintly acrid after-taste. At low temperatures it may be solid or partly solid. If it has solidified, it should be completely melted and mixed before use. Specific gravity 0.910 to 0.915.

Slightly **soluble** in alcohol; miscible with acetone, carbon disulphide, chloroform, ether, and light petroleum. It is **sterilised** by maintaining at 150° for 1 hour. **Store** at a temperature not exceeding 40° in well-filled airtight containers.

Uses. Internally, olive oil is nutrient, demulcent, and mildly purgative. It may also be given by rectal injection (100 to 500 ml warmed to about 32°) to soften impacted faeces. Olive oil in the form of an emulsion has been given as part of a nitrogen-free diet during the treatment of renal failure.

Externally, olive oil is emollient and soothing to inflamed surfaces, and is employed to soften the skin and crusts in eczema and psoriasis, and as a lubricant for massage. It is used to soften ear wax.

Olive oil is used in the preparation of liniments, ointments, plasters, and soaps; it is also used as a vehicle for oily suspensions for injection.

Olive oil has been used to secure acoustic coupling for ultrasound procedures.

Preparations

Oleum Olivae Neutralisatum et Sterilisatum *(Arg. P., Jug. P., Port. P., Span. P.)*. Olive oil warmed with a sufficient quantity of sodium carbonate to neutralise it, then dried, filtered, and sterilised. It is used in the preparation of oily solutions for injection. *Turk. P.* includes a similar preparation.

Olive Oil Emulsion with Methylated Spirit. Olive oil 300 ml, industrial methylated spirit 600 ml, Unemul 100 g, butylated hydroxyanisole (1% in olive oil) 4 ml, water 300 ml. Homogenise. Maize or arachis oil could be used in place of olive oil. For the prevention of bedsores.—W. Swallow, *Pharm. J.*, 1961, *2*, 407.

7364-g

Persic Oil *(U.S.N.F.)*. Oleum Persicorum; Peach or Apricot Kernel Oil.

CAS — 8002-78-6.

Pharmacopoeias. In *Rus.* Also in *U.S.N.F.*
Jap. P. includes Peach Kernel (Persicae Semen) and also Apricot Kernel (Armeniacae Semen).

The fixed oil expressed from the kernels of varieties of *Prunus persica*(peach) or *P. armeniaca* (apricot) (Rosaceae). It is a clear, colourless or pale straw-coloured, almost odourless oil with a bland taste. Specific gravity 0.910 to 0.923. Slightly **soluble** in alcohol; miscible with chloroform, ether, and light petroleum. **Store** in airtight containers.

Persic oil closely resembles almond oil in its general characteristics and it may be used for similar purposes.

7365-q

Poppy-seed Oil. Oleum Papaveris Seminis; Oleum Papaveris; Maw Oil; Huile d'Oeillette.

CAS — 8002-11-7.

The fixed oil expressed from the ripe seeds of the opium poppy, *Papaver somniferum* (Papaveraceae).

It is a pale yellow odourless oil with a faint almond flavour. When spread in a thin film and exposed to air, it forms a hard transparent varnish. Wt per ml about 0.92 g. **Soluble** in carbon disulphide, chloroform, ether, and light petroleum.

Poppy-seed oil is used as a substitute for olive oil for culinary and pharmaceutical purposes. It is also used in the preparation of Iodised Oil Fluid Injection. Commercial grades are used in making soaps, paints, and varnishes.

7366-p

Rape Oil *(B.P.C. 1954)*. Oleum Rapae; Colza Oil; Rapeseed Oil.

CAS — 8002-13-9.

Pharmacopoeias. In *Jap.* and *Pol.*

The fixed oil expressed from the seeds of *Brassica napus* (*Brassica campestris*) var. *oleifera* and certain other species of *Brassica* (Cruciferae). It is a clear yellow to dark yellow somewhat viscous oil with a characteristic odour and a taste which is unpleasant except in the most highly refined varieties. Wt per ml 0.907 to 0.912 g. Practically **insoluble** in alcohol, miscible with chloroform, ether, and light petroleum.

Rape oil is sometimes used in liniments in place of olive oil. It is used in some countries as an edible oil but *animal* studies have shown that it can cause damage to muscle, especially heart muscle. This is thought to be due to the erucic acid ($C_{22}H_{42}O_2$=338.6) content of the oil. The erucic acid content of oils and fats intended for human consumption and of foodstuffs containing oil or fat is restricted in England and Wales under the Erucic Acid in Food Regulations, 1977 (SI 1977: No. 691).

A discussion of the potential cardiotoxicity of rape oil in view of its use as a substitute for olive oil.— *Lancet*, 1974, *2*, 1359.

An investigation into the toxicology of rape oil in Italy where its consumption as a source of edible fat was increasing. As its pathogenicity in humans had not been determined in 1974, the Italian authorities introduced a limit of 15% of erucic acid in seed oil mixtures.— G. L. Gatti and H. Michalek, *Arzneimittel-Forsch.*, 1975, *25*, 1639.

Discussions on the erucic acid content of rape oil and its possible connection with cardiovascular disease.— *Chem. in Br.*, 1978, *14*, 210. Comments and letters.— *ibid.*, 427 and 428.

A discussion of the Spanish toxic-allergic syndrome caused by ingestion of rape oil denatured with aniline and containing acetanilide.— J. M. Tabuenca, *Lancet*, 1981, *2*, 567.

Cirrhosis. Ground rapeseed prevented experimental cirrhosis in *rats*.— M. Alvizouri *et al.* (letter), *Lancet*, 1978, *2*, 951.

7367-s

Safflower Oil

CAS — 8001-23-8.

Pharmacopoeias. Jap. P. includes Safflower, the flower of *Carthamus tinctorius.*

The fixed oil obtained from the seeds (achenes) of the safflower, or false (bastard) saffron, *Carthamus tinctorius*(Compositae). It contains about 75% of linoleic acid and 6 to 7% of saturated fatty acids.

It has similar characteristics to linseed oil (see p.696). It thickens and becomes rancid on prolonged exposure to air. **Soluble** in organic solvents. Wt per ml about 0.92 g.

Uses. Because of its high content of unsaturated fatty acids, safflower oil has been given instead of oils and fats with high concentrations of saturated fatty acids in patients with hypercholesterolaemia, particularly following cardiac infarction, but the value of such treatment has not been established in atherosclerosis or coronary heart disease.

The suggested daily dose is 75 ml of a 65% emulsion given in divided doses (equivalent to about 1900 kJ). This should be accompanied by a regulated diet to prevent weight gain.

Linoleic acid given in the form of safflower oil was effective in remitting the symptoms of 5 patients who developed neurotoxicity while taking low doses of lithium carbonate. Lithium carbonate is believed to inhibit the mobilisation of the linoleic acid metabolite, dihomogammalinolenic acid, and linoleic acid had been given in an attempt to raise concentrations of dihomogammalinolenic acid.— J. Lieb, *Prostaglandins and Medicine*, 1980, *4*, 275.

Proprietary Names

Safflor *(Wisconsin Pharmacal, USA)*.

The proprietary name Obesitol (*Carter Bros*) has been used in Great Britain for safflower oil.

7368-w

Sesame Oil *(B.P., Eur. P., U.S.N.F.)*. Oleum Sesami; Benne Oil; Gingelly Oil; Teel Oil.

CAS — 8008-74-0.

Pharmacopoeias. In *Belg., Br., Chin., Eur., Fr., Ger., Ind., Int., It., Jap., Mex., Neth.*, and *Swiss*. Also in *U.S.N.F.* The *Eur. P.* states that sesame oil is not necessarily suitable for parenteral administration.

The fixed oil obtained from the ripe seeds of *Sesamum indicum* (Pedaliaceae) by expression or extraction and subsequent refining. It is a pale yellow oil almost odourless and with a bland taste. It solidifies to a buttery mass at about −4°. Relative density 0.915 to 0.923.

Practically **insoluble** in alcohol; miscible with carbon disulphide, chloroform, ether, and light petroleum. It is **sterilised** by maintaining at 150° for 1 hour. It is more stable than most other fixed oils. **Store** at a temperature not exceeding 40° in well-filled airtight containers. Protect from light.

Sterilisation. Maximum survival time of *Bacillus subtilis* spores in sesame oil was 1 hour at 140°, and this was modified by the addition of 0.5% phenol to 2 hours at 110°. Benzyl alcohol gave variable results. *B. stearothermophilus* had a limited survival after 1 hour at 150° but none survived 1½ hours; phenol and benzyl alcohol did not significantly reduce the survival time.— R. L. Robison and M. H. Weinswig, *J. pharm. Sci.*, 1967, *56*, 1416.

For a report on the sterilisation of oils used for the preparation of injections, see Arachis Oil, p.695.

Uses. Sesame oil has similar properties to those of olive oil and has been used instead of olive oil in the preparation of liniments, plasters, ointments, and soaps. Because it is relatively stable, it is a useful solvent for certain steroids and other oil-soluble drugs administered in oily solution in capsules or in oily injections.

Acute polyneuropathy associated with the ingestion of sesame oil (gingili oil; jinjili oil) contaminated with tricresyl phosphates.— N. Senanayake and J. Jeyaratnam, *Lancet*, 1981, *1*, 88.

7369-e

Soya Oil. Oleum Sojae; Soybean Oil *(U.S.P.)*; Soja Bean Oil; Soya Bean Oil.

CAS — 8001-22-7.

Pharmacopoeias. In *Chin., Fr., Jap.*, and *U.S.*
Jap. P. specifies oil obtained from seeds of *Glycine max*.

The refined fixed oil expressed from the seeds of the soya plant *Glycine soja*(Leguminosae). It is a pale yellow oil with a faint characteristic odour and a bland taste. Specific gravity 0.916 to 0.922.

Slightly **soluble** in alcohol; miscible with chloroform, ether, and light petroleum. It is **sterilised** by maintaining at 150° for 1 hour. **Store** at a temperature not exceeding 40° in airtight containers. Protect from light.

Soya oil emulsion (Intralipid) for parenteral nutrition was stored for about 2 years at 4°, 20°, and 40°. During storage, the free fatty acid concentration increased and a fall in pH occurred. Gross particles were formed in the emulsion and the toxicity increased with time. All changes were most pronounced in emulsions during storage at 40°.— J. Boberg and I. Håkansson, *J. Pharm. Pharmac.*, 1964, *16*, 641.

The effect of added electrolytes on Intralipid.— W. H. Dawes and M. J. Groves, *Int. J. Pharmaceut.*, 1978, *1*, 141. See also C. R. T. Kawilarnang *et al.*, *J. clin. Hosp. Pharm.*, 1980, *5*, 151.

Adverse Effects. The incidence of immediate side-effects after the infusion of soya oil emulsion appears to be lower than after the administration of cottonseed oil emulsion. Fever or chills have been reported. Pigmentation of tissues after lipid emulsion infusions has also been reported.

The administration of soya oil emulsions for more than a week, or in high dosage, or in patients unable to metabolise infused fat may cause the 'overload syndrome' manifested by bone-marrow depression, anaemia, thrombocytopenia, thrombotic episodes, jaundice, and persistent hyperlipidaemia. The effects are reversible on discontinuing the infusion.

A report of the uptake of infused lipid particles in blood platelets.— T. Hovig and K. A. Grøttum, *Thromb. Diath. haemorrh.*, 1973, *29*, 450.

Two patients experienced major cerebral disorders during Intralipid infusion.— E. H. Jellinek (letter), *Lancet*, 1976, *2*, 967.

Four infants developed pulmonary fat emboli after administration of fractionated soya oil emulsion (Intralipid 20%) for 11 to 18 days; at necroscopy emboli were demonstrated in the lungs, but not in other organs. It was suggested that a transient high rate of infusion could be a causative factor.— A. J. Barson *et al.*, *Archs Dis. Child.*, 1978, *53*, 218.

Fatty infiltration and necrosis of the spleen were found at necroscopy in 12 of 16 patients who had received from 0.5 to 14 litres of Intralipid infusions (10 and/or 20%) during their terminal illnesses.— G. B. Forbes, *J. clin. Path.*, 1978, *31*, 765.

Intravascular fat accumulation was found at necropsy in the lungs of all of 8 very immature infants whose total parenteral nutritional regimen had included Intralipid 20%. Two had been over-infused, but the other 6 had received an average rate less than the recommended maximum for preterm infants and in no case had the plasma been lipaemic on visual examination. Comparison with the lungs of infants who had not received Intralipid before death, indicated a significantly greater concentration of linoleic acid, a marker for Intralipid. Until close biochemical monitoring is shown to reduce the risk of Intralipid pulmonary fat accumulation, the place of Intralipid in total parenteral nutrition for the ill premature infant must be questioned. A prospective controlled study on the safety and benefit of Intralipid 10% in the neonate is being carried out in an effort to resolve the problem.— M. I. Levene *et al.*, *Lancet*, 1980, *2*, 815. Criticism and correction.— I. I. Dainow, *KabiVitrum* (letter), *ibid.*, 1020. Reply.— M. I. Levene *et al.* (letter), *ibid.* Further comment on the hazards of Intralipid in ill neonates.— A. J. Barson (letter), *ibid.*, 1021. See also I. Blumenthal (letter), *ibid.*; D. Gordon (letter), *ibid.*, 1022. Results indicating that pulmonary fat accumulation in very low birth-weight infants is not caused by Intralipid infusion *per se* but may be accentuated by it.— G. E. Andersen *et al.* (letter), *ibid.*, 1981, *1*, 441.

Further reports of lipid deposition following Intralipid infusions: V. D. Black *et al.*, *Pediatrics*, 1978, *62*, 839; D. G. Fagan, *Archs Dis. Childh.*, 1978, *53*, 433; P. E. Wakely and G. Hug (letter), *Lancet*, 1981, *2*, 1416.

From a review of 92 infants including 70 premature infants it was concluded that liver disease was a major complication of total parenteral nutrition.— R. Postuma and C. L. Trevenen, *Pediatrics*, 1979, *63*, 110.

A hyponatraemic hypokalaemic metabolic alkalosis occurred in 3 infants given Neo-Mull-Soy formula (*Syntex, USA*) which was deficient in chloride. Analysis of Neo-Mull-Soy from 4 different lots revealed a chloride concentration of only 1 to 2 mmol per litre compared with the published concentration of 6 mmol per litre.— S. Roy and B. S. Arant (letter), *New Engl. J. Med.*, 1979, *301*, 615. Details of the withdrawal of 2 soy-based infant formulae Neo-Mull-Soy (*Syntex, USA*) and CHO-Free (*Syntex, USA*).— F. Greenberg *et al.* (letter), *Lancet*, 1979, *2*, 462.

Evidence that Intralipid can increase the susceptibility of *mice* to lethal bacterial sepsis, and can also impair human neutrophil chemotaxis *in vitro*. Intralipid may compromise human host defence mechanisms and put patients at risk for invasive bacterial disease.— G. W. Fischer *et al.*, *Lancet*, 1980, *2*, 819. A report of studies in *mice* which do not substantiate the fear that Intralipid causes reticuloendothelial blockade.— J. W. B. Bradfield (letter), *ibid.*, 1138. In conditions chosen to adhere closely to those in clinical practice, Intralipid did not affect the neutrophil function of 10 healthy subjects. Carefully controlled studies are needed to find out whether Intralipid really does impair host defence.— J. Palmblad *et al.* (letter), *ibid.* Further criticism, including mention of studies in patients demonstrating no effect of Intralipid on either the phagocytic or the catabolic function of the reticuloendothelial system.— J. Nordenström *et al.* (letter), *ibid.*, 1139. A recommendation to abandon Intralipid was not made, but it may impair host defences in some situations and patients receiving it should be observed closely for infectious complications.— G. W. Fischer *et al.* (letter), *ibid.*, 1300. *Malassezia* pulmonary vasculitis in an infant on long-term Intralipid therapy.— R. W. Redline and B. B. Dahms, *New Engl. J. Med.*, 1981, *305*, 1395.

Deficiency states. A report of hypophosphataemia developing in 7 patients during Intralipid infusion.— S. J. Tovey *et al.*, *Postgrad. med. J.*, 1977, *53*, 289.

Zinc and copper deficiency were associated with parenteral alimentation in one infant. The addition of zinc sulphate 100 µg per kg body-weight daily to the solution reversed dermatological, behavioural, and neurological changes.— K. N. Sivasubramanian *et al.* (letter), *Lancet*, 1978, *1*, 508.

Hypersensitivity. A report of a specific IgE-antibody response to the allergen Kunitz soybean trypsin inhibitor in a patient with anaphylactic reactions after ingestion of soybean products.— L. A. Moroz and W. H. Yang, *New Engl. J. Med.*, 1980, *302*, 1126.

Generalised pruritic urticaria occurred in a 9-year-old boy an hour after the start of an Intralipid infusion. He had previously received Intralipid for 19 days without ill effect. A skin test proved negative but an urticarial reaction developed when a test dose of 1 ml of Intralipid was given intravenously.— K. R. Kamath *et al.* (letter), *New Engl. J. Med.*, 1981, *304*, 360.

Treatment of Adverse Effects. Immediate reactions to the intravenous administration of soya oil emulsion may be treated by the intravenous administration of a corticosteroid and antihistamine. Treatment with adrenaline 0.5 to 1 ml (0.5 to 1 mg) of a 1 in 1000 solution by subcutaneous or intramuscular injection may be necessary. Heparin may be given, if needed, to aid clearance of fat from the circulation.

Precautions. Soya oil emulsion should not be given to patients with severe liver disease, septicaemia, or hyperlipidaemia, or with other conditions when the ability to absorb or metabolise fat may be impaired.

Soya oil emulsion should be used with caution in neonates with hyperbilirubinaemia because of the risk from bilirubin displaced from binding sites.

Dialysis. A report of 2 cardiac deaths in patients undergoing haemodialysis together with infusion of Intralipid 20%. It was considered that the deaths may have been associated with raised plasma concentrations of free fatty acids. Administration of lipid emulsion for alimentary purposes during haemodialysis had been stopped.— H. Bergrem and T. Leivestad (letter), *Lancet*, 1978, *2*, 1160.

Uses. Emulsions of fractionated soya oil containing 10 or 20% are given by slow intravenous infusion either alone or in conjunction with amino acids as a source of energy. The dose on the first day should not usually exceed the equivalent of 1 g of soya oil per kg body-weight daily, subsequently increased to 2, or, if necessary, 3 g per kg, and treatment is not usually given for more than a week. If longer treatment is required blood clearance of fat should be monitored weekly. The infusion should be started at the rate of 20 drops per minute and then increased slowly to a maximum of 60 drops per minute of a 10% emulsion or to 40 drops per minute of a 20% emulsion.

A suggested dose for infants is 0.5 to 4 g per kg over 24 hours.

Because of its high content of triglycerides of unsaturated fatty acids, soya oil has been given instead of oils and fats with high concentrations of saturated fatty acids to lower blood-cholesterol concentrations in patients with hypercholesterolaemia, particularly following cardiac infarction, but the value of such treatment has not been established in atherosclerosis or coronary heart disease.

Preparations made from whole soya beans, utilising soya oil and soya protein are used as the basis of lactose-free vegetable milks for infant feeding.

Soya oil is used as an edible oil and is also used as a lamp oil and in the manufacture of soaps, paints, and varnishes.

Intralipid infusion was given daily to a total of 180 paediatric patients to supply 40% of their daily energy requirement. The successful use in patients with hyperbilirubinaemia and in those with thrombocytopenia following sepsis or myelosuppression was reported. Cholestasis occurred in 10 patients and transient increases in liver enzyme concentrations during treatment in 4% of patients.— I. T. Cohen *et al.*, *J. pediat. Surg.*, 1977, *12*, 837.

Fatty acid deficiency. Three patients, who developed essential fatty acid deficiency when placed on a low-fat diet after intestinal resection, were successfully treated with Intralipid.— M. Press *et al.*, *Br. med. J.*, 1974, *2*, 247.

Further references: M. C. Riella *et al.*, *Ann. intern. Med.*, 1975, *83*, 786; W. E. Connor, *ibid.*, 895; *Lancet*, 1976, *1*, 1059.

Intravenous nutrition. A brief review of parenteral nutrition with a fat emulsion.— H. Silberman *et al.*, *J. Am. med. Ass.*, 1977, *238*, 1380. See also B. L. McNiff, *Am. J. Hosp. Pharm.*, 1977, *34*, 1080.

Proprietary Preparations

Intralipid 10% *(KabiVitrum, UK)*. An emulsion for intravenous nutrition containing fractionated soya oil 10%, fractionated egg phospholipids 1.2%, and glycerol 2.2% in Water for Injections, providing 4600 kJ per litre. **Intralipid 20%**. A similar preparation containing fractionated soya oil 20%, providing 8400 kJ per litre. Store at 4° to 8°.

7370-b

Sunflower Oil.

Sunflower Oil. Oleum Helianthi; Sunflowerseed Oil; Huile de Tournesol.

CAS — 8001-21-6.

Pharmacopoeias. In *Cz.*, *Fr.*, *Hung.*, and *Roum.*

The fixed oil expressed from the fruits (achenes) of the sunflower, *Helianthus annuus* (Compositae). It is a clear pale yellow oil with a faint characteristic odour and taste. Wt per ml about 0.92 g. Slightly **soluble** in alcohol; miscible with chloroform and ether. It is **sterilised** by maintaining at 150° for 1 hour.

Sunflower oil is used in some countries as a salad oil and margarine oil and as a substitute for olive and arachis oils in pharmaceutical preparations.

The deficiency in essential fatty acids in 3 patients was corrected by the topical application of 230 mg of sunflower oil calculated to contain 120 mg of linoleic acid.— M. Press *et al.*, *Lancet*, 1974, *1*, 597.

Multiple sclerosis. In a double-blind study in 75 patients with multiple sclerosis there was no significant difference in the number of relapses in 36 given two 30-ml doses daily for 2 years of a 50% emulsion of sunflower oil (each 30 ml providing 8.6 g of linoleic acid) and 39 given similar doses of a control emulsion of olive oil, but the severity and duration of relapses was significantly reduced. Platelet adhesiveness was not affected.— J. H. D. Millar *et al.*, *Br. med. J.*, 1973, *1*, 765. A discussion of factors which might affect results.— E. J. Field and B. K. Shenton (letter), *ibid.*, 1975, *1*, 456.

Polyneuritis. Recovery in 2 children with idiopathic polyneuritis (Guillain-Barré syndrome) of 6 and 12 months duration respectively was virtually complete after treatment with a diet containing 30 ml of sunflower oil daily; one child also received 1.5 ml of wheat-germ oil daily. Both children had been treated with no success with prednisolone and one also with cyclophosphamide. A diet with a high content of polyunsaturated fatty acid might be of use in long-term disability after idiopathic polyneuritis and in other autoimmune diseases.— B. D. Bower and E. A. Newsholme, *Lancet*, 1978, *1*, 583.

Preparations

Gallbladder Evacuant. Sunflower oil 50 g, polysorbate '60' 5 g sorbitan mono-oleate 5 g, sucrose 5 g, methyl hydroxybenzoate 100 mg, propyl hydroxybenzoate 100 mg, sorbitol solution 5 g, flavouring q.s., water to 100 ml.—I.L. Higa, *Hosp. Pharmst*, 1964, *17*, 115.

Sunflower oil was formerly marketed in Great Britain under the proprietary name Sunflo Oil (*Savory & Moore*).

7371-v

Hydrogenated Vegetable Oil *(U.S.N.F.)*.

Pharmacopoeias. In *U.S.N.F. Jap.* includes a hydrogenated oil of fish, animal, or vegetable origin.

Refined, bleached, hydrogenated, and deodorised vegetable oil stearins consisting mainly of the triglycerides of stearic and palmitic acids. It is a fine white powder at room temperature. M.p. 61° to 66°.

Practically **insoluble** in water; soluble in chloroform, light petroleum, and hot isopropyl alcohol. **Store** in a cool place in airtight containers.

Hydrogenated vegetable oil is used as a tablet lubricant.

Fluorides and some Fluorine Compounds

7730-l

The principal medicinal use of fluorides is for the prevention of dental caries; for this purpose they may be administered by mouth, applied topically, or used for the fluoridation of water supplies. Some fluorine compounds are used as rodenticides.

7731-y

Fluoroacetamide. Compound 1081.
$FCH_2.CONH_2=77.06$.

CAS — 640-19-7.

A white odourless tasteless powder. Very **soluble** in water; relatively insoluble in organic solvents.

Adverse Effects. As for Sodium Fluoroacetate, p.702.

Uses. Fluoroacetamide is used as a rodenticide. It has also been used to a limited extent as an insecticide.

In Great Britain, the use of fluoroacetamide is restricted to the destruction of rats in ships and in sewers and in specified dock warehouses. When supplied for use as a rodenticide it must contain a distinctive colouring matter.

Fluoroacetamide and Sodium Fluoroacetate as Rodenticides. See *Use of Fluoroacetamide and Sodium Fluoroacetate as Rodenticides; Precautionary Measures,* Ministry of Agriculture, Fisheries and Food, London, HM Stationery Office, 1970.

It was recommended, in view of the extreme hazard to other mammals, that fluoroacetamide and sodium fluoroacetate should only be used by trained pest control operators in areas such as locked warehouses and sewers to which access by unauthorised persons and useful animals could be prevented completely.— Safe Use of Pesticides, Twentieth Report of the WHO Expert Committee on Insecticides, *Tech. Rep. Ser. Wld Hlth Org. No. 513,* 1973.

7732-j

Hydrofluorosilicic Acid. Fluorosilicic Acid; Fluosilicic Acid.
$H_2SiF_6=144.1$.

CAS — 16961-83-4.

It is available commercially as a colourless liquid containing about 30% of H_2SiF_6. Sp. gr. about 1.27. It may precipitate if diluted with less than 20 times its volume of water. **Store** in glass or rubber-lined airtight containers.

Adverse Effects. As for Hydrofluoric Acid, p.785.

Uses. Hydrofluorosilicic acid is used in controlled amounts for the fluoridation of drinking water.

7733-z

Sodium Fluoride *(B.P., U.S.P.).* Sod. Fluor.; Sodii Fluoridum; Natrium Fluoratum.

NaF=41.99.

CAS — 7681-49-4.

Pharmacopoeias. In *Arg., Br., Braz., Cz., Hung., Jug., Nord., Pol., Roum., Swiss,* and *U.S.*

A white odourless powder. Sodium fluoride 2.2 mg is approximately equivalent to 1 mg of fluoride. Each g provides approximately 23.8 mmol (23.8 mEq) of sodium and fluoride. **Soluble** 1 in 25 of water; practically insoluble in alcohol. **Incompatible** with calcium and magnesium salts. Aqueous solutions slowly attack glass. **Store** in airtight containers.

A 0.2% solution of sodium fluoride flavoured with compound orange spirit and saccharin and coloured with amaranth was found to be contaminated when stored for 8 weeks. A similar solution coloured with tartrazine was not contaminated. Preservatives should be used in sodium fluoride solutions.— M. L. Frazer and J. W. Huggonson (letter), *Br. dent. J.,* 1973, *134,* 314.

Adverse Effects. Sodium fluoride is corrosive; when taken by mouth in quantities in excess of about 250 mg it causes salivation, nausea and vomiting, epigastric pain, and diarrhoea; large doses cause thirst, perspiration, paralysis, muscular weakness and clonic convulsions, followed by respiratory and cardiac failure; there may be renal failure; death may occur within 2 to 4 hours.

Chronic fluoride poisoning, manifestations of which include increased density and coarsened trabeculation of bone, may arise from the continued ingestion of fluoride and has occurred in workers handling fluorides and in communities using drinking water containing particularly high concentrations of natural fluorides. Ocular damage has also been reported.

In the controlled amounts (usually 1 ppm in temperate climates) in fluoridated water, fluoride has not been shown to have any side-effects other than the very occasional occurrence of faint white flecks on the teeth. At a concentration of 1.4 to 2 ppm slight light yellow to brownish mottling of the dental enamel occurs in a small proportion of the population. Above 2 ppm brownish spots develop on many teeth in most persons, and above 2.5 ppm the enamel has a darker discoloration and loses its smoothness (dental fluorosis). At 10 ppm, effects on the bones may occur (skeletal fluorosis), though the incidence of senile osteoporosis may be reduced; in some areas skeletal fluorosis may cause crippling deformities.

The fluoridation of water continues to be a subject of considerable controversy. Suggestions that it increases the incidence of chromosome aberrations and cancer have not been substantiated.

Maximum permissible atmospheric concentration of fluoride (calculated as fluorine) 2.5 mg per m^3.

For an extensive review and bibliography of the toxic effects of larger doses of fluoride, with consideration of the effects on dental enamel, skeletal system, kidneys, thyroid, and endocrine system, see *Fluorides and Human Health,* Monograph Series No. 59, Geneva, World Health Organization, 1970, pp. 225–71.

A discussion of chronic fluorosis.— *Br. med. J.,* 1981, *282,* 253.

For clinical reports which refuted suggestions that there was a causal relationship between the fluoride content of domestic water supplies and adverse effects on thyroid function, anaemia in pregnancy, mortality, osteochondritis juvenilis of the spine, mongolism, and peptic ulcer, among other conditions, see The Conduct of the Fluoridation Studies in the United Kingdom and the Results Achieved after Five Years, *Report on Public Health and Medical Subjects No. 105,* London, HM Stationery Office, 1962.

Giant cells were discovered in the bone marrow of a woman taking 150 mg of sodium fluoride daily for osteoporosis and in 2 other patients also taking fluoride. These cells disappeared after fluoride was discontinued.— P. H. Duffey *et al., Ann. intern. Med.,* 1971, *75,* 745, per *Int. pharm. Abstr..* 1972, *9,* 263.

Acne. An acne-like eruption had occurred in several patients during treatment with sodium fluoride.— J. M. Hitch, *J. Am. med. Ass.,* 1967, *200,* 879.

Allergy. Following the use of toothpaste or vitamin preparations containing fluoride, 6 children and 1 adult exhibited reactions which included urticaria, exfoliative dermatitis, atopic dermatitis, stomatitis, and gastro-intestinal and respiratory allergy. Improvement occurred on discontinuing the fluoride preparation.— J. J. Shea *et al., Ann. Allergy,* 1967, *25,* 388, per *J. Am. med. Ass.,* 1967, *201* (Aug. 28), A171.

Risks of allergy from fluoridation of water were considered to be unfounded.— *Lancet,* 1973, *2,* 889.

Carcinogenicity and mutagenicity. Fluoridation and cancer.— J. Yiamouyiannis and D. Burk, *Fluoride,* 1977, *10,* 102.

Analyses showing lack of any association between cancer and fluoridation: P. D. Oldham and D. J. Newell, *Appl. Statist.,* 1977, *26,* 125, per *Abstr. Hyg.,* 1977, *52,* 883; R. Doll and L. Kinlen, *Lancet,* 1977, *1,* 1300. See also L. J. Kinlen *et al.* (letter), *ibid.,* 1980, *2,* 199.

In a 17-year study which included 2469 children with Down's syndrome, no association was found between fluoridation of water supplies and the incidence of children born with Down's syndrome.— H. L. Needleman *et al., New Engl. J. Med.,* 1974, *291,* 821.

Bacteriological and *animal* studies carried out under the auspices of the National Institutes of Health, USA indicated that fluorides did not increase chromosomal aberration and were not considered to be mutagenic.— *Br. dent. J.,* 1977, *143,* 325.

Effects on bones and joints. *Arthritis.* Fluoride was not considered to increase the incidence of arthritis.— *Br. dent. J.,* 1979, *147,* 216. Criticism.— R. V. Mummery (letter), *ibid.,* 1980, *148,* 33.

Skeletal fluorosis. An epidemiological, clinical, and biochemical study of endemic dental and skeletal fluorosis in the Punjab.— S. S. Jolly *et al., Br. med. J.,* 1968, *4,* 427.

Osteoporosis, genu valgum, mottled teeth, and osteosclerosis occurred in 24 patients living in areas of India where the drinking water contained 3.5 to 6 ppm of fluoride.— K. A. V. R. Krishnamachari and K. Krishnaswamy, *Lancet,* 1973, *2,* 877.

Effects on teeth. Mild to very mild mottling of teeth might occur in 10% of children who ingested the equivalent of 2 mg of fluoride per day during the years necessary for calcification of the enamel of the teeth. Exposure to 2 mg of fluoride per day for 16 years was necessary to produce visibly objectionable fluorosis. A single dose of 200 to 500 mg of fluoride was necessary to produce acute symptoms and an acute lethal dose was approximately 2.5 g of fluoride as a single dose.— D. Freeman (letter), *Med. J. Aust.,* 1968, *2,* 38.

A study of mottling in incisor teeth carried out on 2 groups of children (171 and 178) who had received water containing about 0.9 ppm or 0.01 ppm of fluoride throughout their lives indicated that the mottling observed was not due to ingested fluorides and that the incidence of mottling was lower in a community fluoridated to the optimum level (1 ppm) than in a non-fluoridated community.— W. Al-Alousi *et al., Br. dent. J.,* 1975, *138,* 9.

Goitre. Studies of 736 Himalayans from 14 villages demonstrated an association between goitre and the fluoride content and hardness of the water.— T. K. Day and P. R. Powell-Jackson, *Lancet,* 1972, *1,* 1135. Comment.— G. N. Jenkins and J. A. Cooke (letter), *ibid.,* 1293. In another eastern study the incidence of goitre was not related to fluoridation but was associated with the calcium content and was reciprocally related to the iodine content.— T. P. Kuo and S. Chen, *J. Formosan med. Ass.,* 1975, *74,* 489, per *Trop. Dis. Bull.,* 1976, *73,* 107.

Hyperparathyroidism. Five of 20 patients with endemic skeletal fluorosis had concurrent hyperparathyroidism. Clinical findings included mottled discoloration of the teeth, skeletal pain, and restricted and painful joint movements. Radiological and histological features were typical of fluorosis and of hyperparathyroidism. The basis of the association between fluorosis and hyperparathyroidism was not clear, but fluoride might interfere with calcium equilibrium between bone and serum. The fluoride concentration of water from local wells was 10.3 to 13.5 ppm.— S. P. S. Teotia and M. Teotia, *Br. med. J.,* 1973, *1,* 637.

Overdosage. A 25-year-old man who ingested 120 g of a powder containing 97% sodium fluoride developed tetany, multiple episodes of ventricular fibrillation, and oesophageal stricture. Treatment with calcium, potassium, and magnesium salts and frusemide, lignocaine, procainamide, and diazepam enabled the patient to survive.— A. R. Abukurah *et al., J. Am. med. Ass.,* 1972, *222,* 816.

Minimal symptoms in children accidentally exposed to high concentrations of fluoride in drinking water.— R. Hoffman *et al., Pediatrics,* 1980, *65,* 897.

Treatment of Adverse Effects. In acute poisoning, empty the stomach by aspiration and lavage with lime water or a 1% solution of calcium chloride or other calcium salt. Calcium Gluconate Injection, 10 ml of a 10% solution, may be given intravenously to control convulsions and repeated every 4 to 6 hours if needed. Morphine or pethidine may be given by injection, if necessary, to control colic. The circulation should be maintained with infusions of suitable electrolyte solutions. The respiration may require assistance. Haemodialysis has been used.

Discussion of the role of dialysis in the treatment of fluoride poisoning.— J. F. Winchester *et al.*, *Trans. Am. Soc. artif. internal Organs*, 1977, *23*, 762.

A study in *rats* suggested that metabolic alkalosis reduced acute fluoride toxicity and should be used therapeutically.— G. M. Whitford *et al.*, *Toxic. appl. Pharmac.*, 1979, *50*, 31.

Protection of workers. While handling dry fluoride chemicals each worker should be provided with a pair of rubber gloves and preferably with a dust mask. Facilities should be provided for washing the hands and gloves. Chief emphasis, however, should be placed on facilities for preventing the release of dust.— C. R. Cox, *Operation and Control of Water Treatment Processes*, Monograph Series No. 49, Geneva, World Health Organization, 1964.

Precautions. Care should be taken when applying fluorides to teeth or administering fluorides to avoid mottling and allowance should be made for fluorides normally ingested. Changes in the fluoride content of the water supply may affect patients on dialysis not using deionised water.

Topical fluoride preparations were shown to have a deleterious effect on the amalgam of fillings. The durability of such restoration might be reduced.— B. W. Darvell, *Br. dent. J.*, 1977, *142*, 47.

Discussion of the combined intake of fluoride from food, fluoridated dentifrices, water, and supplementary fluoride tablets.— D. E. Leitch (letter), *Pharm. J.*, 1979, *1*, 99.

Osteomalacia developed in a patient with osteoporosis during treatment with sodium fluoride despite the fact that large doses of ergocalciferol were given concurrently.— J. E. Compston *et al.*, *Br. med. J.*, 1980, *281*, 910.

Administration in renal failure. Two patients with impaired renal function developed systemic fluorosis after drinking large quantities of fluoridated water (2.6 and 1.7 ppm respectively) for a number of years.— L. I. Juncos and J. V. Donadio, *J. Am. med. Ass.*, 1972, *222*, 783.

Fears of toxicity from fluoridation of water indicated that risks to patients undergoing dialysis were unfounded.— *Lancet*, 1973, *2*, 889.

Fluoride excretion in patients with impaired renal function might be expected to be normal provided the creatinine clearance was not less than 16 ml per minute. In patients who had undergone renal transplantation fluoride excretion was usually above normal. In patients with chronic renal failure given a 20-mg or 40-mg load of sodium fluoride, plasma-fluoride concentrations rose from a range of about 105 to 325 μg per litre to a range of about 210 to 690 μg per litre.— V. Parsons *et al.*, *Br. med. J.*, 1975, *1*, 128.

An afebrile illness in 8 patients undergoing dialysis, characterised by hypotension, vomiting, nausea, diarrhoea, substernal pain, and pruritus, associated with excess of hydrofluorosilicic acid in the water supply.— R. Anderson *et al.*, *Morb. Mortal.*, 1980, *29*, 134, per *Int. pharm. Abstr.*, 1980, *17*, 997.

Absorption and Fate. Sodium fluoride and other soluble fluorides are readily absorbed from the gastro-intestinal tract. Absorption may be reduced by calcium, magnesium, and aluminium compounds in water or in the diet. Inhaled fluorides are absorbed through the lungs.

Fluoride is a normal component of body fluids and soft tissues and the normal concentration of total fluorides in plasma is 140 to 190 μg per litre, of which about 15 to 20% is in the ionised form. Most of the fluoride in the body is deposited in the bones and teeth. With a normal intake, fluoride is excreted in the urine to maintain a fluoride equilibrium. With a raised intake of fluoride, about one-half is taken up by the skeleton and the remainder rapidly excreted in the urine.

Fluoride diffuses across the placenta; it is present in faeces, sweat, saliva, milk, tears, and hair.

For an extensive review of the absorption, distribution, and excretion of fluorides, see *Fluorides and Human Health*, Monograph Series No. 59, Geneva, World Health Organization, 1970, pp. 75–161. See also *Chronicle Wld Hlth Org.*, 1970, *24*, 271.

A study of the retention of fluoride in 7 patients given fluoride 20 to 45 mg daily for prolonged periods.— H. Spencer *et al.*, *Clin. Chem.*, 1975, *21*, 613.

In areas where the local water supply contained fluoride 1 ppm, breast milk of nursing mothers was considered to provide adequate fluoride for optimum tooth development; extra fluoride given to the mothers might cause mottling of teeth in infants.— R. L. Savage, *Adverse Drug React. Bull.*, 1976, No. 61, 212.

There was no evidence of transfer of fluoride from plasma to breast milk in 5 mothers given 1.5 mg of fluoride as sodium fluoride.— J. Ekstrand *et al.*, *Br. med. J.*, 1981, *283*, 761. Because it had been shown that the fluoride content of breast milk could be increased by raising the daily fluoride intake by amounts larger than 1.5 mg, further studies were required.— K. D. Moudgil (letter), *ibid.*, 1982, *284*, 200.

The pharmacokinetics of sodium fluoride after single and multiple doses. The concentration of fluoride in plasma and in saliva showed a fairly constant relationship, indicating that determination of the saliva-fluoride concentration could be used to estimate the plasma-fluoride concentration.— J. Ekstrand *et al.*, *Eur. J. clin. Pharmac.*, 1977, *12*, 311.

Further references: J. Ekstrand *et al.*, *Clin. Pharmac. Ther.*, 1978, *23*, 329; J. Ekstrand and M. Ehrnebo, *Eur. J. clin. Pharmac.*, 1979, *16*, 211.

Uses. Sodium fluoride is used for the prophylaxis of dental caries in communities where the intake of fluoride from drinking water and food is low. It renders the dentine and enamel of teeth more resistant to acid. A reduction of up to about 60% in the incidence of dental caries has been reported. It may be added to water supplies in temperate regions to give a final concentration of 1 ppm of fluoride, which is fairly critical, since the continued drinking of water containing more than 1.4 ppm during the period of tooth development leads to an increased incidence of mottling of the tooth enamel. In hotter regions, a lower final concentration of about 0.6 ppm may be used.

Where the drinking water is not fluoridated and naturally contains less than 0.3 ppm of fluoride, sodium fluoride may be taken individually dissolved in water or fruit juice. Children up to the age of 2 years may be given 0.55 mg (equivalent to 0.25 mg of fluoride) while children aged 2 to 4 years may be given 1.1 mg (equivalent to 0.5 mg of fluoride), however higher doses have been used. Children older than 4 years may be given 2.2 mg (equivalent to 1 mg of fluoride). If the water naturally contains 0.3 to 0.7 ppm of fluoride, no additional fluoride should be given to children less than 2 years of age and for older children the above doses should be reduced by one-half; if the water contains more than 0.7 ppm of fluoride, supplementation is not recommended.

The value of giving fluoride during pregnancy, to benefit the child, is not established.

Another method of prophylaxis is to apply a 2% solution of sodium fluoride in water to children's teeth, after preliminary cleansing, 3 or 4 times at intervals of several days at 3, 7, 11, and 13 years of age to correspond with tooth eruption. Gel acidified with phosphoric acid and containing up to 2.6% of sodium fluoride has also been used for topical application.

In Great Britain, the Cosmetic Products Regulations 1978 (SI 1978: No. 1354) limit the concentration of sodium fluoride and other fluorides in oral hygiene products to a total fluorine concentration of 0.15%.

Sodium fluoride has also been given to increase bone density and relieve bone pain in patients with various metabolic and neoplastic bone diseases including osteoporosis and osteitis deformans (Paget's disease of bone); many consider this use still to be experimental.

Other fluoride salts that have been used include stannous fluoride (see p.702) and calcium and magnesium fluoride. Hydrofluoric acid is described on p.785.

For an extensive review and bibliography of the effects of fluorides on general and dental health, see *Fluorides and Human Health*, Monograph Series No. 59, Geneva, World Health Organization, 1970, pp. 273–354; *Chronicle Wld Hlth Org.*, 1970, *24*, 271.

For a survey of the methods, costs, and benefits of various methods of supplying fluoride, see G. N. Davies, *Cost and Benefit of Fluoride in the Prevention of Dental Caries*, WHO Offset Publication No. 9, Geneva, World Health Organization, 1974.

Blood preservative. In a concentration of 1%, sodium fluoride was considered the most efficient and suitable preservative for postmortem blood samples, preventing the generation of alcohol in all 16 blood samples tested which had been stored at room temperature for 10 days.— V. D. Plueckhahn and B. Ballard, *Med. J. Aust.*, 1968, *1*, 939.

Bone diseases. *Bone pain.* Bone pain in 9 patients with metastases of prostatic cancer was relieved, usually within 4 weeks, by treatment with sodium fluoride 100 mg daily.— W. P. Scott (letter), *J. Am. med. Ass.*, 1967, *202*, 664.

Myelomatosis. Skeletal fluorosis was induced within 18 months in 8 patients with multiple myeloma following treatment with sodium fluoride 100 to 150 mg daily and calcium lactate 2.7 to 5.4 g daily. Radiological fluorosis developed in 7 of the 8 cases. Five patients showed marked thickening of trabeculae after treatment and 4 who had severe bone pain experienced virtually complete relief of pain.— P. Cohen, *J. Am. med. Ass.*, 1966, *198*, 583; *Br. med. J.*, 1967, *2*, 128.

In a double-blind study for up to 60 months, 150 patients with multiple myeloma were given sodium fluoride 100 mg daily, 200 mg daily, or a placebo, in addition to their antineoplastic therapy. From observation of the progress of the disease it appeared that there was no benefit from sodium fluoride therapy and it could possibly be detrimental.— J. B. Harley *et al.*, *New Engl. J. Med.*, 1972, *286*, 1283 (Acute Leukemia Group B and the Eastern Cooperative Oncology Group,).

In a double-blind study of 24 patients with bone disease resulting from multiple myeloma and who were taking melphalan and prednisone, the effect of sodium fluoride 50 mg twice daily plus calcium carbonate 1 g four times daily was evaluated. After one year of therapy there appeared to be significant increases in bone formation and bone mass compared with the placebo. Bone trabeculae appeared to be thickened on X-ray examination in 6 of 13 treated patients. These changes were not detectable by normal technetium bone scans or bone densitometry determination.— R. A. Kyle *et al.*, *New Engl. J. Med.*, 1975, *293*, 1334.

Osteitis deformans. Reference to the use of sodium fluoride in Paget's disease of bone (osteitis deformans).— J. Haddad, *J. Am. med. Ass.*, 1969, *209*, 1354.

Osteoporosis. Discussions of the use of sodium fluoride in osteoporosis: A. N. Exton-Smith, *Proc. R. Soc. Med.*, 1976, *69*, 931; L. K. Golightly, *Can. J. Hosp. Pharm.*, 1978, *31*, 85; *Med. Lett.*, 1980, *22*, 45.

Fluoride treatment for skeletal disorders should be undertaken only on an investigational basis with careful monitoring.— *J. Am. med. Ass.*, 1978, *240*, 1630 (Ad Hoc Committee, Strategy Workshop for Osteoporosis Research).

Thirty-six patients with osteoporosis were treated with sodium fluoride 40 to 65 mg daily with calcium supplements and, usually, vitamin D; they were followed for 4 to 6 years. Of the 51 new fractures, 23 occurred in the first year of treatment; patients with X-ray evidence of fluoride changes in the vertebrae had a lower incidence of fractures. The regimen should continue to be experimental.— B. L. Riggs *et al.*, *J. Am. med. Ass.*, 1980, *243*, 446. Optimism on the reduction of the numbers of vertebral fractures by sodium fluoride given with conventional therapy in postmenopausal osteoporosis.— *idem*, *New Engl. J. Med.*, 1982, *306*, 446.

Further references: C. Hauswaldt *et al.*, *Dt. med. Wschr.*, 1977, *102*, 1177; H. -P. Kruse *et al.*, *ibid.*, 1978, *103*, 248.

For earlier references to the use of sodium fluoride in osteoporosis, see Martindale 27th Edn, p. 618.

Otosclerosis. Sodium fluoride 40 to 60 mg daily for 1 to 3 years could be used in the treatment of otosclerosis.— G. E. Shambaugh, *J. Lar. Otol.*, 1971, *85*, 301, per D. L. Chadwick, *Practitioner*, 1972, *209*, 460.

Sodium fluoride administered in a dose of 25 mg daily prevented further deterioration in otosclerosis hearing loss.— F. H. Linthicum *et al.*, *J. Am. med. Ass.*, 1973, *224*, 1482.

Further references: H. P. House and F. H. Linthicum, *Archs Otolar.*, 1974, *100*, 427.

Dental caries. Reviews and discussions of the use of fluoride for the prevention of dental caries.— K. R. Powell, *Aust. J. Pharm.*, 1976, *57*, 727; R. S. Levine, *Br. dent. J.*, 1976, *140*, 9; F. J. Hill and R. S. Levine, *ibid.*, 1978, *145*, 240; P. A. Swango, *Pharm. Times*, 1978, *44*, (July), 60.

In a double-blind trial in 434 schoolchildren the daily supervised use for 3 years of a mouth-wash containing 0.05% of sodium fluoride led to a 36% reduction in the incidence of dental caries.— A. J. Rugg-Gunn *et al.*, *Br. dent. J.*, 1973, *135*, 353.

In a group of dentate adults aged 45 years and above whose water supply had contained 1.5 to 2 ppm of fluoride for many years, the incidence of dental caries was 44% less than in a similar group whose water supply contained 0.2 ppm.— D. Jackson *et al.*, *Br. dent. J.*, 1973, *134*, 419.

Acidulated phosphate fluoride (APF; 0.5% fluoride) reduced the solubility of intact enamel surfaces of teeth by 37.7% after 1 or 2 applications. Treatment with stannous fluoride 0.5% reduced the solubility by 25.5% after 1 or 2 applications whilst 0.1% solutions were significantly less effective than 0.5 or 1% solutions. A fresh mixture of acidulated phosphate fluoride (0.5%) and stannous fluoride 0.5% reduced enamel solubility by 55.5% and was significantly more effective than either alone.— P. H. Kleinstub and I. L. Shannon, *Milit. Med.*, 1974, *139*, 722, per *Abstr. Hyg.*, 1975, *50*, 39.

Sodium fluoride added to the growth media in concentrations of up to 10 mmol, reduced peptidoglycan turnover and produced lysis in those bacteria which normally have highly active autolytic systems, such as those involved in plaque formation and caries.— R. J. Lesher *et al.*, *Antimicrob. Ag. Chemother.*, 1977, *12*, 339.

There was a significant reduction in the incidence of dental caries in a double-blind study of 1002 children who used a fluoride toothpaste, a rinse of sodium monofluorophosphate, or both over a 2-year period. Although there was no significant difference between the groups it was considered that combined use of both preparations could be advantageous over their use alone.— F. P. Ashley *et al.*, *Br. dent. J.*, 1977, *143*, 333.

Further references: F. J. Margolis *et al.*, *Am. J. Dis. Child.*, 1975, *129*, 794; J. F. Beal and W. P. Rock, *Br. dent. J.*, 1976, *140*, 307; M. C. Downer *et al.*, *ibid.*, 242; J. J. Murray *et al.*, *ibid.*, 1977, *143*, 11; K. W. Stephen and D. Campbell, *ibid.*, 1978, *144*, 202; E. Newbrun, *Pediatrics*, 1978, *62*, 733, per *Int. pharm. Abstr.*, 1979, *16*, 363; *Br. dent. J.*, 1979, *146*, 51; J. G. Whittle and M. C. Downer, *Br. dent. J.*, 1979, *147*, 67; *Pediatrics*, 1979, *63*, 150 (Committee on Nutrition,); D. Jackson *et al.*, *Br. dent. J.*, 1980, *149*, 231; T. B. Dowell and S. Joyston-Bechal, *Br. dent. J.*, 1981, *150*, 273; K. W. Stephen (letter), *ibid.*, *151*, 40; *Drug & Ther. Bull.*, 1981, *19*, 81.

For earlier references to the use of fluoride for the prevention of dental caries, see Martindale 27th Edn, p. 618.

Fluoridation of drinking water. For information on methods of fluoridation of drinking water, see C. R. Cox, *Operation and Control of Water Treatment Processes*, Monograph Series No. 49, Geneva, World Health Organization, 1964, pp. 183–95.

A study of the continuing effect of fluoridation of water on dental decay in children in the UK confirmed the beneficial effects seen after 5-year studies. However, in Kilmarnock, where fluoridation was discontinued in 1962 after 6 years, the reduction in the incidence of dental decay that had been noted by 1963 was halted, and by 1968 the incidence of decay in children up to 5 years was again almost as bad as that in the control area. After 11 years only 2 patients were reported as having developed symptoms which might have resulted from drinking fluoridated water but double-blind tests did not confirm the connection.— The Fluoridation Studies in the United Kingdom and the Results Achieved after Eleven Years, *Reports on Public Health and Medical Subjects No. 122*, London, HM Stationery Office, 1969.

Water fluoridation reduced the prevalence and incidence of dental caries; the best results occurred in children who had consumed fluoridated water since birth. Only when the natural fluoride intake had been assessed was it possible to calculate the concentration to which the fluoride content of water supplies needed to be adjusted. In temperate areas 1 to 1.2 ppm might be necessary and in tropical areas, because more water was consumed, 0.6 ppm might be adequate.— *Chronicle Wld Hlth Org.*, 1969, *23*, 505.

After an extensive review, the Royal College of Physicians concluded that fluoride, naturally present or added to drinking water at a concentration of 1 mg per litre over the years of tooth formation, substantially reduced dental caries throughout life. In a temperate climate the consumption of water containing 1 mg per litre was safe irrespective of the hardness of the water. By comparison the use of systemic fluoride supplements such as tablets, drops, and fluoridated salt had not been shown to be as effective on a community basis. An examination of common objections to fluoridation disclosed no evidence of harmful effects in the recommended concentration. The discharge of fluoridated water in rivers would have negligible effects on the environment, including the sea. The College recommended fluoridation of water supplies in the United Kingdom where the fluoride level was appreciably below 1 mg per litre.— *Fluoride, Teeth and Health.* A Report and Summary on Fluoride and its Effect on Teeth and Health, Royal College of Physicians of London, Pitman Medical Publishing, 1976. See also P. D. Oldham and D. J. Newell, *Appl. Statist.*, 1977, *26*, 125, per *Abstr. Hyg.*, 1977, *52*, 883.

Alternative fluoridation. Alternatives to fluoridation of drinking water were fluoridation of milk or salt, use of fluoride tablets, use of fluoride-containing dentifrices, and mouth rinsing with fluoride solutions. The main advantages of these methods were that freedom of choice was preserved, the total quantity of fluoride used was much less than that required for fluoridation of water supply, of which less than 1% was used for drinking, and fluoride was directed to the age groups in which it was most effective. Disadvantages of these methods were: they might not be accessible to pre-school children; children might not consume enough salt to receive an adequate fluoride intake; accidental ingestion of tablets by children at home; topical methods must be used continuously; different methods of fluoride application could have an additive effect.— *Br. med. J.*, 1975, *1*, 535.

Preparations

Dental Desensitising Paste. Sodium fluoride 10 g, kaolin 10 g, glycerol to make a paste. This preparation should not be applied to freshly cut tooth surfaces and therefore cannot be used in cavity preparations.— *A.D.T. 1969/70*, 250.

Sodium Fluoride and Phosphoric Acid Gel *(U.S.P.)*. Sodium Fluoride and Orthophosphoric Acid Gel. A gel containing sodium fluoride and phosphoric acid in an aqueous vehicle containing a suitable agent to increase viscosity. Store in airtight plastic containers.

Sodium Fluoride and Phosphoric Acid Topical Solution *(U.S.P.)*. Sodium Fluoride and Orthophosphoric Acid Solution. A solution containing sodium fluoride and phosphoric acid. Store in airtight plastic containers.

Sodium Fluoride Mouthwash *(Orsett Hosp.)*. Sodium fluoride 400 mg, amaranth solution 0.2 ml, benzoic acid solution 2 ml, concentrated raspberry juice 3 ml, freshly distilled water to 100 ml.

Sodium Fluoride Oral Solution *(U.S.P.)*. Sodium Fluoride Solution. A solution containing sodium fluoride. Store in airtight containers. Solutions with a pH below 7.5 should be stored in plastic containers.

Sodium Fluoride Tablets *(U.S.P.)*. Tablets containing sodium fluoride. Store in airtight containers. If they are to be chewed they may be labelled Sodium Fluoride Chewable Tablets.

Solution for Killing Ants. A formula for control of infestation with Pharaoh's ant (*Monomorium pharaonis*) had also been found effective against the common black ant (*Lazius niger*): sodium fluoride 0.8%, honey 6.2%, sucrose 42%, and water 51% all by wt. The resulting syrup was mixed to a mush with sweet cake.— *Pharm. J.*, 1963, *2*, 271.

Proprietary Preparations

En-De-Kay Fluodrops *(Westone, UK: Vestric, UK)*. Paediatric drops containing sodium fluoride 1 mg in each 14-drop dose. **En-De-Kay Fluorinse.** A concentrated mouth-wash containing sodium fluoride 2%. **En-De-Kay Fluotabs 2–4 Years.** Tablets each containing sodium fluoride 1.1 mg **En-De-Kay Fluotabs 4+ Years.** Tablets each containing sodium fluoride 2.2 mg.

En-De-Kay Fluogel *(Westone, UK: Vestric, UK)*. A gel for topical application containing sodium fluoride and hydrofluoric acid providing 1.23% of fluoride, acidified with phosphoric acid, in a flavoured basis.

Fluor-a-day Lac *(Dental Health Promotion, UK)*. Lactose-based scored tablets each containing sodium fluoride 2.2 mg equivalent to 1 mg of fluoride. (Also available as Fluor-a-day in *Canad.*).

Fluorigard *(Hoyt, UK)*. A mouthwash containing sodium fluoride 0.05% and alcohol 6%.

Luride Drops *(Hoyt, UK)*. Paediatric drops containing sodium fluoride 275 µg per drop (equivalent to 125 µg of fluoride). **Luride Lozi-Tabs**. Sodium fluoride, available as fruit-flavoured tablets of 1.1 mg (equivalent to 500 µg of fluoride) and 2.2 mg (equivalent to 1 mg of fluoride). (Also available as Luride in *USA*).

Point-Two *(Hoyt, UK)*. A mouthwash containing sodium fluoride 0.2% and alcohol 6%. (Also available as Point-Two in *USA*).

Zymafluor *(Zyma, UK)*. Sodium fluoride, available as tablets of 550 µg (equivalent to 250 µg of fluoride) and 2.2 mg (equivalent to 1 mg of fluoride). (Also available as Zymafluor in *Belg., Fr., Ger., Ital., Neth., S.Afr., Switz.*).

Some toothpastes containing fluorides are described under Formulas of British Proprietary Medicines.

Other Proprietary Names

Austral.—Denta-Mint Fluoride Mouthwash, Floran Tablets, Flura-tabs, Flurets, F-Tabs, Hifluor, Orofluor; *Belg.*—Fluor; *Canad.*—Flozenges, Fluorinse, Karidium, Oro-Naf, Pedi-Dent, Solu-Flur; *Denm.*—Duraphat, Fluomin, Fluor; *Fr.*—Fluogum, Fluor Oligosol; *Ger.*—Chemifluor, Fluoretten, Mikroplex Fluor, Ossin; *Neth.*—Pharma-Fluor; *Norw.*—AFI-Fluor, Carident, Duraphat, Fluor, Fluortannkrem, Flux; *Spain*—Odontocromil Pasta; *Swed.*—Fludent; *USA*—Fluorigard, Fluoritab, Pediaflor, Phos-flur, Thera-flur.

Preparations containing sodium fluoride were also formerly marketed in Great Britain under the proprietary names Hifluor Gel (*Allied Laboratories*, now *Glaxo*) and Phos-Flur (*Hoyt*).

7734-c

Sodium Fluoroacetate. Compound 1080; Sodium Monofluoroacetate.
$FCH_2.CO_2Na = 100.0$.

CAS — 62-74-8.

A white odourless almost tasteless powder. Very **soluble** in water; relatively insoluble in organic solvents.

Adverse Effects. Sodium fluoroacetate is highly toxic, the lethal dose being about 5 mg per kg body-weight; lower values have also been suggested. Toxic effects are delayed for several hours after absorption by mouth or through the skin and include nausea and vomiting, apprehension, mental confusion, tremors and twitching, cardiac irregularities, and convulsions. Coma may be followed by death from cardiac failure.

Maximum permissible atmospheric concentration 50 µg per m^3.

Treatment of Adverse Effects. Empty the stomach by aspiration and lavage with water. Remove any contaminated clothing and wash the affected skin with soap and water. Saline catharsis has also been recommended. Control convulsions by the intravenous administration of diazepam 5 to 10 mg. Assisted respiration may be required. Monoacetin in a dose of 0.5 ml per kg body-weight by intramuscular injection or by intravenous injection, if diluted with 5 parts of sodium chloride injection, has been suggested as an antidote on the basis of *animal* experiments; as an acetate donor it should be a competitive antagonist to fluoroacetate in the tricarboxylic acid cycle. Acetamide or alcohol may fulfil the same function. Further treatment is symptomatic.

Treatment of fluoroacetate poisoning was largely symptomatic after the stomach had been washed out. A number of substances—acetates, alcohol, monoacetin, and acetamide—had been found to exert a protective action in the laboratory, but their clinical value as antidotes was unproved.— *Br. med. J.*, 1964, *1*, 387.

Uses. Sodium fluoroacetate is a highly effective poison for all kinds of rodents but must be used with great caution because of its toxicity to other animals and to man.

In Great Britain, the use of sodium fluoroacetate is restricted to the destruction of rats in ships and in sewers and in specified dock warehouses. When supplied for use as a rodenticide it must contain a distinctive colouring matter.

Fluoroacetamide and Sodium Fluoroacetate as Rodenticides. See *Use of Fluoroacetamide and Sodium Fluoroacetate as Rodenticides; Precautionary Measures*, Ministry of Agriculture, Fisheries and Food, London, HM Stationery Office, 1970.

It was recommended, in view of the extreme hazard to other mammals, that fluoroacetamide and sodium fluoroacetate should only be used by trained pest control operators in areas such as locked warehouses and sewers to which access by unauthorised persons and useful animals could be prevented completely.— Safe Use of

Pesticides, Twentieth Report of the WHO Expert Committee on Insecticides, *Tech. Rep. Ser. Wld Hlth Org. No. 513,* 1973.

7735-k

Sodium Monofluorophosphate *(U.S.P.).* Sodium Fluorophosphate; MFP Sodium; Natrii Monofluorophosphas.
Na_2PO_3F=143.9.

CAS — 10163-15-2.

Pharmacopoeias. In *Nord.* and *U.S.*

Almost odourless, hygroscopic, colourless crystals or white or slightly grey crystalline powder, with a saline taste. Each g provides 6.9 mmol (6.9 mEq) of fluoride. **Soluble** 1 in 2 of water; practically insoluble in alcohol. A 2% solution in water has a pH of 6.5 to 8. **Store** in airtight containers.

The stability of monofluorophosphate and fluoride ions in dentifrices containing calcium carbonate.— B. Norén and C. Härse, *J. Soc. cosmet. Chem.*, 1974, *25,* 3.

Adverse Effects, Treatment, and Precautions. As for Sodium Fluoride, p.700.

Uses. Sodium monofluorophosphate is used in toothpastes for the prevention of dental caries and is reported to cause less staining than stannous fluoride.

In a double-blind trial in 237 elderly patients given sodium monofluorophosphate equivalent to 25 mg fluoride daily for 5 months for osteoporosis prophylaxis and 223 controls, the fluoride group lost weight while the control group gained weight and exacerbations of arthrosis and fractures were more common in the fluoride group. Plasma concentrations of ionised fluoride of about 10 µmol per litre occurred in some patients and fell only slowly when the dose was reduced or fluoride discontinued. A plasma-fluoride concentration of not more than 3 µmol per litre was suggested in osteoporosis prophylaxis.— J. Inkovaara *et al.*, *Br. med. J.* 1975, *3,* 73.

Dental caries. See under Sodium Fluoride, p.702.

Toothpaste. Sodium monofluorophosphate 0.76% in toothpaste had similar caries-preventing effects to stannous fluoride 0.4% but caused less tooth staining and might prove to be more acceptable.— M. N. Naylor and R. D. Emslie, *Br. dent. J.*, 1967, *123,* 17.

A fluoride toothpaste containing 0.76% of sodium monofluorophosphate and 2% of sodium *N*-lauroylsarcosinate was compared with a control toothpaste in a double-blind trial in 578 children. Use of the fluoride toothpaste for 30 months resulted in an average of 18.9% fewer new decayed, missing, or filled surfaces.— I. J. Møller *et al.*, *Br. dent. J.*, 1968, *124,* 209. Similar results with a silica gel dentifrice containing sodium monofluorophosphate 0.76% and sodium lauryl sulphate in 495 children in a 3 year double-blind study.— A. P. Howat *et al.*, *ibid.*, 1978, *145,* 233.

The addition of sodium fluoride 0.1% to dentifrices containing sodium monofluorophosphate 0.76% enhanced the effectiveness in preventing dental caries, in a double-blind study in 799 children.— H. C. Hodge *et al.*, *Br. dent. J.*, 1980, *149,* 201.

7736-a

Sodium Silicofluoride. Sodium Fluosilicate; Sodium Hexafluorosilicate.
Na_2SiF_6=188.1.

CAS — 16893-85-9.

A fine, white, odourless, granular or crystalline powder, becoming gelatinous when moist.
Soluble 1 in about 200 of water, giving a turbid solution; practically insoluble in alcohol. A saturated solution has a pH of 3.5. Concentrated solutions attack metal and porcelain enamel. **Store** in airtight containers.

Adverse Effects, Treatment, and Precautions. As for Sodium Fluoride, p.700.

Sodium silicofluoride is the sodium salt of hydrofluorosilicic acid (see p.700). It is used in controlled amounts for the fluoridation of drinking water.

7737-t

Stannous Fluoride *(U.S.P.).* Stannosi Fluoridum.
SnF_2=156.7.

CAS — 7783-47-3.

Pharmacopoeias. In *Nord.* and *U.S.*

A white, odourless, hygroscopic, crystalline powder with a bitter saline taste. M.p. about 213°.
Freely **soluble** in water; practically insoluble in alcohol, chloroform, and ether. A 0.4% solution in water has a pH of 2.8 to 3.5. Aqueous solutions decompose within a few hours, with the formation of a white precipitate; they slowly attack glass. **Incompatible** with alkaline substances and oxidising agents. **Store** in airtight containers.

There was a progressive decrease in the amount of soluble fluoride extractable with water or saliva from 3 brands of toothpaste containing stannous fluoride after storage for 30 weeks at 4° to 5°, 19° to 20°, or 35° to 37°. Differences in the stability of the stannous fluoride on storage could not be closely correlated with the calcium content of the pastes. Since each of these pastes had been proved effective clinically, release of soluble fluoride to saliva *in vitro* could not be considered a useful indicator of probable clinical performance. However, the ability to release fluoride was related to age and storage temperature and in view of losses of soluble fluoride of about 40% in 30 weeks at room temperature, cold storage should be used.— R. Duckworth, *Br. dent. J.*, 1968, *125,* 261.

Adverse Effects, Treatment, and Precautions. As for Sodium Fluoride, p.700.

A 3-year-old child died about 3 hours after the topical application of stannous fluoride 4% to non-carious teeth and the accidental ingestion of about half a cup of the solution given as a mouthwash. Five minutes after ingestion the child vomited, developed a convulsive seizure, and went into shock. Cardio-respiratory arrest occurred in the intensive-care unit during a seizure.— L. E. Church, *J. Maryland dent. Ass.*, 1976, *19,* 106, per *Br. dent. J.*, 1976, *141,* 234.

Uses. Stannous fluoride, like sodium fluoride, is used for topical application to the teeth for the prophylaxis of dental caries. After preliminary cleansing of the teeth, a single application is made of a freshly prepared 8% aqueous solution and this application is repeated at intervals of 6 to 12 months.
Toothpastes containing stannous fluoride are also used. Staining of teeth has been noted following the use of stannous fluoride toothpastes.

Dental caries. In a 12-months' controlled study of 1250 children residing in a community whose water supply contained only 0.05 ppm of fluoride, it was found that a significant reduction in dental caries occurred in children subjected to combined treatment with a stannous fluoride prophylactic paste, a topical 8% solution of stannous fluoride, and a stannous fluoride dentifrice; 41% of the children receiving this treatment remained free of caries.— D. Bixler and J. C. Muhler, *J. Am. dent. Ass.*, 1964, *68,* 792, per *Int. pharm. Abstr.*, 1964, *1,* 1529.

Repeated applications of stannous fluoride solutions as 0.1, 2, and 5% solutions to intact dentine produced a cumulative protective effect against the effects of mineral acid. The 2 and 5% solutions were the most effective.— E. Sandoval and I. L. Shannon, *Tex. Rep. Biol. Med.*, 1969, *27,* 111, per *Abstr. Hyg.*, 1969, *44,* 776.

Toothpastes. For favourable reports of the use of toothpastes and dentifrices containing stannous fluoride for the prevention of dental caries, see Martindale 27th Edn, p. 621.

Proprietary Names
Floran Capsules *(Creighton, Austral.)*; Gel-Kam *(Scherer, USA)*; Orostan *(Orapharm, Austral.)*.

Glucagon

7711-s

Glucagon *(B.P., U.S.P.)*. HGF. A polypeptide derived from beef or pork pancreas. His-Ser-Gln-Gly-Thr-Phe-Thr-Ser-Asp-Tyr-Ser-Lys-Tyr-Leu-Asp-Ser-Arg-Arg-Ala-Gln-Asp-Phe-Val-Gln-Trp-Leu-Met-Asn-Thr.
$C_{153}H_{225}N_{43}O_{49}S = 3482.8$.

CAS — 16941-32-5.

Pharmacopoeias. In *Br.* and *U.S.*

A white or faintly coloured, almost odourless and tasteless, crystalline powder. It loses not more than 10% of its weight on drying. Practically **insoluble** in water; soluble in dilute alkalis and acids; practically insoluble in most organic solvents. **Store** at 2° to 8° in airtight containers in which the air has been replaced by nitrogen.

Glucagon is administered as glucagon hydrochloride which is glucagon with hydrochloric acid.

Units. 1.49 units of glucagon, porcine for bioassay, are contained in approximately 1.5 mg, with lactose 5 mg and sodium chloride, in one ampoule of the first International Standard Preparation (1973).

1.49 units of glucagon, porcine for immunoassay, are contained in approximately 1.5 mg, with lactose 5 mg and sodium chloride, in one ampoule of the first International Reference Preparation (1974).

Adverse Effects. Nausea and vomiting are the most frequent side-effects of glucagon. Hypersensitivity reactions and hypokalaemia may also occur.

A continuous infusion of glucagon 45 µg per kg body-weight per hour in conjunction with pentagastrin 6 µg per kg per hour for 4 hours produced diarrhoea in 2 subjects and induced defaecation in another. Diarrhoea also occurred in a patient with Zollinger-Ellison syndrome given glucagon alone. Both hormones might be implicated in the diarrhoea of some intestinal diseases.— G. O. Barbezat *et al.* (letter), *Lancet*, 1972, *1*, 904.

Skin rash attributed to glucagon in one patient and considered to be a manifestation of hyperglucagonaemia.— S. G. Barber and J. D. Hamer (letter), *Lancet*, 1976, *2*, 1138.

A report of diabetic ketoacidosis in a patient with pancreatitis treated with glucagon.— J. Tyler *et al.*, *J. Ir. med. Ass.*, 1977, *70*, 488.

Ventricular or supraventricular extrasystoles in 5 of 22 subjects given glucagon 50 µg per kg body-weight intravenously.— K. Markiewicz *et al.*, *Eur. J. Cardiol.*, 1977, *6*, 449.

Precautions. Glucagon hydrochloride should not be administered in suspected hypoglycaemic emergencies until the diagnosis has been confirmed. It may provoke severe hypertension in patients with phaeochromocytoma. It should be used with care in patients with insulinoma in whom the insulin-releasing effect may cause hypoglycaemia.

Glucagon is not effective in patients with marked depletion of glycogen stores, as in starvation, adrenal insufficiency, or chronic hypoglycaemia.

A diabetic, being treated for hypoglycaemic coma, failed to improve fully on intravenous dextrose and was given an intravenous injection of 1 mg of glucagon. Severe hypoglycaemia immediately followed and the patient became unconscious and showed signs of collapse. She responded to treatment with infusions of dextrose and hydrocortisone. Because glucagon was a strong stimulator of insulin secretion, its use was not recommended in the treatment of hypoglycaemia.— G. Marri *et al.* (letter), *Lancet*, 1968, *1*, 303. In severe hypoglycaemia induced by sulphonylurea drugs the effect of glucagon in stimulating the glucose output of the liver was of greater clinical importance than its stimulant effects on insulin secretion, provided that an adequate amount of dextrose was given.— D. M. Davies (letter), *ibid.*, 1154.

Small pulmonary emboli were found in *dogs* given intravenous infusions of glucagon in doses 4 to 10 times those used to treat cardiac conditions (4 mg per hour in a 70-kg patient). It was recommended that glucagon should not be given by intravenous infusion or repeated intravenous injection until further study had been carried out.— W. I. H. Shedden, *Lilly* (letter), *Lancet*, 1971, *2*, 1421.

Interactions. Alcohol inhibited the glucagon-induced release of insulin but enhanced the glucose-induced release of insulin.— R. Friedenberg *et al.*, *Diabetes*, 1971, *20*, 397, per *Abstr. Wld Med.*, 1971, *45*, 861.

For a report of high doses of glucagon enhancing the anticoagulant effect of warfarin, see Warfarin Sodium, p.779.

Absorption and Fate. Glucagon has a plasma half-life of about 10 minutes. It is inactivated in the liver, kidneys, and plasma.

Uses. Glucagon is a polypeptide which is secreted by the alpha cells of the islets of Langerhans. It is a *hyperglycaemic* agent which mobilises hepatic glycogen so that glucose is released into the blood. It also has lipolytic properties and, under certain conditions, stimulates the secretion of pancreatic insulin. It has a relatively short duration of action. Glucagon is administered as glucagon hydrochloride; doses are usually expressed as glucagon.

In the treatment of insulin hypoglycaemia dextrose is the treatment of choice, by mouth or intravenously (see p.51). If dextrose is not immediately available, glucagon may be given as a 0.1% solution by subcutaneous, intramuscular, or intravenous injection. The usual dose is 0.5 to 1 mg. A response usually occurs in 5 to 20 minutes. After the initial effect, in most patients there is a return to normal or hypoglycaemic levels in 1 to 1.5 hours. In the absence of response 1 or 2 further doses may be given at 20-minute intervals. A suggested dose for children is 25 µg per kg body-weight. After the patient has awakened from hypoglycaemic coma, dextrose or other carbohydrate must be given to prevent a relapse. Dextrose should be given intravenously if the patient does not respond to glucagon.

Glucagon has also been employed to terminate insulin coma in psychiatry, when larger doses of 1 mg or more may be necessary.

Glucagon has a positive inotropic effect on cardiac muscle; it decreases peripheral vascular resistance, increases cardiac index and output, and increases mean arterial pressure; the effect on heart-rate appears to be variable. It has been used as an adjunct in the treatment of refractory heart failure (but see under Precautions). Doses have varied considerably but have usually been within the range 2.5 to 7.5 mg per hour, given by intravenous infusion.

Glucagon reduces the motility of the gastro-intestinal tract and has been used as an adjunct to radiology and endoscopy. The dose required may be 0.2 to 2 mg, usually given intravenously; the effect lasts about 15 minutes; it has also been given intramuscularly.

Reviews and discussions of the physiology and uses of glucagon.—*Glucagon*, P.J. Lefebvre and R.H. Unger (Eds.), Oxford, Pergamon Press, 1972; G. F. Cahill, *New Engl. J. Med.*, 1973, *288*, 157; *Postgrad. med. J.*, 1973, *49*, (Aug.), *Suppl.* 6; J. Lavarenne, *Thérapie*, 1974, *29*, 161; R. P. Eaton *et al.*, *Lancet*, 1974, *2*, 1545; R. C. G. Russell *et al.*, *Br. med. J.*, 1975, *1*, 10; T. H. Maugh, *Science*, 1975, *188*, 920; J. H. Walsh *et al.*, *Ann. intern. Med.*, 1979, *90*, 817; R. H. Unger and L. Orci, *New Engl. J. Med.*, 1981, *304*, 1518 and 1575.

For the use of glucagon in the treatment of excessive beta blockade, see Propranolol Hydrochloride, p.1327.

Administration. In 6 healthy subjects and 6 diabetic patients the effect of glucagon 1 mg given intramuscularly was greater (except initially) and more prolonged than that of the same dose given intravenously. The intramuscular route was the route of choice.— J. R. Taylor *et al.*, *Eur. J. clin. Pharmac.*, 1978, *14*, 125.

Effects on calcium. Glucagon, administered intravenously over 4 hours, significantly reduced the calcium concentration in the serum by about 4.3 and 6.9 µg per ml in healthy persons and in patients with primary hyperparathyroidism respectively. The fall could not be accounted for by increased renal excretion.— S. J. Birge and L. V. Avioli, *J. clin. Endocr. Metab.*, 1969, *29*, 213, per *J. Am. med. Ass.*, 1969, *207*, 2499.

See also under Effects on the Cardiovascular System and under Osteitis Deformans.

Effects on carbohydrate metabolism. Discussions of the role of glucagon in diabetes.— R. S. Sherwin *et al.*, *New Engl. J. Med.*, 1976, *294*, 455; R. Levine, *ibid.*, 494; R. H. Unger and L. Orci, *Archs intern. Med.*, 1977, *137*, 482; P. Felig and R. S. Sherwin, *Ann. intern. Med.*, 1980, *92*, 856. See also A. J. Barnes *et al.*, *New Engl. J. Med.*, 1977, *296*, 1250; H. G. Dammann *et al.* (letter), *Lancet*, 1978, *1*, 1205.

See also under Insulinoma Test.

Hypoglycaemia. Normal blood-glucose concentrations were maintained for 24 hours between injections when zinc glucagon was given at night in a dose of 2.5 to 5 mg to 2 children, aged 2 and 3½ years, with idiopathic hypoglycaemia.— A. L. Rosenbloom, *Am. J. Dis. Child.*, 1966, *112*, 107, per *J. Am. med. Ass.*, 1966, *197*, 654.

Of 100 hypoglycaemic diabetics, 40 responded within 15 minutes to glucagon, 1 mg intramuscularly or intravenously; 1 further patient responded to a second injection 15 minutes later. Of the 59 glucagon-unresponsive patients, 36 became conscious after an initial intravenous injection of dextrose 25 g, 4 after a second dose, and 17 of the remaining 19 responded to mannitol 40 g intravenously, steroids, and oxygen. Two patients died; 1 with pneumococcal meningitis and the other from the effects of 800 units of protamine zinc insulin.— A. C. MacCuish *et al.*, *Lancet*, 1970, *2*, 946.

Zinc glucagon was used successfully in the long-term management of hypoglycaemia in 2 children for 4 years and 1 year respectively. Zinc glucagon was preferred to diazoxide due to the side-effects of the latter.— L. Kollée and L. Monnens (letter), *Lancet*, 1978, *1*, 668. See also L. A. Kollée *et al.*, *Archs Dis. Childh.*, 1978, *53*, 422.

Effects on the cardiovascular system. The effect of glucagon on digital circulation.— G. E. Burch and T. D. Giles, *Clin. Pharmac. Ther.*, 1975, *17*, 409.

A study of the electrophysiological properties of glucagon on human cardiac muscle. The effects of glucagon on the heart were the opposite of those of digitalis; it might therefore be useful in the treatment of digitalis intoxication.— K. Prasad, *Clin. Pharmac. Ther.*, 1975, *18*, 22.

A review of various compounds affecting the heart. Glucagon is reported to possess both inotropic and chronotropic properties and to act probably by increasing intracellular concentrations of cyclic AMP, although an inhibitory effect on membrane ATP-ase allowing an increase in calcium influx has been suggested. These effects are reported not to be influenced by beta-adrenoceptor blockade.— M. J. H. Scallan *et al.*, *Br. J. Anaesth.*, 1979, *51*, 649.

For references to the use of glucagon in the treatment of heart failure, see Martindale 27th Edn, p. 622.

Effects on the gastro-intestinal tract. Glucagon, infused intravenously at the rate of 30 µg per kg body-weight per hour, decreased basal serum-gastrin concentrations and the gastrin response to a meal in healthy subjects and patients with duodenal ulcer. In patients with the Zollinger-Ellison syndrome basal serum-gastrin values were increased and the gastrin response to a meal was not reduced.— H. D. Becker *et al.*, *Gastroenterology*, 1973, *65*, 28, per *Int. pharm. Abstr.*, 1974, *11*, 190. In a study involving 18 healthy male subjects, glucagon 2 mg given within 3 minutes by intravenous injection or 1.64 µg per kg body-weight given over 60 minutes by constant infusion significantly increased gastric mucosal potential difference. Pentagastrin 2 µg per kg given over 60 minutes by infusion significantly reduced potential difference and the effects of each of these hormones could be reversed by administration of the other. At the doses used neither glucagon nor pentagastrin significantly altered the blood concentrations of gastrin or glucagon respectively.— A. Tarnawski *et al.*, *Gut*, 1978, *19*, 1116.

The use of glucagon in ileocolic intussusception.— G. R. Hoy *et al.*, *J. pediat. Surg.*, 1977, *12*, 939.

Glucagon protected volunteers from aspirin-induced gastric mucosal damage.— A. Tarnawski *et al.*, *Gastroenterology*, 1978, *74*, 240.

Further references: *Glucagon in Gastroenterology*, J. Picazo (Ed.), Lancaster, MTP, 1979.

See also Effects on the Oesophagus and Radiography.

Diverticulitis. In 20 patients with acute diverticulitis symptomatic relief was achieved in about 12 hours after the use of glucagon without analgesics or anti-spasmodics, compared with about 4 days in 15 patients previously treated conventionally. The treatment appeared to be specific. Glucagon 1 mg in 10 or 20 ml of diluent was given intravenously every 4 hours for 9 doses; 6 patients received 4.5 mg in 50 ml of diluent by infusion pump over 2 consecutive periods of 18 hours.— O. Daniel *et al.*, *Br. med. J.*, 1974, *3*, 720.

Effects on the liver. Glucagon markedly enhanced the release from the liver of cyclic AMP.— J. E. Liljenquist *et al.*, *J. clin. Invest.*, 1974, *53*, 198, per *J. Am. med. Ass.*, 1974, *228*, 782. A similar report in patients with extrahepatic obstruction.— T. F. Davies *et al.*, *Br. med. J.*, 1976, *1*, 931.

Further references: N. A. Volpicelli, in *Glucagon in Gastroenterology*, J. Picazo (Ed.), Lancaster, MTP, 1979.

Liver-function test. For the use of glucagon, 40 µg per kg body-weight intravenously, to assess liver function, see H. Brunner *et al.*, *Wien. Z. inn. Med.*, 1968, *49*, 409, per *Abstr. Wld Med.*, 1969, *43*, 496.

Blood-sugar concentrations rose by at least 50% when glucagon, 5 µg per kg body-weight, was given intravenously to 20 control subjects, but by only 10% when glucagon was given to 32 patients with hepatic cirrhosis.— H. -J. Schulten and K. Becker, *Z. Gastroent.*, 1969, *7*, 42, per *Abstr. Wld Med.*, 1969, *43*, 667.

Effects on the oesophagus. Studies in volunteers and in *dogs* indicated that glucagon reduced oesophageal sphincter pressure. The elevated sphincter pressure in 10 patients with achalasia was reduced by the intravenous injection of glucagon 60 µg per kg body-weight.— H. M. Jennewein *et al.*, *Gut*, 1973, *14*, 861.

Because of its effect in suppressing gastric secretion and reducing gastric motility, glucagon was used in the conservative treatment of 3 patients with perforation of the oesophagus; 1 mg was given initially over 5 minutes followed by 2 mg every 6 hours by continuous infusion for 4 or 5 days. Only minimal amounts of fluid were detected in the pleural cavities.— R. Pickard (letter), *Br. med. J.*, 1974, *4*, 232.

The use of glucagon intravenously in the management of oesophageal food obstruction.— J. Glauser *et al.*, *JACEP* 1979, *8*, 228.

Gall-stones. Biliary colic was promptly relieved in 26 of 31 patients with cholelithiasis after receiving a single intravenous dose of glucagon 0.2 to 1 mg. Infusion of glucagon 3 to 5 mg daily for 2 to 12 days, resolved stone obstruction of the cystic duct or concrement of the common duct in 6 of 10 patients, and was considered to have facilitated passage of common bile-duct stones in 56 of 61 who underwent endoscopic papillotomy.— F. Paul, in *Glucagon in Gastroenterology*, J. Picazo (Ed.), Lancaster, MTP, 1979.

Reduction of bile duct sphincter pressure by glucagon.— D. L. Carr-Locke and J. A. Gregg, *Clin. Sci.*, 1980, *59*, Sept., 9p.

Growth-hormone deficiency test. A subcutaneous or intramuscular injection of glucagon 1 to 1.5 mg increased the peak serum concentration of growth hormone to 8 ng or more per ml within 2 hours in 33 of 34 persons without apparent pituitary disorder. The maximum value for growth hormone concentration in 21 of 23 patients with clinical pituitary disorders, after stimulation with glucagon, was 4.8 ng per ml. A value of less than 7 ng per ml was suggestive of deficiency.— M. L. Mitchell *et al.*, *New Engl. J. Med.*, 1970, *282*, 539. A rise of less than 5 ng per ml appeared to be abnormal and suggestive of pituitary insufficiency.— J. P. Cain *et al.*, *Can. med. Ass. J.*, 1972, *107*, 617.

The reliability of the glucagon stimulation test for the ability to secrete growth hormone was increased if propranolol was given 2 hours before the test.— C. T. Sawin and M. L. Mitchell (letter), *Br. med. J.*, 1973, *3*, 499.

With rare exceptions plasma-corticosteroid concentrations rose together with growth-hormone concentrations after 1 mg of glucagon given subcutaneously. Absence of response was indicative of corticotrophin deficiency.— *Br. med. J.*, 1973, *4*, 5.

Of 73 children with retarded growth 20 who failed to respond (with growth-hormone concentration greater than 6 ng per ml) to arginine or insulin also failed to respond to propranolol and glucagon; 49 had values of 5 ng per ml initially which rose to 10.9 ng per ml after propranolol and to 20.8 ng per ml after glucagon; 4 who had positive responses had clinical features consistent with growth-hormone deficiency.— J. S. Parks *et al.*, *J. clin. Endocr. Metab.*, 1973, *37*, 85, per *Int. pharm. Abstr.*, 1974, *11*, 291.

Insulinoma test. In 28 healthy subjects peak serum concentrations of immunoreactive insulin (measured at 3- to 5-minute intervals) after the rapid intravenous injection of glucagon 1 mg did not exceed 100 microunits per ml, and exceeded this value in only 1 patient, taking tolbutamide, of 29 patients with hypoglycaemia of varied aetiology. Of 7 patients with proven insulinoma, peak insulin concentrations exceeded 130 microunits per ml in 6; the highest value in the seventh patient (measured at 15-minute intervals) was 93 microunits per ml. A review of other published reports indicated that values above 130 to 160 microunits per ml should be considered positive and values above 100 microunits per ml were suggestive of insulinoma. Samples should be assessed every 5 minutes. False negative results might occur in patients taking diazoxide, hydrochlorothiazide, or phenytoin; false positive results might occur in obese patients or those taking tolbutamide.— D. Kumar *et al.*, *Ann. intern. Med.*, 1974, *80*, 697.

Osteitis deformans. In 4 patients with Paget's disease of bone the infusion of glucagon at a rate of up to 20 mg daily led to a fall in the plasma concentration of alkaline phosphatase and a reduction in the urinary excretion of calcium and hydroxyproline. Bone pain was relieved in 2 patients. The mechanism of action might be a direct effect on bone, stimulation of release of calcitonin, or stimulation of bone pyrophosphates and thus control of bone formation and resorption.— J. R. Condon, *Br. med. J.*, 1971, *4*, 719. Patients with Paget's disease of bone could be maintained, without side-effects, on glucagon 2 to 3 mg subcutaneously once or twice daily.— J. R. Condon (letter), *Br. med. J.*, 1977, *2*, 263.

Pancreatitis. Thirty patients with acute pancreatitis were treated with glucagon intravenously: 1 mg initially, then 1 to 1.5 mg every 4 hours for 24 to 96 hours. Mortality was 7% compared with 22 to 26% in most published series in Britain. The use of glucagon for this condition appeared to be justified.— J. R. Condon *et al.* (letter), *Br. med. J.*, 1972, *1*, 376. See also M. J. Knight *et al.*, *ibid.*, 1971, *2*, 440.

In a controlled pilot study of 15 patients with acute pancreatitis there was a significant reduction in serum-amylase concentration and in pain in the 6 patients given glucagon compared with 9 patients given placebo.— M. W. Waterworth *et al.* (letter), *Lancet*, 1974, *1*, 1231.

Neither glucagon given to 68 patients nor aprotinin given to 66 had any effect on the death-rate of acute pancreatitis when compared with a placebo given to 123 patients. Glucagon was given in a dose of 2 mg intravenously immediately followed by 2 mg by intravenous infusion every 6 hours for 5 days.—MRC Multicentre Trial of Glucagon and Aprotinin, *Lancet*, 1977, *2*, 632. Analysis of the results showed that glucagon or aprotinin did not influence the rate of recovery or the incidence of complications.—MRC Multicentre Trial *Gut*, 1980, *21*, 334.

Further reports of the absence of benefit of glucagon in pancreatitis.— H. K. Dürr *et al.*, *Gut*, 1978, *19*, 175; A. Olazabal and R. Fuller, *Gastroenterology*, 1978, *74*, 489.

Phaeochromocytoma test. The rapid intravenous injection of glucagon hydrochloride (usually 1 mg) to 12 patients with known phaeochromocytoma produced a positive pressor response in 6, the peak being reached usually within 3 minutes. In only 2 patients were circulating catecholamines significantly increased. Blood pressure returned to normal within 15 minutes. No pressor response was obtained in 30 patients without tumour. Side-effects (headache, flushing, nausea, and palpitations) were mild and transient. Four of the 6 patients also responded to the intravenous injection of histamine, usually in a dose of 25 µg; side-effects were more frequent and less mild.— S. G. Sheps and F. T. Maher, *J. Am. med. Ass.*, 1968, *205*, 895. The administration of glucagon could result in excessively high blood pressure, increased heart-rate, and arrhythmias in patients with phaeochromocytoma, and the test should be performed only if clearly indicated.— W. V. Studnitz, *Schweiz. med. Wschr.*, 1970, *100*, 1023, per *J. Am. med. Ass.*, 1970, *213*, 334.

The basis of false-positive glucagon tests for phaeochromocytoma.— O. Kuchel *et al.*, *Clin. Pharmac. Ther.*, 1981, *29*, 687.

Radiography. References to the use of glucagon in radiography.— D. Novak and P. Probst, *Dt. med. Wschr.*, 1973, *98*, 2352; *J. Am. med. Ass.*, 1974, *228*, 1169; R. E. Miller *et al.*, *Radiology*, 1974, *113*, 555; J. C. Meeroff *et al.*, *ibid.*, 5; V. K. Gohel *et al.*, *ibid.*, 1975, *115*, 1; J. T. Ferrucci *et al.*, *Radiology*, 1976, *118*, 466; G. Bertrand *et al.*, *Am. J. Roentg.*, 1977, *128*, 197; L. Kreel, in *Glucagon in Gastroenterology*, J. Picazo (Ed.), Lancaster, MTP, 1979.

Preparations

Glucagon for Injection *(U.S.P.)*. A sterile mixture of glucagon hydrochloride with 1 or more suitable dry diluents; when dissolved in the sterile solvent provided it forms a clear solution with a pH of 2.5 to 3.

Glucagon Injection *(B.P.)*. A sterile solution of glucagon with hydrochloric acid and lactose, prepared by dissolving the contents of a sealed container (Glucagon for Injection) in a suitable solvent which contains a suitable antimicrobial preservative. The solution should be used immediately except in the presence of a bactericide when it may be kept for 7 days if stored at 2° to 8°; it should not be used if a gel or insoluble matter forms. pH of a solution containing 1 unit per ml, 2.5 to 4.

Proprietary Preparations

Glucagon *(Lilly, UK)*. Glucagon hydrochloride, available in vials each containing the equivalent of 1 unit of glucagon with lactose as diluent, supplied with 1-ml vials of solvent, or vials of 10 units with 10-ml vials of solvent. (Also available as Glucagon *Lilly* in *Austral., Canad., Neth., S.Afr., Swed., Switz., USA*).

Glucagon Novo *(Novo, UK: Farillon, UK)*. Glucagon hydrochloride, available in vials of 1 mg, with lactose as diluent, supplied with a disposable syringe containing Water for Injections 1 ml as solvent; or vials of 10 mg, with lactose as diluent, supplied with 10-ml vials of solvent. (Also available as Glucagon *Novo* in *Austral., Belg., Denm., Fr., Ger., Neth., Norw., S.Afr., Spain, Swed., Switz*).

Other Proprietary Names

Glucagone Novo *(Ital.)*; Glukagon Lilly *(Ger.)*.

Glycerol Glycols and Macrogols

1901-y

Glycerol *(B.P., B.P. Vet., Eur. P.).* Glycerolum; Glycerin *(U.S.P.)*; Glicerol. Propane-1,2,3-triol. $C_3H_8O_3$=92.09.

CAS — 56-81-5.

Pharmacopoeias. In all pharmacopoeias examined except *Rus. B.P.* and *Eur. P.* also include Glycerol (85 per cent) which has a range of 84 to 88% of $C_3H_8O_3$; several other pharmacopoeias also specify a similar strength in addition to the most concentrated form which may be described as Anhydrous Glycerin or Concentrated Glycerin.

A clear, colourless, hygroscopic, syrupy liquid, odourless or with a slight odour and with a sweet taste followed by a sensation of warmth; it may contain a small proportion of water. *B.P.* specifies a relative density of 1.258 to 1.263. *U.S.P.* specifies 95 to 101% of $C_3H_8O_3$ and specific gravity of not less than 1.249.

Miscible with water, alcohol, and propylene glycol; slightly soluble in acetone; practically insoluble in chloroform, ether, and fixed and volatile oils. A 10% w/v solution in water is neutral to litmus. A 2.6% w/v solution is iso-osmotic with serum. It may be **sterilised** by maintaining at 150° for 1 hour. **Incompatible** with oxidising agents. **Store** in airtight containers. If kept at low temperatures glycerol may solidify to a mass of crystals. The crystals do not melt until the temperature is raised to about 20°.

Haemolysis. A solution of glycerol in water iso-osmotic with serum (2.6%) caused 100% haemolysis of erythrocytes cultured in it for 45 minutes.— E. R. Hammarlund and K. Pedersen-Bjergaard, *J. pharm. Sci.*, 1961, *50*, 24.

Adverse Effects. Very large doses by mouth can exert systemic effects such as headache, thirst, nausea, and hyperglycaemia. The injection of large doses may induce convulsions, paralysis, haemolysis, and renal failure.

Maximum permissible atmospheric concentration of glycerol mist 10 mg per m^3.

Glycerol had an irritant effect on the gastric mucosa when given at concentrations greater than 40% v/v to *dogs* and *rats*. Sorbitol solution was less irritant, and propylene glycol had almost no irritant effects in equivalent dosage.— R. Staples *et al.*, *J. pharm. Sci.*, 1967, *56*, 398.

A report of glycerol intolerance in a child with a history of hypoglycaemia. Administration by mouth produced euphoria, confusion, drowsiness, nausea, vomiting, and diarrhoea. Intravenous administration produced loss of consciousness, convulsion, and coma within 4 minutes.— N. K. Maclaren *et al.*, *J. Pediat.*, 1975, *86*, 43.

A high serum osmolality was attributed to treatment with glycerol 1 g per kg body-weight every 6 hours in a patient with poorly controlled diabetes, hypertension, ischaemic heart disease, and congestive heart failure who was admitted following a stroke. Withdrawal of the glycerol produced an improvement in osmolality and a reduction in insulin requirements.— B. J. Hurwitz and D. A. Rottenberg (letter), *Lancet*, 1975, *2*, 369. The inability to deal with the glycerol might have been due to the patient's obesity (120 kg body-weight) rather than his diabetes. Also the dose was too high.— A. J. Wade (letter), *ibid.*, 708. The patient only received 400 g daily although 1 g per kg body-weight every 6 hours was prescribed.— B. J. Hurwitz and D. A. Rottenberg (letter), *ibid.*, 933.

A report of temporary hearing loss after a glycerol test.— D. E. Mattox and R. L. Goode, *Archs Otolar.*, 1978, *104*, 359.

Haemolysis. Infusion of glycerol 20% in sodium chloride injection given in doses of 70 g in 30 minutes and 80 g in 60 minutes reduced the intracranial pressure in 2 patients but was associated with severe haemolysis and haemoglobinuria. A third patient given 60 g in 15 minutes had slight evidence of haemolysis.— K. Hägnevik *et al.*, *Lancet*, 1974, *1*, 75.

In a review of 500 patients given glycerol by intravenous infusion no side-effects were seen when 50 g in 500 ml of sodium chloride injection was administered over 6 hours daily for 7 to 10 days. Haemolysis was observed in 4 of 70 patients when the rate of infusion was increased.— K. M. A. Welch *et al.* (letter), *Lancet*, 1974, *1*, 416.

Hypersensitivity. No irritant reactions were seen in 420 consecutive patients with eczema after hypersensitivity testing with glycerol 50%, sorbitol 10%, or xylitol 10% in water. However, a patient who had developed eczema after using a mixture containing glycerol in alcohol after washing her hands showed an allergic reaction to testing with glycerol.— M. Hannuksela and L. Förström, *Contact Dermatitis*, 1976, *2*, 291.

Oxalosis. Crystals of what was considered to be oxalic acid were found in cerebral blood vessels and renal tubules in one patient. Five hours before death he had received a glycerol infusion for what was presumed to be a cerebral infarction and this part of his treatment was considered to be the cause of his oxalosis. Postmortem examination revealed multifocal petechial bleeding in the brain probably associated with a hypertensive crisis and head injury sustained 10 days earlier.— T. Krausz *et al.* (letter), *Lancet*, 1977, *2*, 89.

Precautions. Glycerol should be administered with caution to diabetic patients.

An 82-year-old senile hypertensive woman, given a single dose of glycerol 2.3 g per kg body-weight by mouth for glaucoma, experienced signs which were misdiagnosed as due to cardiac arrest. In a second patient, a 68-year-old woman with diabetes, severe diabetic acidosis was attributed to treatment with glycerol by mouth, also for glaucoma. Such elderly patients were liable to be dehydrated and the effects due to glycerol ingestion on an empty stomach could be acute. Special care must be taken when administering glycerol to elderly diabetic or senile patients.— P. D'Alena and W. Ferguson, *Archs Ophthal., N.Y.*, 1966, *75*, 201.

Glycerol, administered by mouth to a patient with glaucoma who had previously undergone partial gastrectomy, gave rise to severe headache, prostration, and diarrhoea; it was suggested that a reduced dosage be given to post-gastrectomy patients.— A. W. Sollom, *Br. J. Ophthal.*, 1972, *56*, 506.

Nonketotic hyperosmolar hyperglycaemia developed in a 29-year-old diabetic man with chronic renal failure following the repeated use of glycerol by mouth for acute glaucoma. He recovered after treatment with hypotonic sodium chloride, albumin, packed red blood cells, insulin, and bicarbonate. Glycerol should be avoided, where possible, in patients likely to develop nonketotic hyperosmolar hyperglycaemia such as maturity-onset elderly diabetics with severe intercurrent disease that may predispose to fluid deprivation. In those patients in whom glycerol therapy is necessary adequate fluid intake should be maintained.— D. E. Oakley and P. P. Ellis, *Am. J. Ophthal.*, 1976, *81*, 469. A similar report in 2 patients, a 66-year-old nondiabetic man and a 63-year-old woman with insulin-dependent maturity-onset diabetes mellitus; both developed fatal nonketotic hyperosmolar hyperglycaemia following administration of glycerol by nasogastric tube for cerebral oedema.— E. S. Sears, *Neurology, Minneap.*, 1976, *26*, 89.

Absorption and Fate. Glycerol is readily absorbed from the intestine and is metabolised to carbon dioxide and glycogen or is used in the synthesis of body fats.

Ketosis and glycosuria were reduced in 4 insulin-dependent diabetics when glucose in the diet was replaced isocalorically by glycerol, 25 to 50 g four times daily. Glycerol appeared to be metabolised as a carbohydrate without needing insulin.— G. Freund, *Archs intern. Med.*, 1968, *121*, 123.

Uses. When taken by mouth, glycerol is demulcent and mildly laxative. It has an energy value of 18.1 kJ (4.32 kcal) per g. Glycerol is employed as a sweetening agent in mixtures and as an ingredient of some linctuses and pastilles.

Glycerol, by mouth, in doses of 1 to 1.5 g per kg body-weight, usually as a 50% solution, has been used for reducing intra-ocular pressure in glaucoma and before cataract surgery; it has also been found of value in reducing intracranial pressure and has been given by intravenous infusion in sodium chloride injection. Oral administration may be more acceptable if the dose is thoroughly chilled. Alternatively flavouring agents may be used.

When glycerol is given by rectal injection or in suppositories it promotes peristalsis and evacuation of the lower bowel by virtue of its irritant action.

Externally, glycerol is used for its water-retaining and emollient properties in dermatological preparations, toilet creams, and jellies. It absorbs moisture from exposed or inflamed tissues and mucous membranes when applied undiluted. It is employed, in the form of Kaolin Poultice or Magnesium Sulphate Paste, for its hygroscopic action in the treatment of boils, carbuncles, and other inflammatory conditions. Glycerol is used as the solvent vehicle for some ear-drops; it softens wax and has a weak antimicrobial action.

Glycerol is used in non-greasy applications for its humectant properties. In concentrations of 20% and over glycerol is a preservative and has been used in aqueous or non-alcoholic extracts; its antimicrobial action is slight unless it is present in sufficient concentration to dehydrate bacteria.

Sterile glycerol or glycerol-based jellies are used as lubricants for endoscopic instruments.

A review of recent advances in cryobiology including the use of glycerol as a cryoprotectant.— D. E. Pegg, *Practitioner*, 1978, *221*, 543.

The Food Additives and Contaminants Committee recommended that glycerol should continue to be a permitted solvent in food although there should be a maximum permitted concentration of 0.2% for butanetriols which were sometimes present as impurities.— *Report on the Review of Solvents in Food*, FAC/REP/25, Ministry of Agriculture, Fisheries and Food, London, HM Stationery Office, 1978.

Cerebral infarction and raised intracranial pressure. A review of the cerebral dehydrating action of glycerol and of the effects of parenteral administration.— W. W. Tourtellotte *et al.*, *Clin. Pharmac. Ther.*, 1972, *13*, 159.

A discussion of glycerol in the management of acute cerebral infarction.— *Lancet*, 1975, *2*, 1246.

Glycerol, 1 g per kg body-weight 4-hourly by mouth, together with dexamethasone, 4 mg six-hourly by intramuscular injection, was recommended for the treatment of cerebral oedema.— L. J. Hurwitz, *Br. med. J.*, 1969, *3*, 699.

Glycerol 1.2 g per kg body-weight was given every 24 hours by intravenous injection as a 10% solution in dextrose injection or sodium chloride injection or 1.5 g per kg by mouth in 6 divided doses daily to 36 patients with cerebral infarction. Four patients in coma died and of the remaining 32 patients, 30 improved during and after the glycerol. The mean CSF pressure decreased after 4 days' treatment. Six patients with brain tumours and CNS oedema improved when given glycerol. Another 6 with CNS oedema due to anoxic encephalopathy showed no improvement.— J. S. Meyer *et al.*, *Lancet*, 1971, *2*, 993. See also M. Buckell and L. Walsh, *Lancet*, 1964, *2*, 1151.

In a study of 54 patients with acute cerebral infarction, the 29 who were given daily infusions of glycerol 50 g in 500 ml of dextrose 5% in 25% physiological saline improved more rapidly and to a significantly greater extent than did the 25 who received the solution without glycerol: 75% of those given glycerol improved clinically compared with 56% of those given placebo. Treatment for 6 days appeared to be more effective than for 4 days. No benefit was seen in 2 of 5 patients who were given glycerol and survived spontaneous intracerebral haemorrhage.— N. T. Mathew *et al.*, *Lancet*, 1972, *2*, 1327.

A dose of 500 ml of glycerol 10% in sodium chloride injection was infused over 24 hours together with sodium chloride injection or dextrose injection and repeated for 6 days in 30 patients with cerebral infarction. This was compared with dexamethasone 4 mg intramuscularly every 6 hours for 6 days together with the infusions of sodium chloride or dextrose injection in 31 similar patients. Glycerol produced greater neurological and clinical improvement; 67% of those given glycerol improved clinically compared with 33% of those given dexamethasone. There was 1 death in the glycerol group and 6 deaths in the dexamethasone group. Glycerol was considerably superior to dexamethasone although there was still a risk of haemolysis with the 10% solution.— V. Gilsanz *et al.*, *Lancet*, 1975, *1*, 1049. See also R. Guisado and A. I. Arieff (letter), *ibid.*, *2*, 183.

In a double-blind study in 27 patients with stroke less than 6 hours before treatment there was no difference in mortality or improvement in neurological score between 12 treated intravenously with 500 ml of 10% glycerol in dextrose solution over 6 hours on 6 days and 15 treated with dextrose as a placebo.— O. Larsson *et al.*, *Lancet*, 1976, *1*, 832.

Clinical experience indicated that treatment with glycerol 1 g per kg body-weight given by mouth every 6 hours produced symptomatic improvement in patients with raised intracranial pressure despite the reduction in pressure not being sustained throughout all the dose interval. A 4-hourly schedule was evaluated in one patient and found paradoxically to increase further the intracranial pressure.— D. A. Rottenberg *et al.*, *Neurology, Minneap.*, 1977, *27*, 600.

Follow-up 4 months after a placebo-controlled double-blind study involving 51 elderly patients treated 48 hours after the onset of an ischaemic cerebral infarction with glycerol 25 g in 250 ml of a sodium chloride and dextrose solution by intravenous infusion twice daily for 6 days indicated that improvement occurred in patients with a moderate neurological deficit but no improvement occurred in those with a severe disability.— R. Fawer *et al.*, *Stroke*, 1978, *9*, 484.

Diagnosis of Ménière's disease. A single dose of glycerol 1.5 g per kg body-weight by mouth caused a transient reduction of the hearing loss in patients with the early stages of Ménière's disease. No effect occurred in patients with other types of cochlear deafness. Clinically this effect could be used to indicate the reversibility of Ménière's disease and that treatment with diuretic drugs may be of value.— I. Klockhoff and U. Lindblom, *Acta oto-lar.*, 1967, *Suppl.* 224, 449. See also J. M. Snyder, *Archs Otolar.*, 1971, *93*, 155. A theory as to how the test works.— L. Naftalin and K. J. H. Mallett (letter), *Lancet*, 1978, *2*, 103.

See also under Adverse Effects.

Glycerol was capable of improving cochlear function in patients suffering from fluctuating sensorineural hearing loss other than that caused by Ménière's disease and therefore the glycerol test could not be considered to be specific for the diagnosis of Ménière's disease.— D. Celestino and A. Orofino, *J. Lar. Otol.*, 1978, *92*, 467.

Intra-ocular pressure. In a controlled study involving 176 extractions of senile cataract, one-half the patients were given glycerol, about 180 ml of a 50% solution in flavoured physiological saline, and the other half water as a control. In the latter group vitreous loss during surgery was 5 times more frequent than in the glycerol-treated subjects in whom reduced ocular tension was associated with correspondingly reduced risk of vitreous loss.— P. Awasthi *et al.*, *Br. J. Ophthal.*, 1967, *51*, 130. See also T. Jerndal and V. Kriisa, *ibid.*, 1974, *58*, 927.

Liver disease. When glycerol was injected intravenously in a dose of 120 mmol per m^2 of body-surface as a 10% solution in sodium chloride injection over 4 minutes, its metabolism, as shown by glucose and lactate concentrations, was greater in 8 patients with various glycogenoses of the liver than in 9 adults and 13 children used as controls. Injection of glycerol could be used to differentiate between types of glycogenosis.— B. Senior and L. Loridan, *New Engl. J. Med.*, 1968, *279*, 958. A dose of 260 mmol per m^2 body-surface of glycerol by mouth was used in the diagnosis of glycogenoses caused by enzyme deficiencies in 3 patients.— *idem*, 965.

Experience in 5 patients with fulminant hepatic failure showed that glycerol 50 g per 24 hours intravenously as a 10% solution produced no improvement in the encephalopathy. Higher doses might cause intravascular haemolysis.— C. O. Record *et al.*, *Br. med. J.*, 1975, *2*, 540.

Radiation protection. A report of the use of glycerol to protect against radiation. The doses required for protection were near to the toxic doses, but protection by topical application had been demonstrated in *animals*.— *Lancet*, 1969, *1*, 1039.

Use in the ear. Glycerol was often effective in preventing the development of scales on the skin of the meatal canal. Glycerol was as effective as any other preparation for the softening of ear wax.— *Br. med. J.*, 1972, *4*, 623.

Preparations

Creams

Glycerol Cream Oily *(A.P.F.)*. Crem. Glycer. Oleos. Glycerol 20 g, calcium hydroxide solution 32 ml, arachis oil 22 g, wool fat 26 g.

Enemas

Glycerin Enema *(B.P.C. 1949)*. Glycerol, undiluted. *Dose*. 4 to 16 ml rectally.

Eye-drops

Glycerin Ophthalmic Solution *(U.S.P.)*. A sterile anhydrous solution of glycerol containing not less than 98.5% of $C_3H_8O_3$; it may contain one or more suitable antimicrobial preservatives. Store in airtight containers. Protect from light.

Glycerol Eye-drops. Glycerol 15 g, chlorhexidine acetate 5 mg, Water for Injections to 100 ml. Sterilised by autoclaving.—P.L. Jeffs, *Australas. J. Pharm.*, 1962, *43*, 1031.

Jellies

Patch-testing Jelly. Analytical grade glycerol 1.5 g, gelatin 500 mg, water to 4 ml. Known quantities by weight of suspect allergens could be incorporated in this preparation for use in skin tests. Storage at 0° to 4° was sufficient to maintain stability of the base for at least 2 months. The jelly, which was designed to melt at body temperature, was set in a mould, mounted on adhesive tape, and covered, until required, with a protective backing. It had been used for a range of allergens including nickel sulphate, potassium dichromate, neomycin sulphate, framycetin sulphate, and dyes.—W. Frain-Bell and T.M. Macleod, *Br. J. Derm.*, 1967, *79*, 557.

Lotions

Glycerin and Rose Water. Glycerol 2 and rose water 3. An agreeable emollient for the skin.

Ointments

Emollient Ointment *(Leeds Gen. Infirm.)*. Glycerol 20, salicylic acid 2, hydrous wool fat 20, olive oil 20, emulsifying ointment 20, yellow soft paraffin to 100.

Pastilles

Pastille Basis *(B.P.)*. Glycerol 40 g, gelatin 20 g, sucrose 5 g, citric acid monohydrate 2 g, sodium benzoate 200 mg, lemon oil 0.1 ml, amaranth solution 2 ml, freshly boiled and cooled water to 100 g. The rate at which the basis dissolves may be reduced by replacing part of the gelatin with agar; the preparation will then be opalescent.

Pastilles for Dry Mouth. Glycerol 40, gelatin 20, sucrose 5, lemon essence 0.6, sodium benzoate 0.2, citric acid monohydrate 2, amaranth solution 1, water to 100.— P. Dykes *et al.* (letter), *Lancet*, 1960, *2*, 1353.

Solutions

Glycerin Oral Solution *(U.S.P.)*. A solution containing glycerol. pH 5.5 to 7.5. Store in airtight containers.

Suppositories

Glycerol Suppositories *(B.P.)*. Glycer. Suppos.; Glycerin Suppositories. Prepared from gelatin, glycerol, and water. They contain about 70% w/w of glycerol and 14% w/w of gelatin. In tropical and subtropical countries up to 18% w/w of gelatin may be included. Store at a temperature not exceeding 30°.

B.P.C. 1973 permitted the use of this basis for gelatin pessaries.

The usual sizes of glycerol suppositories are: small (1-g mould—for infants), medium (2-g mould), and large (4-g mould).

Several pharmacopoeias include similar formulas. *A.P.F.* has 18% w/w gelatin.

Glycerin Suppositories *(U.S.P.)*. Dissolve sodium stearate 9 g in glycerol 91 g, heated to 120°; add water 5 g, mix, and pour into moulds. Store below 25° in airtight containers.

Several pharmacopoeias include similar formulas.

Glyco-gelatin Gel *(A.P.F.)*. Glyco-gelatin Base; Glyco-gelatin Suppository Base; Glycogelatin Pessary Base. Gelatin 25 g, glycerol 40 g, water to 100 g.

Proprietary Preparations

Glycerol with Sodium Chloride Injection *(Boots, UK)*. A solution for intravenous infusion containing in each litre glycerol 92.63 g and sodium chloride 8.34 g [143 mmol (143 mEq) of sodium and of chloride].

Massé Cream *(Ortho-Cilag, UK)*. Contains glycerol 3% and hydrous wool fat 2% in an emollient basis. For nipple care.

Pricerine *(Unichema, UK)*. A brand of glycerol.

Other Proprietary Names

Babylax *(Ger.)*; Bulboid, Cristal *(both Switz.)*; Glycerotone *(Belg., Fr.)*; Glycilax *(Ger.)*; Glysolax *(Switz.)*.

1902-j

Glycols

Glycols are dihydric alcohols in which the 2 hydroxyl groups are attached to different carbon atoms in a hydrocarbon chain. They occur as almost colourless and odourless liquids with a low vapour pressure. The lower glycols are distinctly hygroscopic, are soluble in water, and are excellent solvents for essential oils, dyes, and a number of gums and resins. Their hygroscopic properties and low evaporation-rate make them valuable as moistening and softening agents for such substances as gelatin, glue, and casein. Some of the glycols, particularly ethylene glycol, are used in antifreeze solutions.

With the exception of propylene glycol, the toxicity of the glycols renders them unsuitable for use in pharmaceutical preparations for internal administration, though they are used to some extent in weak concentrations in the cosmetics industry; they should not be used in preparations to be applied extensively. They are metabolised to carboxylic acids in the body.

The relative toxicity of glycols is reported to increase in the following ascending order: propylene glycol, triethylene glycol, diethylene glycol, ethylene glycol; glycerol is less toxic than propylene glycol. The glycol ethers are reported to be more toxic than their corresponding parent glycols.

1903-z

Diethylene Glycol.

Diglycol; Ethylene Diglycol. 3-Oxapentane-1,5-diol; 2,2′-Oxydiethanol. $C_4H_{10}O_3=106.1$.

CAS — 111-46-6.

A colourless, almost odourless, hygroscopic, syrupy liquid with a sharp sweet taste. Wt per ml about 1.118 g. F.p. −8°; b.p. about 245°. **Miscible** with water, acetone, and alcohol; immiscible with carbon tetrachloride and toluene.

Adverse Effects. The toxic effects of diethylene glycol following ingestion by mouth are depression of the central nervous system and degenerative changes in the kidneys and liver. The symptoms and effects are similar to those produced by ethylene glycol intoxication (see p.708) but the central depression may be less pronounced and hypocalcaemic tetany and metabolic acidosis are reported to occur only rarely.

Poisoning by an elixir of sulphanilamide in which the solvent was 72% diethylene glycol caused 105 deaths.— *J. Am. med. Ass.*, 1937, *109*, 1531; H. O. Calvery and T. G. Klumpp, *Sth. med. J.*, 1939, *32*, 1105.

Seven children, aged 6 to 31 months, died following ingestion of proprietary sedative preparations in which the solvent was found to be diethylene glycol. All of the children exhibited symptoms of hepatomegaly and metabolic acidosis.— M. D. Bowie and D. McKenzie, *S. Afr. med. J.*, 1972, *46*, 931.

Abuse. A 43-year-old man who had ingested about 120 ml of heavy duty brake fluid containing about 70% of diethylene glycol and its ethers developed gastro-intestinal symptoms including haematemesis and melaena, anuria, restlessness, and facial paralysis. After haemodialysis, which was carried out on the 8th day, he became comatose, hypotensive, and apnoeic and died 8 days later. The post mortem showed cerebral and pulmonary oedema, renal cortical necrosis, and hydropic swelling of the renal proximal tubular cells and centrilobular hepatic cells.— D. P. Wilkinson, *Med. J. Aust.*, 1967, *2*, 403.

Treatment of Adverse Effects. The stomach should be emptied by aspiration and lavage. The respiration may require assistance. Haemodialysis may be of value.

Uses. Diethylene glycol is used as a solvent for resins, oils, and many other organic compounds. It has been used in brake fluids and in antifreeze solutions. It is employed as a plasticiser and as a humectant for tobacco, cork, printing ink, and glue.

Diethylene glycol should not be given internally and should not be applied externally in more than small amounts.

Diethylene glycol is not suitable for use as a food additive.— Twenty-third Report of the Joint FAO/WHO Expert Committee on Food Additives, *Tech. Rep. Ser. Wld Hlth Org. No. 648*, 1980.

1904-c

Diethylene Glycol Monoethyl Ether.

Carbitol. 3,6-Dioxaoctan-1-ol; 2-(2-Ethoxyethoxy)ethanol.

$C_6H_{14}O_3=134.2$.

CAS — 111-90-0.

A colourless almost odourless slightly hygroscopic liquid. B.p. 202°. **Miscible** with water and most organic solvents.

Adverse Effects and Treatment. As for Diethylene Glycol.

Applications of ointments and lotions containing 20 to 50% of diethylene glycol monoethyl ether produced no excretion of the ether in the urine or of glucuronic acid above control levels.— J. K. Fellows *et al., J. Pharmac. exp. Ther.*, 1947, *89*, 210.

Studies in *animals* indicated that dangerous effects would be produced in a 70-kg man after drinking about 90 ml of the ether.— P. J. Hanzlik *et al., J. ind. Hyg. Toxicol.*, 1947, *29*, 233.

Abuse. A report of recovery following symptomatic treatment in a 44-year-old alcoholic man after the ingestion of a liquid containing the equivalent of about 150 ml of diethylene glycol monoethyl ether.— O. Brennaas, *Nord. Med.*, 1960, *64*, 1291.

Uses. Diethylene glycol monoethyl ether has been used for determining saponification values of oils. It is a neutral solvent for mineral oil-soap and mineral oil-sulphated oil mixtures, giving fine dispersions in water.

1905-k

Dipropylene Glycol *(B. Vet. C. 1965).* 4-Oxaheptane-2,6-diol; 1,1′-Oxybis(propan-2-ol).

$C_6H_{14}O_3=134.2$.

CAS — 25265-71-8.

A clear colourless liquid with a characteristic odour. Wt per ml 1.02 to 1.03 g. **Miscible** with water, alcohol, chloroform, and ether.

Adverse Effects and Treatment. As for Diethylene Glycol.

Uses. It is used as a solvent in Piperonyl Butoxide Application (see p.841) which is used as an insecticide in veterinary medicine.

1906-a

Ethoxyethanol *(B.P.C. 1949).* Ethylene Glycol Monoethyl Ether. 3-Oxapentan-1-ol; 2-Ethoxyethanol.

$C_4H_{10}O_2=90.12$.

CAS — 110-80-5.

A colourless liquid with a mild, agreeable, fruity odour. Wt per ml 0.93 to 0.932 g. B.p. about 135°. **Miscible** with water, alcohol, chloroform, and ether.

NOTE. Ethoxyethanol is liable to form peroxides and during distillation precautions should be taken against explosion.

Adverse Effects and Treatment. As for Ethylene Glycol. Maximum permissible atmospheric concentration 100 ppm.

Uses. Ethoxyethanol is used in the manufacture of lacquers and printing inks.

1907-t

Ethylene Glycol.

Glycol; Ethylene Alcohol. Ethane-1,2-diol.

$C_2H_6O_2=62.07$.

CAS — 107-21-1.

A colourless, almost odourless, hygroscopic, syrupy liquid with a sweet taste. Wt per ml about 1.114 g. F.p. about −13°; b.p. about 197°. Flash-point 111°. **Miscible** with water, alcohol, acetone, aldehydes, and glycerol.

Adverse Effects. The main toxic effects of ethylene glycol are depression of the central nervous system and nephrotoxicity. A common cause of poisoning is the drinking of antifreeze solutions containing ethylene glycol.

Early symptoms following ingestion by mouth are similar to alcoholic inebriation; nausea, vomiting, abdominal pain, weakness, and muscle tenderness may also be present. Respiratory failure, convulsions, cardiovascular collapse, pulmonary oedema, hypocalcaemic tetany, and severe metabolic acidosis may occur and, without treatment, death may occur in 8 to 24 hours. Acute renal failure usually develops a few days later in patients who survive this period and brain and liver damage can occur. Patients may show only the initial inebriation then develop renal failure after a symptom-free period. The minimum lethal dose in an adult appears to be about 100 ml.

Inhalation of ethylene glycol is not generally regarded as hazardous because of its low vapour pressure but poisoning has occasionally been reported after prolonged industrial exposure.

Maximum permissible atmospheric concentration 10 mg per m^3 particulate and 100 ppm vapour.

Sixteen students inadvertently drank antifreeze solution containing ethylene glycol. Amounts consumed varied from a sip to about 120 ml. The more seriously affected had drunk 30 ml or more. There were 3 stages of the resultant illness. The first was neuromuscular disturbance, with myositis, consequent upon the deposition of calcium oxalate crystals. This came on quickly and was followed by circulatory depression with rapid breathing, cyanosis, and oedema of the lungs. The third stage was renal failure. The 2 most seriously affected students died; each had consumed about 90 to 120 ml.— E. A. Friedman *et al., Am. J. Med.*, 1962, *32*, 891.

Studies in *rats* found that three intermediate metabolic products of ethylene glycol were more toxic than the glycol, causing renal tubular oxalosis. It was suggested that cytotoxicity in the renal tubular epithelium, not oxalate deposition, caused renal failure in man.— K. E. Bove, *Am. J. clin. Path.*, 1966, *45*, 46.

Treatment of Adverse Effects. The stomach should be emptied by aspiration and lavage. Respiration may require assistance and convulsions may be controlled by the intravenous administration of diazepam 5 to 10 mg or, if necessary, a short-acting barbiturate such as thiopentone sodium. Metabolic acidosis should be corrected and hypocalcaemic tetany treated where necessary. Haemodialysis or peritoneal dialysis may be of value. Alcohol has been given since it acts as a competitive inhibitor of ethylene glycol metabolism.

Since ethylene glycol was oxidised to oxalic acid by liver alcohol dehydrogenase, the effects of the glycol could be minimised by administering a large dose of alcohol. W.E.C. Wacker *et al.* (*J. Am. med. Ass.*, 1965, *194*, 1231) had treated 2 patients, 1 of whom had taken about 1 litre of antifreeze solution, with alcohol and peritoneal dialysis. Both survived and oxaluria disappeared in 18 hours. Another patient (P. Flannagan and J.H. Libcke, *Am. J. clin. Path.*, 1964, *41*, 171) treated without alcohol had oxaluria for 5 days. Further clinical studies were required.— A. L. Picchioni, *Am. J. Hosp. Pharm.*, 1966, *23*, 226.

Oliguria which lasted for 50 days occurred in a 65-year-old woman poisoned with ethylene glycol. She was treated with haemodialysis. Renal function gradually improved for 4 months but was not fully restored when the patient was discharged.— J. M. Collins *et al., Archs intern. Med.*, 1970, *125*, 1059.

A 27-year-old male was treated for ethylene glycol intoxication by forced diuresis. Sodium bicarbonate, mannitol, and ethacrynic acid were given. Fluids and alcohol 10 g per hour intravenously were administered for 5 days. The patient was discharged after 9 days with normal pyelogram and urinalysis.— F. Underwood and W. M. Bennett, *J. Am. med. Ass.*, 1973, *226*, 1453.

A 2-year-old child who had ingested about 100 ml of ethylene glycol was unconscious the next morning despite earlier vomiting. He recovered after treatment which included infusion of alcohol, calcium gluconate intravenously, frusemide, diazepam, and peritoneal dialysis which, over 8 days, removed 26.9 g of ethylene glycol and 73 mg of oxalate.— J. A. Vale *et al., Postgrad. med. J.*, 1976, *52*, 598.

The result in a 27-year-old man who had ingested an unknown amount of ethylene glycol suggested that haemoperfusion with coated activated charcoal could be an effective measure to eliminate ethylene glycol from plasma. The patient recovered fully after gastric lavage, the administration of alcohol intravenously, and haemoperfusion. The plasma concentration of ethylene glycol 8 hours after ingestion was 1.4 g per litre compared with 7 mg per litre after 38 hours.— B. Sangster *et al.* (letter), *New Engl. J. Med.*, 1980, *302*, 465.

A pharmacokinetic study in a man who had ingested a potentially lethal amount of ethylene glycol and was treated with alcohol and haemodialysis.— C. D. Peterson *et al., New Engl. J. Med.*, 1981, *304*, 21. Comments and criticisms: C. R. Freed *et al.* (letter), *ibid.*, 976; R. N. Zahlten (letter), *ibid.*, 977; C. D. Peterson *et al.* (letter), *ibid.*; W. E. Harmon and J. A. Sargent (letter), *ibid.*, *305*, 522.

Further references: J. Wolthuis and F. Kalsbeek, *Ned. Tijdschr. Geneesk.*, 1971, *115*, 1224; R. L. Mundy *et al., Toxic. appl. Pharmac.*, 1974, *28*, 320; E. W. Van Stee *et al., ibid.*, *29*, 98.

Precautions.

For the effect of mannitol on estimations of ethylene glycol, see Mannitol, p.604.

Absorption and Fate. Ethylene glycol is metabolised in the kidney and liver. Metabolites, most of which are toxic, include aldehydes, oxalates, formic acid, and lactic acid.

Uses. Ethylene glycol has the general uses of the glycols and is mainly used as a constituent of antifreeze solutions.

Ethylene glycol should not be used in medicinal preparations for internal use nor should it be used in concentrations over 5% in preparations for local application to small areas of skin. In sunscreen lotions and protective creams which are applied to extensive areas it is regarded as a hazard in any concentration.

1908-x

Propylene Glycol *(B.P., B.P. Vet., Eur. P.).*

Propyleneglycolum; Glicol Propilênico; Propilenoglicol. (±)-Propane-1,2-diol.

$CH_3.CHOH.CH_2OH=76.10$.

CAS — 57-55-6; 4254-15-3 (+); 4254-14-2 (−); 4254-16-4 (±).

Pharmacopoeias. In *Aust., Belg., Br., Braz., Cz., Eur., Fr., Ger., Hung., Int., It., Jap., Jug., Neth., Nord., Port., Swiss, Turk.*, and *U.S.*

A clear, colourless, odourless or almost odourless, viscous, hygroscopic liquid with a slightly sweet taste, resembling that of glycerol. *B.P.* specifies relative density of 1.036 to 1.040 and the *U.S.P.* specific gravity of 1.035 to 1.037. B.p. 185° to 189°.

Miscible with water, acetone, alcohol, and chloroform; soluble 1 in 6 of ether; immiscible with light petroleum; it is immiscible with fixed oils but it will dissolve some essential oils. A 2% w/v solution in water is iso-osmotic with serum. It may be **sterilised** by heating in sealed ampoules in an autoclave or by filtration. **Incompatible** with some oxidising agents. **Store** in airtight containers.

Haemolysis. An aqueous solution of propylene glycol iso-osmotic with serum (2%) caused 100% haemolysis of erythrocytes cultured in it for 45 minutes.— E. R. Hammarlund and K. Pedersen-Bjergaard, *J. pharm. Sci.*, 1961, *50*, 24.

Adverse Effects. Probably owing to its rapid breakdown and excretion, propylene glycol is much less toxic than the other glycols. It produces some local irritation on application to mucous membranes and on subcutaneous or intramuscular injections.

Chloramphenicol sodium succinate 5% in Ringer's solution and propylene glycol 10% both caused irreversible deafness when instilled into the middle-ear cavity in *guinea pigs*. It was recommended that propylene glycol should not be used as a solvent for chloramphenicol ear-drops, and that higher concentrations of chloramphenicol should not be used in the middle-ear cavity.— T. Morizono and B. M. Johnstone, *Med. J. Aust.*, 1975, *2*, 634.

For reports of central nervous system toxicity in children associated with the ingestion of preparations containing propylene glycol as the vehicle, see G. Martin and L. Finberg, *J. Pediat.*, 1970, *77*, 877; K. Arulanantham and M. Genel, *ibid.*, 1978, *93*, 515.

Propylene glycol intoxication was accompanied by the development of lactic acidosis and stupor in a patient with uraemic renal disease.— J. C. Cate and R. Hedrick (letter), *New Engl. J. Med.*, 1980, *303*, 1237.

For a report of pain at the injection site and elevation of serum concentration of creatine phosphokinase following injection of a propylene glycol vehicle, see Chlordiazepoxide, p.1507.

Hypersensitivity. Of 38 patients who had been treated topically with preparations containing propylene glycol, 17 reacted to a skin test with a 38% solution of propylene glycol. Of 145 patients who were not known to have received treatment with propylene glycol, 6 reacted to skin tests.— C. Huriez *et al.*, *Bull. Soc. fr. Derm. Syph.*, 1966, *73*, 263.

In 8 patients who developed contact allergy to a corticosteroid ointment, patch tests were performed with the constituents of the vehicle. Positive tests to hexane-1,2,6-triol 5% in water, propylene glycol 10% in water, and stearyl alcohol 20% in soft paraffin occurred in 3, 5, and 5 of the patients respectively. All of the patients had a positive reaction to at least one of the constituents.— I. Pevny and M. Uhlich, *Hautarzt*, 1975, *26*, 252.

A challenge test with propylene glycol given by mouth was made in 38 patients who had previously shown allergic-type epicutaneous test reactions to propylene glycol. Exanthem developed 3 to 16 hours after ingestion in 8 of 10 patients who had had positive reactions to propylene glycol 2% and in 7 of 28 patients who had had positive reactions to propylene glycol 10 to 100%.— M. Hannuksela and L. Förström, *Contact Dermatitis*, 1978, *4*, 41.

Further references: A. A. Fisher *et al.*, *Archs Derm.*, 1971, *104*, 286.

Absorption and Fate. Propylene glycol is absorbed from the gastro-intestinal tract and is converted in the liver to lactate and single carbon compounds. A large proportion is excreted unchanged or as a glucuronide conjugate in the urine.

Uses. Propylene glycol is used as a solvent in the extraction of crude drugs and in the preparation of solutions of alkaloids, volatile oils, steroids, and dyes. It is a useful vehicle for antihistamines, barbiturates, some vitamins, paracetamol, and other substances which are insufficiently soluble in water or unstable in aqueous solution. Preparations made with propylene glycol are less viscous than those made with glycerol. In certain instances it is a better solvent than glycerol, and its power of inhibiting mould growth and fermentation is equal to that of alcohol.

Propylene glycol may be included in spray solutions to stabilise the droplet size. It is used similarly to glycerol in non-greasy applications to prevent drying out. It has also been used as an air disinfectant and is used as a humectant and as a solvent for flavourings in the food industry.

Estimated acceptable daily intake: up to 25 mg per kg body-weight.— Seventeenth Report of the FAO/WHO Expert Committee on Food Additives, *Tech. Rep. Ser. Wld Hlth Org. No. 539*, 1974. For background toxicological information, see *Fd Add. Ser. Wld Hlth Org. No. 5*, 1974.

The Food Additives and Contaminants Committee recommended that propylene glycol be permitted for use as a solvent in food. Reactions might occur between propylene glycol and aldehydes from flavours and such reactions should be avoided.— *Report on the Review of Solvents in Food*, FAC/REP/25, Ministry of Agriculture, Fisheries and Food, London, HM Stationery Office, 1978.

The addition of 10 or 20% propylene glycol to an oil-water system preserved with chlorocresol increased the partitioning of the chlorocresol into the aqueous phase.— Pharm. Soc. Lab. Rep. P/75/24, 1975.

Bactericidal and fungicidal properties. A preparation containing fluocinolone acetonide 10 mg, citric acid 10 mg, and propylene glycol to 100 ml had bactericidal and fungicidal activity against 7 bacterial and 7 fungal organisms. Propylene glycol alone and diluted with normal human serum 10% was actively bactericidal but some activity was lost on dilution to 65%. The use of propylene glycol as a vehicle for dermatological preparations might provide a means of preventing or treating initial or secondary infections.— I. Olitzky, *J. pharm. Sci.*, 1965, *54*, 787.

Skin disorders. A 40 to 60% aqueous solution of propylene glycol with occlusion rapidly cleared scaling skin in ichthyosis. Treatment every 3 to 5 days kept skin free of scales. No toxic reactions occurred.— L. A. Goldsmith and H. P. Baden, *J. Am. med. Ass.*, 1972, *220*, 579.

Twenty patients with tinea versicolor were successfully treated with propylene glycol 50% in water applied twice daily for 2 weeks. Two patients complained of a slight burning sensation of the skin after application.— J. Faergemann and T. Fredriksson, *Acta derm.-vener., Stockh.*, 1980, *60*, 92.

1909-r

Triethylene Glycol. Triglycol. 3,6-Dioxaoctane-1,8-diol; 2,2′-Ethylenedioxydiethanol.

$C_6H_{14}O_4$=150.2.

CAS — 112-27-6.

A colourless, almost odourless, hygroscopic liquid. B.p. about 287°. **Miscible** with water, alcohol, and toluene.

Adverse Effects. It is less toxic than diethylene glycol but more toxic than propylene glycol.

Tests on *monkeys* and *rats* continuously exposed for about 12 to 18 months to atmospheres saturated with triethylene glycol failed to show any differences from animals living in ordinary room conditions. Large groups of industrial workers exposed to partially saturated atmospheres during working hours for years showed no evidence of ill effects due to the vapour.— O. H. Robertson *et al.*, *J. Pharmac. exp. Ther.*, 1949, *91*, 52.

Uses. Triethylene glycol is used for similar purposes to diethylene glycol. It is also employed as an air disinfectant and as a solvent for nitrocellulose.

Air disinfection. After years of study, triethylene glycol was found to be the ideal chemical for aerial disinfection in sterile filling units because it had a high bactericidal potency at reasonable cost and was non-toxic. It was most effective at relative humidities of 30 to 55% and the rate of kill increased with temperature and degree of saturation of air with the vapour.— N. L. Demuth, *Bull. parent. Drug Ass.*, 1966, *20*, 199.

1910-j

Proprietary Preparations of Glycols

Breox PAG *(BP Chemicals, UK: Hythe, UK).* A range of polyalkylene glycols.

1911-z

Hexane-1,2,6-triol.

$C_6H_{14}O_3$=134.2.

CAS — 106-69-4.

A viscous pale yellow liquid; f.p. 32.8°, liable to supercooling; wt per ml about 1.11 g; about half as hygroscopic as glycerol. **Soluble** in water, alcohols, glycols, glycol-ethers, and ketones; practically insoluble in esters, ethers, and aromatic and aliphatic hydrocarbons.

Hexane-1,2,6-triol is used in conjunction with macrogols in ointment and suppository bases.

The following formula produced an ointment basis which was softer than a basis of macrogols alone, had less tendency to become granular, and had a wider compatibility range: macrogol '4000' 34 g, macrogol '400' 50 g, and hexane-1,2,6-triol 16 g.— A. P. Collins and L. C. Zopf, *Am. prof. Pharm.*, 1956, *22*, 691.

A plasticising agent for the macrogols. Suppository bases prepared from a mixture of macrogols with hexane-1,2,6-triol could be easily extruded and compressed to yield products without the layered appearance which sometimes occurred with bases of macrogols alone.— A. P. Collins *et al.*, *Am. prof. Pharm.*, 1957, *23*, 231.

In 8 patients who developed contact allergy to a corticosteroid ointment patch tests were performed with the constituents of the vehicle. Positive tests to hexane-1,2,6-triol 5% in water, propylene glycol 10% in water, and stearyl alcohol 20% in soft paraffin occurred in 3, 5, and 5 of the patients respectively. All of the patients had a positive reaction to at least one of the constituents.— I. Pevny and M. Uhlich, *Hautarzt*, 1975, *26*, 252.

1912-c

Macrogols. Polyethylene Glycols; Polyoxyethylene Glycols; Polyaethylenglycola; Polyäthylenglykole; Polietilenglicoli; Polyoxaetheni.

$CH_2(OH).[CH_2.O.CH_2]_m.CH_2OH$.

CAS — 25322-68-3.

Pharmacopoeias. Macrogols of various molecular weights are included in many pharmacopoeias.

B.P. specifies individual macrogols. *U.S.N.F.* describes Polyethylene Glycol; requires that it be labelled with the average molecular weight; requires that the molecular weight varies from the labelled value by not more than 5%, 10%, and 12.5% respectively for material of nominal molecular weight below 1000, between 1000 and 7000, and above 7000; and gives a viscosity range at about 99° for 44 grades.

NOTE. Some authorities use the general formula $H.(CH_2.O.CH_2)_n.OH$ to describe macrogols. In using this formula the number assigned to *n* for a specified macrogol is 1 more than that of *m* in the general formula $CH_2(OH).[CH_2.O.CH_2]_m.CH_2OH$ which is used to describe the macrogols in this section.

The macrogols are mixtures of condensation polymers of ethylene oxide and water. Those with an average molecular weight of 200 to 700 are liquid; those with an average molecular weight of more than 1000 vary in consistence from soft unctuous to hard wax-like solids. The average molecular weight is indicated by a number in the name; thus macrogol 400 has an average molecular weight of about 400.

The liquid and semi-solid members of the series are hygroscopic; macrogol 200 has a comparative hygroscopicity (glycerol = 100) of 70, but this decreases with increase in molecular weight; macrogol 1540 has a comparative hygroscopicity of 30.

Incompatibilities. The macrogols are incompatible with phenols and may reduce the antimicrobial action of other preservatives, such as the quaternary ammonium compounds. Penicillin and bacitracin are rapidly inactivated by macrogols. Macrogols are also incompatible with iodine, potassium iodide, sorbitol, tannic acid, and with bismuth, mercury, and silver salts. Some plastics, including Polythene, Bakelite, and Celluloid, are attacked by macrogols.

Effect on antimicrobial action of chloroxylenol. The presence of 0.22 to 1.32% macrogol 6000 caused a 60% increase in the minimum inhibitory concentration of chloroxylenol against *Bacillus subtilis* and *Pseudomonas aeruginosa*. Activity against *Aspergillus niger* was unaffected.— M. D. Ray *et al.*, *J. pharm. Sci.*, 1968, *57*, 609.

Haemolysis. Macrogols 200 and 300 were damaging to erythrocytes, and sodium chloride only prevented haemolysis in solutions containing less than 25% and less than 40% respectively. Macrogols 400 and 600 were damaging to erythrocytes at concentrations above 40% but had a protective effect between 10 and 40%. The haemolytic effect appeared to be related to the ability of macrogols 200 and 300 to penetrate erythrocytes.— B. L. Smith and D. E. Cadwallader, *J. pharm. Sci.*, 1967, *56*, 351.

Impurities. Up to 40% of active agent was lost when 1% tripelennamine hydrochloride in macrogol 300 containing 0.1% or more of ethylene oxide as impurity was autoclaved for 30 minutes or kept at room temperature for several days.— P. F. G. Boon and A. W. Mace, *J. Pharm. Pharmac.*, 1968, *20, Suppl.*, 32S.

Traces of peroxides in macrogols used in a corticosteroid cream decreased its stability. The presence of 5 to 10% of water or up to 0.05% of antioxidants such as butylated hydroxytoluene and propyl gallate reduced peroxide concentration, particularly if heated to 60° to 80°.— J. W. McGinity *et al.* (letter), *J. pharm. Sci.*, 1975, *64*, 356.

Incompatibility. Ointment bases containing macrogols or their esters were incompatible with tannic acid, phenol, and salicylic acid, liquefaction usually resulting. These bases also caused discoloration, without affecting the activity, with sulphonamides, chrysarobin, and with mixtures of mercury and salicylic acid. Macrogols rapidly rendered penicillin inactive and discoloured dithranol. Since the glycols had a solvent action on many synthetic materials such as plastics, care must be taken in selecting a suitable packaging material.— F. Neuwald and K. Adams, *Dt. ApothZtg*, 1954, *94*, 1258.

Binding of methyl, propyl, and butyl hydroxybenzoates to macrogol 4000 increased with an increase in temperature. The reverse effect occurred with these perservatives and polysorbate 80.— N. K. Patel and N. E. Foss, *J. pharm. Sci.*, 1964, *53*, 94.

Stability of aqueous ointments. Because macrogols were completely soluble in water, only a limited amount of aqueous liquid could be incorporated into an ointment prepared with these compounds. The reported limit was 3%, but up to 20% of water could be incorporated if 5% of cetyl alcohol was added as a stabiliser.— W. Nixon, *Pharm. J.*, 1951, *2*, 213.

1913-k

Macrogol 200. Polyethylene Glycol 200; PEG 200.

Pharmacopoeias. In *Aust., Fr., Ger., It., Roum.*, and *Swiss.*

A mixture of polycondensation products of ethylene oxide and water, obtained under controlled conditions and represented by the general formula $CH_2(OH).[CH_2.O.CH_2]_m.CH_2OH$, where *m* may be 3. Average molecular weight 190 to 210.

It is a clear, colourless, hygroscopic, viscous liquid with a faint characteristic odour. Wt per ml about 1.127 g. Viscosity, at 100°, about 4 centistokes.

Miscibility and solubility as for Macrogol 300. A 5% solution in water has a pH of 4.5 to 7; a 25% solution is clear and almost colourless. **Store** in airtight containers.

1914-a

Macrogol 300 *(B.P.)*. Liquid Macrogol; Polyethylene Glycol 300; PEG 300.

CAS — 37361-15-2.

Pharmacopoeias. In *Aust., Br., Cz., Fr., Ger., It., Port., Roum.*, and *Swiss. U.S.N.F.* specifies this macrogol under the general monograph on Polyethylene Glycol.

A mixture of polycondensation products of ethylene oxide and water, obtained under controlled conditions, in which *m* in the general formula may be 5 or 6. Average molecular weight 285 to 325.

It is a clear, colourless, hygroscopic, viscous liquid with a faint characteristic odour. Wt per ml 1.12 to 1.13 g. Viscosity, at 25°, 59 to 73 centistokes; viscosity, at about 100°, about 6 centistokes.

Miscible with water, alcohol, acetone, chloroform, and with other glycols; practically insoluble in ether and aliphatic hydrocarbons but soluble in aromatic hydrocarbons. A 5% w/v solution in water has a pH of 4 to 7. Aqueous solutions are **sterilised** by autoclaving or filtration. **Store** in airtight containers.

1915-t

Macrogol 400. Polyethylene Glycol 400; PEG 400.

Pharmacopoeias. In *Arg., Aust., Belg., Braz., Fr., Ger., Hung., It., Jap., Jug., Nord., Pol., Port., Roum., Swiss*, and *Turk. U.S.N.F.* specifies this macrogol under the general monograph on Polyethylene Glycol.

A mixture of polycondensation products of ethylene oxide and water, obtained under controlled conditions, in which *m* in the general formula may be 7 to 9. Average molecular weight 380 to 420.

It is a clear, colourless, slightly hygroscopic, viscous liquid with a faint characteristic odour. F.p. about 3°. Wt per ml about 1.13 g. Viscosity, at about 100°, 6.8 to 8 centistokes.

Miscibility and solubility as for Macrogol 300. A 5% solution in water has a pH of 4.5 to 7.5; a 25% solution is clear and almost colourless. **Store** in airtight containers.

1916-x

Macrogol 600. Polyethylene Glycol 600; PEG 600.

Pharmacopoeias. In *Aust., Braz., Fr., Ger., It.*, and *Roum. U.S.N.F.* specifies this macrogol under the general monograph on Polyethylene Glycol.

A mixture of polycondensation products of ethylene oxide and water, obtained under controlled conditions, in which *m* in the general formula may be 11 to 13. Average molecular weight 570 to 630.

A clear colourless or practically colourless, slightly hygroscopic, viscous liquid with a slight characteristic odour. F.p. about 20°. Wt per ml about 1.13 g. Viscosity, at about 100°, 9.9 to 11.3 centistokes.

Miscibility and solubility as for Macrogol 300. A 5% solution in water has a pH of 4.5 to 7.5; a 25% solution is clear and almost colourless. **Store** in airtight containers.

1917-r

Macrogol 1000. Polyethylene Glycol 1000; PEG 1000.

Pharmacopoeias. In *Aust., Fr., Ger., It.*, and *Roum. U.S.N.F.* specifies this macrogol under the general monograph on Polyethylene Glycol.

A mixture of polycondensation products of ethylene oxide and water, obtained under controlled conditions, in which *m* in the general formula may be 20 to 23. Average molecular weight 950 to 1050.

A white or nearly white wax-like solid. F.p. 30° to 40°. Viscosity, at about 100°, about 16 to 19 centistokes.

Freely **soluble** in water. A 5% solution in water has a pH of 4.5 to 7; a 25% solution is clear and almost colourless.

1918-f

Macrogol 1540 *(B.P.)*. Polyethylene Glycol 1540; PEG 1540.

Pharmacopoeias. In *Br., Hung., Port.*, and *Swiss.* Also in *Aust., Cz., Fr., Ger., It., Pol.*, and *Roum.* under the titles Macrogol 1500 or Polyethylene Glycol 1500. *U.S.N.F.* specifies Polyethylene Glycol 1500 under the general monograph on Polyethylene Glycol.

NOTE. Macrogol 1500 (*Braz. P.* and *Jap. P.*) is a blend of equal parts of macrogols 300 and 1540, with an average molecular weight of 500 to 600 and m.p. 37° to 41°.

A mixture of polycondensation products of ethylene oxide and water, obtained under controlled conditions, in which *m* in the general formula may be 28 to 36. Average molecular weight 1300 to 1600.

A soft creamy-white wax-like solid or free-flowing powder with a faint characteristic odour. F.p. 42° to 46°. Viscosity, at about 100°, 25 to 32 centistokes.

Soluble 1 in 1 of water, 1 in 100 of dehydrated alcohol, and 1 in 3 of chloroform; practically insoluble in ether. A 5% solution in water has a pH of 4 to 7.

1919-d

Macrogol 2000. Polyethylene Glycol 2000; PEG 2000.

Pharmacopoeias. In *Ger., It.*, and *Roum. U.S.N.F.* specifies this macrogol in the general monograph on Polyethylene Glycol.

A mixture of polycondensation products of ethylene oxide and water, obtained under controlled conditions, in which *m* in the general formula may be 40 to 50. Average molecular weight 1800 to 2200.

A white odourless wax-like solid. F.p. 45° to 50°. Viscosity at about 100°, 38 to 49 centistokes. **Soluble** in water; freely soluble in alcohol and chloroform; practically insoluble in ether.

1920-c

Macrogol 3000. Polyethylene Glycol 3000; PEG 3000.

Pharmacopoeias. In *Ger., It., Nord., Roum.*, and *Swiss. U.S.N.F.* specifies this macrogol in the general monograph on Polyethylene Glycol.

A mixture of polycondensation products of ethylene oxide and water, obtained under controlled conditions, in which *m* in the general formula may be 60 to 75. Average molecular weight 2700 to 3300.

It is an almost odourless, creamy-white, hard, wax-like solid or flakes. F.p. 48° to 54°. Viscosity at about 100°, 67 to 93 centistokes.

Soluble 1 in about 2 of water, 1 in about 10 of alcohol, and 1 in about 2 of chloroform; practically insoluble in ether. Solutions are **sterilised** by autoclaving.

1921-k

Macrogol 4000 *(B.P.)*. Hard Macrogol; Polyethylene Glycol 4000; PEG 4000.

Pharmacopoeias. In *Arg., Aust., Belg., Br., Braz., Fr., Ger., Hung., It., Jap., Jug., Pol., Port., Roum.*, and *Swiss. U.S.N.F.* specifies this macrogol in the general monograph on Polyethylene Glycol.

A mixture of polycondensation products of ethylene oxide and water, obtained under controlled conditions, in which *m* in the general formula may be 69 to 84. Average molecular weight 3100 to 3700.

An almost tasteless, creamy-white, hard, wax-like solid or flakes or white free-flowing powder with a faint characteristic odour. F.p. 53° to 56°. Viscosity, at 100°, 76 to 110 centistokes.

Soluble 1 in 3 of water, 1 in 2 of alcohol, and 1 in 2 of chloroform; practically insoluble in ether. A 5% solution in water has a pH of 4.5 to 7.5. **Sterilised** by maintaining at 150° for 1 hour.

1922-a

Macrogol 6000. Polyethylene Glycol 6000; PEG 6000.

Pharmacopoeias. In *Aust., Braz., Fr., Ger., It., Jug., Nord., Port., Roum.*, and *Swiss. Jap.* specifies an average mol. wt of 7300 to 9300. *U.S.N.F.* specifies this macrogol in the general monograph on Polyethylene Glycol.

Fr. P. also includes macrogol 10 000.

A mixture of polycondensation products of ethylene oxide and water, obtained under controlled conditions, in which *m* in the general formula may be 112 to 158. Average molecular weight 5000 to 7000. Mixtures with higher values for *m* are also used.

It is an almost odourless, creamy-white, hard, wax-like solid or flakes or white free-flowing powder. F.p. about 60°. Viscosity, at about 100°, 250 to 390 centistokes.

Soluble 1 in 2 of water and 1 in 2 of chloroform; freely soluble in alcohol; practically insoluble in ether. A 5% solution in water has a pH of 4.5 to 7.5; a 10% solution is clear and almost colourless.

Adverse Effects. Contact dermatitis in patients receiving topical therapy has occasionally been attributed to the presence of macrogols in the preparations.

For a review of the toxicity of macrogols, see T. H. Eickholt and W. F. White, *Drug Stand.*, 1960, *28*, 154.

In a review article on non-aqueous solvents in parenteral products it was pointed out that while macrogols by themselves might be non-toxic, the action of drugs dissolved in them in some cases might be modified and their toxicity increased. A report by W.R. McCabe *et al.* (*Archs intern. Med.*, 1959, *104*, 710) indicated that 7 out of 30 patients given nitrofurantoin intravenously developed severe metabolic acidosis and nephropathy, resulting in 2 deaths; the toxic effects were attributed to macrogol used as the solvent in the injection.— A. J. Spiegel and M. M. Noseworthy, *J. pharm. Sci.*, 1963, *52*, 917.

A brief discussion on the possible carcinogenicity of macrogols.— M. H. Greene and T. I. Young (letter), *Ann. intern. Med.*, 1980, *93*, 781.

Absorption and Fate. Higher molecular weight macrogols are not significantly absorbed from the gastro-intestinal tract. The liquid macrogols of lower molecular weight are absorbed and a large proportion is excreted unchanged in the urine. After injection, higher molecular weight macrogols are quickly excreted unchanged in the urine; the liquid macrogols are excreted more slowly and may be partly metabolised.

References: R. B. Drotman, *Toxic. appl. Pharmac.*, 1980, *52*, 38.

Uses. The macrogols are strongly hydrophilic compounds and are therefore only poor oil-in-water emulsifying agents but they are useful as stabilisers of emulsions. Since they are stable, relatively non-irritant to the skin, and emollient, they are useful as water-miscible bases for ointments. Drugs incorporated in a basis such as macrogol ointment may be more effectively released and absorbed than from a paraffin basis and their concentrations may need to be reduced. Macrogols may be used to facilitate the dispersion of drugs, such as hydrocortisone, sulphur, undecenoic acid, and salicylic acid, which are relatively insoluble in water.

Mixtures of macrogols are used as bases for pessaries and suppositories.

Macrogol 6000 was successfully used as a carrier for the solid dispersion of the 5 poorly water-soluble liquids benzonatate, benzyl benzoate, clofibrate, methyl salicylate, and alpha tocopheryl acetate. The solidified mass containing up to 5 or 10% w/w of the liquid compound, depending on which drug was used, could be pulverised, encapsulated, and tabletted. Complete dissolution of the active ingredients was achieved in 4 to 14 minutes *in vitro*.— W. L. Chiou and L. D. Smith, *J. pharm. Sci.*, 1971, *60*, 125.

Macrogol 6000 could be used to make solid solutions of water-insoluble drugs such as digitoxin, griseofulvin, hydrocortisone acetate, methyltestosterone, and prednisolone acetate. Such solid solutions had greatly improved dissolution rates.— W. L. Chiou and S. Riegelman, *J. pharm. Sci.*, 1971, *60*, 1569.

The use of macrogol 6000 for microencapsulation.— M. A. El-Egakey *et al.*, *Pharmazie*, 1974, *29*, 466.

A study of solid solutions of indomethacin in macrogol 6000. Macrogol 6000 increased the solubility and dissolution rate of indomethacin in water; an optimum being obtained for a mixture containing 15% of indomethacin and 85% of macrogol 6000.— J. L. Ford and M. H. Rubinstein, *Pharm. Acta Helv.*, 1978, *53*, 93.

Metabolic and diagnostic studies. Macrogol 4000 was absorbed in negligible amounts from the gastro-intestinal tract and could therefore be used as a marker for studying the absorption and secretion of water-soluble materials and was a reliable indicator for estimating the volume of intestinal fluid.— E. D. Jacobson *et al.*, *Gastroenterology*, 1963, *44*, 761. See also R. Shields *et al.*, *ibid.*, 1968, *54*, 331.

The use of macrogol 4000 as a faecal marker for calcium, phosphorus, and fatty acids in metabolic balance studies.— R. Wilkinson, *Gut*, 1971, *12*, 654.

Macrogol 600 or 4000 as a probe molecule to investigate intestinal absorption in patients with allergic disorders.— P. G. Jackson *et al.*, *Lancet*, 1981, *1*, 1285.

Suppository bases. The rate of release of salicylate from macrogol suppository bases differed for macrogol 1540 and 6000. However when bases were a mixture of the 2 macrogols the rate favoured that of the higher molecular weight macrogol whatever the percentage composition.— H. W. Puffer and W. J. Crowell, *J. pharm. Sci.*, 1973, *62*, 242.

Suppositories containing macrogol '1000' 65% and macrogol '4000' 35% were retained in the rectum as long as and with fewer minor reactions than suppositories made with a commercial macrogol basis.— S. Stavchansky *et al.*, *Drug Dev. ind. Pharm.*, 1977, *3*, 111.

Tablet coatings. Macrogol 6000 in warm alcoholic solution was a suitable coating material; 25% solutions should be used for the initial coatings and 50% solutions for the later ones in order to build up a suitable thickness. The process was simpler and more rapid than ordinary sugar coatings.— E. H. Gans and L. Chavkin, *J. Am. pharm. Ass., scient. Edn*, 1954, *43*, 483.

1923-t

Preparations of Macrogols

Endotracheal Tube Lubricant. Macrogol '300' 10 g, macrogol '1500' to 100 g. Lignocaine could be dissolved in the preparation.—J.C. Greenleaf and J.W. Hadgraft, *Chemist Drugg.*, 1960, *173*, 179.

Macrogol Ointment *(B.P.)*. Macrogol '300' 65 g, macrogol '4000' 35 g. Store at a temperature not exceeding 25°. *A.P.F.* has equal parts by wt. Mixtures of equal weights of macrogols 300 and 1500 are included in *Cz. P.* and *Ger. P.* and of macrogols 400 and 1540 in *Hung. P.*

Polyethylene Glycol Ointment *(U.S.N.F.)*. Macrogol '400' 60 g, macrogol '3350' 40 g. If a firmer ointment is required up to 10 g of macrogol 400 may be replaced with macrogol 3350. If it is intended to incorporate 6 to 25% of an aqueous solution, replace 5 g of macrogol 3350 with stearyl alcohol.

The name Polyethylene Glycol Ointment is also applied to Macrogol Ointment (*A.P.F.*).

Aust. P. and *Belg. P.* have a similar formula; *Swiss P.* has a similar formula containing 5% cetyl alcohol; *Jap. P.* has a mixture of equal weights.

Suppository Bases

The following bases differed in hardness and water content. They dissolved in water at 37° in 25 to 30 minutes. (1) Macrogol '4000' 33%, macrogol '6000' 47%, and water 20%; (2) macrogol '1540' 33%, macrogol '6000' 47%, and water 20%; (3) macrogol '1540' 33%, macrogol '6000' 47%, and macrogol '400' 20%.— W. H. Hassler and G. J. Sperandio, *J. Am. pharm. Ass., pract. Pharm. Edn*, 1953, *14*, 26.

Of a number of suggested formulas for suppository bases containing macrogols, the following were the best for general use: (a) macrogol '1540' 94% and hexane-1,2,6-triol 6%; and (b) macrogol '1000' 75% and macrogol '4000' 25%.— A. P. Collins *et al.*, *Am. prof. Pharm.*, 1957, *23*, 231.

Massa Polyoxaetheni *(Hung. P.)*. Contains polyoxyl 40 stearate 5 g, macrogol '4000' 5 g, and macrogol '1540' 90 g.

A suggestion for the replacement of Massa Polyoxaetheni (*Hung. P.*) by a base consisting of macrogol 1540 with sorbitan monolaurate 5%.— G. Regdon *et al.*, *Acta pharm. hung.*, 1974, *44*, 97.

Proprietary Preparations of Macrogols

Breox Polyethylene Glycols (formerly known as Carbowax) *(BP Chemicals, UK: Hythe, UK)*. A range of macrogols; grades are available of average molecular weights from 185 to 14 000.

Lutrol E *(BASF, Ger.: Blagden, UK)*. A range of macrogols.

An ointment basis and a cream basis containing macrogols were formerly marketed in Great Britain under the proprietary names Pologol and Pologol Aqueous respectively (*Waterhouse*).

Glycerophosphates and Hypophosphites

1930-a

The compounds described in this section were widely used in tonics but there appears to be little evidence to support this use. They cannot be considered to be a source of phosphorus.

1931-t

Calcium Glycerophosphate *(B.P.C. 1963).*

Calcium Glycerylphosphate; Calcium Glycerinophosphate; Calcium Phosphoglycerate.
$C_3H_7CaO_6P(+xH_2O)$=210.1.

CAS — 27214-00-2 (anhydrous); 126-95-4 (α, anhydrous)

Pharmacopoeias. In *Arg., Aust., Belg., Braz., Fr., It., Mex., Port., Roum., Span.,* and *Swiss.*

A white or creamy-white, odourless, tasteless or slightly bitter hygroscopic powder consisting mainly of hydrated α-glycerophosphate. (For information on the isomers of glycerophosphoric acid, see under Glycerophosphoric Acid, p.712). Preparations containing a large proportion of the sparingly soluble β-glycerophosphate are sometimes made more soluble by the addition of citric acid; such preparations tend to hydrolyse in aqueous solution and to deposit calcium phosphate. Anhydrous calcium glycerophosphate 5.24 g is approximately equivalent to 1 g of calcium. **Soluble** 1 in about 50 of water at 20° and less soluble at higher temperatures, but different samples vary in solubility according to composition; soluble in glycerol; practically insoluble in alcohol and ether. **Incompatible** with mineral acids and with soluble carbonates, phosphates, and sulphates. Solutions decompose when heated. **Store** in airtight containers.

Uses. The glycerophosphates and glycerophosphoric acid were introduced into medicine on the grounds that lecithin contains phosphorus in the form of the glycerophosphate radical and that these compounds would be more easily assimilated by the tissues, particularly by the brain. There is no evidence to support this assumption but the glycerophosphates were widely used in debilitated conditions and in convalescence.

Calcium glycerophosphate has been given in doses of 200 to 600 mg to supplement dietary calcium and phosphorus. Up to 4 g has been given in 24 hours.

When applied topically or ingested, calcium glycerophosphate had been reported to be twice as effective as sodium fluoride in preventing dental caries. It had the added advantage of being less toxic.— B. B. O'Meara (letter), *Lancet*, 1966, *2*, 855.

Four patients with anorexia nervosa who had responded to management in hospital but relapsed when discharged were readmitted and treated additionally with glycerophosphates. Their weight gain was maintained after discharge and eating habits improved.— H. Caplin *et al.* (letter), *Lancet*, 1973, *1*, 319.

Glycerophosphate reduced the molar ratio of cholesterol to bile salts and phospholipids in the hepatic bile of 9 of 10 patients with lithogenic bile. Gall-bladder bile was unaffected.— W. G. Linscheer; K. L. Raheja, *Lancet*, 1974, *2*, 551.

Preparations

For preparations containing Glycerophosphates, see p.713.

1932-x

Calcium Hypophosphite *(B.P.C. 1963).*

$Ca(H_2PO_2)_2$=170.1.

CAS — 7789-79-9.

Pharmacopoeias. In *Port.* and *Span.*

An odourless white powder or lustrous crystals with a nauseous bitter taste. Calcium hypophosphite 4.249 g is approximately equivalent to 1 g of calcium. **Soluble** 1 in 7 of water and 1 in 30 of glycerol; practically insoluble in alcohol. **Incompatible** with oxidising agents. **Store** in airtight containers.

CAUTION. *Hypophosphites are incompatible with chlorates, nitrates, or other oxidising agents, and when triturated or heated with them explosions are liable to occur.*

Uses. The hypophosphites and dilute hypophosphorous acid were used in debilitated conditions and in convalescence. They were also used to provide a dietary supplement of phosphorus but the hypophosphite ion is reported to pass through the body unchanged. Calcium hypophosphite has been given in doses of 200 to 600 mg.

Preparations

Compound Syrup of Hypophosphites *(B.P.C. 1963).* Compound Syrup of Ferric Hypophosphite. Hypophosphites of calcium, manganese, potassium, and iron, with quinine, sucrose, hypophosphorous acid, strychnine hydrochloride (1 mg in 8 ml), and double-strength chloroform water. *Dose.* 4 to 8 ml.

1933-r

Ferric Glycerophosphate *(B.P.C. 1963).* Ferric Glycerylphosphate; Iron Glycerophosphate.

CAS — 1301-70-8; 38455-91-3 (α).

Pharmacopoeias. In *Port.*

Yellow or greenish-yellow odourless and almost tasteless scales, granules, or powder, containing 13 to 16% of Fe together with alkali citrate. Ferric glycerophosphate 6.9 g is approximately equivalent to 1 g of iron. Slowly **soluble** 1 in 2 of water; practically insoluble in alcohol. **Protect** from light.

Uses. Ferric glycerophosphate has been given in doses of 60 to 300 mg for similar purposes to calcium glycerophosphate (see p.712).

1934-f

Ferric Hypophosphite *(B.P.C. 1963).*

Ferrum Hypophosphorosum Oxidatum; Iron Hypophosphite. A complex of variable basicity, containing about 22% of Fe.

CAS — 7783-84-8.

Pharmacopoeias. In *Span.*

A white or greyish-white, odourless, almost tasteless, amorphous powder. Ferric hypophosphite 4.55 g is approximately equivalent to 1 g of iron. **Soluble** 1 in 2300 of water but more soluble in the presence of potassium citrate or hypophosphorous acid. **Incompatible** with oxidising agents (see Caution, under Calcium Hypophosphite, p.712). **Store** in airtight containers.

Uses. Ferric hypophosphite has been given in doses of 60 to 200 mg for similar purposes to calcium hypophosphite (see p.712).

Preparations

Ferric Hypophosphite Solution *(B.P.C. 1963).* Solution of Iron Hypophosphite; Strong Solution of Iron Hypophosphite. A solution prepared from ferric sulphate solution, dilute ammonia solution, citric acid monohydrate, sodium hypophosphite, sodium citrate, and double-strength chloroform water. It contains 8.5 to 10.5% w/v of $Fe(H_2PO_2)_3$. Wt per ml 1.13 to 1.17 g. *Dose.* 0.6 to 2 ml.

1935-d

Glycerophosphoric Acid *(B.P.C. 1963).* Glycerylphosphoric Acid; Monoglycerylphosphoric Acid.
$C_3H_9O_6P$=172.1.

CAS — 27082-31-1; 57-03-4(α); 17181-54-3(β); 5746-57-6(L-α); 1509-81-5(DL-α).

Glycerophosphoric acid is available commercially as a mixture of 3 isomers: the D(+) and L(−) isomers of the α-form (2,3-dihydroxy propylphosphoric acid) and the β-form (2-hydroxy-1-(hydroxymethyl)ethylphosphoric acid).

A clear colourless, odourless liquid with an acid taste, containing a mixture of the α- and β-forms equivalent to 19 to 21% w/v of $C_3H_9O_6P$. The chief constituent is the α-acid. Wt per ml about 1.1 g.

Stronger solutions, namely, 25% w/w (wt per ml about 1.13 g) and 50% w/w (wt per ml about 1.3 g) can also be prepared.

Glycerophosphoric acid has been used in doses of 0.3 to 0.6 ml for similar purposes to calcium glycerophosphate (see p.712).

1936-n

Hypophosphorous Acid *(U.S.N.F., B.P.C. 1963).*

Acidum Hypophosphorosum.
H_3PO_2=66.0.

CAS — 6303-21-5; 14332-09-3.

Pharmacopoeias. In *Ind.* Also in *U.S.N.F.*

A colourless or slightly yellow odourless liquid, containing 30 to 32% w/w of H_3PO_2. Relative density about 1.13. **Store** in airtight containers.

1937-h

Dilute Hypophosphorous Acid *(B.P.C. 1963).*

Acidum Hypophosphorosum Dilutum.

Pharmacopoeias. In *Span.* under the title Acidum Hypophosphorosum.

Contains 10% w/w of H_3PO_2 and may be prepared by mixing 323 g of hypophosphorous acid with 677 g of water. Wt per ml 1.035 to 1.041 g. **Incompatible** with oxidising agents (see Caution, under Calcium Hypophosphite, p.712).

Uses. See Calcium Hypophosphite, p.712.

Dilute hypophosphorous acid has been included in preparations of ferrous salts to retard oxidation.

1938-m

Magnesium Glycerophosphate *(B.P.C. 1963).* Magnesium Glycerylphosphate.
$C_3H_7MgO_6P(+xH_2O)$=194.4.

CAS — 927-20-8 (α, anhydrous).

A white, odourless, amorphous powder with a somewhat bitter taste. It contains a variable amount of water of crystallisation. Anhydrous magnesium glycerophosphate 8 g is approximately equivalent to 1 g of magnesium. **Soluble** 1 in 50 of water containing 0.2 of glycerophosphoric acid. May be rendered more soluble by the addition of citric acid or alkali citrate but the solution deposits magnesium phosphate on standing. **Incompatible** with alkali carbonates.

Uses. Magnesium glycerophosphate has been given in doses of 300 to 600 mg for similar purposes to calcium glycerophosphate (see p.712).

1939-b

Manganese Glycerophosphate *(B.P.C. 1949).* Manganese Glycerylphosphate.
$C_3H_7MnO_6P(+xH_2O)=225.0$.

CAS — 1320-46-3 (anhydrous); 1319-75-1 (hydrate).

A pinkish-white, amorphous, odourless, nearly tasteless powder. **Soluble** 1 in 100 of water; practically insoluble in alcohol; soluble 1 in 5 of a 25% solution of citric acid.

Manganese glycerophosphate has been given in doses of 60 to 300 mg for similar purposes to calcium glycerophosphate (see p.712).

1940-x

Manganese Hypophosphite *(B.P.C. 1963).*
$Mn(H_2PO_2)_2,H_2O=202.9$.

CAS — 10043-84-2 (anhydrous).

Pharmacopoeias. In *Span.*

White or slightly pink, odourless, almost tasteless crystals or granular powder. **Soluble** 1 in 7 of water and 1 in 6 of boiling water; practically insoluble in alcohol. **Incompatible** with oxidising agents (see Caution, under Calcium Hypophosphite, p.712). **Store** in airtight containers.

Manganese hypophosphite has been given in doses of 60 to 300 mg for similar purposes to calcium hypophosphite (see p.712).

1941-r

Potassium Glycerophosphate Solution *(B.P.C. 1963).* Liquor Potassii Glycerophosphatis.

CAS — 1319-69-3 (potassium glycerophosphate).

A colourless, or not more than faintly yellow, odourless, syrupy liquid with a saline taste, containing 48 to 52% w/w of neutral potassium glycerophosphate, mainly α- together with some β-glycerophosphate. (For information on the isomers of glycerophosphoric acid, see under Glycerophosphoric Acid, p.712). Wt per ml about 1.35 g. **Miscible** with water.

Potassium glycerophosphate solution has been given in doses of 0.6 to 2 g for similar purposes to calcium glycerophosphate (see p.712).

1942-f

Potassium Hypophosphite *(B.P.C. 1963).* Kalii Hypophosphis.
$KH_2PO_2=104.1$.

CAS — 7782-87-8.

Pharmacopoeias. In *Span.*

White, odourless, deliquescent crystals or granular powder with a pungent, saline, somewhat bitter taste. **Soluble** 1 in 0.6 of water, 1 in 0.3 of boiling water, 1 in 7.5 of alcohol, and 1 in 3.5 of boiling alcohol. **Incompatible** with oxidising agents (see Caution, under Calcium Hypophosphite, p.712). **Store** in airtight containers.

Potassium hypophosphite has been given in doses of 200 to 600 mg for similar purposes to calcium hypophosphite (see p.712).

1943-d

Sodium Glycerophosphate *(B.P.C. 1949).*

Sodium Glycerylphosphate; Natrium Glycerophosphoricum.
$C_3H_7Na_2O_6P,5\frac{1}{2}H_2O=315.1$.

CAS — 1555-56-2 (α, anhydrous); 819-83-0 (β, anhydrous).

Pharmacopoeias. In *Arg., Aust., Belg., Fr., It., Port., Roum.,* and *Span.* Some specify a mixture of the α- and β-forms with a variable amount of water of crystallisation. (For information on the isomers of glycerophosphoric acid, see under Glycerophosphoric Acid, p.712).

Odourless white monoclinic plates or scales or a white powder with a saline taste. It is hygroscopic. **Soluble** 1 in 2 of water; practically insoluble in alcohol and ether. Solutions in water have a pH of about 9.5. **Store** in airtight containers.

Uses. Sodium glycerophosphate has been given in doses of 300 to 600 mg for similar purposes to calcium glycerophosphate (see p.712).

Preparations

Sodium Glycerophosphate Solution *(B.P.C. 1963).* Liq. Sod. Glycerophosph. A colourless or faintly yellow, odourless, syrupy liquid with a saline taste, containing 48 to 52% w/w of neutral sodium glycerophosphate, mainly α- together with some β-glycerophosphate. Wt per ml about 1.3 g. **Miscible** with water. *Dose.* 0.6 to 2 g.

Proprietary Names

Alfos-OM *(Om, Switz.).*

1944-n

Sodium Hypophosphite *(B.P.C. 1963).* Natrium Hypophosphorosum.
$NaH_2PO_2=87.98$.

CAS — 7681-53-0.

Pharmacopoeias. In *Fr.* and *Port.* In *Belg.* and *Span.* with $1H_2O$.

A white, odourless, granular, deliquescent powder with a bitter nauseous taste. **Soluble** 1 in 1 of water, 1 in 30 of alcohol, and 1 in 2 of glycerol; practically insoluble in ether. **Incompatible** with oxidising agents (see Caution, under Calcium Hypophosphite, p.712). **Store** in airtight containers.

Sodium hypophosphite has been given in doses of 200 to 600 mg for similar purposes to calcium hypophosphite (see p.712).

1945-h

Strychnine Glycerophosphate.
$C_{45}H_{53}N_4O_{10}P,6H_2O=949.0$.

CAS — 1323-31-5 (anhydrous).

A white crystalline powder. **Soluble** 1 in 350 of water and 1 in 310 of alcohol; slightly soluble in chloroform; very slightly soluble in ether.

Strychnine glycerophosphate has been given in doses of 1 to 3 mg for similar purposes to calcium glycerophosphate (see p.712).

1946-m

Preparations containing Glycerophosphates

See also under Sodium Glycerophosphate.

Compound Syrup of Glycerophosphates *(B.P.C. 1963).* Syr. Glycerophosph. Rub. Glycerophosphates of calcium, sodium, potassium, magnesium, and iron, with flavouring, amaranth solution, caffeine, and strychnine hydrochloride (1.6 mg in 8 ml). Store in a cool place. Protect from light. *Dose.* 4 to 8 ml.

Proprietary Preparations containing Glycerophosphates

Calsotone Tablets *(Southon-Horton, UK).* Each contains calcium glycerophosphate 50 mg, ferric glycerophosphate 50 mg, sodium glycerophosphate 50 mg, and ascorbic acid 5 mg. *Dose.*1 tablet thrice daily after meals.

Glykola *(Sinclair, UK).* An elixir containing in each 5 ml calcium glycerophosphate 30 mg, caffeine 20 mg, kola liquid extract 0.12 ml, chloroform spirit 0.12 ml, alcohol (90%) 0.5 ml, and ferric chloride solution 0.01 ml. *Dose.* 5 to 10 ml thrice daily after meals.

Glykola Infans *(Sinclair, UK).* An elixir containing in each 5 ml manganese glycerophosphate 10 mg, kola liquid extract 0.066 ml, compound gentian infusion 1 ml, citric acid monohydrate 40 mg, and ferric chloride solution 0.016 ml. *Dose.* 2.5 to 5 ml diluted with a little water.

Metatone *(Parke, Davis, UK).* A mixture containing in each 5 ml calcium glycerophosphate 45.6 mg, potassium glycerophosphate 45.6 mg, sodium glycerophosphate 22.8 mg, and manganese glycerophosphate 5.7 mg, with thiamine hydrochloride 500 μg (suggested diluent, water). *Dose.* 5 to 10 ml, preferably diluted, twice or thrice daily.

Neuro Phosphates *(Smith Kline & French, UK).* A mixture containing in each 10 ml calcium glycerophosphate 179.3 mg, sodium glycerophosphate 171.4 mg, and strychnine alkaloid (in acid solution) 1.1 mg (suggested diluent, water). *Dose.* 10 ml, with water, twice daily.

Verdiviton Elixir *(Squibb, UK).* Contains in each 15 ml calcium glycerophosphate 110 mg, sodium glycerophosphate 80 mg, potassium glycerophosphate 20 mg, manganese glycerophosphate 10 mg, thiamine mononitrate 2 mg, riboflavine 1 mg, pyridoxine hydrochloride 500 μg, nicotinamide 15 mg, dexpanthenol 1 mg, and cyanocobalamin 15 μg, with alcohol 17% v/v. *Dose.* Adults, 15 ml thrice daily; children, 5 to 10 ml in water.

Vibrona *(Vine Products, UK).* A wine containing glycerophosphoric acid 0.21%, sodium glycerophosphate solution 0.43%, caffeine 0.049%, quinine sulphate 0.0048%, quinidine sulphate 0.00029%, cinchonine sulphate 0.001%, and cinchonidine sulphate 0.0013%.

Virvina *(Merck Sharp & Dohme, UK).* An elixir containing in each 5 ml calcium glycerophosphate 21.5 mg, sodium glycerophosphate 43.5 mg, potassium glycerophosphate 4 mg, manganese glycerophosphate 2.5 mg, thiamine hydrochloride 676 μg, riboflavine 338 μg, pyridoxine hydrochloride 17 μg, and nicotinamide 5 mg, with alcohol 17% v/v. *Dose.* 10 ml thrice daily before meals.

Preparations containing glycerophosphates were also formerly marketed in Great Britain under the proprietary names Biotone (*Biorex*) and Glytona (*Philip Harris*).

Griseofulvin and other Antifungal Agents

2560-c

Antifungal agents in common use include several macrolide antibiotics, griseofulvin, flucytosine, imidazole derivatives, and fatty acids.

The polyene macrolide class of antifungal agents comprises the *tetraenes* (amphotericin A, natamycin, and nystatin) and the *heptaenes* (amphotericin B, candicidin, hachimycin, and hamycin).

The imidazole antifungal agents include clotrimazole, doconazole, econazole, ketoconazole, and miconazole.

The antifungal agents are mainly used in the treatment of infections of the hair, mucous membranes, nails, or by skin organisms of the genera *Candida* (candidiasis), *Epidermophyton, Microsporum,* and *Trichophyton* (tinea; ringworm).

Superficial candidal infection may be treated with local applications of amphotericin, clotrimazole, econazole, miconazole, natamycin, or nystatin, and systemic infections with amphotericin, flucytosine, or miconazole.

In tinea, the principal superficial infections are tinea capitis (tinea tonsurans; head or scalp ringworm), tinea corporis (tinea circinata; body ringworm), tinea cruris (ringworm of the groin; dhobie itch; jock itch), tinea pedis (athlete's foot; ringworm of the feet), and tinea unguium (ringworm of the nails; onychomycosis).

Treatment in these infections is determined by the nature of the infecting organism. Griseofulvin, by mouth, is usually effective in tinea of the body, finger-nails, groin, hands, head, and soles of the feet excepting the toe-clefts; it is variably effective in tinea of the toe-nails and it is not effective in pityriasis versicolor. Local treatments for tinea include fatty acids such as octoic, propionic, and undecenoic acids or their salts, and buclosamide, chlorphenesin, clotrimazole, econazole, fenticlor, haloprogin, miconazole, pecilocin, and tolnaftate. Topical agents are generally not suitable for fungal infections of the hair and nails.

Less common mycoses include infections due to *Aspergillus, Blastomyces, Coccidioides, Cryptococcus, Histoplasma,* and *Paracoccidioides.*

Less common mycoses against which the principal drugs described in this section are used are:

Aspergillosis—amphotericin, natamycin, nystatin
blastomycosis (North American)—amphotericin, hydroxystilbamidine
coccidioidomycosis—amphotericin, miconazole
cryptococcosis—amphotericin, flucytosine, miconazole
favus—griseofulvin
histoplasmosis—amphotericin
paracoccidioidomycosis—amphotericin, miconazole
pityriasis versicolor—clotrimazole, econazole, haloprogin, miconazole, pecilocin, tolnaftate.

Other drugs used in the treatment of fungal infections which are not included in this section include benzoic acid (p.1283), crystal violet (p.560), dequalinium chloride (p.561), potassium iodide (p.866), and salicylic acid (p.277).

Proceedings of a symposium on antifungal therapy.— *Postgrad. med. J.,* 1979, *55,* 583–700. See also *Br. med. J.,* 1980, *280,* 668.

General reviews of the use of antifungal agents.— L. Roller, *Aust. J. Hosp. Pharm.,* 1978, *8,* 103; R. Y. Cartwright, *Br. med. J.,* 1978, *2,* 108; P. H. Jacobs, *Pediat. Clins N. Am.,* 1978, *25,* 357; D. C. E. Speller, *Practitioner,* 1979, *223,* 511; *Med. Lett.,* 1980, *22,* 5.

Reviews of the treatment of systemic fungal infections.— *Med. Lett.,* 1978, *20,* 66; J. E. Edwards *et al., Ann. intern. Med.,* 1978, *89,* 91; G. Rapi and P. Cocchi (letter), *ibid.,* 1979, *90,* 130; G. Medoff and G. S. Kobayashi, *New Engl. J. Med.,* 1980, *302,* 145.

Reviews of the use of topical antifungal preparations.— *Med. Lett.,* 1976, *18,* 101; J. H. S. Pettit, *Drugs,* 1975, *10,* 130; L. E. Millikan, *Postgrad. Med.,* 1976, *60,* 52; *Med. Lett.,* 1979, *21,* 39; P. D. Samman, *Prescribers' J.,* 1980, *20,* 81.

A study of the classification of polyene antibiotics according to chemical structure and biological effects.— J. Kotler-Brajtburg *et al., Antimicrob. Ag. Chemother.,* 1979, *15,* 716.

Nomenclature of fungi pathogenic to man and animals. For the names of pathogenic fungi and the names of fungal diseases recommended by a subcommittee of the British Society for Mycopathology on behalf of the Medical Research Council, see *Med. Res. Coun. Memo, No. 23,* 4th Edn, 1977.

2561-k

Griseofulvin *(B.P., B.P. Vet., Eur. P., U.S.P.).*

Griseofulvinum; Grisófúlvín; Curling Factor. (2*S*,6′*R*)-7-Chloro-2′,4,6-trimethoxy-6′-methylbenzofuran-2-spiro-1′-cyclohex-2′-ene-3,4′-dione.

$C_{17}H_{17}ClO_6$=352.8.

CAS — 126-07-8.

Pharmacopoeias. In *Br., Braz., Chin., Cz., Eur., Fr., Ger., Int., It., Jug., Neth., Nord., Roum., Rus., Swiss, Turk.,* and *U.S.*

An antifungal substance produced by the growth of certain strains of *Penicillium griseofulvum,* or by any other means. It is a white to pale cream-coloured, odourless or almost odourless, tasteless powder. M.p. 217° to 224°. The *B.P.* specifies that the particles of the powder are generally up to 5 μm in maximum dimension, though larger particles, which may occasionally exceed 30 μm, may be present; *U.S.P* describes material with a predominance of particles of the order of 4 μm in diameter.

The *B.P.* specifies 97 to 102% of $C_{17}H_{17}ClO_6$, calculated on the dried substance; the *U.S.P.* specifies not less than 900 μg of $C_{17}H_{17}ClO_6$ per mg.

Very slightly **soluble** in water; soluble 1 in 300 of dehydrated alcohol, 1 in 20 of acetone, 1 in 25 of chloroform, 1 in 250 of methyl alcohol, and 1 in 3 of tetrachloroethane; soluble in dimethylformamide. A solution in dimethylformamide is dextrorotatory. **Store** in airtight containers.

Dissolution. Dissolution of griseofulvin was enhanced in solutions of bile salts.— T. R. Bates *et al., Nature,* 1966, *210,* 1331.

The solubility of griseofulvin in water was increased by the addition of cetomacrogols, macrogols, or Triton X100 to the solvent.— P. H. Elworthy and F. J. Lipscomb, *J. Pharm. Pharmac.,* 1968, *20,* 817. See also *idem,* 923.

References to the use of solid solutions of griseofulvin in macrogols.— W. L. Chiou and S. Riegelman, *J. pharm. Sci.,* 1969, *58,* 1505; *idem,* 1970, *59,* 937; *idem,* 1971, *60,* 1376; W. E. Barrett and J. J. Hanigan, *Curr. ther. Res.,* 1975, *18,* 491; W. E. Barrett and J. R. Bianchine, *ibid.,* 501; W. L. Chiou, *J. pharm. Sci.,* 1977, *66,* 989.

Adverse Effects. Side-effects are usually mild and transient and consist of headache, skin rashes, dryness of the mouth, an altered sensation of taste, and gastro-intestinal disturbances. More severe allergic reactions and angioneurotic oedema, erythema multiforme, exfoliative dermatitis, proteinuria, leucopenia, candidiasis, paraesthesia, photosensitisation, and severe headache have been reported occasionally. Depression, confusion, irritability, and fatigue have also been reported.

Abnormalities of the sexual organs and breasts have occurred, especially in children. There have been a few reports of lupus erythematosus and hepatitis attributed to griseofulvin.

Griseofulvin was embryotoxic and teratogenic in *rats,* and had caused primary hepatic carcinomas in *mice;* the carcinogenic effect was enhanced by the more complete absorption achieved by decreasing particle size of the drug. There was no present evidence of carcinogenicity in man where the latent periods might lie between 10 and 30 years.— *Med. Lett.,* 1976, *18,* 17.

Precautions. Griseofulvin is contra-indicated in patients with porphyria and liver failure.

Griseofulvin may diminish the effects of oral anticoagulants by increasing their rate of metabolism. The effects of griseofulvin may be diminished if a barbiturate is administered concomitantly.

Interactions. References to phenobarbitone decreasing the gastro-intestinal absorption of griseofulvin.— S. Riegelman *et al., J. Am. med. Ass.,* 1970, *213,* 426; I. H. Stockley, *Pharm. J.,* 1972, *2,* 105; F. Jamali and J. E. Axelson, *J. pharm. Sci.,* 1978, *67,* 466.

The response to bromocriptine was blocked in a patient who was also receiving griseofulvin.— G. Schwinn *et al., Eur. J. clin. Invest.,* 1977, *7,* 101.

For details of the inhibition of the anticoagulant activity of warfarin by griseofulvin, see Warfarin Sodium, p.777.

Porphyria. Griseofulvin precipitated porphyria in 2 patients who had been in remission.— A. G. Redeker *et al., J. Am. med. Ass.,* 1964, *188,* 466. A similar report in a 43-year-old woman.— A. Berman and R. L. Franklin, *ibid.,* 1965, *192,* 1005. See also C. J. Watson *et al., Archs Derm.,* 1968, *98,* 451; E. Haneke *et al., Dte GesundhWes.,* 1971, *26,* 404.

Pregnancy and the neonate. Systemic treatment with griseofulvin is best avoided in pregnancy.— W. Mosimann, *Schweiz. med. Wschr.,* 1975, *105,* 257.

Antimicrobial Action. Griseofulvin is an antifungal antibiotic which exerts an inhibitory action *in vitro* against the common dermatophytes, including *Epidermophyton floccosum, Microsporum audouinii, M. canis, Trichophyton mentagrophytes, T. rubrum, T. schoenleinii, T. tonsurans,* and *T. verrucosum.* The inhibitory action has been reported in concentrations of 0.14 to 5 μg per ml though 15 μg per ml or more has on occasion been necessary.

It is inactive against yeasts, such as *Cryptococcus neoformans,* yeast-like fungi such as *Candida albicans,* and against *Aspergillus* spp., *Blastomyces dermatitidis, Coccidioides immitis, Histoplasma capsulatum, Malassezia furfur (Pityrosporum orbiculare), Phialophora compacta, Ph. verrucosa,* and *Sporotrichum schenckii.* It is also inactive against bacteria.

Absorption and Fate. Griseofulvin is irregularly absorbed over a prolonged period from the gastro-intestinal tract. It is deposited in keratin precursor cells and is concentrated in the stratum corneum of the skin and in the nails and hair, thus preventing fungous invasion of newly formed cells. Griseofulvin is metabolised by the liver mainly to 6-demethylgriseofulvin which is excreted in the urine. A large amount of a dose of griseofulvin is excreted unchanged in the faeces and a small amount in the urine; some is excreted in the sweat.

Serum concentrations of griseofulvin have been reported to range from 0.6 to 1.8 μg per ml 4 hours after doses of 0.25 to 1 g. The absorption of griseofulvin is greatly increased by reducing its particle size.

A review of the absorption and fate of griseofulvin.— C. Lin and S. Symchowicz, *Drug Metab. Rev.,* 1975, *4,* 75.

Mean plasma concentrations reached a plateau at about 1.4 to 1.72 μg per ml after several days when a dose of 500 mg of griseofulvin was given daily in 3 formulations. These concentrations exceeded the minimum effective plasma concentration of 1 μg per ml.— S. Symchowicz and B. Katchen, *J. pharm. Sci.,* 1968, *57,* 1383.

A single dose of micronised griseofulvin 0.5 to 1 g resulted in a peak plasma concentration of only 1 to 3 μg per ml which declined to undetectable concentrations after about 72 hours. Absorption occurred over 30 to 40 hours. The average biological half-life was 11 to 14 hours and 6-demethylgriseofulvin was the major metabolite.— T. R. Bates and J. A. L. Sequeira (letter), *J. pharm. Sci.,* 1975, *64,* 709.

Absorption. Higher blood and tissue concentrations of griseofulvin were obtained if the drug was given with a fatty meal or glass of milk. Phenobarbitone and phenytoin given concurrently could reduce the blood and tissue concentrations.— J. M. Beare, *Prescribers' J.*, 1968, *8*, 30.

In 16 subjects given 1 g of griseofulvin in 8 capsules, plasma concentrations were considerably higher than when given the same dose (in the same particle size) as an aqueous suspension. This was possibly explained by a longer transit time in a limited segment of the upper intestinal tract from which absorption occurred. Higher plasma concentrations also occurred in 16 subjects when given 500 mg as two 250-mg capsules than as four 125-mg capsules.— S. Riegelman, *Drug Inform. Bull.*, 1969, *3*, 59.

The absorption of griseofulvin could be increased either by ultramicronisation or by giving microsize (not ultramicrosize) griseofulvin in corn oil emulsion. Emulsions containing 250 mg of microsize griseofulvin with 2, 4, 6, or 12 g of corn oil were evaluated. Optimal absorption occurred with 4 or 6 g of oil.— T. R. Bates *et al.*, *Archs Derm.*, 1977, *113*, 302.

Absorption of griseofulvin from capsules was significantly increased after blending the micronised powder with an alcoholic solution of hydroxypropyl cellulose.— J. T. Fell *et al.*, *J. Pharm. Pharmac.*, 1978, *30*, 479.

Further references: M. Rowland *et al.*, *J. pharm. Sci.*, 1968, *57*, 984; *Med. J. Aust.*, 1973, *2*, 756; T. R. Bates and J. A. Sequeira, *J. pharm. Sci.*, 1975, *64*, 793.

Effect of particle size. Particles of 2.7 µm (surface area 1.5 m^2 per g) were twice as well absorbed as those of 10 µm (0.4 m^2 per g) following administration by mouth.— R. M. Atkinson *et al.*, *Antibiotics Chemother.*, 1962, *12*, 232.

About 45% of a dose of griseofulvin was absorbed from tablets containing micronised material. A solid solution of griseofulvin 10% in macrogol 6000 as capsules or tablets was completely and rapidly absorbed in 2 patients.— W. L. Chiou and S. Riegelman, *J. pharm. Sci.*, 1971, *60*, 1376.

Percutaneous absorption. Some penetration of griseofulvin through the sole of the foot occurred after topical application.— D. D. Munro, *Br. J. Derm.*, 1967, *79*, 637.

Diffusion. *Into skin.* Concentrations of griseofulvin were built up rapidly in the stratum corneum and could be detected within 8 hours. Using palmar skin, concentrations of 16.4, 9.7, and 4.5 ng per mg were found in levels 1, 2 and 3 respectively. Higher concentrations were detected in warm weather than in cool. When griseofulvin was withdrawn concentrations fell more rapidly in skin than in blood.— W. L. Epstein *et al.*, *Archs Derm.*, 1972, *106*, 344, per *J. Am. med. Ass.*, 1972, *221*, 1424.

Excretion. Absorbed griseofulvin was reported to be completely excreted in the urine as the metabolite 6-demethylgriseofulvin. Only about 10% of a dose was absorbed and was excreted within 72 hours.— P. Kabasakalian *et al.*, *J. pharm. Sci.*, 1970, *59*, 595.

Following administration of a single dose of griseofulvin 250 mg, 6-desmethylgriseofulvin and griseofulvic acid were detected in the urine collected 6 hours after administration; however 4-desmethylgriseofulvin, previously reported to be a urinary metabolite, was not detected. The urinary concentration ratio of 6-desmethylgriseofulvin to griseofulvic acid was about 15 to 1.— H. Zia *et al.*, *J. pharm. Sci.*, 1979, *68*, 1335.

Further references: M. C. Meyer and G. Raghow, *J. pharm. Sci.*, 1979, *68*, 1127.

Pregnancy and the neonate. Cord and maternal blood concentrations of griseofulvin in 12 healthy women at term were determined spectrophotofluorometrically between 2½ and 9¼ hours after 500 mg of fine-particle griseofulvin had been administered. In 11 patients, the cord blood concentrations were the same or lower than maternal concentrations, and in all patients the blood concentrations were variable and lower than those usually observed from comparable doses given to non-pregnant individuals. There was no detectable griseofulvin in samples of amniotic fluid obtained from 3 patients who underwent caesarean section.— A. Rubin and D. Dvornik, *Am. J. Obstet. Gynec.*, 1965, *92*, 882.

Uses. Griseofulvin is administered by mouth in the treatment of a variety of fungal infections of the skin, nails, and hair, caused by various species of *Epidermophyton, Microsporum,* and *Trichophyton,* including ringworm, favus, tinea imbricata (Tokelau ringworm), and tinea unguium (onychomycosis). It is considered to be less effective against ringworm of the feet, palms, and nails than against other forms of tinea.

It is ineffective in the treatment of actinomycosis, aspergillosis, blastomycosis, coccidioidomycosis, cryptococcosis, histoplasmosis, chromomycosis, sporotrichosis, nocardiosis, candidiasis, and pityriasis versicolor.

The usual dose of griseofulvin is 0.5 to 1 g daily in single or divided doses; children may be given 10 mg per kg body-weight daily. These recommended doses have been halved when preparations, available in some countries, containing ultramicrocrystalline griseofulvin are used. Griseofulvin is probably best given with or after meals.

For superficial forms of ringworm, treatment needs to be continued for 3 to 6 weeks, and for infections of the nails it may need to be continued for up to 12 months.

Griseofulvin should be reserved for initial treatment of ringworm infection of the scalp or for severe infection of the nails; for other sites griseofulvin should be reserved for the treatment of ringworm resistant to agents used topically.— *Med. Lett.*, 1976, *18*, 17. See also *ibid.*, 101; *ibid.*, 1980, *22*, 5.

A discussion of the antimitotic actions of griseofulvin.— F. E. Samson, *A. Rev. Pharmac. & Toxic.*, 1976, *16*, 143.

In 5 patients with extensive molluscum contagiosum treated with griseofulvin, lesions began to regress within 2 weeks and were cleared in 4 to 6 weeks.— O. P. Singh and A. J. Kanwar (letter), *Archs Derm.*, 1977, *113*, 1615.

For earlier reports of the uses of griseofulvin, see Martindale 27th Edn, pp. 636–7.

Administration. *Topical use.* In a study of 155 patients with superficial tinea infections, topical application of griseofulvin 2% in an ointment basis was more effective than ointment basis alone. Griseofulvin 1% was ineffective and dermatitis necessitating cessation of therapy occurred in 10 of 13 patients treated with griseofulvin 3%.— H. Abdel-Aal, *J. int. med. Res.*, 1977, *5*, 382.

Administration in infants and children. Tinea infections in 2 infants aged about one month were treated successfully with ultrafine griseofulvin 10 mg per kg body-weight daily.— W. L. Weston and E. G. Thorne, *Clin. Pediat.*, 1977, *16*, 601.

Angina pectoris. Results of a double-blind crossover study in 8 ambulant patients with angina pectoris indicated that griseofulvin could prove useful in reducing attacks.— B. N. Paul and B. C. Pakrashi, *Am. Heart J.*, 1966, *71*, 26.

Herpes simplex. A report of the beneficial effect of griseofulvin 2 g daily given for 14 days to patients with herpes progenitalis and herpes labialis.— V. N. Sehgal (letter), *Br. J. vener. Dis.*, 1974, *50*, 80.

Herpes zoster. Cures were ascribed to the administration of large doses of griseofulvin in 14 of 18 patients including 2 of 3 with herpes zoster ophthalmicus. The daily doses ranged from 250 mg (a baby aged 5 months) to 3 g and the length of treatment from 4 to 14 days. Coarse-particle griseofulvin seemed to be better than the micronised forms.— S. D. Randazzo and A. Giardina, *Minerva derm.*, 1965, *40*, 15, per *Bull. Hyg., Lond.*, 1965, *40*, 747. See also J. D. Joubert, *S. Afr. med. J.*, 1978, *54*, 224.

Insecticidal effect. Griseofulvin had a mode of action different from that of conventional insecticides and might be valuable in controlling parasitic arthropods of *animals.*— J. F. Anderson, *J. econ. Ent.*, 1966, *59*, 1476, per *Trop. Dis. Bull.*, 1967, *64*, 1032.

Leprosy. Griseofulvin had a beneficial effect on erythema nodosum leprosum, progressively reducing the size and number of skin lesions, but having little or no effect on nerve pain.— J. Ramos e Silva, *Derm. Int.*, 1968, *7*, 37, per *Trop. Dis. Bull.*, 1969, *66*, 306.

In a controlled study in 43 patients with lepromatous leprosy, griseofulvin was without beneficial effect.— W. H. Kneedler, *Lepr. Rev.*, 1970, *41*, 105.

Lichen planus. In a double-blind study, 12 of 17 patients with lichen planus showed complete regression of lesions after treatment for 4 weeks (6 weeks in 2 patients) with griseofulvin 125 mg four times a day compared with 6 of 17 treated with placebo; the difference was significant.— V. N. Sehgal *et al.*, *Br. J. Derm.*, 1972, *87*, 383.

Raynaud's syndrome. A rise in skin temperature of 1.3° was recorded in 12 patients with Raynaud's disease when given griseofulvin 0.5 to 2 g daily compared to a rise of 0.9° when given placebo.— B. R. Allen, *Lancet,* 1971, *2*, 840.

In a double-blind crossover study in 24 patients with Raynaud's syndrome patient preference (assessed by sequential analysis) was significantly in favour of griseofulvin compared with placebo. The dose was 1 to 2 g daily.— S. Sabri *et al.*, *Postgrad. med. J.*, 1973, *49*, 641.

Further references: C. R. Charles and E. S. Carmick, *Archs Derm.*, 1970, *101*, 331; W. E. S. Hasker (letter), *Lancet*, 1970, *2*, 1136.

Scleroderma. Rapid regression of the symptoms of Raynaud's syndrome and slow but gradual replacement of thickened skin occurred in a 27-year-old woman with progressive scleroderma when treated with griseofulvin; joint lesions deteriorated. Four other patients benefited from treatment with griseofulvin for several months but a fifth patient failed to respond.— M. Giordano (letter), *Lancet*, 1967, *2*, 260. See also G. Pasero *et al.*, *Scand. J. Rheumatol.*, 1975, *4*, *Suppl.* 8, 77.

Tinea capitis. Shaving the scalp was a crucial factor in the effective treatment of scalp ringworm and should be regarded as an essential and routine concomitant to the use of griseofulvin.— J. H. S. Pettit (letter), *J. Am. med. Ass.*, 1967, *199*, 343. Since griseofulvin was rapidly effective in controlling *Microsporum* and *Trichophyton* infections shaving of the head was not required. A daily dose of 500 mg of finely divided griseofulvin for adults and half the dose for children under 10 years of age should clear ringworm of the scalp within one month.— I. B. Sneddon, *Practitioner,* 1972, *208*, 438.

In a boy with monilethrix given griseofulvin 125 mg twice daily for 6 weeks for tinea capitis there was an excellent regrowth of normal scalp hair. Hair growth continued during a second 5 month course of griseofulvin therapy.— J. A. Keipert, *Med. J. Aust.*, 1973, *1*, 1236.

Griseofulvin 500 mg daily by mouth for 6 months produced no objective or subjective improvement in 4 patients with monilethrix.— E. R. Farmer and E. A. Murphy, *Med. J. Aust.*, 1978, *2*, 54. See also J. Keipert (letter), *ibid.*, 328.

Cure-rates of 73.9% at 4 months and 62.3% at 8 months were achieved in 100 children with scalp ringworm given 1.5 g of griseofulvin as a single dose. In a further 134 children given also 30 g of fatty substance the respective cure-rates were 79.8 and 78.1%. There was a high rate of spontaneous cures.— J. De Bruycker *et al.*, *Annls Soc. belge Méd. trop.*, 1974, *54*, 463, per *Trop. Dis. Bull.*, 1975, *72*, 216. A similar report.— D. Beghin and R. Vanbreuseghem, *Annls Soc. belge Méd. trop.*, 1974, *54*, 477, per *Trop. Dis. Bull.*, 1975, *72*, 217.

A 16-year-old girl whose tinea capitis had not responded to griseofulvin 1 g daily for 18 months was cured after receiving cimetidine 300 mg four times daily in association with griseofulvin 1.5 g daily for 2 months. The addition of cimetidine to griseofulvin allowed the patient's cell-mediated immunity to effect a cure.— S. E. Presser and H. Blank (letter), *Lancet*, 1981, *1*, 108.

Preparations

Griseofulvin Capsules *(U.S.P.).* Capsules containing griseofulvin (microsize) 125 or 250 mg. Store in airtight containers.

Griseofulvin Oral Suspension *(U.S.P.).* A suspension containing griseofulvin (microsize) 25 mg per ml; it contains one or more suitable diluents, preservatives, colouring, flavouring, and wetting agents. pH 6.5 to 7.5. Store in airtight containers.

Griseofulvin Tablets *(B.P.).* Tablets containing griseofulvin. They may be film-coated [microparticles].

Griseofulvin Tablets *(U.S.P.).* Tablets containing griseofulvin (microsize) 125, 250, or 500 mg. Store in airtight containers.

Ultramicrosize Griseofulvin Tablets *(U.S.P.).* Tablets containing griseofulvin (ultramicrosize) 125 or 250 mg, dispersed in macrogol 6000.

Proprietary Preparations

Fulcin-125 (known in some countries as Fulcin-S and Neo-Fulcin) *(ICI Pharmaceuticals, UK).* Griseofulvin, available as scored tablets of 125 mg. **Fulcin-500.** Griseofulvin, available as tablets of 500 mg. **Fulcin Oral Suspension.** Contains griseofulvin 125 mg in each 5 ml (suggested diluent, syrup). (Also available as Fulcin in *Austral., Belg., Denm., Ger., Ital., Norw., S.Afr., Spain, Swed., Switz.*).

Grisovin *(Glaxo, UK).* Griseofulvin, available as tablets of 125 and 500 mg. (Also available as Grisovin in *Austral., S.Afr., Swed., Switz.*).

Other Proprietary Names

Austral.—Griseostatin; *Canad.*—Fulvicin U/F, Grisaltin, Grisovin-FP; *Denm.*—Lamoryl; *Fr.*—Fulcine Forte, Griséfuline; *Ger.*—Likuden M; *Greece*—Grisovine; *Israel*—Grifulvin Forte; *Ital.*—Delmofulvina, Grisovina FP; *Mauritania*—Greosin; *Jap.*—Grisovin-FP; *Norw.*—Fungivin, Lamoryl; *Spain*—Greosin; *Swed.*—Lamoryl; *Switz.*—Gris-PEG; *USA*—Fulvicin P/G, Fulvicin-U/F, Grifulvin V, Grisactin, Gris-PEG.

2562-a

Amphotericin *(B.P.)*. Amphotericin B *(U.S.P.)*; Anfotericina B. A mixture of antifungal polyenes produced by the growth of certain strains of *Streptomyces nodosus* or by any other means.
$C_{47}H_{73}NO_{17}$=924.1.

CAS — 1397-89-3.

Pharmacopoeias. In *Br., Braz., Jap.,* and *U.S.*

It occurs as a yellow to orange, odourless or almost odourless, almost tasteless powder. The *B.P.* material is for oral or topical use and contains not less than 750 units of amphotericin per mg and not more than 15% of tetraenes. The *U.S.P.* specifies not less than 750 units per mg and not more than 15% of amphotericin A or, for parenteral use, not more than 5%.

Practically **insoluble** in water, alcohol, acetone, chloroform, ether, and toluene; soluble 1 in 200 of dimethylformamide, 1 in 20 of dimethyl sulphoxide, and 1 in 625 of methyl alcohol; soluble in propylene glycol. A 3% suspension in water has a pH of 6 to 8. In dilute solution it is sensitive to light, and inactivated at low pH.

Store at 2° to 8° in airtight containers. Protect from light. Under these conditions, it does not significantly deteriorate or lose potency for at least 1 year. Amphotericin is precipitated from solution by sodium chloride. Solutions for injection may be diluted with dextrose injection adjusted, if necessary, to a pH above 4.2; they should be used immediately after preparation and protected from light during administration.

Incompatibility has been reported with many drugs including amikacin sulphate, antihistamines, benzylpenicillin, calcium chloride, calcium gluconate, carbenicillin sodium, chlorpromazine hydrochloride, chlortetracycline hydrochloride, corticosteroids (data conflicting), diphenhydramine hydrochloride, dopamine hydrochloride, gentamicin sulphate, heparin (data conflicting), kanamycin sulphate, lignocaine hydrochloride, metaraminol tartrate, methyldopate hydrochloride, nitrofurantoin sodium, oxytetracycline hydrochloride, polymyxin B sulphate, potassium chloride, preservatives, procaine hydrochloride, prochlorperazine mesylate, sodium calciumedetate, sodium chloride, streptomycin sulphate, tetracycline hydrochloride, viomycin sulphate, and vitamins. Solutions of amphotericin in dextrose injection tend to be unstable (see above). It would seem wise not to mix amphotericin with any other drug.

Amphotericin went into colloidal suspension in dextrose solutions and settled out during the period of infusion; higher concentrations thereby entered the blood stream and increased the incidence of chills, fever, nausea, vomiting, and other side-effects.— M. J. Barrash and M. Fort, *Archs intern. Med.*, 1960, *106*, 271.

Precipitation of amphotericin might occur within 6 hours of its addition to dextrose injections sterilised by autoclaving, though not when the dextrose injection was sterilised by filtration. Fine precipitates might not be visible under ordinary lighting conditions. The factor responsible for precipitation appeared to be extracted from unprotected rubber closures during heat sterilisation, since no precipitation occurred in dextrose injections autoclaved in plastic containers, even when the pH fell to 3.8. Many toxic effects observed in patients who had received amphotericin infusions could be attributed to injection of a fine suspension of antibiotic.— G. Bryan, Personal Communication, 1969.

Stability. Amphotericin was a weak amphoteric base. Solubilised amphotericin was precipitated by sodium chloride injection. The drug in solution remained stable for approximately 24 hours at room temperature with minimum loss of potency.— V. T. Andriole and H. M. Kravetz, *J. Am. med. Ass.*, 1962, *180*, 269.

A solution of amphotericin, containing 100 μg per ml in dextrose injection, was stable for up to 6 weeks when stored in darkness at 5° but there was a 2 to 3% loss of potency at 25° in the dark in 3 days or 10 to 16% loss in the light.— J. F. Gallelli, *Am. J. Hosp. Pharm.*, 1967, *24*, 425.

In the presence of phosphate-citrate buffers at 37° the optimum pH for the stability of amphotericin was between pH 6 and 6.5. In incubation studies *in vitro* the activity of amphotericin against *Candida albicans* was less at 30° than at 25° or at 35° and increased at 41°.— J. M. T. Hamilton-Miller, *J. Pharm. Pharmac.*, 1973, *25*, 401.

There was no appreciable loss of activity in reconstituted solutions of amphotericin after exposure to 4 different conditions of light and temperature for up to 8 hours. It was not necessary to protect solutions from light during infusions.— S. Shadomy *et al.*, *Am. Rev. resp. Dis.*, 1973, *107*, 303, per *Int. pharm. Abstr.*, 1974, *11*, 103.

Solutions of amphotericin in dextrose injection became turbid when adjusted to pH 4.7.— R. C. Huber and C. Riffkin, *Am. J. Hosp. Pharm.*, 1975, *32*, 173. A similar report.— C. Riffkin, *ibid.*, 1963, *20*, 21.

Amphotericin injection is stated to be stable for 1 month at temperatures not exceeding 25°.— R. R. Wolfert and R. M. Cox, *Am. J. Hosp. Pharm.*, 1975, *32*, 585.

Units. One unit of amphotericin is contained in 0.001064 mg of the first International Standard Preparation (1963) which contains 940 units per mg.

Adverse Effects. Solutions of amphotericin irritate the venous endothelium and may cause pain and thrombophlebitis at the site of injection. Headache, nausea, vomiting, chills, fever, malaise, muscle and joint pains, rash, anorexia, diarrhoea, and gastro-intestinal cramp may occur. Hypertension, hypotension, cardiac arrhythmias, ventricular fibrillation, cardiac arrest, blurred vision, tinnitus, vertigo, and convulsions have been occasionally reported. Amphotericin is nephrotoxic and abnormal renal function with a rise in blood urea is often observed. This is usually reversible but degeneration of the renal tubules has been reported and is common with high doses in excess of 5 g. Anaemia and hypokalaemia occur frequently. Thrombocytopenia, leucopenia, acute liver failure, and anaphylactic reactions may occur.

Neuropathy with pain, impaired vision, and retention of urine has occurred especially after intrathecal injection.

Topical application may produce local irritation, pruritus, and skin rash.

A general discussion of the side-effects of amphotericin.— J. P. Utz *et al.*, *Ann. intern. Med.*, 1964, *61*, 334.

An evaluation of the side-effects of amphotericin in 15 patients.— H. C. Goodpasture *et al.*, *Ann. intern. Med.*, 1972, *76*, 872.

Complications frequently arose when 21 patients with fungal meningitis were treated with amphotericin by means of subcutaneous reservoirs for intraventricular injections. These included local wound infections at the site of insertion of the reservoir, misplaced catheters, and neurological changes due to the siting of the reservoir resulting in mental deterioration. In 3 cases reservoir insertion was considered a major contributing cause of death.— R. D. Diamond and J. E. Bennett, *New Engl. J. Med.*, 1973, *288*, 186.

An erythematous rash and eosinophilia occurred in a 55-year-old man after he had received a total dose of 1.05 g of amphotericin intravenously.— B. Lorber *et al.* (letter), *Ann. intern. Med.*, 1976, *84*, 54.

Anaemia. References to haemolytic anaemia in patients receiving amphotericin: C. W. Holeman and H. Einstein, *Calif. Med.*, 1963, *99*, 90.

Amphotericin appeared to produce anaemia by inhibition of erythropoietin production rather than by suppressing bone-marrow activity directly.— R. R. MacGregor *et al.*, *Antimicrob. Ag. Chemother.*, 1978, *14*, 270.

Bronchospasm. During an infusion of a 1-mg test dose of amphotericin tachypnoea, dyspnoea, and bronchospasm as well as the expected fever and rigors developed in a 72-year-old man. Relief was obtained with diphenhydramine and hydrocortisone.— H. W. Murray (letter), *New Engl. J. Med.*, 1974, *290*, 693.

Hypokalaemia. Profound muscular weakness, rhabdomyolysis, and myoglobinuria, as well as incomplete renal tubular acidosis and impaired urinary concentrating ability, developed in a 20-year-old man with cryptococcal meningitis who became severely hypokalaemic during treatment with amphotericin. Symptoms first appeared after 40 days' treatment with a dosage of 25 mg daily. Three weeks after amphotericin was started, potassium aspartate was added to the treatment but after 3 weeks this was changed to potassium chloride by mouth and intravenously and the urine concentrating mechanism then improved.— D. J. Drutz *et al.*, *J. Am. med. Ass.*, 1970, *211*, 824.

Nephrotoxicity. A study of 7 patients who developed nephropathy during amphotericin therapy showed that the rise in urea nitrogen concentrations in blood could be arrested by changing to intermittent dosage, but that urinary abnormalities continued. Five patients showed evidence of a distal tubular defect in acid excretion which, superimposed on ischaemia of the kidney, might account for the hypokalaemia and nephrocalcinosis characterising amphotericin nephropathy. Early treatment with adequate doses of alkali might prevent nephrocalcinosis and progressive renal failure.— D. K. McCurdy *et al.*, *New Engl. J. Med.*, 1968, *278*, 124.

Irreversible renal toxicity was considered to be rare with total doses of less than 5 g of amphotericin. Only when the blood-urea concentration reached 1 mg per ml should the nephrotoxicity be considered to be serious.— R. Forgan-Smith and J. H. Darrell (letter), *Br. med. J.*, 1974, *1*, 244. If the blood urea rose above 400 to 500 μg per ml treatment must be stopped or serious renal failure might result.— *Br. med. J.*, 1962, *2*, 603.

A report of amphotericin nephrotoxicity in 2 patients with salt depletion.— J. Feely *et al.* (letter), *Lancet*, 1981, *1*, 1422.

Further references: G. B. Appel and H. C. Neu, *New Engl. J. Med.*, 1977, *296*, 784; G. L. Barbour *et al.*, *Archs intern. Med.*, 1979, *139*, 86.

Neuropathy. *After intrathecal administration.* A 17-year-old girl with coccidioidal meningitis who was treated with injections of amphotericin into the right lateral ventricle and into the cisterna magna suffered injury to the lower brain stem. The patient was later found to have subarachnoid block. Severe neurological impairment was still present 14 months later.— D. C. McCullough and J. C. Harbert, *J. Am. med. Ass.*, 1969, *209*, 558.

A 28-year-old man with coccidioidal meningitis developed acute delirium and EEG abnormalities after intrathecal administration of amphotericin 250 μg. The adverse effects disappeared after amphotericin was withdrawn and 5 days later amphotericin was restarted at a reduced dose of 25 μg and gradually increased to a maintenance dose of 500 μg. Neurological complications appeared to be dose related.— R. E. Winn *et al.*, *Archs intern. Med.*, 1979, *139*, 706, per *Int. pharm. Abstr.*, 1980, *17*, 17.

After intravenous administration. A 62-year-old woman given amphotericin intravenously for aspergillosis of the lung developed a peripheral motor polyneuropathy from which she recovered almost completely within a few weeks after discontinuation of the treatment.— A. Staal *et al.*, *Ned. Tijdschr. Geneesk.*, 1963, *107*, 2276, per *Bull. Hyg., Lond.*, 1964, *39*, 276.

Thrombophlebitis. The administration of buffered infusions of amphotericin to a patient with disseminated histoplasmosis resulted in thrombophlebitis and intense cellulitis. The solution was found to have a pH of 5. During a second course of treatment the infusion was prepared by adding amphotericin and buffering agents (Fungizone) to dextrose injection which had been sterilised by filtration. The infusion was found to have a pH of 6.3 and its infusion was not associated with thrombophlebitis.— A. R. Tanser (letter), *Lancet*, 1966, *1*, 1102. (See also under Pharmaceutical Abstracts, p.716).

Treatment of Adverse Effects. Toxic effects such as fever, nausea, and vomiting may be relieved by aspirin, an antihistamine, and an anti-emetic. To reduce febrile reactions small doses of hydrocortisone may be given intravenously just before or during an infusion of amphotericin; they should not be added to the infusion fluid itself (see Incompatibility, p.716). Heparin has been added to solutions for intravenous injection to reduce the incidence of thrombophlebitis (but see Incompatibility, p.716). Hydrocortisone sodium succinate has been administered concomitantly with amphotericin given by intrathecal injection. Amphotericin is not removed by haemodialysis.

Four patients who had undergone renal transplantation and had fungous infections were successfully treated with amphotericin in total doses of up to 3 g without reduction of their renal function. Mannitol 12.5 g was infused intravenously before and after each dose of amphotericin. It was suggested that patients should also be given sodium bicarbonate to reduce acidosis.— J. J. Olivero *et al.*, *Br. med. J.*, 1975, *1*, 550.

The concurrent administration of mannitol intravenously with each dose of amphotericin to a young woman with mucocutaneous candidiasis and moderate renal insufficiency was effective in reducing the nephrotoxicity of amphotericin.— J. M. Rosch *et al.*, *J. Am. med. Ass.*, 1976, *235*, 1995. Amphotericin 17.5 mg in 3.5 ml was added to 125 ml of a 20% mannitol solution which was diluted with 5% dextrose solution to 1 litre.— *idem*, 1977, *237*, 27.

Mannitol 1 g per kg body-weight did not protect against the nephrotoxicity of amphotericin in a controlled study of 11 patients.— W. E. Bullock *et al.*, *Antimicrob. Ag. Chemother.*, 1976, *10*, 555.

Precautions. To reduce the risk of vein irritation, the rate of intravenous infusion of amphotericin should be slow, and the concentration of solutions should not exceed 100 µg per ml; the injection site should be changed frequently.

Tests of renal function should be performed regularly during treatment and treatment stopped if progressive impairment occurs. Concomitant administration of other nephrotoxic drugs and of antineoplastic agents should be avoided.

The potassium-depleting effect of amphotericin may enhance the effects of muscle relaxants and may increase digitalis toxicity; corticosteroids may enhance the depletion of potassium.

Experience in treating patients over 40 years of age with amphotericin indicated that patients suffering from arteriosclerosis were especially susceptible to the action of amphotericin, with the production of hypertonicity of the sympathetic nervous system. When it was proposed to use this antibiotic in such patients in high dosage, vasodilators or sympatholytics, or both, should be given.— A. Raphael *et al.*, *Revta Ass. méd. bras.*, 1963, *9*, 313, per *Trop. Dis. Bull.*, 1964, *61*, 842.

In a report of the Veterans Administration, Armed Forces Cooperative Study on Histoplasmosis, anorexia, nausea, vomiting, and malaise occurred in more than one-half of a group of men with chronic pulmonary histoplasmosis who were given amphotericin in conjunction with triple sulphonamides. The symptoms were alleviated by withdrawing the sulphonamides. A synergism between the 2 drugs was suggested.— *Am. Rev. resp. Dis.*, 1968, *97*, 96, per *Abstr. Hyg.*, 1968, *43*, 955.

On the third day of treatment with amphotericin a patient with North American blastomycosis went into a coma which lasted for 6 weeks and was caused by adrenal insufficiency.— P. T. Chandler, *Sth. med. J.*, 1977, *70*, 863.

Fatal bone-marrow aplasia occurred in a 32-year-old man with multiple myeloma during treatment with amphotericin and flucytosine for cryptococcal meningitis.— C. S. Bryan and J. A. McFarland, *J. Am. med. Ass.*, 1978, *239*, 1068.

For reference to the immunosuppressant effects of amphotericin, see under Antimicrobial Action.

Interactions. The association of amphotericin and miconazole appeared to be less effective than either drug used alone.— L. P. Schacter *et al.* (letter), *Lancet*, 1976, *2*, 318.

Severe pulmonary reactions occurred in 14 of 22 patients receiving leucocyte transfusions and amphotericin intravenously; 5 patients died. Two of 35 patients receiving leucocyte transfusions without amphotericin suffered respiratory deterioration. Amphotericin should be used cautiously in patients receiving leucocyte transfusions, particularly when leucocyte therapy has been started in the presence of Gram-negative septicaemia. When these therapies are used together, it is advisable to separate the infusion of amphotericin as far as possible from the time of a leucocyte transfusion, to administer amphotericin more slowly than usual, and to be watchful for respiratory deterioration.— D. G. Wright *et al.*, *New Engl. J. Med.*, 1981, *304*, 1185. Comments and different experiences: S. J. Forman *et al.* (letter), *ibid.*, *305*, 584; M. W. DeGregorio *et al.* (letter), *ibid.*, 585. The advice offered by D.G. Wright *et al.* should be followed.— *Lancet*, 1981, *1*, 1405.

See also under Antimicrobial Action.

Pregnancy and the neonate. Systemic treatment with amphotericin is best avoided in pregnancy.— W. Mosimann, *Schweiz. med. Wschr.*, 1975, *105*, 257.

Antimicrobial Action. Amphotericin is a polyene antifungal antibiotic which interferes with the permeability of the cell membrane of sensitive fungi. It is reported to be fungistatic at concentrations achieved clinically. It is active against *Aspergillus fumigatus, Blastomyces dermatitidis, Candida* spp., *Coccidioides immitis, Cryptococcus neoformans, Histoplasma capsulatum, Microsporum audouinii, Paracoccidioides brasiliensis, Rhizopus* spp., *Sporothrix schenckii*, and *Trichophyton* spp. Minimum inhibitory concentrations range from 0.03 to 1 µg per ml for many of these organisms; a concentration of up to 7.3 µg or more per ml has been reported for *Microsporum* and *Trichophyton* spp. *Mucor, Absidia*, and *Basidiobolus spp.* may also be sensitive. It is inactive against bacteria, rickettsias, and viruses but is reported to be effective against *Leishmania* and *Trypanosoma* protozoa.

Amphotericin enhanced the activity *in vitro* of flucytosine, rifampicin, mycophenolic acid glucuronide, tetracycline, and actinomycin D against *Saccharomyces cerevisiae*, probably by increasing their penetration through the fungal cytoplasmic membrane.— C. N. Kwan *et al.*, *Antimicrob. Ag. Chemother.*, 1972, *2*, 61.

Amphotericin was active *in vitro* against *Prototheca* spp. with MICs ranging from 0.09 to 3.12 µg per ml.— E. Segal *et al.*, *Antimicrob. Ag. Chemother.*, 1976, *10*, 75.

Sensitivity studies confirmed amphotericin as the most effective agent against *Naegleria fowleri*. Clotrimazole and miconazole were less active.— R. J. Duma and R. Finley, *Antimicrob. Ag. Chemother.*, 1976, *10*, 370.

Amphotericin increased the activity of macrophages and also increased their supply as well as the supply of precursors.— H. -S. Lin *et al.*, *Antimicrob. Ag. Chemother.*, 1977, *11*, 154.

Twelve strains of *Coccidioides immitis* were uniformly sensitive to amphotericin *in vitro* and *in vivo*. MICs ranged from 0.078 µg per ml at 3 days to 2.5 µg per ml after 15 days' incubation.— M. S. Collins and D. Pappagianis, *Antimicrob. Ag. Chemother.*, 1977, *11*, 1049.

Amphotericin inhibited *in vitro* the ability of neutrophils to reach the site of infection promptly (chemotaxis).— Y. H. Thong and D. Ness (letter), *Lancet* 1977, *2*, 568. Another study *in vitro* suggested that amphotericin might be immunosuppressive.— G. A. Roselle and C. A. Kauffman, *Antimicrob. Ag. Chemother.*, 1978, *14*, 398. Neutrophil viability was reduced after incubation with amphotericin in a medium free from cholesterol and serum. No significant decrease occurred when cholesterol in low-density lipoprotein or serum was added to the medium but neutrophil viability was again reduced on increasing the concentration of amphotericin. It was considered that serum or cholesterol-containing low-density lipoprotein contained a factor which protected neutrophils against the effect of amphotericin.— C. J. Chunn *et al.*, *Antimicrob. Ag. Chemother.*, 1977, *12*, 226.

Good correlation between microdilution and broth dilution techniques was obtained for the susceptibility of 50 clinical isolates of yeast to flucytosine and amphotericin but the microdilution technique was considered to be unsuitable for use with *Cryptococcus neoformans*.— M. F. Mazens *et al.*, *Antimicrob. Ag. Chemother.*, 1979, *15*, 475.

Enhanced activity. References to the increased antifungal activity of amphotericin with *clotrimazole*.— W. H. Beggs *et al.*, *Antimicrob. Ag. Chemother.*, 1976, *9*, 863. With *flucytosine*.— M. Kitahara *et al.*, *Antimicrob. Ag. Chemother.*, 1976, *9*, 915. With *minocycline*.— M. A. Lew *et al.*, *Antimicrob. Ag. Chemother.*, 1978, *14*, 465. With *rifampicin*.— D. Rifkind *et al.*, *Antimicrob. Ag. Chemother.*, 1974, *6*, 783; M. Kitahara *et al.*, *Antimicrob. Ag. Chemother.*, 1976, *9*, 915; W. H. Beggs *et al.*, *J. infect. Dis.*, 1976, *133*, 206; R. M. Bannatyne and R. Cheung, *Curr. ther. Res.*, 1979, *25*, 71; J. E. Edwards *et al.*, *Antimicrob. Ag. Chemother.*, 1980, *17*, 484.

Synergism between tetracycline and amphotericin occurred in experimental amoebic meningoencephalitis in *mice*.— Y. H. Thong *et al.*, *Med. J. Aust.*, 1978, *1*, 663. Amphotericin and minocycline and amphotericin and tetracycline enhanced each other's activity when used together *in vitro* against *Naegleria fowleri*.— K. K. Lee *et al.*, *Antimicrob. Ag. Chemother.*, 1979, *16*, 217.

Several compounds related to phenolic antoxidants including levodopa and dopamine enhanced the inhibitory activity of amphotericin against various species of yeasts *in vitro*.— F. A. Andrews *et al.*, *J. antimicrob. Chemother.*, 1979, *5*, 173. See also W. H. Beggs *et al.*, *Antimicrob. Ag. Chemother.*, 1978, *13*, 266; *idem* (letter), *J. antimicrob. Chemother.*, 1980, *6*, 291 (amphotericin methyl ester).

Further references: G. Medoff and G. S. Kobayashi, *J. Am. med. Ass.*, 1975, *232*, 619.

Resistance. *Candida lusitaniae* associated with an infection in a patient with acute myelogenous leukaemia developed resistance to amphotericin during systemic treatment. The organisms had initially been inhibited by 0.31 µg per ml of amphotericin in yeast nitrogen base agar, but after 20 days it required 30 µg per ml for complete inhibition when incubated for 24 hours.— D. Pappagianis *et al.*, *Antimicrob. Ag. Chemother.*, 1979, *16*, 123.

Further references: J. D. Dick *et al.*, *Antimicrob. Ag. Chemother.*, 1980, *18*, 158.

Absorption and Fate. There is little or no absorption of amphotericin from the gastro-intestinal tract although blood concentrations of up to 500 ng per ml have been detected following administration by mouth. The colloidal form of amphotericin with sodium deoxycholate is reported to be better absorbed but it is also associated wtih an undesirable incidence of gastro-intestinal side-effects. Amphotericin administered intravenously in the colloidal form in a dose of 650 µg per kg body-weight daily has produced peak plasma concentrations of 1.8 to 3.5 µg per ml.

The plasma half-life has been reported to be about 24 hours. Amphotericin is excreted slowly in the urine; traces have been reported to be present 2 months after the completion of treatment.

After a dose of amphotericin, 5 to 40% was excreted in the urine.— C. M. Kunin, *Ann. intern. Med.*, 1967, *67*, 151.

Mean serum concentrations of amphotericin were 1.21, 0.62, and 0.32 µg per ml at 1, 18, and 42 hours respectively after an intravenous infusion. The drug was detected in serum 7 weeks, but not 13 weeks, after treatment.— B. T. Fields *et al.*, *Appl. Microbiol.*, 1970, *19*, 955.

Values for the concentration of amphotericin in serum samples were generally lower when the assay had been carried out on a frozen sample than when an assay had been carried out immediately.— R. M. Bannatyne and R. Cheung, *Antimicrob. Ag. Chemother.*, 1977, *12*, 550.

The elimination half-lives of amphotericin were 14 and 16.5 days in 2 patients (creatinine clearance rates of 28 and 37 ml per minute) who had received long-term therapy with amphotericin.— A. J. Atkinson and J. E. Bennett, *Antimicrob. Ag. Chemother.*, 1978, *13*, 271.

Dialysis. There was no accumulation of amphotericin in an anephric patient given 9 doses of 20 mg intravenously every 24 to 48 hours. Amphotericin was not dialysable with conventional haemodialysis membranes regardless of the degree of binding to plasma proteins.— H. A. Feldman *et al.*, *Antimicrob. Ag. Chemother.*, 1973, *4*, 302.

Only about 3 to 15% of amphotericin was cleared from the blood of 4 patients undergoing haemodialysis. More than 90% was bound *in vitro* to plasma protein; this might account for the poor clearance of amphotericin.— E. R. Block *et al.*, *Ann. intern. Med.*, 1974, *80*, 613.

Diffusion. *Into cerebrospinal fluid.* A 2-year-old boy with meningoencephalitis due to *Naegleria* received amphotericin, 250 µg per kg body-weight in a single intravenous dose daily increased over a week to 1 mg per kg daily. The cerebrospinal fluid concentration of amphotericin after 7 days' treatment was 0.184 µg per ml, and after 11 days had risen to 0.224 µg per ml. In 2 other children exposed to this infection, amphotericin was not detected in CSF after treatment with doses up to 750 µg per kg daily by intravenous injection.— J. Apley *et al.*, *Br. med. J.*, 1970, *1*, 596.

Into saliva. Concentrations of amphotericin in saliva after its application in Orabase.— H. G. De Vries-Hospers and D. Van Der Waaij, *Infection* 1978, *6*, 16, per *Abstr. Hyg.*, 1978, *53*, 742.

Uses. Amphotericin is used for the treatment of severe mycotic infections including North American blastomycosis, candidiasis, coccidioidomycosis, cryptococcosis, and histoplasmosis. It is also used in the treatment of aspergillosis, South American blastomycosis, phycomycosis, and sporotrichosis and has been given for the treatment of American mucocutaneous leishmaniasis. Amphotericin may be used with flucytosine (see p.724) in the treatment of infection such as cryptococcal meningitis.

It is applied topically in concentrations of 3% to treat cutaneous and mucocutaneous infections caused mainly by *Candida* spp.; pessaries and cream are used in the treatment of vaginal candidiasis. Amphotericin is also given by mouth for the suppression of oral or intestinal candidiasis, in doses of up to 800 mg daily. It has sometimes been given with drugs such as tetracycline in an attempt to reduce fungal supra-infection.

A colloidal form of amphotericin with sodium deoxycholate is used for injection and a crystalline form for topical or oral administration. A test dose of 1 mg intravenously is often given before embarking on intravenous therapy. For slow intravenous infusion a solution containing 100 μg of amphotericin per ml in dextrose injection (with a pH greater than 4.2) should be given in an initial daily dose of up to 250 μg per kg body-weight. The dose may be increased gradually to a total of 1 mg per kg daily or 1.5 mg per kg on alternate days. Children have been given similar doses. Severely ill patients may be given 1.5 mg per kg daily; this dose should not be exceeded. If for any reason treatment is interrupted for longer than 7 days, it should be resumed with the lowest initial dose.

Intrathecal injection is used for patients with severe meningitis especially when intravenous therapy has been ineffective. Commencing with 25 μg, the dose may be increased gradually until 500 μg is tolerated without excessive discomfort. A solution containing 250 μg of amphotericin per ml of dextrose injection is used and the dose volume is diluted with cerebrospinal fluid in the syringe before injection. Doses of 0.25 to 1 mg have been administered every 2 or 3 days to a maximum of 15 mg. Doses should be reduced for children.

The water-soluble methyl ester of amphotericin has been tried; it may be less toxic than amphotericin.

Reviews of the action and uses of amphotericin: E. F. Gale, *Br. med. J.*, 1973, *4*, 33; J. E. Bennett, *New Engl. J. Med.*, 1974, *290*, 30; *Med. Lett.*, 1978, *20*, 66; G. Medoff and G. S. Kobayashi, *New Engl. J. Med.*, 1980, *302*, 145.

To reduce the incidence of side-effects during treatment, amphotericin was given intravenously for 10 weeks to 15 patients with systemic mycotic infections in doses gradually increased to those which provided daily peak serum concentrations double those necessary to inhibit the infecting fungus. Until the inhibitory concentration was known, a serum concentration of 1.56 μg per ml was aimed for, and usually was attained with 15 to 50 mg of amphotericin daily. The serum concentration was not allowed to fall below 0.78 μg per ml. Seven patients received less than 1.9 g and only 1 had more than 3 g; the daily dose was about one-half the usual dose. Acute toxic effects were rare and were controlled in all but 1 patient with aspirin and antihistamines. Hypokalaemia in 6 patients was corrected by potassium supplements. Serum concentrations of urea nitrogen rose during treatment in all patients and treatment was withdrawn for 1 or 2 days in 7 patients. Eleven patients followed up for 8 to 45 weeks remained free from infection, while 4 were apparently free at the time of death.— D. J. Drutz *et al.*, *Am. J. Med.*, 1968, *45*, 405, per *Abstr. Wld Med.*, 1969, *43*, 178.

Amphotericin and transfer factor appeared to be successful in treating a patient with a systemic algal infection caused by *Prototheca*.— G. E. Cox *et al.*, *Lancet*, 1974, *2*, 379.

A possible beneficial effect with amphotericin in *Alternaria* maxillary osteomyelitis in one patient.— J. Garu *et al.* (letter), *Ann. intern. Med.*, 1977, *86*, 747.

The production *in vitro* of interferon through induction by poly I. poly C or by a complex of poly I. poly C and a dextran was enhanced from 10 to 100 times by pretreatment of cells with amphotericin or other polyene macrolides.— E. C. Borden *et al.*, *Antimicrob. Ag. Chemother.*, 1978, *13*, 159.

Administration. For patients on maintenance doses of amphotericin, solutions containing 100 μg per ml could be given over a period of 1 hour provided that cardiac monitoring was undertaken during the first infusion.— A. D. Barreuther *et al.* (letter), *Drug Intell. & clin. Pharm.*, 1977, *11*, 368.

Intra-articular use. Reference to the treatment of arthritis caused by *Petriellidium boydii* with intra-articular injections of amphotericin.— G. Hayden *et al.*, *Am. J. Dis. Child.*, 1977, *131*, 927.

Intrathecal use. In mycotic infections involving the CNS, amphotericin might be given intrathecally, by lumbar or cisternal puncture, or into the cerebral ventricles, as well as intravenously. Hydrocortisone sodium succinate, 20 mg dissolved in 5 ml of the patient's spinal fluid, should be injected before giving the amphotericin, also mixed with the patient's CSF, in a final concentration of 100 μg of amphotericin per ml of CSF. Amphotericin given by mouth was effective in preventing relapse in some patients with blastomycosis and coccidioidomycosis of bone, skin, and joints. It was ineffective by mouth in the treatment of cryptococcosis or in preventing relapses.— H. I. Winner, *Prescribers' J.*, 1968, *8*, 36.

The minimum concentration of amphotericin in the serum after a dose of 25 to 105 mg given to patients on alternate days was not significantly different from that following a dose of 5 to 70 mg daily. Peak concentrations were generally higher after the alternate-day regimen, but concentrations did not rise in relation to increased dosage. Intrathecal administration once or twice weekly did not maintain measurable concentrations of amphotericin in the CSF; satisfactory therapy was achieved with daily infusions of 200 to 300 μg into the lateral cerebral ventricle via a subcutaneous reservoir.— D. D. Bindschadler and J. E. Bennett, *J. infect. Dis.*, 1969, *120*, 427, per *Abstr. Wld Med.*, 1970, *44*, 265. See also under Adverse Effects, p.716.

Ocular use. In the treatment of ocular fungous infections subconjunctival injection of amphotericin 125 μg was reasonably well tolerated, but penetration into the eye was not appreciable. Though intra-ocular injection was highly toxic, the eye could tolerate 35 μg in 0.05 ml of solution. For topical use, a 0.3% solution could be prepared in 5% dextrose or purified water.— M. S. Rheins *et al.*, *Br. J. Ophthal.*, 1966, *50*, 533. Although intravitreal injection of amphotericin 5 or 10 μg did not cause clinical or microscopical changes in *rabbits*' eyes, after doses of 25 μg or higher retinal detachment and vitreous opacities were evident within a few days. It was emphasised that even with the lower doses injections should be made into the centre of vitreous as opposed to near the retina.— A. J. Axelrod *et al.*, *Am. J. Ophthal.*, 1973, *76*, 578.

Amphotericin 5 mg given by episcleral injection to 2 patients with endophthalmitis following cataract extraction rapidly reversed their deterioration and produced progressive improvement although there had been no laboratory evidence of fungal infection.— H. F. Allen, *Archs Ophthal., N.Y.*, 1972, *88*, 640, per *J. Am. med. Ass.*, 1972, *222*, 1577.

The successful treatment of candidal endophthalmitis with a single intravitreal injection of amphotericin 5 μg.— G. A. Stern *et al.*, *Archs Ophthal., N.Y.*, 1977, *95*, 89.

Vitrectomy and an intravitreal injection of amphotericin 5 μg, together with repeated intravenous amphotericin and flucytosine by mouth, improved vision in a patient with postnatal candidal endophthalmitis. A similar patient treated with amphotericin intravenously and flucytosine by mouth had not responded to treatment.— H. L. Cantrill *et al.*, *J. Am. med. Ass.*, 1980, *243*, 1163.

Peritoneal use. Reference to the treatment of candidal peritonitis by peritoneal lavage with amphotericin.— R. A. Bortolussi *et al.*, *J. Pediat.*, 1975, *87*, 987.

Administration in renal failure. A report of 5 patients with suspected renal disease and amphotericin-sensitive fungal infections in which amphotericin was not given, or was given in inadequate dosage, for fear of renal damage; 4 of the patients died of their fungal disease.— W. St. C. Symmers, *Br. med. J.*, 1973, *4*, 460.

Data for predicting removal of amphotericin by conventional haemodialysis.— T. P. Gibson and H. A. Nelson, *Clin. Pharmacokinet.*, 1977, *2*, 403.

A maintenance dose of 0.5 mg per kg body-weight daily or 1 mg per kg every 2 days was recommended in renal insufficiency, and 0.5 to 1 mg per kg daily for dialysis patients.— J. S. Cheigh, *Am. J. Med.*, 1977, *62*, 555.

Amphotericin could be given in a usual dosage in renal failure. Concentrations were not affected by haemodialysis.— W. M. Bennett *et al.*, *Ann. intern. Med.*, 1980, *93*, 62.

Further references: P. Sharpstone, *Br. med. J.*, 1977, *2*, 36; G. B. Appel and H. C. Neu, *New Engl. J. Med.*, 1977, *296*, 663.

See also under Absorption and Fate above.

Amoebiasis. A 2-year-old boy with meningoencephalitis due to *Naegleria* amoeba survived for 16 days when treated with amphotericin and sulphadiazine intravenously. Amphotericin, in a daily dose of 250 μg per kg body-weight increased over a week to 1 mg per kg, was infused over 3 to 4 hours, and sulphadiazine, 750 mg, was given 6-hourly. Two other children exposed to the same source of infection who developed mild symptoms recovered after similar treatment.— J. Apley *et al.*, *Br. med. J.*, 1970, *1*, 596.

See also R. J. Duma *et al.*, *Ann. intern. Med.*, 1971, *74*, 923.

Aspergillosis. In 10 patients with aspergilloma of the lung, 5 ml of a paste containing amphotericin 500 mg in 100 ml of basis was injected into the cavity on 4 to 9 occasions at intervals of 7 to 21 days. Aspergilloma regressed in 5 patients of whom 1 died. After treatment, sputum cultures were negative in 7 patients.— P. Karkowka *et al.*, *Tubercle*, 1970, *51*, 184. See also J. L. Hargis *et al.*, *Am. J. Med.*, 1980, *68*, 389.

A report of the successful treatment of invasive *Aspergillus* pneumonia in 2 immunosuppressed patients with blood cancers.— J. E. Pennington, *New Engl. J. Med.*, 1976, *295*, 426. See also J. Aisner *et al.*, *Ann. intern. Med.*, 1977, *86*, 539; B. A. Adelman *et al.* (letter), *Ann. intern. Med.*, 1979, *91*, 323.

Amphotericin by intravenous injection did not appear to be helpful in aspergilloma but some beneficial effects had been reported when amphotericin and sodium iodide were administered via an endobronchial catheter.— *Lancet*, 1977, *1*, 637.

Amphotericin intravenously and flucytosine by mouth were unsuccessful in the treatment of a renal transplant patient with an epidural abscess caused by *Aspergillus fumigatus*.— I. Ingwer *et al.*, *Archs intern. Med.*, 1978, *138*, 153.

Rapid improvement and total eradication of *Aspergillus* pneumonia within 6 months in a patient treated with amphotericin and flucytosine.— S. D. Codish *et al.*, *J. Am. med. Ass.*, 1979, *241*, 2418.

Further references: J. R. Burton *et al.*, *Ann. intern. Med.*, 1972, *77*, 383; K. J. Hammerman *et al.*, *Am. Rev. resp. Dis.*, 1974, *109*, 57.

Blastomycosis. Amphotericin in total doses of 1 to 3.5 g intravenously was successful in the treatment of North American blastomycosis in 18 of 21 men patients. For 1 patient a further course of amphotericin 2 g was necessary to arrest a pulmonary lesion and in 1 patient, where treatment failed, improvement was obtained with hydroxystilbamidine in a total dose of 8 g.— M. W. Kepron, *Can. med. Ass. J.*, 1972, *106*, 243.

A comparison of amphotericin and hydroxystilbamidine in 84 patients with blastomycosis. Amphotericin was considered to be the best treatment for blastomycosis involving any organ other than the lung or skin, when either drug was considered suitable.— J. F. Busey, *Am. Rev. resp. Dis.*, 1972, *105*, 812, per *J. Am. med. Ass.*, 1972, *221*, 522.

Further references: J. C. Chesney *et al.*, *Am. J. Dis. Child.*, 1979, *133*, 1134.

Candidiasis. Two of 3 patients who developed candidal endocarditis, subsequent to treatment for bacterial endocarditis, completely recovered after surgical intervention to remove the gross nidus of infection and treatment with amphotericin. In all patients a solution containing up to 50 mg of amphotericin per 100 ml of lactated Ringer's solution was used to irrigate the aorta and left ventricle. Following replacement of the aortic valve, amphotericin was administered intravenously in doses of up to 50 mg daily on alternate days. One patient, who died, received a total dose of 6.5 g of amphotericin, and the other patients 2.46 g and 1.5 g respectively. In 1 patient, prior administration of Diphenhydramine hydrochloride 50 mg and prochlorperazine 10 mg reduced the side-effects of amphotericin.— J. H. Kay *et al.*, *J. Am. med. Ass.*, 1968, *203*, 621.

Amphotericin was given intravenously in small doses of 10 to 355 mg over 4 to 18 days to 14 patients with severe and disabling candidal infections and was effective in all. No recurrences were observed during follow-up over 2 to 24 months. The only side-effect was transient uraemia in the patient who received the highest dose.— G. Medoff *et al.*, *Archs intern. Med.*, 1972, *130*, 241, per *J. Am. med. Ass.*, 1972, *221*, 1067.

The use of large doses of amphotericin in conjunction with early surgery had reduced the mortality-rate to 20% in patients with candidal endocarditis.— *Br. med. J.*, 1975, *3*, 264.

A report of the treatment of candidal arthritis with amphotericin.— D. G. Poplack and S. A. Jacobs, *J. Pediat.*, 1975, *87*, 989. See also H. W. Murray *et al.*, *Am.J. Med.*, 1976, *60*, 587.

Further references: A. Gauto *et al.*, *Am. J. Surg.*, 1977, *133*, 174; M. A. Keller *et al.*, *Am. J. Dis. Child.*, 1977, *131*, 1260; T. Wegmann *et al.*, *Dt. med. Wschr.*, 1979, *104*, 635.

Candidiasis, cutaneous. Amphotericin and nystatin applied topically were highly and equally effective in a double-blind comparative study in 144 patients with intertriginous candidiasis.— C. Stritzler, *Archs Derm.*, 1966, *93*, 101.

Four patients with chronic mucocutaneous candidiasis, which developed after they were 5 years of age, responded to amphotericin given intravenously in increasing doses up to 40 to 50 mg thrice weekly and maintained for 8 to 10 weeks. Two anergic patients with candidiasis since infancy were treated with amphotericin to clear the mucocutaneous lesions and were then treated with transfer factor.— C. H. Kirkpatrick and T. K. Smith, *Ann. intern. Med.*, 1974, *80*, 310.

Candidiasis, meningeal. Reports of the combined use of amphotericin and flucytosine in the successful treatment of candidal meningitis.— P. J. Chesney *et al.*, *J. Pediat.*, 1976, *89*, 1017; P. J. Chesney *et al.*, *Johns Hopkins med. J.*, 1978, *142*, 155; L. D. Lilien *et al.*, *Pediatrics*, 1978, *61*, 57; S. E. Straus (letter), *Ann. intern. Med.*, 1978, *89*, 574.

Candidiasis, ocular. Amphotericin given intravenously in total doses of 1.7 g and 225 mg was effective in treating candidal endophthalmitis in 2 patients. Flucytosine given to 1 patient was ineffective.— B. R. Meyers *et al.*, *Ann. intern. Med.*, 1973, *79*, 647.

See also under Administration (ocular use), above.

Candidiasis, oral. Amphotericin was applied in a 2% concentration either in an adhesive paste (Orabase) or in an adhesive powder (Orahesive) to oral candidal lesions after meals and before retiring. About 1 g of medication was applied daily, equivalent to about 20 mg of amphotericin. Of 33 patients, there was definite improvement in 28 and slight improvement in 4.— A. H. Kutscher *et al.*, *Oral Surg.*, 1964, *17*, 31, per *Int. pharm. Abstr.*, 1964, *1*, 812.

A study of 8 non-diabetic patients with candidal infections of the mouth resistant to treatment with nystatin or amphotericin showed that all had normal general immune function. The lesions cleared in 4 patients when treatment, continued for up to 6 months, was supplemented by giving folic acid and iron to correct nutritional deficiencies. The remaining 4 patients did not improve and required surgical treatment.— R. M. Mackie *et al.*, *Br. J. Derm.*, 1978, *98*, 343.

Candidiasis, urinary. Amphotericin administered as a continuous bladder irrigation of 50 mg per litre of sterile water for 5 days (1 litre daily) effectively eradicated candidal infection of the bladder in 7 of 10 patients. The other 3 had evidence of disseminated infection and required systemic therapy.— G. J. Wise *et al.*, *J. Am. med. Ass.*, 1973, *224*, 1636.

Candidiasis, vaginal. Amphotericin was effective, clinically and mycologically, in 73% of 63 pregnant patients with vaginal candidiasis and in 86% of 93 non-pregnant patients. Pessaries each containing 50 mg were used at night, usually for 14 days.— A. Ewing, *Br. J. clin. Pract.*, 1967, *21*, 613.

In a double-blind study involving 78 women with vaginal candidiasis, amphotericin gave a much higher cure-rate than natamycin when proprietary pessaries of the 2 drugs were compared.— B. M. Corkill and N. J. McCarthy, *Med. J. Aust.*, 1972, *2*, 33.

Chromomycosis. A pressure-gun method was used to obtain high intralesional concentrations of amphotericin in the treatment of chromomycosis, and produced the most satisfactory results of the methods of local therapy used. The concentrated solutions of the drug required were irritant to tissues and could cause pain, oedema, secondary infection, and thrombosis.— D. A. Whiting, *Br. J. Derm.*, 1967, *79*, 345.

Coccidioidomycosis. A 51-year-old man with disseminated coccidioidomycosis involving both eyes was treated successfully with amphotericin by intravenous, intrathecal, and intraventricular injection. The infection cleared and the chorioretinal lesions healed, leaving hyperpigmentation at the borders.— W. R. Green and J. E. Bennett, *Archs Ophthal.*, *N.Y.*, 1967, *77*, 339, per *J. Am. med. Ass.*, 1967, *199*, (Mar. 20), A213.

An *in vitro* method of measuring the response to amphotericin in patients with disseminated coccidioidomycosis.— K. Borchardt *et al.*, *Archs Derm.*, 1973, *108*, 119, per *J. Am. med. Ass.*, 1973, *225*, 543.

For a report of disseminated coccidioidomycosis responding to treatment with miconazole given intravenously and amphotericin given intrathecally, see Miconazole, p.728.

Cryptococcosis. Amphotericin given in gradually increasing doses to a maximum of 35 mg daily for 16 days (total dose 460 mg) successfully eliminated *Torulopsis glabrata* from an elderly patient.— H. Hahn *et al.*, *J. Am. med. Ass.*, 1968, *203*, 835.

Two patients with ocular infections due to *Cryptococcus neoformans* were successfully treated with intravenously administered amphotericin, 1 to 2 mg per kg bodyweight daily. The duration of treatment was 2 and 4 months respectively; no side-effects occurred.— M. E. Cameron and A. Harrison, *Med. J. Aust.*, 1970, *1*, 935.

Amphotericin applied topically was ineffective in treating an ulcer infected with *Cryptococcus neoformans*.— L. F. Fajardo (letter), *Ann. intern. Med.*, 1973, *78*, 777.

For reports on the use of amphotericin with flucytosine in the treatment of cryptococcal infections, see Flucytosine, p.724.

Cryptococcosis, meningeal. Three patients with meningitis due to *Cryptococcus neoformans* and 1 with meningitis due to *Coccidioides immitis* were treated with amphotericin administered intraventricularly by means of a subcutaneous reservoir and pump. The initial dose of 100 µg in dextrose injection was increased by increments of 100 µg to a maximum of 0.5 to 1 mg, depending on the tolerance of the patient, given once to thrice weekly. Two patients improved after 21 to 74 injections into the reservoir.— P. Witorsch *et al.*, *J. Am. med. Ass.*, 1965, *194*, 699.

A 61-year-old alcoholic with cryptococcal meningitis and an intracranial focal lesion associated with cryptococcosis recovered after intensive treatment with amphotericin alone.— F. L. Sapico (letter), *Lancet*, 1979, *1*, 560.

For reports on the treatment of cryptococcal meningitis with amphotericin and flucytosine, see Flucytosine, p.724.

Histoplasmosis. A study of the dosage of amphotericin in 85 patients with chronic pulmonary histoplasmosis. A small dose of 500 mg given over 3.5 weeks controlled the infection in about 60% of those treated; the failures were cured following retreatment. A relatively large dose of 2.5 g in 17 weeks provided successful treatment but was not tolerated by 29% of the patients.— W. D. Sutcliff, *Am. Rev. resp. Dis.*, 1972, *105*, 60, per *J. Am. med. Ass.*, 1972, *219*, 1657.

Treatment with amphotericin in a total dose of 0.95 g to 5.9 g for histoplasmosis was successful in 6 of 17 patients.— J. W. Smith and J. P. Utz, *Ann. intern. Med.*, 1972, *76*, 557.

Further references: C. L. Giles and H. F. Falls, *Am. J. Ophthal.*, 1968, *66*, 101; G. A. Sarosi *et al.*, *Ann. intern. Med.*, 1971, *75*, 511; A. R. Fosson and W. E. Wheeler, *J. Pediat.*, 1975, *86*, 32; J. U. Egere *et al.*, *J. trop. Med. Hyg.*, 1978, *81*, 225; G. R. Cott *et al.*, *J. Am. med. Ass.*, 1979, *242*, 456.

Leishmaniasis. Reports on the treatment of leishmaniasis with amphotericin.— E. Belfort and R. Medina, *Derm. Venez.*, 1971, *10*, 1121, per *Trop. Dis. Bull.*, 1972, *69*, 496; S. A. P. Sampaio *et al.*, *Int. J. Derm.*, 1971, *10*, 179; P. Yesudian and A. S. Tambiah, *Archs Derm.*, 1974, *109*, 720; M. A. J. Crofts, *J. trop. Med. Hyg.*, 1976, *79*, 111.

Neoplasms. Amphotericin 0.7 to 1.3 mg per kg bodyweight was ineffective in the treatment of inoperable grade III or IV astrocytoma in 6 patients.— F. Colardyn and G. Verdonk (letter), *Lancet*, 1973, *2*, 974.

Amphotericin was added to the treatment regimens of 7 patients with tumours of various tissues. Four patients showed significant tumour regression on the addition of amphotericin 7.5 mg per m^2 body-surface area on day one, 15 mg per m^2 on day 2, and 30 mg per m^2 on days 3 and 4. The antineoplastic drugs were given on days 3 and 4 of this schedule and the programme repeated every 4 weeks. Fever and chills occurred in 6 patients and 2 had bronchospasm and hypotension whilst receiving amphotericin alone. One patient had probable drug-related sinus tachycardia.— C. A. Presant *et al.*, *Ann. intern. Med.*, 1977, *86*, 47.

Phycomycosis. Rhinopulmonary phycomycosis developed in an 8-year-old boy receiving maintenance chemotherapy for acute lymphoblastic leukaemia. Progressive improvement occurred following treatment with amphotericin; the total dose administered was 1.212 g over 7 weeks.— O. B. Eden and J. Santos, *Archs Dis. Childh.*, 1979, *54*, 557.

Further references: G. Medoff and G. S. Kobayashi, *New Engl. J. Med.*, 1972, *286*, 86; B. N. Bogard (letter), *ibid.*, 606; H. C. Pillsbury and N. D. Fischer, *Archs Otolar.*, 1977, *103*, 600; J. E. Ferstenfeld *et al.*, *Postgrad. med. J.*, 1977, *53*, 337; S. P. Hanley, *Postgrad. med. J.*, 1978, *54*, 338; M. B. Succar *et al.*, *Archs Otolar.*, 1979, *105*, 212; M. Henriquez *et al.*, *J. Am. med. Ass.*, 1979, *242*, 1397; B. R. Myers *et al.*, *Archs intern. Med.*, 1979, *139*, 557, per *Int. pharm. Abstr.*, 1979, *16*, 1165.

Preparations

Creams

Amphotericin B Cream *(U.S.P.)*. A cream containing amphotericin 3%.

Eye-drops

Amphotericin Eye-drops. Amphotericin 5 mg per ml in water or dextrose injection 5% with thiomersal 0.01%. The pH of the dextrose solution should be adjusted if necessary to 5.5. There might be some temporary discomfort. For *Candida* and *Fusarium solani* infections.—A. Baker, *J. Hosp. Pharm.*, 1972, *30*, 45.

Injections

Amphotericin B for Injection *(U.S.P.)*. A sterile complex of amphotericin 50 mg and sodium deoxycholate and one or more suitable buffers; the amount of amphotericin A present is not more than 5% of the total amphotericin content. pH of a 1% solution 7.2 to 8. Store at 2 to 8°. Protect from light.

Lotions

Amphotericin B Lotion *(U.S.P.)*. A lotion containing amphotericin 3%. pH 5 to 7.

Lozenges

Amphotericin Lozenges *(B.P.C. 1973)*. Lozenges containing amphotericin. They may contain suitable flavouring. Store in a cool place in airtight containers. Protect from light. *Dose.* 10 mg, four times daily.

Ointments

Amphotericin B Ointment *(U.S.P.)*. An ointment containing amphotericin 3% in a suitable basis.

Proprietary Preparations

Fungilin *(Squibb, UK)*. Amphotericin, available as **Cream** containing 3% in an aqueous cream basis; as **Ointment** containing 3% in Plastibase (a polyethylene and liqud paraffin basis); as **Pessaries** each containing 50 mg in a lactose basis; as **Lozenges** each containing 10 mg; as **Suspension** containing 100 mg in each ml; and as scored **Tablets** of 100 mg. **Fungilin in Orabase.** Contains amphotericin 2% in Orabase, an adhesive basis of gelatin, pectin, and carmellose sodium in Plastibase. For oral lesions. (Also available as Fungilin in *Austral.*, *Denm.*, *Ital.*).

Fungizone Intravenous *(Squibb, UK)*. Amphotericin, available as powder for solution before use, in 20-ml vials each containing 50 mg (50 000 units) together with approximately 41 mg of sodium deoxycholate and sodium phosphate buffer. (Also available as Fungizone in *Austral.*, *Belg.*, *Canad.*, *Fr.*, *Ital.*, *Neth.*, *Norw.*, *S.Afr.*, *Swed.*, *Switz.*, *USA*).

Other Proprietary Names

Amfostat Intravenoso *(Arg.)*; Ampho-Moronal *(Ger., Switz.)*; Funganiline, Fungizona *(Spain)*.

2563-t

Benzoyl Disulphide. Bensulfene. Dibenzoyl disulphide.

$C_{14}H_{10}O_2S_2$=274.4.

CAS — 644-32-6.

Crystals. M.P. 133°. Practically **insoluble** in water; slightly soluble in alcohol.

Benzoyl disulphide is an antifungal agent which has been applied as a 10% cream.

Proprietary Names

Thiocutol *(Rosa-Phytopharma, Fr.)*.

2564-x

Buclosamide. *N*-Butyl-4-chlorosalicylamide; *N*-Butyl-4-chloro-2-hydroxybenzamide.
$C_{11}H_{14}ClNO_2$=227.7.

CAS — 575-74-6.

A white crystalline powder. M.p. about 91°. Practically **insoluble** in water; soluble 1 in 3 of alcohol and ether.

Adverse Effects. Allergic skin reactions and photosensitivity have occurred.

Uses. Buclosamide is an antifungal agent which has been applied topically in concentrations of 10% in the treatment of dermatophytoses, candidal skin infections, and pityriasis versicolor.

Buclosamide was formerly marketed in Great Britain under the proprietary name Jadit (*Hoechst*).

2565-r

Calcium Propionate. Calcium propanoate.
$(C_3H_5O_2)_2Ca$=186.2 (or with $1H_2O$).

CAS — 4075-81-4 (anhydrous); 56744-45-7 (monohydrate).

A white powder with a faint odour of propionic acid. **Soluble** 1 in 4 of water; slightly soluble in alcohol.

Calcium propionate is used in the food industry as a mould inhibitor, see Propionic Acid, p.731.

2566-f

Candicidin *(B.P., U.S.P.).* A mixture of antifungal heptaenes produced by *Streptomyces griseus* and other *Streptomyces* spp.

CAS — 1403-17-4.

Pharmacopoeias. In *Br.* and *U.S.*

It occurs as a yellow to brown powder with a faint acrid odour. The *B.P.* specifies not less than 1850 units per mg and the *U.S.P.* specifies not less than 1000 µg per mg, both calculated on the dried substance. Sparingly to very slightly **soluble** in water; slowly soluble to very slightly soluble in alcohol; slightly to very slightly soluble in acetone and butyl alcohol. A 1% suspension has a pH of 8 to 10. **Protect** from light. The *U.S.P.* recommends storage at 2° to 8° in airtight containers.

Units. One unit of candicidin is contained in 0.0004766 mg of the first International Reference Preparation (1978) which contains 2098 units per mg.

Adverse Effects. Slight irritation has infrequently occurred following vaginal application of candicidin preparations.

Antimicrobial Action. Candicidin is a polyene antibiotic with antifungal actions similar to those of nystatin but is reported to possess greater activity against *Candida* spp.

Uses. Candicidin is poorly absorbed from the gastro-intestinal tract and is used mainly in the treatment of vaginal candidiasis. A vaginal tablet containing 3000 units either as 1.6 or 3 mg is used twice daily for 2 weeks; a vaginal ointment is used similarly.

A brief review of candicidin.— *Aust. J. Pharm.*, 1979, *60*, 402.

Candicidin 100 mg thrice daily was given for at least 5 months to 92 patients with benign prostatic hypertrophy and surgery was avoided in 64 for up to 18 months.— J. G. Keshin, *Int. Surg.*, 1973, *58*, 116, per *Pharm. J.*, 1974, *1*, 75.

Preparations

Candicidin Ointment *(U.S.P.).* An ointment containing candicidin 0.06%. Store at 2° to 8°.

Candicidin Vaginal Tablets *(U.S.P.).* Vaginal tablets containing candicidin 3 mg with suitable binders, diluents, and lubricants. Store at 2° to 8° in airtight containers.

Candeptin *(Pharmax, UK).* Candicidin, available as **Vaginal Ointment** containing 3000 units per 5 g and as **Vaginal Tablets** each containing 3000 units in a basis of starch, lactose, and magnesium stearate. (Also available as Candeptin in *Canad., S.Afr., Swed.*).

Other Proprietary Names

Vanobid *(USA).*

2567-d

Captan. *N*-Trichloromethylthio-3a,4,7,7a-tetrahydrophthalimide.
$C_9H_8Cl_3NO_2S$=300.6.

CAS — 133-06-2.

A white crystalline solid. Practically **insoluble** in water; slightly soluble in chlorinated hydrocarbon solvents. **Incompatible** with alkalis.

Adverse Effects. Allergic reactions have been reported.

Captan was mutagenic in bacteria.— M. J. Ashwood-Smith *et al.* (letter), *Nature* 1972, *240*, 419.

Using the Draize procedure, captan 1% in a cream basis produced sensitisation of the skin in 9 of 205 volunteers.— F. N. Marzulli and H. I. Maibach, *J. Soc. cosmet. Chem.*, 1973, *24*, 399.

For background toxicological data, see 1973 Evaluations of Some Pesticide Residues in Food, *Pestic. Residue Ser. Wld Hlth Org. No. 3*, 1974.

Maximum acceptable daily intake of captan in food: 100 µg per kg body-weight.— Report of the 1973 Joint FAO/WHO Meeting on Pesticide Residues in Food, *Tech. Rep. Ser. Wld Hlth Org. No. 545*, 1974.

Maximum permissible atmospheric concentration of captan: 5 mg per m^3.— Threshold Limit Values 1976, Guidance Note EH 15/76, London, Health and Safety Executive, 1976.

Uses. Captan has antifungal and antibacterial properties. It is used as an agricultural fungicide and has been tried as a bacteriostatic in soaps. It has also been used for the topical treatment of fungal infections of the skin.

References: M. A. Simeray, *Bull. Soc. fr. Derm. Syph.*, 1966, *73*, 337; *Soap chem. Spec.*, 1968, *44*, 240; I. R. Gucklhorn, *Mfg Chem.*, 1970, *41* (Jan), 42.

Proprietary Names

Vancide 89RE *(Vanderbilt, USA).*

2568-n

Chlordantoin. Clodantoin. 5-(1-Ethylpentyl)-3-(trichloromethylthio)hydantoin; 5-(1-Ethylpentyl)-3-(trichloromethylthio)imidazolidine-2,4-dione.
$C_{11}H_{17}Cl_3N_2O_2S$=347.7.

CAS — 5588-20-5.

Chlordantoin has antifungal properties and is used, mainly as a cream containing 1% with benzalkonium chloride, in the treatment of candidiasis of the vagina and vulva.

From patch tests carried out in 413 patients with contact dermatoses, 2 were found to be allergic to chlordantoin.— E. Epstein, *J. Am. med. Ass.*, 1966, *198*, 517.

Proprietary Names

Sporostacin *(Ethnor, Austral.; Ortho, Norw.; Cilag-Chemie, Switz.).*

A preparation containing chlordantoin was formerly marketed in Great Britain under the proprietary name Sporostacin Cream (*Ortho*).

2569-h

Chlormidazole Hydrochloride. Clomidazole Hydrochloride. 1-(4-Chlorobenzyl)-2-methylbenzimidazole hydrochloride.
$C_{15}H_{13}ClN_2,HCl$=293.2.

CAS — 3689-76-7 (chlormidazole); 54118-67-1 (hydrochloride).

Chlormidazole is an antifungal agent which has been used in the treatment of fungal infections of the skin.

Proprietary Names

Fungo-Polycid *(Medinsa, Spain).*

2570-a

Chlorphenesin *(B.P. 1973).* 3-(4-Chlorophenoxy)propane-1,2-diol.
$C_9H_{11}ClO_3$=202.6.

CAS — 104-29-0.

White or pale cream-coloured cyrstals or crystalline aggregates with a slightly phenolic odour and a persistent bitter taste. M.p. 78° to 81°.
Soluble 1 in 200 of water and 1 in 5 of alcohol; soluble in ether; slightly soluble in fixed oils.

Antimicrobial Action. Chlorphenesin is active against some pathogenic fungi, including *Epidermophyton floccosum* and *Trichophyton* spp. and also active against *Candida albicans* and *Trichomonas vaginalis* and against some bacteria.

Uses. Chlorphenesin has antibacterial and antifungal properties. It is used mainly in the prophylaxis and treatment of dermatophytoses of the feet and other sites. It is applied topically as an ointment containing 0.5% and as a dusting-powder containing 1%.
Chlorphenesin carbamate is used as a muscle relaxant.

Chlorphenesin powder 1% applied to the skin and sprinkled in the clothing and bedding, prevented the formation of ammonia and other odours in children suffering from bed wetting.— A. A. Bapty, *Br. med. J.*, 1977, *1*, 514.

Preparations

Chlorphenesin Cream *(B.P.C. 1973).* Chlorphenesin 500 mg, sodium lauryl sulphate 900 mg, white soft paraffin 15 g, cetostearyl alcohol 8.1 g, freshly boiled and cooled water 75.5 g. Add the sodium lauryl sulphate and chlorphenesin dissolved in the water at 50° to the melted oily phase at the same temperature and stir until cold. Store in a cool place in well-closed containers which prevent evaporation and contamination.

Chlorphenesin Dusting-powder *(B.P.C. 1973).* Chlorphenesin 1 g, starch 56 g, zinc oxide 25 g, purified talc, sterilised, 18 g.

Mycil *(Farley, UK).* Chlorphenesin, available as **Ointment** containing 0.5% and as **Powder** containing 1%. (Also available as Mycil in *Austral., Canad., S.Afr.*).

Other Proprietary Names

Kolpicortin-sine *(Switz.)*; Soorphenesin *(Ger.).*

Chlorphenesin was also formerly marketed in Great Britain under the proprietary name Aero-Mycil (*Duncan, Flockhart*).

2571-t

Ciclopirox. 6-Cyclohexyl-1-hydroxy-4-methyl-2-pyridone.
$C_{12}H_{17}NO_2$=207.3.

CAS — 29342-05-0.

2572-x

Ciclopirox Olamine. HOE 296. The 2-aminoethanol salt of ciclopirox.
$C_{14}H_{24}N_2O_3$=268.4.

CAS — 41621-49-2.

M.p. 143°. **Soluble** in water, alcohol, and ether.

Ciclopirox is an antifungal agent which has been used topically in patients with tinea infections and pityriasis versicolor. The olamine salt is also available.

Ciclopirox olamine exhibited a very wide antifungal action with the MIC for 41 dermatophyte and 31 candidal strains ranging between 0.98 and 3.9 µg per ml. It also had an antibacterial action.— W. Dittmar and G. Lohaus, *Arzneimittel-Forsch.*, 1973, *23*, 670. Further refernces: V. N. Sehgal, *Br. J. Derm.*, 1976, *95*, 83; K. Sakurai *et al.*, *Chemotherapy, Basle*, 1978, *24*, 68.

Proprietary Names

Batrafen *(Hoechst, Braz.; Hoechst, Jap.).*

2573-r

Clotrimazole. U.S.P.; Bay b 5097; FB b 5097; Chlortritylimidazol. 1-(α-2-Chlorotrityl)imidazole.
$C_{22}H_{17}ClN_2$=344.8.
CAS — 23593-75-1.

Pharmacopoeias. In *U.S.*

A white to pale yellow crystalline powder. M.p. about 142° with decomposition. Practically **insoluble** in water; freely soluble in alcohol, acetone, chloroform, and methyl alcohol; slightly soluble in ether. **Store** in airtight containers.

Adverse Effects. Gastro-intestinal disturbance and depression occur following ingestion. Neutropenia has been reported. Local reactions including irritation and burning may occur in patients treated topically; contact allergic dermatitis has been reported.

Gastro-intestinal disturbances, frequency of urination, and rashes had occurred in patients treated with clotrimazole.— H. Weuta, *Arzneimittel-Forsch.*, 1974, *24*, 540.

Side-effects reported after the systemic use of clotrimazole included nausea, vomiting, diarrhoea, gastro-intestinal bleeding, cystitis, dysuria, and elevation of hepatic enzymes. Depression, drowsiness, disorientation, and visual hallucinations had occurred, particularly in patients with aspergillosis, and could be a consequence of the lysis of the fungal cells.— P. R. Sawyer *et al.*, *Drugs*, 1975, *9*, 424.

Antimicrobial Action. Clotrimazole is an imidazole antifungal agent which may act on the cell membrane of the fungus. It is effective against a wide variety of fungi including *Epidermophyton, Microsporum*, and *Trichophyton* spp., *Coccidioides immitis, Histoplasma capsulatum, Aspergillus*, and *Candida* spp. These may be inhibited at concentrations of 1 µg per ml *in vitro*; however, up to 6 µg per ml may be required *in vivo*. Other less susceptible fungi include *Cryptococcus neoformans, Malassezia furfur (Pityrosporum orbiculare), Paracoccidioides brasiliensis, Sporothrix schenckii*, and *Allescheria, Madurella*, and *Phialophora* spp. Some strains of *Staphylococcus aureus* and *Streptococcus pyogenes* have been reported to be sensitive. *Trichomonas vaginalis* requires up to 100 µg per ml for inhibition. Clotrimazole is usually fungistatic but in concentrations exceeding 10 µg per ml it may be fungicidal. However, *Candida* spp. have been killed at concentrations of 2 µg per ml.

Detailed studies of the antimicrobial activity of clotrimazole.— M. Plempel and K. Bartmann, *Bayer, Drugs Germ.*, 1972, *15*, 103; R. J. Holt and R. L. Newman, *J. clin. Path.*, 1972, *25*, 1089. See also M. Plempel *et al.*, *Bayer, Postgrad. med. J.*, 1974, *50, Suppl.* 1, 11.

Clotrimazole had significant amoebicidal activity *in vitro* against *Naegleria fowleri*, the causative organism of primary amoebic meningo-encephalitis.— A. Jamieson and K. Anderson (letter), *Lancet*, 1974, *1*, 261.

The activity of clotrimazole against *Candida albicans* was enhanced *in vitro* by anionic surfactants that did not contain an ethylene oxide group and especially by docusate sodium. Surfactants containing this group diminished this activity irrespective of their anionic or nonionic nature.— K. Iwata and H. Yamaguchi, *Antimicrob. Ag. Chemother.*, 1977, *12*, 206.

Clotrimazole in weak inhibitory concentrations enhanced the activity of flucytosine and amphotericin *in vitro* against the yeasts *Candida albicans, C. tropicalis*, and *Torulopsis glabrata*.— W. H. Beggs *et al.*, *Antimicrob. Ag. Chemother.*, 1976, *9*, 863.

Diminished activity. Candidal membrane lipids reduced the activity of clotrimazole and miconazole.— H. Yamaguchi, *Antimicrob. Ag. Chemother.*, 1977, *12*, 16.

The activities of clotrimazole and miconazole *in vitro* against *Candida albicans* were inhibited by egg lecithin. It was considered that this was due to preferential interaction of the drugs with unsaturated phospholipids to form hydrophobic complexes.— H. Yamaguchi, *Antimicrob. Ag. Chemother.*, 1978, *13*, 423.

Enhanced activity. A study *in vitro* demonstrating the synergistic action of clotrimazole and sulphamethoxazole against *Candida albicans* and related species.— W. H. Beggs *et al.*, *Curr. ther. Res.*, 1976, *20*, 623.

Absorption and Fate. Clotrimazole is absorbed from the gastro-intestinal tract. It is metabolised in the liver to inactive compounds and excreted in the faeces and urine. When applied topically clotrimazole penetrates the epidermis but there is little if any systemic absorption. Slight absorption has been reported following the administration of vaginal tablets.

Clotrimazole was given by mouth in a dose of 1.5 g to 7 healthy subjects and 47 patients and peak blood concentrations of up to 1 µg per ml were detected microbiologically at 2 or 4 hours. The half-life was between 3.5 and 5.5 hours. Neither liver nor renal impairment appeared to affect absorption but lower concentrations were detected in 9 patients after gastrectomy. No more than 0.02% of activity was excreted in the urine in 12 hours.— H. P. Menz *et al.*, *Dt. med. Wschr.*, 1973, *98*, 1606.

Following a dose of 1.5 g clotrimazole (^{14}C) given by mouth to 10 subjects, peak serum concentrations of 15 µg per ml of clotrimazole and metabolites were achieved within 3 hours. The major metabolites in the serum were identified as 1-*o*-chlorophenyl-1,1-diphenylmethane and 1-*o*-chlorophenyl-1-*p*-hydroxyphenyl-1-phenylmethane. About 10% of a single dose was excreted in the urine within 24 hours and 25% within 6 days. Two of the subjects were given repeated doses and serum concentrations were found to be cumulative. Measurement of urine concentrations suggested that by 12 days a steady state was reached. There was no systemic absorption following topical administration of a 1% solution or cream. Following the administration of vaginal tablets of 100 mg a serum concentration equivalent to 0.03 µg per ml was detected in 2 patients.— B. Duhm *et al.*, *Bayer, Postgrad. med. J.*, 1974, *50, Suppl.* 1, 13. See also *idem*, *Arzneimittel-Forsch.*, 1972, *22*, 1276; *Drugs Germ.*, 1972, *15*, 99.

Clotrimazole was absorbed from the gastro-intestinal tract and had a biological half-life of about 4 hours. Liver and kidney dysfunction had little influence on serum concentrations or half-life. In long-term therapy doses might have to be increased because of increased metabolism resulting from enzyme induction.— H. Weuta, *Arzneimittel-Forsch.*, 1974, *24*, 540.

Clotrimazole was about 98% bound to serum proteins.— H. Rosenkranz and J. Putter, *Eur. J. Drug Metab. Pharmacokinet.*, 1976, *1*, 73.

Uses. Clotrimazole is applied topically as a 1% cream or solution in the treatment of candidiasis, tinea, and pityriasis versicolor; a 1% powder may be used in conjunction with the cream or solution and has been applied to prevent re-infection. It is given as vaginal tablets of 100 or 200 mg or as a 2% vaginal cream in candidal and trichomonal vaginitis. Clotrimazole has also been administered by mouth.

The proceedings of a symposium on the actions and uses of clotrimazole.— *Postgrad. med. J.*, 1974, *50, Suppl.* 1, 1-108.

A review of the antifungal activity and therapeutic efficacy of clotrimazole.— P. R. Sawyer *et al.*, *Drugs*, 1975, *9*, 424. See also *Med. Lett.*, 1975, *17*, 77; R. J. Holt, *J. cutaneous Pathol.*, 1976, *3*, 45; *Med. Lett.*, 1976, *18*, 101; J. K. Murdoch, *Can. pharm. J.*, 1978, *111*, 255; *Med. Lett.*, 1979, *21*, 39.

In a double-blind study clotrimazole cream 1% was as effective as Whitfield's ointment in the treatment of ringworm, pityriasis versicolor, and erythrasma infections and as effective as nystatin ointment in the treatment of candidal infections.— Y. M. Clayton and B. L. Connor, *Br. J. Derm.*, 1973, *89*, 297.

A clinical evaluation of clotrimazole.— P. H. Spiekermann and M. D. Young, *Archs Derm.*, 1976, *112*, 350.

A report of clotrimazole being of benefit in 10 of 12 patients with active rheumatoid arthritis.— R. Wyburn-Mason (letter), *Lancet*, 1976, *1*, 489. Clotrimazole could not be recommended for rheumatoid arthritis, because of the lack of effect and severe side-effects.— K. Lund-Olesen, *Curr. ther. Res.*, 1977, *21*, 704. See also J. A. Wojtulewski *et al.*, *Ann. rheum. Dis.*, 1980, *39*, 469.

Further references.— *Br. med. J.*, 1978, *2*, 1735.

Candidiasis. In a double-blind comparison involving 43 patients clotrimazole 1% cream was found to be as effective as tolnaftate 1% cream in the treatment of dermatophyte infections. In a further comparison involving 25 patients clotrimazole 1% cream was found to be as effective as nystatin cream 100 000 units per g in the treatment of superficial candidal infections. In the second group 1 patient using clotrimazole and 1 using nystatin complained of severe irritation and discontinued treatment after 2 weeks.— K. Keczkes *et al.*, *Practitioner*, 1975, *214*, 412.

Further references.— N. Zaias; F. Battistini, *Archs Derm.*, 1977, *113*, 307; M. A. Waugh *et al.*, *Br. J. vener. Dis.*, 1978, *54*, 184.

Candidiasis, cutaneous. Chronic mucocutaneous candidiasis in a 11-year-old girl was eventually controlled successfully by the continuous administration of clotrimazole 120 mg per kg body-weight daily by mouth.— S. Leikin *et al.*, *J. Paediat.*, 1976, *88*, 864.

Clotrimazole 60 mg per kg body-weight daily by mouth cleared the lesions of mucocutaneous candidiasis in a woman who had had the condition for 20 years. Topical treatment had not been effective but there had been transient responses to amphotericin. By subsequently taking clotrimazole 2.5 g every 18 days the patient was able to control the candidiasis without stimulating hepatic enzyme induction; gastro-intestinal discomfort was reduced.— R. H. Meade (letter), *Ann. intern. Med.*, 1977, *86*, 314. See also M. M. Ipp *et al.*, *Am. J. Dis. Child.*, 1977, *131*, 305.

Candidiasis, oral. Clotrimazole had a beneficial effect on chronic oral candidiasis when compared with placebo in a double-blind study. Twenty patients, in whom previous treatment with nystatin or crystal violet had been unsuccessful, were given clotrimazole 10 mg troches or placebos which were dissolved in the mouth 5 times daily for 2 weeks. On assessemnt 2 to 7 days after completion of therapy, candida were absent in 9 of 10 patients given clotrimazole compared with only 1 of 10 who received placebo. The treatment was well tolerated. Uncontrolled follow-up studies in 15 of the patients indicated that 1 to 3 clotrimazole troches daily prevented relapse. When treatment was stopped, infection recurred within 2 to 4 weeks.— C. H. Kirkpatrick and D. W. Alling, *New Engl. J. Med.*, 1978, *299*, 1201.

Clotrimazole was administered to a 6-month-old infant with refractory oral candidiasis by crushing a 10-mg troche into 3 ml of a liquid containing methylcellulose (Cologel, *Lilly, USA*) and brushing the mixture on to the oral mucosa or his thumb, which he promptly sucked.— J. M. Montello *et al.* (letter), *New Engl. J. Med.*, 1979, *301*, 1005.

Further references: B. -S. Yap and G. P. Bodey, *Archs intern. Med.*, 1979, *139*, 656.

Candidiasis, vaginal. An evaluation of clotrimazole, administered vaginally, for candidiasis.— *Med. Lett.*, 1976, *18*, 66.

Treatment with clotrimazole as a 100-mg vaginal tablet once daily for 6 days, together with clotrimazole cream applied externally by both patient and partner, was given to 136 patients who developed vaginal candidiasis during pregnancy. The treatment was successful in 84% of women treated during the first trimester, and in 87% and 78% of those treated in the second and third trimester, respectively. Six infected women aborted during pregnancy. Treatment did not appear to have been harmful to the foetus.— W. Frerich and A. Gad, *Curr. med. Res. Opinion*, 1977, *4*, 640.

A report of the successful treatment of candidal vulvovaginitis with a course of two clotrimazole 100-mg pessaries nightly for 3 consecutive nights.— G. Masterton *et al.*, *Br. J. vener. Dis.*, 1977, *53*, 126. See also W. H. Robertson, *J. Am. med. Ass.*, 1980, *244*, 2549.

In a randomised study of 117 patients with vulvovaginal candidiasis, the use of clotrimazole pessaries for 7 days was as effective as their use for 14 days or the application of miconazole nitrate 2% vaginal cream for 14 days.— R. Franklin, *Sth. med. J.*, 1978, *71*, 141. See also W. H. Robertson, *Am. J. Obstet. Gynec.*, 1978, *132*, 321, per *Int. pharm. Abstr.*, 1980, *17*, 737.

Eye infections. Instillation every 4 hours of eye-drops containing clotrimazole 1% in sterilised arachis oil was well tolerated and produced a good response in the treatment of eye infections due to *Aspergillus fumigatus* and *Candida* spp.— A. Baker, *J. Hosp. Pharm.*, 1972, *30*, 45.

Preparations

Clotrimazole Cream *(U.S.P.)*. A cream containing clotrimazole. Store at 2° to 30° in airtight containers.

Clotrimazole Topical Solution *(U.S.P.)*. A solution of clotrimazole in a suitable non-aqueous hydrophilic solvent. Store at 2° to 30° in airtight containers.

Clotrimazole Vaginal Tablets (U.S.P.). Vaginal tablets containing clotrimazole.

Proprietary Preparations

Canesten *(Bayer, UK)*. Clotrimazole, available as **Atomiser Spray** containing 1% in isopropyl alcohol 30%; as **Cream** containing 1%; as **Powder** containing 1%; as **Solution** containing 1% in macrogol 400; as **Vaginal**

Cream containing 2%; and as **Vaginal Tablets** each containing 100 or 200 mg. **Canesten Duopak.** A composite pack of 6 vaginal tablets and cream. (Also available as Canesten in *Austral., Canad., Denm., Ger., Ital., Neth., Norw., S.Afr., Spain, Swed., Switz.*).

Other Proprietary Names
Canastene *(Belg.)*; Empecid *(Arg., Jap.)*; Eparol *(Ger.)*; Gyne-Lotrimin, Lotrimin, Mycelex, Mycelex-G *(all USA)*; Panmicol *(Arg.)*; Trimysten *(Fr.)*.

2574-f

Coparaffinate
CAS — 8001-60-3.

A mixture of water-insoluble isoparaffinic acids, partly neutralised with iso-octyl hydroxybenzyldialkylamines. A viscous, dark brown, oily liquid with a characteristic odour of burnt petroleum. **Miscible** with alcohol and fixed and volatile oils; immiscible with water.

Coparaffinate was formerly used in the form of an ointment (17% with titanium dioxide 4%) for pruritus ani and vulvae and in the treatment of fungal infections of the hands and feet.

2575-d

Diamthazole Hydrochloride. Diamthazole Dihydrochloride; Amycazol Hydrochloride; Amycazolum; Dimazole Hydrochloride; Ro 2-2453. 6-(2-Diethylaminoethoxy)-2-dimethylaminobenzothiazole dihydrochloride.
$C_{15}H_{23}N_3OS,2HCl$=366.3.

CAS — 95-27-2 (diamthazole); 136-96-9 (hydrochloride).

Pharmacopoeias. In *Rus.*

A white hygroscopic crystalline powder. **Soluble** in water, in alcohol, and methyl alcohol; very slightly soluble in chloroform and ether. A 5% solution in water has a pH of about 2.

Adverse Effects. Diamthazole may produce local irritation and sensitisation. Ataxia, tremors, convulsions, and hallucinations have been reported in infants but this may possibly have been due to sucking the fingers or contaminated clothing rather than to percutaneous absorption.

Diamthazole has been found to be a photosensitiser.— J. N. Burry, *Med. J. Aust.*, 1969, *1*, 1226.

Precautions. The use of diamthazole is contra-indicated in children under 6 years. Its use is not recommended during the acute or pyodermic phase of any fungal infection and it should not be applied to mucous membranes.

Uses. Diamthazole has antifungal properties and has been used in a concentration of 5% in the treatment of tinea infections. It has been reported to be effective in cattle ringworm.

Proprietary Names
Asterol *(Roche, Austral.; Roche, Ital.; Roche, Switz.)*; Atelor *(Roche, Arg.)*.

Diamthazole hydrochloride was formerly marketed in Great Britain under the proprietary name Asterol *(Roche)*..

2576-n

Dichlorofluorothiocarbanilide. 3,5-Dichloro-4′-fluorothiocarbanilide.
$C_{13}H_9Cl_2FN_2S$=315.2.

Crystals. M.p. 148°. **Soluble** in ethyl oleate and isopropyl myristate.

Dichlorofluorothiocarbanilide is an antibacterial and antifungal agent which has been used as a 1% ointment, powder, or solution in the treatment of various forms of tinea and pyoderma.

Proprietary Names
Fluonilid *(Pierre Bardin, Arg.; Ascot, Austral.; Continental Pharma, Belg.)*.

2577-h

Doconazole. R 34000. 1-{[4-(Biphenyl-4-yloxymethyl)-2-(2,4-dichlorophenyl)-1,3-dioxolan-2-yl]-methyl}imidazole.
$C_{26}H_{22}Cl_2N_2O_3$=481.4.

CAS — 59831-63-9.

Crystals. M.p. about 156°.

Doconazole is an imidazole antifungal agent.

References: H. B. Levine, *Chest*, 1976, *70*, 755; D. M. Dixon *et al.*, *Chemotherapy, Basle*, 1978, *24*, 364.

Manufacturers
Janssen, Belg.

2578-m

Econazole. SQ 13050. 1-[2,4-Dichloro-β-(4-chlorobenzyloxy)phenethyl]imidazole.
$C_{18}H_{15}Cl_3N_2O$=381.7.

CAS — 27220-47-9.

2579-b

Econazole Nitrate. C-C2470; R 14827; SQ 13050.
$C_{18}H_{15}Cl_3N_2O,HNO_3$=444.7.

CAS — 24169-02-6; 68797-31-9.

A white crystalline powder. Very slightly **soluble** in water; slightly soluble in most organic solvents.

Adverse Effects. Local reactions including burning and irritation may occur when econazole nitrate is applied topically.

Slight burning sensation of the skin occurred in 15 of 92 patients treated with econazole nitrate 1% cream, leading to discontinuation of treatment in 4.— H. Gisslen *et al.*, *Curr. ther. Res.*, 1977, *21*, 681.

Four of 6 subjects taking econazole as a single dose of 2 g by mouth experienced adverse effects including nausea and vomiting (2), mild transitory auditory and visual hallucinations (3), cephalalgia (1), and dizziness (1). However, when the 2 g daily dose was administered in 4 divided doses of 500 mg every 6 hours tolerance was good.— E. Drouhet and B. Dupont, *Mykosen*, 1978, *Suppl.* 1, 192.

Antimicrobial Action. Econazole is an imidazole antifungal agent closely related to miconazole (see p.726) and with similar antifungal and antibacterial activity.

A comparison *in vitro* of the antimicrobial activity of econazole and miconazole. Econazole was more active against filamentous fungi such as *Aspergillus* and *Rhizopus* spp.— G. Schär *et al.*, *Chemotherapy, Basle*, 1976, *22*, 211.

Further references.— D. Thienpont *et al.*, *Arzneimittel-Forsch.*, 1975, *25*, 224; M. Dorn *et al.*, *Münch. med. Wschr.*, 1975, *117*, 687.

Absorption and Fate. Absorption is not significant when econazole nitrate is applied to the skin or vagina. A mean peak plasma concentration of about 3 μg per ml has been reported 2½ hours after a dose of 250 mg of econazole by mouth.

The cutaneous absorption of econazole.— H. Schaefer and G. Stüttgen, *Arzneimittel-Forsch.*, 1976, *26*, 432.

Serum concentrations of econazole after oral and intravenous administration.— E. Drouhet and B. Dupont, *Mykosen*, 1978, *Suppl.* 1, 192.

The vaginal absorption of econazole.— W. Rindt *et al.*, *Arzneimittel-Forsch.*, 1979, *29*, 697.

Further references.— M. Plempel, *Postgrad. med. J.*, 1979, *55*, 662.

Uses. Econazole nitrate is applied topically in a concentration of 1% in the treatment of fungal infections such as candidiasis, pityriasis versicolor, and tinea. Pessaries containing 150 mg of econazole nitrate are used in vaginal candidiasis. Econazole, as the base, has been given by mouth and by intravenous injection.

A detailed review of the actions and uses of econazole nitrate.— R. C. Heel *et al.*, *Drugs*, 1978, *16*, 177. See also R. J. Holt, *J. cutaneous Pathol.*, 1976, *3*, 45.

The antifungal action of econazole.— *Mykosen*, 1978, *Suppl.* 1, 298-345.

Econazole cream 1% was more effective and produced more rapid healing than clotrimazole cream 1% in a double-blind study in 134 patients with various forms of tinea and candidiasis.— T. Fredriksson, *Curr. ther. Res.*, 1979, *25*, 590.

The treatment of trichonocardiosis palmellina with econazole nitrate spray.— H. Krause, *Arzneimittel-Forsch.*, 1978, *28*, 1804.

Further references.— K. J. Schwarz, *Dt. med. Wschr.*, 1975, *100*, 1497; R. Aron-Brunetière *et al.*, *Acta derm.-vener., Stockh.*, 1977, *57*, 77; B. S. Verma, *Curr. ther. Res.*, 1978, *24*, 745; C. A. Quiñones, *Cutis*, 1980, *25*, 386.

Aspergillosis. A 52-year-old woman with pulmonary aspergillosis was successfully treated with econazole. A total of 5.9 g was infused intravenously over 10 days in doses ranging from 200 mg twice daily to 300 mg thrice daily.— D. Hantschke *et al.*, *Mykosen*, 1978, *Suppl.* 1, 230.

Candidiasis, vaginal. In two studies involving 880 patients with vaginal candidiasis there was an overall cure-rate of 93.4% when econazole pessaries of 150 mg were inserted once daily for 3 days; 81 patients were only cured after a second course of treatment. In a few instances, partners were treated with a 1% econazole cream.— J. A. Balmer, *Am. J. Obstet. Gynec.*, 1976, *126*, 436.

Of 59 patients with vaginal candidiasis who received one econazole 150-mg pessary daily for 3 to 5 days, 71% and 90% respectively of those with positive and negative rectal cultures initially responded to treatment. Of 25 similar patients who received one nystatin 100 000-unit pessary daily for 15 days, 64% and 86% respectively responded to treatment.— R. Lambotte *et al.*, *Mykosen*, 1978, *Suppl.* 1, 311.

Further references.— W. Obolensky and F. Maire, *Dt. med. Wschr.*, 1975, *100*, 1730; B. Dogniez *et al.*, *Acta ther.*, 1978, *4*, 119; P. E. R. Rhemrev *et al.*, *J. int. med. Res.*, 1979, *7*, 463; B. S. Verma, *Curr. ther. Res.*, 1979, *26*, 634; B. Fredricsson *et al.*, *ibid.*, 1980, *27*, 309; B. Larsson and A. Kjaeldgaard, *ibid.*, 664; D. Brown *et al.*, *Obstet. Gynec.*, 1980, *56*, 121.

Proprietary Preparations

Ecostatin *(FAIR Laboratories, UK)*. Econazole nitrate, available as **Cream** containing 1%; as **Lotion** containing 1%; as **Pessaries** each containing 150 mg; as **Powder** and **Spray Powder** each containing 1% in a talc basis; and as alcoholic **Spray Solution** containing 1% (Inflammable: keep away from an open flame). **Ecostatin Twin Pack.** A composite pack of 3 pessaries and cream. (Also available as Ecostatin in *Austral., Canad., NZ, S.Afr.*).

Gyno-Pevaryl *(Ortho-Cilag, UK)*. Econazole nitrate, available as pessaries each containing 150 mg. **Gyno-Pevaryl Combipack.** A composite pack of 3 pessaries and cream containing econazole nitrate 1%. (Also available as Gyno-Pevaryl in *Belg., Fr., Ger., Neth., NZ, Norw., S.Afr., Switz.*).

Pevaryl *(Ortho-Cilag, UK)*. Econazole nitrate, available as **Cream**, as **Lotion**, and as **Spray Powder**, each containing 1%. (Also available as Pevaryl in *Austral., Belg., Denm., Fr., Ital., Neth., NZ, Norw., S.Afr., Switz.*).

Other Proprietary Names
Epi-Pevaryl *(Ger.)*; Mycopevaryl *(Swed.)*; Skilar *(Ital.)*.

2580-x

Fenticlor. D 25; HL 1050; Ph 549. 4,4′-Dichloro-2,2′-thiodiphenol.
$C_{12}H_8Cl_2O_2S$=287.2.

CAS — 97-24-5.

A white odourless crystalline powder. M.p. 176°. Practically **insoluble** in water; freely soluble in alcohol. Alcoholic solutions are reported to discolour on exposure to light.

Adverse Effects. Photosensitivity reactions have occurred in patients treated with fenticlor; contact dermatitis has been reported.

References.— J. N. Burry, *Archs Derm.*, 1968, *97*, 497; *idem* (letter), *Br. med. J.*, 1974, *2*, 556.

Antimicrobial Action. Fenticlor is reported to inhibit *Microsporum, Trichophyton* spp., *Candida albicans*, and some bacteria.

Enhanced activity. Phenethyl alcohol enhanced the effect of fenticlor against *Escherichia coli, Staphylococcus aureus*, and *Proteus vulgaris*; the combination also showed antibacterial activity against *Pseudomonas aeruginosa* which fenticlor alone did not possess. Moreover, phenethyl alcohol was a good solvent for fenticlor.— R. M. E. Richards and M. P. Hardie, *J. Pharm. Pharmac.*, 1972, *24, Suppl.*, 90P.

Uses. Fenticlor has been applied topically in concentrations of up to 2% in the treatment of dermatophytic and candidal infections of the skin and mucous membranes.

A review of antimicrobial agents, including fenticlor, used in cosmetics.— I. R. Gucklhorn, *Mfg Chem.*, 1970, *41* (Jan.), 42.

Proprietary Preparations

ADT Spray *(Armour, UK).* An aerosol spray delivering fenticlor 2% in sterilised talc.

Other Proprietary Names

Antimyk *(Ger.).*

2581-r

Fezatione. Fezathione. 3-(4-Methylbenzylideneamino)-4-phenyl-4-thiazoline-2-thione.
$C_{17}H_{14}N_2S_2$=310.4.

CAS — 15387-18-5.

Light yellow crystals or crystalline powder, odourless or with a faint characteristic odour. Practically **insoluble** in water; sparingly soluble in alcohol; freely soluble in chloroform, soluble in acetone. **Store** in airtight containers. Protect from light.

Fezatione is an antifungal agent effective against *Epidermophyton, Microsporum,* and *Trichophyton* spp. It has been used as a solution or ointment containing 2%. Hypersensitivity reactions have been reported.

Proprietary Names

Polyodin *(Takeda, Jap.).*

2582-f

Flucytosine *(B.P., U.S.P.).* 5-FC; Ro 2-9915.

5-Fluorocytosine; 4-Amino-5-fluoropyrimidin-2(1*H*)-one.
$C_4H_4FN_3O$=129.1.

CAS — 2022-85-7.

Pharmacopoeias. In *Br.* and *U.S.*

A white to off-white crystalline powder, odourless or with a slight odour. M.p. 295°. **Soluble** 1 in 67 of water; slightly soluble in alcohol; practically insoluble in chloroform and ether. **Store** in airtight containers. Protect from light.

A solution of flucytosine for intravenous infusion should be stored between 15° and 20°. Precipitation may occur at lower temperatures and decomposition, with the formation of fluorouracil, at higher temperatures.

Adverse Effects. Side-effects of flucytosine include nausea, vomiting, diarrhoea, and skin rashes. Less frequently observed side-effects include confusion, hallucinations, headache, sedation, vertigo, and eosinophilia. Alterations in liver function occur in about 10% of patients and appear to be dose-related and reversible.

Bone-marrow depression, especially leucopenia and thrombocytopenia, is associated with blood concentrations of flucytosine greater than 100 µg per ml. Fatal agranulocytosis and aplastic anaemia have been reported.

Side-effects reported in 17 patients treated with up to 280 mg of flucytosine per kg body-weight included possible nausea and vomiting in 2, possible peripheral neuropathy in 1, and hepatotoxicity in 2. The side-effects were considered less severe than with amphotericin.— P. I. Steer *et al., Ann. intern. Med.*, 1972, *76*, 15.

A fatal colitis-like condition with multiple intestinal perforations and peritonitis occurred in a patient given flucytosine.— E. J. Harder and P. E. Hermans, *Archs intern. Med.*, 1975, *135*, 231. See also D. M. Robertson *et al., Archs Ophthal., N.Y.*, 1974, *91*, 33.

A 60-year-old man developed crystalluria while receiving flucytosine 20 g per day (200 mg per kg body-weight). Reduction of the dosage to 10 g per day resulted in a marked decrease in the excretion of urinary gravel which was shown to be a co-precipitate of flucytosine and uric acid.— K. M. Williams *et al., Med. J. Aust.*, 1979, *2*, 617.

Effect on blood. Leucopenia occurred in 4 of 15 patients receiving flucytosine. All 4 had peak serum-flucytosine concentrations of 125 µg or more per ml and 3 had renal impairment, of whom 1 (with a peak concentration of 500 µg per ml) developed marrow aplasia and died of pseudomonal sepsis. The bone-marrow depression was considered to be dose-related.— C. A. Kauffman and P. T. Frame, *Antimicrob. Ag. Chemother.*, 1977, *11*, 244.

Further references.— R. J. Schlegel *et al., Pediatrics*, 1970, *45*, 926; W. C. Weese and R. W. Schope (letter), *Ann. intern. Med.*, 1972, *77*, 1003; R. Meyer and J. L. Axelrod, *J. Am. med. Ass.*, 1974, *228*, 1573; C. S. Bryan and J. A. McFarland, *J. Am. med. Ass.*, 1978, *239*, 1068.

Treatment of Adverse Effects. Flucytosine may be removed from the body by haemodialysis or peritoneal dialysis.

Precautions. Flucytosine should be administered with care to patients with renal or hepatic impairment or blood disorders. Blood concentrations should be checked regularly especially in patients with renal dysfunction and those also receiving amphotericin or other nephrotoxic drugs; concentrations should generally not exceed 100 µg per ml. Care should be taken in patients receiving other drugs which depress bone marrow. Tests for liver function and blood counts should be carried out routinely in all patients. It should be administered with great care to pregnant patients, especially since flucytosine may be metabolised partly to fluorouracil.

The topical use of flucytosine should be discouraged because of the risk of the development of resistant strains of fungi.

Interactions. Flucytosine has been reported to be competitively inhibited by cytarabine.— R. Y. Cartwright, *Br. med. J.*, 1978, *2*, 108.

For the possible effect of flucytosine in enhancing the activity of gentamicin in renal transplant patients, see Gentamicin Sulphate, p.1171.

See also under Antimicrobial Action, below.

Antimicrobial Action. Flucytosine is an antifungal agent which inhibits *Cryptococcus neoformans* and *Candida* spp. at concentrations of 0.5 to 8 µg per ml. Other sensitive fungi include *Phialophora pedrosoi, Ph. verrucosa, Cladosporium carrionii,* and *Torulopsis glabrata,* but its spectrum of activity is less than that of amphotericin (see p.717).

Resistance has occurred among strains of *Candida* spp. and *Cryptococcus neoformans* during treatment and up to 50% of isolates of *Candida* spp. have been found to be resistant before treatment with flucytosine. Cryptococci are considered to be resistant if the MIC exceeds 12.5 µg per ml and *Candida* spp. if the MIC exceeds 100 µg per ml.

A report of the antifungal activity of flucytosine against *Candida* spp., *Cryptococcus neoformans, Aspergillus* spp., and *Torulopsis glabrata.*— P. I. Steer *et al., Ann. intern. Med.*, 1972, *76*, 15.

Flucytosine was effective against *Acanthamoeba* both *in vitro* and *in vivo* but the amoeba appeared capable of developing resistance.— A. R. Stevens and W. D. O'Dell, *Antimicrob. Ag. Chemother.*, 1974, *6*, 282. Flucytosine was inactive *in vitro* against *Acanthamoeba* spp.— R. J. Duma and R. Finley, *ibid.*, 1976, *10*, 370.

Flucytosine had weak activity *in vitro* against *Prototheca filamenta* and no effect against other species of *Prototheca* tested.— E. Segal *et al., Antimicrob. Ag. Chemother.*, 1976, *10*, 75.

While amphotericin inhibited all of 7 strains of *Aspergillus fumigatus* and all of 6 strains of *A. niger in vitro* at concentrations of up to 2 µg per ml, flucytosine was generally more active against *A. niger* but inhibited only 3 of 7 strains of *A. fumigatus.* Amphotericin and flucytosine had no effect on the activity of each other when used together.— B. A. Lauer *et al., J. antimicrob. Chemother.*, 1978, *4*, 375.

Good correlation between microdilution and broth dilution techniques were obtained for the susceptibility of 50 clinical isolates of yeast to flucytosine and amphotericin but the microdilution technique was considered to be unsuitable for use with *Cryptococcus neoformans.*— M. F. Mazens *et al., Antimicrob. Ag. Chemother.*, 1979, *15*, 475.

Diminished activity. Some purines and pyrimidines inhibited the action of flucytosine against *Aspergillus* spp.— G. E. Wagner and S. Shadomy, *Antimicrob. Ag. Chemother.*, 1977, *11*, 229.

Enhanced activity. Enhanced antifungal activity against *Candida* spp. and *Cryptococcus neoformans* was reported with the combination of amphotericin and flucytosine.— J. W. Smith, *Ann. intern. Med.*, 1973, *78*, 450. Enhanced activity *in vitro* with amphotericin and flucytosine against *Aspergillus.*— M. Kitahara *et al., Antimicrob. Ag. Chemother.*, 1976, *9*, 915.

Clotrimazole in weak inhibitory concentrations enhanced the activity of flucytosine and amphotericin *in vitro* against the yeasts, *Candida albicans, C. tropicalis,* and *Torulopsis glabrata.*— W. H. Beggs *et al., Antimicrob. Ag. Chemother.*, 1976, *9*, 863.

Mode of action. Flucytosine was deaminated intracellularly by susceptible fungi to fluorouracil which was then incorporated into ribonucleic acid.— W. L. Morison *et al., Br. J. Derm.*, 1974, *90*, 445.

Resistance. Reports of resistant strains of *Candida* and cryptococci occurring during treatment with flucytosine.— R. Y. Cartwright *et al.* (letter), *Br. med. J.*, 1972, *2*, 351; R. L. Logan and M. J. Goldberg (letter), *Br. med. J.*, 1972, *3*, 531; R. J. Holt (letter), *Br. med. J.*, 1974, *3*, 523.

Candidal resistance to flucytosine appeared to depend on the presence of a proteinic substance in the cell wall.— S. Montplaisir *et al., Antimicrob. Ag. Chemother.*, 1976, *9*, 1028.

A report of cryptococci resistant to flucytosine in 2 patients. No resistant mutants were isolated from one of the patients when amphotericin was added to the treatment.— D. C. E. Speller *et al., J. clin. Path.*, 1977, *30*, 254.

Absorption and Fate. Flucytosine is absorbed from the gastro-intestinal tract. After doses of 2 g, peak plasma concentrations of 30 to 40 µg per ml have been achieved within 2 to 4 hours; similar concentrations have been achieved but more rapidly, after an intravenous dose. About 90% of a dose is excreted by glomerular filtration and has been recovered unchanged from the urine. It is distributed widely through the body tissues and fluids and diffuses into the CSF. In some species flucytosine is metabolised to fluorouracil; this may also occur in man. Flucytosine may be removed by haemodialysis.

The pharmacokinetics of flucytosine.— J. R. Horn and D. L. Giusti, *Drug Intell. & clin. Pharm.*, 1975, *9*, 180.

The clearance of flucytosine, which was given in a dose of 2 g, was equivalent to that of creatinine in 4 patients undergoing haemodialysis. Only about 3 to 4% of flucytosine was bound to proteins.— E. R. Block *et al., Ann. intern. Med.*, 1974, *80*, 613.

Flucytosine 2 g was given by mouth to 10 healthy subjects and to 40 patients in various stages of renal impairment. The average half-life in the healthy subjects was about 3 hours but this was significantly prolonged with renal dysfunction and reached 85 hours in the 5 patients with no renal function. There was a direct correlation between elimination and creatinine clearance and based on this a dosage schedule was proposed for patients with kidney impairment.— J. Schönebeck *et al., Chemotherapy, Basle*, 1973, *18*, 321.

In 5 patients with normal renal function given 2 g of flucytosine mean peak plasma concentrations of 30 µg per ml were reached in 2 hours; concentrations then gradually fell; 30 to 50% of the dose was recovered in the urine in 8 hours and 63 to 84% in 24 hours. The mean half-life was 5.3 hours. In 5 patients with terminal renal failure, mean peak concentrations of 48 µg per ml were reached at about 6 hours; after 24 hours mean concentrations were 31 µg per ml. The half-life in 10 patients with varying degrees of renal impairment varied from 11.3 to more than 100 hours. Renal clearance of flucytosine was about 75% of creatinine clearance, and about 71% in 4 patients undergoing haemodialysis.— J. K. Dawborn *et al., Br. med. J.*, 1973, *4*, 382.

Further references: R. E. Cutler *et al., Clin. Pharmac. Ther.*, 1978, *24*, 333.

Diffusion. *Into CSF.* Concentrations of flucytosine in the CSF in 5 patients with cryptococcal meningitis were about 75% of those in the serum.— E. R. Block and J. E. Bennett, *Antimicrob. Ag. Chemother.*, 1972, *1*, 476.

Metabolism. Flucytosine did not undergo any detectable metabolism when intravenous doses were given to 8 healthy subjects.— D. N. Wade and G. Sudlow, *Aust. N.Z. J. Med.*, 1972, *2*, 153. See also A. Polak *et al., Chemotherapy, Basle*, 1976, *22*, 137.

Studies in patients with cryptococcal meningitis and healthy subjects indicated that metabolism of flucytosine to fluorouracil occurred in humans. It was considered that fluorouracil might account for some of the toxicity associated with flucytosine.— R. B. Diasio *et al.*, *Antimicrob. Ag. Chemother.*, 1978, *14*, 903.

Uses. Flucytosine is used in the treatment of severe systemic and urinary-tract infections due to susceptible fungi including *Candida* and *Cryptococcus* spp. To reduce the emergence of resistant strains flucytosine may be used with amphotericin (see p.717), especially in the treatment of cryptococcal meningitis. Flucytosine is given by mouth, by the intravenous infusion of a 1% solution over about 20 to 40 minutes, or by intraperitoneal infusion of a 1% solution. A 10% ointment has been used, but see Precautions.

The usual dose by mouth for adults and children is 150 mg per kg body-weight daily in four divided doses. This dose is also used for intravenous or intraperitoneal administration. In some instances daily doses as high as 200 mg per kg or as low as 50 mg per kg have been used.

Reduced doses should be employed in patients with renal impairment; patients with a creatinine clearance of 20 to 40 ml per minute may be given 50 mg per kg every 12 hours and those with a clearance of 10 to 20 ml per minute 50 mg per kg every 24 hours. Where the creatinine clearance is less than 10 ml per minute the initial dose is 50 mg per kg with subsequent doses based on plasma concentrations, which should not exceed 80 µg per ml.

Reviews of the actions and uses of flucytosine.— W. E. Herrell, *Clin. Med.*, 1971, *78* (Feb.), 11; J. P. Utz, *New Engl. J. Med.*, 1972, *286*, 777; *Med. Lett.*, 1972, *14*, 29; N. McCollum, *Drug Intell. & clin. Pharm.*, 1973, *7*, 75; J. E. Bennett, *New Engl. J. Med.*, 1974, *290*, 320; *Drug & Ther. Bull.*, 1975, *13*, 3; H. J. Scholer, *Chemotherapy, Basle*, 1976, *22*, *Suppl.* 1, 103, per *Int. pharm. Abstr.*, 1977, *14*, 293; J. E. Bennett, *Ann. intern. Med.*, 1977, *86*, 319; *Med. Lett.*, 1978, *20*, 66; G. Medoff and G. S. Kobayashi, *New Engl. J. Med.*, 1980, *302*, 145.

Flucytosine was given in doses of 50 to 150 mg per kg body-weight to adults or 4.5 g per m^2 body-surface to children weighing less than 50 kg in the treatment of 22 patients with various fungal infections. The organism was eradicated and symptoms alleviated in 3 of 8 with cryptococcal infections, in 4 of 8 with candidal infections, in 2 of 3 with infections due to *Phialophora* spp., in 1 with infection due to *Torulopsis glabrata*, and in 1 with osteochondritis due to *Aspergillus fumigatus*.— A. G. Vandevelde *et al.*, *Ann. intern. Med.*, 1972, *77*, 43.

Combined treatment with flucytosine and amphotericin was successful in 4 patients with severe deep-seated fungal infections due to *Candida* spp. and *Torulopsis glabrata*.— T. Eilard *et al.*, *J. antimicrob. Chemother.*, 1976, *2*, 239.

Administration in renal failure. Dosage schedules for patients with renal impairment.— D. N. Wade and G. Sudlow, *Aust. N.Z. J. Med.*, 1972, *2*, 153; J. Schönebeck *et al.*, *Chemotherapy, Basle*, 1973, *18*, 321; P. Sharpstone, *Br. med. J.*, 1977, *2*, 36; G. B. Appel and H. C. Neu, *New Engl. J. Med.*, 1977, *296*, 663.

See also under Absorption and Fate.

The normal half-life for flucytosine of 3 to 6 hours was increased to 70 hours in end-stage renal failure. Concentrations were affected by haemodialysis and peritoneal dialysis.— W. M. Bennett *et al.*, *Ann. intern. Med.*, 1977, *86*, 754. See also *idem*, 1980, *93*, 62.

Patients on haemodialysis could be given 25 to 50 mg of flucytosine per kg body-weight every 24 hours.— J. S. Cheigh, *Am. J. Med.*, 1977, *62*, 555.

Data for predicting removal of flucytosine by conventional haemodialysis.— T. P. Gibson and H. A. Nelson, *Clin. Pharmacokinet.*, 1977, *2*, 403.

Aspergillosis. The use of flucytosine in 12 patients with pulmonary and one with meningeal aspergillosis.— G. W. Atkinson and H. L. Israel, *Am. J. Med.*, 1973, *55*, 496, per *J. Am. med. Ass.*, 1974, *227*, 456.

For reports of the use of flucytosine with amphotericin in the treatment of aspergillosis, see Amphotericin, p.718.

Candidiasis. A 10-year-old child with pulmonary candidiasis which had not responded to broad-spectrum antibiotics or to nystatin was successfully treated with flucytosine 100 mg per kg body-weight daily for 6 weeks and with prednisone 1 mg per kg daily for 3 weeks. Diarrhoea and raised serum-transaminase concentrations precluded any increase in flucytosine dosage.— A. Kohlschütter and B. Pelet, *Archs Dis. Childh.*, 1974, *49*, 154. See also B. M. Jenner *et al.*, *Archs Dis. Childh.*, 1979, *54*, 555.

Treatment of candidal arthritis in a 75-year-old patient with amphotericin 335 mg by intravenous injection over 22 days and flucytosine 4 g daily by mouth for at least 4 months resulted in the patient being asymptomatic for 18 months after discontinuation of therapy.— S. A. Imbeau *et al.*, *J. Am. med. Ass.*, 1977, *238*, 1395.

A patient with candidal endocarditis due to *Candida parapsilosis* was given, after valve replacement, amphotericin 70 mg every other day and flucytosine 12 g every day for a 2-month period. No vegetations were seen at surgery 5½ years later.— E. Martin *et al.*, *Ann. intern. Med.*, 1979, *91*, 870.

Further references.— J. F. Warner *et al.*, *Antimicrob. Ag. Chemother.*, 1970, 473; C. O. Record *et al.*, *Br. med. J.*, 1971, *1*, 262; T. Eilard *et al.*, *J. infect. Dis.*, 1974, *130*, 155; M. F. Robinson *et al.*, *Aust. N.Z. J. Med.*, 1975, *5*, 472; M. A. Keller *et al.*, *Am. J. Dis. Child.*, 1977, *131*, 1260; S. M. MacLeod *et al.*, *Drug Intell. & clin. Pharm.*, 1979, *13*, 72.

Candidiasis, meningeal. A report of the treatment of candidal meningo-encephalitis with flucytosine.— L. Nordström *et al.*, *Scand. J. infect. Dis.*, 1977, *9*, 63.

For references to the combined use of flucytosine and amphotericin in the successful treatment of candidal meningitis, see Amphotericin, p.719.

Candidiasis, ocular. Flucytosine was effective in the treatment of endogenous ocular candidiasis in 2 patients and eradicated the disseminated candidiasis in one. The other patient died unexpectedly during treatment.— D. M. Robertson *et al.*, *Archs Ophthal., N.Y.*, 1974, *91*, 33, per *J. Am. med. Ass.*, 1974, *227*, 459.

Candidiasis, urinary. Reports of the treatment of urinary candidiasis with flucytosine.— R. J. Holt and R. L. Newman, *Develop. Med. Child Neurology*, 1972, *14*, *Suppl.* 27, 70; J. Schönebeck *et al.*, *Scand. J. Urol. & Nephrol.*, 1972, *6*, 37; G. J. Wise *et al.*, *J. Urol.*, 1980, *124*, 70.

Candidiasis, vaginal. A 42-year-old woman with long-standing intractable vulval candidiasis responded to treatment with flucytosine 2 g six-hourly for 12.5 days together with topical application of flucytosine cream. There had been no relapse over 9 months.— S. A. Seligman (letter), *Br. med. J.*, 1974, *3*, 173.

Chromomycosis. A patient with chromomycosis which covered a large area on his leg was successfully treated with flucytosine 150 mg per kg body-weight daily by mouth and daily topical occlusive applications. Treatment was continued for 6 months although biopsy specimens were negative for organisms after 2 months.— W. L. Morison *et al.*, *Br. J. Derm.*, 1974, *90*, 445.

Comment, with reports of resistance to flucytosine.— M. A. H. Bayles (letter), *Br. J. Derm.*, 1974, *91*, 715. Reply.— W. L. Morison (letter), *ibid.*

Treatment for 2 to 67 months with flucytosine by mouth cured 16 of 23 patients with chromomycosis. Resistance to flucytosine developed during treatment in 7 patients; it was suggested that resistance is less likely to develop when a dose of 200 mg per kg body-weight daily is given or when lesions are early and well localised. Flucytosine was still considered the treatment of choice. The concomitant topical application of flucytosine in some patients appeared to have no additional therapeutic effect.— C. F. Lopes *et al.*, *Int. J. Derm.*, 1978, *17*, 414.

Cladosporiosis. Flucytosine was effective in *mice* in the treatment of experimentally-induced cladosporiosis using 4 isolates of *Cladosporium bantianum*. Flucytosine might be the first effective treatment for man. It was less effective in sporotrichosis.— E. R. Block *et al.*, *Antimicrob. Ag. Chemother.*, 1973, *3*, 95.

Cryptococcosis. The treatment of cryptococcosis with a combination of flucytosine and amphotericin.— J. P. Utz *et al.*, *J. infect. Dis.*, 1975, *132*, 368. See also *Br. med. J.*, 1978, *1*, 1008; R. A. Tarala and J. D. Smith, *ibid.*, 1980, *281*, 28 (pulmonary cryptococcosis).

Comment and reports on the treatment of cryptococcosis with flucytosine.— *Lancet*, 1979, *2*, 132; P. Tolentino and C. Borrone, *Scand. J. infect. Dis.*, 1976, *8*, 61; J. E. Fusner and K. L. McClain, *J. Pediat.*, 1979, *94*, 599.

Cryptococcosis, meningeal. In a collaborative study of patients with cryptococcal meningitis, treatment with a 6-week course of amphotericin 300 µg per kg body-weight daily and flucytosine 150 mg per kg daily in divided doses every 6 hours was compared with a 10-week regimen of amphotericin alone, 400 µg per kg daily being given for 6 weeks then 800 µg per kg every other day for 4 weeks. Up to 3 intrathecal doses of amphotericin were allowed in either regimen. After 51 courses of treatment 16 of 24 patients were cured or improved by the combination treatment and 11 of 27 by amphotericin alone. Cerebrospinal fluid became sterile more rapidly in patients given the combination. Five patients on each regimen died during treatment. Side-effects attributed to flucytosine occurred in 11 of 34 patients originally randomised to receive the combination therapy and in 6 patients the side-effects were a major factor in the decision to discontinue flucytosine. Nine patients given the combination had leucopenia or thrombocytopenia or both, 3 had diarrhoea, and 3 an erythematous diffuse maculopapular rash. Most of the reactions began 10 to 26 days after starting flucytosine. Nevertheless the combination regimen was considered the treatment of choice in cryptococcal meningitis because of its equivalent or superior efficacy to amphotericin alone, more rapid sterilisation of the CSF, and shorter length of treatment.— J. E. Bennett *et al.*, *New Engl. J. Med.*, 1979, *301*, 126. Comment.— D. R. Graham (letter), *ibid.*, 1451. Reply.— J. E. Bennett (letter), *ibid.*

Further references.— J. S. Watkins *et al.*, *Br. med. J.*, 1969, *3*, 29; M. Roberts *et al.*, *J. Neurosurg.*, 1972, *37*, 229; H. Halkin *et al.*, *Israel J. med. Scis*, 1974, *10*, 1148; J. S. Tobias *et al.*, *Postgrad. med. J.*, 1976, *52*, 305; J. D. Stewart, *E. Afr. med. J.*, 1977, *54*, 684; A. M. Saunders *et al.*, *Br. med. J.*, 1978, *1*, 1030; D. D'A. Webling, *Med. J. Aust.*, 1978, *2*, 336; T. Jimbow *et al.*, *Chemotherapy, Basle*, 1978, *24*, 374.

Ear infections. Flucytosine ointment was used to treat 11 patients with fungal infections of the ear. Nine of the patients were cured.— J. Schönebeck and J. E. Zakrisson, *J. Lar. Otol.*, 1974, *88*, 227.

Eye infections. Fungal infections of the eye susceptible to flucytosine could be treated with 150 to 200 mg per kg body-weight by mouth or with eye-drops containing 1% with thiomersal 0.005%.— A. Baker, *J. Hosp. Pharm.*, 1972, *30*, 45. See also *Br. med. J.*, 1977, *1*, 667.

Leishmaniasis. A patient with cutaneous leishmaniasis whose lesions had been present for 1.5 years was successfully treated with flucytosine 5 g daily for 10 days.— A. Gonzalez-Ochoa and C. M. Collado, *Revta Invest. Salud Publ.*, 1972, *32*, 21, per *Trop. Dis. Bull.*, 1973, *70*, 732.

Pregnancy and the neonate. A 16-year-old girl with cryptococcal meningitis was given flucytosine, 340 g over 11 weeks following the administration of amphotericin, 415 mg over 11 days, in early pregnancy. She developed toxaemia of pregnancy at 34 weeks; despite the earlier use during pregnancy of aspirin, paracetamol, methaqualone, diphenhydramine, and bephenium hydroxynaphthoate she produced a premature and apparently normal infant.— C. R. Philpot and D. Lo, *Med. J. Aust.*, 1972, *2*, 1005.

A young woman aged 22 years who was 3½ months pregnant and with *Candida albicans* septicaemia was successfully treated with a total of 52.6 g of flucytosine. She gave birth to a healthy infant whose progress was uneventful.— J. Schönebeck and E. Segerbrand, *Br. med. J.*, 1973, *4*, 337.

Preparations

Flucytosine Capsules *(U.S.P.)*. Capsules containing flucytosine. Store in airtight containers. Protect from light.

Flucytosine Tablets *(B.P.)*. Tablets containing flucytosine. Protect from light.

Alcobon *(Roche, UK)*. Flucytosine, available as an **Infusion** containing 2.5 g in 250 ml of an aqueous saline solution with 13.8 mmol of chloride per 100 ml, and as scored **Tablets** of 500 mg. (Also available as Alcobon in *NZ, S.Afr.*).

Other Proprietary Names

Ancobon *(USA)*; Ancotil *(Arg., Austral., Canad., Denm., Fr., Ger., Jap., Norw., Swed., Switz.)*.

2583-d

Hachimycin. Trichomycin; Trichomycinum.

An antimicrobial substance produced by the growth of *Streptomyces hachijoensis*.

Approximate molecular formula: $C_{61}H_{84}N_2O_{20}$=1165.3.

CAS — 1394-02-1.

Pharmacopoeias. In *Jap.*

A yellow to yellowish-brown powder; odourless or with a slight characteristic odour. It contains not less than 1000 units per mg. The unit has been defined as 'the amount of hachimycin contained in 1 ml of the minimum hachimycin concentration that inhibits completely the growth of *Candida albicans* No. Yu 1200'.

Practically **insoluble** in water, alcohol, acetone, and methyl alcohol; very soluble in pyridine and solutions of sodium hydroxide; slightly soluble in glacial acetic acid. Hachimycin is **stable** at room temperature for at least 2 years. Aqueous solutions are most stable in phosphate buffer at pH 6.7 to 7 and are best stored below 4°. Solutions are rapidly inactivated by sunlight or ultraviolet light and on heating at 100°.

Antimicrobial Action. Hachimycin is a polyene antibiotic with activity against some pathogenic fungi and yeasts including *Aspergillus* spp., *Candida* spp., *Trichophyton* spp., and against *Trichomonas vaginalis*. There may be cross-resistance with amphotericin and nystatin.

Absorption and Fate. Hachimycin is poorly and irregularly absorbed from the gastro-intestinal tract; blood concentrations of about 0.1 unit per ml have been reported following a dose of 200 000 or 500 000 units.

Uses. Hachimycin is used in the treatment of candidiasis and trichomoniasis. It is used by topical application, as vaginal tablets, and has been given by mouth in doses of 150 000 to 250 000 units daily.

A preliminary study of hachimycin in 70 pregnant women with vulvovaginitis.— A. G. Smith *et al.*, *Am. J. Obstet. Gynec.*, 1963, *87*, 455.

Proprietary Names

Nipotracin *(Ralay, Spain)*; Trichomycin *(Fujisawa, S.Afr.*; *Fujisawa, Jap.)*; Trichomycine *(Syntex, Switz.)*; Tricomicin *(Inibsa, Spain)*.

2584-n

Halethazole. 5-Chloro-2-[4-(2-diethylaminoethoxy)phenyl]benzothiazole.

$C_{19}H_{21}ClN_2OS$=360.9.

CAS — 15599-36-7.

Halethazole is an antibacterial and antifungal agent that was formerly applied topically in the treatment of superficial fungal infections of the skin.

2585-h

Haloprogin.

M 1028. 3-Iodoprop-2-ynyl 2,4,5-trichlorophenyl ether.

$C_9H_4Cl_3IO$=361.4.

CAS — 777-11-7.

A white or pale yellow crystalline powder. M.p. about 114°. Very slightly **soluble** in water; soluble in alcohol.

Adverse Effects. Local reactions occur and include irritation, pruritus, and vesiculation. There may be increased maceration and exacerbation of existing lesions.

Reports of contact dermatitis with preparations of haloprogin being attributed to ethyl sebacate incorporated as a solubiliser H. V. Moss, *Archs Derm.*, 1974, *109*, 572.

A. R. Berlin and F. Miller, *Archs Derm.*, 1976, *112*, 1563.

Antimicrobial Action. Haloprogin is reported to inhibit *Epidermophyton*, *Microsporum*, *Trichophyton*, and *Candida* spp. and *Malassezia furfur (Pityrosporum orbiculare)*.

Absorption and Fate. Following topical application up to 15% of haloprogin may be excreted in the urine within 5 days.

Uses. Haloprogin is used in the treatment of tinea infections and pityriasis versicolor. It is applied topically as a 1% cream or solution.

References to the use of haloprogin in the treatment of fungal skin infections: J. K. Murdoch, *Can. pharm. J.*, 1978, *111*, 255; Y. M. Clayton *et al.*, *Clin. exp. Derm.*, 1979, *4*, 65.

Candidiasis, cutaneous. References: V. H. Carter and S. Olansky, *Archs Derm.*, 1974, *110*, 81; L. F. Montes and H. W. Hermann, *Cutis*, 1978, *21*, 410.

Tinea. In a 4-week comparative study in patients with tinea pedis, 46 of 62 treated with haloprogin and 11 of 20 treated with tolnaftate had negative cultures on completion of treatment. One week later 78% of patients on haloprogin and 41% of those on tolnaftate maintained negative cultures.— V. H. Carter, *Curr. ther. Res.*, 1972, *14*, 307.

Further references: R. Katz and B. Cahn, *Archs Derm.*, 1972, *106*, 837; *Med. Lett.*, 1976, *18*, 101.

Proprietary Names

Halotex *(Westwood, Canad.*; *Westwood, USA)*; Mycanden *(Schering, Arg.*; *Asche, Ger.*; *Schering, S.Afr.)*; Mycilan *(Theraplix, Belg.*; *Théraplix, Fr.)*; Polik *(Jap.)*.

2586-m

Hamycin. A polyene antimicrobial substance produced by the growth of *Streptomyces pimprina*.

CAS — 1403-71-0.

A yellow amorphous powder. Practically **insoluble** in water.

Hamycin has been reported to have antifungal and antitrichomonal properties. It has been administered topically and by mouth in a variety of fungal infections including candidiasis, tinea, blastomycosis, and madura foot.

Separation by high-speed liquid chromatography indicated that hachimycin and hamycin were different antibiotics although minor components could be similar or even identical.— W. Mechlinski and C. P. Schaffner, *J. Chromat.*, 1974, *99*, 619.

Manufacturers

Hindustan Antibiotics, Ind.

2587-b

Hexetidine.

5-Amino-1,3-bis(2-ethylhexyl)perhydro-5-methylpyrimidine.

$C_{21}H_{45}N_3$=339.6.

CAS — 141-94-6.

A viscid oil with faint amine-like odour. Wt per ml about 0.87 g. **Soluble** 1 in 10 000 of water; miscible with alcohol, acetone, chloroform, and macrogols. Hexetidine is inactivated by soaps and alkalis.

Uses. Hexetidine has antibacterial and antiprotozoal actions and is effective against *Candida albicans*.

It is used as a 0.1% solution in mouth and throat infections such as gingivitis, pharyngitis, and tonsillitis. It may also be used for oral hygiene and halitosis.

Hexetidine is used in veterinary practice in the treatment of fungal and bacterial infections of the skin.

Proprietary Preparations

Oraldene *(Warner, UK)*. A solution containing hexetidine 0.1%.

Other Proprietary Names

Buchex *(Arg.)*; Collu-Hextril *(Belg., Fr.)*; Drossadin *(Switz.)*; Duranil *(Arg.)*; Glypesin, Hexoral *(both Ger.)*; Hextril *(Belg., Fr., Neth., Switz.)*; Oraldine *(Spain)*; Oraseptic, Sterisil *(both Ital.)*; Steri/Sol *(Canad.)*.

2588-v

Hydroxystilbamidine Isethionate *(U.S.P.)*.

Oxistilbamidine Isethionate. 2-Hydroxystilbene-4,4′-dicarboxamidine bis(2-hydroxyethanesulphonate).

$C_{16}H_{16}N_4O,2C_2H_6O_4S$=532.6.

CAS — 495-99-8 (hydroxystilbamidine); 533-22-2 (isethionate).

Pharmacopoeias. In *U.S.* which also includes Sterile Hydroxystilbamidine Isethionate.

A fine, yellow, odourless, crystalline powder which decomposes on exposure to light. M.p. about 280°. **Soluble** in water; slightly soluble in alcohol; practically insoluble in ether. A 1% solution in water has a pH of 4 to 5.5. Aqueous solutions deteriorate on storage and should be used immediately after preparation. **Store** in airtight containers. Protect from light.

Incompatibility. A haze or precipitate was observed within an hour when an average dose of hydroxystilbamidine was mixed in dextrose injection with heparin.— J. M. Meisler and M. W. Skolaut, *Am. J. Hosp. Pharm.*, 1966, *23*, 557.

Adverse Effects. The intravenous administration of hydroxystilbamidine isethionate may produce sudden hypotension if administered too rapidly. Dizziness, headache, nausea, vomiting, breathlessness, tachycardia, fainting, incontinence, and oedema can occur. Concentrated solutions may cause thrombophlebitis, particularly in small veins. Generalised pruritus has been reported. It is reported to be irritant when applied topically. Side-effects may be diminished by administering the drug in dilute solution by slow infusion.

Hydroxystilbamidine isethionate could cause progressive malaise, anorexia, nausea, paraesthesia, hepatic dysfunction, headache and rash.— J. E. Bennett, *New Engl. J. Med.*, 1974, *290*, 320.

Precautions. Treatment with hydroxystilbamidine is probably best avoided in patients with impaired hepatic or renal function.

Antimicrobial Action. Hydroxystilbamidine isethionate has antifungal and antiprotozoal properties. It is effective against *Blastomyces dermatitidis* and *Leishmania*.

Uses. Hydroxystilbamidine isethionate is used in the treatment of North American blastomycosis but the incidence of relapse can be high and it is considered less effective than amphotericin (p.717). It is also used in visceral leishmaniasis (kala-azar) and in the American mucocutaneous form. Hydroxystilbamidine isethionate has sometimes been given to patients with multiple myeloma for relief of bone pain.

Hydroxystilbamidine isethionate is usually administered in a dose of 225 or 250 mg daily or on alternate days by intravenous infusion over a period of 2 to 3 hours, the dose being dissolved, immediately before use, in 200 ml of Sodium Chloride Intravenous Infusion or Dextrose Intravenous Infusion 5%. Children may be given 3 to 4.5 mg per kg body-weight daily. To avoid dangerous deterioration of the solution it must be protected from light during its administration. It has sometimes been given intramuscularly in similar doses but these injections are usually painful.

Blastomycosis. Over a period of 11 years, 31 of 53 patients with North American blastomycosis had been successfully treated with hydroxystilbamidine isethionate. Five patients had died while receiving treatment and hepatic toxicity had occurred in 1 patient. A further 12 patients had received amphotericin and treatment was successful in 10. Because of severe toxicity 1 patient was transferred to hydroxystilbamidine with a successful outcome, but in the remaining patient neither drug was successful.— W. R. Lockwood *et al.*, *Am. Rev. resp. Dis.*, 1969, *100*, 314, per *Abstr. Wld Med.*, 1970, *44*, 175.

For a comparative study of the treatment of blastomycosis with amphotericin and hydroxystilbamidine, see Amphotericin, p.718.

Pneumonia. *(Pneumocystis carinii).* Diffuse pneumonitis with an infection of *Pneumocystis carinii* occurred in a 10-year-old boy while being maintained in remission from acute lymphocytic leukaemia with methotrexate. The methotrexate was stopped and he was successfully treated with hydroxystilbamidine intravenously in a dose of 4 mg per kg body weight daily for 13 days.— D. L. Moore *et al.*, *Mayo Clin. Proc.*, 1969, *44*, 162.

Preparations

Sterile Hydroxystilbamidine Isethionate *(U.S.P.)*. Hydroxystilbamidine isethionate suitable for parenteral use. Protect from light.

Manufacturers

Merrell-National, USA.

2589-g

Ketoconazole.

R 41400. *cis*-1-Acetyl-4-{4-[2-(2,4-dichlorophenyl)-2-imidazol-1-ylmethyl-1,3-dioxolan-4-ylmethoxy]phenyl}piperazine. $C_{26}H_{28}Cl_2N_4O_4$=531.4.

CAS — 65277-42-1.

Crystals. M.p. 146°.

Adverse Effects. Gastro-intestinal disturbances, including nausea and vomiting, rash or pruritus, headache, and dizziness have occasionally been reported after administration of ketoconazole.

Toxic hepatitis occurred in one patient given ketoconazole.— J. K. Heiberg and E. Svejgaard, *Br. med. J.*, 1981, *283*, 825. See also A. L. Macnair *et al.*, *Janssen* (letter), *ibid.*, 1058.

Precautions. Concomitant administration of drugs that reduce stomach acidity, such as anticholinergic agents, antacids, and cimetidine, may reduce the absorption of ketoconazole. If indicated, these drugs should be taken not less than 2 hours after ketoconazole.

Absorption and Fate. Ketoconazole is incompletely absorbed from the gastro-intestinal tract; absorption is reduced when stomach acidity is reduced. Peak plasma concentrations of 2.9 to 6.9 μg per ml have been obtained 2 hours after administration of 200 mg by mouth. It is extensively bound to plasma proteins. Penetration into the cerebrospinal fluid is poor following oral administration.

Ketoconazole is extensively metabolised in the body and is excreted in the urine as inactive metabolites and unchanged drug; it is also excreted in the faeces.

Antifungal concentrations of ketoconazole had been obtained in CSF in one patient with meningitis due to *Candida albicans* following a dose of 400 mg twice daily. The patient's condition had remained stable for more than 4 months but it remained to be proved whether this therapy was adequate for *Candida albicans* meningitis.— W. E. Fibbe *et al.* (letter), *J. antimicrob. Chemother.*, 1980, *6*, 681.

Uses. Ketoconazole is an imidazole antifungal agent with activity similar to that of miconazole (see p.726). It has been given by mouth in the treatment of systemic mycotic infections in a dose of 200 mg once or twice daily with meals. A maximum of 400 mg once daily has been used when necessary.

Reviews and discussions of the actions and uses of ketoconazole.— D. Borelli *et al.*, *Postgrad. med. J.*, 1979, *55*, 657; *J. Am. med. Ass.*, 1980, *243*, 12; *ibid.*, *244*, 2019; J. R. Graybill and D. J. Drutz, *Ann. intern. Med.*, 1980, *93*, 921; *Drug & Ther. Bull.*, 1981, *19*, 91; R. C. Heel *et al.*, *Drugs*, 1982, *23*, 1; *Lancet*, 1982, *1*, 319.

A comparison of the antifungal activities *in vitro* of ketoconazole and miconazole.— D. Dixon *et al.*, *J. infect. Dis.*, 1978, *138*, 245.

For the proceedings of a symposium on ketoconazole, see *Rev. infect. Dis.*, 1980, *2*, 519–699.

Reports of the use of ketoconazole: M. P. J. M. Bisschop *et al.*, *Eur. J. Obstet. Gynec. reprod. Biol.*, 1979, *9*, 253 (vaginal candidiasis); A. A. Botter *et al.*, *Mykosen*, 1979, *22*, 274 (skin and nail mycosis); H. M. Rosenblatt *et al.*, *J. Pediat.*, 1980, *97*, 657 (chronic mucocutaneous candidiasis); E. Van Hecke and L. Meysman, *Mykosen*, 1980, *23*, 607 (tinea capitis); L. C. Cucé *et al.*, *Int. J. Derm.*, 1980, *19*, 405 (paracoccidioidomycosis, candidiasis, chromomycosis, lobomycosis, mycetoma); E. A. Petersen *et al.*, *Ann. intern. Med.*, 1980, *93*, 791 (chronic mucocutaneous candidiasis); L. E. Samelson *et al.*, *ibid.*, 838 (*Candida parapsilosis* endocarditis); J. R. Graybill *et al.*, *Archs Derm.*, 1980, *116*, 1137 (chronic mucocutaneous candidiasis); S. S. Hawkins *et al.*, *Ann. intern. Med.*, 1981, *95*, 446 (disseminated histoplasmosis).

Preparations

Nizoral *(Janssen, UK)*. Ketoconazole available as scored tablets of 200 mg.

2590-f

Mepartricin. Methylpartricin; SN654; SPA-S-160. A mixture of the methyl esters of 2 related polyene antibiotics obtained from a strain of *Streptomyces aureofaciens* or by any other means.

CAS — 11121-32-7.

Practically **insoluble** in water.

Studies *in vitro* indicated rapid destruction of mepartricin and SPA-S-222, a water-soluble complex with sodium lauryl sulphate, by simulated gastric juice. In simulated intestinal fluid (pH 7.5), about 10% degradation of mepartricin occurred in 3 hours at 37°; there was about 25% degradation in SPA-S-222 under comparable conditions.— T. Bruzzese *et al.*, *Farmaco, Edn prat.*, 1977, *32*, 422.

Uses. Mepartricin has antifungal and antiprotozoal activity and has been used in candidal and trichomonal infections of the vagina as vaginal tablets containing 25 000 units and as a cream.

A study on the activity *in vitro* of mepartricin on *Trichomonas vaginalis*.— G. Pucci and S. Ripa, *Farmaco, Edn prat.*, 1973, *28*, 293.

Response-rate of 93% in 29 non-pregnant women and 52% in 21 pregnant women with mycotic vulvovaginitis.— G. Bortolozzi, *Minerva ginéc.*, 1973, *25*, 261, per *J. Am. med. Ass.*, 1973, *225*, 331.

More rapid response in 48 patients with vaginal candidiasis than in 25 treated with nystatin.— A. Iannino and P. Testa, *Minerva ginéc.*, 1973, *25*, 284, per *J. Am med. Ass.*, 1973, *225*, 331.

Response in all of 16 patients with candidal infection of the skin treated for 14 to 63 days.— G. Farris, *G. ital. Derm.*, 1973, *108*, 557, per *Abstr. Hyg.*, 1974, *49*, 225.

Further favourable comparisons with nystatin.— A. M. El-Mofty, *G. ital. Derm.*, 1973, *108*, 563, per *Abstr. Hyg.*, 1974, *49*, 225; R. Bruno, *G. ital. Derm.*, 1975, *110*, 23, per *Abstr. Hyg.*, 1975, *50*, 702.

Proprietary Names

Tricandil *(Prospa, Belg.; SPA, Ital.; SPA, Switz.)*.

2591-d

Miconazole.

R 18134. 1-[2,4-Dichloro-β-(2,4-dichlorobenzyloxy)phenethyl]imidazole. $C_{18}H_{14}Cl_4N_2O$=416.1.

CAS — 22916-47-8.

A white crystalline powder. Very slightly **soluble** in water; very soluble in chloroform; soluble in most other organic solvents. Miconazole in a preparation for intravenous use is reported to be stable for up to 24 hours when diluted with Dextrose Intravenous Infusion 5% or Sodium Chloride Intravenous Infusion.

2592-n

Miconazole Nitrate *(B.P., U.S.P.)*.

R 14889. $C_{18}H_{14}Cl_4N_2O,HNO_3$=479.1.

CAS — 22832-87-7.

Pharmacopoeias. In *Br.* and *U.S.*

A white or almost white, odourless or almost odourless, crystalline or microcrystalline powder. M.p. about 182°. Very slightly **soluble** in water and ether; soluble 1 in 140 of alcohol; slightly soluble in chloroform. **Protect** from light.

Adverse Effects. After the intravenous infusion of miconazole, phlebitis, nausea, vomiting, diarrhoea, anorexia, pruritus, rash, febrile reactions, flushes, drowsiness, and hyponatraemia have been reported. Effects on the blood include hyperlipidaemia, aggregation of erythrocytes, anaemia, and thrombocytosis; they may be associated with the injection vehicle which contains Cremophor EL. Transient tachycardia and cardiac arrhythmias have followed the rapid intravenous injection of miconazole. Rare adverse effects include thrombocytopenic purpura, acute psychosis, arthralgia, and anaphylaxis.

Mild gastro-intestinal disturbances may occur when miconazole is taken by mouth.

Local irritation and sensitivity reactions may occur when miconazole nitrate is used topically; contact dermatitis has been reported.

Increased platelet counts and significant normocytic normochromic anaemia occurred in 6 successive patients given miconazole intravenously. Signs appeared after accumulated doses of 1.8 to 12.6 g. Withdrawal of miconazole reversed the thrombocytosis and increased the haemoglobin values in 5.— L. C. Marmion *et al.*, *Antimicrob. Ag. Chemother.*, 1976, *10*, 447.

Extremely high concentrations of serum cholesterol and triglycerides in 2 patients being treated with miconazole intravenously were attributed to the polyethoxylated castor oil (Cremophor EL) in the vehicle.— A. G. Bagnarello *et al.*, *New Engl. J. Med.*, 1977, *296*, 497. A similar report.— H. B. Niell (letter), *ibid.*, 1479.

In 15 patients with severe systemic mycoses treated intravenously with miconazole, several transient haematological and biochemical disturbances were noted in all patients at dosages above 600 mg every 8 hours by infusion; diphenhydramine-controlled pruritus also occurred in 13 patients, and cardiac arrhythmias in one patient who received 800 mg into the inferior vena cava within 2 minutes. Most of the side-effects were probably due to the vehicle but all were reversible and no remaining effects had been noted in the 10 surviving patients, one of whom had completed therapy 36 months previously. Treatment should not be withheld under desperate circumstances.— J. P. Sung and J. G. Grendahl (letter), *New Engl. J. Med.*, 1977, *297*, 786. A study *in vitro* on the vehicle.— N. K. Sheth *et al.* (letter), *ibid.*

Seven patients with haematologic malignancies developed 8 episodes of cardiorespiratory reactions (2 with cardiac arrest, 4 with anaphylactic reactions, and one with respiratory arrest) after receiving miconazole by infusion. None of the patients had had a history of cardiac disease but 5 of the patients had received miconazole diluted in less than 200 ml of fluid.— V. Fainstein and G. P. Bodey, *Ann. intern. Med.*, 1980, *93*, 432.

Treatment of Adverse Effects. The incidence and severity of phlebitis may be reduced by changing the site of infusion of miconazole every 2 to 3 days. Nausea and vomiting may be relieved by giving an antihistamine or anti-emetic drug before infusion, by slowing the rate of infusion, and by avoiding administration at mealtimes.

Precautions. When administered intravenously miconazole should be infused slowly over at least 30 minutes, especially in patients with cardiovascular disorders; blood values should be monitored regularly.

Miconazole given systemically may enhance the activity of anticoagulant or hypoglycaemic drugs.

Miconazole inhibited *in vitro* the ability of neutrophils to reach the site of infection promptly (chemotaxis).— Y. H. Thong and D. Ness (letter), *Lancet*, 1977, *2*, 568. Miconazole had marked immunosuppressive properties which might be undesirable in patients with severe mycotic infections possibly already receiving immunosuppressants.— Y. H. Thong and B. Rowan-Kelly, *Br. med. J.*, 1978, *1*, 149.

The vehicle for miconazole (polyethoxylated castor oil, methyl-and propylhydroxybenzoates, and water) inhibited granulocyte adherence and leukotaxis *in vitro* at concentrations of 0.33% and above. The need to test the vehicle and adjuvants in drug studies was stressed.— C. Lee and E. G. Maderazo, *Antimicrob. Ag. Chemother.*, 1978, *13*, 548.

Interactions. The association of amphotericin and miconazole appeared to be less effective than either drug used alone.— L. P. Schacter *et al.* (letter), *Lancet*, 1976, *2*, 318.

For mention of a possible interaction between nicoumalone and miconazole, see Nicoumalone, p.772.

See also under Antimicrobial Action, below.

Antimicrobial Action. Miconazole is an imidazole antifungal agent and may act by interfering with the permeability of the fungal cell membrane. It has a wide antifungal spectrum and possesses some antibacterial activity. At concentrations of

0.1 to 1 μg per ml it inhibits the dermatophytes, *Epidermophyton floccosum, Microsporum canis, Trichophyton mentagrophytes* and *T. rubrum, Blastomyces dermatitidis, Histoplasma capsulatum, Paracoccidioides brasiliensis, Cryptococcus neoformans, Malassezia furfur (Pityrosporum orbiculare)*, and some *Streptomyces* spp. Concentrations of 1 to 10 μg per ml have been reported to inhibit other dermatophytes and *Candida, Cladosporium,* and *Madurella* spp., *Coccidioides immitis,* and *Sporothrix schenckii.* Other sensitivie fungi include *Phialophora pedrosoi,* and *Aspergillus* and *Nocardia* spp. Sensitive bacteria include staphylococci, streptococci, *Bacillus anthracis*, and *Bacteroides fragilis*.

Studies on the antimicrobial action of miconazole.— J. M. Van Cutsem and D. Thienpont, *Chemotherapy, Basle*, 1972, *17*, 392; M. Refari, *Mykosen*, 1973, *16*, 39; S. Shadomy *et al.*, *J. antimicrob. Chemother.*, 1977, *3*, 147; A. L. Costa *et al.*, *Mykosen*, 1977, *20*, 431.

Miconazole showed varied activity against *Prototheca* spp.; MICs for *P. filamenta* and *P. moriformis* ranged from 0.1 to 1 μg per ml. Strains of *P. stagnora* and *P. wickerhamii* were resistant and although 6 strains of *P. zopfi* were inhibited by miconazole, usually at 10 μg per ml, 3 strains were resistant to its cidal action.— E. Segal *et al.*, *Antimicrob. Ag. Chemother.*, 1976, *10*, 75.

Miconazole was effective *in vitro* against the amoeba *Naegleria fowleri*.— Y. H. Thong *et al.* (letter), *Lancet*, 1977, *2*, 876.

At a concentration of 16 μg per ml miconazole *in vitro* inhibited 11 of 13 strains of *Clostridium difficile* isolated from patients with pseudomembranous colitis or diarrhoea. However, no active drug was detected in the faeces of 2 patients with diarrhoea who received miconazole 250 mg by mouth every 6 hours.— D. W. Burdon *et al.*, *J. antimicrob. Chemother.*, 1979, *5*, 307.

Further references: R. M. Bannatyne and R. Cheung, *Antimicrob. Ag. Chemother.*, 1978, *13*, 1040; T. W. MacFarlane *et al.*, *Br. dent. J.*, 1978, *144*, 199.

Diminished activity. *Cryptococcus neoformans* was inhibited by both amphotericin and miconazole *in vitro* but the activity of miconazole was inhibited and delayed in the presence of serum. The effectiveness of miconazole in cryptococcal meningitis might be limited.— J. R. Graybill *et al.*, *Antimicrob. Ag. Chemother.*, 1978, *13*, 277.

Enhanced activity. Studies *in vitro* indicating synergism between miconazole and sulphamethoxazole against some *Candida albicans* strains.— W. H. Beggs and G. A. Sarosi, *Curr. ther. Res.*, 1977, *21*, 547.

A report of enhanced activity *in vitro* with miconazole and rifampicin against strains of *Candida albicans*.— R. M. Bannatyne and R. Cheung, *Curr. ther. Res.*, 1977, *22*, 869.

Mode of action. A study of yeasts exposed to miconazole suggested that its action involved inhibition of peroxidase and catalase activity.— S. De Nollin *et al.*, *Janssen, Belg.*, *Antimicrob. Ag. Chemother.*, 1977, *11*, 500.

Resistance. Candidal membrane lipids reduced the activity of clotrimazole and miconazole.— H. Yamaguchi, *Antimicrob. Ag. Chemother.*, 1977, *12*, 16.

The development of miconazole resistance in *Candida albicans* causing a urinary-tract infection in a baby.— R. J. Holt and A. Azmi (letter), *Lancet*, 1978, *1*, 50.

Absorption and Fate. Miconazole is incompletely absorbed from the gastro-intestinal tract; peak plasma concentrations of about 1 μg per ml have been achieved 4 hours after a dose of 1 g. By intravenous infusion, doses above 9 mg per kg body-weight usually produce plasma concentrations above 1 μg per ml. Miconazole disappears from the plasma in a triphasic manner; it has a biological half-life of about 24 hours. Over 90% is reported to be bound to plasma proteins. Penetration into the cerebrospinal fluid and sputum is poor but miconazole diffuses well into infected joints.

Miconazole is inactivated in the body and 10 to 20% of an oral or intravenous dose is excreted in the urine, mainly as metabolites, within 6 days; about 50% of an oral dose may be excreted mainly unchanged in the faeces.

Very little miconazole is removed by haemodialysis.

There is little absorption through skin or mucous membranes when miconazole nitrate is applied topically.

Serum concentrations 1 and 12 hours after the intravenous administration of miconazole 1 g to a 50-year-old man with disseminated coccidioidomycosis were 5.1 and 0.9 μg per ml respectively; concentrations in the cerebrospinal fluid were subinhibitory reaching a maximum of 0.26 μg per ml.— P. D. Hoeprich and E. Goldstein, *J. Am. med. Ass.*, 1974, *230*, 1153.

Plasma concentrations achieved in 4 healthy subjects immediately after the intravenous infusion of 522 mg of miconazole over 15 minutes ranged from about 2 to 9 μg per ml. These compared with concentrations ranging from about 3 to 33 μg per ml in 4 patients with severe renal insufficiency and from about 2 to 32 μg per ml in 4 patients on intermittent haemodialysis. Biological half-lives for the 3 groups were similar with means from 24.1 to 25.4 hours.— P. J. Lewi *et al.*, *Eur. J. clin. Pharmac.*, 1976, *10*, 49.

In 4 healthy subjects, mean peak plasma concentrations of 0.37 and 1.16 μg per ml, respectively, were achieved 2 to 4 hours after oral doses of miconazole of 0.522 and 1 g; 27% of the lower dose was absorbed.— J. Boelaert *et al.*, in Chemotherapy Vol. 6, A.M. Geddes and J.D. Williams (Ed.), London, Plenum Press, 1976, p. 165.

Further references: J. Brugmans *et al.*, *Eur. J. clin. Pharmac.*, 1972, *5*, 93.

Uses. Miconazole is administered by intravenous infusion in the treatment of severe systemic fungal infections including candidiasis, coccidioidomycosis, cryptococcosis, and paracoccidioidomycosis. Intravenous doses of miconazole range from 0.2 to 1.2 g thrice daily. Each dose must be diluted in at least 200 ml of Sodium Chloride Intravenous Infusion or Dextrose Intravenous Infusion 5% and infused slowly over 30 to 60 minutes. Children may be given 20 to 40 mg per kg body-weight daily but no more than 15 mg per kg of miconazole should be given at each infusion.

In fungal meningitis, intravenous treatment is supplemented with intrathecal injections of miconazole; an adult dose of 15 to 20 mg has been recommended. An intravenous solution of miconazole has also been used for instillation into the bladder, trachea, and wounds.

Miconazole may be given by mouth in a dose of 250 mg four times daily for the treatment of oral and intestinal candidiasis. It has also been given prophylactically to patients at high risk of opportunistic fungal infections. For the treatment of oral lesions the tablets are dissolved in the mouth; a 2% w/w oral gel may also be used.

Miconazole nitrate is applied as a 2% cream or powder in the treatment of fungal infections of the skin and nails including candidiasis, tinea, and pityriasis versicolor. A 2% cream and pessaries of 100 mg are used in vaginal candidiasis.

Proceedings of a symposium on the experimental and clinical evaluation of miconazole.— *Proc. R. Soc. Med.*, 1977, *70*, *Suppl.* 1, 1–56.

Reviews of the actions and uses of miconazole.— D. A. Stevens, *Am. Rev. resp. Dis.*, 1977, *116*, 801; *Med. Lett.*, 1979, *21*, 31; R. C. Heel *et al.*, *Drugs*, 1980, *19*, 7.

See also R. J. Holt, *J. cutaneous Pathol.*, 1976, *3*, 45; *Med. Lett.*, 1976, *18*, 101; *Br. med. J.*, 1977, *2*, 347; J. K. Murdoch, *Can. pharm. J.*, 1978, *111*, 255; *Med. Lett.*, 1979, *21*, 39.

Miconazole 10 mg per kg body-weight given intravenously every 8 hours failed to control or eradicate infections in 3 patients with destructive arthritis (*Sporothrix schenckii*), meningoencephalitis (*Cryptococcus neoformans*), or disseminated aspergillosis (*Aspergillus fumigatus*). All the organisms were susceptible to miconazole 1.56 μg or less per ml *in vitro*; serum concentrations ranged from 1.35 to 4.35 μg per ml in one patient and concentrations in CSF were undetectable in another patient. Addition of miconazole 15 mg given intraventricularly every 2 to 3 days to the treatment of the patient with meningoencephalitis was without response and failed to increase concentrations of miconazole in the CSF.— J. F. Fisher *et al.*, *Antimicrob. Ag. Chemother.*, 1978, *13*, 965.

In a controlled study of patients undergoing intensive cytotoxic therapy, only 2 of 11 patients given miconazole 500 mg four times daily by mouth developed fungal infections compared with 7 of 14 similar patients given placebo.— H. Brincker, *Acta med. scand.*, 1978, *204*, 123.

Miconazole was successful in treating a 33-year-old woman with a sphenoidal sinus infection which appeared to be due to *Petriellidium boydii*.— J. T. Mader *et al.*, *J. Am. med. Ass.*, 1978, *239*, 2368.

Although the overall response of 40 infants with napkin dermatitis was similar when treatment consisted of the application of either a cream containing miconazole nitrate 2% or the cream basis alone, miconazole was significantly more effective than the basis alone in those infants who had a positive skin culture for bacteria or candida.— R. M. MacKie and E. Scott, *Practitioner*, 1979, *222*, 124.

Miconazole was given in doses of 0.6 to 1.2 g every 8 hours by intravenous infusion to 37 patients who had fungal infections and who were receiving chemotherapy for advanced malignant diseases. Cures were obtained in 9 of 22 patients with *Candida albicans* infections, 3 of 11 with *C. tropicalis* infections, both patients with infections due to *Torulopsis glabrata*, and one patient infected with *C. parapsilosis*. A patient with an unspecified candidal infection failed to respond to treatment.— W. M. Jordan *et al.*, *Antimicrob. Ag. Chemother.*, 1979, *16*, 792.

Administration in renal failure. Miconazole could be given in a usual dosage in renal failure. Concentrations were not affected by haemodialysis or peritoneal dialysis.— W. M. Bennett *et al.*, *Ann. intern. Med.*, 1980, *93*, 62. Renal failure was associated with miconazole 2.4 g daily given intravenously to a renal transplant patient. Renal function improved on reducing the dose. It would therefore seem wise to modify the dosage of miconazole when it is used in patients with chronic renal insufficiency.— K. N. Lai *et al.* (letter), *Lancet*, 1981, *2*, 48.

Candidiasis. In 14 patients with systemic candidiasis, miconazole 200 to 400 mg was given thrice daily intravenously (or occasionally into the site of infection) for 5 to 30 days. Treatment was successful in all the patients. Five of 7 patients with neoplasms, with pyrexia resistant to antibiotics and possibly due to candidal infection, were afebrile within 3 days after receiving miconazole 600 mg daily by intravenous injection.— W. Scheef *et al.* (letter), *Br. med. J.*, 1974, *!*, 78.

A report of the use of miconazole in the treatment of systemic candidiasis in a premature neonate. Therapy was started with a daily dose of 10 mg per kg body-weight in 2 divided doses each given intravenously over 2 hours but after 5 days miconazole was discontinued due to frequent episodes of ventricular tachycardia. About one week later the baby again became ill and miconazole was again given intravenously. However, because of frequent thrombophlebitis miconazole was also given by mouth and thigh abscesses were irrigated with the intravenous preparation. Intravenous therapy was continued for 6 days and the irrigations for 12 days over which time the abcesses healed.— M. Clarke *et al.*, *Br. med. J.*, 1980, *281*, 354.

Further references: M. E. Katz and P. A. Cassileth, *J. Am. med. Ass.*, 1977, *237*, 1124.

Candidiasis, cutaneous. A report of miconazole in the treatment of chronic mucocutaneous candidiasis.— T. J. Fischer *et al.*, *J. Pediat.*, 1977, *91*, 815.

Candidiasis, oral. Reports of the use of miconazole in the treatment of candidiasis of the digestive tract.— E. Svejgaard, *Acta derm.-vener., Stockh.*, 1976, *56*, 303; H. Brincker, *Scand. J. infect. Dis.*, 1976, *8*, 117; G. N. Tytgat *et al.*, *Gastroenterology*, 1977, *72*, 536; B. Roed-Petersen, *Int. J. oral Surg.*, 1978, *7*, 558.

Candidiasis, vaginal. Of 51 women treated for vaginal candidiasis with miconazole cream 2% administered once daily for 2 weeks, 40 were completely cured while symptoms were relieved in 6. The clinical results were better in pregnant than in non-pregnant patients. No side-effects were reported and all childbirths were normal.— F. Peeters *et al.*, *Arzneimittel-Forsch.*, 1973, *23*, 1107.

In a controlled study of 535 pregnant patients with acute candidal vulvovaginitis, treatment with miconazole nitrate as a vaginal cream was significantly more effective than nystatin vaginal tablets in all 3 trimesters of pregnancy.— D. McNellis *et al.*, *Obstet. Gynec.*, 1977, *50*, 674. See also H. C. S. Wallenburg and J. W. Wladimiroff, *Obstet. Gynec.*, 1976, *48*, 491.

Use of medicated tampons containing miconazole 100 mg twice daily for 7 days was considered to be an effective and acceptable method of treatment in 48 women with vaginal candidiasis.— J. Wallin, *Curr. ther. Res.*, 1978, *23*, 661. Cure rates were similar whether treatment was for 3.5 or 7.5 days.— H. Grundsell and L. Djärv, *ibid.*, *24*, 340.

In a multicentre study of 177 women with candidal vulvovaginitis, creams containing miconazole 2 or nystatin 25 000 units per g were considered to be of similar efficacy; both creams were more effective than vaginal tablets containing clotrimazole but this was significant only for miconazole.— E. Svendsen *et al.*, *Curr. ther. Res.*, 1978, *23*, 666. In 74 women with candidal vaginitis treatment with pessaries containing either miconazole 100 mg or nystatin 100 000 units for 14 nights was equally effective; consorts were treated with the appropriate cream.— S. Bentley *et al.*, *Br. J. clin. Pract.*, 1978, *32*, 258.

Efficacy of various schedules of miconazole nitrate in vulvovaginal candidiasis.— S. Rashid and R. S. Morton, *Curr. ther. Res.*, 1980, *27*, 323.

Further references: W. H. Robertson, *Am. J. Obstet. Gynec.*, 1978, *132*, 321; S. R. Mayhew and W. E. Suffield, *Practitioner*, 1979, *222*, 564; S. A. Pasquale *et al.*, *Obstet. Gynec.*, 1979, *53*, 250; C. C. J. Hohner *et al.*, *Curr. ther. Res.*, 1980, *27*, 280; N. Rosedale *et al.*, *ibid.*, 493.

Coccidioidomycosis. Of 10 patients with fungal meningitis caused by *Coccidioides immitis*, 9 of whom had received amphotericin, 5 obtained a beneficial response to miconazole given intravenously in a usual daily dose of 30 mg per kg body-weight and sometimes also intrathecally in a dose of 20 mg on alternate days to twice daily. Three relapsed on discontinuation of therapy but results were considered promising. Side-effects were mild and reversible and a comparative study with amphotericin was indicated.— S. C. Deresinski *et al.*, *Archs intern. Med.*, 1977, *137*, 1180.

An unfavourable response to miconazole given intravenously to 7 patients with coccidioidomycosis. Three patients did not respond to treatment and one required intrathecal amphotericin. Severe side-effects were frequent.— R. D. Meyer *et al.*, *Chest*, 1978, *73*, 825.

A 32-year-old man with disseminated coccidioidomycosis responded dramatically to treatment with miconazole intravenously combined with amphotericin intrathecally. Earlier treatment with amphotericin intravenously and intrathecally or miconazole by both routes had failed.— S. J. Davis and W. H. Donovan, *Chest*, 1979, *76*, 235.

Further references: D. A. Stevens *et al.*, *Am. J. Med.*, 1976, *60*, 191; P. D. Hoeprich *et al.*, *J. Am. med. Ass.*, 1980, *243*, 1923.

Cryptococcosis. A 19-year-old girl with systemic cryptococcosis responded to miconazole 600 mg eight-hourly by intravenous infusion for 4 weeks, then 750 mg thrice daily by mouth for 13 months.— M. E. Morgans *et al.*, *Br. med. J.*, 1979, *2*, 100.

Therapy with miconazole, 400 mg given intravenously every 8 hours for 8 weeks was successful in the treatment of a patient with cryptococcal meningitis complicated by a cerebral cryptococcoma. Complete disappearance of the brain lesion occurred during treatment. The patient's condition had previously failed to respond to 6 weeks of treatment with amphotericin and flucytosine.— L. Weinstein and I. Jacoby, *Ann. intern. Med.*, 1980, *93*, 569.

Paracoccidioidomycosis. A report of dramatic improvements in 6 patients with paracoccidioidomycosis when they were given miconazole intravenously for an average of 32 days. Isolates of *Paracoccidioides brasiliensis* from 2 patients were very sensitive to miconazole *in vitro* and the oral use of miconazole might be possible.— D. A. Stevens *et al.*, *Am. J. trop. Med. Hyg.*, 1978, *27*, 801. See also *Lancet*, 1979, *1*, 368; D. A. Stevens and A. Restrepo-M (letter), *ibid.*, 1301.

No relapses were noted in 9 patients followed up after treatment with miconazole by mouth for paracoccidioidomycosis.— N. Santos-Lima *et al.*, *Revta Inst. Med. trop. S Paulo*, 1978, *20*, 347, per *Trop. Dis. Bull.*, 1979, *76*, 748.

Sporotrichosis. The successful use of miconazole in a patient with pulmonary sporotrichosis.— J. J. Rohwedder and G. Archer, *Am. Rev. resp. Dis.*, 1976, *114*, 403.

Miconazole was not effective in the treatment of a patient with destructive arthritis caused by *Sporothrix schenckii*.— J. F. Fisher *et al.*, *Antimicrob. Ag. Chemother.*, 1978, *13*, 965.

Tinea. In a double-blind study of 30 patients with tinea pedis, treatment with miconazole nitrate 2% cream was more effective than tolnaftate 1% cream and both were more effective than placebo.— R. C. Ongley, *Can. med. Ass. J.*, 1978, *119*, 353.

Further references: S. J. Mandy and T. C. Garrott, *J. Am. med. Ass.*, 1974, *230*, 72; J. C. Gentles *et al.*, *Br. J. Derm.*, 1975, *93*, 79; L. G. Ortiz and C. M. Papa, *Clin. Ther.*, 1978, *1*, 444, per *Int. pharm. Abstr.*, 1979, *16*, 217; J. G. Marks *et al.*, *Archs Derm.*, 1980, *116*, 321.

Preparations

Miconazole Nitrate Cream *(U.S.P.)*. A cream containing miconazole nitrate. Store in airtight containers.

Proprietary Preparations

Daktacort *(Janssen, UK)*. Cream containing miconazole nitrate 2% and hydrocortisone 1%.

Daktarin Cream *(Janssen, UK)*. Contains miconazole nitrate 2%. **Daktarin Intravenous Solution.** Ampoules of 20 ml for the preparation of intravenous infusion solutions, each containing miconazole 200 mg in a vehicle containing Cremophor EL 10%. **Daktarin Oral.** Contains miconazole, available as sugar-free **Gel** containing 125 mg in each 5 ml and as scored **Tablets** of 250 mg. **Daktarin Twin-Pack.** A composite pack of cream and powder each containing miconazole nitrate 2%. (Also available as Daktarin in *Arg., Austral., Belg., Fr., Ital., Neth., S.Afr., Spain, Switz.*).

Dermonistat Cream *(Ortho-Cilag, UK)*. Contains miconazole nitrate 2%.

Gyno-Daktarin *(Janssen, UK)*. Miconazole nitrate, available as **Cream** for vaginal use containing 2%, as **Pessaries** of 100 mg, and as **Tampons** coated with 100 mg. **Gyno-Daktarin Combi-pack.** A composite pack of 14 pessaries and cream. (Also available as Gyno-Daktarin in *Arg., Austral., Belg., Fr., Neth., S.Afr.*).

Monistat *(Ortho-Cilag, UK)*. Miconazole nitrate, available as **Cream** for vaginal use containing 2% and as **Pessaries** of 100 mg. (Also available as Monistat in *Canad., Switz., USA*).

Other Proprietary Names

Albistat *(Belg., Neth.,)*; Andergin *(Ital.)*; Daktar *(Ger., Norw., Swed.)*; Deralbine *(Arg.)*; Epi-Monistat *(Ger.)*; Fungisidin *(Spain)*; Gyno-Daktar, Gyno-Monistat *(both Ger.)*; Micatin *(Canad., USA)*; Micotef *(Ital.)*; Monistat-7 *(Austral., Canad., USA)*.

2593-h

Natamycin *(U.S.P.)*. Pimaricin; Antibiotic A-5283; CL 12625.

An amphoteric antibiotic produced by the growth of *Streptomyces natalensis*.

$C_{33}H_{47}NO_{13}=665.7$.

CAS — 7681-93-8.

Pharmacopoeias. In *U.S.*

A white, odourless, tasteless, crystalline powder. It contains 6 to 9% of water and has a potency of not less than 900 µg per mg calculated on the anhydrous basis.

Very slightly **soluble** in water and alcohol; slightly soluble in methyl alcohol; practically insoluble in acetone, chloroform, and fixed oils; readily soluble in dilute acids and alkalis, forming salts. A 1% aqueous suspension has a pH of 5 to 7.5. **Store** in airtight containers. Protect from light.

Natamycin is stable when dry. A slight discoloration may develop on keeping but this does not affect its activity. Solutions and suspensions at pH 5 to 9 retain their activity for several weeks if protected from air and light. Solutions and suspensions at neutral pH may be heated for short periods at 100° to 110° without appreciable loss of activity.

Adverse Effects. Nausea, vomiting, anorexia, and diarrhoea have occurred after the administration of natamycin by mouth. Topical application of natamycin has sometimes produced mild irritation.

Antimicrobial Action. Natamycin is a polyene antifungal agent with antimicrobial activity similar to that of nystatin (see p.729). In addition it is active against *Trichomonas vaginalis*. The minimum inhibitory concentration of natamycin has been reported to range from 1 to 25 µg per ml.

Of 62 strains of *Candida albicans*, 13 needed 12.5 µg per ml, 12 needed 6.2 µg per ml, and 37 needed 3.1 µg or less per ml of natamycin for inhibition. All 18 strains of other *Candida* spp. tested were sensitive to natamycin, though 3 required a concentration of 50 µg per ml for inhibition. Of 27 strains of *Cryptococcus* belonging to 8 spp., 4 needed 28 µg per ml, 10 needed 12.5 µg per ml, and 13 needed 6.2 µg or less per ml of natamycin for inhibition. For complete inhibition of *Trichophyton* spp., 250 or 500 µg per ml, for *Phialophora* and *Scopulariopsis* spp. 12.5 µg per ml, and for *Cephalosporium* spp. 50 µg per ml of natamycin were necessary.— F. Fegeler *et al.*, *Dt. med. Wschr.*, 1966, *91*, 250, per *Abstr. Wld Med.*, 1966, *40*, 394.

Absorption and Fate. Natamycin is poorly absorbed from the gastro-intestinal tract.

Uses. Natamycin is used for the local treatment of candidiasis, trichomoniasis, and fungal keratitis. It has also been used in aspergillosis.

Natamycin has been given as enteric-coated tablets for the treatment of intestinal candidiasis in a dose of 100 mg three or four times daily. For the treatment of oral candidiasis in infants, 4 drops of a 1% suspension of natamycin may be placed under the tongue after every feed; for older children and adults, 10 drops may be applied to the lesion after each meal.

For inhalation therapy in the treatment of infections of the lungs and respiratory tract caused by susceptible fungi and yeasts, a sterile suspension is administered as an aerosol in a dose equivalent to 2.5 mg of natamycin thrice daily for 4 weeks and then twice daily until sputum cultures are consistently negative for the infecting organism.

For topical application to the skin and nail matrix a 2% cream is used. Vaginal tablets containing natamycin 25 mg in a buffered basis together with a surfactant are used in the treatment of trichomonal and candidal infections of the vagina. One vaginal tablet is inserted nightly for 3 weeks.

A 5% ophthalmic suspension of natamycin is used in the treatment of fungal infections of the eye, including those due to *Fusarium solani*.

Natamycin has been used as a food preservative in some countries.

A review of the properties and uses of natamycin.— W. P. Raab, *Natamycin (Pimaricin)*, Stuttgart, Georg Thieme, 1972.

Estimated acceptable daily intake of natamycin: up to 300 µg per kg body-weight.— Twentieth Report of the Joint FAO/WHO Expert Committee on Food Additives, *Tech. Rep. Ser. Wld Hlth Org. No. 599*, 1976.

Aspergillosis. In 21 patients with bronchopulmonary aspergillosis only 6 of 29 courses of inhalation therapy with solutions of natamycin 1 mg per ml, nystatin 25 000 units per ml, or brilliant green 1 in 5000 or 1 in 10 000 were associated with clinical improvement. Such improvements as were noted could easily have been accounted for by the natural history of the disease.— D. S. McCarthy and D. G. Robertson (letter), *Lancet*, 1968, *1*, 1089.

In 3 patients with bronchopulmonary aspergillosis, the aspergilloma was surgically removed and the cavity irrigated daily with an aqueous suspension of natamycin, 50 mg in 8 ml, for 7 to 8 weeks. Observation for up to 18 months indicated apparent cure. In 3 patients with allergic aspergillosis, aerosol inhalations of natamycin were ineffective.— A. H. Henderson and J. E. G. Pearson, *Thorax*, 1968, *23*, 519.

Further references: G. Edwards and C. J. P. La Touche, *Lancet*, 1964, *1*, 1349.

Candidiasis, vaginal. Fifty patients with candidal vaginitis who were between 14 and 34 weeks pregnant were treated with vaginal tablets containing natamycin 25 mg and benzalkonium chloride 1 mg, once daily for 21 days or more. Forty-seven (94%) were cured and no side-effects were reported.— V. R. Patel, *Practitioner*, 1973, *210*, 701.

For a comparison of natamycin and amphotericin in the treatment of vaginal candidiasis, see Amphotericin, p.719.

Eye infections. A method for preparing eye-drops containing a 5% suspension of natamycin for the treatment of eye infections due to *Aspergillus fumigatus*, *Candida albicans*, or *Fusarium* spp.— A. Baker, *J. Hosp. Pharm.*, 1972, *30*, 45.

A discussion on the use of a 5% ophthalmic suspension of natamycin in the treatment of fungal keratitis, blepharitis, and conjunctivitis.— *Med. Lett.*, 1979, *21*, 79.

Further references: D. B. Jones *et al.*, *Archs Ophthal., N.Y.*, 1972, *88*, 147; E. Newmark *et al.*, *Sth. med. J.*, 1971, *64*, 935; R. K. Forster *et al.*, *Br. J. Ophthal.*, 1975, *59*, 372.

Preparations

Natamycin Ophthalmic Suspension *(U.S.P.)*. A sterile suspension of natamycin 50 mg per ml in a suitable aqueous vehicle; it contains one or more suitable preservatives. pH 6 to 7.5. Store in airtight containers. Protect from light.

Proprietary Preparations

Pimafucin *(Brocades, UK)*. Natamycin, available as a **Cream** containing 2%; as a sterile aqueous **Suspension** containing 1% for oral use, and 2.5% for inhalation as an aerosol; and as **Vaginal Tablets** each containing 25 mg with benzalkonium chloride 1 mg, in a buffered lactose basis. (Also available as Pimafucin in *Austral.*, *Belg.*, *Denm.*, *Ger.*, *Ital.*, *Neth.*, *Norw.*, *S.Afr.*, *Switz.*).

Other Proprietary Names

Natafucin *(Ital.)*; Pimafucine *(Fr.)*.

2594-m

Nifuroxime. 5-Nitro-2-furaldehyde oxime.
$C_5H_4N_2O_4$=156.1.

CAS — 6236-05-1.

A white to pale yellow crystalline powder when fresh. It may become tan in colour on standing and it should not be used if it is darker than a medium tan. It discolours on exposure to direct sunlight and on contact with alkaline materials.
Soluble 1 in 1000 of water and 1 in 25 of alcohol; very soluble in dimethylformamide. **Store** in airtight containers and avoid contact with metals other than stainless steel or aluminium. Protect from light.

Nifuroxime is a fungicide active against a variety of fungi including *Candida albicans*. It was formerly used with furazolidone to treat vaginitis due to *C. albicans* or *Trichomonas vaginalis*.

2596-v

Nystatin *(B.P., B.P. Vet., U.S.P.)*. Nystatinum; Fungicidin; Nistatina. A tetraene antifungal agent.
Approximate molecular formula:
$C_{47}H_{75}NO_{17}$=926.1.

CAS — 1400-61-9.

Pharmacopoeias. In *Br.*, *Braz.*, and *U.S.* which specify not less than 4400 units per mg, *Chin.*, *Cz.*, *Hung.*, *Int.*, and *Jug.* which specify not less than 3000 units per mg, and *Swiss* and *Turk.* which specify not less than 2000 units per mg. *Roum.* specifies not less than 3500 units per mg. *Jap.* does not specify potency.
The *B.P.* also includes Nystatin Dermatological which differs from Nystatin *B.P.* only in that it is not required to pass the test for abnormal toxicity.

A mixture of antifungal polyenes produced by the growth of certain strains of *Streptomyces noursei*, or by any other means. It consists largely of nystatin A_1. It is a yellow to light brown hygroscopic powder with a characteristic odour suggestive of cereals, containing not less than 4400 units per mg of the dried substance.
Very slightly **soluble** in water; sparingly soluble in alcohol, methyl alcohol, *n*-propyl alcohol, and *n*-butyl alcohol; practically insoluble in chloroform and ether; freely soluble in dimethylformamide and formamide. A 3% suspension in water has a pH of 6.5 to 8. **Store** at a temperature not exceeding 5° in airtight containers and protect from light; under these conditions the potency may fall at the rate of about 1% per month.

A report of the temperature stability of nystatin in suppository bases.— A. E. Elkouly *et al.*, *Mfg Chem.*, 1973, *44* (Aug.), 37.

In the presence of phosphate-citrate buffers at 37° the optimum pH for the stability of nystatin was between pH 6.5 and 7 and fell sharply outside this range. In incubation studies *in vitro* the activity of nystatin against *Candida albicans* increased with a decrease in temperature from 41° to 25°.— J. M. T. Hamilton-Miller, *J. Pharm. Pharmac.*, 1973, *25*, 401.

Mention of changes in dissolution-rate and equilibrium solubility of the hydrophobic drug nystatin, brought about by the presence of hydrophilic polymers, povidone and carmellose sodium in the dissolution medium.— *Pharm. J.*, 1978, *2*, 249.

Units. One unit of nystatin is contained in 0.000333 mg of the first International Standard Preparation (1963) which contains 3000 units per mg.

Adverse Effects. Nausea, vomiting, and diarrhoea have occasionally been reported after the oral administration of nystatin. Allergic contact dermatitis has occurred after the topical use of nystatin.

Reference: A. Wasilewski, *Archs Derm.*, 1970, *102*, 216.

Antimicrobial Action. Nystatin is a fungistatic and fungicidal polyene antibiotic but has no antibacterial properties. Its main action is against *Candida* spp. It is also effective against *Coccidioides immitis, Cryptococcus neoformans, Histoplasma capsulatum, Blastomyces dermatidis*, and other yeasts and fungi. Resistance to nystatin may develop.

Nystatin was active *in vitro* against *Prototheca* spp. with MICs ranging from 0.38 to 12.5 µg per ml.— E. Segal *et al.*, *Antimicrob. Ag. Chemother.*, 1976, *10*, 75.

Of 353 yeast strains isolated from clinical material 33 were resistant to flucytosine and 11 resistant to clotrimazole and miconazole. All the strains were sensitive to nystatin and natamycin.— R. Baier and H. Puppel, *Dt. med. Wschr.*, 1978, *103*, 1112.

Diminished activity. The antimicrobial activity of nystatin against *Candida albicans* was almost completely inhibited by the presence of riboflavine phosphate (sodium salt).— M. A. El-Nakeeb *et al.*, *Can. J. pharm. Sci.*, 1976, *11*, 85.

Mode of action. Nystatin was effective by virtue of its ability to cause the yeast cells of *Candida albicans* to lose potassium ions, without which energy metabolism stopped.— L. S. Watt *et al.*, *Antibiotics Chemother.*, 1962, *12*, 173.

Resistance. A report of a strain of *Candida albicans* resistant to nystatin but sensitive to amphotericin.— R. S. Illingworth (letter), *Archs Dis. Childh.*, 1978, *53*, 183.

Further references: J. D. Dick *et al.*, *Antimicrob. Ag. Chemother.*, 1980, *18*, 158.

Absorption and Fate. Nystatin is poorly absorbed from the gastro-intestinal tract. It is not absorbed through the skin or mucous membranes when applied topically.

Uses. Nystatin is used for the local treatment of candidiasis, especially that caused by *Candida albicans*. It may also be given with antibacterial antibiotics as a prophylactic against overgrowth of *Candida*.
For the treatment and prophylaxis of intestinal candidiasis, nystatin is given in doses of 500 000 or 1 000 000 units 3 or 4 times a day. In infants and children a dosage of 100 000 units or more may be given 4 times daily.
For vaginal infections, one or two pessaries containing 100 000 units may be inserted daily and supplemented when necessary by doses by mouth; local treatment may be carried out using a cream. For cutaneous and mucocutaneous lesions, ointment, gel, cream, or dusting powder containing 100 000 units per g may be applied, and for lesions of the mouth, suspensions of a similar strength may be used or tablets allowed to dissolve in the mouth.
An aqueous suspension of finely powdered nystatin 30 000 units per ml has been used as drops in the topical treatment of fungal infections of the eye.

Although a reduction had occurred in the volume of hypertrophied prostates in *dogs* given polyene antifungal agents, a controlled study of 31 patients with prostatic hypertrophy showed no significant differencc between nystatin 1.5 million units daily by mouth for 6 weeks and placebo. One patient given nystatin developed a skin rash.— P. Theodorides *et al.*, *Proc. R. Soc. Med.*, 1972, *65*, 130.

In a pilot study on 13 patients with denture stomatitis, incorporation of nystatin 800 000 units into the denture lining material was as effective as nystatin 500 000 units dissolved on the mouth 4 times daily for 3 weeks in inhibiting colonisation by *Candida*. The 7 patients taking nystatin tablets complained of a bitter taste and 3 complained of nausea.— W. H. Douglas and D. M. Walker, *Br. dent. J.*, 1973, *135*, 55.

Nystatin should be given by aerosol as an aqueous solution of 100 000 units per ml for bronchopulmonary mycoses. An aqueous suspension of 200 000 units per ml or a paste containing 45 000 units per ml could be applied for the local treatment of aspergilloma.— A. Sakula, *Practitioner*, 1974, *212*, 335.

Aspergillosis. A 3-year-old girl with bronchopulmonary aspergillosis was treated with nystatin, 500 000 units by mouth 4 times daily and by inhalation; 1 500 000 units were dissolved in 500 ml of 10% propylene glycol solution and the whole of the solution was vaporised in a mist tent each night. The condition promptly improved, but relapsed during maintenance treatment by mouth. Further inhalation treatment was successful. Nystatin could not be detected in the blood during treatment by mouth, but concentrations of 2.7 to 3.8 units per ml were detected during inhalation treatment.— J. S. Vedder and W. F. Schorr, *J. Am. med. Ass.*, 1969, *209*, 1191.

In 10 patients with aspergilloma of the lung, 5 ml of a paste containing nystatin 45 000 units per ml of basis was injected into the cavity on 5 to 18 occasions at intervals of 7 to 21 days. Five patients expectorated plugs of fungi. Haemoptysis ceased in 6 of 9 patients, fungus balls disappeared in 3 patients and became smaller in 3 more. In all patients sputum cultures became negative after treatment.— P. Krakówka *et al.*, *Tubercle*, 1970, *51*, 184.

For an unfavourable report on the efficacy of nystatin in bronchopulmonary aspergillosis, see Natamycin, p.728.

Candidiasis. Eighty-five infants aged less than 3 months with napkin rash and *Candida albicans* in the faeces were treated with nystatin ointment topically and either nystatin suspension 1 ml four times daily by mouth or a placebo. *C. albicans* was eliminated from about half the treated infants but also disappeared in nearly as great a proportion of those receiving a placebo. Napkin rash cleared in most of the infants in each group; there was slightly less tendency for the rash to recur in the treated group.— P. N. Dixon *et al.*, *Br. J. Derm.*, 1972, *86*, 458.

Prophylactic nystatin therapy had considerably reduced the occurrence of deep candidiasis in patients with leukaemia and other haematological neoplasia.— J. Pizzuto *et al.* (letter), *New Engl. J. Med.*, 1978, *298*, 279. A report of contrary results.— C. J. Williams (letter), *ibid.*, 853. Reply to criticism.— J. Pizzuto *et al.* (letter), *ibid.*, *299*, 661.

Further references: U. Carpentieri *et al.*, *J. Pediat.*, 1978, *92*, 593.

For references to the use of nystatin as part of oral non-absorbable antibiotic regimens given prophylactically to patients with acute leukaemia, see Framycetin Sulphate, p.1166, Gentamicin Sulphate, p.1172, and Neomycin Sulphate, p.1190.

Candidiasis, ocular. Endogenous fungous endophthalmitis due to *Candida albicans* in a 70-year-old man was effectively treated with nystatin, 500 000 units thrice daily, corticosteroids topically, and mydriatics. This regimen cleared the hypopyon in 1 eye within 4 days and the flare and cells in the aqueous of the other in a week. Treatment with nystatin was continued for 3 months and was accompanied by improvement of visual acuity in 1 eye and the resolution of skin ulcers.— A. Tarkkanen *et al.*, *Br. J. Ophthal.*, 1967, *51*, 188.

Candidiasis, oral. A study of 8 non-diabetic patients with candidal infections of the mouth resistant to treatment with nystatin or amphotericin showed that all had normal general immune function. The lesions cleared in 4 patients when treatment, continued for up to 6 months, was supplemented by giving folic acid and iron to correct nutritional deficiencies. The remaining 4 patients did not improve and required surgical treatment.— R. M. Mackie *et al.*, *Br. J. Derm.*, 1978, *98*, 343.

Candidiasis, vaginal. A review of nystatin and other antifungal agents in the treatment of vaginal candidiasis.— *Drug & Ther. Bull.*, 1976, *14*, 75.

In a study in 93 women with vaginal yeast infections, ordinary and effervescent nystatin pessaries were equally effective.— S. Velupillai and R. N. Thin, *Practitioner*, 1977, *219*, 897.

Administration of nystatin in the form of vaginal suppositories was considered to be as effective as administration in the form of vaginal tablets in multicentre studies involving 465 women with vaginal candidiasis.— G. Marion-Landais *et al.*, *Curr. ther. Res.*, 1978, *24*, 739.

Application of 2.5 g of a cream containing nystatin

400 000 units per g once daily was as effective as vaginal tablets containing clotrimazole 100 mg used once daily for 7 days in the treatment of 51 patients with vaginal candidiasis. Nystatin produced earlier subjective relief of symptoms than clotrimazole.— A. Kjaeldgaard *et al.*, *Curr. ther. Res.*, 1979, *26*, 322.

Further references: G. W. Csonka, *Br. J. vener. Dis.*, 1967, *43*, 210; R. Hurley, *Practitioner*, 1975, *215*, 753; *Br. med. J.*, 1976, *1*, 357.

Reports of the comparative efficacy of nystatin and miconazole in the treatment of candidal vaginitis, see Miconazole, p.727.

Eye infections. In the treatment of ocular fungous infections, nystatin was reasonably well tolerated when applied topically in an ointment containing 100 000 units per g, or when 5000 units suspended in 0.5 ml of saline were injected subconjunctivally, though neither route yielded appreciable intra-ocular concentrations. Nystatin, 200 units, could be injected into the vitreous or aqueous chambers, but could cause hyperaemia and leucocytic infiltration lasting for as long as 1 week. Vitreous assays had shown that nystatin concentrations sufficient to inhibit *Aspergillus* (6 to 12 units per ml) persisted for only 24 hours; unfortunately a second intravitreous injection of 200 units given within 36 hours of the first caused vitreous degeneration.— M. S. Rheins *et al.*, *Br. J. Ophthal.*, 1966, *50*, 533.

Two patients with fungal keratitis were successfully treated with eye-drops of nystatin 3000 units per ml.— H. W. Ross and P. R. Laibson, *Am. J. Ophthal.*, 1972, *74*, 438.

See also under Candidiasis, Ocular.

Preparations

Creams

Nystatin Cream *(U.S.P.)*. A cream containing nystatin 100 000 units per g. Store in airtight containers.

Ear-drops

Nystatin Ear Drops *(Middlesex Hosp.)*. Nystatin 100 000 units, propylene glycol to 1 ml. Shelf-life 2 weeks.

Nystatin Ear Drops *(Roy. Nat. T. N. and E. Hosp.)*. Nystatin powder 100 000 units, in any of the following vehicles: water to 1 ml (shelf-life 1 week); alcohol 70% to 1 ml (shelf-life 2 weeks); propylene glycol to 1 ml (shelf-life 2 weeks). All products should be stored in a refrigerator.

Eye-drops

Nystatin Eye Drops *(A.P.F.)*. Nystatin 1 g, sodium chloride 900 mg, chlorhexidine acetate 10 mg, Water for Injections to 100 ml. Prepared aseptically. The eye-drops must be freshly prepared. Store at 2° to 8°, and use within 7 days. Protect from light. The label should include a direction to shake the container.

Insufflations

Nystatin Insufflation *(Roy. Nat. T. N. and E. Hosp.)*. Nystatin powder 100 000 units, povidone (Kollidon K30 grade) to 1 g.

Lotions

Nystatin Lotion *(U.S.P.)*. A lotion containing nystatin 100 000 units per ml. pH 5.5 to 7.5. Store at 15° to 30° in airtight containers.

Mixtures

Nystatin Mixture *(B.P.C. 1973)*. Nystatin Suspension. A suspension of nystatin in a suitable flavoured vehicle, prepared freshly by dispersing granules of the dry mixed ingredients in the specified volume of water. Store in a cool place and use within 1 week of preparation. Loses not more than 20% potency in a week at 15°. The mixture should not be diluted; doses less than 5 ml should be measured in a graduated pipette.

Mouth-washes

Nystatin Mouth-wash *(St. Bart.'s Hosp.)*. Nystatin suspension (equivalent to 100 000 units) 1 ml, sterile methylcellulose solution 9 ml. The methylcellulose solution contains methylcellulose '20' 3 g, methyl hydroxybenzoate 100 mg, and water to 100 ml. The admixture is made immediately before use. *Dose.* 10 ml.

Ointments

Nystatin Ointment *(B.P.C. 1973)*. A dispersion of nystatin, of specified particle size, in a polyethylene mineral oil gel basis or other suitable anhydrous basis.

Nystatin Ointment *(U.S.P.)*. An ointment containing nystatin 100 000 units per g.

Pessaries

Nystatin Pessaries *(B.P.C. 1973, A.P.F.)*. Pessaries containing nystatin.

Nystatin Vaginal Tablets *(U.S.P.)*. Vaginal tablets containing nystatin 100 000 units, with suitable binders, diluents, and lubricants. Store in airtight containers. Protect from light.

Powders

Nystatin Topical Powder *(U.S.P.)*. A dry powder consisting of nystatin and purified talc. It contains nystatin 100 000 units per g.

Suspensions

Nystatin Oral Suspension *(U.S.P.)*. A suspension of nystatin 100 000 units per ml; it contains suitable preservatives, dispersing, flavouring, and suspending agents. pH 4.5 to 6 or, if it contains glycerol, 6 to 7.5. Store in airtight containers. Protect from light.

Tablets

Nystatin Tablets *(B.P.)*. Tablets containing nystatin. They are sugar-coated. Store at a temperature not exceeding 25°; under these conditions they may be expected to retain their potency for not less than 3 years.

Nystatin Tablets *(U.S.P.)*. Tablets containing nystatin 500 000 units; they may be coated. For oral use only. Store in airtight containers. Protect from light.

Proprietary Preparations

Multilind *(FAIR Laboratories, UK: Squibb, UK)*. Nystatin, available as ointment containing 100 000 units per g, with zinc oxide 5%.

Nyspes *(DDSA Pharmaceuticals, UK)*. Nystatin, available as pessaries each containing 100 000 units.

Nystadermal *(Squibb, UK)*. A cream containing in each g nystatin 100 000 units and triamcinolone acetonide 1 mg in a vanishing cream basis. For inflammatory conditions accompanied by candidal infection.

Nystaform *(Dome/Hollister-Stier, UK)*. Preparations containing nystatin 100 000 units per g and clioquinol 1%, available as **Cream** and as **Ointment** in a water-repellent basis. For bacterial and candidal infections.

Nystaform-HC *(Dome/Hollister-Stier, UK)*. **Cream** containing in each g nystatin 100 000 units, clioquinol 30 mg, and hydrocortisone 5 mg. For infected dermatoses. **Lotion** containing in each ml nystatin 100 000 units, clioquinol 30 mg, and hydrocortisone 5 mg, in a hydrophilic basis. For intertriginous candidal or mixed infections. **Ointment** containing in each g nystatin 100 000 units, clioquinol 30 mg, and hydrocortisone 10 mg, in a water-repellent basis. For napkin rash with candidal and/or tineal infection and for other infected dermatoses.

Nystan *(Squibb, UK)*. Nystatin, available as **Sterile Powder** in vials of 500 000 units; as **Non-Sterile Powder** in bottles of 3 000 000 units; as **Cream** containing 100 000 units per g in a vanishing cream basis; as **Dusting Powder** containing 100 000 units per g in purified talc; as **Gel** containing 100 000 units per g; as **Ointment** containing 100 000 units per g in Plastibase (a polyethylene and liquid paraffin basis); as **Pessaries** each containing 100 000 units with lactose 950 mg; as **Vaginal Cream** containing 100 000 units in each 4 g in an aqueous cream basis; as **Suspension Ready Mixed** containing 100 000 units per ml; and as **Tablets** of 500 000 units. **Nystan Triple Pack.** A composite pack of 28 Nystavescent pessaries, 42 tablets, and gel.

Nystatin-Dome *(Dome/Hollister-Stier, UK)*. Nystatin, available as oral suspension containing 100 000 units per ml.

Nystavescent *(Squibb, UK)*. Nystatin, available as effervescent pessaries of 100 000 units.

Timodine *(Lloyd-Hamol, Reckitt & Colman Pharm., UK)*. Cream containing nystatin 100 000 units per g, with hydrocortisone 0.5%, benzalkonium chloride solution 0.2%, and dimethicone '350' 10%, in a vanishing cream basis. For bacterial and candidal infections of the skin.

NOTE. The name Timodyne is used as a proprietary name for mefexamide.

Other Proprietary Names

Arg.—Micostatin, Nilstat; *Austral.*—Diastatin, Mycostatin, Nilstat; *Belg.*—Gyno-Nilstat, Nilstat; *Canad.*—Mycostatin, Nadostine, Nilstat, Nyaderm; *Denm.*—Mycostatin; *Fr.*—Mycostatine; *Ger.*—Biofanal, Candio-Hermal, Moronal; *Ital.*—Mycostatin; *Neth.*—Candio-Hermal; *Norw.*—Mycostatin; *S.Afr.*—Canstat, Fungistatin, Mycostatin; *Spain*—Mycostatin; *Switz.*—Candio-Hermal, Mycostatin; *USA*—Candex, Korostatin, Mycostatin, Nilstat.

2597-g

Octoic Acid *(B.P.C. 1954)*. Caprylic Acid. Octanoic acid.

$CH_3.(CH_2)_6.CO_2H = 144.2$.

CAS — 124-07-2.

A clear colourless liquid or a white crystalline mass with a characteristic odour and an acid taste. Wt per ml about 0.91 g. F.p. not lower than 15°.

Practically **insoluble** in cold water; sparingly soluble in hot water; miscible with alcohol; soluble in most organic solvents and in glacial acetic acid.

Octoic acid has antifungal activity against species of *Trichophyton* and *Candida*. It was formerly used in the form of its sodium and zinc salts in dusting-powders and ointments.

2598-q

Pecilocin. An antifungal substance produced by the growth of *Paecilomyces varioti* Bainier var. *antibioticus*. 1-[(2*E*,4*E*,6*Z*,8*R*)-8-Hydroxy-6-methyldodeca-2,4,6-trienoyl]pyrrolidin-2-one.

$C_{17}H_{25}NO_3 = 291.4$.

CAS — 19504-77-9.

A colourless oil with an aromatic odour. Slightly **soluble** in water; soluble in alcohol and propylene glycol.

Antimicrobial Action. Pecilocin exerts an inhibitory effect on the growth of *Blastomyces*, *Cryptococcus*, *Epidermophyton*, *Microsporum*, and *Trichophyton* spp. It has no effect on *Candida albicans* or pathogenic bacteria.

Uses. Pecilocin is used in the treatment of various tinea infections. It has also been used in pityriasis versicolor. It is employed in the form of an ointment containing 3000 units per g; a solution containing 1500 units per ml is available in some countries.

References: G. Holti *et al.*, *Br. J. Derm.*, 1966, *78*, 661; R. R. Wethered, *Br. J. Derm.*, 1967, *79*, 352; C. Harris and C. M. Philpot, *Br. J. clin. Pract.*, 1969, *23*, 449.

Proprietary Preparations

Variotin Ointment *(Leo, UK)*. Contains pecilocin 3000 units per g in a bland basis. (Also available as Variotin in *Denm.*, *Neth.*).

Other Proprietary Names

Leofungine *(Fr.)*; Supral *(Ger.)*.

2599-p

Pentalamide. 2-*n*-Amyloxybenzamide. *O*-Pentylsalicylamide; 2-Pentyloxybenzamide.

$C_{12}H_{17}NO_2 = 207.3$.

CAS — 5579-06-6.

A white crystalline powder. M.p. about 86°. Sparingly **soluble** in water; readily soluble in alcohol, acetone, chloroform, ether, and other organic solvents.

Pentalamide was formerly applied topically, usually in conjunction with other antifungal or antiseptic agents for controlling fungal infections of the skin.

3000-z

Pentamycin. A polyene antibiotic obtained from *Streptomyces pentaticus*.

CAS — 6834-98-6.

A slightly yellow amorphous or crystalline powder. Practically **insoluble** in water; very slightly soluble in alcohol; slightly soluble in methyl alcohol; soluble in dimethylformamide and pyridine.

Pentamycin is an antifungal agent with activity *in vitro* against *Candida* and *Trichophyton* spp. It is also active against *Trichomonas vaginalis* and has been used as vaginal tablets containing 2 mg, sometimes with kanamycin, in the treatment of vaginitis.

Manufacturers
Nikken, Jap.

3001-c

Propionic Acid *(B.P.C. 1954).* Propanoic acid.
$C_2H_5.CO_2H$=74.08.

CAS — 79-09-4.

A colourless or slightly yellow liquid with a characteristic odour. Wt per ml about 0.995 g. **Miscible** with water, alcohol, chloroform, and ether.

Uses. Propionic acid is an antifungal agent effective against *Epidermophyton, Microsporum,* and *Trichophyton* spp. It has been used locally, as an ointment or dusting-powder, usually in the form of its calcium, sodium, or zinc salts.

Propionic acid and its calcium, sodium, and potassium salts are used in the baking and dairy industries as inhibitors of moulds.

Under the Preservatives in Food Regulations 1979 (SI 1979: No. 752) and Preservatives in Food (Scotland) Regulations 1979 [SI 1979: No. 1073 (S.96)], flour confectionery and Christmas pudding may contain not more than 1 g per kg and bread not more than 3 g per kg (calculated on the weight of flour) of propionic acid or its sodium, calcium, or potassium salts.

The use of propionic acid and its calcium, potassium, and sodium salts in food was limited only by good manufacturing practice.— Seventeenth Report of the Joint FAO/WHO Expert Committee on Food Additives, *Tech. Rep. Ser. Wld Hlth Org. No. 539,* 1974.

For background toxicological information, see *Fd Add. Ser. Wld Hlth Org. No. 5,* 1974.

3002-k

Pyrrolnitrin. 52230. An antifungal antibiotic isolated from *Pseudomonas pyrrocinia.* 3-Chloro-4-(3-chloro-2-nitrophenyl)pyrrole.
$C_{10}H_6Cl_2N_2O_2$=257.1.

CAS — 1018-71-9.

Yellow to yellowish-brown, odourless, tasteless crystals or crystalline or amorphous powder. M.p. about 126°. Slightly **soluble** in water; freely soluble in alcohol and chloroform; very soluble in acetone, ether, and ethyl acetate.

Pyrrolnitrin has antifungal activity against *Trichophyton* and other spp. and has been used topically, at concentratons of up to 1%, in the treatment of conditions due to susceptible organisms. Erythema and skin eruptions may occur.

Pyrrolnitrin has antifungal activity *in vitro* against *Candida, Torulopsis,* some *Aspergillus* spp., *Madurella mycetomi, Histoplasma, Coccidiodes, Blastomyces,* and others.— R. Vanbreuseghem and C. De Vroey, *Farmaco, Edn Prat.,* 1977, *32,* 617.

Further references: R. S. Gordee and T. R. Matthews, *Appl. Microbiol.,* 1969, *17,* 690; A. V. Reynolds, *J. Pharm. Pharmac.,* 1979, *31, Suppl.,* 29P.

Proprietary Names
Micutrin *(Seber, Belg.; ISF, Ital.; Seber, Spain);* Pyroace *((Jap.)).*

3003-a

Salicylanilide. *N*-Phenylsalicylamide; 2-Hydroxy-*N*-phenylbenzamide.
$C_{13}H_{11}NO_2$=213.2.

CAS — 87-17-2.

Odourless white or slightly pink crystals. M.p. 136° to 138°. **Soluble** in water; freely soluble in alcohol, chloroform, and ether. **Protect** from light.

Salicylanilide is an antifungal agent which is particularly effective against *Microsporum audouinii.* It has been employed as an ointment in the treatment of tinea capitis (ringworm of the scalp). Concentrations stronger than 5% are irritant to the skin and should not be used.

A series of brominated salicylanilides is discussed under Bromsalans (see p.551). Trichlorosalicylanilide (see p.732) is a chlorinated derivative.

3004-t

Sodium Octoate *(B.P.C. 1954).* Sodium Caprylate. Sodium octanoate.
$C_8H_{15}NaO_2$=166.2.

CAS — 1984-06-1.

A white crystalline powder. **Soluble** in water; sparingly soluble in alcohol. A 10% solution in water has a pH of 8 to 10.

Sodium octoate has the antifungal properties of octoic acid (p.730). It was formerly employed in the form of solution, powder, or ointment, usually in concentrations of 5 to 10% either alone or with other octoates.

3005-x

Sodium Propionate *(B.P. Vet., U.S.N.F.).* Sodium propanoate.
$C_3H_5NaO_2$=96.06.

CAS — 137-40-6.

Pharmacopoeias. In *Fr.* and *Nord.* Also in *U.S.N.F.*

Colourless crystals or white granular powder; odourless or with a slight odour. Hygroscopic at relative humidities above 60% and deliquescent above 70%.

Soluble 1 in 1 of water, 1 in 0.65 of boiling water, and 1 in 24 of alcohol; practically insoluble in chloroform and ether. Solutions are **sterilised** by autoclaving. **Incompatible** with ferric salts. **Store** in airtight containers.

Sodium propionate has the antifungal properties of propionic acid (p.731) and has been used topically in concentrations of 5 or 10% alone or together with other propionates, octoates, or other antimycotics. Eye-drops containing 5% of sodium propionate have been used in the topical treatment of ophthalmic infections.

Sodium propionate is also used in veterinary medicine and as a mould inhibitor in the food industry.

Proprietary Names
C_3 *(Thilo, Ger.).*

3006-r

Sulbentine. Sulbentinum; Dibenzthion. 3,5-Dibenzyl-tetrahydro-2*H*-1,3,5-thiadiazine-2-thione.
$C_{17}H_{18}N_2S_2$=314.5.

CAS — 350-12-9.

Sulbentine is an antifungal and antibacterial agent applied topically in the form of a 3% ointment, gel, tincture, or nail varnish or a 1% powder for treating fungal infections of the skin and nails; suppositories containing 20 mg have been used in the treatment of anogenital mycotic infections.

References: L. Ziprkowski, *Derm. Int.,* 1965, *4,* 169, per *Abstr. Hyg.,* 1968, *43,* 313.

Proprietary Names
Fungiplex *(Hermal, Ger.; Bruschettini, Ital.; Hermal, Swed.; Hermal, Switz.);* Mycoplex *(Alcon-Couvreur, Belg.);* Refungine *(Hermal, Neth.).*

3007-f

Ticlatone. FER 1443. 6-Chloro-1,2-benzisothiazolin-3-one.
C_7H_4ClNOS=185.6.

CAS — 70-10-0.

Ticlatone is an antifungal agent. It has been used as an ointment, powder, or spray containing 0.5%, and as a tincture containing 0.1% in the treatment of skin infections.

Proprietary Names
Landromil *(Wander, S.Afr.; Wander, Switz.).*

3008-d

Tolciclate. K 9147; KC 9147. *O*-(1,2,3,4-Tetrahydro-1,4-methano-6-naphthyl) *m,N*-dimethylthiocarbanilate.
$C_{20}H_{21}NOS$=323.5.

CAS — 50838-36-3.

A white crystalline powder. Practically **insoluble** in water; soluble in many organic solvents.

Tolciclate is an antifungal agent with activity against *Epidermophyton, Microsporum,* and *Trichophyton* spp. It has been used as a 1% cream, lotion, or ointment, or as a 0.5% powder in the treatment of various tinea infections and in pityriasis versicolor.

Tolciclate had a fungistatic activity *in vitro* comparable to that of tolnaftate.— I. de Carneri, *Arzneimittel-Forsch.,* 1976, *26,* 769.

Tolciclate was more active *in vitro* than clotrimazole or miconazole against 14 strains of *Trichophyton* spp., 6 strains of *Microsporum* spp., and 2 strains of *Epidermophyton floccosum.*— A. Bianchi *et al., Antimicrob. Ag. Chemother.,* 1977, *12,* 429.

Reports of the clinical use of tolciclate: L. C. Cucè *et al., J. int. med. Res.,* 1980, *8,* 144; C. Intini *et al., Pharmatherapeutica,* 1980, *2,* 439.

Proprietary Names
Tolmicen *(Carlo Erba, Ital.).*

3009-n

Tolnaftate *(B.P., U.S.P.).* *O*-2-Naphthyl *m,N*-dimethylthiocarbanilate.
$C_{19}H_{17}NOS$=307.4.

CAS — 2398-96-1.

Pharmacopoeias. In *Br.* and *U.S.*

A white to creamy-white powder, odourless or with a slight odour. M.p. 109° to 113°. Practically **insoluble** in water; soluble 1 in 4000 of alcohol, 1 in 9 of acetone, 1 in 3 of chloroform, and 1 in 55 of ether; soluble in macrogol 400. **Store** in airtight containers.

Adverse Effects. Skin reactions including irritation and pruritus may occur; contact dermatitis has been reported.

Antimicrobial Action. Tolnaftate inhibits the growth of *Epidermophyton, Microsporum, Trichophyton* spp., and *Malassezia furfur (Pityrosporum orbiculare),* but is not active against *Candida* spp. or bacteria.

Studies *in vitro* of the comparative activity of undecenoic acid and tolnaftate against fungi usually present in tinea pedis infections.— L. P. Amsel *et al., J. pharm. Sci.,* 1979, *68,* 384.

Uses. Tolnaftate is an antifungal agent used topically as a 1% solution, powder, or cream in the treatment of various forms of tinea and of pityriasis versicolor. Infections due to *Trichophyton rubrum* may relapse and a second course of treatment may be required. It has been used with nystatin when candidal infections are present.

Tolnaftate is not considered suitable for deep infections in nail beds or hair follicles but it may be applied concomitantly with a systemic agent.

Erythrasma. Eight patients with erythrasma benefited from treatment with tolnaftate, 1% solution in macrogol 400. AFter 2 to 3 weeks' treatment the scaly eruption had disappeared and the bright red fluorescence to ultraviolet light was no longer present.— S. Ayres and R. Mihan, *Archs Derm.,* 1968, *97,* 173, per *J. Am. med. Ass.,* 1968, *203* (Feb. 26), A309.

Tinea. A double-blind comparison showed tolnaftate 1% cream and zinc undecenoate ointment to be equally effective in 54 patients with ringworm due to *Epidermophyton floccosum, Trichophyton mentagrophytes,* or *T. rubrum.* An apparent advantage of tolnaftate was lack of irritant effect.— S. O. B. Roberts and R. H. Champion, *Practitioner,* 1967, *199,* 797.

The overall incidence of tinea infections fell from 8.5 to 2.1% from 1969–73 in users of a swimming bath following the routine issue of sachets of tolnaftate (Tinaderm) powder. The incidence of verruca over the same period fell from 4.8 to 1.2% though the relevance of the use of tolnaftate was not known.— J. C. Gentles *et al.*, *Br. med. J.*, 1974, *2*, 577.

Further references: *Med. Lett.*, 1976, *18*, 101.

For a report of miconazole being more effective than tolnaftate in patients with tinea pedis, see Miconazole Nitrate, p.728.

Preparations

Tolnaftate Cream *(U.S.P.)*. A cream containing tolnaftate. Store in airtight containers.

Tolnaftate Gel *(U.S.P.)*. A gel containing tolnaftate. Store in airtight containers.

Tolnaftate Powder *(U.S.P.)*. A powder containing tolnaftate. Store in airtight containers.

Tolnaftate Topical Aerosol Powder *(U.S.P.)*. A suspension of tolnaftate in suitable propellents in a pressurised container. Store at a temperature not exceeding 40°.

Tolnaftate Topical Solution *(U.S.P.)*. Tolnaftate Solution. A solution containing tolnaftate. Store in airtight containers.

Proprietary Preparations

Tinaderm *(Kirby-Warrick, UK)*. Preparations containing tolnaftate 1%, available as **Cream**, as **Powder**, and as **Solution**. **Tinaderm-M.** Cream containing tolnaftate 1% and nystatin 100 000 units per g. For fungal infections of the skin. (Also available as Tinaderm in *Arg., Austral., Ital., S.Afr., Spain*).

Other Proprietary Names

Aftate *(USA)*; Focusan *(Swed.)*; Sporiderm, Sporiline *(both Fr.)*; Tinacidin *(Austral.)*; Tinactin *(Canad., Switz., USA)*; Tonoftal *(Ger.)*.

3010-k

Triacetin *(U.S.P.)*. Glyceryl Triacetate. 1,2,3-Propanetriol triacetate.
$C_9H_{14}O_6$=218.2.

CAS — 102-76-1.

A clear colourless somewhat oily liquid with a slight fatty odour and a bitter taste. *U.S.P.* specifies specific gravity 1.152 to 1.158. **Soluble** 1 in 15 of water; slightly soluble in carbon disulphide; miscible with alcohol, chloroform, and ether. **Store** in airtight containers and avoid contact with metal.

Triacetin is reported to possess fungistatic properties based on the liberation of acetic acid. It is applied topically in the treatment of superficial fungal infections, usually as a solution, cream, or dusting-powder, in concentrations of 15 to 33%.

Use in food. The Food Additives and Contaminants Committee recommended that the mono-, di-, and triacetates of glycerol be temporarily permitted for use as solvents in food. Further studies on hydrolysis and toxicity were required.— *Report on the Review of Solvents in food*, FAC/REP/25, Ministry of Agriculture, Fisheries and Food, London, HM Stationery Office, 1978.

Proprietary Names

Enzactin *(Ayerst, Austral.; Ayerst, Ital.; Ayerst, USA)*; Fungacetin *(Harvey, Switz.; Blair, USA)*.

3011-a

Trichlorosalicylanilide. 3′,4′,5-Trichlorosalicylanilide; 5-Chloro-*N*-(3,4-dichlorophenyl)-2-hydroxybenzamide.
$C_{13}H_8Cl_3NO_2$=316.6.

CAS — 642-84-2.

An off-white to yellowish powder, discolouring on exposure to light.

Trichlorosalicylanilide is an antiseptic that has been used in toilet soap and for the treatment of localised fungal infections of the skin in the form of lotions and ointments at concentrations of up to 5%.

3012-t

Undecenoic Acid *(B.P., Eur. P.)*. Acidum Undecylenicum; Undecylenic Acid *(U.S.P.)*; 10-Hendecenoic Acid. It consists mainly of undec-10-enoic acid.

$C_{11}H_{20}O_2$=184.3.

CAS — 112-38-9.

Pharmacopoeias. In *Arg., Aust., Belg., Br., Braz., Chin., Cz., Eur., Fr., Ger., Ind., Int., It., Neth., Nord., Swiss*, and *U.S.*

A colourless or pale yellow liquid or a white to very pale yellow crystalline mass with a characteristic odour. F.p. 21° to 24°. Relative density 0.910 to 0.913.

Practically **insoluble** in water; freely soluble in alcohol, chloroform, ether, and fixed and volatile oils. **Store** in airtight containers. Protect from light.

Antimicrobial Action. Undecenoic acid is active against some pathogenic fungi, including *Epidermophyton, Trichophyton,* and *Microsporum* spp.

Uses. Undecenoic acid has antifungal properties and is applied topically in the prophylaxis and treatment of dermatophytic infections of superficial areas. It is used as the acid or the zinc or calcium salts.

It is applied to the skin in concentrations of 2 to 10%, sometimes in conjunction with zinc undecenoate, in ointments, emulsions, and dusting-powders. Concentrations greater than 1% may cause irritation if applied to mucous membranes. As with other fatty acids, its antifungal activity is greatest at acid pH.

Undecenoic acid is an effective insect repellent but its disagreeable odour is difficult to mask.

Copper undecenoate is used in veterinary practice.

Proprietary Preparations

Mycota Spray *(Crookes Products, UK)*. Aerosol spray solution containing undecenoic acid 2.5% and dichlorophen 0.25%.

For Mycota Cream and Powder, see p.732.

Other Proprietary Names

Caldesene, Cruex *(both calcium undecenoate) (both USA)*; Decylon *(Neth.)*; Pedzyl *(Switz.)*.

Proprietary Preparations of Related Compounds

Rewocid DU 185 *(Rewo, UK)*. A brand of undec-10-enoic acid polydiethanolamide. **Rewocid SBU 185.** A brand of the sodium salt of the sulphosuccinate monoester of undec-10-enoic acid monoethanolamide. **Rewocid U 185.** A brand of undec-10-enoic acid monoethanolamide.

Synogist *(Maltown, UK: Farillon, UK)*. A shampoo containing 4% of the disodium salt of the sulphosuccinate monoester of undec-10-enoic acid monoethanolamide ($C_{17}H_{27}NaNO_8$ = 396.4).

Other Proprietary Names

Arrow Fusscrème *(undecenoic acid monoethanolamide) (Switz.)*.

3013-x

Zinc Propionate. Zinc propanoate.
$(C_3H_5O_2)_2Zn$=211.5 (or with 1 H_2O).

CAS — 557-28-8.

A white crystalline powder. **Soluble** 1 in 4 of water and 1 in 40 of alcohol. **Store** in airtight containers.

For the uses of zinc propionate, see under Propionic Acid, p.731.

3014-r

Zinc Undecenoate *(B.P., Eur. P.)*. Zinc Undecylenate *(U.S.P.)*; Zinci Undecylenas; Undecilinato de Zinco. Zinc undec-10-enoate.

$(C_{11}H_{19}O_2)_2Zn$=431.9.

CAS — 557-08-4.

Pharmacopoeias. In *Arg., Aust., Br., Braz., Chin., Cz., Eur., Fr., Ger., Ind., Neth., Nord., Swiss,* and *U.S.*

A fine white or almost white powder with a characteristic odour. M.p. 116° to 121°. Practically **insoluble** in water and alcohol; soluble in boiling alcohol; slightly soluble in chloroform; very slightly soluble in ether. **Protect** from light.

Uses. Zinc undecenoate has antifungal properties similar to those of undecenoic acid and is used similarly in the treatment of superficial dermatophytoses.

It is applied to the skin in concentrations of up to 20%, often in conjunction with undecenoic acid, in ointments and dusting-powders.

Preparations

Compound Undecylenic Acid Ointment *(U.S.P.)*. Zinc undecenoate 18 to 22% and undecenoic acid 4.5 to 5.5% in a suitable ointment basis. Store at a temperature not exceeding 30° in airtight containers.

Pomatum Undecylenici *(F.N. Belg.)*. Zinc undecenoate 20 g, undecenoic acid 5 g, macrogol '1500' 70 g, propylene glycol 5 g.

Zinc Undecenoate Dusting-powder *(B.P.C. 1973)*. Conspersus Zinci Undecenoatis. Zinc undecenoate 10 g, undecenoic acid 2 g, pumilio pine oil 0.5 ml, starch 50 g, sterilised light kaolin to 100 g. *A.P.F.* has zinc undecenoate 10 g, undecenoic acid 2 g, sterilised light kaolin or light kaolin (natural) 38 g, and starch 50 g.

Zinc Undecenoate Ointment *(B.P. 1973, A.P.F.)*. Zinc Undecen. Oint.; Ung. Zinc. Undecen. Zinc undecenoate 20% and undecenoic acid 5% in emulsifying ointment.

Proprietary Preparations

Mycota Cream *(Crookes Products, UK)*. Contains zinc undecenoate 20% and undecenoic acid 5% in a water-miscible basis.

Mycota Powder *(Crookes Products, UK)*. Contains zinc undecenoate 20% and undecenoic acid 2% in an absorbent basis.

Tineafax Ointment *(Warner, UK)*. Contains zinc undecenoate 8%, zinc naphthenate 8%, mesulphen 8%, methyl salicylate 2.5%, terpineol 2.5% and chlorocresol 0.1% in a penetrating basis. For ringworm infections of the skin.

Tineafax Powder *(Warner, UK)*. Contains zinc undecenoate 10%. (Also available as Tineafax Powder in *Austral.*).

Other Proprietary Names

Pelsano *(Switz.)*.

Haemostatics

1710-g

Haemostatic substances in clinical use include those applied topically to bleeding surfaces to accelerate the coagulation of the blood. They are useful to control capillary oozing and venous bleeding but should not be expected to control bleeding from arteries or veins when there is appreciable pressure at the bleeding point from within the bleeding vessel. Some such as oxidised cellulose, absorbable gelatin sponge, and calcium alginate may be absorbed.

Aminocaproic acid and tranexamic acid inhibit fibrinolysis and are used systemically in certain haemorrhagic states. Other systemic haemostatics include aprotonin and ethamsylate. Other substances not described in this section but which act as haemostatics when applied topically include adrenaline (p.4), alum (p.283), noradrenaline (p.21), and iron salts (p.872). Certain blood preparations (thrombin, fibrinogen, fibrin foam, and preparations containing thromboplastin—see under Blood Preparations, p.321) are also employed as local haemostatics.

Physiological considerations underlying the use of haemostatics.— D. Ogston and A. S. Douglas, *Drugs,* 1971, *1,* 228.

A discussion of haemostasis, haemorrhage and thrombosis.— D. Ogston and A. S. Douglas, *Br. med. J.,* 1974, *3,* 787.

For a critical review of several general haemostatic agents and recommendations for studies to determine the clinical efficacy of systemic haemostatic agents, see M. Verstraete, *Haemostatic Drugs, A Critical Appraisal,* The Hague, Martinus Nijhoff, 1977.

For a short discussion on the use of antifibrinolytic agents, see G. D. O. Lowe and D. H. Lawson, *Am. J. Hosp. Pharm.,* 1978, *35,* 414.

Haemorrhage due to specific bleeding disorders should be treated where possible by correcting the defect—for example, by transfusion of a missing clotting factor, fresh frozen plasma, or fresh platelets, or administration of vitamin K. In the absence of a correctable defect local measures to arrest bleeding should be tried first. Only if these fail or are impracticable should the use of haemostatic drugs be considered.— *Br. med. J.,* 1980, *280,* 1305.

1711-q

Adrenalone Hydrochloride. Adrenalonium Chloratum; Adrenoni Hydrochloridum. 3′,4′-Dihydroxy-2-methylaminoacetophenone hydrochloride.

$C_9H_{11}NO_3HCl(+xH_2O)=217.7$.

CAS — 99-45-6 (adrenalone); 62-13-5 (hydrochloride, anhydrous).

Pharmacopoeias. In *Swiss.*

A white odourless, crystalline powder or colourless crystals with a bitter and faintly acid taste. **Soluble** 1 in 8 of water and 1 in 45 of alcohol (94%); slightly soluble in acetone; practically insoluble in chloroform and ether. **Incompatible** with alkalis, sulphates, and iron salts. A 4.24% solution in water is iso-osmotic with serum. **Store** in airtight containers. Protect from light.

Adrenalone hydrochloride has been used as a local haemostatic and vasoconstrictor.

Proprietary Names

Stryphnonasal *(Nadrol, Ger.)*; Stryphnon *(Hauser, Denm.)*.

1712-p

Aminocaproic Acid *(B.P., U.S.P.).* Epsilon Aminocaproic Acid; CY 116; EACA; JD 177. 6-Aminohexanoic acid.

$C_6H_{13}NO_2=131.2$.

CAS — 60-32-2.

Pharmacopoeias. In *Br., Chin., Nord.,* which also includes an injection grade, *Roum.,* and *U.S.*

Odourless or almost odourless, colourless crystals or white crystalline powder with a bitter taste. M.p. about 204° with decomposition. **Soluble** 1 in 1.5 of water and 1 in 450 of methyl alcohol; freely soluble in solutions of acids and alkalis; slightly soluble in alcohol; practically insoluble in chloroform and ether. A 20% solution in water has a pH of 7.5 to 8. A 3.52% solution in water is iso-osmotic with serum. Solutions for injections are **sterilised** by filtration. **Incompatible** with laevulose infusion. **Store** in airtight containers.

Adverse Effects. Aminocaproic acid may cause diarrhoea, headache, hypotension, dizziness, pruritus, erythema, skin rash, nausea, heartburn, conjunctival suffusion, nasal stuffiness, diuresis, and muscle pain and weakness.

It may stabilise thrombi once they have formed. Intrarenal obstruction has occurred in patients, especially haemophiliacs, given aminocaproic acid for haematuria.

Rapid intravenous injection may cause hypotension, bradycardia, or arrhythmia.

For reports of muscle weakness, myoglobinuria, and rhabdomyolysis in patients receiving aminocaproic acid, see K. Korsan-Bengsten *et al., Acta med. scand,* 1969, *185,* 341; J. R. Bennett, *Postgrad. med. J.,* 1972, *48,* 440; R. A. Rizza *et al.* (letter), *J. Am. med. Ass.,* 1976, *236,* 1845; A. R. MacKay *et al., J. Neurosurg.,* 1978, *49,* 597; R. J. M. Lane *et al., Postgrad. med. J.,* 1979, *55,* 282; C. W. Britt *et al., Archs Neurol., Chicago,* 1980, *37,* 187.

Glomerular capillary thrombosis in a patient given aminocaproic acid.— D. T. Purtilo *et al.* (letter), *Lancet,* 1975, *1,* 755.

An acute delirious state in one patient was associated with aminocaproic acid.— A. J. Wysenbeek *et al.* (letter), *Lancet,* 1978, *1,* 221. See also *idem, Clin. Toxicol.,* 1979, *14,* 93.

A report of dizziness, weakness, and a grand mal seizure associated with administration of a 6-g infusion of aminocaproic acid in a 32-year-old man with mild haemophilia. No neurological sequelae developed in the subsequent 14 months after treatment.— S. E. Feffer *et al., J. Am. med. Ass.,* 1978, *240,* 2468.

A report of cerebral thrombosis, associated with the use of aminocaproic acid, in 2 patients.— E. P. Hoffman and A. H. Koo, *Radiology,* 1979, *131,* 687.

Acute renal failure and acute massive muscle necrosis occurred in a 20-year-old patient after 7 weeks of therapy with aminocaproic acid 30 g daily for a subarachnoid haemorrhage. Renal function recovered after 4 weeks, and 3 months later muscle power in all limbs was almost normal.— C. K. Biswas *et al., Br. med. J.,* 1980, *281,* 115.

Inhibition of ejaculation. Six reports of dry ejaculation in haemophilic patients associated with ingestion of aminocaproic acid. The effect had so far been completely reversible and was assumed to be harmless, but patients should be warned of its possible occurrence to allay any subsequent anxiety.— B. E. Evans and L. M. Aledort (letter), *New Engl. J. Med.,* 1978, *298,* 166.

Precautions. Aminocaproic acid should be given in reduced doses to patients with impaired renal function and its use is contra-indicated in patients with severe impairment. Its use is not advised in patients with intravascular coagulation. It is not recommended for bleeding into body cavities.

The risk of clotting may be increased in patients taking oral contraceptives and in those with underlying thrombotic states. It should be used with care in haemophiliacs being treated for haematuria.

Heparin was considered safer than aminocaproic acid for treating hypofibrinogenaemic bleeding after intra-uterine death of the foetus. The inhibition of secondary fibrinolysis by aminocaproic acid was theoretically hazardous in intravascular coagulation and might fail to remove fibrin from blood vessels, bringing about acute renal failure.— R. G. Lerner and W. G. Slate (letter), *New Engl. J. Med.,* 1966, *275,* 1382.

Absorption and Fate. Aminocaproic acid is readily absorbed from the gastro-intestinal tract and peak plasma concentrations are reached within 2 hours. It is widely distributed throughout the body fluids and diffuses across the placenta. It is rapidly excreted in the urine mainly unchanged, the greater part of a single dose being eliminated within 12 hours.

The elimination half-life of aminocaproic acid ranged from 61 to 102 minutes.— H. Kaller, *Naunyn-Schmiedebergs Arch. exp. Path. Pharmak.,* 1967, *256,* 160.

After repeated administration of aminocaproic acid 100 mg per kg body-weight by mouth or intravenously it was considered that antifibrinolytic activity would be maintained in serum for about 3 hours, in body tissues for about 6 hours and in urine for up to 24 hours.— L. Andersson *et al., Ann. N.Y. Acad. Sci.,* 1968, *146,* 642.

Further references.— G. P. McNicol *et al., J. Lab. clin. Med.,* 1962, *59,* 15; A. J. Johnson *et al., Thromb. Diath. haemorrh.,* 1962, *7,* 203.

Uses. Aminocaproic acid is an antifibrinolytic agent. It acts principally by inhibiting plasminogen activators which have fibrinolytic properties and to a lesser degree by inhibiting plasmin. It is used in the treatment of severe haemorrhage associated with excessive fibrinolysis. However, by inhibiting fibrinolysis it may interfere with the normal mechanism for maintaining the patency of blood vessels, and its use may be dangerous in the presence of an underlying thrombosing state, which, in some haemorrhagic states, can occur at the same time as excessive fibrinolysis.

Aminocaproic acid is used in the treatment of haemorrhage with fibrinolysis occurring in some forms of surgery, including surgery of the prostate and urinary tract, and in haematuria, as well as in haemorrhage caused by the administration of plasminogen activators such as streptokinase and urokinase. It has also been given in haemorrhage due to obstetric complications, in selected cases of menorrhagia, in neoplasms such as metastatic carcinoma of the prostate and leukaemia, in hepatic cirrhosis, and in angioneurotic oedema. It is of little value in controlling spontaneous haemorrhage due to coagulation defects or where there is loss of vascular integrity, but may be used with coagulation factor concentrates before dental extraction in patients with congenital bleeding disorders.

Aminocaproic acid may be given by mouth or by slow intravenous infusion diluted with sodium chloride injection, dextrose injection, or compound sodium chloride injection. An initial dose of 5 g is followed by 1 to 1.25 g every hour to maintain a plasma concentration of about 130 µg per ml. Alternatively 3 to 6 g has been given 4 to 6 times daily.

The usual dose by intravenous infusion for severe haematuria following prostatectomy and surgery of the urinary tract is 4 to 5 g in the first hour followed by 1 g per hour for about 8 hours or until bleeding has been controlled. A 0.5% solution may be used as a bladder irrigation for postoperative haemorrhage from the bladder. After dental extraction in haemophiliacs a sterile 10% solution may be used to rinse the sockets, and plugs moistened with the solution may be inserted into the sockets.

Aminocaproic acid was considered to be an effective haemostatic agent when used in menorrhagia, when given before prostatectomy and when given before dental extractions with coagulation factor concentrates to patients with congenital bleeding disorders.— M. Verstraete, *Haemostatic Drugs, A Critical Appraisal,* The Hague, Martinus Nijhoff, 1977, p. 118.

A review of the actions and uses of aminocaproic acid.— J. D. Griffin and L. Ellman, *Semin. Thromb. Hemost.,* 1978, *5,* 27.

Allergy. Aminocaproic acid was used to prevent allergic reactions to iodine preparations used in pyelography.— D. Kimche *et al., Harefuah,* 1968, *74,* 15, per *Int. pharm. Abstr.* 1968, *5,* 544.

Angioneurotic oedema. In a double-blind crossover

study, 5 patients with hereditary angioneurotic oedema were given courses of either aminocaproic acid 16 g daily in divided doses, or a placebo, each course lasting 30 days. Four of the 5 patients had attacks of angio-oedema during each placebo course but no clinically important attacks during the aminocaproic acid course. Reduction of the dose lessened weakness and fatigue, which were the main side-effects noted by patients.— M. M. Frank *et al., New Engl. J. Med.*, 1972, *286*, 808. Of a further 15 patients who received aminocaproic acid for periods of 6 months to 5 years 13 responded to treatment. About 25% of patients might experience muscle discomfort with 15 g daily. Lower doses of 8 to 10 g daily were considered effective but adults did not usually respond to a daily dose of less than 7 g.— *idem, Ann. intern. Med.*, 1976, *84*, 580. A caution on prophylactic use for dental procedures.— *idem* (letter), *New Engl. J. Med.*, 1977, *296*, 1235.

The dose of aminocaproic acid was assessed in 9 patients with hereditary angioneurotic oedema. Children under 11 years of age tolerated 3 g daily and patients over 11 years of age were able to take 6 g daily without side-effects. However, 3 of the most severely affected patients still experienced some attacks.— C. M. Gwynn, *Archs Dis. Childh.* 1974, *49*, 636.

A 6-year-old boy with hereditary angioneurotic oedema was progressing satisfactorily on aminocaproic acid 3 g six-hourly.— B. Thalayasingham (letter), *Lancet*, 1976,, *1*, 299.

Congenital heart disease. Aminocaproic acid, 4 g initially in adults and 2 g in children followed hourly by 0.75 to 1 g in adults and 250 to 500 mg in children, reduced fibrinolytic activity in 4 patients with cyanotic congenital heart disease. The same hourly dose was given by intravenous infusion in dextrose injection preoperatively, during surgery, and for 6 hours postoperatively.— H. R. Gralnick, *Lancet*, 1970, *1*, 1204.

Epistaxis. Aminocaproic acid or tranexamic acid, given intravenously, had been used successfully in epistaxis when recumbency, sedation, and external compression had failed.— R. H. Hardy (letter), *Br. med. J.*, 1974, *2*, 224.

Haematuria. Haematuria in 22 patients with sickle-cell disorders subsided in about 2 days after treatment with aminocaproic acid. Treatment should be limited to those patients whose haematuria is either unusually severe or prolonged.— W. D. Black *et al., Archs intern. Med.*, 1976, *136*, 678. See also R. Vega *et al., J. Urol.*, 1971, *105*, 522.

Haemophilia. The administration of aminocaproic acid 0.5 to 1 g per kg body-weight daily by mouth or intravenously for 4 weeks reduced the need for cryoprecipitated plasma concentrates or fresh frozen plasma in 46 patients with haemophilia A or B who underwent synovectomy.— E. Starti *et al., New Engl. J. Med.*, 1972, *287*, 198.

References to use in haemophiliacs following dental extractions.— P. N. Walsh *et al., Br. J. Haemat.*, 1971, *20*, 463; J. J. Corrigan, *J. Pediat.*, 1972, *80*, 124; H. L. Needleman *et al., J. Am. dent. Ass.*, 1976, *93*, 586.

Haemorrhage. Aminocaproic acid, 16 g daily by mouth, reduced the mean daily blood loss from a secondary tumour deposit in the arm from 216 ml to 135 ml in a 70-year-old woman with a giant cell carcinoma of the lung. When increased to 24 g daily, the daily blood loss fell to 18 ml. The tumour was rich in plasminogen activator, but only minor fibrinolytic abnormalities were found in the systemic circulation.— J. F. Davidson *et al., Br. med. J.* 1969, *1*, 88.

A review of the use of aminocaproic acid for the bleeding associated with intra-uterine devices.— *Drug & Ther. Bull.*, 1972, *10*, 78.

The pre-insertion menstrual loss in 56 women about to be fitted with the Lippes D intra-uterine device was about 43 ml. In 28 of the women it rose to 121 ml decreasing to 82 ml by the eighth period. In 28 women given aminocaproic acid 3 g four times daily for 7 days after insertion, then a similar dose during menstruation, blood loss rose to 54 ml—significantly less than in the controls. Blood loss in 35 other women already fitted with intra-uterine devices fell from 100 to 41 to 50 ml when given aminocaproic acid during menstruation.— J. M. Kasonde and J. Bonnar, *Br. med. J.*, 1975, *4*, 17. See also *idem*, 21.

Secondary haemorrhage occurred in 1 of 32 patients with traumatic hyphema who were treated with aminocaproic acid 100 mg per kg body-weight every 4 hours for 5 days compared with 9 of 27 similar patients who received a placebo. It was recommended that treatment with aminocaproic acid should begin as early as possible in the first 24 hours of the initial hyphema.— E. R. Crouch and M. Frenkel, *Am. J. Ophthal.*, 1976, *81*, 355.

A beneficial response to aminocaproic acid in 6 patients with severe bleeding following renal biopsy. The average dose was 9.6 g daily and the mean duration of treatment was 17.3 days. One patient experienced persistent clots in the bladder and ureter.— E. Savdie *et al., Br. J. Urol.*, 1978, *50*, 8.

Intracranial. In 20 patients with aneurysmal subarachnoid haemorrhage aminocaproic acid was given, 4 g every 4 hours by mouth or 1 g every hour by intravenous infusion, until surgery. Two patients died, 1 from pulmonary embolism. There were no recurrent haemorrhages within 6 weeks of the initial haemorrhage.— G. Corkill, *Med. J. Aust.*, 1974, *1*, 468.

Aminocaproic acid 4 g every 4 hours did not appear to reduce the incidence of rebleeding from intracranial aneurysms. Increasing the dose to 3 g every 2 hours was associated in 5 of 9 patients with a second subarachnoid haemorrhage. Extensive muscle necrosis was observed in 1 patient given the lower dose. In view of the toxic effects of aminocaproic acid it was considered that this use was not justified.— M. D. M. Shaw and J. D. Miller (letter), *Lancet*, 1974, *2*, 847.

Aminocaproic acid 6 g six times daily by mouth or intravenously was given to 83 patients with spontaneous subarachnoid haemorrhage; 82 similar patients acted as controls. Only 3 patients (one of whom died) in the aminocaproic acid group suffered recurrence of haemorrhage, whereas in the control group 22 suffered recurrence and 10 died. Nausea, vomiting, and slight diarrhoea occurred in 10% of the patients given aminocaproic acid; 3 patients required intravenous administration to control diarrhoea. The incidence of deep-vein thrombosis was the same in both groups, and one patient in each group died of pulmonary embolism.— U. M. Chowdhary *et al., Lancet*, 1979, *1*, 741. Severe criticism.— A. R. Wintzen and J. van Rossum (letter), *ibid.*, 1084.

Lepra reactions. For a favourable report of the use of aminocaproic acid in reducing lepra reactions in 12 patients with nodular leprosy, see G. Tarabini-Castellani, *Revta Leprol. Fontilles*, 1967, *6*, 745, per *Trop. Dis. Bull.*, 1968, *65*, 998. A similar report in erythema nodosum leprosum in 2 patients.— Y. Malfart and M. Ducloux, *Bull. Soc. méd. Afr. noire Langue franç.*, 1970, *15*, 300, per *Lepr. Rev.*, 1971, *42*, 293.

Menstrual disorders. In a trial in 215 women with menorrhagia, aged 17 to 51 years, the effects of aminocaproic acid, tranexamic acid, ovulation inhibitors, methylergometrine maleate, and curettage on blood loss were studied. Aminocaproic acid, given to 172 women during 246 periods in doses of 18 g daily for the first 3 days then 12, 9, 6, and 3 g daily during the following days, reduced blood loss by 42.5%. Tranexamic acid given to 85 patients during 205 periods in doses of 6 g daily for the first 3 days, then 4, 3, 2, and 1 g daily, reduced blood loss by 49.7%. Ovulation inhibitors given to 164 women during 284 periods reduced blood loss by 53.7%. Methylergometrine maleate in 82 patients and curettage performed on 78 patients did not significantly reduce menstrual blood loss. A number of women received more than one treatment concomitantly. Side-effects occurring in 91 of 172 women receiving aminocaproic acid and 36 of 85 receiving tranexamic acid were nausea, dizziness, diarrhoea, headache, abdominal pain, and allergic manifestations. Side-effects with tranexamic acid were usually slight.— L. Nilsson and G. Rybo, *Am. J. Obstet. Gynec.*, 1971, *110*, 713.

Rheumatoid arthritis. Of 16 patients with rheumatoid arthritis given aminocaproic acid 10 g daily by mouth for 25 days, 5 showed considerable improvement and 8 some improvement. Of 7 patients with advanced disease given aminocaproic acid 2.5 g four times daily by intravenous injection for 10 days, 3 showed marked improvement. Three of 4 patients with scleroderma also benefited from oral treatment.— G. Gaspardy *et al., Revue Rhum. Mal. osteo-artic.*, 1968, *35*, 531, per *Abstr. Wld Med.*, 1969, *43*, 378.

Surgery. Aminocaproic acid 20 g daily given for 30 hours controlled post-operative bleeding due to systemic fibrinolysis following prostatectomy. Bleeding in a second patient was similarly controlled by aminocaproic acid 8 g daily together with aprotinin, 50,000 units per hour for 18 hours.— E. F. O'Sullivan and J. G. Joyce, *Med. J. Aust.*, 1972, *2*, 1165.

Of 62 patients over 50 years of age undergoing prostatectomy, 30 were given 6 g of aminocaproic acid by mouth and 12 g intravenously over an 18-hour perioperative period and 32 were untreated and used as controls. One death occurred in each group but no significant difference was found between the 2 groups in the incidence of deep-vein thrombosis.— I. C. Gordon-Smith *et al., Br. J. Surg.*, 1972, *59*, 522.

Thrombasthenia. Aminocaproic acid 5 g pre-operatively and 5 g thrice daily for 10 days could help promote haemostasis in patients with thrombasthenia undergoing surgery. After dental extractions 5 g could be given daily for 5 days.— P. Barkhan, *Br. med. J.*, 1974, *2*, 376.

Thrombocytopenia. Aminocaproic acid, given orally or parenterally, controlled mucosal bleeding in 13 of 14 patients with amegakaryocytic thrombocytopenia. Doses ranged from 2 to 24 g daily, and therapy was continued for up to 13 months.— F. H. Gardner and R. E. Helmer, *J. Am. med. Ass.*, 1980, *243*, 35.

Ulcerative colitis. In 11 patients with ulcerative colitis given aminocaproic acid, 6 g four times daily for 7 days, rectal bleeding cleared within 48 hours in 6, was reduced in 2, and remained unchanged in 2. Treatment was discontinued in 1 patient due to severe nausea and faintness.— R. H. Salter and A. E. Read, *Gut*, 1970, *11*, 585.

In a double-blind crossover study in 13 patients with ulcerative colitis there was no significant reduction in gastro-intestinal blood loss with either aminocaproic acid or placebo.— N. A. G. Mowat *et al., Am. J. dig. Dis.*, 1973, *18*, 959, per *J. Am. med. Ass.*, 1974, *227*, 1193.

Preparations

Aminocaproic Acid Injection *(B.P. 1973)*. A sterile solution in Water for Injections, adjusted to pH 6.6 with dilute hydrochloric acid.

Aminocaproic Acid Injection *(U.S.P.)*. A sterile solution of aminocaproic acid in Water for Injections. pH 6 to 7.6.

Aminocaproic Acid Syrup *(U.S.P.)*. A syrup containing aminocaproic acid. pH 6.1 to 6.6. Store in airtight containers.

Aminocaproic Acid Tablets *(U.S.P.)*. Tablets containing aminocaproic acid. Store in airtight containers.

Proprietary Preparations

Epsikapron *(KabiVitrum, UK)*. Aminocaproic acid, available as **Effervescent Powder 50%** in sachets containing aminocaproic acid 3 g, and as **Syrup** containing 300 mg per ml (suggested diluent, syrup). (Also available as Epsikapron in *S.Afr., Swed., Switz.*).

Other Proprietary Names

Amicar *(Austral., Canad., S.Afr., USA)*; Capracid *(Ital.)*; Capralense *(Fr.)*; Caprolisin *(Ital.)*; Capramol *(Belg., Fr., Ital., Switz.)*; Caproamin Fides *(Spain)*; Ekaprol *(Austral.)*; Epsamon *(Switz.)*; Hemocaprol *(Fr., Spain, Switz.)*; Ipsilon *(Arg.)*.

1713-s

Aminomethylbenzoic Acid.

PAMBA; α-Amino-*p*-toluic Acid. 4-Aminomethylbenzoic acid.

$C_8H_9NO_2=151.2$.

CAS — 56-91-7.

Pharmacopoeias. In *Chin.* which specifies the monohydrate.

A colourless, odourless, microcrystalline powder with a faintly bitter taste. Slowly **soluble** in cold water; soluble 1 in 25 of boiling water.

Aminomethylbenzoic acid has similar actions and uses to aminocaproic acid (see above). Up to 50% of a dose by mouth is reported to be excreted unchanged in the urine in 24 hours; there is evidence of some metabolism to an inactive acetyl compound. Up to 2 g by mouth or 600 mg by intramuscular or slow intravenous injection has been given daily in divided doses.

Aminomethylbenzoic acid was given to 15 women with menorrhagia in a dose of 3 to 4 g daily for 4 to 7 days. Menstrual blood loss was reduced by a mean of 36%.— L. Nilsson and G. Rybo, *Am. J. Obstet. Gynec.*, 1971, *110*, 713.

Further references: I. S. Menon, *Br. J. clin. Pract.*, 1967, *21*, 405; L. Anderson *et al., Arzneimittel-Forsch.*, 1971, *21*, 424; M. Verstraete, *Haemostatic Drugs, A Critical Appraisal*, The Hague, Martinus Nijhoff, 1977, p. 127.

Proprietary Names

Gumbix *(Kali-Chemie, Ger.)*.

1714-w

Aprotinin.

Bayer A 128, Riker 52G; RP 9921. A straight-chain polypeptide proteinase inhibitor derived from bovine lung tissue. It consists of about 58 amino-acid residues and has a molecular weight of about 6500.

CAS — 9004-04-0.

Aprotinin has been reported to be **incompatible** with corticosteroids, heparin, nutrient solutions containing amino acids or fat emulsions, and tetracyclines.

Units. Potency is expressed in terms of kallidinogenase inactivator units. One unit inactivates about 500 ng of trypsin, and is contained in 140 ng of the pure substance. Potency is also expressed in terms of trypsin inactivation.

Adverse Effects. Nausea and vomiting, diarrhoea, muscle pains, and blood-pressure changes have occurred. Allergic reactions such as erythema, urticaria, and bronchospasm have occasionally been reported.

Consumptive coagulopathy occurred in 2 patients with pancreatitis treated with aprotinin. Three cases of disseminated intravascular coagulation had been already reported.— M. L. Lewis (letter), *Br. med. J.*, 1974, *3*, 741.

Anaphylactic shock. A report of severe anaphylaxis associated with administration of aprotinin.— G. Proud and J. Chamberlain (letter), *Lancet*, 1976, *2*, 48.

Pancreatitis. In patients who had operations in the vicinity of the pancreas, the incidence of mild to severe pancreatitis was 22% in 49 patients who had been given aprotinin 100 000 units intravenously during surgery and then 200 000 units daily for 2 days, compared with 10% in 50 patients given a placebo.— D. B. Skinner *et al.*, *J. Am. med. Ass.*, 1968, *204*, 945. See also M. Siegel and M. Werner, *Dt. med. Wschr.*, 1965, *90*, 1712, per F. Clark, *Adverse Drug React. Bull.*, 1977, Oct., 232.

Absorption and Fate. After intravenous injection or infusion aprotinin is reported to have a calculated elimination half-life of about 150 minutes. It is excreted in the urine in an inactive form.

Uses. Aprotinin inhibits proteolytic enzymes including chymotrypsin, kallidinogenase, and trypsin. It also inhibits plasmin and some plasminogen activators which have fibrinolytic properties.

It has been used in the treatment of acute pancreatitis, although there is some doubt about its efficacy, and in the treatment of haemorrhage due to hyperfibrinolysis. For the treatment of acute pancreatitis 500 000 kallidinogenase inactivating units are given immediately by slow intravenous injection at a rate not exceeding 100 000 units per minute, followed by 200 000 units by intravenous infusion every 4 hours.

For prophylaxis before surgery in patients with hyperfibrinolysis, 200 000 units may be given pre-operatively by slow intravenous injection and 200 000 units by continuous intravenous infusion or slow intravenous injection during the operation and every 4 hours postoperatively.

In the treatment of haemorrhage due to hyperfibrinolysis up to 500 000 units may be given immediately by slow intravenous injection followed by 50 000 units per hour by continuous intravenous infusion until haemorrhage is controlled. In disseminated intravascular coagulation with secondary hyperfibrinolysis, dosages up to 1 000 000 units or more may be necessary.

A brief review on the actions and uses of aprotinin.— M. Verstraete, *Haemostatic Drugs, A Critical Appraisal*, The Hague, Martinus Nijhoff, 1977, p. 108.

The properties and assay methods of aprotinin.— Aprotinin, in *Pharmaceutical Enzymes*, R. Ruyssen and A. Lauwers (Ed.), Gent, E. Story-Scientia, 1978, pp. 227–241.

Under controlled dietary conditions, aprotinin 500 000 units administered intravenously over 8 hours to 4 patients with an established ileostomy failed to reduce the output of trypsin and chymotrypsin.— D. M. Goldberg *et al.*, *Gut*, 1970, *11*, 697.

Aprotinin was administered by inhalation to patients with chronic obstructive respiratory disease. It had a favourable effect on the course of the disease and was well tolerated.— B. Rasche *et al.*, *Arzneimittel-Forsch.*, 1975, *25*, 110.

The use of aprotinin in the treatment of post-traumatic shock-lung syndrome.— J. C. McMichan *et al.*, *Medsche Welt, Stuttg.*, 1976, *27*, 2331.

Aprotinin 500 000 units by intraperitoneal application significantly reduced the incidence of post-operative mechanical ileus in 78 children who underwent surgery for perforated appendicitis with suppurating peritonitis, compared with 118 similar children who underwent surgery alone.— S. Perovic *et al.*, *J. int. med. Res.*, 1978, *6*, 89.

Resistance to subcutaneously injected insulin was successfully treated by concomitant injection of aprotinin.— W. A. Müller *et al.* (letter), *Lancet*, 1980, *1*, 1245. A report of a diabetic patient with massive resistance to subcutaneous insulin whose control was not improved by aprotinin treatment, and who subsequently developed anaphylaxis on repeated exposure to the drug.— J. C. Pickup *et al.* (letter), *ibid.*, *2*, 93.

For a report of the use of aprotinin with aminocaproic acid in the control of postoperative bleeding, see Aminocaproic Acid, above.

Myocardial infarction. The use of aprotinin as an adjunct in the treatment of myocardial infarction.— B. Andréka *et al.*, *Therapia hung.*, 1976, *24*, 98.

Further references: F. A. Ceceña-Seldner and J. Villarreal, *Angiology*, 1980, *31*, 488.

Osteoarthritis and rheumatoid arthritis. Improvement was noted in 25 of 28 patients with osteoarthritis or monarthritis who were given intra-articular injections of aprotinin 25 000 units, but in only 4 of 10 with rheumatoid arthritis.— N. Thumb *et al.*, *Wien. Z. inn. Med.*, 1970, *51*, 7, per *Abstr. Wld Med.*, 1970, *44*, 549.

Further references: G. Riffat *et al.*, *Rhumatologie*, 1970, *22*, 19.

Pancreatitis. In a double-blind study of 105 patients with acute pancreatitis 53 patients received aprotinin 200 000 units by intravenous infusion every 6 hours for 5 days. Aprotinin reduced the overall mortality and appeared to modify the severity of the illness when compared with the controls. Also the rise in mortality with increasing age observed in the controls was diminished in the treated group.— J. E. Trapnell *et al.*, *Br. J. Surg.*, 1974, *61*, 177. Comment.— C. W. Imrie and L. H. Blumgart (letter), *Br. med. J.*, 1974, *3*, 626.

Neither glucagon given to 68 patients nor aprotinin given to 66 had any effect on the death-rate of acute pancreatitis when compared with a placebo given to 123 patients. Aprotinin was given in a dose of 500 000 units intravenously immediately followed by 300 000 units by intravenous infusion every 6 hours for 5 days.— MRC Multicentre Trial of Glucagon and Aprotinin, *Lancet*, 1977, *2*, 632. Criticism of the design of the study.— N. Back (letter), *ibid.*, 1978, *2*, 370. Further analysis of the data indicated that neither aprotinin nor glucagon influenced the rate of recovery or incidence of complications in surviving patients.— MRC Multicentre Trial, *Gut*, 1980, *21*, 334.

In a double-blind study involving 161 patients with primary acute pancreatitis there was no significant difference between the overall mortality-rate in patients who received aprotinin and those who received a placebo.— C. N. Imrie *et al.*, *Gut*, 1977, *18*, A957. Similar results in 43 patients.— G. Storck and B. Persson, *Nord. Med.*, 1968, *79*, 651, per *J. Am. med. Ass.*, 1968, *205* (July 1), A170.

Aprotinin was used successfully to treat 2 patients with acute pancreatitis associated with pregnancy. One patient who was 14 weeks pregnant received aprotinin 500 000 units and then 100 000 units hourly for 5 days. Delivery at 40 weeks was uncomplicated and the infant had no abnormalities. The other patient received 50 000 units every hour for 3 days after developing acute pancreatitis which occurred 8 weeks after termination of pregnancy.— C. R. J. Woodhouse, *Br. J. clin. Pract.*, 1977, *31*, 79.

In a double-blind placebo-controlled study in 50 patients aprotinin therapy of high dosage and short duration (2 million units initially repeated after 4 hours) conferred no advantage in the management of patients with primary acute pancreatitis.— C. W. Imrie *et al.*, *Gut*, 1980, *21*, A457.

Further references: *Drug & Ther. Bull.*, 1974, *12*, 90; S. Banks *et al.*, *Drugs*, 1977, *13*, 373.

See also under Adverse Effects.

Pregnancy and the neonate. For the use of aprotinin, in daily doses of 0.5 to 1.5 million units by intravenous infusion, in the treatment of the dead foetus syndrome in 4 patients, see G. W. Pfeifer, *Dt. med. Wschr.*, 1968, *93*, 479, per *J. Am. med. Ass.*, 1968, *204* (Apr. 8), A207.

Use of aprotinin was recommended in the treatment of uterine atony that might accompany disseminated intravascular coagulation and hyperfibrinolysis following accidental haemorrhage in the late stages of pregnancy. A dose of 1 million units should be given intravenously with 500 000 units every 2 hours thereafter until delivery is achieved. Uterine activity could be expected to return in 3 to 4 hours after the first dose with delivery occurring 2 to 4 hours later. Caesarean section was indicated if delivery was not imminent within 7 hours of the first dose. Hydrocortisone could be given for the prophylaxis of the shock-lung syndrome.— G. Sher, *S. Afr. med. J.*, 1975, *49*, 1383.

Urticaria. Aprotinin 100 000 units every other day for 30 to 45 days cured or improved 42 of 52 patients with various types of urticaria refractory to other treatment. Failure to respond was noted mainly in patients with acute urticaria. In a further double-blind study of 20 patients with chronic urticaria 13 were completely cured and 4 improved.— N. Berova *et al.*, *Br. J. Derm.*, 1974, *90*, 431.

Proprietary Preparations

Trasylol *(Bayer, UK)*. Aprotinin, available as an injection containing 20 000 kallidinogenase inactivating units per ml, in ampoules of 5 and 10 ml. (Also available as Trasylol in *Arg., Austral., Belg., Canad., Denm., Ger., Ital., Neth., Norw., S.Afr., Spain, Swed., Switz.*).

Other Proprietary Names

Antagosan *(Fr., Ger., Ital., Jap.)*; Antikrein *(Jap.)*; Gordox *(Hung.)*; Iniprol *(Fr.)*; Kir *(Ital.)*; Midran *(S.Afr.)*; Onquinin, Repulson, Trazinin *(all Jap.)*; Tzalol *(Ital.)*; Zymofren *(Fr.)*.

1715-e

Calcium Alginate

(B.P.C. 1973). Calc. Algin.

CAS — 9005-32-7 (alginic acid); 9005-35-0 (calcium alginate).

Pharmacopoeias. In *Fr.*

It consists chiefly of the calcium salt of alginic acid, a polyuronic acid composed of residues of D-mannuronic and L-guluronic acids; it may contain a small proportion of sodium alginate to give a product more easily absorbed by body tissues. It is an odourless or almost odourless, tasteless, white to pale yellowish-brown powder or fibres. It loses not more than 22% of its weight on drying.

Practically **insoluble** in water, alcohol, chloroform, and ether; soluble in dilute solutions of sodium citrate, sodium bicarbonate, and in sodium chloride solution. It is **sterilised** by autoclaving. **Incompatible** with alkalis and alkali salts. **Store** in airtight containers.

Uses. Calcium alginate is used as an absorbable haemostatic. It is slowly absorbed by body tissues but large pieces may not be completely absorbed. Calcium alginate fibres are prepared in a form resembling gauze or wool and when applied to bleeding surfaces they act as a matrix for coagulation and swell to a gel-like mass.

Alginate dressings are used to pack sinuses, fistulas, and bleeding tooth sockets, to cover or pack wounds and burns, and in the treatment of epistaxis. Alginate dressings may be removed by the application of a sterile 3% sodium citrate solution, followed after a few minutes by washing with sterile water.

Estimated acceptable daily intake of calcium alginate: up to 25 mg, as alginic acid, per kg body-weight.— Seventeenth Report of the FAO/WHO Expert Committee on Food Additives, *Tech. Rep. Ser. Wld Hlth Org. No. 539*, 1974.

Proprietary Preparations

See under Sodium Alginate, p.961.

1716-l

Carbazochrome. Adrenochrome Monosemicarbazone. 5,6-Dihydro-3-hydroxy-1-methylindoline-5,6-dione 5-semicarbazone.
$C_{10}H_{12}N_4O_3$=236.2.

CAS — 69-81-8.

An oxidation product of adrenaline. Yellowish-red or red odourless crystals or crystalline powder. M.p. about 222° with decomposition. Very slightly **soluble** in water and alcohol; practically insoluble in ether. **Store** in airtight containers.

Carbazochrome has been used similarly to the more soluble carbazochrome salicylate.

Proprietary Names
Adcal, Adedolon, Adnamin, Adorzon, Adozon *(all Jap.)*; Adrenocron *(Climax, Arg.)*; Adrenoxyl *(base or dihydrate) (Labaz, Belg.; Labaz, Fr.; Nordmark-Werke, Ger.; Labaz, Neth.)*; Adrezon *(Jap.)*; Cromadren Zambeletti *(Craveri, Arg.)*; Cromosil *(Zambeletti, Ital.)*; Cromoxin *(R. Rius, Spain)*.

1717-y

Carbazochrome Salicylate. A complex of carbazochrome with sodium salicylate.

CAS — 13051-01-9.

A fine, orange-red, odourless crystalline powder with a sweetish saline taste. **Soluble** in water and alcohol. A 10% solution in water has a pH of about 7.

Uses. Carbazochrome salicylate, a soluble form of carbazochrome has been used in doses equivalent to 5 to 10 mg of carbazochrome intramuscularly or by mouth every 2 hours in the prophylaxis and treatment of capillary bleeding, but its efficacy has not been established. It is contra-indicated in patients with salicylate hypersensitivity and should not be given by intravenous injection.

Reports on absence of efficacy.— E. R. Dykes and R. Anderson, *J. Am. med. Ass.*, 1961, *177*, 716; M. J. Inwood *et al.* (letter), *Can. med. Ass. J.*, 1972, *107*, 112; E. J. Diefenbach, *Obstet. Gynec., N.Y.*, 1972, *39*, 357.

A review of the literature suggested that carbazochrome salicylate modestly reduced bleeding time, but most controlled studies had not shown significant clinical effect. The belief of several experienced surgeons that carbazochrome played an important role in reducing postoperative haemorrhage needed support from valid controlled studies.— M. Verstraete, *Haemostatic Drugs, A Critical Appraisal*, The Hague, Martinus Nijhoff, 1977, p. 59.

Proprietary Names
Adrenosem Salicylate *(Beecham, USA)*.

1718-j

Carbazochrome Sodium Sulphonate. Carbazochrome Sodium Sulfonate. Sodium 5,6-dihydro-1-methyl-6-oxo-5-semicarbazonoindoline-2-sulphonate.
$C_{10}H_{11}N_4NaO_5S$=322.3.

CAS — 51460-26-5.

Orange to yellow, almost odourless and tasteless, fine needle-like crystals. M.p. 227° to 228° with decomposition. **Soluble** 1 in 67 of cold water; slightly soluble in alcohol; practically insoluble in chloroform and ether.

Carbazochrome sodium sulphonate has been used similarly to carbazochrome salicylate in doses of up to 30 mg every 2 to 4 hours; 10 mg has been given by intramuscular and 10 to 50 mg by intravenous injection several times daily.

Proprietary Names
Adenaron, Adona (AC-17), Adrechros, Auzei, Blockel, Carbazon, Chichina, Donaseven, Olinate, Ranobi-V, Shiketsumin, Tazin *(all Jap.)*; Adona *(ISF, Ital.; Tanabe, Switz.)*; Emex *(Archifar, Ital.; Archifar, Switz.)*; Hubercrom *(Hubber, Spain)*.

1719-z

Oxidised Cellulose *(B.P.)*. Oxidized Cellulose *(U.S.P.)*; Cellulosum Oxidatum; Cellulosic Acid.

CAS — 9032-53-5.

Pharmacopoeias. In *Br., It.,* and *U.S.*

A sterile polyanhydroglucuronic acid, prepared by the oxidation of a suitable form of cellulose. It occurs as white or creamy-white gauze, lint, or knitted material, with a faint odour and an acid taste. It loses not more than 15% of its weight on drying. The *B.P.* specifies not less than 16% and not more than 22% of carboxyl, calculated with reference to the dried substance. *U.S.P.* specifies 16 to 24% of carboxyl.
Soluble in aqueous solutions of alkali hydroxides; practically insoluble in acids and water. It cannot be satisfactorily resterilised and if a portion only of the contents of a container is used on any one occasion, strict aseptic precautions must be taken to avoid contamination. **Store** in a cool place in containers sealed to exclude micro-organisms. Protect from light.

Adverse Effects. Foreign body reactions have occurred and there have been reports of intestinal and urethral obstruction. Headache, burning, stinging, and sneezing have been reported after use of oxidised cellulose in epistaxis and other rhinological procedures and stinging has been reported after application to surface wounds.

Precautions. Oxidised cellulose should not be used as a surface dressing, except for immediate control of bleeding, as it inhibits epithelialisation; it is also contra-indicated in bone surgery since it delays callus formation and may result in the formation of cysts. Silver nitrate or other escharotic chemicals should not be applied prior to use as cauterisation might inhibit absorption of oxidised cellulose.

In 2 patients the use of small amounts of oxidised cellulose around the optic nerve caused pressure, due to swelling, and rapid loss of vision. In 1 patient rapid removal led to recovery of vision.— F. J. Otenasek and R. J. Otenasek, *J. Neurosurg.*, 1968, *29*, 209, per *J. Am. med. Ass.*, 1968, *205* (Sept. 9), A205.

Uses. Oxidised cellulose is an absorbable haemostatic the action of which is dependent on the formation of a coagulum consisting of salts of polyanhydroglucuronic acid and haemoglobin; the fibres in the material are also reported to provide reinforcement for the fibrin mesh. When applied to a bleeding surface, it swells to form a brown gelatinous mass that is gradually absorbed by the tissues, usually within 2 to 7 days. Complete absorption of large amounts of such material may take 6 weeks or more. However, absorption may be inhibited when oxidised cellulose is applied to areas that have been cauterised chemically. Despite this absorption, removal of oxidised cellulose should be considered once haemostasis is achieved especially if it is used in orthopaedic procedures such as laminectomy or around the optic nerve.
Oxidised cellulose is employed in surgery as an adjunct in the control of moderate bleeding where suturing or ligation is impracticable or ineffective; it should not be used to control haemorrhage from large arteries. Oxidised cellulose is used as a sutured implant or temporary packing, especially in abdominal, urological, and gynaecological surgery. In a clean wound it may be enclosed without drainage, but this is a dangerous procedure in the presence of contamination or infection. It should be packed loosely as tight packing, especially within rigid cavities, may cause necrosis.
Oxidised cellulose is also used as a temporary packing to control secondary haemorrhage in adenoidectomy and tonsillectomy, and for packing tooth sockets.
Oxidised cellulose should be used as the dry material as its haemostatic effect is reduced by moistening. Because of its acid character, it inactivates thrombin, so that if used with thrombin solution it should first be neutralised with sodium bicarbonate solution. Oxidised cellulose inactivates penicillin.

Preparations
Oxidized Regenerated Cellulose *(U.S.P.)*. Sterile oxidised cellulose prepared from regenerated cellulose. It occurs as off-white knitted material with a faint odour. It loses not more than 15% of its weight on drying. It contains not less than 18% and not more than 21% of carboxyl, calculated with reference to the dried substance. It is used similarly to Oxidised Cellulose.

Oxycel *(Associated Hospital Supply, UK)*. Oxidised cellulose, available as sterile 8-ply gauze pads. (Also available as Oxycel in *Austral., Belg., Neth., Norw., S.Afr.*).

Surgicel *(Ethicon, UK)*. Oxidised cellulose, available as sterile gauze. (Also available as Surgicel in *Fr., Ital., USA*).

1720-p

Ethamsylate. Cyclonamine; Etamsylate; E-141; MD-141. Diethylammonium 2,5-dihydroxybenzenesulphonate.
$C_{10}H_{17}NO_5S$=263.3.

CAS — 2624-44-4.

Pharmacopoeias. In *Chin.*

A white, odourless, crystalline powder with a slightly saline taste. M.p. 127° to 130°. Freely **soluble** in water; soluble in alcohol, acetone, and chloroform; practically insoluble in ether. A solution in water has a pH of 6.5.

Adverse Effects. Nausea, headache, and skin rash have occurred.

Hypotension. All of 8 consecutive patients developed transient hypotension (a fall of 25 to 85 mmHg) when given ethamsylate 500 to 750 mg intravenously over 30 to 40 seconds while under general anaesthesia.— L. Langdon (letter), *Br. med. J.*, 1977, *1*, 1472. Comment.— B. Watson, *Delandale* (letter), *ibid.*, 1664.

Precautions. High-molecular-weight plasma expanders may be given after but not before ethamsylate.

Absorption and Fate. Ethamsylate is absorbed from the gastro-intestinal tract and when given by this route it produces an effect within 1 hour. It is excreted unchanged mainly in the urine; some appears in the faeces and bile.

Uses. Ethamsylate is a systemic haemostatic agent. Its precise mode of action is unknown. Its use has been suggested for the prophylaxis and control of haemorrhages due to the rupture of small blood vessels in surgery and in clinical conditions such as haematemesis, haematuria, and menorrhagia.
It is administered by mouth or by intramuscular or intravenous injection. The prophylactic dose is 750 to 1000 mg either intramuscularly with the premedication or intravenously at the induction of anaesthesia. The therapeutic dose is initially 750 to 1000 mg by injection, followed by a maintenance dose of 500 mg by injection or by mouth every 4 to 6 hours. The suggested dose for children is 250 mg by mouth or 500 to 750 mg by intramuscular or intravenous injection in the same schedule as for adults.

Of 12 patients who underwent strictly controlled hypotensive surgery on the pterygoid space and middle ear, ethamsylate, 500 mg by intravenous injection, was effective in reducing capillary bleeding in 4. The curtailment of blood loss occurred suddenly from 10 to 15 minutes after the injection.— C. H. Boyd (letter), *Br. J. Anaesth.*, 1969, *41*, 465.

The effect of ethamsylate on blood loss during and after transurethral resection for enlargement of the prostate was studied in 87 patients, the first 46 being studied on a single-blind basis and the last 41 in a double-blind manner. Analysis was carried out on 76 of the patients with a benign condition who were regarded as a single group, since trends were the same in those studied either in a single-blind or double-blind manner. Patients received ethamsylate 1 g intravenously during induction of anaesthesia and 250 mg intramuscularly every 4 hours postoperatively, while controls received equal volumes of sodium chloride injection. Mean or median blood loss at operation was 17 ml in treated patients compared with 72 ml in the controls and the median postoperative blood loss was 38 and 103 ml respectively.— J. M. Symes *et al.*, *Br. J. Urol.*, 1975, *47*, 203.

A review of ethamsylate; it appeared to be effective in primary menorrhagia and possibly effective in prostatectomy, dental extraction, and adenotonsillectomy. Evidence of efficacy in menorrhagia associated with the use of an IUD was contradictory. Possible interaction with other drugs should be studied.— M. Verstraete, *Haemostatic Drugs, A Critical Appraisal,* The Hague, Martinus Nijhoff, 1977, p. 26.

In a double-blind study in 42 patients undergoing vaginal surgery ethamsylate 750 mg intravenously immediately after the induction of general anaesthesia produced a modest, but not significant, reduction in estimated blood loss, fever, and haematoma formation compared with placebo, but the incidence of deep-vein thrombosis was significantly increased.— M. F. Vere *et al.*, *Br. med. J.*, 1979, *2*, 528.

Further references: T. Hypher and R. Carpenter, *Br. J. Ophthal.*, 1968, *52*, 375.

Menstrual disorders. In a study in 11 women with intra-uterine devices there was no evidence that ethamsylate 500 mg four times daily reduced excessive menstrual blood loss.— J. M. Kasonde and J. Bonnar, *Br. med. J.*, 1975, *4*, 21.

Ethamsylate 500 mg four times daily for 10 days for each of 2 consecutive periods starting 5 days before the expected onset of menstruation reduced menstrual blood loss when compared with placebo in 9 patients with primary menorrhagia and 13 with menorrhagia associated with an intra-uterine contraceptive device. The reduction in the first group was from 124 to 67 ml and in the second group from 65 to 54 ml. There was no change in tampon usage or in the duration of menstrual flow.— R. F. Harrison and S. Campbell, *Lancet*, 1976, *2*, 283.

Further references.— G. Jaffé and A. Wickham, *J. int. med. Res.*, 1973, *1*, 127.

Pregnancy and the neonate. Reduction in the incidence of periventricular haemorrhage in very low birth-weight babies given ethamsylate 100 µg per kg body-weight intramuscularly within 2 hours of birth and thereafter every 6 hours for 4 days.— M. E. I. Morgan *et al.*, *Lancet*, 1981, *2*, 830.

Tonsillectomy. In a double-blind study in 100 children undergoing adenotonsillectomy one group received 500 mg of ethamsylate by mouth on the night before operation, 500 mg by mouth 4 hours before operation, and 250 mg intravenously immediately after induction of anaesthesia. The second group received placebo. There was no difference in mean blood loss between the groups but the frequency of secondary haemorrhage was significantly lower in the ethamsylate group.— Y. R. Arora and M. L. M. Manford, *Br. J. Anaesth.*, 1979, *51*, 557.

Further references: A. J. Gray and W. A. Noble, *Br. J. Anaesth.*, 1966, *38*, 827.

Proprietary Preparations

Dicynene *(Delandale, UK).* Ethamsylate, available as **Injections** containing 125 mg per ml, in ampoules of 2 ml, and 500 mg per ml, in disposable syringes of 2 ml, and as **Tablets** of 250 and 500 mg.

Other Proprietary Names

Aglumin *(Jap.)*; Altodor *(Ger.)*; Antihemorragico Fortuny *(Spain)*; Dicinone *(Spain)*; Dicynone *(Fr., Ital., Switz.)*; Eselin *(Ital.)*; Hemo 141 *(Spain)*; Impedil *(Arg.)*.

1721-s

Absorbable Gelatin Film *(U.S.P.)*.

Pharmacopoeias. In *U.S.*

A sterile, light amber, transparent, pliable film which becomes rubbery when moistened. Practically **insoluble** in water, but slowly digested by solutions of pepsin. **Store** in containers sealed to exclude micro-organisms.

Absorbable gelatin film has actions similar to Absorbable Gelatin Sponge (below) and is used in ophthalmic surgery and for repairs to the dura and pleural membranes. From 8 days to 6 months are required for complete absorption.

Ophthalmic surgery. An absorbable gelatin film was used in 100 ophthalmic operations for scleral buckling. It was absorbed over 2 to 5 months.— H. N. Jacklin *et al.*, *Archs Ophthal., N.Y.*, 1968, *79*, 286, per *J. Am. med. Ass.*, 1968, *203* (Mar. 11), A206. See also *J. Am. med. Ass.*, 1966, *196*, 1033. Ray, G.S. *et al Archs Ophthal., N.Y.*, 1975, *93*, 799; L. M. King *et al.*, *ibid.*, 807.

Proprietary Names

Espongostan Film *(Leo, Spain)*; Gelfilm *(Upjohn, Austral.; Upjohn, Ger.; Upjohn, USA)*.

1722-w

Absorbable Gelatin Sponge *(B.P., U.S.P.)*.

Spongia Gelatini Absorbenda; Gelatin Sponge; Gelatin Foam.

Pharmacopoeias. In *Br.*, *Chin.*, *Ind.*, *It.*, and *U.S.*

A sterile, light, white or almost white, tough, finely porous sponge-like material; it is rapidly wetted by kneading with moistened fingers. The *B.P.* specifies that it takes up not less than 30 times its weight of water at 20°; the *U.S.P.* specifies no less than 35 times its weight. It may be prepared by whisking a warmed solution of gelatin to a foam of uniform porosity, drying, cutting the dried material into pieces of the required size and shape, packing in the final container, and **sterilising** by maintaining at 150° for 1 hour. It cannot be satisfactorily resterilised and if a portion only of the contents of a container is used on any one occasion, strict aseptic precautions must be taken to avoid contamination.

Practically **insoluble** in water, but readily digested by solutions of pepsin. **Store** in containers sealed to exclude micro-organisms.

Precautions. Absorbable gelatin sponge is contra-indicated in aural surgery where it might come into contact with fluid from the inner ear. Its use is best avoided in ophthalmic surgery where the vitreous or aqueous humour is exposed. If used in the presence of infection it should be removed once bleeding is controlled.

In a retrospective study of 265 stapedectomies, total cochlear hearing loss developed in 20 ears in which absorbable gelatin sponge or fat had been used as an oval window seal; the incidence was twice as high in those using gelatin sponge. Absorbable gelatin sponge was considered to contain 0.367% formaldehyde and studies in *animals* showed that formaldehyde destroyed the organ of Corti and outer hair cells.— P. M. Shenoi, *Proc. R. Soc. Med.*, 1973, *66*, 193.

Uses. Absorbable gelatin sponge is capable of absorbing many times its weight of blood. When it is applied to a bleeding surface a clot is rapidly formed which adheres to the tissues, permitting formation of fibrin plugs at the capillary ends. It is not antigenic and may be left in a wound; absorption is usually complete within 4 to 6 weeks.

It may be used either dry or moistened with sterile physiological saline or a sterile solution of an antibiotic; by soaking in thrombin solution (100 units per ml) before application the clotting time may be accelerated. If it is to be used in the moistened condition, a piece of sponge is soaked in the chosen medium, squeezed to remove air and excess solution, moulded to the required shape, and then applied with firm pressure to the bleeding point or area until it adheres.

Absorbable gelatin sponge is effective in the control of capillary oozing and venous bleeding but should not be used to control haemorrhage from arteries or veins where there is appreciable intravascular pressure. It may be used in a variety of surgical procedures (but see Precautions). It should be packed loosely in any cavities to prevent expansion damaging surrounding tissues.

Embolisation of the hepatic artery using absorbable gelatin sponge produced symptomatic relief from hepatic carcinoid metastases in 2 patients.— D. J. Allison *et al.* (preliminary communication), *Lancet*, 1977, *2*, 1323.

A specially prepared sterile treated gelatin powder (Gelfoam powder) had been reported to be more effective than absorbable gelatin sponge in stimulating granulation in the treatment of small ulcers.— M. R. Sather *et al.*, *Drug Intell. & clin. Pharm.*, 1977, *11*, 162.

The temporary occlusion of blood vessels with absorbable gelatin sponge to reduce regional blood flow. Small fragments of sponge soaked and suspended in normal saline or contrast medium are loaded 1 or 2 at a time into a 1-ml or 3-ml syringe and injected through the angiographic catheter into the vessel to be embolised. The gelatin sponge may be rendered radiopaque.— C. A. Athanasoulis, *New Engl. J. Med.*, 1980, *302*, 1117.

Proprietary Preparations

Sterispon *(Allen & Hanburys, UK).* A brand of absorbable gelatin sponge.

Other Proprietary Names

Fibrospuma Esponja *(Spain)*; Gelfoam *(Austral., Belg., Ger., S.Afr., Switz., USA)*; Spongostan *(Belg., S.Afr.)*.

1723-e

Metacresolsulphonic Acid-Formaldehyde. *m*-Cresolsulphonic acid-formaldehyde condensation product. Dihydroxydimethyldiphenylmethanedisulphonic acid polymer; Methylenebis(hydroxytoluenesulphonic acid) polymer. Polycresolsulfonate.
$(C_{15}H_{16}O_8S_2)_n$.

Soluble in water forming colloidal solutions. A 5% solution in water has a pH of about 1.

Metacresolsulphonic acid-formaldehyde is a local haemostatic and antiseptic. A solution containing about 40% or a 1 in 10 dilution of such a solution is used as a styptic, in the treatment of protozoal infections of the genito-urinary tract, and in the treatment and desloughing of burns and surfacc ulcer wounds; a 5.7% lotion is used in the treatment of skin conditions.

Negatan diluted 1 to 10 might be used to control pain and bleeding when applied to mouth ulcers occurring during acute leukaemia.— R. A. Kyle and J. E. Maldonado, *Mayo Clin. Proc.*, 1966, *41*, 383.

Proprietary Names

Albocresil *(Byk Liprandi, Arg.)*; Albothyl *(Byk Gulden, Ger.)*; Lotagen *(Byk, Neth.)*; Negatan *(Savage, USA)*; Negatol *(Valpan, Fr.; Byk Gulden, Spain)*; Nelex *(Byk Gulden, Denm.; Byk Gulden, Norw.; Byk Gulden, Swed.)*; Negaderm *(Byk Gulden, Ital.)*.

1724-l

Naftazone. 1,2-Naphthoquinone 2-semicarbazone.
$C_{11}H_9N_3O_2$=215.2.

CAS — 15687-37-3.

Brown to red crystals. M.p. 185° to 187°. Slightly **soluble** in water; soluble in alcohol and in acetone.

Naftazone is a haemostatic agent which appears to increase capillary resistance and not affect clotting-time. It has been suggested for use in the prophylaxis and treatment of various conditions of venous insufficiency and capillary haemorrhage and has been given in doses of 2.5 to 5 mg thrice daily by mouth or 100 to 300 µg daily by intramuscular or intravenous injection.

For a study indicating that naftazone produced beneficial results in the control of bleeding during and after tooth extraction, see A. Lambert and J. Abravanel, *Acta stomatol. belg.*, 1970, *67*, 365.

In a double-blind controlled study in 40 patients undergoing prostatectomy, 20 received naftazone to control bleeding and 20 received a placebo. Naftazone 4 mg was administered by mouth the evening before surgery and treatment was continued with intramuscular and intravenous injections of 100 to 200 µg before and during surgery. The mean blood loss of 604 ml in the control group was reduced to 314 ml in the treated group and the volumes of blood transfused were 600 and 342 ml respectively.— O. Charles and B. Coolsaet, *Annls Urol.*, 1972, *6*, 209.

Out of a group of 100 patients with diabetic retinopathy, 50 received naftazone 2 mg thrice daily for 15 months and 50 acted as controls. At the final ophthalmic examination 24 patients had improved in the treatment group and 3 in the control group; 5 and 28 patients respectively had deteriorated during the study.— R. Deuil, *Gaz. méd. Fr.*, 1972, *79*, 1917.

Some improvement was obtained in 315 of 396 patients with various varicose conditions after taking naftazone 5 to 10 mg thrice daily for at least one month. Side-effects included gastric pain, nausea, generalised pruritus, and rashes.— I. Berson, *Praxis*, 1977, *66*, 180.

The haemostatic effect of naftazone appeared to be similar to that of carbazochrome.— M. Verstraete, *Haemostatic Drugs, A Critical Appraisal*, The Hague, Martinus Nijhoff, 1977, p. 54.

Proprietary Names

Karbinone *(Du Bled, Belg.)*; Mediaven *(Syntex, Switz.)*.

Naftazone was formerly marketed in Great Britain under the proprietary name Haemostop Injection (*Consolidated Chemicals*).

1725-y

Russell's Viper Venom

Pharmacopoeias. In *Ind.*

The dried sterile venom obtained from the poison glands of *Vipera russelli* (Viperidae). *Ind. P.* allows also venom from other species of *Viperae*.

Soluble in water. **Store** between 2° and 10° when it may be expected to retain its potency for at least 5 years. A solution in water is stable for about 7 days.

Russell's viper venom is a local haemostatic which rapidly activates prothrombin. It has been applied as a 1 in 10 000 solution in the treatment of haemorrhage following tonsillectomy or dental surgery, and in the treatment of external wounds suffered by haemophiliacs. It is used for the assay of coagulation factors.

1726-j

Tranexamic Acid.

Acidum Tranexamicum; AMCA; *trans*AMCHA; CL 65336. *trans*-4-(Aminomethyl)cyclohexanecarboxylic acid. $C_8H_{15}NO_2$=157.2.

CAS — 1197-18-8.

Pharmacopoeias. In *Chin.* and *Nord.*

A white odourless crystalline powder. **Soluble** 1 in 6 of water; very slightly soluble in alcohol; practically insoluble in chloroform and ether. **Incompatible** with benzylpenicillin.

Adverse Effects and Precautions. These are similar to those of Aminocaproic Acid, p.733, but the incidence of side-effects is reported to be less.

Intracranial thrombosis in 2 patients given tranexamic acid.— E. Rydin and P. O. Lundberg (letter), *Lancet*, 1976, *2*, 49. Thrombosis and fatal cerebral infarction associated with tranexamic acid in one patient. The thrombus formed on a localised patch of indolent arteritis which might have been induced by her treatment.— D. Davies and D. A. Howell (letter), *ibid.*, 1977, *1*, 49.

Absorption and Fate. Tranexamic acid is rapidly absorbed from the gastro-intestinal tract. Up to 40% of a dose by mouth and 90% of a dose by intravenous injection is excreted in the urine within 24 hours. It diffuses across the placenta.

In healthy subjects given a single dose of tranexamic acid 10 to 15 mg per kg body-weight, 91% of the dose was recovered in the urine within 24 hours when given intravenously and 38.5% when given by mouth. The serum half-life after intravenous injection was considered to be 1 to 3 hours. It was considered that after repeated doses of 10 mg per kg given intravenously or 20 mg per kg given by mouth, adequate antifibrinolytic activity was maintained in serum for 7 to 8 hours, in body-tissues for up to 17 hours, and in urine for up to 48 hours.— L. Andersson *et al.*, *Ann. N.Y. Acad. Sci.*, 1968, *146*, 642.

Following intravenous administration, plasma concentrations of tranexamic acid show an initial rapid decay, a second decay with a half-life of 1.3 to 2 hours and a third with a half-life of 9 to 18 hours.— H. Kjellman, *Kabi, Swed.*, per M. Verstraete, *Haemostatic Drugs, A Critical Appraisal*, The Hague, Martinus Nijhoff, 1977, p. 140.

Further references: H. Kaller, *Naunyn-Schmiedebergs Arch. exp. Path. Pharmak.*, 1967, *256*, 160; F. Cormack *et al.*, *Lancet*, 1973, *1*, 1207; O. Eriksson *et al.*, *Eur. J. clin. Pharmac.*, 1974, *7*, 375.

Pregnancy and the neonate. Serum concentrations of tranexamic acid in 12 healthy pregnant women who received an infusion of 10 mg per kg body-weight 5 to 25 minutes before undergoing caesarean section ranged from 10 to 53 µg per ml at delivery; serum concentrations in the infant's cord ranged from less than 4 µg per ml to 31 µg per ml.— S. Kullander and I. M. Nilsson, *Acta obstet. gynec. scand.*, 1970, *49*, 241.

Uses. Tranexamic acid has the actions and uses of aminocaproic acid (see p.733) but is reported to be about 10 times more potent. The suggested dose is 0.5 to 1 g given 2 to 3 times daily by slow intravenous injection over a period of at least 5 minutes or 1 to 1.5 g given by mouth 2 to 3 times daily. Dosage should be reduced in patients with renal failure.

The pharmacology, toxicity, and use of tranexamic acid.— J. Kjellman and M. Schannong, *Nord. Med.*, 1970, *83*, 166, per *Int. pharm. Abstr.*, 1972, *9*, 93. See also M. Verstraete, *Haemostatic Drugs, A Critical Appraisal*, The Hague, Martinus Nijhoff, 1977, p. 132.

The beneficial use of tranexamic acid 500 mg thrice daily in the treatment of 1 patient with severe autoimmune disease considered to be systemic lupus erythematosus.— G. Nymand and J. Dyerberg (letter), *Lancet*, 1975, *2*, 546.

Encapsulation of tumour cells with fibrin and inhibition of growth of a metastasising ovarian carcinoma was found in a patient who had been treated for almost 2 years with heparin, tranexamic acid 4 to 6 g daily, and cyclophosphamide intermittently during the first year.— B. Åstedt *et al.*, *J. Am. med. Ass.*, 1977, *238*, 154. See also H. Soma *et al.*, *Acta obstet. gynec. scand.*, 1980, *59*, 285.

A description and family history of a Japanese man suffering from haemorrhagic diathesis due to α_2-plasmin-inhibitor deficiency (Miyasato disease) which benefited from admistration of tranexamic acid.— K. Koie *et al.*, *Lancet*, 1978, *2*, 1334.

Administration in renal failure. Following a study of 28 patients with chronic renal disease this dosage scheme was recommended for tranexamic acid: 10 mg per kg body-weight given intravenously, twice daily to patients with a serum-creatinine concentration of 120 to 250 nmol per ml, every 24 hours to patients with a concentration of 250 to 500 nmol per ml, and every 48 hours to patients with a concentration of 500 nmol or more per ml.— L. Andersson *et al.*, *Urol. Res.*, 1978, *6*, 83.

Angioneurotic oedema. A discussion on the diagnosis and management of hereditary angioneurotic oedema.— R. P. Ward-Booth, *Br. dent. J.*, 1979, *146*, 211. See also C. Scully (letter), *ibid.*, 301.

Seven of 18 patients did not suffer attacks of hereditary angioneurotic oedema whilst taking tranexamic acid 1 g thrice daily, although the attacks recurred during treatment with a placebo. Four patients had attenuated attacks, 6 patients did not complete both drug and placebo studies, and 1 patient showed no improvement. The side-effects were minimal and all patients except the 1 failure continued on a reduced dosage of 1 g daily.— A. L. Sheffer *et al.*, *New Engl. J. Med.*, 1972, *287*, 452.

Tranexamic acid 1 g given every 6 hours for 48 hours before surgery and for 48 hours postoperatively enabled 14 patients with angioneurotic oedema to undergo dental and surgical procedures. Eight of the patients had experienced 1 or more attacks of angioneurotic oedema after previous dental extractions without prophylactic therapy.— A. L. Sheffer *et al.*, *J. Allergy & clin. Immunol.*, 1977, *60*, 38.

Response of 2 patients with idiopathic angioneurotic oedema, with normal C1 esterase inhibitor concentrations, to tranexamic acid.— R. A. Thompson and D. D. Felix-Davies, *Br. med. J.*, 1978, *2*, 608.

A report on experience of treating 21 patients with hereditary angioneurotic oedema over 3½ years. Continuous administration of tranexamic acid 1.5 to 2 g daily has abolished all but the most trivial symptoms. Danazol 300 mg daily is equally successful in abolishing attacks. Premenopausal women and males are given tranexamic acid and postmenopausal women are given danazol. The only side-effect has been slight and transient weight gain with danazol. There had been 2 successful uncomplicated pregnancies and 2 more are under supervision; tranexamic acid was continued after the first trimester in all. All patients with hereditary angioneurotic oedema should be offered one or other of these treatments.— P. Naish and J. Barratt (letter), *Lancet*, 1979, *1*, 611. Further comment. If oral surgery is required, tranexamic acid a week before surgery and a week postoperatively seems to be satisfactory.— P. Ward-Booth (letter), *ibid.*

Haemophilia. Dental extraction was performed on 32 occasions in 28 patients with classical haemophilia or Christmas disease. All received factor VIII or IX equivalent to 1 litre of plasma before extraction and tetracycline 250 mg four times daily. In 14 given tranexamic acid 1 g thrice daily for 5 days starting 2 hours before extraction, the mean blood loss was 61.2 ml (range 1 to 749 ml) compared with 84.1 ml (range 4 to 323 ml) in those receiving a placebo in a double-blind trial. The difference was significant. Two of the treated patients needed further transfusions of plasma compared with 11 of the placebo group. There were no side-effects.— C. D. Forbes *et al.*, *Br. med. J.*, 1972, *2*, 311.

Dental extraction was performed on 51 occasions in 19 patients with haemophilia and 3 with Christmas disease. No prior transfusions of factor VIII were given. Tranexamic acid 1.5 g every 6 hours was started half an hour before extraction and continued until the patient left hospital. Haemorrhage occurred on 5 occasions in 3 patients requiring transfusions of blood and/or cryoprecipitate. Two patients complained of mild diarrhoea. Tranexamic acid was as effective as aminocaproic acid and caused fewer side-effects.— R. W. H. Tavenner, *Br. med. J.*, 1972, *2*, 314.

Further references: G. Bjorlin and I. M. Nilsson, *Oral Surg.*, 1973, *36*, 482.

Haemorrhage. Tranexamic acid reduced the increased menstrual blood loss by about 71% in a double-blind controlled study of 65 women with recently inserted intra-uterine contraceptive devices. The dose which started at the onset of menstrual bleeding was 1.5 g four times daily for 5 days, followed if necessary by 1 g thrice daily for a further 5 days.— L. Weström and L. P. Bengtsson, *J. reprod. Med.*, 1970, *5*, 154.

In a controlled study of 150 patients with upper gastro-intestinal haemorrhage, treatment with tranexamic acid 1.5 g every 8 hours for 7 days was judged to be no more effective overall in the 76 patients treated compared to the 74 who received placebo. When patients with bleeding due to hiatus hernia or oesophageal varices were excluded, treatment failed in 7 of 62 patients given tranexamic acid compared to 17 of 63 given placebo.— F. Cormack *et al.*, *Lancet*, 1973, *1*, 1207.

In a double-blind study, 103 patients with upper gastro-intestinal haemorrhage received tranexamic acid 1 g by intravenous injection and 1 g by mouth 8-hourly for 2 days, then 1 g by mouth 8-hourly for 3 days, and 97 patients were given a placebo. Seven patients in the treated group required surgery, compared to 21 of the controls.— J. C. Biggs *et al.*, *Gut*, 1976, *17*, 729.

Discussion of the use of tranexamic acid for acute gastric haemorrhage.— *Br. med. J.*, 1977, *2*, 1565.

Further references: H. O. Österberg *et al.*, *Acta chir. scand.*, 1977, *143*, 463.

Intracranial. Following a preliminary study with aminocaproic acid in patients with recurrent subarachnoid haemorrhage, tranexamic acid 12 g in 24 hours was given to 182 patients. In the first 14 days only 22 patients suffered further haemorrhage and 14 died.— D. Uttley and A. E. Richardson (letter), *Lancet*, 1974, *2*, 1080.

In a double-blind multicentre controlled study in 51 patients with subarachnoid haemorrhage, tranexamic acid 4 g given daily by intravenous infusion or injection for 10 days did not improve mortality or rebleeding-rates compared with placebo after a 3-month follow-up.— J. van Rossum *et al.*, *Ann. Neurol.*, 1977, *2*, 242.

There were 3 deaths (all from bleeding) in 25 patients with ruptured intracranial haemorrhage treated with tranexamic acid for 6 weeks compared with 11 (10 from bleeding) in 25 patients not given tranexamic acid. Survival-rates in those not undergoing surgery were 13 of 16 (81%) and 8 of 19 (42%) respectively. The dose of tranexamic acid was 6 g daily, intravenously for the first 7 days, then by mouth. It appeared that prolonged antifibrinolysis might permanently improve the natural history of ruptured aneurysms.— R. S. Maurice-Williams, *Br. med. J.*, 1978, *1*, 945. Criticism.— J. van Rossum and A. R. Wintzen (letter), *ibid.*, 1978, *2*, 568. Reply.— R. S. Maurice-Williams (letter), *ibid.*, 831.

Menstrual disorders. In a double-blind study involving 16 women with menorrhagia, for which no organic cause had been found, treatment with tranexamic acid, 1 g four times daily, for the first 4 days of menstruation significantly decreased menstrual blood loss. Side-effects were negligible.— S. T. Callender *et al.*, *Br. med. J.*, 1970, *4*, 214.

See also under Aminocaproic Acid, p.734.

Pregnancy and the neonate. The successful use of tranexamic acid in a patient with abruptio placentae.—

B. Åstedt and I. M. Nilsson, *Br. med. J.*, 1978, *1*, 756.

Surgery. Tranexamic acid reduced operative and postoperative bleeding in 10 children who underwent re-implantation of ureters compared with bleeding in 12 similar children who received a placebo. Tranexamic acid 15 mg per kg body-weight was given thrice daily by mouth the day before operation; on the day of the operation 10 mg per kg was given intravenously immediately before operation with a further dose in the evening. Treatment with 15 mg per kg given twice daily by mouth was continued for 7 days post-operatively. Of the children who received tranexamic acid 6 passed large blood clots in the urine.— J. S. Rö *et al.*, *J. pediat. Surg.*, 1970, *5*, 315.

Mean blood losses following cervical conization were 23 ml in 22 women who received tranexamic acid 4.5 g daily for 12 days compared with 79 ml in 23 women who received a placebo.— G. Rybo and H. Westerberg, *Acta obstet. gynec. scand.*, 1972, *51*, 347.

There was significant reduction of blood loss during and after tonsillectomy in 40 patients who received tranexamic acid compared with 40 similar patients who acted as controls. Later bleeding which occurred in about 28% of the patients who received tranexamic acid and in about 68% of those in the control group lasted for a mean of 2 and 5.6 hours respectively.— G. Castelli and E. Vogt, *Schweiz. med. Wschr.*, 1977, *107*, 780, per *J. Am. med. Ass.*, 1977, *238*, 1974.

Urticaria. Tranexamic acid 1 g was no more effective than a placebo when given thrice daily in a 9-week double-blind study to 17 patients with chronic urticaria and slightly depressed C1 esterase inhibitor concentrations.— G. Laurberg, *Acta derm.-vener., Stockh.*, 1977, *57*, 369.

Tranexamic acid 1 g given 4 times daily reduced the frequency and severity of attacks in 2 patients with intractable chronic urticaria. The effect was maintained when the dose was reduced to 500 mg twice daily.— D. Tant (letter), *Br. med. J.*, 1979, *1*, 266.

Proprietary Preparations

Cyklokapron *(KabiVitrum, UK)*. Tranexamic acid, available as **Injection** containing 100 mg per ml, in ampoules of 5 ml; as **Syrup** containing 500 mg in each 5 ml; and as scored **Tablets** of 500 mg. (Also available as Cyklokapron in *Denm.*, *Ger.*, *Neth.*, *Norw.*, *S.Afr.*, *Swed.*, *Switz.*).

Other Proprietary Names

Arg.—Cyclokapron; *Belg.*—Cyclokapron; *Fr.*—Exacyl, Frénolyse; *Ger.*—Anvitoff, Ugurol; *Ital.*—Amcacid, Tranex, Ugurol; *Jap.*—Carxamin, Hexapromin, Hexatron, Tranexan, Transamin, Trasmalon, Trasmalon-G; *Spain*—Amchafibrin, Amstat; *Switz.*—Anvitoff.

Halothane and other General Anaesthetics

3100-t

General anaesthetics are administered either by inhalation or by intravenous or occasionally intramuscular injection. Those administered by inhalation and described in this section include: chloroform, cyclopropane, enflurane, ether, fluroxene, halothane, methoxyflurane, nitrous oxide,trichloroethylene.

With the potent inhalation anaesthetics accurate control of the delivered vapour concentrations is essential.

Anaesthetic agents administered parenterally produce a short period of unconsciousness, the duration of which varies according to the amount of drug given and its mode of metabolism; varying degrees of analgesia are produced.

Anaesthetic agents given parenterally include: alphaxalone, etomidate, ketamine hydrochloride, methohexitone sodium, propanidid, sodium oxybate, sodium thiamylal, thiopentone sodium.

Adverse Effects of General Anaesthetics. Adverse effects which may occur during general anaesthesia include involuntary muscle movements, hiccup, coughing, bronchospasm, laryngospasm, hypotension, cardiac arrhythmias, respiratory depression, emergence reactions, and postoperative nausea and vomiting.

Malignant hyperpyrexia has occasionally been reported with some general anaesthetics; suxamethonium has also been given in many of the cases. The condition is familial and is often fatal. It is characterised by a rapid rise in body temperature usually accompanied by muscle rigidity. There may be cardiovascular changes, acidosis, and increases in serum-enzyme concentrations.

Concern has been expressed about the possible danger to anaesthetists and other operating theatre personnel from exposure to subanaesthetic concentrations of anaesthetic gases. There have been reports of fatigue; headache; impairment of memory and motor function; an increased incidence of hypertension and liver disorders; an increase in infertility, spontaneous abortion (affecting not only female personnel but the wives of male personnel), still-births, low birth-weight, congenital malformations (offspring of wives also affected), and development disorders. Other possible effects reported include an effect on the immune response and an increased incidence of cardiac arrhythmias, gall-bladder disease, lumbar disk disease, migraine, neoplasms, peptic ulcer, renal disease, and ulcerative colitis. Reports are not unanimous and the ultimate role of anaesthetic gases remains to be established.

For a report of postanaesthetic morbidity in 408 out-patients, see A. Fahy and M. Marshall, *Br. J. Anaesth.*, 1969, *41*, 433; A. Fahy *et al.*, *ibid.*, 439.

Anaesthetics and the immune response.— E. C. Moudgil and A. G. Wade, *Br. J. Anaesth.*, 1976, *48*, 31. See also P. G. Duncan and B. F. Cullen, *Anesthesiology*, 1976, *45*, 522; P. G. Duncan *et al.*, *Anesthesiology*, 1976, *45*, 661; J. Watkins, *Br. J. Hosp. Med.*, 1980, *23*, 583.

Discussions of hypersensitivity and other adverse reactions to intravenous anaesthetic agents.— J. W. Dundee, *Br. J. Anaesth.*, 1976, *48*, 57; J. Watkins *et al.*, *Br. J. Anaesth.*, 1976, *48*, 881; J. Watkins *et al.* (letter), *Br. med. J.*, 1977, *2*, 1084; R. S. J. Clarke *et al.*, *Proc. R. Soc. Med.*, 1977, *70*, 782; J. G. Whitwam, *Br. J. Anaesth.*, 1978, *50*, 677; *Br. med. J.*, 1978, *2*, 648.

A review of the toxicity of inhalation anaesthetic agents.— E. N. Cohen, *Br. J. Anaesth.*, 1978, *50*, 665.

A discussion on the effects of anaesthetics on the cardiovascular system, liver, and kidney.— S. H. Ngai, *New Engl. J. Med.*, 1980, *302*, 564.

Cardiac arrhythmias. The dose of adrenaline required to produce cardiac arrhythmias was less during anaesthesia with chloroform, cyclopropane, halothane, methoxyflurane, and trichloroethylene than it was during anaesthesia with ether or nitrous oxide or in the unanaesthetised patient. Adrenaline could safely be given with halothane and trichloroethylene so long as the adrenaline was in a concentration of 1 in 100 000 to 1 in 200 000 and the dose in adults did not exceed 10 ml of a 1 in 100 000 solution given in a 10-minute period or 30 ml in an hour.— R. L. Katz and G. J. Katz, *Br. J. Anaesth.*, 1966, *38*, 712.

A comparison was made of 5 standard dental anaesthetic techniques and the occurrence of cardiac arrhythmias, in 644 patients ranging from 2 to 69 years old. Arrhythmias were most frequent with halothane (33%) and trichloroethylene (31%), less frequent with vinyl ether (20.5%) and methoxyflurane (21%), and did not occur with intravenous intermittent methohexitone. All arrhythmias ceased within seconds of the termination of anaesthesia and surgery. Since halothane was the only agent to provide anaesthesia of acceptable quality, it was suggested that methohexitone be used to induce anaesthesia which would then be maintained with halothane.— W. Ryder and D. Townsend, *Br. J. Anaesth.*, 1974, *46*, 760.

A discussion of cardiac arrest related to anaesthesia in infants and children.— M. R. Salem *et al.*, *J. Am. med. Ass.*, 1975, *233*, 238.

Further references: R. L. Katz, *Bull. N.Y. Acad. Med.*, 1967, *43*, 1106.

Dental surgery. Sixteen deaths had occurred during or after dental anaesthesia and 11 of them were in young and healthy persons. The usual cause of such deaths was anaesthesia in the upright position; dental patients should be treated lying down.— J. G. Bourne (letter), *Lancet*, 1970, *1*, 525. For a report of the treatment of cardiorespiratory arrest during dental anaesthesia, see J. S. Robinson, *Br. dent. J.*, 1970, *128*, 323. Comments.— J. G. Bourne (letter), *ibid.*, 475; J. S. Robinson (letter), *ibid.*

A brief account of medical risks and dental anaesthetics.— I. Laws, *Practitioner*, 1975, *214*, 365.

The management of collapse under general dental anaesthesia.— E. R. Perks, *Br. dent. J.*, 1977, *143*, 196 and 235.

A review of emergencies in the dental surgery and their treatment.— J. A. Thornton, *Practitioner*, 1978, *220*, 759. See also E. H. Seward, *ibid.*, 766.

See also above under Cardiac Arrhythmias.

Effect on body temperature. In susceptible *pigs*, procaine blocked the initiation of the hyperpyrexial syndrome induced by halothane and by suxamethonium chloride. In 5 *pigs* with the established syndrome, procaine relaxed the rigor and 2 survived. On the basis of these results and the known biochemical changes occurring in the syndrome the following regimen for treatment was proposed: discontinuance of anaesthetic agents, rapid correction of acidosis, active body cooling, procaine intravenously (30 to 40 mg per kg body-weight initially followed by 200 μg per kg per minute until rigor relaxed), support of circulation with isoprenaline under ECG control, and correction of hyperkalaemia.— G. G. Harrison, *Br. med. J.*, 1971, *3*, 454. See also *ibid.*, 441; L. W. Hall *et al.*, *ibid.*, 1972, *2*, 145.

Malignant hyperthermia due to anaesthetics was linked to the presence of muscle disease. Symptoms suggesting underlying muscle disease should be investigated. Symptoms of a myopathy occurring in young boys and associated with malignant hyperthermia were described.— J. O. King and M. A. Denborough, *J. Pediat.*, 1973, *83*, 37.

Suggestions that vitamin E might increase the risk of malignant hyperpyrexia have not been substantiated.— P. James (letter), *Br. med. J.*, 1979, *1*, 200.

Further references: F. R. Ellis *et al.*, *Br. med. J.*, 1972, *3*, 559; *Br. med. J.*, 1973, *1*, 249; G. Owen and R. J. Kerry, *Br. med. J.*, 1974, *4*, 75; D. A. Bloom *et al.*, *J. pediat. Surg.*, 1976, *11*, 185; D. Bennett *et al.*, *Br. J. Anaesth.*, 1977, *49*, 979; P. J. Halsall *et al.*, *ibid.*, 1979, *51*, 949.

For the use of dantrolene sodium in the treatment of malignant hyperpyrexia, see Dantrolene Sodium, p.990.

For the use of procaine in the treatment of malignant hyperpyrexia, see Procaine Hydrochloride, p.922.

Fatalities. During the 5-year period 1969 to 1974 the causes of 232 deaths in South Australia associated with anaesthesia were examined. The anaesthetic agent or technique was claimed to be responsible to a substantial degree for the death in 36 cases.— Anaesthetics Mortality Committee (S.A.), *Med. J. Aust.*, 1976, *1*, 4.

The frequency of death to which anaesthesia contributed in 240 483 anaesthetics administered over 10 years (1967–76) at a hospital in Cape Town was 0.22 per 1000 anaesthetics. This compared with a frequency of 0.33 per 1000 in the previous 10 years. The deaths were responsible for 2.2% of the total mortality from surgery.— G. G. Harrison, *Br. J. Anaesth.*, 1978, *50*, 1041.

Discussions and studies of deaths associated with the use of anaesthetics: *Br. med. J.*, 1979, *1*, 703; R. W. D. Nickalls (letter), *ibid.*, 958; D. M. Moir, *Br. J. Anaesth.*, 1980, *52*, 1; M. Hovi-Viander, *ibid.*, 483.

Hazard to user. Some selected references: D. L. Bruce and M. J. Bach, *Br. J. Anaesth.*, 1976, *48*, 871; A. A. Spence *et al.*, *J. Am. med. Ass.*, 1977, *238*, 955 and 2144; P. O. D. Pharoah *et al.*, *Lancet*, 1977, *1*, 34; A. A. Spence and R. P. Knill-Jones, *Br. J. Anaesth.*, 1978, *50*, 713; P. J. Tomlin, *Br. med. J.*, 1979, *1*, 779; M. P. Vessey and J. F. Nunn, *Br. med. J.*, 1980, *281*, 696.

Precautions for General Anaesthetics. Patients with impaired function of the adrenal cortex, such as those who are being treated or have recently been treated with corticosteroids, may experience hypotension with the stress of anaesthesia. Treatment with corticosteroids, pre-operatively and postoperatively, may be necessary—see Corticosteroids, p.451.

Diabetics, particularly those with a severe unstable condition, may require adjustment to their diet or therapy prior to anaesthesia.

In patients being treated for hypertension, change in therapy may be necessary to provide better control during anaesthesia—see Antihypertensive Agents, p.136. Patients being treated for cardiac arrhythmias should be anaesthetised with special care. For a discussion of beta-adrenoceptor blocking therapy and anaesthesia, see p.1324. Sensitisation of the myocardium to beta-adrenergic stimulation occurs with some anaesthetics and ventricular fibrillation may occur if adrenaline or some other sympathomimetic agents are administered concomitantly, see Adrenaline, p.2.

Serious effects may follow the use of some drugs administered as adjuncts to anaesthesia in patients taking, or having recently taken, some antidepressants, see Amitriptyline Hydrochloride, p.112 and Phenelzine Sulphate, p.128.

Discussions of awareness during anaesthesia: *Lancet*, 1973, *2*, 1305; *Br. med. J.*, 1980, *280*, 811.

Changes in plasma potassium induced by intravenous induction agents.— I. M. Bali *et al.*, *Br. J. Anaesth.*, 1973, *45*, 1238.

Reviews of possible interactions between anaesthetics and other drugs: *Med. Lett.*, 1974, *16*, 19; A. W. Grogono, *Br. J. Anaesth.*, 1974, *46*, 613; A. W. Grogono and J. L. Seltzer, *Drugs*, 1980, *19*, 279; T. N. Calvey, *Prescribers' J.*, 1980, *20*, 14.

A study in 12 patients with forced expiratory volumes in 1 second (FEV_1) of less than 1 litre (less than 50% of the predicted value) undergoing surgery on 15 occasions showed no special anaesthetic or recovery problems for those with mild hypoxaemia, but hypercapnia ($PaCO_2$ more than 50 mmHg) often indicated a need for postoperative assisted respiration.— J. S. Milledge and J. F. Nunn, *Br. med. J.*, 1975, *3*, 670.

Anaesthetics or the drugs used during anaesthesia could interfere with investigations of hormones in plasma and tissue obtained during surgery.— E. N. Cole *et al.* (letter), *Lancet*, 1976, *2*, 1416.

Anaesthesia and surgery in patients with hypertension and ischaemic heart disease.— C. Prys-Roberts, *Ann. R. Coll. Surg.*, 1976, *58*, 465.

In a study in 587 patients who had previously had myocardial infarction 4 of 15 receiving anaesthesia and surgery within 3 months of their infarction had a further infarction (all died); 2 of 18 receiving anaesthesia and surgery within 3 and 6 months had a reinfarction (1 died); after 6 months the reinfarction-rate stabilised at 4 to 5%. Hypertension, hypotension during surgery, and lengthy thoracic or upper abdominal surgical procedures were predisposing factors.— P. A. Steen *et al.*, *J. Am. med. Ass.*, 1978, *239*, 2566. See also *Lancet*, 1978, *2*, 1350; *Br. med. J.*, 1980, *281*, 341.

Anaesthesia in multiple sclerosis.— C. Barnford *et al.*, *Can. J. neurol. Sci.*, 1978, *5*, 41.

A discussion of the effect of liver disease on drugs used in anaesthesia.— *Br. med. J.*, 1978, *1*, 1374.

Effect on driving. From a double-blind study in healthy students it was considered that patients should not drive for at least 2 hours after propanidid anaesthesia, 8 hours after alphaxalone with alphadolone, and 24 hours after methohexitone or thiopentone.— K. Korttila *et al.*, *Anesthesiology*, 1975, *43*, 291. Recommendation of a period of 24 hours or 'a night's sleep' before driving after general anaesthesia.— P. J. F. Baskett and M. D. Vickers (letter), *Lancet*, 1979, *1*, 490. Recommendation against driving for 48 hours.— J. Havard (letter), *Br. med. J.*, 1979, *1*, 687; G. S. Routh (letter), *Lancet*, 1979, *1*, 673.

Porphyria. The successful anaesthetic and analgesic management of a patient with acute intermittent porphyria who required caesarean section. The safety of the use of various agents in porphyria is briefly discussed.— S. C. Allen and G. A. D. Rees, *Br. J. Anaesth.*, 1980, *52*, 835.

Sickle-cell anaemia. Local analgesia should be used for dental procedures in patients with sickle-cell anaemia, whenever possible, to avoid a haemolytic crisis which might occur due to hypoxia during general anaesthesia.— J. S. Robinson, *Br. dent. J.*, 1970, *128*, 165.

A simple regimen for anaesthesia in sickle-cell disorders.— K. A. Oduro and J. F. Searle, *Br. med. J.*, 1972, *4*, 596. A plea for the use of dextrose and sodium bicarbonate to reduce sickling.— H. Lehmann (letter), *ibid.*, 1973, *1*, 290.

The effects of cyclopropane, fluroxene, halothane, and methoxyflurane on sickle-cell anaemia were studied in 19 patients. No deaths occurred nor was there any toxicity attributed to the anaesthetics. There was a considerable reduction in sickling in arterial and especially venous blood during anaesthesia. Some patients continued to show some improvement after recovery; sickling in the other patients returned to preanaesthetic states. Ventilation was slightly increased and oxygen inspiration greatly increased during anaesthesia.— A. L. Maduska *et al.*, *Anesth. Analg. curr. Res.*, 1975, *54*, 361.

Experience of administering general anaesthesia on 284 occasions to 200 patients with sickle-cell disease suggested that careful anaesthetic technique and selective, not routine, blood transfusion was associated with minimal morbidity and mortality.— J. Homi *et al.*, *Br. med. J.*, 1979, *1*, 1599.

Preparation for General Anaesthesia. Treatment is often given as premedication prior to the induction of anaesthesia to diminish some of the side-effects of the anaesthetic and to assist the induction process. Atropine or a similiar antisialogogue may be given to reduce the increased bronchial and salivary secretions and to reduce vagal predominance sometimes shown as bradycardia and hypotension. Sedatives and tranquillisers are often given to reduce anxiety and apprehension. Narcotic analgesics are commonly used if pain is present.

A review of drugs used for premedication.— *Med. Lett.*, 1973, *15*, 71.

Uses of General Anaesthetics. General anaesthetics depress the central nervous system and produce loss of consciousness. An ideal anaesthetic agent would produce unconsciousness, analgesia, and muscle relaxation suitable for all surgical procedures and be metabolically inert and rapidly eliminated. No single agent in safe concentrations fulfils all these requirements and it is customary to employ a number of agents to produce the required surgical conditions. A typical anaesthetic sequence is: induction with a short-acting barbiturate, such as thiopentone; intubation after the use of suxamethonium chloride, maintenance of unconsciousness with an inhalation anaesthetic, such as halothane vaporised with nitrous oxide and oxygen; and supplementary analgesia obtained by injection of such drugs as morphine, pethidine, or phenoperidine. If muscle relaxation is required a skeletal muscle relaxant, such as tubocurarine, is injected. If unconsciousness is not required, adequate conditions for some surgical procedures can be obtained with local anaesthetic techniques (see p.901) or by the injection of analgesics in conjunction with tranquillisers (see p.1001).

A review of the effects of anaesthetics on carbohydrate metabolism.— R. S. J. Clarke, *Br. J. Anaesth.*, 1973, *45*, 237.

A review of the effects of anaesthetics on endogenous hormones.— T. Oyama, *Br. J. Anaesth.*, 1973, *45*, 276.

Brief reviews of advances in anaesthesia: R. S. J. Clarke, *Practitioner*, 1976, *217*, 611; P. K. Barnes, *ibid.*, 1980, *224*, 1045.

In a total of 41 patients recovery after dental or minor surgery (as assessed by 11 motor and cognitive tests) was most rapid after short exposure to halothane in 70 to 80% nitrous oxide in oxygen, and was progressively longer after methohexitone, long exposure to halothane and nitrous oxide, and diazepam intravenously.— G. D. Gale, *Br. J. Anaesth.*, 1976, *48*, 691.

A report of a symposium on neurosurgical anaesthesia.— *Br. J. Anaesth.*, 1976, *48*, 717–804.

The use of anaesthesia in the elderly: M. T. S. Roberts, *Drugs*, 1976, *11*, 200; D. G. White, *Br. J. Hosp. Med.*, 1980, *24*, 145.

The problems of anaesthesia in injured patients.— F. J. M. Walters and M. R. Nott, *Br. J. Anaesth.*, 1977, *49*, 707.

A short review of the use of anaesthetics in day-case surgery.— T. W. Ogg, *Br. med. J.*, 1980, *281*, 212.

A brief discussion on steroid anaesthetic agents.— C. Prys-Roberts and J. Sear, *Br. J. Anaesth.*, 1980, *52*, 363.

For the proceedings of a symposium on anaesthesia and the eye, see *Br. J. Anaesth.*, 1980, *52*, 641–703.

Comment on anaesthesia used during the termination of pregnancy.— I. S. Grant, *Br. J. Anaesth.*, 1980, *52*, 711.

Pregnancy and the neonate. Solubility coefficients of anaesthetics in maternal and foetal blood.— C. P. Gibbs *et al.*, *Anesthesiology*, 1975, *43*, 100.

For a brief discussion of the effect of general anaesthetics in the newborn, see D. R. Cook, *Drugs*, 1976, *12*, 212.

Brief discussions of the use of nitrous oxide, trichloroethylene, and methoxyflurane for analgesia in labour.— D. B. Scott, *Br. J. Anaesth.*, 1977, *49*, 11; M. Rosen, *Br. J. Anaesth.*, 1979, *51*, *Suppl.* 1, 115.

From a study of 920 neonates whose mothers had received epidural or general anaesthesia, with or without pethidine, epidural anaesthesia was considered preferable, and the dose of pethidine should be reduced to a minimum.— R. Hodgkinson *et al.*, *Can. Anaesth. Soc. J.*, 1978, *25*, 405.

3101-x

Halothane *(B.P., Eur. P., U.S.P.)*.

Halothanum; Alotano; Phthorothanum. 2-Bromo-2-chloro-1,1,1-trifluoroethane.

$CHBrCl.CF_3$=197.4.

CAS — 151-67-7.

Pharmacopoeias. In *Br.*, *Braz.*, *Chin.*, *Cz.*, *Eur.*, *Fr.*, *Ger.*, *It.*, *Jap.*, *Jug.*, *Neth.*, *Nord.*, *Rus.*, *Swiss*, and *U.S.*

A colourless, mobile, heavy, non-inflammable liquid with a characteristic chloroform-like odour and a sweet burning taste. It contains 0.01% w/w of thymol as a preservative. Distillation range 49° to 51°. Relative density 1.872 to 1.877.

Soluble 1 in 400 of water; miscible with dehydrated alcohol, chloroform, ether, trichloroethylene, and fixed and volatile oils. Halothane is soluble in rubber. In the presence of moisture it reacts with many metals. **Store** at a temperature not exceeding 25° in airtight containers. Protect from light. On prolonged exposure to ultraviolet radiation halothane decomposes with the formation of halogens and halogen acids.

Thermal decomposition of halothane with the release of halogens might occur if mixtures of halothane and oxygen were in contact with ignition sources having a temperature above 270°.— T. A. Brown and G. Morris, *Br. J. Anaesth.*, 1966, *38*, 164.

A report of explosion during halothane anaesthesia. Providing the necessary static discharge was produced it appeared that an explosion with halothane could occur. Earthing of the anaesthetic machines should be considered.— T. W. May, *Br. med. J.*, 1976, *1*, 692.

The diffusion of halothane through rubber and plastic tubes; a contribution to atmospheric pollution.— D. H. Enderby *et al.*, *Br. J. Anaesth.*, 1977, *49*, 561.

The adsorption of halothane by 4 different grades of charcoal.— D. H. Enderby *et al.*, *Br. J. Anaesth.*, 1977, *49* 567.

Adverse Effects. Halothane has a depressant action on the cardiovascular system and reduces blood pressure. Signs of overdosage are bradycardia and profound hypotension. Cardiac arrhythmias and respiratory depression may occur. Halothane increases the sensitivity of the heart to beta-adrenergic activity.

Hepatic dysfunction, hepatitis, and necrosis have been reported following the use of halothane and have been reported to be more frequent following repeated use. Malignant hyperpyrexia has been reported (see also under Suxamethonium Chloride, p.995).

In the USA the FDA considered that there was sufficient evidence to cause concern about the carcinogenic and teratogenic potential of halogenated inhalational anaesthetic preparations.— J. W. C. Fox (letter), *lancet*, 1976, *1*, 1024.

A report of skin sensitivity in a nurse exposed to halothane vapour.— R. Bodman (letter), *Br. J. Anaesth.*, 1979, *51*, 1092.

Cardiovascular effects. Halothane significantly depressed left ventricular function in healthy subjects.— B. E. Filner and J. S. Karliner, *Anesthesiology*, 1976, *45*, 610.

The development of cardiac arrhythmia in children during halothane anaesthesia.— W. Silver *et al.* (letter), *J. Am. med. Ass.*, 1976, *236*, 2602.

For earlier reports of the effects of halothane on cardiovascular function, see Martindale 27th Edn, p. 687.

Effect on body temperature. There was a greater and more frequent fall in body temperature in a group of 25 children anaesthetised with halothane, nitrous oxide, and oxygen than in 21 children anaesthetised with ketamine.— D. R. Engelman and C. H. Lockhart, *Anesth. Analg. curr. Res.*, 1972, *51*, 98.

Fatal malignant hyperpyrexia occurred in a patient after anaesthesia with halothane and suxamethonium.— M. A. Denborough *et al.*, *Lancet*, 1970, *1*, 1137.

Death due to malignant hyperthermia in a 30-year-old man following anaesthesia with thiopentone and suxamethonium, and maintenance with halothane, nitrous oxide, and oxygen.— R. K. Parikh and W. H. S. Thomson, *Br. J. Anaesth.*, 1972, *44*, 742.

A report of malignant hyperthermia in a 19-month-old boy who was anaesthetised with halothane and then received suxamethonium.— B. Peltz and J. Carstens, *Anaesthesia*, 1975, *30*, 346.

A discussion of malignant hyperpyrexia.— M. A. Denborough, *Med. J. Aust.*, 1977, *2*, 757.

For a comparison of the hyperthermic effects of ether and halothane, see Ether, p.748.

Headache. The incidence of postoperative headache after dental surgery was significantly higher in a group of 25 patients in which thiopentone-induced anaesthesia was maintained with nitrous oxide, oxygen, and halothane, with controlled ventilation, than in a comparable group in which halothane was omitted. Halothane had been shown to produce increased cerebral blood flow due to vasodilatation, with a subsequent rise in cerebrospinal fluid pressure, and these effects might be responsible for the headache. In a third group, in whom nitrous oxide, oxygen, and halothane were used with spontaneous respiration, the incidence of headache was even higher but might have been due to other causes.— M. F. Tyrrell and S. A. Feldman, *Br. J. Anaesth.*, 1968, *40*, 99.

The incidence of headache in the first 6 postoperative hours was studied in 536 patients who had been given 1 of 4 premedication regimens and then anaesthetised with halothane and nitrous oxide with oxygen. The incidence was highest (32.8%) in those premedicated with atropine 600 µg and lowest (8.9%) in those given atropine 600 µg, pethidine 50 to 100 mg, and promethazine 25 mg. In general, the incidence of headache was highest in patients anaesthetised for longer periods.— A. F. M. Zohairy, *Br. J. Anaesth.*, 1969, *41*, 972.

Kidney damage. Urinary oxalate crystals were detected in 6 of 14 patients given halothane.— R. E. Tobey and R. J. Clubb, *J. Am. med. Ass.*, 1973, *223*, 649.

Postoperative renal failure with increased blood urea and creatinine concentrations, which started 11 days after she was given halothane, oxygen, and nitrous oxide anaesthesia for an aortofemoral bypass operation, was reported in a 65-year-old woman; she required weekly dialysis for the following 10 months. The clinical and pathological findings resembled those of methoxyflurane nephrotoxicity.— J. R. Cotton *et al.*, *Archs Path.*, 1976, *100*, 628.

Liver damage. Liver damage has been reported on many occasions in patients anaesthetised with halothane. When a large survey of over 800,000 anaesthetised patients was carried out in the USA by the National Halothane Study (*J. Am. med. Ass.*, 1966, *197*, 775) halothane was found to be no more toxic to the liver than the other anaesthetics but there was an increase in the incidence of hepatic necrosis in patients given further anaesthesia within weeks and this increase was higher with halothane than the other anaesthetics. In 1974 the Committee on Safety of Medicines of the U.K. reported (see *Pharm. J.*, 1974, *1*, 16) that between 1964 and 1972, it had received 130 reports of jaundice following anaesthesia and that halothane had been involved in all patients. The Committee also stated that it agreed with the findings of W.H.W. Inman and W.W. Mushin (*Br. med. J.*, 1974, *1*, 5) whose analysis of the 130 reports showed that 20 patients exposed to halothane on one occasion developed jaundice in a mean of 11.7 days and 7 died from hepatic failure; 49 exposed on 2 occasions developed jaundice in a mean of 6.7 days and 26 died; 29 exposed on 3 occasions developed jaundice in a mean of 4.6 days and 17 died; 12 of 16 exposed on 4 or more occasions developed jaundice in a mean of 5.3 days and 10 of the 16 died. There were also 16 patients with incomplete anaesthetic histories of whom 6 died. Inman and Mushin considered that there was strong evidence that repeated exposure, especially within a short period, increased the risk of jaundice. This analysis and the conclusions were not universally accepted.

A Working Party set up by the MRC accepted (*Br. J. Anaesth.*, 1976, *48*, 1037) that unexplained jaundice might occur on rare instances after repeated exposure to halothane but noted that there was insufficent evidence to state that any other general anaesthetic might be safer in a patient who had been exposed to halothane. J. McEwan (*Br. J. Anaesth.*, 1976, *48*, 1065) reported smaller changes in liver-function tests in 41 patients who had previously had multiple halothane anaesthesia when they were again submitted to halothane anaesthesia than when they were submitted to non-halothane anaesthesia. W.H.W. Inman and W.W. Mushin (*Br. med. J.*, 1978, *2*, 1455) analysed reports of a further 137 patients with jaundice after halothane; considering all the patients the conclusions were broadly comparable with those they had previously reported. Mortality increased with increasing age.

While it is not possible to distinguish hepatitis after halothane from viral hepatitis, most authorities accept that halothane may cause hepatitis, that the incidence is low, and that halothane should not be given to a patient who has experienced hepatitis after an earlier exposure. But a suggestion by S. Sherlock (*Lancet*, 1978, *2*, 364) that halothane should not be used for minor surgery was widely criticised.

The mechanism by which halothane may cause hepatitis remains unresolved; suggestions include an immunological mechanism, oxidative or reductive metabolites, the role of enzyme-inducing agents, and hypoxia.

A 51-year-old woman who required multiple operations for bladder carcinoma remained clinically well after 3 exposures to halothane in 30 days, despite a finding of halothane-induced hepatitis as part of a routine study of reactions to blood transfusions. She was subsequently admitted as an emergency and required surgery which, on the clinical judgement of the anaesthetist, again called for halothane anaesthesia. She made a good recovery without becoming jaundiced.— R. J. Kirkham; M. A. Nassim (letter), *Lancet*, 1978, *2*, 889.

Halothane hepatitis in 3 pairs of closely related women.— R. H. Hoft *et al.*, *New Engl. J. Med.*, 1981, *304*, 1023. See also M. J. Cousins *et al.* (letter), *Br. med. J.*, 1981, *283*, 1334.

Further references: J. Dundee and R. C. Gray (letter), *Br. med. J.*, 1974, *2*, 174; R. Wright *et al.*, *Lancet*, 1975, *1*, 817; J. Trowell *et al.*, *Lancet*, 1975, *1*, 821; B. Walton *et al.*, *Br. med. J.*, 1976, *1*, 1171; P. J. Allen and J. W. Downing, *Br. J. Anaesth.*, 1977, *49*, 1035; *Br. med. J.*, 1977, *1*, 532; M. J. Cousins, *Drugs*, 1980, *19*, 1; *Br. med. J.*, 1980, *280*, 1197; J. L. Dienstag, *New Engl. J. Med.*, 1980, *303*, 102.

For a comparison of the incidence of abnormal liver enzyme values following anaesthesia with halothane or enflurane, see under Liver Damage in Enflurane, p.747.

Poisoning. A 48-year-old woman who ingested halothane 250 ml with suicidal intent recovered after intensive therapy including artificial ventilation. No hepatitis occurred and hepatic function was normal over a period of 4 months. A second patient who ingested a similar amount also recovered.— I. Curelaru *et al.*, *Br. J. Anaesth.*, 1968, *40*, 283.

For a report of suicide by ingestion of halothane, see J. A. E. Spencer and N. M. Green, *J. Am. med. Ass.*, 1968, *205*, 702.

A 16-year-old girl who mistakenly received halothane, 2.5 ml intravenously, had severe pulmonary oedema and right-heart failure. She recovered with oxygen administered by positive-pressure ventilation.— J. Sutton *et al.* (letter), *Lancet*, 1971, *1*, 345.

Three young hospital workers died after inhaling halothane illicitly. Postmortem examinations showed pulmonary oedema in all 3 and blood levels of 0.36%, 0.15%, and 0.5%. Death was probably due to cardiac arrhythmias.— J. D. Spencer *et al.*, *J. Am. med. Ass.*, 1976, *235*, 1034.

Hepatitis developed in 3 hospital workers following illicit inhalation of halothane. The effects appeared to be slowly reversible in 2 workers, although the third worker who had been sniffing halothane for over a year and who had consumed about 1.25 litres in the previous month died following cardiac arrhythmia.— H. G. Kaplan *et al.*, *Ann. intern. Med.*, 1979, *90*, 797.

Treatment of Adverse Effects. Bradycardia may be controlled by the intravenous injection of 300 to 600 µg of atropine. Hypotension associated with bradycardia occurring during anaesthesia may be controlled by reducing the dosage of halothane or by the intravenous injection of atropine. In severe hypotension the circulation should be maintained with infusions of plasma or suitable electrolyte solutions, or with phenylephrine, methoxamine, or mephentermine. Respiratory depression should be treated by reducing the concentration of halothane and by assisted respiration. Both blood pressure and respiratory minute volume increase quickly if the concentration of halothane administered is decreased. Cardiac arrhythmias are usually controlled by stopping halothane and administering oxygen. Beta-adrenoceptor blocking agents may be of value in the more serious cases.

For the use of dantrolene sodium in the treatment of malignant hyperpyrexia, see Dantrolene Sodium, p.990.

For the use of procaine in the treatment of malignant hyperpyrexia, see Procaine Hydrochloride, p.922.

Precautions. Halothane reduces muscle tone in the pregnant uterus and generally its use is not recommended in obstetrics because of the increased risk of postpartum haemorrhage. Halothane should not be used for patients with cardiac arrhythmias.

It is generally considered advisable not to administer halothane to patients who have shown signs of liver damage or fever after previous halothane anaesthesia. Routine premedication with atropine 300 to 600 µg by subcutaneous or intramuscular injection has been recommended to reduce vagal tone and to prevent bradycardia and severe hypotension. Assisted ventilation may be advisable to reduce the risk of respiratory depression, but care must then be taken to avoid forcing high concentrations of halothane into the lungs.

Adrenaline and most other sympathomimetic agents, except possibly in very dilute solution for the control of local haemorrhage, should be avoided during halothane anaesthesia since they can produce cardiac arrhythmias—see Adrenaline, p.2; methoxamine or phenylephrine may be administered cautiously. The effects of non-depolarising muscle relaxants such as gallamine and tubocurarine are enhanced by halothane and if required they should be given in reduced dosage. Antibiotics such as streptomycin that possess neuromuscular blocking activity should also be used with caution. Morphine increases the depressant effects of halothane on respiration and its use during anaesthesia may be followed by post-operative nausea and vomiting. Chlorpromazine also enhances the depressant effect of halothane.

See also Precautions for General Anaesthetics, p.740.

The depression of phagocytosis in patients anaesthetised with halothane and nitrous oxide.— A. Doenicke and W. Kropp, *Br. J. Anaesth.*, 1976, *48*, 1191.

Halothane had an adverse effect on a PO_2 electrode, causing an upward drift in readings.— I. H. S. Douglas *et al.* (letter), *Lancet*, 1978, *2*, 1370.

The effects of drugs, including halothane, on driving.— T. Seppala *et al.*, *Drugs*, 1979, *17*, 389.

Increased cerebrospinal pressure. The use of volatile anaesthetic agents in patients with intracranial space-occupying lesions might cause considerable rises in cerebrospinal fluid pressures even when controlled ventilation was employed.— J. Barker *et al.* (letter), *Br. J. Anaesth.*, 1968, *40*, 307.

In patients with intracranial space-occupying lesions, anaesthesia with halothane, trichloroethylene, or methoxyflurane increased intracranial pressure by a mean of 239 mm of water. The greatest rise occurred in patients with frontal lesions.— W. B. Jennett *et al.*, *Lancet*, 1969, *1*, 61.

Interactions. Sodium bicarbonate, given to induce metabolic alkalosis, decreased total peripheral resistance during halothane anaesthesia and might lead to severe hypotension.— J. A. Kaplan *et al.*, *Anesthesiology*, 1975, *42*, 550.

A study in *dogs* suggesting that frusemide may adversely influence renal function when administered during halothane anaesthesia.— K. M. Leighton *et al.*, *Can. Anaesth. Soc. J.*, 1976, *23*, 48.

Absorption and Fate. Halothane is absorbed on inhalation. It has a relatively low solubility in blood and the arterial tension only slowly reaches the alveolar tension. Halothane reaches the highly vascular tissues in concentrations approaching those in arterial blood; it is more soluble in the neutral fats of adipose tissue than in the phospholipids of brain cells. The blood/gas partition coefficient is low. Halothane is excreted unchanged through the lungs and a variable amount is metabolised by the liver. Bromide concentrations in serum may possibly be sufficient to exert a pharmacological effect. Urinary metabolites include trifluoroacetic acid and bromide and chloride salts. It diffuses across the placenta.

Halothane given to 9 patients produced an initial rise in blood-bromide concentrations followed by a reduction. After recovery the patients showed another higher and more prolonged rise. Eight of the patients were given 1.5% halothane and at the end of 20 minutes' anaesthesia they had blood concentrations of halothane ranging from 50.5 to 106.5 µg per ml. At recovery 10 minutes later the range was 22 to 30 µg per ml. Traces were still detectable after 44 hours.— M. M. Atallah and I. C. Geddes, *Br. J. Anaesth.*, 1973, *45*, 464.

Metabolism of halothane in obesity.— S. R. Young *et al.*, *Anesthesiology*, 1975, *42*, 451. See also R. A. Saraiva *et al.*, *Anaesthesia*, 1977, *32*, 240.

Identification of trifluoroacetic acid, *N*-trifluoroacetyl-2-aminoethanol, and *N*-acetyl-*S*-(2-bromo-2-chloro-1,1-difluoroethyl)-L-cysteine as urinary metabolites of halothane.— E. N. Cohen *et al.*, *Anesthesiology*, 1975, *43*, 392.

The metabolism of halothane, enflurane, and methoxyflurane was studied in 22 surgical patients. Anaesthesia was carried out with either halothane 0.93% (5 patients), enflurane 1.3% (5), or methoxyflurane 0.31% (6), all in conjunction with nitrous oxide in oxygen. A control group (6) were given nitrous oxide in oxygen with pancuronium bromide. Serum concentration of inorganic fluoride was highest in the methoxyflurane group and 2 hours after induction of anaesthesia was 13.18 µmol per litre compared with 2.62 µmol per litre in the halothane group and 7.29 µmol per litre in the enflurane group. On the day of operation a mean excess of 6.226 mmol of fluoride, mostly organic, was excreted in the urine by those who had received halothane, 0.627 mmol was excreted by the enflurane group, and 10.978 mmol by the methoxyflurane group. The amounts of anaesthetic expired unchanged were halothane 72.8%, enflurane 79.3%, and methoxyflurane 34.8% whereas the amounts excreted in the urine as fluoride-containing metabolites were 17.7%, 2.3%, and 46.3% respectively of the total amounts absorbed.— T. Sakai and M. Takaori, *Br. J. Anaesth.*, 1978, *50*, 785.

A study of the time-course formation of the 2 reductive metabolites of halothane, 2-chloro-1,1,1-trifluoroethane and 2-chloro-1,1-difluoroethylene, in the breath of 4 patients.— G. K. Gourlay *et al.*, *Br. J. Anaesth.*, 1980, *52*, 331.

Isobutene concentrations in the breath of patients receiving halothane were significantly greater than in patients receiving ketamine or diazepam.— V. Hempel *et al.*, *Br. J. Anaesth.*, 1980, *52*, 989.

Further references: D. C. Sawyer *et al.*, *Anesthesiology*,

1971, *34*, 230; H. F. Cascorbi *et al.*, *Ann. N.Y. Acad. Sci.*, 1971, *179*, 244; D. A. Blake *et al.*, *Anaesthesiology*, 1972, *36*, 152.

Pregnancy and the neonate. Halothane reached the foetal circulation within 2 minutes of the commencement of maternal anaesthesia. Initial studies had suggested that it had little depressant effect upon the newborn, but a greater incidence of depression had been reported after caesarean section under halothane anaesthesia than in a comparable group of infants born under thiopentone, nitrous oxide, and suxamethonium anaesthesia.— F. Moya and V. Thorndike, *Clin. Pharmac. Ther.*, 1963, *4*, 628.

Uses. Halothane is a volatile anaesthetic administered by inhalation. It is not inflammable and is not explosive when mixed with oxygen at normal atmospheric pressure. It is not irritant to the skin and mucous membranes and does not produce necrosis when spilt on tissues. It suppresses salivary, mucous, bronchial, and gastric secretions and is reported to dilate the bronchioles.

Halothane may be given by any of the usual inhalation methods but specially designed apparatus is recommended to provide close control over the concentration of inhaled vapour.

Anaesthesia may be induced with 2 to 3% v/v of halothane in oxygen or mixtures of nitrous oxide and oxygen. It takes about 5 minutes to attain full surgical anaesthesia and there is little or no excitement in the induction period. The more usual practice is to induce anaesthesia with thiopentone or other intravenous agents before administering halothane with oxygen. Anaesthesia is maintained with concentrations of 0.5 to 1.5% v/v and recovery, which is dependent on the concentration used and the duration of anaesthesia, is usually rapid. Shivering may occur during recovery; restlessness is an indication for postoperative analgesia.

Adequate muscle relaxation is only achieved with deep anaesthesia so suxamethonium may be given to increase muscular relaxation if necessary. Neostigmine (see p.1035) should not be used to reverse the effects of non-depolarising muscle relaxants unless it is preceded by an injection of atropine, since the effects of halothane and neostigmine on the heart may produce severe bradycardia.

A study in 62 healthy adults suggested that a mixture of 67% of nitrous oxide and 33% oxygen was a suitable vehicle for light halothane anaesthesia, provided respiratory depression was avoided by assisted respiration.— J. E. Graber *et al.*, *Anesth. Analg. curr. Res.*, 1966, *45*, 484.

A drop of pineapple essence to the mask before anaesthesia was found to counteract the sweet odour of halothane and unpleasant odours of the anaesthetic mask tubing.— A. W. Diamond (letter), *Lancet*, 1967, *2*, 1155.

The minimum alveolar concentration of halothane for anaesthesia to prevent a muscular response to a skin incision in 50% of persons was 0.765%.— L. J. Saidman *et al.*, *Anesthesiology*, 1967, *28*, 994.

For discussions of the use of halothane in controlled hypotension during surgery, see G. E. H. Enderby, *Postgrad. med. J.*, 1974, *50*, 572; A. P. Adams, *Br. J. Anaesth.*, 1975, *47*, 777.

The influence of halothane on plasma concentrations of vasopressin during cardiopulmonary bypass.— P. Simpson and M. Forsling, *Br. J. Anaesth.*, 1976, *48*, 265.

Cardiovascular responses to nitrous oxide during halothane anaesthesia.— G. E. Hill *et al.*, *Anesth. Analg. curr. Res.*, 1978, *57*, 84, per *J. Am. med. Ass.*, 1978, *240*, 297.

Analgesia. Halothane 0.35% and nitrous oxide 30% had similar analgesic effects in 9 subjects. Halothane 0.25% had no analgesic effect.— I. T. Houghton *et al.*, *Br. J. Anaesth.*, 1973, *45*, 1105.

Caesarean section. In 15 women undergoing caesarean section anaesthesia was maintained with 50% nitrous oxide in oxygen with a supplement of 0.65% halothane. Mean maternal arterial concentrations and umbilical-vein concentrations of halothane were 60.3 and 21.3 μg per ml respectively; it was likely that there was some inhibition of uterine activity. In 5 further patients given a supplement of 0.2% halothane concentrations were 15.6 and 8μg per ml respectively; there was little likelihood of inhibition of uterine activity. There was no evidence of awareness in any of the women.— I. P. Latto and B. A. Waldron, *Br. J. Anaesth.*, 1977, *49*, 371.

Dental surgery. Of 92 patients attending an outpatient department for dental extractions under general anaesthesia 53 received halothane (group A) and 39 fentanyl (group B). Patients in group A were anaesthetised with thiopentone followed by alcuronium 10 to 15 mg and anaesthesia maintained with halothane 0.5% in nitrous oxide 66% in oxygen. Patients in group B were anaesthetised with fentanyl followed by thiopentone and alcuronium and anaesthesia maintained with nitrous oxide 66% in oxygen. The frequency of arrhythmia attributed to surgery was 5% in both groups. It was suggested that alcuronium, a non-depolarising muscle relaxant, might prevent ventricular arrhythmia in patients receiving halothane.— V. J. E. Thomas *et al.*, *Br. J. Anaesth.*, 1978, *50*, 1243.

Proprietary Preparations

Fluothane *(ICI Pharmaceuticals, UK)*. A brand of halothane. (Also available as Fluothane in *Austral., Canad., Denm., Ger., Ital., Neth., Norw., S.Afr., Switz., USA*).

Halothane *(May & Baker, UK)*. Available in bottles of 250 ml.

Other Proprietary Names

Fluopan *(S.Afr.)*; Halovis *(Ital.)*; Rhodialothan *(Ger.)*; Somnothane *(Canad.)*.

3102-r

Alphadolone Acetate. Alfadolone Acetate; GR 2/1574. 3α,21-Dihydroxy-5α-pregnane-11,20-dione 21-acetate.

$C_{23}H_{34}O_5$=390.5.

CAS — 14107-37-0 (alphadolone); 23930-37-2 (acetate).

A white or almost white odourless crystalline powder. M.p. 175° to 181°. Practically **insoluble** in water; freely soluble in acetone and chloroform.

Alphadolone acetate is used to enhance the solubility of alphaxalone. It possesses some anaesthetic properties and is considered to be about half as potent as alphaxalone.

3103-f

Alphaxalone. Alfaxalone; GR2/234. 3α-Hydroxy-5α-pregnane-11,20-dione.

$C_{21}H_{32}O_3$=332.5.

CAS — 23930-19-0.

NOTE. CT 1341 and alphadione describe an aqueous solution of alphadolone acetate 0.3% and alphaxalone 0.9% with sodium chloride 0.25% and 20% of polyoxyethylated castor oil (Cremophor EL).

A white or almost white, odourless, crystalline powder. M.p 165° to 171°. Practically **insoluble** in water; freely soluble in acetone and chloroform.

Adverse Effects. Administration of a preparation of alphaxalone with alphadolone acetate may cause thrombophlebitis, transient flushing, hypotension, short periods of apnoea, muscle twitching, and occasionally convulsions. Cough, hiccup, salivation, laryngospasm, and shivering may occur.

Hypersensitivity reactions may occur and are characterised by erythema, cyanosis, bronchospasm, hypotension, facial oedema, profuse sweating, and cardiac arrhythmias. The possible role of the solvent cannot be excluded. Fatalities have occurred.

In a survey of adverse reactions to intravenous anaesthetics 86 of 100 consecutive reports were attributed to the intravenous induction agent. Types of reaction reported were histaminoid (19), histaminoid with bronchospasm (33), bronchospasm (12), cardiovascular collapse(11), delayed histaminoid (6), and clonic contractions (5). Alphaxalone with alphadolone was responsible for 70 of the reactions, thiopentone for 12, and propanidid for 4. There were 4 deaths all of which followed histaminoid-with-bronchospasm reactions after injection of thiopentone. The overall incidence of reactions to alphaxalone was estimated at 1 in 11 000 to 1 in 19 000.— R. S. J. Clarke *et al.*, *Br. J. Anaesth.*, 1975, *47*, 575.

In a retrospective survey of adverse reactions to intravenous anaesthetic induction agents 20 reactions involving the use of alphaxalone with alphadolone were noted. There were 10 histaminoid reactions, 3 involving cardiac arrest, and 4 occurring after the use of only 0.5 ml of the commercial injection; 4 patients had generalised convulsions and 3 had muscular rigidity; 2 patients had apnoea and 1 bronchospasm. The incidence of reactions was estimated at 1 in 930 and was unacceptable.— J. M. Evans and J. A. M. Keogh, *Br. med. J.*, 1977, *2*, 735.

A study in 90 healthy women in the first trimester of pregnancy undergoing therapeutic abortion using different types of anaesthesia indicated that anaesthesia with Althesin was characterised by pronounced blood loss, particularly in the ninth and tenth week of pregnancy. Blood loss was less in patients who received thiopentone and significantly less in those who received only local anaesthesia.— B. R. Møller *et al.*, *Acta obstet. gynec. scand.*, 1979, *58*, 481.

The recorded frequency of adverse reactions to alphaxalone with alphadolone acetate (Althesin), propanidid, and Stesolid MR (diazepam) has suggested that the common solvent, Cremophor, is responsible for the adverse reactions.— M. S. Hüttel *et al.*, *Br. J. Anaesth.*, 1980, *52*, 77.

A study indicating that the possibility of an adverse reaction is more than 30 times greater with alphaxalone with alphadolone acetate than with thiopentone.— D. Beamish and D. T. Brown, *Br. J. Anaesth.*, 1981, *53*, 55.

Cardiovascular effects. In 12 patients about to undergo anaesthesia, injections of Cremophor EL, the solubilising agent used with alphaxalone and alphadolone acetate, produced a transient fall in blood pressure and a rise in pulse-rate which were significant when the dose reached 20 ml.— T. M. Savage *et al.*, *Br. J. Anaesth.*, 1973, *45*, 515.

In 42 patients undergoing cardiac surgery, anaesthesia was induced by incremental intravenous doses of alphaxalone and alphadolone acetate (23 patients) or thiopentone (19 patients). Both anaesthetics produced an equally smooth induction and mean induction doses were 0.028 ml per kg body-weight and 2.5 mg per kg respectively. Cardiovascular effects were similar, with a significant decrease in arterial pressure, but alphaxalone produced a more pronounced fall in cardiac output than thiopentone, over which it had no advantage.— J. N. Broadley and P. A. Taylor, *Br. J. Anaesth.*, 1974, *46*, 687.

A preparation of alphaxalone and alphadolone acetate, in a dose of 0.075 ml per kg body-weight intravenously at 0.5 ml per second, was used to induce anaesthesia, subsequently maintained with halothane, in 100 healthy male patients undergoing oral surgery. A protective effect against cardiac arrhythmias was noted but there was marked sinus tachycardia after induction.— J. P. Alexander, *Br. J. Anaesth.*, 1974, *46*, 770.

A study of many parameters of cardiorespiratory function in 24 patients with heart disease given 2 repeated doses of alphaxalone with alphadolone or of ketamine. Contrary to previous reports alphaxalone caused little change in heart-rate, while ketamine caused an increase of 14% in the cardiac index, probably reflecting limited myocardial reserve. Both agents caused a considerable increase in $PaCO_2$, possibly partly due to premedication. The second dose of alphaxalone with alphadolone produced similar effects to the first dose while the second dose of ketamine tended to depress the cardiovascular system.— T. M. Savage *et al.*, *Br. J. Anaesth.*, 1976, *48*, 1071.

A report of dose-related cardiovascular effects of continuous infusions of alphaxalone with alphadolone acetate.— J. W. Sear and C. Prys-Roberts, *Br. J. Anaesth.*, 1979, *51*, 867.

Hyperlipidaemia. An unusual hyperlipidaemia occurred in a 33-year-old man given alphaxalone with alphadolone by continuous infusion for 7 days for sedation; the solvent, Cremophor EL, was probably responsible; there was disappearance of the α-lipoprotein band and the appearance of a densely staining abnormal band in the β-lipoprotein region. The lipoprotein pattern was similar to that seen in dogs given a surfactant [Triton] which, over a few months, produced arteriosclerosis.— A. R. W. Forrest *et al.* (letter), *Br. med. J.*, 1977, *2*, 1357.

Hypersensitivity. Following administration of alphaxolone and alphadolone acetate a 40-year-old woman exhibited involuntary movements of the arms and was apnoeic for about 15 seconds. After surgery she suddenly went into respiratory and cardiac arrest. Despite resuscitation she required assisted ventilation and died 8 days later without regaining consciousness. Death was considered to be due to bronchopneumonia following prolonged and irreversible cerebral anoxia related to hypersensitivity to alphaxalone and alphadolone.— P. Vanezis, *Practitioner*, 1979, *222*, 249.

Of 22 patients who developed hypersensitivity reactions to alphaxalone with alphadolone acetate, 17 had received the drug on at least one previous occasion, while 5 had no known previous exposure. Nine of the 17 patients had severe clinical reactions, involving cardiovascular collapse; and , of these, eight had already received the anaesthetic within the previous 2 months. Of the 5 who reacted on first exposure, only one had severe symptoms.— S. G. Radford *et al.* (letter), *Br. med. J.*, 1980, *281*, 60.

Further reports of hypersensitivity.— T. R. Austin *et al.* (letter), *Br. med. J.*, 1973, *2*, 661; A. N. Crowther (letter), *ibid.*, 775; T. E. J. Healy (letter), *Lancet*, 1973, *2*, 975; J. W. Dundee *et al.*, *Br. med. J.*, 1974, *1*, 63; J. Kessell and E. S. K. Assem (letter), *Br. J. Anaesth.*, 1974, *46*, 209; D. G. Tweedie and P. M. Ordish (letter), *ibid.*, 244; J. M. Watt, *Br. med. J.*, 1975, *3*, 205; G. C. Steel (letter), *Br. J. Anaesth.*, 1976, *48*, 50; M. Fisher (letter), *ibid.*, 1977, *49*, 87; J. Watkins *et al.*, *Br. med. J.*, 1978, *1*, 1180; S. M. Hart (letter), *Br. J. Anaesth.*, 1978, *50*, 1169.

Overdose. A 43-year-old woman was inadvertently given 48 ml of a preparation of alphaxalone with alphadolone acetate, 35 ml of which was given over 2 minutes. She had a rectal temperature of 31° after surgery, was awake 12 hours later, and experienced no nausea, no cyanosis, no change in the ECG, and no hypotension.— N. B. Bøggild-Madsen and T. Cargnelli, *Can. Anaesth. Soc. J.*, 1978, *25*, 245.

Pregnancy and the neonate. In infants delivered by caesarean section foetal metabolic acidosis was significantly greater after anaesthesia with alphaxalone and alphadolone than with thiopentone.— J. W. Downing (letter), *Br. J. Anaesth.*, 1976, *48*, 393.

Precautions. Alphaxalone with alphadolone acetate is contraindicated in patients with liver failure and in those who have previously shown hypersensitivity reactions. Premedication with hyoscine alone has been reported to increase the incidence of unwanted muscle movements. The jaw muscles are relaxed during anaesthesia and require support.

There was no interaction between alphaxalone with alphadolone acetate and pancuronium, suxamethonium, or tubocurarine.— E. M. W. Bradford *et al.*, *Br. J. Anaesth.*, 1971, *43*, 940.

Induction of anaesthesia with alphaxalone and alphadolone acetate produced fewer excitatory and respiratory side-effects than induction with methohexitone. Atropine and diazepam were suitable premedicants. Hyoscine increased the incidence of muscle movements with both anaesthetics.— R. S. J. Clarke *et al.*, *Br. J. Anaesth.*, 1972, *44*, 845.

The fall in blood pressure following the injection of alphaxalone, 450 to 540 µg per kg body-weight with alphadolone acetate, was more marked in the group of 6 patients aged 21 to 55 years who received premedication with atropine sulphate 20 µg per kg than in the similar groups given 10 µg per kg or sodium chloride injection 2 ml prior to minor gynaecological operations. The increase in pulse-rate due to atropine was not affected further by administration of alphaxalone. A further study on 12 patients aged 31 to 58 years undergoing various surgical procedures, in whom anaesthesia was maintained with nitrous oxide, oxygen, intravenous infusion with alphaxalone at the rate of 18 to 45 µg per kg per minute, and inhalation of methoxyflurane, 0.5%, showed no evidence of interaction between alphaxalone and methoxyflurane but there was 1 case of cardiac dysrhythmia.— D. Campbell *et al.*, *Postgrad. med. J.*, 1972, *48* (June), *Suppl.*, 123.

In 7 subjects alphaxalone with alphadolone significantly reduced cerebral blood flow, the cerebral metabolic-rate for oxygen, and arterial PO_2, and increased cerebral vascular reistance, when compared with 13 controls.— A. Sari *et al.*, *Br. J. Anaesth.*, 1976, *48*, 545.

Absorption and Fate. Both alphaxalone and alphadolone acetate are rapidly and widely distributed following injection. They are metabolised in the liver and excreted in the urine; animal studies have also demonstrated excretion in the faeces. There is evidence of enterohepatic circulation. Up to 50% of alphaxalone may be bound to plasma proteins. Alphaxalone crosses the placenta.

In 5 patients with normal renal and hepatic function given radioactive alphaxalone (with alphadolone) intravenously peak concentrations fell rapidly over 2 minutes, followed by a plateau effect for 2 to 100 minutes, and then slow clearance up to 17 hours; 59% of the dose was recovered in the urine in 24 hours and 80% in 5 days. In 5 patients undergoing cholecystectomy initial clearance was slightly slower; alphaxalone appeared in bile within 10 minutes; 38% of the dose was recovered in the urine in 24 hours, 56% in 5 days, and 15% in the bile in about 2 days (13% in 24 hours). In 5 patients undergoing haemodialysis initial clearance was slightly delayed, but the anaesthetic effect was not prolonged; some radioactivity remained in the plasma at 17 hours; it was assumed that excretion was via the bile and faeces.— L. Strunin *et al.*, *Br. J. Anaesth.*, 1977, *49*, 609.

Pharmacokinetics of alphaxalone/alphadolone (Althesin).— M. E. Simpson, *Br. J. Anaesth.*, 1978, *50*, 1231. See also M. M. Ghoneim and K. Korttila, *Clin. Pharmacokinet.*, 1977, *2*, 344.

Plasma concentrations of alphaxalone during continuous infusion of alphaxalone with alphadolone acetate.— J. W. Sear and C. Prys-Roberts, *Br. J. Anaesth.*, 1979, *51*, 861.

Uses. Alphaxalone is used with alphadolone acetate as a general anaesthetic. Both compounds are administered intravenously in a solution containing 9 mg of alphaxalone and 3 mg of alphadolone acetate per ml and doses are often expressed in terms of the volume of this solution. The preparation has little analgesic activity and an anti-analgesic affect has been demonstrated. There may be good muscle relaxation but relaxants may be required especially if small doses are used. It is more potent than the other injectable general anaesthetics.

Induction is rapid and occurs in 1 arm/brain circulation time. A dose of 0.05 ml of the preparation per kg body-weight produces about 7 minutes of anaesthesia; recovery is usually prompt.

Alphaxalone with alphadolone acetate is used for the induction of anaesthesia or for anaesthesia for short procedures. It is administered by slow intravenous injection (10 seconds per ml) in a dose of 0.05 to 0.075 ml per kg body-weight (450 to 675 µg per kg of alphaxalone with 150 to 225 µg per kg of alphadolone acetate). Anaesthesia may be maintained by further incremental doses or by the infusion of 10 to 20 ml of the preparation per hour administered as a 10% dilution in sodium chloride injection or dextrose injection.

Reviews of the actions and uses of alphaxalone with alphadolone acetate: *Pharm. J.*, 1972, *2*, 10; A. R. Hunter, *Practitioner*, 1973, *211*, 476; *Drug & Ther. Bull.*, 1973, *11*, 51; R. N. Brogden *et al.*, *Drugs*, 1974, *8*, 87.

The proceedings of a symposium on alphaxalone with alphadolone acetate.— *Postgrad. med. J.*, 1972, *48* (June), *Suppl.* See also *Lancet*, 1972, *1*, 888.

Induction times of alphaxalone with alphadolone and of thiopentone were found to be dose-dependent except when alphaxalone was used following premedication with promethazine, 50 mg in addition to atropine and pethidine. In a study involving 240 patients alphaxalone/alphadolone acetate 30 µl per kg body-weight and thiopentone 3 mg per kg were considered equipotent, but alphaxalone/alphadolone acetate 90 µl per kg was equivalent to thiopentone 7 mg per kg. The incidence of falling asleep was higher when promethazine was used but some patients on the lower doses required an additional dose of anaesthetic; premedication with promethazine was also found to increase motor responses to painful stimuli when alphaxalone was used. The incidence of motor reactions was greater with thiopentone 7 mg per kg than with thiopentone 5 mg per kg, and greater with alphaxalone 630 µg per kg than with 450 µg per kg.— T. Tammisto *et al.*, *Br. J. Anaesth.*, 1973, *45*, 100.

From a comparative study in 150 patients of recovery from anaesthesia induced with alphaxalone/alphadolone, thiopentone, and methohexitone, it was concluded that alphaxalone/alphadolone was suitable for use in outpatients, recovery being more rapid than with thiopentone. There was no relapse into sleep, unlike methohexitone (4%) and thiopentone (18%). The incidence of nausea and vomiting was lowest with alphaxalone/alphadolone and highest with thiopentone. Five patients who received alphaxalone/alphadolone became very emotional during recovery.— I. W. Carson *et al.*, *Br. J. Anaesth.*, 1975, *47*, 358.

The speed of onset of anaesthesia with alphaxalone/alphadolone was assessed in 190 female patients. An average dose of 81 µl per kg body-weight induced sleep in 88% of patients within 11 seconds. On the basis of previous work (R.S.J. Clarke *et al.*, *Br. J. Anaesth.*, 1968, *40*, 593) alphaxalone/alphadolone 60 to 80 µl per kg was considered to be equipotent with thiopentone 4 mg per kg and methohexitone 1.2 mg per kg.— I. W. Carson *et al.*, *Br. J. Anaesth.*, 1975, *47*, 512.

Absence of effect on plasma-cortisol and plasma-thyroxine concentrations.— T. Oyama *et al.*, *Br. J. Anaesth.*, 1975, *47*, 837.

The effects of anaesthesia with alphaxalone and alphadolone acetate and of surgery on blood-sugar concentration and plasma concentrations of insulin, free fatty acids, cortisol, and growth hormone were assessed in 36 patients, including 6 diabetics, who underwent minor, body surface, and abdominal surgery. Plasma-free fatty acid concentrations were increased significantly during anaesthesia alone and during minor surgery in 4 patients. There were no other significant changes and the hyperglycaemic response in diabetic patients did not differ significantly from that in non-diabetics.— S. Mehta and P. Burton, *Br. J. Anaesth.*, 1975, *47*, 863.

Plasma-luteinising hormone concentrations increased significantly in 10 male patients during anaesthesia with alphaxalone and alphadolone acetate but decreased steadily after recovery from anaesthesia. Plasma-testosterone concentrations decreased during anaesthesia with a further reduction on the first postoperative day.— T. Oyami *et al.*, *Br. J. Anaesth.*, 1975, *47*, 1093.

A study in 32 patients with chronic liver disease who underwent major surgery concluded that alphaxalone with alphadolone acetate could be substituted safely for thiopentone as an induction agent.— M. E. Ward *et al.*, *Br. J. Anaesth.*, 1975, *47*, 1199. But see Precautions.

Alphaxalone/alphadolone acetate infusion was used to induce sleep in patients undergoing major gynaecological surgery performed under extradural analgesia. Operating conditions were satisfactory in all patients and postoperative recovery was smooth and uncomplicated. The infusion could cause transient depression of breathing if given very rapidly and in extreme cases apnoea could result.— G. R. Park and J. Wilson, *Br. J. Anaesth.*, 1978, *50*, 1219.

Studies had been carried out in animals and in human subjects on alphaxalone with alphadolone acetate as an anaesthetic under conditions of saturation diving. It appeared to be acceptable clinically.— C. R. Dundas (letter), *Lancet*, 1979, *1*, 378.

For a comparison of the hypotensive effects of thiopentone, methohexitone, and alphaxalone in patients with cardiac disease, see Thiopentone Sodium, p.759.

Cardioversion. In 52 patients anaesthetised on 64 occasions for cardioversion with either alphaxalone 387 µg per kg body-weight with alphadolone, or with thiopentone, alphaxalone was not considered superior to thiopentone, although with care it could be used for cardioversion.— J. Heinonen *et al.*, *Br. J. Anaesth.*, 1973, *45*, 49.

Cataract extraction. Alphaxalone, 450 µg per kg body-weight, with alphadolone acetate, produced a marked fall in intra-ocular tension and was suitable for induction of anaesthesia in 36 of 37 patients undergoing cataract extraction. There was no increase in bleeding during the operation. Postoperative nausea occurred in 2 patients.— R. M. M. Fordham *et al.*, *Postgrad. med. J.*, 1972, *48* (June), *Suppl.*, 129.

Dental surgery. Alphaxalone with alphadolone acetate was used as the sole anaesthetic agent in 99 dental out-patients. The average induction dose was 4.12 ml and in 13 patients this alone was adequate. Incremental doses of 1 to 2 ml were injected as necessary in other patients, the first increment being given an average 2.2 minutes after the start of induction in 78 patients. In 42 patients the mean time for recovery of consciousness was 4 minutes 42 seconds. Muscle tremor was the most frequent side-effect.— W. N. Rollason *et al.*, *Br. J. Anaesth.*, 1974, *46*, 881.

Alphaxalone with alphadolone acetate was given on 52 occasions to patients undergoing conservative dental treatment; the initial dose was 2.5 ml, increased by increments of 0.5 ml to a mean of 5.4 ml, and compared with a single dose of diazepam (mean dose 15.3 mg). Jaw tremor, hand tremor, or shivering occurred in about half the patients, and verbal contact was lost at many sessions. Recovery was more rapid after alphaxalone with alphadolone and thrombophlebitis less troublesome; it could be satisfactorily used in subanaesthetic doses for sedation.— R. A. Dixon *et al.*, *Br. J. Anaesth.*, 1976, *48*, 431.

Electroconvulsive therapy. Alphaxalone with alphadolone acetate was suitable for out-patients undergoing ECT but was less suitable than barbiturates for narcohypnosis.— J. Cooper, *Postgrad. med. J.*, 1972, *48* (June), *Suppl.*, 115. See also E. I. Foley *et al.*, *ibid.*, 112.

Epilepsy. Refractory status epilepticus in 3 patients was relieved by the infusion of alphaxalone with alphadolone acetate. The procedure suggested was an initial bolus injection of 1 to 3 ml followed by the infusion of a 1 in 20 dilution at the rate of 40 to 50 ml per hour.— L. S. Chin *et al.*, *Anaesth. & intensive Care*, 1979, *7*, 50.

Neurosurgery. In 9 patients with intracranial space-occupying lesions who were undergoing neurosurgery, anaesthesia was induced with either thiopentone or methohexitone and maintained with nitrous oxide, oxygen, and fentanyl. Alphaxalone 450 µg per kg body-weight with alphadolone given not less than 20 minutes later caused a fall in blood pressure which was not considered responsible for the accompanying fall in intracranial pressure of 10 minutes duration. Alphaxalone was considered useful in neurosurgery in patients with intracranial compression.— J. M. Turner *et al.*, *Br. J. Anaesth.*, 1973, *45*, 168.

Sedation. In a study in 30 patients undergoing intensive care the intravenous infusion of a preparation of alphaxalone and alphadolone acetate provided satisfactory sedation for 86% of the total time; it provided light sleep, permitted rapid variation in the degree of sedation, and permitted rapid recovery when needed, for example for neurological assessment. Analgesics and muscle relaxants were given concomitantly as required. The anaesthetic was given diluted with 5 volumes of dextrose injection by constant infusion pump and the dose was titrated to maintain the required degree of sedation. Treatment lasted for from 1.5 to 480 hours with total doses ranging from 3 ml to 4.367 litres. There was a slight initial increase in heart-rate; while there was no evidence to suggest depression of ventilation, caution would be needed in patients with shock; there was no evidence of tachyphylaxis; minor side-effects included muscle twitching (13 episodes), hiccup (10), nausea (8), salivation (5), and flushing of the skin (2).— M. A. E. Ramsey *et al.*, *Br. med. J.*, 1974, *2*, 656.

Use in children. Alphaxalone with alphadolone acetate and methohexitone were compared as induction agents given by intravenous injection in 2 age groups. In the 2 to 10-year-old group (54 children), the mean minimum sleep dose was 0.07 ml per kg body-weight of alphaxalone with alphadolone compared with 1.1 mg per kg of methohexitone. In the 10 to 16-year-old group (72 children) the mean doses were 0.05 ml per kg and 1.2 mg per kg respectively. With alphaxalone and alphadolone, involuntary muscle movement was commoner and more severe; unlike methohexitone, the injection was painless and the dose volume small.— P. J. Keep and M. L. M. Manford, *Br. J. Anaesth.*, 1974, *46*, 685.

A comparison of the effects of alphadolone with alphaxalone, of ketamine, and of thiopentone, with and without pethidine, in 157 children undergoing otolaryngological surgery.— L. Saarnivarra, *Br. J. Anaesth.*, 1977, *49*, 363.

Proprietary Preparations

Althesin *(Glaxo, UK)*. An iso-osmotic solution containing in each ml alphaxalone 9 mg and alphadolone acetate 3 mg, with polyoxyethylated castor oil (Cremophor EL) 20%, in ampoules of 5 and 10 ml. (Also available as Althesin in *Denm.*, *Ital.*).

Other Proprietary Names of Mixtures of Alphaxalone and Alphadolone Acetate

Alfatesin *(Neth., Norw.)*; Alfatésine *(Fr.)*; Alfathesin *(Austral.)*; Alphadione *(Jap.)*.

3104-d

Chloroform *(B.P.)*. Chlorof.; Chloroformum; Chloroformium Anesthesicum; Chloroformum pro Narcosi. Trichloromethane.

$CHCl_3$=119.4.

CAS — 67-66-3.

Pharmacopoeias. In *Arg.*, *Aust.*, *Belg.*, *Br.*, *Chin.*, *Fr.*, *Ger.*, *Hung.*, *Ind.*, *Int.*, *Jug.*, *Mex.*, *Nord.*, *Pol.*, *Port.*, *Rus.*, *Span.*, *Swiss*, and *Turk.* Also in *U.S.N.F.*

Some pharmacopoeias include a grade of chloroform, with less stringent standards, which may be taken by mouth but which must not be used as an anaesthetic.

A colourless mobile volatile liquid with a characteristic odour and a sweet burning taste. It contains 1 to 2% v/v of ethyl alcohol; the *U.S.N.F.* specifies 0.5 to 1% v/v. Not inflammable. B.p. about 61°. Wt per ml 1.474 to 1.479 g. The addition of the small percentage of alcohol greatly retards the gradual oxidation which occurs when chloroform is exposed to air and light and which results in its becoming contaminated with the very poisonous carbonyl chloride (phosgene) and with chlorine; the alcohol also serves to decompose any carbonyl chloride that may have been formed.

Soluble 1 in 200 of water; miscible with dehydrated alcohol, ether, fixed and volatile oils, light petroleum, and most other organic solvents. **Store** at a temperature not exceeding 30° in airtight containers with glass stoppers or other suitable closures. Protect from light.

Stability. There was a loss of about 30% of chloroform from 2-litre samples of Chloroform Water and Double-strength Chloroform Water in bulk containers opened regularly during a study period of 28 days. Once the containers had been opened the contents should be used entirely or discarded within 10 days. Examination of smaller lots likely to be dispensed showed that there would be an acceptable amount of chloroform present for up to 14 days when patients opened their containers thrice daily. If the medicines were to be taken twice or once daily then this period would extend to 3 and 4 weeks respectively.— Pharm. Soc. Lab. Rep. P/75/11, 1975.

There was little loss of chloroform from non-sedimented mixtures (e.g. Paediatric Ferrous Sulphate Mixture) stored in filled unopened bulk containers for more than 4 weeks. There could be a 10% reduction in chloroform content after 7 to 9 days if the containers were opened at regular intervals, and a 30 to 40% reduction after 28 days. In freshly prepared mixtures containing sediments (e.g. Magnesium Trisilicate Mixture) the initial concentration of chloroform in the liquid phase was found to be considerably less than the theoretical concentrations, possibly due to sorption of chloroform by the insoluble powders. Further losses could be expected in regularly opened containers. Studies on the antimicrobial effectiveness of chloroform in aqueous mixtures and suspensions was required.— Pharm. Soc. Lab. Rep. P/75/25, 1975.

Chloroform 0.1 to 0.5% was an effective bactericide against small inocula of *Staphylococcus aureus*, *Escherichia coli*, and *Pseudomonas aeruginosa;* against large inocula chloroform 0.1% was effective against *Ps. aeruginosa*, but higher concentrations were needed against the other organisms. Spores of *Bacillus pumilus* were not killed. From a study of chloroform losses from chloroform water and from 6 typical *B.P.C.* mixtures under various conditions of storage the following shelf-lives were recommended: chloroform solutions and non-sedimented mixtures could be stored in well-closed well-filled containers for 2 months at ambient temperatures; when stored in partially-filled containers periodically opened the shelf-life should not exceed 2 weeks; sedimented mixtures could be stored for 2 months in well-closed well-filled containers, but because loss of chloroform could be expected in containers periodically opened such mixtures should be prepared as required or packed in their final containers; for chloroform-containing mixtures in the home a shelf-life of 2 weeks was suggested.— M. Lynch *et al.*, *Pharm. J.*, 1977, *2*, 507.

Storage. The Pharmaceutical Society's Department of Pharmaceutical Sciences found that PVC bottles softened and distorted rapidly when filled with Chloroform and Morphine Tincture. Free chloroform produced softening, even in low concentrations; this was associated with loss by permeation. Alcoholic solutions of chloroform produced no physical effect. In Chloroform Water stored at room temperature migration of chloroform was slight in 4 weeks, increased after 7 weeks, and after 9 weeks the content of chloroform had fallen to less than 20%. PVC bottles should not be used for storing or dispensing Chloroform and Morphine Tincture, aqueous mixtures containing more than 5% thereof, mixtures or dispersions in which chloroform was present in excess of its aqueous solubility, aqueous mixtures containing chloroform and high concentrations of electrolytes, or Chloroform Water or mixtures containing it if the period of use would exceed 6 weeks.— *Pharm. J.*, 1973, *1*, 100.

Adverse Effects. Chloroform is hepatotoxic and nephrotoxic. It depresses respiration and produces hypotension. Cardiac output is reduced and arrhythmias may develop. Poisoning leads to respiratory depression and cardiac arrest; it may take 6 to 24 hours after a dose before appearance of delayed symptoms characterised by abdominal pain, vomiting, and, at a later stage, jaundice.

Liquid chloroform is irritant to the skin and mucous membranes and may cause burns if spilt on them.

In the UK the Medicines (Chloroform Prohibition) Order 1979 (SI 1979: No. 382), which came into operation on 28 March 1980, prohibits, subject to exceptions, the supply of medicinal products containing more than 0.5% (w/w or v/v as appropriate) of chloroform. Exceptions include supply by a doctor or dentist, or in accordance with his prescription, to a particular patient, supply for external use, and supply for anaesthetic purposes.

In the USA the FDA have banned the use of chloroform in medicines and cosmetics, because of reported carcinogenicity in *animals*.

The sale within or import into England and Wales and Scotland of food containing any added chloroform is prohibited by the Chloroform in Food Regulations 1980 (SI 1980: No. 36) and the Chloroform in Food (Scotland) Regulations 1980 [SI 1980: No. 289 (S.25)].

Maximum permissible atmospheric concentration 10 ppm.

The Food Additives and Contaminants Committee was in full agreement with the recommendation of the Carcinogenesis Sub-Committee which, after reviewing data which demonstrated that chloroform was a carcinogenic risk to *animals*, concluded that where chloroform had no clearly demonstrable benefit to man or where a suitable alternative could be used it should be excluded from food, cosmetics, and medicines. The Sub-Committee had no epidemiological data showing that chloroform was harmful to man.— *Report on the Review of Solvents in Food,* FAC/REP/25, Ministry of Agriculture, Fisheries and Food, London, HM Stationery Office, 1978.

Chloroform is not suitable for use as a food additive.— Twenty-third Report of Joint FAO/WHO Expert Committee on Food Additives, *Tech. Rep. Ser. Wld Hlth Org. No. 648*, 1980.

Treatment of Adverse Effects. Respiratory depression should be treated with assisted respiration. In severe hypotension the circulation should be maintained with infusions of plasma or suitable electrolyte solutions, or phenylephrine, methoxamine, or mephentermine.

Precautions. Chloroform should not be administered to patients with renal, hepatic, or cardiovascular disease, diabetes mellitus, or severe anaemia.

It is best avoided in patients with acute septic conditions and in patients who are undernourished.

Adrenaline and most other sympathomimetic agents should not be used during chloroform anaesthesia; methoxamine or phenylephrine may be administered cautiously.

See also Precautions for General Anaesthetics, p.740.

Absorption and Fate. Chloroform is readily absorbed by inhalation; equilibrium of concentrations in blood and in brain is rapidly achieved. It is highly soluble in adipose tissue. The blood/gas partition coefficient is high and most of the inhaled chloroform is slowly eliminated through the lungs; a small amount is metabolised. Chloroform readily diffuses across the placenta.

Adequate surgical anaesthesia was obtained with a mean chloroform concentration in arterial blood of about 160 µg per ml.— N. Poopalasingam and J. P. Payne, *Br. J. Anaesth.*, 1975, *47*, 632.

The uptake and elimination of chloroform was rapid in 16 patients studied during general anaesthesia. The pattern of recovery after anaesthesia with chloroform did not differ significantly from that seen after the use of halothane.— N. Poobalasingham and J. P. Payne, *Br. J. Anaesth.*, 1978, *50*, 325.

Uses. Chloroform is an anaesthetic administered by inhalation. It possesses good analgesic and muscle relaxant properties. Because of its toxicity chloroform is seldom used as an anaesthetic and other safer agents are preferable. Concentrations of 2 to 4% of the vapour have been used for induction and 1 to 2% for maintenance of anaesthesia. Adequate premedication is necessary to reduce the risk of ventricular fibrillation.

Chloroform is used as a carminative and as a flavouring agent and preservative. For these purposes it is usually employed as Chloroform Spirit or Chloroform Water but doubts have been cast on the safety of the long-term use of chloroform in mixtures and toothpastes.

Externally, chloroform has a rubefacient action and is used, in liniments, as a counter-irritant.

Chloroform is also used as a solvent for resins, alkaloids, fats, fixed and volatile oils, gutta percha, and rubber.

Herpes. In a controlled study in 41 patients with herpes labialis chloroform, applied topically for 10 minutes once daily for 3 days, reduced the time for scab formation, compared with a placebo, but did not affect the time to healing. The routine use of chloroform could not be recommended.— C. A. Taylor *et al.*, *Archs Derm.*, 1977, *113*, 1550.

Solvent for gallstones. Large residual cholesterol stones were successfully removed from the bile ducts of 2 patients by instillation of 5 ml of chloroform warmed to 40°. In 1 case 2 instillations were necessary.— B. K. H. Semb *et al.*, *Acta chir. scand.*, 1974, *140*, 469.

Preparations

Emulsions

Chloroform Emulsion *(B.P.C. 1963)*. Emuls. Chlorof. Chloroform 5 ml, quillaia liquid extract 0.1 ml, tragacanth mucilage 5 ml, water to 100 ml. *Dose.* 0.3 to 2 ml. It is equivalent in content of chloroform to Chloroform Spirit.

A preliminary study indicated that polysorbate 20 and docusate sodium were both worthy of further investigation as alternatives to quillaia liquid extract in Chloroform Emulsion (*B.P.C. 1963*). The results also suggested that improved emulsions could be produced either by increasing the proportion of tragacanth mucilage to about 10% or by using carmellose sodium. Further studies were necessary to confirm the optimum concentrations of suspending agents.— Pharm. Soc. Lab. Rep. P/79/3, 1979.

Spirits

Chloroform Spirit *(B.P.)*. Chloric Ether. Chloroform 5% v/v in alcohol (90%). Store at a temperature not exceeding 25°.

Tinctures

Chloroform and Morphine Tincture *(B.P.)*. Chlorof. and Morph. Tinct.; Chlorodyne; Tinct. Chlorof. et Morph. Chloroform 12.5 ml, morphine hydrochloride 229 mg, alcohol (90%) 12.5 ml, liquorice liquid extract 12.5 ml, treacle of commerce 12.5 ml, water 5 ml, anaesthetic ether 3 ml, peppermint oil 0.1 ml, syrup to 100 ml. It contains the equivalent of 0.157 to 0.191% w/v of anhydrous morphine. A 0.6-ml dose contains about 0.075 ml of chloroform and about 1.374 mg of morphine hydrochloride. Store in airtight containers.

For chlorodyne dependence, see under Morphine, p.1018.

Waters

Chloroform Water *(B.P.)*. Chlorof. Water; Aq. Chlorof. Chloroform 0.25% v/v in freshly boiled and cooled water.

Most pharmacopoeias have 0.5% w/w. Electrolytes are apt to cause deposition of chloroform from aqueous solutions.

Concentrated Chloroform Water *(B.P.C. 1959)*. Chloroform Water Concentrated *(A.P.F.)*; Aq. Chlorof. Conc. Chloroform 10 ml, alcohol (90%) 60 ml, water to 100 ml. *Dose.* 0.4 to 0.8 ml. Diluted with 39 times its volume of water it yields a preparation of equivalent strength to Chloroform Water.

Double-Strength Chloroform Water *(B.P.)*. Aqua Chloroformi Duplex; Aq. Chlorof. Dup. Chloroform 0.5% v/v in freshly boiled and cooled water.

3105-n

Cyclopropane *(B.P., U.S.P.)*. Cycloprop.; Trimethylene.

C_3H_6=42.08.

CAS — 75-19-4.

Pharmacopoeias. In *Arg., Aust., Br., Braz., Cz., Ind., It., Mex., Nord., Rus., Swiss, Turk.,* and *U.S.*

A colourless inflammable gas with a characteristic odour and pungent taste supplied compressed in metal cylinders. B.p. about −34.5°.

Very **soluble** in alcohol, chloroform, and ether; soluble in fixed oils; 1 vol. measured at normal temperature and pressure dissolves, at 20°, in 2.85 vol. of water.

Store in metal cylinders in a special room which should be cool and free from inflammable materials. The cylinder should be painted orange; the name or chemical symbol of the gas should be stencilled in paint on the shoulder of the cylinder and clearly and indelibly stamped on the cylinder valve.

CAUTION. *Mixtures of cyclopropane with oxygen or air at certain concentrations are explosive. Cyclopropane should not be used in the presence of an open flame or of any electrical apparatus liable to produce a spark. Precautions should be taken against the production of static electrical discharge.*

The incompatibility of cyclopropane with flexible plastic or rubber tubing.— A. Bracken, *British Oxygen* (letter), *Br. J. Anaesth.*, 1976, *48*, 52. See also J. E. MacKenzie (letter), *Pharm. J.*, 1977, *1*, 38.

Adverse Effects. A fairly wide margin of safety exists between the anaesthetic and toxic concentrations of cyclopropane.

Cyclopropane depresses respiration to a greater extent than many other anaesthetic agents. It may cause bronchospasm if surgical stimulation occurs under light anaesthesia; laryngospasm may occur. Cardiac arrhythmias, particularly associated with hypercarbia, may occur. Cyclopropane increases the sensitivity of the heart to beta-adrenergic activity. Tachycardia gives warning of overdosage.

Postoperative nausea and vomiting are frequent although less severe than with ether. Severe postoperative fall in blood pressure occasionally occurs and also varying degrees of collapse of the lung. Postoperative headache is more common than with other anaesthetics. Cyclopropane has a tendency to increase haemorrhage. Priapism has been reported.

Blood flow to the kidney and liver may be impaired during cyclopropane anaesthesia.

Adverse effects of cyclopropane on renal function.— S. Deutsch *et al.*, *Anesthesiology*, 1967, *28*, 547.

Subjective and objective changes in mental performances were noted in 18 healthy persons after profound and prolonged cyclopropane anaesthesia.— F. M. James, *Anesthesiology*, 1969, *30*, 264, per *J. Am. med. Ass.*, 1969, *207*, 2125.

Cardiac arrhythmias. A study in 47 elderly patients with cardiovascular disease indicated that such patients had a lower tendency to cardiac arrhythmias during cyclopropane anaesthesia than young healthy adults. Arrhythmias occurred less frequently when anaesthesia was induced with thiopentone. Rapid intravenous injection of 150 mg of thiopentone caused the disappearance of arrhythmias in 6 of 8 patients.— M. J. Strong *et al.*, *Anesthesiology*, 1968, *29*, 295.

Cardiac arrhythmias developed in 901 of 5013 patients during anaesthesia; the incidence of arrhythmias was significantly greater during cyclopropane anaesthesia than with halothane. Occurrence of arrhythmias increased with the age of the patient and was more frequent during induction of anaesthesia, in patients intubated, and in patients receiving digitalis.— P. E. Vanik and H. S. Davis, *Anesth. Analg. curr. Res.*, 1968, *47*, 299.

Liver damage. A study was made of 3 patients who had liver disturbance after cyclopropane; in 1 patient anaesthesia was induced with thiopentone. Within 5 days, the first patient developed jaundice which increased during the next 3 weeks and then regressed over a 2-month period. The second patient also developed jaundice within 5 days, died 3 days later from pulmonary embolism, and showed a subacute hepatitis at post mortem. The third patient developed, from the second day after the operation, a slight fever, nausea, and vomiting. She died 19 days later and showed interstitial subacute hepatitis and parenchymatous liver degeneration at post mortem.— K. -Å. Bennike and J. O. Hagelsten (letter), *Lancet*, 1964, *2*, 255.

Over 800 000 anaesthetic administrations were analysed during a 4-year period in the USA in the National Halothane Study. About 147 000 of the procedures involved the use of cyclopropane which was found to be associated with the highest rate of massive hepatic necrosis and the highest crude mortality-rate when compared with halothane, ether, nitrous oxide with barbiturates, and combinations of these anaesthetics.— *J. Am. med. Ass.*, 1966, *197*, 775.

Treatment of Adverse Effects. As for Halothane, p.742.

Precautions. Cyclopropane should be used with caution in patients with bronchial asthma and cardiovascular disorders.

Pre-operation sedation with respiratory depressants should be used with caution. Adrenaline and most other sympathomimetic agents should not be used during cyclopropane anaesthesia; methoxamine or phenylephrine may be administered cautiously. As with halothane (p.742) routine premedication with atropine may be advisable to reduce vagal tone. The effects of non-depolarising muscle relaxants are enhanced and they should be used in reduced doses.

It has been suggested that cyclopropane and gallamine be not given concomitantly because of the possibility of ventricular arrhythmias.

See also Precautions for General Anaesthetics, p.740.

In a study of the effect of cyclopropane on carbohydrate and fat metabolism in 20 patients there was an increase in blood-glucose and cortisol concentrations during anaesthesia and surgery and decrease in plasma concentrations of free fatty acids. The hyperglycaemic effect of cyclopropane did not appear to be related to growth-hormone or insulin concentrations.— T. Oyama and T. Takazawa, *Anesth. Analg. curr. Res.*, 1972, *51*, 389.

Absorption and Fate. Cyclopropane is readily absorbed on inhalation. It has a relatively low solubility in adipose tissue. The blood/gas coefficient is low and with anaesthesia of short duration most of the inhaled cyclopropane is eliminated through the lungs in a few minutes. It diffuses across the placenta and may cause respiratory depression in the neonate.

A study of the pulmonary equilibration of cyclopropane in infants and children indicated that less cyclopropane might be absorbed into the adipose tissue of the infants.— H. Rackow and E. Salanitre, *Br. J. Anaesth.*, 1974, *46*, 35.

Uses. Cyclopropane is an anaesthetic administered by inhalation. It is non-irritant and induction and recovery are rapid. It has analgesic properties but it may not produce adequate muscle relaxation with the lighter planes of anaesthesia.

It is usually administered with oxygen; a concentration of 4% of cyclopropane in oxygen produces analgesia, 8% produces light anaesthesia, and 20 to 25% produces surgical anaesthesia. Prolonged administration of concentrations of about 40% causes respiratory failure. It may be employed in obstetrics; it does not depress uterine activity but can cause respiratory depression in the neonate.

The usual signs of anaesthetic overdosage, such as pupillary changes, cannot be relied upon with cyclopropane; slowing of the heart to 50 beats or less per minute or definite tachycardia shows the need to decrease the concentration of cyclopropane. Because of the risk of explosion, the usual method of administration is by means of a closed circuit. Premedication with atropine is desirable. Thiopentone is frequently given with cyclopropane to provide smoother induction.

The minimum alveolar concentration of cyclopropane for anaesthesia to prevent a muscular response to a skin incision in 50% of persons was 9.2%.— L. J. Saidman *et al.*, *Anesthesiology*, 1967, *28*, 994.

Cyclopropane, 10 to 30% in oxygen, following narcobarbital given intravenously to induce sleep, was preferred for the maintenance of anaesthesia in 100 patients undergoing renal transplantation. One patient had cardiac arrest during the operation, but this was not attributed to cyclopropane or to the suxamethonium used for intubation. None of the cardiac arrhythmias known to occur with cyclopropane were seen.— D. D. Hansen *et al.*, *Br. J. Anaesth.*, 1972, *44*, 584.

In a study of 15 patients given cyclopropane there was a reduction in blood viscosity, the haematocrit, and fibrinogen concentration. The plasma-protein concentration was decreased.— F. Magora *et al.*, *Br. J. Anaesth.*, 1974, *46*, 343.

Pregnancy and the neonate. In a prospective study 589 patients undergoing caesarean section were anaesthetised with cyclopropane. A concentration of 40% was administered for 2 to 3 minutes then anaesthesia was maintained with 7.5%. Cyclopropane did not cause depression in the neonate or influence the frequency of respiratory distress syndrome. The frequency of awareness during operation was 1.5% but it was thought that it could be avoided if the concentration was increased to 10%.— M. B. Kristoffersen, *Br. J. Anaesth.*, 1979, *51*, 227.

Proprietary Preparations

Cyclopropane *(ICI Pharmaceuticals, UK: BOC Medishield, UK)*. A brand of cyclopropane.

3106-h

Enflurane *(U.S.P.)*. Compound 347; Methylflurether. 2-Chloro-1,1,2-trifluoroethyl difluoromethyl ether.

$C_3H_2ClF_5O$=184.5.

CAS — 13838-16-9.

Pharmacopoeias. In *U.S.*

A colourless volatile liquid with a pleasant ethereal odour. Not inflammable. Relative density 1.516 to 1.519. B.p. 55.5° to 57.5°. **Store** at a temperature not exceeding 40° in airtight containers. Protect from light.

Adverse Effects. Nausea, vomiting, hiccup, and shivering may occasionally occur. Hypotension, respiratory depression, and cardiac arrhythmias have been reported. Enflurane has a stimulant effect on the CNS and increased motor activity, and convulsions, have occurred. Asthma and bronchospasm have been reported. There have been reports of elevated serum-fluoride concentrations but renal damage appears to be rare. There have been changes in measurements of hepatic enzymes.

Acute asthma in an anaesthetist on 6 occasions 8 to 12 hours after administering enflurane.— R. S. Schwettmann and C. L. Casterline, *Anesthesiology*, 1976, *44*, 166.

Effect on body temperature. Malignant hyperpyrexia occurred in a patient anaesthetised for the second time in 6 months with enflurane.— T. -H. Pan *et al.*, *Anesth. Analg. curr. Res.*, 1975, *54*, 47.

Effect on the EEG. The EEG activity observed in 8 patients given enflurane at various concentrations correlated with the pCO_2. Spike discharge activity was observed at alveolar concentrations greater than 2.5%; this effect was increased by hyperventilation and suppressed by carbon dioxide.— M. H. Lebowitz *et al.*, *Anesth. Analg. curr. Res.*, 1972, *51*, 355.

The effect on the EEG pattern in children with dyskinesia was eliminated with low concentrations of enflurane.— G. Faggioni and M. B. Noccioli, *Minerva anest.*, 1974, *40*, 469.

Seizure activity in 2 patients 6 and 8 days after enflurane anaesthesia.— W. W. Ohm *et al.*, *Anesthesiology*, 1975, *42*, 367.

See also under Uses.

Further references: M. Kruczek *et al.*, *Anesthesiology*, 1980, *53*, 175.

Kidney damage. A report of possible nephrotoxicity due to enflurane in a patient with severe renal disease.— R. W. Loehning and R. I. Mazze, *Anesthesiology*, 1974, *40*, 203.

In 50 patients anaesthetised with enflurane the only appreciable change found in renal studies was cloudy urine and albuminuria persisting for up to 10 days.— C. L. Graves and N. H. Downs, *Anesth. Analg. curr. Res.*, 1974, *53*, 898.

Renal failure associated with a high serum-fluoride concentration in a 66-year-old man after enflurane anaesthesia.— J. H. Eichhorn *et al.*, *Anesthesiology*, 1976, *45*, 557.

A study of fluoride kinetics after enflurane anaesthesia in healthy and anephric patients and in patients with poor renal function. Although the 24-hour values of fluoride ion were significantly higher after administration of enflurane than before in the anephric and low-creatinine clearance patients this difference disappeared after one dialysis; there was no significant clinical difference. There was no significant difference among the 3 groups of patients in relation to maximum inorganic fluoride ion concentration or the time to the peak value. In no patients did the serum concentrations of inorganic fluoride reach the threshold for subclinical toxicity of 50 µmol per litre.— R. Carter *et al.*, *Clin. Pharmac. Ther.*, 1976, *20*, 565.

In 10 patients undergoing surgery and given enflurane 0.5 to 2.5%, a peak mean blood-enflurane concentration of 95 µg per ml was achieved after 30 minutes. The mean concentration of inorganic fluoride in serum rose from 5.3 to 16 µmol per litre after 2 hours of anaesthesia and fell within 4 days to less than initial values. The peak urinary excretion of inorganic fluoride of 200 µmol a day on the first postoperative day was approaching normal by the 4th day. In 20 further patients significant changes in concentrations of glucose, phosphate, aspartate aminotransferase (SGOT) and in the white-blood-cell count were not considered attributable to enflurane. Enflurane appeared unlikely to cause nephrotoxicity in patients with normal hepatic and renal function.— I. M. Corall *et al.*, *Br. J. Anaesth.*, 1977, *49*, 881.

Liver damage. A 62-year-old diabetic woman with cirrhosis of the liver died with a hepatorenal syndrome and massive hepatic necrosis 20 days after an operation during which she received enflurane.— L. van der Reis *et al.*, *J. Am. med. Ass.*, 1974, *227*, 76. This episode was not incompatible with acute viral hepatitis superimposed on chronic liver disease leading to necrosis.— W. L. Higgins (letter), *ibid.*, *228*, 158. Further comment.— M. Shirley *et al.* (letter), *ibid.*; A. DelPizzo (letter), *ibid.*; T. S. Morley (letter), *ibid.*, 159.

Another report of liver damage associated with enflurane.— J. K. Denlinger *et al.*, *Anesthesiology*, 1974, *41*, 86.

In 49 black African women exposed to enflurane on up to 3 occasions prior to radium therapy for carcinoma of the cervix there was a significant increase in total serum-bilirubin concentrations 24 hours after a second exposure in 20 patients, but values compatible with clinical jaundice were not attained. Enflurane was a reasonable alternative to halothane when multiple exposures were required.— P. J. Allen and J. W. Downing, *Br. J. Anaesth.*, 1977, *49*, 1035.

Abnormal enzyme values in 8 of 59 patients after repeated enflurane anaesthesia, compared with 25 of 68 after repeated halothane anaesthesia.— J. W. Dundee *et al.* (letter), *Br. med. J.*, 1979, *1*, 265. See also J. P. H. Fee *et al.*, *Br. J. Anaesth.*, 1979, *51*, 1133. Criticisms: L. Strunin, *ibid.*, 1097; *Lancet*, 1980, *1*, 24; J. A. Lewis (letter), *ibid.*, 198; M. Johnstone (letter), *ibid.*, 422. Replies: J. P. H. Fee *et al.* (letter), *ibid.*, 361; R. Wright and O. E. Eade, *ibid.*, 545.

Precautions. Enflurane should not be administered to patients with convulsive disorders. As with halothane, enflurane sensitises the myocardium to the effects of adrenaline and most other sympathomimetic agents. The effects of non-depolarising muscle relaxants such as gallamine and tubocurarine are enhanced, and recovery from such effects may be slower than with other commonly used anaesthetics. High concentrations may cause uterine relaxation.

Possible induction of hepatic microsomal enzymes by enflurane.— M. L. Berman *et al.*, *Anesthesiology*, 1976, *44*, 496.

Absorption and Fate. Enflurane is readily absorbed on inhalation. The blood/gas coefficient is low. It is mostly excreted unchanged through the lungs; small amounts are excreted in the urine as fluorinated metabolites.

Metabolism and renal effects of enflurane.— M. J. Cousins *et al.*, *Anesthesiology*, 1976, *44*, 44.

For a comparison of the metabolism of halothane, enflurane, and methoxyflurane, see Halothane, p.742.

Uses. Enflurane is a volatile anaesthetic administered by inhalation. It has anaesthetic actions similar to those of halothane (see p.743).

It is administered using a vaporiser to achieve control of the concentration of inhaled vapour. Anaesthesia may be induced with up to 4% v/v in oxygen or oxygen and nitrous oxide and may be maintained by 0.5 to 3% v/v. To avoid excitement a short-acting barbiturate or other intravenous induction agent has been recommended before the inhalation of enflurane. Although enflurane is reported to possess muscle relaxant properties, muscle relaxants may be required. Postoperative analgesia may be necessary.

Reviews: *J. Am. med. Ass.*, 1973, *225*, 898; C. Prys-Roberts, *Br. J. Anaesth.*, 1977, *49*, 845; G. W. Black *et al.*, *Br. J. Anaesth.*, 1979, *51*, 627. See also *Acta anaesth. scand.*, 1979, *Suppl.* 71.

In a comparison in 100 patients enflurane was as satisfactory as halothane as a primary inhalation anaesthetic in patients with chronic obstructive pulmonary disease.— R. Rodriguez and M. I. Gold, *Anesth. Analg. curr. Res.*, 1976, *55*, 806.

In 120 patients aged 10 to more than 60 years in whom anaesthesia was induced intravenously enflurane 1 to 3% was adequate for the maintenance of anaesthesia. In 16 of 30 children aged less than 10 years who inhaled enflurane in nitrous oxide 70% in oxygen, concentrations of 2.5% or more were needed and in some infants under 2 years 5% enflurane was inadequate. Induction in 10 children was achieved in a mean of 2.3 minutes compared with 3.3 minutes for halothane. Recovery was generally rapid. A reduction of about 10% in mean arterial pressure and frequent respiratory depression were largely counteracted by the stimulus of surgery. Muscular relaxation was such that neuromuscular blocking agents were often not required. There were no consistent changes in heart-rate or rhythm and no arrhythmias were observed on the ECG in 12 children given about 10 ml of adrenaline 1: 400 000 for haemostasis.— G. W. Black *et al.*, *Br. J. Anaesth.*, 1977, *49*, 875.

The influence of airway resistance and ventilatory pattern on Pa CO_2 during enflurane anaesthesia.— W. M. Wahba, *Br. J. Anaesth.*, 1979, *51*, 123.

The effects of enflurane anaesthesia and surgery on endocrine function in man.— T. Oyama *et al.*, *Br. J. Anaesth.*, 1979, *51*, 141.

Enflurane 3% anaesthesia was used in 2 patients to activate epileptogenic foci as an aid to surgical treatment.— D. C. Flemming *et al.*, *Anesthesiology*, 1980, *52*, 431, per *Int. pharm. Abstr.*, 1980, *17*, 931.

Herpes. The use of enflurane in the topical treatment of recurrent herpes simplex.— W. F. Willis (letter), *Archs Derm.*, 1978, *114*, 1096.

Ophthalmic surgery. It was concluded from a study in 20 patients that enflurane 1% decreased intra-ocular pressure significantly and could be used in ophthalmic anaesthesia instead of halothane which, in this study, failed to alter mean intra-ocular pressure significantly and produced varying effects in individual patients.— J. C. Runciman *et al.*, *Br. J. Anaesth.*, 1978, *50*, 371.

Phaeochromocytoma. Use in a patient with phaeochromocytoma.— J. F. Kreul *et al.*, *Anesthesiology*, 1976, *44*, 265.

Pregnancy and the neonate. Amnesia, absence of foetal depression, and absence of excessive bleeding in 50 women given enflurane for caesarean section.— A. J. Coleman and J. W. Downing, *Anesthesiology*, 1975, *43*, 354.

Use in children. In a comparative study in 104 infants and children induction and recovery were significantly shorter with enflurane (52 patients) than with halothane (52). Quality of recovery was similar in both groups.— M. J. M. Govaerts and M. Sanders, *Br. J. Anaesth.*, 1975, *47*, 877.

Use in the elderly. From a study of the outcome of surgery in 500 patients over 80 years of age, enflurane appeared to be a safe general anaesthetic for sick, elderly patients.— J. L. Djokovic and J. Hedley-Whyte, *J. Am. med. Ass.*, 1979, *242*, 2301.

Proprietary Preparations

Ethrane *(Abbott, UK)*. A brand of enflurane. (Also available as Ethrane in *Austral.*, *Belg.*, *Canad.*, *Ger.*, *Ital.*, *Neth.*, *Switz.*).

Other Proprietary Names

Efrane *(Denm., Norw., Swed.)*; Inhelthran *(Arg.)*.

3107-m

Anaesthetic Ether *(B.P., Eur. P.)*. Anaesth.

Ether; Aether Anaesthecicus; Diethyl Ether; Ether; Ether Anesthesicus; Aether ad Narcosin; Aether Purissimus; Aether pro Narcosi; Éter Purísimo.

$(C_2H_5)_2O$=74.12.

CAS — 60-29-7.

Pharmacopoeias. In all pharmacopoeias examined. *Rus.* also includes Aether Medicinalis, which is intended for oral administration (max. daily dose, 1 ml) and for use in topical applications; it has a slightly higher wt per ml and a wider boiling range (34° to 36°).

Diethyl ether to which an appropriate quantity of a non-volatile antoxidant may have been added. It contains not more than 0.2% of water. Ether *U.S.P.* contains 96 to 98% of $(C_2H_5)_2O$, the remainder consisting of alcohol and water. It is slowly oxidised by the action of air and light, with the formation of peroxides. Propyl gallate and hydroquinone are among the substances used as stabilisers. A clear, colourless, volatile, inflammable, and very mobile liquid with a characteristic odour and a sweet burning taste. Relative density 0.714 to 0.716. B.p. 34° to 35°. Flash-point about −29° (closed-cup test).

Soluble 1 in 10 to 12 of water; miscible with alcohol, chloroform, light petroleum, and fixed and volatile oils. Anaesthetic ether for injection may be **sterilised** by filtration. **Store** in a cool place in dry airtight containers. Protect from light. Ether remaining in a partly used container may deteriorate rapidly.

CAUTION. *Ether is very volatile and inflammable and mixtures of its vapour with oxygen, nitrous oxide, or air at certain concentrations are explosive. It should not be used in the presence of an open flame or any electrical apparatus liable to produce a spark. Precautions should be taken against the production of static electrical discharge.*

The Pharmaceutical Society's Department of Pharmaceutical Sciences found that free ether, even in low concentrations, caused softening of PVC bottles and was associated with loss by permeation.— *Pharm. J.*, 1973, *1*, 100.

Adverse Effects. Ether has an irritant action on the mucous membrane of the respiratory tract; it stimulates salivation and increases bronchial secretion. Laryngeal spasm may occur. Ether causes vasodilatation which may lead to a severe fall in blood pressure and it reduces blood flow to the kidneys; it also increases capillary bleeding. The bleeding time is unchanged but the prothrombin time may be prolonged; leucocytosis occurs after ether anaesthesia. Alterations in kidney and liver function have been reported.

Convulsions occasionally occur in children or young adults under deep ether anaesthesia.

Recovery is slow from prolonged ether anaesthesia and postoperative vomiting commonly occurs.

Acute overdosage of ether is characterised by respiratory failure and cardiac arrest.

Dependence on ether or ether vapour has been reported. Prolonged contact with ether spilt on any tissue produces necrosis.

Maximum permissible atmospheric concentration 400 ppm.

An intra-arterial injection was made in error in an attempt to determine the venous circulation time by the injection of a mixture of 0.5 ml of ether and 0.5 ml of saline. Immediate pain in the arm and hand ensued and later there was oedema and cyanosis. There was no thrombosis of the large arteries but the soft tissue pressure occluded the vessels so that ischaemia and gangrene developed.— H. King and D. B. Hawtof, *J. Am. med. Ass.*, 1963, *184*, 241.

Effect on body temperature. Anaesthetic ether could cause malignant hyperthermia in genetically predisposed individuals.— M. E. Pembrey, *Practitioner*, 1974, *213*, 647.

In a study of 70 children anaesthetised with either halothane or ether, rectal temperatures rose in relation to the duration of anaesthesia and were more pronounced with ether. Skin temperatures decreased progressively with both anaesthetics and again this was more pronounced with ether. There was a decrease in pCO_2 with ether but not halothane and carbon dioxide accumulation was not considered to be a cause of the increases in body temperature.— H. Naito *et al.*, *Anesthesiology*, 1974, *41*, 237.

Precautions. Ether anaesthesia is contra-indicated in patients with diabetes mellitus, impaired kidney function, and severe liver disease. Its use is not advisable in hot and humid conditions for patients with fever as convulsions are liable to occur, particularly in children and in patients who have been given atropine.

Ether enhances the action of non-depolarising muscle relaxants to a greater degree than most other anaesthetics. See also Precautions for General Anaesthetics, p.740.

Muscle relaxation following anaesthesia with ether was attributed mainly to depression of the central nervous system. The effect of suxamethonium was enhanced in 50% of patients when given during ether anaesthesia and the action of tubocurarine was prolonged.— R. L. Katz, *Anesthesiology*, 1966, *27*, 52.

Absorption and Fate. Ether is readily absorbed on inhalation. The blood/gas partition coefficient is high and most of the inhaled ether is slowly eliminated through the lungs; a small amount is metabolised. Ether readily crosses the placenta.

A comparative study of 5 subjects who underwent general surgery under ether anaesthesia compared with 5 similar subjects in whom other agents replaced ether, indicated that some metabolism of ether to acetaldehyde occurred.— H. Aune *et al.* (letter), *Lancet*, 1978, *2*, 97.

Uses. Ether is an anaesthetic administered by inhalation; it was one of the first successful anaesthetic agents, and is considered to have a wide margin of safety, although it has now been replaced by the halogenated anaesthetic agents such as halothane. It possesses a respiratory stimulant effect in all but the deepest planes of anaesthesia and there are only minor cardiovascular changes during light planes of anaesthesia. Ether also possesses good muscle relaxant properties.

Premedication with atropine is usually required to inhibit troublesome bronchial and salivary secretions.

The concentration of ether in the inspired air used to induce anaesthesia is generally from 10 to 20% by volume, though it may be desirable to exceed this concentration on occasions. Light anaesthesia may be maintained with concentrations of up to 5% but deep anaesthesia may require up to 10%.

It is administered on an open mask or by semi-closed or closed methods. When ether is used alone in this way it requires a long time for the induction of anaesthesia, thus prolonging the stage of excitement so it is common practice to premedicate the patient and to employ mixtures of ether with other anaesthetics such as nitrous oxide.

Given by mouth, ether exerts a narcotic action somewhat similar to that of alcohol. In the stomach it is reputed to have a carminative action and has been administered in mixtures.

For the measurement of the circulation time (arm to lung time), 0.15 ml of anaesthetic ether has been mixed with 0.15 ml of sodium chloride injection and rapidly injected into the antecubital vein. Normally the patient noticed the odour of ether after 3 to 8 seconds, but this interval was prolonged in cases of right-sided heart failure.

The minimum alveolar concentration of ether for anaesthesia to prevent a muscular response to a skin incision in 50% of persons was 1.92%.— L. J. Saidman *et al.*, *Anesthesiology*, 1967, *28*, 994.

Obstructed urinary balloon catheters could be removed by distending the bladder with 200 to 300 ml of sterile water, injecting 2 to 5 ml of anaesthetic ether down the inflation tube to burst the balloon, and withdrawing the catheter.— D. J. Arwade (letter), *Br. med. J.*, 1973, *1*, 359.

Instillation of ether into the ears of 8 patients with myiasis due to maggots allowed removal of the parasite. Turpentine oil used similarly was less effective and caused local pain.— R. Sharan and D. K. Isser, *J. Lar. Otol.*, 1978, *92*, 705.

Hiccups. Instillation of 1 ml of ether into a nostril stopped the hiccup reflex in 26 of 27 anaesthetised patients.— J. A. Moses *et al.*, *Anesth. Analg. curr. Res.*, 1970, *49*, 367.

Solvent for gallstones. Ether was used to dissolve residual common duct stones in 2 patients following cholecystectomy and implantation of a catheter in the common bile duct. Papaverine 100 mg was given by mouth thrice daily, followed after an hour by the instillation of 5 or 6 ml of a mixture of ether 4 ml and alcohol 2 ml into the catheter. Stones were cleared in 1 week and 6 weeks respectively in the 2 patients.— C. L. N. Robinson, *Can. med. Ass. J.*, 1966, *95*, 1205. A warning on the indiscriminate use of ether.— G. K. Thomas, *ibid.*, 1967, *96*, 162. Care and the use of papaverine were stressed.— C. L. N. Robinson, *ibid.*, 163.

Status asthmaticus. The rectal administration of anaesthetic ether to a man in severe status asthmaticus not responding to standard treatment resulted in prompt improvement and an uneventful recovery. He was given 100 ml of a 65% solution of ether in warm olive oil.— F. W. Wittman (letter), *Br. med. J.*, 1966, *2*, 172.

Ether relaxed bronchial constriction; given as a 5% suspension in saline by intravenous injection it could assist respiration in patients with status asthmaticus unresponsive to other treatment.— L. O. Mountford (letter), *Br. med. J.*, 1973, *1*, 47.

Use in food. The Food Additives and Contaminants Committee recommended that ether be permitted for use as a solvent in food provided that it was stabilised with butylated hydroxytoluene at a maximum concentration in the solvent of 20 ppm. They recommended the use of ether on a temporary basis if it was stabilised with pyrogallol at a maximum concentration in the solvent of 3 ppm. Further toxicity studies were required when pyrogallol or other stabilisers not previously evaluated were used.— *Report on the Review of Solvents in Food*, FAC/REP/25, Ministry of Agriculture, Fisheries and Food, London, HM Stationery Office, 1978.

Preparations

Compound Ether Spirit *(B.P.C. 1949)*. Sp. Aether. Co.; Hoffmann's Anodyne. The simple spirit is called Hoffmann's Anodyne in some countries. Anaesthetic ether 13.75 ml, alcohol (90%) 195 ml, sulphuric acid 90 ml, water 3.75 ml, and sodium bicarbonate q.s. to neutrality. Preparation involves a distillation process. *Dose.* 4 to 6 ml single; 1.3 to 2.6 ml for repeated doses.

Ether Spirit *(B.P.C. 1973)*. Sp. Aether.; Hoffmann's Drops; Aether Alcoholisatus. Anaesthetic ether 33 ml, alcohol (90%) to 100 ml. Store in a cool place in airtight containers. Protect from light. This preparation is inflammable. Keep away from an open flame.

A similar spirit, with varying proportions of the 2 ingredients, is included in many pharmacopoeias. *Dose.* 1 to 4 ml (*B.P. 1953*).

3108-b

Ethyl Chloride *(B.P., U.S.P.)*. Ethyl Chlor.;

Ethylis Chloridum; Chlorethyl; Hydrochloric Ether; Monochlorethane; Aethylium Chloratum; Cloruro de Etilo. Chloroethane.

C_2H_5Cl=64.51.

CAS — 75-00-3.

Pharmacopoeias. In *Arg., Aust., Belg., Br., Chin., Cz., Hung., Ind., Int., It., Jug., Mex., Nord., Pol., Port., Roum., Rus., Span., Swiss, Turk.*, and *U.S.*

At ordinary temperatures and pressures ethyl chloride is gaseous but condenses, when slightly compressed, into a colourless, mobile, inflammable, very volatile liquid with a pleasant ethereal odour and a burning taste; it is usually supplied in the liquid form. If prepared from Industrial Methylated Spirit it contains a small variable proportion of methyl chloride. Relative density, at 0°, about 0.921. B.p. 12° to 13°. Flash-point −50° (closed-cup test).

Soluble about 1 in 200 of water; miscible with

alcohol, chloroform, and ether. It is neutral to litmus. **Store** in a cool place. Protect from light.

CAUTION. *Ethyl chloride is highly inflammable and mixtures of the gas with 5 to 15% of air are explosive.*

Adverse Effects, Treatment, and Precautions. As for Chloroform, p.745.

Laryngeal spasm may follow general anaesthesia with ethyl chloride, particularly when high doses are used.

Maximum permissible atmospheric concentration 1,000ppm.

Absorption and Fate. Ethyl chloride is rapidly absorbed on inhalation and is rapidly eliminated, mainly through the lungs.

Uses. Ethyl chloride is an anaesthetic which has been administered by inhalation. Both induction and recovery are rapid but an adequate depth of anaesthesia is difficult to maintain and it has largely been superseded by anaesthetics with a greater margin of safety.

On account of its low boiling-point and the intense cold produced by evaporation, ethyl chloride has been used as a local anaesthetic in minor surgery but this procedure is not generally recommended. It has also been used topically for the relief of pain in sprains and myalgias and for the treatment of cutaneous larva migrans (creeping eruption).

Haemorrhoids. Spraying of prolapsed haemorrhoids with ethyl chloride facilitated the reduction of strangulation.— C. P. Broad, *Lancet*, 1968, *1*, 729.

Local anaesthesia. When used as a local anaesthetic, ethyl chloride produced numbness preceded by pain. The numbness was superficial and evanescent and was inadequate for the incision of inflamed hypersensitive tissues.— *Lancet*, 1968, *2*, 1394.

Preparations

Ethyl Chloride, Bengué *(Bengué, UK)*. A brand of ethyl chloride.

3109-v

Ethylene *(B.P. 1948)*. Aethylenum; Olefiant Gas; Etileno.

C_2H_4=28.05.

CAS — 74-85-1.

Pharmacopoeias. In *Arg.*

A colourless inflammable gas somewhat lighter than air with a faint sweetish odour and taste.

One vol. measured at normal temperature and pressure dissolves, at 25°, in 9.2 vol. of water and in 0.5 vol. of alcohol, and, at 15.5°, in 0.05 vol. of ether.

CAUTION. *Mixtures with oxygen, air, or nitrous oxide at certain concentrations are explosive. Ethylene should not be used in the presence of an open flame or of any electrical apparatus liable to produce a spark. Precautions should be taken against the production of static electrical discharge.*

Uses. Ethylene is an inhalation anaesthetic that has similar actions to and is more potent than nitrous oxide. However, it is now seldom used because of its explosive nature.

With adequate pre-operative medication, concentrations of up to 90% with 10% oxygen have been employed for induction and a concentration of 80% or less for maintenance.

Mixtures containing 3 to 80% of oxygen are explosive. Mixtures of ethylene and nitrous oxide are violently explosive and should never be used.

3110-r

Etomidate. R 16659; R 26490 *(sulphate)*. *R*-(+)-Ethyl 1-(α-methylbenzyl)imidazole-5-carboxylate.

$C_{14}H_{16}N_2O_2$=244.3.

CAS — 33125-97-2.

A white or yellowish crystalline or amorphous powder. M.p. about 67°.

Adverse Effects. Coughing, hiccup, and excitement may occur in patients who have not received premedication. Apnoea has been reported. Laryngospasm is rare; skin rash and skin flushing have occasionally occurred. Nausea and vomiting may occur postoperatively.

Involuntary myoclonic muscle movements, sometimes severe, are common, but may be reduced by the prior injection of fentanyl.

A high incidence of pain on injection was associated with the original aqueous solution of etomidate sulphate. Thrombophlebitis has occasionally occurred. The incidence of pain is lower with the newer formulations in macrogols or propylene glycol, and may be reduced by giving the injection into a large vein in the arm, rather than into the hand.

In 14 patients given etomidate 200 µg per kg body-weight intravenously, anaesthesia was induced in 10 seconds and lasted for 6 to 8 minutes. There was a slight reduction (8.5%) in mean arterial pressure, a negligible increase (2.8%) in heart-rate, and no significant effect on the mean pulmonary artery pressure. Cardiac output and stroke volume were lowered by 7.6 and 10% respectively and peripheral vascular resistance was lowered by 3.8%.— K. Rifat *et al.*, *Can. Anaesth. Soc. J.*, 1976, *23*, 492.

In 48 patients in whom anaesthesia was induced with thiopentone 4 mg per kg body-weight or etomidate (as sulphate) 300 µg per kg there was a reduction of 15 mmHg systolic pressure after thiopentone and 5 mmHg after etomidate; diastolic pressure was not affected; the changes were not significant. Slight myoclonia occurred in 25% of those given etomidate, and severe myoclonia in 8%; no severe myoclonia occurred after premedication with fentanyl or diazepam. Hypoventilation occurred in 25% of those given etomidate, and transient apnoea in 16%.— J. M. Gooding and G. Corssen, *Anesth. Analg. curr. Res.*, 1976, *55*, 286.

In 30 patients premedicated with diazepam and atropine apnoea lasting for about 30 seconds occurred in 12 after receiving etomidate (as sulphate) 300 µg per kg body-weight; 8 of 30 given papaveretum and hyoscine as premedication became apnoeic. The respiratory-rate was significantly increased in the diazepam group but not in the papaveretum group; there was a transient depression of minute volume in the papaveretum group. Etomidate might be of value in obstetric anaesthesia, but involuntary muscle movements might be a limiting factor.— M. Morgan *et al.*, *Br. J. Anaesth.*, 1977, *49*, 233.

A randomised comparison in 120 patients of the effects of etomidate 300 µg per kg body-weight and thiopentone 3.5 mg per kg. Pain on injection occurred in 43.3 and 1.7% of patients respectively, with 5 and 3 patients experiencing thrombophlebitis. [The solvent for etomidate was not specified.] Myoclonic movements occurred in 28% of those given etomidate and were severe in about a third; in several they resembled generalised convulsive seizures but no epileptiform discharges were seen in the EEGs of 10 patients studied. There were no myoclonic movements after thiopentone. Seven patients developed tonic movements after etomidate and one after thiopentone. Apnoea occurred in 8 given etomidate and 25 given thiopentone. There was a slight initial reduction in respiration-rate after etomidate, followed by an increase, compared with a greater initial reduction after thiopentone. There were no significant differences between etomidate and thiopentone in respect of slight increases in pulse-rate and slight reductions in blood pressure. No arrhythmias were seen.— M. M. Ghoneim and T. Yamada, *Anesth. Analg. curr. Res.*, 1977, *56*, 479.

In 50 patients anaesthetised with etomidate 300 µg per kg body-weight in a macrogol basis, the incidence of involuntary muscle movement was 18%, and that of pain on injection 4%. Cardiovascular stability was maintained.— J. G. B. Hendry *et al.*, *Anaesthesia*, 1977, *32*, 996. A similar report.— B. van Dijk, *Anaesthetist*, 1978, *27*, 60.

Three formulations of etomidate injection were evaluated in 143 unpremedicated patients undergoing minor gynaecological surgery. The preparations compared were: an aqueous 0.15% solution of the sulphate, a 0.2% solution of etomidate in macrogol, and a 0.2% solution of etomidate in propylene glycol. Injections of 300 µg per kg body-weight [form unspecified] were given at either 2 mg or 1 mg per second. Pain occurred in about 30% of all patients with no significant difference between formulations or injection-rates. Excitatory effects occurred in about 80% of all patients during induction and were significantly more frequent than those previously reported with methohexitone, regardless of formulation or speed of injection. Recovery from all 3 formulations was rapid although vomiting frequently occurred. Etomidate was not considered to be a satisfactory induction agent when used alone.— M. Zacharias *et al.*, *Br. J. Anaesth.*, 1978, *50*, 925.

In a study in 500 patients the frequency of phlebitis, thrombosis, and thrombophlebitis following intravenous administration of etomidate was governed by injection formulation and dose used and was not related to pain on injection. The frequency was greatest (23.1%) with the propylene glycol formulation compared with 10.8% for the aqueous formulation and 7.7% for the macrogol formulation.— M. Zacharias *et al.*, *Br. J. Anaesth.*, 1979, *51*, 779.

Pain on injection and involuntary muscle movements were considered to be still unacceptably severe in 5% of 43 patients given fentanyl 2.5 µg per kg body-weight or diazepam 125 µg per kg intravenously before administration of etomidate 300 µg per kg (dissolved in propylene glycol 35%) to induce anaesthesia.— K. Korttila *et al.*, *Br. J. Anaesth.*, 1979, *51*, 1151.

Of more than 100 patients, none reported pain when etomidate was injected into the antecubital fossa over an average time of 10 seconds. Premedication had been diazepam and droperidol by mouth and injection of etomidate had been preceded by fentanyl 1 µg per kg body-weight.— N. T. M. Jack (letter), *Br. J. Anaesth.*, 1980, *52*, 843.

Absorption and Fate. After injection, etomidate is rapidly redistributed to other body tissues. Plasma concentrations decrease rapidly for about 30 minutes and then more slowly; traces are still detectable after 6 hours; metabolites, chiefly of hydrolysis, are more slowly excreted. Etomidate is extensively (about 76%) bound to plasma protein; metabolites are less extensively bound. About 75% of a dose is excreted in the urine in 24 hours.

In 4 patients given etomidate sulphate 300 µg per kg body-weight plasma concentrations suggested a 3-compartment pharmacokinetic model. Mean half-lives were: distribution, 2.8 minutes; intermediate, 32.1 minutes; elimination, 3.9 hours. The apparent volume of distribution suggested considerable tissue uptake.— J. J. Ambre *et al.*, *Fedn Proc.*, 1977, *36*, 997. See also M. J. Van Hamme, *Anesthesiology*, 1978, *49*, 274.

Etomidate was found to be 75.1%, 56.6%, and 55.8% bound to plasma proteins *in vitro* when added to plasma samples from healthy subjects, patients with renal failure, and patients with hepatic cirrhosis respectively; the amount of binding was proportional to the serum albumin concentration. Administration of etomidate in a usual dosage to patients with renal failure or hepatic disease might possibly produce an abnormal response.— R. Carlos *et al.*, *Clin. Pharmacokinet.*, 1979, *4*, 144.

Further references: M. M. Ghoneim and K. Korttila, *Clin. Pharmacokinet.*, 1977, *2*, 344.

Uses. Etomidate is administered intravenously for complete anaesthesia of short duration. It has no analgesic activity. Anaesthesia is rapidly induced and may last for 6 to 8 minutes with a single usual dose.

Etomidate appears to have only slight effects on blood pressure, heart-rate, or respiration.

The usual dose is 300 µg per kg body-weight given slowly, preferably into a large vein in the arm, followed by further individual doses of 100 to 200 µg per kg as required. Narcotic analgesics as premedication reduce myoclonic movements. A muscle relaxant is necessary if intubation is required.

Anaesthesia has been maintained by the infusion of etomidate; a suggested dose is 10 to 40 µg per kg per minute; adequate analgesia is required.

Etomidate is available as a concentrated solution for the preparation of infusion solutions.

A brief review of etomidate in anaesthesia.— J. W. Dundee, *Br. J. Anaesth.*, 1979, *51*, 641.

Etomidate was not considered to release histamine when given intravenously.— A. Doenicke *et al.*, *Br. J. Anaesth.*, 1973, *45*, 1097.

A brief report of experience in 3000 patients.— J. Van De Walle *et al.*, *Acta anaesth. belg.*, 1976, *27*, *Suppl.*, 139.

Selective anaesthesia of one cerebral hemisphere was effectively carried out by injecting etomidate 20 µg per kg body-weight into the internal carotid artery. Intra-arterial injection was considered harmless.— Z. Kalenda (letter), *Lancet*, 1976, *2*, 1143.

Reduction of cerebral blood flow by etomidate.— J. Van Aken and G. Rolly, *Acta anaesth. belg.*, 1976, *27*, *Suppl.*, 175. See also A. M. Renou *et al.*, *Br. J. Anaesth.*, 1978, *50*, 1047.

In 40 patients in whom anaesthesia was induced by etomidate 300 µg per kg body-weight, intra-ocular pressure was significantly reduced from a mean of 15.52 mmHg to a mean of 10.51 mmHg.— C. E. Famewo and C. O. Odugbesan, *Can. Anaesth. Soc. J.*, 1978, *25*, 130.

A multinational evaluation of etomidate sulphate (in phosphate buffer) for induction of anaesthesia in 4452 patients.— V. Schuermans *et al.*, *Anaesthesist*, 1978, *27*, 52.

Results of a study in 10 patients with intracranial lesions requiring craniotomy indicated that etomidate could be used for the induction of anaesthesia in patients with intracranial space-occupying lesions without increasing intracranial pressure or seriously reducing cerebral perfusion pressure.— E. Moss *et al.*, *Br. J. Anaesth.*, 1979, *51*, 347.

Further references.— M. Morgan *et al.*, *Lancet*, 1975, *1*, 955; A. Holdcroft *et al.*, *Br. J. Anaesth.*, 1976, *48*, 199; G. S. Ingram *et al.*, *Br. J. clin. Pharmac.*, 1976, *3*, 356; M. Zindler, *Acta anaesth. belg.*, 1976, *27*, *Suppl.*, 143; K. Rifat *et al.*, *Annls Anesthesiol. fr.*, 1976, *17*, 1217; J. du Cailar *et al.*, *ibid.*, 1223; R. J. Fragen *et al.*, *Anesth. Analg. curr. Res.*, 1976, *55*, 730; D. Patschke *et al.*, *Can. Anaesth. Soc. J.*, 1977, *24*, 57; S. Urdinovic, *J. int. med. Res.*, 1978, *6*, 452; M. P. Colvin *et al.*, *Br. J. Anaesth.*, 1979, *51*, 551; M. Delrue *et al.*, *Curr. ther. Res.*, 1980, *27*, 699; L. Daehlin and L. Gran, *ibid.*, 706; A. Criado *et al.*, *Br. J. Anaesth.*, 1980, *52*, 803.

Comparison with methohexitone. Comparison with methohexitone in 200 patients.— J. Dubois-Primo *et al.*, *Acta anaesth. belg.*, 1976, *27*, *Suppl.*, 187.

Comparison with thiopentone. Etomidate was superior to thiopentone as an induction agent in 296 patients undergoing various minor surgical procedures. Return to awareness postoperatively was more rapid when etomidate was given.— J. J. C. Oudenaarden, *Curr. med. Res. Opinion*, 1979, *6*, 30.

Electroconvulsive therapy. Successful use as an induction agent prior to electroconvulsive therapy.— T. M. O'Carroll *et al.*, *Anaesthesia*, 1977, *32*, 868. See also B. Kay, *Br. J. Anaesth.*, 1976, *48*, 213.

Gynaecological procedures. Etomidate 300 µg per kg body-weight was used to induce anaesthesia in 396 women undergoing minor gynaecological operations. Pain on injection was significantly reduced by fast injection and pethidine premedication and with macrogol and propylene glycol formulations compared with aqueous solution. Excitatory phenomena were reduced by premedication with diazepam or pethidine. Recovery from anaesthesia was quick but nausea and vomiting were common in all groups including those receiving premedication. Patient acceptability was high.— M. Zacharias *et al.*, *Br. J. Anaesth.*, 1979, *51*, 127.

Open-heart surgery. Elevation of systolic blood pressure and a reduction in cardiac index after etomidate, suxamethonium, and intubation in patients undergoing open-heart surgery were probably due to the short action of etomidate and to the absence of analgesic effect.— B. Thomas *et al.*, *Acta anaesth. belg.*, 1976, *27*, *Suppl.*, 167.

Pregnancy and the neonate. In a study in 60 women undergoing caesarean section etomidate 300 µg per kg body-weight or thiopentone 3.5 mg per kg body-weight was used for induction of anaesthesia. The clinical status of the newborn was considered superior with etomidate.— J. W. Downing *et al.*, *Br. J. Anaesth.*, 1979, *51*, 135. A similar report.— P. J. C. Houlton *et al.*, *S.Afr. med. J.*, 1978, *54*, 773.

Urology. A report of the use of etomidate in 200 patients undergoing urological procedures.— N. W. Lees and J. G. B. Hendry, *Anaesthesia*, 1977, *32*, 592.

Use in children. In 198 children given etomidate buffered injection (pH 3.3) for the induction of anaesthesia induction was considered good in 118 and fair in 77. Myoclonia occurred in 10% of patients and pain in 27%. Pain was not relieved by the addition of lignocaine 1 mg to the injection. A few patients had increases or decreases in systolic blood pressure. ECG changes were unlikely to be due to etomidate. Pain on injection did not occur in 20 patients given injections of 0.3% etomidate sulphate in 20% aqueous solution of Cremophor EL.— B. Kay, *Br. J. Anaesth.*, 1976, *48*, 207.

Proprietary Preparations

Hypnomidate *(Janssen, UK)*. Etomidate, available as an **Injection** containing 2 mg per ml in an aqueous vehicle containing propylene glycol 35%, in ampoules of 10 ml, and as **Concentrate** containing etomidate hydrochloride equivalent to etomidate 125 mg per ml, in ampoules of 1 ml, for preparing infusions. (Also available as Hypnomidate in *Aust.*, *Belg.*, *Ger.*, *Neth.*, *S.Afr.*, *Switz.*).

Other Proprietary names

Hypnomidat *(Denm.)*.

3111-f

Fluroxene. (2,2,2-Trifluoroethoxy)ethylene; 2,2,2-Trifluoroethyl vinyl ether.
$C_4H_5F_3O$=126.1.

CAS — 406-90-6.

A clear, almost colourless, inflammable, volatile liquid with a mild ethereal odour. Wt per ml about 1.13 g. B.p. about 43°. **Soluble** 1 in 220 of water; miscible with alcohol, acetone, ether, and most halogenated solvents. **Store** below 40° in airtight containers. Protect from light.

CAUTION. *Fluroxene is very volatile and inflammable and mixtures of its vapour with oxygen or air at certain concentrations are explosive. It should not be used in the presence of an open flame or any electrical apparatus liable to produce a spark. Precautions should be taken against the production of static electrical discharge.*

Adverse Effects. Fluroxene depresses the myocardium but the effect may be masked by concomitant sympathetic stimulation; it does not appear to sensitise the myocardium to the effects of catecholamines. As the depth of anaesthesia is increased there is respiratory depression and a fall in arterial pressure. Postoperative nausea and vomiting are common following prolonged deep anaesthesia. The bleeding time is prolonged during anaesthesia. There have been several reports of hepatotoxicity in patients receiving fluroxene.

Uses. Fluroxene is an anaesthetic which has been administered by inhalation. It possesses good analgesic but poor muscle relaxant properties and is less inflammable than ether. Both induction and recovery are rapid. Fluroxene may be administered with oxygen or a nitrous oxide and oxygen mixture by a closed or semi-closed method. Anaesthesia may be induced with 6 to 15% v/v and maintained with 3 to 8% v/v. If administered with 75% nitrous oxide and 25% oxygen, concentrations of up to 2% may be adequate.

3112-d

Hydroxydione Sodium Succinate. Sodium 3,20-dioxo-5α-pregnan-21-yl succinate.
$C_{25}H_{35}NaO_6$=454.5.

CAS — 303-01-5 (hydroxydione); 53-10-1 (sodium succinate).

A white crystalline solid. Readily **soluble** in water; soluble in acetone and chloroform. **Incompatible** with salts of pethidine, tubocurarine, and suxamethonium.

Hydroxydione sodium succinate is a steroid formerly given in doses of 0.5 to 1.5 g intravenously for the induction of anaesthesia.

Proprietary Names

Viadril G *(Pfizer, Fr.)*.

3113-n

Isoflurane.

Compound 469. 1-Chloro-2,2,2-trifluoroethyl difluoromethyl ether.
$C_3H_2ClF_5O$=184.5.

CAS — 26675-46-7.

A volatile liquid with a characteristic odour. B.p. about 49°.

Adverse Effects and Precautions. Isoflurane depresses respiration to a greater extent than halothane but it produces less cardiac depression. The effects of the non-depolarising muscle relaxants such as tubocurarine are enhanced to a greater extent by isoflurane than by other anaesthetics. It does not appear to sensitise the myocardium to the effect of catecholamines.

There was greater neuromuscular blockade with gallamine, pancuronium, and suxamethonium in 36 patients anaesthetised with isoflurane than in 36 patients anaesthetised with halothane.— R. D. Miller *et al.*, *Anesthesiology*, 1971, *35*, 509.

A comparison of the toxicity of isoflurane, ether, fluroxene, and halothane.— W. C. Stevens *et al.*, *Can. Anaesth. Soc. J.*, 1973, *20*, 357, per *J. Am. med. Ass.*, 1973, *225*, 80.

In 12 subjects isoflurane caused no seizure activity in the EEG.— D. L. Clark *et al.*, *Anesthesiology*, 1973, *39*, 261.

Isoflurane and halothane caused a similar depression of respiration in a study of 32 healthy surgical patients who had also received nitrous oxide and morphine.— C. J. France *et al.*, *Br. J. Anaesth.*, 1974, *46*, 117.

Intra-anaesthetic depression of renal blood flow, glomerular filtration-rate, and urine flow were similar in patients anaesthetised with halothane or isoflurane. Postanaesthetic renal function was normal in both groups.— R. I. Mazze *et al.*, *Anesthesiology*, 1974, *40*, 536.

Uses. Isoflurane is a volatile anaesthetic administered by inhalation. It is an isomer of enflurane and is considered to produce smooth induction and emergence. Isoflurane is reported to possess good analgesic properties.

A review: E. I. Eger, *Anesthesiology*, 1981, *55*, 559. See also H. W. Linde and M. H. M. Dykes, *J. Am. med. Ass.*, 1981, *245*, 2335; A. R. Hunter, *Practitioner*, 1973, *211*, 476.

The cardiovascular effects of isoflurane during surgery.— C. L. Graves *et al.*, *Anesthesiology*, 1974, *41*, 486.

Absence of significant biotransformation.— D. A. Holaday *et al.*, *Anesthesiology*, 1975, *43*, 325.

In 7 elderly patients given isoflurane 0.75 increased to 1.5% in 70% nitrous oxide and oxygen blood pressure, peripheral resistance, end-systolic volume, the rate of left-ventricular pressure development, tension time index, and myocardial oxygen consumption fell; there were no changes in other haemodynamic parameters. The main disadvantage of isoflurane was hypotension.— J. Tarnow *et al.*, *Br. J. Anaesth.*, 1976, *48*, 669.

Proprietary Names

Forane *(Ohio Medical, USA)*.

NOTE. The name Forane has also been applied to an aerosol propellent.

3114-h

Ketamine Hydrochloride *(U.S.P.)*.

CI 581; CL 369. (±)-2-(2-Chlorophenyl)-2-methylaminocyclohexanone hydrochloride.
$C_{13}H_{16}ClNO,HCl$=274.2.

CAS — 6740-88-1 (ketamine); 1867-66-9 (hydrochloride).

Pharmacopoeias. In *Chin.* and *U.S.*

A white crystalline powder with a slight characteristic odour. M.p. 258° to 261°. Ketamine hydrochloride 1.15 mg is approximately equivalent to 1 mg of ketamine base. **Soluble** 1 in 4 of water, 1 in 14 of alcohol, 1 in 60 of dehydrated alcohol and chloroform, and 1 in 6 of methyl alcohol; practically insoluble in ether. A 10% solution has a pH of 3.5 to 4.1. **Incompatible** with soluble barbiturates.

Adverse Effects. Emergence reactions are common during recovery from ketamine anaesthesia and include vivid often unpleasant dreams, confusion, hallucinations, irrational behaviour, and increased muscle tone. Children and elderly patients appear to be slightly less sensitive than other adult patients. The incidence is reported to be lower after intramuscular than after intravenous injection. Blood pressure and heart-rate may be temporarily increased by ketamine but hypotension, arrhythmias, and bradycardia have occurred rarely.

The respiration may be depressed, especially during too rapid intravenous injection. Apnoea and laryngospasm have occurred. Diplopia and nystagmus may occur. Nausea and vomiting, dizziness, and headache may arise during recovery from ketamine anaesthesia. Transient skin rashes and pain at the site of injection have occasionally been reported.

A 33-year-old woman developed progressive polyneuropathy shortly after she was given ketamine 150 mg for the removal of a benign breast cyst. The Guillain-Barré syndrome might be a complication of this drug.— M. Cherington (letter), *Lancet*, 1970, *2*, 569.

A 3-year-old boy developed profuse salivation and total

respiratory obstruction after an intramuscular injection of ketamine 10 mg per kg body-weight. Atropine was now routinely given as premedication and resuscitative facilities were immediately available.— C. K. Davies (letter), *Br. med. J.*, 1972, *4*, 178.

Abuse. Hallucinations, dizziness, diplopia, horizontal nystagmus, and disconjugate eye movements might occur in patients following illicit ingestion of ketamine.— L. L. Shaffer (letter), *J. Am. med. Ass.*, 1974, *229*, 763.

Cardiovascular effects. Renin was not responsible for hypertension occurring after the use of ketamine.— E. D. Miller *et al.*, *Anesthesiology*, 1975, *42*, 503.

A study in 12 patients indicated that the cardiovascular stimulant effect of ketamine was due to enhanced sympathoneuronal and sympatho-adrenal activity.— E. Appel *et al.*, *Eur. J. clin. Pharmac.*, 1979, *16*, 91.

Reports on the absence of cardiovascular effects: D. C. Nettles *et al.*, *Anesth. Analg. curr. Res.*, 1973, *52*, 59.

Convulsions. Abnormal EEG recordings were observed in 9 patients with epilepsy given ketamine in doses of 0.5 to 4 mg per kg body-weight. Behaviour changes included unconsciousness and tonic and clonic motor activity.— T. Ferrer-Allado *et al.*, *Anesthesiology*, 1973, *38*, 333.

There were no seizures recorded during ketamine anaesthesia in 23 patients with epilepsy. Specific paroxysmal discharges were activated more by natural sleep than by ketamine.— G. G. Celesia *et al.*, *Neurology, Minneap.*, 1974, *24*, 386.

Of 19 brain-damaged patients with epilepsy who were anaesthetised with ketamine, 10 had seizures during or after anaesthesia, whereas seizures occurred in 1 of 20 similar patients receiving thiopentone sodium. Those patients who had seizures whilst receiving ketamine had a higher base-line seizure frequency than those who had no seizures.— J. A. Madsen *et al.*, *Neurology, Minneap.*, 1974, *24*, 386.

Effect on body temperature. A report of malignant hyperthermia possibly associated with ketamine in 2 patients.— J. V. Mogensen *et al.* (letter), *Lancet*, 1974, *1*, 461. See also S. Roervik and J. Stovner (letter), *ibid.*, 1974, *2*, 1384; D. E. Lees and T. MacNamara, *Anesthesiology*, 1977, *47*, 390.

Ketamine had no effect on plasma creatine phosphokinase activity in 10 of 11 healthy subjects.— H. Y. Meltzer *et al.* (letter), *Lancet*, 1975, *1*, 1195.

Effect on the eye. When given to 46 patients of various ages with no ophthalmological disturbance, ketamine hydrochloride caused a mild but significant increase in intra-ocular pressure, which was not related to changes in blood pressure.— G. Corssen and J. E. Hoy, *J. Pediat. Ophthal.*, 1967, *4*, 20.

Three patients suffered temporary blindness lasting about 25 minutes after operations in which they had been anaesthetised with ketamine in doses of 150 mg, 125 mg, and 125 mg.— J. Fine *et al.*, *Anesth. Analg. curr. Res.*, 1974, *53*, 72.

Ketamine 2 mg per kg body-weight had no significant effect on intra-ocular pressure in 20 patients.— M. Peuler *et al.*, *Anesthesiology*, 1975, *43*, 575.

Hazard to respiration. See below under Precautions.

Psychic disturbance. A 29-year-old woman developed psychosis after an intravenous injection of ketamine 300 mg; the condition was still present a year later.— B. D. Johnson (letter), *Br. med. J.*, 1971, *4*, 428. A 23-year-old woman with a history of psychosis was anaesthetised on 6 occasions, with ketamine up to 260 mg during a 90-minute operation, without adverse effect. Premedication was necessary, excessive dosage should be avoided, and post-operative sedation was probably advisable.— S. M. Laird and M. Sage (letter), *ibid.*, 1972, *1*, 246.

Ketamine produced a high incidence of illusions in a study of 48 subjects. This incidence was higher than that with thiopentone with nitrous oxide and halothane whereas there was no difference in postoperative anxiety.— J. M. Garfield *et al.*, *Anesthesiology*, 1972, *36*, 329.

Further references: J. W. D. Knox *et al.*, *Br. J. Anaesth.*, 1970, *42*, 875; B. B. Collier, *Anaesthesia*, 1972, *27*, 120; J. Fine and S. C. Finestone, *Anesth. Analg. curr. Res.*, 1973, *52*, 428; A. Perel and J. T. Davidson, *Anaesthesia*, 1976, *31*, 1081; E. F. Meyers and P. Charles, *Anesthesiology*, 1978, *49*, 39; *Br. J. Anaesth.*, 1980, *52*, 967.

Treatment of Adverse Effects. Emergence delirium may be controlled by tranquillisers. Assisted ventilation may be required for severe respiratory depression.

Droperidol administered before or following surgery reduced the postoperative central effects of ketamine in a study of 75 patients but had no effect on the incidence of side-effects during anaesthesia. Pentobarbitone had no effect on ketamine side-effects either during or after anaesthesia.— M. S. Sadove *et al.*, *Anesth. Analg. curr. Res.*, 1971, *50*, 526.

The unpleasant postoperative sequelae of ketamine could be effectively treated by the administration of diazepam 1 mg per 6 kg body-weight at the end of surgery.— D. L. Coppel and J. W. Dundee (letter), *Br. med. J.*, 1972, *1*, 805.

In a study of 300 patients anaesthetised with ketamine, chlorpromazine 10 mg intravenously or placebo was administered prior to induction and diazepam 5 mg, droperidol 5 mg, or placebo was administered intravenously after anaesthesia. Chlorpromazine with diazepam was most effective in reducing emergence reactions. Droperidol had no beneficial effect.— P. H. Erbguth *et al.*, *Anesth. Analg. curr. Res.*, 1972, *51*, 693.

Droperidol 75 µg per kg body-weight alone or with fentanyl 0.375 µg per kg reduced the incidence of emergence reactions following ketamine anaesthesia and also decreased the induced tachycardia and hypertension in a controlled study of 214 patients undergoing abortions. Diazepam 150 µg per kg and thiopentone 1.5 mg per kg had no effect on ketamine side-effects.— L. Becsey *et al.*, *Anesthesiology*, 1972, *37*, 536.

Increases in intracranial pressure were observed in 7 patients with intracranial lesions when they were undergoing ketamine anaesthesia on 11 occasions. The increase could be reversed rapidly by administration of thiopentone.— H. M. Shapiro *et al.*, *Br. J. Anaesth.*, 1972, *44*, 1200. See also below under Precautions.

In a study of 59 patients receiving ketamine for anaesthesia amantadine was considered to be superior to diazepam in reducing emergence reactions.— G. Lucca *et al.*, *Br. J. clin. Pract.*, 1975, *29*, 15.

Lorazepam 4 mg intravenously 1 hour before surgery under ketamine anaesthesia virtually abolished unpleasant dreams and severe emergence delirium in 45 patients but had no effect on other complications of ketamine.— J. K. Lilburn *et al.*, *Br. J. Anaesth.*, 1976, *48*, 1125.

When assessed for control of emergence delirium and reduction of unpleasant dreams in 255 patients anaesthetised with ketamine 2 mg per kg body-weight and increments as required for short minor operations, lorazepam 4 mg, flunitrazepam 1.5 mg or a combination of droperidol 5 mg and fentanyl 0.1 mg given intravenously 10 minutes before anaesthesia, had greater beneficial effects than diazepam, pentobarbitone, hydroxyzine, pethidine or promethazine. However, the combination of droperidol and fentanyl caused a high incidence of respiratory depression. Lorazepam 4 mg was also effective when given to 35 patients 30 to 40 minutes before anaesthesia. Experience in treating a further 120 patients justified the recommendation that lorazepam 4 mg given intravenously at least 30 minutes before ketamine-induced anaesthesia was a reliable method of controlling emergence sequelae.— J. K. Lilburn *et al.*, *Br. J. clin. Pharmac.*, 1977, *4*, 641 P.

Labetalol given in an initial dose of 1 mg per kg body-weight was considered to be promising in the control of the cardio-stimulatory effects of ketamine. However, patients were unduly sensitive to blood loss and bronchospasm was precipitated in an asthmatic patient.— J. W. Dundee *et al.*, *Br. J. clin. Pharmac.*, 1977, *4*, 658P.

In a double-blind study of adverse reactions after anaesthesia solely with ketamine, 135 women were allocated to 1 of 4 groups and given premedication with pentobarbitone or droperidol, intravenously or intramuscularly. Adverse emergence reactions were not prevented and there was a high incidence of visual disturbance in all groups. Patients who received pentobarbitone intravenously did not recall unpleasant dream-like experiences and those given droperidol intravenously had the shortest recovery time. Pentobarbitone protected against the increase in arterial systolic pressure associated with ketamine and droperidol protected against the initial increase of heart-rate after ketamine administration.— E. M. Figallo *et al.*, *Br. J. Anaesth.*, 1977, *49*, 1159.

A favourable report of the use of diazepam to prevent emergence reactions.— S. P. Kothary and E. K. Zsigmond, *Clin. Pharmac. Ther.*, 1977, *21*, 108.

Precautions. Ketamine hydrochloride is contra-indicated in patients with hypertension. It is best avoided in patients with eclampsia and should be used with caution in patients with a history of convulsive disorders or psychiatric disease. Ketamine should not be given to patients with increased intra-ocular or CSF pressure or intracranial space-occupying lesions. Alternative anaesthetics should be considered for patients with penetrating wounds of the eye. Patients should be intubated to avoid the risk of aspiration. Verbal, tactile, and visual stimuli should be kept to a minimum during recovery in an attempt to reduce the risk of emergence reactions.

See also Precautions for General Anaesthetics, p.740.

Ketamine enhanced the depressant effects of barbiturates and narcotic analgesics and anaesthetising abusers of such drugs might produce potentially fatal respiratory depression which might not always be immediately obvious after surgery.— E. Bloomquist (letter), *J. Am. med. Ass.*, 1971, *218*, 1301.

The duration of sleep produced by ketamine was significantly prolonged in patients receiving diazepam, hydroxyzine, or quinalbarbitone for premedication. This effect was considered to be due to a decreased rate of metabolism of ketamine.— J. N. Lo and J. F. Cumming, *Anesthesiology*, 1975, *43*, 307.

Increases in ventricular fluid pressure in hydrocephalic children during ketamine anaesthesia.— R. S. Crumrine *et al.*, *Anesthesiology*, 1975, *42*, 758.

The chronotropic and inotropic effects of ketamine were prevented by halothane.— M. Johnstone, *Anaesthesia*, 1976, *31*, 873. See also A. V. Bidwai *et al.*, *Anesth. Analg. curr. Res.*, 1975, *54*, 588.

Pulmonary vascular resistance rose by 42% and pulmonary arterial pressure by 47% in 16 patients given ketamine 2.2 mg per kg body-weight. Intrapulmonary shunting increased by 22% but was barely significant. Pulmonary hypertension might be a relative contra-indication to the use of ketamine.— J. M. Gooding *et al.*, *Anesth. Analg. curr. Res.*, 1977, *56*, 813.

For the enhancement of the effect of tubocurarine by ketamine, see Tubocurarine Chloride, p.999.

Effect on CSF pressure. Ketamine was not recommended as an anaesthetic in neurosurgical procedures because it produced greatly increased intrathecal pressures which could be dangerous in certain neurosurgical and neuroradiological situations.— J. Evans *et al.* (letter), *Lancet*, 1971, *1*, 40. Comments.— G. H. Wilson, *ibid.*, 243.

Ketamine, 1 to 1.3 mg per kg body-weight, given rapidly as a single intravenous injection, caused a slight rise in intrathecal pressure in some patients undergoing lumbar surgery, and marked increases in 6 of 9 patients with known intracranial space-occupying lesions. The rise in blood pressure associated with ketamine was also greater in these patients.— J. M. Gibbs, *Br. J. Anaesth.*, 1972, *44*, 1298.

Measurements in 8 patients given ketamine showed an increase in the CSF pressure accompanied by an increase in the cerebral blood flow. The increased pressure was abolished by hypocarbia.— A. Sari *et al.*, *Anesth. Analg. curr. Res.*, 1972, *51*, 560.

Further references: A. E. Gardner *et al.*, *Anesth. Analg. curr. Res.*, 1972, *51*, 741.

Hazard to respiration. Depression of the laryngeal-closure reflex occurred in 7 patients anaesthetised with ketamine. It was suggested that endotracheal intubation should be used to prevent the risk of silent aspiration.— P. A. Taylor and R. M. Towey, *Br. med. J.*, 1971, *2*, 688.

The use of contrast medium on the tongue had shown aspiration into the lungs in 1 of 10 children anaesthetised with ketamine given intramuscularly. The use of ketamine for anaesthesia in burn dressings (where starvation was undesirable) had been abandoned.— M. Sage and S. M. Laird (letter), *Br. med. J.*, 1972, *4*, 670.

A report of aspiration pneumonitis in a child anaesthetised with ketamine.— B. H. Penrose, *Anesth. Analg. curr. Res.*, 1972, *51*, 41.

Aspiration with subsequent respiratory problems occurred in 3 patients anaesthetised with ketamine for surgery in the nasal or oral cavity. Ketamine was contra-indicated as an anaesthetic for such procedures.— W. M. Bryant, *Plastic reconstr. Surg.*, 1973, *51*, 562.

Hypoxia from ketamine; oxygen and assisted respiration should be used during ketamine anaesthesia.— E. K. Zsigmond *et al.*, *Anesth. Analg. curr. Res.*, 1976, *55*, 311.

Absorption and Fate. Ketamine appears to be rapidly distributed in the body tissues following parenteral administration. It diffuses into the

CSF. Most of the dose is excreted in the urine as conjugated metabolites. The estimated half-life is about 2 hours. It crosses the placenta.

The pharmacokinetics of ketamine.— M. M. Ghoneim and K. Korttila, *Clin. Pharmacokinet.*, 1977, *2*, 344.

Further references: J. Idvall *et al.*, *Br. J. Anaesth.*, 1979, *51*, 1167.

Uses. Ketamine hydrochloride produces dissociative anaesthesia characterised by catalepsy, amnesia, and marked analgesia which may persist into the recovery period. There is often an increase in muscle tone and the patient's eyes may remain open for all or part of the period of anaesthesia. It may be administered by intravenous or intramuscular injection.

Induction is slower than with the barbiturate anaesthetics or propanidid. A dose equivalent to 2 mg of ketamine per kg body-weight given intravenously usually produces surgical anaesthesia within 30 seconds and lasting for 5 to 10 minutes; an intramuscular dose equivalent to 10 mg of ketamine per kg usually produces surgical anaesthesia within 3 to 4 minutes lasting for 12 to 25 minutes.

Ketamine is used for anaesthesia for diagnostic or short surgical operations, for the induction of anaesthesia to be maintained with other agents, and as a supplementary anaesthetic for use with nitrous oxide and oxygen. However, its undesirable effects during recovery may preclude its use in adults in all but a few procedures such as cardiac catheterisation and conditions where repeated anaesthesia is required. Intravenous injections in the usual doses equivalent to 1 to 4.5 mg of ketamine per kg body-weight must be given over 60 seconds to prevent respiratory depression. Doses of 6.5 to 13 mg per kg body-weight may be given intramuscularly. Administration should be preceded by atropine or other suitable anticholinergic agent. Additional analgesia is required in procedures involving visceral pain pathways.

Reviews of the actions and uses of ketamine hydrochloride: *Br. med. J.*, 1971, *2*, 666; *Drug & Ther. Bull.*, 1971, *9*, 75; J. G. Bovill *et al.*, *Lancet*, 1971, *1*, 1285; *Med. Lett.*, 1977, *19*, 58; A. O. Lotfy, *J. int. med. Res.*, 1978, *6*, 61.

Ketamine produced good anaesthesia in 87 elderly poor-risk patients undergoing various surgical procedures. All patients experienced a rise in diastolic and systolic blood pressure. There were 5 deaths, none associated with anaesthesia.— P. H. Lorhan and M. Lippman, *Anesth. Analg. curr. Res.*, 1971, *50*, 448.

In a study of 15 patients, ketamine did not reduce the blood viscosity or fibrinogen concentration. There was an increase in the haematocrit.— F. Magora *et al.*, *Br. J. Anaesth.*, 1974, *46*, 343.

Ketamine was a reversible inhibitor of plasma cholinesterase at concentrations slightly larger than those in clinical use.— F. T. Schuh, *Br. J. Anaesth.*, 1975, *47*, 1315.

The use of physostigmine might permit the analgesic action of ketamine to be used without its unpleasant psychological effects.— H. G. R. Balmer and S. R. Wyte, *Br. J. Anaesth.*, 1977, *49*, 510. The combined use of ketamine and physostigmine was not advised because of the risk of convulsions.— A. Houghton (letter), *ibid.*, 1978, *50*, 81.

The effect of ketamine on plasma concentrations of luteinising hormone, testosterone, and cortisol.— T. Oyama *et al.*, *Br. J. Anaesth.*, 1977, *49*, 983.

There was no awareness of intubation in 39 patients given ketamine 2 mg per kg body-weight intravenously followed immediately by suxamethonium 1 mg per kg.— I. A. R. Dunnett, *Br. J. Anaesth.*, 1977, *49*, 491.

Successful use in a patient with acute intermittent porphyria.— S. F. Rizk *et al.*, *Anesthesiology*, 1977, *46*, 305.

Asthma. A 5-year-old child with a history of bronchial asthma was wheezing when given ketamine. After a dose of 75 mg given intramuscularly the wheezing cleared rapidly but started again as anaesthesia lightened. Increasing the depth of anaesthesia produced further relief.— E. K. Betts and C. E. Parkin, *Anesth. Analg. curr. Res.*, 1971, *50*, 420.

Ketamine hydrochloride protected asthmatic patients against bronchospasm during induction and reduced or abolished bronchospasm precipitated by other anaesthetics.— G. Corssen *et al.*, *Anesth. Analg. curr. Res.*, 1972, *51*, 588.

In 9 of 10 patients with pulmonary dysfunction or moderate or severe bronchospasm airway resistance was dramatically reduced after the administration of ketamine.— F. C. Huber *et al.*, *Sth. med. J.*, 1972, *65*, 1176.

Burns. Ketamine had been used for the anaesthetic management of severely burnt children with good results. It caused little nausea or vomiting and was tolerated as well by burnt children as by healthy children.— R. D. Wilson *et al.*, *Anesth. Analg. curr. Res.*, 1967, *46*, 719.

In a study of 62 patients anaesthetised with ketamine prior to burns surgery it was found that for patients weighing under 35 kg an intramuscular injection of ketamine, 4 mg per kg body-weight, was sufficient as an initial dose. Further injections of 2 mg per kg were then given intermittently during the operation. The use of pethidine premedication for patients weighing over 35 kg who received ketamine by intermittent intravenous injection was considered to lessen unpleasant psychic effects of the drug.— M. Sage and S. M. Laird, *Postgrad. med. J.*, 1972, *48*, 156.

A favourable report on the use of ketamine for anaesthesia during the dressing of burns. An initial dose of 2 mg per kg body-weight was given intravenously, with atropine, followed by 4 mg per kg intramuscularly, with further doses as needed; a dose of 1 mg per kg was given intravenously at the end of the procedure.— C. M. Ward and A. W. Diamond, *Postgrad. med. J.*, 1976, *52*, 222.

Further references: F. W. Roberts, *Anaesthesia*, 1967, *22*, 23; F. W. Roberts and W. F. Thompson, *Med. J. Aust.*, 1968, *1*, 128.

Convulsions. Ketamine given intramuscularly or intravenously controlled the seizures in 3 children with severe febrile convulsions unresponsive to anticonvulsants.— R. W. Davis and G. C. Tolstoshev (letter), *Med. J. Aust.*, 1976, *2*, 465.

See also below under Eclampsia.

Eclampsia. Ketamine successfully controlled epileptic seizures in 2 patients with eclampsia.— F. S. Rucci and G. Caroli (letter), *Br. J. Anaesth.*, 1974, *46*, 546.

Electroconvulsive therapy. A comparison of ketamine 2.2 mg per kg body-weight given intravenously, thiopentone 4.5 mg per kg also given intravenously, and ketamine 4.4 mg per kg given intramuscularly with hyaluronidase to patients undergoing ECT.— C. L. Brewer *et al.*, *Br. J. Psychiat.*, 1972, *120*, 679. Comment.— C. D. Green (letter), *ibid.*, 1973, *122*, 123.

Gynaecological procedures. Ketamine was used successfully as the sole anaesthetic for uterine curettage or therapeutic abortion in 272 patients and was also used followed by nitrous oxide and oxygen in a further 50 patients. It was considered especially suitable for therapeutic abortions due to its contracting effect on the uterus and the minimal bleeding it caused. The choice of premedication influenced recovery times and reactions; diazepam 143 µg per kg body-weight with hyoscine 400 µg or atropine 600 µg was considered to be the best premedication.— S. Galloon, *Can. Anaesth. Soc. J.*, 1971, *18*, 600. See also *idem*, *Can. Anaesth. Soc. J.*, 1973, *20*, 141, per *J. Am. med. Ass.*, 1973, *224*, 1312.

Analgesia was good in 74% and fair in 20% of 50 patients undergoing tubal ligation who were anaesthetised with ketamine. Premedication consisted of pethidine 50 mg and atropine 400 µg, both given intravenously.— I. Azar and E. Ozomek, *Anesth. Analg. curr. Res.*, 1973, *52*, 39.

An investigation into possible mechanisms of action for the contractile effect of ketamine on uterine tone.— M. L. Forsling *et al.*, *Br. J. Pharmac.*, 1973, *49*, 152P.

In a study of patients undergoing termination of pregnancy or caesarean section, ketamine produced uterine contractions equal to ergometrine in the first trimester of pregnancy but produced no significant effect at term.— J. N. Oats *et al.*, *Br. J. Anaesth.*, 1979, *51*, 1163.

Further references: W. H. Hervey and R. F. Hustead, *Anesth. Analg. curr. Res.*, 1972, *51*, 647.

Hiccup. Ketamine given intravenously in a dose of 400 µg per kg body-weight had been used to control hiccup occurring during surgery and in the recovery room.— T. R. Shantha, *Anesth. Analg. curr. Res.*, 1973, *52*, 822.

Pregnancy and the neonate. A study of ketamine as an obstetric anaesthetic in 18 non-pregnant and 14 pregnant subjects. Doses in the pregnant group were 1.5 or 2.2 mg per kg body-weight for priming followed by infusions of 80 and 110 µg per kg body-weight per minute respectively. Non-pregnant subjects received only the higher doses. There was reduced clearance in the pregnant patients. Side-effects included a 30 to 40% increase in diastolic and systolic blood pressure, increased pulse-rate and respiration, salivation, nausea, and vivid dreams. No undesirable effects were observed in the foetus.— B. Little *et al.*, *Am. J. Obstet. Gynec.*, 1972, *113*, 247.

In a study in 60 obstetric patients, patient acceptance favoured methoxyflurane compared with ketamine, each with nitrous oxide. Apgar scores of the infants were comparable.— M. L. Krantz, *Anesth. Analg. curr. Res.*, 1974, *53*, 890.

There were reports of reduced Apgar scores in infants after maternal ketamine anaesthesia; if used for delivery the total dose should not exceed 0.55 mg per kg body-weight.— S. Galloon, *Anesthesiology*, 1976, *44*, 522.

Further references: P. Chodoff and J. G. Stella, *Anesth. Analg. curr. Res.*, 1966, *45*, 527.

Open-heart surgery. Use for induction of anaesthesia in 14 patients undergoing open-heart surgery.— A. P. F. Jackson *et al.*, *Br. J. Anaesth.*, 1978, *50*, 375.

Pain. Ketamine 500 µg per kg body-weight intravenously thrice daily provided effective postoperative analgesia in a 59-year-old man.— T. R. Austin (letter), *Br. med. J.*, 1976, *2*, 943. Some patients experienced clouding of consciousness, excitement, and a bizarre feeling of detachment.— J. A. Thornton *et al.* (letter), *ibid.*, 1074.

Further references: I. Yusuke, *Anaesthesia*, 1974, *29*, 222.

Use in children. Children with cerebral leukaemia requiring intrathecal medication were satisfactorily anaesthetised within 5 to 10 minutes for periods of 10 to 20 minutes by ketamine hydrochloride 2.5 to 10 mg per kg body-weight given intramuscularly with atropine 300 µg for children weighing under 40 kg or 600 µg for heavier children. The children recovered fully within 1 to 3 hours. Side-effects included vomiting in 4 children, one of whom developed laryngospasm. A dose of 5 mg per kg was found to be adequate to produce anaesthesia in children aged 2 to 15 years requiring marrow aspiration and lumbar puncture.— J. Q. Matthias and P. J. Knapton (letter), *Lancet*, 1972, *1*, 388. A dose of 2 mg per kg body-weight of ketamine hydrochloride with 10 µg per kg of atropine was found to be sufficient to produce satisfactory anaesthesia for lumbar puncture and marrow aspiration in 45 children.— S. R. Keilty and J. M. Bridges (letter), *ibid.*, 631. See also A. T. Meadows *et al.* (letter), *ibid.*; R. H. A. Campbell *et al.*, *Archs Dis. Childh.*, 1978, *53*, 262.

Ketamine, 5 mg per kg body-weight by intramuscular injection or 2 mg per kg by intravenous injection was considered suitable for the sedation of 10 children prior to radiotherapy. Tolerance to the dose developed in 7 children after a few weeks and higher doses were required for subsequent treatments.— J. A. Bennett and J. A. Bullimore, *Br. J. Anaesth.*, 1973, *45*, 197.

Following a study of ketamine in 91 children undergoing heart surgery it was considered to be a useful anaesthetic for paediatric cardiac surgery especially in seriously ill children with severely reduced cardiac reserve where the depressant effects of other anaesthetics might be intolerable.— R. W. Vaughan and C. R. Stephen, *Sth. med. J.*, 1973, *66*, 1226, per *Int. pharm. Abstr.*, 1974, *11*, 632.

In 29 children, aged 1 month to 6 years, undergoing herniorrhaphy and given ketamine 11 mg per kg body-weight intramuscularly, about three-quarters of those less than 1 year old needed supplementation with 1.1 mg per kg intravenously to prevent movement.— C. H. Lockhart and W. L. Nelson, *Anesthesiology*, 1974, *40*, 507.

Ketamine hydrochloride 2 mg per kg body-weight by slow intravenous injection, followed by atropine 200 to 300 µg through the same needle, was successfully used for anaesthesia on 100 occasions in 61 children who underwent medical procedures including lumbar punctures, aspirations, and skin dressings. Strange dreams occurred in 4 children and 2 brief convulsions in 1 child but there were no serious complications.— E. Elliott *et al.*, *Archs Dis. Childh.*, 1976, *51*, 56.

Ketamine did not provide adequate anaesthesia for pneumoencephalography in a 10-week-old child with agenesis of the corpus callosum. Associated neurological defects were considered to be the most likely reason for this failure.— I. F. Russell, *Br. J. Anaesth.*, 1979, *51*, 983. A similar report in a 14-week-old child with neurological disturbances.— S. M. Willatts (letter), *Br. J. Anaesth.*, 1980, *52*, 840.

Further references: D. V. Catton, *Can. Anaesth. Soc. J.*, 1973, *20*, 227; R. W. Fynn, *Br. J. Anaesth.*, 1974, *46*, 699; *Lancet*, 1976, *1*, 1335.

Preparations

Ketamine Hydrochloride Injection *(U.S.P.)*. A sterile solution in Water for Injections. pH 3.5 to 5.5. Potency is expressed in terms of the equivalent amount of ketamine. Protect from light.

Ketalar *(Parke, Davis, UK)*. Ketamine hydrochloride, available as injections containing the equivalent of 10 mg of ketamine per ml, in vials of 20 ml; the equivalent of 50 mg per ml, in vials of 10 ml; and the equivalent of 100 mg per ml, in vials of 5 ml. The contents of the 20-ml vials are iso-osmotic with serum and the 10-ml and 5-ml vials contain benzethonium chloride 0.01%. (Also available as Ketalar in *Arg., Austral., Belg., Canad., Denm., Fr., Ital., Neth., Norw., S.Afr., Swed., Switz., USA*).

Other Proprietary Names

Ketaject *(USA)*; Ketanest *(Ger.)*.

3115-m

Methohexitone.

Methohexital *(U.S.P.)*. α-(±)-5-Allyl-1-methyl-5-(1-methylpent-2-ynyl)barbituric acid.

$C_{14}H_{18}N_2O_3$=262.3.

CAS — 151-83-7; 18652-93-2.

Pharmacopoeias. In *U.S.*

A white to faintly yellowish-white crystalline odourless powder. M.p. 92° to 96° with a range not exceeding 3°. Very slightly **soluble** in water; slightly soluble in alcohol, chloroform, and dilute alkalis.

3116-b

Methohexitone Sodium.

Sodium Methohexital; Compound 25398; Enallynymalnatrium.

$C_{14}H_{17}N_2NaO_3$=284.3.

CAS — 309-36-4.

Pharmacopoeias. U.S. includes Methohexital Sodium for Injection.

A white odourless crystalline substance. **Soluble** in water. **Incompatible** with clindamycin phosphate, metocurine iodide, hyoscine hydrobromide, pentazocine lactate, silicones, suxamethonium chloride, thiamine hydrochloride, tubocurarine chloride, compound sodium lactate injection, and acidic substances.

Solutions in Water for Injections are **stable** for at least 6 weeks at room temperature; solutions in dextrose or sodium chloride injections are stable only for about 24 hours.

Significant uptake of methohexitone sodium by polyvinyl chloride was demonstrated when aqueous solutions were exposed to plastic strips. This uptake increased with time.— P. Moorhatch and W. L. Chiou, *Am. J. Hosp. Pharm.*, 1974, *31*, 72.

Incompatibility. Methohexitone sodium 5% injection gave a precipitate with atropine sulphate injection; injections should be given in opposite arms.— J. Mokrzycki and G. Phillips (letter), *Br. dent. J.*, 1968, *125*, 432.

A haze developed over 3 hours when methohexitone sodium 2 g per litre was mixed with methicillin sodium 4 g per litre or prochlorperazine mesylate 100 mg per litre in dextrose injection, with amiphenazole hydrochloride 600 mg per litre in sodium chloride injection, or with mustine hydrochloride 40 mg per litre in dextrose injection or sodium chloride injection. An immediate precipitate occurred when methohexitone sodium was mixed with lignocaine hydrochloride 2 g per litre in dextrose injection or with chlorpromazine hydrochloride 200 mg per litre, kanamycin sulphate 4 g per litre, oxytetracycline hydrochloride 1 g per litre, promazine hydrochloride 200 mg per litre, promethazine hydrochloride 100 mg per litre, or with tetracycline hydrochloride 1 g per litre in dextrose injection or sodium chloride injection. A yellow colour occurred and a precipitate developed over 3 hours when methohexitone sodium was mixed with hydralazine hydrochloride 80 mg per litre in dextrose injection or sodium chloride injection. Crystals were produced when methohexitone sodium was mixed with methyldopate hydrochloride 1 g per litre in sodium chloride injection, but a haze developed when they were mixed in dextrose injection. Crystals were produced when methohexitone sodium was mixed with Strong Vitamins B and C Injection for intravenous use, 4 pairs of ampoules per litre, in dextrose injection or with streptomycin sulphate 4 g per litre in sodium chloride injection.— B. B. Riley, *J. Hosp. Pharm.*, 1970, *28*, 228.

Adverse Effects, Treatment, and Precautions. As for Thiopentone Sodium, p.759.

Abnormal muscle movements, coughing, sneezing, hiccuping, and laryngospasm occur more often with methohexitone than with thiopentone. Hyoscine and some phenothiazines, especially promethazine, have been reported to increase the incidence of abnormal muscle movements.

Cardiovascular effects. A study in 12 patients with supraventricular arrhythmias suggested that methohexitone had a depressant effect on myocardial contractility.— D. J. Rowlands *et al., Br. J. Anaesth.*, 1967, *39*, 554.

For a comparison of the cardiovascular effects of propanidid and methohexitone, see Propanidid, p.757.

Epilepsy. Methohexitone should not be used for dental anaesthesia in children with a history of epilepsy because it was a convulsant and might precipitate status epilepticus under anaesthesia. Propanidid might be more satisfactory for such patients. Status epilepticus had occurred in 2 patients.— V. Goldman, *Br. dent. J.*, 1966, *121*, 468 and 544. See also V. Goldman (letter), *Br. dent. J.*, 1969, *126*, 109; W. Ryder (letter), *ibid.*, 343.

Absorption and Fate. As for Thiopentone Sodium, p.759.

Methohexitone sodium has a lower oil/water partition coefficient than thiopentone sodium and it is not absorbed by fatty tissues to the same extent. It is metabolised more rapidly than thiopentone. About 73% of a dose is reported to be bound to plasma proteins and about 20% to red blood-cells. Methohexitone sodium is reported to cross the placenta.

After clinical doses of methohexitone only about 500 ng per ml was found in urine.— I. Sunshine *et al., Br. J. Anaesth.*, 1966, *38*, 23.

In 4 healthy subjects given methohexitone sodium 3 mg per kg body-weight over 1 hour there was an early rapid reduction in the plasma-methohexitone concentration representing rapid tissue localisation and a later more gradual reduction reflecting elimination or sequestration; the mean half-life of the later phase was 97 minutes.— D. D. Breimer, *Br. J. Anaesth.*, 1976, *48*, 643.

The pharmacokinetics of methohexitone.— M. M. Ghoneim and K. Korttila, *Clin. Pharmacokinet.*, 1977, *2*, 344.

Pregnancy and the neonate. Methohexitone sodium rapidly crossed the placenta, equilibrium between foetal and maternal blood being reached within 2 or 3 minutes.— F. Moya and B. E. Smith, *Anesthesiology*, 1965, *26*, 465.

Uses. Methohexitone is a barbiturate which is administered intravenously as the sodium salt for the induction of general anaesthesia or the production of complete anaesthesia of short duration. It has little muscle relaxant activity and is anti-analgesic. It is about 3 times as potent as thiopentone sodium (p.759) and has similar actions and uses.

Induction is rapid, occurring in one arm/brain circulation time. Recovery starts in about 3 minutes but sleepiness may persist for some time. It is a useful anaesthetic for minor operative procedures which do not require muscle relaxation. It may, however, be employed with skeletal muscle relaxants.

Methohexitone sodium is injected intravenously for induction of anaesthesia as a 1% solution in a dose of 50 to 120 mg at the rate of approximately 1 ml every 5 seconds. For intermittent administration in the maintenance of general anaesthesia, 20 to 40 mg may be given at intervals as required, e.g. every 4 to 7 minutes. Methohexitone sodium may also be administered as a 0.1 or 0.2% solution by continuous intravenous drip for the maintenance of general anaesthesia.

Light anaesthesia for conservative dentistry has been induced and maintained by methohexitone but the procedure has not gained general acceptance because of side-effects.

Methohexitone sodium has also been administered by intramuscular injection and rectally.

A review: J. G. Whitwam, *Br. J. Anaesth.*, 1976, *48*, 617.

Light methohexitone anaesthesia resulted in a mean increase of 89.2% in the flow-rate of peripheral blood in the leg in 8 patients without cardiovascular disease, and 45.1% in 10 patients with peripheral arterial disease. In 4 of 5 patients who had vascular disease and in whom lumbar sympathectomy had been performed, there was a mean decrease of 24.5% in flow-rate; the other patient showed an increase of 17%.— J. A. Dormandy and J. Bullough, *Br. J. Anaesth.*, 1969, *41*, 656.

Endotracheal intubation could be successfully carried out by inducing anaesthesia with methohexitone followed by diazepam up to 10 mg both given intravenously to patients in the supine position. This technique usually eliminated the need for suxamethonium.— M. W. PHudson (letter), *Br. med. J.*, 1974, *4*, 345.

For a comparison of the hypotensive effects of thiopentone, methohexitone, and alphaxalone with alphadolone in patients with cardiac disease, see Thiopentone Sodium, p.759.

Comparative potency. A comparison of the narcotic potency of methohexitone and propanidid. Methohexitone was 5.2 times as potent as propanidid in all the doses used. Equipotent doses of both drugs produced the same duration of anaesthesia.— T. H. Howells *et al., Br. J. Anaesth.*, 1967, *39*, 31.

Electroconvulsive therapy. Methohexitone was compared with thiopentone, each being used in a series of about 500 cases of ECT. Other medication, such as atropine and suxamethonium, was the same in both groups. The dosage of thiopentone was 100 to 200 mg by slow intravenous injection over 20 to 30 seconds, as a 2.5% solution. Methohexitone was given intravenously in 5 seconds as a 5% solution in a dose ranging from 30 to 60 mg. Methohexitone was clinically superior and caused fewer abnormalities than thiopentone in the ECG after the convulsions. Thiopentone caused even more frequent cardiac arrhythmias in patients with cardiac disease than in those without.— F. M. Pitts *et al., New Engl. J. Med.*, 1965, *273*, 353.

In 220 patients submitted to ECT with a graded electrical stimulus and anaesthetised with methohexitone, there were fewer increases in blood pressure and less dental or oral trauma than in patients submitted to conventional ECT. Methohexitone was given as a 1% solution in a dose of 1 mg per kg body-weight to a maximum of 100 mg. Atropine 600 µg was given concomitantly.— A. E. Delilkan, *Br. J. Anaesth.*, 1969, *41*, 884.

Epilepsy. Methohexitone in incremental doses ranging from 5 to 100 mg intravenously elicited active high-voltage spike discharges in 18 and less pronounced activation in 4 of 25 patients with psychomotor epilepsy. This technique was considered superior to other activating methods in patients with temporal lobe epilepsy.— L. Musella *et al., Neurology, Minneap.*, 1971, *21*, 594. See also J. Gumpert *et al.* (letter), *Lancet*, 1969, *2*, 110.

In a study of 41 patients with epilepsy, methohexitone activation demonstrated no more effectiveness than sleep and was considered to have little value in the diagnosis of epilepsy.— G. G. Celesia and R. E. Paulsen, *Archs Neurol., Chicago*, 1972, *27*, 361.

Phobia. References to the use of methohexitone sodium in systematic desensitisation of phobic symptoms: D. E. I. Friedman and J. T. Silverstone, *Lancet*, 1967, *1*, 470; N. J. Yorkston *et al., ibid.*, 1968, *2*, 651; H. G. S. Sergeant and N. J. Yorkston, *ibid.*, 653; J. Penman (letter), *ibid.*, 731; D. Friedman and T. Silverstone (letter), *ibid.*, 833; A. B. Mawson, *ibid.*, 1970, *1*, 1084; Z. Hussain (letter), *ibid.*, 1291; D. E. Friedman and M. S. Lipsedge, *Br. J. Psychiat.*, 1971, *118*, 87.

Pregnancy and the neonate. In 12 mothers given methohexitone 1.4 mg per kg body-weight intravenously for induction of anaesthesia prior to caesarean section and 14 mothers given 1 mg per kg, there was no difference in maternal status, awareness, or pH, pCO_2 or pO_2 of the cord blood, but the infants in the low-dose group had less need of assisted respiration, a shorter mean time to regular respiration, better Apgar scores, and better 'Apgar minus colour' scores than those in the high-dose group.— A. Holdcroft *et al., Br. med. J.*, 1974, *2*, 472. See also *idem, Br. J. Anaesth.*, 1973, *45*, 1237.

Preparations

Methohexital Sodium for Injection *(U.S.P.)*. A sterile freeze-dried mixture of methohexitone sodium and anhydrous sodium carbonate as a buffer prepared from an aqueous solution of methohexitone, sodium hydroxide, and sodium carbonate (anhydrous or monohydrate). pH of a 5% solution 10.6 to 11.6.

Methohexitone Injection *(B.P.)*. A sterile solution of a mixture of 100 parts by weight of methohexitone sodium (α-form) and 6 parts by weight of dried sodium carbonate in Water for Injections free from carbon dioxide. It is prepared by dissolving the contents of a sealed container (Methohexitone Sodium for Injection) in the requisite amount of Water for Injections free from carbon dioxide. pH of a 5% solution 11 to 11.6. It should be freshly prepared and used within 24 hours; solutions that are cloudy should not be used.

Brietal Sodium *(Lilly, UK)*. Methohexitone sodium with anhydrous sodium carbonate for solution before use, available in 10-ml vials of 100 mg, in 50-ml vials containing 500 mg, in 17.5-ml vials containing 2.5 g, in 250-ml vials containing 2.5 g, and in 35-ml vials containing 5 g. (Also available as Brietal Sodium in *Austral., Belg., Canad., Neth., Switz.*, as Brietal-Sodium in *S.Afr., Swed.*, and as Brietal in *Denm., Norw.*).

Other Proprietary Names

Brevimytal Natrium *(Ger.)*; Brevital Sodium *(USA)*.

3117-v

Methoxyflurane *(B.P., U.S.P.)*. 2,2-Dichloro-1,1-difluoro-1-methoxyethane; 2,2-Dichloro-1,1-difluoroethyl methyl ether.

$C_3H_4Cl_2F_2O$=165.0.

CAS — 76-38-0.

Pharmacopoeias. In *Br., Braz., Chin., Cz.,* and *U.S.*

A clear, almost colourless, non-inflammable mobile liquid with a characteristic fruity odour and a sweet burning taste. The *B.P.* specifies 0.01% w/w of butylated hydroxytoluene as an antoxidant; the *U.S.P.* permits a suitable stabiliser. B.p. 103.5° to 107.5°. Wt per ml 1.423 to 1.427 g.

Soluble 1 in 500 of water; miscible with alcohol, acetone, chloroform, ether, and oils. It is soluble in rubber. Stable to light, air, and moisture, but the presence of butylated hydroxytoluene may cause a brown colour to develop slowly on exposure to light. **Store** in a cool place in airtight containers. Protect from light.

Adverse Effects. Methoxyflurane depresses the cardiovascular system and hypotension may occur. It is reported not to sensitise the myocardium to catecholamines to any considerable extent. Respiratory depression is slight with low doses but assisted respiration is necessary when deep anaesthesia is achieved.

Methoxyflurane impairs renal function in a dose-related manner due to the effect of the released fluoride on the distal tubule and may cause polyuric or oliguric renal failure. There have been occasional reports of hepatic dysfunction, jaundice, and hepatic necrosis. Headache has been reported by some patients. Bronchospasm, laryngospasm, gastro-intestinal side-effects, and emergence delirium have been observed.

The subjective visual and auditory alterations associated with nitrous oxide and methoxyflurane were not confirmed by objective testing in 11 subjects.— P. J. Tomlin *et al., Br. J. Anaesth.*, 1973, *45*, 719.

Abuse. A 27-year-old nurse suffered from progressive renal disease and painful diffuse and multifocal periostitis which had developed as a probable consequence of intermittent self-exposure to methoxyflurane possibly over a 9-year period.— P. J. Klemmer and N. M. Hadler, *Ann. intern. Med.*, 1978, *89*, 607.

Fatal hepatitis after repeated sniffing of methoxyflurane.— K. -W. Min *et al., Sth. med. J.*, 1977, *70*, 1363.

Effect on body temperature. Methoxyflurane could cause malignant hyperthermia in genetically predisposed individuals.— M. E. Pembrey, *Practitioner*, 1974, *213*, 647.

Kidney damage. *For reports and discussions of the renal toxicity of methoxyflurane, see Martindale 27th Edn,* p. 704.

Liver damage. Fatal hepatic necrosis, probably caused by methoxyflurane, occurred in a 51-year-old woman 10 days after anaesthesia with thiopentone, nitrous oxide, methoxyflurane, and oxygen. Anaesthesia had been induced 14 weeks earlier using the same agents; on both occasions it was prolonged.— F. P. Becker (letter), *Lancet*, 1970, *2*, 719.

A review of 24 patients with hepatitis induced by methoxyflurane.— P. H. Joshi and H. O. Conn, *Ann. intern. Med.*, 1974, *80*, 395.

Further reports.— N. C. Klein and G. H. Jeffries, *J. Am. med. Ass.*, 1966, *197*, 1037; M. W. Lischner *et al., Archs intern. Med.*, 1967, *120*, 725; D. Rubinger *et al., Anesthesiology*, 1975, *43*, 593; B. -E. Dahlgren and B. H. Goodrich, *Br. J. Anaesth.*, 1976, *48*, 145; B. -E. Dahlgren, *Br. J. Anaesth.*, 1977, *49*, 1271; N. M. Kalkay, *N.Y. St. J. Med.*, 1977, *77*, 2265.

Treatment of Adverse Effects. As for Halothane, p.742.

Precautions. Methoxyflurane is contra-indicated in the presence of kidney or liver impairment. It is best avoided in patients with toxaemia of pregnancy or requiring renal vascular surgery. It is also advisable to monitor kidney function following methoxyflurane anaesthesia, especially with large doses and in obese patients. It has been reported to increase the cerebrospinal pressure and its use in the presence of space-occupying lesions is best avoided. The concomitant use of tetracycline increases the risk of kidney damage and methoxyflurane should not be used in patients taking tetracycline or other potentially nephrotoxic compounds.

It is advisable not to administer methoxyflurane to patients who have shown signs of liver damage or fever after previous methoxyflurane anaesthesia. It is also recommended that at least 1 month should pass between successive procedures using methoxyflurane.

The effects of non-depolarising muscle relaxants, such as gallamine and tubocurarine, are enhanced by methoxyflurane and if required they should be given in reduced dosage. The respiratory effects of morphine are also enhanced. The concomitant use of enzyme-inducing agents, such as barbiturates, may enhance the metabolism of methoxyflurane. There is significant absorption of methoxyflurane by the rubber in anaesthetic circuits. Polyvinyl chloride plastics are partially soluble in methoxyflurane.

See also Precautions for General Anaesthetics, p.740.

Administration of adrenaline to 100 patients who were anaesthetised with methoxyflurane suggested that not more than 10 ml of local anaesthetic containing 1 in 100 000 of adrenaline should be given in the first 10 minutes and not more than 30 ml in 1 hour. It was important to ensure adequate ventilation.— J. F. Arens, *Anesth. Analg. curr. Res.*, 1968, *47*, 391.

Reduced serum-cholinesterase activity associated with methoxyflurane.— R. J. Polahniuk and M. Cumming, *Anesthesiology*, 1977, *47*, 520.

Absorption and Fate. Methoxyflurane is absorbed on inhalation. The blood/gas coefficient is high. It is very soluble in adipose tissue and excretion may be slow. Some methoxyflurane undergoes metabolism releasing fluoride. Methoxyflurane crosses the placenta.

After inhalation, methoxyflurane was stored in the body for up to 12 days. Two subjects exhaled 29 and 35% respectively of unchanged methoxyflurane, and in other subjects 7 to 21% was metabolised to carbon dioxide, fluoride ion, and dichloroacetic acid. A larger fraction was dechlorinated and oxidised to methoxyfluoroacetic acid, which was excreted in the urine.— D. A. Holaday *et al., Anesthesiology*, 1970, *33*, 579. See also R. I. Mazze *et al., ibid.*, 1971, *35*, 247.

The mean peak serum-fluoride concentration in 13 children 24 hours after low-dose methoxyflurane anaesthesia was 21.6 μmol per litre compared with a previously-reported concentration of 43.9 μmol per litre in adults. Possible explanations included slower metabolism, increased renal clearance, greater storage in bone, and more rapid elimination.— R. K. Stoelting and C. Peterson, *Anesthesiology*, 1975, *42*, 26.

The metabolism of methoxyflurane in obese patients.— S. R. Young *et al., Anesthesiology*, 1975, *42*, 451.

In 12 patients inhaling methoxyflurane 0.24% for a mean of 138 minutes, a mean of 19% was recovered in exhaled air. Urinary excretion of organic fluorine, fluoride, and oxalic acid was 29, 7.7, and 7.1% respectively.— N. Yoshimura *et al., Anesthesiology*, 1976, *44*, 372.

For a comparison of the metabolism of halothane, enflurane, and methoxyflurane, see Halothane, p.742.

Pregnancy and the neonate. Anaesthesia for 43 healthy parturient women was induced by methoxyflurane, nitrous oxide, and oxygen, and the methoxyflurane blood concentrations estimated in the maternal arterial and in the umbilical venous and arterial cord blood. It was found that methoxyflurane (as with ether, cyclopropane, and halothane) diffused across the placenta early and in significant amounts. As the duration of anaesthesia increased the delivered concentration of methoxyflurane was reduced as an adequate light plane of anaesthesia was attained. This reduction was reflected in the fall in maternal arterial and umbilical venous methoxyflurane concentrations.— E. S. Siker *et al., Br. J. Anaesth.*, 1968, *40*, 588.

When methoxyflurane-air was used for obstetric analgesia in 64 women, low methoxyflurane-blood concentrations were achieved which were not associated with neonatal depression. With surgical planes of anaesthesia, high concentrations occurred in foetal and maternal blood.— R. B. Clark *et al., Br. J. Anaesth.*, 1970, *42*, 286.

Blood concentrations of methoxyflurane were measured in 16 women in labour who were using intermittent self-administered inhalation analgesia. The expected accumulation did not occur, as the mothers tended to inhale less methoxyflurane as labour progressed, thus maintaining a fairly even concentration. Umbilical vein concentrations were less than those in the mother.— I. P. Latto *et al., Br. J. Anaesth.*, 1972, *44*, 391.

For reports of fluoride concentrations in neonates after exposure to methoxyflurane, see R. B. Clark *et al., Anesthesiology*, 1976, *45*, 88; O. S. Cuasay *et al., Anesth. Analg. curr. Res.*, 1977, *56*, 646; B. -E. Dahlgren, *Acta pharm. suec.*, 1978, *15*, 211.

Uses. Methoxyflurane is a potent volatile anaesthetic administered by inhalation. In recommended concentrations it is not inflammable, or explosive when mixed with oxygen. Methoxyflurane possesses good analgesic properties. It also possesses muscle relaxant properties but these are only significant at concentrations that produce deep anaesthesia so it is common practice to administer a muscle relaxant with methoxyflurane when required.

Because of its low vapour pressure, induction is slow. Anaesthesia may be induced with 1.5 to 3% of methoxyflurane usually in nitrous oxide and oxygen. A concentration of 3% should be maintained for not more than 5 minutes and then progressively reduced to the lowest concentration that will maintain adequate anaesthesia; a concentration of 0.2 to 0.4% may be sufficient. The production of deep anaesthesia with methoxyflurane is not recommended, and a maximum of 4 hours exposure at a concentration of 0.25% (or the equivalent at other concentrations) is suggested.

Recovery from anaesthesia is prolonged but may be shortened by discontinuing the administration of methoxyflurane before the end of surgery allowing 10 minutes for each hour of exposure. Analgesia extends to recovery or beyond.

In obstetrics 0.5% with a mixture of nitrous oxide and oxygen is used for anaesthesia and 0.35% in air for intermittent analgesia, without affecting uterine contractions. Concentrations of up to 0.8% are used to provide analgesia in a variety of situations.

The minimum alveolar concentration of methoxyflurane for anaesthesia to prevent a muscular response to a skin incision in 50% of persons was 0.16%.— L. J. Saidman *et al., Anesthesiology*, 1967, *28*, 994.

The intra-ocular pressure was effectively reduced in 30 patients during the first 30 minutes of arousal from methoxyflurane anaesthesia as well as during light or moderate anaesthesia.— A. Schettini *et al., Can. Anaesth. Soc. J.*, 1968, *15*, 172.

In a study of the effect of methoxyflurane on the splanchnic circulation of 12 healthy subjects there was a 50% reduction in splanchnic blood flow and a 30% reduction in hepatic venous oxygen tension with an end-expired concentration of 0.2%. These effects were considered to be due to arterial hypotension and constriction of the hepatic artery.— M. Libonati *et al.*,

Anesthesiology, 1973, *38*, 466.

Burns. The use of methoxyflurane as an analgesic was tested on 60 occasions in 10 patients requiring burns dressings. Good results were obtained when methoxyflurane 0.5% in air was inhaled from a Pentec vaporiser (Cyprane) for 5 minutes before a dressing commenced and until 10 to 15 minutes before the end of the treatment. The concentration of methoxyflurane was increased to 0.7% for short periods if required. Drowsiness was noted on 3 occasions and nausea by 2 patients.— M. A. Marshall and H. P. L. Ozorio, *Br. J. Anaesth.*, 1972, *44*, 80.

Methoxyflurane analgesia was given to 88 patients, ranging in age from 4 months to 82 years, who required burns dressings. A modified Cyprane vaporiser gave the best results. Patients received 0.9% methoxyflurane mixed with air for 10 minutes before treatment and a lower concentration, 0.3% to 0.5%, during treatment. Methoxyflurane was tolerated by all except 3 patients and no toxic effects were noted even when repeated administrations were required.— K. J. Packer, *Postgrad. med. J.*, 1972, *48*, 128.

Dental surgery. Methoxyflurane was as effective as halothane when used for dental anaesthesia in 254 children. Recovery was much more tranquil than with halothane. An induction time of 75 seconds for methoxyflurane 1% with a mixture of nitrous oxide 85% and oxygen 15% was adequate in all cases.— W. A. Allen, *Br. dent. J.*, 1968, *124*, 133. This low proportion of oxygen was used only for purposes of comparison with halothane. When intravenous induction was used, a 35 to 50% oxygen mixture was satisfactory.— *idem*, 201. The results claimed were very similar to those obtained with a mixture of nitrous oxide 80% and oxygen 20% alone, and methoxyflurane or halothane should rarely be necessary as a supplement.— P. Butler, *ibid.*, 295.

Methoxyflurane, at a concentration of at least 1.5%, with nitrous oxide was considered a suitable anaesthetic for use in major oral surgery because it gave a prolonged period of recovery and produced good sedation, analgesia, and tolerance of an endotracheal tube.— V. Goldman and P. B. Hardwick, *Br. J. Anaesth.*, 1969, *41*, 323.

Inhalation sedation for conservative dentistry was used successfully in 24 extremely anxious patients with either nitrous oxide 25% or methoxyflurane 0.35%.— D. H. Edmunds and M. Rosen, *Br. dent. J.*, 1975, *139*, 398.

Effect on respiration. In 6 healthy adults specific airways conductance was increased by a mean of 20.3% after breathing methoxyflurane 0.35% for 1½ minutes. Methoxyflurane should receive favourable consideration for use in obstetric analgesia in women with a history of asthma.— R. B. Douglas and S. M. Forsey (letter), *Br. med. J.*, 1973, *4*, 106.

Pregnancy and the neonate. The Central Midwives Board had decided that methoxyflurane might now be administered without supervision by midwives using the Cardiff inhaler.— *Br. med. J.*, 1970, *3*, 413.

Use in children. Methoxyflurane was administered, by a Cardiff Penthrane inhaler giving 0.35% methoxyflurane in air, on 94 occasions to 36 children aged 4 months to 13 years for burns dressings and minor painful ward procedures lasting from 10 minutes to 2½ hours. Preoperative starvation was not required. Fair to very good analgesia was obtained on all but 6 occasions, and for these improvement was obtained by giving trimeprazine tartrate 1½ hours before using methoxyflurane.— S. Firn, *Br. J. Anaesth.*, 1972, *44*, 517.

Proprietary Preparations

Penthrane *(Abbott, UK)*. A brand of methoxyflurane. (Also available as Penthrane in *Austral., Canad., Denm., Ger., Norw., Switz., USA*).

Other Proprietary Names

Pentrane *(Arg., Ital.)*.

3118-g

Narcobarbital.

Enibomal. 5-(2-Bromoallyl)-5-isopropyl-1-methylbarbituric acid.

$C_{11}H_{15}BrN_2O_3$=303.2.

CAS — 125-55-3.

A white powder. Slightly **soluble** in water; soluble 1 in 20 of alcohol; soluble in acetone, chloroform, ether, and solutions of alkalis.

Narcobarbital is a barbiturate which has been administered intravenously as an anaesthetic. It was usually given as a 10% solution of the sodium derivative in doses of 5 to 10 ml (0.5 to 1 g).

3119-q

Nitrous Oxide

(B.P., Eur. P., U.S.P.). Nitrogenii Monoxidum; Nitrogenii Oxidum; Dinitrogen Oxide; Laughing Gas; Nitrogen Monoxide; Oxydum Nitrosum; Distickstoffmonoxid; Protoxyde d'Azote; Stickoxydul; Nitrogenium Oxydulatum; Oxyde Nitreux; Azoto Protossido.

N_2O=44.01.

CAS — 10024-97-2.

Pharmacopoeias. In *Arg., Aust., Belg., Br., Braz., Chin., Cz., Eur., Fr., Ger., Hung., Ind., Int., It., Jap., Mex., Neth., Nord., Pol., Rus., Swiss, Turk.*, and *U.S.*

A colourless gas, heavier than air, odourless or almost odourless and tasteless; it supports combustion. It is supplied compressed in metal cylinders. One vol. measured at normal temperature and pressure dissolves, at 20°, in about 1.5 vol. of water; freely soluble in alcohol and chloroform; soluble in ether and in oils.

Store in metal cylinders at a temperature not exceeding 36° in a special room free from inflammable materials. The whole cylinder should be painted blue; the name or chemical symbol of the gas should be stencilled in paint on the shoulder of the cylinder and clearly and indelibly stamped on the cylinder valve.

Storage. Cylinders of Entonox (50% nitrous oxide and 50% oxygen) delivered in cold weather should be stored in a horizontal position at 5° or more for at least 24 hours before use, as the gas might not contain adequate quantities of oxygen if the cylinder has been cooled and then allowed to warm up in a vertical position.— A. Bracken *et al.*, *Br. med. J.*, 1968, *3*, 715.

For a 50% mixture of nitrous oxide and oxygen the maximum condensation temperature, the critical pressure, and the critical temperature were found to be −5.5°, 138 atmospheres, and −30° respectively. Thus no liquid would form in a cylinder containing 50% nitrous oxide and 50% oxygen under any pressure conditions as long as storage was at a temperature above −5.5°.— G. B. Broughton, *Br. J. Anaesth.*, 1969, *41*, 193.

Adverse Effects. The main complications following the use of nitrous oxide are those due to varying degrees of hypoxia. Prolonged administration has been followed by depression of the bone marrow.

Hearing acuity was reduced in a few patients after anaesthesia with nitrous oxide for adenotonsillectomy.— J. E. Waun *et al.*, *Anesthesiology*, 1967, *28*, 846.

Raised intracranial pressure occurred in 12 patients with intracranial disorders during 14 anaesthetic inductions with nitrous oxide. Since intubation could increase intracranial pressure nitrous oxide might be best given after intubation.— H. T. Hendriksen and P. B. Jörgensen, *Br. J. Anaesth.*, 1973, *45*, 486. Increased intracranial pressure in a patient anaesthetised with nitrous oxide 5 days after pneumoencephalography.— A. Artru *et al.*, *Anesthesiology*, 1978, *49*, 136. A study in 3 patients with head injuries indicated that nitrous oxide (12 administrations) exacerbated the increases in intracranial pressure occurring during chest physiotherapy. In 9 further patients with head injuries nitrous oxide (16 administrations) increased intracranial pressure during mechanical ventilation. Nitrous oxide should be avoided in spontaneously breathing patients with head injuries during transport and admission to hospital.— E. Moss and D. G. McDowall, *Br. J. Anaesth.*, 1979, *51*, 757.

Gastric regurgitation was studied in 152 surgical patients and found to depend on the site of operation, the position of the patient, and the type of anaesthesia. There was a significantly greater incidence during anaesthesia using nitrous oxide than that using halothane and nitrous oxide.— H. Turndorf *et al.*, *Anesth. Analg. curr. Res.*, 1974, *53*, 700.

In the USA, the FDA considered that there was sufficient evidence to cause concern about the carcinogenic and teratogenic potential of nitrous oxide.— J. W. C. Fox (letter), *Lancet*, 1976, *1*, 1024.

Continuous exposure to nitrous oxide 0.5% in air caused foetal death, skeletal malformations, and prenatal growth retardation in *rats*.— E. Vieira, *Br. J. Anaesth.*, 1979, *51*, 283.

Abuse. Brief discussions of the abuse of nitrous oxide: *J. Am. med. Ass.*, 1978, *239*, 2425; *FDA Drug Bull.*, 1980, *10*, 15.

For reports of neuropathy after abuse of nitrous oxide, see p.755.

Bone-marrow depression. In a prospective study of patients undergoing cardiac bypass surgery, all of 8 who received a mixture of nitrous oxide 50% and oxygen 50% continuously for 24 hours suffered megaloblastic changes in their bone marrow and abnormal deoxyuridine suppression tests (indicative of abnormal vitamin B_{12} metabolism). Of 9 similar patients who received the nitrous oxide and oxygen mixture during the operation only (for 5 to 12 hours), 3 had mildly megaloblastic erythropoiesis, and 2 of these and 1 other patient had abnormal deoxyuridine suppression tests. In a further 5 similar patients who did not receive nitrous oxide the bone marrows were normoblastic and deoxyuridine suppression tests normal. Administration of hydroxocobalamin before and after the operation to one patient in the first group did not prevent the megaloblastic changes.— J. A. L. Amess *et al.*, *Lancet*, 1978, *2*, 339. Discussion and comment.— *ibid.*, 613; J. A. L. Amess *et al.* (letter), *ibid.*, 740; M. E. J. Beard and J. W. Hamer (letter), *ibid.*, 795; J. C. Linnell *et al.* (letter), *ibid.*, 1372; J. F. Nunn and I. Chanarin, *Br. J. Anaesth.*, 1978, *50*, 1089.

Cardiovascular effects. Alterations in heart activity associated with nitrous oxide given alone or with other agents: A. G. Tolas, *J. oral Surg.*, 1967, *25*, 54; W. N. Rollason, *Br. med. J.*, 1969, *2*, 180; C. Fisch *et al.*, *J. Am. med. Ass.*, 1969, *208*, 1839; J. H. Eisele and N. T. Smith, *Anesth. Analg. curr. Res.*, 1972, *51*, 956; R. W. McDermott and T. H. Stanley, *Anesthesiology*, 1974, *41*, 89; J. A. Hulf *et al.* (letter), *Br. med. J.*, 1975, *1*, 511; R. K. Stoelting *et al.*, *Anesthesiology*, 1975, *42*, 319; D. G. Lappas *et al.*, *ibid.*, *43*, 61; G. E. Hill *et al.*, *Anesth. Analg. curr. Res.*, 1978, *57*, 84; J. Wynne *et al.*, *J. Am. med. Ass.*, 1980, *243*, 1440.

Contamination with higher oxides of nitrogen. Poisoning, with symptoms of cyanosis, hypotension, and methaemoglobinaemia, occurred in 2 patients anaesthetised with nitrous oxide contaminated with nitric oxide. One patient died. A patient at another hospital died after being similarly poisoned.— J. Clutton-Brock, *Br. J. Anaesth.*, 1967, *39*, 388.

Further references: *Lancet*, 1966, *2*, 628 and 739; *ibid.*, 1967, *1*, 581; *ibid.*, 1967, *2*, 930; *Br. J. Anaesth.*, 1967, *39*, 343 to 448; *Br. med. J.*, 1967, *3*, 191.

Treatment . The effects of inhaling the higher oxides of nitrogen should be treated in the following order of priority; administer 100% oxygen by assisted respiration if necessary; give an initial dose of 2 mg per kg bodyweight of methylene blue for methaemoglobinaemia and titrate further doses against methaemoglobin remaining in the blood; treat chemical pneumonitis by endobronchial instillation or inhalation of a nebulised solution of 50 mg of hydrocortisone in 50 ml of a 1.3% solution of sodium bicarbonate; give 100 mg of hydrocortisone by intravenous injection every 6 to 8 hours for a week and then gradually reduce the dose, and give antibiotics prophylactically; correct derangement of acid-base equilibrium with intravenous sodium bicarbonate. Increased airway resistance should be treated with inhalations of 1% isoprenaline solution and intermittent positive-pressure ventilation should be used in cases of respiratory failure. Severe hypotension should be countered with pressor agents. The use of dimercaprol, which specifically antagonised the effects of the oxides of nitrogen, was suggested.— C. Prys-Roberts, *Br. J. Anaesth.*, 1967, *39*, 432.

Effect on body temperature. An 11-year-old girl whose father had died from malignant hyperpyrexia after anaesthesia herself developed malignant hyperpyrexia, with a rise in body temperature at a rate of 6° per hour, after anaesthesia which included diazepam, thiopentone, nitrous oxide, and oxygen. The temperature fell equally rapidly after dexamethasone intravenously; a dose of 1 to 2 mg per kg body-weight was suggested in preference to procaine. As thiopentone was suspected she was later given anaesthesia with nitrous oxide and oxygen alone and again experienced hyperpyrexia. Thiopentone was later given uneventfully.— F. R. Ellis *et al.*, *Br. med. J.*, 1974, *4*, 270. Precautions had been taken to avoid contamination with halothane.— *idem* (letter), 1975, *1*, 575.

Nitrous oxide and thiopentone had been used to anaesthetise more than 150 susceptible *pigs* without precipitating malignant hyperpyrexia.— J. N. Lucke *et al.* (letter), *Br. med. J.*, 1975, *1*, 454.

Neuropathy. A report of severe neurological symptoms

in 15 patients (all but 1 of whom were dentists) following prolonged heavy exposure to nitrous oxide associated with professional use, self-administration, or both. Initial symptoms were usually numbness or tingling in the hands or legs. Later symptoms included: Lhermitte sign (12), numbness of trunk (10), impairment of equilibrium or gait (12), inability to walk unassisted (7), impotence (7), sphincter impairment (4), mental changes (7), dysarthria (2), impairment of smell or taste (1). Ten patients had to stop work. Symptoms resembled those of subacute combined degeneration of the spinal cord, and it was considered possible that nitrous oxide interfered with the action of vitamin B_{12} on the nervous system. All improved on stopping exposure to nitrous oxide and regained the ability to walk unaided but 6 followed a relapsing course associated with re-exposure to nitrous oxide. Administration of corticosteroids to 6 and vitamin B_{12} to 4 did not appear to influence the extent of recovery.— R. B. Layzer, *Lancet*, 1978, *2*, 1227.

Neuropathy in 2 patients after abuse of nitrous oxide.— M. A. Nevins (letter), *J. Am. med. Ass.*, 1980, *244*, 2264.

Psychic disturbance. Six patients experienced more or less severe psychotic sensations during anaesthesia with nitrous oxide and oxygen for caesarean section. Similar effects did not occur in 11 other patients anaesthetised with a barbiturate.— H. Bergström and K. Bernstein (preliminary communication), *Lancet*, 1968, *2*, 541.

Treatment of Adverse Effects. As for Chloroform, p.745.

Precautions. Hypoxic anaesthesia is dangerous and nitrous oxide should always be administered with oxygen. Nitrous oxide diffuses into gas-filled body cavities and care is essential when using it in patients with abdominal distension, pneumothorax, or similar cavities in the pericardium or peritoneum, and in patients during or after air encephalography. Oxygen should be administered during emergence from prolonged anaesthesia with nitrous oxide to prevent diffusion hypoxia where the alveolar oxygen concentration is diminished. See also Precautions for General Anaesthetics, p.740.

Nitrous oxide diffused into latex rubber endotracheal tube cuffs in considerable amounts. Any resultant over expansion of the cuffs could cause upper-airway obstruction and trauma in intubated patients.— T. H. Stanley *et al.*, *Anesthesiology*, 1974, *41*, 256.

In 5 healthy adults specific airways conductance was reduced by a mean of 26% after the inhalation of 10 breaths of Entonox (nitrous oxide and oxygen, equal parts).— R. B. Douglas *et al.* (letter), *Br. med. J.*, 1974, *2*, 277.

Depression by nitrous oxide of the hypoxic ventilatory response.— O. Yacoub *et al.*, *Anesthesiology*, 1976, *45*, 385.

Two of 10 subjects anaesthetised with nitrous oxide 50% in oxygen and undergoing simulated dental procedures inhaled contrast medium placed on the back of the tongue; nitrous oxide differed little from other anaesthetic techniques in suppressing pharyngeal and laryngeal reflexes.— J. Rubin *et al.*, *Br. J. Anaesth.*, 1977, *49*, 1005.

Profound hypotension due to peripheral vasodilatation after the concomitant use of diazepam intravenously and nitrous oxide for the induction of anaesthesia.— R. B. Falk *et al.*, *Anesthesiology*, 1978, *49*, 149.

Awareness during anaesthesia. There had been reports of awareness during nitrous oxide/oxygen anaesthesia. There was no evidence of awareness in a study in 138 patients, some of whom received diazepam or pethidine as premedication.— G. Agarwal and S. S. Sikh, *Br. J. Anaesth.*, 1977, *49*, 835.

Effect on driving. A slight but quantified impairment in driving ability was found up to 30 minutes following 15 minutes' inhalation of nitrous oxide/oxygen mixtures.— D. G. Moyes *et al.* (letter), *Br. med. J.*, 1979, *1*, 1425.

Hazard to user. In studies in healthy subjects reaction times, after exposure for 1.5 hours, were not affected by nitrous oxide in concentrations up to 8% in air, but were significantly affected by nitrous oxide 12% in air.— R. H. Allison *et al.*, *Br. J. Anaesth.*, 1979, *51*, 177.

A discussion on the hazards of nitrous oxide exhaust from cryosurgical probes.— *J. Am. med. Ass.*, 1979, *242*, 2379.

Blood concentrations of nitrous oxide in theatre personnel.— J. R. Krapez *et al.*, *Br. J. Anaesth.*, 1980, *52*, 1143.

Absorption and Fate. Nitrous oxide is rapidly absorbed on inhalation. The blood/gas partition coefficient is low and most of the inhaled nitrous oxide is rapidly eliminated through the lungs though small amounts diffuse through the skin.

The mean arterial concentration of nitrous oxide was 201 mg per litre in 15 women breathing 50% nitrous oxide and oxygen as required during labour. This was equivalent to breathing 26.4% nitrous oxide until equilibrium between the inspired concentration and the blood was attained.— I. P. Latto *et al.*, *Br. J. Anaesth.*, 1973, *45*, 1029.

The pharmacokinetics of nitrous oxide in 2 subjects.— W. D. A. Smith *et al.*, *Br. J. Anaesth.*, 1974, *46*, 3.

The transfer of nitrous oxide into body air cavities.— E. S. Munson, *Br. J. Anaesth.*, 1974, *46*, 202.

Pregnancy and the neonate. Studies of the transplacental diffusion of nitrous oxide.— Marx. G.F. *et al.*, *Anesthesiology*, 1970, *32*, 429; D. M. Hay, *Br. J. Obstet. Gynaec.*, 1978, *85*, 299.

The uptake and elimination of nitrous oxide by the newborn.— D. J. Steward and R. E. Creighton, *Can. Anaesth. Soc. J.*, 1978, *25*, 215.

Uses. Nitrous oxide is an anaesthetic administered by inhalation. It is a weak anaesthetic but has strong analgesic properties. It produces little muscle relaxation.

When administered without air or oxygen nitrous oxide would produce deep anaesthesia in about 1 minute but signs of hypoxia would occur, therefore in practice such a procedure is not performed. Induction is usually carried out with 20% of oxygen and maintenance with at least 30%. It is usually employed only for induction and as a vehicle for or as an adjuvant to other anaesthetics.

Nitrous oxide 50% with oxygen is widely used for analgesia especially in obstetrics. Mixtures of nitrous oxide with air (gas and air) are rarely used now for analgesia.

It should not be used for more than 24 hours because of the risk of bone-marrow depression.

For the use of nitrous oxide in the measurement of regional blood flow, see D. G. McDowall, *Br. J. Anaesth.*, 1969, *41*, 761.

Light anaesthesia with nitrous oxide appeared to protect normal cells from the effects of cytarabine without altering the response of tumour cells.— D. L. Bruce *et al.*, *Cancer Res.*, 1970, *30*, 1803. *Animal* studies had not demonstrated nitrous oxide to have any enhancing effect on the action of cytostatic drugs.— D. Marinković (letter), *Lancet*, 1978, *2*, 998.

A discussion on the use of nitrous oxide as an aerosol propellent.— *Mfg Chem.*, 1972, *43*, (Dec.), 33.

The effect of nitrous oxide on the cerebral blood flow and EEG during halothane anaesthesia.— T. Sakabe *et al.*, *Br. J. Anaesth.*, 1976, *48*, 957.

Analgesia. The self-administration of a 50/50 mixture of nitrous oxide and oxygen by patients in ambulances led to complete or partial relief of pain without worsening of the patient's condition. No patient with impaired consciousness, maxillofacial or oral injuries, or who was drunk received this treatment. There were no undesirable side-effects, and there was a reduction in anxiety.— P. J. F. Baskett and A. Withnell, *Br. med. J.*, 1970, *2*, 41. See also E. R. Thal *et al.*, *J. Am. med. Ass.*, 1979, *242*, 2418. Comment.— R. N. Hindin (letter), *ibid.*, 1980, *244*, 769. Reply.— S. J. Montgomery *et al.*, *ibid.*

In the relief of pain during minor but painful procedures, self-administration of an equal mixture of nitrous oxide and oxygen (Entonox) by patients on 237 occasions, supervised by specially trained staff, was a safe and satisfactory procedure, almost completely free from undesirable side-effects.— P. J. F. Baskett and J. A. Bennett, *Br. med. J.*, 1971, *2*, 509. Similar results in 91 patients. Adverse effects included drowsiness, dizziness, tingling of fingers and toes, disorders of smell or taste and nausea. The use of nitrous oxide and oxygen was not recommended in association with head injuries and when consciousness was impaired; maxillo-facial injuries; the very young and the very old; pneumothorax; the 'bends' and heavy sedation including the effects of alcohol.— R. A. A. Johnson, *Practitioner*, 1979, *222*, 681.

In 7 subjects the stepwise increase in the concentration of nitrous oxide caused a progressive rise in the pain threshold to levels higher than those achieved when the highest concentration was administered from the start. The inhalation of a constant concentration produced a maximum effect in about 10 minutes, the effect of 50% nitrous oxide being only marginally greater than that of 33%.— J. G. Whitwam *et al.*, *Br. J. Anaesth.*, 1976, *48*, 425.

In a study in 40 patients given nitrous oxide 25% in oxygen for 15 minutes postoperatively or methadone 6 mg intravenously in 2-mg increments, nitrous oxide was equipotent with methadone 4 mg in terms of analgesia.— D. G. Dalrymple and G. D. Parbrook, *Br. J. Anaesth.*, 1976, *48*, 593.

Asthma. An asthmatic attack in a 10-year-old dental patient was terminated by the administration of a 50/50 mixture of nitrous oxide and oxygen.— V. Rice (letter), *Br. dent. J.*, 1970, *128*, 476.

Cardiac infarction. In a double-blind study of 81 patients, inhalation of nitrous oxide with oxygen in equal proportions was only marginally better than placebo in providing initial analgesia.— F. Kerr *et al.*, *Lancet*, 1975, *1*, 1397.

A double-blind trial in 69 patients and a clinical study in 42 patients showed that the administration of nitrous oxide in concentrations of 35% with oxygen 60% effectively relieved the pain of acute cardiac infarction.— P. L. Thompson and B. Lown, *J. Am. med. Ass.*, 1976, *235*, 924.

Further references: F. Kerr *et al.*, *Lancet*, 1972, *1*, 63; J. Wynne *et al.*, *Circulation*, 1977, *56*, *Suppl.* 3, 8.

Cryoanalgesia. Fifteen patients who underwent thoracotomy obtained better postoperative relief of pain with cryoanalgesia than 9 similar patients who received either intercostal blocks with long-acting local anaesthetics or no nerve block therapy at all. Pain relief in the cryoanalgesia group lasted for about 2 to 3 weeks, with full return of sensation occurring in all patients by the 30th postoperative day. No adverse effects were noted during follow-up over 6 months. The principle of the technique is the formation of an ice-ball (temperature −60°) at the tip of the cryoprobe by means of rapid expansion of nitrous oxide through a micropore outlet. Cells at the site of nerve-freezing are destroyed, but perineural collagen, which provides a scaffolding for regenerating capillaries, axons and Schwann cells, and intraneural connective tissue, are preserved.— J. Katz *et al.*, *Lancet*, 1980, *1*, 512.

Dental surgery. A discussion on the use of nitrous oxide with oxygen sedation in dentistry.— S. J. E. Lindsay and G. J. Roberts, *Br. dent. J.*, 1979, *147*, 206. Comments: G. H. Bard (letter), *ibid.*, 293; F. H. Heighway Bates (letter), *ibid.*, 294.

A mixture containing nitrous oxide 50%, oxygen 43%, and carbon dioxide 7% (to stimulate ventilation) was given with halothane to over 500 dental patients aged 3 to 65 years. The required depth of anaesthesia was reached more rapidly than previously observed without the addition of carbon dioxide and recovery was also rapid. No premedication was required.— J. Davies *et al.*, *Br. J. Anaesth.*, 1975, *47*, 603.

Inhalation sedation for conservative dentistry was used successfully in 24 extremely anxious patients with either nitrous oxide 25% with oxygen and air or methoxyflurane 0.35% vaporised with compressed air.— D. H. Edmunds and M. Rosen, *Br. dent. J.*, 1975, *139*, 398.

Studies in 65 children (4 to 17 years) indicated that administration of oxygen and nitrous oxide gas mixtures (in the range 80% oxygen to 20% nitrous oxide and 30% oxygen to 70% nitrous oxide) to severely anxious dental patients enabled them to co-operate and to allow dental treatment to be carried out. No patients became unconscious during treatment and the effects on the cardiovascular and respiratory systems were minimal.— G. J. Roberts *et al.*, *Br. dent. J.*, 1979, *146*, 177.

Further references.— D. M. O'Mullane *et al.*, *Br. dent. J.*, 1978, *145*, 364.

Laparoscopy. A fall in cardiac output accompanied by an increase in mean arterial pressure and in heart-rate occurred in 8 patients and an increase in central venous pressure in 7 during peritoneal cavity insufflation with nitrous oxide for laparoscopy. Release of nitrous oxide from the abdomen was followed by return of cardiac output to former levels within 12 minutes in the 7 patients in whom it was measured.— R. L. Marshall *et al.*, *Br. J. Anaesth.*, 1972, *44*, 1183.

The use of nitrous oxide with narcotic analgesics for anaesthetising out-patients for laparoscopy.— J. I. Fishburne *et al.*, *Anesth. Analg. curr. Res.*, 1974, *53*, 1.

Pregnancy and the neonate. A comparison was made of the results of administering nitrous oxide 50 or 70% in oxygen for obstetric analgesia in 501 mothers. Both concentrations provided a similar relief from pain, but the number of mothers with normal deliveries who lost consciousness was slightly but significantly higher in those receiving nitrous oxide 70%. It was concluded that 50% nitrous oxide in oxygen could be safely used by midwives in domiciliary and hospital practice, without supervision.—Report to the MRC of the Committee on Nitrous Oxide and Oxygen Analgesia in Midwifery, *Br. med. J.*, 1970, *1*, 709.

In a comparison of nitrous oxide 50% with oxygen, pethidine, and pethidine with nitrous oxide and oxygen in 663 women in labour, nitrous oxide produced a higher incidence of pain relief than pethidine although the total number of patients (less than half) receiving satisfactory analgesia was disturbingly low.— A. Holdcroft and M. Morgan, *J. Obstet. Gynaec. Br. Commonw.*, 1974, *81*, 603.

For an account of analgesia and anaesthesia during labour, see J. S. Crawford, *Practitioner*, 1974, *212*, 677.

Use in children. For 49 burnt children under 12 years old, the use of nitrous oxide 50% with oxygen together with droperidol 100 to 200 µg per kg body-weight and phenoperidine hydrochloride 30 to 50 µg per kg was found to provide sufficient analgesia to allow dressings to be changed without undue discomfort to the patients.— P. J. F. Baskett, *Postgrad. med. J.*, 1972, *48*, 138.

Proprietary Preparations

Entonox *(BOC Medishield, UK)*. A mixture of equal volumes of nitrous oxide and oxygen.

3120-d

Propanidid *(B.P.)*. FBA 1420. Propyl 4-diethylcarbamoylmethoxy-3-methoxyphenylacetate.

$C_{18}H_{27}NO_5=337.4$.

CAS — 1421-14-3.

Pharmacopoeias. In *Br.*

A pale greenish-yellow hygroscopic viscous liquid with a slight odour. B.p. about 210°. Very slightly **soluble** in water; miscible with alcohol, chloroform, and ether. A 5% solution in water can be prepared by adding 16% of a butyl alcohol extract of polyoxyethylated castor oil (Micellophor).

Solutions of propanidid and methohexitone sodium were immediately compatible, but because the pH difference was considerable, degradation of the propanidid preparation rapidly occurred. Such a mixture should under no circumstances be used.— D. Whitfield, *Personal Communication*, 1967.

Adverse Effects. Involuntary muscle movements and hiccup may occur during induction. Hyperventilation is common and is followed by hypoventilation or possibly by apnoea. Hypotension has been reported and may be severe. Cardiac arrest has occurred. There is a greater incidence of thrombo-embolic phenomena with propanidid than with thiopentone or methohexitone. Allergic reactions may occur in patients and anaesthetists; the precise role of the solubilising agent is not clear. Nausea and vomiting may be frequent complications during recovery.

The recorded frequency of adverse reactions to alphaxalone with alphadolone acetate (Althesin), propanidid, and Stesolid MR (diazepam) has suggested that the common solvent, Cremophor, is responsible for the adverse reactions.— M. S. Hüttel *et al.*, *Br. J. Anaesth.*, 1980, *52*, 77.

Allergic reactions and hypersensitivity. Reports of allergic reactions or hypersensitivity.— D. Miloschewsky and M. Červenková (letter), *Br. J. Anaesth.*, 1970, *42*, 833; K. J. Turner *et al.*, *Br. J. Anaesth.*, 1972, *44*, 211; W. Lorenz *et al.*, *Br. J. Anaesth.*, 1972, *44*, 355; C. A. N. Jarvis (letter), *ibid.*, 989; I. B. Sneddon and R. C. Glew, *Practitioner*, 1973, *211*, 321; J. W. Dundee *et al.*, *Br. med. J.*, 1974, *1*, 63; A. Baraka and S. Steir, *J. Am. med. Ass.*, 1980, *243*, 1745.

Cardiovascular effects. The comparative cardiovascular effects of propanidid 7.5 mg per kg body-weight and methohexitone 2.4 mg per kg were investigated in 10 healthy adult males. The initial increase in heart-rate was greater and fell to normal more rapidly with propanidid than with methohexitone. The average period of hyperventilation during administration was 26 seconds after methohexitone and 44 seconds after propanidid.— A. Bernhoff *et al.*, *Br. J. Anaesth.*, 1972, *44*, 2.

Precautions. Propanidid should not be administered to patients known to be hypersensitive. It should be given with caution to patients with acute alcoholism, severe anaemia, cardiovascular disorders, and impaired renal function. The effects of suxamethonium may be prolonged. See also Precautions for General Anaesthetics, p.740.

An elderly man with a history of myocardial infarction and angina pectoris experienced hypotension and delayed recovery after propanidid 400 mg intravenously; this was believed to be the result of poor circulation due to myocardial depression. Extreme care was necessary when propanidid was given to patients with extensive myocardial disease.— J. Gjessing (letter), *Br. J. Anaesth.*, 1969, *41*, 1012.

A haemolytic crisis, thought to be a splenic infarction, occurred in a 39-year-old Ghanaian patient 4 minutes after he received propanidid 500 mg by intravenous injection. Earlier tests had shown normal haemoglobin levels, but on recovery he was found to be a sickle-cell trait carrier.— T. H. Howells *et al.*, *Br. J. Anaesth.*, 1972, *44*, 975.

A 32-year-old woman weighing 52 kg who had taken chlordiazepoxide 10 mg twice daily for 18 months lost consciousness after only 100 mg of a 500-mg dose of propanidid had been injected intravenously. The operation proceeded and recovery was uneventful.— J. A. O. Magbagbeola (letter), *Br. J. Anaesth.*, 1975, *47*, 161.

In 20 patients in whom anaesthesia was induced with propanidid 7 mg per kg body-weight, followed by suxamethonium 1 mg per kg, mean serum-potassium concentrations fell from about 4.1 mmol per litre to about 3.9 mmol per litre two minutes after induction and to about 3.7 mmol per litre 4 minutes after induction. In 20 given methohexitone 1 mg per kg and suxamethonium values fell from about 4.3 mmol per litre to about 4.05 mmol per litre after 2 minutes and reverted almost to their original value after 4 minutes.— I. Pulay (letter), *Br. J. Anaesth.*, 1976, *48*, 1029.

Absorption and Fate. When given intravenously propanidid is rapidly metabolised by esterases, mainly in the liver and plasma; the inactive metabolites are rapidly eliminated in the urine. Propanidid is bound to plasma proteins and diffuses across the placenta.

The concentration of propanidid in serum depended on the rate of injection. When a dose of 7 mg per kg body-weight was given over 5 seconds, mean serum concentrations decreased from 14.9 µg per ml after 1 minute to zero after 15 minutes. When the same dose was given over 20 seconds mean serum concentrations decreased from 13.6 µg per ml after 1 minute to zero after 25 minutes. Propanidid diffused across the placenta; concentrations in the umbilical vein increased with the dose given and were inversely related to the concentration of cholinesterase activity in maternal blood. Propanidid was bound to serum proteins.— A. Doenicke *et al.*, *Br. J. Anaesth.*, 1968, *40*, 415. Criticisms of the findings and conclusions.— J. S. Crawford (letter), *ibid.*, 713.

The pharmacokinetics of propanidid.— M. M. Ghoneim and K. Korttila, *Clin. Pharmacokinet.*, 1977, *2*, 344.

Uses. Propanidid is administered intravenously for complete anaesthesia of short duration or for induction of general anaesthesia. It is a eugenol derivative and is less potent than thiopentone. It is reported to possess local anaesthetic activity. Propanidid has little analgesic activity but it has not been shown to be anti-analgesic. It is not a muscle relaxant although the effects of suxamethonium may be prolonged.

Induction is rapid, occurring in 1 arm/brain circulation time, and recovery starts in 3 to 4 minutes.

The usual dose is 5 to 7 mg per kg body-weight, usually administered as a 5% solution (up to 10 mg per kg may sometimes be required). Smaller doses of about 3 to 4 mg per kg should be used in elderly patients; for debilitated patients dosage should be adjusted according to response and may be reduced to 2 mg per kg. Children and adolescents may need 7 to 10 mg per kg. It has been recommended that the injection period must not be less than 30 seconds and should amount to approximately 60 seconds in poor-risk patients.

The dose of propanidid may be repeated to a maximum total of 1.5 to 2 g for adults if it is necessary to prolong the duration of anaesthesia; if further prolongation is needed transition to another anaesthetic agent is recommended.

A review: S. M. Conway and D. B. Ellis, *Br. J. Anaesth.*, 1970, *42*, 249.

Blind nasotracheal intubation was successfully performed in 64 of 72 patients during propanidid-induced hyperventilation. In 49 of these patients only one dose of propanidid 5 mg per kg body-weight intravenously over 15 seconds was required. The remaining 15 required a further 2.5 mg per kg.— A. O. Oyegunle, *Br. J. Anaesth.*, 1975, *47*, 379. A similar report.— J. A. H. Davies, *ibid.*, 1972, *44*, 528.

In a prospective study 400 patients underwent induction of anaesthesia with 1 of 4 regimens. Muscle fasciculations were significantly less after induction with propanidid 100 to 500 mg intravenously followed by suxamethonium 350 µg per kg body-weight and lignocaine 750 µg per kg injected intravenously together than with methohexitone 1.5 mg per kg followed by suxamethonium 750 µg per kg intravenously.— E. N. S. Fry, *Br. J. Anaesth.*, 1975, *47*, 723.

For an unfavourable comparison of propanidid with diazepam or thiopentone for anaesthesia prior to DC cardioversion, see R. Orko, *Br. J. Anaesth.*, 1976, *48*, 257.

Cardiac arrhythmias. Lasting reversion to sinus rhythm followed within 15 to 30 seconds of an intravenous injection of 300 to 500 mg of propanidid in 9 patients with acute or paroxysmal cardiac arrhythmias. The treatment was unsuccessful in 125 patients with atrial fibrillation. Its use was suggested in paroxysmal supraventricular tachycardia and atrial flutter refractory to some other treatments, and when counter-shock therapy was not available.— K. Bachmann *et al.*, *Dt. med. Wschr.*, 1967, *92*, 1264.

Experience with 50 patients undergoing anal dilation under anaesthesia induced by propanidid, nitrous oxide, and halothane with ECG monitoring, suggested that propanidid protected the heart from most reflex arrhythmias.— R. E. C. Collins *et al.*, *Br. med. J.*, 1973, *2*, 457.

Propanidid controlled cardiac rhythm disturbances in 2 of 7 patients; it seemed that propanidid might be of benefit in certain arrhythmias.— R. J. Vecht *et al.*, *Br. med. J.*, 1975, *4*, 143. Criticism.— S. Homsek (letter), *Br. med. J.*, 1976, *1*, 398.

Pregnancy and the neonate. Propanidid was used successfully for the induction of anaesthesia in 81 women undergoing caesarean section. Of the 81 infants, 63 cried at birth, 13 within 1 minute, 3 within 2 minutes and 2 after a longer period. When propanidid used for induction in 28 women and thiopentone used in 54 women were compared, no infants in the propanidid group and 4 in the thiopentone group suffered respiratory depression.— L. Gran and J. M. Maltau, *Anaesthetist*, 1971, *20*, 247.

For 175 women undergoing caesarean section, propanidid 400 to 600 mg was administered into an intravenous infusion of compound sodium lactate injection over 15 to 20 seconds and anaesthesia maintained by means of further injections of propanidid, 200 mg every 3 minutes. Of 145 questioned on the day after, 1 recorded painful recall due to faulty management, 6 awareness, and 6 unpleasant dreams. Among the 178 infants delivered 30 showed mild and 19 severe foetal depression at 1 minute after delivery, and 4 mild and 7 severe depression 5 minutes after delivery. A shorter interval between induction and delivery was advantageous to the infant.— J. W. Downing *et al.*, *Br. J. Anaesth.*, 1972, *44*, 1069.

Proprietary Preparations

Epontol *(Bayer, UK)*. Propanidid, available as an injection containing 5%, with polyoxyethylated castor oil (Micellophor) 16%, in ampoules of 10 ml. (Also available as Epontol in *Austral., Fr., Ger., Ital., Neth., Norw., Spain, Swed., Switz.*).

Other Proprietary Names

Fabantol *(S.Afr.)*; Fabontal *(Arg.)*.

3121-n

Sodium Oxybate. Sodium Gamma-hydroxybutyrate; Wy 3478. Sodium 4-hydroxybutyrate.

$C_4H_7NaO_3=126.1$.

CAS — 502-85-2.

A white crystalline hygroscopic powder with a

saline taste. **Soluble** in water. A 24% solution in water has a pH of about 9.5. **Incompatible** with dextromoramide, promethazine, and thiopentone sodium.

Adverse Effects. Side-effects with sodium oxybate include abnormal muscle movements during the induction period and nausea and vomiting. Occasional emergence delirium has been reported. Bradycardia frequently occurs. Respiration may be slowed during induction and Cheyne-Stokes respiration has been reported to occur in the postoperative period.

Precautions. Sodium oxybate should be administered with caution in patients with severe hypertension, bradycardia, conditions associated with defects of cardiac conduction, epilepsy, and alcoholic delirium. It should be given in reduced doses to the elderly. Sodium oxybate enhances the effects of narcotic analgesics and skeletal muscle relaxants. See also Precautions for General Anaesthetics, p.740.

Uses. Sodium oxybate has anaesthetic properties and when injected intravenously produces unconsciousness, but little analgesia, for about 90 minutes. It may be used to produce complete anaesthesia, but is generally employed to produce basal anaesthesia and may be used with nitrous oxide and oxygen or with a narcotic analgesic such as pethidine. Skeletal muscle relaxants may be necessary. Because its effects are not evident for 5 to 10 minutes after injection it has been given with thiopentone sodium to hasten induction.

An anticholinergic should be given for premedication. A solution of sodium oxybate equivalent to 20% of the acid is administered slowly by intravenous injection, usually in a dose of 60 mg per kg body-weight; further smaller doses may be required in long procedures. In the elderly, 50 mg per kg is adequate and in children up to 100 mg per kg may be necessary.

After premedication with papaveretum or pethidine and either atropine or hyoscine, anaesthesia was induced in 50 patients with 50 to 70 mg per kg body-weight of sodium oxybate and 100 mg of thiopentone. In 44 patients maintenance was with nitrous oxide and oxygen (with a supplementary agent in 14) and in 6 the hypnotic effects of sodium oxybate were supplemented with analgesics. The average duration of sleep was 168 minutes. Postoperative nausea and vomiting occurred in 52% of patients and Cheyne-Stokes respiration in 28%.— P. J. Appleton and J. M. B. Burn, *Anesth. Analg. curr. Res.*, 1968, *47*, 164.

Sodium oxybate, 60 mg per kg body-weight, was not satisfactory as a principal anaesthetic in microsurgery of the larynx. Used in 93 patients, a delay in loss of consciousness of up to 8 minutes occurred, together with manifestations of cerebral stimulation.— W. H. J. Cole, *Med. J. Aust.*, 1970, *1*, 372.

Sodium oxybate by mouth in doses ranging from 1.8 to 10.2 g daily was ineffective in controlling the symptoms of parkinsonism in 9 patients.— P. S. Papavasiliou *et al.* (letter), *J. Am. med. Ass.*, 1973, *224*, 130.

Sodium oxybate 1 to 3 g given nightly by mouth was an effective hypnotic in 5 patients with insomnia.— M. Mamelak *et al.* (letter), *Lancet*, 1973, *2*, 328.

Ophthalmic surgery. From a study in 168 patients it was considered that sodium oxybate 40 to 50 mg per kg body-weight with methohexitone 1 mg per kg with local anaesthesia produced a light level of unconsciousness suitable for ophthalmic surgery. In comparison with conventional general anaesthesia, better operation conditions were obtained in that the eye was soft and not congested.— I. Smith *et al.*, *Br. J. Ophthal.*, 1972, *56*, 429.

The intra-ocular pressure of 45 patients during sodium oxybate narcosis was lowered by 10 to 40% of the pre-induction level and immediately pre-operatively the pressure was lower than that of patients under general anaesthesia.— A. M. Wyllie *et al.*, *Br. J. Ophthal.*, 1972, *56*, 436.

Proprietary Names

Gamma-OH *(Egic, Fr.; Egic, Neth.)*; Somsanit *(Köhler, Ger.)*.

3128-p

Sodium Thiamylal.

Sodium 5-allyl-5-(1-methylbutyl)-2-thiobarbiturate.

$C_{12}H_{17}N_2NaO_2S = 276.3$.

CAS — 77-27-0 (thiamylal); 337-47-3 (sodium thiamylal).

3122-h

Sodium Thiamylal for Injection.

Thiamylal Sodium for Injection *(U.S.P.)*. A sterile mixture of sodium thiamylal with anhydrous sodium carbonate as a buffer.

Pharmacopoeias. In *U.S.*

A pale yellow hygroscopic powder with a disagreeable odour. **Soluble** in water. A 5% solution in water has a pH of 10.7 to 11.5.

Adverse Effects, Treatment, and Precautions. As for Thiopentone Sodium, p.759.

Allergic reactions and hypersensitivity. A 44-year-old man developed bronchial spasm, facial oedema, urticaria, and shock after induction of anaesthesia with sodium thiamylal. A skin test 2 weeks later confirmed the allergic reaction.— D. S. Thompson *et al.*, *Anesthesiology*, 1973, *39*, 556.

Absorption and Fate. As for Thiopentone Sodium, p.759.

Pregnancy and the neonate. Sodium thiamylal rapidly crossed the placenta, equilibrium between foetal and maternal blood being reached within 2 or 3 minutes.— F. Moya and B. E. Smith, *Anesthesiology*, 1965, *26*, 465.

Uses. Sodium thiamylal is a barbiturate which is administered intravenously for the production of complete anaesthesia of short duration or for the induction of general anaesthesia. It is possibly slightly more potent than thiopentone sodium and has similar actions and uses. It is also used as a supplement to local anaesthetics during regional and spinal anaesthesia. It may be employed with skeletal muscle relaxants.

It is given as a 2.5% solution, an initial injection of 3 to 6 ml being sufficient to produce short periods of anaesthesia. During induction the rate of injection should be 1 ml every 5 seconds, additional injections of 0.5 to 1 ml being made intermittently as required with the needle remaining in the vein. The maximum total dose should not exceed 1 g (40 ml). A continuous intravenous infusion of a 0.3% solution has also been used for maintenance. It has been administered rectally. Anaesthesia may be induced in 20 to 60 seconds with recovery occurring within 10 to 30 minutes.

Proprietary Names

Surital *(Parke, Davis, Canad.; Parke, Davis, USA)*.

3123-m

Thialbarbitone Sodium

(B.P.C. 1963). Thialbarbital Sodium; Natrium Cyclohexenylallylthiobarbituricum; Thiohexallymalnatrium. Sodium 5-allyl-5-(cyclohex-2-enyl)-2-thiobarbiturate.

$C_{13}H_{15}N_2NaO_2S = 286.3$.

CAS — 467-36-7 (thialbarbitone); 3546-29-0 (thialbarbitone sodium).

Pharmacopoeias. In *Aust.* and *Jug.*

A pale yellow hygroscopic powder with a somewhat alliaceous odour. Very **soluble** in water and alcohol; slightly soluble in chloroform; practically insoluble in ether. A 2.5% solution in water has a pH of about 10.5. Solutions for injection are prepared by dissolving, immediately before use, the sterile contents of a sealed container in the requisite amount of Water for Injections. **Store** in a cool place in airtight containers. Protect from light.

Thialbarbitone sodium is a barbiturate which has been administered intravenously, in doses of 0.2 to 1 g, for the production of complete anaesthesia of short duration or for the induction of general anaesthesia.

3124-b

Thiopentone Sodium

(B.P., B.P. Vet., Eur. P.). Thiopent. Sod.; Soluble Thiopentone; Thiopental Sodium; Thiopentalum Natricum; Thiopentalum Natricum cum Natrii Carbonate; Penthiobarbital Sodique; Thiopentobarbitalum Solubile; Thiomebumalnatrium cum Natrii Carbonate; Natrium Isopentylaethylthiobarbituricum (cum Natrio Carbonico). A mixture of 100 parts of thiopentone sodium with 6 parts of anhydrous sodium carbonate. Sodium 5-ethyl-5-(1-methylbutyl)-2-thiobarbiturate.

$C_{11}H_{17}N_2NaO_2S = 264.3$.

CAS — 76-75-5 (thiopentone); 71-73-8 (thiopentone sodium).

NOTE. The name thiopental sodium has been applied to thiopentone sodium with or without sodium carbonate; the name thiobarbital has been applied to thiopentone and has also been used to describe a barbiturate of different composition.

Pharmacopoeias. In *Aust., Belg., Br., Chin., Cz., Eur., Fr., Ger., Ind., Int., Jug., Neth., Nord., Pol., Rus., Swiss,* and *Turk.* (all with anhydrous sodium carbonate).

In *Arg., Braz., Jap.,* and *U.S.* without admixture with anhydrous sodium carbonate (Thiopental Sodium).

In *Arg., Ind., It., Jap., Nord., Swiss,* and *U.S.* as a sterile mixture for injection (Thiopental Sodium for Injection; Thiopentone Injection; Thiopentalum Solubile ad Injectionem).

A white to yellowish-white to pale greenish hygroscopic powder with a characteristic alliaceous odour and a bitter taste. **Soluble** 1 in 1.5 of water; partly soluble in alcohol; practically insoluble in ether and light petroleum. A 5% solution in water is strongly alkaline. A 3.5% solution of sodium 5-ethyl-5-(1-methylbutyl)-2-thiobarbiturate is iso-osmotic with serum. Solutions for injection are prepared by dissolving, immediately before use, the sterile contents of a sealed container in the requisite amount of Water for Injections. **Incompatible** with acids, acidic salts, and oxidising agents, and with amikacin sulphate, cefapirin sodium, clindamycin phosphate, and pentazocine lactate. Solutions decompose on standing and precipitation occurs on boiling. **Store** in airtight containers.

For a report of latex and polyvinyl chloride tubing adsorbing thiopentone, see Chlorpromazine Hydrochloride, p.1509.

Effect of gamma-irradiation. The colour of thiopentone sodium deepened and an odour developed on irradiation. A solution of the irradiated material showed numerous fine white insoluble particles. The ultraviolet absorption of the irradiated material and the potency were also affected.— *The Use of Gamma Radiation Sources for the Sterilisation of Pharmaceutical Products*, London, ABPI, 1960.

Incompatibility. Thiopentone sodium solution 2.5% was incompatible when 3 ml was mixed with the following injection solutions: chlorpromazine hydrochloride 50 mg in 2 ml, dimenhydrinate 50 mg in 1 ml, diphenhydramine hydrochloride 50 mg in 1 ml, ephedrine sulphate 50 mg in 1 ml, methylamphetamine hydrochloride 15 mg in 0.75 ml, morphine sulphate 16.2 mg in 1 ml, pethidine hydrochloride 100 mg in 2 ml, procaine hydrochloride 100 mg in 100 ml, prochlorperazine edisylate 10 mg in 2 ml, promethazine hydrochloride 100 mg in 4 ml, and sodium bicarbonate 3.75 g in 50 ml. A precipitate of thiopentone acid might appear in a 2.5% solution in about 11 days in dextrose injection stored at 5° or 2.5 days at 25°, in about 117 days in Water for Injections at 5° or 60 days at 25°, and in about 120 days in sodium chloride injection at 5° or 53 days at 25°.— R. W. Jones *et al.*, *Am. J. Hosp. Pharm.*, 1961, *18*, 700.

Thiopentone sodium 250 mg was 'physically incompatible' with arginine glutamate 2.5 g, metaraminol 20 mg, penicillin 2 million units, plasmin 200 mg, promazine 100 mg, sulphafurazole 400 mg, or tetracycline 50 mg in 100 ml of dextrose injection.— R. D. Dunworth and F. R. Kenna, *Am. J. Hosp. Pharm.*, 1965, *22*, 190.

There was loss of clarity when intravenous solutions of thiopentone sodium were mixed with those of hydromorphone hydrochloride, diphenhydramine hydrochloride, dimenhydrinate, ephedrine sulphate, insulin, narcotic salts, noradrenaline acid tartrate, procaine hydrochloride, prochlorperazine maleate, protein hydrolysate, sodium bicarbonate, or suxamethonium chloride; also (in dextrose injection) benzylpenicillin, metaraminol tartrate, promazine hydrochloride, promethazine hydrochloride, sulphafurazole diethanolamine, or tetracycline hydrochloride; thiopentone was also incompatible with lactated Ringer's injection and 10% dextrose with sodium chloride injection.— J. A. Patel and G. L. Phillips, *Am. J. Hosp. Pharm.*, 1966, *23*, 409.

A precipitate formed within 1 hour when thiopentone sodium was mixed with 10% dextrose or 10% invert sugar in saline or water, or with 10% laevulose solutions.— E. A. Parker, *Am. J. Hosp. Pharm.*, 1969, *26*, 653.

Stability of solution. Thiopentone sodium, 2 g per litre, had good chemical stability in dextrose injection, sodium chloride injection, 5% dextrose in sodium chloride injection, multi-electrolyte solution, or Water for Injections for up to 48 hours at room temperature, but in this period solutions of pH above 10 attacked the glass containers.— E. A. Parker, *Am. J. Hosp. Pharm.*, 1967, *24*, 434.

Adverse Effects. As for Phenobarbitone, p.812.
Coughing, sneezing, laryngeal spasm, or bronchospasm may occur, particularly during induction with thiopentone sodium. The intravenous injection of concentrated solutions such as 5% may result in thrombophlebitis. Extravasation may cause tissue necrosis. Intra-arterial injection causes burning pain and may cause prolonged blanching of the forearm and hand and gangrene of digits. Hypersensitivity reactions have been reported. A serious danger arising during anaesthesia with thiopentone is respiratory depression, and means for treating respiratory failure should always be at hand. Cardiac arrhythmias associated with hypercarbia or hypoxia may occur; thiopentone depresses cardiac output and often causes an initial fall in blood pressure, and overdosage may result in circulatory failure. Postoperative vomiting is infrequent but there may be persistent drowsiness, confusion, and amnesia. Headache has been reported with the barbiturate anaesthetics.

Thiopentone did not reduce the blood viscosity or the fibrinogen concentration in a study of 15 patients. There was some reduction in the haematocrit.— F. Magora *et al.*, *Br. J. Anaesth.*, 1974, *46*, 343.

In a retrospective survey of adverse reactions to intravenous anaesthetic induction agents there were 6 reactions to thiopentone; 3 were histaminoid with cardiac arrest in 2, 2 involved hypotension and cardiac arrest, and 1 involved jaw rigidity, laryngospasm, and cyanosis. The incidence was estimated at 1 in 14 000.— J. M. Evans and J. A. M. Keogh, *Br. med. J.*, 1977, *2*, 735.

A study of the respiratory effects of thiopentone.— L. Daehlin and L. Gran, *Curr. ther. Res.*, 1980, *27*, 706.

Allergic reactions and hypersensitivity. References: T. L. Fisher, *Can. med. Ass. J.*, 1968, *99*, 854; K. P. Barjenbruch and J. R. Jones, *Anesth. Analg. curr. Res.*, 1972, *51*, 113, per *J. Am. med. Ass.*, 1972, *219*, 1660; J. W. Dundee *et al.*, *Br. med. J.*, 1974, *1*, 63; H. J. Lewi and T. V. Taylor (letter), *Br. med. J.*, 1977, *2*, 1480; M. Fisher (letter), *Br. J. Anaesth.*, 1977, *49*, 87; A. D. Baxter, *Anaesthesia*, 1978, *33*, 349; A. C. Baldwin, *ibid.*, 1979, *34*, 333; J. Dolovich, *Can. med. Ass. J.*, 1980, *123*, 292; M. S. Etter *et al.*, *Anesthesiology*, 1980, *52*, 181.

Cardiovascular effects. The cardiovascular effects of bolus or incremental administration of thiopentone.— J. L. Seltzer *et al.*, *Br. J. Anaesth.*, 1980, *52*, 527.

Effect on body temperature. Thiopentone and nitrous oxide had been used to anaesthetise more than 150 susceptible *pigs* without precipitating malignant hyperpyrexia.— J. N. Lucke *et al.* (letter), *Br. med. J.*, 1975, *1*, 454.

Treatment of Adverse Effects. As for Phenobarbitone, p.812.
Intra-arterial injection may be treated by injecting a solution of procaine into the artery and also by the administration of heparin and anticoagulants by mouth until the circulation has been re-established. The pain may be controlled by sympathetic block. Vasodilators are often administered intra-arterially although their effectiveness in this situation is disputed. Perivenous injection may be treated by immediate infiltration of the area with hyaluronidase dissolved in a 0.5 or 1% solution of procaine hydrochloride or in sodium chloride injection.

Precautions. Thiopentone sodium should be administered only by experienced anaesthetists, and it should not be given to out-patients who have to return home unaccompanied. It should only be administered to patients in the recumbent or semi-recumbent position because of danger of cerebral damage following hypotension. Apparatus for inflating the lungs with air or oxygen and for establishing a clear airway should be available.
Care is necessary when thiopentone sodium is administered to a patient with a full stomach and in operations on the upper air passages.
It is contra-indicated in respiratory obstruction, status asthmaticus, severe shock, dystrophia myotonica, and porphyria.
Thiopentone sodium alone should not be used for peroral endoscopy since laryngeal spasm may cause grave anoxia. It may also precipitate acute circulatory failure in patients with constrictive pericarditis or with gross dyspnoea due to diseases of the heart or lungs. It should be given cautiously to patients with asthma. Doses of thiopentone sodium should be greatly reduced in shock and dehydration, severe anaemia, hyperkalaemia, toxaemia, myxoedema and other metabolic disorders, or in severe hepatic or renal disease. Reduced doses are also required in the elderly. Thiopentone sodium should be used with caution in patients with cardiovascular disease, adrenocortical insufficiency, or with increased intracranial pressure.
Difficulty may be experienced in producing anaesthesia with the usual doses in patients accustomed to taking alcohol or some drugs; additional anaesthetic agents may be necessary. Care is required when anaesthetising patients being treated with phenothiazine tranquillisers since there may be increased hypotension. Reduced doses may be required in patients receiving sulphafurazole.
See also Precautions for General Anaesthetics, p.740.

Barbiturates used intravenously as anaesthetics decreased cerebrospinal fluid pressure.— T. Takahashi *et al.*, *Br. J. Anaesth.*, 1973, *45*, 179.

Significantly less thiopentone was needed to induce anaesthesia following premedication with hyoscine and morphine, than after atropine, diazepam, and pethidine. Furthermore 37 patients taking digoxin and a diuretic required significantly less thiopentone than 37 patients who did not receive this treatment. It was noted that 21 patients who underwent operation for valvular heart disease required only 60% of the thiopentone dose required by patients undergoing operations on limbs.— F. Andreasen and J. H. Christensen, *Br. J. clin. Pharmac.*, 1977, *4*, 640P.

Awareness during anaesthesia. There was awareness of intubation in 1 of 38 patients given thiopentone 3 mg per kg body-weight intravenously followed immediately by suxamethonium 1 mg per kg.— I. A. R. Dunnett, *Br. J. Anaesth.*, 1977, *49*, 491.

Enhancement of effect. Enhancement of the effect of thiopentone by sulphafurazole.— S. I. Csögör and S. F. Kerek, *Br. J. Anaesth.*, 1970, *42*, 988.

Absorption and Fate. When administered intravenously thiopentone sodium may reach effective concentrations in the brain within 30 seconds. Redistribution to other tissues, particularly fat, occurs and concentrations in the brain and plasma are reduced. Thiopentone is bound to plasma albumin. Thiopentone is metabolised in the body, chiefly in the liver, at a very slow rate. It readily diffuses across the placenta.

The biological half-life of thiopentone was 16 hours.— W. A. Ritschel, *Drug Intell. & clin. Pharm.*, 1970, *4*, 332.

The pharmacokinetics of thiopentone sodium.— M. M. Ghoneim and K. Korttila, *Clin. Pharmacokinet.*, 1977, *2*, 344. See also P. Duvaldestin, *ibid.*, 1981, *6*, 61.

Pharmacokinetics of thiopentone during anaesthesia with enflurane and nitrous oxide.— M. M. Ghoneim and M. J. Van Hamme, *Br. J. Anaesth.*, 1978, *50*, 1237.

Pregnancy and the neonate. Neonatal depression rarely followed maternal anaesthesia with thiopentone in 31 infants delivered vaginally, but occurred in 5 of 6 infants delivered by caesarean section.— M. Finster *et al.*, *Am. J. Obstet. Gynec.*, 1966, *95*, 621.

Prolonged thiopentone half-life in pregnancy.— D. J. Morgan *et al.*, *Anesthesiology*, 1981, *54*, 474.

Protein binding. The degree of protein binding of thiopentone was increased as the plasma concentration of thiopentone decreased below about 6 µg per ml. The plasma concentration of thiopentone was decreased by the administration of dextran, chiefly due to volume expansion.— P. G. Dayton *et al.*, *Biochem. Pharmac.*, 1967, *16*, 2321.

The amount of unbound thiopentone was 28% in 10 healthy subjects, 53% in 10 patients with hepatic disease, and about 55% in patients with renal disease.— M. M. Ghoneim and H. Pandya, *Anesthesiology*, 1975, *42*, 545. See also F. Andreasen, *Acta pharmac. tox.*, 1973, *32*, 417.

The amount of free (unbound) thiopentone in normal serum was about 52 to 57%; in serum from patients with kwashiorkor, with a reduced albumin concentration, the amount of free thiopentone was about 65 to 68%. In kwashiorkor serum more thiopentone was bound to other protein fractions; the significance of this secondary binding was not clear.— N. Buchanan and L. A. van der Walt, *Br. J. Anaesth.*, 1977, *49*, 247.

Uses. Thiopentone sodium is a barbiturate which is administered intravenously for the induction of general anaesthesia or for the production of complete anaesthesia of short duration. It has poor analgesic and muscle relaxant properties. Small doses have been shown to be anti-analgesic and lower the pain threshold.
Thiopentone sodium is administered intravenously as a 2.5% or occasionally as a 5% solution, the usual dose for inducing anaesthesia being 100 to 150 mg injected over 10 to 15 seconds; if unconsciousness has not occurred within 30 seconds a further 100 to 150 mg may be given. For longer operations additional injections of 50 to 100 mg may be given as required; concentrations of 0.2 to 0.4% have sometimes been used by continuous intravenous infusion.
Recovery is usually rapid after moderate doses, but the patient may remain sleepy or confused for several hours. Large doses or repeated smaller doses may markedly delay recovery. Rapid injection gives a more pronounced effect and is followed by a more rapid recovery than slow injection. There is no stage of excitement with thiopentone anaesthesia. Its use should be preceded by atropine or similar agent to depress vagal reflexes and mucous secretions. Morphine or pethidine may be given to enhance the poor analgesic effects of thiopentone. Muscle relaxants may be required and should be administered separately.
Thiopentone sodium has been given rectally as a solution, suspension, or suppositories for basal anaesthesia in a dose of about 30 to 40 mg per kg body-weight; its effects were usually observed within 15 minutes. Doses of 20 mg per kg have been used to supplement phenothiazine premedication.
If anaesthesia with thiopentone has to be repeated within 36 hours, smaller doses should be given because the previous dose will not have been fully metabolised. Tolerance to thiopentone rapidly develops.
Thiopentone sodium is used for the control of convulsions, including drug-induced convulsions, but diazepam (see p.1523) is often preferred.

Thiopentone 4 mg per kg body-weight, methohexitone 1.5 mg per kg, and alphaxalone 450 µg per kg with alphadolone acetate each lowered the blood pressure to the same degree in 20 heavily premedicated patients with cardiac disease.— S. M. Lyons and R. S. J. Clarke, *Br. J. Anaesth.*, 1972, *44*, 575.

Thiopentone given in bolus doses significantly reduced the average intracranial pressure from 40 to 22 mmHg when given on 21 occasions to 13 patients with elevated intracranial pressure or with episodes of intracranial hypertension during the surgical procedure.— H. M. Shapiro *et al.*, *Br. J. Anaesth.*, 1973, *45*, 1057.

A report of the recovery of a 26-month-old boy after a period of cold water submersion and cerebral ischaemic anoxia of approximately 45 minutes' duration. Treatment included deep barbiturate hypothermic coma using thiopentone sodium 25 mg per kg body-weight daily in 10 divided doses.— D. R. Derbyshire and R. G. Clark (letter), *Lancet*, 1980, *2*, 637.

Prolongation of thiopentone anaesthesia by probenecid.— S. Kaukinen *et al.*, *Br. J. Anaesth.*, 1980, *52*, 603.

For the use of thiopentone in cardioversion, see Diazepam p.1524.

Electroconvulsive therapy. Thiopentone 4 mg per kg body-weight and propanidid 7 mg per kg by intravenous injection were considered to be equally suitable as induction agents for ECT after consideration of the results of psychological tests, waking times, talking times, and incidence of side-effects in a controlled study on 23 patients. There was some decrease in waking and talking times, and some improvement of psychological performance after propanidid compared with thiopentone.— A. L. Naftalin *et al.*, *Br. J. Anaesth.*, 1969, *41*, 506.

Neurosurgery. In 166 patients undergoing neurosurgery, anaesthesia was induced with sufficient thiopentone to abolish eyelash reflex; then in addition to nitrous oxide and oxygen anaesthesia, thiopentone sodium was administered by continuous intravenous infusion at a rate dependent on the dose already received during induction. Anaesthesia was maintained until dural closure was begun. Blood-thiopentone concentrations determined in 7 patients were between 5 and 7.6 μg per ml. No tendency to produce thombosis was noted. Of 47 patients for whom postoperative data was available, 25 were awake when removed from the operating table, and postoperative restlessness was noted in 4.— A. R. Hunter, *Br. J. Anaesth.*, 1972, *44*, 506.

Status epilepticus. Of 117 patients with status epilepticus treated by thiopentone infusion, only 2 required the infusion to be continued for longer than 72 hours. Initially 25 to 100 mg was given by slow intravenous injection until convulsions ceased and then usually about 1 g by slow intravenous drip was required during the first 12 hours. No side-effects or difficulty of management was encountered. Results with lignocaine and phenytoin were not very successful.— A. S. Brown and J. M. Horton, *Br. med. J.*, 1967, *1*, 27.

Further references: M. Partinen *et al.*, *Br. med. J.*, 1981, *282*, 520.

Preparations

Thiopental Sodium for Injection *(U.S.P.)*. A sterile mixture of thiopental sodium *U.S.P.* and anhydrous sodium carbonate. pH of an 8% solution 10.2 to 11.2.

Thiopentone Injection *(B.P.)*. Thiopentone Sodium Injection. A sterile solution of thiopentone sodium in Water for Injections, prepared by dissolving the sterile contents of a sealed container (Thiopentone Sodium for Injection) in the requisite amount of Water for Injections. The injection should be freshly prepared and used within 24 hours.

Proprietary Preparations

Intraval Sodium *(May & Baker, UK)*. Thiopentone sodium, available as powder for preparing injections, in ampoules of 0.5 and 1 g, and in vials of 2.5 and 5 g. (Also available as Intraval Sodium in *Austral.* and as Intraval-Sodium in *S.Afr.*).

Pentothal *(Abbott, UK)*. Thiopentone sodium, available as powder for preparing injection, in ampoules of 0.5 and 1 g. **Pentothal Rectal Suspension**. Contains thiopentone sodium *U.S.P.* 40% with sodium carbonate as a buffer in a basis of light liquid paraffin and dimethyldioctadecyl ammonium bentonite, supplied in a disposable plastic (Abbo-Sert) syringe graduated for a total dosage of 2 g of thiopentone sodium in increments of 100 mg. (Also available as Pentothal or Pentothal Sodium in *Arg., Austral., Belg., Canad., Ital., Switz., USA*).

Other Proprietary Names

Farmotal *(Ital.)*; Hypnostan *(Fin.)*; Leopental *(Denm.)*; Nesdonal *(Belg., Neth.)*; Pentothal-Natrium *(Denm., Norw.)*; Thio-Barbityral *(Switz.)*; Tiobarbital *(Spain)*; Trapanal *(Ger.)*.

3125-v

Tribromoethyl Alcohol *(B.P. 1953)*. Tribromoethanol; Tribromoethanolum. 2,2,2-Tribromoethanol.
$C_2H_3Br_3O$=282.8.

CAS — 75-80-9.

Pharmacopoeias. In *Int., Nord.,* and *Turk.*

A white crystalline powder with a slightly aromatic odour and taste. M.p. 79° to 81°.
Soluble 1 in 39 of water; very soluble in amylene hydrate and light petroleum; soluble in alcohol, chloroform, and ether. It decomposes on exposure to light and moist air. Aqueous solutions should not be heated above 40° and should preferably be prepared immediately before use. **Store** in airtight containers. Protect from light.

Adverse Effects. Tribromoethyl alcohol, in the usual anaesthetic doses, causes an early but temporary fall in blood pressure which lasts about 10 to 15 minutes. Occasionally, as with hypertensive patients, the blood pressure falls rapidly. Full anaesthetic doses depress respiration and large doses cause respiratory paralysis and depress cardiac function. Large doses also impair liver function and in persons with liver disease the effect may occur with smaller doses.
Solutions which have decomposed, with the formation of dibromacetaldehyde, are highly irritant.

Pregnancy and the neonate. Bromethol appeared to be profoundly depressant to the foetus; infants had remained relatively inactive for up to 4 days after its use for basal maternal anaesthesia.— J. B. E. Baker, *Pharmac. Rev.*, 1960, *12*, 37.

Uses. Tribromoethyl alcohol has been used as a basal anaesthetic and to control patients with eclampsia, tetanus, and other convulsive disorders. It was administered rectally.
Tribromoethyl alcohol was used in the form of Bromethol (see below) which was administered as a 2.5% solution freshly prepared in warm distilled water. Solutions were tested before use by adding 0.1 ml of 0.1% congo red solution to 5 ml of the diluted solution. The Bromethol being tested was fit to be used if the indicator remained bright red or orange.
The usual dose was about 80 to 100 mg of tribromoethyl alcohol per kg body-weight. Elderly and debilitated patients were given not more than 70 mg per kg.

Preparations

Bromethol *(B.P. 1953, Nord. P.)*. Tribromethanol Solution; Tribromoethyl Alcohol Solution. Tribromoethyl alcohol 66.7% w/w in amylene hydrate; 1 ml contains 1 g of tribromoethyl alcohol. Store in dry airtight containers. Protect from light. It is rapidly decomposed by moisture. *Dose.* 0.075 to 0.1 ml per kg body-weight, by rectal injection. CAUTION. *Bromethol is inflammable and volatile; care must be taken not to employ it near an open flame.*

Bromethol was formerly marketed in Great Britain under the proprietary name Avertin (*Winthrop*).

3126-g

Trichloroethylene *(B.P., Eur. P.)*. Trichlorethylene; Trichlorethylenum; Trichloroethylenum.

$CHCl:CCl_2$=131.4.

CAS — 79-01-6.

Pharmacopoeias. In *Aust., Br., Cz., Eur., Fr., Ger., Hung., Ind., Int., It., Jug., Neth., Nord.,* and *Turk.*

A clear, colourless or pale blue, mobile liquid with a chloroform-like odour and a sweet burning taste. It contains thymol 0.01% w/w as a preservative and may contain not more than 0.001% w/w of a suitable blue colouring matter to distinguish it from chloroform. Relative density 1.464 to 1.470. B.p. 85° to 88°. Practically **insoluble** in water; miscible with dehydrated alcohol, chloroform, ether, fixed and volatile oils, and most other organic solvents. It decomposes in light in the presence of air with the formation of hydrochloric acid; in the presence of heat and alkali dichloroacetylene is formed. **Store** in a cool place in airtight containers. Protect from light.

Stability. Trichloroethylene was stable for long periods provided that it was stored in a cool place, in the closed, light-proof containers in which it was supplied. It was readily decomposed by strong light or by contact with hot surfaces. For example, when left in a clear glass bottle for 3 weeks, it was found to have undergone considerable decomposition with the formation of phosgene and hydrochloric acid. In an anaesthetic apparatus it should be placed in a tinted bottle; it should be changed every few days, and should never be used if it has been exposed for a long or unknown period to the action of light.— *Br. med. J.*, 1959, *2*, 103.

Adverse Effects. Trichloroethylene increases the rate and decreases the depth of respiration and may be followed by apnoea. The heart-rate may be slowed, and the sensitivity of the heart to beta-adrenergic activity increased, possibly with arrhythmias. Trichloroethylene anaesthesia may be followed by nausea, vomiting, headache, and confusion. It may depress liver and kidney function.
In industry, exposure to high concentrations of trichloroethylene vapour has caused acute poisoning and fatalities have occurred, though temporary unconsciousness is a more common manifestation. Chronic poisoning arising from the industrial use of trichloroethylene may result in cardiotoxicity and neurological impairment especially of the first and fifth cranial nerves. Blindness may develop. Liver necrosis has been reported. Prolonged contact with trichloroethylene can cause dermatitis, eczema, burns, and conjunctivitis.
Dependence of the barbiturate-alcohol type has been reported in medical personnel and factory workers who regularly inhale trichloroethylene vapour.
Maximum permissible atmospheric concentration 100 ppm.

A brief review of the toxicity of trichloroethylene.— *Br. med. J.*, 1974, *4*, 525.

A 16-year-old girl who took 400 to 500 ml of trichloroethylene developed coma, respiratory difficulty, muscle spasm, hyperreflexia, severe vomiting, and tachycardia. She recovered with tracheotomy, dextrose infusions, additional potassium, and mechanical respiration; there was no residual damage.— H. Warembourg *et al.*, *Lille méd.*, 1964, *9*, 192.

A comparison of the blood losses from operation wounds of the conjunctiva during anaesthesia with trichloroethylene and halothane. The loss was significantly greater in patients anaesthetised with trichloroethylene.— F. R. Ellis, *Br. J. Anaesth.*, 1966, *38*, 941.

Acute liver damage developed in 3 teenagers who inhaled a commercial cleaning fluid containing trichloroethylene and was associated with renal tubular necrosis in 2 of them.— R. D. Baerg and D. V. Kimberg, *Ann. inter. Med.*, 1970, *73*, 713.

Diseases resembling vinyl chloride disease had been noted after exposure to trichloroethylene.— N. Rowell, *Practitioner*, 1977, *219*, 820.

Industrial poisoning. Reports of industrial poisoning with trichloroethylene: C. F. Gutch *et al.*, *Ann. intern. Med.*, 1965, *63*, 128; P. H. Buxton and M. Hayward, *J. Neurol. Neurosurg. Psychiat.*, 1967, *30*, 511, per *Abstr. Wld Med.*, 1968, *42*, 474; A. B. S. Mitchell and B. G. Parsons-Smith, *Br. med. J.*, 1969, *1*, 422; M. Bauer and S. F. Rabens, *Archs Derm.*, 1974, *110*, 886; R. T. Gun *et al.*, *Med. J. Aust.*, 1978, *1*, 535.

Treatment of Adverse Effects. As for Chloroform, p.745.

When rapid breathing developed during anaesthesia with trichloroethylene, it could be controlled better with pethidine than with pentazocine.— V. K. N. Unni *et al.*, *Br. J. Anaesth.*, 1972, *44*, 692.

Precautions. Trichloroethylene is contra-indicated in disease of the heart and is best avoided in patients with liver disease. It has been reported to increase the cerebrospinal pressure and a contra-indication in space-occupying lesions of the brain has been suggested.
Trichloroethylene should not be used in a closed-circuit apparatus because the heat produced by the action of carbon dioxide and water vapour on the soda lime causes the trichloroethylene to react with the soda lime to form dichloroacetylene, which may cause cranial nerve paralysis and possibly death.

Adrenaline and most other sympathomimetic agents, except possibly in very dilute solution for the control of haemorrhage, should not be used during trichloroethylene anaesthesia (see Adrenaline, p.2); methoxamine or phenylephrine may be administered cautiously. There may be severe reduction in cardiac output in patients undergoing beta-blockade.

See also Precautions for General Anaesthetics, p.740.

When trichloroethylene was administered so that there was a continuous flow of fresh gases the temperature of the soda lime never rose above room temperature and a temperature of 60°, at which dichloroacetylene was increasingly formed, was not reached. Present-day soda lime did not reach a temperature of much above 40° in use.— E. L. Lloyd (letter), *Br. med. J.*, 1969, *2*, 118. Trichloroethylene did not decompose until a temperature of 400° was exceeded, except in the presence of alkali. Anaesthetic tragedies occurred following the use of trichloroethylene in closed circuit with soda lime; the decomposition occurred more rapidly at increased temperatures.— A. B. S. Mitchell and B. G. Parsons-Smith, *ibid.*, 516.

Alcohol, but not meprobamate or thonzylamine, enhanced the central nervous depressant effects of trichloroethylene.— R. K. Ferguson and R. J. Vernon, *Archs envir. Hlth*, 1970, *20*, 462.

Pethidine given to 11 patients anaesthetised with thiopentone and maintained with trichloroethylene, nitrous oxide, and oxygen reduced increases in respiratory-rate but was associated with a slowing of the mean pulse-rate to 63 beats per minute, a fall in blood-pH, a moderate rise in pCO_2, with considerable individual variation, and with prolongation of recovery time. One patient did not recover consciousness and died. A similar group of 11 patients who did not receive pethidine showed tachypnoea during the operation, but no change in acid/base balance, and recovered rapidly at the end of anaesthesia.— A. S. Buchan and H. W. Bauld, *Br. J. Anaesth.*, 1973, *45*, 93.

Alcohol produced vasodilatation of the superficial skin vessels in 6 of 7 subjects repeatedly exposed to trichloroethylene.— R. D. Stewart *et al.*, *Archs envir. Hlth*, 1974, *29*, 1.

Alcohol intolerance occurred in a man exposed to trichloroethylene. Complete relief of symptoms occurred after removal of trichloroethylene from the plant.— S. Pardys and M. Brotman (letter), *J. Am. med. Ass.*, 1974, *229*, 521.

Administration of trichloroethylene vapour 1% for 15 minutes produced a highly significant reversible rise in intra-ocular pressure and central venous pressure in all of 8 patients. Trichloroethylene was generally not suitable for use in intra-ocular surgery or in patients with glaucoma.— M. H. Al-Abrak and J. R. Samuel, *Br. J. Ophthal.*, 1975, *59*, 107.

Absorption and Fate. Trichloroethylene is rapidly absorbed on inhalation. It is highly soluble in adipose tissue. The blood/gas partition coefficient is relatively high. Most of the inhaled trichloroethylene is slowly eliminated through the lungs; some is metabolised. It diffuses across the placenta.

Reports showed that trichloroethylene was metabolised in man, the metabolites being trichlorethanol and trichloroacetic acid. The former was the principal metabolite; the latter could be detected in urine for up to 48 hours after anaesthesia.— B. R. Brown and L. D. Vandam, *Ann. N.Y. Acad. Sci.*, 1971, *179*, 235.

Chloral hydrate was a transient metabolite of trichloroethylene.— W. J. Cole *et al.*, *J. Pharm. Pharmac.*, 1975, *27*, 167.

The pharmacokinetics of trichloroethylene after skin exposure compared with inhalation exposure; absorption through the skin would be minimal in normal industrial use.— A. Sato and T. Nakajima, *Br. J. ind. Med.*, 1978, *35*, 43.

Pregnancy and the neonate. Trichloroethylene rapidly appeared in foetal blood after administration to the mother, reaching the maternal concentration within 6 minutes, and exceeding it after 16 minutes. Prolonged administration might result in neonatal depression.— F. Moya and V. Thorndike, *Clin. Pharmac. Ther.*, 1963, *4*, 628.

Uses. Trichloroethylene is a weak volatile anaesthetic administered by inhalation. It is a potent analgesic but a poor muscle relaxant. There is little superficial oozing from cut tissues. It is not inflammable.

Trichloroethylene is used mainly in short surgical procedures where light anaesthesia with good analgesia is required, as in obstetrics, and is often mixed with air, or with nitrous oxide and oxygen. Anaesthesia is usually induced with thiopentone or nitrous oxide. Owing to its low volatility it is unsuitable for administration on an open mask and is usually given by semi-open apparatus (see also Precautions).

A concentration of about 0.5 to 2% of the vapour is required to produce light anaesthesia. To produce analgesia during childbirth a concentration of 0.35 to 0.5% of trichloroethylene in air is recommended. It may be given by an inhaler designed for self-administration and there is little depression of uterine muscle when it is used in analgesic concentrations.

Trichloroethylene has also been used for the relief of pain in trigeminal neuralgia and for the prevention and treatment of attacks of angina of effort, 1 ml being inhaled from a crushable glass ampoule with the patient in a reclining position.

Trichloroethylene is used in industry in a less pure form as a solvent for oils and fats, for degreasing metals, and for dry cleaning.

Pregnancy and the neonate. A study of obstetric anaesthesia in 405 patients compared the use of trichloroethylene and methoxyflurane, both 0.1% vapour, in an oxygen and nitrous oxide mixture. There was no difference in the well-being of the infants and no difference in the mothers in the incidence of nausea, vomiting, and headache. Awareness was increased with trichloroethylene. It was concluded that trichloroethylene could be substituted for methoxyflurane, which was potentially nephrotoxic.— J. S. Crawford and P. Davies, *Br. J. Anaesth.*, 1975, *47*, 482.

The effect of trichloroethylene 0.2% or methoxyflurane 0.2% was studied in 358 patients undergoing caesarean section and the results compared with those of a previous study using 0.1% of either agent. The incidence of awareness and unpleasant dreams was halved in those receiving trichloroethylene 0.2% and doubled in those receiving methoxyflurane 0.2%. The incidence of nausea and vomiting was reduced for both anaesthetics with the 0.2% concentration. No changes in infant status attributable to the anaesthetics were detected.— J. S. Crawford *et al.*, *Br. J. Anaesth.*, 1976, *48*, 661.

Use in food. The Food Additives and Contaminants Committee recommended that trichloroethylene be temporarily permitted for use as a solvent in food and recommended a maximum concentration of use in food as consumed of 5 ppm. Recommended additives to trichloroethylene were either triethylamine at a maximum concentration in the solvent of 380 ppm or thymol at a maximum concentration in the solvent of 100 ppm. Further toxicity studies were required. Reactions might occur between trichloroethylene and soya bean protein and such reactions should be avoided.— *Report on the Review of Solvents in Food*, FAC/REP/25, Ministry of Agriculture, Fisheries and Food, London, HM Stationery Office, 1978.

Preparations

Triklone *(ICI Mond, UK)*. A brand of trichloroethylene available in different grades; for dry-cleaning purposes.

Trilene *(ICI Pharmaceuticals, UK)*. Trichloroethylene, stabilised by the addition of thymol 0.01% and coloured with a blue dye. (Also available as Trilene in *Austral.*, *Neth.*, *S.Afr.*).

3127-q

Vinyl Ether *(B.P., U.S.P.)*. Aether Vinylicus; Ether Vinylicus; Divinyl Ether; Divinyl Oxide; Éter Vinílico. $(CH_2{:}CH)_2O = 70.09$.

CAS — 109-93-3.

Pharmacopoeias. In *Br.*, *Braz.*, *Ind.*, *Int.*, *Nord.*, and *U.S.*

Divinyl ether, to which has been added about 4% v/v of dehydrated alcohol and not more than 0.01% of phenyl-α-naphthylamine or other suitable stabiliser. *U.S.P.* specifies not more than 0.025% of a suitable preservative.

It is a clear, colourless, inflammable liquid with a characteristic odour, and often with a purplish fluorescence derived from the stabiliser. Flash-point below −30° (closed-cup test). Wt per ml 0.77 to 0.778 g. B.p. 28° to 31°.

Soluble 1 in 100 of water; miscible with alcohol, acetone, chloroform, and ether. When shaken with water the aqueous layer is neutral to litmus. On exposure to air and light it decomposes into formaldehyde and formic acid, ultimately polymerising to a jelly; the rate of decomposition is retarded by the presence of a stabiliser. **Store** in a cool place in airtight containers of not more than 200-ml capacity. Protect from light. It should not be used if the container has been opened longer than 48 hours.

CAUTION. *Vinyl ether is very volatile and inflammable and mixtures of its vapour with oxygen, nitrous oxide, or air at certain concentrations are explosive. It should not be used in the presence of an open flame or any electrical apparatus liable to produce a spark. Precautions should be taken against the production of static electrical discharge.*

Adverse Effects. Even after premedication with atropine, salivation is more frequent with vinyl ether than with other anaesthetics. Convulsions during vinyl ether anaesthesia have been reported. Overdosage is usually indicated by respiratory depression. Necrosis of the liver has followed prolonged or repeated anaesthesia with vinyl ether and is probably aggravated by hypoxia. Renal damage has also been reported.

Uses. Vinyl ether is a potent volatile anaesthetic administered by inhalation. It has about 4 times the potency of ether and has comparable effects although it is less irritating to the respiratory tract. It is analgesic but produces variable and unreliable muscle relaxation. It is not used for long operations because of the risk of liver necrosis.

It has been used for short operations or as an induction anaesthetic. Concentrations required for anaesthesia vary but up to 8% may be required for induction and 2 to 4% for maintenance. Concentrations of 10% can rapidly produce respiratory arrest. One part of vinyl ether with 3 parts of ether forms a mixture giving a vapour of constant composition.

Preparations

Vinycombinum *(Nord. P.)*. A mixture of vinyl ether 25% w/w and anaesthetic ether 75% w/w.

Proprietary Names

Vinéther *(Robert et Carrière, Fr.)*; Vinydan *(Lundbeck, Denm.; Byk Gulden, Ger.)*.

Vinyl ether was formerly marketed in Great Britain under the proprietary name Vinesthene *(May & Baker)*.

Heparin and other Anticoagulants

4800-s

Anticoagulants may be divided into direct anticoagulants such as heparin and indirect anticoagulants such as the coumarin and indanedione derivatives. Heparin inhibits the activity of activated factor X, inhibits the formation of thrombin from prothrombin, and inhibits the formation of fibrin from fibrinogen. The coumarins and indanediones depress the hepatic vitamin K-dependent synthesis of coagulation factors II (prothrombin), VII, IX, and X. Whereas heparin inhibits the coagulation of blood both *in vivo* and *in vitro*, the coumarins and indanediones have no action *in vitro*. There is a delay before the indirect anticoagulants take effect, even after intravenous administration.

Coumarin derivatives include: cumetharol, p.770, dicoumarol, p.770, ethyl biscoumacetate, p.771, nicoumalone, p.772, phenprocoumon, p.773, warfarin potassium, p.774, warfarin sodium, p.775.

Indanedione derivatives include: anisindione, p.770, bromindione, p.770, diphenadione, p.771, fluorindione, p.772, phenindione, p.773.

Ethyl biscoumacetate, nicoumalone, and phenindione have an intermediate duration of action, dicoumarol, phenprocoumon, and warfarin sodium are long-acting, and diphenadione has a very long action; its effects last for up to 20 days.

Coagulation Tests. Various methods have been used for assessing defects of coagulation and the effects of anticoagulants. The *whole blood clotting time (Lee-White) test* measures the time taken for blood to clot in glass tubes. In the *activated clotting time test* clotting is accelerated by contact with diatomite. The *one-stage prothrombin time test (Quick)* measures the time required for the coagulation of plasma in the presence of thromboplastin and calcium; it is sensitive to reduced activity of factors II, VII, and X. Rigorous control of the thromboplastin is essential. The result is expressed in seconds compared with a control plasma or as prothrombin ratio (the factor by which the control value is extended; results should be expressed by reference to a standard thromboplastin). The *prothrombin and proconvertin test* and *Thrombotest* are variants of the one-stage prothrombin time test. The *partial thromboplastin time test* is not extensively used, but the *activated partial thromboplastin time test (kaolin-cephalin clotting time)* is extensively used; it measures the time required for the coagulation of platelet-free plasma in the presence of kaolin, thromboplastin, and calcium; it is sensitive to reduced activity of factors V, VIII, IX, and X. The *thromboplastin generation test* is used to demonstrate deficiency of specific clotting factors. The *recalcification time (calcium clotting time) test* measures the time required for the formation of a clot when calcium is added to citrated plasma; it is sensitive to all plasma coagulation factors except calcium. Addition of an activator in the *activated recalcification test* reduces the time required for clotting. *The factor Xa inhibitor assay* is used for the measurement of heparin concentrations and is sensitive to low concentrations of heparin. The *protamine titration test* measures the concentration of heparin in blood or plasma by titration with protamine sulphate.

Numerous other tests and variations of the above tests have also been used.

For the control of heparin treatment the whole blood clotting time (Lee-White time) is usually maintained at 2 to 3 times the pre-treatment figure, or the activated partial thromboplastin time is maintained at 1.5 to 2.5 times its normal value. The factor Xa inhibitor assay is also used. For the control of treatment with oral anticoagulants the Quick one-stage prothrombin time test is commonly used; the prothrombin time is usually maintained at 2 to 2.5 times the control value.

Discussions and comparisons of coagulation tests.— R. A. O'Reilly and P. M. Aggeler, *Pharmac. Rev.*, 1970, *22*, 35; P. K. Ray and T. A. Harper, *J. Lab. clin. Med.*, 1971, *77*, 901; A. S. Gallus and J. Hirsh, *Drugs*, 1976, *12*, 41.

An activated plasma recalcification test.— D. T. Hunter and J. L. Allensworth, *J. clin. Path.*, 1967, *20*, 244.

From a study in 103 patients on long-term oral anticoagulant therapy, the activated partial thromboplastin clotting test was considered a more valuable test for control compared with the corresponding prothrombin ratio.— R. D. Eastham, *Br. med. J.*, 1968, *2*, 337.

An evaluation of the one-stage prothrombin time test for monitoring anticoagulant therapy, and a comparison with the two-stage prothrombin assay, the thromboplastin generation test, and Thrombotest.— P. W. Boyles, *Clin. Pharmac. Ther.*, 1970, *11*, 251.

A comparison of the activated partial prothrombin time test and 2 activated whole blood coagulation time tests.— J. E. Congdon *et al.*, *J. Am. med. Ass.*, 1973, *226*, 1529.

The measurement of heparin based on the potentiation of anti-factor Xa.— K. W. E. Denson and J. Bonnar, *Thromb. Diath. haemorrh.*, 1973, *30*, 471.

Advice from the British Anticoagulant Control Panel of the British Committee for Standardization in Haematology on laboratory methods of controlling anticoagulant doses.— E. K. Blackburn, *Prescribers' J.*, 1977, *17*, 73.

The need for uniformity in the thromboplastins used in the prothrombin time tests.— B. Bain *et al.*, *Med. J. Aust.*, 1978, *2*, 459. Discussion.— B. Firkin, *Med. J. Aust.*, 1978, *2*, 472.

An assessment of the risk of haemorrhage from oral anticoagulants.— J. C. Forfar, *Br. Heart J.*, 1979, *42*, 128.

The Use of Anticoagulants. Anticoagulants are used in the prophylaxis and treatment of thrombo-embolic occlusive vascular disease such as venous thrombosis, pulmonary embolism, and myocardial infarction, and in the prophylaxis of thrombosis during extracorporeal circulation and in patients with prosthetic heart valves.

In acute myocardial infarction anticoagulants may be of benefit by reducing thrombo-embolic complications in high-risk patients.

In the long-term management of patients who have had a myocardial infarction the value of anticoagulant therapy is obscure, though some studies have indicated a reduction in the incidence of re-infarction and in the mortality-rate in certain categories of male patients. Some authorities consider the use of anticoagulants justified in patients considered to be poor risks.

Anticoagulants should be used with care in patients taking drugs likely to produce haemorrhage or with disorders associated with haemorrhage.

Plasmin (p.655), streptokinase (p.656), and urokinase (p.660) are also used in the treatment of thrombo-embolic disorders.

An extensive review, with 683 references, of factors involved in the use of oral anticoagulants, including data on blood coagulation, clotting, laboratory control, physiological and genetic factors, the absorption and fate of anticoagulants, and the effects of other drugs.— R. A. O'Reilly and P. M. Aggeler, *Pharmac. Rev.*, 1970, *22*, 35.

Other reviews and discussions of the use of anticoagulants.— A. S. Gallus and J. Hirsh, *Drugs*, 1976, *12*, 41 and 132; C. R. M. Prentice, *Prescribers' J.*, 1976, *16*, 116; M. J. Mackie and A. S. Douglas, *Br. J. Hosp. Med.*, 1976, *16*, 118; A. Breckenridge, *Br. med. J.*, 1976, *1*, 419; D. H. Lawson and G. D. O. Lowe, *Am. J. Hosp. Pharm.*, 1977, *34*, 1225; L. Poller, *Practitioner*, 1978, *221*, 211; A. Fenech *et al.*, *Drugs*, 1979, *18*, 48.

A series of papers on haemostasis.— *Br. med. Bull.*, 1977, *33*, 183–288.

A series of papers on thrombosis.— *Br. med. Bull.*, 1978, *34*, 101–207.

Myocardial infarction. A detailed retrospective and prospective review of anticoagulants in coronary heart disease.— J. R. A. Mitchell, *Lancet*, 1981, *1*, 257. Comments.— L. Poller (letter), *ibid.*, 668; T. W. Meade and S. G. Thompson (letter), *ibid.*, 717; A. S. Douglas and G. P. McNicol (letter), *ibid.*

A review of the secondary prevention in survivors of myocardial infarction. Long-term anticoagulant treatment is indicated in patients who are at special risk from thrombo-embolic complications but for other patients the evidence from controlled trials is not entirely consistent.—Joint Recommendations by the International Society and Federation of Cardiology Scientific Councils on Arteriosclerosis, Epidemiology and Prevention, and Rehabilitation, *Br. med. J.*, 1981, *282*, 894.

A multicentre study of 710 patients who had been admitted to hospital with myocardial infarction and had received anticoagulants, and of 597 others who had not received anticoagulants, indicated lower death-rates for the treated group, both during hospital stay and during a follow-up period of at least 5 years. The two groups were disparate in several characteristics which might have affected the results, and statistical adjustments were applied to allow for this. After adjustment, the death-rates for patients in hospital were 18% and 31% for the treated and untreated groups respectively. The death-rates after 3 years, again adjusted for other variables, were 25% for the treated group and 31% for the untreated group, calculated from approximately 90% of those who were discharged from hospital.— M. Szklo *et al.*, *J. Am. med. Ass.*, 1979, *242*, 1261. Comment.— A. Selzer (letter), *ibid.*, 1980, *243*, 1629. Reply.— M. Szklo *et al.* (letter), *ibid.*

Results of a long-term randomised double-blind study in patients over 60 years of age who had had a myocardial infarction indicated that continuation of intensive and stable oral anticoagulant therapy substantially reduced the risk of recurrent myocardial infarction and thereby of cardiac death. Of 439 patients over 60 years of age who had received nicoumalone or phenprocoumon since their primary myocardial infarction the 2-year total mortality was 7.6% compared with 13.4% of 439 in the placebo group. In the anticoagulant-treated group the 2-year incidence of recurrent myocardial infarction was 5.7% compared with 15.9% in the placebo group.—Report of the Sixty Plus Reinfarction Study Research Group, *Lancet*, 1980, *2*, 989. Comment.— M. F. Oliver (letter), *ibid.*, 1981, *1*, 101. Reply.— J. G. P. Tijssen (letter), *ibid.* Further comment.— I. Graham *et al.* (letter), *ibid.*, 1981, *1*, 223.

Thrombo-embolic disorders. A review of the treatment of thrombosis of veins of the lower extremities.— R. Adar and E. W. Salzman, *New Engl. J. Med.*, 1975, *292*, 348.

A review of the uses of anticoagulants in thrombo-embolic disorders.— A. S. Gallus and J. Hirsh, *Drugs*, 1976, *12*, 41 and 132.

See also Myocardial Infarction, above.

Further references: *Lancet*, 1981, *2*, 1396.

Artificial heart valves. Permanent treatment with anticoagulants was now recommended for patients with Starr-Edwards heart valves; dipyridamole or aspirin would further reduce the incidence of embolism.— *Br. med. J.*, 1978, *1*, 1505.

In patients with prosthetic heart valves undergoing non-cardiac surgery, anticoagulation could be interrupted and restored rapidly after surgery.— R. E. Katholi *et al.*, *Am. Heart J.*, 1978, *96*, 163.

Pregnancy and the neonate. Discussions on the use of anticoagulants for coagulation disorders in pregnancy.— C. W. G. Redman, *Postgrad. med. J.*, 1979, *55*, 367; *Br. med. J.*, 1979, *1*, 1661; M. C. Macnaughton, *Prescribers' J.*, 1979, *19*, 52.

Warfarin was not recommended for venous thrombo-embolism in pregnancy. Heparin could be given intravenously in a dose of about 40 000 units in 24 hours for 5 days followed by heparin subcutaneously in a dose of about 10 000 units twelve-hourly. Control was necessary because heparin requirements changed as pregnancy progressed; treatment should continue for 6 weeks after delivery. Heparin was given subcutaneously for prophylaxis to all pregnant women with an adequate history of thrombo-embolism. Warfarin could be given when the puerperium had passed. Subcutaneous heparin was not adequate for more than a few days in women with prosthetic heart valves; warfarin was given, accepting the risk to the foetus, till 37 to 38 weeks of gestation and again 1 week after delivery.— M. de Swiet,

Drugs, 1979, *18*, 478.

A discussion of the use of anticoagulants during pregnancy in patients with heart-valve prostheses.— *Br. med. J.*, 1977, *1*, 1047.

Stroke and transient ischaemic attacks. See under Heparin, p.766 and Warfarin Sodium, p.781.

Withdrawal of anticoagulant therapy. In a study of 223 men with ischaemic heart disease who received anticoagulants (usually phenindione) for up to 14 weeks, there was no evidence that stopping anticoagulants abruptly was especially hazardous compared with gradual termination.— D. E. Sharland, *Br. med. J.*, 1966, *2*, 392. Similar results in 115 patients who had taken phenindione. However, the incidence of thrombo-embolic episodes and deaths was significantly greater in patients whose therapy was withdrawn than in those in whom it was continued. Results showed that there was less risk when phenindione was withdrawn before, rather than after, 2 years of treatment.— V. R. Kamath and M. G. Thorne, *Lancet*, 1969, *1*, 1025.

4801-w

Heparin Calcium *(B.P.)*. Calcium Heparinate.

CAS — 9005-49-6 (heparin); 37270-89-6 (calcium salt).

Pharmacopoeias. In *Br.*

A preparation containing the calcium salt of a sulphated polysaccharide acid present in mammalian tissues, and having the characteristic property of delaying the clotting of shed blood. It is prepared from the lungs of oxen [Heparin Calcium (Lung)], or the intestinal mucosa of oxen, pigs, or sheep [Heparin Calcium (Mucous)]. When dried, Heparin Calcium (Lung) contains not less than 110 units per mg and Heparin Calcium (Mucous) contains not less than 130 units per mg. The *B.P.* requires that the source of the material be stated on the label.

A white or creamy-white moderately hygroscopic powder. It loses not more than 8% of its weight when dried. **Soluble** in water (1 in less than 5) and saline solutions, forming clear, colourless, or straw-coloured solutions. A solution in water is dextrorotatory. A 1% solution in water has a pH of 5 to 7. Solutions are **sterilised** by filtration. **Incompatibility.** See Heparin Sodium (below). **Store** in containers sealed to exclude micro-organisms and, as far as possible, moisture.

4802-e

Heparin Sodium *(B.P., U.S.P.)*. Heparin; Heparinum; Heparinum Natricum; Soluble Heparin; Sodium Heparin; Eparina.

CAS — 9041-08-1.

Pharmacopoeias. In *Arg., Aust., Br., Braz., Chin., Cz., Hung., Ind., Int., It., Jap., Jug., Pol., Roum., Turk.,* and *U.S.*

A preparation containing the sodium salt of a sulphated polysaccharide acid present in mammalian tissues, and having the characteristic property of delaying the clotting of shed blood. It is prepared from the lungs of oxen [Heparin (Lung); Heparin Sodium (Lung)] or the intestinal mucosa of oxen, pigs, or sheep [Heparin (Mucous); Heparin Sodium (Mucous)]. The *B.P.* requires that, when dried, Heparin Sodium (Lung) contains not less than 110 units per mg and Heparin Sodium (Mucous) contains not less than 130 units per mg. The *U.S.P.* requires that heparin sodium derived from lungs contains not less than 120 *U.S.P.* units (see p.763) per mg, and not less than 140 *U.S.P.* units per mg when derived from other tissues. The *B.P.* and *U.S.P.* require that the source of the material be stated on the label.

A white or creamy-white, odourless or almost odourless, moderately hygroscopic powder. It loses not more than 8% of its weight when dried. **Soluble** in water (1 in 2.5) and saline solution, forming clear, colourless, or straw-coloured solutions. A solution in water is dextrorotatory. A 1% solution in water has a pH of 6 to 8. Solutions are **sterilised** by filtration. **Store** in containers sealed to exclude micro-organisms and, as far as possible, moisture.

Reviews of the chemistry and pharmacology of heparin.— J. Ehrlich and S. S. Stivala, *J. pharm. Sci.*, 1973, *62*, 517; *Heparin: Structure, Function, and Clinical Implications*, R.A. Bradshaw and S. Wessler (Ed.), London, Plenum Press, 1975; W. W. Coon, *Clin. Pharmac. Ther.*, 1978, *23*, 139; T. W. Barrowcliffe *et al.*, *Br. med. Bull.*, 1978, *34*, 143.

The adsorption of heparin on to activated charcoal.— D. O. Cooney, *Clin. Toxicol.*, 1977, *11*, 569.

Analysis of 32 commercial samples of heparin sodium (*U.S.P.*) and sterile solutions of heparin sodium (*U.S.P.*) indicated that the average molecular weight was 9000 to 12 000 daltons with only minor differences between the heparins extracted from beef lung and porcine intestinal mucosa. A correlation was observed between the average molecular weight and the anticoagulant activity *in vitro*.— H. J. Rodriguez and A. J. Vanderwielen, *J. pharm. Sci.*, 1979, *68*, 588.

Heparin: Structure, Cellular Functions, and Clinical Applications, N.M. McDuffie (Ed.), London, Academic Press, 1979.

Activity in solution. The following drugs were found to have no significant effect, *in vitro*, on the anticoagulant activity of heparin: ampicillin sodium, cloxacillin sodium, potassium chloride, hydrocortisone sodium succinate, isoprenaline hydrochloride, cephalothin sodium, lignocaine hydrochloride, tetracycline hydrochloride, benzylpenicillin, a proprietary injection containing vitamins of the B group, and one containing vitamins B and C. Sodium chloride and dextrose did not affect the activity of heparin, which was also unaffected at pH 3.2 and at pH 9.2. All the tests were carried out immediately after admixture with heparin, and again after the mixture had been stored for 24 hours.— E. D. Hodby *et al.*, *Can. med. Ass. J.*, 1972, *106*, 562.

A report of the rise in anticoagulant activity of heparin in autoclaved dextrose injection for 5 hours following admixture; after this time activity returned to the expected level.— W. Anderson *et al.*, *J. Pharm. Pharmac.*, 1979, *31*, *Suppl.*, 55P. Further studies on the dextrose effect.— W. Anderson and J. E. Harthill, *ibid.*, 1982, *34*, 90.

Effect of gamma-irradiation. Freeze-dried heparin in sealed glass tubes showed a loss in potency of 1.6% at 25 000 Gy and 23 to 26% at 250 000 Gy. A solution of heparin containing 5000 units per ml, preserved with chlorocresol 0.15%, lost 22% of its potency at 25 000 Gy and 84% at 250 000 Gy.— *The Use of Gamma Radiation Sources for the Sterilisation of Pharmaceutical Products*, London, ABPI, 1960.

Inactivation. When 1 unit of heparin and about 2 mg of ascorbic acid were added to 1 ml of blood the anticoagulant effect of both substances was markedly decreased.— C. A. Owen *et al.*, *Mayo Clin. Proc.*, 1970, *45*, 140.

Incompatibility. Incompatibility has been reported between heparin and amikacin sulphate, cephaloridine, daunorubicin hydrochloride, doxorubicin hydrochloride, erythromycin gluceptate, erythromycin lactobionate, gentamicin sulphate, hyaluronidase, hydroxyzine hydrochloride, hydrocortisone sodium succinate, kanamycin sulphate, narcotic analgesics, novobiocin sodium, polymyxin B sulphate, prochlorperazine, promazine hydrochloride, promethazine hydrochloride, streptomycin sulphate, tobramycin sulphate, viomycin sulphate, and, depending on the diluent, with cephalothin sodium and vancomycin hydrochloride. Compatibility and incompatibility have been reported with ampicillin sodium, benzylpenicillin, dimenhydrinate, methicillin sodium, oxytetracycline hydrochloride, sulphafurazole diethanolamine, and tetracycline hydrochloride. References.— R. Misgen, *Am. J. Hosp. Pharm.*, 1965, *22*, 92; J. A. Patel and G. L. Phillips, *Am. J. Hosp. Pharm.*, 1966, *23*, 409; J. M. Meisler and M. W. Skolaut, *Am. J. Hosp. Pharm.*, 1966, *23*, 557; M. Edward, *Am. J. Hosp. Pharm.*, 1967, *24*, 440; E. A. Parker, *Am. J. Hosp. Pharm.*, 1969, *26*, 655; B. B. Riley, *J. Hosp. Pharm.*, 1970, *28*, 228; J. Jacobs *et al.*, *J. clin. Path.*, 1973, *26*, 742.

There was no precipitate when solutions containing gentamicin 10 mg per litre and heparin 1000 units per litre were mixed. The precipitate formed when concentrated solutions were mixed appeared to redissolve on dilution.— J. R. Koup and L. Gerbracht (letter), *Drug Intell. & clin. Pharm.*, 1975, *9*, 388. Further study showed considerable loss of anticoagulant activity in solutions in which a precipitate had formed and been redissolved.— J. R. Koup and L. Gerbracht (letter), *Drug Intell. & clin. Pharm.*, 1975, *9*, 568.

Species difference. Suggestions of differing activity, dependent on the species from which heparin was obtained (E. Goldberg *et al.* (letter), *Lancet*, 1972, *1*, 789; E. Novak *et al.*, *Clin. Med.*, 1972, *79* (July), 22; *J. Am. med. Ass.*, 1974, *227*, 481) have not been generally substantiated.

Absence of species difference. References.— F. Gomez-Perez, *J. clin. Pharmac.*, 1972, *12*, 413; M. P. T. Gillett and E. M. M. Besterman (letter), *Lancet*, 1973, *2*, 1204; B. J. Baltes *et al.*, *Clin. Pharmac. Ther.*, 1973, *14*, 287; F. G. McMahon *et al.*, *Clin. Pharmac. Ther.*, 1975, *17*, 79; A. K. Jain *et al.*, *Curr. ther. Res.*, 1977, *22*, 427; R. F. Bedford and T. E. O'Brien, *Am. J. Hosp. Pharm.*, 1977, *34*, 936.

Stability of solutions. Heparin Injection *B.P.* preserved with chlorocresol 0.15% was stable within the pH range of 7 to 8 for up to 15 years if stored at 4°, for over 7 years at room temperature (approximately 18°), and for 6 to 8 years at 37°. The stability was markedly reduced below pH 6. Heparin should not be kept mixed for any length of time with dextrose solutions owing to their low pH.— J. Pritchard, *J. Pharm. Pharmac.*, 1964, *16*, 487.

Heparin, 20 000 units per litre, was chemically stable for up to 72 hours at room temperature in various intravenous fluids.— E. A. Parker, *Am. J. Hosp. Pharm.*, 1967, *24*, 434.

The pH of dextrose injection rose from 4.1 to 5.95 and of laevulose injection 5% from 3.67 to 4.14 when 2 ml of heparin injection, 5000 units per ml, was added. Heparin would be completely stable at room temperature and stable for at least 72 hours respectively in these solutions.— J. W. Hadgraft (letter), *Lancet*, 1970, *2*, 1254.

Heparin 20 or 40 units per ml in dextrose injection or sodium chloride injection was stable at 27° for 48 hours.— J. F. Mitchell *et al.*, *Am. J. Hosp. Pharm.*, 1976, *33*, 540.

A report of 65% loss of heparin in 5 hours in dextrose injection.— *Chemist Drugg.*, 1977, *208*, 389.

Units. 1370 units of heparin are contained in approximately 8 mg in one ampoule of the third International Standard Preparation (1973) of heparin sodium.

U.S.P. units are usually equivalent to international units. For heparin, however, the *U.S.P.* states that the units are not equivalent. In the collaborative assay (*Bull. Wld Hlth Org.*, 1970, *42*, 129) of the material now accepted as the international standard and of the *U.S.P.* and other reference standards the interlaboratory variation using the same assay methods was considerably greater than the mean variation between the *U.S.P.* and international units.

There were claims that the *U.S.P.* unit of heparin was 10 to 15% more potent than the international unit.—Council on Thrombosis of the American Heart Association, *Circulation*, 1977, *55*, 423A.

Results of collaborative assay showed that, with 2 commonly used assay procedures, separate international standards for lung and mucous heparin were not needed.— Twenty-first Report of WHO Expert Committee on Biological Standardization, *Tech. Rep. Ser. Wld Hlth Org. No. 413*, 1969. See also *Lancet*, 1970, *1*, 1215.

Adverse Effects. Complications of therapy are bleeding in various sites and, rarely, febrile or allergic reactions. Slight epistaxis, occasional red cells in the urine, and bruising are signs of overdosage. Transient alopecia may occur. Thrombocytopenia and osteoporosis with spontaneous fractures have been reported.

An extensive review of the side-effects of heparin, heparinoids, and their antagonists.— W. W. Coon and P. W. Willis, *Clin. Pharmac. Ther.*, 1966, *7*, 379.

Systemic reactions occurred in 2 patients and local reactions in 7 after the injection of chlorocresol-preserved heparin (*Weddel*). Sensitivity to the preservative was considered responsible; only 1 of the patients showed sensitivity to preservative-free heparin from the same manufacturer.— B. W. Hancock and A. Naysmith, *Br. med. J.*, 1975, *3*, 746.

SGPT values were not affected in 19 patients undergoing haemodialysis and given heparin up to 10 000 units before or during the procedure.— J. G. Salway and G. S. Walker, *Br. med. J.*, 1976, *2*, 919.

Femoral neuropathy during anticoagulant therapy.— M. R. Young and J. W. Norris, *Neurology, Minneap.*, 1976, *26*, 1173.

Necrosis at the site of injection developed in 2 patients given heparin sodium subcutaneously and in a third who had also received warfarin sodium.— J. C. Hall *et al.*, *J. Am. med. Ass.*, 1980, *244*, 1831. See also A. M. Jackson and A. V. Pollock, *Br. med. J.*, 1981, *283*, 1087.

Femoral neuropathy in a 50-year-old woman with myocardial infarction was associated with the administration of heparin.— N. G. Kounis and G. E. Karatzas, *Practitioner*, 1980, *224*, 741.

Abuse. A 24-year-old woman developed bleeding complications as a result of self-administration of large doses of heparin. On the first occasion she administered 'several hundred mg' of heparin by intramuscular injection and the haemorrhage rapidly cleared without treatment. On the second occasion she injected 700 mg of heparin; the bleeding was more severe but quickly responded to 50 mg of protamine sulphate by intravenous injection.— C. M. Martin *et al.*, *J. Am. med. Ass.*, 1970, *212*, 475.

Haemorrhage. A review of 4325 autopsies revealed 30 cases of adrenal haemorrhage; 9 patients had been taking anticoagulants—heparin or heparin and dicoumarol; a further case was reported from the author's experience.— E. Amador, *Ann. intern. Med.*, 1965, *63*, 559, per *Med. J. Aust.*, 1966, *1*, 682. A report of 4 further cases of adrenal insufficiency due to adrenal haemorrhage.— G. I. Portnay *et al.* (letter), *Ann. intern. Med.*, 1974, *81*, 115. Another report of acute adrenocortical insufficiency considered to be associated with anticoagulant treatment with heparin.— S. Ahmad (letter), *J. Am. med. Ass.*, 1979, *241*, 2703.

Heparin was administered to 97 patients, in 3 instances to keep intravenous infusions running, but in most cases to treat deep venous thrombosis or pulmonary embolism. Adverse reactions occurred in 18 of 56 women (32%) and in 6 of 41 men (15%), and were attributed to bleeding in 23 and to increased prothrombin time in 1 of the group. The increased toxicity of heparin in women appeared to be limited to those older than 60.— H. Jick *et al.*, *New Engl. J. Med.*, 1968, *279*, 284.

Of 76 patients with venous thrombo-embolisms treated with heparin 7500 units intravenously initially then with 5000 units every 4 hours or 30 000 units daily by continuous infusion, 24 suffered haemorrhagic complications and in 10 the bleeding was severe. There was no difference in incidence between the intermittent or continuous schedules.— M. J. Mant *et al.* (preliminary communication), *Lancet*, 1977, *1*, 1133.

In a study in 175 patients undergoing surgery haemorrhagic complications occurred in 27% of those given heparin 5000 units before surgery and twice daily for 5 days postoperatively, compared with 7.5% in those given heparin postoperatively and 1.4% in a control group.— H. L. Pachter and T. S. Riles, *Ann. Surg.*, 1977, *186*, 669.

In a double-blind study in 60 patients undergoing transurethral prostatectomy there was no significant difference in operative blood loss between those given heparin calcium prophylactically and those not given heparin, but postoperative blood loss was approximately doubled in those given heparin.— N. H. Allen *et al.*, *Br. med. J.*, 1978, *1*, 1326. Criticism of the assessment of blood loss.— R. G. Faber (letter), *Br. med. J.*, 1978, *1*, 1700.

Major gastro-intestinal bleeding in 1.2% and minor gastro-intestinal bleeding in 8.3% of 575 patients exposed to heparin.— H. Jick and J. Porter, *Lancet*, 1978, *2*, 87.

Factors predisposing to bleeding during heparin therapy.— A. M. Walker and H. Jick, *J. Am. med. Ass.*, 1980, *244*, 1209. See also T. H. Spaet, *ibid.*, 1243.

Further reports and references.— F. S. Morrison and H. A. Wurzel, *Am. J. Cardiol.*, 1964, *13*, 329, per *Int. pharm. Abstr.*, 1964, *1*, 427; P. E. Cianci and R. L. Piscatelli, *J. Am. med. Ass.*, 1969, *210*, 1100; D. Prager and T. Kowalyshyn (letter), *Lancet*, 1969, *2*, 800; M. Rosen (letter), *Med. J. Aust.*, 1972, *1*, 660; T. R. Browne and S. H. Wray, *Am. J. Ophthal.*, 1973, *76*, 981, per *Drug Intell. & clin. Pharm.*, 1974, *8*, 204; R. McWilliam *et al.* (letter), *Lancet*, 1974, *2*, 286; E. Salzman *et al.*, *New Engl. J. Med.*, 1975, *292*, 1046; R. S. Bone *et al.*, *Am. J. med. Sci.*, 1976, *272*, 197; R. A. Rostand *et al.*, *Sth. med. J.*, 1977, *70*, 1128.

Osteoporosis. Spontaneous fractures of ribs and vertebrae occurred in 6 of 10 patients receiving 15 000 units or more of heparin daily for 6 months or more. This did not occur in 107 patients given 10 000 units or less daily. Parathyroid dysfunction was not present in any of the 6 patients and 5 of them improved when they were given a coumarin derivative instead of heparin. Three of them resumed heparin therapy on a dosage of 10 000 units daily.— G. C. Griffith *et al.*, *J. Am. med. Ass.*, 1965, *193*, 91.

Osteoporosis developed in 2 of 21 patients treated with calcium heparin in an average dose of 20 000 units daily for an average of 2 years. In one the pre-existing signs of osteoporosis were aggravated and the other was simultaneously receiving corticosteroids.— A. Kher *et al.*, *Nouv. Presse méd.*, 1973, *2*, 1585.

After 11 months of treatment with heparin 6000 to 10 000 units every 6 hours a 15-year-old boy developed compression fractures of the thoracic vertebrae and other changes consistent with osteoporosis. It was thought to have been induced by heparin.— J. P. Sackler and L. Liu, *Br. J. Radiol.*, 1973, *46*, 548.

A report of severe osteopenia in a 22-year-old woman given heparin for thrombosis for 8 weeks before term and for 4 weeks after delivery of a healthy infant which she breast fed. The heparin was discontinued when X-rays disclosed gross thoracolumbar spinal osteoporosis with compression fractures. Her serum concentrations of 25-hydroxyvitamin D and 24,25-dihydroxyvitamin D were normal, indicating an adequate vitamin D intake and exposure to sun. The serum concentrations of 1,25-dihydroxyvitamin D were, however, well below normal on 2 separate determinations. Although the mechanism for the heparin-induced osteopenia remains unclear, the rational measure to prevent this rare complication of heparin treatment would seem to be to prescribe calcitriol or alfacalcidol routinely to patients on long-term treatment with high doses of heparin.— D. Aarskog *et al.* (letter), *Lancet*, 1980, *2*, 650. See also J. W. Squires and L. W. Pinch, *J. Am. med. Ass.*, 1979, *241*, 2417; P. H. Wise and A. J. Hall, *Br. med. J.*, 1980, *281*, 110.

Pregnancy and the neonate. A 32-year-old woman in the 32nd week of pregnancy had severe abdominal pain and uterine contractions on 2 occasions after the intravenous injection of heparin. The contractions were attributed to the heparin.— K. Shaker *et al.* (letter), *Br. med. J.*, 1974, *4*, 408.

A literature review of the use of heparin in pregnancy showed that pregnancy ended in still-birth in about 1 in 8 cases and in premature delivery in 1 in 5.— R. M. Pauli and J. G. Hall (letter), *Lancet*, 1979, *2*, 144.

See also under Osteoporosis, above.

Thrombocytopenia. In a study of 52 patients who had received heparin by continuous intravenous infusion for at least 5 consecutive days, 16 patients developed thrombocytopenia 2 to 10 days after starting therapy. The platelet count returned to normal when heparin therapy was withdrawn. The thrombocytopenia was not dose-related.— W. R. Bell *et al.*, *Ann. intern. Med.*, 1976, *85*, 155.

Severe thrombocytopenia occurred in 2 patients given heparin subcutaneously every 12 hours; in 1 patient the heparin-induced bleeding was fatal.— W. Hrushesky (letter), *Lancet*, 1977, *2*, 1286.

The results of a randomised double-blind study in 149 patients given one of 3 heparin preparations demonstrated that bovine-lung heparin was associated with a significantly greater incidence of thrombocytopenia than were intestinal-mucosa preparations. Patients received conventional continuous intravenous heparin therapy on at least 4 consecutive days and thrombocytopenia developed in 13 of 50 given bovine-lung heparin and in 8 of 99 given intestinal-mucosa heparin.— W. R. Bell and R. M. Royall, *New Engl. J. Med.*, 1980, *303*, 902. Differing results from a study of 200 patients who received intestinal-mucosa heparin intravenously in full dosage or subcutaneously in low dosage. Overall only 0.3% of patients developed persistent thrombocytopenia.— J. Olin and R. Graor (letter), *ibid.*, 1981, *304*, 609. Comment.— W. R. Bell and R. M. Royall (letter), *ibid.*

Factors influencing heparin-associated thrombocytopenia.— H. C. Godal, *Thromb. Haemostasis*, 1980, *43*, 222.

Further reports and references.— G. R. Rhodes *et al.*, *Surgery Gynec. Obstet.*, 1973, *136*, 409, per *Int. pharm. Abstr.*, 1974, *11*, 88; J. Fratantoni *et al.*, *Blood*, 1975, *45*, 395; R. B. Babcock *et al.*, *New Engl. J. Med.*, 1976, *295*, 237; W. R. Bell, *ibid.*, 276; M. M. Stevenson (letter), *ibid.*, 1200; P. C. Galle *et al.*, *Obstet. Gynec.*, 1978, *52*, *Suppl.*, 9S; A. A. Trowbridge *et al.*, *Am. J. Med.*, 1978, *65*, 277; D. N. Kapsch *et al.*, *Surgery, St Louis*, 1979, *86*, 148; I. D. Malcolm *et al.*, *Can. med. Ass. J.*, 1979, *120*, 1086; P. J. Powers *et al.*, *J. Am. med. Ass.*, 1979, *241*, 2396; *ibid.*, 2424; T. S. Rector *et al.*, *Am. J. Hosp. Pharm.*, 1979, *36*, 1561; D. B. Cines *et al.*, *New Engl. J. Med.*, 1980, *303*, 788.

Treatment of Adverse Effects. Slight haemorrhage due to overdosage can usually be treated by withdrawing the drug. Severe bleeding may be reduced by the administration of protamine sulphate (see p.390).

Precautions. Heparin is contra-indicated in patients with haemorrhagic diseases or acute or potential bleeding sites, including haemophilia, postoperative oozing of blood, subacute bacterial endocarditis, gastric or duodenal ulcer, and threatened abortion, and in patients with advanced renal or hepatic disease, jaundice, or severe hypertension. Menstruation, unless excessive, is not a contra-indication to the use of heparin.

Heparin should be used with care in conjunction with oral anticoagulants or agents, such as aspirin and dipyridamole, which affect platelet function, and with dextran injections.

Suggested interactions with antihistamines, digitalis, nicotine, probenecid, quinine, and tetracyclines do not appear to be clinically significant.

A review of 2 years' experience with heparin in a coronary care unit showed that elderly women were particularly susceptible to bleeding episodes.— W. V. R. Vieweg *et al.*, *J. Am. med. Ass.*, 1970, *213*, 1303.

Elevated serum aminotransferase concentrations occurred in 10 of 14 patients given heparin 10 000 units 6-hourly for 10 to 21 days. Values returned to normal when treatment ended. Such rises should be recognised when serum aminotransferase values were used for diagnostic purposes.— M. Sonnenblick *et al.*, *Br. med. J.*, 1975, *3*, 77.

Heparin inhibited ristocetin-induced platelet aggregation in patients undergoing cardiopulmonary bypass.— Y. Pekcelen and S. Inceman (letter), *Br. med. J.*, 1975, *4*, 101.

Heparin for intravenous use should be given by infusion and its administration reduced slowly to reduce the risk of hypercoagulability occurring after heparin clearance.— A. Ur (letter), *Lancet*, 1976, *1*, 959.

Interference by heparin of the measurement of serum-gentamicin concentrations by the luciferase method.— L. Nilsson, *Antimicrob. Ag. Chemother.*, 1980, *17*, 918.

Effect on antithrombin III. Reduced blood concentrations of antithrombin III were associated with heparin in a study of 24 patients. This effect appeared to require the continuous presence of heparin in blood for long periods. One patient with hereditary deficiency of antithrombin III experienced a further reduction in this enzyme's binding capacity. This paradoxical effect of heparin reducing anticoagulant enzyme activity might explain the thrombotic episodes experienced by some patients receiving heparin.— E. Marciniak and J. P. Gockerman, *Lancet*, 1977, *2*, 581.

A report in 1 patient of symptoms suggestive of rethrombosis occurring immediately after heparin was stopped and when antithrombin III activity was reduced.— R. A. Fisken *et al.* (letter), *Lancet*, 1977, *2*, 1231.

Patients on intermittent haemodialysis might also experience reduction in antithrombin III activity when receiving heparin.— K. A. Jorgensen and E. Stoffersen (letter), *Lancet*, 1977, *2*, 1231.

There might be some justification for the custom of starting warfarin therapy for deep-vein thrombosis a few days before stopping heparin since warfarin raised antithrombin III activity which might otherwise become dangerously low.— J. R. O'Brien and M. D. Etherington (letter), *Lancet*, 1977, *2*, 1232.

A study demonstrating increased antithrombin III concentrations in patients with extensive deep-vein thrombosis given heparin subcutaneously, but reduced concentrations in similar patients given heparin intravenously. The reason is not understood but these findings may be clinically important if subcutaneous heparin proves to be more effective in controlling thrombo-embolic process.— V. V. Kakkar *et al.* (letter), *Lancet*, 1980, *1*, 103. Conflicting results with subcutaneous heparin.— P. J. Green (letter), *ibid.*, 374.

Further references.— *Lancet*, 1978, *1*, 538; A. Ur (letter), *ibid.*, 874.

Effect on serum lipids. Heparin 1 mg per kg bodyweight given to 30 healthy subjects aged 20 to 40, 40 to 60, and 80 or more years produced a maximum increase in free fatty acid concentrations in serum within 15 minutes and this increase was more pronounced in those aged 20 to 60 years.— M. Rubegni *et al.* (letter), *Lancet*, 1974, *2*, 903.

A study in 15 patients with coronary artery disease showed that heparin-induced elevation of the concentration of free fatty acids did not increase myocardial oxygen extraction at rest or during pacing and did not accentuate signs of ischaemia during pacing.— G. R. Dagenais and B. Jalbert, *Circulation*, 1977, *56*, 315. See also W. J. Rogers *et al.*, *Am. J. Cardiol.*, 1977, *40*, 365.

Heparin increased lipoprotein lipase activity and concentrations of circulating free fatty acids; even small amounts could cause a reduction in the plasma protein binding of a number of drugs.— M. Wood and A. J. J. Wood (letter), *Br. med. J.*, 1979, *2*, 611.

Bolus injection of 2500 units of porcine mucosal heparin in 27 patients being evaluated for angina, undergoing cardiac catheterisation, was associated with significant increases in plasma concentrations of free fatty acids and thromboxane B_2, although there was no correlation between these 2 values. Thus, the use of heparin anticoagulation to prevent coronary thrombosis in patients with angina pectoris or myocardial infarction seems to have the potential for adversely influencing coronary flow.— R. I. Lewy *et al.* (letter), *Lancet*, 1979, *2*, 97. See also R. T. Jung *et al.*, *Postgrad. med. J.*, 1980, *56*, 330.

Recent studies have demonstrated that the true extent of plasma lipolysis induced by heparin may have been greatly overestimated.— R. A. Riemersma *et al.* (letter), *Lancet*, 1981, *2*, 471.

Effect on thyroid. Bolus doses of 10 000 units of heparin administered intravenously to 7 healthy euthyroid subjects increased serum concentrations of free triiodothyronine by a mean of 48% in 6 subjects and serum concentrations of free thyroxine by a mean of 173% in all 7 subjects. There was no resultant effect on the serum concentration of thyrotrophin. Further investigation was suggested to establish if the raised concentrations produced any direct tissue effects.— J. E. Thomson *et al.* (letter), *Br. J. clin. Pharmac.*, 1977, *4*, 701.

In 16 euthyroid subjects there was a significant impairment of the thyrotrophin response to thyrotrophin-releasing hormone 24 hours after starting intravenous therapy with heparin compared with the response 7 days after the continuous infusion of heparin or after treatment with warfarin for 7 days. It was suggested that the known transient rise in free thyroid hormones, which was produced by heparin, had suppressed the release of thyrotrophin from the pituitary.— J. E. Thomson *et al.*, *Br. J. clin. Pharmac.*, 1978, *6*, 239.

Interactions. There was a 40% incidence of gastro-intestinal bleeding in 40 patients who received ethacrynic acid intravenously and heparin, compared with 14% in 117 given ethacrynic acid alone.— D. Slone *et al.*, *J. Am. med. Ass.*, 1969, *209*, 1668.

The effect of heparin on the pharmacokinetics of digoxin in terminal renal failure.— W. J. F. van der Vijgh and P. L. Oe, *Int. J. clin. Pharmac. Biopharm.*, 1977, *15*, 560.

Of 12 patients with fractures of the hip who received heparin 5000 units subcutaneously every 12 hours and aspirin 600 mg twice daily rectally before operation and by mouth after operation, 8 had serious bleeding complications. This association of heparin and aspirin should not be used for prophylaxis against deep-vein thrombosis in such patients.— H. S. Yett *et al.* (letter), *New Engl. J. Med.*, 1978, *298*, 1092.

For the effect of heparin on the plasma binding of diazepam, see Diazepam, p.1522.

Resistance. Heparin insensitivity after prolonged total parenteral nutrition.— F. J. Forster, *J. Am. med. Ass.*, 1980, *244*, 271.

Absorption and Fate. After injection heparin is extensively bound to plasma proteins. It does not cross the placenta or appear in the milk of nursing mothers.

A review of the clinical pharmacokinetics of heparin.— J. W. Estes, *Clin. Pharmacokinet.*, 1980, *5*, 204.

In 10 subjects with normal renal function the mean half-life of heparin was about 36.8 minutes after a dose of 0.6 unit per ml of blood volume and about 22.7 minutes after 0.3 unit per ml; this indicated that the anticoagulant half-life of heparin was dose dependent. In 13 subjects with chronic renal failure the mean half-life was about 47.5 minutes after 0.6 unit per ml and 32.6 minutes after 0.3 unit per ml.— P. J. Perry *et al.*, *Clin. Pharmac. Ther.*, 1974, *16*, 514.

In 6 patients with cirrhosis of the liver the mean half-life of heparin was 117.8 minutes compared with 74 minutes in 6 healthy subjects—a significant difference.— A. N. Teien, *Thromb. Haemostasis*, 1977, *38*, 701.

Mean half-lives of heparin: in 17 healthy subjects, 107 minutes; in 14 patients with thrombophlebitis 106 minutes; in 12 patients with renal disease, 110 minutes; in 11 patients with pulmonary embolism, 80 minutes; in 7 patients with liver disease, 80 minutes.— T. L. Simon *et al.*, *Br. J. Haemat.*, 1978, *39*, 111.

In 15 healthy subjects peak plasma-heparin concentrations after 5000 units of heparin calcium subcutaneously occurred at 3 hours compared with 1.6 hours when they received the same dose of heparin sodium 2 days earlier or later. The maximum heparin concentrations achieved were not significantly different. In 12 subjects given heparin calcium and heparin sodium prepared by the same manufacturer from different batches of heparin, the times to peak concentrations were not significantly different but the mean peak concentration after heparin sodium (0.25 unit per ml) was significantly greater than that after heparin calcium (0.115 unit per ml); significant difference persisted and the partial thromboplastin times (kaolin) were significantly more prolonged over 7 hours. In 12 subjects given heparin sodium and heparin calcium prepared by the same manufacturer from the same batch of heparin (the heparin sodium had about 5% greater activity when assayed), the peak concentration after heparin sodium was slightly but not significantly earlier, and the peak concentration was significantly greater at 1 hour, but not at 2 hours or later.— J. Low and J. C. Biggs, *Thromb. Haemostasis*, 1978, *40*, 397.

Apparent discrepancies in published values for the half-life of heparin are due to differing methods of dealing with the experimental data. The expression 'half-life' should be qualified in the case of heparin, so as to make clear precisely what has been measured.— T. J. McAvoy, *Clin. Pharmac. Ther.*, 1979, *25*, 372.

No significant difference was found between equi-unit doses of 4 preparations of heparin.— F. Bender *et al.*, *Clin. Pharmac. Ther.*, 1980, *27*, 224.

Further references.— D. P. Thomas *et al.*, *Thromb. Res.*, 1976, *9*, 241.

Uses. Heparin is an anticoagulant which inhibits clotting of blood *in vitro* and *in vivo*. It is considered to act by enhancing the effect of antithrombin III (an alpha-2 globulin; heparin cofactor) in plasma. Heparin and antithrombin III inhibit the activity of activated factor X, inhibit the formation of thrombin from prothrombin, and thus inhibit the formation of fibrin from fibrinogen. The effect of heparin on antithrombin III is considered to be of particular significance in relation to low-dose prophylactic heparin therapy. Other coagulation factors are also affected but to a lesser degree.

Heparin is ineffective when given by mouth and is usually given intravenously, either by intermittent injection or by continuous infusion. An infusion pump may be used to measure accurately the dose administered by infusion. Given intravenously, heparin has a rapid but transient action and its effect on the clotting time depends on the dose given. It has no effect on a clot *in vitro*, but there is a more rapid resolution of a clot in a heparinised patient than in an untreated one, and heparin prevents further clotting. It is also given subcutaneously usually for low-dose prophylactic therapy.

In the treatment of venous thrombosis a common practice is to give an initial intravenous injection of up to 12 500 units of heparin, followed by doses of 5000 to 10 000 units every 4 hours to keep the clotting time, tested not less than 3 hours after the last injection, at 2 to 3 times the pre-treatment figure, or to keep the activated partial prothrombin time at 1.5 to 2.5 times the control value. For infusion, 10 000 to 20 000 units of heparin is given in dextrose injection or sodium chloride injection over 12 hours and continued as necessary. Heparin may also be given subcutaneously in a dose of 10 000 units 8-hourly or 15 000 units 12-hourly, after an initial intravenous loading dose.

A test dose of 1000 units may be given to patients with a history of allergy.

A suggested initial dose for children is 50 units per kg body-weight by infusion, followed by 100 units per kg every 4 hours according to the clotting time.

In myocardial infarction a slower-acting anticoagulant such as warfarin sodium is usually given by mouth simultaneously with initial heparin injections, and the heparin is discontinued after 36 to 48 hours when the other anticoagulant has taken effect.

Heparin has been given by deep intramuscular injection in an emergency but intramuscular injection may lead to haematoma formation.

A number of studies have shown that the incidence of postoperative deep-vein thrombosis and pulmonary embolism is reduced in many types of surgery by the prophylactic subcutaneous administration of heparin sodium or heparin calcium; results in the emergency treatment of hip fractures in the elderly, in hip and knee joint replacement, and in open prostatectomy have not generally been encouraging. Many authorities accept the value of such prophylaxis in patients over 40 years of age who are free from disorders of haemostasis, though some controversy continues. The usual dose is 5000 units subcutaneously into the abdominal wall 2 hours before surgery and repeated every 8 to 12 hours for 7 days or longer if the patient is not then mobile. Many authorities consider that the risk of haemorrhage is not appreciably increased and that laboratory control is not needed. Because of the dangers of haemorrhage into the eye or brain such prophylaxis is not generally used in ophthalmic or neurological surgery.

Long-acting forms of heparin have been used, for instance using Pitkin's menstruum (see p.954), by intramuscular or deep subcutaneous injection but the rate of absorption from these preparations is unpredictable.

If blood transfusions are required during anticoagulant therapy, 3 units of heparin per ml may be added to the transfused blood in addition to the dose already being administered. Heparin is used in extracorporeal blood circuits and in locks giving access to veins.

Heparin has been used in the treatment of fat embolism and coagulation defects associated with disseminated intravascular coagulation.

Heparin, 1 unit per ml, has been added to intravenous solutions to prevent intravascular thrombosis.

Heparin calcium or heparin sodium may be used for subcutaneous injections for prophylaxis in surgery; heparin sodium is used for larger subcutaneous doses and for intravenous use.

Heparin magnesium has also been used subcutaneously. Heparin lithium and heparin strontium are used as *in vitro* anticoagulants.

Reviews, discussions, and symposia on the actions and uses of heparin.— *Curr. ther. Res.*, 1975, *18*, 1; L. B. Jaques, *Pharmac. Rev.*, 1979, *31*, 99; V. V. Kakkar, *Prescribers' J.*, 1979, *19*, 35; T. H. Spaet, *J. Am. med. Ass.*, 1980, *244*, 1243.

A cholesterol gall-stone disappeared after 10 days of continuous infusion, via a T-tube, of 50 000 units of heparin given every 12 hours in 500 ml of sodium chloride injection. This treatment was ineffective in a second patient who subsequently responded to conventional therapy.— A. Iseil and D. L. Crosby (letter), *Lancet*, 1975, *1*, 583.

Heparin in sodium chloride injection was given to irrigate the common duct to 43 patients with gall-stones and in 31 the gall-stones disappeared.— B. Gardner *et al.*, *Am. J. Surg.*, 1975, *130*, 293.

Dissolution of radiolucent bile-duct calculi, retained after surgery, in 19 of 26 patients after infusion into the T-tube of sodium cholate 15 to 20 g in 1 litre of saline alternating with or combined with heparin 20 000 units in 1 litre of saline for 24 hours.— L. A. Christiansen *et al.*, *Scand. J. Gastroenterol.*, 1977, *12*, 337.

The use of heparin-agarose beads for the extracorporeal removal of low-density lipoprotein from the plasma.— P.-J. Lupien *et al.*, *Lancet*, 1976, *1*, 1261.

Adjunct to intravenous infusions. In a double-blind study of 151 patients, the addition of 1000 units of beef-lung heparin to each litre of fluid given intravenously reduced the frequency of thrombophlebitis at infusion sites.— H. W. Daniell, *J. Am. med. Ass.*, 1973, *226*, 1317. See also R. W. Schafermeyer (letter), *J. Am. med. Ass.*, 1974, *228*, 695.

In a study in 20 patients there was less thrombus formation in those with indwelling Teflon radial arterial catheters than in those with heparin-impregnated polyethylene catheters.— J. B. Downs *et al.*, *Archs Surg., Chicago*, 1974, *108*, 671, per *J. Am. med. Ass.*, 1974, *228*, 1050.

Heparin solutions used to fill and flush a heparin lock should be standardised.— E. N. Deeb and P. I. DiMattia (letter), *New Engl. J. Med.*, 1976, *294*, 448. Comment.— J. G. Marshall (letter), *ibid.*, 957. A double-blind study in healthy subjects demonstrated that Bacteriostatic Sodium Chloride Injection (*U.S.P.*) containing 3.3, 16.5, or 132 units of heparin was superior to saline alone in maintaining function; no side-effects attributable to heparin were noted. The optimal concentration of heparin was not known but a 1-ml flush with any concentration within the range studied was adequate. Intracutaneous injection of 0.1 ml of the maintenance solution was, moreover, an effective and safe way to reduce the discomfort of venepuncture.— N. H. G. Holford *et al.* (letter), *ibid.*, 1977, *296*, 1300.

In a study in 59 patients the intravenous administration of heparin 2000 units daily significantly increased the time during which an intravenous cannula was left at one site, chiefly by preventing clotting in and around the needle tip. Thrombophlebitis was not significantly affected.— J. R. Stradling, *Br. med. J.*, 1978, *2*, 1195.

In 80 patients receiving parenteral nutrition via an indwelling central venous catheter the incidence of sepsis was reduced in those given infusate to which had been added heparin 1 unit per ml; the tip of the catheter was infected in 1 of 40 given heparin compared with 9 of 40 controls. It was suggested that heparin prevented the formation of a fibrin sleeve at the catheter tip.— M. J. Bailey, *Br. med. J.*, 1979, *1*, 1671.

Administration. A discussion of the administration and monitoring of heparin.— *Med. Lett.*, 1977, *19*, 31.

Comment on the possible use of intrapulmonary heparin for the prevention of deep-vein thrombosis.— *Lancet*, 1980, *1*, 910.

The intrapulmonary administration of heparin by inhalation was assessed in healthy subjects and *animals* and considered to be safe and effective. This method produced a prolonged effect with single doses providing anticoagulant activity for up to 2 weeks. It was estimated that effective doses would be above 8 mg per kg body-weight. An initial dose of 15 to 20 mg per kg might be desirable followed by 12 mg per kg once a week or 15 to 20 mg per kg every 2 weeks.— L. B. Jaques *et al.*, *Lancet*, 1976, *2*, 1157.

In a clinical trial in 41 patients the use of continuous heparin therapy appeared to be safer with regard to haemorrhagic complications than the use of intermittent therapy.— R. L. Glazier and E. B. Crowell, *J. Am. med. Ass.*, 1976, *236*, 1365.

The incidence of major bleeding was 8% in 72 patients given heparin 4-hourly, the dose being adjusted according to the activated partial thromboplastin time (APTT), 10% in 68 patients given heparin 4-hourly in a fixed dose, and 1% in 69 patients given heparin by continuous infusion, the dose being adjusted according to the APTT.— D. Deykin, *Drugs*, 1977, *13*, 46.

The successful administration of heparin 5000 units subcutaneously by jet injection.— J. Black *et al.*, *Br. med. J.*, 1978, *2*, 95.

In a randomised study major bleeding episodes were not significantly more common in 40 patients treated intermittently with heparin than in 40 treated by continuous infusion.— J. R. Wilson and J. Lampman, *Am. Heart J.*, 1979, *97*, 155.

Administration in renal failure. Heparin could be given in usual doses to patients with renal failure. Concentrations of heparin were not affected by haemodialysis.— W. M. Bennett *et al.*, *Ann. intern. Med.*, 1980, *93*, 286.

Angioneurotic oedema. Heparin was reported to enhance the inhibitory action of antithrombin III which inhibited kallikrein. Plasma from patients with angioneurotic oedema had little neutralising activity against kallikrein and as therapeutic concentrations of heparin increased this activity, heparin might be useful in controlling acute attacks of hereditary angioneurotic oedema.— R. W. Colman (letter), *Ann. intern. Med.*, 1976, *85*, 399.

Burns. Heparin administered intravenously or subcutaneously in doses of 20 000 to 80 000 units initially, followed by 10 000 to 60 000 units four-hourly for 22 to 60 hours or applied topically (20 000 to 480 000 units 2 to 4 times a day) to 7 patients with deep second- and third-degree burns relieved pain and prevented extension of the burn area. No side-effects occurred and there was enhanced revascularisation, granulation, and re-epithelialisation.— M. J. Saliba *et al.*, *J. Am. med. Ass.*, 1973, *225*, 261.

Diagnosis of cystic fibrosis. There was an increased uptake of heparin in the lymphocytes of 14 patients with cystic fibrosis and 16 parents and siblings compared with healthy unrelated controls. This might aid the differentiation of cystic fibrosis families.— J. A. Robertson *et al.* (preliminary communication), *Lancet*, 1974, *1*, 1256.

Disseminated intravascular coagulation. Discussion of the pathogenesis, pathology, and diagnosis of disseminated intravascular coagulation (DIC) and of the clinical conditions which might be associated with DIC. Heparin might form a part of treatment. Reports suggested that it might be of value in DIC associated with amniotic-fluid embolism, reactions due to incompatible transfusions, metastatic carcinoma, acute leukaemia, septic abortion and other septicaemias, heat stroke, the dead-foetus syndrome, and purpura fulminans; beneficial effects in acute liver failure had not been confirmed; heparin was ineffective in the DIC which occurred after many snake bites. Very large doses of heparin might be required.— A. A. Sharp, *Br. med. Bull.*, 1977, *33*, 265.

Reports of the use of heparin in conditions associated with disseminated intravascular coagulation.—In thrombotic microangiopathy (thrombotic thrombocytopenic purpura).— K. D. Allanby *et al.*, *Lancet*, 1966, *1*, 237; R. G. Luke *et al.*, *ibid.*, 1970, *2*, 750.

In 5 children with cyanotic congenital heart disease.— L. H. Dennis *et al.*, *Lancet*, 1967, *1*, 1088.

In purpura fulminans.— D. L. Cram and R. L. Soley, *Br. J. Derm.*, 1968, *80*, 323.

In cryofibrinogenaemia.— D. M. Komp and M. H. Donaldson, *New Engl. J. Med.*, 1968, *279*, 1439.

In microangiopathic haemolytic anaemia.— M. C. Brain *et al.*, *Br. J. Haemat.*, 1968, *15*, 603, per *Abstr. Wld Med.*, 1969, *43*, 437.

In thrombotic thrombocytopenic purpura.— J. H. Richardson and B. T. Smith, *J. Am. med. Ass.*, 1968, *203*, 518; E. J. VanSlyck *et al.*, *J. Am. med. Ass.*, 1969, *209*, 768; P. J. Fiddes and R. Penny, *Australas. Ann. Med.*, 1970, *19*, 350, per *Int. pharm. Abstr.*, 1972, *9*, 198.

In acute haemolysis.— P. G. Hattersley (letter), *J. Am. med. Ass.*, 1969, *209*, 1720.

In the defibrination syndrome.— R. Lerner *et al.*, *Am. J. Obstet. Gynec.*, 1967, *97*, 373, per *Int. pharm. Abstr.*, 1967, *4*, 1065; H. Leiba *et al.*, *Harefuah*, 1970, *78*, 229, per *J. Am. med. Ass.*, 1970, *212*, 1094.

In scorpion stings in *dogs*.— C. S. Devi *et al.*, *Br. med. J.*, 1970, *1*, 345.

In purpura fulminans.— D. L. Dudgeon *et al.*, *Archs Surg., Chicago*, 1971, *103*, 351, per *Clin. Med.*, 1972, *79* (Dec.), 34; N. A. Nagi and A. R. A. Al-Hasso, *Postgrad. med. J.*, 1974, *50*, 750.

In hepatic failure and serum hepatitis.— M. O. Rake *et al.*, *Lancet*, 1971, *2*, 1215.

In renal failure.— I. Timor-Tritsch *et al.*, *Br. med. J.*, 1970, *4*, 221.

In toxaemia of pregnancy.— R. Brehm and H. Janisch, *Dt. med. Wschr.*, 1972, *97*, 418, per *J. Am. med. Ass.*, 1972, *220*, 743. See also P. W. Howie *et al.*, *Br. J. Obstet. Gynaec.*, 1975, *82*, 711 (absence of effect), per *Int. pharm. Abstr.*, 1977, *14*, 333.

After bite by a saw-scaled viper.— H. J. Weiss *et al.*, *Am. J. Med.*, 1973, *54*, 653, per *J. Am. med. Ass.*, 1973, *225*, 650.

In respiratory failure following multiple trauma.— M. Schamaun *et al.*, *Schweiz. med. Wschr.*, 1973, *103*, 941, per *J. Am. med. Ass.*, 1973, *225*, 1146.

In meningococcal purpura.— P. Gerard *et al.*, *J. Pediat.*, 1973, *82*, 780, per *J. Am. med. Ass.*, 1973, *225*, 654; J. Hunter, *Archs Dis. Childh.*, 1973, *48*, 233, per *Int. pharm. Abstr.*, 1974, *11*, 392.

In abruptio placentae.— T. R. Martin *et al.*, *Can. med. Ass. J.*, 1974, *110*, 1159.

In heat stroke.— J. S. Perchick *et al.*, *J. Am. med. Ass.*, 1975, *231*, 480. Comment.— *ibid.*, 496. Another report.— C. J. Cornell *et al.* (letter), *Ann. intern. Med.*, 1974, *81*, 702. A contrary view.— S. Shibolet and Z. Farfel (letter), *ibid.*, *82*, 857.

Absence of effect in acute renal failure.— E. A. Ribes *et al.*, *Br. med. J.*, 1975, *3*, 745.

Effect in severe cirrhosis of the liver.— M. Coleman *et al.*, *Ann. intern. Med.*, 1975, *83*, 79.

In leukaemia.— H. R. Gralnick *et al.*, *Am. J. Med.*, 1972, *52*, 167, per *J. Am. med. Ass.*, 1972, *220*, 740; U. Gafter *et al.*, *Harefuah*, 1977, *92*, 212, per *J. Am. med. Ass.*, 1977, *238*, 269.

In septicaemia.— V. Gurewich and B. Lipinski, *Am. J. med. Sci.*, 1977, *274*, 83, per *Int. pharm. Abstr.*, 1978, *15*, 1226.

Absence of value in meningitis.— J. T. MacFarlane *et al.*, *Br. med. J.*, 1977, *2*, 1522.

In acute promyelocytic leukaemia.— A. J. Collins *et al.*, *Archs intern. Med.*, 1978, *138*, 1677.

Associated with abdominal aortic aneurysm.— C. J. Diskin and A. B. Weitberg, *Archs intern. Med.*, 1980, *140*, 263.

Haemolytic-uraemic syndrome. A review of the use of heparin in the haemolytic-uraemic syndrome.— W. Proesmans and R. Eeckles, *J. Pediat.*, 1974, *85*, 142, per *Br. med. J.*, 1974, *4*, 533.

Eight children, aged 6½ weeks to 6½ years, with the haemolytic-uraemic syndrome received heparin intravenously, 100 units per kg body-weight initially, then 4-hourly in a dose to maintain the whole-blood clotting time at 20 to 30 minutes. Five also received peritoneal dialysis. Heparin was given until the onset of diuresis which occurred in 5 to 18 days in 5 patients. Treatment was successful in 5 patients, 1 child developed myocarditis, 1 had a kidney removed, and 1 died of septicaemia.— G. S. Gilchrist *et al.*, *Lancet*, 1969, *1*, 1123.

In 3 children, aged 11, 7, and 1 year, with the haemolytic-uraemic syndrome, heparin in an initial dose of 100 units per kg was given intravenously, followed by a dosage adjusted to maintain the blood-clotting time between 20 and 30 minutes. In 2 patients who survived, renal biopsy specimens showed widespread glomerular disease, but only occasional thrombi. Heparin was considered to prevent further intrarenal thrombosis, allowing removal of existing thrombi by the normal fibrinolytic process.— M. W. Moncrieff and E. F. Glasgow, *Br. med. J.*, 1970, *3*, 188. Criticisms.— A. R. Clarkson *et al.* (letter), *ibid.*, 463.

In 30 children with the haemolytic-uraemic syndrome mortality was 40% in 10 treated with heparin to keep the coagulation time at 3 times its initial value and 30% in 20 who did not receive heparin. Further evaluation was required.— M. Vitacco *et al.*, *J. Pediat.*, 1973, *83*, 271, per *Int. pharm. Abstr.*, 1974, *11*, 390.

Nine of 10 women with the haemolytic-uraemic syndrome post partum or following treatment with oestrogens who recovered useful renal function had received regular injections of heparin compared with 12 of 27 others who either died or survived with damaged kidneys.— *Lancet*, 1976, *1*, 943.

Results of a study involving 9 children with the haemolytic-uraemic syndrome indicating that the rate of recovery of patients who had received peritoneal dialysis was unaffected by the use of heparin.— M. G. Coulthard, *Archs Dis. Childh.*, 1980, *55*, 393.

Migraine. In 9 of 12 patients with migraine, the pain was terminated when an intravenous injection of heparin, 150 to 175 mg, was given shortly after the beginning of the attack.— *J. Am. med. Ass.*, 1969, *209*, 853. See also E. Thonnard-Neumann, *Headache*, 1973, *13*, 49, per *J. Am. med. Ass.*, 1973, *225*, 1724.

Myocardial infarction. Of 24 patients given no anticoagulants after myocardial infarction, 7 developed thromboses, as detected by the radioactive fibrinogen test, within the next 2 weeks. In 24 given heparin 5000 units intravenously initially then 20 000 units every 12 hours by continuous intravenous infusion pump for 14 days, there were no thromboses.— A. J. Handley *et al.*, *Br. med. J.*, 1972, *2*, 436.

In a controlled study of 50 patients with myocardial infarction, 23% of the patients given heparin 5000 units intravenously followed by 7500 units subcutaneously repeated every 12 hours for 7 days developed thromboses compared with 29% of the control patients.— A. J. Handley, *Lancet*, 1972, *2*, 623.

A deep-vein leg thrombosis was detected in 2 of 63 patients who were treated within 12 hours of a myocardial infarction with heparin 5000 units given subcutaneously every 12 hours for 10 days. In a group of matched controlled patients, 11 of 64 had evidence of deep-vein thrombosis.— C. Warlow *et al.*, *Lancet*, 1973, *2*, 934.

Subcutaneous administration of heparin calcium, 20 000 to 25 000 units initially followed by 10 000 to 12 500 units every 12 hours, was as effective as intravenous infusion of heparin sodium 30 000 to 40 000 units per day in reducing the incidence of venous thrombosis in patients who had suffered a recent myocardial infarction.— W. R. Pitney *et al.*, *Med. J. Aust.*, 1974, *1*, 38.

The effect of heparin on the ECG and enzymes values in patients with myocardial infarction.— M. J. Saliba *et al.*, *Am. J. Cardiol.*, 1976, *37*, 605.

The incidence of deep-vein thrombosis (assessed by the fibrinogen uptake test) after myocardial infarction was 2 of 37 in patients given low-dose-heparin subcutaneously compared with 14 of 41 not given heparin; 3 (possibly 5) of the controls developed pulmonary embolism compared with none in the heparin group. Of the controls 3 of the 14 who developed thrombosis were smokers compared with 17 of 27 who did not develop thrombosis. Heparin should be given routinely to non-smokers after myocardial infarction.— P. A. Emerson and P. Marks, *Br. med. J.*, 1977, *1*, 18. The dose was 5000 units intravenously and 7500 units subcutaneously as soon as possible, then 7500 units subcutaneously every 12 hours for 10 days.— P. A. Emerson (letter), *ibid.*, 838.

Results indicating that intravenous heparin was of benefit in preventing myocardial infarction in patients with the intermediate coronary syndrome.— A. M. Telford and C. Wilson, *Lancet*, 1981, *1*, 1225.

Further references.— A. N. Nicolaides *et al.*, *Br. med. J.*, 1971, *1*, 432; P. Marks and D. Teather, *Practitioner*, 1978, *220*, 425; H. Arnesen *et al.*, *Acta med. scand.*, 1980, *207*, 21.

Neoplasms. Heparin did not prevent tumour growth but antineoplastic agents were more effective when given after anticoagulant therapy. Patients with metastatic disease and hyperfibrinogenaemia were initially resistant to heparin.— E. G. Elias *et al.*, *J. surg. Oncol.*, 1973, *5*, 189, per *J. Am. med. Ass.*, 1973, *224*, 264. See also *idem*, *Cancer*, 1975, *36*, 129, per *J. Am. med. Ass.*, 1975, *234*, 114.

Renal failure. Rapid improvement in urine output followed continuous heparin infusions in 6 patients with oliguric renal failure due to glomerulonephritis or obstructive lesions in the arterioles and glomeruli. The initial dose was 15 000 to 20 000 units every 12 hours, and thereafter the dose was adjusted to maintain the coagulation time above 25 minutes. If necessary, treatment was continued for up to 6 weeks and further treatment was given with phenindione and dipyridamole for several months. Steroids or immunosuppressive drugs, or both, were given in addition. Two patients died but the others were well 2 to 9 months after starting treatment.— P. Kincaid-Smith *et al.*, *Lancet*, 1968, *2*, 1360.

In 5 patients with accelerated hypertension, 7 with chronic or progressive proliferative glomerulonephritis, and 3 with rejection episodes following renal transplantation, heparin was beneficial in reducing the fibrinogen catabolic-rate in some patients in the hypertensive and rejection groups but not in the patients with glomerulonephritis. All patients had some increase in glomerular filtration-rate. After an initial intravenous dose of 10 000 units, heparin was given by infusion at the rate of 20 000 units every 12 hours for at least 4 days.— E. N. Wardle and P. R. Uldall, *Br. med. J.*, 1972, *4*, 135. See also J. S. Cameron, *Br. med. J.*, 1972, *4*, 217.

Heparin administered intravenously in doses of 75 to 100 mg every 12 hours for 2 to 3 weeks relieved cutaneous itching in patients with advanced renal failure.— H. Yatzidis *et al.* (letter), *J. Am. med. Ass.*, 1972, *222*, 1183.

The use of quadruple therapy with prednisolone, azathioprine or cyclophosphamide, dipyridamole, and heparin followed by warfarin in the treatment of 15 patients with rapidly progressing glomerulonephritis. Six with anuria or severe oliguria did not benefit; the remainder improved.— C. B. Brown *et al.*, *Lancet*, 1974, *2*, 1166.

Further references.— M. Rathaus and J. L. Bernheim (letter), *Archs intern. Med.*, 1979, *139*, 251.

See also Haemolytic-uraemic Syndrome, above.

Thrombo-embolic disorders. From a study of 162 patients treated for venous thrombo-embolism it was suggested that in order to prevent recurrent embolism the maintenance dose of heparin should be sufficient to maintain the activated partial thromboplastin time at between 1.5 and 2.5 times control values.— D. Basu *et al.*, *New Engl. J. Med.*, 1972, *287*, 324. See also *ibid.*, 355.

Three groups each of about 70 patients with thrombo-embolic disorders were given heparin according to the following regimens: one group by intermittent intravenous injection every four hours, the dose adjusted on the basis of partial thromboplastin time; the second by intermittent injection, 75 to 125 units per kg body-weight every 4 hours; and the third, continuous infusion, the dose again based on the partial thromboplastin time. The occurrence of major bleeding episodes was not significantly different in the first 2 groups (8 and 10%) but occurred in only 1% of the third group. Mortality-rates were not different and there was 1 pulmonary embolism in each group.— E. W. Salzman *et al.*, *New Engl. J. Med.*, 1975, *292*, 1046.

In a 10-year study 407 patients with all grades of thrombophlebitis apart from the severe acute form with fever and/or leucocytosis were treated as outpatients with self-administered subcutaneous doses of heparin as well as with mechanical therapy. Treatment was started with a dose of 20 000 *U.S.P.* units with the aim of achieving a clotting time of 20 to 30 minutes. When this was achieved the dose was gradually reduced and withdrawn as long as this figure was maintained. Thereafter anticoagulation was continued with aspirin 1.2 to 2.4 g daily. The duration of heparin therapy, which was an indication of effectiveness, ranged from 1 month to 9 years and for 78% of patients was 6 months or less; 73% remained free of recurrence.— R. M. Stillman *et al.*, *Surgery Gynec. Obstet.*, 1977, *145*, 193. See also *Lancet*, 1977, *2*, 963.

See also above under Disseminated Intravascular Coagulation and Myocardial Infarction.

For a comparison of the effects of warfarin sodium and heparin in preventing the recurrence of venous thrombo-embolism, see Warfarin Sodium, p.781.

For the role of streptokinase and other forms of enzyme therapy in thrombo-embolic disorders, including comparisons with heparin, see Strepkokinase, p.657.

See also under Use in Surgery.

Pregnancy and the neonate. Experience in 22 pregnancies in 19 women showed that self-administered heparin could be safely used subcutaneously for the prophylaxis of thrombo-embolism. The dose ranged from 4000 to 24 000 units daily at the beginning of treatment to 10 000 to 30 000 units daily at the end of pregnancy.— G. Spearing *et al.*, *Br. med. J.*, 1978, *1*, 1457. See also H. F. Baskin *et al.*, *Am. J. Obstet. Gynec.*, 1977, *129*, 590; V. V. Kakkar and P. G. Bentley (letter), *Br. med. J.*, 1978, *2*, 124.

Two cousins belonging to a family with hereditary anti-thrombin deficiency developed pregnancy-associated thrombosis which was successfully treated with long-term subcutaneous administration of heparin.— P. Brandt and S. Stenbjerg (letter), *Lancet*, 1979, *1*, 100.

For references to the use of heparin in conditions associated with disseminated intravascular coagulation in pregnancy, see under Disseminated Intravascular Coagulation, above.

See also under the section in Anticoagulants, p.762.

Stroke. Heparin calcium 5000 units was given subcutaneously every 8 hours for 14 days to 16 elderly patients admitted with a diagnosis of stroke occurring within 48 hours and was associated with a significant reduction in deep-vein thrombosis. The incidence of thrombosis in 16 control patients was 75% and in the treated group 12.5%. There were 3 deaths in the treated and 5 in the control group.— S. T. McCarthy *et al.* (preliminary communication), *Lancet*, 1977, *2*, 800. No benefit was seen in a series of 25 patients with nonhaemorrhagic acute stroke given heparin calcium 5000 units every 12 hours for at least 14 days.— O. J. S. Buruma *et al.* (letter), *ibid.*, 1978, *1*, 160 and 500.

Further references.— P. Millac and K. Wood (letter), *Br. med. J.*, 1975, *3*, 595.

Use in radiography. An intra-arterial injection of heparin 3000 to 7000 units at the start of percutaneous coronary arteriography by the percutaneous femoral method greatly reduced the morbidity and mortality previously associated with this method.— W. J. Walker *et al.*, *New Engl. J. Med.*, 1973, *288*, 826.

In a randomised study in 400 patients undergoing trans-femoral angiography the incidence of mild or major haematoma was similar in those given heparin 45 units per kg body-weight into the abdominal aorta, with small amounts (about 250 units) for flushing of the catheter, compared with those receiving only heparin for flushing (about 750 units). There were no occlusions of the femoral artery in those receiving systemic heparin, compared with 2 in the control group, and the incidence of thrombus at the entry site was reduced; delayed bleeding was significantly increased.— R. Antonovic *et al.*, *Am. J. Roentg.*, 1976, *127*, 223.

A suggestion that a 'heparin flush' might prevent post-venographic thrombophlebitis.— R. D. Arndt *et al.*, *Radiology*, 1979, *130*, 249. See also F. Laerum *et al.* (letter), *Lancet*, 1980, *1*, 1141.

Evidence that heparin bonding reduces thrombogenicity of pulmonary-artery catheters.— P. F. Hoar *et al.*, *New Engl. J. Med.*, 1981, *305*, 993.

Use in surgery. Discussions of the use of low doses of heparin to prevent deep-vein thrombosis.— S. Wessler, *J. Am. med. Ass.*, 1976, *236*, 389; *Med. Lett.*, 1977, *19*, 71; *Drug & Ther. Bull.*, 1977, *15*, 21; N. L. Browse, *Ann. R. Coll. Surg.*, 1977, *59*, 138; E. M. Matt and U. F. Gruber, *Fortschr. Med.*, 1977, *95*, 669; J. R. A. Mitchell, *Br. med. J.*, 1979, *1*, 1523.

A report by the Council on Thrombosis of the American Heart Association on the use of heparin for the prevention of venous thrombo-embolism in surgery.— *Circulation*, 1977, *55*, 423A. Comment.— H. L. Pachter and T. S. Riles (letter), *ibid.*, *56*, 327.

In a controlled double-blind study of 78 patients undergoing major surgery, 17 of 39 given a placebo developed deep-vein thrombosis postoperatively compared with 3 of 39 patients given heparin calcium 5000 units subcutaneously 2 hours before surgery and every 12 hours thereafter for 7 days. A further 133 patients with conditions predisposing to thrombo-embolism were treated with the same dose of heparin calcium before and after surgery and 13 developed thrombosis. Emergency operations were carried out on 50 patients with fractured neck of the femur who were also given heparin calcium, but 20 of these developed thromboses. Haemorrhage during and after surgery was a problem in 3 patients.— V. V. Kakkar *et al.*, *Lancet*, 1972, *2*, 101.

No haemorrhage occurred in 22 patients undergoing major hip surgery given heparin 10 000 units subcutaneously the night before surgery and 2500 units every 6 hours after surgery until discharge. When 1330 patients undergoing major surgery, including surgery for hip fractures in 70 patients, were treated similarly, the incidence of fatal pulmonary embolism fell from 4 to 0.0014%.— J. G. Sharnoff *et al.* (letter), *Lancet*, 1972, *2*, 488.

Heparin calcium 5000 units subcutaneously pre-operatively then thrice daily for 7 or 10 days did not significantly reduce the incidence of deep-vein thrombosis in a controlled study of 100 patients aged 60 to 80 years who had undergone hip-replacement surgery.— W. G. J. Hampson *et al.*, *Lancet*, 1974, *2*, 795.

Heparin calcium 5000 units was given subcutaneously to 45 patients 2 hours before major hip surgery and then every 8 hours until the patient was mobile. Deep-vein thrombosis was detected in 8 of the patients (17.7%) compared with 18 of 46 similar patients (39.1%) who had received no heparin and acted as controls.— P. M. Mannucci *et al.* (letter), *Lancet*, 1974, *2*, 1143. See also G. K. Morris *et al.*, *ibid.*, 1974, *2*, 797.

In a multi-centre trial of 386 patients undergoing major surgery, 128 were given heparin sodium 2500 units subcutaneously 2 hours before operation then 5000 units twice daily until the 7th day, and 130 were given infusions of 500 ml of dextran 70 over 4 hours, the infusion being started in the anaesthetic room with further infusions of 500 ml on the 1st and 2nd days after surgery. The remaining 128 patients acted as controls. The incidence of deep-vein thrombosis diagnosed by radio-iodine scanning was 12% in the heparin group, 25% in the dextran group, and 37% in the control group.— *Lancet*, 1974, *2*, 118.

In 79 patients undergoing bladder or prostate surgery there was no difference in the overall incidence of deep-vein thrombosis between those given heparin calcium, those treated by electrical stimulation of calf muscle during surgery, and controls. In 194 patients undergoing laparotomy heparin calcium significantly reduced thrombosis; electrical stimulation reduced the overall incidence of thrombosis only in patients without malignant disease. The dose of heparin calcium was 5000 units 2 hours before surgery, then every 8 hours till the end of the sixth postoperative day or until the patient was fully mobile.— I. L. Rosenberg *et al.*, *Br. med. J.*, 1975, *1*, 649. Criticism.— F. S. A. Doran, *ibid.*, 1975, *2*, 442.

In an international multicentre study of 4121 patients over 40 years of age undergoing major surgery, 2045 were given heparin calcium 5000 units subcutaneously 2 hours pre-operatively and every 8 hours thereafter for 7 days, or longer if necessary until the patient was ambulant, and 2076 acted as controls for assessment of the effect of heparin on pulmonary embolism, deep-vein thrombosis, and operative and postoperative bleeding and haematoma. The incidence of fatal pulmonary embolism was significantly less in the heparin (2) than in the control group (16). Deep-vein thrombosis was diagnosed clinically in 39 of the heparin and 81 of the control group. Scanning using ^{125}I-fibrinogen in 1292 patients also revealed a statistical superiority for heparin. Of the 2045 patients given heparin 70 withdrew from treatment mainly due to blood loss or haematoma. Blood loss during surgery was excessive in 182 of those given heparin and 126 of the controls and haematomas occurred in 158 and 117 patients respectively. A detailed study of the transfusion requirements and haemoglobin concentration in 731 heparin and 744 control patients showed no significant difference between the 2 groups. This heparin schedule could now be recommended for prophylaxis against venous thrombo-embolism for use on a large scale in high-risk patients undergoing major surgery.— *Lancet*, 1975, *2*, 45. See also *ibid.*, 63. Criticism from one of the centres (Basle) on the definition of fatal pulmonary embolism and on the above recommendations applying to all types of major surgery. The centre extended its study to observe the effects of heparin, dextran 40, and xanthinol nicotinate in 318 patients. Xanthinol nicotinate was soon dropped from the study for lack of effect. Infusions of 500 ml of dextran 40 during surgery, at the end of surgery, and on the first and second postoperative days did not reduce deaths from pulmonary embolism which was more broadly defined than in the multicentre study; 4 patients in the control group died compared with 6 in the heparin group and 1 in the dextran group. Heparin did reduce deep-vein thrombosis during the first postoperative week and although it caused more side-effects it was more effective than dextran 40.— U. F. Gruber *et al.*, *ibid.*, 1977, *1*, 207. Because of inconsistencies in the data supplied by this centre, the results of the multicentre study were reanalysed excluding patients from Basle. This exclusion did not influence the findings or their significance.— *ibid.*, 567.

Heparin 5000 units reduced blood viscosity in 18 healthy subjects and in 16 surgical patients given the anticoagulant pre- and postoperatively. This effect might be involved in heparin's prophylactic effect against thrombo-embolisms.— A. Erdi *et al.* (preliminary communication), *Lancet*, 1976, *2*, 342. Criticism. In a study of 26 patients, heparin had not significantly affected blood or plasma viscosity even when given intravenously in large doses. Temperature also affected the viscosity of blood and plasma.— A. Girolami and G. Cella (letter), *ibid.*, 909.

In a study in 176 elderly patients with fracture of the femoral neck heparin 5000 units subcutaneously every 8 hours for 10 days slightly reduced the incidence of deep-vein thrombosis, but the reduction was not statistically significant. There was no reduction in thrombosis in those treated with dipyridamole, dipyridamole plus aspirin, or flurbiprofen.— G. K. Morris and J. R. A. Mitchell, *Br. med. J.*, 1977, *1*, 535.

The routine use of heparin 5000 units every 8 or 12 hours for patients undergoing surgery was discontinued in one hospital because of the incidence of significant postoperative bleeding. Prophylaxis with heparin would be used in selected high-risk patients.— B. J. Britton *et al.* (letter), *Lancet*, 1977, *2*, 604. Criticism.— V. V. Kakkar (letter), *Lancet*, 1977, *2*, 1236.

Heparin 5000 units subcutaneously given 8-hourly to 12 patients before mastectomy was associated with increased wound drainage, increased delay in discharge, and a greater fall in haemoglobin after surgery when compared with 12 patients not given heparin. The only patient to develop a proven pulmonary embolus was in the heparin group.— J. G. Mosley (letter), *lancet*, 1978, *1*, 161.

In a double-blind prospective study heparin, 5000 units subcutaneously the evening before surgery and every 12 hours thereafter for 7 days or until earlier discharge, was given to 643 patients aged over 40 years and undergoing elective surgery lasting 1 hour or longer; placebo injections were given to 653 similar patients. There was a significant difference in thrombo-embolic complications with 16 occurring within 7 days in the placebo group and only 4 in the heparin group, leading to 3 and 1 deaths respectively from a pulmonary embolus. When the heparin injections were stopped after 7 days the incidence of thrombo-embolic complications became identical between the 2 groups.— J. Kiil *et al.*, *Lancet*, 1978, *1*, 1115.

In a double-blind study heparin sodium 5000 *U.S.P.* units subcutaneously before surgery then 12-hourly for 2 weeks or until discharge did not reduce the incidence of acute pulmonary embolism in 78 patients undergoing surgery for hip fracture or hip replacement or in 94 patients undergoing above-knee amputation; a similar apparent lack of effect in 40 patients undergoing below-knee amputation did not yet warrant conclusions, because of the low incidence of pulmonary embolism.— J. W. Williams *et al.*, *Ann. Surg.*, 1978, *188*, 468.

In 100 patients undergoing intracranial surgery the incidence of deep-vein thrombosis was 6% in 50 given heparin calcium, usually 5000 units, 2 hours before surgery then every 8 hours for 7 days, compared with 34% in 50 controls. The 5000-unit dose of heparin was reduced if, at prior testing, a plasma-heparin concentration of 0.18 or more units per ml was achieved 3 hours after administration.— D. Cerrato *et al.*, *J. Neurosurg.*, 1978, *49*, 378.

Of 25 patients with a fractured neck of the femur given heparin calcium 100 units per kg body-weight subcutaneously every 8 hours for 2 weeks none developed deep-vein thrombosis compared with 12 of 25 similar patients given a placebo. Four patients in the heparin group did however develop a deep-vein thrombosis within one week of stopping treatment.— A. Xabregas *et al.*, *Med. J. Aust.*, 1978, *1*, 620.

In a randomised study in 81 patients undergoing open urological procedures the incidence of deep-vein thrombosis was not reduced by heparin sodium 5000 units 2 hours before surgery and continued 12-hourly during hospitalisation, compared with a control group; the incidence was reduced by external pneumatic compression.— N. P. Coe *et al.*, *Surgery, St Louis*, 1978, *83*, 230.

Evaluation of the first 100 patients treated prophylactically with heparin subcutaneously before and after abdominal surgery showed that the overall incidence of deep-vein thrombosis was significantly reduced compared with 99 control patients; benefit was limited to calf-vein thrombosis; femoral or ileofemoral thrombosis and pulmonary embolism were not reduced. Routine heparin prophylaxis could not be recommended for all surgical procedures in patients over 40 years of age. The study continued.—Groote Schuur Hospital Thromboembolus Study Group, *Br. med. J.*, 1979, *1*, 1447. Criticisms.— M. Adiseshiah (letter), *Br. med. J.*, 1979, *1*, 1707; R. S. Stubbs (letter), *Br. med. J.*, 1979, *1*, 1707; V. V. Kakkar (letter), *Br. med. J.*, 1979, *2*, 127; C. Prentice *et al.* (letter), *Br. med. J.*, 1979, *2*, 128; R. H. Fell (letter), *Br. med. J.*, 1979, *2*, 129.

In a multicentre study 1993 patients undergoing general, gynaecological, urological, or orthopaedic surgery were allocated to receive infusions of dextran '70' 6% in saline (500 ml pre-operatively, postoperatively, and on the first postoperative day) and 1991 to receive heparin sodium (5000 units pre-operatively and 8-hourly to a total of 21 injections). Fatal pulmonary embolism occurred in 6 patients in each group (sole cause and contributory cause in 5 and 1, and 3 and 3 respectively); only 2 of those receiving heparin had received an adequate course. Allergic reactions were more common with dextran (22 versus 3) and haemorrhage with heparin (94 versus 6).— U. F. Gruber *et al.*, *Br. med. J.*, 1980, *280*, 69.

A study indicating that ultra-low-dose intravenous heparin (1 unit per kg body-weight per hour for 3 to 5 days) is a convenient method of preventing deep-vein thrombosis in the early postoperative period and is as effective as existing methods. It avoids the complications of haemorrhage, injection-site haematoma formation, circulatory overloading, and anaphylaxis. The study was double-blind and involved 45 patients given heparin sodium 1 unit per kg per hour by constant infusion pump immediately after induction of anaesthesia and continued for as long as the patient required intravenous fluid, within the limits of 2 to 5 days. The control group comprised 50 patients given infusions of physiological saline. Small wound haematomas occurred in 2 patients on heparin and 1 on saline.— D. Negus *et al.*, *Lancet*, 1980, *1*, 891. Comment.— *ibid.*, 907. A report of results agreeing that small intravenous doses of heparin are enough to reverse hypercoagulability. However, part of the hypercoagulation of surgery seems to be caused by the use of intravenous fluids given during and after operation.— S. B. Janvrin *et al.* (letter), *ibid.*, 1302. Comments on the mode of action of low doses of heparin.— H. Engelberg (letter), *ibid.*, 1303; J. M. Ham (letter), *ibid.*, *2*, 36; J. R. O'Brien (letter), *ibid.*, 420; L. B. Jaques *et al.* (letter), *ibid.*, 1369.

A method for identifying pre-operatively patients with a high risk of developing deep-vein thrombosis.— A. J. Crandon *et al.*, *Br. med. J.*, 1980, *281*, 343. A study limiting the use of prophylactic low-dose heparin therapy to those patients identified as being at high risk of developing deep-vein thrombosis postoperatively provided results similar to other studies where the whole population was treated. It was suggested that this method saved many patients from being treated unnecessarily.— *idem*, 345. Comment.— J. D. Hamer (letter), *ibid.*, 745.

Further references on heparin reducing the incidence of thrombosis following surgery.— H. T. Williams, *Lancet*, 1971, *2*, 950; I. C. Gordon-Smith *et al.*, *Lancet*, 1972, *1*, 1133; A. N. Nicolaides *et al.*, *Lancet*, 1972, *2*, 890; G. Lahnborg *et al.*, *Lancet*, 1974, *1*, 329; I. G. Smith *et al.* (letter), *Lancet*, 1974, *2*, 286; S. Sagar *et al.*, *Br. med. J.*, 1975, *4*, 257; A. S. Gallus *et al.*, *J. Am. med. Ass.*, 1976, *235*, 1980.

For a report of the use of heparin calcium to reduce the incidence of deep-vein thrombosis in patients undergoing vaginal or abdominal surgery, see Nicoumalone, p.772.

Use in surgery with other drugs. In a double-blind study in patients undergoing thoracic or abdominal surgery 63 received aspirin 500 mg (as lysine acetylsalicylate 900 mg) intravenously and a placebo subcutaneously on the evening before surgery then twice daily for a week, 57 received a placebo intravenously and heparin 5000 units subcutaneously, and 57 received aspirin plus heparin. Calf thrombosis occurred in 16, 6, and 5 patients respectively, and thigh thrombosis (considered a high risk for the development of pulmonary embolism) occurred in 3, 5, and nil patients respectively. Pulmonary embolism occurred in 2 patients in the heparin group.— D. Loew *et al.*, *Thromb. Res.*, 1977, *11*, 81.

In 15 patients undergoing hip-joint surgery the incidence of deep-vein thrombosis was 60%; in 30 given heparin calcium 5000 units thrice daily subcutaneously it was 30%; in 30 also given lysine acetylsalicylate it was 27%; in 38 given heparin 7500 units thrice daily it was 11%.— T. H. Schöndorf, *Dt. med. Wschr.*, 1978, *103*, 1877.

In a randomised study the incidence of deep-vein thrombosis in 50 patients undergoing abdominal surgery and given heparin calcium, 5000 units subcutaneously 2 hours before surgery and then 8-hourly for 7 days or longer, was 4% compared with 20% in 50 given dihydroergotamine mesylate 500 µg subcutaneously before surgery and then 12-hourly; the difference was significant. The incidence was 4% in 48 further patients given heparin calcium 5000 units, compared with 6% in 49 given heparin 2500 units per dose plus dihydroergotamine; the difference was not significant. The incidence was 52% in 50 patients undergoing hip surgery and given heparin in 5000-unit doses for 10 to 14 days compared with 20% in 50 given heparin in 5000-unit doses plus dihydroergotamine; the difference was significant and such combined treatment was considered of value.— V. V. Kakkar *et al.*, *J. Am. med. Ass.*, 1979, *241*, 39.

Preparations of Heparin Calcium and Heparin Sodium

Anticoagulant Heparin Solution *(U.S.P.)*. A sterile solution of heparin sodium in sodium chloride injection, containing 75 *U.S.P.* units of heparin in each ml. It may be buffered but contains no antibacterial agents. pH 5 to 7.5.

For use in the proportion of 30 ml of solution to each 500 ml of whole blood.

Heparin Injection *(B.P.)*. A sterile solution of heparin calcium or heparin sodium in Water for Injections, adjusted to pH 5 to 8 by the addition of a suitable alkali. Store at a temperature not exceeding 25°, preferably in glass containers sealed by fusion of the glass. It may contain a bactericide; if kept in containers sealed by rubber closures, a satisfactory concentration of bactericide may not be maintained for more than 3 years. The label specifies the type of heparin present. If it contains no bactericide, any portion not used immediately should be discarded.

Similar injections are included in several other pharmacopoeias.

Heparin Lock Flush Solution *(U.S.P.)*. A sterile solution of heparin sodium rendered iso-osmotic with blood by the addition of not more than 1% of sodium chloride; it may contain a suitable stabiliser. pH 5 to 7.5. For the maintenance of patency of intravenous injection devices.

Heparin Sodium Injection *(U.S.P.)*. A sterile solution of heparin sodium in Water for Injections. pH 5 to 7.5.

Proprietary Preparations of Heparin Calcium and Heparin Sodium

Calciparine *(Labaz Sanofi, UK)*. Heparin calcium, available in disposable syringes each containing 5000 units in approximately 0.2 ml. For subcutaneous injection. (Also available as Calciparine in *Austral.*, *Canad.*, *Fr.*, *S.Afr.*, *Switz.*).

Hepacort Plus *(Rona, UK)*. **Cream** containing in each g heparin sodium 1000 units and hydrocortisone acetate 1 mg, for superficial phlebitis and varicose conditions; and **Suppositories** each containing heparin sodium 2000 units and hydrocortisone acetate 2 mg, for pruritic and inflamed conditions of the anus and rectum.

Heparin Retard Injection *(Boots, UK)*. Contains heparin sodium 10 000 units per ml in a modified Pitkin's menstruum, in ampoules of 2 ml. For intramuscular or deep subcutaneous injection.

Hep-Rinse *(Leo, UK)*. Heparin sodium, available as a sterile solution containing 100 units per ml, with chlorbutol 0.5%, in ampoules of 2 ml. For the maintenance of patency of intravenous injection devices.

Hepsal *(Weddel, UK)*. Heparin sodium, available as a sterile solution containing 10 units per ml, with sodium chloride 0.9%, in ampoules of 5 ml. For the maintenance of patency of intravenous injection devices.

Minihep *(Leo, UK)*. Heparin sodium, available as an injection containing 25 000 units per ml, with chlorbutol 0.4%, in single-dose ampoules of 0.2 ml. For subcutaneous injection.

Minihep Calcium *(Leo, UK)*. Heparin calcium, available as an injection containing 25 000 units per ml, in single-dose ampoules of 0.2 ml. For subcutaneous injection.

Uniparin *(Weddel, UK)*. Heparin sodium, available as an injection containing 25 000 units per ml, in single-dose syringes of 0.2 ml. For subcutaneous injection. (Also available as Uniparin in *Austral.*).

Proprietary Preparations of other Heparinoid Substances

Anacal *(Luitpold-Werk, UK: Farillon, UK)*. **Ointment** containing in each g a heparinoid 2 mg, prednisolone 1.5 mg, lauromacrogol '400' 50 mg, and hexachlorophane 5 mg, and **Suppositories** each containing a heparinoid 4 mg, prednisolone 1 mg, lauromacrogol '400' 50 mg, and hexachlorophane 5 mg. For haemorrhoids and ano-rectal disorders.

Reference.— M. J. Clyne, *Practitioner*, 1977, *218*, 706.

Hirudoid Cream *(Luitpold-Werk, UK: Farillon, UK)*. Contains in each 100 g a heparinoid 300 mg (equivalent to 25 000 units of heparin). For topical anticoagulant and anti-inflammatory therapy. **Hirudoid Gel.** Contains the same active ingredients in a gel basis. (Also available as Hirudoid in *Ger., Neth., Norw., S.Afr., Spain, Switz.*).

For reports of the use of Hirudoid, see B. S. S. Acharya, *Practitioner*, 1973, *211*, 371; H. Tronnier, *Clin. Trials J.*, 1973, *10*, 91; M. Fateh, *ibid.*, 122; P. P. Mehta *et al.*, *Br. med. J.*, 1975, *3*, 614.

Movelat Cream (known in certain countries as Mobilat Ointment) *(Luitpold-Werk, UK: Farillon, UK)*. Contains in each 100 g a heparinoid 200 mg, adrenal extract (total corticosteroid content 2%) 1 g, and salicylic acid 2 g. For inflammatory and arthritic conditions. **Movelat Gel.** Contains the same active ingredients in a gel basis.

In a controlled study in 97 patients the application of Movelat thrice daily over the cannula site reduced, by about half, the incidence of thrombophlebitis in patients receiving intravenous infusions expected to last 48 hours or longer.— C. R. J. Woodhouse, *Br. med. J.*, 1979, *1*, 454.

Further references.— B. L. Bisley *et al.*, *Br. J. clin. Pract.*, 1972, *26*, 477.

Other Proprietary Names of Heparin Calcium and Heparin Sodium

Arg.— Liquemine; *Austral.*—Caprin, Pularin; *Belg.*—Calparine, Liquemine, Pularine; *Canad.*—Hepalean, Lipo-Hepin; *Denm.*—Noparin; *Fr.*—Liquémine, Percase; *Ger.*—Calciparin, Hämocura, Liquemin, Praecivenin, Thrombareduct, Thrombophob, Thrombo-Vetren, Vetren; *Ital.*—Calciparina, Chemyparin, Clearane, Croneparina, Disebrin, Eparinoral, Eparinovis, Liquemin; *Jap.*—Hepacarin, Heparinin, Panheprin; *Neth.*—Calparine, Liquemin, Thromboliquine; *S.Afr.*— Pularin; *Spain*—Darkinal; *Swed.*—Thrombophob; *Switz.*—HepaGel, Liquemin, Thrombophob; *USA*—Hep-Lock, Heprinar, Lipo-Hepin, Liquaemin Sodium, Panheprin.

Other Proprietary Names of Other Heparinoids

Hemeran *(Switz.)*; Heparilene, Mesarin *(both Spain)*.

Proprietary Names of Other Heparin Salts

Cuthéparine *(heparin magnesium) (Fr., Switz.)*.

A preparation containing heparin was also formerly marketed in Great Britain under the proprietary name Contusol Lotion (*Barclay & Sons*).

The proprietary names Pularin-Ca and Pularin (*Evans Medical*) were formerly used in Great Britain for heparin calcium and heparin sodium respectively.

4803-l

Acetonyliodobenzylhydroxycoumarin. 3-(α-Acetonyl-*p*-iodobenzyl)-4-hydroxycoumarin; 4-Hydroxy-3-[1-(4-iodophenyl)-3-oxobutyl]coumarin.

$C_{19}H_{15}IO_4$=434.2.

CAS — 5543-62-4.

Acetonyliodobenzylhydroxycoumarin is an oral anticoagulant which has been used in initial doses of 6 mg with maintenance doses of 2 to 4 mg daily.

4804-y

Ancrod.

An active enzymatic principle derived from the venom of the Malayan pit-viper (*Agkistrodon rhodostoma* = *Calloselasma rhodostoma*). It is a glycoprotein with a molecular weight of about 30 000.

CAS — 9046-56-4.

Units. 55 units are contained in 16.90 mg with lactose and albumin in one ampoule of the first International Reference Preparation (1976).

The international unit corresponds to the earlier Twyford unit.

Adverse Effects. Localised oedema and erythema may occur at the site of injections administered through a catheter. Haemorrhage may occur, particularly from recent surgical wounds. Urticaria has been reported. Some patients have shown resistance to a second course of treatment, particularly after intramuscular injections. Some patients have experienced headache.

Platelet aggregation induced by adenosine diphosphate was significantly reduced in 7 patients during the first 24 hours of treatment with ancrod by intravenous injection. Forty-eight hours after starting treatment, aggregation was no longer inhibited. Concentrations of the degradation products of fibrinogen increased and then decreased similarly; in 4 patients the greatest inhibition occurred at the time of the peak concentration of degradation products. Impaired platelet aggregation might inhibit deposition of fibrin in blood vessels but might increase the risk of haemorrhage in conditions where bleeding was a hazard.— C. R. M. Prentice *et al.*, *Lancet*, 1969, *1*, 644.

Treatment of Adverse Effects. Haemorrhage usually responds to withdrawal of ancrod. If severe it may be treated by an antiserum, each ml of which is sufficient to neutralise 70 units of ancrod. An initial dose of 0.2 ml is given subcutaneously, followed in the absence of untoward reaction after 30 minutes by 0.8 ml intramuscularly; in the absence of untoward reaction 1 ml is then given intravenously 30 minutes later. In emergency the intramuscular dose may be omitted in the absence of untoward reaction to the subcutaneous dose. In life-threatening haemorrhage it may be necessary to give the serum intravenously without prior test doses but with adrenaline, antihistamines, and corticosteroids available against the possibility of anaphylactic shock. Fibrinogen 5 g or 1 litre of fresh blood or plasma should also be given to restore the fibrinogen concentration.

Precautions. As for Heparin, p.764.

Ancrod should not be given to patients with thrombocytopenia, coronary thrombosis, severe infections, septicaemia, or disseminated intravascular coagulation. It should be used cautiously in patients with cardiovascular disorders that may be complicated by defibrination and in uraemia and renal colic. Dextran injections or aminocaproic acid should not be given concomitantly. Ancrod should not be given during pregnancy.

Absorption and Fate. Ancrod is partially bound to plasma proteins. About half of a radioactive dose is eliminated from the plasma in 3 to 5 hours.

Uses. Ancrod reduces the blood-concentration of fibrinogen by the cleavage of microparticles of fibrin which are rapidly removed from the circulation by fibrinolysis or phagocytosis. It reduces blood viscosity but has no effect on established thrombi. Haemostatic concentrations of fibrinogen are normally restored in about 12 hours and normal concentrations in 10 to 20 days.

It is used in the treatment of thrombotic disorders including retinal vein occlusion and deep-vein thrombosis and to prevent thrombosis after surgery.

The usual initial dose is 2 to 3 units per kg body-weight in 50 to 500 ml of sodium chloride injection given over 4 to 12 hours (usually 6 to 8 hours) to permit physiological elimination of the microparticles. Maintenance doses of 2 units per kg are given every 12 hours by slow intravenous injection or by infusion, usually for about 7 days. The blood-fibrinogen concentration should be monitored daily; should it have risen to near normal values the next dose should be given by intravenous infusion as for the initial dose.

For the prevention of deep-vein thrombosis after hip surgery 4 units per kg have been given by subcutaneous injection postoperatively, followed by 1 unit per kg daily for 4 days.

Discussions of the role of ancrod in anticoagulant therapy.— D. Ogston and A. S. Douglas, *Drugs*, 1971, *1*, 228; *Drug & Ther. Bull.*, 1977, *15*, 87.

Reports of resistance to ancrod.— W. R. Pitney *et al.*, *Lancet*, 1969, *1*, 79; N. C. Thomson *et al.*, *Br. J. clin. Pract.*, 1976, *30*, 232. See also K. E. Chan (letter), *Lancet*, 1969, *1*, 425.

It was reported that ancrod did not provoke the platelet membrane changes required for clot retraction.— G. de Gaetano and M. B. Donati (letter), *Lancet*, 1974, *1*, 464.

Plasma fibrinogen concentrations were persistently high in 2 infants with necrotising enterocolitis. If persistent hyperfibrinogenaemia is a characteristic of necrotising enterocolitis, fibrinogen-lowering agents, such as defibrinating enzymes, like ancrod, may be of value.— L. Pickart (letter), *Lancet*, 1980, *1*, 770.

Myocardial infarction. Since a correlation had been found between the development of thrombo-embolism following myocardial infarction and a plasma-fibrinogen concentration of 7.5 mg per ml (R.M. Fulton and K. Duckett, *Lancet*, 1976, *2*, 1161) treatment with ancrod might be considered as this would reduce the fibrinogen concentration.— A. A. Sharp (letter), *Lancet*, 1977, *2*, 251.

Sickle-cell disease. In a controlled trial in 33 patients with painful sickle-cell crises there was no detectable difference between 16 treated with ancrod and 17 not so treated.— D. R. W. Haddock *et al.*, *J. trop. Med. Hyg.*, 1973, *76*, 274, per *Trop. Dis. Bull.*, 1974, *71*, 537. A similar negative report in 5 children.— J. R. Mann *et al.*, *Lancet*, 1972, *1*, 934. A contrary report.— H. M. Gilles *et al.*, *Lancet*, 1968, *2*, 542.

Thrombo-embolic disorders. Complete clinical resolution was achieved in 12 of 18 patients with deep-vein thrombosis treated with ancrod.— W. R. Pitney *et al.*, *Am. Heart J.*, 1970, *80*, 144, per *Drugs*, 1971, *2*, 167.

Neither ancrod, 140 units in 12 hours then 70 units every 12 hours for 96 hours, nor heparin 2500 units hourly for the same period had any significant effect on the thromboses in the leg veins of all 30 patients studied.— J. A. Davies *et al.*, *Lancet*, 1972, *1*, 113.

In 15 patients with peripheral arterial occlusions treated with ancrod, blood-fibrinogen concentrations fell by 96% and blood viscosity by 20 to 35%. Blood flow in the lower leg and foot increased by about 8.5%, pain ceased in 10 of 13 limbs, and small necrotic areas healed rapidly.— H. Ehringer, *Dt. med. Wschr.*, 1973, *98*, 2298, per *J. Am. med. Ass.*, 1974, *227*, 964.

Ancrod 4 units per kg body-weight daily for 6 days followed by 8 units per kg twice weekly for 4 weeks was given by subcutaneous injection to 15 patients with stable intermittent claudication. There was an 85% fall in plasma-fibrinogen concentration during the first week but after 7 weeks this had returned to its pretreatment value. There was also a temporary reduction in whole-blood viscosity. Objective signs of clinical improvement matched these changes.— J. A. Dormandy *et al.* (preliminary communication), *Lancet*, 1977, *1*, 625.

Ancrod given for 7 days was used to achieve initial defibrination in 27 patients with deep-vein thrombosis. Adequate defibrination was maintained by the use of heparin together with warfarin, phenformin, and ethyloestrenol for about 3 months. No recurrences of thrombosis had occurred during a 2-year-follow up. Nine patients complained of headache during administration of ancrod.— N. G. Kounis and W. H. Evans, *Practitioner*, 1979, *222*, 420.

Further references: N. G. Kounis and W. H. Evans (letter), *Br. med. J.*, 1977, *1*, 290; G. Lowe *et al.* (letter), *Br. med. J.*, 1977, *1*, 509.

For a comparison of ancrod, heparin, and streptokinase in the treatment of deep-vein thrombosis, see Streptokinase, p.657.

Retinal vein occlusion. In 8 patients with occlusion of the central retinal vein, defibrination was induced by an intravenous infusion over 4 hours of ancrod, 1 unit per kg body-weight in 500 ml of dextrose injection, then with the same dose in 20 ml of sodium chloride injection every 12 hours for 7 days.— R. E. Bowell *et al.*, *Lancet*, 1970, *1*, 173.

Use in surgery. Twenty-three patients undergoing surgery for fracture of the neck of the femur, a procedure associated with a high incidence of deep-vein thrombosis, were treated with low-dose ancrod and the results compared with 24 similar patients. Ancrod, given for 72 hours after surgery, reduced the fibrinogen concentration of the blood and the effect persisted to the eighth day. Three patients in the control group died from pulmonary embolism and there were 3 more non-fatal cases; there was 1 non-fatal case of pulmonary embolism in the ancrod group. The incidence of deep-vein thrombosis was not significantly different. Initially the dose of ancrod was 0.5 unit per kg body-weight over 12 hours; after the first 10 patients this was increased to 1 unit per kg over the first 12 hours, then 0.5 unit per kg per 12 hours.— W. W. Barrier *et al.*, *Br. med. J.*, 1974, *4*, 130.

In a double-blind placebo-controlled study 55 patients received subcutaneous injections of ancrod (280 units initially followed by 70 units on the 4 subsequent days) after operation for fractured neck of femur; 55 similar patients received placebo injections. Bilateral ascending venography or necropsy carried out 6 to 16 days after surgery revealed no deep-vein thrombosis in 29 of 53 patients in the ancrod group and 14 of 52 in the placebo group. The incidence of total and bilateral deep-vein thrombosis was significantly lower in the ancrod group, the difference being even more marked if only major deep-vein thromboses were included. No complications were associated with ancrod therapy.— G. D. O. Lowe *et al., Lancet*, 1978, *2*, 698.

Use in haemodialysis. In an investigation of 4 patients undergoing intermittent haemodialysis, ancrod reduced the deposition of fibrin and leucocytes on the cuprophane membrane. The procedure involved in initiating and maintaining defibrination with ancrod was more complicated than administering heparin by constant infusion, and urea elimination appeared to be less.— G. H. Hall *et al., Br. med. J.*, 1970, *4*, 591.

Proprietary Preparations

Arvin *(Berk Pharmaceuticals, UK).* Ancrod, available as an injection containing 70 units per ml, in ampoules of 1 ml. Store at 4° to 10°.

NOTE. 1-ml ampoules of antiserum specific against ancrod are available from *Berk Pharmaceuticals.*

4805-j

Anisindione. 2-(4-Methoxyphenyl)indan-1,3-dione.

$C_{16}H_{12}O_3$=252.3.

CAS — 117-37-3.

A white or creamy-white tasteless powder, odourless or with a slight sweet odour. M.p. 152° to 158°. Practically **insoluble** in water; soluble in ether, methyl alcohol, and sodium hydroxide solution; very slightly soluble in hydrochloric acid. **Store** in airtight containers.

Adverse Effects. Anisindione may cause dermatitis. An early sign of overdosage is mild bleeding.

Treatment of Adverse Effects. As for Warfarin Sodium, p.775.

Precautions. As for Phenindione, p.773.

For a report of the anticoagulant effect of anisindione being enhanced by *paracetamol*, see Warfarin Sodium, p.779.

Uses. Anisindione is an indanedione anticoagulant with actions and uses similar to those of warfarin sodium (see p.780). The full therapeutic effect is usually obtained about 36 hours after administration and the prothrombin depression may persist for up to 3 days after cessation of therapy.

The usual initial dose is 300 mg on the first day, 200 mg on the second day, and 100 mg on the third. The usual maintenance dose is 75 to 100 mg daily, but may range from 25 to 250 mg daily.

During treatment with anisindione the urine may be coloured pink.

Proprietary Names

Miradon *(Schering, USA)*; Unidone *(Unilabo, Fr.).*

4806-z

Bromindione. *p*-Bromindione. 2-(4-Bromophenyl)indan-1,3-dione.

$C_{15}H_9BrO_2$=301.1.

CAS — 1146-98-1.

Bromindione is an indanedione anticoagulant with actions and uses similar to those of phenindione. It has been given in maintenance doses of 2 to 4 mg.

Clinical reports: A. J. Seaman, *J. Am. med. Ass.*, 1961, *177*, 712; M. M. Singer *et al., ibid.*, 1962, *179*, 150; I. M. Vigran, *Curr. ther. Res.*, 1967, *9*, 372.

Proprietary Names

Fluidane *(Métadier, Fr.).*

4807-c

Clorindione. Chlorphenindione; G 25 766. 2-(4-Chlorophenyl)indan-1,3-dione.

$C_{15}H_9ClO_2$=256.7.

CAS — 1146-99-2.

Clorindione is an indanedione anticoagulant with actions and uses similar to those of phenindione (see p.773). It has been given in initial doses of 16 to 20 mg with maintenance doses of 2 to 4 mg daily.

Clinical reports: L. Poller and P. K. O'Brien, *Br. med. J.*, 1962, *1*, 1666; A. Stacher, *Wien. med. Wschr.*, 1964, *114*, 150.

Proprietary Names

Indalitan *(Ciba-Geigy, Switz.).*

4808-k

Cumetharol. Coumetarol. 3,3′-(2-Methoxyethylidene)bis(4-hydroxycoumarin).

$C_{21}H_{16}O_7$=380.4.

CAS — 4366-18-1.

Cumetharol is an orally administered anticoagulant with actions and uses similar to those of warfarin sodium (see p.775). The suggested dose was 200 to 250 mg daily for 3 days with maintenance doses of 100 to 200 mg daily.

Proprietary Names

Dicoumoxyl *(Labaz, Fr.).*

4809-a

Cyclocoumarol *(B.P.C. 1963).* Cyclocumarol. 3,4-Dihydro-2-methoxy-2-methyl-4-phenylpyrano[3,2-*c*]-chromen-5(2*H*)-one.

$C_{20}H_{18}O_4$=322.4.

CAS — 518-20-7.

Cyclocoumarol is an oral anticoagulant which has been used in doses of 100 to 200 mg initially with subsequent doses in accordance with the patient's needs.

4810-e

Dextran Sulphate *(B.P. 1958).* Dextran Sulphate Sodium. The sodium salt of sulphuric acid esters of dextran, containing not less than 10 units per mg.

CAS — 9042-14-2.

Dextran sulphate is an anticoagulant resembling heparin in its action. It was formerly used for the same purposes as heparin. Doses of 5000 to 15 000 units have been given.

In vitro studies on thrombin activity showed that dextran sulphates with a high molecular weight and high sulphur content inhibit thrombin activity directly and do not act via antithrombin III unlike heparin which may depend upon the presence of this factor to exert its anticoagulant effects.— K. Suzuki and S. Hashimoto, *J. clin. Path.*, 1979, *32*, 439.

Proprietary Names

Dextrarine *(Egic, Belg.*; *Egic, Switz.)*; Lipemol (as potassium salt) *(Rocador, Spain)*; MDS *(Jap.).*

4811-l

Dicoumarol *(B.P.C. 1954).* Dicoumarolum; Dicumarol *(U.S.P.)*; Bishydroxycoumarin; Dicumarinum; Melitoxin. 3,3′-Methylenebis(4-hydroxycoumarin).

$C_{19}H_{12}O_6$=336.3.

CAS — 66-76-2.

Pharmacopoeias. In *Braz., Int., Jug., Mex., Nord., Pol., Rus., Swiss, Turk.*, and *U.S.*

A white or creamy-white crystalline powder with a faint pleasant odour and a slightly bitter taste. The *U.S.P.* specifies the particle size. M.p. about 290°.

Practically **insoluble** in water, alcohol, and ether; slightly soluble in chloroform; freely soluble in solutions of alkali hydroxides. **Protect** from light.

When tablets of dicoumarol were reformulated to a larger size, to facilitate administration of a half-dose when required, some stabilised patients required larger doses, though disintegration-times of the new tablet were satisfactory. After investigation had shown that availability was dependent upon particle size, the tablets were again reformulated and some patients developed haemorrhage.— E. Lozinski (letter), *Can. med. Ass. J.*, 1960, *83*, 177.

The solubility of dicoumarol in water was increased by more than 20 times in the presence of 1% of povidone.— M. J. Cho *et al., J. pharm. Sci.*, 1971, *60*, 720.

Adverse Effects. As for Warfarin Sodium, p.775.

Effect on liver. The cause of the rise in serum-aminotransferase concentrations which might occur during treatment with dicoumarol was obscure. The rise in serum-lactic dehydrogenase concentrations in some patients given dicoumarol might be as great as that produced by an acute myocardial infarction.— F. Clark, *Adverse Drug React. Bull.*, 1977, Oct., 232.

Haemorrhage. Reports of haemorrhage.— I. F. Duff and W. H. Shull, *J. Am. med. Ass.*, 1949, *139*, 762; L. T. Wright and M. Rothman, *J. Am. med. Ass.*, 1951, *145*, 844; A. R. Nourizadeh and F. W. Pitts, *J. Am. med. Ass.*, 1965, *193*, 623; V. Sreerama *et al., Can. med. Ass. J.*, 1973, *108*, 305.

Pregnancy and the neonate. For details of embryopathy associated with coumarin anticoagulants, see Warfarin, p.775.

Treatment of Adverse Effects. As for Warfarin Sodium, p.775.

A 33-year-old woman who had taken dicoumarol in an attempt to secure abortion was found on examination to have a 20-week pregnancy and a plasma-dicoumarol concentration of 21 μg per ml. She was given phytomenadione, 20 mg by intramuscular injection, to control bleeding. Pregnancy continued to full-term and a healthy infant was born.— N. S. T. De Jager *et al., Can. med. Ass. J.*, 1972, *107*, 50.

Precautions. As for Warfarin Sodium, p.776.

Marked variations in anticoagulant response were recorded when dicoumarol 150 mg was given to healthy volunteers who had earlier been shown to metabolise the drug at similar rates and to attain comparable blood concentrations. Differences in the affinities of their dicoumarol receptor sites were postulated as a possible explanation, and illustrated by a clinical report of a patient with marked sensitivity to coumarin anticoagulants, presumably for that reason.— H. M. Solomon and J. J. Schrogie, *Clin. Pharmac. Ther.*, 1967, *8*, 65.

Dicoumarol could interfere with the Schack and Waxler spectrophotometric assay for plasma-theophylline concentrations to give significantly lowered results.— L. E. Matheson *et al., Am. J. Hosp. Pharm*, 1977, *34*, 496.

The daily maintenance dose of dicoumarol was significantly reduced in patients aged between 61 to 70 years of age compared with those between 50 and 60 years of age. There was a significant relationship between the dose of dicoumarol required and the weight of the patient.— S. Husted and F. Andreasen, *Br. J. clin. Pharmac.*, 1977, *4*, 559.

Interactions, absence of effect. Absence of effect of *aluminium hydroxide*.— J. J. Ambre and L. J. Fischer, *Clin. Pharmac. Ther.*, 1973, *14*, 231.

For the absence of effect of *benziodarone* on dicoumarol, see Warfarin Sodium, p.778.

An apparent enhancement of the effect of dicoumarol in 2 patients when given *tolbutamide* was not substantiated by laboratory studies or studies in 3 further patients.— H. Chaplin and M. Cassell, *Am. J. med. Sci.*, 1958, *235*, 706.

In 4 healthy subjects given dicoumarol and *tolbutamide* various pharmacokinetics parameters were affected; these opposing effects generally resulted in no change in anticoagulant effect.— E. Jähnchen *et al., Eur. J. clin. Pharmac.*, 1976, *10*, 349.

Interactions, diminished effect. Fatal haemorrhage in a patient taking dicoumarol was attributed to hypoprothrombinaemia induced by the discontinuation of *chloral hydrate* (which was found to provoke the metabolic breakdown of dicoumarol). The ability of chloral hydrate to stimulate the metabolism of dicoumarol was demonstrated in an animal study, and also observed in another patient who had received both the drugs concomitantly.— S. A. Cucinell *et al.*, *J. Am. med. Ass.*, 1966, *197*, 366.

In 6 patients taking dicoumarol the Quick index rose from 38 to 55% over 18 days when *ethchlorvynol* 1 g daily was given concomitantly.— S. A. Johansson, *Acta med. scand.*, 1968, *184*, 297, per *Pharm. J.*, 1973, *1*, 395.

The anticoagulant response to dicoumarol was diminished in 3 of 4 subjects after 1 cycle of *oral contraceptives*. The prothrombin time (of plasma stored in plastic tubes) was shortened in about half of 42 women taking oral contraceptives.— J. J. Schrogie *et al.*, *Clin. Pharmac. Ther.*, 1967, *8*, 670.

In 6 persons receiving a constant daily dose (40 to 160 mg) of dicoumarol, the serum concentration of dicoumarol fell when *phenytoin* 300 mg daily was given concomitantly for 7 days—from 29 µg per ml on the fifth day of phenytoin treatment to 21 µg per ml 5 days after phenytoin was withdrawn. The prothrombin-proconvertin (PP) concentration rose from 20 to 50% from the third to the eighth day after phenytoin was withdrawn. In 2 of 4 persons receiving dicoumarol 60 mg daily and phenytoin 300 mg daily for a week, then 100 mg daily for 5.5 weeks, the serum concentration of dicoumarol fell from 20 to 5 µg per ml. The PP concentration rose from 20 to 70%. Values returned to normal in about 3.5 and 5.5 weeks respectively after phenytoin was withdrawn. The other 2 persons showed similar falls in serum concentrations of dicoumarol but only slight rises in PP concentrations. There was no correlation between blood concentrations of phenytoin and changes in half-life of dicoumarol given intravenously.— J. M. Hansen *et al.*, *Acta med. scand.*, 1971, *189*, 15. See also under Warfarin Sodium, Enhanced Effect.

In 12 patients taking dicoumarol the whole blood clotting time was significantly reduced from a mean of 28.1 minutes to 23.9 and 22 minutes, 2 and 4 hours respectively after the administration of *prednisone* 10 mg.— J. Menczel and F. Dreyfuss, *J. Lab. clin. Med.*, 1960, *56*, 14. See also under Enhanced Effect.

Interactions, enhanced effect. In 6 healthy men the mean half-life (51 ± 9 hours) of dicoumarol rose significantly (152.5 ± 72.6) after treatment for 2 weeks with *allopurinol* 2.5 mg per kg twice daily.— E. S. Vesell *et al.*, *Ann. N.Y. Acad. Sci.*, 1971, *179*, 752.

In 4 patients taking dicoumarol, the administration of *chloramphenicol* 2 g daily caused a considerable rise in the half-life of dicoumarol.— L. K. Christensen and L. Skovsted, *Lancet*, 1969, *2*, 1397.

Enhancement by *clofibrate* or *dextrothyroxine* in 10 and 8 subjects respectively.— J. J. Schrogie and H. M. Solomon, *Clin. Pharmac. Ther.*, 1967, *8*, 70.

Plasma-dicoumarol concentrations were increased in healthy subjects given *magnesium hydroxide*.— J. J. Ambre and L. J. Fischer, *Clin. Pharmac. Ther.*, 1973, *14*, 231.

Enhancement by *norethandrolone* in 7 subjects.— J. J. Schrogie and H. M. Solomon, *Clin. Pharmac. Ther.*, 1967, *8*, 70.

In 6 healthy men the mean half-life (35.3 ± 5.3 hours) of dicoumarol after a single dose of 4 mg per kg body-weight rose significantly (105.7 ± 54.2 hours) after treatment for 8 days with *nortriptyline* 200 µg per kg thrice daily.— E. S. Vesell *et al.*, *Ann. N.Y. Acad. Sci.*, 1971, *179*, 752.

For a report of the anticoagulant effect of dicoumarol being enhanced by *paracetamol*, see Warfarin Sodium, p.779.

In males with myocardial infarction treated with *prednisone* the amount of dicoumarol needed to achieve a therapeutic index was on the average a total of 1.11 g during the first 12 days compared with 1.3 g in those not receiving prednisone—a significant difference.— J. Sievers *et al.*, *Cardiologia*, 1964, *45*, 65. See also under Diminished Effect.

A 42-year-old woman well controlled on dicoumarol developed haematuria 16 days after *stanozolol* 5 mg twice daily was added to her treatment. A second patient needed reduction in dosage of dicoumarol.— C. W. Howard *et al.* (letter), *Br. med. J.*, 1977, *1*, 1659.

Interactions, effect on other drugs. For the effect of dicoumarol in increasing the half-life of chlorpropamide and tolbutamide, see Chlorpropamide, p.853 and Tolbutamide, p.860.

Absorption and Fate. Dicoumarol is irregularly absorbed from the gastro-intestinal tract and is extensively bound to plasma protein. It crosses the placenta and appears in breast milk. It is metabolised in the liver and is excreted in the urine, mainly as metabolites.

The half-life of dicoumarol in 5 healthy persons given 2 mg per kg body-weight as a single dose was 18 to 30 hours, and 38 to 68 hours after a single dose of 4 mg per kg; in 3 of the subjects given 2 mg per kg daily for 6 days the half-life was 80 to 144 hours.— E. S. Vesell and J. G. Page, *J. clin. Invest.*, 1968, *47*, 2657, per E. S. Vesell *et al.*, *Ann. N.Y. Acad. Sci.*, 1971, *179*, 752.

Dicoumarol was bound to plasma proteins to the extent of 99%.— R. A. O'Reilly and P. M. Aggeler, *Pharmac. Rev.*, 1970, *22*, 35.

In 10 volunteers given dicoumarol 250 mg absorption, judged by the area (AUC) under the time/concentration curve, was variable, but was increased by a mean of 85% when taken with food compared with the value when taken fasting. The interindividual variation in AUC was reduced from about 6-fold fasting to less than 3-fold when taken with food.— A. Melander and E. Wåhlin, *Eur. J. clin. Pharmac.*, 1978, *14*, 441.

Uses. Dicoumarol is an orally administered anticoagulant with actions and uses similar to those of warfarin sodium (see p.780). Development of the therapeutic effect takes from 36 to 72 hours and the effect may persist for 5 days or more after discontinuing therapy. The initial dose of dicoumarol is usually 200 to 300 mg with a daily maintenance dose of 25 to 150 mg.

Because of its slow onset and long duration of action and the unpredictability of response, dicoumarol has been largely replaced by warfarin sodium.

The incidence of embolism was 0.7% in 137 patients with mitral-valve lesions and atrial fibrillation given dicoumarol for an average of 3 years, 8.3% in 48 given dicoumarol for short periods, and 2.8% in 178 not given an anticoagulant.— F. Loogen *et al.*, *Dt. med. Wschr.*, 1972, *97*, 1845.

Alcoholism. Dicoumarol therapy benefited 20 of 23 chronic alcoholics with organic brain damage, enabling them to take care of themselves and reducing the need for long-term nursing.— A. C. Walsh (letter), *J. Am. med. Ass.*, 1972, *220*, 1359.

Thrombo-embolic disorders. *Use in surgery.* The incidence of deep-vein thrombosis (34.4%) in 61 patients undergoing surgery for fracture of the neck of the femur and given dicoumarol prophylactically was not significantly different from that (36.5%) in 74 similar patients given injections of dextran 70 prophylactically.— A. Bronge *et al.*, *Acta chir. scand.*, 1971, *137*, 29, per *Abstr. Wld Med.*, 1971, *45*, 507.

Preparations

Dicumarol Capsules *(U.S.P.)*. Capsules containing dicoumarol. The *U.S.P.* requires 60% dissolution in 30 minutes.

Dicumarol Tablets *(U.S.P.)*. Tablets containing dicoumarol.

Proprietary Names

Apekumarol *(Ferrosan, Swed.)*; Dicumol *(ACF, Neth.)*; Dufalone *(Frosst, Canad.)*.

4812-y

Diphenadione *(U.S.P.)*. Diphacinone. 2-(Diphenylacetyl)indan-1,3-dione.

$C_{23}H_{16}O_3$=340.4.

CAS — 82-66-6.

Pharmacopoeias. In *U.S.*

Odourless yellow crystals or crystalline powder. M.p. 144° to 150°. Practically **insoluble** in water; soluble 1 in less than 100 of alcohol and chloroform; slightly soluble in acetone; soluble in ether and glacial acetic acid; very slightly soluble in methyl alcohol. **Store** in airtight containers. Protect from light.

Adverse Effects. Diphenadione appears to cause fewer side-effects than phenindione. Nausea has been reported. Early signs of overdosage are mild bleeding and the presence of erythrocytes in the urinary deposit.

Treatment of Adverse Effects. As for Warfarin Sodium, p.775.

Precautions. As for Phenindione, p.773.

For a report of the action of *benziodarone* in enhancing the effect of diphenadione, see Warfarin Sodium, p.778.

Uses. Diphenadione is an indanedione anticoagulant with actions and uses similar to those of warfarin sodium (see p.780). Full therapeutic effect is usually obtained within 48 to 72 hours after administration of the initial dose and prothrombin depression may persist for as long as 20 days after cessation of therapy.

The usual dose is 20 to 30 mg on the first day and 10 to 15 mg on the second day; thereafter adjusted according to the response of the patient. The average daily maintenance dose is usually 2.5 to 5 mg.

During treatment with diphenadione the urine may be coloured pink.

Diphenadione is also used as a rodenticide.

Preparations

Diphenadione Tablets *(U.S.P.)*. Tablets containing diphenadione. Store in airtight containers.

4813-j

Ethyl Biscoumacetate *(B.P.C. 1968)*. Ethyl Biscoumac.; Ethylis Biscoumacetas; Aethylis Biscoumacetas; Ethyldicoumarol; Neodicumarinum. Ethyl bis(4-hydroxycoumarin-3-yl)acetate.

$C_{22}H_{16}O_8$=408.4.

CAS — 548-00-5.

Pharmacopoeias. In *Arg.*, *Int.*, *It.*, *Jug.*, *Rus.*, and *Turk.*

A white to yellowish-white, odourless, fine crystalline powder with a persistent bitter taste. There are two forms, one melts at about 155° and the other at about 180°.

Very slightly **soluble** in water; soluble in alcohol, chloroform, and ether; soluble 1 in 40 of acetone; readily soluble in aqueous solutions of alkali hydroxides.

Of the 2 polymorphic crystal forms of ethyl biscoumacetate, form II was more suitable for use in pharmaceuticals because of its greater stability.— R. Cameroni *et al.*, *Farmaco, Edn prat.*, 1977, *32*, 125.

Adverse Effects and Treatment. As for Warfarin Sodium, p.775.

Precautions. As for Warfarin Sodium, p.776. Increased resistance to insulin is reported to have occurred in a few patients with severe diabetes during treatment with ethyl biscoumacetate.

Interactions, diminished effect. An increased dose of ethyl biscoumacetate was required in a patient while being treated with *corticotrophin*.— J. B. Chatterjea and L. Salomon, *Br. med. J.*, 1954, *2*, 790. See also under Interactions, Enhanced Effect, below.

An increased dose of ethyl biscoumacetate was required in a patient while being treated with *cortisone*.— J. B. Chatterjea and L. Salomon, *Br. med. J.*, 1954, *2*, 790.

The prothrombin time was reduced and the half-life of ethyl biscoumacetate was reduced when *glutethimide* 500 mg daily was given for 10 days. The pattern was consistent in many observations.— F. E. van Dam *et al.* (letter), *Lancet*, 1966, *2*, 1027.

Interactions, enhanced effect. In 5 adults the clearance of ethyl biscoumacetate from the plasma, after an intravenous dose of 10 mg per kg body-weight, was significantly retarded when *benziodarone* 600 mg daily was given for 6 days.— M. Verstraete *et al.*, *Archs int. Pharmacodyn. Thér.*, 1968, *176*, 33.

Haemorrhage in a patient given ethyl biscoumacetate and *corticotrophin* concomitantly. In *rabbits* haemorrhagic deaths were more frequent in those given dicoumarol and corticotrophin than in those given dicoumarol alone.— H. van Cauwenberge and L. B. Jaques, *Can. med. Ass. J.*, 1958, *79*, 536. See also under Interactions, Diminished Effect, above.

The half-life in serum of ethyl biscoumacetate was prolonged in 4 healthy men when *methylphenidate* was given for 3 to 5 days previously.— L. K. Garrettson *et al.*, *J. Am. med. Ass.*, 1969, *207*, 2053.

In 4 healthy subjects given *methylphenidate*, 10 mg twice daily for 4 days, there was no significant difference in prothrombin time or the half-life of ethyl biscoumacetate after a single dose of 20 mg per kg body-weight, before, 1 day after, or 8 days after methylphenidate.— D. E. Hague *et al.*, *Clin. Pharmac. Ther.*, 1971, *12*, 259.

Haemorrhage in 2 patients taking ethyl biscoumacetate also given *tienilic acid*.— M. Detilleux *et al.*, *Nouv. Presse méd.*, 1976, *5*, 2395.

Hemiplegia in a patient taking ethyl biscoumacetate was attributed to the replacement of his previous diuretic with *tienilic acid*.— H. Portier *et al.*, *Nouv. Presse méd.*, 1977, *6*, 468.

Absorption and Fate. Ethyl biscoumacetate is readily absorbed from the gastro-intestinal tract and is extensively bound to plasma proteins.

Ethyl biscoumacetate has been reported to appear in only small amounts in breast milk.

Ethyl biscoumacetate was readily absorbed from the gastro-intestinal tract; about 90% was bound to plasma albumin. Plasma concentrations declined at an average of about 25% per hour, but there was wide individual variation. Small doses were metabolised more rapidly than larger doses. Ethyl biscoumacetate was found in the faeces of 1 of 8 persons studied.— B. B. Brodie *et al.*, *J. Pharmac. exp. Ther.*, 1952, *106*, 453.

Ethyl biscoumacetate was almost completely metabolised in the body. An important metabolite was a hydroxylated compound, free of anticoagulant activity, which was formed in the liver and excreted into the bile and reabsorbed into the blood before being excreted in the urine.— J. J. Burns *et al.*, *J. Pharmac. exp. Ther.*, 1953, *108*, 33.

In 4 healthy men, the half-life of ethyl biscoumacetate was 2 to 3.5 hours.— L. K. Garrettson *et al.*, *J. Am. med. Ass.*, 1969, *207*, 2053.

The plasma half-life of ethyl biscoumacetate was 2 hours; it was bound to plasma proteins to the extent of 90%.— R. A. O'Reilly and P. M. Aggeler, *Pharmac. Rev.*, 1970, *22*, 35.

Uses. Ethyl biscoumacetate is an orally administered anticoagulant with actions and uses similar to those of warfarin sodium (see p.780). Maximum therapeutic effect is obtained in about 24 hours and prothrombin times usually return to normal within 48 hours of discontinuing treatment.

The usual dose is 1.2 g daily in divided doses for the first 2 or 3 days and subsequently 300 to 600 mg daily.

Preparations

Ethyl Biscoumacetate Tablets *(B.P.C. 1968)*. Tablets containing ethyl biscoumacetate.

Proprietary Names

Stabilène *(Auclair, Fr.)*; Tromexan *(Geigy, Arg.; Geigy, Belg.; Ciba-Geigy, Switz.)*; Tromexane *(Geigy, Fr.)*; Tromexano *(Padro, Spain)*.

Ethyl biscoumacetate was formerly marketed in Great Britain under the proprietary name Tromexan (*Geigy*).

4814-z

Ethylidene Dicoumarin. Ethylidene Dicoumarol. 3,3′-Ethylidenebis(4-hydroxycoumarin).

$C_{20}H_{14}O_6$=350.3.

CAS — 1821-16-5.

Ethylidene dicoumarin is an orally administered anticoagulant which has been used in initial doses of 500 mg with maintenance doses of 100 to 300 mg daily.

Proprietary Names

Pertrombon *(Gerot, Belg.)*.

4815-c

Fluorindione. Fluindione; LM 123. 2-(4-Fluorophenyl)indan-1,3-dione.

$C_{15}H_9FO_2$=240.2.

CAS — 957-56-2.

Fluorindione is an orally administered anticoagulant with actions and uses similar to those of phenindione (see p.773). It has been given in doses of 20 mg daily for 4 days with subsequent doses in accordance with the patients's needs.

An 80-mg loading dose of fluorindione reduced the prothrombin level to 37% in 24 hours; the effect lasted for 48 hours. The mean elimination half-life of fluorindione was 31 hours; about 94% was bound to plasma proteins.— J. -P. Tillement *et al.*, *Eur. J. clin. Pharmac.*, 1975, *8*, 271.

Proprietary Names

Préviscan *(Nativelle, Fr.)*.

4816-k

Leech *(B.P.C. 1954)*. Hirudo; Sangsue; Blutegel; Sanguessugas; Sanguisuga.

Pharmacopoeias. In *Chin.*, *Hung.*, *Port.*, and *Swiss.*

Leeches are fresh-water annelids; the speckled or German leech and the green or Hungarian leech are varieties of *Hirudo medicinalis*, and the five-striped or Australian leech is *H. quinquestriata* (Hirudinidae).

Leeches should be stored in unglazed earthenware pans, half-filled with soft water, and having pebbles, turf, or moss and charcoal on the bottom; the pans should be covered with muslin and kept in a shady place at a temperature between 10° and 20°.

Leeches have been used as an alternative to venesection and for withdrawing blood from inflamed and congested areas. The buccal secretion of the leech contains the anticoagulant hirudin. The part to be bitten is cleansed, moistened with sugar solution, and the leech applied by means of a leech glass or perforated pill box. About 6 ml of blood is withdrawn by each leech and does not coagulate since it is mixed with the hirudin of the buccal secretion.

Should bleeding continue after the removal of the leeches, it may be arrested with a styptic or by the pressure of a pad of cotton wool fixed over the skin puncture.

4817-a

Nicoumalone *(B.P.)*. Acenocumarin; Acenocoumarol; G 23350. 4-Hydroxy-3-[1-(4-nitrophenyl)-3-oxobutyl]coumarin.

$C_{19}H_{15}NO_6$=353.3.

CAS — 152-72-7.

Pharmacopoeias. In *Br.* and *Braz.*

An almost white to buff-coloured odourless or almost odourless powder with a slightly sweet taste and a bitter after-taste. M.p. about 198°. Practically **insoluble** in water and ether; soluble 1 in 400 of alcohol, 1 in 200 of chloroform; soluble in ethyl acetate and in solutions of alkali hydroxides. **Protect** from light.

Adverse Effects. As for Warfarin Sodium, p.775.

Usual therapeutic doses of nicoumalone slightly interfered with colour vision.— J. Laroche and C. Laroche, *Annls pharm. Fr.*, 1977, *35*, 173.

Treatment of Adverse Effects and Precautions. As for Warfarin Sodium, p.775.

Interactions, absence of effect. Absence of interaction with *diclofenac sodium*.— F. Michot *et al.*, *J. int. med. Res.*, 1975, *3*, 153.

Interactions, diminished effect. The anticoagulant effect of nicoumalone was reduced in a patient taking Gon tablets (nicotinamide and *acetomenaphthone*) concomitantly.— G. E. Heald and L. Poller (letter), *Br. med. J.*, 1974, *1*, 455.

In 18 patients under treatment with nicoumalone it was necessary to increase the dose of nicoumalone during and after 7 days' treatment with *rifampicin*.— F. Michot *et al.*, *Schweiz. med. Wschr.*, 1970, *100*, 583, per *Int. pharm. Abstr.*, 1971, *8*, 740.

Interactions, enhanced effect. For a report of *benziodarone* enhancing the effect of nicoumalone, see Warfarin Sodium, p.778.

For a report of *cimetidine* enhancing the effect of nicoumalone, see Warfarin Sodium, p.778.

A clinically significant increase in prothrombin time was reported in 3 of 6 patients given nicoumalone and *diflunisal* concomitantly.— K. F. Tempero *et al.*, *Br. J. clin. Pharmac.*, 1977, *4*, 31S.

Mention of possible enhancement of the effect of nicoumalone by *miconazole* in 1 patient.— *Proc. R. Soc. Med.*, 1977, *70*, *Suppl.* 1, 52.

Increased prothrombin time in a woman given *nalidixic acid* in addition to nicoumalone.— I. Potasman and H. Bassan (letter), *Ann. intern. Med.*, 1980, *92*, 571.

The mean prothrombin-time ratio was 1.5 in 11 women taking nicoumalone and studied over 144 woman-months; the mean dose of nicoumalone was 2.53 [mg]. When the same women and one other were studied over 230 woman-months while taking *oestrogen/progestogen contraceptives* (orally in 11) the mean prothrombin-time ratio was 1.67 and the mean dose of nicoumalone was 2.05 [mg]. The differences were statistically significant though the prothrombin-time ratios were usually within the normal range and the clinical effects were slight.— E. de Teresa *et al.*, *Br. med. J.*, 1979, *2*, 1260.

Severe haematuria and subcutaneous bleeding occurred in a 35-year-old man stabilised on nicoumalone when *oxymetholone* 100 mg daily was added to his treatment.— J. C. de Oya *et al.* (letter), *Lancet*, 1971, *2*, 259.

Ecchymoses in a patient taking nicoumalone when given *tienilic acid*.— A. Grand *et al.*, *Nouv. Presse méd.*, 1977, *6*, 2691.

Absorption and Fate. Nicoumalone is readily absorbed from the gastro-intestinal tract. It crosses the placenta and appears in breast milk. It is rapidly excreted, largely unchanged, in the urine.

The plasma half-life of nicoumalone was 24 hours.— R. A. O'Reilly and P. M. Aggeler, *Pharmac. Rev.*, 1970, *22*, 35.

The elimination half-life of nicoumalone was about 8.5 hours in 2 healthy subjects; almost 99% was bound to serum proteins *in vitro*. Aminoacetamido, and 2 alcohol metabolites were identified in plasma, all of which were shown to be active in *mice*, suggesting that the anticoagulant activity of nicoumalone was partly due to its metabolites.— W. Dieterle *et al.*, *Ciba-Geigy, Switz.*, *Eur. J. clin. Pharmac.*, 1977, *11*, 367.

Uses. Nicoumalone is an orally administered anticoagulant with actions and uses similar to those of warfarin sodium (see p.780). The maximum therapeutic effect is usually obtained within 36 to 48 hours and the prothrombin time returns to normal within about 48 hours of administration of the last dose.

The usual dose on the first day is 8 to 12 mg, on the second day 4 to 8 mg, and with a maintenance dose ranging from 1 to 8 mg depending on the prothrombin level. Higher doses have been given and it may be given as a single daily dose.

Whereas *R*(+)-nicoumalone produced an increase in the prothrombin time in 4 healthy subjects, *S*(−)-nicoumalone was ineffective in 3 subjects. The *R*(+) enantiomer of nicoumalone was considered to be the pharmacologically active component of nicoumalone.— T. Meinertz *et al.* (letter), *Br. J. clin. Pharmac.*, 1978, *5*, 187.

Myocardial infarction. For a study of nicoumalone in the prevention of recurrent myocardial infarction, see under the section in Anticoagulants, p.762.

Thrombo-embolic disorders. Use in surgery. In a randomised study in 145 women undergoing major vaginal or abdominal surgery the incidence of deep-vein thrombosis was significantly reduced by nicoumalone (incidence 3 of 48 patients) or heparin calcium (3 of 49), compared with a control group given placebo (11 of 48); when patients with malignancy were excluded the effect of nicoumalone, but not of heparin calcium, remained significant. Nicoumalone was given for 14 days, commencing at least 5 days before surgery, in a dose designed to maintain the pre-operative thromboplastin ratio (based on the British comparative thromboplastin) between 2 and 2.5; in the 3 patients who developed thrombosis this objective had not been achieved even though the partial thromboplastin time seemed adequately prolonged. Heparin calcium 5000 units was given subcutaneously twice daily for 7 days commencing 2 hours before surgery. Haemorrhage was not a major problem.— D. A. Taberner *et al.*, *Br. med. J.*, 1978, *1*, 272.

Preparations

Nicoumalone Tablets *(B.P.)*. Tablets containing nicoumalone.

Sinthrome *(Geigy, UK)*. Nicoumalone, available as tablets of 1 mg and scored tablets of 4 mg.

Other Proprietary Names

Sintrom *(Arg., Austral., Belg., Canad., Fr., Ger., Ital., Neth., Spain, Switz.)*.

4818-t

Phenindione *(B.P., U.S.P.).* Phenylinium; Fenindiona; Phenylindanedione. 2-Phenylindan-1,3-dione.

$C_{15}H_{10}O_2$=222.2.

CAS — 83-12-5.

Pharmacopoeias. In *Arg., Br., Braz., Ind., Rus., Turk.,* and *U.S.*

Soft, almost odourless, tasteless, white or creamy-white or pale yellow crystals or crystalline powder. M.p. 148° to 151°. Very slightly **soluble** in water; soluble 1 in 100 to 125 of alcohol, 1 in 6.5 of chloroform, and 1 in 110 of ether, forming yellow to red solutions; soluble 1 in 100 of 0.1M sodium hydroxide solution. **Store** in airtight containers.

The dissolution-rate of 4 brands of phenindione tablets varied from 0.08 to 2.2 mg per litre per minute. It was considered that *in vivo* the amount of phenindione available from 50-mg tablets would be about 2, 13, 13, and 45 mg respectively for the 4 brands. Three of the samples disintegrated in not more than 12 minutes.— G. B. Engel, *Australas. J. Pharm.,* 1966, *47,* S22.

The disintegration and dissolution of experimental phenindione tablets.— D. Ganderton *et al., Pharm. Acta Helv.,* 1967, *42,* 152.

A contaminant of phenindione tablets, 3-benzylidenephthalide, was a potentially immunogenic substance. As phenindione did not react irreversibly with proteins *in vitro* it was suggested that the contaminant might account for allergic reactions to phenindione.— H. Bundgaard, *Acta pharm. suec.,* 1975, *12,* 333.

Adverse Effects. Phenindione may cause haemorrhage from almost any organ of the body. Other side-effects include skin rashes, pruritus, pyrexia, diarrhoea, vomiting, and sore throat and may be early symptoms of hypersensitivity to phenindione.

The hypersensitivity reaction, which has occurred in many patients, usually occurs a few weeks after starting therapy and may lead to stomatitis, ulcerative colitis, liver and kidney damage, exfoliative dermatitis, agranulocytosis, leucopenia, eosinophilia and a leukaemoid syndrome. Deaths have occurred in persons sensitive to phenindione. Other toxic effects include alopecia, conjunctivitis, and paralysis of ocular accommodation.

A brownish-yellow discolouration of the fingernails, fingers, and palms of the hands has been reported in persons handling phenindione.

Early signs of overdosage are mild bleeding from the gums or elsewhere and the presence of erythrocytes in the urinary deposit.

Phenindione had been reported to cause aplastic anaemia.— R. H. Girdwood, *Drugs,* 1976, *11,* 394.

Phenindione could cause taste abnormalities.— I. P. Griffith, *Practitioner,* 1976, *217,* 907.

Usual therapeutic doses of phenindione slightly interfered with colour vision.— J. Laroche and C. Laroche, *Annls pharm. Fr.,* 1977, *35,* 173.

Ileus. Abdominal distension with diminished or absent bowel sounds was reported in 3 patients being treated with phenindione. One patient with complete ileus died. In 2 of the patients the condition improved when phenindione was withdrawn but when phenindione treatment was restarted in 1 of them distension again developed.— I. S. Menon (letter), *Lancet,* 1966, *1,* 1421. Paralytic ileus in another patient.— A. G. Nash (letter), *ibid.,* 1966, *2,* 51.

Neuropathy. Two cases of apparent phenindione-induced neuropathy; it was considered that spontaneous haemorrhages into the nerve sheaths, due to an unknown local factor, resulted in ischaemic neuritis of the nerve and caused the palsy in both cases.— T. N. Mehrotra, *Br. med. J.,* 1967, *3,* 218.

Pregnancy and the neonate. Congenital malformations including hypoplasia of the nasal bones occurred in 3 infants whose mothers had received warfarin or phenindione during the first trimester of pregnancy. Other effects included stippling of epiphyses and bones.— J. M. Pettifor and R. Benson, *J. Pediat.,* 1975, *86,* 459.

Treatment of Adverse Effects. As for Warfarin Sodium, p.775.

Precautions. As for Warfarin Sodium, p.776.

Since phenindione and other indanediones are more toxic than the coumarin derivatives they are generally reserved for patients who cannot take warfarin and other coumarin derivatives.

There are few specific reports but the anticoagulant effect of phenindione and other indanediones appears to be less affected than the coumarin derivatives (see Warfarin Sodium p.776) by the concomitant administration of other drugs. On theoretical grounds a range of interactions similar to that for warfarin sodium has been suggested by various authorities.

Phenindione should be used with caution in patients taking drugs liable to cause haemorrhage.

Interactions, absence of effect. For the absence of effect of *benziodarone* on phenindione, see Warfarin Sodium, p.778.

No untoward hypoprothrombinaemia had occurred in an anticoagulant clinic of about 1000 patients, generally taking phenindione, when *co-trimoxazole* was, when needed, added to their treatment.— J. de Swiet (letter), *Br. med. J.,* 1975, *3,* 491.

Phenindione was about 70% bound to plasma albumin *in vitro* at a concentration of 20 µg per ml and the degree of binding was not changed by *phenylbutazone.* There was significant displacement of coumarins under similar conditions. This could explain why there were no reports of interactions between indanediones and phenylbutazone.— J. P. Tillement *et al., Eur. J. clin. Pharmac.,* 1973, *6,* 15.

Interactions, diminished effect. A report of a *dimethicone* additive used in cooking oil associated with a diminished effect of warfarin and phenindione.— J. M. Talbot and B. W. Meade (letter), *Lancet,* 1971, *1,* 1292.

The anticoagulant effects of daily maintenance doses of 50 mg of phenindione taken by a 45-year-old man were diminished when he was given treatment with *haloperidol* 3 mg twice daily.— D. P. Oakley and H. Lautch (letter), *Lancet,* 1963, *2,* 1231.

Interactions, enhanced effect. For the enhancement of phenindione by *cimetidine,* see Warfarin Sodium, p.778.

The dose of phenindione had to be reduced in 4 men when *clofibrate* was given concomitantly.— M. F. Oliver *et al., Lancet,* 1963, *1,* 143.

There was a slight increase in sensitivity to anticoagulants in 10 of 14 patients (12 taking phenindione, 2 dicoumarol) when *corticotrophin* was given concomitantly.— A. J. Hellem and J. H. Solem, *Acta med. scand.,* 1954, *150,* 389.

When a 59-year-old man was being changed from treatment with phenindione to fibrinolytic therapy with phenformin and *ethyloestrenol* he experienced heavy subcutaneous haemorrhage and a succeeding superficial venous thrombosis. It was suggested that interaction between ethyloestrenol and phenindione was probably responsible.— D. W. Vere and G. R. Fearnley (letter), *Lancet,* 1968, *2,* 281.

Of 1158 reports of adverse reactions submitted to the Australian Drug Evaluation Committee between October 1965 and December 1968, five related to suspected interaction. Phenindione was involved in 3, its effect being enhanced by *indomethecin* in 1 and by *paracetamol* in 2 instances.— M. J. Rand, *Australas. J. Pharm.,* 1971, *52,* S17.

In 4 patients under treatment with phenindione prothrombin values of 20 to 33% fell to values of about 10 to 15% when *phenyramidol,* 0.8 to 1.6 g daily, was given concomitantly.— S. A. Carter, *New Engl. J. Med.,* 1965, *273,* 423.

The increase in the prothrombin time in 16 patients given phenindione 50 mg and *sulphaphenazole* 500 mg was significantly greater than that in 12 patients given phenindione alone.— D. R. Varma *et al.* (letter), *Br. J. clin. Pharmac.,* 1975, *2,* 467.

Absorption and Fate. Phenindione is absorbed from the gastro-intestinal tract. It diffuses across the placenta and appears in breast milk. A metabolite of phenindione is excreted in the urine.

A woman breast fed her baby while she was taking phenindione 50 mg each morning, and 50 mg alternating with 25 mg at night. The baby developed prothrombin deficiency and a large right inguinal hernia. After surgery, a large scrotal haematoma developed; cessation of breast feeding, blood transfusions, and 2 daily doses each of 1 mg of vitamin K led to recovery.— H. B. Eckstein and B. Jack (letter), *Lancet,* 1970, *1,* 672.

Uses. Phenindione is an orally administered anticoagulant with actions and uses similar to those of warfarin sodium (see p.780) but with a higher incidence of severe adverse effects so that it is now rarely employed. Maximum therapeutic effect is obtained within 36 to 48 hours and prothrombin times return to normal about 48 hours after stopping therapy.

The usual initial dose of phenindione is 200 mg as a single dose or in 2 divided doses on the first day (higher initial doses have been recommended by some authorities), 100 mg on the second day, and then maintenance doses of 25 to 150 mg daily, given in 2 divided doses at 12-hour intervals.

Phenindione has been used in conjunction with dipyridamole in glomerulonephritis and after renal transplantation.

During treatment with phenindione the urine is sometimes coloured orange or pink; disappearance of the colour when the urine is acidified distinguishes it from haematuria.

Phenindione was unsuitable for use in new patients because of its serious and occasionally fatal toxic effects, but might be used in patients also receiving an oral hypoglycaemic agent or phenytoin. Patients long stabilised on phenindione could safely continue.— *Drug & Ther. Bull.,* 1972, *10,* 25.

For the use of phenindione and dipyridamole in patients with renal allografts, see under Dipyridamole, p.1619.

Withdrawal of phenindione therapy. See under Withdrawal of Anticoagulant Therapy, p.763.

Preparations

Phenindione Tablets *(B.P., Ind. P.).* Phenylindanedione Tablets. Tablets containing phenindione. Store in airtight containers.

Phenindione Tablets *(U.S.P.).* Tablets containing phenindione.

Dindevan *(Duncan, Flockhart, UK).* Phenindione, available as scored tablets of 10, 25, and 50 mg. (Also available as Dindevan in *Austral., Denm., S.Afr.*).

Other Proprietary Names

Danilone *(Canad.);* Emandione *(Ital.);* Hedulin *(USA);* Pindione *(Belg., Fr., Ital., Switz.);* Trombantin *(Norw.).*

4819-x

Phenprocoumon *(U.S.P.).* Phenylpropylhydroxycoumarin. 4-Hydroxy-3-(1-phenylpropyl)coumarin.

$C_{18}H_{16}O_3$=280.3.

CAS — 435-97-2.

Pharmacopoeias. In *U.S.*

A fine white crystalline powder, odourless or with a slight odour. M.p. 177° to 181°. Practically **insoluble** in water; soluble in chloroform, methyl alcohol, and solutions of alkali hydroxides.

Adverse Effects and Treatment. As for Warfarin Sodium, p.775.

Cutaneous necrosis in 6 patients, due to phenprocoumon, appeared to be due to hypersensitivity.— C. H. Viets and D. Gebauer, *Dt. med. Wschr.,* 1967, *92,* 1767, per *J. Am. med. Ass.,* 1967, *202* (Oct. 23), A252.

A report of finger necrosis after 5 days' treatment with phenprocoumon.— G. Schott, *Dte GesundhWes.,* 1974, *29,* 498, per *Int. pharm. Abstr.,* 1975, *12,* 194.

A woman who had twice previously developed jaundice while taking phenprocoumon developed jaundice and parenchymal liver damage when, after some years, phenprocoumon was again given.— W. den Boer and E. A. Loeliger (letter), *Lancet,* 1976, *1,* 912. Two cases of phenprocoumon-associated hepatitis.— G. Slagboom and E. A. Loeliger, *Archs intern. Med.,* 1980, *140,* 1028.

In a 35-year-old man who had taken phenprocoumon 90 to 105 mg and piribedil 400 mg with suicidal intent, the half-life of phenprocoumon was 6.8 days; when cholestyramine 4 g was given thrice daily for 10 days from about the 7th day the half-life was reduced to 3.5 days. Cholestyramine reduced the absorption of phenprocoumon and hastened its elimination by interrupting enterohepatic recycling.— T. Meinertz *et al., Br. med. J.,* 1977, *2,* 439.

Precautions. As for Warfarin Sodium, p.776.

The absorption of phenprocoumon was unaffected by pretreatment with metformin but the elimination half-life was 123 hours in diabetic patients treated with a dietary regimen compared with 85 hours in patients treated with metformin.— E. E. Ohnhaus, *Br. J. clin. Pharmac.*, 1974, *1*, 341P.

The daily maintenance dose of phenprocoumon was significantly reduced in patients aged between 61 to 70 years of age compared with those between 50 and 60 years of age. There was also a relationship between the dose of phenprocoumon and plasma-albumin concentration.— S. Husted and F. Andreasen, *Br. J. clin. Pharmac.*, 1977, *4*, 559.

Interactions, absence of effect. In a double-blind study in 30 patients on long-term phenprocoumon treatment, the partial thromboplastin time was shortened during treatment for 3 weeks with *aspirin* 1.5 g [daily], but the one-stage prothrombin time was not affected and the dose of phenprocoumon remained unchanged.— P. Barth *et al.*, *Dt. med. Wschr.*, 1972, *97*, 1854.

For the absence of effect of *benziodarone* on the dose requirement of phenprocoumon, see Warfarin Sodium, p.778. For a report of benziodarone enhancing the effect of phenprocoumon, see below.

The fluorescence intensity, *in vitro*, (indicating binding) of phenprocoumon in the presence of human serum albumin was not significantly affected by *clofibrate*.— M. Otagiri *et al.*, *J. Pharm. Pharmac.*, 1980, *32*, 478.

Absence of effect in 19 patients taking phenprocoumon and *ibuprofen* 200 mg thrice daily.— D. Thilo *et al.*, *J. int. med. Res.*, 1974, *2*, 276. Similar findings in 24 patients.— M. J. Boekhout-Mussert and E. A. Loeliger, *ibid.*, 279. See also under Interactions, Diminished Effect, below.

Absence of effect of *insulin* on phenprocoumon concentrations in 15 patients.— P. Heine *et al.*, *Eur. J. clin. Pharmac.*, 1976, *10*, 31.

In a double-blind trial in 60 patients *mianserin* up to 60 mg daily had no significant effect on the anticoagulant activity of phenprocoumon.— H. Kopera *et al.*, *Eur. J. clin. Pharmac.*, 1978, *13*, 351.

Nitrazepam had no effect on the anticoagulant actions of phenprocoumon in a double-blind study in 22 patients.— R. Bieger *et al.*, *Clin. Pharmac. Ther.*, 1972, *13*, 361.

Absence of effect of *pindolol* on phenprocoumon in a double-blind study.— H. Vinazzer, *Int. J. clin. Pharmac. Biopharm.*, 1975, *12*, 458.

Absence of effect of *tolbutamide, glibenclamide,* or *glibornuride* on phenprocoumon concentrations in 31 patients.— P. Heine *et al.*, *Eur. J. clin. Pharmac.*, 1976, *10*, 31.

Interactions, diminished effect. In 6 subjects the effect of phenprocoumon 30 mg intravenously was significantly reduced during treatment with *cholestyramine* 12 g daily. Phenprocoumon appeared to undergo extensive enterohepatic recycling which could be interrupted by cholestyramine.— T. Meinertz *et al.*, *Clin. Pharmac. Ther.*, 1977, *21*, 731.

The fluorescence intensity, *in vitro*,(indicating binding) of phenprocoumon in the presence of human serum albumin was enhanced by *fenoprofen*.— M. Otagiri *et al.*, *J. Pharm. Pharmac.*, 1980, *32*, 478.

The fluorescence intensity, *in vitro*, (indicating binding) of phenprocoumon in the presence of human serum albumin was enhanced by *ibuprofen*.— M. Otagiri *et al.*, *J. Pharm. Pharmac.*, 1980, *32*, 478. See also under Interactions, Absence of Effect, above.

A report of 2 patients whose requirements for phenprocoumon were doubled when *rifampicin* was taken concomitantly but returned to normal after it was stopped.— R. J. Boekhout-Mussert *et al.*, *J. Am. med. Ass.*, 1974, *229*, 1903.

A report in 3 patients receiving tuberculostatic agents and phenprocoumon confirming the diminished effect of phenprocoumon induced by *rifampicin*.— H. Held, *Dt. med. Wschr.*, 1979, *104*, 1311.

See also under Nicoumalone, p.772, and Warfarin Sodium, p.778 for *rifampicin* diminishing anticoagulant activity.

Interactions, enhanced effect. Enhancement of the effect of phenprocoumon by *allopurinol* in 2 patients, with haematuria in 1; in both patients the effect was considerably delayed.— E. Jähnchen *et al.*, *Klin. Wschr.*, 1977, *55*, 759.

In 9 of 29 patients stabilised on phenprocoumon, the mean weekly dose of 17.9 mg of phenprocoumon was reduced to 14.7 mg when *benziodarone* 300 mg daily was taken, and to 9 mg when benziodarone 600 mg daily was taken, reverting to 18.4 mg when benziodarone was withdrawn. Benziodarone alone had no effect on prothrombin time. Amiodarone had no comparable effect.— M. Verstraete *et al.*, *Archs int. Pharmacodyn. Thér.*, 1968, *176*, 33.

Enhancement of the effect of phenprocoumon by *bezafibrate*.— R. Zimmerman *et al.*, *Dt. med. Wschr.*, 1977, *102*, 509.

For enhancement of the effect of a coumarin derivative by amiodarone, see Warfarin, p.778.

In 10 patients taking phenprocoumon and *diazepam* the dose of phenprocoumon needed to be increased by 0.7 mg daily (32%) when diazepam was withdrawn.— C. Schunter *et al.*, *Klin. Wschr.*, 1978, *56*, 305.

In a double-blind study 20 patients stabilised on phenprocoumon were given in addition *glafenine* 200 mg or a placebo thrice daily for 4 weeks. Thrombotest values were prolonged by glafenine during the second and third weeks of the study, and returned to their previous values during the fourth. Plasma concentrations of phenprocoumon did not change significantly, suggesting that displacement from binding sites was not involved.— J. K. Boeijinga and W. J. F. van der Vijgh, *Eur. J. clin. Pharmac.*, 1977, *12*, 291. A study reporting absence of effect of *glafenine* with indanedione derivatives, ethyl biscoumacetate, and nicoumalone.— C. Raby, *Thérapie*, 1977, *32*, 293.

A 58-year-old man who was receiving *methyltestosterone* as replacement therapy showed high sensitivity to phenprocoumon.— S. Husted *et al.*, *Eur. J. clin. Pharmac.*, 1976, *10*, 209.

For a report of the anticoagulant effect of phenprocoumon being enhanced by *paracetamol*, see Warfarin Sodium, p.779.

Absorption and Fate. Phenprocoumon is readily absorbed from the gastro-intestinal tract.

The plasma half-life of phenprocoumon was 6.5 days.— R. A. O'Reilly and P. M. Aggeler, *Pharmac. Rev.*, 1970, *22*, 35.

Phenprocoumon was bound to plasma proteins to the extent of 99%.— J. Koch-Weser and E. M. Sellers, *New Engl. J. Med.*, 1971, *285*, 487.

In 4 patients with acute myocardial infarction the half-life of phenprocoumon was 2.7 to 5.5 days, and 2.8 to 7.0 days in 5 patients with chronic cardiovascular disease.— S. Husted and F. Andreasen, *Eur. J. clin. Pharmac.*, 1977, *11*, 351.

Investigations *in vitro* into the binding of phenprocoumon to human serum albumin using fluorescence spectroscopy. Results indicated that the affinity for the *S*(−)-enantiomer of phenprocoumon is greater than the affinity for the *R*(+)-enantiomer for both the first and second binding site on crystalline human serum albumin and that the racemic form, the commercial form of phenprocoumon, had intermediate behaviour.— M. Otagiri *et al.*, *J. Pharm. Pharmac.*, 1980, *32*, 478.

Uses. Phenprocoumon is an orally administered anticoagulant with actions and uses similar to those of warfarin sodium (see p.780). The full therapeutic effect is obtained about 48 hours after administration and it takes from 7 to 14 days after cessation of treatment for the prothrombin level to return to normal.

The usual dose on the first day is from 15 to 21 mg, on the second day from 9 to 12 mg, and on the third day from 0.75 to 9 mg, depending on the prothrombin time. The maintenance dose usually ranges from 0.75 to 4.5 mg daily.

S(−)-phenprocoumon was a more potent anticoagulant than *R*(+)-phenprocoumon; the pharmacokinetic differences were mainly a result of different distributions.— E. Jähnchen *et al.*, *Clin. Pharmac. Ther.*, 1976, *20*, 342.

Myocardial infarction. For a study of phenprocoumon in the prevention of recurrent myocardial infarction, see under the section on Anticoagulants, p.762.

Preparations

Phenprocoumon Tablets *(U.S.P.)*. Tablets containing phenprocoumon.

Proprietary Names

Liquamar *(Organon, USA)*; Marcoumar *(Roche, Belg.; Roche, Denm.; Roche, Neth.; Roche, Switz.)*; Marcumar *(Roche, Canad.; Roche, Ger.)*.

Phenprocoumon was formerly marketed in Great Britain under the proprietary name Marcoumar (*Roche*).

4820-y

Sodium Iodoheparinate. Iodohéparinate de Sodium. A derivative of heparin.

Sodium iodoheparinate 1 mg is stated to be equivalent to 100 units of heparin.

Sodium iodoheparinate is an anticoagulant with actions and uses similar to those of heparin (see p.763). It is given intravenously in doses of 200 to 600 mg daily. In smaller doses and as sublingual tablets it is given in atherosclerotic disorders. It is also used topically as a 2.5% ointment and a 1.5% eye lotion.

Proprietary Names

Dioparine *(Biosédra, Fr.; Biosedra, Switz.)*.

4821-j

Sodium Pentosan Polysulphate. Sodium Xylanpolysulphate. A synthetic sulphated polyanion with heparin-like properties. Preparations with a molecular weight of about 2000 and about 4000 appear to be used.

CAS — 37319-17-8.

Sodium pentosan polysulphate reduces thrombogenesis and has fibrinolytic properties; its anticoagulant effect is much less than that of heparin. It is used in the prevention and treatment of thrombo-embolic disorders. Doses of 100 mg have been given intramuscularly. It has also been given by mouth and used topically as a 0.5 or 1.5% ointment.

A double-blind study was carried out on 12 patients with thrombophilia and hyperdyslipidaemia who were given sodium pentosan polysulphate by mouth and intramuscularly. There was increased fibrinolytic activity, a reduction in platelet aggregation, and a decrease in cholesterol and triglycerides, accompanied by an increase in lipoprotein-lipase.— G. Frandoli *et al.*, *Arzneimittel-Forsch.*, 1972, *22*, 759.

In a controlled trial the incidence of deep-vein thrombosis was 9% in those treated with calcium heparinate, 15% in those treated with sodium pentosan polysulphate, and 51% in controls.— S. Joffe, *Archs Surg., Chicago*, 1976, *111*, 37, per *J. Am. med. Ass.*, 1976, *235*, 216.

In 6 patients with primary hyperlipidaemias (Fredrickson types IIb, IV, and V) and 10 healthy subjects given sodium pentosan polysulphate (SP 54, mol. wt 2000) 75 mg thrice daily by mouth or 100 mg thrice daily rectally no effect on serum-lipid concentrations was observed. In a further 11 patients and 5 healthy subjects given a single dose (Depot Thrombocid, mol. wt 4000) of 300 mg intramuscularly a 50% decrease in serum-triglyceride concentration occurred after 6 hours returning to pre-treatment values after 24 hours. No lasting effect on serum lipids was observed in 5 patients given Depot Thrombocid 300 mg weekly for 3 weeks. Side-effects included haemorrhagic diatheses, hair loss, and thrombocytopenia.— H. Greten *et al.*, *Dt. med. Wschr.*, 1978, *103*, 204.

Further references: G. Turazza *et al.*, *Arzneimittel-Forsch.*, 1973, *23*, 654; M. Loos and V. W. Rahlfs, *Arzneimittel-Forsch.*, 1976, *26*, 584; M. Raff *et al.*, *Münch. med. Wschr.*, 1977, *119*, 817.

Proprietary Names

Fibrase *(Smith Kline & French, Ital.)*; Fibrocid *(Lacer, Spain)*; Hémoclar *(Clin-Comar-Byla, Fr.)*; SP 54 *(Bene-Chemie, Ger.)*; Tavan-SP 54 *(Noristan, S.Afr.)*; Thrombocid *(Bene-Chemie, Ger.; Lacer, Spain)*.

4822-z

Warfarin Potassium *(U.S.P.)*.

Potassium Warfarin; Warfarinum Kalicum.

$C_{19}H_{15}KO_4$=346.4.

CAS — 2610-86-8.

Pharmacopoeias. In *Jap.* and *U.S.*

A white odourless crystalline powder with a slightly bitter taste; it is discoloured by light. It loses not more than 10% of its weight on drying. **Soluble** 1 in 1.5 of water and 1 in 1.9 of alcohol;

very slightly soluble in chloroform and ether; freely soluble in acetone and methyl alcohol. A 1% solution in water has a pH of 7.2 to 8.3. **Protect** from light.

Warfarin potassium has properties and uses similar to those of warfarin sodium (below).

Preparations

Warfarin Potassium Tablets *(U.S.P.)*. Tablets containing warfarin potassium. Potency is expressed in terms of anhydrous warfarin potassium. Store in airtight containers. Protect from light.

Proprietary Names

Athrombin-K *(Purdue Frederick, Canad.; Purdue Frederick, USA)*.

4823-c

Warfarin Sodium *(B.P., U.S.P.)*. Warfarin Sod.; Warfarinum Natricum; Sodium Warfarin.

The sodium salt of 4-hydroxy-3-(3-oxo-1-phenylbutyl)coumarin.

$C_{19}H_{15}NaO_4$=330.3.

CAS — 81-81-2 (warfarin); 129-06-6 (sodium salt).

The *B.P.*, *Braz. P.*, and *U.S.P.* permit also the use of the crystalline clathrate with isopropyl alcohol, containing 4.3 to 8.3% w/w of isopropyl alcohol.

NOTE. Commercial warfarin sodium is racemic.

Pharmacopoeias. In *Br.*, *Braz.*, *Int.*, *Nord.*, *Turk.*, and *U.S. Nord.* also includes an injection grade.

A white odourless amorphous or crystalline powder with a slightly bitter taste; it is discoloured by light.

Soluble 1 in less than 1 of water and alcohol; slightly soluble in chloroform and ether. A 1% solution in water has a pH of 7.2 to 8.3 and a 5% solution is not more than slightly opalescent. A 6.1% solution is iso-osmotic with serum. **Store** in airtight containers. Protect from light.

Incompatibility has been reported with adrenaline hydrochloride, amikacin sulphate, cyanocobalamin, metaraminol tartrate, oxytocin, promazine hydrochloride, tetracycline hydrochloride, and vancomycin hydrochloride.

There was loss of clarity when intravenous solutions of warfarin sodium were mixed with those of adrenaline hydrochloride, cyanocobalamin, metaraminol tartrate, promazine hydrochloride, or tetracycline hydrochloride in dextrose injection, or ammonium chloride, invert sugar, laevulose, or lactated Ringer's injections.— J. A. Patel and G. L. Phillips, *Am. J. Hosp. Pharm.*, 1966, *23*, 409.

Absorption of warfarin sodium increasing with time occurred when solutions in water were exposed to polyvinyl chloride infusion bags. Absorption was greater when dextrose injection was the diluent.— P. Moorhatch and W. L. Chiou, *Am. J. Hosp. Pharm.*, 1974, *31*, 72.

Adverse Effects. The major risk from warfarin therapy is of haemorrhage from almost any organ of the body. Other adverse effects occasionally reported include alopecia, fever, nausea, vomiting, diarrhoea, hypersensitivity reactions, priapism, and, rarely, skin reactions and necrosis. Early signs of overdosage are mild bleeding from the gums or elsewhere and the presence of erythrocytes in the urinary deposit.

A foetal warfarin syndrome has been described.

An abnormal form of prothrombin was detected in the plasma taken 12 hours after the first dose of warfarin in 3 patients; this increased until the proportion of abnormal to normal prothrombin was greater at 48 to 84 hours. In a healthy subject given one dose of warfarin 15 mg the abnormal form first appeared at 8 hours and reached a maximum between 24 and 48 hours.— M. Brozović and L. Gurd (letter), *Lancet*, 1971, *2*, 427. See also *idem*, *Br. J. Haemat.*, 1973, *24*, 579.

Spontaneous unilateral kidney rupture occurred in 2 patients who were treated with warfarin sodium. Nephrectomy was performed but only 1 patient survived.— I. Luna *et al.*, *J. Urol.*, 1973, *109*, 788.

Warfarin sodium could cause orange discoloration of the urine.— R. B. Baran and B. Rowles, *J. Am. pharm. Ass.*, 1973, *NS13*, 139.

A report of eosinophilia associated with the administration of warfarin sodium in a 70-year-old man.— D. Hall and K. Link (letter), *New Engl. J. Med.*, 1981, *304*, 732.

Abuse. A report of the abuse of warfarin.— R. Gelfand and G. Mitani, *J. nerv. ment. Dis.*, 1979, *167*, 447.

Effect on liver. Sign of liver cell necrosis in 2 patients regressed only when anticoagulants (warfarin and dicoumarol) were withdrawn.— N. Rehnquist, *Acta med. scand.*, 1978, *204*, 335.

Intrahepatic cholestasis following warfarin therapy; the patient recovered on withdrawal of warfarin.— D. B. Jones *et al.*, *Postgrad. med. J.*, 1980, *56*, 671.

Haemorrhage. A 23-year-old man, who soaked bread in a 0.5% solution of warfarin for periods of 30 minutes on 10 occasions in 24 days, developed gross haematuria 2 days after the last exposure. Other symptoms were haematoma and bleeding from the nose, lips, and mucous membranes. It was considered that the warfarin was absorbed percutaneously.— B. Fristedt and N. Sterner, *Archs envir. Hlth*, 1965, *11*, 205, per *Bull. Hyg., Lond.*, 1966, *41*, 30.

There was one case of major and 14 of minor gastro-intestinal haemorrhage in 423 patients treated with warfarin alone.— H. Jick and J. Porter, *Lancet*, 1978, *2*, 87.

Other reports of haemorrhage. Haemorrhagic pancreatitis.— R. R. Larsen *et al.*, *N.Y. St. J. Med.*, 1962, *62*, 2397. Spontaneous haemarthrosis in 3 patients.— G. E. McLaughlin *et al.*, *J. Am. med. Ass.*, 1966, *196*, 1020. Haemorrhage from the bowel wall in 3 elderly patients taking warfarin sodium or diphenadione.— S. T. Killian and E. J. Heitzman, *J. Am. med. Ass.*, 1967, *200*, 591. Intrathoracic haemorrhage in 2 patients given heparin and warfarin sodium.— H. B. Simon *et al.*, *J. Am. med. Ass.*, 1969, *208*, 1830. Haemopericardium in 3 patients.— R. L. Miller, *J. Am. med. Ass.*, 1969, *209*, 1362. Salivary-gland haemorrhage.— S. P. Glasser *et al.* (letter), *Am. Heart J.*, 1971, *82*, 282, per *Int. pharm. Abstr.*, 1972, *9*, 746. Haemothorax.— M. T. Diamond and S. C. Fell, *N.Y. St. J. Med.*, 1973, *73*, 691. Intramural haematoma.— N. F. Hacker, *Med. J. Aust.*, 1973, *2*, 220. Intramural haemorrhage in the ileum and ascending colon.— J. E. Hale, *Postgrad. med. J.*, 1975, *51*, 107. Hepatic rupture.— M. H. Roberts and F. R. Johnston, *Archs Surg., Chicago*, 1975, *110*, 1152. Haemarthrosis of the knee joint.— J. H. Wild and N. J. Zvaifler, *Arthritis Rheum.*, 1976, *19*, 98. Intraperitoneal haemorrhage from a ruptured corpus luteum.— J. R. Krause and R. Amores, *Sth. med. J.*, 1976, *69*, 1220. Retinal haemorrhage leading to blindness.— K. Maddox (letter), *Med. J. Aust.*, 1977, *1*, 420. Haemorrhagic corpus luteum.— K. P. Wong and P. G. Gillett, *Can. med. Ass. J.*, 1977, *116*, 388. Haematuria.— Y. F. Dajani (letter), *New Engl. J. Med.*, 1977, *297*, 222. Oesophageal haematoma.— R. F. Smart and A. R. Stone, *N.Z. med. J.*, 1978, *87*, 176. Corpus-luteum haemorrhage in 6 patients.— D. D. Tresch *et al.*, *Ann. intern. Med.*, 1978, *88*, 642. Rupture of the liver.— H. Dizadji *et al.*, *Archs Surg., Chicago*, 1979, *114*, 734. Haemobilia.— J. C. Goldsmith *et al.*, *Sth. med. J.*, 1979, *72*, 748.

See also under Pregnancy and the Neonate, below.

Pregnancy and the neonate. In a review of warfarin embryopathy 27 cases were exposed between the 6th and 9th weeks of pregnancy; 7 died in infancy and 6 had significant disability. Of 13 further infants exposed in the 2nd and 3rd trimester of pregnancy 6 had embryopathy and had CNS abnormalities not attributable to haemorrhage. Exposure in the first trimester was associated with embryopathy while exposure in the 2nd or 3rd trimesters was associated with an increased incidence of CNS defects. An analysis of all published reports of the use of coumarin anticoagulants during pregnancy suggested that 1 in 6 of such pregnancies resulted in live-born infants with embryopathy, CNS manifestations, or haemorrhage, while 1 in 6 resulted in still-birth or spontaneous abortion.— R. M. Pauli and J. G. Hall (letter), *Lancet*, 1979, *2*, 144.

Discussions of warfarin embryopathy.— J. Warkany, *Teratology*, 1976, *14*, 205; R. W. Smithells, *Br. med. Bull.*, 1976, *32*, 27; W. L. Shaul and J. G. Hall, *Am. J. Obstet. Gynec.*, 1977, *127*, 191; R. M. Hill and L. Stern, *Drugs*, 1979, *17*, 182.

Foetal fatalities associated with warfarin.— W. A. Epstein, *J. Mt Sinai Hosp.*, 1959, *26*, 562, per *Clin. Pharmac. Ther.*, 1961, *2*, 458; G. H. Mahairas and A. B. Weingold, *Am. J. Obstet. Gynec.*, 1963, *85*, 234; S. J. Fillmore and E. McDevitt, *Ann. intern. Med.*, 1970, *73*, 731, per *Clin. Med.*, 1972, *79* (Mar.), 33.

An infant died of haemorrhage on the third day after birth even though the mother's warfarin therapy had been discontinued 7 days before delivery and the infant had been given 1 mg of vitamin K at birth.— E. Ikonen *et al.* (letter), *Lancet*, 1970, *2*, 1252. An infant with a large head caused by bilateral subdural haemorrhage was born to a woman who had received warfarin during pregnancy; the infant died 3 hours after birth.— M. J. Robinson *et al.*, *Br. med. J.*, 1980, *281*, 35.

An infant exposed to warfarin in the first trimester of pregnancy was considered normal until 5 months of age when delay in psychomotor development was noted. He was found to have primary brain malformation (agenesis of the corpus callosum), very mildly affected facial features, and possible optic atrophy. In an analysis of all published reports of foetal warfarin exposure for at least 5 days and up to 32 weeks of gestation 16 of 115 were live-born with abnormalities and 15 of 115 represented foetal wastage. Exposure throughout pregnancy was associated with the foetal warfarin syndrome of severe nasal hypoplasia, stippled epiphyses, optic atrophy, microcephaly, and mental retardation. Exposure for at least a month was associated with microcephaly and optic atrophy without the facial or bone defects.— W. Holzgreve *et al.* (letter), *Lancet*, 1976, *2*, 914.

Asplenia with cardiac, gastro-intestinal, and liver defects were reported in an infant whose mother had received warfarin and heparin during the first 6 weeks of pregnancy.— D. R. Cox *et al.* (letter), *Lancet*, 1977, *2*, 1134.

A report of abnormal development in a child born after a 31-week gestation to a woman who had taken warfarin throughout pregnancy.— R. E. Stevenson *et al.*, *J. Am. med. Ass.*, 1980, *243*, 1549.

Reports of the foetal warfarin syndrome (chondrodysplasia punctata).— I. J. Kerber *et al.*, *J. Am. med. Ass.*, 1968, *203*, 223; M. H. Becker *et al.*, *Am. J. Dis. Child.*, 1975, *129*, 356; W. L. Shaul *et al.*, *ibid.*, 360; J. M. Pettifor and R. Benson, *J. Pediat.*, 1975, *86*, 459; S. Sherman and B. D. Hall (letter), *Lancet*, 1976, *1*, 692; M. Carson and M. Reid (letter), *ibid.*, 1356; R. M. Pauli *et al.*, *J. Pediat.*, 1976, *88*, 506; E. M. Richman and J. E. Lahman, *ibid.*, 509; M. Barr and A. R. Burdi, *Teratology*, 1976, *14*, 129; A. Abbott *et al.*, *Br. med. J.*, 1977, *1*, 1639; K. O. Raivio *et al.*, *Acta paediat. scand.*, 1977, *66*, 735; M. J. Robinson *et al.* (letter), *Med. J. Aust.*, 1978, *1*, 157; M. F. Smith and M. D. Cameron (letter), *Lancet*, 1979, *1*, 727; M. Baillie *et al.*, *Br. J. Ophthal.*, 1980, *64*, 633; M. F. Whitfield, *Archs Dis. Childh.*, 1980, *55*, 139.

Skin disorders and necrosis. Bilateral breast necrosis, disseminated intravascular coagulation, and micro-angiopathic haemolytic anaemia developed in a 59-year-old woman 4 days after anticoagulant therapy had been changed from heparin (8 days) to warfarin sodium 2.5 mg daily. Mastectomy was performed.— M. DiCato and L. Ellman (letter), *Ann. intern. Med.*, 1975, *83*, 233. A similar report.— J. P. Lacy and R. R. Goodin (letter), *ibid.*, *82*, 381.

Extensive dermal gangrene followed administration of inappropriately high loading doses of warfarin in 2 patients with compromised hepatic function. Subsequently small doses of warfarin were re-introduced without further lesions.— C. A. Hardisty, *Postgrad. med. J.*, 1978, *54*, 123.

A pruritic rash on the legs, trunk, and upper arms of a 52-year-old man was associated with treatment with warfarin sodium. The patient tolerated dicoumarol.— P. Kwong *et al.*, *J. Am. med. Ass.*, 1978, *239*, 1884.

The risk of the development of warfarin necrosis of the skin during anticoagulant therapy might be reduced by the now more usual practice of commencing treatment with small incremental doses of warfarin sodium 10 mg over 2 or 3 days rather than a large loading dose of 40 mg.— J. D. Kirby and R. L. Brearley (letter), *Br. J. Derm.*, 1978, *98*, 707.

Further references to skin discoloration and necrosis in patients taking warfarin.— E. D. Vaughan *et al.* (letter), *J. Am. med. Ass.*, 1969, *210*, 2283; E. D. Everett and E. L. Overholt, *Archs Derm.*, 1969, *100*, 588, per *J. Am. med. Ass.*, 1969, *210*, 1115; C. E. Davis *et al.*, *Ann. Surg.*, 1972, *175*, 647, per *Practitioner*, 1972, *209*, 393; R. G. Moses and J. R. Warren, *Med. J. Aust.*, 1973, *2*, 76; M. Di Cato, *Postgrad. Med.*, 1975, *58*, 133; J. D. Kirby and P. J. Marriott, *Br. J. Derm.*, 1976, *94*, 97; M. Schnider and C. R. D'Souza, *Can. J. Surg.*, 1976, *19*, 64; P. A. Faraci *et al.*, *Surgery Gynec. Obstet.*, 1978, *146*, 695.

Treatment of Adverse Effects. Mild bleeding due to overdosage of warfarin sodium is usually adequately controlled by discontinuing the drug. Phytomenadione 2 to 20 mg by mouth is usually effective in treating the effects of overdosage.

Severe hypoprothrombinaemia may be treated by the slow intravenous injection of 2.5 to 20 mg of phytomenadione. In rare cases, 50-mg doses have been given. The dose of phytomenadione should be the smallest needed to control bleeding, particularly if anticoagulant treatment is to continue. Infusions of whole blood, plasma, or suitable concentrates of appropriate coagulation factors may also be given.

In 6 healthy volunteers, considerable variation occurred in the response of phytomenadione to counter the anticoagulant effects of warfarin administered either at the same time or 48 hours earlier.— P. D. Zieve and H. M. Solomon, *J. Lab. clin. Med.*, 1969, *73*, 103.

Skin necrosis due to coumarin therapy was a rare but potentially lethal complication which usually developed within 3 to 10 days of starting treatment. Until haemorrhagic infarcts occurred the lesions were reversible. Treatment included phytomenadione if the prothrombin time was prolonged and heparin 35 000 units daily in 3 divided doses for at least 3 or 4 days.— R. M. Nalbandian *et al.*, *Obstet. Gynec., N.Y.*, 1971, *38*, 395, per *Int. pharm. Abstr.*, 1972, *9*, 344.

A woman who had suffered warfarin-induced skin necrosis developed early signs of oral anticoagulant necrosis on receiving phenindione. Immediate intravenous administration of heparin abolished the skin changes over the next 3 hours; no vitamin K was given.— J. M. Boss and R. Summerly (letter), *Br. J. Derm.*, 1979, *100*, 617.

A prothrombin complex concentrate (Prothromplex) provided quicker, more controlled, but less sustained reversal of coumarin overdosage than phytomenadione.— D. A. Taberner *et al.*, *Br. med. J.*, 1976, *2*, 83.

The successful treatment with phytomenadione of a woman who took warfarin 250 mg and an unknown number of tablets containing carisoprodol, phenacetin, and caffeine. It was emphasised that account must be taken of the rapid turnover of phytomenadione compared with the slow elimination of warfarin when treating warfarin overdosage.— T. D. Bjornsson and T. F. Blaschke (letter), *Lancet*, 1978, *2*, 846 and 1164. A valid estimate of the turnover-rate of vitamin K_1 in man was not yet possible. Repeated doses of phytomenadione should be given in massive warfarin overdosage, but this did not necessarily apply to complete or partial reversal of the anticoagulant effect in patients on therapeutic doses of warfarin, where single small doses of phytomenadione were often sufficient.— M. J. Shearer and P. Barkhan (letter), *Lancet*, 1979, *1*, 266.

Repeated infusions of fresh frozen plasma maintained partial reversal of massive warfarin overdosage in 2 patients with prosthetic heart valves in whom complete anticoagulant reversal was undesirable.— F. Toolis *et al.*, *Br. med. J.*, 1981, *283*, 581.

Precautions. Warfarin sodium and other anticoagulants should be administered with great caution to patients with impaired liver or kidney function or severe hypertension and also in any condition where there is a risk of serious haemorrhage, such as haemorrhagic blood dyscrasias, haemophilia, ulcerative disorders, threatened abortion, subacute bacterial endocarditis, in the presence of extensive surgical wounds, and after recent surgery to the eye or CNS. It should be given with care during menstruation. Warfarin should not be used immediately after parturition or surgery. Because of the risk of foetal damage and haemorrhage it is not generally recommended during pregnancy. Use in breast-feeding is discussed under Absorption and Fate, p.780.

The response to anticoagulant therapy may be altered by many factors, including varying individual response, genetic factors, pregnancy, hepatic or renal function, other concomitant diseases, decreased synthesis or absorption of vitamin K, enhanced or diminished metabolism, protein binding, and concomitant drug therapy.

The effects of coumarin anticoagulants are *diminished* by barbiturates, cholestyramine, glutethimide, phenazone, rifampicin, and vitamin K, and may be diminished by griseofulvin. There have been occasional reports of a diminished effect with carbamazepine, chlorthalidone, dichloralphenazone, dimethicone, and ethchlorvynol.

The effects of coumarin anticoagulants are *enhanced* in most patients by oxyphenbutazone or phenylbutazone, and are enhanced in some patients by anabolic agents (especially 17-alkyl compounds), some aminoglycoside antibiotics, aspirin in large doses, azapropazone, benziodarone, chloral hydrate (diminished effect also reported) or triclofos, chloramphenicol, cimetidine, clofibrate, dextrothyroxine (and, probably to a lesser degree, other thyroid preparations), diflunisal, disulfiram, mefenamic acid, metronidazole, paracetamol in large doses, phenyramidol, and quinidine.

There have been occasional reports of an enhanced effect with allopurinol, aminosalicyclic acid, co-trimoxazole and some sulphonamides, disopyramide, ethacrynic acid, feprazone, glafenine, glucagon, indomethacin, isoniazid, magnesium hydroxide, methylphenidate, nalidixic acid, phenformin, sulindac, sulphinpyrazone, tienilic acid, and the tricyclic antidepressants amitriptyline and nortriptyline.

On theoretical grounds the effects of coumarin anticoagulants might be enhanced by contrast media, liquid paraffin, propylthiouracil and other thiouracils, quinine, and tetracyclines, but there appear to be no clinical reports.

Absence of interaction has been reported for bumetanide, chlorothiazide, diclofenac, frusemide, hydrochlorothiazide, insulin, meprobamate, methaqualone, mianserin, naproxen, pindolol, tolbutamide, and, apart from isolated cases, for the benzodiazepine tranquillisers and ibuprofen.

There are conflicting reports of the effects of corticosteroids and oral contraceptives.

It is often possible to give anticoagulants concomitantly with other drugs provided the effect is monitored and the dose of anticoagulant is adjusted, if necessary, on commencing or discontinuing the second drug.

A patient with Graves' disease exhibited sensitivity to warfarin when he was hyperthyroid.— A. G. Vagenakis *et al.*, *Johns Hopkins med. J.*, 1972, *131*, 69, per *J. Am. med. Ass.*, 1972, *221*, 1576. A similar report.— T. Self *et al.*, *J. Am. med. Ass.*, 1975, *231*, 1165.

Decreased anticoagulant sensitivity was observed by the author in himself whenever he experienced a migraine attack.— P. Narasimhan (letter), *Lancet*, 1974, *2*, 1143.

A 72-year-old man with impaired hepatic ability to metabolise theophylline was unusually sensitive to warfarin, needing none for 5 days, and a 2-mg dose sufficing for 10 days.— M. H. Jacobs and R. M. Senior, *Am. Rev. resp. Dis.*, 1974, *110*, 342, per *Drugs*, 1975, *9*, 381.

Warfarin could interfere with the Schack and Waxler spectrophotometric assay for plasma-theophylline concentrations to give significantly lowered results.— L. E. Matheson *et al.*, *Am. J. Hosp. Pharm.*, 1977, *34*, 496.

Factors affecting interindividual differences in the response to oral anticoagulants.— A. M. Breckenridge, *Drugs*, 1977, *14*, 367.

The ingestion of leafy vegetables or other foods high in vitamin K would not affect the dose requirements of warfarin provided the intake of those foods was consistent.— *J. Am. med. Ass.*, 1977, *237*, 1871.

Warfarin in therapeutic doses interfered with tissue factor generation and so with the skin test reactivity used to assess the integrity of the cell-mediated immune system, and in the diagnosis of specific diseases.— R. L. Edwards and F. R. Rickles, *Science*, 1978, *200*, 541.

Grossly impaired warfarin metabolism was associated with iron-deficiency anaemia in a 24-year-old woman.— D. P. Nicholls and A. M. M. Shepherd (letter), *Lancet*, 1978, *2*, 215.

Comparable effect of warfarin in 34 diabetic and 33 non-diabetic patients.— T. H. Self *et al.* (letter), *J. Am. med. Ass.*, 1978, *239*, 2239.

A retrospective study of 98 patients who underwent coronary by-pass surgery indicated that warfarin or aspirin taken up to 7 days pre-operatively could significantly increase the degree of mediastinal bleeding during the first 3 or 4 hours following surgery. Mean mediastinal blood loss in the 9 patients who had received heparin was no different from the 64 patients in the control group. It was recommended that warfarin or aspirin should be withdrawn at least 7 days before coronary by-pass surgery.— M. Torosian *et al.*, *Ann. intern. Med.*, 1978, *89*, 325.

Interactions. For reviews of drugs affecting the response to warfarin sodium and other anticoagulants, see R. A. O'Reilly and P. M. Aggeler, *Pharmac. Rev.*, 1970, *22*, 35; A. I. Sandler, *Drug Intell. & clin. Pharm.*, 1970, *4*, 146; *Br. med. J.*, 1971, *4*, 128; J. Koch-Weser and E. M. Sellers, *New Engl. J. Med.*, 1971, *285*, 487 and 547; *Drug & Ther. Bull.*, 1972, *10*, 25; I. H. Stockley, *Pharm. J.*, 1973, *1*, 339; *Am. J. Hosp. Pharm.*, 1973, *30*, 705; D. Bernstein, *Drug Intell. & clin. Pharm.*, 1974, *8*, 172; A. Breckenridge, *Br. J. clin. Pharmac.*, 1974, *1*, 285; S. M. MacLeod and E. M. Sellers, *Drugs*, 1976, *11*, 461; G. S. Avery, *Drugs*, 1977, *14*, 132; F. B. Davis *et al.*, *Archs intern. Med.*, 1977, *137*, 197; *Med. Lett.*, 1979, *21*, 5; M. L'E. Orme and M. J. Serlin, *Adverse Drug React. Bull.*, 1980, Apr., 292.

The half-life of warfarin sodium, following a single dose of 40 mg by mouth, was 26.5 hours in 15 heavy drinkers compared with 41 hours in 11 control subjects.— *J. Am. med. Ass.*, 1968, *206*, 1709.

The prothrombin time rose in 1 of 10 patients stabilised on warfarin given *alcohol* about 240 ml daily for 2 weeks.— J. A. Udall, *Clin. Med.*, 1970, *77* (Aug.), 20.

In a patient taking warfarin who had taken *alcohol* (about 50 ml of whisky) daily, plasma concentrations of warfarin fell and the Thrombotest value changed when alcohol was withdrawn. When challenged with alcohol the concentration in plasma rose and epistaxis occurred.— A. Breckenridge and M. Orme, *Ann. N.Y. Acad. Sci.*, 1971, *179*, 421.

Alcohol 30 to 100 g had no significant effect on the prothrombin times of 41 volunteers receiving chronic anticoagulant therapy with coumarins.— J. Koch-Weser and E. M. Sellers, *New Engl. J. Med.*, 1971, *285*, 547.

In a 6-month study of 277 patients taking anticoagulants, usually warfarin, the frequency of dose changes was used to assess the stability of control in patients taking other drugs; on this basis the following might enhance the anticoagulant effect—antimicrobial agents including cephalosporins, phenformin, clofibrate, tricyclic antidepressants including imipramine, chlorpromazine, anabolic steroids, and allopurinol; barbiturates might diminish the effect.— J. R. B. Williams *et al.*, *Q. J. Med.*, 1976, *45*, 63.

Interactions, absence of effect. Absence of effect of *aluminium hydroxide* on the absorption of warfarin.— J. J. Ambre and L. J. Fischer, *Clin. Pharmac. Ther.*, 1973, *14*, 231.

Absence of effect of *bumetanide* in 11 subjects.— C. M. Nilsson *et al.*, *J. clin. Pharmac.*, 1978, *18*, 91.

In 5 patients stabilised on warfarin, *chlordiazepoxide* 5 or 10 mg thrice daily had no effect on plasma-warfarin concentrations or Thrombotest values. In 2 of the 5 patients the urinary excretion of 6β-hydroxycortisol, a measure of liver microsomal enzyme activity, was increased.— M. Orme *et al.*, *Br. med. J.*, 1972, *3*, 611. A similar report.— J. B. Whitfield *et al.*, *Br. med. J.*, 1973, *1*, 316.

Absence of effect of *chlordiazepoxide* with unspecified coumarin anticoagulants.— P. P. deCarolis and M. L. Gelfand, *J. clin. Pharmac.*, 1975, *15*, 557.

See also under Interactions, Diminished Effect, below.

Absence of effect with *chlorothiazide*.— D. S. Robinson and D. Sylwester, *Ann. intern. Med.*, 1970, *72*, 853.

For the absence of effect of *clofibrate in vitro* on anticoagulant activity, see Phenprocoumon, p.774. But see also under Interactions, Enhanced Effect, below.

In 4 patients stabilised on warfarin, *diazepam* 5 mg thrice daily had no effect on plasma-warfarin concentrations or Thrombotest values.— M. Orme *et al.*, *Br. med. J.*, 1972, *3*, 611. A similar report.— J. B. Whitfield *et al.*, *Br. med. J.*, 1973, *1*, 316.

Absence of effect of *diazepam* with unspecified coumarin anticoagulants.— P. P. deCarolis and M. L. Gelfand, *J. clin. Pharmac.*, 1975, *15*, 557.

For the absence of effect of *diclofenac sodium* on a coumarin anticoagulant, see Nicoumalone, p.772.

Digoxin had no effect on plasma-warfarin concentrations in patients on long-term warfarin treatment.— A. Breckenridge and M. Orme, *Ann. N.Y. Acad. Sci.*, 1971, *179*, 421.

Studies in healthy subjects given warfarin and *fenbufen* indicating that the minor, nonsignificant prolongations of coagulation tests are unlikely to be clinically significant.— J. P. Savitsky *et al.*, *Clin. Pharmac. Ther.*, 1980, *27*, 284.

Administration of *flunitrazepam* to 20 patients receiving long-term therapy with coumarin anticoagulants had no effect on prothrombin levels.— J. Dry *et al.* (letter), *Thérapie*, 1976, *31*, 805.

Absence of effect of *frusemide* in 11 healthy subjects.— C. M. Nilsson *et al.*, *J. clin. Pharmac.*, 1978, *18*, 91.

Hydrochlorothiazide had no effect on plasma-warfarin concentrations in patients on long-term warfarin treatment.— A. Breckenridge and M. Orme, *Ann. N.Y. Acad. Sci.*, 1971, *179*, 421.

Absence of effect in 50 patients taking warfarin and *ibuprofen* 0.6 to 1.2 g daily.— L. Goncalves, *J. int. med. Res.*, 1973, *1*, 180. Double-blind studies in 36 subjects showed that administration of *ibuprofen* in doses of 1.2 to 2.4 g daily during administration of warfarin 7.5 mg daily for 14 days did not alter the degree of hypoprothrombinaemia caused by warfarin.— J. A. Penner and P. H. Abbrecht, *Curr. ther. Res.*, 1975, *18*, 862.

Studies on the displacement of albumin-bound warfarin by anti-inflammatory agents *in vitro* indicating that *ibuprofen* appeared not to be involved in a clinically significant interaction with warfarin.— J. C. McElnay and P. F. D'Arcy, *J. Pharm. Pharmac.*, 1980, *32*, 709.

For the absence of effect of *ibuprofen* on anticoagulant activity, see also under Phenprocoumon, p.774.

See also under Interactions, Diminished Effect and Interactions, Enhanced Effect, below.

Double-blind studies in healthy subjects indicated that the anticoagulant effect of warfarin sodium was neither enhanced nor reduced by *indomethacin*.— E. S. Vesell *et al.*, *J. clin. Pharmac.*, 1975, *15*, 486.

Studies on the displacement of albumin-bound warfarin by anti-inflammatory agents *in vitro* indicating that *indomethacin* appeared not to be involved in a clinically significant interaction with warfarin.— J. C. McElnay and P. F. D'Arcy, *J. Pharm. Pharmac.*, 1980, *32*, 709.

For *indomethacin* enhancing anticoagulant activity, see Interactions, Enhanced Effect, below and under Phenindione, p.773.

Studies on the displacement of albumin-bound warfarin by anti-inflammatory agents *in vitro* indicating that *ketoprofen* appeared not to be involved in a clinically significant interaction with warfarin.— J. C. McElnay and P. F. D'Arcy, *J. Pharm. Pharmac.*, 1980, *32*, 709.

Absence of effect of *magnesium hydroxide*.— J. J. Ambre and L. J. Fischer, *Clin. Pharmac. Ther.*, 1973, *14*, 231.

But see under Dicoumarol, p.771.

Studies on the displacement of albumin-bound warfarin by anti-inflammatory agents *in vitro* indicating that *mefenamic acid* appeared not to be involved in a clinically significant interaction with warfarin.— J. C. McElnay and P. F. D'Arcy, *J. Pharm. Pharmac.*, 1980, *32*, 709. See also under Interactions, Enhanced Effect, below.

The mean prothrombin time in 9 patients taking warfarin was unchanged when *meprobamate* 1.6 g daily was given concomitantly.— J. A. Udall, *Curr. ther. Res.*, 1970, *12*, 724.

In 8 patients stabilised on long-term therapy with warfarin sodium, prothrombin times were slightly reduced when *meprobamate* 2.4 g daily was added to their treatment, but the effect was not clinically different from that in 9 patients given warfarin and placebo.— L. Gould *et al.*, *J. Am. med. Ass.*, 1972, *220*, 1460.

Absence of effect of *meprobamate* with unspecified coumarin anticoagulants.— P. P. deCarolis and M. L. Gelfand, *J. clin. Pharmac.*, 1975, *15*, 557.

For the absence of effect of *mianserin* on anticoagulant activity, see under Phenprocoumon, p.774.

Absence of effect of *methaqualone*.— J. B. Whitfield *et al.*, *Br. med. J.*, 1973, *1*, 316.

Studies in healthy subjects showed no evidence of a clinically important alteration of either the pharmacokinetics or anticoagulant activity of racemic warfarin by the usual therapeutic doses of *naproxen*.— A. Jain *et al.*, *Clin. Pharmac. Ther.*, 1979, *25*, 61. See also J. T. Slattery *et al.*, *ibid.*, 51.

Studies on the displacement of albumin-bound warfarin by anti-inflammatory agents *in vitro* indicating that *naproxen* appeared not to be involved in a clinically significant interaction with warfarin.— J. C. McElnay and P. F. D'Arcy, *J. Pharm. Pharmac.*, 1980, *32*, 709.

In 3 patients stabilised on warfarin *nitrazepam* 10 mg at night had no effect on plasma-warfarin concentrations or Thrombotest values.— M. Orme *et al.*, *Br. med. J.*, 1972, *3*, 611. Further similar reports.— A. Breckenridge and M. Orme, *Ann. N.Y. Acad. Sci.*, 1971, *179*, 421; J. B. Whitfield *et al.*, *Br. med. J.*, 1973, *1*, 316.

See also under Phenprocoumon, p.774, for the absence of effect of *nitrazepam* on anticoagulant activity.

For the absence of effect of *pindolol* on anticoagulant activity, see Phenprocoumon, p.774.

Absence of effect of *psyllium* on warfarin.— D. S. Robinson *et al.*, *Clin. Pharmac. Ther.*, 1971, *12*, 491.

In healthy subjects *sulindac* had no significant effect on the hypoprothrombinaemia induced by warfarin but in 1 patient with a potassium-losing renal tubular defect, sulindac markedly increased the warfarin-induced hypoprothrombinaemia.— J. P. Loftin and E. S. Vesell, *J. clin. Pharmac.*, 1979, *19*, 733. See also under Interactions, Enhanced Effect, below.

A retrospective survey of 224 patients with diabetes indicated that the effects of warfarin and dicoumarol were not enhanced or diminished by *tolbutamide*.— R. L. Poucher and T. J. Vecchio, *J. Am. med. Ass.*, 1966, *197*, 1069.

See also under Dicoumarol, p.770, and Phenprocoumon, p.774 for the absence of effect of *tolbutamide* on anticoagulant activity.

Many interactions have been suggested for which there appear to be no reports to suggest clinical significance. Such interactions include those between oral anticoagulants and the following: acetohexamide, acetylcholine, adrenaline, antihistamines (except the H_2-receptor antagonist, cimetidine), atropine, bile salts, carbenoxolone sodium, carisoprodol, activated charcoal, chlorbutol, chlormezanone, chloroquine, chlorphenesin, cyclamates, dextrans, ethotoin, glyceryl trinitrate, guaiphenesin, guanethidine, mersalyl sodium, mephenytoin, methyldopa, methocarbamol, methyprylone, monoamine oxidase inhibitors, narcotic analgesics, nitrofurantoin, nicotinamide, paraldehyde, phentolamine, primidone, probenecid, propranolol, protamine, proteolytic enzymes, purgatives, reserpine, riboflavine, tolazoline, tybamate, vitamin A, vitamin D, and xanthines.

Interactions, diminished effect. For the effect of *acetomenaphthone* diminishing anticoagulant activity, see under Nicoumalone, p.772.

The administration of *ascorbic acid* for a cold shortened the prothrombin time in a 52-year-old woman who was receiving warfarin sodium.— G. Rosenthal (letter), *J. Am. med. Ass.*, 1971, *215*, 1671. *Ascorbic acid* 1 g daily for 2 weeks did not significantly shorten the prothrombin time in 5 patients on warfarin therapy.— R. Hume *et al.* (letter), *ibid.*, 1972, *219*, 1479. A 70-year-old woman who had been consuming approximately 16 g of *ascorbic acid* daily was resistant to warfarin therapy. Only when the dose of warfarin sodium was increased to 25 mg daily did a significant increase in prothrombin time occur.— E. C. Smith *et al.* (letter), *ibid.*, *221*, 1166. A study in 19 patients stabilised on warfarin sodium therapy in doses ranging from 1.5 to 7.5 mg daily indicated that no clinically significant antagonism of the hypoprothrombinaemic action of warfarin occurred when doses of *ascorbic acid* 3, 5, and 10 g were given concurrently for 7-day periods although falls in total plasma warfarin of 2 to 40% were noted.— C. L. Feetam *et al.*, *Toxic. appl. Pharmac.*, 1975, *31*, 544.

In vitro the absorption of warfarin sodium was reduced by 6.9% by *bismuth carbonate*.— J. C. McElnay *et al.* (letter), *Br. med. J.*, 1978, *2*, 1166.

Serum-warfarin concentrations were reduced and plasma-prothrombin-proconvertin values increased in 2 patients when given *carbamazepine*. The half-life of warfarin in blood was reduced in 2 of 3 patients given carbamazepine.— J. M. Hansen *et al.*, *Clin. Pharmac. Ther.*, 1971, *12*, 539.

Prothrombin time increased following withdrawal of *carbamazepine* in a 56-year-old man receiving warfarin 6 mg daily and carbamazepine 300 to 600 mg daily and he subsequently required only 4 mg of warfarin daily. Following re-introduction of carbamazepine some months later his warfarin requirement increased to 5.5 mg daily over a period of 5 weeks. It was suggested that this interaction was probably due to increased warfarin metabolism produced by carbamazepine.— J. R. Y. Ross and L. Beeley, *Br. med. J.*, 1980, *280*, 1415.

The anticoagulant action of warfarin was antagonised by normal sedative doses of *chloral hydrate*.— S. A. Cucinell *et al.*, *J. Am. med. Ass.*, 1966, *197*, 366.

Concentrations of warfarin fell significantly in 4 of 5 patients on long-term warfarin treatment given *chloral hydrate* 1 g daily, but Thrombotest values remained stable.— A. Breckenridge and M. Orme, *Ann. N.Y. Acad. Sci.*, 1971, *179*, 421.

See also under Dicoumarol, p.770 for *chloral hydrate* diminishing anticoagulant activity.

See also under Interactions, Enhanced Effect, below, for *chloral hydrate* enhancing the anticoagulant activity of warfarin.

One of 2 patients given *chlordiazepoxide* 15 mg daily had a fall in warfarin concentration.— A. Breckenridge and M. Orme, *Ann. N.Y. Acad. Sci.*, 1971, *179*, 421. See also under Interactions, Absence of Effect, above.

In 6 healthy subjects given a single dose of warfarin sodium the hypoprothrombinaemia was significantly reduced when the dose of warfarin was repeated with the addition of *chlorthalidone* 100 mg daily. The plasma-warfarin concentration remained stable, and the haematocrit was significantly increased. The decreased response to warfarin was probably due to a concentration of circulating clotting factors during diuresis.— R. A. O'Reilly *et al.*, *Ann. N.Y. Acad. Sci.*, 1971, *179*, 173.

The anticoagulant activity of warfarin and its serum concentrations were reduced in 6 subjects given *cholestyramine* 12 g in 3 divided doses starting either before or at the same time as warfarin 40 mg.— D. S. Robinson *et al.*, *Clin. Pharmac. Ther.*, 1971, *12*, 491.

In 5 healthy subjects treatment with *cholestyramine* about 12 g daily reduced the biological half-life of warfarin from a mean of 1.98 to 1.34 days and increased the rate of elimination of warfarin. The total activity of warfarin per dose was reduced by cholestyramine in all the subjects. It was suggested that warfarin underwent enterohepatic recycling which could be interrupted by cholestyramine.— E. Jähnchen *et al.*, *Br. J. clin. Pharmac.*, 1978, *5*, 437.

See also under Phenprocoumon, p.774 for *cholestyramine* diminishing anticoagulant activity.

For the effect of *corticosteroids* in diminishing or enhancing anticoagulant activity, see under Dicoumarol, (prednisone) p.771, and Ethyl Biscoumacetate (corticotrophin), p.771.

For the effect of *danazol* in reducing clotting time, see p.1409.

Plasma concentrations of warfarin fell significantly with a change in Thrombotest values in 5 patients taking warfarin who were given *dichloralphenazone* 1.3 g daily (equivalent to 1 g of chloral hydrate).— A. Breckenridge and M. Orme, *Ann. N.Y. Acad. Sci.*, 1971, *179*, 421. A significant fall in plasma concentrations of warfarin occurred in patients taking warfarin sodium and who were also given *dichloralphenazone* or phenazone.— J. B. Whitfield *et al.*, *Br. med. J.*, 1973, *1*, 316.

A *dimethicone* additive used in cooking oil was associated with a diminished effect of warfarin and phenindone.— J. M. Talbot and B. W. Meade (letter), *Lancet*, 1971, *1*, 1292.

Prothrombin activity in a 45-year-old man taking warfarin sodium was reduced when griseofulvin 1 g daily was given concomitantly and was further reduced when *ethchlorvynol* 500 mg daily was added to the regimen.— S. I. Cullen and P. M. Catalano, *J. Am. med. Ass.*, 1967, *199*, 582. See also Dicoumarol, p.771 for *ethchlorvynol* diminishing anticoagulant activity.

For the effect of *fenoprofen* in diminishing anticoagulant activity *in vitro*, see under Phenprocoumon, p.774.

Pretreatment of 10 healthy volunteers with *glutethimide* 1 g reduced plasma-warfarin concentrations at 24, 48, and 72 hours and reduced the half-life by nearly 50%. *Chloral betaine* 1.74 g had less effect. Phenobarbitone and glutethimide interfered with the hypoprothrombinaemic effect of warfarin; chloral betaine and placebo did not.— M. G. MacDonald *et al.*, *Clin. Pharmac. Ther.*, 1969, *10*, 80. In 10 patients stabilised on warfarin 17.5 to 77.5 mg weekly mean prothrombin times were significantly reduced from 18.8 to 16.1 seconds when *glutethimide* 500 mg was given daily at night.— J. A. Udall, *Curr. ther. Res.*, 1975, *17*, 67.

See also under Ethyl Biscoumacetate, p.771 for *glutethimide* reducing anticoagulant activity.

Griseofulvin depressed the anticoagulant activity of warfarin in 3 of 4 patients. This was restored to normal levels when the griseofulvin was stopped.— S. I. Cullen and P. M. Catalano, *J. Am. med. Ass.*, 1967, *199*, 582.

The prothrombin time fell in 4 of 10 patients stabilised on warfarin given *griseofulvin* 1 g daily for 2 weeks.— J. A. Udall, *Clin. Med.*, 1970, *77* (Aug.), 20.

For the effect of *haloperidol* on diminishing anticoagulant activity, see under Phenindione, p.773.

For the effect of *ibuprofen* in diminishing anticoagulant activity, see under Phenprocoumon, p.774. See also under Interactions, Absence of Effect, above and Interactions, Enhanced Effect, below.

The effect of warfarin was diminished in a farmer after exposure to the *insecticides* toxaphene and gamma benzene hexachloride.— W. H. Jeffery *et al.*, *J. Am. med. Ass.*, 1976, *236*, 2881.

In vitro the absorption of warfarin sodium was reduced by 19.4% by *magnesium trisilicate*.— J. C. McElnay *et al.* (letter), *Br. med. J.*, 1978, *2*, 1166.

When *mercaptopurine* was given on 2 occasions to a patient receiving warfarin the dose of warfarin had to be increased to cope with the increased Thrombotest.— A. S. D. Spiers and R. S. Mibashan (letter), *Lancet*, 1974, *2*, 221.

For the effect of *oral contraceptives* in diminishing anticoagulant activity, see under Dicoumarol, p.771. See also Enhanced Effect under Nicoumalone, p.772.

Concentrations of warfarin fell significantly with a change in Thrombotest values in 5 patients given *phen-*

azone 600 mg daily; this was attributed to induction of enzyme activity.— A. Breckenridge and M. Orme, *Ann. N.Y. Acad. Sci.*, 1971, *179*, 421. A significant fall in plasma concentration of warfarin occurred in patients taking warfarin sodium and who were also given dichloralphenazone or *phenazone*. The plasma concentration of gamma-glutamyl transpeptidase (a measure of liver enzyme activity) was increased, approximately proportionately.— J. B. Whitfield *et al.*, *Br. med. J.*, 1973, *1*, 316.

For the effect of *phenytoin* in diminishing anticoagulant activity, see under Dicoumarol, p.771. See also Interactions, Enhanced Effect, below.

The anticoagulant effect of warfarin was diminished when a patient began to use a liquid nutrition preparation which contained *phytomenadione*.— R. A. O'Reilly and D. A. Rytand (letter), *New Engl. J. Med.*, 1980, *303*, 160. See also M. Lee *et al.* (letter), *Ann. intern. Med.*, 1981, *94*, 140.

Studies in 10 healthy subjects showed that *rifampicin* reduced the prothrombin time and plasma-warfarin concentrations following the administration of warfarin by mouth or intravenous injection. The interaction was considered to be due to rifampicin enhancing the elimination of warfarin from the body.— R. A. O'Reilly, *Ann. intern. Med.*, 1974, *81*, 337. A similar report in 18 patients.— F. Michot *et al.*, *Schweiz. med. Wschr.*, 1970, *100*, 583, per *Pharm. J.*, 1973, *1*, 339. Further references.— J. A. Romankiewicz and M. Ehrman, *Ann. intern. Med.*, 1975, *82*, 224; R. A. O'Reilly, *ibid.*, *83*, 506.

See also under Nicoumalone, p.772, and Phenprocoumon, p.774 for *rifampicin* diminishing anticoagulant activity.

A study into the interaction between *spironolactone* and warfarin. It was concluded that the interaction results from the diuresis induced by spironolactone leading to concentration of clotting factors and decreased anticoagulant effect.— R. A. O'Reilly, *Clin. Pharmac. Ther.*, 1980, *27*, 198.

Interactions, enhanced effect. In 6 healthy subjects usual doses of *allopurinol* had no significant influence on the elimination-rate of warfarin in the group as a whole, although an apparent inhibitory effect was observed in some individuals. No significant changes were observed in the steady-state plasma concentrations of warfarin in 2 patients during administration of allopurinol. Administration to most patients on anticoagulant therapy was unlikely to alter dosage requirements but, because of wide individual variability, warfarin requirements might be reduced in a few patients.— M. D. Rawlins and S. E. Smith, *Br. J. Pharmac.*, 1973, *48*, 693.

A patient receiving digitalis, diuretics, and heparin was also given warfarin. Heparin was discontinued 4 days later and on the next day allopurinol and indomethacin were given for hyperuricaemia. Six days later the prothrombin time had increased to 42.2 seconds. *Allopurinol* and *indomethacin* were considered to enhance the action of warfarin.— T. H. Self *et al.* (letter), *Lancet*, 1975, *2*, 557.

In a study of 8 healthy subjects *allopurinol* had no significant effect on warfarin.— S. M. Pond *et al.*, *Aust. N.Z. J. Med.*, 1975, *5*, 324.

For *allopurinol* enhancing other anticoagulants, see also under Dicoumarol, p.771 and Phenprocoumon, p.774.

A 71-year-old man who received *aminosalicylic acid* 12 g daily with isoniazid and pyridoxine had greatly increased prothrombin times (17.8 to 130 seconds over 20 days) when his usual dose of warfarin was increased from 2.5 to 5 mg.— T. H. Self (letter), *J. Am. med. Ass.*, 1973, *223*, 1285.

A report of *amiodarone* enhancing the effect of warfarin sodium in 9 patients. Amiodarone was discontinued after a few months in 4 of the patients but its potentiating effect on the activity of warfarin persisted for another 1½ to 4 months.— U. Martinowitz *et al.* (letter), *New Engl. J. Med.*, 1981, *304*, 671. See also A. Rees *et al.*, *Br. med. J.*, 1981, *282*, 1756; M. J. Serlin *et al.* (letter), *ibid.*, *283*, 58.

Report, without detail, of clinically significant interaction between the tricyclic antidepressant *amitriptyline* and warfarin.— J. Koch-Weser, *Clin. Pharmac. Ther.*, 1973, *14*, 139.

See also abstract below relative to nortriptyline.

There was no significant increase in the prothrombin time in 10 patients stabilised on warfarin when also given *aspirin* 3 g daily for 2 weeks.— J. A. Udall, *Clin. Med.*, 1970, *77* (Aug.), 20. There was no significant difference in prothrombin activity between healthy subjects given a single dose of warfarin and the same subjects when given a single dose of warfarin plus *aspirin* 1.95 g daily for several days before and after the warfarin. In 4 of 11 healthy subjects given an anticoagulant (usually warfarin 5 to 7.5 mg daily) prothrombin activity was reduced to 28 to 38% and was further reduced when aspirin 1.95 g daily was given concomitantly. In 4 subjects given warfarin and aspirin 3.9 g daily prothrombin activity was further reduced and all 4 had mild haemorrhage. Cutaneous bleeding time was increased in subjects given warfarin when aspirin 1.95 g was given concomitantly, platelet adhesiveness was not affected, and platelet aggregation was reduced in some parameters. Anticoagulants given alone in a dose sufficient to cause a reduction to about 35% of prothrombin activity did not affect bleeding time, platelet adhesiveness, or platelet aggregation.— R. A. O'Reilly *et al.*, *Ann. N.Y. Acad. Sci.*, 1971, *179*, 173.

Interaction with *salicylates* in 4 patients with loss of control.— K. J. Starr and J. C. Petrie, *Br. med. J.*, 1972, *4*, 133. See also under Phenprocoumon, p.774 for a report of *aspirin* not affecting anticoagulant activity.

A 59-year-old woman who had taken warfarin for about 6 years developed a gastric ulcer treated for about 4 months with Caved-(S) and antacids; she was also taking digoxin, frusemide, spironolactone, and allopurinol. She developed haematemesis 4 days after *azapropazone* 300 mg four times daily was added to her treatment; the prothrombin ratio was increased from about 2.8 to 15.7 and the prothrombin time to 220 seconds.— P. R. Powell-Jackson, *Br. med. J.*, 1977, *1*, 1193.

Marked enhancement of the effect of warfarin occurred in 3 patients given *azapropazone*. In 2 healthy subjects the prothrombin time was increased when azapropazone was added to the stabilised dose of warfarin.— A. E. Green *et al.* (letter), *Br. med. J.*, 1977, *1*, 1532.

The binding of warfarin to human serum albumin was reduced in the presence of *azapropazone*.— J. C. McElnay and P. F. D'Arcy (letter), *Br. med. J.*, 1977, *2*, 773. See also *idem*, *J. Pharm. Pharmac.*, 1980, *32*, 709.

In 15, 7, 9, and 8 patients respectively the dose of warfarin sodium, nicoumalone, ethyl biscoumacetate, and diphenadione was reduced by 46, 25, 17, and 42% when *benziodarone* 300 to 600 mg daily was given concomitantly. The dose of phenprocoumon, dicoumarol, phenindione, and clorindione was not affected.— K. Pyörälä *et al.*, *Acta med. scand.*, 1963, *173*, 385.

See also under Ethyl Biscoumacetate, p.771 and Phenprocoumon, p.774 for *benziodarone* enhancing anticoagulant activity.

An elevated prothrombin time in a 49-year-old man stabilised on warfarin was possibly due to his receiving *benzylpenicillin* 24 million units daily for endocarditis; concomitant treatment included digoxin, diuretics, paracetamol, and, for 1 day, streptomycin.— M. A. Brown *et al.*, *Can. J. Hosp. Pharm.*, 1979, *32*, 18.

Three healthy physicians were given warfarin; when stable prothrombin times were achieved *chloral hydrate* in 1-g daily doses was given concomitantly. Plasma-warfarin concentrations fell but the prothrombin times increased.— E. M. Sellers and J. Koch-Weser, *New Engl. J. Med.*, 1970, *283*, 827.

Warfarin *in vitro* was displaced from human albumin by trichloroacetic acid, a metabolite of chloral hydrate. In volunteers given a single dose of warfarin before and after treatment with *chloral hydrate* there was no consistent change in hypoprothrombinaemia. Persons regularly taking warfarin experienced an enhanced effect when given chloral hydrate. These different effects could be explained by the double effect of displacing warfarin from binding sites—increase of free warfarin and more rapid elimination. Of 500 patients taking warfarin, 237 also received chloral hydrate, 52 for at least 3 days. Of these 52 patients 13 experienced significant enhancement of effect (assessed by computer analysis), 27 experienced no enhancement, and in 12 evaluation was not possible.— E. M. Sellers and J. Koch-Weser, *Ann. N.Y. Acad. Sci.*, 1971, *179*, 213.

No significant differences in prothrombin times, plasma-warfarin concentrations, or daily warfarin requirement occurred in 17 subjects receiving long-term warfarin treatment when they were given *chloral hydrate* or an equivalent amount of *chloral betaine* concomitantly.— P. F. Griner *et al.*, *Ann. intern. Med.*, 1971, *74*, 540, per *Int. pharm. Abstr.*, 1971, *8*, 555.

The course of therapy with warfarin was observed in 134 adult hospital patients, 67 of whom also received *chloral hydrate*. On days 2 to 4 of treatment the dose of warfarin necessary to maintain a satisfactory prothrombin time was lower in those receiving chloral hydrate but from the 5th day the necessary doses of warfarin were similar whether or not the patient also received chloral hydrate.—Boston Collaborative Drug Surveillance Program, *New Engl. J. Med.*, 1972, *286*, 53.

A review of interactions between anticoagulants and *chloral hydrate*.— *Lancet*, 1972, *1*, 524.

In 5 of 8 subjects given warfarin 25 mg initially then 5 mg daily for 5 days, warfarin activity was increased when *chloral hydrate* 1 g was taken at night. The mean prothrombin time in the 8 patients while taking chloral hydrate was significantly greater than when taking placebo. In 10 subjects given a constant dose of warfarin there was no significant difference in the prothrombin time during ingestion of chloral hydrate 500 mg daily for 4 weeks compared with 4 weeks before and after such ingestion. A review of the literature showed no report of haemorrhage. Minor enhancement during the initation of warfarin treatment was not important because the dose would then be carefully monitored. The effect was not considered clinically significant.— J. A. Udall, *Ann. intern. Med.*, 1974, *81*, 341.

Prolongation of the prothrombin time to 51.5 seconds in a 17-year-old man stabilised on warfarin was attributed to a single dose of 3 g of *chloral hydrate*.— R. E. Galinsky *et al.* (letter), *Ann. intern. Med.*, 1975, *83*, 286.

See also under Interactions, Diminished Effect, above for reports of *chloral hydrate* reducing the anticoagulant activity of warfarin.

Massive gastro-intestinal haemorrhage and low prothrombin concentrations developed in 3 patients who had been given respectively *chloramphenicol* and tetracycline, chloramphenicol and procaine penicillin, and chloramphenicol, tetracycline, and procaine penicillin.— A. P. Klippel and B. Pitsinger, *Archs Surg., Chicago*, 1968, *96*, 266.

See also under Dicoumarol, p.771 for *chloramphenicol* enhancing anticoagulant activity.

A preliminary report of a study demonstrating that administration of *cimetidine* 1 g daily to subjects receiving a stable dose of warfarin, might raise the blood-clotting ratio and prothrombin time by about 20%. These results had been confirmed by a small number of clinical reports. The mechanism of the interaction was unknown. Patients receiving concurrent anticoagulant and cimetidine therapy should be monitored carefully and might need a reduced dose of warfarin or other oral anticoagulant.— A. C. Flind, *Smith Kline & French* (letter), *Lancet*, 1978, *2*, 1054.

Cimetidine 200 mg thrice daily and 400 mg at night was given to 4 patients receiving warfarin, 1 receiving nicoumalone, and 1 receiving phenindione. Prolongation of prothrombin time occurred in all patients (more than doubled in 2 patients), being induced more rapidly in those taking nicoumalone and phenindione than in those taking warfarin. The enhancement of the effect of warfarin was subsequently confirmed in 7 healthy subjects. Studies on the effect of cimetidine on the half-life of phenazone suggested that the basis of the interaction was probably inhibition of drug metabolism.— M. J. Serlin *et al.*, *Lancet*, 1979, *2*, 317.

Further reports of *cimetidine* enhancing warfarin activity.— D. Hetzel *et al.* (letter), *Lancet*, 1979, *2*, 639; B. A. Silver and W. R. Bell, *Ann. intern. Med.*, 1979, *90*, 348; B. A. Wallin *et al.* (letter), *Ann. intern. Med.*, 1979, *90*, 993.

The prothrombin time rose in 2 of 10 patients stabilised on warfarin when given *clofibrate* 2 g daily for 2 weeks. The remaining 8 tolerated clofibrate without effect for 4 weeks.— J. A. Udall, *Clin. Med.*, 1970, *77* (Aug.), 20.

Interaction with *clofibrate* in 4 patients with loss of control.— K. J. Starr and J. C. Petrie, *Br. med. J.*, 1972, *4*, 133.

The action of warfarin was significantly enhanced in patients taking *clofibrate*. Age increased the action of warfarin in patients given clofibrate but not in others.— R. D. Eastham (letter,), *Lancet*, 1973, *1*, 1450.

The effect of *clofibrate* in enhancing the anticoagulant action of warfarin was studied in 8 healthy subjects. The rate of elimination and the half-life of warfarin were unchanged and there was no significant displacement from plasma proteins. It was considered that the interaction was due to an enhancement of effect on the clotting factors dependent on vitamin K.— S. M. Pond *et al.*, *Aust. N.Z. J. Med.*, 1975, *5*, 324.

Enhancement by *clofibrate* of the effect of $S(-)$-warfarin in 3 of 4 patients; absence of effect with $R(+)$-warfarin.— T. D. Bjornsson *et al.*, *J. Pharmacokinet. Biopharm.*, 1977, *5*, 495.

Evidence to suggest that the enhanced effect of warfarin by *clofibrate* is not a pure pharmacokinetic displacement interaction since the concentration of free warfarin in plasma is unaltered, but that the underlying mechanism of the interaction must be of a pharmacodynamic nature.— T. D. Bjornsson *et al.*, *J. Pharmac. exp. Ther.*, 1979, *210*, 316.

See also under Dicoumarol, p.771 and Phenindione, p.773 for *clofibrate* enhancing anticoagulant activity.

But see also under Interactions, Absence of Effect, above.

For changes in clotting function in patients given *colaspase*, see Colaspase, p.198.

For a report of the prolongation of prothrombin times by *contrast media*, see p.436.

For conflicting reports of *corticotrophin*, diminishing or enhancing anticoagulant activity, see Ethyl Biscoumacetate, p.771.

The anticoagulant effects of warfarin, as measured by the prothrombin ratio, were enhanced by *co-trimoxazole* in 6 of 20 patients given both drugs.— C. Hassall *et al.* (letter), *Lancet*, 1975, *2*, 1155.

A 39-year-old woman well controlled on warfarin for 4 years suffered haematemesis after taking *co-trimoxazole* for 2 weeks. No effect was observed in 4 other patients taking warfarin.— W. J. Tilstone *et al.*, *Postgrad. med. J.*, 1977, *53*, 388.

A further report of enhancement with *co-trimoxazole*.— J. K. Errick and P. W. Keys, *Am. J. Hosp. Pharm.*, 1978, *35*, 1399.

Prothrombin time in 8 healthy subjects, following warfarin 1.5 mg per kg body-weight as a single dose, was significantly increased when *co-trimoxazole* 480 mg four times daily was given for 7 days before, and several days after, the administration of the same dose of warfarin. No significant differences were found in the warfarin plasma-clearance values, indicating that the drug interaction had occurred at the warfarin receptor sites.— R. A. O'Reilly and C. H. Motley, *Ann. intern. Med.*, 1979, *91*, 34.

In a crossover study in 8 healthy subjects of the interaction between *co-trimoxazole* and the enantiomorphs of warfarin, marked augmentation of both the plasma concentrations of warfarin and hypoprothrombinaemia occurred with *S*-warfarin and co-trimoxazole; none occurred with *R*-warfarin.— R. A. O'Reilly, *New Engl. J. Med.*, 1980, *302*, 33.

See also abstracts below relative to other sulphonamides.

Dextropropoxyphene (in Distalgesic tablets) was considered to have enhanced the anticoagulant effect of warfarin causing haematuria in 2 patients.— M. Orme *et al.*, *Br. med. J.*, 1976, *1*, 200. A further report in 1 patient.— R. V. Jones (letter), *ibid.*, 460.

Dextrothyroxine given to 11 patients receiving long-term therapy with warfarin sodium enhanced the anticoagulant effect and produced a prolongation of the prothrombin time during the first 4 weeks. In 4 of the 11 patients the concentration of prothrombin and factor VII was reduced.— J. C. Owens *et al.*, *New Engl. J. Med.*, 1962, *266*, 76. A further case report.— H. M. Solomon and J. J. Schrogie, *Clin. Pharmac. Ther.*, 1967, *8*, 797.

See also under Dicoumarol, p.771 for *dextrothyroxine* enhancing anticoagulant activity.

In vitro, warfarin was displaced from albumin by *diazoxide*.— E. M. Sellers and J. Koch-Weser, *Ann. N.Y. Acad. Sci.*, 1971, *179*, 213.

A study of concomitant administration of warfarin and *diflunisal* indicating loss of anticoagulant effect on stopping diflunisal.— M. J. Serlin *et al.*, *Br. J. clin. Pharmac.*, 1980, *9*, 287P.

For the effect of *diflunisal* enhancing anticoagulant activity, see under Nicoumalone, p.772.

A 58-year-old man was stabilised on digoxin, frusemide, potassium supplements, warfarin, and disopyramide following myocardial infarction. A fall in the prothrombin time and an increase in the required dose of warfarin when *disopyramide* was withdrawn suggested the possibility of an interaction.— E. Haworth and A. K. Burroughs, *Br. med. J.*, 1977, *2*, 866.

Reports of enhancement of warfarin by *disulfiram*.— E. Rothstein (letter), *J. Am. med. Ass.*, 1968, *206*, 1574; E. S. Vesell *et al.*, *Clin. Pharmac. Ther.*, 1971, *12*, 785; E. Rothstein (letter), *J. Am. med. Ass.*, 1972, *221*, 1052; R. A. O'Reilly, *Ann. intern. Med.*, 1973, *78*, 73; R. A. O'Reilly, *Clin. Pharmac. Ther.*, 1981, *29*, 332 (mode of interaction).

The prothrombin time of a 77-year-old woman receiving warfarin was prolonged when she was given *erythromycin*.— W. R. Bartle (letter), *Archs intern. Med.*, 1980, *140*, 985.

In vitro, warfarin was displaced from albumin by *ethacrynic acid*.— E. M. Sellers and J. Koch-Weser, *Ann. N.Y. Acad. Sci.*, 1971, *179*, 213.

Report, without detail, of clinically significant interaction between warfarin and *ethacrynic acid*.— J. Koch-Weser, *Clin. Pharmac. Ther.*, 1973, *14*, 139.

A 38-year-old woman taking warfarin sodium about 10 mg daily experienced 2 episodes of increased prothrombin time after *ethacrynic acid* in doses of 150 to 300 mg daily.— R. J. Petrick *et al.*, *J. Am. med. Ass.*, 1975, *231*, 843.

For the possible effect of *ethyloestrenol* enhancing anticoagulant activity, see under Phenindione p.773.

Elevation of mean prothrombin time (up to 38.4 seconds) in 5 patients stabilised on warfarin and given *feprazone* 400 mg daily concomitantly.— S. Chierichetti *et al.*, *Curr. ther. Res.*, 1975, *18*, 568.

In 8 of 9 patients being treated with warfarin sodium, the prothrombin time was prolonged threefold to twelvefold when *glucagon*, in a total dose exceeding 50 mg was given over at least 2 days. In 11 other patients, glucagon in total doses of less than 30 mg over one or two days did not affect the action of warfarin sodium.— J. Koch-Weser, *Ann. intern. Med.*, 1970, *72*, 331.

A study *in vitro* indicating that *ibuprofen* in doses estimated at 600 mg four times daily would increase unbound warfarin in serum by only 10%; doubling this would cause appreciable displacement of warfarin and could be expected to cause enhancement of anticoagulant effect.— J. T. Slattery and G. Levy (letter), *J. pharm. Sci.*, 1977, *66*, 1060. See also under Interactions, Absence of Effect and Interactions, Diminished Effect, above.

Report, without detail, of clincially significant interactions between *indomethacin* and warfarin.— J. Koch-Weser, *Clin. Pharmac. Ther.*, 1973, *14*, 139. See also T. H. Self *et al.* (letter), *Lancet*, 1975, *2*, 557.

See also under Phenindione, p.773 for *indomethacin* enhancing anticoagulant activity.

But see also Interactions, Absence of Effect, above.

A 35-year-old patient with bleeding gums, bloody urine, and right flank pain and tenderness had been receiving a maintenance dose of warfarin 10 mg daily and isoniazid 300 mg daily. Ten days before admission to hospital he had accidentally begun to take 600 mg daily of isoniazid. Interaction between *isoniazid* and warfarin was suggested.— A. R. Rosenthal *et al.*, *J. Am. med. Ass.*, 1977, *238*, 2177.

For the effect of *magnesium hydroxide* in enhancing anticoagulant activity, see under Dicoumarol, p.771.

The dose of warfarin had to be reduced by 0 to 25% when *meclofenamate sodium* was given concomitantly.— F. D. Baragar and T. C. Smith, *Curr. ther. Res.*, 1978, *23, Suppl.* 4S, S51.

In 12 healthy subjects given warfarin sodium 2.5 to 15 mg daily to produce prothrombin concentrations of 17.5 to 23.5%, prothrombin concentrations were further reduced by a mean of 3.49% when *mefenamic acid* 2 g daily was given concomitantly.— E. L. Holmes, *Ann. phys. Med.*, 1966, *8, Suppl.*, 36. See also under Interactions, Absence of Effect, above.

For conflicting reports of the effect of *methylphenidate* on anticoagulant activity, see under Ethyl Biscoumacetate, p.771.

For a report of *methyltestosterone* enhancing anticoagulant activity, see under Phenprocoumon, p.774.

In 8 healthy subjects concomitant administration of *metronidazole* enhanced the anticoagulant effect of racemic warfarin. The interaction could be reduced or even avoided by using *R*(+)-warfarin.— R. A. O'Reilly, *New Engl. J. Med.*, 1976, *295*, 354.

Excessive bruising with subcutaneous haemorrhage in the legs and a prothrombin time increased to 147 seconds were reported in a 31-year-old woman on maintenance therapy with warfarin a week after she had completed a 10-day course of treatment with *metronidazole*; she was also taking dextropropoxyphene occasionally.— F. J. Kazmier, *Mayo Clin. Proc.*, 1976, *51*, 782.

A 55-year-old woman controlled on warfarin developed a purpuric rash and the prothrombin time rose to 45 seconds a few days after starting treatment with *nalidixic acid*, 500 mg four times daily.— B. I. Hoffbrand (letter), *Br. med. J.*, 1974, *2*, 666.

See also under Nicoumalone, p.772 for *nalidixic acid* enhancing anticoagulant activity.

The prothrombin time rose in 6 of 10 patients stabilised on warfarin given *neomycin* 2 g daily for 3 weeks.— J. A. Udall, *Clin. Med.*, 1970, *77* (Aug.), 20.

For a report of *norethandrolone* enhancing anticoagulant activity, see Dicoumarol, p.771.

Amitriptyline or *nortriptyline* had no effect on the plasma half-life of warfarin. In some patients the half-life of dicoumarol was increased, but the effect was not consistent.— S. M. Pond *et al.*, *Clin. Pharmac. Ther.*, 1975, *18*, 191.

See also under Dicoumarol for *nortriptyline* enhancing anticoagulant activity.

Reduced anticoagulant tolerance occurred in 6 patients given *oxymetholone* 15 mg daily in addition to their anticoagulant (warfarin and phenindione) treatment. One patient developed subcutaneous bleeding and another haematuria.— R. G. M. Longridge *et al.* (letter), *Lancet*, 1971, *2*, 90. A similar report in 5 patients.— B. H. B. Robinson (letter), *ibid.*, 1971, *1*, 1356. See also M. S. Edwards and J. R. Curtis (letter), *ibid.*, 1971, *2*, 221.

See also under Nicoumalone for *oxymetholone* enhancing anticoagulant activity.

Intrapulmonary bleeding occurred in a man taking warfarin when he was given *oxyphenbutazone* as well.— N. Kaplinsky *et al.* (letter), *J. Am. med. Ass.*, 1980, *243*, 513.

In a double-blind trial in 112 patients who were being treated with warfarin sodium, dicoumarol, phenprocoumon, or anisindione, *paracetamol* 650 mg four times daily significantly increased the prothrombin time.— A. M. Antlitz *et al.*, *Curr. ther. Res.*, 1968, *10*, 501.

Paracetamol 650 mg, followed after 4 hours by a further similar dose, had no effect on the prothrombin time in 10 patients taking oral anticoagulants.— A. M. Antlitz and L. F. Awalt, *Curr. ther. Res.*, 1969, *11*, 360.

There was no significant increase in the prothrombin time in 10 patients stabilised on warfarin when also given *paracetamol* 3.25 g daily for 2 weeks.— J. A. Udall, *Clin. Med.*, 1970, *77* (Aug.), 20.

Continued ingestion of *liquid paraffin* (mineral oil) could significantly reduce the absorption of vitamin K.— *J. Am. med. Ass.*, 1968, *204*, 937.

Severe haematuria and increased fibrinolysis occurred in a patient who had been taking warfarin 12 mg daily and was given *phenformin* 50 mg daily.— T. J. Hamblin (letter), *Lancet*, 1971, *2*, 1323.

Enhancement of warfarin by *phenylbutazone*.— M. J. Eisen, *J. Am. med. Ass.*, 1964, *189*, 64; B. I. Hoffbrand and D. A. Kininmonth (letter), *Br. med. J.*, 1967, *2*, 838; P. M. Aggeler *et al.*, *New Engl. J. Med.*, 1967, *276*, 496; J. A. Udall, *Clin. Med.*, 1970, *77* (Aug.), 20; S. Chierichetti *et al.*, *Curr. ther. Res.*, 1975, *18*, 568.

Prolongation of the prothrombin time in 6 patients taking warfarin or dicoumarol and *phenyramidol* 0.8 to 1.6 g daily.— S. A. Carter, *New Engl. J. Med.*, 1965, *273*, 423.

See also under Phenindione, p.773 for *phenyramidol* enhancing anticoagulant activity.

Prothrombin time was increased in 2 patients taking maintenance doses of warfarin, when they were also given *phenytoin*.— J. M. Nappi (letter), *Ann. intern. Med.*, 1979, *90*, 852. But for *phenytoin* diminishing anticoagulant activity, see Dicoumarol, p.771.

For a report of hypoprothrombinaemia in a patient taking *propylthiouracil*, see Propylthiouracil, p.358.

In 3 patients with stable prothrombin times during treatment with warfarin, severe hypoprothrombinaemia occurred when *quinidine* 0.8 to 1.4 g daily was added to their treatment.— J. Koch-Weser, *Ann. intern. Med.*, 1968, *68*, 511, per *Abstr. Wld Med.*, 1968, *42*, 761.

There was no significant increase in the prothrombin time in 10 patients stabilised on warfarin when also given *quinidine* 800 mg daily for 2 weeks.— J. A. Udall, *Clin. Med.*, 1970, *77* (Aug.), 20.

Haemorrhage in a patient taking warfarin was possibly due to the concomitant administration of *quinidine*.— A. B. Gazzaniga and D. R. Stewart, *New Engl.*, *J. Med.*, 1969, *280*, 711.

For the effect of *stanozolol* in enhancing anticoagulant activity, see under Dicoumarol.

Reduced requirement of warfarin in a 72-year-old man might have been due to concomitant administration of *sulindac*.— S. A. Carter (letter), *Lancet*, 1979, *2*, 698.

Enhancement of warfarin by *sulindac* in 2 patients.— J. R. Y. Ross and L. Beeley (letter), *Lancet*, 1979, *2*, 1075. See also under Interactions, Absence of Effect.

Enhancement of warfarin by *sulphafurazole* in 1 patient.— T. H. Self *et al.*, *Circulation*, 1975, *52*, 528.

Another report of the enhanced effect of warfarin by *sulphafurazole* in 1 patient.— L. J. Sioris *et al.*, *Archs intern. Med.*, 1980, *140*, 546.

Sulphamethizole appeared to inhibit the hepatic metabolism of warfarin.— B. Lumholtz *et al.*, *Clin. Pharmac. Ther.*, 1975, *17*, 731.

For the effect of *sulphamethoxazole* on enhancing anticoagulant activity, see under *co-trimoxazole*, above.

Warfarin was displaced from human albumin by *sulphaphenazole*.— H. M. Solomon and J. J. Schrogie, *Biochem. Pharmac.*, 1967, *16*, 1219, per E. M. Sellers and J. Koch-Weser, *Ann. N.Y. Acad. Sci.*, 1971, *179*, 213.

See also under Phenindione, p.773 for *sulphaphenazole* enhancing anticoagulant activity.

A 63-year-old man stabilised on warfarin 8 mg daily developed melaena and generalised haemorrhage a week after starting *sulphinpyrazone* 200 mg four times daily.— D. Mattingly *et al.* (letter), *Br. med. J.*, 1978, *2*, 1786.

The prothrombin time in a 53-year-old man stabilised on warfarin was prolonged from 18 to 56 seconds, a week after he began taking *sulphinpyrazone* 800 mg daily.— J. W. Davis and L. E. Johns (letter), *New Engl. J. Med.*, 1978, *299*, 955.

On 6 occasions the administration of warfarin 10 to 15 mg to patients taking *sulphinpyrazone* had been associated with an enhanced anticoagulant effect. In one patient this interaction provoked life-threatening haematemesis and melaena.— R. R. Bailey and J. Reddy (letter), *Lancet*, 1980, *1*, 254.

A report of 3 patients in whom the anticoagulant effects of warfarin were enhanced by *sulphinpyrazone*.— A. Gallus and D. Birkett (letter), *Lancet*, 1980, *1*, 535.

A further report.— M. Weiss (letter), *Lancet*, 1979, *1*, 609.

Initial enhancement of the effect of warfarin by *sulphinpyrazone*, but subsequent antagonism.— G. G. Nenci *et al.*, *Br. med. J.*, 1981, *282*, 1361.

Massive gastro-intestinal haemorrhage and low prothrombin concentrations developed in 3 patients who had been given respectively chloramphenicol and *tetracycline*, chloramphenicol and procaine penicillin, and chloramphenicol, tetracycline, and procaine penicillin.— A. P. Klippel and B. Pitsinger, *Archs Surg., Chicago*, 1968, *96*, 266.

For a report of reduced prothrombin activity in 14 patients given *tetracycline*, see Tetracycline Hydrochloride, p.1217.

A comment that *tienilic acid* demonstrated some competition with warfarin, and that some patients had required a reduction of their anticoagulant dose.— *Postgrad. med. J.*, 1979, *55*, *Suppl.* 3, 67.

See also under Ethyl Biscoumacetate and Nicoumalone.

Studies *in vitro* indicated that warfarin would not be significantly displaced from serum protein binding sites by *tienilic acid* under the usual therapeutic conditions.— J. T. Slattery and G. Levy, *J. pharm. Sci.*, 1979, *68*, 393.

The mean prothrombin time increased in 7 subjects given *triclofos* after having been stabilised on warfarin, and in 3 the dose of warfarin had to be reduced. Concentrations of factors II and X fell within 9 hours of triclofos being ingested.— E. M. Sellers *et al.*, *Clin. Pharmac. Ther.*, 1972, *13*, 911.

Prolongation of the prothombin time and haemorrhage on 2 occasions when *vitamin E* was taken by a patient stabilised on warfarin, digoxin, and clofibrate.— J. J. Corrigan and F. I. Marcus, *J. Am. med. Ass.*, 1974, *230*, 1300. See also J. J. Schrogie (letter), *J. Am. med. Ass.*, 1975, *232*, 19.

Absorption and Fate. Warfarin sodium is readily absorbed from the gastro-intestinal tract and is reported to have been absorbed through the skin. It is extensively bound to plasma proteins and its plasma half-life is about 40 hours. It crosses the placenta. Warfarin is not now considered to occur in significant quantities in breast milk, though some authorities suggest careful observation of the infant. It is metabolised in the liver and is excreted in the urine, mainly as metabolites.

A review of the clinical pharmacokinetics of oral anticoagulants.— J. G. Kelly and K. O'Malley, *Clin. Pharmacokinet.*, 1979, *4*, 1. A discussion of the clinical relevance of pharmacokinetic studies.— G. Tognoni *et al.*, *Clin. Pharmacokinet.*, 1980, *5*, 105.

Absorption and plasma concentrations. Similar pharmacokinetic parameters after the oral or intravenous administration of warfarin.— P. B. Andreasen and E. S. Vesell, *Clin. Pharmac. Ther.*, 1974, *16*, 1059.

The effect of acute viral hepatitis on the disposition and effect of warfarin.— R. L. Williams *et al.*, *Clin. Pharmac. Ther.*, 1976, *20*, 90.

Successful use of warfarin in a man with short-bowel syndrome substantiated high absorption in the proximal intestine.— J. F. Mitchell *et al.*, *Am. J. Hosp. Pharm.*, 1977, *34*, 171.

In 7 healthy subjects given a single dose of warfarin 15 mg a mean peak plasma concentration of 1.8 µg per ml occurred 1 hour after administration. The elimination half-life from plasma was about 50 hours.— S. Hanna *et al.*, *Endo, USA*, *J. pharm. Sci.*, 1978, *67*, 84.

Pharmacokinetics and pharmacodynamics of warfarin at steady state.— P. A. Routledge *et al.*, *Br. J. clin. Pharmac.*, 1979, *8*, 243.

Half-life. In a patient resistant to warfarin and phenindione, the half-life of warfarin was 6.5 hours, compared with the normal half-life of about 44 hours.— R. J. Lewis *et al.*, *Am. J. Med.*, 1967, *42*, 620.

The plasma half-life of warfarin was 44 hours; it was bound to plasma proteins to the extent of 97%.— R. A. O'Reilly and P. M. Aggeler, *Pharmac. Rev.*, 1970, *22*, 35. See also J. -P. Tillement *et al.*, *Eur. J. clin. Pharmac.*, 1973, *6*, 15.

In 4 patients with impaired renal function the mean half-life of warfarin was about 30 hours, compared to 45 hours in 5 normal subjects.— K. Bachmann *et al.*, *J. clin. Pharmac.*, 1977, *17*, 292.

Isomers. Serum half-lives of the 2 enantiomers of warfarin, determined in 4 normal individuals given a single dose of 100 mg of one of these together with 50 mg of vitamin K were between 34.9 and 64.2 hours (mean 45.4) for (*R*)-warfarin and between 23.5 and 51.6 hours (mean 33) for (*S*)-warfarin. These values were considered to be unaffected by the administration of vitamin K, used to decrease the anticoagulant effect of warfarin in volunteers.— D. S. Hewick and J. McEwen, *J. Pharm. Pharmac.*, 1973, *25*, 458.

(*R*)-Warfarin was oxidised to 6-hydroxywarfarin and reduced to (*R,S*)-alcohol while (*S*)-warfarin was largely oxidised to 6- and 7-hydroxywarfarin.— A. Breckenridge, *Br. J. clin. Pharmac.*, 1974, *1*, 285.

The concurrent administration of phenobarbitone altered the pattern of elimination and thus the plasma half-life of *R*(+)- as well as *S*(−)-warfarin.— M. Orme and A. Breckenridge (letter), *New Engl. J. Med.*, 1976, *295*, 1482. Confirmation of these findings. The stereoselective interactions with warfarin now included co-trimoxazole as well as metronidazole and phenylbutazone.— R. A. O'Reilly (letter), *ibid.*

The effects of racemic warfarin and of *S*(−)-warfarin (levowarfarin) were enhanced by metronidazole, phenylbutazone, and co-trimoxazole while *R*(+)-warfarin (dextrowarfarin) was not affected.— *J. Am. med. Ass.*, 1977, *238*, 574.

Further references.— N. Refsum *et al.*, *Meddr norsk farm. Selsk.*, 1978, *40*, 105, per *Int. pharm. Abstr.*, 1978, *15*, 1132; L. B. Wingard and G. Levy (letter), *Br. J. clin. Pharmac.*, 1978, *6*, 434; G. Levy *et al.*, *J. pharm. Sci.*, 1978, *67*, 867; M. Otagiri *et al.*, *Int. J. Pharmaceut.*, 1979, *2*, 283; C. Hignite *et al.*, *Clin. Pharmac. Ther.*, 1980, *28*, 99.

Metabolism. The metabolites of warfarin in man included 7-hydroxywarfarin, 6-hydroxywarfarin, and 2 warfarin alcohols with half-lives of 33 and 12 hours respectively.— R. J. Lewis and W. F. Trager, *Ann. N.Y. Acad. Sci.*, 1971, *179*, 205.

Pregnancy and the neonate. *Excretion in breast milk.* Plasma-warfarin concentrations in 6 nursing mothers taking warfarin 5 to 12 mg daily ranged from 0.48 to 1.8 µg per ml. Since the concentration of warfarin in either breast milk or infant plasma remained below a detectable concentration of 25 ng per ml it was considered that there was no contra-indication to breast-feeding by mothers taking warfarin.— J. D. Baty *et al.*, *Br. J. clin. Pharmac.*, 1976, *3*, 969P.

Warfarin was not detected in the breast milk of 6 women taking warfarin nor in the breast milk or infants' plasma of 7 women taking warfarin and breast-feeding their infants.— M. L'E. Orme *et al.*, *Br. med. J.*, 1977, *1*, 1564.

Protein binding. A review of the protein binding of coumarin anticoagulants in disease states.— K. Bachmann and R. Shapiro, *Clin. Pharmacokinet.*, 1977, *2*, 110.

A decrease was found in the plasma-binding capacity of elderly people for warfarin.— M. J. Hayes *et al.*, *Br. J. clin. Pharmac.*, 1975, *2*, 69.

In 31 patients with cardiovascular disease warfarin was 98.11 to 99.56% bound to serum proteins.— A. Yacobi *et al.*, *Clin. Pharmac. Ther.*, 1976, *19*, 552.

Protein binding of warfarin and its enantiomers.— A. Yacobi and G. Levy, *J. Pharmacokinet. Biopharm.*, 1977, *5*, 123.

Genetic control of interindividual variations in racemic warfarin binding to plasma and albumin of twins.— G. Wilding *et al.*, *Clin. Pharmac. Ther.*, 1977, *22*, 831.

Warfarin binding in kwashiorkor.— N. Buchanan and L. A. Van der Walt, *Am. Heart J.*, 1977, *93*, 128.

A study *in vitro* of plasma protein binding of warfarin in patients undergoing renal transplantation.— I. Odar-Cederlof, *Clin. Pharmacokinet.*, 1977, *2*, 147.

Uses. Warfarin sodium is an anticoagulant which depresses the hepatic vitamin K-dependent synthesis of coagulation factors II (prothrombin), VII, IX, and X. It is equally effective either orally or intravenously, and may also be given intramuscularly. The therapeutic effect begins to develop in 12 to 18 hours, reaches a maximum in 36 to 48 hours, and may persist for 5 to 6 days.

Warfarin sodium is employed for the same general purposes as heparin (see p.765). It is, however, slower in action than heparin, and if an immediate effect on blood coagulation is required, heparin should be given intravenously or subcutaneously to cover the first 36 to 48 hours.

Warfarin sodium is used in the prevention and treatment of venous thrombosis or pulmonary embolism, and in patients with prosthetic heart valves, rheumatic valvular disease, atrial fibrillation, and transient ischaemic attacks. It is used similarly to heparin for the prevention of postoperative deep-vein thrombosis. The role of anticoagulants in myocardial infarction remains to be established.

Dosage must be determined according to the prothrombin activity of the blood; it is usual to maintain the prothrombin time at 2 to 2½ times normal; some authorities recommend a slightly higher ratio in the treatment of established thrombosis. The prothrombin time is checked daily or every other day initially, then less frequently. Initial doses of 30 to 50 mg have been given, with smaller doses for the old or frail, but some authorities favour a more gradual approach with initial doses of 10 to 15 mg daily. Subsequent maintenance doses usually range from 3 to 12 mg daily.

Warfarin sodium is a potent rodenticide and is widely used for this purpose, though the development of resistance to warfarin has been reported in *rats*.

Reports of clinical resistance to warfarin.— J. Zager *et al.* (letter), *Ann. intern. Med.*, 1973, *78*, 775; D. B. Barnett and B. W. Hancock, *Br. med. J.*, 1975, *1*, 608.

Investigations in 7 healthy male volunteers and 4 male patients who were completing a course of racemic warfarin for deep-vein thrombosis indicated that (*S*)-warfarin was a more potent anticoagulant than (*R*)-warfarin.— A. Breckenridge *et al.*, *Clin. Pharmac. Ther.*, 1974, *15*, 424.

Studies on the optical enantiomorphs of warfarin in 10 healthy subjects.— R. A. O'Reilly, *Clin. Pharmac. Ther.*, 1974, *16*, 348.

Oral anticoagulants elevated concentrations of antithrombin III.— E. Marciniak *et al.*, *Blood*, 1974, *43*, 219.

Continuous treatment with warfarin sodium 2.5 to 5 mg daily was effective in the management of skin lesions some of which were gangrenous in a 56-year-old man. Cryofibrinogenaemia might have caused thrombosis leading to skin infarctions.— G. V. Ball and L. N. Goldman, *Ann. intern. Med.*, 1976, *85*, 464.

There might be some justification for the custom of starting warfarin therapy for deep-vein thrombosis a few days before stopping heparin since warfarin raised antithrombin III activity which might otherwise become dangerously low.— J. R. O'Brien and M. D. Etherington (letter), *Lancet*, 1977, *2*, 1232.

Racemic warfarin sodium and the *S*(−)- but not the *R*(+)-enantiomer showed antimetastatic activity in *mice*. The *R*(+)-enantiomer showed little or no anticoagulant activity.— A. Poggi *et al.* (letter), *Lancet*, 1978, *1*, 163.

A report of a Mexican study which showed that administration of warfarin to *cattle* in intramuscular doses of 5 mg per kg body-weight did not harm them but rendered their blood toxic to the vampire bat, *Desmodus rotundus* causing it to bleed to death. This was an approach preferable to one being considered whereby vampires were caught, painted with anticoagulants, then returned to their roosts to be licked clean by their soon-to-be-doomed companions.— *Lancet*, 1979, *2*, 649.

Administration in renal failure. Warfarin could be given in usual doses to patients in renal failure.— W. M. Bennett *et al.*, *Ann. intern. Med.*, 1980, *93*, 286.

Dementia. In a pilot study warfarin sodium seemed effective in controlling increasing senile dementia in 7 patients whose average age was 83.4 years.— *J. Am. med. Ass.*, 1972, *220*, 1065.

Dose. In 91 patients receiving long-term treatment the dose of warfarin required to maintain an optimum anticoagulant effect was increased in patients with elevated concentrations of cholesterol but was not related to serum-triglyceride concentrations. The half-life of warfarin sodium varied widely in 37 patients but was not related to serum-cholesterol or triglyceride concentrations.— K. Pyörälä *et al.*, *Acta med. scand.*, 1968, *183*, 437, per *Abstr. Wld Med.*, 1968, *42*, 923.

The frequency of unduly prolonged prothrombin time and of untoward bleeding episodes during the initiation of warfarin therapy had been reduced by beginning treatment with daily doses of 10 to 15 mg of warfarin sodium until the required prolongation of the bleeding time had been achieved. This regimen was preferable to the loading dose technique.— D. Deykin, *New Engl. J. Med.*, 1970, *283*, 691.

There was a linear relationship between the logarithm of the Thrombotest response to a loading dose of 10 mg of warfarin daily for 3 successive days and the maintenance dose required to achieve an anticoagulant Thrombotest response of 8 to 12%. This was expressed by the regression equation: maintenance dose $=7.60\times\log_{10}$ Thrombotest -3.33. A range of maintenance doses for different Thrombotest results had been calculated and these values or the equation could be used within certain limitations to predict maintenance dose requirements of warfarin.— P. A. Routledge *et al.* (preliminary communication), *Lancet*, 1977, *2*, 854. In a study of 22 patients, when assessed by the prothrombin-time ratio, the response to a standard loading dose of warfarin was found to be a poor predictor of maintenance dose requirements.— G. W. Morrison (letter), *ibid.*, 1979, *1*, 167. In 32 patients the relationship had proved a useful, if rough, guide.— P. J. Green (letter), *ibid.*, 829.

Anticoagulant control as indicated by the percentage of Thrombotest values outside a defined range was studied in 139 patients, of whom 109 received warfarin and 30 phenindione. Anticoagulant control did not seem to vary with age for patients aged 40 to 70 years, nor with sex. Thrombotest values, however, tended to be lower for the 60 to 69 years age group and these patients also received a lower average daily dose of warfarin, supporting the suggestion of increased sensitivity of the elderly. Anticoagulant control was significantly affected by duration of treatment; in the first 6 months of treatment 40% of Thrombotest values indicated poor control, decreasing to 16% in the 18 to 24th month of treatment but remaining relatively stable thereafter.— A. M. M. Shepherd *et al.*, *Postgrad. med. J.*, 1978, *54*, 784.

The urinary excretion of γ-carboxyglutamic acid was reduced in patients receiving warfarin when compared with healthy control subjects. Estimation of urinary γ-carboxyglutamic acid may be useful in control of anticoagulant therapy.— R. J. Levy and J. B. Lian, *Clin. Pharmac. Ther.*, 1979, *25*, 562.

Dose in the elderly. There was no significant correlation between the patient's age and the dose of warfarin needed to maintain the activated partial thromboplastin time between 50 and 70 seconds, but 25 patients with mitral valve disease required significantly less warfarin than did 255 patients who had had venous or intracranial thrombosis, or myocardial infarction.— R. D. Eastham (letter), *Br. med. J.*, 1973, *2*, 554.

A retrospective survey of 177 hospital patients receiving warfarin showed than anticoagulant control varied with age of the patient but not with sex or indication for anticoagulation.— K. O'Malley *et al.*, *Br. J. clin. Pharmac.*, 1977, *4*, 309. An increased sensitivity in old age was confirmed in a study of 4 young and 4 elderly patients.— A. M. M. Shepherd *et al.*, *ibid.*, 315.

The daily maintenance dose of warfarin was significantly reduced in patients aged between 61 to 70 years of age compared with those between 50 and 60 years of age.— S. Husted and F. Andreasen, *Br. J. clin. Pharmac.*, 1977, *4*, 559.

A study in 15 patients taking warfarin and whose ages ranged from 33 to 78 years indicated that the therapeutic effects of warfarin were associated with lower plasma-warfarin concentrations and reduced dosage in elderly patients.— D. M. Davies *et al.*, *Br. J. clin. Pharmac.*, 1977, *4*, 636P.

Myocardial infarction. In 500 patients with definite myocardial infarction, after an initial loading dose of warfarin 40 mg by mouth, the dose was reduced to maintain the Thrombotest between 5 and 10%. Thrombo-embolic complications occurred in 17 patients and haemorrhagic complications in 8, including melaena in 3, haematuria in 3 (1 had renal calculi), and bruising of the skin in 2. The initial dose of warfarin was reduced in a few cases when warranted.— S. J. Jachuck, *Br. J. clin. Pract.*, 1973, *27*, 341.

Neoplasms. Thirty patients with lymphoma or chronic leukaemia, receiving busulphan, chlorambucil, or cyclophosphamide, were given warfarin when their disease became resistant. The dose of warfarin was adjusted to double the prothrombin time. Twenty-one patients responded and the dose of antineoplastic agent required to maintain remission was reduced to 25% of the pre-warfarin dose.— R. D. Thornes (letter), *Br. med. J.*, 1972, *1*, 110.

In a controlled trial in 128 patients with neoplasms the 2-year survival-rate was doubled when warfarin was added to their treatment. Best results were achieved in postmenopausal patients with breast cancer.— R. D. Thornes, *Cancer*, 1975, *35*, 91.

Coumarin anticoagulants had an anticancer effect that might not be related to their anticoagulant effect but to their vitamin-K inhibition.— P. Hilgard (letter), *Lancet*, 1977, *2*, 403.

Longer survival in lung cancer patients given warfarin in addition to standard therapy.— L. R. Zacharski *et al.*, *J. Am. med. Ass.*, 1981, *245*, 831.

Pregnancy and the neonate. For advice on the management of pulmonary embolism in pregnancy, see under the section on Anticoagulants, p.762. See also Heparin, p.766.

Renal transplantation. For the use of warfarin in patients receiving cadaveric renal transplants, see A. D. Barnes *et al.*, *Transplantn Bull.*, 1974, *17*, 491.

For a favourable report of the use of warfarin and dipyridamole in patients with renal allografts, see Dipyridamole, p.1619.

Thrombo-embolic disorders. In a study of 68 patients with acute deep-vein thrombosis, patients were treated with continuous intravenous heparin for 14 days and were then randomised to receive either warfarin sodium by mouth (33 patients) or low-dose heparin subcutaneously (35). Warfarin sodium, 10 mg daily initially and subsequently adjusted according to the prothrombin time, was begun 4 days before the heparin was stopped whereas heparin, in a fixed dose of 5000 units subcutaneously every 12 hours, was started on day 14. Treatment continued for 12 weeks in patients with proximal-vein thrombosis and for 6 weeks in those with calf-vein thrombosis; follow-up lasted for about 7 months. Recurrent venous thrombo-embolism occurred in 9 of 19 patients (47%) with proximal-vein thrombosis given heparin compared with none of 17 similar patients who received warfarin. No patients with calf-vein thrombosis had a recurrence of thrombosis during the study. There were bleeding complications in 7 of the 33 patients taking warfarin, 4 of whom required blood transfusions, but in none of those receiving heparin.— R. Hull *et al.*, *New Engl. J. Med.*, 1979, *301*, 855. Comments.— S. Wessler and S. N. Gitel, *ibid.*, 889; W. M. Miller and C. A. Medbery (letter), *ibid.*, 1980, *302*, 752; D. L. Clarke-Pearson (letter), *ibid.*; A. F. Barker (letter), *ibid.*, 753. Reply.— R. Hull *et al.* (letter), *ibid.*

See also under Myocardial Infarction, above.

Artificial heart valves. The use of anticoagulants appeared to result in a marked reduction in thrombo-embolism after prosthetic heart-valve replacement. Of 111 patients 93 were treated with warfarin sodium and only 5 experienced subsequent embolic episodes; of the remaining 18 patients 8 developed systemic embolisms.— H. L. Gadboys *et al.*, *J. Am. med. Ass.*, 1967, *202*, 282. See also I. Sakashita *et al.*, *Jap. Heart J.*, 1978, *19*, 324.

Stroke. From a survey of the literature and from personal experience, guidelines were developed for the treatment of transient ischaemic attacks. Suitable patients might be submitted to endarterectomy. Other patients with attacks of less than 2 months' duration were given warfarin (to maintain the prothrombin time at a ratio of 1.5 to 2) for 3 months, followed by aspirin. Patients with attacks of more than 2 months' duration were treated with aspirin 650 mg twice daily unless recent changes in attacks made an initial course of warfarin advisable. Aspirin was continued until the patient had been free of attacks for a year. No treatment was advised for patients who had been free of attacks for a year.— B. A. Sandok *et al.*, *Mayo Clin. Proc.*, 1978, *53*, 665.

Patients who received anticoagulant therapy for the treatment of transient ischaemic attacks had a poorer prognosis than those receiving other treatments including antiplatelet aggregation.— A. F. Haerer *et al.*, *J. Am. med. Ass.*, 1977, *238*, 142.

A prospective epidemiological study of anticoagulants in stroke and transient ischaemic attacks, including factors associated with a high risk of bleeding.— A. Terént and B. Andersson, *Acta med. scand.*, 1980, *208*, 359.

Further references.— L. J. Hurwitz, *Br. med. J.*, 1969, *3*, 699; *Drug & Ther. Bull.*, 1978, *16*, 5.

Use in surgery. A discussion of the use of warfarin in the prevention of venous thrombo-embolism during surgery.— G. P. Clagett and E. W. Salzman, *New Engl. J. Med.*, 1974, *290*, 93.

The incidence of thrombo-embolic episodes after surgery in 336 high-risk patients treated with warfarin was 1.7%, compared with 1% in low-risk untreated patients and 10% in high-risk untreated patients. Haemorrhage occurred in 29 treated patients and 6 patients died, but in only 1 patient was anticoagulant treatment considered to be involved.— D. B. Skinner and E. B. Salzman, *Surgery Gynec. Obstet.*, 1967, *125*, 741.

In a study of 227 patients undergoing total hip replacement the prophylactic efficacy of warfarin and injection of dextran 40 against venous thrombo-embolism was similar.— W. H. Harris *et al.*, *J. Am. med. Ass.*, 1972, *220*, 1319.

Warfarin sodium was compared with heparin and heparin with hydrocortisone in 300 patients undergoing total hip replacement. There was a lower incidence of thrombo-embolic complications (4.6%) in the 108 patients given warfarin than in those given the heparin schedules (9.9 to 12.9%) but the difference was only significant when warfarin was compared with the schedule in which heparin was given to 31 patients 2 hours pre-operatively then every 12 hours postoperatively.— M. A. Ritter and C. W. Hamilton, *Ann. Surg.*, 1975, *181*, 896.

Warfarin sodium was given in an initial loading dose within 24 hours of admission in a controlled study of 160 elderly patients with fractures of the neck of the femur; treatment was continued on the 3rd day for 3 months or until mobility. The frequency of deep-vein thrombosis was significantly less in the treated than in the control patients but there was no significant difference in mortality. Radiographic scanning which was possible in all but 11 patients showed evidence of venous thrombosis in 23 of 75 treated and 50 of 74 control patients. Pulmonary embolisms caused the death of 6 control patients; there was no evidence of pulmonary embolism in the treated patients. Despite the lack of significant difference in mortality-rates prophylactic anticoagulation for patients with hip fractures was considered beneficial for all but the very elderly infirm patient with intercurrent disease.— G. K. Morris and J. R. A. Mitchell, *Lancet*, 1976, *2*, 869.

In 128 patients undergoing total hip replacement the incidence of calf deep-vein thrombosis (assessed by the fibrinogen uptake test) was similar (above 50%) in 58 treated with warfarin, in 51 treated with infusions of dextran 70, and in 19 treated with heparin. There was no pulmonary embolism in those given warfarin, a 4% incidence in those given dextran 70, and a 15.8% incidence in those given heparin. The use of warfarin was advocated.— H. M. Barber *et al.*, *Postgrad. med. J.*, 1977, *53*, 130.

A controlled study in 50 patients who had undergone coronary-artery bypass surgery indicated that anticoagulant treatment with warfarin or antiplatelet treatment with aspirin and dipyridamole, starting on the third postoperative day and continuing for 6 months, failed to improve the patency of the grafts.— G. A. Pantely *et al.*, *New Engl. J. Med.*, 1979, *301*, 962. A suggestion that treatment should be started earlier.— I. D. Goldberg and M. B. Stemerman (letter), *ibid.*, 1980, *302*, 865. The dosage of aspirin was inappropriate.— L. Klotz (letter), *ibid.*, 866. Comment on an earlier study on the effects of aspirin and dipyridamole in similar patients.— S. J. Phillips *et al.* (letter), *ibid.* Criticism of the study.— H. B. Barner (letter), *ibid.* Reply.— G. A. Pantely *et al.* (letter), *ibid.*

Withdrawal of anticoagulant therapy. Absence of rebound hypercoagulability.— R. B. Van Cleve, *J. Am. med. Ass.*, 1966, *196*, 1156; P. Côté *et al.*, *Can. med. Ass. J.*, 1977, *117*, 1281; J. H. Tinker and S. Tarhan, *J. Am. med. Ass.*, 1978, *239*, 738.

Preparations

Warfarin Sodium for Injection *(U.S.P.)*. A sterile freeze-dried mixture of warfarin sodium and sodium chloride; it may contain a suitable buffer. Protect from light.

Warfarin Sodium Tablets *(U.S.P.)*. Tablets containing warfarin sodium. Potency is expressed in terms of anhydrous isopropyl alcohol-free warfarin sodium. Store in airtight containers. Protect from light.

Warfarin Tablets *(B.P.)*. Tablets containing warfarin sodium. Potency is expressed in terms of anhydrous isopropyl alcohol-free warfarin sodium. The *B.P.* requires 70% dissolution in 45 minutes. Protect from light.
Store in airtight containers.

Proprietary Preparations

Marevan *(Duncan, Flockhart, UK)*. Warfarin sodium,

available as scored tablets of 1, 3, and 5 mg. (Also available as Marevan in *Austral., Belg., Denm., Norw., S.Afr.*).

Warfarin *(WB Pharmaceuticals, UK: Boehringer Ingelheim, UK).* Warfarin sodium, available as scored tablets of 1, 3, and 5 mg.

Other Proprietary Names

Coumadan Sodico *(Arg.)*; Coumadin *(Austral., Canad., Ger., Ital., S.Afr., USA)*; Coumadine *(Belg., Fr.)*; Panwarfin *(USA)*; Waran *(Swed.)*; Warfilone, Warnerin *(both Canad.)*.

4824-k

Warfarin-Deanol. MD 6134. The 2-dimethylaminoethanol salt of warfarin.

$C_{19}H_{16}O_4,C_4H_{11}NO$=397.5.

CAS — 3324-63-8.

Warfarin-deanol is an oral anticoagulant which has been used in doses of 5 to 10 mg daily.

Hydrochloric Acid and some other Acids

1300-e

The acids described in this section are used clinically for the removal of warts or the correction of metabolic alkalosis. Some are used to produce effervescent drinks or in pharmaceutical manufacturing processes. Acids with other actions, e.g. vitamins or diuretics, are described in their relevant sections.

1301-l

Hydrochloric Acid *(B.P.)*. Acidum Hydrochloricum Concentratum *(Eur. P.)*; Concentrated Hydrochloric Acid; Acidum Hydrochloricum; Salzsäure.

HCl=36.46.

CAS — 7647-01-0.

Pharmacopoeias. In *Arg., Belg., Br., Chin., Eur., Fr., Ger., Ind., Int., It., Jap., Mex., Neth., Nord., Port., Roum., Span.,* and *Turk.* (all specify approximately 35 to 38%). *U.S.N.F.* specifies 36.5 to 38%. The following specify 25%: *Cz., Jug.,* and *Rus. Swiss* has Acidum Chloratum 25% or 37%. *Aust.* has Acidum Hydrochloricum Concentratum (not less than 35%), and Acidum Hydrochloricum (20%). *Hung.* has Acidum Hydrochloricum Concentratissimum (36 to 39%) and Acidum Hydrochloricum Concentratum (25%). The impure acid of commerce is known as Spirits of Salt and as Muriatic Acid.

A clear colourless fuming aqueous solution of hydrogen chloride with a pungent odour, containing 35 to 38% w/w of HCl. Relative density about 1.18. When distilled, it yields a constant-boiling mixture, boiling at about 110°, containing about 20% w/w of HCl.

Incompatible with alkalis, alkaline carbonates, metallic oxides, and with salts of silver, mercury, and lead. **Store** below 30° in stoppered containers of glass or other inert material.

Adverse Effects. Hydrochloric acid is highly irritant and corrosive. Severe pain, violent vomiting, and haematemesis occur almost as soon as the acid is swallowed and there is a rapid fall in blood pressure. Viscid white or blood-stained foamy mucus and shreds of tissue appear in the mouth, the mucus later becoming yellow or brownish. The vomit contains altered blood, shreds of mucosa, and food remains, and often has a characteristic 'coffee-grounds' appearance. Suffocation may occur owing to the irritant fumes.

Maximum permissible atmospheric concentration (of hydrogen chloride) 5 ppm.

Treatment of Adverse Effects. Aspiration and lavage or emetics must *not* be used. Emergency measures should consist of diluting the acid and relieving pain. Large amounts of water or milk should be drunk instantly for dilution; magnesium oxide, milk of magnesia, lime water, or aluminium hydroxide mixture may be given for neutralisation. Carbonates should be avoided if possible as the gas liberated enhances the risk of gastric perforation. Milk, white of egg, olive oil, or other demulcents may also be used. Morphine sulphate 10 mg can be given by injection for the relief of pain. Alleviate shock. Corticosteroids may be administered to reduce inflammation and prevent oesophageal stricture formation.

Acid burns of the skin should be flooded immediately with water and the washing continued for at least 15 minutes. Any affected clothing should be removed while flooding is being carried out. For burns in the eye, the lids should be kept open and the eye flushed with a steady stream of water for 15 or more minutes. A few drops of a local anaesthetic solution will relieve lid spasm and facilitate irrigation.

Neutralisation with weak alkalis for acid ingestion is considered inappropriate due to the exothermic reaction that occurs when these agents are administered. Soap solution is also no longer considered appropriate because of the tendency towards emesis that occurs in 50 to 60% of patients following its ingestion. Most paediatric surgeons preferred not to use olive oil, white of egg, or liquid paraffin since they interfere with oesophagoscopy or in the case of white of egg may induce emesis.— B. H. Rumack (letter), *J. Am. Coll. emergency Physns,* 1979, *8* (Mar.), 124. Criticism of the extrapolation of a study *in vitro*, but support for the concept of the rapid administration of diluents as the single most important factor in preventing long-term sequelae.— K. I. Maull (letter), *ibid.*

Uses. Hydrochloric acid is an escharotic, but is less corrosive than sulphuric or nitric acid. It is used medicinally only in the diluted form.

1302-y

Dilute Hydrochloric Acid *(B.P., Eur. P.)*. Acidum Hydrochloricum Dilutum; Diluted Hydrochloric Acid *(U.S.N.F.)*; Verdünnte Salzsäure.

Pharmacopoeias. In *Arg., Br., Chin., Eur., Fr., Ger., Hung., Ind., Int., It., Jap., Jug., Mex., Neth., Pol., Roum., Span., Swiss,* and *Turk.* (all approximately 10% w/w); in *Aust.* (7% w/w); in *Belg.* (7 to 7.6%); in *Cz.* (11% w/w); and in *Rus.* (8.3% w/w). Also in *U.S.N.F.*

It contains 9.5 to 10.5% w/w of HCl and may be prepared by mixing hydrochloric acid 274 g with water 726 g. Relative density about 1.05. **Store** below 30° in a stoppered container of glass or other inert material.

Uses. Dilute hydrochloric acid has been used in conditions of achlorhydria, a dose of 2 to 5 ml diluted with 200 to 250 ml of cold water being sipped through a straw during the course of a meal. Not more than 20 ml of dilute hydrochloric acid should be given over 24 hours.

Dilute hydrochloric acid has occasionally been used in the management of metabolic alkalosis, given by intravenous infusion, diluted with water or appropriate infusion fluids.

Achlorhydria. Dilute hydrochloric acid was considered to be ineffective in the treatment of achlorhydria.— S. Buchs, *Dt. med. Wschr.,* 1971, *96,* 1925, per *Germ. Med.,* 1972, *2,* 64. See also *Med. Lett.,* 1972, *14,* 56.

Alkalosis. An account of the intravenous infusion of diluted hydrochloric acid through a central venous catheter for the treatment of severe refractory metabolic alkalosis in 8 patients. The infusion should be given over a period of 6 to 24 hours and, during therapy, repeated measurements of pH, blood gas analysis, plasma electrolyte, and blood urea nitrogen should be carried out at intervals of 4 to 6 hours. The acid should preferably be given in an iso-osmotic solution which is prepared by adding 150 ml of 1M hydrochloric acid to 1 litre of sterile water [providing H^+ 150 mmol and Cl^- 150 mmol in 1 litre]. In most cases, alkalosis can be corrected after infusion of 1 to 2 litres over 24 hours.— G. M. Abouna *et al., Surgery, St Louis,* 1974, *75,* 194. Comment.— *Lancet,* 1974, *1,* 720. Correction to comment.— C. Sanderson (letter), *ibid.,* 933.

A woman with metabolic alkalosis following profuse vomiting for 24 hours benefited initially from the intravenous infusion over 18 hours of 300 mmol of hydrogen ion, given as an 0.1 M solution of hydrochloric acid.— S. E. Williams, *Br. med. J.,* 1976, *1,* 1189.

The successful use of hydrochloric acid by intravenous infusion in 4 patients with alkalosis unresponsive to conventional therapy. The rate of infusion should not exceed 0.2 mmol (hydrogen ion) per kg body-weight per hour in dextrose injection; it should be given through a central venous catheter and the acid-base state should be monitored every 6 to 12 hours.— L. I. G. Worthley, *Br. J. Anaesth.,* 1977, *49,* 811.

Severe metabolic alkalosis secondary to gastric hypersecretion was reversed in 2 patients with dilute hydrochloric acid by intravenous infusion followed by cimetidine 200 mg every 4 hours intravenously at a rate of 100 mg per hour (increasing to 600 mg four-hourly after 48 hours in one patient) together with electrolyte replacement.— B. J. Rowlands *et al., Postgrad. med. J.,* 1978, *54,* 118.

Further references to the use of dilute hydrochloric acid given intravenously in the treatment of alkalosis.— F. X. M. Beach and E. S. Jones, *Postgrad. med. J.,* 1971, *47,* 516; D. J. Martin (letter), *Drug Intell. & clin. Pharm.,* 1976, *10,* 231; R. Whang, *J. Am. med. Ass.,* 1979, *242,* 2015.

Diagnosis of reflux oesophagitis. In 48 patients with symptoms of reflux oesophagitis, the result of an acid perfusion test were significantly related to the symptom pattern and to endoscopic abnormality, but not to radiological evidence of reflux. In the acid perfusion test 0.15 M sodium chloride solution was perfused into the oesophagus at the rate of 10 ml per minute for 10 minutes, followed by 0.1 M hydrochloric acid at the same rate for 15 minutes or until typical symptoms were produced; the rate of perfusion was increased to 20 ml per minute for a further 15 minutes before the result was considered negative. After relief of symptoms by the perfusion of 0.1 M sodium bicarbonate the test was repeated for confirmation. The acid perfusion test was considered to be a useful procedure in patients with symptoms that were difficult to assess. A clear positive result would strongly support the diagnosis of reflux oesophagitis.— G. E. Sladen *et al., Br. med. J.,* 1975, *1,* 71.

Heartburn. For the use of hydrochloric acid in heartburn in pregnancy, see Antacids, p.71.

1303-j

Betaine Hydrochloride *(B.P.C. 1949)*. Trimethylglycine Hydrochloride. (Carboxymethyl)trimethylammonium hydroxide inner salt hydrochloride.

$C_5H_{11}NO_2,HCl$=153.6.

CAS — 107-43-7 (betaine); 590-46-5 (hydrochloride).

Pharmacopoeias. In *Aust., Hung., Jug.,* and *Port.*

Colourless crystals or white crystalline powder with not more than a slight odour. **Soluble** 1 in 2 of water and 1 in 20 of alcohol (90%); practically insoluble in chloroform and ether. A 10% solution in water has a pH of 1 to 1.5. **Incompatible** with alkalis and silver salts.

When dissolved in water, betaine hydrochloride hydrolyses and almost 25% of its weight of hydrochloric acid is formed.

Betaine hydrochloride has been given in doses of 60 to 500 mg, dissolved in water, in the treatment of hypochlorhydria. A wide variety of betaine salts have been used in various countries, mainly for gastro-intestinal disturbances.

Proprietary Preparations of Betaine Hydrochloride and some other Betaine Salts

Acidol Pepsin *(Sterling Research, UK)*. Tablets each containing betaine hydrochloride 388 mg and pepsin 97 mg. For achlorhydria. *Dose.* 1 to 3 dissolved in a tumblerful of water and taken through a straw, thrice daily, preferably after meals. (Also available as Acidol-Pepsin in *Austral.*).

Some other proprietary preparations containing betaine hydrochloride are described under Potassium Chloride, p.631.

Other Proprietary Names of some other Betaine Salts

Somatyl *(aspartate)(Fr., Ital.)*; Stea-16 *(cyclobutyrol salt)(Belg.)*.

1304-z

Acetic Acid (6 per cent) *(B.P.)*. Dilute Acetic Acid; Diluted Acetic Acid *(U.S.N.F.)*.

CAS — 64-19-7.

Pharmacopoeias. In *Br., Cz.,* and *Ind.*; also in *U.S.N.F.* (all 6%). In *Aust.* (11.5 to 12.2%), and *It.* and *Port.* (10%). See also under Acetic Acid (33 per cent).

Contains 5.7 to 6.3% w/w of $C_2H_4O_2$. It may be prepared by diluting 18.2 g of Acetic Acid (33 per cent) with 81.8 g of water. Wt per ml about 1.005 g.

Worcester Sauce, stated to contain a high concentration of acetic acid, garlic and spices, might have caused renal damage and calculi in 2 patients who took large quantities for prolonged periods.— K. J. Murphy, *Lancet*, 1967, *2*, 401.

Uses. It may be given diluted in the treatment of poisoning by alkalis. Well diluted, it is used as a soothing application to inflamed joints and as a cooling lotion to the skin in cases of fever. A solution containing not less than 4% w/v of acetic acid ($C_2H_4O_2$) in water, with colouring, is known as artificial vinegar or non-brewed condiment. Vinegar is a product of a fermentation process.

In the treatment of patients with black or brown hairy tongues subsequent to treatment with antibiotics by mouth, the use of vinegar to clean the tongue once or twice a day for a week appeared to be effective.— L. Taylor (letter), *Br. med. J.*, 1971, *1*, 115.

Bee and jelly-fish stings. Rubbed well at the point of the sting with a mixture of a teaspoonful of salt and an equal quantity of vinegar, relief was instantaneous and no inflammation resulted.— J. F. Gow, *Br. med. J.*, 1949, *2*, 1064.

1305-c

Acetic Acid (33 per cent) *(B.P.)*. Acetic Acid.

CAS — 64-19-7.

Pharmacopoeias. In *Br.* and *Ind.* (33%), *Aust.* (33.7 to 35.5%), *Chin.* (36 to 37%), *Jap.* (30 to 32%), and *Pol.* (30%). In the following under the title or synonym Acidum Aceticum Dilutum: *Belg.*, *Jug.*, *Pol.*, *Roum.*, *Swiss* (all 30%), *Hung.* (20%), and *Span.* (36%). Also in *U.S.N.F.* (36 to 37%).

A clear colourless liquid with a pungent odour and sharply acid taste, containing 32.5 to 33.5% w/w of $C_2H_4O_2$. It may be prepared by diluting 1 part by weight of glacial acetic acid with 2 parts by weight of water or by suitably diluting a pure commercial acid. Wt per ml 1.040 to 1.042 g. **Miscible** with water, alcohol, and glycerol. Solutions are **sterilised** by autoclaving. **Store** in airtight containers.

Uses. Acetic acid is considered to have a mild expectorant action. It is administered by mouth as oxymel or squill oxymel and it is an ingredient of some linctuses. Applied externally it has an irritant action and is used in liniments.

Acetic acid possesses antibacterial activity and concentrations of 5% may be bactericidal. It is reported to be effective against bacteria of the *Haemophilus* and *Pseudomonas* spp. and against *Candida* and *Trichomonas*. Solutions have been applied to the skin and used in vaginal douches. Acetic acid is also reported to be spermicidal.

For the possible use of acetic acid in conjunction with moderate heat treatment in the preparation of concentrated haemodialysis solutions, see E. Sandell *et al.*, *Acta pharm. suec.*, 1972, *9*, 147.

The use of acetic acid and acetates in food was limited only by good manufacturing practice.— Seventeenth Report of the Joint FAO/WHO Expert Committee on Food Additives, *Tech. Rep. Ser. Wld Hlth Org. No. 539*, 1974. For background toxicological information, see *Fd Add. Ser. Wld Hlth Org. No. 5*, 1974.

Buffers. For formulas of acetate buffers from pH 3.6 to 5.6, see G. E. Schumacher, *Am. J. Hosp. Pharm.*, 1966, *23*, 628.

Disinfection of equipment. Bacteraemia due to *Bacillus cereus* occurred in 5 patients undergoing haemodialysis and was associated with contamination of the dialysis equipment despite sterilisation with acetic acid 3%. No contamination occurred with formaldehyde sterilisation.— J. R. Curtis *et al.*, *Lancet*, 1967, *1*, 136.

The incidence of bacterial contamination of inhalation-therapy equipment decreased from 84 to 10% during a 4-year period of daily decontamination with a 0.25% acetic acid solution. Also the incidence of Gram-negative bacillary necrotising pneumonia at autopsy was reduced from 7.9% during the time before use of acetic acid to about 2% during the last 2 years of the study.— A. K. Pierce *et al.*, *New Engl. J. Med.*, 1970, *282*, 528.

Pseudomonal infections. Twice daily dressings with a solution containing 5% of acetic acid [$C_2H_4O_2$] eliminated *Pseudomonas aeruginosa* from infected burns and wounds by the 7th day of treatment in 7 of 10 patients. In a control group dressings with either chlorhexidine or Chlorinated Lime and Boric Acid Solution eliminated *Pseudomonas* infection in only 1 of 10 patients. Acetic acid did not appear to be effective against other organisms; *Staphylococcus aureus* and *Proteus* actually increased in quantity in many of the wounds during treatment. Applications of acetic acid produced stinging but the pain, though immediately unpleasant, did not continue.— I. Phillips *et al.*, *Lancet*, 1968, *1*, 11.

Urinary-tract infections. Tests *in vitro* of the antibacterial action of a variety of bladder irrigation solutions on urinary-tract pathogens showed that 0.25% acetic acid added to a sodium acetate buffer was twice as effective as a 0.25% solution of acetic acid in purified water. The sodium acetate buffer consisted of sodium acetate 2.1%, polysorbate '80' 0.5%, and glacial acetic acid Q.S. to yield a solution of pH 5.— R. H. Parker and P. D. Hoeprich, *Antimicrob. Ag. Chemother.*, 1962, 26.

Use in ear. Instillation, after swimming, of acetic acid 5% in isopropyl alcohol (85%) could be used to prevent otitis externa associated with swimming ('swimmer's ear').— E. H. Jones, *Laryngoscope, St Louis*, 1971, *81*, 731, per D. L. Chadwick, *Practitioner*, 1972, *209*, 460.

The instillation of acetic acid ear-drops was as effective as topical antibiotics in the treatment of chronic suppurative otitis media, achieving a cure-rate of about 40% in both sets of patients. The use of acetic acid plus antibiotics gave a cure-rate of 50%.— M. K. Malik *et al.*, *J. Lar. Otol.*, 1975, *29*, 837.

Further references: D. Heilig *et al.*, *Curr. ther. Res.*, 1979, *26*, 862.

Preparations

Acetic Acid Ear Drops *(A.P.F.)*. Acetic acid (33 per cent) 3 ml, freshly boiled and cooled water to 100 ml.

Acetic Acid 2% in Spirit Drops *(Roy. Nat. T. N. and E. Hosp.)*. Acetic acid (33 per cent) 2 ml, industrial methylated spirit 50 ml, water to 100 ml. Ear-drops. Shelf-life 6 months.

Acetic Acid Irrigation *(A.P.F.)*. Acetic acid (33 per cent) 6 ml, Water for Injections to 100 ml. Sterilised by autoclaving.

Acetic Acid Irrigation *(U.S.P.)*. A sterile solution of glacial acetic acid 0.2375 to 0.2625% w/v in Water for Injections. pH 2.8 to 3.4.
For bladder irrigation.

Acetum *(Port. P.)*. Acetum Vini; Vinaigre Officinal; Vinagre. White wine vinegar containing about 8% of acetic acid.

Proprietary Preparations

Aci-jel *(Ortho-Cilag, UK)*. A vaginal jelly (buffered to pH4) containing glacial acetic acid 0.92%.

1306-k

Glacial Acetic Acid *(B.P.)*. Glac. Acet. Acid; Concentrated Acetic Acid; Acide Acetique Cristallisable; Eisessig; Etanoico; Konzentrierte Essigsäure.

$CH_3.CO_2H$=60.05.

CAS — 64-19-7.

Pharmacopoeias. In *Arg.*, *Br.*, *Chin.*, *Ger.*, *Ind.*, and *Jap.*; in *Aust.*, *Belg.*, *Hung.*, *Jug.*, *Pol.*, and *Roum.* (all not less then 96%); in *Nord.* (not less than 96.5%); in *Cz.*, *It.*, *Port.*, *Span.*, and *Swiss* (not less than 98%); in *Mex.* and *U.S.* (all not less than 99.5%). The title Acidum Aceticum is used in *Arg.*, *Belg.*, *Mex.*, *Pol.*, *Port.*, *Roum.*, and *Span.*

A translucent crystalline mass or a clear colourless liquid with a pungent odour. It contains not less than 99% w/w of $C_2H_4O_2$. It crystallises when cooled to about 10° and does not completely remelt until warmed to about 15°. Wt per ml 1.048 to 1.051 g. B.p. about 117°. F.p. not lower than 14.8°. Flash-point about 44° (open cup).

Miscible with water, alcohol, chloroform, ether, glycerol, and most fixed and volatile oils. **Store** in airtight containers.

Adverse Effects. The ingestion of glacial acetic acid leads to severe pain in the mouth, throat, and abdomen, and to the formation of white plaques and ulcers on mucous membranes. Vomiting, haematemesis, and diarrhoea may occur. Hoarseness, rapid and shallow respiration, circulatory collapse, and a low body temperature may develop.

Maximum permissible atmospheric concentration 10 ppm.

Treatment of Adverse Effects. As for Hydrochloric Acid, p.783.

Uses. It has been applied as an escharotic to corns and warts, but causes great pain if in contact with the surrounding skin.

An aromatic preparation of glacial acetic acid was formerly used as a type of smelling salts.

Preparations

Aromatic Vinegar *(B.P.C. 1934)*. Acid. Acet. Aromat.; Gewürzessig. Oils of bergamot 2.5, cinnamon 1.25, clove 10, lavender 5, orange 5, and thyme 2.5, and glacial acetic acid to 100, all by vol. Intended for use as a restorative and stimulant in fainting, by inhalation of the vapour. *F.N. Belg.* includes a similar preparation.

1307-a

Citric Acid *(B.P., Eur. P.)*. Acidum Citricum; Citronensäure. 2-Hydroxypropane-1,2,3-tricarboxylic acid.

$C_6H_8O_7$=192.1.

CAS — 77-92-9.

NOTE. Citric acid was formerly known as anhydrous citric acid.

Pharmacopoeias. In *Br.*, *Eur.*, *Fr.*, *Ger.*, *Jap.*, *Jug.*, *Neth.*, and *Nord. It.*, *Swiss*, and *U.S.* also allow the monohydrate.

Odourless or almost odourless, colourless crystals or white crystalline powder with a strongly acid taste. M.p. about 153°. It absorbs insignificant amounts of moisture at 25° at relative humidities of about 25 to 50% and significant amounts at 50 to 75%, with formation of the monohydrate in the upper part of the range; substantial amounts of moisture are absorbed under damper conditions.

Solubility as for citric acid monohydrate. **Store** in airtight containers.

1308-t

Citric Acid Monohydrate *(B.P., Eur. P.)*. Acidum Citricum Monohydricum; Hydrous Citric Acid; Acido del Limón.

$C_6H_8O_7,H_2O$=210.1.

CAS — 5949-29-1.

Pharmacopoeias. In all pharmacopoeias examined except *Braz.*, *Int.*, and *Rus. It.*, *Swiss*, and *U.S.* also allow citric acid.

Odourless or almost odourless colourless crystals or white crystalline powder with a strongly acid taste, obtained from lemon juice, which contains as much as 7 to 9%, or the juice of other citrus fruits, or prepared from glucose by the growth of species of *Aspergillus*. It loses water at 75°, becoming anhydrous at 135°, and fusing at about 153°. At relative humidities lower than about 65%, it effloresces at 25° and the anhydrous acid is formed at humidities below about 40%; at relative humidities between about 65 and 75% it absorbs insignificant amounts of moisture, but above this substantial amounts are absorbed.

Soluble 1 in less than 1 of water, 1 in 1.5 of alcohol, 1 in 2 of glycerol, and 1 in 30 of ether. A 7% solution is approximately equal in acidity to lemon juice. A 5.52% solution is iso-osmotic with serum.

Solutions are **sterilised** by autoclaving. Aqueous solutions generally develop fungous growths on standing. **Store** in a cool place in airtight containers.

Adverse Effects. Citric acid ingested frequently or in large quantities may cause erosion of the teeth and have a local irritant action.

Erosion of teeth. In 4 patients erosion of the enamel of the incisor teeth was caused by drinking pure lemon juice in 2 patients and by raw lemons in the other 2. The pH of bottled pure juice was 2.65, that of juice diluted 1 teaspoonful to a tumblerful of water pH 2.85, and fresh lemon juice had a pH of 2.56. Any liquid with a pH below 3.5 was a potential source of damage to the teeth.— D. N. Allan, *Br. dent. J.*, 1967, *122*, 300.

Absorption and Fate. Citric acid is absorbed from the gastro-intestinal tract and is oxidised in the body to carbon dioxide and water.

Uses. Citric acid may be employed in a 1% solution as a cooling drink to relieve thirst in fever; it is preferably given as lemon or lime juice. It is used in effervescing mixtures, the acid being added to an alkaline mixture at the time of administration. The following are the proportions necessary to form approximately neutral mixtures with 10 parts of citric acid monohydrate; ammonium bicarbonate 7.5 parts, magnesium carbonate 7 parts, potassium bicarbonate 14.5 parts, sodium bicarbonate 12 parts.

Citric acid monohydrate is used in the preparation of effervescent granules, the water of hydration present being sufficient for preparing the mass prior to granulation.

Citric acid monohydrate is used as a synergist to enhance the effectiveness of antoxidants; this action is probably due to its property of forming complexes with the traces of heavy metals which often accelerate autoxidation reactions.

Weak solutions of citric acid monohydrate have been used for treating alkali burns but copious rinsing with water is preferable.

A review of the uses and efficacy of citric acid, the monohydrate, isopropyl citrate, and stearyl citrate as synergists to antoxidants.— *Fd Add. Ser. Wld Hlth Org. No. 3*, 1972.

The use of citric acid and its calcium, potassium, and sodium salts in food was limited only by good manufacturing practice.— Seventeenth Report of the Joint FAO/WHO Expert Committee on Food Additives, *Tech. Rep. Ser. Wld Hlth Org. No. 539*, 1974. For background toxicological information, see *Fd Add Ser. Wld Hlth Org. No. 5*, 1974.

The Food Additives and Contaminants Committee recommended that, on the grounds of safety, citric acid could continue to be used as a stabiliser for solvents used in food.— *Report on the Review of Solvents in Food*, FAC/REP/25, Ministry of Agriculture, Fisheries and Food, London, HM Stationery Office, 1978.

Buffer. For formulas of citrate buffers from pH 2.5 to 6.5, see G. E. Schumacher, *Am. J. Hosp. Pharm.*, 1966, *23*, 628.

Hyperammonaemia. Citric acid, 3 g daily, had been claimed to be of value in hyperammonaemia, probably because it caused acidification of the urine and increased elimination of ammonia.— *Lancet*, 1969, *2*, 196.

Renal calculus. Discussions on the use of preparations containing citric acid to dissolve renal calculi: D. Rennie, *New Engl. J. Med.*, 1979, *300*, 361; *Br. med. J.*, 1979, *1*, 1746.

New renal stones were completely dissolved in 4 of 6 patients suffering from recurrent stones composed of struvite ($MgNH_4PO_4$) or apatite ($CaPO_4$) or both, by irrigation with Hemiacidrin, a mixture of citric and gluconic acids, magnesium hydroxycarbonate, magnesium acid citrate, and calcium carbonate (Renacidin), through percutaneous nephrostomy tubes. Partial dissolution was achieved in the other 2 patients. Perfusion of up to 120 ml of hemiacidrin per hour for 7 to 30 days provided continuous lavage of the surface of the stones. Less than 10 days' perfusion was necessary in 4 kidneys. On several occasions irrigation had to be stopped temporarily because of flank pain and low-grade fever. Calcium oxalate stones, the most common type of calculi, are insoluble in hemiacidrin.— S. P. Dretler *et al.*, *New Engl. J. Med.*, 1979, *300*, 341. Criticism.— M. I. Resnick and W. H. Boyce (letter), *ibid.*, 1488. Reply.— S. P. Dretler *et al.* (letter), *ibid.*

Further references: K. Somasundaram and H. B. Eckstein, *Br. med. J.*, 1966, *2*, 91; G. Kierfield, *Dt. med. Wschr.*, 1968, *93*, 1547, per *J. Am. med. Ass.*, 1968, *205* (Sept. 9), A202.

See also under Solution G, p.785.

Test of secretin production. The poor secretin response to duodenal instillation of 5 ml of citric acid monohydrate 0.5 M could be used as a test of duodenal endocrine function. There was significantly less response to citric acid monohydrate in 6 children with active coeliac disease than in 6 children with treated coeliac disease or 15 healthy children.— S. R. Bloom *et al.*, *Gut*, 1976, *17*, 812.

Use of disinfectants on farms. In Great Britain, citric acid 1 in 500 of water is an approved disinfectant for foot-and-mouth disease under the Diseases of Animals (Approved Disinfectants) Order 1978 (SI 1978: No. 32), as amended (SI 1978: No. 934).

Preparations

Citric Acid Eye Lotion *(A.P.F.)*. Collyr. Acid. Cit.; Acid Eye Lotion. Citric acid monohydrate 1 g, sodium chloride 600 mg, Water for Injections to 100 ml. Sterilised by autoclaving. To be applied freely, undiluted, in the treatment of alkali burns.

Citric Acid Eye Lotion *(B.P.C. 1963)*. Citric acid monohydrate 2 g, sodium chloride 1.14 g, water, freshly boiled and cooled, to 100 ml. To be diluted with an equal volume of warm water before use. For alkali in the eyes.

Amended formula. Citric acid monohydrate 1.7 g, sodium chloride 1 g, distilled water to 100 ml.—*Compendium of Past Formulae 1933 to 1966*, London, The National Pharmaceutical Union, 1969.

Lemon Mouthwash *(St. Thomas' Hosp.)*. Citric acid monohydrate 675 mg, terpeneless lemon oil 0.0015 ml, glycerol 15 ml, concentrated chloroform water 2.5 ml, water to 100 ml. Dilute with an equal quantity of warm water before use.

Solution G. Suby's G Solution. Citric acid monohydrate 3.225 g, magnesium oxide 384 mg, anhydrous sodium carbonate 437 mg, water to 100 ml. pH about 4. Used by retrograde introduction in 7 patients with urinary calculi; partial or complete dissolution of the stones resulted in 6 cases.—H.J. Suby and F. Albright, *New Engl. J. Med.*, 1943, *228*, 81. Solution G remains in use today.—D. Rennie, *ibid.*, 1979, *300*, 361.

Proprietary Preparations

Renacidin *(Guardian, USA: Farillon, UK)*. A white powder for preparing irrigating solutions; a 10% solution is stated to contain, immediately after autoclaving, gluconic acid 0.2 to 0.3%, gluconolactone 0.07 to 0.1%, citric acid 0.3 to 0.6%, magnesium acid citrate 5.3 to 5.9%, magnesium acid gluconate 0.3 to 0.6%, complex gluconocitrates of magnesium 0.5 to 1.2%, magnesium bicarbonate 0.6 to 0.8%, and calcium bicarbonate 0.1 to 0.2%. For the prevention of calcification of indwelling urethral catheters and to promote the solution of renal calculi.

1309-x

Formic Acid *(B.P.C. 1934)*. Aminic Acid; Ameisensäure.

CH_2O_2=46.03.

CAS — 64-18-6.

Pharmacopoeias. In *Aust.* and *Pol.*

A colourless liquid with a pungent odour, containing about 25% w/w of CH_2O_2. Wt per ml about 1.05 g. **Miscible** with water and with alcohol.

Formic acid resembles acetic acid in its actions but is more irritating and pungent. The acid and its sodium and calcium salts are used as preservatives in food. They were formerly used, as was the calcium salt, as diuretics. Ferric formate was used as a haematinic. Solutions containing about 60% formic acid are marketed for the removal of lime scales from kettles.

Maximum permissible atmospheric concentration (of CH_2O_2) 5 ppm.

A 2-year-old boy slowly recovered after swallowing an unknown amount of a kettle descaler containing 60% of formic acid. The most serious complication was severe laryngeal stridor, and tracheostomy and gastrostomy became necessary.— *Practitioner*, 1968, *200*, 179.

Estimated acceptable daily intake: up to 3 mg per kg body-weight.— Seventeenth Report of the Joint FAO/WHO Expert Committee on Food Additives, *Tech. Rep. Ser. Wld Hlth Org. No. 539*, 1974. For background toxicological information, see *Fd Add. Ser. Wld Hlth Org. No. 5*, 1974. Ethyl formate could be included in the acceptable daily intake for formic acid.— Twenty-third Report of Joint FAO/WHO Expert Committee on Food Additives, *Tech. Rep. Ser. Wld Hlth Org. No. 648*, 1980..

A report of 3 patients who swallowed descaling agents containing 40 or 55% formic acid. The major complications included the local effects on the oropharynx, oesophagus, and stomach, metabolic acidosis, derangement of blood-clotting mechanisms with intravascular coagulation or haemolysis, and the acute onset of respiratory and renal failure. All 3 patients died betwen 5 to 14 days after admission to hospital. It was suggested that intense therapy should include from the outset exchange transfusion, infusion of clotting factors, high dose corticosteroids, respiratory assistance, and peritoneal or haemodialysis with parenteral nutrition.— R. B. Naik *et al.*, *Postgrad. med. J.*, 1980, *56*, 451.

1310-y

Fumaric Acid *(U.S.N.F.)*. Allomalenic Acid; Boletic Acid. *trans*-Butenedioic acid.

$C_2H_2(CO_2H)_2$=116.1.

CAS — 110-17-8.

Pharmacopoeias. In *U.S.N.F.*

White odourless granules or crystalline powder. M.p. about 301°. Slightly **soluble** in water and ether; soluble in alcohol; very slightly soluble in chloroform.

Fumaric acid is used as an acidifier and flavouring agent; 50 to 3600 ppm is used in foods.

1311-j

Hydrofluoric Acid *(B.P.C. 1934)*. Fluohydric Acid; Fluoric Acid.

HF=20.01.

CAS — 7664-39-3.

A solution of hydrogen fluoride in water, adjusted to contain 40% w/w of HF. It is a clear colourless liquid with a pungent odour. It attacks glass strongly and must be **stored** in plastic bottles or in bottles coated internally with ceresin or hard paraffin.

Crude hydrofluoric acid of various strengths up to 55% w/w is available for technical purposes. The crude acid contains sulphuric, sulphurous, and fluorosilicic acids; it may be purified by redistillation.

Adverse Effects. As for Hydrochloric Acid, p.783. Although the corrosive effects of hydrofluoric acid tend to predominate absorption may produce systemic fluoride poisoning described under Sodium Fluoride, p.700.

The pain from burns may be delayed, so that the patient does not know he has been burned until some hours later, when the area begins to smart; intense pain then sets in and this may persist for several days. Destruction of tissue proceeds under the toughened coagulated skin, so that the ulcers extend deeply, heal slowly, and leave a scar.

Solutions of less than 5%, if speedily removed, have little effect on human skin, but even 1% solutions if left for a long enough period may lead to deep necrosis. Solutions above 30% produce immediate pain.

The fumes of hydrofluoric acid are highly irritant.

Maximum permissible atmospheric concentration (hydrogen fluoride) 3 ppm.

The use of a 1% solution of hydrofluoric acid for cleaning windows was a health hazard and weakened the glass.— A. G. Phillips (letter), *Lancet*, 1966, *1*, 601. See also G. MacBain and C. White (letter), *ibid.*, 312.

A study of the excretion of fluoride in the urine of 20 workers in the glass industry indicated that there was a direct correlation between the atmospheric concentrations of hydrofluoric acid they were exposed to and their urinary excretion of fluoride. The total urinary fluoride excretion was between 10 and 60% of the inhaled intake. As the atmospheric concentration of hydrofluoric acid increased there appeared to be a decrease in the amount of fluoride excreted in the urine. Analysis of post-shift urine samples was considered to be a suitable method for monitoring workers exposed to hydrofluoric acid but the results depended on the form of the inhalation so that studies in the aluminium industry (fluoride containing dust) could not be compared with those in the glass industry (gaseous hydrofluoric acid).— A. Zober *et al.*, *Int. Archs occup. environ. Hlth*, 1977, *40*, 13, per *Abstr. Hyg.*, 1977, *52*, 1388.

A report of chronic intoxication in an industrial worker who had been exposed to hydrogen fluoride vapour over a period of 10 years. Symptoms of the disease were identical with those of preskeletal fluoride intoxication and included pains in bones, mental impairment, faecal incontinence, cough and dyspnoea, and osteoarthritis. Bone biopsy 4 years after exposure had ceased revealed a fluoride concentration of 1125 ppm compared with the usual adult concentration of 300 to 500 ppm.— G. L. Waldbott and J. R. Lee, *Clin. Toxicol.*, 1978, *13*, 391.

Treatment of Adverse Effects. For the treatment of hydrofluoric acid burns in the eye, immediate flooding of the eye with water for at least 15 minutes is recommended.

Skin burns should be washed by flooding with water for at least 15 minutes, after which magnesium oxide paste (heavy magnesium oxide 1, glycerol 1.5 or 2) is applied. Alternatively, soak the affected area in alcohol and ice for at least 1 hour before applying magnesium oxide paste. Subsequently, Calcium Gluconate Injection 10% should be injected, under local anaesthesia if necessary, into and under the coagulum formed, in sufficient quantity to raise a wheal under the whole of the burned area. Washing with quaternary ammonium compounds has also been recommended.

Hydrofluoric acid appears to pass through finger- and toe-nails without causing any apparent damage; nails will therefore have to be removed to be able to treat the underlying tissues.

Benzethonium chloride might be absorbed in toxic quantities from the surface of hydrofluoric acid burns and the total dosage should therefore be limited.— *Br. med. J.*, 1972, *1*, 45. See also *ibid.*, 1971, *3*, 526.

The safe handling of hydrofluoric acid in dental laboratories.— E. Rosenstiel, *Br. dent. J.*, 1974, *136*, 413.

The application of calcium gluconate gel was at least as effective as calcium gluconate injection as the first treatment of hydrofluoric acid burns. It had been used by ICI Mond Division for 43 liquid splashes and 10 vapour burns since 1971. Benzalkonium chloride solution 0.003% was too irritant for the eyes and it was recommended that only water or saline be used for irrigation of the eyes, followed by the instillation of a few drops of sterile calcium gluconate solution 10%.— T. D. Browne, *J. Soc. occup. Med.*, 1974, *24*, 80, per *Abstr. Hyg.*, 1974, *49*, 1075.

1312-z

Lactic Acid *(B.P., Eur. P.).* Acidum Lacticum; Milchsäure. 2-Hydroxypropionic acid.

$C_3H_6O_3$=90.08.

CAS — 50-21-5; 79-33-4 (+); 10326-41-7 (−); 598-82-3 (±).

Pharmacopoeias. In all pharmacopoeias examined except *Rus.*

A colourless or slightly yellow, viscous hygroscopic liquid, which is odourless or has a slight but not unpleasant odour and a mildly acid taste in dilute aqueous solution. It consists of a mixture of lactic acid, its condensation products such as lactoyl lactic acid and other polylactic acids, and water. The condensation products slowly revert to lactic acid on dilution with water. In most cases lactic acid is in the form of the racemate (*RS*-lactic acid), but in some cases the (+)-(*S*)-isomer is predominant. It contains the equivalent of 88 to 92% w/w of $C_3H_6O_3$. Relative density about 1.2. *U.S.P.* specifies a mixture of lactic acid and lactoyl lactic acid equivalent to 85 to 90% w/w of $C_3H_6O_3$.

Miscible with water, alcohol, and ether; immiscible with carbon disulphide, chloroform, and light petroleum. A 2.3% solution in water is iso-osmotic with serum. Solutions are *sterilised* by autoclaving or by filtration. **Incompatible** with oxidising agents. **Store** in airtight containers.

Adverse Effects and Treatment. As for Hydrochloric Acid, p.783.

Administration of insufficiently diluted acid to infants produces oesophageal corrosion and stricture.

Reports of deaths of 3 premature infants following administration of an acid milk mixture containing an excess of lactic acid causing acute haemorrhagic and gangrenous gastritis.— E. J. Young and R. P. Smith, *J. Am. med. Ass.*, 1944, *125*, 1179.

There was evidence that neonates had difficulty in metabolising D-(−)-lactic acid and this isomer and the racemate should not be used in foods for infants less than 3 months old.— Seventeenth Report of the FAO/WHO Expert Committee on Food Additives, *Tech. Rep. Ser. Wld Hlth Org. No. 539*, 1974. For background toxicological information, see *Fd Add. Ser. Wld Hlth Org. No. 5*, 1974.

For a report of severe metabolic acidosis, due to D-lactic acid, in a patient who took tablets containing *Lactobacillus acidophilus*, see under Lactic-acid-producing Organisms, p.786.

Absorption and Fate. Lactic acid is readily absorbed from the gastro-intestinal tract and is slowly converted to bicarbonate in the circulation.

Uses. Lactic acid is used in the preparation of Compound Sodium Lactate Intravenous Infusion and of other solutions containing sodium lactate which are given by intravenous injection in the treatment of acidosis. It has a less rapid action than sodium bicarbonate. See also under Sodium Lactate in the section on Sodium Salts, p.640.

Lactic acid has also been given in the form of lactic acid milk, made by adding, drop by drop, 5 to 7 ml of lactic acid to a litre of cold whole milk which is vigorously stirred to prevent the formation of clots. Lactic acid milk may check the vomiting but not the diarrhoea of infantile gastro-enteritis; it has also been used for infant feeding when breast milk was not available.

A 0.5 to 2% solution of lactic acid is used as a vaginal douche in the treatment of leucorrhoea, or pessaries containing 5% lactic acid are used.

Lactic acid is also used as a food preservative.

In studies in 299 women, use of hand lotions containing sodium lactate 10% or lactic acid 10% adjusted to pH 4, for 2 weeks, resulted in less hand skin dryness and flaking than use of control lotions. Lactic acid products were more effective than sodium lactate products.— J. D. Middleton, *J. Soc. cosmet. Chem.*, 1974, *25*, 519.

Neonatal staphylococcal infections. The frequency and distribution of organisms were similar in the nasal and cord areas of newborn babies washed with either a 3% hexachlorophane solution or a soap containing lactic acid. No infants developed skin infections or bacterial septicaemia.— J. C. McHattie *et al.*, *Can. med. Ass. J.*, 1974, *110*, 1248.

Stingray wounds. For the treatment of stingray wounds the affected area should be immersed in a warm solution of lactic acid 0.5 to 1% and this procedure repeated for 3 to 5 days. The wound should then heal in about 5 days with minimal disability.— J. Hartmann (letter), *J. Am. med. Ass.*, 1966, *197*, 153.

Warts. A study of 389 patients in 2 centres showed that the application of a mixture of salicylic acid 1 part and lactic acid 1 part in flexible collodion 4 parts (SAL paint) was as effective as that of liquid nitrogen or of a combination of both in the treatment of hard warts. The percentage cures were 67, 69, and 78 respectively and the differences were not statistically significant. No recurrences were reported 6 months after treatment with SAL paint in 46 of 50 patients in a general practice. Other studies indicated that SAL paint cured 45% of patients with mosaic plantar warts and it was no less effective than preparations containing fluorouracil 5%, idoxuridine 5%, a 10% buffered solution of glutaraldehyde, or a paint prepared to contain 40% of an adduct of benzalkonium chloride and bromine (Callusolve 40).— M. H. Bunney *et al.*, *Br. J. Derm.*, 1976, *94*, 667.

Preparations

Lactic Acid Irrigation *(B.P.C. 1963).* Lactic acid 0.63 ml, water to 100 ml.

Lactic Acid Pessaries *(B.P.).* Pessaries containing lactic acid in a Glycerol Suppositories type mass. Store at a temperature not exceeding 30°. *A.P.F.* has pessaries of 4 to 5 g containing 5% w/w in Glyco-gelatin Gel.

Proprietary Names

Lacta-Gynecogel *(Therapeutica, Belg.)*; pHygiene *(Owen, Canad.)*; Tampovagan c. acid. lact. *(AGM, Ger.)*; Tonsillosan *(Spitzner, Ger.)*.

NOTE. The name Tonsillosan has also been used in some countries for a preparation containing dequalinium chloride.

A preparation containing lactic acid was formerly marketed in Great Britain under the proprietary name Tampovagan Lactic Acid (*Norgine*).

1313-c

Lactic-acid-producing Organisms

Lactic-acid-producing organisms were introduced as a therapeutic agent by Metchnikoff with the idea of acidifying the intestinal contents and thus preventing the growth of putrefactive organisms. The organism chosen by him for this purpose was *Lactobacillus bulgaricus*, which occurs in naturally soured milk, but many workers found it difficult to produce a growth of this organism in the intestines and preferred *L. acidophilus* which is an inhabitant of the human intestine. Yogurt is a common preparation of lactic-acid-producing organisms.

Lactobacillus preparations have been used in the treatment of gastro-intestinal disorders but there is little evidence to support this use.

Adverse effects. Severe metabolic acidosis and neurological manifestations occurred in a 30-year-old man with short-bowel syndrome after he began taking *Lactobacillus acidophilus* tablets to reduce his diarrhoea. D-Lactic acid was responsible for the acidosis and the source was considered to be bacterial fermentation in the colon since after long-term treatment with neomycin by mouth the acidosis and neurological dysfunction were resolved.— M. S. Oh *et al.*, *New Engl. J. Med.*, 1979, *301*, 249.

Migraine. A tablet preparation of *Lactobacillus acidophilus* in doses of 150 to 225 million organisms daily was successful in 8 of 10 patients with migraine who had failed to respond to other treatments.— E. Ask-Upmark (letter), *Lancet*, 1966, *2*, 446. A similar report in 9 of 16 patients with migraine.— J. Braham (letter), *Br. med. J.*, 1969, *3*, 533.

Vaginitis. The twice daily intravaginal injection of yogurt 3 ml for 1 week, followed by twice weekly injection for 2 weeks, decreased the volume of vaginal discharge and signs of vaginitis and gave subjective improvement in 25 women when they were examined 3 weeks after finishing treatment.— K. D. Gunston and P. F. Fairbrother, *S. Afr. med. J.*, 1975, *49*, 675, per *Practitioner*, 1975, *215*, 8.

Patients with chronic candidal vulvovaginitis had had some amelioration of symptoms after self-medication with preparations containing viable *Lactobacillus acidophilus* cultures.— T. E. Will (letter), *Lancet*, 1979, *2*, 482. Confirmation that *Lactobacillus acidophilus* is of value in the treatment of vaginal candidiasis. Treatment with a freeze-dried preparation of *Lactobacillus acidophilus* (Enpac) together with natural yoghurt containing the live bacillus has proved very effective. Administration of the lactobacillus, incidentally, appeared to alleviate symptoms of eczema in 3 women.— B. Sandler (letter), *ibid.*, 791.

Buttermilk. The acidulous milk which remains after the butter has been churned out. It contains protein 3, fat 0.5, sugar 4.8, and water 91%.

Koumiss (Artificial). Dissolve dextrose 12.5 g in water 100 ml and add yeast 1.1 g and cows' milk 100 ml. Place in a litre bottle and fill up with milk; cork and wire. Keep cool and shake frequently during 4 days.

Yogurt. Yoghourt; Yoghurt. Raise milk to boiling point, remove from heat, and allow a skin to form on top. While still too hot to be held conveniently inoculate by allowing some previous yogurt, thinned with sterile water, if necessary, to slip down the edge of the container all round the rim. Cover and maintain at blood heat until the next day.

Proprietary Preparations Containing Lactic-acid-producing Organisms

Enpac *(Aplin & Barrett, UK)*. A powder containing freeze-dried cells of strains of *L. acidophilus* which are resistant to benzylpenicillin and synthetic penicillins, streptomycin, chlortetracycline, tetracycline, oxytetracycline, neomycin, erythromycin, chloramphenicol, lincomycin, and kanamycin, incorporated in a nutrient medium. It is stated that by replacing the normal intestinal lactobacilli with these antibiotic-resistant strains, side-effects arising from the destruction of the normal intestinal flora during treatment with antibiotics are minimised; also used in disorders due to abnormal intestinal flora. *Dose.* 3 g (1 teaspoonful) in cold or tepid milk or water 4 times daily, preferably in intervals between administration of the antibiotic; the powder should be given during the full course of antibiotic treatment and continued for 2 or 3 days thereafter. (Also available as Enpac in *Austral.*, *Switz.*).

Hepatic encephalopathy. Enpac, given in a daily dose of 20 to 40 g, produced an improvement in EEG and clinical status in 5 out of 7 patients with chronic hepatic encephalopathy on long-term neomycin. A fall in blood-ammonia occurred in 3 out of 5 patients tested.— A. E. Read *et al.*, *Br. med. J.*, 1966, *1*, 1267.

Flar Capsules *(Consolidated Chemicals, UK)*. Each contains lactic acid bacilli, resistant to antibiotics and sulphonamides, 5000 million, thiamine hydrochloride 5 mg, riboflavine 500 µg, pyridoxine hydrochloride 500 µg, nicotinamide 20 mg, sodium pantothenate 7.5 mg, inositol 20 mg, folic acid 200 µg, cyanocobalamin 5 µg, and crude dried liver extract equivalent to 20 g of fresh liver. For gastro-enteritis and other inflammatory conditions of the gastro-intestinal tract, with or without antibiotic or chemotherapeutic drugs. *Dose.* 1 to 2 capsules before meals.

Uniflor *(Aplin & Barrett, UK)*. Tablets containing a freeze-dried strain of *L. acidophilus* not resistant to antibiotics, incorporated in a nutrient medium. For gastro-intestinal disorders where antibiotics are not being administered. *Dose.* 2 to 4 tablets daily, to be sucked or chewed, which may be increased to 12 daily. Infants may take half the adult dose. (Also available as Uniflor in *Austral.*).

Other Proprietary Names of Preparations Containing Lactic-acid-producing Organisms

Arg.— Acidofilofago, Entero Vacuna, Lacto Lemos, Lactophilus; *Spain*— Lacto Level; *Switz.*— Tapo, Ventrux Acido; *USA*— Bacid, DöFus, Lactinex, Novaflor.

1314-k

Maleic Acid *(B.P.)*. Toxilic Acid. *cis*-Butenedioic acid.

$C_2H_2(CO_2H)_2$=116.1.

CAS — 110-16-7.

Pharmacopoeias. In *Br.* and *Fr.*

A white odourless crystalline powder with a strongly acid taste. M.p. 132° to 140°. **Soluble** 1 in 1.5 of water, 1 in 2 of alcohol, and 1 in 12 of ether.

Maleic acid is used in the preparation of Ergometrine Injection *B.P.* and Ergometrine and Oxytocin Injection *B.P.*

1315-a

Malic Acid. Apple Acid; Hydroxysuccinic Acid. Hydroxybutanedioic acid.

$C_4H_6O_5$=134.1.

CAS — 6915-15-7; 636-61-3 (+); 97-67-6 (−); 617-48-1 (±).

Pharmacopoeias. In *Ind.*

An acid present in apples, pears, and many other fruits. It occurs as colourless, odourless, deliquescent crystals. M.p. about 99°. Freely **soluble** in water; soluble 1 in 2 of alcohol and of ether and 1 in 1 of methyl alcohol.

The action of malic acid is similar to that of tartaric acid and it has been used in effervescent saline preparations. It is a permitted food additive.

1316-t

Monochloroacetic Acid. Chloroacetic Acid.

$CH_2Cl.CO_2H$=94.5.

CAS — 79-11-8.

A colourless or white deliquescent crystalline powder. **Soluble** about 4 in 1 of water; soluble in alcohol, chloroform, and ether.

Monochloroacetic acid is used as an escharotic for plantar and mosaic warts. For plantar warts, the surrounding parts are usually protected with soft paraffin or collodion and monochloroacetic acid crystals or a saturated solution is applied to the wart which may be excised 2 days later. Mosaic warts are lightly swabbed with monochloroacetic acid and then covered with a salicylic acid plaster; the treatment is repeated weekly after debridement.

Use of a saturated solution of monochloroacetic acid for the removal of plantar warts.— W. D. Watts, *Chiropodist*, 1968, *23*, 454, per *Practitioner*, 1969, *202*, 180.

1317-x

Morrhuic Acid *(B.P.C. 1949)*.

An amber-coloured oily liquid with a fishy odour and taste, consisting of that fraction of the fatty acids of cod-liver oil which is liquid at 15°. Wt per ml 0.907 to 0.912 g. When cooled at 10° for 30 minutes, no solid matter separates. Practically **insoluble** in water; soluble in alcohol, carbon tetrachloride, chloroform, and ether. **Store** in well-filled airtight containers.

Adverse Effects. Severe allergic reactions have occurred following administration of sodium morrhuate injection.

Uses. Morrhuic acid is used in the preparation of sodium morrhuate injection. Doses of 0.5 to 5 ml of a 5% solution of sodium morrhuate have been give as a sclerosing agent in the treatment of varicose veins but the sensitivity of the patient should be tested with a small preliminary dose.

Sodium morrhuate injection had been given by intra-synovial injection in 76 joints of 33 patients with rheumatoid arthritis or osteoarthritis. The dose was 4 to 6 ml for a knee, 2 ml for elbow, wrist, or shoulder, and 0.3 to 0.4 ml for smaller joints. There was increased mobility and less pain in 97.3% of the joints, but there were relapses in 4 patients.— D. Niculescu *et al.*, *Z. Rheumaforsch.*, 1970, *29*, 27, per *Abstr. Wld Med.*, 1970, *44*, 696.

Preparations

Morrhuate Sodium Injection *(U.S.P.)*. A sterile solution of the sodium salts of the fatty acids of cod-liver oil containing 46.5 to 53.5 mg of sodium morrhuate in each ml. It may contain up to 0.5% of a suitable antimicrobial agent and not more than 3% of ethyl or benzyl alcohol. Solid matter may form on standing; the injection must not be used if such solid does not dissolve completely on warming.

1318-r

Nitric Acid *(B.P., U.S.N.F.)*. Nit. Acid; Azotic Acid; Aqua Fortis; Salpetersäure.

HNO_3=63.01.

CAS — 7697-37-2.

Pharmacopoeias. In *Br.* and *Mex.* (both approximately 70%). In *Belg.* (64 to 66%), *Port.* (not less than 63%), *Span.* (63.64%), and *Swiss* (Acidum Nitricum 65%; 64 to 66%). *Aust.* has Acidum Nitricum Concentratum (64.3 to 66.4%) and Acidum Nitricum (31.1 to 32.2%). Also in *U.S.N.F.* (69 to 71%).

A clear, colourless or almost colourless, fuming liquid, with a characteristic irritating odour, containing 69 to 71% w/w of HNO_3. Wt per ml about 1.41 g. When distilled it forms a constant-boiling mixture, boiling at 120.5°, containing 68% w/w of HNO_3. **Store** in airtight containers.

Adverse Effects and Treatment. As for Hydrochloric Acid, p.783.

Fumes of nitrogen oxides tend to attack the lower rather than the upper respiratory tract, unless the patient is exposed to very high concentrations. There may be methaemoglobinaemia. Nitric acid stains the skin yellow.

Maximum permissible atmospheric concentration (HNO_3) 2 ppm.

Corrosive jejunitis due to ingestion of nitric acid.— J. T. Adams and J. Skucas, *Am. J. Surg.*, 1980, *140*, 282.

For a detailed regimen of treatment for the effects of inhalation of the vapours of nitric acid and the higher oxides of nitrogen, see under Nitrous Oxide, p.755.

Uses. Nitric Acid has a powerful corrosive action and has been used to remove warts, but it should be applied with caution. It is used in the preparation of Strong Ferric Chloride Solution *B.P.C. 1973*.

1319-f

Oleic Acid *(B.P., U.S.N.F.)*. Acidum Oleicum; Ölsäure.

CAS — 112-80-1 ($C_{18}H_{34}O_2$).

Pharmacopoeias. In *Arg.*, *Aust.*, *Br.*, *Braz.*, *Hung.*, *Ind.*, *Mex.*, *Pol.*, *Span.*, and *Swiss.* Also in *U.S.N.F.*

A colourless to pale brown oily liquid with a characteristic lard-like odour and taste. On exposure to air it darkens in colour and the odour and taste become more pronounced.

It consists chiefly of (*Z*)-octadec-9-enoic acid [$CH_3.(CH_2)_7.CH{:}CH.(CH_2)_7.CO_2H$ = 282.5] and also contains some stearic and palmitic acids, with traces of iron. Wt per ml 0.889 to 0.895 g. Congealing point about 4° to 10°.

Practically **insoluble** in water; very soluble in alcohol, chloroform, ether, light petroleum, and fixed and volatile oils. Most metallic oxides dissolve in an excess of oleic acid forming solutions of metal oleates; they are soluble in fats. Oleic acid also reacts with alkalis to form soaps. **Store** in well-filled airtight containers and avoid contact with metals. Protect from light.

Uses. Oleic acid forms soaps with alkaline substances and has been used in ointments to assist the absorption by the skin of medicaments such as alkaloids and metallic oxides. It must not be used in eye ointments.

Proprietary Preparations

Priolene 6986 *(Unichema, UK)*. A brand of oleic acid.

1320-z

Oxalic Acid *(B.P.C. 1934)*.

$HO_2C.CO_2H,2H_2O$=126.1.

CAS — 144-62-7 (anhydrous); 6153-56-6 (dihydrate).

Colourless, transparent, efflorescent crystals. **Soluble** 1 in 12 of water, 1 in 3 of alcohol, 1 in 100 of ether, and 1 in 6 of glycerol; practically insoluble in chloroform and light petroleum.

Adverse Effects. In dilute solution the acid and its salts are toxic owing to withdrawal of ionisable calcium from the blood and tissues. Strong solutions of the acid are corrosive. In acute poisoning from ingestion there is local irritation and corrosion of the mouth, oesophagus, and stomach, with pain and vomiting, followed shortly by muscular tremors, convulsions, and collapse. Death may occur within a few minutes. After apparent recovery acute renal failure may occur from blocking of the renal tubules by calcium oxalate crystals.

Maximum permissible atmospheric concentration 1 mg per m^3.

A 16-year-old girl was accidentally given 1.2 g of sodium oxalate intravenously. She died after 5 minutes, but the heart function was restored by cardiac massage and maintained for 4 days without restoration of consciousness. Postmortem examination showed tubular necrosis of the kidneys, with calcium oxalate crystals in the lumen and epithelium of the tubules. Ganglion cells throughout the central nervous system were necrosed. This finding was attributed to blocking of glycogenolysis by the oxalate.— I. Dvoracova, *Arch. Tox.*, 1966, *22*, 63, per *Pharm. J.*, 1968, *1*, 212.

Treatment of Adverse Effects. Give a dilute solution of any soluble calcium salt to precipitate the oxalate and if mucosal corrosion has not occurred carefully empty the stomach by aspiration and lavage using large quantities of diluted lime water or dilute solutions of other calcium salts. It is advisable to leave about 100 ml of the solution in the stomach. Calcium Gluconate Injection 10% should be given intravenously in doses of 10 to 20 ml to prevent tetany. Morphine sulphate 10 mg may be given by injection for the relief of pain. The circulation should be maintained with infusions of plasma or other suitable electrolyte solutions. If renal function is not impaired, 4 to 5 litres of fluid should be given daily to prevent crystalluria.

Uses. Oxalic acid is used for removing ink stains, cleaning leather and metals, and for removing the colour from calico printing.

The use of oxalic acid, its esters, and alkaline salts in cosmetics and toiletries is restricted in Great Britain under the Cosmetic Products Regulations 1978 (SI 1978: No. 1354).

1321-c

Phosphoric Acid *(B.P.)*. Phosph. Acid; Concentrated Phosphoric Acid *(Eur. P.)*; Acidum Phosphoricum Concentratum; Orthophosphoric Acid; Phosphorsäure; Acido Fosfórico.

H_3PO_4=98.00.

CAS — 7664-38-2.

Pharmacopoeias. In *Br.*, *Eur.*, *Fr.*, *Ger.*, *It.*, *Neth.*, and *Swiss* (85 to 90%); in *Arg.* and *Ind.* (approximately 87 to 90%); in *Aust.*, *Hung.*, *Mex.*, *Port.*, and *Span.* (approximately 85 to 88%); in *Belg.* (82 to 84%); and in *Roum.* (50%). Also in *U.S.N.F.* (85 to 88%).

Odourless, clear, colourless, corrosive, syrupy liquid containing 85 to 90% w/w of H_3PO_4. Relative density about 1.7. When heated it loses water and is converted finally to metaphosphoric acid, HPO_3, which on cooling forms a transparent glassy mass.

Miscible with water or alcohol with evolution of heat. The concentrated acid attacks porcelain when heated in it. When stored at a low temperature it may solidify, forming a mass of colourless crystals which do not melt until the temperature reaches 28°. **Store** in airtight glass containers.

Adverse Effects and Treatment. As for Hydrochloric Acid, p.783.

Maximum permissible atmospheric concentration (H_3PO_4) 1 mg per m^3.

Uses. Phosphoric acid in concentrations of 0.01% may be used to remove traces of copper, iron, and nickel during the refining of edible oils and fats.

1322-k

Dilute Phosphoric Acid *(B.P., Eur. P.)*. Acidum Phosphoricum Dilutum; Diluted Phosphoric Acid *(U.S.N.F.)*.

Pharmacopoeias. In *Arg.*, *Br.*, *Eur.*, *Fr.*, *Ger.*, *It.*, *Ind.*, *Neth.*, *Pol.*, *Roum.*, *Span.*, and *Swiss* (all approximately 10%); in *Aust.* (9.1 to 9.54%); in *Belg.* (12%). Also in *U.S.N.F.*

It contains 9.5 to 10.5% w/w of H_3PO_4, and may be prepared by mixing phosphoric acid 116 g with water 884 g. Wt per ml 1.051 to 1.057 g. **Store** in airtight containers.

Incompatible with alkalis, with many compounds of aluminium, calcium, and iron, and with salts of silver, lead, and mercury.

Uses. It has been given in doses of 0.25 to 5 ml, well diluted, with vegetable bitters, to stimulate the secretion of gastric juice.

Estimated acceptable total daily dietary phosphorus load: up to 70 mg per kg body-weight, attention being given to the reverse relationship with calcium intake.— Seventeenth Report of the FAO/WHO Expert Committee on Food Additives, *Tech. Rep. Ser. Wld Hlth Org. No. 539*, 1974. For background toxicological information, see *Fd Add. Ser. Wld Hlth Org. No. 5*, 1974.

Use of disinfectants on farms. In Great Britain, a technical grade of orthophosphoric acid 1 in 330 of water is an approved disinfectant for foot-and-mouth disease under the Disease of Animals (Approved Disinfectants) Order 1978 (SI 1978: No. 32), as amended (SI 1978: No. 934).

1323-a

Ricinoleic Acid *(B.P. 1948)*.

A yellow or yellowish-brown viscous liquid with a characteristic odour and taste, consisting of a mixture of fatty acids obtained by the hydrolysis of castor oil. Wt per ml 0.94 to 0.943 g. Practically **insoluble** in water; soluble in alcohol and ether.

Ricinoleic acid forms soaps with alkalis or triethanolamine which, in solution, are more stable than the corresponding soaps prepared from other fatty acids. It has been used as a spermicide in some proprietary contraceptive creams and jellies.

1324-t

Stearic Acid *(B.P.C. 1973)*. Stearinsäure; Acido Esteárico.

CAS — 57-11-4 (stearic acid); 57-10-3 (palmitic acid).

Pharmacopoeias. In *Arg.*, *Aust.*, *Belg.*, *Braz.*, *Chin.*, *Cz.*, *Fr.*, *Hung.*, *Ind.*, *It.*, *Jap.*, *Jug.*, *Nord.*, *Pol.*, *Port.*, *Roum.*, *Span.*, and *Swiss.* Also in *U.S.N.F.*

U.S.N.F. also includes Purified Stearic Acid containing not less than 90% stearic acid and not less than 96% of stearic and palmitic acids. Congealing point 66° to 69°.

White, almost tasteless, greasy, flaky crystals or hard masses, odourless or with a slight odour suggesting tallow, consisting of a mixture of fatty acids, chiefly stearic and palmitic acids. *U.S.N.F.* specifies not less than 40% of stearic acid, not less than 40% of palmitic acid, and not less than 90% of stearic and palmitic acids. It may be powdered by sprinkling with alcohol during trituration. M.p. not below 54°. It may contain a suitable antoxidant, such as 0.005% of butylated hydroxytoluene. It is sometimes wrongly called 'stearine' in commerce.

Practically **insoluble** in water; soluble 1 in 15 of alcohol, 1 in 2 of chloroform, and 1 in 3 of ether.

The pure acid, $C_{17}H_{35}.CO_2H$ = 284.5, occurs in white shining flaky crystals or as a hard somewhat glossy solid, melting at 69.3°.

Uses. Stearic acid is used as a lubricant in making compressed tablets and as an enteric coating for pills and tablets. When partly neutralised with alkalis or triethanolamine it forms a creamy basis with 5 to 15 times its weight of aqueous liquid and this is sometimes used as the basis of vanishing creams. Free stearic acid in such creams may produce a pearly appearance on standing. After being neutralised and dissolved by heat in glycerol or alcohol, stearic acid will solidify when cold with at least 10 times its weight of liquid.

For the experimental use of stearic acid as a coating or basis for sustained-release tablets, see A. A. Kassem *et al.*, *Mfg Chem.*, 1973, *44* (Mar.), 43.

Preparations

Cremor Ammonii Stearatis *(F.N. Belg.)*. Ammonium Stearate Cream; Glyceritum Ammonii Stearatis. Stearic acid 17 g, dilute ammonia solution (*Belg. P.*) 3 g, water 11 g, and glycerol 69 g.

Stearic Acid Paste *(B.P.C. 1954)*. Past. Acid. Stear.; Unscented Vanishing Cream. A non-greasy preparation containing partially saponified stearic acid. Stearic acid 20 g, potassium hydroxide 0.5 g, alcohol (90%) 5 ml, borax 1.5 g, and water 73 ml. Add the potassium hydroxide, dissolved in the alcohol, to the melted stearic acid followed by a boiling solution of the borax in the water; stir thoroughly and allow to stand for 12 hours. Store in containers which prevent loss of moisture.

Unguentum Stearini *(Hung. P.)*. Stearic acid 10 g, cetostearyl alcohol 4.5 g, sodium lauryl sulphate 0.5 g, solutio conservans (*Hung. P.*) 1 g, sorbitol 3.5 g, glycerol 10 g, distilled water to 100 g.

Proprietary Preparations

Pristerene 4900, 4901, and 4968 *(Unichema, UK)*. Brands of stearic acid.

Other Proprietary Names

Emersol 132 *(USA)*.

1325-x

Sulphuric Acid *(B.P.)*. Sulfuric Acid *(U.S.N.F.)*; Acid. Sulph. Conc.; Oil of Vitriol; Schwefelsäure.

H_2SO_4=98.07.

CAS — 7664-93-9.

Pharmacopoeias. In *Aust.* (Acidum Sulfuricum Concentratum), *Br.*, *Ind.*, *Nord.*, *Port.*, *Span.*, and *Swiss* (all approximately 95%). Also in *U.S.N.F.*

A colourless corrosive liquid of oily consistence. Much heat is evolved when sulphuric acid is added to water. It contains not less than 95% w/w of H_2SO_4. Wt per ml about 1.84 g. Concentrated oil of vitriol of commerce, 'COV', contains about 95 to 98% w/w, and brown oil of vitriol, 'BOV', contains 75 to 85% w/w of H_2SO_4. Nordhausen or fuming sulphuric acid, 'Oleum', is sulphuric acid containing SO_3; battery or accumulator acid is sulphuric acid diluted with distilled water to a specific gravity of 1.2 to 1.26. **Store** in airtight containers.

CAUTION. *When sulphuric acid is mixed with other liquids, it should always be added slowly, with constant stirring, to the diluent.*

Adverse Effects and Treatment. As for Hydrochloric Acid, p.783.

Maximum permissible atmospheric concentration 1 mg per m^3.

The first treatment of sulphuric acid burns was to wash the skin with water as quickly as possible. If available, a sterile buffer solution containing potassium dihydrogen phosphate 30 g and disodium hydrogen phosphate 220 g per litre (pH 6.8 to 7) could be applied locally. It could also be used as a mouth-wash and for irrigating the eyes.— *Br. med. J.*, 1973, *4*, 228.

Preparations

Acidum Sulfuricum Spirituosum *(Port. P.)*. Aqua Rabel; Elixir Acidum Haller; Rabel Water. Sulphuric acid 25 g and alcohol 75 g.

Aromatic Sulphuric Acid *(B.P.C. 1934, Ind. P.)*. Acid. Sulph. Aromat.; Elixir of Vitriol. Sulphuric acid 7 ml, ginger tincture 25 ml (*Ind. P.* has strong ginger tincture 5 ml), cinnamon spirit 1.5 ml (*Ind. P.* has cinnamon oil 0.15 ml), alcohol (90%) to 100 ml. It is used for the same purposes as Dilute Sulphuric Acid. *Dose.* 0.3 to 1.2 ml.

1326-r

Dilute Sulphuric Acid *(B.P.)*. Acid. Sulph. Dil.; Verdünnte Schwefelsäure.

Pharmacopoeias. In *Br.*, *Ind.*, *Span.*, and *Swiss* (all approximately 10%); in *Aust.* (9.1 to 9.4%) and in *Pol.* (16%).

It contains 9.5 to 10.5% w/w of H_2SO_4. Wt per ml 1.062 to 1.072 g. **Incompatible** with alkalis and carbonates; it precipitates barium, calcium, lead, and silver from solutions of their salts.

Uses. Dilute sulphuric acid has been used as an astringent in diarrhoea and it has occasionally been prescribed in mixtures with vegetable bitters to stimulate appetite. It has been given in doses of 0.3 to 5 ml well diluted and administered through a glass tube to avoid injury to the teeth.

1327-f

Tartaric Acid *(B.P., Eur. P., U.S.N.F.)*. Tart. Acid; Acidum Tartaricum; Tartrique (Acide); Weinsäure. (+)-L-Tartaric acid; (+)-L-2,3-Dihydroxybutanedioic acid.

$C_4H_6O_6$=150.1.

CAS — 87-69-4.

Pharmacopoeias. In *Arg., Aust., Belg., Br., Braz., Cz., Eur., Fr., Ger., Hung., Int., It., Jap., Jug., Mex., Neth., Nord., Pol., Port., Roum., Span., Swiss,* and *Turk.* Also in *U.S.N.F.*

Colourless crystals or a white or almost white crystalline powder, odourless or almost odourless, with a strongly acid taste. It absorbs insignificant amounts of moisture at relative humidities up to about 65%, but at relative humidities above about 75% it is deliquescent.

Soluble in less than 1 of water, 1 in 2.5 of alcohol, 1 in 4 of glycerol, 1 in 250 of ether, and 1 in 1.7 of methyl alcohol; practically insoluble in chloroform. A solution in water is dextrorotatory. A 3.9% solution in water is iso-osmotic with serum. Solutions are **sterilised** by autoclaving. **Store** in airtight containers.

Adverse Effects. Strong solutions of tartaric acid are mildly irritant and if ingested undiluted may cause gastro-enteritis.

Treatment of Adverse Effects. Give freely calcium hydroxide or magnesium hydroxide, stirred in water.

Absorption and Fate. Tartaric acid is absorbed from the gastro-intestinal tract but up to 80% of an ingested dose is probably destroyed by micro-organisms in the lumen of the intestine before absorption occurs. Absorbed tartaric acid is excreted unchanged in the urine.

Uses. Tartaric acid is used in the preparation of effervescent powders, granules, and tablets, as an ingredient of cooling drinks, and as a saline purgative. If not neutralised, it must be taken well diluted. The following are the proportions necessary to form approximately neutral mixtures with 10 parts of tartaric acid; ammonium bicarbonate 11 parts, magnesium carbonate 6.5 parts, potassium bicarbonate 13.25 parts, sodium bicarbonate 11.25 parts. Tartaric acid is an ingredient of Compound Effervescent Powder *B.P.C. 1973*, p.643.

Estimated acceptable daily intake: up to 30 mg per kg body-weight.— Seventeenth Report of the FAO/WHO Expert Committee on Food Additives, *Tech. Rep. Ser. Wld Hlth Org. No. 539*, 1974. The existing specifications were confirmed.— Twenty-first Report of the Joint FAO/WHO Expert Committee on Food Additives, *Tech. Rep. Ser. Wld Hlth Org. No. 617*, 1978.

For background toxicological information, see *Fd Add. Ser. Wld Hlth Org. No. 5*, 1974.

The use of metatartaric acid is permitted in wine under the Miscellaneous Additives in Food Regulations 1980 (SI 1980: No. 1834) for England and Wales and the Miscellaneous Additives in Food (Scotland) Regulations 1980 [SI 1980: No. 1889 (S. 176)]. Metatartaric acid is defined as consisting chiefly of a mixture of polyesters obtained by the controlled dehydration of L-(+)-tartaric acid, together with unchanged L-(+)-tartaric acid.

1328-d

Trichloroacetic Acid *(B.P., Eur. P., U.S.P.)*. Trichloroacet. Acid; Trichloracetic Acid; Acidum Trichloraceticum; Trichloressigsäure.

$CCl_3.CO_2H$=163.4.

CAS — 76-03-9.

Pharmacopoeias. In *Aust., Br., Eur., Fr., Ger., Hung., Jap., Neth., Nord., Pol., Port., Span., Swiss,* and *U.S.*

Colourless, very deliquescent crystals, or crystalline masses, with a slight or pungent characteristic odour. B.p. about 195°. M.p. 55° to 57°. **Soluble** 9 in 1 of water; very soluble in alcohol, chloroform, and ether. **Store** at 15° to 30° in airtight containers.

Adverse Effects and Treatment. As for Hydrochloric Acid, p.783.

Maximum permissible atmospheric concentration 1 ppm.

Uses. Trichloroacetic acid is caustic and astringent. It is used as a quick escharotic for warts. It is applied as a strong solution, prepared by adding 10% by weight of water; the surrounding parts are usually protected with soft paraffin or collodion. It does not cause inflammation but produces a white slough which peels off in 1 or 2 days. A 10% aqueous solution has been used for application to corneal warts; it is applied by means of an orange stick, a piece of cotton wool being held against the margin of the eyelid to soak up excess acid. As an astringent, a 0.1 to 1% solution may be applied for hyperhidrosis.

A saturated solution of trichloroacetic acid could be used to treat acne scars.— *Br. med. J.*, 1972, *2*, 461.

A report of the use of trichloroacetic acid as a 50% solution in the treatment of filtering blebs occurring after cataract extraction.— J. R. Gehring and E. C. Ciccarelli, *Am. J. Ophthal.*, 1972, *74*, 622.

Hydrocyanic Acid and Cyanides

7750-c

Included in this section are hydrocyanic acid and potassium sodium cyanide which are used under controlled conditions for the eradication of pests. Weak solutions of hydrocyanic acid in various forms were formerly used for the treatment of nausea and vomiting.
Some cyanide salts with industrial applications are also described.

7751-k

Stronger Hydrocyanic Acid *(B.P.C. 1934).*

Stronger Hydrocyanic Acid Solution *(B. Vet. C. 1965)*; Acid. Hydrocyan. Fort.; Scheele's Hydrocyanic Acid; Scheele's Prussic Acid.

CAS — 74-90-8 (hydrocyanic acid).

An aqueous solution containing 4% w/w of hydrogen cyanide, HCN = 27.03. A colourless liquid with a characteristic odour. Wt per ml about 0.99 g. **Store** in a cool place in airtight glass-stoppered bottles. Protect from light.

CAUTION. *Hydrocyanic acid and its vapour are intensely poisonous.*

Adverse Effects. Cyanides interfere with the oxygen uptake of cells by inhibition of cytochrome oxidase, an enzyme necessary for cellular oxygen transport.
Poisoning by cyanides may occur from inhalation of the vapour, ingestion, or absorption through the skin. Poisoning may also occur from cyanide-containing plants or fruits.
When large doses of hydrocyanic acid are taken, unconsciousness occurs within a few seconds and death within 5 minutes. With smaller toxic doses the symptoms, which occur within a few minutes, may include constriction of the throat, nausea, vomiting, confusion, giddiness, staggering, headache, dilated pupils, foaming at the mouth, hypotension, tachycardia, palpitation, hyperpnoea then dyspnoea, unconsciousness, and violent convulsions, death occurring within 15 minutes to an hour. The characteristic smell of bitter almonds may not be obvious. Cyanosis is not prominent. Similar but usually slower effects occur with cyanide salts.
The fatal dose of hydrocyanic acid (HCN) for man is about 50 mg and of the cyanides about 250 mg.
Maximum permissible atmospheric concentration of HCN 10 ppm.

For a review of chronic neurotoxicity caused by cyanides in foods, see *Lancet*, 1969, *2*, 942.

The toxicological and clinical aspects of cyanide metabolism.— R. G. H. Baumeister *et al.*, *Arzneimittel-Forsch.*, 1975, *25*, 1056.

Brief discussion of the danger of cyanide poisoning from the use of Cymag which releases HCN and is used for gassing rabbits and rodents.— *Br. med. J.*, 1978, *2*, 1141.

Possible cyanide neurotoxicity from plant and environmental sources.— A. G. Freeman (letter), *Br. med. J.*, 1981, *282*, 1321.

Treatment of Adverse Effects. Treatment must be given rapidly if it is to prove effective in cyanide poisoning. Immediate diagnosis can often be made by the characteristic cyanide odour of the breath but this is not always detectable. Remove the patient to fresh air; remove contaminated clothing; wash splashed material from the skin. Give amyl nitrite inhalations for 10 to 30 seconds every 2 to 3 minutes. A second capsule may be used. If necessary maintain the respiration to aid the inhalations. In definite cyanide poisoning, inject as soon as possible 300 mg of dicobalt edetate intravenously over about 1 minute as 20 ml of a 1.5% solution (see p.382), followed, with the same needle, by 50 ml of dextrose injection 50%. The dose may be repeated if necessary and followed by a further injection of dextrose; a third dose of dicobalt edetate may be given if required. Dicobalt edetate acts by forming a stable complex with the cyanide ion.
In Great Britain dicobalt edetate is recommended as the first choice by the Health and Safety Executive. Alternatively, the following older method may be used either as the initial treatment or subsequent to the unsuccessful use of dicobalt edetate: inject as soon as possible 10 ml of sodium nitrite injection (3%) intravenously at the rate of 2.5 to 5 ml per minute; using the same needle and vein continue with an injection of 12.5 g of sodium thiosulphate (50 ml of a 25% solution or 25 ml of a 50% solution) administered over a period of about 10 minutes. Sodium nitrite converts haemoglobin to methaemoglobin, which competes with cytochrome oxidase for cyanide with the formation of cyanmethaemoglobin which slowly dissociates as cyanide is converted to thiocyanate; sodium thiosulphate aids the conversion or inactivation of cyanide. If toxic symptoms recur, the injections of nitrite and thiosulphate may be repeated at half the initial doses. Oxygen should be given. Hypotension may be treated with a pressor agent such as metaraminol. *No case should be considered hopeless until it is certain that the heart has completely stopped.*
If cyanide has been ingested, one of the above procedures should be instituted and the stomach then emptied by aspiration and lavage up to 300 ml of a 25% solution of sodium thiosulphate may be left in the stomach.
As well as the preparation of dicobalt edetate described on p.382 a Cyanide Emergency Kit is available in Great Britain from *Cuxson and Gerrard.*

Reviews and discussions of cyanide poisoning and its treatment: R. P. Smith and R. E. Gosselin, *A. Rev. Pharmac. & Toxic.*, 1976, *16*, 189; M. Davis, *Topics Ther.*, 1978, *4*, 54; G. E. Burrows *et al.*, *Toxic. appl. Pharmac.*, 1978, *45*, 359; A. T. Proudfoot, *Prescribers' J.*, 1979, *19*, 183.

A discussion on cyanide antidotes. The use of hydroxocobalamin was not considered practicable. Dicobalt edetate remained the antidote of choice.— *Lancet*, 1977, *2*, 1167. The need for careful clinical evaluation to establish the reality of cyanide poisoning.— D. D. Bryson (letter), *ibid.*, 1978, *1*, 92.

A 21-year-old man admitted unconscious to hospital developed pulmonary oedema and acidosis, and was treated with oxygen, frusemide, intravenous fluids, sodium bicarbonate, and potassium chloride. Nine hours after administration it was discovered that the patient had taken potassium cyanide—capsules containing 200 mg were discovered and the patient stated that he had taken 3 capsules; the blood-cyanide concentration 12 and 22 hours after admission was 2 and 1.6 µg per ml respectively. Because of the delay no specific treatment was given; the acidosis was shown to be lactic acidosis and the patient recovered uneventfully. The value of nitrite/thiosulphate was questioned; oxygen and hydroxocobalamin with or without thiosulphate was suggested.— D. L. Graham, *Archs intern. Med.*, 1977, *137*, 1051. See also C. Berlin, *ibid.*, 993.

A patient survived self-poisoning with potassium cyanide 413 mg due to aggressive supportive therapy which included the intracardiac injection of adrenaline, oxygen 100%, correction of the acidosis, and blood volume replacement. He also received mannitol and practolol but no dicobalt edetate. The peak blood-cyanide concentration 60 minutes after ingestion was 3.8 µg per ml. This was higher than the usual fatal concentration of 3 µg per ml.— A. C. Edwards and I. D. Thomas (letter), *Lancet*, 1978, *1*, 92.

Absorption and Fate. Hydrocyanic acid is readily absorbed when inhaled or taken by mouth. It may be absorbed through the skin from aqueous solutions. Cyanide salts and compounds are more slowly absorbed from the gastro-intestinal tract.

Uses. Cyanides have various industrial applications. Hydrocyanic acid is used as a gas for the eradication of rabbits, rodents, and some other pests.

7752-a

Dilute Hydrocyanic Acid *(B.P.C. 1954).* Dilute Prussic Acid; Acido Cianídrico Diluído.

Pharmacopoeias. In *Port.*

A colourless aqueous solution with a characteristic odour, containing 2% w/w of HCN. Wt per ml about 0.997 g. **Incompatible** with soluble salts of silver, mercury, and iron. **Store** in a cool place in well-closed glass-stoppered bottles. Protect from light.

Adverse Effects and Treatment. As for Stronger Hydrocyanic Acid.

Uses. Dilute hydrocyanic acid was formerly used to allay vomiting.

Maximum acceptable daily intake of hydrogen cyanide: 50 µg per kg body-weight.— Report of the 1972 Joint FAO/WHO Meeting on Pesticide Residues in Food, *Tech. Rep. Ser. Wld Hlth Org. No. 525*, 1973.

7753-t

Bitter Almond *(B.P.C. 1934).* Amygdala Amara; Amande Amère; Bittere Mandel; Almendra Amarga; Amêndoas Amargas.

CAS — 8013-76-1 (bitter almond oil).

Pharmacopoeias. In *Jug.*, *Port.*, and *Span.*

The dried ripe seeds of ***Prunus dulcis*** var. ***amara.*** (=*Amygdalus communis* var. *amara*) (Rosaceae). ***Prunus dulcis*** may also be known as *Prunus amygdalus.* It contains about 50% of fixed oil and 3 to 4% of amygdalin, and yields 0.5 to 0.8% of essential oil containing 4 to 7% of hydrogen cyanide, HCN.

Adverse Effects and Treatment. As for Stronger Hydrocyanic Acid, p.790.

Uses. Bitter almond is a source of almond oil and has been used in demulcent skin lotions and for the preparation of waters containing 0.1% of hydrogen cyanide.

Preparations

Bitter Almond Water. Aqua Amygdalae Amarae; Benzaldehyde Cyanhydrin Solution. A water usually adjusted to contain 0.1% of hydrogen cyanide, HCN. In *Aust. P.*, which states that it may be used when Aqua Laurocerasi (Cherry-laurel Water) is prescribed. Also in *Port. P.* It is prepared either from bitter almond by distillation, or from benzaldehyde cyanhydrin.
Jap. P. includes a similar water under the title Aqua Armeniacae (Apricot Kernel Water) which may be prepared either by steam distillation of apricot kernels from which the fixed oil has previously been removed or from benzaldehyde cyanhydrin. It is adjusted to contain 0.1% of HCN.

7754-x

Benzaldehyde Cyanhydrin. Mandelonitrile; Nitrilo Amigdálico; Nitrilofeniloglicólico.
$C_6H_5.CH(OH)CN = 133.1$.

CAS — 532-28-5.

Pharmacopoeias. In *Arg.*, *Aust.*, and *Port.*

A yellow oily liquid with an odour resembling that of benzaldehyde. Wt per ml about 1.12 g. Practically **insoluble** in water; soluble in alcohol, chloroform, and ether. **Store** in airtight containers. Protect from light.

Benzaldehyde cyanhydrin has been used for making bitter almond water.

7755-r

Cherry-laurel *(B.P.C. 1949).* Laurocerasus; Cherry-laurel Leaves; Laurier-Cerise; Kirschlorbeerblatt; Loureiro-cerejeira.

Pharmacopoeias. In *Arg., Belg., Fr., Port., Span.,* and *Swiss.*

The fresh leaves of *Prunus laurocerasus* (Rosaceae), collected as soon as they are fully grown.

Uses. Cherry-laurel is used for the preparation of Cherry-laurel Water, which has been used as a flavouring agent and in nausea and vomiting.

Preparations

Cherry-laurel Water *(B.P.C. 1949).* Aqua Laurocerasi. Distilled from cherry-laurel in the presence of sodium chloride and standardised to contain 0.1% of HCN. Store in a cool place in well-filled containers. Protect from light. *Swiss P.* requires this to be dispensed when Bitter Almond Water is prescribed. *Dose.* 2 to 8 ml. A similar preparation is included in some pharmacopoeias..

7756-f

Potassium Cyanide *(B.P.C. 1934).* Pot. Cyanid.; Kalium Cyanatum; Cyanure de Potasse.
KCN=65.12.

CAS — 151-50-8.

White crystals, fused masses, or sticks, deliquescent and decomposing on exposure to air and moisture. **Soluble** 1 in 2.5 of water, 1 in 100 of alcohol (90%), and 1 in 2 of glycerol.

CAUTION. *This substance is intensely poisonous.*

Adverse Effects and Treatment. As for Stronger Hydrocyanic Acid,p.790.

Uses. Potassium cyanide is used for similar purposes to sodium cyanide.

7757-d

Potassium Ferricyanide.
$K_3Fe(CN)_6$=329.2.

CAS — 13746-66-2.

Ruby-red crystals. Very **soluble** in water; slightly soluble in alcohol. Solutions must be freshly prepared.

Potassium ferricyanide is used as an analytical reagent and as a reducing agent in photography. It is an ingredient of Sodium Thiosulphate and Potassium Ferricyanide Eye Lotion, *A.P.F.,* which is used in the treatment of silver nitrate burns.

A simple screening test in which potassium ferricyanide solution was used to check the ingestion of prescribed iron.— A. M. Afifi *et al., Br. med. J.,* 1966, *1,* 1021.

7758-n

Potassium Sodium Cyanide *(B.P.C. 1949).* Pot. et Sod. Cyanid.; Potassium Cyanide Double Salt.

White deliquescent cubical crystals or white opaque fused masses with an odour of hydrocyanic acid. **Soluble** 1 in 2.5 of water; partly soluble in alcohol.

CAUTION. *This substance is intensely poisonous.*

Adverse Effects and Treatment. As for Stronger Hydrocyanic Acid, p.790.

Uses. Potassium sodium cyanide has similar industrial uses to sodium cyanide.
It is also used by entomologists for killing insects. For this purpose the salt is usually broken into small pieces, and a layer, about 2 cm deep, is placed at the bottom of a wide-mouthed bottle provided with an airtight lid; plaster of Paris cream is poured over the cyanide to form a level floor and allowed to set; the bottle constantly contains a poisonous vapour.

Destruction of wasps' nests. The use of cyanide gassing powders for the destruction of wasps in houses was illegal except under the conditions prescribed by the Hydrogen Cyanide (Fumigation of Buildings) Regulations, 1951. Cyanide was no more effective than carbon tetrachloride, dicophane, and rotenone.— Wasps, *Advis. Leafl. Minist. Agric. Fish. Fd, No. 451,* London, HM Stationery Office, 1965.

7759-h

Sodium Cyanide. Cianeto de Sódio.
NaCN=49.01.

CAS — 143-33-9.

White granules or fused masses with an odour of hydrocyanic acid. Very **soluble** in water; slightly soluble in alcohol.

CAUTION. *This substance is intensely poisonous.*

Adverse Effects and Treatment. As for Stronger Hydrocyanic Acid,p.790.

Uses. Sodium cyanide is used industrially for extracting gold and silver from ores, for case-hardening metals, and in electroplating and photographic processes.

Hypnotics and Sedatives

4000-d

Hypnotics and sedatives depress the central nervous system. Hypnotics are used to produce sleep and sedatives to relieve anxiety and restlessness in the waking patient without inducing sleep. There is no sharp distinction between the 2 effects and the same drug may have both actions depending on the method of use and the dose employed. High doses may depress sufficiently to produce coma.

Insomnia may result from a variety of causes and may therefore necessitate treatment other than with hypnotics. When a hypnotic is required the attitude of the patient should be directed towards its short-term use only. In general, it may be expected to act within half-an-hour to provide sleep lasting about 8 hours. Hypnotics generally have no analgesic action and unless an analgesic is given wakefulness and excitement may occur in the presence of pain. Some hypnotics are also used as anticonvulsants.

Normal physiological sleep is composed of 2 alternating phases: non-dreaming, orthodox, or 'slow wave' (EEG) and rapid-eye-movement (REM) or paradoxical sleep, in which most dreaming takes place. Orthodox sleep can itself be divided into 4 stages, from drowsiness to profound sleep.

Most hypnotics reduce the duration and intensity of REM sleep. When the hypnotic is withdrawn there is a rebound phenomenon and extra dreaming takes place. Changes in the brain after prolonged use or even a single overdose of some hypnotics produce tolerance and may take weeks or months to be reversed (see also under Dependence, p.792). Sleep induced by hypnotics may not be as restful as normal sleep.

The choice of a suitable hypnotic depends on the onset and duration of action required, the period of treatment, the personality and age of the patient, and whether pain is present.

The 3 main types of hypnotics and sedatives described in this section are the barbiturates, benzodiazepines, and other non-barbiturate hypnotics such as chloral hydrate. Many other substances have sedative and hypnotic effects or side-effects. Such drugs include alcohol (p.38), antihistamines (see pp.1294-5), bromides (p.338), general anaesthetics (p.741), hyoscine (p.303), and narcotic analgesics (p.1001).

Pharmacology of Sleep, R.L. Williams and I. Karacan (Ed.), London, John Wiley, 1976.

Further references: *Med. Lett.*, 1976, *18*, 89; *Postgrad. med. J.*, 1976, *52*, 1–58.

The barbiturates have many disadvantages as hypnotics, including tolerance, liability to abuse and severe withdrawal effects, hang-over and other prolonged effects, interference with metabolism of other drugs, enhancement by alcohol, and severe toxic effects in overdosage. They are being replaced by less toxic hypnotic agents, in particular, the benzodiazepines.

All barbiturates depress the central nervous system and their effect and duration of action is a function of the dose given and the rate of elimination by the patient. The sleep produced by standard doses of all barbiturates formerly classified as long-acting and intermediate-acting lasts about 8 hours, hence this classification is not considered valid. However, in terms of repeated doses, the risk of a cumulative effect is greatest for those with a very long half-life, such as barbitone and phenobarbitone which are not generally used for hypnosis; although in the case of phenobarbitone in the treatment of epilepsy, this long half-life facilitates the desired even concentration in the plasma throughout 24 hours. The elimination half-lives of most former standard barbiturate hypnotics such as butobarbitone and pentobarbitone can also lead to cumulation on repeated nightly ingestion. Only a few with very short half-lives such as heptabarbitone and hexobarbitone might be considered suitable for true nightly hypnosis without concomitant daytime sedation.

Barbiturates mainly used for producing anaesthesia or controlling convulsions were formerly termed 'very short-acting'. This ability to produce anaesthesia of short duration following intravenous administration is a function of their redistribution from the brain to other tissues rather than a characteristic of their hypnotic action. They are described under the section on general anaesthetics (see p.740).

Problems associated with barbiturates and guidelines for their withdrawal.— *Drug & Ther. Bull.*, 1976, *14*, 7 and 11. See also under Phenobarbitone, Dependence, p.812.

A detailed review of the clinical pharmacokinetics of hypnotics. Of the barbiturates, in appropriate dosage, hexobarbitone, heptabarbitone, and cyclobarbitone can probably produce a satisfactory plasma concentration profile of the intermittent type during nightly administration. Only if daytime sedation is required might the other compounds be chosen. In contrast to the free acids, barbiturate salts are readily absorbed, although food may delay absorption. Elimination of some barbiturates may be remarkably retarded in liver disease, and in renal disease the accumulation of pharmacologically active polar metabolites should be considered.— D. D. Breimer, *Clin. Pharmacokinet.*, 1977, *2*, 93. See also L. C. Mark, *Clin. Pharmac. Ther.*, 1969, *10*, 287.

Recommendations of the Committee on the Review of Medicines on barbiturate preparations, other than phenobarbitone and agents used in anaesthesia and epilepsy.— *Br. med. J.*, 1979, *2*, 719. Comment.— *Drug & Ther. Bull.*, 1980, *18*, 9.

Further references: *Am. J. Hosp. Pharm.*, 1976, *33*, 333; F. Solomon *et al.*, *New Engl. J. Med.*, 1979, *300*, 803.

The benzodiazepines such as nitrazepam and flurazepam are often the preferred hypnotics because of their relatively low incidence of adverse effects, abuse, and interactions. Other benzodiazepines which may also be used as hypnotics are described in the section on Tranquillisers, p.1504.

Other non-barbiturate hypnotics are sometimes used. They depress the central nervous system but differ widely in dosage and duration of action, and some have a wider margin of safety than the barbiturates.

The following are included in this group: carbromal, p.795, chloral hydrate, p.796, dichloralphenazone, p.799, ethchlorvynol, p.800, ethinamate, p.801, glutethimide, p.802, methaqualone, p.805, methyprylone, p.807, paraldehyde, p.809, and triclofos sodium, p.818.

Chloral hydrate and its derivatives such as dichloralphenazone and triclofos tend to be used especially in children and elderly patients. The irritant effect of chloral hydrate on the stomach and its unpleasant taste are disadvantages.

Ten patients who had been taking hypnotic drugs regularly for periods ranging from months to years had as great or greater difficulty in falling asleep and staying asleep as control insomniac patients. However, ineffective hypnotics should not be abruptly withdrawn, because of withdrawal phenomena. Since the importance of particular stages of sleep was unknown, the superiority of hypnotics could not yet be defined from the presence or absence of sleep-stage alteration.— A. Kales *et al.*, *J. Am. med. Ass.*, 1974, *227*, 513. See also I. Oswald, *Br. med. J.*, 1979, *1*, 1167.

Review of the benzodiazepines.— Committee on the Review of Medicines, *Br. med. J.*, 1980, *280*, 910.

Dependence. Dependence of the barbiturate-alcohol type is liable to occur in susceptible patients given any of the sedatives and hypnotics in this section. It is characterised by a strong need to continue taking the drug, a tendency to increase the dose, a psychic dependence on the effects of the drug, and a physical dependence on the effects of the drug for the maintenance of homoeostasis, with a characteristic abstinence syndrome on withdrawal.

The detrimental effects of hypnotic dependence arise particularly from the persistence of effects such as ataxia, dysarthria, mental impairment and confusion, and poor judgement.

Withdrawal symptoms are similar to those of alcohol abstinence and are characterised after several hours by apprehension and weakness, followed by anxiety, headache, dizziness, tremors, and vomiting and then by nausea, abdominal cramps, insomnia, and tachycardia. Orthostatic hypotension and convulsions may develop after a day or two, sometimes leading to status epilepticus. Hallucinations and delirium tremens may develop after several days followed by a deep sleep before the symptoms disappear.

The time at which symptoms develop varies with the duration of action of the drug used. Symptoms may be dramatically reversed by the administration of almost any sedative and this should be followed by the slow withdrawal of the sedative over a period of days or weeks.

For an extensive review of dependence on hypnotics and sedatives, see H. Isbell and T. L. Chrusciel, *Dependence Liability of 'Non-narcotic' Drugs*, Geneva, World Health Organization, 1970; *idem, Bull. Wld Hlth Org.*, 1970, *43, Suppl.*

A review with an extensive bibliography, of the acute and chronic toxicity of barbiturates, and of tolerance, withdrawal syndrome, and dependence following their use.— Amphetamines, Barbiturates, LSD and Cannabis, their Use and Misuse, *Reports on Public Health and Medical Subjects No. 124*, London, HM Stationery Office, 1970.

The diagnosis and treatment of abuse of CNS depressants.— *Med. Lett.*, 1977, *19*, 13.

See also under Phenobarbitone, Dependence, p.812.

4001-n

Acetylcarbromal. Acecarbromal; Acetcarbromal. *N*-Acetyl-*N'*-(2-bromo-2-ethylbutyryl)urea.
$C_9H_{15}BrN_2O_3$=279.1.

CAS — 77-66-7.

Almost odourless, colourless crystals or white crystalline powder with a slightly bitter taste. **Soluble** 1 in 1000 of water; soluble in alcohol, chloroform, and ether. It is decomposed by boiling water. **Protect** from light.

Acetylcarbromal is a light sedative which was claimed to have less hypnotic effect than carbromal; it was given in doses of 250 to 500 mg thrice daily.

Proprietary Names

Abasin *(Bayer, Ger.)*; Sedamyl *(Riker, USA)*.

NOTE. Abacin is used as a proprietary name for co-trimoxazole.

4002-h

Acetylglycinamide-Chloral Hydrate. AGAC; AGAK.
$C_6H_{11}Cl_3N_2O_4$=281.5.

A complex of chloral hydrate and *N*-acetylglycinamide containing about 60% of chloral hydrate.

White odourless crystals. **Soluble** in water.

Acetylglycinamide-chloral hydrate is used as a hypnotic, in doses of 1.7 g at night (equivalent to 1 g of chloral hydrate). It is also used as a sedative.

Proprietary Names

Ansopal *(Gobbi-Novag, Arg.; Ferrosan, Swed.)*.

4003-m

Allobarbitone *(B.P.C. 1959).* Allobarbital; Diallylbarbitone; Diallylmalonylurea; Diallymalum. 5,5-Diallylbarbituric acid.
$C_{10}H_{12}N_2O_3$=208.2.

CAS — 52-43-7.

Pharmacopoeias. In *Aust., Cz., Hung., It., Jap., Pol., Port.,* and *Swiss.*

A white odourless crystalline powder with a slightly bitter taste. M.p. about 173°. **Soluble** 1 in 700 of water, 1 in 15 of alcohol, and 1 in 20 of ether; soluble in solutions of alkalis.

Allobarbitone is a barbiturate (see p.792) that has been used as a hypnotic in doses of 100 to 200 mg at night, and as a sedative in doses of 30 mg three or four times daily.

4004-b

Amylene Hydrate *(B.P. 1953).* Amyleni Hydras; Tertiary Amyl Alcohol; Dimethylethyl Carbinol; Aethyldimethylmethanolum; Hidrato de Amileno. 2-Methylbutan-2-ol.
$C_5H_{12}O$=88.15.

CAS — 75-85-4.

Pharmacopoeias. In *Arg., Aust., Int., Nord.,* and *Turk.* Also in *U.S.N.F.*

A clear, colourless, volatile liquid with a characteristic camphoraceous odour and a pungent burning taste. Specific gravity 0.803 to 0.807. Boiling point 97° to 103°. Flash-point 19.4° (closed-cup test).
Soluble 1 in 10 of water; miscible with alcohol, chloroform, ether, glycerol, and fixed oils. A 10% v/v solution in water is neutral to litmus. **Store** in airtight containers. Protect from light.

Amylene hydrate has been used as a hypnotic in doses of 2 to 4 ml at night. It is used as a solvent for tribromoethyl alcohol, see Bromethol, p.760.

Preparations

Mixtura Amyleni Hydratis *(Nord. P.).* Amylene Hydrate Mixture. Amylene hydrate 10 g, diluendum glycyrrhizae (*Nord. P.*)(a liquid extract of liquorice) 6 g, and water 84 g.

4005-v

Amylobarbitone *(B.P.).* Amylobarb.; Amobarbitalum; Amobarbital *(U.S.P.)*; Pentymalum. 5-Ethyl-5-isopentylbarbituric acid.
$C_{11}H_{18}N_2O_3$=226.3.

CAS — 57-43-2.

Pharmacopoeias. In *Arg., Br., Chin., Cz., Fr., Hung., Ind., Int., It., Jap., Nord., Port.,* and *U.S.*

A white odourless crystalline powder with a slightly bitter taste. M.p. 155° to 161° with a range of not more than 3°. At 25° it absorbs insignificant amounts of moisture at relative humidities up to about 90%.
Soluble 1 in 1500 of water, 1 in 5 of alcohol, 1 in 20 of chloroform, and 1 in 6 of ether; soluble in aqueous solutions of alkali hydroxides and carbonates. A saturated solution in water has a pH of about 5.6. **Incompatibilities** as for phenobarbitone (see p.811).

4006-g

Amylobarbitone Sodium *(B.P., Eur. P.).*

Amylobarb. Sod.; Amobarbitalum Natricum; Amobarbital Sodium *(U.S.P.)*; Barbamylum; Pentymalnatrium; Sodium Amobarbital; Soluble Amylobarbitone. Sodium 5-ethyl-5-isopentylbarbiturate.
$C_{11}H_{17}N_2NaO_3$=248.3.

CAS — 64-43-7.

Pharmacopoeias. In *Arg., Br., Braz., Chin., Eur., Fr., Ger., Ind., Int., It., Neth., Roum., Rus., Swiss,* and *U.S. Jap.* and *U.S.* also include a sterile form.

A white, odourless, hygroscopic, granular powder with a bitter taste. M.p. about 156°. It loses not more than 5% of its weight on drying. **Soluble** 1 in less than 1 of water and 1 in 2 of alcohol; practically insoluble in chloroform and ether. A 10% solution in water has a pH of 9.6 to 10.4. A 3.6% solution is iso-osmotic with serum. Solutions for injection are prepared aseptically in Water for Injections free from carbon dioxide and should be used immediately after preparation.
Incompatible with acids, acidic salts such as ammonium bromide, acidic syrups such as lemon syrup, and with chloral hydrate (see also p.796). Amylobarbitone may be precipitated from mixtures containing amylobarbitone sodium. This precipitation is dependent upon the concentration and the pH. At a concentration of 30 mg of amylobarbitone sodium in 10 ml, precipitation occurs at pH 8.9 and below. Corresponding figures for other concentrations are: 60 mg, pH 9.2; 100 mg, pH 9.4; 200 mg, pH 9.6. Solutions in water decompose on standing. **Store** in airtight containers.

Incompatibility. There was loss of clarity when intravenous solutions of amylobarbitone sodium were mixed with dimenhydrinate, diphenhydramine hydrochloride, hydrocortisone sodium succinate, hydroxyzine hydrochloride, insulin, narcotic analgesics, noradrenaline acid tartrate, procaine hydrochloride, streptomycin sulphate, tetracycline hydrochloride, or vancomycin hydrochloride.— J. A. Patel and G. L. Phillips, *Am. J. Hosp. Pharm.*, 1966, *23*, 409.

Stability of solutions. A 10% solution of amylobarbitone sodium in water lost 1.8% of its strength in 5 days at 20°, 3.7% in 14 days, 5.6% in 32 days, and 15.1% in 90 days. When heated at 100°, a 10% solution lost 4.2% of its strength in 10 minutes, 6.2% in 20 minutes, and 17.9% in 1 hour.— H. Nuppenau, *Dansk Tidsskr. Farm.*, 1954, *28*, 261.

Dependence. Prolonged use of amylobarbitone may lead to dependence of the barbiturate-alcohol type (see p.792).

Plasma-cortisol concentrations were higher in 30 chronic alcoholic patients after 9 or more hours of alcohol abstinence than in control subjects. When the alcoholic patients were given alcohol or enough amylobarbitone to reproduce the same clinical response there was a fall in plasma-cortisol concentrations which was not observed with diazepam.— J. Merry and V. Marks, *Lancet*, 1972, *2*, 990.

Adverse Effects, Treatment, and Precautions. As for Phenobarbitone, p.812.

Administration in the elderly. Investigations in 2 groups of healthy adult male subjects indicated that the rate of hydroxylation of amylobarbitone sodium decreased with age.— R. E. Irvine *et al.*, *Br. J. clin. Pharmac.*, 1974, *1*, 41.

Effects on driving performance. Amylobarbitone sodium, given in five 30-mg doses over 36 hours, significantly affected low-speed tests of driving ability; alcohol given concomitantly had little effect. There was no correlation between performance and the objective and subjective effects of medication.— T. A. Betts *et al.*, *Br. med. J.*, 1972, *4*, 580.

Controlled tests of cognitive function showed that amylobarbitone and, to a lesser extent, hydroxyamylobarbitone impaired performance.— K. Balasubramanian *et al.*, *Br. J. Pharmac.*, 1972, *45*, 360.

Effects on the skin. Amylobarbitone was strongly suspected of being responsible for fixed drug eruptions in 2 patients.— J. A. Savin, *Br. J. Derm.*, 1970, *83*, 546.

Effects on thyroid-function tests. Amylobarbitone sodium in doses of 30 mg thrice daily for 4 weeks was shown to have no effect on tests of thyroid function and therefore need not be withdrawn before such tests were carried out.— S. D. Slater, *Br. J. clin. Pract.*, 1972, *26*, 463.

Pregnancy and the neonate. Following intramuscular injection of amylobarbitone sodium 200 mg to mildly hypertensive women in labour 0.7 to 3.5 hours before delivery, the plasma half-life of amylobarbitone was 2.5 times as long in the neonates as in the mothers.— B. Krauer *et al.*, *Clin. Pharmac. Ther.*, 1973, *14*, 442. A similar distribution of half-lives was noted in 7 of 10 neonates whose mothers had also received amylobarbitone or phenobarbitone chronically for hypertension during pregnancy. There was no evidence of induction of amylobarbitone hydroxylation possibly because the foetal liver microsomes were not inducible by barbiturates in the doses used or because they had already been induced by other substances such as maternal hormones. Two apparently healthy children had very considerably longer half-lives (about 86 and 118 hours) and in one initially lethargic child the plasma-amylobarbitone concentration did not change significantly throughout the study-period.— G. H. Draffan *et al.*, *Clin. Pharmac. Ther.*, 1976, *19*, 271.

For a report suggesting an association between congenital malformations and exposure to amylobarbitone in pregnancy, see Phenobarbitone, p.814.

Absorption and Fate. See under Phenobarbitone, p.814.

About 40 to 60% of amylobarbitone is bound to plasma proteins. It has a half-life of about 20 hours which is considerably extended in neonates. It is metabolised in the liver; up to about 50% is excreted in the urine as 3′-hydroxyamylobarbitone and up to about 30% as *N*-hydroxyamylobarbitone, less than 1% appearing unchanged; up to about 5% is excreted in the faeces.

Distribution. Monitoring of saliva-amylobarbitone concentrations.— T. Inaba and W. Kalow, *Clin. Pharmac. Ther.*, 1975, *18*, 558.

Metabolism and excretion. Following administration of radioactively labelled amylobarbitone to 2 healthy subjects 79 to 92% was recovered in the urine in 6 days, and only 4 to 5% in the faeces. Unchanged drug was practically absent from both urine and faeces, and less than 50% of the dose was identified as 3′-hydroxyamylobarbitone. A second main metabolite was identified as *N*-hydroxyamylobarbitone and found to account for up to 30% of the dose.— B. K. Tang *et al.*, *Drug Metab. & Disposit.*, 1975, *3*, 479.

5-(3′-Carboxybutyl)-5-ethylbarbituric acid appeared to be a significant urinary metabolite of amylobarbitone.— W. Baldeo *et al.* (letter), *J. Pharm. Pharmac.*, 1977, *29*, 254.

Further references: R. I. Freudenthal and F. I. Carroll, *Drug Metab. Rev.*, 1973, *2*, 265; T. Inaba *et al.*, *Clin. Pharmac. Ther.*, 1976, *20*, 439; W. Kalow *et al.*, *Clin. Pharmac. Ther.*, 1979, *26* 766 (racial differences in metabolism).

Uses. Amylobarbitone is a barbiturate (see p.792) that is used as a hypnotic and sedative. As a hypnotic it is usually given in doses of 100 to 200 mg at night. As a sedative it may be given in doses of 15 to 50 or 60 mg two to four times daily; higher doses of up to 600 mg daily have been given to patients under supervision in psychiatric hospitals. A more rapid onset of effect is obtained with the sodium salt.

Amylobarbitone sodium may also be given by intramuscular injection, when oral administration is not possible or for the emergency control of status epilepticus (it is not suitable for the routine control of grand mal epilepsy); no more than 500 mg should be given intramuscularly and no more than 5 ml should be injected at any one site. Under close hospital supervision, in emergency, it may also be given by intravenous injection as a 5 to 10% solution at a rate not exceeding 1 ml per minute in a dose of 0.3 to 1 g. Subcutaneous injections may cause tissue necrosis.

For the effect of amylobarbitone sodium on anxiety, the ability to concentrate, various stages of sleep, and plasma concentrations of growth hormone and corticosteroids, see O. O. Ogunremi *et al.*, *Br. med. J.*, 1973, *2*, 202.

Administration in hepatic failure. Metabolism of amylobarbitone, after intravenous injection of 3.23 mg per kg body-weight, was compared in 10 healthy subjects and 10 patients with chronic liver disease. Of the patients with hepatic disorders, 5 had low serum-albumin concentrations and showed reduced serum binding of amylobarbitone and impaired metabolism: the other 5 had normal serum-albumin concentrations and showed no abnormality in amylobarbitone metabolism. No differences in clinical response were observed between the groups.— G. E. Mawer *et al.*, *Br. J. Pharmac.*, 1972, *44*, 549.

See also under Precautions for Phenobarbitone, p.813.

Tinnitus. A study demonstrating the beneficial effect of amylobarbitone in tinnitus.— I. Donaldson, *J. Lar. Otol.*, 1978, *92*, 123, per *Lancet*, 1979, *1*, 1124.

Preparations of Amylobarbitone and Amylobarbitone Sodium

Capsules

Amobarbital Sodium Capsules *(U.S.P.)*. Capsules containing amylobarbitone sodium. Store in airtight containers.

Amylobarbitone Sodium Capsules *(B.P.)*. Amylobarb. Sod. Caps.; Amobarbital Sodium Capsules; Soluble Amylobarbitone Capsules. Capsules containing amylobarbitone sodium. Store at a temperature not exceeding 30°.

Elixirs

Amobarbital Elixir *(U.S.P.)*. Amylobarbitone Elixir. An elixir containing amylobarbitone with alcohol 26 to 30%. Store in airtight containers.

Amylobarbitone Elixir *(A.P.F.)*. Amylobarbitone 25 mg, alcohol (90%) 2 ml, glycerol 1.5 ml, aromatic syrup 1 ml, water to 5 ml. *Dose.* 5 to 10 ml.

Injections

Amylobarbitone Injection *(B.P.)*. Amylobarb. Inj.; Amylobarbital Injection; Amylobarbitone Sodium Injection. A sterile solution of amylobarbitone sodium in Water for Injections free from carbon dioxide, prepared by dissolving, immediately before use, the sterile contents of a sealed container (Amylobarbitone for Injection) in the requisite amount of Water for Injections free from carbon dioxide. pH of a 10% solution not more than 11.

Sterile Amobarbital Sodium *(U.S.P.)*. Amylobarbitone sodium suitable for parenteral use.

Tablets

Amobarbital Tablets *(U.S.P.)*. Tablets containing amylobarbitone. The *U.S.P.* requires 70% dissolution in 30 minutes.

Amylobarbitone Sodium Tablets *(B.P.)*. Amylobarb. Sod. Tab.; Soluble Amylobarbitone Tablets; Amobarbital Sodium Tablets. Tablets containing amylobarbitone sodium.

Store in airtight containers.

Amylobarbitone Tablets *(B.P.)*. Amylobarb. Tab.; Amobarbital Tablets. Tablets containing amylobarbitone.

Proprietary Preparations of Amylobarbitone and Amylobarbitone Sodium

Amytal *(Lilly, UK)*. Amylobarbitone, available as tablets of 15, 30, 50, and 100 mg and as scored tablets of 200 mg. (Also available as Amytal in *Austral., Belg., Canad., Ital., Neth., USA*).

Sodium Amytal *(Lilly, UK)*. Amylobarbitone sodium, available as **Ampoules** of 250 and 500 mg of powder for preparing injections; as **Capsules** of 60 and 200 mg; and as **Tablets** of 60 and 200 mg. (Also available as Sodium Amytal or Amytal Sodium in *Austral., Belg., Canad., Ital., Neth., S.Afr., USA*).

Other Proprietary Names of Amylobarbitone and Amylobarbitone Sodium

Austral.—Amal, Amylbarb, Amylobeta, Neur-Amyl; *Fr.*—Eunoctal; *Ger.*—Stadadorm; *Ital.*—Etamyl; *Norw.*—Amycal; *Spain*—Isoamitil Sedante.

Preparations containing amylobarbitone were also formerly marketed in Great Britain under the proprietary names Amylomet (*Woodward*) and Gerisom (*Winthrop*).

4007-q

Aprobarbitone. Aprobarbital; Allylisopropylmalonylurea; Allypropymal. 5-Allyl-5-isopropylbarbituric acid. $C_{10}H_{14}N_2O_3$=210.2.

CAS — 77-02-1.

Pharmacopoeias. In *Nord.*

A fine, white, odourless, crystalline powder with a slightly bitter taste. M.p. about 142°. **Soluble** 1 in 350 of water, 1 in 2.5 of alcohol, 1 in 40 of chloroform, and 1 in 5 of ether; soluble in aqueous solutions of alkali hydroxides and carbonates. A saturated solution in water is acid to litmus.

Aprobarbitone is a barbiturate (see p.792) that has been used as a hypnotic in doses of 40 to 160 mg at night and as a sedative in doses of 20 to 40 mg thrice daily.

N-Hydroxyaprobarbitone was shown to be only a minor metabolite of aprobarbitone.— J. N. T. Gilbert *et al., J. Pharm. Pharmac.*, 1978, *30*, 173.

Proprietary Names

Alurate *(Roche, USA)*.

4008-p

Apronal. Apronalide; Allylisopropylacetylurea. *N*-(2-Isopropylpent-4-enoyl)urea. $C_9H_{16}N_2O_2$=184.2.

CAS — 528-92-7.

Pharmacopoeias. In *Nord.*

Colourless, odourless, tasteless crystals or white crystalline powder. **Soluble** 1 in 4000 of water, 1 in 50 of alcohol, 1 in 45 of chloroform, and 1 in 100 of ether.

Adverse Effects. Marked idiosyncrasy with purpura or thrombocytopenic purpura ending in death has been reported.

Causation of purpura.— R. R. A. Coombs, *Br. J. Derm.*, 1969, *81, Suppl.* 3, 2.

Administration of apronal exacerbated experimental porphyria in *rats* but the validity of the tests must depend on clinical observation.— A. A. -B. Badawy (letter), *Lancet*, 1978, *1*, 1361.

Uses. Apronal was formerly used as a mild hypnotic and sedative. It was given in doses of 250 to 500 mg at night with a maximum in 24 hours of 750 mg.

4009-s

Barbitone *(B.P.C. 1963, Eur. P.)*.
Barb.; Barbitalum; Barbital; Diethylmalonylurea; Malonal; Diemalum. 5,5-Diethylbarbituric acid. $C_8H_{12}N_2O_3$=184.2.

CAS — 57-44-3.

Pharmacopoeias. In *Arg., Aust., Belg., Chin., Eur., Fr., Ger., Hung., It., Jap., Jug., Mex., Neth., Nord., Pol., Port., Roum., Rus., Span., Swiss,* and *Turk.*

Odourless colourless crystals or white crystalline powder with a slightly bitter taste. M.p. 188° to 192°.

Soluble 1 in 160 of water, 1 in 13 of boiling water, 1 in 15 of alcohol, 1 in 6 of acetone, 1 in 75 of chloroform, and 1 in 40 of ether; soluble in ethyl acetate and solutions of alkali carbonates and hydroxides and ammonia.

4010-h

Barbitone Sodium *(B.P. 1973)*.
Soluble Barbitone; Barbital Sodium; Barbitalum Natricum; Diemalnatrium. Sodium 5,5-diethylbarbiturate. $C_8H_{11}N_2NaO_3$=206.2.

CAS — 144-02-5.

Pharmacopoeias. In *Arg., Aust., Fr., Hung., Ind., Int., It., Pol., Roum., Rus., Span., Swiss,* and *Turk.*

A white odourless crystalline powder with a bitter taste. M.p. about 190°. It absorbs insignificant amounts of moisture at 25° at relative humidities up to 80%.

Soluble 1 in 5 of water and 1 in 600 of alcohol; practically insoluble in chloroform and ether. A 5% solution in water is alkaline to litmus. A solution in water slowly decomposes, the rate of decomposition increasing with rise in temperature. A 3.12% solution is iso-osmotic with serum. Solutions for injection are prepared aseptically in Water for Injections free from carbon dioxide and should be used immediately after preparation. **Incompatibilities** as for phenobarbitone sodium, p.811. It should preferably be given alone. **Store** in airtight containers.

Stability in solution. A 10% solution in water lost 2% of its strength in 10 days at 20°, 3.2% in 20 days, 8.1% in 40 days, and 15.1% in 80 days. When heated at 100°, a 10% solution lost 11% of its strength in 30 minutes and 34.7% in 2 hours.— H. Nuppenau, *Dansk Tidsskr. Farm.*, 1954, *28*, 261.

Dependence. Prolonged use of barbitone may lead to dependence of the barbiturate-alcohol type (see p.792).

Adverse Effects, Treatment, and Precautions. As for Phenobarbitone, p.812.

Pregnancy and the neonate. Barbitone sodium appeared in foetal blood within 2 or 3 minutes of administration to the mother; blood concentrations comparable with those of the mother persisted for up to 15 hours.— C. E. Flowers, *Obstet. Gynec.*, 1957, *9*, 332.

Quantities of barbitone excreted in breast milk were enough to produce marked sedation in the infant.— T. E. O'Brien, *Am. J. Hosp. Pharm.*, 1974, *31*, 844.

Absorption and Fate. See under Phenobarbitone, p.814.

Barbitone is not significantly metabolised in the body. It is not very lipid-soluble and is only slightly bound to plasma proteins. It is slowly excreted in the urine over several days.

Uses. Barbitone is a barbiturate (see p.792) that has been used mainly as a hypnotic in doses of 300 to 600 mg about an hour before bedtime. Owing to its slow rate of excretion there is a special risk of a cumulative action. Sodium barbitone has been preferred for its more rapid onset of action following administration by mouth; it was also formerly given by intramuscular injection as a 10% solution and rectally as a 5% solution.

Preparations

Barbitone Sodium Tablets *(B.P. 1973)*. Barb. Sod. Tab.; Barbital Sodium Tablets; Soluble Barbitone Tablets. Tablets containing barbitone sodium. Store in airtight containers.

Proprietary Names

Dormileno *(Faes, Spain)*.

A preparation containing barbitone was formerly marketed in Great Britain under the proprietary name Somnytic Tablets (*Philip Harris*).

4011-m

Benzobarbitone. Benzobarbital; Benzonal; Benzonalum. 1-Benzoyl-5-ethyl-5-phenylbarbituric acid. $C_{19}H_{16}N_2O_4$=336.3.

CAS — 744-80-9.

Pharmacopoeias. In *Int.* and *Rus.*

A white crystalline powder. M.p. 134° to 137°. Very slightly **soluble** in water; sparingly soluble in alcohol; freely soluble in chloroform; soluble in ether; soluble 1 in 15 of methyl alcohol. **Protect** from light.

Benzobarbitone is a barbiturate (see p.792) that has been used in the treatment of epilepsy.

Preparations

Tabulettae Benzonali *(Rus. P.)*. Tablets each containing benzobarbitone 100 mg. Protect from light.

4012-b

Benzoclidine Hydrochloride. Oxylidinum. Quinuclidin-3-yl benzoate hydrochloride. $C_{14}H_{17}NO_2,HCl$=267.8.

CAS — 16852-81-6 (benzoclidine); 7348-26-7 (hydrochloride).

Pharmacopoeias. In *Rus.*

A white odourless crystalline powder. M.p. about 248°. Freely *soluble* in water; soluble in alcohol; practically insoluble in acetone and ether. **Store** in airtight containers. Protect from light.

Benzoclidine hydrochloride is a sedative and antihypertensive. The usual dose is 20 mg by mouth or by subcutaneous or intramuscular injection as a 2 or 5% solution; up to 200 to 300 mg daily has been given.

4013-v

Bromvaletone *(B.P.C. 1949)*. Bromisoval; Bromisovalerylurea; Bromisovalum; Bromvalerylurea; Bromylum. *N*-(2-Bromo-3-methylbutyryl)urea. $C_6H_{11}BrN_2O_2$=223.1.

CAS — 496-67-3.

Pharmacopoeias. In *Aust., Cz., Ger., Hung., Jap., Neth., Nord., Pol., Roum., Rus., Span.,* and *Swiss.*

Small, white, almost odourless and tasteless, acicular or

scale-like crystals which sublime on heating. M.p. about 150°. **Soluble** 1 in 500 of water, 1 in 15 of alcohol, 1 in 6 of chloroform, and 1 in 25 of ether; soluble in solutions of alkali hydroxides.

Bromvaletone has actions and uses similar to those of carbromal (see p.795). The usual dose as a hypnotic is 600 to 900 mg; as a sedative, 300 mg.

Proprietary Names
Bromural *(Knoll AG, Austral.; Knoll, Ger.; Knoll, Neth.).*

4014-g

Butalbital *(U.S.P.).* Alisobumalum; Allylbarbituric Acid; Itobarbital. 5-Allyl-5-isobutylbarbituric acid.
$C_{11}H_{16}N_2O_3$=224.3.

CAS — 77-26-9.

NOTE. The name Butalbital has also been applied to talbutal (p.817), the s-butyl analogue.

Pharmacopoeias. In *U.S.*

A white odourless crystalline powder with a slightly bitter taste. M.p. 138° to 141°. Slightly **soluble** in cold water; soluble in boiling water; freely soluble in alcohol, chloroform, and ether; soluble in aqueous solutions of alkali hydroxides and carbonates. A saturated solution is acid to litmus.

Butalbital is a barbiturate (see p.792) that has been used as a hypnotic in doses of 200 mg at night, and as a sedative in doses of 50 to 100 mg three or four times daily.

A study of the metabolism of butalbital.— J. N. T. Gilbert *et al., Eur. J. Drug Metab. Pharmacokinet.,* 1977, *2,* 69.

4015-q

Butobarbitone *(B.P., Eur. P.).* Butobarb.; Butethal; Butobarbital *(distinguish from Butabarbital);* Butobarbitalum. 5-Butyl-5-ethylbarbituric acid.
$C_{10}H_{16}N_2O_3$=212.2.

CAS — 77-28-1.

Pharmacopoeias. In *Br., Eur., Fr., Ger., Hung., It., Neth.,* and *Swiss.*

Colourless crystals or white crystalline, almost odourless, powder with a slightly bitter taste. M.p. 122° to 127°. It absorbs insignificant amounts of moisture at 25° at relative humidities up to about 90%.
Soluble 1 in 250 of water, 1 in 1 of alcohol, 1 in 3 of chloroform, and 1 in 10 of ether; soluble in aqueous solutions of alkali hydroxides and carbonates and ammonia, forming salts. A saturated solution in water is acid to litmus.

Dependence. Prolonged use of butobarbitone may lead to dependence of the barbiturate-alcohol type (see p.792).

Adverse Effects, Treatment, and Precautions. As for Phenobarbitone, p.812.

Butobarbitone was responsible for a fixed drug eruption in 3 patients and was strongly suspected in 2 further cases.— J. A. Savin, *Br. J. Derm.,* 1970, *83,* 546.

A 28-year-old conscious woman, who later stated that she had taken butobarbitone 6 g in the 3 previous days, had vertical gaze paralysis suggestive of brain lesions. Recognition of such paralysis in barbiturate poisoning might obviate unnecessary neurological investigation.— R. H. Edis and F. L. Mastaglia, *Br. med. J.,* 1977, *1,* 144.

Absorption and Fate. See under Phenobarbitone, p.814.
Butobarbitone is inactivated in the liver mainly by hydroxylation; small amounts are excreted in the urine as unchanged drug. It has been reported to have a half-life of about 40 hours and to be about 26% bound to plasma proteins.

A kinetic study of urinary excretion in 2 healthy subjects; results for butobarbitone and its 3′-hydroxyl, 3′-oxo, and 3-acid metabolites. The half-life of butobarbitone was estimated as 50.2 hours in one subject and 55.5 hours in the other.— J. N. T. Gilbert *et al., J. Pharm. Pharmac.,* 1974, *26, Suppl.,* 16P.

Following administration of butobarbitone 200 mg to 5 healthy subjects, half-lives of 33.6 to 41.5 hours were measured. Nightly administration of 50 to 200 mg for several days to 4 of the subjects led to substantial accumulation; the half-lives decreased by about 20 to 25% probably due to enzyme induction. Repeated administration of butobarbitone should be avoided, and occasional use restricted to hospital in-patients in whom daytime sedation is required.— D. D. Breimer, *Eur. J. clin. Pharmac.,* 1976, *10,* 263.

Further references: J. N. T. Gilbert and J. W. Powell, *Eur. J. Drug Metab. Pharmacokinet.,* 1976, *1,* 188 (enzyme induction).

Uses. Butobarbitone is a barbiturate (see p.792) that is used as a hypnotic and sedative. As a hypnotic it is usually given in doses of 100 to 200 mg at night. It has been given rectally as suppositories containing 200 or 300 mg.

Preparations

Butobarbitone Tablets *(B.P.).* Butobarb. Tab. Tablets containing butobarbitone.

Soneryl *(May & Baker, UK).* Butobarbitone, available as scored tablets of 100 mg. (Also available as Soneryl in *Austral., Belg., Canad., Denm., Fr., Neth., S.Afr., Switz.)*

Other Proprietary Names
Sonabarb *(Austral.).*

Preparations containing butobarbitone were also formerly marketed in Great Britain under the proprietary names Butomet (*Woodward*), and Dolalgin, Sonergan, and Sonalgin (*May & Baker*).

4016-p

Butylchloral Hydrate *(B.P.C. 1949).* Croton-Chloral Hydrate; Trichlorobutylidene Glycol. 2,2,3-Trichlorobutane-1,1-diol.
$C_4H_7Cl_3O_2$=193.5.

CAS — 76-40-4.

Pearly-white crystalline scales with a pungent but not acrid odour resembling that of chloral hydrate, and a pungent bitter taste. M.p. about 78°.
Soluble 1 in 40 of water, 5 in 3 of alcohol (forming an alcoholate), 1 in 20 of chloroform, 1 in 1 w/w of glycerol, 1 in 20 of olive oil, and 1 in 2 of ether. A solution in water is neutral or slightly acid to litmus. **Incompatible** with alkalis and alkaloids; with alcohol the butylchloral alcoholate may crystallise out.

Butylchloral hydrate is a hypnotic with actions similar to those of chloral hydrate (see below); it has been given in doses of 0.3 to 1.2 g at night.

4017-s

Capuride. McN-X-94. *N*-(2-Ethyl-3-methylvaleryl)urea.
$C_9H_{18}N_2O_2$=186.3.

CAS — 5579-13-5.

Capuride has been used as a hypnotic in doses of 400 mg at night.

Peak plasma concentrations were noted 1 to 2 hours after administration of radioactively labelled capuride to 6 healthy subjects. Nearly 80% of the radioactivity was excreted in the urine over the 144-hour study period and only about 2% in the faeces.— P. C. Johnson *et al., Clin. Pharmac. Ther.,* 1972, *13,* 377.

Hypnosis. Studies on the use of capuride as a hypnotic agent.— J. Katz *et al., Curr. ther. Res.,* 1970, *12,* 255; F. J. Tornetta, *Anesth. Analg. curr. Res.,* 1970, *49,* 862; A. G. Silverman and R. Okun, *J. clin. Pharmac.,* 1971, *11,* 215.

4018-w

Carbromal *(B.P.).* Bromadal; Bromodiethylacetylurea; Karbromal; Uradal. *N*-(2-Bromo-2-ethylbutyryl)urea.
$C_7H_{13}BrN_2O_2$=237.1.

CAS — 77-65-6.

Pharmacopoeias. In *Arg., Aust., Belg., Br., Ger., Hung., Mex., Nord., Pol., Port., Rus., Span.,* and *Swiss.*

A white, odourless or almost odourless, tasteless, crystalline powder. M.p. 117° to 120°. **Soluble** 1 in 3000 of water, 1 in 18 of alcohol, 1 in 2 of chloroform, and 1 in 25 of ether. A saturated solution in water is neutral to litmus. **Incompatible** with acids and alkalis.

Dependence. Prolonged use of carbromal may lead to dependence of the barbiturate-alcohol type (see p.792).

Abuse of bromureide preparations.— W. Poser *et al., Dt. med. Wschr.,* 1974, *99,* 2489.

Adverse Effects. Carbromal in doses greatly in excess of the therapeutic range may cause acute adverse effects similar to those described under phenobarbitone (see p.812) and deaths have been recorded. Continuous use of carbromal over long periods may give rise to symptoms of chronic toxicity resembling bromism, including severe mental depression, irritability, and slurring of speech. Skin eruptions including non-thrombocytopenic purpura, have been reported.

Reversible cataracts were seen in a man who had taken half or one Carbrital capsule every night continuously for 5 years. The condition appeared to have been due to the carbromal and cleared up on stopping administration of the drug.— R. Crawford, *Br. med. J.,* 1959, *2,* 1231.

Five alcoholic patients suffered some or all the following symptoms after taking excessive doses of bromureide preparations: confusion, disorientation, agitation, tearfulness, nystagmus, slurred speech, and ataxic gait.— P. Wilkinson *et al., Med. J. Aust.,* 1969, *1,* 1352. See also D. V. Schapira (letter), *Can. med. Ass. J.,* 1976, *115,* 116.

Extrapyramidal effects were noted in 2 children suffering from carbromal overdosage.— R. Schydlo, *Klin. Pediat.,* 1974, *186,* 257.

Effects on the skin. For reports of skin eruptions due to carbromal in 4 patients, and in 1 patient associated with cross-sensitivity with meprobamate, see W. C. Peterson and K. P. Manick, *Archs Derm.,* 1967, *95,* 40.

Treatment of Adverse Effects and Precautions. As for Phenobarbitone, p.812. See also under Bromides, p.338.

A review of the treatment of 121 patients with bromureide poisoning all but 5 of whom survived.— B. Grabensee *et al., Dt. med. Wschr.,* 1972, *97,* 1911.

Six of 7 patients who had ingested an estimated 26 to 60 g of carbromal and in whom routine gastric lavage had been unsuccessful survived after gastroscopic lavage had been performed until the stomach appeared free of tablet mass.— H. -J. Marsteller and R. Gugler (letter), *New Engl. J. Med.,* 1977, *296,* 1003.

Absorption and Fate. Carbromal is readily absorbed from the gastro-intestinal tract and is partly metabolised to 2-ethylbutyrylurea and bromide ion.

Excretion of bromine in the urine after therapeutic and suicidal doses of carbromal.— H. Schütz and Y. D. Ha, *Arzneimittel-Forsch.,* 1975, *25,* 432.

Uses. Carbromal has been used to treat mild insomnia in doses of 0.3 to 1 g at night.

Preparations

Carbromal Tablets *(B.P.C. 1973).* Tablets containing carbromal.

Proprietary Names
Adalin *(Bayer, Ger.);* Diacid *(Daro, Neth.);* Mirfudorm *(Diabetylin, Ger.);* Neo-diacid *(Daro, Neth.).*

4019-e

Chloral Betaine *(B.P. 1963).* The adduct formed by chloral hydrate, $CCl_3.CH(OH)_2$, and betaine, $C_5H_{11}NO_2$.
$C_7H_{12}Cl_3NO_3,H_2O$=282.6.

CAS — 2218-68-0.

A white or almost white crystalline powder with a bitter taste and a faint, penetrating, slightly acrid odour resembling that of chloral hydrate. It contains 56 to 59.5% of $CCl_3.CH(OH)_2$. M.p. about 124° with decomposition. Chloral betaine 1.74 g is approximately equivalent to 1 g of chloral hydrate.

Soluble 1 in 1 of water and 1 in 4 of alcohol; practically insoluble in chloroform and ether. It is decomposed by caustic alkalis with the liberation of chloroform. **Store** in airtight containers.

Adverse Effects, Treatment, and Precautions. As for Chloral Hydrate, p.796.

Chloral betaine has been reported to cause less gastric irritation than chloral hydrate.

Uses. Chloral betaine has actions similar to those of chloral hydrate (see p.797) and it is used for the same purposes. The usual hypnotic dose is 0.87 to 1.74 g (equivalent to 0.5 to 1 g of chloral hydrate) at night, but doses of up to 3.5 g may be necessary. The usual sedative dose is 870 mg twice or thrice daily.

Reports on the hypnotic activity of chloral betaine.— R. C. B. Aitken *et al.*, *Clin. Trials J.*, 1965, *2*, 65, per *Abstr. Wld Med.*, 1965, *38*, 308; H. Jick *et al.*, *J. Am. med. Ass.*, 1969, *209*, 2013.

4020-b

Chloral Hydrate *(B.P., B.P. Vet., Eur. P., U.S.P.)*.

Chloral Hydr.; Chlorali Hydras; Chloral; Kloralhydrat. 2,2,2-Trichloroethane-1,1-diol. $C_2H_3Cl_3O_2$=165.4.

CAS — 302-17-0.

Pharmacopoeias. In all pharmacopoeias examined.

Colourless or white crystals with a pungent but not acrid odour and a pungent bitter caustic taste. It volatilises slowly on exposure to air and it liquefies between 50° and 58°.

Soluble 1 in 0.3 of water, 1 in 0.2 of alcohol, 1 in 3 of chloroform, 1 in less than 1 of ether, 1 in 0.5 of glycerol, and in fixed and volatile oils. A 10% solution in water has a pH of 3.5 to 4.4.

Incompatible with alkalis, alkaline earths, alkali carbonates, soluble barbiturates, borax, tannin, iodides, oxidising agents, permanganates, and alcohol (chloral alcoholate may crystallise out). It forms a liquid mixture when triturated with many organic compounds, such as camphor, menthol, phenazone, phenol, thymol, and quinine salts. **Store** in a cool place in airtight containers. Protect from light.

NOTE. Aqueous solutions are liable to develop mould growth.

Stability of solutions. Aqueous solutions of chloral hydrate decomposed rapidly when exposed to ultraviolet light, with the formation of hydrochloric acid, trichloroacetic acid, and formic acid. Under ordinary storage conditions decomposition was slow; a 1% solution lost about 5% of its strength after storage at room temperature for 20 weeks.— P. W. Dankwortt, *Arch. Pharm. Berl.*, 1942, *280*, 197.

No loss of active constituent or detectable deterioration of the container occurred when Chloral Syrup or Paediatric Chloral Elixir were stored for 8 weeks in polyvinyl chloride bottles.— *Pharm. J.*, 1973, *1*, 100.

The bioavailability of chloral hydrate was lower from oily vehicles than from a hydrophilic macrogol basis *in vivo*.— D. D. Breimer *et al.*, *Pharm. Weekbl. Ned.*, 1973, *108*, 1101, per *Pharm. J.*, 1974, *1*, 337.

Dependence. Prolonged use of chloral hydrate may lead to dependence of the barbiturate-alcohol type (see p.792).

A 45-year-old woman with a history of barbiturate dependence became dependent upon chloral hydrate, taking doses of up to 10 g daily. She was admitted to hospital and suffered no ill effects on abrupt withdrawal, but to minimise the risk of symptoms such as delirium tremens it would probably be better to treat such a patient with low doses of chloral hydrate for at least a week.— C. B. Stone and R. Okun, *Clin. Toxicol.*, 1978, *12*, 377.

Adverse Effects. Chloral hydrate has an unpleasant taste and is corrosive to skin and mucous membranes unless well diluted. In therapeutic doses side-effects include gastric irritation, light-headedness, ataxia, nightmares, excitement, and confusion (sometimes with paranoia). Cardiac arrhythmias have been reported, but respiratory depression does not seem to be a problem. Hangover is less common than with barbiturates. Allergic reactions include skin rashes, which may occur within hours or several days of administration and eosinophilia. Leucopenia may occur. The effects of acute overdosage resemble acute barbiturate intoxication (see Phenobarbitone, p.812). In addition the irritant effect may cause initial vomiting, and gastric necrosis leading to strictures. Cardiac arrhythmias have been reported. Jaundice may follow liver damage, and kidney damage is associated with albuminuria.

Chronic ingestion of high doses is associated with gastritis, skin rashes, peripheral vasodilatation, hypotension, and myocardial depression. Renal damage may occur. Sudden withdrawal may produce symptoms similar to delirium tremens

In a drug surveillance programme, 1618 patients received chloral hydrate as a hypnotic, usually in doses of 0.5 to 1 g. In 1130 patients evaluated the response was considered good in 70.9%. Side-effects, which were reversible, occurred in 2.3% of patients and included gastro-intestinal symptoms (10 patients), CNS depression (20), and skin rash (5). In 1 patient the prothrombin time was increased; in 1 patient hepatic encephalopathy seemed to worsen; and bradycardia developed in 1 patient.— S. Shapiro *et al.*, *J. Am. med. Ass.*, 1969, *209*, 2016. In a Boston Collaborative Drug Surveillance Program side-effects occurred in approximately 2% of 5435 patients who received chloral hydrate. Three reactions were described as life-threatening.— R. R. Miller and D. J. Greenblatt, *J. clin. Pharmac.*, 1979, *19*, 669.

Overdosage. A 6-year-old boy awoke from a deep sleep 18 hours after taking 8 g of chloral hydrate and was subsequently well.— R. H. S. Mindham (letter), *Br. med. J.*, 1968, *3*, 187.

Cardiac and respiratory arrest occurred in a 22-month-old boy immediately after aspiration of a dose of chloral hydrate elixir. The child recovered after receiving immediate cardiac massage and oxygen.— D. M. Granoff *et al.*, *Am. J. Dis. Child.*, 1971, *122*, 170.

A 25-year-old woman who ingested 20 g of chloral hydrate developed initial respiratory failure, hypotension, hypothermia, and pulmonary oedema, and was deeply unconscious. Massive gastric necrosis with generalised peritonitis was found, followed by complete obstruction at the oesophago-gastric junction.— I. D. A. Vellar *et al.*, *Br. J. Surg.*, 1972, *59*, 317. See also G. J. Gleich *et al.*, *J. Am. med. Ass.*, 1967, *201*, 266.

Of 76 cases of chloral hydrate poisoning reported to the National Poisons Information Service 47 were severe. Of 39 adults 12 had cardiac arrhythmias including 5 with cardiac arrest. Anti-arrhythmic drugs such as lignocaine were recommended unless obviously contra-indicated. In prolonged coma haemoperfusion through charcoal, or haemodialysis, was recommended.— H. M. Wiseman and G. Hampel (letter), *Br. med. J.*, 1978, *2*, 960. See also A. J. Marshall, *ibid.*, 1977, *2*, 994.

Treatment of Adverse Effects. As for Phenobarbitone, p.812.

Demulcents such as liquid paraffin may be given to relieve gastric and oesophageal irritation. Lignocaine has been reported to control cardiac arrhythmias. Forced diuresis or dialysis may be beneficial in severe poisoning.

A 38-year-old woman who had taken about 38 g of chloral hydrate was successfully treated with haemodialysis; lignocaine was used initially to control arrhythmias, and dopamine to maintain blood pressure.— N. E. Stalker *et al.*, *J. clin. Pharmac.*, 1978, *18*, 136.

Precautions. Chloral hydrate should not be used in patients with marked hepatic or renal impairment or severe cardiac disease and its use is best avoided in the presence of gastritis. It should be used with caution in patients susceptible to porphyria.

Chloral hydrate and similar sedatives cause drowsiness and patients receiving them should not take charge of vehicles or machinery where loss of attention could lead to accidents. These effects are enhanced by the simultaneous administration of depressants of the central nervous system such as alcohol (the 'Mickey Finn' of detective fiction), barbiturates, and other sedatives. A vasodilator reaction has also occurred after concomitant administration with alcohol.

It has been suggested on theoretical grounds that its effects may be enhanced if monoamine oxidase inhibitors are given concurrently but the validity of any reported interactions has been questioned. Chloral hydrate has been reported to shorten the half-life and to enhance the effects of coumarin anticoagulants. Chloral hydrate is reported not to induce liver enzymes.

Asthma. Chloral hydrate, 20 mg per kg body-weight, appeared to depress respiration more in 6 asthmatic patients than in 6 controls and it was suggested that higher doses might be dangerous in asthmatics.— J. A. Aldrete and K. H. Itkin, *J. Allergy*, 1969, *43*, 342.

Interactions. Alcohol. In a controlled study of 5 healthy subjects, alcohol 500 mg per kg body-weight, given after chloral hydrate 15 mg per kg, increased and prolonged the plasma-trichloroethanol concentrations and reduced plasma concentrations of trichloroacetic acid. In turn chloral hydrate increased the absorption of alcohol leading to more rapidly achieved and higher blood concentrations in the first 30 minutes.— E. M. Sellers *et al.*, *Clin. Pharmac. Ther.*, 1972, *13*, 37. The heart-rate of these subjects was increased when given alcohol after having received chloral hydrate 15 mg per kg daily for 7 days, the last dose being given 12 hours before the alcohol. Systolic pressure was increased at 1 hour and decreased at 3 hours, motor performance was reduced when alcohol was taken after chloral hydrate, and auditory vigilance impaired. One subject had a vasodilator reaction with palpitations, anxiety, and flushing; although similar to the 'acetaldehyde syndrome' the blood-alcohol concentration was only half that found after alcohol alone, which had caused no reaction.— *idem*, 50.

Other references to a disulfiram-like reaction following concomitant ingestion of alcohol and chloral hydrate: *J. Am. med. Ass.*, 1958, *167*, 273; Z. Bardodej, *Ceska farm.*, 1965, *14*, 478.

Frusemide. For reports of cardiovascular effects in patients treated with chloral hydrate and frusemide, see Frusemide, p.597.

Glucose. Chloral hydrate may produce false positive results in some tests for glucose.— M. Lubran, *Med. Clins N. Am.*, 1969, *53*, 211.

Steroids. The administration of chloral hydrate could interfere with measurements of urinary 17-hydroxycorticosteroids.— J. M. Rosenberg and I. S. Kampa, *Drug Intell. & clin. Pharm.*, 1973, *7*, 33.

Urea. Chloral hydrate could interfere technically with chemical estimations for urea in the blood to produce erroneous raised results.— *Drug & Ther. Bull.*, 1972, *10*, 69. See also *Med. Lett.*, 1971, *13*, 82.

Warfarin. For reports on the effect of chloral hydrate on warfarin, see Warfarin Sodium, p.777.

Pregnancy and the neonate. Maternally administered chloral hydrate lowers the bilirubin concentrations of the infants.— J. H. Drew and W. H. Kitchen, *J. Pediat.*, 1976, *89*, 657.

Chloral hydrate was reported to enter breast milk in amounts sufficient to cause minimal sedation after large feeds.— R. L. Savage, *Adverse Drug React. Bull.*, 1976, Dec., 212. See also J. B. Bernstine, *J. Obstet. Gynaec. Br. Commonw.*, 1956, *63*, 228; J. B. Bernstine *et al.*, *Am. J. Obstet. Gynec.*, 1957, *73*, 801.

Absorption and Fate. Chloral hydrate is rapidly absorbed from the stomach and starts to act within 30 minutes. It is widely distributed throughout the body. It is metabolised to trichloroethanol and trichloroacetic acid in the erythrocytes, liver, and other tissues and excreted partly in the urine as trichloroethanol and its glucuronide (urochloralic acid) and as trichloroacetic acid. Significant amounts are also excreted in the bile.

Trichloroethanol is also an active hypnotic and with chloral it passes into the cerebrospinal fluid, into milk, and through the placenta to the foetus.

Studies on the absorption of chloral hydrate and chloral betaine following oral and rectal administration.— M. Simpson and E. L. Parrott, *J. pharm. Sci.*, 1980, *69*, 227.

Metabolism and excretion. In a comparative study 7 healthy subjects were given chloral hydrate 15 mg per kg body-weight and triclofos 22.5 mg per kg. Peak plasma concentrations of trichloroethanol were 8.5 μg per ml after a single dose of chloral hydrate and 8.2 μg per ml after a single dose of triclofos, no unchanged chloral hydrate or triclofos being detected. The plasma half-lives of trichloroacetic acid and trichloroethanol were 67.2 and 8.2 hours, and the plasma protein binding was 94% and 35% respectively. The pattern of urinary metabolites was similar for both drugs with 7.1% of the chloral hydrate dose and 4.6% of the triclofos dose being recovered as trichloroethanol glucuronide, trichloroethanol, and trichloroacetic acid. After 24 hours less than 12% of each drug was recovered in the urine and it was considered that biliary excretion is probably an important elimination route. Following administration of either drug for 7 days, plasma concentrations of trichloroacetic acid greater than 80 μg per ml were obtained.— E. M. Sellers *et al.*, *Clin. Pharmac. Ther.*, 1973, *14*, 147.

Uses. Chloral hydrate is a hypnotic and sedative with properties similar to those of the barbiturates; therapeutic doses have little effect on respiration and blood pressure.

Externally, chloral hydrate has a rubefacient action and was formerly employed as an anodyne and counter-irritant.

Chloral hydrate is usually administered to adults and children as Chloral Mixture and to infants as Paediatric Chloral Elixir. Gelatin capsules with chloral hydrate dissolved in a suitable vehicle also provide a method of administration. It has also been dissolved in a bland fixed oil and given by enema or as suppositories.

It should not be given as tablets or pills as these concentrated forms may damage the mucous membrane of the alimentary tract.

The usual hypnotic dose is 0.5 to 2 g at night and as a sedative 250 mg is given thrice daily, up to a max. single or daily dose of 2 g. It should be taken well diluted with water or milk. Children usually tolerate chloral well and 30 to 50 mg per kg body-weight daily may be given to a maximum single dose of 1 g as a hypnotic. A suggested sedative dose in children is 8 mg per kg thrice daily.

Administration in the elderly. No relationship between clinical toxicity and age had been noted for chloral hydrate.— D. J. Greenblatt *et al.*, *Clin. Pharmac. Ther.*, 1977, *21*, 355.

Preparations

Capsules

Chloral Hydrate Capsules *(U.S.P.).* Capsules containing chloral hydrate. Store in airtight containers.

Elixirs

Chloral Hydrate Elixir *(Guy's Hosp.).* Chloral hydrate 1 g, raspberry syrup 2 ml, glycerol 2 ml, concentrated anise water 0.15 ml, chloroform spirit 0.25 ml, saccharin sodium 5 mg, citric acid monohydrate 75 mg, water to 10 ml. *Dose.* 5 to 20 ml.

Paediatric Chloral Elixir *(B.P.).* Elixir Chloralis pro Infantibus; Chloral Elixir Paediatric. Chloral hydrate 200 mg, black currant syrup 1 ml, water 0.1 ml, syrup to 5 ml. It should be recently prepared. When a dose less than, or not a multiple of, 5 ml is prescribed the elixir should be diluted to 5 ml, or a multiple, with syrup. Such dilutions must be freshly prepared and not used more than 2 weeks after issue.

Mixtures

Chloral Mixture *(B.P.).* Chloral Hydrate Mixture. Chloral hydrate 1 g, syrup 2 ml, water to 10 ml. It should be recently prepared. When a dose which is not a multiple of 5 ml is prescribed, the mixture should be diluted to a multiple of 5 ml with a mixture of 1 vol. of syrup and 4 vol. of water. Such dilutions must be freshly prepared and not used more than 2 weeks after issue. *Dose.* 5 to 20 ml, well diluted with water.

When protected from light Chloral Mixture was stable for at least 12 weeks at room temperature. Benzoic acid was a suitable preservative.— Pharm. Soc. Lab. Rep. P/77/15, 1977. Chloral Mixture preserved with benzoic acid and protected from light was stable for 48 weeks at 25°.— Pharm. Soc. Lab. P/78/6, 1978. Microbiological studies indicated that unpreserved Chloral Mixture was very rapidly bactericidal and sporicidal, and the inclusion of benzoic acid as an additional preservative appeared to be unnecessary.— Pharm. Soc. Lab. Rep. P/78/3, 1978.

Chloral Mixture *(A.P.F.).* Mist. Chloral.; Chloral Hydrate Mixture. Chloral hydrate 1 g, orange syrup 1 ml, concentrated chloroform water 0.25 ml, water to 10 ml. *Dose.* 10 to 20 ml well diluted with water.

Chloral Mixture CF *(A.P.F.).* Chloral Hydrate Mixture for Children. Chloral hydrate 250 mg, orange syrup 2 ml, concentrated chloroform water 0.1 ml, water to 5 ml. *Dose.* As a daytime sedative for children weighing 20 kg, 5 ml three or four times daily.

Syrups

Chloral Hydrate Syrup *(U.S.P.).* A syrup containing chloral hydrate. Store in airtight containers. Protect from light.

Chloral Syrup *(B.P.C. 1968).* Syr. Chloral. Chloral hydrate 1 g, water 1 ml, syrup to 5 ml. It should be recently prepared. *Dose.* 2.5 to 10 ml.

NOTE. This preparation is twice the strength of Chloral Mixture *B.P.*.

Proprietary Preparations

Noctec *(Squibb, UK).* Chloral hydrate, available as capsules each containing 500 mg in solution. (Also available as Noctec in *Austral., Canad., USA*).

Other Proprietary Names

Austral.—Chloradorm, Chloralix, Dormel, Elix-Nocte; *Belg.*—Somnox; *Canad.*—Chloralex, Chloralvan, Novochlorhydrate; *Ger.*—Chloraldurat; *Neth.*—Chloraldurat; *Switz.*—Chloraldurat, Medianox; *USA*—Aquachloral, Rectules.

Preparations containing chloral hydrate were also formerly marketed in Great Britain under the proprietary name Nohaesa (*Camden*, now *Norgine*).

4021-v

Chloralformamide *(B.P.C. 1949).* Chloralamide; Chloramide. *N*-(2,2,2-Trichloro-1-hydroxyethyl)formamide.
$C_3H_4Cl_3NO_2 = 192.4$.

CAS — 515-82-2.

Colourless, odourless, shining crystals with a slightly bitter taste. M.p. about 120°. **Soluble** 1 in 20 of water, 1 in 2 of alcohol, and 1 in 12 of glycerol; soluble in acetone and ether. It hydrolyses when heated with water above 60°. **Incompatible** with alkalis, yielding chloroform, ammonia, and the corresponding formate.

Chloralformamide is a hypnotic slower and less predictable in its action than chloral hydrate but less irritating to the stomach. It should not be given in hot liquids. It has been given in doses of 1 to 3 g at night.

4022-g

Chloralose. Alphachloralose; α-Chloralose; Glucochloral. 1,2-*O*-(2,2,2-Trichloroethylidene)-α-D-glucofuranose.
$C_8H_{11}Cl_3O_6 = 309.5$.

CAS — 15879-93-3.

White odourless anhydrous needles with a disagreeable bitter taste. M.p. about 186°. **Soluble** 1 in 170 of water and 1 in 33 of alcohol; slightly soluble in chloroform and ether.

Chloralose has been used as a hypnotic in doses of 100 to 500 mg but its action is very variable and it may cause vomiting, paralysis, tremors, and bradycardia. It is chiefly employed for surgical anaesthesia in laboratory animals and as a rodenticide for mice.

The use of chloralose (Alphakil) as a rodenticide.— P. B. Cornwell, *Pharm. J.*, 1969, *1*, 74.

Proprietary Names

Somio *(Dergo, Belg.).*

4023-q

Chlorhexadol. Chloralodol; Chloralodolum. 2-Methyl-4-(2,2,2-trichloro-1-hydroxyethoxy)pentan-2-ol.
$C_8H_{15}Cl_3O_3 = 265.6$.

CAS — 3563-58-4.

Pharmacopoeias. In *Nord.*

Colourless crystals or white crystalline powder with an odour of chloral hydrate and a bitter taste. M.p. about 100°. Chlorhexadol 1.6 g is approximately equivalent to 1 g of chloral hydrate. **Soluble** 1 in 0.4 of alcohol, 1 in 8 of chloroform, and 1 in 20 of ether. When suspended in water it hydrolyses with the release of chloral hydrate. **Store** in airtight containers. Protect from light.

Chlorhexadol has the actions of Chloral Hydrate, p.796. It was given as a hypnotic in doses of 0.8 to 1.6 g at night and as a sedative in doses of 400 mg morning and midday.

Proprietary Names

Mechloral *(Dumex, Denm.)*; Mecoral *(Dumex, Norw.).*

Chlorhexadol was formerly marketed in Great Britain under the proprietary name Medodorm (*Medo-Chemicals*).

4024-p

Chlormethiazole Edisylate.

Chlormethiazole Ethanedisulphonate; Clomethiazole Edisylate. 5-(2-Chloroethyl)-4-methylthiazole ethane-1,2-disulphonate.
$C_{14}H_{22}Cl_2N_2O_6S_4 = 513.5$.

CAS — 533-45-9 (chlormethiazole); 1867-58-9 (edisylate).

A white crystalline powder with a characteristic odour which becomes more distinct and rather unpleasant when exposed to heat. Freely **soluble** in water and warm alcohol; sparingly soluble in warm acetone; practically insoluble in ether. High concentrations in water have an acid reaction. Solutions should be **stored** in a cool place.

Incompatibility. Chlormethiazole 8 g per litre in dextrose 4% injection reacted with plastic giving sets.— S. Lingam *et al.*, *Br. med. J.*, 1980, *280*, 155.

Dependence. Use of chlormethiazole may produce dependence of the barbiturate-alcohol type (see p.792). The risk of dependence appears to be associated with prolonged use in alcoholic patients.

A man who had been given chlormethiazole for the treatment of alcoholism appeared to have transferred his dependence to chlormethiazole; he was taking 40 to 50 tablets daily.— A. Foster (letter), *Br. med. J.*, 1977, *1*, 1355. See also K. Kryspin-Exner and R. Mader, *Wien. med. Wschr.*, 1971, *121*, 811.

Warnings on the risk of using chlormethiazole in ambulant alcoholic patients are timely but should not be taken out of context. Experience over 15 years at the St Bernard's Hospital Alcoholic Unit has not only confirmed the findings of many observers that chlormethiazole is an extremely valuable drug in the treatment and prophylaxis of severe alcohol withdrawal syndromes (including delirium tremens) but has also indicated that when used in patients for a limited period only (usually no more than 6 or 7 days) the risk of dependence is extremely low. It should be stressed that the risk of chlormethiazole dependence is a real one when it is given indiscriminately for lengthy use in unstable alcoholics treated as outpatients but seems very low when it is used in the withdrawal phase of alcoholism in the correct way, and equally so when used in sections of the population not prone to dependence.— M. M. Glatt (letter), *Br. med. J.*, 1978, *2*, 894. See also *idem*, 1976, *2*, 582; *idem*, 1977, *2*, 1088.

A report on 5 patients who were considered to have become physically dependent on chlormethiazole, taken by 4 of them in doses of up to about 5 to 10 g daily. Withdrawal symptoms included suicidal depression and an acute psychotic state.— M. A. Hession *et al.*, *Lancet*, 1979, *1*, 953. The doses prescribed in the first patients were far in excess of the recommended dosage. The criticisms made should more appropriately be levelled at other hypnotics rather than chlormethiazole which is rarely associated with withdrawal symptoms when used in the correct dosage.— A. N. Exton-Smith and A. E. McLean (letter), *ibid.*, 1093. Similar severe criticisms.— S. K. Majundar (letter), *ibid.*, 1093 and 1254; M. M. Glatt (letter), *ibid.*, 1093; C. J. Scott (letter), *ibid.*, 1094.

Adverse Effects. Chlormethiazole edisylate may cause sneezing a few minutes after taking a dose. Gastro-intestinal disturbances (dyspepsia, nausea, and vomiting) have followed administration of the tablets. Conjunctival irritation, transient hypotension, and increased bronchial secretions have also been reported. Mild superficial phlebitis often follows intravenous infusion and thrombophlebitis has occasionally been reported.

Allergy. A 48-year-old woman developed a severe allergic reaction 12 hours after being started on chlormethiazole by mouth for alcohol-withdrawal symptoms.— A. A. Khan, *Br. med. J.*, 1976, *2*, 1105. A 56-year-old man taking chlormethiazole for alcoholism developed a pruritic allergic rash.— N. A. Halstead and J. S. Madden (letter), *ibid.*, 1563. Both reactions followed the use of capsules which contained tartrazine; this might have been responsible.— G. R. Weeks (letter), *ibid.*, 1977, *1*, 290.

Effects on the heart. Cardiac arrest in 2 chronic alcoholics might have been associated with chlormethiazole infusion.— G. T. McInnes *et al.*, *Postgrad. med. J.*, 1980, *56*, 742.

Effects on the lungs. Pulmonary complications following high doses of chlormethiazole given intravenously for delirium tremens.— R. Schiessel and P. Sporn, *Anaesthesist*, 1974, *23*, 59.

Effects on mental state. Alpha coma (normally associated with a poor prognosis in structural brain damage) was noted in 3 patients given chlormethiazole for alcohol-withdrawal states. Withdrawal of the chlormethiazole was accompanied by complete recovery, indicating that such a finding in association with drug intoxication need not imply that secondary hypoxic brain damage has occurred.— W. M. Carroll and F. L. Mastiglia, *Br. med. J.*, 1977, *2*, 1518.

Overdosage. A report of suicide by chlormethiazole poisoning in 5 alcoholic men being treated for depression with chlormethiazole; at least 2 of the men had also ingested alcohol.— J. M. Horder, *Br. med. J.*, 1978, *1*, 693.

A report of chlormethiazole poisoning on 16 occasions in 13 patients, some of whom had also taken other drugs and alcohol. There was increased salivation on 7 occasions; otherwise the clinical features were those of barbiturate poisoning. The highest plasma-chlormethiazole concentration was 36 µg per ml, with the highest value in a conscious patient 11.5 µg per ml. All the patients survived following intensive supportive treatment as for barbiturate poisoning.— R. N. Illingworth *et al.*, *Br. med. J.*, 1979, *2*, 902.

Pregnancy and the neonate. Severe depression with hypotonia, hypoventilation, or apnoea was reported to have occurred in the immediate neonatal period in 13 infants among 21 born to mothers treated for toxaemia of pregnancy. All the mothers had received chlormethiazole edisylate 4 to 24 g by intravenous infusion, and 12 of the affected infants came from a group of 14 mothers who also received diazoxide as intravenous boluses of 75 to 150 mg to control hypertension. Adverse reactions were not considered to be related to the doses used.— R. A. Johnson, *Br. med. J.*, 1976, *1*, 943.

Ten of 16 babies whose mothers were given chlormethiazole for pre-eclampsia were sleepy compared with only one of 15 whose mothers were given hydralazine. Nine of the chlormethiazole infants required gavage feeding compared with 4 in the hydralazine group.— C. Wood and P. Renou (letter), *Med. J. Aust.*, 1978, *2*, 73.

Treatment of Adverse Effects. As for Phenobarbitone, p.812. The patient's airway should be maintained where necessary and an aspirator should always be close at hand.

Precautions. Chlormethiazole causes drowsiness and patients receiving it should not take charge of vehicles or machinery where loss of attention could lead to accidents. These effects are enhanced by the simultaneous administration of depressants of the central nervous system such as alcohol, barbiturates, and other sedatives and by phenothiazines and butyrophenones.

The safety of chlormethiazole in elderly patients and in chronic bronchitis is questionable since it might produce hypothermia and respiratory depression.— R. N. Illingworth *et al.*, *Br. med. J.*, 1979, *2*, 902. Absence of respiratory complications after wide use of chlormethiazole.— R. W. Morris (letter), *ibid.*, 1219. Criticism.— R. N. Illingworth *et al.* (letter), *ibid.*, 1980, *280*, 47.

Sinus bradycardia developed in an 84-year-old woman taking propranolol for hypertension 3 hours after she took a second dose of chlormethiazole 192 mg. Her pulse-rate increased on discontinuation of propranolol and chlormethiazole and later stabilised when she took propranolol with haloperidol.— *Med. J. Aust.*, 1979, *2*, 553.

In 5 children with status epilepticus resistant to diazepam thrombophlebitis occurred when they were given chlormethiazole intravenously; all experienced fever (severe in 3) and severe headache. These problems indicated the need for care, and the desirability of limiting the duration of the injection.— S. Lingam *et al.*, *Br. med. J.*, 1980, *280*, 155.

Administration in hepatic failure. Studies in 8 patients with advanced cirrhosis of the liver and in 6 healthy men showed that the amount of unmetabolised chlormethiazole reaching the circulation after an oral dose was about 10 times higher in the patients than in the controls. Low concentrations in the controls were related to extensive first-pass metabolism in the liver.— P. J. Pentikäinen *et al.*, *Br. med. J.*, 1978, *2*, 861. See also *idem*, *Eur. J. clin. Pharmac.*, 1980, *17*, 275.

Cardiac arrest (fatal in one patient) in 2 patients with chronic alcoholism given infusions of chlormethiazole.— G. T. McInnes *et al.* (letter), *Br. med. J.*, 1979, *2*, 1218. It was not proven that the arrhythmias were due to chlormethiazole D. B. Scott (letter), *ibid.*, 1437.

Absorption and Fate. Chlormethiazole is rapidly absorbed from the gastro-intestinal tract, peak plasma concentrations appearing about 15 to 45 minutes after oral administration. It is widely distributed in the body, and extensively metabolised, probably by first-pass metabolism in the liver with only small amounts appearing unchanged in the urine. It crosses the placenta.

Absorption. A study in 10 healthy subjects indicated more rapid and complete absorption of chlormethiazole after capsules than after tablets. Degree and speed of absorption increased even further after the oral solution.— M. Fischler *et al.*, *Acta pharm. suec.*, 1973, *10*, 483. See also E. P. Frisch and B. Ortengren, *Acta psychiat. scand.*, 1966, *42*, *Suppl.* 192, 35.

Metabolism and excretion. A study of the pharmacokinetics of chlormethiazole following intravenous infusion in 6 healthy subjects. Unlike earlier workers a biphasic decay was found for the plasma concentrations, with half-lives of 0.54 and 4.05 hours. Hepatic metabolism is probably the main process of elimination of chlormethiazole and in 3 subjects studied less than 5% was found unchanged in the urine. A significant first-pass effect of chlormethiazole was predicted with the systemic availability of an orally administered dose being about 15%.— R. G. Moore *et al.*, *Eur. J. clin. Pharmac.*, 1975, *8*, 353.

A study of the pharmacokinetics of chlormethiazole and 2 metabolites after administration by mouth to young adult and old subjects. Reduced plasma binding and higher plasma concentrations were noted in the elderly.— R. L. Nation *et al.*, *Eur. J. clin. Pharmac.*, 1977, *12*, 137. See also *idem*, 1976, *10*, 407.

Urinary metabolites of chlormethiazole.— M. Ende *et al.*, *Arzneimittel-Forsch.*, 1979, *29*, 1655.

The pharmacokinetics of chlormethiazole in the elderly.— E. J. Triggs, in *Drugs and the Elderly*, J. Crooks and I.H. Stevenson (Ed.), London, Macmillan Press, 1979, pp. 117–131.

Further references: D. B. Scott *et al.*, *Br. J. Anaesth.*, 1980, *52*, 541.

Pregnancy and the neonate. Intravenous administration of a 0.8% solution of chlormethiazole edisylate at a rate of 20 ml per minute was found in 19 pregnant women at term to give plasma concentrations in maternal blood of 4.7 to 22.4 µg per ml of chlormethiazole and concentrations of 4.5 to 16.9 µg in the umbilical vein.— G. M. Duffus *et al.* (preliminary communication), *Lancet*, 1968, *1*, 335.

A study of maternal and neonatal concentrations of chlormethiazole following the use of chlormethiazole edisylate in the treatment of 4 patients with pre-eclampsia. After breast-feeding started, chlormethiazole was detectable in only 3 of 27 serial blood samples from babies and the concentrations were 18, 9, and 6 ng per g. The highest calculated amount of chlormethiazole ingested at a single breast feed was 37.2µg.— M. E. Tunstall *et al.*, *Br. J. Obstet. Gynaec.*, 1979, *86*, 793.

See also Adverse Effects.

Uses. Chlormethiazole edisylate is a hypnotic and sedative with anticonvulsant effects. It is used in confusion, agitation, and restlessness, particularly of geriatric psychosis, in sleep disorders in the elderly, and in the treatment of acute alcohol and drug withdrawal symptoms. It is also used in status epilepticus and toxaemia of pregnancy.

Chlormethiazole as Heminevrin (*Astra*) has been used as tablets containing 500 mg of edisylate, as well as capsules containing 192 mg of chlormethiazole base (equivalent in effect to 500 mg of edisylate in the tablets), and as syrup containing 250 mg of edisylate in 5 ml, or as a 0.8% intravenous infusion of the edisylate. As a result of differences in the bioavailability of these different preparations, not only was 500 mg of the edisylate in the tablets equivalent to 192 mg of the base in the capsules, but it was also equivalent to only 250 mg (5 ml) of the edisylate in the syrup. For further details see under Preparations, below.

The usual hypnotic dose of chlormethiazole is 384 mg of the base in capsules (2 capsules), which is equivalent to 500 mg of the edisylate in syrup (10 ml); this was equivalent to 1 g of the edisylate as tablets (2 tablets). Corresponding doses for daytime sedation are 192 mg of the base (1 capsule) or 250 mg of the edisylate in syrup (5 ml) given thrice daily; this was equivalent to 500 mg of the edisylate as tablets (1 tablet) given thrice daily.

The usual dosage for treatment of alcohol and drug withdrawal states is 576 mg of the base (3 capsules) or 750 mg of the edisylate in syrup (15 ml) given every 6 hours for 2 days, followed by 384 mg of the base (2 capsules) or 500 mg of the edisylate in syrup (10 ml) given every 6 hours for 3 days, followed by 192 mg of the base (1 capsule) or 250 mg of the edisylate in syrup (5 ml) given every 6 hours for 4 days; equivalent doses of the edisylate as tablets were 1.5 g (3 tablets), 1 g (2 tablets), and 500 mg (1 tablet) given according to the same frequency. Treatment should be carried out in hospital, and administration for longer than 9 days is not recommended (see Dependence).

For pre-eclamptic toxaemia an initial infusion of 30 to 50 ml of a 0.8% solution of the edisylate is given at the rate of 60 drops per minute until the patient is drowsy, then reduced to a rate of about 10 to 15 drops per minute. An infusion of 40 to 100 ml of the 0.8% solution may be given over 5 to 10 minutes to control convulsions in status epilepticus. Thereafter an intravenous infusion may be required according to the patient's response. Either of these 2 regimens may also be used for acute alcohol withdrawal symptoms and delirium tremens but, owing to the short half-life of chlormethiazole, the rapid infusion method must be followed either by a further intravenous infusion of 0.8% solution or by oral therapy with the capsules. Close supervision is essential during intravenous infusions to avoid the risk of overdose.

Administration in the elderly. References to the use of chlormethiazole for the hypnosis and sedation of elderly subjects: M. Bergener and K. Neller, *Acta psychiat. scand.*, 1966, *42*, *Suppl.* 192, 187; N. Zgaga, *Wien. med. Wschr.*, 1971, *121*, 646; M. S. Pathy, *Curr. med. Res. Opinion*, 1975, *2*, 648; A. Harenko, *ibid.*, 657; H. W. ter Haar, *Pharmatherapeutica*, 1977, *1*, 563; R. V. Magnus, *Clin. Ther.*, 1978, *1*, 387, per *Int. pharm. Abstr.*, 1979, *16*, 210; O. Dehlin *et al.*, *Clin. Ther.*, 1978, *2*, 41, per *Int. pharm. Abstr.*, 1980, *17*, 511; R. S. Briggs *et al.*, *Br. med. J.*, 1980, *280*, 601. Criticisms: I. Oswald and K. Adam (letter), *ibid.*, 860; A. F. Macklon *et al.* (letter), *ibid.*, 861; C. G. Swift *et al.* (letter), *ibid.*, 1322.

Hemiballismus. Chlormethiazole [edisylate] in a concentration of 0.8% was given by continuous intravenous infusion to an 80-year-old patient with severe hemiballismus. Within 5 minutes of the rapid infusion of 100 ml all involuntary movements ceased. The infusion was continued until the patient had received 800 ml over 14 hours. There was no recurrence of the involuntary movements after the infusion was stopped.— P. Mestitz (letter), *Br. med. J.*, 1975, *4*, 169.

Alcohol and drug withdrawal. In a double-blind study in 97 alcoholic patients with symptoms from the recent withdrawal of alcohol, chlormethiazole [edisylate as tablets] in a dosage of respectively 2, 5, 3.5, 2.5, 1.5, 1, and 0.5 g on each of the 7 days after admission, was compared with placebo. During the trial period almost all of the individual symptoms, particularly psychiatric symptoms, improved more rapidly in the treated group. The incidence of sedation was 53% in the treated group compared with 25% in the placebo group. Overall assessment on the first, second, and third days showed an improvement in respectively 50, 67, and 71% of the patients given chlormethiazole, and respectively 22, 27, and 41% of patients given the placebo. There was no evidence that chlormethiazole was contra-indicated in depression. Side-effects included a sneezing reflex in 11 given chlormethiazole. In view of the possible risk of dependence, chlormethiazole should not be continued beyond 6 days.— M. M. Glatt *et al.*, *Br. med. J.*, 1965, *2*, 401.

Further studies and reports: Proceedings of a Symposium (Astra), June 1965, *Acta psychiat. scand.*, 1966, *42, Suppl.* 192; S. D. McGrath, *Br. J. Addict.*, 1975, *70, Suppl.* 1, 80; A. P. Parada (letter), *Am. J. Psychiat.*, 1975, *132*, 1225.

For the use of chlormethiazole with diphenoxylate in the treatment of diamorphine dependence, see Diphenoxylate Hydrochloride, p.1011.

Anaesthesia. In 5 healthy adults, 1 to 2 g of chlormethiazole [edisylate] was infused over about 8 minutes (a rate 2 to 3 times greater than recommended) to produce unconsciousness. Cardiac output, mean arterial pressure, central venous pressure, and respiration showed no significant changes; heart-rate increased by an average of about 48%. Chlormethiazole might be of value to produce sedation in patients undergoing intensive care.— J. Wilson *et al.*, *Br. J. Anaesth.*, 1969, *41*, 840.

Chlormethiazole [edisylate] as a 0.8% solution, caused local pain when given by rapid infusion (20 ml per minute) prior to fibre-endoscopic examination of the upper gastro-intestinal tract. It was ineffective as a sedative in 5 of 25 patients compared with only 1 of 50 given diazepam 5 mg per minute intravenously.— E. J. Galizia *et al.*, *Br. J. Anaesth.*, 1975, *47*, 402.

Convulsions. In 9 episodes of status epilepticus, unresponsive to diazepam, in 8 patients the condition responded on 7 occasions to the infusion of chlormethiazole [edisylate] 500 to 700 mg per hour, without serious impairment of consciousness or depression of respiration.— P. K. P. Harvey *et al.*, *Br. med. J.*, 1975, *2*, 603.

Review: *Drug & Ther. Bull.*, 1976, *14*, 89.

Hyperprolactinaemia. In 16 chronic alcoholics treatment with chlormethiazole significantly reduced serum-prolactin concentrations. It might be valuable in treating hyperprolactinaemia.— S. K. Majumdar *et al.*, *Br. med. J.*, 1978, *2*, 1266.

Mania. A report of beneficial effects with chlormethiazole [edisylate as tablets] in manic patients, using a dose of 6 to 10 g daily. The optimum dose had to be carefully determined for each patient and, because it was rapidly excreted, doses had to be given at intervals not exceeding 4 hours.— M. J. Hackett and R. F. Chatfield (letter), *Lancet*, 1967, *2*, 716.

Toxaemia of pregnancy. A 0.8% solution of chlormethiazole given by intravenous infusion was found to be useful in the management of pre-eclamptic toxaemia in labour. The infusion was started at 60 drops per minute for 5 to 10 minutes until the patient was well sedated; a maintenance dose of 15 drops per min was given and the dose was increased if the patient was restless and reduced again when the desired degree of sedation had been achieved. Pain during labour was treated with pethidine and nitrous oxide and oxygen, and hypertension occurring after treatment with chlormethiazole was treated with a continuous infusion of protoveratrine in dextrose injection. Oxytocin, intravenously, was used when contractions were not satisfactory. Of 34 patients with moderate pre-eclampsia and 16 with severe pre-eclampsia who were treated with chlormethiazole, all babies were born alive but 3 died in the neonatal period, giving a perinatal mortality-rate of 6%. Superficial phlebitis at the injection site occurred in all patients.— G. M. Duffus *et al.* (preliminary communication), *Lancet*, 1968, *1*, 335.

Further references: T. Varda, *J. Obstet. Gynaec. Br. Commonw.*, 1972, *79*, 513, per *Practitioner*, 1972, *209*, 587.

Proprietary Preparations of Chlormethiazole and Chlormethiazole Edisylate

Heminevrin *(Astra, UK)*. Chlormethiazole edisylate, available as **Infusion** containing 8 mg per ml and as **Syrup** containing 250 mg in each 5 ml (to be taken in water or fruit juice). **Heminevrin Capsules** each contain chlormethiazole base 192 mg (equivalent in effect to 500 mg of chlormethiazole edisylate) in arachis oil. (Also available as Heminevrin in *Denm., Norw., S.Afr., Swed.*).

Based on plasma levels of chlormethiazole in man, one Heminevrin tablet containing 500 mg chlormethiazole edisylate is considered to be clinically equivalent to one Heminevrin capsule containing 192 mg chlormethiazole base in arachis oil or 5 ml Heminevrin syrup containing 250 mg chlormethiazole edisylate.— A. K. Watson, *Astra, Personal Communication*, 1979.

Other Proprietary Names of Chlormethiazole and Chlormethiazole Edisylate

Distraneurin *(Ger.)*; Distraneurine *(Belg., Spain)*; Hemineurin *(Arg., Austral.)*; Héminevrine *(Fr.)*.

4025-s

Cyclobarbitone *(B.P. 1958)*. Cyclobarbital; Ethylhexabital; Hexemalum. 5-(Cyclohex-1-enyl)-5-ethylbarbituric acid.

$C_{12}H_{16}N_2O_3$=236.3.

CAS — 52-31-3.

NOTE. The name ciclobarbital has been applied to hexobarbitone.

Pharmacopoeias. In *Aust., Braz., Hung., Ind., It., Jap., Jug., Pol.,* and *Roum.*

A white odourless crystalline powder with a slightly bitter taste. M.p 171° to 175°. **Soluble** 1 in 800 of water, 1 in 4 of alcohol, 1 in 20 of chloroform, and 1 in 15 of ether; soluble in solutions of alkali hydroxides and carbonates. A saturated solution in water is acid to litmus. **Protect** from light.

NOTE. Since it has been shown that cyclobarbitone gradually decomposes on storage (see S. Åhlander, below), the more stable cyclobarbitone calcium is now usually preferred and has replaced cyclobarbitone in the British Pharmacopoeia.

Stability. Samples 4 years old showed more than 20% decomposition (bromometric titration) and cyclobarbitone tablets showed considerable loss in strength after 1 to 4 years' storage. The decomposition was in the cyclohexene ring and was accompanied by the formation of peroxides. Cyclobarbitone calcium and hexobarbitone did not decompose on storage.— S. Åhlander, *Svensk farm. Tidskr.*, 1956, *60*, 249.

4026-w

Cyclobarbitone Calcium *(B.P., Eur. P.)*. Cyclobarb. Calc.; Cyclobarbitalum Calcicum; Cyclobarbital Calcium; Hexemalcalcium. Calcium 5-(cyclohex-1-enyl)-5-ethylbarbiturate.

$(C_{12}H_{15}N_2O_3)_2Ca$=510.6.

CAS — 143-76-0.

Pharmacopoeias. In *Aust., Br., Cz., Eur., Fr., Ger., Int., It., Neth., Nord.,* and *Swiss.*

A white or slightly yellowish, almost odourless, crystalline powder with a persistent bitter taste. **Soluble** 1 in 100 of water; very slightly soluble in alcohol; practically insoluble in chloroform and ether. A saturated solution in water is alkaline to litmus. **Store** in airtight containers.

Dependence. Prolonged use of cyclobarbitone may lead to dependence of the barbiturate-alcohol type (see p.792).

Adverse Effects, Treatment, and Precautions. As for Phenobarbitone, p.812.

Absorption and Fate. See under Phenobarbitone, p.814.

Cyclobarbitone is metabolised in the liver and only about 2 to 7% is excreted unchanged.

In a crossover study of the pharmacokinetics of cyclobarbitone calcium in 6 healthy subjects, 2 tablet formulations and an aqueous solution were compared. After oral administration of a 300-mg dose of the tablets peak plasma concentrations were obtained in 20 to 180 minutes. Absorption was most rapid with the aqueous solution but, contrary to expectations, bioavailability was lowest. In 4 of the subjects the half-lives of 8 to 11 hours were sufficiently short for a hypnotic agent, but in the other 2 subjects the half-lives of 15 to 17 hours were too long for its rational use in the treatment of insomnia.— D. D. Breimer and M. A. C. M. Winten, *Eur. J. clin. Pharmac.*, 1976, *9*, 443. See also D. D. Breimer (letter), *J. pharm. Sci.*, 1975, *64*, 1576.

A ketonic oxidation product (corresponding to 3-oxocyclobarbitone) was detected in the urine of subjects given cyclobarbitone by mouth.— R. Bouche *et al.*, *J. pharm. Sci.*, 1978, *67*, 1019.

Uses. Cyclobarbitone is a barbiturate (see p.792). It is used as a hypnotic and sedative. As a hypnotic it is usually given in doses of 200 to 400 mg at night.

Preparations of Cyclobarbitone Calcium

Cyclobarbitone Tablets *(B.P. 1973)*. Cyclobarb. Tab.; Cyclobarbital Calcium Tablets. Tablets containing cyclobarbitone calcium. Store in airtight containers.

Phanodorm *(Winthrop, UK)*. Cyclobarbitone calcium, available as tablets of 200 mg. (Also available as Phanodorm in *Denm., Ger., Neth., Swed.*).

Other Proprietary Names of Cyclobarbitone Calcium

Ami-nal, Cyclosedal *(both Belg.)*; Fanodormo Calcico *(Spain)*; Panodorm-Calcium *(Ital.)*; Phanodorme Calcium *(Belg.)*; Prodorm *(Norw.)*.

Cyclobarbitone calcium was also formerly marketed in Great Britain under the proprietary name Rapidal (*Medo-Chemicals*). A preparation containing cyclobarbitone calcium was formerly marketed under the proprietary name Cyclomet (*Woodward*).

4027-e

Cyclopentobarbitone. Cyclopentobarbital; Cyclopentenylallyl Barbituric Acid. 5-Allyl-5-(cyclopent-2-enyl)barbituric acid.

$C_{12}H_{14}N_2O_3$=234.3.

CAS — 76-68-6.

Crystals with a bitter taste. M.p. 139° to 140°. Slightly **soluble** in cold water; more soluble in hot water; freely soluble in alcohol and other organic solvents.

Cyclopentobarbitone is a barbiturate (see p.792) that has been used as a hypnotic in doses of 100 to 200 mg at night.

Proprietary Names

Cyclopal *(Siegfried, Ger.; Siegfried, Switz.)*.

4028-l

Dichloralphenazone *(B.P.)*. A complex of chloral hydrate and phenazone.

$C_{15}H_{18}Cl_6N_2O_5$=519.0.

CAS — 480-30-8.

Pharmacopoeias. In *Br.*

A white microcrystalline powder with a slight odour characteristic of chloral hydrate and a taste which is at first saline and then acrid. M.p. 64° to 67°.

Soluble 1 in 10 of water, 1 in 1 of alcohol, and 1 in 2 of chloroform; soluble in dilute acids. It is decomposed by dilute alkalis, liberating chloroform. **Store** in airtight containers.

In aqueous solution it dissociates into chloral hydrate and phenazone.

Dependence. Prolonged use of dichloralphenazone may lead to dependence of the barbiturate-alcohol type (see p.792).

Adverse Effects. As for Chloral Hydrate, p.796. See also Phenazone, p.272.

It is less likely than chloral hydrate to cause gastric irritation.

Allergy. A 66-year-old man suffered anaphylaxis 15 minutes after taking one tablet of dichloralphenazone; symptoms included pruritus, rash, peri-orbital oedema, chest pain, atrial fibrillation, and absence of recordable blood pressure; he recovered after treatment with hydrocortisone, promethazine, and oxygen. He had suffered a similar occurrence after taking dichloralphenazone about 14 years earlier; it had then been considered vasovagal syncope.— S. Perl, *Br. med. J.*, 1977, *2*, 1187.

A 55-year-old man given 2 tablets of dichloralphenazone developed severe bronchospasm and a widespread bullous skin eruption.— D. G. Limb (letter), *Br. med. J.*, 1977, *2*, 1480.

Effects on the skin. A report of a fixed drug eruption to dichloralphenazone.— J. Verbov (letter), *Br. J. Derm.*, 1972, *86*, 438.

Treatment of Adverse Effects. As for Chloral Hydrate, p.796.

Precautions. As for Chloral Hydrate, p.796 and Phenazone, p.272.

Dichloralphenazone is contra-indicated in patients with acute intermittent porphyria.

For a report of the effect of dichloralphenazone on plasma concentrations of warfarin, see Warfarin Sodium, p.777.

Absorption and Fate. Dichloralphenazone dissociates to form phenazone (see p.272) and chloral hydrate (see p.796).

Pregnancy and the neonate. The concentration of the active metabolite, trichloroethanol, in the milk of a lactating mother taking 1.3 g of dichloralphenazone at night was 60 to 80% of that in the plasma.— J. H. Lacey (letter), *Br. med. J.*, 1971, *4*, 684.

Uses. Dichloralphenazone has the actions of chloral and phenazone and is used similarly to chloral hydrate (see p.797) as a hypnotic and sedative. It may have slight antipyretic and analgesic actions.

The usual hypnotic dose is 0.65 to 1.95 g at night. It has been used as a sedative in doses of 650 mg twice or thrice daily. A suggested hypnotic dose for children is: up to 1 year of age 112 to 225 mg, 1 to 5 years 225 to 450 mg, 6 to 12 years 450 to 900 mg; this dose may be halved for a sedative dose.

Preparations

Dichloralphenazone Elixir *(B.P.)*. A solution of dichloralphenazone in a suitable flavoured vehicle, which may be coloured. When a dose less than, or not a multiple of 5 ml is prescribed, the mixture should be diluted to 5 ml, or a multiple, with syrup. Such dilutions must be freshly prepared and not used more than 2 weeks after issue. Store at a temperature not exceeding 25° in well-filled airtight containers. Protect from light.

Dichloralphenazone Tablets *(B.P.)*. Tablets containing dichloralphenazone. The tablets are flavoured with peppermint oil; they may be film-coated.
Store in airtight containers.

Proprietary Preparations

Paedo-Sed *(Pharmax, UK)*. A syrup containing in each 5 ml dichloralphenazone 200 mg and paracetamol 100 mg (suggested diluent, syrup). Sedative and analgesic for paediatric use. *Dose.* Children up to 6 months, 2.5 ml; 6 to 12 months, 5 ml; 1 to 4 years, 10 ml; over 4 years, 15 to 20 ml three or four times daily.

Welldorm *(Smith & Nephew Pharmaceuticals, UK)*. Dichloralphenazone, available as **Elixir** containing 225 mg in each 5 ml (suggested diluent, syrup); and as **Tablets** of 650 mg.

Other Proprietary Names

Bonadorm *(Austral.)*; Chloralol *(Canad.)*; Restwel *(S.Afr.)*.

4029-y

Ectylurea. Ectylcarbamide. *N*-(2-Ethylisocrotonoyl)urea.
$C_7H_{12}N_2O_2$=156.2.

CAS — 95-04-5.

A white crystalline powder. Practically **insoluble** in water; very slightly soluble in warm alcohol and in ether; soluble 1 in 30 of warm propylene glycol.

Adverse Effects and Precautions. Ectylurea may cause skin rashes and, occasionally, jaundice. It is contra-indicated in liver disease.

Uses. Ectylurea has been used as a sedative in treating simple anxiety and tension in doses of 150 to 300 mg three or four times daily.

4030-g

Estazolam. D-40TA. 8-Chloro-6-phenyl-4*H*-1,2,4-triazolo[4,3-*a*]-1,4-benzodiazepine.
$C_{16}H_{11}ClN_4$=294.7.

CAS — 29975-16-4.

A white to slightly yellowish, odourless, crystalline powder with a bitter taste. Practically **insoluble** in water; freely soluble in chloroform; soluble in methyl alcohol; sparingly soluble in acetone.

Estazolam is a hypnotic with actions and uses similar to those of nitrazepam (see p.807). It is given in a dose of 1 to 2 mg at night.

Actions and uses of estazolam.— *Drugs Today*, 1976, *12*, 353. Study in 1139 subjects.— T. Momose *et al.*, *Curr. ther. Res.*, 1976, *19*, 277. Effects on the sleep pattern of healthy subjects.— H. Isozaki *et al.*, *ibid.*, *20*, 493.

Effects on respiration. Carbon dioxide narcosis in association with estazolam administration.— *Jap. med. Gaz.*, 1978, *15* (Jan. 20), 12.

Proprietary Names

Domnamid *(Lundbeck, Denm.)*; Eurodin *(Takeda, Jap.)*; Nuctalon *(Cassenne-Takeda, Fr.)*.

4031-q

Ethchlorvynol *(B.P. 1973, U.S.P.)*. β-Chlorovinyl Ethyl Ethynyl Carbinol. 1-Chloro-3-ethylpent-1-en-4-yn-3-ol.
C_7H_9ClO=144.6.

CAS — 113-18-8.

Pharmacopoeias. In *U.S.*

A colourless to yellow, slightly viscous liquid with a characteristic pungent odour and a pungent and slightly bitter taste. Wt per ml about 1.072 g. It darkens on exposure to air and light. Practically **insoluble** in water; miscible with alcohol, acetone, chloroform, ether, and most other organic solvents. **Store** in airtight containers and avoid contact with metals. Protect from light.

Dependence. Prolonged use of ethchlorvynol may lead to dependence of the barbiturate-alcohol type (see p.792). Withdrawal symptoms have been reported when doses of 1 g daily were abruptly discontinued.

Ethchlorvynol withdrawal symptoms (including convulsions, hypertonicity, and hyperreflexia) occurred in a 67-year-old man who had taken the drug in a dose increased from 1 to at least 1.25 g daily over about 5 months.— H. T. Abuzahra and M. Rossdale (letter), *Br. med. J.*, 1968, *2*, 433.

Withdrawal symptoms in a neonate.— B. H. Rumack and P. A. Walravens, *Pediatrics*, 1973, *52*, 714.

Further reports of dependence and withdrawal symptoms: M. D. Blumenthal and M. J. Reinhart, *J. Am. med. Ass.*, 1964, *190*, 154; J. B. Aycrigg, *Am. J. Psychiat.*, 1964, *120*, 1201; C. F. Essig, *J. Am. med. Ass.*, 1966, *196*, 714; A. Flemenbaum and B. Gunby, *Dis. nerv. Syst.*, 1971, *32*, 188.

Reports of abuse by intravenous injection: F. L. Glauser *et al.*, *Ann. intern. Med.*, 1976, *84*, 46; P. Van Swearingen (letter), *ibid.*, 614. See also under Adverse Effects (below).

Adverse Effects. Side-effects include nausea, vomiting, gastric discomfort, after-taste, dizziness, headache, hang-over, blurred vision, facial numbness, and hypotension. Skin rashes, urticaria, and occasionally, thrombocytopenia and cholestatic jaundice have also been reported as has toxic amblyopia. Idiosyncratic reactions include excitement, prolonged hypnosis, severe muscular weakness, and syncope without marked hypotension.

Acute overdosage is characterised by prolonged deep coma, respiratory depression, hypothermia, hypotension, and relative bradycardia.

Chronic intoxication causes incoordination, tremors, ataxia, confusion, slurred speech, hyperreflexia, diplopia, peripheral neuropathy, and generalised muscle weakness. Pulmonary oedema has followed abuse by intravenous injection.

Effects on the blood. A report of fatal thrombocytopenia associated with ethchlorvynol.— E. S. Jacobson, *Ann. intern. Med.*, 1972, *77*, 73.

Effects on the eyes. Toxic amblyopia occurred in a patient who received ethchlorvynol 0.5 to 1 g at night for about 3 months. Treatment consisted of cyanocobalamin injections of 1 mg daily for 10 days. Recovery was complete 6 months after withdrawal of ethchlorvynol.— W. M. Haining and G. W. Beveridge, *Br. J. Ophthal.*, 1964, *48*, 598.

A report of unusual nystagmus occurring after ethchlorvynol use.— A. H. Ropper (letter), *J. Am. med. Ass.*, 1975, *232*, 907.

Effects on the lungs. A report of 2 subjects with rapid-onset severe non-haemodynamic pulmonary oedema following intravenous injection of the contents of ethchlorvynol capsules. This effect was reproduced in *dogs* and it was established that the polyethylene glycol vehicle was not responsible. Pulmonary oedema might be secondary to the direct effects of ethchlorvynol on the alveolar capillary membrane.— F. L. Glauser *et al.*, *Ann. intern. Med.*, 1976, *84*, 46. See also P. Van Swearingen (letter), *ibid.*, 614; T. H. Self *et al.*, *Drug Intell. & clin. Pharm.*, 1979, *13*, 96.

Overdosage. Six patients took ethchlorvynol with suicidal intent. Overdosage was characterised by deep, often prolonged coma, hypothermia, marked respiratory depression, and hypotension without compensatory tachycardia. Complications included peripheral neuropathy and severe pneumonia. Haemodialysis was more effective than peritoneal dialysis or forced diuresis.— B. P. Teehan *et al.*, *Ann. intern. Med.*, 1970, *72*, 875.

Recovery after taking 200 to 250 capsules of ethchlorvynol 500 mg. Haemodialysis for 14 hours removed 14 g of ethchlorvynol. Severe pancytopenia developed on the 15th day but there was no bleeding or infection.— J. C. Klock (letter), *ibid.*, 1974, *81*, 131.

Treatment of Adverse Effects. As for Phenobarbitone, p.812.

Dialysis may be of value in the treatment of severe poisoning with ethchlorvynol.

The slow removal of ethchlorvynol from the body seen after therapeutic doses and overdosage may reflect localisation in adipose and other tissues rather than a slow rate of biotransformation.— P. F. Gibson and N. Wright, *J. pharm. Sci.*, 1972, *61*, 169.

A review of studies and reports on the removal of ethchlorvynol.— J. F. Winchester *et al.*, *Trans. Am. Soc. artif. internal Organs*, 1977, *23*, 762. See also T. N. Tozer *et al.*, *Am. J. Hosp. Pharm.*, 1974, *31*, 986.

Dialysis. A patient who had taken approximately 40 g of ethchlorvynol was treated successfully by haemodialysis using an oil dialysant.— L. T. Welch *et al.*, *Clin. Pharmac. Ther.*, 1972, *13*, 745.

Other reports: J. S. Hyde *et al.*, *Clin. Pediat.*, 1968, *7*, 739 (peritoneal dialysis); A. Hume *et al.*, *Clin. Res.*, 1970, *18*, 62 (lipid haemodialysis).

Haemoperfusion. Beneficial results with charcoal haemoperfusion in ethchlorvynol poisoning.— M. C. Gelfand *et al.*, *Trans. Am. Soc. artif. internal Organs*, 1977, *23*, 599.

Three patients, who had ingested 12 to 22 g of ethchlorvynol, were successfully treated by haemoperfusion utilising Amberlite XAD-4 resin.— R. I. Lynn *et al.*, *Ann. intern. Med.*, 1979, *91*, 549. Comment.— N. L. Benowitz *et al.* (letter), *ibid.*, 1980, *92*, 435. Reply.— A. S. Kliger (letter), *ibid.*

Further references: S. L. Dua *et al.* (letter), *Ann. intern. Med.*, 1980, *92*, 436; N. Benowitz *et al.*, *Clin. Pharmac. Ther.*, 1980, *27*, 236.

Precautions. Ethchlorvynol is contra-indicated in patients with porphyria, and caution is needed in hepatic or renal failure. The effect of ethchlorvynol may be enhanced by alcohol, barbiturates, and other central nervous system depressants. It has been reported to decrease the effects of coumarin anticoagulants, and delirium has followed concomitant use with tricyclic antidepressants.

Absorption and Fate. Ethchlorvynol is readily absorbed from the gastro-intestinal tract and extensively metabolised in the liver. It has a biphasic plasma half-life with a rapid initial phase and a very prolonged terminal phase owing to extensive tissue redistribution.

Studies in healthy subjects indicated that ethchlorvynol is rapidly absorbed following oral administration, and extensively metabolised with only traces of unchanged drug appearing in the urine. The metabolic half-life is a rather rapid 5.6 hours, but it disappears from plasma with a rapid α-phase and a much slower β-phase owing to extensive tissue redistribution.— L. M. Cummins *et al.*, *J. pharm. Sci.*, 1971, *60*, 261. See also P. F. Gibson and N. Wright, *ibid.*, 1972, *61*, 169.

Ethchlorvynol is 35 to 50% bound to plasma proteins.— W. M. Bennett *et al.*, *Ann. intern. Med.*, 1980, *93*, 286.

Administration in renal failure. A single dose of ethchlorvynol 500 mg given to 9 normal subjects produced a rapid rise in plasma-ethchlorvynol concentration to about 4.2 μg per ml in 2 hours, followed by a fall to about 2.4 and 1.6 μg per ml at 4 and 6 hours after administration respectively. In 8 anephric patients on maintenance dialysis, the peak plasma concentration of about 3.9 μg per ml at 2 hours was maintained with little fall and was about 3.7 μg per ml 6 hours after administration.— J. K. Dawborn *et al.*, *Med. J. Aust.*, 1972, *2*, 702.

See also under Uses.

Uses. Ethchlorvynol has mild hypnotic effects and some anticonvulsant properties. The usual hypnotic dose is 500 mg at night but doses ranging from 0.25 to 1 g have been given. It has also been employed as a sedative in doses of 100 or 200 mg two or three times daily. Administration with milk was recommended to avoid dizziness or ataxia caused by ethchlorvynol's rapid onset of effect of 15 to 30 minutes.

Following a study of ethchlorvynol as a hypnotic in 4 young insomniac patients it was concluded that side-effects militate against its use. One subject suffered severe headache, another experienced confusion and stuttering; the other 2 had feelings of tiredness, occasional headache, loss of concentration, and dizziness. There were also significant withdrawal effects.— D. F. Kripke *et al.*, *Psychopharmacology*, 1978, *56*, 221.

Administration in renal failure. Ethchlorvynol could be given in a usual dosage to patients with renal failure. Concentrations of ethchlorvynol in plasma were affected by haemodialysis.— W. M. Bennett *et al.*, *Ann. intern. Med.*, 1980, *93*, 286.

See also under Absorption and Fate.

Preparations

Ethchlorvynol Capsules *(B.P. 1973)*. Capsules containing ethchlorvynol. Protect from light.

Ethchlorvynol Capsules *(U.S.P.)*. Capsules containing ethchlorvynol. Store in airtight containers. Protect from light.

Proprietary Names

Placidyl *(Abbott, Canad.; Abbott, USA)*.

Ethchlorvynol was formerly marketed in Great Britain under the proprietary names Arvynol (*Pfizer*) and Serenesil (*Abbott*).

4032-p

Ethinamate *(U.S.P.)*. 1-Ethynylcyclohexyl carbamate.

$C_9H_{13}NO_2$=167.2.

CAS — 126-52-3.

Pharmacopoeias. In *U.S.*

A white almost odourless powder with a slightly bitter taste. M.p. 94° to 98°. **Soluble** 1 in 400 of water, 1 in about 3 of alcohol, 1 in 50 of light petroleum, 1 in 4.6 of propylene glycol, and 1 in 140 of sesame oil; freely soluble in chloroform and ether. A saturated solution in water has a pH of about 6.5. **Store** in airtight containers.

Dependence. Prolonged use of ethinamate may lead to dependence of the barbiturate-alcohol type (see p.792).

Two patients dependent on ethinamate.— C. H. Ellinwood *et al.*, *New Engl. J. Med.*, 1962, *266*, 185.

Withdrawal of ethinamate had been followed by agitation, syncopal episodes, tremulousness, and hyperactive reflexes. Major convulsions, disorientation, delusions, and hallucinations had also been reported.— C. F. Essig, *J. Am. med. Ass.*, 1966, *196*, 714.

Adverse Effects. Gastro-intestinal discomfort, excitement in children, and skin rashes have been reported. Rarely, thrombocytopenic purpura and hypersensitivity with fever have occurred.

Treatment of Adverse Effects. As for Phenobarbitone, p.812.

Dialysis may be of value in the treatment of severe poisoning with ethinamate.

Precautions. Ethinamate causes drowsiness and patients receiving it should not take charge of vehicles or machinery where loss of attention could lead to accidents. These effects are enhanced by the simultaneous administration of depressants of the central nervous system such as alcohol, barbiturates, and other sedatives.

Absorption and Fate. Ethinamate is rapidly absorbed from the gastro-intestinal tract and extensively metabolised in the body, partly by hydroxylation in the liver; only small amounts appear unchanged in the urine. It has a short half-life.

After administration of ethinamate 1 g by mouth to 8 healthy subjects the maximum blood concentrations occurred in 6 after about 60 minutes. The biological half-life was 135 minutes.— J. M. Clifford *et al.*, *Clin. Pharmac. Ther.*, 1974, *16*, 376.

Ethinamate 1 g was administered as tablets to 12 subjects. The mean peak plasma concentration was about 9.6 μg per ml. The biological half-life in plasma was calculated to be about 2 hours. Excluding one subject with a very low value mean 24-hour recovery from urine for the major metabolite *trans*-4-hydroxyethinamate was about 35%.— J. W. Kleber *et al.*, *J. pharm. Sci.*, 1977, *66*, 992.

Uses. Ethinamate has mild sedative and hypnotic properties and is used mainly as a hypnotic. It has been reported to induce sleep in about 20 minutes and to have an effect lasting about 4 hours. The usual dose is 0.5 to 1 g at night.

Preparations

Ethinamate Capsules *(U.S.P.)*. Capsules containing ethinamate. Store in airtight containers.

Proprietary Names

Valamin *(Asche, Ger.)*; Valmid *(Dista, USA)*.

4033-s

Ethylbutylethylmalonylamide. Ethyl 2-carbamoyl-2-ethyl-3-methylvalerate.

$C_{11}H_{21}NO_3$=215.3.

Ethylbutylethylmalonylamide has been used as a sedative in doses of 400 to 600 mg daily in divided doses.

4034-w

Flunitrazepam. Ro 05-4200. 5-(2-Fluorophenyl)-1,3-dihydro-1-methyl-7-nitro-2*H*-1,4-benzodiazepin-2-one.

$C_{16}H_{12}FN_3O_3$=313.3.

CAS — 1622-62-4.

A pale yellow crystalline solid. Sparingly **soluble** in water; readily soluble in alcohol.

Dependence. Prolonged use of flunitrazepam may lead to dependence of the barbiturate-alcohol type (see p.792). It has a low liability for abuse.

Psychiatric complications of flunitrazepam abuse.— S. H. Teo *et al.*, *Singapore med. J.*, 1979, *20*, 270.

For reference to intense rebound insomnia associated with abrupt withdrawal of benzodiazepines with a relatively short duration of action, see Nitrazepam, p.807.

Adverse Effects, Treatment, and Precautions. As for Nitrazepam, p.807.

Effects on mental state. A study in 12 healthy subjects indicated that flunitrazepam 1 or 2 mg significantly altered the EEG up to 18 hours after administration, and motor impairment 12 hours after administration.— A. J. Bond and M. H. Lader, *Br. J. clin. Pharmac.*, 1975, *2*, 143.

Porphyria. A study in *rats* indicating that flunitrazepam may be liable to induce porphyria in susceptible subjects.— G. H. Blekkenhorst *et al.*, *Br. J. Anaesth.*, 1980, *52*, 759.

Absorption and Fate. Flunitrazepam is readily absorbed from the gastro-intestinal tract. About 77 to 80% is bound to plasma proteins. It is extensively metabolised in the liver and excreted mainly in the urine as metabolites. Both major metabolites, the 7-amino derivative and the *N*-demethyl derivative, are active. Flunitrazepam crosses the placental barrier and is excreted in breast milk.

The mean terminal exponential half-life of flunitrazepam following administration of a single 2-mg dose to 8 healthy subjects was 13.5 hours; a half-life of 19.2 hours was obtained in a further 6 subjects following variable repeated doses.— H. G. Boxenbaum *et al.*, *J. Pharmacokinet. Biopharm.*, 1978, *6*, 283.

A terminal half-life of between 20 and 36 hours on prolonged administration of flunitrazepam.— E. Wickstrøm *et al.*, *Eur. J. clin. Pharmac.*, 1980, *17*, 189.

Concentrations of flunitrazepam in umbilical-vein and -artery plasma were lower than those in maternal venous plasma about 11 to 15 hours after administration of flunitrazepam 1 mg to 14 pregnant women; concentrations in amniotic fluid were lower still. Concentrations in breast milk after a single 2-mg dose were considered to be too low to produce clinical effects in breast-feeding infants but accumulation in the milk might occur after repeated administration.— J. Kanto *et al.*, *Curr. ther. Res.*, 1979, *26*, 539.

Further references: J. P. Cano *et al.*, *Arzneimittel-Forsch.*, 1977, *27*, 2383.

Uses. Flunitrazepam is a benzodiazepine derivative with hypnotic properties similar to those of nitrazepam (p.808). As a hypnotic it is usually given in doses of 1 to 2 mg at night. It is also used for some anaesthetic procedures.

Reviews: M. A. K. Mattila and H. M. Larni, *Drugs*, 1980, *20*, 353. See also *Aust. J. Pharm.*, 1979, *60*, 246.

Anaesthesia. In 3 studies in a total of 220 subjects or patients flunitrazepam, in doses of 2 to 6 mg intravenously, exerted its maximum effect 1 to 1.5 minutes after injection; some patients were not asleep after doses equivalent to 100 μg per kg body-weight. Tremor, hypertonus, or involuntary muscle movements occurred in 11 patients; cough, hiccup, or laryngospasm occurred in 61 patients, and transient marked respiratory depression in 5; arterial hypotension in many patients did not cause concern; all these effects were more common in those who did not receive opiates as premedication. Prolonged drowsiness was not uncommon. Venous sequelae (in 21% of subjects) were similar to those observed after diazepam. Although flunitrazepam was considered to be 10 times more potent than diazepam it was too unreliable to be used as a routine induction agent.— J. W. Dundee *et al.*, *Br. J. Anaesth.*, 1976, *48*, 551.

Of 43 patients given a single intravenous dose of flunitrazepam 1 to 2 mg two had thrombosis 7 to 10 days later. The incidence was lower than in those given diazepam.— J. E. Hegarty and J. W. Dundee, *Br. med. J.*, 1977, *2*, 1384. See also H. Mikkelsen *et al.*, *Br. J. Anaesth.*, 1980, *52*, 817.

In a double-blind study the induction of anaesthesia by flunitrazepam in 48 patients was comparable with the effect of alphaxalone and alphadolone in 49 patients. The maintenance of anaesthesia was considered superior in the flunitrazepam group. Transient erythema occurred in 4 patients given flunitrazepam, postoperative respiratory depression in 8, and laryngospasm on extubation in 2. The dose of flunitrazepam was 50 μg per kg body-weight with a supplementary dose of 10 μg per kg if needed and an additional dose of 10 μg per kg at incision.— M. A. K. Mattila *et al.*, *Br. J. Anaesth.*, 1977, *49*, 1041.

In a study of 92 patients undergoing bronchoscopy flunitrazepam 10 μg per kg body-weight intravenously had a greater amnesic effect than diazepam 125 μg per kg. When the doses were doubled the effects of the 2 drugs were comparable. Mean serum-concentrations of flunitrazepam 2 hours after injection were 25 and 58 ng per ml respectively for the 2 doses.— K. Korttila *et al.*, *Br. J. Anaesth.*, 1978, *50*, 281.

In a double-blind study in 142 children undergoing routine surgery, flunitrazepam was compared with diazepam as premedication. The drugs were given by mouth 90 minutes before operation and atropine was not given. Flunitrazepam was associated with greater sedation before operation and less vomiting after operation and a greater frequency of amnesia before and immediately after operation. Flunitrazepam, 1, 1.5, or 2 mg, or diazepam, 10, 15, or 20 mg, was given, according to body-weight, to children weighing 31 to 40 kg, 41 to 50 kg, or more than 50 kg respectively.— F. J. Richardson and M. L. M. Manford, *Br. J. Anaesth.*, 1979, *51*, 313.

Flunitrazepam 1 mg or diazepam 10 mg intravenously was given, as an adjunct to general anaesthesia, immediately before operation to 90 female patients undergoing abdominal surgery. The quality of anaesthesia was better and the need for supplementary doses of pethidine lower in the flunitrazepam group. Flunitrazepam appeared to have a greater amnesic action than diazepam. Recovery was equally good in both groups.— M. A. K. Mattila *et al.*, *Br. J. Anaesth.*, 1979, *51*, 329.

In 20 women undergoing total abdominal hysterectomy, anaesthesia was induced by flunitrazepam 30 µg per kg body-weight given intravenously and maintained using ketamine. No patients experienced emergence phenomena associated with ketamine and no patients had retrograde amnesia. Only 2 patients reported dreaming.— P. J. C. Houlton and J. W. Downing, *S. Afr. med. J.* 1978, *54*, 1048.

The use of flunitrazepam 20 µg per kg body-weight as a premedicant in children undergoing otolaryngological surgery.— L. Lindgren *et al.*, *Br. J. Anaesth.*, 1980, *52*, 283.

Further reports and studies on flunitrazepam in anaesthesia: M. J. Ungerer and F. R. Erasmus, *S. Afr. med. J.*, 1973, *47*, 787; C. Pearce, *Br. J. Anaesth.*, 1974, *46*, 877; K. Korttila, *Arzneimittel-Forsch.*, 1975, *25*, 1303; A. Mortasawi, *Opusc. med.*, 1975, *20*, 229, per *Int. pharm. Abstr.*, 1976, *13*, 883; I. Freuchen *et al.*, *Curr. ther. Res.*, 1976, *20*, 36; W. A. W. McGowan *et al.*, *Br. J. Anaesth.*, 1980, *52*, 447; L. Lindgren *et al.*, *Br. J. Anaesth.*, 1979, *51*, 321; C. G. Male *et al.*, *ibid.*, 1980, *52*, 429.

Hypnotic effect. In a double-blind study of 160 healthy subjects who took fosazepam 40, 60, or 80 mg, lorazepam 2.5 or 5 mg, or flunitrazepam 1 or 2 mg, flunitrazepam was considered to be the most effective hypnotic and lorazepam more effective than fosazepam.— J. W. Dundee *et al.* (letter), *Br. J. clin. Pharmac.*, 1977, *4*, 706.

Flunitrazepam 2 mg produced a quicker onset of sleep and fewer awakenings than nitrazepam 5 mg or aprobarbitone 100 mg when taken by 147 patients before retiring. Duration of sleep obtained with each of the drugs was identical but flunitrazepam produced a hangover or drowsiness the following morning in about 20% of patients.— I. Freuchen *et al.*, *Curr. ther. Res.*, 1978, *23*, 90.

Further reports and studies on the hypnotic effect of flunitrazepam: E. O. Bixler *et al.*, *J. clin. Pharmac.*, 1977, *17*, 569; I. Hindmarch *et al.*, *Br. J. clin. Pharmac.*, 1977, *4*, 229; U. J. Jovanović, *J. int. med. Res.*, 1977, *5*, 77; H. Hartelius *et al.*, *Acta psychiat. scand.*, 1978, *58*, 1; A. N. Nicholson and B. M. Stone, *Br. J. clin. Pharmac.*, 1980, *9*, 187; H. Bertel, *S. Afr. med. J.*, 1980, *57*, 769.

Proprietary Names

Darkene *(Sigurtà, Ital.)*; Narcozep *(Roche, Fr.)*; Primun *(Labinca, Arg.)*; Rohipnol *(Roche, Spain)*; Rohypnol *(Roche, Arg.; Roche, Austral.; Roche, Belg.; Roche, Denm.; Roche, Fr.; Roche, Neth.; Roche, Norw.; Roche, S.Afr.; Roche, Switz.)*; Roipnol *(Roche, Ital.)*; Valsera *(Polifarma, Ital.)*.

4035-e

Flurazepam Monohydrochloride.

7-Chloro-1-(2-diethylaminoethyl)-5-(2-fluorophenyl)-1,3-dihydro-2*H*-benzodiazepin-2-one hydrochloride.

$C_{21}H_{23}ClFN_3O,HCl$=424.4.

CAS — 17617-23-1 (flurazepam); 36105-20-1 (monohydrochloride).

Flurazepam monohydrochloride 32.8 mg is approximately equivalent to 30 mg of flurazepam.

4036-l

Flurazepam Hydrochloride *(U.S.P.)*.

Ro 5-6901; Flurazepam Dihydrochloride.

$C_{21}H_{23}ClFN_3O,2HCl$=460.8.

CAS — 1172-18-5.

Pharmacopoeias. In *U.S.*

An off-white to yellow, odourless or almost odourless, crystalline powder. M.p. about 212° with decomposition. Flurazepam hydrochloride 30 mg is approximately equivalent to 25.3 mg of flurazepam. **Soluble** 1 in 2 of water, 1 in 4 of alcohol, 1 in 90 of chloroform, 1 in 3 of methyl alcohol, and 1 in 69 of isopropyl alcohol; very slightly soluble in ether and light petroleum. A solution in water is acid to litmus. **Store** in airtight containers. Protect from light.

Dependence. Prolonged use of flurazepam may lead to dependence of the barbiturate-alcohol type (see p.792). It has a low liability for abuse.

Adverse Effects, Treatment, and Precautions. As for Nitrazepam, p.807.

Comment on the pronounced cumulative effects of flurazepam.— I. Oswald, *Br. med. J.*, 1979, *1*, 1167.

Administration in the elderly. The frequency of reported toxicity due to flurazepam increased with age in a study from the Boston Collaborative Drug Surveillance Program involving 2542 patients in hospital for medical treatment, more than 40% of whom were over 60 years of age. None of the side-effects was serious and most related to residual drowsiness. Of patients aged under 60 years, 1.9% experienced unwanted effects whereas of those aged 80 or over toxicity reached 7.1%. Higher doses increased the frequency of adverse reactions this effect being most marked in the elderly; of patients aged 70 years or more who received an average dose of 30 mg or more, 39% experienced side-effects whereas at doses under 15 mg daily side-effects occurred in no more than 2% regardless of age.— D. J. Greenblatt *et al.*, *Clin. Pharmac. Ther.*, 1977, *21*, 355.

Administration in renal failure. Five patients on maintenance haemodialysis developed encephalopathy attributed to flurazepam and diazepam.— L. Taclob and M. Needle, *Lancet*, 1976, *2*, 704.

Effects on the liver. Reports of cholestatic jaundice following the use of flurazepam: M. H. Fang *et al.*, *Ann. intern. Med.*, 1978, *89*, 363; R. Reynolds *et al.*, *Can. med. Ass. J.*, 1981, *124*, 893.

Absorption and Fate. Flurazepam is fairly readily absorbed from the gastro-intestinal tract. It is rapidly metabolised and the metabolites and very little unchanged drug are excreted in the urine.

The metabolism of flurazepam was studied in 4 healthy male volunteers given 30 mg daily for 2 weeks. A hydroxyethyl metabolite was present in the blood shortly after administration. The *N*-desalkyl metabolite, the major metabolite in the blood, had a half-life ranging from 47 to 100 hours. Steady-state concentrations were reached after 7 to 10 days and were approximately 5 to 6 times greater than those observed on day 1.— S. A. Kaplan *et al.*, *J. pharm. Sci.*, 1973, *62*, 1932.

Further references: M. A. Schwartz and E. Postma, *J. pharm. Sci.*, 1970, *59*, 1800; J. A. F. de Silva and N. Strojny, *ibid.*, 1971, *60*, 1303; J. A. F. de Silva *et al.*, *ibid.*, 1974, *63*, 1837.

A review of the therapeutic activity of drug metabolites including those of flurazepam.— D. E. Drayer, *Clin. Pharmacokinet.*, 1976, *1*, 426.

A study in 3 patients indicating that following administration by mouth some metabolism of flurazepam occurred in the small bowel mucosa.— W. A. Mahon *et al.*, *Clin. Pharmac. Ther.*, 1977, *22*, 228.

Kinetics and clinical effects of flurazepam in young and elderly non-insomniac adults.— D. J. Greenblatt *et al.*, *Clin. Pharmac. Ther.*, 1981, *30*, 475.

Uses. Flurazepam is a benzodiazepine derivative with hypnotic properties similar to those of nitrazepam (see p.808). In the USA flurazepam is given in doses of 15 to 30 mg of the dihydrochloride (flurazepam hydrochloride) at night. In the UK it is given as the monohydrochloride in doses equivalent to 15 to 30 mg of flurazepam at night.

Reviews of the action, uses, and adverse effects of flurazepam: *Drug & Ther. Bull.*, 1974, *12*, 35; *Med. Lett.*, 1975, *17*, 29; D. J. Greenblatt *et al.*, *Clin. Pharmac. Ther.*, 1975, *17*, 1; *idem, Ann. intern. Med.*, 1975, *83*, 237.

Anaesthesia. Flurazepam 1 to 1.5 mg per kg body-weight was suitable for the induction of anaesthesia maintained by halothane, oxygen, and nitrous oxide. There was a slight fall in systolic blood pressure in some patients and occasional transient apnoea.— E. Domenichini *et al.*, *Curr. ther. Res.*, 1973, *15*, 534.

Hypnotic effect. Sleep laboratory studies of flurazepam in 23 insomniac patients. Although sleep was significantly improved on the first night of administration increased benefit occurred on the second and third nights after build-up of metabolites.— A. Kales *et al.*, *Clin. Pharmac. Ther.*, 1976, *19*, 576.

Some other reports and studies on the hypnotic activity of flurazepam: J. Kales *et al.*, *Clin. Pharmac. Ther.*, 1971, *12*, 691; A. M. Zimmerman, *Curr. ther. Res.*, 1971, *13*, 18; Boston Collaborative Drug Surveillance Program, *J. clin. Pharmac.*, 1972, *12*, 217; J. A. Meyer and K. Z. Kurland, *Milit. Med.*, 1973, *138*, 471; D. J. Greenblatt *et al.*, *Ann. intern. Med.*, 1975, *83*, 237; A. Kales *et al.*, *Clin. Pharmac. Ther.*, 1975, *18*, 356; M. R. Salkind and T. Silverstone, *Br. J. clin. Pharmac.*, 1975, *2*, 223; A. Pines *et al.*, *Practitioner*, 1976, *217*, 281; I. Saario and M. Linnoila, *Acta pharmac. tox.*, 1976, *38*, 382; I. Feinberg *et al.*, *Science*, 1977, *198*, 847; M. Viukari *et al.*, *Acta psychiat. scand.*, 1978, *57*, 27; J. D. Frost and M. R. DeLucchi, *J. Am. Geriat. Soc.*, 1979, *27*, 541; M. Linnoila *et al.*, *J. clin. Pharmac.*, 1980, *20*, 117.

Preparations of Flurazepam Monohydrochloride and Hydrochloride

Flurazepam Hydrochloride Capsules *(U.S.P.)*. Capsules containing flurazepam hydrochloride. The *U.S.P.* requires 75% dissolution in 20 minutes. Store in airtight containers. Protect from light.

Dalmane *(Roche, UK)*. Flurazepam monohydrochloride, available as capsules each containing the equivalent of 15 or 30 mg of flurazepam.

NOTE. Dalmane *(Roche, Austral.; Roche, Canad.; Roche, USA)* contains 15 and 30 mg of flurazepam hydrochloride.

Other Proprietary Names of Flurazepam Monohydrochloride and Hydrochloride

Arg.—Fordrim, Natam, Somlan; *Belg.*— Niotal; *Denm.*—Dalmadorm; *Ger.*—Dalmadorm; *Ital.*—Dalmadorm, Felison, Flunox, Midorm AR, Remdue, Valdorm; *Jap.*—Benozil, Dalmate, Insumin; *Neth.*—Dalmadorm; *Norw.*—Dalmadorm; *S.Afr.*—Dalmadorm; *Spain*—Dormodor; *Switz.*—Dalmadorm.

4037-y

Glutethimide *(B.P., U.S.P.)*.

Glutethimidum. 2-Ethyl-2-phenylglutarimide; 3-Ethyl-3-phenylpiperidine-2,6-dione.

$C_{13}H_{15}NO_2$=217.3.

CAS — 77-21-4.

Pharmacopoeias. In *Belg.*, *Br.*, *Chin.*, *Cz.*, *Int.*, *Jug.*, *Pol.* (which also includes the monohydrate), and *U.S.*

Odourless colourless crystals or white crystalline powder with a bitter taste. M.p. 85° to 89°. Practically **insoluble** in water; soluble 1 in 5 of alcohol, 1 in less than 1 of chloroform, and 1 in 12 of ether; freely soluble in acetone and ethyl acetate; soluble in methyl alcohol; slightly soluble in light petroleum. A saturated solution in water is acid to litmus. **Store** in airtight containers. Protect from light.

Stability. Hydrolysis of glutethimide was a base-catalysed first-order reaction. At pH 5 the chemical half-life was 28.3 years at 25° and 1.02 months at pH 8, with decreasing stability at higher pH. Hydrolysis to 4-ethyl-4-phenylglutaramic acid occurred, and the use of the water-soluble glutethimide hydrochloride was suggested.— J. W. Wesolowski *et al.*, *J. pharm. Sci.*, 1968, *57*, 811.

Dependence. Prolonged use of glutethimide may lead to dependence of the barbiturate-alcohol type (see p.792).

Abuse. A warning of the hazards associated with the abuse of glutethimide in a combination termed 'loads'.— J. J. Sramek and A. Khajawall (letter), *New Engl. J. Med.*, 1981, *305*, 231.

Dependence. Manifestations of glutethimide withdrawal had been reported to include nausea, vomiting, abdominal cramping, tachycardia, sweating, fever, agitation, and tremulousness. Major reactions included convulsions, or delirium, or both, characterised by confusion, disorientation, and hallucinations. The lowest dosages reported to have been followed by abstinence convulsions were 2.5 g and 5 g daily in 2 patients who had taken the drug for 3 months and 'several weeks' respectively.— C. F. Essig, *J. Am. med. Ass.*, 1966, *196*, 714. Further report in 1 patient.— C. A. Shamoian and A.

K. Shapiro (letter), *ibid.*, 1969, *207*, 1919.

Facial grimacing and a catatonia-like psychosis in a 37-year-old woman might have been due to glutethimide withdrawal in association with antihistamine administration.— M. I. Good, *Am. J. Psychiat.*, 1976, *133*, 1454.

For other reports of dependence on glutethimide, see F. A. Johnson and H. C. Van Buren, *J. Am. med. Ass.*, 1962, *180*, 1024; E. D. Luby and E. F. Domino, *ibid.*, *181*, 46; J. N. DiGiacomo and C. L. King, *Int. J. Addict.*, 1970, *5*, 279.

Neonatal dependence. Neonatal withdrawal symptoms in an infant born to a mother addicted to diamorphine and glutethimide initially responded to chlorpromazine. Recurrence on the tenth day might have been due to glutethimide withdrawal.— M. Reveri *et al.*, *Clin. Pediat.*, 1977, *16*, 424.

Adverse Effects. In therapeutic doses side-effects include nausea, excitement, hang-over, blurred vision, and occasional skin rashes. Acute hypersensitivity reactions, blood disorders and exfoliative dermatitis have been reported in rare instances.

Overdosage with glutethimide produces symptoms similar to those of barbiturate overdosage (see p.812) including the presence of bullae, but there are considerable fluctuations in the depth of coma and wakefulness. Sudden apnoea and convulsions may occur with signs of raised intracranial pressure and severe hypotension, and persistent acidosis may develop. Anticholinergic effects such as mydriasis, dryness of the mouth, paralytic ileus, and urinary bladder atony often occur. Irregular absorption and storage in fat depots may complicate treatment.

Chronic ingestion of high doses of glutethimide is associated with impaired memory, inability to concentrate, impaired gait, ataxia, tremors, hyporeflexia, and slurring of speech; convulsions may also occur. Sudden withdrawal may produce symptoms ranging from nervousness and anxiety to grand mal convulsions.

Effects on the blood. Significant methaemoglobinaemia occurred in a patient with glutethimide intoxication.— L. Filippini, *Schweiz. med. Wschr.*, 1965, *95*, 1618.

A man aged 47, estimated to have taken 100 to 400 mg daily of glutethimide for 5 years, had megaloblastic anaemia and a haemoglobin value of 41%. Following drug withdrawal, he was given 20 mg of folic acid thrice daily. Within 7 days the haemoglobin rose to 80% and subsequently the dosage of folic acid was reduced to 15 mg daily. Haematological and other examinations indicated that the anaemia was probably due to glutethimide.— D. Pearson (letter), *Lancet*, 1965, *1*, 110.

Effects on the nervous system. A woman who had taken increasingly large doses of glutethimide (up to 5 g daily) for about 5 years developed peripheral neuropathy and cerebral impairment, which persisted after the drug had been withdrawn.— R. Nover, *Clin. Pharmac. Ther.*, 1967, *8*, 283.

Three patients developed peripheral neuritis and cerebellar ataxia following prolonged glutethimide ingestion in doses varying from 0.75 to 4 g daily.— D. C. Haas and A. Marasigan, *J. Neurol. Neurosurg. Psychiat.*, 1968, *31*, 561.

A patient who took glutethimide about 15 to 22.5 g by mouth in a suicide attempt recovered with conventional support therapy. In the absence of cerebral ischaemia or hypoxaemia secondary to cardiopulmonary depression, complete clinical recovery from glutethimide-induced coma appeared to be possible no matter how severe the presenting neurological and EEG signs.— R. R. Myers and J. J. Stockard, *Clin. Pharmac. Ther.*, 1975, *17*, 212.

Treatment of Adverse Effects. As for Phenobarbitone, p.812.

Gastric lavage with a mixture of equal parts of castor oil and water may be used as glutethimide is fat-soluble and large doses are only slowly absorbed; 50 ml of castor oil should be left in the stomach on completion of lavage.

Episodes of apnoea, associated with raised intracranial pressure, are prevented by intravenous infusion of mannitol 20% over 20 minutes followed by 500 ml of dextrose injection over the next 4 hours. Special attention should also be paid to correction of acidosis.

Forced diuresis is ineffective and hazardous, and dialysis is generally considered to be of no real value. Dialysis against purified soya oil has been suggested; because of release from fat storage depots such a procedure should be continued after the patient has become conscious. Haemoperfusion has also been tried.

Adsorption. For comment on the *in vitro* adsorption of glutethimide by activated charcoal, see p.79.

Catharsis. A 29-year-old woman, who had been deeply comatose for 48 hours following ingestion of 13 g of glutethimide, was given 30 ml of castor oil by nasogastric tube and during the next 9 hours there was a marked cathartic effect and she awoke.— J. M. Baron and D. L. Tritch (letter), *J. Am. med. Ass.*, 1970, *211*, 1012.

Dialysis. A study of 39 patients who had taken overdoses of glutethimide showed that there was no correlation between the concentration of glutethimide in the blood and the severity of their symptoms or their clinical progress. Five of 17 severely poisoned patients were treated by haemodialysis, which was not considered to have been of value. Treatment should include the giving of a purgative to remove unabsorbed glutethimide.— J. A. Chazan and J. J. Cohen, *J. Am. med. Ass.*, 1969, *208*, 837.

Thirty of 31 patients with acute glutethimide poisoning were successfully treated by gastric lavage followed by intensive supportive therapy. It was concluded that haemodialysis was not essential in the management of severely poisoned patients and advocates of haemodialysis were criticised.— N. Wright and P. Roscoe, *J. Am. med. Ass.*, 1970, *214*, 1704. Similar reports: J. A. Chazan and S. G. Garella, *Archs intern. Med.*, 1971, *128*, 215.

A report of a woman with glutethimide intoxication in whom peritoneal dialysis and haemodialysis were considered to be beneficial.— A. I. Özdemir and A. M. Tannenberg, *N.Y. St. J. Med.*, 1972, *72*, 2076.

Reports and comments on lipid dialysis: *J. Am. med. Ass.*, 1966, *198* (Oct. 17), A45; L. H. King *et al.*, *ibid.*, 1970, *211*, 652.

Haemoperfusion. Some reports on removal of glutethimide by means of charcoal or resin haemoperfusion: T. M. S. Chang *et al.*, *Can. med. Ass. J.*, 1973, *108*, 429; J. A. Vale *et al.*, *Br. med. J.*, 1975, *1*, 5; A. M. Martin *et al.* (letter), *ibid.*, 392; J. L. Rosenbaum *et al.*, *Archs intern. Med.*, 1976, *136*, 263.

Precautions. Glutethimide is contra-indicated in patients with porphyria.

Glutethimide causes drowsiness and patients receiving it should not take charge of vehicles or machinery where loss of attention could lead to accidents. These effects are enhanced by the simultaneous administration of depressants of the central nervous system such as alcohol, barbiturates, and other sedatives. Absorption of glutethimide is also markedly enhanced by concomitant administration of alcohol. Like the barbiturates glutethimide induces microsomal hepatic enzymes, and it can thus cause increased metabolism of coumarin anticoagulants and other drugs, with reduced effect. Chronic administration of glutethimide may also enhance vitamin D metabolism.

Rises in serum and lipoprotein cholesterol concentrations associated with enzyme induction occurred in 6 healthy subjects who received glutethimide 500 mg daily for 21 days. Triglyceride concentrations were unchanged.— C. H. Bolton *et al.*, *Br. J. clin. Pharmac.*, 1980, *9*, 285P.

Interactions. *Alcohol.* Interaction of glutethimide and phenobarbitone with alcohol.— G. P. Mould *et al.*, *J. Pharm. Pharmac.*, 1972, *24*, 894.

Calcium and vitamin D. An elderly woman who ingested 18.75 g of glutethimide developed prolonged hypocalcaemia with an isolated episode of severe hypocalcaemia. She eventually recovered after about 7 weeks.— J. A. Crawshaw, *Practitioner*, 1968, *200*, 739.

A 53-year-old woman whose diet contained marginally adequate amounts of vitamin D and who had taken glutethimide 500 mg at night for 10 years developed osteomalacia. Study showed that this was due to increased enzymatic metabolism of cholecalciferol caused by glutethimide. Nitrazepam did not appear to have this effect.— R. H. Greenwood *et al.*, *Br. med. J.*, 1973, *1*, 643.

Steroids. Glutethimide affected the estimation of urinary 17-oxosteroids and 17-oxogenic-steroids.— *Adverse Drug React. Bull.*, 1972, June, 104.

Absorption and Fate. Glutethimide is irregularly absorbed from the gastro-intestinal tract and extensively metabolised in the liver. It has a biphasic plasma half-life probably owing to tissue redistribution and storage in fat depots. It crosses the placental barrier and traces are found in breast milk.

Absorption and excretion. Following oral administration of glutethimide 500 mg to 6 healthy subjects absorption was irregular with peak plasma-glutethimide concentrations of 2.85 to 7.05 µg per ml being achieved after 1 to 6 hours. In 4 of the 6 subjects decline after the peak was biphasic with initial half-lives of 2.7 to 4.3 hours and subsequent half-lives of 5.1 to 22 hours. Plasma protein binding of glutethimide was about 50%; little unmetabolised drug was excreted in the urine of 3 subjects studied. Mean glutethimide concentrations in the breast milk of 13 nursing mothers given 500 mg were 0.27, 0.27, 0.22, 0.12, and 0.04 µg per ml at 8, 12, 16, 20, and 23 hours respectively but in 32 of the 90 samples analysed no glutethimide was detected. Maternal and neonatal plasma concentrations were found to be similar when 4 women were given 1 g of glutethimide about 2 hours before parturition.— S. H. Curry *et al.*, *Clin. Pharmac. Ther.*, 1971, *12*, 849. See also *idem*, *Br. J. clin. Pharmac.*, 1977, *4*, 109.

Metabolism. Glutethimide was completely metabolised in the body and excreted mainly in the bile; there was considerable intestinal reabsorption, which consequently prolonged its action.— L. E. Hollister, *Clin. Pharmac. Ther.*, 1966, *7*, 142. Little unmetabolised glutethimide was detected in the bile of *dogs* and 5 patients undergoing biliary drainage who were given glutethimide. It was considered that the enterohepatic circulation had no significant effect on the absorption or excretion of glutethimide.— C. Charytan, *ibid.*, 1970, *11*, 816.

Two young women who went into coma after ingesting glutethimide woke after 24 hours, went back into a coma 12 hours later, and woke again about 40 hours after ingesting the drug. Concentrations of glutethimide in the serum rose and fell in correlation with the patients' states of consciousness; with a serum concentration of over 20 µg per ml the patients were asleep. Enterohepatic recirculation and other causes were suggested in explanation of the second peak concentration of glutethimide in the serum.— W. J. Decker *et al.* (letter), *Lancet*, 1970, *1*, 778.

Identification of the hydroxy metabolite of glutethimide as an active metabolite.— J. J. Ambre and L. J. Fischer, *Drug Metab. & Disposit.*, 1974, *2*, 151. Metabolism of glutethimide.— W. G. Stillwell, *Res. Commun. chem. Path. Pharmac.*, 1975, *12*, 25.

The active metabolite of glutethimide, 4-hydroxy-2-ethyl-2-phenylglutarimide, was possibly a major contributory factor in the coma induced by glutethimide overdosage. The long duration of coma, which appeared to be unrelated to the half-life of glutethimide, might be due to the accumulation of this metabolite.— A. R. Hansen *et al.*, *New Engl. J. Med.*, 1975, *292*, 250.

A catechol metabolite.— B. D. Andresen *et al.*, *Res. Commun. chem. Path. Pharmac.*, 1976, *14*, 259. See also *idem*, *J. pharm. Sci.*, 1979, *68*, 283.

Uses. Glutethimide is a piperidinedione hypnotic and sedative. It has been reported to act in about 30 minutes to induce sleep lasting 4 to 8 hours. The usual dose is 250 to 500 mg at night; some sources have recommended one repeat dose during the night if necessary.

The severe toxic effects from overdosage and dependence potential made glutethimide unsuitable as an alternative to the barbiturates.— *Br. med. J.*, 1976, *1*, 1424.

Administration in renal failure. Glutethimide could be given in usual doses to patients with renal failure, but should be avoided in patients with a glomerular filtration-rate of less than 10 ml per minute. Concentrations of glutethimide were not affected by haemodialysis or peritoneal dialysis.— W. M. Bennett *et al.*, *Ann. intern. Med.*, 1977, *86*, 754. See also *idem*, 1980, *93*, 286.

Preparations

Glutethimide Capsules *(U.S.P.)*. Capsules containing glutethimide.

Glutethimide Tablets *(B.P.)*. Tablets containing glutethimide. Protect from light.

Glutethimide Tablets *(U.S.P.)*. Tablets containing glutethimide.

Proprietary Preparations

Doriden *(Ciba, UK)*. Glutethimide, available as scored tablets of 250 mg. (Also available as Doriden in

Austral., Canad., Denm., Ger., Ital., Neth., Norw., Spain, Switz., USA).

Other Proprietary Names
Doridene *(Belg.)*; Doridène *(Fr.)*; Dorimide *(USA)*; Glimid *(Pol.)*.

4038-j

Heptabarbitone. Heptabarb.; Heptabarbital (distinguish from Heptobarbitalum). 5-(Cyclohept-1-enyl)-5-ethylbarbituric acid.
$C_{13}H_{18}N_2O_3$=250.3.

CAS — 509-86-4.

A white odourless crystalline powder with a slightly bitter taste. M.p. 167° to 171°. Very slightly **soluble** in water; soluble 1 in 30 of alcohol, 1 in 20 of acetone, and 1 in 75 of chloroform; soluble in solutions of alkali hydroxides.

Dependence. Prolonged use of heptabarbitone may lead to dependence of the barbiturate-alcohol type (see p.792).

Adverse Effects, Treatment, and Precautions. As for Phenobarbitone, p.812.

Absorption and Fate. See under Phenobarbitone, p.814.
It is metabolised in the liver by oxidation and hydroxylation and the metabolites are excreted in the urine.

After a dose of 300 or 400 mg of heptabarbitone at night three metabolites were excreted in the urine, mostly within the first 24 hours. They were the 3′-oxo- and 3′-hydroxy-derivatives and another hydroxy derivative.— J. N. T. Gilbert *et al., J. Pharm. Pharmac.*, 1974, *26*, 123.

Heptabarbitone 6.6 mg per kg body-weight was given by mouth to 6 healthy subjects. The maximum blood concentration was obtained after an average of 6 hours although there was considerable variation, a maximum concentration occurring after only 1 hour in 1 subject. No heptabarbitone could be detected in the blood of any of the subjects after 60 hours; the calculated biological half-life was about 9.7 hours.— J. M. Clifford *et al., Clin. Pharmac. Ther.*, 1974, *16*, 376.

Uses. Heptabarbitone is a barbiturate (see p.792) that is used as a hypnotic and sedative. As a hypnotic it is usually given in doses of 200 to 400 mg at night. As a sedative it is given in doses of 50 to 100 mg three or four times daily.

Proprietary Preparations

Medomin *(Geigy, UK)*. Heptabarbitone, available as scored tablets of 200 mg. (Also available as Medomin in *Canad., Ger., Neth., Switz.*).

Other Proprietary Names
Medapan *(Swed.)*;Medomina *(Spain)*; Medomine *(Belg., Fr.)*.

4039-z

Hexapropymate. L 2103; Propinylcyclohexanol Carbamate. 1-(Prop-2-ynyl)cyclohexyl carbamate.
$C_{10}H_{15}NO_2$=181.2.

CAS — 358-52-1.

Hexapropymate is given by mouth as a hypnotic in doses of 400 mg at night, doses of 400 to 800 mg at night have also been recommended; it is also given rectally as suppositories in doses of 300 to 600 mg an hour before bedtime. It is contra-indicated with alcohol.

Overdosage. A 28-year-old man who had ingested about 16 g of hexapropymate was unconscious, hypotensive, hypothermic, and cyanosed; corneal, gag, and cough reflexes were absent and there were abnormalities in the ECG; lactic acidosis was present. He recovered slowly after gastric lavage, assisted ventilation, rewarming, and intravenous fluids.— G. Robbins and A. K. Brown, *Br. med. J.*, 1978, *1*, 1593.

Proprietary Names
Biradon *(Osiris, Arg.)*; Merinax *(Labaz, Belg.*; *Labaz, Fr.*; *Sigmatau, Ital.*; *Labaz, Neth.*; *Labaz, Spain*; *Labaz, Switz.)*; Modirax *(Mekos, Swed.)*.

4040-p

Hexobarbitone *(Eur. P., B.P.C. 1959)*. Hexobarbitalum; Hexobarbital *(U.S.P.)*; Enimal; Methexenyl; Methyl-cyclohexenylmethyl-barbitursäure; Methylhexabarbital; Ciclobarbital; Enhexymalum. 5-(Cyclohex-1-enyl)-1,5-dimethylbarbituric acid.
$C_{12}H_{16}N_2O_3$=236.3.

CAS — 56-29-1.

Pharmacopoeias. In *Aust., Cz., Eur., Fr., Ger., Hung., Int., It., Jug., Neth., Nord., Pol., Rus., Swiss, Turk.*, and *U.S.*

Odourless colourless crystals or a white crystalline powder, tasteless or slightly bitter. M.p. 144° to 148°. **Soluble** 1 in 3000 of water, 1 in 250 of boiling water, 1 in 45 of alcohol, 1 in 4 of chloroform, and 1 in 80 of ether; soluble in acetone, methyl alcohol, and solutions of alkali hydroxides, practically insoluble in solutions of alkali carbonates. A saturated solution in water is neutral to methyl red. **Store** in airtight containers.

4041-s

Hexobarbitone Sodium *(B.P.C. 1959)*.
Soluble Hexobarbitone; Sodium Hexobarbital; Hexobarbitalum Natricum; Hexenalum; Enhexymalnatrium; Narcosanum Solubile. Sodium 5-(cyclohex-1-enyl)-1,5-dimethylbarbiturate.
$C_{12}H_{15}N_2NaO_3$=258.3.

CAS — 50-09-9.

Pharmacopoeias. In *Aust., Belg., Hung., Int., Jug., Nord., Pol., Rus., Swiss*, and *Turk.*

A white, odourless, very hygroscopic powder with a bitter taste. It discolours on exposure to air. Very **soluble** in water, alcohol, methyl alcohol, and acetone; soluble in chloroform; very slightly soluble in ether. A solution in water is strongly alkaline (pH 10.5 to 12) and slowly decomposes; it absorbs carbon dioxide which causes the separation of hexobarbitone crystals. A 3.88% solution in water is iso-osmotic with serum. Solutions for injection are prepared by dissolving, immediately before use, the sterile contents of a sealed container in the requisite amount of Water for Injections free from carbon dioxide. **Store** in glass containers sealed by fusion of the glass.

Stability of solutions. A 10% solution of hexobarbitone sodium in water lost 4.2% of its strength in 1 day at 20°, 7.3% in 2 days, 13.2% in 4 days, and 21.3% in 8 days.— H. Nuppenau, *Dansk Tidsskr. Farm.*, 1954, *28*, 261.

Dependence. Prolonged use of hexobarbitone may lead to dependence of the barbiturate-alcohol type (see p.792).

Adverse Effects, Treatment, and Precautions. As for Phenobarbitone, p.812. See also Thiopentone Sodium, p.759.

Administration in hepatic failure. Hexobarbitone sodium was given by intravenous infusion in doses equivalent to 2.97 to 7.32 mg of free acid per kg body-weight to 13 patients with acute hepatitis. The elimination half-life was 490 minutes for these patients compared with 261 minutes for controls from an earlier study (D.D. Breimer *et al., J. Pharmacokinet. Biopharm.*, 1975, *3*, 1). There was a reduction in clearance in the hepatitis patients but no difference between them and the controls in the volume of distribution at steady state. Values improved but had still not returned to normal in 6 patients who were given hexobarbitone sodium when they had recovered from the hepatitis.— D. D. Breimer *et al., Clin. Pharmac. Ther.*, 1975, *18*, 433. Similar reports.— E. Richter *et al., Dt. med. Wschr.*, 1972, *97*, 254; W. Zilly *et al., Klin. Wschr.*, 1973, *51*, 346.

Interactions. Barbiturates. Treatment of *rats* with phenobarbitone for several days caused enzyme induction in liver microsomes so that the metabolism of a subsequent dose of hexobarbitone or zoxazolamine was increased to such a degree that the pharmacological effects of these drugs were almost completely abolished.— J. J. Burns and A. H. Conney, *Proc. R. Soc. Med.*, 1965, *58*, 955.

Absorption and Fate. See under Phenobarbitone, p.814 and Thiopentone Sodium, p.759.
It is metabolised in the liver by *N*-demethylation and oxidation.

The mean plasma half-life of (±)-hexobarbitone 400 mg given by mouth to 5 healthy subjects was 4 hours, compared with 4.6 hours for (+)-hexobarbitone, and 1.4 hours for (−)-hexobarbitone which caused very little central depressive effect. Hardly any unchanged hexobarbitone was present in urine or faeces.— D. D. Breimer and J. M. Van Rossum (letter), *J. Pharm. Pharmac.*, 1973, *25*, 762.

Circadian fluctuations of pharmacokinetic parameters after oral administration of hexobarbitone.— P. Altmayer *et al., Arzneimittel-Forsch.*, 1979, *29*, 1422. See also *idem*, 1633.

Uses. Hexobarbitone is a barbiturate (see p.792) that is used as a hypnotic and sedative. As a hypnotic it is usually given in doses of 250 to 500 mg at night. As a sedative it is given in doses of 250 mg up to thrice daily. Hexobarbitone sodium was formerly used similarly to thiopentone sodium (see p.759). For inducing anaesthesia the dose was 3 to 5 ml of a 10% solution intravenously. If used for complete anaesthesia the injection was continued at the rate of 1 ml in 15 seconds until the rquired depth was obtained; a total dose of 10 ml (1 g) was usually regarded as maximum.

Preparations of Hexobarbitone

Hexobarbital Tablets *(U.S.P.)*. Tablets containing hexobarbitone.

Hexobarbitone Tablets *(B.P.C. 1954)*. Tablets containing hexobarbitone.

Evidorm *(Winthrop, UK)*. Scored tablets each containing hexobarbitone 250 mg and cyclobarbitone calcium 100 mg. For insomnia. *Dose.* 1 or 2 tablets at bedtime.

Other Proprietary Names of Hexobarbitone and Hexobarbitone Sodium
Citopan *(Norw.)*; Evipan, Evipan-Natrium (both *Ger.)*; Noctivane *(Fr.)*; Sombulex *(USA)*.

Hexobarbitone sodium was also formerly marketed in Great Britain under the proprietary name Cyclonal Sodium (*May & Baker*).

4042-w

Ibomal. Bromoaprobarbitone; Propallylonal; Isopropyl-bromallyl-barbitursäure. 5-(2-Bromoallyl)-5-isopropylbarbituric acid.
$C_{10}H_{13}BrN_2O_3$=289.1.

CAS — 545-93-7.

A white crystalline powder with a slightly bitter taste. M.p. 179° to 182°. Very slightly **soluble** in water; soluble in alcohol; slightly soluble in ether; soluble with salt formation in aqueous solutions of alkalis.

Ibomal is a barbiturate (see p.792) used as a hypnotic in doses of 100 to 400 mg at night.

Proprietary Names
Noctal *(Cassella-Riedel, Ger.)*.

4043-e

Ibrotamide. Ibrotal. 2-Bromo-2-ethyl-3-methylbutyramide.
$C_7H_{14}BrNO$=208.1.

CAS — 466-14-8.

Crystals. M.p. 51°. **Soluble** in many organic solvents and in oils.

Ibrotamide has been used as a hypnotic and sedative. As a hypnotic it was given in doses of 400 to 600 mg at night, and as a sedative in doses of 200 mg up to three times daily.

4077-r

Lormetazepam.
Wy-4082. 7-Chloro-5-(2-chlorophenyl)-1,3-dihydro-3-hydroxy-1-methyl-2*H*-1,4-benzodiazepin-2-one.
$C_{16}H_{12}Cl_2N_2O_2$=335.2.

CAS — 848-75-9.

Lormetazepam is a hypnotic with actions and uses similar to those of nitrazepam (see p.807). It is given in a dose of 1 to 2 mg at night, with half these doses for elderly patients.

References: I. Oswald and K. Adam, *Br. med. J.*, 1980, *281*, 1039; M. Hümpel *et al.*, *Clin. Pharmac. Ther.*, 1980, *28*, 673; D. Kampf *et al.*, *ibid.*, 1981, *30*, 77; *Drug & Ther. Bull.*, 1982, *20*, 3.

Proprietary Preparations

Noctamid *(Schering, UK)*. Lormetazepam, available as scored tablets of 0.5 and 1 mg.

4044-l

Mecloqualone. W 4744. 3-(2-Chlorophenyl)-2-methylquinazolin-4(3*H*)-one.
$C_{15}H_{11}ClN_2O$=270.7.

CAS — 340-57-8.

Mecloqualone is a hypnotic that has been given in doses of 150 to 300 mg at night.

Clinical study in 40 geriatric patients.— S. Sugarman, *Clin. Med.*, 1969, *76* (Aug.), 30.

Metabolism and renal excretion of mecloqualone were studied in 45 volunteers after a single dose of 150 mg by mouth. About 2 to 3% of mecloqualone was excreted unchanged in the urine, and 95% underwent hydroxylation in the body. Four hydroxylated metabolites and 3 other metabolites were identified.— P. Daenens and M. Van Boven, *Arzneimittel-Forsch.*, 1974, *24*, 195.

Proprietary Names

Nubarène *(Diamant, Fr.)*.

4045-y

Methaqualone *(B.P., U.S.P.)*.
2-Methyl-3-*o*-tolylquinazolin-4(3*H*)-one; Methachalonum.
$C_{16}H_{14}N_2O$=250.3.

CAS — 72-44-6.

Pharmacopoeias. In *Br.*, *Chin.*, *Cz.*, *Nord.*, and *U.S.*

An odourless, white or almost white, crystalline powder with a bitter taste. M.p. 114° to 117°. Practically **insoluble** in water; soluble 1 in 12 of alcohol, 1 in 1 of chloroform, and 1 in 50 of ether. **Store** in airtight containers. Protect from light.

4046-j

Methaqualone Hydrochloride *(U.S.P.)*.
Methaqualoni Chloridum; QZ 2; TR 495.
$C_{16}H_{14}N_2O,HCl$=286.8.

CAS — 340-56-7.

Pharmacopoeias. In *Nord.* and *U.S.*

A white odourless crystalline powder with a bitter taste. M.p. about 250° with decomposition. Methaqualone hydrochloride 200 mg is approximately equivalent to 175 mg of methaqualone. **Soluble** 1 in 65 of water, 1 in 31 of alcohol, and 1 in 13 of chloroform; practically insoluble in ether; soluble in acetone, soluble 1 in about 70 of M hydrochloric acid. **Store** in airtight containers. Protect from light.

Dependence. Abuse of methaqualone, particularly when taken in conjunction with diphenhydramine, has been reported and prolonged use may lead to dependence of the barbiturate-alcohol type (see p.792).

Addiction to methaqualone was recorded in a 47-year-old man who had taken increasing doses over a period of 4 years until he reached a dose of sixty 150-mg tablets daily. Delirium tremens was noted on withdrawal of methaqualone and dramatic improvement resulted from administration of thioridazine in doses up to 800 mg daily.— R. B. L. Ewart and R. G. Priest, *Br. med. J.*, 1967, *3*, 92.

In 3 subjects who had taken 1.5 to 2 g of methaqualone daily for several months abrupt cessation of the drug resulted in severe withdrawal symptoms, including grand mal seizure in 1 patient. Methaqualone was used when diamorphine was not available.— M. Swartzburg *et al.*, *Archs gen. Psychiat.*, 1973, *29*, 46.

Reviews of the misuse of methaqualone.— F. A. Whitlock, *Drugs*, 1973, *6*, 167; D. S. Inaba *et al.*, *J. Am. med. Ass.*, 1973, *224*, 1505; E. F. Pascarelli, *ibid.*, 1512 and 1521.

Further reports: J. S. Madden (letter), *Br. med. J.*, 1966, *1*, 676; R. de Alarcon (letter), *ibid.*, 1969, *1*, 122 and 319; D. R. Benady (letter), *ibid.*, 577; J. A. H. Forrest and R. A. Tarala, *ibid.*, 1973, *4*, 136; M. C. Gerald and P. M. Schwirian, *Archs gen. Psychiat.*, 1973, *28*, 627; N. L. Rock and H. Silsby (letter), *J. Am. med. Ass.*, 1974, *230*, 1389.

Adverse Effects. Side-effects of treatment with methaqualone or its hydrochloride in therapeutic doses include headache, 'hangover', dizziness, drowsiness, anorexia, nausea and gastro-intestinal discomfort, transient paraesthesia, dry mouth, restlessness, and sweating. Skin reactions have also been reported. Aplastic anaemia may occur rarely but the association is not proven.

Dependence and tolerance may develop and overdosage with suicidal or abusive intent has become increasingly common. In most cases, a preparation containing methaqualone 250 mg and diphenhydramine hydrochloride 25 mg (Mandrax) has been used but the diphenhydramine does not appear to contribute significantly to the toxicity.

The symptoms of mild acute poisoning are the same as those of the barbiturates and most other hypnotics (see p.812). Severe overdosage results in delirium, coma, restlessness, tachycardia, and hypertonia, hyperreflexia, and myoclonus, which may progress to convulsions. Cardiac and respiratory depression occurs less frequently than with acute barbiturate poisoning. Pulmonary and cutaneous oedema, cardiac and hepatic damage, renal insufficiency, and bleeding may occur with severe poisoning. Spontaneous vomiting and increased secretions are common and may lead to pneumonitis or respiratory obstruction.

Effects on the blood. Agranulocytosis in an elderly man was associated with methaqualone.— F. Azizi (letter), *Ann. intern. Med.*, 1974, *81*, 268.

Effects on the eyes. Keratitis occurred in 2 subjects dependent on methaqualone.— F. C. Rodger (letter), *Br. J. Ophthal.*, 1973, *57*, 712.

Effects on the nervous system. Polyneuropathy occurred in 7 patients who had taken methaqualone 250 to 500 mg daily for up to 2 years. Improvement was seen in 4 patients 2 to 5 months after withdrawal of the drug.— J. Finke and U. Spiegelberg, *Nervenarzt*, 1973, *44*, 104. A discussion on the possible association between methaqualone and neuropathy.— *Br. med. J.*, 1973, *3*, 307.

Other reports: P. Marks, *Practitioner*, 1974, *212*, 721; P. Marks and J. Sloggem, *Am. J. med. Sci.*, 1976, *272*, 323.

Effects on the skin. Methaqualone in conjunction with diphenhydramine was strongly suspected of being responsible for a fixed drug eruption in 1 patient.— J. A. Savin, *Br. J. Derm.*, 1970, *83*, 546. See also G. W. Csonka, *Br. J. vener. Dis.*, 1973, *49*, 316.

Overdosage. Of 28 cases of poisoning due to tablets containing methaqualone 250 mg and diphenhydramine hydrochloride 25 mg (Mandrax) admitted to the Edinburgh Poisoning Treatment Centre, 19 were mildly poisoned and 9 more severely poisoned. All were treated by intensive supportive therapy and subsequently recovered. The most striking clinical features in the severe cases were pyramidal signs (marked hypertonia, increased tendon reflexes, and myoclonia). Four of the 9 showed impairment of cardiovascular function. Plasma-methaqualone concentrations on admission ranged from 2 to 20 µg per ml, in all except 1 case in which the concentration was below the limit of detection. It was considered that plasma concentrations greater than 30 µg per ml, corresponding to 20 tablets ingested, were indicative of dangerous poisoning in patients who had not become habituated. The diphenhydramine component of Mandrax did not appear to contribute significantly to its toxicity.— A. A. H. Lawson and S. S. Brown (letter), *Br. med. J.*, 1966, *2*, 1455.

A 54-year-old man who ingested about 25 Mandrax tablets lost consciousness but following treatment he regained consciousness by the fourth day. Neurological sequelae included hallucinations and agitation which disappeared at the end of a month.— P. M. Ford and C. A. Birt (letter), *Br. med. J.*, 1967, *2*, 112.

A 38-year-old woman became deeply unconscious, hypotensive, and required mechanically assisted respiration after taking about 180 tablets of Mandrax. An ECG showed flat T-waves and a prolonged Q-T interval. Hypotension responded to treatment with metaraminol, and spontaneous respiration and tendon-reflexes returned after haemodialysis. An EEG taken 2 days after the drug was ingested was flat except for irregular bilateral spike complexes appearing at intervals of 1 to 8 seconds. Though the woman had many fits during the first few days, she made a slow recovery and 13 days after admission to hospital the EEG record was almost normal.— M. R. Wallace and E. Allen (letter), *Lancet*, 1968, *2*, 1247.

Although lack of respiratory depression has been proposed as characteristic of methaqualone poisoning, respiratory arrest and 36 hours of apnoea developed in a 21-year-old woman following overdosage with methaqualone.— R. E. Johnstone *et al.*, *Ohio St. med. J.*, 1971, *67*, 1018.

A woman who was a frequent drug abuser took a single dose of 9 g of methaqualone. She had no response to painful stimuli, exaggerated deep tendon reflexes, shivering and muscle twitching, and bilateral ankle clonus. After 16 hours muscle overactivity increased and could not be controlled by diazepam. She was given tubocurarine 12 mg, followed by 2 further doses at hourly intervals. Response to painful stimuli returned after 26 hours and the patient was conscious after 40 hours.— R. T. Abboud *et al.*, *Chest*, 1974, *65*, 204.

A 73-year-old man who had taken about 7 g of methaqualone (as Mandrax) and who was unconscious for 7 days developed severe peripheral motor and sensory neuropathy with numbness, tingling, and weakness of the legs.— K. Constantinidis, *Br. med. J.*, 1975, *2*, 370.

Treatment of Adverse Effects. As for Phenobarbitone, p.812.

The use of forced diuresis is not effective and may increase the risk of pulmonary oedema. Haemodialysis may remove small amounts of methaqualone but is only of value in very severely poisoned patients. Analeptics are contra-indicated.

A report of the successful conservative management of 116 patients with Mandrax poisoning.— H. Matthew *et al.*, *Br. med. J.*, 1968, *2*, 101.

Dialysis. A patient with poisoning due to tablets each containing methaqualone 250 mg and diphenhydramine hydrochloride 25 mg (Mandrax) was successfully treated by haemodialysis and supportive measures. The blood-methaqualone concentration was reduced from 105 µg per ml before haemodialysis to 58 µg per ml at the end of 6 hours' haemodialysis.— D. T. Caridis (letter), *Br. med. J.*, 1966, *2*, 1655. See also D. T. Caridis *et al.*, *Lancet*, 1967, *1*, 51. See also J. P. W. Young, *Roussel* (letter), *Br. med. J.*, 1967, *1*, 301.

Other reports: A. T. Proudfoot *et al.*, *Scott. med. J.*, 1968, *13*, 232; A. E. Wallace (letter), *Lancet*, 1968, *2*, 1247; T. M. S. Chang *et al.*, *Trans. Am. Soc. artif. internal Organs*, 1973, *19*, 87.

Precautions. Methaqualone should be used with caution in patients with impaired hepatic function. Its use should be avoided during pregnancy and in patients with epilepsy. It causes drowsiness and patients being treated with it should not take charge of vehicles or machinery where loss of attention could lead to accidents. These effects are enhanced by the simultaneous administration of depressants of the central nervous system such as alcohol, barbiturates, and other sedatives. Methaqualone may moderately induce microsomal hepatic enzymes.

Interactions. *Alcohol.* In a study on 12 subjects who received methaqualone 500 mg with diphenhydramine hydrochloride 50 mg at night followed by 3 single doses of alcohol 500 mg per kg body-weight at 24, 48, and 72 hours it was shown that residual levels of methaqualone reacted with alcohol 72 hours later. This resulted in greater subjective mental and physical sedation and impairment of cognitive tasks.— S. Roden *et al.* (letter),

Br. J. clin. Pharmac., 1977, *4*, 245.

Anticholinergics. Within 2 days of starting treatment for depression with methaqualone and diphenhydramine hydrochloride (Mandrax) and thioridazine, 10 patients had side-effects including nasal bleeding, swelling, furring, fissuring, and discoloration of the tongue, excessive dryness of the mouth, and a feeling of light-headedness akin to depersonalisation. The effects were considered to be due to heightened anticholinergic activity due to interaction between the drug treatments. Six of the patients were also given imipramine and amitriptyline. When the methaqualone and diphenhydramine preparation was stopped the side-effects disappeared within 1 to 4 days.— A. Kessell and A. G. Williams (letter), *Lancet*, 1967, *2*, 612. See also A. Kessell *et al.*, *Med. J. Aust.*, 1967, *2*, 1195.

Diphenhydramine. Studies *in vitro* demonstrated that diphenhydramine inhibited the metabolism of methaqualone by *rat* liver homogenate. This inhibition of conversion of methaqualone to an inactive metabolite may account for the enhanced effect claimed by drug abusers when the two drugs are taken together.— K. W. Hindmarsh *et al.*, *J. pharm. Sci.*, 1978, *67*, 1547.

Steroids. Methaqualone taken as Mandrax tablets was found to interfere with tests for urinary steroids in 1 patient, giving spuriously high values.— K. Wiener and C. H. Foot (letter), *Br. med. J.*, 1976, *1*, 1072.

Pregnancy and lactation. As the administration of methaqualone to pregnant *rats* had increased the incidence of cleft palate in the offspring, it was suggested that the use of methaqualone in women of child-bearing age should be avoided.— CanadaFood and Drug Directorate, *Pharm. J.*, 1970, *2*, 720.

See also under Absorption and Fate.

Absorption and Fate. Methaqualone is readily absorbed from the gastro-intestinal tract and extensively metabolised, mainly by hydroxylation, in the liver. It has a biphasic plasma half-life and is extensively bound to plasma protein. It is excreted in the urine and faeces; about 2% is excreted in the urine unchanged.

In normal fasting subjects absorption of methaqualone base was rapid and peak plasma concentrations were reached within 2 hours; absorption of the hydrochloride was significantly faster. The drug was strongly protein bound at plasma concentrations up to those in severe acute overdosage and was largely excluded from red cells. The major route of metabolism in man involved relatively non-specific hydroxylation of the tolyl substituent and little unchanged drug was excreted either after therapeutic doses or after overdosage.— S. S. Brown and S. Goenechea, *Clin. Pharmac. Ther.*, 1973, *14*, 314. Methaqualone hydrochloride 300 mg was given by mouth to 7 healthy subjects. The maximum blood concentration occurred after an average of 3 hours and the concentration diminished in a biphasic manner. The biological half-lives were calculated to be about 50 minutes for the first component and 16 hours for the second. Methaqualone was detected in the plasma after 34 hours but not after 40 hours.— J. M. Clifford *et al.*, *ibid.*, 1974, *16*, 376.

Methaqualone was still detected in the blood of a healthy subject 17 days after the commencement of a 5-day administration period of methaqualone 250 mg and diphenhydramine hydrochloride 25 mg each night. The study had been terminated prematurely after 5 days because the subject had become too confused and drowsy.— M. E. Williams *et al.*, *J. clin. Pharm.*, 1976, *1*, 63.

Estimation of a 74-hour terminal half-life for methaqualone.— H. d'A. Heck *et al.*, *J. Pharmacokinet. Biopharm.*, 1978, *6*, 111.

Further references: G. Alván *et al.*, *Eur. J. clin. Pharmac.*, 1973, *6*, 187; *idem*, 1974, *7*, 449; R. K. Nayak *et al.*, *J. Pharmacokinet. Biopharm.*, 1974, *2*, 107; O. Ericsson and B. Danielsson, *Drug Metab. & Disposit.*, 1977, *5*, 497, per *Int. pharm. Abstr.*, 1978, *15*, 1090.

Pregnancy and lactation. Inactive metabolites of methaqualone were possibly excreted in the milk of lactating mothers.— J. J. Rowan (letter), *Pharm. J.*, 1976, *2*, 184.

Studies in *mice* established that methaqualone crossed the placenta.— N. S. Shah *et al.*, *Toxic. appl. Pharmac.*, 1977, *40*, 497.

See also under Precautions.

Uses. Methaqualone is a hypnotic and sedative. The usual hypnotic dose is 150 to 300 mg at night and the usual sedative dose 75 mg up to 4 times daily. It has also been given in conjunction with diphenhydramine hydrochloride for an enhanced hypnotic effect.

Methaqualone hydrochloride, which is more rapidly absorbed than methaqualone is given in a roughly equivalent hypnotic dose of 200 to 400 mg at night and sedative dose of 100 mg up to 4 times daily.

Administration in renal failure. Methaqualone could be given in usual doses to patients with renal failure. Concentrations of methaqualone were affected by haemodialysis.— W. M. Bennett *et al.*, *Ann. intern. Med.*, 1980, *93*, 286.

Anaesthesia. Methaqualone used as a 10% solution in propylene glycol was found to be suitable as a sole anaesthetic for short surgical procedures of about 10 minutes duration.— R. C. Saxena *et al.*, *Br. J. Anaesth.*, 1972, *44*, 83.

Further study: W. Norris and A. B. M. Telfer, *Br. J. Anaesth.*, 1969, *41*, 874 (premedication).

Hypnotic effect. Reports and studies on the use of methaqualone, either alone or with diphenhydramine hydrochloride, for sleep induction: P. A. Coldrey, *Practitioner*, 1963, *190*, 368; I. Haider, *Br. J. Psychiat.*, 1968, *114*, 465; A. J. Dresner *et al.*, *Clin. Trials J.*, 1973, *10*, 113; W. Sargant (letter), *Br. med. J.*, 1973, *2*, 716; R. G. Borland *et al.*, *Br. J. clin. Pharmac.*, 1975, *2*, 131.

Preparations of Methaqualone and Methaqualone Hydrochloride

Methaqualone Hydrochloride Capsules *(U.S.P.).* Capsules containing methaqualone hydrochloride. The *U.S.P.* requires 60% dissolution in 60 minutes.

Methaqualone Tablets *(U.S.P.).* Tablets containing methaqualone. The *U.S.P.* requires 70% dissolution in 20 minutes.

Proprietary Names of Methaqualone and Methaqualone Hydrochloride

Cateudyl *(Covor, Belg.)*; Dormogen *(Cz.)*; Mequelon *(Frosst, Canad.)*; Mequin *(Lemmon, USA)*; Metakvalon *(DAK, Denm.)*; Methasedil *(Cooper, Switz.)*; Nobadorm *(Streuli, Switz.)*; Normi-Nox *(Herbrand, Ger.*; *Herbrand, Switz.)*; Parest *(Parke, Davis, USA)*; Pro Dorm *(Schürholz, Ger.)*; Quāālude *(Lemmon, USA)*; Rebuso *(Montpellier, Arg.)*; Revonal *(Merck, Belg.*; *Cascan, Ger.*; *E. Merck, Neth.*; *E. Merck, Swed.)*; Rouqualone *(Rougier, Canad.)*; Sedalone *(Nordic, Canad.)*; Sindesvel *(York, Arg.)*; Sleepinal *(Medichem, Austral.)*; Sopor *(American Critical Care, USA)*; Sovelin *(Weiders, Norw.)*; Sovinal *(ND & K, Denm.)*; Toquilone *(Serumwerk, Belg.*; *Medichemie, Switz.)*; Torinal *(Med. y Prod. Quím., Spain)*; Triador *(Trianon, Canad.)*; Tualone *(ICN, Canad.)*; Vitalone *(Sabex, Canad.)*.

Methaqualone was formerly marketed in Great Britain under the proprietary names Melsed (*Boots*) and Revonal (*E.Merck*). Methaqualone hydrochloride was formerly marketed under the proprietary name Melsedin (*Boots*). A preparation containing methaqualone and diphenhydramine hydrochloride was formerly marketed under the proprietary name Mandrax (*Roussel*).

4047-z

Metharbitone. Metharbital *(U.S.P.)*; Endiemal. 5,5-Diethyl-1-methylbarbituric acid.
$C_9H_{14}N_2O_3$=198.2.

CAS — 50-11-3.

Pharmacopoeias. In *U.S.*

A white or almost white crystalline powder with a faint aromatic odour. M.p. 151° to 155°.

Soluble 1 in 830 of water, 1 in 23 of alcohol, and 1 in 40 of ether. A saturated solution in water has a pH of about 6. **Store** in airtight containers.

Metharbitone is demethylated in the liver to barbitone (p.794). It has been given in the treatment of epilepsy in usual doses of 100 mg once to thrice daily.

Preparations

Metharbital Tablets *(U.S.P.).* Tablets containing metharbitone. Store in airtight containers.

Proprietary Names

Gemonil *(Abbott, NZ*; *Abbott, USA)*.

4048-c

Methylpentynol *(B.P.C. 1968).* Meparfynol; Methylparafynol. 3-Methylpent-1-yn-3-ol.
$C_6H_{10}O$=98.14.

CAS — 77-75-8.

A colourless or pale yellow liquid with a characteristic odour and an unpleasant burning taste. Wt per ml 0.865 to 0.873 g. B.p. about 120°. **Soluble** 1 in 10 of water; miscible with organic solvents and fixed oils. **Incompatible** with oxidising agents. **Store** in a cool dry place.

Adverse Effects and Precautions. Gastric irritation may occur. Repeated doses may provoke liver and skin reactions. High doses produce effects resembling those of alcohol.

Treatment of Adverse Effects. As for Phenobarbitone, p.812.

Uses. Methylpentynol is a hypnotic and sedative. It is given in doses of 0.5 to 1 g at night to induce sleep; sedative doses range from 250 to 500 mg.

Pregnancy and the neonate. Methylpentynol was excreted in the milk of lactating mothers in amounts too small to affect the baby.— J. J. Rowan (letter), *Pharm. J.*, 1976, *2*, 184.

Proprietary Names

Allotropal *(Heyl, Ger.)*; Oblivon *(Nicholas, Switz.)*.

Methylpentynol was formerly marketed in Great Britain under the proprietary names Insomnol Elixir (*Medo-Chemicals*) and Oblivon (*Nicholas*).

4049-k

Methylpentynol Carbamate. Mepentamate. 3-Methylpent-1-ynyl carbamate.
$C_7H_{11}NO_2$=141.2.

CAS — 302-66-9.

A white powder. M.p. 53° to 56°. **Soluble** 1 in less than 200 of water, 1 in 1 of alcohol, 1 in 60 of arachis oil, 1 in 2 of chloroform, and 1 in 22 of ethyl oleate.

Methylpentynol carbamate has the actions and uses of methylpentynol but has a longer duration of action. As a hypnotic it is given in doses of 200 to 400 mg at night, and as a sedative in doses of 200 mg thrice daily.

Proprietary Names

N-Oblivon *(Latema, Belg.*; *Latéma, Fr.)*; Olosed *(Prodotti Erma, Ital.)*; Vereden *(Nagel, Ital.)*.

Methylpentynol carbamate was formerly marketed in Great Britain under the proprietary name Oblivon-C (*Nicholas*).

4050-w

Methylphenobarbitone *(B.P., Eur. P.).* Methylphenobarbitalum; Mephobarbital *(U.S.P.)*; Phemitone; Enphenemalum. 5-Ethyl-1-methyl-5-phenylbarbituric acid.
$C_{13}H_{14}N_2O_3$=246.3.

CAS — 115-38-8.

Pharmacopoeias. In *Aust., Belg., Br., Eur., Fr., Ger., It., Jug., Neth., Nord., Pol., Port., Swiss*, and *U.S.*

Odourless colourless crystals or a white crystalline powder with a slightly bitter taste. M.p. 176° to 181°. Practically **insoluble** in water; soluble 1 in 240 of alcohol, 1 in 40 of chloroform, and 1 in 200 of ether; soluble in solutions of ammonia and alkali hydroxides and carbonates. A saturated solution in water is acid to litmus.

Dependence. Prolonged use of methylphenobarbitone may lead to dependence of the barbiturate-alcohol type (see p.792).

Adverse Effects, Treatment, and Precautions. As for Phenobarbitone, p.812.

Absorption and Fate. Methylphenobarbitone is incompletely absorbed from the gastro-intestinal tract. It is demethylated to phenobarbitone in the liver.

Uses. Methylphenobarbitone has the actions and uses of phenobarbitone (see p.814) and has been given as a sedative in doses of 30 to 100 mg three or four times daily. It is given as an anticonvulsant in usual doses of 400 to 600 mg daily; change-over from phenobarbitone to methylphenobarbitone should be effected gradually and the plasma-phenobarbitone monitored for equivalence if necessary.

The dose of methylphenobarbitone required to produce a given plasma-phenobarbitone concentration tended to decrease progressively with age in a study of 123 patients. In patients over 14 years of age, females tended to require higher doses than males to achieve the same plasma concentrations. The relationship between plasma-phenobarbitone concentration and methylphenobarbitone dose was not affected by phenytoin, carbamazepine, or sulthiame.— M. J. Eadie *et al.*, *Br. J. clin. Pharmac.*, 1977, *4*, 541.

Preparations

Mephobarbital Tablets *(U.S.P.)*. Tablets containing methylphenobarbitone.

Methylphenobarbitone Tablets *(B.P.C. 1963)*. Phemitone Tablets. Tablets containing methylphenobarbitone.

Prominal *(Winthrop, UK)*. Methylphenobarbitone, available as tablets of 30, 60, and 200 mg. (Also available as Prominal in *Austral., Belg., Ital., Spain*).

Other Proprietary Names

Mebaral *(Canad., USA)*; Prominalette *(Ital.)*.

4051-e

Methylsulphonal *(B.P.C. 1949)*. Sulphonethylmethane; Trional. 2,2-Bis(ethylsulphonyl)butane.
$C_8H_{18}O_4S_2$=242.3.

CAS — 76-20-0.

Methylsulphonal is a hypnotic with a stronger action than sulphonal (see p.817). It was formerly given in doses of 0.3 to 1.2 g at night but is no longer used because of its toxicity.

4052-l

Methyprylone

Methyprylone *(B.P.)*. Methypryl.; Methyprylon *(U.S.P.)*; Ro 1-6463. 3,3-Diethyl-5-methylpiperidine-2,4-dione.
$C_{10}H_{17}NO_2$=183.2.

CAS — 125-64-4.

Pharmacopoeias. In *Br.* and *U.S.*

A white or almost white crystalline powder with a slight characteristic odour and a burning taste with a bitter after-taste. M.p. 74° to 77.5°. **Soluble** 1 in 11 to 14 of water, 1 in 0.7 of alcohol, 1 in 0.6 of chloroform, and 1 in 3.5 of ether. **Store** in airtight containers. Protect from light.

Dependence. Prolonged use of methyprylone may lead to dependence of the barbiturate-alcohol type (see p.792).

Methyprylone withdrawal had been reported to cause confusion, restlessness, excitement, sweating, and polyuria. Generalised convulsions and auditory and visual hallucinations had also occurred. Psychotic behaviour was precipitated in a patient who had discontinued the daily use of 4.8 g of methyprylone, and death had been reported after withdrawal of methyprylone in a patient who had been taking 7.5 to 12 g daily for about 18 months.— C. F. Essig, *J. Am. med. Ass.*, 1966, *196*, 714. See also *idem*, *Clin. Pharmac. Ther.*, 1964, *5*, 334.

Reports of dependence: G. R. Jensen, *N.Z. med. J.*, 1960, *59*, 431; H. Berger, *J. Am. med. Ass.*, 1961, *177*, 13.

Adverse Effects. At therapeutic doses drowsiness, dizziness, ataxia, headache, paradoxical excitation, skin rashes, nausea, vomiting, and diarrhoea have been reported. There have been rare unconfirmed reports of leucopenia.

Symptoms of overdosage are similar to those of phenobarbitone (see p.812). Pulmonary oedema and prolonged hypotension may be prominent; there may be hyperactivity and convulsions.

Effects on the blood. A possible association between bone-marrow suppression and ingestion of methyprylone was reported in 2 sisters.— G. D. McLaren *et al.*, *J. Am. med. Ass.*, 1978, *240*, 1744.

Effects on the liver. A report of liver damage associated with overdosage of methyprylone.— T. A. Loludice *et al.*, *Am. J. dig. Dis.*, 1978, *23*, *Suppl.*, 33S, per *Int. pharm. Abstr.*, 1978, *15*, 1163.

Overdosage. A woman became unconscious for 28 hours after taking 40 tablets, each containing methyprylone 200 mg. She then suffered insomnia, delirium, and increased paradoxical sleep. The latter declined to normal over a period of several weeks.— I. Haider and I. Oswald, *Br. med. J.*, 1970, *2*, 318.

Coma with bullae and sweat gland necrosis had been noted following a suicide attempt with methyprylone.— A. J. Varma *et al.*, *Archs intern. Med.*, 1977, *137*, 1207.

Treatment of Adverse Effects. As for Phenobarbitone, p.812.

In severe intoxication, treatment with haemodialysis or peritoneal dialysis may be of value.

Treatment of methyprylone overdosage with supportive therapy alone.— D. N. Bailey and P. I. Jatlow, *Clin. Toxicol.*, 1973, *6*, 563.

Dialysis. A report of the successful use of peritoneal dialysis to treat a 16-year-old girl with methyprylone intoxication.— R. A. Polin *et al.*, *J. Pediat.*, 1977, *90*, 831. Criticism.— J. M. Collins (letter), *ibid.*, 1978, *92*, 519. Reply.— R. A. Polin and C. E. Pippinger (letter), *ibid.*, 520.

Further reports of peritoneal dialysis and haemodialysis in severe methyprylone poisoning: G. Xanthaky *et al.*, *J. Am. med. Ass.*, 1966, *198*, 1212; J. M. Mandelbaum and N. M. Simon, *ibid.*, 1971, *216*, 139. See also M. Yudis *et al.*, *Ann. intern. Med.*, 1968, *68*, 1301; T. M. S. Chang *et al.*, *Can. med. Ass. J.*, 1973, *108*, 429; A. S. Pancorbo *et al.*, *J. Am. med. Ass.*, 1977, *237*, 470.

Precautions. Methyprylone causes drowsiness and patients receiving it should not take charge of vehicles or machinery where loss of attention could lead to accidents. These effects are enhanced by the simultaneous administration of depressants of the central nervous system such as alcohol, barbiturates, and other sedatives. Like the barbiturates methyprylone induces microsomal hepatic enzymes, it may thus cause increased metabolism of other drugs and may be contra-indicated in porphyria.

Absorption and Fate. Methyprylone is absorbed from the gastro-intestinal tract and extensively metabolised in the liver. About 60% of a dose is excreted in the urine as metabolites, together with about 3% of unchanged methyprylone. A short half-life has been reported but it may be considerably prolonged in overdosage.

Uses. Methyprylone, which like glutethimide is a piperidinedione derivative, is a hypnotic and sedative. It has been reported to act in 15 minutes to an hour to induce sleep lasting 5 to 8 hours. The usual dose is 200 to 400 mg at night. It has been used as a sedative in doses of 50 to 100 mg up to 4 times daily.

Preparations

Methyprylon Capsules *(U.S.P.)*. Capsules containing methyprylone. Store in airtight containers. Protect from light.

Methyprylon Tablets *(U.S.P.)*. Tablets containing methyprylone. Store in airtight containers. Protect from light.

Methyprylone Tablets *(B.P.)*. Tablets containing methyprylone. The tablets may be sugar-coated. If not sugar-coated protect from light.

Proprietary Preparations

Noludar *(Roche, UK)*. Methyprylone, available as scored tablets of 200 mg. (Also available as Noludar in *Belg., Canad., Denm., Ger., S.Afr., Switz., USA*).

4053-y

Nealbarbitone *(B.P. 1968)*. Nealbarb.; Alneobarbital; Nealbarbital; Neallymalum. 5-Allyl-5-neopentylbarbituric acid.
$C_{12}H_{18}N_2O_3$=238.3.

CAS — 561-83-1.

A white or slightly cream-coloured powder with a very slight odour and a bitter taste. M.p. 155° to 157°. **Soluble** 1 in 5000 of water, 1 in 4 of alcohol, 1 in 80 of chloroform, and 1 in 5 of ether; soluble in aqueous solutions of alkalis.

Nealbarbitone is a barbiturate (see p.792) that has been used as a hypnotic in doses of up to 200 mg at night, and as a sedative in doses of up to 60 mg thrice daily.

The metabolism of nealbarbitone.— J. N. T. Gilbert *et al.*, *J. Pharm. Pharmac.*, 1974, *26*, 119.

Preparations

Nealbarbitone Tablets *(B.P. 1968)*. Tablets containing nealbarbitone.

Nealbarbitone was formerly marketed in Great Britain under the proprietary name Censedal *(May & Baker)*.

4054-j

Nitrazepam

Nitrazepam *(B.P., Eur. P.)*. Ro 4-5360; Ro 5-3059. 1,3-Dihydro-7-nitro-5-phenyl-2*H*-1, 4-benzodiazepin-2-one.
$C_{15}H_{11}N_3O_3$=281.3.

CAS — 146-22-5.

Pharmacopoeias. In *Br., Braz., Cz., Eur., Fr., Ger., Neth.*, and *Nord.*

A yellow, odourless or almost odourless, tasteless, crystalline powder. M.p. 226° to 230°. Practically **insoluble** in water; soluble 1 in 120 of alcohol, 1 in 45 of chloroform, and 1 in 900 of ether. **Store** in airtight containers. Protect from light.

Dependence. Prolonged use of nitrazepam may lead to the development of dependence of the barbiturate-alcohol type (see p.792). It has a low liability for abuse.

Analysis of data from sleep laboratory evaluations of flunitrazepam, nitrazepam, and triazolam, and presentation of a hypothesis of benzodiazepine receptors to explain rebound withdrawal. Abrupt withdrawal of benzodiazepines with a relatively short duration of action may result in an intense form of rebound insomnia owing to a lag in the production and replacement of endogenous benzodiazepine-like compounds.— A. Kales *et al.*, *Science*, 1978, *201*, 1039. Comment.— A. N. Nicholson, *Br. J. clin. Pharmac.*, 1980, *9*, 223. For data concerning the presence of specific benzodiazepine receptors in the brain, see H. Möhler and T. Okada, *ibid.*, 1977, *198*, 849. See also under Diazepam, p.1519.

For reports, reviews, and comments on misuse of or dependence on the benzodiazepines, see Diazepam, p.1519.

Adverse Effects. Drowsiness, hang-over, and light-headedness have been reported on the day following a hypnotic dose of nitrazepam. Confusion has been reported in elderly patients. Excessive secretion of mucus and saliva may occur in children given high doses.

Overdosage does not usually produce serious side-effects.

See also Diazepam, p.1520.

Adverse reactions to nitrazepam were studied by the Boston Collaborative Drug Surveillance Program in 2111 hospital in-patients who received nitrazepam mainly for insomnia. Central nervous system (CNS) depression (drowsiness, fatigue, confusion, and ataxia) occurred in 49 patients, CNS stimulation (nightmares, hallucinations, insomnia and agitation) in 15, cutaneous reactions (rash and pruritus) in 5, and headache and gastro-intestinal disturbances in 3. The frequency of side-effects caused by CNS depression or stimulation were generally greater at higher doses of nitrazepam and those caused by CNS depression were also more frequent in elderly patients.— D. J. Greenblatt and M. D. Allen, *Br. J. clin. Pharmac.*, 1978, *5*, 407.

Acroparaesthesia. In a 55-year-old woman tingling and numbness of the hands was correlated with the ingestion of nitrazepam.— H. MacLean (letter), *Br. med. J.*, 1973, *1*, 488.

Effects on respiration. In 3 elderly patients with respiratory failure, carbon-dioxide narcosis developed when nitrazepam was given for night sedation. Breathing was improved in 2 by oxygen and injections of nikethamide; the third required only vigorous physical stimulation.— T. J. H. Clark *et al.*, *Lancet*, 1971, *2*, 737.

In 6 patients with chronic obstructive bronchitis and ventilatory failure, the forced vital capacity and forced expiratory volume in 1 second were significantly reduced 2 hours after 10 mg of nitrazepam given by mouth, compared with a placebo. There was a tendency for pO_2 to fall and pCO_2 to rise. In 1 patient studied for 4 hours there were major changes in blood-gas tensions. Nitrazepam was contra-indicated in patients with severe chronic obstructive bronchitis.— J. Gaddie *et al.*, *Br. med. J.*, 1972, *2*, 688.

In 5 patients with respiratory failure given nitrazepam 5 to 10 mg at night, respiratory depression was increased; the mean capillary pCO_2 rose from 53 to 79 mmHg.— A. Pines (letter), *Br. med. J.*, 1972, *3*, 352.

Normal doses of nitrazepam could be fatal in patients with raised carbon dioxide concentrations due to chronic obstructive lung disease.— D. G. Model (letter), *Lancet*, 1974, *1*, 224.

Gout. A 40-year-old Chinese man with a history of gout had acute attacks on 5 occasions after taking nitrazepam 10 mg; attacks were also precipitated by diazepam 5 mg, chlordiazepoxide 15 mg, and Mandrax.— C. O. Leng (letter), *Br. med. J.*, 1975, *2*, 561.

Overdosage. A 23-year-old man took 180 mg of nitrazepam. Five hours later he felt slightly sleepy but held a rational conversation. Two abnormalities were: coarse, sustained, bilateral nystagmus with a rotatory element elicited on lateral gaze; and incoordination of the lower limbs and ataxia. Abdominal reflexes were absent. After 2 days, the speech was clear and the nystagmus had ceased. The ataxia cleared after 7 days.— K. D. Bardhan (letter), *Lancet*, 1969, *1*, 1319.

Two women each took about 200 mg of nitrazepam. After the overdosage both patients, when conscious, suffered restlessness and increased rapid-eye-movement sleep.— I. Haider and I. Oswald, *Br. med. J.*, 1970, *2*, 318.

A 24-year-old woman who had ingested 100 tablets of nitrazepam recovered uneventfully after having been unconscious for 36 hours. While unconscious she had tense bullae on the left side of her face and body. They subsequently healed leaving considerable scarring.— C. M. Ridley, *Br. med. J.*, 1971, *3*, 28. See also M. J. Boyce and P. Mason (letter), *Lancet*, 1972, *2*, 874.

The effects of acute poisoning from self-administered overdosage of a variety of hypnotic drugs were compared in 1176 patients. In the 102 who had taken nitrazepam, coma was shallow and lasted for a maximum of 12 hours, in contrast to the findings from the other hypnotics.— H. Matthew *et al.*, *Practitioner*, 1972, *208*, 254. See also *idem*, *Br. med. J.*, 1969, *3*, 23.

Alpha coma (normally associated with poor prognosis in structural brain damage) was noted in a 41-year-old man after an overdose of nitrazepam. He made a complete recovery indicating that such a finding in association with drug intoxication need not imply that secondary hypoxic brain damage has occurred.— W. M. Carroll and F. L. Mastiglia, *Br. med. J.*, 1977, *2*, 1518.

A report of death by suicide of a 55-year-old man following ingestion of alcohol and nitrazepam; chronic bronchitis was considered to have been a major contributory factor in the death.— J. M. Torry, *Practitioner*, 1977, *217*, 648.

Treatment of Adverse Effects. There is no specific treatment. In recent severe overdosage with the benzodiazepines the stomach should be emptied by aspiration and lavage. Recovery usually follows symptomatic treatment. Dialysis is of no value. For general guidelines to the symptomatic therapy of central nervous system depressants, see Phenobarbitone, p.812.

See also under Diazepam, p.1521.

Precautions. Nitrazepam should be used with caution in patients with chronic obstructive lung disease or respiratory failure. Elderly subjects may be more susceptible to nitrazepam.

Nitrazepam causes drowsiness and patients receiving it should not take charge of vehicles or machinery where loss of attention could lead to accidents. These effects are enhanced by the simultaneous administration of depressants of the central nervous system such as alcohol.

There have been reports that, unlike the barbiturates, nitrazepam does not generally cause induction of hepatic microsomal enzymes.

See also Diazepam, p.1521.

A study indicating that usual therapeutic doses of nitrazepam slightly interfere with colour vision.— J. Laroche and C. Laroche, *Annls pharm. fr.*, 1977, *35*, 173.

Administration in the elderly. A characteristic syndrome occurred in elderly patients taking nitrazepam 5 mg at night. Symptoms included the unmasking of earlier cerebral damage, mental confusion, symptoms of postural hypotension, ataxia, and incontinence, and could appear after nitrazepam had been taken for some time; symptoms subsided rapidly when nitrazepam was withdrawn.— J. G. Evans and E. H. Jarvis (letter), *Br. med. J.*, 1972, *4*, 487. Scepticism.— F. Wells (letter), *ibid.*, 1973, *4*, 235.

Several elderly patients taking nitrazepam (usually 7.5 mg at night) reported vivid nightmares often related to earlier traumatic experiences.— F. Taylor (letter), *Br. med. J.*, 1973, *1*, 113.

An 86-year-old woman developed hypothermia after administration of nitrazepam 5 mg. After recovery she was mistakenly given another 5-mg dose of nitrazepam and again developed hypothermia.— M. Impallomeni and R. Ezzat (letter), *Br. med. J.*, 1976, *1*, 223.

In a double-blind study the plasma-nitrazepam concentration was not significantly different 12, 36, and 60 hours after a 10-mg dose in 10 healthy young persons (less than 40 years) and 10 elderly persons (over 69 years). The elderly made more errors in a simple psychomotor test 12 and 36 hours after the dose but the time taken to complete the test was not significantly different in the 2 groups. Subjectively subjects in both groups felt less alert 12 and 36 hours after the dose. Differences between the 2 groups were probably due to variations in the effects on the brain with the ageing brain perhaps having an increased sensitivity to nitrazepam.— C. M. Castleden *et al.*, *Br. med. J.*, 1977, *1*, 10.

Effects on mental state. A double-blind crossover study in 10 healthy young men showed that when taken before going to bed nitrazepam, 5 or 10 mg, or amylobarbitone sodium, 100 or 200 mg, provided a good night's sleep but impaired ability to perform card-sorting tests for up to 13 hours. Both doses of nitrazepam slowed motor performance and the higher doses of both nitrazepam and amylobarbitone sodium significantly slowed ability to make decisions. EEG studies showed that delayed hypnotic effects were more pronounced with nitrazepam than with amylobarbitone sodium.— A. Malpas *et al.*, *Br. med. J.*, 1970, *2*, 762. A similar report in 10 patients.— A. J. Walters and M. H. Lader (letter), *Nature*, 1971, *229*, 638. A similar comparison of the residual effects of nitrazepam, flurazepam hydrochloride, and pentobarbitone sodium on human performance.— R. G. Borland and A. N. Nicholson, *Br. J. clin. Pharmac.*, 1975, *2*, 9.

A double-blind study in 10 light and 10 sound sleepers showed that when taken at bedtime nitrazepam 2.5 or 5 mg improved vigilance performance in light sleepers the morning after treatment. Nitrazepam 10 mg impaired performance of several tests in both light and sound sleepers.— A. W. Peck *et al.*, *Br. J. clin. Pharmac.*, 1977, *4*, 101.

Pregnancy and the neonate. The floppy-infant syndrome in one neonate and sedation in another were associated with the maternal use of nitrazepam. The mother of the first child also took diazepam and this too was implicated.— A. N. P. Speight (letter), *Lancet*, 1977, *2*, 878. See also under Absorption and Fate.

Absorption and Fate. Nitrazepam is fairly readily absorbed from the gastro-intestinal tract, although there is some individual variation. It has a biphasic half-life probably owing to tissue redistribution, and is extensively bound to plasma proteins. It is metabolised in the liver, mainly by nitroreduction and acetylation (which is reported to be subject to genetic polymorphism). It is excreted in the urine in the form of its metabolites with only small amounts of a dose appearing unchanged. Up to about 20% of an oral dose is found in the faeces. It crosses the placental barrier and traces are found in breast milk.

Absorption and metabolism. After administration of nitrazepam 10 mg by mouth to volunteers, absorption varied from 53 to 94%. Maximum plasma concentrations were reached within 2 hours.— J. Rieder, *Arzneimittel-Forsch.*, 1973, *23*, 212.

When 9 healthy subjects took nitrazepam 5 mg, absorption was usually fairly rapid, but with some intersubject variation. A mean initial peak plasma concentration of 37.1 ng per ml (range 28.2 to 45.0 ng per ml) was obtained after a mean of 81 minutes (range 30 to 240 minutes). In most subjects there was a subsequent rapid decrease in plasma-nitrazepam concentration until 4 hours after taking the dose, followed by a slight increase to produce a second peak after 6 to 8 hours. The mean elimination half-life was 30 hours (range 18 to 36 hours).— D. D. Breimer *et al.* (letter), *Br. J. clin. Pharmac.*, 1977, *4*, 709. See also S. H. Curry *et al.*, *ibid.*, 109.

In 6 healthy subjects given a single 5-mg dose of nitrazepam the mean serum concentration of nitrazepam and active metabolites was 7.4 ng per ml 72 hours after administration.— P. Hunt *et al.*, *J. Pharm. Pharmac.*, 1979, *31*, 448.

Further references: J. Rieder and G. Wendt, Pharmacokinetics and Metabolism of the Hypnotic Nitrazepam, in *The Benzodiazepines*, S. Garattini *et al.* (Ed.), New York, Raven Press, 1973, p. 99.

Acetylation. The polymorphic acetylation of nitrazepam.— A. K. M. Karim and D. A. P. Evans, *J. med. Genet.*, 1976, *13*, 17.

Distribution. A study in 38 neurological patients indicated that nitrazepam is eliminated considerably more slowly from the CSF than from the plasma. Its β-phase half-life was found to be about 68 hours in the CSF compared with 27 hours in plasma. Whereas the CSF concentration after 2 hours was only 8% of that in plasma, after 36 hours it was nearly 16%.— L. Kangas *et al.*, *Acta pharmac. tox.*, 1977, *41*, 74.

Administration in the elderly. The serum half-life (β-phase) of nitrazepam was 24.2 and 39.6 hours respectively in 25 healthy subjects aged 21 to 38 years who took nitrazepam 5 mg daily for 14 days and 12 hospitalised elderly patients aged 66 to 89 years who took nitrazepam 5 mg daily for 2 months. Peak serum-nitrazepam concentrations were 39.9 and 21.8 ng per ml respectively in the young and the old group, and the volumes of distribution were 2.4 and 4.8 litres per kg body-weight respectively. The immobility of the older patients and their diseases were considered to be responsible for the differences.— E. Iisalo *et al.*, *Br. J. clin. Pharmac.*, 1977, *4*, 646P.

See also under Precautions.

Pregnancy and the neonate. In early pregnancy a lower concentration of nitrazepam was found in foetal plasma than in maternal plasma, but as pregnancy progressed placental transfer of nitrazepam increased so that in late pregnancy foetal and maternal concentrations were not significantly different.— L. Kangas *et al.*, *Eur. J. clin. Pharmac.*, 1977, *12*, 355.

Uses. Nitrazepam is a benzodiazepine hypnotic with actions similar to those of diazepam. It is reported to act in 30 to 60 minutes to produce sleep lasting for 6 to 8 hours. Because of its relative freedom from toxic effects in usual doses or in overdose and from interactions with other drugs it may be preferred to barbiturates and to some non-barbiturate hypnotics.

As a hypnotic the usual dose is 5 to 10 mg at night. Doses of 2.5 to 5 mg at night have been suggested for children, and these may also be more suitable for elderly patients.

Nitrazepam has also been used in epilepsy, notably for myoclonic seizures.

Anaesthesia. Nitrazepam 10 mg was the most effective of several premedicants in reducing the vasoconstrictive reaction to fear pre-operatively in a study in 350 patients. Droperidol 20 mg by mouth enhanced the sedative effect. Reactions to droperidol were suppressed by nitrazepam.— M. Johnstone, *Br. J. Anaesth.*, 1971, *43*, 380. Nitrazepam 10 mg and droperidol 20 mg by mouth 2 hours before induction of ketamine anaesthesia in 100 patients suppressed the dreams, mental agitation, and muscular catatonia sometimes precipitated during recovery from ketamine.— *Anaesth. & intensive Care*, 1972, *1*, 70.

In a study of premedication with nitrazepam, 61 patients given 5 mg on the night before operation and 2.5 mg the next morning slept better and were more sedated and less apprehensive than 60 similar patients who received no premedication. There was however no significant correlation between plasma concentrations of nitrazepam and the quality of sleep or the degree of sedation, apprehension, excitement, or headache.— L. Kangas *et al.*, *Br. J. Anaesth.*, 1977, *49*, 1153.

Further references: W. Norris and A. B. M. Telfer, *Br. J. Anaesth.*, 1969, *41*, 877; M. James and A. Fisher,

Anaesthesia, 1970, *25*, 364; A. Pakkanen *et al.*, *Br. J. Anaesth.*, 1980, *52*, 1009.

Convulsions. Nitrazepam was given as an anticonvulsant to 24 infants, aged 1 to 18 months, with infantile spasms, including 22 with hypsarrhythmia. In 13 there was complete control of spasms with a dose of 0.6 to 1 mg per kg body-weight daily, in 6 there was temporary improvement followed by relapse, and in 5 there was no effect. Side-effects in 14 infants included hypersecretion of mucus and saliva in 7, drowsiness in 6, and difficulty in swallowing in 4. Hypersecretion occurred with doses as low as 700 µg per kg daily.— E. Völzke *et al.*, *Epilepsia*, 1967, *8*, 64.

In a double-blind crossover study comparing the anticonvulsant effects of nitrazepam and diazepam in 9 children with myoclonic seizure disorders, initial doses of 5 to 10 mg and 10 to 20 mg respectively were given daily in addition to phenobarbitone 30 to 60 mg and adjusted over periods of 6 months to an average of 18 and 40 mg respectively. Assessed by incidence of seizures and by EEG, the drugs were equally effective in producing at least 50% improvement in 5 patients, transient improvement in 2, and no improvement in 2. Side-effects included occasional drowsiness, hypotonia, and drooling with both drugs and bronchopneumonia in 3 while on high doses of diazepam.— J. M. Killian and G. H. Fromm, *Develop. Med. Child Neurology*, 1971, *13*, 32.

Further references: W. G. Peterson, *Neurology, Minneap.*, 1967, *17*, 878; J. W. Lance, *Med. J. Aust.*, 1968, *1*, 113; N. Sörensen and R. Dreyer, *Medsche Welt, Stuttg.*, 1970, *33*, 1407; J. E. Jan *et al.*, *Can. med. Ass. J.*, 1971, *104*, 571.

Hypnotic effect. A double-blind study in 25 patients compared the length of sleep following the administration of nitrazepam 10 mg, nitrazepam 5 mg, methyprylone 200 mg, quinalbarbitone sodium 100 mg, or placebo. One capsule was given at 10 pm and the patients were observed throughout the night. The drugs were all significantly more hypnotic than the placebo but differed little between themselves, except that nitrazepam had a slightly longer duration of action. The major side-effect was drowsiness in the morning. This was more marked with nitrazepam 10 mg and 3 patients were withdrawn from the trial through drowsiness and agitation the day after taking the drug. The patients had, on average, 1 hour more sleep after taking the drugs than after the placebo.— W. H. le Riche *et al.*, *Can. med. Ass. J.*, 1966, *95*, 300.

In 10 subjects (mean age 57 years) nitrazepam 5 mg at night for 10 weeks significantly prolonged sleep. There was no tolerance, but when the drug was withdrawn sleep was temporarily worse than before treatment. Slow-wave sleep was reduced by nitrazepam but secretion of growth hormone, thought to be important for restorative function, was not impaired.— K. Adam *et al.*, *Br. med. J.*, 1976, *1*, 1558.

Further references: A. G. Fraser and F. G. G. Shepherd, *Practitioner*, 1966, *196*, 829; I. Haider, *Br. J. Psychiat.*, 1968, *114*, 337; T. Andersen and O. Lingjaerde, *Br. J. Psychiat.*, 1969, *115*, 1393; H. Matthew *et al.*, *Br. med. J.*, 1969, *3*, 23; J. M. Bordeleau *et al.*, *Dis. nerv. Syst.*, 1970, *31*, 318; R. Mea.es *et al.*, *Med. J. Aust.*, 1972, *1*, 266; M. W. Johns, *Drugs*, 1975, *9*, 448.

Preparations

Nitrazepam Capsules *(B.P.)*. Capsules containing nitrazepam. Store at a temperature not exceeding 30°.

Nitrazepam Tablets *(B.P.)*. Tablets containing nitrazepam. Protect from light.

Proprietary Preparations

Mogadon *(Roche, UK)*. Nitrazepam, available as **Capsules** and scored **Tablets** of 5 mg. (Also available as Mogadon in *Arg., Austral., Belg., Denm., Fr., Ger., Ital., Neth., Norw., S.Afr., Spain, Switz.*).

Nitrados *(Berk Pharmaceuticals, UK)*. Nitrazepam, available as scored tablets of 5 mg.

Remnos *(DDSA Pharmaceuticals, UK)*. Nitrazepam, available as scored tablets of 5 and 10 mg.

Somnite *(Norgine, UK)*. Nitrazepam, available as scored tablets of 5 mg.

Surem *(Galen, UK)*. Nitrazepam, available as capsules of 5 mg.

Unisomnia *(Unigreg, UK: Vestric, UK)*. Nitrazepam, available as scored tablets of 5 mg.

Other Proprietary Names

Arg.—Relact, Sindepres; *Austral.*—Dormicum; *Denm.*—Apodorm, Dumolid, Pacisyn; *Ital.*—Mitidin, Persopir, Prosonno, Quill, Sonnolin; *Norw.*—Apodorm, Paxisyn; *S.Afr.*—Arem, Hypnotin, Noctene; *Spain*—Hipsal, Pelson; *Swed.*—Apodorm, Dumolid.

Nitrazepam was also formerly marketed in Great Britain under the proprietary name Somnased (*Duncan, Flockhart*).

4055-z

Paraldehyde *(B.P., Eur. P.)*. Paraldehydum; Paracetaldehyde. The trimer of acetaldehyde; 2,4,6-Trimethyl-1,3,5-trioxane.

$(C_2H_4O)_3=132.2$.

CAS — 123-63-7.

Pharmacopoeias. In *Arg., Aust., Br., Eur., Fr., Ger., Hung., Ind., It., Neth., Nord., Span., Swiss, Turk.*, and *U.S.*

A clear colourless or pale yellow liquid with a strong characteristic odour and a disagreeable taste. The *B.P.* specifies that it contains a suitable amount of an antoxidant; the *U.S.P.* permits a suitable stabiliser. Relative density 0.993 to 0.996. F.p. 10° to 12°. Not more than 10% distils below 123° and not less than 95% below 126°.

Soluble 1 in 9 of water, less soluble in boiling water; miscible with alcohol, chloroform, ether, and volatile oils. A 3.65% solution in water is iso-osmotic with serum. It may be **sterilised** by filtration; contact with rubber should be avoided. **Store** in a cool place in small well-filled airtight containers, in complete darkness, avoiding contact with cork. The *U.S.P.* specifies that it must not be used more than 24 hours after opening the container.

Because of its solvent action upon rubber, polystyrene, and styrene-acrylonitrile copolymer, paraldehyde should not be administered in plastic syringes made with these materials.

At low temperature it solidifies to form a crystalline mass. If it solidifies, the whole should be liquefied and mixed before use.

CAUTION. *Paraldehyde decomposes on storage, particularly after the container has been opened. The administration of partly decomposed paraldehyde is dangerous. It must not be used if it has a brownish colour or a sharp penetrating odour of acetic acid.*

An aqueous solution of paraldehyde iso-osmotic with serum (3.65%) caused 97% haemolysis of erythrocytes cultured in it for 45 minutes.— C. Sapp *et al.*, *J. pharm. Sci.*, 1975, *64*, 1884.

Solubility in water and saline. In water: at 20°, 1 in 9; at 30°, 1 in 10; and at 37° 1 in 11.5. In 0.9% sodium chloride solution: at 20°, 1 in 9.5; at 30°, 1 in 11; and at 37°, 1 in 12.5.— Pharm. Soc. Lab. Rep. No. 856, 1962.

Dependence. Prolonged use of paraldehyde may lead to dependence of the barbiturate-alcohol type (see p.792), especially in alcoholics.

Adverse Effects. Paraldehyde decomposes on storage and deaths from corrosive poisoning have followed the use of such material. Paraldehyde has an unpleasant taste and imparts a smell to the breath; it may cause skin rashes.

Oral and rectal administration of paraldehyde may cause gastric or rectal irritation. Intramuscular administration is painful and associated with sterile abscesses and nerve damage. Intravenous administration is extremely hazardous since it may cause pulmonary oedema and haemorrhage, and cardiac dilatation; thrombophlebitis is also associated with intravenous administration.

Overdosage results in rapid laboured breathing owing to damage to the lungs by paraldehyde and to acidosis. Nausea and vomiting may follow an overdose by mouth. Hepatic and renal damage may occur.

A patient with chronic tuberculosis died from corrosion of the upper air passages and subsequent bronchopneumonia 2 days after taking paraldehyde in water. The paraldehyde was old stock and contained 40% glacial acetic acid and excess oxidants.— *Br. med. J.*, 1954, *2*, 1114; A. S. Curry, *ibid.*, 1962, *1*, 687.

Pulmonary oedema was associated with paraldehyde given intravenously to a 2-year-old child with aplastic anaemia.— S. H. Sinal and J. E. Crowe, *Pediatrics*, 1976, *57*, 158.

Severe proctitis with stricture, and an excoriating rash affecting the buttocks and peri-anal area, were judged to have resulted from a paraldehyde enema given 4 days previously.— J. H. Stanley, *J. Am. med. Ass.*, 1980, *243*, 1749.

Overdosage. A report of acidosis in association with overdosage of paraldehyde.— L. S. Beier *et al.*, *Ann. intern. Med.*, 1963, *58*, 155.

Treatment of Adverse Effects. As for Phenobarbitone, p.812.

Attention should be paid to the possibility of acidosis. Hydrocortisone may be given intravenously to reduce hepatic and renal damage.

Precautions. Paraldehyde should not be given to patients with gastric disorders and it should be used with caution, if at all, in patients with bronchopulmonary disease or hepatic impairment. It should not be given rectally in the presence of colitis.

Old paraldehyde must never be used. It must be well diluted before oral or rectal administration; if it is deemed essential to give paraldehyde intravenously it must be well diluted and given very slowly with extreme caution (see also Adverse Effects and Uses). Intramuscular injections may be given undiluted but plastic syringes must be avoided and care should be taken to avoid nerve damage.

Paraldehyde causes drowsiness and persons receiving it should not take charge of vehicles or machinery where loss of attention could lead to accidents. These effects are enhanced by simultaneous administration of depressants of the central nervous system such as alcohol, barbiturates, and other sedatives. Paraldehyde should not be administered to patients receiving disulfiram.

Interactions. *Alcohol.* A report on the deaths of 9 patients following administration of paraldehyde to treat acute alcohol intoxication. Preliminary *animal* studies confirmed a synergistic action between alcohol and paraldehyde.– S. Kaye and H. B. Haag, *Toxic. appl. Pharmac.*, 1964, *6*, 316.

Disulfiram. A study in *animals* of the enhancing effect of disulfiram on paraldehyde-induced sedation.— M. L. Keplinger and J. A. Wells, *Fedn Proc. Fedn Am. Socs exp. Biol.*, 1956, *15*, 445.

Steroids. Paraldehyde affected the estimation of urinary 17-oxo-steroids and 17-oxogenic-steroids.— *Adverse Drug React. Bull.*, 1972, June, 104.

Absorption and Fate. Paraldehyde is readily absorbed when given by mouth, rectally, or intramuscularly and is distributed throughout the tissues. About 80% of a dose is metabolised in the liver probably to acetaldehyde, which is oxidised to acetic acid. A very high proportion is excreted unchanged through the lungs; only small amounts appear in the urine. It crosses the placental barrier.

A constant proportion of about 7% of an oral dose was exhaled within 4 hours as unchanged paraldehyde and no metabolites were detected.— D. W. Lang and H. H. Borgstedt, *Toxic. appl. Pharmac.*, 1969, *15*, 269.

Pregnancy and lactation. Many hours after an initial dose of paraldehyde, the average concentration in the foetal circulation was almost equal to that in the maternal blood. The odour of paraldehyde was detectable in the breath of the newborn for 2 or 3 days after birth. It was considered that when given in sufficient dosage to cause amnesia, paraldehyde would cause neonatal depression in a large percentage of infants.— F. Moya and V. Thorndike, *Am. J. Obstet. Gynec.*, 1962, *84*, 1778.

Uses. Paraldehyde is a hypnotic and sedative with anticonvulsant effects. Following oral administration it is reported to act in 10 to 15 minutes to induce sleep lasting 4 to 8 hours.

The usual hypnotic dose by mouth or intramuscularly is 10 ml at night, and the usual sedative dose is 5 ml thrice daily. Oral doses must be well diluted to avoid gastric irritation and not more than 5 ml of an intramuscular dose should be injected into any one site. Similar doses have also been given rectally diluted with oil or water; higher doses were formerly given rectally as a basal anaesthetic.

Paraldehyde has also been used intramuscularly for the emergency treatment of epilepsy but the pain associated with its use, its tendency to react with plastic syringes, and the risk associated with deterioration, militate against its use. A suggested dose for children is 0.1 to 0.15 ml per kg body-weight.

Paraldehyde has also been given by intravenous infusion, diluted with several volumes of sodium chloride injection but severe untoward effects have been associated with its use by this route. Excitement, cough, and apnoea may occur, with pulmonary haemorrhage and oedema (see also Adverse Effects and Precautions). A suggested dose is 0.15 ml per kg body-weight.

Paraldehyde was recommended as the sedative for patients with tetanus as it did not embarrass the circulatory and respiratory systems. Doses of up to 12 ml every 4 hours by stomach tube as a 10% solution or by intramuscular injection had been given.— L. Cole and H. Youngman, *Lancet*, 1969, *1*, 1017. See also *idem* (letter), *Br. med. J.*, 1969, *3*, 474. An alternative view.— B. H. Bonnlander (letter), *J. Am. med. Ass.*, 1968, *20*5 187.

The traditional paediatric dose [for status epilepticus] of paraldehyde 1 ml per year of age might be satisfactory in the first 2 or 3 years of life, but could be excessive in the older child.— R. A. Shanks (letter), *Br. med. J.*, 1978, *2*, 1086. In older children it would be better to use 0.15 ml per kg body-weight.— D. P. Addy (letter), *ibid.* See also H. B. Valman, *Br. med. J.*, 1980, *280*, 1113.

Discussions and tests on the use of plastic syringes.— V. I. Fenton-May and F. Lee (letter), *Br. med. J.*, 1978, *2*, 1166; D. P. Addy *et al.* (letter), *ibid.*, 1434.

Preparations

Paraldehyde Draught *(B.P.C. 1973).* Paraldehyde 4 ml, syrup 8 ml, liquorice liquid extract 3 ml, water to 50 ml. It should be freshly prepared. *Dose.* 50 ml.

Batches of Paraldehyde Draught, prepared with paraldehyde from 4 different suppliers, after storage at room temperature for 4 months showed a 15- to 40-fold increase in acidity.—Pharm. Soc. Lab. Rep., *Pharm. J.*, 1956, *2*, 341.

Paraldehyde Enema *(B.P.C. 1973).* Paraldehyde 10 ml, sodium chloride solution to 100 ml. It must be freshly prepared. It contains 0.5 ml of paraldehyde in 5 ml. *Dose.* 5 ml per kg body-weight, to a maximum of 300 ml, by rectal injection.

Paraldehyde Injection *(B.P.).* Sterile paraldehyde which has been sterilised by filtration; it contains no added antimicrobial preservatives. Store at a temperature not exceeding 25° in complete darkness in ampoules sealed by fusion of the glass. Plastic syringes should not be used for administering this injection, and contact with rubber should be avoided.

Paraldehyde Mixture *(A.P.F.).* Paraldehyde Draught. Paraldehyde 10 ml, liquorice liquid extract 10 ml, water to 100 ml. *Dose.* 20 to 80 ml. It should be recently prepared and stored below 25°. Separation occurs below 5° and above 25°.

Nord. P. has paraldehyde 10 g, menthol 10 mg, alcohol 20 g, acacia mucilage 30 g, liquorice liquid extract 5 g, and water 35 g..

Sterile Paraldehyde *(U.S.P.).* Paraldehyde suitable for parenteral use. Store at a temperature not exceeding 25°. Protect from light.

Proprietary Names

Paral *(O'Neal, USA).*

4056-c

Pentobarbitone *(B.P., Eur. P.).*

Pentobarbitalum; Pentobarbital *(U.S.P.)*; Mébubarbital; Mebumal. 5-Ethyl-5-(1-methylbutyl)barbituric acid.

$C_{11}H_{18}N_2O_3$=226.3.

CAS — 76-74-4.

Pharmacopoeias. In *Br., Eur., Fr., Ger., It., Neth., Nord., Span.,* and *U.S.*

Odourless or almost odourless, colourless crystals or a white or almost white crystalline powder. M.p. 127° to 133°. A polymorphic form may occur, with a m.p. of about 115°; it gradually reverts to the more stable form on heating at about 110°.

Very slightly **soluble** in water and carbon tetrachloride; soluble 1 in 4.5 of alcohol, 1 in 4 of chloroform, and 1 in 10 of ether; very soluble in acetone and methyl alcohol. **Store** in airtight containers.

4057-k

Pentobarbitone Calcium.

Pentobarbital Calcium. Calcium 5-ethyl-5-(1-methylbutyl)barbiturate.

$(C_{11}H_{17}N_2O_3)_2Ca$=490.6.

Pharmacopoeias. In *Jap. P.*

A fine, white, odourless, crystalline powder with a slightly bitter taste. Sparingly **soluble** in water; slightly soluble in alcohol; paractically insoluble in ether. A saturated solution in water has a pH of about 9.5. **Store** in airtight containers.

4058-a

Pentobarbitone Sodium *(B.P., B.P. Vet., Eur. P.).*

Pentobarb. Sod.; Ethaminal Sodium; Pentobarbitalum Natricum; Mebumalnatrium; Pentobarbital Sodium *(U.S.P.)*; Sodium Pentobarbital; Soluble Pentobarbitone; Aethaminalum-Natrium. Sodium 5-ethyl-5-(1-methylbutyl)barbiturate.

$C_{11}H_{17}N_2NaO_3$=248.3.

CAS — 57-33-0.

Pharmacopoeias. In *Arg., Br., Braz., Cz., Eur., Fr., Ger., Ind., It., Mex., Neth., Rus., Swiss,* and *U.S.*

A white, hygroscopic, crystalline powder or granules, odourless or with a slight characteristic odour, with a slightly bitter taste. Very **soluble** in water and alcohol; practically insoluble in ether. A 10% solution in water has a pH of 9.6 to 11 and slowly decomposes. Solutions for injection are prepared aseptically in Water for Injections free from carbon dioxide and should be used immediately after preparation. **Incompatibilities** as for phenobarbitone sodium (p.811). Incompatibility has been reported with cephaloridine, cephazolin sodium, clindamycin phosphate, and pentazocine lactate. **Store** in airtight containers.

Effect of gamma-irradiation. The colour of pentobarbitone sodium deepened on irradiation. Solutions of irradiated material were opalescent and had developed a slight odour.— *The Use of Gamma Radiation Sources for the Sterilisation of Pharmaceutical Products,* London, ABPI, 1960.

Incompatibility. Fluopromazine hydrochloride injection was incompatible with pentobarbitone sodium.— C. Riffkin, *Am. J. Hosp. Pharm.*, 1963, *20*, 19.

There was loss of clarity when intravenous solutions of pentobarbitone sodium were mixed with those of chlorpheniramine maleate, dimenhydrinate, diphenhydramine hydrochloride, ephedrine sulphate, erythromycin gluceptate, hydrocortisone sodium succinate, hydroxyzine hydrochloride, insulin, narcotic salts, noradrenaline acid tartrate, oxytetracycline hydrochloride, phenytoin sodium, prochlorperazine maleate, promazine hydrochloride (in dextrose injection), promethazine hydrochloride, protein hydrolysate, sodium bicarbonate, streptomycin sulphate, suxamethonium chloride, tetracycline hydrochloride, or vancomycin hydrochloride.— J. A. Patel and G. L. Phillips, *Am. J. Hosp. Pharm.*, 1966, *23*, 409.

Pentobarbitone sodium was reported to be incompatible with cephalothin sodium, chlorpromazine hydrochloride, diphenhydramine hydrochloride, and prochlorperazine hydrochloride.— J. M. Meisler and M. W. Skolaut, *Am. J. Hosp. Pharm.*, 1966, *23*, 557.

Dependence. Prolonged use of pentobarbitone sodium may lead to dependence of the barbiturate-alcohol type (see p.792). It is commonly abused by addicts.

Consumption of up to 12 capsules daily of pentobarbitone sodium and carbromal (Carbrital) over a period of 5 years caused megaloblastic anaemia and bromism in a 59-year-old man.— S. D. Slater, *Br. J. clin. Pract.*, 1974, *28*, 97.

Adverse Effects, Treatment, and Precautions. As for Phenobarbitone, p.812.

Administration in children. A report of toxic encephalopathy noted in 7 children, over a period of several years, following administration of suppositories containing pentobarbitone sodium and mepyramine maleate. In 3 children the dose was within the manufacturer's recommendations.— J. F. Schwartz and J. H. Patterson, *Am. J. Dis. Child.*, 1978, *132*, 37.

Administration in the elderly. No relationship between clinical toxicity and age has been noted for pentobarbitone.— D. J. Greenblatt *et al.*, *Clin. Pharmac. Ther.*, 1977, *21*, 355.

Administration in hepatic failure. Prolongation of the half-life of pentobarbitone in patients with cirrhosis.— F. W. Ossenberg *et al.*, *Digestion*, 1973, *8*, 448.

Further references: H. Held *et al.*, *Klin. Wschr.*, 1970, *48*, 565.

Administration in renal failure. Results calculated from single-dose studies of pentobarbitone in 11 healthy subjects and 9 uraemic patients suggested that pentobarbitone elimination is normal in renal failure; the plasma half-lives were shortened in some patients possibly owing to low apparent volumes of distribution.— M. M. Reidenberg *et al.*, *Clin. Pharmac. Ther.*, 1976, *20*, 67.

Effects on respiration. Pentobarbitone and quinalbarbitone were shown to produce respiratory depression when given in low and high doses of 60 and 180 mg, and 70 and 210 mg respectively to 6 healthy subjects. From calculations based on the displacement of the respiratory response curve 70 mg of quinalbarbitone was approximately equivalent to 100 mg of pentobarbitone.— C. R. Brown *et al.*, *J. clin. Pharmac.*, 1973, *13*, 28.

There was significant depression of the ventilatory response to hypoxia 30 minutes after the administration of pentobarbitone 2 mg per kg body-weight intramuscularly in 5 of 10 healthy subjects. It was suggested that dosage should be related to maximal oxygen uptake rather [illegible] body-weight.— C. A. Hirshman *et al.*, *Br. J. Ana[illegible].*, 1975, *47*, 963.

Interactions. *Corynebacterium parvum.* During evaluations of a vaccine of killed suspensions of *Corynebacterium parvum*, intravenous injections of *C. parvum* into *mice* rendered them lethally sensitive to normal safe anaesthetic doses of pentobarbitone. Caution was recommended when both preparations might be used in man.— B. Mosedale and M. A. Smith, *Wellcome* (letter), *Lancet*, 1975, *1*, 168.

Overdosage. Muscle necrosis and calcification occurred in a 35-year-old man during the course of severe acute renal failure due to intoxication with pentobarbitone. The calcification virtually disappeared by the end of 3 months.— J. G. Clark and M. D. Sumerling, *Br. med. J.*, 1966, *2*, 214.

Pregnancy and the neonate. Doses of up to 300 mg of pentobarbitone administered intravenously to the mother before delivery had no appreciable effect upon the clinical condition of the infants at birth. By contrast doses of 600 to 750 mg had been followed by moderate to severe neonatal depression in 40% of the infants, with delay in the establishment of normal respiration.— F. Moya and V. Thorndike, *Clin. Pharmac. Ther.*, 1963, *4*, 628.

Absorption and Fate. See under Phenobarbitone, p.814.

Pentobarbitone is extensively bound to tissue proteins. It is largely metabolised in the liver, mainly by hydroxylation, and the metabolites are excreted in the urine.

Following intravenous administration of pentobarbitone sodium 50 mg to 5 healthy subjects pentobarbitone was noted to have a distribution phase (α phase) of about 4 hours, and elimination occurred with a harmonic mean β-phase half-life of about 50 hours. This suggested that for pentobarbitone the body has a central plasma compartment and one or more extravascular compartments. Following oral administration of pentobarbitone, absorption was found to be considerably delayed, but not reduced, by food.— R. B. Smith *et al.*, *J. Pharmacokinet. Biopharm.*, 1973, *1*, 5. Findings in 7 healthy subjects of an average β-phase half-life of only 22.3 hours following intravenous administration of pentobarbitone sodium 100 mg. After oral administration the half-life was about the same. A more detailed knowledge of pentobarbitone pharmacokinetics was needed to explain the deviation from the findings of R.B. Smith *et al.* (above). Of pentobarbitone in the central compartment of the body only about 13% was present in the blood, where about 4% was in the plasma water, 5% was bound to plasma protein, and 4% was distributed to blood cells. Pentobarbitone appeared to undergo extensive tissue binding in both the central and peripheral compartments.— M. Ehrnebo, *J. pharm. Sci.*, 1974, *63*, 1114.

Following oral administration to healthy subjects, capsules containing pentobarbitone sodium 100 mg were totally absorbed, with an absorption half-life of 0.35 hours. Absorption was slower following rectal administration of suppositories, and varied considerably according to the suppository basis.— J. T. Doluisio *et al.*, *J. pharm. Sci.*, 1978, *67*, 1586.

Uses. Pentobarbitone is a barbiturate (see p.792) that is used as a hypnotic and sedative. As a hypnotic it is usually given in doses of 100 to 200 mg at night, and about 30 mg has been given 3 or 4 times daily as a sedative. Similar doses may be given of the sodium or calcium salt.

Pentobarbitone has been used for premedication in anaesthetic procedures but its use for these purposes has largely been superseded by other agents, such as the benzodiazepines. It has also been used as an anticonvulsant.

A report of the use of pentobarbitone in the treatment of submersion hypothermia.— A. W. Conn, *Can. med. Ass. J.*, 1979, *120*, 397.

Anaesthesia. References to pentobarbitone in anaesthesia: N. B. Jorgensen, *Br. dent. J.*, 1967, *122*, 202; W. J. Murray *et al.*, *J. Am. med. Ass.*, 1968, *203*, 327; T. Oyama *et al.*, *Anesth. Analg. curr. Res.*, 1969, *48*, 367; S. M. Lyons *et al.*, *Br. J. Anaesth.*, 1975, *47*, 630.

Hypnotic effect. In a drug surveillance programme, 453 patients received pentobarbitone as a hypnotic, usually in doses of 50 to 100 mg. In 320 patients evaluated, the response was considered good in 79.4%. Side-effects, which were reversible, occurred in 5.1% of patients and included CNS depression (20 patients), skin rash (1), nightmares (1), and drug fever (1).— S. Shapiro *et al.*, *J. Am. med. Ass.*, 1969, *209*, 2016.

The effects of pentobarbitone on the sleep of 8 former opiate addicts.— D. C. Kay *et al.*, *Clin. Pharmac. Ther.*, 1972, *13*, 221.

Intracranial hypertension. A technique for the management of patients with intracranial hypertension, using intravenous pentobarbitone as a sedative.— L. F. Marshall *et al.*, *Neurosurgery*, 1978, *2*, 100.

Preparations of Pentobarbitone and its Salts

Capsules

Pentobarbital Sodium Capsules *(U.S.P.)*. Capsules containing pentobarbitone sodium. Store in airtight containers.

Pentobarbitone Capsules *(B.P.)*. Pentobarb. Caps.; Pentobarbitone Sodium Capsules; Pentobarbital Sodium Capsules; Soluble Pentobarbitone Capsules. Capsules containing pentobarbitone sodium. Store at a temperature not exceeding 30°.

Elixirs

Pentobarbital Elixir *(U.S.P.)*. An elixir containing pentobarbitone, with alcohol 16 to 20%. Store in airtight containers.

Pentobarbital Sodium Elixir *(U.S.P.)*. Pentobarbitone sodium 400 mg, glycerol 45 ml, alcohol 15 ml, orange oil 0.075 ml, caramel 200 mg, syrup 15 ml, dilute hydrochloric acid 0.6 ml, water to 100 ml. Store in airtight containers.

Injections

Pentobarbital Sodium Injection *(U.S.P.)*. A sterile solution of pentobarbitone sodium (or an equivalent amount of pentobarbitone for adjustment of the pH) in a suitable solvent. pH 9 to 10.5.

Tablets

Pentobarbitone Tablets *(B.P.)*. Pentobarb. Tab.; Pentobarbitone Sodium Tablets; Pentobarbital Sodium Tablets; Soluble Pentobarbitone Tablets. Tablets containing pentobarbitone sodium.
Store in airtight containers.

Proprietary Preparations of Pentobarbitone and its Salts

Nembutal *(Abbott, UK)*. Pentobarbitone sodium, available as capsules of 100 mg. (Also available as Nembutal in *Austral., Belg., Denm., Fr., Ger., Ital., Neth., Switz.*, and as Nembutal Sodium in *Canad., USA.* Nembutal Elixir (*Abbott, USA*) contains pentobarbitone.).

Other Proprietary Names of Pentobarbitone and its Salts

Arg.— Embutal; *Austral.*— Penbon, Pentone, Petab; *Canad.*— Nova-Rectal, Pentogen; *Ger.*— Neodorm Repocal; *Jap.*— Schlafen; *S.Afr.*— Sopental; *Spain*— Insom Rapido; *Switz.*— Repocal.

A preparation containing pentobarbitone sodium and carbromal was formerly marketed in Great Britian under the proprietary name Carbrital (*Parke, Davis*).

4059-t

Perlapine. HF-2333; AW 142333. 6-(4-Methylpiperazin-1-yl)morphanthridine; 6-(4-Methylpiperazin-1-yl)-11*H*-dibenz[*b,e*]azepine.
$C_{19}H_{21}N_3$=291.4.

CAS — 1977-11-3.

Practically odourless tasteless crystals.

Adverse Effects. Hang-over, dizziness, dry mouth and dyspepsia.

Uses. Perlapine is a hypnotic that has been given in doses of 10 mg at night, an hour before retiring.

Following administration of 20 mg by mouth to human subjects, perlapine was almost completely absorbed. It was detected in the blood after 20 minutes and peak concentrations were reached after 3 hours. It was mainly excreted in the urine with only 1 to 2% appearing as unchanged drug. The pharmacokinetics were not affected by daily administration of 20 mg for 28 days.— T. Flage, *Drugs Today*, 1975, *11*, 76.

Further references: S. R. Allen and I. Oswald, *Psychopharmacologia*, 1973, *32*, 1.

Proprietary Names
Hypnodin *(Takeda, Jap.)*.

4060-l

Phenobarbitone *(B.P., B.P. Vet., Eur. P.)*.

Phenobarb.; Phenobarbitalum; Phenobarbital *(U.S.P.)*; Phenylethylbarbituric Acid; Phenylethylmalonylurea; Phenemalum; Fenobarbital. 5-Ethyl-5-phenylbarbituric acid.
$C_{12}H_{12}N_2O_3$=232.2.

CAS — 50-06-6.

Pharmacopoeias. In all pharmacopoeias examined except *Ind.*

Colourless crystals or a white odourless crystalline powder with a slightly bitter taste. It may exhibit polymorphism. M.p. 174° to 178°.

Soluble 1 in 1000 of water, 1 in 10 of alcohol, 1 in 40 of chloroform, 1 in 40 of ether; soluble in aqueous solutions of alkali carbonates and hydroxides and ammonia. A saturated solution in water has a pH of about 5.

Incompatibilities. The barbiturates and thiobarbiturates do not contain a carboxyl group but their aqueous solutions are acid to litmus and they are able to form metal derivatives. The acids are weaker acids than carbon dioxide in solution, so that the free acids may be precipitated from solutions of their metal derivatives by carbon dioxide, other stronger acids, and acid salts, including alkaloidal salts.

Incompatibility. Phenobarbitone formed a complex of reduced solubility with macrogol 4000. Dissolution and absorption of phenobarbitone from tablets containing macrogol 4000 were reduced.— P. Singh *et al.*, *J. pharm. Sci.*, 1966, *55*, 63.

Solubility. Information on the solubility of phenobarbitone in solvent mixtures was available from the following sources: G. M. Krause and J. M. Cross, *J. Am. pharm. Ass., scient. Edn*, 1951, *40*, 137 (for alcohol-glycerol-water mixtures); R. A. Anderson, *Australas. J. Pharm.*, 1949, *30*, 96 (for alcohol-water mixtures); A. Urdang and E. E. Leuallen, *J. Am. pharm. Ass., scient. Edn*, 1956, *45*, 525; C. F. Peterson and R. E. Hopponen, *J. Am. pharm. Ass., scient. Edn*, 1953, *42*, 540 (for propylene glycol-alcohol-water mixtures); N. C. Zacharias, *Can. pharm. J.*, 1951, *84*, 608 (for alcohol-water and alcohol-glycerol-water mixtures).

A study of the solubility of several barbiturates in water-alcohol mixtures.— T. L. Breon and A. N. Paruta, *J. pharm. Sci.*, 1970, *59*, 1306.

Solubilisation of barbiturates with macrogol stearates.— M. W. Gouda *et al.*, *J. pharm. Sci.*, 1970, *59*, 1402.

Stability. The kinetics of hydrolysis of barbituric acid and some of its derivatives in neutral and alkaline solutions.— E. R. Garrett *et al.*, *J. pharm. Sci.*, 1971, *60*, 1145.

4061-y

Phenobarbitone Sodium *(B.P., B.P. Vet.)*.

Phenobarb. Sod.; Phenobarbitalum Natricum; Phenobarbital Sodium *(U.S.P.)*; Sodium Phenylethylbarbiturate; Soluble Phenobarbitone; Phenemalnatrium; Fenobarbital Sódico. Sodium 5-ethyl-5-phenylbarbiturate.
$C_{12}H_{11}N_2NaO_3$=254.2.

CAS — 57-30-7.

Pharmacopoeias. In *Arg., Aust., Belg., Br., Braz., Cz., Ger., Hung., Ind., Int., It., Jap., Jug., Mex., Nord., Pol., Roum., Span., Swiss, Turk.*, and *U.S. Jap.* and *U.S.* also include a sterile form.

A white odourless hygroscopic powder, granules, or flakes with a bitter taste. M.p. about 175°. It loses not more than 7% of its weight when dried. In moist air it absorbs carbon dioxide, liberating phenobarbitone.

Soluble 1 in 3 of water and 1 in 25 of alcohol; practically insoluble in chloroform and ether. A 10% solution in water has a pH of 9.2 to 10.2 and slowly decomposes. A 3.95% solution in water is iso-osmotic with serum. Solutions in propylene glycol and water are **sterilised** by maintaining at 98° to 100° for 30 minutes.

Incompatible with ammonium salts, acids, and acidic substances, and with chloral hydrate. Phenobarbitone may be precipitated from mixtures containing phenobarbitone sodium. This precipitation is dependent upon the concentration and the pH, and also on the presence of other solvents such as alcohol and glycerol. At a concentration of 30 mg of phenobarbitone sodium in 10 ml of water, precipitation occurs at pH 7.5 and below. Corresponding figures for other concentrations are: 60 mg, pH 7.9; 100 mg, pH 8.3; and 200 mg, pH 8.6. **Store** in airtight containers.

Aqueous solutions of the sodium derivatives of barbiturates are alkaline and if acid stronger than the barbituric acid is added precipitation occurs when the proportion of free acid in the solution is in excess of its solubility. The solubility of a barbiturate is therefore dependent upon the pH of the solution. Aqueous solutions of the alkali-metal and alkaline-earth derivatives are strongly alkaline, and will liberate ammonia from ammonium salts and decompose chloral to chloroform. As the acids are amide in nature, they are hydrolysed fairly rapidly in alkaline solution, the reaction being accelerated by elevated temperatures, and some alkali-metal derivatives in solution decompose on standing. In view of the instability of soluble barbiturates in solution all mixtures containing them should be freshly prepared.

Incompatibility of phenobarbitone sodium. Incompatibility has been reported with cephalothin sodium, chlorpromazine hydrochloride, clindamycin phosphate, dimenhydrinate, diphenhydramine hydrochloride, ephedrine sulphate, erythromycin gluceptate, hydralazine hydrochloride, hydrocortisone sodium succinate, hydroxyzine hydrochloride, insulin, kanamycin sulphate, metaraminol tartrate, narcotic salts, oxytetracycline hydrochloride, pentazocine lactate, phenytoin sodium, procaine hydrochloride, prochlorperazine salts, promazine hydrochloride, promethazine hydrochloride, propiomazine hydrochloride, streptomycin sulphate, suxamethonium chloride, tetracycline hydrochloride, thiamine hydrochloride, tripelennamine hydrochloride, and vancomycin hydrochloride; many of these incompatibilities may be explained on the basis of pH.

References: R. Misgen, *Am. J. Hosp. Pharm.*, 1965, *22*, 92; J. A. Patel and G. L. Phillips, *ibid.*, 1966, *23*, 409; J. MMeisler and M. W. Skolaut, *ibid.*, 557; B. B. Riley, *J. Hosp. Pharm.*, 1970, *28* 228.

Precipitates formed between solutions of phenobarbitone sodium and salts of weak bases were usually attributed to the lowered pH of the solutions resulting in the precipitation of phenobarbitone. But precipitates were sometimes still formed when the pH was within the solubility of the parent acid. Examples were the reactions between phenobarbitone sodium and calcium chloride, magnesium sulphate, diphenhydramine hydrochloride, and codeine phosphate; the precipitates formed were considered to be complexes of the weak base with phenobarbitone.— V. H. Bruin and W. H. Oliver, *Australas. J. Pharm.*, 1957, *38*, 226.

It was recommended that when phenobarbitone sodium and ephedrine hydrochloride were prescribed together in solution, each should be separately dissolved and the solutions diluted before mixing, in order to prevent the formation of a slowly dissolving precipitate.— N. E. Bateman and M. D. Graham, *Australas. J. Pharm.*, 1967, *48*, S68.

Incompatibility of sodium salts of barbiturates. The precipitation of free barbiturates from mixtures containing their sodium derivatives usually depended on the proportion of barbiturates present and on the final pH of the mixture. It was often very difficult to predict the final pH of the mixture. If the mixture was obviously acid, then the solubility of the barbiturate could be taken as that of the free acid and it was simple to decide whether precipitation was likely. If the mixture was slightly alkaline, however, precise determination of pH might be necessary.— G. Smith, *Pharm. J.*, 1961, *2*, 495.

Stability of phenobarbitone sodium solutions. A 10% solution in water lost 2% of its strength in 5 days at 20°, 3% in 10 days, 6.1% in 20 days, and 10.7% in 50 days. When heated at 100°, a 10% solution lost 6.5% of its strength in 10 minutes, 10.7% in 30 minutes, and 17% in 1 hour.— H. Nuppenau, *Dansk Tidsskr. Farm.*, 1954, *28*, 261. A 5% solution in water lost none of its phenobarbitone content in 25 days at 5°, 2% at 15°, and 14% at 30°. A 10% solution lost 5.9% at 5°, 6.4% at 15°, and 17.8% at 30°. A 20% solution lost 3.6% at 5°, 4.1% at 15°, and 13% at 30°.— W. J. O'Reilly and S. E. Wright, *J. Pharm. Pharmac.*, 1954, *6*, 253. A 20% solution of phenobarbitone sodium in 60% v/v propylene glycol showed no loss in strength during 35 days' storage at room temperature. A 10% solution in 50% v/v alcohol showed a 1% loss at 10 days and a 3% loss at 35 days.— *idem*, *Australas. J. Pharm.*, 1954, *35*, 135.

Stability of sodium salts of barbiturates. The stabilising effect of propylene glycol, macrogol 400, alcohol, and glycerol on solutions of the sodium derivatives of amylobarbitone, aprobarbitone, barbitone, pentobarbitone, and phenobarbitone were investigated. Both the glycols as well as alcohol produced definite stabilisation of approximately equal degree and the effect increased as the proportion of glycol was increased. Glycerol had considerably lower stabilising properties. Solutions in pure propylene glycol and macrogol 400 showed no alteration in concentration after heating at 100° for 24 hours, nor were any signs of deterioration established in solutions stored for 1 year at 20° and 4°.— S. Linde, *Svensk farm. Tidskr.*, 1961, *7*, 181.

Dependence. Prolonged use of phenobarbitone may lead to dependence of the barbiturate-alcohol type (see p.792).

Studies in *animals* indicated that enzyme induction is not responsible for the development of tolerance to phenobarbitone.— J. Caldwell *et al.*, *Br. J. Pharmac.*, 1978, *62*, 438P.

A retrospective study of the development of psychiatric illness in 51 male drug abusers. At the end of 6 years, 6 of 11 patients who used stimulants (mainly amphetamine or methylphenidate by the end of the study) had been diagnosed as schizophrenic; 8 of 14 patients who used depressants (mainly barbiturates, benzodiazepines, and sedative hypnotics) had anxiety and depression and 5 had attempted suicide. Very little psychological change was apparent in 26 patients who abused opiates.— A. T. McLellan *et al.*, *New Engl. J. Med.*, 1979, *301*, 1310. Comment.— H. G. Pope, *ibid.*, 1341.

Neonatal dependence. An infant born to a 21-year-old woman who had been taking anticonvulsants, including phenobarbitone, was initially hypotonic and unable to suck, then overactive, subject to high-pitched crying, jitteriness, and feeding difficulties. The symptoms abated when phenobarbitone was given and gradually withdrawn. A review of case histories showed that of 53 infants born to barbiturate-treated epileptic mothers 9 were jittery and 19 had feeding difficulties.— I. Blumenthal and S. Lindsay, *Postgrad. med. J.*, 1977, *53*, 157.

Further references: M. M. Desmond *et al.*, *J. Pediat.*, 1972, *80*, 190; *Br. med. J.*, 1972, *4*, 63; M. J. Erith (letter), *ibid.*, 1975, *3*, 40; R. M. Hill *et al.*, *Am. J. Dis. Child.*, 1977, *131*, 546.

Withdrawal. Apart from their use in anaesthetics and epilepsy there are no medical reasons why barbiturates should be prescribed today. No patient who has not received them before should be prescribed barbiturates, and attempts should be made to stop the prescription of barbiturates for chronically dependent subjects. To avoid withdrawal symptoms any alternative to a barbiturate should be gradually substituted over a period of up to 3 months. A benzodiazepine such as diazepam or nitrazepam is the best alternative. One effective substitution scheme involves replacement of 100 mg of barbiturate by 5 mg of diazepam at a rate of one dose weekly enabling the changeover from barbitone 200 mg at night to diazepam 10 mg at night to be spread over 13 weeks. This changeover is almost imperceptible and most patients are prepared to accept the substitution at a rate of diazepam 10 mg for barbiturate 200 mg weekly, taking 7 or 8 weeks in all. After a stabilising period on the benzodiazepine, it too should be withdrawn, using a similarly slow technique but with no substitute drug.— *Drug & Ther. Bull.*, 1976, *14*, 7 and 11.

Further references: D. E. Smith and D. R. Wesson, *J. Am. med. Ass.*, 1970, *213*, 294; *idem*, *Archs gen. Psychiat.*, 1971, *24*, 56.

Adverse Effects. In therapeutic doses the side-effects of barbiturates are mild and include respiratory depression, sedation, and occasional allergic reactions, particularly affecting the skin (where an incidence of 1 to 3% has been reported for phenobarbitone). The skin rashes are most commonly of the maculopapular type, sometimes scarlatiniform; fixed-drug eruptions are commonly associated with barbiturates, and photosensitivity may occur. Purpura, exfoliative dermatitis, erythema multiforme (the Stevens-Johnson syndrome), and toxic epidermal necrolysis have occasionally been reported.

Nystagmus and ataxia may occur with excessive doses, and 'hang-over' with impaired judgement often follows a hypnotic dose of barbiturate. Paradoxical excitement, restlessness, and confusion may occur in the elderly or in the presence of pain; irritability and hyperexcitability may occur in children. Folate deficiency has developed during chronic administration of phenobarbitone for epilepsy, and hypoprothrombinaemia has occurred in infants of mothers who have received phenobarbitone during pregnancy. Hepatitis and cholestasis have been associated with barbiturate administration.

Barbiturate overdosage is a frequent cause of acute poisoning and death; the toxic effects of overdosage include prolonged coma, respiratory depression, and cardiovascular depression, with hypotension and shock leading to renal failure. Absent bowel sounds are a sign of severe poisoning, their return sometimes heralding further absorption of any remaining barbiturate in the gastro-intestinal tract, with resultant relapse. Hypothermia is common, with associated pyrexia during recovery. Characteristic erythematous or haemorrhagic blisters (bullae) occur in about 6% of patients. Death is usually due to respiratory and circulatory failure.

The chronic effects of the barbiturates on neurological and psychic functions closely resemble those of alcohol and symptoms of chronic poisoning include disorientation, mental confusion, ataxia, dizziness, depression, and skin rashes.

Continued use of barbiturates, even in therapeutic doses, may result in psychic or physical dependence. Abrupt withdrawal of the drug may result in a severe abstinence syndrome which includes grand mal seizures and delirium (see Dependence, p.792). Withdrawal of the drug in these cases should be cautious and gradual. Tolerance to the hypnotic effects of barbiturates may also occur after prolonged administration.

Owing to their extreme alkalinity necrosis has followed subcutaneous injection of sodium salts of barbiturates. Intravenous injections can be hazardous and cause hypotension, shock, laryngospasm, and apnoea.

There was a myth that unintentional overdose with barbiturates could occur when a patient took a dose, forgot about it, and took another dose until intoxication occurred.— T. L. Dorpat, *Archs gen. Psychiat.*, 1974, *31*, 216.

Effects on blood and circulation. For a review of the haemodynamic effects of some barbiturates, see C. M. Conway and D. B. Ellis, *Br. J. Anaesth.*, 1969, *41*, 534.

A 31-year-old man dependent on diamorphine and methadone developed swelling, redness, and cyanosis of the limb down to the fingers after the injection into the arm of a barbiturate preparation. He had muscle contracture which was unresolved 12 months later. A further patient suffered blanching of the arm and hand and the loss of all or part of 3 fingers and part of the thumb after the intra-arterial injection of barbiturate.— R. Pollard, *Br. med. J.*, 1973, *1*, 784.

Effects on the kidneys. Mention of acute interstitial nephritis as an occasional side-effect of phenobarbitone.— J. R. Curtis, *Br. med. J.*, 1977, *2*, 242.

Effects on the liver. A review of phenobarbitone-induced hepatic dysfunction.— W. E. Evans *et al.*, *Drug Intell. & clin. Pharm.*, 1976, *10*, 439.

Further references: H. W. Aiges *et al.*, *J. Pediat.*, 1980, *97*, 22.

Effect on mental state. Studies of the cognitive and behavioural effects of phenobarbitone in children: S. M. Wolf and A. Forsythe, *Pediatrics*, 1978, *61*, 728 (hyperactivity), per *Int. pharm. Abstr.*, 1979, *16*, 467; C. S. Camfield *et al.*, *J. Pediat.*, 1979, *95*, 361 (impairment of memory concentration and general comprehension). Criticism.— M. A. Fishman, *ibid.*, 403; C. J. Bacon *et al.*, *Archs Dis. Childh.*, 1981, *56*, 836 (behavioural effects).

Effects on the muscles. An increase in serum-concentrations of creatine phosphokinase and aminotransferases found in patients who had taken overdoses of hypnotics probably resulted from skeletal muscle injury.— N. Wright *et al.*, *Br. med. J.*, 1971, *3*, 347.

Effects on the skin. A review of skin reactions to barbiturates and other hypnotics.— J. Almeyda and A. Levantine, *Br. J. Derm.*, 1972, *86*, 313.

See also under Overdosage (below).

Overdosage. A 25-year-old woman regained consciousness 96 hours after ingestion of phenobarbitone 8 g. Blood-phenobarbitone concentrations fell only slowly. Restlessness, rapid-eye-movement sleep, and insomnia increased over 19 days after the overdosage. Three other patients who took overdoses of sodium amylobarbitone, butobarbitone, and pentobarbitone showed increasing restlessness, increasing rapid-eye-movement sleep, and decreasing sleep duration until disappearance of drug-induced EEG fast activity.— I. Haider and I. Oswald, *Br. med. J.*, 1970, *2*, 318.

A patient developed chorea and torsion dystonia during recovery from an apparent overdose of phenobarbitone.— S. L. Lightman, *Postgrad. med. J.*, 1978, *54*, 114.

Bullous lesions. Reports and comments on bullous lesions associated with barbiturate intoxication: G. W. Beveridge and A. A. H. Lawson, *Br. med. J.*, 1965, *1*, 835; *Lancet*, 1972, *1*, 733.

Shoulder-hand syndrome. Reports and comments on the possible association of the shoulder-hand syndrome with phenobarbitone treatment, usually in epilepsy: J. K. van der Korst *et al.*, *Ann. rheum. Dis.*, 1966, *25*, 553; *Br. med. J.*, 1967, *2*, 130; D. N. Golding (letter), *ibid.*, 572; A. D. Desai and H. M. Dastur, *ibid.*, *4*, 173.

Stomatitis. A report associated with barbiturates.— S. Kennett, *Oral Surg.*, 1968, *25*, 351.

Treatment of Adverse Effects. Avoidance of analeptic therapy, and the introduction of intensive nursing care directed at monitoring and maintaining the physical well-being of the unconscious patient while the drug is being detoxified in the body, has resulted in a considerable decline in the number of deaths from poisoning by barbiturates and other hypnotics. The aims in treating poisoning with barbiturates are thus to maintain respiration, treat shock, and prevent further absorption of the drug.

A clear airway should be maintained and oxygen and assisted respiration provided if necessary. Although analeptics should generally be avoided, a single dose of nikethamide may be given in emergency while other measures to aid respiration are being prepared.

Severe hypotension and shock may respond to placing the patient in the supine position with the feet raised. Failing this, cautious administration of not more than 2 or 3 doses of metaraminol 2.5 mg intravenously at intervals of 20 minutes to raise the systolic pressure to not more than 100 mmHg may be required. Failing this, the intravenous infusion of dextran 40 injection or plasma is indicated, but care must be taken not to overload the circulation. Additional therapy includes provision of oxygen, and correction of acidaemia, cardiac arrhythmias, and congestive heart failure. Hydrocortisone 100 mg every six hours may be beneficial.

If the barbiturate has been taken by mouth, the stomach should be emptied by aspiration and lavage with warm water through a wide-bore tube, leaving the stomach empty at the end of the procedure.

General care involves intensive nursing and includes: half-hourly turning, physiotherapy, and respiratory suction; correction of dehydration with alternate infusions of dextrose injection and sodium chloride injection; and correction of acid-base and electrolyte status, as necessary. Bullous lesions should be treated as superficial burns. Hypothermia, if severe, may also require treatment. In the absence of dehydration, intravenous infusion is unnecessary in the first 12 hours; bladder catheterisation should be avoided unless essential; prophylactic antibiotics should not be given.

Only in severely poisoned patients who continue to deteriorate despite supportive treatment is more active removal of barbiturate from the body indicated. The hazards of these more active measures, which include forced diuresis, peritoneal dialysis, haemodialysis, and haemoperfusion, generally outweigh any purported benefits.

Forced diuresis is only applicable to drugs that are excreted in useful quantities in the urine, either unmetabolised or in the form of an active metabolite. Most barbiturates are converted to inactive metabolites in the liver and only barbitone, phenobarbitone, and possibly butobarbitone are excreted unchanged in the urine in significant amounts. The elimination of phenobarbitone may also be hastened by rendering the urine alkaline. Regimens of forced alkaline diuresis comprise the administration of dextrose injection and sodium chloride injection together with infusions of sodium bicarbonate (1.26%) to maintain the urinary pH above 7.5. Supplements of potassium chloride are given, and osmotic diuretics such as mannitol 5% may be given in association with frusemide. It is essential that the blood chemistry be carefully controlled and adjustments to the fluid and electrolyte balance be made when necessary.

The benefits of peritoneal dialysis and haemodialysis are similarly limited by the properties of the drug, including its molecular weight, the degree of ionisation, its protein- or lipid-binding properties, the relative pH of blood and dialysate, and its toxicity relative to its blood concentration. Of the barbiturates, barbitone and phenobarbitone are more effectively dialysed since they are less protein-bound, less lipid-soluble, and are not extensively metabolised. Trometamol or albumen have been added to peritoneal dialysis fluids to increase recovery.

Newer methods of drug removal include ion-exchange and charcoal haemoperfusion which have some advantages over haemodialysis but which introduce other hazards, see p.79.

In the conscious patient, vomiting may be induced by administration of ipecacuanha (see p.690) but this is not always wholly effective and, if absorbed, may exacerbate the depressant action of the barbiturate; salt solution, apomorphine, and copper sulphate solution should not be used to induce vomiting. Activated charcoal (see p.79) has been administered to reduce absorption of the barbiturate but should not be used before administration of ipecacuanha since it nullifies the emetic effect. Administration of a purgative such as sodium sulphate 30 g in 250 ml of water has also been advocated.

References: H. Matthew and A. A. H. Lawson, *Treatment of Common Acute Poisonings*, 4th Edn, London, Churchill Livingstone, 1979.

Reviews and reports of barbiturate intoxication and treatment: H. Matthew and A. A. H. Lawson, *Q. J. Med.*, 1966, *35*, 539; J. Hadden *et al.*, *J. Am. med. Ass.*, 1969, *209*, 893; H. Matthew, *Clin. Toxicol.*, 1975, *8*, 495; J. M. Goodman *et al.*, *West. J. Med.*, 1976, *124*, 179.

Adsorption. For studies of the adsorptive capacity of oral activated charcoal for phenobarbitone, see under Activated Charcoal, p.79.

Aspiration and lavage. It was recommended that gastric aspiration and lavage should be performed: (a) in patients suffering from barbiturate poisoning who ingested the drug within 4 hours, unless it could be definitely established that fewer than 10 tablets or capsules were taken; (b) if the patient was unconscious and the time of ingestion was not known.— H. Matthew *et al.*, *Br. med. J.*, 1966, *1*, 1333.

In a detailed study of 26 cases of acute barbiturate poisoning it was concluded that gastric lavage was of no value unless carried out within 8 to 10 hours of swallowing the drug.— A. Premel-Cabic *et al.*, *Thérapie*, 1973, *28*, 977.

Dialysis. Some reports on the use of dialysis to treat barbiturate poisoning: H. A. Lee and A. C. Ames, *Br. med. J.*, 1965, *1*, 1217; R. F. Lash *et al.*, *J. Am. med. Ass.*, 1967, *201*, 269; A. C. Kennedy *et al.*, *Lancet*, 1969, *1*, 995.

Diuresis. A favourable report on forced alkaline diuresis in 110 patients with severe barbiturate overdosage.— A. L. Linton *et al.*, *Lancet*, 1967, *2*, 377. Criticism.— H. Matthew and A. A. H. Lawson (letter), *ibid.*, 559. Reply.— A. L. Linton *et al.* (letter), *ibid.*, 677.

Other reports and studies on the beneficial effects of forced diuresis in barbiturate intoxication: H. A. Bloomer, *J. Lab. clin. Med.*, 1966, *67*, 898; G. E. Mawer and H. A. Lee, *Br. med. J.*, 1968, *2*, 790.

Haemoperfusion. A technique of pumping the blood over an anion-exchange resin column was successfully used to treat barbiturate poisoning in *dogs* who were given lethal doses of phenobarbitone sodium. The resin column contained Amberlite IRA '900', 860 g in the chloride cycle, 120 g in the bicarbonate cycle, and 120 g in the lactate cycle. Perfusion of the blood over the resin at 100 ml per minute for 2 hours lowered the serum-phenobarbitone concentration from 170 µg per ml to between 52 and 78 µg per ml.— T. F. Nealon *et al.*, *J. Am. med. Ass.*, 1966, *197*, 118. See also under Activated Charcoal, p.80.

Comment on the role of haemoperfusion in acute intoxication with hypnotic drugs.— *Lancet*, 1979, *2*, 1116.

Precautions. Phenobarbitone and other barbiturates should be administered cautiously to the elderly; reduced dosage should be employed until tolerance is assessed. They should be used with care in patients with impaired hepatic or renal function and are contra-indicated when the impairment is severe. They are also contra-indicated in patients with acute intermittent porphyria, and in hyperkinetic children. Care is needed when barbiturates are given to patients with severe respiratory insufficiency.

The number of tablets prescribed at any one time should be limited, particularly in patients of unbalanced personality, as barbiturates are frequently used in suicidal attempts.

In the presence of severe pain, barbiturates may fail to exert their hypnotic action and may cause wakefulness, excitement, and delirium unless accompanied by an analgesic.

Phenobarbitone and other barbiturates cause drowsiness and patients receiving them should not take charge of vehicles or machinery where loss of attention could cause accidents.

Soluble salts of barbiturates are given parenterally and as these tend to be alkaline care should be taken to avoid extravasation.

The effects of phenobarbitone and other barbiturates are enhanced by concurrent administration of other sedatives, monoamine oxidase inhibitors, and some tranquillisers, and may be enhanced by anticholinesterases, sodium valproate, sulphonylurea antidiabetics, and tricyclic antidepressants.

The concomitant administration of barbiturates and alcohol may produce very serious respiratory depression and a lowering of the lethal dose of the barbiturate. The effects of other depressants of the central nervous system such as anaesthetics, antihistamines, and narcotic analgesics may also be enhanced by barbiturates. The effects of phenothiazines may be initially enhanced and subsequently diminished. The effects of phenobarbitone may be diminished by rendering the urine alkaline and possibly by reserpine and folic acid.

Phenobarbitone and other barbiturates may also enhance the activity of methotrexate, cyclophosphamide, and sulphonylureas, as well as the toxic effects of tricyclic antidepressants.

Phenobarbitone and other barbiturates increase the rate of metabolism of many drugs by induction of drug-metabolising enzymes in liver microsomes. This may result in a reduction in activity. Drugs affected include carbamazepine, coumarin anticoagulants, doxycycline, folic acid, phenylbutazone, phenazone, phenytoin, corticosteroids and other steroid hormones. The activity of griseofulvin may be reduced if it is given by mouth with phenobarbitone.

Variations, in identical and fraternal twins, in the plasma concentration of phenazone when phenobarbitone was given concomitantly suggested that the induction of enzymes by phenobarbitone was genetically controlled.— E. S. Vesell *et al.*, *Ann. N.Y. Acad. Sci.*, 1971, *179*, 752.

The effect of phenobarbitone on hepatic drug-metabolising enzymes and urinary D-glucaric acid excretion.— D. S. Lecamwasam *et al.*, *Br. J. clin. Pharmac.*, 1975, *2*, 257.

Administration in the elderly. Barbiturates might precipitate accidental hypothermia in the elderly and they should be used with care, especially in winter, for patients who were not under regular medical supervision, and the dosage should be kept to the minimum.— Amulree, *Abstr. Wld Med.*, 1968, *42*, 333.

Barbiturate usage appeared to be a major factor in producing nocturnal falls resulting in femoral fracture in elderly patients. Of 98 patients suffering nocturnal falls 93% were taking barbiturates compared with 6% of 217 suffering morning falls and none of 75 suffering afternoon falls. Of 97 taking barbiturates 37 had mental status scores below the minimum level considered necessary for living alone; after withdrawal of barbiturates only 1 had a score below that level.— J. B. Macdonald and E. T. Macdonald, *Br. med. J.*, 1977, *2*, 483.

Administration in hepatic failure. A 57-year-old mentally deficient epileptic man who was on long-term phenobarbitone and primidone therapy developed toxic blood concentrations in association with acute hepatitis. He became comatose and required resuscitation.— K. E. L. McColl *et al.* (letter), *Lancet*, 1978, *1*, 1201.

Administration in renal failure. Of 39 patients who had received regular haemodialysis for 4 years or longer, pathological fractures and histological evidence of osteomalacia were significantly more common in those taking barbiturates. Of 58 renal transplant recipients surveyed after 1 year, 7 had osteomalacia; 4 of these 7 had been taking phenobarbitone and phenytoin and 1 had been taking amylobarbitone (having previously received phenytoin while on haemodialysis). It was considered that agents such as barbiturates and phenytoin that induced hepatic microsomal enzymes should probably be avoided where possible in patients with chronic renal failure and after transplantation.— A. M. Pierides *et al.*, *Br. med. J.*, 1976, *1*, 190.

Interactions. A review of drug interactions involving hypnotics and sedatives.— S. R. Brown and E. A. Hartshorn, *Drug Intell. & clin. Pharm.*, 1976, *10*, 570.

For reports, in addition to those given below, on the effects of phenobarbitone on the adverse effects, metabolism, excretion, and therapeutic effects of various drugs, see under the precautions for carbamazepine, chlorpromazine, clonazepam, corticosteroids, cyclophosphamide, desipramine hydrochloride, digitoxin, doxycycline hydrochloride, methyldopa, phenazone, phenytoin sodium, and warfarin sodium.

Alcohol. The Committee on Safety of Drugs suggested that patients be warned not to take alcohol while under treatment with drugs affecting the CNS, in particular, barbiturates and antihistamines.— *Chemist Drugg.*, 1968, *190*, 524.

Calcium. For reference to the effect of phenobarbitone on serum-calcium concentrations, see under Vitamin D (below).

Chloramphenicol. Serum concentrations of phenytoin and phenobarbitone in a previously stabilised patient were increased when he took chloramphenicol concomitantly. Subsequent monitoring revealed a similar effect when chloramphenicol was taken with phenobarbitone alone.— J. R. Koup *et al.*, *Clin. Pharmac. Ther.*, 1978, *24*, 571.

For the effect of phenobarbitone on serum-concentrations of chloramphenicol, see under Chloramphenicol, p.1138.

Coumarin anticoagulants. The mean serum-phenobarbitone concentration in 4 subjects taking phenobarbitone 50 mg thrice daily rose from 17 to 28 µg per ml when dicoumarol was given concomitantly.— J. M. Hansen *et al.* (preliminary communication), *Lancet*, 1966, *2*, 265.

For a review of the effects of barbiturates on coumarin anticoagulants, see J. Koch-Weser and E. M. Sellers, *New Engl. J. Med.*, 1971, *85*, 549.

Frusemide. Serum-phenobarbitone concentrations were raised in 8 of 10 epileptic patients taking phenobarbitone and additional anticonvulsants when given frusemide 40 mg thrice daily for 4 weeks. This might have been the cause of drowsiness in 5 of 14 patients, 3 of whom had to discontinue frusemide.— S. Ahmad *et al.*, *Br. J. clin. Pharmac.*, 1976, *3*, 621.

Glucose. Phenobarbitone should be used with caution in patients with diabetes mellitus since it could interact to lower blood-glucose concentrations.— *Drug & Ther. Bull.*, 1973, *11*, 5.

Methsuximide. For the effect of methsuximide on phenobarbitone, see Phenytoin, p.1239.

Paracetamol. Combined overdosage of barbiturates and paracetamol is particularly dangerous since the barbiturate cannot be metabolised in the presence of paracetamol-induced liver damage.— L. F. Prescott, *Adv. Med. Topics Ther.*, 1975, *1*, 21.

Phenytoin. Phenytoin might interfere with estimations of barbiturates in the blood.— J. Millhouse, *Adverse Drug React. Bull.*, 1974, Dec., 164.

Phenobarbitone induces the enzymes which metabolise phenytoin but because both phenobarbitone and phenytoin compete for the same enzymes the metabolism of phenytoin may be inhibited rather than enhanced; the plasma concentration of phenobarbitone may be increased by phenytoin.— *Drug & Ther. Bull.*, 1976, *14*, 13. See also under Precautions for Phenytoin, p.1239.

Pyridoxine. Pyridoxine reduced serum-phenobarbitone concentrations in 5 patients.— O. Hansson and M. Sillanpaa (letter), *Lancet*, 1976, *1*, 256.

Quinidine. For the effect of phenobarbitone on quinidine, see Quinidine, p.1371.

Sulthiame. Serum concentrations of phenobarbitone were enhanced when sulthiame was given concomitantly.— O. V. Olesen and O. N. Jensen, *Dan. med. Bull.*, 1969, *16*, 154, per A. Richens and G. W. Houghton (letter), *Lancet*, 1973, *2*, 1442.

Sulthiame might interfere with estimations of barbiturates in the blood.— J. Millhouse, *Adverse Drug React. Bull.*, 1974, Dec., 164.

Theophylline. For the effect of phenobarbitone on the disposition of theophylline, see under Aminophylline, p.343.

Thiopentone. Epileptics on heavy doses of phenobarbitone and phenytoin might be sensitive to the depressant effects of thiopentone and methohexitone on respiration because their barbiturate detoxifying mechanisms were saturated.— *Lancet*, 1967, *1*, 991.

Valproate. Phenobarbitone requirements were significantly reduced in 11 of 13 epileptic patients on addition of sodium valproate. Phenobarbitone concentrations in the blood significantly increased in the other 2 patients who remained on a constant dose.— B. J. Wilder *et al.*, *Neurology, Minneap.*, 1978, *28*, 892.

Evidence for inhibition of phenobarbitone metabolism by valproate.— I. M. Kapetanović *et al.*, *Clin. Pharmac. Ther.*, 1981, *29*, 480.

Serum concentrations of phenobarbitone were measured in 7 epileptic patients who had been given sodium valproate in addition to their usual anticonvulsant therapy. A significant rise was noted.— A. Richens and S. Ahmad, *Br. med. J.*, 1975, *4*, 255.

For a suggestion that concomitant administration of phenobarbitone may enhance sodium valproate-associated liver damage, see Sodium Valproate, p.1256.

Further references: J. Bruni *et al.*, *Neurology, N.Y.*, 1980, *30*, 94; I. H. Patel *et al.*, *Clin. Pharmac. Ther.*, 1980, *27*, 515.

Vitamin D. Phenobarbitone could interfere biologically with chemical estimations for calcium in the blood to produce erroneous lowered results.— *Drug & Ther. Bull.*, 1972, *10*, 69.

Investigations in *rats* and *dogs* did not demonstrate that the activity of vitamin D was affected by phenobarbitone.— T. Balazs *et al.*, *Toxic. appl. Pharmac.*, 1974, *29*, 47. Further studies in *rats* giving similar results.— R. Burt *et al.*, *J. clin. Pharmac.*, 1976, *16*, 393.

Serum-alkaline-phosphatase and urinary hydroxyproline concentrations were increased early in treatment with phenobarbitone in a study of 36 children requiring prolonged anticonvulsant treatment. There were no obvious bone changes and a dose of ergocalciferol 200,000 units did not reverse the changes. However 4000 units of ergocalciferol daily for 2 months delayed the emergence of rickets or corrected latent rickets. Phenobarbitone was considered to be associated with the development of rickets.— D. Liakakos *et al.*, *J. Pediat.*, 1975, *87*, 291.

In 21 patients taking barbiturates for conditions other than epilepsy serum-calcium concentrations were significantly lower than in 31 patients taking diazepam or nitrazepam, or 28 controls. The clinical significance was not clear, but vitamin-D metabolism might be affected and the possibility of osteomalacia in such patients should be considered.— R. E. Young *et al.*, *Postgrad. med. J.*, 1977, *53*, 212. See also *idem* (letter), *Br. med. J.*, 1977, *2*, 700.

For reports of vitamin-D deficiency and osteomalacia in patients taking anticonvulsants including phenobarbitone, see under Phenytoin Sodium, p.1236.

Xylose. A report of reduced xylose absorption in 15 subjects after a short course of phenobarbitone.— M. J. Kendall and L. Beeley (letter), *Br. med. J.*, 1974, *3*, 471.

Pregnancy and the neonate. Of 836 mothers of congenitally malformed infants 27 had used barbiturates during the first trimester of pregnancy, compared with 12 in 836 controls. The case : control incidence ratio of 2.25 was significant; when families with a history of congenital malformation were excluded the ratio (2) was no longer significant.— G. Greenberg *et al.*, *Br. med. J.*, 1977, *2*, 853.

Of 50 282 children born to mothers monitored by the Collaborative Perinatal Project, 2413 were found to have been exposed to barbiturates, and possibly other drugs, at some time during the first 4 months of the pregnancy. Some suggestion of association between barbiturate exposure and cardiovascular malformations was noted with amylobarbitone and quinalbarbitone producing the stronger associations. The findings require independent confirmation before any conclusions can be made.— O. P. Heinonen *et al.*, *Birth Defects and Drugs in Pregnancy*, Littleton MA, Publishing Sciences Group, 1977, p. 335.

A report of increased risk of brain tumours in children exposed to barbiturates *in utero* or in early childhood.— E. Gold *et al.*, *J. natn. Cancer Inst.*, 1978, *61*, 1031.

For a general comment on epilepsy and pregnancy, for references to surveys on the incidence of congenital malformations in the infants of epileptic women, and for a study demonstrating an increased incidence of a vitamin K responsive coagulation defect in the infants of mothers given barbiturates, see Phenytoin, p.1238.

For reference to foetal head growth retardation in the children of epileptic mothers given phenobarbitone during pregnancy, see Carbamazepine, p.1246.

Absorption and Fate. Barbiturates are readily absorbed from the gastro-intestinal tract and most act within 30 minutes of ingestion, although the relatively lipid-insoluble barbitone and phenobarbitone may require an hour or longer. The sodium salts are a little more rapid in action. Barbiturates diffuse across the placenta and may be excreted in the milk of nursing mothers.

The duration of action of barbiturates depends on their rate of inactivation in the liver and rate of excretion unchanged in the urine. Barbitone and phenobarbitone are mainly excreted unchanged in the urine but most of the other barbiturates are inactivated, mainly by hydroxylation, in the liver though a variable proportion is excreted unchanged.

Phenobarbitone is only about 40% bound to plasma proteins, is not very lipid-soluble, and is only partly metabolised in the liver. About 25% or more of a dose is excreted in the urine unchanged. It has a plasma half-life of up to about 75 hours in children and 100 hours in adults; this is increased in the elderly, in overdosage, and in renal or hepatic disease. Small amounts have been reported to be excreted in the bile. Its excretion is increased in high-volume alkaline urine.

Absorption. In a double-blind study in 41 healthy subjects, phenobarbitone sodium 150 mg or quinalbarbitone sodium 150 mg produced more rapid and deeper impairment of performance in mental and physical tests than phenobarbitone or quinalbarbitone, probably resulting from a more rapid absorption of the sodium salts.— L. C. Epstein and L. Lasagna, *J. Pharmac. exp. Ther.*, 1968, *164*, 433.

There was no significant difference in serum concentration when equivalent doses of phenobarbitone were given by mouth or by intramuscular injection. Peak serum concentrations occurred 1 to 3 hours after administration, and the elimination half-life was about 90 hours.— C. T. Viswanathan *et al.*, *J. clin. Pharmac.*, 1978, *18*, 100.

Evaluation of phenobarbitone sodium given intramuscularly to 11 and by mouth to 16 children, all of whom had experienced febrile convulsions, showed the intramuscular route to be of little value in the therapeutic management of such children.— J. L. Pearce *et al.*, *Pediatrics*, 1977, *60*, 569. A study of the absorption of phenobarbitone following intramuscular administration of single doses in infants.— A. Bracket-Liermain *et al.*, *J. Pediat.*, 1975, *87*, 624.

Distribution. Phenobarbitone was bound to serum albumin mainly in its ionised form, as were amylobarbitone and pentobarbitone.— J. -O. Brånstad and U. Meresaar, *Acta pharm. suec.*, 1972, *9*, 129.

There was significant correlation between brain and plasma concentrations of phenobarbitone in 8 patients with epilepsy undergoing temporal lobectomy.— F. Vajda *et al.*, *Clin. Pharmac. Ther.*, 1974, *15*, 597.

Monitoring of saliva-phenobarbitone concentrations.— C. E. Cook *et al.*, *Clin. Pharmac. Ther.*, 1975, *18*, 742. See also M. Danhof and D. D. Breimer, *Clin. Pharmacokinet.*, 1978, *3*, 39.

Serum protein binding of phenobarbitone in 220 patients varied between 20% and 75% with a mean of 47.4%.— H. Walther and F. P. Meyer, *Int. J. clin. Pharmac. Biopharm.*, 1979, *17*, 392, per *Int. pharm. Abstr.*, 1980, *17*, 426.

Metabolism and excretion. The serum half-life of phenobarbitone in 6 children ranged from 37 to 73 hours which is lower than that reported for adults.— L. K. Garrettson *et al.*, *Clin. Pharmac. Ther.*, 1970, *11*, 674.

A quantitative determination of phenobarbitone and its main metabolites in the urine.— N. Kållberg *et al.*, *Eur. J. clin. Pharmac.*, 1975, *9*, 161. See also M. P. Whyte and A. S. Dekaban, *Drug Metab. & Disposit.*, 1977, *5*, 63.

Pregnancy and the neonate. In 32 mothers regularly taking phenobarbitone or primidone, the concentration of phenobarbitone found in the serum of the umbilical cord after parturition was 95% of the level in the mother's serum. The rate of elimination of phenobarbitone in newborn infants varied from 1% to 20% daily.— J. C. Melchior *et al.*, *Lancet*, 1967, *2*, 860.

A study of phenytoin and phenobarbitone clearance during pregnancy.— K. I. Mygind *et al.*, *Acta neurol. scand.*, 1976, *54*, 160.

In neonates up to 4 weeks of age, the elimination half-life of phenobarbitone was significantly longer than in older infants. This was considered to be due to slower renal elimination in neonates, rather than reduced metabolism in the liver.— G. Heimann and E. Gladtke, *Eur. J. clin. Pharmac.*, 1977, *12*, 305. See also L. O. Boréus *et al.*, *Acta paediat. scand.*, 1978, *67*, 193.

In a study of 14 patients the plasma clearance of phenytoin, phenobarbitone, and carbamazepine was generally increased during pregnancy and immediately after delivery although there were considerable individual fluctuations.— M. Dam *et al.*, *Clin. Pharmacokinet.*, 1979, *4*, 53.

Further references: W. Pitlick *et al.*, *Clin. Pharmac. Ther.*, 1978, *23*, 346; L. O. Boreus *et al.*, *J. Pediat.*, 1978, *93*, 695; L. N. Rossi *et al.*, *Acta paediat. scand.*, 1979, *68*, 431.

For a study of the concentrations of anticonvulsant drugs, including phenobarbitone, in serum and breast milk in lactating women, see under Phenytoin, p.1241.

See also under Dependence and Precautions.

Uses. Phenobarbitone is a barbiturate (see p.792) used as a hypnotic and sedative and as an anticonvulsant in the treatment of epilepsy. It is especially of value in the treatment of patients with grand mal seizures or psychomotor attacks. Sudden withdrawal of phenobarbitone from an epileptic patient should be avoided as it may precipitate a conditon of status epilepticus.

The usual hypnotic dose of phenobarbitone is 100 mg at night and the usual sedative dose is 15 to 30 mg three or four times daily. In general, more recently developed and safer drugs, such as the benzodiazepines, are now preferred for the purposes of sedation and sleep induction.

The usual anticonvulsant dose of phenobarbitone is 30 to 60 mg twice or thrice daily. Young children may be given 1 to 2 mg per kg body-weight thrice daily. Plasma-phenobarbitone concentrations required for the control of epilepsy are usually about 10 to 30 µg per ml, with a minimum of 15 µg per ml being required to control febrile convulsions. Doses of about 200 mg of phenobarbitone sodium, repeated after 6 hours if necessary, may be given intramuscularly for the emergency control of convulsions. Children may be given 3 to 5 mg per kg intramuscularly, but doubts have been expressed as to the efficacy of phenobarbitone by the intramuscular route in emergency, owing to the delay in achieving adequate blood concentrations. Phenobarbitone sodium has also been given, slowly and well diluted, by intravenous injection but the intravenous route is hazardous. Subcutaneous injections may cause tissue necrosis.

Phenobarbitone stimulates the enzymes in hepatic microsomes responsible for the metabolism of some drugs and normal body constituents including bilirubin. For this reason phenobarbitone has been used to reduce hyperbilirubinaemia in neonatal jaundice.

The dose of phenobarbitone required to produce a given plasma-phenobarbitone concentration tended to decrease progressively with age in a study of 121 patients. In children under 5 years of age, boys tended to require higher doses than girls to achieve the same plasma concentrations. The relationship between plasma-phenobarbitone concentration and phenobarbitone dose was not affected by phenytoin, carbamazepine, or sulthiame.— M. J. Eadie *et al.*, *Br. J. clin. Pharmac.*, 1977, *4*, 541.

Administration in hepatic failure. A study of the disposition of phenobarbitone in patients with cirrhosis of the liver and acute viral hepatitis compared with healthy subjects. It might be reasonable to choose phenobarbitone as a sedative in patients with liver disease, but until results of long-term studies were known blood-phenobarbitone concentrations should be monitored periodically in patients with severe liver disease undergoing long-term phenobarbitone therapy.— J. Alvin *et al.*, *J. Pharmac. exp. Ther.*, 1975, *192* 224.

See also under Precautions.

Administration in renal failure. The usual phenobarbitone half-life of 36 to 96 hours was increased to 117 hours in end-stage renal failure. The interval between doses should be extended from 8 hours to 8 to 16 hours in patients with a glomerular filtration-rate of less than 10 ml per minute. Concentrations of phenobarbitone were affected by haemodialysis and peritoneal dialysis.— W. M. Bennett *et al.*, *Ann. intern. Med.*, 1980, *93*, 286.

See also under Precautions.

Convulsions. For detailed comments on the role of the different anticonvulsants in epilepsy, see Phenytoin, p.1243.

Febrile convulsions. In a study completed by 161 children without known neurological disorder who suffered their first febrile convulsion between the ages of 6 months and 3 years, regular treatment with phenobarbitone did not appear to prevent the convulsions. Of 88 who received phenobarbitone therapy 10 had further convulsions during a 6-month study period compared with 14 of 73 control children; of the 88 only 49 took the phenobarbitone regularly and 4 had convulsions.— J. Z. Heckmatt *et al.*, *Br. med. J.*, 1976, *1*, 559. Criticism.— S. M. Wolf and A. B. Forsythe (letter), *ibid.*, 1277. A reply.— J. Z. Heckmatt *et al.*, *ibid.*

In a study of 355 children seen after their first febrile convulsion continuous treatment with phenobarbitone 3 to 4 mg per kg body-weight daily increased at the time of any fever was more effective in preventing convulsions than intermittent treatment or a placebo.— S. M. Wolf *et al.*, *Pediatrics*, 1977, *59*, 378.

Absorption of phenobarbitone from the intramuscular route was inconsistent and would be unlikely to arrest an established convulsion within a critical time period.— J. L. Pearce *et al.*, *Pediatrics*, 1977, *60*, 569.

A placebo-controlled study of phenobarbitone and phenytoin in the prophylaxis of febrile convulsions. Results indicated that for children who have a first seizure before 14 months of age phenobarbitone, at plasma concentrations above 15 mg per litre, is effective. Behavioural disturbance in children taking phenobarbitone was not a serious problem.— C. J. Bacon *et al.*, *Lancet*, 1981, *2*, 600 and 704. Criticism.— J. B. P. Stephenson (letter), *ibid.*, 1051.

For the role of anticonvulsants in the treatment and prevention of febrile convulsions in children, see also Diazepam, p.1525.

Haemolytic disease of newborn. Phenobarbitone, in doses of approximately 2 mg per kg body-weight, reduced the number of exchange transfusions required by 30 infants with rhesus haemolytic disease to 21, compared with 40 required by 30 control infants. No neonatal mortality occurred in the treated group, but 2 infants in the control group died as a direct result of haemolytic disease or exchange transfusion.— G. P. McMullin *et al.*, *Lancet*, 1970, *2*, 949. Comments and criticisms.— W. Walker (letter), *ibid.*, 1089. A reply.— G. P. McMullin (letter), *ibid.*, 1194.

Hypnotic effect. Report of EEG studies in volunteers to determine the effect of barbiturates on sleep.— J. I. Evans *et al.*, *Br. Med. J.*, 1968, *4*, 291.

Discussions on the use of barbiturates and other similar hypnotics.— *J. Am. med. Ass.*, 1974, *230*, 1440; *Drug & Ther. Bull.*, 1976, *14*, 7 and 11.

Intraventricular haemorrhage. The possible role of phenobarbitone in the prevention of intraventricular haemorrhage in preterm infants.— S. M. Donn *et al.*, *Lancet*, 1981, *2*, 215. Comments and criticisms.— R. W. I. Cooke *et al.* (letter), *ibid.*, 414; P. L. Hope *et al.* (letter), *ibid.*, 527; H. S. Schub *et al.* (letter), *ibid.*, 869.

Jaundice. Four patients with jaundice and generalised itching due to chronic intrahepatic cholestasis were treated with phenobarbitone in a daily dose of 180 mg. Total bilirubin concentrations in plasma were substantially reduced, generally within the first week or 2 of treatment, and the patients noted a striking decrease in itching and an improvement in general well-being. In each case the jaundice was reduced. Drowsiness and lethargy were experienced by all the patients but were controlled by reducing the dosage. One patient was maintained on a dose of 90 mg of phenobarbitone daily and 2 patients were controlled on 120 mg; daily doses were divided and given at noon and at bedtime. Phenobarbitone was considered to lower plasma-bilirubin concentrations by stimulating the enzymes in liver microsomes.— R. P. H. Thompson and R. Williams, *Lancet*, 1967, *2*, 646.

A 9-month-old boy with complete extrahepatic biliary atresia obtained a striking decrease in the symptoms of pruritus and excoriation during 3 months' treatment with phenobarbitone. Initially, a dose of 10 mg was given thrice daily but was later increased to 40 mg daily. Though the patient's general condition improved the clinical jaundice persisted.— M. D. Cunningham *et al.* (letter), *Lancet*, 1968, *1*, 1089. See also R. P. H. Thompson and R. Williams (letter), *Lancet*, 1970, *2*, 466; L. G. Linarelli *et al.*, *J. Pediat.*, 1973, *83*, 291.

Phenobarbitone 120 to 250 mg daily was given to 15 patients with various cholestatic disorders (primary biliary cirrhosis, sclerosing cholangitis, intrahepatic biliary hypoplasia, and cholestatic hepatitis) for 1 to 5 months. Serum bilirubin and bile acid concentrations were reduced and there was relief from pruritus in most patients except those with cholestatic hepatitis. Hepatic clearance of sulphobromophthalein and rose bengal sodium (^{131}I) was enhanced in some patients and there was a significant increase in serum alkaline phosphatase concentration in 12 patients. One patient withdrew because of a skin rash.— J. R. Bloomer and J. L. Boyer, *Ann. intern. Med.*, 1975, *82*, 310.

Further references: M. J. Kreek and M. H. Sleisenger, *Lancet*, 1968, *2*, 73; I. Matsuda and A. Takase, *ibid.*, 1969, *2*, 1006; I. J. Ertel and W. A. Newton, *Pediatrics*, 1969, *44*, 43; M. Black and S. Sherlock, *Lancet*, 1970, *1*, 1359; M. M. Thaler and R. Schmid, *Pediatrics*, 1971, *47*, 807; H. L. Sharp and B. L. Mirkin, *J. Pediat.*, 1972, *81*, 116; W. Braun *et al.*, *Schweiz. med. Wschr.*, 1972, *102*, 1769; J. Espinoza *et al.*, *Am. J. Obstet. Gynec.*, 1974, *119*, 234; M. Shani *et al.*, *Gastroenterology*, 1974, *67*, 303.

Jaundice, neonatal. In a controlled study, treatment of pregnant women with phenobarbitone sodium, 30 to 120 mg daily, for 2 weeks or more prior to delivery significantly lowered serum-bilirubin concentrations in the infants. The maximum mean serum-bilirubin concentration was 25 µg per ml for infants whose mothers had taken phenobarbitone and occurred on the second day of life. The comparable figure in the control group was 57 µg per ml and was reached on the third day of life.— H. M. Maurer *et al.*, *Lancet*, 1968, *2*, 122.

Phenobarbitone treatment for neonatal jaundice was most effective when the mother was given 50 to 150 mg of phenobarbitone daily for at least 3 days before delivery and the infant was given 5 mg intramuscularly on 7 to 10 occasions during the first 3 days after birth.— D. Trolle, *Lancet*, 1968, *2*, 705.

Treatment with phenobarbitone, 8 mg per kg body-weight daily in 2 divided doses every 12 hours for 6 consecutive doses, failed to show any significant clinical or chemical response in 52 full-term infants with icterus neonatorum. It was assumed that once unconjugated bilirubin was present in the blood of neonates, treatment with phenobarbitone was ineffective.— M. D. Cunningham *et al.*, *Lancet*, 1969, *1*, 550.

Chinese babies with jaundice due to ABO incompatibility, glucose-6-phosphate dehydrogenase deficiency, cephalhaematoma, and non-specific causes during the first 2 weeks after birth were given phenobarbitone, 5 mg eight-hourly, for 2 to 7 days until jaundice subsided or the serum-bilirubin concentration fell below 100 µg per ml; phenobarbitone, 6 mg per kg body-weight daily in 3 equally divided doses, was given to babies under 2.5 kg. Only 4 of 93 babies treated with phenobarbitone, but 53 of 117 untreated babies, required an exchange transfusion.— C. Y. Yeung and C. E. Field, *Lancet*, 1969, *2*, 135.

In a comparative study, 44 newborn infants were given phenobarbitone 5 mg every 8 hours for an average of 3.5 days, the mothers of a further 44 received phenobarbitone 30 mg every night for an average of 2 weeks before delivery, and a control group of 45 were not treated. There were significantly less hyperbilirubinaemia in treated infants, and treating the infant was more effective than treating the mother, possibly because of the low dose and short course given to the latter.— C. Y. Yeung *et al.*, *Pediatrics*, 1971, *48*, 372.

Blue fluorescent light was more effective than phenobarbitone in reducing hyperbilirubinaemia in 75 mainly Negro, low birth-weight infants.— O. S. Valdes *et al.*, *J. Pediat.*, 1971, *79*, 1015. A similar result in 6 sets of premature identical twins.— M. G. Blackburn *et al.*, *Pediatrics*, 1972, *49*, 110.

A study of phenobarbitone in neonates suggesting a possible additional therapeutic benefit of increased blood sugar concentrations.— C. Y. Yeung, *Archs Dis. Childh.*, 1972, *47*, 246.

Only 8 of 221 neonates born to mothers given phenobarbitone 15 mg four times daily starting at 36 weeks' gestation, developed significant jaundice, whereas 39 of 239 control infants did so.— C. R. Thomas, *Obstet. Gynec.*, 1976, *47*, 304.

Further references: C. Y. Yeung and V. Y. Yu, *Pediatrics*, 1971, *48*, 556; D. Gmyrek *et al.*, *Dte Gesundh-Wes.*, 1972, *27*, 2221; T. F. Halpin *et al.*, *Obstet. Gynec.*, 1972, *40*, 85; H. W. Kintzel *et al.*, *Schweiz. med. Wschr.*, 1972, *102*, 1339; T. Meloni *et al.*, *J. Pediat.*, 1973, *82*, 1048; J. -P. Babin *et al.*, *Thérapie*, 1974, *29*, 399.

Narcotic withdrawal. Phenobarbitone has been employed to control neonatal withdrawal symptoms, especially irritability and insomnia. A dose of 5 to 10 mg per kg body-weight per 24 hours, given in 3 or 4 divided portions is usually sufficient. This dose is maintained for 10 to 40 days and tapered off over 1 to 3 weeks.— R. G. Harper and G. B. Edwards, *Drug Abuse in Pregnancy and Neonatal Effects*, J. L. Rementeria (Ed.), Saint Louis, C.V. Mosby, 1977, p. 103.

Further references: R. M. Hill and M. M. Desmond, *Pediat. Clins N. Am.*, 1963, *10*, 67; E. J. Kahn *et al.*, *J. Pediat.*, 1969, *75*, 495; A. M. Reddy *et al.*, *Pediatrics*, 1971, *48*, 353.

Preparations of Phenobarbitone and its Salts

Elixirs

Phenobarbital Elixir *(U.S.P.)*. An elixir containing phenobarbitone and alcohol 12 to 15%. *U.S.P. XVIII* (1970) gave the following formula: phenobarbitone 400 mg, orange oil 0.075 ml, amaranth solution 1 ml, alcohol 15 ml, glycerol 45 ml, syrup 15 ml, water to 100 ml. Store in airtight containers. Protect from light.

Phenobarbitone Elixir *(A.P.F.)*. Phenobarbitone 15 mg, alcohol (90%) 2 ml, glycerol 1.5 ml, aromatic syrup 1 ml, water to 5 ml. *Dose*. 5 to 10 ml.

Phenobarbitone Elixir *(B.P.)*. Phenobarbitone 30 mg, compound orange spirit 0.24 ml, compound tartrazine solution 0.1 ml, alcohol (90%) 4 ml, glycerol 4 ml, water to 10 ml. Protect from light. When a dose less than, or not a multiple of, 5 ml is prescribed the elixir should be diluted to 5 ml, or a multiple, with syrup. Such dilutions must be freshly prepared and not used more than 2 weeks after issue.

The presence of alcohol or some other solvent is essential if phenobarbitone is to remain in solution. Attention is also drawn to the instability of aqueous solutions of phenobarbitone.— W. Lund and M. Lynch (letter), *Pharm. J.*, 1978, *1*, 211.

Injections

Phenobarbital Sodium Injection *(U.S.P.)*. A sterile solution of phenobarbitone sodium (or an equivalent amount of phenobarbitone to adjust the pH) in a suitable solvent. pH 9.2 to 10.2.

Phenobarbitone Injection *(B.P.)*. Phenobarb. Inj.; Phenobarbitone Sodium Injection. A sterile solution of phenobarbitone sodium in a mixture of propylene glycol 90% v/v and Water for Injections 10%. It may contain up to 0.02% of disodium edetate. Sterilised by heating at 98° to 100° for 30 minutes. pH 10 to 11. If intended for intravenous injection it should be diluted to at least 10 times its volume with Water for Injection before use.

Sterile Phenobarbital Sodium *(U.S.P.)*. Sterile phenobarbitone sodium suitable for parenteral use.

Tablets

Phenobarbitone and Theobromine Tablets *(B.P.C. 1973)*. Each contains phenobarbitone 30 mg and theobromine 300 mg. Store in airtight containers. Protect from light. *Dose*. 1 or 2 tablets.

Phenobarbitone Sodium Tablets *(B.P.)*. Phenobarb. Sod. Tab.; Phenobarbital Sodium Tablets*(U.S.P.)*; Soluble Phenobarbitone Tablets. Tablets containing phenobarbitone sodium.
Store in airtight containers.

Phenobarbitone Tablets *(B.P.)*. Phenobarb. Tab.; Phenobarbital Tablets *(U.S.P.)*. Tablets containing phenobarbitone.

Proprietary Preparations of Phenobarbitone and its Salts

Luminal *(Winthrop, UK)*. Phenobarbitone, available as tablets of 15, 30, and 60 mg. (Also available as Luminal in *Arg., Belg., Ger., Spain, Switz., USA*. Luminal in *Canad.* and Luminal Sodium in *USA* contain phenobarbitone sodium).

Parabal *(Sinclair, UK)*. Tablets each containing phenobarbitone sodium dihydroxyaluminiumaminoacetate 250 mg (equivalent, on a molecular basis, to phenobarbitone 10 mg and claimed to be therapeutically equivalent to phenobarbitone 60 mg). Sedative.

Phenobarbitone Spansule *(Smith Kline & French, UK)*. Phenobarbitone, available as sustained-release capsules of 60 and 100 mg.

Theominal *(Winthrop, UK)*. Tablets each containing phenobarbitone 30 mg and theobromine 300 mg.

Other Proprietary Names of Phenobarbitone and its Salts

Arg.— Luminaletas; *Austral.*— Maliasin *(propylhexedrine salt)*; *Belg.*— Gardenal, Luminalettes; *Canad.*— Gardenal, Nova-Pheno; *Fr.*— Gardénal; *Ger.*— Luminaletten, Phenaemal, Phenaemaletten, Seda-Tablinen; *Ital.*— Gardenale, Luminale, Luminalette, Sedofèn, Tequil *(tetraethylammonium salt)*; *Norw.*— Fenemal; *S.Afr.*— Gardenal; *Spain*— Fenilcal *(calcium salt)*, Gardenal, Lumcalcio *(calcium salt)*, Luminaletas; *Swed.*— Fenemal; *Switz.*— Aphenylbarbit, Aphenyletten, Lumen, Luminaletten, Mephabarbital; *USA*— Sedadrops, Solfoton.

Phenobarbitone and phenobarbitone sodium were also formerly marketed in Great Britain under the proprietary names Gardenal and Gardenal Sodium (both *May & Baker*). Preparations containing phenobarbitone or phenobarbitone sodium were also formerly marketed under the proprietary names Becosed Elixir (*Norton*), Beplete, (*Wyeth*), Phenomet (*Woodward*), and Theogardenal (*May & Baker*).

4062-j

Phenylmethylbarbituric Acid. Heptobarbitalum *(distinguish from Heptabarbital)*. 5-Methyl-5-phenylbarbituric acid.
$C_{11}H_{10}N_2O_3$=218.2.

CAS — 76-94-8.

Pharmacopoeias. In *Cz.*

A white crystalline powder with a slightly bitter taste. M.p. about 226°. Very slightly **soluble** in water; soluble 1 in 60 of alcohol; soluble in ether and aqueous solutions of alkalis. A saturated solution in water is acid to litmus.

Phenylmethylbarbituric acid has been used similarly to phenobarbitone as an anticonvulsant in epilepsy in doses of 200 mg twice daily.

A report of disseminated intravascular coagulation associated with toxic epidermal necrolysis (Lyell's syndrome) in a 7-year-old boy treated with phenylmethylbarbituric acid.— J. Kvasnička *et al.*, *Br. J. Derm.*, 1979, *100*, 551.

4063-z

Phetharbital. Phenetharbital; Phenidiemal; *N*-Phenylbarbitone. 5,5-Diethyl-1-phenylbarbituric acid.
$C_{14}H_{16}N_2O_3$=260.3.

CAS — 357-67-5.

Phetharbital is a barbiturate (see p.792) reported to have a less depressant effect than phenobarbitone. It was used as an anticonvulsant and has been given in the treatment of unconjugated hyperbilirubinaemia.

Convulsions. For reference to the use of phetharbital as an anticonvulsant, see J. G. Millichap *et al.*, *Neurology, Minneap.*, 1960, *10*, 575.

Jaundice. In a double-blind crossover study, 11 patients with mild unconjugated hyperbilirubinaemia received tablets of phenobarbitone 60 mg or phetharbital 600 mg for periods of 4 weeks, with a 6-week interval between periods. Both drugs had a similar effect in reducing plasma bilirubin. Phetharbital was preferred by 7 patients and sleepiness was complained of by only 1 patient in this group compared with 6 while taking phenobarbitone. Symptoms of nausea and abdominal pain were not consistently relieved. In severe unconjugated hyperbilirubinaemia, phetharbital caused a significant fall in plasma bilirubin when given in a dosage of up to 1.2 g daily. Withdrawal of either drug caused a return of plasma bilirubin to original concentrations.— J. Hunter *et al.*, *Br. med. J.*, 1971, *2*, 497.

4064-c

Proxibarbal. D_1H; HH184. 5-Allyl-5-(2-hydroxypropyl)barbituric acid.
$C_{10}H_{14}N_2O_4$=226.2.

CAS — 2537-29-3.

Proxibarbal is a barbiturate (see p.792) that has been used as a sedative in doses of 300 to 600 mg daily.

Proxibarbal 100 mg thrice daily for 1 month, twice daily for a 2nd, and once daily for a 3rd month was given to 5 patients with hereditary allergies to dairy produce, meat, eggs, fish, and drugs with an aromatic ring structure. Within 2 months food and drug allergy was completely and urticaria considerably alleviated without undue sedation. Asthma did not improve. The time taken for the patients' serum to destroy histamine was reduced from 6 to 1 hour and urinary-histamine excretion returned to normal. Its mode of action was unclear, but might be based on enzyme induction.— F. G. Sulman (letter), *Lancet*, 1977, *1*, 1206.

Further references: A. Zador, *Gyogyszereink*, 1970, *20*, 16 (vascular headaches).

Proprietary Names

Axeen *(Hommel, Ger.; Bonomelli-Hommel, Ital.; Hommel, Switz.)*; Centralgol *(Valpan, Fr.)*; Ipronal *(Biosedra, Arg.)*.

4065-k

Pyrithyldione. Nu 903; Didropyridinium. 3,3-Diethylpyridine-2,4(1*H*,3*H*)-dione.
$C_9H_{13}NO_2$=167.2.

CAS — 77-04-3.

Pyrithyldione is a hypnotic given in doses of 200 to 400 mg at night.

Proprietary Names

Persedon *(Roche, Belg.; Roche, Ger.; Roche, Swed.; Roche, Switz.)*.

4066-a

Quinalbarbitone.

Secobarbital *(U.S.P.)*; Meballymal. 5-Allyl-5-(1-methylbutyl)barbituric acid.
$C_{12}H_{18}N_2O_3$=238.3.

CAS — 76-73-3.

Pharmacopoeias. In *Braz.* and *U.S.*

A white odourless amorphous or crystalline powder with a slightly bitter taste. Very slightly **soluble** in water; freely soluble in alcohol, ether, and solutions of fixed alkali hydroxides and carbonates; soluble in chloroform. A saturated solution in water has a pH of about 5.6. **Store** in airtight containers.

4067-t

Quinalbarbitone Sodium *(B.P., Eur. P.)*.

Quinalbarb. Sod.; Secobarbitone Sodium; Secobarbitalum Natricum; Secobarbital Sodium *(U.S.P.)*; Meballymalnatrium. Sodium 5-allyl-5-(1-methylbutyl)barbiturate.
$C_{12}H_{17}N_2NaO_3$=260.3.

CAS — 309-43-3.

Pharmacopoeias. In *Arg., Br., Braz., Chin., Eur., Fr., Ger., Ind., Int., It., Neth., Swiss,* and *U.S. U.S.* also includes Sterile Secobarbital Sodium.

A white odourless hygroscopic powder with a bitter taste. **Soluble** 1 in 3 of water and 1 in 5 of alcohol; practically insoluble in chloroform and ether. A 10% solution in water has a pH of 9.7 to 10.5 and decomposes on standing. A 3.9% solution is iso-osmotic with serum.

Incompatibilities as for phenobarbitone sodium (see p.811). **Store** in airtight containers.

Incompatibility. There was loss of clarity when intravenous solutions of quinalbarbitone sodium were mixed with those of diphenhydramine hydrochloride, ephedrine sulphate, erythromycin gluceptate, hydrocortisone sodium succinate, insulin, narcotic salts, noradrenaline acid tartrate, phenytoin sodium, procaine hydrochloride, streptomycin sulphate, tetracycline hydrochloride, or vancomycin hydrochloride.— J. A. Patel and G. L. Phillips, *Am. J. Hosp. Pharm.*, 1966, *23*, 409.

Dependence. Prolonged use of quinalbarbitone sodium may lead to dependence of the barbiturate-alcohol type (see p.792). Quinalbarbitone has been commonly abused.

A report of barbiturate withdrawal syndrome in an infant exposed to quinalbarbitone *in utero* and again at 4 months.— W. A. Bleyer and R. E. Marshall, *J. Am. med. Ass.*, 1972, *221*, 185.

Adverse Effects, Treatment, and Precautions. As for Phenobarbitone, p.812.

Abuse. Volkmann's ischaemic contracture in 3 patients resulted from the inadvertent intra-arterial injection of quinalbarbitone, 50 or 100 mg in tap water.— N. R. Morgan *et al.*, *J. Am. med. Ass.*, 1970, *212*, 476.

A 2-year-old boy who suffered repeated deep comas without obvious explanation had been subjected to administration of quinalbarbitone and amylobarbitone (Tuinal).— J. Lorber (letter), *Lancet*, 1978, *2*, 680.

Administration in the elderly. No relationship between clinical toxicity and age had been noted for quinalbarbitone.— D. J. Greenblatt *et al.*, *Clin. Pharmac. Ther.*, 1977, *21*, 355.

Effects on mental state. A 200-mg dose of quinalbarbitone at night would increase the frequency of drowsy spells on the following day for periods of up to 14 hours after ingestion.— *Br. med. J.*, 1969, *3*, 253.

A report on the incidence of quinalbarbitone use among youthful assaultive and sexual offenders. Quinalbarbitone was considered by the miscreants to increase aggression.— J. R. Tinklenberg and K. M. Woodrow, *Res. Publ. Ass. nerv. ment. Dis.*, 1974, *52*, 209.

Effects on respiration. Pentobarbitone and quinalbarbitone as sodium salts were shown to produce respiratory depression when given in low and high doses of 60 and 180 mg, and 70 and 210 mg respectively to 6 healthy volunteers. From calculations based on the displacement of the respiratory response curve 70 mg of quinalbarbitone was approximately equivalent to 100 mg of pentobarbitone.— C. R. Brown *et al.*, *J. clin. Pharmac.*, 1973, *13*, 28.

Interactions. *Steroids.* Quinalbarbitone affected the estimation of urinary 17-oxo-steroids and 17-oxogenic steroids.— *Adverse Drug React. Bull.*, 1972, June, 104.

Pregnancy and the neonate. For a report suggesting an association between congenital malformations and exposure to quinalbarbitone in pregnancy, see Phenobarbitone, p.814.

Absorption and Fate. See under Phenobarbitone, p.814.
Quinalbarbitone is extensively bound to tissue proteins. It is largely metabolised in the liver, mainly by hydroxylation, and the metabolites are excreted in the urine.

Quinalbarbitone (as free acid) 3.3 mg per kg bodyweight was given by mouth to 6 healthy subjects. The maximum blood concentration was obtained after an average of 3 hours and in all 6 quinalbarbitone was detected in the blood after 108 hours; the calculated biological half-life was 28.9 hours.— J. M. Clifford *et al.*, *Clin. Pharmac. Ther.*, 1974, *16*, 376.

A study of the metabolism of quinalbarbitone following administration of quinalbarbitone sodium 200 or 300 mg to 6 healthy subjects. No unchanged drug was detected in the urine.— J. N. T. Gilbert *et al.*, *J. Pharm. Pharmac.*, 1975, *27*, 343.

Pregnancy and the neonate. Quinalbarbitone sodium was detected in foetal cord blood within 1 minute of intravenous administration to the mother of 200 to 300 mg; equilibrium was reached within 3 to 5 minutes with the foetal concentration 70% of that of the mother. Of 76 infants, 90% showed little or no depression at birth.— F. Moya and V. Thorndike, *Clin. Pharmac. Ther.*, 1963, *4*, 628.

Uses. Quinalbarbitone is a barbiturate (see p.792) that is used as a hypnotic and sedative. As a hypnotic it is usually given in doses of 50 to 100 mg at night but occasionally 200 mg may be required; 30 to 50 mg has been given 3 or 4 times daily as a sedative. Similar doses may be given of the sodium salt.
Quinalbarbitone has been used for premedication in anaesthetic procedures but its use for these purposes has largely been superseded by other agents, such as the benzodiazepines.

Administration in renal failure. Quinalbarbitone could be given in usual doses to patients with renal failure. Concentrations of quinalbarbitone were not affected by haemodialysis or peritoneal dialysis.— W. M. Bennett *et al.*, *Ann. intern. Med.*, 1980, *93*, 286.

Hypnotic effect. In a drug surveillance programme 462 patients received quinalbarbitone as a hypnotic, usually in doses of 50 to 100 mg. In 336 patients evaluated the response was considered good in 80.9%. CNS depression occurred in 2.6% of patients.— S. Shapiro *et al.*, *J. Am. med. Ass.*, 1969, *209*, 2016.

Preparations of Quinalbarbitone and Quinalbarbitone Sodium

Capsules

Quinalbarbitone Capsules *(B.P.)*. Quinalbarb. Caps.; Quinalbarbitone Sodium Capsules. Capsules containing quinalbarbitone sodium. Store at a temperature not exceeding 30°.

Secobarbital Sodium Capsules *(U.S.P.)*. Capsules containing quinalbarbitone sodium. Store in airtight containers.

Elixirs

Secobarbital Elixir *(U.S.P.)*. Quinalbarbitone Elixir. Quinalbarbitone 0.417 to 0.461% w/v in a suitable flavoured vehicle. It contains 10 to 14% of alcohol. Store in airtight containers.

Injections

Secobarbital Sodium Injection *(U.S.P.)*. Quinalbarbitone Sodium Injection. A sterile solution of quinalbarbitone sodium in a suitable solvent. pH 9 to 10.5. Store at 2° to 8°. Protect from light.

Sterile Secobarbital Sodium *(U.S.P.)*. Quinalbarbitone sodium suitable for parenteral use.

Tablets

Quinalbarbitone Tablets *(B.P.)*. Quinalbarb. Tab.; Quinalbarbitone Sodium Tablets. Tablets containing quinalbarbitone sodium. The tablets are sugar-coated.

Proprietary Preparations of Quinalbarbitone and Quinalbarbitone Sodium

Seconal Sodium *(Lilly, UK)*. Quinalbarbitone sodium, available as capsules of 50 and 100 mg. (Also available as Seconal Sodium in *Austral., Belg., Canad., Neth., S.Afr., Switz., USA* and as Seconal-Natrium in *Norw.*).

Tuinal *(Lilly, UK)*. Quinalbarbitone sodium and amylobarbitone sodium in equal parts, available as capsules of 100 mg. For insomnia. *Dose.* 100 to 200 mg at bedtime.

Other Proprietary Names of Quinalbarbitone and Quinalbarbitone Sodium

Dormona *(Switz.)*; Imménoctal *(Fr.)*; Immenox *(Ital.)*; Proquinal, Quinbar *(both Austral.)*; Secogen *(Canad.)*; Seconal *(USA)*; Sedonal Natrium *(Denm.)*; Seral *(Canad.)*.

4068-x

Secbutobarbitone *(B.P.)*. Secbutobarbital; Butabarbital. 5-*sec*-Butyl-5-ethylbarbituric acid.

$C_{10}H_{16}N_2O_3$=212.2.

CAS — 125-40-6.

Pharmacopoeias. In *Br.*

A fine, white, odourless, microcrystalline powder with a bitter taste. M.p. 165° to 168°.
Soluble 1 in 1400 of water, 1 in 12 of alcohol, and 1 in 30 of chloroform and ether; soluble in aqueous solutions of alkali hydroxides and carbonates. A saturated solution in water is acid to litmus.

4069-r

Secbutobarbitone Sodium. Butabarbital Sodium *(U.S.P.)*; Butabarbitone Sodium *(distinguish from Butobarbitone)*; Sodium Butabarbital; Secumalnatrium. Sodium 5-*sec*-butyl-5-ethylbarbiturate.

$C_{10}H_{15}N_2NaO_3$=234.2.

CAS — 143-81-7.

Pharmacopoeias. In *U.S.*

A white powder with a bitter taste. **Soluble** 1 in 2 of water, and 1 in 7 of alcohol; very slightly soluble in chloroform; practically insoluble in ether. A 10% solution in water has a pH of 9.5 to 10.6. **Store** in airtight containers.

Dependence. Prolonged use of secbutobarbitone sodium may lead to dependence of the barbiturate-alcohol type (see p.792).

Adverse Effects, Treatment, and Precautions. As for Phenobarbitone, p.812.

Absorption and Fate. See under Phenobarbitone, p.814.
Secbutobarbitone is probably largely metabolised in the liver. The metabolites are excreted in the urine together with small amounts of unchanged drug. Larger amounts of unchanged drug may be excreted in the urine following overdosage.

A study of the urinary excretion of secbutobarbitone in 3 male volunteers. From 5 to 9% of the drug was excreted unchanged and 24 to 34% was excreted as a terminal carboxylic acid; small amounts of 2 other metabolites were also found.— J. N. T. Gilbert *et al.*, *J. Pharm. Pharmac.*, 1975, *27*, 923.

Uses. Secbutobarbitone is a barbiturate (see p.792) that is used as a hypnotic and sedative. As a hypnotic it is usually given in doses of 50 to 100 mg at night, as a sedative 15 to 30 mg has been given 3 or 4 times daily. Similar doses may be given of the sodium salt.

Preparations of Secbutobarbitone and Secbutobarbitone Sodium

Butabarbital Sodium Capsules *(U.S.P.)*. Capsules containing secbutobarbitone sodium.

Butabarbital Sodium Elixir *(U.S.P.)*. An elixir containing secbutobarbitone sodium, with alcohol. Store in airtight containers.

Butabarbital Sodium Tablets *(U.S.P.)*. Tablets containing secbutobarbitone sodium.

Proprietary Names of Secbutobarbitone and Secbutobarbitone Sodium

Buticaps *(McNeil, USA)*; Butisol Sodium *(Ethnor, Austral.; McNeil, Canad.; McNeil, USA)*; Neo-Barb *(Neo, Canad.)*.

4070-j

Sulphonal *(B.P. 1948)*. 2,2-Bis(ethylsulphonyl)propane.
$C_7H_{16}O_4S_2$=228.3.

CAS — 115-24-2.

Pharmacopoeias. In *Port.*

Odourless, colourless, almost tasteless crystals or white powder. M.p. about 126°. **Soluble** 1 in 450 of water, 1 in 80 of alcohol, 1 in 3 of chloroform, and 1 in 90 of ether.

Sulphonal was formerly used as a hypnotic but is no longer considered suitable for this purpose owing to its toxicity. It has a very slow onset of action (requiring 6 hours) and was only slowly excreted, so that successive doses had a cumulative effect. Symptoms of chronic poisoning included headache, vertigo, hallucinations, confusion, depression, gastric disturbances, liver damage, and haematoporphyrinuria from destruction of haemoglobin.

4071-z

Talbutal *(U.S.P.)*. 5-Allyl-5-*sec*-butylbarbituric acid.
$C_{11}H_{16}N_2O_3$=224.3.

CAS — 115-44-6.

Pharmacopoeias. In *U.S.*

A white crystalline powder with a slightly bitter taste; it may have a slight odour of caramel. It occurs in 2 polymorphic forms with m.p. about 108° and 111°.
Soluble 1 in 500 of water, 1 in 1 of alcohol, 1 in 2 of chloroform, and 1 in 40 of ether; soluble in glacial acetic acid, acetone, and solutions of alkali hydroxides and carbonates. A saturated solution in water is acid to litmus. **Store** in airtight containers.

Talbutal is a barbiturate (see p.792) that has been used as a hypnotic in doses of 120 mg at night, and as a sedative in doses of 30 to 50 mg twice or thrice daily.

Preparations

Talbutal Tablets *(U.S.P.)*. Tablets containing talbutal. Store in airtight containers.

Proprietary Names

Lotusate *(Winthrop, USA)*.

4072-c

Temazepam. 3-Hydroxydiazepam; ER 115; K-3917; SaH 47-603; Wy 3917. 7-Chloro-1,3-dihydro-3-hydroxy-1-methyl-5-phenyl-2*H*-1,4-benzodiazepin-2-one.

$C_{16}H_{13}ClN_2O_2$=300.7.

CAS — 846-50-4.

Dependence. Prolonged use of temazepam may lead to dependence of the barbiturate-alcohol type (see p.792). It has a low liability for abuse.

A report of dependence on temazepam.— L. Ratna, *Br. med. J.*, 1981, *282*, 1837.

Adverse Effects, Treatment, and Precautions. As for Nitrazepam, p.807.

Absorption and Fate. Temazepam is fairly readily absorbed from the gastro-intestinal tract, although there is some individual variation. It has a biphasic half-life probably owing to tissue redistribution. It is excreted in the urine in the form of its conjugate together with small amounts of the demethylated derivative, oxazepam, also in conjugated form.

Following administration of three 10-mg capsules of temazepam to each of 4 healthy subjects, temazepam was rapidly absorbed with peak plasma concentrations obtained within 2 hours in all 4 subjects. On the basis of urinary excretion the amount absorbed varied considerably, ranging from 51.1% to 84.8%. The decline in plasma concentrations was at least biphasic, suggesting extensive distribution in tissues. The rapid phase had a half-life of 2 to 3 hours, reflecting distribution in the tissues and the slow phase had a half-life of 15 to 20 hours representing the apparent elimination of the drug from plasma. Following rectal administration of 30-mg suppositories absorption was slow with more inter-subject variation, and lower peak plasma concentrations were achieved. Following administration of the capsules, conjugates of temazepam and its demethylated metabolites, oxazepam, were detected in the urine in the ratio of twenty to one. No oxazepam could be detected in the plasma after administration of the suppositories.— L. M. Fuccella *et al.*, *Int. J. clin. Pharmac.*, 1972, *6*, 303.

Results of a crossover study in 6 healthy subjects demonstrated that temazepam is more rapidly absorbed from soft than from hard gelatin capsules. Following repeated administration of temazepam 20 mg each night for 7 days, the mean half-life of 5.87 hours was not significantly longer than that of 5.28 hours obtained after the first administration. Following morning administration, however, the mean half-life was significantly longer, being 8.35 hours, suggesting a possible circadian rhythm in the rate of metabolism of temazepam.— L. M. Fuccella *et al.*, *Eur. J. clin. Pharmac.*, 1977, *12*, 383.

Further references: H. J. Schwarz, *Br. J. clin. Pharmac.*, 1979, *8*, *Suppl.* 1, 23S; L. M. Fuccella, *ibid.*, 31S; P. Bittencourt *et al.*, *ibid.*, 37S; A. Huggett *et al.* (letter), *Br. med. J.*, 1981, *282*, 475.

Uses. Temazepam is a benzodiazepine derivative (and a metabolite of diazepam) with hypnotic properties similar to those of nitrazepam (p.808). As a hypnotic it is given in a usual dose of 10 to 30 mg at night; up to 60 mg may sometimes be required.

Reviews of temazepam.— *Drug & Ther. Bull.*, 1978, *16*, 21; R. C. Heel, *Drugs*, 1981, *21*, 321.

For the proceedings of a symposium on temazepam and related 1,4-benzodiazines and their effects on sleep and on performance, see *Br. J. clin. Pharmac.*, 1979, *8*, *Suppl.* 1, 1S–84S.

References: C. Maggini *et al.*, *Arzneimittel-Forsch.*, 1969, *19*, 1647; P. Sarteschi *et al.*, *ibid.*, 1972, *22*, 93; I. Hindmarch, *ibid.*, 1975, *25*, 1836; *idem*, 1976, *26*, 2113; B. M. Stone, *Br. J. clin. Pharmac.*, 1976, *3*, 543; R. G. Priest *et al.*, *J. int. med. Res.*, 1976, *4*, 145; L. K. Fowler, *ibid.*, 1977, *5*, 295; *idem*, 297; E. O. Bixler *et al.*, *J. clin. Pharmac.*, 1978, *18*, 110; T. V. A. Harry and P. A. Johnson, *Curr. med. Res. Opinion*, 1978, *5*, 476; A. N. Nicholson and B. M. Stone, *Br. J. clin. Pharmac.*, 1978, *5*, 352P; R. S. W. Middleton, *J. int. med. Res.*, 1978, *6*, 121; R. S. Briggs *et al.*, *Br. med. J.*, 1980, *280*, 601; I. Oswald and K. Adam (letter), *ibid.*, 860; A. F. Macklon *et al.* (letter), *ibid.*, 861; C. G. Swift *et al.* (letter), *ibid.*, 1322; J. G. Douglas *et al.*, *Br. J. Anaesth.*, 1980, *52*, 811; B. J. Pleuvry *et al.*, *ibid.*, 901; T. V. A. Harry and A. N. Latham (letter), *Br. J. clin. Pharmac.*, 1980, *9*, 618.

Proprietary Preparations

Euhypnos *(Farmitalia Carlo Erba, UK).* Temazepam, available as capsules of 10 mg. **Euhypnos Forte.** Temazepam, available as capsules of 20 mg. (Also available as Euhypnos in *Austral.*).

Normison *(Wyeth, UK).* Temazepam, available as capsules of 10 and 20 mg. (Also available as Normison in *S.Afr.*).

Other Proprietary Names

Cerepax, Lenal, Levanxene (all *Arg.*); Levanxol (*Belg., Ital., Neth., S.Afr., Spain*); Maeva (*Ital.*); Restoril (*Canad., USA*).

4073-k

Triazolam.
Clorazolam; U-33030. 8-Chloro-6-(2-chlorophenyl)-1-methyl-4*H*-1,2,4-triazolo-[4,3-*a*]-1,4-benzodiazepine.

$C_{17}H_{12}Cl_2N_4$=343.2.

CAS — 28911-01-5.

A white or pale yellow crystalline powder. Poorly **soluble** in water; soluble in alcohol. **Protect** from light.

Dependence. Prolonged use of triazolam may lead to dependence of the barbiturate-alcohol type (see p.792). It has a low liability for abuse.

For reference to intense rebound insomnia associated with abrupt withdrawal of benzodiazepines with a relatively short duration of action, see Nitrazepam, p.807.

Adverse Effects, Treatment, and Precautions. As for Nitrazepam, p.807.

A report of a syndrome (adverse mental effects) associated with triazolam administration, with special reference to a close study of 25 patients.— C. van der Kroef (letter), *Lancet*, 1979, *2*, 526. This report in 25 patients is contrary to the massive amount of data collected elsewhere.— N. MacLeod and C. H. Kratochvil, *Upjohn* (letter), *ibid.*, 638. Further severe criticism, and doubt as to the validity of the conclusion, and alarm at the inappropriate use of the term 'syndrome'.— F. J. Ayd *et al.* (letter), *ibid.*, 1018.

Effects on the liver. Fatal intrahepatic cholestasis possibly associated with triazolam.— I. Cobden *et al.*, *Postgrad. med. J.*, 1981, *57*, 730.

Absorption and Fate. Triazolam is rapidly and nearly completely absorbed from the gastro-intestinal tract. It has a biphasic half-life with a reported mean apparent half-life of 3.4 hours for the initial phase and 7.8 hours for the terminal phase. It is reported to be extensively bound to plasma proteins. It is excreted in the urine in the form of its metabolites with only small amounts appearing unchanged.

In a study of triazolam tablets and a liquid formulation in healthy subjects, the bioavailability of the tablets was rapid and, relative to the liquid formulation, complete. The average half-life for absorption was 8 minutes with peak concentrations being achieved an average of 42 minutes after dosing.— C. M. Metzler *et al.*, *Clin. Pharmac. Ther.*, 1977, *21*, 111.

Further references: F. S. Eberts *et al.*, *Clin. Pharmac. Ther.*, 1981, *29*, 81.

Uses. Triazolam is a benzodiazepine derivative with hypnotic properties similar to those of nitrazepam (p.808). As a hypnotic it is given in doses of 250 µg at night; initial doses of 125 µg at night have been suggested for elderly subjects, increased to 250 µg if necessary.

A clinical review of benzodiazepines in general and triazolam in particular.— *Br. J. clin. Pharmac.*, 1981, *11*, 3S.

Hypnotic effect. Reports and studies on triazolam: B. Matta *et al.*, *Curr. ther. Res.*, 1974, *16*, 958; W. Veldkamp *et al.*, *J. clin. Pharmac.*, 1974, *14*, 102; A. Sunshine, *Clin. Pharmac. Ther.*, 1975, *17*, 573; K. Rickels *et al.*, *ibid.*, 1975, *18*, 315; P. Lomen and O. I. Linet, *J. int. med. Res.*, 1976, *4*, 55; J. Roth *et al.*, *ibid.*, 59; D. Bossier, *Acta ther.*, 1977, *3*, 257; J. C. Chatwin and W. L. Johns, *Curr. ther. Res.*, 1977, *21*, 207; A. Kales *et al.*, *J. clin. Pharmac.*, 1977, *17*, 207; R. L. Reeves, *ibid.*, 319; L. F. Fabre *et al.*, *ibid.*, 402; R. I. H. Wang, *J. int. med. Res.*, 1977, *5*, 184; L. F. Fabre and C. M. Metzler, *Clin. Ther.*, 1978, *1*, 339; R. B. Knapp *et al.*, *Curr. ther. Res.*, 1978, *23*, 230; K. K. Okama, *ibid.*, 381; N. P. V. Nair and G. Schwartz, *ibid.*, 388; L. Verguts *et al.*, *Acta ther.*, 1978, *4*, 5; A. J. Bowen, *J. int. med. Res.*, 1978, *6*, 337; K. K. Okawa and G. S. Allen, *ibid.*, 343; J. A. Lipani, *Curr. ther. Res.*, 1978, *24*, 397; P. R. Sundaresan *et al.*, *Clin. Pharmac. Ther.*, 1979, *25*, 391; R. Deberdt, *Curr. ther. Res.*, 1979, *26*, 1005; M. R. B. Keighley *et al.*, *Br. med. J.*, 1980, *281*, 829; A. N. Singh and B. Saxena, *Curr. ther. Res.*, 1980, *27*, 627; A. N. Nicholson and B. M. Stone, *Br. J. clin. Pharmac.*, 1980, *9*, 187; H. Bertel, *S.Afr. med. J.*, 1980, *57*, 769; K. D. Shugars *et al.*, *Clin. Ther.*, 1980, *2*, 390; V. Pegram *et al.*, *J. int. med. Res.*, 1980, *8*, 224.

Proprietary Preparations

Halcion *(Upjohn, UK).* Triazolam, available as scored tablets of 125 or 250 µg. (Also available as Halcion in *Belg., Canad., Denm., S.Afr., Switz.*).

4074-a

Triclofos Sodium *(B.P.).*
Sodium Triclofos. Sodium hydrogen 2,2,2-trichloroethyl phosphate.

$C_2H_3Cl_3NaO_4P$=251.4.

CAS — 306-52-5 (triclofos); 7246-20-0 (sodium salt).

Pharmacopoeias. In *Br.*

A white or almost white, odourless, hygroscopic powder with a saline taste. **Soluble** 1 in 2 of water and 1 in 250 of alcohol; practically insoluble in ether. A 2% solution in water is clear and has a pH of 3 to 4.5. Aqueous solutions are **incompatible** with salts of heavy metals, calcium, magnesium, and alkaloids. **Store** in airtight containers.

Dependence. Prolonged use may lead to dependence of the barbiturate-alcohol type (see p.792).

Adverse Effects, Treatment, and Precautions. As for Chloral Hydrate, p.796.

Triclofos sodium is not corrosive to skin and mucous membranes.

Interactions. Warfarin. For a report of the anticoagulant action of warfarin being enhanced by triclofos sodium, see Warfarin Sodium, p.780.

Overdosage. A 47-year-old woman who took 100 triclofos tablets (50 g) was deeply unconscious and hypothermic; reflexes were absent and she was hypotensive. After intravenous fluids she recovered consciousness on the third day.— J. M. Orwin and H. G. Schroeder (letter), *Br. med. J.*, 1968, *3*, 187.

Absorption and Fate. Triclofos sodium is rapidly hydrolysed to trichloroethanol. For the distribution and fate of trichloroethanol, see Chloral Hydrate, p.796.

Uses. Triclofos sodium has hypnotic and sedative actions similar to those of chloral hydrate (see p.797) but it is more palatable and relatively free from the tendency to cause gastric irritation.

The usual adult dose as a hypnotic is 1 g (equivalent to 600 mg of chloral hydrate) at night, but up to 2 g may be necessary in some patients, and the usual dose as a daytime sedative is 500 mg once or twice daily. A suggested hypnotic dose for children up to 1 year of age is 25 to 30 mg per kg body-weight; children aged 1 to 5 years may be given single doses of 250 to 500 mg, and children aged 6 to 12 years may be given single doses of 0.5 to 1 g.

Anaesthesia. Premedication with triclofos or diazepam was satisfactory in 130 of 200 children although there was less disturbance of behaviour in the operating room in children given triclofos.— J. D. Boyd and M. L. M. Manford, *Br. J. Anaesth.*, 1973, *45*, 501.

Further references: E. O. Henschel *et al.*, *Curr. ther. Res.*, 1967, *9*, 453; J. G. Millichap, *Am. J. Dis. Child.*, 1972, *124*, 526; L. Lindgren *et al.*, *Br. J. Anaesth.*, 1980, *52*, 283.

Hypnotic effect. A review of triclofos for the treatment of insomnia.— *Med. Lett.*, 1972, *14*, 78.

Further references: S. G. F. Matts (letter), *Br. med. J.*, 1962, *1*, 1835; D. T. Pearson (letter), *ibid.*, *2*, 1130; H. Caplan *et al.*, *Practitioner*, 1964, *192*, 122; C. F. Rolland, *ibid.*, 123; W. Turner, *ibid.*, 125; R. J. Rushton, *ibid.*, 126; C. R. Brown *et al.*, *J. clin. Pharmac.*, 1972, *12*, 306.

Preparations

Triclofos Elixir *(B.P.).* Triclofos Syrup. A solution of triclofos sodium in a suitable flavoured vehicle which may be coloured. Store at a temperature not exceeding 25°. When a dose less than, or not a multiple of, 5 ml is prescribed, the elixir should be diluted to 5 ml, or a multiple, with syrup. Such dilutions must be freshly prepared and not used more than 2 weeks after issue.

Triclofos Tablets *(B.P.).* Tablets containing triclofos sodium. They are film-coated.
Store in airtight containers.

Proprietary Names

Triclos *(Merrell-National, USA)*; Tricloryl *(Glaxo, S.Afr.)*.

NOTE. Triclose is a proprietary name for azanidazole.

Triclofos sodium was formerly marketed in Great Britain under the proprietary name Tricloryl (*Glaxo*).

4075-t

Vinbarbitone.
Vinbarbital; Butenemal. 5-Ethyl-5-(1-methylbut-1-enyl)barbituric acid.

$C_{11}H_{16}N_2O_3$=224.3.

CAS — 125-42-8.

A white powder with a characteristic odour and a bitter taste. M.p. 160° to 163°. Very slightly **soluble** in water; soluble in alcohol; sparingly soluble in ether.

Vinbarbitone is a barbiturate (see p.792) that has been used as a hypnotic in doses of 100 to 200 mg at night and as a sedative in doses of 25 to 50 mg four times daily. Similar doses of the sodium salt have been given by mouth or by injection.

Pregnancy and the neonate. Reports of neonatal depression following obstetric use: F. F. Nyberg *et al.*, *Obstet. Gynec.*, 1958, *11,* 184; B. Batt, *Am. J. Obstet. Gynec.*, 1968, *102,* 591.

4076-x

Vinylbitone. Vinylbital; Butyvinal; Vinymalum. 5-(1-Methylbutyl)-5-vinylbarbituric acid.
$C_{11}H_{16}N_2O_3$=224.3.

CAS — 2430-49-1.

Vinylbitone is a barbiturate (see p.792) that has been used as a hypnotic in doses of 100 to 200 mg at night. It has also been given rectally as suppositories.

In 6 healthy subjects given vinylbitone 150 mg by mouth or 200 mg rectally peak plasma concentrations of 2.2 to 3.9 and 1.8 to 3.3 µg per ml occurred 1 to 2 and 2 to 6 hours respectively after administration. Sleepiness consistently occurred when the plasma concentration of vinylbitone was 2 to 2.5 µg per ml. The mean half-life of absorption was 14.4 and 38.4 minutes after administration by mouth and rectally respectively and the half-life of elimination varied from 17.6 to 33.5 hours but was not dependent on the method of administration. In 3 subjects about 1.6% of the administered dose was excreted in the urine as unchanged vinylbitone.— D. D. Breimer and A. G. de Boer, *Arzneimittel-Forsch.*, 1976, *26,* 448. See also R. Preuss and D. Müller, *ibid.*, 1968, *18,* 412; M. Geldmacher-von Mallinckrodt *et al.*, *ibid.*, 1971, *21,* 939.

Proprietary Names
Bykonox *(Byk, Belg.; Byk, Neth.)*; Optanox *(Valpan, Fr.)*; Speda *(Byk Gulden, Ger.)*; Suppoptanox *(Valpan, Fr.)*.

Idoxuridine and some other Antiviral Agents

1680-c

The drugs described in this section are used in the treatment of viral infection or for providing protection, usually for a brief period only, against infection. They do not provide an alternative to immunisation for the long-term prophylaxis of infection—for details of such treatment see the section on Vaccines and other Immunological Products, p.1586. Other drugs used in the treatment of viral infection discussed elsewhere include amantadine hydrochloride (p.890), cytarabine (p.203), and levamisole (p.95). Immunoglobulins are also used in the treatment of viral infections and are described in the section on Blood Preparations, p.321.

Reviews of virus diseases and their treatment: B. E. Juel-Jensen, *Practitioner*, 1974, *213*, 508; D. G. James, *ibid.*, 1976, *217*, 602.

Reviews of antiviral agents and their actions and uses: *Drug & Ther. Bull.*, 1974, *12*, 13; T. H. Maugh, *Science*, 1976, *192*, 128; T. -W. Chang and D. R. Snydman, *Drugs*, 1979, *18*, 354; R. A. Buchanan, *Can. med. Ass. J.*, 1979, *120*, 7; M. S. Hirsch and M. N. Swartz, *New Engl. J. Med.*, 1980, *302*, 903 and 949.

Herpes simplex. In the majority of 80 subjects with recurrent herpes simplex labialis the natural healing process began within 24 hours of the onset of symptoms suggesting that studies involving therapy started up to 48 hours after the onset of symptoms might contain false results. Prompt initiation of therapy involving medication kept at home could potentially alter the course of the disease since, contrary to previous reports, viral replication did not appear to be maximum at the initial onset of the lesion. A subgroup of patients with severe symptoms and a prolonged course were most likely to derive benefit because therapy was more likely to precede the natural healing process.— S. L. Spruance *et al.*, *New Engl. J. Med.*, 1977, *297*, 69.

A discussion of genital herpes and its treatment.— *Br. med. J.*, 1980, *280*, 1335.

Herpes zoster. Brief discussions on the treatment of varicella-zoster infections.— *Br. med. J.*, 1976, *2*, 1466; *ibid.*, 1979, *1*, 5.

Pregnancy and the neonate. A brief discussion on the problems of using antiviral agents in the neonate.— P. Brunell, *J. Pediat.*, 1975, *86*, 317.

Resistance. A brief discussion on viral resistance to antiviral agents.— J. McGill, *J. antimicrob. Chemother.*, 1977, *3*, 284.

1681-k

Idoxuridine *(B.P., U.S.P.)*. IDU; 5 IDUR; SKF 14287. 2′-Deoxy-5-iodouridine.

$C_9H_{11}IN_2O_5$=354.1.

CAS — 54-42-2.

Pharmacopoeias. In *Br.*, *Chin.*, *Jap.*, and *U.S.*

Odourless or almost odourless, tasteless, colourless crystals or a white crystalline powder from which iodine vapour is liberated on heating.

Soluble 1 in 500 of water, 1 in 400 of alcohol, and 1 in 230 of methyl alcohol; practically insoluble in chloroform and ether. A solution in sodium hydroxide is dextrorotatory. A 0.1% solution in water has a pH of about 6. Aqueous solutions are most stable at pH 2 to 6; they should be freshly prepared and stored in a refrigerator. Some decomposition products such as iodouracil are more toxic than idoxuridine and reduce its antiviral activity. **Store** in airtight containers. Protect from light.

Solution for intravenous injection. *For details of the preparation of intravenous injections of idoxuridine, see Martindale 27th Edn, p. 912.*

Stability. Idoxuridine was stable under all storage conditions when dry. A 0.1% ophthalmic solution was stable for 1 year when stored at room temperature and 5°, but to maintain optimum stability, refrigeration was suggested. Aqueous solutions were more stable in acid than in alkaline solution. They were sensitive to light and should be stored in amber bottles. There was about 50% decomposition if they were autoclaved for 20 minutes at 121°.— L. J. Ravin and J. J. Gulesich, *J. Am. pharm. Ass.*, 1964, *NS4*, 122.

The degradation of idoxuridine in acetate and phosphate buffers at various pH values.— E. R. Garrett *et al.*, *Chem. pharm. Bull., Tokyo*, 1965, *13*, 1113.

Heating a solution of idoxuridine 0.1% in either 0.9% sodium chloride solution or borate buffer of pH 7.5 at 100° for 30 minutes resulted in a loss of 12.6 and 18.1% respectively of idoxuridine. The loss during autoclaving for 30 minutes was about 65% in both solutions. Stability during storage seemed greater at acid pH than at alkaline pH.— E. T. Backer and J. van de Langerijt, *Pharm. Weekbl. Ned.*, 1966, *101*, 489.

The breakdown products of idoxuridine in aqueous media were toxic in cell cultures in very low concentrations. Iodouracil also appeared to be irritating or toxic to the cornea and to inhibit the antiviral activity of idoxuridine.— *Pharm. J.*, 1972, *1*, 338.

Adverse Effects. Adverse effects, which occur occasionally when idoxuridine is applied to the eyes, include irritation, pain, pruritus and inflammation or oedema of the eyes or eyelids. Photophobia may develop. Occlusion of the lachrymal duct has been reported. Excessive use may damage the corneal epithelium.

Hypersensitivity reactions have been reported following the administration of idoxuridine to the eyes and to the skin. Adverse effects after intravenous administration of idoxuridine may be severe and fatalities have occurred. Bone marrow depression with leucopenia and thrombocytopenia have been common with doses used. Hepatotoxic effects including jaundice have occurred. Other systemic adverse effects include glossitis, stomatitis, alopecia, and gastro-intestinal disturbances.

References to the toxicity of idoxuridine given intravenously: A. R. M. Upton (letter), *Br. med. J.*, 1972, *2*, 226; C. G. Geary, *Postgrad. med. J.*, 1973, *49*, 413; D. C. Nolan *et al.*, *Ann. intern. Med.*, 1973, *78*, 243. See also under Herpes Simplex Encephalitis in Uses.

Effect on corneal wound healing. Studies in *rabbits* indicated that although idoxuridine and trifluridine did not retard closure of corneal epithelial wounds they produced toxic changes in regenerating epithelium. Vidarabine phosphate significantly retarded wound closure and produced vascularisation of the corneal stratum. Stromal wound strength was reduced by idoxuridine and trifluridine but significantly increased by vidarabine.— C. S. Foster and D. Pavan-Langston, *Archs Ophthal., N.Y.*, 1977, *95*, 2062.

Hypersensitivity. A report of allergic contact dermatitis in 2 patients using an ophthalmic ointment containing idoxuridine. Patch tests with idoxuridine 1% in soft paraffin were positive for both patients.— P. E. Osmundsen, *Contact Dermatitis*, 1975, *1*, 251.

Allergic contact dermatitis developed in 4 patients following topical treatment for herpes simplex infections with an ointment containing idoxuridine 0.5% or a 5% solution in dimethylacetamide. One patient also displayed a reaction to an ophthalmic preparation of hyoscine hydrobromide he was also using. Studies indicated that the patients showed a delayed cutaneous hypersensitivity to idoxuridine rather than to its degradation products. Patch testing indicated the relationship between the structure of pyrimidine compounds and their antigenic cross-sensitivity.— R. B. Amon *et al.*, *Archs Derm.*, 1975, *111*, 1581.

Jaundice. A 60-year-old man with herpes simplex encephalitis received idoxuridine, 30 g intravenously in divided doses over 8 days. Rapid impairment of liver function occurred, which partially regressed on cessation of the drug. Biochemical abnormalities and histological findings at necropsy suggested cholestatic jaundice due to the idoxuridine.— A. D. Dayan and P. D. Lewis (letter), *Lancet*, 1969, *2*, 1073.

Pregnancy and the neonate. Idoxuridine applied topically to the eye in doses similar to those used clinically was teratogenic to *rabbits*, causing exophthalmic-like deformities and malformed forelegs.— M. Itoi *et al.*, *Archs Ophthal., N.Y.*, 1975, *93*, 46.

Treatment of Adverse Effects. It has been suggested that an intravenous injection containing 50 mg of thymidine may partially reverse the systemic effects of idoxuridine.

Precautions. Idoxuridine should be used with caution in conditions where there is also deep ulceration involving the stromal layers of the cornea, as delayed healing has resulted in corneal perforation. Prolonged topical use should be avoided. Corticosteroids should be applied with caution in patients also receiving idoxuridine. Boric acid preparations should not be applied to the eye in patients also receiving ocular preparations of idoxuridine as irritation ensues.

Parenteral therapy with idoxuridine is discouraged generally and is contra-indicated in pregnant patients. Caution is recommended in treating pregnant patients with topical preparations of idoxuridine in dimethyl sulphoxide.

Activation of viruses in human tumours by idoxuridine and dimethyl sulphoxide.— S. E. Stewart *et al.*, *Science*, 1972, *175*, 198.

The abnormal epithelium in patients with dry eye was sensitive to idoxuridine and could be damaged during treatment of herpes simplex keratitis.— *Drug & Ther. Bull.*, 1974, *12*, 81.

Absorption and Fate. Idoxuridine is rapidly metabolised in the body to iodouracil, uracil and iodide which are rapidly excreted in the urine. Concentrations of idoxuridine in serum, cerebrospinal fluid, and urine after intravenous injection are dependent on the rate of administration. The metabolites have no antiviral activity. Idoxuridine is not significantly bound to plasma proteins.

Concentrations of idoxuridine in serum, urine and cerebrospinal fluid after intravenous infusion.— A. M. Lerner and E. J. Bailey, *J. clin. Invest.*, 1972, *51*, 45.

Further references: D. R. Clarkson *et al.*, *J. Pharmac. exp. Ther.*, 1967, *157*, 581.

Uses. Idoxuridine is an antiviral agent which acts by blocking the uptake of thymidine into the deoxyribonucleic acid (DNA) of the virus and inhibits replication of viruses such as adenovirus, cytomegalovirus, herpes simplex (*Herpesvirus hominis*), varicella-zoster or herpes zoster (*Herpesvirus varicellae*), and vaccinia. It has no action against latent forms of the virus. It does not inhibit RNA viruses such as influenza virus or poliovirus.

It is used in the treatment of superficial herpes simplex keratitis (dendritic keratitis) of recent origin. Healing usually occurs within 7 days but if there is no improvement after this, alternative treatment is indicated. To minimise recurrences, treatment should be continued for 3 to 5 days after healing is complete.

The dose of a 0.1% ophthalmic solution is 1 drop hourly during the day and every 2 hours at night. When improvement occurs the intervals between doses may be doubled. A 0.5% ointment can be used similarly every 4 hours with the last treatment at bedtime, but absorption from a solution is more reliable. Although viral DNA is more susceptible than the DNA in the corneal cells, prolonged administration may affect the corneal cells with consequent damage. Treatment should therefore not be continued for more than 21 days or given more often than every hour.

Solutions of idoxuridine 5 to 40% in dimethyl sulphoxide are applied locally 4 times daily for 3 to 7 days in the treatment of cutaneous herpes simplex, genital herpes, and herpetic whitlows, with variable response since resistance may develop. Idoxuridine has been applied in the treatment of herpes infections of the mouth; forms used have included a 0.1% aqueous mouthwash.

Idoxuridine is also used in the treatment of herpes zoster lesions by local application of 5 to 40% solutions in dimethyl sulphoxide. The solution may be applied 4 times daily for 4 days. Treatment should start within 2 to 3 days of the appearance of vesicles.

Idoxuridine has been given intravenously as an infusion in the treatment of herpes simplex encephalitis and some other systemic viral diseases but is now considered to be ineffective and too toxic to justify its use.

Reviews and discussions on the use of idoxuridine in viral infections: H. Ashton *et al.*, *Br. J. Derm.*, 1971, *84*, 496; L. Weinstein and T. Chang, *New Engl. J. Med.*, 1973, *289*, 725; B. E. Juel-Jensen, *Br. med. J.*, 1973, *1*, 406; *Drug & Ther. Bull.*, 1975, *13*, 13; C. Stuart-Harris, *J. antimicrob. Chemother.*, 1976, *2*, 112; J. Verbov, *ibid.*, 1979, *5*, 126; *Br. med. J.*, 1979, *1*, 5; *ibid.*, 1980, *280*, 1335; *Lancet*, 1980, *1*, 1337.

The development and therapeutic uses of topical preparations of idoxuridine 5%.— R. P. R. Dawber, *Scott. med. J.*, 1977, *22*, 310.

Cytomegalovirus infection. References to the use of idoxuridine by intravenous infusion in the treatment of congenital cytomegalovirus infections: A. F. Conchie *et al.*, *Br. med. J.*, 1968, *4*, 162; R. F. House *et al.* (letter), *Lancet*, 1973, *1*, 39.

Herpes simplex. In a double-blind controlled study in 16 patients, the average expected duration of attacks of herpes was reduced by 6.3 days with a 5% solution of idoxuridine in dimethyl sulphoxide, and by 4.1 days by dimethyl sulphoxide alone. These solutions were used in 10 and 11 attacks respectively, each solution being applied thrice daily for 3 days.— F. O. MacCallum and B. E. Juel-Jensen, *Br. med. J.*, 1966, *2*, 805.

In 4 patients with herpes simplex and a history of associated erythema multiforme, treatment with idoxuridine 5% in dimethyl sulphoxide led to prompt resolution of the lesions but did not prevent the recurrence of erythema multiforme. A fifth patient had no recurrence of herpes or of erythema multiforme.— R. P. R. Dawber (letter), *Br. med. J.*, 1972, *4*, 300.

In a double-blind study 53 patients with recurrent genital herpes were treated with topical applications of idoxuridine 20% in dimethyl sulphoxide, idoxuridine 5% in dimethyl sulphoxide or dimethyl sulphoxide alone. Both treatments with idoxuridine were superior to dimethyl sulphoxide alone and lesions treated with idoxuridine 20% healed more rapidly and shed virus for a shorter period than those treated with idoxuridine 5%. There was no significant difference in the recurrence-rate of lesions for the different groups in 34 patients who were followed up for up to 2 years.— J. D. Parker, *J. antimicrob. Chemother.*, 1977, *3*, *Suppl.* A, 131.

Encephalitis. Discussions on the use of idoxuridine in the treatment of herpes simplex encephalitis: *Lancet*, 1975, *1*, 1324; M. Longson, *J. antimicrob. Chemother.*, 1977, *3*, *Suppl.* A, 115.

Two double-blind studies of the use of idoxuridine 100 mg per kg body-weight injected daily in the treatment of herpes simplex virus encephalitis were terminated prematurely due to the high mortality-rate and severe toxicity in patients receiving the drug. Six of 8 patients with proved or probable herpes simplex virus encephalitis died, despite receiving a full course of therapy with idoxuridine. Myelosuppression was also evident in 6 patients who received idoxuridine and leucopenia developed in 5 and thrombocytopenia in 6. Herpes simplex virus (*Herpesvirus hominis*) was isolated from the brain in all of 4 patients who were examined at post mortem and in 2 where quantitative data were available, the quantity of virus was equal to or greater than before treatment.— Boston Interhospital Virus Study Group and the NIAID-Sponsored Cooperative Antiviral Clinical Study, *New Engl. J. Med.*, 1975, *292*, 599.

Further references: B. R. Silk and A. P. C. H. Roome (letter), *Lancet*, 1970, *1*, 411; D. C. Nolan *et al.*, *New Engl. J. Med.*, 1970, *282*, 10; B. Goldman *et al.* (letter), *Lancet*, 1970, *2*, 155; M. A. Fishman *et al.*, *Am. J. Dis. Child.*, 1971, *122*, 250, per *Int. pharm. Abstr.*, 1972, *9*, 235; D. C. Nolan *et al.*, *Ann. intern. Med.*, 1973, *78*, 243; M. Rappel, *Postgrad. med. J.*, 1973, *49*, 419; T. C. Hall *et al.*, *Postgrad. med. J.*, 1973, *49*, 429; C. B. Lauter *et al.*, *Proc. Soc. exp. Biol. Med.*, 1975, *150*, 23, per *Abstr. Hyg.*, 1976, *51*, 1309; O. Paulsen, *Scand. J. infect. Dis.*, 1977, *9*, 85, per *Abstr. Hyg.*, 1979, *54*, 452.

Keratitis . Ultraviolet light enhanced the effect of idoxuridine in the treatment of superficial herpes simplex keratitis. However, the treatment was not recommended as there was a higher recurrence-rate compared with idoxuridine therapy alone; the patients also experienced considerable pain after phototherapy and there was a greater risk of stromal keratitis.— R. Daniel and A. Karseras, *Br. J. Ophthal.*, 1972, *56*, 604.

For a comparative study of the efficacy of idoxuridine and trifluridine in herpes simplex keratitis, see Trifluridine, p.825.

For comparative studies of the efficacy of idoxuridine and vidarabine in herpes simplex keratitis, see Vidarabine, p.827.

Herpes zoster. In herpes zoster ophthalmicus the skin of the forehead and eyelids should be treated with gauze dressings soaked in a 40% solution of idoxuridine in dimethyl sulphoxide. The gauze should not be thrown away between dressings but resoaked. Dimethyl sulphoxide should not be applied to the eye as it was toxic to the lens, and treatment of *the eye* consisted of prednisolone sodium phosphate 0.5% eye-drops hourly together with atropine sulphate 1% eye-drops twice daily if there was a suspected anterior uveitis. To be effective the treatment must be started in the very early stages of the infection, and must be given in hospital under the care of an ophthalmologist. The efficacy of the treatment was still under review and should be regarded as unproven.— P. G. Watson, *Practitioner*, 1973, *211*, 829.

A report of the successful use of idoxuridine with corticosteroids in the treatment of 2 patients with herpes zoster dendritic keratitis. A further patient was successfully treated with steroids alone.— D. Pavan-Langston and J. P. McCulley, *Archs Ophthal., N.Y.*, 1973, *89*, 25.

In a double-blind trial in 118 patients with herpes zoster, the period of vesiculation, the healing time, and the duration of pain were all significantly reduced by the application 2-hourly or 4-hourly for 4 days of 5% or 25% idoxuridine in dimethyl sulphoxide (from a 10-ml supply) compared with the use of dimethyl sulphoxide alone. There was no significant difference between 2-hourly and 4-hourly application, or between 5% or 25% solution. A garlic-like taste was noticed by 17 patients, tenderness and erythema by 3, and whealing in 2 with dermographia. Treatment was not recommended for children or pregnant women.— R. Dawber, *Br. med. J.*, 1974, *2*, 526. Criticism. Double-blind trials recently carried out established that 40% idoxuridine in dimethyl sulphoxide was significantly superior to 20% or 5%; 35% solution appeared to be as effective as 40%. More than 1000 patients had been treated with 40 or 35% solution; analysis of 300 cases showed pain of 7 days' duration or less in 95.9%, 4 days or less in 79.6%, and 2 days or less in 45%.— B. E. Juel-Jensen and F. O. MacCallum (letter), *ibid.*, 1974, *3*, 41.

A double-blind random-selection comparison of the therapeutic effects of idoxuridine 40% in dimethyl sulphoxide or idoxuridine 5% in dimethyl sulphoxide showed no apparent difference between the 2 concentrations of idoxuridine with regard to side-effects or benefits in the treatment of herpes zoster. In 17 of the 50 patients in the study the skin lesions healed more rapidly than would have been expected without treatment; in 47 of the patients where pain was a feature of the attack 26 obtained relief more rapidly than expected. Side-effects included transient stinging or burning in 29 patients, and acute sensitivity to idoxuridine in 1.— J. R. Simpson, *Practitioner*, 1975, *215*, 226.

In a double-blind study 100 patients with acute herpes zoster received treatment with idoxuridine 40% in dimethyl sulphoxide or one of the following ointments: a basis of macrogol; a basis with dimethyl sulphoxide 60%; a basis with idoxuridine 5% and dimethyl sulphoxide 60%, or a basis with idoxuridine 40% and dimethyl sulphoxide 60%. Treatment with any of the ointments was without any positive effect and although the effect of idoxuridine in solution was statistically significant, it was only slightly better than the ointments with respect to healing and there was no apparent effect on pain and sensitivity. However, analysis revealed that the age of the patient correlated with the duration of pain and with delayed healing, that rapid healing was influenced by the duration of pain, and that herpes zoster in the trigeminal area healed more quickly than in other areas. It was suggested that treatment with idoxuridine should be re-evaluated and these variables taken into account.— K. E. Wildenhoff *et al.*, *Scand. J. infect. Dis.*, 1979, *11*, 1. Results of a double-blind randomised study comparing idoxuridine in dimethyl sulphoxide with dimethyl sulphoxide alone and with saline, again showed that trigeminal zoster (in 42 patients) healed faster than thoracic zoster (in 80 patients). Patients with thoracic zoster, however, experienced pain significantly longer before the eruption of the skin lesions, which might explain the apparent therapeutic failure of idoxuridine in thoracic zoster.— V. Esmann and K. E. Wildenhoff (letter), *Lancet*, 1980, *2*, 474.

Further references: B. E. Juel-Jensen *et al.*, *Br. med. J.*, 1970, *4*, 776.

Orf. Idoxuridine 35% in dimethyl sulphoxide applied as a wet dressing for 4 to 5 days cleared lesions of orf, the DNA virus becoming undetectable on electron microscopy; a 5% solution of idoxuridine could be used if stronger solutions could not be obtained.— B. E. Juel-Jensen (letter), *J.R. Coll. gen. Pract.*, 1977, *27*, 57.

Vaccinial keratitis. For a brief mention of the use of idoxuridine in 4 patients with ocular vaccinia, see A. G. R. Rennie *et al.*, *Lancet*, 1974, *2*, 273.

Warts. Idoxuridine 20% in a cream basis applied under occlusion was a possible effective treatment of warts resistant to other methods of treatment. Neither hydroxyurea 25% in dimethyl sulphoxide nor idoxuridine 40% in dimethyl sulphoxide was effective.— W. L. Morison, *Br. J. Derm.*, 1975, *92*, 97.

Preparations

Idoxuridine Eye Drops *(B.P.)*. A sterile solution of idoxuridine in water. When intended for use on more than one occasion they also contain a suitable antimicrobial preservative. Store below 8° and avoid freezing. Do not use continuously for more than 21 days. Do not use more than one month after first opening the container.

Idoxuridine Ophthalmic Ointment *(U.S.P.)*. A sterile ointment containing 0.45 to 0.55% of idoxuridine in a soft paraffin basis. Store in a cool place.

Idoxuridine Ophthalmic Solution *(U.S.P.)*. A sterile aqueous solution containing 0.09 to 0.11% of idoxuridine; it may contain suitable buffers, stabilisers, and antimicrobial agents. pH 5 to 7.5. Store at 2° to 8° in airtight containers. Protect from light.

Proprietary Preparations

Dendrid *(Alcon, UK: Farillon, UK)*. Idoxuridine, available as eye-drops containing 0.1%. (Also available as Dendrid in *Arg.*, *Switz.*).

Herpid *(WB Pharmaceuticals, UK: Boehringer Ingelheim, UK)*. Idoxuridine, available as solution containing 5% in dimethyl sulphoxide.

Idoxene *(Spodefell, UK)*. Idoxuridine, available as eye ointment containing 0.5%.

Iduridin *(Ferring, UK: Nordic, UK)*. Idoxuridine, available as solution containing 5% or 40% in dimethyl sulphoxide. (Also available as Iduridin in *Denm.*, *Ger.*, *Neth.*, *Norw.*, *Swed.*).

Kerecid *(Smith Kline & French, UK)*. Idoxuridine, available as **Eye-drops** containing 0.1% with thiomersal 0.002% and as **Ophthalmic Ointment** containing 0.5%.

Ophthalmadine *(Sas, UK)*. Idoxuridine, available as **Eye-drops** containing 0.1% and as **Eye Ointment** containing 0.5%.

Other Proprietary Names

Cheratil *(Ital.)*; Collyre 'V' P.O.S. *(Switz.)*; Herpetil *(Ital.)*; Herpidu *(Norw., Switz.)*; Herplex *(Arg., Austral., Belg., Canad., Neth., S.Afr., USA)*; Idulea *(Arg.)*; Idustatin '5' *(Ital.)*; Iduviran *(Fr., Switz.)*; Stoxil *(Austral., Canad., S.Afr., USA)*; Synmiol *(Ger.)*; Virexen, Virucida (both *Spain)*; Virunguent, Vistaspectran (both *Ger.)*; Zostrum *(Eire, Ger.)*.

Idoxuridine was also formerly marketed in Great Britain under the proprietary name Herplex (*Allergan*).

1682-a

Acyclovir. Wellcome 248U; Acycloguanosine. 9-(2-Hydroxyethoxymethyl)guanine; 2-Amino-1,9-dihydro-9-(2-hydroxyethoxymethyl)purin-6-one.
$C_8H_{11}N_5O_3$=225.21.

CAS — 59277-89-3.

Crystals. M.p. 257°.

The antiviral activity of acyclovir is dependent upon conversion, by viral thymidine kinase, to the active triphosphate compound which then appears selectively to inhibit herpes virus DNA polymerase enzyme. It is active against herpesviruses but has no activity against viruses such as vaccinia, some adenoviruses and RNA viruses. Resistance *in vitro* has been reported.

Acyclovir as the sodium salt has been given intravenously in doses of up to 10 mg per kg body-weight every 8 hours in the treatment of herpesvirus infections in immunosuppressed patients. Acyclovir has also been used as an ophthalmic ointment in the treatment of herpes simplex keratitis.

Reviews and discussions on acyclovir.— J. S. Oxford, *J. antimicrob. Chemother.*, 1979, *5*, 333; N. Kappagoda, *Med. J. Aust.*, 1979, *1*, 557; M. S. Hirsch and M. N. Swartz, *New Engl. J. Med.*, 1980, *302*, 949.

Studies of the antiviral activity of acyclovir *in vitro* and in *animals*.— G. B. Elion *et al.*, *Proc. natn. Acad. Sci. U.S.A.*, 1977, *74*, 5716; H. J. Schaeffer *et al.*, *Nature*, 1978, *272*, 583; H. E. Kaufman *et al.*, *Antimicrob. Ag. Chemother.*, 1978, *14*, 842; P. Collins and D. J. Bauer, *J. antimicrob. Chemother.*, 1979, *5*, 431; H. J. Field *et al.*, *Antimicrob. Ag. Chemother.*, 1979, *15*, 554; C. S. Crumpacker *et al.*, *ibid.*, 642; R. J. Klein *et al.*, *ibid.*,

723; N. -H. Park *et al., ibid.*, 775; M. G. Falcon and B. R. Jones, *Br. J. Ophthal.*, 1979, *63*, 422; H. Shiota *et al., ibid.*, 425; D. J. Bauer *et al., ibid.*, 429; K. O. Smith *et al., Antimicrob. Ag. Chemother.*, 1980, *17*, 144; E. A. Boulter *et al., Br. med. J.*, 1980, *280*, 681.

In a double-blind study 12 patients with dendritic corneal ulcers were treated by minimal wiping debridement followed by application of 3% acyclovir eye ointment 5 times daily for 7 days; 12 similar patients received debridement followed by application of a placebo ointment. Within 7 days of debridement there were 7 recurrences in the placebo group and none in the acyclovir group. Brisk healing rates occurred in a further 4 patients with dendritic ulcers treated with 3% acyclovir ointment alone. No side-effects associated with acyclovir topical therapy were noted in any of the 16 patients treated.— B. R. Jones *et al.* (preliminary communication), *Lancet*, 1979, *1*, 243.

Acyclovir 5 mg per kg body-weight every 8 hours intravenously appeared to be highly effective in a 14-year-old immunosuppressed boy with probable viral pneumonia.— J. M. Goldman *et al.* (letter), *Lancet*, 1979, *1*, 820.

Acyclovir successfully controlled recurrent herpetic lesions in the mouth and both nostrils of an 11-year-old boy undergoing chemotherapy for acute lymphoblastic leukaemia; the lesions were resistant to topical idoxuridine therapy. He was initially given acyclovir 2.5 mg per kg body-weight intravenously every 8 hours for 5 days and the lesions dried after 6 doses. Recurrences were treated again with intravenous therapy and subsequently with topical therapy alone (application of 5% acyclovir ointment 4 to 5 times daily). No adverse effects were noted.— A. O'Meara *et al.* (letter), *Lancet*, 1979, *2*, 1196.

A report of the results of an uncontrolled study involving acyclovir therapy for herpesvirus infections, in 23 immunosuppressed patients with malignant disease. Acyclovir was usually given by intravenous bolus injection over 2 minutes, at a dose of 5 mg per kg body-weight, every 8 hours for 5 days. Two patients with reduced renal function were given a twice daily dosage, and a third was treated for 2 days only. All of 7 patients with localised herpes zoster experienced pain relief within 24 hours of starting treatment; no new skin lesions occurred after 24 hours of treatment and those which formed during the first 24 hours did not usually vesiculate; in no patient did the lesions become disseminated; best results were obtained when treatment was started within 4 days of onset, with arrest of progression of the rash and very slight scarring. Similar good results were also obtained in 7 of 8 patients with disseminated varicella zoster, and in 6 with localised herpes simplex (5 perioral and 1 ocular; healing of lesions starting within 12 to 24 hours of the first injection, and crusting being complete within 3 days in all of the oral infections). In 2 patients believed to have herpes simplex dissemination, pneumonitis in one cleared radiologically in 3 days and fever in the second resolved in 2 days. The only side-effect noted was the possibility of impairment of renal function by acyclovir in 2 patients; in both patients treatment was continued at a lower dosage and additional fluids were given, and blood urea and creatinine concentrations had improved before the completion of 5 days' treatment. Trough plasma concentrations following a dose of 5 mg per kg every 8 hours were 0.14 to 1.84 μg per ml (0.6 to 8.2 μmol per litre) in 6 patients with normal renal function, and in a patient with impaired renal function, 4.73 to 12.84 μg per ml (21 to 57 μmol per litre), although there was no evidence of toxicity.— P. J. Selby *et al., Lancet*, 1979, *2*, 1267. Transient renal impairment in 2 patients given acyclovir; both patients had been adequately hydrated.— M. G. Harrington *et al.* (letter), *ibid.*, 1981, *2*, 1281.

A favourable report of the use of acyclovir in a patient with very severe chicken-pox.— J. W. M. van der Meer *et al.* (letter), *Lancet*, 1980, *2*, 473. Two leukaemic children treated with acyclovir for early chicken-pox subsequently developed recurrent atypical varicella virus skin infection, probably associated with the leukaemia chemotherapy.— M. H. van Weel-Sipman *et al.* (letter), *ibid.*, 1981, *1*, 147.

Effective treatment with acyclovir in transplant patients with herpes simplex infections.— C. D. Mitchell *et al., Lancet*, 1981, *1*, 1389; S. Chou *et al., ibid.*, 1392.

Prophylaxis of herpes-simplex-virus infection with acyclovir; latent infection does not appear to be eradicated.— R. Saral *et al., New Engl. J. Med.*, 1981, *305*, 63.

Treatment of herpes zoster with acyclovir.— N. A. Peterslund *et al., Lancet*, 1981, *2*, 827.

Absorption and fate. Mean peak plasma concentrations of acyclovir, given as the sodium salt to 14 patients with advanced malignancies by intravenous infusion over 1 hour in doses of 0.5, 1.0, 2.5 and 5 mg per kg body-weight, were 1.44, 2.73, 3.36 and 7.59 μg per ml (6.4, 12.1, 14.9 and 33.7 μmol per litre) at the end of the infusion and had fallen to 135, 270, 338 and 923 ng per ml (0.6, 1.2, 1.5 and 4.1 μmol per litre) six hours later. The disposition of acyclovir in plasma showed a biexponential decay with the half-life of the slow phase ranging from 2.0 to 3.8 hours (5 hours in 1 patient). The drug was detectable in plasma for at least 18 hours after the infusion. Between 30–69% of the drug was excreted unchanged within 72 hours with the majority being excreted within 8 hours after the end of the infusion. 9-Carboxymethoxymethylguanine was identified as a metabolite. Acyclovir was 22 to 33% bound to plasma proteins. There was no indication of toxicity in any of the patients.— P. de Miranda *et al., Clin. Pharmac. Ther.*, 1979, *26*, 718. See also P. J. Selby *et al., Lancet*, 1979, *2*, 1267; P. de Miranda *et al., Clin. Pharmac. Ther.*, 1981, *30*, 662.

Proprietary Preparations

Zovirax *(Wellcome, UK)*. Acyclovir, available as eye ointment containing 3%. **Zovirax I.V.** consists of acyclovir sodium available as powder for preparing infusion solutions, in vials containing the equivalent of acyclovir 250 mg.

1683-t

Interferons.

Low-molecular-weight glycoproteins produced in human or animal cells following exposure chiefly to viruses.

CAS — 9008-11-1.

So far there are three main types of interferon known by various names.

Interferon-α (IFN-α) also known as Le interferon, type I; it may be derived from leucocytes:

Interferon-β (IFN-β) also known as F interferon, type I; it may be derived from fibroblasts:

Interferon-γ (IFN-γ) also known as interferon, type II or IIF or immune; it is derived from immunologically stimulated T lymphocytes.

The cell source may be indicated when specifying the interferon, for instance by using Hu for human and Mu for mouse.

Production and purification.— M. Azuma *et al., Antimicrob. Ag. Chemother.*, 1978, *13*, 566; F. Klein *et al., ibid.*, 1979, *15*, 420; A. Billiau *et al., ibid.*, *16*, 49; S. Nagata *et al., Nature*, 1980, *284*, 316.

Stability. Whereas human interferon β (fibroblast) induced by complexed poly I. poly C or by Newcastle disease virus was similarly inactivated in various human body fluids; human interferon α (leucocyte) induced by Newcastle disease virus has been reported to be more stable in these fluids and was considered to have a greater potential for human use.— T. C. Cesario, *Curr. ther. Res.*, 1978, *24*, 153.

Units. 5000 units of human interferon α (leucocyte) are contained in one ampoule of the first International Reference Preparation (1978).

10 000 units of human interferon β (fibroblast) are contained in one ampoule of the first International Reference Preparation (1978).

International Reference Preparations (1978) are also available for chick, mouse and rabbit interferon.

Recommendations relating to interferon standards.— *J. biol. Stand.*, 1979, *7*, 383.

Adverse Effects and Precautions. It is not clear whether the adverse effects obtained with human interferon after parenteral use are due to interferon or to contaminating proteins in the preparations used, although the increasing use of pure material indicates that interferon can produce adverse effects. Pyrexia, shivering, malaise, fatigue, pain and erythema at the site of injection and hair loss are amongst the most common adverse effects following injection. Myelosuppression with leucopenia and thrombocytopenia have also occurred. Other adverse effects reported include transient hypotension, elevations in serum aminotransferases, anorexia, nausea and vomiting.

It has been reported that aspirin or indomethacin might reduce interferon activity.

Restoration of bone-marrow function following marrow transplantation was delayed in 3 patients given a human interferon preparation. In a 4th patient also given interferon the transplant failed to take. Laboratory results showed an inhibition of granulocyte colony growth by human leucocyte interferon. It was considered that interferon was contra-indicated in patients with severe bone-marrow insufficiency and should not be given to marrow transplant patients before the graft was fully functional.— C. Nissen *et al.* (letter), *Lancet*, 1977, *1*, 203.

A warning that human interferon administration could be associated with transmission of slow viruses.— G. Wadell (letter), *New Engl. J. Med.*, 1977, *296*, 1295.

There was no antiviral interaction between interferon and arabinosides.— Y. J. Bryson and L. H. Kronenberg, *Antimicrob. Ag. Chemother.*, 1977, *11*, 299.

Intramuscular injections of human interferon β (fibroblasts) did not always produce detectable serum concentrations. It was considered that this form of interferon might be inactivated in the circulation.— V. G. Edy *et al.* (letter), *Lancet*, 1978, *1*, 451.

Absorption and Fate. Interferons are inactive following oral administration. They are absorbed from subcutaneous or intramuscular sites, and are generally given intramuscularly. Some forms are inactivated in muscle tissue and must be given intravenously. They are not absorbed following topical administration. Interferons have been variously reported to have serum half-lives ranging from 2 to 6 hours. They are readily inactivated in body fluids, such as saliva, serum and urine, and do not readily penetrate into the cerebrospinal fluid.

Uses. Interferons possess antiviral properties. They inhibit the growth of many viruses, probably by inducing the production of antiviral proteins, and are potentially useful in the treatment of viral infections. As they also interfere with cell growth and affect the immune system, interferons are being investigated for cancer therapy.

Reviews and discussions on interferons.— S. E. Grossberg, *New Engl. J. Med.*, 1972, *287*, 13, 79, and 122; D. H. Metz, *Adv. Drug Res.*, 1975, *10*, 101; *Br. med. J.*, 1977, *1*, 64; F. Assaad *et al., Bull. Wld Hlth Org.*, 1978, *56*, 229; T. C. Merigan, *New Engl. J. Med.*, 1979, *300*, 42; T. -W. Chang and D. R. Snydman, *Drugs*, 1979, *18*, 354; M. Ho, *Med. J. Aust.*, 1979, *2*, 11; M. S. Hirsch and M. N. Swartz, *New Engl. J. Med.*, 1980, *302*, 949; G. M. Scott and D. A. J. Tyrrell, *Br. med. J.*, 1980, *280*, 1558. Correction.— *ibid.*, *281*, 695.

A symposium on the interferon system.— *Tex. Rep. Biol. Med.*, 1977, *35*, 1–573.

Findings suggesting that the transient drop in high-density lipoprotein cholesterol which can occur in viral infections may be mediated by interferon. Attention should be paid, in future studies, to the possible relation between interferon treatment and cardiovascular disease.— K. Cantell *et al.* (letter), *New Engl. J. Med.*, 1980, *302*, 1032.

Auto-immune disorders. A study indicating that interferon is produced in patients with immunologically active diseases such as systemic lupus erythematosus, rheumatoid arthritis, scleroderma, and Sjögren's syndrome.— J. J. Hooks *et al., New Engl. J. Med.*, 1979, *301*, 5. In a double-blind study, partially purified human interferon α (leucocyte) 3 000 000 units subcutaneously daily, from Monday to Friday for 8 weeks, in addition to their usual therapy, was given to 3 patients with active rheumatoid arthritis. Control injections of albumin were given to 3 similar patients. Interferon was not noted to have any beneficial effect; if further trials are planned a much longer treatment period seems necessary. One patient in the interferon group discontinued therapy owing to rising transaminase values and slight transaminase elevations were seen in the other 2 noted retrospectively to have received interferon. All of the patients in the interferon group had a transient fever reaction found to coincide with the start of treatment; no local reactions were noted. Interferon may cause more side-effects in patients with rheumatoid arthritis than in those with tumours.— A. Kajander *et al.* (letter), *Lancet*, 1979, *1*, 984. See also *J. Am. med. Ass.*, 1980, *243*, 20.

Cancer. Reviews and comments on the use of interferon in cancer.— *J. Am. med. Ass.*, 1978, *239*, 1946; E. C. Borden, *Ann. intern. Med.*, 1979, *91*, 472; T. J. Priestman, *Cancer Treat. Rev.*, 1979, *6*, 223; *Lancet*, 1979, *1*,

1171; B. J. Culliton and W. K. Waterfall, *Br. med. J.*, 1979, *2*, 195; J. Lister, *New Engl. J. Med.*, 1980, *303*, 741; K. Sikora, *Br. med. J.*, 1980, *281*, 855.

Studies on the use of interferon in cancer.— I. S. Christophersen *et al.*, *Acta med. scand.*, 1978, *204*, 471; T. C. Merigan *et al.*, *New Engl. J. Med.*, 1978, *299*, 1449 (lymphoma); T. Sawada *et al.*, *Cancer Treat. Rep.*, 1979, *63*, 2111 (neuroblastoma); K. Ideström *et al.*, *Acta med. scand.*, 1979, *205*, 149 (myeloma); H. Mellstedt *et al.* (preliminary communication), *Lancet*, 1979, *1*, 245 (myeloma); J. Treuner *et al.* (letter), *Lancet*, 1980, *1*, 817 (nasopharyngeal carcinoma); J. U. Gutterman *et al.*, *Ann. intern. Med.*, 1980, *93*, 399 (breast cancer; myeloma; lymphoma); T. J. Priestman, *Lancet*, 1980, *2*, 113; D. Ikič *et al.*, *ibid.*, 1981, *1*, 1022 (breast cancer; bladder cancer; melanoma); *idem*, 1025 (cancer of the head and neck); *idem*, 1027 (cervical carcinoma).

Organ and tissue transplantation. Preliminary results of a double-blind controlled study in 41 patients undergoing renal transplantation suggested that a prophylactic course of human interferon α (leucocyte) delayed the shedding of cytomegalovirus and decreased the incidence of viraemia after transplantation when compared with placebo, whereas treatment with antithymocyte globulin was associated with an increase in the severity of cytomegalovirus infection. Effects on herpes simplex infection were less striking but the trend was similar. The first 2 patients received interferon intramuscularly immediately before transplantation and then every other day but, because of haematological toxicity, subsequent patients received a dose on the day of transplantation, on the next day, and then twice weekly for a total of 15 doses. Injections were discontinued if the white cell count fell below 3000 per ml or the platelet count below 80 000 per ml, until they improved. Patients also received standard immunosuppression with azathioprine and prednisone and about half were given antithymocyte globulin. Seven patients given interferon and 2 patients given placebo had leucopenia or thrombocytopenia or both.— S. H. Cheeseman *et al.*, *New Engl. J. Med.*, 1979, *300*, 1345. Study of these patients also indicated that increasing immunosuppression with antithymocyte globulin increased excretion of Epstein-Barr virus but this was partially reversed in patients also receiving interferon.— S. H. Cheeseman *et al.*, *Ann. intern. Med.*, 1980, *93*, 39.

Further studies and reports of the use of interferon in patients receiving organ and tissue transplants.— W. Weimar *et al.*, *Eur. J. clin. Invest.*, 1978, *8*, 255; J. D. Meyers *et al.*, *J. infect. Dis.*, 1980, *141*, 555.

Viral infections. Interferon appeared to act indirectly by binding to specific cell-surface receptors and inducing the production of cellular enzymes that block viral reproduction.— F. Dianzani and S. Baron, *Tex. Rep. Biol. Med.*, 1977, *35*, 297. See also *Nature*, 1977, *267*, 486.

Studies *in vitro* and in *animals* into the antiviral activity of interferon.— B. Postic and J. N. Dowling, *Antimicrob. Ag. Chemother.*, 1977, *11*, 656 (cytomegalovirus); E. R. Kern *et al.*, *ibid.*, 1978, *13*, 344 (cytomegalovirus); G. Volckaert-Vervliet *et al.*, *J. gen. Virol.*, 1978, *41*, 459 (measles), per *Abstr. Hyg.*, 1979, *54*, 582.

Mechanisms of interferon induced transfer of viral resistance between *animal* cells.— J. E. Blalock and S. Baron, *J. gen. Virol.*, 1979, *42*, 363, per *Abstr. Hyg.*, 1979, *54*, 573.

Studies and reports of the use of interferon either alone or as an adjunct in the management of various viral infections.— T. C. Merigan *et al.*, *Lancet*, 1973, *1*, 563 (influenza; used as nasal spray); L. Åhström *et al.* (letter), *Lancet*, 1974, *1*, 166 (prophylaxis in compromised patients); *J. Am. med. Ass.*, 1974, *227*, 1244 (herpes zoster; influenza; rhinovirus); G. S. Turner, *Immun. Infekt.*, 1977, *5*, 208 (rabies), per *Abstr. Hyg.*, 1979, *54*, 593; R. T. D. Emond *et al.*, *Br. med. J.*, 1977, *2*, 541 (Ebola virus); G. M. Scott *et al.*, *J. biol. Stand.*, 1978, *6*, 73 (vaccinia); A. M. Arvin *et al.*, *Antimicrob. Ag. Chemother.*, 1978, *13*, 605 (varicella); S. B. Greenberg *et al.*, *ibid.*, *14*, 596 (nasal viruses); V. I. Reznik *et al.*, *Vop. Virus.*, 1978, *6*, 732; G. M. Scott and G. W. Csonka, *Br. J. vener. Dis.*, 1979, *55*, 442 (genital warts); J. Kovanen *et al.*, *Br. med. J.*, 1980, *280*, 902 (Creutzfeldt-Jakob disease).

Hepatitis. In a double-blind study administration of human interferon α (leucocyte) did not appear to have any beneficial effect in 8 patients with chronic HBsAg-positive hepatitis when compared with 8 similarly affected control patients who received albumin as placebo. The interferon was given in a dose of 12×10^6 reference units daily by intramuscular injection in the first week, this dose being subsequently halved each week until discontinuation after the sixth week. The only effect on the hepatitis was a transient reduction in DNA-polymerase activity, without apparent clinical significance. Side-effects included chills and/or fever in all of the 8 patients after the first injection and one patient had increasing hair loss. Leucocytes decreased significantly during the first 3 weeks of treatment and 6 patients developed leucopenia; thrombocytes also decreased significantly after the first week of treatment.— W. Weimar *et al.*, *Lancet*, 1980, *1*, 336. Better results have been obtained with much higher doses (400 to 900 million units) and patients must be treated for 4 to 6 months and followed-up for 6 to 12 months.— T. C. Merigan *et al.* (letter), *ibid.*, 422. Comment.— W. Weimar and H. Schellekens (letter), *ibid.*, 590.

Further reports, comments and studies on interferon in hepatitis.— H. B. Greenberg *et al.*, *New Engl. J. Med.*, 1976, *295*, 517; *ibid.*, 562; J. Desmyter *et al.*, *Lancet*, 1976, *2*, 645; W. Weimar *et al.* (letter), *ibid.*, 1977, *2*, 1282; A. J. Zuckerman *et al.*, *ibid.*, 1978, *2*, 652; J. G. C. Kingham *et al.*, *Gut*, 1978, *19*, 91; B. Hafkin *et al.*, *Antimicrob. Ag. Chemother.*, 1979, *16*, 781; V. Damjanovic and W. Brumfitt, *J. antimicrob. Chemother.*, 1980, *6*, 11.

Herpes simplex. Human interferon α (leucocyte) significantly reduced the reactivation of latent herpes simplex infection when compared with placebo in a double-blind study in 37 patients, with a history of herpes infection, who underwent an operation on the trigeminal root, a procedure associated with reactivation. Human interferon α 70 000 units per kg body-weight daily was given intramuscularly morning and evening for 5 days starting on the day before operation. Total reactivation occurred in 9 of 19 patients given interferon compared with 15 of 18 given placebo. The interferon was generally well-tolerated but 5 patients became feverish on the first day and one had to withdraw from the study. Serum-aminotransferase concentrations were raised in the interferon group post-operatively.— G. J. Pazin *et al.*, *New Engl. J. Med.*, 1979, *301*, 225. Follow-up 3 weeks after surgery revealed recurrence in some patients who had remained asymptomatic throughout the initial period of observation. A subsequent survey of patients involved in the study suggested that a single course of treatment of a recurrent herpes simplex infection, with interferon, does not itself cure latency in the neural ganglions.— H. W. Haverkos *et al.* (letter), *ibid.*, 1980, *303*, 699.

Further studies of the use of interferon in the treatment of herpes simplex infections.— K. Kobza *et al.* (letter), *Lancet*, 1975, *1*, 1343 (disseminated and keratitis); O. Palin *et al.* (letter), *ibid.*, 1976, *1*, 1187 (keratitis); R. Sundmacher *et al.* (letter), *ibid.*, 1406 (keratitis); B. R. Jones *et al.* (preliminary communication), *ibid.*, *2*, 128 (keratitis); A. Khan and N. O. Hill, *Ann. Allergy*, 1980, *44*, 289 (labial).

For reference to the beneficial effect of high potency interferon in association with trifluridine in dendritic keratitis, see Trifluridine, p.825.

Herpes zoster. Three randomised double-blind controlled studies in 90 patients with cancer assessed the effect of human interferon α (leucocyte) given intramuscularly at doses between 42 000 and 510 000 units per kg body-weight daily in the treatment of early localised herpes zoster infections. At the highest dose early treatment prevented cutaneous dissemination completely and reduced the spread of infection within the primary dermatome. Visceral complications were also reduced among interferon recipients. Post-herpetic neuralgia was less severe at the higher doses. Fever and bone-marrow suppression occurred at all doses and there was mild transient granulocytopenia at the highest dose.— T. C. Merigan *et al.*, *New Engl. J. Med.*, 1978, *298*, 981. Comments and criticisms.— M. S. Hirsch, *ibid.*, 1022; W. Weimar and H. Schellekens (letter), *ibid.*, 1979, *300*, 923. A reply.— T. C. Merigan (letter), *ibid.*, 924. See also *Lancet*, 1978, *2*, 84.

Some Manufacturers

Abbott, USA; Parke, Davis, USA; Searle, UK; Wellcome, UK.

Various national organisations also produce interferons.

1684-x

Methisazone *(B.P.).*

Metisazone; *N*-Methylisatin β-Thiosemicarbazone; AN 5051; 33-T-57. 1-Methylindoline-2,3-dione 3-thiosemicarbazone.

$C_{10}H_{10}N_4OS = 234.3$.

CAS — 1910-68-5.

Pharmacopoeias. In *Br.*

A very fine orange-yellow powder with a slightly bitter taste. M.p. about 248° with decomposition. Practically **insoluble** in water; soluble 1 in 25 of acetone, 1 in 800 of chloroform, and 1 in 2000 of methyl alcohol; soluble in warm dilute solutions of alkali hydroxides and in hot glacial acetic acid. **Protect** from light.

Freshly prepared methisazone occurred as orange-yellow fluffy microneedles. It was used pharmaceutically as an ultra-fine powder. On standing, the milled powder slowly developed outgrowths or 'whiskers', which showed that the powder was unsuitable for pharmaceutical use. In solution, a short exposure to light caused a reversible change, possibly isomerisation, but irreversible decomposition occurred on prolonged exposure to light.— J. C. Deavin and D. H. Mitchell, *J. Pharm. Pharmac.*, 1965, *17*, 56S.

A discussion of the properties of methisazone and of the problems of formulating suspensions and tablets; 2 formulas are quoted.— A. Axon, *Wellcome*, *J. mond. Pharm.*, 1972, *15*, 221.

A study of the crystal modification of methisazone by grinding; there appeared to be at least 2 polymorphic forms of methisazone.— K. C. Lee and J. A. Hersey, *J. Pharm. Pharmac.*, 1977, *29*, 249.

Adverse Effects. Nausea and vomiting are common side-effects during treatment with methisazone. Anorexia and diarrhoea may also occur. Skin rashes and alopecia have been reported. Fluid retention may occur for a few hours after administration of methisazone.

Treatment of Adverse Effects. Anti-emetic agents may be used in controlling nausea and vomiting.

Precautions. Methisazone is contra-indicated in patients with impaired liver function except in smallpox contacts and in vaccination complications.

Alcohol taken concomitantly may enhance the side-effects.

Absorption and Fate. Methisazone is irregularly absorbed from the gastro-intestinal tract and serum concentrations achieved are variable. Peak serum concentrations occur after 4 to 7 hours and the drug is not detectable in the serum after 10 to 12 hours. Methisazone is extensively metabolised in the body and is excreted in the urine as metabolites and unchanged drug.

Uses. Methisazone is an antiviral agent which appears to act by preventing viral replication, probably by inhibiting viral protein synthesis. It is active against the poxviruses and has been used in the prophylaxis of smallpox and alastrim (variola minor) although smallpox vaccination provides better long-term protection.

Methisazone may be considered for mass administration in conjunction with vaccination in the event of an epidemic of smallpox ever occurring again. The adult prophylactic dose is 3 g by mouth in the morning and a second dose 12 hours later, and children of 3 to 10 years of age may be given one-half the dose; younger children need one-quarter the dose. The irritant effect of methisazone upon the stomach may be reduced if it is taken after meals.

Methisazone has also been given to prevent complications following vaccination and has been used in the treatment of eczema vaccinatum and vaccinia gangrenosa. An initial dose of 200 mg per kg body-weight is given followed by 50 mg per kg every 6 hours for 8 doses. The dosage may be repeated after 7 days, if necessary. For reports on the eradication of smallpox, see under Smallpox Vaccine, p.1607.

Reviews of the use of methisazone.— C. Stuart-Harris, *Br. med. J.*, 1971, *1*, 387; *Med. Lett.*, 1971, *13*, 77; D. J. Bauer, *Proc. R. Soc. Med.*, 1971, *64*, 544; *idem*, *Br. med. J.*, 1973, *3*, 275; L. Weinstein and T. Chang, *New Engl. J. Med.*, 1973, *289*, 725; *Drug & Ther. Bull.*, 1974, *12*, 13; T. -W. Chang and D. R. Snydman, *Drugs*, 1979, *18*, 354.

Methisazone inhibited growth of some strains of rhinovirus in test cultures.— J. M. Z. Gladych *et al.* (letter), *Nature*, 1969, *221*, 286.

Chicken-pox. Methisazone was ineffective for the prophylaxis of chicken-pox.— D. Reed *et al.*, *J. Am. med. Ass.*, 1966, *195*, 586; A. K. Sinha, *Br. J. clin. Pract.*, 1971, *25*, 177.

Eczema vaccinatum. A baby subject to infantile eczema developed eczema vaccinatum after both parents had been vaccinated. Treatment with antibiotics and vaccinial hyperimmune gamma globulin did not have any beneficial effects. Methisazone was given in doses of 250 mg every 6 hours and the child ultimately recovered.— W. Turner *et al.* (preliminary communication), *Br. med. J.*, 1962, *1*, 1317. For a similar report, see D. Mainwaring (letter), *ibid.*, 1412.

Methisazone, given in the form of a syrup for 48 hours, was successful in treating 2 children, aged 5 months and 4½ years, suffering from eczema vaccinatum. The initial dose was 200 mg per kg body-weight and subsequent doses were 50 mg per kg. Treatment was given 6-hourly to 1 child but it was given inadvertently to the other at 4-hourly intervals. Both children were given hyperimmune vaccinial antiserum intramuscularly at the same time as the first dose of methisazone.— B. R. Adels and T. E. Oppé, *Lancet*, 1966, *1*, 18.

Molluscum contagiosum. Methisazone in a dose of 1.5 g initially followed by 700 mg every 6 hours for 8 doses, was ineffective in the treatment of molluscum contagiosum in a 2½-year-old girl with atopic dermatitis. Existing lesions were not cured, but no new lesions appeared.— L. M. Solomon and P. Telner, *Can. med. Ass. J.*, 1966, *95*, 978.

Prevention of vaccination complications. Methisazone was considered superior to immunoglobulin injection in protecting children against the complications of primary smallpox vaccination as a result of a comparative study involving 55 children, aged 2½ to 9 years. Four days after vaccination, when the vesicle was beginning to develop, the children were given either methisazone, 100 mg per kg body-weight followed by a dose of 50 mg per kg daily for 3 to 6 days, or immunoglobulin injection with a haemagglutination inhibition titre of 320, in a single intramuscular injection of 3 ml of a 15% solution. Of the 26 children given methisazone, 17 had clinical contra-indications to vaccination including eczema, tuberculosis, and asthma; similar contra-indications were present in 15 of the 29 children given immunoglobulin injection. The severity and the total duration of the reaction were significantly reduced in the methisazone group; 3 patients given methisazone had mild complications compared with 7 treated with immunoglobulin injection. No case of eczema vaccinatum occurred.— B. Jaroszyńska-Weinberger and J. Mészáros, *Lancet*, 1966, *1*, 948.

In a study in East Africa the incidence of complications of vaccination among children up to 12 years of age suffering from kwashiorkor, yaws, and various skin diseases considered to be contra-indications to the use of smallpox vaccine was 17 among 279 (6.1%) children given methisazone 300 to 600 mg daily for 4 days beginning 4 days after vaccination compared with 55 among 298 (18.5%) children in a control group.— I. D. Ladny, *Zh. Mikrobiol. Épidem. Immunobiol.*, 1974, *1*, 46, per *Abstr. Hyg.*, 1974, *49*, 505.

Smallpox. Studies, with favourable and unfavourable results, of the use of methisazone in the prophylaxis of smallpox and alastrim.— D. J. Bauer *et al.*, *Lancet*, 1963, *2*, 494; D. J. Bauer, *Ann. N.Y. Acad. Sci.*, 1965, *130*, 110; L. A. R. Do Valle *et al.*, *Lancet*, 1965, *2*, 976; A. R. Rao *et al.*, *Indian J. med. Res.*, 1969, *57*, 477 and 484; D. J. Bauer *et al.*, *Am. J. Epidem.*, 1969, *90*, 130; G. G. Heiner *et al.*, *ibid.*, 1971, *94*, 435.

Vaccinia. A child of 4½ with intractable eczema was accidentally vaccinated and developed vaccinia and numerous primary lesions. He was given immunoglobulin but still showed evidence of toxicity. Twelve days later he was given methisazone in a dosage of 2 g daily for 7 days and showed rapid improvement.— A. J. E. Barlow (letter), *Br. med. J.*, 1962, *1*, 1144. A similar report.— O. Hansson and B. Vahlquist (letter), *Lancet*, 1963, *2*, 687.

Two courses of treatment with methisazone together with surgical intervention were necessary for the healing of a vaccinial lesion caused by the vaccination of a man with diabetes and lymphosarcoma despite the administration of immune serum globulin 20 hours after vaccination. The patient was also receiving cyclophosphamide and steroids. Numbness and tingling in fingers and toes and red urine were reported when methisazone was given.— R. G. Douglas *et al.*, *Archs intern. Med.*, 1972, *129*, 980, per *Abstr. Hyg.*, 1972, *47*, 1013.

Methisazone used alone or with antivaccinia immunoglobulin injection was the recommended drug of first choice in the treatment of vaccinia virus infections.— *Med. Lett.*, 1980, *22*, 5.

Preparations

Methisazone Mixture *(B.P.)*. Methisazone Suspension. A suspension of methisazone, of specified particle size, in a suitable syrupy vehicle. It contains 6 g of methisazone in 30 ml. Protect from light.

Proprietary Names

Marboran *(Wellcome, Switz.)*.

Methisazone was formerly marketed in Great Britain under the proprietary name Marboran (*Wellcome*).

1685-r

Ribavirin. Virazole; ICN 1229; RTC. 1-β-D-Ribofuranosyl-1*H*-1,2,4-triazole-3-carboxamide.
$C_8H_{12}N_4O_5$=244.2.

CAS — 36791-04-5.

Adverse Effects and Precautions. Adverse effects reported during treatment with ribavirin have included headache, abdominal cramps, fatigue, reversible anaemia and elevation of bilirubin concentrations. Ribavirin has been reported to be teratogenic in *animals*; it should not be given to pregnant patients.

Animal toxicity including teratogenicity.— L. H. Kilham and V. H. Ferm, *Science*, 1977, *195*, 413; F. Assaad *et al.*, *Bull. Wld Hlth Org.*, 1978, *56*, 229.

Absorption and Fate. Ribavirin is rapidly absorbed following oral administration producing peak blood concentrations within 60 to 90 minutes. It is phosphorylated in the liver and other tissues to produce active metabolites. It is excreted chiefly in the urine.

Uses. Ribavirin is an antiviral agent which inhibits viral replication. Its mechanism of action is not yet fully understood but may be due to the inhibitory effects of its phosphate metabolites on viral nucleic acid and protein synthesis. It is active *in vitro* against a wide range of both DNA and RNA viruses including influenza virus type A and B, parainfluenza virus, rubella, rhinovirus, coxsackie, herpes simplex (*Herpesvirus hominis*), adenovirus, cytomegalovirus, and vaccinia.

It has been given in doses of up to 1 g daily in divided doses in the treatment of influenza, viral hepatitis, and herpesvirus infections but its efficacy remains to be established.

Reviews and discussions on ribavirin.— F. Assaad *et al.*, *Bull. Wld Hlth Org.*, 1978, *56*, 229; T. -W. Chang and D. R. Snydman, *Drugs*, 1979, *18*, 354; R. W. Sidwell *et al.*, *Pharmac. Ther.*, 1979, *6*, 123; T. -W. Chang and R. C. Heel, *Drugs*, 1981, *22*, 111.

Antiviral action. Ribavirin triphosphate selectively inhibited influenza virus RNA polymerase. Ribavirin and its monophosphate had no effect on the polymerase.— B. Eriksson *et al.*, *Antimicrob. Ag. Chemother.*, 1977, *11*, 946.

Treatment with ribavirin prolonged the survival time of *mice* that had developed an autoimmune disease with glomerulonephritis similar to that found in human systemic lupus erythematosus; the titre of antibodies to DNA was reduced and proteinuria reversed by treatment in these *mice*. Ribavirin appeared to be more effective than other antiviral agents tested.— L. W. Klassen *et al.*, *Science*, 1977, *195*, 787.

A study in HeLa cells indicated that ribavirin inhibited cellular synthesis of deoxyribonucleic acid first and then ribonucleic acid and protein synthesis with increasing concentrations. The inhibition of cellular macromolecular synthesis was reversible even after prolonged treatment with ribavirin.— A. Larsson *et al.*, *Antimicrob. Ag. Chemother.*, 1978, *13*, 154.

Further studies on the antiviral action of ribavirin.— R. W. Sidwell *et al.*, *Science*, 1972, *177*, 705; G. P. Khare *et al.*, *Antimicrob. Ag. Chemother.*, 1973, *3*, 517; R. W. Sidwell *et al.*, *Chemotherapy, Basle*, 1975, *21*, 205; C. W. Potter *et al.*, *Nature*, 1976, *259*, 496; E. Katz *et al.*, *J. gen. Virol.*, 1976, *32*, 327, per *Abstr. Hyg.*, 1977, *52*, 1336; G. H. Scott *et al.*, *Antimicrob. Ag. Chemother.*, 1978, *13*, 284; J. R. McCammon and V. W. Riesser, *ibid.*, 1979, *15*, 356; M. J. Browne, *ibid.*, 747; S. Z. Wilson *et al.*, *ibid.*, 1980, *17*, 642.

Hepatitis. In 13 patients with chronic hepatitis B virus infection, given ribavirin usually 800 mg daily for 21 days, the failure of treatment to cause disappearance of surface antigen from the serum suggested that treatment was not likely to be effective. One patient, and a 14th patient, developed transient mild intravascular haemolysis.— M. C. Kew and H. C. Seftel (letter), *Br. med. J.*, 1977, *1*, 904.

Ribavirin 800 mg daily for 4 weeks, could not be shown to be beneficial in the treatment of 6 patients with chronic hepatitis B.— S. Jain *et al.*, *J. antimicrob. Chemother.*, 1978, *4*, 367.

In a double-blind placebo-controlled study, ribavirin, 100 mg given every 6 hours for 10 days produced beneficial results in the treatment of acute viral hepatitis.— P. A. Ayrosa-Galvão and I. O. Castro, *Ann. N.Y. Acad. Sci.*, 1977, *284*, 278.

Further studies of the use of ribavirin in the treatment of viral hepatitis type A.— C. B. Zuniga *et al.*, *Revta Ass. méd. bras.*, 1974, *20*, 386; H. Fernandez-Zertuche and R. Diaz-Perches, *Ann. N.Y. Acad. Sci.*, 1977, *284*, 284.

Influenza. Ribavirin suppressed signs and symptoms of artificially induced influenza type B in 15 healthy subjects who received ribavirin 600 mg daily for 2 days before challenge and 8 days after, but its effectiveness was marginal compared with that of placebo in 15 similar subjects. There was no difference between the frequencies of isolation of virus or the antibody responses in the 2 groups.— Y. Togo and E. A. McCracken, *J. infect. Dis.*, 1976, *133, Suppl.*, A109.

Ribavirin 200 mg given thrice daily for 10 days did not affect the development of artificially induced influenza type A illness in a comparative study with amantadine and placebo involving 29 healthy subjects. Signs and symptoms of influenza, febrile response, and viral excretion from the nose were not suppressed in subjects receiving ribavirin although there was a slight lowering of serum-antibody titres. Treatment with amantadine significantly reduced development of illness, titres of antibody and febrile responses. Ribavirin was also ineffective in a further 18 similar subjects.— A. Cohen *et al.*, *J. infect. Dis.*, 1976, *133, Suppl.*, A114.

In a double-blind placebo controlled study in 45 children (8 to 16 years of age) with influenza type A_2, ribavirin 100 mg thrice daily for 5 days markedly reduced the clinical symptoms of the disease 24 hours after the initiation of therapy. Recoverable virus and specific serum antibody titre were also significantly reduced in the ribavirin treated group.— F. Salido-Rengell *et al.*, *Ann. N.Y. Acad. Sci.*, 1977, *284*, 272.

Ribavirin 1 g taken daily in four divided doses for 5 days prevented the occurrence of moderate to severe symptoms and fever to a greater extent than placebo in 24 healthy subjects who became ill after intranasal inoculation with influenza type A virus. Four of the 14 subjects who received ribavirin had elevated serum concentrations of bilirubin which returned to normal within 4 weeks of the end of the study.— C. R. Magnussen *et al.*, *Antimicrob. Ag. Chemother.*, 1977, *12*, 498.

Lassa fever. Six of 10 rhesus *monkeys* infected with Lassa fever virus died, whereas of 4 similar *monkeys* treated with ribavirin, given by intramuscular injection in a dose of 50 mg per kg body-weight initially followed by 10 mg per kg thrice daily from the fifth to the eighteenth day after virus inoculation, none died. A further 4 *monkeys* given identical doses of ribavirin from immediately after inoculation until the eighteenth day also survived and the early appearance of detectable viraemia was prevented.— E. L. Stephen and P. B. Jahrling (letter), *Lancet*, 1979, *1*, 268.

Proprietary Names

Vilona, Viramid, Virazole (all Latin America: *ICN, USA*).

1686-f

Rimantadine Hydrochloride. α-Methyl-1-adamantane-methylamine Hydrochloride; EXP-126. 1-(1-Adamantyl)ethylamine hydrochloride; 1-(Tricyclo[3.3.1.$1^{3,7}$]-dec-1-yl)ethylamine hydrochloride.
$C_{12}H_{21}N,HCl$=215.8.

CAS — 13392-28-4 (rimantadine); 1501-84-4 (hydrochloride).

Adverse Effects. Vomiting, nightmares and anxiety have been reported.

Uses. Rimantadine hydrochloride is an antiviral agent with actions similar to those of amantadine hydrochloride (see p.890); it has been given in doses of 150 to 200 mg twice daily for prophylaxis against infection with influenza type A virus.

Antiviral action. Studies of the action of rimantadine *in vitro* against influenza type A virus.— G. A. Galegov *et al.* (letter), *Lancet*, 1979, *1*, 269; W. C. Koff and V. Knight, *Proc. Soc. exp. Biol. Med.*, 1979, *160*, 246.

Influenza. Rimantadine hydrochloride reduced the incidence and severity of artificially induced influenza of the Asian type in a double-blind study involving 55 subjects. It was given in 200-mg doses twice daily for 11 days, starting about 26 hours before the subjects were inoculated with virus. The drug was well tolerated by the patients with 3 exceptions: these experienced vomiting, nightmares and possibly hallucinations, and anxiety with acroparaesthesia, respectively.— A. T. Dawkins *et al.*, *J. Am. med. Ass.*, 1968, *203*, 1095. For a similar report, see S. Rabinovichi *et al.*, *Am. J. med. Sci.*, 1969, *257*, 328, per *Abstr. Wld Med.*, 1969, *43*, 905.

Rimantadine hydrochloride 150 mg, amantadine hydrochloride 100 mg, or a placebo, was given twice daily for 10 days to 95 patients with influenza due to type A virus. The duration of fever in the 3 groups was 19 hours, 23 hours, and 45 hours respectively, and overall clinical improvement was more rapid in those taking the drugs than the placebo. There were no side-effects. Serological conversion occurred in 35 of 48 taking the placebo, 21 of 24 taking rimantadine, and 19 of 23 taking amantadine.— W. L. Wingfield *et al.*, *New Engl. J. Med.*, 1969, *281*, 579.

Further references.— V. F. Krylov *et al.*, *Vop. Virus*, 1976, *2*, 186; N. P. Obrosova-Serova *et al.*, *Vop. Virus*, 1977, *3*, 295; J. R. LaMontagne and G. J. Galasso, *J. infect. Dis.*, 1978, *138*, 928, per *Abstr. Hyg.*, 1980, *55*, 258.

Manufacturers
Endo, USA.

1687-d

Stallimycin Hydrochloride. Distamycin A Hydrochloride; F.I. 6426. *N*″-(2-Amidinoethyl)-4-formamido-1,1′,1″-trimethyl-*N*,4′:*N*′,4″-ter[pyrrole-2-carboxamide] hydrochloride.
$C_{22}H_{27}N_9O_4,HCl = 517.97$.

CAS — 636-47-5 (stallimycin); 6576-51-8 (hydrochloride).

Stallimycin hydrochloride is an antibiotic derived from *Streptomyces distallicus*. A yellowish white crystalline powder. M.p. 184° to 187°. Very slightly **soluble** in water; soluble in alcohol and methyl alcohol.

Adverse Effects. Hypersensitivity reactions may occur after topical application of stallimycin hydrochloride.

Precautions. Preparations containing stallimycin hydrochloride should not be applied to the conjunctiva. They should be applied with care to patients with kidney or liver impairment.

Uses. Stallimycin hydrochloride is an antibiotic with antiviral activity against DNA containing viruses such as adenoviruses, herpesviruses and vaccinia. It has been used in the form of a 1% cream, ointment or paste for cutaneous or mucocutaneous infections produced by herpes simplex, herpes zoster and vaccinia viruses.

Some arrest in the further development of maculopapular lesions of varicella was achieved in 32 of 35 children treated with a 1% ointment of stallimycin hydrochloride applied thrice daily for 5 days.— D. Bassetti, *G. Mal. infett. parassit.*, 1968, *20*, 827, per *Abstr. Hyg.*, 1969, *44*, 1231. A favourable report of its use in 2 children with severe herpes zoster.— D. Bassetti, *G. Mal. infett. parassit.*, 1969, *21*, 849, per *Abstr. Hyg.*, 1970, *45*, 1176.

'Good' to 'excellent' results from the use of a 1% ointment of stallimycin hydrochloride in 30 patients with chicken-pox, 7 with herpes zoster, and 9 of 10 with vaccinia.— A. De Vriendt and I. Weemaes, *G. Mal. infett. parassit.*, 1972, *24*, 63, per *Abstr. Hyg.*, 1972, *47*, 1013.

Proprietary Names
Herperal *(Farmitalia, Ital.)*.

1688-n

Trifluridine. Trifluorothymidine; F_3TDR; F_3T. ααα-Trifluorothymidine; 2′-Deoxy-5-trifluoromethyluridine.
$C_{10}H_{11}F_3N_2O_5 = 296.2$.

CAS — 70-00-8.

M.p. 190°.

The stability of trifluridine in pharmaceutical preparations.— H. J. Nestler and E. R. Garrett, *J. pharm. Sci.*, 1968, *57*, 1117.

The preparation of a stable formulation of trifluridine eye-drops. Dry and moist heat were shown to be unsuitable for the sterilisation of trifluridine eye-drops and such preparations must be sterilised by filtration.— M. G. Lee *et al.*, *J. clin. Pharm.*, 1978, *3*, 179.

Adverse Effects. Adverse effects occurring after the use of trifluridine in the eyes are similar to those for idoxuridine (p.820) but have been reported to occur less frequently.

Trifluridine applied topically to the eye in doses similar to those used clinically was not teratogenic to *rabbits*.— M. Itoi *et al.*, *Archs Ophthal., N.Y.*, 1975, *93*, 46.

For the effects of trifluridine on corneal wound healing, see under Adverse Effects in Idoxuridine, p.820.

Uses. Trifluridine is an antiviral agent which is active against herpes simplex (*Herpesvirus hominis*). It is used similarly to idoxuridine (p.820) and vidarabine (p.826) in the treatment of herpetic keratitis. One drop of a 1% ophthalmic solution is instilled into the eye every 2 hours up to a maximum of 9 times daily until complete re-epithelialisation has occurred. Treatment is then reduced to one drop every 4 hours for a further 7 days. It has also been used as a 2% ophthalmic ointment.

Reviews and discussions on the uses of trifluridine.— *Drugs Today*, 1977, *13*, 381; C. Heidelberger and D. H. King, *Pharmac. Ther.*, 1979, *6*, 427; *Med. Lett.*, 1980, *22*, 46.

Herpes simplex keratitis. In a double-blind study in 40 patients with herpes simplex virus ulcers of the cornea treatment failures were significantly lower after the use of trifluridine 1% than after the use of idoxuridine 0.1%. The mean time to healing was significantly reduced from 8.2 to 6.3 days.— P. C. Wellings *et al.*, *Am. J. Ophthal.*, 1972, *73*, 932, per *J. Am. med. Ass.*, 1972, *221*, 1177.

In a single-blind study, 40 patients with active herpes simplex corneal ulcers were treated with either 1% trifluridine or 0.1% idoxuridine eye-drops. There was no significant difference between the rates of healing in the 2 groups but significantly more eyes healed successfully within 14 days with trifluridine (96%) compared with idoxuridine (75%). All of 8 eyes treated with trifluridine and corticosteroids together healed, but one eye treated with idoxuridine and corticosteroids failed to heal; numbers were too small for statistical analysis. Of a further 15 similar patients who had had previous treatment failures with idoxuridine or vidarabine, 87% of eyes healed using trifluridine.— D. Pavan-Langston and C. S. Foster, *Am. J. Ophthal.*, 1977, *84*, 818.

The average healing time of dendritic herpetic keratitis that had been unresponsive to 10 days of topical treatment with idoxuridine or vidarabine was 6.1 days in 10 patients who were treated with a 1% ophthalmic solution of trifluridine. Patients were treated for a minimum of 14 days, regardless of healing time. Recurrences occurred within 7 days of stopping treatment in 2 patients. Trifluridine was generally well tolerated except in 1 patient who developed a reversible diffuse punctate epithelial keratitis after 22 days of treatment.— R. A. Hyndiuk *et al.*, *Archs Ophthal., N.Y.*, 1978, *96*, 1839.

Eleven patients with dendritic keratitis obtained a beneficial response (mean healing time: 2.9 days) to daily application of 5 drops of trifluridine 1% in association with 2 drops of an interferon preparation containing 30 million units per ml. There was no significant difference between 15 patients who received the trifluridine with albumin (mean healing time: 5.7 days) and those who received it with an interferon preparation containing only 1 million units per ml (mean healing time: 5.3 days).— R. Sundmacher *et al.* (letter), *Lancet*, 1978, *2*, 687.

For studies indicating that trifluridine is as effective as vidarabine in the treatment of herpetic keratitis, see under Herpetic Keratitis in Vidarabine, p.827.

Proprietary Names
Bephen *(Thilo, Ger.)*; TFT *(Mann, Neth.)*; Triherpine *(Lux.)*; Viroptic *(Wellcome, USA)*.

1689-h

Tromantadine Hydrochloride. D41. *N*-1-Adamantyl-2-(2-dimethylaminoethoxy)acetamide hydrochloride; 2-(2-Dimethylaminoethoxy)-*N*-(tricyclo[3.3.1.1^{3,7}]dec-1-yl)acetamide hydrochloride.
$C_{16}H_{28}N_2O_2,HCl = 316.9$.

CAS — 53783-83-8 (tromantadine); 41544-24-5 (hydrochloride).

Adverse Effects. Contact dermatitis has been reported following the topical use of tromantadine hydrochloride.

Of 240 patients with herpes simplex treated with a gel containing tromantadine hydrochloride 1%, 20 showed local irritation. Patch testing confirmed that this was due to contact dermatitis to tromantadine in 12 of the patients. None of the patients tested was sensitive to the gel base.— D. Fanta and P. Mischer, *Contact Dermatitis*, 1976, *2*, 282.

Further references.— P. Mischer and D. Fanta, *Hautarzt*, 1978, *29*, 337.

Uses. Tromantadine hydrochloride is a derivative of amantadine (see p.890) used for its antiviral activity. It is applied as a 1% gel in the treatment of herpes simplex infections of the skin and eye.

References to the use of tromantadine in the treatment of herpes simplex infections.— S. Borelli and H. Gehrken, *Praxis*, 1976, *65*, 108; D. Fanta, *Wien. med. Wschr.*, 1976, *126*, 315; E. J. Feuerman, *Harefuah*, 1977, *93*, 73; M. P. Ahumada, *Therapie Gegenw.*, 1977, *116*, 100.

Proprietary Names
Viru-Merz *(Merz, Ger.; Merz, Neth.; Merz, Switz.)*.

1690-a

Vidarabine. Adenine Arabinoside; Ara-A; CI 673. 9-β-D-Arabinofuranosyladenine monohydrate.
$C_{10}H_{13}N_5O_4,H_2O = 285.3$.

CAS — 5536-17-4 (anhydrous); 24356-66-9 (monohydrate).

Pharmacopoeias. U.S. includes Sterile Vidarabine.

A white to off-white crystalline powder. M.p. 260° to 270°. **Soluble** 1 in about 2200 of water; slightly soluble in dimethylformamide. A solution in dimethylformamide is laevorotatory. **Store** in airtight containers.

A study of the physical properties of vidarabine formate indicated that it was at least 60 times more soluble in water than vidarabine and did not appear to be subject to enzymatic deamination. The formate therefore possesses useful features as a prodrug for vidarabine in the formulation of an intravenous preparation.— A. J. Repta *et al.*, *J. pharm. Sci.*, 1975, *64*, 392.

Adverse Effects. Adverse effects following the application of vidarabine to the eyes are similar to those of idoxuridine (p.820) but the incidence and severity has been reported to be lower.

Gastro-intestinal disturbances are the most common adverse effects following intravenous administration of vidarabine and include nausea, vomiting, diarrhoea, anorexia, and weight loss. Effects on the central nervous system such as dizziness, tremor, weakness, ataxia, confusion, psychosis, hallucinations, abnormal electro-encephalogram, and encephalopathy have also occurred. Haematological changes induced by vidarabine have included decreases in haemoglobin concentrations or haematocrit. Megaloblastosis, reticulocytopenia, leucopenia, and thrombocytopenia have also been reported.

Other side-effects occurring occasionally after the intravenous administration of vidarabine have included malaise, pruritus, rash, haematemesis, thrombophlebitis and pain at the site of injection, constipation, and elevation in bilirubin concentrations.

Vidarabine has been reported to be teratogenic,, carcinogenic and mutagenic in some species of *animals*.

Seven patients with herpesvirus infections were given intravenous injections of vidarabine of 10 or 20 mg per kg body-weight daily with one of the patients receiving a course at both dosage levels. Haematologic changes associated with vidarabine treatment occurred most often in patients with concomitant underlying chronic diseases, were most frequent with the higher dose, and were limited to patients who also had decreases in haemoglobin concentrations. All 5 patients receiving 20 mg per kg daily had decreases in haemoglobin of more than 2 g per 100 ml, whereas only 1 of 3 patients who received 10 mg per kg had a similar reduction. The number of neutrophils, white blood cells, and platelets did not decrease during treatment, even in patients who had low counts before treatment. Two patients, who had received the same chemotherapy for Hodgkin's disease and were treated with vidarabine 20 mg per kg daily for disseminated herpes zoster infection, developed a transient motor aphasia resembling akinetic mutism. The condition resolved on cessation of therapy with vidarabine.— C. B. Lauter *et al.*, *J. infect. Dis.*, 1976, *134*, 75.

Forty-two patients with compromised immunity and complications of infections due to herpesviruses were evaluated for adverse effects to intravenous treatment with vidarabine. Patients received either a placebo or vidarabine in a daily dosage of 10, 15 or 20 mg per kg body-weight for 4 to 10 days; one patient received vidarabine 30 mg per kg. Six forms of reversible adverse effects were observed: nausea and vomiting, weight loss, weakness (often with impaired ambulation), megaloblastosis in erythroid series in bone marrow, tremors 5 to 7 days after the start of therapy (including tremors in one patient with an abnormal EEG that was consistent with toxic metabolic encephalopathy) and thombophlebitis at the site of injection. The incidence of side-effects was generally greater in patients who received 20 mg per kg daily.— A. H. Ross *et al.*, *J. infect. Dis.*, 1976, *133, Suppl.*, A192.

Adverse effects in 15 patients with chronic hepatitis B treated with vidarabine (12 also received human leucocyte interferon concomitantly) included gastro-intestinal symptoms, weakness or fatigue, myalgia, reversible granulocytopenia and thrombocytopenia, jaw pain, tremor, ataxia, difficulty in walking, and neurological effects with EEG changes mimicking metabolic encephalopathy. The patient with the most severe neurological effects also had a transient compromise in renal function. Close monitoring of liver function, renal function, neurological status and haematologic values should be undertaken during treatment with vidarabine.— S. L. Sacks *et al.* (letter), *J. Am. med. Ass.*, 1979, *241*, 28.

A patient with disseminated herpes zoster developed a syndrome of inappropriate secretion of antidiuretic hormone and hyponatraemia secondary to the administration of vidarabine.— E. Ramos *et al.*, *Antimicrob. Ag. Chemother.*, 1979, *15*, 142.

For the effects of vidarabine on corneal wound healing, see under Adverse Effects in Idoxuridine, p.820.

Further references.— B. Hafkin *et al.*, *Antimicrob. Ag. Chemother.*, 1979, *16*, 781 (lymphocytopenia).

Precautions. Vidarabine should not be administered intramuscularly or subcutaneously; it may be given intravenously but rapid administration is not advised. Give with care to patients with impaired renal function or cerebral oedema, indeed caution is recommended in all patients at risk from fluid overload.

Two patients with chronic lymphocytic leukaemia who were receiving allopurinol daily developed severe neurotoxicity on the fourth day of treatment with vidarabine. Xanthine oxidase has a role in the degradation of vidarabine and inhibition of this enzyme by allopurinol could increase concentrations of hypoxanthine arabinoside, the major metabolite of vidarabine.— H. M. Friedman and T. Grasela (letter), *New Engl. J. Med.*, 1981, *304*, 423.

Absorption and Fate. Following intravenous administration vidarabine is rapidly metabolised, principally by deamination to hypoxanthine arabinoside, although a smaller proportion may be phosphorylated to phosphate nucleotides. Peak plasma concentrations of 6 µg and 0.4 µg per ml have been obtained for hypoxanthine arabinoside and vidarabine respectively at the end of a 12-hour infusion of 10 mg of vidarabine per kg body-weight. The plasma half-life for hypoxanthine arabinoside appears to be about 3.5 hours.

Hypoxanthine arabinoside is widely distributed in tissues, with the highest concentrations being detected in kidney, liver, and spleen and lower concentrations in brain and skeletal muscle. It diffuses into the cerebrospinal fluid to give concentrations about one-third to one-half of those in plasma.

Excretion is principally through the kidney with about 40 to 50% of a dose appearing in the urine as hypoxanthine arabinoside within 24 hours and 1 to 3% as unchanged drug.

Twenty-five samples of aqueous humour were obtained from 21 patients during routine cataract surgery. Each patient had used a 3% vidarabine ointment pre-operatively every 6 hours for a total of 8 doses. Vidarabine could not be detected in any of the samples but varying concentrations of hypoxanthine arabinoside from 0.02 µg per ml (the lower limit of sensitivity of the assay) to 0.28 µg per ml were found.— R. H. Poirier *et al.*, in *Adenine Arabinoside: An Antiviral Agent*, D. Pavan-Langston *et al.* (Ed.), New York, Raven Press, 1975, p. 307.

Vidarabine was given for 5 days in a daily dose of 10 mg per kg body-weight by slow intravenous infusion over 12 hours to 5 immunosuppressed patients with herpes zoster. Vidarabine appeared to be rapidly deaminated since virtually all of the drug present in plasma and urine was in the form of hypoxanthine arabinoside with a peak mean plasma concentration of about 3 µg per ml occurring at the end of each infusion. There was no indication of drug accumulation. Mean urinary excretion in 24 hours ranged from 1.94 to 2.39% for vidarabine and from 40.8 to 49.5% for hypoxanthine arabinoside.— R. A. Buchanan *et al.*, *Clin. Pharmac. Ther.*, 1980, *27*, 690.

Further references.— A. J. Glazko *et al.*, in *Adenine Arabinoside: An Antiviral Agent*, D. Pavan-Langston *et al.* (Ed.), New York, Raven Press, 1975, p. 111; R. J. Whitley *et al.*, *New Engl. J. Med.*, 1977, *297*, 289.

Uses. Vidarabine is an antiviral agent which inhibits viral DNA synthesis. Its exact mechanism of action is not yet known but it appears that the phosphorylated form of vidarabine and to a lesser extent of hypoxanthine arabinoside inhibits viral DNA polymerase. In spite of the rapid deamination of vidarabine it has a broad spectrum of activity against DNA viruses but is primarily active against herpesviruses and some poxviruses. With few exceptions it does not inhibit RNA viruses.

Vidarabine is used topically in the treatment of herpes simplex keratitis in the form of a 3% ophthalmic ointment and can be used when there has been no response to treatment with idoxuridine or when ocular toxicity or hypersensitivity to idoxuridine has occurred. The ointment is applied 5 times daily until corneal re-epithelialisation has occurred then twice daily for a further 7 days to prevent recurrence. If there is no improvement within 7 days or if there is no complete healing within 21 days, other forms of therapy should be considered. Severe conditions or conditions which have not healed with idoxuridine treatment may take longer to respond.

Vidarabine is also used intravenously in the treatment of encephalitis due to herpes simplex (*Herpesvirus hominis*) but does not appear to alter morbidity and neurological sequelae in the already comatose patient. A suggested dose is 15 mg per kg body-weight daily for 10 days; this is infused at a constant rate over a period of 12 to 24 hours. As each mg of vidarabine requires at least 2.22 ml of intravenous fluid for complete solubilisation large quantities of fluids are infused in order to administer the daily dose. The more soluble phosphate salt of vidarabine has been used to try and overcome this problem.

Vidarabine has also been given intravenously in a dose of 10 mg per kg daily in the treatment of herpes zoster infections, especially in immunosuppressed patients.

Reviews and discussions on the use of vidarabine in the treatment of viral infections.— *Br. med. J.*, 1976, *2*, 1466; M. Deshpande, *Can. pharm. J.*, 1978, *111*, 108; T. -W. Chang and D. R. Snydman, *Drugs*, 1979, *18*, 354; R. A. Buchanan, *Can. med. Ass. J.*, 1979, *120*, 7; M. S. Hirsch and M. N. Swartz, *New Engl. J. Med.*, 1980, *302*, 903; *Lancet*, 1980, *1*, 1337; R. J. Whitley *et al.*, *Drugs*, 1980, *20*, 267.

For the proceedings of a symposium on vidarabine, see *Adenine Arabinoside: An Antiviral Agent*, D. Pavan-Langston *et al.* (Ed.), New York, Raven Press, 1975.

Antiviral action. Coformycin, an inhibitor of adenosine deaminase, enhanced the activity of vidarabine by preventing deamination to the less active metabolite hypoxanthine arabinoside. There was no effect on the selectivity of vidarabine.— P. M. Schwartz *et al.*, *Antimicrob. Ag. Chemother.*, 1976, *10*, 64.

A review of the mechanism of the lethal action of vidarabine on viruses indicated that it was due to its conversion to its aranucleoside triphosphate that appeared to act by relatively specific inhibition of DNA synthesis and possibly by incorporation into cell or virus DNA.— S. S. Cohen, *Cancer*, 1977, *40*, 509.

Further studies of the antiviral action and activity of vidarabine.— F. A. Miller *et al.*, *Antimicrob. Ag. Chemother.*, 1968, 136; R. W. Sidwell *et al.*, *ibid.*, 148; J. L. Schardein and R. W. Sidwell, *ibid.*, 155; B. J. Sloan *et al.*, *ibid.*, 161; G. J. Dixon *et al.*, *ibid.*, 172; S. M. Kurtz *et al.*, *ibid.*, 180; F. A. Miller *et al.*, *ibid.*, 1969, 192; M. Coker-Vann and R. Dolin, *J. infect. Dis.*, 1977, *135*, 447, per *Abstr. Hyg.*, 1978, *53*, 1247; W. E. G. Müller *et al.*, *Ann. N.Y. Acad. Sci.*, 1977, *284*, 34.

Cytomegalovirus infection. A report of clinical improvements in some infants and adults given vidarabine intravenously for the treatment of cytomegalovirus infections including CNS involvement, disseminated congenital infection, pneumonitis and mononucleosis.— J. V. Baublis *et al.*, in *Adenine Arabinoside: An Antiviral Agent*, D. Pavan-Langston *et al.* (Ed.), New York, Raven Press, 1975, p. 247.

Two patients with acute cytomegalovirus encephalitis were successfully treated with vidarabine 15 mg per kg body-weight daily for 10 days given intravenously. One patient also received dexamethasone 4 mg every 6 hours by intravenous injection. No serious toxic reactions to vidarabine were reported at this dosage.— C. A. Phillips *et al.*, *J. Am. med. Ass.*, 1977, *238*, 2299.

Hepatitis. For a brief discussion on the use of vidarabine in the treatment of viral hepatitis, see V. Damjanovic and W. Brumfitt, *J. antimicrob. Chemother.*, 1980, *6*, 11.

Vidarabine 15 mg per kg body-weight was administered daily to 2 patients with chronic hepatitis B in 2 courses of 9 to 14 days separated by 20 and 42 days respectively. In one patient there was a rapid decrease in Dane particle DNA polymerase during both courses of treatment followed by an increase when treatment ceased. There was no significant change in complement-fixation titre of surface antigen. In the second patient DNA polymerase was undetectable after the first course and remained undetectable 12 months after discontinuation of therapy; the titre of surface antigen was also significantly reduced.— R. B. Pollard *et al.*, *J. Am. med. Ass.*, 1978, *239*, 1648.

In 4 patients positive for hepatitis B surface antigen, DNA polymerase activity was reduced during treatment with vidarabine 10 mg per kg body-weight daily by infusion in 2 litres of dextrose injection 5% for 5 days in each of 2 weeks. The role of vidarabine in chronic liver disease remained to be established but it was considered that infectivity would be reduced.— R. G. Chadwick *et al.*, *Br. med. J.*, 1978, *2*, 531.

Further references.— M. F. Bassendine *et al.*, *Gut*, 1978, *19*, A991; *idem*, 1979, *20*, A906.

Herpes simplex. Stomatitis, due to herpes simplex (*Herpesvirus hominis*) type 1 (HSV) and unresponsive to idoxuridine in 10 patients responded to treatment with vidarabine; virus was still detected in half the patients after treatment but there was no clinical recurrence. Concomitant genital lesions due to HSV type 2 in 3 patients responded more slowly. Two of 6 infants with disseminated herpes simplex infections treated early survived, and a third survived with severe brain damage. The only side-effect was nausea.— L. T. Ch'ien *et al.*, *J. infect. Dis.*, 1973, *128*, 658, per *Abstr. Hyg.*, 1974, *49*, 508.

The application of vidarabine 3% in a basis of soft paraffin 60% and liquid paraffin 40% did not modify the clinical course or viral titre of herpes progenitalis in 15 episodes when compared with a placebo in a double-blind study. Possibly this lack of effect was due to limited diffusion into the lesion which might be improved by use of a more soluble form or a different vehicle.— E. L. Goodman *et al.*, *Antimicrob. Ag. Chemother.*, 1976, *8*, 693. Similar results.— H. G. Adams *et al.*, *J. infect. Dis.*, 1976, *133, Suppl.*, A151; A. L. Hilton *et al.*, *Br. J. vener. Dis.*, 1978, *54*, 50.

Vidarabine monophosphate, used topically as a 10% cream, was found to be ineffective when compared with placebo in the treatment of recurrent herpes simplex labialis in a collaborative double-blind study of 233 patients. Inadequate penetration of the skin might be responsible for this failure.— S. L. Spruance *et al.*, *New Engl. J. Med.*, 1979, *300*, 1180.

Vidarabine 3% in a water-miscible gel basis applied 6 times daily for 7 days was significantly more effective than placebo in reducing lesion size in 70 patients with recurrent herpes simplex labialis who were evaluated over 12 months, but there was no statistical difference between the vidarabine and placebo groups in episode frequency or lesion duration. Treatment during the tingling stage accelerated development of the lesion. The most effective time to apply vidarabine appeared to be during the prevesiculation stage of development.— N. H. Rowe *et al.*, *Oral Path.*, 1979, *47*, 142.

Encephalitis. Reviews and discussions of the use of vidarabine in the treatment of herpes simplex encephalitis.— *J. Am. med. Ass.*, 1977, *238*, 1121; *Med. Lett.*, 1979, *21*, 17.

In a National Institute of Allergy and Infectious Diseases Collaborative Antiviral Study, of 18 patients with virologically confirmed herpes simplex encephalitis who received vidarabine 15 mg per kg body-weight daily (by intravenous infusion over a period of 12 hours) for 10 days, 5 died compared with 7 of 10 who received placebo; this was a reduction in mortality from 70 to 28%. In the active group 7 patients recovered to lead reasonably normal lives compared with 2 in the placebo group. Early therapy prior to coma was needed for a beneficial effect but, although no acute drug toxicity had been noted, should be preceded by brain biopsy to avoid unnecessary prolongation of treatment of non-responsive encephalitides.— R. J. Whitley *et al.*, *New Engl. J. Med.*, 1977, *297*, 289. Criticisms; further controlled studies were needed.— I. R. Tager (letter), *ibid.*, 1289; J. C. Gluckman (letter), *ibid.* Reply.— R. J. Whitley *et al.* (letter), *ibid.*, 1290. Results of an uncontrolled study in 132 patients confirmed the beneficial effect of vidarabine in herpes simplex encephalitis and emphasised the need for brain biopsy in diagnosis.— *idem*, 1981, *304*, 313.

Four of 5 patients with biopsy confirmed herpes simplex encephalitis survived more than 12 months after intravenous treatment with vidarabine but some degree of neurological impairment was noted in all the patients. Four of the patients had been comatose when vidarabine therapy was instituted. Three of the patients had shown a progressive improvement since. No apparent toxicity attributable to vidarabine was found.— L. H. Taber *et al.*, *Archs Neurol., Chicago*, 1977, *34*, 608.

No improvement in a 7-year-old child in terminal coma with subacute sclerosing panencephalitis given vidarabine as the 5′-phosphate in sodium chloride injection at a concentration of 37.5 mg per ml by intravenous and intrathecal injections for 10 days.— H. E. Webb *et al.* (letter), *Lancet*, 1977, *2*, 978.

Clinical improvement occurred in 2 infants with herpes simplex encephalitis, 1 of whom had relapsed after cytarabine therapy, given vidarabine 15 mg per kg body-weight as a 12-hourly intravenous infusion for 7 days. Although both infants survived CNS damage was apparent. A further infant given only cytarabine had died.— G. M. Maxwell *et al.*, *Med. J. Aust.*, 1978, *1*, 181.

A plea for caution in the use of vidarabine for the treatment of herpes encephalitis.— T. -W. Chang (letter), *New Engl. J. Med.*, 1979, *300*, 796.

Postinfectious encephalomyelitis occurred in a 28-year-old man about 2 weeks after he had been treated successfully for herpes simplex encephalitis with vidarabine 15 mg per kg body-weight daily by slow intravenous infusion for 10 days. Biopsy of brain tissue did not demonstrate reactivation of the infection and a second course of vidarabine was of no benefit.— H. Koenig *et al.*, *New Engl. J. Med.*, 1979, *300*, 1089.

Vidarabine was the recommended drug of first choice in the treatment of herpes simplex encephalitis.— *Med. Lett.*, 1980, *22*, 5.

Keratitis. Discussions and reviews of the use of vidarabine in the treatment of herpetic keratitis.— *J. Am. med. Ass.*, 1974, *230*, 189; J. I. McGill *et al.*, *Trans. ophthal. Soc. U.K.*, 1975, *95*, 246; *Med. Lett.*, 1977, *19*, 42; *Drug & Ther. Bull.*, 1979, *17*, 43.

In a study of 54 patients with ocular herpes simplex, there was no significant difference between the healing time of ulcers of 27 eyes treated with vidarabine 3% ointment (12.4 days) and 24 eyes treated with idoxuridine 0.5% ointment (11.5 days). Visual acuity was improved in more patients treated with vidarabine and was considered to be due to smoother epithelial healing rather than to any differences in stromal scarring. In a further study vidarabine was used successfully in 49 of 57 patients who had had severe allergy or toxic reaction to idoxuridine, or had no improvement or deterioration of herpetic ulcers while receiving idoxuridine therapy; the mean healing time was 10.6 days. Except for one patient, who had redness and irritation and punctate keratitis there were no adverse reactions in these patients during therapy lasting up to 192 days.— D. Pavan-Langston, *Am. J. Ophthal.*, 1975, *80*, 495.

In a double-blind study vidarabine 3.3% ointment or trifluridine 1% eye-drops were used 5 times daily to treat 102 patients with dendritic or amoeboid ulcers of the cornea due to herpes simplex (*Herpesvirus hominis*). The frequency of treatment was reduced to thrice daily applications when the epithelial defect healed and the total treatment was given for a maximum of 14 days. The dendritic ulcers of only 1 of 87 patients failed to heal and this was in a patient treated with vidarabine. The mean time required to heal was not significantly different for the 2 groups being 5.13 days for vidarabine and 5.75 days for trifluridine. Recurrence or recrudescence of epithelial herpetic disease occurred in 10 patients treated with vidarabine and in 4 treated with trifluridine, but was considered to be due to the arbitrary choice of the length of treatment after initial healing. In the 15 patients with amoeboid ulcers, trifluridine appeared to be more effective than vidarabine.— D. J. Coster *et al.*, *J. infect. Dis.*, 1976, *133*, *Suppl.*, A173. See also J. P. Travers and A. Patterson, *J. int. med. Res.*, 1978, *6*, 102. Similar results were obtained in 63 patients treated with 2% trifluridine ointment or 3% vidarabine ointment but the mean healing times were 11.14 days and 10.54 days respectively. The difference in the healing times between this study and that of D.J. Coster *et al.* may have been due to the criteria used to decide healing.— O. P. Van Bijsterveld and H. Post, *Br. J. Ophthal.*, 1980, *64*, 33.

Vidarabine 3% ointment was used to treat 2 groups of patients with active herpes simplex keratitis who had either had toxic or hypersensitivity reactions to idoxuridine or had failed to respond to idoxuridine. Of 35 patients without initial stromal involvement 34 healed with a mean healing time of 21 days. Of 21 patients who had developed active epithelial keratitis during corticosteroid therapy for active stromal keratitis or uveitis, 11 had complete re-epithelialisation after 14 days, 2 failed to heal, and the remainder healed in 21 to 48 days. There was no recurrence of active herpes simplex in 26 patients from both groups who had required concomitant vidarabine and corticosteroid therapy.— D. M. O'Day *et al.*, *Am. J. Ophthal.*, 1976, *81*, 642.

In a double-blind study of 169 patients with herpetic keratitis, vidarabine and idoxuridine were equally effective in terms of improvement of lachrymation, photophobia and sensitivity, and in the degree and rate of healing. However, vidarabine improved distant visual acuity in significantly more patients than idoxuridine. Of a further 116 patients who had failed to respond to idoxuridine therapy or had exhibited allergic or toxic reactions to idoxuridine, 91 had re-epithelialisation within 4 weeks of commencing treatment with vidarabine.— D. Pavan-Langston and R. A. Buchanan, *Trans. Am. Acad. Ophthal. Oto-lar.*, 1976, *81*, 813.

Further references.— D. Pavan-Langston and C. H. Dohlman, *Am. J. Ophthal.*, 1972, *74*, 81; R. A. Hyndiuk *et al.*, *ibid.*, 1975, *79*, 655.

Herpes zoster. Discussions on the use of vidarabine in the treatment of disseminated herpes zoster particularly in immunosuppressed patients.— R. Dolin *et al.*, *Ann. intern. Med.*, 1978, *89*, 375; A. W. Hopefl, *Drug Intell. & clin. Pharm.*, 1979, *13*, 255.

In 14 patients with zoster, new lesions ceased to appear within 4 days of infusion of vidarabine 5 to 20 mg (usually 10 mg) per kg body-weight over 6 hours daily. Favourable results were obtained in 6 of 9 patients with varicella. Haemoglobin concentrations fell by 3 g per 100 ml in 3 patients.— M. T. Johnson *et al.*, *J. infect. Dis.*, 1975, *131*, 225, per *Abstr. Hyg.*, 1975, *50*, 1168.

From a randomised controlled crossover collaborative study by the National Institute of Allergy and Infectious Diseases of a total of 87 patients with active herpes zoster, it was reported that although there was rapid healing with a placebo, the clearance of virus from vesicles, the cessation of new vesicle formation, and the time to total pustulation were significantly improved when vidarabine 10 mg per kg body-weight was given daily, by slow intravenous injection over 12 hours, for the first 5 days of treatment. The treatment was of particular value when given within the first 6 days of the disease to young patients with reticuloendothelial neoplasms.— R. J. Whitley *et al.*, *New Engl. J. Med.*, 1976, *294*, 1193. See also *J. Am. med. Ass.*, 1976, *236*, 13.

A 37-year-old immunosuppressed woman with a renal transplant developed varicella pneumonia and did not improve on administration of hyperimmune anti-varicella immunoglobulin injection. She was given vidarabine 10 mg per kg body-weight (infused in 500 ml of dextrose-saline over 4 to 6 hours) daily for 5 days and within 2 days had made a remarkable recovery.— E. L. Teare and J. A. Cohen (letter), *Lancet*, 1979, *1*, 873.

Further references.— B. Juel-Jensen, *J. antimicrob. Chemother.*, 1976, *2*, 261, per *Abstr. Hyg.*, 1977, *52*, 90; P. A. M. Walden *et al.* (letter), *Br. med. J.*, 1977, *1*, 378.

Encephalitis. A 3-year-old child with viral encephalitis associated with increased titres of antibodies to varicella zoster (*Herpesvirus varicella*) improved dramatically within 2 days of receiving vidarabine monophosphate 15 mg per kg body-weight. Another child with severe encephalitis associated with cytomegalovirus made a slow recovery under treatment with vidarabine monophosphate. Further controlled clinical studies with vidarabine appear to be justified.— G. T. Werner and O. Sauer (letter), *Lancet*, 1979, *1*, 1040.

Smallpox. In a double-blind study in 20 patients with smallpox there was no significant benefit from the infusion of vidarabine 20 mg per kg body-weight daily for 7 days.— J. P. Koplan *et al.*, *J. infect. Dis.*, 1975, *131*, 34, per *Abstr. Hyg.*, 1975, *50*, 1045.

Vaccinia. Rapid resolution of a vaccinial lesion of the eye of a 5-year-old boy was felt to be largely due to topical application of 3% vidarabine eye ointment.— P. Gatenby (letter), *Lancet*, 1979, *1*, 676. See also D. Pavan-Langston and C. H. Dohlman, *Am. J. Ophthal.*, 1972, *74*, 81.

Preparations

Sterile Vidarabine *(U.S.P.)*. Sterile vidarabine monohydrate; it has a potency equivalent to 845 to 985 µg of anhydrous vidarabine per mg. Store in airtight containers.

Vidarabine Ophthalmic Ointment *(U.S.P.)*. Contains vidarabine 30 mg per g. Store at 15° to 30°.

Proprietary Preparations

Vira-A *(Parke, Davis, UK)*. Vidarabine, available as eye ointment containing 3%. **Vira-A Parenteral**. Vidarabine, available as an injection containing 200 mg per ml, in vials of 5 ml. (Also available as Vira-A in *Austral., Canad., USA*).

1691-t

Xenazoic Acid. Xenalamine; Xenalmine. 4-[2-(Biphenyl-4-yl)-1-ethoxy-2-oxoethylamino]benzoic acid. $C_{23}H_{21}NO_4$=375.4.

CAS — 1174-11-4.

Xenazoic acid has been reported to have antiviral properties and has been tried in the prevention and treatment of influenza and in the treatment of chicken-pox, measles, and other viral infections. Jaundice has developed during treatment.

Insect Repellents

2550-j

The principal insect repellents described in this section are dibutyl phthalate, dimethyl phthalate, and diethyltoluamide. Other effective insect repellents not in this section include benzyl benzoate (see p.833), which is not readily removed from clothes by washing, and undecenoic acid (see p.732), which has an odour that is difficult to mask.

Complete protection against biting insects requires the frequent application of repellents to the skin. Clothing also requires treatment; repellents which are used on the skin may also be applied to clothing, with the exception of certain synthetic fabrics such as rayon, but repellents used on clothing may not be suitable for use on the skin. Effective repellents for clothing include benzyl benzoate, butylethylpropanediol, dibutyl phthalate, and diethyltoluamide. The frequency of application may be reduced by using insect repellents such as benzyl benzoate or dibutyl phthalate which are not readily removed by water.

Plastics may be softened by insect repellents.

A report of a symposium on insects and disease and papers on factors concerned with the attraction and repulsion of insects, the evaluation and use of mosquito repellents, and the possible development of systemic insect repellents for human use.— *J. Am. med. Ass.*, 1966, *196,* 236–266.

The most effective tick repellents approved on toxicological grounds for civilian use included butopyronoxyl, diethyltoluamide, dimethyl phthalate, and benzyl benzoate. Undecenoic acid was more effective but its odour could not readily be masked. These agents afforded 80 to 99% protection when used on clothing. Diethyltoluamide and benzyl benzoate were the most effective agents against fleas and afforded 90 to 99% protection when used on clothing. Diethyltoluamide could also be applied to the skin. Diethyltoluamide, dimethyl phthalate, and ethohexadiol, applied to skin or clothing, were effective against chiggers (the larvae of *Trombicula* [harvest-bugs] and similar mites) and against mosquitoes. Benzyl benzoate might be applied to clothing for this purpose. Diethyltoluamide 25% in lanolin had been used as a leech repellent.— H. K. Gouck, *Archs Derm.*, 1966, *93,* 112.

For recommendations of the most suitable repellents for many common biting insects, see Insecticide Resistance and Vector Control, Seventeenth Report of the Expert Committee on Insecticides, *Tech. Rep. Ser. Wld Hlth Org. No. 443,* 1970.

2551-z

Butopyronoxyl. Indalone. Butyl 3,4-dihydro-2,2-dimethyl-4-oxo-2*H*-pyran-6-carboxylate.
$C_{12}H_{18}O_4$=226.3.

CAS — 532-34-3.

A yellow to pale reddish-brown liquid with a characteristic aromatic odour. Wt per ml about 1.055 g. Practically **insoluble** in water and glycerol; miscible with alcohol, chloroform, ether, and glacial acetic acid. **Store** in airtight containers. Protect from light.

Butopyronoxyl is an insect repellent which is effective against ticks, but it may be mildly irritating to the skin. It has been used mainly in conjunction with dimethyl phthalate and ethohexadiol.

For an assessment of butopyronoxyl as an insect repellent see p.828.

2552-c

Butylethylpropanediol.
$C_9H_{20}O_2$=160.3.

Butylethylpropanediol is an insect repellent used for the treatment of clothing. It should not be applied directly to the skin. It is effective against blackflies, mosquitoes, and other biting Diptera.

2553-k

Dibutyl Phthalate *(B.P. 1963).* DBP; Butyl Phthalate. Dibutyl benzene-1,2-dicarboxylate.

$C_{16}H_{22}O_4$=278.3.

CAS — 84-74-2.

Pharmacopoeias. In *Ind.*

A clear, colourless or faintly yellow, somewhat viscous liquid; it is odourless or has not more than a faint odour. Wt per ml about 1.045 g. B.p. about 330°. **Soluble** 1 in 2500 of water; miscible with most organic solvents.

Adverse Effects. Dibutyl phthalate has low toxicity but occasional hypersensitivity has been reported. Ingestion may cause CNS depression. Maximum permissible atmospheric concentration 5 mg per m^3.

Uses. Dibutyl phthalate has properties similar to those of dimethyl phthalate (see p.828). It is slightly less effective than dimethyl phthalate as an insect repellent but it is more effective against the trombidid mite, the vector of scrub typhus.

It is less volatile and less easily removed by washing then dimethyl phthalate, and its chief use is for the impregnation of clothing. Application of about 30 ml per set of clothes, rubbed in by hand, may give protection for up to 2 weeks.

2554-a

Diethyltoluamide *(B.P., U.S.P.).* Deet. *NN*-Diethyl-*m*-toluamide.

$C_{12}H_{17}NO$=191.3.

CAS — 134-62-3.

Pharmacopoeias. In *Br.* and *U.S.*

A colourless or faintly yellow liquid, odourless or with a faint pleasant odour. Wt per ml 0.997 to 1 g. Practically **insoluble** in water and glycerol; miscible with alcohol, carbon disulphide, chloroform, ether, isopropyl alcohol, and propylene glycol. **Store** in airtight containers.

Adverse Effects and Precautions. Occasional hypersensitivity has been reported. Diethyltoluamide should not be applied near the eyes, to mucous membranes, to broken skin or to areas of skin flexion as irritation or blistering may occur.

A 35-year-old woman developed contact urticaria (considered to be an immediate-type hypersensitivity) after application of diethyltoluamide; this was confirmed by patch testing.— H. I. Maibach and H. L. Johnson, *Archs Derm.*, 1975, *111,* 726.

A 5-year-old child with a deficiency of ornithine carbamoyltransferase who sprayed herself lavishly with a 15% solution of diethyltoluamide developed a fatal toxic encephalopathy; the clinical picture resembled Reye's syndrome.— H. M. C. Heick *et al., J. Pediat.* 1980, *97,* 471, per *Lancet,* 1981, *1,* 368.

Further references: J. Gryboski *et al., New Engl. J. Med.*, 1961, *264,* 289; S. I. Lamberg and J. A. Mulrennan, *Archs Derm.*, 1969, *100,* 582.

Uses. Diethyltoluamide is an insect repellent which is effective against blackflies, harvest-bugs or chiggers, midges, mosquitoes, ticks, and fleas. It has also been used as a repellent against leeches. It may be applied as a 50 to 75% solution in alcohol or isopropyl alcohol to skin and clothing. When applied to the skin it is effective for several hours.

A study of the protective efficacy of diethyltoluamide solution against *Aedes aegypti* indicated that the minimum effective dose ranged from 50 to 77 µg per cm^2 of skin.— C. N. Smith, *J. Am. med. Ass.*, 1966, *196,* 236.

Diethyltoluamide was found to be the most effective repellent against *Aedes aegypti* and *A. taeniorhynchus* and better than standard repellents against *Stomoxys calcitrans, Chrysops atlanticus, Culicoides canithorax,* and *Mansonia* spp.It had also been reported to be superior in low concentrations against *Anopheles quadrimaculatus* and various species of *Aedes.* Its meta-isomer was the most active.— I. H. Gilbert, *J. Am. med. Ass.*, 1966, *196,* 253.

Vanillin significantly prolonged the protection time of diethyltoluamide. It was considered that vanillin mixed with some insect repellents could provide protection against mosquito bites for almost 24 hours.— A. A. Khan *et al., Mosquito News,* 1975, *35,* 223, per *Trop. Dis. Bull.*, 1975, *72,* 834.

For an assessment of diethyltoluamide as an insect repellent, see p.828.

Preparations

Diethyltoluamide Topical Solution *(U.S.P.).* A solution containing diethyltoluamide in alcohol or isopropyl alcohol. Store in airtight containers.

Autan *(Bayer, UK).* Preparations containing diethyltoluamide available as **Gel** containing 15%; as pressurised **Spray** containing 28.368%; and as a **Stick** containing 33%.

Diethyltoluamide was formerly marketed in Great Britain under the proprietary name Metadelphene (*Hercules*).

2555-t

Dimethyl Phthalate *(B.P.).* DMP; Methyl Phthalate. Dimethyl benzene-1,2-dicarboxylate.

$C_{10}H_{10}O_4$=194.2.

CAS — 131-11-3.

Pharmacopoeias. In *Br.* and *Nord.*

A colourless or faintly coloured liquid, odourless or with not more than a faint odour. Wt per ml 1.186 to 1.192 g. B.p. about 280° with decomposition.

Soluble 1 in 250 of water; miscible with alcohol, ether, and most organic solvents. **Protect** from light. Contact with plastic materials should be avoided.

Adverse Effects. Dimethyl phthalate may cause temporary smarting and should not be applied near the eyes or to mucous membranes. Ingestion may cause CNS depression.

Maximum permissible atmospheric concentration 5 mg per m^3.

Uses. Dimethyl phthalate is an insect repellent which is effective against blackflies, harvest-bugs or chiggers, mosquitoes, midges, mites, ticks, and fleas. It is usually applied to the skin as a cream or lotion containing at least 40% of dimethyl phthalate; weaker preparations are not effective. When applied to the skin it is active for 3 to 5 hours and for much longer periods when used to impregnate clothing, though for this purpose dibutyl phthalate is usually preferred as it is less volatile and less easily removed by washing.

Dimethyl phthalate should not be allowed to come into contact with synthetic fibres such as rayon or with plastic spectacle frames.

Wide-mesh head veils, which had been soaked in dimethyl phthalate and then wrung out and hung in the open air, afforded complete protection against mosquito bites for 5 to 6 days.— *Ministry of Health Memorandum on Measures for the Control of Mosquito Nuisances in Great Britain,* London, HM Stationery Office, 1961.

A study of the protective efficacy of dimethyl phthalate against *Aedes aegypti* indicated that the minimum effective dose ranged from about 1.15 to 1.32 mg per cm^2 of the skin but 1 subject required more than 3.5 mg per cm^2.— C. N. Smith, *J. Am. med. Ass.*, 1966, *196,* 236.

For an assessment of dimethyl phthalate as an insect repellent, see p.828.

Preparations

Dimethyl Phthalate Application *(A.P.F.).* Mosquito-repellent Cream. Dimethyl phthalate 40 ml, emulsifying wax 4 g, triethanolamine 5 ml, stearic acid 10 g, freshly boiled and cooled water to 100 g.

Mosquito Repellent Cream. Dimethyl phthalate 100 ml, Lanette Wax SX 5 g, triethanolamine 9 ml, oleic acid

27 ml, and water 100 ml.— *Ministry of Health Memorandum on Measures for the Control of Mosquito Nuisances in Great Britain,* London, HM Stationery Office, 1961.

Proprietary Names
Affel *(Fr.).*

Dimethyl phthalate was formerly marketed in Great Britain under the proprietary name Sketofax (*Wellcome*).

2556-x

Ethohexadiol. Ethylhexanediol; Rutgers 612. 2-Ethylhexane-1,3-diol.

$C_8H_{18}O_2$=146.2.

CAS — 94-96-2.

A clear colourless oily liquid which is odourless or has only a slight odour. Wt per ml about 0.94 g. **Soluble** 1 in 50 of water; miscible with alcohol, chloroform, ether, isopropyl alcohol, and propylene glycol. **Store** in airtight containers.

Adverse Effects. As for Dimethyl Phthalate p.828.

Uses. Ethohexadiol is an insect repellent which is effective against blackflies, harvest-bugs or chiggers, and mosquitoes. It may be applied topically to the skin and to clothing. It is stated to be especially effective when used in conjunction with dimethyl phthalate and butopyronoxyl.

A study of the protective efficacy of ethohexadiol against *Aedes aegypti* indicated that the minimum effective dose ranged from about 80 to 280 µg per cm² of skin.— C. N. Smith, *J. Am. med. Ass.*, 1966, *196,* 236.

No synergistic effect had been found between ethohexadiol and diethyltoluamide.— I. H. Gilbert, *J. Am. med. Ass.*, 1966, *196,* 253.

For an assessment of ethohexadiol as a repellent for harvest-bugs or chiggers, see p.828.

Insecticides and some other Pesticides

3560-n

The *insecticides* or *pesticides* in current use may be classified into several groups, namely, *chlorinated insecticides* (p.830) such as dicophane (p.835) and gamma benzene hexachloride (p.837), *organophosphorus insecticides* (p.832) such as malathion (p.838) and metriphonate (p.839), and organic *insecticides of natural origin* such as pyrethrum (p.841). The synthetic pyrethroids are structurally similar to the pyrethrins and have a wide range of actions. Other groups include the *carbamates* (p.830) and the *dinitrophenols* (p.830).

Pesticides are also classified according to their toxicity and both voluntary and legal measures control their use. Many insecticides are also effective *acaricides*. Those commonly used for this purpose include benzyl benzoate (p.833), gamma benzene hexachloride (p.837), and monosulfiram (p.840).

Molluscicides are described on p.833; *rodenticides* are described on p.833.

Permissible atmospheric concentrations.— *Threshold Limit Values 1980*, Guidance Note EH15/80, London, Health and Safety Executive, 1980.

Recommended maximum acceptable daily intakes of pesticides.— Pesticide Residues in Food, Report of the 1976 Joint FAO/WHO Meeting, *Tech. Rep. Ser. Wld Hlth Org. No. 612*, 1977. See also *Tech. Rep. Ser. Wld Hlth Org. No. 525*, 1973; *ibid., No. 545*, 1974; *ibid., No. 574*, 1975; *ibid., No. 592*, 1976.

References on the safe use of insecticides: *Pesticides Safety Precautions Scheme*, London, Ministry of Agriculture, Fisheries and Food; *Review of the Present Safety Arrangements for the Use of Toxic Chemicals in Agriculture and Food Storage*, London, HM Stationery Office, 1967; *Safe Use of Pesticides*, Third Report of the WHO Expert Committee on Vector Biology and Control, *Tech. Rep. Ser. Wld Hlth Org. No. 634*, 1979; *Safe Use of Pesticides in Public Health*, Sixteenth Report of the WHO Expert Committee on Insecticides, *Tech. Rep. Ser. Wld Hlth Org. No. 356*, 1967; Twentieth Report, *Tech. Rep. Ser. Wld Hlth Org. No. 513*, 1973; *Poisonous Chemicals on the Farm*, Health and Safety Executive, London, HM Stationery Office, 1978; *Approved Products for Farmers and Growers*, London, Ministry of Agriculture, Fisheries and Food.

General references: *Application and Dispersal of Pesticides*, Eighteenth Report of the WHO Expert Committee on Insecticides, *Tech. Rep. Ser. Wld Hlth Org. No. 465*, 1971; *Bull. Wld Hlth Org.*, 1971, *44*, 1–424; The Use of Viruses for the Control of Insect Pests and Disease Vectors, Report of a Joint FAO/WHO Group on Insect Viruses, *Tech. Rep. Ser. Wld Hlth Org. No. 531*, 1973; Chemical and Biochemical Methodology for the Assessment of Hazards of Pesticides for Man, Report of a WHO Scientific Group, *Tech. Rep. Ser. Wld Hlth Org. No. 560*, 1975; *Chemistry and Specifications of Pesticides*, Second Report of the WHO Expert Committee on Vector Biology and Control, *Tech. Rep. Ser. Wld Hlth Org. No. 620*, 1978; *Specifications for Pesticides used in Public Health*, 5th Edn, Geneva, WHO, 1979.

Nomenclature. In *Martindale*, the nomenclature used for insecticides generally follows (1) the British Approved Names, where these exist, (2) the British Standard Recommended Common Names for Pesticides (BS 1831: 1969 as updated), and (3) the names issued by the International Organisation for Standardisation (ISO).

Resistance to Insecticides. Resistance by disease vectors is a problem with the common groups of insecticides and has extended to cover the newer groups, including the pyrethroids, hormone mimics, and other insect development inhibitors. Also most if not all vector groups are now involved.

References: *Insecticide Resistance and Vector Control*, Thirteenth Report of the WHO Expert Committee on Insecticides, *Tech. Rep. Ser. Wld Hlth Org. No. 265*, 1963; *Insecticide Resistance and Vector Control*, Seventeenth Report of the WHO Expert Committee on Insecticides, *Tech. Rep. Ser. Wld Hlth Org. No. 443*, 1970; *Resistance of Vectors and Reservoirs of Disease to Pesticides*, Twenty-second Report of the WHO Expert Committee on Insecticides, *Tech. Rep. Ser. Wld Hlth Org. No. 585*, 1976.

Insecticides in the Body and Diet. Insecticides can be absorbed during application, by consumption of treated products, or by accidental contamination and they may be stored or retained in the tissues. International regulations and controls operate to reduce the risk to both public and user. In the UK there appears to be no evidence that the legitimate use of authorised insecticides produces toxic residues in the diet or that toxic concentrations accumulate. The adverse effects of groups or individual insecticides are discussed below.

Conclusions from investigations into the use of dicophane, aldrin, benzene hexachloride, camphechlor, chlordane, dieldrin, endosulfan, endrin, gamma benzene hexachloride, heptachlor, and TDE included the denunciation of statements that these compounds were severe liver poisons. There was no proof that dicophane caused injury while stored in the fat of human beings or animals, and dicophane and dieldrin could not be condemned as presenting a carcinogenic hazard to man. Nevertheless, it was recommended that accumulative contamination of the environment by the more persistent organochlorine pesticides be curtailed and restrictions on their use be imposed. The most important of these appeared to be that the use of aldrin and dieldrin in fertiliser mixtures and in dips and sprays for sheep should cease as soon as this could be arranged, that products containing aldrin, dieldrin, and heptachlor for garden use should no longer be available, and that endosulfan and endrin should be available for certain commercial uses only.— *Review of the Persistent Organochlorine Pesticides*—Report (February 1964) and Supplementary Report (July 1964) by the Advisory Committee on Pesticides and other Toxic Chemicals, London, HM Stationery Office, 1964.

Organochlorine compounds, especially dicophane, TDE, aldrin, and dieldrin, were more widely present in the environment than had previously been demonstrated. Residues in food of dicophane and its derivatives, aldrin, dieldrin, and benzene hexachloride appeared in general to be declining; dietary levels of dicophane and benzene hexachloride were well below the maximum acceptable daily intakes; the level of dieldrin was near the acceptable maximum which however incorporated large safety factors. Recommendations, if implemented, should result in a reduced use of dicophane in agriculture and horticulture. Withdrawal of some recommended uses of aldrin, camphechlor, chlordane, dieldrin, endosulfan, endrin, and heptachlor was advised where they were no longer required, where resistance was developing, or when satisfactory alternatives were available. The presence in the environment of organochlorine compounds was undesirable, but there was no evidence of adverse effects on man and no case for the complete withdrawal of any of the compounds.— *Further Review of Certain Persistent Organochlorine Pesticides Used in Great Britain*, Report by the Advisory Committee on Pesticides and other Toxic Chemicals, London, HM Stationery Office, 1969.

Residues in the body. Analyses of 101 samples of human abdominal fat collected post mortem from residents of Somerset showed mean values of 2.85 ppm for dicophane, 0.19 ppm for benzene hexachloride, and 0.34 ppm for dieldrin.— W. Cassidy *et al.*, *Mon. Bull. Minist. Hlth*, 1967, *26*, 2.

In 44 post mortems, the highest concentration of dicophane and other chlorinated insecticides was found in patients with emaciation, carcinoma, or focal or generalised liver disorders.— L. J. Casarett *et al.*, *Archs envir. Hlth*, 1968, *17*, 306, per *J. Am. med. Ass.*, 1968, *205* (Sept. 23), A167.

The geometric mean concentrations of dieldrin, dicophane and its metabolites, and gamma benzene hexachloride in 201 samples of renal fat obtained at necropsy from January 1969 to March 1971 were 0.12, 1.9, and 0.24 ppm respectively. For dieldrin and dicophane and its metabolites this represented a decline of about 30% and 20% respectively from values reported for 1965/7. For children under 5 the decline was about 50%.— D. C. Abbott *et al.*, *Br. med. J.*, 1972, *2*, 553. See also *idem*, 1968, *3*, 146.

For data concerning the concentration of chlorinated insecticide residues in 241 autopsy specimens in Japan, see A. Curley *et al.* (letter), *Nature*, 1973, *242*, 338.

Residues in the diet. A study of organochlorine pesticide residues in the average diet in England and Wales during 1966–67 showed that the daily intake of gamma benzene hexachloride, dieldrin, and dicophane was 6.6, 6.6, and 20.6 µg per person respectively. The WHO acceptable daily intake was 875, 7, and 700 µg respectively, so that the daily intake of dieldrin was very near the limit of acceptability.— D. C. Abbott *et al.*, *J. Sci. Fd Agric.*, 1969, *20*, 245.

In 1969, the acceptable daily intake concentrations of the following insecticides were not being exceeded: chlorobenzilate, chloropropylate, coumaphos, crufomate, dimethoate, diphenyl, fenchlorphos, hydrogen cyanide, and parathion. However, the concentrations of heptachlor and phosphamidon were borderline, and there was a potential for the acceptable daily intake to be exceeded with azinphos-methyl, chlordane, diazinon, dicofol, endosulfan, lindane, malathion, and a greater potential with carbaryl, dicophane, dieldrin, dioxathion, ethion, and parathionmethyl.— Report of the 1969 Joint FAO/WHO Meeting, *Tech. Rep. Ser. Wld Hlth Org. No. 458*, 1970.

A study of food consumption indicated that the acceptable daily intake of most pesticides would not be exceeded. However, the following compounds could exceed the limit and required further study: chlordane, dichlorvos, endrin, fentin compounds, heptachlor, malathion, carbaryl, diazinon, hexachlorobenzene, and quintozene. Also the acceptable daily intakes of dicophane, dieldrin, fenthion, omethoate, and piperonyl butoxide might well be exceeded. When the effects of processing and cooking were taken into account in foods containing carbaryl, dicophane, and malathion, the concentrations of all 3 were considerably reduced although only with malathion was the concentration reduced below the acceptable daily intake.— *Pesticide Residues in Food*, Report of the 1971 Joint FAO/WHO Meeting, *Tech. Rep. Ser. Wld Hlth Org. No. 502*, 1972.

Calculations were made on the potential daily intakes of residues of 12 pesticides using food-intake figures from 5 countries. These calculations showed that with good agricultural practice there was theoretically no possibility that the acceptable daily intakes (ADIs) for 8 would be exceeded; these were: acephate, captafol, cartap, diphenylamine, edifenphos, paraquat, pirimicarb, and thiometon. For dialifos the ADI could be exceeded up to 4 times in one or more countries. For carbofuran, methamidophos, and pirimiphos-methyl the ADIs could be exceeded by 5 to 13 times in the 5 countries.— *Pesticide Residues in Food*, Report of the 1976 Joint FAO/WHO Meeting, *Tech. Rep. Ser. Wld Hlth Org. No. 612*, 1977.

Further references: *Off. J.E.E.C.*, 1976, *19*, L340, 26; *Pesticides Residues in Food: 1977 Evaluations*, FAO Plant Production and Protection Paper 10sup., Rome, 1978.

3561-h

Carbamate Insecticides

The carbamate insecticides and pesticides include: aldicarb, allyxycarb, aminocarb, bendiocarb, butacarb, butocarboxim, butoxycarboxim, carbanolate, carbaryl, carbofuran, decarbofuran, dimetilan, dioxacarb, ethiofencarb, fenethacarb, formetanate, formparanate, isoprocarb, methiocarb, methomyl, mexacarbate, pirimicarb, promecarb, propoxur, thiocarboxime.

Adverse Effects of Carbamate Insecticides. As for Organophosphorus Insecticides, p.832.

The carbamates are cholinesterase inhibitors, differing from the organophosphorus insecticides in that the inhibition they produce is generally less intense and more rapidly reversible. Symptoms of poisoning develop rapidly thus minimising the likelihood of prolonged exposure.

The related thiocarbamates or dithiocarbamates such as cartap, ferbam, mancozeb, maneb, metham, nabam, thiram, zineb, and ziram are considered to be less toxic. They are also related to disulfiram (p.579) and thus could produce a similar reaction with alcohol.

A 17-year-old youth was found unconscious after drinking what was later established to be a 22% solution of mexacarbate. He was believed to have drunk 250 ml or less and had vomited. He had bilateral pinpoint pupils, an irregular heart-beat, marked pulmonary oedema, sinus bradycardia with recurrent heart failure, and died 4 to 4½ hours after the incident.— G. A. Reich and J. O. Welke, *New Engl. J. Med.*, 1966, *274*, 1432.

A farmer suffered sweating, headache, and anorexia after spraying methomyl from an ultra-low-volume handsprayer. He was treated with atropine and had recovered after a week.— Smith D.M., *Practitioner*, 1977, *218*, 877.

Acute renal failure in a 62-year-old man, associated with exposure to maneb.— A. Koizumi *et al.*, *J. Am. med. Ass.*, 1979, *242*, 2583.

Treatment of Adverse Effects. If carbamates have been ingested the stomach should be emptied by aspiration and lavage or by inducing emesis. Contaminated clothing should be removed and the skin washed with soap and water. Symptoms of toxicity should be treated with atropine in doses of 1 or 2 mg. Pralidoxime or other oximes should *not* be given. The respiration may require assistance.

Symptoms of poisoning by carbamates disappeared much more rapidly than with organophosphorus compounds and atropine was often not necessary. Doses of 1 to 2 mg of atropine sulphate could be given to adults by intramuscular or intravenous injection and repeated when necessary. Overdosage with atropine should be avoided, particularly in children, and pralidoxime and other oximes should not be given. Inhibition of cholinesterases by carbamates was rapid in the early stages but production of severe inactivation of enzyme was difficult as the rate of reactivation of enzyme approached that of inactivation. No 'ageing' effect like that with organophosphorus insecticides had been seen.— Sixteenth Report of WHO Expert Committee on Insecticides, *Tech. Rep. Ser. Wld Hlth Org. No. 356*, 1967.

3562-m

Chlorinated Insecticides

The chlorinated insecticides and pesticides include: aldrin, benzoximate, bromocyclen, camphechlor, captafol, captan, chlorbenside, chlorbicyclen, chlordane, chlordecone, chlordimeform, chlorfenethol, chlorfenson (ovex), chlorfensulphide, chlorobenzilate, chloromebuform, chloropropylate, DDT (dicophane), *pp'*-DDT, dicofol, dieldrin, dienochlor, diflubenzuron, endosulfan, endrin, fenazaflor, fenson, fluorbenside, folpet, gamma benzene hexachloride, HCH (benzene hexachloride), HEOD, HHDN, heptachlor, isobenzan, isodrin, kelevan, methoxychlor (methoxy-DDT), quintozene, TDE, tetradifon (chlorodifon), tetrasul.

Adverse Effects of Chlorinated Insecticides. Chlorinated insecticides form a very wide group and the toxicity of individual members varies widely. Aldrin, dieldrin, and endrin are considered to be the members that commonly cause poisoning. In general these insecticides produce symptoms consistent with central nervous system stimulation. They may be absorbed through the respiratory and gastro-intestinal tracts and through the skin, and whatever its route this absorption is facilitated by oily substances. Poisoning has occurred through the accidental ingestion, inhalation, or percutaneous absorption of various preparations containing these substances, although it has been reported that poisoning following percutaneous absorption is rare with this group.

Symptoms of acute poisoning include vomiting and diarrhoea, paraesthesia, excitement, giddiness, and fatigue, followed by tremors, convulsions, coma, and possibly pulmonary oedema. Liver, kidney, and myocardial toxicity and hypothermia have been reported. Respiration may be accelerated initially, and later depressed. Symptoms may be complicated by the effects of the solvent.

Early symptoms of chronic poisoning are headache, loss of appetite, muscular weakness, fine tremors, and an apprehensive mental state.

Chlorinated insecticides have been reported to enhance microsomal hepatic enzyme activity. This contributes to interactions with steroid hormones. For effects arising from the ingestion of chlorinated insecticides in the diet, see Insecticides in the Body and Diet, p.830.

For further information on the toxic effects of chlorinated insecticides, see under Dicophane (p.835), Benzene Hexachloride (p.833), Dieldrin (p.836), and Gamma Benzene Hexachloride (p.837).

Polychlorinated biphenyl (PCB) and terphenyl compounds were formerly used as insecticides in many countries, but because of their toxicity they now have only a few industrial applications. They are stored in body fat and not readily excreted except in breast milk and possibly through the placenta; because of this and because of accidental contamination in Japan, they remain a cause for concern. The related polybrominated biphenyl compounds (PBB) which have no insecticidal uses have also been absorbed by the public following accidental contamination of cattle feeds in Michigan.

Evidence was considered concerning the possible carcinogenic potential of 12 chlorinated compounds: aldrin, Aramite [2-(4-t-butylphenoxy)-1-methylethyl 2-chloroethyl sulphite], benzene hexachloride, chlorobenzilate, dicophane, dieldrin, endrin, heptachlor, methoxychlor, mirex (a dodecachloropentacyclodecane), quintozene, and Strobane (chlorinated terpene isomers). All except aldrin, endrin, heptachlor, and methoxychlor produced tumours in *mice*. Data on carcinogenicity in man were either absent or inadequate to permit conclusions to be drawn.— *IARC Monographs on the Evaluation of Carcinogenic Risk of Chemicals to Man*, Vol. 5, Lyon, International Agency for Research on Cancer, 1974.

See also general references above.

Hepatotoxicity. Liver disease in 8 chemical workers was attributed to contact with dicophane and/or gamma benzene hexachloride in the course of their work; none had a history of hepatitis, diabetes, or alcoholism; in 4 patients the disease progressed to complete cirrhosis. The diet of patients with any liver disorder should be free from pesticide residues.— W. Schüttman, *Arch. Gewerbepath. Gewerbehyg.*, 1968, *24*, 193, per *Abstr. Hyg.*, 1969, *44*, 260.

Impotence and infertility. Four of 5 workers became impotent following intensive use of various herbicides and pesticides. The condition was reversed when contact with the chemicals ceased and methyltestosterone therapy was given.— M. L. E. Espir *et al.*, *Br. med. J.*, 1970, *1*, 423. Impotence in agricultural workers following exposure to chlorinated hydrocarbon insecticides might have been due to an enhanced metabolism of testosterone leading to a relative deficiency of this hormone.— A. W. Peck (letter), *ibid.*, 690.

Discussion of reduced fertility.— *Lancet*, 1978, *2*, 79.

Poisoning and exposure. Aldrin. Symptoms in 6 of 12 men exposed to aldrin.— G. Kazantzis *et al.*, *Br. J. ind. Med.*, 1964, *21*, 46, per *Bull. Hyg., Lond.*, 1964, *39*, 503.

Camphechlor. A 9-month-old child suffered convulsions and died from respiratory arrest after acute exposure to a preparation containing camphechlor 13.8% and dicophane 7.04%. Cerebral oedema was evident at post mortem. The relative concentrations of camphechlor and dicophane in the brain and liver were 10:1 and in the kidney 3:1. Camphechlor was considered to be the principal cause of death and appeared to be more readily absorbed than dicophane.— E. C. Haun and C. Cueto, *Am. J. Dis. Child.*, 1967, *113*, 616, per *J. Am. med. Ass.*, 1967, *200* (May 8), A245. For a similar report in 3 children, see L. C. McGee *et al.*, *J. Am. med. Ass.*, 1952, *149*, 1124.

NOTE. Toxaphene is a preparation of camphechlor.

Chlordane. Convulsions associated with chlordane in individual patients: J. Stranger and G. Kerridge, *Med. J. Aust.*, 1968, *1*, 267; A. Curley and L. K. Garrettson, *Archs envir. Hlth*, 1969, *18*, 211; F. D. Aldrich and J. H. Holmes, *Archs envir. Hlth*, 1969, *19*, 129.

Megaloblastic anaemia in one patient.— B. Furie and S. Trubowitz, *J. Am. med. Ass.*, 1976, *235*, 1720.

There was no reported evidence for chlordane or other pesticides causing chronic monocytic leukaemia.— I. S. Collins and W. A. Crawford (letter), *Med. J. Aust.*, 1976, *1*, 762.

A report of 5 cases of neuroblastoma associated with chlordane exposure pre- or postnatally and of 3 cases of aplastic anaemia and 3 of acute leukaemia all associated with chlordane.— P. F. Infante *et al.*, *Scand. J. Work Environ. & Hlth*, 1978, *4*, 137, per *Abstr. Hyg.*, 1978, *53*, 772. One case of neuroblastoma developing about 2.5 years after prenatal exposure to chlordane.— P. F. Infante and W. A. Newton (letter), *New Engl. J. Med.*, 1975, *293*, 308.

Chlordimeform. Nine of 22 workers who packaged chlordimeform became severely ill with symptoms including abdominal pain, penile discharge, cystitis and haematuria. The illness lasted 1 week to 2 months.— D. S. Folland *et al.*, *J. Am. med. Ass.*, 1978, *239*, 1052.

Endosulfan. Convulsions in 9 men handling endosulfan.— T. S. Ely *et al.*, *J. occup. Med.*, 1967, *9*, 35, per *Bull. Hyg., Lond.*, 1967, *42*, 1079.

Endrin. Acute endrin poisoning with epileptiform convulsions and frothing at the mouth developed suddenly in 3 people after eating bread made of contaminated flour. The convulsions were succeeded by a period of semiconsciousness and vomiting. All 3 made full spontaneous recoveries, in 2 cases within 24 hours.— Y. Coble *et al.*, *J. Am. med. Ass.*, 1967, *202*, 489.

For a report of 874 cases of poisoning, including 26 fatalities, arising from the contamination of flour by endrin, see D. E. Weeks, *Bull. Wld Hlth Org.*, 1967, *37*, 499.

Of 13 children poisoned with endrin from various sources 6 died. Autopsy in 4 showed congestion of the brain and meninges, congestion and oedema of the lungs, pleural haemorrhage, and congestion of the liver.— M. Karplus, *Harefuah*, 1971, *81*, 113, per *Int. pharm. Abstr.*, 1972, *9*, 344.

The US Environmental Protection Agency reported that endrin has caused birth defects in laboratory *animals* and may pose the same danger in humans. It was not suspected as a human cancer agent. Acute hazards from skin contact with certain endrin formulations were not proven. The Agency proposed that use should continue in the US on a restricted basis.— *J. Am. med. Ass.*, 1979, *241*, 353.

Treatment of Adverse Effects. Ingested material should be removed by aspiration and lavage. Contaminated clothing should be removed and the skin washed with soap and water. A saline purgative may be given. Convulsions may be controlled with diazepam. Assisted respiration may be needed.

Milk and oily substances should not be given, nor should adrenaline since it may precipitate arrhythmias in a heart sensitised by chlorinated insecticides.

Chlordane. A patient swallowed about 90 g of chlordane. Vomiting was induced and magnesium sulphate given by mouth. A grand mal seizure occurred and haemoperfusion over charcoal was started 4 hours later and continued for 4 hours. Body concentrations of chlordane were reduced and the patient recovered.— E. F. Nielsen (letter), *Lancet*, 1978, *1*, 506.

Chlordecone. Administration of cholestyramine over a period of 5 months was associated with a significant increase in the rate of disappearance of chlordecone from the blood of 7 of 12 workers exposed to toxic concentrations as against a significant increase in only 1 of 11 similar subjects given placebo. Cholestyramine was considered to prevent the reabsorption of chlordecone which is excreted chiefly in the bile and eliminated in the faeces. The results indicated that cholestyramine is a practical treatment for subjects exposed to large quantities of chlordecone and possibly to other lipophilic toxins.— W. J. Cohn *et al.*, *New Engl. J. Med.*, 1978, *298*, 243.

3563-b

Dinitrophenol and Related Insecticides

The dinitrophenol derivatives used as insecticides and acaricides include: binapacryl, DNOC (dinitrocresol), dinex, dinobuton, dinocap, dinocap-6, dinocton, dinopenton, dinoprop, dinosam, dinoseb, dinosulfon, dinoterbon.

Adverse Effects of Dinitrophenol and Related Insecticides. These substances may be absorbed by inhalation, by accidental ingestion, or by absorption through the skin. They are cumulative poisons, causing an increase in the metabolic rate, which may lead to death in a manner resembling heat stroke.

Yellow discoloration of the sclera, skin, and hair indicates absorption of significant quantities and may precede onset of symptoms. Mild poisoning is usually accompanied by copious sweating and thirst; nevertheless, patients often feel well, owing to the increased metabolic rate.

More severe poisoning is shown by profuse and continuous sweating, fatigue, nausea, abdominal pain, restlessness, and loss of weight. Late symptoms include an increase in rate and depth of respiration, tachycardia, and a raised temperature. Death may occur from respiratory and circulatory failure.

The toxic and lethal concentrations in the air of DNOC and related compounds were estimated to be respectively 36 and 100 µg per litre.— E. N. Burkatskaya, *Gig. Sanit.*, 1965, *30*, 34, per *Bull. Hyg., Lond.*, 1965, *40*, 599.

Treatment of Adverse Effects. Ingested material should be removed by aspiration and lavage. Contaminated clothing should be removed and the skin washed with soap and water. Treatment is symptomatic and its most important aspect is probably rest and the prevention of body heat accumulation. Cold packs, alcohol sponges, and cold water enemas are indicated. Fluids and salts lost by the excessive sweating must be replaced; assisted respiration and oxygen may be required. Atropine should *not* be given.

3564-v

Organophosphorus Insecticides

The organophosphorus insecticides include: acephate, amidithion, amiton, athidathion, azinphos-ethyl, azinphos-methyl, azothoate, bromophos, bromophos-ethyl, butonate, carbophenothion, chlorfenvinphos, chlormephos, chlorphoxim, chlorprazophos, chlorpyrifos, chlorpyrifos-methyl, chlorthiophos, coumaphos, coumithoate, crotoxyphos, crufomate, cyanofenphos, cyanophos, cyanthoate, demephion, demephion-O, demephion-S, demeton, demeton-methyl, demeton-O, demeton-O-methyl, demeton-S, demeton-S-methyl, demeton-S-methyl sulphone, dialifos, diazinon (dimpylate), dichlofenthion, dichlorvos, dicrotophos, dimefox, dimethoate, dioxathion, disulfoton, endothion, ethion, ethoate-methyl, ethoprophos, etrimfos, fenchlorphos (ronnel), fenitrothion, fensulfothion, fenthion, fonofos, formothion, fospirate, heptenophos, iodofenphos, isofenphos, leptophos, lythidathion, malathion, mazidox, mecarbam, mecarphon, menazon, mephosfolan, methacrifos, methamidophos, methidathion, methocrotophos, mevinphos, mipafox, monocrotophos, morphothion, naled, omethoate, oxydemeton-methyl, oxydisulfoton, parathion, parathion-methyl, phenkapton, phenthoate, phorate, phosalone, phosfolan, phosmet, phosnichlor, phosphamidon, phoxim, phoxim-methyl, pirimiphos-ethyl, pirimiphos-methyl, propetamphos, prothidathion, prothoate, quinalphos, quinothion, quintiofos, schradan, sophamide, sulfotep, temephos, TEPP (ethylpyrophosphate), terbufos, tetrachlorvinphos, thiometon, thionazin, triazophos, trichloronate, trichlorphon (metriphonate), vamidothion.

Adverse Effects of Organophosphorus Insecticides. Organophosphorus insecticides are potent cholinesterase inhibitors and are very toxic.

Exposure to the vapour or to particulate material may cause miosis, sometimes unequal, hyperaemia of the conjunctiva, dimness of vision, rhinorrhoea, frontal headache, bronchoconstriction, increased bronchial secretion, cough, nausea, vomiting, and fasciculation and sweating at the site of contact.

Toxic effects may include anorexia, abdominal cramps, nausea, vomiting, diarrhoea, incontinence, eye changes, weakness, dyspnoea, bronchospasm, lachrymation, increased salivation and sweating, bradycardia, hypotension or hypertension due to asphyxia, cyanosis, and muscular twitching of the eyelids, tongue, face, and neck, possibly progressing to convulsions. Central nervous system symptoms include restlessness, anxiety, dizziness, drowsiness, tremor, ataxia, depression, confusion, and coma. Death may occur from depression of the respiratory or cardiovascular system.

Neuropathy appears to be a rare problem with the organophosphorus insecticides now in use. Repeated exposure may have a cumulative effect though the organophosphorus insecticides are, in contrast to the chlorinated insecticides, rapidly metabolised and excreted and are not appreciably stored in body tissues.

For further information on the toxic effects of organophosphorus insecticides, see under Dichlorvos (p.835), Malathion (p.838), and Metriphonate (p.839).

Poisoning and exposure. A review of poisoning by organophosphorus insecticides and recommended treatment.— T. Namba, *Bull. Wld Hlth Org.*, 1971, *44*, 289.

Chromosome abnormalities were temporarily increased in patients with organophosphorus poisoning.— T. van Bao *et al.*, *Egészségtudomány*, 1974, *18*, 348, per *Abstr. Hyg.*, 1975, *50*, 350.

A short review of contact dermatitis associated with the use of organophosphorus pesticides.— R. J. G. Rycroft, *Br. J. Derm.*, 1977, *97*, 693.

Organophosphorus poisoning in a 50-year-old man with maturity-onset diabetes resulted in lowered blood-glucose concentrations which rose again after treatment with atropine and pralidoxime.— S. K. Samantray (letter), *Med. J. Aust.*, 1978, *1*, 443.

Carbophenothion. There were no fatalities in 19 cases of carbophenothion poisoning among workers on a sugar-cane estate in Trinidad. In 9 cases whole-blood cholinesterase concentrations were between 25 and 62.5% of normal. Seven of the 19 required treatment.— C. E. D. Hearn, *Br. J. ind. Med.*, 1961, *18*, 231, per *Bull. Hyg., Lond.*, 1961, *36*, 1113.

Food poisoning in 7 members of a family after eating food contaminated with carbophenothion.— J. J. Older and R. L. Hatcher, *J. Am. med. Ass.*, 1969, *209*, 1328.

Coumaphos. Acute pancreatitis associated in one patient with acute coumaphos poisoning.— P. G. Moore and O. F. James, *Postgrad. med. J.*, 1981, *57*, 660.

Demeton-S-methyl and disulfoton. A 48-year-old man developed headaches, nausea, dizziness, anorexia, and reduced mental ability after exposure to demeton-S-methyl and disulfoton in the course of his work, despite strict observance of safety regulations.— I. H. Redhead, *Lancet*, 1968, *1*, 686. Comment.— G. C. Fryer (letter), *ibid.*, 1153.

Demeton-S-methyl and phosphamidon. Ten farmers suffered symptoms of organophosphorus poisoning of varying severity after emergency use of demeton-S-methyl in ultra-low-volume handsprayers to control a sudden outbreak of aphid infestation; another 2 suffered symptoms after its use in tractors with booms, and a further 2 after helicopter spraying operations using phosphamidon as well as demeton-S-methyl. Symptoms were sweating, anorexia, nausea, vomiting, diarrhoea, and prostration. Cramps, muscle twitching, diplopia, and a feeling of inebriation occurred in more severe cases; 1 patient suffered opisthotonus (tetanic spasm) and another had alarming nightmares amounting almost to hallucinations. Treatment was with atropine, pralidoxime, and bathing; it was considered that fatalities had only been avoided by the prompt action of medical personnel.— D. M. Smith, *Practitioner*, 1977, *218*, 877.

Diazinon. Twenty-five patients poisoned with diazinon showed stupor, restlessness, tachypnoea, tachycardia, and hypertension in addition to usual symptoms. Twenty-three survived; post-mortem examination of the other 2 showed diffuse hyperaemia, cloudy swelling of the tubular epithelium, and haemorrhage in the kidneys.— G. S. Mutalik *et al.*, *J. Indian med. Ass.*, 1962, *38*, 67.

Acute short-term psychosis developed in a person handling diazinon.— R. A. J. Conyers and L. E. Goldsmith, *Med. J. Aust.*, 1971, *1*, 27.

Acute poisoning from diazinon contaminated oatmeal in 8 members of 2 related families.— E. R. Reichert *et al.*, *Clin. Toxicol.*, 1977, *11*, 5, per *Trop. Dis. Bull.*, 1978, *75*, 2.

Dichlofenthion. Five patients took dichlofenthion in suicide attempts and 2 died. Initial symptoms were mild or delayed with severe cholinergic reactions not occurring until 40 to 48 hours after ingestion. In the 3 survivors the cholinergic reactions lasted for 5 to 48 days and in 1 of them almost total inhibition of cholinesterase continued for 66 days. Residues of dichlofenthion were present for up to 75 days. The partition coefficient of dichlofenthion in fat was only exceeded by leptophos and was 20 times greater than that of parathion.— J. E. Davies *et al.*, *Archs envir. Hlth*, 1975, *30*, 608, per *J. Am. med. Ass.*, 1975, *234*, 982.

Methidathion. See below under Treatment of Adverse Effects.

Mevinphos. Mevinphos, unlike parathion, was soluble in lipids as well as water. It was consequently more rapidly transported after absorption and produced a more rapid onset of symptoms from which recovery was also correspondingly faster.— H. Van Raalte, *Archs Mal. prof. Méd. trav.*, 1962, *23*, 132, per *Bull. Hyg., Lond.*, 1962, *37*, 713.

A report of 3 patients with reduced blood-cholinesterase concentrations after absorption of mevinphos and of 1 patient with poisoning by mevinphos.— A. Bell *et al.*, *Med. J. Aust.*, 1968, *1*, 178.

A report of marked fibrinolysis in a patient with mevinphos poisoning and of marked hypercoagulability in a second patient.— J. H. Holmes *et al.*, *Archs envir. Hlth*, 1974, *29*, 84, per *Abstr. Hyg.*, 1974, *49*, 940.

Dermal poisoning from mevinphos and parathion in one agricultural worker.— E. R. Reichert *et al.*, *Clin. Toxicol.*, 1978, *12*, 33.

Monocrotophos. Twenty-eight hours after a 19-year-old man splashed himself with monocrotophos liquid emulsion concentrate he suffered muscular weakness and blurred vision, chest pain, and blackouts. After 38 hours, he was sweating, lethargic, and vague, he suffered dry retching, his pupils were constricted, and salivation was increased. An improvement was obtained after giving atropine 1.2 mg intramuscularly, then pralidoxime 1 g intravenously, followed by a further 1.2 mg of atropine, with 500 mg of pralidoxime the next day. All acute symptoms had cleared after 3 days. A final 500 mg of pralidoxime was given on the eighth day after exposure.— R. E. Simson *et al.*, *Med. J. Aust.*, 1969, *2*, 1013.

Parathion. Following the ingestion of even a few drops of parathion, death was essentially instantaneous. Report of 5 fatal cases of parathion poisoning.— E. Handal (letter), *Br. med. J.*, 1960, *2*, 1161.

An 8-week-old girl developed severe respiratory symptoms 2 hours after her room had been sprayed with parathion. She recovered after being given atropine intravenously. Regeneration of cholinesterase in red cells proceeded much more rapidly than anticipated.— R. W. Mackey, *Am. J. Dis. Child.*, 1966, *111*, 321, per *Med. J. Aust.*, 1966, *2*, 657. For a similar report, see Z. Hruban *et al.*, *J. Am. med. Ass.*, 1963, *184*, 590.

For a report of 2 outbreaks of food-poisoning, in Qatar and Saudi Arabia, involving 280 persons and 78 fatalities, arising from the contamination of flour by parathion, see D. E. Weeks, *Bull. Wld Hlth Org.*, 1967, *37*, 499.

In 2 cases of accidental poisoning with an insecticide mixture, a 5-year-old boy ingested about 500 mg of parathion, 85 mg of chlordane, and 187 mg of diazinon and an 8-year-old girl ingested about 1.4 g of parathion, 254 mg of chlordane, and 559 mg of diazinon. The girl developed cardiac and respiratory arrest and died about 17 hours after ingestion despite prompt treatment including cardiac massage, gastric lavage, and administration of atropine sulphate and pralidoxime chloride. In both patients, the onset of symptoms was rapid and quickly progressed to coma and convulsions. The boy recovered.— A. E. DePalma *et al.*, *J. Am. med. Ass.*, 1970, *211*, 1979.

In men spraying parathion absorption was greatest through the skin but inhalation was more hazardous. *p*-Nitrophenol persisted in the urine for up to 10 days after exposure.— W. F. Durham *et al.*, *Archs envir. Hlth*, 1972, *24*, 381, per *J. Am. med. Ass.*, 1972, *220*, 1386.

The estimated lethal dose of parathion for adults was 20 mg. The oral LD50 for *rats* ranged from 6 to 30 mg per kg body-weight.— *Bulletin of the National Clearinghouse for Poison Control Centers*, Nov.-Dec., 1972.

Parathion-methyl. A report of erythema multiforme after exposure to parathion-methyl.— R. K. Bhargava *et al.* (letter), *Archs Derm.*, 1977, *113*, 686.

TEPP. Symptoms of organophosphorus poisoning developed following exposure to air laden with an insecticidal dust containing 1% of TEPP. In 14 people shortness of breath occurred within 30 to 60 minutes of exposure.— G. E. Quinby and G. M. Doornink, *J. Am. med. Ass.*, 1965, *191*, 1.

Treatment of Adverse Effects. Rapid treatment is essential. Ingested materials should be removed by aspiration and lavage. Contaminated clothing should be removed and the skin, including any areas contaminated by vomiting or hypersecretion, washed with soap and water for at least 10 minutes. Contamination of the eye is treated by washing of the conjunctiva. Assisted respiration and oxygen may be needed and the patient should be treated with atropine and pralidoxime—see Pralidoxime Chloride, p.389. A short acting barbiturate may be given to control convulsions (but see abstract, below). The patient should be observed for signs of deterioration due to delayed absorption. Morphine and phenothiazines must *not* be given nor must aminophylline.

It was suggested that metaraminol might be given in doses of 10 mg in conjunction with atropine. Repeated intake of barbiturates could increase the metabolic conversion of parathion to its highly toxic metabolite, paraoxon; this was because of an increased formation of the appropriate converting enzymes.— W. J. R. Taylor *et al.*, *Can. med. Ass. J.*, 1965, *93*, 966.

Massive poisoning with methidathion in one patient. Treatment is discussed; as methidathion is slowly metabolised to its more toxic oxygen analogue patients should be hospitalised and monitored closely for at least one week, even when poisoning is mild.— U. Teitelman *et al.*, *Clin. Toxicol.*, 1975, *8*, 277, per *Int. pharm. Abstr.*, 1976, *13*, 881.

Animal studies suggesting that pretreatment with carbamates might protect against poisoning by organophosphates including those such as soman which does not respond to therapy with atropine and pralidoxime. Pretreatment with carbamates did not reduce the efficacy of atropine and pralidoxime in oxime-sensitive organophosphates.— J. J. Gordon *et al.*, *Toxic. appl. Pharmac.*, 1978, *43*, 207.

3565-g

Larvicides

Larvicides are being used increasingly, especially in onchocerciasis control. Temephos is in use; other organophosphorus compounds are being investigated.

3566-q

Molluscicides

Molluscicides are used for the control of freshwater snails which are the intermediate hosts of schistosomes. Many compounds have been used effectively including niclosamide (p.100) and trifenmorph (p.842). Inorganic and organic compounds containing copper, organotin compounds which can be incorporated into rubber, and vegetable drugs containing saponins have also been used.

For further information on the use of molluscicides, see *Molluscicides in Schistosomiasis Control*, T.C. Cheng, (Ed.), London, Academic Press, 1974.

3567-p

Rodenticides

In addition to warfarin many other coumarin or indanedione anticoagulants are used as rodenticides, including brodifacoum, chlorophacinone, coumachlor, fumarin (coumafuryl), coumatetralyl (racumin), dicoumarol, diphacinone (diphenadione, p.771) and pindone.

Other compounds used as rodenticides include chloralose (p.797), crimidine (a convulsant), dicophane (p.836), endrin, fluoroacetamide (p.700), gamma benzene hexachloride (p.837), norbormide (p.840), phosacetim (an organophosphorus compound), red squill (p.693), sodium fluoroacetate (p.702), strychnine (p.320), zinc phosphide (p.842), and aluminium phosphide. Ergocalciferol (p.1662) is also used as a rodenticide either alone or with warfarin.

The use of the following is not recommended: antu (1-naphthylthiourea), arsenic trioxide, gophacide (an organophosphorus compound), phosphorus, and thallium sulphate.

Insecticide Resistance and Vector Control, Seventeenth Report of the WHO Expert Committee on Insecticides, *Tech. Rep. Ser. Wld Hlth Org. No. 443*, 1970.

Anticoagulant rodenticides in current use.— E. W. Bentley, *Bull. Wld Hlth Org.*, 1972, *47*, 275.

Acute rodenticides in current use.— N. G. Gratz, *Bull. Wld Hlth Org.*, 1973, *48*, 469.

Ecology and Control of Rodents of Public Health Importance, Report of a WHO Scientific Group, *Tech. Rep. Ser. Wld Hlth Org. No. 553*, 1974.

Further references: *Br. med. J.*, 1975, *2*, 105; A. P. Meehan, *Rentokil, Chemist Drugg.*, 1978, *209*, 3; F. P. Barrett, *Sorex, ibid.*, 357.

3568-s

Benzene Hexachloride *(B. Vet. C. 1965).*

BHC; Benzeni Hexachloridum; HCH; Hexachlorocyclohexane; Technical Benzene Hexachloride.
$C_6H_6Cl_6$=290.8.

CAS — 319-84-6 (α); 319-85-7 (β); 58-89-9 (γ); 319-86-8 (δ); 6108-10-7 (ε).

A mixture of the several isomers of 1, 2, 3, 4, 5, 6-hexachlorocyclohexane, containing not less than 12% of the gamma-isomer. Benzene hexachloride has 5 known isomers all with the composition $C_6H_6Cl_6$ and designated alpha, beta, gamma, delta, and epsilon; of these only the gamma-isomer (see Gamma Benzene Hexachloride, p.837) is outstandingly active as an insecticide. Benzene hexachloride occurs as white to light brown granules, flakes, or powder, with a characteristic musty odour. It is practically **insoluble** in water and its solubility in organic solvents depends upon the proportions of the various isomers present.

Adverse Effects and Treatment. As for Chlorinated Insecticides, p.831.

Benzene hexachloride is reported to be more toxic than the pure γ-isomer.

Benzene hexachloride is reported to be extremely toxic to fish; dip or spray residues should not be allowed to drain into streams or ponds.

The lethal dose of benzene hexachloride for man had been estimated as 200 mg per kg body-weight.— H. Kneidel, *Zentbl. ArbMed. ArbSchutz*, 1963, *13*, 33, per *Bull. Hyg., Lond.*, 1963, *38*, 909.

Of 10 adults and children who consumed food contaminated with about 4% of benzene hexachloride, 3 died within 7 hours. It was concluded that the adults had consumed 300 mg per kg body-weight of the gamma-isomer alone. Profuse emesis in the 7 survivors had probably prevented serious illness.— R. W. W. Kay *et al.*, *Ghana med. J.*, 1964, *3*, 72, per *Bull. Hyg., Lond.*, 1965, *40*, 139.

Following the ingestion of biscuits found on a rubbish tip which had been sprayed the previous night with a tip dressing containing 4% benzene hexachloride, of which only 0.5% was the gamma-isomer, an 8-year-old boy developed vomiting and drowsiness. His condition deteriorated and he was treated with an intravenous infusion of 500 ml of mannitol 10% to combat presumed cerebral oedema. His level of consciousness then improved. Grand mal convulsions were treated with an intramuscular injection of paraldehyde 5 ml and dexamethasone intravenously. He was fully recovered within 72 hours.— B. G. P. Macnamara (letter), *Br. med. J.*, 1970, *3*, 585.

Residues in the body and diet. As the activity of benzene hexachloride was due to its content of gamma isomer but the alpha and beta isomers were found most often in food intake studies, technical benzene hexachloride should be replaced by gamma benzene hexachloride or alternative pesticides wherever possible. No acceptable daily intake could be specified.— 1973 Evaluations of some Pesticide Residues in Food, *Pestic. Residue Ser. Wld Hlth Org. No. 3*, 1974.

See also p.830.

Uses. Benzene hexachloride has been used in veterinary dips and sprays.

3569-w

Benzyl Benzoate *(B.P., U.S.P.).*

Benzyl Benz.; Benzylis Benzoas; Benzoesäurebenzylester; Benzoato de Bencilo.
$C_6H_5.CO.O.CH_2.C_6H_5$=212.2.

CAS — 120-51-4.

Pharmacopoeias. In *Arg., Aust., Br., Braz., Chin., Cz., Fr., Hung., Ind., Int., It., Jap., Jug., Mex., Neth., Nord., Pol., Port., Span., Swiss, Turk.,* and *U.S.*

Colourless crystals or a clear colourless oily liquid with a faintly aromatic odour and a sharp burning taste. The *B.P.* specifies f.p. not below 17° but it is liable to become supercooled; the *U.S.P.* specifies not below 18°. B.p. about 320°. Wt per ml 1.116 to 1.120 g. Practically **insoluble** in water and glycerol; miscible with alcohol, acetone, chloroform, carbon disulphide, ether, and fixed and volatile oils. **Incompatible** with alkalis. **Store** at a temperature not exceeding 40° in well-filled airtight containers. Protect from light.

Adverse Effects and Treatment. Benzyl benzoate is irritant to the eyes and mucous membranes and it may be irritant to the skin. Hypersensitivity reactions have been reported. When ingested, benzyl benzoate may cause stimulation of the CNS and convulsions. Poisoning should be treated by inducing emesis or by gastric lavage; anticonvulsants may be needed.

Residues in the body and diet. The Food Additives and Contaminants Committee recommended that benzyl benzoate be temporarily permitted for use as a solvent in food and recommended a maximum concentration of use in food as consumed of 40 ppm. Further toxicity studies were required.— *Report on the Review of Solvents in Food*, FAC/REP/25, Ministry of Agriculture, Fisheries and Food, London, HM Stationery Office, 1978.

Estimated acceptable daily intake of the benzyl/benzoic moiety: up to 5 mg per kg body-weight.— Twenty-third Report of Joint FAO/WHO Expert Committee on Food Additives, *Tech. Rep. Ser. Wld Hlth Org. No. 648*, 1980.

Precautions. Benzyl benzoate should not be allowed to come into contact with the eyes.

Uses. Benzyl benzoate is an acaricide and is used in the treatment of scabies. The patient is first scrubbed with soap in a hot bath to open up the burrows, and immediately after drying Benzyl Benzoate Application is applied over the whole body surface from the neck down; a second application is made on the following day. Alternatively 3 applications may be made at 12-hourly intervals. Clothing and bedding should be changed to prevent reinfestation.

Benzyl benzoate has also been used as a pediculicide.

Benzyl benzoate is used as an insect repellent. It is usually applied to clothing and remains effective when the clothing is washed once or twice. Garments may be treated by the application of a 5% solution of benzyl benzoate in a volatile solvent until they become thoroughly wet.

Benzyl benzoate is used as a solubilising agent in the preparation of oily injections.

Scabies. Scabies could be effectively treated by Benzyl Benzoate Application, 1% cream or lotion of gamma benzene hexachloride, 25% solution of monosulfiram diluted immediately before use with about 3 vol. of water, or by crotamiton lotion or ointment. Benzyl benzoate might occasionally cause dermatitis. Sulphur Ointment was also effective but could cause dermatitis. The technique involved a hot bath with gentle rubbing of the affected areas, drying, and the application from the chin to the soles of the feet of the treatment which was allowed to dry; the patient then retired. The application was repeated on the following day and washed off on the third day. All members of the household and close contacts were treated concomitantly, and treatment was given even in the presence of secondary infection.— *Scabies,* Department of Health and Social Security, London, 1970. See also M. Garretts, *Prescribers' J.,* 1972, *12,* 32; F. A. Ive, *Br. med. J.,* 1973, *4,* 475.

Half-strength Benzyl Benzoate Application could be used to treat infants with scabies; 3 applications were recommended. Burrows above the neck should be treated with crotamiton.— J. Verbov, *Practitioner,* 1978, *220,* 779.

Use as an insect repellent. Benzyl benzoate alone or in conjunction with dibutyl phthalate was the best insect repellent for chiggers and one of the best repellents for fleas. It was applied to clothing and its action persisted after washing.— *Insecticide Resistance and Vector Control,* Seventeenth Report of the WHO Expert Committee on Insecticides, *Tech. Rep. Ser. Wld Hlth Org. No. 443,* 1970.

For another assessment of the value of benzyl benzoate as a repellent for ticks, fleas, and chiggers, see under Insect Repellents, p.828.

Preparations

Benzyl Benzoate Application *(B.P., A.P.F., Ind. P.).* Benzyl benzoate 25 g, emulsifying wax 2 g, freshly boiled and cooled water to 100 ml.

Two of 6 samples of Benzyl Benzoate Application were deficient in benzyl benzoate. Variations in viscosity were found in 5 samples and could affect spreading and the amount applied to the body. It was suggested that a more stable, uniform, and acceptable product should be formulated.— J. A. Baker *et al., Pharm. J.,* 1967, *2,* 565.

Benzyl Benzoate Lotion *(U.S.N.F.).* Benzyl benzoate 25 ml, triethanolamine 500 mg, oleic acid 2 g, and water 75 ml. pH 8.5 to 9.2. Store in airtight containers.

Linimentum Benzyli Benzoatis *(Nord. P.).* Benzyl benzoate 33 g, propyl alcohol 24 g, potash soap spirit 43 g.

Proprietary Preparations

Ascabiol *(May & Baker, UK).* Benzyl benzoate, available as an emulsion containing 25%. For scabies and pediculosis. (Also available as Ascabiol in *Austral.* and *S.Afr.*).

Other Proprietary Names

Antiscabiosum Mago *(Ger.)*; Benzemul *(Austral.)*; Scabanca *(Canad.)*.

3570-m

Carbaryl. Carbaril; OMS-29. 1-Naphthyl methylcarbamate.

$C_{12}H_{11}NO_2$=201.2.

CAS — 63-25-2.

A white crystalline solid. Practically **insoluble** in water; soluble in most polar organic solvents.

Adverse Effects and Treatment. As for Carbamate Insecticides, p.830.

Experimental ingestion of 250 mg has caused moderately severe poisoning.

Maximum permissible atmospheric concentration 5 mg per m^3.

Although several cases of poisoning had occurred, symptoms usually subsided by the time medical observation was obtained and were gone in 3 to 4 hours, whether or not atropine was given.— *Safe Use of Pesticides in Public Health,* Sixteenth Report of the WHO Expert Committee on Insecticides, *Tech. Rep. Ser. Wld Hlth Org. No. 356,* 1967.

Twelve pesticides, including 5 organophosphates, 3 chlorinated hydrocarbons, 2 carbamates, and 2 herbicides all penetrated the skin. The least absorbed was *diquat* and the greatest absorption was with *carbaryl.*— R. J. Feldmann and H. I. Maibach, *Toxic. appl. Pharmac.,* 1974, *28,* 126.

For the speed of absorption of carbaryl from various body sites, see Malathion, p.838.

Residues in the body and diet. Maximum acceptable daily intake of carbaryl: 10 µg per kg body-weight. Further studies were desirable to elucidate the effects of carbaryl on renal function.— Report of the 1976 Joint FAO/WHO Meeting on Pesticide Residues in Food, *Tech. Rep. Ser. Wld Hlth Org. No. 612,* 1977. For background toxicological data, see 1973 and 1975 Evaluations of some Pesticide Residues in Food, *Pestic. Residue Ser. Wld Hlth Org. No. 3,* 1974; *ibid., No. 5,* 1976.

Uses. Carbaryl is a carbamate insecticide which is also used for the treatment of pediculosis capitis. Carbaryl has been used for the control of bedbugs, body lice, fleas, mosquitoes, and ticks and mites.

Proprietary Preparations

Carylderm *(Napp, UK).* Carbaryl, available as **Lotion** containing 0.5% in an alcoholic basis (Inflammable: keep away from an open flame) and as **Shampoo** containing 1%.

Derbac Shampoo *(Bengué, UK).* Contains carbaryl 0.5%.

Suleo Shampoo *(Jeyes, UK).* A cream shampoo containing carbaryl 0.5%.

Other Proprietary Names

Sevin.

3571-b

Clenpyrin. Clenpirin; FBb6896. 1-Butyl-2-(3,4-dichlorophenylimino)pyrrolidine; *N*-(1-Butylpyrrolidin-2-ylidene)-3,4-dichloroaniline.

$C_{14}H_{18}Cl_2N_2$=285.2.

CAS — 27050-41-5.

A chlorinated insecticide used in veterinary medicine.

3572-v

Crufomate. 4-*tert*-Butyl-2-chlorophenyl methyl methylphosphoramidate.

$C_{12}H_{19}ClNO_3P$=291.7.

CAS — 299-86-5.

White crystals or (technical) a yellow oil. Practically **insoluble** in water and light petroleum; readily soluble in acetone.

An organophosphorus veterinary anthelmintic and insecticide. Maximum permissible atmospheric concentration 5 mg per m^3.

Maximum acceptable daily intake of crufomate for man 100 µg per kg body-weight.— Report of the 1972 Joint FAO/WHO Meeting on Pesticide Residues in Food, *Tech. Rep. Ser. Wld Hlth Org. No. 525,* 1973. For background toxicological data, see 1972 Evaluations of some Pesticide Residues in Food, *Pestic. Residue Ser. Wld Hlth Org. No. 2,* 1973..

3573-g

Cythioate. *OO*-Dimethyl *O*-(4-sulphamoylphenyl) phosphorothioate.

$C_8H_{12}NO_5PS_2$=297.3.

CAS — 115-93-5.

An organophosphorus compound (see p.832) given by mouth for the control of fleas, mange mites, and ticks on dogs and cats.

3574-q

Derris *(B.P. Vet.).* Tuba Root; Aker-tuba.

CAS — 83-79-4 (rotenone).

The dried rhizome and roots of *Derris elliptica, D. malaccensis* (Leguminosae), and other species of *Derris,* containing not less than 4% of rotenone. Derris has a slight aromatic odour with a bitter taste causing a persistent sensation of numbness in the mouth and throat.

Rotenone is readily oxidised in the presence of alkali, and materials of this nature should be avoided in preparing sprays, dips, or dusts of derris. **Store** at a temperature not exceeding 25° in airtight containers. Derris, in powder, should be protected from light.

When derris is demanded lonchocarpus may be supplied; when lonchocarpus is demanded derris may be supplied.

3575-p

Prepared Derris *(B. Vet. C. 1965).* Derris Praeparata.

Finely powdered derris or lonchocarpus (see p.838), or a mixture of the 2, adjusted to contain 4 to 6% of rotenone. **Store** in a cool place in airtight containers. Protect from light.

Adverse Effects. Powdered derris is irritant to the eyes and mucosa. Derris appears to be reasonably harmless in man although it has been reported that convulsions and stupor may occur if the powder is inhaled. It is extremely toxic to fish; residues must not be allowed to drain into streams or ponds.

Uses. Derris is an agricultural and horticultural insecticide and larvicide, its action being due to the presence of rotenone and other resins. Its action is more rapid but less persistent than dicophane and less rapid but more persistent than pyrethrum.

3576-s

Dichlorophenoxyacetic Acid. 2,4-D.

2,4-Dichlorophenoxyacetic acid.

$C_8H_6Cl_2O_3$=221.0.

CAS — 94-75-7.

A white powder with a slight phenolic odour. Very slightly **soluble** in water; soluble in aqueous solutions of alkalis and in alcohols; practically insoluble in petroleum oils.

Adverse Effects. Clinical reports of poisoning appear to be rare and show no consistent pattern. After ingestion dichlorophenoxyacetic acid or its salts may cause vomiting, abdominal cramps, diarrhoea, anorexia, muscle weakness, myotonia, and excessive salivation. Other symptoms include ataxia, mental confusion, incoordination, tachycardia, hypotension, alterations in body temperature, peripheral neuropathy, convulsions, and coma.

Death from ventricular fibrillation has occurred after the ingestion of 6 g, yet in another patient recovery followed ingestion of 7 g.

Maximum permissible atmospheric concentration 10 mg per m^3.

Report of a fatality following ingestion of not less than 6 g.— K. Neilsen *et al., Acta pharmac. tox.,* 1965, *22,* 244.

Recovery after the ingestion of 7 g.— P. Berwick, *J. Am. med. Ass.,* 1970, *214,* 1114.

Reversible lung involvement following ingestion by a patient of 40 ml of a weedkiller containing potassium salts of chlorophenoxyacetic and propionic acids (Verdone). Other symptoms included drowsiness, tremors, loss of bladder sensation, haematemesis, and haematuria.— M. K. Davies and R. T. Jung (letter), *Lancet,* 1976, *2,* 370.

Malignant lymphoma of the histiocytic type in one patient exposed to dichlorophenoxyacetic acid and in 6 exposed to dichlorophenoxyacetic and trichlorophenoxyacetic acids.— L. Hardell (letter), *Lancet,* 1979, *1,* 55.

Residues in the body and diet. Maximum acceptable daily intake of dichlorophenoxyacetic acid: 300 µg per kg body-weight.— Report of the 1975 Joint FAO/WHO Meeting on Pesticide Residues in Food, *Tech. Rep. Ser. Wld Hlth Org. No. 592,* 1976. For background toxicological data, see 1971 and 1974 Evaluations of some Pesticide Residues in Food, *Pestic. Residue Ser. Wld Hlth Org. No. 1,* 1972; *ibid., No. 4,* 1975.

Five male subjects took a single dose of 5 mg of dichlorophenoxyacetic acid per kg body-weight without any detectable clinical effects. Peak plasma concentrations of 25 µg per ml were achieved at 4 hours. Excretion appeared to be by first-order kinetics with about 82% of the dose excreted unchanged and about 13% excreted as conjugates. The average half-life was 11.6 hours. There was no evidence to suggest that repeated administration would cause accumulation.— M. W. Sauerhoff *et al.*, *Toxicology*, 1977, *8*, 3, per *Int. pharm. Abstr.*, 1978, *15*, 510.

Blood and urine analyses were carried out on a patient who had ingested about 100 ml of a mixture of dichlorophenoxyacetic and dichloromethoxybenzoic acids. Predicted biological half-lives for dichlorophenoxyacetic acid were 59 and 17 hours and for the other acid 15 and 17 hours.— J. F. Young and T. J. Haley, *Clin. Toxicol.*, 1977, *11*, 489, per *Int. pharm. Abstr.*, 1979, *16*, 427.

Treatment of Adverse Effects. Ingested material should be removed by aspiration and lavage. Contaminated clothing should be removed and the skin washed with soap and water. Further treatment is symptomatic.

For comment on the *in vitro* adsorption of dichlorophenoxyacetic acid by activated charcoal, see p.79.

Uses. Dichlorophenoxyacetic acid is a selective systemic weedkiller widely used in cereals and other crops. It is used as alkyl amine or alkyl ester derivatives, often with other herbicides.

3577-w

Dichlorvos. DDVP; OMS-14; SD 1750.

2,2-Dichlorovinyl dimethyl phosphate.

$C_4H_7Cl_2O_4P=221.0$.

CAS — 62-73-7.

A colourless to amber liquid with an aromatic odour. **Soluble** about 1 in 100 of water and about 1 in 40 of kerosene; miscible with most organic solvents. It is slowly hydrolysed in the presence of moisture. **Store** in airtight containers.

Adverse Effects and Treatment. As for Organophosphorus Insecticides, p.832.

Maximum permissible atmospheric concentration 0.1 ppm (1 mg per m^3).

Contact dermatitis in 4 patients.— P. C. Cronce and H. S. Salden, *J. Am. med. Ass.*, 1968, *206*, 1563.

In wards kept free from insects by Vapona strips containing dichlorvos, there was a moderate decrease in plasma concentrations of cholinesterase in patients exposed continuously to an atmospheric concentration in excess of 100 µg per m^3 and in patients with impaired liver function. Cholinesterase in red cells was not affected. There was no effect on cholinesterase in plasma or red cells from the use of garments stored in cupboards containing Vapona strips.— G. Cavagna *et al.*, *Archs envir. Hlth*, 1969, *19*, 112, per *J. Am. med. Ass.*, 1969, *209*, 580. No adverse effect from such strips used in the home.— J. S. Leary *et al.*, *Archs envir. Hlth*, 1974, *29*, 308, per *J. Am. med. Ass.*, 1974, *230*, 1338.

The Department of Health had rejected a suggestion that insecticidal strips containing dichlorvos should carry a general warning label. The matter had been considered on several occasions by the Advisory Committee on Pesticides which had taken into account the US labelling requirement prohibiting use in rooms where infants, ill patients, or the aged were confined or in areas where food was prepared or served.— *Community Med.*, 1972, *127*, 133.

In 13 factory workers exposed to dichlorvos (mean atmospheric concentration 700 µg per m^3) during working hours for 8 months, there was some depression of cholinesterase activity in plasma and red blood-cells, but there were no clinical effects or other haematological changes.— M. Menz *et al.*, *Archs envir. Hlth*, 1974, *28*, 72, per *Abstr. Hyg.*, 1974, *49*, 661.

A 54-year-old pest control operator whose clothing became contaminated with dichlorvos developed erythema and bullae on areas of the skin exposed to dichlorvos. He also complained of tiredness and constipation and had blood-cholinesterase concentrations 36% of normal. He recovered with conservative treatment.— J. A. Bisby and G. R. Simpson, *Med. J. Aust.*, 1975, *2*, 394.

Five children with aplastic anaemia and one with acute lymphoblastic leukaemia had been exposed to dichlorvos with propoxur; one of the children had also been exposed to a pyrethrin. A seventh child with aplastic anaemia had been exposed to malathion.— J. D. Reeves *et al.* (letter), *Lancet*, 1981, *2*, 300. Criticism of a causal relationship.— H. G. S. v. Raalte and J. D. Jansen, *Shell Research, Neth* (letter), *ibid.*, 811.

Residues in the body and diet. Maximum acceptable daily intake: 4 µg per kg body-weight.— Report of the 1974 Joint FAO/WHO Meeting on Pesticide Residues in Food, *Tech. Rep. Ser. Wld Hlth Org. No. 574*, 1975.

Uses. Dichlorvos is an organophosphorus insecticide of short persistence, effective against a wide range of insects. It is used in the form of impregnated strips or blocks which slowly release vapour. Impregnated animal collars may contain dichlorvos. It is also used for the extermination of insects in aircraft (disinsection).

Helminth infestation. Single doses of dichlorvos, 6 or 12 mg per kg body-weight, administered 2 hours before breakfast as a polyvinyl chloride resin formulation to adults with various helminth infestations gave the following cure-rates assessed up to a month after treatment: hookworm infestation, 77 to 100%; roundworm (*Ascaris*) infestation, 72 to 100%; whipworm (*Trichuris*) infestation, 85 to 94%; hookworm/whipworm and hookworm/roundworm mixed infestation, 68 to 97%; and triple infestation, 62 to 67%. Some depression of plasma-cholinesterase activity occurred and slight depression of red-cell cholinesterase activity; in other respects the treatment was well tolerated.— W. A. Cervoni *et al.*, *Am. J. trop. Med. Hyg.*, 1969, *18*, 912, per *J. Am. med. Ass.*, 1970, *211*, 694. A similar report.— A. Peña Chavarría *et al.*, *Am. J. trop. Med. Hyg.*, 1969, *18*, 907, per *J. Am. med. Ass.*, 1970, *211*, 694. See also A. Davis, *Drug Treatment in Intestinal Helminthiases*, Geneva, World Health Organization, 1973.

Proprietary Preparations

Defest *(Ashe, UK)*. Spray containing iodofenphos and dichlorvos. For use against fleas and other household pests. Not for use on animals.

3578-e

Dicophane *(B.P. 1973)*. DDT; Chlorophenothane; Dichlorodiphenyltrichloroethane; Chlorphenothanum; Clofenotanum; Dichophanum; Clorofenotano. 1,1,1-Trichloro-2,2-bis(4-chlorophenyl)ethane.

$C_{14}H_9Cl_5=354.5$.

CAS — 50-29-3.

Pharmacopoeias. In *Arg.* and *Pol.* (both not less than 96% $C_{14}H_9Cl_5$), *Aust.* (not less than 98%), *Br.* and *Turk.* (not less than 70%), *Ind.* (not less than 75%), *Swiss* (not less than 95%), *Nord.* (not less than 99%), and *Span.* (not less than 80%).

White or nearly white crystals, small granules, flakes, or powders; odourless or with a slight aromatic odour. Crystallising-point not less than 89°. It contains 9.5 to 11.5% of hydrolysable chlorine and not less than 70% of 1,1,1-trichloro-2,2-bis(4-chlorophenyl)ethane, also varying quantities of an isomer, 1,1,1-trichloro-2-(2-chlorophenyl)-2-(4-chlorophenyl)ethane and the carbinol resulting from condensation of 1 molecular proportion of chlorobenzene with chloral hydrate. Practically **insoluble** in water; soluble 1 in 50 of alcohol, 1 in 6 of boiling alcohol, 1 in 2.5 of acetone, 1 in 5 of benzyl benzoate, 1 in 2 of carbon tetrachloride, 1 in 3.5 of chloroform, 1 in 4 of dimethyl phthalate, 1 in 4 of ether, 1 in 20 of kerosene, and 1 in 10 of most fixed oils. The greater the purity of dicophane the lower its solubility in alcohol. **Store** in airtight containers. Protect from light.

Solubility. Figures for the solubility of commercial dicophane at 0°, 15° and 25° in 16 solvents.— W. Mitchell, *Pharm. J.*, 1950, *1*, 278.

Standard for efficiency of aerosols. A British Standards Specification for the insecticidal efficiency of aerosols containing dicophane and pyrethrins against flies (BS 4172: 1967) is published by the British Standards Institution.

Adverse Effects and Treatment. As for Chlorinated Insecticides, p.831.

Dicophane enhances microsomal hepatic enzyme activity.

Maximum permissible atmospheric concentration 1 mg per m^3.

A 13-year-old Mexican was admitted to hospital with anaemia, bleeding, high fever, and unconsciousness. His home had been sprayed with dicophane every other day for 4 months preceding admission and repeatedly for the past 2 years. Laboratory investigation showed low haemoglobin, low reticulocytes, low white-cell count, and diminished platelets. He started to recover after transfusions of packed red blood-cells, and prednisone and tetracycline. But spraying of the hospital room with a 10% solution of dicophane provoked an allergic reaction; he slowly deteriorated and died about 30 hours later. Post-mortem examination showed hypocellularity of the bone marrow and massive bleeding in the lungs.— L. Sanchez-Medal *et al.*, *New Engl. J. Med.*, 1963, *269*, 1365.

The estimated oral LD50 of dicophane for man was 300 to 500 mg per kg body-weight.— H. Kneidel, *Zentbl. ArbMed. ArbSchutz*, 1963, *13*, 33, per *Bull. Hyg., Lond.*, 1963, *38*, 909.

It appeared, from a study of available information on accidental or intentional ingestion of dicophane, that the single oral dose that would cause poisoning in man was about 10 mg per kg body-weight.— G. E. Quinby *et al.*, *Nature*, 1965, *207*, 726.

Twenty-four volunteers ingested technical or *pp'*-DDT, up to 35 mg daily, for 21.5 months and were observed for a further 25.5 months (16 for up to 5 years). There was no laboratory or clinical evidence of injury. Storage of DDT and of [the ethylene compound] DDE and excretion of [the acetic acid compound] DDA was proportional to the dose. The fat of those receiving the highest dose of the technical compound contained 105 to 619 ppm of DDT. The average dose was 555 times that of the average intake of DDT-related compounds and 1250 times the average intake of *pp'*-DDT.— W. J. Hayes *et al.*, *Archs envir. Hlth*, 1971, *22*, 119, per *Abstr. Wld Med.*, 1971, *45*, 629.

Severe scrotal pain followed the local use of Dicophane Application for pubic lice in 2 patients.— *Lancet*, 1972, *1*, 498. A further report.— A. S. Clark (letter), *ibid.*, 590.

Dicophane was carcinogenic in *mice*.— *Br. med. J.*, 1972, *3*, 542.

There was no evidence of liver disease or abnormalities in liver-function tests in 31 chemical workers who in the course of their work had ingested the equivalent of 3.6 to 18 mg of DDT daily for 16 to 25 years. Serum concentrations of DDT and its metabolites in 10 patients were 20 times greater than in the normal population.— E. R. Laws *et al.*, *Archs envir. Hlth*, 1973, *27*, 318, per *Abstr. Hyg.*, 1974, *49*, 470. For a report of chronic liver disease due to industrial exposure to dicophane and gamma benzene hexachloride, see Chlorinated Insecticides, p.831.

A discussion of the distribution and toxicity of dicophane.— T. H. Jukes, *J. Am. med. Ass.*, 1974, *229*, 571. Criticism.— C. F. Wurster (letter), *ibid.*, 1975, *231*, 463. See also *Nature*, 1972, *237*, 417, 420, and 422.

Dicophane had been reported to cause aplastic anaemia.— R. H. Girdwood, *Drugs*, 1976, *11*, 394.

Further references: DDT and its Derivatives, *Environmental Health Criteria 9*, WHO, Geneva, 1979.

Residues in the body and diet. Maximum conditional acceptable daily intake of dicophane: 5 µg per kg body-weight.— Report of the 1972 Joint FAO/WHO Meeting on Pesticide Residues in Food, *Tech. Rep. Ser. Wld Hlth Org. No. 525*, 1973.

Absorption and Fate. Dicophane may be absorbed after ingestion or inhalation or through the skin from solutions in organic solvents. Dicophane is stored in the body, particularly in body fat, and is very slowly eliminated. It crosses the placenta and appears in breast milk. It is metabolised in the body to the ethylene derivative (DDE); the acetic acid derivative (DDA) also appears in the urine.

The rate of metabolism and degradation of dicophane in mammals was slow but appreciable and the concentration in body fat reflected the rate of intake; it was not totally cumulative. Dicophane was metabolised only to a slight extent, if at all, in cold-blooded creatures and predators might suffer from ingesting increasing quantities. Dicophane, however, was cheap and its use had contributed to the reduction of disease. Despite its extensive use in agriculture no death attributable to dicophane had occurred and no syndrome of poisoning was recognisable even among workers heavily exposed for more than 20 years.— *Br. med. J.*, 1969, *4*, 446. A further reference: O. G. Fitzhugh, *Can. med. Ass. J.*, 1966, *94*, 598.

A subject who took technical dicophane (77% *pp'*-DDT and 23% *op'*-DDT) at the rate of 20 mg per day for 183 days excreted the compounds at the rate of 3.1 and 1.1 mg daily when administration ceased. This rate was far in excess of the estimated dietary intake of 16 to 199 µg daily in America.— D. P. Morgan and C. C. Roan (letter), *Nature*, 1972, *238*, 221.

Serum concentrations of dicophane and its metabolite were lower in 117 patients in a mental hospital given various schedules of phenobarbitone, phenytoin, tranquillisers, and other sedatives than in 46 patients not given drugs. The lowest serum-dicophane concentrations occurred in the 15 given phenytoin and phenobarbitone concomitantly.— M. Watson *et al.*, *Clin. Pharmac. Ther.*, 1972, *13*, 186. See also J. E. Davies *et al.*, *Lancet*, 1969, *2*, 7.

Pregnancy and lactation. Concentrations of dicophane in human milk: G. E. Quinby *et al.*, *Nature*, 1965, *207*, 726; G. J. Miller and J. A. Fox, *Med. J. Aust.*, 1973, *2*, 261; D. J. Wilson *et al.*, *Am. J. Dis. Child.*, 1973, *125*, 814; A. Rappl and W. Waiblinger, *Dt. med. Wschr.*, 1975, *100*, 228 and 235.

Dicophane and its metabolite were present in maternal blood in all of 152 pregnant women, in cord blood in 70, and in amniotic fluid in 42. The concentrations of dicophane and its metabolite were higher in Negro than in Caucasian women. In 12 women in whom the vernix caseosa and placenta were assayed, the metabolite of dicophane was present in all specimens and dicophane in 12 and 3 specimens respectively. Chlorinated hydrocarbons were present in the products of conception at 4 weeks' gestation but the effect on the foetus was unknown. Because microsomal enzymatic metabolism of oestrogens and progesterone in the liver was enhanced by chlorinated hydrocarbons, premature labour was theoretically possible.— J. A. O'Leary *et al.*, *Am. J. Obstet. Gynec.*, 1970, *107*, 65.

Uses. Dicophane is a chlorinated insecticide and larvicide. It is a stomach and contact poison and retains its activity for long periods under a variety of conditions. It does not have the immediate lethal effect of derris and pyrethrum. Fleas and body lice may be eliminated by applications of dicophane.

Because of the extreme persistence of dicophane, concern in respect of its effect in the environment, and the problem of resistance, the widespread use of dicophane is now generally discouraged and limited to those applications for which there is no effective or suitable alternative.

After considering the known and speculative hazards of dicophane, the Committee on Occupational Toxicology of the AMA recommended that the indiscriminate use of dicophane was to be deplored, that its use be continued for the control of agricultural pests if no adequate alternative was available, that its local use should be limited or discontinued if its use had created a real hazard to wildlife, that tolerances established by the FDA be stringently enforced, and that education be continued so that dicophane and other pesticides be used with adequate caution.—AMA Committee on Occupational Toxicology, *J. Am. med. Ass.*, 1970, *212*, 1055. See also T. H. Jukes, *ibid.*, 1974, *229*, 571.

In order to maintain and extend malaria eradication programmes dicophane should remain available. Its withdrawal from public health use could lead to great problems, and expose considerable populations to outbreaks of endemic and epidemic malaria. It was considered that the liver tumours found in *mice* given dicophane did not provide an adequate basis for recommending the withdrawal of dicophane where its use could be life-saving and where any possible risk to man would be outweighed by the benefits arising from its controlled use.— Safe Use of Pesticides, Twentieth Report of the WHO Expert Committee on Insecticides, *Tech. Rep. Ser. Wld Hlth Org. No. 513*, 1973. Liver tumours had not been produced in any other species tested and the limited epidemiological evidence available in man, including intermittent exposure over 30 years, gave no evidence that dicophane might be a human carcinogen.— Pesticide Residues in Food, *Tech. Rep. Ser. Wld Hlth Org. No. 574*, 1975.

Vector control. The use of dicophane preparations had led to considerable progress towards the elimination of the vectors of sandfly fever and of tick-borne encephalitis, but dicophane was of little value against *Hyalomma plumbeum*, the vector of Crimean haemorrhagic fever. Chlorofos and carbaryl were effective against *Hyalomma*. A new low-volume technique of application of malathion from aircraft had shown promise against mosquitoes and their larvae.— *Arboviruses and Human Disease*, Report of a WHO Scientific Group, *Tech. Rep. Ser. Wld Hlth Org. No. 369*, 1967.

For the use of dicophane in the control of vectors of disease, see *Insecticide Resistance and Vector Control*, Seventeenth Report of the WHO Expert Committee on Insecticides, *Tech. Rep. Ser. Wld Hlth Org. No. 443*, 1970.

Indoor spraying with dicophane to control transmission of malaria was not a significant risk to human health or wildlife and was essential to maintain control of malaria. The outdoor use of dicophane should be avoided and chemicals which were biologically degradable should be substituted where possible.— *Chronicle Wld Hlth Org.*, 1971, *25*, 201.

Malaria transmission in irrigated areas of the north-eastern region of Afghanistan was sustained by *Anopheles hyrcanus*, which was strongly resistant to dicophane, and *A. pulcherrimus* which was still largely susceptible and seemed to be deterred from entering houses sprayed with dicophane. Studies in one area where dicophane had not been applied for 2 consecutive years indicated that dicophane still played an important role in reducing malaria transmission in the area, although it could not interrupt transmission. A deterioration in the epidemiological situation could be expected if dicophane was withdrawn.— E. Onori *et al.*, *Trans. R. Soc. trop. Med. Hyg.*, 1975, *69*, 236.

Bat control. An account of the conditions under which dicophane could be used in the USA for the control of bats.— L. F. Wells and K. F. Girard, *New Engl. J. Med.*, 1977, *297*, 390.

Preparations

Dicophane Application *(B.P.C. 1973).* Applic Dicophan.; DDT Application. Dicophane 2 g, emulsifying wax 4 g, xylene of commerce 15 ml, citronella oil 0.5 ml, water to 100 ml. About 15 ml is rubbed into the hair and roots of the hair and the head must not be washed during the next 24 hours. The application does not kill parasites immediately; some may persist for a few days. This preparation should not be applied to the genital area.

Dicophane Dusting-powder *(B.P.C. 1973).* Conspersus Dicophani; DDT Dusting-powder. Dicophane 10 g, calcium carbonate 10 g, and sterilised light kaolin or light kaolin (natural) 80 g.

Emulsio Clofenotani *(Dan. Disp.).* Dicophane Emulsion. Dicophane 500 mg, chloroform 1.5 g, turpentine oil 2 g, potash soap spirit 3 g, and water 93 g.

Spiritus Clofenotani *(Nord. P.).* DDT Spirit. Dicophane 2 g, acetone 18 g, and alcohol 80 g.

Proprietary Preparations

Esoderm *(Priory Laboratories, UK).* **Lotion** containing dicophane 1% and gamma benzene hexachloride 1% in isopropyl alcohol. (Inflammable: keep away from an open flame). For pediculosis capitis and scabies. **Shampoo** containing dicophane 1%, gamma benzene hexachloride 1%, ti-tree oil, wool fat, and a sulphonated alcohol. For pediculosis capitis.

Other Proprietary Names

Ivoran *(Denm.).*

3579-l

Dieldrin *(B. Vet. C. 1965).* Technical Dieldrin.

CAS — 60-57-1 (HEOD).

A light-tan flaky crystalline solid with a characteristic odour, consisting mainly of (1*R*,4*S*,5*S*,8*R*)-1,2,3,4,10,10-hexachloro-6,7-epoxy-1,4,4a,5,6,7,8,8a-octahydro-1,4:5,8-dimethanonaphthalene (HEOD), $C_{12}H_8Cl_6O$ = 380.9. Dieldrin contains about 85% HEOD, the remaining 15% being mainly chlorinated organic compounds related to HEOD.

Practically **insoluble** in water; soluble, at 25°, 1 in 4 of alcohol, 1 in 40 of carbon tetrachloride, 1 in 1 of methyl alcohol, and in most aromatic hydrocarbons.

Adverse Effects and Treatment. As for Chlorinated Insecticides, p.831.

Dieldrin is more toxic than dicophane and is readily absorbed through the skin. Fish are highly susceptible to dieldrin and pollution of streams must be avoided. Birds are also susceptible and dressed seeds may be regarded as a source of poisoning which is thought to have caused considerable losses to bird life; dogs and other animals feeding on the carcasses of poisoned birds may also be affected.

Maximum permissible atmospheric concentration 250 µg per m³.

The lethal dose of dieldrin in man was estimated as 65 mg per kg body-weight and its oral toxicity was 3 to 5 times greater than that of dicophane. Symptoms of intoxication had occurred after as little as 10 mg per kg body-weight by mouth. Dieldrin was less than twice as toxic by ingestion as by skin absorption and its acute dermal toxicity in xylene was about 40 times that of dicophane. Dermal rather than respiratory exposure was the major source of occupational poisoning in man. Mild intoxication caused headache, blurred vision, dizziness, nausea, sweating, involuntary movements, insomnia, and bad dreams. Deeper forms of intoxication included all the above together with convulsions and short periods of coma. Intoxication had been seen among industrial workers handling the substance and among workers using it as an insecticidal spray. Many cases of mild chronic intoxication among the latter had been reported.—Committee on Toxicology of AMA, *J. Am. med. Ass.*, 1960, *172*, 2077.

A skin reaction developed in 288 of 1209 men following the use of socks impregnated with dieldrin for moth-proofing.— *Pharmacy Dig.*, 1965, *28*, 262.

Thirteen volunteers were given dieldrin by mouth for 18 months; in 9 of them the daily dose ranged from 10 to 211 µg. None showed evidence of ill health and results of clinical and laboratory investigations remained within the normal range and showed no significant change. The average concentration of dieldrin in fat was 156 times that in the blood.— C. G. Hunter and J. Robinson, *Archs envir. Hlth*, 1967, *15*, 614, per *J. Am. med. Ass.*, 1967, *202* (Nov. 27), A165.

The Environmental Protection Agency of the USA had recommended a ban on further production of aldrin and dieldrin because liver tumours had been produced in *mice*; similar tumours could be produced in mice on normal diets. There was no reason for the authorities in the UK to follow the USA action.— *Br. med. J.*, 1975, *1*, 170.

Further reports of toxic effects: W. J. Hayes, *Publ. Hlth Rep., Wash.*, 1957, *72*, 1087; T. B. Patel and V. N. Rao, *Br. med. J.*, 1958, *1*, 919; T. E. Fletcher *et al.*, *Bull. Wld Hlth Org.*, 1959, *20*, 15; T. G. Schwär, *J. forens. Med.*, 1965, *12*, 142; I. Picton-Robinson (letter), *Br. med. J.*, 1967, *1*, 630; L. K. Garrettson and A. Curley, *Archs envir. Hlth*, 1969, *19*, 814.

Residues in the body and diet. Maximum acceptable daily intake of dieldrin or aldrin: 0.1 µg per kg body-weight.— Report of the 1974 Joint FAO/WHO Meeting on Pesticide Residues in Food, *Tech. Rep. Ser. Wld Hlth Org. No. 574*, 1975.

Uses. Dieldrin is a chlorinated insecticide which is effective after ingestion or contact. Formerly used as a sheep dip, its use in Great Britain is now limited to a few specified purposes. It has also been used for residual spraying against mosquitoes and other vectors in the control of insect-borne diseases. The development of resistant strains has been reported in insect species that are normally susceptible to dieldrin.

Dieldrin had a residual half-life in the blood of about 80 days.— G. R. Simpson and D. J. Penney, *Med. J. Aust.*, 1974, *1*, 258.

Vector control. For the use of dieldrin in the control of vectors of diseases, see *Insecticide Resistance and Vector Control*, Seventeenth Report of the WHO Expert Committee on Insecticides, *Tech. Rep. Ser. Wld Hlth Org. No. 443*, 1970.

3580-v

Dinitrophenol. 2,4-Dinitrophenol.

$C_6H_4N_2O_5$=184.1.

CAS — 51-28-5.

Yellow crystals; sparingly **soluble** in water and readily soluble in alcohol, chloroform, and ether.

Dinitrophenol was formerly used in the treatment of obesity. It has also been used as a selective weedkiller and insecticide. It has the adverse effects described under Dinitrophenol and Related Insecticides. Fatalities have occurred following its use.

3581-g

Dioxathion *(B.P. Vet.).* Dioxation. It consists mainly of *cis* and *trans* isomers of *SS'*-1,4-dioxane-2,3-diyl bis(*OO*-diethyl phosphorodithioate). $C_{12}H_{26}O_6P_2S_4$=456.5.

CAS — 78-34-2.

A dark amber-coloured liquid with an odour characteristic of sulphides. Wt per ml at 25° 1.24 to 1.27 g. Practically **insoluble** in water; miscible with alcohol, acetone, and xylene. **Store** at a temperature not exceeding 25°.

CAUTION. *Dioxathion is very toxic when inhaled, swallowed, or spilled on the skin. It can be removed from the skin by washing with soap and water. Contaminated material should be immersed in a 2% aqueous solution of sodium hydroxide for several hours.*

Adverse Effects and Treatment. As for Organophosphorus Insecticides, p.832.

Maximum acceptable daily intake of dioxathion: 1.5 µg per kg body-weight.— Report of the 1972 Joint FAO/WHO Meeting on Pesticide Residues in Food, *Tech. Rep. Ser. Wld Hlth Org. No. 525,* 1973.

Uses. Dioxathion is an agricultural insecticide and acaricide. It has been used for the control of cattle ticks but it is also active against lice and hornfly of cattle, against ticks, lice, keds, and blowfly of sheep, and against some external parasites of goats and pigs.

3582-q

Diphenylamine.
$C_{12}H_{11}N$=169.2.

CAS — 122-39-4.

Pharmacopoeias. In *Nord.*

A white crystalline powder with a mild characteristic odour and taste. M.p. 54° to 55°. Practically **insoluble** in water; soluble 1 in 5 of alcohol (90%); very soluble in chloroform and ether. **Incompatible** with iron and silver salts. **Protect** from light.

Diphenylamine has been used as a veterinary larvicide for topical application for the prevention and treatment of screw-worm (*Callitroga americana*) infestations in livestock. It is approved for use in Great Britain as a scald inhibitor for apples and pears at concentrations not exceeding 10 ppm. Maximum permissible atmospheric concentration 10 mg per m^3.

Maximum acceptable daily intake of diphenylamine for man: 20 µg per kg body-weight. Further work with special attention to the formation of Heinz bodies was desirable.— Report of the 1976 Joint FAO/WHO Meeting on Pesticide Residues in Food, *Tech. Rep. Ser. Wld Hlth Org. No. 612,* 1977.

3583-p

Diquat. 9,10-Dihydro-8a,10a-diazoniaphenanthrene ion; 1,1'-Ethylene-2,2'-bipyridyldiylium ion.
$C_{12}H_{12}N_2$=184.2.

CAS — 2764-72-9.

3584-s

Diquat Dibromide.
$C_{12}H_{12}Br_2N_2$=344.0.

CAS — 85-00-7.

Diquat is a contact herbicide used usually as the dibromide in agriculture and horticulture. It has similar adverse effects to those of paraquat (see p.840). Diquat dichloride also appears to be used. Maximum permissible atmospheric concentration 500 µg per m^3.

A non-fatal case of poisoning by diquat.— D. G. Oreopoulos and J. McEvoy, *Postgrad. med. J.,* 1969, *45,* 635, per *Abstr. Hyg.,* 1970, *45,* 43.

Death of a young man after ingesting diquat. Post-mortem findings included oesophageal and gastric necrosis, oedema and bleeding of the lungs, but no lung proliferation.— H. Schönborn *et al., Arch. Tox.,* 1971, *27,* 204, per P. Cooper (letter), *Pharm. J.,* 1972, *2,* 566.

Residues in the body and diet. Maximum acceptable daily intake of diquat as the dichloride: 5 µg per kg body-weight.— Report of the 1976 Joint FAO/WHO Meeting on Pesticide Residues in Food, *Tech. Rep. Ser. Wld Hlth Org. No. 612,* 1977.

For background toxicological data, see 1972 Evaluations of some Pesticide Residues in Food, *Pestic. Residue Ser. Wld Hlth Org. No. 2,* 1973.

Proprietary Names
Aquacide *(Chipman, UK)*; Reglone *(ICI Plant Protection, UK).*

Present in Pathclear *(ICI Plant Protection, UK)*; Weedol *(ICI Plant Protection, UK).*

3585-w

Fenchlorphos. ENT 23 284; Ronnel. *OO*-Dimethyl *O*-(2,4,5-trichlorophenyl)phosphorothioate.
$C_8H_8Cl_3O_3PS$=321.5.

CAS — 299-84-3.

A colourless crystalline powder. Practically **insoluble** in water; readily soluble in most organic solvents. M.p. 40° to 42°. **Incompatible** with alkalis.

Fenchlorphos is an organophosphorus insecticide effective against flies and animal ectoparasites.

Proprietary Names
Nankor *(Dow Corning, USA)*; Trolene *(Dow Corning, USA).*

3586-e

Fenthion *(B.P. Vet.).* Bayer 29493; S 752. *OO*-Dimethyl *O*-4-methylthio-*m*-tolylphosphorothioate.
$C_{10}H_{15}O_3PS_2$=278.3.

CAS — 55-38-9.

A yellowish-brown almost odourless oily liquid. Practically **immiscible** with water; miscible with alcohol and chloroform.

An organophosphorus insecticide (see p.832). In veterinary practice it is used for the control of warble fly and lice on cattle.

Proprietary Names
Tiguvon *(Bayer, UK; Ciba-Geigy Agrochemicals, UK).*

3587-l

Gamma Benzene Hexachloride *(B.P.).* Gamma-BHC; Benhexachlor; Hexicide; Lindane *(U.S.P.)*; HCH; Gamma-HCH; 666.
1α,2α,3β,4α,5α,6β-Hexachlorocyclohexane.
$C_6H_6Cl_6$=290.8.

CAS — 58-89-9.

Pharmacopoeias. In *Arg., Aust., Br., Braz., Ind., Nord., Pol.,* and *U.S.*

A white tasteless crystalline powder with a slight musty odour. Crystallising-point not less than 112°. Practically **insoluble** in water; soluble 1 in 19 of dehydrated alcohol, 1 in 2 of acetone, 1 in 3.5 of chloroform, 1 in 5.5 of ether, and in other organic solvents; slightly soluble in ethylene glycol. **Protect** from light.

Adverse Effects and Treatment. As for Chlorinated Insecticides, p.830.

Gamma benzene hexachloride enhances microsomal hepatic enzyme activity. There has been some concern over the application of higher than normal concentrations of gamma benzene hexachloride to the skin in the treatment of scabies and pediculosis; children are considered to be particularly at risk.

Maximum permissible atmospheric concentration 500 µg per m^3.

A review of the toxicity of gamma benzene hexachloride. It should not be applied after a hot soapy bath; application for less than 24 hours might be effective; a concentration of less than 1% might be sufficient, especially for excoriated skin; the 1% preparation should be used with extreme caution, if at all, in pregnancy, in very small infants, in the presence of massive excoriation; retreatment should not take place before 8 days and then only if infection could be demonstrated.— L. M. Solomon *et al., Archs Derm.,* 1977, *113,* 353.

Use of an algorithm, or logical flow chart, to investigate the quality of evidence in reported cases of adverse drug reactions to a 1% solution of gamma benzene hexachloride. It was concluded that a 1% solution of gamma benzene hexachloride is an extraordinarily safe preparation when used according to instructions. Publicity about its toxicity appears to be unjustified, arising from physicians who confused the insecticide with the drug, or who submitted reports of reactions that fail to fulfil operational criteria for the diagnosis of adverse drug reaction. Only 6 probable and no definite cases of toxicity could be confirmed for the drug, despite the use of over 24 million applications during the past 17 years.— M. S. Kramer *et al., Clin. Pharmac. Ther.,* 1980, *27,* 149.

Neuro-ocular manifestations of chronic poisoning with gamma benzene hexachloride.— S. B. Khare *et al., J. Ass. Physns India,* 1977, *25,* 215.

Reports of poisoning with gamma benzene hexachloride: B. Lee *et al.* (letter), *J. Am. med. Ass.,* 1976, *236,* 2846; B. Lee and P. Groth (letter), *Pediatrics,* 1977, *59,* 643; Z. M. Munk and A. Nantel, *Can. med. Ass. J.,* 1977, *117,* 1050; M. Wheeler, *West. J. Med.,* 1977, *127,* 518.

Aplastic anaemia. Fatal aplastic anaemia occurred following exposure to fumes of gamma benzene hexachloride from a vaporiser. An 8-year-old girl had been exposed to the fumes for about 2 hours daily for 2 years and a 52-year-old man for 8 to 15 hours weekly for about 3 months. Neither patient responded to blood transfusions or treatment with prednisone or methyltestosterone.— J. P. Loge, *J. Am. med. Ass.,* 1965, *193,* 110. Another report on 6 patients.— I. West, *Archs envir. Hlth,* 1967, *15,* 97.

In 40 persons exposed in their work to gamma benzene hexachloride the concentration in blood was 0.0119 ppm compared with 0.0001 ppm in 40 persons not so exposed. In the exposed groups the creatinine concentration and the counts of erythrocytes, total white cells, and polymorphonuclear leucocytes were significantly higher; all other parameters were within the normal range. No evidence was found that gamma benzene hexachloride had any toxic effect on the bone marrow at these concentrations.— T. H. Milby and A. J. Samuels, *J. occup. Med.,* 1971, *13,* 256, per *Abstr. Hyg.,* 1972, *47,* 21.

Residues in the body and diet. Maximum acceptable daily intake of gamma benzene hexachloride: 10 µg per kg body-weight.— Report of the 1975 Joint FAO/WHO Meeting on Pesticide Residues in Food, *Tech. Rep. Ser. Wld Hlth Org. No. 592,* 1976.

For background toxicological data, see 1973 and 1974 Evaluations of some Pesticide Residues in Food, *Pestic. Residue Ser. Wld Hlth Org. No. 3,* 1974; *ibid., No. 4,* 1975.

The absorption of gamma benzene hexachloride by infants and children following the application of a 1% lotion.— C. M. Ginsburg *et al., J. Pediat.,* 1977, *91,* 998.

Uses. Gamma benzene hexachloride is an insecticide, larvicide, and acaricide. It has a more rapid action than dicophane and is effective in lower concentrations but as it is more volatile it has much less residual action. It is used against agricultural pests and house flies.

Topically, a 0.2% alcoholic solution or a 0.1% application is used against head lice and a 1% emulsion is employed in the treatment of scabies. Some authorities consider that alternative treatment should be used in infants, children and perhaps pregnant women.

The development of resistant strains has been reported in species of insects, including lice, that are normally susceptible.

Four of 14 patients with atopic dermatitis and positive scratch tests to house dust and house dust mites were relieved of their symptoms for 4 months after treatment with a 1% o/w emulsion of gamma benzene hexachloride left on the skin for 24 hours and repeated after 3 days.— M. Alani and N. Hjorth, *Acta allerg.,* 1970, *25,* 41, per *Clin. Med.,* 1972, *79* (Jan.), 34.

Pediculosis. In the treatment of body lice with a 1% powder of gamma benzene hexachloride a second application was required 7 to 10 days after the first. This rendered the insecticide unsatisfactory for mass delousing of migrant populations. Resistance to gamma benzene hexachloride was less widespread than resistance to dicophane.— M. M. Cole *et al.*, *Soap chem. Spec.*, 1960, *36* (May), 101.

A cream, lotion, or shampoo containing 1% of gamma benzene hexachloride had been effective in patients with *Phthirus pubis* infestation. Creams and lotions were massaged into the affected area and washed off after 24 hours. The shampoo was lathered in for 4 minutes, washed out, and the hair rubbed dry and combed. One application was usually sufficient, but with heavy infestation the process might have to be repeated 2 or 3 times at 4-day intervals.— A. B. Ackerman, *New Engl. J. Med.*, 1968, *278*, 950.

A single treatment with 1% gamma benzene hexachloride shampoo in 83 patients completely eliminated infestation by *Pediculosis capitis* and *Phthirus pubis*.— L. Wexler, *Clin. Med.*, 1968, *75* (Aug.), 28.

Head lice usually responded to a single thorough application to the scalp of a 2% solution of gamma benzene hexachloride in a detergent basis. There was evidence of true resistance to the insecticide in some areas and malathion was currently recommended for treatment of resistant strains. For pubic lice a single application of a 1% cream was usually effective and gamma benzene hexachloride powder was used for dusting the clothing and bedding of patients with body lice.— F. A. Ive, *Br. med. J.*, 1973, *4*, 475.

Gamma benzene hexachloride was considered to be completely ovicidal to head, body and pubic lice when properly applied once only in a 1% concentration. Resistance was not considered to be a problem.— A. J. Singer, *Br. med. J.*, 1977, *2*, 1608.

Further references: *Med. Lett.*, 1977, *19*, 18.

See also above under Adverse Effects.

Scabies. During the course of a year 22 patients had been treated for infestation with the mite *Sarcoptes scabiei* var. *canis*, contracted from pet dogs. A single application of gamma benzene hexachloride cream, applied over the whole body and left on for 24 hours, was usually effective.— E. B. Smith and T. F. Claypoole, *J. Am. med. Ass.*, 1967, *199*, 59.

A 1% shampoo was effective in the treatment of scabies; it was applied to the whole body for 30 minutes on 2 successive evenings. Mild pruritus might persist for 7 to 10 days.— J. R. Haydon and R. M. Caplan, *Archs Derm.*, 1971, *103*, 168, per *Clin. Med.*, 1973, *80* (Feb.), 30.

Further references: A. B. Cannon and M. E. McRae, *J. Am. med. Ass.*, 1948, *138*, 557; B. H. E. James (letter), *Br. med. J.*, 1972, *1*, 178; R. J. G. Rycroft and C. D. Calnan, *Br. med. J.*, 1977, *2*, 303; *Med. Lett.*, 1977, *19*, 18.

See also under Adverse Effects, above and under Benzyl Benzoate, p.833.

Vector control. For the use of gamma benzene hexachloride in the control of vectors of disease, see *Insecticide Resistance and Vector Control*, Seventeenth Report of the WHO Expert Committee on Insecticides, *Tech. Rep. Ser. Wld Hlth Org. No. 443*, 1970.

Preparations

Gamma Benzene Hexachloride Application *(B.P.)*. Gamma benzene hexachloride 100 mg (or a suitable quantity), emulsifying wax 4 g, xylene of commerce 15 ml, lavender oil 1 ml, freshly boiled and cooled water to 100 ml.

A.P.F. also has a similar preparation containing 0.1% gamma benzene hexachloride.

Gamma Benzene Hexachloride Cream *(B.P.)*. Contains gamma benzene hexachloride in a suitable basis. It may be prepared to the following formula: gamma benzene hexachloride 1 g (or a suitable quantity), cetomacrogol emulsifying wax 14 g, liquid paraffin 8 g, freshly boiled and cooled water to 100 g.

Gamma Benzene Hexachloride Cream Aqueous *(A.P.F.)*. Gamma benzene hexachloride 1 g, xylene of commerce 10 ml, emulsifying wax 10 g, spike lavender oil 1 ml, freshly boiled and cooled water to 100 ml.

Lindane Cream *(U.S.P.)*. Gamma Benzene Hexachloride Cream. Gamma benzene hexachloride in a suitable cream basis. pH of a 20% dilution 8 to 9. Store in airtight containers.

Lindane Lotion *(U.S.P.)*. Gamma Benzene Hexachloride Lotion. Gamma benzene hexachloride in a suitable aqueous vehicle. pH 6.5 to 8.5. Store in airtight containers.

Proprietary Preparations

Derbac Soap *(Bengué, UK)*. Contains gamma benzene hexachloride 1% and cresol 0.779%.

Lorexane *(ICI Pharmaceuticals, UK)*. Gamma benzene hexachloride, available as **Concentrate** containing 1%; as **Cream** containing 1% in a vanishing cream basis; as **Dusting-powder** containing 0.6%; and as **Lorexane No. 3**, a cream shampoo containing 2% in a detergent basis. (Also available as Lorexane in *Austral.*).

Quellada Lotion *(Stafford-Miller, UK)*. Contains gamma benzene hexachloride 1% in a water-miscible basis. **Quellada Application P.C.** Contains gamma benzene hexachloride 1% in a shampoo basis. (Also available as Quellada in *Austral.*, *S.Afr.*).

Other Proprietary Names

Belg.—Lencid; *Canad.*—GBH, Kwellada; *Denm.*—Hexicid; *Fin.*—Desantin; *Fr.*—Aphtiria, Élentol; *Ger.*—Jacutin; *Greece*—Kwellada; *Neth.*—Jacutin; *Norw.*—Hexicid; *Port.*—Desantin; *S.Afr.*—Skabex; *Switz.*—Atan, Jacutin, Kwellada; *USA*—Gamene, Kwell.

3588-y

Isobornyl Thiocyanoacetate.

Terpinyl Thiocyanoacetate. Isoborn-2-yl thiocyanatoacetate.
$C_{13}H_{19}NO_2S=253.4$.

CAS — 115-31-1.

A yellow oily liquid with a terpene-like odour. Practically **insoluble** in water; very soluble in alcohol, chloroform, and ether.

Isobornyl thiocyanoacetate is used in the treatment of pediculosis. It is irritant to the eyes and mucous membranes. It should not be applied to the skin for longer than 10 minutes.

Proprietary Names

Bornex *(Wyeth, Canad.)*.

3589-j

Lonchocarpus

(B.P. Vet.). Cube Root; Timbo; Barbasco.

CAS — 83-79-4 (rotenone).

The dried root of *Lonchocarpus utilis, L. urucu*, and other species of *Lonchocarpus* (Leguminosae), containing not less than 4% of rotenone.

Lonchocarpus has a slight odour with a taste slight at first, becoming acrid and producing an unpleasant numbing sensation in the mouth and throat.

Rotenone is readily oxidised in the presence of alkali and materials of this nature should be avoided in preparations of lonchocarpus. **Store** at a temperature not exceeding 25° in airtight containers. Lonchocarpus, in powder, should be protected from light.

When lonchocarpus is demanded derris may be supplied; when derris is demanded lonchocarpus may be supplied.

Uses. Lonchocarpus is used for the same purposes as derris (see p.834).

3590-q

Malathion.

Carbofos; Compound 4047; OMS-1. Diethyl 2-(dimethoxyphosphinothioylthio)succinate.
$C_{10}H_{19}O_6PS_2=330.4$.

CAS — 121-75-5.

A colourless to light amber liquid with a characteristic odour. Very slightly **soluble** in water; miscible with many organic solvents.

Adverse Effects and Treatment. As for Organophosphorus Insecticides, p.832.

Malathion is one of the safer organophosphorus insecticides.

Maximum permissible atmospheric concentration 10 mg per m^3.

A 42-year-old woman took at least 120 ml of a 50% malathion spray, corresponding to 1 g per kg bodyweight. She became unconscious and developed hypersecretion and cyanosis but recovered after treatment.— A. R. Goldin *et al.*, *New Engl. J. Med.*, 1964, *271*, 1289. Similar reports of recovery after treatment.— W. J. Crowley and T. R. Johns, *Archs Neurol., Chicago*, 1966, *14*, 611; P. W. M. Windsor, *Practitioner*, 1968, *200*, 600; I. Mathewson and E. A. Hardy, *Anaesthesia*, 1970, *25*, 265; N. Gadoth and A. Fisher, *Ann. intern. Med.*, 1978, *88*, 654.

A fatality.— *Br. med. J.*, 1966, *1*, 304.

In a modified 'repeated-insult' patch test, 25% 'technical' malathion was found to produce extreme sensitisation of the skin.— A. M. Kligman, *J. invest. Derm.*, 1966, *47*, 393.

After a city in Texas had been sprayed with 95% malathion at the rate of 21.2 mg per m^2, 119 volunteers were questioned about symptoms of exposure 24 and 72 hours after spraying. Six patients complained but there was no correlation between symptoms and changes in plasma cholinesterase. Some of the symptoms were considered to be psychogenic. The spraying entailed a 'negligible risk' to health and effectively controlled mosquitoes.— A. L. Gardner and R. E. Iverson, *Archs envir. Hlth*, 1968, *16*, 823, per *Abstr. Wld Med.*, 1969, *43*, 164.

The speed of absorption of malathion, parathion, and carbaryl was dependent on the site of contact. In ascending order of speed of absorption: the forearm and skin of the palm; the dorsum of the hand and abdominal skin; follicle-rich skin of the scalp, jaw angle, forehead, and post-aural region; axillary skin; scrotal skin.— H. I. Maibach *et al.*, *Archs envir. Hlth*, 1971, *23*, 208, per *Pharm. J.*, 1972, *1*, 177.

Chlorine was reported to inactivate malathion; patients should not go swimming for one week after treatment.— M. Tamblyn, *Br. med. J.*, 1977, *2*, 1292.

Among 7500 field workers exposed to malathion during malaria control operations in Pakistan, poisoning occurred in probably more than 2500, of whom 5 died. Poisoning was attributed to the presence of other organophosphorus compounds as impurities in some batches of malathion powder. Isomalathion was implicated as the main cause of increased toxicity.— Chemistry and Specifications of Pesticides, Second Report of the WHO Expert Committee on Vector Biology and Control, *Tech. Rep. Ser. Wld Hlth Org. No. 620*, 1978. See also E. L. Baker *et al.*, *Lancet*, 1978, *1*, 31.

Residues in the body and diet. Maximum acceptable daily intake: 20 μg per kg body-weight.— Report of the 1972 Joint FAO/WHO Meeting on Pesticide Residues in Food, *Tech. Rep. Ser. Wld Hlth Org. No. 525*, 1973.

For background toxicological data, see 1973 Evaluations of some Pesticide Residues in Food, *Pestic. Residue Ser. Wld Hlth Org. No. 3*, 1974.

Uses. Malathion is an organophosphorus insecticide active both as a stomach and as a contact poison and effective against a wide range of insects. It is applied in concentrations of 0.5% or 1% in the treatment of pediculosis. Residual spraying of malathion has proved effective against mosquitoes and houseflies.

Malathion is also used as an agricultural and horticultural pesticide. The development of resistant strains has been reported in species of insects that are normally susceptible.

Malathion had been widely used as a space spray against adult mosquitoes and as a larvicide in the USA. Its safety in use as a 1% dust for louse control was confirmed and it could be used in public health measures when it was needed, provided suitable precautions were observed.— Sixteenth Report of WHO Expert Committee on Insecticides, *Tech. Rep. Ser. Wld Hlth Org. No. 356*, 1967.

Pediculosis. In 106 children (29 boys, 77 girls) with head infestation probably resistant to gamma benzene hexachloride and treated with malathion, the success-rate in boys was 100% and in girls 89.6%; in the 8 girls who did not respond there was doubt as to whether treatment had been properly undertaken in 4.— J. Maguire and A. J. McNally, *Community Med.*, 1972, *128*, 374.

Two applications, 1 week apart, of malathion lotion was the recommended treatment for head lice which were resistant to gamma benzene hexachloride and dicophane; malathion was lethal to both insects and eggs.— J. S. Pegum, *Practitioner*, 1972, *209*, 453.

A shampoo preparation of malathion 1% was as effective as a lotion containing malathion 0.5% in treating children with head lice.— S. Preston and L. Fry, *R. Soc. Hlth J.*, 1977, *97*, 291.

Vector control. For the use of malathion in the control of vectors of disease, see *Insecticide Resistance and Vector Control,* Seventeenth Report of the WHO Expert Committee on Insecticides, *Tech. Rep. Ser. Wld Hlth Org. No. 443,* 1970. See also *Asian J. infect. Dis.,* 1978, *2,* 112, per *Trop. Dis. Bull.,* 1979, *76,* 995.

Proprietary Preparations

Derbac Liquid *(Bengué, UK).* Contains malathion 0.5%, in an aqueous basis.

Prioderm Lotion *(Napp, UK).* Malathion, available as an alcoholic solution containing 0.5%. (Inflammable: keep away from an open flame). **Prioderm Shampoo.** Contains malathion 1% in a cream shampoo basis. (Also available as Prioderm in *Neth., NZ*).

Other Proprietary Names

Noury Hoofdlotion *(Neth.).*

3591-p

Metaldehyde.

A polymer of acetaldehyde.
$(C_2H_4O)_x$.

CAS — 9002-91-9.

A white crystalline solid, burning readily and subliming at 100°.

Adverse Effects. Symptoms of poisoning by metaldehyde include vomiting and diarrhoea, fever, drowsiness, convulsions, and coma. Death from respiratory failure may occur within 48 hours. Kidney and liver damage may occur.

Treatment of Adverse Effects. The stomach should be emptied by aspiration and lavage. Appropriate supportive treatment should be instituted.

A 20-month-old infant who swallowed an unknown quantity of metaldehyde was treated within half an hour by gastric lavage and an intravenous infusion of dextrose in saline. On the third day, tremor, hypertonia, increased tendon reflexes, and irritability developed. The intravenous infusion was resumed and phenobarbitone and bicarbonate by mouth were given and the symptoms resolved by the fifth day.— *Practitioner,* 1968, *200,* 319.

Uses. Metaldehyde is a molluscicide used in pellets against slugs and snails. It is also reported to be an ingredient of some firelighters.

'Meta' is compressed metaldehyde which has been used as a solid fuel burning with a non-luminous carbon-free flame.

3592-s

Methoprene.

ZR-515. Isopropyl 11-methoxy-3,7,11-trimethyldodeca-2(*E*),4(*E*)-dienoate.
$C_{19}H_{34}O_3$=310.5.

CAS — 40596-69-8.

An amber liquid. Practically **insoluble** in water; soluble in most organic solvents.

Methoprene is a juvenoid insecticide which mimics the action of insect juvenile hormones causing death by preventing the transformation of larva to pupa, if applied at the appropriate period of sensitivity.

Proprietary Names
Altocid *(Zoecon, USA).*

3593-w

Methylchlorophenoxyacetic Acid.

MCPA. 4-Chloro-2-methylphenoxyacetic acid.
$C_9H_9ClO_3$=200.6.

CAS — 4841-22-9.

A white crystalline solid. Very slightly **soluble** in water.

A selective weedkiller with similar actions to dichlorophenoxyacetic acid (p.834).

It is usually used as the amine, potassium, or sodium salts.

Death after the ingestion of 440 mg per kg body-weight.— R. D. Popham and D. M. Davies, *Br. med. J.,* 1964, *1,* 677.

Death after the ingestion of 250 mg per kg body-weight.— H. R. M. Johnson and O. Koumides, *Br. med. J.,* 1965, *2,* 629.

Malignant lymphoma of the histiocytic type in one patient exposed to methylchlorophenoxyacetic acid.— L. Hardell (letter), *Lancet,* 1979, *1,* 55.

3594-e

Metriphonate

(B. Vet. C. 1965). Metrifonate; Trichlorfon; Trichlorphon. Dimethyl 2,2,2-trichloro-1-hydroxyethylphosphonate.
$C_4H_8Cl_3O_4P$=257.4.

CAS — 52-68-6.

Pharmacopoeias. In *Cz.*

A white or pale yellow crystalline powder with a characteristic musty odour. Setting-point not less than 73.5°.

Soluble 1 in 7 of water; soluble in alcohols, in hydrocarbons such as xylenes and methylnaphthalenes, and in chlorinated hydrocarbons such as trichloroethylene. Solutions should be prepared immediately before use. Metriphonate is unstable in alkaline solution.

CAUTION. *Metriphonate is very toxic when inhaled, swallowed, or spilled on the skin. It can be removed from the skin by washing with soap and water. Contaminated material should be immersed in a 2% aqueous solution of sodium hydroxide for several hours.*

Adverse Effects and Treatment. As for Organophosphorus Insecticides, p.832.

When used medicinally it may cause nausea, vomiting, abdominal pain, headache, and vertigo.

A summary of toxicological and pharmacological information on metriphonate.— B. Holmstedt *et al., Arch. Tox.,* 1978, *41,* 3.

Studies in 28 patients showed that a single dose of 10 mg of metriphonate per kg body-weight caused an initial depression of blood cholinesterase but that concentrations returned to normal within 2 weeks; a second dose given 15 days after the first to 15 patients caused a similar effect. Atropine, given in a dose of 600 µg subcutaneously to 6 boys with a mean weight of 52 kg, did not modify the effect on serum-cholinesterase concentrations.— D. M. Forsyth and C. Rashid, *Lancet,* 1967, *1,* 130.

Symptoms of poisoning due to metriphonate in an adult were relieved by a single injection of atropine. Repeated applications of metriphonate to the skin caused a fall of about one-half in cholinesterase activity in red cells and plasma.— B. Svetlicic and K. Wihelm, *Arh. Hig. Rada,* 1968, *19,* 241, per *Int. pharm. Abstr.,* 1969, *6,* 629.

Plasma cholinesterase was completely inhibited and erythrocyte cholinesterase inhibited by 40 to 60% in children with urinary schistosomiasis after treatment with metriphonate in doses of 7.5, 10, and 12.5 mg per kg body-weight for up to 3 doses at 14-day intervals.— P. Pleština *et al., Bull. Wld Hlth Org.,* 1972, *46,* 747.

Further references: V. P. Jamnadas and J. E. P. Thomas, *Cent. Afr. J. Med.,* 1979, *25,* 130.

Residues in the body and diet. Temporary maximum acceptable daily intake of metriphonate: 5 µg per kg body-weight. Further work was required on carcinogenicity and further studies were desirable on the spontaneous conversion of metriphonate to dichlorvos and on the possible intermediaries involved.— Report of the 1975 Joint FAO/WHO Meeting on Pesticide Residues in Food, *Tech. Rep. Ser. Wld Hlth Org. No. 592,* 1976.

For background toxicological data, see 1971 Evaluations of some Pesticide Residues in Food, *Pestic. Residue Ser. Wld Hlth Org. No. 1,* 1972.

Uses. Metriphonate is an organophosphorus insecticide used in agriculture and horticulture and as a veterinary anthelmintic. As an insecticide it is effective against a wide range of ectoparasites, either by direct application or by oral administration. As a veterinary anthelmintic it is effective against certain nematodes in ruminants but it has no action against flukes or tapeworms. Its activity is of short duration as it is rapidly metabolised within the body and it is not persistent on the skin; dichlorvos is a metabolite.

Metriphonate has also been used in the treatment of human helminth infections, especially those due to *Schistosoma haematobium.*

In a study in the Congo, metriphonate was given as an anthelmintic, usually in a dose of 15 mg per kg body-weight, repeated once after 24 hours. Of 625 children with hookworm (*Ancylostoma*) infestation, 91% were cleared with this dosage but with half this dosage only about 70% of 42 adults were cleared. Of 1209 children with roundworm (*Ascaris*) infestation, 66 to 86% were cleared, as were 75 to 88% with whipworm (*Trichuris*) infestation. Of 54 patients with rectal schistosomiasis treated with metriphonate 17 mg per kg body-weight for 4 days, 70% were negative on stool examination 11 days afterwards, but this dropped to 40% after 80 days, as a result of either relapse or reinfection. Two or 3 applications of a 20% cream in a water-soluble basis cured 10 children with creeping eruption refractory to other methods.— J. Cerf *et al., Am. J. trop. Med. Hyg.,* 1962, *11,* 514, per *Trop. Dis. Bull.,* 1963, *60,* 41.

Onchocerciasis. In 19 patients with *Onchocerca volvulus* infestations treated with metriphonate 7.5 to 15 mg per kg body-weight at fortnightly intervals for 4 to 16 doses, 25 of 65 nodules had become smaller and 2 had disappeared. Of worms removed from nodules after treatment about 75% were non-motile compared with about 25% in controls. Eggs and microfilariae showed degenerative changes. Skin snips taken before and after 4 doses showed a 71 to 100% reduction in microfilarial count. Side-effects included pruritus, adenopathy, fever, and eosinophilia.— M. Salazar-Mallén *et al., Ann. trop. Med. Parasit.,* 1971, *65,* 393, per *Trop. Dis. Bull.,* 1972, *69,* 660.

In 7 patients with *Onchocerca volvulus* infestation given metriphonate 10 mg per kg body-weight daily for 6 consecutive days, with atropine sulphate, microfilariae disappeared from the skin in 4 and remained absent for at least 3 weeks. In 2 further patients there was transitory disappearance of microfilariae.— M. Salazar-Mallén *et al., Revta Inst. Med. trop. S Paulo,* 1971, *13,* 363, per *Trop. Dis. Bull.,* 1972, *69,* 420.

Metriphonate had a moderate action against *Onchocerca volvulus* but no action against *Wuchereria bancrofti.*— D. E. Abaru and J. E. McMahon, *Tropenmed. Parasit.,* 1978, *29,* 175, per *Trop. Dis. Bull.,* 1979, *76,* 1031.

Further references: H. Fuglsang and J. Anderson, *Tropenmed. Parasit.,* 1978, *29,* 168, per *Trop. Dis. Bull.,* 1979, *76,* 1031.

Schistosomiasis. Of 115 children with *Schistosoma haematobium* infestation treated with metriphonate 7.5 mg per kg body-weight repeated once after 3 weeks, 89 were adequately followed; 48 appeared to be cured while an 80% reduction in the number of eggs in the urine occurred in the others. Single-dose administration made the treatment worth while.— S. Diallo and P. Druilhe, *Bull. Soc. méd. Afr. noire Langue franç.,* 1973, *18,* 574, per *Trop. Dis. Bull.,* 1974, *71,* 1035.

Urinary schistosomiasis in 50 patients was treated with metriphonate usually 10 mg per kg body-weight, generally repeated after 15 days. Of 49 evaluated at 14 days 18 were still passing live ova; the respective figures for those evaluated at 3 and 6 months were 1 of 18 and 1 of 12.— M. Gentilini *et al., Bull. Soc. Path. exot.,* 1973, *66,* 299, per *Trop. Dis. Bull.,* 1974, *71,* 160.

A cure-rate of 43.6% and an overall reduction in egg-count of 94.5% was achieved in 39 children with *Schistosoma haematobium* infestation treated with metriphonate 7.5 mg per kg body-weight repeated on 2 occasions at 4-weekly intervals.— S. Reddy *et al., Ann. trop. Med. Parasit.,* 1975, *69,* 73, per *Trop. Dis. Bull.,* 1975, *72,* 630.

Metriphonate 7.5 mg per kg body-weight given every 2 weeks for 3 doses produced a cure in 60% of children infected with *Schistosoma haematobium.* The same dose given every 4 weeks was considered to be effective in preventing infection in an endemic area.— J. M. Jewsbury *et al., Ann. trop. Med. Parasit.,* 1977, *71,* 67, per *Trop. Dis. Bull.,* 1977, *74,* 521.

Further references: M. Saif *et al., J. Egypt. med. Ass.,* 1973, *56,* 527, per *Trop. Dis. Bull.,* 1975, *72,* 153; I. Farahmandian *et al., Iran. J. publ. Hlth,* 1974, *3,* 23, per *Trop. Dis. Bull.,* 1975, *72,* 154; A. H. S. Omer and C. H. Teesdale, *Ann. trop. Med. Parasit.,* 1978, *72,* 145, per *Trop. Dis. Bull.,* 1979, *76,* 86; R. N. H. Pugh, *Ann. trop. Med. Parasit.,* 1978, *72,* 495, per *Trop. Dis. Bull.,* 1979, *76,* 480.

Vector control. For the use of metriphonate in the control of vectors of disease, see *Insecticide Resistance and Vector Control,* Seventeenth Report of the WHO Expert Committee on Insecticides, *Tech. Rep. Ser. Wld Hlth Org. No. 443,* 1970.

Proprietary Names

Bilarcil *(Bayer, Ger.).*

3595-l

Monosulfiram *(B.P., B.P. Vet.)*. Sulfiram; Sulfiramum. Tetraethylthiuram monosulphide.
$C_{10}H_{20}N_2S_3$=264.5.

CAS — 95-05-6.

Pharmacopoeias. In *Aust.* and *Br.*

A yellow or yellowish-brown, soft crystalline powder with a sulphurous odour and a bitter taste, containing about 36% of organically combined sulphur. F.p. 28.5° to 32°. Practically **insoluble** in water, acids, and alkalis; soluble 1 in 3 of alcohol; freely soluble in acetone, chloroform, ether, and most other organic solvents; sparingly soluble in liquid paraffin. *Store* in a cool place. Protect from light.

Adverse Effects. An erythematous rash has occasionally been reported. Ingestion of the alcoholic solutions causes symptoms similar to those caused by disulfiram (see p.579) and alcohol.

A healthy man being treated with a solution of monosulfiram for scabies developed skin swelling, flushing, sweating, and severe tachycardia when he took alcohol.— S. Gold (letter), *Lancet*, 1966, *2*, 1417.

A 47-year-old woman developed toxic epidermal necrolysis 3½ hours after application of monosulfiram solution to her body. She recovered following treatment with triamcinolone. She had some years previously had a skin hypersensitivity to thiram (a rubber vulcanising accelerator).— P. W. M. Copeman, *Br. med. J.*, 1968, *1*, 623.

Uses. Monosulfiram is a parasiticide which is active against fleas, lice, ticks, and certain mites. It is also an effective fungicide.

A 25% alcoholic solution is used in the treatment of scabies. This solution is diluted with 2 or 3 parts of water immediately before use; such dilution produces a fine suspension which is not stable. After a hot bath, the diluted preparation is applied over the whole of the body, with the exception of the face and scalp, rubbed well in and allowed to dry. If necessary the treatment may be repeated daily for 2 or 3 days. The soap is used in place of toilet soap for controlling the spread of scabies, especially in closed communities such as schools and hospitals.

Monosulfiram has been used in veterinary medicine in certain types of mange.

Preparations

Monosulfiram Solution *(B.P.)*. A solution of monosulfiram in alcohol (or industrial methylated spirit) containing a suitable dispersing agent. Crystals which may deposit at low temperatures may be redissolved by warming. Flammable: keep away from an open flame.

Tetmosol *(ICI Pharmaceuticals, UK)*. Monosulfiram, available as a 25% alcoholic **Solution** (inflammable: keep away from an open flame) and as a 5% medicated **Soap.** (Also available as Tetmosol in *Austral.*).

3596-y

Naphthalene. Naphthalin.
$C_{10}H_8$=128.2.

CAS — 91-20-3.

Pharmacopoeias. In *Port.*

Colourless transparent scales with a characteristic odour and an aromatic taste. Practically **insoluble** in water; soluble 1 in 1.5 of chloroform, 1 in 8 of olive oil, and in alcohol.

Adverse Effects and Treatment. There may be headache, nausea and vomiting, diarrhoea, profuse perspiration, optic neuritis, dysuria, haematuria, acute haemolytic anaemia, coma, and convulsions. Doses as low as 2 g have proved fatal to the small child. Treatment is symptomatic and includes emptying the stomach by aspiration and lavage. Blood transfusions may be required.

Maximum permissible atmospheric concentration 10 ppm.

For reports of haemolytic anaemia due to naphthalene in patients with a deficiency in glucose-6-phosphate dehydrogenase, see *Chronicle Wld Hlth Org.*, 1974, *28*, 25.

Uses. Naphthalene is used in lavatory deodorant discs and in old-fashioned mothballs. It was formerly used as an anthelmintic and was applied in the treatment of pediculosis and scabies.

3597-j

Norbormide. McN-1025. 5-[α-Hydroxy-α-(2-pyridyl)benzyl]-7-[α-(2-pyridyl)benzylidene]-8,9,10-trinorborn-5-ene-2,3-dicarboximide.
$C_{33}H_{25}N_3O_3$=511.6.

CAS — 991-42-4.

A white or off-white crystalline powder consisting of a mixture of stereoisomers. Practically **insoluble** in water, alcohol, and ether; very slightly soluble in chloroform; soluble in oils.

A selective rodenticide effective against most species of rats, in which it produces extreme irreversible peripheral vasoconstriction, but not very toxic to mice or other rodents. The concentration in baits is usually 0.5 to 1%.

The pharmacology of norbormide.— A. P. Roszkowski, *J. Pharmac. exp. Ther.*, 1965, *149*, 288.

A brief review of the use of norbormide.— N. G. Gratz, *Bull. Wld Hlth Org.*, 1973, *48*, 469.

Norbormide was considered to be one of the safest rodenticides and its use was endorsed. It was reported to have low toxicity to other mammals; the LD50 for *rabbits* was around 1 g per kg body-weight and *dogs* had been fed a dietary concentration of 1% without harm.— *Safe Use of Pesticides*, Twentieth Report of the WHO Expert Committee on Insecticides, *Tech. Rep. Ser. Wld Hlth Org. No. 513*, 1973.

3598-z

Orthodichlorobenzene. 1,2-Dichlorobenzene.
$C_6H_4Cl_2$=147.0.

CAS — 95-50-1.

A heavy inflammable colourless liquid with a characteristic odour.

Orthodichlorobenzene is used as an insecticide and as a wood and furniture preservative.

It irritates the skin and may cause dermatitis; it is severely irritant to the eyes; lens opacities have occurred. Inhalation of the vapour may cause drowsiness and nasal irritation. Maximum permissible atmospheric concentration 50 ppm.

3599-c

Paradichlorobenzene *(B.P.C. 1949)*. Dichlorbenzol. 1,4-Dichlorobenzene.
$C_6H_4Cl_2$=147.0.

CAS — 106-46-7.

Colourless shining crystals with a characteristic odour; slowly volatile in air. M.p. 53° to 54°. Liquefies when mixed with camphor, phenol, salol, etc. Practically **insoluble** in water; soluble in most organic solvents. **Store** in airtight containers.

Paradichlorobenzene is an insecticide used against moths and furniture beetles.

The adverse effects of the vapour are similar to those of orthodichlorobenzene (see above) but are less pronounced.

Maximum permissible atmospheric concentration 75 ppm.

Allergy. A 69-year-old man developed allergic purpura complicated by acute glomerulonephritis after sitting in a chair which had been treated with paradichlorobenzene crystals earlier in the day.— R. M. Nalbandian and J. F. Pearce, *J. Am. med. Ass.*, 1965, *194*, 828.

Proprietary Preparations

Santochlor *(Monsanto, UK)*. A brand of paradichlorobenzene.

3600-c

Paraquat. 1,1′-Dimethyl-4,4′-bipyridyldiylium ion.
$C_{12}H_{14}N_2$=186.3.

CAS — 4685-14-7.

3601-k

Paraquat Dichloride.
$C_{12}H_{14}Cl_2N_2$=257.2.

CAS — 1910-42-5.

A white crystalline solid. Very **soluble** in water. Hydrolysed by alkalis.

Adverse Effects. Concentrated solutions of paraquat may cause irritation of the skin, inflammation, and possibly blistering; cracking and shedding of the nails; and delayed healing of cuts and wounds. It is not significantly absorbed from the skin. A few fatalities have occurred following skin contact but these appear to have been associated with prolonged contact and concentrated solutions.

Splashes in the eye cause severe inflammation, which may be delayed for 12 to 24 hours, corneal oedema, reduced visual acuity, and extensive superficial stripping of the corneal and conjunctival epithelium, which usually slowly heals. Inhalation of dust or spray may cause nasal bleeding.

When ingested paraquat is irritant to mucous membranes and may cause burning of the mouth and throat, difficulty in swallowing, vomiting, abdominal discomfort, and diarrhoea. Delayed symptoms which occur after ingestion of large doses include renal and hepatic failure and most importantly lung changes which include congestion, oedema, haemorrhage, and alveolar thickening and fibrosis. There have been many fatalities; a dose of 2 or 3 g may be expected to be fatal if not treated.

Maximum permissible atmospheric concentration 500 µg per m^3.

Reviews of paraquat poisoning.— *Lancet*, 1971, *2*, 1018; *Med. J. Aust.*, 1974, *2*, 800; J. F. Dasta, *Am. J. Hosp. Pharm.*, 1978, *35*, 1368; T. J. Haley, *Clin. Toxicol.*, 1979, *14*, 1.

Rapidly progressive normochromic anaemia developed within a few days in 5 patients who had taken paraquat, and was accompanied by isolated aplastic anaemia.— J. Lautenschlager *et al.*, *Dt. med. Wschr.*, 1974, *99*, 2348.

Fatalities following cutaneous contact with paraquat: F. Jaroš (letter), *Lancet*, 1978, *1*, 275; M. Newhouse *et al.*, *Archs Derm.*, 1978, *114*, 1516; J. J. J. Waight, *J. Am. med. Ass.*, 1979, *242*, 472.

Seven men who died from paraquat poisoning had paraquat excretion-rates of 1 mg or more per hour in urine in the first 24 hours after ingestion, compared with much lower rates in most of 9 less severely poisoned patients who survived. The excretion-rate in urine was not, however, considered a reliable prediction of survival.— N. Wright *et al.*, *Br. med. J.*, 1978, *2*, 396.

Plasma-paraquat concentrations were measured in 79 patients suffering from paraquat poisoning. It was found that patients whose plasma concentrations did not exceed 2.0, 0.6, 0.3, 0.16, and 0.1 mg per litre at 4, 6, 10, 16, and 24 hours after ingestion, survived. Minimally poisoned patients should be protected from unnecessary treatment.— A. T. Proudfoot *et al.*, *Lancet*, 1979, *2*, 330. A report of 2 patients with plasma-paraquat concentrations greatly in excess of the critical values, who survived after charcoal haemoperfusion. They were haemoperfused with acrylic-hydrogel-coated activated charcoal for an average of 8 hours daily for 2 to 3 weeks.— S. Okonek *et al.* (letter), *ibid.*, 1980, *2*, 589. A report of a further patient who survived paraquat poisoning despite blood concentrations well above the limit for an expected fatal result. The implications are that active treatment should be given to all patients.— J. D. R. Rose (letter), *ibid.*, 924.

Problems in interpreting kidney-function tests in paraquat poisoning.— D. B. Webb and C. G. Davies (letter), *Lancet*, 1981, *1*, 1424.

Further references to poisoning with paraquat: K. Funke *et al.*, *Dtc GesundhWes.*, 1976, *31*, 2143; C. D. Ward *et al.* (letter), *Lancet*, 1976, *1*, 1247; P. Ackrill *et al.*, *Br. med. J.*, 1978, *1*, 1252; K. E. Powell, *Bull. Nat.*

Clearinghouse Poison Control Centers, Spring, 1978; M. I. Fow, *ibid.*

Residues in the body and diet. Maximum acceptable daily intake of paraquat dichloride: 2 µg per kg body-weight.— Report of the 1976 Joint FAO/WHO Meeting on Pesticide Residues in Food, *Tech. Rep. Ser. Wld Hlth Org. No. 612*, 1977.

For background toxicological data, see 1972 Evaluations of some Pesticide Residues in Food, *Pestic. Residue Ser. Wld Hlth Org. No. 2*, 1973.

Treatment of Adverse Effects. Following contact with paraquat contaminated clothing should be removed and the skin washed with soap and water. The eyes, if splashed, should be irrigated and treated with antibiotics to control infection. After regrowth of corneal and conjunctival epithelium, corticosteroids may be necessary to promote resolution of granulation tissue.

There is no specific treatment for paraquat poisoning and there is some controversy surrounding most routine procedures. In Great Britain, doctors are invited to refer patients immediately to the nearest centre organised by the National Poisons Information Service.

Prompt treatment of poisoning is essential. Despite paraquat's caustic nature vomiting should be induced immediately and this should be followed as soon as possible by gastric aspiration and lavage in hospital. One litre of a suspension of Fuller's earth 15% may be left in the stomach; a suspension of bentonite 7% may be used but is considered to adsorb less paraquat. Mannitol (200 ml of a 20% solution) or a saline purgative such as magnesium sulphate is often given with the adsorbent. Haemodialysis is commonly used although there are reports that neither peritoneal dialysis nor haemodialysis is effective. Haemoperfusion is also employed as is forced diuresis although the latter procedure is hazardous in patients who develop pulmonary oedema and renal failure. Oxygen appears to enhance the pulmonary toxicity of paraquat and tends not to be given despite the patient's need for assisted respiration. A hypoxic nursing environment has been suggested. Patients may require analgesics and fluid and electrolyte replacement.

Immunosuppressants, ascorbic acid, dexpropranolol, superoxide dismutase, and plasmaphaeresis have been tried or suggested in the treatment of paraquat poisoning but their value is still to be confirmed.

Reviews and discussions on the treatment of paraquat poisoning: *Lancet*, 1976, *1*, 1057; A. T. Proudfoot and L. F. Prescott, Poisoning with Paraquat, Salicylate and Paracetamol, in *Recent Advances in Intensive Therapy*, No. 1, I.M. Ledingham (Ed.), London, Churchill Livingstone, 1977, 217; J. F. Winchester *et al.*, *Trans. Am. Soc. artif. internal Organs*, 1977, *23*, 762; J. F. Dasta, *Am. J. Hosp. Pharm.*, 1978, *35*, 1368.

Some reports on the treatment of paraquat poisoning: D. B. Galloway and J. C. Petrie, *Postgrad. med. J.*, 1972, *48*, 684; T. D. Lewis, *Med. J. Aust.*, 1974, *2*, 814; J. A. Laithwaite (letter), *Br. med. J.*, 1975, *1*, 266; P. D. Thomas *et al.*, *Med. J. Aust.*, 1977, *2*, 564. See also D. P. Dearnaley and M. F. R. Martin (letter), *Lancet*, 1978, *1*, 162. Criticism: J. Miller *et al.* (letter), *ibid.*, 875.

See also above under Adverse Effects.

Uses. Paraquat is a contact herbicide widely used as the dichloride in agriculture and horticulture. Liquid concentrates are supplied in the UK only to approved users.

Proprietary Names

Dextrone X *(Chipman, UK)*; Gramoxone *(ICI Plant Protection, UK)*.

Present in Dexcuron *(Chipman, UK)*; Pathclear *(ICI Plant Protection, UK)*; Weedol *(ICI Plant Protection, UK)*.

3602-a

Phenothrin. 3-Phenoxybenzyl (1*RS*)-*cis, trans*-chrysanthemate.

$C_{23}H_{26}O_3$=350.5.

CAS — 26002-80-2.

A colourless liquid. Practically **insoluble** in water; miscible with most organic solvents.

Phenothrin is a pyrethroid insecticide with actions and uses similar to those of pyrethrum flower (see p.841); pyrethroids are claimed to be faster acting and less toxic to mammals.

References: V. I. Vashkov *et al.*, *J. Hyg. Epidem. Microbiol. Immun.*, 1978, *22*, 361, per *Trop. Dis. Bull.*, 1979, *76*, 1035.

Proprietary Names

Sumithrin *(Sumitomo, Jap.: British Traders & Shippers, UK)*.

3603-t

Piperonyl Butoxide *(B.P. Vet.)*. 5-[2-(2-Butoxyethoxy)ethoxymethyl]-6-propyl-1,3-benzodioxole.

$C_{19}H_{30}O_5$=338.4.

CAS — 51-03-6.

A yellow or pale brown oily liquid with a faint characteristic odour and a slightly bitter taste. Wt per ml 1.05 to 1.065 g.

Very slightly **soluble** in water; miscible with alcohol, chloroform, ether, petroleum oils, and liquefied aerosol propellents such as dichlorodifluoromethane, dichlorotetrafluoroethane, and trichlorofluoromethane.

Residues in the body and diet. Maximum acceptable daily intake of piperonyl butoxide: 30 µg per kg body-weight.— Report of the 1972 Joint FAO/WHO Meeting on Pesticide Residues in Food, *Tech. Rep. Ser. Wld Hlth Org. No. 525*, 1973. For background toxicological data, see 1972 Evaluations of some Pesticide Residues in Food, *Pestic. Residue Ser. Wld Hlth Org. No. 2*, 1973.

Uses. Piperonyl butoxide is an active acaricide and has some insecticidal activity. It enhances the actions of the pyrethrins.

Preparations

Piperonyl Butoxide Application *(B.P. Vet.)*. Piperonyl butoxide 5 g, butyl aminobenzoate 2 g, and dipropylene glycol 93 g.

3604-x

Pyrethrum Flower *(B.P. Vet.)*. Pyrethri Flos; Insect Flowers; Dalmatian Insect Flowers; Chrysanthème Insecticide; Insektenblüten; Piretro.

CAS — 8003-34-7 (pyrethrum); 121-21-1 (pyrethrin I); 121-29-9 (pyrethrin II); 25402-06-6 (cinerin I); 121-20-0 (cinerin II).

Pharmacopoeias. In *Arg.*, *Aust.*, *Fr.*, and *Ind.*

The dried flowerheads of *Chrysanthemum cinerariaefolium* (Compositae), containing not less than 1% of pyrethrins of which not less than one-half consists of pyrethrin I.

Pyrethrum flower should be **stored** in a cool place in well-filled containers, protected from light, and should not be kept for more than 2 years. Extracts of pyrethrum, when similarly stored, are much more stable than pyrethrum flower.

Pyrethrum flower owes its insecticidal properties to 2 groups of esters. One group consists of pyrethrin I and cinerin I, both of which have chrysanthemic acid (chrysanthemum monocarboxylic acid) as their acid component. The second group of esters consists of pyrethrin II and cinerin II, both of which have pyrethric acid (monomethyl ester of chrysanthemum dicarboxylic acid) as their acid component. The 2 groups of esters are generally present in approximately equal amounts.

As the assays for pyrethrin I and pyrethrin II are based respectively on the total chrysanthemic acid and the total pyrethric acid the determinations also include cinerin I and cinerin II so that the content of 'pyrethrins' is in effect the content of pyrethrins and cinerins.

Adverse Effects. Pyrethrum is irritant to the eyes and mucosa. Hypersensitivity reactions have been reported.

Maximum permissible atmospheric concentration 5 mg per m^3.

Hypersensitivity pneumonitis due to pyrethrum in 1 patient.— J. E. Carlson and J. W. Villaveces, *J. Am. med. Ass.*, 1977, *237*, 1718.

Another report of hypersensitivity.— J. C. Mitchell *et al.*, *Br. J. Derm.*, 1972, *86*, 568.

Residues in the body and diet. Maximum acceptable daily intake of pyrethrins: 40 µg per kg body-weight.— Report of the 1974 Joint FAO/WHO Meeting on Pesticide Residues in Food, *Tech. Rep. Ser. Wld Hlth Org. No. 574*, 1975. For background toxicological data, see 1972 Evaluations of some Pesticide Residues in Food, *Pestic. Residue Ser. Wld Hlth Org. No. 2*, 1973.

Uses. Pyrethrum flower is mainly used for the preparation of Pyrethrum Extract.

Pyrethrum is rapidly toxic to many insects. It has no appreciable effect on insects as a stomach poison but acts by contact. Pyrethrum has a much quicker knock-down effect than dicophane or gamma benzene hexachloride, but it is less persistent and less stable. Its action can be enhanced by certain substances such as piperonyl butoxide and bucarpolate (the piperonylic acid ester of the monobutyl ether of diethylene glycol) and this synergistic effect is frequently utilised in pyrethrum preparations, which may include dicophane and gamma benzene hexachloride to combine a quick knock-down with a prolonged effect. Pyrethrins with piperonyl butoxide have been used in the treatment of pediculosis.

Pyrethrum is widely used in domestic and agricultural insecticidal sprays and dusting-powders.

Pyrethrum: its sources, cultivation, and applications in insecticides.— *Soap Perfum. Cosm.*, 1966, *39*, 213.

For the use of pyrethrum in the control of vectors of disease, see *Insecticide Resistance and Vector Control*, Seventeenth Report of the WHO Expert Committee on Insecticides, *Tech. Rep. Ser. Wld Hlth Org. No. 443*, 1970.

Preparations

Compound Pyrethrum Spray *(B.P. Vet.)*. Pyrethrum extract 380 mg, piperonyl butoxide 760 mg, and deodorised kerosene 98.86 g.

Pyrethrum Aerosol. The formulation of the Pyrethrum Board of Kenya: decolorised pyrethrum extract (23.5% pyrethrins) 1.7% w/w, sulfoxide ($C_{18}H_{28}O_3S$ = 324.5) 2% w/w, isopropyl myristate 2.4% w/w, deodorised base-oil (Shellsol T) 13.9% w/w, Freon 11 and 12 of each equal parts 80% w/w. The preparation had an effective knock-down effect and was lethal to houseflies and mosquitoes resistant to DDT. In comparative tests it was shown to be preferable to the WHO Reference Standard Aerosol and Aerosol G-1492 of the United States Department of Agriculture.—J.U. McGuire *et al.*, *Bull. Wld Hlth Org.*, 1966, *34*, 151.

Pyrethrum Dusting-powder *(B.P. Vet.)*. Conspersus Pyrethri. Pyrethrum extract 1.6 g, chloroform q.s., diatomite, in fine powder, 30 g, talc, in fine powder, 68.4 g. Dissolve the pyrethrum extract in the chloroform and spray the solution on the diatomite and talc while mixing; sift and mix.

Pyrethrum Extract *(B.P. Vet.)*. A dark olive-green or brown viscous liquid (or if decolorised, a pale amber-coloured liquid). It is prepared by exhausting pyrethrum flower, in coarse powder, by percolation with a suitable hydrocarbon solvent; the solvent is then removed from the percolate, which is concentrated at a low temperature. The extract is adjusted to contain 25% w/w of total pyrethrins of which not less than one-half consists of pyrethrin I. Store in well-filled containers, protected from light.

Pyrethrum Solution *(Ind. P.)*. An extract of pyrethrum flower in kerosene, containing 1% of total pyrethrins.

3605-r

Pyrimithate *(B. Vet. C. 1965).* ICI 29,661. *O*-2-Dimethylamino-6-methylpyrimidin-4-yl *OO*-diethyl phosphorothioate.
$C_{11}H_{20}N_3O_3PS$=305.3.

CAS — 5221-49-8.

A deep straw-coloured liquid with a characteristic pungent odour. Practically **insoluble** in water; miscible with alcohol, chloroform, and methyl alcohol; very slightly soluble in light petroleum. **Store** in airtight containers. Protect from light.

CAUTION. *Pyrimithate is very toxic when inhaled, swallowed, or spilled on the skin. It can be removed from the skin by washing with soap and water. Contaminated material should be immersed in a 2% aqueous solution of sodium hydroxide for several hours.*

An organophosphorus pesticide used in veterinary medicine for the dipping of sheep and for the control of 'fly strike' and of lice, keds, and sheep ticks.

3606-f

Rotenone. Rotenonum. (−)-1,2,12,12a-Tetrahydro-2-isopropenyl-8,9-dimethoxy-6a*H*-furo[2,3-*h*][1]benzopyrano[3,4-*b*][1]benzopyran-6-one.
$C_{23}H_{22}O_6$=394.4.

CAS — 83-79-4.

Pharmacopoeias. In *Nord.*

Colourless to brownish crystals, or a white to brownish-white, odourless, tasteless, crystalline powder. Practically **insoluble** in water; soluble 1 in 300 of alcohol, 1 in 12 of acetone, 1 in 3 of chloroform, and 1 in 200 of ether. **Incompatible** with alkalis and oxidising agents. **Store** in airtight containers. Protect from light.

Maximum permissible atmospheric concentration 5 mg per m^3.

Rotenone is the principal active insecticidal constituent of derris (see p.834) and of lonchocarpus (see p.838).

A short communication on polymorphic and solvated forms of rotenone.— L. Borka, *Acta pharm. suec.*, 1974, *11*, 413.

3607-d

Sabadilla. Cevadilla; Caustic Barley; Cevadilha.

CAS — 62-59-9 (cevadine).

Pharmacopoeias. In *Port.*

The dried ripe seeds of *Schoenocaulon officinale* (Liliaceae), containing several alkaloids of which the most important is cevadine (crystalline veratrine). The name veratrine is given to the mixed alkaloids.

Sabadilla was formerly used as a parasiticide, especially for pediculosis capitis.

3608-n

Staphisagria *(B.P.C. 1949).* Stavesacre Seeds; Paparraz.

CAS — 8047-63-0.

Pharmacopoeias. In *Port.*

The dried ripe seeds of *Delphinium staphisagria* (Ranunculaceae), containing about 30% of fixed oil and 1% of alkaloids, the most important of which is delphinine.

Staphisagria was formerly used in the form of a lotion or ointment to destroy pediculi.

3609-h

Temephos. Temefos. *OO'*-(Thiodi-*p*-phenylene) *OOO'O'*-tetramethyl bis(phosphorothioate).
$C_{16}H_{20}O_6P_2S_3$=466.5.

CAS — 3383-96-8.

A brown viscous liquid. Practically **insoluble** in water.

Temephos is an organophosphorus insecticide effective against the larvae of mosquitoes and other insects. It is also effective against lice and fleas.

The use of temephos for the control of guinea worm.— *Chronicle Wld Hlth Org.*, 1980, *34*, 159.

Manufacturers
American Cyanamid, USA.

3610-a

Tetramethrin. 4,5,6,7-Tetrahydrophthalimidomethyl (1*RS*)-*cis,trans*-chrysanthemate.
$C_{19}H_{25}NO_4$=331.4.

CAS — 7696-12-0.

A white crystalline powder with a slight odour. M.p. 60° to 80°. Practically **insoluble** in water; soluble in alcohol and methyl alcohol; freely soluble in acetone and chloroform.

Tetramethrin is a pyrethroid insecticide with actions and uses similar to those of pyrethrum flower (see p.841) but it is claimed to be faster acting and less toxic to mammals. It is usually used in conjunction with a synergist such as piperonyl butoxide.

References: V. Rupeš *et al., Čslká Epidem. Mikrobiol. Imunol.*, 1976, *25*, 345; V. I. Vashkov *et al., J. Hyg. Epidem. Microbiol. Immun.*, 1978, *22*, 361, per *Trop. Dis. Bull.*, 1979, *76*, 1035.

Proprietary Names
Neo-Pynamin *(Sumitomo, Jap.: British Traders & Shippers, UK).*

3611-t

Trichlorophenoxyacetic Acid. 2,4,5-T. 2,4,5-Trichlorophenoxyacetic acid.
$C_8H_5Cl_3O_3$=255.5.

CAS — 35915-18-5.

A white crystalline solid. Very slightly **soluble** in water; soluble in alcohol, acetone, and ether.

Trichlorophenoxyacetic acid is a selective weedkiller with similar actions to dichlorophenoxyacetic acid (see p.834). It is usually used in ester formulations. It was used as a defoliating agent in the Vietnam conflict.

Maximum permissible atmospheric concentration 10 mg per m^3. The content of TCDD which may be formed during production should be less than 1 ppm.

The fate of trichlorophenoxyacetic acid following oral administration to man.— P. J. Gehring *et al., Toxic. appl. Pharmac.*, 1973, *26*, 352.

In all EEC states except Italy the content of TCCD in trichlorophenoxyacetic acid was limited to less than 0.1 ppm; its use was banned in Italy since 1970; a temporary suspension was being considered in France; it was not prohibited in the USA.— *Off. J.E.E.C.*, 1976, *19*, C276, 31. Reviews carried out in France, Germany, and the UK indicated that when properly applied for the purpose intended herbicides containing trichlorophenoxyacetic acid complying with this limit of TCDD can be used without risk to human or animal health and with minimal risk to the environment.— *ibid.*, 1977, *20*, C162, 28.

Excessive urine concentrations of trichlorophenoxyacetic acid in exposed council and forestry workers fell dramatically following the introduction of the use of protection clothing to prevent absorption through exposed skin.— G. R. Simpson *et al., Med. J. Aust.*, 1978, *2*, 536.

Malignant lymphoma of the histiocytic type in 6 patients exposed to dichlorophenoxyacetic and trichlorophenoxyacetic acids.— L. Hardell (letter), *Lancet*, 1979, *1*, 55.

Pregnancy and the neonate. There was laboratory evidence of the teratogenicity of trichlorophenoxyacetic acid or its contaminants in *rats, mice*, and *chickens.*— *Lancet*, 1970, *1*, 609. There was no evidence of a teratogenic effect in rhesus *monkeys.*— W. H. Dougherty *et al., Toxic. appl. Pharmac.*, 1973, *25*, 442.

Analysis of data on infants with neural tube defects over a 10-year period in New South Wales yielded a linear correlation between the previous year's Australian usage of trichlorophenoxyacetic acid and the annual New South Wales combined birth-rate of anencephaly and meningomyelocele. Although this cannot be taken as direct evidence of any causal association, further retrospective analyses, together with careful evaluation of prospective avoidance trials, may be informative.— B. Field and C. Kerr (letter), *Lancet*, 1979, *1*, 1341.

A call for balance in considering the dangers of trichlorophenoxyacetic acid.— *Lancet*, 1979, *2*, 1114. A call for an emergency ban on trichlorophenoxyacetic acid pending an investigation of its toxicity.— *New Scient.*, 1980, *85*, 558.

Use of trichlorophenoxyacetic acid in Hungary has not been associated with an increase in congenital malformations.— H. F. Thomas (letter), *Lancet*, 1980, *2*, 214.

3612-x

Trifenmorph. WL 8008. *N*-Tritylmorpholine.
$C_{23}H_{23}NO$=329.4.

CAS — 1420-06-0.

An off-white to yellow powder. Practically **insoluble** in water; soluble 1 in about 100 of alcohol and methyl alcohol, 1 in about 20 of ether, and 1 in about 10 of acetone; freely soluble in chloroform and tetrachloroethylene.

Uses. Trifenmorph is a molluscicide used for the control of snail vectors of schistosomiasis.

The susceptibility of various fish to trifenmorph.— C. J. Shiff *et al., Bull. Wld Hlth Org.*, 1967, *36*, 500.

For a series of papers on trifenmorph, see *Bull. Wld Hlth Org.*, 1967, *37*, 1–78.

The decreasing effectiveness with time of aqueous solutions of trifenmorph as a molluscicide.— L. S. Ritchie and L. A. Berríos-Durán, *Bull. Wld Hlth Org.*, 1969, *40*, 471.

No residues were found in plants treated for schistosomiasis control.— K. I. Beynon *et al., Bull. Wld Hlth Org.*, 1972, *46*, 761.

Application as granules.— B. Gilbert *et al., Bull. Wld Hlth Org.*, 1973, *49*, 377.

Results of a large-scale field trial indicated that a concentration of trifenmorph of 15 µg per litre was adequate to give 100% mortality of *Bulinus truncatus* over 7.5 days; it was possible that a lower concentration would be equally satisfactory.— M. A. Amin *et al., Bull. Wld Hlth Org.*, 1976, *54*, 573.

Trifenmorph was effective in the control of fascioliasis.— H. J. Over *et al., Tijdschr. Diergeneesk.*, 1977, *102*, 304, per *Abstr. Hyg.*, 1977, *52*, 1261.

Proprietary Names
Frescon *(Shell Chemicals).*

3613-r

Zinc Phosphide.
Zn_3P_2=258.1.

CAS — 1314-84-7.

A steel-grey crystalline powder. Practically **insoluble** in water and alcohol; decomposed by acid. **Incompatible** with acidic vegetable extracts.

Zinc phosphide is employed in pastes as a rat poison. The adverse effects following the ingestion of zinc phosphide are probably due to the release of phosphine and include nausea and vomiting, dyspnoea, bradycardia, pulmonary oedema, and circulatory collapse. Gastric lavage with a 3 to 5% solution of sodium bicarbonate has been suggested with the intention of minimising the conversion. Ingestion of phosphine causes severe reactions which include shock, oliguria, acidosis, tetany, convulsions, and coma.

Aluminium phosphide is also used as a rodenticide.

Zinc phosphide was an effective rodenticide and its uses was endorsed. When moist it released phosphine gas which had a garlic-like odour repulsive to man and domestic animals but not apparently to *rats.* It was highly toxic to *poultry.*— *Safe Use of Pesticides*, Twentieth Report of the WHO Expert Committee on Insecticides, *Tech. Rep. Ser. Wld Hlth Org. No. 513*, 1973.

Insulin and other Antidiabetic Agents

7200-s

Diabetes mellitus is a state of chronic hyperglycaemia, which may be due to insulin deficiency or to factors that diminish or oppose insulin activity and which in turn may be due to environmental and/or genetic factors. This results in disturbances of metabolism of carbohydrate, fat, and protein. The long-term complications include an increased incidence of retinopathy and cataract, progressive renal disease, neuropathy, heart disease, ischaemic foot disease, cerebrovascular disease, and an increased risk of infection.

Blood-glucose Concentrations. According to the World Health Organization (*Tech. Rep. Ser. Wld Hlth Org. No. 646,* 1980) in adults random blood-glucose concentrations (venous plasma) of or above 2 mg per ml (about 11.1 mmol per litre) or fasting concentrations of or above 1.4 mg per ml (about 7.8 mmol per litre) are considered diagnostic of diabetes mellitus. A fasting concentration of or above 1.4 mg per ml and/or a concentration of or above 2 mg per ml 2 hours after a glucose load of 75 g is similarly diagnostic. A fasting concentration below 1.4 mg per ml and a concentration between 1.4 and 2 mg per ml after a glucose load represents 'impaired glucose tolerance'. Patients with impaired glucose tolerance should be periodically re-examined or, if pregnant, treated as if diabetic. The above values would be about 0.15 mg per ml (about 0.8 mmol per litre) lower after a 50-g glucose load and about the same amount higher after a 100-g glucose load. Whole-blood values are generally about 15% lower than venous-plasma values; capillary whole-blood values are intermediate.

Good diabetic control requires the monitoring of the patient's blood-glucose concentrations. Analysis of blood samples using laboratory procedures gives the most accurate control. Approximate figures may be obtained by the use of test strips; reflectance meters are available to help with the interpretation of colour changes produced by the blood on test strips. Some approximation of blood-glucose status may be achieved by estimating concentrations of glucose in the urine using reagent tablets or test strips.

A discussion of proposed new criteria for the assessment of diabetes and impaired glucose tolerance. The expression 'impaired glucose tolerance' would replace the confusing terms of chemical, borderline, subclinical, asymptomatic, and latent diabetes.— *Br. med. J.*, 1980, *281*, 1512. Criticism.— J. V. Zammit Maempel (letter), *ibid.*, 1981, *282*, 481. A defence.— R. J. Jarrett (letter), *ibid.*, 990.

A summary of current concepts of the nature of insulin-dependent diabetes mellitus.— G. F. Cahill and H. O. McDevitt, *New Engl. J. Med.*, 1981, *304*, 1454.

References to the measurement of glycosylated haemoglobin, HbA_1, especially HbA_{1c}, for the assessment of blood-glucose control over a period of weeks.— R. J. Koenig *et al.*, *New Engl. J. Med.*, 1976, *295*, 417; K. H. Gabbay, *ibid.*, 443; J. Ditzel and J. -J. Kjaergaard, *Br. med. J.*, 1978, *1*, 741; *Br. med. J.*, 1978, *1*, 1373; R. D. G. Leslie *et al.*, *Lancet*, 1978, *2*, 958; D. M. Fraser *et al.*, *Br. med. J.*, 1979, *1*, 979; E. A. M. Gale *et al.* (letter), *Lancet*, 1979, *2*, 1240; R. D. Eastham (letter), *Br. med. J.*, 1980, *280*, 116; G. Boden *et al.*, *Ann. intern. Med.*, 1980, *92*, 357.

References to home monitoring of blood-glucose concentrations, including reference to Eyetone, Reflomat, Glucochek, Hypocount, Glucometer, and Gem meters.— M. A. Preece and R. G. Newall, *Br. med. J.*, 1977, *2*, 152; R. White *et al.* (letter), *Br. med. J.*, 1977, *2*, 894; P. H. Sönksen *et al.*, *Lancet*, 1978, *1*, 729; S. Walford *et al.*, *ibid.*, 732; *ibid.*, 757; S. Howe-Davies *et al.*, *Br. med. J.*, 1978, *2*, 596; L. J. Borthwick and I. S. Ross (letter), *Lancet*, 1979, *1*, 924; B. A. Elliott (letter), *Lancet*, 1979, *1*, 1410; I. Peacock *et al.*, *Br. med. J.*, 1979, *2*, 1333; J. L. Day *et al.* (letter), *Lancet*, 1979, *2*, 39; R. Worth *et al.* (letter), *Lancet*, 1979, *2*, 742; P. M. Lawson *et al.* (letter), *ibid.*; E. de Nobel *et al.* (letter), *ibid.*, 1365; D. J. Webb *et al.*, *Br. med. J.*, 1980, *280*, 362; *Lancet*, 1980, *2*, 187; R. T. Jung *et al.* (letter), *Lancet*, 1980, *2*, 1203; M. Cohen *et al.* (letter), *Br. med. J.*, 1981, *282*, 742; *Drug & Ther. Bull.*, 1981, *19*, 31.

Treatment. For infants and children, treatment is mainly with insulin, the oral hypoglycaemic agents being used only in exceptional cases. Insulin is usually the initial therapy for young adults who are not obese. For adults and the elderly, the initial treatment is dietary control, and for the elderly obese patient this will often suffice. In patients with diabetes which is not controlled by diet, oral hypoglycaemic agents may be given to reduce the blood-sugar concentration. Some patients do not respond to oral hypoglycaemic agents (primary failure) and some, initially responsive, relapse (secondary failure); treatment with insulin may then be necessary. Insulin may also be necessary during illness and infection, in accidental or surgical trauma, and in pregnancy.

Reviews of diabetes mellitus and its treatment.— H. D. Breidahl *et al.*, *Drugs*, 1972, *3*, 79; *idem*, 204; T. D. R. Hockaday, *Practitioner*, 1974, *213*, 535; J. R. Turtle, *Med. J. Aust.*, 1974, *1*, 925; B. L. Furman, *Pharm. J.*, 1979, *1*, 353; WHO Expert Committee on Diabetes Mellitus, *Tech. Rep. Ser. Wld Hlth Org. No. 646*, 1980.

The management of diabetes during pregnancy, surgery, or other illness.— J. M. Malius and M. J. Sulway, *Br. J. Hosp. Med.*, 1972, *7*, 201. The management of the obese patient with diabetes mellitus.— B. F. Clarke and L. J. P. Duncan, *ibid.*, 219. Metabolic disorders in diabetes mellitus.— R. Fraser, *Br. med. J.*, 1972, *4*, 591. Diabetes mellitus in the elderly.— M. F. Green, *ibid.*, 1974, *1*, 232. The management of diabetes in the young.— J. M. Court, *Drugs*, 1976, *11*, 128.

Of 200 women with diabetes 76 considered that the control of their diabetes changed with menstruation; effects ranged from hypoglycaemia to hyperglycaemia with ketoacidosis.— C. H. Walsh and J. M. Malins, *Br. med. J.*, 1977, *2*, 177.

Discussions on the complications of diabetes and of the value of good control of blood glucose.— M. D. Siperstein *et al.*, *New Engl. J. Med.*, 1977, *296*, 1060; F. J. Ingelfinger, *New Engl. J. Med.*, 1977, *296*, 1228; A. I. Winegrad and D. A. Greene, *ibid.*, 1978, *298*, 1250; R. Bressler, *Drugs*, 1979, *17*, 461; R. J. Jarrett and H. Keen (letter), *Lancet*, 1980, *2*, 30.

The role of acetylator status in diabetes.— A. W. Burrows *et al.*, *Br. med. J.*, 1978, *1*, 208.

High-density lipoprotein concentrations in patients with various types of diabetes.— A. L. Kennedy *et al.*, *Br. med. J.*, 1978, *2*, 1191. See also J. M. Sosenko *et al.*, *New Engl. J. Med.*, 1980, *302*, 650.

A report on 7 diabetic patients whose insulin treatment was either unnecessary or actually harmful.— H. Kromann *et al.*, *Br. med. J.*, 1981, *283*, 1386.

Dietary control. The dose of insulin or oral hypoglycaemic agent might need to be reduced in patients on a high-fibre diet.— E. W. Pomare, *Drugs*, 1977, *14*, 213. See also H. C. R. Simpson *et al.*, *Lancet*, 1981, *1*, 1.

It is no longer necessary to limit patients with maturity-onset diabetes to a low-carbohydrate diet.— R. W. Simpson *et al.*, *Br. med. J.*, 1979, *1*, 1753.

Further references: *Drug & Ther. Bull.*, 1979, *17*, 85.

Pregnancy and the neonate. A comprehensive approach to the control of diabetes in pregnancy involved identification, rigid control of glucose concentrations, adequate surveillance of mother and foetus, and the timing and mode of delivery. Using this approach the perinatal mortality-rate had been reduced from 13.5 to 4.2% and the incidence of macrosomia (large for gestational age) in the infants from 30.9 to 17.7%.— M. T. Gyves *et al.*, *Am. J. Obstet. Gynec.*, 1977, *128*, 606.

Comment on metabolic control and diabetes in pregnancy.— N. Freinkel, *New Engl. J. Med.*, 1981, *304*, 1357.

Insulin Preparations. Insulin is an amphoteric pancreatic protein giving soluble salts with weak acids or alkalis. It is inactivated by proteolytic enzymes and is ineffective by mouth.

Insulin Injection is an acidic solution of crystalline insulin containing a small amount of zinc, and may be given by subcutaneous, intramuscular, or intravenous injection. Neutral Insulin Injection is a similar neutral solution and may be used similarly.

In order to prolong the duration of effect, insulin has been used as a complex with other proteins. Protamine Zinc Insulin Injection is a complex of insulin with an excess of protamine and zinc; Globin Zinc Insulin Injection is a complex of insulin with globin and zinc; Isophane Insulin Injection is a complex with a minimum quantity of protamine and zinc. Protamine Zinc Insulin Injection and Isophane Insulin Injection contain phosphate buffers.

Insulin Zinc Suspensions contain insoluble zinc compounds of insulin, prepared in amorphous or crystalline forms, dependent upon the conditions of manufacture or admixture, with consequent varying duration of effect. These suspensions have the advantage of freedom from added protein, with consequent reduced risk of allergic reaction, and have largely replaced Protamine Zinc Insulin Injection, Globin Zinc Insulin Injection, and Isophane Insulin Injection.

Biphasic Insulin Injection is a buffered neutral suspension of crystalline insulin in a solution of crystalline insulin and has therefore both a prompt and a prolonged action.

Highly Purified Insulins. Conventional insulins may be separated into: *component a*, comprising material of high molecular weight; *component b*, comprising pro-insulin, intermediates, and a dimer; and *component c*, comprising insulin, arginine insulin, the ethyl ester of insulin, and desamidoinsulin.

The development of antibodies and fat dystrophy are believed to be associated with contaminant material. It is generally agreed that *component a* is antigenic, and most of the factors other than insulin in *components b* and *c* have been incriminated, though reports are not unanimous. It is generally agreed that beef insulin is more antigenic than pork insulin, probably due to the closer chemical relationship between human and pork insulins than between human and beef insulins.

Purified or highly purified (HP) insulins may include: *single-species* or *monospecies* (usually pork) insulin; *single-peak* insulin, representing *component c; pro-insulin-freed* insulin (beef or beef and pork insulin); *'rarely immunogenic (RI)'* insulin, pork insulin of low pro-insulin content prepared by chromatography and ion exchange; *single-component* insulin; and *monocomponent* insulin, beef or pork insulin freed by a series of chromatographic procedures from most other insulin-like material. Most of these insulins are commercially available in various countries. Insulin structurally identical with human insulin, produced by chemical manipulation of insulin from animal sources, is commercially available; 'human' insulin produced by recombinant DNA technology is in production. The code (emp) is used to designate human insulin produced by enzymatic modification of insulin obtained from the pancreas of the pig; the code (crb) has been proposed to designate human insulin produced by recombinant DNA technology from protein chains obtained from genetically-modified bacteria.

The highly purified insulins are indicated in patients with fat atrophy or insulin resistance. They may also be of value in patients with insulin allergy, although reactions have occurred with these insulins. There appears to be little reason to change treatment to these highly purified insulins when patients with stable uncomplicated diabetes are well controlled by ordinary insulin.

The possible nomenclature of insulins with special reference to human insulin.— P. Turner and D. H. Calam, *Lancet*, 1981, *2*, 918.

Reviews and discussions of purified insulins.— P. H.

Sönksen, *Adv. Med.*, 1977, *13*, 402; *Drug & Ther. Bull.*, 1977, *15*, 18; *Lancet*, 1977, *1*, 128; R. Tattersall, *Prescribers' J.*, 1978, *18*, 8; K. G. M. M. Alberti and M. Nattrass, *Diabetologia*, 1978, *15*, 77; P. J. Watkins, *Br. med. J.*, 1979, *1*, 1548; I. Caterson, *Drugs*, 1979, *17*, 289; *Lancet*, 1979, *1*, 363.

Radio-immunoassay of commercially available insulin preparations demonstrated considerable quantities of pancreatic glucagon, pancreatic polypeptide, vasoactive intestinal peptide, and somatostatin in the conventional insulin preparations whereas the highly purified or monocomponent insulins appeared effectively hormone-free, their only detectable contaminant being vasoactive intestinal peptide. Of 448 insulin-dependent diabetics who had not received highly purified or monocomponent insulin 280 had pancreatic polypeptide antibodies, 28 had vasoactive intestinal peptide antibodies, 25 had glucagon antibodies, and 2 had somatostatin antibodies. None of 22 insulin-dependent diabetics who had received only monocomponent insulin, 180 maturity-onset diabetics who had not received insulin, and 125 healthy control subjects had antibodies.— S. R. Bloom *et al.*, *Lancet*, 1979, *1*, 14.

Demonstration in a small number of intensively studied healthy subjects, of the safety and efficacy of a human insulin preparation produced in *Escherichia coli* by recombinant DNA technology.— H. Keen *et al.* (preliminary communication), *Lancet*, 1980, *2*, 398. A report of studies in which fully synthetic human insulin had the same hypoglycaemic effects as natural extracted human and pig insulin. Moreover, only some patients with known allergy to insulin showed a positive skin test to synthetic insulin.— A. Teuscher and P. Diem (letter), *ibid.*, 1186. Further references: R. S. Baker, *Lancet*, 1981, *2*, 1139.

In 6 healthy subjects (previously given somatostatin) human insulin, produced by conversion from porcine insulin and purified to monocomponent standards, had effects comparable to those of monocomponent porcine insulin on plasma-concentrations of glucose, insulin, C-peptide, and intermediate metabolites.— D. R. Owens *et al.*, *Br. med. J.*, 1981, *282*, 1264.

Reports of reactions to purified insulins.— N. Minars *et al.*, *J. Allergy & clin. Immunol.*, 1975, *56*, 411; R. A. Goldman *et al.*, *J. Am. med. Ass.*, 1976, *236*, 1148; C. Reisner *et al.* (letter), *Br. med. J.*, 1978, *2*, 56; D. Q. Borsey and D. N. S. Malone, *Postgrad. med. J.*, 1979, *55*, 199; J. P. Simmonds *et al.*, *Br. med. J.*, 1980, *281*, 355; J. M. Goldman and H. C. Brynildsen, *Br. med. J.*, 1980, *281*, 1494.

Lipoatrophy in a patient treated exclusively with monocomponent insulin.— G. R. Jones *et al.*, *Br. med. J.*, 1981, *282*, 190.

Favourable reports of the use of purified insulins.— L. Ferland and R. M. Ehrlich, *J. Pediat.*, 1975, *86*, 741; P. Daggett *et al.*, *Br. J. Derm.*, 1977, *96*, 439; P. Daggett *et al.*, *Practitioner*, 1977, *218*, 563; N. K. Griffin *et al.*, *Archs Dis. Childh.*, 1979, *54*, 123; A. D. Wright *et al.*, *Br. med. J.*, 1979, *1*, 25; J. G. Devlin *et al.*, *Postgrad. med. J.*, 1979, *55*, *Suppl.* 2, 14.

For further references to purified insulins, see Martindale 27th Edn, p. 797.

Units. The international unit of insulin is the activity contained in 0.04167 mg of the fourth International Standard Preparation (1958). The standard preparation is a mixture of 52% bovine and 48% porcine insulin, containing 24 units per mg.

Three international units of *human* insulin are contained in approximately 130 µg (with sucrose 5 mg) in one ampoule of the first International Reference Preparation for Immunoassay (1974).

Collaborative assay of the European Pharmacopoeia Biological Reference Preparation for Insulin; a potency of 24 international units per mg was assigned.— D. R. Bangham *et al.*, *J. biol. Stand.*, 1978, *6*, 301.

Oral Hypoglycaemic Drugs. The drugs used orally in the management of diabetes mellitus are mainly of 2 types: *the sulphonylureas*, which include acetohexamide (p.851), chlorpropamide (p.852), glibenclamide (p.854), glibornuride (p.854), gliclazide (p.855), glipizide (p.855), gliquidone (p.855), glisoxepide (p.856), tolazamide (p.858), and tolbutamide (p.859), and *the biguanides*, which include metformin (p.856) and phenformin (p.857). Glymidine (p.856) is a sulphonamidopyrimidine derivative.

Reviews and discussions of the use of oral hypoglycaemic drugs.— *Drug & Ther. Bull.*, 1977, *15*, 37; J. M. Stowers and L. J. Borthwick, *Drugs*, 1977, *14*, 41; S. -W. Shen and R. Bressler, *New Engl. J. Med.*, 1977, *296*, 493; *idem*, 787; *idem*, *297*, 396; P. J. Watkins, *Prescribers' J.*, 1977, *17*, 76; J. M. Foy, *Pharm. J.*, 1978, *2*, 94; F. J. Timoney, *Postgrad. med. J.*, 1979, *55*, *Suppl.* 2, 22; P. Taft, *Drugs*, 1979, *17*, 134; *Drug & Ther. Bull.*, 1981, *19*, 49.

Of 62 diabetic patients who originally could not be adequately controlled on diet alone and who were taking oral hypoglycaemic agents (phenformin, phenformin plus sulphonylurea, or sulphonylurea alone), 19 (31%) were still adequately controlled 6 months after their medication had been replaced by a placebo. This suggested that the dosage of oral hypoglycaemic agents could periodically be re-assessed and possibly discontinued.— A. M. Tomkins and A. Bloom, *Br. med. J.*, 1972, *1*, 649.

Guidelines for the use of oral hypoglycaemic drugs.—Council on Scientific Affairs of the American Medical Association, *J. Am. med. Ass.*, 1980, *243*, 2078.

7201-w

Insulin *(B.P., U.S.P.)*.

CAS — 9004-10-8.

Pharmacopoeias. In *Br.* and *U.S. Cz.*, *Ger.*, *Pol.*, and *Span.* have amorphous or crystalline insulin with not less than 23 (*Cz.*), not less than 22 (*Ger.* and *Pol.*), and not less than 18 (*Span.*) units per mg. Also in *Chin.*

The specific antidiabetic principle of the pancreas of the healthy pig or ox, appropriately purified. It complies with a limit test for related proteins and peptides. It loses not more than 10% of its weight on drying and contains not less than 26 units per mg of insulin. The *B.P.* specifies a zinc content of 0.3 to 0.6% while the *U.S.P.* specifies 0.27 to 1.08%, both calculated on the dried basis. The *B.P.* material is crystalline single-peak insulin substantially free of pro-insulin.

A white or almost white crystalline powder. Slightly **soluble** in water; practically insoluble in alcohol, chloroform, and ether; soluble in dilute solutions of mineral acids and, with degradation, in solutions of alkali hydroxides.

Store below 8° in airtight containers. The label states the animal source of the insulin.

The insulin injections of the *B.P.* may be prepared from insulin of lower potency than the above.

7202-e

Insulin Injection *(B.P., Eur. P., U.S.P.)*. Insulin Inj.; Insulini Injectio; Insulini Solutio Iniectabilis; Insulin Hydrochloride; Ordinary Insulin; Regular Insulin; Soluble Insulin; Unmodified Insulin.

Pharmacopoeias. In *Arg.*, *Aust.*, *Belg.*, *Br.*, *Chin.*, *Cz.*, *Eur.*, *Fr.*, *Ger.*, *Hung.*, *Ind.*, *Int.*, *It.*, *Jap.*, *Jug.*, *Mex.*, *Neth.*, *Nord.*, *Pol.*, *Port.*, *Roum.*, *Rus.*, *Swiss*, *Turk.*, and *U.S.* The number of units per ml where specified varies from 5 to 500.

A sterile solution of the specific antidiabetic principle of the mammalian pancreas. It may be prepared by dissolving crystalline insulin containing not less than 23 units per mg (calculated on the dried basis) in Water for Injections containing a suitable substance to render the injection iso-osmotic with blood, hydrochloric acid to adjust the pH to 3 to 3.5, and a suitable bactericide. *U.S.P.* specifies a sterile, acidified or neutral solution of Insulin *U.S.P.* containing 40, 80, 100, or 500 units per ml as well as 1.4 to 1.8% w/v of glycerol and 0.1 to 0.25% of phenol or cresol. The pH of the acidified injection is 2.5 to 3.5 while that of the neutral injection is 7 to 7.8.

Insulin Injection is a colourless or almost colourless, or straw-coloured liquid practically free from solid matter which deposits on standing. It contains not more than 40 µg of zinc for each 100 units of insulin. It is **sterilised** by filtration and kept in multidose glass containers. **Store** at 2° to 8° and avoid freezing; under these conditions it may be expected to retain its potency for not less than 2 years; the rate of deterioration increases rapidly when stored at temperatures above 10°.

The label states the animal source or sources of the insulin.

The use of coloured labels or packs should not be relied upon for the identification of the type or strength of insulin preparations.

Adsorption. Measurement of insulin concentration by radioimmunoassay showed that insulin was rapidly adsorbed by glass or polyvinyl chloride infusion bottles, 42 to 52% being adsorbed 5 minutes after addition to infusion solutions containing insulin 30 units per litre. About 55% of the remaining insulin was adsorbed by the giving set. The addition of albumin 1 ml or plasma protein fraction 60 ml reduced adsorption in the infusion bottle to about 30%.— C. Petty and N. L. Cunningham, *Anesthesiology*, 1974, *40*, 400. See also S. M. Genuth, *J. Am. med. Ass.*, 1973, *223*, 1348.

The percentage recovery of insulin, 20 units in 500 ml, from varying diluents and in varying containers was measured after delivery through a paediatric giving set; mean recovery over 8 hours was 22% from saline in plastic; 31% from saline in glass; 68% from saline and 2% albumin in glass; 88% from 3.5% polygeline in glass; and 99% from 3.5% polygeline in plastic. Further study showed that polygeline 0.5 to 3.5% was effective in preventing significant adsorption.— E. W. Kraegen *et al.*, *Br. med. J.*, 1975, *3*, 464.

Solutions of amino acids and protein hydrolysates in dextrose injections failed to deliver about 44 to 47% of added insulin and the use of a polyvinyl chloride delivery system caused an even greater loss. The addition of albumin or electrolytes and vitamins reduced the adsorption of the insulin on to the delivery systems.— S. S. Weber *et al.*, *Am. J. Hosp. Pharm.*, 1977, *34*, 353.

Initial adsorption of insulin by in-line membrane filters used during routine intravenous infusion.— N. J. Goldberg and S. R. Levin (letter), *New Engl. J. Med.*, 1978, *298*, 1480.

Further references: S. Weisenfeld *et al.*, *Diabetes*, 1968, *17*, 766; P. Semple *et al.* (letter), *Br. med. J.*, 1975, *4*, 228; L. Peterson *et al.*, *Diabetes*, 1976, *25*, 72, per *J. Am. med. Ass.*, 1976, *235*, 1385; J. Kristoffersen *et al.*, *Norsk farm. Tidsskr.*, 1977, *85*, 220, per *Int. pharm. Abstr.*, 1977, *14*, 994.

Incompatibility. There was loss of clarity when intravenous solutions of insulin were mixed with those of amylobarbitone sodium, chlorothiazide sodium, nitrofurantoin sodium, novobiocin sodium, pentobarbitone sodium, phenobarbitone sodium, phenytoin sodium, sodium bicarbonate, sulphadiazine sodium, sulphafurazole diethanolamine, or thiopentone sodium.— J. A. Patel and G. L. Phillips, *Am. J. Hosp. Pharm.*, 1966, *23*, 409.

Insulin Syringes. A British Standard (BS 1619: 1962) specifies requirements for hypodermic syringes for insulin injection. The Standard specifies syringes of the all-glass and of the metal-and-glass types, mounted with the Luer conical fitting (6% taper), of 1 and 2 ml total graduated capacity. The 1-ml syringes are graduated into 20 scale intervals of 0.05 ml and the 2-ml syringes are graduated into 40 scale intervals of 0.05 ml. Marking with the BSI certification mark is a requirement of the Standard.

A pre-set insulin syringe, for use by blind patients, is available.

Consideration should be given to the use of disposable syringes which are now readily available.

Disturbingly high contamination of non-disposable syringes and needles and insulin vials.— J. Dankert and N. M. Drayer (letter), *Lancet*, 1978, *1*, 1256.

Thirty diabetic patients used 76 disposable syringes for periods of 1 to 8 weeks per syringe. Of 60 syringes cultured 59 yielded no pathogens. The syringes were replaced in their package and refrigerated until next used.— A. Greenough *et al.*, *Br. med. J.*, 1979, *1*, 1467. For a discussion see *Br. med. J.*, 1981, *282*, 340. See also P. G. F. Swift and J. R. Hearnshaw (letter), *ibid.*, 1323.

Bilateral abscesses of the thigh in a diabetic patient associated with the use of surgical spirit instead of industrial methylated spirit for the storage of insulin syringes.— D. A. Leigh and G. W. Hough, *Br. med. J.*, 1980, *281*, 541.

Units. See p.844.

Adverse Effects. Overdosage with insulin causes hypoglycaemia, especially if the patient omits to eat an adequate amount of food containing carbohydrate or has been engaged in unusual exercise.

The early symptoms, such as weakness, hunger, giddiness, pallor, sweating, a sinking feeling in the stomach, palpitations, irritability, nervousness, headache, and tremor, resemble those of sympathetic stimulation. Later symptoms are either depression or euphoria, inability to concentrate, drowsiness, lack of judgement and self-control, and amnesia. Other symptoms are hemiplegia, ataxia, tachycardia, diplopia, and paraesthesia. If untreated, hypoglycaemia may lead to convulsions and coma.

In the pre-coma state the Babinski reflex is often present. The pupils are often dilated but still respond to light, but later the pupils become constricted and no longer react to light. Respiration may be shallow and rapid.

Patients in hypoglycaemic (insulin) coma must be carefully differentiated from patients in hyperglycaemic (diabetic) coma (see below).

The speed of onset of hypoglycaemia varies with the preparation of insulin used. Symptoms are likely to appear at any time when the blood-sugar concentration falls below 600 to 700 μg per ml. Convulsions occur if the blood-sugar concentration falls below 350 μg per ml. In untreated diabetics who have become accustomed to blood-sugar concentrations higher than normal, symptoms of hypoglycaemia may occur at higher concentrations. A few patients may develop hypoglycaemic coma without significant prior symptoms.

Non-specific local reactions at the site of injection and allergic reactions, such as skin rashes, urticaria, pruritus, and angioneurotic oedema, may occasionally occur. Allergic reactions may occur less frequently with the highly purified insulins. Atrophy of fat or induration and hypertrophy sometimes occurs at the site of injection, but is not a problem with the highly purified insulins.

Distinction between Insulin Coma and Diabetic Coma

In insulin coma: (1) skin usually pale and moist, but may be normal in colour; moist tongue; (2) breath does not smell of acetone; (3) respiration as in normal sleep; (4) ocular tension normal; (5) urine usually free of sugar; but may contain sugar if the bladder has not been emptied for some hours; (6) urine does not usually contain acetoacetic acid but may do so if the bladder has not been emptied for some hours; (7) blood sugar below 700 μg per ml and may be as low as 400 μg per ml; (8) full rapid pulse; (9) normal or raised blood pressure; (10) brisk reflexes; (11) normal CO_2-combining power.

In diabetic coma: (1) dry skin, usually flushed; dry tongue; (2) breath smells of acetone; (3) laboured respirations; (4) lowered ocular tension; (5) urine always contains large amounts of sugar; (6) urine always contains large amounts of acetoacetic acid; (7) blood sugar is over 2 mg per ml and may even exceed 10 mg per ml; (8) weak rapid pulse; (9) lowered blood pressure; (10) diminished reflexes; (11) reduced CO_2-combining power.

The insulin-obesity syndrome was common and involved obesity in patients receiving more than 50 units daily, severe hypoglycaemia, and hunger.— C. R. Bemiller *et al.*, *Milit. Med.*, 1973, *138*, 85, per *Int. pharm. Abstr.*, 1973, *10*, 824.

A report of the development of cancer at the site of a long-term insulin injection.— E. Eisenbud and R. M. Walter, *J. Am. med. Ass.*, 1975, *233*, 985.

Hypomagnesaemia was found in 7 of 13 patients after the injection of insulin for pituitary-function assessment tests.— R. Lindsay, *Curr. med. Res. Opinion*, 1976, *4*, 296.

A 31-year-old man developed generalised oedema about 7 days after being started on insulin; the condition responded to bumetanide and he later tolerated insulin. The condition was considered a rare example of insulin oedema.— N. R. Bleach *et al.*, *Br. med. J.*, 1979, *2*, 177. Reference to further cases of fluid retention.— J. R. Lawrence and M. G. Dunnigan (letter), *Br. med. J.*, 1979, *2*, 445.

Insulin lipoatrophy was common in patients with allergy and was often associated with hypertrophy.— R. Bressler, *J. Am. med. Ass.*, 1980, *244*, 78.

Abuse. An account of factitious hypoglycaemia in 7 subjects owing to abuse of insulin injections.— J. A. Scarlett *et al.*, *New Engl. J. Med.*, 1977, *297*, 1029. Hypoglycaemia in a 27-year-old woman owing to surreptitious injection of insulin.— H. F. Safrit and C. W. Young (letter), *ibid.*, 1978, *298*, 515.

Allergy. Acute systemic allergic reactions to insulin were diagnosed in 5 patients by the presence of urticaria or angioneurotic oedema or both, which subsided within 24 hours after insulin was withdrawn. Two patients were successfully desensitised to insulin and 3 were treated with oral hypoglycaemic agents.— P. Lieberman *et al.*, *J. Am. med. Ass.*, 1971, *215*, 1106.

Two diabetic patients were allergic to the zinc in their insulin preparations.— M. N. Feinglos and B. V. Jegasothy, *Lancet*, 1979, *1*, 122.

In a 72-year-old woman with ketoacidaemia, due to uncontrolled diabetes, an anaphylactic reaction occurred immediately after intravenous administration of insulin 8 units. Extensive intracutaneous testing with highly purified insulins revealed an allergy of the immediate type against the insulin molecule itself.— W. Bachmann *et al.*, *Dt. med. Wschr.*, 1979, *104*, 1014.

Further reports of allergic reactions to insulin: N. Lamkin *et al.*, *J. Allergy & clin. Immunol.*, 1976, *58*, 213; L. A. Witters *et al.*, *Am. J. Med.*, 1977, *63*, 703; R. D. deShazo *et al.*, *J. Allergy & clin. Immunol.*, 1977, *59*, 161.

Cardiac arrhythmias. Of 96 patients undergoing the Hollander test, 36 developed cardiac arrhythmias; in 20 patients the arrhythmias were judged to be serious. The test, to determine the completeness of vagotomy, involved the intravenous injection of insulin and the measurement of gastric secretion in response to hypoglycaemia. The arrhythmias were believed to be due to hypokalaemia and the release of catecholamines.— *J. Am. med. Ass.*, 1969, *210*, 2005.

In a study of 7 diabetic subjects with no evidence of neuropathy intravenous injection of insulin was found to cause an increase in heart-rate which might be a compensatory response to maintain cardiac output. A separate study had shown that insulin injected subcutaneously might lower blood pressure after both morning and evening injections in diabetics with autonomic neuropathy. Routine daily insulin injections might cause circulatory stress with a consequent long-term effect on the cardiovascular system in insulin-dependent diabetics.— M. M. Page *et al.*, *Br. med. J.*, 1976, *1*, 430.

Hyperglycaemia. A study into rebound hyperglycaemia or the Somogyi effect.— E. A. M. Gale *et al.*, *Lancet*, 1980, *2*, 279. Comment on the problem of diabetic control at night.— *ibid.*, 297.

Hypoglycaemia. In a study involving 11 insulin-dependent diabetic subjects, leg exercise accelerated insulin absorption from a subcutaneous injection site in the leg, whereas it had no effect on insulin absorption from the arm and reduced it from the abdomen.— V. A. Koivisto and P. Felig, *New Engl. J. Med.*, 1978, *298*, 79. Most exercise involved many muscle groups and increased absorption was still likely. Patients who developed hypoglycaemia were advised to take extra carbohydrate before exercise rather than decrease the insulin dose.— B. Zinman *et al.* (letter), *ibid.*, 1202.

A study in 39 insulin-dependent diabetic subjects indicated that a high proportion suffered nocturnal hypoglycaemia although their diabetes was considered to be poorly controlled. Seventeen had blood-glucose values below 2 mmol per litre for 3 hours or more.— E. A. M. Gale and R. B. Tattersall, *Lancet*, 1979, *1*, 1049. See also P. Schwandt *et al.* (letter), *ibid.*, 1979, *2*, 261; R. F. Smith *et al.* (letter), *ibid.*, 634.

Measurement of the cortisol:creatinine ratio in overnight urine samples for the assessment of possible nocturnal hypoglycaemia; in patients with a raised ratio a reduction in the dose of insulin was possible.— C. M. Asplin *et al.*, *Br. med. J.*, 1980, *280*, 357. The test was unreliable in children.— B. A. Darlow *et al.* (letter), *Lancet*, 1980, *2*, 266.

See also under Abuse, above and Overdosage, below.

Overdosage. Hypoglycaemia due to insulin overdosage in the treatment of diabetic acidosis could cause serious brain damage, including mental deficiency, spasticity, and fits.— *Br. med. J.*, 1972, *1*, 5.

A report of a woman who developed severe hypoglycaemic coma and barbiturate-type blisters after the self-administration of insulin in an estimated dose of 800 units.— L. W. Raymond and A. B. Cohen (letter), *Lancet*, 1972, *2*, 764.

Of 4 diabetics who attempted suicide by insulin overdosage with up to 3000 units, 3 recovered uneventfully whilst the other showed marked mental impairment.— F. I. R. Martin *et al.*, *Med. J. Aust.*, 1977, *1*, 58.

Hypoglycaemia associated with chronic overdosage with insulin in a study in 101 children.— A. L. Rosenbloom and B. P. Giordano, *Am. J. Dis. Child.*, 1977, *131*, 881.

A 59-year-old woman suffered hypoglycaemic coma after a decubitus ulcer was sprayed with 1 to 2 ml of Insulin Injection 80 units per ml instead of 20 units per ml.— D. R. Coid, *Br. med. J.*, 1977, *2*, 1063.

Transient recurrent hepatomegaly associated with hypoglycaemia occurred in a 12-year-old diabetic girl as a result of insulin overdoses.— J. Asherov *et al.*, *Archs Dis. Childh.*, 1979, *54*, 148. A similar report.— R. Dershewitz *et al.*, *Am. J. Dis. Child.*, 1976, *130*, 998.

Pregnancy and the neonate. Hypoglycaemia, severe in 17 cases, occurred during the first 6 hours of life in 25 of 34 infants born to diabetic mothers who received insulin. Clinical features were only present in 2.— F. I. R. Martin *et al.*, *Archs Dis. Childh.*, 1975, *50*, 472.

Congenital malformation occurred in 17 of 117 babies born to diabetic mothers taking insulin at the time of conception. This was significantly greater than the incidence of 5 of 117 control babies. There was no difference in the incidence between controls and 31 infants whose mothers were managed by diet or oral hypoglycaemic agents or 57 infants whose mothers' diabetic condition was diagnosed or became apparent during pregnancy.— R. E. Day and J. Insley, *Archs Dis. Childh.*, 1976, *51*, 935.

Treatment of Adverse Effects. To treat hypoglycaemia dextrose or 3 or 4 lumps of sucrose should be taken at once with water and may be repeated in 10 to 15 minutes if needed.

If coma occurs, up to 50 ml of a 50% solution of dextrose should be given intravenously, or dextrose or sucrose may be given by stomach tube. If dextrose is not immediately available, glucagon, 0.5 to 1 mg by subcutaneous, intramuscular, or intravenous injection, can be used to produce a return to consciousness; 1 or 2 further doses may be given at 20-minute intervals if required. If the patient fails to respond to glucagon the use of dextrose intravenously is essential. Dextrose should then be given by mouth.

The treatment of hypoglycaemic crises.— S. R. Newmark *et al.*, *J. Am. med. Ass.*, 1975, *231*, 185.

Precautions. Differing immunological responses to bovine and porcine insulin have been reported, and hypoglycaemia has been reported in patients changing from bovine to porcine insulin. Care is recommended to avoid the inadvertent change from insulin of one species to another. Care may also be necessary if changing to a highly purified insulin.

The hypoglycaemia induced by insulin may be diminished transiently by adrenaline and by infections and may be enhanced by alcohol, monoamine oxidase inhibitors, and propranolol or other beta-adrenoceptor blocking agents. Propranolol may mask symptoms of hypoglycaemia.

In diabetic patients with therapeutically induced hypopituitary function, blood-sugar concentrations did not rise during fasting to the extent that they did before pituitary ablation. In treating such patients, allowances should be made for this effect in addition to their increased sensitivity to insulin; in many cases the morning dose of insulin injection could be omitted and in patients with greatly reduced pituitary function blood-sugar control was achieved with isophane insulin before breakfast and insulin injection before supper.— N. W. Oakley *et al.*, *Lancet*, 1967, *1*, 523.

Hypercoagulation associated with hyperinsulinism might be a contra-indication to the use of insulin in ischaemic heart disease.— W. Martin and V. Tilsner (letter), *Lancet*, 1973, *1*, 380.

Insulin decreased the urinary excretion of sodium in 5 patients in whom sodium intake was maintained constant; this effect should be considered in patients with cardiac or renal failure.— C. D. Saudek *et al.*, *Diabetes*, 1974, *23*, 240, per *J. Am. med. Ass.*, 1974, *228*, 1328.

Provocation of postural hypotension by insulin in diabetic autonomic neuropathy.— M. M. Page and P. J. Watkins, *Diabetes*, 1976, *25*, 90.

Insulin-induced weakness in hypokalaemic myopathy.— R. L. Ruff, *Ann. Neurol.*, 1979, *6*, 139.

Studies in 8 insulin-dependent diabetic men indicated that a sauna accelerated insulin absorption from the subcutaneous injection site and that 2 hours after the sauna mean blood-glucose concentration was significantly lower than on the control day.— V. A. Koivisto,

Br. med. J., 1980, *280*, 1411. Comment.— H. J. Cüppers *et al.* (letter), *Br. med. J.*, 1980, *281*, 307; V. A. Koivisto (letter), *Br. med. J.*, 1980, *281*, 621.

Evidence that smoking reduces absorption of insulin from subcutaneous tissues.— P. Klemp *et al.*, *Br. med. J.*, 1982, *284*, 237.

Interactions. *Absence of effect.* Absence of effect of *sulphinpyrazone* on insulin requirements in 19 patients.— M. A. G. Pannebakker *et al.*, *J. int. med. Res.*, 1979, *7*, 328.

A prospective 8-month study involving 50 insulin-treated diabetic patients receiving *beta-adrenoceptor blocking agents* and 100 insulin-treated diabetic controls found a similar incidence of loss of consciousness resulting from hypoglycaemia in both groups. It was concluded that beta-blockers are generally safe to use in insulin-treated diabetics and that hypoglycaemic unconsciousness resulting from their use is rare.— A. H. Barnett *et al.*, *Br. med. J.*, 1980, *280*, 976. For *propranolol* enhancing the action of insulin, see below.

Diminished effect. In some diabetic patients the administration of *dextrothyroxine* necessitated larger doses of hypoglycaemic agents.— *J. Am. med. Ass.*, 1969, *208*, 1014.

Possible reduction of the effect of insulin by *tricyclic antidepressants*.— *J. Am. med. Ass.*, 1978, *240*, 423.

Appreciable increase in the insulin requirement of a diabetic with ketoacidosis during treatment with *dobutamine;* hypotension, acidosis, and infection were considered to have played only a small part.— S. M. Wood *et al.*, *Br. med. J.*, 1981, *282*, 946.

For the effects of thiazide diuretics on the dose requirements of hypoglycaemic agents, see Chlorpropamide, p.853.

Enhanced effect. References to the effect of insulin being enhanced by other drugs: J. Reid and T. D. Lightbody, *Br. med. J.*, 1959, *1*, 897 (aspirin); J. Landon *et al.*, *Metabolism*, 1963, *12*, 924 (methandienone); A. J. Cooper and K. M. G. Keddie, *Lancet*, 1964, *1*, 1133 (mebanazine); L. Wickström and K. Pettersson, *ibid.*, 1964, *2*, 995 (mebanazine); J. B. Miller (letter), *Br. med. J.*, 1966, *2*, 1007 (oxytetracycline); E. A. Abramson *et al.*, *Lancet*, 1966, *2*, 1386 (propranolol); E. A. Abramson and R. A. Arky, *Diabetes*, 1968, *17*, 141 (propranolol; see above for absence of effect), per *J. Am. med. Ass.*, 1968, *204* (May 6), A265; P. I. Adnitt, *Diabetes*, 1968, *17*, 628 (phenelzine), per *J. Am. med. Ass.*, 1968, *206*, 1821; R. A. Arky *et al.*, *J. Am. med. Ass.*, 1968, *206*, 575 (alcohol); L. Baker *et al.*, *J. Pediat.*, 1969, *75*, 19 (Sotalol).

For the possible enhancement of the effect of insulin by *guanethidine*, see Guanethidine Monosulphate, p.146.

Warning to drivers. It is an offence to drive when under the influence of a drug *to such an extent as to be incapable of having proper control of the vehicle.* For the purposes of the Road Traffic Act insulin has been judged to be a 'drug'.

References to insulin-dependent diabetes and driving.— B. Clarke *et al.*, *Br. med. J.*, 1980, *281*, 586; B. M. Frier *et al.*, *Lancet*, 1980, *1*, 1232.

Absorption and Fate. Insulin is rapidly inactivated when given by mouth. Following parenteral administration it is metabolised mainly in the kidney and liver and a small amount is excreted in the urine.

Insulin was normally filtered at the glomerulus and then almost completely reabsorbed or destroyed at the proximal tubule. In healthy individuals the amount of insulin in the urine did not exceed 1.5% of the load filtered at the glomerulus. In patients with severely impaired renal tubular function, the urinary clearance of insulin approached the glomerular filtration-rate.— M. J. Chamberlain and L. Stimler, *J. clin. Invest.*, 1967, *46*, 911, per *J. Am. med. Ass.*, 1967, *200* June 19, A245.

The plasma half-life of insulin was 4 to 5 minutes; the half-life after subcutaneous injection was about 4 hours and after intramuscular injection about 2 hours.— K. G. M. M. Alberti *et al.*, *Lancet*, 1973, *2*, 515.

The kinetics of the metabolism of monocomponent human insulin.— D. P. Frost *et al.*, *Postgrad. med. J.*, 1973, *49*, *Suppl.* 7, 949.

The role of the kidney in the metabolism of insulin.— F. Aun *et al.*, *Postgrad. med. J.*, 1975, *51*, 622.

Studies in 5 subjects, given 10 units of monocomponent Neutral Insulin Injection subcutaneously, suggested that absorption was increased by exercise.— P. Dandona *et al.*, *Br. med. J.*, 1978, *1*, 479. See also V. R. Soman *et al.*, *New Engl. J. Med.*, 1979, *301*, 1200. See also under Adverse Effects, p.845.

The concentration of insulin in ocular fluids.— S. S. Feman *et al.*, *Am. J. Ophthal.*, 1978, *85*, 387.

A comparative study of subcutaneous, intramuscular, and intravenous administration of human insulin derived from porcine insulin.— D. R. Owens *et al.*, *Lancet*, 1981, *2*, 118.

Further references: H. P. J. Bennett and C. McMartin, *Pharmac. Rev.*, 1978, *30*, 247; K. Kølendorf *et al.*, *Clin. Pharmac. Ther.*, 1979, *25*, 598.

Pregnancy and the neonate. The half-life of bovine insulin 0.1 units per kg body-weight in normal and pregnant women was similar—about 8.5 minutes.— R. L. Burt and I. W. F. Davidson, *Obstet. Gynec., N.Y.*, 1974, *43*, 161, per *Int. pharm. Abstr.*, 1975, *12*, 364.

The placental transfer of radioactive human insulin in 4 diabetics and 4 healthy mothers was negligible.— S. C. Kalhan *et al.*, *J. clin. Endocr. Metab.*, 1975, *40*, 139, per *J. Am. med. Ass.*, 1975, *233*, 97.

Protein binding. In a study of the effect of insulin antibodies on free and total plasma-insulin concentrations it was found that insulin-dependent diabetic patients with high insulin-binding capacity tended to have high total but low free plasma-insulin concentrations. It was considered that bound insulin was not necessarily inactive as dissociation could take place.— A. B. Kurtz *et al.*, *Lancet*, 1977, *2*, 56.

The protein binding of insulin was reported to be about 10 times higher in insulin-treated diabetics than in healthy subjects.— J. J. Vallner, *J. pharm. Sci.*, 1977, *66*, 447.

Resistance to Insulin. Insulin-binding antibodies develop in most patients being treated with insulin but their presence is generally without a significant effect on insulin requirements. Very occasionally, the daily insulin requirement increases considerably, even up to several thousand units. In patients with marked resistance to insulin, excessive formation of antibody usually occurs.

Lack of response may also be due to deficient absorption from injection sites.

The use of highly purified insulins is associated with a reduced concentration of antibodies and these preparations are indicated in patients resistant to insulin.

Discussions of insulin resistance.— R. M. Elenbaas and P. J. Forni, *Am. J. Hosp. Pharm.*, 1976, *33*, 491; J. S. Flier *et al.*, *New Engl. J. Med.*, 1979, *300*, 413.

A 55-year-old man with maturity-onset diabetes was resistant to pork insulin but responsive to tolbutamide 2 g daily.— M. Rendell *et al.*, *Ann. intern. Med.*, 1979, *90*, 195.

Diabetes mellitus in a 40-year-old woman was resistant to treatment with insulin; 10 000 units daily corrected ketosis but not glycosuria. Plasma exchange produced dramatic but short-lived reductions in antibody titre. Insulin binding and receptor affinity were similarly improved but the effect was almost completely lost in the 2 to 3 days between exchanges. Definite improvement in metabolic control only occurred after the 7th plasma exchange and because of the transient effect, immunosuppressant drugs should also be given to deplete existing antibodies and inhibit their synthesis.— M. Muggeo, *New Engl. J. Med.*, 1979, *300*, 477.

An adult patient had 2 episodes of resistance to insulin. The patient's serum-binding capacity for insulin was greatly increased during the first episode, but hardly increased at all during the second.— B. A. Leatherdale *et al.*, *Postgrad. med. J.*, 1980, *56*, 38.

The use of aprotinin to overcome resistance to subcutaneous insulin.— G. R. Friedenberg *et al.*, *New Engl. J. Med.*, 1981, *305*, 363. Discussion, including emphasis on the hazards: J. C. Pickup *et al.* (letter), *ibid.*, 1413; S. Colagiuri and H. Grunstein (letter), *ibid.;* M. Berger *et al.* (letter), *ibid.*, 1414; G. R. Freidenberg *et al.* (letter), *ibid.*

Further references to insulin resistance: E. P. Paulsen *et al.*, *Diabetes*, 1979, *28*, 640.

Uses. Insulin is the hormone, secreted by the beta cells of the islets of Langerhans of the pancreas, which regulates carbohydrate metabolism. In a normal person, with a daily output of about 50 units of insulin, the fasting blood-sugar concentration is maintained in the region of 0.7 to 1.1 mg per ml (about 3.9 to 6.1 mmol per litre); a store of glucose, as glycogen, is maintained in the liver and muscles. As the blood-sugar concentration falls, the liver glycogen is mobilised and converted into glucose which passes into the blood.

In diabetes mellitus, insulin is generally deficient, the blood-sugar concentration rises, and when the renal threshold for sugar is exceeded, glycosuria occurs; in addition, glycogen is not stored in the liver, and lipolysis may be increased. Oxidation of the fat results in the formation of ketone bodies, such as acetone and acetoacetic acid, and β-hydroxybutyric acid, which appear in the urine. Diabetes mellitus is defined on p.843.

When administered parenterally, insulin causes a fall in the blood-sugar concentration and prevents the formation of ketone bodies.

Insulin is used for the treatment of insulin-sensitive diabetes mellitus unresponsive to diet alone. It is usually administered subcutaneously but may be given intramuscularly or, for very rapid effect, intravenously. When given as Insulin Injection it is quickly absorbed from the site of injection and markedly lowers the blood-sugar concentration. The effect begins in about 30 minutes, reaches its maximum in about 4 hours, and lasts 6 to 8 hours.

Injections are usually given twice a day, just before breakfast and the evening meal; a third dose may be necessary before the midday meal. The number of injections required can be reduced by the simultaneous injection of a long-acting insulin before breakfast.

The dosage of insulin depends upon the severity of the diabetes and will vary from patient to patient. The amount necessary may range from 10 to 100 units or more a day but the minimum amount necessary to maintain a normal concentration of blood-sugar on a diet of adequate energy value must be determined for each patient individually. Larger doses are necessary during illness and infection, in accidental or surgical trauma, in emotional stress, and in pregnancy.

While the required maintenance dose of insulin is being established, blood-glucose estimations are advisable so that the necessary adjustments can be made to the dose. Once stabilisation has been achieved, however, tests for glucose in the urine may be adequate.

Insulin Injection is often administered with Protamine Zinc Insulin Injection. The latter, however, contains an excess of protamine which reacts with soluble insulin and thus reduces the amount of soluble insulin available for immediate effect. Insulin Injection has also been given with Isophane Insulin Injection. Because of variations in pH, admixture with insulin zinc suspensions is not recommended.

Insulin is essential for the treatment of *diabetic ketoacidosis,* with or without coma, but the precipitating cause, such as acute infection, must be sought and treated. Treatment includes rehydration, the administration of insulin and potassium, if necessary the partial correction of acidosis by bicarbonate and of hypotension by volume expanders, and must be adjusted to the needs of the individual patient. Adequate fluid replacement is essential; 1 litre or more of sodium chloride injection may be given per hour for the first hour or two, followed by about 500 ml per hour; six litres or more may be required in the first 24 hours. Some authorities give alternate volumes of sodium chloride injection and half-strength sodium chloride injection. Insulin is given as Insulin Injection or Neutral Insulin Injection. Typical doses for severely ill patients are 10 to 20 units intravenously, followed by intravenous infusion at a rate of about 6 units per hour. In less severely ill patients insulin may be given intramuscularly in an initial dose of 12 to 20 units followed by about 6 units hourly. The considerably larger bolus intravenous doses previously used are now less common. Potassium, up to 200 mmol in the first 24 hours, is given, usually starting from the second hour. Some authorities give the first 30 mEq as phosphate to correct hypophosphataemia. When the blood-glucose concentration has fallen to about 2.7 mg per ml it is necessary to give dextrose, as dextrose injection 5% or dextrose 4% in sodium chloride injection 0.18%, with continued insulin, to correct ketosis. In the treatment of hyperosmolar nonketotic coma treatment is broadly similar except that the initial hydrating fluid is commonly half-strength sodium chloride injection.

Insulin is used as a test of pituitary function and the stimulant effect of insulin on gastric secretion is used as a test for the completeness of vagotomy.

Insulin was formerly used in the hypoglycaemic shock therapy of schizophrenia and anxiety states.

Highly purified insulin preparations are described on p.843.

The mixing of insulin injections.— *Drug & Ther. Bull.*, 1971, *9*, 27 and 44; A. D. B. Harrower *et al.*, *Practitioner*, 1975, *214*, 228.

The hypoglycaemic response to fish insulin in 16 normal and obese subjects and in 1 patient with an insulinoma.— R. C. Turner and P. C. Johnson, *Lancet*, 1973, *1*, 1483. See also R. C. Turner and E. Harris, *ibid.*, 1974, *2*, 188; R. C. Turner *et al.*, *ibid.*, 1976, *1*, 1252.

A hypothesis on the mode of action of insulin.— A. H. Kissebah *et al.*, *Lancet*, 1975, *1*, 144.

Insulin injection was associated with improved growth, increased activity, and subjective improvement in 2 children with type I glycogen-storage disease.— O. Dulac *et al.* (letter), *Lancet*, 1978, *1*, 107.

Administration. Discussion of insulin-delivery systems, including 'closed-loop' systems ('artificial pancreas') and 'open-loop' systems for continuous intravenous or subcutaneous infusion.— *Lancet*, 1979, *1*, 1275; J. C. Pickup and H. Keen, *Diabetologia*, 1980, *18*, 1; *Lancet*, 1980, *1*, 1005; P. J. Watkins, *Br. med. J.*, 1980, *280*, 350; R. A. Rizza *et al.*, *New Engl. J. Med.*, 1980, *303*, 1313; P. Felig and W. V. Tamborlane, *Ann. intern. Med.*, 1980, *93*, 627.

Discussion of the proposed introduction of insulin in one strength only—100 units per ml.— J. M. Moss and J. A. Galloway, *J. Am. med. Ass.*, 1977, *238*, 1823; *FDA Drug Bull.*, 1978, *8*, 32.

Comment on the hazards of introducing U-100 insulin and the plans for the safe introduction of U-100 and the phased withdrawal of U-40 and U-80.— C. Hardwick *et al.* (letter), *Lancet*, 1979, *2*, 1083; *idem*, *Br. med. J.*, 1979, *2*, 1363.

Intramuscular administration. Control of severe brittle diabetes in 5 of 6 patients by continuous intramuscular infusion of insulin; they appeared to have impaired absorption of insulin given subcutaneously.— J. C. Pickup *et al.*, *Br. med. J.*, 1981, *282*, 347.

Intranasal administration. A report on the safety and efficacy of intranasal insulin in healthy subjects and insulin-dependent diabetics.— A. E. Pontiroli *et al.*, *Br. med. J.*, 1982, *284*, 303.

Intraperitoneal administration. Intraperitoneal administration of insulin in certain ketoacidotic patients.— R. H. Greenwood *et al.* (letter), *Lancet*, 1979, *2*, 312. In end-stage renal failure.— C. T. Flynn and J. A. Nanson (letter), *ibid.*, 591. See also A. Balducci *et al.*, *Br. med. J.*, 1981, *283*, 1021.

Intravenous administration. In 6 patients with insulin requirements of 120 to 3000 units daily, diabetic control was improved by the use of intravenous infusions of insulin in doses of 50 to 63 units daily. It was considered that there was a defect in absorption from subcutaneous tissue.— P. Dandona *et al.*, *Lancet*, 1978, *2*, 283.

See also under Diabetes Mellitus, below.

Jet injection. A comparison of the administration of insulin by jet injection and by conventional syringe. R. Worth *et al.*, *Br. med. J.*, 1980, *281*, 713.

Subcutaneous infusion. Favourable reports of continuous subcutaneous insulin infusion (CSII).— J. C. Pickup *et al.*, *Lancet*, 1979, *1*, 1255 (metabolic effects); W. V. Tamborlane *et al.*, *Lancet*, 1979, *1*, 1258 (metabolic effects); W. V. Tamborlane *et al.*, *New Engl. J. Med.*, 1979, *300*, 573; J. M. Potter *et al.*, *Br. med. J.*, 1980, *280*, 1099; V. A. Koivisto *et al.*, *Br. med. J.*, 1981, *282*, 778.

Cautionary comment on continuous subcutaneous insulin infusion.— R. C. Turner *et al.* (letter), *Lancet*, 1979, *2*, 481; P. Felig *et al.* (letter), *New Engl. J. Med.*, 1979, *301*, 1004.

Details of satisfactory results in 6 insulin-requiring diabetic subjects using long-term continuous subcutaneous insulin infusion at home.— J. C. Pickup *et al.*, *Lancet*, 1979, *2*, 870. Patient reaction to continuous subcutaneous infusion of insulin.— J. C. Pickup *et al.*, *Br. med. J.*, 1981, *282*, 766.

Improved growth in 2 adolescents given insulin subcutaneously by infusion pump.— W. V. Tamborlane *et al.*, *New Engl. J. Med.*, 1981, *305*, 303.

Improved metabolic control and arrest or reversal of some of the features associated with diabetic microangiopathy.— Steno Study Group, *Lancet*, 1982, *1*, 121.

Further references: J. C. Pickup *et al.* (letter), *New Engl. J. Med.*, 1979, *301*, 267; F. J. Service *et al.* (letter), *ibid.*; R. B. Tattersall and E. A. M. Gale (letter), *ibid.*, 268; P. Felig *et al.* (letter), *ibid.*; W. V. Tamborlane *et al.*, *Diabetes*, 1979, *28*, 785; A. Pietri *et al.*, *ibid.*, 1980, *29*, 668; L. S. Lieberman *et al.* (letter), *New Engl. J. Med.*, 1980, *303*, 940; J. D. Nelson *et al.*, *Lancet*, 1980, *1*, 1383.

Rectal administration. Studies in *dogs* on the absorption of insulin from a suppository.— M. Shichiri *et al.*, *J. Pharm. Pharmac.*, 1978, *30*, 806. See also M. S. Mesekha *et al.*, *Farmatsiya, Mosk.*, 1978, *27*, 11, per *Int. pharm. Abstr.*, 1979, *16*, 1020.

Administration in renal failure. Insulin was reported to be 5% bound to plasma proteins. The normal half-life of 2 hours after subcutaneous injection was prolonged in end-stage renal failure. Doses should be reduced to 75% in patients with a glomerular filtration-rate (GFR) of 10 to 50 ml per minute, and to 50% in those with a GFR of less than 10 ml per minute, according to the blood-glucose concentrations.— W. M. Bennett *et al.*, *Ann. intern. Med.*, 1980, *93*, 286.

See also under Intraperitoneal Administration, above.

Burns. Insulin 200 to 600 units daily given intravenously in 50% dextrose solution, reduced the nitrogen and potassium losses of severely burnt patients to levels which could be replaced by a normal diet.— P. Hinton *et al.*, *Lancet*, 1971, *1*, 767. Comments and criticisms.— W. P. T. James *et al.* (letter), *ibid.*, 1078.

A study in 22 patients with severe trauma ranging from burns to head injury, all of whom required parenteral nutrition, confirmed that insulin had a specific protein-sparing effect in catabolic patients which is independent of the type of energy source given. Insulin was given with large doses of glucose and might be useful in such patients to prevent excessive protein catabolism, especially when renal function is impaired.— A. M. J. Woolfson *et al.*, *New Engl. J. Med.*, 1979, *300*, 14. Comment.— H. N. Munro, *ibid.*, 41.

Diabetes mellitus. A discussion of the prevention and management of emergencies in the treatment of diabetes.— J. M. Stowers, *Prescribers' J.*, 1973, *13*, 61.

Treatment of 4 consecutive patients with severe uncontrolled diabetes mellitus demonstrated that small bolus injections of 5 units given intravenously every hour were effective. Fluid replacement and potassium supplementation, if required, were also carried out.— N. Clumeck *et al.* (letter), *Lancet*, 1975, *2*, 416.

The mechanism of action of insulin in diabetic patients.— P. M. Brown *et al.*, *Br. med. J.*, 1978, *1*, 1239.

The successful use of an intravenous insulin delivery system to reverse florid diabetic retinopathy in a 24-year-old woman with very unstable, insulin-dependent diabetes.— K. Irsigler *et al.* (letter), *Lancet*, 1979, *2*, 1068.

A brief discussion of the use of insulin in the management of diabetes.— A. Bloom, *Postgrad. med. J.*, 1979, *55*, *Suppl.* 2, 27.

The importance of the timing of the morning injection of insulin for the control of postprandial hyperglycaemia in diabetic children.— A. L. Kinmonth and J. D. Baum, *Br. med. J.*, 1980, *280*, 604.

The 24-hour metabolic profiles in 15 diabetic children receiving insulin injections once daily (Monotard and Actrapid) or twice daily (Semitard and Actrapid) indicated that by conventional standards mean diabetic control was adequate on both regimens but neither regimen provided physiological diabetic control. It was suggested that specific modifications to the regimens may help to produce more normal profiles.— G. A. Werther *et al.*, *Br. med. J.*, 1980, *281*, 414. See also N. K. Griffin *et al.*, *Archs Dis. Childh.*, 1980, *55*, 112.

Further references: University Group Diabetes Program, *J. Am. med. Ass.*, 1978, *240*, 37.

In pregnancy. Discussions of the control of diabetes in pregnancy.— N. L. Essex *et al.*, *Br. med. J.*, 1973, *4*, 89; *Drug & Ther. Bull.*, 1978, *16*, 3; F. P. Vince, *Practitioner*, 1978, *220*, 279; R. E. Robinson, *Postgrad. med. J.*, 1979, *55*, 358; *Lancet*, 1980, *1*, 633.

A study of the management of the pregnant diabetic, at home, in hospital, and with or without glucose meters.— S. M. Stubbs *et al.*, *Lancet*, 1980, *1*, 1122. See also K. Teramo *et al.* (letter), *ibid.*, 1410.

References to the use of infusions of insulin during labour.— J. M. Steel (letter), *Br. med. J.*, 1977, *1*, 1537; K. G. M. M. Alberti *et al.* (letter), *ibid.*, 1977, *2*, 266; M. Nattrass *et al.*, *ibid.*, 1978, *2*, 599; N. L. Essex *et al.* (letter), *ibid.*, 1978, *2*, 962; J. D. Yeast *et al.*, *Am. J. Obstet. Gynec.*, 1978, *131*, 861.

Further references to the treatment of diabetes in pregnancy: G. D. Roversi *et al.*, *Am. J. Obstet. Gynec.*, 1979, *135*, 567.

In surgery. Discussions and reviews of the use of insulin in the control of diabetes mellitus, with special reference to use during surgery.— *Br. med. J.*, 1972, *4*, 98; K. G. M. M. Alberti and D. J. B. Thomas, *Br. J. Anaesth.*, 1979, *51*, 693.

The intravenous injection of insulin, by mini-pump, during minor surgery.— A. H. Barnett *et al.*, *Br. med. J.*, 1980, *280*, 78.

Further references: U. Taitelman *et al.*, *J. Am. med. Ass.*, 1977, *237*, 658.

Diabetic ketoacidosis. Reviews and discussion of the treatment of diabetic ketoacidosis and of hyperosmolar nonketotic coma.— S. R. Newmark *et al.*, *J. Am. med. Ass.*, 1975, *231*, 185; D. J. Chisholm, *Med. J. Aust.*, 1976, *2*, 494; *Drug & Ther. Bull.*, 1976, *14*, 77; *Br. med. J.*, 1977, *1*, 405; A. C. MacCuish, *Recent Advances in Intensive Therapy*, No. 1, I.M. Ledingham (Ed.), London, Churchill Livingstone, 1977; R. A. Kreisberg, *Ann. intern. Med.*, 1978, *88*, 681; J. Sheldon, *Practitioner*, 1979, *222*, 333; R. Bienia and I. Ripoll, *J. Am. med. Ass.*, 1979, *241*, 510; M. Nattrass, *Prescribers' J.*, 1980, *20*, 91.

Episodes of 'euglycaemic diabetic ketoacidosis' [plasma bicarbonate of 10 mmol or less per litre, without excessive hyperglycaemia; blood glucose less than 3 mg per ml] occurred in 17 young insulin-dependent patients on 37 occasions. Treatment consisted of correction of dehydration and electrolyte loss and re-establishment of carbohydrate metabolism. Fluid and electrolytes should therefore be given in 5% (or even 10%) dextrose solution with adequate doses of insulin. Bicarbonate was necessary only in 12 episodes in 4 patients.— J. F. Munro *et al.*, *Br. med. J.*, 1973, *2*, 578.

Twelve children with severe diabetic crisis were treated on 14 occasions by rehydration and the intramuscular injection of insulin, 0.25 unit per kg body-weight initially then 0.1 unit per kg body-weight hourly until the plasma-glucose concentration had fallen below 2 mg per ml. The mean time for the relief of hyperglycaemia was 5 hours (range 2 to 8 hours). Sodium bicarbonate was given intravenously when required, and potassium chloride under ECG control.— J. Moseley, *Br. med. J.*, 1975, *1*, 59.

Further reports and references to the use of insulin in ketoacidosis: K. G. M. M. Alberti *et al.*, *Lancet*, 1973, *2*, 515; N. G. Soler *et al.*, *Lancet*, 1975, *2*, 1221; T. J. Hannan and G. M. Stathers, *Med. J. Aust.*, 1976, *1*, 11; N. Clumeck *et al.*, *Br. med. J.*, 1976, *2*, 394; A. E. Kitabchi *et al.*, *Ann. intern. Med.*, 1976, *84*, 633; P. N. Malleson, *Archs Dis. Childh.*, 1976, *51*, 373; M. M. Martin and A. A. Martin, *J. Pediat.*, 1976, *89*, 560; D. Heber *et al.*, *Archs intern. Med.*, 1977, *137*, 1377; R. S. Sherwin, *ibid.*, 1361; B. F. Clarke *et al.*, *Br. med. J.*, 1977, *2*, 1395; G. A. Edwards *et al.*, *J. Pediat.*, 1977, *91*, 701; E. S. Lightner *et al.*, *Pediatrics*, 1977, *60*, 681; J. N. Fisher *et al.*, *New Engl. J. Med.*, 1977, *297*, 238; R. D. G. Leslie and J. D. Mackay, *Br. med. J.*, 1978, *2*, 1343; J. A. Lutterman *et al.*, *Diabetologica*, 1979, *17*, 17; K. Onur *et al.*, *J. Pediat.*, 1979, *94*, 307; H. S. Sacks *et al.*, *Ann. intern. Med.*, 1979, *90*, 36; P. Fort *et al.*, *J. Pediat.*, 1980, *96*, 36.

Hepatitis. References to the possible use of insulin and glucagon in hepatitis.— M. Farivar *et al.*, *New Engl. J. Med.*, 1976, *295*, 1517; S. Sherlock, *ibid.*, 1535; *Lancet*, 1978, *2*, 244; K. H. Usadel (letter), *New Engl. J. Med.*, 1979, *300*, 1223.

Hyperlipidaemia. Severe hypertriglyceridaemia responding to insulin and nicotinic acid therapy.— S. R. Smith, *Postgrad. med. J.*, 1981, *57*, 511.

Myocardial infarction. For reports of the use of insulin, dextrose, and potassium chloride in the treatment of myocardial infarction, see under Potassium Chloride, p.630.

Occlusive vascular disease. References to the use of insulin in occlusive vascular disease.— C. Bonessa and L. Cremonini, *Minerva med., Roma*, 1966, *57*, 2027, per *Abstr. Wld Med.*, 1967, *41*, 43; P. A. Majid *et al.*, *Lancet*, 1972, *2*, 937.

Pancreatitis. Acute pancreatitis was treated in 20 patients by the intravenous infusion of dextrose injection containing 20 units of insulin per litre, at a rate of 300 to 400 ml in the first hour. There was a smaller reduction in blood-glucose concentrations compared with matched controls and 15 patients were free from pain within a few hours.— D. Hallberg and N. O. Theve, *Acta chir. scand.*, 1974, *140*, 138, per H. Ellis, *Postgrad. med. J.*, 1975, *51*, 121.

Test of gastric innervation. The Hollander test for the completeness of vagotomy was used in 182 patients after vagotomy; the dose of insulin was 20 units intravenously or, later, 0.25 unit per kg body-weight, and was designed to reduce the blood-sugar concentration to less than 450 µg per ml. The incidence of incomplete vagotomy in males was 38% and in females 18%. It was suggested that it was necessary to apply different criteria, of increased gastric acid secretion, to males and females.— J. Spencer *et al.*, *Gut*, 1969, *10*, 307. The Hollander test after vagotomy was too unreliable and the dose of insulin was too high.— S. J. Stempien (letter), *ibid.*, 695.

The dose of insulin required to elicit the maximum gastric acid response without producing hypoglycaemia, which depressed the effect, was 0.2 unit per kg body-weight.— J. H. Baron *et al.*, *Gut*, 1969, *10*, 1046.

Insulin was given by continuous infusion on 26 occasions to 12 healthy volunteers. At a rate of 0.04 unit per kg body-weight per hour, a mean acid output of 28.3 mmol per hour was achieved with minimal symptoms of hypoglycaemia. The results were reproducible and were suggested as being suitable for evaluation to replace the Hollander test for completeness of vagotomy.— D. C. Carter *et al.*, *Br. med. J.*, 1972, *2*, 202.

Mean gastric secretion, corrected for duodenal reflux and pyloric loss, half to 2 hours after the intravenous injection of insulin 0.2 unit per kg body-weight was 215 ml per hour in 29 pre-operative patients. Of 71 who had had vagotomy 54 had a secretion of less than 116 ml per hour and none of these had recurrent ulcers; of 17 secreting more than 116 ml per hour 9 had recurrent ulcers and 4 recurrent symptoms. Estimation of basal secretion was not necessary.— R. G. Faber *et al.*, *Gut*, 1974, *15*, 347.

The measurement of insulin-stimulated gastric secretion for predicting the liability to relapse of patients with duodenal ulcer after treatment with cimetidine.— N. K. Maybury and D. L. Carr-Locke, *Br. J. Surg.*, 1980, *67*, 315.

Tests of pituitary function. Experience with 4 healthy subjects and 20 patients with hypothalamic or pituitary disease suggested that the insulin test, the protirelin test, and the gonadorelin test could be given concomitantly for the evaluation of hypothalamic-pituitary function. The dose of insulin was 0.05 to 0.3 unit per kg body-weight, of protirelin 200 to 500 µg, and of gonadorelin 100 µg.— P. Harsoulis *et al.*, *Br. med. J.*, 1973, *4*, 326.

Insulin-induced hypoglycaemia was not associated with a rise in plasma concentrations of arginine vasopressin in 3 patients with cranial diabetes insipidus whereas there was a rise in 10 patients with unimpaired posterior pituitary function. The differences in response might be used for a test of posterior pituitary function.— P. H. Baylis and D. A. Heath (preliminary communication), *Lancet*, 1977, *2*, 428.

The sequential use of insulin and levodopa to promote release of growth hormone.— E. O. Reiter *et al.*, *Am. J. Dis. Child.*, 1977, *131*, 189. See also R. Collu *et al.*, *Pediatrics*, 1978, *61*, 242.

Further references to the effects of insulin on growth hormone: P. H. Sönksen *et al.*, *Lancet*, 1972, *2*, 155; A. P. Hansen (letter), *Lancet*, 1972, *2*, 432; R. G. Wilson *et al.*, *Lancet*, 1972, *2*, 1283.

For a comparison of the effects of pyrogen, lypressin, and insulin on pituitary-adrenal function, see Pyrogens, p.1671.

Wounds. A deeply pitted scar following influenza vaccination was completely resolved in 82 days by injection of insulin, and had remained normal for 7 months. Monocomponent insulin 4 units was injected subcutaneously, in approximately equal amounts into each quadrant of the pit, thrice daily. There was no evidence of hypoglycaemia.— F. R. Amroliwalla, *Br. med. J.*, 1977, *1*, 1389.

Other reports of the topical use of insulins: T. N. Paul, *Lancet*, 1966, *2*, 574; G. Csapó and M. Hódi (letter), *ibid.*, 1466; P. Hodgson and H. Mowat, *J. Hosp. Pharm.*, 1967, *24*, 319; J. Balassa, *Med. J. Aust.*, 1967, *2*, 604; J. E. Lopez and B. Mena (letter), *Lancet*, 1968, *1*, 1199; S. R. Van Ort and R. M. Gerber, *Nurs. Res.*, 1977, *25*, 9.

Manufacturers

Boots, UK; Evans Medical, UK; Weddel, UK; Wellcome, UK.

Proprietary Names

Regular Iletin *(Lilly, USA)*.

7204-y

Biphasic Insulin Injection *(B.P.)*. Biphasic Insulin.

CAS — 8063-29-4.

Pharmacopoeias. In *Br.*

A sterile buffered suspension of crystals of bovine insulin, containing not less than 23 units per mg (calculated on the dried basis), in a solution of porcine insulin of similar potency. It is a white suspension, in which the majority of the particles are crystalline having a maximum dimension greater than 10 µm but rarely exceeding 40 µm, having a pH of 6.6 to 7.2, and iso-osmotic with blood. It contains 27.5 to 37.5 µg of zinc for each 100 units of insulin, and a suitable bactericide. A quarter of the insulin is present in soluble form; it complies with a test for prolongation of insulin effect. **Store** in multidose glass containers as for Insulin Injection.

The label states the animal source or sources of the insulin.

Units. See p.844.

Adverse Effects. As for Insulin Injection, p.844.

Treatment of Adverse Effects. As for Insulin Injection (see p.845), but when the patient has recovered consciousness and is able to swallow, frequent glucose drinks and a slowly digestible form of carbohydrate such as bread should be given until the action of the biphasic insulin has ceased.

Precautions. As for Insulin Injection, p.845.

CAUTION. *Biphasic insulin should never be given intravenously and is not suitable for the emergency treatment of diabetic ketoacidosis.*

Uses. Biphasic Insulin Injection combines the properties of a quick-acting insulin with the prolonged action of the crystalline component. The effect begins about 30 minutes after subcutaneous injection, reaches a maximum after 4 to 12 hours, and lasts 18 to 22 hours.

It is usually given, subcutaneously, half an hour before breakfast and half an hour before the evening meal. The second dose is usually 30 to 50% of the morning dose. In mild diabetes a single daily dose may be sufficient. Before a dose is withdrawn the vial should be shaken gently. It may be mixed with Neutral Insulin Injection for a greater initial hypoglycaemic effect, but should not be mixed with other insulins. The dose is adjusted to suit the patient's needs, and is usually 20 to 80 units or more daily.

Rapitard insulin was used in the management of 132 diabetic children. Almost all children who had changed from either isophane or semilente insulin twice daily required a substantial increase in insulin dose on Rapitard. Control was not satisfactory in 18 children.— J. M. Court and G. C. Amies, *Med. J. Aust.*, 1973, *2*, 5.

Blood-glucose concentrations after Rapitard MC.— M. Neubauer *et al.*, *Dt. med. Wschr.*, 1979, *104*, 384.

Proprietary Preparations

Rapitard MC *(Novo, UK: Farillon, UK)*. Biphasic Insulin Injection prepared from monocomponent beef and pork insulins (see p.843), containing 40 or 80 units per ml, in vials of 10 ml.

7205-j

Desphenylalanine Insulin. Insulin Defalan. Insulin modified by the removal of the terminal phenylalanine from the amino-acid chain.

CAS — 11091-62-6 (porcine); 51798-72-2 (bovine).

Uses. The removal of phenylalanine from the amino-acid chain alters the antigenicity. Desphenylalanine insulin is used similarly to soluble insulin, and in conjunction with other insulins for prolonged effect.

References: I. Caterson, *Drugs*, 1979, *17*, 289; F. D. Peters *et al.*, *Dt. med. Wschr.*, 1979, *104*, 973.

Pregnancy and the neonate. The use of desphenylalanine insulin in 7 pregnant diabetics. All the patients produced normal infants.— F. D. Peters, *Dt. med. Wschr.*, 1979, *104*, 973.

Proprietary Names

Optisulin *(Hoechst, Ger.)*.

7206-z

Globin Zinc Insulin Injection *(B.P., U.S.P.)*. GZI; Globin Zinc Insulin; Globin Insulin; Globin Insulin with Zinc.

CAS — 9004-21-1.

Pharmacopoeias. In *Arg., Br., Cz., Ind., Port., Swiss,* and *U.S.*

The *B.P.* specifies a sterile preparation of mammalian insulin in the form of a complex obtained by the addition of a suitable globin and zinc chloride. It is prepared from crystalline insulin containing not less than 23 units per mg (calculated on the dried basis). The *U.S.P.* specifies a sterile solution of Insulin *U.S.P.* modified by the addition of zinc chloride and globin obtained from globin hydrochloride prepared from beef blood. It contains 40, 80, or 100 units per ml.

An almost colourless liquid, substantially free from turbidity and from matter which deposits on standing, having a pH of 3 to 3.8 and iso-osmotic with blood. It contains for each 100 units of insulin 3.6 to 4 mg of globin and 250 to 350 µg of zinc. It also contains a suitable bactericide. The *U.S.P.* specifies 0.2 to 0.26% phenol or 0.15 to 0.2% cresol; *U.S.P.* also specifies 1.3 to 1.7% w/v of glycerol and a suitable bactericide. **Store** in multidose glass containers at 2° to 8° and avoid freezing.

The label states the animal source or sources of the insulin.

Units. See p.844.

Adverse Effects. As for Insulin Injection, p.844.

Hypoglycaemia is most likely to occur in the late afternoon or early evening in patients receiving Globin Zinc Insulin Injection before breakfast.

Allergic reactions to the globin may also occur though globin zinc insulin produces fewer cutaneous and allergic reactions than protamine zinc insulin.

Treatment of Adverse Effects. As for Insulin Injection (see p.845), but once the patient has recovered consciousness and is able to swallow, frequent glucose drinks and a slowly digestible form of carbohydrate such as bread should be given until the action of the globin zinc insulin has ceased.

Precautions. As for Insulin Injection, p.845.

CAUTION. *Globin zinc insulin should never be given intravenously and is not suitable for the emergency treatment of diabetic ketoacidosis.*

Uses. Globin Zinc Insulin Injection produces effects similar to those of Insulin Injection (see p.846), but it has a delayed action which is intermediate between that of Insulin Injection and Protamine Zinc Insulin Injection. The effect of a subcutaneous injection begins within 2 hours, reaches a maximum in 6 to 12 hours, and lasts for 18 to 24 hours.

It is given subcutaneously preferably 30 minutes before breakfast. In severe cases, 2 injections a day may be necessary. Soluble insulin is sometimes given with globin zinc insulin. Redistribution of the carbohydrate intake may be necessary, about one-fifth of the total daily allowance being taken at breakfast and two-fifths each at the midday and the evening meals. Alternatively, or in addition, a light carbohydrate meal may be taken in the afternoon.

Manufacturers

Boots, UK; Evans Medical, UK; Wellcome, UK.

7209-a

Insulin Zinc Suspension *(B.P., U.S.P.)*.

Insulini Zinci Suspensio Iniectabilis Mixta *(Eur. P.)*; Insulini cum Zinco Suspensio Composita; IZS; Insulin Lente; Insulin Zinc Suspension (Mixed).

CAS — 8049-62-5.

Pharmacopoeias. In *Arg., Aust., Br., Eur., Fr., Ger., Ind., Int., It., Jap., Neth., Port., Rus., Swiss, Turk.*, and *U.S.*

The *B.P.* specifies a sterile buffered suspension of mammalian insulin in the form of a complex obtained by the addition of zinc chloride. The insulin is in a form insoluble in water. It may be prepared by mixing about 3 volumes of Insulin Zinc Suspension (Amorphous) and about 7 volumes of Insulin Zinc Suspension (Crystalline). The *U.S.P.* describes a sterile suspension of Insulin *U.S.P.* modified by the addition of zinc chloride in a manner such that the solid phase of the suspension consists of crystalline and amorphous insulin in a ratio of 7:3. It contains 40, 80, or 100 units per ml.

It is a white suspension in which the majority of particles are crystals with a maximum dimension greater than 10 μm but rarely exceeding 40 μm; a considerable proportion have no uniform shape and do not exceed 2 μm in maximum dimension. pH 6.9 to 7.5. It complies with a test for prolongation of insulin effect, and with a limit test for insulin in solution. **Store** in multidose glass containers at 2° to 8° and avoid freezing. The label states the animal source or sources of the insulin.

7210-e

Insulin Zinc Suspension (Amorphous) *(B.P., Eur. P.)*.

Insulini cum Zinco (Amorphi) Suspensio; Insulini Zinci Amorphi Suspensio Iniectabilis; Amorph. IZS; Amorphous IZS; Insulin Semilente; Prompt Insulin Zinc Suspension *(U.S.P.)*.

Pharmacopoeias. In *Aust., Br., Eur., Fr., Ger., Ind., Int., It., Jap., Neth., Port., Rus., Swiss, Turk.*, and *U.S.*

The *B.P.* specifies a sterile buffered suspension of mammalian insulin in the form of a complex obtained by the addition of zinc chloride. The insulin is in a form insoluble in water. It is prepared from crystalline insulin containing not less than 23 units per mg (calculated on the dried basis).

It is a white or almost colourless suspension in which the particles have no uniform shape and rarely exceed 2 μm in maximum dimension. It has a pH 6.9 to 7.5 and is iso-osmotic with blood. It contains a suitable bactericide. Preparations containing 40 or 80 units per ml contain respectively not more than 0.0095% and 0.014% of zinc. It shows little or no retardation or prolongation of insulin effect, and complies with a limit test for insulin in solution.

The *U.S.P.* describes a sterile suspension of Insulin *U.S.P.* in buffered Water for Injections, modified by the addition of zinc chloride in a manner such that the solid phase of the suspension is amorphous. It contains 40, 80, or 100 units per ml. It also contains sodium acetate 0.15 to 0.17%, sodium chloride 0.65 to 0.75%, methyl hydroxybenzoate 0.09 to 0.11%, and, for each 100 units of insulin, 120 to 250 μg of zinc. pH 7.2 to 7.5.

Store in multidose glass containers at 2° to 8° and avoid freezing. The label states the animal source or sources of the insulin.

7211-l

Insulin Zinc Suspension (Crystalline) *(B.P., Eur. P.)*.

Insulini cum Zinco (Crystallisati) Suspensio; Insulini Zinci Crystallisati Suspensio Iniectabilis; Cryst. IZS; Crystalline IZS;Insulin Ultralente; Extended Insulin Zinc Suspension *(U.S.P.)*.

Pharmacopoeias. In *Aust., Br., Eur., Fr., Ger., Ind., Int., It., Jap., Neth., Port., Rus., Swiss, Turk.*, and *U.S.*; some do not specify the animal source.

The *B.P.* specifies a sterile buffered suspension of bovine insulin in the form of a complex obtained by the addition of zinc chloride. The insulin is in a crystalline form insoluble in water. It is prepared from crystalline insulin containing not less than 23 units per mg (calculated on the dried basis).

It is a white or almost colourless suspension in which the particles are crystalline, the majority of the crystals having a maximum dimension greater than 10 μm but rarely exceeding 40 μm. It has a pH of 6.9 to 7.5 and is iso-osmotic with blood. It contains a suitable bactericide. Preparations containing 40 or 80 units per ml contain respectively not more than 0.0095% and 0.014% of zinc. It complies with a test for prolongation of insulin effect, and with a limit test for insulin in solution.

The *U.S.P.* describes a sterile suspension of Insulin *U.S.P.* containing 40, 80, or 100 units per ml. It also contains sodium acetate 0.15 to 0.17%, sodium chloride 0.65 to 0.75%, methyl hydroxybenzoate 0.09 to 0.11%, and, for each 100 units of insulin, 120 to 250 μg of zinc. pH 7.2 to 7.5. **Store** in multidose glass containers at 2° to 8° and avoid freezing. The label states the animal source or sources of the insulin.

Reports of needle plugging with insulin crystals.— N. M. O'Mullane and P. L. Robinson (letter), *Lancet*, 1978, *2*, 165; K. J. Gurling (letter), *ibid.*, 267; A. M. Powell (letter), *ibid.*; P. D. Neufeld (letter), *ibid.*, 681.

A study of the effect of a single freezing and thawing of several commercially available insulin suspensions indicated that although the biological and chemical properties of the suspensions were not altered the marked increase in the rate of sedimentation and the aggregated crystals, which may not readily pass through a syringe needle, may make it difficult to obtain reproducible doses of insulin from suspensions which have been frozen.— D. T. Graham and A. R. Pomeroy, *Int. J. Pharmaceut.*, 1978, *1*, 315.

Units. See p.844.

Adverse Effects. As for Insulin Injection, p.844.

The 3 types of insulin zinc suspension may give rise to hypoglycaemic attacks at various times of the day according to the type of preparation used. Because they are free of foreign protein, insulin zinc suspensions are less likely to produce local and allergic reactions than Protamine Zinc Insulin and Globin Zinc Insulin.

Treatment of Adverse Effects. As for Insulin Injection, p.845.

Once the patient has recovered consciousness and is able to swallow, frequent glucose drinks and a slowly digestible form of carbohydrate such as bread should be given until the action of insulin has ceased.

Precautions. As for Insulin Injection, p.845.

CAUTION. *Insulin zinc suspensions should never be given intravenously and are not suitable for the emergency treatment of diabetic ketoacidosis.*

Uses. Insulin zinc suspensions are suspensions of insulin, in an insoluble form with zinc chloride, the duration of effect depending upon the relative proportions of amorphous and crystalline insulin particles present.

The effect of Insulin Zinc Suspension (Amorphous) begins about one hour after subcutaneous injection, reaches a maximum in about 6 hours, and lasts about 12 to 16 hours.

The effect of Insulin Zinc Suspension (Crystalline) begins in about 4 to 6 hours after subcutaneous injection, reaches a maximum in about 10 to 18 hours, and lasts for 30 to 36 hours.

These preparations are freely miscible with each other, without affecting the absorbability of the different particles. Mixtures may therefore be prepared which will control the blood-sugar concentration by means of a single daily injection.

Insulin Zinc Suspension (containing 7 parts of crystalline and 3 parts of amorphous insulin zinc suspension) gives suitable control for the average diabetic. The effect begins within about 2 hours, reaches a maximum in about 8 to 12 hours, and lasts for about 30 hours. The onset of action of the usual morning dose may be sufficiently rapid to control the rise of blood-sugar concentration after breakfast. Diabetics needing insulin may often be satisfactorily controlled by a single daily injection of this preparation; a small proportion need the addition of Insulin Zinc Suspension (Amorphous) or Insulin Zinc Suspension (Crystalline) for the optimum control.

Insulin zinc suspensions are administered by subcutaneous injection, usually 30 to 45 minutes before breakfast. The dosage varies according to the condition of the patient. With uncomplicated diabetes of moderate severity, an initial dose of 10 to 16 units is given before breakfast and the dose gradually increased by 4 units a day until the blood-sugar concentration and glycosuria are satisfactorily controlled. The total daily dose is usually between 20 and 100 units daily. Before a dose is withdrawn, the vial should be shaken gently; vigorous shaking may cause excessive frothing. Severe hyperglycaemia is first brought under control with Insulin Injection and an insulin zinc suspension is then substituted in the same or slightly larger daily dosage.

When a patient who has been receiving Protamine Zinc Insulin is changed to Insulin Zinc Suspension, an increase in the dose of about 20% will probably be required. When transferring from other insulin preparations to Insulin Zinc Suspension, the carbohydrate intake may have to be readjusted.

Insulin zinc suspensions may, if necessary, be mixed with Neutral Insulin Injection immediately before injection but should not be mixed with other insulins.

In a crossover study in 15 diabetic children there were no significant differences in control between those treated once daily with Insulin Zinc Suspension and Neutral Insulin Injection and twice daily with Insulin Zinc Suspension (Amorphous) and Neutral Insulin Injection; all were monocomponent insulins.— G. A. Werther and J. D. Baum (letter), *Br. med. J.*, 1978, *2*, 52.

Proprietary Preparations

Human Monotard *(Novo, UK: Farillon, UK)*. Insulin Zinc Suspension prepared from human insulin (emp) (see p.843), containing 40 or 80 units per ml, available in vials of 10 ml.

Hypurin Lente *(Weddel, UK)*. Insulin Zinc Suspension prepared from beef insulin, purified to remove component *a* and reduce the content of component *b* (see p.843), containing 40 or 80 units per ml, available in vials of 10 ml.

Lentard MC *(Novo, UK: Farillon, UK)*. Insulin Zinc Suspension prepared from monocomponent amorphous pork and crystalline beef insulin (see p.843), containing 40 or 80 units per ml, in vials of 10 ml.

Monotard MC *(Novo, UK: Farillon, UK)*. Insulin Zinc Suspension prepared from monocomponent pork insulin (see p.843), containing 40 or 80 units per ml, available in vials of 10 ml. The duration of effect is somewhat shorter than for conventional Insulin Zinc Suspension.

Neulente *(Wellcome, UK)*. Insulin Zinc Suspension prepared from beef insulin, purified virtually to remove component *a* and pro-insulin and to minimise the content of desamidoinsulin (see p.843), containing 40 or 80 units per ml, available in vials of 10 ml.

Semitard MC *(Novo, UK: Farillon, UK).* Insulin Zinc Suspension (Amorphous) prepared from monocomponent pork insulin (see p.843), containing 40 or 80 units per ml, available in vials of 10 ml.

Ultratard MC *(Novo, UK: Farillon, UK).* Insulin Zinc Suspension (Crystalline) prepared from monocomponent beef insulin (see p.843), containing 40 or 80 units per ml, in vials of 10 ml.

Insulin Zinc Suspensions are also marketed in Great Britain by *Boots, Evans Medical, Weddel,* and *Wellcome.*

Other Proprietary Names

Lente Iletin, Semilente Iletin, Ultralente Iletin *(all USA).*

7207-c

Isophane Insulin Injection *(B.P., U.S.P.).*

Isophane Protamine Insulin Injection *(Eur. P.)*; Insulini Isophani Protaminati Suspensio Iniectabilis; Isophane Insulin; Isophane Insulin Suspension; Isophane Insulin (NPH); NPH Insulin.

CAS — 53027-39-7.

Pharmacopoeias. In *Arg., Br., Eur., Fr., Ger., It., Jap., Neth., Swiss,* and *U.S.*

The *B.P.* specifies a sterile buffered suspension of mammalian insulin in the form of a complex obtained by the addition of a suitable protamine. It is prepared from crystalline insulin containing not less than 23 units per mg (calculated on the dried basis).

It is a white suspension of rod-shaped crystals, most of which have a dimension not less than 5 μm and rarely exceeding 60 μm; free from large aggregates. It has a pH of 6.9 to 7.5 and is iso-osmotic with blood.

It contains for each 100 units of insulin 300 to 600 μg of protamine sulphate and not more than 40 μg of zinc, a suitable bactericide, and sodium phosphate as a buffering agent. It complies with a test for prolongation of insulin effect, and with a limit test for insulin in solution.

The *U.S.P.* describes a sterile suspension of zinc-insulin crystals and protamine sulphate in buffered Water for Injections, combined in a manner such that the solid phase of the suspension consists of crystals composed of insulin, protamine, and zinc. It contains 40, 80, or 100 units per ml. It is free from more than traces of amorphous material. It contains either glycerol 1.4 to 1.8% w/v, metacresol 0.15 to 0.17%, and phenol 0.06 to 0.07%; or glycerol 1.4 to 1.8% w/v and phenol 0.2 to 0.25%; it also contains sodium phosphate 0.15 to 0.25% and, for each 100 units of insulin, 10 to 40 μg of zinc. pH 7.1 to 7.4. It complies with a limit test for insulin in solution.

Store in multidose glass containers at 2° to 8° and avoid freezing. The label states the animal source or sources of the insulin.

Units. See p.844.

Adverse Effects. As for Insulin Injection, p.844.

Hypoglycaemia is most likely to occur in the afternoon or in the evening in patients receiving isophane insulin early before breakfast. Allergic reactions to the protamine may also occur.

Treatment of Adverse Effects. As for Insulin Injection (see p.845), but when the patient has recovered consciousness and is able to swallow, frequent glucose drinks and a slowly digestible form of carbohydrate such as bread should be given until the action of the isophane insulin has ceased.

Precautions. As for Insulin Injection, p.845.

CAUTION. *Isophane insulin should never be given intravenously and is not suitable for the emergency treatment of diabetic ketoacidosis.*

Uses. Isophane Insulin Injection is a suspension of insulin with protamine and zinc. It contains no excess of protamine. Isophane insulin in many respects resembles protamine zinc insulin, but its duration of action is shorter. After subcutaneous injection the effect begins within 2 hours, reaches a maximum in about 10 hours, and lasts for 18 to 28 hours. A single daily injection given before breakfast is often sufficient. Alternatively, two-thirds of the dose may be given in the morning and the remainder in the late afternoon. Before a dose is withdrawn the vial should be gently shaken.

Isophane insulin may be given together with Insulin Injection when the combined effect of quick-acting and slow-acting insulin is required. It may also be given if required, with Neutral Insulin Injection. When used in such mixtures it has the advantage over protamine zinc insulin that it does not affect the rapid action of the soluble insulins. Redistribution of carbohydrate intake may be necessary as for Globin Zinc Insulin Injection (see p.848).

Proprietary Preparations

Hypurin Isophane *(Weddel, UK).* Isophane Insulin Injection prepared from beef insulin, purified to remove component *a* and reduce the content of component *b* (see p.843), containing 40 or 80 units per ml, available in vials of 10 ml.

Initard 50/50 *(Nordisk-UK, UK: Leo, UK).* A mixture of Isophane Insulin Injection (Insulatard, see below) 50% and Neutral Insulin Injection (Velosulin, see p.850) 50%.

Insulatard *(Nordisk-UK, UK: Leo, UK).* Isophane Insulin Injection prepared from pork insulin, purified by gel chromatography and ion-exchange chromatography, containing 40 or 80 units per ml, available in vials of 10 ml.

Mixtard 30/70 *(Nordisk-UK, UK: Leo, UK).* A mixture of Isophane Insulin Injection (Insulatard, see above) 70% and Neutral Insulin Injection (Velosulin, see p.850) 30%.

Neuphane *(Wellcome, UK).* Isophane Insulin Injection prepared from beef insulin, purified virtually to remove component *a* and pro-insulin and to minimise the content of desamidoinsulin (see p.843), containing 40 or 80 units per ml, available in vials of 10 ml.

Isophane Insulin Injection is also marketed in Great Britain by *Boots* and *Evans Medical.*

Other Proprietary Names

NPH Iletin *(USA).*

7203-l

Neutral Insulin Injection *(B.P.).* Neutral Insulin.

Pharmacopoeias. In *Br.* and *Cz. U.S.* describes a neutral insulin injection under the title Insulin Injection.

A sterile buffered solution of bovine or porcine insulin of potency not less than 23 units per mg (calculated on the dried basis), having a pH of 6.6 to 8 and iso-osmotic with blood. It is a colourless liquid free from turbidity and foreign matter; traces of a very fine deposit may develop on storage. It contains not more than 20 μg of zinc per 100 units of insulin, and a suitable bactericide. **Store** in multidose glass containers as for Insulin Injection.

The label states the animal source or sources of the insulin.

Neutral Insulin Injection was more stable at room temperature than Insulin Injection prepared from the same material; degradation reactions were similar but slower. Mixtures of either with long-acting insulins had similar activity despite changes of pH.— R. L. Jackson *et al., Diabetes,* 1972, *21,* 235, per *J. Am. med. Ass.,* 1972, *220,* 1795.

Neutral Insulin Injection retained its potency for 18 months at room temperature.— A. W. Hopefl (letter), *Am. J. Hosp. Pharm.,* 1975, *32,* 1084. A similar comment.— R. C. Barger (letter), *ibid.,* 1089.

Units. See p.844.

Adverse Effects, Treatment, and Precautions. As for Insulin Injection, p.844.

Uses. Neutral Insulin Injection produces effects similar to those of Insulin Injection (see p.846) but the onset of action is slightly more rapid. It may be given alone or with biphasic insulin or isophane insulin. When mixed with protamine zinc insulin the immediate effects of Neutral Insulin Injection may be diminished by reaction with the excess protamine.

Neutral Insulin Injection may be used in the emergency treatment of diabetic ketoacidosis and hyperosmolar nonketotic coma.

Reports of the use of Neutral Insulin Injection in severe hyperglycaemia.— W. Kidson *et al., Br. med. J.,* 1974, *2,* 691; L. V. Campbell *et al., Med. J. Aust.,* 1976, *2,* 519.

The use of Neutral Insulin Injection by continuous subcutaneous injection.— J. C. Pickup *et al., Br. med. J.,* 1978, *1,* 204.

Pregnancy and the neonate. The use of Neutral Insulin Injection and dextrose, by infusion, in pregnancy.— T. E. T. West and C. Lowy, *Br. med. J.,* 1977, *1,* 1252.

Proprietary Preparations

Actrapid MC *(Novo, UK: Farillon, UK).* Neutral Insulin Injection prepared from monocomponent pork insulin (see p.843), containing 40 or 80 units per ml, available in vials of 10 ml.

Human Actrapid *(Novo, UK: Farillon, UK).* Neutral Insulin Injection prepared from human insulin (emp) (see p.843), containing 40 or 80 units per ml, available in vials of 10 ml.

Hypurin Neutral *(Weddel, UK).* Neutral Insulin Injection prepared from beef insulin, purified to remove component *a* and reduce the content of component *b* (see p.843), containing 40 or 80 units per ml, available in vials of 10 ml.

Neusulin *(Wellcome, UK).* Neutral Insulin Injection prepared from beef insulin, purified virtually to remove component *a* and pro-insulin and to minimise the content of desamidoinsulin (see p.843), containing 40 or 80 units per ml, available in vials of 10 ml.

Nuso Neutral Insulin *(Boots, UK; Evans Medical, UK; Wellcome, UK).* Neutral Insulin Injection, containing 40 or 80 units of beef insulin per ml, available in vials of 10 ml.

Velosulin *(Nordisk-UK, UK: Leo, UK).* Neutral Insulin Injection prepared from pork insulin, purified by gel chromatography and ion-exchange chromatography, containing 40 or 80 units per ml, available in vials of 10 ml. Patients transferred from beef or beef/pork insulins may require smaller doses.

7208-k

Protamine Zinc Insulin Injection *(B.P., Eur. P., U.S.P.).*

Insulini Zinci Protaminati Injectio; Insulini Zinci Protaminati Suspensio Iniectabilis; PZI; Protamine Zinc Insulin; Injectio Insulini Protaminati cum Zinco.

CAS — 9004-17-5.

Pharmacopoeias. In *Arg., Aust., Belg., Br., Chin., Eur., Fr., Ger., Hung., Ind., Int., It., Jap., Jug., Neth., Pol., Port., Roum., Rus., Swiss, Turk.,* and *U.S.*

The *B.P.* specifies a sterile buffered suspension of mammalian insulin in the form of a complex obtained by the addition of a suitable protamine and zinc chloride. It is prepared from crystalline insulin containing not less than 23 units per mg (calculated on the dried basis). A white suspension having a pH of 6.9 to 7.5, and iso-osmotic with blood. It contains for each 100 units of insulin 1 to 1.7 mg of protamine sulphate, a quantity of zinc chloride equivalent to 200 μg of zinc, 10 to 11 mg of sodium phosphate, and a suitable bactericide. It complies with a test for prolongation of insulin effect, and with a limit test for insulin in solution.

The *U.S.P.* describes a sterile suspension of Insulin *U.S.P.* in buffered Water for Injections, modified by the addition of zinc chloride and protamine sulphate. It contains 40, 80, or 100 units per ml and is free, after moderate agitation, from large particles. It contains glycerol 1.4 to 1.8% w/v and either cresol 0.18 to 0.22% or phenol 0.22 to 0.28%; it also contains sodium phosphate 0.15 to 0.25% and, for each 100 units of insulin,

1 to 1.5 mg of protamine and 150 to 250 µg of zinc. pH 7.1 to 7.4.
Store in multidose glass containers at 2° to 8° and avoid freezing. The label states the animal source or sources of the insulin.

Units. See p.844.

Adverse Effects. As for Insulin Injection, p.844. Hypoglycaemia is most likely to occur insidiously during the night or early morning in patients receiving protamine zinc insulin before breakfast. Allergic reactions to the protamine may also occur.

Treatment of Adverse Effects. As for Insulin Injection, p.845, but when the patient has recovered consciousness and is able to swallow, glucose drinks and a slowly digestible form of carbohydrate such as bread should be continued until the more prolonged action of protamine zinc insulin has ceased.

Precautions. As for Insulin Injection, p.845.

CAUTION. *Protamine zinc insulin should never be given intravenously and is not suitable for the emergency treatment of diabetic ketoacidosis.*

Uses. Protamine Zinc Insulin Injection allows a slow but steady absorption of insulin throughout the day but it may cause late and insidious hypoglycaemia. After an injection of protamine zinc insulin the blood-sugar concentration begins to fall in about 4 hours, the maximum effect is obtained in 15 to 20 hours, and the effect persists for 24 to 36 hours.
It is usually administered 30 to 60 minutes before breakfast and is often given with a dose of Insulin Injection to provide insulin in the period until the Protamine Zinc Insulin Injection is absorbed. A redistribution of carbohydrate intake may be necessary, less being taken at breakfast and more for tea and supper.
The dose of Protamine Zinc Insulin Injection is modified to suit the patient and usually varies between 10 and 100 units, though more than 80 units should rarely be given on account of the severe nocturnal hypoglycaemic attacks which may result. It should be given subcutaneously; intramuscular injections may be painful. Before a dose is withdrawn the vial should be shaken gently.
When changing from soluble insulin to protamine zinc insulin, the initial dose of protamine zinc insulin should be from two-thirds to the same number of units, given in a single dose before breakfast. Severe hyperglycaemia should be treated with soluble insulin until the protamine zinc insulin has begun to exert its full effect.
Protamine Zinc Insulin Injection contains an excess of protamine which, when mixed with Insulin Injection or Neutral Insulin Injection, reacts with soluble insulin and thus reduces the amount of soluble insulin available for immediate effect.

Proprietary Preparations

Hypurin Protamine Zinc *(Weddel, UK).* Protamine Zinc Insulin Injection prepared from beef insulin, purified to remove component *a* and reduce the content of component *b* (see p.843), containing 40 or 80 units per ml, available in vials of 10 ml.

Protamine Zinc Insulin Injection is also marketed in Great Britain by *Boots, Evans Medical, Weddel,* and *Wellcome.*

Other Proprietary Names
Protamine, Zinc & Iletin *(USA).*

7212-y

Sulphated Insulin. A modified insulin prepared by the action of sulphuric acid on bovine insulin.

Sulphated insulin has been reported to be of value in the treatment of patients with diabetes resistant to other insulins.

References: P. J. Moloney *et al., J. new Drugs,* 1964, *4,* 258; J. A. Little and J. H. Arnott, *Diabetes,* 1966, *15,* 457, per *Abstr. Wld Med.,* 1967, *41,* 62; A. Goldschmied and L. Laurian (letter), *Lancet,* 1968, *2,* 405; S. J. Hopkins, *Chemist Drugg.,* 1970, *193,* 28.

7213-j

Acetohexamide *(U.S.P.).* 1-(4-Acetylbenzenesulphonyl)-3-cyclohexylurea.
$C_{15}H_{20}N_2O_4S = 324.4.$

CAS — 968-81-0.

Pharmacopoeias. In *Jap.* and *U.S.*

A white, almost odourless, crystalline powder. M.p. 182.5° to 187°. Practically **insoluble** in water and ether; soluble 1 in 230 of alcohol and 1 in 210 of chloroform; soluble in pyridine and dilute solutions of alkali hydroxides.

Adverse Effects. As for Chlorpropamide, p.852.

Effects on the liver. A 58-year-old man with diabetes mellitus was given chlorothiazide 500 mg and acetohexamide 500 mg daily. Three weeks later, jaundice developed and liver biopsy revealed acute parenchymal disease with large numbers of eosinophils in the portal areas. Liver function improved after 5 weeks, but a second liver biopsy 6½ months later showed inactive postnecrotic cirrhosis. Further treatment with the 2 drugs for 2 weeks produced no toxic reaction. The nature of the liver lesions suggested that acetohexamide rather than chlorothiazide was responsible for the lesion.— M. J. Goldstein and A. J. Rothenberg, *New Engl. J. Med.,* 1966, *275,* 97.

Overdosage. A 16-year-old girl who had ingested fifty 250-mg tablets of acetohexamide was opisthotonic, unresponsive to stimuli except corneal light reflex, and had tonic and clonic seizures continuously. Her blood pressure was 90/20 mmHg and heart-rate was 80 beats per minute. The blood-glucose concentration on admission to hospital was less than 200 µg per ml. Coma persisted despite blood-glucose concentrations of 2 mg per ml or more after the intravenous administration of dextrose. The patient gradually recovered after treatment with dexamethasone, metaraminol, noradrenaline, and assisted respiration.— D. L. Cowen *et al.* (letter), *J. Am. med. Ass.,* 1967, *201,* 141.

Treatment of Adverse Effects. Hypoglycaemia should be treated as for Insulin Injection, p.845.

In a 42-year-old patient with chronic renal disease and azotaemia, prolonged hypoglycaemia after one 500 mg dose of acetohexamide failed to respond to repeated injections of dextrose injection 50% but responded promptly to peritoneal dialysis.— W. T. Lampe, *Archs intern. Med.,* 1967, *120,* 239, per *Int. pharm. Abstr.,* 1967, *4,* 1415.

Precautions. As for Chlorpropamide, p.852.
The safety of acetohexamide in pregnancy is not established.

In 2 diabetic patients with impaired renal function, hypoglycaemia occurred after treatment with acetohexamide and persisted for 3 and 8 days respectively after acetohexamide was stopped.— R. W. Alexander, *Diabetes,* 1966, *15,* 362, per *J. Am. med. Ass.,* 1966, *197* (July 11), A225.

Inadvertent administration of acetohexamide to 3 patients instead of acetazolamide.— R. Ritch *et al.* (letter), *J. Am. med. Ass.,* 1977, *238,* 1628.

Interactions. *Enhanced effect.* The hypoglycaemic effect of an injection of acetohexamide 500 mg was enhanced in 9 patients given phenylbutazone 100 mg four times daily for a week. Phenylbutazone was considered to delay the renal excretion of hydroxyhexamide, the active metabolite of acetohexamide.— J. B. Field *et al., New Engl. J. Med.,* 1967, *277,* 889.

Absorption and Fate. Acetohexamide is readily absorbed from the gastro-intestinal tract and is extensively bound to plasma proteins. It is rapidly metabolised to hydroxyhexamide which also has hypoglycaemic activity. The plasma half-life of acetohexamide is about 1.3 hours and of its metabolite about 5 hours. About 80% of a dose is excreted in the urine within 24 hours, largely as metabolites.

The mean peak plasma concentrations of acetohexamide after administration of 750 mg to 8 subjects of 3 different tablet formulations were about 28, 40, and 44 µg per ml two hours after administration. About a third of the acetohexamide dose was recovered from 8-hour urine samples largely as hydroxyhexamide.— J. W. Kleber *et al., J. pharm. Sci.,* 1977, *66,* 635.

Uses. Acetohexamide is a sulphonylurea with actions and uses similar to those of chlorpropamide (see p.853). The peak effect occurs in about 3 hours and the effect lasts for 12 hours or more. Patients with mild diabetes may be given 250 mg daily before breakfast, increased by 250 to 500 mg daily every 5 to 7 days as needed. For patients with moderately severe diabetes a loading dose may be given; 1.5 g on the first day, 1 g on the second day, and 500 mg on the third day. Maintenance doses may range from 0.25 to 1.5 g daily. Doses in excess of 1 g may be taken in 2 divided doses, before the morning and evening meals. Elderly patients may require smaller doses. If the patient has previously been having more than 20 units of insulin daily, this dosage should be gradually reduced.
Acetohexamide may be given concomitantly with a biguanide.

Acetohexamide 1 g was approximately equivalent in hypoglycaemic effect to tolbutamide 2.25 g or chlorpropamide 500 mg.— D. A. D. Montgomery *et al., Br. med. J.,* 1964, *1,* 868.

Acetohexamide had no antidiuretic effect but enhanced diuresis after water load in 7 subjects.— A. M. Moses *et al., Ann. intern. Med.,* 1973, *78,* 541.

Administration in renal failure. The dosage interval of acetohexamide should be increased from 12 hours in normal patients to 24 hours in those with mild renal failure; it should be avoided in those with moderate or severe renal failure.— P. Sharpstone, *Br. med. J.,* 1977, *2,* 36.

Acetohexamide was reported to be 65 to 90% bound to plasma proteins. The normal half-life was increased in end-stage renal failure. Acetohexamide should be avoided in patients with a glomerular filtration-rate of less than 50 ml per minute.— W. M. Bennett *et al., Ann. intern. Med.,* 1980, *93,* 286.

See also under Precautions.

Preparations

Acetohexamide Tablets *(U.S.P.).* Tablets containing acetohexamide. The *U.S.P.* requires 50% dissolution in 60 minutes.

Dimelor *(Lilly, UK).* Acetohexamide, available as scored tablets of 500 mg. (Also available as Dimelor in *Arg., Austral., Belg., Canad., Ital., S.Afr.*).

Other Proprietary Names
Dymelor *(USA)*; Gamadiabet, Metaglucina *(both Spain)*; Ordimel *(Neth., Swed.).*

7214-z

Buformin Hydrochloride. BS 5892; DBV *(buformin)*; W37 *(buformin)*. 1-Butylbiguanide hydrochloride.
$C_6H_{15}N_5,HCl = 193.7.$

CAS — 692-13-7 (buformin); 1190-53-0 (hydrochloride).

Adverse Effects and Treatment. As for Phenformin Hydrochloride, p.857.
The incidence of lactic acidosis is considered to be lower than with phenformin.

Absorption and Fate. Buformin hydrochloride is readily absorbed from the gastro-intestinal tract.

In 6 female diabetics given radioactive buformin hydrochloride 100 mg the mean peak plasma concentration was 370 ng per ml about 2.5 hours after administration. After 24 hours 64% of the administered dose had been excreted (36% urinary, 28% faecal) and after 72 hours a total of 80% had been excreted.— H. Gutsche *et al., Arzneimittel-Forsch.,* 1976, *26,* 1227.

Further references: F. Ritzl *et al., Arzneimittel-Forsch.,* 1978, *28,* 1184.

Uses. Buformin hydrochloride is a biguanide with actions and uses similar to those of phenformin hydrochloride (see p.858). It is given, often as a sustained release preparation, in doses of 100 to 300 mg daily.

In 100 diabetic patients in whom treatment with sulphonylurea compounds had resulted in late failure, treatment with buformin in an average dose of 150 mg daily resulted in improved control in 55.— H. Schmechel, *Dte GesundhWes.*, 1968, *23*, 301, per *Int. pharm. Abstr.*, 1969, *6*, 43.

The use of a tosylate derivative for prolonged action.— P. Singer and H. Thoelke, *Dte GesundhWes.*, 1973, *28*, 995, per *Int. pharm. Abstr.*, 1973, *10*, 895.

Proprietary Names

Diabrin *(US Vitamin, Arg.)*; Silubin Retard *(Grünenthal, Belg.*; *Grünenthal, S.Afr.*; *Medinsa, Spain*; *Grünenthal, Switz.)*; Sindiatil *(Bayer, Ital.)*.

7215-c

Carbutamide. Glybutamide; BZ 55; U 6987. 1-Butyl-3-sulphanilylurea.

$C_{11}H_{17}N_3O_3S$=271.3.

CAS — 339-43-5.

Pharmacopoeias. In *Fr.*, *It.*, *Nord.*, and *Swiss.*

A tasteless, almost odourless, white, crystalline powder. Practically **insoluble** in water, chloroform, and ether; soluble in alcohol, acetone, and in dilute acids and alkalis.

Carbutamide is a sulphonylurea with similar actions and uses to chlorpropamide (see below) but which is more toxic. It has been given in single daily doses of 0.5 to 1 g.

Proprietary Names

Biouren *(Nessa, Spain)*; Carbutil *(Lopez-Brea, Spain)*; Diabetin *(Diasan, Switz.)*; Diabetoplex *(Vaillant, Ital.)*; Diabutan *(Streuli, Switz.)*; Dia-Tablinen *(Sanorania, Ger.)*; Dibefanil *(Mepha, Switz.)*; Dicarbul *(Grossmann, Switz.)*; Glucidoral *(Servier, Fr.)*; Glucofren *(Cophar, Switz.)*; Insoral *(see also under Phenformin Hydrochloride) (Valeas, Ital.)*; Invenol *(Hoechst, Ger.)*; Nadisan *(Boehringer, Arg.*; *Boehringer Mannheim, Belg.*; *Boehringer Mannheim, Ger.*; *Boehringer Mannheim, Spain*; *Boehringer Mannheim, Swed.*; *Boehringer Mannheim, Switz.)*.

7216-k

Chlorpropamide *(B.P., B.P. Vet., U.S.P.)*.

Chlorpropam.; Chlorglypropamide; P607. 1-(4-Chlorobenzenesulphonyl)-3-propylurea.

$C_{10}H_{13}ClN_2O_3S$=276.7.

CAS — 94-20-2.

Pharmacopoeias. In *Br.*, *Braz.*, *Chin.*, *It.*, *Jap.*, *Jug.*, *Nord.*, *Rus.*, *Swiss*, and *U.S.*

A white, odourless or almost odourless, almost tasteless, crystalline powder. M.p. 126° to 130°. Practically **insoluble** in water; soluble 1 in 12 of alcohol, 1 in 5 of acetone, 1 in 9 of chloroform, and 1 in 200 of ether; soluble in solutions of alkali hydroxides.

Adverse Effects. Mild effects include nausea, vomiting, epigastric pain, dizziness, weakness, and paraesthesia. Sensitivity reactions with fever, eosinophilia, jaundice, skin rashes, and blood disorders, including leucopenia, thrombocytopenia, aplastic anaemia, and agranulocytosis have occurred. Intolerance to alcohol, characterised by facial flushing, may also occur. Side-effects occur more frequently after chlorpropamide than after tolbutamide.

Prolonged hypoglycaemia has been reported following the ingestion of chlorpropamide.

Sixty-one reports of reactions to chlorpropamide had been received by the Committee on Safety of Drugs; 25 related to skin reactions including the Stevens-Johnson syndrome, exfoliative dermatitis, eczema, photodermatitis, erythema nodosum, and purpuric and papular rashes. Blood disorders included aplastic anaemia (3), agranulocytosis (2), pancytopenia (3), leucopenia (4), thrombocytopenia (5), and haemolytic anaemia (2). Liver damage occurred in 8 patients.— E. L. Harris, *Br. med. J.*, 1971, *3*, 29.

Abuse. A report of hypoglycaemia in a 30-year-old nurse following the self-administration of chlorpropamide.— K. G. M. M. Alberti *et al.*, *Br. med. J.*, 1972, *1*, 87.

Hypoglycaemia in 2 patients following surreptitious ingestion of chlorpropamide tablets.— R. M. Jordan *et al.*, *Archs intern. Med.*, 1977, *137*, 390.

Blood disorders. A 63-year-old woman who had been taking chlorpropamide 375 mg daily for about 7 weeks developed marrow aplasia and died.— L. L. R. White, *Br. med. J.*, 1962, *1*, 691.

Chlorpropamide induced immune haemolytic anaemia in a 61-year-old man. The antibody present in the patient's serum was found to react *in vitro* with other sulphonylureas, but not with sulphafurazole.— G. L. Logue *et al.*, *New Engl. J. Med.*, 1970, *283*, 900.

An analysis of blood dyscrasias reported to the Swedish Adverse Drug Reaction Committee for the 5-year period 1966–70 showed that agranulocytosis attributable to sulphonylureas had been reported on 2 occasions. It was estimated that reported figures represented one-third of the true frequency.— L. E. Böttiger and B. Westerholm, *Br. med. J.*, 1973, *3*, 339. A further report.— S. C. Tucker *et al.*, *J. Am. med. Ass.*, 1977, *238*, 422.

Red blood cell aplasia in an elderly patient taking chlorpropamide 1 g daily.— A. T. Planas *et al.*, *Archs intern. Med.*, 1980, *140*, 707. Red blood cell aplasia, hypoglycaemic coma, and cholestatic jaundice in a woman taking chlorpropamide.— M. J. Gill *et al.*, *ibid.*, 714.

Cardiovascular effects. For varied reports of the effects of oral hypoglycaemic agents on the cardiovascular system, see Tolbutamide, p.859.

Effects on electrolytes. A case-report of hyponatraemia and inappropriate antidiuretic hormone secretion in a patient taking chlorpropamide.— P. Nisbet (letter), *Br. med. J.*, 1977, *1*, 904. See also P. N. Weissman *et al.*, *New Engl. J. Med.*, 1971, *284*, 65; *Lancet*, 1971, *1*, 386; A. Ravina (letter), *ibid.*, 1973, *2*, 203.

Four patients with diabetes mellitus given chlorpropamide developed water intoxication. The syndrome of inappropriate secretion of antidiuretic hormone should be considered when a diabetic patient taking chlorpropamide presents with symptoms of drowsiness, headache, anorexia, nausea, vomiting, depression, and confusion.— D. V. Hamilton, *Practitioner*, 1978, *220*, 469.

In 25 patients with diabetes mellitus chlorpropamide 125 to 750 mg daily had no effect on mean fasting concentrations of antidiuretic hormone; chlorpropamide 62.5 mg intravenously had no effect in 9 healthy subjects.— R. Huupponen *et al.* (letter), *Br. med. J.*, 1980, *281*, 1354.

Effects on the liver. Hepatitis with fever and exfoliative dermatitis occurred in a diabetic woman taking chlorpropamide 250 mg daily. Granulomas with eosinophilic infiltrations were found in the liver and bone marrow. This was probably an allergic reaction.— L. A. Rigberg *et al.*, *J. Am. med. Ass.*, 1976, *235*, 409.

Cholestatic jaundice after an overdose of chlorpropamide.— B. M. Frier and W. K. Stewart, *Clin. Toxicol.*, 1977, *11*, 13.

Effects on the skin. Stevens-Johnson syndrome and neutropenia in a woman given chlorpropamide.— T. M. Kanefsky and S. J. Medoff, *Archs intern. Med.*, 1980, *140*, 1543.

Facial flushing. In 234 diabetics not dependent on insulin, chlorpropamide-alcohol flushing was common; it was rare in 60 insulin-dependent diabetics and in 60 controls. Flushing was considered to be a dominant inherited trait.— R. D. G. Leslie and D. A. Pyke, *Br. med. J.*, 1978, *2*, 1519. See also D. A. Pyke and R. D. G. Leslie, *ibid.*, 1521.

Results of a study in 291 non-insulin-dependent diabetic subjects indicated that patients not experiencing chlorpropamide-alcohol flush are genetically susceptible to the development of diabetic retinopathy whereas those who do experience this interaction are not.— R. D. G. Leslie *et al.*, *Lancet*, 1979, *1*, 997. Of 291 diabetics taking chlorpropamide 191 experienced facial flushing when taking alcohol, 12 suffered breathlessness, and 5 wheezing; tests showed these 5 to have asthma. Tests in 3 suggested that the asthma was mediated by endogenous peptides with opiate-like activity; in 2 patients it was blocked by naloxone and in 1 it was precipitated by an enkephalin analogue.— *idem*, *Br. med. J.*, 1980, *280*, 16.

A study involving 220 non-insulin-dependent diabetic patients indicated that those who flush in response to chlorpropamide and alcohol are significantly less likely to develop macrovascular disease than those who do not flush.— A. H. Barnett and D. A. Pyke, *Br. med. J.*, 1980, *281*, 261.

A study completed by 23 chlorpropamide-treated patients with non-insulin-dependent diabetes mellitus demonstrated that aspirin can block the chlorpropamide-alcohol flush that occurs in such patients on drinking alcohol. It is suggested that the chlorpropamide-alcohol flush may have a prostaglandin step in its mechanism which can be blocked by aspirin.— C. R. Strakosch *et al.*, *Lancet*, 1980, *1*, 394.

Data suggesting that endogenous opioids may be implicated in the chlorpropamide-alcohol flush.— S. Medbak *et al.*, *Br. med. J.*, 1981, *283*, 937.

Further references: D. B. Jefferys *et al.* (letter), *Lancet*, 1979, *2*, 1195; N. G. Soler and G. H. Motl, *ibid.*, 1299; R. J. A. Butland *et al.* (letter), *Br. med. J.*, 1980, *281*, 387; J. Köbberling and M. Weber (letter), *Lancet*, 1980, *1*, 538; A. H. Barnett *et al.*, *ibid.*, *2*, 164; N. E. de Silva *et al.*, *ibid.*, 1981, *1*, 128; A. H. Barnett and D. A. Pyke (letter), *ibid.*, 222.

Hypoglycaemia. Studies in 6 patients with chlorpropamide-induced hypoglycaemia suggested that the condition was related to inhibition of glycogenolysis by the liver rather than to chlorpropamide or insulin concentrations in serum.— H. M. M. Frey and B. Rosenlund, *Diabetes*, 1970, *19*, 930, per *Abstr. Wld Med.*, 1971, *45*, 606.

During a period of 5 years 13 patients with an average age of 70 years were treated for severe hypoglycaemic reactions to chlorpropamide. All were comatose and required prolonged infusions of dextrose, 3 had renal impairment, 1 developed coronary insufficiency, and 2 died.— R. J. Schen (letter), *Lancet*, 1973, *1*, 1121.

Overdosage. A nondiabetic woman died 7.5 days after ingesting 10 g of chlorpropamide, despite vigorous treatment. An unusual aspect was the occurrence of polyuria on the 3rd day.— A. De Troyer *et al.* (letter), *Lancet*, 1975, *2*, 514.

Pregnancy and the neonate. Perinatal foetal deaths occurred in 16 of 25 pregnancies in women given chlorpropamide. In all other pregnancies in diabetic women, whether treated with diet alone, insulin, or tolbutamide, the perinatal death-rate was about 20%. All the chlorpropamide deaths were associated with doses of 500 mg daily. In 3 patients where the dose was only 250 mg daily no deaths occurred. The high death-rate did not appear to be related to congenital abnormalities. It was suggested that doses should be limited to 250 mg daily or less and that the drug should be withdrawn and insulin substituted 10 days before delivery. It was not advocated that chlorpropamide should be avoided in all women of child-bearing age.— W. P. U. Jackson and G. D. Campbell (letter), *Br. med. J.*, 1963, *2*, 1652.

In a study of 19 women treated with chlorpropamide 200 mg or more daily for all or part of their pregnancy with a total range of 5.25 to 105 g there were no teratogenic effects. There were 2 intra-uterine deaths and 1 neonatal death. The poor clinical condition of some infants was considered to be due to inadequate control of the diabetes rather than to chlorpropamide. In practice a dose of 100 mg of chlorpropamide was adequate and safe in mild diabetes mellitus in pregnancy; severer cases were treated with insulin rather than higher doses of chlorpropamide.— H. W. Sutherland *et al.*, *Archs Dis. Childh.*, 1974, *49*, 283. See also *Lancet*, 1974, *2*, 32.

Treatment of Adverse Effects. Hypoglycaemia should be treated as for Insulin Injection, p.845. The patient should be observed over 3 to 5 days in case hypoglycaemia recurs.

For reports of diazoxide being used in the treatment of chlorpropamide-induced hypoglycaemia, see p.144.

Precautions. Chlorpropamide is contra-indicated in diabetes mellitus complicated by fever, trauma, or gangrene, and in patients with impaired renal or hepatic function or serious impairment of thyroid or adrenal function. Chlorpropamide is contra-indicated in pregnancy.

A disulfiram-like reaction may occur in patients taking alcohol during treatment with chlorpropamide.

The hypoglycaemic effects of chlorpropamide and other sulphonylureas may be enhanced by chloramphenicol, clofibrate or halofenate, cyclophosphamide, dicoumarol, monoamine oxidase inhibitors, phenylbutazone, propranolol and other beta-adrenergic blocking agents, and some sulphonamides. The hypoglycaemic effects may be diminished by adrenaline, corticosteroids, and diuretics.

Propranolol may mask symptoms of hypoglycaemia.

A patient with angina pectoris, nocturnal angina, and diabetes mellitus experienced alleviation of various symptoms and no longer experienced nocturnal angina when chlorpropamide was withdrawn from his treatment schedule. It was suggested that chlorpropamide should be withdrawn in patients with nocturnal angina and other signs of congestive heart failure.— C. F. Strauss (letter), *Ann. intern. Med.*, 1973, *78*, 454.

A 72-year-old diabetic on chlorpropamide 250 mg twice daily developed hypoglycaemic coma postoperatively 60 hours after his last pre-operative dose. On the day of surgery isophane insulin was substituted for chlorpropamide. Because of the prolonged effect of chlorpropamide special vigilance was needed for 4 days postoperatively in patients who underwent emergency surgery.— R. J. Schen and A. S. Khazzam, *Br. J. Anaesth.*, 1975, *47*, 899.

Interactions. Reviews of the agents diminishing or enhancing the effects of the hypoglycaemic agents.— I. H. Stockley, *Pharm. J.*, 1971, *2*, 37; J. M. Hansen and L. K. Christensen, *Drugs*, 1977, *13*, 24.

For reference to facial flushing on concomitant intake of *alcohol* and chlorpropamide, see under Adverse Effects (above).

Diminished effect. In a group of 82 patients with maturity-onset diabetes with or without hypertension or cardiovascular disease treated with diet, insulin, or oral hypoglycaemic agents (acetohexamide, chlorpropamide, tolbutamide, or phenformin) the mean blood-sugar concentrations rose significantly when *trichlormethiazide* (usually 4 mg daily) or *chlorothiazide* (usually 500 mg daily) was added to their treatment. No patient on diet needed insulin or an oral hypoglycaemic agent and 1 patient on an oral hypoglycaemic agent needed insulin. The dose of oral hypoglycaemic agent was increased in 4 of about 40 patients, and that of insulin in 2 of about 27 patients.— P. C. Kansal *et al.*, *Sth. med. J.*, 1969, *62*, 1374.

Increased dose requirements of chlorpropamide in a patient taking *rifampicin*.— T. H. Self and T. Morris, *Chest*, 1980, *77*, 800.

Enhanced effect. In 5 diabetics poorly controlled with sulphonylurea treatment, tolerance to glucose was improved when *mebanazine* 20 mg daily was given for 5 weeks.— P. I. Adnitt, *Diabetes*, 1968, *17*, 628, per *J. Am. med. Ass.*, 1968, *206*, 1821.

See also under Insulin, p.846.

Since *salicylic acid, phenylbutazone, ethionamide*, and *aminosalicylic acid* lowered blood-sugar concentrations they were associated with severe hypoglycaemic reactions in patients being treated with sulphonylureas including chlorpropamide.— E. Schulz, *Arch. Klin. Med.*, 1968, *214*, 135.

A patient who had taken chlorpropamide 375 mg daily for 2 years had a hypoglycaemic attack 3 months after starting *dicoumarol* treatment. In patients taking both drugs the half-life of chlorpropamide was increased from about 40 hours to about 90 hours.— M. Kristensen and J. M. Hansen, *Acta med. scand.*, 1968, *183*, 83, per *Med. J. Aust.*, 1969, *1*, 29.

The half-life of chlorpropamide was increased by *dicoumarol* and by *sulphaphenazole*.— M. Kristensen and L. K. Christensen, *Acta diabetol. latin.*, 1969, *6*, *Suppl.* 1, 116.

The half-life of chlorpropamide (normal 30 to 36 hours) was increased in 5 patients with normal renal function to 40, 60, 82, 116, and 146 hours when *chloramphenicol* 1.5 to 3 g daily was given concomitantly.— B. Petitpierre and J. Fabre (letter), *Lancet*, 1970, *1*, 789.

Of severe hypoglycaemic episodes in 88 patients taking sulphonylureas (chlorpropamide, tolbutamide, acetohexamide, carbutamide), 33 in patients without renal impairment were associated with the concomitant administration of *sulphonamides, pyrazolone* derivatives, *salicylates, coumarin* derivatives, *sympatholytic agents, diuretics*, or *rauwolfia* preparations.— W. Berger, *Schweiz. med. Wschr.*, 1971, *101*, 1013.

Severe hypoglycaemia occurred in a 77-year-old man taking chlorpropamide and phenformin when he was given *sulphafurazole*, 1 g four times daily.— H. S. G. Tucker and J. I. Hirsch (letter), *New Engl. J. Med.*, 1972, *286*, 110.

The mean half-life of chlorpropamide was 35.6 hours; it was increased after the simultaneous administration of *chloramphenicol, probenecid*, or *nicoumalone*, and was probably prolonged by *allopurinol* and *clofibrate*.— B. Petitpierre *et al.*, *Int. J. clin. Pharmac.*, 1972, *6*, 120, per *Int. pharm. Abstr.*, 1975, *12*, 419.

A study *in vitro* showed that binding of chlorpropamide, acetohexamide, and tolbutamide to plasma albumin was inhibited by phenylbutazone and sulphaphenazole. The binding of chlorpropamide was also inhibited by sodium salicylate, aspirin, sulphadimethoxine, and sulphafurazole, but acetohexamide and tolbutamide were affected to a lesser extent. These findings could explain the enhancement of the hypoglycaemic action of the sulphonylureas by the other drugs.— J. Judis, *J. pharm. Sci.*, 1972, *61*, 89.

The ability of various anticoagulants to displace chlorpropamide, tolbutamide, and acetohexamide from human serum albumin *in vitro* at pH 7.4 was in the following decreasing order: ethyl biscoumacetate, anisindione, nicoumalone, and phenprocoumon.— J. Judis, *J. pharm. Sci.*, 1973, *62*, 232.

Enhancement of the effect of phenformin with a sulphonylurea during treatment with halofenate.— D. J. Kudzma and S. J. Friedberg, *Diabetes*, 1977, *26*, 291.

Two of 13 patients taking chlorpropamide had hypoglycaemic episodes when halofenate 1 g daily was added to their treatment.— L. H. Krut *et al.*, *S.Afr. med. J.*, 1977, *51*, 348.

Improved diabetic control in a Pakistani woman taking chlorpropamide after eating curries containing karela (*Momordica charantia*).— M. Aslam and I. H. Stockley (letter), *Lancet*, 1979, *1*, 607. See also C. S. Pitchumoni (letter), *ibid.*, 924; K. Shah and E. Hickman (letter), *ibid.*, 925.

Hypoglycaemia in a woman taking chlorpropamide and metformin, possibly induced by the addition of *fenclofenac*.— P. A. Allen and R. T. Taylor (letter), *Br. med. J.*, 1980, *281*, 1642.

Absorption and Fate. Chlorpropamide is readily absorbed from the gastro-intestinal tract and is extensively bound to plasma proteins. The half-life in plasma is about 35 hours. About 80 to 90% of a dose is excreted, partly unchanged, in the urine within 4 days.

Chlorpropamide was metabolised in man to *p*-chlorobenzenesulphonylurea and *p*-chlorobenzenesulphonamide which were excreted in the urine. Other unidentifiable metabolites were also formed. The proportion of chlorpropamide metabolised varied in different individuals on long-term therapy.— P. M. Brotherton *et al.*, *Clin. Pharmac. Ther.*, 1969, *10*, 505.

In a study of the pharmacokinetics of chlorpropamide, 2 additional metabolites, 2-hydroxychlorpropamide, and β-hydroxychlorpropamide, were identified.— J. A. Taylor, *Clin. Pharmac. Ther.* 1972, *13*, 710.

In a crossover study, 6 healthy subjects were given a 250-mg tablet of one of three brands of chlorpropamide; after 6 hours, the serum concentration for 2 brands was over 26 μg per ml, but in the third brand was only 12.5 μg per ml.— A. M. Munro and P. G. Welling, *Eur. J. clin. Pharmac.*, 1974, *7*, 47.

Uses. Chlorpropamide, a sulphonylurea, is an orally active hypoglycaemic agent which reduces the blood-sugar concentration. It probably acts by stimulating insulin secretion, as it has no action on muscle-glucose metabolism when given alone. It is only effective in the presence of functioning islet tissue. Maximum blood concentrations after a single dose are reached in 2 to 4 hours and the effect lasts at least 24 hours.

Chlorpropamide is used in the treatment of mild or moderately severe uncomplicated maturity-onset diabetes mellitus unresponsive to diet alone but it is unsuitable for diabetic patients with ketonuria or diabetic ketosis. It should not be used to replace dietary therapy in the obese and is unsuitable for juvenile, growth-onset, or unstable ('brittle') diabetes.

The initial dose is 250 to 500 mg daily reduced to a maintenance level as soon as possible in order to avoid hypoglycaemic attacks. Adjustments of 50 to 100 mg to the daily dose may be made every 3 to 5 days. The usual maintenance dose is 100 to 375 mg daily. Elderly patients may require smaller doses. The maximum effect of chlorpropamide may not be evident for 4 to 7 days and it may take several weeks to achieve adequate control. It is preferable to give chlorpropamide with breakfast or before breakfast; it should not be given in the evening without food. In patients inadequately controlled on 500 mg, phenformin 50 to 100 mg daily or metformin 1 to 3 g daily may be given concomitantly.

If the patient is taking less than 20 units of insulin daily it is usually possible to change to chlorpropamide without admission to hospital. For patients receiving more than 40 units of insulin daily, insulin should be reduced by 50% during the first few days of chlorpropamide therapy. During insulin withdrawal the urine should be tested for sugar and ketones at least thrice daily. After some weeks or months, chlorpropamide fails to control diabetes in some patients who then require insulin therapy. Insulin therapy may also be necessary in periods of stress such as illness or infection, and in accidental or surgical trauma.

Chlorpropamide, in doses of 100 to 500 mg daily, is used in the treatment of diabetes insipidus.

Pancreatic beta-cell activity was studied in 30 patients with maturity-onset diabetes at various stages of treatment with chlorpropamide and in 6 healthy controls. There was an increased output of insulin by the beta-cells in newly treated patients but this effect was transient and was not observed in patients who had been previously treated. It was considered that the main hypoglycaemic action of chlorpropamide was extrapancreatic.— A. J. Barnes *et al.*, *Lancet*, 1974, *2*, 69.

Administration in renal failure. The dosage interval of chlorpropamide should be increased from 24 hours in normal patients to 36 hours in those with mild renal failure; it should be avoided in those with moderate and severe renal failure.— P. Sharpstone, *Br. med. J.*, 1977, *2*, 36.

Chlorpropamide was reported to be 60 to 90% bound to plasma proteins. The normal half-life of 35 hours was prolonged in end-stage renal failure. Its use should be avoided in patients with a glomerular filtration-rate of less than 50 ml per minute. Concentrations of chlorpropamide were not affected by peritoneal dialysis.— W. M. Bennett *et al.*, *Ann. intern. Med.*, 1980, *93*, 286.

Diabetes insipidus. Ten of 13 patients with vasopressin-sensitive diabetes insipidus had a reduced diuresis after being given chlorpropamide 350 to 500 mg. Alcohol antagonised the effect of chlorpropamide which was dependent on residual circulating concentrations of antidiuretic hormone.— M. Miller and A. M. Moses, *J. clin. Endocr. Metab.*, 1970, *30*, 488, per *Drugs*, 1971, *1*, 494.

Chlorpropamide 150 to 400 mg was given to 17 patients with vasopressin-sensitive diabetes insipidus: urine volume was reduced by 8 to 67% and the osmolality of the urine was increased. Treatment was most effective in 11 patients in whom the disorder was secondary to a known intracranial disorder and least effective in 6 patients with idiopathic diabetes insipidus in whom antidiuretic hormone was probably absent. Hypoglycaemia was a limiting factor to long-term treatment in about half the patients.— R. M. Ehrlich and S. W. Kooh, *Pediatrics*, 1970, *45*, 236, per *Drugs*, 1971, *1*, 494.

Chlorpropamide in doses ranging from 100 to 500 mg daily was used to treat diabetes insipidus in 8 children aged 3 to 13 years. Treatment was successful in 5.— A. L. Rosenbloom, *Curr. ther. Res.*, 1971, *13*, 671.

Five of 8 patients with diabetes insipidus treated for 2 to 6 years with chlorpropamide had peak concentrations of immunoreactive insulin 4 to 5 times higher than in controls, due to hypertrophy of the beta-cells.— A. E. Meinders *et al.*, *J. clin. Endocr. Metab.*, 1974, *38*, 539, per *J. Am. med. Ass.*, 1974, *229*, 226.

Evidence to suggest that the mechanism of action of long-term therapy with chlorpropamide in diabetes insipidus is unlikely to be a direct action on the pituitary or hypothalamus resulting in release of antidiuretic hormone.— M. C. Champion *et al.*, *Br. med. J.*, 1980, *281*, 645 and 1250.

Diabetes mellitus. Lack of correlation between chlorpropamide dose, serum concentration, and blood-glucose concentrations in diabetic patients.— A. Melander *et al.*, *Br. med. J.*, 1978, *1*, 142.

In 7 of 9 children with juvenile-onset chemical diabetes, abnormal glucose tolerance was reversed after treatment with chlorpropamide. Six achieved and maintained highly significant reversal of carbohydrate intolerance.— W. J. Mutch and J. M. Stowers, *Lancet*, 1980, *1*, 1158.

Effects on serum lipids. Reports of the effects of sulphonylureas on serum-lipid concentrations.— *Clin. Sci. & mol. Med.*, 1978, *54*, 37p; G. D. Calvert *et al.*, *Lancet*, 1978, *2*, 66; G. M. Shenfield *et al.*, *Practitioner*, 1979, *222*, 111.

Preparations

Chlorpropamide Tablets *(B.P.)*. Tablets containing chlorpropamide. The *B.P.* requires 70% dissolution in 45 minutes.

Chlorpropamide Tablets *(U.S.P.)*. Tablets containing chlorpropamide.

Proprietary Preparations

Diabinese *(Pfizer, UK)*. Chlorpropamide, available as scored tablets of 100 and 250 mg. (Also available as Diabinese in *Arg., Austral., Belg., Canad., Ital., Neth., Norw., S.Afr., Spain, Switz., USA*).

Glymese *(DDSA Pharmaceuticals, UK)*. Chlorpropamide, available as scored tablets of 250 mg.

Melitase *(Berk Pharmaceuticals, UK).* Chlorpropamide, available as scored tablets of 100 and 250 mg.

Other Proprietary Names

Bioglumin, Clordiabet, Clordiasan, Cloro-Hipoglucina, Diabet, Glucosulfina *(all Spain)*; Catanil, Diabetasi, Diabexan, Diatron, Gliconorm, Melisar, Normoglig *(all Ital.)*; Chloromide *(Canad.)*; Chloronase *(Canad., Ger., Neth., Norw.)*; Diabenal *(Norw.)*; Diabetal, Diabines *(both Swed.)*; Diabetoral *(Ger.)*; Diabinèse *(Fr.)*; Insulase *(USA)*; Mellinese *(Denm., Ital.)*; Nogluc *(Arg.)*; Novopropamide, Stabinol *(both Canad.)*; Promide *(Austral.)*.

7217-a

Glibenclamide *(B.P.)*.

Glyburide; Glybenclamide; Glycbenzcyclamide; HB 419; U 26 452. 1-{4-[2-(5-Chloro-2-methoxybenzamido)ethyl]benzenesulphonyl}-3-cyclohexylurea.

$C_{23}H_{28}ClN_3O_5S$=494.0.

CAS — 10238-21-8.

NOTE. The name glibornuride has frequently but erroneously been applied to glibenclamide.

Pharmacopoeias. In *Br., Braz.,* and *Nord.*

A white or almost white, odourless or almost odourless, tasteless, crystalline powder. M.p. 172° to 174°.

Practically **insoluble** in water and ether; soluble 1 in 330 of alcohol, 1 in 36 of chloroform, and 1 in 250 of methyl alcohol. **Protect** from light.

Adverse Effects and Treatment. As for Chlorpropamide, p.852.

Five patients with diabetes suffered severe hypoglycaemia and 1 died after treatment with 5 mg daily of glibenclamide. Another, who had received up to 15 mg of glibenclamide daily, also died from severe hypoglycaemia.— H. Gottesbüren *et al.* (letter), *Lancet*, 1970, *2*, 576.

A 67-year-old man who had received glibenclamide 20 to 30 mg [daily] for 4 weeks developed an extensive maculopapular rash, cholestatic jaundice, eosinophilia, a prolonged prothrombin time, pneumonia, and renal failure. He died 22 days after the onset of the reaction.— B. Clarke *et al., Diabetes*, 1974, *23*, 739, per *Int. pharm. Abstr.*, 1975, *12*, 342.

Nocturia occurred in about 90% of 49 patients taking glibenclamide.— K. M. Shaw *et al.* (letter), *Br. med. J.*, 1977, *1*, 1415.

Allergy. Cross allergy between glisoxepide, glibenclamide, frusemide, and probenecid in a 55-year-old diabetic man.— B. Ummenhofer and D. Djawari, *Dt. med. Wschr.*, 1979, *104*, 514.

Overdosage. In a 16-year-old girl in coma after taking 50 glibenclamide tablets with suicidal intent, consciousness was rapidly restored after the infusion of dextrose, but the blood-glucose concentration 64 hours after ingestion did not exceed 600 µg per ml despite almost continuous infusion of dextrose.— S. Marigo *et al., Acta diabetol. latin.*, 1972, *9*, 688.

A 30-month-old boy who had ingested a small number of 5-mg tablets of glibenclamide was admitted to hospital 48 hours later with severe hypoglycaemia. He recovered after intensive treatment but 12 months later had persisting third nerve paralysis, optic involvement, and epilepsy.— D. O. Sillence and J. M. Court (letter), *Br. med. J.*, 1975, *3*, 490.

Precautions. As for Chlorpropamide, p.852.

The safety of glibenclamide in pregnancy is not established.

Interactions. Glibenclamide is less susceptible to displacement from protein binding by acidic drugs than tolbutamide or chlorpropamide.— K. F. Brown and M. J. Crooks, *Biochem. Pharmac.*, 1976, *25*, 1175, per *Int. pharm. Abstr.*, 1976, *13*, 950.

Absorption and Fate. Glibenclamide is readily absorbed from the gastro-intestinal tract and is extensively bound to plasma proteins. It is excreted in the faeces and, as metabolites, in the urine.

Glibenclamide was bound to plasma proteins to the extent of 99%.— W. Heptner *et al., Acta diabetol. latin.*, 1969, *6*, *Suppl.* 1, 105.

The peak serum concentration was reached in 4 hours after a dose of 5 mg of glibenclamide in normal subjects. No accumulation occurred even after repeated doses. The biological half-life was estimated at 5 to 7 hours.— S. K. Bhatia *et al., Br. med. J.*, 1970, *2*, 570.

In 2 healthy volunteers glibenclamide 5 mg was completely absorbed, following a lag-time of 30 to 60 minutes, and reached a peak plasma-concentration in 2 hours. Its metabolites were excreted in approximately equal amounts in the urine and faeces.— L. M. Fuccella *et al., J. clin. Pharmac.*, 1973, *13*, 68.

Studies in 6 diabetic patients suggested that although glibenclamide did not accumulate in the blood, it tended to accumulate in a deep body compartment from which it was released over a period of days. This could explain why hypoglycaemic episodes had occurred 2 days after glibenclamide withdrawal.— L. Balant *et al., Eur. J. clin. Pharmac.*, 1977, *11*, 19.

Further references: L. Balant *et al., Eur. J. clin. Pharmac.*, 1975, *8*, 63; G. Sartor *et al., Diabetologia*, 1980, *18*, 17.

Uses. Glibenclamide is a sulphonylurea with similar actions and uses to chlorpropamide (see p.853). After a single dose of glibenclamide the blood-sugar concentration falls within 3 hours and a reduced concentration may persist for about 15 hours. The usual initial dose is 5 mg daily, with or immediately after the first principal meal, adjusted every 7 days by increments of 2.5 or 5 mg daily up to about 15 mg daily. Elderly patients may require smaller doses. Some patients are better controlled by the concomitant administration of a biguanide compound.

A few patients controlled on insulin may be controlled with glibenclamide. Small doses of insulin may be replaced immediately; larger doses should be reduced and replaced gradually.

The pharmacology and toxicology of glibenclamide.— *Arzneimittel-Forsch.*, 1969, *19*, 1326–1494.

For reviews of glibenclamide, see *Drugs*, 1971, *1*, 116; A. Marble, *ibid.*, 109.

Improved glucose tolerance in patients with maturity-onset diabetes persisted through 6 months' treatment with glibenclamide but increases in plasma insulin and the insulin-glucose ratio decreased significantly. Glibenclamide possibly acted by a mechanism other than increased insulin secretion.— J. M. Feldman and H. E. Lebovitz, *Diabetes*, 1971, *20*, 745, per *J. Am. med. Ass.*, 1972, *219*, 243. See also W. C. Duckworth *et al., J. clin. Endocr. Metab.*, 1972, *35*, 585, per *J. Am. med. Ass.*, 1973, *223*, 97.

Diabetes insipidus. Glibenclamide had no antidiuretic effect but enhanced diuresis after water load in 14 subjects.— A. M. Moses *et al., Ann. intern. Med.*, 1973, *78*, 541.

Glibenclamide 20 mg daily significantly increased free water excretion in 5 patients with pituitary diabetes insipidus. In 2 patients given 1 or 2 g of clofibrate a dose-related antidiuretic effect was produced, which was significantly inhibited by glibenclamide.— J. P. Radó and L. Szende, *J. clin. Pharmac.*, 1974, *14*, 290.

Raised plasma concentrations of antidiuretic hormone in a 30-year-old woman were not affected by treatment with glibenclamide.— P. L. Yap *et al., Br. med. J.*, 1977, *1*, 1137.

Diabetes mellitus. *For references to the use of glibenclamide in the treatment of diabetes mellitus, see Martindale, 27th Edn,* p. 813.

Effects on platelets. Possible beneficial effect on platelet aggregation.— L. J. Klaff *et al., S.Afr. med. J.*, 1979, *56*, 247.

Preparations

Glibenclamide Tablets *(B.P.).* Tablets containing glibenclamide.

Daonil *(Hoechst, UK).* Glibenclamide, available as scored tablets of 5 mg. **Semi-Daonil.** Scored tablets each containing glibenclamide 2.5 mg. (Also available as Daonil, Hemi-Daonil, or Semi-Daonil in *Alg., Arg., Austral., Belg., Denm., Fr., Ital., Morocco, Neth., Norw., S.Afr., Spain, Swed., Switz., Tun.*).

Euglucon *(Cassenne, UK).* Glibenclamide, available as tablets of 2.5 mg and as scored tablets of 5 mg. (Also available as Euglucon or Semi-Euglucon in *Arg., Austral., Belg., Canad., Denm., Ger., Ital., Neth., Norw., S.Afr., Spain, Swed., Switz.*).

Other Proprietary Names

Adiab, Gliben *(both Ital.)*; Diaβeta *(Canad.)*; Euglucan, Miglucan *(both Fr.)*; Gilemal *(Hung.)*; Glidiabet, Glucolon *(both Spain)*; Pira *(Arg.)*.

7218-t

Glibornuride.

Ro6-4563. 1-[(2*S*,3*R*)-2-Hydroxyborn-3-yl]-3-tosylurea; 1-[(2*S*,3*R*)-2-Hydroxyborn-3-yl]-3-*p*-tolylsulphonylurea.

$C_{18}H_{26}N_2O_4S$=366.5.

CAS — 26944-48-9.

NOTE. The name glibornuride has frequently but erroneously been applied to glibenclamide.

Adverse Effects, Treatment, and Precautions. Skin reactions and gastro-intestinal disturbances have been reported. It would appear reasonable to expect any of the side-effects described under chlorpropamide, p.852, and to apply similar precautions.

The plasma half-life of glibornuride was 3 times longer in 2 non-diabetic patients with severe renal disease than in healthy volunteers.— G. Rentsch *et al., Schweiz. med. Wschr.*, 1972, *102*, 650, per *J. Am. med. Ass.*, 1972, *220*, 1638.

The elimination half-life of glibornuride was not affected by the concomitant administration of *phenylbutazone*. It was slightly prolonged by *phenprocoumon* and prolonged by one-half by *sulphaphenazole*.— W. Eckhardt *et al., Arzneimittel-Forsch.*, 1972, *22*, 2212.

Absorption and Fate. Glibornuride is readily absorbed from the gastro-intestinal tract. The half-life is about 8 hours. It is extensively metabolised; the metabolites have little or no hypoglycaemic activity.

The metabolism of glibornuride was mainly by oxidation. Six metabolites with insignificant hypoglycaemic activity had been identified in the urine.— F. Bigler *et al., Arzneimittel-Forsch.*, 1972, *22*, 2191.

After oral administration, glibornuride was rapidly absorbed from the gastro-intestinal tract. About 95% was bound to plasma proteins and the average plasma half-life was 8.2 hours. Metabolism occurred mainly in the liver, 60 to 72% of metabolites being excreted by the kidneys and 23 to 33% by the bile into the faeces.— G. Rentsch *et al., Arzneimittel-Forsch.*, 1972, *22*, 2209.

Uses. Glibornuride is a sulphonylurea with actions and uses similar to those of chlorpropamide (see p.853). The usual initial dose is 12.5 mg taken with breakfast; this may be gradually increased, if necessary, up to 50 mg. If a higher dose (up to 75 mg daily) is required, it is recommended that 50 mg be taken in the morning and the remainder in the evening. A biguanide may be given concomitantly if necessary.

The pharmacology of glibornuride.— *Arzneimittel-Forsch.*, 1972, *22*, 2154–2222.

Diabetes mellitus. Four of 7 newly diagnosed patients with diabetes were excellently controlled on glibornuride 12.5 to 75 mg daily. Of 23 refractory to other antidiabetic agents 9 had improved control on glibornuride 100 mg daily. Of the 17 patients unresponsive to glibornuride 3 were controlled on glibenclamide and the remainder required insulin.— A. W. Logie and J. M. Stowers, *Br. med. J.*, 1975, *3*, 514.

It was considered that the relatively short duration of action, the metabolism to inactive substances, and the possible low incidence of hypoglycaemia made glibornuride a suitable oral hypoglycaemic agent for the treatment of elderly patients. Glibornuride did not appear to be more effective than other sulphonylureas.— *Drug & Ther. Bull.*, 1976, *14*, 41.

Comparison of glibornuride with glibenclamide.— E. F. Mogensen *et al., Curr. ther. Res.*, 1976, *19*, 559. A double-blind crossover study of glibenclamide and glibornuride in 28 maturity-onset diabetics indicated that glibornuride has an antidiabetic activity approximately equal to that of glibenclamide but may be associated with increased reduction in body-weight.— R. G. A. van Wayjen and A. van den Ende, *Acta ther.*, 1978, *4*, 101.

Further references: N. Zollner *et al., Dt. med. Wschr.*, 1972, *97*, 1083; C. J. Fox *et al., J.R. Soc. Med.*, 1978, *71*, 899; E. W. Schmitt and J. Nijssen, *Med. Welt.*, 1978, *29*, 1170.

Proprietary Preparations

Glutril *(Roche, UK).* Glibornuride, available as scored tablets of 25 mg. (Also available as Glutril in *Denm., Fr., Ger., S.Afr., Swed., Switz.*).

Other Proprietary Names

Glitrim *(Spain)*; Gluborid *(Ger., Neth., Switz.)*; Glutrid *(Arg.)*.

7219-x

Glicetanile Sodium. Glydanile Sodium; Glidanile Sodium; SH 1051. The sodium salt of 5′-chloro-2-{4-[*N*-(5-isobutylpyrimidin-2-yl)sulphamoyl]phenyl}-2′-methoxyacetanilide.
$C_{23}H_{24}ClN_4NaO_4S$=511.0.

CAS — 24455-58-1 (glicetanile); 24428-71-5 (sodium salt).

A sulphonamidopyrimidine derivative which has been used as a hypoglycaemic agent in doses of 10 to 20 mg daily.

Metabolism.— E. Gerhards *et al.*, *Arzneimittel-Forsch.*, 1976, *26*, 278.

Manufacturers
Schering, Ger.

7220-y

Gliclazide.
S 1702; SE 1702. 1-(3-Azabicyclo[3.3.0]oct-3-yl)-3-tosylurea; 1-(3-Azabicyclo[3.3.0]oct-3-yl)-3-*p*-tolylsulphonylurea.
$C_{15}H_{21}N_3O_3S$=323.4.

CAS — 21187-98-4.

A crystalline solid. M.p. about 181°.

Adverse Effects, Treatment, and Precautions. Skin reactions, headache, and gastro-intestinal disturbances have been reported with gliclazide. It would appear reasonable to expect any of the side-effects described under chlorpropamide, p.852, and to apply similar precautions.

Absorption and Fate. Gliclazide is readily absorbed from the gastro-intestinal tract; varying rates of absorption have been reported. It is extensively bound to plasma proteins. The half-life is about 10 to 12 hours. Gliclazide is extensively metabolised in the liver; less than 5% of a dose appears unchanged in the urine.

Uses. Gliclazide is a sulphonylurea with actions and uses similar to those of chlorpropamide (see p.853). The usual initial dose is 40 to 80 mg daily, gradually increased, if necessary, up to 320 mg daily. It is suggested that the higher doses should be related to the main meals of the day. A biguanide may be given concomitantly if necessary.

A report of a symposium, including reports of the effect of gliclazide on platelet aggregation, coagulation factors, and fibrinolysis.— *Gliclazide and the Treatment of Diabetes*, H. Keen *et al.*(Ed.), London, Royal Society of Medicine, 1980.

A study indicating that the beneficial effects of gliclazide on platelet aggregation seem likely to be due to its hypoglycaemic action rather than to any direct effect on haemostatic function.— R. C. Paton *et al.*, *Br. med. J.*, 1981, *283*, 1018.

Diabetes mellitus. In a 12-month study of 45 patients with maturity-onset diabetes gliclazide 80 to 240 mg daily produced adequate control of blood-glucose concentrations; a biguanide was also required in 6 patients. Platelet adhesiveness was significantly reduced.— Z. Rubinjoni *et al.*, *Curr. med. Res. Opinion*, 1978, *5*, 625.

Diabetic retinopathy. In a group of 135 patients with diabetic retinopathy treated with gliclazide, 38 initially had intact retinas, 52 had angiographic evidence of retinopathy, and 45 clinical evidence. In a control group treated with other antidiabetic agents the respective numbers were 37, 60, and 29. After treatment for an average of 18 months deterioration occurred in 36 and 51 patients respectively (26.7 and 40.5%) and amelioration in 26 and 12 (19.3 and 9.5%).— Y. Barre *et al.*, *Gaz. méd. Fr.*, 1975, *82*, 167.

Proprietary Preparations

Diamicron *(Servier, UK).* Gliclazide, available as scored tablets of 80 mg. (Also available as Diamicron in *Austral., Fr., Ital., Neth., S.Afr., Spain*).

Other Proprietary Names

Dramion *(Ital.)*.

7221-j

Gliflumide. SH 3.1168; ZK 28200. (−)-(*S*)-*N*-(5-Fluoro-2-methoxy-α-methylbenzyl)-2-[4-(5-isobutylpyrimidin-2-ylsulphamoyl)phenyl]acetamide.
$C_{25}H_{29}FN_4O_4S$=500.6.

CAS — 35273-88-2.

A sulphonamidopyrimidine compound which has been used as a hypoglycaemic agent.

Of 26 patients with maturity-onset diabetes, treated with tolbutamide, glibenclamide, or glibenclamide with a biguanide, 22 were controlled by gliflumide; 3 to 10 mg (usually 5 mg) daily was equivalent to 15 mg of glibenclamide. Hypoglycaemia in 7 possibly reflected a delayed onset and prolonged duration of action.— L. Blumenbach *et al.*, *Int. J. clin. Pharmac.*, 1975, *12*, 141.

Effect on platelet aggregation.— C. Sholz *et al.*, *Arzneimittel-Forsch.*, 1975, *25*, 38; W. Losert *et al.*, *ibid.*, 170.

Manufacturers
Schering, Ger.

7222-z

Glipizide.
Glydiazinamide; CP 28720; K 4024. 1-Cyclohexyl-3-{4-[2-(5-methylpyrazine-2-carboxamido)ethyl]benzenesulphonyl}urea.
$C_{21}H_{27}N_5O_4S$=445.5.

CAS — 29094-61-9.

A white odourless powder. M.p. about 205°. Practically **insoluble** in water, alcohol, and chlorinated solvents; sparingly soluble in acetone.

Adverse Effects, Treatment, and Precautions. Skin reactions, headache, and gastro-intestinal disturbances have been reported with glipizide. It would appear reasonable to expect any of the side-effects described under chlorpropamide, p.852, and to apply similar precautions.

Absorption and Fate. Glipizide is absorbed from the gastro-intestinal tract; peak concentrations occur in 1 to 2 hours. It is extensively bound to plasma proteins. It is excreted chiefly in the urine, 64 to 87% of a dose being recovered in 24 hours, largely as inactive metabolites.

In a comparison of the absorption of glipizide and glibenclamide given to 2 healthy volunteers, glipizide was rapidly absorbed, after a lag-time of 20 to 30 minutes, and reached a higher plasma concentration than was obtained with the same dose of glibenclamide. Peak plasma-concentrations of glipizide were found 1 hour after administration of 5 mg by mouth. Glipizide was 98% bound to plasma proteins and very little unchanged drug was excreted in the urine. The 2 main metabolites were hydroxycyclohexyl derivatives which were rapidly excreted in the urine with 11% of the dose excreted in the faeces. The plasma half-life of glipizide was 3 to 4 hours.— L. M. Fuccella *et al.*, *J. clin. Pharmac.*, 1973, *13*, 68.

The mean half-life of glipizide in 4 subjects with normal renal function was 3.7 hours; in 2 patients with impaired renal function it was 6 to 12 hours.— L. Balant *et al.*, *Diabetologia*, 1973, *9*, *Suppl.*, 331.

A comparison of the pharmacokinetics of glipizide and glibenclamide in man.— L. Balant *et al.*, *Eur. J. clin. Pharmac.*, 1975, *8*, 63.

Uses. Glipizide is a sulphonylurea with actions and uses similar to those of chlorpropamide (see p.853).

The peak effect on the blood-sugar concentration occurs in about 2 hours; the hypoglycaemic effect lasts for about 6 hours. The usual initial dose is 2.5 to 5 mg daily adjusted every 3 to 5 days by increments of 2.5 to 5 mg daily up to about 30 mg daily if necessary. Doses of 10 mg or more daily should be given in 2 or 3 divided doses with the principal meals. Elderly patients may require smaller doses. A few patients controlled on insulin may be controlled with glipizide. Small doses of insulin may be replaced immediately; larger doses should be reduced and replaced gradually.

Glipizide may be taken concomitantly with a biguanide.

A report of a symposium on glipizide.— *Curr. med. Res. Opinion*, 1975, *3*, *Suppl.* 1, 1–84.

Reviews of glipizide.— *Drug & Ther. Bull.*, 1975, *13*, 83; R. N. Brogden *et al.*, *Drugs*, 1979, *18*, 329.

Diabetes mellitus. A comparison of glipizide and glibenclamide.— G. Vailati *et al.*, *J. clin. Pharmac.*, 1975, *15*, 60.

A comparison of glipizide and chlorpropamide.— M. S. Bandisode and B. R. Boshell, *Hormone metab. Res.*, 1976, *8*, 88.

A comparison of glipizide and glibenclamide.— G. Blohmé and J. Waldenström, *Acta med. scand.*, 1979, *206*, 263.

A comparison of glipizide and tolbutamide.— S. E. Fineberg and S. H. Schneider, *Diabetologia*, 1980, *18*, 49.

Further references to the use of glipizide in diabetes mellitus: A. Emanueli *et al.*, *Arzneimittel-Forsch.*, 1972, *22*, 1881; A. Johannessen and S. E. Fagerberg, *Diabetologia*, 1973, *9*, *Suppl.*, 339; G. Persson, *ibid.*, 348; A. Masbernard *et al.*, *ibid.*, 356; I. De Leeuw *et al.*, *ibid.*, 364; H. F. J. Lahon and R. D. Manu, *J. int. med. Res.*, 1973, *1*, 608; A. Adetuyibi and O. O. Ogundipe, *Curr. ther. Res.*, 1977, *21*, 479; L. K. Fowler, *Curr. med. Res. Opinion*, 1978, *5*, 418.

Proprietary Preparations

Glibenese *(Pfizer, UK).* Glipizide, available as scored tablets of 5 mg. (Also available as Glibenese in *Belg., Denm., Ger., Neth., Spain, Swed., Switz.*).

Minodiab *(Farmitalia Carlo Erba, UK).* Glipizide, available as scored tablets of 5 mg. (Also available as Minodiab in *Arg., Spain*).

Other Proprietary Names

Glibénèse *(Fr.)*; Mindiab *(Denm., Swed.)*; Minidiab *(Belg., Fr., Ital.)*.

7223-c

Gliquidone.
ARDF 26. 1-Cyclohexyl-3-{4-[2-(3,4-dihydro-7-methoxy-4,4-dimethyl-1,3-dioxo-2(1*H*)-isoquinolyl)ethyl]benzenesulphonyl}urea.
$C_{27}H_{33}N_3O_6S$=527.6.

CAS — 33342-05-1.

A white or slightly yellow crystalline substance. M.p. about 178°. Practically **insoluble** in water; soluble in acetone and chloroform; slightly soluble in alcohol and methyl alcohol.

Adverse Effects, Treatment, and Precautions. There have been reports of skin reactions and gastro-intestinal disturbances with gliquidone. It would appear reasonable to expect any of the side-effects described under chlorpropamide, p.852, and to apply similar precautions.

Absorption and Fate. Gliquidone is readily absorbed from the gastro-intestinal tract and is extensively bound to plasma proteins. It is extensively metabolised in the liver by hydroxylation and demethylation (the metabolites have no significant hypoglycaemic effect) and is eliminated chiefly in the faeces via the bile; less than 5% of a dose is excreted via the kidneys.

Uses. Gliquidone is a sulphonylurea with actions and uses similar to those of chlorpropamide (see p.853).

The hypoglycaemic effect starts within an hour and the optimum effect lasts for 2 to 3 hours. The dose is adjusted to the needs of the patient; most patients respond to doses of 45 to 60 mg daily in 2 or 3 divided doses. Single doses above 60 mg and daily doses above 180 mg are not recommended. Gliquidone may be given concomitantly with a biguanide if necessary.

References: P. Bottermann, *Dt. med. Wschr.*, 1975, *100*, 1733, per *J. Am. med. Ass.*, 1975, *234*, 443; Z. Kopitar, *Arzneimittel-Forsch.*, 1975, *25*, 1455; Z. Kopitar and F.-W. Koss, *ibid.*, 1933.

Proprietary Preparations

Glurenorm *(Winthrop, UK).* Gliquidone, available as scored tablets of 30 mg. (Also available as Glurenorm in *Ger., Neth.*).

Other Proprietary Names
Glurenor *(Arg., Spain).*

7224-k

Glisoxepide. BS 4231; Bay b 4231; FB b 4231; RP 22410. 1-(Perhydroazepin-1-yl)-3-{4-[2-(5-methylisoxazole-3-carboxamido)ethyl]benzenesulphonyl}urea.
$C_{20}H_{27}N_5O_5S$=449.5.

CAS — 25046-79-1.

Adverse Effects, Treatment, and Precautions. As for Chlorpropamide, p.852.

Toxicology in *animals*.— D. Tettenborn, *Arzneimittel-Forsch.*, 1974, *24*, 409.

In 2258 patients treatment with glisoxepide was discontinued in 26 because of side-effects including allergic skin reactions (5), gastro-intestinal disturbances (16), elevated serum-transaminase values (1), pruritus vulvae (1), and dizziness (1).— N. H. K. Kiesselbach *et al.*, *Arzneimittel-Forsch.*, 1974, *24*, 447.

Cross allergy between glisoxepide, glibenclamide, frusemide, and probenecid in a 55-year-old diabetic man.— B. Ummenhofer and D. Djawari, *Dt. med. Wschr.*, 1979, *104*, 514.

Uses. Glisoxepide is a sulphonylurea with actions and uses similar to those of chlorpropamide (see p.853). The usual dose is 4 to 16 mg daily in divided doses.

Pharmacology of glisoxepide.— W. Puls *et al.*, *Arzneimittel-Forsch.*, 1974, *24*, 375.

Diabetes mellitus. In trials involving 2734 patients treated with glisoxepide 54% of those treated for at least 3 months achieved 'good' control and 72% at least 'satisfactory' control; 11% discontinued treatment because of inadequate control. The daily dose ranged from 2 to 16 mg. Mild hypoglycaemia occurred in 7% of the patients. Mean body-weight fell in all patients, together with serum-lipid concentrations and blood pressure in those in whom these values were initially elevated.— L. Blumenbach *et al.*, *Arzneimittel-Forsch.*, 1974, *24*, 437. A further report with similar results.— L. Blumenbach *et al.*, *Arzneimittel-Forsch.*, 1976, *26*, 931.

Studies in 8 maturity-onset diabetics indicated that glisoxepide 8 mg by mouth would produce plasma concentrations with sufficient β-cytotropic activity for a therapeutic response of at least 8 hours.— H. Gutsche and W. Losert, *Arzneimittel-Forsch.*, 1977, *27*, 1719.

Further references: E. Haupt *et al.*, *Arzneimittel-Forsch.*, 1974, *24*, 418; W. Birk and P. Petrides, *ibid.*, 425.

Proprietary Names
Glisepin *(Bayer, Ital.)*; Glucoben *(Farmades, Ital.)*; Pro-Diaban *(Bayer, Ger.; Schering, Ger.).*

7225-a

Glybuzole. AN 1324; RP 7891; TH 1395; Désaglybuzole. *N*-(5-*tert*-Butyl-1,3,4-thiadiazol-2-yl)benzenesulphonamide.
$C_{12}H_{15}N_3O_2S_2$=297.4.

CAS — 1492-02-0.

Glybuzole is an oral hypoglycaemic agent with a structure distinct from that of the sulphonylureas, biguanides, or sulphonamidopyrimidines. It has been given in initial doses of 500 mg daily, with maintenance doses of 250 to 750 mg daily.

Proprietary Names
Gludease *(Jap.).*

7226-t

Glyclopyramide. 1-(4-Chlorobenzenesulphonyl)-3-(pyrrolidin-1-yl)urea.
$C_{11}H_{14}ClN_3O_3S$=303.8.

CAS — 631-27-6.

A white odourless tasteless crystalline powder. M.p. about 198°. Practically **insoluble** in water and chloroform; very slightly soluble in alcohol, acetone, and ether; freely soluble in dilute alkaline solutions.

Uses. Glyclopyramide is a sulphonylurea with actions and uses similar to those of chlorpropamide (see p.852). The usual dose is 125 to 500 mg daily.

Proprietary Names
Deamelin-S *(Jap.).*

7227-x

Glycyclamide. K 386; Glycyclamidum; Tolcyclamide. 1-Cyclohexyl-3-tosylurea; 1-Cyclohexyl-3-*p*-tolylsulphonylurea.
$C_{14}H_{20}N_2O_3S$=296.4.

CAS — 664-95-9.

Pharmacopoeias. In *Roum.*

A white or yellowish-white crystalline powder. M.p. 170° to 176°. Practically **insoluble** in water and ether; readily soluble in alcohol and acetone.

Glycyclamide is a sulphonylurea with actions and uses similar to those of chlorpropamide (see p.852). It is used in doses of 0.5 to 1.5 g daily.

Proprietary Names
Diaborale *(Carlo Erba, Ital.).*

7228-r

Glymidine. Glycodiazine; Glidiazine Sodique; Sodium Glymidine; SH 717. The sodium salt of *N*-[5-(2-methoxyethoxy)pyrimidin-2-yl]benzenesulphonamide.
$C_{13}H_{14}N_3NaO_4S$=331.3.

CAS — 3459-20-9.

A white crystalline powder. M.p. about 223°. **Soluble** in water; slightly soluble in alcohol.

Adverse Effects. Gastro-intestinal disturbances have been reported and, more rarely, allergic skin reactions, leucopenia, and thrombocytopenic purpura. Hypoglycaemia may occur.

The use of an antihistamine to control allergic skin reactions may increase their severity in some patients.

Treatment of Adverse Effects. Hypoglycaemia should be treated as for Insulin Injection, p.845.

Precautions. Glymidine should not be given to patients with severe impairment of hepatic or renal function. It is reported to reduce the tolerance to alcohol. The safety of glymidine in pregnancy is not established.

Absorption and Fate. Glymidine is readily absorbed from the gastro-intestinal tract. It is extensively bound to plasma proteins. It is excreted in the urine chiefly as metabolites.

The demethylated metabolite of glymidine had hypoglycaemic activity comparable with that of glymidine.— M. Kramer *et al.*, *Arzneimittel-Forsch.*, 1964, *14*, 377.

Glymidine was demethylated and subsequently oxidised to the corresponding carboxylic acid. After an oral dose of 0.5 to 2 g, 83 to 95% was excreted in the urine chiefly as metabolites; about 6% of a dose was excreted in the faeces.— E. Gerhards *et al.*, *Arzneimittel-Forsch.*, 1964, *14*, 394.

Glymidine 12 mg per kg body-weight by intravenous infusion was eliminated more slowly in 14 of 29 patients with acute or chronic liver disease. In these 14 the half-life ranged from 5.7 to 27.3 hours. In 18 healthy persons the half-life was between 2.6 and 5.6 hours. In 2 of the 14 patients it was eliminated more quickly after active symptoms of liver disease disappeared.— H. Held *et al.*, *Arzneimittel-Forsch.*, 1973, *23*, 1801.

Uses. Glymidine is an oral hypoglycaemic agent which is not related to the biguanides or to the sulphonylureas. It is only effective in the presence of functioning islet tissue. After a single dose of glymidine, the blood-sugar concentration falls within about 30 minutes and the reduced concentration is maintained for up to 12 hours. It is used in the treatment of maturity-onset diabetes. It is unsuitable for diabetic patients with ketonuria or diabetic ketosis.

The suggested initial dose of glymidine is 1 to 1.5 g daily with breakfast for a few days; if necessary an additional 500 mg may be given later in the day.

Glymidine may be given concomitantly with a sulphonylurea.

Proprietary Preparations

Gondafon *(Schering, UK).* Glymidine, available as tablets of 500 mg. (Also available as Gondafon in *Austral., Belg., Ital., Neth., S.Afr., Swed., Switz.*).

Other Proprietary Names
Lycanol *(Austral., Swed.)*; Redul *(Ger.).*

7229-f

Metahexamide. Glyhexylamide. 1-(3-Amino-*p*-tolylsulphonyl)-3-cyclohexylurea.
$C_{14}H_{21}N_3O_3S$=311.4.

CAS — 565-33-3.

Adverse Effects, Treatment, and Precautions. As for Chlorpropamide, p.852. A high incidence of adverse effects, including liver damage, has been reported.

Uses. Metahexamide is a sulphonylurea with actions and uses similar to those of chlorpropamide (see p.853). The usual dose is 100 to 200 mg daily.

Proprietary Names
Isodiane *(Servier, Fr.).*

7230-z

Metformin Chlorophenoxyacetate. Metformin 4-chlorophenoxyacetate.
$C_4H_{11}N_5,C_8H_7ClO_3$=315.8.

A biguanide derivative with actions and uses similar to those of metformin hydrochloride (see p.856). It is given in doses of 1 to 1.5 g daily.

Proprietary Names
Glucinan *(Anphar-Rolland, Fr.).*

7231-c

Metformin Hydrochloride *(B.P.)*. LA 6023.

1,1-Dimethylbiguanide hydrochloride.
$C_4H_{11}N_5,HCl$=165.6.

CAS — 657-24-9 (metformin); 1115-70-4 (hydrochloride).

Pharmacopoeias. In *Br., Nord.*, and *Roum.*

A white, almost odourless, hygroscopic, crystalline powder with a bitter taste. M.p. about 225°. **Soluble** 1 in 2 of water and 1 in 100 of alcohol; practically insoluble in chloroform and ether. **Store** in airtight containers.

Adverse Effects. As for Phenformin Hydrochloride, p.857.

Lactic acidosis has been reported, but the incidence is considered to be lower than after phenformin.

The risk of lactic acidosis associated with the use of metformin was calculated to be one-fiftieth of that associated with the use of phenformin. Of the 23 cases reported in the literature most occurred in patients with some predisposing factor.— P. J. Phillips (letter), *Br. med. J.*, 1978, *1*, 239.

Some case reports and references: E. G. Lebacq and A. Tirzmalis (letter), *Lancet*, 1972, *1*, 314; P. J. Phillips *et al.* (letter), *Br. med. J.*, 1977, *1*, 234; R. Assan *et al.*, *Diabetologia*, 1977, *13*, 211; W. D. Alexander and J. Marples (letter), *Lancet*, 1977, *1*, 191; T. Korhonen *et al.*, *Eur. J. clin. Pharmac.*, 1979, *15*, 407; P. Biron, *Can. med. Ass. J.*, 1980, *123*, 11.

Treatment of Adverse Effects. As for Phenformin Hydrochloride, p.857.

Precautions. As for Phenformin Hydrochloride, p.857.

Abnormally low absorption of vitamin B_{12} occurred in 21 of 71 diabetic patients receiving metformin for more than 2 years, and haemoglobin concentrations were also significantly lower in these patients. After stopping metformin for 7 to 28 days absorption became normal in 6 of 7 patients. All patients receiving long-term metformin therapy should have estimations of serum vitamin B_{12} annually.— G. H. Tomkin *et al.*, *Br. med. J.*, 1971, *2*, 685.

Megaloblastic anaemia due to vitamin B_{12} malabsorption in a 58-year-old woman was associated with long-term treatment with metformin.— T. S. Callaghan *et al.*, *Br. med. J.*, 1980, *280*, 1214.

Absorption and Fate. Metformin hydrochloride is incompletely absorbed from the gastro-intestinal tract and is excreted, unchanged, in the urine.

The mean half-life of metformin after intravenous administration to 5 healthy subjects was 1.52 hours. After administration by mouth 37.6% of a dose was recovered in the urine after 48 hours. Metformin was not protein-bound in plasma or metabolised.— C. R. Sirtori *et al.*, *Clin. Pharmac. Ther.*, 1978, *24*, 683.

About 90% of a dose of metformin 1.5 g given to a healthy subject was eliminated unchanged over 8 days. Half appeared in the urine and half in the faeces.— M. S. Lennard *et al.* (letter), *Br. J. clin. Pharmac.*, 1978, *6*, 183.

Metformin kinetics in healthy subjects and in patients with diabetes mellitus.— G. T. Tucker *et al.*, *Br. J. clin. Pharmac.*, 1981, *12*, 235.

Further references: C. Casey *et al.*, *Br. J. clin. Pharmac.*, 1979, *8*, 382P; P. J. Pentikäinen *et al.*, *Eur. J. clin. Pharmac.*, 1979, *16*, 195; C. G. Swift *et al.*, *Br. J. clin. Pharmac.*, 1979, *8*, 406P.

Uses. Metformin hydrochloride is a biguanide with actions and uses similar to those of phenformin hydrochloride (see p.858).

The initial dose is 500 mg thrice daily or 850 mg twice daily with meals, gradually increased if necessary to a maximum of 3 g daily.

It may be given concomitantly with a sulphonylurea.

Glucose tolerance in 6 slightly obese patients with diabetes was markedly improved during treatment with metformin 2 g daily for 10 days; the decrease of plasma-glucagon concentration after glucose ingestion was not affected by metformin, but the usual peak concentrations of growth hormone and cortisol were significantly lower.— D. Giugliano *et al.*, *Farmaco, Edn prat.*, 1979, *34*, 32. See also L. Hausmann and R. Schubotz, *Arzneimittel-Forsch.*, 1975, *25*, 668.

Diabetes mellitus. A 47-year-old woman in whom phenformin induced lactic acid acidosis was able to substitute metformin with no recurrence of this condition.— A. M. Tomkins *et al.*, *Postgrad. med. J.*, 1972, *48*, 386.

In a study in 189 patients with non-obese maturity-onset diabetes mellitus of recent onset, not controlled by diet alone, diabetic control was comparable in those treated with metformin or chlorpropamide for a year. The mean respective doses were 2 g (range 1 to 3 g) and 284 mg (range 100 to 375 mg) daily. Patients aged 40 to 59 years lost a mean of 2.1 kg body-weight on metformin or gained a mean of 3.6 kg on chlorpropamide; there was a similar difference in older patients. At the end of a year 61 patients were crossed to the other drug with continued satisfactory control. Side-effects with metformin were not a major problem if a small dose was given initially. For patients under weight and with severe symptoms a sulphonylurea was indicated; for patients near correct weight at risk of hypoglycaemia or hypersensitivity metformin might be preferred.— B. F. Clarke and I. W. Campbell, *Br. med. J.*, 1977, *2*, 1576.

Metformin as a single daily dose was as effective as divided doses in reduction of blood-glucose concentrations in 45 obese diabetics.— G. M. Shenfield *et al.*, *Practitioner*, 1977, *219*, 745.

Following biguanide withdrawal from 118 subjects with maturity-onset diabetes, taking biguanides either alone or in association with sulphonylureas, the mean fasting blood-glucose concentration and the mean urinary-glucose excretion both increased. There were no changes in blood lipid concentrations or in body-weight. These results indicate that biguanides effectively lower blood-glucose concentrations in most patients with maturity-onset diabetes. The hypoglycaemic effect does not depend on body-weight, fasting blood-glucose concentration, or duration of diabetes or of biguanide treatment. Although there was a progressive decrease in the systolic and diastolic blood pressures of the patients after withdrawal, these findings should be interpreted with caution, and unless further evidence on the cardiovascular risks of biguanides is presented, it appears that metformin, which has been reported to be associated with a relatively small risk of lactic acidosis, can still be a useful adjunct to the treatment of maturity-onset diabetes inadequately controlled by dietary regimen and sulphonylureas.— O. Siitonen *et al.*, *Lancet*, 1980, *1*, 217.

Pregnancy and the neonate. Use of metformin in pregnancy.— E. J. Coetzee and W. P. U. Jackson, *Diabetologia*, 1979, *16*, 241.

Fibrinolytic effects. Increased fibrinolysis associated with metformin: G. R. Fearnley *et al.*, *Lancet*, 1968, *2*, 1004.

A comparison of serum-cholesterol concentrations in patients taking a sulphonylurea or metformin.— G. M. Shenfield *et al.*, *Practitioner*, 1979, *222*, 111.

Preparations

Metformin Tablets *(B.P.)*. Tablets containing metformin hydrochloride; they may be film-coated. The *B.P.* requires 70% dissolution in 45 minutes.

Glucophage *(Rona, UK)*. Metformin hydrochloride, available as tablets of 500 and 850 mg. (Also available as Glucophage in *Austral., Belg., Canad., Denm., Fr., Ger., Ital., Neth., Norw., S.Afr., Swed., Switz.*).

Other Proprietary Names

Diaberit, Diabetosan, Glucadal, Mellitin, Metiguanide *(all Ital.)*; Diabex SR *(Austral.)*; Glufagos *(Spain)*; Islotin *(Arg.)*; Orabet *(Denm.)*; Stagid (as embonate) *(Fr.)*.

Metformin hydrochloride was also formerly marketed in Great Britain under the proprietary name Metiguanide (*Farmitalia Carlo Erba*).

7232-k

Phenformin Hydrochloride *(B.P.)*.

Fenformina Cloridrato; Phenethylbiguanide Hydrochloride. 1-Phenethylbiguanide hydrochloride.

$C_{10}H_{15}N_5,HCl = 241.7$.

CAS — 114-86-3 (phenformin); 834-28-6 (hydrochloride).

Pharmacopoeias. In *Br., Braz.*, and *Nord.*

A white or almost white, odourless, crystalline powder with a bitter taste. M.p. 176° to 179°. **Soluble** 1 in 8 of water and 1 in 15 of alcohol; practically insoluble in chloroform, ether, and light petroleum. A 2.5% solution in water has a pH of 6 to 7.

Adverse Effects. Anorexia, nausea, vomiting, and diarrhoea, are not uncommon; occasionally, a metallic taste, loss of weight, weakness, lassitude, or skin rashes may occur.

Lactic acidosis, possibly heralded by vomiting, abdominal pain, hyperventilation, and diminished consciousness, may occur. An increase in the anion gap (see p.618) not accounted for by uraemia, ketonaemia, or salicylate poisoning, is highly suggestive of lactic acidosis; the mortality-rate is about 50%.

Recurrent acute pancreatitis occurred in a patient with maturity-onset diabetes controlled by insulin and phenformin 50 mg twice daily.— H. Wilde (letter), *Ann. intern. Med.*, 1972, *77*, 324. See also H. S. Chase and G. R. Mogan, *Ann. intern. Med.*, 1977, *87*, 314.

Cardiovascular effects. Studies in patients with maturity-onset diabetes showed that treatment with phenformin 100 mg daily was no more effective in reducing cardiovascular complications than diet alone or diet with insulin therapy. Mortality from all causes and from cardiovascular causes was higher in the phenformin group than in the other groups and the use of phenformin in the trial had been stopped.— G. L. Knatterud *et al.*, *University Group Diabetes Program*, *J. Am. med. Ass.*, 1971, *217*, 777. Criticism.— H. S. Seltzer (letter), *ibid.*, 594. Comment.— *Med. Lett.*, 1972, *14*, 1. In follow-up of 160 patients treated with phenformin mean initial systolic blood pressure of 138 mmHg rose over a period of about 5½ years to a mean of 148.7 mmHg. Mean diastolic pressure rose over the same period from 82.1 to 85.1 mmHg. The percentage of patients becoming hypertensive during the study was greater in those treated with phenformin than in the other treatment groups. Mean heart-rate rose from 68.2 to 75.7 beats per minute.—University Group Diabetes Program, *Diabetes*, 1975, *24*, *Suppl.* I, 65. The evidence was not strong enough to warrant abandoning the use of phenformin in appropriate cases.— *Br. med. J.*, 1975, *3*, 724. Comment on the accuracy of the data.— G. Dunea, *ibid.*, 1978, *2*, 1215.

There was no difference in the mortality-rates during a 5-year study of 83 patients aged between 25 and 50 years who had recently had a myocardial infarction and were given continuous phenformin treatment together with a controlled diet and of 54 similar patients given only the diet.— M. Tzagournis and R. Reynertson, *Ann. intern. Med.*, 1972, *76*, 587.

Further references: N. W. Rodger, *Can. med. Ass. J.*, 1976, *115*, 379; P. Biron, *ibid.*, 380.

For the Report of the Committee for the Assessment of Biometric Aspects of Controlled Trials of Hypoglycaemic Agents, see Tolbutamide (p.859).

Lactic acidosis. Reviews and discussions.— R. I. Misbin, *Ann. intern. Med.*, 1977, *87*, 591; *Br. med. J.*, 1977, *2*, 1436; R. D. Cohen, *Topics Ther.*, 1978, *4*, 191; R. D. Cohen, *Adverse Drug React. Bull.*, 1978, June, 248; R. D. Cohen, *Br. J. Hosp. Med.*, 1980, *23*, 577.

Of 8 patients who died from phenformin-induced lactic acidosis 6 were in coma when admitted to hospital; in none of the 8 had the correct diagnosis been considered before admission. One patient had impaired renal function before phenformin had been commenced and intermittent proteinuria and diabetic retinopathy was suggestive of nephropathy in another. Five had hypertension (controlled in 3) before phenformin was given and one became hypertensive. Regular screening was not practicable and phenformin should no longer be used in the treatment of diabetes.— E. A. M. Gale and R. B. Tattersall, *Br. med. J.*, 1976, *2*, 972.

The Swedish Adverse Drug Reaction Committee had received 50 reports (assessed as 'probable' or 'not excluded') of lactic acidosis associated with the use of phenformin in the period 1965–77; there were 19 fatalities. One similar report had been received in respect of metformin. During the period 1975–77, when the usage of the 2 drugs was comparable, there had been 13 reports of lactic acidosis (6 fatal) in respect of phenformin and one report in respect of metformin.— U. Bergman *et al.*, *Br. med. J.*, 1978, *2*, 464.

Twenty-four patients with biguanide-induced lactic acidosis were reported to the Adverse Drug Reaction Register of the Finnish National Board of Health from 1974 to 1977. Of them 23 had received phenformin and 1 metformin.— T. Korhonen *et al.*, *Eur. J. clin. Pharmac.*, 1979, *15*, 407.

Further references: P. J. Phillips *et al.* (letter), *Br. med. J.*, 1977, *1*, 234; L. A. Conlay and J. E. Lowenstein, *Ann. intern. Med.*, 1977, *87*, 312; C. G. Berbatis *et al.*, *Aust. J. Hosp. Pharm.*, 1978, *8*, 60; M. Nattrass and K. G. M. M. Alberti, *Diabetologia*, 1978, *14*, 71; D. Luft *et al.*, *ibid.*, 75; A. Czyzyk *et al.*, *ibid.*, 89; A. K. Waters *et al.*, *ibid.*, 95.

For earlier references to phenformin-induced lactic acidosis, see Martindale 27th Edn, p. 816.

Overdosage. Following the ingestion of about thirty 50-mg sustained-release capsules of phenformin, a 44-year-old woman developed nausea and vomiting and became unconscious. The blood-glucose concentration 24 hours after ingestion was less than 250 µg per ml. Despite an improvement in her condition after intravenous injection of dextrose 50%, severe acidosis was confirmed and only partly responded to 1250 mmol (1250 mEq) of bicarbonate. Pulmonary oedema subsequently developed and the patient died 30 hours after ingestion of phenformin. The liver was found to contain 8% of the administered dose. The blood-phenformin concentration at necropsy was 3 µg per ml.— J. P. Bingle *et al.*, *Br. med. J.*, 1970, *3*, 752. See also M. B. Davidson *et al.*, *New Engl. J. Med.*, 1966, *275*, 886.

A 30-year-old man who had taken phenformin 300 to 400 mg daily as sustained-release capsules for 6 months (2 to 2.5 times the maximum recommended dose) experienced massive haematemesis consequent on anorexia, loss of weight, and low epigastric pain. He was treated with blood transfusions, phenformin was withdrawn, and insulin started. After 5.5 weeks, he was well, free from gastric pain, and had gained 6.1 kg in weight. His symptoms were attributed to phenformin overdosage.— N. R. T. Pashley and R. H. Felix (letter), *Br. med. J.*, 1972, *1*, 112.

Treatment of Adverse Effects. In the treatment of lactic acidosis sodium bicarbonate (not lactate) is given promptly by infusion to correct the acidosis; it may be necessary to give diuretics to avoid sodium overload. Insulin has been given, with dextrose; while there have been favourable reports the rationale is not universally accepted. Such treatment will however relieve associated ketonaemia. There have been reports of the successful use of peritoneal dialysis or haemodialysis.

Of 18 diabetic patients with lactic acidosis 15 had received phenformin, 10 had renal impairment, 8 had liver disease, and 12 died. Those who recovered had received large doses of sodium bicarbonate, blood, frusemide and/or peritoneal dialysis, and insulin in moderate doses of 20 to 100 units.— R. Assan *et al.*, *Diabetes*, 1975, *24*, 791.

Six diabetic patients with phenformin-induced lactic acidosis were successfully treated by haemodialysis.— P. -H. Althoff *et al.*, *Dt. med. Wschr.*, 1978, *103*, 61.

For the use of dichloroacetate in lactic acidosis, see Sodium Dichloroacetate, p.1754.

Precautions. Phenformin hydrochloride should not be given to patients with impaired hepatic or renal function, cardiovascular collapse, congestive heart failure, acute myocardial infarction, or other conditions leading to hypotension or to hypoxaemia. It should not be given to patients with diabetes mellitus complicated by acidosis, infection, or gangrene, or during surgery or pregnancy.

Alcohol should be avoided by patients being treated with phenformin.

Of 24 patients who had taken phenformin for not less than 3 years in a mean dose of 102.4 mg [daily], 11 had impaired absorption of vitamin B_{12} though serum concentrations of vitamin B_{12} were not affected. Similar malabsorption with reduced serum concentrations of vitamin B_{12} had been reported (G.H. Tomkin *et al.*, *Br. med. J.*, 1971, *2*, 685). Reduced absorption of vitamin B_{12} might be related to the reported mode of action of biguanides in reducing the absorption of glucose. It was recommended that patients on long-term treatment with phenformin or metformin should have serum concentrations of vitamin B_{12} checked annually.— G. H. Tomkin, *Br. med. J.*, 1973, *3*, 673.

Precipitation of phenformin-induced lactic acidosis by tetracycline in a 76-year-old patient.— A. Aro *et al.*, *Lancet*, 1978, *1*, 673. See also C. K. Tashima (letter), *Br. med. J.*, 1971, *4*, 557.

For a report of haematuria and increased fibrinolysis in a patient given warfarin and phenformin, see Warfarin Sodium, p.779.

Absorption and Fate. Phenformin hydrochloride is readily absorbed from the gastro-intestinal tract and is excreted, partly metabolised, in the urine within about 24 hours.

About a third of a dose of phenformin was metabolised to hydroxyphenethylbiguanide.— R. Beckmann, *Ann. N.Y. Acad. Sci.*, 1968, *148*, 820, per G. H. Tomkin, *Br. med. J.*, 1973, *3*, 673.

Studies on the urinary disposition of phenformin and its metabolite, 4-hydroxyphenformin, in 1 healthy subject indicated the existence of a significant first-pass effect.— N. S. Oates *et al.*, *J. Pharm. Pharmac.*, 1980, *32*, 731.

Evidence of genetic polymorphism in the metabolism of phenformin.— R. R. Shah *et al.* (letter), *Lancet*, 1980, *1*, 1147.

Data suggesting that impaired ability to hydroxylate phenformin may be only one among several factors involved in the development of lactic acidosis during phenformin treatment.— B. -E. Wiholm *et al.* (letter), *Lancet*, 1981, *1*, 1098.

Further references: H. Mehnert, *Acta diabetol. latin.*, 1969, *6*, *Suppl.* 1, 137; D. Alkalay *et al.*, *J. clin. Pharmac.*, 1975, *15*, 446.

Uses. Phenformin hydrochloride is a biguanide derivative which is given by mouth in the treatment of diabetes mellitus. The precise mode of action is not clear. Phenformin is used only in the treatment of maturity-onset diabetes not responsive to diet alone or to diet plus treatment with a sulphonylurea. In some countries it is no longer used. It has no significant hypoglycaemic effect in non-diabetic subjects. It may be used alone or in conjunction with another oral hypoglycaemic agent such as a sulphonylurea or with insulin.

The hypoglycaemic effect of phenformin hydrochloride lasts 4 to 5 hours. It is usually given in initial doses of 25 mg, often as sustained-release capsules, in the morning and evening and this dosage may be increased if necessary by increments of 25 mg at intervals of 2 to 3 days. The daily dose should not generally exceed 100 mg.

During stabilisation on phenformin, the urine must be tested frequently for sugar and ketones and the fasting blood sugar should also be estimated.

Phenformin hydrochloride is reported to enhance fibrinolytic activity.

Diabetes mellitus. For reference to biguanide therapy in diabetes mellitus, see Metformin, p.857.

Fibrinolytic effects. Increased fibrinolysis associated with phenformin usually given with ethyloestrenol: G. R. Fearnley *et al.*, *Lancet*, 1968, *2*, 1004; E. Fiaschi *et al.*, *Arzneimittel-Forsch.*, 1969, *19*, 638; G. R. Fearnley *et al.*, *Lancet*, 1969, *1*, 910; *idem*, 1971, *1*, 723; I. K. Brown *et al.*, *ibid.*, 774.

Behçet's syndrome. A man with Behçet's syndrome featuring deep-vein thrombosis and extensive ulceration, unresponsive to phenindione, was given, in addition, phenformin hydrochloride 50 mg twice daily as a long-acting preparation and ethyloestrenol 2 mg four times daily. Within 4 months, the patient's condition was improved, the ulcers were completely healed, and there were no further pulmonary embolic episodes. His fibrinolytic activity remained normal or greater than normal, and prothrombic activity required no change in phenindione dosage.— W. J. Cunliffe and I. S. Menon, *Lancet*, 1969, *1*, 1239.

The satisfactory treatment of another patient with Behçet's syndrome with phenformin and ethyloestrenol or stanozolol.— W. J. Cunliffe *et al.* (letter), *Br. med. J.*, 1973, *2*, 486.

Malignant atrophic papulosis. A patient with malignant atrophic papulosis treated with phenformin 50 mg twice daily and ethyloestrenol 2 mg four times daily had relief of pruritus within a month and no new lesions appeared. Treatment continued and about a year later the existing lesions were smaller.— T. J. Delaney and M. M. Black, *Br. med. J.*, 1975, *3*, 415.

Myocardial infarction. In a study of 48 patients who had survived a myocardial infarction and were given phenformin 50 mg twice daily in conjunction with ethyloestrenol 4 mg twice daily for 3 years, low fibrinolytic activity was observed in 21 patients which was increased and maintained in 20 by the treatment; plasma-fibrinogen concentrations were reduced in 32. Side-effects including anorexia or nausea in 14, weight-loss and folic acid deficiency in 1, were attributed to phenformin, and sodium retention in about 20 was attributed to ethyloestrenol.— R. Chakrabarti and G. R. Fearnley, *Lancet*, 1972, *2*, 556.

For controversy regarding the cardiovascular effects of phenformin, see under Adverse Effects (above).

Raynaud's syndrome. Four patients who suffered from Raynaud's syndrome in winter became free from symptoms after treatment with sustained-release capsules of phenformin 50 mg twice daily together with ethyloestrenol 4 mg twice daily.— G. R. Fearnley and R. Chakrabarti (letter), *Lancet*, 1969, *2*, 906.

In 22 patients with Raynaud's syndrome, who received phenformin hydrochloride and ethyloestrenol, 1 patient with progressive systemic sclerosis treated for 15 months, showed excellent improvement, and 5 patients treated for up to 4 to 12 months responded satisfactorily. In 9 patients there was no effect after 2 to 4 months and in 7 therapy was stopped because of side-effects which included gastro-intestinal upset, diarrhoea, and amenorrhoea.— I. S. Menon and W. J. Cunliffe (letter), *Lancet*, 1969, *2*, 1135.

Thrombo-embolic disorders. Although phenformin 50 mg given in conjunction with ethyloestrenol 4 mg twice daily had a fibrinolytic action in a study of 95 patients undergoing surgery, the treatment had no effect on the incidence of postoperative deep-vein thrombosis.— D. P. Fossard *et al.*, *Lancet*, 1974, *1*, 9. Surgery increased fibrinogen concentrations.— R. Chakrabarti (letter), *ibid.*, 868.

Further references: I. M. Nilsson *et al.*, *Br. med. J.*, 1974, *4*, 365.

Vasculitis. In a double-blind study 12 patients with cutaneous vasculitis of at least 6 months' duration were treated for 3 months at a time with a placebo, phenformin 50 mg twice daily (as a sustained-release preparation) and ethyloestrenol 2 mg four times daily, or phenformin and stanozolol 5 mg twice daily; 7 showed clinical response during treatment with active medication; this was associated with improvement in impaired fibrinolytic activity. There was no change in the concentration of fibrinogen-fibrin-related antigen.— B. Dodman *et al.*, *Br. med. J.*, 1973, *2*, 82. See also W. J. Cunliffe, *Lancet*, 1968, *1*, 1226.

A 20-year-old woman with a 15-year history of widespread livedo reticularis with painful ulceration obtained relief of pain within a month of starting therapy with phenformin 50 mg and ethyloestrenol 2 mg, each taken 3 times daily; all ulceration disappeared and the reticulated pattern considerably faded after 6 months. A year later the ulcers recurred within a month of discontinuing therapy. Many similar patients had subsequently benefited from this treatment.— R. S. W. Basler and H. E. Jones (letter), *New Engl. J. Med.*, 1978, *298*, 281.

Preparations

Phenformin Tablets *(B.P.)*. Tablets containing phenformin hydrochloride.

Dibotin *(Winthrop, UK)*. Phenformin hydrochloride, available as sustained-release **Capsules** of 25 or 50 mg and as scored **Tablets** of 25 mg.

Other Proprietary Names

DBI *(Arg., Belg.)*; Cronoformin, Diabenide (both *Ital.)*; Dipar *(S.Afr., Spain)*; Glucopostin *(Arg., S.Afr.)*; Insoral *(Austral., S.Afr.)* (see also under Carbutamide); Normoglucina *(Arg.)*.

Phenformin hydrochloride was also formerly marketed in Great Britain under the proprietary names Dipar (*Hoechst*) and Meltrol (*Berk Pharmaceuticals*).

7233-a

Tolazamide *(U.S.P.)*. U 17 835. 1-(Perhydroazepin-1-yl)-3-tosylurea; 1-(Perhydroazepin-1-yl)-3-*p*-tolylsulphonylurea.

$C_{14}H_{21}N_3O_3S=311.4$.

CAS — 1156-19-0.

Pharmacopoeias. In *U.S.*

A white to off-white crystalline powder, odourless or with a slight odour. M.p. 161° to 169° with decomposition. Very slightly **soluble** in water; slightly soluble in alcohol; soluble in acetone; freely soluble in chloroform.

Adverse Effects, Treatment, and Precautions. As for Chlorpropamide, p.852.

Jaundice developed in a 62-year-old man with diabetes within a month of starting tolazamide 500 mg daily.— D. H. Van Thiel *et al.*, *Gastroenterology*, 1974, *67*, 506.

Allergy to tolazamide might induce or activate systemic lupus erythematosus.— D. Alarcón-Segovia, *Drugs*, 1976, *12*, 69.

Pseudoinsulinoma syndrome in a woman who had been taking tolazamide in mistake for tolmetin.— D. A. Ahlquist *et al.*, *Ann. intern. Med.*, 1980, *93*, 281.

Absorption and Fate. Tolazamide is relatively slowly absorbed from the gastro-intestinal tract. Some of its metabolites have hypoglycaemic activity. The biological half-life of tolazamide and its metabolites is about 7 hours. About 85% of a dose is excreted in the urine, chiefly as metabolites.

In a subject given tolazamide 2 g the major urinary metabolite was 1-(hexahydroazepin-1-yl)-3-p-carboxyphenylsulphonylurea.— A. A. Forist and R. W. Judy, *J. Pharm. Pharmac.*, 1974, *26*, 565.

Uses. Tolazamide is a sulphonylurea with actions and uses similar to those of chlorpropamide (see p.853).

The peak effect on the blood-sugar concentration occurs in 4 to 6 hours and lasts for 10 hours or more.

The usual initial dose is 100 to 250 mg daily given as a single dose with breakfast, increased at weekly intervals by 100 to 250 mg if necessary. Doses of 500 mg or more daily may be given in divided doses. Up to 1 g may be given daily. Elderly patients may require smaller doses.

Doses of insulin of more than 40 units should be replaced gradually; the suggested equivalent dose is about 100 mg of tolazamide for 20 units of insulin.

Tolazamide may be given concomitantly with a biguanide.

Tolazamide had no antidiuretic effect but enhanced diuresis after water load in 13 subjects.— A. M. Moses *et al.*, *Ann. intern. Med.*, 1973, *78*, 541.

Diabetes mellitus. References to the use of tolazamide in diabetes mellitus: G. Kanzler *et al.*, *Arzneimittel-Forsch.*, 1968, *18*, 1345; G. Vogel and E. Krummel, *ibid.*, 1969, *19*, 1128; J. R. Turtle, *Br. med. J.*, 1970, *3*, 606; J. Sheldon (letter), *ibid.*, 1970, *4*, 246; M. C. Balodimos and A. Marble, *Curr. ther. Res.*, 1971, *13*, 6.

Preparations

Tolazamide Tablets *(U.S.P.)*. Tablets containing tolazamide. Store in airtight containers.

Tolanase *(Upjohn, UK)*. Tolazamide, available as scored tablets of 100 and 250 mg.

Other Proprietary Names

Diabewas *(Ital., Spain, Switz.)*; Norglycin *(Ger.)*; Tolinase *(Austral., Belg., Neth., Spain, Swed., Switz., USA)*; Tolisan *(Denm.)*.

7234-t

Tolbutamide *(B.P., B.P. Vet., Eur. P., U.S.P.).* Tolbut.; Tolbutamidum; Butamidum; Tolglybutamide; D 860; U 2043. 1-Butyl-3-tosylurea; 1-Butyl-3-*p*-tolylsulphonylurea.
$C_{12}H_{18}N_2O_3S$=270.3.

CAS — 64-77-7.

Pharmacopoeias. In *Arg., Belg., Br., Braz., Chin., Cz., Eur., Fr., Ger., Ind., Int., It., Jap., Jug., Neth., Nord., Pol., Roum., Rus., Swiss, Turk.*, and *U.S.*

A white or almost white, almost odourless, crystalline powder with a slightly bitter taste. M.p. 126° to 132°. Practically **insoluble** in water; soluble 1 in 10 of alcohol and 1 in 3 of acetone; soluble in chloroform, dilute mineral acids, and dilute solutions of alkali hydroxides; slightly soluble in ether.

Stability in tablets. Tolbutamide tablets exposed at a temperature of 70° and 75% relative humidity lost up to 47% of their potency after 45 days. Decomposition products were *p*-toluenesulphonamide and *n*-butylamine.— K. K. Kaistha and W. N. French, *J. pharm. Sci.*, 1968, *57*, 459.

Adverse Effects and Treatment. As for Chlorpropamide, p.852.

Mortality from cardiovascular causes has been reported by the University Group Diabetes Program to be higher in patients receiving tolbutamide than in patients receiving insulin. While this has been accepted by the FDA, the study has been the subject of intense and continued criticism.

Post-mortem findings showed that there was no significant difference in the incidence of myocardial infarction, cerebral vascular accidents, diabetic retinopathy, nephropathy, neoplasms, thyroid disease, or peptic ulcer in 55 diabetic patients who had taken a sulphonylurea compound, usually tolbutamide, for an average of 45.7 months, in 55 patients treated with insulin, and in 19 patients treated with diet alone.— M. C. Balodimos *et al., Diabetes*, 1968, *17*, 503, per *Abstr. Wld Med.*, 1969, *43*, 52.

Reactions to tolbutamide reported to the Committee on Safety of Drugs included 7 cases of rash including eczema and macular erythema, aplastic anaemia (2), jaundice (1), and a syndrome resembling acute systemic lupus erythematosus.— E. L. Harris, *Br. med. J.*, 1971, *3*, 29.

Diffuse lung disease, with eosinophilia, developed in a 59-year-old man given tolbutamide 1 g daily for 18 months; the condition regressed almost completely within 3 weeks when tolbutamide was withdrawn.— G. F. Ascherl *et al., Milit. Med.*, 1976, *141*, 851.

Abuse. Hypoglycaemic coma occurred in a 15-year-old boy following ingestion of 3 tablets of tolbutamide for psychotropic effect.— D. R. Miller *et al.* (letter), *New Engl. J. Med.*, 1977, *297*, 339.

Blood disorders. Reports of pancytopenia associated with tolbutamide I. Chapman and Wan Ho Cheung, *J. Am. med. Ass.*, 1963, *186*, 595; K. J. Traumann, *Dt. med. Wschr.*, 1975, *100*, 250, per *J. Am. med. Ass.*, 1975, *232*, 873.

Tolbutamide-induced haemolytic anaemia.— P. Malacarne *et al., Diabetes*, 1977, *26*, 156. See also G. J. Pavlic, *J. Am. med. Ass.*, 1966, *197*, 57; G. W. G. Bird *et al., Br. med. J.*, 1972, *1*, 728.

Cardiovascular effects. Of 270 survivors from a first acute cardiac infarction 178, free from overt diabetes, were studied for 12 to 66 months (mean 3 years) while taking tolbutamide up to 1 g daily (95 patients) or a placebo (83). There were 13 deaths in the tolbutamide group and 16 in the placebo group; in the first 18 months mortality was significantly reduced in the tolbutamide group—7 and 15 respectively; the mean survival-time was 6 months for those of the placebo group who died and 18 months for those of the tolbutamide group. In 27 of the 29 fatalities death was associated with supraventricular ectopic beats, atrial fibrillation, or treatment with digitalis.— J. Paasikivi, *Acta med. scand.*, 1970, *Suppl.*, 507.

In a long-term double-blind study 823 patients with newly diagnosed diabetes mellitus, free from cardiovascular disease limiting life expectancy to less than 5 years, were treated with insulin in standard or varying dosage, tolbutamide, or a placebo; 654 had completed 5 years of follow-up. Poor blood-glucose control was achieved in 28.3%, 11.6%, 25.6%, and 40.7% respectively. The most uniform control was achieved with the variable insulin dose. There was no significant difference in the incidence of non-fatal events or overall deaths, but the incidence of deaths from cardiovascular causes was significantly greater with tolbutamide than with the other groups. The percentage of deaths from cardiovascular causes in the tolbutamide group remained higher when analysed for groups with or without risk factors, and treatment with tolbutamide was discontinued. Oral hypoglycaemic agents should be used with more caution than in the past—when serious dieting had not afforded control and when the patient was unwilling or unable to administer insulin.—University Group Diabetes Program, *J. Am. med. Ass.*, 1971, *218*, 1400. Criticism.— *Lancet*, 1971, *1*, 171; W. E. Herrell, *Clin. Med.*, 1971, *78* (June), 13; H. S. Seltzer (letter), *J. Am. med. Ass.*, 1971, *218*, 594. The FDA recommended that the use of tolbutamide and the other sulphonylurea type agents, acetohexamide, chlorpropamide, and tolazamide, should be limited to those patients with symptomatic adult-onset non-ketotic diabetes mellitus which could not be adequately controlled by diet or weight loss alone and in whom the addition of insulin was impractical or unacceptable. The oral hypoglycaemic agents were not recommended in the treatment of chemical or latent diabetes, in suspected diabetes, or in pre-diabetes, and were contra-indicated in patients with keto-acidosis.— *J. Am. med. Ass.*, 1971, *215*, 108. The Committee on Safety of Drugs would not ban the use of tolbutamide and other oral antidiabetic drugs at present, even though the FDA had indicated that the number of deaths from cardiovascular disease was significantly greater in patients treated with tolbutamide.— *Lancet*, 1971, *1*, 171. The Biometric Society had been charged by the National Institutes of Health to assess the UGDP and other controlled trials of oral hypoglycaemic drugs. Only the UGDP study and the Bedford study (*Acta diabetol. latin.*, 1971, *8*, *Suppl.* 1, 444) provided sufficient mortality data for evaluation. The Bedford study claimed no greater death-rate for those taking tolbutamide and a protective effect for those with mild or moderate disease; adjustment of the data for variables did not alter the basic conclusion that death-rates did not differ significantly. Criticisms which had been made of the UGDP study were not generally such as to invalidate the conclusions. The omission of a history of smoking was regrettable. A difference in death-rate remained after adjustment for variables. Fresh statistical analysis showed an excess mortality, both cardiovascular and total, for women; the data did not support that conclusion for men, possibly because of the smaller numbers. Suspicions of mortality due to tolbutamide and phenformin raised by the UGDP could not be dismissed.—Report of the Committee for the Assessment of Biometric Aspects of Controlled Trials of Hypoglycaemic Agents, *J. Am. med. Ass.*, 1975, *231*, 583. Comment.— *ibid.*, 624; *Lancet*, 1975, *2*, 489. A committee of 9 experts in diabetes appointed by the Canadian Diabetic Association unanimously agreed that the data provided by the University Group Diabetes Program, re-assessed by the Biometric Society, did not provide sufficient evidence to consider tolbutamide harmful if used in proper doses in suitably selected patients.— A. M. Fisher (letter), *Can. med. Ass. J.*, 1975, *113*, 364. An FDA team completed an audit of the UGDP study. While there were errors and discrepancies between the data file and the published reports, these did not invalidate the findings of increased cardiovascular mortality in the tolbutamide and phenformin groups.— *FDA Drug Bull.*, 1978, *8*, 34.

In a retrospective study covering 1958–70, the incidence of myocardial infarctions in 670 female patients with maturity-onset diabetes was 1.52 per 100 patient-years for those treated by diet, 2.14 per 100 patient-years for those treated with insulin, and 3.06 per 100 patient-years for those given oral antidiabetic treatment. The incidence of deaths from cerebrovascular accidents was 1.07, 2.01, and 1.81 respectively.— D. R. Hadden *et al., Lancet*, 1972, *1*, 335.

In a prospective study of 186 male and female patients from the time of diagnosis of maturity-onset diabetes in 1965 to 1971, the incidence of myocardial infarctions of 19.7% (14 of 71) in those given oral antidiabetic treatment was significantly greater than the incidence of 9.5% (11 of 115) in those treated by diet.— D. Boyle *et al., Lancet*, 1972, *1*, 338. Comment.— R. J. Jarrett and H. Keen (letter), *ibid.*, 492; P. A. Nicholson (letter), *ibid.*, 632.

In a study of 184 diabetic patients with myocardial infarctions admitted to coronary-care units, there were no deaths in the 27 patients whose diabetes was mild enough to be controlled by diet alone compared with 21 deaths in 90 patients receiving oral hypoglycaemic agents and 12 deaths in 67 receiving insulin. After 5 days the patients were transferred to the wards and during the next 25 days the mortalities increased to 4 of the 27 patients treated by diet, 36 of the 90 on oral hypoglycaemics, and 25 of the 67 on insulin. Primary ventricular fibrillation occurred in 12% of the patients receiving oral hypoglycaemics compared with 3% of those on insulin.— N. G. Soler *et al., Lancet*, 1974, *1*, 475.

Further references: *Drug & Ther. Bull.*, 1977, *15*, 37; S.-W. Shen and R. Bressler, *New Engl. J. Med.*, 1977, *296*, 787; *J. Am. med. Ass.*, 1979, *241*, 17; C. Kilo *et al., J. Am. med. Ass.*, 1980, *243*, 450; A. M. Sackler, *J. Am. med. Ass.*, 1980, *243*, 1435.

Effects on electrolytes. Reports of hyponatraemia associated with the use of tolbutamide.— V. V. Gossain *et al., Postgrad. med. J.*, 1976, *52*, 720; B. A. Darlow, *Postgrad. med. J.*, 1977, *53*, 223.

Effects on the liver. A 48-year-old woman developed jaundice during treatment with tolbutamide. Treatment with tolbutamide was continued for 12 months and the patient died. Post-mortem examination showed cholestasis, cholangiolitis, and cholangitis.— D. H. Gregory *et al., Archs Path.*, 1967, *84*, 194, per *J. Am. med. Ass.*, 1967, *201* (Aug. 14), A175.

A 69-year-old man who had taken tolbutamide 500 mg daily for 4 years was given thioridazine for 3 days, then pethidine and dexamphetamine 5 times in a 2-week period. Three days later he developed jaundice which regressed when tolbutamide was withdrawn and recurred when tolbutamide was again given.— J. V. Ananth *et al.* (letter), *Can. med. Ass. J.*, 1970, *103*, 1194.

Hypothyroidism. An elderly diabetic gradually developed signs of hypothyroidism during treatment with tolbutamide 500 mg daily. When treatment with tolbutamide was replaced by insulin the patient's general condition improved and signs of hypothyroidism disappeared.— J. Scharf *et al.* (letter), *Lancet*, 1968, *1*, 250. Other similar reports: C. D. Burda (letter), *ibid.*, 1965, *2*, 1016; G. L. Schless (letter), *J. Am. med. Ass.*, 1966, *195*, 1073.

Of 200 diabetic patients who had been treated with tolbutamide for 1 to 7 years none was clinically hypothyroid but 3% had thyroid hypofunction. The hypothyroidism did not appear to be related to the length of treatment with tolbutamide.— I. Portioli and F. Rocchi (letter), *Lancet*, 1969, *1*, 681.

Overdosage. Tolbutamide 25 to 30 g was taken by a non-diabetic woman with suicidal intent. Hypoglycaemic coma occurred with permanent brain damage and death 5 months later.— J. Lazner, *Med. J. Aust.*, 1970, *1*, 327.

Pregnancy and the neonate. A 16-year-old diabetic girl who had taken tolbutamide 500 mg daily for 16 months gave birth to a child with multiple congenital deformities. The possibility of tolbutamide having a teratogenic effect could not be excluded and the avoidance of sulphonylurea administration during pregnancy was advocated.— Y. Larsson and G. Sterky, *Lancet*, 1960, *2*, 1424.

Treatment with tolbutamide was successful in controlling diabetes in 74 of 97 pregnant women. The incidence of foetal and neonatal loss (7.2%) and of congenital defects (3.1%) were comparable with the incidence in diabetics generally.— H. Dolger *et al., J. Mt Sinai Hosp.*, 1969, *36*, 471, per *J. Am. med. Ass.*, 1970, *211*, 531.

Precautions. As for Chlorpropamide, p.852.

Tolbutamide had been reported to aggravate porphyria.— *Br. med. J.*, 1972, *3*, 603.

Interactions. Acute administration of *alcohol* was reported to increase the half-life of tolbutamide, while chronic administration reduced the half-life.— E. M. Sellers and M. R. Holloway, *Clin. Pharmacokinet.*, 1978, *3*, 440.

Absence of effect. Absence of effect of *sulindac* on tolbutamide.— J. R. Ryan *et al., Clin. Pharmac. Ther.*, 1977, *21*, 231.

Absence of effect of *naproxen* on tolbutamide.— G. Sachse *et al., Arzneimittel-Forsch.*, 1979, *29*, 835.

Absence of significant effect of *naproxen* on blood glucose or on tolbutamide pharmacokinetics in healthy subjects.— B. Whiting *et al., Br. J. clin. Pharmac.*, 1981, *11*, 295.

Diminished effect. The fall in blood-glucose concentration was significantly reduced when *propranolol* 150 µg per kg body-weight was injected intravenously 5 minutes before the injection of 1 g of tolbutamide in 11 healthy fasting subjects. This might be due to beta-receptor blockade in the granules of the β-cells of the islets of Langerhans or to a decreased splanchnic blood flow reducing the access to the pancreas of the tolbutamide.— O. de Divitiis *et al.* (letter), *Lancet*, 1968, *1*, 749.

An African patient with diabetes mellitus, controlled satisfactorily by tolbutamide 1 g thrice daily, had a paradoxical elevated blood-sugar concentration when she was also given phenylbutazone for 1 week; blood sugar did not return to normal for 16 weeks. A similar effect was noted in 2 other patients.— S. K. Owusu and K. Ocran (letter), *Lancet*, 1972, *1*, 440.

Serum concentrations of tolbutamide were decreased by 49% and the half-life by 43% in 16 patients also given *rifampicin*.— E. K. G. Syvälahti *et al.* (letter), *Lancet*, 1974, *2*, 232.

Chlorpromazine and *phenytoin* each might reduce the antidiabetic effect of tolbutamide due to enzyme induction.— R. M. Pearson and C. W. H. Havard, *Br. J. Hosp. Med.*, 1974, *12*, 812.

For the effect of tolbutamide on phenytoin, see p.1240.

Enhanced effect. Hypoglycaemia occurred in 3 diabetic patients controlled with tolbutamide when *sulphaphenazole* was given concomitantly. Clinical experiments showed that a 2-g daily dose of sulphaphenazole caused a threefold to fivefold increase in the serum concentrations of tolbutamide. The half-life of tolbutamide in the blood also rose from 4 to 17 hours.— L. K. Christensen *et al.*, *Lancet*, 1963, *2*, 1298.

Two patients taking tolbutamide developed hypoglycaemia when given *sulphafurazole* in addition; the outcome was fatal in 1 patient. One of the patients was also given chloramphenicol and the patient who died had chronic uraemia.— J. S. Soeldner and J. Steinke, *J. Am. med. Ass.*, 1965, *193*, 398. In 4 healthy volunteers the half-life of tolbutamide was increased fivefold to sixfold when *sulphaphenazole* was given concomitantly. No similar effect occurred after the administration of sulfadoxine, sulphadimethoxine, sulphafurazole, or sulphamethoxazole.— U. C. Dubach *et al.*, *Schweiz. med. Wschr.*, 1966, *96*, 1483, per *Abstr. Wld Med.*, 1967, *41*, 215.

In 8 healthy volunteers the half-life of tolbutamide after an intravenous dose of 1 g was increased from 4.9 hours to 17.5 hours after treatment for a week with *dicoumarol*. In 4 diabetic patients taking 500 mg of tolbutamide daily, the plasma concentration of tolbutamide was increased and the hypoglycaemic effect enhanced when dicoumarol was given concomitantly. No enhancement of hypoglycaemic effect occurred when 2 volunteers and 3 patients were given phenindione.— M. Kristensen and J. M. Hansen, *Diabetes*, 1967, *16*, 211, per *Abstr. Wld Med.*, 1967, *41*, 879.

In healthy volunteers the half-life of tolbutamide after intravenous injection was increased from about 7 hours to 18 hours after treatment with *phenyramidol* and to 24 hours after treatment with *dicoumarol*. Phenyramidol and dicoumarol inhibited enzymatic metabolism of tolbutamide in the liver.— H. M. Solomon and J. J. Schrogie, *Metabolism*, 1967, *16*, 1029, per *J. Am. med. Ass.*, 1968, *203* (Jan. 8), A214.

Since *salicylic acid, phenylbutazone, ethionamide*, and *aminosalicylic acid* lowered blood-sugar concentrations they were associated with severe hypoglycaemic reactions in patients being treated with sulphonylureas, including tolbutamide.— E. Schulz, *Arch. klin. Med.*, 1968, *214*, 135.

In patients taking tolbutamide 500 mg thrice daily the administration of *chloramphenicol* 2 g daily caused a twofold rise in the concentration of tolbutamide in serum, and the half-life of tolbutamide was prolonged. Chloramphenicol, 3 g and 1.5 g intravenously, prolonged the half-life of tolbutamide from 5 to 8¾ hours and from 4¾ to 7 hours respectively.— L. K. Christensen and L. Skovsted, *Lancet*, 1969, *2*, 1397. See also J. M. Hansen and M. Kristensen, *Dan. med. Bull.*, 1965, *12*, 181.

In 4 patients the half-life of tolbutamide was increased from 3.75 hours to 22 hours when *sulphaphenazole* was given concomitantly; in 5 patients it was increased from 4.75 hours to 37.5 hours or 32.75 hours when the methyl and ethyl derivatives respectively were given concomitantly. *Sulphadiazine* caused a slight increase from 3.5 hours to 5.5 hours in tolbutamide half-life in 4 patients; and *sulphadimethoxine* caused a reduction in half-life from 5 hours to 2.75 hours in 5 patients. *Sulphafurazole* and *sulphamethoxypyridazine* had no effect. *Phenylbutazone* caused an increase in tolbutamide half-life from 4.5 to 10.5 hours in 6 healthy subjects and *oxyphenbutazone* caused an increase in half-life from 4.75 hours to 12 hours in 5 subjects. *Dicoumarol* caused an increase in half-life from 5 hours to 17.5 hours in 8 subjects, and had caused hypoglycaemic coma. *Phenindione* had no effect.— M. Kristensen and L. K. Christensen, *Acta diabetol. latin.*, 1969, *6*, *Suppl.* 1, 116.

Severe hypoglycaemia was precipitated in 2 patients taking tolbutamide when *phenylbutazone* was given concomitantly.— E. L. Harris, *Br. med. J.*, 1971, *3*, 29. See also L. A. Dent and S. G. Jue, *Drug Intell. & clin. Pharm.*, 1976, *10*, 711.

In 8 patients with maturity-onset diabetes *methysergide maleate* 2 mg six-hourly for 8 doses had no effect on the plasma-glucose response to tolbutamide 1 g intravenously but the plasma-insulin response was increased by a mean of 39.3%.— J. A. Baldridge *et al.*, *Diabetes*, 1974, *23*, 21.

Studies in 4 diabetics indicated that *phenylbutazone* interacted with tolbutamide to reduce its urinary excretion.— K. -F. Ober, *Eur. J. clin. Pharmac.*, 1974, *7*, 291. See also J. M. Hansen *et al.*, *Lancet*, 1966, *2*, 265.

Sulphamethizole appeared to inhibit the hepatic metabolism of tolbutamide.— B. Lumholtz *et al.*, *Clin. Pharmac. Ther.*, 1975, *17*, 731.

In a placebo-controlled trial the hypoglycaemic effect of tolbutamide was enhanced in 6 volunteers previously given *halofenate* 1 g daily for 12 days. Six of 9 diabetic patients controlled with sulphonylureas with or without phenformin required a reduction in dose of these drugs when they were also taking halofenate; 2 patients on insulin and 2 on carbohydrate-controlled diets were not affected by halofenate.— A. K. Jain *et al.*, *New Engl. J. Med.*, 1975, *293*, 1283.

In 6 previously untreated patients with mild clinical diabetes the hypoglycaemic response to 1 g of tolbutamide intravenously was enhanced after 7 days of treatment with clofibrate.— C. Ferrari *et al.* (letter), *New Engl. J. Med.*, 1976, *294*, 1184.

The half-life of tolbutamide in healthy subjects was increased significantly by the administration of *sulphaphenazole, phenylbutazone*, or *oxyphenbutazone* for up to 7 days in 2, 8, and 2 patients respectively.— S. M. Pond *et al.*, *Clin. Pharmac. Ther.*, 1977, *22*, 573.

Mean fasting plasma-glucose concentrations were significantly reduced in 3 diabetic patients taking tolbutamide (1 was also taking phenformin) when given halofenate 0.5 to 1.5 g [daily] for 48 to 96 weeks.— E. B. Feldman *et al.*, *J. clin. Pharmac.*, 1978, *18*, 241.

In 10 patients the mean half-life of tolbutamide, after a 3-g dose, was significantly increased from 7.18 to 8.87 hours when *methyldopa* 1 g daily was given for 7 days.— B. Gachályi *et al.*, *Int. J. clin. Pharmac.*, 1980, *18*, 133.

Hypoglycaemia in a woman given *azapropazone* in addition to her tolbutamide therapy.— P. B. Andreasen *et al.*, *Br. J. clin. Pharmac.*, 1981, *12*, 581.

Absorption and Fate. Tolbutamide is readily absorbed from the gastro-intestinal tract and is extensively bound to plasma proteins. Tolbutamide is metabolised in the liver and the metabolites, chiefly 1-butyl-3-*p*-carboxyphenylsulphonylurea, are excreted in the urine; up to 75% of a dose is recovered in 24 hours.

Tolbutamide 12 mg per kg body-weight by intravenous infusion was eliminated more quickly (half-life 2.2 to 5 hours) in 9 patients with acute hepatitis than in 10 otherwise healthy patients (half-life about 7 hours). In 3 patients, tolbutamide was eliminated more slowly once symptoms of acute hepatitis had abated. Protein binding of tolbutamide was decreased in 12 patients with jaundice.— H. Held *et al.*, *Arzneimittel-Forsch.*, 1973, *23*, 1801. Despite previous reports, a study in 5 subjects during and again after apparent recovery from viral hepatitis indicated that dosage alterations for tolbutamide and drugs similarly metabolised were not necessary to maintain a constant plasma concentration of unbound drug.— R. L. Williams *et al.*, *Clin. Pharmac. Ther.*, 1977, *21*, 301.

In 9 patients with maturity-onset diabetes, previously untreated, the mean plasma half-life of tolbutamide was 5.7 and 5.3 hours respectively before and after 2 weeks' treatment with tolbutamide 1 to 1.5 g daily.— D. R. Redman *et al.*, *Diabetes*, 1973, *22*, 210, per *J. Am. med. Ass.*, 1973, *224*, 644.

Following administration of tolbutamide 1 g intravenously to 3 male diabetic patients a linear relationship was noted between salivary-tolbutamide and plasma-tolbutamide concentrations.— S. B. Matin *et al.*, *Clin. Pharmac. Ther.*, 1974, *16*, 1052.

Tolbutamide had been found in breast milk and could cause hypoglycaemia in suckling infants.— R. L. Savage, *Adverse Drug React. Bull.*, 1976, Dec., 212.

Studies *in vitro* indicated that the unbound fraction of tolbutamide in elderly subjects (range 61 to 87 years) was increased by about 25% compared to a younger group (range 23 to 57 years).— A. K. Miller *et al.*, *J. pharm. Sci.*, 1978, *67*, 1192.

Uses. Tolbutamide is a sulphonylurea with actions and uses similar to those of chlorpropamide (see p.853).

After a single dose of tolbutamide, the maximum effect on blood-sugar concentrations occurs in about 5 hours and the effect lasts for 8 to 10 hours.

A suggested initial dose of tolbutamide is 3 g on the first day, 2 g on the second day, and 1 g on the third day, or 1 to 1.5 g daily, followed by a maintenance dose which is usually 0.5 to 1.5 g daily but may range from 0.25 to 3 g daily. The total daily dose may be taken either in the morning with breakfast or in divided doses during the day. When given in divided doses, gastric irritation is reduced. Elderly patients may require smaller doses.

If the patient is taking less than 20 units of insulin daily, this may be discontinued when treatment with tolbutamide is started. Larger doses of insulin should be decreased gradually and frequent estimation should be made of sugar and ketones in the urine.

Tolbutamide may be given concomitantly with a biguanide.

Tolbutamide increased the linear growth-rate in patients with achondroplasia.— *J. Am. med. Ass.*, 1973, *226*, 617. Glucose-tolerance tests had been normal in a large number of patients with achondroplasia and there was no reason to believe that tolbutamide would be effective.— R. M. Blizzard and V. A. McKusick (letter), *ibid.*, 1974, *228*, 1368.

Administration in renal failure. The dosage interval of tolbutamide should be increased from 8 hours in normal patients to 12 hours in those with severe renal failure.— P. Sharpstone, *Br. med. J.*, 1977, *2*, 36.

Tolbutamide could be given in usual doses to patients with renal failure. Concentrations of tolbutamide were not affected by haemodialysis.— W. M. Bennett *et al.*, *Ann. intern. Med.*, 1980, *93*, 286.

Cirrhosis of the liver. In a double-blind study in 50 patients with cirrhosis of the liver who were treated with tolbutamide, the only significant improvements were increased appetite and an increase in the albumin fraction in the serum. Hypoglycaemia occurred in 20% of the patients.— P. D. Gulati *et al.*, *Am. J. dig. Dis.*, 1967, *12*, 42, per *J. Am. med. Ass.*, 1967, *199* (Mar. 6), A221.

Five of 11 patients with steatosis of the liver showed major improvement after treatment with tolbutamide.— H. Sarles *et al.*, *Am. J. dig. Dis.*, 1968, *13*, 35, per *J. Am. med. Ass.*, 1968, *203*, (Mar. 4), A222.

See also under Absorption and Fate.

Diabetes mellitus. Lack of correlation between tolbutamide dose, serum concentrations, and blood-glucose concentrations.— A. Melander *et al.*, *Br. med. J.*, 1978, *1*, 142.

Preparations

Sterile Tolbutamide Sodium *(U.S.P.)*. Tolbutamide sodium suitable for parenteral use. Potency is expressed in terms of the equivalent amount of tolbutamide.

Tolbutamide Tablets *(B.P.)*. Tablets containing tolbutamide. The *B.P.* requires 70% dissolution in 45 minutes.

Tolbutamide Tablets *(U.S.P.)*. Tablets containing tolbutamide. The *U.S.P.* requires 70% dissolution in 30 minutes.

Proprietary Preparations

Pramidex *(Berk Pharmaceuticals, UK)*. Tolbutamide, available as scored tablets of 500 mg.

Rastinon *(Hoechst, UK)*. Tolbutamide, available as scored tablets of 500 mg. **Rastinon Injection.** A solution containing tolbutamide sodium equivalent to tolbutamide 50 mg per ml, in ampoules of 20 ml. (Also available as Rastinon in *Austral., Belg., Denm., Ger., Ital., Neth., Norw., S.Afr., Spain, Switz.*).

Other Proprietary Names

Aglicem, Fordex *(both Spain)*; Aglycid, Diabeton Metilato, Neo-Insoral, Proinsul *(all Ital.)*; Arcosal *(Denm.)*; Artosin *(Arg., Austral., Belg., Ger., Neth., S.Afr., Spain, Swed.)*; Diaben *(Arg.)*; Diasulfon *(Switz.)*; Dolipol *(Alg., Fr., Morocco, Tun.)*; Guabeta N *(Ger.)*; Insilange-D, Nigloid *(both Jap.)*; Chembutamide, Mellitol, Mobenol, Neo-Dibetic, Novobutamide, Oramide, Tolbutone *(all Canad.)*; Oribetic *(USA)*; Orinase *(Canad., USA)*; Tolbet *(Neth.)*.

7235-x

Tolbutamide Sodium *(U.S.P.)*. Sodium Tolbutamide. The sodium salt of 1-butyl-3-tosylurea.
$C_{12}H_{17}N_2NaO_3S$=292.3.

CAS — 473-41-6.

Pharmacopoeias. In *U.S.* which also includes Sterile Tolbutamide Sodium.

A white or off-white, almost odourless, crystalline powder with a slightly bitter taste. Tolbutamide sodium 1.08 g is approximately equivalent to 1 g of tolbutamide. Freely **soluble** in water; soluble in alcohol and chloroform; very slightly soluble in ether. A 5% solution in water has a pH of 8.5 to 9.8. **Store** in airtight containers.

Adverse Effects, Treatment, and Precautions. As for Tolbutamide, p.859, although these effects and precautions should be interpreted in the light of the diagnostic rather than therapeutic use of tolbutamide sodium.

The intravenous injection of tolbutamide sodium may cause severe hypoglycaemia, particularly in patients with insulin-secreting tumours. Too rapid injection may cause a transient sensation of heat in the vein.

Uses. Tolbutamide sodium is given by intravenous injection as an aid to the diagnosis of suspected diabetes in patients with abnormal glucose tolerance. In healthy adults the intravenous injection over about 3 minutes of the equivalent of 1 g of tolbutamide produces a rapid and marked fall in blood-sugar concentrations, gradually returning to normal. In healthy subjects the blood-sugar concentration 20 minutes after the injection is usually 74% or less of the initial fasting value; a value of 85% to 89% is suggestive of diabetes and a value of 90% or more or 77% or more at 30 minutes is diagnostic.

Tolbutamide sodium has also been used to differentiate between hyperinsulinaemia due to tumours of the islet cells of the pancreas or to hepatic or functional disorders. Patients with tumours usually respond with marked and sustained hypoglycaemia.

Studies in 4 diabetics, 2 obese non-diabetics, and 4 healthy controls showed that the intravenous administration of 1 g of tolbutamide was followed within 5 minutes by increased plasma-insulin concentration. In 5 of these subjects the peak concentrations were reached within 1 to 2½ minutes. The findings suggested that sampling for insulin assays should start immediately after the injection of tolbutamide sodium.— D. Maingay *et al.*, *Lancet*, 1967, *1*, 361.

Diagnosis of diabetes. References: R. S. Swerdloff *et al.*, *Diabetes*, 1967, *16*, 161, per *Abstr. Wld Med.*, 1967, *41*, 794; R. M. Ehrlich and J. M. Martin, *J. Pediat.*, 1967, *71*, 485.

Diagnosis of insulinoma. References: S. S. Fajans and J. W. Conn, *J. Lab. clin. Med.*, 1959, *54*, 811; R. V. Randall, *Mayo Clin. Proc.*, 1966, *41*, 390; M. G. Schotland *et al.*, *Pediatrics*, 1967, *39*, 838, per *Abstr. Wld Med.*, 1968, *42*, 154; F. J. Service *et al.*, *Mayo Clin. Proc.*, 1976, *51*, 417.

Test of gastric innervation. References: S. J. Stempien *et al.*, *Am. J. dig. Dis.*, 1968, *13*, 643, per *Abstr. Wld Med.*, 1969, *43*, 27.

Preparations

See under Tolbutamide.

Iodine and Iodides

4570-e

Iodine, as a solution, is used as a disinfectant and antiseptic as are other iodine compounds such as the iodophores.

Iodine and inorganic iodide salts are used in the treatment of various thyroid disorders. The salts are used as expectorants although there is doubt concerning their efficacy for this purpose.

4571-l

Iodine *(B.P., B.P. Vet., Eur. P., U.S.P.).* Iod.; Iodum; Jodum; Yodo.
I_2=253.809.

CAS — 7553-56-2.

Pharmacopoeias. In all pharmacopoeias examined.

Greyish-violet or bluish-black brittle plates or small crystals, with a metallic sheen, a distinctive penetrating irritant odour, and an acrid taste. It is slowly volatile at room temperature and when heated it is completely volatilised to violet-coloured vapours which may be condensed as a bluish-black crystalline sublimate.

Soluble 1 in 3500 of water, 1 in 8 of alcohol, 1 in 6 of carbon disulphide, 1 in 45 of carbon tetrachloride, 1 in 30 of chloroform, 1 in 5 of ether, and 1 in 125 of glycerol; very readily soluble in strong aqueous solutions of iodides. A solution in alcohol, ether, or aqueous solutions of iodides is reddish-brown; in chloroform, carbon tetrachloride, or carbon disulphide it is violet-coloured.

Incompatible with alkalis and alkali carbonates, alkaloids, ammonia, chloral hydrate, phenol, sodium thiosulphate, soluble lead and mercury salts, starch, tannin, and vegetable astringents; with turpentine oil and most essential oils it forms explosive mixtures; with acetone it forms a pungent irritating compound. **Store** in glass-stoppered bottles or in glass or earthenware containers with well-waxed bungs.

A short review of interactions of iodine with solvents and surfactants.— K. J. Morgan and R. A. Anderson, *Aust. J. pharm. Sci.*, 1974, *NS3*, 110.

Solubility. A report on the solubility of iodine in glycols, glycol-water and glycerol-water mixtures.— A. Osol and C. C. Pines, *J. Am. pharm. Ass., scient. Edn*, 1952, *41*, 634.

The solubility of iodine in a 10% aqueous solution of cetomacrogol was about 1% w/v at 20° and increased linearly with increases in the cetomacrogol concentration and the temperature.— W. B. Hugo and J. M. Newton, *J. Pharm. Pharmac.*, 1963, *15*, 731. Report on the antibacterial properties of such solutions.— W. B. Hugo and J. M. Newton, *J. Pharm. Pharmac.*, 1964, *16*, 189.

A complex was formed in aqueous and non-aqueous solutions of iodine in cetomacrogol.— G. Henderson and J. M. Newton, *Pharm. Acta Helv.*, 1966, *41*, 228.

Stability of solutions. The stability of alcoholic solutions of iodine increased as the iodide/free iodine ratio increased and, for a given concentration of iodide, with increased strength of alcohol. Degradation of iodine was associated with a fall in pH which might come down to pH 2.— S. K. Baveja and R. D. Singla, *Indian J. Pharm.*, 1967, *29*, 275.

Adverse Effects. Continued administration of iodine and iodides may lead to mental depression, nervousness, insomnia, sexual impotence, and myxoedema. Hyperthyroidism has been reported. Goitre has occurred in patients taking iodides and in infants born to mothers taking iodides.

Iodism or hypersensitivity may occur acutely or after prolonged administration and is characterised by severe coryza, headache, pain and swelling in the salivary glands, lachrymation, weakness, conjunctivitis, fever, laryngitis, and bronchitis. Skin reactions (iododerma) may vary from mild erythema and acneform eruptions to urticaria and suppurative or haemorrhagic rashes. The topical application of iodine solutions may produce allergic reactions; goitre and exacerbation of acne may occur in children and adolescents. Inhalation of iodine vapour is very irritating to mucous membranes.

The symptoms of acute poisoning from ingestion of iodine are mainly due to its corrosive effects on the gastro-intestinal tract; a disagreeable metallic taste, vomiting, abdominal pain, and diarrhoea occur. If the stomach contains starch the vomit is coloured blue. Anuria may occur 1 to 3 days later or death may be due to circulatory failure, oedema of the glottis resulting in asphyxia, aspiration pneumonia, or pulmonary oedema. Oesophageal stricture may occur if the patient survives the acute stage. The fatal dose is usually about 2 or 3 g. The prognosis is generally favourable.

Maximum permissible atmospheric concentration 0.1 ppm.

Effects on the blood. Thrombocytopenia had been associated with treatment with iodine.— M. G. Wilson, *Am. J. Obstet. Gynec.*, 1962, *83*, 818.

Effects on electrolytes. Serum acid-base disturbances observed in a 56-year-old woman who had ingested a large unknown quantity of a solution containing iodine 5% and potassium iodide 10% might be related to the production of a lactic acidosis due to the iodine/iodide intoxication.— R. F. Dyck *et al.*, *Can. med. Ass. J.*, 1979, *120*, 704.

Effects on the eye. Iodides could cause amblyopia, green vision, keratitis, hypopyon, iridocyclitis, topical dermatitis of the lens, retinal haemorrhage which might lead to retinal degeneration and optic neuritis, the risk of precipitating malignant exophthalmos and ophthalmoplegia, iritis, and intraocular haemorrhage.— H. I. Silverman, *Am. J. Optom.*, 1972, *49*, 335.

The lachrymatory effects of iodine in industrial methylated spirits were due not only to acetone but to other ketones. In 3 samples acetophenone was present to the extent of 0.015 to 0.021%. A solution containing iodine in absolute alcohol containing acetophenone 0.015% gave rise to lachrymatory vapours when warmed; no such effect occurred with absolute alcohol alone.— F. G. R. Prior (letter), *Pharm. J.*, 1974, *2*, 370.

Effects on the heart. Within 12 hours of ingestion of about 600 ml of a potassium iodide solution (15 g iodide), a man developed swelling of the mouth, neck, and face. Short bursts of ventricular tachycardia and ventricular bigeminy plus ectopic atrial beats were noted on admission to hospital. Cardiac rhythm was normal after 10 days.— D. D. Tresch *et al.*, *Archs intern. Med.*, 1974, *134*, 760.

Effects on the skin. Results from a study using a modified 'repeated-insult' patch test indicated that iodine well deserved its reputation as a contact sensitiser.— A. M. Kligman, *J. invest. Derm.*, 1966, *47*, 393.

Iodides induced typical attacks of generalised pustular psoriasis in 2 patients who had this disease recurrently. Salicylates also appeared to have a similar effect. By the strict avoidance of both, prolonged remissions were achieved.— W. B. Shelley, *J. Am. med. Ass.*, 1967, *201*, 1009.

Iodides could cause acneform eruptions, bullous eruptions, tumour-like lesions, eruptions resembling erythema multiforme, and eruptions resembling erythema nodosum.— R. L. Baer and H. Harris, *J. Am. med. Ass.*, 1967, *202*, 710.

Fungating, suppurative abscesses appeared on the face and hands of an elderly woman within 6 days of receiving potassium iodide for chronic bronchitis. The lesions rapidly worsened but biopsies revealed no micro-organisms. On discontinuation of potassium iodide the lesions immediately began to heal. The patient had received potassium iodide 15 months earlier with no adverse effects.— F. Khan *et al.*, *New Engl. J. Med.*, 1973, *289*, 1018.

Blistering of the skin occurred in 2 patients after the use of an acetone-containing plastic spray dressing and an occlusive dressing over skin treated with Weak Iodine Solution.— J. Morgan-Hughes and R. A. Bray (letter), *Br. med. J.*, 1978, *2*, 639. The effect on the skin was likely to be due to an irritant compound formed from the reaction of iodine with acetone.— E. Powell (letter), *ibid.*, 1500. The essential factor was occlusion of the skin. The use of an acetone-containing plastic spray dressing alone over iodine-prepared skin did not constitute a hazard.— J. G. B. Howes and P. Kirwan (letter), *ibid.*, 1979, *1*, 487.

Further references: T. G. Baumgartner, *Am. J. Hosp. Pharm.*, 1976, *33*, 601.

Effects on the thyroid. Thyroid pain in 4 patients after normal doses of potassium iodide. The symptoms subsided within 2 or 3 days of stopping administration.— H. T. Edmunds (letter), *Br. med. J.*, 1955, *1*, 354.

Goitre and hypothyroidism. Of 5 patients with asthma and bronchitis who had taken about 300 to 500 g of potassium iodide annually for 7 to 15 years, 4 became hypothyroid, 3 having goitres weighing about 40 g and 1 a goitre weighing 80 g. The fifth patient remained euthyroid and had a goitre weighing about 40 g. All became clinically euthyroid when iodide medication was stopped and the goitres subsided within 1 to 2 months. Patients receiving a high dosage of iodine should stop taking it for 2 to 4 weeks several times a year.— H. Frey, *Acta endocr., Copenh.*, 1964, *47*, 105.

Two patients developed goitre after taking preparations containing iodine for 4 and 12 years respectively. It appeared that the critical factor in the development of iodine goitre was a persistently high concentration of iodide within the thyroid, inhibiting thyroid synthesis.— I. P. C. Murray and R. D. H. Stewart, *Lancet*, 1967, *1*, 922. See also *ibid.*, 939.

Hypothyroidism was reported in a 2-year-old child who had been treated with potassium iodide 500 mg daily in divided doses for the treatment of rhinitis with recurrent bouts of wheezing, starting at 6 months of age. Although during treatment with thyroxine the child became clinically euthyroid, mental retardation was still evident 2 years later.— N. D. Barnes *et al.*, *Ann. Allergy*, 1975, *35*, 305.

Further references: A. Parrow, *Nord. Med.*, 1966, *76*, 1003; R. S. Chapman and R. A. Main, *Br. J. Derm.*, 1967, *79*, 103; D. K. Weaver *et al.*, *Archs Surg., Chicago*, 1969, *98*, 183; T. Dolan and L. Gibson, *J. Pediat.*, 1971, *79*, 684; H. Bürgi *et al.*, *Schweiz. med. Wschr.*, 1972, *102*, 837.

Hyperthyroidism. Hyperthyroidism and goitre in a 38-year-old woman who had taken a preparation of seaweed for over 2 years and estimated to be equivalent to a daily intake of 1 to 2 mg of iodine.— K. Liewendahl and A. Gordin, *Acta med. scand.*, 1974, *196*, 237.

Epidemics of thyrotoxicosis in northern Tasmania were associated with iodised bread to combat goitre, and the use of iodine-containing disinfectants on dairy farms. It was considered that the iodine concentrations of food should be monitored regularly and that the addition of iodine to common foods should be more strictly controlled.— J. C. Stewart and G. I. Vidor, *Br. med. J.*, 1976, *1*, 372. See also J. C. Stewart *et al.*, *Aust. N.Z. J. Med.*, 1971, *1*, 203.

Bronchial asthma was complicated in one patient by hyperthyroidism induced by an iodine-containing expectorant. Asthmatic patients should not take such expectorants since the complications could be very serious and the benefits of iodine in expectorants were questionable.— B. Thorsteinsson and C. Kirkegaard (letter), *Lancet*, 1977, *2*, 294.

Reversible thyrotoxicosis in a 33-year-old woman appeared to be associated with ingestion of large doses of potassium iodide for control of asthma.— D. R. Gutknecht (letter), *New Engl. J. Med.*, 1977, *296*, 1236. Comment on the paradoxical development of myxoedema associated with high doses of potassium iodide. High doses might be associated with hypothyroidism, whereas in predisposed individuals repeated low doses might be associated with hyperthyroidism.— H. Herxheimer (letter), *ibid.*, *297*, 171.

Pregnancy and the neonate. Of 50 282 children born to mothers monitored by the Collaborative Perinatal Project 489 were found to have been exposed to iodides, and possibly other drugs, at some time during the first 4 months of pregnancy. Four of 5 children with eye or ear malformations had cataract and this suggestion of possible teratogenicity needed independent confirmation.— O. P. Heinonen *et al.*, *Birth Defects and Drugs in Pregnancy*, Littleton MA, Publishing Sciences Group, 1977, p. 401.

Goitre and hypothyroidism. Eight infants were born with congenital goitre and hypothyroidism due to maternal ingestion during pregnancy of 12 to 1650 mg of elemental iodine daily contained in expectorants and cough suppressants for asthma and bronchitis; several of these preparations were available without prescription. It was recommended that iodine-containing preparations should not be used during pregnancy and that they should cease to be available without prescription.— F. Carswell *et al.*, *Lancet*, 1970, *1*, 1241.

For further reports of goitre and hypothyroidism occurring in infants, including some fatalities, following the administration of iodides to the mothers during pregnancy, see M. P. Galina *et al.*, *New Engl. J. Med.*, 1962, *267*, 1124; C. S. Livingstone (letter), *Br. med. J.*, 1966, *2*, 50; K. P. Dawson (letter), *ibid.*, 1970, *2*, 112; J. Ayromlooi, *Obstet. Gynec.*, 1972, *39*, 818; C. Courpotin *et al.*, *Nouv. Presse méd.*, 1977, *6*, 4189.

Iodides in breast milk could possibly cause hypothyroidism or goitre in infants.— *Med. Lett.*, 1974, *16*, 26. See also T. E. O'Brien, *Am. J. Hosp. Pharm.*, 1974, *31*, 844; R. L. Savage, *Adverse Drug React. Bull.*, 1976, Dec., 212.

Five of 30 neonates studied in an intensive care unit developed goitre and hypothyroidism after frequent applications of an iodine-alcohol solution for topical disinfection. All recovered after treatment with lyophilised thyroid extract.— J. P. Chabrolle and A. Rossier, *Archs Dis. Childh.*, 1978, *53*, 495.

Hyperthyroidism. A thyrotoxic infant was born to a woman receiving maintenance treatment with thyroxine sodium for hypothyroidism. The thyrotoxicosis could have been due to the transplacental passage of iodine from a preparation containing 3.6% of sodium iodide (Elixir Sibec) taken by the mother for asthma.— J. A. Thomson and I. D. Riley, *Lancet*, 1966, *1*, 635. Comments.— W. Singer (letter), *ibid.*, 1041. A reply.— J. A. Thomson and I. D. Riley, *ibid.*, 1160.

Treatment of Adverse Effects. In acute iodine poisoning copious draughts of milk and starch mucilage should be given and the stomach emptied by aspiration and lavage with dilute starch mucilage or a 1% solution of sodium thiosulphate. The use of gastric lavage with activated charcoal has also been suggested. Electrolyte and water losses should be replaced and the circulation should be maintained. Pethidine 100 mg or morphine sulphate 10 mg may be given for pain. A tracheostomy may become necessary.

The symptoms of iodism usually subside rapidly when administration of iodine or iodides is discontinued. Fluids and sodium chloride injection may be given to hasten elimination.

It has been suggested that haemodialysis may reduce excessively elevated serum-iodine concentrations.

For comment on the *in vitro* adsorption of iodine by activated charcoal, see p.79.

Precautions. Caution is necessary if preparations containing iodine or iodides are taken for prolonged periods, and such preparations should not be taken regularly during pregnancy or lactation, or given to children. Iodides may aggravate or even initiate the eruption of dermatitis herpetiformis.

Solutions of iodine applied to the skin should not be covered with occlusive dressings. The administration of preparations containing iodine or iodides interferes with tests of thyroid function.

The Committee of Drugs of the American Academy of Pediatrics reviewed the toxicity of iodides used for the treatment of asthma and other pulmonary disorders and recommended: 1) iodides should be used as expectorants in the lowest possible doses, for the shortest time, and only when a response is obtained and less toxic substances are ineffective; 2) iodides should not be used as expectorants in pregnancy and should be withdrawn or the dose reduced during breast-feeding; 3) they should not be used as expectorants in adolescents because of their acneform and thyroid effects; 4) they should not be used as expectorants in patients with goitre.— *Pediatrics*, 1976, *57*, 272.

Of 126 subjects who received numerous doses of potassium iodide 500 mg during metabolic studies 4 repeatedly developed sensitivity reactions after iodide administration. These 4 subjects were found to exhibit hypocomplementaemia and dermal vasculitis associated with chronic urticaria or systemic lupus erythematosus and it was suggested that these clinical features may indicate iodide sensitivity.— J. G. Curd *et al.*, *Ann. intern. Med.*, 1979, *91*, 853. Comment.— R. Bookman (letter), *ibid.*, 1980, *92*, 712. Reply.— J. G. Curd *et al.* (letter), *ibid.*

Interference with laboratory estimations. Potassium iodide could interfere technically with chemical estimations for protein-bound iodine to provide erroneous raised results.— *Drug & Ther. Bull.*, 1972, *10*, 69.

When a 2% solution of iodine in 70% alcohol was painted over an area of skin 25 cm by 18 cm, total serum-iodine levels were raised in samples taken 30 minutes and 1 day after painting the skin, but were back to normal after 1 week. Application of tincture of iodine to the skin might interfere with tests of thyroid function.— T. S. Reeve *et al.*, *Med. J. Aust.*, 1973, *1*, 891.

It was reported that the administration of iodides could interfere with measurements of urinary 17-hydroxycorticosteroids.— J. M. Rosenberg and I. S. Kampa, *Drug Intell. & clin. Pharm.*, 1973, *7*, 33.

Absorption and Fate. Iodine is slightly absorbed when applied to the skin. When taken by mouth it is rapidly converted to iodide and is stored in the thyroid gland as thyroglobulin. Iodides diffuse across the placenta. They are excreted mainly in the urine, with smaller amounts appearing in the faeces, saliva, sweat, and milk.

Uses. Iodine is an essential trace element in the human diet. Deficiency of iodine leads to development of goitre and in many countries culinary salt is iodised mainly with iodides. The minimum daily requirement for an adult is about 100 µg.

Iodine and iodides are used in conjunction with antithyroid agents (see under Carbimazole, p.356) in the pre-operative treatment of thyrotoxicosis. The patient is rendered euthyroid with an antithyroid agent and iodine or iodides are then added to the therapy for about 10 to 12 days before subtotal thyroidectomy. The usual dose of Aqueous Iodine Solution for this purpose is 0.1 to 0.3 ml in milk or water thrice daily. This produces a gland of firm texture suitable for operation and avoids the increased vascularity and friability of the gland with increased risk of haemorrhage which may result from the use of an antithyroid agent alone. Treatment with iodine or iodides may be continued postoperatively for a few days to avert thyrotoxic crises although this is not always considered necessary. Aqueous Iodine Solution has been used alone in pre-operative treatment but its sole use for this purpose is no longer considered to be entirely satisfactory.

In the immediate treatment of thyrotoxic crisis larger doses of 2 to 3 ml daily of Aqueous Iodine Solution may be given.

Iodine has a powerful bactericidal action and is used for disinfecting unbroken skin before operation. Iodine is also active against fungi and viruses. It is generally employed as Weak Iodine Solution or as a 2% solution of iodine in 75% industrial methylated spirit. The industrial methylated spirit should be free from acetone, with which iodine forms an irritant and lachrymatory compound. Iodine may also be employed as the weak solution for the first-aid treatment of small wounds and abrasions, but it is rapidly inactivated by combining with tissue substances and so delays healing. It has been applied topically in the treatment of herpes simplex.

A 2% solution in glycerol has been used for application to mucous membranes and Compound Iodine Paint has been used as a throat paint in pharyngitis and follicular tonsillitis. Iodine ointments are applied as counter-irritants in rheumatism and tenosynovitis.

When iodine combines chemically it is decolorised and so-called colourless iodine preparations do not have the disinfectant properties of iodine.

Iodine stains the skin a deep reddish-brown; the stain can readily be removed by dilute solutions of alkalis or sodium thiosulphate.

Organic compounds of iodine are used as X-ray contrast media, see p.434.

The antibacterial activity of mixtures of iodine and *N*-alkyl betaines.— J. M. Newton and P. G. Hugbo, *Pharm. Acta Helv.*, 1968, *43*, 349.

After the application of 0.5% iodine tincture, basal cell carcinoma had a characteristic glister which was diagnostic; of 127 lesions histologically proven, 122 were identified by the iodine test.— D. Mahler, *Br. J. Derm.*, 1971, *85*, 239.

The iodine test for the detection of neoplasms of the cervix and vagina was of no value. In 257 women whose mothers had taken stilboestrol during pregnancy, non-staining areas, reputedly diagnostic for neoplasms, were detected in 214 women none of whom was shown to have a cervical or vaginal neoplasm.— E. C. Sandberg and J. C. Hebard, *Am. J. Obstet. Gynec.*, 1977, *128*, 364.

Inorganic iodine solutions were more effective as anti-plaque agents than solutions of povidine-iodine and another iodophore (Wescodyne). It was considered that topical application of inorganic iodine solutions might be useful in controlling dental caries and actinomyces-associated periodontal disease.— J. M. Tanzer *et al.*, *Antimicrob. Ag. Chemother.*, 1977, *12*, 107.

Amoebiasis. Aqueous solution of iodine, 200 ppm, could be used to remove amoebic cysts from uncooked fruits and vegetables.— W. P. Stamm, *Lancet*, 1970, *2*, 1355.

Cretinism. Comments on endemic goitre and cretinism.— *Lancet*, 1979, *2*, 1165.

A controlled study of the use of iodised oil intramuscularly in the prevention of endemic cretinism was carried out on a population of 8000 in New Guinea. Follow-up over 4 years revealed 26 endemic cretins out of 534 children born to mothers who did not receive iodised oil, and 7 endemic cretins out of 498 children born to mothers who had received iodised oil. Severe iodine deficiency in the mother seemed to produce neurological damage during foetal development.— P. O. D. Pharoah *et al.*, *Lancet*, 1971, *1*, 308. A controlled follow-up study involving 5 of the villages in the original trial, carried out under double-blind conditions, indicated that 115 ostensibly normal children born to mothers who had received iodine were significantly faster and more accurate in tests of manual function than 79 similar children born to control mothers who had received saline; a further 14 children (13 from the control group) who were found to be cretins were excluded from the analysis. These results indicate that children whose mothers have a severe dietary deficiency of iodine are at risk, not only of endemic cretinism, but also of subclinical deficits which put them at a developmental disadvantage.— K. J. Connolly *et al.*, *ibid.*, 1979, *2*, 1149.

Disinfection of skin. A 1% solution of iodine in 70% alcohol and 0.5% chlorhexidine gluconate in 70% alcohol were equally effective in reducing resident skin flora by about 80% and in removing superficial *Pseudomonas aeruginosa*, though some patients were sensitive to iodine. Less effective disinfectants were 70% alcohol, Aqueous Iodine Solution, aqueous 0.5% chlorhexidine solution, and undecoylium chloride-iodine.— E. J. L. Lowbury *et al.*, *Br. med. J.*, 1960, *2*, 1039. See also *ibid.*, 1969, *2*, 462.

Estimation, by 3 different techniques, of the bacterial population of abdominal skin before and after disinfection indicated that virtually all non-sporing bacteria could be eliminated by swabbing for 30 seconds with 1.5% iodine in 70% alcohol.— S. Selwyn and H. Ellis, *Br. med. J.*, 1972, *1*, 136.

The virucidal activities of several antimicrobial liquids and foams were determined against rhinoviruses when applied to the hands. Solutions containing iodine 1% in water were most effective and were virucidal when applied immediately after contamination. Foams containing hexachlorophane 0.23% (w/v) with alcohol 58% (v/v) or benzalkonium chloride 0.2% with alcohol 50% (w/w) were less effective and alcohol alone or in a mixture with benzyl alcohol was the least effective preparation.— J. O. Hendley *et al.*, *Antimicrob. Ag. Chemother.*, 1978, *14*, 690.

Disinfection of water. The effectiveness of iodine 0.4 ppm in disinfecting swimming pools.— O. E. Byrd *et al.*, *Publ. Hlth Rep., Wash.*, 1963, *78*, 393.

For the iodination of public water supplies for control of waterborne viruses, see S. L. Chang, *Bull. Wld Hlth Org.*, 1968, *38*, 401.

Studies in 22 persons showed that after 1 month's use of a swimming pool disinfected with iodine, absorption of iodine was insufficient to modify the uptake of radioactive iodine or the serum concentration of protein-bound iodine. Effective bacteriological control of community water supplies was obtained using 1 ppm of iodine; the uptake of iodine-131 was reduced in users of such a supply.— W. C. Thomas *et al.*, *Archs environ. Hlth*, 1969, *19*, 124.

Human dietary requirements. The British Medical Association in 1950 recommended the daily intake of 100 µg of iodine for adults, and 150 µg for children, adolescents, and pregnant and nursing women. The amounts were unlikely to be reached without iodisation of salt. Young children and adolescents were unlikely to benefit from amounts in excess of 300 μg daily, and 150 μg daily appeared reasonable. A similar amount, if consumed daily by women during child-bearing years, would be adequate during pregnancy. More data was needed before firm recommendations could be made.— Recommended Intakes of Nutrients for the United Kingdom, *Reports on Public Health and Medical Subjects No. 120*, London, HM Stationery Office, 1969.

Protein-rich mixtures used as supplementary foods should contain 28 μg of iodine per 419 kJ.— Report of a WHO Expert Group on Trace Elements in Human Nutrition, *Tech. Rep. Ser. Wld Hlth Org. No. 532*, 1973, 55.

Supplements to dietary iodine were urgently needed if the mean excretion rate of iodine in the urine fell to below 20 μg in 24 hours, or below 20 μg per g of creatinine excreted.— J. B. Stanbury *et al.*, *Chronicle Wld Hlth Org.*, 1974, *28*, 220.

The US National Research Council made the following recommendations for daily dietary allowances of iodine: infants up to 6 months, 40 μg; 6 to 12 months, 50 μg; children 1 to 3 years, 70 μg; 4 to 6 years, 90 μg; 7 to 10 years, 120 μg; children over 11 years and adults, 150 μg; in pregnancy 175 μg; in lactation 200 μg.— *Recommended Dietary Allowances*, 9th Edn, Washington, The National Research Council, 1980.

Preparations

Glycerins

Compound Iodine Glycerin *(Jap. P.)*. Glycerin. Iod. Comp. Iodine 1.2 g, potassium iodide 2.4 g, glycerol 90 ml, mentha water 4.5 ml, liquified phenol 0.5 ml, water to 100 ml. Protect from light.

Dental Iodine Glycerin *(Jap. P.)*. Glycerin. Iod. Dent. Iodine 10 g, potassium iodide 8 g, zinc sulphate 1 g, glycerol 35 ml, water to 100 ml. Protect from light.

Iodine Glycerin *(B.P.C. 1923)*. Glycerinum Iodi; Iodo-glycerin Solution; Morton's Fluid. Iodine 2.28 g, potassium iodide 6.86 g, water 5 ml, glycerol to 100 ml. It has been used as an injection (2 ml) into tumours and as an application to the skin.

A similar preparation (2% w/w of iodine) is included in *Dan. Disp.* and *Port. P.*

Injections

Intravenous Injection of Iodine. Aqueous Iodine Solution (Lugol's Solution) 2 ml, sodium chloride injection to 10 ml. For slow intravenous injection in thyrotoxic crisis.

As free iodine crystals occurred in autoclaved solutions, sterilisation of Intravenous Injection of Iodine by filtration was suggested.— Pharm. Soc. Lab. Rep. No. P/68/11, 1968.

Iodine Injection. Fiale Iodo-iodurate 1° *(It. P.)*. Iodine 1 g, potassium iodide 2 g, Water for Injections to 100 ml. Sterilise in 1-ml ampoules by maintaining at 100° for 30 minutes. Protect from light. *Dose.* 1 to 2 ml daily by intramuscular injection. Fiale Iodo-iodurate 2° (*It. P.*) contains the same solution in 2-ml ampoules.

Insufflations

Iodine and Boric Acid Insufflation *(B.P.C. 1949)*. ABI; Insuff. Iod. et Acid. Boric.; Powder of Boric Acid and Iodine. Iodine 1% in boric acid. An aural insufflation used in the treatment of chronic otitis media.

Iodine Insufflation *(A.P.F.)*. Iodine 0.8, potassium iodide 0.4, anaesthetic ether 10, and lactose, in fine powder, 98.8. Store below 25°.

Ointments

Iodine Ointment *(B.P.C. 1949)*. Ung. Iod. Iodine 4 g, potassium iodide 4 g, water 4 ml, and yellow simple ointment 88 g. The free iodine content may decrease on storage.

Non-staining Iodine Ointment *(B.P.C. 1968)*. Unguentum Iodi Denigrescens; Ung. Iod. Denig. Iodine 5% w/w in arachis oil and yellow soft paraffin. Store in a cool place in containers which prevent evaporation.

Non-staining Iodine Ointment with Methyl Salicylate *(B.P.C. 1968)*. Ung. Iod. Denig. c. Methyl. Sal. Methyl salicylate 5% v/w in non-staining iodine ointment. Store in a cool place in containers which prevent evaporation.

Strong Iodine Ointment *(B. Vet. C. 1965)*. Iodine 10, wool fat 55, yellow soft paraffin 17.5, potassium iodide 7.5, water 10. Dissolve the iodine and potassium iodide in the water and add slowly, with stirring, to the melted wool fat and yellow soft paraffin. Stir until cold. Contact with metal or plastics should be avoided. It has been used in ringworm in cattle.

Paints

Compound Iodine Paint *(B.P.C. 1968)*. Iodine Compound Paint; Pig. Iod. Co.; Mandl's Paint. Iodine 1.25 g, potassium iodide 2.5 g, water 2.5 ml, peppermint oil 0.4 ml, alcohol (90%) 4 ml, glycerol to 100 ml. It should be well shaken before use. Store in a cool place in airtight containers.

A.P.F. (Iodine Paint Compound) has a similar formula with peppermint spirit 4 ml.

Iodine Paint *(St. Thomas' Hosp.)*. Pig. Iod. Iodine 2 g, potassium iodide 2 g, water 25 ml, industrial methylated spirit acetone-free to 100 ml. For pre-operative preparation of the skin.

Pastes

Rozental's Iodine Paste. Stated to consist of iodine 3, rectified alcohol 20, paraffin 30, and chloroform 150. Applied topically in the treatment of inflammatory diseases of the peripheral nervous system and muscles.—N.I. Andrejashkin, *Klin. Med., Mosk.*, 1961, *42*, 79.

Solutions and tinctures

Aqueous Iodine Solution *(B.P.)*. Aqueous Iod. Soln.; Iodine Aqueous Solution; Compound Iodine Solution; Lugol's Solution; Strong Iodine Solution *(U.S.P.)*. Iodine 5 g, potassium iodide 10 g, water to 100 ml. It contains in 1 ml 50 mg of free iodine and about 130 mg of total iodine. Store in airtight containers, the materials of which are resistant to iodine.

A similar preparation is included in several other pharmacopoeias.

NOTE. Lugol's Solution (*Fr. P. 1965*) contains 1% w/w of iodine—see Soluté Iodo-Ioduré Fort.

Decolorised Iodine Solution *(B.P.C. 1934)*. Liq. Iod. Decol.; Decolorised Tincture of Iodine. Dissolve, with gentle heat, iodine 2.86 g in alcohol (90%) 27.5 ml, add strong ammonia solution 6.25 ml, keep the mixture in a warm place until decolorised, and then add alcohol (90%) to produce 100 ml.

Iodine Disclosing Solution. (1) Iodine 7.7 g, zinc iodide 2.3 g, potassium iodide 2.3 g, glycerol 49 g, water 38.7 ml. (2) Iodine 8.9 g, zinc iodide 2.7 g, potassium iodide 2.7 g, glycerol 42.9 g, water 42.8 ml.—*A.D.T.* 1975, 204.

Iodine Tincture *(U.S.P.)*. Iodine 2 g, sodium iodide 2.4 g, alcohol 50 ml, water to 100 ml. Store in airtight containers.

Iodine Topical Solution *(U.S.P.)*. Iodine Solution. Iodine 2 g, sodium iodide 2.4 g, water to 100 ml. Store at a temperature not exceeding 35° in airtight containers. Protect from light.

Phenolated Iodine Solution *(U.S.N.F. XI)*. Boulton's Solution; Carbolized Iodine Solution; French Mixture. Strong iodine solution (*U.S.P.*) [aqueous iodine solution (*B.P.*)] 1.5 ml, liquefied phenol 0.6 ml, glycerol 16.5 ml, water to 100 ml; expose to sunlight, or heat at a temperature not exceeding 70°, in a strong tightly stoppered bottle, until the solution becomes colourless or faintly yellow. It has been used undiluted as an antiseptic mouth-wash.

Suggested modification. Strong iodine solution (*U.S.P.*) 1.5 ml, liquefied phenol 0.6 ml, glycerol 16.5 ml, sodium bicarbonate 30 mg, sodium acid phosphate 400 mg, water to 100 ml. Mix the sodium bicarbonate, liquefied phenol, and strong iodine solution in a large flask and shake until the iodine colour has disappeared. Add the glycerol, 50 ml of water, and the sodium acid phosphate; dissolve and make up to volume with water. This product was quick and convenient to prepare and was at least as effective as the *U.S.N.F.* XI preparation.— G. Levy *et al.*, *Drug Stand.*, 1960, *28*, 129.

Schiller's Iodine. Iodine 333.3 mg, potassium iodide 666.6 mg, water to 100 ml. For the diagnosis of cancer of the cervix. (However, see above).

Simple Iodine Solution *(B.P.C. 1959)*. Liq. Iod. Simp. Iodine 9% w/v in alcohol. Store in a cool place in well-closed glass-stoppered bottles. It is liable to alteration in strength on storage. Simple Iodine Solution contains about 10% w/w of iodine and it is therefore the same strength as Teinture d'Iode (*Fr. P. 1908*).

Soluté Iodo-Ioduré Fort *(Fr. P. 1965)*. Soluté dit de Lugol; Lugol's Solution. Iodine 1 g, potassium iodide 2 g, water to 100 g.

NOTE. A solution to this formula is used under the title Lugol's Iodine for Bacteriological Staining.

Strong Iodine Solution *(B.P. 1958)*. Strong Iod. Soln; Liq. Iod. Fort.; Strong Iodine Tincture; Linimentum Iodi. Iodine 10 g, potassium iodide 6 g, water 10 ml, alcohol (90%) to 100 ml. Store in well-closed glass-stoppered bottles.

Teinture d'Iode *(Fr. P. 1908)*. Tincture of Iodine *(*French Codex*)*; French Tincture of Iodine. Iodine 10% w/w in alcohol. This is the preparation usually intended when 'French Tincture of Iodine' is ordered in Great Britain; Simple Iodine Solution, *B.P.C. 1959*, which is the same strength, should be supplied.

Weak Iodine Solution *(B.P.)*. Weak Iod. Soln; Liq. Iod. Mit.; Iodine Tincture; Tinct. Iod. Mit. Iodine 2.5 g, potassium iodide 2.5 g, water 2.5 ml, alcohol (90%) to 100 ml. It contains in 1 ml 25 mg of free iodine and about 44 mg of total iodine. Store in airtight containers, the materials of which are resistant to iodine.

A similar preparation is included in most other pharmacopoeias, the specified strength of iodine varying between 2 and 7%.

Proprietary Preparations

Iodex Plain *(Menley & James, UK)*. A non-staining ointment containing iodine 4% in a basis of soft paraffin. **Iodex with Wintergreen.** A non-staining ointment containing iodine 4% with methyl salicylate 5%. (Also available as Iodex in Switz.).

Other Proprietary Names

Iodosan *(Ital.)*; Jodosan *(Norw.)*; Mikroplex Jod *(Ger.)*.

4572-y

Ammonium Iodide *(B.P.C. 1934)*. Ammonii Iodidum; Ammonii Iodetum; Ammonium Iodatum.

NH_4I = 144.9.

CAS — 12027-06-4.

Pharmacopoeias. In *Port.*

A white deliquescent crystalline powder, becoming yellow on exposure to air and light; it has a sharply saline taste.

Soluble 1 in 1 of water, 1 in 4 of alcohol, and 1 in 1.5 of glycerol. Solutions in water are neutral or acid to litmus. **Store** in airtight containers. Protect from light.

Ammonium iodide has actions and uses similar to those of potassium iodide and was formerly used in doses of 120 to 400 mg.

4573-j

Calcium Iodide *(B.P.C. 1934)*.

CaI_2 = 293.9.

CAS — 10102-68-8.

A white deliquescent mass or powder with a bitter taste; it becomes yellow on exposure to air and light. **Soluble** in water and alcohol. **Store** in airtight containers. Protect from light.

Calcium iodide has actions and uses similar to those of potassium iodide and has been used in doses of up to 320 mg.

A preparation containing calcium iodide was formerly marketed in Great Britain under the proprietary name Calcidrine (*Abbott*).

4574-z

Calcium Iodobehenate. Calciiodinum; Calcium Iodbehenicum; Calcium Monoiodobehenate; Saiodinum.

CAS — 1319-91-1.

Pharmacopoeias. In *Rus.*

A white or yellowish powder consisting mainly of calcium 13 (or 14)-iododocosanoate, $(C_{21}H_{42}I.CO_2)_2Ca$ = 971.0, and containing not less than 23.5% of iodine. It is unctuous to the touch and is odourless or has a slight fatty odour.

Practically **insoluble** in water; very slightly soluble in alcohol and ether; freely soluble in warm chloroform. **Protect** from light.

Calcium iodobehenate has actions and uses similar to those of potassium iodide and has been used in doses of 500 mg.

4575-c

Dilute Hydriodic Acid *(B.P.C. 1949)*. Acid. Hydriod. Dil.

CAS — 10034-85-2 (hydrogen iodide).

A clear colourless odourless liquid containing 10% w/w of hydrogen iodide, HI = 127.9, with 0.3% w/w of hypophosphorous acid, H_3PO_2, added to prevent discoloration on keeping. Wt per ml about 1.1 g. **Incompatible** with alkalis and oxidising agents. **Store** in well-closed glass-stoppered bottles. Protect from light.

Dilute hydriodic acid has the general properties of iodine in weak combination. It was usually administered as Hydriodic Acid Syrup.

Preparations

Hydriodic Acid Syrup *(B.P.C. 1949)*. Syr. Acid. Hydriod. Dilute hydriodic acid 10 ml, water 5 ml, and syrup to 100 ml. *Dose.* 2 to 4 ml.

4576-k

Iodinated Glycerol. Iodopropylidene Glycerol. An isomeric mixture of iodinated dimers of glycerol, $C_6H_{11}IO_3$ = 258.1. It contains about 50% of organically bound iodine.

CAS — 5634-39-9.

A pale yellow liquid with a pungent bitter after-taste. **Soluble** in chloroform, ether, and ethyl acetate. **Protect** from light.

Adverse Effects, Treatment, and Precautions. As for Iodine, p.862.

Uses. Iodinated glycerol is used as an expectorant in bronchitis and bronchial asthma in doses of 60 mg four times daily with fluids.

Proprietary Preparations

Organidin *(WB Pharmaceuticals, UK: Boehringer Ingelheim, UK)*. Elixir containing in each 5 ml iodinated glycerol 60 mg and alcohol 1.25 ml (suggested diluent, equal parts of glycerol and water).

Other Proprietary Names

Mucorama Rectal Infantil *(Spain)*.

4577-a

Iodoform *(B.P.C. 1954)*. Formène Tri-iodé. Tri-iodomethane.

CHI_3=393.7.

CAS — 75-47-8.

Pharmacopoeias. In *Arg., Aust., Belg., Fr., It., Jug., Pol., Port., Rus., Span.,* and *Swiss.*

Shining lemon-yellow crystals or powder, somewhat unctuous to the touch, with a characteristic, persistent, penetrating odour and disagreeable taste. Slightly volatile at room temperature. M.p. 115°; at higher temperatures it decomposes with loss of iodine.

Practically **insoluble** in water; soluble 1 in 60 of alcohol, 1 in 3 of carbon disulphide, 1 in 13 of chloroform, 1 in 8 of ether, 1 in 100 of glycerol, 1 in 35 of olive oil; soluble in other fixed and volatile oils, and in flexible collodion. **Incompatible** with alkalis, oxidising agents, lead, silver, and mercury salts. **Store** in a cool place in airtight containers. Protect from light.

To cover its odour it may be mixed with coumarin 1 in 50, or with menthol, phenol, or thymol, or with oils of anise, eucalyptus, geranium, peppermint, rosemary, or sassafras, about 1 or 2%.

Adverse Effects. Symptoms of systemic toxicity, as described under Iodine (see p.862), sometimes occur on prolonged or extensive application to wounds. As a precaution not more than 2 g should usually be applied as a wound dressing. Some persons are hypersensitive to iodoform and even small quantities applied locally may cause an erythematous rash.

Severe poisoning, which may be fatal, is characterised by headache, somnolence, delirium, and rapid feeble pulse.

Maximum permissible atmospheric concentration 0.6 ppm.

Uses. Iodoform has a marked anaesthetic action when applied to mucous membranes. It slowly releases elemental iodine when applied to the tissues and has a mild disinfectant action. It was formerly used extensively as a wound dressing but is not very effective.

Compound Iodoform Paint has been used as a protective covering and to hold gauze dressings and radium needles in position.

Bismuth Subnitrate and Iodoform Paste (BIPP) has been applied to wounds and abscesses, the area to be treated being cleaned and smeared with the paste. Sterile gauze impregnated with the paste has also been used for packing cavities after oral and otorhinological surgery.

Preparations

B.I.P.P. Gauze *(Roy. Nat. T. N. and E. Hosp.)*. Sterile ribbon gauze impregnated with a sterile paste consisting of iodoform 40%, bismuth subnitrate 20%, and liquid paraffin 40%.

Bismuth Subnitrate and Iodoform Paste *(B.P.C. 1954)*. Past. Bism. Subnit. et Iodof.; BIPP; Bismuth and Iodoform Paste. Bismuth subnitrate 1, iodoform 2, sterilised liquid paraffin 1, by wt, prepared aseptically. Store in a cool place in sterilised collapsible tubes. Prolonged or extensive application may give rise to iodoform poisoning.

Adverse effects. Open leg ulcers in a Malay child aged 13 months were treated with the paste. They healed but oedema and pain increased. After 9 weeks, X-ray examination showed dense transverse bands of metallic bismuth deposited in metaphyseal growth areas of long bones.— H. N. Krige, *S. Afr. med. J.*, 1963, *37,* 1005.

Two reactions to dental dressings with Bismuth Subnitrate and Iodoform Paste occurred in which crystals of bismuth subnitrate were considered to be the cause rather than the iodoform.— W. A. Miller and G. S. Taylor, *Br. dent. J.*, 1968, *124,* 420.

Symptoms compatible with iodoform toxicity occurred in 1 patient and raised iodine concentrations in 2 further patients following the packing of cavities with gauze impregnated with Bismuth Subnitrate and Iodoform Paste. In a further patient who received a pack soaked in Compound Iodoform Paint no signs of iodoform toxicity were observed. It was suggested that Bismuth Subnitrate and Iodoform Paste was satisfactory for packing small operative cavities but for large cavities Compound Iodoform Paint pastes were safer.— A. F. F. O'Connor *et al., J. Lar. Otol.*, 1977, *91,* 903.

Compound Iodoform Paint *(B.P.C. 1954)*. Pig. Iodof. Co.; Iodoform Varnish; Whitehead's Varnish. Prepared from iodoform 10 g, benzoin 10 g, prepared storax 7.5 g, tolu balsam 5 g, and solvent ether to 100 ml.

4578-t

Iodophores

Iodophores are carriers of iodine and are usually complexes of iodine with certain types of surfactants with detergent properties. It is possible for iodine to be taken up in chemical combination by high molecular weight surfactants and water-soluble polymers. The surfactants may be nonionic, cationic, or anionic, but generally the most efficient and stable iodophores are compounds of nonionic surfactants.

Though the iodine in an iodophore is held in loose chemical combination, part of the iodine is available and retains its bactericidal activity. Iodophores may solubilise up to 25% by weight of iodine of which about 80% may be released as available iodine when a concentrated solution is diluted.

Solutions of an iodophore are more stable than solutions of iodine which lose strength by volatilisation and there is no precipitation on dilution of an iodophore solution. The stability of the majority is not affected by changes in pH. As the available iodine is taken up, the colour of the solution changes from amber to pale yellow.

Unlike the hypochlorites, solutions of iodophores can be formulated with acid and the bactericidal action of most of them is enhanced by lowering the pH. Increases in temperature increase the bactericidal action of iodophores, but above 43° they break down with the liberation of iodine.

Stability of solutions. Use-dilutions of an iodophore preparation (Wescodyne) containing 150 ppm available iodine and 0.05% sodium nitrite lost their typical brown colour after standing for a few days and were found to lose 24% potency in 24 hours or 42% in 48 hours at 35°. Similar dilutions without sodium nitrite were more stable and lost 9.2% potency after 3 weeks at 35°.— R. J. Abrahams and H. J. Derewicz, *Am. J. Hosp. Pharm.*, 1968, *25,* 192.

Uses. Solutions of iodophores are employed in pre-operative skin disinfection and for disinfecting blankets and some instruments. Stains of iodophores on skin and natural fabrics may be removed by washing with soap and water. The iodophores described in this section are Povidone-Iodine (see p.867) and Undecoylium Chloride-Iodine (see p.868).

Disinfection of skin. There was no significant difference in the incidence of wound infections when an iodophore and hexachlorophane were used as surgical hand scrubs.— J. J. White and A. Duncan, *Surgery Gynec. Obstet.*, 1972, *135,* 890.

The effectiveness of iodophores against both Gram-negative and Gram-positive organisms was an advantage over hexachlorophane, but they did not persist in the skin to provide cumulative, continuing antibacterial activity. Like alcohol, iodophores could cause excessive dryness of the skin with repeated use.— *Med. Lett.*, 1976, *18,* 85. Iodophores were active against both Gram-negative and Gram-positive bacteria and did not require repeated application for maximum effectiveness. They were considered to be less bactericidal but less irritant than aqueous or alcoholic solutions of iodine.— *ibid.*, 1977, *19,* 83.

Studies involving 95 women in active labour necessitating continuous epidural analgesia indicated that skin disinfection of the catheter site with an iodophore (Prepodyne) was superior to that with a benzalkonium chloride preparation.— E. Abouleish *et al., Anesthesiology*, 1977, *46,* 351.

For other reports, see Povidone-Iodine, p.867.

Uses of disinfectants on farms. For a list of disinfectants, including iodophores, and their rate of dilution approved for use in Great Britain in foot-and-mouth disease, swine vesicular disease, fowl pest, and tuberculosis in animals, see The Diseases of Animals (Approved Disinfectants) Order 1978 (SI 1978: No. 32), as amended (SI 1978: No. 934; SI 1979: No. 37).

A list of proprietary iodophore preparations approved for the cleansing and disinfecting of milk containers and appliances is contained in Circular FSH 8/78, Ministry of Agriculture, Fisheries and Foods, London, HM Stationery Office, 1978.

Virus disinfection. For the disinfection of materials in contact with lassa fever virus, see *Memorandum on Lassa Fever*, Dept of Health and Social Security, London, HM Stationery Office, 1976.

Recommendations for precautions in medical care of, and in handling materials from, patients with transmissible virus dementia (Creutzfeldt-Jakob disease).— D. C. Gajdusek *et al., New Engl. J. Med.*, 1977, *297,* 1253.

For the use of iodophores in the disinfection of fabrics exposed to smallpox virus, see Disinfectants, General, p.548.

Proprietary Preparations

Faringets *(Winthrop, UK)*. Lozenges each containing 4 mg of miristalkonium iodine chloride (myristyl benzalkonium iodine chloride; benzyldimethyltetradecylammonium chloride-iodine complex; $C_{23}H_{42}ClI_2N$=621.9). For minor infections of the throat. *Dose.* 1 or 2 lozenges to be sucked slowly every 4 hours; not more than 6 in 24 hours.

Steribath *(Stuart, UK)*. An antiseptic solution containing an iodophore (complexed with a nonoxynol) and providing 4.5% of available iodine; available in 14-ml sachets for addition to the bath.

Vanodine *(Evans Vanodine, UK)*. A bactericidal and fungicidal detergent solution containing available iodine 1.92% w/v (in the form of an iodine-poloxamer complex 18.7%). For the control of foot infections in swimming baths and changing rooms. Dilute 1 vol. in 100 vol. of water for use.

Other Proprietary Names

SeptoDyne *(USA)*.

4579-x

Potassium Iodide *(B.P., B.P. Vet., Eur. P., U.S.P.)*. Pot. Iod.; Potassii Iodidum; Kalii Iodidum; Kalii Iodetum; Kalii Jodidum; Kalium Iodatum; Kalium Jodatum; Potassium (Iodure de); Iodeto de Potássio.
KI=166.0.

CAS — 7681-11-0.

Pharmacopoeias. In all pharmacopoeias examined except *Chin.*

Odourless, colourless, transparent or somewhat opaque crystals or white granular powder with a slightly bitter saline taste. It is slightly hygroscopic in moist air. Each g represents 6 mmol (6 mEq) of potassium and of iodide.

Soluble 1 in 0.7 of water, 1 in 23 of alcohol, 1 in 75 of acetone, 1 in 2.5 of methyl alcohol, and 1 in 2 of glycerol. Solutions in water are neutral or alkaline to litmus. A 2.59% solution in water is iso-osmotic with serum. When potassium iodide is dissolved in water to form a strong solution, there is a marked fall in the temperature of the solution; when sodium iodide is dissolved, there is a marked rise in temperature. Solutions in water may be faintly alkaline and become yellowish in colour on standing, especially when exposed to light, owing to the liberation of a trace of free iodine. Iodine readily dissolves in an aqueous solution of potassium iodide, forming a dark brown solution containing potassium tri-iodide. Certain iodides, such as mercuric iodide, which are insoluble in water, also dissolve in an aqueous solution, double iodides being formed. A slightly alkaline solution keeps better than an acid one. Solutions are **sterilised** by autoclaving or by filtration.

Incompatible with salts of iron, bismuth, copper, lead, and mercury, potassium chlorate and other oxidising agents, mineral acids, strychnine hydrochloride, quinine sulphate, and other alkaloidal salts. **Store** in airtight containers. Protect from light.

When mixtures containing potassium iodide, sodium bicarbonate or other alkaline substance, and alcohol were stored for prolonged periods, iodoform was produced from the free iodine released by atmospheric oxidation.— J. C. Barfield and H. S. Grainger, *Pharm. J.*, 1952, *2,* 263.

Incompatibility. Solutions containing potassium iodide 3% with chlorhexidine acetate 0.01% were autoclaved for 30 minutes at 115°. A white crystalline precipitate developed after 5 days. A precipitate also developed in solutions not autoclaved.— Pharm. Soc. Lab. Rep., P/73/13, 1973.

Masking the taste. Glycyrrhiza syrup was more effective than aromatic elixir, syrup of cinnamon, or simple syrup, in masking the taste of a concentrated solution of potassium iodide. The stability of the potassium iodide was greatest in the presence of glycyrrhiza syrup and least in the presence of simple syrup.— M. David and C. L. Huyck, *Am. J. Hosp. Pharm.*, 1958, *15,* 586.

Stability of solutions. To prevent discoloration of potassium iodide solutions, the addition of ascorbic acid 0.018% was suggested.— *Australas. J. Pharm.*, 1965, *46,* 12.

Adverse Effects, Treatment, and Precautions. As for Iodine, p.862.

Potassium iodide should not generally be given in pulmonary tuberculosis as it may convert a dormant into an active disease.

Absorption and Fate. Potassium iodide is readily absorbed from the gastro-intestinal tract. It diffuses across the placenta. It is excreted mainly in the urine, with smaller amounts appearing in the faeces, saliva, sweat, and milk.

Uses. Potassium iodide may be used for the prophylaxis and treatment of simple goitre, which is endemic in districts where the diet is deficient in iodides. It is usually given for this purpose as iodised salt, commercial forms of which may contain 0.01% potassium iodide or potassium iodate.

It is used similarly to Aqueous Iodine Solution in the pre-operative treatment of thyrotoxicosis (see under Iodine, p.863). Some authorities recommend a dose of 150 mg daily in divided doses; other authorities consider a smaller dose, such as 15 mg daily in divided doses, to be sufficient.

Potassium iodide may be given by mouth in doses of 150 mg before the administration of iodine radionuclides to saturate the thyroid when uptake of radio-iodine by the thyroid is not desired. Potassium iodide is also given for about 3 weeks after radio-iodine.

Potassium iodide is also used in the treatment of cutaneous lymphatic sporotrichosis. It is usually given in a gradually increasing dosage up to the limit of tolerance and should be continued for at least 1 month after the disappearance or stabilisation of the lesions. Potassium iodide was also formerly used in the treatment of actinomycosis, blastomycosis, and the later stages of syphilis.

Potassium iodide in doses of 250 to 500 mg has been used as an expectorant in the belief that bronchial secretion is increased by reflex stimulation of the gastric mucosa but there is little evidence to show that it is effective.

Potassium iodide is usually administered in mixtures or in solution, freely diluted, since concentrated solutions have an irritant action on the gastric mucosa. Its use should be avoided in children (see Iodine, p.863).

Potassium iodide is not appreciably absorbed percutaneously so topical preparations cannot be expected to have any effect on the thyroid.

In veterinary medicine potassium iodide is used in the treatment of actinobacillosis of *cattle.*

Erythema nodosum responded to potassium iodide 360 to 900 mg daily in 24 of 28 patients and nodular vasculitis in 16 of 17.— E. J. Schulz and D. A. Whiting, *Br. J. Derm.*, 1976, *94,* 75.

A lymphocutaneous infection in a 72-year-old man initially considered to be sporotrichosis but later found to be due to *Nocardia brasiliensis* responded well to treatment with a saturated solution of potassium iodide in a dose of 60 drops thrice daily. The patient received potassium iodide therapy for 8 weeks and on follow-up 5 months later showed no recurrence of the lesions.— G. Mitchell *et al.*, *Am. Rev. resp. Dis.*, 1975, *112,* 721.

Bronchitis. Viscous hypersecretion leading to mucous plugging of bronchi could be reduced with potassium iodide and corticosteroids. In optimum dosage, potassium iodide was effective within 12 to 24 hours, but corticosteroids reduced hypersecretion only within 2 to 3 weeks.— H. Herxheimer (letter), *Br. med. J.*, 1969, *2,* 246.

In 89 patients with chronic obstructive pulmonary disease, tablets containing potassium iodide 135 mg and nicotinamide hydriodide 25 mg effectively reduced viscosity of mucus, decreased difficulty in expectorating, and increased the volume of sputum. Dosage was 2 tablets thrice daily after meals. Four other patients had poor response and 4 were withdrawn because of side-effects.— H. H. Pelz, *Clin. Med.*, 1973, *80* (Apr.), 18.

Further references: C. Bernecker, *Acta allerg.*, 1969, *24,* 216.

Goitre. A significant reduction in the prevalence of endemic goitre among schoolchildren in Tasmania was achieved after 16 years' prophylactic treatment with potassium iodide. Dosage was generally 10 mg weekly in tablet form.— F. W. Clements *et al.*, *Bull. Wld Hlth Org.*, 1968, *38,* 297. See also J. C. Stewart and G. I. Vidor, *Br. med. J.*, 1976, *1,* 372.

Further references: M. Ranke *et al.*, *Dt. med. Wschr.*, 1979, *104,* 132.

Hyperthyroidism. Supplementary treatment with potassium iodide given to patients after treatment for thyrotoxicosis was considered to have no effect on relapse-rate.— N. C. Thalassinos and T. R. Fraser, *Lancet*, 1971, *2,* 183.

Pre-operative use. Preliminary results suggesting that potassium iodide with propranolol may be the treatment of choice in the pre-operative preparation of patients with Graves' disease. Ten women with Graves' disease took propranolol 80 mg every 8 hours for a mean of 40 days pre-operatively and continued until the end of the fifth postoperative day, particular care being taken to ensure that the last dose before operation was not omitted. Potassium iodide 60 mg thrice daily was taken for 10 days pre-operatively and produced a marked fall in serum concentrations of thyroid hormone in all patients. At operation all patients were clinically euthyroid with a resting pulse-rate of less than 90 per minute; there were no complications. There is a possibility of a secondary rise in thyroid hormone concentrations if potassium iodide is taken for longer than 10 days.— C. M. Feek *et al.*, *New Engl. J. Med.*, 1980, *302,* 883. Comments and criticisms: C. H. Emerson and M. M. S. El-Zaheri (letter), *ibid.*, *303,* 527; J. Feely, *ibid.*, 528.

See also under Propranolol, p.1333.

Iodised salt. In 23 countries which had legislation requiring the use of iodised salt in strengths ranging from 1 in 130 000 to 1 in 10 000 in part or the whole of the country, the incidence of endemic goitre had been reduced by 42 to 95%.— F. W. Lowenstein, *Am. J. publ. Hlth*, 1967, *57,* 1815.

Recommended additions of potassium or sodium iodides or of their corresponding iodates, for the prevention of endemic goitre, were of concentrations varying between 1 in 25 000 and 1 in 50 000; 1 in 10 000 was considered to be higher than was generally required, and 1 in 100 000 might be insufficient.— J. B. Stanbury *et al.*, *Chronicle Wld Hlth Org.*, 1974, *28,* 220.

Further references: R. de León Méndez, *Boln Of. sanit. pan-am.*, 1966, *61,* 1; A. Steck *et al.*, *Schweiz. med. Wschr.*, 1972, *102,* 829; K. P. Chen *et al.*, *J. Formosan med. Ass.*, 1976, *75,* 471.

Phycomycosis. A 25-year-old patient with subcutaneous phycomycosis in the left thigh was successfully treated with potassium iodide, 450 mg thrice daily, for 4 months.— A. M. El Hassan *et al.*, *Trans. R. Soc. trop. Med. Hyg.*, 1970, *64,* 134. See also S. Kelly *et al.*, *ibid.*, 1980, *74,* 396.

Sporotrichosis. A 40-year-old man with primary pulmonary sporotrichosis due to *Sporothrix schenckii* responded satisfactorily to treatment with potassium iodide and griseofulvin. The potassium iodide was given as a saturated solution in as high a dosage as the patient could tolerate. After 2 months' treatment, griseofulvin 500 mg daily was added to the regimen for a further 2 months. After discharge, the patient was maintained on 15 drops of saturated potassium iodide solution thrice daily for a month or 2 to prevent relapse.— R. D. Trevathan and S. Phillips, *J. Am. med. Ass.*, 1966, *195,* 965.

A report in 2 children of skin lesions considered to be due to *Sporothrix schenkii* responding well to treatment with potassium iodide by mouth and local application of tincture of iodine. The infecting organism could not be demonstrated in 1 patient, but the presence of *Leishmania donovanii* was excluded in both.— S. A. Gumaa, *Trans. R. Soc. trop. Med. Hyg.*, 1978, *72,* 637.

Further references: J. W. Chandler *et al.*, *Am. J. Dis. Child.*, 1968, *115,* 368; D. D. Munro, *Br. J. Derm.*, 1968, *80,* 478; F. T. Becker and H. R. Young, *Minn. Med.*, 1970, *53,* 851; P. J. Lynch and F. Botero, *Am. J. Dis. Child.*, 1971, *122,* 325; E. R. Orr and H. D. Riley, *J. Pediat.*, 1971, *78,* 951.

Thyroid blocking. Although most references reported the use of potassium iodide 150 mg or sodium iodide 100 mg 24 hours before and daily for 3 weeks after the ^{125}I-fibrinogen test, potassium iodide 400 mg by mouth was as effective if given at the same time as the fibrinogen injection and 200 mg daily given for 3 weeks.— K. Forsberg (letter), *Br. med. J.*, 1974, *1,* 392.

A study providing guidelines for stable iodide prophylaxis in the event of exposure to radioactive iodine in a radiation emergency.— E. Sternthal *et al.*, *New Engl. J. Med.*, 1980, *303,* 1083.

Thyrotoxic crisis. A suggestion that iodides and propranolol may be used for the treatment of thyrotoxic crisis in labour. It was considered that treatment with iodides for this brief period only was unlikely to affect the foetus.— G. N. Burrow, *New Engl. J. Med.*, 1978, *298,* 150.

Preparations

Liniments

Potassium Iodide with Soap Liniment *(B.P.C. 1949)*. Lin. Pot. Iod. c. Sap. A solid liniment prepared from potassium iodide 15 g, curd soap 20 g, glycerol 10 ml, lemon oil 1 ml, and water 100 ml. It contains about 10.5% w/w of KI.

Mixtures

Ammoniated Potassium Iodide Mixture *(B.P.C. 1973)*. Potassium Iodide and Ammonia Mixture. Potassium iodide 150 mg, ammonium bicarbonate 150 mg, liquorice liquid extract 1 ml, double-strength chloroform water 5 ml, water to 10 ml. It should be recently prepared. *Dose.* 10 to 20 ml.

Potassium Iodide and Ephedrine Mixture *(A.P.F.)*. Potassium iodide 250 mg, ephedrine hydrochloride 10 mg, ammonium bicarbonate 100 mg, liquorice liquid extract

0.5 ml, concentrated chloroform water 0.25 ml, water to 10 ml. *Dose.* 10 to 30 ml.

Potassium Iodide and Ephedrine Mixture CF *(A.P.F.).* Potassium Iodide and Ephedrine Mixture for Children. Potassium iodide 100 mg, ephedrine hydrochloride 10 mg, stramonium tincture 0.2 ml, aromatic ammonia spirit 0.1 ml, liquorice liquid extract 0.2 ml, concentrated chloroform water 0.1 ml, water to 5 ml. *Dose.* 5 to 10 ml.

Potassium Iodide and Stramonium Mixture Compound *(A.P.F.).* Potassium iodide 250 mg, stramonium tincture 0.5 ml, lobelia ethereal tincture 0.5 ml, aromatic ammonia spirit 0.5 ml, liquorice liquid extract 0.5 ml, concentrated chloroform water 0.25 ml, water to 10 ml. *Dose.* 10 to 20 ml.

Potassium Iodide Mixture *(A.P.F.).* Mist. Pot. Iod. Potassium iodide 250 mg, ammonium bicarbonate 100 mg, liquorice liquid extract 0.5 ml, concentrated chloroform water 0.25 ml, water to 10 ml. *Dose.* 10 to 30 ml.

Potassium Iodide Mixture *(Jap. P.).* Potassium iodide 500 mg, sodium bicarbonate 2 g, bitter tincture 2 ml, water to 100 ml.

Potassium Iodide Mixture CF *(A.P.F.).* Potassium Iodide Mixture for Children. Potassium iodide 100 mg, liquorice liquid extract 0.25 ml, aromatic ammonia spirit 0.1 ml, concentrated chloroform water 0.1 ml, water to 5 ml. *Dose.* 5 to 10 ml.

Solutions

Potassium Iodide Oral Solution *(U.S.P.).* Potassium Iodide Solution. Potassium iodide 100 g, water to 100 ml. If the solution is not to be used within a short time, 50 mg of sodium thiosulphate is added to each 100 ml. Crystals of potassium iodide may form during storage. Store in airtight containers. Protect from light.

Tablets

Potassium Iodide Tablets *(U.S.P.).* Tablets containing potassium iodide. Store in airtight containers.

Proprietary Names

Jodetten *(Winzer, Ger.)*; Pherajod *(Kanoldt, Ger.)*; Pima *(Fleming, USA)*; SSKI *(Upsher-Smith, USA)*; Solvejod *(Draco, Swed.)*.

Eye-drops containing potassium iodide and calcium chloride were formerly marketed in Great Britain under the proprietary name Chibret Iodo-chloride Collyrium *(Chibret, Fr.)*.

4580-y

Povidone-Iodine *(U.S.P.).* Polyvidone-Iodine; Polyvinylpyrrolidone-Iodine Complex; PVP-Iodine.

CAS — 25655-41-8.

Pharmacopoeias. In *U.S.*

A complex of iodine with povidone, containing 9 to 12% of available iodine calculated on the dried basis. It occurs as a yellowish-brown amorphous hygroscopic powder with a slight characteristic odour. It loses not more than 8% of its weight on drying.

Soluble in water and alcohol; practically insoluble in acetone, carbon tetrachloride, chloroform, ether, and light petroleum. A 10% solution in water has a pH of 1.5 to 2.5. **Store** in airtight containers.

Incompatibility. A mixture of equal parts of povidone-iodine solution and hydrogen peroxide 3% exploded about 100 minutes after dispensing. It was suggested that iodine had accelerated the decomposition of the peroxide thus liberating oxygen and the explosion had been caused by the inadvertent tightening of the cap on the bottle.— E. Dannenberg and J. Peebles (letter), *Am. J. Hosp. Pharm.*, 1978, *35*, 525.

Stability of solutions. A study on the stability on storage of aqueous solutions of povidone-iodine buffered to about pH 6.— H. L. M. Cox, *Pharm. Weekbl. Ned.*, 1977, *112*, 1174.

Adverse Effects. Local irritation and sensitivity may occur following topical administration of povidone-iodine.

Systemic effects including metabolic acidosis, hypernatraemia, and renal impairment may follow the application of povidone-iodine to severe burns or to large areas otherwise denuded of skin.

Following the introduction of a regimen in patients undergoing abdominal hysterectomy using povidone-iodine pessaries pre-operatively and the spraying of wounds with a povidone-iodine spray containing 5% available iodine after the closure of the peritoneal cavity, the incidence of postoperative pyrexia, tachycardia, and urinary retention increased.— E. de Valera and J. Vaughan, *J. Ir. med. Ass.*, 1978, *71*, 162.

Allergy. From patch tests carried out in 413 patients with contact dermatoses, 1 was found to be allergic to povidone-iodine.— E. Epstein, *J. Am. med. Ass.*, 1966, *198*, 517.

Effects on electrolytes. Severe metabolic acidosis occurred in 2 patients (a 30-year-old man and a 72-year-old woman with 75% and 35% burns respectively) whose burns were treated topically with povidone-iodine every 8 or 12 hours. Serum-iodine concentrations were markedly elevated. It was suggested that iodophores should not be applied topically to burns greater than 20% of the body surface.— J. Pietsch and J. L. Meakins, *Lancet*, 1976, *1*, 280.

Severe hypernatraemia and acidosis occurred in a patient with second-degree burns who was treated topically with povidone-iodine. Three similar cases had been observed. This hazard should be considered especially when treating second-degree burns.— C. Scoggin *et al.* (letter), *Lancet*, 1977, *1*, 959.

Effects on the thyroid. A 21-year-old woman with impaired renal function developed reversible hyperthyroidism during the second week of treatment of first-and second-degree burns to the dorsa of both hands with povidone-iodine; delayed iodine excretion might have been involved.— J. R. Fisher (letter), *New Engl. J. Med.*, 1977, *297*, 171.

A report of hypothyroidism in a neonate following topical administration to a surgical wound of a povidone-iodine ointment.— A. Wuilloud *et al.*, *Z. kinderchir.*, 1977, *20*, 181.

Precautions. Povidone-iodine should not be used on patients with non-toxic nodular colloid goitre. Application to large areas of broken skin should be avoided as excessive absorption of iodine may occur.

Absorption of povidone-iodine may interfere with tests of thyroid function.

A report of iodine absorption resulting from irrigation of the peritoneal cavity with 550 ml of a 10% solution of povidone-iodine. The intraperitoneal use of this preparation should be limited.— C. F. Strife *et al.* (letter), *Lancet*, 1977, *1*, 1265. The dose used would provide 5.5 g of available iodine, over 10 times what was considered to be an effective dose.— O. J. A. Gilmore (letter), *ibid.*, 1977, *2*, 37.

Dental use. There was no significant change in the mean wet-weight of plaque in 16 healthy subjects who had used a 0.5% aqueous solution of povidone-iodine as a mouth-wash four times daily for 14 days. However, there was a significant increase in the total serum iodide, protein bound iodide, total thyroxine and free thyroxine index. It was recommended that the use of povidone-iodine in a mouth-wash be restricted to acute situations and that it should not be used over prolonged periods. Brown staining of the teeth occurred in 5 subjects.— M. M. Ferguson *et al.*, *Br. dent. J.*, 1978, *144*, 14.

For a comparison of solutions of povidone-iodine, another iodophore, and inorganic iodine used as anti-plaque agents, see iodine, p.863.

Interference with diagnostic tests. Urine contaminated with povidone-iodine gave a false-positive result for urinary occult blood tested with reagent strips.— R. Said, *J. Am. med. Ass.*, 1979, *242*, 748.

Pregnancy and the neonate. Studies involving 40 neonates indicated that topical application of povidone-iodine to the umbilical cord and the surrounding area of normal intact skin resulted in significantly increased plasma-iodine concentrations. Although no alteration in thyroid function was observed it was suggested that until further information was available caution should be exercised in the prolonged use of povidone-iodine in neonates.— S. P. Pyati *et al.*, *J. Pediat.*, 1977, *91*, 825.

A suggestion that vaginitis in pregnant women should not be treated with povidone-iodine because of the possible development of iodine-induced goitre and hypothyroidism in the foetus and neonate due to vaginal absorption of iodine.— H. Vorherr *et al.*, *J. Am. med. Ass.*, 1980, *244*, 2628.

Uses. Povidone-iodine is an iodophore (see p.865) which slowly liberates inorganic iodine in contact with the skin and mucous membranes. It is used similarly to iodine (see p.863) and is employed for the treatment of contaminated wounds, pre-operative preparation of the skin and vagina, infections of the mouth, herpes infections, oral and vaginal candidiasis, vaginal trichomoniasis, acne vulgaris, and other pyogenic or seborrhoeic infections of the scalp or skin. It has also been used in the treatment of eczematoid ringworm.

The antiseptic activity of povidone-iodine is reduced by alkalis. Preparations containing 0.4 to 1% of available iodine are used for application to the skin and solutions containing up to 1% of available iodine for application to the mouth and oral mucosa.

Stains on synthetic fabrics may be removed by washing and rinsing in dilute ammonia.

In a clinical study, 95% of patients treated with povidone-iodine aerosol (Betadine) prior to application of plaster casts had no skin irritation or scaling when the cast was removed. Although dimethicone cream afforded some protection, only 10% of the patients in this group and 3% of the control group had no scaling, roughness, or irritation.— G. L. Mouzas, *Br. J. clin. Pract.*, 1973, *27*, 216.

Povidone-iodine solution (1% available iodine) was effective against *Mycobacterium tuberculosis* in a modified Kelsey-Sykes capacity test.— P. J. McDonald *et al.*, *Med. J. Aust.*, 1974, *2*, 41.

For the use of povidone-iodine as a pre-operative vaginal disinfectant, see A. D. Haeri *et al.*, *S. Afr. med. J.*, 1976, *50*, 1984; N. G. Osborne and R. C. Wright, *Obstet. Gynec.*, 1977, *50*, 148.

The use of a mixture of equal parts of povidone-iodine ointment 10% (Betadine) and honey for the treatment of abrasions and varicose ulcers.— N. Lawrence (letter), *J. R. Coll. gen. Pract.*, 1976, *26*, 843.

Good or excellent symptomatic relief was reported by 20 elderly patients with decubitus and stasis ulcers treated with povidone-iodine solution and ointment thrice daily.— A. Gilgore, *Curr. ther. Res.*, 1978, *24*, 843.

Evidence to suggest that rectal antisepsis with povidone-iodine 10% solution before transrectal prostatic biopsy reduces the risk of contamination and the incidence of bacteraemia.— M. Rees *et al.*, *Br. med. J.*, 1980, *281*, 650. See also E. C. Ashby *et al.*, *ibid.*, 1978, *2*, 1263.

Acne. References: A. L. Hudson, *Clin. Trials J.*, 1973, *10* (1), 23; E. J. Brown, *Br. J. clin. Pract.*, 1977, *31*, 218; S. A. Khan, *ibid.*, 1979, *33*, 289.

Cervical erosions. Sixty-eight women with cervical erosions were treated with povidone-iodine pessaries, 400 mg or hydrargaphen pessaries 10 mg each night for up to 4 months. Of the 34 patients in each group 20 responded well to treatment with povidone-iodine, with 5 defaulting, and 17 responded to hydrargaphen, with 3 defaulting. The difference between the 2 preparations used was not considered to be significant, but toxicity associated with the absorption of mercury during extended therapy with hydrargaphen should be considered.— J. P. Todd, *Br. J. clin. Pract.*, 1979, *33*, 47.

Disinfection of contact lenses. An account of the kinetics of a transient iodine-disinfecting system using povidone-iodine and sodium formate for hydrophilic contact lenses.— J. K. Andrews *et al.*, *J. Pharm. Pharmac.*, 1977, *29*, *Suppl.*, 65P.

Disinfection of equipment. Mention of the use of a povidone-iodine solution in the disinfection of a fibreoptic bronchoscope.— H. J. Weinstein *et al.*, *Am. Rev. resp. Dis.*, 1977, *116*, 541.

Disinfection of skin. A study of postoperative clostridial infection in 2 patients suggested that povidone-iodine, which had good sporicidal activity on artificially contaminated skin, proved much less effective than might have been expected in freeing the skin from *Clostridium welchii*.— M. T. Parker, *Br. med. J.*, 1969, *3*, 671.

Clostridium welchii was isolated from 81 of 100 skin samples taken from the anal cleft or hips of 100 patients. Cultures of samples taken from 60 of these patients after application of a gauze compress soaked in povidone-iodine solution were negative.— S. E. Drewett *et al.*, *Lancet*, 1972, *1*, 1172.

After studies in *rats* had shown that povidone-iodine aerosol (Disadine DP) did not irritate the wound, 101 patients undergoing 'clean' non-abdominal surgery were studied. In 48 the wound was sprayed for 10 seconds prior to closure. There were 2 cases of wound infection in the controls and none in the povidone-iodine group. Povidone-iodine was a suitable alternative to antibiotics for use in wounds.— O. J. A. Gilmore *et al.*, *Postgrad. med. J.*, 1977, *53*, 122.

Povidone-iodine sprayed onto the wound after closing the peritoneum and after inserting skin sutures was no more effective than no treatment in preventing wound infections following abdominal surgery, the incidence of infection being 15 of 38 patients in the povidone-iodine group and 16 of 38 in the control group. Two intramuscular doses of tobramycin 160 mg with lincomycin 600 mg significantly reduced wound infection.— R. B. Galland *et al.*, *Lancet*, 1977, *2*, 1043. Povidone-iodine had been shown to be effective in preventing wound infection without producing bacterial resistance.— O. J. A. Gilmore (letter), *ibid.*, 1284.

Of 166 hospital out-patients, with superficial wounds suitable for primary suture, sprayed with povidone-iodine, only 10 (6%) were noted to have a wound infection at review 6 days later, whereas of 154 similar control patients 22 (14%) had an infection.— W. J. Morgan (letter), *Lancet*, 1978, *1*, 769.

Further references: E. J. L. Lowbury *et al.*, *Br. med. J.*, 1964, *2*, 531; *ibid.*, 1969, *2*, 328; G. A. J. Ayliffe and E. J. L. Lowbury, *ibid.*, 333; O. J. A. Gilmore *et al.*, *Lancet*, 1973, *1*, 220; A. V. Pollock and M. Evans, *Br. J. Surg.*, 1975, *62*, 292; *Lancet*, 1976, *1*, 73; O. J. A. Gilmore, *Ann. R. Coll. Surg.*, 1977, *59*, 93; P. Keller and E. Rubinstein, *Curr. ther. Res.*, 1978, *24*, 673; J. K. Gosnold, *Practitioner*, 1979, *223*, 271; W. J. Morgan, *Br. J. clin. Pract.*, 1979, *33*, 109.

For further reports of the use of povidone-iodine in skin disinfection, see under Disinfectants, p.548, and Chlorhexidine Gluconate Solution, p.556.

See also under Iodophores, p.865.

Herpes. A favourable report of the use of povidone-iodine in the treatment of 10 patients with herpes simplex infection of the external genitalia.— E. G. Friedrich and T. Masukawa, *Obstet. Gynec.*, 1975, *45*, 337.

Good results following the use of povidone-iodine, as a 10% alcoholic solution, in the treatment of 34 patients with herpes simplex or herpes zoster.— P. Woodbridge, *J. int. med. Res.*, 1977, *5*, 378.

Further references: J. Bullough, *Curr. med. Res. Opinion*, 1979, *6*, 175.

Vaginitis. Favourable results were obtained in 74 women with candidal vaginitis, 4 out of 5 with trichomonal vaginitis, and 13 out of 14 with candidal-trichomonal vaginitis who were treated daily for 1 to 4 weeks with povidone-iodine (Betadine) as a vaginal gel at bedtime and a douche next morning.— J. J. Ratzan, *Calif. Med.*, 1969, *110*, 24.

Following twice-daily insertion of pessaries containing povidone-iodine 200 mg for 14 days, 29 of 41 women with vaginitis were relieved of symptoms and 25 were bacteriologically cured. There were no replapses in 18 who returned for re-examination after 3 months.— P. G. Harris, *Practitioner*, 1972, *209*, 828.

Preparations

Povidone-Iodine Solution *(B.P.)*. An aqueous solution of povidone-iodine containing 0.85 to 1.2% of available iodine. pH 3 to 5.5.

Povidone-Iodine Topical Aerosol Solution *(U.S.P.)*. Povidone-Iodine Aerosol. A solution of povidone-iodine under nitrogen in a pressurised container. Store at a temperature not exceeding 40°.

Povidone-Iodine Topical Solution *(U.S.P.)*. Povidone-Iodine Solution. A solution of povidone-iodine; it may contain a small amount of alcohol. pH not more than 6. Store in airtight containers.

Proprietary Preparations

Betadine *(Napp, UK)*. Preparations containing povidone-iodine, available as **Aerosol Spray** containing 5% w/v [equivalent to 0.5% of available iodine]; as **Alcoholic Solution** containing 10% w/v; as **Antiseptic Paint** containing 10% w/v in an alcoholic solution; as **Antiseptic Solution** containing 10% w/v; as **Gargle and Mouthwash** containing 1% w/v; as **Ointment** containing 10% w/w in a water-soluble basis; as **Scalp and Skin Cleanser** containing 7.5% w/v, with surfactant; as **Shampoo** containing 4% w/v, with surfactant and lanolin; as **Skin Cleanser** containing 4% w/v, with surfactant; as **Skin Cleanser Foam** containing 7.5% w/v; as **Surgical Scrub** containing 7.5% w/v, with non-ionic surfactants; as **Vaginal Gel** containing 10% w/w; as **Vaginal Pessaries** each containing 200 mg; and as **VC Kit** comprising **Betadine VC Concentrate** containing 10% w/v, supplied with a measuring bottle and vaginal applicator. (Also available as Betadine in *Austral., Canad., Fr., Neth., S.Afr., Spain, Switz., USA*).

Disadine DP *(Stuart, UK)*. An aerosol dry powder spray containing povidone-iodine 0.5% [equivalent to 0.05% of available iodine]. (Also available as Disadine DP in *S.Afr.*).

Pevidine *(Berk Pharmaceuticals, UK)*. Povidone-iodine, available as **Solution** containing 1% of available iodine and as **Surgical Scrub** containing 0.75% of available iodine, with surfactant.

PV-I (1%) Aural Insufflation *(Roy. Nat. T. N. and E. Hosp.)*. Povidone-iodine 10 g and povidone (Kollidon K 30) 90 g.

Videne *(Beta Medical Products, UK)*. Povidone-iodine, available as **Disinfectant Solution** and **Disinfectant Tincture** each containing 1% of available iodine and as **Surgical Scrub** containing 0.75% of available iodine in a detergent basis.

Other Proprietary Names

Arg.— Betiadine, Pervinox; *Austral.*— Savlon Dry; *Belg.*— Iso-Betadine; *Canad.*— Bridine, Proviodine; *Denm.*— Isobetadine; *Ger.*— Betaisodona; *Ital.*— Jodocur; *Jap.*— Neojodin; *S.Afr.*— Nutradine; *Spain*— Topionic; *USA*— Efodine, Final Step, Frepp, Isodine, Polydine.

4581-j

Sodium Iodide *(B.P., B.P. Vet., Eur. P., U.S.P.)*. Sod. Iod.; Sodii Iodidum; Natrii Iodidum; Natrii Iodetum; Natrii Jodidum; Natrium Iodatum; Sodium (Iodure de); Iodeto de Sódio.

$NaI = 149.9$.

CAS — 7681-82-5.

Pharmacopoeias. In all pharmacopoeias examined except *Chin.*

Colourless crystals or white odourless crystalline powder with a saline slightly bitter taste. It must be crystallised at a temperature above 20° otherwise the dihydrate is obtained. It is deliquescent in moist air and decomposes, becoming yellow in colour due to the liberation of iodine. Each g represents 6.7 mmol (6.7 mEq) of sodium and of iodide.

Soluble 1 in about 0.6 of water, 1 in 2 of alcohol, 1 in 1 of glycerol, and in acetone. A 2.37% solution is iso-osmotic with serum. When sodium iodide is dissolved in water to form a strong solution, there is a marked rise in the temperature of the solution; when potassium iodide is dissolved, there is a marked fall in temperature. Solutions are **sterilised** by autoclaving or by filtration. **Incompatibilities** are the same as for potassium iodide (see p.866). Aqueous solutions gradually become coloured on exposure to light and air due to the liberation of iodine. **Store** in airtight containers. Protect from light.

Incompatibility. There was loss of clarity when intravenous solutions of sodium iodide were mixed with those of narcotic salts, noradrenaline acid tartrate, or procaine hydrochloride.— J. A. Patel and G. L. Phillips, *Am. J. Hosp. Pharm.*, 1966, *23*, 409.

Adverse Effects, Treatment, and Precautions. As for Iodine, p.862.

Sodium iodide should generally not be given in pulmonary tuberculosis as it may convert a dormant into an active disease.

Absorption and Fate. As for Potassium Iodide, p.866.

Uses. Sodium iodide is used similarly to potassium iodide (see p.866).

For the prophylaxis of endemic goitre it may be given in doses of not more than 0.5 to 1 mg daily, 5 to 10 mg once a week, or 200 mg daily for 10 days twice a year.

Sodium iodide is used similarly to Aqueous Iodine Solution in the pre-operative treatment of thyrotoxicosis (see under Iodine, p.863). Some authorities recommend a dose of 150 mg daily in divided doses; other authorities consider a smaller dose, such as 15 mg daily in divided doses, to be sufficient.

In the immediate treatment of thyrotoxic crisis sodium iodide may be given by slow intravenous injection in doses of about 1 g.

Sodium iodide in doses of 250 to 500 mg has been used as an expectorant in the belief that bronchial secretion is increased by reflex stimulation of the gastric mucosa but there is little evidence to show that it is effective.

In veterinary medicine sodium iodide is used in the treatment of actinobacillosis and actinomycosis of *cattle.*

Hyperthyroidism. Seventeen patients with hyperthyroidism were given 1 mg of iodine, as sodium iodide, daily by mouth for several weeks. Twelve showed clinical and biochemical signs of improvement which was, however, temporary for many. But a dosage of 2 mg effected improvement, at least for a time, in all of a further 13 patients, and a dosage of 4 mg in 2 more patients acted similarly. The drug seemed to be without action on 11 euthyroid persons given 1 to 20 mg of iodine daily for 3 to 36 weeks.— R. Volpé and M. W. Johnston, *Ann. intern. Med.*, 1962, *56*, 577.

Thyroid blocking. Mention of the use of sodium iodide 100 mg intravenously followed by 100 mg twice daily by mouth for 28 days to block the uptake of iodine by the thyroid gland in the ^{125}I-fibrinogen uptake test.— G. K. Morris and J. R. A. Mitchell, *Br. med. J.*, 1977, *1*, 264.

Thyrotoxic crisis. The use of sodium iodide in hyperthyroid crises.— S. R. Newmark *et al.*, *J. Am. med. Ass.*, 1974, *230*, 592.

Preparations

Injectabile Natrii Jodidi *(Nord. P.)*. Sodium Iodide Injection. A 5% solution in Water for Injections.
Roum. P. includes a similar 10% injection.

Proprietary Names

Aminojod *(DAK, Denm.)*; Davurresolutivo *(Davur, Spain)*.

4582-z

Undecoylium Chloride-Iodine. A complex of iodine with the quaternary compound acylcolaminoformylmethylpyridinium chloride, the acyl group of which is a mixture containing 8 to 14 carbon atoms but principally a 10 to 11 carbon chain.

$\{CH_3.[CH_2]_n.CO.O.[CH_2]_2.NH.CO.CH_2.N^+C_5H_5\}Cl^-.I_2$, where n = 6 to 12.

CAS — 1338-54-1.

Soluble in water.

Undecoylium chloride-iodine is an iodophore (see p.865) which liberates iodine when in contact with skin or mucous membranes. It has similar uses to povidone-iodine.

For a comparison of undecoylium chloride-iodine with other agents in the disinfection of the skin, see Iodine, p.863.

Ion-exchange Resins

5000-p

Ion-exchange resins are synthetic inert organic polymers consisting of a hydrocarbon network to which ionisable groups are attached and they have the property of being able to exchange their labile ions for ions present in the solution with which they are in contact. The resins may be divided into 2 classes: cation exchangers, in which the ionisable group is acidic, e.g. sulphonic, carboxylic, or phenol groups, and anion exchangers, in which the ionisable group is basic, e.g. quaternary ammonium or amine groups.

For many purposes, ion-exchange resins may be regarded as insoluble acids or bases, the salts of which are also insoluble. Cation exchangers in the acid (or hydrogen) form may be neutralised by bases and regenerated with acids, and their salts (e.g. sodium, potassium, and ammonium forms) used for the exchange of cations. Anion exchangers behave analogously; in the base (or hydroxyl) form they may be neutralised by acids and regenerated with alkalis, and their salts used for the exchange of anions.

The ability of a resin to exchange one ion for another depends largely on its differing affinity for the various ions and the concentrations of the ions in solution. Cation-exchange resins tend to have affinity in decreasing order for calcium, magnesium, potassium, ammonium, sodium, and hydrogen ions.

Cholestyramine and colestipol hydrochloride anion-exchange resins are described under the section on Clofibrate and other Lipid Regulating Agents, p.408.

Adverse Effects. As cation-exchange resins are not totally selective, electrolyte disturbances may occur and adequate biochemical control should be maintained throughout treatment.

Anorexia, nausea, vomiting, constipation, and occasionally diarrhoea may develop. Large doses in elderly patients may cause faecal impaction.

For the adverse effects of the main anion-exchange resins in clinical use, see Cholestyramine, p.411.

Precautions. Because of the danger of producing uncompensated acidosis with preparations containing the hydrogen or ammonium resin these should not be employed in the presence of severely impaired renal function or diabetes mellitus. Preparations containing the calcium resin can cause calcium overloading and should not be given to patients with renal failure or hypercalcaemia. Preparations containing the sodium resin can cause sodium overloading and should be given cautiously to patients with renal failure, severe hypertension, or congestive heart failure. Cation-exchange resins should also be used with caution in patients receiving digitalis preparations since the adverse effects of digitalis may be enhanced in the presence of hypokalaemia.

Alkalosis has been reported after the concurrent administration of sodium resins and cation-donating antacids and laxatives.

See also under Cholestyramine, p.411.

Water retention of several years duration in a woman was found to be due to the raised sodium content of her drinking water. The original water which had been quite hard had been passed through an ion-exchange water softener which exchanged sodium ions for cations in the water.— W. D. Kumler (letter), *Am. Pharm.*, 1979, *NS19* (Jan.), 5.

Uses of Ion-exchange Resins. CLINICAL USES. Ion-exchange resins, administered by mouth, exchange their ions with those present in the gastro-intestinal tract and hence effect changes in the electrolyte balance of the plasma.

Cation-exchange resins in the calcium and sodium forms (see Calcium Polystyrene Sulphonate, p.870, and Sodium Polystyrene Sulphonate, p.870) are used in the treatment of hyperkalaemia associated with anuria or severe oliguria. The aluminium form has been used similarly (see Aluminium Polystyrene Sulphonate). Since their action may not be evident for some hours they are not suitable where rapid correction of severe hyperkalaemia is required and other measures should be used. Treatment should be stopped as soon as the serum-potassium concentration falls to 5 mmol per litre.

Cation-exchange resins have been used in the ammonium form to reduce the absorption of sodium from the gastro-intestinal tract in cardiovascular disease, cirrhosis of the liver, and pre-eclamptic toxaemia. Depletion of plasma potassium may be prevented by including a proportion of resin in the potassium form (see Ammonium Polystyrene Sulphonate, p.869).

The average adult dose of the cation-exchange resins is 15 g up to four times daily, the dose being adjusted to meet individual needs. Cation-exchange resins are also administered as enemas in the treatment of hyperkalaemia.

Cation-exchange resins should not be employed unless adequate laboratory facilities are available to follow the serum-electrolyte pattern.

Weak anion-exchange resins have been used as antacids for the control of symptoms in the treatment of peptic ulcer. They appear to be as effective for this purpose as the more commonly used antacids but their unpalatability detracts from their usefulness. See under Polyamine-methylene Resin (p.870).

Cholestyramine and colestipol hydrochloride (see pp.411-2) exchange chloride ions for the anions of bile salts and so prevent the normal reabsorption of these salts.

Polymeric compounds have been used in haemoperfusion for the treatment of poisoning, but in general these act mainly by adsorption and not by ion-exchange. For a discussion of haemoperfusion in the treatment of poisoning, see p.79.

Haemoperfusion through a mixture of Amberlite IR-120 (cationic) resins was performed on 3 patients in hepatic coma with hyperammonaemia. The resin mixture consisted of 4 forms of Amberlite IR-120, the sodium form 380.3 mmol, potassium form 18.15 mmol, calcium form 164 mmol, and magnesium form 11.8 mmol. In all cases perfusion lowered the blood-ammonium concentration considerably without affecting the blood concentration of sodium, potassium, calcium, or magnesium. However all patients subsequently relapsed.— J. S. Juggi, *Med. J. Aust.*, 1973, *1*, 926.

The bilirubin content of the blood of a jaundiced patient was reduced by a third by haemoperfusion through a blood-compatible anion-exchange resin.— U. M. Lopukhin *et al.* (letter), *Lancet*, 1975, *2*, 461.

PROLONGATION OF DRUG ACTION. Ion-exchange resins are used to form chemical complexes (resinates) with certain drugs in order to prolong absorption from the gastro-intestinal tract and thus extend the drug action. The method has been used for basic drugs, such as ephedrine, and for acidic drugs, such as the barbiturates. The rate of release of drugs from ion-exchange resins depends on the diameter of the resin-beads, on the degree of cross-linking within the resin, and on the strength of the resin. For effective prolongation of drug action, the resin complex is usually administered as tablets.

Ion-exchange resins have also been employed to prolong the release of drugs from ointments.

Resin complexes are sometimes useful in disguising the taste of bitter drugs and in reducing the nausea produced with some irritant drugs. They are also used as disintegrating agents in tablets.

PURIFICATION OF WATER. Ion-exchange resins are used to purify water by removal of the ionised impurities. Purified water is obtained by passing potable water through 2 columns containing a strong cation-exchange resin and a strong anion-exchange resin respectively, or through a single column containing a mixture of the 2 resins. When the cation-exchange resin is used in the acid (or hydrogen) form the cations in the water are replaced by hydrogen ions to form the corresponding acids of the salts in water. Carbonic acid formed decomposes to some extent to form carbon dioxide and water. Other acids may either undergo complete adsorption on to the anion-exchange resin or exchange anions with the resin and strongly basic anion resins may be required for the exchange of some acids. If the anion-exchange resin is used in the hydroxyl form water will be formed during this process.

The anion exchanger may be regenerated by sodium hydroxide solution and the cation exchanger by hydrochloric acid.

The main disadvantages of deionisation methods are that non-ionised and colloidal materials present in the feed water are not removed. Micro-organisms may multiply in ion-exchange columns, but their growth can be minimised by using the column continuously and regenerating regularly after a thorough backwashing.

The limitations of ion-exchange methods for the preparation of purified water, with special emphasis on bacteriological aspects.— J. M. Prickett *et al.*, *Australas. J. Pharm.*, 1971, *52*, S89. See also A. Budziszewski, *Arch. Immunol. & Ther. exp.*, 1973, *21*, 357.

For the use of ozone as a bactericide in large-scale water deionisation, see S. A. Nazarey *et al.*, *Bull. parent. Drug Ass.*, 1974, *28*, 70.

OTHER USES. Ion-exchange resins are widely used in various industrial processes to remove electrolyte impurities. They are also employed in the recovery and purification of biological materials, metals, solvents, and reagents, as catalysts, and in chemical analysis.

5001-s

Aluminium Polystyrene Sulphonate. The aluminium form of a cation-exchange resin.

CAS — 52808-31-8.

Aluminium polystyrene sulphonate is a cation-exchange resin and has the properties and uses described under Ion-exchange Resins, p.869; it has been used in the treatment of hyperkalaemia.

For the preparation and use of aluminium polystyrene sulphonate, see K. S. Chugh *et al.* (preliminary communication), *Lancet*, 1968, *2*, 952.

Raised serum concentrations of aluminium were found in 6 of 20 patients with advanced hyperkalaemic renal failure, taking 45 g or more of aluminium resin daily. It was recommended that aluminium resins and salts should be avoided in renal failure until the effects of hyperaluminaemia were determined.— G. M. Berlyne *et al.*, *Lancet*, 1970, *2*, 494.

5002-w

Ammonium Polystyrene Sulphonate. The ammonium form of a cation-exchange resin.

Ammonium polystyrene sulphonate is a cation-exchange resin and has the properties and uses described under Ion-exchange Resins, p.869. It has been used as a mixture with the potassium resin to reduce absorption of sodium ions from the gastro-intestinal tract. Each gram exchanges up to 1.2 mmol (1.2 mEq) of sodium.

5003-e

Azuresin *(B.P.C. 1973).* Azure A Carbacrylic Resin.

CAS — 8050-34-8 (azuresin); 531-53-3 (azure A).

A carbacrylic cation-exchange resin containing about 6% of 3-amino-7-dimethylaminophenothiazin-5-ium chloride (azure A).

Moist, irregular, dark blue or purple granules with a slightly pungent odour containing 18 to 35% moisture. When dried it contains 50 to 70 mg of the dye per g. **Store** in airtight containers.

Uses. Azuresin has been used in doses of 2 g usually in conjunction with a stimulant to gastric secretion for the detection without intubation of free hydrochloric acid in the gastric juice. In the presence of free acid in the stomach the dye component of the resin is displaced by hydrogen ions and is subsequently excreted in the urine, to which it imparts a green or blue colour. The amount of dye present in the urine is determined by matching the colour against that of control urine containing a known amount of the dye. The incidence of false positive and false negative results may be increased by conditions which result in decreased gastro-intestinal absorption or renal excretion.

Azuresin was formerly marketed in Great Britain with caffeine and sodium benzoate under the proprietary name Diagnex Blue (*Squibb*).

5004-l

Calcium Polystyrene Sulphonate.

The calcium form of a cation-exchange resin.

CAS — 37286-92-3.

A buff-coloured fine powder. Practically **insoluble** in water.

Adverse Effects and Precautions. As for Ion-exchange Resins, p.869.

An elderly man with a recent cardiac infarction was given calcium polystyrene sulphonate to control hyperkalaemia. He died from cardiac arrest. Necropsy also showed bronchopneumonia with large numbers of angular fragments considered to be inhaled calcium polystyrene sulphonate.— A. J. Chaplin and P. R. Millard, *Br. med. J.*, 1975, *3*, 77.

Hypercalcaemia. Significant hypercalcaemia occurred in 5 of 8 patients with chronic renal failure being treated with calcium polystyrene sulphonate, 60 g twice weekly, in addition to twice-weekly 12-hour dialysis with a dialysate calcium concentration of 1.5 mmol per litre. Serum-calcium concentrations in all the patients fell to within the normal limits when treatment with calcium polystyrene sulphonate was stopped.— M. Papadimitriou *et al.*, *Lancet*, 1968, *2*, 948. A further 5 of 10 patients treated with cation-exchange resin in the calcium form developed hypercalcaemia. The aluminium form of the resin might be better.— L. H. Sevitt and O. M. Wrong, *ibid.*, 950.

Calcium resins in a dose of 30 to 60 g daily had been used in about 100 patients without hypercalcaemia occurring. Doses of 15 to 45 g of calcium resin would provide 0.6 to 1.8 g of free calcium ions, an amount unlikely to be the sole cause of hypercalcaemia in patients with renal failure.— G. M. Berlyne (letter), *Lancet*, 1968, *2*, 1190.

Uses. Calcium polystyrene sulphonate has the properties and uses described under Ion-exchange Resins, p.869. It is used in the treatment of hyperkalaemia and may be used as an alternative to the resin in the sodium form in patients who cannot tolerate an increase in their sodium load. Each gram exchanges about 1.3 mmol (1.3 mEq) of potassium.

It is administered by mouth, in a dose of up to 15 g three or four times daily, as a suspension in water or syrup. A suggested dose for children is up to 1 g per kg body-weight daily in divided doses, reduced to a maintenance dose of 500 mg per kg. It should not be given in fruit juices that have a high potassium content.

When oral administration is difficult, calcium polystyrene sulphonate may be administered rectally as an enema. The usual daily dose is 30 g in 200 ml of an aqueous basis containing methylcellulose 1%.

Proprietary Preparations

Calcium Resonium *(Winthrop, UK)*. A brand of calcium polystyrene sulphonate. (Also available as Calcium Resonium in *Ger.*).

Other Proprietary Names

Kalimate *(Jap.)*; Kayexalate Calcium *(Belg., Fr., USA)*; Resonium Calcium *(Canad., Denm., Norw., Swed., Switz.)*; Sorbisterit *(Neth.)*.

5005-y

Carbacrylamine Resins. A mixture of 87.5% of cation-exchange resin (polyacrylic carboxylic resin, two-thirds in hydrogen form and one-third in potassium form), and 12.5% of anion-exchange resin (polyamine-methylene resin).

An almost odourless, light buff-coloured, free-flowing powder. Practically **insoluble** in water, alcohol, ether, dilute acids, and dilute alkalis.

Carbacrylamine resins have the properties and uses described under Ion-exchange Resins, p.869. The mixture has been used in doses of 16 g taken thrice daily to reduce absorption of sodium ions from the gastro-intestinal tract. A proportion of anion-exchange resin is included to counteract acidosis caused by the hydrogen form of the cation-exchange resin. Each gram exchanges about 1 mmol (1 mEq) of sodium.

5006-j

Polacrilin Potassium *(U.S.N.F.)*. The potassium salt of a synthetic unifunctional low-crosslinked carboxylic cation-exchange resin prepared from methacrylic acid and divinylbenzene.

Pharmacopoeias. In *U.S.N.F.*

It loses not more than 10% of its weight on drying; the dried material contains 20.6 to 25.1% of potassium.

Polacrilin potassium is used as a tablet disintegrant.

Proprietary Preparations

Amberlite IRP-88 *(Rohm & Haas, UK)*. A brand of polacrilin potassium. **Amberlite IRP-64** and **IRP-64M**. Brands of polacrilin.

5007-z

Polyamine-methylene Resin. A weak anion-exchange resin in the basic form.

CAS — 9009-14-7.

An almost odourless, light amber, granular, free-flowing powder. Practically **insoluble** in water and alcohol.

Polyamine-methylene resin acts as an acid adsorbent and has been used in doses of 0.5 to 1 g taken every 2 hours as an antacid in the treatment of peptic ulcer. It should only be used where symptoms are directly related to hyperchlorhydria.

5008-c

Polycarbophil *(U.S.P.)*. A synthetic hydrophilic resin of the polycarboxylic acid type, a copolymer of acrylic acid, loosely cross-linked with divinyl glycol.

CAS — 9003-97-8.

Pharmacopoeias. In *U.S.*

White to creamy-white granules with a characteristic, ester-like odour. Practically **insoluble** in water, dilute acids, dilute alkalis, and common organic solvents. A mixture of 1 g of polycarbophil and 100 ml of water has a pH of not more than 4. **Store** in airtight containers.

Polycarbophil swells in water and has a marked binding capacity for water and bile-salts. It has been used in doses of up to 6 g daily in the treatment of diarrhoea and as a bulk laxative. It is pharmacologically inert and is not absorbed from the gastro-intestinal tract.

Calcium polycarbophil (AHR-3260B) has no water-binding capacity and can therefore be made up in a palatable aqueous suspension; in the stomach, the calcium is replaced by hydrogen ions from the gastric acid to form polycarbophil.

A suspension containing calcium polycarbophil was considered to be more effective than a suspension containing kaolin and pectin in the treatment of 224 children with nonspecific diarrhoea. Control of diarrhoea was obtained within 48 hours in 91 of 127 children who took calcium polycarbophil and in 45 of 97 children who took kaolin and pectin. Both preparations were well tolerated.— M. L. Rutledge, *Curr. ther. Res.*, 1978, *23*, 443.

5009-k

Sodium Polystyrene Sulphonate.

Sodium Polystyrene Sulfonate *(U.S.P.)*. A cation-exchange resin prepared in the sodium form.

Pharmacopoeias. In *U.S.*

An odourless, tasteless, golden brown, fine powder containing not more than 10% of water. Practically **insoluble** in water.

Laboratory tests showed that breakdown of the sodium polystyrene sulphonate in Resonium-A did not occur on autoclaving a suspension for 1 hour at 121°.— E. Bretherton, *Winthrop*, personal communication, 1967.

Adverse Effects and Precautions. As for Ion-exchange Resins, p.869.

Uses. Sodium polystyrene sulphonate is a cation-exchange resin and has the properties and uses described under Ion-exchange Resins, p.869. It is used in the treatment of hyperkalaemia. Each gram exchanges about 3.1 mmol (3.1 mEq) of potassium *in vitro*, and about 1 mmol (1 mEq) *in vivo*.

It is administered by mouth, in a usual dose of 15 g three or four times daily, as a suspension in water or syrup. A suggested dose for children is up to 1 g per kg body-weight daily in divided doses, reduced to a maintenance dose of 500 mg per kg. It should not be given in fruit juices that have a high potassium content and may reduce the exchange-capacity of the resin.

When oral administration is difficult, sodium polystyrene sulphonate may be administered rectally as an enema. The usual dose is 30 g given once or twice daily in 150 to 200 ml of an aqueous vehicle containing sorbitol or methylcellulose 1%.

Metabolic acidosis in a 43-year-old man was reversed when sodium polystyrene sulphonate, 90 g daily, was given in conjunction with magnesium hydroxide mixture 90 ml daily. It appeared that, in the gastro-intestinal tract, magnesium polystyrene sulphonate and sodium chloride were formed and, as gastric acidity was neutralised, sodium bicarbonate in the small intestine was reabsorbed leading to metabolic alkalosis.— P. C. Fernandez and P. J. Kovnat, *New Engl. J. Med.*, 1972, *286*, 23. A similar report.— E. T. Schroeder, *Gastroenterology*, 1969, *56*, 868.

Preparations

Sodium Polystyrene Sulphonate Granules (Lime-flavoured) *(Roy. Free Hosp.)*. Granules prepared from sodium polystyrene sulphonate (Resonium A) 100 g, citric acid monohydrate 4 g, and powdered sucrose 50 g, and then sprayed with 8 ml of Soluble Lime Essence No. 1 *(Bush)*.— C.W. Barrett *et al.*, *Pharm. J.*, 1965, *1*, 378. Shelf-life 1 year. Store in a cool place.

Sodium Polystyrene Sulphonate Suspension. Sodium polystyrene sulphonate 25%, carmellose, medium viscosity, 0.5%, Veegum regular grade 0.3%, water q.s.— G.E. Schumacher and H. Haskill, *Am. J. Hosp. Pharm.*, 1969, *26*, 650.

A formula used in some hospitals: sodium polystyrene sulphonate 25 g, sorbitol 25 g, propylene glycol 2 ml, Veegum Regular 1 g, wild cherry syrup 0.1 ml, methyl hydroxybenzoate 100 mg, propyl hydroxybenzoate 20 mg, saccharin sodium 20 mg, water to 100 ml.

Proprietary Preparations

Resonium A *(Winthrop, UK)*. Sodium polystyrene sulphonate, available as a flavoured powder. (Also available as Resonium A in *Aust., Austral., Fin., Ger., Neth., Switz.*).

Other Proprietary Names
Kayexalate *(Ital., USA)*; Kayexalate Sodium *(Belg., Fr.)*; Resonium *(Denm., Iceland, Norw., Swed.)*.

5025-k

Proprietary Preparations of Some Other Ion-exchange Resins with Pharmaceutical Applications

Amberlite *(Rohm & Haas, UK)*. A range of ion-exchange resins. Those with pharmaceutical applications are available in 2 particle size ranges: 100 to 500 mesh and finer than 325 mesh (the suffix M indicates the finer particle size), and include anion-exchange resins of the polyamine type, **Amberlite IRP-58** and **IRP-58M;** cation-exchange resins of the sulphonated polystyrene type, **Amberlite IRP-69** and **IRP-69M.** There is also a large range of Amberlite ion-exchange resins for water conditioning and industrial applications.

Iron and Iron Salts

5030-j

Iron is an essential constituent of the body, being necessary for haemoglobin formation and for the oxidative processes of living tissues. The body contains about 4 g of iron of which 65 to 70% is present as haemoglobin. Most of the remainder is present in storage form, either as ferritin or haemosiderin in the reticuloendothelial system. A further 4% is present as myoglobin with smaller amounts occurring in haem-containing enzymes or in plasma bound to transferrin.

Iron is absorbed chiefly in the duodenum and jejunum, absorption being aided by the acid secretion of the stomach and being more readily effected when the iron is in the ferrous state. Only about 5 to 10% of the iron ingested in food is normally absorbed but the 15 to 20 mg of iron in the average Western diet each day is usually sufficient to maintain normal adults in iron equilibrium. Absorption is increased in conditions of iron deficiency and is decreased if the body stores are overloaded.

Good dietary sources of iron include meat, fish, legumes, and some leafy vegetables, but some products such as eggs which have a high iron content also contain phosphates and phytates which inhibit absorption by the formation of unabsorbable complexes. Absorption is also decreased by antacids, tetracyclines, and tea. Absorption of iron may be increased in the presence of ascorbic or succinic acids.

Iron oxides and hydroxides are used as colouring agents.

Human Requirements. Apart from haemorrhage, iron is lost from the body in the urine, faeces, nails, hair, skin, and sweat, but the total loss is small. In healthy men and non-menstruating women the loss is replaced by the absorption of about 1 mg of iron daily; about 2 mg needs to be absorbed daily by menstruating women. In childhood and adolescence, the need is proportionately greater because of growth. In pregnancy and lactation 3 mg or more must be absorbed daily.

For discussions of iron intake and requirements, see *Lancet*, 1971, *2*, 475; *Br. med. J.*, 1972, *2*, 728; W. H. Crosby, *New Engl. J. Med.*, 1977, *297*, 543; *Med. Lett.*, 1978, *20*, 45; B. S. N. Rao, *Br. med. Bull.*, 1981, *37*, 25.

The daily intake of iron of breast fed infants up to the age of 4 months was considered to be adequate. Recommended daily intake of iron in individuals who obtained more than 25% of calories from foods of animal origin: infants 5 to 12 months, 4 mg; children, 1 to 12 years, 5 mg; boys, 13 to 16 years, 9 mg; girls, 13 to 16 years, 12 mg; men and non-menstruating women, 5 mg; menstruating women, 14 mg. For the prevention of anaemia during pregnancy and lactation in populations with and without body iron stores, daily supplements of 30 to 60 and 120 to 240 mg of iron respectively were required. In addition about 500 µg daily of folic acid was required. Supplementation with both iron and folic acid should start not later than the second trimester of pregnancy and should continue until the end of lactation.—Report of a WHO Group of Experts on Nutritional Anaemias, *Tech. Rep. Ser. Wld Hlth Org. No. 503*, 1972.

The following daily intake of iron was recommended for infants: normal full-term infants by the age of 3 months, 1 mg per kg body-weight; infants of low birth-weight or deficient in iron, by the age of 2 months, 2 mg per kg; neither dose to exceed a maximum of 15 mg daily.— Canadian Paediatric Society, *Can. med. Ass. J.*, 1972, *106*, 259 (Recommendations of the Nutrition Committee). See also *Pediatrics*, 1969, *43*, 134 (Report of the Committee on Nutrition of the American Academy of Pediatrics).

In a survey of 1000 healthy children, aged from 6 to 36 months, in Sydney, the mean dietary intake of iron was 6.3 mg per day, yet only 31 children suffered from iron-deficiency anaemia. The bioavailability of iron from mixtures of various foods could account for the finding that the average haemoglobin level for all the children was 12.3 g per 100 ml blood.— V. A. Lovric *et al.*, *Med. J. Aust.*, 1972, *1*, 11.

A discussion of iron losses during blood donation. It was considered that iron supplements were not usually necessary for subjects giving blood every 6 months.— *Lancet*, 1975, *1*, 1174.

Provided that the iron status of the mother during pregnancy is satisfactory, the infant is born with stores of iron in the body which together with the iron present in human milk, can satisfy iron requirements for the first 4 to 6 months. Recommended daily intakes of iron: infants up to 1 year, 6 mg; boys and girls, 1 to 2 years, 7 mg; 3 to 4 years, 8 mg; 5 to 8 years, 10 mg; 9 to 17 years, 12 mg; men over 18 years, 10 mg; women 18 to 55 years, 12 mg; over 55 years, 10 mg; during pregnancy, 13 mg; during lactation, 15 mg. The recommended intake of iron may not be sufficient for about 10% of girls and women with large menstrual losses.— *Reports on Health and Social Subjects No. 15*, London, HM Stationery Office, 1979 (Report by the Committee on Medical Aspects of Food Policy).

The US National Research Council made the following recommendations for daily dietary allowances of iron: infants up to 6 months, 10 mg; children 6 months to 3 years, 15 mg; 4 to 10 years, 10 mg; males 11 to 18 years, 18 mg; over 18 years, 10 mg; females 11 to 50 years, 18 mg; over 50 years, 10 mg; in pregnancy the increased requirement could not be met by the iron content of the diet nor by the existing iron stores of many women and the use of 30 to 60 mg of supplemental iron was recommended; in lactation the iron needs were not substantially different from those of nonpregnant women but it was advisable to continue supplementation of the mother for 2 to 3 months after parturition.— *Recommended Dietary Allowances*, 9th Edn, Washington, The National Research Council, 1980.

See also Parenteral Nutrition under Therapy with Iron and Iron Salts, p.874.

Fortification of food. For a review of the use and suitability of various iron compounds for the iron fortification of food, see Control of Nutritional Anaemia with Special Reference to Iron Deficiency, Report of an IAEA/USAID/WHO Joint Meeting, *Tech. Rep. Ser. Wld Hlth Org. No. 580*, 1975.

A discussion on the fortification of food with iron and the prevention of iron deficiency.— *Lancet*, 1980, *1*, 1117.

For a spray-mixing method of fortifying common salt with iron in order to counteract iron-deficiency anaemia in developing countries, see R. Suwanik *et al.* (letter), *Lancet*, 1978, *2*, 1101.

Addition to bread. In England and Wales, The Bread and Flour Regulations 1963 (SI 1963: No. 1435), as amended (SI 1972: No. 1391), require all flour to contain not less than 1.65 mg of iron per 100 g, and to ensure this, iron is added to lower-extraction flours. The Regulations permit the use of ferric ammonium citrate, ferrous sulphate, and iron powder, for which specifications are laid down.

References.— P. C. Elwood *et al.*, *Clin. Sci.*, 1971, *40*, 31; *Med. Lett.*, 1972, *14*, 81; *J. Am. med. Ass.*, 1972, *220*, 855; W. H. Crosby, *J. Am. med. Ass.*, 1978, *239*, 2026 and 2760.

Addition to infant food. Iron-fortified milk formulas were recommended for infants until at least 12 months old.— *Pediatrics*, 1971, *47*, 786.

The need for iron-fortified formulas for infants.— *Med. Lett.*, 1971, *13*, 65. See also C. W. Woodruff, *J. Am. med. Ass.*, 1978, *240*, 657.

Criticism of the policy of addition of iron to foods, especially baby foods.— T. C. Washburn (letter), *J. Am. med. Ass.*, 1973, *224*, 530.

The addition of iron to infant food was considered hazardous because of antagonism between iron and vitamin E. Infant foods were generally deficient in vitamin E.— S. Ayres (letter), *J. Am. med. Ass.*, 1973, *225*, 527.

Protein-rich mixtures used as supplementary foods should contain 2.7 mg of iron per 419 kJ.— Report of a WHO Expert Group on Trace Elements in Human Nutrition, *Tech. Rep. Ser. Wld Hlth Org. No. 532*, 1973, 55.

There was good evidence that fortified infant cereals could improve nutrition. From studies in adults on the absorption of iron from various cereals it appeared advisable for infant formulas to include both an absorbable iron salt and ascorbic acid with an iron to ascorbic acid ratio of at least 1 to 10.— Report of an IAEA/USAID/WHO Joint Meeting, *Tech. Rep. Ser. Wld Hlth Org. No. 580*, 1975.

In a double-blind study serum-iron concentrations were significantly higher in infants given an iron-fortified artificial milk formula than in those who received a similar unfortified formula. Not all haematological indices showed significant differences.— A. T. Lammi *et al.*, *Med. J. Aust.*, 1975, *1*, 441.

In a study involving 8 adults who received 5 different types of milk, iron absorption was greater from human milk than from simulated human milk or 2 commercial formulas. Breast milk alone might be sufficient to supply all the iron requirements for the first 6 months of life.— J. A. McMillan *et al.*, *Pediatrics*, 1977, *60*, 896.

Absorption of iron from a test dose given to 45 healthy full-term infants about 6 to 7 months of age was significantly greater in infants in whom breast feeding had been the only source of milk than in those infants whose source of iron had been cow's milk from the age of 2 months. Values for mean corpuscular volume, transferrin saturation, and serum ferritin were also significantly greater in breast-fed infants. Routine administration of supplementary iron may not be necessary in term infants, who continue to be breast fed, especially if iron fortified foods are included in the diet after 3 to 5 months of age.— V. M. Saarinen *et al.*, *J. Pediat.*, 1977, *91*, 36.

Iron deficiency is a serious nutritional problem in the USA and a dietary intake of 2.1 g of iron over the first year of life would regularly prevent iron-deficiency anaemia. The possibility of adverse effects from iron supplementation in breast-fed infants appeared to be remote.— S. J. Fomon and R. G. Strauss (letter), *New Engl. J. Med.*, 1978, *299*, 1471.

Further references.— P. Lanzkowsky (letter), *New Engl. J. Med.*, 1978, *298*, 343; V. Y. H. Yu, *Med. J. Aust.*, 1978, *1*, 22.

Therapy with Iron and Iron Salts. Iron and iron salts should only be given for the treatment or prophylaxis of iron deficiency anaemias. They should not be given for the treatment of other types of anaemia except where iron deficiency is also present. Iron-deficiency anaemias are most often the result of severe or chronic haemorrhage, nutritional deficiency, pregnancy, or parasitic infestation, or more rarely they may result from malabsorption of iron from the diet. Iron-deficiency anaemias respond readily to iron therapy but the underlying cause of the anaemia should be determined and treated. Iron therapy should be continued after the haemoglobin concentration has returned to normal, to replenish the body stores of iron. With therapy by mouth, the haemoglobin concentration may take up to 10 weeks to reach normal values and 3 to 6 months' treatment may be necessary to replenish iron stores. Failure to respond to oral iron after 3 weeks of therapy may be indicative of non-compliance, continued blood loss with inadequate replacement of iron, malabsorption, wrong diagnosis, or other complicating factors and the treatment should be reassessed.

Compounds of iron are used in the treatment of microcytic anaemia, including simple achlorhydric anaemia, simple anaemia of pregnancy, the nutritional anaemia of infants, anaemia due to excessive haemorrhage, and anaemia associated with infections and malignant disease. Folic acid is often given with iron during the last trimester of pregnancy to prevent the development of a folate-deficiency megaloblastic anaemia.

Preparations of iron are administered either by mouth or by intramuscular or intravenous injection. Soluble ferrous salts are the most effective by mouth; the ferric salts are relatively ineffective. Large doses of iron are necessary to relieve iron deficiency; the daily oral dosage of the soluble salts should contain 100 to 200 mg of iron.

In the treatment of macrocytic anaemia, preparations of iron given alone are of no value but they may be of value as a supplement to cyanocobalamin therapy whenever the reserves of iron are depleted and the increase in haemoglobin does not parallel the rise in the number of red blood-cells. The addition of small doses of copper and manganese to iron compounds does not appear to aid the formation of haemoglobin.

The oral administration of iron preparations sometimes produces gastro-intestinal irritation with nausea, vomiting and diarrhoea. These side-effects occur in about 15% of patients and are related to the amount of elemental iron taken rather than the type of preparation. Side-effects may be reduced by administration immediately after food or by beginning therapy with a small dose and increasing gradually. Continued administration may produce constipation. Sustained release or enteric coated products are claimed to produce fewer side-effects but this may only reflect the lower availability of iron from these preparations. Oral liquid preparations may blacken the teeth and should be drunk through a straw. The faeces of patients taking iron salts may be coloured black.

Parenteral iron is rarely necessary because oral iron produces such satisfactory results. Parenteral iron should be used only for patients who do not respond to oral iron, for patients requiring a rapid effect such as those with severe hypochromic anaemia in advanced pregnancy, for patients who cannot be relied upon to take oral medication regularly, and in those with genuine intolerance. Iron Dextran Injection is given by intravenous infusion or intramuscular injection, and Iron Sorbitol Injection by intramuscular injection.

Iron overload, with increased storage of iron in the tissues (haemosiderosis), may occur as a result of excessive oral and parenteral therapy or multiple blood transfusions. Patients mistakenly given iron therapy when not suffering from iron-deficiency anaemia are also at risk as are those with pre-existing iron storage or absorption diseases.

Externally, some iron salts are powerfully astringent and styptic, ferric chloride being most commonly used for these purposes.

The hazards and use of iron preparations.— R. G. Coombe, *Aust. J. Pharm.*, 1976, *57*, 395.

Iron-metabolism disorders and their treatment.— R. L. C. Cumming, *Practitioner*, 1978, *221*, 184. See also A. S. Prasad, *Trace Elements and Iron in Human Metabolism*, Chichester, John Wiley, 1978.

The range and efficacy of oral iron preparations.— *Drug & Ther. Bull.*, 1979, *17*, 33.

Absorption and fate. In 16 healthy adults absorption of iron was significantly higher in females than in males, and correlated with plasma-iron concentration, total iron-binding capacity, and, particularly, with the degree of transferrin saturation.— I. N. Kuhn *et al.*, *J. Lab. clin. Med.*, 1968, *71*, 715.

In subjects eating Western diets, the percentage of iron absorbed was about 6% in normal males, 14% in normal females, and 20% in iron-deficient subjects. Even in iron-deficient subjects the percentage of iron absorbed from cereal diets was very much less.— Report of a WHO Group of Experts on Nutritional Anaemias, *Tech. Rep. Ser. Wld Hlth Org. No. 503*, 1972.

The mean serum concentration of ferritin in 21 patients with iron-deficiency anaemia was 5 ng per ml (range 1 to 12 ng) and in 8 patients with haemochromatosis it was 2646 ng per ml (range 940 to 4240 ng). These values were compared with values of 69.2 ng per ml (range 6 to 186 ng) and 34.8 ng per ml (range 3 to 162 ng) in healthy men and women respectively.— A. Jacobs *et al.*, *Br. med. J.*, 1972, *4*, 206.

A review of the role of transferrin and other plasma proteins in the absorption and transfer of iron in the body.— E. H. Morgan, *Med. J. Aust.*, 1972, *3*, 322.

Studies in 45 healthy subjects demonstrated that the absorption of iron was related to serum-ferritin concentrations.— G. O. Walters *et al.* (letter), *Lancet*, 1973, *2*, 1216.

The internal regulation of iron absorption.— I. Cavill *et al.* (letter), *Nature*, 1975, *256*, 328.

A prospective study of serum-ferritin concentrations and bone marrow iron stores in 248 unselected patients indicated that the finding of normal concentrations of serum-ferritin did not exclude the possibility of iron deficiency in patients with hepatitis, neoplastic diseases, or inflammatory conditions such as glomerulonephritis.— M. A. M. Ali *et al.*, *Can. med. Ass. J.*, 1978, *118*, 945. See also P. L. McGinnis *et al.* (letter), *ibid.*, 1979, *120*, 1204.

Raised serum-ferritin concentrations found in 58 of 76 black patients with primary liver cancer were thought to be due mainly to the production and secretion of specific isoferritins by the tumour.— M. C. Kew *et al.*, *Gut*, 1978, *19*, 294.

Transfusional iron overload and increased intestinal absorption of iron are serious complications of thalassaemia. Studies in 5 patients with transfusion-dependent thalassaemia major and one with thalassaemia intermedia, all of whom had had splenectomies, demonstrated that as the haemoglobin concentration fell, iron absorption increased. The nucleated red cell count accurately predicted the percentage of iron absorbed. Tea produced a 41 to 95% inhibition of iron absorption; the effect was apparently specific for non-haem iron and could be especially useful in the management of patients with thalassaemia intermedia who might absorb large amounts of dietary iron.— P. A. de Alarcon *et al.*, *New Engl. J. Med.*, 1979, *300*, 5.

In a study of 32 probands with haemochromatosis and 174 family members, serum ferritin was a more satisfactory determinant of heterozygous carriers of the disease than was serum iron. Ferritin concentrations distinguished more clearly between heterozygous and homozygous subjects and in the latter they were generally elevated. The presence of fibrosis, and especially cirrhosis, was associated with markedly elevated serum-ferritin concentrations.— C. Beaumont *et al.*, *New Engl. J. Med.*, 1979, *301*, 169.

For a discussion and comments on the possible use of a radio-immunoassay of serum-ferritin concentrations to replace measurements of serum iron and total iron-binding capacity in the assessment of iron status, see *Lancet*, 1979, *1*, 533; J. R. Beck *et al.* (letter), *ibid.*, 1080; G. Lindstedt *et al.* (letter), *ibid.*, 1980, *1*, 205; M. Worwood (letter), *ibid.*, 375.

Absorption in children. In healthy children below 6 months of age 2.2% of orally administered iron was absorbed. Absorption rose to 13.3% in children between 6 months and 2 years of age and to 25% in those between 2 and 14 years. Absorption was increased in children with blood loss or on iron-deficient diets.— S. Doctor *et al.*, *Münch. med. Wschr.*, 1968, *110*, 2860.

The mean absorption of iron-59 measured in 19 children during 20 febrile episodes due either to illness or to diphtheria, tetanus, and pertussis immunisation was 15.1% compared with 41.2% during 22 afebrile episodes.— C. H. Beresford *et al.*, *Lancet*, 1971, *1*, 568.

Effect of drugs. Laevulose, in a 50:1 molar excess with respect to elemental iron, was found markedly to enhance iron absorption. Dextrose did not have the same effect. Laevulose formed a chelate with iron and it was suggested that the iron-laevulose chelate complex was absorbed significantly better than inorganic iron.— P. S. Davis and D. J. Deller, *Gut*, 1967, *8*, 198.

There was a possibility that salicylates contributed to iron-deficiency anaemia by the formation of an iron-salicylate chelate complex.— D. J. Deller *et al.*, *Gut*, 1967, *8*, 524.

The absorption of iron was studied in 44 persons, most of whom had iron-deficiency anaemia, after medication with ferrous fumarate or ferrous sulphate with and without the addition of ascorbic or succinic acids. Succinic acid caused increased absorption of iron from solutions of ferrous fumarate but not from tablets of ferrous fumarate or sulphate. Ascorbic acid caused increased absorption of ferrous fumarate from tablets, but absorption was not greater than from ferrous sulphate alone. The addition of both ascorbic acid and succinic acid to tablets of ferrous sulphate did not significantly increase absorption of iron.— S. T. Callender and G. T. Warner, *Br. med. J.*, 1969, *4*, 532.

Iron absorption from a 50- to 66-mg dose of ferrous iron measured 14 days after administration by the iron-59 whole body retention test was not significantly affected by the presence of succinate, docusate, fumarate, aspartate, ascorbate, or folate in people with normal or depleted iron stores. Slow-release preparations of ferrous sulphate had half the effect on haemoglobin regeneration of simple preparations and were not improved by addition of ascorbic acid. Simple ferrous sulphate was considered to be well tolerated and the best absorbed, most effective, and least expensive iron preparation available.— H. C. Heinrich *et al.*, *Arzneimittel-Forsch.*, 1972, *22*, 1091.

The absorption of iron from solutions of ferric chloride or ferrous sulphate plus ascorbic acid, bread, rice meal, or uncooked haemoglobin was significantly inhibited when they were ingested with tea, whether the tea contained milk or not. No inhibition was noted if the haemoglobin was cooked. The effect, which was ascribed to the formation of insoluble iron tannate complexes, might contribute to the pathogenesis of iron deficiency if the diet consisted largely of vegetable food stuffs.— P. B. Disler *et al.*, *Gut*, 1975, *16*, 193.

Studies *in vitro* on the interaction between antacids and oral haematinics indicated that at usual hydrogen ion concentrations the proportion of soluble iron was reduced by most antacids except aluminium hydroxide.— J. F. Coste *et al.*, *Curr. ther. Res.*, 1977, *22*, 205.

A brief review of drugs which may interfere with tests for serum iron concentrations and iron-binding capacity.— P. P. Sher, *Drug Ther.*, 1977, *1*, 63.

For further studies on the effect of ascorbic acid on the absorption of ferrous sulphate, see p.878.

Effect of gastric juice. Iron, as inorganic ferric or ferrous salts, could form complexes in gastric juice which were soluble when the pH was raised and enabled the iron to be in a form suitable for absorption in the small intestine.— A. Jacobs and P. M. Miles, *Gut*, 1969, *10*, 226.

Anaemia of pregnancy. Pregnant women with anaemia and in their second trimester of pregnancy were divided into 3 groups and received either the equivalent of 100 mg of elemental iron with folic acid 300 µg (184 patients), or iron only (76 patients), or folic acid only (22 patients), daily for 6 weeks. Another group of 219 pregnant women received a placebo. At examination 2 to 3 weeks after the end of therapy there had been a rise in the haemoglobin concentration of more than 0.5 g per 100 ml in 90% (166) of the patients who had received iron with folic acid and a similar rise was seen in 26% (20) and 27% (6) of the patients who had received only iron or only folic acid respectively. A fall in the haemoglobin concentration was seen in about 6.5%, 25%, and 23% of the patients respectively. Over 70% of the patients who received placebo had a gradually falling haemoglobin concentration during the study.— G. Izak *et al.*, *Scand. J. Haemat.*, 1973, *11*, 236.

In a WHO sponsored collaborative study of the effects of iron supplementation completed by 647 pregnant women in India, treatment with one of the following regimens was given for 10 to 12 weeks from the 26th week of pregnancy: group 1, placebo; group 2, cyanocobalamin and folic acid; groups 3, 4, 5 and 6, as for group 1 plus 30, 60, 120 and 240 mg of elemental iron respectively as ferrous fumarate; group 7, 120 mg of elemental iron as ferrous fumarate. Iron and folic acid 5 mg were given daily by mouth for 6 days per week and cyanocobalamin 100 µg was given by injection every 2 weeks. Groups 2 to 6 inclusive also received folic acid and cyanocobalamin for the 4 weeks prior to the study. The mean haemoglobin concentration rose significantly in all the groups given iron but declined in the groups given no iron. The women who received folic acid and cyanocobalamin in addition to iron had a greater rise in mean haemoglobin concentration than those given an equivalent amount of iron without further supplementation. In each group receiving iron the rise in haemoglobin tended to be greatest in those with the lowest initial haemoglobin concentration. The best results were seen in groups 6 and 5 where 90% of 84 and 81% of 115 women respectively had a rise in their haemoglobin concentration of more than 0.1 g per 100 ml. However, at the end of the study 56% of the women in groups 5 and 6 had a final haemoglobin concentration below 11 g per 100 ml.— S. K. Sood *et al.*, *Q.J. Med.*, 1975, *44*, 241.

A survey of haemoglobin concentrations in pregnancy over about 30 years indicated that prophylaxis with iron and folic acid should continue.— J. M. Scott *et al.*, *Br. med. J.*, 1975, *1*, 259.

In 35 pregnant women with β-thalassaemia trait, 21 of 22 who underwent bone-marrow biopsy at 32 weeks' gestation had absent iron stores; serum-iron concentrations and total iron-binding capacity were not reliable in assessing iron deficiency in such patients. In 18 such patients given iron supplements for less than 12 weeks mean initial haemoglobin concentrations of 11.1 g per 100 ml fell to 9.6 g per 100 ml in the third trimester, compared with no fall (10.8 to 10.7 g per 100 ml) in 16 given iron supplements for more than 12 weeks.— U. M. Hegde *et al.*, *Br. med. J.*, 1975, *3*, 509.

A discussion of the doubtful need for added iron in pregnancy in developed countries.— *Br. med. J.*, 1978, *2*, 1317. Comments.— *ibid.*, 1493 and 1494; M. Jolliffe (letter), *ibid.*, 1571; *ibid.*, 1576.

Recommendations on the use of iron and folic acid in anaemia of pregnancy.— M. C. Macnaughton, *Prescribers' J.*, 1979, *19*, 52. See also M. H. Hall, *Br. med. J.*, 1974, *2*, 661; *Lancet*, 1974, *2*, 1429.

Haemodialysis. Unless they received 10 units of transfused blood in a year, patients with chronic renal failure who were undergoing maintenance dialysis should be given the equivalent of 2 g yearly of elemental iron by injection to prevent iron depletion.— M. S. Edwards *et al.*, *Lancet*, 1970, *2*, 491.

A study of 28 haemodialysis patients with depleted bone-marrow iron stores, indicated that administration of iron supplements by mouth or intravenously improved their anaemia and reduced their blood transfusion requirements. It was recommended that iron supplements should be routinely given to these patients with regular monitoring of body-iron stores. Administration by mouth may be safer on a long-term basis.— R. J. Winney *et al.*, *Proc. Eur. Dialysis Transplant Ass.*, 1977, *14*, 184.

Study of serum-ferritin concentrations, as a measure of marrow-iron stores, in 61 patients on maintenance haemodialysis suggested that a daily dose of 60 mg Fe was adequate for maintenance in most patients on flat-board dialysis.— A. M. Cotterill *et al.*, *Br. med. J.*, 1979, *1*, 790 and 1052.

Further references: J. W. Eschbach *et al.*, *Ann. intern. Med.*, 1977, *87*, 710; P. A. Parker *et al.*, *Nephron*, 1979, *23*, 181; L. E. Human, *J. Am. med. Ass.*, 1980, *244*, 371.

Infection. In children with severe kwashiorkor and low serum-transferrin concentrations an increase in serum iron following treatment with iron compounds, particularly during the first week, might encourage bacterial infection, ultimately leading to death. Consideration should be given to the appropriate time at which iron therapy should be instituted in these patients.— H. McFarlane *et al.*, *Br. med. J.*, 1970, *4*, 268.

Low plasma-transferrin concentrations in neonates, especially when premature, necessitated caution in the administration of iron, since this might lead to increased transferrin saturation and thereby reduce transferrin's anti-infective activity.Parenteral iron produced a greater degree of saturation and was not given to neonates. Oral iron was not given to breast-fed infants to avoid saturation of the lactoferrin in breast milk.— P. H. Scott *et al.*, *Archs Dis. Childh.*, 1975, *50*, 796.

Iron given by mouth or intramuscularly improved the reduced immune response in a study of 23 anaemic children. The altered immune response in anaemia was considered to be due primarily to iron deficiency.— P. Bhaskaram *et al.* (letter), *Lancet*, 1977, *1*, 1000.

From a review of the literature up to 1976 it appeared that the inflammatory response, when assessed by skin reactivity, was diminished in patients with iron deficiency. It was concluded that in many clinical situations iron imbalance was related to susceptibility to infections but an increased susceptibility to the type of infection expected in immunodeficiency had not been clearly documented in iron deficiency. Many conditions characterised by marked iron overload were associated with increased susceptibility to infection.— R. G. Strauss, *Am. J. clin. Nutr.*, 1978, *31*, 660.

A discussion on chronic mucocutaneous candidiasis and the possible role of iron deficiency.— *Lancet*, 1978, *1*, 1026. See also J. M. Higgs and R. S. Wells, *Br. J. Derm.*, 1972, *86*, *Suppl.* 8, 88.

In 137 iron-deficient Somali nomads the incidence of infection was significantly increased in 71 given iron supplements for 30 days compared with those given a placebo. Infections tended to occur in the latter part of treatment, as iron deficiency was relieved, and included activation of quiescent malaria, brucellosis, and tuberculosis.— M. J. Murray *et al.*, *Br. med. J.*, 1978, *2*, 1113.

For reports of an increased incidence of sepsis in neonates receiving iron dextran injections, see Iron Dextran Injection p.880.

Further references: *Lancet*, 1974, *2*, 325; E. D. Weinberg, *J. Am. med. Ass.*, 1975, *231*, 39.

Iron overload. A discussion of iron metabolism with special reference to iron overload.— M. Barry, *Gut*, 1974, *15*, 324. See also A. Jacobs, *Semin. Hematol.*, 1977, *14*, 89.

Iron-deficiency anaemia. For reviews of the treatment of iron-deficiency anaemias, see R. W. Beal, *Drugs*, 1971, *2*, 190 and 207; J. R. D. Matthews and T. P. Casey, *ibid.*, 1973, *6*, 244; G. O. Walters, *Practitioner*, 1974, *212*, 493; J. H. Dagg, *Br. med. J.*, 1974, *2*, 494; C. W. Woodruff, *Pediat. Clins N. Am.*, 1977, *24*, 85; S. J. Baker, *Bull. Wld Hlth Org.*, 1978, *56*, 659.

In 80 women treated for severe iron-deficiency anaemia the average rate of increase in haemoglobin concentration was as follows: 250 mg per 100 ml daily after ferrous sulphate, ferrous gluconate, or ferrous fumarate given in doses providing 180 to 220 mg of iron daily; 280 mg daily per 100 ml daily after intramuscular iron dextran providing 250 mg of iron; and 330 mg per 100 ml daily after intravenous saccharated iron oxide providing 200 mg of iron.— J. A. Pritchard, *J. Am. med. Ass.*, 1966, *195*, 717.

In a study in 75 children between 6 and 36 months with iron deficiency without anaemia, there was a significant weight gain in children who received 6 mg of elemental iron per kg body-weight daily for 3 months compared with those who received placebo.— A. T. Lammi and V. A. Lovric, *Med. J. Aust.*, 1973, *2*, 541.

Mean serum-ferritin concentration (a reflection of iron stores) was 6.5 µg per litre in 26 patients with iron-deficiency anaemia, rose to 30.5 µg per litre when haemoglobin concentrations reached normal after treatment with oral iron preparations, and rose to 60.1 µg per litre after a further 2 months' treatment. In 12 given Iron Dextran Injection by total-dose infusion, initial values of 5.7 µg per litre rose to 144 µg per litre 7 months after treatment. The study supported the practice of continuing to give oral iron for 2 months after normalisation of haemoglobin concentration.— D. P. Bentley and A. Jacobs, *Br. med. J.*, 1975, *2*, 64.

Of 200 patients with recurrent oral ulceration 33 had iron deficiency; replacement treatment led to resolution in 6 patients and improvement in 7.— F. F. Nally and G. C. Blake (letter), *Br. med. J.*, 1975, *3*, 308.

A study in patients with iron deficiency indicated that those with chronic active ulcerative colitis absorbed iron given by mouth as readily as those without colitis.— I. G. Barrison *et al.*, *Br. med. J.*, 1981, *282*, 1514.

Slow-release preparations. A study of 474 women with iron-deficiency anaemia showed little difference between slow-release preparations of iron and conventional tablets.— P. C. Elwood and G. Williams, *Practitioner*, 1970, *204*, 812. Slow-release preparations produced lower serum concentrations of iron than conventional preparations.— E. J. Middleton *et al.*, *New Engl. J. Med.*, 1966, *274*, 136. See also E. Beutler and G. Meerkreebs (letter), *ibid.*, 1152; H. Dietzfelbinger and W. Kaboth, *Dt. med. Wschr.*, 1979, *104*, 742.

In a semi-blind trial in 85 anaemic patients there was a better rise in haemoglobin concentrations at 4 weeks in patients treated with ferrous sulphate 160 mg (Slow Fe) once daily than twice daily or in patients treated with ferrous sulphate 525 mg and ascorbic acid 500 mg daily. At 16 weeks there was little significant difference between the 3 regimens. There was a relatively low incidence of side-effects with all 3 treatments.— *Practitioner*, 1973, *210*, 566 (Report No. 181 of the General Practitioner Research Group).

Owing to the risk of intestinal obstruction, sustained-release preparations such as Ferro-Gradumet, Ferrograd C, Ferrograd-folic, and Irofol C, where the drug is released in transit, but the matrix ghost is often eliminated intact, should not be prescribed in patients with Crohn's disease or other intestinal disease in which strictures may form.— J. L. Shaffer *et al.* (letter), *Lancet*, 1980, *2*, 487.

Leprosy. Reduced serum-iron concentrations in leprotic patients were not due to true lack of iron in the body (tissue iron deficiency) but were probably partly a toxic effect of the disease. Administration of multivitamin preparations and other measures directed at improving the nutritional status of the leprotic patient might be preferable to routine administration of iron supplements.— T. Shwe *et al.*, *Lepr. Rev.*, 1976, *47*, 287.

Pagophagia. In 19 of 25 patients with lack of iron who were persistently consuming excessive quantities of ice, the administration of iron by mouth or by injection, in doses less than those necessary to correct the lack of iron, resolved the condition in from 1 to 14 days; the response was more rapid after iron by injection.— C. A. Coltman, *J. Am. med. Ass.*, 1969, *207*, 513. Comments.— *ibid.*, 552.

Parenteral nutrition. Balance studies of 9 elements including iron, during complete intravenous feeding of small premature infants.— B. E. James and R. A. MacMahon, *Aust. paediat. J.*, 1976, *12*, 154.

Restless leg syndrome. Rapid relief from symptoms of the restless leg syndrome followed treatment with iron by mouth in 3 patients in whom the condition was associated with iron-deficiency anaemia.— W. B. Matthews (letter), *Br. med. J.*, 1976, *1*, 898.

5031-z

Iron *(B.P.C. 1973)*. Ferrum.

Fe=55.847.

CAS — 7439-89-6.

Pharmacopoeias. In *Arg.*, *Belg.*, *Hung.*, *Pol.*, *Port.*, and *Span.*, most of which specify iron filings or powder.

Iron wire of about 0.3 mm in diameter; it is free from rust and has a dull metallic lustre, becoming bright when freshly scratched. Practically **insoluble** in water and alcohol; almost completely soluble in dilute mineral acids. **Store** in airtight containers.

Iron wire has been used in the preparation of some solutions and syrups.

A 66-year-old toolmaker suffered allergic contact dermatitis due to exposure to iron.— R. L. Baer, *J. Allergy & clin. Immunol.*, 1973, *51*, 35.

5032-c

Reduced Iron *(B.P.C. 1949, B. Vet. C. 1965)*. Ferrum Redactum; Ferrum Pulveratum Hydrogenio Paratum; Quevenne's Iron; Fer Réduit; Reduziertes Eisen; Hierro Reducido; Ferro Ridotto.

Pharmacopoeias. In *Arg.*, *Aust.*, *Belg.*, *Braz.*, *Hung.*, *It.*, *Pol.*, *Port.*, *Roum.*, and *Rus.*, containing varying amounts of iron.

A fine greyish-black powder, free from metallic lustre and gritty particles, containing not less than 80% of metallic iron. Practically **insoluble** in water and alcohol; almost completely soluble in dilute mineral acids. **Incompatible** with tannin and metallic salts. **Store** in airtight containers.

Uses. Reduced iron has the actions and uses of iron salts (p.872). It is a form of iron used for food fortification. It has also been used in doses of 60 to 600 mg in the treatment of iron-deficiency anaemias. In veterinary medicine, it has been used for the prevention of piglet anaemia.

5033-k

Dextriferron. Dextriferron Injection; Iron Dextrin Injection; Iron-Dextrin Complex.

CAS — 9004-51-7.

A sterile, colloidal, clear, dark brown solution, iso-osmotic with serum, prepared from a complex of ferric hydroxide with partially hydrolysed dextrin in Water for Injections. The average molecular weight of the complex is about 230 000. The solution contains the equivalent of 20 mg of elemental iron per ml. pH about 7.6. Wt per ml 1.062 to 1.072 g.

Adverse Effects. Following injection, flushing, nausea and an unpleasant taste, headache, abdominal pain, and transient diarrhoea have been reported. Later side-effects include stiffness, chills, and fever. Allergic reactions, sometimes severe, have been reported. Injection outside the vein may cause inflammation and permanent discoloration of the skin. See also Iron Dextran Injection, p.880.

Reports of allergic reactions to dextriferron.— A. S. Blazar and M. G. del Riego, *Obstet. Gynec.*, 1962, *20*, 156; A. J. Morris (letter), *Lancet*, 1970, *2*, 774.

Treatment of Adverse Effects and Precautions. As for Iron Dextran Injection, p.880.

Uses. Dextriferron has been used in the treatment of iron-deficiency anaemia where oral therapy is ineffective or impracticable.

It is given by slow intravenous injection at a rate not exceeding 2.5 ml per minute. Total dosage is calculated according to the haemoglobin concentration of the blood. The usual initial adult dose is 30 to 40 mg of iron (1.5 to 2 ml), gradually increased over subsequent days. Not more than 100 mg of iron (5 ml) should be given in 1 injection. The total calculated dose is given over several days and it has been suggested that the total dose of iron should not exceed 2 g.

Dextriferron should not be given intramuscularly.

Proprietary Names

Astrafer *(Astra, Austral.)*; Ferrigen *(Astra, Swed.)*; Ferrum Hausmann *(see also under Ferrous Fumarate, Iron Polymaltose, and Saccharated Iron Oxide) (Asta, Ger.)*.

Dextriferron was formerly marketed in Great Britain under the proprietary name Astrafer IV (*Astra*).

5034-a

Ferric Ammonium Citrate *(B.P. 1973).*

Ferr. Ammon. Cit.; Iron and Ammonium Citrate; Ferricum Citricum Ammoniatum. A complex ammonium ferric citrate containing about 21.5% of iron, about 1.2 g in 6 g.

CAS — 1185-57-5.

Pharmacopoeias. In *Arg., Chin., Ind., It., Mex., Port.,*and *Span.* (Fe content varying from 16 to 22.5%).

Thin, deliquescent, dark red, transparent scales or brown shiny granular powder, with an astringent taste.
Soluble 2 in 1 of water; practically insoluble in alcohol and in ether. **Incompatible** with mineral acids, alkali carbonates, and vegetable astringents. **Store** in airtight containers. Protect from light.

NOTE. Aqueous solutions of ferric ammonium citrate are liable to grow moulds; chloroform or some other suitable preservative should be added.

Adverse Effects, Treatment, and Precautions. As for Ferrous Sulphate, p.878. It is considered to be relatively free from astringent properties and local irritant effects.

Uses. Ferric ammonium citrate has the actions and uses of iron salts (see p.872) and is given in doses of up to 6 g daily.
Aqueous solutions containing up to 50% of the salt are given as mixtures, with the addition of chloroform water (see above). Mixtures should be well diluted with water before taking and a straw should be used to prevent discoloration of the teeth.

Preparations

Ferric Ammonium Citrate Mixture *(A.P.F.).* Mist. Ferr. et Ammon. Cit.; Iron and Ammonium Citrate Mixture. Ferric ammonium citrate 1.5 g, syrup 1 ml, concentrated chloroform water 0.25 ml, water to 10 ml. *Dose.* 10 to 20 ml.

Ferric Ammonium Citrate Mixture *(B.P.C. 1973).* Mist. Ferr. et Ammon. Cit.; Iron and Ammonium Citrate Mixture. Ferric ammonium citrate 2 g, double-strength chloroform water 5 ml, water to 10 ml. It should be recently prepared. *Dose.* 10 ml.

Ferric Ammonium Citrate Solution. A 1 in 2 solution is commercially available.

Paediatric Ferric Ammonium Citrate Mixture *(B.P.C. 1973).* Mist. Ferr. et Ammon. Cit. pro Inf.; Ferric Ammonium Citrate Mixture Paediatric; Paediatric Iron and Ammonium Citrate Mixture. Ferric ammonium citrate 400 mg, compound orange spirit 0.01 ml, syrup 0.5 ml, double-strength chloroform water 2.5 ml, water to 5 ml. It should be recently prepared. *Dose.* Children, up to 1 year, 5 ml; 1 to 5 years, 10 ml. To be taken well diluted with water.

Proprietary Preparations

Lexpec Iron *(R.P. Drugs, UK).* Liquid containing ferric ammonium citrate 200 mg in each 5 ml. Stated to be suitable for children intolerant to sugar.

5035-t

Green Ferric Ammonium Citrate *(B.P.C. 1954).*

Ferri et Ammonii Citras Viridis.

Green deliquescent scales or granular powder, containing 14 to 16% of Fe.
Soluble 2 in 1 of water; practically insoluble in alcohol. Solutions are **sterilised** by autoclaving or by filtration. **Store** in airtight containers. Protect from light.

Green ferric ammonium citrate has been used similarly to ferric ammonium citrate in doses of 1 to 4 g.

5036-x

Ferric Chloride *(B.P.C. 1949).*

Ferr. Perchlor.; Iron Perchloride; Iron Sesquichloride; Iron Trichloride; Ferrum Sesquichloratum.
$FeCl_3,6H_2O$=270.3.

CAS — 7705-08-0 (anhydrous); 10025-77-1 (hexahydrate).

Pharmacopoeias. In *Aust., Cz., Hung., Port., Span.,* and *Swiss.*

An orange-coloured, very deliquescent, crystalline mass with a slight odour of hydrochloric acid and an astringent metallic taste. It contains about 60% of $FeCl_3$.
Readily **soluble** in water, alcohol, ether, and glycerol. **Incompatible** with astringent infusions, with alkalis, alkaloids, iodides, salicylates, silver salts, tannic acid, and acacia mucilage. **Store** in airtight containers. Protect from light.

Adverse Effects, Treatment, and Precautions. As for Ferrous Sulphate, p.878. Local application of ferric chloride or iron salts may cause permanent discoloration of the skin.

Uses. Ferric chloride has the general properties of iron salts (see p.872) but is exceptionally astringent. It has been used mainly by local application for its styptic and astringent properties.

Recurrent nasal and tooth-socket bleeding was successfully cauterised by the application of strong ferric chloride solution.— *Br. med. J.,* 1974, *2,* 616.

Preparations

Gargles

Ferric Chloride Gargle *(B.P.C. 1963).* Garg. Ferr. Perchlor. Ferric chloride solution 3.13 ml, potassium chlorate 3.43 g, glycerol 6.25 ml, water to 100 ml. It must be freshly prepared. To be diluted with twice its volume of warm water before use.

Loss of potassium chlorate in Ferric Chloride Gargle occurred on storage. After 1 month at room temperature, the loss was 4.4% from a full bottle of white glass and 11% from a partly-filled winchester of white glass. Possible explanations were: (a) glycerol was oxidised by potassium chlorate and (b) hydrochloric acid in the ferric chloride solution was oxidised to form chlorine, chlorine dioxide, and potassium chloride.— *Pharm. J.,* 1961, *2,* 187 (Pharm. Soc. Lab. Rep.).

Solutions

Dialysed Iron Solution *(B.P.C. 1949).* Liq. Ferr. Dialysat. A colloidal solution of ferric hydroxide containing the equivalent of 3 to 4% w/v of Fe, and not more than 0.7% w/v of chloride, calculated as Cl, and prepared from Strong Ferric Chloride Solution. Store in a warm place. *Dose.* 0.6 to 2 ml. Dialysed Iron Solution has been used as a non-astringent haematinic.

Ferric Chloride Solution *(B.P.C. 1973).* Liquor Ferri Perchloridi. Strong ferric chloride solution 25 ml, water to 100 ml. It contains 15% w/v of $FeCl_3$, equivalent to about 5% w/v of Fe. *Dose.* 0.3 to 1 ml.

Gerhardt's Reagent *(D.T.F.).* A 10% solution of ferric chloride.

Strong Ferric Chloride Solution *(B.P.C. 1973).* Liquor Ferri Perchloridi Fortis; Liq. Ferr. Perchlor. Fort. An aqueous solution containing 60% w/v of $FeCl_3$.

A preparation containing dialysed iron was formerly marketed in Great Britain under the proprietary name Colliron (*Duncan, Flockhart*).

5037-r

Red Ferric Oxide *(U.S.N.F.).*

Fe_2O_3=159.7.

CAS — 1309-37-1.

Pharmacopoeias. In *Port. Chin.* includes Ferri Oxydum Rubrum. Also in *U.S.N.F. B.P.C. 1949* included Red Precipitated Ferric Oxide (Ferri Carb.; Ferri Subcarb.; Red Hydrated Iron Oxide) prepared by the oxidation of precipitated ferrous carbonate, and yielding not less than 80% of Fe_2O_3 on ignition.

A fine red powder which loses not more than 1% of its weight on ignition and contains 97 to 100.5% of Fe_2O_3, calculated on the ignited basis. **Soluble** in hydrochloric acid.

Red ferric oxide is used mainly for tinting calamine.

5038-f

Yellow Ferric Oxide *(U.S.N.F.).*

CAS — 51274-00-1.

Pharmacopoeias. In *U.S.N.F.*

A fine yellow powder which loses not more than 13% of its weight on ignition, and contains not less than 97% of Fe_2O_3 calculated on the ignited basis. **Soluble** in hydrochloric acid.

Yellow ferric oxide is used mainly for tinting pharmaceutical preparations.

Estimated acceptable daily intake of iron oxides and hydrated iron oxides: up to 500 µg per kg body-weight. Ferric oxide is less available as a source of biologically active iron than are other forms of iron.— Twenty-third Report of Joint FAO/WHO Expert Committee on Food Additives, *Tech. Rep. Ser. Wld Hlth Org. No. 648,* 1980.

5039-d

Ferric Quinine Citrate *(B.P.C. 1954).*

Ferr. et Quinin. Cit.; Iron and Quinine Citrate; Ferrum Citricum Chiniatum.

CAS — 8053-35-8.

Pharmacopoeias. In *Aust.* and *Ind.*; *Aust.* contains 9 to 10% of anhydrous quinine and 21 to 26.5% of iron.

A complex ammonium quinine ferric citrate, containing 14.5 to 15.5% of anhydrous quinine and 12 to 14% of iron. It occurs as greenish-yellow deliquescent scales or granular powder with a bitter chalybeate taste.
Soluble 2 in 1 of water. **Incompatible** with alkalis, alkali carbonates and citrates, and vegetable astringents, also with phosphoric acid (ferric phosphate may be precipitated) unless considerably diluted before mixing. **Store** in airtight containers. Protect from light.

Ferric quinine citrate has been used in 'tonic' preparations in doses of 0.3 to 1 g. It may be administered in mixtures flavoured with lemon or orange syrup or chloroform water.

5040-c

Ferric Sodium Citrate.

Sodium Ferric Citrate.

CAS — 52031-09-1.

Ferric sodium citrate is an ingredient of Ferrlecit 100, see p.879.

5041-k

Ferric Sulphate Solution *(B.P.C. 1963).*

Liq. Ferr. Persulph.

Pharmacopoeias. Span. includes an aqueous solution containing 10% w/w of Fe.

An aqueous solution prepared by oxidising ferrous sulphate with sulphuric and nitric acids. It contains 14 to 15% w/v of ferric iron calculated as Fe. **Protect** from light.

Ferric sulphate solution was used for preparing Ferric Hypophosphite Solution.

5042-a

Ferrocholinate.

Iron Choline Citrate Chelate.

CAS — 1336-80-7.

A chelate prepared by reacting equimolecular quantities of freshly precipitated ferric hydroxide with choline dihydrogen citrate, containing 12 to 13% of iron.

Ferrocholinate has been used similarly to the iron salts (see p.872). The suggested dose for adults was 330 to 660 mg thrice daily.

5043-t

Ferropolimaler. Iron Polymalether.

CAS — 54063-44-4.

The iron(II) salt of a maleic acid polymer with methyl vinyl ether, $(C_7H_8FeO_5)_n$.

Ferropolimaler has been used in the treatment of iron-deficiency anaemia.

Proprietary Names

Tetucur *(Jap.)*.

5044-x

Ferrous Aspartate.

$C_8H_{12}FeN_2O_8,4H_2O=392.1$.

A greenish-white odourless powder with a chalybeate taste, containing 14.2% of iron. Very **soluble** in water.

Ferrous aspartate has the actions and uses of iron salts (see p.872), and has been used in doses of 350 mg.

Proprietary Names

Ferofer *(Sigmatau, Ital.)*; Ferroglobine *(Veride, Belg.)*; Spartocine *(UCB, Arg.; UCB, Belg.; UCB, Ger.; Infal, Spain)*.

5055-d

Ferrous Carbonate. Ferri Carbonas; Carbonato de Hierro. It consists chiefly of ferrous carbonate with variable proportions of ferric hydroxide and ferroso-ferric oxide.

$FeCO_3=115.9$.

CAS — 563-71-3 ($FeCO_3$).

Pharmacopoeias. In *Span.*

A yellowish-green amorphous solid. Practically **insoluble** in water and alcohol. **Incompatible** with acids and oxidising agents. **Store** in colourless hermetically sealed containers exposed to light.

Preparations of ferrous carbonate tend to be made from ferrous sulphate and a carbonate.

5056-n

Saccharated Ferrous Carbonate *(B.P.C. 1959)*. Ferr. Carb. Sacch.; Saccharated Iron Carbonate; Carbonate de Fer Sucré; Zuckerhaltiges Eisenkarbonat.

CAS — 1335-56-4.

Ferrous carbonate, which may be partly oxidised, mixed with liquid glucose. It contains not less than 24% of ferrous iron equivalent to not less than 49.8% of $FeCO_3$. It contains in 2 g about 500 mg of ferrous iron.

An olive-brown, slightly hygroscopic powder with a feebly chalybeate taste. Partly **soluble** in water; soluble with effervescence in dilute hydrochloric acid. **Incompatible** with tannin, acids, and acid salts. **Store** in airtight containers.

Saccharated ferrous carbonate has the actions and uses of ferrous sulphate (see p.877) and is claimed to be less astringent than most iron salts. It has been used in doses of 0.6 to 2 g.

Preparations

Ferrous Carbonate Capsules *(B.P.C. 1959)*. Caps. Ferr. Carb. Each contains not less than the equivalent of 55 mg of $FeCO_3$. *Dose.* 1 to 6 capsules.

Ferrous Carbonate Pills *(B.P.C. 1959)*. Pil. Ferr. Carb.; Blaud's Pills; Iron Pills. Each contains not less than the equivalent of 58 mg of $FeCO_3$. *Dose.* 1 to 6 pills.

Ferrous Carbonate Tablets *(B.P.C. 1959)*. Tab. Ferr. Carb.; Blaud's Tablets; Iron Tablets. Each contains not less than the equivalent of 54 mg of $FeCO_3$. *Dose.* 1 to 6 tablets.

Proprietary Preparations

Triple Iron Pill Dellipsoids D 23 *(Pilsworth, UK)*. Tablets each containing iron equivalent to 1 g of Blaud's Pill.

Other Proprietary Names

Abofer *(Denm.)*; Ingoferron *(Ger.)*.

5054-f

Ferrous Fumarate *(B.P., U.S.P.)*. Ferr. Fumar.

$C_4H_2FeO_4=169.9$.

CAS — 141-01-5.

Pharmacopoeias. In *Br., Neth., Nord.,* and *U.S.*

A fine reddish-orange to reddish-brown powder, odourless or with a slight odour and a slightly astringent taste; 200 mg contains about 65 mg of iron. Slightly **soluble** in water; very slightly soluble in alcohol.

Adverse Effects, Treatment, and Precautions. As for Ferrous Sulphate, p.878.

Uses. Ferrous fumarate has the actions and uses of iron salts (see p.872) and is used in the treatment of iron-deficiency anaemia. The usual dose is 200 mg thrice daily for an adult.

The dose for children up to 1 year of age is 35 mg; 1 to 5 years, 70 mg; and 6 to 12 years, 140 mg, all thrice daily.

In iron-deficient women whose anaemia had been treated, 10 mg of iron daily, taken as ferrous fumarate, prevented a fall in the mean haemoglobin concentration. A 30-mg dose had a greater effect, but 5 mg did not produce a significantly different effect from that of a placebo.— P. C. Elwood *et al., Lancet*, 1970, *2*, 175.

Preparations

Ferrous Fumarate Mixture *(B.P.C. 1973)*. A suspension of ferrous fumarate in a suitable coloured flavoured vehicle. When a dose less than 5 ml is prescribed, the mixture should be diluted to 5 ml with syrup. Such dilutions must be freshly prepared and not used more than 2 weeks after issue. Protect from light.

Ferrous Fumarate Tablets *(B.P.)*. Ferr. Fumar. Tab. Tablets containing ferrous fumarate. They may be film-coated. Store in airtight containers.

Ferrous Fumarate Tablets *(U.S.P.)*. Tablets containing ferrous fumarate. Store in airtight containers.

Proprietary Preparations

Co-Ferol *(Cox Continental, UK)*. Tablets each containing ferrous fumarate 120 mg and folic acid 200 µg. For the prevention of anaemia in pregnancy. *Dose.* 1 tablet twice daily.

Ferrocap *(Consolidated Chemicals, UK)*. Sustained-release capsules each containing ferrous fumarate 330 mg and thiamine hydrochloride 5 mg. For iron-defiency anaemia. **Ferrocap F-350**. Capsules each containing ferrous fumarate 330 mg and folic acid 350 µg. For the prevention of anaemia in pregnancy. *Dose.* 1 capsule of Ferrocap or Ferrocap F-350 daily.

Fersaday *(Glaxo, UK)*. Ferrous fumarate, available as tablets each containing the equivalent of 100 mg of Fe.

Fersamal *(Glaxo, UK)*. Ferrous fumarate, available as **Syrup** containing the equivalent of 45 mg of Fe in each 5 ml (suggested diluent syrup), and as **Tablets** each containing the equivalent of 65 mg of Fe. (Also available as Fersamal in *Arg., Austral., Canad.*).

Folex-350 *(Rybar, UK)*. Tablets each containing ferrous fumarate 308 mg and folic acid 350 µg. For the prevention of megaloblastic anaemia in pregnancy. *Dose.* 1 tablet daily.

Galfer Capsules *(Galen, UK)*. Each contains ferrous fumarate equivalent to 100 mg of ferrous iron. For iron-deficiency anaemia. **Galfer FA Capsules.** Each contains, in addition, folic acid 350 µg. For the prevention of anaemia in pregnancy. *Dose.* 1 capsule daily.

Galfer-Vit *(Galen, UK)*. Capsules each containing ferrous fumarate 305 mg, nicotinamide 10 mg, pyridoxine hydrochloride 4 mg, riboflavine 2 mg, sodium ascorbate 56 mg, and thiamine mononitrate 2 mg. For iron-deficiency anaemia. *Dose.* 1 or 2 capsules daily before food.

Givitol *(Galen, UK)*. Capsules each containing ferrous fumarate 250 mg, folic acid 500 µg, nicotinamide 10 mg, pyridoxine hydrochloride 1 mg, riboflavine 2 mg, sodium ascorbate 56 mg, and thiamine mononitrate 2 mg. For the prevention of iron and folate deficiency in pregnancy. *Dose.* 1 or 2 capsules daily before food.

Plancaps *(Unimed, UK)*. Ferrous fumarate, available as capsules of 290 mg.

Pregaday *(Glaxo, UK)*. Tablets each containing ferrous fumarate equivalent to 100 mg of Fe and folic acid 350 µg. For the prevention of iron-deficiency and megaloblastic anaemias in pregnancy. *Dose.* 1 or 2 tablets daily.

Tifolic *(Ticen, Eire)*. Capsules each containing ferrous fumarate 300 mg and folic acid 300 µg. For the prevention of anaemia in pregnancy. *Dose.* 1 capsule daily.

Other Proprietary Names

Austral.—Bramiron, Fumiron; *Belg.*—Ferrone, Ferumat, Soparon; *Canad.*—Feroton, Ferrofume, Hematon, Novofumar, Palafer; *Denm.*—Erco-Fer; *Fr.*—Fumafer; *Ger.*—Ferrokapsul, Ferrum Hausmann (see also under Dextriferron, Iron Polymaltose, and Saccharated Iron Oxide); *Ital.*—Ferromikron; *Neth.*—Ferumat; *Norw.*—Neo-Fer; *Swed.*—Erco-Fer, Fumafer; *Switz.*—Ercofer; *USA*—Fem Iron, Feostat, Fumasorb, Hemocyte, Ircon, Laud-Iron, Span-FF, Toleron.

Preparations containing ferrous fumarate were also formerly marketed in Great Britain under the proprietary names Norfer (*Norton*) and Pregamal (*Glaxo*).

5058-m

Ferrous Gluconate *(B.P., Eur. P., U.S.P.)*.

Ferr. Glucon.; Ferrosi Gluconas; Eisen(II)-Gluconat.

$C_{12}H_{22}FeO_{14},2H_2O=482.2$.

CAS — 299-29-6 (anhydrous); 12389-15-0 (dihydrate).

Pharmacopoeias. In *Arg., Aust., Br., Braz., Eur., Fr., Ger., Ind., Int., It., Jug., Neth., Pol., Swiss, Turk.,* and *U.S.*

Grey powder or granules with a green or yellow tint with a slight odour resembling that of burnt sugar and a taste which is saline at first and then slightly chalybeate. It contains not less than 12.25% of iron calculated on the dried material; about 70 mg in 600 mg of the dihydrate.

Slowly **soluble** 1 in 10 of water, but more readily soluble on warming; practically insoluble in alcohol. A 10% solution in water has a pH of 3.7 to 6. **Store** in airtight containers. Protect from light.

Stability of solutions. Aqueous solutions were less stable than solid ferrous gluconate and oxidation occurred most rapidly in neutral or alkaline solutions. Solutions were incompatible with ascorbic acid, glycine , and pyridoxine. Solutions in citrate buffer solution, pH 3.5 to 4.5, might be sterilised by filtration and kept in ampoules under nitrogen or carbon dioxide.— G. B. Stone, *J. Am. pharm. Ass., scient. Edn*, 1950, *39*, 16.

To minimise oxidation, solutions of ferrous gluconate should be dispensed in small well-closed containers, and the maximum concentration compatible with the formation of a stable solution should be used (10% was suggested). If the solution was to be stored in the dark about 7.5% of dextrose should be included and this should be increased to 20% if the preparation was to be stored in the light. Storage in darkness resulted in some increase in ferric iron content, especially in partly filled containers; storage in the light resulted in a slight increase in ferrous iron due to reduction of ferric iron initially present, but ferrous oxalate was also formed and might be deposited.— C. A. Johnson and J. A. Thomas, *J. Pharm. Pharmac.*, 1954, *6*, 1037.

Adverse Effects, Treatment, and Precautions. As for Ferrous Sulphate, p.878.

Uses. Ferrous gluconate has the actions and uses of iron salts (see p.872) and is used for the treatment of iron-deficiency anaemia. The usual initial dose is 1.2 to 1.8 g daily in divided doses followed by a maintenance dose of 600 mg daily. Children of 6 to 12 years may be given 300 mg thrice daily.

Preparations

Capsules

Ferrous Gluconate Capsules *(U.S.P.)*. Capsules containing ferrous gluconate. Store in airtight containers.

Elixirs

Ferrous Gluconate Elixir *(U.S.P.)*. An elixir containing ferrous gluconate, with alcohol 6.3 to 7.7%. pH 3.4 to 3.8. Store in airtight containers. Protect from light.

Mixtures

Ferrous Gluconate Mixture CF *(A.P.F.)*. Ferrous Gluconate Mixture for Children. Ferrous gluconate 200 mg, dextrose 500 mg, orange syrup 1 ml, citric acid monohydrate 25 mg, concentrated chloroform water 0.1 ml, water to 5 ml. Protect from light. *Dose.* Children weighing 12 to 15 kg, 5 ml thrice daily.

Solutions

Ferrous Gluconate Solution. Ferrous gluconate 6 g, citric acid monohydrate 300 mg, methyl hydroxybenzoate 100 mg, propyl hydroxybenzoate 20 mg, peppermint oil 0.01 ml, sorbitol solution 40 ml, water to 100 ml.—G.E. Schumacher, *Am. J. Hosp. Pharm.*, 1967, *24*, 378.

Tablets

Ferrous Gluconate Tablets *(B.P.).* Ferr. Glucon. Tab. Tablets containing ferrous gluconate. The tablets are film-coated or sugar-coated. Store in airtight containers.

Ferrous Gluconate Tablets *(U.S.P.).* Tablets containing ferrous gluconate. Store in airtight containers.

Proprietary Preparations

Feravol-F *(Carlton Laboratories, UK).* Tablets each containing ferrous gluconate 300 mg and folic acid 3 mg. For anaemias associated with folic acid deficiency. *Dose.* 1 tablet thrice daily.

Feravol-G *(Carlton Laboratories, UK).* **Syrup** containing in each 5 ml ferrous gluconate 300 mg and thiamine hydrochloride 1 mg, and **Tablets** each containing ferrous gluconate 300 mg, thiamine hydrochloride 400 µg, riboflavine 1 mg, ascorbic acid 9 mg, with a trace of copper. For iron-deficiency anaemia. *Dose.* 5 ml of syrup or 1 tablet thrice daily after food.

Ferfolic *(Sinclair, UK).* Tablets each containing ferrous gluconate 250 mg, folic acid 5 mg, thiamine hydrochloride 3 mg, nicotinamide 10 mg, riboflavine 1 mg, and ascorbic acid 10 mg. **Ferfolic-SV**. Tablets each containing ferrous gluconate 250 mg, folic acid 5 mg, and ascorbic acid 10 mg. For the prevention and treatment of anaemia associated with folic acid deficiency. *Dose.* 1 tablet of Ferfolic or Ferfolic-SV thrice daily.

Fergluvite *(Sinclair, UK).* Tablets each containing ferrous gluconate 250 mg, thiamine hydrochloride 3 mg, nicotinamide 10 mg, riboflavine 1 mg, and ascorbic acid 10 mg. For hypochromic and microcytic anaemias. *Dose.* 1 tablet thrice daily.

Fergon *(Winthrop, UK).* Ferrous gluconate, available as tablets of 300 mg. (Also available as Fergon in *Austral., Canad., USA*).
The name Fergon is also applied in *Spain* to cephalexin.

Ferrous Gluconate Dellipsoids D 28 *(Pilsworth, UK).* Tablets each containing ferrous gluconate 200 mg and thiamine hydrochloride 1 mg. For iron-deficiency anaemia. *Dose.* 1 or 2 tablets 4 times daily after meals.

Sidros *(Potter & Clarke, UK).* Tablets each containing ferrous gluconate 300 mg and ascorbic acid 30 mg. For the prevention and treatment of iron-deficiency anaemia. *Dose.* 1 or 2 tablets twice or thrice daily after food.

Other Proprietary Names

Austral.—Ferro-G, Fersin, Glucohaem; *Canad.*—Fertinic, Novoferrogluc; *Spain*—Ferronicum, Hierro Laquifal; *Switz.*—Glucoferron; *USA*—Ferralet, Simron.

A preparation containing ferrous gluconate was also formerly marketed in Great Britain under the proprietary name Ferlucon (*Duncan, Flockhart*).

5059-b

Ferrous Glycine Sulphate. Ferrous Aminoacetosulphate.

CAS — 14729-84-1.

A chelate of ferrous sulphate and glycine containing about 40 mg of ferrous iron in each 225 mg.

Ferrous glycine sulphate is used as a source of iron. The usual dose is the equivalent of 75 to 150 mg of iron daily.

Proprietary Preparations

Fe-cap *(MCP Pharmaceuticals, UK).* Capsules each containing ferrous glycine sulphate 565 mg (equivalent to 100 mg Fe). **Fe-cap C**. Capsules each containing ferrous glycine sulphate 565 mg and ascorbic acid 300 mg. For iron-deficiency anaemia. **Fe-cap folic**. Capsules each containing ferrous glycine sulphate 450 mg (equivalent to 80 mg Fe) and folic acid 350 µg. For the prophylaxis of iron and folic acid deficiencies in pregnancy. *Dose.* 1 capsule of Fe-cap C or Fe-cap folic daily.

Ferrocontin *(Napp, UK).* Ferrous glycine sulphate, available as sustained-release tablets each containing the equivalent of 100 mg of Fe. For iron-deficiency anaemia. **Ferrocontin Folic**. Sustained-release tablets each containing, in addition, folic acid 500 µg. For the prevention of anaemia in pregnancy. *Dose.* 1 tablet daily.

Gastrovite *(MCP Pharmaceuticals, UK).* Tablets each containing ferrous glycine sulphate 225 mg (equivalent to 40 mg of ferrous iron), calcium gluconate 100 mg, ascorbic acid 15 mg, and ergocalciferol 200 units. For the prophylaxis and treatment of iron and calcium deficiencies. *Dose.* 1 tablet thrice daily.

Kelferon *(MCP Pharmaceuticals, UK).* Ferrous glycine sulphate, available as tablets of 225 mg (equivalent to 40 mg of ferrous iron).

Kelfolate Tablets *(MCP Pharmaceuticals, UK).* Each contains ferrous glycine sulphate 225 mg and folic acid 150 µg. For the prevention of anaemia in pregnancy. *Dose.* 2 tablets daily.

Plesmet *(Coates & Cooper, UK).* Syrup containing in each 5 ml ferrous glycine sulphate equivalent to 25 mg of Fe (suggested diluent, syrup). (Also available as Plesmet in *Austral.*).

Other Proprietary Names

Ferro-Chel *(Austral.)*; Ferro Sanol *(Ger.)*; Ferrosanol *(Switz.)*; Glycifer *(Denm., Swed.)*.

A preparation containing ferrous glycine sulphate was also formerly marketed in Great Britain under the proprietary name Jectoral (*Astra*).

5060-x

Ferrous Lactate *(B.P.C. 1949).* Ferr. Lact.; Iron Lactate.
$C_6H_{10}FeO_6,3H_2O = 288.0$.

CAS — 5905-52-2 (anhydrous); 6047-24-1 (trihydrate).

Pharmacopoeias. In *Pol.* and *Span.*

Greenish-white crystals or crystalline powder with a characteristic odour and sweet, mildly chalybeate taste. **Soluble** 1 in 40 of water and 1 in 12 of boiling water; freely soluble in alkali citrate solutions with the formation of a green colour; practically insoluble in alcohol. A 2% solution in water is slightly acid to litmus. **Store** in airtight containers. Protect from light.

Ferrous lactate has the actions and uses of iron salts (see p.872). It has been used in doses providing up to 150 mg of iron daily.

Proprietary Names
Ferro Drops *(Parke, Davis, S.Afr.)*.

5061-r

Ferrous Oxalate. Iron Protoxalate; Ferrum Oxalicum Oxydulatum.
$C_2FeO_4,2H_2O = 179.9$.

CAS — 516-03-0 (anhydrous); 6047-25-2 (dihydrate).

Pharmacopoeias. In *Arg., Belg., Fr.,* and *Port.*

A yellow amorphous or crystalline odourless powder. Practically **insoluble** in water and alcohol; soluble in dilute mineral acids. **Incompatible** with alkalis and oxidising agents. **Store** in airtight containers. Protect from light.

Ferrous oxalate has the actions and uses of iron salts (see p.872). It has been used in the treatment of iron-deficiency anaemia in doses of 100 to 200 mg.

5062-f

Ferrous Succinate *(B.P.).* Ferr. Succin.

$C_4H_4FeO_4 = 171.9$.

CAS — 10030-90-7.

Pharmacopoeias. In *Br.*

A basic salt; it is a brownish-yellow to brown amorphous almost tasteless powder with a slight odour, containing 34 to 36% of ferrous iron; about 70 mg in 200 mg. Practically **insoluble** in water and alcohol; soluble in dilute mineral acids. **Store** in airtight containers. Protect from light.

Adverse Effects, Treatment, and Precautions. As for Ferrous Sulphate, p.878.
Ferrous succinate is claimed to cause fewer gastro-intestinal side-effects than ferrous sulphate.

Recovery of 2 women who had ingested ferrous succinate equivalent to 2 and 11 g respectively of Fe, after treatment with desferrioxamine and, in 1 patient, partial exchange transfusion.— F. Eriksson *et al.*, *Acta med. scand.*, 1974, *196*, 231.

Uses. Ferrous succinate has the actions and uses of iron salts (see p.872). Doses of up to 600 mg daily in divided doses are given in the treatment of iron-deficiency anaemia; 200 mg daily has been used for prophylaxis.

After taking ferrous succinate 330 mg with multivitamins the absorption in normal subjects was 5.2 mg Fe, in subjects with latent iron deficiency 9.9 mg Fe, and in subjects with manifest iron deficiency 34 mg Fe. No significant increase in the iron absorption-rate was observed in women taking oral contraceptives and not suffering from iron deficiency.— E. Zillessen *et al.*, *Arzneimittel-Forsch.*, 1977, *27*, 1606.

Preparations

Ferrous Succinate Capsules *(B.P.).* Capsules containing ferrous succinate. Store at a temperature not exceeding 30°. Protect from light.

Ferrous Succinate Tablets *(B.P.).* Ferr. Succin. Tab. Tablets containing ferrous succinate. They may be sugar-coated. Store in a cool place. Protect from light.

Proprietary Preparations

Ferromyn *(Calmic, UK).* Ferrous succinate, available as **Elixir** containing 106 mg in each 5 ml (suggested diluent, syrup) and as **Tablets** of 100 mg. For iron-deficiency anaemia. **Ferromyn B. Elixir** (suggested diluent, syrup) containing in each 5 ml and **Tablets** each containing ferrous succinate 106 mg, nicotinamide 10 mg, riboflavine 1 mg, and thiamine hydrochloride 1 mg. For deficiency of iron and B-group vitamins. **Ferromyn S.** Tablets each containing ferrous succinate 106 mg and succinic acid 110 mg. For iron-deficiency anaemia. **Ferromyn S Folic.** Tablets each containing, in addition, folic acid 100 µg. For anaemia of pregnancy. *Dose.* 1 tablet of Ferromyn B, Ferromyn S, or Ferromyn S Folic thrice daily; 5 ml of Ferromyn B Elixir thrice daily. (Also available as Ferromyn in *Austral., Denm., Swed.*).

Ferrous Succinate Compound Dellipsoids D 30 *(Pilsworth, UK).* Tablets each containing ferrous succinate 150 mg, ascorbic acid 5 mg, copper sulphate 2.5 mg, and manganese sulphate 2.5 mg. For iron-deficiency anaemia. *Dose.* 1 or 2 tablets thrice daily.

Other Proprietary Names

Cerevon *(Canad.)*; Kepler *(Malaysia, Nigeria, Singapore)*; Mediron *(Denm.)*; Succifer *(Ger.)*.

5063-d

Ferrous Sulphate *(B.P., B.P. Vet., Eur. P.).*

Ferr. Sulph.; Ferrous Sulfate *(U.S.P.)*; Ferrosi Sulfas; Iron(II) Sulphate Heptahydrate; Iron Sulphate; Ferrum Sulfuricum Oxydulatum; Eisen(II)-Sulfat; Ferreux (Sulfate).
$FeSO_4,7H_2O = 278.0$.

CAS — 7720-78-7 (anhydrous); 7782-63-0 (heptahydrate).

NOTE. Crude ferrous sulphate is known as Green Vitriol or Green Copperas.

Pharmacopoeias. In all pharmacopoeias examined except *Jug., Roum.,* and *Rus.*

Odourless bluish-green crystals or granules or a pale green crystalline powder with an astringent, metallic taste, containing about 60 mg of iron in 300 mg. It is efflorescent in dry air; on exposure to moist air it is oxidised and becomes brown in colour due to the formation of basic ferric sulphate. It loses 6 molecules of water of crystallisation at 38°; basic sulphates are formed at higher temperatures. A 5% solution in water has a pH of 3 to 4.

Completely or almost completely **soluble** 1 in 1.5 of water, 1 in 0.5 of boiling water; soluble 1 in 4 of glycerol; practically insoluble in alcohol. Aqueous solutions rapidly oxidise. **Incompatible** with alkalis, benzoates, phosphates, and oxidising agents. **Store** in airtight containers.

Dextrose (40%) and dextrose (40%) with hypophosphorous acid (0.2%) were efficient in stabilising solutions of ferrous sulphate (2.2%), containing 0.02% of butyl hydroxybenzoate, and exposed to air at room temperature over a period of 6 months. The addition of hypophosphorous acid alone did not retard oxidation.— C. L. Huyck, *Am. J. Pharm.*, 1941, *113*, 189.

A study of the rate of dissolution in water and simulated gastric juice of ferrous sulphate from tablets of 12 formulations.— C. E. Blezek *et al.*, *Am. J. Hosp. Pharm.*, 1970, *27*, 533.

Adverse Effects. Therapeutic doses of iron may cause gastro-intestinal discomfort, diarrhoea, and vomiting. These side-effects have been reported to occur in up to 20% or more of patients treated and are related to the amount of elemental iron taken rather than the type of preparation. Although iron is better absorbed between meals, side-effects can be reduced by taking it with, or immediately after, food. Continued administration may sometimes cause constipation.

Large doses of ferrous sulphate may have irritant and corrosive effects on the gastro-intestinal mucosa and necrosis and perforation may occur; stricture formation may subsequently follow. Symptoms, which may not appear for several hours, include epigastric pain, diarrhoea, vomiting, and haematemesis. Circulatory failure may follow if the diarrhoea and haemorrhage are severe. Hours or days later, after apparent recovery, metabolic acidosis, convulsions, and coma may occur. If the patient survives, symptoms of acute liver necrosis may develop and may lead to death due to hepatic coma.

Maximum permissible atmospheric concentration of soluble iron salts: 1 mg per m^3 as Fe.

It was considered that reduction of the recommended dosage of iron salts from 200 mg of iron to 100 mg daily would reduce almost entirely the side-effects suffered by 15% of the patients receiving the higher dose.— T. H. Bothwell, *Med. J. Aust.*, 1972, *2*, 433.

Ulceration and swelling of the hypopharynx and cervical oesophagus occurred in an 89-year-old woman after a single ferrous sulphate tablet became lodged in the hypopharynx.— T. R. Abbarah *et al.*, *J. Am. med. Ass.*, 1976, *236*, 2320.

A report of neutropenia associated with iron therapy. There was a significant reduction in neutrophils in 100 anaemic women receiving iron compared with 100 healthy female controls. There was an expected increase in neutrophils in 100 women with iron-deficient anaemia not receiving iron.— T. Hamblin and T. Simmonds (letter), *Lancet*, 1976, *2*, 310.

Ferrous salts could cause black discoloration of the urine.— J. Karlstrand, *J. Am. pharm. Ass.*, 1977, *NS17*, 735.

Further references: G. Perman, *Acta med. scand.*, 1967, *182*, 281; K. J. Murphy, *Med. J. Aust.*, 1968, *1*, 1051; L. W. Powell (letter), *ibid.*, *2*, 91.

Overdosage. A woman who ingested 3 to 4.5 g of ferrous sulphate suffered nausea, vomiting, generalised weakness, and mild tachycardia. Treatment with gastric lavage, intravenous fluids, and desferrioxamine mesylate 1 g initially followed by 500 mg twelve hours later, was followed by gradual improvement.— M. K. Wallack and A. Winkelstein, *J. Am. med. Ass.*, 1974, *229*, 1333. See also S. Lavender and J. A. Bell, *Br. med. J.*, 1970, *2*, 406.

A 17-year-old pregnant woman suffered hypotension, hypoglycaemia, metabolic acidosis, tissue necrosis, a bleeding diasthesis, and renal impairment after ingestion of ferrous sulphate 29.25 g. About 30 hours after ingestion exchange transfusion was performed but the patient spontaneously aborted a 16-week-old foetus and she died 80 hours after admission to hospital. Postmortem examination revealed haemorrhagic necrosis of the liver, oesophageal and gastric ulceration, subendocardial haemorrhage, pulmonary congestion, and cerebral oedema.— A. S. Manoguerra, *Am. J. Hosp. Pharm.*, 1976, *33*, 1088.

Overdosage in children. The ingestion of 3 g of ferrous sulphate had caused death in a small child. Poisoning in children was characterised by 3 phases: first, vomiting possibly within 30 minutes, pallor, shock, haematemesis, melaena, circulatory collapse, and coma; secondly, a period of clinical improvement followed by hepatic, metabolic, and cerebral injury with renewed restlessness, collapse, convulsions, coma, jaundice, fever, leucocytosis, lowered pH of the blood, depressed serum bicarbonate, and occasionally an abnormal EEG; thirdly, in patients who survived, gastritis, and, about 3 to 6 weeks later, symptoms of upper gastro-intestinal obstruction. Hepatic and cerebral functions recovered.— *Lancet*, 1961, *1*, 869.

A 21-month-old child who ingested ferrous sulphate 1.5 to 3 g, phenobarbitone 150 to 300 mg, and methylamphetamine 75 to 150 mg, died 42 hours later despite intensive supportive care and treatment with desferrioxamine.— D. J. Greenblatt *et al.*, *Clin. Pediat.*, 1976, *15*, 835.

A 16-month-old child died of acute liver failure 5 days after ingesting about 15 g of ferrous sulphate. Hypoglycaemia developed on day 2 and during the last 3 days the child had further recurrent episodes of hypoglycaemia with signs of liver and pancreatic damage.— F. J. deCastro *et al.*, *Clin. Toxicol.*, 1977, *10*, 287.

Further references: W. A. Gleason *et al.*, *J. Pediat.*, 1979, *95*, 138.

Photosensitivity. A 26-year-old woman developed severe photosensitivity with symptoms of erythropoietic protoporphyria associated with iron therapy. The effects were reversible.— H. Baker, *Proc. R. Soc. Med.*, 1971, *64*, 610.

Treatment of Adverse Effects. In acute poisoning the procedure described under desferrioxamine (see p.381) should be followed. If desferrioxamine is not available, empty the stomach immediately by emesis and lavage using a 1 to 5% solution of sodium bicarbonate, and leave about 300 ml of the solution in the stomach.

Fluid loss should be replaced by the intravenous administration of compound sodium lactate injection or sodium chloride and dextrose injection. Exchange transfusion may be necessary in severe cases.

In treating iron poisoning, speed is essential to block absorption of iron from the alimentary tract. A dose of as little as 1 g should be considered toxic in children

A study over a 10-year period of the treatment of acute iron poisoning in children.— D. S. Fischer *et al.*, *J. Am. med. Ass.*, 1971, *218*, 1179.

A review of the treatment of acute iron poisoning in 29 children.— V. A. Green, *Clin. Toxicol.*, 1971, *4*, 245.

Severe electrolyte imbalance occurred in a 2-year-old boy following gastric lavage with a total of 1380 ml of a hyperosmotic sodium phosphate enema given in the treatment of acute iron poisoning. It might be advisable to avoid liberal use of such solutions until a safe maximum volume can be established or to use a 5% solution of sodium bicarbonate. Close monitoring of electrolytes and acid-base status is an essential part of the management of acute iron ingestion.— L. Bachrach *et al.*, *J. Pediat.*, 1979, *94*, 147.

Precautions. Ferrous sulphate and other iron salts should not be given to patients receiving repeated blood transfusions or to patients with anaemias not produced by iron deficiency unless iron deficiency is also present. Care should be taken when given to patients with iron-storage or iron-absorption diseases, haemoglobinopathies, or existing gastro-intestinal disease.

The absorption of iron salts and tetracylines is diminished when they are taken concomitantly by mouth. If treatment with both drugs is required, the iron salt should be administered 3 hours before or 2 hours after the tetracycline. The absorption of iron salts is also decreased in the presence of antacids or when taken with tea. Iron salts appear to reduce the effects of penicillamine.

Mixtures containing iron salts should be well diluted with water and swallowed through a straw to prevent discoloration of the teeth.

Iron therapy with ferrous sulphate 600 mg daily for iron-deficient anaemia was ineffective in 3 patients also taking cimetidine 1 g daily. Reducing the cimetidine dose to 400 mg daily and maintaining the iron dose corrected the blood picture.— R. Esposito (letter), *Lancet*, 1977, *2*, 1132. It was unlikely that cimetidine would interfere with the absorption of iron in the ferrous form since this form is readily absorbed without the need for endogenous gastric acid or exogenous ascorbic acid.— F. Rosner (letter), *ibid.*, 1978, *1*, 95.

Absorption and Fate. Ferrous sulphate is irregularly and incompletely absorbed from the gastro-intestinal tract, absorption being usually increased in conditions of iron deficiency—see under Iron and Iron Salts, p.872.

Peak plasma-iron concentrations in 6 healthy subjects occurred about 2 hours after receiving capsules containing ferrous sulphate equivalent to 96, 140, or 163 mg of iron. The amount of iron absorbed increased with the increasing amount of iron administered. When 163 mg of iron was administered in 3 divided doses every 2 hours it was estimated that only 68% of the iron was as available as a similar single dose.— E. J. Middleton *et al.*, *New Engl. J. Med.*, 1966, *274*, 136.

Serum-iron concentrations 4 hours after taking 1 g of ascorbic acid together with 200 mg of ferrous sulphate were higher in 40 non-anaemic fasting subjects than when ferrous sulphate was given alone. Ascorbic acid 50 mg had no significant effect on iron absorption.— P. C. Lee *et al.*, *Can. med. Ass. J.*, 1967, *97*, 181.

A slow-release tablet containing 525 mg of ferrous sulphate and the equivalent of 500 mg of ascorbic acid given once daily to 45 patients with iron-deficiency anaemia, was marginally more effective than a comparable tablet without ascorbic acid. Two patients reported side-effects with the treatment.— M. C. G. Israëls and A. V. Simmons, *Lancet*, 1967, *1*, 1297.

Peak serum concentrations of iron in 15 healthy fasting subjects occurred about 2 to 3 hours after administration of ferrous sulphate (equivalent to 100 mg elemental iron) as capsules or as sustained-release capsules also containing ascorbic acid and sodium bicarbonate.— B. B. Gaitondé *et al.*, *Indian J. med. Res.*, 1972, *60*, 1674.

There was no significant difference between the absorption of iron from Ferrous Sulphate Tablets and from Slow-Fe in healthy persons, in anaemia, following gastrectomy, or in coeliac disease. The absorption of iron was enhanced by ascorbic acid given concomitantly.— I. M. Baird *et al.*, *Br. med. J.*, 1974, *4*, 505.

A review on the bioavailability of ferrous sulphate from various preparations.— W. L. Chiou, *J. Am. pharm. Ass.*, 1977, *NS17*, 377.

Uses. Ferrous sulphate has the general properties of iron salts (see p.872) and is one of the most widely used iron salts in the treatment of iron-deficiency anaemia. It is usually given in the form of tablets prepared with the dried salt.

The usual initial therapeutic dose is 600 to 900 mg daily in divided doses, followed by a maintenance dose of 300 mg daily. Up to 1.8 g daily has been given. Children under 1 year of age may be given 60 mg thrice daily; children 1 to 5 years, 120 mg thrice daily; and children 6 to 12 years, 300 mg twice daily.

Anaemia of pregnancy. Routine administration of elemental iron in a dosage of at least 105 mg daily from the 24th week to term corrected the anaemia of pregnancy in about 80% of patients. Given in this dosage, no difference was found between ferrous sulphate and ferrous gluconate with regard to gastro-intestinal side-effects.— D. N. S. Kerr and S. Davidson, *Lancet*, 1958, *2*, 483.

In a study in 146 women 26 of 40 not receiving iron and 28 of 60 receiving iron had no stainable intracellular iron at the end of the trial. It was concluded that ferrous sulphate providing 60 mg of Fe daily was not adequate as a supplement during pregnancy.— A. F. Fleming *et al.*, *Med. J. Aust.*, 1974, *2*, 429.

Iron-deficiency anaemia. Iron, as ferrous sulphate 180 mg daily, given to 47 preterm infants with a low birth-weight failed to increase their serum-iron concentrations or to prevent iron-deficiency anaemia in over half of the group.— B. Brozović *et al.*, *Archs Dis. Childh.*, 1974, *49*, 386.

In a study in 14 patients in a residential hospital there was no difference in acceptability (as assessed by the percentage of medication taken) between 9 oral iron preparations, including 3 sustained-release preparations, except in respect of ferrous calcium citrate and ferrous gluconate elixir. Acceptability was dependent more on the number of tablets to be taken than on the content of elemental iron. Ferrous Sulphate Tablets were equally acceptable before or after meals.— A. B. S. Mitchell, *Postgrad. med. J.*, 1974, *50*, 702.

Polycythaemia vera. Proliferation of megakaryocytes in the bone marrow and an increase of platelets to normal concentrations were reported during 4 cycles of treatment with ferrous sulphate in a 67-year-old man with polycythaemia vera who had previously been treated also with cyclophosphamide.— H. Scher and R. Silber (letter), *Ann. intern. Med.*, 1976, *84*, 571.

Preparations

Ferrous Sulfate Oral Solution *(U.S.P.)*. A solution containing ferrous sulphate. pH 1.8 to 2.2. Store in airtight containers. Protect from light.

Ferrous Sulfate Syrup *(U.S.P.)*. Ferrous sulphate 400 mg, citric acid monohydrate 21 mg, peppermint spirit 0.02 ml, sucrose 8.25 g, water to 10 ml. Store in airtight containers.

Ferrous Sulphate Mixture *(B.P.C. 1973)*. Ferrous sulphate 300 mg, ascorbic acid 20 mg, orange syrup 0.5 ml, double-strength chloroform water 5 ml, freshly boiled and cooled water to 10 ml. It should be recently prepared. *Dose*. 10 ml. To be taken well diluted with water.

If tap water is used in the preparation of this mixture, discoloration may occur.

A.P.F. has a similar mixture with concentrated chloroform water 0.25 ml, water to 10 ml.

Discoloration occurred in Ferrous Sulphate Mixture (*B.P.C. 1973*) after 7 days' storage at room temperature regardless of whether it was stored in daylight or in darkness. When the ascorbic acid concentration was increased to 0.3% no discoloration occurred in samples stored for 39 days in daylight. Use of ascorbic acid concentrations above 0.3% resulted in yellow-brown discoloration, especially in samples stored in daylight, presumably due to a breakdown product of ascorbic acid.— Pharm. Soc. Lab. Rep., P/75/15, 1975.

For a report of incompatibility when Ferrous Sulphate Mixture *B.P.C. 1973* was prepared with or diluted with syrup preserved with hydroxybenzoates, see under Sucrose, p.61.

Ferrous Sulphate Mixture CF *(A.P.F.)*. Ferrous Sulphate Mixture for Children. Ferrous sulphate 100 mg, ascorbic acid 5 mg, orange syrup 1 ml, concentrated chloroform water 0.1 ml, water to 5 ml. *Dose*. 5 ml well diluted with water for a child weighing 10 to 12 kg.

Paediatric Ferrous Sulphate Mixture *(B.P.)*. Ferrous Sulphate Mixture Paediatric. Ferrous sulphate 60 mg, ascorbic acid 10 mg, orange syrup 0.5 ml, double-strength chloroform water 2.5 ml, water to 5 ml. It should be recently prepared. To be taken well diluted with water.

If tap water is used in the preparation of this mixture, discoloration may occur.

Proprietary Preparations

See under Dried Ferrous Sulphate (below).

5064-n

Dried Ferrous Sulphate *(B.P.)*. Dried Ferr. Sulph.; Dried Ferrous Sulfate *(U.S.P.)*; Ferrosi Sulfas Exsiccatus; Exsiccated Ferrous Sulphate.

CAS — 13463-43-9.

Pharmacopoeias. In *Arg., Aust., Br., Ind., Int., Mex., Swiss, Turk.*, and *U.S.*

Ferrous sulphate deprived of part of its water of crystallisation by drying at 40°. A greyish-white to buff-coloured powder with a metallic astringent taste. The *B.P.* specifies 80 to 90% of $FeSO_4$; the *U.S.P.* specifies 86 to 89% of $FeSO_4$, as hydrates. Dried ferrous sulphate contains about 60 mg of iron in 200 mg.

Slowly but almost completely **soluble** in freshly boiled and cooled water; practically insoluble in alcohol. **Store** in airtight containers.

Discoloration. For a report of interactions between iron and adjuvants used in tableting, see M. Bornstein *et al.*, *J. pharm. Sci.*, 1968, *57*, 1653.

Dried ferrous sulphate has the actions and uses described under Ferrous Sulphate (see p.877). It is mainly used for the administration of ferrous sulphate in tablets.

The usual initial therapeutic dose is 400 to 600 mg daily in divided doses, followed by a maintenance dose of 200 mg daily. Up to 1.2 g daily has been given. Children 6 to 12 years may be given 200 mg twice daily.

Preparations

Compound Ferrous Sulphate Tablets *(B.P.C. 1973)*. Ferrous Sulphate Compound Tablets. Each contains dried ferrous sulphate equivalent to 170 mg of $FeSO_4$, copper sulphate 2.5 mg, and manganese sulphate 2.5 mg. The tablets may be coated and coloured. Store in airtight containers. Protect from light. *Dose*. 1 or 2 tablets.

Ferrous Sulfate Tablets *(U.S.P.)*. Tablets containing ferrous sulphate or dried ferrous sulphate. Potency is expressed in terms of $FeSO_4,7H_2O$. Store in airtight containers.

Ferrous Sulphate Tablets *(B.P.)*. Ferr. Sulph. Tab.; Dried Ferrous Sulphate Tablets; Exsiccated Ferrous Sulphate Tablets. Tablets containing dried ferrous sulphate. They may be film-coated or sugar-coated; sugar-coated tablets are supplied unless otherwise stated.
Store in airtight containers.

Proprietary Preparations Containing Ferrous Sulphate and Dried Ferrous Sulphate

Anorvit *(Cox Continental, UK)*. Tablets each containing dried ferrous sulphate 200 mg, ascorbic acid 10 mg, and acetomenaphthone 2 mg. For iron-deficiency anaemia. *Dose*. 2 tablets thrice daily with or immediately after meals.

FEAC *(Robins, UK)*. Tablets each containing dried ferrous sulphate 150 mg for sustained release and, in a separate layer, ascorbic acid 150 mg, nicotinamide 25 mg, pyridoxine hydrochloride 2.5 mg, riboflavine 5 mg, and thiamine mononitrate 7.5 mg. For iron-deficiency anaemia. *Dose*. 1 tablet twice daily.

Fefol Spansule *(Smith Kline & French, UK)*. Sustained-release capsules each containing dried ferrous sulphate 150 mg and folic acid 500 µg. For the prevention of iron and folic acid deficiencies during pregnancy. **Fefol-Vit Spansule**. Capsules containing, in addition, ascorbic acid 50 mg, calcium pantothenate 2.17 mg, nicotinamide 10 mg, pyridoxine hydrochloride 1 mg, riboflavine 2 mg, and thiamine mononitrate 2 mg. For use in pregnancy complicated by inadequate diet. *Dose*. 1 Fefol Spansule or Fefol-Vit Spansule daily.

Feospan Spansule *(Smith Kline & French, UK)*. Sustained-release capsules each containing dried ferrous sulphate 150 mg.

Feravol *(Carlton Laboratories, UK)*. **Syrup** containing in each 5 ml and **Tablets** each containing ferrous sulphate 200 mg, ascorbic acid 9 mg, riboflavine 1 mg, and thiamine hydrochloride 400 µg. For iron-deficiency anaemia. *Dose*. 5 ml of syrup or 1 tablet thrice daily.

Ferraplex B *(Bencard, UK)*. Tablets containing dried ferrous sulphate 167 mg, copper carbonate 400 µg, ascorbic acid 8 mg, thiamine hydrochloride 500 µg, riboflavine 1 mg, nicotinamide 5 mg, and dried brewers' yeast 292 mg. For iron-deficiency anaemia. *Dose*. 1 or 2 tablets thrice daily during or after meals.

Ferrlecit 100 *(Wade, UK)*. Tablets each containing dried ferrous sulphate 165 mg, ferric sodium citrate 150 mg, and ascorbic acid 50 mg. For iron-deficiency anaemia. *Dose*. 1 or 2 tablets daily with meals.

Ferrograd C *(Abbott, UK)*. Filmtabs (film-coated tablets) each containing in a porous plastic basis for slow release dried ferrous sulphate 325 mg and, in a separate layer, sodium ascorbate equivalent to 500 mg of ascorbic acid. For iron-deficiency anaemia. *Dose*. 1 tablet daily before a meal.

Ferrograd Folic *(Abbott, UK)*. Filmtabs (film-coated tablets) each containing in a porous plastic basis for slow release dried ferrous sulphate 325 mg, and, in a separate layer, folic acid 350 µg. For the prevention of iron and folate deficiency in pregnancy. *Dose*. 1 tablet daily before food.

A report of a woman with Crohn's disease in whom intestinal obstruction was precipitated by the accumulation of unabsorbed matrices of Ferrograd-folic behind a stenosed terminal ileum.— J. L. Shaffer *et al.* (letter), *Lancet*, 1980, *2*, 487.

Ferro-Gradumet *(Abbott, UK)*. Filmtabs (film-coated tablets) each containing in a porous plastic basis for slow release dried ferrous sulphate 325 mg. *Dose*. 1 tablet daily before food. (Also available as Ferro-Gradumet in *Austral., Switz.*).

A report of the entrapment of 98 plastic matrices of Ferro-Gradumet tablets in a patient with neoplastic colonic stricture.— M. Spigelman and R. W. McNabb, *Br. med. J.*, 1971, *4*, 534.

Jejunal diverticular perforation in a 74-year-old woman appeared to be due to Ferro-Gradumet; the remains of a tablet were lodged in the perforation and the neighbouring tissues were heavily stained with iron.— C. J. H. Ingoldby, *Br. med. J.*, 1977, *1*, 949. See also A. B. Alaily, *ibid.*, 1974, *1*, 103.

Fesovit Spansule *(Smith Kline & French, UK)*. Capsules each containing dried ferrous sulphate 150 mg for sustained-release, with ascorbic acid 50 mg, calcium pantothenate 2.17 mg, nicotinamide 10 mg, pyridoxine hydrochloride 1 mg, riboflavine 2 mg, and thiamine mononitrate 2 mg. For iron-deficiency anaemia associated with inadequate nutrition. *Dose*. 1 or 2 capsules daily.

Folicin *(Paines & Byrne, UK)*. Tablets each containing dried ferrous sulphate 170 mg, copper sulphate 2.5 mg, manganese sulphate 2.5 mg, and folic acid 2.5 mg. *Dose*. 1 or 2 tablets thrice daily.

Folvron Tablets *(Lederle, UK)*. Each contains dried ferrous sulphate 194 mg and folic acid 1.7 mg. For the prevention and treatment of iron-deficiency amaemia. *Dose*. 1 tablet thrice daily after meals.

Iberet 500 *(Abbott, UK)*. Filmtabs (film-coated tablets) each containing in a porous plastic basis for slow release dried ferrous sulphate 325 mg, and, in a separate layer, calcium pantothenate 10 mg, nicotinamide 30 mg, pyridoxine hydrochloride 5 mg, riboflavine 6 mg, sodium ascorbate equivalent to ascorbic acid 500 mg, and thiamine mononitrate 6 mg. For iron-deficiency anaemia. *Dose*. 1 tablet daily before food.

Iberol *(Abbott, UK)*. Filmtabs (film-coated tablets) each containing ferrous sulphate 325 mg, sodium ascorbate equivalent to ascorbic acid 75 mg, and vitamins of the B complex in the form of liver fraction 2 (*U.S.N.F. XI*) 100 mg with thiamine mononitrate 3 mg, nicotinamide 15 mg, riboflavine 3 mg, and pyridoxine hydrochloride 1.5 mg. For iron-deficiency and nutritional anaemias. *Dose*. 2 tablets daily.

Irofol C *(Abbott, UK)*. Tablets each containing dried ferrous sulphate 325 mg in a porous plastic basis for slow release and, in a separate layer, folic acid 350 µg and sodium ascorbate equivalent to ascorbic acid 500 mg. For the prevention of anaemia in pregnancy. *Dose*. 1 tablet daily before food.

Iron and Yeast Dellipsoids D 1 *(Pilsworth, UK)*. Tablets each containing dried ferrous sulphate 200 mg, dried yeast 200 mg (providing about 75 µg of thiamine hydrochloride), copper sulphate 1.25 mg, and manganese sulphate 1.25 mg. For iron-deficiency anaemia. *Dose*. 1 or 2 tablets 3 times daily after meals.

Iron Dellipsoids D 3 *(Pilsworth, UK)*. Tablets each containing dried ferrous sulphate 200 mg, copper sulphate 2.5 mg, and manganese sulphate 2.5 mg.

Ironorm *(Wallace Mfg Chem., UK: Farillon, UK)*. **Capsules** each containing dried ferrous sulphate 195 mg, liver fraction 130 mg, concentrated intrinsic factor 10 mg, thiamine hydrochloride 1 mg, riboflavine 2 mg, cyanocobalamin 5 µg, ascorbic acid 15 mg, nicotinamide 10 mg, and folic acid 1.7 mg. For iron-deficiency anaemia. *Dose*. 1 capsule thrice daily. **Drops** containing ferrous sulphate equivalent to 25 mg of ferrous iron in each ml, in stabilised solution.

Pregfol *(Wyeth, UK)*. Capsules each containing dried ferrous sulphate 270 mg and folic acid 500 µg. For anaemia of pregnancy. *Dose*. Prophylaxis, 1 capsule daily; treatment, 1 capsule thrice daily.

Pregnavite Forte *(Bencard, UK)*. Tablets containing in each daily dose of 3 tablets dried ferrous sulphate 252 mg, vitamin A 4000 units, ergocalciferol 400 units, thiamine hydrochloride 1.5 mg, riboflavine 1.5 mg, pyridoxine hydrochloride 1 mg, nicotinamide 15 mg, ascorbic acid 40 mg, and calcium carbonate 450 mg. **Pregnavite Forte F.** Contains, in addition, folic acid 360 µg in each daily dose of 3 tablets. For iron and vitamin supplementation during pregnancy.

Slow-Fe *(Ciba, UK)*. Sustained-release tablets each containing dried ferrous sulphate 160 mg. For iron-deficiency anaemia. **Slow-Fe Folic.** Sustained-release tablets containing, in addition, folic acid 400 µg. For the prevention of anaemia in pregnancy. *Dose*. 1 tablet daily. (Also available as Slow-Fe in *Austral., Canad.*).

Tonic Dellipsoids D 2 *(Pilsworth, UK)*. Tablets each containing dried ferrous sulphate 125 mg, dried yeast 125 mg, calcium gluconate 200 mg, vitamin D 250 units, strychnine hydrochloride 200 µg, copper sulphate 1.25 mg, and manganese sulphate 1.25 mg. *Dose*. 1 or 2 tablets thrice daily after meals.

Other Proprietary Names

Arg.— Fer-in-Sol, Siderblut; *Austral.*— Feritard, Fespan; *Belg.*— Fer-in-Sol, Fero-Gradumet, Tardyferon; *Canad.*— Fer-in-Sol, Fesofor, Novoferrosulfa; *Denm.*— Ferro, Ferro-Retard; *Ger.*— Ferro-O_2, Ferro 66 *(ferrous chloride)*, Ferro 66 DL, Ferrophor *(see also under Saccharated Iron Oxide)*; *Ital.*— Eryfer, Ferro-Grad; *Jap.*— Feroretard, Tetucur-S; *Neth.*— Fero-Gradumet, Ferro 66 *(ferrous chloride)*, Ferrofer, Microfer, Plexafer, Resoferon, Tardyferon; *Norw.*— Duroferon, Ferromax, Ferro-Retard; *S.Afr.*— Ferrosan, Fesofor; *Spain*— Fero-Gradumet; *Swed.*— Duroferon; *USA*— Feosol, Fer-in-Sol, Fero-Gradumet, Mol-Iron.

Dried ferrous sulphate was also formerly marketed in Great Britain under the proprietary name Toniron (*Medo-Chemicals*). Preparations containing ferrous sulphate or dried ferrous sulphate were also formerly marketed under the proprietary names Pholrexone (*Philip Harris*) and Plastules (*Wyeth*).

5065-h

Ferrous Tartrate. Ferrosi Tartras.
$C_4H_4FeO_6,2\frac{1}{2}H_2O = 249.0$.

CAS — 2944-65-2 (anhydrous).

Pharmacopoeias. In *Nord.*

A yellowish-green odourless and almost tasteless powder, containing about 22% of ferrous iron. **Soluble** 1 in 600 of water; practically insoluble in alcohol, chloroform, and ether; soluble in dilute acids. **Incompatible** with oxidising agents. **Store** in airtight containers. Protect from light.

Ferrous tartrate has the actions and uses of iron salts (see p.872). It has been used in daily doses of up to 450 mg in the treatment of iron-deficiency anaemia.

Proprietary Names
Ferroplex *(DAK, Denm.).*

5066-m

Iron Dextran Injection *(B.P.)*. Iron-Dextran Complex.

CAS — 9004-66-4.

Pharmacopoeias. In *Br.* (5%), *Chin.* (2.5%), and *U.S.*

A sterile, dark brown, slightly viscous, colloidal solution containing a complex of ferric hydroxide with dextrans of weight average molecular weight between 5000 and 7500. It contains about 5% (50 mg per ml) of iron. pH 5.2 to 6.5. The *U.S.P.* does not specify the strength, specifies dextrans of low molecular weight, and permits up to 0.5% of phenol as a preservative. It is **sterilised** by autoclaving or filtration.

The structure of iron dextran complex. The molecular weight of the complex was about 73 000.— J. S. G. Cox *et al., Fisons, J. Pharm. Pharmac.*, 1972, *24*, 513.

Incompatibility. A haze which developed over 3 hours was produced when iron dextran 400 mg per litre was mixed with oxytetracycline hydrochloride 1 g per litre in sodium chloride injection, and a crystalline precipitate occurred when iron dextran was mixed with sulphadiazine sodium 4 g per litre in dextrose injection and sodium chloride injection.— B. B. Riley, *J. Hosp. Pharm.*, 1970, *28* 228.

Adverse Effects. Severe allergic reactions, sometimes fatal, have occurred after the administration of Iron Dextran Injection. There may be headache, nausea, vomiting, fever, dyspnoea, changes in heart-rate, and circulatory collapse. There may also be arthralgia, myalgia, lymphadenopathy, and encephalopathy with convulsions. Intramuscular injection is associated with pain and staining at the site of injection; intravenous injection is associated with thrombophlebitis although the incidence may be reduced by administering Iron Dextran Injection in sodium chloride injection rather than dextrose injection.

A discussion of the adverse effects of iron given parenterally.— *Med. Lett.*, 1977, *19*, 35.

Hypersensitivty. Iron dextran, in the recommended dose, was given to 10 anaemic patients with active rheumatoid arthritis by total-dose infusion, in 500 to 1000 ml of dextrose injection containing hydrocortisone 25 mg, over 8 to 12 hours. One patient had an immediate allergic reaction, and in the other 9 patients there was generally a transient exacerbation of their joint pains, swelling, and stiffness accompanied by a feeling of general malaise, low-grade fever, and a rise in ESR. These effects could be due to a delayed hypersensitivity reaction. Intravenous infusion of iron dextran was a potentially dangerous treatment in rheumatoid arthritis. To detect patients liable to allergic reaction, a test dose of 2 ml should be given, followed by total-dose infusion, initially begun very slowly, with frequent checks of blood pressure.— K. N. Lloyd and P. Williams, *Br. med. J.*, 1970, *2*, 323.

The Boston Collaborative Drug Surveillance Program monitored consecutively 32 812 medical in-patients. Drug-induced anaphylaxis occurred in 1 of 169 patients given iron dextran.— J. Porter and H. Jick, *Lancet*, 1977, *1*, 587.

Further references: A. Goldberg, *Prescribers' J.*, 1967, *6*, 101; M. Soots and G. D. Hart (letter), *Br. med. J.*, 1970, *4*, 54.

Neoplasms. Eight cases of sarcoma after intramuscular injection of Iron Dextran Injection or Iron Sorbitol Injection had been reported. In 1 instance the time interval excluded iron from implication. Histological re-examination excluded sarcoma in 2 further cases. In contrast to experimental iron-induced sarcoma there was no common histological pattern in the 5 valid cases. If iron was responsible an increased incidence of sarcoma would by now be expected; no such increase was evident. The association was therefore considered to be remote.— K. Weinbren *et al., Br. med. J.*, 1978, *1*, 683.

For further clinical reports and discussions on the purported association between the development of soft tissue sarcomas and intramuscular injections of iron preparations, see A. E. MacKinnon and J. Bancewicz, *Br. med. J.*, 1973, *2*, 277; P. Grasso (letter), *ibid.*, 667; G. Greenberg, *ibid.*, 1976, *1*, 1508; J. B. Metcalfe (letter), *ibid.*, *2*, 233; G. Greenberg (letter), *ibid.*, 234; A. G. Robertson and W. C. Dick, *ibid.*, 1977, *1*, 946; M. B. McIllmurray and M. J. S. Langman, *ibid.*, 1978, *2*, 864.

Treatment of Adverse Effects. Allergic reactions to Iron Dextran Injection should be treated with adrenaline, possibly in association with antihistamine and corticosteroid therapy. For detailed recommendations concerning the management of anaphylaxis, see Adrenaline, p.4.

Precautions. Iron Dextran Injection is contra-indicated in patients with severe liver damage, acute kidney infection, or a history of hypersensitivity to the preparation. Iron Dextran Injection is not recommended during early pregnancy or in patients receiving other iron therapy or transfusions of blood. It should not be used to treat anaemias other than those associated with iron deficiency. Care should be taken when treating patients with iron-storage diseases or haemoglobinopathies.

A test dose should be given before administration of a full therapeutic dose and emergency measures for the treatment of allergic reactions should be available. Patients should be kept under observation for at least 1 hour after administration of a test dose or following intravenous infusion. Iron Dextran Injection should be administered with caution to patients with a history of allergy or asthma and the total-dose infusion method is contra-indicated in these patients. Repeated parenteral administration can lead to a form of iron overload. Patients with rheumatoid arthritis may experience a worsening of symptoms when given the infusion of Iron Dextran Injection.

Iron Dextran Injection formulated with phenol as a preservative is intended for administration by the intramuscular route only.

Anaphylactoid reactions had occurred after a total-dose infusion of iron dextran in 500 ml of saline over several hours. Such reactions could be minimised if all patients with a history of allergy were excluded, an antihistamine was given by mouth half an hour before treatment, the infusion was started at a rate of 10 drops per minute for 15 to 30 minutes, and the rate then increased to 45 drops per minute, completing the infusion over 4 to 8 hours.— J. Richmond, *Prescribers' J.*, 1967, *7*, 43.

Calcification. Calcification of the soft tissues of the thighs occurred in a 21-year-old man with uraemia within 5 days of the completion of a 6-day course of Iron Dextran Injection; the condition was unresponsive to treatment with aluminium hydroxide and the patient died. The condition was considered to be an example of calciphylaxis in which calcification could occur after the administration of a 'challenger' during a critical period after sensitisation. Sensitising agents included dihydrotachysterol, vitamin D derivatives, and parathyroid; iron dextran was a 'challenger'. Iron dextran should be given with caution to patients with a history of uraemia who might be sensitised by a high concentration of parathyroid hormone in the blood.— J. K. H. Rees and G. A. Coles, *Br. med. J.*, 1969, *2*, 670.

Infection. Because of reports of an increased incidence of sepsis due to *Escherichia coli* in infants given Iron Dextran Injection, studies were carried out *in vitro* on blood samples from 7 infants given 1 ml of Iron Dextran Injection on 2 consecutive days. The response of neutrophils to chemotactic stimulus was significantly reduced as were the bacteriostatic properties of sera against *E. coli*. It was considered that Iron Dextran Injection was contra-indicated for the prevention of iron deficiency in early infancy.— D. M. O. Becroft *et al., Archs Dis. Childh.*, 1977, *52*, 778.

During a 5-year period the mean incidence of neonatal sepsis in Polynesian neonates was 11 per 1000 births compared with 0.6 per 1000 for European neonates. The years of high incidence appeared to be confined to periods when intramuscular injections of iron dextran were given. Administration of iron had been stopped and subsequent analysis inidcated that the incidence of neonatal sepsis over the 5-year period was 17 per 1000 in those who had received iron and 2.7 per 1000 in those who had not. The data suggested that injections of iron dextran might impair the immunity of the treated infants, making them more susceptible to sepsis produced by *Escherichia coli*.— D. M. J. Barry and A. W. Reeve, *Pediatrics*, 1977, *60*, 908.

Absorption and Fate. Iron Dextran Injection is readily absorbed after intramuscular injection and maximum plasma concentrations are achieved within 24 to 48 hours. The dextran fraction is removed in the liver and metabolised or excreted. The iron is transported in the plasma by transferrin and incorporated into haemoglobin or stored as ferritin and haemosiderin.

Preliminary studies in babies born of mothers given infusions of iron dextran in the later stages of pregnancy suggested that iron dextran or excess iron did not cross the placenta once maternal serum-iron concentrations had returned to normal. In 2 patients given iron-dextran infusions within a fortnight of delivery, foetal serum-iron concentrations were found to exceed physiological levels; the excess iron was present as iron dextran, suggesting that a small proportion had diffused across the placenta.— J. S. G. Cox *et al., Fisons* (letter), *Lancet*, 1966, *1*, 821.

In 6 patients with severe iron-deficiency anaemia given up to 2.55 g of iron as iron dextran by total-dose infusion, the drug was cleared from the plasma within 8 to 10 days, chiefly by the liver. The plasma half-life was 2.3 to 3 days. In 5 of the patients 50% of the iron was incorporated into haemoglobin within 24 to 32 days.— J. K. Wood *et al., Br. J. Haemat.*, 1968, *14*, 119.

Iron Dextran Injection, injected into the buttocks or lateral aspect of the thighs of patients with iron-deficiency anaemia and healthy subjects, was principally absorbed within the first 72 hours after injection; absorption continued more slowly for 28 days. There was wide individual variation in absorption which did not appear to be related to the presence or absence of iron deficiency or to the concentration of haemoglobin. Absorption was also more rapid and complete from the thigh. There was no significant excretion of iron in the faeces or urine.— G. Will, *Br. J. Haemat.*, 1968, *14*, 395.

Compared with healthy subjects, the utilisation of iron from iron dextran for haemoglobin formation at 14 days was impaired in patients with uraemia, rheumatoid arthritis, and malignant diseases in whom stainable iron was present in the bone marrow.— A. G. Davies *et al., Br. med. J.*, 1971, *1*, 146.

Serum-iron concentrations and total iron-binding capacity were studied in 22 pregnant patients given their total dose of iron as an infusion of iron dextran. The mean serum half-life of iron dextran was calculated as 42 hours. The increase in serum-iron concentration and the decrease in total iron-binding capacity were sustained in patients infused close to delivery but this was often not the case when given before the 30th week of pregnancy.— A. B. Duke *et al., J. Obstet. Gynaec. Br. Commonw.*, 1974, *81*, 895.

Uses. Iron Dextran Injection is used in the treatment of iron-deficiency anaemia where oral therapy is ineffective or impracticable.

It may be given by deep intramuscular injection into the upper outer quadrant of the buttock; to prevent leakage along the injection track, the subcutaneous tissue is drawn to one side before the needle is inserted.

Total dosage is calculated according to the haemoglobin concentration, allowance being made for additional iron to replenish iron stores; in an adult weighing 70 kg, approximately 45 mg of iron is needed for each 1% deficiency in the concentration of haemoglobin. The volume and number of injections required to provide the total dosage is related to the condition of the patient, the usual initial adult dose being 1 ml (50 mg) on the first day, then 2 ml (100 mg) daily or at longer intervals; the dose may be increased up to 5 ml (250 mg).

The suggested dosage per injection for children is: less than 4 kg body-weight, up to 0.5 ml (25 mg); 4 to 10 kg, up to 1 ml (50 mg); over 10 kg, up to 2 ml (100 mg).

Iron Dextran Injection is also administered intravenously by total-dose infusion (TDI), the total dose, calculated according to the haemoglobin concentration, being given by slow intravenous infusion over 6 to 8 hours, preferably in sodium chloride injection.

It is advisable to stop oral administration of iron probably at least 24 hours before giving Iron Dextran Injection; other parenteral forms of iron should also be withdrawn probably for at least several days beforehand.

Studies in 36 patients with severe iron-deficiency anaemia showed that the intravenous administration of Iron Dextran Injection was followed by an appreciable rise in gastric acid output in patients under 30 years of age and in patients with an acid output of 5 to 15 mmol per hour.— H. G. Desai *et al.*, *Gut*, 1968, *9*, 91. See also W. D. Stone, *ibid.*, 99.

A short review of Iron Dextran Injection in the treatment of anaemia in patients with rheumatoid arthritis.— A. G. Mowat, *Prescribers' J.*, 1975, *15*, 107. For a study on the role of iron in rheumatoid disease, see D. R. Blake *et al.*, *Lancet*, 1981, *2*, 1142.

A report of the effectiveness and toxicity of iron dextran injections given intravenously to 481 people over a period of 8 years.— R. D. Hamstra *et al.*, *J. Am. med. Ass.*, 1980, *243*, 1726.

Candidiasis. Of 31 patients with chronic mucocutaneous candidiasis, 23 had evidence of iron deficiency. Four with a haemoglobin concentration greater than 12 g per 100 ml were treated, in a controlled trial, with Iron Dextran Injection by total-dose infusion, followed by ferrous fumarate 200 mg thrice daily for 2 months; 3 showed definite clinical improvement in their candidiasis. Eight further patients were treated with iron, usually with improvement in their candidiasis, though iron stores were not consistently replenished.— J. M. Higgs and R. S. Wells, *Br. J. Derm.*, 1972, *87, Suppl.* 8, 88.

Haemodialysis. Iron dextran was shown to be of use for the anaemia of chronic renal failure in patients on maintenance dialysis.— R. A. Carter *et al.*, *Br. med. J.* 1969, *3*, 206.

In 44 patients undergoing haemodialysis serum-ferritin concentrations correlated closely with bone-marrow iron stores; estimation was more convenient than bone-marrow biopsy. Maintenance therapy of Iron Dextran Injection 100 mg on alternate weeks, with folic acid, cyanocobalamin, and vitamin supplements provided more iron than was needed in most patients.— S. Hussein *et al.*, *Br. med. J.*, 1975, *1*, 546.

Proprietary Preparations

Imferon *(Fisons, UK)*. Iron Dextran Injection, available in ampoules of 2, 5, and 20 ml. (Also available as Imferon in *Austral., Belg., Canad., Denm., Neth., S.Afr., USA*).

Ironorm Injection *(Wallace Mfg Chem., UK: Farillon, UK)*. Iron Dextran Injection, available in ampoules of 2 ml.

Other Proprietary Names

Chromagen-D *(USA)*; Imferdex *(Switz.)*; Iron Hy-Dex *(S.Afr.)*; Irotran *(USA)*.

Proprietary Preparations of Similar Compounds

Direx *(Andard-Mount, UK)*. An iron-dextran complex prepared from low-molecular-weight dextran in which the aldehyde groups are condensed with glycerol, available as a solution containing the equivalent of 50 mg of iron per ml, in ampoules of 2 and 5 ml.

Niferex *(Tillotts, UK)*. Preparations containing a polysaccharide-iron complex, available as **Elixir** containing the equivalent of 100 mg of Fe in each 5 ml and as **Tablets** each containing the equivalent of 50 mg of Fe. (Also available as Niferex in *Spain*).

5067-b

Saccharated Iron Oxide. Ferrum Oxydatum Saccharatum; Oxyde de Fer Sucré; Eisenzucker.

CAS — 8047-67-4.

Pharmacopoeias. In *Aust.* and *Swiss.*

A reddish-brown odourless powder with a slightly chalybeate taste, containing about 2.9% of iron. Very **soluble** in water; soluble in dilute alcohol. **Incompatible** with acids. **Protect** from light.

Adverse Effects. Adverse effects following the parenteral administration of saccharated iron oxide are headache, dizziness, flushing of the face, nausea and vomiting, pains in the back and legs, dyspnoea, bronchospasm, and fever. Discomfort or pain is sometimes felt at the site of injection.

Excessive dosage may also give rise to severe, sometimes fatal, reactions. See also Iron Dextran Injection, p.880.

A 69-year-old man died 30 minutes after receiving 5 ml of an intravenous injection containing 100 mg of saccharated iron oxide. It was recommended that the initial dose should not exceed 25 mg.— D. W. Barritt and G. C. Swain, *Br. med. J.*, 1953, *1*, 379.

Treatment of Adverse Effects and Precautions. As for Iron Dextran Injection, p.880.

Uses. Saccharated iron oxide has been given in doses of 0.6 to 3 g by mouth in the treatment of iron-deficiency anaemia. It was also formerly given by intravenous injection in the form of a 2% solution containing the equivalent of 100 mg Fe in 5 ml but because of the high incidence of adverse reactions it has been largely replaced.

Estimated acceptable daily intake of iron oxides and hydrated iron oxides: up to 500 µg per kg body-weight. Ferric oxide is less available as a source of biologically active iron than are other forms of iron.— Twenty-third Report of Joint FAO/WHO Committee on Food Additives, *Tech. Rep. Ser. Wld Hlth Org. No. 648*, 1980.

Proprietary Names

Anemicid *(Jap.)*; Egmofer *(Omegin, Ger.)*; Ferrophor *(see also under Dried Ferrous Sulphate) (TAD, Ger.)*; Ferrum Hausmann *(see also under Dextriferron, Ferrous Fumarate, and Iron Polymaltose) (Manzoni, Ital.; Spain)*; Macofer *(Hausmann, Norw.)*.

5068-v

Iron Phosphate *(B.P.C. 1973)*. Iron Phos.; Ferri Phosphas.

A mixture of hydrated ferrous phosphate and ferric phosphate and some hydrated oxides of iron. It is a slate-blue amorphous powder, darkening on exposure to air owing to oxidation. It contains not less than 16% of ferrous iron, calculated as Fe. equivalent to not less than 47.9% of $Fe_3(PO_4)_2,8H_2O$. Practically **insoluble** in water; soluble in hydrochloric acid. **Store** in airtight containers.

Adverse Effects, Treatment, and Precautions. As for Ferrous Sulphate, p.878.

Uses. Iron phosphate has the actions and uses of iron salts (see p.872) and has been included in 'tonic' preparations. Doses of up to 2 g have been used.

An iron phosphate (Ferrum Phosphoricum; Ferr. Phos.) is used in homoeopathic medicine.

Preparations

Compound Ferrous Phosphate Syrup *(B.P.C. 1968)*. Syr. Ferr. Phos. Co.; Chemical Food; Parrish's Food; Parrish's Syrup. Phosphates of iron, calcium, potassium, and sodium, with cochineal and orange-flower water, in syrup. It contains 0.4 to 0.45% w/v of Fe (about 45 mg in 10 ml). Store in well-filled airtight containers. *Dose.* 2.5 to 10 ml.

Ferrous Phosphate, Quinine, and Strychnine Syrup *(B.P.C. 1968)*. Syr. Ferr. Phos. c. Quinin. et Strych.; Easton's Syrup; Syrupus Trium Phosphatum; Ferrous Phosphate with Quinine and Strychnine Syrup. Iron phosphate with quinine and strychnine in syrup, glycerol, and water. It contains the equivalent of 91 mg of anhydrous ferrous phosphate or 43 mg of iron, quinine sulphate 74 mg, and strychnine hydrochloride 1.5 mg in 5 ml. Store in well-filled airtight containers. Protect from light. *Dose.* 2.5 to 5 ml.

Ferrous Phosphate, Quinine, and Strychnine Tablets *(B.P.C. 1973)*. Tab. Ferr. Phosph. c. Quinin. et Strych.; Easton's Tablets; Tablettae Trium Phosphatum. Prepared in 2 strengths: *Formula A* contains iron phosphate 200 mg, quinine sulphate 50 mg, and strychnine hydrochloride 100 µg; *Formula B* contains iron phosphate 100 mg, quinine sulphate 25 mg, and strychnine hydrochloride 50 µg. They may be coated. Unless otherwise specified, Formula A tablets are supplied. *Dose.* 1 tablet.

5069-g

Soluble Iron Pyrophosphate *(B.P.C. 1949, B. Vet. C. 1965)*. Ferr. Pyrophosph. Solub.; Soluble Ferric Pyrophosphate; Sodio-citro-ferric Pyrophosphate.

Transparent green odourless scales with an acid, slightly saline taste, containing not less than 10% of iron. Freely **soluble** in water; practically insoluble in alcohol. Solutions in water are fairly stable and are miscible with solutions of hypophosphites, with malt extract, and with cod-liver oil emulsions.

Soluble iron pyrophosphate has the actions and uses of iron salts (see p.872) and has been used in doses of 500 mg.

In veterinary medicine, it has been used for the prevention of piglet anaemia.

5070-f

Iron Sorbitol Injection *(B.P.)*. Iron-Sorbitol-Citric Acid Complex; Inj. Ferr. Sorbitol.; Iron Sorbitex Injection *(U.S.P.)*.

CAS — 1338-16-5.

Pharmacopoeias. In *Br.* and *U.S.*

A sterile, brown, colloidal solution containing a complex of ferric iron, sorbitol, and citric acid, stabilised with dextrin and sorbitol. The average molecular weight of the complex is less than 5000. The solution contains about 5% (50 mg per ml) of Fe. pH 7.2 to 7.9. Wt per ml 1.17 to 1.19 g. The *U.S.P.* does not specify the strength. It is **sterilised** by autoclaving. **Store** at 15° to 30° and avoid freezing or low temperatures.

In Iron Sorbitol Injection, atoms of ferric iron probably linked together molecules of citrate and sorbitol to form an aggregate, the particles generally being about 2 µm in diameter. This was much smaller than in iron dextran which had aggregates of 3 to 4 µm in diameter. These size differences might affect distribution of the complexes in the body after injection.— M. Hall and C. R. Ricketts (letter), *J. Pharm. Pharmac.*, 1968, *20*, 662.

Adverse Effects, Treatment, and Precautions. As for Iron Dextran Injection, p.880. There may be a metallic taste or a loss of taste.

Three patients with the malabsorption syndrome were treated with intramuscular injections of iron sorbitol. One patient, who received 100 mg of iron as iron sorbitol, developed symptoms including severe chest pain, profuse sweating, and heavy breathing, and died shortly afterwards. Toxic symptoms developed in the second patient after each of 3 injections, and she died 3 hours after the onset of ventricular tachycardia followed by asystole. In the third patient, nausea, chest pain, and dizziness followed the sixth injection of iron sorbitol. A further dose 2 weeks later caused a more severe reaction from which she recovered, but a complete atrioventricular block developed, and 1 year later a second-degree atrioventricular block persisted.— P. Karhunen *et al.*, *Br. med. J.*, 1970, *2*, 521.

A patient developed signs and symptoms of myocardial damage following an intramuscular injection of iron sorbitol.— P. Eliasen and A. Bendtsen, *Ugeskr. Laeg.*, 1976, *138*, 1522.

Absorption and Fate. Iron Sorbitol Injection is readily absorbed after intramuscular injection, maximum plasma concentrations being achieved in about 2 hours. About 30% of a dose is excreted in the urine within 24 hours.

References: S. Lindvall and N. S. E. Andersson, *Br. J. Pharmac.*, 1961, *17*, 358.

Uses. Iron Sorbitol Injection is used in the treatment of iron-deficiency anaemia where oral therapy is ineffective or impracticable. It is more rapidly absorbed from the site of injection than Iron Dextran Injection.

It is given by deep intramuscular injection into the upper outer quadrant of the buttock; to prevent leakage along the injection track, the subcutaneous tissue is drawn to one side before the needle is inserted.

Total dosage is calculated according to the haemoglobin concentration of the blood. The volume and number of injections required to provide the total dosage is related to the condition of the patient, the recommended adult dose per injection being the equivalent of 1.5 mg of iron per kg body-weight daily. A similar dose has been given to children over 3.5 kg in weight.

It is advisable to stop oral administration of iron for at least 24 hours before giving Iron Sorbitol Injection and to stop administration of other injectable iron preparations for a week beforehand. After an injection, the urine may become dark on standing.

Iron Sorbitol Injection should not be administered intravenously.

As a haematinic for intramuscular use iron sorbitol was stable and neither haemolytic nor apt to prolong the blood-clotting time. Compared with iron dextran, absorption from the site of injection was quicker, diffusion similar, and excretion more rapid. The increased rate of absorption was due to its low molecular weight, its stability in tissue fluids, and its passage into the blood stream both directly and through the lymphatics. Iron dextran was absorbed by the lymphatics alone.— S. Lindvall and N. S. E. Andersson, *Br. J. Pharmac.*, 1961, *17*, 358.

A short review of Iron Sorbitol Injection in the treatment of anaemia in patients with rheumatoid arthritis.— A. G. Mowat, *Prescribers' J.*, 1975, *15*, 107.

Proprietary Preparations

Jectofer *(Astra, UK)*. Iron Sorbitol Injection, available in ampoules of 2 ml. (Also available as Jectofer in *Austral., Canad., Denm., Fr., Ger., Neth., Norw., Switz.*).

Other Proprietary Names

Yectofer *(Spain)*.

5071-d

Sodium Ironedetate.

Ferric Monosodium Edathamil. The monohydrated iron chelate of the monosodium salt of ethylenediamine-*NNN′N′*-tetra-acetic acid.

$C_{10}H_{12}FeN_2NaO_8,H_2O=385.1.$

CAS — 15708-41-5 (anhydrous).

A yellow or pale brown hygroscopic powder with a faint odour and a saline taste. **Soluble** 1 in 12 of water; very slightly soluble in alcohol; practically insoluble in chloroform and ether.

Adverse Effects, Treatment, and Precautions. As for Ferrous Sulphate, p.878.

Uses. Sodium ironedetate is used in the treatment of iron-deficiency anaemia, see iron salts (p.872). Small doses are used initially, gradually increasing to a suggested maintenance dose for an adult of the equivalent of 55 mg of iron thrice daily. Children may be given one-quarter to one-half the adult dose.

Proprietary Preparations

Sequestrene Fe3 *(Ciba-Geigy, UK)*. A brand of sodium ironedetate, technical grade.

Sytron *(Parke, Davis, UK)*. A sugar-free mixture containing in each 5 ml sodium ironedetate equivalent to 27.5 mg of iron (suggested diluent, water).

Other Proprietary Names

Ferrostrane *(Fr.)*; Ferrostrene *(Switz.)*; Irostrene *(Norw., Swed.)*.

Levodopa and some other Dopaminergic Agents

4540-v

Dopamine is a key neurotransmitter in the central nervous system; in particular, striatal dopamine depletion is associated with the clinical condition of parkinsonism. Dopamine also inhibits prolactin release from the pituitary and is believed to be the prolactin-release inhibiting factor (PRIF or PIF); its deficiency here is associated with conditions characterised by hyperprolactinaemia, for example, the galactorrhoea-amenorrhoea syndrome.

Accordingly, agents which replenish central dopamine or which themselves can act as stimulants of dopamine receptors (dopamine agonists), may alleviate the symptoms of parkinsonism, hyperprolactinaemia, and related disorders.

Dopaminergic agents described in this section are:

1. levodopa, which is converted into dopamine in the body, and which, unlike dopamine itself, can penetrate the blood-brain barrier hence supplying a source of dopamine to the brain;
2. peripheral decarboxylase inhibitors which have no antiparkinsonian action of their own but enhance the action of levodopa; they include benserazide, p.892, and carbidopa, p.896.
3. the aporphines, apomorphine (p.891) and *N*-propylnoraporphine (p.897) which are structurally related to dopamine and act as dopaminergic agonists, i.e. stimulants of dopamine receptors;
4. the adamantanamines, amantadine (p.890) and memantine (p.897) which may provoke release of dopamine from nerve endings;
5. the semisynthetic polypeptide ergot alkaloid, bromocriptine (p.893) which acts as a dopaminergic agonist, and the non-peptide ergot derivative (or ergoline), lergotrile (p.897);
6. the dopamine-β-hydroxylase inhibitor, fusaric acid (p.897), which prevents the conversion of dopamine into noradrenaline.

The non-ergot dopamine agonist, piribedil (p.897) has also been tried in parkinsonism. Other drugs used include Atropine and other Anticholinergic Agents (see p.289).

The aetiology and natural history of Parkinson's disease.— J. M. S. Pearce, *Br. med. J.*, 1978, *2*, 1664.

Further reviews: K. R. Hunter, *Adv. Med. Topics Ther.*, 1976, *2*, 115; M. O. Thorner, *Adv. Med.*, 1977, *13*, 99; M. M. Cohen and R. T. Scheife, *Am. J. Hosp. Pharm.*, 1977, *34*, 531; A. J. Lees, *Br. J. Hosp. Med.*, 1977, *18*, 336.

4541-g

Levodopa *(B.P., U.S.P.).* Levodopum; Dopa; L-Dopa; Laevo-dopa; Dihydroxyphenylalanine. (−)-3-(3,4-Dihydroxyphenyl)-L-alanine.
$C_9H_{11}NO_4$=197.2.

CAS — 59-92-7.

Pharmacopoeias. In *Br., Braz., Chin., Cz., Jap., Neth., Nord.,* and *U.S.*

A white or slightly cream-coloured, odourless, almost tasteless, crystalline powder. It darkens on exposure to air and light. M.p. about 275° with decomposition.

Soluble 1 in 300 of water; soluble in aqueous solutions of mineral acids and alkali carbonates; practically insoluble in alcohol, chloroform, and ether. A 1% suspension in water has a pH of 4.5 to 7. Aqueous solutions are readily oxidised in air and light. **Store** at a temperature not exceeding 40° in airtight containers. Protect from light.

Adverse Effects. Nausea and anorexia commonly occur during treatment with levodopa, and may be accompanied by vomiting early in treatment, particularly if the dosage is increased too rapidly. Less common side-effects include abdominal pain, constipation, diarrhoea, and dysphagia; dyspepsia and gastro-intestinal bleeding have been reported in patients with a history of gastric ulcer.

The commonest cardiovascular effect is postural hypotension, which is usually asymptomatic but may be associated with faintness and dizziness. There may be palpitations and flushing, often accompanied by excess sweating. Cardiac arrhythmias, particularly atrial and ventricular ectopic beats, have been reported and hypertension has occasionally occurred.

Psychiatric symptoms include agitation, anxiety, elation, and insomnia, or sometimes drowsiness and depression. More severe effects include aggression, paranoid delusions, hallucinations, suicidal behaviour, and unmasking of dementia.

Involuntary movements are very common at the optimum dose required to control Parkinson's disease, and usually start in the mouth, jaws, or tongue. Abnormal limb movements often develop after several months and severe choreoathetoid movements may also occur. Oculogyric crises may rarely be exacerbated and muscle twitching and blepharospasm occur occasionally. Headache, peripheral neuropathy, and widening of the palpebral fissures have occurred.

Polyuria, incontinence, and difficulty in micturition may occur. Slight miosis has been noted; blurred vision, mydriasis, diplopia, and glaucoma are rare.

Uncommon effects include transient rises in tests for liver function and blood urea nitrogen, abnormal respiratory movements, hoarseness, loss of hair, skin rashes, priapism, activation of latent Horner's syndrome, weight changes, and rarely leucopenia or haemolytic anaemia.

Some of the adverse effects are related to the use of anticholinergic agents, to increased mobility, or to unmasking of underlying conditions as parkinsonism improves.

Of 32 patients treated with levodopa for parkinsonism, 25 suffered marked side-effects as follows: nausea 22, including vomiting in 7, treatment having to be stopped in 6; postural hypotension 6; faintness and dizziness 2; early mild depression 3; hallucinations 2; increased libido 3 (2 male, 1 female); deep-calf thrombosis 1; urticarial skin rash 1.— C. Mawdsley, *Br. med. J.*, 1970, *1*, 331.

In 22 patients with parkinsonism treated with levodopa, side-effects were nausea 59% (particularly in the early stages of treatment); anorexia 36%; vomiting 23%; constipation 14%; dizziness 18%; hallucinations 18%; hyperkinesis 9%; choreoathetosis 23%. The average tolerated dose was 3 g daily.— M. J. T. Peaston and J. R. Bianchine, *Br. med. J.*, 1970, *1*, 400.

A study of clinical laboratory abnormalities in 974 patients receiving levodopa.— F. McDowell, *Clin. Pharmac. Ther.*, 1971, *12*, 335.

A study of patients who had received levodopa for more than 2 years revealed a syndrome of subtle mental changes, persistence of stereotyped movements, and hypotonic akinetic episodes (with occasional gait ataxia). The duration of effectiveness of each dose appeared to have fallen over the 2 years from about 4 to about 2 hours.— A. Barbeau (letter), *Lancet*, 1971, *1*, 395. The syndrome also occurred in patients receiving combined therapy of levodopa and benserazide for more than 12 months.— A. Barbeau *et al.*, *Can. med. Ass. J.*, 1972, *106*, 1169.

Side-effects reported in a trial of levodopa included nausea, vomiting, anorexia, involuntary movements, laryngeal stridor, transient dizziness, hallucinations, postural hypotension, and the development of brown body fluids.— V. Dallos *et al.*, *Postgrad. med. J.*, 1972, *48*, 354.

The major adverse effects of levodopa were dyskinesia in 75% of patients and psychiatric disturbances in 25%. Nausea and vomiting in 40 to 50% were gradually tolerated and hypotension in 25 to 30% was generally asymptomatic.— D. B. Calne and J. L. Reid, *Drugs*, 1972, *4*, 49.

Following adminstration of levodopa 75 to 300 mg per kg body-weight daily to beagle *dogs* for 1 year toxic effects were readily reversible on discontinuation.— R. A. Levin *et al.*, *Toxic. appl. Pharmac.*, 1977, *41*, 211.

A discussion on patterns of dystonia experienced in response to levodopa by a group of 87 patients with parkinsonism. In 11 patients the response after discontinuing levodopa lasted from 3 to 5 days. The 'on-off' effect was experienced by 39 patients; there was a rapid response to a dose but this response wore off within 1 to 4 hours. The remainder of the group showed a combination of the 2 effects. Five of the patients showing a short duration response had maximum improvement when the plasma-levodopa concentration was above 2 μg per ml, and had 2 phases of dystonia; in the 34 other patients the response occurred while the plasma concentration of levodopa was above 1 μg per ml, and they had a single phase of dystonia. The effectiveness of levodopa was enhanced in 2 patients by giving glucose with or soon after the dose of levodopa. There was evidence in 1 patient that improvement without dystonia in patients showing short duration response could be achieved by giving levodopa 50 mg with carbidopa 5 mg at hourly intervals instead of levodopa 500 mg with carbidopa 50 mg at 2-hourly intervals.— M. D. Muenter *et al.*, *Mayo Clin. Proc.*, 1977, *52*, 163. See also under Akinesia and Dyskinesia. Related abstracts and comments are also under Absorption and Fate, and Uses.

Akinesia. Akinesia paradoxica ('start hesitation') occurred in 6 of 51 patients on levodopa. All 6 patients had been receiving the drug continuously for over 2 years but the only significant difference between them and the other 45 patients was their superior response to levodopa therapy. Reduction in dosage resulted in disappearance of the side-effect in 5 of the 6 patients with no loss of drug efficacy. 'Start hesitation' could be confused with a worsening of the disease or tolerance to the action of levodopa.— L. M. Ambani and M. H. Van Woert, *New Engl. J. Med.*, 1973, *288*, 1113.

Diuresis. Administration of levodopa 1 to 2 g to 7 patients with idiopathic or postencephalitic Parkinson's disease produced significant increments in renal plasma flow, glomerular filtration rate, and sodium and potassium excretion. The natriuretic effects of levodopa might be of value in congestive heart disease, and could also contribute to the orthostatic hypotension commonly noted in patients receiving levodopa.— G. D. Finlay *et al.*, *New Engl. J. Med.*, 1971, *284*, 865.

Diuresis was provoked in a 32-year-old woman weighing 150 kg, after administration of levodopa 500 mg but not after administration of placebo.— M. F. Banasiak *et al.* (letter), *New Engl. J. Med.*, 1977, *296*, 1122. Comment. Levodopa-induced diuresis is probably due to generation of dopamine since levodopa does not exhibit cardiovascular actions when it is administered after a decarboxylase inhibitor.— L. I. Goldberg (letter), *ibid.*, *297*, 112.

Administration of levodopa to 3 patients with hypokalaemia increased excretion of potassium and sometimes also of sodium. This effect was not noted in 5 normokalaemic patients. Administration of a peripheral dopa decarboxylase inhibitor stopped this kaliuretic effect.— A. K. Granerus *et al.*, *Acta med. scand.*, 1977, *201*, 291.

Dyskinesia. Severe dyskinesias lasting for 0.5 to 1 hour with pains and a burning sensation in the feet and legs, a rapid pulse, and rise in blood pressure (termed diphasic dyskinesia) occured in 12 of 400 patients at least 3 hours after a dose of levodopa and towards the end of the dose interval. The phenomenon invariably occurred in patients who also had the more frequent orofacial dyskinesias, observed at the time of maximum levodopa-induced motility when blood-levodopa concentrations were high.— A. Barbeau (letter), *Lancet*, 1975, *1*, 756. A further report of dyskinesias during levodopa therapy.— E. S. Tolosa *et al.* (letter), *ibid.*, 1381.

Further references: C. H. Markham, *Clin. Pharmac. Ther.*, 1971, *12*, 340; D. B. Calne and J. L. Reid, *Drugs*, 1972, *4*, 49; T. N. Chase *et al.*, *Archs Neurol., Chicago*, 1973, *29*, 328.

Effects on the blood. A report of acute non-haemolytic anaemia and a skin rash occurring in 1 patient during treatment with levodopa.— I. Alkalay and T. Zipoli, *Ann. Allergy*, 1977, *39*, 191.

Haemolytic anaemia. Of 365 patients on a mean daily dosage of 4.04 g of levodopa over a period of 10 to 902 days, 32 developed a positive direct Coombs' test but there were no cases of haemolytic anaemia.— C. Joseph, *New Engl. J. Med.*, 1972, *286*, 1401.

Levodopa did not cause haemolysis in Chinese patients with glucose 6-phosphate dehydrogenase deficiency. These observations do not support the hypothesis that favism, which is found in Mediterranean and Chinese people, is due to the levodopa content of fava beans.— T. K. Chan *et al.*, *Br. med. J.*, 1976, *2*, 1227.

References to patients developing haemolytic anaemia following administration of levodopa: G. C. Cotzias and P. S. Papavasiliou (letter), *J. Am. med. Ass.*, 1969, *207*, 1353; M. C. Territo *et al.*, *ibid.*, 1973, *226*, 1347; D. C. Moir *et al.* (letter), *Br. J. clin. Pharmac.*, 1975, *2*, 173; F. D. Lindström *et al.*, *Ann. intern. Med.*, 1977, *86*, 298; R. M. Bernstein, *Br. med. J.*, 1979, *1*, 1461.

Thrombocytopenia. A 63-year-old man developed thrombocytopenia after long-term levodopa and procyclidine therapy. Thrombocytopenia was attributed to levodopa and was amenable to prednisone therapy.— W. M. Wanamaker *et al.*, *J. Am. med. Ass.*, 1976, *235*, 2217.

Effects on the eyes. In 25 patients treated with levodopa for post-encephalitic parkinsonism, 5 who were initially subject to frequent oculogyric crises obtained a remission lasting from 2 weeks to 5 months. Recurrence of the crises then occurred. These were mild and infrequent at first, but later became more severe and frequent. One patient, who previously had not had oculogyric crises, developed severe crises in the fourth month of therapy with levodopa.— O. W. Sacks and M. Kohl (letter), *Lancet*, 1970, *2*, 215.

In 10 of 11 patients with Parkinson's disease who were receiving levodopa 1 to 6.8 g daily, the pupillary diameter was significantly decreased 4 hours after a dose. The miotic effect might reflect decreased peripheral sympathetic activity following partial noradrenaline depletion at sympathetic nerve endings, or be a central sympatholytic action.— A. S. D. Spiers *et al.*, *Br. med. J.*, 1970, *2*, 639. See also M. I. Weintraub *et al.*, *New Engl. J. Med.*, 1970, *283*, 120.

Effects on the heart. Four of 20 patients with parkinsonism and heart disease, who were being treated with levodopa in a maximum dose of 5.5 g daily, developed cardiac changes which might have been related to levodopa. One patient had a recurrence of angina, 2 developed dysrhythmias (1 required treatment with practolol), and the other died 8 weeks after the beginning of levodopa therapy, possibly from myocardial infarction.— K. R. Hunter *et al.*, *Lancet*, 1971, *1*, 932.

An account of the cardiovascular actions of levodopa. Ventricular arrhythmia was a risk in patients with myocardial irritability or ischaemia.— L. I. Goldberg and T. L. Whitsett, *Clin. Pharmac. Ther.*, 1971, *12*, 376. See also *idem*, *J. Am. med. Ass.*, 1971, *218*, 1921.

See also under Diuresis (above).

Effects on mental state. Over a 6-year treatment period mental symptoms increased in frequency in 100 patients with parkinsonism treated with levodopa. Dementia was found in about a third of the patients throughout the treatment period and was considered to reflect prolongation of the course of the illness rather than to be a direct effect of levodopa. Agitated confusion became increasingly frequent and involved about 60% of the patients; unlike dementia it was alleviated by withdrawal of levodopa.— R. D. Sweet *et al.*, *Neurology, Minneap.*, 1976, *26*, 305.

Further references and reviews on mental changes associated with levodopa therapy: *Br. med. J.*, 1974, *2*, 1; C. Moskovitz *et al.*, *Am. J. Psychiat.*, 1978, *135*, 669.

Dementia. In patients with dementia and parkinsonism levodopa did not influence the extrapyramidal disorder in either clinical context, but profound depression, worsening of the dementia, and hallucinosis could occur at low dose levels.— J. Pearce (letter), *Br. med. J.*, 1974, *2*, 445. See also S. M. Wolf and R. L. Davis, *Archs Neurol., Chicago*, 1973, *29*, 276.

Depression. Of 153 patients with idiopathic parkinsonism, 61 had signs of dementia, 57 (37%) had depression, and 20 had acute psychoses. None of those with dementia or depression had taken levodopa. Of 110 patients treated with levodopa 27 (24%) had depression. Thus levodopa did not appear to cause depression and might even prevent its appearance.— G. G. Celesia and W. M. Wanamaker, *Dis. nerv. Syst.*, 1972, *33*, 577. Comment.— *Br. med. J.*, 1973, *2*, 67. See also M. Riklan *et al.*, *J. nerv. ment. Dis.*, 1973, *157*, 452.

Hallucinations. A patient developed delusions and hallucinations when levodopa was temporarily withdrawn.— R. B. Jenkins and R. H. Groh, *Lancet*, 1970, *2*, 177. See also R. L. Weinmann (letter), *J. Am. med. Ass.*, 1972, *221*, 1054.

Mania. In 7 of 12 depressed patients with Parkinson's disease treatment with levodopa brought about a remission of depression in the same degree as the improvement of motor function. Two experienced mood elevation out of proportion to motor improvement and 1 became hypomanic.— C. P. O'Brien *et al.*, *Archs gen. Psychiat.*, 1971, *24*, 61. See also D. L. Murphy *et al.*, *Am. J. Psychiat.*, 1973, *130*, 79.

Effects on respiration. Levodopa therapy induced respiratory disturbances in 12 patients, and respiratory and phonatory tics in 8 of 25 patients with postencephalitic parkinsonism; the effects were either immediate or delayed for up to 9 months after treatment with levodopa had commenced. All 20 patients also suffered tachypnoea, bradypnoea, and asymmetrical movement of both sides of the chest, paradoxical diaphragmatic movements, and reversal of inspiratory and expiratory phases.— O. W. Sacks *et al.* (letter), *Lancet*, 1970, *1*, 1006.

Further references: A. -K. Granerus *et al.*, *Acta med. scand.*, 1974, *195*, 39.

Effects on skin and hair. Two women who were given levodopa, up to 3 g daily, developed diffuse alopecia in addition to nausea, mental agitation, and involuntary choreiform movements.— A. Marshall and M. J. Williams (letter), *Br. med. J.*, 1971, *2*, 47.

Repigmentation of hair occurred in a white-bearded man after being treated with levodopa 1.5 g daily for 8 months.— K. M. Grainger (letter), *Lancet*, 1973, *1*, 97.

See also Melanoma, under Precautions.

Endocrine effects. A 66-year-old woman with parkinsonism became febrile and had a very low plasma-cortisol concentration after taking levodopa 250 mg four times a day gradually increased to 2.5 g daily. Her temperature and plasma cortisol returned to normal 4 days after withdrawing levodopa but on challenging with a dose of 250 mg thrice daily the symptoms recurred.— S. R. Greenberg (letter), *New Engl. J. Med.*, 1972, *286*, 375.

Postmenopausal bleeding occurred in varying degrees in 12 of 47 women treated with levodopa.— J. Wajsbort (letter), *New Engl. J. Med.*, 1972, *286*, 784.

For the effects on growth hormone see under Uses (below).

Gastro-intestinal lesions. A 56-year-old man developed acute melaena, necessitating surgery and pyloroplasty, 5 weeks after discharge from hospital after being stabilised on levodopa 2 g daily for parkinsonism. Five other cases of gastro-intestinal haemorrhage were recorded in the literature.— D. Riddoch (letter), *Br. med. J.*, 1972, *1*, 53.

Gout. Three patients treated for parkinsonism with levodopa developed elevated serum concentrations of uric acid, with gout occurring in 2. On cessation of levodopa therapy the serum concentrations returned to normal and did not increase when levodopa 4 g daily was again administered.— H. Honda and R. W. Gindin, *J. Am. med. Ass.*, 1972, *219*, 55.

Further references: M. Al-Hujaj and H. Schönthal (letter), *New Engl. J. Med.*, 1971, *285*, 859; S. Jonas (letter), *ibid.*, 1488; W. J. Paladine (letter), *ibid.*, 1972, *286*, 376; D. B. Calne and J. Fermaglich, *Postgrad. med. J.*, 1976, *52*, 232.

Lupus. A lupus syndrome occurred in a 62-year-old man treated for 2 months with levodopa and benserazide.— G. Massarotti *et al.* (letter), *Br. med. J.*, 1979, *2*, 553.

Myoclonus. A report of nocturnal myoclonic attacks induced by levodopa in 6 parkinsonian patients. Similar attacks were also induced by bromocriptine.— J. Vardi *et al.*, *J. Neurol.*, 1978, *218*, 35.

Treatment of Adverse Effects. Reduction of the dosage of levodopa causes the reversal of many side-effects, particularly dyskinesias and mental effects. Nausea may be diminished by taking levodopa after meals, and by taking an anti-emetic such as cyclizine hydrochloride shortly before each dose of levodopa. Orthostatic hypotension may respond to the use of elastic stockings.

If overdosage occurs the stomach should be emptied by aspiration and lavage. Hypotension may require cautious administration of intravenous fluids, and if arrhythmias develop anti-arrhythmic therapy may be necessary. Pyridoxine has been given to reverse some toxic effects of levodopa, but see also under Precautions (below).

The administration of dopamine-receptor blocking agents, such as pimozide or phenothiazines, has been suggested as a logical antidote to levodopa.

A single intravenous dose of 10 mg of pyridoxine was effective in relieving, within 30 minutes, torsion dystonia due to levodopa in a 51-year-old man.— H. D. Jameson (letter), *J. Am. med. Ass.*, 1970, *211*, 1700.

Concomitant administration of lithium carbonate controlled levodopa-induced manic tendencies in a 69-year-old man.— R. S. Ryback and R. S. Schwab, *New Engl. J. Med.*, 1971, *285*, 788.

If hazardous cardiac arrhythmias occurred levodopa should be discontinued; peripheral decarboxylase inhibitors or beta-adrenoceptor blocking agents might possibly reduce their frequency. Levodopa therapy should also be discontinued if delusions occurred and if necessary a tranquilliser could be administered; thioridazine was the least likely to exacerbate parkinsonism. It was advisable to give pilocarpine eye-drops to any patient receiving levodopa who had a family history of glaucoma.— D. B. Calne *et al.*, *Clin. Med.*, 1971, *78* (Feb), 21.

Metoclopramide in doses of 30 to 80 mg daily reduced or prevented the gastro-intestinal side-effects of levodopa.— D. Tarsy *et al.* (letter), *Lancet*, 1975, *1*, 1244.

For a report of disulfiram controlling hypertension and hyperkinesia induced by levodopa, see Disulfiram, p.580.

Hypotension. Postural hypotension produced by levodopa in a woman with parkinsonism was controlled by propranolol.— R. C. Duvoisin (letter), *Br. med. J.*, 1970, *3*, 47. Criticism.— R. G. Shanks (letter), *ibid.*, 403.

Six patients with severe levodopa-induced postural hypotension were treated with fludrocortisone acetate, initially 50 µg daily, increasing by 50 µg weekly until symptoms were relieved. The highest maintenance dose was 200 µg.— M. M. Hoehn, *Archs Neurol., Chicago*, 1975, *32*, 50.

For the use of etilefrine in the treatment of postural hypotension during levodopa therapy, see Etilefrine Hydrochloride, p.13.

Precautions. Levodopa is contra-indicated in patients with severe psychotic disorders or closed-angle glaucoma. It should be used with caution in patients with cardiovascular, endocrine, hepatic, pulmonary, or renal disease and in patients with psychiatric disturbances, open-angle glaucoma, or a history of gastric or duodenal ulceration. Levodopa with benserazide should be used with caution in patients with a history of osteoporosis. It is advisable to carry out periodic evaluations of hepatic, haematological, renal, and cardiovascular functions in patients receiving levodopa therapy.

There are recommendations that levodopa should not be given to patients with a history of malignant melanoma nor to patients with malignant melanoma or skin disorders suggestive of malignant melanoma. However, the association between the use of levodopa and activation of this neoplasm is only suspected.

Its use should be avoided during pregnancy if possible as foetal abnormalities have been reported in *animals* given high doses. Levodopa should not be given with benserazide or carbidopa during pregnancy. Levodopa should not be given to nursing mothers.

Levodopa may cause discoloration of the urine and other body fluids. Patients who benefit from levodopa therapy should be warned to resume normal activities gradually to avoid the risk of injury.

Supplements of pyridoxine lead to increased concentrations of pyridoxal-5-phosphate, the coenzyme involved in the decarboxylation of levodopa to dopamine; hence pyridoxine has been reported to enhance the peripheral metabolism of levodopa to dopamine leaving less available to cross the blood-brain barrier for central conversion to dopamine; pyridoxine therefore inhibits the action of levodopa but this can be stopped by concurrent administration of a peripheral decarboxylase inhibitor.

The effects of levodopa are also diminished by butyrophenones, phenothiazine derivatives, reserpine, or tetrabenazine, and are enhanced by amantadine and decarboxylase inhibitors such as benserazide and carbidopa; they may also be enhanced by anticholinergic agents such as atropine, and also by amphetamine.

Administration of levodopa with monoamine oxidase inhibitors may cause dangerous hypertension; it is suggested that levodopa should not be given within 14 days of stopping a monoamine oxidase inhibitor. Concurrent administration of levodopa with guanethidine, methyldopa, and other antihypertensive agents may cause increased hypotension.

Cardiac arrhythmias due to levodopa may be augmented by anaesthetic agents such as cyclopropane or halothane and it has been recommended that levodopa therapy should be discontinued at least 8 hours prior to surgery; sympathomimetic agents such as adrenaline or isoprenaline may also enhance the cardiac side-effects of levodopa. Beta-adrenoceptor blocking agents such as propranolol may enhance the action of levodopa on tremor and diminish the cardiac side-effects. In some patients the administration of antacids with levodopa may enhance the gastro-intestinal absorption of levodopa.

Absorption. Patients with achlorhydria absorbed levodopa more rapidly and might become toxic on doses that most people were able to tolerate satisfactorily.— L. Rivera-Calimlim *et al.*, *Eur. J. clin. Invest.*, 1971, *1*, 313. The presence or absence of achlorhydria as indicated by the azuresin diagnostic test did not influence the effectiveness of levodopa in the treatment of parkinsonism in 93 patients.— R. Jenkins *et al.* (letter), *J. Am. med. Ass.*, 1973, *223*, 81.

Cardiovascular disease. Levodopa was used in the treatment of 40 patients with parkinsonism and heart disease but excluding those with increasing angina, cardiac infarction within the last year, transient cerebral ischaemia, and postural hypotension. Dosage (under ECG control) was 250 mg thrice daily initially, increased by 250 mg daily every 2 or 3 days to an optimum dosage or the maximum tolerated dosage. Anti-arrhythmic drugs were given to a few patients. Angina improved and then worsened in 1 patient, and a second patient died from myocardial infarction after 31 months' treatment with levodopa. The remaining patients were satisfactorily controlled. With this regimen it was considered that heart disease was not a contra-indication to therapy with levodopa.— R. B. Jenkins *et al.*, *Br. med. J.*, 1972, *3*, 512.

See also under Uses.

Diabetes mellitus. In a study over 1 year of 23 patients with parkinsonism, levodopa was found to stimulate the release of human growth hormone 2 to 3 hours after the dose was given. There was also some decrease in glucose tolerance in all patients, associated with a delayed hypersecretion of insulin. It was suggested that patients who received levodopa over a long period should be observed carefully for the development of diabetes mellitus or acromegaly.— C. R. Sirtori *et al.*, *New Engl. J. Med.*, 1972, *287*, 729. See also M. H. Van Woert and P. S. Mueller, *Clin. Pharmac. Ther.*, 1971, *12*, 360; L. Rivera-Calimlim and J. R. Bianchine, *Metabolism*, 1972, *21*, 611; M. H. Van Woert *et al.*, *J. Endocr.*, 1973, *59*, 523.

Plasma-glucagon concentrations increased after a single dose of levodopa 500 mg by mouth. Maximum increase occurred after 30 minutes.— E. J. Rayfield *et al.*, *New Engl. J. Med.*, 1975, *293*, 589.

Increased libido. Seven of 19 patients reported activation of sexual behaviour at some point during levodopa therapy.— M. B. Bowers *et al.*, *Am. J. Psychiat.*, 1971, *127*, 1691. See also A. Gisselmann, *Nouv. Presse méd.*, 1973, *2*, 1616.

A 12-year-old boy with epilepsy given levodopa 75 mg thrice daily for behavioural disorders improved. Higher doses elicited strong hypersexual behaviour. After 10 months he had hypergenitalism. The patient's external genitalia stopped growing after withdrawal of levodopa and the behavioural disorders returned.— J. J. Korten *et al.* (letter), *J. Am. med. Ass.*, 1973, *226*, 355.

Interactions. Observations on 25 patients with parkinsonism suggested that ampicillin, antacids, barbiturates, chlorpropamide, cyclizine, dexamphetamine, dichloralphenazone, digoxin, diuretics, general anaesthetics, insulin, paracetamol, prednisolone, phenindione, sulphadimidine, thyroxine, and tricyclic antidepressants could safely be used in association with levodopa. Benzodiazepines caused a temporary change in parkinsonian status and guanethidine could be used in a greatly reduced dose. Monoamine oxidase inhibitors and pyridoxine should not be used with levodopa.— K. R. Hunter *et al.*, *Lancet*, 1970, *2*, 1283.

Levodopa could cause chemical interference in laboratory tests for catecholamines, blood or urine creatinine, uric acid, and glucose.— *Med. Lett.*, 1971, *13*, 82.

Plasma-phenazone half-lives were unaffected by levodopa, slightly prolonged by carbidopa, and significantly prolonged by a slightly lower dose of levodopa in conjunction with the same dose of carbidopa. This suggested an inhibition of drug metabolising enzymes.— E. S. Vesell *et al.* (letter), *Lancet*, 1971, *2*, 370. Prolonged treatment with levodopa in *animals* increased the drug-metabolising activity of the liver.— P. Arvela *et al.* (letter), *ibid.*, 1972, *1*, 439.

For a review of interactions between levodopa and other drugs, see J. R. Bianchine and L. Sungapridakul, *Drugs*, 1973, *6*, 364.

Amino acids. Fourteen patients with parkinsonism, under treatment with levodopa, were placed on a dietary regimen low in L-methionine for 8 days; 7 were given methionine 4.5 g daily and 7 received placebo. Patients taking L-methionine regressed in respect of gait, bradykinesia, tremor, and rigidity; the effect ceased when L-methionine was withdrawn.— L. A. Pearce and L. D. Waterbury, *Neurology, Minneap.*, 1974, *24*, 640.

A low-protein diet appeared to even out the differences in control of neurological symptoms between morning and afternoon in patients receiving levodopa for parkinsonism. Five patients with moderate neurological instability became more stable when maintained on a low-protein diet for 2 months to 1 year and some reduction in their levodopa dosage was necessary. A high-protein diet was found to block the effects of levodopa in some patients.— I. Mena and G. C. Cotzias, *New Engl. J. Med.*, 1975, *292*, 181.

Concurrent administration with levodopa limited the intestinal absorption of phenylalanine. Although no signs of amino-acid deficiency have been noted in parkinsonian patients treated over 1 to 2 years, this inhibition might have clinical significance, especially in patients with a low intake of protein.— A. -K. Granerus *et al.*, *Proc. Soc. exp. Biol. Med.*, 1971, *137*, 942. See also J. R. Bianchine *et al.*, *Ann. N.Y. Acad. Sci.*, 1971, *179*, 126.

Blood concentrations of levodopa were lower after concurrent administration with tryptophan than after administration alone.— W. -U. Weitbrecht and K. Weigel, *Dt. med. Wschr.*, 1976, *101*, 20.

Antacids. In a 58-year-old man with parkinsonism, therapy with levodopa, up to 5 g daily, did not lead to clinical improvement. He was found to have a reduced rate of absorption of levodopa due to delayed gastric emptying. Administration of an antacid, taken 30 minutes before each 3-g dose of levodopa, resulted in objective and subjective improvement.— L. Rivera-Calimlim *et al.*, *Br. med. J.*, 1970, *4*, 93.

An antacid (Mylanta) given before, with, or before and with a dose of levodopa 1 g to 8 patients (3 with Parkinson's disease) had no long-term effect on the plasma-dopa concentrations. However, there was significant reduction to the urinary excretion of dopa, dopamine, and homovanillic acid during the first 2 hours after levodopa administration when antacid was administered before levodopa. Administration of antacid with levodopa did not give a lower effective dose of levodopa in the 3 patients with parkinsonism.— A. S. Leon and H. E. Spiegel, *J. clin. Pharmac.*, 1972, *12*, 263.

Anticholinergic agents. Of 34 patients with parkinsonism who had been receiving anticholinergic therapy for several years and levodopa in stable dosage for at least 2 months concomitantly, only 11 were able to tolerate gradual or abrupt withdrawal of anticholinergic drugs for more than 8 weeks. Resumption was necessary due to subjective increases in slowness, tremor, and hypersalivation. Side-effects were more severe if anticholinergic drugs were withdrawn abruptly, and slow withdrawal was recommended. There was an apparent synergism between levodopa and anticholinergic drugs.— R. C. Hughes *et al.*, *Br. med. J.*, 1971, *2*, 487.

Studies in 6 healthy subjects, 6 patients with parkinsonism, and *rats* demonstrated than benzhexol reduced plasma concentrations of levodopa probably by reducing gastro-intestinal absorption.— S. Algeri *et al.*, *Eur. J. Pharmac.*, 1976, *35*, 293.

Further references: R. L. Golden *et al.* (letter), *J. Am. med. Ass.*, 1970, *213*, 628; A. S. Leon *et al.*, *ibid.*, 1971, *218*, 1924.

Bananas. A patient vomited liquorice-coloured material whenever he took banana and levodopa. The colour change could be reproduced experimentally.— H. A. Garfinkel (letter), *Br. med. J.*, 1972, *1*, 312.

Diazepam. Reversible deterioration was observed in 3 patients with parkinsonism when they were given diazepam in addition to levodopa.— J. Wodak *et al.*, *Med. J. Aust.*, 1972, *2*, 1277.

Isoniazid. Isoniazid might enhance the effects of levodopa.— J. P. Morgan (letter), *Ann. intern. Med.*, 1980, *92*, 434.

Melanostatin. The actions of levodopa were enhanced by melanostatin.— A. Barbeau (preliminary communication), *Lancet*, 1975, *2*, 683. See also A. J. Kastin and A. Barbeau, *Can. med. Ass. J.*, 1972, *107*, 1079.

Metoclopramide. In a study of 11 healthy subjects given levodopa 15 mg per kg body-weight and metoclopramide 10 mg, peak plasma concentration of levodopa occurred 20 minutes after administration and was higher than that produced by levodopa alone at 60 minutes. Although the amount of levodopa absorbed in both cases was similar, plasma concentrations fell more quickly after levodopa and metoclopramide and it was suggested that more frequent dosing might be necessary when the drugs were used together. Neither carbidopa nor benserazide reduced the rate of elimination of levodopa from plasma.— J. G. L. Morris *et al.*, *Br. J. clin. Pharmac.* 1976, *3*, 983.

Further references: D. M. Berkowitz and R. W. McCallum, *Clin. Pharmac. Ther.*, 1980, *27*, 414.

Monoamine oxidase inhibitors. In a 57-year-old man with idiopathic parkinsonism given phenelzine 15 mg thrice daily for 10 days, administration of levodopa 50 mg caused a marked rise in blood pressure without any change in pulse-rate, but 25 mg did not change the blood pressure. Phentolamine, 9 mg by intravenous injection, was used to control the hypertensive effect of the higher dose of levodopa. Monoamine oxidase inhibitors should be withdrawn from all patients with parkinsonism before levodopa was given, an interval of at least 1 month being recommended.— K. R. Hunter *et al.*, *Br. med. J.*, 1970, *3*, 388.

Interactions of levodopa with inhibitors of monoamine oxidase and L-aromatic aminoacid decarboxylase.— P. F. Teychenne *et al.*, *Clin. Pharmac. Ther.*, 1975, *18*, 273.

Papaverine. In a 71-year-old woman with Parkinson's disease which was controlled moderately well with levodopa and carbidopa, addition of papaverine hydrochloride 100 mg once daily to her regimen lead to a gradual deterioration in her condition. After withdrawal of papaverine the patient regained her usual response to levodopa. A similar response to papaverine was observed in 4 other patients.— R. C. Duvoisin, *J. Am. med. Ass.*, 1975, *231*, 845. See also D. M. Posner (letter), *ibid.*, *233*, 768.

Phenylbutazone. The action of levodopa was antagonised by phenylbutazone in one patient.— J. Wodak *et al.*, *Med. J. Aust.*, 1972, *2*, 1277.

Phenytoin. Phenytoin decreased the therapeutic effects of levodopa in patients with parkinsonism and patients with chronic manganese poisoning. It also reduced the levodopa-induced choreiform movements but increased the chorea and mental agitation of Huntington's chorea, indicating that these 2 movements were not mediated by the same mechanism.— J. S. Mendez *et al.*, *Archs Neurol., Chicago*, 1975, *32*, 44.

Pyridoxine. It was considered that the long-term administration of levodopa together with a diet low in pyridoxine could produce a serious vitamin deficiency state, as pyridoxine in the form of pyridoxal phosphate combined with dopamine and levodopa thus inactivating the pyridoxine.— M. H. Van Woert (letter), *J. Am. med. Ass.*, 1972, *219*, 1211. The amount of pyridoxine in the diet was insufficient to influence levodopa therapy. The possible adverse effects of levodopa on pyridoxine metabolism had not been noted in over 700 patients but could not be excluded.— M. D. Yahr and R. C. Duvoisin (letter), *ibid.*, *220*, 861.

A study involving 4 healthy subjects and 5 parkinsonian patients indicated that pyridoxine might enhance levodopa metabolism in patients chronically treated with levodopa but not in healthy subjects.— J. R. Bianchine *et al.*, *Ann. intern. Med.*, 1973, *78*, 830. See also T. H. Hsu *et al.*, *Proc. Soc. exp. Biol. Med.*, 1973, *143*, 578. Pyridoxine 100 mg was adminstered by intravenous injection to 8 patients with parkinsonism treated for 2 to 4 years with levodopa and to 8 controls, 4 of whom had parkinsonism. The increase in plasma and erythrocyte pyridoxal phosphate concentrations was greater in the levodopa-treated patients than controls. This suggested an enhanced metabolic synthesis of the coenzyme in long-term levodopa-treated patients which would protect against pyridoxine deficiency but would also result in a decreased effect from levodopa.— H. Mars, *Neurology, Minneap.*, 1975, *25*, 263.

Sympathomimetics. Sympathomimetic amines such as adrenaline or isoprenaline might enhance the cardiac side-effects of levodopa and concurrent administration should be avoided. Patients receiving levodopa might be more susceptible to ventricular arrhythmias due to anaesthetic agents such as cyclopropane or halothane. These agents should probably not be used in patients within 6 hours of ingesting levodopa.— L. I. Goldberg and T. L. Whistett, *Clin. Pharmac. Ther.*, 1971, *12*, 376.

There was no change in pressor sensitivity to tyramine or noradrenaline in 9 patients taking levodopa or levodopa in conjunction with carbidopa.— J. Reid *et al.*, *Clin. Pharmac. Ther.*, 1972, *13* 400.

Thioxanthenes. The butyrophenones and thioxanthenes appear to block post-synaptic dopamine receptors in a manner very similar to that of the phenothiazines and should be avoided.— R. Hausner (letter), *New Engl. J. Med.*, 1976, *295*, 1538.

Tricyclic antidepressants. Imipramine reduced the excretion of levodopa metabolites and might reduce gastro-intestinal absorption of levodopa.— F. S. Messiha and J. P. Morgan, *Biochem. Pharmac.*, 1974, *23*, 1503, per *Int. pharm. Abstr.*, 1975, *12*, 351.

A report of hypertensive crisis, possibly drug-related, in a patient taking amitriptyline, levodopa with carbidopa, and metoclopramide concomitantly.— D. S. Rampton, *Br. med. J.*, 1977, *2*, 607.

Melanoma. An association between initiation of levodopa therapy and growth of melanoma. Levodopa should be used with caution in patients with melanomas or other pigmented lesions.— A. N. Lieberman and J. L. Shupack, *Neurology, Minneap.*, 1974, *24*, 340. See also: J. L. Skibba *et al.*, *Archs Path.*, 1972, *93*, 556; R. Happle, *Fortschr. Med.*, 1974, *92*, 1065; J. E. Berstein *et al.*, *Archs Derm.*, 1980, *116*, 1041.

A survey of 1099 patients with primary cutaneous melanoma showed that only 1 patient had taken levodopa. It was considered that levodopa therapy was not an important factor in the induction of malignant melanoma.— A. J. Sober and M. M. Wick, *J. Am. med. Ass.*, 1978, *240*, 554.

Overactivity. Patients who achieved mobility after successful treatment of their parkinsonism with levodopa were likely to indulge in harmful overactivity. Such patients were liable to be osteoporotic, and 3 cases were reported where activity had led to hip fracture.— J. Greenberg (letter), *New Engl. J. Med.*, 1969, *281*, 621. See also O. W. Sacks *et al.* (letter), *J. Am. med. Ass.*, 1970, *213*, 2270.

Absorption and Fate. Levodopa is absorbed from the gastro-intestinal tract and is widely distributed in the tissues, including the central nervous system. It has a plasma half-life of about 1 hour and is mainly converted by decarboxylation to dopamine, a proportion of which is converted to noradrenaline. Up to 30% is converted to 3-*O*-methyldopa which has a half-life of about 9 to 22 hours. About 80% of levodopa is excreted in the urine within 24 hours in the form of metabolites, mainly as homovanillic acid (13 to 29% or more) and dihydroxyphenylacetic acid. Less than 1% is excreted unchanged. It is secreted in milk.

Levodopa is so rapidly decarboxylated in the gastro-intestinal tract and the liver that very little unchanged levodopa is available to cross the blood-brain barrier for central conversion into dopamine. The dopamine produced by peripheral decarboxylation cannot cross the blood-brain barrier to achieve its therapeutic aim but its peripheral action is responsible for many of the side-effects of levodopa. Hence, the value of peripheral decarboxylase inhibitors which permit a considerably higher proportion of levodopa to enter the brain, so that much lower doses provide the same therapeutic effect, at the same time as they block peripheral production of dopamine with its attendant side-effects.

Response to levodopa varies considerably between patients and in the same patient at different stages of the disease. The many causes for this variation are still the subject of investigation, and have been linked with multiple factors including fluctuating plasma concentrations, the influence of metabolites, and variations in receptor sensitivity.

Studies in 9 patients with parkinsonism showed that peak serum concentrations of levodopa occurred 1 to 2 hours after a dose was taken and two-thirds of the dose was excreted as metabolites in the urine in 8 hours.— M. J. T. Peaston and J. R. Bianchine, *Br. med. J.*, 1970, *1*, 400.

In 6 patients with parkinsonism and acid gastric juice (pH 1.1 to 2.1) gastric emptying time was 183 minutes and the time to peak serum concentrations of levodopa after a 500-mg dose was 90 minutes; in 3 patients with neutral gastric juice the respective times were 30 minutes and 60 minutes; in 3 patients who had undergone total gastrectomy the peak serum concentration was reached in 30 minutes; and in 4 patients given levodopa directly into the duodenum the peak concentration was reached in 15 minutes. A patient unresponsive to levodopa responded promptly to intraduodenal administration and continued to respond when gastric emptying was hastened by reducing the gastric acidity to pH 4 with magnesium and aluminium hydroxides. Anticholinergic drugs in high dosage might decrease gastric motility and delay and decrease the absorption of levodopa.— J. R. Bianchine *et al.*, *Ann. N.Y. Acad. Sci.*, 1971, *179*, 126. See also R. Pocelinko *et al.*, *Clin. Pharmac. Ther.*, 1972, *13*, 149.

Absorption and metabolism of levodopa by the human stomach.— L. Rivera-Calimlim *et al.*, *Eur. J. clin. Invest.*, 1971, *1*, 313.

Intermittent control of parkinsonism in 3 patients given levodopa by mouth was considered to be due to the fluctuating plasma concentrations. When given by constant intravenous infusion steady plasma concentrations and an even control of the symptoms were obtained.— A. C. Woods *et al.* (letter), *Lancet*, 1973, *1*, 1391. See also L. E. Claveria *et al.*, *Br. med. J.*, 1973, *2*, 641.

A patient with parkinsonism, controlled for 9 months with levodopa 5.5 to 6 g daily failed to respond regularly and predictably to treatment despite adjustments of the dose between 5 and 7 g. The degree of disability coincided with low plasma-levodopa concentrations. Increasing the dose to 9.5 g daily brought some control and at 11 g symptoms were almost completly controlled at which dose, despite fluctuating concentrations, the plasma-levodopa value never fell below 1.13 µg per ml.— E. S. Tolosa *et al.* (letter), *Lancet*, 1973, *1*, 942.

Further references to fluctuations in the plasma concentrations of levodopa: E. S. Tolosa *et al.*, *Neurology, Minneap.*, 1975, *25*, 177; C. D. Marsden and J. D. Parkes, *Lancet* 1976, *1*, 292.

The great variation in the optimal dose of levodopa tolerated by different patients did not correlate with differences in rate of absorption or clearance of levodopa. It was likely that differences in optimal therapeutic dosage reflected differences in receptor sensitivity to dopamine. Concurrent administration with anticholinergic agents or amantadine was not associated with any significant differences in levodopa or 3-*O*-methyldopa concentrations.— S. Bergmann *et al.*, *Br. J. clin. Pharmac.*, 1974, *1*, 417.

A study indicating that a high protein dietary regimen can block the effects of levodopa in some patients with Parkinson's disease.— I. Mena and G. C. Cotzias, *New Engl. J. Med.*, 1975, *292*, 181. See under Precautions (above) for more details.

Further references to the effects of diet on levodopa: M. H. Van Woert, *Clin. Pharmac. Ther.*, 1971, *12*, 360.

A report of the transport of levodopa into the brain undergoing competition with the other aromatic amino acids phenylalanine, trytophan, tyrosine, and histidine. This might account for the variability in response.— P. M. Daniel *et al.* (letter), *Lancet*, 1976, *1*, 95.

A detailed review of the available pharmacokinetic data involving levodopa, especially as it relates to therapeutic response of parkinsonian patients. Following administration of levodopa by mouth many factors affect plasma concentrations, including protein intake, gastric emptying time, pyridoxine ingestion, and dopa decarboxylase activity. Other variables affect the rate of uptake by the brain from the blood. Nevertheless, plasma-levodopa concentrations generally correlate with dosage, and also in many parkinsonian patients, with therapeutic response. Accordingly, correlation of clinical response with plasma-levodopa concentrations can provide valuable information in some cases. Although not firmly established, CSF concentrations of homovanillic acid, a major metabolite of levodopa, may have some value in predicting response to levodopa. Concentrations of homovanillic acid or levodopa in body fluids may also correlate closely with certain adverse effects, such as abnormal involuntary movements, gastric discomfort, and psychiatric disturbances. A clearer understanding of the pharmacokinetics of levodopa may improve the clinical management of parkinsonism.— J. R. Bianchine and G. M. Shaw, *Clin. Pharmacokinet.*, 1976, *1*, 313. See also K. R. Hunter, *Adv. Med. Topics Ther.*, 1976, *2*, 115.

Levodopa 50 mg in 200 ml of sodium chloride injection was given intravenously over 20 minutes to 5 patients with Parkinson's disease. A mean peak plasma-levodopa concentration of 890 ng per ml occurred at the end of the infusion and plasma concentrations subsequently decreased rapidly with levodopa being almost undetectable in the plasma after 200 minutes. The mean terminal half-life was 39 minutes. The plasma concentration of total dopamine increased with time and reached a mean peak value of 180 ng per ml 50 minutes after the start of the infusion. The concentrations then decreased more slowly compared to the elimination of levodopa and were approximately 33% of peak concentrations 200 minutes after the start of the infusion. Levodopa was excreted in the urine over 8 hours as total levodopa, total dopamine, total 3,4-dihydroxyphenylacetic acid, and total homovanillic acid, which represented 2.5%, 11.2%, 11.8%, and 29.6% of the dose respectively. In a further 6 patients with Parkinson's disease given a single dose of levodopa 1 g by mouth a mean peak plasma-levodopa concentration of about 1.9 µg per ml occurred about 1 hour after administration with a mean peak concentration for total dopamine of about 1.3 µg per ml occurring after about 2 hours. Levodopa was excreted in the urine over 24 hours as total levodopa, total dopamine, total 3,4-dihydroxyphenylacetic acid, and total homovanillic acid, which represented 0.58%, 13.5%, 15.1%, and 18.2% of the dose respectively. Calculations indicated that following oral administration the absolute bioavailability and total amount absorbed were about 33% and 88% respectively.— K. Sasahara *et al.*, *J. pharm. Sci.*, 1980, *69*, 261.

Further references to attempts to elucidate and prevent fluctuations in response to levodopa: F. L'hermitte *et al.*, *Archs Neurol., Chicago*, 1978, *35*, 261 (dosage adjustments); A. -K. Granérus, *Acta med. scand.*, 1978, *203*, 75 (causal factors).

Metabolites. 3-*O*-Methyldopa, a metabolite of levodopa that penetrates the blood-brain barrier, has no therapeutic effect in parkinsonism.— D. B. Calne *et al.*, *Clin. Pharmac. Ther.*, 1973, *14*, 386. Three patients with parkinsonism who did not respond to levodopa and who developed involuntary movements on concurrent administration of a decarboxylase inhibitor, had unusually high plasma concentrations of 3-*O*-methyldopa.— L. Rivera-Calimlim *et al.*, *Archs Neurol., Chicago*, 1977, *34*, 228. See also C. Feuerstein *et al.*, *Acta neurol. scand.*, 1977, *56*, 508; D. K. Reilly *et al.*, *Clin. Pharmac. Ther.*, 1980, *28*, 278.

Identification of tetrahydropapaveroline and salsolinol in the urine of patients receiving levodopa.— M. Sandler *et al.*, *Nature*, 1973, *241*, 439.

An investigation in 6 patients indicated that conjugated dopamine appeared to accumulate in plasma during levodopa therapy.— G. M. Tyce *et al.*, *Clin. Pharmac. Ther.*, 1974, *16*, 782.

A new class of tetrahydroisoquinoline alkaloids, norlaudanosolinecarboxylic acids, were identified in the urine of patients with parkinsonism who were receiving levodopa.— C. J. Coscia *et al.*, *Nature*, 1977, *269*, 617.

Uses. Levodopa, a naturally occurring amino acid, is the immediate precursor of the synaptic neurotransmitter substance dopamine. Unlike dopamine, levodopa readily enters the central nervous system and has been used in the treatment of conditions, such as Parkinson's disease, which may result from depletion of dopamine in the brain.

Over 65% of patients with Parkinson's disease are benefited by levodopa. The improvement is maintained only while treatment is continued, and is gradually lost after a period of years, probably as the disease progresses. Arteriosclerotic, idiopathic, and postencephalitic parkinsonism respond to levodopa, but there is a higher incidence of side-effects in the postencephalitic form.

Levodopa has also been used to control the neurological symptoms of chronic manganese poisoning, which resemble those of parkinsonism. It is not generally beneficial in drug-induced parkinsonism.

Treatment of parkinsonism should commence with small doses of levodopa gradually increased to the maximum tolerated dose. If severe side-effects occur the dosage should be gradually decreased to the maximum tolerated dose.

A suggested initial dosage for patients in hospital is 0.25 to 1 g daily in 4 or 5 divided doses after meals, increased by 0.5 to 1 g daily at intervals of 3 to 4 days. Out-patients may be given an initial dosage of 250 mg daily in 2 divided doses, increased to 125 mg four or five times daily after one week and subsequently increased at weekly invervals by 375 mg daily. The usual dose range is 2.5 to 8 g daily; maximum improvement may take up to 6 months or longer to occur.

Concomitant administration of an inhibitor of decarboxylase at peripheral sites, such as benserazide, p.893 or carbidopa, p.896, enables the dose of levodopa to be reduced and may diminish some side-effects; it may also provide a more rapid response at the start of therapy. See also under Absorption and Fate.

Sudden fluctuations in the degree of benefit (the 'on-off' effect) develop after about the first 2 years of treatment. The underlying mechanism of this has not been elucidated and attempts to control it by various means, such as dosage adjustment, have been largely unsuccessful.

Administration. Levodopa was absorbed from a suppository and restored an elderly patient's ability to take her medication by mouth.— B. L. Beasley *et al.* (letter), *New Engl. J. Med.*, 1973, *289*, 919.

Beneficial results with a sustained-release preparation of levodopa.— B. Eckstein *et al.* (letter), *Lancet*, 1973, *1*, 431. No practical advantage.— G. Curzon *et al.* (letter), *ibid.*, 781.

Use of enteric-coated tablets.— B. Gilligan and R. Hancock, *Med. J. Aust.*, 1975, *2*, 824.

With amantadine. In 12 patients with parkinsonism, who had been treated with optimal doses of levodopa (0.75 to 5 g daily) for over 8 months, no significant increase in benefit was obtained when amantadine was added in doses of 100 mg daily for 3 days, followed by 100 mg twice daily for 4 days. A further 12 patients who had been treated with amantadine, 200 to 500 mg daily for 3 to 6 months, improved when levodopa was added in doses of 4 g daily.— R. B. Godwin-Austen *et al.*, *Lancet*, 1970, *2*, 383.

Of 77 patients with parkinsonism taking amantadine, 19 who had initial good to excellent responses were studied over an average period of 21 months. All patients maintained their original improvement. A further 37 who either had only slight to moderate responses with amantadine or whose parkinsonism was not sufficiently controlled with levodopa received amantadine with levodopa. All patients showed improvement. When amantadine was replaced by a placebo, there was marked deterioration.— L. R. Zeldowicz and J. Huberman, *Can. med. Ass. J.*, 1973, *109*, 588.

Further reports: G. Scotti (letter), *Lancet*, 1970, *1*, 1394; C. Fieschi *et al.* (letter), *ibid.*, *2*, 154; K. R. Hunter *et al.* (letter), *ibid.*, 566; P. Millac *et al.* (letter), *ibid.*, 720; J. E. Walker *et al.*, *Clin. Pharmac. Ther.*, 1972, *13*, 28; R. B. Bauer and J. T. McHenry, *Neurology, Minneap.*, 1974, *24*, 715, per *J. Am. med. Ass.*, 1974, *230*, 1344.

With anticholinergic agents. A double-blind crossover study of 16 parkinsonian patients receiving maximum tolerated doses of levodopa showed that greater benefit was conferred by concomitant orphenadrine hydrochloride therapy than by placebo R. K. Whyte *et al.*, *Eur. J. clin. Pharmac.*, 1971, *4*, 18.

Addition of anticholinergic agents after 6 months of levodopa therapy had adverse effects in 7 patients who were moderately or severely demented.— G. A. Broe and F. I. Caird, *Med. J. Aust.*, 1973, *1*, 630.

In a double-blind study of 30 patients with parkinsonism benzhexol hydrochloride had no specific value for control of the major features of parkinsonism in patients receiving treatment with levodopa. Adverse reactions that occurred during treatment with levodopa were not related to concurrent benzhexol therapy.— W. E. Martin *et al.*, *Neurology, Minnneap.*, 1974, *24*, 912.

Further references: N. Shomrat *et al.*, *Curr. ther. Res.*, 1978, *24*, 403; H. Hökendorf *et al.*, *J. int. med. Res.*, 1979, *7*, 19.

With apomorphine. Apomorphine injections decreased bradykinesia in parkinsonian patients whether or not they were also receiving levodopa. The side-effects of levodopa and apomorphine were not additive, the 'awakening effect', involuntary movements, and nausea due to levodopa being reduced by apomorphine, whereas the sedative effect and the nausea due to apomorphine were diminished by levodopa.— S. E. Düby *et al.*, *Archs Neurol., Chicago*, 1972, *27*, 474.

With benserazide. A detailed review on the use of benserazide with levodopa.— R. M. Pinder *et al.*, *Drugs*, 1976, *11*, 329.

A study of 60 patients aged 37 to 80 years suffering from parkinsonism showed that treatment with levodopa together with benserazide was better tolerated than levodopa alone. While no cardiac arrhythmias were encountered among patients taking both drugs, involuntary movements occurred during the course of treatment at an earlier stage than with levodopa alone.— A. Barbeau *et al.*, *Can. med. Ass. J.*, 1972, *106*, 1169.

After 1 year and 4 years of treatment with levodopa and benserazide, respectively 8 and 15 of 17 patients with Parkinson's disease had gained more than 10% in body-weight. It was considered that alleviation by benserazide of levodopa-induced gastro-intestinal side-effects had unmasked a levodopa-induced gain in weight.— M. Gasparini and H. Spinnler (letter), *Med. J. Aust.*, 1975, *2*, 617.

Further references: R. Tissot *et al.*, *Presse méd.*, 1969, *77*, 619; A. Barbeau *et al.*, *Clin. Pharmac. Ther.*, 1971, *12*, 353; J. Wajsbort *et al.*, *Wien. med. Wschr.*, 1971, *121*, 741; J. Görlich and E. Markus, *Dt. med. Wschr.*, 1972, *97*, 1246; A. Barbeau, *Adv. Neurol.*, 1973, *2*, 173; J. J. Eisenlohr and W. Gehlen, *Münch. med. Wschr.*, 1974, *116*, 1353; G. Gauthier *et al.*, *Eur. Neurol.*, 1974, *11*, 133; W. Birkmayer *et al.*, *Wien. med. Wschr.*, 1974, *124*, 340; E. M. Miller and L. Wiener, *Neurology, Minneap.*, 1974, *24*, 482; P. Rondot *et al.*, *Thérapie*, 1975, *30*, 653; G. Campanella *et al.*, *Eur. J. clin. Pharmac.*, 1977, *11*, 255.

With bromocriptine. For the administration of bromocriptine with levodopa, see Bromocriptine, p.896.

With carbidopa. Reviews on the use of levodopa with carbidopa.— *Med. Lett.*, 1976, *18*, 117; R. M. Pinder *et al.*, *Drugs*, 1976, *11*, 329.

Carbidopa 50 mg four times a day was given with levodopa to 40 patients with parkinsonism until the optimum dose of levodopa was achieved, usually at 7 weeks; improvement occurred in most patients in the first week with significant reductions in total disability shown at 2 weeks. Patients were allocated to continue to take carbidopa and levodopa or levodopa and placebo. At the end of a year there was no significant difference in total disability between the 16 patients still taking both drugs and the 18 taking levodopa and placebo. However, the average daily dose of levodopa in the first group was 900 mg compared with 2.6 g in the second group where the patients had had to increase their doses. The incidence of nausea and vomiting was also much less in those in the first group in contrast to the incidence of abnormal involuntary movement which was greater in the first group.— C. D. Marsden *et al.*, *Lancet*, 1973, *2*, 1459.

There was definite or moderate improvement in 49% and 27% respectively of 111 patients with parkinsonism after treatment with levodopa for 9 months. The response-rates fell to 19% and 25% respectively after 2 years' treatment. Seventy-three of the 111 treated for 2 years were then given levodopa with carbidopa in addition. The response rate rose from 19% to 38% after 16 weeks. Of 24 patients not previously treated with levodopa and given levodopa with carbidopa, 54% were definitely improved at 20 weeks and 17% moderately so.— E. Critchley, *Postgrad. med. J.*, 1975, *51*, 619.

Further references: D. B. Calne *et al.*, *Br. med. J.*, 1971, *3*, 729; J. R. Bianchine *et al.*, *Clin. Pharmac. Ther.*, 1972, *13*, 584; D. B. Calne *et al.*, *Br. J. Pharmac.*, 1972, *44*, 162; T. N. Chase and A. M. Watanabe, *Neurology, Minneap.*, 1972, *22*, 384; P. S. Papavasiliou *et al.*, *New Engl. J. Med.*, 1972, *286*, 8; H. Mars, *Archs Neurol., Chicago*, 1973, *28*, 91; C. H. Markham *et al.*, *ibid.*, 1974, *31*, 128, per *J. Am. med. Ass.*, 1974, *229*, 861; E. M. Holden *et al.*, *Neurology, Minneap.*, 1974, *24*, 263; *Lancet*, 1973, *1*, 979; *Br. med. J.*, 1974, *4*, 250; *Drug & Ther. Bull.*, 1974, *12*, 83; G. L. Glasgow *et al.*, *Aust. N.Z. J. Med.*, 1974, *4*, 373, per *Int. pharm. Abstr.*, 1975, *12*, 497; A. Lieberman *et al.*, *Neurology, Minneap.*, 1975, *25*, 911, per *J. Am. med. Ass.*, 1976, *235*, 219; J. Wajsbort *et al.*, *Curr. med. Res. Opinion*, 1978, *5*, 695; U. K. Rinne and P. Mölsä, *Neurology, Minneap.*, 1979, *29*, 1584; M. M. Hoehn, *Archs Neurol., Chicago*, 1980, *37*, 146.

With carbidopa and pyridoxine. Pyridoxine accelerated the systemic metabolism of levodopa thereby decreasing its availability to brain parenchyma. Carbidopa given with levodopa prevented the loss of effect produced by exogenous pyridoxine.— H. Mars, *Archs Neurol., Chicago*, 1974, *30*, 444, per *J. Am. med. Ass.*, 1974, *228*, 1447. See also G. C. Cotzias and P. S. Papavasiliou (letter), *J. Am. med. Ass.*, 1971, *215*, 1504; M. D. Yahr and R. C. Duvoisin (letter), *ibid.*, *216*, 2141; S. Fahn, *Neurology, Minneap.*, 1974, *24*, 431, per *J. Am. med. Ass.*, 1974, *229*, 356.

With fludrocortisone. In a patient with Shy-Drager syndrome levodopa and fludrocortisone given concomitantly produced a greater symptomatic improvement than either alone.— J. A. Steiner *et al.*, *Med. J. Aust.*, 1974, *2*, 133.

See also under Treatment of Adverse Effects.

With methyldopa. Methyldopa 125 to 750 mg given daily in conjunction with levodopa 1 to 8 g daily to 22 patients with parkinsonism who were no longer being managed satisfactorily with levodopa alone caused an improvement in 14 and deterioration in 5. After 20 weeks 7 of the 14 continued to benefit from methyldopa. The side-effects of levodopa were not reduced.— R. D. Sweet *et al.*, *Clin. Pharmac. Ther.*, 1972, *13*, 23. See also D. O. Marsh *et al.*, *J. Neurol. Neurosurg. Psychiat.*, 1963, *26*, 505; *Br. med. J.*, 1964, *1*, 997; J. Fermaglich and T. N. Chase (letter), *Lancet*, 1973, *1*, 1261.

For a study indicating that hypertensive patients taking levodopa could be given methyldopa, in hospital, see Methyldopa, p.154.

With propranolol. In a study of 25 patients with parkinsonism, propranolol reduced the tremors. When propranolol was given with levodopa the response was better than when either drug was given alone.— P. Kissel *et al.* (letter), *Lancet*, 1974, *1*, 403.

Propranolol enhanced the rise in plasma-growth-hormone concentrations observed after the administration of levodopa.— F. Camanni and F. Massara (letter), *Lancet*, 1974, *1*, 942.

With tiapride. Administration of tiapride with levodopa, reduced levodopa-induced dyskinesias in 9 of 10 patients with Parkinson's disease. Seven of the patients required an increase in their levodopa dosage to combat tiapride-induced deterioration of their parkinsonism, but in 5 of these the increase did not result in further levodopa-induced dyskinesia. Overall, 7 of the 10 patients therefore obtained improved mobility following administration of tiapride in association with levodopa.— P. Price *et al.* (letter), *Lancet*, 1978, *2*, 1106. Experience with tiapride and sulpiride had shown that even small doses may aggravate end-of-dose deterioration (the wearing-off effect), the evoked bradykinesia taking several weeks to wear off despite prompt cessation of the drug. If further clinical studies provide more convincing evidence of clinical value this must be balanced against the hazards of irreversibly aggravating parkinsonism and inducing tardive dyskinesias.— A. J. Lees *et al.*, *ibid.*, 1205.

With tryptophan. Levodopa was given to 40 patients with parkinsonism in a dose of 750 mg daily increasing by 150 mg every 3 days to a maximum, controlled by the toxicity, which varied from 0.9 to 3.8 g daily, either with a placebo or, in the case of 22 patients, with tryptophan 2 g thrice daily. All patients showed neurological improvement irrespective of the use of tryptophan; however, the group who were given tryptophan had a small but significant decrease in the Hamilton rating scale for depression and a significant increase in a scale which measured available energy, interpreted as drive. Physiotherapy and occupational therapy assessments showed that significant improvement occurred only in patients treated with levodopa and tryptophan; no patient showed any improvement in speech.— A. Coppen *et al.*, *Lancet*, 1972, *1*, 654. Comment.— A. Nistri (letter), *ibid.*, 905. A favourable report in 9 patients.— E. M. Miller and H. A. Nieburg, *Dis. nerv. Syst.*, 1974, *35*, 20.

See also Interactions (Amino Acids), p.885, and Depression (below).

Administration in the elderly. Providing the dosage was low elderly parkinsonian patients should be given levodopa as a first choice. A suitable dose is: levodopa 50 mg once or twice daily, in association with a decarboxylase inhibitor, increased by a similar amount every 4 or 5 days until a satisfactory response has been obtained or side-effects occur.— F. I. Caird and J. Williamson (letter), *Lancet*, 1978, *1*, 986. See also J. Wener *et al.*, *J. Am. Geriat. Soc.*, 1976, *24*, 185.

Further references: M. A. Evans *et al.*, *Eur. J. clin. Pharmac.*, 1980, *17*, 215.

Administration in heart disease. The administration of levodopa in a dose of 1 or 2 g to 7 patients with Parkinson's disease, 4 of whom had not previously received the drug and 3 who had been treated with it for at least 3 months, produced a significant increase in glomerular filtration-rate, renal plasma flow, and sodium and potassium excretion. Sodium and potassium excretion also increased in 3 patients with congestive heart failure and 1 with essential hypertension after a dose of 0.75 to 1 g of levodopa. The natriuretic effect persisted for more than 150 minutes. It was suggested that levodopa might be of value in the treatment of congestive heart failure.— G. D. Finlay *et al.*, *New Engl. J. Med.*, 1971, *284*, 865.

Four of 89 patients with parkinsonism given amantadine 100 to 600 mg daily in addition to levodopa and 2 of 64 similar patients on levodopa 0.5 to 8 g daily developed angina pectoris, dyspnoea, pulmonary congestion, or venous distension in the neck during treatment. However all 6 were elderly and 5 had some cardivascular disorders. The amantadine and levodopa were continued and the signs of cardiac failure were effectively treated with diuretics and digoxin. The benefits of antiparkinsonian therapy were greater than the risk of inducing cardiac problems. Treatment should not be withheld in parkinsonian patients with heart disease.— J. D. Parkes *et al.* (letter), *Lancet*, 1977, *1*, 904.

Administration in renal failure. Levodopa could be given in usual doses to patients with renal failure.— W. M. Bennett *et al.*, *Ann. intern. Med.*, 1980, *93*, 286.

Anorexia nervosa. Four of 6 patients with anorexia nervosa gained weight when treated with levodopa. Three sustained their improvement and attained normal weight.— A. J. Johanson and N. J. Knorr (letter), *Lancet*, 1974, *2*, 591.

Further references: K. A. Halmi and B. S. Sherman, *Psychopharmac. Bull.*, 1977, *13*, 63.

Anoxia. Levodopa 50 mg daily by mouth in 2 divided doses had beneficial effects on anoxia-induced neurological damage in 6 neonates.— G. Blancher and J. Chassevent (letter), *Thérapie*, 1975, *30*, 613.

Benedikt's syndrome. The tremor of a patient with Benedikt's syndrome was relieved by treatment with levodopa in increasing doses up to 1 g thrice daily.— T. Fujieda *et al.* (letter), *Br. med. J.*, 1974, *1*, 456.

Bronchitis. A 56-year-old man with long-standing chronic bronchitis and severe bronchospasm was relieved of dyspnoea after commencing levodopa for parkinsonism.— H. G. Jeffs (letter), *Br. med. J.*, 1974, *1*, 454. See also K. K. Nakano *et al.*, *Archs intern. Med.*, 1972, *130*, 346; F. Oppel, *Dt. med. Wschr.*, 1975, *100*, 1461.

Chorea. In an attempt to identify persons with presymptomatic Huntington's chorea, levodopa was given for 10 weeks to 28 young adults who were symptomless children of patients with definite Huntington's chorea. The dose was increased to a maximum of 2.5 g daily, or 800 mg in some who were also given benserazide 200 mg daily. Twenty-four subjects in the same age range were given the same dose and used as controls. No abnormal movements were observed in the control group whereas half the group at risk developed chorea, which disappeared when the levodopa was discontinued. The result suggested that possibly these subjects had the gene for Huntington's chorea.— H. L. Klawans *et al.*, *New Engl. J. Med.*, 1972, *286*, 1332. Thirty patients at risk of developing Huntington's chorea have been followed up to 8 years and 5 of the 10 in whom transient chorea had developed after exposure to levodopa now have the disease as well as 1 of 20 patients who originally had no chorea when given levodopa. The hypothesis that patients in whom levodopa-related chorea develops are at higher risk for Huntington's disease appears to be true but the predictive value of the test can only be determined after a longer follow-up.— H. L. Klawans *et al.* (letter), *ibid.*, 1980, *302*, 1090. Comment on the levodopa provocative test for Huntington's disease and a belief that it should not be used.— S. Fahn (letter), *ibid.*, *303*, 884. A similar comment.— C. D. Marsden (letter), *Br. med. J.*, 1980, *281*, 871.

Although levodopa normally exacerbates Huntington's chorea, in 2 patients both psychiatric and neurological symptoms greatly improved after levodopa therapy. In both patients the CSF concentrations of homovanillic acid had been markedly depressed, and were increased by levodopa therapy. There may be an unexplained variety of the disease.— G. Loeb *et al.*, *J. Neurol. Neurosurg. Psychiat.*, 1976, *39*, 958. Similar reports: B. K. Tan *et al.* (letter), *Lancet*, 1972, *1*, 903; G. Schenk and H. J. Leijnse-Ybema, *ibid.*, 1974, *1*, 364; P. A. Low *et al.*, *Med. J. Aust.*, 1974, *1*, 393.

Dementia. In an 8-week double-blind crossover study in 14 patients with senile dementia there was a significant increase in the intellectual rating scale while under treatment with levodopa 875 mg daily but negligible changes in behaviour rating scales.— C. Lewis *et al.*, *Br. med. J.*, 1978, *1*, 550. While the small gains in intellectual performance had, in general, been maintained the clinical relevance was doubtful. Levodopa was not yet recommended for routine treatment.— K. Johnson *et al.* (letter), *ibid.*, 1625.

Further references: D. A. Drachman and S. Stahl (letter), *Lancet*, 1975, *1*, 809.

See also under Effects on Mental Performance (below).

Depression. Symptoms of depression were reversed in a 56-year-old woman following treatment with levodopa by mouth. As the dose was gradually increased from 1 to 7 g daily her condition improved; she deteriorated when the dosage was reduced.— W. E. Bunney *et al.* (letter), *Lancet*, 1969, *1*, 885.

In a controlled double-blind study against a placebo, relatively large doses of levodopa and tryptophan given to depressed patients were not associated with enough clinical improvement to allow them to leave hospital.— J. Mendels *et al.*, *Archs gen. Psychiat.*, 1975, *32*, 22. See also N. Matussek *et al.* (letter), *Lancet*, 1970, *2*, 660.

Different responses of growth hormone and prolactin to levodopa were observed in patients with depression or manic depression classified as unipolar or bipolar.— P. W. Gold *et al.* (letter), *Lancet*, 1976, *2*, 1308. Findings at variance.— J. Mendlewicz *et al.* (letter), *ibid.*, 1977, *1*, 652.

Dystonia musculorum deformans. A group of 20 patients with dystonia musculorum deformans underwent surgical treatment with an average response of good to excellent and a relapse-rate of 15%. Another 15 patients who had been given levodopa received the same surgical treatment where the average response was only fair to good and the relapse-rate was 70%.— I. S. Cooper (letter), *Lancet*, 1972, *2*, 1317.

A 15-year-old girl with severe generalised dystonia responded rapidly to treatment with levodopa 250 mg six times daily. After 18 months this was reduced to 250 mg five times daily and at 30 months the patient still maintained her response.— A. H. Rajput (letter), *Lancet*, 1973, *1*, 432. A similar report.— T. Hongladarom (letter), *ibid.*, 1114. See also *J. Am. med. Ass.*, 1969, *208*, 2266.

Effects on mental performance. Controlled tests for mental changes carried out on 33 patients with parkinsonism treated with levodopa indicated that despite continued improvement in motor function there was deterioration in intellectual activity.— M. I. Botez and A. Barbeau (letter), *Lancet*, 1973, *2*, 1028.

Verbal communication was improved in 9 of 10 patients receiving neuroleptic medication when levodopa 1 or 2 g daily was added to the regimen; the speed of response was increased in 8 of the 10 patients.— J. A. Yaryura-Tobias *et al.* (letter), *Nature*, 1971, *234*, 224. See also G. G. Marsh *et al.*, *J. Neurol. Neurosurg. Psychiat.*, 1971, *34*, 209; A. W. Loranger *et al.*, *Archs gen. Psychiat.*, 1972, *26*, 163; A. Violon *et al.*, *Acta psychiat. belg.*, 1972, *72*, 168; K. K. Nakano *et al.*, *Neurology, Minneap.*, 1973, *23*, 865; F. P. Bowen *et al.*, *ibid.*, 1101; M. Riklan *et al.*, *J. nerv. ment. Dis.*, 1973, *157*, 452; G. G. Marsh and C. H. Markham, *J. Neurol. Neurosurg. Psychiat.*, 1973, *36*, 925; D. J. de L. Horne, *Psychopharmacologia*, 1974, *36*, 175; R. Halgin *et al.*, *J. nerv. ment. Dis.*, 1977, *164*, 268.

Effects on nails. A 78-year-old woman who had received levodopa for 12 months noticed an increase in growth and hardness of her nails and, on questioning, 11 of 85 women also receiving levodopa had noticed an improvement in their nails.— E. Miller (letter), *New Engl. J. Med.*, 1973, *288*, 916.

Galactorrhoea-amenorrhoea syndrome. Levodopa 500 mg thrice daily was administered for 6 to 9 months to 11 patients with galactorrhoea and amenorrhoea of 1 to 20 years' duration. Menstrual cycles resumed in 9 patients, 4 ovulated, and 2 became pregnant; galactorrhoea disappeared in 7 patients, diminished in 3, and remained unchanged in 1.— A. Zárate *et al.*, *Fert. Steril.*, 1973, *24*, 340.

Testing with levodopa or protirelin alone was of no predictive value in distinguishing between those patients with galactorrhoea and amenorrhoea produced by pituitary tumours and those with galactorrhoea-amenorrhoea due to other causes.— A. E. Boyd *et al.*, *Ann. intern. Med.*, 1977, *87*, 165.

Further references: M. Edmonds *et al.*, *Can. med. Ass. J.*, 1972, *107*, 534; M. T. Buckman *et al.*, *J. clin. Endocr. Metab.*, 1973, *36*, 911; A. Zárate *et al.*, *J. clin. Endocr. Metab.*, 1973, *37*, 855; D. Ayalon *et al.*, *Obstet. Gynec.*, 1974, *44*, 159.

Growth-hormone secretion tests. Levodopa was administered to 21 children in a dose of 250 mg per 1.73 m^2 body-surface thrice daily with meals for 48 hours followed by 500 mg per 1.73 m^2 in the morning of the third day on an empty stomach. Growth hormone concentrations increased in 20 of the children to concentrations comparable with those observed during insulin provocation. The use of levodopa as a diagnostic agent for growth hormone reserve in children was considered as reliable as and less dangerous than the insulin tolerance test.— B. A. Porter *et al.*, *Am. J. Dis. Child.*, 1973, *126*, 589.

Ingestion of levodopa 500 mg per 1.73 m^2 body-surface concurrently with propranolol 750 µg per kg body-weight (to a maximum of 40 mg) induced a significant increase of more than 5 ng per ml in plasma-growth hormone concentrations in 17 children and adolescents with short stature. Six subjects who failed to respond had abnormal responses to at least 2 other stimulatory tests and of a further 10 subjects suffering from various disorders 2 who failed to respond had a pituitary or hypothalamic disorder. Children with a previous history of asthma or heart disease were excluded and all subjects were kept recumbent during the test; a few patients experienced nausea but no vomiting. The test was considered reliable, safe, and easy to perform.— R. Collu *et al.*, *Pediatrics*, 1975, *56*, 262. The advantages of administration with a decarboxylase inhibitor.— F. O. Fevang *et al.*, *Acta paediat. scand.*, 1977, *66*, 81.

Sequential use of insulin and levodopa to provoke pituitary secretion of growth hormone. Each of the normal children responded to at least one test.— E. O. Reiter *et al.*, *Am. J. Dis. Child.*, 1977, *131*, 189.

Studies on the effect of levodopa on plasma concentrations of growth hormone in various disease states: C. F. Colucci *et al.* (letter), *Br. med. J.*, 1973, *4*, 420 (arteriosclerotic hemiplegia); J. D. Parkes *et al.*, *Br. J. clin. Pharmac.*, 1977, *4*, 343 (narcolepsy); M. K. Jones *et al.*, *ibid.*, 1978, *5*, 425 (breast cancer).

Further references: A. Hayek and J. D. Crawford, *J. clin. Endocr. Metab.*, 1972, *34*, 764; A. W. Root and R. D. Russ, *J. Pediat.*, 1972, *81*, 808; T. Lin and J. R. Tucci, *Ann. intern. Med.*, 1974, *80*, 464; R. Collu *et al.*, *Pediatrics*, 1978, *61*, 242; P. R. Blackett *et al.*, *Sth. med. J.*, 1979, *72*, 842.

Hepatic encephalopathy. Of 6 patients with chronic, usually longstanding, hepatic encephalopathy resistant to conventional treatment, 3 gained significant improvement and 1 possible improvement after treatment with levodopa in a mean dose of 2.1 g daily. The EEG was not signficantly affected, and gastro-intestinal side-effects were a limiting factor.— M. Lunzer *et al.*, *Gut*, 1974, *15*, 555.

Although large doses of levodopa may be followed by increased responsiveness in hepatic encephalopathy the effect is very short-lasting and cannot be recommended as a form of therapy. One explanation for the effect is that it flushes away false neurotransmitter substances.— I. M. Murray-Lyon and P. N. Trewby, Hepatic Failure, in *Recent Advances in Intensive Therapy*, No. 1, I.M. Ledingham (Ed.), London, Churchill Livingstone, 1977, p. 125.

Coma, induced by the injection of ammonium chloride in *rats*, could be prevented by the administration of levodopa. This was probably the result of a peripheral effect of dopamine on renal function, with increased excretion of ammonia and urea, rather than a central action.— L. Zieve *et al.*, *Gut*, 1979, *20*, 28.

Further references: J. D. Parkes *et al.* (preliminary communication), *Lancet*, 1970, *2*, 1341; A. Sarrazin *et al.*, *Presse méd.*, 1971, *79*, 2226, per *Practitioner* 1972, *208*, 310; M. Stefanini and E. N. Hetherington (letter), *J. Am. med. Ass.*, 1972, *220*, 1247; O. Abramsky and Z. Goldschmidt, *Surgery, St Louis*, 1974, *75*, 188, per *J. Am. med. Ass.*, 1974, *228*, 784; P. A. Contoyiannis *et al.* (letter), *Br. med. J.*, 1975, *1*, 272; D. V. Datta *et al.*, *Am. J. med. Sci.*, 1976, *272*, 95; T. Chajek *et al.*, *Postgrad. med. J.*, 1977, *53*, 262; F. Savery and E. B. Uy, *Curr. ther. Res.*, 1977, *22*, 143.

Hypotension. A 58-year-old man with idiopathic orthostatic hypotension responded well to a regimen of levodopa given in alternating doses of 100 mg or 50 mg, at hourly intervals together with tranylcypromine, 2.5 mg every 5 hours. His blood pressure remained controlled with this treatment, rigidity of his neck was reduced, and he no longer exhibited tremors of wrists and ankles, but he still suffered from urinary bladder incontinence and dysfunction due to impairment of preganglionic sympathetic nerve fibres.— J. Sharpe *et al.*, *Can. med. Ass. J.*, 1972, *107*, 296.

See also Precautions.

Increased libido. Four of 7 male parkinsonian patients reported increased libido during administration of levodopa. Hormonal factors appeared to be involved.— E. Brown *et al.*, *Am. J. Psychiat.*, 1978, *135*, 1552.

See also Precautions.

Malignant neoplasms. Seven postmenopausal women with breast cancer failed to respond to treatment with levodopa 250 mg every 4 hours daily increased to 500 mg four times daily, but 3 of the 7 had significant tumour regression when given conjugated oestrogens 1.25 mg four times daily in conjuction with levodopa. None of the patients had responded to earlier oestrogen therapy.— B. A. Stoll (letter), *Lancet*, 1972, *1*, 431. Comment.— A. N. Papaioannou (letter), *ibid.*, *2*, 226.

Use of levodopa to predict responses to endocrine therapy of patients with advanced breast cancer.— G. H. Sasaki *et al.*, *Ann. Surg.*, 1976, *183*, 392. See also R. P. Dickey *et al.*, *New Engl. J. Med.*, 1972, *286*, 843; J. P. Minton and R. P. Dickey, *Surgery Gynec. Obstet.*, 1973, *136*, 971.

References to levodopa-induced relief of metastatic bone pain in various cancers: J. P. Minton and R. P. Dickey (letter), *Lancet*, 1972, *1*, 1069 (breast cancer); D. W.

Nixon (letter), *New Engl. J. Med.*, 1975, *292*, 647 (prostatic carcinoma, hypernephroma, lymphoma); G. J. Tolis (letter), *ibid.*, 1352 (breast cancer); J. P. Minton *et al.* (letter), *ibid.*, 1976, *294*, 340 (prostatic carcinoma); W. E. Farnsworth and M. J. Gonder, *Urology*, 1977, *10*, 33 (prostatic carcinoma).

Manganese poisoning. Neurological signs and symptoms of chronic manganese poisoning were relieved or abolished in 7 of 8 patients by levodopa, given initially in a dose of 100 mg six times daily, slowly increased to an optimal dose of up to 8 g daily. Rigidity, hypotonia, and postural reflex disturbances were mainly affected. In 1 patient weakness, hypotonia, tremor, and hypokinesia were aggravated. This patient responded to treatment with DL-5-hydroxytryptophan, up to 3 g daily.— I. Mena *et al.*, *New Engl. J. Med.*, 1970, *282*, 5.

Further references: H. A. Rosenstock *et al.*, *J. Am. med. Ass.*, 1971, *217*, 1354; W. Schunk, *Dte Gesundh-Wes.*, 1976, *31*, 1847.

Migraine. A 48-year-old woman with a history of monthly migraine attacks was given levodopa 1 g daily when she developed Parkinson's disease. No migraine attacks occurred for 7 months and her neurological recovery on levodopa 2.5 g daily was good. When the drug was replaced by a placebo the attacks returned.— J. L. Antunes *et al.* (letter), *Lancet*, 1970, *2*, 928.

In a preliminary study of 6 patients, levodopa in doses up to 500 mg four times daily either alone or with benserazide had no effect on migraine.— H. J. Hansen and E. Dupont (letter), *Lancet*, 1972, *1*, 97.

Myoclonus. One patient with postanoxic action myoclonus was successfully treated with levodopa in doses of up to 2 g daily. Diazepam and clonazepam were also given but the latter had no effect on the myoclonic jerks. Levodopa had no effect in 2 patients with myoclonus epilepsy and 1 with facial myoclonus whereas clonazepam produced a good response.— G. Minoli and G. Tredici (letter), *Lancet*, 1974, *2*, 472.

Obesity. For a total of 24 days, 5 obese woman received a low-energy dietary regimen together with levodopa gradually increased over 7 days to a total of 4 g daily; 11 similar women acted as controls and received the dietary regimen alone. In the levodopa group the expected adaptive fall in resting metabolic rate did not occur although the expected fall in serum-tri-iodothyronine concentration was no different from that in the control group. A slight increase in weight loss was noted in the levodopa group. If levodopa can prevent a long-term decline in energy expenditure it may be a useful adjunct to slimming dietary regimens.— P. S. Shetty *et al.* (preliminary communication), *Lancet*, 1979, *1*, 77.

Phenylketonuria. Levodopa 150 mg with carbidopa 12.5 mg and 5-hydroxytryptophan 40 mg daily produced improvement in a child with phenylketonuria not due to a phenylalanine-hydroxylase deficiency.— K. Bartholomé and D. J. Byrd (letter), *Lancet*, 1975, *2*, 1042.

Panencephalitis. Six of 10 children with subacute sclerosing panencephalitis responded to daily treatment with levodopa alone or with carbidopa and sometimes with nialamide 25 to 50 mg. All 6 who were in the early stage of the disease were still free of symptoms when followed-up at 2 to 3 months.— B. Halikowiski and M. Piotropawlowska-Weinert (letter), *Lancet*, 1977, *2*, 1033.

Parkinsonism. Reviews of drugs, including levodopa, used in the treatment of parkinsonism.— D. B. Calne and J. L. Reid, *Drugs*, 1972, *4*, 49; O. Hornykiewicz, *Br. med. Bull.*, 1973, *29*, 172; G. Selby, *Drugs*, 1976, *11*, 61; J. R. Bianchine, *New Engl. J. Med.*, 1976, *295*, 814; K. R. Hunter, *Adv. Med. Topics Ther.*, 1976, *2*, 115; *idem*, *Prescribers' J.*, 1976, *16*, 101; R. B. Godwin-Austen, *Postgrad. med. J.*, 1977, *53*, 729; W. R. Millington and M. A. Vance, *Hosp. Pharmst*, 1977, *12*, 377; G. M. Stern and A. J. Lees, *Practitioner*, 1977, *219*, 537; *Med. Lett.*, 1979, *21*, 37; J. L. Marx, *Science*, 1979, *203*, 737; *Br. med. J.*, 1981, *282*, 417. See also: *The Treatment of Parkinsonism with L-Dopa*, J. Marks (Ed.), Lancaster, Medical and Technical Publishing, 1974; *The Clinical Uses of Levodopa*, G. Stern (Ed.), Lancaster, Medical and Technical Publishing, 1975.

Slowly increasing doses of levodopa were given to 28 patients with parkinsonism. Initially 100 mg was given thrice daily, with an increase of 200 to 300 mg daily every 2 to 4 days until an optimal dose with minimal side-effects was reached. Improvement was very marked in 10 patients, marked in 10, moderate in 4, and slight in the remaining 4. The usual sequence of improvement of parkinsonian signs was akinesia, rigidity, and finally tremor. Walking, dysphagia, aphonia, articulation, diaphoresis, lachrymation, posture, salivation, seborrhoea, ankle oedema, and facial expression were usually strikingly improved, but not in any regular order. In 10 of 12 patients with dysuria, this symptom improved.— G. C. Cotzias *et al.*, *New Engl. J. Med.*, 1969, *280*, 337.

In 20 patients with idiopathic parkinsonism, the effects of levodopa, given in addition to previous therapy for parkinsonism, were compared with a placebo. The initial dosage of levodopa was 250 mg thrice daily, then increased gradually to a maximum tolerated daily dosage of 1 to 8 g (mean 3 g) over 2 to 12 weeks, then maintained at the maximum for 6 to 12 weeks. Under double-blind conditions, patients received placebo instead of levodopa 6, 8, 10, and 12 weeks after reaching the maximum tolerated dosage. Improvement after levodopa was impressive in 50% of the patients, and less benefit was obtained in 25%; of the remaining 25%, several suffered a deterioration when the placebo was stopped.— D. B. Calne *et al.*, *Lancet*, 1969, *2*, 973.

Benefit to 22 parkinsonian patients followed treatment with levodopa, 500 mg daily increased by 500 mg daily to a total of 4 g daily in 4 divided doses or until the emergence of side-effects (chiefly nausea), when the dosage was reduced by 1 g daily to a suitable level. Previous medication with other drugs for parkinsonism was continued unchanged. The average tolerated daily dose was 3 g. About 50% improvement of disabilities was achieved in about 40 days and 60% after 100 days. Response was greater in younger patients or when the disease was less severe or of short duration. Out-patient treatment should be carefully supervised over several months, with gradual increments in doses.— M. J. T. Peaston and J. R. Bianchine, *Br. med. J.*, 1970, *1*, 400.

In a double-blind crossover study, 31 patients with parkinsonism received levodopa for 10 weeks in a dosage increasing by 1 g each week up to a maximum daily dosage of 6 g and the same daily dosage then maintained if possible. Involuntary movements were most severe in those deriving most benefit from the treatment. Marked or moderate improvement occurred in 27 patients with maximum benefit evident in bradykinesia, rigidity and associated features, and tremor. Side-effects included nausea, vomiting or anorexia, involuntary movements, and hypotension. An altered mental state and speech deterioration occurred in a few patients.— R. C. Hughes *et al.*, *Br. med. J.*, 1971, *1*, 7.

Signficant functional improvement in walking, climbing, and hand movement occurred in 18 patients with parkinsonism when measured 3 to 5 months after starting treatment with levodopa 0.75 to 3 g daily. Measurement at an average interval of 13.3 months later when the patients were still taking levodopa showed no change in walking and climbing but continued improvement in hand function.— K. M. Grainger (letter), *Lancet*, 1973, *1*, 209.

After 3 months' treatment with levodopa 120 of 174 patients with parkinsonism gained a pronounced to moderate response. After 2 years 79 patients were still taking levodopa and in 51 this response was sustained, but by the end of 3 years only 20 of the 50 patients on levodopa continued to have a sustained response.— K. R. Hunter *et al.*, *Lancet*, 1973, *2*, 929.

In a long-term study of 126 patients with parkinsonism who were treated with levodopa for 12 to 36 months, there was maximal response after 6 months but 13.6% continued to improve after 12 months, all of them with a short history of disease. Treatment was considered satisfactory by relatives of two-thirds of the patients and 92% had benefit after 12 months. Nausea and vomiting decreased while involuntary movements increased and had occurred in 80% of patients. There were serious mental disturbances in 26% and akinesia paradoxica in 12%.— J. Presthus and R. Holmsen, *Acta neurol. scand.*, 1974, *50*, 774.

In a prospective study of levodopa in the treatment of 100 patients with Parkinson's disease 47 were still receiving levodopa after 5 years. Improvement was maximal at ½ to 1 year; thereafter there was moderate worsening of symptoms but functional rating was still better at 5 years than before treatment in 34 of the 47. Dose-related side-effects included nausea and anorexia which were maximal at 6 months whereas abnormal involuntary movements, impaired postural reflexes, and mental changes increased with time as did rapid alterations in motor performance ('on-off' effect). This latter effect became refractory to dosage adjustment. Postural hypotension also occurred. During the 5-year period 32 patients died. Levodopa remained the single most effective symptomatic treatment for Parkinson's disease.— R. D. Sweet and F. H. McDowell, *Ann. intern. Med.*, 1975, *83*, 456.

An account of the success and problems of long-term levodopa therapy in Parkinson's disease. About 85% of people obtain useful and even dramatic benefit from initial levodopa therapy and maintain a stable level of improved function over the next few years, despite progression of the disease. After 2 or 3 years of treatment disability begins to return in many patients, either as insidious deterioration or as increasingly severe fluctuations in function ('on-off' phenomena). After 5 years of treatment about two-thirds of patients will have had some loss of initial benefit, probably due to continued progression of the underlying disease rather than because of the treatment.— C. D. Marsden and J. D. Parkes, *Lancet*, 1977, *1*, 345.

Long-term clinical and sociological studies: E. Singer, *J. chron. Dis.*, 1974, *27*, 581; A. Barbeau, *Archs Neurol., Chicago*, 1976, *33*, 333; L. Battistin *et al.*, *Acta neurol. scand.*, 1978, *57*, 186; C. Joseph *et al.*, *Ann. Neurol.*, 1978, *3*, 116.

For comparisons of amantadine and levodopa in parkinsonism, see Amantadine Hydrochloride, p.891.

Juvenile parkinsonism. Reports on the treatment of juvenile parkinsonism with levodopa: W. E. Martin *et al.*, *Archs Neurol., Chicago*, 1971, *25*, 494; A. W. Kilroy *et al.*, *ibid.*, 1972, *27*, 350; K. K. Sachdev *et al.*, *ibid.*, 1977, *34*, 244.

Schizophrenia. Addition of levodopa to the usual medication of schizophrenic patients was of doubtful value. Of 94 patients, 21 showed some improvement, 69 were unchanged, and 4 became worse.— C. Ogura *et al.*, *Curr. ther. Res.*, 1976, *20*, 308.

Further references: M. Campbell *et al.*, *Curr. ther. Res.*, 1976, *19*, 70; P. E. Garfinkel and H. C. Stancer, *Can. pyschiat. Ass. J.*, 1976, *21*, 27.

Skin disorders. *Acne.* Levodopa, up to 1 g thrice daily, had no effect on the seborrhoea of 7 patients with acne vulgaris.— J. L. Burton *et al.* (letter), *Lancet*, 1971, *2*, 370. A similar report.— J. A. Cotterill *et al.*, *ibid.*, *1*, 1271.

In patients with parkinsonism receiving levodopa 2 to 5 g daily there was a significant reduction in sebum excretion-rate (SER) in 11 patients with initial seborrhoea, but no significant reduction in SER in the 8 patients with a normal initial SER.— J. L. Burton *et al.*, *Br. J. Derm.*, 1973, *88*, 475. See also L. C. Parish (letter), *New Engl. J. Med.*, 1970, *283*, 879.

Psoriasis. Nine patients with psoriasis were given levodopa 100 mg thrice daily after meals, increased after 2 weeks to 600 mg daily, in conjunction with benserazide 50 mg thrice daily. Assessment at 4 months showed excellent improvement in 3, good in 4, and satisfactory in 2. Two patients who withdrew from the study experienced nausea, somnolence, and dizziness.— J. -M. Giroux *et al.* (letter), *Lancet*, 1972, *2*, 333.

Conflicting reports: A. Barbeau and J. -M. Giroux (letter), *Lancet*, 1972, *1*, 204; J. -M. Devoitille *et al.* (letter), *Lancet*, 1973, *1*, 619; F. Savery *et al.*, *Curr. ther. Res.*, 1976, *20*, 130.

Vitiligo. In a study of 16 patients the twice daily application of a topical preparation containing levodopa 10 or 20% for a period of 8 to 20 weeks during August to January had no appreciable effect on vitiligo.— H. Woolfson and O. A. Finn (letter), *Lancet*, 1972, *1*, 598.

Almost complete repigmentation occurred in 2 and partial repigmentation in another 2 of 7 patients with vitiligo treated for 3 to 8 months with levodopa 125 mg daily increased over 4 to 6 weeks to 1.5 g daily in conjunction with ultraviolet light treatment 3 times a week.— S. K. Goolamali (letter), *Lancet*, 1973, *1*, 675.

Supranuclear palsy. A 75-year-old man who had had the palsy for 2 years was given levodopa in doses increasing daily by 500-mg increments. His condition improved with 6 g daily, but he became depressed after 2 days.Amitriptyline was added and improvement resumed after 2 weeks. A 69-year-old woman showed no improvement after treatment for 51 days with levodopa.— A. Wagshul and R. B. Daroff (letter), *Lancet*, 1969, *2*, 105. See also J. R. Mendell *et al.*, *ibid.*, 1970, *1*, 593.

Reports of unsuccessful treatment with levodopa: J. J. Gilbert and R. G. Feldman (letter), *Lancet*, 1969, *2*, 494; O. W. Sacks (letter), *ibid.*, 591; R. Jenkins (letter), *ibid.*, 742; M. Gross (letter), *ibid.*, 1359; I. M. Donaldson, *Aust. N.Z. J. Med.*, 1973, *3*, 413.

Torticollis. Of 17 patients with torticollis given levodopa, 6 improved but 3 of them regressed when a placebo was substituted. Prolonged follow-up after levodopa treatment was reinstated showed that only 1 patient maintained the initial improvement. Amantadine up to 200 mg daily produced temporary improvement in 1 of 9 of the patients who had not responded to levodopa. Tetrabenazine up to 150 mg daily produced similar improvement in 1 of the 9, while haloperidol up to 3 mg daily produced sustained improvement within 48 hours in 1 of 6 of the non-responders.— K. M. Shaw *et al.* (letter), *Lancet*, 1972, *1*, 1399.

Preparations

Levodopa and Carbidopa Tablets *(B.P.).* Tablets containing levodopa and carbidopa. The content of carbidopa is expressed in terms of anhydrous carbidopa.

Levodopa Capsules *(B.P.).* L-Dopa Capsules. Capsules containing levodopa. Store at a temperature not exceeding 30°.

Levodopa Capsules *(U.S.P.).* Capsules containing levodopa. Store at a temperature not exceeding 40° in airtight containers. Protect from light.

Levodopa Tablets *(B.P.).* L-Dopa Tablets. Tablets containing levodopa.

Levodopa Tablets *(U.S.P.).* Tablets containing levodopa. Store at a temperature not exceeding 40° in airtight containers. Protect from light.

Proprietary Preparations

Berkdopa *(Berk Pharmaceuticals, UK).* Levodopa, available as scored tablets of 500 mg.

Brocadopa *(Brocades, UK).* Levodopa, available as **Capsules** of 125, 250, and 500 mg and as scored **Tablets** of 500 mg. **Brocadopa Temtabs.** Levodopa, available as scored sustained-release tablets of 500 mg. (Also available as Brocadopa in *Fr., Ger.*).

Larodopa *(Roche, UK).* Levodopa, available as scored tablets of 500 mg. (Also available as Larodopa in *Arg., Austral., Belg., Canad., Demn., Fr., Ger., Ital., Neth., Norw., S.Afr., Switz., USA*).

Madopar 62.5 (known as Prolopa in *Canad.* and Madopark in *Swed.*) *(Roche, UK).* Capsules each containing levodopa 50 mg and benserazide hydrocholoride equivalent to benserazide 12.5 mg. **Madopar 125.** Capsules each containing levodopa 100 mg and benserazide hydrochloride equivalent to benserazide 25 mg. **Madopar 250.** Capsules each containing levodopa 200 mg and benserazide hydrochloride equivalent to benserazide 50 mg. For parkinsonism.

Sinemet-110 *(Merck Sharp & Dohme, UK).* Scored tablets each containing levodopa 100 mg and carbidopa equivalent to anhydrous carbidopa 10 mg. **Sinemet-275.** Scored tablets each containing levodopa 250 mg and carbidopa equivalent to anhydrous carbidopa 25 mg. For parkinsonism.

Sinemet Plus *(Merck Sharp & Dohme, UK).* Scored tablets each containing levodopa 100 mg and carbidopa equivalent to anhydrous carbidopa 25 mg. For parkinsonism.

Other Proprietary Names

Arg.— Doparkine; *Austral.*— Levopa, Syndopa; *Belg.*— Eldopal; *Canad.*— Levopa; *Ital.*— Dopaidan; *Jap.*— Doparl, Dopasol, Dopaston; *Neth.*— Eldopal, Levopa, Rigakin; *Norw.*— Eldopar; *Spain*— Dopalfher, Maipedopa, Novedopa; *Swed.*— Dopastral; *Switz.*— Eldopatec; *USA*— Bendopa, Dopar.

Levodopa was also formerly marketed in Great Britain under the proprietary names Levopa (*Arco, Switz.*) and Veldopa (*Smith & Nephew Pharmaceuticals*).

4542-q

Amantadine Hydrochloride *(U.S.P.).*

1-Adamantanamine Hydrochloride; EXP-105-1. Tricyclo[3.3.1.1^{3,7}]dec-1-ylamine hydrochloride. $C_{10}H_{17}N,HCl = 187.7$.

CAS — 768-94-5 (amantadine), 665-66-7 (hydrochloride).

Pharmacopoeias. In *Chin.* and *U.S.*

A white or almost white odourless crystalline powder with a bitter taste.

Soluble 1 in 2.5 of water, 1 in about 5 of alcohol, 1 in 18 of chloroform, and 1 in 70 of macrogol 400. A 20% solution in water has a pH of 3 to 5.5.

Adverse Effects. Most side-effects associated with amantadine therapy are dose-related and relatively mild. They may be reversed by withdrawing therapy but many resolve despite continuation.

The most common side-effects are livedo reticularis and ankle oedema; nervous excitement, confusion, difficulty in concentration, dizziness or lightheadedness, orthostatic hypotension, urinary retention, slurred speech, ataxia, depression, insomnia, and lethargy may also occur; nausea, anorexia, vomiting, dry mouth, constipation, tremors, skin rash, and visual disturbances have occasionally been reported. More serious side-effects may include congestive heart failure, psychosis, and leucopenia.

Hallucinations and feelings of detachment have occurred. These effects appear to be dose-related and disappear upon withdrawal of the drug. Doses of about 4 times the recommended dose have caused convulsions.

About 10% of healthy volunteers have mild reactions to an initial single dose of 100 mg of amantadine and 10 to 15% to a single dose of 200 mg. Although the incidence of reactions in healthy volunteers decreased with continuous doses at the same level, side-effects occurred on average in 3 to 7% of healthy adults.— F. Assaad *et al., Bull. Wld Hlth Org.*, 1978, *56*, 229.

Effects on the eyes. Sudden loss of vision occurred in a 67-year-old man who had been taking amantadine 200 mg daily for several weeks. Improvement of visual acuity occurred gradually after discontinuation of amantadine.— J. T. Pearlman *et al.* (letter), *J. Am. med. Ass.*, 1977, *237*, 1200. See also *idem, Archs Neurol., Chicago*, 1977, *34*, 199.

Effects on the heart. Side-effects reported in a study of amantadine hydrochloride included paroxysmal supraventricular tachycardia responsive to dosage reduction.— V. Dallos *et al., Postgrad. med. J.*, 1972, *48*, 354.

Congestive heart failure associated with amantadine occurred in a patient who had been receiving combined treatment with amantadine, levodopa, and orphenadrine for 4 years.— J. A. Vale and K. S. Maclean (letter), *Lancet*, 1977, *1*, 548.

Effects on mental state. Coloured lilliputian hallucinations with amantadine.— R. W. Harper and B. U. Knothe, *Med. J. Aust.*, 1973, *1*, 444.

Hallucinations and delirium in 13 elderly patients, 12 of whom had Parkinson's disease, during amantadine therapy.— J. U. Postma and W. van Tilburg, *J. Am. Geriat. Soc.*, 1975, *23*, 212.

Livedo reticularis. The occurrence of livedo reticularis in 36 of 40 patients with Parkinson's disease who received amantadine hydrochloride, 100 to 400 mg daily, for 2 to 12 months, usually with anticholinergic drugs and sometimes with levodopa, might have been a physiological response provoked by a widespread dilatation of the dermal vessels following depletion of catecholamine stores in peripheral nerve terminals. Some patients developed ankle oedema as well.— D. I. Vollum *et al., Br. med. J.*, 1971, *2*, 627. A similar report.— C. N. Shealy *et al., J. Am. med. Ass.*, 1970, *212*, 1522.

Treatment of Adverse Effects. If overdosage occurs the stomach should be emptied by aspiration and lavage. In particular, symptoms of excessive central stimulation with convulsions and psychosis should be treated appropriately. Anti-arrhythmic agents may also be required.

Bladder catheterisation may be required. Elimination of amantadine has been reported to be increased in acid urine. For comments on forced diuresis in drug overdosage, see Phenobarbitone, p.812.

A patient with postencephalitic parkinsonism who had taken an estimated 2.8 g of amantadine in a suicide attempt suffered an acute toxic psychosis with disorientation, visual hallucinations, and aggresive behaviour. Convulsions did not occur, possibly because he had been receiving phenytoin which was continued. Urinary retention and mild dilatation of the pupils occurred suggesting that amantadine might have anticholinergic or sympathetic properties. The patient was treated with hydration and chlorpromazine and recovered in 4 days.— S. Fahn *et al., Archs Neurol.*, 1971, *25*, 45.

Following administration of amantadine to control extrapyramidal symptoms associated with haloperidol therapy for psychosis, a 67-year-old man became disorientated and agitated, and developed visual hallucinations, slurred speech, ataxia, myoclonus, dry mucous membranes, urinary retention and elevated blood urea nitrogen and creatinine. Therapy was discontinued and 1-mg doses of physostigmine were given which rapidly reversed the delirium and myoclonus for periods of 1 or 2 hours, a total of 9.5 mg being required to control symptoms during the initial 24 hours. His condition returned to the base-line psychiatric, renal, and neurological status within 48 hours. The mechanism of action of physostigmine in the control of amantadine-induced delirium is unclear.— D. E. Casey (letter), *New Engl. J. Med.*, 1978, *298*, 516.

Dialysis. Amantadine accumulated in the blood of 2 patients with parkinsonism who had decreased kidney function. Concentrations were reduced by haemodialysis in 1 patient to 64% and by peritoneal dialysis in both patients to 60% and 76% respectively of initial values. Frequently repeated dialysis might be required for complete removal of amantadine.— T. S. Ing *et al., Can. med. Ass. J.*, 1976, *115*, 515. Evidence of extremely poor total body clearance of amantadine in patients with renal failure; only a small fraction of the total body store was removed by haemodialysis.— L. -S. Soung *et al., Ann. intern. Med.*, 1980, *93*, 46.

Precautions. Amantadine should not be given to patients with a history of epilepsy or gastric or duodenal ulceration. Care should be taken in elderly patients with cerebral arteriosclerosis and in patients being treated with stimulants of the central nervous system, such as amphetamine. It should also be used with caution in patients with cardiovascular, hepatic, or renal disorders and in patients with recurrent eczema or psychosis.

Amantadine may enhance the effects of anticholinergic agents such as benzhexol, benztropine, and orphenadrine and the dose of these drugs should be reduced when amantadine is given concomitantly. Treatment with amantadine should not be stopped abruptly.

Administration in renal failure. Confusion, nightmares, hallucinations, and restlessness occurred in a patient with negligible renal function when given amantadine 200 mg daily. Two other patients with diminished renal function also showed similar effects.— T. S. Ing *et al.* (letter), *New Engl. J. Med.*, 1974, *291*, 1257. Similar reports: K. F. W. Armbruster *et al., Nephron*, 1974, *13*, 183; J. U. Postma and W. Van Tilburg, *J. Am. Geriat. Soc.*, 1975, *23*, 212; R. L. Borison, *Am. J. Psychiat.*, 1979, *136*, 111; T. S. Ing *et al., Can. med. Ass. J.*, 1979, *120*, 695.

Interactions. *With anticholinergic agents.* Amantadine given with benzhexol or orphenadrine might cause hallucinations and doses of these drugs might need to be reduced during amantadine therapy.— V. Dallos *et al., Br. med. J.*, 1970, *4*, 24.

Pregnancy and the neonate. A report of a complex cardiovascular lesion in an infant; the mother had taken amantadine hydrochloride 100 mg daily for the first 3 months of pregnancy.— J. J. Nora *et al.* (letter), *Lancet*, 1975, *2*, 607.

Absorption and Fate. Amantadine hydrochloride is readily absorbed from the gastro-intestinal tract, and maximum concentrations in the blood appear after 1 to 4 hours. It is mainly excreted unchanged in the urine. It is also excreted in milk.

In a study of the effect of amantadine hydrochloride on the metabolic processes of the liver, no significant difference was found in the plasma half-life of phenazone in 6 subjects.— K. O'Malley *et al.* (letter), *Lancet*, 1972, *1*, 685.

Following administration of amantadine 100 mg twice daily to physically healthy schizophrenic subjects, plasma concentrations after 7 days ranged from 0.12 to 1.12 µg per ml.— D. J. Greenblatt *et al., J. clin. Pharmac.*, 1977, *17*, 704.

Further references: P. Biandrate *et al., J. Chromat.*, 1972, *74*, 31; R. M. Rizzo *et al., Eur. J. clin. Pharmac.*, 1973, *5*, 226; F. Y. Aoki *et al., Clin. Pharmac. Ther.*, 1979, *26*, 729.

Some estimations of the half-life of amantadine: W. E. Bleidner *et al., J. Pharmac. exp. Ther.*, 1965, *150*, 484 (9 to 15 hours); M. Rizzo *et al., Eur. J. clin. Pharmac.*, 1973, *5*, 226 (21.8 hours); C. Montanari *et al., ibid.*, 1975, *8*, 349 (about 34 hours in elderly subjects); G. M. Pacifici *et al., Br. J. clin. Pharmac.*, 1976, *3*, 883 (10 to 28.5 hours).

Uses. Amantadine hydrochloride is an antiviral agent which probably inhibits penetration of the virus into the host cell. It has no virucidal actions. It is used prophylactically against infection with influenza type A2 virus but is of no value in preventing infection with other types of influenza virus. In this context, it has been reported that amantadine does not appear to suppress antibody response, and accordingly there are no specific contra-indications to its administration in subjects who have recently received Influenza Vaccine. It has also been used to ameliorate symptoms when administered during the early stages of influenza due to type A2 virus and it has been tried in the treatment of herpes zoster.

Amantadine may augment dopaminergic activity and is used in the treatment of parkinsonism, usually in conjunction with other therapy. It may improve hypokinesia and rigidity but usually has less effect on tremor.

The usual dose is 100 mg twice daily and in influenza treatment should be given for 5 to 7 days. For the prophylaxis of influenza the same dose is given for as long as protection from infection is required (usually 7 to 10 days). In herpes zoster treatment may be given for 14 days, and for a further 14 days if postherpetic pain continues.

A suggested dose for children aged 1 to 9 years is 4 to 8 mg per kg body-weight daily in divided doses, up to a maximum of 150 mg daily.

In parkinsonism, treatment is usually started with 100 mg daily and is increased to 100 mg twice daily, after a week. Doses up to 400 mg daily have occasionally been used.

A report of *animal* studies which failed to provide evidence that the antiparkinsonian effect of amantadine is related to an action on dopaminergic mechanisms.— F. Brown and P. H. Redfern, *Br. J. Pharmac.*, 1976, *58*, 561.

Administration. Studies on the anti-viral effect of amantadine administered by aerosol.— V. Knight *et al.*, *Antimicrob. Ag. Chemother.*, 1979, *16*, 572; F. G. Hayden *et al.*, *ibid.*, 644.

Administration in renal failure. Recommendations for giving amantadine in reduced dosage and at increased dosage intervals in patients with renal failure.— W. M. Bennett *et al.*, *Ann. intern. Med.*, 1980, *93*, 286. Evidence of extremely poor total body clearance of amantadine in patients with renal failure; only a small fraction of the total body store was removed by haemodialysis.— L. -S. Soung *et al.*, *ibid.*, 46.

See also under Precautions.

Further references: V. W. Horadam *et al.*, *Ann. intern. Med.*, 1981, *94*, 454.

Chorea. Three of 13 patients with choreiform movements improved markedly with amantadine 100 or 200 mg daily and 6 gained marginal improvement.— M. W. Gray *et al.* (letter), *Lancet*, 1975, *2*, 132.

Dementia. In a crossover study 20 elderly patients with signs of mental deterioration showed slight improvement after treatment with amantadine 100 mg twice daily for 15 days, compared to a placebo.— S. M. Chierichetti *et al.*, *Curr. ther. Res.*, 1977, *22*, 158.

Depression. In a controlled study of 34 patients with depression, 14 of 18 given amantadine 100 or 200 mg daily for 4 weeks improved compared with 6 of 16 given placebo.— S. Vale *et al.* (letter), *Lancet*, 1971, *2*, 437.

Four elderly depressed patients were treated for 3 weeks with amantadine 100 mg daily gradually increased over 10 days to 300 mg daily. No benefit was observed but there was a progressive increase in motor restlessness, anxiety, and outbursts of violent and aggressive behaviour, associated with plasma-amantadine concentrations of about 800 ng per ml.— M. Rizzo and P. L. Morselli (letter), *Br. med. J.*, 1972, *3*, 50. See also M. Rizzo *et al.*, *Eur. J. clin. Pharmac.*, 1973, *5*, 226.

Down's syndrome. An infant with Down's syndrome was given amantadine hydrochloride in graduated doses from about 2 weeks of age. Up to the age of 9 months the child had developed within normal limits in motor, speech, personal, and social activities. On days when the child did not receive amantadine there was loss of muscular tone, increased floppiness, and excessive drooling.— G. White (letter), *Med. J. Aust.*, 1974, *2*, 184.

Herpes zoster. In a double-blind study in general practice (99 doctors) in 100 patients with herpes zoster there was no significant difference between treatment with amantadine hydrochloride [100 mg] twice daily and placebo in respect of crusting of lesions, skin healing, and new lesions. There was no significant difference in the duration of pain up to 28 days, though fewer patients taking amantadine had pain lasting more than 28 days; patients with pain lasting more than 28 days (taking either amantadine or placebo) were significantly older.— A. W. Galbraith, *Br. med. J.*, 1973, *4*, 693.

Influenza. Reviews on the role of amantadine in the prophylaxis and treatment of influenza.— *Br. med. J.*, 1976, *1*, 1552; P. C. Hoffmann *et al.*, *Ann. intern. Med.*, 1977, *87*, 725; L. A. Liesenberg and S. K. Shimomura, *Drug Intell. & clin. Pharm.*, 1978, *12*, 362; *Med. Lett.*, 1978, *20*, 25; C. Stuart-Harris, *J. antimicrob. Chemother.*, 1978, *4*, 295; T. -W. Chang and D. R. Snydman, *Drugs*, 1979, *18*, 354; *Ann. intern. Med.*, 1980, *92*, 256; *Med. Lett.*, 1980, *22*, 91; M. S. Hirsch and M. N. Swartz, *New Engl. J. Med.*, 1980, *302*, 903.

In a double-blind study in 404 volunteers, 206 were given amantadine 100 or 200 mg daily for 11 days and 198 received a placebo. Amantadine was found to be 51% effective in preventing the development of artificially induced A2 influenza and 73 to 92% effective in preventing the more severe forms of A2 influenza. In those subjects who developed A2 influenza in spite of amantadine therapy, symptoms were milder and lasted a shorter time than in subjects who received a placebo. Amantadine did not appear to have any effect against influenza B virus. No benefit was observed when amantadine was withheld until symptoms of influenza developed.— A. A. Smorodintsev *et al.*, *J. Am. med. Ass.*, 1970, *213*, 1448.

In a double-blind controlled study of 153 patients with influenza, the mean duration of fever was significantly less in the 72 who received amantadine in a dose of 100 mg twice daily for adults, 100 mg daily for children aged 10 to 15, and a proportionally lower dose for children between 2 and 10 years, than in the 81 given placebo. There were no changes in other symptoms or in circulating influenza antibodies.— A. W. Galbraith *et al.*, *Lancet*, 1971, *2*, 113. See also *idem*, 1969, *2*, 1026.

In a double-blind study in the winter 1971–72 of 65 patients with influenza type A2, amantadine produced a faster relief from symptoms than a placebo although the duration of fever was not reduced. Antibody responses showed amantadine did not depress the immunological response to infection.— A. W. Galbraith *et al.*, *J. R. Coll. gen. Pract.*, 1973, *23*, 34.

Recovery from uncomplicated influenza type A was more rapid in patients receiving amantadine hydrochloride 100 mg twice daily for 7 days than those receiving a placebo. Amantadine also improved peripheral airways function.— J. W. Little *et al.*, *Ann. intern. Med.*, 1976, *85*, 177.

Further references: H. A. Wendel *et al.*, *Clin. Pharmac. Ther.*, 1966, *7*, 38; O. Kitamoto, *Jap. J. Tuberc. Chest Dis.*, 1971, *17*, 1; C. McLaren and C. W. Potter, *Lancet*, 1973, *1*, 1157; J. M. O'Donoghue *et al.*, *Am. J. Epidem.*, 1973, *97*, 276; A. W. Galbraith, *J. antimicrob. Chemother.*, 1975, *1*, *Suppl.*, 81; A. S. Monto *et al.*, *J. Am. med. Ass.*, 1979, *241*, 1003; H. J. Rose, *J. R. Coll. gen. Pract.*, 1980, *30*, 619.

Manganese poisoning. A report of the treatment of the neurological symptoms of chronic manganese poisoning with levodopa and amantadine.— W. Schunk, *Dte Gesundh Wes.*, 1976, *31*, 1847.

Multiple sclerosis. Noticeable progress and improvement during a period of 2 years occurred in a patient with multiple sclerosis after receiving amantadine 100 mg twice daily for 9 days subsequently increased to 300 mg daily.— M. Schapira, *J. R. Coll. gen. Pract.*, 1974, *2*, 411, per *Pharm. J.*, 1974, *2*, 457.

Panencephalitis. Amantadine usually with sedatives or anticonvulsants given to 6 children with subacute sclerosing panencephalitis was considered to have stabilised the disease process in 5. Mental function and neurological signs were not reversed even when treatment was begun within 1 month of the onset of illness.— R. H. A. Haslam *et al.*, *Neurology, Minneap.*, 1969, *19*, 1080.

Parkinsonism. For reviews of drugs, including amantadine, used in parkinsonism, see D. B. Calne and J. L. Reid, *Drugs*, 1972, *4*, 49; J. R. Bianchine, *New Engl. J. Med.*, 1976, *295*, 814; K. R. Hunter, *Adv. Med. Topics Ther.*, 1976, *2*, 115; *idem*, *Prescribers' J.*, 1976, *16*, 101; R. B. Godwin-Austen, *Postgrad. med. J.*, 1977, *53*, 729; W. R. Millington and M. A. Vance, *Hosp. Pharmst*, 1977, *12*, 377; G. M. Stern and A. J. Lees, *Practitioner*, 1977, *219*, 537.

Comparison with levodopa. Amantadine hydrochloride was given with or without levodopa to 351 patients in doses of 200 mg daily for more than 60 days. Of those taking amantadine alone, 48% had a favourable response to treatment whereas 79% taking amantadine with levodopa responded favourably. There was a reduction in efficacy between 30 and 60 days of use. Commonly occurring side-effects were confusion, disorientation, depression, nervousness, insomnia, dizziness, lightheadedness, and abdominal complaints.— R. S. Schwab *et al.*, *J. Am. med. Ass.*, 1972, *222*, 792.

A 8-week study to compare the effects of levodopa and amantadine, completed by 55 patients, with a slightly higher proportion of those on amantadine withdrawing, indicated that levodopa was the more effective drug.— V. Dallos *et al.*, *Postgrad. med. J.*, 1972, *48*, 354.

Further references: J. D. Parkes *et al.*, *Postgrad. med. J.*, 1971, *47*, 116; C. Mawdsley *et al.*, *Clin. Pharmac. Ther.*, 1972, *13*, 575; S. Fahr and W. P. Isgreen, *Neurology, Minneap.*, 1975, *25*, 695.

For clinical reports of the administration of amantadine hydrochloride in conjunction with levodopa in the treatment of parkinsonism, see Levodopa, p.887.

Drug-induced parkinsonism. Amantadine 200 mg daily, administered in a double-blind crossover study to 15 patients with drug-induced extrapyramidal symptoms poorly controlled by anticholinergic agents, produced marked improvement in rigidity and tremor without any evident side-effects. Hypokinesia and vegetative disturbances also improved.— G. M. Pacifici *et al.*, *Br. J. clin. Pharmac.*, 1976, *3*, 883.

In schizophrenic patients with drug-induced extrapyramidal symptoms given amantadine 100 mg twice daily, improvement in rigidity was the only symptom which correlated with plasma concentrations of amantadine.— D. J. Greenblatt *et al.*, *J. clin. Pharmac.*, 1977, *17*, 704.

Further references: E. M. Merrick and P. P. Schmitt, *Curr. ther. Res.*, 1973, *15*, 552; J. Ananth *et al.*, *Int. J. clin. Pharmac. Biopharm* 1975, *11*, 323; A. DiMascio *et al.*, *Archs gen. Psychiat.*, 1976, *33*, 599; R. M. Allen, *Curr. ther. Res.*, 1977, *22*, 914; A. J. Gelenberg and M. R. Mandel, *Archs gen. Psychiat.*, 1977, *34*, 947; A. J. Gelenberg, *Curr. ther. Res.*, 1978, *23*, 375.

Postoperative use. Amantadine 150 mg was more effective than diazepam 10 to 20 mg in reducing the side-effects of ketamine anaesthesia.— G. P. Lucca *et al.*, *Br. J. clin. Pract.*, 1975, *29*, 15.

Torticollis. Amantadine 100 mg twice daily for a month had no beneficial effect on spasmodic torticollis in a double-blind placebo-controlled crossover study involving 10 patients.— H. H. West, *Neurology, Minneap.*, 1977, *27*, 198.

For other reports of the use of amantadine in the treatment of torticollis, see Levodopa, p.889 and Haloperidol, p.1534.

Tremor. In a study of essential tremor, 15 of 26 patients found amantadine was beneficial compared with 6 of 12 given chlordiazepoxide, and 5 of 14 given placebo. Alcohol helped 19 of 25 patients. Mephenesin used intermittently was effective in 2 patients.— E. Critchley, *J. Neurol. Neurosurg. Psychiat.*, 1972, *35*, 365.

Warts. In 23 of 35 patients given amantadine, 100 or 200 mg daily for 3 to 7 days prior to removal of eruptive warts by means of surgery or caustic solutions, no relapse occurred. A definitive cure was obtained in 7 of 23 control patients who received local treatment only.— E. G. Jung and A. Grafe, *Dt. med. Wschr.*, 1971, *96*, 1863.

Preparations

Amantadine Hydrochloride Capsules *(U.S.P.)*. Capsules containing amantadine hydrochloride. Store in airtight containers.

Amantadine Hydrochloride Syrup *(U.S.P.)*. A syrup containing amantadine hydrochloride. Store in airtight containers.

Proprietary Preparations

Symmetrel *(Geigy, UK)*. Amantadine hydrochloride, available as **Capsules** of 100 mg and as **Syrup** containing 50 mg in each 5 ml. (Also available as Symmetrel in *Austral., Canad., Denm., Ger., Neth., Norw., S.Afr., Switz., USA*).

Other Proprietary Names

Amantan *(Belg.)*; Amazolon *(Jap.)*; Antadine *(Austral., NZ, S.Afr.)*; Contenton (as sulphate) *(Ger., Switz.)*; Mantadan *(Ital.)*; Mantadix *(Belg., Fr.)*; PK-Merz (as sulphate) *(Ger.)*; Protexin *(Spain)*; Solu-Contenton *(Ger.)*; Trivaline (as sulphate) *(Fr.)*; Virofral *(Swed.)*; Virosol *(Arg.)*.

4543-p

Apomorphine Hydrochloride *(B.P., B.P. Vet., Eur. P., U.S.P.)*.

Apomorph. Hydrochlor.; Apomorphinae Hydrochloridum; Apomorphini Hydrochloridum; Chloretum Apomorphicum; Apomorphinum Chloratum. 6aβ-Aporphine-10,11-diol hydrochloride hemihydrate; (6a*R*) 5,6,6a,7-Tetrahydro-6-methyl-4*H*-dibenzo[*de,g*]-quinoline-10,11-diol hydrochloride hemihydrate. $C_{17}H_{17}NO_2,HCl,\frac{1}{2}H_2O=312.8$.

CAS — 58-00-4 (apomorphine); 314-19-2 (hydrochloride, anhydrous); 41372-20-7 (hydro-

chloride, hemihydrate).

Pharmacopoeias. In all pharmacopoeias examined except *Braz., Jap.,* and *Roum. Port.* specifies anhydrous; *Rus.* and *Swiss* have ¾H_2O.

White or greyish-white, odourless, glistening crystals or microcrystalline powder, becoming green on exposure to light and air. **Soluble** 1 in 50 of water and 1 in 20 of water at 80°; soluble 1 in 50 of alcohol; very slightly soluble in ether; practically insoluble in chloroform. A solution in water prepared with the aid of hydrochloric acid, or in dimethyl sulphoxide, is laevorotatory. A 1% solution in water has a pH of 4.5 to 5.5. Solutions in water are colourless when freshly prepared but they readily decompose and become green on exposure to light and air; the change takes place more rapidly in alkaline solution and may be retarded by the addition of dilute hydrochloric acid or sodium metabisulphite and by keeping in an oxygen-free atmosphere. Solutions for injection should be free from dissolved air and should contain 0.1% of sodium metabisulphite; they are sterilised by distributing in ampoules, replacing the air with nitrogen or other suitable gas, sealing immediately and autoclaving. **Incompatible** with alkalis, iodides, tannin, iron salts, and oxidising agents. **Store** in small airtight containers. Protect from light.

CAUTION. *Apomorphine hydrochloride must be rejected if it at once gives an emerald-green colour when 1 part is shaken with 100 parts of water.*

Adverse Effects. Administration of apomorphine may cause both stimulation and depression of the central nervous system. Persistent vomiting may occur leading to acute circulatory failure, coma, and death. Although drowsiness generally occurs, euphoria, restlessness, and tremors have also been reported. Respiratory depression follows large or repeated doses. Azotaemia has been associated with the high doses required for parkinsonism.

Allergy. Allergic reactions developed in 2 persons in contact with apomorphine powder.— I. Dahlquiest, *Contact Dermatitis*, 1977, *3*, 349.

Treatment of Adverse Effects. Excessive vomiting may be stopped by administration of a narcotic antagonist such as naloxone.

References: R. Tarala and J. A. H. Forrest (letter), *Br. med. J.*, 1973, *2*, 550.

Precautions. Apomorphine should be used with extreme caution in children, debilitated patients, or those with cardiac decompensation, and in persons prone to nausea and vomiting. If vomiting does not result from the first dose of apomorphine a second dose should *not* be given. It should not be used in patients with respiratory or central nervous system depression, or in patients suffering from the effects of corrosive poisons.

The effectiveness of apomorphine as an emetic is diminished by drugs that depress the vomiting centre which in turn may enhance its central depressant effects.

The antiparkinsonian effects of dopaminergic agents can be antagonised by reserpine, phenothiazines, and butyrophenones (see Levodopa, p.884).

Uses. The chief effect of apomorphine is emesis which it produces within a few minutes of administration and which is preceded by nausea and salivation. It has been given subcutaneously as a single dose of 100 µg per kg body-weight for adults and 70 µg per kg for children, for the induction of emesis in acute non-corrosive poisoning (a glass of water being given before the injection). This practice is considered dangerous owing to the risk of inducing protracted vomiting and shock, although some sources have advocated its use together with administration of an antagonist, such as naloxone, at the end of productive vomiting. Some sources have also recommended the intramuscular route for apomorphine administration.

When apomorphine is administered by mouth its emetic action is not dependable. In small doses by mouth it has been reported to act as an expectorant and has been used for this purpose in acute bronchitis.

Apomorphine is structurally related to dopamine and has been used to control the symptoms of parkinsonism.

For a discussion of the pharmacology of apomorphine, chiefly in *animals*, see B. A. Callingham, *Pharm. J.*, 1973, *2*, 71.

Alcoholism. A 70% success reported in the use of the Dent apomorphine treatment (J.Y. Dent *Anxiety and its Treatment*, 3rd Edn, London, Skeffington, 1955) in 87 alcoholics; for 5 to 20 days patients had 2- or 3-hourly apomorphine injections and immediately drank alcohol/water (50/50) copiously.— N. H. Moynihan, *Practitioner*, 1965, *195*, 223. See also *Br. med. J.*, 1977, *1*, 759.

Further references: H. Beil and A. Trojan, *Br. J. Addict. Alcohol*, 1977, *72*, 129; S. B. Jensen *et al.*, *ibid.*, 325; V. Borg and T. Weinholdt, *Curr. ther. Res.*, 1980, *27*, 170.

Asthma. For formulas of preparations for the administration of apomorphine hydrochloride in the treatment of asthma, see R. J. Engelhardt *et al.*, *J. Am. pharm. Ass.*, 1968, *NS 8*, 198.

Chorea. Although apomorphine would have been expected to worsen Huntington's chorea, single intramuscular doses of apomorphine hydrochloride 1 to 4 mg caused a marked decrease in abnormal involuntary movements in 4 sufferers. This effect was blocked by prior administration of haloperidol or sulpiride which suggested that Huntington's chorea is mediated by a special kind of dopamine receptor.— G. U. Corsini *et al.*, *Archs Neurol., Chicago*, 1978, *35*, 27.

Further references: J. Braham and I. Sarova-Pinhas (letter), *Lancet*, 1973, *1*, 432; E. S. Tolosa (letter), *J. Am. med. Ass.*, 1974, *229*, 1579.

Dyskinesia and torticollis. Apomorphine had a paradoxically beneficial effect in a group of patients with movement disorders (mainly tardive dyskinesia). It also slightly alleviated spasmodic torticollis.— E. S. Tolosa, *Archs Neurol., Chicago*, 1978, *35*, 459.

Emesis in acute poisoning. Apomorphine has no valid place as an emetic, because of the dangers of toxicity.— *Br. med. J.*, 1977, *2*, 977.

Clinical trial of a stable solution of apomorphine hydrochloride containing sodium metabisulphite as an antoxidant. Apomorphine hydrochloride 70 µg per kg body-weight was given subcutaneously to 20 children who had ingested toxic substances; 11 also accepted charcoal by mouth. All the children but one (who had taken an anti-emetic) vomited within 3 to 12 minutes. All the children suffered lethargy, especially those who had taken sedatives or hypnotics, and 4 of the 20 also suffered mild respiratory depression. Both the lethargy and the respiratory depression responded well to naloxone hydrochloride 20 µg per kg, repeated in 10 minutes in 12 of the children, and a third time in 6 of the children.— F. J. deCastro *et al.*, *Clin. Toxicol.*, 1978, *12*, 65.

Further reports, and comparative studies on the use of apomorphine to produce emesis in the treatment of acute poisoning: F. A. Berry and M. A. Lambdin, *Am. J. Dis. Child.*, 1963, *105*, 160; A. H. Abdallah and A. Tye, *Am. J. Dis. Child.*, 1967, *113*, 571; D. G. Corby *et al.*, *Pediatrics*, 1968, *42*, 361; W. C. MacLean, *J. Pediat.*, 1973, *82*, 121; O. Jonas and N. Smyth, *Med. J. Aust.*, 1975, *1*, 534.

Growth hormone effects. Doses of 0.75 and 1.5 mg of apomorphine hydrochloride increased the serum concentration of growth hormone in healthy subjects and although the higher dose produced a greater increase it also produced nausea.— S. Lal *et al.* (letter), *Lancet*, 1972, *2*, 661.

Further references: J. T. La Rosa *et al.*, *Am. J. Med.*, 1977, *63*, 909.

Parkinsonism. In 13 patients with parkinsonism whose tremor had been unresponsive to levodopa 4 to 8 g daily, apomorphine 0.5 to 2 mg injected subcutaneously in a single dose caused cessation of tremor in 8, a reduction in 3, and no effect in 2 patients. Beneficial responses began within 5 to 10 minutes, lasting usually from 1 to 2 hours. Nausea and vomiting appeared in 4 patients, and syncope occurred twice.— J. Braham *et al.* (letter), *Br. med. J.*, 1970, *3*, 768.

Doses of apomorphine required to control the symptoms of parkinsonism (up to 1400 mg daily by mouth) caused a high incidence of azotaemia. Although this appeared to be reversible it precluded further study of apomorphine in parkinsonism.— G. C. Cotzias *et al.*, *New Engl. J. Med.*, 1976, *294*, 567.

In a double-blind study of 4 patients with moderately severe Parkinson's disease domperidone 100 µg per kg body-weight given intramuscularly 60 minutes before apomorphine 20 µg per kg intramuscularly, markedly reduced apomorphine-induced side-effects compared with control injections of saline. Administration of apomorphine with saline was associated with nausea, sedation, drowsiness, hypotension, yawning, and pallor, whereas administration with domperidone was only associated with yawning. The apomorphine-induced improvement in parkinsonian symptoms (mean improvement 33.8%) was enhanced by prior administration of domperidone to a mean improvement of 43.3%. This further improvement was due to a reduction in akinesia, possibly as a result of less drowsiness and fewer side-effects.— G. U. Corsini *et al.* (preliminary communication), *Lancet*, 1979, *1*, 954.

For the use of injections of apomorphine with orally administered levodopa for the treatment of parkinsonism, see Levodopa, p.887.

Schizophrenia. Double-blind studies in 18 schizophrenic patients who had psychotic symptoms even when treated with neuroleptics, showed apomorphine given subcutaneously was better than a placebo in reducing these symptoms.— C. A. Tamminga *et al.*, *Science*, 1978, *200*, 567. See also *Am. Pharm.*, 1978, *NS18*, (Feb.), 44.

Drug-induced extrapyramidal effects. The dyskinetic-dystonic extrapyramidal reactions which occurred in 13 patients with schizophrenia given haloperidol 2 mg or more intramuscularly thrice daily were controlled within 15 minutes in 7 who were given apomorphine 5 mg intramuscularly. Five of the 6 patients given a control injection suffered the extrapyramidal effects for more than 3 hours.— R. Gessa *et al.* (letter), *Lancet*, 1972, *2*, 981. See also Dyskinesia and Torticollis (above).

Use in surgery. A study of the use of apomorphine as an alternative to the use of stomach tube to empty the stomachs of patients in labour prior to the induction of general anaesthesia. The apomorphine was used as follows; 3 mg of apomorphine was diluted in 10 ml of sodium chloride injection or Water for Injections, and the solution was injected intravenously at the rate of 1 ml (300 µg) every 15 seconds with the patient sitting up holding a vomit bowl; when the patient retched or vomited the injection was stopped. After a short time atropine 600 µg or hyoscine 600 µg was injected intravenously, and 20 ml of Magnesium Trisilicate Mixture *B.P.C. 1973* given by mouth. The apomorphine technique was used in 43 patients and 37 had a stomach tube passed. Apomorphine was found to be much more pleasant for the patients and just as effective as the stomach tube, but neither method guaranteed an empty stomach and nor did the absence of vomiting with apomorphine guarantee an empty stomach; no deleterious effects were noted on the infants.— J. D. Holdsworth, *J. int. med. Res.*, 1978, *6*, *Suppl.* 1, 26. Discussion, including comments on the hazards of intravenous atropine, and emphasis that the danger of the acid aspiration cannot be guaranteed to be removed.— *ibid.*, 30–32. Further comment.— J. S. Crawford (letter), *Lancet*, 1979, *2*, 353.

Preparations

Apomorphine Hydrochloride Tablets *(U.S.P.)*. Tablets containing apomorphine hydrochloride. Store in airtight containers. Protect from light.

Apomorphine Injection *(B.P. 1973)*. Apomorph. Inj.; Apomorphine Hydrochloride Injection. A sterile solution in Water for Injections free from dissolved air and containing 0.15% of sodium metabisulphite as an antoxidant. pH 3 to 4. It may decompose on keeping. A solution which has become green should be rejected. Protect from light.

Many other pharmacopoeias include a similar injection.

4544-s

Benserazide Hydrochloride. Serazide Hydrochloride; Ro 4-4602. DL-Serine 2-(2,3,4-trihydroxybenzyl)hydrazide hydrochloride; DL-2-Amino-3-hydroxy-2′-(2,3,4-trihydroxybenzyl)propionohydrazide hydrochloride.

$C_{10}H_{15}N_3O_5,HCl=293.7$.

CAS — 322-35-0 (benserazide); 14919-77-8

(hydrochloride).

A crystalline solid. M.p. about 95°. Benserazide hydrochloride 28.5 mg is approximately equivalent to 25 mg of benserazide.

Benserazide is highly soluble in water; it is unstable in neutral, alkaline, or strongly acidic medium.— D. E. Schwartz and R. Brandt, *Arzneimittel-Forsch.*, 1978, *28*, 302.

Precautions. Benserazide should not be given to patients under 25 years of age, or during pregnancy. It should be given with caution in patients with a history of osteoporosis. Pyridoxine does not inhibit the response to levodopa in patients also receiving benserazide.

For a toxicological study of developmental derangements of the *rat* skeleton after administration of benserazide, see K. Schärer, *Beitr. Pathol.*, 1974, *152*, 127.

Further references: E. Theiss and K. Schärer, in *Monoamines Noyaux Gris Centraux et Syndrome de Parkinson*, J. de Ajuriaguerra and G. Gauthier (Eds), Geneva, Georg, 1971, p. 497; W. H. Ziegler *et al.*, *ibid.*, p. 505.

Absorption and Fate. Benserazide is rapidly but incompletely absorbed from the gastro-intestinal tract. It is primarily metabolised in the gut and is rapidly excreted in the urine in the form of metabolites. It does not cross the blood-brain barrier.

Pharmacokinetic and metabolic studies of benserazide in *animals* and man. Following oral administration to parkinsonian patients benserazide was rapidly absorbed to the extent of about 58%, simultaneous administration of levodopa tending to increase slightly this absorption. It was rapidly excreted in the urine in the form of metabolites, 70 to 77% being excreted within 6 hours, and up to 90% within 12 hours. Benserazide is predominantly metabolised in the gut and appears to protect levodopa against decarboxylation primarily in the gut, but also in the rest of the organism, mainly by way of its metabolite trihydroxybenzylhydrazine.— D. E. Schwartz *et al.*, *Eur. J. clin. Pharmac.*, 1974, *7*, 39; D. E. Schwartz and R. Brandt, *Arzneimittel-Forsch.*, 1978, *28*, 302.

Uses. Benserazide hydrochloride is a peripheral inhibitor of decarboxylase with actions and uses similar to those of carbidopa (below). It is usually given with levodopa in the ratio of 1 part of benserazide base to 4 parts of levodopa.

The suggested initial dose is benserazide 25 mg with levodopa 100 mg twice daily, increased by steps of 25 and 100 mg respectively at intervals of 3 or 4 days. The usual dose range is levodopa 400 to 800 mg with benserazide 100 to 200 mg daily in divided doses; it is rarely necessary to exceed 1 g of levodopa and 250 mg of benserazide.

Patients already receiving levodopa should omit therapy for a day before starting benserazide with levodopa. The initial dose of levodopa given with benserazide should be about 15% of the dose previously being taken.

Parkinsonism. A detailed review of levodopa and decarboxylase inhibitors, including details of pharmacokinetics, therapeutic trials, adverse effects, interactions, and the long-term role of such therapy. Decarboxylase inhibitors like benserazide and carbidopa increase intestinal absorption of levodopa and enhance its plasma concentrations, facilitate its passage into the brain and as a consequence, alter the intracerebral distribution of derived catecholamines. One of the outstanding advantages of adding benserazide or carbidopa to levodopa is the lowered dose of levodopa required to produce equivalent therapeutic benefit. All studies have recorded a decrease, usually of the order of 60 to 80%. Retrospective comparison of the relative therapeutic efficacies of associations of levodopa with either benserazide or carbidopa suggest that the two treatments are identical.— R. M. Pinder *et al.*, *Drugs*, 1976, *11*, 329.

For reports of the clinical use of benserazide with levodopa, see Levodopa, p.886.

Schizophrenia. In a double-blind study involving 32 schizophrenic patients benserazide in doses of 450 mg daily was a less effective antipsychotic agent than chlorpromazine. Higher doses might be more effective.— G. Chouinard *et al.*, *Int. Pharmacopsychiat.*, 1977, *12*, 1.

Proprietary Preparations

Benserazide is an ingredient of Madopar, p.890.

4545-w

Bromocriptine. CB 154; Bromocryptine; 2-Bromoergocryptine; 2-Bromo-alpha-ergocryptine. 2-Bromo-12′-hydroxy-5′α-isobutyl-2′-isopropylergotaman-3′,6′,18-trione.

$C_{32}H_{40}BrN_5O_5$=654.6.

CAS — 25614-03-3.

4546-e

Bromocriptine Mesylate. Bromocriptine Methanesulphonate.

$C_{32}H_{40}BrN_5O_5,CH_4O_3S$=750.7.

CAS — 22260-51-1.

A yellowish-white crystalline powder. Bromocriptine mesylate 2.87 mg is approximately equivalent to 2.5 mg of bromocriptine. **Protect** from light.

Adverse Effects. Nausea is the most common side-effect but vomiting, dizziness, and postural hypotension may also occur. Syncope has followed initial doses of bromocriptine.

Other side-effects reported include headache, leg cramps, nasal congestion, bradycardia, sedation, hallucinations, depression and mania, dryness of the mouth, constipation, diarrhoea, palpitations, peripheral vasospasm, and prolonged severe hypotension. Dyskinesias have occurred in patients suffering from parkinsonism. Gastro-intestinal bleeding has been reported in acromegalic patients. Psychosis occurs particularly at the high dosage required to treat parkinsonism; altered liver-function tests have also been reported.

The side-effects of bromocriptine could be divided into those which occurred at the outset of treatment and those which occurred when patients were established on high doses. Any patient given a sufficiently large initial dose might develop nausea, vomiting, and postural hypotension. Micturition syncope had also been reported. Normal subjects were the most sensitive to these initiating side-effects, patients with hyperprolactinaemia and acromegaly less so, while side-effects were virtually unknown in women immediately post partum. Side-effects found during continuous therapy were rare when the daily dose was less than 20 mg and included mild constipation, muzziness, nasal congestion, cramps in the legs at night, and dystonic reactions in the parkinsonian patients. Cardiac dysrhythmias had also occurred occasionally when high doses were given.— *Br. med. J.*, 1975, *4*, 667.

Side-effects might include a metallic taste, erythematous and swollen ankles, burning discomfort of the eyes, and diplopia. With doses of 100 mg daily cardiac dysrhythmias could occur.— *Drug & Ther. Bull.*, 1976, *14*, 33.

Of 92 patients with parkinsonism treated with high doses of bromocriptine, 29 suffered adverse effects requiring discontinuation. They were: psychiatric (8), erythromelalgia (red, tender, warm oedematous lower extremities) (7), nausea (3), dizziness (3), exacerbation of angina (2), and diplopia (1), nasal congestion (1), sedation (1), fractured femur (1), gastro-intestinal bleeding (aspirin being taken concomitantly) (1), and abnormal liver-function tests (1). Nausea and dizziness frequently occurred early in treatment and were transient, usually responding to temporary dosage reduction, whereas erythromelalgia and psychiatric reactions (which were similar to those associated with levodopa but more florid and longer-lasting) tended to occur later and at higher doses, erythromelalgia being less likely with dosages below 100 mg daily. Increased transaminase concentrations occurred in a total of 6 patients suggesting that liver-function tests should be carried out during long-term bromocriptine therapy.— D. B. Calne *et al.*, *Lancet*, 1978, *1*, 735.

Effects on the cardiovascular system. Reversible pallor of fingers and toes, induced by cold and not associated with pain during recovery, was reported in 36% of 45 acromegalic patients who were receiving bromocriptine 20 to 60 mg daily from 1 to 12 months.— J. A. H. Wass *et al.* (letter), *Lancet*, 1976, *1*, 1135. See also R. C. Duvoisin (letter), *ibid.*, 1976, *2*, 204.

Bromocriptine in doses of up to 75 mg daily had a significant and prolonged hypotensive effect in a study of 28 patients with parkinsonism; 3 discontinued bromocriptine because of hypotensive symptoms and 6 because of other side-effects. It was recommended that cardiovascular function should be monitored in patients receiving bromocriptine, particularly in high doses.— J. K. Greenacre *et al.*, *Br. J. clin. Pharmac.*, 1976, *3*, 571.

Syncope occurred in 2 patients on the first day of bromocriptine treatment. The first patient fainted twice at the beginning of each of two cycles of treatment with bromocriptine 2.5 mg daily. The second time she fainted while driving a car. Patients should be warned of syncope and should not drive, at least during the first day of treatment.— I. A. Brosens (letter), *Lancet*, 1977, *2*, 244. A shock syndrome attributed to bromocriptine in one patient.— F. Maneschi *et al.* (letter), *ibid.*, 462.

A 33-year-old man with acromegaly and hypopituitarism developed severe hypotension after receiving his first dose of bromocriptine (2.5 mg daily with hydrocortisone 20 mg daily). The hypotension recurred following a second 2.5 mg dose but after administration solely of hydrocortisone 20 mg daily for a week he tolerated the bromocriptine with only a slight drop in blood pressure. Acromegalic patients with hypopituitarism should receive at least 1 week of glucocorticoid therapy before the first dose of bromocriptine.— D. C. Linch *et al.* (letter), *Lancet*, 1978, *2*, 320. See also N. M. O'Mullane *et al.* (letter), *ibid.*, 1976, *2*, 1358.

Studies in 18 normotensive patients with parkinsonism, Huntington's chorea, or the Shy-Drager syndrome given bromocriptine indicated that the lowering of blood pressure was not produced by alpha-blockade but rather through a central or peripheral inhibition of noradrenaline release.— M. G. Ziegler *et al.*, *Clin. Pharmac. Ther.*, 1979, *25*, 137.

Further references: D. G. Kissner and J. C. Jarrett (letter), *New Engl. J. Med.*, 1980, *302*, 749; D. Parkes (letter), *ibid.*

Effects on the eyes. A 22-year-old man with hypothalamic hyperprolactinaemia developed myopia on receiving bromocriptine therapy. The myopia resolved on withdrawal of the bromocriptine.— R. S. Manor *et al.* (letter), *Lancet*, 1981, *1*, 102.

Effects on the gastro-intestinal tract. Of 96 patients receiving bromocriptine 6 developed peptic ulcers; 3 had severe bleeding.— J. A. H. Wass *et al.* (letter), *Lancet*, 1976, *2*, 851.

The influence of bromocriptine on gastric-acid output was studied in 9 healthy subjects and although the increases that occurred were not significant they might explain the gastro-intestinal side-effects of bromocriptine. Bromocriptine might need to be used with caution in patients with a history of peptic ulceration.— G. O. Cowan (letter), *Lancet*, 1977, *1*, 425. Bromocriptine 5 mg had no effect on serum-gastrin concentrations in 6 healthy women. In a second study bromocriptine did not influence the basal gastric acid secretion in 6 subjects but the response to a submaximal dose of pentagastrin was higher after bromocriptine than placebo suggesting that there might be some effect on gastric acid secretion.— R. Caldara *et al.* (letter), *ibid.*, 902. Results of a study in 11 subjects with no history of gastro-intestinal disease indicated that bromocriptine does not appear to increase gastrin release to the extent that it could significantly enhance gastric acid secretion.— P. Reding *et al.* (letter), *ibid.*, 1978, *1*, 1202.

The gastro-intestinal side-effects experienced by 2 women taking bromocriptine were markedly reduced when they abstained from alcohol.— J. Ayres and M. N. Maisey (letter), *New Engl. J. Med.*, 1980, *302*, 806.

Effects on mental state. Post-partum mania in a 27-year-old woman might have been due to bromocriptine which had been taken for 7 days.— D. N. Vlissides *et al.* (letter), *Br. med. J.*, 1978, *1*, 510. A further possible case of bromocriptine-induced mania.— N. M. Brook and I. B. Cookson (letter), *ibid.*, 790. A review of bromocriptine in parkinsonism. The psychological symptoms resulting from bromocriptine may occur with a low dosage of 2.5 to 5 mg daily. Instead of the mild nocturnal hallucinosis, day-time depression, or transient psychosis that characterised levodopa toxicity, bromocriptine produces a severe psychosis in which the patient is violent and aggressive, suffering from intense delusions which are often hostile and violent. Complete withdrawal may still leave a residue of severe psychotic illness persisting for one to three weeks.— I. Pearce and J. M. S. Pearce, *ibid.*, 1402.

Comments on the mechanisms of bromocriptine-induced hallucinations.— D. A. Goodkin (letter), *New Engl. J. Med.*, 1980, *302*, 1479; D. Parkes (letter), *ibid.*

Further references: M. Serby *et al.*, *Am. J. Psychiat.*, 1978, *135*, 1227.

Effects on the respiratory tract. Pleuropulmonary changes in 2 patients receiving long-term therapy with bromocriptine alone and 5 receiving long-term bromocriptine therapy in association with levodopa could have been drug-associated, although none of the cases represents a clear-cut drug-induced effect.— U. K. Rinne (letter), *Lancet*, 1981, *1*, 44. Comment.— P. Krupp, *Sandoz, Switz.* (letter), *ibid.* A report of a parkinsonian patient on bromocriptine therapy who may have had a similar adverse reaction.— P. A. LeWitt and D. B. Calne (letter), *ibid.* Further comment.— G. M. Besser and J. A. H. Wass (letter), *ibid.*, 323.

Effects on the skin and hair. Increased loss of hair was noted by women receiving bromocriptine. It did not progress to alopecia, even after treatment for 3 years.— I. Blum and S. Leiba (letter), *New Engl. J. Med.*, 1980, *303*, 1418.

Malignant neoplasms. A 100-week study in *rats* given bromocriptine had shown progression of endometrial changes to malignant tumours in some. [*Sandoz*, personal communication to authors.] No cytological or histological evidence of endometrial neoplasia, metaplasia, or hyperplasia, or cervical abnormalities were found in 88 women who had taken bromocriptine for up to 6 years. Annual gynaecological assessment was recommended.— G. M. Besser *et al.*, *Br. med. J.*, 1977, *2*, 868. In 200 male and 200 female *rats* bromocriptine decreased mortality, peri-arteritis, chronic nephropathy, and mammary and adrenal tumours; the incidence of uterine tumours was however increased. While the ageing process in *rats* differed from that in women regular gynaecological assessment of women was desirable until evidence showed it to be unnecessary.— R. W. Griffith, *Sandoz, Switz.* (letter), *ibid.*, 1605.

Treatment of Adverse Effects. Reduction of the dosage of bromocriptine, followed in a few days by a more gradual increase, causes the reversal of many side-effects. Nausea may be diminished by taking bromocriptine with food. If overdosage occurs the stomach should be emptied by aspiration and lavage. Hypotension may require cautious administration of intravenous fluids.

Precautions. Patients with hypogonadism and galactorrhoea should be investigated for the possibility of a pituitary tumour before treatment with bromocriptine. Treatment of women with the galactorrhoea-amenorrhoea syndrome results in ovulation; such patients should be advised to use contraceptive measures other than an oral contraceptive. Visual fields should be checked in patients who become pregnant. Acromegalic patients should be checked for symptoms of peptic ulcer before therapy and should immediately report symptoms of gastro-intestinal discomfort during therapy.

For patients on long-term therapy liver-function checks have been recommended, and annual gynaecological examinations have been suggested for women.

Bromocriptine has been administered concurrently to patients receiving phenothiazines and has effectively lowered raised prolactin concentrations apparently without interfering with the psychotropic effect. The antiparkinsonian effects of dopaminergic agents can, however, be antagonised by reserpine, phenothiazine, and the butyrophenones (see Levodopa, p.884). There may be decreased tolerance of alcohol.

Contra-indications to bromocriptine therapy were considered to include: psychiatric and hepatic disease, severe angina, and myocardial infarction.— D. B. Calne *et al.*, *Lancet*, 1978, *1*, 735.

Interactions. With butyrophenones. Pretreatment with pimozide reduced the growth hormone response to bromocriptine.— F. Dammacco *et al.*, *Hormone metab. Res.*, 1976, *8*, 247.

With griseofulvin. The response to bromocriptine was blocked in a patient who was also receiving griseofulvin.— G. Schwinn *et al.*, *Eur. J. clin. Invest.*, 1977, *7*, 101.

With levodopa. A 47-year-old woman with a 5-year history of parkinsonism, being treated with levodopa, benzhexol, and amantadine, had her levodopa replaced by bromocriptine. Levodopa with carbidopa was subsequently added to the regimen and the bromocriptine gradually withdrawn due to development of an erythematous rash on the legs, leg swelling, and tenderness. Two days after complete withdrawal of bromocriptine the patient developed a persisting psychosis. Dosage alterations should be made with great caution when levodopa with carbidopa and bromocriptine were administered concomitantly.— S. Lipper (letter), *Lancet*, 1976, *2*, 571.

Pregnancy and the neonate. In 19 children born to mothers in whom ovulation had been induced by bromocriptine no numerical or structural chromosomal anomalies which might be ascribed to the maternal use of bromocriptine could be demonstrated.— L. A. Schellekens *et al.*, *Arzneimittel-Forsch.*, 1977, *27*, 2151.

Of 10 women who had conceived after bromocriptine therapy for infertility, one aborted early in pregnancy, one had a premature delivery and 6 had signs of cervical incompetence. Of these 6 who were sutured, 2 went to term, 3 delivered prematurely, and 1 was still pregnant.— O. Jürgensen and H. -D. Taubert (letter), *Lancet*, 1977, *2*, 203. No evidence of cervical incompetence or premature delivery associated with bromocriptine in 43 patients.— A. Singer *et al.* (letter), *ibid.*, 503. Delivery was normal in a patient who continued taking bromocriptine until the 19th week of pregnancy. The neonate was healthy and mature.— G. Modena and I. Portioli (letter), *ibid.*, 558.

Pregnancy occurred in 1 patient after 485 days' therapy with bromocriptine. A dose of 35 mg daily was maintained until the 33rd week when labour followed premature rupture of the foetal membranes. The infant was normal.— T. Espersen and J. Ditzel (letter), *Lancet*, 1977, *2*, 985.

A study of 448 completed pregnancies in women who had taken bromocriptine during early pregnancy (the majority for hyperprolactinaemic conditions and 70 for pituitary tumours). There were 369 live births, 49 (10.9%) spontaneous and 21 induced abortions and a further 9 induced abortions due to: 3 extra-uterine pregnancies, 3 intra-uterine deaths, 2 premature deliveries and one hydatidiform mole. Malformations occurred in 11 infants but no specific type was more common than another. Twin pregnancies occurred in 1.9% of the pregnancies and premature deliveries in 10.1%. It was considered that the uses of bromocriptine to restore fertility was not associated with an increased risk of abortion, multiple pregnancy or the occurrence of malformations in the infants.— R. W. Griffith *et al.*, *Br. J. clin. Pharmac.*, 1978, *5*, 227. Of 805 previously infertile women in whom pregnancy was achieved with the aid of bromocriptine treatment, 137 were diagnosed as having pituitary tumours. Of 116 patients who completed pregnancy, tumour-related complications occurred in 9, with visual field impairment in 8, and severe headache in 1. Craniotomy was necessary in 2 patients and reinstitution of bromocriptine produced remission of symptoms in 1 patient. Surgery or irradiation of pituitary tumours should be considered for patients contemplating pregnancy.— *idem*, 1979, *7*, 393.

A short review of published data on the potential human teratogenicity of bromocriptine, and a report of work in *animals*. At present there is no reason to attribute a teratogenic effect to bromocriptine.— R. L. Elton and H. M. Langrall (letter), *Ann. intern. Med.*, 1979, *91*, 791. See also W. P. Maclay (letter), *Br. med. J.*, 1980, *280*, 862.

Isolated reports of maternal complications: R. S. Corbey *et al.*, *Obstet. Gynec.*, 1977, *50*, *Suppl.* 1, 69S (visual); A. D. R. Ogborn, *Br. J. Obstet. Gynaec.*, 1977, *84*, 717 (hydatidiform mole).

Withdrawal. Transient galactorrhoea and hyperprolactinaemia occurred in a young woman after withdrawal of bromocriptine therapy for Parkinson's disease. Investigations failed to reveal any underlying lesion, such as a prolactinoma, that may have been masked by the administration of bromocriptine and it was suggested the effects were due to a rebound phenomenon.— B. Pentland and J. S. A. Sawers, *Br. med. J.*, 1980, *281*, 716.

Absorption and Fate. Bromocriptine is incompletely absorbed from the gastro-intestinal tract, metabolised in the liver, and mainly excreted in the bile. It has been reported to be 90 to 96% bound to serum albumin.

In a study involving 10 patients with Parkinson's disease, single doses of bromocriptine 12.5, 25, 50, and 100 mg resulted in very variable peak plasma concentrations ranging from 1.3 to 5.3, 1.4 to 3.5, 2.6 to 19.7, and 6.5 to 24.6 ng per ml respectively, 30 to 210 minutes (mean 102 minutes) after dosage. After 4 hours plasma concentrations were about 75% of the peak values. Clinical improvement was evident within 30 to 90 minutes of a dose with peak effect at about 130 minutes and in most patients improvement persisted throughout the 4-hour study period. Peak clinical response, peak fall in blood pressure, and peak rise in plasma concentrations of growth hormone occurred about 30, 60, and 70 minutes respectively after peak plasma-bromocriptine concentrations but there was no significant relationship between them. There was however a significant relationship between plasma concentrations and concurrent changes in clinical response compared with pretreatment scores. Dyskinesias occurred within 90 to 180 minutes of dosage in 5 of 10 patients. Metoclopramide 60 mg given 30 minutes before bromocriptine had no consistent effect on plasma-bromocriptine concentrations.— P. Price *et al.*, *Br. J. clin. Pharmac.*, 1978, *6*, 303.

Further references: S. Flechter *et al.*, *Curr. ther. Res.*, 1979, *25*, 540; M. L. Friis *et al.*, *Eur. J. clin. Pharmac.*, 1979, *15*, 275.

Uses. Bromocriptine is a dopaminergic agonist; it inhibits release of prolactin (see p.1275) by the pituitary and prolactin concentrations in plasma fall.

For the prevention of puerperal lactation it is given by mouth as the mesylate in a dose equivalent to 2.5 mg of bromocriptine on the day of delivery followed by 2.5 mg twice daily for 14 days. For the suppression of lactation it is given in a dose of 2.5 mg daily for 2 to 3 days subsequently increased to 2.5 mg twice daily for 14 days.

Bromocriptine is used in the treatment of hypogonadism and galactorrhoea syndromes and infertility in both men and women. The usual dose is the equivalent of 1.25 mg of the base at night increased to 2.5 mg at night after 2 to 3 days, subsequently increased in steps of 1.25 to 2.5 mg at intervals of 2 to 3 days to 2.5 mg twice daily; dosage may then be increased in similar steps at intervals of 2 to 3 days thereafter. Most patients respond to 7.5 mg daily but up to 30 mg daily may be required.

Bromocriptine is used as an adjunct to surgery and radiotherapy to reduce growth hormone concentrations in plasma in acromegalic patients. The usual dose is the equivalent of 1.25 mg of the base at night increased to 2.5 mg at night after 2 to 3 days, subsequently increased in steps of 1.25 to 2.5 mg at intervals of 2 to 3 days to 2.5 mg twice daily; dosage may then be increased in steps of 2.5 mg daily at intervals of 2 to 3 days as follows: 2.5 mg every eight hours, 2.5 mg every six hours, 5 mg every six hours.

Bromocriptine is used in cyclical benign breast and menstrual disorders. The usual dose is the equivalent of 1.25 mg of the base at night increased to 2.5 mg at night after 2 to 3 days, subsequently increased in steps of 1.25 to 2.5 mg at intervals of 2 to 3 days to 2.5 mg twice daily.

Bromocriptine is used in Parkinson's disease. The usual dose is the equivalent of 1.25 mg of the base at night increased to 2.5 mg at night after 2 to 3 days, subsequently increased in steps of 1.25 to 2.5 mg at invervals of 2 to 3 days to 2.5 mg twice daily; dosage may then be increased in steps of 2.5 mg every 2 to 3 days to 30 to 40 mg daily; dosage may then be further increased in steps of 10 mg every 2 to 3 days. Most patients respond to 40 to 100 mg daily, but up to 300 mg daily has been used. Transfer from levodopa to bromocriptine should be made gradually.

Bromocriptine should be taken with food.

Studies in *rats* supported the conclusion that bromocriptine acted by stimulating dopamine receptors in the CNS but unlike apomorphine its action depended upon intact catecholamine stores.— A. M. Johnson *et al.*, *Br. J. Pharmac.*, 1976, *56*, 59.

Further references to *animal* studies: D. M. Loew *et al.*, *Postgrad. med. J.*, 1976, *52*, *Suppl.* 1, 40; E. Flückiger *et al.*, *ibid.*, 57.

Bromocriptine: A Clinical and Pharmacological Review, M.O. Thorner *et al.* (Ed.), New York, Raven, 1980.

Reviews and reports on the actions and uses of bromocriptine: *Br. med. J.*, 1977, *1*, 863; A. J. Lees, *Br. J. Hosp. Med.*, 1977, *18*, 336; *Med. Lett.*, 1977, *19*, 103; D. Parkes, *Adv. Drug Res.*, 1977, *12*, 247; M. O. Thorner, *Adv. Med.*, 1977, *13*, 99; *Med. J. Aust.*, 1978, *2*, *Suppl.* 3, 3; *Drugs*, 1979, *17*, 313; D. Parkes, *New Engl. J. Med.*, 1979, *301*, 873; R. F. Spark and G. Dickstein, *Ann. intern. Med.*, 1979, *90*, 949; J. Kellett and H. G. Friesen, *ibid.*, 980; M. O. Thorner *et al.* (letter), *ibid.*, *91*, 652.

Acromegaly. Of 73 patients with acromegaly 71 experienced improvement after treatment for 3 to 25 months with bromocriptine 10 to 20 mg daily, increased if necessary to 60 mg daily. Improvement included reduced sweating, decreased hand, foot, and finger size, relief of headache, and increased libido. Mean growth-hormone concentrations and growth-hormone concentrations during a glucose-tolerance test generally fell and glucose tolerance was improved in 20 of 23 diabetic patients. Serum-prolactin concentrations fell. Nausea, vomiting, and hypotension could usually be controlled by gradual increase in dosage, given with food; constipation occurred in about half the patients. Dry mouth, alcohol intolerance, leg cramp, and hyperkinesia also occurred. Digital vasospasm induced by cold occurred in 29 patients. The aetiology of peptic ulcer in 4 patients was not clear.— J. A. H. Wass *et al.*, *Br. med. J.*, 1977, *1*, 875.

A double-blind placebo-controlled crossover study in 18 patients did not confirm earlier reports of a beneficial effect of bromocriptine in acromegaly.— J. Lindholm *et al.*, *New Engl. J. Med.*, 1981, *304*, 1450. Criticism of the study.— M. O. Thorner *et al.* (letter), *ibid.*, *305*, 1092. Reply.— J. Lindholm *et al.*, *ibid.*

Further references: A. Liuzzi *et al.*, *J. clin. Endocr. Metab.*, 1974, *38*, 910; V. K. Summers *et al.*, *ibid.*, 1975, *40*, 904; M. O. Thorner *et al.*, *Br. med. J.*, 1975, *1*, 299; E. E. Müller *et al.* (letter), *Lancet*, 1975, *1*, 468; J. Kobberling *et al.*, *Dt. med. Wschr.*, 1975, *100*, 1540; Y. Sachdev *et al.*, *Lancet*, 1975, *2*, 1164; M. O. Thorner and G. M. Besser, *Postgrad. med. J.*, 1976, *52*, *Suppl.* 1, 71; G. Benker *et al.*, *Hormone metab. Res.*, 1976, *8*, 291; C. Lucke *et al.*, *Dt. med. Wschr.*, 1976, *101*, 1756; J. Cassar *et al.*, *Metabolism*, 1977, *26*, 539; R. N. Corston and R. B. Godwin-Austen (letter), *Br. med. J.*, 1980, *280*, 254.

See also under Pituitary Tumours, below.

Administration in renal failure. Bromocriptine could be given in usual doses to patients with renal failure.— W. M. Bennett *et al.*, *Ann. intern. Med.*, 1980, *93*, 286.

See also under Renal Disorders, below.

Alzheimer's disease. Bromocriptine, up to 20 mg daily, failed to benefit 9 patients with early presenile dementia presumed to have Alzheimer's disease.— P. Phuapradit *et al.* (letter), *Br. med. J.*, 1978, *1*, 1052.

Anorexia nervosa and obesity. Elevated growth-hormone concentrations during a glucose-tolerance test were reduced in 8 patients with anorexia nervosa during treatment with bromocriptine 10 mg daily; there was no significant change in body-weight but further study was merited. There were no significant changes in growth-hormone concentrations or body-weight in 9 patients with refractory obesity; further study was not justified.— A. D. B. Harrower *et al.*, *Br. med. J.*, 1977, *2*, 156. See also *idem*, 264.

Further references: A. D. B. Harrower, *Br. J. Hosp. Med.*, 1978, *20*, 672.

Asthma. Evidence that bromocriptine is ineffective in asthma.— K. M. Christensen *et al.*, *Thorax*, 1979, *34*, 284.

Chorea. A double-blind placebo-controlled crossover study of bromocriptine in 6 patients with Huntington's chorea and involuntary movements of moderate severity. No significant effect was noted with doses of up to 40 mg daily and those above 45 mg daily caused exacerbation of the involuntary movements.— R. Kartzinel *et al.*, *Archs Neurol.*, *Chicago*, 1976, *33*, 517.

Findings of a beneficial effect of bromocriptine in Huntington's chorea especially in mildly affected patients. Increasing the dose above 10 mg daily produced no further change.— L. Frattola *et al.*, *Acta neurol. scand.*, 1977, *56*, 37.

Cushing's disease. The use of bromocriptine in Nelson's syndrome and Cushing's disease.— S. W. J. Lamberts and J. C. Birkenhänger (letter), *Lancet*, 1976, *2*, 811.

Further references: A. L. Kennedy and D. A. D. Montgomery (letter), *Br. med. J.*, 1977, *1*, 1083; J. Marek *et al.* (letter), *Lancet*, 1977, *2*, 653.

Dystonia. Clinical improvement occurred in a woman and a 9-year-old girl with dystonia when they took 'high' doses of bromocriptine (60 mg and 30 mg daily, respectively). Lower doses had no clinical effect and beneficial effects were lost when they received placebo treatment. A further patient had no change in facial dystonia during treatment with 'low' or 'high' doses of bromocriptine.— S. M. Stahl and P. A. Berger, *Lancet*, 1981, *2*, 745.

Galactorrhoea-amenorrhoea syndrome. Reviews of bromocriptine in obstetrics and gynaecology: *Lancet*, 1977, *2*, 804; H. S. Jacobs and C. S. Wright, *Br. J. Hosp. Med.*, 1978, *20*, 652; S. J. Judd, *Drugs*, 1978, *16*, 167.

Bromocriptine restored ovulation in patients with pituitary tumours, amenorrhoea, and hyperprolactinaemia as long as gonadotrophin function was demonstrable. Patients with functional secondary amenorrhoea and hyperprolactinaemia also responded to bromocriptine.— H. Jacobs and S. Franks (letter), *Br. med. J.*, 1975, *2*, 141.

A report of 13 pregnancies in 12 women with infertility treated with bromocriptine 2.5 mg at night initially and increasing to 5 to 7.5 mg daily at intervals of 3 to 7 days. Five patients with suspected pituitary tumours received prior irradiation to prevent swelling of the pituitary. In 10 pregnancies which had come to term there were no multiple pregnancies and the infants were normal. One patient with a pituitary tumour was induced in the 38th week of pregnancy after developing a visual-field defect; this disappeared after delivery.— M. O. Thorner *et al.*, *Br. med. J.*, 1975, *4*, 694. A study of pregnancies in amenorrhoeic women with pituitary tumours after induction of ovulation with various agents including bromocriptine. Of 16 pregnancies in 12 women given bromocriptine 12 went to term. Visual-field defects due to tumour enlargement occurred in 1 patient and severe headache in another. Re-institution of treatment with bromocriptine might be the best treatment for tumour complications.— T. Bergh *et al.*, *ibid.*, 1978, *1*, 875. A favourable report of 2 patients who received bromocriptine during pregnancy. Bromocriptine seems to be a promising non-surgical approach to the management of these tumours.— B. H. Yuen (letter), *Lancet*, 1978, *2*, 1314. Pregnancy occurred on 92 occasions in 76 women with hyperprolactinaemia treated with bromocriptine; 31 had radiological evidence suggesting a pituitary tumour; radiotherapy prior to conception was considered safe and effective in preventing tumour enlargement during pregnancy.— M. O. Thorner *et al.*, *Br. med. J.*, 1979, *2*, 771.

Menstruation returned in 9 of 18 women with secondary amenorrhoea found to have normal serum-prolactin concentrations and in 6 of 14 others who were hyperprolactinaemic, during treatment with bromocriptine 2.5 mg twice daily; in most patients normal cycles did not continue when treatment ceased. Serum-prolactin concentrations fell in all patients, but in 2 patients they were still at above normal values after treatment for 12 and 19 weeks respectively.— M. Seppälä *et al.*, *Lancet*, 1976, *1*, 1154. No clear difference was found between the response of 14 women with normoprolactinaemic amenorrhoea given bromocriptine, and that of 19 similar women given placebo.— P. G. Crosignani *et al.*, *Br. J. Obstet. Gynaec.*, 1978, *85*, 773.

Bromocriptine 1.25 mg increased to 2.5, or in one patient 5 mg daily induced ovulation in 14 of 19 women with anovulation following oral-contraceptive withdrawal and without altered prolactin concentrations.— H. J. van der Steeg and H. J. T. C. Bennink, *Lancet*, 1977, *1*, 502.

Further references: P. M. Lutterbeck *et al.*, *Br. med. J.*, 1971, *3*, 228; G. M. Besser *et al.*, *ibid.*, 1972, *3*, 669; E. Del Pozo and A. Audibert (letter), *New Engl. J. Med.*, 1972, *287*, 723; M. O. Thorner *et al.*, *Br. med. J.*, 1974, *2*, 419 (in men); M. Seppälä *et al.*, *ibid.*, 1975, *2*, 305; D. F. Child *et al.*, *ibid.*, 1975, *4*, 87; J. E. Tyson *et al.*, *Obstet. Gynec.*, 1975, *46*, 1; W. H. Utian *et al.*, *Br. J. Obstet. Gynaec.*, 1975, *82*, 755; T. Aono *et al.*, *Fert. Steril.*, 1976, *27*, 341 (acromegalic patient); R. P. Dickey and S. C. Stone, *Obstet. Gynec.*, 1976, *48*, 84; G. Tolis and F. Naftolin, *Am. J. Obstet. Gynec.*, 1976, *126*, 426; H. J. T. C. Bennink *et al.* (letter), *Lancet*, 1976, *1*, 1177; D. W. Morrish and P. M. Crockford (letter), *ibid.*, *2*, 851; D. A. Perry-Keene *et aL.*, *Med. J. Aust.*, 1976, *2*, 602; R. F. Spark *et al.*, *Ann. intern. Med.*, 1976, *84*, 532; Y. Floersheim-Shachar and P. J. Keller, *Fert. Steril.*, 1977, *28*, 1158; E. A. Lenton *et al.*, *Br. med. J.*, 1977, *2*, 1179; C. M. March *et al.*, *Fert. Steril.*, 1977, *28*, 521; A. M. Mroueh and T. M. Siler-Khodr, *Am. J. Obstet. Gynec.*, 1977, *127*, 291; R. J. Pepperell *et al.*, *Br. J. Obstet. Gynaec.*, 1977, *84*, 58; R. H. Wiebe *et al.*, *Fert. Steril.*, 1977, *28*, 426; J. S. E. Dericks *et al.*, *Contraception*, 1978, *17*, 79; R. A. Vaidya *et al.*, *Fert. Steril.*, 1978, *29*, 632; D. Mühlenstedt *et al.*, *Int. J. Fert.*, 1978, *23*, 213; E. A. Cowden and J. A. Thomson (letter), *Lancet*, 1979, *1*, 613; A. D. Noble (letter), *ibid.*, 1079; P. Lehtovirta *et al.*, *Int. J. Fert.*, 1979, *24*, 57.

Hepatic encephalopathy. A 56-year-old cirrhotic man with portasystemic encephalopathy who had become incapable of independent existence obtained dramatic improvement and was able to return to part-time work after administration of bromocriptine 1.25 mg at night with food increased every third day to a maximum of 15 mg daily. He relapsed within 5 days of placebo substitution and improved within 7 days of reintroduction of bromocriptine.— M. Y. Morgan *et al.*, *New Engl. J. Med.*, 1977, *296*, 793. Beneficial results in a double-blind crossover study involving 6 patients.— *idem*, *Gut*, 1978, *19*, A453. See also *idem*, *Gastroenterology*, 1980, *78*, 663. Contrary findings.— M. Uribe *et al.*, *Gastroenterology*, 1979, *76*, 1347.

Hypertension. A discussion on the hypotensive actions of bromocriptine.— M. J. Lewis, *Br. J. Hosp. Med.*, 1978, *20*, 661.

In a study of 19 young men with essential hypertension and 8 normotensive controls, significantly higher plasma-prolactin concentrations were found in the hypertensive men and these correlated with plasma-renin activity. Of 14 of the patients treated with bromocriptine 5 to 15 mg twice daily for 4 weeks, all 9 with high plasma-prolactin concentrations had a reduction in blood pressure. The 5 patients without marked increases in prolactin had a reduced response.— K. O. Stumpe *et al.*, *Lancet*, 1977, *2*, 211. Bromocriptine in doses up to 10 to 30 mg daily given for at least 3 months to hypertensive patients being treated with methyldopa produced a further significant reduction in blood pressure in 9 patients and in serum-prolactin concentrations in 6. The side-effects of methyldopa appeared to be reduced.— M. J. Lewis and A. H. Henderson (letter), *ibid.*, 562.

A report of a 57-year-old hypertensive man with primary aldosteronism secondary to bilateral adrenal hyperplasia, in whom bromocriptine did not consistently suppress aldosterone production or manifest a significant hypotensive effect.— M. J. Hogan *et al.* (letter), *Lancet*, 1980, *2*, 89.

Impotence. Bromocriptine had no effect on impotence in a simple study on 15 men.— A. J. Cooper and E. Merck (letter), *Lancet*, 1977, *2*, 567. Another report of bromocriptine being ineffective in impotence in a double-blind study of 30 patients.— B. Ambrosi *et al.* (letter), *ibid.*, 987.

Bromocriptine 2.5 mg twice daily reduced plasma-prolactin concentrations and improved sexual function in 7 men on home dialysis. A further 8 men were unable to complete the study owing to hypotension which occurred one hour after ingestion. Other side-effects reported were nausea (7), vomiting (4), diplopia (1), and loss of appetite (8).— J. Bommer *et al.*, *Lancet*, 1979, *2*, 496.

Inhibition of lactation. Bromocriptine 2.5 mg twice daily for 14 days given immediately after delivery to 32 patients was more effective in suppressing lactation than quinestrol 4 mg as a single dose given to 28 patients or placebo given to 27 patients.— S. Walker *et al.*, *Lancet*, 1975, *2*, 842. A similar report. In several patients bromocriptine was effective in suppressing established lactation.— L. Varga *et al.*, *Br. med. J.*, 1972, *2*, 743.

A reminder that puerperal lactation is a physiological state and advice that such a powerful drug as bromocriptine be used for its inhibition only when more conservative measures are inadequate.— *Br. med. J.*, 1977, *1*, 189.

In 36 women with puerperal breast engorgement given a single dose of bromocriptine 2.5 mg, significant relief occurred in 28, a second dose was required by 6, and 2 patients failed to respond. Bromocriptine 2.5 mg thrice daily for 3 days then 2.5 mg twice for 11 days reduced temperature, and relieved pain and tension within 24 hours in 25 of 26 with breast inflammation.— F. Peters and M. Breckwoldt, *Dt. med. Wschr.*, 1977, *102*, 1754.

Rebound lactation occurred in 8 of 20 women given bromocriptine 5 mg daily for 14 days for inhibition of puerperal lactation.— E. K. Steenstrup and O. R. Steenstrup, *Curr. ther. Res.*, 1977, *21*, 327.

Further references: S. Walker, *Br. J. clin. Pharmac.*, 1975, *2*, 368P; I. Cooke *et al.*, *Postgrad. med. J.*, 1976, *52*, *Suppl.* 1, 75; F. D. Peters and V. M. Roemer, *Br. J. Obstet. Gynaec.*, 1977, *84*, 531; B. H. Yuen *et al.*, *Can. med. Ass. J.*, 1977, *117*, 919.

Male infertility. Eight oligospermic men with slight hyperprolactinaemia were treated with bromocriptine 2.5 mg daily. Three showed immediate intolerance and treatment was withdrawn. The other 5 achieved a 5- to 10-fold increase in sperm production within 4 to 7 weeks and an equally rapid increase in serum-testosterone concentration where this had been reduced. Serum-prolactin concentrations fell as did serum-gonadotrophin concentrations. Three wives became pregnant. Three azoospermic men were also treated and similar hormone responses were achieved but there was no sperm production and normal gonadal function was not achieved.— K. Saidi *et al.* (letter), *Lancet*, 1977, *1*, 250.

Results of a double-blind controlled study indicated that bromocriptine was ineffective in the treatment of oligospermia.— O. Hovatta *et al.*, *Clin. Endocr.*, 1979, *11*, 377.

Further references: G. D. Montanari and A. Volpe (letter), *Lancet*, 1978, *1*, 160.

Malignant neoplasms. A report of beneficial results with bromocriptine and medroxyprogesterone in advanced hormone-dependent breast cancer.— A. Mussa *et al.*, *Minerva med.*, *Roma*, 1977, *68*, 2233.

Mania. Treatment with bromocriptine 5 mg thrice daily was effective in 48 hours, and without side-effects, for the treatment of severe mania in 2 patients with long-standing manic-depressive psychosis for whom phenothiazines and lithium carbonate were contra-indicated.— C. Dorr and K. Sathananthan (letter), *Br. med. J.*, 1976, *1*, 1342.

A beneficial result was obtained in 3 of 4 manic patients given bromocriptine 5 mg thrice daily in association with chlorpromazine, haloperidol and/or lithium carbonate.— B. M. Saran and S. Acharya (letter), *Am. J. Psychiat.*, 1977, *134*, 702. Comment.— R. H. Gerner *et al.* (letter), *ibid.*, 703.

A double-blind study completed by 20 women failed to show any benefit from bromocriptine in mania.— A. H. W. Smith *et al.*, *Br. med. J.*, 1980, *280*, 86.

Mastalgia. A short review of the drugs used, including bromocriptine, in breast pain.— *Br. med. J.*, 1981, *282*, 505.

In a double-blind crossover study in 10 patients with severe mastalgia associated with diffuse fibrocystic disease of the breast, pain was relieved in 8 and reduced in 2 while receiving bromocriptine 2.5 mg daily for a week then twice daily for 7 weeks. Pain recurred when bromocriptine was withdrawn except in one patient; a placebo had no analgesic effect.— M. Blichert-Toft *et al.*, *Br. med. J.*, 1979, *1*, 237. Comment that patients with mastalgia should be divided into cyclical and non-cyclical groups as only the former are likely to respond to bromocriptine.— R. E. Mansel *et al.* (letter), *ibid.*, 619.

Further references: B. V. Palmer and J. C. M. P. Monteiro (letter), *Br. med. J.*, 1977, *1*, 1083; R. E. Mansel *et al.* (letter), *ibid.*, 1356; J. Martin-Comin *et al.*, *Obstet. Gynec.*, 1976, *48*, 703; R. E. Mansel *et al.*, *Br. J. Surg.*, 1978, *65*, 724; A. C. V. Montgomery *et al.*, *J.R. Soc. Med.*, 1979, *72*, 489.

Parkinsonism. A review of the role of bromocriptine in Parkinson's disease. Bromocriptine 3.5 to 10 mg daily is about equivalent to levodopa 100 mg plus a decarboxylase inhibitor.— *Lancet*, 1978, *1*, 754.

Further general reviews and comments on the role of bromocriptine in Parkinson's disease: *Br. med. J.*, 1976, *1*, 1169; I. Pearce and J. M. S. Pearce, *ibid.*, 1978, *1*, 1402; G. Stern and A. Lees, *Br. J. Hosp. Med.*, 1978, *20*, 666.

Of 92 patients with parkinsonism treated with bromocriptine, 48 had continued to obtain a beneficial response, some for up to 30 months. Thirteen of the 48 were taking bromocriptine alone and in the other 35 it had been added to levodopa therapy, permitting an average reduction in levodopa dosage of 41%. It was noted that patients most likely to benefit from bromocriptine therapy are those with prominent dyskinesia or 'on-off' reactions. Therapy was discontinued in the other 44 patients: 4 died for reasons apparently unconnected with bromocriptine therapy, 8 obtained no net benefit, 3 did not comply, and 29 suffered adverse effects.— D. B. Calne *et al.*, *Lancet*, 1978, *1*, 735. Comment.— *ibid.*, 754.

Of 40 previously untreated idiopathic parkinsonian patients given bromocriptine in doses of up to 120 mg daily for 1 to 3 years only 18 derived benefit at 1 year and at 2 years only 5 continued to derive sustained benefit comparable to that with levodopa; the 13 who deteriorated subsequently responded to levodopa; none of the 40 had 'on-off' oscillations. No definite value was note in 30 levodopa failures, 12 patients with chronic post-encephalitic disease, or 33 disabled patients receiving maximum tolerated doses of levodopa. Although bromocriptine could permit levodopa to be reserved for later use in a minority of patients with idiopathic symptoms, probably delaying the onset of 'on-off' symptoms, it was not of benefit in most patients, and concurrent administration with levodopa offered little advantage.— K. M. Shaw *et al.* (letter), *Lancet*, 1978, *1*, 1255. See also A. J. Lees *et al.*, *Archs Neurol., Chicago*, 1978, *35*, 503.

A report on patients in whom bromocriptine had been given successfully with levodopa.— H. P. Ludin *et al.* (letter), *Lancet*, 1978, *2*, 578.

Further references: D. B. Calne *et al.*, *Br. med. J.*, 1974, *4*, 442; *idem*, *Lancet*, 1974, *2*, 1355; P. F. Teychenne *et al.*, *Lancet*, 1975, *2*, 473; A. J. Lees *et al.* (letter), *ibid.*, 709; A. G. Debono *et al.* (letter), *ibid.*, 987; D. B. Calne *et al.*, *Postgrad. med. J.*, 1976, *52*, *Suppl.* 1, 81; A. G. Debono *et al.*, *Br. J. clin. Pharmac.*, 1976, *3*, 977; J. D. Parkes *et al.* (letter), *Lancet*, 1976, *1*, 483; R. Kartzinel *et al.*, *ibid.*, *2*, 272; A. Lieberman *et al.*, *Neurology, Minneap.*, 1976, *26*, 405; A. Lieberman *et al.*, *New Engl. J. Med.*, 1976, *295*, 1400; R. B. Godwin-Austen and N. Smith, *J. Neurol. Neurosurg. Psychiat.*, 1977, *40*, 479; T. A. Caraceni *et al.*, *ibid.*, 1142; U. Grøn, *Acta neurol. scand.*, 1977, *56*, 269; O. Kristensen and E. Hansen, *ibid.*, 274; U. K. Rinne *et al.*, *Archs Neurol., Chicago*, 1977, *34*, 626; S. Fahn *et al.*, *Neurology, Minneap.*, 1979, *29*, 1077; A. J. Lees and G. M. Stern (letter), *Lancet*, 1980, *2*, 215; M. Hallett (letter), *ibid.*, 1981, *1*, 616.

Pituitary tumours. Reviews and discussions on the role of bromocriptine in pituitary tumours: *Br. med. J.*, 1980, *281*, 338; N. T. Zervas and J. B. Martin, *New Engl. J. Med.*, 1980, *302*, 210.

Bromocriptine was given to 11 men with prolactin-secreting pituitary tumours, some of whom had already undergone surgery and radiotherapy. Their potency was improved and persistent elevated serum-prolactin concentrations were markedly reduced; 4 became asymptomatic when treated with bromocriptine alone. In 2 similar patients who had previously undergone surgery and radiotherapy, testosterone replacement therapy failed to correct impotence until their persistent hyperprolactinaemia had been reduced by bromocriptine.— J. N. Carter *et al.*, *New Engl. J. Med.*, 1978, *299*, 847.

Results in 69 patients with prolactin-secreting or growth-hormone-secreting pituitary tumours, treated with bromocriptine with or without pituitary irradiation, indicated that bromocriptine can reduce the size of prolactinomas, and also of adenomas, associated with acromegaly. Evidence of tumour shrinkage was seen in 14 of the 69, and 5 of these 14 had received no pituitary irradiation.— J. A. H. Wass *et al.*, *Lancet*, 1979, *2*, 66. Similar reports of the regression of pituitary tumours after treatment with bromocriptine.— L. G. Sobrinho *et al.* (letter), *Lancet*, 1978, *2*, 257; B. Corenblum (letter), *ibid.*, 786; A. M. Landolt *et al.* (letter), *ibid.*, 1979, *1*, 1082; S. R. George *et al.*, *Am. J. Med.*, 1979, *66*, 697; A. M. McGregor *et al.*, *New Engl. J. Med.*, 1979, *300*, 291; S. L. Aronoff *et al.* (letter), *ibid.*, 1391; T. Bergh *et al.* (letter), *ibid.*; K. von Werder *et al.* (letter), *ibid.*

Long-term treatment with bromocriptine failed to stop the growth of eosinophilic pituitary adenomas in 3 female patients with mild acromegaly, despite the reduction of plasma concentrations of growth hormone to normal and substantial clinical improvement.— I. S. Salti and N. Istfan (letter), *New Engl. J. Med.*, 1979, *301*, 386.

Further references: K. Mashiter *et al.* (letter), *Lancet*, 1977, *2*, 197.

Premenstrual syndrome. A double-blind crossover study comparing bromocriptine 2.5 mg twice daily and a placebo in 17 women with premenstrual symptoms, who acted as their own controls, showed that taking bromocriptine from the 10th day of the cycle until menstruation for 2 cycles relieved symptoms in the 10 women who completed both cycles. Further longer studies from which 8 of 42 women and 2 of 45 women withdrew, mainly because of side-effects, confirmed the value of bromocriptine for relief of the premenstrual syndrome.— L. J. Benedek-Jaszmann and M. D. Hearn-Sturtevant, *Lancet*, 1976, *1*, 1095.

In a double-blind crossover study in 13 patients bromocriptine 2.5 mg daily for 10 days before menstruation had no significant effect on symptoms of the premenstrual syndrome.— K. Ghose and A. Coppen, *Br. med. J.*, 1977, *1*, 147.

In most of 12 patients with idiopathic oedema administration of bromocriptine was of little value but in 2 it had a dramatic effect.— C. R. W. Edwards *et al.* (letter), *Lancet*, 1979, *2*, 94. Administration of bromocriptine to 7 patients with idiopathic oedema produced definite symptomatic improvement in 2, and a significant decrease in the excessive diurnal weight gains, in a third. The changes were not, however, dramatic and frequent side-effects limited the usefulness of the drug.— R. G. Dent and O. M. Edwards (letter), *ibid.*, 355.

Further references to bromocryptine being used to treat the premenstrual syndrome: J. M. Hockaday *et al.*, *Headache*, 1976, *16*, 109; A. N. Andersen *et al.*, *Br. J. Obstet. Gynaec.*, 1977, *84*, 370; J. J. Graham *et al.*, *Med. J. Aust.*, 1978, *2*, *Suppl.* 3, 18; A. N. Andersen and J. F. Larsen, *Drugs*, 1979, *17*, 383.

Renal disorders. In 4 patients with chronic renal failure mean growth-hormone concentrations rose after treatment with bromocriptine; glucose tolerance and insulin response were not affected.— J. A. Kanis *et al.*, *Br. med. J.*, 1976, *1*, 879.

Schizophrenia. In a pilot study in 2 schizophrenia patients, negative symptoms were not reversed by the dopamine agonist bromocriptine which, like levodopa, should supplement any dopamine deficiency and/or reverse a dopamine-receptor denervation hypersensitivity.— D. J. King (letter), *Br. J. clin. Pharmac.*, 1978, *6*, 541.

Torticollis. Relief from spasmodic torticollis occurred in 1 patient (also taking levodopa) of 10 given bromocriptine in doses increased gradually from 2.5 mg daily; the effective dose was 80 mg daily.— A. Lees *et al.* (letter), *Br. med. J.*, 1976, *1*, 1343. No benefit with bromocriptine in patients with spasmodic torticollis.— J. Juntunen *et al.*, *Archs Neurol., Chicago*, 1979, *36*, 449.

Urinary incontinence. Beneficial results using bromocriptine in the treatment of the unstable bladder. Of 24 patients who began treatment 14 appeared to benefit.— D. J. Farrar and J. L. Osborne, *Br. J. Urol.*, 1976, *48*, 235. A study indicating that bromocriptine is of little value in the treatment of the unstable bladder. Of 18 patients with unstable bladders given bromocriptine 2.5 mg twice daily only 2 noted moderate improvement in their symptoms.— K. P. J. Delaere *et al.*, *ibid.*, 1978, *50*, 169.

Further references: P. H. Abrams and M. Dunn, *Br. J. Urol.*, 1979, *51*, 24.

Proprietary Preparations

Parlodel *(Sandoz, UK)*. Bromocriptine mesylate, available as **Capsules** each containing the equivalent of 10 mg of bromocriptine and as scored **Tablets** each containing the equivalent of 2.5 mg. (Also available as Parlodel in *Arg., Austral., Belg., Canad., Denm., Fr., Ital., Jap., Neth., Norw., S.Afr., Switz., USA*).

Other Proprietary Names

Pravidel *(Ger., Swed.)*.

4547-l

Carbidopa *(B.P., U.S.P.)*. (−)-L-α-Methyldopa Hydrazine; MK 486. (−)-L-2-(3,4-Dihydroxybenzyl)-2-hydrazinopropionic acid monohydrate.

$C_{10}H_{14}N_2O_4,H_2O = 244.2$.

CAS — 28860-95-9 (anhydrous); 38821-49-7 (monohydrate).

NOTE. The synonym MK485 has been used for the racemic mixture.

Pharmacopoeias. In *Br.* and *U.S.*

A white or creamy-white, odourless or almost odourless powder. M.p. about 210° with decomposition. **Soluble** 1 in 500 of water and 1 in 5000 of alcohol; slightly soluble in methyl alcohol; freely soluble in 3M hydrochloric acid; practically insoluble in alcohol, acetone, chloroform, and ether. A 1% suspension in water has a pH of 4 to 6. A solution in aluminium chloride solution is laevorotatory. **Protect** from light.

Precautions. The use of carbidopa and levodopa should be avoided during pregnancy.

Pyridoxine does not inhibit the response to levodopa in patients also receiving carbidopa.

For reference to treatment with L-5-hydroxytryptophan and carbidopa unmasking a scleroderma-like illness, see 5-Hydroxytryptophan, p.1718.

Absorption and Fate. Carbidopa is rapidly but incompletely absorbed from the gastro-intestinal tract. It is rapidly excreted in the urine both unchanged and in the form of metabolites. It does not cross the blood-brain barrier. It crosses the placenta and is excreted in milk.

Pharmacokinetic and metabolic studies of carbidopa in *animals* and man. Following oral administration to human subjects carbidopa was rapidly but incompletely absorbed and about 50% was subsequently excreted in the urine, with about 30% of this as unchanged drug. Turnover was rapid, with virtually all the unchanged carbidopa appearing in the urine within 7 hours; traces of metabolites were still detected after 72, 96, and 120 hours. Little difference was noted between metabolism by parkinsonian and by healthy subjects, except that more appeared in the faeces of the healthy subjects (47% as against 35%); poor faecal recovery from parkinsonian patients might reflect their tendency to constipation. An investigation was made into the various metabolites and it was concluded that the loss of the hydrazine functional group represents the major metabolic pathway.— S. Vickers *et al.*, *Fedn Proc.*, 1971, *30*, 336; *idem*, *Drug Metab. & Disposit.*, 1974, *2*, 9; *idem*, *J. med. Chem.*, 1975, *18*, 134.

Uses. Carbidopa inhibits the peripheral decarboxylation of levodopa to dopamine and as, unlike levodopa, it does not cross the blood-brain barrier, effective brain concentrations of dopamine are produced with lower doses of levodopa. At the same time reduced peripheral formation of dopamine reduces peripheral side-effects notably, nausea and vomiting, and cardiac arrhythmias.

It is given with levodopa to enable a lower dosage of the latter to be used and a more rapid response to be obtained, and to decrease side-effects. It is usually given in the ratio of 1 part of carbidopa to 10 parts of levodopa.

The suggested initial dose is the equivalent of anhydrous carbidopa 12.5 mg with levodopa 125 mg once or twice daily, increased by steps of 12.5 and 125 mg respectively daily or on alternate days. The usual dose range is levodopa 0.75 to 1.5 g with carbidopa 75 to 150 mg daily in divided doses. There is no advantage in increasing carbidopa beyond 200 mg daily, though extra levodopa may be given rarely.

Patients already receiving levodopa should omit therapy for a day before starting carbidopa with levodopa. The initial dose of levodopa when given with carbidopa should be about 20% of the dose previously being taken.

Studies on the metabolic effects of carbidopa: P. E. Garfinkel *et al.*, *Archs gen. Psychiat.*, 1976, *33*, 1462; S. G. Ball and M. R. Lee, *Br. J. clin. Pharmac.*, 1977, *4*, 115; P. E. Garfinkel *et al.*, *Neurology, Minneap.*, 1977, *27*, 443.

Parkinsonism. A detailed review of levodopa and decarboxylase inhibitors, including details of pharmacokinetics, therapeutic trials, adverse effects, interactions, and the long-term role of such therapy. Decarboxylase inhibitors like benserazide and carbidopa increase intestinal absorption of levodopa and enhance its plasma concentrations, facilitate its passage into the brain and, as a consequence, alter the intracerebral distribution of derived catecholamines. One of the outstanding advantages of adding benserazide or carbidopa to levodopa is the lowered dose of levodopa required to produce equivalent therapeutic benefit. All trials have recorded a decrease, usually of the order of 60 to 80%. Retrospective comparison of the relative therapeutic efficacies of associations of levodopa with either benserazide or carbidopa suggest that the two treatments are identical.— R. M. Pinder *et al.*, *Drugs*, 1976, *11*, 329. Mention of the use of carbidopa as a single agent.— *FDA Drug Bull.*, 1979, *9*, 29.

For reports of the clinical use of carbidopa with levodopa, see Levodopa, p.887.

Adverse effects. No unwanted effects had been attributed to the carbidopa in tablets containing levodopa with carbidopa (Sinemet); dyskinesia and hallucinations were more common during treatment with Sinemet because nausea and vomiting were reduced and higher effective doses were usually possible.— *Drug & Ther. Bull.*, 1974, *12*, 83. Psychosis developed in 2 patients on changing from levodopa therapy alone to levodopa with carbidopa. The symptoms subsided on resuming treatment with levodopa alone.— J. T. -Y. Lin and D. K. Ziegler, *Neurology, Minneap.*, 1976, *26*, 699.

For a report of levodopa in conjunction with carbidopa exhibiting an inhibitory effect on drug metabolism, see Levodopa, p.885.

Proprietary Preparations

Carbidopa is an ingredient of Sinemet, p.890.

4548-y

Fusaric Acid. 5-Butylpicolinic Acid. 5-Butylpyridine-2-carboxylic acid.
$C_{10}H_{13}NO_2$=179.2.

CAS — 536-69-6.

Fusaric acid is an inhibitor of dopamine-β-hydroxylase, the enzyme responsible for conversion of dopamine into noradrenaline. It is believed to have both central and peripheral actions, and has been reported to have an apparent biological half-life of about 19 hours. It has been studied for its antihypertensive properties, and has been used in doses of 50 to 150 mg thrice daily in various dyskinesias.

The clinical pharmacology of fusaric acid.— R. J. Matta and G. F. Wooten, *Clin. Pharmac. Ther.*, 1973, *14*, 541. See also T. Nagatsu *et al.*, *Experientia*, 1972, *28*, 779.

Animal studies: M. M. Bonnay *et al.*, *Biochem. Pharmac.*, 1974, *23*, 2770.

A review of dopamine-β-hydroxylase together with details of the action of the dopamine-β-hydroxylase inhibitor, fusaric acid.— I. J. Kopin *et al.*, *Ann. intern. Med.*, 1976, *85*, 211.

Amphetamine and narcotic addiction. Fusaric acid suppressed craving and withdrawal symptoms in one patient dependent upon amphetamine and another dependent upon morphine; it was given in doses of 250 mg daily gradually increased to 1000 to 1200 mg daily.— J. Pozuelo, *Cleveland Clin. Q.*, 1976, *43*, 89.

Dyskinesias. Fusaric acid did not reduce the severity of parkinsonism in 9 otherwise untreated patients, nor did it have any consistent effect on the ability of levodopa to ameliorate the symptoms of parkinsonism.— T. N. Chase, *Neurology, Minneap.*, 1974, *24*, 637.

In an open study involving 15 psychogeriatric patients, fusaric acid was given in initial doses of 50 mg thrice daily gradually increased to 150 mg thrice daily over a period of 3 weeks. It effectively relieved oro-facial dyskinesia and tremor, and improved psychotic symptoms. It was less effective in relieving rigidity and had no effect on akinesia, dystonic spasms, and anxiety. Akathisia was exacerbated in 2 patients, and developed in one during treatment.— M. Viukari and M. Linnoila, *Acta psychiat. scand.*, 1977, *56*, 57.

4549-j

Lergotrile Mesylate. 83636; 79907 *(lergotrile)*. (2-Chloro-6-methylergolin-8β-yl)acetonitrile methanesulphonate.
$C_{17}H_{18}ClN_3,CH_4O_3S$=395.9.

CAS — 36945-03-6 (lergotrile); 51473-23-5 (mesylate).

Lergotrile mesylate is a dopaminergic agonist, structurally related to bromocriptine (p.893). It was studied in the galactorrhoea-amenorrhoea syndrome and in parkinsonism, but findings of undue toxicity halted extensive investigation. In particular, it is hepatotoxic; it also commonly causes orthostatic hypotension and mental changes. The significance of genital tumours in *rats* was not evaluated in other species. In the galactorrhoea-amenorrhoea syndrome it was given in doses of 3 to 6 mg daily and in parkinsonism in doses of up to 50 to 150 mg daily.

The pharmacology of lergotrile.— H. Corrodi *et al.*, *J. Pharm. Pharmac.*, 1973, *25*, 409.

The clinical pharmacokinetics of lergotrile.— A. Rubin *et al.*, *Clin. Pharmac. Ther.*, 1978, *23*, 272.

Further references: P. G. Guerzon and O. H. Pearson, *Clin. Res.*, 1974, *22*, 632A (breast cancer); A. N. Lieberman *et al.*, *Neurology, Minneap.*, 1975, *25*, 459; *idem*, *Lancet*, 1976, *2*, 515 (parkinsonism); D. L. Kleinberg *et al.*, *New Engl. J. Med.*, 1977, *296*, 589 (galactorrhoea-amenorrhoea); H. L. Klawans *et al.*, *Neurology, Minneap.*, 1978, *28*, 699 (parkinsonism); W. Leebaw *et al.*, *Acta endocr., Copenh.*, 1978, *87*, 12 (acromegaly); M. Serby *et al.*, *Am. J. Psychiat.*, 1978, *135*, 1227 (lergotrile-induced mental changes in parkinsonism); B. M. Sherman *et al.*, *Fert. Steril.*, 1978, *29*, 291 (galactorrhoea-amenorrhoea); P. F. Teychenne *et al.*, *Ann. Neurol.*, 1978, *3*, 319 (parkinsonism).

Manufacturers
Lilly, USA.

4550-q

Memantine. D145; 3,5-Dimethyl-1-adamantanamine. 3,5-Dimethyltricyclo[3.3.1.1^{3,7}]dec-1-ylamine.
$C_{12}H_{21}N$=179.3.

CAS — 19982-08-2.

Memantine is a derivative of amantadine that has been tried in the treatment of parkinsonism.

The pharmacology of memantine.— B. Costall and R. J. Naylor, *Psychopharmacologia*, 1975, *43*, 53.

Parkinsonism. Rigor, tremor, and motor drive in 12 patients with parkinsonism improved after receiving memantine 40 mg by intravenous infusion.— P. -A. Fischer *et al.*, *Arzneimittel-Forsch.*, 1977, *27*, 1487.

Manufacturers
Merz, Ger.

4551-p

Piribedil. ET 495; EU 4200. 2-(4-Piperonylpiperazin-1-yl)pyrimidine.
$C_{16}H_{18}N_4O_2$=298.3.

CAS — 3605-01-4.

A white crystalline powder. M.p. about 97°. Practically **insoluble** in water; soluble in chloroform.

Piribedil is a non-ergot dopamine receptor agonist. It has been used in the treatment of parkinsonism in doses of up to 300 mg daily. It has also been used in the treatment of circulatory disorders in usual doses of 80 to 100 mg daily by mouth, or 3 to 6 mg daily by intramuscular injection or slow intravenous infusion. Its adverse effects include nausea and vomiting, dizziness, mental effects, drowsiness, hypothermia, and dyskinesias.

The pharmacology of piribedil.— H. Corrodi *et al.*, *Eur. J. Pharmac.*, 1972, *20*, 195. Further references: U. K. Rinne *et al.*, *Archs Neurol., Chicago*, 1977, *34*, 626 (dopamine-receptor activation).

The metabolism of piribedil.— P. Jenner *et al.* (letter), *J. Pharm. Pharmac.*, 1973, *25*, 749.

Cardiovascular actions. In a single-blind placebo-controlled crossover study in 10 subjects with healthy arterial systems, increases in skin temperature occurred in all subjects within 75 minutes of taking piribedil 60 mg, and more slowly following the administration of piribedil 50 mg in a sustained-release preparation.— J. Huys *et al.*, *Curr. med. Res. Opinion*, 1977, *4*, 654.

Further references: J. C. Milliken *et al.*, *Minerva med., Roma*, 1976, *67*, 1662.

Mental disorders. Piribedil 60 mg daily by mouth controlled manic episodes in 2 patients.— R. M. Post *et al.* (letter), *Lancet*, 1976, *1*, 203.

Of 11 patients with moderate to severe depression given piribedil (mean dose 175 mg daily) 9 showed improvement, 1 deteriorated, and 1 became manic. Transient and mild nausea occurred in 8 patients and heightened sexual feeling in 6.— R. M. Post *et al.*, *Archs gen. Psychiat.*, 1978, *35*, 609.

Parkinsonism. A review of alternatives to levodopa, including piribedil.— *Br. med. J.*, 1976, *1*, 1169.

In a 4-week double-blind crossover study of piribedil in 20 parkinsonian patients 7 improved by more than 25% after receiving piribedil and 3 of these by more than 50%. After the completion of the study 8 patients continued to receive piribedil with satisfactory results. The dose of piribedil was 40 mg daily initially increased by 20 mg on alternate days to a maximum of 300 mg daily. Side-effects in this study and in 12 patients in a prior study were similar to those of levodopa and included nausea (10), dyskinesia (9), confusion or agitation (8), dyspnoea and fluid retention (1), drowsiness (9), and a transient rise in alkaline phosphatase (1).— R. D. Sweet *et al.*, *Clin. Pharmac. Ther.*, 1974, *16*, 1077.

Piribedil, initially 60 mg and increasing to 240 mg daily or until side-effects appeared, was given to 10 patients with idiopathic parkinsonism. Eight patients were withdrawn because of side-effects or lack of effect. Side-effects included mental symptoms (5), neurological symptoms (1), increased alkaline phosphatase activity (1), and increased transaminase activity (1).— J. Engel *et al.*, *Eur. J. clin. Pharmac.*, 1975, *8*, 223.

Further references: T. N. Chase *et al.*, *Archs Neurol., Chicago*, 1974, *30*, 383; J. S. Feigenson *et al.*, *Neurology, Minneap.*, 1976, *26*, 430; J. L. Truelle *et al.*, *Nouv. Presse méd.*, 1977, *6*, 2987.

Drug-induced parkinsonism. Poor results with piribedil in the control of drug-induced parkinsonism. Side-effects were common and included headache and vomiting.— R. H. S. Mindham *et al.*, *Br. J. Psychiat.*, 1977, *130*, 581.

Proprietary Names
Trivastal *(Euthérapie, Fr.*; *Pharmacodex, Ger.*; *Servier, Spain*; *Servier, Switz.)*; Trivastan *(Servier, Ital.)*.

4552-s

***N*-Propylnoraporphine.** NPA; Win 28928. 6-Propylnoraporphine-10,11-diol; 5,6,6a,7-Tetrahydro-6-propyl-4*H*-dibenzo[*de,g*]quinoline-10,11-diol.
$C_{19}H_{21}NO_2$=295.4.

CAS — 18426-20-5.

NOTE. The synonym NPA has also been applied to naptalam, a herbicide; the name NPA-Acid has been applied to an arsenical coccidiostat.

N-Propylnoraporphine is a dopamine agonist which is a derivative of apomorphine. It has been used with levodopa in the treatment of parkinsonism.

Reviews of alternatives to levodopa, including *N*-propylnoraporphine.— *Br. med. J.*, 1976, *1*, 1169; *Lancet*, 1976, *1*, 786.

Doses of apomorphine that controlled the symptoms of parkinsonism also caused a high incidence of uraemia, whereas *N*-propylnoraporphine, in optimal doses of 10 to 15 mg six times daily, gave improvement in 9 of 10 patients without inducing uraemia in any. Increasing the dose to a total of 500 mg daily produced uraemia in 2 of the patients. In these and some additional patients studied, maximal improvement was sustained for only 3 weeks. Better control was obtained when treatment included suboptimal doses of carbidopa plus levodopa.— G. C. Cotzias *et al.*, *New Engl. J. Med.*, 1976, *294*, 567.

Manufacturers

Winthrop, USA.

Lignocaine and other Local Anaesthetics

7600-h

The local anaesthetics are compounds which produce insensitivity by preventing or diminishing the conduction of sensory nerve impulses near to the site of their application or injection. The effects are reversible. As local anaesthetics are most often used to produce loss of pain without loss of nervous control, it has been suggested that they might more appropriately be described as local analgesics.

Local anaesthetics are generally of 2 chemical types: the older compounds are esters, usually of *p*-aminobenzoic acid; the more recent compounds are amides. The esters are less stable and more readily metabolised than the amides.

Local anaesthetics of the ester type include: amethocaine, p.908, benzocaine, p.909, cocaine, p.914, procaine, p.921.

Local anaesthetics of the amide type include: bupivacaine, p.910, cinchocaine, p.913, etidocaine, p.917, lignocaine, p.902, mepivacaine, p.918, prilocaine, p.920.

Other drugs with local anaesthetic actions include aerosol propellents, some antihistamines, some beta-adrenoceptor blocking agents, some anticholinergic agents, some anti-arrhythmic agents, benzyl alcohol, chlorbutol, menthol, and phenol.

Adverse Effects of Local Anaesthetics. Side-effects apparent after local anaesthesia may be due to the anaesthetic or to errors in technique or may be the result of blockade of the sympathetic nervous system. Local anaesthetics may have systemic adverse effects as a result of the raised plasma concentrations which ensue when the rate of absorption into the circulation exceeds the rate of breakdown, for example, after excessive dosage or accidental intravenous injection or by absorption of large amounts through mucous membranes or damaged skin or from highly vascular areas.

Allergic reactions to local anaesthetics are rare and generally limited to agents of the ester type. Idiosyncrasy to local anaesthetics has been reported. Vasovagal attacks may be associated with local anaesthesia. Local use, particularly repeated application to the skin, is more likely than systemic administration to give rise to allergic reactions.

The systemic toxicity of local anaesthetics mainly involves the central nervous system and the cardiovascular system. Excitation of the CNS may be manifested by yawning, restlessness, excitement, nervousness, dizziness, tinnitus, nystagmus, blurred vision, nausea and vomiting, muscle twitching and tremors, and convulsions. Numbness of the tongue and perioral region is an early sign of systemic toxicity. Excitation may be transient and followed by depression with drowsiness, respiratory failure, and coma. There may be simultaneous effects on the cardiovascular system with myocardial depression and peripheral vasodilatation resulting in hypotension and bradycardia; arrhythmias and cardiac arrest may occur. Hypotension often accompanies spinal and epidural anaesthesia; inappropriate positioning of the patient may be a contributory factor for women in labour.

Some local anaesthetics cause methaemoglobinaemia.

Foetal intoxication has occurred following the use of local anaesthetics in labour, either as a result of the transplacental diffusion or after accidental injection of the foetus.

Reviews of adverse reactions to local anaesthetics: J. Adriani, *J. Am. med. Ass.*, 1966, *196*, 405; P. J. Verrill, *Practitioner*, 1975, *214*, 380; M. H. Alper, *New Engl. J. Med.*, 1976, *295*, 1432; B. G. Covino, *Anesth. Analg. curr. Res.*, 1978, *57*, 387; R. H. de Jong, *J. Am. med. Ass.*, 1978, *239*, 1166.

Deaths associated with the use of local anaesthetics.— J. L. Christie, *J. forens. Sci.*, 1976, *21*, 671.

A report of 3 deaths associated with paracervical anaesthesia for first trimester abortion. In the first 2 patients the deaths were associated with lignocaine overdosage and possible intravascular injection, but the third might have been associated with intolerance to mepivacaine. A further 2 deaths have been reported since 1972. Paracervical anaesthesia should only be given when resuscitative drugs and equipment and staff skilled in their use are available.— D. A. Grimes and W. Cates, *New Engl. J. Med.*, 1976, *295*, 1397. Comments.— R. H. de Jong (letter), *ibid.*, 1977, *296*, 760; C. L. Berman and R. A. Jaffin, *ibid.*; M. L. Schwartz, *ibid.* Reply.— D. A. Grimes and W. Cates (letter), *ibid.* Discussions on the dangers of paracervical block.— M. H. Alper, *New Engl. J. Med.*, 1976, *295*, 1432; *Lancet*, 1977, *1*, 131.

Findings in *mice* that solutions compounded from local anaesthetics with different pharmacological properties are less toxic than the sum of the toxicities of the component drugs. In particular, bupivacaine was rendered less toxic when mixed with either chloroprocaine or lignocaine.— R. H. de Jong and J. D. Bonin, *Toxic. appl. Pharmac.*, 1980, *54*, 501.

Allergy and effects on the skin. Allergic reactions to local anaesthetics are uncommon and hypotension during dental anaesthesia is usually a vasovagal response and is associated with bradycardia. Reactions are more likely to occur with the ester type of local anaesthetic, such as amethocaine, benzocaine, and procaine, than with the amide type, such as lignocaine, mepivacaine, and prilocaine, although they have been reported with lignocaine. The vasovagal response is unrelated to the type of anaesthetic used and may be prevented by premedication with atropine sulphate 600 µg intravenously or with a sedative such as diazepam.— *Br. med. J.*, 1980, *280*, 1360. See also *ibid.*, *281*, 211.

A 19-year-old woman died following injection of 5 to 6 ml of a 2% solution of cinchocaine hydrochloride. She had previously been found to be sensitised to a 2% injection of procaine hydrochloride but not to a 0.2% injection of cinchocaine.— *Br. med. J.*, 1952, *2*, 672.

Further references to allergic reactions with local anaesthetics: J. A. Aldrete and D. A. Johnson, *Anesth. Analg. curr. Res.*, 1970, *49*, 173; R. D. deShazo and H. S. Nelson, *J. Allergy clin. Immunol.*, 1979, *63*, 387 (patients with a history of hypersensitivity to local anaesthetics).

Topical use. Twenty cases of dermatitis resulted from application of ointments containing local anaesthetics. Most patients were sensitive to amethocaine or cinchocaine. In some cases sensitivity developed within 1 or 2 weeks of using the ointment and in others it did not occur for over a year.— H. Wilson, *Practitioner*, 1966, *197*, 673. See also J. K. Morgan, *Br. J. clin. Pract.*, 1968, *22*, 261.

Apart from lignocaine, local anaesthetics should not be applied to the skin because of the real danger of their causing contact dermatitis. Sensitised patients may subsequently develop a widespread eruption when similar drugs are given systemically. The use of strong sensitisers such as benzocaine and amethocaine in lozenges and throat sprays may also sensitise patients.— J. Verbov, *Practitioner*, 1979, *222*, 400.

References to sensitivity reactions associated with surface anaesthesia: S. K. Gupta, *Br. med. J.*, 1959, *1*, 695 (during bronchoscopy and bronchography); J. H. Eckersley *et al.*, *Lancet*, 1960, *2*, 526 (pessaries).

Effects on the blood. Patients with normal haemoglobin values were given, with adrenaline, 500 mg of lignocaine (14 patients), 300 mg of prilocaine (18 patients), 600 mg of prilocaine (25 patients), or 1.2 g of procaine (10 patients). In all groups the methaemoglobin concentration usually reached a peak 4 to 6 hours after administration, and expressed as a percentage of total haemoglobin the mean peak concentrations were 0.8, 1.9, 5.3, and 1.2% in the respective groups. (In normal individuals methaemoglobin values range from 0.2 to 1.2%). In a few patients who had received 600 mg of prilocaine, cyanosis developed and was reversed within 15 to 20 minutes by methylene blue 1 mg per kg bodyweight.— M. Hjelm and M. H. Holmdahl (letter), *Lancet*, 1965, *1*, 53.

Methaemoglobinaemia was associated with the use of a topical anaesthetic spray, Cetacaine [containing benzocaine, butyl aminobenzoate, and amethocaine], in 2 patients.— W. W. Douglas and V. F. Fairbanks, *Chest*, 1977, *71*, 587.

Effects on the eyes. *Topical use.* Severe contact keratitis can develop from the prolonged use of topical anaesthetics in the eye. Local anaesthetics are known to inhibit the rate of movement of corneal epithelial cells migrating to cover wounds.— R. P. Burns and I. Gipson (letter), *J. Am. med. Ass.*, 1978, *240*, 347.

See also Precautions (below).

Effects on the nervous system. A review of the neurological complications following epidural anaesthesia.— J. E. Usubiaga, *Int. Anesth. Clin.*, 1975, *13*, 1.

Reports of facial paralysis following local dental anaesthesia and its successful treatment with prednisolone.— I. B. Tiwari and T. Keane, *Br. med. J.*, 1970, *1*, 798; G. Parsons-Smith and J. M. N. Roberts (letter), *Br. med. J.*, 1970, *4*, 745.

A unilateral Horner's syndrome has occurred many times (possibly 1%) after epidural and caudal analgesia.— D. V. Thomas (letter), *Br. J. Anaesth.*, 1976, *48*, 611. See also L. E. S. Carrie and J. Mohan (letter), *ibid.*

Further reports on the adverse effects of local anaesthetics on the nervous system: Y. I. Kim *et al.*, *Anesthesiology*, 1975, *43*, 370 (massive spinal block with hemicranial palsy after a test dose for extradural analgesia); S. D. Woerth *et al.*, *Anesthesiology*, 1977, *47*, 380 (total spinal anaesthesia due to inadvertent dural puncture); E. J. Fox *et al.*, *Neurology, Minneap.*, 1979, *29*, 379 (myoclonus following spinal anaesthesia); J. Stone and L. B. Kaban, *Oral Surg.*, 1979, *48*, 29 (trismus following local anaesthetic injection).

Pregnancy and the neonate. *Effects on the foetus.* Of 50 282 children born to mothers monitored by the Collaborative Perinatal Project, 2165 were found to have been exposed to local anaesthetics, and possible other drugs, at some time during the first 4 months of the pregnancy. No association between malformations and local anaesthetic exposure was detected.— O. P. Heinonen *et al.*, *Birth Defects and Drugs in Pregnancy*, Littleton MA, Publishing Sciences Group, 1977, p. 357.

Effects on the neonate. The neonatal depressant effect of local anaesthetics given in obstetrics.— *Lancet*, 1974, *1*, 1090.

Local-regional anaesthesia administered during childbirth had an effect on newborn behaviour. Three-day-old infants showed greater irritability and decreased motor maturity. Mepivacaine could be detected in infants' blood up to 24 hours, and lignocaine up to 8 hours, after birth.— K. Standley *et al.*, *Science*, 1974, *186*, 634. See also under Bupivacaine Hydrochloride, p.911.

There are conflicting views on whether epidural anaesthesia during labour is associated with neonatal jaundice. Although S.R. Gould *et al.* (*Br. med. J.*, 1974, *3*, 228) found that bupivacaine had no significant effect on neonatal serum-bilirubin concentrations and P.R. Bromage (*Lancet*, 1979, *1*, 669) has insisted that allegations associating epidural anaesthesia with neonatal jaundice are unfounded, other workers (N. Campbell *et al.*, *Br. med. J.*, 1975, *2*, 548; P.J. Lewis and L.A. Friedman, *Lancet*, 1979, *1*, 669; B. Wood *et al.*, *Archs Dis. Childh.*, 1979, *54*, 111) have reported that epidural anaesthesia is associated with an increased frequency of neonatal jaundice.

Further references to the effects of local anaesthesia on the neonate: W. E. Dodson, *Pediat. Clins N. Am.*, 1976, *23*, 399; D. H. Ralston and S. M. Shnider, *Anesthesiology*, 1978, *48*, 34.

Effects on the mother. Of 100 pregnant patients at term given bupivacaine 0.5% for continuous caudal block for routine vaginal delivery, 63 required bladder catheterisation post partum and of these 15 required catheterisation on two or more occasions. This compared with 22 of 100 women given chloroprocaine. When a similar study was carried out with lignocaine and mepivacaine, the incidence of catheterisation was 34 and 42% respectively. The incidence of catheterisation appeared to decrease as the duration of effect of the local anaesthetic decreased. This effect was not considered to outweigh the advantage of bupivacaine's prolonged action.— L. D. Bridenbaugh, *Anesthesiology*, 1977, *46*, 357.

Assisted respiration had not been necessary in about 1300 patients given epidural analgesia for labour.— J. S. Crawford (letter), *Br. med. J.*, 1977, *2*, 1475.

A report of orthostatic hypotension persisting for many weeks after epidural analgesia for delivery.— R. S. Briggs *et al.*, *Br. med. J.*, 1978, *1*, 892. There was maternal hypotension in one of 49 women given 1 litre of compound sodium lactate injection over 10 to 15 minutes immediately before induction of lumbar epidural analgesia with bupivacaine, and foetal heart-rate abnormalities after block in 6, compared with 15 and 18 respectively in 53 similar women not given a fluid load.— K. M. Collins *et al.*, *Br. med. J.*, 1978, *2*, 1460. A study involving 50 women given continuous lumbar epidural analgesia during labour and 50 control women indicated that there was no significant difference in the magnitude of postural hypotension in the early puerperium between the 2 groups. It was suggested that long-term postural hypotension after epidural analgesia occurs only in exceptional cases and that transient postural hypotension after delivery is no more common in patients who have received epidural analgesia than in others.— E. Moss and R. Macdonald, *Br. med. J.*, 1980, *281*, 22.

Comment on maternal deaths attributable to anaesthesia.— D. M. Moir, *Br. J. Anaesth.*, 1980, *52*, 1.

Treatment of Adverse Effects. Absorption of local anaesthetics from subcutaneous or intramuscular injections may be reduced, if necessary, by applying a tourniquet. When systemic reactions to local anaesthetics occur steps should be taken to maintain the circulation and respiration and to control convulsions. A patent airway must be established and oxygen given, together with assisted ventilation if necessary. The circulation should be maintained with infusions of plasma or suitable electrolyte solutions. Vasopressor agents such as ephedrine, metaraminol, and methoxamine have been suggested in the treatment of marked hypotension although their use is accompanied by a risk of CNS excitation. Vasopressors should not be given to patients receiving oxytocic drugs. Convulsions may be controlled by the intravenous administration of diazepam or a short-acting barbiturate such as thiopentone sodium. It should be remembered that anticonvulsant treatment may also depress respiration and the circulation. The muscle relaxant suxamethonium, together with endotracheal intubation and artificial respiration, has been used when convulsions persist.

Methaemoglobinaemia may be treated by the intravenous administration of a 1% solution of methylene blue in a dose of 1 to 4 mg per kg body-weight.

Treatment of hypotension or other depressant effects of local anaesthetics should include: establishment of a patent airway and administration of 100% oxygen; lowering the patient's head and trunk; giving intravenous fluids and, for a marked or unresponsive hypotension, pressor agents.— Z. W. Gramling, *Clin. Med.*, 1967, *74* (Jan.), 49.

Treatment of collapse due to local dental anaesthesia.— E. R. Perks, *Br. dent. J.*, 1977, *143*, 307.

Hyperexcitability following intravenous regional anaesthesia with bupivacaine in a 15-year-old boy was treated with two intravenous injections of diazepam 10 mg given 12 minutes apart, followed by sedation with 100 mg of chlorpromazine given intravenously in 25-mg increments.— A. M. Henderson, *Br. med. J.*, 1980, *281*, 1043. A view that systemic reactions to local anaesthetics are treated far more effectively with 50-mg increments of thiopentone.— J. A. W. Wildsmith *et al.* (letter), *ibid.*, 1287.

For reference to the treatment of neonates injected accidentally with mepivacaine during labour, see Mepivacaine Hydrochloride, p.918.

Precautions for Local Anaesthetics. The use of local anaesthetics is contra-indicated in patients with known hypersensitivity. It may be possible to avoid reactions by using a local anaesthetic of the alternative chemical type. Small doses have been given as a test for hypersensitivity but the results are not necessarily reliable. Facilities for resuscitation should be available when local anaesthetics are administered. Local anaesthetics should only be given cautiously to patients with epilepsy, impaired cardiac conduction or respiratory function, or with liver damage; patients with myasthenia gravis are particularly susceptible to the effects of local anaesthetics. The ester type of local anaesthetic is contra-indicated in patients with low plasma-cholinesterase concentrations or in those receiving anticholinesterases. Techniques such as epidural anaesthesia should not be employed in patients with cerebrospinal diseases. Doses should generally be reduced in elderly and debilitated patients and in children.

The risk of adverse effects from the absorption of local anaesthetics may be reduced by the inclusion of adrenaline to produce vasoconstriction but the lowest effective concentration of adrenaline should be used. Solutions containing adrenaline should not, however, be used for producing anaesthesia in appendages such as digits, because the profound ischaemia that follows may lead to gangrene. Prilocaine and mepivacaine do not require the addition of a vasoconstrictor and can be used in these cases. If local anaesthetics containing adrenaline are given for caudal, epidural, or paracervical block during labour the use of an oxytocic drug post partum may lead to severe hypertension. For details of the precautions to be observed when local anaesthetics containing adrenaline or noradrenaline are needed in patients receiving monoamine oxidase inhibitors, some volatile anaesthetics, and some other drugs, see p.2 and p.21 respectively.

The effect of local anaesthetics may be reduced if the injection is made into an inflamed or infected area with a low tissue pH. The cornea may be damaged by prolonged application of anaesthetic eye-drops and ointment, and the anaesthetised eye should be protected from dust and bacterial contamination.

The application of local anaesthetics to the skin for prolonged periods or to extensive areas should be avoided.

Effects on driving. Minimum times during which driving is not recommneded after outpatient anaesthesia with the following local anaesthetics: lignocaine 500 mg with adrenaline intramuscularly, no limitations; dental local anaesthesia, 1 hour; lignocaine (plain) 200 mg intramuscularly, 1 to 1.5 hours; bupivacaine (plain) 1.3 mg per kg body-weight intramuscularly, 2 to 4 hours; etidocaine (plain) 2.6 mg per kg intramuscularly, 2 to 4 hours.— K. Korttila, *Mod. Problems Pharmacopsychiat.*, 1976, *11*, 91.

Effects on the eyes. Damage to the cornea and symptoms which included loss of visual acuity, oedema, and hypopyon had been reported following repeated use in the eye of preparations of amethocaine, butacaine, oxybuprocaine, and proxymetacaine.— *Lancet*, 1968, *2*, 1068.

Further references to corneal damage with local anaesthetics: H. J. Meyer, *Dt. med. Wschr.*, 1965, *90*, 1676; D. L. Epstein and D. Paton, *New Engl. J. Med.*, 1968, *279*, 396.

Interference with diagnostic tests. Traces of some local anaesthetics used for lumbar puncture reacted in varying degrees and produced erroneous results with reagents used in the determination of the protein content of cerebrospinal fluid.— S. L. Burgee (letter), *Am. J. Hosp. Pharm.*, 1968, *25* (May), 34.

Malignant hyperpyrexia. A woman with a history of frequent hypersensitivity reactions of the skin developed malignant hyperpyrexia, from which she recovered, when she underwent epidural anaesthesia with lignocaine and bupivacaine in association with adrenaline.— J. Klimanek *et al.*, *Anaesth. Resusc. intens. Ther.*, 1976, *4*, 143. Findings from a study in *swine* suggested that amide-linked local anaesthetics in conventional dosage are safe to use in patients known to be genetically susceptible to malignant hyperpyrexia.— G. G. Harrison and D. F. Morrell, *Br. J. Anaesth.*, 1980, *52*, 385.

Reports of symptoms of malignant hyperpyrexia associated with local anaesthesia in patients with a personal or family history of malignant hyperpyrexia: J. D. Katz and L. B. Krich, *Can. Anaesth. Soc. J.*, 1976, *23*, 285 (spinal anaesthesia with amethocaine and procaine); R. K. Wadhwa, *Anesthesiology*, 1977, *46*, 63 (spinal anaesthesia with amethocaine).

Porphyria. Although the safe use of extradural, caudal, and pudendal blocks has been reported in porphyria, general anaesthesia was considered to be the most suitable technique for caesarean section in a patient with acute intermittent porphyria.— S. C. Allen and G. A. D. Rees, *Br. J. Anaesth.*, 1980, *52*, 835.

Pregnancy and the neonate. The incidence of foetal malposition in 211 mothers with vertex presentation and epidural analgesia (bupivacaine 0.5%) was 21.3% compared with 6.2% in 275 similar mothers not receiving epidural analgesia. The incidence of instrumental delivery was 59.3 and 10.6% respectively.— I. J. Hoult *et al.*, *Br. med. J.*, 1977, *1*, 14. Criticism, with an admission that the incidence of forceps delivery was increased 3- to 4-fold after epidural block.— B. Hibbard *et al.* (letter), *ibid.*, 286. The assisted-delivery rate increased from 14 to 30% between 1970 and 1975 and was associated with an increase from 4 to 58% in epidural analgesia.— J. McQueen and L. Mylrea (letter), *ibid.*, 640. An increase in assisted delivery was not associated exclusively with increased epidural analgesia; more active management of labour was also involved.— S. Bakhoum *et al.* (letter), *ibid.*, 641.

An extensive review of foetal heart-rate changes following paracervical block. Suggested prophylactic measures included low strength, low volume, and the absence of adrenaline; a superficial injection site; and the avoidance of bupivacaine; the prophylactic use of magnesium sulphate appeared unwarranted.— L. A. Cibils and J. J. Santonja-Lucas, *Am. J. Obstet. Gynec.*, 1978, *130*, 73.

For comparisons of the effects of maternally-administered pethidine and epidural bupivacaine or chloroprocaine on neonates, see Pethidine Hydrochloride, p.1026.

Tolerance. A report of the Sixth Multidiscipline Research Forum of the AMA. Variations in tolerance to local anaesthetics might be due to disturbances in acid-base balance, electrolyte balance, the presence of other drugs, and differences in body temperature. The dose which produced irreversible cardiac arrest was reduced by metabolic acidosis; respiratory acidosis or alkalosis had a similar effect but cardiac resuscitation was possible. The presence of infection or central nervous system stimulants in non-convulsive doses lowered the doses of local anaesthetics which might cause excitation.— R. Zeppernick *et al.*, *J. Am. med. Ass.*, 1966, *196*, 582.

When 329 epidural injections of 2% solutions of lignocaine, mepivacaine, or prilocaine, with or without adrenaline 1:200 000, were given to 140 patients, in successive injections, each dose of anaesthetic was 25 to 30% less effective than its predecessor. Anaesthetic response was greater in older than younger subjects, and greatly increased by the addition of adrenaline. Augmentation of anaesthesia was obtained if successive injections were given after an interval of less than 10 minutes.— P. R. Bromage *et al.*, *J. clin. Pharmac.*, 1969, *9*, 30.

Absorption and Fate. Most local anaesthetics are readily absorbed from subcutaneous injection sites, through mucous membranes, and through damaged skin. They exert their effects in the form of the non-ionised base. Anaesthetics of the ester type are hydrolysed by esterases in the plasma and liver. As there is little esterase in the spinal fluid, the effect of spinal anaesthetics lasts until the drug is absorbed into the blood. Metabolism of amide-type anaesthetics takes place in the liver and, in some cases, kidneys.

A review of the clinical pharmacokinetics of local anaesthetics.— G. T. Tucker and L. E. Mather, *Clin. Pharmacokinet.*, 1979, *4*, 241.

Following peridural administration of lignocaine, mepivacaine, or prilocaine, the drugs were taken up very rapidly by the blood and then appeared in the spinal fluid. It appeared that the amount of local anaesthetic in the spinal fluid was directly related to the blood concentrations of the specific agent. The lower blood concentrations of prilocaine than of lignocaine and mepivacaine indicated a more rapid distribution and/or metabolism of prilocaine.— P. C. Lund and B. G. Covino, *J. clin. Pharmac.*, 1967, *7*, 324.

Further references to the pharmacokinetics of local anaesthetics: G. T. Tucker and L. E. Mather, *Br. J. Anaesth.*, 1975, *47*, 213 (amide-type); R. N. Boyes, *ibid.*, 225 (metabolism of amide-type agents); R. L. Eyres *et al.*, *Anaesth. & intensive Care*, 1978, *6*, 243 (plasma concentrations in children).

Pregnancy and the neonate. Reviews of the pharmacokinetics of local anaesthetics during childbirth: C. A. DiFazio, *Br. J. Anaesth.*, 1979, *51*, *Suppl.* 1, 29S (metabolism); R. L. Nation, *Clin. Pharmacokinet.*, 1980, *5*, 340; P. L. Morselli *et al.*, *Clin. Pharmacokinet.*, 1980, *5*, 485 (neonates and infants).

Prilocaine appeared to diffuse across the placenta more than did lignocaine and mepivacaine; the diffusion of bupivacaine was lower still. Route of administration and maternal blood concentration of anaesthetic did not affect diffusion, but there was an inverse relationship between the diffusion and the degree of protein binding.— B. G. Covino, *New Engl. J. Med.*, 1972, *206*, 1035.

The metabolic clearance of local anaesthetics is markedly reduced in premature neonates.— L. F. Prescott, *Prescribers' J.*, 1978, *18*, 50.

Further references to the placental transfer of local anaesthetics: W. U. Brown *et al.*, *Anesthesiology*, 1975, *42*, 698, per *Int. pharm. Abstr.*, 1977, *14*, 498; G. Garstka and H. Stoeckel, *Prakt. Anaesth.*, 1978, *13*, 1.

Uses of Local Anaesthetics. Local anaesthetics act by preventing transmission of impulses along nerve fibres and at nerve endings; depolarisation and ion-exchange are inhibited. The effects are reversible. The lipid-soluble anaesthetic base must penetrate the lipoprotein nerve sheath before it can act. In general, loss of pain (analgesia) occurs before loss of sensory and autonomic function (anaesthesia) and loss of motor function (paralysis). The effectiveness of an anaesthetic depends on the concentration attained at the nerve fibre. There is a latent period before the onset of action which varies according to the agent used and the method of administration.

The activity of local anaesthetics is greater at neutral or slightly alkaline pH values than at acid values as the active base is less ionised. However they are generally administered as acidic solutions of the water-soluble hydrochloride salts. Formulations employing the carbonated base rather than the hydrochloride have also been used. When adrenaline is added, a solution of about pH 3 is necessary to ensure stability.

The smallest effective dose and the lowest effective concentration should be used. Smaller doses are needed in elderly and debilitated patients and in children. Meticulous attention to technique is essential particularly in nerve block and spinal procedures. In spinal anaesthesia sterility of the injection and equipment must be meticulously preserved. Injections for central nerve block, such as epidural or caudal block, and spinal anaesthesia should not contain preservatives.

Local anaesthetics may be administered in many different ways, some compounds being more suitable than others for a particular route of administration. The agents described in this chapter vary in their potency and speed of onset and duration of action. For example, lignocaine, cinchocaine, and etidocaine have a rapid onset of action; mepivacaine and prilocaine may be slower in onset of action; and bupivacaine may be slower still. When classified according to their duration of action chloroprocaine and procaine are short-acting; lignocaine, cocaine, mepivacaine, and prilocaine are intermediate-acting; and amethocaine, bupivacaine, cinchocaine, and etidocaine are long-acting. The effect is sometimes prolonged by the addition of a vasoconstrictor and solutions containing adrenaline 1 in 200 000 are generally advocated. The total amount of adrenaline injected should not exceed 500 µg although some consider that the maximum dose should be 200 µg.

Surface or **topical anaesthesia** blocks the sensory nerve endings in the skin or mucous membranes, but to reach these structures the drug must have good powers of penetration. Many of the local anaesthetics are effective surface anaesthetics, a notable exception being procaine hydrochloride. There are a number of special uses of topical anaesthesia including anaesthetising the cornea during ophthalmological procedures and the throat and larynx before intubation and bronchoscopy. Great care is necessary when employing local anaesthetics to anaesthetise the urethra; if trauma has occurred, rapid absorption of the drug may occur and give rise to serious adverse effects. Absorption from the respiratory tract is also rapid and care is essential to avoid administering a toxic dose.

The local anaesthetics mainly used for surface anaesthesia are amethocaine, benzocaine, cocaine, lignocaine, and prilocaine. In ophthalmological procedures amethocaine, cocaine, oxybuprocaine, and proxymetacaine are used.

Infiltration anaesthesia is produced by injection of an anaesthetic agent into and around the field of operation. The drug must not be absorbed too rapidly otherwise the anaesthesia will wear off too quickly for practical use; many of the synthetic local anaesthetics require the addition of a vasoconstrictor, such as a small amount of adrenaline. If adrenaline is added to such drugs a larger total dose may be given. In dentistry, infiltration anaesthesia is extensively used.

Chloroprocaine, etidocaine, lignocaine, mepivacaine, prilocaine, and procaine are the compounds mainly used for infiltration anaesthesia.

Regional nerve block anaesthesia may include field block, peripheral nerve block, and central nerve block. In *field block* anaesthesia sensory nerve paths are blocked by subcutaneous injection of local anaesthetic close to nerves around the area to be anaesthetised. *Peripheral nerve block* anaesthesia involves injection into or around a peripheral nerve or plexus supplying the part to be anaesthetised; motor fibres may be blocked as well as sensory fibres. Examples of this type of block include brachial plexus block, intercostal nerve block, paracervical block, and pudendal block. Adrenaline is often added as a vasoconstrictor but it must not be used when producing a nerve block in an appendage, as gangrene may occur.

Epidural anaesthesia (*extradural* or *peridural anaesthesia*) is a form of *central nerve block*. Continuous epidural anaesthesia is employed in obstetrics, local anaesthetic being introduced by means of a cannula into the extradural space in the lumbar region in order to block the roots of sensory nerves supplying the uterus and lower birth canal; lignocaine or bupivacaine are the agents generally used. In *caudal anaesthesia* an epidural injection is made through the sacral hiatus.

For regional nerve block the compounds mainly used are bupivacaine, chloroprocaine, etidocaine, lignocaine, mepivacaine, prilocaine, and procaine.

Spinal or **subarachnoid anaesthesia** is another special form of regional anaesthesia; it is produced by injecting a solution of a suitable drug within the spinal theca, intrathecally, causing temporary paralysis of the nerves with which it comes into contact. The addition of adrenaline is usually avoided because of the danger of restricting the blood supply to the spinal cord.

The somatic level at which anaesthesia occurs depends on the specific gravity of the anaesthetic solution used and the positioning of the patient. **Hypobaric solutions** are lighter than the cerebrospinal fluid and rise, thus producing anaesthesia of thoracic structures in a suitably positioned patient. **Isobaric solutions** have about the same specific gravity as the cerebrospinal fluid and produce their effect at about the level of the intrathecal injection.

Hyperbaric solutions are heavier than the cerebrospinal fluid and thus exert their effects at levels lower than the site of injection. They are used mainly for operations on the lower limbs and the perineum.

For spinal anaesthesia, amethocaine, cinchocaine, lignocaine, mepivacaine, and prilocaine have been used.

In **intravenous regional anaesthesia** a dilute solution of local anaesthetic is injected into a suitable limb vein after application of a tourniquet, in order to produce anaesthesia distal to it. Arterial flow must remain occluded and adrenaline should not be used. Lignocaine and bupivacaine have been used for this technique.

In **intravenous analgesia,** local anaesthetics have been injected by continuous infusion to produce a general analgesia but the technique is potentially dangerous and seldom employed.

Reviews and discussions on the actions and uses of local anaesthetics: B. Löfström, *Br. J. Anaesth.*, 1970, *42*, 194; B. G. Covino, *New Engl. J. Med.*, 1972, *286*, 975 and 1035; *Br. J. Anaesth.*, 1975, *47*, *Suppl.*, 163–333; *Drug & Ther. Bull.*, 1976, *14*, 17; J. Adriani and M. Naraghi, *A. Rev. Pharmac. & Toxic.*, 1977, *17*, 223; J. M. Kidd *et al.*, *Aust. J. Hosp. Pharm.*, 1977, *7*, 73 (in children); L. E. Mather and M. J. Cousins, *Drugs*, 1979, *18*, 185.

Further reports on local anaesthetics: J. Adriani, *Clin. Pharmac. Ther.*, 1960, *1*, 645 (clinical pharmacology); J. Adriani *et al.*, *Clin. Pharmac. Ther.*, 1964, *5*, 49 (a method of testing the effectiveness of surface anaesthesia); B. J. Urban, *Anesthesiology*, 1973, *39*, 496 (changing site of action after spinal and epidural anaesthesia).

Action. Reviews on the mode of action of local anaesthetics: G. Strichartz, *Anesthesiology*, 1976, *45*, 421; R. H. de Jong, *J. Am. med. Ass.*, 1977, *238*, 1383.

Administration. The lack of an association between the dose of local anaesthetics of the amide-type (bupivacaine, etidocaine, and mepivacaine) and the patients' age, sex, weight, height, or underlying disease.— D. C. Moore *et al.*, *Anesthesiology*, 1977, *47*, 263.

Anaesthesia in the eye. Local anaesthetics might generally be used once in eye injuries. Amethocaine might be used to relieve the pain of arc eye.— P. A. Gardiner, *Br. med. J.*, 1978, *2*, 1347.

A discussion on the technique of local anaesthesia in the eye.— E. D. Allen and A. R. Elkington, *Br. J. Anaesth.*, 1980, *52*, 689.

Caudal block. Analysis of the spread of analgesia after caudal injection in 3 groups totalling 152 children showed a linear relationship between the spread of analgesia and age. A regression line for predicting dose requirements was developed.— O. Schulte-Steinberg and V. W. Rahlfs, *Br. J. Anaesth.*, 1977, *49*, 1027.

Segmented dose requirements for caudal anaesthesia in children up to the age of 7 years were better based on body-weight than on age.— M. Takasaki *et al.*, *Anesthesiology*, 1977, *47*, 527.

Further references to caudal block: S. Z. Hassan, *Anesth. Analg. curr. Res.*, 1977, *56*, 686 (in infants).

Epidural block. The effects of concentration of local anaesthetic on epidural block for surgery were assessed in a double-blind study of 60 patients. Increasing the concentration of bupivacaine from 0.5 to 0.75% and of etidocaine from 1 to 1.5% appeared to offer significant clinical advantages since there was a more rapid onset of sensory analgesia and motor blockade, a greater frequency of adequate analgesia, a greater depth of motor block, and a longer duration of effect. There was no significant advantage when the concentration of prilocaine was increased from 2 to 3%.— D. B. Scott *et al.*, *Br. J. Anaesth.*, 1980, *52*, 1033.

For a report of minimal ventilatory changes in 7 patients given thoracic epidural anaesthesia with mepivacaine, see G. S. McCarthy, *Br. J. Anaesth.*, 1976, *48*, 243.

In obstetrics. Reviews and discussions on epidural anaesthesia in obstetrics.— *Drug & Ther. Bull.*, 1976, *14*, 9; D. B. Scott, *Br. J. Anaesth.*, 1977, *49*, 11; A. B. W. Taylor *et al.*, *Br. med. J.*, 1977, *2*, 370; J. S. Crawford, *Br. med. J.*, 1979, *1*, 72.

A comparison of lignocaine, prilocaine, bupivacaine, and amethocaine for the production of epidural anaesthesia in 433 obstetric patients showed that lignocaine 1% in carbonated solution gave the lowest incidence of unblocked segments, and carbonated prilocaine the next lowest; both were preferable to lignocaine or prilocaine hydrochlorides. Amethocaine gave the highest incidence of failures and was considered unsuitable for obstetric patients.— P. R. Bromage, *Br. J. Anaesth.*, 1972, *44*, 676. In groups of about 80 to 90 patients undergoing epidural analgesia for delivery the mean times to onset of analgesia were: 10.2 minutes for bupivacaine 0.5%; 11.6 minutes for bupivacaine 0.5% with adrenaline 1 in 200 000; 8.4 minutes for carbonated lignocaine 2%; and 8.7 minutes for carbonated lignocaine 2% with adrenaline 1 to 200 000. Duration of analgesia was, respectively, about 120, 145, 85, and 125 minutes; the duration of analgesia fell in the 4th group after repeated doses. Unblocked segments were present in about 7% of patients in each group and unilateral block in 5 to 12%. Complete analgesia in the first stage of labour occurred in 80, 77, 56, and 61% of patients. Postpartum difficulty with urination was common.— D. D. Moir *et al.*, *Br. J. Anaesth.*, 1976, *48*, 129. Further references to the use of carbonated solutions of local anaesthetics for epidural block: P. R. Bromage, *Can. med. Ass. J.*, 1967, *97*, 1377; P. R. Bromage *et al.*, *Br. J. Anaesth.*, 1967, *39*, 197.

In a study of the effects of anaesthesia on the adrenocortical response to caesarean section, maternal plasma cortisol concentrations were found to increase significantly in patients receiving general anaesthesia whereas concentrations did not change significantly in those receiving epidural anaesthesia. The method of anaesthesia did not influence the cortisol response of the foetus.— Y. Namba *et al.*, *Br. J. Anaesth.*, 1980, *52*, 1027.

Further references to the effects of epidural anaesthesia

on the response to surgical stress: A. Engquist *et al.*, *Br. J. Anaesth.*, 1976, *48*, 903; M. R. Brandt *et al.*, *Br. med. J.*, 1978, *1*, 1106; J. Rem *et al.*, *Lancet*, 1980, *1*, 283; P. Whelan and P. J. Morris (letter), *ibid.*, 828.

Further references to epidural anaesthesia in obstetrics: J. W. Scanlon *et al.*, *Anesthesiology*, 1974, *40*, 121 (neurobehavioural responses of newborn infants); D. G. Littlewood *et al.*, *Br. J. Anaesth.*, 1977, *49*, 75 (a comparison of lignocaine, bupivacaine, and etidocaine); A. I. Hollmen *et al.*, *Anesthesiology*, 1978, *48*, 350 (neurological activity of neonates); C. Carlsson *et al.*, *Br. J. Anaesth.*, 1980, *52*, 827 (in patients who had previously undergone caesarean section); J. S. Crawford, *Br. J. Anaesth.*, 1980, *52*, 821 (lumbar epidural block for caesarean section); J. A. Spinnato *et al.*, *New Engl. J. Med.*, 1981, *304*, 1215 (chloroprocaine for elective caesarean section in a patient with Eisenmenger's syndrome).

Pain. In a double-blind study of 28 patients with myofascial pain, local injections of physiological saline tended to achieve better pain relief than mepivacaine 0.5%.— F. A. Frost *et al.*, *Lancet*, 1980, *1*, 499. A reminder that it could have been the needling itself that alleviated the pain.— K. Lewit (letter), *ibid.*, 1034.

A view that strapping is a simpler and more effective method of alleviating the pain of broken ribs than the injection of local anaesthetics.— K. Norcross (letter), *Lancet*, 1980, *1*, 589. Long-acting local anaesthetics are of help in controlling the pain of broken ribs. The action of bupivacaine, the only long-acting local anaesthetic now available is between 16 and 18 hours which is inadequate for simple rib fractures.— H. D. W. Powell (letter), *Lancet*, 1980, *1*, 1032.

Local infiltration of lignocaine 1.5% or physiological saline into pericranial tender spots were both found to have a beneficial effect on attacks of common migraine.— P. Tfelt-Hansen *et al.* (letter), *Lancet*, 1980, *1*, 1140. See also K. M. Hay, *Practitioner*, 1979, *222*, 827.

Paracervical block. A recommended technique for paracervical block involved the injection of 10 ml of a lignocaine solution at a concentration of no more than 1% into either side of the cervical-vaginal junction. The needle point should be just below the mucosa surface.— J. Slome (letter), *Lancet*, 1977, *1*, 260. Paracervical block was achieved by the use of a modified jet injector using only one-fifth of the dose of anaesthetic needed for needle and syringe techniques.— R. McKenzie and W. L. Shaffer, *Am. J. Obstet. Gynec.*, 1978, *130*, 317.

See also Adverse Effects, p.899.

Pregnancy and the neonate. A study of 241 newborn infants revealed that obstetric anaesthesia or analgesia had no effect on alterations in body-weight during the first 5 days of life.— E. Abouleish *et al.*, *Br. J. Anaesth.*, 1978, *50*, 569.

See also Epidural Block in Obstetrics (above).

Regional anaesthesia, intravenous. In regional intravenous analgesia for surgery of the limbs, prilocaine and mepivacaine caused fewer side-effects than lignocaine when injected intravenously in doses of 3 mg per kg body-weight.— J. A. Lowson (letter), *Med. J. Aust.*, 1968, *2*, 149.

Regional nerve block. A review of the use of local anesthetics for regional analgesia in labour.— A. Hollmen, *Br. J. Anaesth.*, 1979, *51*, *Suppl.* 1, 17S.

Plasma concentrations of lignocaine, bupivacaine, etidocaine, and prilocaine after interscalene *brachial plexus block*. Prilocaine without adrenaline was considered to be the safest agent for this procedure. Bupivacaine with adrenaline was a suitable alternative if a longer block was required. If etidocaine were to be used its concentration should be 0.75% or more; the addition of adrenaline would give a very long block.— J. A. W. Wildsmith *et al.*, *Br. J. Anaesth.*, 1977, *49*, 461.

The effect of *intercostal nerve blockade* on lung function during operation and on analgesia following thoracotomy was assessed in 138 patients. Three groups of 46 patients received either bupivacaine 0.5% with adrenaline 1 in 200 000 or lignocaine 2% with adrenaline 1 in 200 000 or no injection. Neither injection improved lung function, and sustained pain relief postoperatively was not achieved.— J. E. Galway *et al.*, *Br. J. Anaesth.*, 1975, *47*, 730. For a study demonstrating that cryoanalgesia provides better relief of post-thoracotomy pain than intercostal nerve blocks with long-acting local anaesthetics, see Nitrous Oxide, p.756.

Further references to regional nerve block anaesthesia: G. T. Tucker *et al.*, *Anesth. Analg. curr. Res.*, 1972, *51*, 579, per *Drug. Intell. & clin. Pharm.*, 1973, *7*, 93; B. G. Covino, *Anaesthetist*, 1980, *29*, 33.

See also Caudal Block, Epidural Block, and Paracervical Block (above).

Spinal anaesthesia. A discussion of the advantages of spinal anaesthesia.— D. B. Scott and J. T. Thorburn, *Br. J. Anaesth.*, 1975, *47*, 421.

Local spinal anaesthesia for hip replacement resulted in reduced blood loss and reduced deep-vein thrombosis.— J. R. Loudon *et al.* (letter), *Br. med. J.*, 1978, *1*, 1550. See also J. Thorburn *et al.*, *Br. J. Anaesth.*, 1980, *52*, 1117.

A report on the use of spinal analgesia with cinchocaine, lignocaine, or prilocaine in 443 patients undergoing various obstetric procedures, excluding caesarean section. A success-rate of 94.8% was achieved and the re-introduction of spinal analgesia into British obstetric anaesthetic practice is advocated.— J. S. Crawford, *Br. J. Anaesth.*, 1979, *51*, 531.

Further references to spinal anaesthesia: D. H. Robertson *et al.*, *Anaesthesia*, 1978, *33*, 913.

7602-b

Lignocaine.

Lidocaine *(U.S.P.)*; Lidocainum. 2-Diethylaminoaceto-2′,6′-xylidide.
$C_{14}H_{22}N_2O$=234.3.

CAS — 137-58-6.

Pharmacopoeias. In *Braz., Hung., Int., It., Jap., Roum., Swiss,* and *U.S.*

A white to slightly yellow crystalline powder with a characteristic odour. It is stable in air. M.p. 66° to 69°.

Practically **insoluble** in water; very soluble in alcohol and chloroform; freely soluble in ether; soluble in oils. **Store** in airtight containers.

7601-m

Lignocaine Hydrochloride

(B.P.). Lignoc. Hydrochlor.; Lidocaine Hydrochloride *(Eur. P., U.S.P.)*; Lidocaini Hydrochloridum.
$C_{14}H_{22}N_2O,HCl,H_2O$=288.8.

CAS — 73-78-9 (anhydrous); 6108-05-0 (monohydrate).

Pharmacopoeias. In *Arg., Aust., Belg., Br., Braz., Chin., Eur., Fr., Ger., Hung., Ind., Int., It., Jug., Neth., Nord., Pol., Port., Swiss, Turk.,* and *U.S.*

A white crystalline odourless powder with a slightly bitter numbing taste. M.p. 74° to 79°. **Soluble** 1 in 0.7 of water, 1 in 1.5 of alcohol, 1 in 40 of chloroform; practically insoluble in ether. A 0.5% solution in water has a pH of 4 to 5.5. A 4.42% solution in water is iso-osmotic with serum. Solutions are **sterilised** by autoclaving or by filtration.

Carbonated solutions. For a report on the preparation of carbonated solutions of prilocaine and lignocaine, see Prilocaine Hydrochloride, p.920.

Incompatibility. Lignocaine hydrochloride caused precipitation of amphotericin.— D. A. Whiting, *Br. J. Derm.*, 1967, *79*, 345.

An immediate precipitate occurred when lignocaine hydrochloride 2 g per litre was mixed with *methohexitone sodium* 2 g per litre, and a crystalline precipitate occurred with *sulphadiazine sodium* 4 g per litre in dextrose injection.— B. B. Riley, *J. Hosp. Pharm.*, 1970, *28*, 228.

For reference to possible incompatibility between lignocaine hydrochloride and *ampicillin sodium*, see Ampicillin Sodium, p.1091.

Stability of solutions. Injections of lignocaine with adrenaline were sometimes followed by oedematous swellings at the site of the injection. These were attributed to the release of heavy metal ions, particularly copper, from the metal parts of the syringe which came in contact with the acid solution.— *Br. dent. J.*, 1959, *106*, 47.

Lignocaine, bupivacaine, and mepivacaine as bases, exhibited decreased solubility in phosphate buffer with increasing temperature. It was suggested that possible precipitation of the base of these local anaesthetics from the hydrochloride salt may occur at the site of injection due to an increase in pH of the base to the tissue pH or due to a lowering of free base solubility at body temperature relative to ambient temperature.— N. I. Nakano, *J. pharm. Sci.*, 1979, *68*, 667.

For a report on the stability of injections containing lignocaine hydrochloride and adrenaline, see Adrenaline, p.2.

Adverse Effects and Treatment. As for Local Anaesthetics, p.899.

Concentrations of lignocaine hydrochloride below 0.5% have about the same toxicity as similar concentrations of procaine hydrochloride, but stronger solutions of lignocaine hydrochloride are relatively more toxic. Drowsiness, lassitude, and amnesia have been reported with therapeutic doses of lignocaine.

A survey by the Boston Collaborative Drug Surveillance Program of the use and toxicity of lignocaine given intravenously to 750 patients with a mean age of 65 years for the treatment of cardiac arrhythmias. Treatment was started within 48 hours of admission in 77% of patients and adverse reactions were reported in 47 patients (6.3%) as follows: CNS disturbances, 31 patients; cardiovascular disturbances, 8; CNS and cardiovascular reactions, 4; phlebitis at the injection site, 3; and rash, 1. Twelve reactions were considered life-threatening. The majority of adverse effects were reported within the first 2 days of therapy and were more frequent in elderly patients, in those who died, and in those with long hospitalisations. Diagnoses of acute myocardial infarction or congestive heart failure, and low body-weight were also associated with a higher frequency of unwanted effects. Patients with serious underlying disease or with diminished hepatic clearance of lignocaine appear to be predisposed to adverse effects.— H. J. Pfeifer *et al.*, *Am. Heart J.*, 1976, *92*, 168.

Toxicity in patients given lignocaine after admission to a coronary care unit consisted mainly of mild CNS effects and was noted in 26 of 50 patients. All 6 patients with serum-lignocaine concentrations above 5.9 µg per ml had signs of toxicity. Concentrations were measured by gas chromatography and direct measurement by enzyme immunoassay which was found to be accurate and much faster than gas chromatography.— K. Buckman *et al.*, *Clin. Pharmac. Ther.*, 1980, *28*, 177. See also N. L. Benowitz and W. Meister, *Clin. Pharmacokinet.*, 1978, *3*, 177.

Allergy and effects on the skin. A 17-year-old girl developed a rash after the third injection of lignocaine in 10 days for dental anaesthesia; the reaction was confirmed by an intradermal test and by inflammation of the nostril and lachrymation following the insertion into the nostril of a pledget of cotton wool soaked in the anaesthetic. This procedure might be useful for diagnosis.— J. P. Rood, *Br. dent. J.*, 1973, *135*, 411.

A report of generalised exfoliative dermatitis in 1 patient after injections of 2% lignocaine hydrochloride as a dental anaesthetic.— H. Hofman *et al.*, *Archs Derm.*, 1975, *111*, 266.

Further reports of allergic reactions with lignocaine.— N. Ravindranathan, *Br. dent. J.*, 1975, *138*, 101; J. E. Fish and V. I. Peterman, *Respiration*, 1979, *37*, 201 (inhaled lignocaine); S. Fregert *et al.*, *Contact Dermatitis*, 1979, *5*, 185 (topical lignocaine).

Effects on the blood. A 26-year-old primigravida with severe labour pain was given a continuous epidural block with 1.5% of lignocaine, receiving prior to delivery a total of 1.8 g over 8.25 hours. Nine hours later she was distinctly cyanosed and *methaemoglobinaemia* was confirmed. Cyanosis disappeared a few hours after the intravenous injection of 15 ml of 1% methylene blue. She had received, in addition, 500 mg of aspirin, 500 mg of phenacetin, and 16 mg of codeine phosphate after delivery.— D. Burne and A. Doughty (letter), *Lancet*, 1964, *2*, 971. Acute *methaemoglobinaemia* was induced on 2 occasions firstly when a spray containing benzocaine (and also butyl aminobenzoate and amethocaine: Cetacaine), and later 4% lignocaine, was used to anaesthetise the pharynx of a 28-year-old man.— W. J. O'Donohue *et al.*, *Archs intern. Med.*, 1980, *140*, 1508.

A report of acute *thrombocytopenic purpura* associated with the administration of lignocaine.— M. Stefanini and M. N. Hoffman, *Am. J. med. Sci.*, 1978, *275*, 365.

Effects on bones. Lignocaine, 40 mg with or without adrenaline, was inadvertently introduced into the sacral marrow of 3 adults and 1 infant, who weighed 8 kg, during initiation of caudal anaesthesia, without giving rise to toxic symptoms.— R. G. McGown, *Br. J. Anaesth.*, 1972, *44*, 613.

Effects on the ears. Lignocaine with adrenaline, used by injection for ear-canal anaesthesia or applied directly into the middle ear, could cause severe vertigo lasting 6 to 9 hours.— F. B. Simmons *et al.*, *Archs Otolar.*, 1973, *98*, 42.

Effects on the eyes. A study indicating that usual therapeutic doses of lignocaine slightly interfere with colour vision.— J. Laroche and C. Laroche, *Annls pharm. fr.*, 1977, *35*, 173.

Effects on the heart. Refractory cardiac arrest developed in 2 patients with diminished cardiac output when they were given lignocaine 50 mg intravenously. Both patients had experienced a previous cardiac arrest which had responded to treatment.— J. R. Wagner and A. R. Hunter (letter), *Lancet*, 1972, *1*, 967.

In an 88-year-old woman with congestive heart failure, the sinus rhythm was replaced by junctional rhythm when she received therapeutic doses of lignocaine. Sinus rhythm returned when external cardiac massage was applied but the patient did not recover from cardiogenic shock.— T. O. Cheng and K. Wadhwa, *J. Am. med. Ass.*, 1973, *223*, 790. Permanent asystole occurred in a woman who had received an intracardiac injection of 1 or 2 ml of lignocaine 1%.— G. J. Hill (letter), *ibid.*, *224*, 401.

Further reports of adverse effects on the heart with lignocaine in patients with cardiac disease.— C. T. Lippestad and K. Forfang, *Br. med. J.*, 1971, *1*, 537 (cessation of sinus node activity); R. M. Jeresaty *et al.*, *Chest*, 1972, *61*, 683; R. Zelis, *ibid.*, 599 (sinus bradycardia with sino-atrial arrest and atrioventricular junction escape rhythm); S. T. Sinatra and R. M. Jeresaty, *J. Am. med. Ass.*, 1977, *237*, 1356 (accelerated atrioventricular conduction); D. E. Manyari-Ortega and F. J. Brennan, *Chest*, 1978, *74*, 227 (sinus bradycardia and asystole).

Effects on the nervous system. The Boston Collaborative Drug Surveillance Program monitored consecutively 32 812 medical inpatients. Drug-induced convulsions occurred in 4 of 1229 patients given lignocaine. The convulsion after the intravenous injection of lignocaine in 1 patient with myocardial infarction might have contributed to death.— J. Porter and H. Jick, *Lancet*, 1977, *1*, 587.

Local irritant effect. The incidence of thrombophlebitis was about 50% in 30 patients with ventricular tachyarrhythmias given dextrose plus lignocaine infusions compared with 8.4% in 83 who received dextrose infusions only.— K. Nordell *et al.*, *Acta med. scand.*, 1972, *192*, 263.

Overdosage. Two patients collapsed after using urethral anaesthetic jelly; about 225 mg of lignocaine as a 2% preparation was used in 1 case.— V. W. Dix and G. C. Tresidder (letter), *Lancet*, 1963, *1*, 890. A recommendation that lignocaine jelly should not be used for urethral anaesthesia in quantities of more than 15 ml or strengths greater than 1%.— J. T. Flynn and J. P. Blandy, *Br. med. J.*, 1980, *281*, 928. A view that 50 ml of 2% lignocaine gel can be used provided that the patient has no history of allergy to local anaesthetics.— K. Axelsson *et al.*, *ibid.*, 1981, *282*, 153.

A 54-year-old woman, accidentally given a 1-g bolus injection of lignocaine instead of 50 mg, became asystolic and apnoeic within seconds of the injection. Grand mal seizures were eventually controlled with diazepam. Her blood pressure could not be recorded until dopamine and sodium chloride infusions were begun; over the next 5 hours the patient was successfully taken off dopamine and the respirator.— F. Finkelstein and J. Kreeft (letter), *New Engl. J. Med.*, 1979, *301*, 50. For similar reports, see P. P. Mayer (letter), *Br. med. J.*, 1972, *3*, 291; B. Burlington and C. R. Freed (letter), *J. Am. med. Ass.*, 1980, *243*, 1036 (fatal overdose).

Convulsions and respiratory arrest occurred in a 22-month-old child after she accidentally swallowed 20 to 25 ml of a lignocaine hydrochloride 2% viscous solution which had been prescribed for stomatitis. The patient was resuscitated successfully and her convulsions were controlled with intravenous diazepam.— R. I. Sakai and J. E. Lattin, *Am. J. Dis. Child.*, 1980, *134*, 323.

CNS toxicity in an elderly woman after swallowing 30 ml of a 4% solution of lignocaine for topical use.— R. J. Fruncillo *et al.* (letter), *New Engl. J. Med.*, 1982, *306*, 426.

Pregnancy and the neonate. *Effects on the foetus.* Of 12 foetuses whose mothers were given paracervical block with the equivalent of 173 mg of lignocaine base 3 developed bradycardia and 3 tachycardia.— W. A. Liston *et al.*, *Br. J. Anaesth.*, 1973, *45*, 750. There was no change in foetal heart-rate when 30 patients in labour were given continuous paracervical block with lignocaine 1% without adrenaline.— K. S. Amankwah and J. M. Esposito, *Am. J. Obstet. Gynec.*, 1972, *112*, 50.

In 10 patients given paracervical block maximum mean maternal and foetal blood concentrations of lignocaine occurred within 9 to 10 minutes. Foetal bradycardia occurred in 2 patients, associated in 1 with an elevated foetal lignocaine concentration. Foetal bradycardia did not occur in the 1 instance in which the foetal lignocaine concentration exceeded the maternal concentration. There was 1 instance of foetal acidosis. Apgar scores were good. There was some indication that the metabolite : lignocaine ratio was higher in the foetuses.— R. H. Petrie *et al.*, *Am. J. Obstet. Gynec.*, 1974, *120*, 791.

Effects on the neonate. A report of lignocaine intoxication in a newborn infant following accidental injection of the foetal scalp during maternal episiotomy.— W. Y. Kim *et al.*, *Pediatrics*, 1979, *64*, 643.

Effects on the mother. Segments of uterine artery contracted *in vitro* in the presence of lignocaine at a concentration of 20 μg or more per ml; such concentrations could occur during paracervical block. Vasoconstriction might explain bradycardia during paracervical block.— C. P. Gibbs and S. C. Noel, *Br. J. Anaesth.*, 1977, *49*, 409.

Precautions. As for Local Anaesthetics,p.900.

In general lignocaine should not be given to patients with hypovolaemia, heart block or other conduction disturbances, bradycardia, or cardiac decompensation or hypotension not due to treatable tachyarrhythmias. It should be given with caution in other cardiac conditions. Lignocaine is metabolised in the liver and must be given with caution to patients with hepatic insufficiency. The plasma half-life of lignocaine may be prolonged in conditions which reduce hepatic blood flow such as cardiac and circulatory failure.

Administration in cardiac disorders. In a 40-year-old woman who was given lignocaine intravenously, atrial flutter with 2 : 1 atrioventricular block, possibly due to digitalis intoxication, was converted to 1 : 1 conduction. Intravenous lignocaine should not be used in atrial flutter with block unless there is overwhelming evidence of digitalis intoxication.— A. R. Adamson and F. H. N. Spracklen, *Br. med. J.*, 1968, *2*, 223.

Lignocaine is not the agent of choice for ventricular premature contractions arising in the presence of heart block because of the danger of inducing extreme bradycardia.— F. H. Cohen and H. E. Cohen (letter), *New Engl. J. Med.*, 1968, *278*, 626.

Lignocaine should not be given for ventricular arrhythmias following myocardial infarction if the systolic blood pressure is less than 80 mmHg and if the heart-rate is less than 50 beats per minute.— L. McDonald *et al.*, *Practitioner*, 1969, *202*, 238.

The use of lignocaine for ventricular arrhythmias not associated with myocardial infarction could be hazardous, especially in patients with hypoxia. Lignocaine might depress the cough reflex, thereby increasing pooling of secretions, and possibly lead to more severe hypoxia and arrhythmias.— J. J. Adler (letter), *New Engl. J. Med.*, 1973, *288*, 1303.

A study in 53 patients with atrial flutter or fibrillation indicated that there may be potentially serious clinical effects associated with an increased ventricle-rate if lignocaine is given intravenously to patients with atrial arrhythmias.— D. T. Danahy and W. S. Aronow, *Am. Heart J.*, 1978, *95*, 474.

There was limited risk of serious sinus bradyarrhythmia in patients without sinus node disease when given lignocaine, but lignocaine produced slight but significant lengthening of sino-atrial conduction time in patients with sino-atrial dysfunction; this might explain reports of serious sinus bradycardia and sinus arrest after lignocaine.— R. C. Dhingra, *Circulation*, 1978, *57*, 448.

Further references to lignocaine in cardiac disorders.— V. Aravindakshan *et al.*, *Am. J. Cardiol.*, 1977, *40*, 177.

See also Cardiac Arrhythmias under Uses.

Administration in hepatic insufficiency. Reports of adverse effects with lignocaine in patients with impaired liver-function.— R. Selden and A. A. Sasahara (letter), *New Engl. J. Med.*, 1968, *278*, 626; G. R. Schwartz (letter), *New Engl. J. Med.*, 1968, *278*, 626; D. C. Harrison, *ibid.*, 627.

See also under Uses (below).

Interactions. In smokers the systemic bioavailability of lignocaine was decreased secondary to a marked increase in clearance after oral administration, reflecting an induction of drug-metabolising activity.— P. -M. Huet and J. Lelorier, *Clin. Pharmac. Ther.*, 1980, *28*, 208.

Anti-arrhythmic agents. Transient delirium and hallucinations in a 66-year-old man were possibly due to a synergistic effect between lignocaine and *procainamide*.— M. Ilyas *et al.* (letter), *Lancet*, 1969, *2*, 1368.

Sino-atrial arrest occurred in a man with heart block complicating inferior infarction when *phenytoin* was given intravenously following the intravenous administration of lignocaine.— R. A. Wood, *Br. med. J.*, 1971, *1*, 645. Although the concomitant administration of *phenytoin*, intravenously or intramuscularly, or of *procainamide*, by mouth or intravenously, had no effect on plasma concentrations of lignocaine in patients receiving continuous intravenous infusions, there was a high incidence of CNS toxicity during the concomitant use of lignocaine and phenytoin.— E. Karlsson *et al.*, *Eur. J. clin. Pharmac.*, 1974, *7*, 455.

A prolonged Q-T interval, atrioventricular block, and ventricular fibrillation in a woman who had received lignocaine 8.16 g and *disopyramide* 900 mg in 29 hours.— M. T. Rothman, *Br. med. J.*, 1980, *280*, 922.

Anticholinergic agents. Concurrent administration of *atropine* (600 μg intramuscularly) and lignocaine (400 mg by mouth) delayed the time to reach the peak plasma-lignocaine concentration; inhibition of gastric emptying by atropine probably delayed absorption of lignocaine.— K. K. Adjepon-Yamoah *et al.*, *Eur. J. clin. Pharmac.*, 1974, *7*, 397.

Anticonvulsants. After an intravenous injection plasma concentrations of lignocaine were lower in 7 epileptic patients taking various anticonvulsants, including *phenytoin*, *benzodiazepines*, and *barbiturates*, than in 6 healthy subjects.— J. Heinonen *et al.*, *Acta anaesth. scand.*, 1970, *14*, 89. See also E. Perucca and A. Richens, *Br. J. clin. Pharmac.*, 1979, *8*, 21.

For interactions between lignocaine and *phenytoin*, see Anti-arrhythmic Agents (above).

Antihypertensive agents. For the effect of lignocaine with adrenaline on *debrisoquine*, see Debrisoquine Sulphate, p.142.

Barbiturates. All of 6 *dogs* became apnoeic and 4 died when given pentobarbitone intravenously while receiving an infusion of lignocaine.— J. LeLorier, *Toxic. appl. Pharmac.*, 1978, *44*, 657.

See also Anticonvulsants (above).

Beta-adrenoceptor blocking agents. A study demonstrating that, in healthy subjects, both prolonged infusion of lignocaine and co-administration of *propranolol* reduce the plasma clearance of lignocaine. It may be necessary to reduce the dosage of lignocaine when propranolol is given concomitantly and to reduce the rate of infusion when lignocaine is given for prolonged periods.— H. R. Ochs *et al.*, *New Engl. J. Med.*, 1980, *303*, 373. Two reports of the concomitant administration of propranolol possibly enhancing the toxicity of lignocaine.— C. F. Graham *et al.* (letter), *ibid.*, 1981, *304*, 1301.

Muscle relaxants. For references to lignocaine enhancing the effects of muscle relaxants, see Suxamethonium Chloride, p.997, and Tubocurarine Chloride, p.999.

Sympathomimetic agents. Experimental studies indicating that *isoprenaline* will increase total body clearance of lignocaine and reduce plasma-lignocaine concentrations by increasing hepatic blood flow whereas *noradrenaline* will have the opposite effect by decreasing hepatic blood flow.— N. Benowitz *et al.*, *Clin. Pharmac. Ther.*, 1974, *16*, 99.

Interference with diagnostic tests. In 9 healthy young men the intramuscular administration of lignocaine hydrochloride 10% elevated some serum-enzyme values which are useful in the diagnosis of acute myocardial infarction. However, only creatine phosphokinase (CPK) values rose above the normal range and subsequent isoenzyme assay of CPK and lactic dehydrogenase was able to identify the elevations as originating from skeletal rather than cardiac muscle.— J. C. Zener and D. C. Harrison, *Archs intern. Med.*, 1974, *134*, 48. In a study in 12 patients intramuscular injections of lignocaine caused a three-fold increase in serum-creatine phosphokinase concentrations in 50% of subjects but no significant changes in serum glutamic oxaloacetic transaminase (SGOT) concentrations.— I. Kronborg *et al.* (letter), *Med. J. Aust.*, 1975, *1*, 635.

Porphyria. From studies in *rats* it is suggested that lignocaine should not be given to patients with porphyria.— R. K. Parikh and M. R. Moore, *Br. J. Anaesth.*, 1978, *50*, 1099.

Absorption and Fate. Lignocaine is readily absorbed from the gastro-intestinal tract, from mucous membranes, and through damaged skin. It is rapidly absorbed from injection sites including muscle. After an intravenous dose plasma concentrations decline rapidly with a half-life of about 10 minutes; the elimination half-life is about 2 hours. Anti-arrhythmic plasma concentrations are reported to range from about 1.5 to

6 µg per ml. Lignocaine is rapidly distributed into the heart, brain, kidneys, and other tissues with a high blood flow and is then redistributed to muscle and adipose tissue. It diffuses across the placenta a few minutes after injection.

Lignocaine undergoes first-pass metabolism in the liver and bioavailability is low after administration by mouth. It is rapidly de-ethylated to the active metabolite monoethylglycinexylidide and then hydrolysed by amidases to various compounds, including glycinexylidide which has reduced activity but a longer elimination half-life and may accumulate to potentially toxic concentrations. Less than 10% of a dose is excreted unchanged via the kidneys. The metabolic products are excreted in the urine.

See also under Local Anaesthetics, p.900.

A review of the clinical pharmacokinetics of lignocaine.— N. L. Benowitz and W. Meister, *Clin. Pharmacokinet.*, 1978, *3*, 177.

In 10 healthy adults given a bolus intravenous injection of lignocaine 50 mg the mean half-life in plasma was 7 minutes with a mean half-life of 108 minutes for elimination. After a 100-mg dose in 5 subjects these values were 8.8 and 92 minutes respectively. Less than 4% of unchanged lignocaine was excreted in the urine in 24 hours.— M. Rowland *et al.*, *Ann. N.Y. Acad. Sci.*, 1971, *179*, 383.

Following the intravenous administration of 50 mg of lignocaine as a bolus to a group of normal subjects and patients with *heart failure*, *kidney disease*, or *liver disease*, the 8 patients with heart failure showed a significant reduction in volume of distribution and plasma clearance which suggested that lignocaine dosage should be reduced in such patients. The 8 patients with liver disease showed a significant decrease in plasma clearance and prolongation of the dominant phase of the half-life which also indicated that dosage should be reduced. No similar changes were seen in the 6 patients with kidney disease.— P. D. Thomson *et al.*, *Ann. intern. Med.*, 1973, *78*, 499.

After administration by mouth the half-life of lignocaine was prolonged in 19 of 21 patients with chronic liver disease; the mean half-life for the 21 was 6.6 hours compared with 1.4 hours for healthy subjects.— J. A. H. Forrest *et al.*, *Br. med. J.*, 1977, *1*, 1384. See also K. K. Adjepon-Yamoah *et al.*, *Br. med. J.*, 1974, *4*, 387; R. L. Williams *et al.*, *Clin. Pharmac. Ther.*, 1976, *20*, 290; P. -M. Huet and J. LeLorier, *Clin. Pharmac. Ther.*, 1980, *28*, 208.

The mean elimination half-life of lignocaine was 3.22 hours in 12 patients with uncomplicated *myocardial infarction* after they had received an intravenous bolus injection of lignocaine 1 mg per kg body-weight followed by an intravenous infusion of 20 µg per kg per minute for between 25 and 60 hours. It was recommended that even in patients without cardiac or hepatic failure the rate of infusion of lignocaine should be reduced by one half after the first 24 hours to compensate for the decrease in the rate of elimination.— J. LeLorier *et al.*, *Ann. intern. Med.*, 1977, *87*, 700. See also L. Rydén *et al.*, *Am. Heart J.*, 1975, *89*, 470; R. A. Zito *et al.*, *Am. Heart J.*, 1977, *94*, 292.

Although there was no change in plasma-clearance, lignocaine hydrochloride 50 mg given as a bolus intravenous injection, had a longer half-life in 6 *elderly* subjects than in 4 young subjects with mean ages of 65 years and 24 years respectively. Lignocaine distribution was different in the elderly group who had an increased apparent volume of distribution and reduced 24-hour recovery of its major metabolite.— R. L. Nation *et al.*, *Br. J. clin. Pharmac.*, 1977, *4*, 439.

Further references to the pharmacokinetics of lignocaine: S. W. Klein *et al.*, *Can. med. Ass. J.*, 1968, *99*, 472; K. K. Adjepon-Yamoah *et al.*, *Br. J. Anaesth.*, 1973, *45*, 143; A. H. Hayes, *Clin. Pharmac. Ther.*, 1974, *16*, 201; J. R. Patterson *et al.*, *Am. Rev. resp. Dis.*, 1975, *112*, 53; G. Cheymol *et al.*, *Thérapie*, 1976, *31*, 149.

Absorption. Determination of plasma concentrations of lignocaine after application as an aerosol to either the vagina, perineal skin, or for episiotomy repair in 22 women showed that lignocaine was absorbed from the intact mucous membrane and skin as well as from damaged tissue. The highest plasma concentration of lignocaine recorded was 1.2 µg per ml.— J. Thomas *et al.*, *Br. J. Anaesth.*, 1969, *41*, 442.

Lignocaine, 500 mg by mouth after an overnight fast, caused dizziness when blood concentrations exceeded 10 µg per ml. Concentrations exceeding 5 µg per ml, an optimum therapeutic concentration, lasted for 2.5 hours. When given with food this blood concentration was maintained for 4.5 hours. After 250 mg, blood concentrations did not exceed 10 µg per ml, and concentrations exceeding 5 µg per ml persisted for less than 2 hours. Ventricular arrhythmias in 4 patients were successfully treated with lignocaine given by mouth.— P. I. Parkinson *et al.*, *Br. med. J.*, 1970, *2*, 29. Transient toxic symptoms occurred in subjects receiving lignocaine by mouth at much lower plasma concentrations than had been observed with intravenous administration. It might be that a metabolite of lignocaine formed in the liver was responsible for these effects.— D. B. Scott and D. G. Julian (letter), *ibid.*, 297. See also R. N. Boyes *et al.*, *Clin. Pharmac. Ther.*, 1971, *12*, 105.

After the intramuscular injection of lignocaine hydrochloride 200 mg, effective concentrations were reached in 15 to 20 minutes and were maintained for at least 60 minutes.— V. Bernstein *et al.*, *J. Am. med. Ass.*, 1972, *219*, 1027.

A mean plasma concentration of 6.48 µg per ml was reached in 15 minutes when lignocaine 400 mg was given to produce intercostal block, compared with 4.27 µg per ml reached in 20 minutes when the same amount of lignocaine was used to produce epidural block. The concentration of lignocaine in an injection did not affect the maximum plasma concentration reached but increasing the speed of administration produced a slightly higher plasma concentration which could be critical for intravenous injections given for the treatment of myocardial infarctions.— D. B. Scott *et al.*, *Br. J. Anaesth.*, 1972, *44*, 1040.

Peak plasma concentrations of about 1 µg per ml were recorded after peri-oral injection of 80 mg of lignocaine hydrochloride. Lignocaine was absorbed systemically from the injection site for about 2 hours.— H. Cannell and A. H. Beckett, *Br. dent. J.*, 1975, *139*, 242.

Findings in 6 healthy subjects suggested that it may be possible to reduce drug loss resulting from first-pass metabolism of lignocaine after administration by mouth, by using the rectal route. Mean bioavailability of lignocaine hydrochloride administered rectally as an aqueous solution was about twice that of a similar oral dose given in hard gelatin capsules. Mean elimination half-lives from plasma were 90 and 101 minutes respectively after oral and rectal administration.— A. G. de Boer *et al.*, *Clin. Pharmac. Ther.*, 1979, *26*, 701. See also A. H. Beckett *et al.*, *Br. J. clin. Pharmac.*, 1978, *6*, 442P.

Further reports of the absorption of lignocaine after administration by various routes: D. A. Pelton *et al.*, *Can. Anaesth. Soc. J.*, 1970, *17*, 250 (laryngotracheal administration using a 20% spray); O. Viegas and R. K. Stoelting, *Anesthesiology*, 1975, *43*, 491 (laryngotracheal administration); R. B. Smith (letter), *Anesthesiology*, 1976, *44*, 269 (tracheal administration); P. Kálmán *et al.*, *Therapia hung.*, 1977, *25*, 24 (oral administration); S. Nattel *et al.*, *New Engl. J. Med.*, 1979, *301*, 418 (subcutaneous injection).

For a comparative study of serum concentrations following maxillary buccal infiltrations of mepivacaine hydrochloride or lignocaine hydrochloride, see Mepivacaine Hydrochloride, p.918.

Metabolism. Glycinexylidide (GX) was identified in the plasma and urine of patients given lignocaine intravenously.— J. M. Strong *et al.*, *Clin. Pharmac. Ther.*, 1973, *14*, 67. A study of the pharmacological activity, metabolism, and pharmacokinetics of GX in *mice*. GX was estimated to have 26% of the antiarrhythmic potency of lignocaine and 27% of the potency of monoethylglycinexylidide, with respect to plasma concentrations. In 2 healthy subjects GX, at plasma concentrations comparable to those found in patients, produced symptoms of headache and impaired concentration but cardiovascular toxicity was not seen. The elimination phase half-life for GX was about 10 hours and renal excretion accounted for 58% of GX elimination. Further metabolism, in part to a conjugate of xylidine and to *p*-OH xylidine glucuronide, was noted.— *idem*, 1975, *17*, 184.

The blood concentrations of lignocaine and its active metabolite monoethylglycinexylidide (MEGX) were measured in 31 patients, and higher concentrations of MEGX were found in those with congestive heart failure. In 3 patients who were studied intensively the elimination half-life of MEGX was considered to be similar to that of lignocaine. In 1 patient who experienced CNS toxicity the MEGX concentration probably contributed to the reaction although the contribution of other metabolites of lignocaine could not be discounted.— H. Halkin *et al.*, *Clin. Pharmac. Ther.*, 1975, *17*, 669.

Of several metabolites identified in urine after administration of lignocaine hydrochloride by mouth to 3 healthy subjects, 4-hydroxy-2,6-dimethylaniline accounted for 63.5% of the administered dose and unchanged lignocaine 1.95%.— S. D. Nelson *et al.*, *J. pharm. Sci.*, 1977, *66*, 1180.

A rapid and sensitive method for assaying lignocaine and its 2 known active metabolites, monoethylglycylxylidide (MEGX) and glycylxylidide (GX), in 3 patients.— P. K. Narang *et al.*, *Clin. Pharmac. Ther.*, 1978, *24*, 654.

In a study of the metabolism of lignocaine to the active metabolites monoethylglycinexylidide (MEGX) and glycinexylidide (GX) after epidural anaesthesia for labour or caesarean section, MEGX appeared in maternal plasma within about 13 minutes of the administration of lignocaine and GX within about 1 hour. Both the foetus and the neonate appeared capable of metabolising lignocaine.— B. R. Kuhnert *et al.*, *Clin. Pharmac. Ther.*, 1979, *26*, 213.

Further references to the metabolism of lignocaine: J. Lelorier *et al.*, *Clin. Res.*, 1975, *28*, 609-a, per G. Caille *et al.*, *J. pharm. Sci.*, 1977, *66*, 1383.

Pregnancy and the neonate. Lignocaine, given intravenously to the mother before delivery, rapidly rose in concentration in arterial blood and the concentration then declined with half-lives of 30 seconds and 30 minutes. Lignocaine appeared in foetal blood within minutes of the injection but only reached concentrations of 55% of those in the mother; half-lives were similar to those in the mother.— S. M. Shnider and E. L. Way, *Anesthesiology*, 1968, *29*, 944.

In 13 women given epidural injections of lignocaine, 5.1 to 8 mg per kg body-weight, mostly with adrenaline 1 in 250 000, maternal plasma concentrations at delivery ranged from 1.1 to 4.68 µg per ml and umbilical venous plasma concentrations from 0.6 to 2.2 µg per ml. In 7 women given repeated epidural injections of lignocaine 1% in total doses of 2.6 to 18.5 mg per kg, in some cases with adrenaline, maternal plasma concentrations ranged from 1.48 to 4.52 µg per ml and umbilical venous plasma concentrations from 0.72 to 4.28 µg per ml at delivery.— J. Thomas *et al.*, *Br. J. Anaesth.*, 1968, *40*, 965. See also B. S. Epstein *et al.*, *Anesth. Analg. curr. Res.*, 1968, *47*, 223.

The mean maternal venous plasma concentration of lignocaine in mothers given epidural anaesthesia with lignocaine 1.5% and adrenaline 1 in 200 000 for caesarean section was 2.79 µg per ml at delivery compared with 1.70 µg per ml (cord plasma) in the neonates. Of the total amount of lignocaine and metabolites excreted in the urine of the neonates 50% appeared as unchanged lignocaine in the first 12 hours and 23% in the next 12 hours, thus demonstrating that lignocaine metabolism does occur in the newborn.— W. L. Blankenbaker *et al.*, *Anesthesiology*, 1975, *42*, 325. In premature neonates lignocaine had a mean half-life of 3.16 hours and was mainly excreted as unchanged lignocaine, but in healthy adults the mean half-life was about 1.80 hours and lignocaine was mainly eliminated as metabolites.— G. W. Mihaly *et al.*, *Eur. J. clin. Pharmac.*, 1978, *13*, 143. See also Metabolism (above).

The mean maximum arterial lignocaine concentrations in infants born to multiparous mothers receiving continuous or intermittent extradural or paracervical analgesia were 0.29, 0.29, and 0.23 µg per ml respectively while corresponding concentrations in infants born to primiparous mothers were 0.43, 0.29, and 0.38 µg per ml.— L. -E. Bratteby *et al.*, *Br. J. Anaesth.*, 1979, *51*, *Suppl.* 1, 41S.

Further references to the pharmacokinetics of lignocaine in neonates: J. Thomas *et al.*, *Clin. exp. Pharmac. Physiol.*, 1978, *5*, 257.

Protein binding. Plasma protein-binding of local anaesthetics was found to be related inversely to total drug concentrations. The following mean values for binding, determined by ultrafiltration at plasma concentrations of 5 µg of base per ml in 6 subjects, are reported: lignocaine, 51.2%; mepivacaine, 65.9%; and bupivacaine, 84.7%. The binding figure for lignocaine is much lower than those reported by E. Eriksson (*Acta chir. scand.*, 1966, *Suppl.* 358, 1) and S.M. Shnider and E.L. Way (*Anesthesiology*, 1968, *29*, 944).— G. T. Tucker *et al.*, *Anesthesiology*, 1970, *33*, 287.

Further references to the protein binding of lignocaine:— P. J. McNamara *et al.* (letter), *J. pharm. Sci.*, 1980, *69*, 749 (increased binding in the serum of cigarette smokers); P. A. Routledge *et al.*, *Clin. Pharmac. Ther.*, 1980, *27*, 347; P. A. Routledge *et al.*, *Br. J. clin. Pharmac.*, 1981, *11*, 245 (sex-related differences).

Uses. As for Local Anaesthetics, p.901.

Lignocaine is a local anaesthetic of the amide type and is widely used by injection and for local application to mucous membranes. It has a rapid onset of action when injected and rapidly spreads through surrounding tissues. It has a more intense action and its effects are more prolonged than those of procaine but shorter than those of bupivacaine or prilocaine.

The speed of onset and duration of action of lignocaine are increased by the addition of a vasoconstrictor and absorption into the circulation from the site of injection is reduced. Solutions containing adrenaline 1 in 200 000 or less may be employed; higher concentrations are seldom necessary though solutions containing adrenaline 1 in 80 000 are used in dentistry. The total amount of adrenaline injected should not exceed 500 µg; some consider that the total dose should not exceed 200 µg. The total dose of lignocaine hydrochloride for anaesthesia should not exceed 200 mg (3 mg per kg body-weight); some consider that the total dose should not exceed 300 mg (4.5 mg per kg). When given with adrenaline the total dose should not exceed 500 mg (7 mg per kg). Children should receive smaller amounts of lignocaine, generally in lower concentrations, than adults.

Solutions containing 0.5 to 1% of lignocaine hydrochloride may be used for infiltration in volumes of 1 to 60 ml; a 0.25% solution has been used when larger volumes are required.

For peripheral and central regional nerve block 1 to 2% solutions of lignocaine hydrochloride are employed, often with adrenaline 1 in 200 000. Adrenaline should not be used for digits, ears, nose, penis, or scrotum because of the risk of tissue necrosis.

A hyperbaric solution of 1.5 or 5% of lignocaine hydrochloride and 7.5% dextrose has been used for spinal anaesthesia. A 0.5% solution without adrenaline may be used for intravenous regional anaesthesia of the limbs.

In dentistry, a 2% solution with adrenaline 1 in 100 000 or 1 in 80 000 is generally used. The gums may be anaesthetised by inunction of a 5% cream.

Lignocaine differs from procaine in being a useful surface anaesthetic. The base is used in creams, ointments, suppositories, and sprays, and the hydrochloride in solutions and gels. A 2 to 4% solution without adrenaline produces insensitivity of the cornea, without mydriasis, although agents such as oxybuprocaine or proxymetacaine are preferred. The mouth, throat, and upper gastro-intestinal tract may be anaesthetised with a 2% viscous solution with a maximum dose of 600 mg daily in divided doses. Ano-genital pruritus and painful haemorrhoids may be relieved with suppositories or a 5% ointment or cream. A 2% gel may also be applied prior to cystoscopy or catheterisation providing no trauma exists in the urethra, and a 4% spray may be used to anaesthetise the pharynx, larynx, and trachea before bronchoscopy.

Lignocaine is a class I anti-arrhythmic agent (see p.1370). It reduces cardiac irritability and is given intravenously, with ECG monitoring, to control ventricular arrhythmias following myocardial infarction or general anaesthesia, during cardiac catheterisation and open-heart surgery, or after overdosage with digoxin or a sympathomimetic agent. Lignocaine is widely used as the treatment of choice for ventricular premature contractions (ventricular ectopic beats, ventricular extrasystoles), in patients with myocardial infarction, but its value in preventing the more dangerous ventricular fibrillation is less certain. It is administered as the hydrochloride, usually in doses of 50 to 100 mg as a 1 or 2% solution by slow intravenous injection over 2 minutes. It may be necessary to repeat the dose after 5 to 10 minutes. The loading dose is usually followed by an 0.1 or 0.2% infusion in dextrose injection of 1 to 4 mg per minute for 12 to 48 hours. In the emergency management of patients with acute myocardial infarction doses of 300 mg may be given by intramuscular injection into the deltoid muscle.

Lignocaine hydrochloride has been given by intravenous infusion in the treatment of refractory status epilepticus.

Action. In a double-blind study of the vasoactivity of bupivacaine hydrochloride 0.125, 0.25, and 0.5% and lignocaine hydrochloride 0.5, 1, and 2%, given intradermally to healthy subjects, vasoconstriction was seen more frequently at low concentrations and vasodilation at high concentrations. The duration of action of lignocaine was unaffected by concentration whereas the effect of bupivacaine was more prolonged at a concentration of 0.5%.— C. Aps and F. Reynolds, *Br. J. Anaesth.*, 1976, *48*, 1171.

Administration. A reminder that solutions of lignocaine hydrochloride deposited around fractured ends of bone may be absorbed almost as rapidly as from an intravenous injection.— V. Goldman (letter), *Br. med. J.*, 1963, *2*, 184.

In 10 healthy men given 10 ml of 2% lignocaine or 2 ml of 10% lignocaine by intramuscular injection into the thigh, there was no significant difference in blood concentrations achieved. There were no local reactions to the 10% solution and its smaller volume was of potential benefit.— P. Jebson, *Br. med. J.*, 1971, *3*, 566.

Intrapleural administration. The discomfort caused by intrapleural instillation of tetracycline in a woman with pleural effusions was drastically reduced by adding 15 ml of a 1% lignocaine hydrochloride solution to the tetracycline solution.— G. N. Fox (letter), *J. Am. med. Ass.*, 1979, *242*, 1362. Following the occurrence of severe chest pain in a patient given a mixture of tetracycline and lignocaine intrapleurally the technique has been amended and 15 to 30 ml of a 1% lignocaine hydrochloride solution, followed by 20 ml of physiological saline, is instilled intrapleurally 30 minutes before the tetracycline. During this 30 minutes the patient is rotated through various positions in order to anaesthetise the pleura fully before instillation of the sclerosing agent.— R. G. Harbecke (letter), *ibid.*, 1980, *244*, 1899.

Administration in cardiac insufficiency. See under Cardiac Arrhythmias (below), Absorption and Fate (above), and Precautions (above).

Administration in hepatic insufficiency. A study of the disposition of lignocaine in 6 subjects during and after recovery from acute viral hepatitis demonstrated that lignocaine disposition might be impaired in patients with acute hepatic dysfunction but provided no guideline by which the changes could be predicted.— R. L. Williams *et al.*, *Clin. Pharmac. Ther.*, 1976, *20*, 290.

See also Absorption and Fate (above) and Precautions (above).

Administration in renal insufficiency. Data for predicting removal of lignocaine and glycinexylidide by conventional haemodialysis.— T. P. Gibson and H. A. Nelson, *Clin. Pharmacokinet.*, 1977, *2*, 403.

Normal half-lives for lignocaine of 1.2 to 2.2 hours are reported to be increased to 1.3 to 3 hours in end-stage renal failure. It can be given in usual doses to patients with renal failure. Lignocaine is not removed by haemodialysis.— W. M. Bennett *et al.*, *Ann. intern. Med.*, 1980, *93*, 286. See also K. A. Collinsworth *et al.*, *Clin. Pharmac. Ther.*, 1975, *18*, 59; J. S. Cheigh, *Am. J. Med.*, 1977, *62*, 555; P. Sharpstone, *Br. med. J.*, 1977, *2*, 36.

Anaesthesia in the ear. A report on anaesthesia of the tympanic membrane using the technique of iontophoresis. With the patient's head on one side the external meatus was filled with a warmed, freshly prepared solution of 2% lignocaine with adrenaline 1 in 2000. A low amperage direct current from a positive electrode was then used to drive positive lignocaine ions into the tympanic membrane and produce complete anaesthesia. The main indications for this technique have been in outpatient myringotomy and transtympanic electrocochleography.— R. T. Ramsden *et al.*, *J. Lar. Otol.*, 1977, *91*, 779. A similar technique was used successfully to anaesthetise the tympanic membrane in 39 patients with serous otitis media and 11 patients with Ménière's disease.— M. Hasegawa *et al.*, *Clin. Otolar.*, 1978, *3*, 63.

For reference to lignocaine in the ear causing severe vertigo, see under Effect on the Ears in Adverse Effects (p.902).

Antibacterial activity. A report on the antibacterial activity of lignocaine *in vitro*.— N. Wimberley *et al.*, *Chest*, 1979, *76*, 37.

Biliary calculi. Retained biliary calculi were successfully removed in 6 of 10 patients. Propantheline bromide was given intramuscularly 30 minutes before flushing the bile ducts with 1 litre of sodium chloride injection containing 40 ml of 1% lignocaine hydrochloride solution. Three washouts were given at daily intervals.— P. B. Catt *et al.*, *Ann. Surg.*, 1974, *180*, 247.

Cardiac arrhythmias. Reviews on anti-arrhythmic drugs, including lignocaine: M. Thomas, *Adv. Med. Topics Ther.*, 1977, *3*, 1; *Med. Lett.*, 1978, *20*, 113; J. L. Anderson *et al.*, *Drugs*, 1978, *15*, 271; R. W. F. Campbell, *Prescribers' J.*, 1978, *18*, 1; *Lancet*, 1979, *1*, 193; A. A. J. Adgey and S. W. Webb, *Br. J. Hosp. Med.*, 1979, *21*, 356; H. W. Moses and P. N. Yu, *J. clin. Pharmac.*, 1980, *20*, 598; L. H. Opie, *Lancet*, 1980, *1*, 861.

References to the use of lignocaine in the Wolff-Parkinson-White syndrome: M. E. Josephson *et al.*, *Ann. intern. Med.*, 1976, *84*, 44; E. K. Chung, *Am. J. Med.*, 1977, *62*, 252.

For reference to lignocaine in the classification of anti-arrhythmic agents, see Quinidine and some other Anti-arrhythmic Agents, p.1370.

Action. Lignocaine reduced the maximum rate of depolarisation of cardiac muscle in patients with normal serum-potassium concentrations; it was ineffective in patients with low serum-potassium concentrations, in whom the dose response curve appeared to be shifted so that higher doses of lignocaine would be required to produce the same effect.— E. M. V. Williams, *Adv. Drug Res.*, 1974, *9*, 69.

Further references to studies on the cardiac action of lignocaine: M. E. Josephson *et al.*, *Am. Heart J.*, 1972, *84*, 778; J. C. Roos and A. J. Dunning, *Am. Heart J.*, 1975, *89*, 686; T. R. Engel *et al.*, *Clin. Pharmac. Ther.*, 1976, *19*, 515; H. Boudoulas *et al.*, *Chest*, 1977, *71*, 170; A. Fleckenstein, *A. Rev. Pharmac. Toxic.*, 1977, *17*, 149; M. A. Martin *et al.*, *Br. J. clin. Pharmac.*, 1980, *10*, 237.

Administration. A pharmacokinetic approach to the clinical use of lignocaine intravenously. Single 50- or 100-mg loading doses of lignocaine hydrochloride may fail to maintain therapeutic plasma concentrations in the first hour of therapy and it is suggested that two bolus doses of 100 mg separated by 20 to 30 minutes or rapid infusion of the total loading dose over 15 to 60 minutes will achieve and maintain adequate concentrations.— D. J. Greenblatt *et al.*, *J. Am. med. Ass.*, 1976, *236*, 273.

On theoretical grounds, it is unnecessary to taper the dose of lignocaine infusion after control of arrhythmias.— P. R. Reid, *J. clin. Pharmac.*, 1976, *16*, 162. After control of arrhythmias, administration for 24 hours, with gradual tapering of the dose, is customary to prevent recurrence.— J. L. Anderson *et al.*, *Drugs*, 1978, *15*, 271.

Recommendations for lignocaine dosage regimens based on pharmacokinetic studies and indications for the measurement of blood concentrations.— N. L. Benowitz and W. Meister, *Clin. Pharmacokinet.*, 1978, *3*, 177.

Indocyanine green plasma clearance, a measure of hepatic blood flow, could be correlated with lignocaine plasma clearance in 26 patients, half of them with congestive heart failure, who had received a 24-hour infusion of lignocaine. Patients with heart failure had significantly higher plasma-lignocaine concentrations than those without (6.8 µg compared with 2.9 µg per ml) despite a lower infusion rate and their lignocaine plasma clearance was also significantly reduced. Indocyanine green clearance could be used to determine optimal infusion-rates and thus avoid subtherapeutic or toxic plasma concentrations.— R. A. Zito and P. R. Reid, *New Engl. J. Med.*, 1978, *298*, 1160. Comment.— P. Goldman and J. A. Ingelfinger, *ibid.*, 1193. Conflicting results and the view that indocyanine green is not helpful in predicting lignocaine dosage requirements in post-myocardial infarction patients.— N. D. S. Bax *et al.* (letter), *ibid.*, *299*, 662. The guidelines only appear adequate during the first 24 hours of lignocaine administration.— J. LeLorier (letter), *ibid.* Reply.— P. R. Reid; R. A. Zito (letter), *ibid.*, 663.

A study demonstrating that it may be necessary to reduce the rate of infusion when lignocaine is given for prolonged periods.— H. R. Ochs *et al.*, *New Engl. J. Med.*, 1980, *303*, 373.

See also under Plasma Concentrations (below).

Cardiac resuscitation. Recommendations concerning lignocaine, at the National Conference on Standards for Cardiopulmonary Resuscitation and Emergency Cardiac Care held in May 1973. Lignocaine raises the fibrillation threshold and exerts its antidysrhythmic effect by increasing the electrical stimulation threshold of the ventricle during diastole. In usual therapeutic doses, there is no significant change in myocardial contractility, systemic arterial pressure, or absolute refractory period. This drug is particularly effective in depressing irritability where successful defibrillation repeatedly reverts to ventricular fibrillation. It is also particularly effective in the control of multifocal premature ventricular beats and episodes of ventricular tachycardia. It should be given in a slow intravenous bolus dose of 50 to 100 mg and may be repeated if necessary. It may be followed by a continuous infusion of 1 to 3 mg per minute, usually not exceeding 4 mg per minute. Lignocaine is of no value in asystole. Where prompt establishment of an intravenous lifeline is not possible, lignocaine 50 to 100 mg per 10 ml sterile distilled water (0.5 to 1%) can be effective when instilled directly into the tracheobronchial tree through an endotracheal tube.— American Heart Association and the National Academy of Sciences-National Research Council, *J. Am. med. Ass.*, 1974, *227, Suppl.*, 833–868.

See also Adrenaline, p.5.

Myocardial infarction. The *prophylactic* use of lignocaine to prevent primary ventricular fibrillation in patients with myocardial infarction has been widely debated. Some studies have indicated a reduction in the incidence of fibrillations but not necessarily in mortality-rate whereas others have been unable to show any beneficial effect. Many cardiologists recommend prophylaxis in patients with suspected infarction (*Med. Lett.*, 1978, *20*, 113), others are less certain (*Lancet*, 1979, *1*, 193; A.A.J. Adgey and S.W. Webb, *Br. J. Hosp. Med.*, 1979, *21*, 356; L.H. Opie, *Lancet*, 1980, *1*, 861). In an evaluation of 15 randomised trials D.A. DeSilva *et al.* (*Lancet*, 1981, *2*, 855) considered that lignocaine treatment does provide prophylaxis and that the failure of most trials to demonstrate such an effect is due to small sample sizes and inadequate treatment protocols. On the other hand B.L. Pentecost *et al.* (*Br. Heart J.*, 1981, *45*, 42), after a survey of 3 two-year treatment periods involving 1483 patients, have concluded that myocardial infarction damage, not lignocaine prophylaxis appears to be the main determinant of death or survival.

In a controlled study in 82 patients with myocardial infarction and varying ventricular ectopic activity, there was no difference in the incidence of ventricular tachycardia, fibrillation, and mortality in patients given lignocaine or placebo.— M. P. Chopra *et al.*, *Br. med. J.*, 1971, *3*, 668. Lignocaine 200 mg administered intramuscularly to 103 patients who had recently experienced a myocardial infarction and then administered as an infusion of 2 mg per minute for 48 hours to 92 of the patients, had no effect on ventricular extrasystoles when compared with 100 control patients. Both ventricular tachycardia and fibrillation occurred more frequently in the treated group although the difference was not significant.— S. Darby *et al.*, *Lancet*, 1972, *1*, 817. An intramuscular injection of lignocaine 300 mg, given within 6 hours of the onset of symptoms of myocardial infarction, was ineffective in preventing primary ventricular fibrillations within 1 hour of injection, in a double-blind placebo-controlled study in 300 patients.— K. I. Lie *et al.*, *Am. J. Cardiol.*, 1978, *42*, 486. Further reports indicating that routine prophylaxis with lignocaine in patients with acute myocardial infarction is of no benefit: K. P. O'Brien *et al.*, *Med. J. Aust.*, 1973, *2*, *Suppl.* 1, 36; W. Bleifield *et al.*, *Eur. J. clin. Pharmac.*, 1973, *6*, 119.

In a double-blind study of 212 patients, less than 70 years of age, with acute myocardial infarction, 107 were given a bolus injection of 100 mg of lignocaine followed by an intravenous infusion of lignocaine 3 mg per minute. The infusion was started within 6 hours of onset of symptoms and continued for 48 hours. No ventricular fibrillations occurred in the treated patients although 46 experienced occasional ventricular extrasystoles. In the control group 11 had fibrillations. Side-effects, including drowsiness and dizziness, were noted in 16 patients given lignocaine, 12 of whom were over 60 years of age, and necessitated halving the rate of infusion in 7 patients.— K. I. Lie *et al.*, *New Engl. J. Med.*, 1974, *291*, 1324. In a double-blind study of 269 patients an intramuscular injection of lignocaine 300 mg administered before admission to hospital and as soon after onset of symptoms as possible appeared to reduce the incidence of early deaths in patients with myocardial infarction.— P. A. Valentine *et al.*, *New Engl. J. Med.*, 1974, *291*, 1327. An intravenous injection of 100 mg of lignocaine hydrochloride followed by an intramuscular injection of 300 mg is reported to give adequate protection to patients with acute myocardial infarction during transportation to hospital.— J. M. Barber *et al.*, *Br. Heart J.*, 1977, *39*, 1361. Further reports of the beneficial prophylactic effect of lignocaine in patients with myocardial infarction: S. Bellet *et al.*, *Am. J. Cardiol.*, 1971, *27*, 291 (lignocaine 300 mg intramuscularly); A. Pitt *et al.*, *Lancet*, 1971, *1*, 612 (lignocaine by intravenous infusion); V. Bernstein *et al.*, *J. Am. med. Ass.*, 1972, *219*, 1027 (lignocaine 200 mg intramuscularly); M. C. O. Fehmers and A. J. Dunning, *Am. J. Cardiol.*, 1972, *29*, 514 (lignocaine 250 mg intramuscularly); M. G. Wyman and L. Hammersmith, *Am. J. Cardiol.*, 1974, *33*, 661 (lignocaine by intravenous bolus and infusion); P. Schonherr *et al.*, *Dte GesundhWes.*, 1976, *31*, 56, per *Int. pharm. Abstr.*, 1976, *13*, 888; J. B. Singh and S. L. Kocot, *Am. Heart J.*, 1976, *91*, 430.

Further references to the prophylactic use of lignocaine in acute myocardial infarction: D. C. Harrison, *Circulation*, 1978, *58*, 581; J. W. Noneman and J. F. Rogers, *Medicine, Baltimore*, 1978, *57*, 501.

After a study of 24 patients with a primary diagnosis of acute myocardial infarction without gross circulatory disturbance the following regimen for lignocaine therapy was recommended: an initial bolus injection of lignocaine 75 to 100 mg intravenously followed by intravenous infusion at a rate of 4 mg per minute for 30 minutes, 2 mg per minute for 2 hours, and 1 mg per minute thereafter. Studies in 12 patients who had undergone cardiothoracic surgery indicated that in patients who had had cardiac surgery and were likely to have decreased cardiac output and hepatic dysfunction, the initial bolus followed by infusion of 1 mg per minute could be adequate; the risk of toxicity with prolonged infusion would be greater in these patients.— C. Aps *et al.*, *Br. med. J.*, 1976, *1*, 13.

In a study of 13 patients with myocardial infarction or cardiac failure given lignocaine hydrochloride 100 mg intravenously as a bolus injection followed by 1.3 or 1.4 mg per minute for up to 46 hours, the mean plasma half-life was increased to 4.3 hours in patients with cardiac infarction and 10.2 hours in those with cardiac failure. One patient developed cardiogenic shock and appeared unable to eliminate lignocaine. Severe toxicity might be expected within a few hours in patients with cardiac failure infused at rates of 4 mg per minute or above. It was considered advisable to use 2 mg per minute for such patients and to halve the rate after 24 hours if the arrhythmias were being controlled. Plasma concentrations should be monitored in patients with cardiogenic shock and in these patients rates of 4 mg per minute or more would lead to possibly fatal and irreversible toxicity within 12 hours.— L. F. Prescott *et al.*, *Br. med. J.*, 1976, *1*, 939.

The intravenous injection of 100 mg of lignocaine over 3 minutes followed immediately by the intramuscular administration of 300 mg produced plasma concentrations (mean 6.3 µg per ml) of lignocaine within 1 minute in 9 patients seen within 12 hours of the onset of symptoms of acute myocardial infarction. Ventricular ectopic beats were markedly reduced within 15 minutes and a maximum effect was maintained for about 90 minutes although there was still a significant effect at 3 hours when the mean plasma concentration was 1.7 µg per ml. This schedule might be of value in the prehospital treatment of early myocardial infarction especially if combined with an antiarrhythmic agent such as disopyramide or mexiletine that might be given by mouth.— D. J. Sheridan *et al.*, *Lancet*, 1977, *1*, 824. Disopyramide on its own was considered to be preferable to a 2-drug regimen in early uncomplicated infarction.— J. W. Ward (letter), *ibid.*, 1006. A better method of administration to avoid side-effects might be to administer lignocaine intramuscularly in 2 doses an hour apart. The second peak plasma concentration would be reduced and the effective plasma concentration prolonged.— F. Reynolds and C. Aps (letter), *ibid.*, 1202.

An infusion schedule based on kinetic data was compared with several more standard infusion-rates in an attempt to achieve adequate plasma concentrations of lignocaine in the first hour of treatment after myocardial infarction. Satisfactory concentrations were generally achieved in 6 patients given 75 mg of lignocaine intravenously followed by an infusion of 10 mg per minute for 20 minutes and 1.5 mg per minute thereafter.— N. P. S. Campbell *et al.*, *Br. Heart J.*, 1978, *40*, 1371.

Further references to the treatment of myocardial infarction with lignocaine: D. E. Jewitt *et al.*, *Lancet*, 1968, *1*, 266 (lignocaine appeared to facilitate cardioversion of ventricular fibrillation); M. G. Wyman *et al.*, *Am. J. Cardiol.*, 1978, *41*, 313.

Plasma concentrations. The plasma half-life of lignocaine is greatly prolonged in patients with cardiac failure due to myocardial infarction, and in cardiogenic shock metabolism of lignocaine virtually ceases.— L. F. Prescott, *Prescribers' J.*, 1978, *18*, 50. Adjustment of the rate of infusion of lignocaine will prevent toxicity and can be achieved by measuring steady-state plasma concentrations.— J. C. Mucklow, *Adverse Drug React. Bull.*, 1978, Dec., 260. The therapeutic range of plasma-lignocaine concentrations is 1.5 to 6 µg per ml although in practice plasma concentrations are considered to be of limited value.— A. Richens and S. Warrington, *Drugs*, 1979, *17*, 488.

A report of the determination of serum-lignocaine concentrations in the coronary care unit using a rapid enzyme immunoassay technique.— S. M. Deglin *et al.*, *J. Am. med. Ass.*, 1980, *244*, 571. See also B. E. Pape *et al.*, *Clin. Chem.*, 1978, *24*, 2020.

Increased lignocaine binding was associated with the rise in alpha-1-acid glycoprotein after myocardial infarction and suggests that the use of total plasma-lignocaine concentrations to monitor therapy after myocardial infarction is likely to be misleading.— P. A. Routledge *et al.*, *Ann. intern. Med.*, 1980, *93*, 701.

Caudal block. Of 201 patients with chronic or acute backache 59 achieved a very good response (complete or almost complete relief from pain and improvement in straight leg raising lasting more than 18 months) after epidural analgesia and 54 achieved a good response (4 to 18 months). Lignocaine hydrochloride 0.5% about 40 ml was injected via the caudal approach and was followed by methylprednisolone acetate 80 mg and, more recently, hydrocortisone sodium succinate 50 mg in addition. Patients were recommended to pass urine before leaving hospital since urinary retention is a possible side-effect of epidural injection.— R. K. Sharma, *Postgrad. med. J.*, 1977, *53*, 1.

Cough. Severe intractable cough was relieved for periods of between 1 and 6 weeks in 4 patients after the inhalation of 400 mg of lignocaine administered by nebuliser as 4 ml of a 10% solution in saline.— P. Howard *et al.*, *Br. J. Dis. Chest*, 1977, *71*, 19. Intractable cough was relieved similarly in 3 cancer patients. The lignocaine was preceded by the inhalation of 2 to 5 mg of a salbutamol. Inhalations of lignocaine were needed at intervals of 5 to 7 days.— C. J. Stewart and T. J. Coady (letter), *Br. med. J.*, 1977, *1*, 1660.

Dental use. Given alone lignocaine has a mild vasodilator effect and, injected into the vascular tissues of the mouth, is quickly absorbed so that its local anaesthetic action is frequently transient or inadequate for dental purposes. Where it is desired to avoid the additional use of adrenaline or other vasoconstrictors, prilocaine hydrochloride 4% or mepivacaine hydrochloride 3% are to be preferred.— N. M. Ross (letter), *J. Am. med. Ass.*, 1967, *201*, 334.

A technique of regional nerve block for maxillary permanent molars, using about 1.5 ml of an injection of lignocaine hydrochloride 2% with adrenaline 1 in 80 000.— A. K. Adatia, *Br. dent. J.*, 1976, *140*, 87.

Lignocaine hydrochloride 2% given intraosseously in a dose of no more than 20 mg over 30 seconds with adrenaline 1 in 80 000 produced plasma-lignocaine concentrations comparable with intravenous administration in 2 subjects. Since higher doses or faster administration could produce sudden large increases in circulating lignocaine concentrations and since the adrenaline produced side-effects without vasoconstriction it was recommended that in dentistry the volume injected should be restricted and that the technique should only be used when unavoidable.— H. Cannell and P. D. Cannon, *Br. dent. J.*, 1976, *141*, 48.

A study involving 37 patients with acutely painful teeth indicated that a 5% solution of lignocaine with adrenaline 1 in 80 000 was preferable to a 2% solution for infiltration or inferior alveolar block.— D. J. Eldridge and J. P. Rood, *Br. dent. J.*, 1977, *142*, 129. See also J. P. Rood, *Br. dent. J.*, 1976, *140*, 413.

Dialysis pruritus. In a preliminary study lignocaine 200 mg in 100 ml of physiological saline given during dialysis as an infusion through the arterial line of the artificial kidney over a 20-minute period provided some relief of itching to all of 20 patients with persistent severe pruritus during haemodialysis; none responded to physiological saline alone. In a subsequent double-blind study 8 of 10 patients obtained relief of pruritus following lignocaine therapy whereas only 1 of 6 did so after saline placebo.— L. Tapia *et al.*, *New Engl. J. Med.*, 1977, *296*, 261.

Dumping syndrome. Lignocaine hydrochloride 2% viscous solution in doses of 15 ml thrice daily an hour before meals prevents the dumping syndrome by dampening the mechanical shock of food ingestion.— A. A. Concon (letter), *Lancet*, 1981, *1*, 1429.

Epidural block. Blood loss during major vaginal surgery was reduced to about one-third when lignocaine hydrochloride was used for epidural analgesia, compared with the loss under general anaesthesia. Hypotension was only partly responsible for reduced bleeding.— D. Moir, *Br. J. Anaesth.*, 1968, *40*, 233.

Dose requirements for epidural analgesia with lignocaine 2% with adrenaline 1 in 200 000 were at a maximum in the age range 16 to 22 and fell linearly for younger and older patients. Because the degree of segmental spread increased in patients below 10 and over 80 years of age, doses are best administered to these patients in fractions at 10-minute intervals.— P. R. Bromage, *Br. J. Anaesth.*, 1969, *41*, 1016.

The cardiovascular effects of lignocaine, with or without adrenaline, in epidural block in patients under light general anaesthesia.— D. B. Scott *et al.*, *Br. J. Anaesth.*, 1977, *49*, 917.

There was no evidence of significant plasma accumulation of lignocaine in 6 patients given lignocaine 400 mg epidurally (as 2% solution) before surgery followed by 4 doses of 200 mg at 1-hour intervals for postoperative pain relief.— G. T. Tucker *et al.*, *Br. J. Anaesth.*, 1977, *49*, 237.

See also under Caudal Block (above).

In obstetrics. Maternal and foetal blood concentrations of lignocaine were determined in 42 patients after epidural injection of 20 ml of 2% lignocaine with adrenaline 1 in 250 000 (24 patients) and without adrenaline (18 patients). The mean maternal plasma concentrations were 2.62 and 3.43 µg per ml respectively. Cord plasma concentrations were not significantly different between the 2 groups at any time intervals. The addition of adrenaline increased the safety of the procedure for the mother but not to the same degree for the foetus.— J. Thomas *et al.*, *Br. J. Anaesth.*, 1969, *41*, 1029.

Of 1533 nulliparous patients, 1000 were given an epidural block using lignocaine 1% with adrenaline 1 : 200 000 during labour and delivery. Freedom from pain was achieved in 61.2 and 70.8% during labour and delivery respectively, with satisfactory relief of pain in a further 29.9 and 15.9%. There was no evidence of an increase in forceps delivery. Some patients had headache because of dural puncture. Some degree of hypotension occurred in 7.9% of patients receiving the block. There was no evidence of decreased Apgar scores or increased foetal mortality.— N. Potter and R. D. Macdonald, *Lancet*, 1971, *1*, 1031.

In 9 healthy women placental blood flow was not significantly reduced by extradural analgesia with lignocaine prior to caesarean section.— R. Jouppila *et al.*, *Br. J. Anaesth.*, 1978, *50*, 275.

Epilepsy. Status epilepticus in one patient was controlled by an intravenous bolus injection of lignocaine hydrochloride 30 mg after treatment with diazepam, phenobarbitone, and phenytoin had failed.— W. P. Zmyslowski (letter), *J. Am. med. Ass.*, 1976, *236*, 2173. Lignocaine has generally been ineffective in controlling status epilepticus.— S. Schneider (letter), *ibid.*, 2174.

A report of the succesful control of epileptic convulsions in 4 patients using conventional anticonvulsant therapy and lignocaine, given intravenously. The preferred method for the administration of lignocaine is considered to be as an intravenous infusion of 200 to 300 mg per hour, in adults, to achieve a blood concentration of 2 to 5 µg per ml.— L. J. Lemmen *et al.*, *J. Am. med. Ass.*, 1978, *239*, 2025.

Further references to the use of lignocaine as an anticonvulsant: H. H. Morris, *Sth. med. J.*, 1979, *72*, 1564.

Hyperhidrosis. A eutectic mixture of 5% lignocaine (base) and 5% prilocaine (base) had a greater inhibitory effect on adrenaline-induced sweating in 12 healthy subjects than 10% lignocaine alone, 10% prilocaine alone, or placebo. When compared with placebo a striking inhibition of sweating was seen in the majority of 17 patients with hyperhidrosis when about 2 to 3 ml of the eutectic mixture was applied as an emulsion for 1 hour under an occlusive dressing on one hand and axilla. The effect persisted for up to 6 hours. However, the treatment was less effective when used daily at home.— L. Juhlin *et al.*, *Acta derm.-vener., Stockh.*, 1979, *59*, 556.

Infiltration anaesthesia. Comment that a 0.5% rather than a 1% solution of lignocaine is generally adequate for the production of local anaesthesia by infiltration, the only apparent disadvantage being the shorter mean duration of anaesthesia reported for the weaker solution—75 minutes against 127 minutes.— G. Bashein (letter), *New Engl. J. Med.*, 1980, *302*, 122.

Intubation. Intubation was achieved in 12 conscious patients by the following procedure: compound sodium lactate injection intravenously; phenoperidine and droperidol to reduce pain and allay apprehension; puncture of cricothyroid membrane (after infiltration with lignocaine) and rapid injection into the trachea of 1.5 ml of lignocaine 4%; 4% lignocaine swabs progressively to anaesthetise the tongue, fauces, uvula, and soft palate; liberal spraying of vocal cords with 4% lignocaine; intubation; proceeding to anaesthesia and surgery. Light sedation was necessary to avoid restlessness and straining, and atropine to reduce salivation and for its effect on the vagus.— J. A. T. Duncan, *Br. J. Anaesth.*, 1977, *49*, 619.

Further references to the use of lignocaine in intubation: J. K. Denlinger *et al.*, *Anesthesiology*, 1974, *41*, 409.

Mouth ulcers. A viscous preparation containing lignocaine 0.5%, diluted 1 to 5 with water, might be used just before eating to relieve the pain of oral ulceration such as might occur during treatment for leukaemia with folic acid antagonists.— R. A. Kyle and J. E. Maldonado, *Mayo Clin. Proc.*, 1966, *41*, 383.

Pain. Based on experience of more than 1000 patients with craniocervical injuries and symptoms of nerve entrapment, treatment consisted of the injection of 1 or 2% alcohol in 3 to 5 ml of 2% lignocaine with 2 ml of a depot preparation of methylprednisolone acetate; diazepam and phenylbutazone were also given. Weekly injections cleared 60% of the symptoms in 6 weeks and 90% in 12 weeks.— R. Cilento (letter), *Br. med. J.*, 1972, *4*, 789.

The most useful treatment for temporomandibular joint disorders, often difficult to diagnose, appeared to be the intra-articular injection of 1 ml of 2% lignocaine; complete relief might occur after 3 to 5 injections.— C. W. Norris and K. Eakins, *Laryngoscope, St. Louis*, 1974, *9*, 1466, per *Practitioner*, 1975, *214*, 316.

A report that perurethral instillation of lignocaine gel immediately after cystoscopy under general anaesthesia ensures analgesia during the painful 24 to 48-hour period which follows this procedure.— D. Blatchley (letter), *Br. med. J.*, 1977, *1*, 1416.

Pain associated with translumbar aortography can be eliminated by adding 2 ml of 2% lignocaine per 40 ml of contrast medium to be injected intra-arterially.— R. S. Dossetor (letter), *Br. med. J.*, 1978, *2*, 127. For further reports on the intra-arterial use of lignocaine as an analgesic during angiography, see I. J. Gordon and J. L. Westcott, *Radiology*, 1977, *124*, 43; D. F. Guthaner *et al.*, *Am. J. Roentg.*, 1977, *128*, 737; W. C. Widrich *et al.*, *Radiology*, 1977, *124*, 37; Y. Ben-Menachem, *Am. J. Roentg.*, 1978, *130*, 360; R. L. Eisenberg *et al.*, *Radiology*, 1978, *127*, 109; W. C. Widrich *et al.*, *Radiology*, 1978, *129*, 371.

The direct injection of lignocaine into metastatic bone lesions has been used to control intractable bone pain in 9 cancer patients. Complete pain relief was achieved in 5 patients after the intralesional injection of 2 to 3 ml of a 2% lignocaine solution. On the return of pain these 5 patients were re-injected with a suspension of 1 part lignocaine 2% to 2 parts procaine penicillin 600 mg per ml in volumes of up to 6 ml. Pain relief lasting from 3 to 4 days was achieved in 4 of the patients and for 24 hours in the fifth. Lesions of the spine should not be treated in this way.— J. I. Zweig *et al.*, *J. Am. med. Ass.*, 1980, *244*, 2445.

Regional anaesthesia, intravenous. Complete regional anaesthesia was achieved in 47 of 50 children, and partial anaesthesia (some discomfort) in 2, with simple forearm fractures or elbow dislocations. With a tourniquet around the upper arm lignocaine 4 mg per kg body-weight was given intravenously in a concentration of 0.5%. There were no complications.— B. FitzGerald, *Br. J. Anaesth.*, 1976, *48*, 485.

Further references to intravenous regional anaesthesia with lignocaine: T. B. Scarff, *Surg. Neurol.*, 1974, *2*, 225, per *J. Am. med. Ass.*, 1974, *230*, 629.

Regional nerve block. In 421 patients requiring surgery of the hand, all soft tissue to be operated upon was slowly infiltrated with the minimum amount of a solution containing lignocaine 0.5% and adrenaline 1 in 200 000. A fine low-intensity cautery for complete haemostasis was essential. The procedure eliminated the need for tourniquets or for general anaesthesia, though in some children the latter supplemented the procedure. There were no ischaemic complications.— H. A. Johnson, *J. Am. med. Ass.*, 1967, *200*, 990.

In 30 patients requiring haemodialysis, vasodilatation following brachial plexus block with lignocaine hydrochloride 1% and adrenaline 1 in 200 000 facilitated the insertion of intravenous cannulas of adequate size; leakage was slight subsequently.— B. J. Urban *et al.*, *J. Am. med. Ass.*, 1967, *199*, 889.

The recommended average dose of lignocaine hydrochloride for regional anaesthesia was 300 mg as 0.5% solution, 250 mg as 1% solution, and 200 mg as 2% solution. The maximum dose should not exceed 300 mg. When adrenaline was added, the respective figures were 500, 450, and 400 mg, with a maximum of 500 mg.— L. Eisenberg, *J. Am. med. Ass.*, 1968, *206*, 2531.

Blocking of the medial and lateral plantar nerves at the ankle by the use of 3 to 6 ml of lignocaine 1% with adrenaline 1 in 200 000 was successful in establishing anaesthesia prior to curetting plantar warts.— W. G. R. M. Laurie (letter), *Br. med. J.*, 1972, *3*, 116.

Further references to regional nerve block with lignocaine: P. R. Bromage and M. Gertel, *Anesthesiology*, 1972, *36*, 479 (supraclavicular brachial block); C. R. Wheeless, *Obstet. Gynec.*, 1972, *39*, 767 (partial salpingectomy).

See also Caudal Block and Epidural Block (above).

Respiratory disorders. If conventional treatment of acute and chronic obstructive pulmonary disease was ineffective, lignocaine hydrochloride given initially as a bolus intravenously followed by an infusion over the next 12 to 24 hours, might be effective, and bronchodilator therapy could be gradually discontinued.— A. Manheim (letter), *J. Am. med. Ass.*, 1972, *220*, 1500.

Lignocaine given intravenously suppressed the cough reflex and facilitated bronchography.— F. R. Smith and P. C. Kundahl, *Chest*, 1973, *63*, 427.

References to the effect of lignocaine by aerosol on increased respiratory resistance: R. W. Loehning *et al.*, *Anesthesiology*, 1976, *44*, 306; E. B. Weiss and A. V. Patwardhan, *Chest*, 1977, *72*, 429.

See also Cough (above).

Spinal anaesthesia. The potency ratio of amethocaine to lignocaine for spinal anaesthesia is 1 : 6.79.— C. W. White *et al.*, *Br. J. Anaesth.*, 1966, *38*, 185.

Chronic low back pain in 46 patients was diagnosed as of organic origin in 27 by successive subarachnoid injections of 5, 25, and 50 mg of lignocaine in sodium chloride injection to produce differential spinal blockade.— M. A. Brothers and D. C. Finlayson, *Can. Anaesth. Soc. J.*, 1968, *15*, 478.

Stings. The stings from fish with venomous spines, including weevers, short-spined cottus, spiny dogfish, and stingray, may be treated by infiltration with lignocaine 1%.— D. A. Warrell, *Prescribers' J.*, 1979, *19*, 190.

Surface anaesthesia. In a double-blind study in 215 infants, the analgesic effect of a teething solution containing 0.3% lignocaine hydrochloride and 0.3% benzyl alcohol appeared to be better than a control solution. In all the infants the control solution had some analgesic effect.— M. H. Seward, *Br. dent. J.*, 1969, *127*, 457.

Local anaesthesia over the site of minor operations had been induced in over 8000 patients, without adverse effect, by the application under occlusive dressings of 30% lignocaine cream.— H. M. Lubens *et al.*, *Am. J. Dis. Child.*, 1974, *128*, 192.

Endoscopy was performed in more than 1000 patients with no medication other than the use of lignocaine throat spray.— W. S. C. Chao (letter), *Br. med. J.*, 1975, *1*, 97.

In 6 patients the mean maximum plasma-lignocaine concentration was 1.03 µg per ml after the endotracheal application of ten 10-mg metered doses of lignocaine; in 5 patients paralysed with suxamethonium the maximum concentration of lignocaine following the application of 100 mg was 1.6 µg per ml. These values were below those at which toxicity was likely to occur.— D. B. Scott *et al.*, *Br. J. Anaesth.*, 1976, *48*, 899.

Comment on the use of topical anaesthesia for endoscopy. With the advent of the fibreoptic bronchoscope, topical anaesthesia of the larynx and trachea can be achieved by injecting the agent down the bronchoscope itself.— *Lancet*, 1980, *2*, 1064.

Further references to the use of lignocaine before endoscopy: R. K. Stoelting, *Anesthesiology*, 1977, *47*, 381.

For a view that unlike the procaine series of local anaesthetics, lignocaine only rarely sensitises and is a useful antipruritic drug topically, see Antihistamines, p.1294.

See also Intubation (above) and for urethral anaesthesia see under Overdosage in Adverse Effects (p.903).

Thrombo-embolisms, prophylaxis. A 2% solution of lignocaine was given as a bolus intravenous injection over 5 minutes in a dose of 1 mg per kg body-weight 2 hours before anaesthesia to 28 patients undergoing elective hip surgery. Lignocaine infusion was then continued for 6 days at a rate of 2 mg per minute. Deep-vein thrombosis occurred in 11 of 14 control patients postoperatively; in 8 patients thigh veins were involved. There were 6 calf-vein thromboses in the 28 treated patients during the period of lignocaine administration. However, when lignocaine was discontinued another 9 patients developed thromboses and in 6 the thigh veins were involved. More prolonged prophylaxis might be desirable. There was no toxicity or hypersensitivity.— E. D. Cooke *et al.* (preliminary communication), *Lancet*, 1977, *2*, 797.

Tinnitus. Lignocaine significantly reduced tinnitus when assessed audiometrically and subjectively in a double-blind crossover study in 32 patients. Lignocaine 2% was given intravenously in a dose of 1.5 mg per kg body-weight and was compared with an equal volume of sodium chloride injection.— F. W. Martin and B. H. Colman, *Clin. Otolaryngol.*, 1980, *5*, 3.

Further references to the use of intravenous lignocaine in tinnitus: P. S. Melding *et al.*, *J. Lar. Otol.*, 1978, *92*, 115; J. J. Shea and M. Harell, *Laryngoscope, St. Louis*, 1978, *88*, 1477.

For the use of lignocaine to predict those patients with tinnitus who may respond to carbamazepine or phenytoin therapy, see Carbamazepine, p.1248.

Vasectomy. An injection of 10 ml of 1% lignocaine solution into each vas at the time of vasectomy hastened sterility.— B. B. Errey (letter), *Med. J. Aust.*, 1977, *1*, 642.

Venepuncture. Prior intradermal injection of 0.1 ml of lignocaine reduced the pain of venepuncture compared with prior intradermal injection of 0.1 ml of isotonic saline used as control.— G. Sultany *et al.* (letter), *New Engl. J. Med.*, 1975, *293*, 830. The saline control was not a placebo; intradermal saline gave better results than lignocaine because there was no initial burning sensation.— L. C. Mark (letter), *ibid.*, 1976, *294*, 614. Intradermal saline injection was not painless and could be difficult in patients with thin skin.— A. M. Smith (letter), *ibid.*, 1013. A study in healthy subjects confirming the good results with Mark's technique.— N. H. G. Holford *et al.* (letter), *ibid.*, 1977, *296*, 1300.

A view that when it is necessary to use glucose or other irritant intravenous solutions, infusion phlebitis can be minimised by the administration of 2 ml of a 1 or 2% solution of lignocaine or procaine.— G. T. Watts (letter), *Br. med. J.*, 1977, *2*, 462.

Preparations of Lignocaine and Lignocaine Hydrochloride

Lidocaine Hydrochloride and Epinephrine Injection *(U.S.P.)*. A sterile solution prepared from lignocaine or lignocaine hydrochloride and adrenaline with the aid of hydrochloric acid in Water for Injections. It contains not more than 1 in 50 000 of adrenaline. pH 3.3 to 5.5.

Lidocaine Hydrochloride Injection *(U.S.P.)*. A sterile solution of lignocaine hydrochloride in Water for Injections, or of lignocaine in Water for Injections prepared with the aid of hydrochloric acid. pH 5 to 7.

Lidocaine Hydrochloride Jelly *(U.S.P.)*. Lignocaine hydrochloride in a suitable sterile water-soluble viscous basis. pH 6 to 7. Store in airtight containers.

Lidocaine Ointment *(U.S.P.)*. Contains lignocaine in a suitable hydrophilic ointment basis. Store in airtight containers.

Lidocaine Topical Aerosol *(U.S.P.)*. Lidocaine Aerosol. A solution of lignocaine in a suitable flavoured vehicle with suitable propellents in a pressurised container equipped with a metered-dose valve.

Lignocaine and Adrenaline Injection *(B.P.)*. Lignocaine and Adren. Inj. A sterile solution containing lignocaine hydrochloride and adrenaline acid tartrate in Water for Injections containing the equivalent of 0.1% of sulphur dioxide. Sterilised by autoclaving. pH 3 to 4.5. Protect from light.

Lignocaine and Adrenaline Injection in 10-ml ampoules could be autoclaved at 134° for 3.75 minutes up to 6 times without loss of adrenaline.— T. R. Lowther and J. King, *J. Hosp. Pharm.*, 1973, *31*, 218.

Lignocaine Eye Drops *(A.P.F.)*. Lignocaine hydrochloride 4 g, chlorhexidine acetate 10 mg, Water for Injections to 100 ml. Sterilised by autoclaving.

Lignocaine Gel *(B.P.C. 1973)*. Lignocaine Hydrochloride Gel. A sterilised solution of lignocaine hydrochloride in a suitable water-miscible basis containing chlorhexidine gluconate or a mixture of the sodium salts of methyl hydroxybenzoate and propyl hydroxybenzoate. Sterilised by autoclaving. Store in sealed sterilised collapsible tubes.

Lignocaine Hydrochloride Injection *(B.P.)*. Lignocaine Injection. A sterile solution in Water for Injections. Sterilised by autoclaving.

Proprietary Preparations of Lignocaine and Lignocaine Hydrochloride

Instillagel *(Farco-Pharma, Ger.: Rimmer, UK)*. Sterile gel containing lignocaine hydrochloride 2% and chlorhexidine gluconate solution 0.25%. For urethral, vaginal, and rectal surface anaesthesia and for instrument lubrication.

Laryng-O-Jet *(IMS, UK)*. A cartridge assembly designed for laryngo-tracheal anaesthesia containing a sterile solution of lignocaine hydrochloride 4%.

Lidocaton *(Pharmaton, Switz.: Ash Dental, UK)*. Lignocaine hydrochloride, available as 2% solution for injection in cartridges of 2.2 ml; also 2% with adrenaline 1 in 80 000 in cartridges of 2.2 ml.

Lidothesin *(Pharmaceutical Mfg, UK)*. Lignocaine hydrochloride, for injection, available as solutions of the following strengths: 0.5% in ampoules of 2, 5, and 10 ml, vials of 20 and 50 ml, and dental cartridges of 2.2 ml; 1% in ampoules of 2, 5, and 10 ml, vials of 20 and 50 ml, and dental cartridges of 2.2 ml; 1.5% in vials of 20 ml; 2% in ampoules of 2, 5, 10, and 20 ml, vials of 20 and 50 ml, and dental cartridges of 2.2 ml; also 0.5% with adrenaline 1 in 200 000 in vials of 20 and 50 ml and dental cartridges of 2.2 ml; 1% with adrenaline 1 in 100 000 in ampoules of 5 and 10 ml, and vials of 20 and 50 ml; 2% with adrenaline 1 in 100 000 in ampoules of 2, 5, and 10 ml, and vials of 20 and 50 ml; and 2% with adrenaline or noradrenaline 1 in 80 000 in dental cartridges of 2.2 ml.

Lidothesin *(Pharmaceutical Mfg, UK)*. **1% Antiseptic Gel.** A sterile preparation containing lignocaine hydrochloride 1% and chlorhexidine gluconate solution 0.25% in a water-miscible lubricant basis. For urethral, vaginal, and rectal surface anaesthesia and for instrument lubrication. **2% Antiseptic Gel** is also available. **Solution.** Contains lignocaine hydrochloride 4%.

Lidothesin 5% Plain *(Pharmaceutical Mfg, UK)*. Lignocaine hydrochloride, available as a solution containing 50 mg per ml, in ampoules of 10 ml, for dilution to 500 ml for intravenous infusion. Protect from light.

Lignocaine in Dextrose Injection *(Travenol, UK)*. A solution for intravenous injection containing lignocaine hydrochloride 0.1% or 0.2% and anhydrous dextrose 5%. For prevention and control of ventricular arrhythmias.

Lignostab *(Boots, UK)*. Lignocaine hydrochloride, available as an injection containing 2% in dental cartridges of 2 ml. **Lignostab-A** contains lignocaine hydrochloride 2% with adrenaline 1 in 80 000. **Lignostab-A '100'** contains lignocaine hydrochloride 2% with adrenaline 1 in 100 000. **Lignostab-N** contains lignocaine hydrochloride 2% with noradrenaline 1 in 80 000.

Minims Lignocaine and Fluorescein *(Smith & Nephew Pharmaceuticals, UK)*. Sterile eye-drops containing lignocaine hydrochloride 4% and fluorescein sodium 0.25% in single-use disposable applicators.

NOTE. The code LIG FLN is permitted in Great Britain for single-dose eye-drops of lignocaine and fluorescein.

Neo-Lidocaton 2% *(Pharmaton, Switz.: Ash Dental, UK)*. Solution for injection, containing lignocaine hydrochloride 2%, noradrenaline 1 in 50 000, and vasopressin 0.25 units per ml, in cartridges of 2.2 ml. **Neo-Lidocaton Forte 3%** contains the above ingredients but with lignocaine hydrochloride 3%.

Oral-B Dental Gel *(Cooper, UK)*. Contains lignocaine 0.6%, cetylpyridinium chloride 0.02%, menthol 0.06%, and cineole 0.1%. For painful conditions of the oral mucosa.

Uro-Jet *(IMS, UK)*. A cartridge assembly containing lignocaine gel 2%, designed for urethral instillation.

Xylocaine *(Astra, UK)*. Anhydrous lignocaine hydrochloride, for use by injection, available as solutions in the following strengths: 0.5% in ampoules of 10 ml and vials of 20 and 50 ml; 1% in ampoules of 2 and 10 ml, and vials of 20 and 50 ml; 1.5% in ampoules of 25 ml; 2% in cartridges of 2 ml, ampoules of 5 ml, and vials of 20 and 50 ml; also with adrenaline 1 in 200 000, 0.5% in vials of 50 ml, 1% in ampoules of 10 ml, and vials of 20 and 50 ml and 2% in vials of 20 and 50 ml; 2% with adrenaline 1 in 80 000 in cartridges of 2 ml. Vial and cartridge packs of these preparations contain methyl hydroxybenzoate 0.1%; all packs containing adrenaline contain sodium metabisulphite 0.055%. (Also available as Xylocaine in *Austral., Belg., Canad., Fr., Jap., Neth., Switz., USA*).

Xylocaine *(Astra, UK)*. Lignocaine hydrochloride, for ophthalmic use, available as **4% Eye Drops** containing anhydrous lignocaine hydrochloride 4%.

Xylocaine *(Astra, UK)*. Lignocaine hydrochloride, for topical use, available as **Antiseptic Gel,** a sterile preparation containing anhydrous lignocaine hydrochloride 2% and chlorhexidine gluconate solution 0.25% v/v; as **Gel,** a sterile preparation containing anhydrous lignocaine hydrochloride 2%; as **Ointment** containing lignocaine (base) 5% in water-miscible basis; as an aerosol **Spray** containing lignocaine (base) 8 g, cetylpyridinium chloride 8 mg, menthol 40 mg, cineole 24 mg, and vehicle (polyethylene glycol and alcohol) and propellent to 82 g, and delivering lignocaine 10 mg in each spray dose; as **Xylocaine 4% Topical,** an aqueous solution containing anhydrous lignocaine hydrochloride 4%; and as **Xylocaine Viscous Solution,** containing anhydrous lignocaine hydrochloride 2%, for surface analgesia of the upper digestive tract.

Xylocard 100 mg *(Astra, UK)*. Anhydrous lignocaine hydrochloride, available as a solution containing 20 mg per ml, in disposable syringes of 5 ml for slow intravenous bolus injection. **Xylocard 1 g.** Anhydrous lignocaine hydrochloride, available as a solution containing 200 mg per ml, in disposable syringes of 5 ml for dilution to 500 ml for intravenous infusion. **Xylocard 2 g.** Anhydrous lignocaine hydrochloride, available as a solution containing 200 mg per ml in disposable syringes of 10 ml, for dilution to 500 ml for intravenous infusion. (Also available as Xylocard in *Austral., Belg., Canad., Fr., Neth., Norw.*).

Xylodase *(Astra, UK)*. A cream containing lignocaine (base) 5% and hyaluronidase 0.015%, in a water-miscible basis.

Xyloproct *(Astra, UK)*. **Ointment** containing in each g lignocaine 50 mg, aluminium acetate 35 mg, zinc oxide 180 mg, and hydrocortisone acetate 2.75 mg, and **Suppositories** each containing lignocaine 60 mg, aluminium acetate 50 mg, zinc oxide 400 mg, and hydrocortisone acetate 5 mg. For haemorrhoids and other ano-rectal conditions.

Xylotox *(Pharmaceutical Mfg, UK)*. Lignocaine hydrochloride, for injection, available as a solution containing the equivalent of lignocaine 2% in dental cartridges of 2.2 ml, and 2% with adrenaline or noradrenaline 1 in 80 000 in dental cartridges of 1.8 or 2.2 ml. (Also available as Xylotox in *Austral., Neth., S.Afr., Switz.*).

Xylotox *(Pharmaceutical Mfg, UK)*. Preparations for topical use available as **Jelly** containing lignocaine hydrochloride 2%; as **Ointment** containing lignocaine (base) 5% in a water-miscible basis; as **Extra Paste** containing lignocaine (base) 5% and amethocaine hydrochloride 2%; as **Normal Paste** containing lignocaine (base) 5%; as **Spray** containing lignocaine (base) 10% in a non-alcoholic antibacterial vehicle in an aerosol container delivering in each metered dose lignocaine (base) 10 mg; and as **Xylotox 4%** containing lignocaine hydrochloride 4% with adrenaline 1 in 50 000.

Xylotox Oral *(Pharmaceutical Mfg, UK)*. A solution of lignocaine hydrochloride 2% in a viscous basis. For surface anaesthesia of the upper digestive tract.

Other Proprietary Names

Arg.—Xylocaina; *Austral.*—Leostesin, Nurocain, Sarnacaine; *Canad.*—Democaine; *Denm.*—Leostesin, Xylocain; *Ger.*— Neo-Novutox, Xylocain; *Ital.*—Luan, Ortodermina; *Norw.*—Leostesin, Xylocain; *S.Afr.*—Leostesin, Peterkaien, Remicane, Remicard; *Switz.*—Cito-Optadren, Lidocaton, Rapidocaine, Xylesin; *USA*—Anestacon, Lida-Mantle, Lidopen, Ultracaine.

7603-v

Amethocaine.

Tetracaine *(U.S.P.)*. 2-Dimethylaminoethyl 4-butylaminobenzoate.

$C_{15}H_{24}N_2O_2$=264.4.

CAS — 94-24-6.

Pharmacopoeias. In *U.S.*

A white or light yellow waxy solid. M.p. 41° to 46°. Very slightly **soluble** in water; soluble 1 in 5 of alcohol and 1 in 2 of chloroform and ether. **Store** in airtight containers. Protect from light.

7604-g

Amethocaine Hydrochloride *(B.P.)*.

Tetracaine Hydrochloride *(Eur. P., U.S.P.)*; Tetracaini Hydrochloridum; Tetracainii Chloridum; Dicainum.

$C_{15}H_{24}N_2O_2$,HCl=300.8.

CAS — 136-47-0.

Pharmacopoeias. In *Arg., Aust., Br., Braz., Chin., Cz., Eur., Fr., Ger., Hung., Ind., Int., It., Jap., Jug., Mex., Neth., Nord., Pol., Port., Rus., Swiss, Turk.*, and *U.S.*
U.S. also includes Sterile Tetracaine Hydrochloride; *Nord.* also includes Amethocaine Nitrate.

A white, odourless, hygroscopic, crystalline powder with a slightly bitter numbing taste. It melts at about 148° or may occur in either of 2 polymorphic forms which melt at about 134° and 139° respectively. Mixtures of the forms may melt within the range 134° to 147°.

Soluble 1 in 7.5 of water, 1 in 40 of alcohol, and 1 in 30 of chloroform; soluble in glycerol; practically insoluble in acetone and ether. A 1% solution in water has a pH of 4.5 to 6.5. Solutions are **sterilised** by autoclaving, by maintaining at 98° to 100° for 30 minutes with a bactericide, or by filtration. **Incompatible** with alkalis, iodides, and inorganic mercury and silver salts. **Store** in airtight containers. Protect from light. Aqueous solutions should be discarded if discoloured or cloudy.

Incompatibility. In aqueous solutions of amethocaine hydrochloride approximately 20% was bound in the presence of polysorbate 80 in a concentration of 5%, and in a concentration of 10% approximately 30% became bound to the polysorbate.— A. R. Hurwitz *et al.*, *J. pharm. Sci.*, 1963, *52*, 893.

Preservative for eye-drops. Benzalkonium chloride 0.01% was a suitable preservative for amethocaine hydrochloride eye-drops sterilised by filtration.— M. Van Ooteghem, *Pharm. Tijdschr. Belg.*, 1968, *45*, 69.

Prolonged effect. Local anaesthetic effects of 0.15 and 0.25% injections of amethocaine hydrochloride with adrenaline 1 in 200 000 were prolonged by replacing sodium chloride injection with dextran 6% in sodium chloride injection as the basis for the injection.— M. A. Chinn and K. Wirjoatmadja (letter), *Lancet*, 1967, *2*, 835.

Further references to the prolongation of the effect of amethocaine.— A. M. Kuiantseva *et al.*, *Farmatsiya, Mosk.*, 1977, *26*, 22; L. A. Tsvykh, *Farmatsiya, Mosk.*, 1979, *28*, 24.

Stability of solutions. The presence of sodium chloride very slightly reduced the rate of hydrolysis of amethocaine hydrochloride and of procaine hydrochloride; this was attributed to the slight reduction of pH of solutions by sodium chloride. However, the presence of sodium chloride reduced by about 50% the time in which the appearance of colour occurred.— R. E. Thomas and M. Woodward, *Australas. J. Pharm.*, 1963, *44*, S90.

The stability of solutions of amethocaine hydrochloride did not appear to be affected by the addition of dextrose.— N. Harb, *J. Hosp. Pharm.*, 1969, *26*, 44.

Sterilisation. Aqueous solutions of amethocaine hydrochloride could be sterilised by heating with a bactericide at 98° to 100° for 30 minutes and ampoules could be sterilised in an autoclave without serious decomposition. Repeated and prolonged autoclaving however was undesirable. Injections of amethocaine hydrochloride containing electrolytes should be prepared aseptically.— P. Chalaresunthornvatee and R. E. Thomas, *Australas. J. Pharm.*, 1961, *42*, 800.

Amethocaine hydrochloride in 1% solution at pH 5.6 hydrolysed to the extent of 3.5% after autoclaving at 115° for 30 minutes. In a similar solution adjusted initially to pH 4 it hydrolysed to the extent of less than 1%.— D. A. Norton, *J. Hosp. Pharm.*, 1967, *48*, 328.

Adverse Effects and Treatment. As for Local Anaesthetics, p.899.

Allergy. A 62-year-old man was given an amethocaine lozenge to suck half an hour before his throat was anaesthetised prior to bronchoscopy. He showed no reaction to the lozenge but while ½ to 1 ml of a solution of amethocaine hydrochloride was being sprayed on the throat he went into convulsions and died within 3 minutes.— *Br. med. J.*, 1955, *1*, 610.

Precautions. As for Local Anaesthetics, p.900.

Amethocaine is hydrolysed in the body to *p*-aminobenzoic acid and may inhibit the action of sulphonamides.

Absorption and Fate. See under Local Anaesthetics, p.900.

Uses. As for Local Anaesthetics, p.901.

Amethocaine is a potent local anaesthetic of the ester type. Its local anaesthetic action is greater than that of lignocaine and it is used in lower concentrations, though its systemic toxicity is several times greater. Amethocaine has vasodilator properties; the risk of adverse effects can be reduced by the addition of adrenaline to delay absorption.

Amethocaine is mainly used as a surface anaesthetic. It is 5 to 10 times more potent than cocaine but its action is more prolonged. A 0.5 to 2% solution of amethocaine hydrochloride has been used for surface anaesthesia but lignocaine hydrochloride is safer and is generally preferred. Up to 8 ml of a 0.5% solution has been used as a throat spray before endoscopy; lozenges containing 60 mg have also been used.

In ophthalmology, a 0.25 to 1% solution is employed; stronger solutions may damage the cornea. A 0.5% eye ointment of amethocaine is also used. A 0.5% ointment or a 1% cream is used in painful conditions of the anus or rectum.

Amethocaine hydrochloride will provide spinal anaesthesia for 2 to 3 hours or more and is injected in doses of 5 to 20 mg, usually as a 0.5% solution. Hyperbaric solutions containing 5% of dextrose and hypobaric solutions are used.

Spinal anaesthesia. References to spinal anaesthesia with amethocaine.— A. P. Winnie, *J. Am. med. Ass.*, 1969, *207*, 1663 (lower incidence of hypotension and mortality with patients induced in the supine position than in the lateral position); B. Root (letter), *ibid.*, *208*, 1192 (criticism); T. Kallos and T. C. Smith, *Anesth. Analg. curr. Res.*, 1972, *51*, 766 (hypobaric); H. Rosenberg, *Anesthesiology*, 1976, *45*, 682 (hypobaric); D. T. Brown *et al.*, *Br. J. Anaesth.*, 1980, *52*, 589 (comparison of hyperbaric, isobaric, and hypobaric solutions).

Preparations Containing Amethocaine and Amethocaine Hydrochloride

Amethocaine Eye Drops *(A.P.F.)*. Amethocaine hydrochloride 1 g, boric acid 1.5 g, sodium metabisulphite 100 mg, phenylmercuric nitrate 2 mg, Water for Injections to 100 ml. Sterilised by autoclaving.

Amethocaine Eye Drops *(B.P.)*. Guttae Amethocainae; AME. A sterile solution of amethocaine hydrochloride in water. When intended for use on more than one occasion they contain the equivalent of not more than 0.1% of sulphur dioxide and 0.002% of phenylmercuric acetate or nitrate; such drops should not be used more than one month after first opening the container. Protect from light.

This solution is adversely affected by alkali.

F.N. Belg. has Oculoguttae Tetracaini Hydrochloridi containing phenylmercuric borate.

Amethocaine Lollipops. To granulated sugar 150 g and potassium acid tartrate 500 mg, add water 50 ml, and heat to 154°. Add amethocaine hydrochloride 900 mg, soluble essence of lemon 0.5 ml, green colour solution 2 ml, and water 5 ml. Pour into starch moulds. The quantity given was sufficient for 30 lollipops. For use before bronchoscopy.—T.D. Whittet *et al.*, *Chemist Drugg.*, 1951, *156*, 731.

Sterile Tetracaine Hydrochloride *(U.S.P.)*. Amethocaine hydrochloride suitable for parenteral use. A 1% solution has a pH of 5 to 6.

Tetracaine Hydrochloride Cream *(U.S.P.)*. Amethocaine hydrochloride in a suitable water-miscible basis. Potency is expressed in terms of the equivalent amount of amethocaine. pH 3.2 to 3.8.

Tetracaine Hydrochloride Injection *(U.S.P.)*. A sterile solution of amethocaine hydrochloride in Water for Injections. pH 3.2 to 6. Store at 2° to 8°. It should not be used if it contains crystals or is cloudy or discoloured.

Tetracaine Hydrochloride Ophthalmic Solution *(U.S.P.)*. A sterile aqueous solution of amethocaine hydrochloride. It may contain suitable antimicrobial and thickening agents. pH 3.7 to 6. Store in airtight containers. Protect from light. It should not be used if it contains crystals or is cloudy or discoloured.

Tetracaine Hydrochloride Topical Solution *(U.S.P.)*. An aqueous solution of amethocaine hydrochloride containing a suitable antimicrobial agent. pH 4.5 to 6. Store in airtight containers. Protect from light. It should not be used if it contains crystals or is cloudy or discoloured.

Tetracaine Ointment *(U.S.P.)*. Amethocaine in a suitable ointment basis.

Tetracaine Ophthalmic Ointment *(U.S.P.)*. A sterile eye ointment containing amethocaine 0.45 to 0.55% in white soft paraffin.

Proprietary Preparations Containing Amethocaine and Amethocaine Hydrochloride

Anethaine Cream *(Farley, UK)*. Contains amethocaine hydrochloride 1% in a vanishing cream basis. (Also available as Anethaine in *S.Afr.*).

Biosone GA Dental Paste *(Biorex, UK)*. Contains amethocaine hydrochloride 2%, cinchocaine 2%, enoxolone 1%, and neomycin sulphate 0.5%, in a basis of Polythene and hydrocarbons. For dry socket.

Locan *(Duncan, Flockhart, UK)*. Cream containing amethocaine 0.8%, amylocaine 1%, and cinchocaine 0.4%, in a non-greasy basis. Antipruritic.

Minims Amethocaine Hydrochloride *(Smith & Nephew Pharmaceuticals, UK)*. Sterile eye-drops containing amethocaine hydrochloride 0.5 or 1%, in single-use disposable applicators. (Also available as Minims Amethocaine Hydrochloride in *Austral.*).

Other Proprietary Names

Contralgine *(Belg.)*; Decicain *(Austral.)*; Lubricante Urologico Miro *(Spain)*; Pantocain *(Denm., Ger.)*; Pontocaine Hydrochloride *(USA)*.

7605-q

Amylocaine Hydrochloride *(B.P.C. 1949)*. Amylocain. Hydrochlor.; Amyleinii Chloridum; Chlorhydrate d'Amyléine. 1-Dimethylaminomethyl-1-methylpropyl benzoate hydrochloride.

$C_{14}H_{21}NO_2,HCl = 271.8$.

CAS — 644-26-8 (amylocaine); 532-59-2 (hydrochloride).

Pharmacopoeias. In *Belg.*, *Fr.*, *Port.*, *Roum.*, and *Span.*

A white odourless crystalline powder with a bitter numbing taste. M.p. 177° to 179°.

Soluble 1 in 2 of water and 1 in 3 of dehydrated alcohol; readily soluble in methyl alcohol; practically insoluble in ether. A 5% solution in water is faintly acid to litmus. A 4.98% solution in water is iso-osmotic with serum. Solutions are **sterilised** by heating with a bactericide or by filtration. **Incompatible** with alkalis, iodides, and mercury and silver salts. **Protect** from light.

Haemolysis. An aqueous solution of amylocaine hydrochloride iso-osmotic with serum (4.98%) caused 100% haemolysis of erythrocytes cultured in it for 45 minutes.— E. R. Hammarlund and K. Pedersen-Bjergaard, *J. pharm. Sci.*, 1961, *50*, 24.

Amylocaine hydrochloride is a local anaesthetic of the ester type and was formerly used as a surface anaesthetic in ophthalmology.

The general actions of local anaesthetics are described on p.899.

A preparation containing amylocaine hydrochloride was formerly marketed in Great Britain under the proprietary name Phenolaine Eye Drops (*Phenolaine Co.*).

7606-p

Aptocaine Hydrochloride. 2-(Pyrrolidin-1-yl)propiono-*o*-toluidide hydrochloride.

$C_{14}H_{20}N_2O,HCl = 268.8$.

CAS — 19281-29-9 (aptocaine); 19281-32-4 (hydrochloride).

Aptocaine hydrochloride is a local anaesthetic.

The general actions of local anaesthetics are described on p.899.

Identification of metabolites of aptocaine and some related compounds.— A. H. Beckett and W. Vutthikongsirigool, *J. Pharm. Pharmac.*, 1976, *28*, 54P.

As judged by intradermal injection aptocaine hydrochloride had a duration of action similar to that of mepivacaine and longer-lasting than bupivacaine, lignocaine, or prilocaine. Aptocaine had vasoconstrictor activity and 1 or 2% solutions appeared likely to be of use in dental anaesthesia.— F. Reynolds *et al.*, *Br. J. Anaesth.*, 1976, *48*, 347.

Manufacturers

Pharmaceutical Mfg, UK.

7607-s

Benzamine Hydrochloride *(B.P.C. 1954)*. Beta-eucaine Hydrochloride; Eucaine Hydrochloride. 2,2,6-Trimethyl-4-piperidyl benzoate hydrochloride.

$C_{15}H_{21}NO_2,HCl = 283.8$.

CAS — 500-34-5 (benzamine); 555-28-2 (hydrochloride).

Benzamine hydrochloride is a local anaesthetic formerly used for surface anaesthesia. The lactate has also been used.

The general actions of local anaesthetics are described on p.899.

7608-w

Benzocaine *(B.P., Eur. P., U.S.P.)*.

Benzocainum; Ethylis Aminobenzoas; Ethyl Aminobenzoate; Anaesthesinum; Éthoforme; Anesthamine. Ethyl 4-aminobenzoate.

$C_9H_{11}NO_2 = 165.2$.

CAS — 94-09-7.

Pharmacopoeias. In *Arg.*, *Aust.*, *Br.*, *Braz.*, *Chin.*, *Eur.*, *Fr.*, *Ger.*, *Hung.*, *Ind.*, *Int.*, *It.*, *Jap.*, *Jug.*, *Mex.*, *Neth.*, *Pol.*, *Roum.*, *Rus.*, *Span.*, *Swiss*, *Turk.*, and *U.S.*

Colourless crystals or a white odourless crystalline powder with a slightly bitter numbing taste. M.p. 88° to 92°.

Soluble 1 in 2500 of water, 1 in 8 of alcohol, 1 in 2 of chloroform, and 1 in 4 of ether; soluble in liquid paraffin and dilute acids. **Store** in airtight containers. Protect from light.

The presence of benzocaine *N*-glucoside as an impurity in benzocaine lozenges.— D. L. Simmons *et al.*, *Can. J. pharm. Sci.*, 1970, *5*, 85.

The rate of release of benzocaine was greater from water-soluble bases than other bases and was usually dependent upon the concentration of drug in the basis.— J. W. Ayres and P. A. Laskar, *J. pharm. Sci.*, 1974, *63*, 1402.

Studies *in vitro* with human stratum corneum indicated that the release of benzocaine from various macrogol ointments was dependent on the macrogol composition. Ointments containing relatively large proportions of lower molecular weight macrogols might retard benzocaine release.— A. A. Belmonte and W. Tsai, *J. pharm. Sci.*, 1978, *67*, 517.

Diffusion through polyethylene. Benzocaine diffused slowly through polyethylene (Polythene). When benzocaine suppositories were stored in polyethylene containers with walls 0.7 mm in thickness, it was possible to detect benzocaine on the outside of the containers after storage at about 24° for about 5 months.— O. Weis-Fogh, *Arch. Pharm. Chemi*, 1961, *68*, 736.

Incompatibility. Benzocaine was incompatible with citric acid, corn syrup, and natural cherry flavour, 3 of 11 excipients in a throat lozenge formulation; this resulted in an 80% loss of potency. The primary aromatic amine grouping, not the ester linkage, of benzocaine was considered to be the cause of the incompatibility.— P. Kabasakalian *et al.*, *J. pharm. Sci.*, 1969, *58*, 45.

Stability in solutions. The rate of hydrolysis of benzocaine in aqueous solution could be reduced to less than one-fifth by the addition of 2.5% of caffeine which formed a water-soluble complex with benzocaine.— T. Higuchi and L. Lachman, *J. Am. pharm. Ass., scient. Edn*, 1955, *44*, 521.

At a concentration (3%) in excess of their critical micelle concentrations, 4 nonionic surfactants, poloxamer, lauromacrogol, tyloxapol, and a propylene oxide-ethylenediamine-ethylene oxide polymer (Tetronic 908, *Wyandotte*), enhanced the stability of benzocaine in an alkaline solution by up to 4 times. The half-life of homatropine was only increased by up to 60%.— P. B. Sheth and E. L. Parrott, *J. pharm. Sci.*, 1967, *56*, 983.

Further references.— J. L. Lach and W. A. Pauli, *Drug Stand.*, 1959, *27*, 104.

Adverse Effects and Treatment. As for Local Anaesthetics, p.899.

Methaemoglobinaemia has been reported in infants following the topical application of benzocaine.

Allergy and effects on the skin. Of 887 persons with dermatitis or eczema submitted to patch testing with benzocaine 5% in yellow soft paraffin, 5.9% gave a positive reaction.— E. Rudzki and D. Kleniewska, *Br. J. Derm.*, 1970, *83*, 543. Of 4000 patients subjected to patch testing in 5 European clinics 3.3% of males and 4.5% of females showed positive reactions to benzocaine 5% in soft paraffin.— H. Bandmann *et al.*, *Archs Derm.*, 1972, *106*, 335.

Effects on the blood. Reports of *methaemoglobinaemia* occurring in infants after absorption of benzocaine.— H. de C. Peterson, *New Engl. J. Med.*, 1960, *263*, 454; J. R. Hughes, *J. Pediat.*, 1965, *66*, 797; P. L. Townes *et al.*, *Am. J. Dis. Child.*, 1977, *131*, 697.

For a report of methaemoglobinaemia being associated with the use of benzocaine in an adult, see Lignocaine Hydrochloride, p.902.

Precautions. As for Local Anaesthetics, p.900.

Benzocaine is hydrolysed in the body to *p*-aminobenzoic acid and may inhibit the action of sulphonamides. It should not be used in infants.

Absorption and Fate. See under Local Anaesthetics, p.900.

Uses. As for Local Anaesthetics, p.901.

Benzocaine is a surface anaesthetic of the ester type. It is comparatively non-irritant and has a low systemic toxicity. It may be given by mouth to relieve the pain of gastric ulcer or gastric carcinoma.

Benzocaine lozenges or compound benzocaine lozenges, allowed to dissolve slowly in the mouth, are used to prevent nausea and vomiting during the taking of dental impressions and the passing of instruments for bronchoscopy, laryngoscopy, or gastroscopy. These lozenges may also be used to relieve the pain arising from lacerations of the tongue or cheek, acute pharyngitis, tonsillectomy, or carcinoma of the mouth.

As an insufflation, or as a 2% solution in equal parts of alcohol and water, benzocaine may be used for the relief of painful throat affections. In concentrations of 5 to 10% it is employed in ointments or dusting-powders as a local analgesic application to ulcerated surfaces, burns, or wounds, or for the relief of intractable pruritus. Suppositories containing up to 200 mg have been used.

Benzocaine absorbs ultraviolet light and has been used in sunscreen creams and lotions.

Obesity. Despite the inclusion of benzocaine in some over-the-counter appetite suppressants there is no good evidence of its value in obesity.— *Med. Lett.*, 1979, *21*, 65.

Preparations

Creams

Benzocaine Cream *(U.S.P.)*. Benzocaine in a suitable cream basis. Store at a temperature not exceeding 30° in airtight containers. Protect from light.

Emulsions

Benzocaine and Paraffin Emulsion *(Roy. Marsden Hosp.)*. Benzocaine, in fine powder, 200 mg, liquid paraffin emulsion to 10 ml. To be swallowed slowly, undiluted.

Lozenges

Benzocaine Lozenges. Lozenges prepared by compression, each containing benzocaine 10 mg.

Compound Benzocaine Lozenges *(B.P.C. 1973)*. Benzocaine Compound Lozenges; Trochisci Benzocainae Compositi; Compound Benzocaine Tablets. Each lozenge weighs about 1 g and contains benzocaine 100 mg and menthol 3 mg.

Mixtures

For a sore throat mixture containing benzocaine, see Aspirin, p.243..

Ointments

Benzocaine and Adrenaline Ointment *(A.P.F.)*. Ung. Benzocain. et Adrenal.; Anaesthetic Adrenaline Ointment. Benzocaine 5 g, adrenaline solution 10 ml, wool fat 15 g, liquid paraffin 20 g, and yellow soft paraffin 50 g. It should be recently prepared and dispensed in a collapsible tube with a rectal applicator.

Benzocaine Ointment *(U.S.P.)*. Benzocaine in a suitable ointment basis. Store at a temperature not exceeding 30° in airtight containers. Protect from light.

Compound Benzocaine Ointment *(B.P.C. 1973)*. Benzocaine Compound Ointment; Unguentum Benzocainae Compositum. Benzocaine 10% in equal parts of hamamelis ointment and zinc ointment. Store in containers which prevent evaporation.

Trituratio Benzocaini *(Dan. Disp.)*. Benzocaine 33.3 g, liquid paraffin 13.3 g, and yellow soft paraffin 53.4 g.

Suppositories

Benzocaine and Adrenaline Suppositories *(A.P.F.)*. Benzocaine 5 g, adrenaline 100 mg, boric acid 200 mg, freshly boiled and cooled water 5 ml, theobroma oil or other suitable fatty basis to 100 g. Pour into 1-g moulds. They should be wrapped individually in metal foil or stored and supplied in an airtight container. Store below 25°.

Proprietary Preparations

AAA Mouth and Throat Spray *(Armour, UK)*. Contains benzocaine 1.5% and cetalkonium chloride 0.0413% in a metered aerosol delivering in each dose benzocaine 1.5 mg and cetalkonium chloride 40 µg.

Dermogesic (known is some countries as Caligesic) *(Merck Sharp & Dohme, UK)*. An ointment containing benzocaine 3%, calamine 8%, and hexylated *m*-cresol ($C_{13}H_{20}O$ = 192.3) 0.05% in a vanishing cream basis. For pruritic conditions.

Intralgin *(Riker, UK)*. Gel containing benzocaine 2% and salicylamide 5% in an alcoholic vehicle. For strains, sprains, and rheumatic conditions.

Medilave Gel *(Martindale Pharmaceuticals, UK)*. Contains benzocaine 1% and cetylpyridinium chloride 0.01% in a water-immiscible protective basis. For painful conditions of the oral mucosa.

Nestosyl *(Bengué, UK)*. Ointment containing benzocaine 2%, butyl aminobenzoate 2%, resorcinol 2%, zinc oxide 10%, and hexachlorophane 0.1%. For haemorrhoids, minor wounds, and pruritus.

Other Proprietary Names

Americaine *(USA)*; Anaesthesin *(Ger.)*.

Preparations containing benzocaine were also formerly marketed in Great Britain under the proprietary names Dermoplast (*Ayerst*) and RBC (*Rybar*).

7609-e

Bupivacaine Hydrochloride *(B.P., U.S.P.)*.

AH 2250; LAC-43; Win 11 318. (±)-(1-Butyl-2-piperidyl)formo-2′,6′-xylidide hydrochloride monohydrate.

$C_{18}H_{28}N_2O,HCl,H_2O$ = 342.9.

CAS — 2180-92-9 (bupivacaine); 18010-40-7 (hydrochloride, anhydrous); 14252-80-3 (hydrochloride, monohydrate).

Pharmacopoeias. In *Br.* and *U.S.*

A white odourless crystalline powder with a bitter taste. M.p. about 248° to 250° with decomposition.

Soluble 1 in 25 of water and 1 in 8 of alcohol; slightly soluble in acetone, chloroform, and ether. A 1% solution in water has a pH of 4.5 to 6. A 5.38% solution in water is iso-osmotic with serum. Solutions are **sterilised** by autoclaving or by filtration. **Store** in airtight containers.

When commercial ampoules containing bupivacaine and adrenaline (Marcaine) were autoclaved the contents turned yellow and emitted a foul odour.— B. C. DeLeo *et al.*, *Anesthesiology*, 1974, *40*, 297.

Comment on the mixing of bupivacaine with other local anaesthetics. Equal volumes of bupivacaine 0.75% and chloroprocaine 3% will produce a strongly acid mixture of pH 3.7. A mixture of equal volumes of bupivacaine 0.75% and lignocaine 2% has a pH of 6.5 and so about 20 times more uncharged bupivacaine is available than when mixed with chloroprocaine. If the administration of a local anaesthetic mixture is to be repeated it may be preferable to mix bupivacaine with lignocaine.— J. B. Brodsky and J. G. Brock-Utne (letter), *Br. J. Anaesth.*, 1978, *50*, 1269.

Haemolysis. An aqueous solution of bupivacaine hydrochloride iso-osmotic with serum (5.38%) caused 83% haemolysis of erythrocytes cultured in it for 45 minutes.— C. Sapp *et al.*, *J. pharm. Sci.*, 1975, *64*, 1884.

Stability of solutions. For reference to the decreased solubility of bupivacaine in phosphate buffer with increasing temperature and its possible precipitation at the site of injection, see Lignocaine Hydrochloride, p.902.

Adverse Effects and Treatment. As for Local Anaesthetics, p.899.

Foetal bradycardia has been reported following paracervical block with bupivacaine during labour and may require the administration of atropine sulphate intravenously.

For an evaluation of the toxicity of bupivacaine, see under Regional Nerve Block in Uses (below).

Effects on the heart. Cardiac arrest occurring in 6 patients during regional anaesthesia with bupivacaine or etidocaine, probably as a result of inadvertent intravascular injection, was not preceded by hypoxia and it appeared that even prompt oxygenation and blood pressure support might not prevent arrest. Marked cardiovascular depression may occur with bupivacaine or etidocaine at plasma concentrations only slightly above those for CNS toxicity.— G. A. Albright, *Anesthesiology*, 1979, *51*, 285.

Effects on the nervous system. Reports of convulsions after the accidental intravascular injection of bupivacaine.— D. W. Ryan, *Br. J. Anaesth.*, 1973, *45*, 907; H. Yamashiro, *Anesthesiology*, 1977, *47*, 472; J. S. DeVore and R. Asrani, *Anesthesiology*, 1978, *48*, 386; W. C. Korevaar *et al.*, *Anesth. Analg.*, 1979, *58*, 329.

Hyperexcitability in a 15-year-old boy following intravenous regional anaesthesia with bupivacaine 95 mg.— A. M. Henderson, *Br. med. J.*, 1980, *281*, 1043.

Pregnancy and the neonate. Effects on the foetus. Bupivacaine 0.5% with adrenaline 1 in 200 000 was used during labour in 118 women in an assessment of paracervical nerve block anaesthesia. Haemorrhage occurred during insertion of the needle in 17% of the women who received continuous block anaesthesia, 2 perinatal deaths occurred following single paracervical block, and overall there was an 11% incidence of foetal bradycardia. It was suggested that amide-type local anaesthetics should not be used for single paracervical block and that the use of continuous paracervical block should be discontinued.— P. J. Murphy *et al.*, *Br. med. J.*, 1970, *1*, 526.

The risk of foetal bradycardia associated with paracervical block was considerable with the use of 20 ml of bupivacaine 0.5%. An injection of 20 ml of bupivacaine 0.25% could provide analgesia lasting up to 3 hours. More prolonged analgesia without foetal bradycardia followed injection of 14 ml of bupivacaine 0.5% with adrenaline 1 in 200 000.— F. C. R. Picton (letter), *Br. med. J.*, 1970, *2*, 49.

Further reports of foetal bradycardia as a complication of paracervical block with bupivacaine.— F. C. R. Picton (letter), *Br. med. J.*, 1968, *2*, 561; C. Ruoss and J. M. Beazley (letter), *Br. med. J.*, 1968, *2*, 622; M. J. Yates (letter), *Br. med. J.*, 1968, *2*, 699; D. B. Whitehouse (letter), *ibid.*, 764; K. Teramo and O. Widholm (letter), *Br. J. Anaesth.*, 1969, *41*, 1013; E. Abouleish, *Br. J. Anaesth.*, 1976, *48*, 481 (following caudal analgesia).

Decreased visual skills and alertness but increased muscle tone, in some cases lasting several weeks, in the infants of mothers given high doses of bupivacaine.— D. B. Rosenblatt *et al.*, *Br. J. Obstet. Gynaec.*, 1981, *88*, 407.

Precautions. As for Local Anaesthetics, p.900.

During prolonged epidural block with bupivacaine, venous stasis and pressure sores may develop.

A report of prolonged block of about 72 hours' duration following the use of 18 ml of bupivacaine 0.5% for extradural analgesia of a patient in labour.— G. V. Pathy and M. Rosen, *Br. J. Anaesth.*, 1975, *47*, 520.

Interactions. Bupivacaine is highly bound to plasma proteins. *Desipramine, pethidine, phenytoin,* and *quinidine* increased the amount of unbound bupivacaine in plasma *in vitro*.— M. M. Ghoneim and H. Pandya, *Br. J. Anaesth.*, 1974, *46*, 435. Criticism.— G. T. Tucker and L. E. Mather (letter), *ibid.*, 1975, *47*, 1029.

Absorption and Fate. Bupivacaine is extensively bound to plasma proteins. Foetal concentrations are lower than maternal concentrations. It is metabolised in the liver and is rapidly removed from the blood.

See also Local Anaesthetics, p.900.

Bupivacaine hydrochloride was administered by epidural injection to 12 patients in a dose of 150 mg with adrenaline 1 in 200 000, to 5 without adrenaline, and in a dose of 225 mg with adrenaline to a further 6. Mean peak plasma concentrations of bupivacaine were 1.14, 1.26, and 2.33 µg per ml respectively and occurred 20 minutes after administration; elimination half-lives were 2.8, 2.4, and 3.6 hours. In 5 of the patients given 150 mg of bupivacaine hydrochloride with adrenaline a peak CSF concentration of 30.6 µg per ml was achieved 30 minutes after administration.— G. R. Wilkinson and P. C. Lund, *Anesthesiology*, 1970, *33*, 482.

Peak plasma-bupivacaine concentrations of 4.5, 2.61, and 3.45 µg per ml were achieved in 3 subjects given bupivacaine hydrochloride 130, 102, and 104 mg respectively by slow intravenous injection. About 91 to 96% was bound to plasma protein and only 4.02 to 10.2% of the dose was excreted unchanged in the urine.— L. E. Mather *et al.*, *Clin. Pharmac. Ther.*, 1971, *12*, 935.

The absorption of bupivacaine hydrochloride, bupivacaine hydrochloride with adrenaline, and carbonated bupivacaine given during epidural blockade.— T. N. Appleyard *et al.*, *Br. J. Anaesth.*, 1974, *46*, 530.

Half-lives reported after the intravenous injection of bupivacaine were: α, 0.045 hours; β, 0.46 hours; and γ, 3.5 hours.— G. T. Tucker and L. E. Mather, *Br. J. Anaesth.*, 1975, *47*, 213.

Arterial and venous plasma concentrations of bupivacaine after epidural and intercostal nerve blocks.— D. C. Moore *et al.*, *Anesthesiology*, 1976, *45*, 39. See also *idem*, *Anesth. Analg. curr. Res.*, 1976, *55*, 763.

Pregnancy and the neonate. Maternal protein bound approximately twice as much bupivacaine as foetal protein at a drug concentration in the range of 0.05 to 5 µg per ml.— L. E. Mather *et al.*, *J. Pharm. Pharmac.*, 1971, *23*, 359. Studies *in vitro* indicated that plasma alpha-1-lipoproteins had a high affinity for bupivacaine. As foetal plasma contains little alpha-1-lipoprotein, the binding capacity for bupivacaine would be reduced, which probably contributes to the higher concentration of bupivacaine in maternal plasma at delivery.— L. E. Mather and J. Thomas, *ibid.*, 1978, *30*, 653.

Following pudendal block plasma-bupivacaine concentrations at delivery ranged from 115 to 329 ng per ml (mean 215) in 11 mothers and from 28 to 82 ng per ml (mean 50) in umbilical blood.— P. Belfrage *et al.*, *Br. J. Anaesth.*, 1973, *45*, 1067.

Six women were given bupivacaine 30 to 45 mg during labour. The maternal β-phase half-life was 1.25 hours compared with 25 hours for the neonate. It was suggested that neonates were less able to metabolise bupivacaine.— J. Caldwell *et al.*, *Br. J. clin. Pharmac.*, 1976, *3*, 956P.

In a study involving a total of 31 women in labour who received bupivacaine epidurally before delivery, maternal venous plasma concentrations of bupivacaine were significantly higher than the umbilical venous plasma concentrations but no correlation was found between the ratio of foetal to maternal concentrations of bupivacaine and the time from the last dose to delivery. No significant difference was noted between unbound bupivacaine concentrations in umbilical and maternal plasma but the fraction of unbound bupivacaine was greater in the foetal plasma than in the maternal plasma.— J. Thomas *et al.*, *Clin. Pharmac. Ther.*, 1976, *19*, 426. See also P. Belfrage *et al.*, *Am. J. Obstet. Gynec.*, 1975, *121*, 360.

The neonatal elimination of bupivacaine was studied in the infants of 19 women given doses of 25 to 185 mg epidurally during labour. Maternal plasma concentrations reached 300 ng per ml and the ratio of cord to maternal concentrations was 0.59. Bupivacaine was eliminated from 11 infants in 24 hours and from all 19 in 30 hours.— L. V. Cooper *et al.*, *Archs Dis. Childh.*, 1977, *52*, 638.

Further references to the pharmacokinetics of bupivacaine in pregnancy and the neonate.— J. M. Beazley *et al.*, *Obstet. Gynec.*, 1972, *39*, 2; C. E. Blogg and B. R. Simpson (letter), *Lancet*, 1974, *1*, 1283; R. Magno *et al.*, *Acta anaesth. scand.*, 1976, *20*, 141; J. W. Scanlon *et al.*, *Anesthesiology*, 1976, *45*, 400; R. Jouppila *et al.*, *Annls Chir. Gynaec. Fenn.*, 1978, *67*, 190; G. A. McGuinness *et al.*, *Anesthesiology*, 1978, *49*, 270; R. L. Nation, *Clin. Pharmacokinet.*, 1980, *5*, 340.

Protein binding. Bupivacaine was reported to be 84% bound to plasma proteins.— B. G. Covino, *Anesthesiology*, 1971, *35*, 158.

For reference to the protein binding of bupivacaine, see Lignocaine Hydrochloride, p.904.

Uses. As for Local Anaesthetics, p.901.

Bupivacaine hydrochloride is a long-acting local anaesthetic of the amide type, similar to lignocaine and mepivacaine but about 4 times more potent. Onset of action and depth of anaesthesia are similar to those of lignocaine hydrochloride but the effects of bupivacaine last longer. It is used mainly for regional nerve blocks, particularly epidural block, when a prolonged effect is required.

Doses of bupivacaine are expressed in terms of the anhydrous hydrochloride.

For regional nerve blocks, bupivacaine is used as a 0.25 or 0.5% solution alone or with adrenaline 1 in 400 000 or 1 in 200 000 respectively. The usual dose is about 10 to 40 ml of 0.25% solution or about 15 to 30 ml of 0.5% solution. For nerve block of finger or toe, about 2 to 10 ml of 0.25% or 2 to 6 ml of 0.5% solution without adrenaline is employed. For surgical procedures, lumbar epidural block may be induced by doses of 15 to 20 ml of 0.25 or 0.5% solution with or without adrenaline; for caudal block 15 to 40 ml of 0.25% solution or 15 to 25 ml of 0.5% solution with or without adrenaline may be used. Somewhat smaller doses are used to produce analgesia in labour.

A 0.75% solution is used in single doses for the production of epidural block and for retrobulbar block in ophthalmic surgery.

Bupivacaine hydrochloride 0.5% solution without adrenaline, diluted to 0.2% with sodium chloride injection, may be given in a dose of 1.5 mg per kg body-weight for intravenous regional anaesthesia.

The maximum recommended dose of bupivacaine hydrochloride is 2 mg per kg body-weight in any 4-hour period, equivalent to 25 to 30 ml of 0.5% solution in adults of average weight.

A brief evaluation of bupivacaine.— *Med. lett.*, 1977, *19*, 4.

Action. Solutions of the L(−) and D(+) isomers of bupivacaine were given intradermally in a range of concentrations (0.002 to 0.25%) to 17 healthy subjects. Both isomers had a vasodilator effect at the highest concentrations whereas the L(−) isomer was significantly more vasoconstrictive at intermediate concentrations. The longer duration of analgesic action of L(−) bupivacaine was thought to be due to a difference in vasoactivity and was reflected in a higher apparent potency *in vivo*.— C. Aps and F. Reynolds, *Br. J. clin. Pharmac.*, 1978, *6*, 63.

For a study on the vasoactivity of bupivacaine, see Lignocaine Hydrochloride, p.905.

Caudal block. In 75 patients who had previously undergone caesarean section or other abdominal surgery, caudal anaesthesia was successfully induced in 71 and 66 were delivered vaginally, with the judicious use of oxytocin in 25. The integrity of scars was monitored by digital assessment and by constant observation of pulse-rate and blood pressure. Caudal anaesthesia was induced by the use of 20 ml of bupivacaine 0.5% with adrenaline 1 in 200 000. The duration of effect of each 20-ml dose was 3 hours.— F. P. Meehan *et al.*, *Br. med. J.*, 1972, *2*, 740.

See also Regional Nerve Block (below).

Epidural block. Factors affecting the spread of local anaesthetic solutions in the extradural space were studied. Extradural analgesia was performed on 334 occasions using bupivacaine 0.75% solution 10 ml, 15 ml, or 20 ml, injected at a rate of 1 ml per second using a technique in which site of injection, bevel direction of needle, and position of the patient were all standardised. Arteriosclerosis in 18 patients had no effect on the spread of 15 ml of bupivacaine solution when compared with 70 patients without evidence of cardiac or vascular disease. There was a slight correlation between height of the patient and the level of analgesia. With increasing age there was a small increase in the spread of bupivacaine. The number of segments blocked was not directly related to the volume of anaesthetic solution injected.— E. M. Grundy *et al.*, *Br. J. Anaesth.*, 1978, *50*, 805.

Further references to epidural block with bupivacaine hydrochloride.— M. J. Watt *et al.*, *Anaesthesia*, 1968, *23*, 331 (comparison with lignocaine); P. R. Bromage, *Can. Anaesth. Soc. J.*, 1969, *16*, 37 (comparison with amethocaine, lignocaine, and mepivacaine); P. O. Bridenbaugh *et al.*, *Anesthesiology*, 1976, *45*, 560 (comparison with etidocaine); G. B. Drummond and D. G. Littlewood, *Br. J. Anaesth.*, 1977, *49*, 999; W. S. Nimmo *et al.*, *Br. J. Anaesth.*, 1978, *50*, 559; D. T. Brown *et al.*, *Br. J. Anaesth.*, 1980, *52*, 419 (a lack of benefit with carbonated bupivacaine when compared with the hydrochloride).

In obstetrics. A review of 923 women who had undergone lumbar epidural block with bupivacaine and adrenaline before or during labour showed that only 6% of them received no beneift. The optimum dose appeared to be 8 ml of bupivacaine 0.5% solution, which was effective for about 2 hours. The persistence of sensory and motor nerve block after delivery was decreased when the concentration of bupivacaine in the final dose, given 1 hour before delivery, was reduced to 0.25%.— J. S. Crawford, *Br. J. Anaesth.*, 1972, *44*, 66. See also *idem*, *Practitioner*, 1974, *212*, 677. A standard dose of 10 ml of bupivacaine 0.25% plain was given by epidural injection to 80 patients about to undergo surgical induction of labour. A unilateral block occurred in 17 patients, 9 of whom were given an additional 5 ml of either 0.25% or 0.5% bupivacaine plain. Of 72 patients only 1 found the induction painful.— N. G. Caseby, *Br. J. Anaesth.*, 1974, *46*, 747.

Plasma-bupivacaine concentrations were significantly reduced by adrenaline in a study of 70 mothers undergoing epidural block during delivery. It was considered that, using bupivacaine 0.5%, doses of up to 320 mg could be given without adrenaline before there was any risk of systemic toxicity.— F. Reynolds *et al.*, *Br. J. Anaesth.*, 1973, *45*, 1049. In a study of extradural analgesia in 8 women in labour there were no significant cardiovascular effects when bupivacaine 0.5%, with or without adrenaline 5 µg per ml, was used. It was concluded that since adrenaline might cause anterior spinal artery thrombosis and inhibit the force of uterine contractions the plain solution should be used for all but the longest labours.— I. M. Corall *et al.*, *Br. J. Anaesth.*, 1975, *47*, 1297.

Bupivacaine 0.125% with adrenaline 1 in 400 000 was

used in 500 patients for epidural block analgesia during the first and second stage of labour. A 10-ml dose was repeated every 45 to 90 minutes, as required, and 15 ml given at the start of the second stage. In most cases there was complete pain relief within 15 minutes of the first injection and 93% of the deliveries were painless. In 71.4% of patients a total dose of less than 60 mg bupivacaine was necessary and 96% required less than 100 mg. The duration of epidural block was less than 6 hours in 91% of patients. Hypotension occurred in 21 mothers.— G. Vanderick *et al.*, *Br. J. Anaesth.*, 1974, *46*, 838. A study in 598 receiving epidural analgesia with 0.125% bupivacaine with adrenaline 1: 200 000 during labour did not shown any prolongation of labour.— J. C. Phillips *et al.*, *Am. J. Obstet. Gynec.*, 1977, *129*, 316. See also A. Bleyaert *et al.*, *Anesthesiology*, 1979, *51*, 435 (bupivacaine 0.125% with adrenaline 1 in 800 000).

There was no significant decrease in uterine activity in 16 patients given 34 top-up doses of bupivacaine for lumbar epidural analgesia during delivery.— J. C. Schellenberg, *Am. J. Obstet. Gynec.*, 1977, *127*, 26.

In a comparison of 50 twin pregnancies in which analgesia was provided by lumbar epidural block (bupivacaine 0.5% with adrenaline 1 in 400 000) with 92 twin pregnancies in which analgesia was provided by pethidine and promethazine, with nitrous oxide and oxygen, there were no differences in the length of the 1st and 2nd stages of labour, the number of assisted deliveries, the number of breech presentations, Apgar scores, or perinatal mortality. Epidural block was considered preferable.— A. R. L. Weekes *et al.*, *Br. med. J.*, 1977, *2*, 730. Experience suggesting that lumbar epidural anaesthesia, using bupivacaine 0.25 to 0.5% is a safe form of analgesia for the delivery of twins.— F. M. James *et al.*, *Am. J. Obstet. Gynec.*, 1977, *127*, 176. See also J. S. Crawford, *Br. J. Obstet. Gynaec.*, 1975, *82*, 929; O. E. Jaschevatzky *et al.*, *Br. J. Obstet. Gynaec.*, 1977, *84*, 327; D. W. Watson and G. O. Downey, *Anesthesiology*, 1980, *52*, 259.

Segmental epidural analgesia during the first stage of labour was produced in 8 women with a 4 ml-dose of bupivacaine 0.5% solution; a further 10 patients received 4 ml of bupivacaine 0.5% with adrenaline 1 in 200 000. Placental blood flow was not impaired when measured 15 to 20 minutes after the onset of analgesia. There were no instances of maternal hypotension or abnormal changes in foetal heart-rate.— R. Jouppila *et al.*, *Br. J. Anaesth.*, 1978, *50*, 563.

In a double-blind study in 80 patients bupivacaine 0.125%, 0.25%, and 0.5% and lignocaine 2% all with and without adrenaline 1 in 200 000 were compared with regard to efficacy, time of onset, and duration of analgesia during extradural nerve block in the first stage of labour. Bupivacaine 0.25% and 0.5% with adrenaline and lignocaine 2% with adrenaline were most effective, while bupivacaine 0.5% was the most effective of the plain solutions.— D. G. Littlewood *et al.*, *Br. J. Anaesth.*, 1979, *51*, *Suppl.* 1, 47S.

References to the effects of epidural anaesthesia with bupivacaine on the foetus and neonate.— P. Donnai and A. D. Nicholas, *Br. J. Obstet. Gynaec.*, 1975, *82*, 360; J. W. Scanlon *et al.*, *Anesthesiology*, 1976, *45*, 400. See also under Pregnancy and the Neonate in Adverse Effects (above).

Further references to epidural block with bupivacaine in labour.— A. M. Duthie *et al.*, *Anaesthesia*, 1968, *23*, 20; F. M. James and P. Davies, *Am. J. Obstet. Gynec.*, 1976, *126*, 195; A. Matouskova, *Acta obstet. gynec. scand.*, 1979, *Suppl.* 83, 1; C. F. Goodfellow and C. Studd, *Br. J. clin. Pract.*, 1979, *33*, 287.

See also Regional Nerve Block (below).

Ergotism. For reference to the unsuccessful use of epidural block with bupivacaine in an attempt to control vasospasm due to ergotism, see P. K. Andersen *et al.*, *New Engl. J. Med.*, 1977, *296*, 1271.

Pain. Nerve blocks were carried out successfully on 27 patients with intractable post-herpetic neuralgia, neoplastic pain, and orthopaedic pain using bupivacaine 0.25% with adrenaline 1 in 400 000. All patients reported immediate relief from pain. After one day 18 still had relief, at 7 days 13 were free from pain, and at 21 days 12 were still free.— J. G. Hannington-Kiff, *Lancet*, 1971, *2*, 1392.

Postoperative extradural analgesia by intermittent injection of bupivacaine (0.5% with adrenaline 1 in 200 000) or continuous infusion (0.125 to 0.25%) for 48 hours following thoracotomy, was attempted in 20 patients. At 10 days 47% of 15 evaluable patients stated that they had been pain-free in the 48 hours after operation and only 7% complained of severe pain. Drowsiness occurred in 7 patients; 5 were on continuous infusion of bupivacaine 0.25%. Hypotension was noted in all patients blocked successfully and in 1 patient abandonment of the block was necessary. There was urinary retention in all of 9 men on continuous infusion and in 3 of 8 on intermittent bupivacaine.— D. P. G. Griffiths *et al.*, *Br. J. Anaesth.*, 1975, *47*, 48.

Further references to bupivacaine in the relief of pain.— R. J. Defalque, *Anesth. Analg. curr. Res.*, 1974, *53*, 841; J. Dinley and R. A. Dickson, *J. Bone Jt Surg.*, 1976, *58*, 356 (bupivacaine by instillation in orthopaedic surgery); H. M. Perkins and P. R. Hanlon, *Archs Surg., Chicago*, 1978, *113*, 253 (epidural bupivacaine in cutaneous herpes zoster); R. Rosenblatt *et al.*, *Anesthesiology*, 1979, *51*, 565 (continuous axillary analgesia for traumatic hand injury); T. W. Ogg, *Br. med. J.*, 1980, *281*, 212 (caudal analgesia with bupivacaine after painful anal or penile surgery).

Paracervical block. Reports on the use of bupivacaine for paracervical block in labour.— H. Stockhausen, *Dt. med. Wschr.*, 1967, *92*, 2217, per *J. Am. med. Ass.*, 1968, *203* (Jan. 8), A208; F. C. R. Picton, *Br. J. clin. Pract.*, 1969, *23*, 162; P. J. Meis *et al.*, *Obstet. Gynec.*, 1978, *52*, 545; J. A. Read and F. C. Miller, *Obstet. Gynec.*, 1979, *53*, 166.

Regional anaesthesia, intravenous. A suggestion that in order to increase the safety of intravenous regional anaesthesia with bupivacaine an intravenous needle or cannula should first be placed in an unoccluded limb, and that after injection re-inflation of the tourniquet should be considered at the first signs of toxicity.— M. Futter (letter), *Br. med. J.*, 1980, *281*, 1427.

Studies of intravenous regional anaesthesia with bupivacaine hydrochloride in patients with various pain syndromes indicated that 200 mg, as 40 ml of a 0.5% solution, may be the optimal dose for producing safe and prolonged intravenous regional anaesthesia.— F. Magora *et al.*, *Br. J. Anaesth.*, 1980, *52*, 1123; *idem*, 1131.

Regional nerve block. An evaluation of the tissue and systemic toxicity of bupivacaine based on a review of its use in 7688 regional nerve block procedures indicated that bupivacaine has a wide margin of safety and that its toxic dosage had not yet been established. It was considered that doses of up to at least 225 mg of bupivacaine with adrenaline 1 in 200 000 for single-dose epidural block and up to at least 400 mg with adrenaline 1 in 320 000 or less for peripheral nerve block may be safely used in adults when necessary for rapid establishment of surgical anaesthesia, for complete motor blockade, and for prolonged duration of anaesthesia.— D. C. Moore *et al.*, *Acta anaesth. scand.*, 1977, *21*, 109.

A detailed review of the use of bupivacaine hydrochloride for regional nerve block (caudal, epidural, and peripheral) with guidelines on dosage. Of 11 080 procedures performed from 1966 through 1976 using 0.25, 0.5, or 0.75% solutions, with and without adrenaline, 6599 were for surgical, 3496 were for obstetrical, and 985 were for diagnostic and therapeutic procedures. Solutions containing adrenaline were used in 9304 procedures and a dose of 250 µg of adrenaline was seldom exceeded. Sensory anaesthesia of the integumentary and musculoskeletal systems occurred with all strengths of bupivacaine hydrochloride but only the 0.75% solution eliminated traction reflexes from the pelvic viscera. In epidural or caudal block, onset of sensory anaesthesia was noted in 4 to 10 minutes with 0.25 and 0.5% solutions and maximum sensory anaesthesia in 15 to 35 minutes; results were similar in peripheral nerve block. In epidural or caudal block using a 0.75% solution onset of sensory anaesthesia occurred in 3 to 5 minutes and was at a maximum in 10 to 30 minutes. The degree of motor blockade varied with technique and concentration and usually occurred 4 to 8 minutes after sensory anaesthesia; following caudal and epidural block maximum motor blockade in the lower extremities might take up to 60 minutes. Using the single-injection epidural or caudal block techniques for intra-abdominal surgery, including caesarean section and back surgery, profound muscle relaxation in the abdomen and back occurred consistently only with the 0.75% solution. Bupivacaine was well tolerated apart from the following adverse effects: total spinal anaesthesia following caudal block in one patient who recovered completely and systemic toxicity resulting from unrecognised intravascular injections in 13 patients and from absorption in 2 patients; there were no untoward sequelae.— D. C. Moore *et al.*, *Anesth. Analg. curr. Res.*, 1978, *57*, 42.

Further references to regional nerve block with bupivacaine.— P. R. Bromage and M. Gertel, *Anesthesiology*, 1972, *36*, 479 (supraclavicular brachial block); D. C. Moore, *Br. J. Anaesth.*, 1975, *47*, 284 (bupivacaine 0.25 or 0.5% was the anaesthetic of choice in intercostal nerve block); D. F. Pricco, *J. oral Surg.*, 1977, *35*, 126; L. Wiklund and A. Berlin-Wahlen, *Acta anaesth. scand.*, 1977, *21*, 521 (comparison with etidocaine).

See also Caudal Block, Epidural Block, and Paracervical Block (above).

Shoulder-hand syndrome. Stellate ganglion block using bupivacaine might be of value in severe cases of shoulder-hand syndrome.— D. Woolf, *Practitioner*, 1974, *213*, 176. For reference to the use of intravenous regional anaesthesia with bupivacaine in patients with shoulder-hand syndrome, see F. Magora *et al.*, *Br. J. Anaesth.*, 1980, *52*, 1123.

Tinnitus. For a report of the use of bupivacaine as 6 ml of a 0.25% solution with hyaluronidase 1000 units, in the induction of stellate ganglion block in the treatment of Ménière's disease and for the symptomatic relief of tinnitus, see J. W. Warrick, *Br. J. Anaesth.*, 1969, *41*, 699. See also P. Adlington and J. Warwick, *J. Lar. Otol.*, 1971, *85*, 159.

Preparations

Bupivacaine and Adrenaline Injection *(B.P.)*. Bupivacaine and Adren. Inj. A sterile solution of bupivacaine hydrochloride and adrenaline acid tartrate in Water for Injections containing the equivalent of not more than 0.1% of sulphur dioxide. Sterilised by autoclaving. Potency is expressed in terms of anhydrous bupivacaine hydrochloride. pH 3 to 5.5. Protect from light.

Bupivacaine Hydrochloride and Epinephrine Injection *(U.S.P.)*. A sterile solution of bupivacaine hydrochloride and adrenaline in Water for Injections. Potency is expressed in terms of anhydrous bupivacaine hydrochloride; it contains not more than 1 in 100 000 of adrenaline. pH 3.3 to 5.5.

Bupivacaine Hydrochloride Injection *(B.P.)*. Bupivacaine Hydrochlor. Inj. A sterile solution of bupivacaine hydrochloride in Water for Injections. Sterilised by autoclaving. Potency is expressed in terms of anhydrous bupivacaine hydrochloride. pH 5 to 7.5.

Bupivacaine Hydrochloride Injection *(U.S.P.)*. A sterile solution of bupivacaine hydrochloride in Water for Injections. Potency is expressed in terms of anhydrous bupivacaine hydrochloride. pH 4 to 6.5.

Proprietary Preparations

Marcain Plain *(Duncan, Flockhart, UK)*. Bupivacaine hydrochloride, available as an injection containing the equivalent of anhydrous bupivacaine hydrochloride 0.25, 0.5, or 0.75% in ampoules of 10 ml. **Marcain with Adrenaline.** Injections containing the equivalent of anhydrous bupivacaine hydrochloride 0.25 or 0.5% with adrenaline 1 in 400 000 and 1 in 200 000 respectively, in ampoules of 10 ml. (Also available as Marcain in *Austral.*, *Denm.*, *Norw.*, *Swed.*).

Other Proprietary Names

Carbostesin *(Ger., Switz.)*; Duracaine *(Arg.)*; Marcaina *(Ital.)*; Marcaine *(Belg., Canad., Neth., USA)*.

7610-b

Butacaine Sulphate *(B.P.C. 1968)*. Butacain. Sulph.; Butacaine Sulfate *(U.S.P.)*. 3-Dibutylaminopropyl 4-aminobenzoate sulphate.

$(C_{18}H_{30}N_2O_2)_2,H_2SO_4=711.0$.

CAS — 149-16-6 (butacaine); 149-15-5 (sulphate).

Pharmacopoeias. In *Braz.*, *Ind.*, *Turk.*, and *U.S.*

A white or almost white, almost odourless, very hygroscopic crystalline powder with a slightly bitter numbing taste. M.p. about 100°.

Soluble 1 in 1.5 of water, 1 in 2 of alcohol, 1 in 2.5 of chloroform, and 1 in 2000 of ether; slightly soluble in acetone; practically insoluble in methyl isobutyl ketone. A 1% solution in water has a pH of 6 to 7. Solutions are **sterilised** by maintaining at 98° to 100° for 30 minutes with a bactericide or by filtration. **Store** in airtight containers. Protect from light.

Incompatibility. Butacaine sulphate was incompatible with bromides, chlorides, and bactericides such as chlorocresol. It was compatible with phenylmercuric acetate 0.001%.— R. Laird and G. S. Rolph, *Pharm. J.*, 1953, *2*, 113.

Adverse Effects, Treatment, and Precautions. As for Local Anaesthetics, p.899.

Allergy and effects on the skin. In a modified 'repeated-insult' patch test, 25% butacaine sulphate was found to produce moderate sensitisation of the skin.— A. M. Kligman, *J. invest. Derm.*, 1966, *47*, 393.

Uses. Butacaine sulphate is a surface anaesthetic of the ester type with effects similar to those of cocaine, but its action is more rapid in onset and more prolonged. It does not dilate the pupil and does not affect accommodation; it is less likely to damage the cornea than

cocaine.
A 2% solution has been used for surface anaesthesia of the eye, nose, and throat.

Antibacterial activity. Butacaine sulphate 1% in 0.9% sodium chloride solution was found to have some antimicrobial action *in vitro*, particularly against *Escherichia coli*. The addition of butacaine sulphate enhanced the bactericidal activity of benzalkonium chloride, chlorocresol, and of methyl hydroxybenzoate.— M. A. El-Nakeeb and A. Farouk, *Can. J. pharm. Sci.*, 1976, *11*, 58.

Preparations

Butacaine Sulfate Topical Solution *(U.S.P.)*. Butacaine Sulfate Solution. A sterile aqueous solution of butacaine sulphate. pH 5 to 6.5. Store in airtight containers. Protect from light.

7611-v

Butanilicaine Phosphate. 2-Butylamino-6′-chloroaceto-*o*-toluidide dihydrogen phosphate.
$C_{13}H_{19}ClN_2O,H_3PO_4=352.8$.

CAS — 3785-21-5 (butanilicaine); 2081-65-4 (phosphate).

Butanilicaine phosphate is a local anaesthetic of the amide type with the general actions described under Local Anaesthetics, p.899. It has a rapid onset of action and short duration of analgesia. It has been used as a 0.5 or 1% solution for infiltration or nerve block anaesthesia, and as a 3% solution in dentistry.

Proprietary Names
Hostacain *(also as hydrochloride) (Hoechst, Ger.; Hoechst, Spain).*

7612-g

Butethamine Hydrochloride. Ibylcaini Chloridum. 2-Isobutylaminoethyl 4-aminobenzoate hydrochloride.
$C_{13}H_{20}N_2O_2,HCl=272.8$.

CAS — 2090-89-3 (butethamine); 553-68-4 (hydrochloride).

Odourless, small, white crystals or white crystalline powder with a bitter numbing taste. M.p. 193° to 197°. **Soluble** in water, alcohol, and chloroform; practically insoluble in ether. A 1% solution in water has a pH of about 5.

Butethamine hydrochloride is a local anaesthetic of the ester type which was formerly used in dentistry.
The general actions of local anaesthetics are described on p.899.

7613-q

Butyl Aminobenzoate *(B.P. Vet.)*. Butamben *(U.S.P.)*; Butoforme. Butyl 4-aminobenzoate.
$C_{11}H_{15}NO_2=193.2$.

CAS — 94-25-7.

Pharmacopoeias. In *U.S.*

A white, odourless, tasteless, crystalline powder. M.p. 57° to 59°.
Soluble 1 in 7000 of water, 1 in 3 of alcohol, and 1 in 2 of ether; soluble in chloroform, liquid paraffin, fixed oils, and dilute acids. It slowly hydrolyses when boiled with water. **Protect** from light.

Adverse Effects, Treatment, and Precautions. As for Local Anaesthetics, p.899.
Skin reactions to butyl aminobenzoate may occur.

Uses. Butyl aminobenzoate is a local anaesthetic of the ester type and has been used for surface anaesthesia (see p.901), usually in concentrations of 1 or 2% and in conjunction with other local anaesthetics, in creams, ointments, sprays, and suppositories. It may also be an ingredient in certain injections, for example, erythromycin ethylsuccinate injection.
Butyl aminobenzoate picrate is applied as a 1% ointment for the relief of pruritus and pain due to minor burns.
Isobutyl aminobenzoate (isobutamben) is under investigation.

Proprietary Names
Butesin Picrate *(picrate) (Abbott, USA).*

7614-p

Carticaine Hydrochloride. 40 045; Hoe 045; Carticain Hydrochloride. Methyl 4-methyl-3-(2-propylaminopropionamido)thiophene-2-carboxylate hydrochloride.
$C_{13}H_{20}N_2O_3S,HCl=320.8$.

CAS — 23964-58-1 (carticaine); 23964-57-0 (hydrochloride).

A white odourless crystalline powder. M.p. about 175°. **Soluble** in water and alcohol.

Carticaine hydrochloride is a local anaesthetic of the amide type and has the general actions described under Local Anaesthetics, p.899. It has been used as 1 or 2% solution with adrenaline for infiltration anaesthesia and nerve block; a 4% solution with adrenaline has been used in dentistry.

References to carticaine hydrochloride: A. Den Hertog, *Eur. J. Pharmac.*, 1974, *26*, 175 (pharmacology in *animals*); K. Strasser *et al.*, *Z. Geburtsh. Perinatol.*, 1977, *181*, 118 (placental transfer); S. Kaukinen *et al.*, *Ann. clin. Res.*, 1978, *10*, 191 (spinal anaesthesia).

Proprietary Names
Ultracain *(Hoechst, Ger.)*; Ultracain D-S *(with adrenaline) (Hoechst, Ger.; Hoechst, Neth.).*

NOTE. Ultracaine (*USA*) contains lignocaine hydrochloride.

7615-s

Chloroprocaine Hydrochloride *(U.S.P.)*.
2-Diethylaminoethyl 4-amino-2-chlorobenzoate hydrochloride.
$C_{13}H_{19}ClN_2O_2,HCl=307.2$.

CAS — 133-16-4 (chloroprocaine); 3858-89-7 (hydrochloride).

Pharmacopoeias. In *U.S.*

A white odourless crystalline powder with a numbing taste. M.p. 173° to 176°.
Soluble 1 in 20 of water and 1 in 100 of alcohol; very slightly soluble in chloroform; practically insoluble in ether. Solutions in water are acid to litmus. Discoloured solutions should not be used.

Adverse Effects, Treatment, and Precautions. As for Local Anaesthetics, p.899.
The toxicity of chloroprocaine hydrochloride is less than that of procaine hydrochloride.

Absorption and Fate. Chloroprocaine is hydrolysed rapidly in the circulation by plasma cholinesterase.
See also under Local Anaesthetics, p.900.

In 7 healthy subjects given chloroprocaine 250 mg by constant-rate intravenous infusion over 30 or 60 minutes no intact chloroprocaine could be detected in the plasma. Studies in the 4 subjects given the drug over 30 minutes demonstrated the presence of a metabolite, 2-chloro-4-aminobenzoic acid, in the plasma, and 1 hour after discontinuation of the infusion up to 65% of the administered dose had been excreted in the urine, chiefly as a conjugate of this metabolite. In 2 pregnant women given about 800 mg of chloroprocaine for obstetric epidural anaesthesia no intact chloroprocaine was detected in the maternal or umbilical blood and the low ratios of foetal to maternal concentrations of the metabolite indicated that the placental transfer of this compound was very limited.— J. E. O'Brien *et al.*, *J. pharm. Sci.*, 1979, *68*, 75.

Uses. As for Local Anaesthetics, p.901.
Chloroprocaine hydrochloride is a local anaesthetic of the ester type with properties similar to those of procaine hydrochloride (p.921) but it has a more rapid action and is about twice as potent.
It is used for infiltration and regional nerve block, including paracervical block and epidural or caudal anaesthesia, as a 0.5 to 3% solution, if necessary with adrenaline 1 in 200 000 to delay absorption and reduce toxicity. For infiltration anaesthesia, up to 100 ml of a 0.5% solution has been used. For peripheral nerve block up to 40 ml of a 2% solution may be injected; for digital block 3 to 4 ml of a 1% solution without adrenaline is used. For caudal and epidural anaesthesia the usual dose is 15 to 25 ml of a 2 or 3% solution. Chloroprocaine is not an effective surface anaesthetic.

Chloroprocaine hydrochloride, in a dose of 12 ml of a 1% solution containing adrenaline 1 in 200 000, was used for 261 paracervical blocks in 211 patients during childbirth. Apgar scores were depressed in 11 of 213 infants and no foetal deaths were related to chloroprocaine. In 6 of 104 foetuses monitored abnormal heart-rate patterns were recorded *in utero* but none had a depressed Apgar score at birth. In 172 blocks pain relief was excellent in 83%, partially effective in 5%, and ineffective in 12%.— D. W. Freeman and N. I. Arnold, *J. Am. med. Ass.*, 1975, *231*, 56.

Further references to the use of chloroprocaine.— R. G. Strauss *et al.*, *Am. J. Obstet. Gynec.*, 1979, *133*, 891 (prolongation of paracervical block by the addition of dextran); Y. R. Park and D. W. Eastwood, *Anesthesiology*, 1980, *52*, 439 (the effect of dextrose on the gravitational spread of epidural anaesthesia).

Preparations

Chloroprocaine Hydrochloride Injection *(U.S.P.)*. A sterile solution in Water for Injections. pH 2.7 to 4.

Proprietary Names
Nesacaine *(Pennwalt, USA).*

7616-w

Cinchocaine *(B.P.C. 1973)*. Cincainum; Dibucaine *(U.S.P.)*. 2-Butoxy-*N*-(2-diethylaminoethyl)cinchoninamide; 2-Butoxy-*N*-(2-diethylaminoethyl)quinoline-4-carboxamide.
$C_{20}H_{29}N_3O_2=343.5$.

CAS — 85-79-0.

Pharmacopoeias. In *Nord.* and *U.S.*

A white to off-white, somewhat hygroscopic powder, odourless or with a slight characteristic odour. M.p. 62° to 65.5°.
Soluble 1 in 4600 of water, 1 in less than 1 of alcohol and of chloroform, and 1 in 1.4 to 1.5 of ether; soluble in light petroleum, liquid paraffin, and mineral acids; soluble 1 in 30 of arachis oil. Oily solutions for injection are prepared aseptically. It darkens on exposure to light. **Store** in airtight containers. Protect from light.

7617-e

Cinchocaine Hydrochloride *(B.P.)*. Dibucaine Hydrochloride *(U.S.P.)*; Cincaini Chloridum; Dibucainium Chloride; Percainum; Sovcainum.
$C_{20}H_{29}N_3O_2,HCl=379.9$.

CAS — 61-12-1.

NOTE. This compound was originally marketed under the name Percaine, but accidents occurred owing to the confusion of this name with procaine.

Pharmacopoeias. In *Arg., Aust., Br., Braz., Cz., Fr., Ind., Jap., Nord., Port., Rus., Swiss,* and *U.S.*

Fine, white, odourless, hygroscopic colourless crystals or white to off-white crystalline powder, with a slighly bitter taste. M.p. 95° to 100°.
Soluble 1 in 0.5 of water; freely soluble in alcohol and acetone; soluble in chloroform; practically insoluble in ether and oils. A 2% solution in water has a pH of 5 to 6. Solutions are **sterilised**

by autoclaving or by filtration. **Incompatible** with alkalis, iodides, and mercury and silver salts. It darkens on exposure to light. **Store** in airtight containers. Protect from light.

Sterilisation. Solutions of pH 4.5 to 6 were sterilised by heating in an autoclave at 120° for 20 minutes. Below pH 4.5, hydrolysis occurred much more rapidly and above pH 6 the base might be precipitated.— J. Mørch, *Dansk Tidsskr. Farm.*, 1953, *27*, 173.

Repeated autoclaving to sterilise the outside surface of ampoules used with lumbar puncture sets did not cause deterioration provided that the total time of heating at 115° did not exceed about 2 hours.— T. D. Whittet, *Anaesthesia*, 1954, *9*, 271.

Adverse Effects, Treatment, and Precautions. As for Local Anaesthetics, p.899.

Allergy and effects on the skin. From patch tests, 4 of 413 patients with contact dermatoses were found to be allergic to cinchocaine.— E. Epstein, *J. Am. med. Ass.*, 1966, *198*, 517.

A report of a photosensitivity reaction to cinchocaine.— T. Horio, *Archs Derm.*, 1979, *115*, 986.

Absorption and Fate. Like other local anaesthetics of the amide type, cinchocaine is metabolised in the liver.

See also under Local Anaesthetics, p.900.

Uses. As for Local Anaesthetics, p.901.

Cinchocaine is a local anaesthetic of the amide type which is suitable for surface or spinal anaesthesia. It is several times more toxic than lignocaine by injection or cocaine by local application but its local anaesthetic action is greater and it can therefore be used in lower concentrations. It has a more prolonged action than lignocaine.

Cinchocaine has vasodilator properties; the risk of adverse effects may be reduced by the inclusion of adrenaline to delay absorption. Analgesia may be preceded by irritation.

For surface anaesthesia cinchocaine has been used, as the base or hydrochloride, in concentrations of 0.1 to 2%. Suppositories containing 11 mg of the hydrochloride have been used.

For spinal anaesthesia up to 2 ml of a hyperbaric solution of cinchocaine hydrochloride 0.25% and dextrose 5% may be injected. A hypobaric injection containing 0.067% (1 in 1500) in 0.5% sodium chloride and an isobaric injection of 0.1% in cerebrospinal fluid have also been used.

A report of the beneficial effects of regional nerve block with cinchocaine 0.15% in the treatment of muscular atrophy.— Y. Terauchi (letter), *Lancet*, 1976, *2*, 477.

Preparations of Cinchocaine and Cinchocaine Hydrochloride

Cinchocaine Mouth-wash *(Roy. Marsden Hosp.)*. Cinchocaine hydrochloride 0.2, water to 100. To be used diluted with an equal quantity of warm water.

Cinchocaine Suppositories *(B.P.C. 1973)*. Supp. Cinchocain. Suppositories containing cinchocaine hydrochloride in theobroma oil or other suitable fatty basis. About 1.5 g of cinchocaine hydrochloride displaces 1 g of theobroma oil. Store in a cool place.

Dibucaine Cream *(U.S.P.)*. Cinchocaine in a suitable cream basis. Store in airtight containers. Protect from light.

Dibucaine Hydrochloride Injection *(U.S.P.)*. A sterile solution of cinchocaine hydrochloride in Water for Injections. pH 4.5 to 7. Protect from light.

Dibucaine Ointment *(U.S.P.)*. Cinchocaine in a suitable ointment basis. Store in airtight containers. Protect from light.

Dibucaine Suppositories *(U.S.P.)*. Suppositories containing cinchocaine. Store at a temperature not exceeding 30°. Protect from light.

Proprietary Preparations of Cinchocaine and Cinchocaine Hydrochloride

Nupercainal Ointment *(Ciba, UK)*. Contains cinchocaine hydrochloride 1.1%. (Also available as Nupercainal in *Belg., Canad., Denm., Ital., Switz.,USA*).

Nupercaine *(Ciba, UK)*. Cinchocaine hydrochloride, available as **Cream** containing 1.1% in a water-miscible basis and as 1 in 200 **Heavy Spinal Solution** with dextrose 6%, in ampoules of 3 ml. (Also available as Nupercaine in *Austral., S.Afr.*, and *USA*).

Other Proprietary Names

Cincain *(Denm., Swed.)*; Cinkain *(Denm.)*; Percainal *(Spain)*.

Cinchocaine was also formerly marketed in Great Britain under the proprietary name Dermacaine Cream (*Medo-Chemicals*).

7618-l

Coca *(B.P.C. 1934)*. Coca Leaves; Hoja de Coca.

Pharmacopoeias. In *Arg., Fr., Port.*, and *Span.*

The dried leaves of *Erythroxylum coca* (Bolivian or Huanuco leaf) or of *E. truxillense* (Peruvian or Truxillo leaf) (Erythroxylaceae), indigenous to Bolivia and Peru and cultivated in Java.

The total alkaloid content varies from 0.5 to 1.5%. Truxillo and Java leaf contain more, but only about half is cocaine. The alkaloid content of Bolivian leaf is 70 to 80% cocaine. Coca is frequently valued on its ecgonine content since commercial cocaine is obtained synthetically from ecgonine.

Coca was formerly employed, usually in the form of an elixir or liquid extract, as a cerebral and muscle stimulant and for the relief of gastric pain, nausea, and vomiting, but has no valid place in modern medicine. In Bolivia and Peru the leaf is chewed to relieve hunger and fatigue.

The deleterious effects of the wide-spread habit of chewing of coca leaves in Peru. The majority of users consume 30 to 50 g of coca a day.— V. Zapata-Ortiz, *Int. J. Addict.*, 1970, *5*, 287. See also A. A. Buck *et al.*, *Bull. Narcot.*, 1970, *22* (4), 23; J. C. Negrete, *Bull. Pan. Am. Hlth Org.*, 1978, *12*, 211 (lasting brain function changes associated with chronic coca leaf chewing); *Lancet*, 1979, *1*, 963.

A report of the syndromes produced by coca paste smoking.— F. R. Jerí *et al.*, *Bull. Narcot.*, 1978, *30*, No. 3, 1.

7619-y

Cocaine *(B.P., U.S.P.)*. Cocaina; Methyl Benzoylecgonine. (1*R*,2*R*,3*s*,5*S*)-2-Methoxycarbonyltropan-3-yl benzoate.

$C_{17}H_{21}NO_4$=303.4.

CAS — 50-36-2.

Pharmacopoeias. In *Br., Ind., It., Mex., Port., Span., Swiss, Turk.*, and *U.S.*

Colourless odourless crystals or white crystalline powder with a bitter numbing taste obtained from the leaves of *Erythroxylum coca* and other spp. of *Erythroxylum*, or by synthesis. M.p. 96° to 98°. It is slightly volatile.

Soluble 1 in 600 of water, 1 in 7 of alcohol, 1 in 30 of arachis oil, 1 in 10 of castor oil, 1 in about 0.5 of chloroform, 1 in 4 of ether, 1 in 80 to 120 of liquid or soft paraffin, 1 in 4 of oleic acid, 1 in 12 of olive oil, 1 in 2 of warm anhydrous wool fat; soluble in acetone, light petroleum, and volatile oils; practically insoluble in glycerol. A solution in diluted hydrochloric acid is laevorotatory. A saturated solution in water is alkaline to phenolphthalein. Sterile oily solutions are prepared aseptically. **Protect** from light.

In the preparation of oily solutions of cocaine only a mild degree of heat should be used.

7620-g

Cocaine Hydrochloride *(B.P., Eur. P., U.S.P.)*. Cocaine Hydrochlor.; Cocaini Hydrochloridum; Cocainium Chloride; Chloridrato de Cocaína.

$C_{17}H_{21}NO_4$,HCl=339.8.

CAS — 53-21-4.

Pharmacopoeias. In all pharmacopoeias examined.

Odourless hygroscopic colourless crystals or white crystalline powder with a bitter sharp numbing taste. M.p. about 197° with decomposition. Cocaine hydrochloride 1.12 g is approximately equivalent to 1 g of cocaine.

Soluble 1 in 0.5 of water, 1 in 3.5 to 4.5 of alcohol, 1 in 15 to 18 of chloroform, 1 in 3 of glycerol; practically insoluble in ether and fixed oils. A solution in water is laevorotatory. A 6.33% solution is iso-osmotic with serum. Solutions are **sterilised** by maintaining at 98° to 100° for 30 minutes with a bactericide or by filtration. **Incompatible** with alkali hydroxides and carbonates, mercuric chloride, iodides, tannic acid, and soluble silver salts. It is incompatible with borax but a clear aqueous solution may be made by dissolving equal weights of borax and boric acid and adding the cocaine hydrochloride in solution. Solutions of cocaine hydrochloride are liable to develop fungous growths and should contain a preservative. **Store** in airtight containers. Protect from light.

Compatibility. At the concentrations likely to be encountered in ophthalmic practice, cocaine hdyrochloride was compatible with zinc sulphate.—Pharm. Soc. Lab. Rep., *Pharm. J.*, 1960, *2*, 454.

Haemolysis. An aqueous solution of cocaine hydrochloride iso-osmotic with serum (6.33%) caused 47% haemolysis of erythrocytes cultured in it for 45 minutes.— E. R. Hammarlund and K. Pedersen-Bjergaard, *J. pharm. Sci.*, 1961, *50*, 24.

Preservative for eye-drops. Benzalkonium chloride 0.01% or chlorhexidine gluconate 0.02% were suitable preservatives for cocaine hydrochloride eye-drops sterilised by filtration.— M. Van Ooteghem, *Pharm. Tijdschr. Belg.*, 1968, *45*, 69.

Stability of solutions. Aqueous solutions containing cocaine hydrochloride 5% and phenol 0.5% remained clear and colourless for a year at 0° to 4°, room temperature, and 37°. A fall in pH from 4.6 to 3.9, 2.7, and 2.1 respectively suggested chemical change; such solutions should therefore be stored in a cool place.— Pharm. Soc. Lab. Rep. P/75/14, 1975.

Dependence. Drug dependence of the cocaine type is a state arising from the repeated administration of cocaine or an agent with cocaine-like properties; it is characterised by an overwhelming need to continue taking the drug and by a psychic dependence on the drug. Tolerance does not develop but repeated use at short intervals may result in an intense toxic reaction. There is no physical dependence and therefore no characteristic withdrawal syndrome, though depression and delusions may persist for some time.

It is abused as snuff, which causes ulceration and perforation of the nasal septum on prolonged use, by mouth, and by intravenous injection of the hydrochloride. It may be injected with diamorphine or morphine to control the excitatory effects. Cocaine base has been smoked.

Cocaine dependence may give rise to psychotic states and hallucinations, digestive disorders, nausea, loss of appetite, emaciation, formication, impotence, sleeplessness, tremors and convulsions. Deaths have occurred following the illicit use of cocaine.

For treatment of dependence the drug should be withdrawn abruptly and any withdrawal symptoms treated symptomatically.

Cocaine is now one of the most widely used drugs of abuse in the USA although powders may often be contaminated with other substances such as mannitol, lignocaine, or sugars. It is most commonly 'snorted' into the nose but is also active by mouth and has been smoked in pipes or cigarettes. Some users may inject the drug intravenously. Psychotic reactions similar to those seen with amphetamines have occurred and large doses can cause convulsions and death.— *Med. Lett.*, 1979, *21*, 18. Intravenous cocaine and the smoking of cocaine base produce extreme compulsive use.— *ibid.*, 1980, *22*, 73.

When injected or inhaled cocaine produced a condition of hyperstimulation, of short duration, characterised by overalertness, euphoria, and feelings of great power. Heavy users had been known to inject cocaine intravenously every 10 minutes. Cocaine delayed ejaculation. In consistent users depression might occur when cocaine was withdrawn. Heavy use led to weight loss, insomnia, and anxiety. Oversuspiciousness and paranoid thinking with hallucinations were not uncommon. Violent behaviour might occur. Increases in the heart-rate, blood pressure, and respiration were the result of sympathetic stimulation. Overdosage produced tremors, convulsions, and delirium.— S. Cohen, *J. Am. med. Ass.*, 1975, *231*, 74.

A report of laboratory-controlled studies of the comparative effects of cocaine, dexamphetamine, and saline in 12 subjects with a history of illicit drug use. Cocaine 16 mg was generally rated as similar to an average illicit dose; 24 and 32 mg as the highest ever taken. Several identified their response to intravenous injection of dexamphetamine as being the same as that to illicit cocaine; this was not surprising as illicit cocaine is frequently heavily adulterated with dexamphetamine. The cardiovascular effects of cocaine were of short duration and usually limited to sinus tachycardia; a second injection of 32 mg within 150 minutes did not appear to enhance toxicity.— W. H. Fennel *et al.* (letter), *New Engl. J. Med.*, 1976, *295*, 960.

A growing trend towards the smoking of cocaine alkaloid or 'free base' had been detected. The clinical signs associated with such abuse included mydriasis, anorexia, hyperactivity, insomnia, weight loss, and rapid pulse. Depending on dose and personality there might be progression to manic-like euphoria, depressive-like dysphoria, or schizophrenic-like paranoid psychosis. These manifestations of cocaine smoking were very rare when cocaine was used intranasally.— R. K. Siegel (letter), *New Engl. J. Med.*, 1979, *300*, 373.

Comment on the use of cocaine substitutes.— R. K. Siegel (letter), *New Engl. J. Med.*, 1980, *302*, 817.

References to toxicity associated with the abuse of cocaine.— A. Benchimol *et al.*, *Ann. intern. Med.*, 1978, *88*, 519 (palpitations and accelerated ventricular rhythm); R. K. Siegel, *Am. J. Psychiat.*, 1978, *135*, 309 (hallucinations); C. V. Wetli and R. K. Wright, *J. Am. med. Ass.*, 1979, *241*, 2519 (deaths in 24 subjects after the oral, nasal, or intravenous use of cocaine).

Adverse Effects. As for Local Anaesthetics, p.899.

Symptoms of central nervous stimulation and sympathetic overactivity are very marked in overdosage with cocaine. A single dose of 1.2 g may be fatal, but some persons have a cocaine idiosyncrasy and death from cardiovascular failure may occur quite suddenly after doses of only 20 mg. Excessive concentrations should not be used as, in addition to risks of systemic toxicity following absorption, they may produce lasting local damage.

See also Dependence (above).

Effects on the ears. Cocaine, applied to the middle ear, caused severe vertigo, nausea, and vomiting. It should not be used to assist in the removal of foreign bodies from the external canal.— B. H. Senturia, *J. Am. med. Ass.*, 1968, *206*, 1802.

Effects on the eyes. Repeated use of cocaine eye-drops caused clouding of the cornea.— M. D. Vickers, *Prescribers' J.*, 1968, *8*, 75.

Effects on the skin. Circinate bluish atrophic scars in a 79-year-old woman were attributed to the use, many years earlier, of cocaine, and were considered due to vasoconstriction, tissue toxicity, and local infection.— H. S. Yaffee, *Cutis*, 1968, *4*, 286.

Treatment of Adverse Effects. As for Local Anaesthetics, p.900.

If an overdose of cocaine has been taken by mouth, empty the stomach by lavage and aspiration using a 0.02% (*very pale pink*) solution of potassium permanganate. Activated charcoal has been suggested to delay absorption.

For convulsions, diazepam or a short-acting barbiturate such as thiopentone sodium may be given intravenously. Assisted respiration may be required.

A view that propranolol hydrochloride should be used to treat overdose with cocaine and related sympathomimetic agents. A 1-mg dose administered intravenously at one-minute intervals up to a total dose of 8 mg was effective and safe in over 50 cases. There was an almost instantaneous titration toward reversal of cardiopressor effects and hypertension, tachycardia, and tachypnoea were resolved. Constant cardiovascular monitoring is vital and the problem of hyperpyrexia must be dealt with.— R. T. Rappolt *et al.* (letter), *New Engl. J. Med.*, 1976, *295*, 448. See also *idem* (letter), *Lancet*, 1976, *2*, 640; *idem*, *Clin. Toxicol.*, 1977, *10*, 265. Studies on the illicit use of cocaine indicated that the cardiovascular effects of cocaine were of short duration and usually limited to sinus tachycardia. It was considered that subjects under the influence of cocaine did not require acute intervention and that if toxic cardiovascular or thermal signs persisted agents other than cocaine might be responsible.— W. H. Fennell *et al.* (letter), *New Engl. J. Med.*, 1976, *295*, 960. Further criticism; any beneficial effects of propranolol in the acute treatment of 'casual' overdosage with cocaine should not be extrapolated to potentially lethal cases of cocaine poisoning. Of 5 *dogs* pretreated with propranolol and subsequently given a lethal dose of cocaine all died whereas of 6 pretreated with chlorpromazine hydrochloride all survived. Chlorpromazine prevented the cocaine-induced changes in cardiovascular function and antagonised the increase in body temperature and the decline in arterial pH whereas propranolol did not.— J. D. Catravas *et al.* (letter), *ibid.*, 1977, *297*, 1238. Results in *monkeys* also suggested that chlorpromazine would be the best agent to use in the management of severe cocaine toxicity. Propranolol appeared to sensitise the animals to the convulsant effects of cocaine administered intravenously.— M. M. Guinn *et al.*, *Toxic. appl. Pharmac.*, 1978, *45*, 355.

A 31-year-old man swallowed 6 packages of cocaine each containing 5 g and had blood concentrations of 3.6 µg per ml rising to 5.2 µg per ml after one of the packages had burst *in situ*. Magnesium citrate as a laxative was ineffective in removing the packages. Four hours after receiving ipecac syrup *U.S.P.* 30 ml and before emesis, toxic symptoms included disorientation, euphoria, and loss of consciousness. Seizures required treatment with diazepam, phenytoin, and pancuronium. Additional therapy included dopamine. Within 3 hours the patient's blood pressure and urine output returned to normal. The remainder of the packages were removed intact. The patient recovered but experienced loss of recent memory and disorientation.— C. A. Suarez *et al.*, *J. Am. med. Ass.*, 1977, *238*, 1391.

Precautions. As for Local Anaesthetics, p.900.

Since some patients have a marked sensitivity to cocaine the administration of a test dose before use on mucous membranes has been suggested. Ophthalmic preparations of cocaine should not be applied to the eyes for prolonged periods as damage to the cornea may occur not only from the local action of cocaine, but also from loss of the protective eyelid reflexes.

Patients receiving cocaine for surface anaesthesia should be monitored for possible cardiovascular effects. Cocaine and adrenaline enhance each other's sympathomimetic effects and should preferably not be used in association.

Cocaine should be used with great caution in patients with hypertension, cardiovascular disease, or thyrotoxicosis.

Interactions. Cocaine was absorbed to a variable extent when it was sprayed on to mucous membranes of a patient taking a sympathomimetic such as amphetamine. It was more likely to cause cardiac arrhythmias or convulsions.— D. R. Laurence, *Prescribers' J.*, 1963, *3*, 48.

Cocaine was reported to block the uptake of endogenous or exogenous noradrenaline. Interaction was theoretically possible with methyldopa, tricyclic antidepressants, monoamine oxidase inhibitors, chlorpromazine, reserpine, guanethidine, adrenaline, and alpha- and beta-adrenoceptor blocking agents.— R. B. Smith, *Archs Otolar.*, 1973, *98*, 139.

In view of the dangerous potential interaction between cocaine and catecholamines the mixture of dry cocaine powder moistened with adrenaline solution ('Cocaine mud') was unsafe.— E. N. Willey (letter), *J. Am. med. Ass.*, 1977, *238*, 1813.

Absorption and Fate. Cocaine may be slowly absorbed because of the vasoconstriction it produces, but absorption occurs from all sites of application, including mucous membranes and the gastro-intestinal tract, and may be enhanced when there is inflammation. It is hydrolysed by plasma esterases and some is demethylated in the liver; a small proportion is excreted unchanged in the urine.

See also under Local Anaesthetics, p.900.

An addict taking cocaine hydrochloride 120 mg and diamorphine 180 mg, as hydrochloride, intravenously daily excreted 1 to 9% of the cocaine unchanged and about 35 to 55% as benzoylecgonine in the urine.— F. Fish and W. D. C. Wilson, *J. Pharm. Pharmac.*, 1969, *21, Suppl.*, 135S. In 4 addicts taking cocaine, urine-cocaine concentrations were 91, 76, 42, and 2 ng per ml respectively with corresponding urine-benzoylecgonine concentrations of 1.6, 1.5, 1.8, and 1.8 µg per ml respectively.— S. P. Jindal and P. Vestergaard, *J. pharm. Sci.*, 1978, *67*, 811. The metabolism of cocaine was studied in 2 healthy subjects given 10 mg of radioactively-labelled cocaine by mouth. The results indicated that esterases play a major role and the hydrolysis product ecgonine methyl ester accounted for 49% of the total radioactivity in the urine of subject 1 and 32% in subject 2; subject 1 also had greater plasma cholinesterase activity. *N*-demethylation of cocaine also took place in the liver or intestinal wall or both but it appeared that only a small fraction is converted to norcocaine in man.— T. Inaba *et al.*, *Clin. Pharmac. Ther.*, 1978, *23*, 547. The hydrolysis of cocaine *in vitro* by human hepatic and plasma enzymes (esterases) yielded, ecgonine methyl ester. Norcocaine yielded norecgonine methyl ester when treated in the same way. Benzoylecgonine, a major hydrolytic metabolite of cocaine was not produced from either compound by the action of these enzymes.— D. J. Stewart *et al.*, *Clin. Pharmac. Ther.*, 1979, *25*, 464.

In 13 surgical patients peak plasma concentratons of cocaine were reached in from 15 to 60 minutes after the application as a vasoconstrictor of cocaine hydrochloride solution 10%, in doses of 1.5 mg per kg body-weight, to the nasal mucosa before intubation; cocaine was detectable in the nose 3 hours later, and persisted in the plasma for 6 hours in some patients. Diazepam and morphine sulphate had also been given as premedication to patients in the study.— C. Van Dyke *et al.*, *Science*, 1976, *191*, 859.

Studies in 4 healthy subjects used to the effects of cocaine showed that the mean peak plasma concentrations after oral administration of cocaine hydrochloride 2 mg per kg body-weight were 104 to 424 ng per ml, reached in about 1 to 1½ hours, and decreasing gradually over the following 4 to 5 hours. Following intranasal administration of a similar dose as 10% solution, mean peak plasma concentrations were 61 to 408 ng per ml reached 1 to 2 hours after use and decreasing over the next 2 to 3 hours.— C. Van Dyke *et al.*, *Science*, 1978, *200*, 211.

Studies in 10 subjects with a known history of cocaine dependence showed a positive relationship between the peak plasma concentration, increase in heart-rate and the amount of cocaine hydrochloride given either intravenously or intranasally. The peak plasma concentration was reached in 30 to 60 minutes after intranasal administration and fell gradually over the next hour. In all patients the heart-rate returned to pre-drug values before the elimination of cocaine from plasma was complete.— J. I. Javaid *et al.*, *Science*, 1978, *202*, 227.

Further references.— M. J. Kogan *et al.*, *Analyt. Chem.*, 1977, *49*, 1965; D. L. von Minden and N. A. D'Amato, *Analyt. Chem.*, 1977, *49*, 1974 (determinations of benzoylecgonine and cocaine in biological fluids); P. Wilkinson *et al.*, *Clin. Pharmac. Ther.*, 1980, *27*, 386 (pharmacokinetics after intranasal and oral administration).

Uses. Cocaine is a surface anaesthetic (see p.901) of the ester type but, because of systemic adverse effects and the danger of causing dependence its use is now almost entirely restricted to surgery of the ear, nose, and throat, and occasionally to ophthalmic surgery. Cocaine also blocks the uptake of catecholamines at adrenergic nerve endings and potentiates the action of endogenous and exogenous catecholamines. Its sympathomimetic actions cause tachycardia, peripheral vasoconstriction, hypertension, and mydriasis. The use of cocaine in association with drugs such as adrenaline should be avoided.

When applied to mucous membranes, surface anaesthesia develops in about 5 to 10 minutes and persists for 20 minutes or longer depending on the concentration of cocaine used and on the vascularity of the tissue.

When instilled into the eye, cocaine causes blanching of the sclera, dilates the pupil, and anaesthetises the superficial structures of the eye. At first, however, the instillation may be painful. The mydriasis may be enhanced by the addition of atropine or homatropine. Cycloplegia has been reported with cocaine.

Systemically, cocaine stimulates the cerebral cortex and gives rise to a feeling of well-being and exhilaration; fatigue is overcome and capacity for work increased. Repeated use of cocaine may lead to dependence (see above).

Cocaine hydrochloride is used for the administration of cocaine in aqueous solutions. For ophthalmic use, cocaine hydrochloride has been employed in solutions containing 1 to 4%, alone or with homatropine hydrobromide. Cocaine alkaloid has been used in oily eye-drops.

Solutions containing 5 to 10% of cocaine hydrochloride have been used as sprays for the nose and throat, and concentrations of up to 20% have been used on the larynx. It has been recommended that no more than 100 mg should be applied to mucous membranes in adults.

Cocaine is used in conjunction with diamorphine or morphine for the relief of severe pain, especially in terminal illness (see p.1009 and p.1020).

Cocaine solutions should never be administered by injection for local, regional, or spinal anaesthesia; other local anaesthetics are equally effective and much safer.

A review of the biochemical pharmacology of cocaine.— J. Caldwell and P. S. Sever, *Clin. Pharmac. Ther.*, 1974, *16*, 625.

Reviews and discussions on the use and abuse of cocaine.— *Br. med. J.*, 1979, *1*, 971; D. J. Egan and D. O. Robinson, *Int. J. Addict.*, 1979, *14*, 231; L. M. Haddad, *J. Am. Coll. emergency Physns*, 1979, *8*, 374; K. Pearman, *J. Lar. Otol.*, 1979, *93*, 1191.

The effects of cocaine on depressed patients.— F. K. Goodwin *et al.*, *Am. J. Psychiat.*, 1974, *131*, 511, per *Int. pharm. Abstr.*, 1975, *12*, 349.

See also under Dependence (above).

Nose bleeds. In severe nose bleeds a 2.5 to 10% solution of cocaine, sprayed onto the nasal mucosa, helps to stop the bleeding by vasoconstriction. It also anaesthetises the mucosa so that any later manoeuvre that may be necessary can be performed without discomfort.— H. Ludman, *Br. med. J.*, 1981, *282*, 967.

Surface anaesthesia. The view that a 25% paste of cocaine hydrochloride suspended in soft paraffin is an effective and safe local anaesthetic for the nasal mucosa when used very sparingly.— R. P. E. Barton and R. F. E. Gray, *J. Lar. Otol.*, 1979, *93*, 1201.

Cocaine hydrochloride did not exert any clinically significant sympathomimetic effect when a 10% solution was applied to the nasal mucosa before intubation in a study of 18 patients undergoing coronary artery surgery, under general anaesthesia with nitrous oxide, halothane, and pancuronium bromide.— P. G. Barash *et al.*, *J. Am. med. Ass.*, 1980, *243*, 1437.

Preparations of Cocaine and Cocaine Hydrochloride

Eye Preparations

Atropine and Cocaine Eye Ointment *(B.P.C. 1968)*. See p.292.

Cocaine, Adrenaline and Zinc Eye Drops *(A.P.F.)*. BCAZ Eye Drops. Cocaine hydrochloride 500 mg, boric acid 3 g, glyercol 1.5 ml, adrenaline solution 10 ml, zinc sulphate 250 mg, chlorbutol 500 mg, sodium metabisulphite 50 mg, Water for Injections to 100 ml. Sterilised by autoclaving. Protect from light.

Cocaine and Adrenaline Eye Drops *(A.P.F.)*. BCA Eye Drops. Cocaine hydrochloride 500 mg, boric acid 3 g, glycerol 1.5 ml, adrenaline solution 10 ml, chlorbutol 500 mg, sodium metabisulphite 50 mg, Water for Injections to 100 ml. Sterilised by autoclaving. Protect from light.

Cocaine and Homatropine Eye-drops *(B.P.C. 1973)*. Guttae Cocainae et Homatropinae. A sterile solution containing cocaine hydrochloride 2% and homatropine hydrobromide 2%, with chlorhexidine acetate 0.01%, in water. The solution is sterilised by filtration or by maintaining at 98° to 100° for 30 minutes. It is adversely affected by alkali.

A.P.F. (Homatropine and Cocaine Eye Drops) has cocaine hydrochloride 2%, homatropine hydrobromide 2%, boric acid 0.5%, chlorhexidine acetate 0.01%, in Water for Injections; sterilised by autoclaving.

Cocaine and Homatropine Lamellae *(B.P.C. 1963)*. Lamellae containing cocaine hydrochloride and homatropine hydrobromide.

Cocaine and Mercuric Chloride Oily Eye-drops *(B.P.C. 1959)*. Gutt. Cocain. et Hydrarg. Perchlor. Oleos. Cocaine 500 mg, mercuric chloride 33 mg, dehydrated alcohol 1 ml, and castor oil 95 g. Protect from light and do not use if marked precipitation has occurred.

NOTE. Cocaine and Mercuric Chloride Oily Eye-drops have been known as Factory Eye-drops. Current regulations in Great Britain require that factory first-aid boxes contain an 'approved eye ointment'—sulphacetamide eye ointment 6 or 10%. See also Sodium Bicarbonate, p.635.

The crystals which formed on standing consisted of benzoylecgonine and were produced by hydrolysis of the cocaine. The conditions necessary for maximum stability were the use of a good quality castor oil having a low acid value, a dry container, absence of water in the alcohol, and use of little or no heat.— W. Forster, *Pharm. J.*, 1936, *2*, 83.

Cocaine Eye Drops Strong *(A.P.F.)*. Cocaine hydrochloride 5 g, chlorhexidine acetate 10 mg, Water for Injections to 100 ml. Sterilised by autoclaving.

Cocaine Eye Drops Weak *(A.P.F.)*. Cocaine hydrochloride 1 g, sodium chloride 700 mg, chlorhexidine acetate 10 mg, Water for Injections to 100 ml. Sterilised by autoclaving. To be supplied when Cocaine Eye Drops *A.P.F.* are requested.

Cocaine Eye-drops *(B.P.C. 1973)*. Guttae Cocainae; CCN. A sterile solution containing up to 5% of cocaine hydrochloride in water. The solution also contains either phenylmercuric acetate or nitrate 0.002%, or chlorhexidine acetate 0.01%; it is sterilised by filtration or by maintaining at 98° to 100° for 30 minutes. This solution is adversely affected by alkali.

A study of the stability of cocaine hydrochloride in aqueous solution. It was concluded that the formulation and methods of preparation recommended by the *B.P.C. 1973* are acceptable in respect of the chemical stability of the alkaloid, that the assay should be replaced by the method used in the present study, and that the eye-drops should be stored at 5° with a 6-month shelf-life.— J. B. Murray and H. I. Al-Shora. *J. clin. Pharm.*, 1978, *3*, 1.

Homatropine and Cocaine Eye Drops *(A.P.F.)*. See Cocaine and Homatropine Eye Drops, above.

Pastes

Cocaine Paste *(King's Coll. Hosp.)*. Cocaine hydrochloride 25 g, suprarenal (*B.P.C. 1934*) 5 g, chlorbutol 1 g, liquid paraffin 40 ml, white soft paraffin to 100 g.

Pasta Cocainae Composita *(Univ. Coll. Hosp.)*. Cocaine hydrochloride 25 g, suprarenal (*B.P.C. 1934*) 5 g, chlorbutol 1 g, liquid paraffin 60 ml, white soft paraffin to 100 g. Mill the product thoroughly. Shelf-life one year.

Solutions

Bonain's Anaesthetic Mixture *(F.N. Belg.)*. Bonain's Solution; Cocaine Anaesthetic Mixture. Cocaine hydrochloride, phenol, and menthol, equal parts. The crystals are ground together to form a liquid mixture. A local anaesthetic for use in ear, nose, and throat surgery.

Cocaine Hydrochloride Tablets for Topical Solution *(U.S.P.)*. Solution-tablets containing cocaine hydrochloride. Protect from light.

Cocaine Solution *(Roy. Nat. T. N. and E. Hosp.)*. Cocaine hydrochloride 10 g, chlorocresol 100 mg, amaranth solution 2 ml, water to 100 ml.

7621-q

Cyclomethycaine Sulphate *(B.P.)*.

Cyclomethycaine Sulfate (*U.S.P.*). 3-(2-Methylpiperidino)propyl 4-cyclohexyloxybenzoate hydrogen sulphate.

$C_{22}H_{33}NO_3,H_2SO_4$=457.6.

CAS — 139-62-8 (cyclomethycaine); 50978-10-4 (sulphate).

Pharmacopoeias. In *Br.* and *U.S.*

A white odourless crystalline powder with a bitter numbing taste. M.p. 162° to 165.5°. **Soluble** 1 in 50 of water, 1 in 50 of alcohol, and 1 in about 227 of chloroform; slightly soluble in dilute mineral acids. Solutions may be **sterilised** by autoclaving or by filtration.

Adverse Effects, Treatment, and Precautions. As for Local Anaesthetics, p.899.

Allergy and effects on the skin. From patch tests, 5 of 413 patients with contact dermatoses were found to be allergic to cyclomethycaine sulphate.— E. Epstein, *J. Am. med. Ass.*, 1966, *198*, 517.

Uses. Cyclomethycaine sulphate has been used as a surface anaesthetic (see p.901) in concentrations of 0.5 to 1% in abrasions and superficial skin irritation, burns, pruritus ani and vulvae, haemorrhoids and anal fissure, cracked nipples, and before cystoscopy providing there is not trauma. Analgesia occurs within 5 to 10 minutes and lasts for 4 to 8 hours. Cyclomethycaine is not suitable for injection or for anaesthesia of the ear, eye, nose, or throat, and should not be used on extensive areas of broken or burnt skin.

Preparations

Cyclomethycaine Sulfate Cream *(U.S.P.)*. Cyclomethycaine sulphate in a suitable cream basis. Store in airtight containers.

Cyclomethycaine Sulfate Jelly *(U.S.P.)*. Cyclomethycaine sulphate in a water-soluble viscous basis. A 10% dilution has a pH of 4.8 to 5.8. Store in airtight containers.

Cyclomethycaine Sulfate Ointment *(U.S.P.)*. Cyclomethycaine sulphate in a suitable ointment basis. Store in airtight containers.

Cyclomethycaine Sulfate Suppositories *(U.S.P.)*. Suppositories containing cyclomethycaine sulphate. Store at 2° to 8°.

Proprietary Names

Surfacaine *(Lilly, USA)*.

7622-p

Dimethisoquin Hydrochloride *(U.S.P.)*.

Chinisocaine Hydrochloride; Dimethisoquinium Chloride; Quinisocaine Hydrochloride. 2-(3-Butyl-1-isoquinolyloxy)-*NN*-dimethylethylamine hydrochloride.

$C_{17}H_{24}N_2O,HCl$=308.9.

CAS — 86-80-6 (dimethisoquin); 2773-92-4 (hydrochloride).

Pharmacopoeias. In *U.S.*

A white to off-white odourless crystalline powder with a bitter numbing taste. M.p. 144° to 148°. **Soluble** 1 in 8 of water, 1 in 3 of alcohol, and 1 in 2 of chloroform; very slightly soluble in ether. A 1% solution in water has a pH of 3.5 to 5.5. **Protect** from light.

Adverse Effects, Treatment, and Precautions. As for Local Anaesthetics, p.899.

Dimethisoquin hydrochloride should not be applied to extensive areas, to bleeding haemorrhoids, or near the eyes.

Uses. Dimethisoquin hydrochloride is a surface anaesthetic (see p.901) and has been employed as a lotion or ointment in a concentration of 0.5% which is stated to be effective for 2 to 4 hours. It has been used for the relief of pruritus, skin irritation, and mild sunburn.

Preparations

Dimethisoquin Hydrochloride Lotion *(U.S.P.)*. A lotion containing dimethisoquin hydrochloride. Store in airtight containers. Protect from light.

Dimethisoquin Hydrochloride Ointment *(U.S.P.)*. An ointment containing dimethisoquin hydrochloride. Store in airtight containers. Protect from light.

Proprietary Names

Haenal *(Stroschein, Ger.)*; Isochinol *(Chemipharm, Ger.; Chemipharm, Switz.)*; Pruralgan *(Pharmacia, Ger.)*; Pruralgin *(Pharmacia, Norw.; Pharmacia, Switz.)*; Quotane *(Smith Kline & French, Austral.; Bellon, Belg.; Smith Kline & French, Canad.; Bellon, Fr.; Bellon, Neth.; Smith Kline & French, S.Afr.; Smith Kline & French, USA)*.

Dimethisoquin hydrochloride was formerly marketed in Great Britain under the proprietary name Quotane (*Smith, Kline & French*).

7623-s

Diperodon *(U.S.P.)*.

Diperocaine. 3-Piperidinopropylene bis(phenylcarbamate) monohydrate.

$C_{22}H_{27}N_3O_4,H_2O$=415.5.

CAS — 101-08-6 (anhydrous); 51552-99-9 (monohydrate).

Pharmacopoeias. In *U.S.*

A white to cream-coloured powder with a characteristic odour. Practically **insoluble** in water; soluble 1 in 3 of alcohol, 1 in 10 of chloroform, 1 in 4 of ether, and 1 in 1 of methyl alcohol.

7624-w

Diperodon Hydrochloride.

Diperocaine Hydrochloride.

$C_{22}H_{27}N_3O_4,HCl$=433.9.

CAS — 537-12-2.

An odourless white crystalline powder with a bitter numbing taste. M.p. about 198°. **Soluble** 1 in 100 of water; soluble in alcohol; slightly soluble in acetone and ethyl acetate; practically insoluble in ether.

Adverse Effects, Treatment, and Precautions. As for Local Anaesthetics, p.899.

Uses. Diperodon is a local anaesthetic which has been used as the base or hydrochloride for surface anaesthe-

sia. A 1% cream or ointment has been applied to the skin or rectally.
The general actions of local anaesthetics are described on p.901.

Preparations

Diperodon Ointment *(U.S.P.)*. Diperodon in a suitable ointment basis. Potency is expressed in terms of anhydrous diperodon. Store in airtight containers.

Proprietary Names

Diothane Ointment *(Merrell-National, USA)*.

7625-e

Dyclonine Hydrochloride *(U.S.P.)*. Dyclocaini Chloridum. 4′-Butoxy-3-piperidinopropiophenone hydrochloride. $C_{18}H_{27}NO_2,HCl=325.9$.

CAS — 586-60-7 (dyclonine); 536-43-6 (hydrochloride).

Pharmacopoeias. In *U.S.*

White crystals or white crystalline powder, with a slight odour. M.p. 173° to 178°. **Soluble** 1 in 60 of water, 1 in 24 of alcohol, and 1 in 2.3 of chloroform; soluble in acetone; practically insoluble in ether and hexane. A 1% solution in water has a pH of 4 to 7. **Store** in airtight containers. Protect from light.

Dyclonine hydrochloride is a local anaesthetic. It is absorbed through the skin and mucous membranes and is used as a 0.5 or 1% aqueous solution for application to the skin and to anaesthetise mucous membranes. It may cause irritation at the site of application.
The general actions of local anaesthetics are described on p.899.

A viscous preparation containing dyclonine 0.5%, diluted 1 to 5 with water, might be used just before eating to relieve the pain of oral ulceration in patients with leukaemia.— R. E. Kyle and J. E. Maldonado, *Mayo Clin. Proc.*, 1966, *41*, 383.

Preparations

Dyclonine Hydrochloride Topical Solution *(U.S.P.)*. Dyclonine Hydrochloride Solution. A sterile aqueous solution of dyclonine hydrochloride; it may contain suitable stabilisers and antimicrobial agents. pH 3 to 5. Store in airtight containers. Protect from light.

Proprietary Names

Dyclone *(Dow, USA)*.

7626-l

Etidocaine Hydrochloride. W-19053.

(±)-2-(*N*-Ethylpropylamino)butyro-2′,6′-xylidide hydrochloride.
$C_{17}H_{28}N_2O,HCl=312.9$.

CAS — 36637-18-0 (etidocaine); 36637-19-1 (hydrochloride).

Adverse Effects, Treatment, and Precautions. As for Local Anaesthetics, p.899.

Relative toxicities of etidocaine, bupivacaine, and lignocaine, when given intravenously, were assessed in a double-blind study in 5 subjects. At an infusion-rate of 10 mg per minute mean toxic threshold doses for bupivacaine and etidocaine were 112 and 236 mg respectively. At 20 mg per minute etidocaine had a mean toxic threshold dose of 161 mg and was at least 1.55 times as toxic as lignocaine. All toxicity was related to the CNS.— D. B. Scott, *Br. J. Anaesth.*, 1975, *47*, 56.

Effects on the heart. For a report of cardiac arrest, not preceded by hypoxia, in patients given etidocaine, see Bupivacaine Hydrochloride, p.910.

Absorption and Fate. Etidocaine is rapidly absorbed into the circulation after epidural injection and is extensively bound to plasma proteins. It crosses the placenta. Etidocaine is metabolised in the liver and the metabolites are excreted in the urine.
See also under Local Anaesthetics, p.900.

A comparative study of the pharmacokinetics of etidocaine and bupivacaine given intravenously to 6 healthy subjects. At similar doses (25 or 50 mg) etidocaine disappeared much more quickly from the plasma and gave significantly lower concentrations than bupivacaine.— D. B. Scott *et al.*, *Br. J. Anaesth.*, 1973, *45*, 1010.

Half-lives reported after the intravenous injection of etidocaine were: α, 0.036 hour; β, 0.31 hour; and γ, 2.6 hours.— G. T. Tucker and L. E. Mather, *Br. J. Anaesth.*, 1975, *47*, 213.

The concentration of etidocaine in the umbilical vein (UV) was 0.07 to 0.45 μg per ml compared with 0.25 to 1.3 μg per ml in maternal (M) arterial or venous plasma. The UV:M ratio was lower for etidocaine than for bupivacaine, mepivacaine, lignocaine, or prilocaine.— P. J. Poppers, *Br. J. Anaesth.*, 1975, *47*, 322.

In a study on the disposition of etidocaine following epidural administration, there were no significant differences between pregnant and non-pregnant women except during delivery when the fraction of unbound etidocaine in plasma increased. Following administration during labour the placental transfer of etidocaine was rapid and the cord/maternal venous blood concentration ratio was nearly always less than 1 (mean 0.342). Measurable concentrations of mono-dealkylated metabolites of etidocaine, 2-*N*-propylamino-2′-butyroxylidide (PABX) and 2-*N*-ethylamino-2′-butyroxylidide (EABX), were detectable in maternal blood within 5 minutes and in cord blood within 30 minutes.— D. J. Morgan *et al.*, *Eur. J. clin. Pharmac.*, 1977, *12*, 359.

The pharmacokinetics and metabolism of etidocaine in the neonates of mothers who had received epidural injections during labour. In 5 neonates the mean elimination half-life of etidocaine was 6.42 hours and half-lives of the metabolites PABX, EABX, and 2-amino-2′-butyroxylidide (ABX) were 8.15, 8.60, and 13.3 hours respectively.— D. Morgan *et al.*, *Eur. J. clin. Pharmac.*, 1978, *13*, 365.

Further references to the pharmacokinetics of etidocaine.— P. C. Lund *et al.*, *Anesthesiology*, 1975, *42*, 497 (blood concentrations); M. Stanton-Hicks *et al.*, *Anesthesiology*, 1975, *42*, 398 (blood concentrations); D. Morgan *et al.*, *Clin. exp. Pharmac. Physiol.*, 1977, *4*, 210 (metabolism); J. A. W. Wildsmith *et al.*, *Br. J. Anaesth.*, 1977, *49*, 461 (plasma concentrations after brachial plexus block); R. L. Nation, *Clin. Pharmacokinet.*, 1980, *5*, 340 (during childbirth).

Uses. As for Local Anaesthetics, p.901.
Etidocaine hydrochloride is a local anaesthetic of the amide type. It is more potent than lignocaine, with a similarly rapid onset and a longer duration of action.
Etidocaine is used for infiltration anaesthesia and regional nerve block, usually with adrenaline 1 in 200 000. A 0.5% solution of etidocaine hydrochloride is used for infiltration and a 0.5 or 1% solution for peripheral nerve block. The maximum dose should not generally exceed 300 mg, or 400 mg when given with adrenaline. The total amount of adrenaline injected should not exceed 500 μg.
When given by epidural injection etidocaine hydrochloride produces a profound degree of motor blockade and abdominal muscle relaxation. Up to 300 mg may be injected as a 1 or 1.5% solution for lumbar epidural block prior to surgery, including caesarean section. Lower doses of up to 200 mg as a 0.5 or 1% solution are suggested for epidural anaesthesia during labour. For caudal anaesthesia up to 300 mg as a 0.5 or 1% solution may be given.

Bupivacaine 0.5% had a longer duration of analgesia than etidocaine 0.5% but less than that of etidocaine 1%.— M. Morgan and W. J. Russell, *Br. J. Anaesth.*, 1975, *47*, 586.

Further references to the actions and uses of etidocaine.— P. C. Lund *et al.*, *Anesth. Analg. curr. Res.*, 1973, *52*, 482; B. Paradis and L. Fournier, *Can. Anaesth. Soc. J.*, 1975, *22*, 70; *Br. J. Anaesth.*, 1975, *47, Suppl.*, 164–333;; *Med. Lett.*, 1977, *19*, 4.

Epidural block. In an evaluation of the extradural block produced by etidocaine the duration of block with a 1% solution was similar to that with bupivacaine 0.5%. Etidocaine caused motor paralysis more frequently than bupivacaine, especially when adrenaline was added.— A. R. Abdel-Salam *et al.*, *Br. J. Anaesth.*, 1975, *47*, 1081.
In a double-blind study the duration of effect of etidocaine 1.5% for epidural analgesia was longer than that of 1% and motor block was more intense. The addition of adrenaline 1 in 200 000 did not increase the duration of analgesia but increased motor block.— F. P. Buckley *et al.*, *Br. J. Anaesth.*, 1978, *50*, 171.

The quality of spinal epidural anaesthesia was assessed in 246 patients using etidocaine 1 or 1.5%, bupivacaine 0.5%, and lignocaine 1.5 or 2%. All solutions contained adrenaline 1 in 200 000. A 2-ml test dose was injected 3 minutes before the therapeutic dose. The first sacral segment (S1) was most difficult to block, with an overall failure-rate of 17.53%; this could be due to the large diameter of the S1 nerve root. Etidocaine 1.5% (40 patients) was the only anaesthetic completely to block the S1 segment in all patients and its use was associated with fewer complaints from patients.— A. Galindo *et al.*, *Br. J. Anaesth.*, 1975, *47*, 41.

A double-blind crossover comparison in 5 healthy men of the effects of epidural block at L2 by etidocaine 1.5% or bupivacaine 0.75%, both with adrenaline, yielded the following mean data: spread of sensory analgesia to 4 segments above and below injection site in 13 and 22 minutes respectively; 2-segment regression in 180 and 260 minutes; caudal spread of analgesia more extensive with etidocaine; onset of motor blockade in 5.8 and 10 minutes; regression in motor blockade in 306 and 238 minutes; comparable cardiovascular changes; maximum arterial concentration 1.52 μg per ml at 14 minutes and 1.35 μg per ml at 20 minutes respectively. There appeared to be fast and slow half-lives of 20 minutes and 8 hours for both drugs.— M. Stanton-Hicks *et al.*, *Br. J. Anaesth.*, 1976, *48*, 575.

There was no evidence of significant plasma accumulation of etidocaine in 5 patients given etidocaine hydrochloride 200 mg epidurally (as 1% solution) before surgery followed by 4 doses of 100 mg at 2-hour intervals for postoperative pain relief. Prolonged block in some patients suggested local accumulation.— G. T. Tucker *et al.*, *Br. J. Anaesth.*, 1977, *49*, 237.

Further references to epidural block with etidocaine.— P. O. Bridenbaugh *et al.*, *Anesth. Analg. curr. Res.*, 1973, *52*, 407; D. C. Moore *et al.*, *Anesth. Analg. curr. Res.*, 1974, *53*, 690; D. C. Moore *et al.*, *Anesth. Analg. curr. Res.*, 1975, *54*, 250 (caudal anaesthesia); P. O. Bridenbaugh *et al.*, *Anesthesiology*, 1976, *45*, 560; T. M. Murphy *et al.*, *Br. J. Anaesth.*, 1976, *48*, 893.

In obstetrics. In a double-blind randomised study 100 patients were given a single varying dose of either bupivacaine or etidocaine by extradural injection during the surgical induction of labour. Etidocaine had a quicker onset of action than bupivacaine but its duration of action was shorter and it produced a greater degree of muscle weakness. It was not the drug of choice for use during labour.— G. Phillips, *Br. J. Anaesth.*, 1975, *47*, 1305.

A favourable report of the use of 25 ml of etidocaine 1% with or without adrenaline for epidural block in caesarean delivery in 81 patients. The ratio of the pooled umbilical arterial plus venous blood concentration to maternal venous blood concentration was low at about 0.38 for plain solution and 0.28 for solution containing adrenaline. A dose of 20 ml of 1% etidocaine with adrenaline was probably adequate; 214 patients had now been treated.— P. C. Lund *et al.*, *Br. J. Anaesth.*, 1977, *49*, 457.

Regional nerve block. In a double-blind study of ulnar nerve block in 10 subjects etidocaine 0.25% and lignocaine 1%, both with adrenaline 1 in 200 000, had a similar rapid onset and similar duration of action. Etidocaine 0.5% and lignocaine 1%, both with adrenaline, produced analgesia lasting 583 and 262 minutes and motor block lasting 653 and 294 minutes, respectively. Etidocaine 0.5% and lignocaine 1%, both without adrenaline, produced analgesia lasting 320 and 165 minutes and motor block lasting 358 and 139 minutes, respectively.— P. J. Poppers *et al.*, *Anesthesiology*, 1974, *40*, 13.

Proprietary Names

Duranest *(Astra, Ger.; Astra, USA)*.

7627-y

Euprocin Hydrochloride. Isopentylhydrocupreine Dihydrochloride; Isoamylhydrocupreine Dihydrochloride. (9*R*)-10,11-Dihydro-6′-(3-methylbutoxy)cinchonan-9-ol dihydrochloride monohydrate.
$C_{24}H_{34}N_2O_2,2HCl,H_2O=473.5$.

CAS — 1301-42-4 (euprocin); 18984-80-0 (hydrochloride, anhydrous).

Euprocin hydrochloride is a local anaesthetic with some bactericidal action formerly used as a 0.1% solution in ear-drops. Serious toxic symptoms, including disturbance of vision and blindness, have followed internal administration.
The general actions of local anaesthetics are described on p.899.

7628-j

Fomocaine. Fomocainum. 4-[3-(α-Phenoxy-*p*-tolyl)propyl]morpholine.
$C_{20}H_{25}NO_2$=311.4.

CAS — 17692-39-6.

Fomocaine is a local anaesthetic which has been used for surface anaesthesia as a 4% cream or ointment.
The general actions of local anaesthetics are described on p.899.

Fomocaine had antiarrhythmic properties in *animals*.— N. Reuter *et al.*, *Arzneimittel-Forsch.*, 1975, *25*, 1900.

Proprietary Names
Erbocain *(Heilit, Ger.)*.

7629-z

Hexothiocaine Hydrochloride. 2-Diethylaminoethyl 4-amino-2-hexyloxythiobenzoate hydrochloride.
$C_{19}H_{32}N_2O_2S,HCl$=389.0.

CAS — 13957-60-3 (hexothiocaine).

Hexothiocaine hydrochloride is a local anaesthetic which has been used for surface anaesthesia as a 0.01% ointment.
The general actions of local anaesthetics are described on p.899.

7630-p

Hexylcaine Hydrochloride *(U.S.P.)*. Hexylcainium Chloride. 2-Cyclohexylamino-1-methylethyl benzoate hydrochloride.
$C_{16}H_{23}NO_2,HCl$=297.8.

CAS — 532-77-4 (hexylcaine); 532-76-3 (hydrochloride).

Pharmacopoeias. In *U.S.*

A white powder with a slight aromatic odour and a bitter taste. M.p. 182° to 184°. **Soluble** 1 in 17 of water; freely soluble in alcohol and chloroform; practically insoluble in ether. A 5% solution in water has a pH of 4 to 6. **Store** in airtight containers.

Adverse Effects, Treatment, and Precautions. As for Local Anaesthetics, p.899.
Tissue irritation and necrosis has followed the parenteral administration of hexylcaine hydrochloride.

Effects on the nervous system. Convulsions occurred on 5 of 200 occasions in which hexylcaine was used for extradural anaesthesia.— P. C. Lund *et al.*, *Br. J. Anaesth.*, 1975, *47*, *Suppl.*, 313.

Uses. Hexylcaine hydrochloride is a local anaesthetic of the ester type which is used for surface anaesthesia (see p.901). The onset and duration of action of hexylcaine is about the same as for lignocaine. A solution containing up to 5% has been used.

Preparations

Hexylcaine Hydrochloride Injection *(U.S.P.)*. A sterile solution in Water for Injections with or without the addition of dextrose. pH 3 to 5.

Hexylcaine Hydrochloride Topical Solution *(U.S.P.)*. Hexylcaine Hydrochloride Solution. A solution of hexylcaine hydrochloride. pH 3 to 5. Store in airtight containers.

Proprietary Names
Cyclaine *(Merck Sharp & Dohme, USA)*.

7631-s

Isobucaine Hydrochloride *(U.S.P.)*. 2-Isobutylamino-2-methylpropyl benzoate hydrochloride.
$C_{15}H_{23}NO_2,HCl$=285.8.

CAS — 14055-89-1 (isobucaine); 3562-15-0 (hydrochloride).

Pharmacopoeias. In *U.S.*

A white odourless crystalline powder. M.p. 182° to 185°. **Soluble** 1 in 1 of water, 1 in 8 of alcohol, and 1 in 6 of chloroform; sparingly soluble in isopropyl alcohol; very slightly soluble in ether. A 2% solution in water has a pH of about 6. **Incompatible** with alkalis.

Isobucaine hydrochloride is a local anaesthetic of the ester type with the general actions described under Local Anaesthetics, p.899. It has been used in dentistry as a 2% solution with adrenaline.

Preparations

Isobucaine Hydrochloride and Epinephrine Injection *(U.S.P.)*. A sterile solution of isobucaine hydrochloride and adrenaline in Water for Injections.

7632-w

Leucinocaine Mesylate. 2-Diethylamino-4-methylpentyl 4-aminobenzoate methanesulphonate.
$C_{18}H_{32}N_2O_5S$=388.5.

CAS — 92-23-9 (leucinocaine); 135-44-4 (mesylate).

A white to slightly yellow crystalline powder. **Soluble** 1 in 3 of water; soluble in alcohol.

Leucinocaine mesylate is a local anaesthetic of the ester type and has been used as a 0.3 or 5% solution for injection. A 5% ointment of leucinocaine has been used topically.
The general actions of local anaesthetics are described on p.899.

7633-e

Mepivacaine Hydrochloride *(U.S.P.)*. Mepivacaini Chloridum. (1-Methyl-2-piperidyl)formo-2′,6′-xylidide hydrochloride.
$C_{15}H_{22}N_2O,HCl$=282.8.

CAS — 96-88-8 (mepivacaine); 1722-62-9 (hydrochloride).

Pharmacopoeias. In *Braz.*, *Nord.*, and *U.S.*

A white odourless crystalline powder with a slightly bitter numbing taste. M.p. 255° to 262° with decomposition.
Freely **soluble** in water and methyl alcohol; soluble 1 in 10 of alcohol; very slightly soluble in chloroform; practically insoluble in ether. A 2% solution in water has a pH of about 4.5. A 4.6% solution is iso-osmotic with serum. Solutions are **sterilised** by autoclaving or by filtration. **Incompatible** with alkalis. **Store** in airtight containers. Protect from light.

Stability of solutions. For reference to the decreased solubility of mepivacaine in phosphate buffer with increasing temperature and its possible precipitation at the site of injection, see Lignocaine Hydrochloride, p.902.

Adverse Effects, Treatment, and Precautions. As for Local Anaesthetics, p.899.
Foetal bradycardia has followed paracervical block with mepivacaine during labour.

In an analysis of 30 885 regional anaesthesias with mepivacaine, given with and without vasoconstrictors, systemic reactions were seen on only 74 occasions and were not related to dose. The presence of adrenaline or noradrenaline did not diminish the frequency of systemic reactions, a number of which could be attributed to the vasoconstrictor. A mortality study did not indicate late toxic reactions.— K. G. Dhunér, *Acta anaesth. scand.*, 1972, *Suppl.* 48, 23. See also *idem*, 3.

An observation in *animals* that L(+)-mepivacaine is less toxic than the D(−)-isomer.— G. Åberg, *Acta pharmac. tox.*, 1972, *31*, 273.

Allergy. Death in a patient following administration of mepivacaine for paracervical anaesthesia might have been due to mepivacaine intolerance.— D. A. Grimes and W. Cates, *New Engl. J. Med.*, 1976, *295*, 1397.

Pregnancy and the neonate. *Effects on the foetus and neonate.* Apnoea, bradycardia, persisting despite adequate oxygenation, and convulsions within minutes of birth were reported in 4 infants whose mothers were given, ineffectually, 20 to 25 ml of 1.5% mepivacaine during labour, for caudal anaesthesia. Two infants died but in the other 2 exchange transfusion was considered to be life-saving.— J. C. Sinclair *et al.*, *New Engl. J. Med.*, 1965, *273*, 1173.

Bradycardia occurred in 3 of 15 infants whose mothers had received 300 mg of mepivacaine for paracervical block. Peak maternal blood concentrations 10 to 20 minutes after the injection were 4.7 to 17.2 μg per ml (average 8.5 μg per ml). Peak foetal blood concentrations within 30 minutes ranged from 3.4 to 15 μg per ml, bradycardia being associated with 12.8 μg per ml or more. The highest concentration not associated with bradycardia was 7.3 μg per ml.— H. R. Gordon, *New Engl. J. Med.*, 1968, *279*, 910. Changes in foetal heart-rate had been observed in 30% of more than 1000 cases where paracervical block had been induced by mepivacaine. After 200 mg of mepivacaine, the mean arterial blood concentration in 13 patients reached 2.3 μg per ml, while foetal scalp blood concentrations averaging 4 μg per ml had accompanied bradycardia. Where no bradycardia had occurred, foetal blood concentrations had averaged 1 μg per ml.— S. M. Shnider *et al.* (letter), *New Engl. J. Med.*, 1968, *279*, 947.

A characteristic syndrome including neonatal depression, seizures, often associated with apnoea and beginning before 6 hours of age, and other neurological findings was seen at birth in 7 infants who had been injected accidentally with mepivacaine during paracervical and/or pudendal block. Promotion of urinary excretion appeared to be the treatment of choice; only small amounts of mepivacaine were recovered by exchange transfusion or by gastric lavage or drainage. Although the infants were critically ill on the first day of life their outcome was generally good and the 6 survivors were subsequently free of seizures and neurologically and developmentally normal.— L. S. Hillman *et al.*, *J. Pediat.*, 1979, *95*, 472.

Further references to neonatal toxicity following the use of mepivacaine for paracervical block during labour.— J. B. Rosefsky and M. E. Petersiel, *New Engl. J. Med.*, 1968, *278*, 530; L. S. James *et al.* (letter), *ibid.*, 1072; A. Vasicka *et al.*, *Obstet. Gynec.*, 1971, *38*, 500; D. Chase and J. P. Brady, *J. Pediat.*, 1977, *90*, 127.

Absorption and Fate. After epidural and paracervical injection, mepivacaine is rapidly absorbed into the circulation. It diffuses across the placenta. Mepivacaine is rapidly metabolised in the liver and less than 10% of a dose is reported to be excreted unchanged in the urine. Several metabolites are also excreted via the kidneys and include glucuronide conjugates of hydroxy compounds and an *N*-demethylated compound, 2′,6′-pipecoloxylidide (PPX).
See also under Local Anaesthetics, p.900.

In 70 surgical patients given mepivacaine hydrochloride 500 mg for epidural or caudal anaesthesia or for nerve block, peak plasma concentrations (of base) were generally 2 to 5 μg per ml, but were considerably higher after intercostal nerve block without adrenaline.— G. T. Tucker *et al.*, *Anesthesiology*, 1972, *37*, 277.

Half-lives reported after the intravenous injection of mepivacaine were: α, 0.012 hour; β, 0.12 hour; and γ, 1.9 hours.— G. T. Tucker and L. E. Mather, *Br. J. Anaesth.*, 1975, *47*, 213.

A comparative study in 5 healthy subjects of serum concentrations obtained following maxillary buccal infiltrations of 36 mg of mepivacaine hydrochloride or lignocaine hydrochloride, administered as 2% solutions. A mean peak serum concentration of 400 ng per ml was achieved 30 minutes after injection of mepivacaine and of 310 ng per ml 15 minutes after injection of lignocaine; there was considerable intersubject variation. Although mepivacaine has been considered to have inherent vasoconstrictor activity it was not apparent in this study.— W. M. Goebel *et al.*, *Br. dent. J.*, 1980, *148*, 261. Comments.— H. Cannell (letter), *ibid.*, *149*, 125; J. P. Rood (letter), *ibid.*; A. Cowan (letter), *ibid.*

Further references to the pharmacokinetics of mepivacaine.— H. O. Morishima *et al.*, *Anesthesiology*, 1966, *27*, 147; D. F. Gomez (letter), *Lancet*, 1969, *2*, 1079; W. U. Brown *et al.*, *Anesthesiology*, 1975, *42*, 698.

For a comparison of the pharmacokinetics of mepivacaine and prilocaine, see Prilocaine Hydrochloride, p.920.

Pregnancy and the neonate. In 19 women given mepivacaine for epidural anaesthesia during labour mean maternal blood concentration was 2.2 μg per ml; the corresponding foetal concentration was 1.6 μg per ml.— A. O. Lurie and J. B. Weiss, *Am. J. Obstet. Gynec.*, 1970, *106*, 850.

Between 0.7 and 5.5 mg of mepivacaine, calculated as the hydrochloride, and its metabolites were recovered over a 30-hour period from urine of neonates whose mothers had been given mepivacaine hydrochloride 250 to 580 mg for epidural block during labour. There was a higher ratio of mepivacaine to its metabolites in neonatal urine than in the urine of adult subjects also given mepivacaine.— P. Meffin *et al.*, *Clin. Pharmac. Ther.*, 1973, *14*, 218.

Mepivacaine diffused into the amniotic fluid and concentrations of 1.8 μg per ml were detected in samples at delivery.— W. U. Brown *et al.*, *Anesthesiology*, 1977,

47, 384.

In a comparison of the pharmacokinetics of mepivacaine hydrochloride given subcutaneously to 4 premature male neonates and intravenously to 6 healthy men, mean terminal phase half-lives were 8.69 and 3.17 hours respectively. Total plasma clearance and hepatic blood clearance were significantly smaller in the neonates but renal plasma clearance was significantly greater and about 43% of the dose was excreted unchanged in the neonates compared with 3.5% in the adults. In the neonates 11.4% of the dose was excreted in the urine over 48 hours as the *N*-demethylated metabolite (PPX) whereas the excretion of 3-hydroxy and 4-hydroxy mepivacaine (free and conjugated) was negligible; this compares with about 2% as PPX and about 15% and 12% as 3-hydroxy and 4-hydroxy mepivacaine reported in adults by P. Meffin *et al. (Clin. Pharmac. Ther.,* 1973, *14,* 218).— R. G. Moore *et al., Eur. J. clin. Pharmac.,* 1978, *14,* 203.

Further references to the pharmacokinetics of mepivacaine in pregnancy and the neonate.— R. L. Nation, *Clin. Pharmacokinet.,* 1980, *5,* 340 (in childbirth).

Protein binding. Mepivacaine was reported to be 65% bound to plasma proteins.— B. G. Covino, *Anesthesiology,* 1971, *35,* 158.

For reference to the protein binding of mepivacaine, see Lignocaine Hydrochloride, p.904.

Uses. As for Local Anaesthetics, p.901.

Mepivacaine hydrochloride is a local anaesthetic of the amide type used for infiltration, peripheral nerve block, and epidural anaesthesia. It has a potency and time of onset similar to lignocaine but may have a slightly longer duration of action. Mepivacaine does not have vasodilator properties and the addition of a vasoconstrictor is not generally necessary. Its use has therefore been advocated where local anaesthetics containing adrenaline are contra-indicated.

An adult dose of mepivacaine hydrochloride should not generally exceed 400 mg and the total dose in 24 hours should not exceed 1 g. Adrenaline 1 in 200 000 has been added to control bleeding in vascular areas.

Up to 40 ml of a 1% solution or 80 ml of a 0.5% solution is used for infiltration and up to 20 ml of a 1 to 2% solution for peripheral nerve block. For epidural or caudal anaesthesia 150 to 400 mg is given as a 1 to 2% solution. Solutions containing 2% of mepivacaine hydrochloride with adrenaline 1 in 200 000 or 3% plain solution are used in dentistry.

For spinal anaesthesia, a 4% hyperbaric solution has been used.

It has also been used as a surface anaesthetic but other local anaesthetics such as lignocaine are more effective.

Maximum recommended total doses of mepivacaine for continuous extradural analgesia during labour were 12 mg per kg body-weight in the non-obese and 12 mg per kg lean body-weight in the obese.— R. B. Clark *et al., Br. J. Anaesth.,* 1975, *47,* 1283.

For earlier reports on the use of mepivacaine hydrochloride, see Martindale 27th Edn, pp. 874–5.

Preparations

Injectabile Mepivacain-Adrenalini *(Nord. P.).* A sterile solution containing mepivacaine hydrochloride 10 mg and adrenaline 5 µg in each ml.

Mepivacaine Hydrochloride and Levonordefrin Injection *(U.S.P.).* A sterile solution of mepivacaine hydrochloride and levonordefrin in Water for Injections. pH 3.3 to 5.5.

Mepivacaine Hydrochloride Injection *(U.S.P.).* A sterile solution of mepivacaine hydrochloride in Water for Injections. pH 4.5 to 6.8.

Proprietary Preparations

Chlorocain 3% *(Pharmaceutical Mfg, UK).* Mepivacaine hydrochloride for injection, available as a solution containing 30 mg per ml, in dental cartridges of 2.2 ml.
Chlorocain 4% Hyperbaric. Mepivacaine hydrochloride, available as a solution containing 40 mg per ml, with anhydrous dextrose 95 mg per ml, in ampoules of 2 ml, for spinal anaesthesia.

Other Proprietary Names

Carbocain *(Denm., Norw., Swed.)*; Carbocaina *(Ital.)*; Carbocaine *(Austral., Canad., S.Afr., USA)*; Meaverin, Mepivastesin *(Ger.)*; Scandicain *(Ger., Spain, Switz.)*; Scandicaine *(Belg., Neth.).*

7634-l

Meprylcaine Hydrochloride *(U.S.P.).* Meprylcaini Chloridum. 2-Methyl-2-propylaminopropyl benzoate hydrochloride.

$C_{14}H_{21}NO_2,HCl=271.8$.

CAS — 495-70-5 (meprylcaine); 956-03-6 (hydrochloride).

Pharmacopoeias. In *U.S.*

A white odourless crystalline powder. M.p. 150° to 153°. **Soluble** 1 in 6 of water, 1 in 5 of alcohol, 1 in 3 of chloroform, and 1 in 12 of ether; slightly soluble in acetone. A 2% solution in water has a pH of about 5.7.

Meprylcaine hydrochloride is a local anaesthetic of the ester type, with the general actions described under Local Anaesthetics, p.899. A 2% solution with adrenaline has been employed in dentistry.

Preparations

Meprylcaine Hydrochloride and Epinephrine Injection *(U.S.P.).* A sterile solution of meprylcaine hydrochloride and adrenaline in Water for Injections. Protect from light.

7635-y

Metabutethamine Hydrochloride. Metabutethaminium Chloride. 2-Isobutylaminoethyl 3-aminobenzoate hydrochloride.

$C_{13}H_{20}N_2O_2,HCl=272.8$.

CAS — 4439-25-2 (metabutethamine); 553-58-2 (hydrochloride).

A white odourless crystalline powder. M.p. 181° to 184°. **Soluble** in water; soluble in alcohol, acetone, and chloroform. A 2% solution in water has a pH of about 6.

Metabutethamine, the *m*-isomer of butethamine, is a local anaesthetic of the ester type which was formerly used as the hydrochloride in dentistry.

The general actions of local anaesthetics are described on p.899.

7636-j

Metabutoxycaine Hydrochloride. Metabutoxycainium Chloride. 2-Diethylaminoethyl 3-amino-2-butoxybenzoate hydrochloride.

$C_{17}H_{28}N_2O_3,HCl=344.9$.

CAS — 3624-87-1 (metabutoxycaine); 550-01-6 (hydrochloride).

A white odourless crystalline powder. M.p. 117° to 120°. Very **soluble** in water and alcohol; soluble in acetone and chloroform; very slightly soluble in ether. A 2% solution in water has a pH of about 5.5.

Metabutoxycaine hydrochloride is a local anaesthetic which was formerly used in dentistry.

The general actions of local anaesthetics are described on p.899.

7637-z

Orthocaine *(B.P. 1953).* Methylium Aminooxybenzoicum. Methyl 3-amino-4-hydroxybenzoate.

$C_8H_9NO_3=167.2$.

CAS — 536-25-4.

Pharmacopoeias. In *Span.*

A white or faintly yellow, odourless, tasteless, crystalline powder. M.p. 141° to 143°. Slightly **soluble** in water; soluble 1 in 7 of alcohol, and 1 in 50 of ether; readily soluble in solutions of alkali hydroxides.

Orthocaine is a local anaesthetic of the ester type formerly used for surface anaesthesia. It has caused irritation and necrosis.

The general actions of local anaesthetics are described on p.899.

7638-c

Oxethazaine. Oxetacaine; Wy 806. 2,2′-(2-Hydroxyethylimino)bis[*N*-(αα-dimethylphenethyl)-*N*-methylacetamide].

$C_{28}H_{41}N_3O_3=467.7$.

CAS — 126-27-2.

A white crystalline powder with a bitter taste. M.p. about 104°. Practically **insoluble** in water; soluble in alcohol and in dilute acids.

Oxethazaine is a surface anaesthetic of the amide type which is stated to have a prolonged action after a somewhat slow onset and to be poorly absorbed from mucous membranes. It is administered by mouth in conjunction with antacids for the symptomatic relief of oesophagitis. It is an ingredient of Mucaine, p.73.

The general actions of local anaesthetics are described on p.899.

Clinical reports: E. L. Posey, *Am. J. Gastroent.,* 1963, *40,* 425, per *Abstr. Wld Med.,* 1964, *35,* 151; G. V. Balmforth *et al., Br. med. J.,* 1964, *1,* 355; S. J. Carne, *ibid.,* 907; M. Korhon, *Prakt. Lék.,* 1967, *47,* 726, per *Int. pharm. Abstr.,* 1968, *5,* 960. See also *Prescribers' J.,* 1963, *2,* 126; *ibid., 3,* 40; J. Adriani *et al., Clin. Pharmac. Ther.,* 1964, *5,* 49; J. F. Pontes *et al., Curr. ther. Res.,* 1975, *18,* 315.

Proprietary Names

Emoren (as hydrochloride)*(IFI, Ital.).*

7639-k

Oxybuprocaine Hydrochloride. Benoxinate Hydrochloride *(U.S.P.).* 2-Diethylaminoethyl 4-amino-3-butoxybenzoate hydrochloride.

$C_{17}H_{28}N_2O_3,HCl=344.9$.

CAS — 99-43-4 (oxybuprocaine); 5987-82-6 (hydrochloride).

Pharmacopoeias. In *U.S.*

White or off-white crystals or crystalline powder, odourless or with a slight characteristic odour, and with a saline numbing taste. M.p. about 158°.

Soluble 1 in 0.8 of water, 1 in 2.6 of alcohol, and 1 in 2.5 of chloroform; practically insoluble in ether. Solutions in water are neutral to litmus.

Incompatibility. An ophthalmic solution of oxybuprocaine was incompatible with fluorescein solution, a dense precipitate forming on mixing. This was due to the presence of chlorhexidine acetate and could be avoided by using the following solution: oxybuprocaine hydrochloride 0.4%, sodium chloride 0.8%, phenylmercuric nitrate 0.002%, water to 100%; sterilised by autoclaving. For applanation tonometry, 3 parts of this solution were mixed aseptically with 1 part of 0.5% fluorescein sodium solution.— P. J. Fenton, *Br. J. Ophthal.,* 1965, *49,* 205; *idem* (letter), 504.

Adverse Effects, Treatment, and Precautions. As for Local Anaesthetics, p.899.

Effects on the eyes. Repeated topical application of oxybuprocaine resulted in keratitis and serious corneal lesions of the eye in 3 patients. One patient also developed allergic eczema of the eyelids and fingers.— H. E. Henkes and T. N. Waubke, *Br. J. Ophthal.,* 1978, *62,* 62.

Absorption and Fate. See under Local Anaesthetics, p.900.

Uses. Oxybuprocaine hydrochloride is a surface anaesthetic (see p.901) of the ester type and has about the same systemic toxicity as amethocaine hydrochloride (p.909) but is less irritant when applied to the conjunctiva in similar concentrations.

It is an effective surface anaesthetic when used as a 0.4% solution in short ophthalmological procedures. One drop instilled into the conjunctival sac anaesthetises the surface sufficiently to allow tonometry after 60 seconds, and 3 drops at 90-second intervals produces sufficient anaesthesia after 5 minutes for a foreign body to be removed from the corneal epithelium, or for incision of a Meibomian cyst through the conjunctiva. The sensitivity of the cornea is normal again after about 1 hour. The solution has no effect on

the pupil; it has a bacteriostatic action.
It has also been used as a 1% solution for surface anaesthesia of the ear, nose, and throat.

Preparations

Benoxinate Hydrochloride Ophthalmic Solution *(U.S.P.)*. A sterile solution of oxybuprocaine hydrochloride in water. pH 3 to 6. Store in airtight containers.

NOTE. The code BNX is permitted in Great Britain for single-dose eye-drops of oxybuprocaine.

Alcon Opulets Benoxinate *(Alcon, UK: Farillon, UK)*. Sterile eye-drops containing oxybuprocaine hydrochloride 0.4%, available in single-use disposable applicators.

Minims Benoxinate Hydrochloride *(Smith & Nephew Pharmaceuticals, UK)*. Sterile eye-drops containing oxybuprocaine hydrochloride 0.4%, available in single-use disposable applicators. (Also available as Minims Benoxinate Hydrochloride in *Austral.*).

Other Proprietary Names

Cébésine *(Fr.)*; Conjuncain *(Ger.)*; Novesin *(Switz.)*; Novesina *(Ital.)*; Novesine *(Austral., Belg., Fr., Ger., Neth.)*; Oftalmocaina *(Arg.)*; Poen Caina *(Arg.)*.

7640-w

Phenacaine Hydrochloride *(U.S.P.)*. Phenacainium Chloride; Phenetidylphenacetin Hydrochloride. *NN'*-Bis(4-ethoxyphenyl)acetamidine hydrochloride monohydrate.
$C_{18}H_{22}N_2O_2,HCl,H_2O=352.9$.

CAS — 101-93-9 (phenacaine); 620-99-5 (hydrochloride, anhydrous); 6153-19-1 (hydrochloride, monohydrate).

Pharmacopoeias. In *U.S.*

White odourless crystals with a slightly bitter numbing taste. M.p. not below 190°. **Soluble** 1 in 50 of water; freely soluble in alcohol and chloroform; practically insoluble in ether. Solutions are **sterilised** by autoclaving or by filtration. **Incompatible** with alkalis and alkali carbonates. Solutions should be kept in alkali-free containers.

Phenacaine hydrochloride is a local anaesthetic with the general actions described under Local Anaesthetics, p.899. It has been used as a surface anaesthetic for the eye in the form of a 1% aqueous solution or as a 1 or 2% eye ointment.

Proprietary Names
Holocaine *(City Chemical Corp., USA)*.

7641-e

Piperocaine Hydrochloride *(B.P. 1963)*. Piperocaini Hydrochloridum; Piperocainium Chloride. 3-(2-Methylpiperidino)propyl benzoate hydrochloride.
$C_{16}H_{23}NO_2,HCl=297.8$.

CAS — 136-82-3 (piperocaine); 24561-10-2 (hydrochloride).

Pharmacopoeias. In *Int.*

Odourless small white crystals or white crystalline powder with a slightly bitter numbing taste. M.p. 172° to 175°. **Soluble** 1 in 1.5 of water and 1 in 4.5 of alcohol; soluble in chloroform; practically insoluble in ether and fixed oils. Solutions in water are acid to litmus (pH about 6). Solutions are **sterilised** by filtration. **Store** in airtight containers. Protect from light.

Piperocaine hydrochloride is a local anaesthetic of the ester type and has the general actions described under Local Anaesthetics, p.899. A 2 to 10% solution may be used for surface anaesthesia in the nose and throat and a 2 to 4% solution to anaesthetise the untraumatised urethra in cystoscopy or catheterisation. A 0.5 to 1% solution has been used for infiltration anaesthesia and a 0.5 to 2% solution for regional nerve block.

Proprietary Names
Metycaine Hydrochloride *(Lilly, USA)*.

7642-l

Pramoxine Hydrochloride *(U.S.P.)*. Pramocaine Hydrochloride; Pramoxinium Chloride. 4-[3-(4-Butoxyphenoxy)propyl]morpholine hydrochloride.
$C_{17}H_{27}NO_3,HCl=329.9$.

CAS — 140-65-8 (pramoxine); 637-58-1 (hydrochloride).

Pharmacopoeias. In *U.S.*

A white or almost white crystalline powder with a numbing taste; it may have a faint aromatic odour. M.p. 170° to 174°.
Freely **soluble** in water and alcohol; soluble 1 in 35 of chloroform; very slightly soluble in ether. A 1% solution in water has a pH of about 4.5. **Store** in airtight containers.

Pramoxine hydrochloride is a surface anaesthetic which is used on the skin and less delicate mucous membranes. It is irritant and initial pain may occur. It should not be used for the nose or eyes or by injection, and should not be used for bronchoscopy or gastroscopy.
As a 1% cream or jelly pramoxine hydrochloride is used to relieve surface pain and pruritus and is also used prior to endotracheal endoscopy and proctoscopy.
The general actions of local anaesthetics are described on p.899.

Preparations

Pramoxine Hydrochloride Cream *(U.S.P.)*. Pramoxine hydrochloride in a suitable water-miscible basis. Store in airtight containers.

Pramoxine Hydrochloride Jelly *(U.S.P.)*. A jelly containing pramoxine hydrochloride. Store in airtight containers.

Proprietary Names
Proctofoam/non steroid *(Reed & Carnrick, USA)*; Tronothane *(Abbott, Canad.; Abbott, Fr.; Abbott, Switz.; Abbott, USA)*.

7643-y

Prilocaine Hydrochloride *(B.P., U.S.P.)*.

Propitocaine Hydrochloride; L67. 2-Propylaminopropiono-*o*-toluidide hydrochloride.
$C_{13}H_{20}N_2O,HCl=256.8$.

CAS — 721-50-6 (prilocaine); 1786-81-8 (hydrochloride).

Pharmacopoeias. In *Br.* and *U.S.*

A white odourless crystalline powder with a bitter numbing taste. M.p. 166° to 169°.
Soluble 1 in 5 of water, 1 in 6 of alcohol, and 1 in 175 of chloroform; very slightly soluble in acetone; practically insoluble in ether. A 2% solution in water has a pH of about 4.6. Solutions are **sterilised** by autoclaving or by filtration. Prolonged contact of solutions of prilocaine hydrochloride with metal surfaces should be avoided. **Store** in airtight containers.

Carbonated solutions. Carbonate salts of prilocaine and lignocaine were prepared to give 1.72% and 1.74% solutions respectively of the bases and were sealed in ampoules at a pressure of 600 to 700 mmHg of carbon dioxide. Opened ampoules lost carbon dioxide relatively slowly and its partial pressure fell from 700 to 500 mmHg in 40 minutes. In use, the ampoules were opened and the contents aspirated immediately through a wide-bore needle.— P. R. Bromage, *Can. med. Ass. J.*, 1967, *97*, 1377. See also *idem, Acta anaesth. scand.*, 1965, *Suppl.* xvi, 55.

Adverse Effects and Treatment. As for Local Anaesthetics, p.899.
Methaemoglobinaemia and cyanosis, attributed to the metabolite *o*-toluidine, may occur particularly when doses of prilocaine hydrochloride exceed 600 mg.

Effects on the blood. Prilocaine was given as a local anaesthetic to 124 patients in doses ranging from 0.4 to 2.1 g without evidence of toxicity of the central nervous system. However, all the patients receiving more than 900 mg became cyanosed owing to the formation of methaemoglobin, and in 10 patients given 1 to 1.8 g by epidural infusion the maximum amount of methaemoglobin recorded 4 to 8 hours after the start ranged from 0.9 to 3.4 g per 100 ml. The cyanosis had disappeared by the morning and in 3 patients given methylene blue intravenously in a dosage of 1 mg per kg body-weight, cyanosis disappeared within 30 minutes. There was no evidence of erythrocyte destruction.— D. B. Scott *et al., Lancet*, 1964, *2*, 728.

A mother who had received prilocaine shortly before delivery gave birth to an infant who became deeply cyanosed for several hours and developed methaemoglobinaemia. These symptoms disappeared within a few hours when ascorbic acid 200 mg intramuscularly was administered.— D. M. J. Barry (letter), *N.Z. med. J.*, 1972, *76*, 451.

Further reports of methaemoglobinaemia associated with prilocaine.— D. J. Daly *et al., Br. J. Anaesth.*, 1964, *36*, 737; M. Hjelm and M. H. Holmdahl, *Acta anaesth. scand.*, 1965, *9*, 99; P. J. Poppers *et al., Am. J. Obstet. Gynec.*, 1966, *95*, 630; C. R. Climie *et al., Br. J. Anaesth.*, 1967, *39*, 155; W. E. Spoerel *et al., Can. Anaesth. Soc. J.*, 1967, *14*, 1; R. I. Mazze, *Anesth. Analg. curr. Res.*, 1968, *47*, 122; K. E. Trudnowski, *Bull. Mason Clin.*, 1968, *22*, 33, per *Clin. Med.*, 1968, *75* (Nov.), 81; P. I. Bridenbaugh *et al., Anesth. Analg. curr. Res.*, 1969, *48*, 824; J. F. Arens and A. E. Carrera, *Anesth. Analg. curr. Res.*, 1970, *49*, 219.

Precautions. As for Local Anaesthetics, p.900.
The use of prilocaine should be avoided in patients with anaemia or congenital or acquired methaemoglobinaemia.

Prilocaine had no place in obstetrics or neonatal practice.— G. R. Ford and T. M. Agnew, *N.Z. med. J.*, 1972, *76*, 104, per *Drug Intell. & clin. Pharm.*, 1973, *7*, 94.

Absorption and Fate. Prilocaine hydrochloride is absorbed more slowly than lignocaine because of its slight vasoconstrictor action, but its half-life in blood is less than that of lignocaine. Amidases in the liver and also in the kidneys metabolise prilocaine directly. One metabolite excreted in the urine is *o*-toluidine, and it is believed to cause the methaemoglobinaemia observed after large doses. Prilocaine crosses the placenta and during prolonged epidural anaesthesia may produce methaemoglobinaemia in the foetus.
See also under Local Anaesthetics, p.900.

Reports of comparative studies in which plasma concentrations after lignocaine injections were greater than those after similar injections of prilocaine.— D. B. Scott *et al., Br. J. Anaesth.*, 1972, *44*, 1040; J. A. W. Wildsmith *et al., Br. J. Anaesth.*, 1977, *49*, 461.

After the intravenous injection of 250 mg of prilocaine hydrochloride or mepivacaine hydrochloride in 5 healthy male subjects, plasma concentrations of prilocaine were substantially less than those of mepivacaine and mean elimination half-lives were 93 and 125 minutes respectively, although there was considerable intersubject variation. Total body clearance of prilocaine was consistently greater than that for mepivacaine.— G. R. Arthur *et al., Br. J. Anaesth.*, 1979, *51*, 481.

Further references.— P. J. Poppers and M. Finster, *Anesthesiology*, 1968, *29*, 1134 (transplacental diffusion of prilocaine and methaemoglobinaemia).

Uses. As for Local Anaesthetics, p.901.
Prilocaine hydrochloride is a local anaesthetic of the amide type which is used for surface, infiltration, and nerve block. It has a similar potency to lignocaine and has been reported to be 40% less toxic; the onset of action may be slower. It has less vasodilator activity than lignocaine and can be used without adrenaline or with a maximum of 1 in 200 000 of adrenaline. Without adrenaline it has a greater duration of action than lignocaine but the addition of adrenaline produces a comparable prolonged action for both anaesthetics. The maximum adult dosage of prilocaine hydrochloride is 400 mg, or 600 mg in solutions with adrenaline.
A 4% solution is used for surface anaesthesia of mucous membranes in bronchoscopy and minor surgery of the mouth, nose, and throat. A 0.5 or 1% solution is used for infiltration anaesthesia. In dentistry, 3% solutions with adrenaline 1 in 300 000 or felypressin 0.03 unit per ml and a 4% plain solution are used.
For peripheral nerve block, 0.5 to 3% solutions are used. Epidural and caudal blocks are usually produced with 1 to 3% solutions. A 5% hyperbaric solution has been used for spinal analgesia.
Prilocaine hydrochloride has also been used for intravenous regional anaesthesia.

For reports of 34 papers and discussions on most aspects of prilocaine, see *Citanest, An International Conference*, Santos, Brazil, 1964, S. Wiedling (Ed.), *Acta anaesth. scand.*, 1965, *Suppl.* 16.

A technique had been developed for performing postpartum tubal ligation under local anaesthesia. The patient was prepared for the possibility of general anaesthesia, given pethidine 100 mg intramuscularly, and diazepam 10 mg intravenously (increased during surgery if needed); 20 ml of 1% prilocaine hydrochloride was infiltrated to produce anaesthesia. Of 208 patients, 3 required general anaesthesia. Preliminary assessment of a prospective study was encouraging.— A. Dey and G. Mackay (letter), *Br. med. J.*, 1974, *3*, 252.

Dental use. In a comparison of the analgesic effects in infiltration and block analgesia of prilocaine 4% and lignocaine 2% with 1 in 80 000 adrenaline, prilocaine 4% was found to give a higher frequency of successful analgesia with a shorter time of onset.— G. Brown and N. L. Ward, *Br. dent. J.*, 1969, *126*, 557.

If a patient receiving tricyclic antidepressants required the injection of a local anaesthetic with a vasoconstrictor during dental treatment, the use of a solution containing prilocaine 3% and felypressin 0.03 units per ml was acceptable and did not risk the precipitation of a dangerous hypertensive episode.— V. Goldman (letter), *Br. med. J.*, 1971, *1*, 175.

Hyperhidrosis. For a report on the use of prilocaine with lignocaine in the treatment of hyperhidrosis, see Lignocaine Hydrochloride, p.907.

Regional anaesthesia, intravenous. Prilocaine hydrochloride 0.5% was used for regional intravenous anaesthesia in 42 operations on limbs. Average time of onset was 6 minutes and sensation returned in about 3 minutes after release of the tourniquet.— S. N. Jacobs and V. R. Keep, *Med. J. Aust.*, 1965, *2*, 956.

Preparations

Prilocaine Hydrochloride Injection *(U.S.P.)*. A sterile solution in Water for Injections. pH 6 to 7.

Citanest *(Astra, UK)*. Prilocaine hydrochloride, available as solutions for injection in the following strengths: 0.5% in vials of 20 and 50 ml; 1% in vials of 20 and 50 ml. The above solutions contain also sodium chloride and methyl hydroxybenzoate. **Citanest 3% with Adrenaline** contains prilocaine hydrochloride 3% with adrenaline 1 in 300 000, together with methyl hydroxybenzoate and sodium chloride, available in cartridges of 2 ml. **Citanest 3% with Octapressin** contains in each ml prilocaine hydrochloride 30 mg and felypressin 0.03 units, in cartridges of 2 ml. **Citanest 4%** contains prilocaine hydrochloride 4%, in cartridges of 2 ml. (Also available as Citanest in *Austral., Belg., Denm., Fr., Swed., USA*).

Other Proprietary Names

Xylonest *(Ger.)*.

7644-j

Procaine Hydrochloride *(B.P., Eur. P., U.S.P.)*.

Procainii Chloridum; Procaini Hydrochloridum; Novocainum; Ethocaine Hydrochloride; Procainium Chloride; Allocaine; Syncaine. 2-Diethylaminoethyl 4-aminobenzoate hydrochloride.

$C_{13}H_{20}N_2O_2$,HCl=272.8.

CAS — 59-46-1 (procaine); 51-05-8 (hydrochloride).

Pharmacopoeias. In all pharmacopoeias examined. *U.S.* also includes Sterile Procaine Hydrochloride. *Ind. P.* and *Port. P.* apply the title Procaine to the hydrochloride; *Swiss P.* includes the base, hydrochloride, and nitrate.

Colourless odourless crystals or a white crystalline powder with a slightly bitter saline numbing taste. M.p. 153° to 158°.

Soluble 1 in 1 of water, 1 in 25 of alcohol, and 1 in 30 of dehydrated alcohol; slightly soluble in chloroform; practically insoluble in ether. A 2% solution in water has a pH of 5 to 6.5. A 5.05% solution in water is iso-osmotic with serum. Solutions are **sterilised** by autoclaving or by filtration. **Incompatible** with alkalis, benzylpenicillin, iodine, mercury salts, potassium dichromate, potassium permanganate, silver salts, and tannic acid; with silver salts, procaine nitrate may be used. **Protect** from light.

Procaine hydrochloride decomposes mainly by hydrolysis, the reaction being catalysed by hydroxyl ions. The hydrolysis reaction obeys first-order reaction kinetics and though slight hydrolysis occurs on autoclaving at 115° for 30 minutes, it would appear reasonable to sterilise procaine solutions by this method. An oxidation reaction may also occur on very prolonged heating. The procaine hydrolyses to form *p*-aminobenzoic acid and decarboxylation of this acid occurs with the formation of aniline; the aniline rapidly oxidises to produce a coloured solution.

Effect of gamma-irradiation. Procaine hydrochloride powder became yellow at 25 000 Gy and pale brown at 250 000 Gy and solutions of the treated materials were coloured but clear. There was no significant loss of potency even at 250 000 Gy.— *The Use of Gamma Radiation Sources for the Sterilisation of Pharmaceutical Products*, London, ABPI, 1960.

Procaine hydrochloride was slightly discoloured, but no decomposition was apparent after irradiation with 25 000 Gy.— G. Hortobagyi *et al.*, *Radiosterilization of Medical Products*, Vienna, International Atomic Energy Agency, 1967, p. 25.

Haemolysis. A solution of procaine hydrochloride in water iso-osmotic with serum (5.05%) caused 91% haemolysis of erythrocytes cultured in it for 45 minutes.— E. R. Hammarlund and K. Pedersen-Bjergaard, *J. pharm. Sci.*, 1961, *50*, 24.

Incompatibility. There was loss of clarity when intravenous solutions of procaine hydrochloride were mixed with *aminophylline, amylobarbitone sodium, chlorothiazide sodium, magnesium sulphate, nitrofurantoin sodium, novobiocin sodium, phenobarbitone sodium; phenytoin sodium, quinalbarbitone sodium, sodium bicarbonate, sodium iodide, sulphadiazine sodium, sulphafurazole diethanolamine, or thiopentone sodium.*— J. A. Patel and G. L. Phillips, *Am. J. Hosp. Pharm.*, 1966, *23*, 409.

Procaine hydrochloride caused precipitation of amphotericin.— D. A. Whiting, *Br. J. Derm.*, 1967, *79*, 345.

Polyvinyl chloride discoloration. An enema solution containing procaine hydrochloride 150 mg, methyl hydroxybenzoate 100 mg, and water to 100 ml showed no decomposition of procaine to *p*-aminobenzoic acid after 2 months' storage at 20°, with or without previous heating at 98° to 100° for 30 minutes. However, the polyvinyl chloride (non-toxic grade) bags in which the enema solution had been dispensed were stained yellow in patches.— G. Smith and P. H. Cox, *Pharm. J.*, 1964, *1*, 241.

Preservative for eye-drops. Benzalkonium chloride 0.01% or chlorhexidine gluconate 0.02% were suitable preservatives for procaine hydrochloride eye-drops sterilised by filtration.— M. Van Ooteghem, *Pharm. Tijdschr. Belg.*, 1968, *45*, 69.

Prolonged effect. A report on the effects of povidone on the duration of action of procaine hydrochloride.— L. A. Tsvykh, *Farmatisiya, Mosk.*, 1979, *28*, 24.

Stability of solutions. On storage of solutions containing procaine hydrochloride and glucose, the formation of procaine-*N*-glucoside caused a decrease in local anaesthetic activity. Storage at high temperatures produced the smallest amount of glucoside. Solutions should be prepared at a temperature near 100° and sterilised by heat.— K. Ikeda, *Pharm. Bull., Tokyo*, 1957, *5*, 101, per *Am. J. Hosp. Pharm.*, 1958, *15*, 78.

Adverse Effects and Treatment. As for Local Anaesthetics, p.899.

Though procaine is one of the least toxic local anaesthetics, as little as 10 mg has provoked a fatal reaction in hypersensitive patients.

Allergy and effects on the skin. In a modified 'repeated-insult' patch test, 25% procaine hydrochloride was found to produce mild sensitisation of the skin.— A. M. Kligman, *J. invest. Derm.*, 1966, *47*, 393. Of 600 persons with dermatitis or eczema submitted to patch testing with 2% aqueous solution of procaine hydrochloride, 4.8% gave a positive reaction.— E. Rudzki and D. Kleniewska, *Br. J. Derm.*, 1970, *83*, 543.

Severe hypotension leading to death developed in 1 patient following the infusion of 600 mg of procaine for malignant hyperthermia.— D. MacLachlan and A. L. Forrest (letter), *Lancet*, 1974, *1*, 355.

Further references to allergic reactions with procaine.— L. Förström *et al.*, *Dermatologica*, 1977, *154*, 367 (generalised skin reactions associated with the topical or parenteral use of Gerovital—preparations containing procaine hydrochloride).

Effects on the eyes. The presumed intra-arterial injection of procaine, given for dental nerve block in 3 patients with uncommon vascular patterns, was considered to have caused transient blindness in 2 and isolated external ocular muscle paresis in the other.— P. L. Blaxter and M. J. A. Britten, *Br. med. J.*, 1967, *1*, 681.

Overdosage. A 39-year-old man was accidentally given 4 g instead of 950 mg of procaine hydrochloride intravenously following administration of thiopentone, hexafluorenium, and suxamethonium chloride. Mydriasis, pupils unreactive to light, arterial hypertension, sinus tachycardia, and deepening and widening of the S-waves on the ECG were noted immediately and lasted for several minutes. A peak blood concentration of procaine of 96 µg per ml was reached, which then slowly decreased. Artificial respiration with 100% oxygen resulted in spontaneous recovery without any sequelae.— J. A. Wikinski *et al.*, *J. Am. med. Ass.*, 1970, *213*, 621.

Precautions. As for Local Anaesthetics, p.900.

Procaine is hydrolysed in the body to *p*-aminobenzoic acid and may inhibit the action of sulphonamides. There is cross-sensitivity between procaine and procainamide.

Views on the use of procaine for local anaesthesia in patients who have had procainamide-induced systemic lupus erythematosus. E.L. Dubois considered that, in view of the lack of specific information, it might be safer to use a general anaesthetic whereas D. Alarcón-Segovia thought that the short-term use of procaine derivatives were permissible in such patients. S.L. Lee also felt that procaine could be used but suggested a single test dose 48 hours before the contemplated surgery.— *J. Am. med. Ass.*, 1977, *238*, 2201.

Interactions. *Anticholinesterases.* Since procaine is hydrolysed by plasma cholinesterase it should not be used in the presence of anticholinesterase drugs.— M. de Swiet, *Prescribers' J.*, 1979, *19*, 59.

Diuretics. Evidence that concomitant administration of *acetazolamide* extends the plasma half-life of procaine.— R. Calvo *et al.*, *Clin. Pharmac. Ther.*, 1980, *27*, 179.

Muscle relaxants. For references to procaine enhancing the effects of muscle relaxants, see Suxamethonium Chloride, p.997, and Tubocurarine Chloride, p.999.

Absorption and Fate. After absorption, procaine is rapidly hydrolysed by plasma cholinesterase to *p*-aminobenzoic acid and diethylaminoethanol; some may also be metabolised in the liver. About 80% of the *p*-aminobenzoic acid is excreted unchanged or conjugated in the urine. About 30% of the diethylaminoethanol is excreted in the urine, the remainder being metabolised in the liver.

See also under Local Anaesthetics, p.900.

Intravenous infusions of 10, 15, and 20 mg per kg body-weight of procaine produced arterial-blood concentrations of 12.5, 16, and 28 µg per ml respectively 5 minutes after injection, but they declined rapidly. Concentrations of procaine in cerebrospinal fluid increased during the 10 minutes after injection and then declined. Cerebrospinal fluid concentrations 5 minutes after intravenous injection of doses of 10, 15, and 20 mg per kg of procaine were 7.2, 9.5, and 16.5 µg per ml respectively.— J. E. Usubiaga *et al.*, *Br. J. Anaesth.*, 1967, *39*, 943.

The serum half-life of procaine was prolonged in newborn infants, patients with liver disease, and in some uraemic patients.— M. M. Reidenberg *et al.*, *Clin. Pharmac. Ther.*, 1972, *13*, 279.

Further references.— J. E. Usubiaga *et al.*, *Am. J. Obstet. Gynec.*, 1968, *100*, 918.

Uses. As for Local Anaesthetics, p.901.

Procaine is a local anaesthetic of the ester type. Because of its poor penetration of intact mucuous membranes, it is useless for surface application and has been chiefly used by injection although in general it has been replaced by lignocaine and other local anaesthetics of the amide type. Its action is prompt but rather transitory and as it has a vasodilator action adrenaline 1 in 200 000 is usually added to solutions for injection to prolong the effect. The total amount of adrenaline should not exceed 500 µg. For infiltration anaesthesia 0.25 to 1% solutions of procaine hydrochloride may be used. A 1 to 2% solution of procaine hydrochloride may be used for peripheral nerve block and for caudal or epidural anaesthesia. In dental practice, procaine has largely been replaced by lignocaine.

For spinal anaesthesia procaine hydrochloride

may be given, usually as a 5% solution in sodium chloride injection, Water for Injections, or cerebrospinal fluid; to increase its specific gravity for hyperbaric injection, 5% of dextrose may be added.

Procaine hydrochloride has been given for its reputed effect in the rejuvenation of senile patients but its value is not established. It has also been used in the treatment of malignant hyperpyrexia.

Action. Procaine was reported to be a strong prostaglandin antagonist and weak agonist.— M. S. Manku and D. F. Horrobin, *Lancet*, 1976, *2*, 1115.

Arterial spasm. Arterial spasm associated with the withdrawal of the catheter, needle, or cannula used in angiography was minimised by the intra-arterial injection of 5 to 10 ml of 1% procaine; too rapid injection could cause transient cortical irritation.— A. C. Ng and R. E. Miller, *Am. J. Roentg.*, 1971, *111*, 791.

Blood disorders. References to the anti-sickling effect of procaine hydrochloride.— R. Baker *et al.*, *Biochem. biophys. Res. Commun.*, 1974, *59*, 548; J. Palek *et al.*, *Blood*, 1977, *50*, 155.

Dental use. In a patient with hypersensitivity to lignocaine, procaine was a satisfactory alternative dental anaesthetic and was used on several occasions.— J. P. Rood, *Br. dent. J.*, 1973, *135*, 411.

Infiltration anaesthesia. Caesarean section was performed on 62 patients at full term using local infiltration anaesthesia. A total dose of 20 ml of procaine 2% solution was sufficient, anaesthesia beginning midway between umbilicus and symphysis pubis, then under the anterior rectus sheath. One patient died 4 days after the operation, probably from pulmonary embolism, and another required general anaesthesia; the remainder had no complications.— A. Hai-Khan (letter), *Lancet*, 1970, *2*, 719.

Malignant hyperpyrexia. Caffeine caused contracture of human skeletal muscle and this was used to simulate the muscle rigidity of malignant hyperpyrexia. Halothane *in vitro* increased the caffeine contracture and in a patient with genetic susceptibility caused contracture in the absence of caffeine. Reversal of contracture by procaine supported the use of procaine in malignant hyperpyrexia.— R. F. W. Moulds and M. A. Denborough, *Br. med. J.*, 1972, *4*, 526.

Treatment of malignant hyperpyrexia occurring after suxamethonium or halothane included oxygen, sodium bicarbonate, procaine, and mannitol intravenously, and active cooling. The loading dose of procaine hydrochloride was 30 to 40 mg per kg body-weight intravenously as a 1% solution, followed by 200 µg per kg per minute under ECG control.— J. E. S. Relton *et al.*, *Can. Anaesth. Soc. J.*, 1972, *19*, 200. Procaine 3.5 g infused in 500-mg portions per 5 minutes, given after other treatment including bicarbonate, relieved the symptoms of malignant hyperpyrexia in a 15-year-old boy following thiopentone and suxamethonium. Response might be related to sequence of treatment.— B. Höivik and J. Stovner (letter), *Lancet*, 1975, *2*, 185.

The blood concentrations of procaine that had been shown *in vitro* to be required for the control of malignant hyperpyrexia would not be safely achieved in clinical practice.— G. M. Hall and D. Lister (letter), *Lancet*, 1974, *1*, 208. From studies *in vitro* on muscle from patients susceptible to malignant hyperpyrexia it was concluded that procaine was not the drug of choice in the treatment of hyperpyrexic episodes induced by halothane anaesthesia.— I. M. C. Clarke and F. R. Ellis, *Br. J. Anaesth.*, 1975, *47*, 17.

Regional nerve block. The recommended average dose of procaine hydrochloride for regional anaesthesia was 800 mg as 0.5% solution, 700 mg as 1% solution, and 600 mg as 2% solution, but the maximum dose should not exceed 1 g.— L. Eisenberg, *J. Am. med. Ass.*, 1968, *206*, 2531.

Venepuncture. The prompt use of elevation, warmth, and the local injection of procaine or hyaluronidase has been recommended in the management of extravasation during treatment with intravenous infusions.— *Lancet*, 1978, *2*, 419.

'H3' (Aslan's Treatment of Old Age). Professor Anna Aslan and her colleagues at the Parhon Institute of Geriatrics, Bucharest, in a series of papers (1956 et seq.), claimed remarkable beneficial results in a wide range of disorders, including the rejuvenation of senile patients, from the intramuscular injection of a 2% solution of procaine, buffered at pH 4.3. This solution, which Aslan called 'H3', was injected in 5-ml doses thrice weekly in a series of 12 injections with a 10-day interval between each course, the treatment being continued more or less indefinitely. The remarkable claims for this treatment were not supported by any scientifically valid evidence or by subsequent trials carried out by other workers.

References.— A. Aslan, *Ther. Umsch. med. Biblphie*, 1956, *13*, 165; C. I. Parhon and A. Aslan, *Rev. Sci. méd. Buc.*, 1957, No. 2, 5, per *Br. med. J.*, 1959, *1*, 872; *Br. med. J.*, 1959, *2*, 1163, 1175, and 1317; T. O'Connell and F. Ofner, *Med. J. Aust.*, 1961, *1*, 514; S. R. Fee and A. N. G. Clark, *Br. med. J.*, 1961, *2*, 1680; J. A. W. Berryman *et al.*, *ibid.*, 1683; J. Hirsh, *ibid.*, 1684; V. A. Kral *et al.*, *Can. med. Ass. J.*, 1962, *87*, 1109; *J. Am. med. Ass.*, 1962, *180*, 965; R. F. Long and S. S. Gislason, *J. Neuropsychiat.*, 1964, *5*, 186, per *Abstr. Wld Med.*, 1964, *36*, 125; G. Sakalis *et al.*, *Curr. ther. Res.*, 1974, *16*, 59.

Gerovital H3 (GH3), an injection consisting of a 2% procaine hydrochloride solution with small amounts of benzoic acid, potassium metabisulphite, and sodium phosphate has been claimed to retard the ageing process but although many uncontrolled studies have described great benefits from the use of GH3, controlled studies have failed to demonstrate any improvement in the physical or mental status of elderly patients with cerebral arteriosclerosis or chronic degenerative disorders, including senile dementia. It has been suggested that procaine acts as a monoamine oxidase inhibitor and W.W.K. Zung *et al.* (*Psychosomatics*, 1974, *15*, 127) found GH3 to be a superior antidepressant to placebo. However in further studies reported by I. Zwerling *et al.* (*J. Am. Geriat. Soc.*, 1975, *23*, 355) and E.J. Olsen *et al.* (*J. Geront.*, 1978, *33*, 514), GH3 did not relieve depression.— *Med. Lett.*, 1979, *21*, 4.

Further references to the use of procaine in ageing.— J. P. Hracovec, *Proc. Ann. Meet. Geront. Soc. U.S.*, 1972, 31, per A. Comfort (letter), *Lancet*, 1973, *1*, 1193; M. D. MacFarlane (letter), *Lancet*, 1972, *2*, 337; A. Comfort (letter), *Lancet*, 1973, *1*, 1193; E. Arriola and S. Shimomura, *Drug Intell. & clin. Pharm.*, 1978, *12*, 42.

Preparations

Procaine and Adrenaline Injection *(B.P.)*. Strong Procaine and Adrenaline Injection. A sterile solution of procaine hydrochloride 2%, Adrenaline Solution 2% v/v, with sodium chloride 0.5%, chlorocresol 0.1%, and sodium metabisulphite 0.1% in Water for Injections. Sterilise by maintaining at 98° to 100° for 30 minutes. pH 3 to 4.5. Protect from light. The injection contains adrenaline 1 in 50 000.

Procaine and Phenylephrine Hydrochlorides Injection *(U.S.P.)*. A sterile solution of procaine hydrochloride and phenylephrine hydrochloride in Water for Injections. pH 3 to 5.5.

Procaine and Tetracaine Hydrochlorides and Levonordefrin Injection *(U.S.P.)*. A sterile solution of procaine hydrochloride, amethocaine hydrochloride, and levonordefrin in Water for Injections. pH 3.5 to 5.

Procaine Hydrochloride and Epinephrine Injection *(U.S.P.)*. A sterile solution of procaine hydrochloride and adrenaline hydrochloride in Water for Injections. It contains not more than 1 in 50 000 of adrenaline. pH 3 to 5.5.

Procaine Hydrochloride Injection *(U.S.P.)*. A sterile solution of procaine hydrochloride in Water for Injections. pH 3 to 5.5.

Solutio Višněvski 0.25% et 0.5% *(Cz. P.)*. Procaine hydrochloride 250 or 500 mg, sodium chloride 500 mg, potassium chloride 7.5 mg, calcium chloride hexahydrate 12.5 mg, 0.1 N hydrochloric acid 0.7 ml, Water for Injections to 100 ml. Sterilised by autoclaving. pH 3.2 to 4.5.

Sterile Procaine Hydrochloride *(U.S.P.)*. Procaine hydrochloride suitable for parenteral use.

Proprietary Names

Gero H3 Aslan *(Phoenix, Arg.; Chefaro, Ger.)*; Novocain *(Vandos, Austral.; Winthrop, Canad.; Hoechst, Ger.; Breon, USA)*; Recorcaina *(Recordati, Ital.)*; Syntocaine *(Sintetica, Switz.)*; Venocaina *(Organon, Spain)*.

Procaine hydrochloride was formerly marketed in Great Britain under the proprietary name Novutox (*Willows Francis* now *Pharmaceutical Mfg*).

7645-z

Propanocaine Hydrochloride. 467D₃. 3-Diethylamino-1-phenylpropyl benzoate hydrochloride.
$C_{20}H_{25}NO_2,HCl = 347.9$.

CAS — 493-76-5 (propanocaine); 1679-79-4 (hydrochloride).

Propanocaine hydrochloride is a local anaesthetic which has been used topically at a strength of 1.5% in ointments for the treatment of pruritus and other skin disorders.

The general actions of local anaesthetics are described on p.899.

7646-c

Propoxycaine Hydrochloride *(U.S.P.)*. Propoxycainium Chloride. 2-Diethylaminoethyl 4-amino-2-propoxybenzoate hydrochloride.
$C_{16}H_{26}N_2O_3,HCl = 330.9$.

CAS — 86-43-1 (propoxycaine); 550-83-4 (hydrochloride).

Pharmacopoeias. In *U.S.*

A white odourless crystalline powder. M.p. 146° to 151°. It discolours on prolonged exposure to light and air.

Soluble 1 in 2 of water, 1 in 10 of alcohol, and 1 in 80 of ether; practically insoluble in acetone and chloroform. A 2% solution in water has a pH of about 5.4. **Protect** from light.

Adverse Effects, Treatment, and Precautions. As for Local Anaesthetics, p.899.

Propoxycaine is reported to be 8 to 10 times more toxic than procaine.

Uses. Propoxycaine hydrochloride is a local anaesthetic of the ester type which has been used as 0.5% solution for infiltration and nerve block (see p.901) and to prolong and deepen the anaesthesia produced by procaine; 0.4% has been added to a 2% solution of procaine hydrochloride.

Preparations

Propoxycaine and Procaine Hydrochlorides and Norepinephrine Bitartrate Injection *(U.S.P.)*. A sterile solution of propoxycaine hydrochloride, procaine hydrochloride, and noradrenaline acid tartrate in Water for Injections. pH 3.5 to 5.

Propoxycaine and Procaine Hydrochlorides and Levonordefrin Injection *(U.S.P.)*. A sterile solution of propoxycaine hydrochloride, procaine hydrochloride, and levonordefrin in Water for Injections. pH 3.5 to 5.

7647-k

Proxymetacaine Hydrochloride *(B.P.C. 1973)*.

Proparacaine Hydrochloride *(U.S.P.)*. 2-Diethylaminoethyl 3-amino-4-propoxybenzoate hydrochloride.
$C_{16}H_{26}N_2O_3,HCl = 330.9$.

CAS — 499-67-2 (proxymetacaine); 5875-06-9 (hydrochloride).

Pharmacopoeias. In *U.S.*

A white or faintly buff-coloured, odourless or almost odourless, crystalline powder. M.p. 178° to 185° with a range of not more than 2°. **Soluble** 1 in 30 of water, and 1 in 50 of alcohol; soluble in methyl alcohol; practically insoluble in ether. A 1% solution in water has a pH of 5.5 to 6.1. Solutions are **sterilised** by filtration in an atmosphere of nitrogen or other inert gas. Solutions are **incompatible** with alkalis and fluorescein sodium. Proxymetacaine hydrochloride discolours on heating or exposure to air, and solutions exposed to air become yellow and then dark brown with some loss of potency. Such solutions should not be used. **Store** in airtight containers in which the atmosphere has been replaced by nitrogen or other inert gas.

Adverse Effects, Treatment, and Precautions. As for Local Anaesthetics, p.899.

Allergy and effects on the skin. An ophthalmologist developed dermatitis with fissuring of the finger tips after using proxymetacaine solution.— C. March and M. A. Greenwood, *Archs Ophthal., N.Y.*, 1968, *79*, 159, per *J. Am. med. Ass.*, 1968, *203* (Feb. 5), A162.

A skin reaction occurred in a woman with the Stevens-Johnson syndrome after ophthalmic anaesthesia with proxymetacaine hydrochloride.— B. Ward *et al.*, *Am. J. Ophthal.*, 1978, *86*, 133.

Effects on the eyes. A warning against the regular use of proxymetacaine hydrochloride in solutions for insertion of contact lenses. Such ophthalmic drugs are stated to be toxic to the corneal epithelium and likely to result in sloughing of corneal epithelial cells. The use of an ice-cold bland ophthalmic solution is advised instead.— W. G. Sampson, *J. Am. med. Ass.*, 1967, *200*, 905.

Absorption and Fate. See under Local Anaesthetics, p.900.

Uses. Proxymetacaine hydrochloride is a surface anaesthetic (see p.901) of the ester type and is used in ophthalmology. It is slightly more potent than amethocaine in equal concentrations and only rarely causes irritation or mydriasis. Instillation of 1 or 2 drops of a 0.5% solution permits tonometry in about 20 seconds; anaesthesia lasts about 15 minutes. For cataract extraction 1 drop is instilled every 5 to 10 minutes to a total of 5 to 7 applications. Proxymetacaine is suitable for most ophthalmic applications and drug sensitivity is rare.

Preparations

Proparacaine Hydrochloride Ophthalmic Solution *(U.S.P.)*. A sterile aqueous solution of proxymetacaine hydrochloride. pH 3.5 to 6. Store in airtight containers. After opening the container, store at 2° to 8°. Protect from light.

Proxymetacaine Eye-drops *(B.P.C. 1973)*. PROX. A sterile solution containing 0.52% of proxymetacaine hydrochloride, with suitable preservatives, in water. It may contain glycerol. Protect from light. After opening the container, store at 2° to 10° and avoid freezing.

Ophthaine *(Squibb, UK)*. Proxymetacaine hydrochloride, available as eye-drops containing 0.5% with chlorbutol 0.2%, benzalkonium chloride 0.01%, and glycerol. Store in a refrigerator. (Also available as Ophthaine in *Austral., Canad., USA*).

Other Proprietary Names

Alcaine *(Austral., Canad., Norw., Switz., USA)*; Kéracaine *(Fr.)*; Ophthetic *(Austral., Canad., USA)*; Piloptic *(Ger.)*.

7648-a

Pyrrocaine Hydrochloride. EN 1010. Pyrrolidin-1-ylaceto-2′,6′-xylidide hydrochloride.
$C_{14}H_{20}N_2O,HCl=268.8$.

CAS — 2210-77-7 (pyrrocaine); 2210-64-2 (hydrochloride).

A white odourless crystalline powder. M.p. 200° to 204°. **Soluble** 1 in 1.5 of water and 1 in 12 of alcohol; soluble in isopropyl alcohol; practically insoluble in chloroform and ether.

Pyrrocaine hydrochloride is a local anaesthetic of the amide type which was formerly used for infiltration and nerve block anaesthesia in dentistry.

The general actions of local anaesthetics are described on p.899.

References: E. K. Zsigmond and R. L. Patterson, *Anesth. Analg. curr. Res.*, 1969, *48*, 66.

7649-t

Tolycaine Hydrochloride. Methyl 2-(2-diethylaminoacetamido)-*m*-toluate hydrochloride.
$C_{15}H_{22}N_2O_3,HCl=314.8$.

CAS — 3686-58-6 (tolycaine); 7210-92-6 (hydrochloride).

A white crystalline powder. M.p. about 140°. **Soluble** in water.

Tolycaine hydrochloride is a local anaesthetic formerly used as a 3% solution with adrenaline and noradrenaline.

The general actions of local anaesthetics are described on p.899.

7650-l

Trimecaine Hydrochloride. Trimecainium Chloratum. 2-Diethylamino-2′,4′,6′-trimethylacetanilide hydrochloride.
$C_{15}H_{24}N_2O,HCl=284.8$.

CAS — 616-68-2 (trimecaine); 1027-14-1 (hydrochloride).

Pharmacopoeias. In *Cz.*

A white crystalline powder. M.p. about 140°. **Soluble** in water.

Trimecaine hydrochloride is a local anaesthetic which has been used in the USSR and eastern Europe for similar purposes to lignocaine hydrochloride in solutions containing 0.5 to 2%, with adrenaline if necessary.

The general actions of local anaesthetics are described on p.899.

Lysergide and other Hallucinogenic Agents

5010-w

This group of drugs is termed variously psychodysleptics, psychotomimetics, psychotogens, psychodelics, or, more usually but often inappropriately, hallucinogens. The characteristic feature of these substances is their ability to induce states of altered perception, mood, or thought. Changes in visual perception are often the most significant. There may be personality changes.

The hallucinogenic agents described in this section are not generally used therapeutically.

Reviews of hallucinogenic drugs: A. Hofmann, *Indian J. Pharm.*, 1963, *25*, 245; R. A. Sandison, *Practitioner*, 1964, *192*, 30; S. Cohen, *Ann. Rev. Pharmac.*, 1967, *7*, 301; N. R. Farnsworth, *Science*, 1968, *162*, 1086; A. M. Walshe, *Australas. J. Pharm.*, 1968, *49*, 588; R. E. Schultes, *Bull. Narcot.*, 1969, *21* (July-Sept.), 3; *idem*, *Science*, 1969, *163*, 245; H. Kalant *et al.*, *Pharmac. Rev.*, 1971, *23*, 135; *Pharm. J.*, 1971, *2*, 239; P. Brawley and J. C. Duffield, *Pharmac. Rev.*, 1972, *24*, 31; H. Osmond, *Practitioner*, 1973, *210*, 112; L. E. Hollister, in *Handbook of Psychopharmacology*, Vol. 11, L.L. Iversen *et al.* (Ed.), London, Plenum Press, 1978, p. 389.

Adverse effects and treatment. The diagnosis and treatment of acute reactions to hallucinogens. Patients should be treated in a quiet place and given reassurance that the effects will subside. When sedation is required diazepam or a barbiturate should be given. Phenothiazines are also effective but should not be given if anticholinergic substances have also been taken. A withdrawal syndrome does not occur.— *Med. Lett.*, 1977, *19*, 13. See also *idem*, 1980, *22*, 73.

Recurring panic attacks which developed after use of hallucinogenic agents might be related to induced changes in temporal lobe functioning. Generally attacks resolve slowly provided the patient avoids further contact with the relevant substance.— D. Jacobs (letter), *Br. med. J.*, 1979, *2*, 49.

Dependence. For a review of dependence on hallucinogenic agents, see H. Isbell and T. L. Chrusciel, *Dependence Liability of 'Non-narcotic' Drugs*, Geneva, World Health Organization, 1970; *idem*, *Bull. Wld Hlth Org.*, 1970, *43*, *Suppl.* See also Nineteenth Report of WHO Expert Committee on Drug Dependence, *Tech. Rep. Ser. Wld Hlth Org. No. 526*, 1973; Evaluation of Dependence Liability and Dependence Potential of Drugs, *Tech. Rep. Ser. Wld Hlth Org. No. 577*, 1975.

Interactions. A review of interactions of lysergide and mescaline with drugs used clinically.— R. J. Wyatt *et al.*, *Ann. N.Y. Acad. Sci.*, 1976, *281*, 456.

5011-e

Lysergide. Lysergic Acid Diethylamide; LSD; LSD 25. (+)-*NN*-Diethyl-D-lysergamide; (6a*R*,9*R*)-*NN*-Diethyl-4,6,6a,7,8,9-hexahydro-7-methylindolo[4,3-*fg*]quinoline-9-carboxamide. $C_{20}H_{25}N_3O$=323.4.

CAS — 50-37-3.

A colourless, tasteless, odourless, crystalline substance related to ergometrine. It is normally used as the water-soluble tartrate.

Aqueous solutions are stable for about 1 week at 0° in the dark when exposed to air. At room temperature or in daylight solutions deteriorate within 24 hours of being exposed to air. **Incompatible** with free chlorine or other halogens, so that solutions should be diluted before use with *purified water*, not tap water.

Adverse Effects. There is considerable variation in individual reaction to lysergide. Disorders of visual perception are among the first and most constant reactions to lysergide. Subjects may be hypersensitive to sound. Extreme alterations of mood, depression, distortion of body image, depersonalisation, disorders of thought and time sense, and synaesthesias may be experienced. Anxiety, often amounting to panic, may occur. A prolonged toxic psychosis may be induced. The effects of lysergide may recur months after ingestion of lysergide; the recurrence or 'flashback' may be spontaneous or induced by alcohol, other drugs, stress, or injection.

The subjective effects of lysergide may be preceded or accompanied by somatic effects which are mainly sympathomimetic in nature and include mydriasis, tremor, hyperreflexia, fever, salivation, piloerection, and ataxia. There may be nausea and vomiting and variable effects on heart-rate and blood pressure.

Tolerance develops to the effects of lysergide after several days and may be lost over a similar period. There is cross-tolerance between lysergide, mescaline, and psilocybin and psilocin, but not to amphetamine or to cannabis.

Physical dependence on lysergide does not seem to occur.

Descriptions of the adverse reactions of lysergide: W. A. Frosch *et al.*, *New Engl. J. Med.*, 1965, *273*, 1235; J. T. Ungerleider *et al.*, *J. Am. med. Ass.*, 1966, *197*, 389; T. H. Bewley, *Br. med. J.*, 1967, *3*, 28; R. G. Smart and K. Bateman, *Can. med. Ass. J.*, 1967, *97*, 1214; R. Denson, *Can. med. Ass. J.*, 1967, *97*, 1222; S. Hamzepour, *Br. J. clin. Pract.*, 1968, *22*, 436; R. Clayton, *Br. med. J.*, 1968, *1*, 163; N. Malleson, *Br. J. Psychiat.*, 1971, *118*, 229; T. Bewley, *Br. med. J.*, 1975, *2*, 318.

For reviews of the toxic effects of lysergide, see S. Mårtens *et al.*, *Läkartidningen*, 1967, *64*, 1856; *Lancet*, 1967, *2*, 504; *ibid.*, 929; *The Amphetamines and Lysergic Acid Diethylamide (LSD)*, London, HM Stationery Office, 1970; Amphetamines, Barbiturates, LSD and Cannabis, their Use and Misuse, *Reports on Public Health and Medical Subjects No. 124*, London, HM Stationery Office, 1970; A. A. Baker, *Lancet*, 1970, *1*, 714.

Chromosomal aberrations. Lysergide has been reported to increase chromosomal abnormalities *in vitro* in cell culture (M.M. Cohen *et al.*, *Science*, 1967, *155*, 1417). Studies of chromosomal damage in man following ingestion of lysergide have yielded contradictory results. In some studies a significant increase in chromosomal abnormalities has been reported in patients who had taken lysergide (S. Irwin and J. Egozcue, *Science*, 1967, *157*, 313; J. Nielsen *et al.*, *Br. med. J.*, 1968, *2*, 801; J. Nielsen *et al.* (letter), *Nature*, 1968, *218*, 488; J. Nielsenet *al.*, *Br. med. J.*, 1969, *3*, 634). Other studies have indicated that lysergide had no significant effect on chromosomal abnormalities (J.-H. Tjio *et al.*, *J. Am. med. Ass.*, 1969, *210*, 849; J.M. Aase *et al.*, *Lancet*, 1970, *2*, 100; K.W. Dumars, *Pediatrics*, 1971, *47*, 1037; J.T. Robinson *et al.*, *Br. J. Psychiat.*, 1974, *125*, 238).

Reviews of the effects of lysergide on chromosomes (N.I. Dishotsky *et al.*, *Science*, 1971, *172*, 431; P.J. Balson, *Adverse Drug React. Bull.*, 1972, Dec. 116; S.Y. Long, *Teratology*, 1972, *6*, 75; H. Tuchmann-Duplessis, *Monographs on Drugs, Vol. 2, Drug Effects on the Fetus*, G.S. Avery (Ed.), London, Adis, 1975, p. 158) have concluded that chromosomal damage *in vivo* cannot be attributed to lysergide and that claims for teratogenic, mutagenic, or carcinogenic action of lysergide have not been substantiated.

Pregnancy and the neonate. The frequency of spontaneous abortions (15%) and premature births (7%) in 121 pregnancies following infrequent low doses of medically administered lysergide were within the normal ranges. The incidence of spontaneous abortions (37%) was above average for 27 pregnancies where lysergide was taken under both medical and non-medical conditions. In both groups there were more abortions when the mother or mother and father received lysergide than when only the father received lysergide. Congenital abnormalities were reported in 14 infants and some of these were minor. In all 14 lysergide was limited to medical use and the dosage range was 75 to 250 µg.— W. H. McGlothlin *et al.*, *J. Am. med. Ass.*, 1970, *212*, 1483.

There was no strong evidence of dysmorphogenic action by lysergide in *animals* or man.— H. Tuchmann-Duplessis, *Monographs on Drugs, Vol. 2, Drug Effects on the Fetus*, G.S. Avery (Ed.), London, Adis, 1975, p. 158. See also J. L. Schardein, *Drugs as Teratogens*, Cleveland, CRC, 1976, p. 129.

Ocular malformations in infants associated with maternal ingestion of lysergide during pregnancy.— C. C. Chan *et al.*, *Archs Ophthal., N.Y.*, 1978, *96*, 282.

Further reports of congenital abnormalities associated with lysergide: C. B. Jacobson and C. M. Berlin, *J. Am. med. Ass.*, 1972, *222*, 1367; B. Bogdanoff *et al.*, *Am. J. Dis. Child.*, 1972, *123*, 145; D. J. Apple and T. O. Bennett, *Archs Ophthal., N.Y.*, 1974, *92*, 301.

See also under Chromosomal Aberrations.

Psychosis. In studies on 19 patients who were admitted to mental hospitals with psychoses resulting from ingestion of lysergide, it was found that 6 had become psychotic after a single dose, although in 2 the onset of symptoms was delayed; of the other patients, 2 had become psychotic after 2 and 6 doses respectively and 11 were long-term users. Common symptoms included thought disorders, auditory hallucinations, disturbed behaviour, and paranoid delusions. Although similar to schizophrenia, detailed study revealed diagnostic differences. Chlorpromazine combined with ECT was the treatment of choice. Because of the danger of recurrent visual disturbances, patients should be warned not to drive.— K. Dewhurst and J. A. Hatrick, *Practitioner*, 1972, *209*, 327.

Further reports: J. A. Hatrick and K. Dewhurst, *Lancet*, 1970, *2*, 742; P. Reich and R. B. Hepps, *J. Am. med. Ass.*, 1972, *219*, 869; B. H. Fookes (letter), *Lancet*, 1972, *1*, 1074; A. Klepfisz and J. Racy, *J. Am. med. Ass.*, 1973, *223*, 429.

Treatment of Adverse Effects. Diazepam 15 to 30 mg by mouth or by intravenous injection or chlorpromazine 50 to 100 mg by mouth or by intramuscular injection have been given to treat acute panic reactions. Lysergide-induced psychosis has also been treated with chlorpromazine.

References: T. H. Bewley, *Br. med. J.*, 1967, *3*, 603; B. O'Neil, *Can. pharm. J.*, 1968, *101*, 62; R. M. Levy (letter), *Lancet*, 1971, *1*, 1297; B. E. W. Barnett (letter), *ibid.*, 1971, *2*, 270; W. H. Anderson and J. E. O'Malley (letter), *J. Am. med. Ass.*, 1972, *220*, 1244; J. A. H. Forrest and R. A. Tarala, *Br. med. J.*, 1973, *4*, 136.

Precautions. It is suggested that treatment with lysergide should not be given during the early stages of pregnancy.

The effects of lysergide may be enhanced by reserpine.

A report of chlorpromazine inducing psychosis in patients who had received lysergide.— C. J. Schwartz, *Can. med. Ass. J.*, 1971, *105*, 241.

Interactions of lysergide with drugs used clinically.— R. J. Wyatt *et al.*, *Ann. N.Y. Acad. Sci.*, 1976, *281*, 456.

Absorption and Fate. Lysergide is readily absorbed from the gastro-intestinal tract. It is metabolised in the liver and is excreted in the bile.

Uses. Lysergide has a doubtful therapeutic role and has been used mainly as an adjunct to psychotherapy. Doses of 100 to 750 µg by mouth have been used. The effects of a dose may last for 12 to 24 hours.

Lysergide had an enormous number of physiological, biochemical, and behavioural effects. In the central nervous system it acted primarily to block synapses. The behavioural changes it induced had been found to correlate well with alterations in intracellular serotonin concentrations. Its potential medical applications included alcoholism, psychoneuroses, sexual deviancy, autism in children, and psychopathies, but data regarding its value in such conditions were often inadequate. Lysergide might achieve analgesia in terminal disease. For most of these purposes 100 to 750 µg had been given by mouth, but occasionally 1 to 3 mg might be given or 50 to 500 µg injected intravenously.— D. B. Louria, *New Engl. J. Med.*, 1968, *278*, 435.

Experiments in *cats* and *rats* indicated that lysergide-like psychotomimetics might act by antagonism of serotonin in the lower brain stem rather than by stimulation of serotonin receptors.— P. B. Bradley and I. Briggs, *Br. J. Pharmac.*, 1974, *50*, 345.

A review of the biochemical pharmacology of lysergide.— J. Caldwell and P. S. Sever, *Clin. Pharmac. Ther.*, 1974, *16*, 625. See also L. Pieri *et al.*, *Nature*, 1978, *272*, 278.

Alcoholism. Reports on the use of lysergide as an adjunct in the treatment of chronic alcoholism.— R. G. Smart *et al.*, *Q. J. Stud. Alcohol*, 1966, *27*, 469; L. E. Hollister *et al.*, *Am. J. Psychiat.*, 1969, *125*, 1352; A. Ludwig *et al.*, *Am. J. Psychiat.*, 1969, *126*, 59; F. G. Johnson, *Am. J. Psychiat.*, 1969, *126*, 481; W. N. Pahnke *et al.*, *J. Am. med. Ass.*, 1970, *212*, 1856.

Analgesic action. A study of the analgesic action of lysergide.— E. C. Kast and V. J. Collins, *Anesth. Analg. curr. Res.*, 1964, *43*, 285.

Psychotherapy. Use of lysergide in psychotherapy.— A. K. Busch and W. C. Johnson, *Dis. nerv. Syst.*, 1950, *11*, 241; E. F. W. Baker, *Can. med. Ass. J.*, 1964, *91*, 1200; D. Turns and H. C. B. Denber, *Arzneimittel-Forsch.*, 1966, *16*, 251; H. Leuner, *ibid.*, 253; W. N. Pahnke *et al.*, *Int. Z. klin. Pharmak.*, 1971, *4*, 446, per *Int. pharm. Abstr.*, 1972, *9*, 348.

5012-l

Bufotenine. Mappine; *NN*-Dimethylserotonin; 5-Hydroxy-*NN*-dimethyltryptamine. 3-(2-Dimethylaminoethyl)indol-5-ol.
$C_{12}H_{16}N_2O=204.3$.

CAS — 487-93-4.

An indole alkaloid obtained from the seeds and leaves of *Piptadenia peregrina* and *P. macrocarpa* (Mimosaceae). It was first isolated from the skin glands of toads (*Bufo* spp.) and has also been isolated from species of *Amanita* (Agaricaceae).
Almost **insoluble** in water; freely soluble in alcohol; less soluble in ether; soluble in dilute acids and alkalis.

Bufotenine is stated to have hallucinogenic properties. It is inactive when given by mouth.

Cohoba Snuff. A hallucinogenic snuff prepared from the seeds and leaves of *Piptadenia peregrina*. The plant has been found to contain bufotenine, dimethyltryptamine, *N*-methyltryptamine, and 5-methoxy-*NN*-dimethyltryptamine.— A. Hofmann, *Indian J. Pharm.*, 1963, *25*, 245. See also *Pharm. J.*, 1957, *2*, 420.

5013-y

Dimethyltryptamine. DMT. 3-(2-Dimethylaminoethyl)indole.
$C_{12}H_{16}N_2=188.3$.

CAS — 61-50-7.

An active principle obtained from the seeds and leaves of *Piptadenia peregrina* (Mimosaceae) and other South American plants.

Dimethyltryptamine produces effects which are similar to those of lysergide, but of shorter duration. It is inactive when taken by mouth.

References: A. Hofmann, *Indian J. Pharm.*, 1963, *25*, 245; D. R. Rubin (letter), *J. Am. med. Ass.*, 1967, *201*, 143; J. R. Unwin, *Can. med. Ass. J.*, 1968, *98*, 402.

5014-j

DOM. 2,5-Dimethoxy-4-methylamphetamine. 2,5-Dimethoxy-4,α-dimethylphenethylamine.
$C_{12}H_{19}NO_2=209.3$.

CAS — 15588-95-1.

DOM is chemically related to amphetamine and mescaline. It is reported to have hallucinogenic properties and to be the active principle of the hallucinogenic preparation known as STP. (STP has also been used as a synonym for DOM.)
DOM produces sympathetic stimulation with dilatation of the pupils, increased reflexes, tremor, and increased pulse-rate and blood-pressure.

References: S. H. Snyder *et al.*, *Science*, 1967, *158*, 669; *Br. med. J.*, 1967, *3*, 570; *J. Am. med. Ass.*, 1968, *204* (June 24), A29; J. R. Unwin, *Can. med. Ass. J.*, 1968, *98*, 402; L. P. Solursh and W. R. Clement, *ibid.*, 407; S. H. Snyder *et al.*, *Am. J. Psychiat.*, 1968, *125*, 113; G. F. Phillips and R. J. Mesley, *J. Pharm. Pharmac.*, 1969, *21*, 9; H. Weingartner *et al.*, *J. clin. Pharmac.*, 1971, *11*, 103.

5015-z

Harmaline. 3,4-Dihydroharmine.
$C_{13}H_{14}N_2O=214.3$.

CAS — 304-21-2.

An alkaloid obtained from peganum, the dried seeds of *Peganum harmala* (Zygophyllaceae). It has also been found together with harmine in the South American hallucinogenic drink 'caapi'—see below under Harmine.

5016-c

Harmine. 7-Methoxy-1-methyl-9*H*-pyrido[3,4-*b*]indole.
$C_{13}H_{12}N_2O=212.3$.

CAS — 442-51-3.

An alkaloid obtained from peganum, the dried seeds of *Peganum harmala* (Zygophyllaceae).
Harmine is identical with an alkaloid known as banisterine or telepathine obtained from *Banisteria caapi* (Malpighiaceae) and with the alkaloid, yageine, from *Haemadictyon amazonicum* (Apocynaceae).

A hallucinogenic drink which is known in the Western Amazonian regions as 'caapi' (Brazil and Colombia), 'Yagé' (Colombia), and 'ayahuasca' (Ecuador, Peru, and Bolivia), is made basically from the same or closely related plants of the family Malpighiaceae. The main active principles are harmine and harmaline.

References: A. Hofmann, *Indian J. Pharm.*, 1963, *25*, 245; D. H. Aarons *et al.*, *J. pharm. Sci.*, 1977, *66*, 1244.

5017-k

Mescaline. 3,4,5-Trimethoxyphenethylamine.
$C_{11}H_{17}NO_3=211.3$.

CAS — 54-04-6.

An alkaloid obtained from the cactus *Lophophora williamsii* (=*Anhalonium williamsii*=*A. lewinii*) (Cactaceae), which grows in the northern regions of Mexico. The cactus is known in those areas by the Aztec name 'peyote' or 'peyotl' and dried slices of the cactus are called 'mescal buttons'. Both Mexican and North American Indians have used peyotl in religious ceremonies on account of its hallucinogenic activity.

Mescaline produces effects similar to those produced by lysergide, but it is less potent. It has occasionally been used in psychiatry.

Effects of mescaline in man.— A. Hofmann, *Indian J. Pharm.*, 1963, *25*, 254.

Pharmacological studies of mescaline *in vitro*.— E. Clemente and V. de P. Lynch, *J. pharm. Sci.*, 1968, *57*, 72.

A detailed review of the chemistry, biogenesis, and biological effects of 42 constituents of peyote.— G. J. Kapadia and M. B. E. Fayez, *J. pharm. Sci.*, 1970, *59*, 1699.

An investigation of the use of peyote among Navajo Indians.— R. L. Bergman, *Am. J. Psychiat.*, 1971, *128*, 695.

A study of 57 Huichol Indians with an individual and cultural tradition of peyote ingestion and 60 controls indicated that ingestion of peyote was not associated with abnormalities in lymphocyte chromosomes.— D. L. Dorrance *et al.*, *J. Am. med. Ass.*, 1975, *234*, 299. See also *ibid.*, 313.

5018-a

Ololiuqui

CAS — 2889-26-1 (isoergine); 478-94-4 (ergine); 2390-99-0 (chanoclavine); 548-43-6 (elymoclavine); 602-85-7 (lysergol).

The seeds of *Rivea corymbosa* or *Ipomoea tricolor* (=*I. violacea*) both convolvulaceous plants similar to the common 'morning glory', *Ipomoea purpurea*. The brown seeds of *R. corymbosa* are known as 'badoh' and the black seeds of *I. tricolor* as 'badoh negro', the former containing 0.01% of alkaloid and the latter 0.05%.

Ololiuqui has hallucinogenic properties and is considered to be sacred by some Mexican Indians. Alkaloidal fractions contain at least 5 closely related individual components, viz. D-isolysergic acid amide (isoergine), D-lysergic acid amide (ergine), chanoclavine, elymoclavine, and lysergol.
The name 'ololiuqui' has been erroneously applied to seeds of *Datura metel* (Solanaceae).

Pharmacology of ololiuqui.— A. Hofmann, *Indian J. Pharm.*, 1963, *25*, 245.

Reports of adverse effects following ingestion of morning glory seeds.— A. L. Ingram, *J. Am. med. Ass.*, 1964, *190*, 1133; P. J. Fink *et al.*, *Archs gen. Psychiat.*, 1966, *15*, 209.

Following press reports in 1966 that 'morning glory' seeds were being purchased and used for their hallucinogenic properties, an investigation initiated in the laboratories of the Pharmaceutical Society of Great Britain showed that of the many species sold by seedsmen under the name 'morning glory', only those of *Ipomoea violacea* contained lysergic acid derivatives and presumably had hallucinogenic properties.— K. R. Capper, Lysergic Acid Derivatives in Morning Glory Seeds, *The Pharmacological and Epidemiological Aspects of Adolescent Drug Dependence*, C.W.M. Wilson, Oxford, Pergamon Press, 1968.

5019-t

Psilocin. 4-Hydroxy-*NN*-dimethyltryptamine. 3-(2-Dimethylaminoethyl)indol-4-ol.
$C_{12}H_{16}N_2O=204.3$.

CAS — 520-53-6.

An indole alkaloid obtained from the mushroom *Psilocybe mexicana* (Agaricaceae).

Psilocin possesses hallucinogenic properties similar to those of lysergide, but they are of shorter duration.
The properties of psilocin are similar to those of psilocybin.

5020-l

Psilocybin. 4-Phosphoryloxy-*NN*-dimethyltryptamine. 3-(2-Dimethylaminoethyl)indol-4-yl dihydrogen phosphate.
$C_{12}H_{17}N_2O_4P=284.3$.

CAS — 520-52-5.

The main indole alkaloid present in the mushroom *Psilocybe mexicana* (Agaricaceae), which grows in certain parts of Mexico. Psilocybin is also present in the mushrooms *Stropharia cubensis* and *Conocybe* spp.

Psilocybin has hallucinogenic properties similar to those of lysergide. In the body, psilocybin is immediately converted to psilocin.

Effects of psilocybin on mental state.— A. Hofmann, *Indian J. Pharm.*, 1963, *25*, 245. See also R. Růžičková *et al.*, *Čslká Psychiat.*, 1967, *63*, 158; R. Fischer *et al.* (letter), *Nature*, 1968, *218*, 296; C. Hyde *et al.*, *Br. J. Psychiat.*, 1978, *132*, 602; C. Benjamin, *Br. med. J.*, 1979, *1*, 1319.

A controlled study showed that a dose of 10 mg of psilocybin given to 22 healthy adults prolonged reaction time and increased heart-rate, pupil size, and blood pressure. In 4, EEG tracings showed that visual symptoms were associated with changes in the visual cortex.— R. R. Rynearson *et al.*, *Mayo Clin. Proc.*, 1968, *43*, 191.

Psilocybin was identified in mushrooms of the *Gymnopilus* spp. Poisoning had occurred in 2 individuals after ingestion of *Gymnopilus validipes*.— G. M. Hatfield *et al.*, *Lloydia*, 1978, *41*, 140.

The clinical toxicology of *Psilocybe semilanceata* (magic mushroom; liberty cap): N. R. Peden *et al.*, *Postgrad. med. J.*, 1981, *57*, 543; A. D. Harries and V. Evans, *ibid.*, 571.

Metals and some Metallic Salts

5260-v

The therapeutic and toxicological properties of metals stem from their physical and chemical properties which in turn are associated with their atomic structure. Thus, the behaviour of sodium, potassium, calcium, and magnesium (see under Electrolytes, p.618) is dominated by their property of forming electrovalent or ionic compounds so that they behave as free ions in the body. Heavy metals such as bismuth (p.927), gold (p.932), lead (p.935), mercury (p.937), and silver (p.940) have the alternative property of forming stable covalent or coordinate compounds so that they enter into complexes with proteins. It is for this reason that their toxicological properties frequently outweigh any real or postulated beneficial effect and some heavy metals and their salts have become of toxicological, rather than therapeutic, interest.

Some metals such as copper (p.930), manganese (p.937), and zinc (p.943) and others mentioned elsewhere (e.g. cobalt) are constituents of enzymes and are accordingly essential trace elements (see also under Amino Acids and Nutritional Agents, p.47); unlike iron (p.872) they are needed in such small amounts that their deficiency is rare or unknown. Barium (p.926) is highly toxic in the form of its soluble salts owing to its ability to form ions able to mimic those of calcium, but the physical properties of its insoluble salts (see Barium Sulphate, p.434) confer upon it merit as a contrast medium. Metals such as aluminium (p.926) and tin (p.943) are generally poorly absorbed and are themselves usually non-toxic so that they have important uses in the packaging of food.

Metals and their alloys are sometimes used, e.g. in dentistry (gold, mercury, silver) and in heart-valve and orthopaedic prostheses (e.g. nickel). In general few problems are encountered but allergy can occur.

5261-g

Aluminium. Aluminum.

Al=26.98154.

CAS — 7429-90-5.

A malleable and ductile soft silvery-white metal, becoming coated with a thin layer of oxide. It is attacked slowly by organic acids in the presence of sodium chloride and by hydrochloric acid, and more rapidly by solutions of alkali hydroxides and mercurials.

Adverse Effects. Intestinal absorption of aluminium is very slight and any aluminium absorbed is quickly excreted by healthy kidneys. It has been suggested, however, that osteomalacia and encephalitis occurring in patients undergoing haemodialysis might be associated with the aluminium content of the water supplies. For the side-effects of aluminium salts, see under Aluminium Hydroxide Mixture, p.72.

Maximum permissible atmospheric concentration 10 mg per m^3.

Culinary utensils. The usual dietary intake of aluminium obtained from food, water, and foods prepared in aluminium cooking utensils, which has been estimated to be 10 to 100 mg daily, is considered to be insufficient to cause phosphate deficiency. FDA scientists have reported that there is no evidence that aluminium utensils and wrappings are unsafe.— N. Selvey, *J. Am. med. Ass.*, 1977, *238*, 1567. See also G. A. Trapp and J. B. Cannon (letter), *New Engl. J. Med.*, 1981, *304*, 172.

Dialysis. Subsequent to a study by M.M. Platts *et al.* (*Br. med. J.*, 1977, *2*, 657) who noted dialysis encephalopathy in 11 and spontaneous fractures in 21 of 202 patients undergoing home dialysis, J.R. McDermott *et al.* (*Lancet*, 1978, *1*, 901) indicated that there was a significantly higher mean brain concentration of aluminium in 7 patients with dialysis encephalopathy than in 12 nondemented patients undergoing dialysis. Like J.A. Flendrig *et al.* (*Lancet*, 1976, *1*, 1235) who attributed dialysis dementia in 6 patients to aluminium contamination of the dialysate, they considered the aluminium content of the dialysate to be implicated. Their observations agreed with those of the European Dialysis and Transplant Association (C. Jacobs *et al.*, *Proc. Eur. Dialysis Transplant Ass.*, 1977, *14*, 51) who found no correlation between ingestion of aluminium hydroxide and dialysis dementia, but J.R. McDermott *et al.* nevertheless considered that it would be premature to exonerate aluminium hydroxide completely since over long periods of time aluminium hydroxide might make an important contribution to the body load. They also noted in 2 patients that restoration of renal function by transplantation did not readily remove aluminium from brain tissue and recommended that efforts should be made to reduce and monitor the aluminium content of dialysis fluid.

From an epidemiological study carried out on 1293 patients undergoing intermittent haemodialysis in 18 dialysis centres in Great Britain, I.S. Parkinson *et al.* (*Lancet*, 1979, *1*, 406) found a striking association between dialysate aluminium content, dialysis encephalopathy, and fracturing dialysis osteodystrophy or histologically proven osteomalacia. There seemed little doubt that dialysis encephalopathy was associated with a high concentration of aluminium in the dialysate. The findings also suggested that aluminium might be the major cause of fracturing osteodystrophy and histologically proven dialysis osteomalacia. It was suggested that the aluminium content of the dialysate should probably be below 50 µg per litre and, more likely, below 20 µg per litre. This figure of 50 µg per litre was considered too high by P. Gilli *et al.* (*Lancet*, 1980 *2*, 742) for peritoneal dialysis; data subsequently obtained by K.C. Hodge *et al.* (*Lancet*, 1981, *2*, 803) led to these authors proposing a limit of 15 µg per litre.

Analysis of questionnaires, returned to the Registry of the European Dialysis and Transplant Association, giving details of dialysis dementia in 150 patients treated in 65 dialysis centres in Europe in 1976 and 1977. Allowance being made for non-returned questionnaires, the prevalence of dialysis dementia was estimated to be about 600 per 100 000 patients.—Registration Committee of the European Dialysis and Transplant Association, *Lancet*, 1980, *2*, 190.

Uses. Aluminium foil has been used as a dressing for burns. Aluminium is used in industry for collapsible tubes, in the foil packing of tablets, and as extruded aluminium screw-cap cans. Aluminium salts are used as antacids, astringents, and antiperspirants.

Aluminium foil adsorbed *Staphylococcus aureus* and *Pseudomonas aeruginosa* from aqueous suspension but failed to adsorb or kill *Escherichia coli* and *Proteus vulgaris*.— T. J. Bradley *et al.*, *J. Pharm. Pharmac.*, 1965, *17*, 98S.

5262-q

Aluminium Powder *(B.P.)*. Alumin. Pdr.; Pulvis Aluminii.

Pharmacopoeias. In *Arg.* and *Br.*

Aluminium powder is an odourless or almost odourless, silvery-grey powder. It consists mainly of metallic aluminium in very small flakes, usually with an appreciable quantity of aluminium oxide. It is lubricated with stearic acid during manufacture and this lubricant protects the metal from oxidation during subsequent storage. It contains not less than 86% of Al, calculated with reference to the substance freed from lubricant and volatile matter. *Arg. P.* allows oleic or stearic acid as the lubricant and contains not less than 95% Al.

Practically **insoluble** in water and alcohol; almost completely soluble, with evolution of hydrogen, in dilute acids and solutions of alkali hydroxides. **Store** in airtight containers.

WARNING. *The Council of the Pharmaceutical Society of Great Britain advises pharmacists not to supply materials likely to be used for making fireworks, including aluminium powder, to children under any circumstances, and recommends that aluminium powder should be sold only to persons who are, or appear to be, 18 years of age or over.*

Adverse Effects. As for Aluminium (above).

Uses. Aluminium powder has been used for dusting the skin around an ileostomy, caecostomy, or colostomy to prevent irritation due to proteolytic or irritant discharges. The skin is dried and freed from grease and repeated applications of the powder made until a thick film adheres. Alternatively, Compound Aluminium Paste may be employed; the paste is applied thickly round the fistula or sinus in order to prevent the discharge from coming in contact with the skin.

Aluminium powder has been used as a dressing for burns, tropical ulcers, and indolent wounds.

Vaginitis. All vaginal pathogens produced vaginal hypoacidity which could be corrected by the instillation of micronised aluminium powder; 466 patients with trichomonal and 100 with candidal infection had responded to this treatment.— K. J. Karnaky (letter), *Am. J. Obstet. Gynec.*, 1977, *129*, 929.

Preparations

Compound Aluminium Paste *(B.P.)*. Baltimore Paste. Aluminium powder 2, zinc oxide 4, and liquid paraffin 4, by wt.

5263-p

Barium.

Ba=137.33.

CAS — 7440-39-3.

A soft highly reactive silvery-white metal; the finely divided form ignites spontaneously in air.

With the exception of the sulphate (see p.434), which is insoluble and thus not absorbed and is used as a contrast medium, barium is not used internally in therapeutics owing to its toxic effects; it stimulates all muscle, striated, smooth, and cardiac.

Adverse Effects. The symptoms of barium poisoning include vomiting, colic, and diarrhoea, with slow irregular pulse, hypertension, hypokalaemia, convulsive tremors, and muscular paralysis. Death from cardiac or respiratory failure may occur within one to many hours. A fatal dose of the chloride may be as low as 1 g but larger doses have been tolerated.

Maximum permissible atmospheric concentration 500 µg per m^3 of soluble barium compounds.

For the hazards of inhaling barium sulphate, see p.434.

Of over 100 patients who ate sausage contaminated with barium carbonate 19 required hospital admission. Symptoms included: diarrhoea, vomiting, general weakness, dryness of the mouth, paralysis, tightness in the throat, dysarthria, and headaches; other symptoms were muscle twitching, testicular tenderness, urinary retention, and gastro-intestinal haemorrhage. Two severely affected patients had hypokalaemia with associated ECG changes.— Z. Lewi and Y. Bar-Khayim, *Lancet*, 1964, *2*, 342. Two severely affected patients suffered flaccid paralysis in all 4 extremities, associated with hypokalaemia. One recovered dramatically after intravenous injection of potassium chloride; the other responded initially but subsequently died, post-mortem examination revealing haemorrhagic gastritis and duodenitis, cardiac haemorrhage, and pulmonary oedema.— D. Diengott *et al.*, *ibid.*, 343.

The prolonged contact of barium-containing contraceptive devices with cervical cells presented a potential cancer risk in susceptible individuals.— J. E. Ayre and J. LeGuerrier, *Ann. N.Y. Acad. Sci.*, 1967, *141*, 414.

Acute renal failure associated with barium chloride poisoning.— S. F. Wetherill *et al.*, *Ann. intern. Med.*, 1981, *95*, 187.

Treatment of Adverse Effects. A solution of 30 g of sodium or magnesium sulphate in 250 ml of water should be given immediately by mouth to precipitate barium as the insoluble sulphate; this may be repeated in 1 hour. Gastric lavage may be carried out, especially after recent ingestion; a 2 to 5% solution of sodium or magnesium sulphate has been recommended as the lavage solution and this should be used until the return is clear.

In severe poisoning assisted respiration may be necessary; hypokalaemia, muscle paralysis, and cardiac arrhythmias should be counteracted by administration of potassium, if necessary intravenously; diuresis to enhance excretion of barium ions can be promoted by infusion of sodium chloride injection, augmented by a diuretic, such as frusemide.

Injection of atropine has been recommended to relieve the pain of intestinal colic or, if necessary, morphine may be given. Glyceryl trinitrate has been suggested to counter hypertension and cardiac pain, and sodium or magnesium sulphate has been injected intravenously with the reported aim of systemically precipitating insoluble barium sulphate.

A rapid severe fall in plasma-potassium concentrations was associated with barium poisoning. One patient who had taken a large dose of barium chloride was successfully treated with sodium sulphate 30 g by mouth and 30 g intravenously to precipitate the barium, potassium infusions, artificial respiration, and sodium bicarbonate. An infusion of 25 mmol of potassium appeared to be sufficient to balance the hypokalaemic action of the absorbed barium that had not been precipitated. An immediate bolus injection of 50 to 75 mmol might be given in severe cases.— J. Berning (letter), *Lancet*, 1975, *1*, 110.

A brief discussion on potassium in the management of barium poisoning.— R. P. Smith and R. E. Gosselin, *A. Rev. Pharmac. & Toxic.*, 1976, *16*, 189.

See also Barium Sulphide (below).

5264-s

Barium Sulphide *(B. Vet. C. 1953).* Barii Sulphidum; Sulphurated Baryta; Baryta Sulphurata *(B.P.C. 1934).*

CAS — 21109-95-5 (BaS).

A grey or yellow powder consisting of a mixture of barium sulphide (BaS = 169.4) and barium sulphate. In moist air it is converted into barium carbonate and thiosulphate, hydrogen sulphide being evolved. Partly **soluble** in water, with decomposition, giving barium hydroxide and hydrosulphide. **Store** in airtight containers.

Adverse Effects and Treatment. As for Barium, above.

A 26-year-old man ingested a facial depilatory (Magic Shave), containing 15.8 g of barium sulphide. Despite ipecacuanha-induced vomiting he developed progressive paralysis after 3 hours. He was treated with oxygen, assisted respiration, sodium bicarbonate intravenously, magnesium sulphate by nasogastric tube, gastric lavage, diuresis (infusing a total of 6.5 litres of sodium chloride injection over 19 hours, augmented by frusemide 40 mg intravenously initially and repeated thrice over the 19 hours), and correction of profound hypokalaemia, a total of 260 mmol (260 mEq) of potassium being given over 19 hours. Correction of the hypokalaemia, diuresis, and assisted respiration were considered to have contributed greatly to his survival, the diuresis being considered as indispensable as the potassium.— D. B. Gould *et al.*, *Archs intern. Med.*, 1973, *132*, 891.

Uses. It has been applied externally as a depilatory although it is very poisonous.

5265-w

Bismuth.
Bi=208.9804.

CAS — 7440-69-9.

A silvery-white crystalline brittle metal with a pinkish tinge.

Bismuth and its salts were once widely used in the treatment of syphilis and yaws.

Adverse Effects. The effects of acute bismuth intoxication include gastro-intestinal disturbance, anorexia, headache, malaise, skin reactions, discoloration of mucous membranes, and mild jaundice. A blue line of the gums, the 'bismuth line', may persist for years. If albuminuria or stomatitis occurs bismuth should be immediately withdrawn as serious ulcerative stomatitis or renal failure may result. Renal failure may be reversible if treated early but anuria and death have occurred.

Owing to limited gastro-intestinal absorption, administration of insoluble bismuth compounds by mouth does not usually give rise to acute toxic effects, but a reversible neurological syndrome characterised by deterioration of mental ability, confusion, tremor, and impaired coordination has occurred in colostomy and ileostomy patients taking bismuth subgallate by mouth over long periods. Also, intestinal bacteria may reduce bismuth subnitrate to nitrite and so cause nitrite poisoning with sufficiently large doses.

Adverse reactions reported to the Australian Drug Evaluation Committee by patients with colostomies and ileostomies taking bismuth subgallate by mouth were: an unwell feeling, lack of energy, peculiar sensation in the fingers and toes, and after a period of months or years, deterioration of mental ability, loss of concentration, impaired ability to read and write, and muscle twitching. Patients might become bedridden, incontinent, confused, and disorientated. In all patients full recovery occurred within a few weeks of discontinuing bismuth subgallate therapy.— A. W. Morrow (letter), *Med. J. Aust.*, 1973, *1*, 912.

A chronic organic brain syndrome in 2 patients was considered to be caused by the bismuth content of a cosmetic cream containing bismuth and mercury. Both patients had been using this cream for many years.— G. Krüger *et al.*, *Lancet*, 1976, *2*, 485.

An epidemiological study of intoxication by bismuth salts in France. Of 294 patients identified, 16 had died. It was considered that this was not a usual toxicological occurrence but might be associated with a bacterial factor which could convert the ingested bismuth salt into a more toxic form.— G. Martin-Bouyer, *Thérapie*, 1976, *31*, 683.

Bismuth-induced osteoarthropathies.— A. Gaucher *et al.*, *Med. J. Aust.*, 1979, *1*, 129.

Other references to systemic toxicity following oral or topical administration of bismuth salts.— R. Burns *et al.*, *Br. med. J.*, 1974, *1*, 220; J. F. Robertson, *Med. J. Aust.*, 1974, *1*, 887; Australian Drug Evaluation Committee, *ibid.*, 1974, *2*, 664; G. L. Coffey and J. W. Graham (letter), *ibid.*, 885; V. Supino-Viterbo *et al.*, *J. Neurol. Neurosurg. Psychiat.*, 1977, *40*, 748.

Nephrotoxicity. Kidney damage developed in a 19-year-old girl after the ingestion of 21 tablets of bismuth sodium triglycollamate; aminoaciduria and decreased phosphate and glucose reabsorption implied selective proximal tubular involvement. Renal function was restored by treatment with dimercaprol.— A. W. Czerwinski and H. E. Ginn, *Am. J. Med.*, 1964, *37*, 969.

Other reports of reversible renal failure following oral or intramuscular administration of bismuth sodium triglycollamate.— J. D. Gryboski and S. P. Gotoff, *New Engl. J. Med.*, 1961, *265*, 1289; R. Urizar and R. L. Vernier, *J. Am. med. Ass.*, 1966, *198*, 187; R. E. Randall *et al.* (letter), *Ann. intern. Med.*, 1972, *77*, 481.

Treatment of Adverse Effects. Severe bismuth intoxication may be treated with dimercaprol (see p.383).

Induction of acidosis by administration of ammonium chloride has been claimed to promote mobilisation of bismuth from tissue depots and increase the rate of urinary excretion.

Dialysis. *In vitro* studies indicated that severe neurological symptoms of bismuth intoxication were liable to occur above a threshold blood concentration of 200 ng per ml. Initial studies indicated that bismuth occurred in the blood in 2 forms: strongly bound up to about 200 to 400 ng per ml and weakly bound and easily dialysable above that concentration. Haemodialysis might therefore be beneficial where concentrations were very high.— P. Allain *et al.*, *Thérapie*, 1976, *31*, 703.

Precautions. Renal and hepatic disease and septic conditions of the mouth are contra-indications to the parenteral use of bismuth preparations.

If bismuth salts are given by mouth then high doses and prolonged administration should be avoided, especially in subjects with chronic ulceration of the gastro-intestinal tract or who have undergone colostomies. Caution has been recommended in constipation. It has also been recommended that the concomitant use of alcohol should be avoided.

Absorption and Fate. The rate of absorption of bismuth from an intramuscular injection depended on the salt used, its solubility in tissue fluids, and the injection vehicle. Bismuth salts could be absorbed within hours from aqueous solutions but could take weeks to be absorbed from an oily suspension. Absorbed bismuth salts permeate the body fluids and tissues and are excreted mainly in the urine, but some bismuth is retained in the tissues. It is deposited in the metaphyses of young bones and bismuth can pass the placenta into the foetus. Soluble bismuth salts are absorbed from the gastro-intestinal tract; excretion in the urine is rapid. The more insoluble bismuth salts are only slightly absorbed and are excreted in the faeces which may be turned black by bismuth sulphide.

Pregnancy and lactation. Relatively insoluble bismuth compounds appeared to be concentrated in the placenta. Soluble compounds rapidly diffused across the placenta and were detectable in foetal blood.— H. E. Thompson *et al.*, *Am. J. Syph.*, 1941, *25*, 725.

Uses of Bismuth Salts. Bismuth and certain of its salts are active against treponemes. They were formerly given mainly by injection, alone or with other agents, in the treatment of syphilis but were superseded by antibiotic therapy.

Some insoluble salts of bismuth have been given by mouth for their protective and antacid action, for their mildly astringent action in diarrhoea, and for their supposed antiseptic effect; in general their value remains doubtful.

Certain insoluble salts of bismuth have been employed topically for their protective action on mucous membranes and raw surfaces and for their weakly astringent and supposed antiseptic properties, but there is little confirmation of their value.

Bismuth compounds are in general incompatible with iodides, the insoluble brown bismuth triiodide being formed.

Reviews of bismuth salts.— K. L. Stemmer, *Pharmac. Ther.*, 1976, *1*, 153; M. Wesolowski, *Arzneimittel-Forsch.*, 1978, *28*, 372.

5266-e

Precipitated Bismuth *(B.P.C. 1959).* Precip. Bism.
Bi=208.9804.

A dull grey powder consisting of finely divided metallic bismuth. Practically **insoluble** but readily diffusible in water; soluble in nitric acid. **Store** in completely filled airtight containers or in containers in which the air has been replaced by nitrogen.

Adverse Effects, Treatment, and Precautions. See Bismuth, above.

Uses. Precipitated bismuth was used, usually with other agents, in the treatment of syphilis and yaws. It has been given in doses of 100 to 200 mg, intramuscularly, as an aqueous suspension. When injected intramuscularly it is slowly absorbed, possibly as a protein compound.

5267-l

Bibrocathol. Bibrocathin; Bibrokatol; Bismuth Tetrabrompyrocatechinate; Tetrabromopyrocatechol Bismuth. 4,5,6,7-Tetrabromo-2-hydroxy-1,3,2-benzodioxabismole. $C_6HBiBr_4O_3$=649.7.

CAS — 6915-57-7.

Pharmacopoeias. In *Nord.*

A yellow, odourless, and almost tasteless powder. Practically **insoluble** in water, chloroform, and ether; slightly soluble in alcohol. **Incompatible** with ferric salts, oxidising agents, and strong acids and alkalis. **Store** in airtight containers. Protect from light.

Bibrocathol has been used as a 5% eye ointment in the treatment of blepharitis.

Proprietary Names

Noviform *(Dispersa, Ger.; Heyden, Ger.; Heyden, Swed.; Chauvin-Blache, Switz.).*

5268-y

Bismuth Aluminate.

$Bi_2(Al_2O_4)_3,10H_2O$=952.0.

CAS — 12284-76-3 (anhydrous).

A very light powder. Practically **insoluble** in water.

Adverse Effects, Treatment, and Precautions. As for Bismuth, p.927.

Uses. Bismuth aluminate has been used as an antacid.

References: P. R. Bateson, *J. Pharm. Pharmac.*, 1958, *10,* 123; S. G. F. Matts *et al.*, *Br. med. J.*, 1965, *1,* 753; J. A. Rider, *Curr. ther. Res.*, 1968, *10,* 109.

Proprietary Preparations

Bislumina *(MCP Pharmaceuticals, UK).* Suspension containing bismuth aluminate 750 mg in each 5 ml. For peptic ulcer and dyspepsia. *Dose.* 5 to 10 ml half an hour before meals thrice daily and at bedtime.

5269-j

Bismuth and Ammonium Citrate *(B.P.C. 1949).* Bism. et Ammon. Cit.; Bismuth-ammonium Citrate.

CAS — 25530-63-6.

Odourless, shining, semi-opaque scales or white powder with a metallic taste, containing the equivalent of 46 to 50% of Bi_2O_3.

Slowly **soluble** in water; slightly soluble in alcohol. **Store** in airtight containers. Protect from light.

Adverse Effects, Treatment, and Precautions. As for Bismuth, p.927; it is somewhat astringent and irritant.

Uses. Bismuth and ammonium citrate was formerly used as an antacid. It has been given in doses of 120 to 300 mg.

Proprietary Preparations of Related Compounds

De-Nol *(Brocades, UK).* Contains in each 5 ml tri-potassium di-citrato bismuthate equivalent to 120 mg of Bi_2O_3 in an ammonia-containing buffered solution. For gastric and duodenal ulcers. *Dose.* 5 ml diluted with 15 ml of water thrice daily half an hour before food and 2 hours after the last meal. (Also available as De-Nol in *Austral.*).

Reviews and evaluations of tri-potassium di-citrato bismuthate.— R. N. Brogden *et al.*, *Drugs*, 1976, *12,* 401. See also M. J. S. Langman, *Drugs*, 1977, *14,* 105; J. Poulantzas *et al.*, *Br. J. clin. Pract.*, 1978, *32,* 147.

Studies on the use of tri-potassium di-citrato bismuthate for gastric and duodenal ulcers.— P. R. Salmon, *Postgrad. med. J.*, 1975, *51 Suppl.* 5, 26; D. R. Shreeve, *ibid.*, 33; M. G. Moshal, *ibid.*, 36; B. E. Boyes *et al.*, *ibid.*, 29; G. P. Coughlin *et al.*, *Med. J. Aust.*, 1977, *1,* 294; S. P. Lee and G. I. Nicholson, *ibid.*, 808.

Other Proprietary Names of Related Compounds

Duosol *(tri-potassium di-citrato bismuthate) (Cooper, Switz.)*; Ulcerone *(tri-potassium di-citrato bismuthate) (De-Nol, S.Afr.).*

5270-q

Bismuth Hydroxide. Hydrated Bismuth Oxide; Bismuth Oxyhydrate; Hidróxido de Bismuto.

BiO_2H=242.0.

Pharmacopoeias. In *Span.*

A white, amorphous, odourless, tasteless powder containing the equivalent of about 96% of Bi_2O_3. Practically **insoluble** in water; soluble in acids and in a mixture of glycerol and sodium hydroxide solution. **Protect** from light.

Adverse Effects, Treatment, and Precautions. As for Bismuth, p.927.

Uses. Bismuth hydroxide has been used as an antacid. Intramuscular injections were formerly used in the treatment of syphilis.

The yellow, partly hydrated, bismuth oxide is also known as Bismuth Hydroxide.

Preparations

Milk of Bismuth *(U.S.P.).* Bismuth Cream; Bismuth Magma. A thick, odourless, almost tasteless, white, aqueous suspension which separates on standing and contains bismuth hydroxide and bismuth subcarbonate equivalent to 5.2 to 5.8% of Bi_2O_3. Store in airtight containers. Protect from freezing.

5271-p

Bismuth Oxide. Bismuth Trioxide.

Bi_2O_3=466.0.

CAS — 1304-76-3.

A dull yellow powder. Practically **insoluble** in water.

Adverse Effects, Treatment, and Precautions. As for Bismuth, p.927.

Uses. Bismuth oxide has been used in ointments for ano-rectal disorders.

Proprietary Preparations

Anugesic-HC Cream *(Warner, UK).* Contains bismuth oxide 0.875%, resorcinol 0.87%, Peru balsam 1.8%, zinc oxide 12.33%, benzyl benzoate 1.2%, pramoxine hydrochloride 1%, and hydrocortisone acetate 0.5%. For haemorrhoids and other ano-rectal disorders.

For Anugesic-HC Suppositories, see p.929.

Anusol Cream *(Warner, UK).* Contains bismuth oxide 2.14%, resorcinol 0.875%, Peru balsam 1.8%, benzyl benzoate 1.2%, and zinc oxide 10.75%, in a water-miscible basis. For haemorrhoids and other ano-rectal disorders. For other Anusol Preparations, see p.929.

5272-s

Bismuth Oxychloride *(B.P.C. 1963).* Bism. Oxychlor.; Bismuth Subchloride; Bismuthum Oxychloratum.

CAS — 7787-59-9.

A basic salt of varying composition, containing 80% of Bi and not less than 12.5% of Cl. It is an odourless, tasteless, white or nearly white, amorphous or minutely crystalline powder.

Practically **insoluble** in water; soluble in mineral acids. **Protect** from light.

Adverse Effects, Treatment, and Precautions. As for Bismuth, p.927.

Uses. Bismuth oxychloride was formerly injected intramuscularly as an aqueous suspension in doses of 100 to 200 mg in the treatment of syphilis and yaws. It has been given by mouth in a dose of 0.6 to 2 g for its supposed protective action on the mucous membranes and has been used as suppositories or ointment (5%) in the treatment of haemorrhoids. It has also been used as a pearling agent in tablets and cosmetics.

5273-w

Bismuth Oxyiodide. Bismuth Subiodide; Bismuthyl Iodide.

BiOI=351.9.

CAS — 7787-63-5.

A yellowish-red powder. Practically **insoluble** in water.

Adverse Effects, Treatment, and Precautions. As for Bismuth, p.927.

Uses. Bismuth oxyiodide has been used as a substitute for iodoform.

Preparations

EDP *(Evans Medical, UK).* Evans Dermal Powder. A dusting-powder containing bismuth oxyiodide 4.18%, thymol iodide 1.14%, chlorbutol 5.22%, and formalinised gelatin 3.98%, with magnesium borate, magnesium carbonate, magnesium stearate, and sterilised talc. For minor skin disorders.

5274-e

Bismuth Oxyiodogallate *(B.P.C. 1954).* Bismuth Oxyiodosubgallate; Bijogalum; Wismutoxyjodidgallat.

CAS — 138-58-9.

Pharmacopoeias. In *Nord.* and *Swiss.*

A bulky, greyish or greyish-green, odourless, tasteless powder, darkening on exposure to moist air. It contains about 40% of Bi and at least 20% of I. Practically **insoluble** in water, alcohol, chloroform, and ether; soluble with decomposition in solutions of alkali hydroxides and mineral acids. **Incompatible** with oxidising agents. **Store** in airtight containers. Protect from light.

Bismuth oxyiodogallate is not astringent or irritant when applied locally. It has been used for its supposed protective action as a dusting-powder or ointment and as suppositories for haemorrhoids.

5275-l

Bismuth Salicylate *(B.P. 1953).* Bismuthi Subsalicylas; Basic Bismuth Salicylate; Bismuth Oxysalicylate; Bismuth Subsalicylate; Basisches Wismutsalicylat.

CAS — 14882-18-9.

Pharmacopoeias. In *Arg., Aust., Belg., Hung., Int., It., Mex., Neth., Nord., Port., Roum., Span., Swiss,* and *Turk.*

A basic salt of varying composition, corresponding approximately to $C_6H_4(OH).CO_2(BiO)$ and containing about 58% of Bi. It is a white or nearly white, odourless, tasteless, microcrystalline powder.

Practically **insoluble** in water, alcohol, chloroform, ether, and glycerol. Sterile suspensions in oil are prepared aseptically with a suitable oil previously heated at 150° for 1 hour.

Incompatible with mineral acids and iron salts. It is partly dissociated in contact with water or alcohol and it is decomposed, with effervescence, by alkali bicarbonates. **Protect** from light.

Adverse Effects, Treatment, and Precautions. As for Bismuth, p.927, and Sodium Salicylate, p.279.

Uses. Bismuth salicylate has been given intramuscularly in the treatment of syphilis and yaws in weekly doses of 60 to 200 mg. It has been given by mouth in doses of 0.6 to 2 g; following oral administration it is converted to bismuth carbonate and sodium salicylate in the small intestine before excretion in the faeces. See also Uses of Bismuth Salts, p.927.

Proprietary Names

Spiromak *(Valeas, Ital.)*; Vismut *(DAK, Denm.).*

5276-y

Bismuth Sodium Tartrate *(B.P.C. 1963).* Bism. Sod. Tart.; Sodium Bismuthyltartrate; Sodium Tartrobismuthate; Bismuthi Natrii Tartras.

CAS — 31586-77-3.

NOTE. This is the neutral compound; it must be distinguished from Acid Bismuth Sodium Tartrate (*B.P.C. 1949*) which was described in the *B.P.C. 1934* as Bismuth Sodium Tartrate.

Pharmacopoeias. In *Ind.*

A white powder or yellowish scales, odourless or with a very faint odour of burnt sugar. It contains 35 to 42% of Bi. **Soluble** 1 in less than 1 of water; practically insoluble in alcohol, chloroform, and ether. A 10% solution in water has a pH of 5.4 to 7. A 8.91% solution is iso-osmotic with serum. Solutions in water are **sterilised** by autoclaving or by filtration. Sterile suspensions in oil are prepared aseptically with a suitable oil previously maintained at 150° for 1 hour. **Protect** from light.

Adverse Effects, Treatment, and Precautions. As for Bismuth, p.927.

Uses. Bismuth sodium tartrate has been given intramuscularly in the treatment of syphilis and yaws in doses of 60 to 200 mg. See also Uses of Bismuth Salts, p.927. The injections exert a diuretic effect.

5277-j

Acid Bismuth Sodium Tartrate *(B.P.C. 1949).* Soluble Bismuth Tartrate.

NOTE. This substance was described in the *B.P.C. 1934* as Bismuth Sodium Tartrate. It is the acid compound and is unsuitable for injection. It must be distinguished from Bismuth Sodium Tartrate *B.P.C. 1963.*

A white odourless powder or scales with an acid astringent taste. It contains 38 to 44% of Bi and consists of a mixture of bismuth and sodium tartrates with an excess of tartaric acid. Slowly **soluble** in water, giving a strongly acid solution. **Protect** from light.

Adverse Effects, Treatment, and Precautions. As for Bismuth, p.927.

Uses. Acid bismuth sodium tartrate was formerly employed, usually in conjunction with pepsin, for digestive disorders. It has been given in doses of 120 to 300 mg.

5278-z

Bismuth Sodium Triglycollamate. A double salt of bismuthyl sodium triglycollamate, $C_6H_7BiNNaO_7$ and disodium triglycollamate, $C_6H_7NNa_2O_6$ (1:3).
$C_{24}H_{28}BiN_4Na_7O_{25}$=1142.4.

CAS — 5798-43-6.

A white crystalline odourless powder with a somewhat salty taste containing about 18% of Bi. Very **soluble** in water; practically insoluble in alcohol, acetone, and ether. A 2% solution in water has a pH of 7 to 8.

Adverse Effects, Treatment, and Precautions. As for Bismuth, p.927. There have been several reports of renal failure in patients taking bismuth sodium triglycollamate.

Uses. Bismuth sodium triglycollamate has been used by mouth in the treatment of syphilis. See also Uses of Bismuth Salts, p.927. It has been given in doses of 400 to 800 mg thrice daily.

5279-c

Bismuth Subcarbonate *(B.P., Eur. P.).* Bismuth Carbonate; Bism. Carb.; Bismuthi Subcarbonas; Bismutylum Carbonicum; Basic Bismuth Carbonate; Bismuth Oxycarbonate; Basisches Wismutkarbonat; Carbonato de Bismutila.

CAS — 5892-10-4 (anhydrous); 5798-45-8 (hemihydrate).

Pharmacopoeias. In *Arg., Aust., Belg., Br., Chin., Cz., Eur., Fr., Ger., Ind., Int., Jug., Mex., Neth., Nord., Pol., Port., Roum., Span., Swiss,* and *Turk.*

A basic salt of varying composition, approximating to $(BiO)_2CO_3,\frac{1}{2}H_2O$. It contains the equivalent of 80 to 82.5% of Bi.
It is a white or creamy-white, odourless, tasteless powder. The bulk density varies considerably; the light varieties need no suspending agent. If a suspending agent is required, acacia should not be used; tragacanth is suitable.
Practically **insoluble** in water, alcohol, ether, and neutral organic solvents; completely soluble in mineral acids with effervescence. **Protect** from light.

Adverse Effects, Treatment, and Precautions. As for Bismuth, p.927.

Uses. Bismuth subcarbonate has been given as an antacid in doses of 0.6 to 2 g. It has also been applied topically in mild skin conditions.

Preparations

Compound Bismuth Lozenges *(B.P.).* Trochisci Bismuthi Compositi. Each contains bismuth subcarbonate 150 mg, calcium carbonate 300 mg, heavy magnesium carbonate 150 mg, rose oil, of commerce, 0.00006 ml, in a basis of acacia and sucrose. Protect from light.

Bismuth Carbonate Paste *(Roy. Nat. T. N. and E. Hosp.).* Bismuth subcarbonate 25% and liquid paraffin 75%. To prepare **Bismuth Carbonate Rolls** the paste is evenly spread on to ribbon gauze strips which are then rolled, packed in plastic containers, and sterilised by irradiation.

Compound Bismuth Oral Powder *(B.P.).* Compound Bismuth Powder; Pulv. Bism. Co. Bismuth subcarbonate 1, calcium carbonate 3, heavy magnesium carbonate 3, and sodium bicarbonate 1.

Proprietary Names
Bismicron *(Cochard, Belg.).*

Bismuth subcarbonate was formerly marketed in Great Britain under the proprietary name Lac Bismuth *(Philip Harris).*

5280-s

Bismuth Subgallate *(B.P.).* Bism. Subgall.; Bismuth Oxygallate; Basic Bismuth Gallate; Dermatol; Basisches Wismutgallat.

CAS — 99-26-3.

Pharmacopoeias. In *Arg., Aust., Belg., Br., Ger., Hung., Ind., It., Jap., Jug., Neth., Pol., Port., Roum., Rus., Span., Swiss,* and *Turk.*

A citron-yellow odourless or almost odourless tasteless powder containing, when dried, 46 to 52% of Bi; it loses not more than 7% of its weight when dried.
Practically **insoluble** in water, dehydrated alcohol, and ether; freely soluble in hot mineral acids with decomposition and in solutions of alkali hydroxides forming clear yellow solutions which rapidly become dark red. **Incompatible** with alkaline sulphur compounds and iron salts. **Store** in airtight containers. Protect from light.

Adverse Effects, Treatment, and Precautions. As for Bismuth, p.927.

Uses. Bismuth subgallate has been employed as a dusting-powder in some skin disorders, and as suppositories in the treatment of haemorrhoids. It was formerly given for its supposed astringent properties in the treatment of diarrhoea, dysentery, and ulcerative colitis, in doses of 0.6 to 2 g. It has been administered by mouth to help control the odour and consistency of stool in patients with a colostomy or ileostomy. See also Uses of Bismuth Salts, p.927.

Preparations

Bismuth Subgallate Suppositories *(B.P.).* Supp. Bism. Subgall. Suppositories containing bismuth subgallate in theobroma oil or other suitable fatty basis. About 3 g of bismuth subgallate displaces 1 g of theobroma oil. Store at a temperature not exceeding 20°.

Compound Bismuth Subgallate Suppositories *(B.P.).* Co. Bismuth Subgallate Suppos.; Bismuth Subgallate Compound Suppositories; Supp. Bism. Subgall. Co.; Compound Bismuth and Resorcin Suppositories. Each contains bismuth subgallate 200 mg, castor oil 60 mg, resorcinol 60 mg, zinc oxide 120 mg, in a suitable fatty basis such as theobroma oil sufficient to fill a 1-g mould. About 1 g of theobroma oil is displaced by bismuth subgallate 3 g, castor oil 1 g, resorcinol 1.5 g, or zinc oxide 5 g. Store at a temperature not exceeding 20°.
A.P.F. describes a similar preparation; it contains Peru balsam 60 mg but no castor oil.

Proprietary Preparations

Anugesic-HC Suppositories *(Warner, UK).* Each contains bismuth subgallate 59 mg, bismuth oxide 24 mg, Peru balsam 49 mg, zinc oxide 296 mg, benzyl benzoate 33 mg, pramoxine hydrochloride 27 mg, and hydrocortisone acetate 5 mg. For haemorrhoids and other ano-rectal disorders. *Dose.* 1 suppository night and morning. For Anugesic-HC Cream, see p.928..

Anusol *(Warner, UK).* **Ointment** containing bismuth subgallate 2.25%, bismuth oxide 0.87%, Peru balsam 1.87%, and zinc oxide 10.75%. **Suppositories** each containing bismuth subgallate 59 mg, bismuth oxide 24 mg, Peru balsam 49 mg, and zinc oxide 296 mg. For haemorrhoids and other ano-rectal disorders. *Dose.* 1 suppository night and morning. For Anusol Cream, see p.928.

Anusol-HC *(Warner, UK).* **Ointment** containing the same ingredients as Anusol Ointment with hydrocortisone acetate 0.25%, benzyl benzoate 1.25%, and resorcinol 0.87%. **Suppositories** each containing the same ingredients as Anusol Suppositories with hydrocortisone acetate 10 mg, benzyl benzoate 33 mg, and resorcinol 24 mg. For haemorrhoids and other ano-rectal disorders. *Dose.* 1 suppository night and morning.

Bismodyne *(Loveridge, UK: Typharm, UK).* **Ointment** containing bismuth subgallate 2%, hexachlorophane 0.5%, lignocaine 0.5%, and zinc oxide 7.5%. **Suppositories** each containing bismuth subgallate 150 mg, hexachlorophane 2.5 mg, lignocaine 10 mg, and zinc oxide 120 mg. For haemorrhoids. *Dose.* 1 suppository night and morning.

Other Proprietary Names
Dermatol *(Ger., Neth.).*

Preparations containing bismuth subgallate were also formerly marketed in Great Britain under the proprietary names Anorm *(Norma)* and BFI *(Merck Sharp & Dohme).*

5281-w

Bismuth Subnitrate *(B.P.C. 1973).* Bism. Subnit.; Bismuthi Subnitras; Basic Bismuth Nitrate; Bismuth Oxynitrate; Bismuthyl Nitrate; Magistery of Bismuth; White Bismuth; Bismuth (Nitrate Basique de) Lourd; Basisches Wismutnitrat; Nitrato de Bismutilo; Subazotato de Bismuto.

CAS — 1304-85-4.

Pharmacopoeias. In *Arg., Aust., Cz., Fr., Ger., Hung., Int., It., Jap., Jug., Mex., Pol., Port., Roum., Rus., Span., Swiss, Turk.,* and *U.S. Fr.* also includes Bismuth (Nitrate Basique de) Léger (Bismuthi Subnitras Levis) which is described as a variable mixture of bismuth hydroxide, carbonate, and subnitrate, containing 73.5 to 80% of Bi.

A white, odourless or almost odourless, tasteless, micro-crystalline powder, approximating to the formula $6Bi_2O_3,5N_2O_5,9H_2O$, and containing 71 to 75% of Bi. *U.S.P.* includes Bismuth Subnitrate, a basic salt which contains the equivalent of not less than 79% of Bi_2O_3 calculated in the dried basis.
Practically **insoluble** in water, alcohol, and most organic solvents; readily soluble in dilute nitric and hydrochloric acids. A suspension in water is slightly acid to litmus.
Incompatible with carbonates and bicarbonates, iodides, tannin, and sulphur. If a mixture containing bismuth subnitrate and a carbonate or bicarbonate is prescribed, the two reacting salts should be rubbed together with warm water until the effervescence subsides before the mixture is completed. The addition of a gum as a suspending agent should be avoided because gummy substances cause the insoluble salt to cohere and form indiffusible masses. **Protect** from light.

Adverse Effects, Treatment, and Precautions. As for Bismuth, p.927.
Bismuth subnitrate may be reduced by intestinal bacteria to nitrite thereby causing methaemoglobinaemia and symptoms of nitrite poisoning. If methaemoglobinaemia occurs it should be treated with methylene blue (see p.385).

Absorption and Fate. Absorption of bismuth has occurred after administration of bismuth subnitrate by mouth or in body cavities or fistulas. The nitrate may be reduced by intestinal bacteria to nitrite, thereby causing methaemoglobinaemia.

Uses. Bismuth subnitrate is more astringent than other bismuth salts. It has been used in the form of Bismuth Subnitrate and Iodoform Paste (BIPP) as a wound dressing (see Iodoform p.865); the paste may give rise to iodoform poisoning.
Internally, bismuth subnitrate was formerly used as an antacid.
It has been given in doses of 0.3 to 1.2 g.

Preparations

Compound Bismuth Subnitrate Cream *(Middlesex Hosp.).* Paremanol. Bismuth subnitrate 1, arachis oil 3, hydrous wool fat 3, and yellow soft paraffin 3. Shelf-life 1 year. For the treatment of radiotherapy burns.
A similar preparation known as Paramenol Ointment is manufactured at *Bristol Roy. Infirm.*

Bismuth Subnitrate and Iodoform Paste. BIPP. See under Iodoform, p.865.

Proprietary Preparations

Roter Tablets *(Roterpharma, UK: Squibb, UK).* Each contains bismuth subnitrate 300 mg, light magnesium carbonate 400 mg, sodium bicarbonate 200 mg, and frangula bark 25 mg. For peptic ulcer. *Dose.* 2 tablets thrice daily after meals. NOTE. The name Roter is also applied to a preparation of ephedrine.

References: R. Sezer *et al.*, *Br. J. clin. Pract.*, 1975, *29*, 227.

Stomachic Dellipsoids D20 *(Pilsworth, UK)*. Coated elliptical tablets each containing bismuth subnitrate 200 mg, magnesium hydroxide 250 mg, and belladonna dry extract 20 mg. For hyperacidity and peptic ulcer. *Dose.* 1 tablet 3 or 4 times daily before meals.

Other Proprietary Names
Bismufilm, Bismuth Tulasne pur *(both Switz.)*.

A preparation containing bismuth subnitrate was also formerly marketed in Great Britain under the proprietary name Frangula Compound Tablets, Woolley (*Vestric*).

5282-e

Bismuth Tribromphenate *(B.P.C. 1949)*. Bromphenol Bismuth; Bismutum Tribromophenylicum; Brompheno-bis; Xeroformium. Bismuth derivative of 2,4,6-tri-bromophenol.
$C_{12}H_5Bi_3Br_6O_6$=1351.5.

Pharmacopoeias. In *Aust.*, *Jug.*, *Port.*, *Rus.*, *Span.*, and *Swiss.*

A yellow, almost odourless, tasteless neutral powder containing about 50% of Bi. Practically **insoluble** in water, alcohol, chloroform, and ether. It is decomposed by acids and alkalis. **Protect** from light.

Adverse Effects, Treatment, and Precautions. As for Bismuth, p.927.

Uses. Bismuth tribromphenate has been claimed to have antiseptic and analgesic properties and has been used as a substitute for iodoform as a dusting-powder or dressing. It was formerly given by mouth in the treatment of gastro-intestinal disorders in doses of 0.3 to 1 g.

A technique of burn management using bismuth tribromphenate ointment.— A. Anastassiadis (letter), *Lancet*, 1973, *2*, 45.

Antimycotic action. Bismuth tribromphenate was found to inhibit the growth *in vitro* of dermatophytes at concentrations between 1 in 20 000 and 1 in 100 000 and of yeasts at concentrations between 1 in 2000 and 1 in 10 000.— K. Ito and H. Reith, *Bull. pharm. Res. Inst., Takatsuki*, 1961, May, No. 32,, per *Bull. Hyg., Lond.*, 1963, *38*, 296.

Proprietary Names
Xeroform *(Heyden, Ger.)*.

5283-l

Quinine Iodobismuthate *(B.P.C. 1949)*. Bismuth Quinine Iodide; Yodobismutato de Quinina.

CAS — 8048-94-0.

Pharmacopoeias. In *Arg.*, *Belg.*, *Mex.*, *Port.*, and *Span.*

A double salt of bismuth iodide and quinine hydriodide containing about 23% of Bi, 57% of I, and 18% of quinine. It is a fine red odourless powder.
Practically **insoluble** in water, fixed oils, and most organic solvents. Sterile suspensions in oil are prepared aseptically with a suitable oil previously maintained at 150° for 1 hour. It decomposes slowly when moist. **Protect** from light.

Adverse Effects, Treatment, and Precautions. As for Bismuth, p.927.

Uses. Quinine iodobismuthate has been injected intramuscularly or subcutaneously in the treatment of syphilis and yaws in doses of 100 to 300 mg. See also Uses of Bismuth Salts, p.927.

Proprietary Names
Bijogadol III *(Neopharmed, Ital.)*.

5284-y

Copper.

Cu=63.546.

CAS — 7440-50-8.

A reddish-coloured metal with a bright lustre; it is malleable and ductile.

Copper is a constituent of all animal tissues. The total body content in adults is about 100 to 150 mg with the highest concentrations in the brain, kidneys, heart, liver, and pancreas; over 90% of copper in the plasma is associated with the alpha-2-globulin, caeruloplasmin. Copper is essential for the metabolism of iron in the synthesis of haemoglobin and is a component of several enzymes.

Adverse Effects. Chronic copper poisoning in man has not been identified with certainty; raised tissue concentrations of copper are associated with tissue injury in hepatolenticular degeneration (Wilson's disease).

Metal fume fever with nausea, dyspnoea, and chest pain follows inhalation of copper-containing dusts; the extent to which this is an effect of copper is uncertain. For details of the acute toxicity of soluble copper salts see under Copper Sulphate (below).

Maximum permissible atmospheric concentration: copper dusts and mists 1 mg per m^3; copper fume 200 µg per m^3.

Maximum daily load of copper as copper sulphate: up to 500 µg per kg body-weight.— Fourteenth Report of the Joint FAO/WHO Expert Committee on Food Additives, *Tech. Rep. Ser. Wld Hlth Org. No. 462*, 1971. Estimated maximum daily body load of copper from all sources: up to 500 µg per kg body-weight.— Seventeenth Report of the Joint FAO/WHO Expert Committee on Food Additives, *Tech. Rep. Ser. Wld Hlth Org. No. 539*, 1974. For background toxicological information, see *Fd Add. Ser. Wld Hlth Org. No. 5*, 1974.

Allergy. Reports of dermatitis associated with copper allergy.— C. H. Paine (letter), *Lancet*, 1968, *2*, 520 (water pipes); E. I. Saltzer and J. W. Wilson, *Archs Derm.*, 1968, *98*, 375 (jewellery); V. P. Barranco, *Archs Derm.*, 1972, *106*, 386 (intra-uterine contraceptive device); G. G. Dhir *et al.*, *Ann. Allergy*, 1977, *39*, 204 (alcohol colorant).

Culinary utensils. Reports of acute copper poisoning resulting from use of copper utensils.— *Morb. Mortal.*, 1974, *23*, 407, per *Abstr. Hyg.*, 1975, *50*, 112; *Morb. Mortal.*, 1975, *24*, 99, per *Abstr. Hyg.*, 1975, *50*, 484.

Dialysis. For a discussion of haemolysis and other toxic effects of copper arising during haemodialysis through the use of tap water with a high copper content for the preparation of dialysis solutions, see W. H. Lyle (letter), *New Engl. J. Med.*, 1967, *276*, 1209.

Further references to copper toxicity and dialysis: W. J. Klein *et al.*, *Archs intern. Med.*, 1972, *129*, 578; W. H. Lyle *et al.*, *Lancet*, 1976, *1*, 1324.

See also under Water, p.1669.

Green hair. A report of 2 children who developed green hair. Copper absorbed from swimming pools was considered to be responsible, the source being either copper piping or a copper-containing algicide.— R. M. Lampe *et al.*, *J. Am. med. Ass.*, 1977, *237*, 2092.

Treatment of Adverse Effects. Excess copper may be removed by chelating agents such as penicillamine (see p.387); sodium calciumedetate (see p.391) has also been suggested.

Precautions. Copper should not be used in patients with hepatolenticular degeneration (Wilson's disease).

The biological half-life of copper was about 26 days in normal persons and about 131 days in homozygote patients and 59 days in heterozygote patients with Wilson's disease.— S. O'Reilly *et al.*, *J. nucl. Med.*, 1969, *10*, 143, per *J. Am. med. Ass.*, 1969, *208*, 389.

Absorption and Fate. Copper is absorbed from the gastro-intestinal tract; bile is a major route of excretion. Sulphides and soluble phytates may affect absorption of copper.

For a comprehensive review of copper deficiency, metabolism, human requirements, and toxicity, see Report of a WHO Expert Group on Trace Elements in Human Nutrition, *Tech. Rep. Ser. Wld Hlth Org. No. 532*, 1973, 15. See also F. W. Alexander, *Archs Dis. Childh.*, 1974, *49*, 589 (metabolism in children).

Uses. Copper has a contraceptive effect when present in the uterus. It is added to some intra-uterine contraceptive devices permitting reduction in their size with concomitant reduction in the associated side-effects such as pain and bleeding; owing to their smaller size copper-containing intra-uterine contraceptive devices are used in nulliparous women.

Copper supplements (usually administered in the form of the sulphate) are occasionally required in malnourished infants or in patients receiving total parenteral nutrition.

Copper bracelets are worn as a folk remedy for rheumatic disorders; there is no good evidence to justify such a practice.

Copper (Cuprum Metallicum; Cuprum Met.) is used in homoeopathic medicine.

A review of the actions of copper as a trace element covering the effects of deficiency and excess, its pharmacokinetics and briefly its toxicity.— R. E. Burch *et al.*, *Clin. Chem.*, 1975, *21*, 501.

Contraception. A detailed review of the copper intra-uterine device. Addition of copper to the intra-uterine device permitted the use of a small device with consequent reduction in the frequency of pain, bleeding, and expulsion. Such a device could also be used in nulliparous women. Copper absorption was negligible but uterine perforation usually called for removal of copper devices since inflammation and adhesions might form around the metal. The device might act by inhibiting implantation, possibly as a result of sterile inflammation. *Animal* studies by S.K. Saksena and M.J.K. Harper (*Fert. Steril.*, 1974, *25*, 121) had demonstrated some loss of contraceptive action on administration of the anti-inflammatory agent, indomethacin.— G. Oster and M. P. Salgo, *New Engl. J. Med.*, 1975, *293*, 432.

Other reviews and studies.— *Drug & Ther. Bull.*, 1973, *11*, 65; J. Newton *et al.*, *Br. med. J.*, 1974, *3*, 447; *ibid.*, 1974, *4*, 181; W. A. Nebel *et al.*, *Am. J. Obstet. Gynec.*, 1976, *126*, 586; J. Kemp, *Med. J. Aust.*, 1976, *2*, 295; B. W. Simcock, *ibid.*, 297; *Lancet*, 1977, *1*, 1239; *Med. Lett.*, 1980, *22*, 86.

Calcification and corrosion. For studies and reports on incrustation of intra-uterine copper devices, some associating this with a higher pregnancy-rate after 2 years, and others refuting this finding and suggesting that the elution of copper remained adequate for considerably longer, see J. Newton *et al.*, *Br. med. J.*, 1977, *1*, 197; C. Gosden *et al.*, *ibid.*, 202; E. Chantler *et al.*, *ibid.*, *2*, 288; I. Sivin (letter), *ibid.*, 387; J. Guillebaud (letter), *ibid.*, 705; M. Cohen, *Searle* (letter), *ibid.*, 1087; J. F. Miller and M. Elstein (letter), *ibid.*, 1289; R. D. Archer *et al.* (letter), *Lancet*, 1977, *2*, 458; R. H. Davis (letter), *ibid.*, 762; K. M. Lewis *et al.*, *Contraception*, 1977, *15*, 93, per *Int. pharm. Abstr.*, 1977, *14*, 1046.

Diabetes. A study in 11 diabetic women which indicated that the presence of a copper intra-uterine device did not significantly increase the fibrinolytic activity of the endometrium, might explain the reportedly less reliable contraceptive effect of copper intra-uterine devices in diabetic women.— B. Larsson *et al.*, *Contraception*, 1977, *15*, 711, per *Int. pharm. Abstr.*, 1977, *14*, 1196.

Infection. A study in 296 women with copper intra-uterine devices compared with 632 non-users, revealed no association between the device and an increased frequency of pelvic inflammatory disease. Removal offered no advantage to women receiving chemotherapy for pelvic inflammatory disease.— B. Larsson and M. Wennergren, *Contraception*, 1977, *15*, 143, per *Int. pharm. Abstr.*, 1977, *14*, 1031.

A review of the risk of pelvic infection associated with intra-uterine contraceptive devices.— *Br. med. J.*, 1976, *2*, 717. Comment.— M. S. Buckingham *et al.* (letter), *ibid.*, 942. Conflicting reports on the inhibition of gonococci by copper.— B. Fiscina *et al.*, *Am. J. Obstet. Gynec.*, 1973, *116*, 86; W. N. Spellacy *et al.*, *Fert. Steril.*, 1974, *25*, 772; L. Cohen and G. Thomas, *Br. J. vener. Dis.*, 1974, *50*, 364.

Deficiency. Trace elements, including details of copper requirements and the manifestations of deficiency have been reviewed by D.D. Ulmer (*New Engl. J. Med.*, 1977, *297*, 318). Although acquired copper deficiency is exceedingly rare it was observed in a premature infant by R.A. Al-Rashid and J. Spangler (*New Engl. J. Med.*, 1971, *285*, 841), and in 61 of 173 severely malnourished infants by G.C. Graham and A. Cordano (*Johns Hopkins med. J.*, 1969, *124*, 139). Copper deficiency in 2 patients receiving long-term parenteral nutrition was reported by W.M. Dunlap *et al.* (*Ann. intern. Med.*, 1974, *80*, 470) and subsequently in another patient by R.W. Vilter *et al.* (*New Engl. J. Med.*, 1974, *291*, 188). W.M. Dunlap *et al.* estimated that copper supplements should be given by mouth or parenterally in an initial dose of 1.25 mg elemental copper (about 5 mg copper sulphate) daily followed by a maintenance dose of 0.4 mg elemental copper (1.6 mg copper sulphate) daily. In premature infants receiving long-term intravenous feeding B.E. James and R.A. MacMahon (*Aust. paediatr. J.*, 1976, *12*, 154) have reported copper requirements to be 50 μg of copper per kg body-weight daily. A minimum daily intake of 80 μg of copper per kg body-weight has been suggested (*Wld Hlth Org. Tech. Rep. Ser. No. 532*, 1973); this would provide an acceptable margin of safety against copper deficiency in infants and young children whereas 50 μg per kg might not. Older children would be adequately protected by a daily intake of 40 μg per kg and adult males by 30 μg per kg. Attempts made to counter genetic copper deficiency (Menkes' kinky-hair syndrome) by intravenous and subcutaneous infusion of copper as the sulphate or the acetate (A.S. Dekaban and J.K. Steusing *Lancet*, 1974, *2*, 1523; A.D. Garnica and S.R. Fletcher, *ibid.*, 1975, *2*, 659; H. Wehinger *et al. ibid.*, 1975, *1*, 1143) have been disappointing but a more encouraging initial result was reported by W.D. Grover and M.C. Scrutton (*J. Pediat.*, 1975, *86*, 216).

A review of studies of human copper deficiency.— G. G. Graham and A. Cordano, Copper Deficiency in Human Subjects, *Trace Elements in Human Health and Disease*, Vol. 1, A.S. Prasad and D. Oberleas (Ed.), London, Academic Press, 1976, p. 363.

Other references: M. S. Lawson *et al.*, *Archs Dis. Childh.*, 1977, *52*, 62; A. S. Prasad, *Trace Elements and Iron in Human Metabolism*, Chichester, John Wiley, 1978.

Parenteral nutrition. For reference to findings of low concentrations of copper in parenteral solutions, see Zinc, p.945.

Pregnancy and the neonate. The incidence of developmental defects was not increased in the infants of 157 women who elected to remain pregnant after conceiving with a copper intra-uterine device in place, and who retained the device throughout pregnancy. Compared with 118 similar women whose devices were expelled or extracted the incidence of spontaneous abortion was almost doubled and the prematurity-rates were quadrupled.— H. J. Tatum *et al.*, *Am. J. Obstet. Gynec.*, 1976, *126*, 869.

Rheumatism. Complexes of copper with salicylates appeared to have an enhanced anti-arthritic action in *animals*.— J. R. J. Sorenson (letter), *J. Pharm. Pharmac.*, 1977, *29*, 450.

5285-j

Copper Sulphate *(B.P. Vet., B.P.C. 1973).*

Copper Sulph.; Cupri Sulphas; Cupr. Sulph.; Cupric Sulfate *(U.S.P.)*; Cuivre (Sulfate de); Kupfersulfat; Sulfato de Cobre. Copper (II) sulphate pentahydrate.

$CuSO_4,5H_2O=249.7$.

CAS — 7758-98-7 (anhydrous); 7758-99-8 (pentahydrate).

Crude copper sulphate is sometimes known as 'blue copperas', 'blue stone', and 'blue vitriol'.

Pharmacopoeias. In *Arg., Aust., Belg., Fr., Hung., Ind., Jap., Jug., Mex., Nord., Pol., Port., Rus., Span., Swiss,* and *U.S.*

Blue crystals or crystalline odourless or almost odourless powder with an astringent taste. It slowly effloresces in air. The exsiccated salt is nearly white.

Soluble 1 in 3 of water, 1 in 0.5 of boiling water, and 1 in 500 of alcohol; soluble 1 in 3 of glycerol. A 5% solution in water has a pH of 3.8. A 6.85% solution is iso-osmotic with serum. Solutions are **sterilised** by autoclaving or by filtration. **Incompatible** with alkalis and phosphates. **Store** in airtight containers.

Incompatibility. Copper sulphate solutions were incompatible with betanaphthol, propylene glycol, sulphathiazole, and triethanolamine, owing to the formation of chelates; the pH usually needed to be above 7 for the reaction to proceed.— G. B. Engel, *Pharm. J. N.Z.*, 1958, *20*, No. 3, 19.

Copper sulphate 2% was incompatible with phenylmercuric nitrate 0.004% and benzalkonium chloride 0.02% when heated at 98° to 100° for 30 minutes.— M. Williamson, *Australas. J. Pharm.*, 1957, *38*, 240.

Benzalkonium chloride 0.01% or phenylmercuric borate 0.005% were suitable preservatives for copper sulphate eye-drops sterilised by filtration.— M. Van Ooteghem, *Pharm. Tijdschr. Belg.*, 1968, *45*, 69.

Adverse Effects. The ingestion of a large quantity of copper sulphate is rapidly followed by nausea and vomiting, a metallic taste, and a burning sensation in the oesophagus and stomach. Colic and bloody diarrhoea may follow, with convulsions, hypotension and coma. Renal damage may occur with acute kidney necrosis; jaundice may be associated with liver injury and haemolysis.

Owing to its emetic action, fatal poisoning is rare, but death may occur after as little as 1 g.

Acute poisoning. A report of 11 patients who had ingested an estimated 1 to 50 g of copper sulphate; they suffered nausea and vomiting, with epigastric pain in 5, diarrhoea in 5, hypotension in 2, haematemesis or melaena in 10, pallor in 10, jaundice in 8, delirium in 3, and coma in 2. All had intravascular haemolysis and 10 developed oliguria or anuria. Five patients died despite gastric lavage, intravenous fluids, mannitol, diuretics, and dialysis.— K. S. Chugh *et al.*, *Postgrad. med. J.*, 1977, *53*, 18.

Further references: H. K. Chuttani *et al.*, *Am. J. Med.*, 1965, *39*, 849; K. S. Chugh *et al.*, *Ann. intern. Med.*, 1975, *82*, 226.

Following emetic use. A 44-year-old woman given 10 ml of a 10% copper sulphate solution as an emetic failed to vomit and gastric lavage was performed. Her condition deteriorated and she died 6 days later with respiratory, renal, and hepatic failure, haemolytic anaemia, and gastro-intestinal haemorrhage. A three-quarter gastrectomy performed 3 years earlier might have contributed to increased absorption of copper sulphate.— R. S. Stein *et al.* (letter), *J. Am. med. Ass.*, 1976, *235*, 801.

Following topical application. The application of copper sulphate crystals to granulations of burns on 7 occasions during 9 weeks induced jaundice, haemolytic anaemia, and oliguria in a 5½-year-old girl.— N. A. Holtzman *et al.*, *New Engl. J. Med.*, 1966, *275*, 347.

Lung damage. Pathological lung changes in vineyard workers using copper sulphate sprays included blue spots on the surface of the lung, histiocytes and granulomas in the septa, fibro-hyaline nodules, and desquamated macrophages. All lesions contained particles of copper. In chronic conditions there were massive opacities in the lungs or respiratory insufficiency due to progressive diffuse fibrosis.— T. G. Villar *et al.*, *Lyon méd.*, 1974, *10*, 605, per *Practitioner*, 1974, *213*, 281. See also J. C. Pimentel and A. P. Menezes, *Am. Rev. resp. Dis.*, 1975, *111*, 189.

Treatment of Adverse Effects. The stomach should be emptied by aspiration and lavage, and demulcents such as milk, or white of egg, should be given freely. Morphine or pethidine may be given to relieve pain, and fluid and electrolyte balance should be corrected. Chelating agents such as penicillamine (see p.387) or sodium calciumedetate (see p.391) should be given.

Recovery of an 18-month-old boy after taking a solution containing about 3 g of copper sulphate. He was treated with lavage, dimercaprol injection, and edetic acid; he subsequently received penicillamine 250 mg daily for a month.— F. M. Walsh *et al.*, *Am. J. Dis. Child.*, 1977, *131*, 149.

Dialysis. Peritoneal dialysis appeared to be effective in the treatment of copper sulphate poisoning accompanied by haemolytic anaemia and renal failure in a 2-year-old boy.— D. E. C. Cole (letter), *Br. med. J.*, 1978, *1*, 50.

Precautions. As for Copper (above).

Uses. Copper sulphate and other soluble salts of copper have an astringent action on mucous surfaces and in strong solutions they are corrosive.

A 0.1% solution of copper sulphate has been used for gastric lavage in phosphorus poisoning; it must be removed promptly to avoid copper poisoning. Topical application of a 1% solution is of value for phosphorus burns of the skin.

Traces of copper sulphate have sometimes been administered in conjunction with iron in the treatment of microcytic anaemias but do not significantly enhance the absorption or utilisation of iron. Copper deficiency in subjects receiving total parenteral nutrition has been treated with copper sulphate in initial doses of 5 mg daily (equivalent to about 1.25 mg of elemental copper) and subsequent maintenance doses of 1.6 mg (equivalent to 0.4 mg of elemental copper).

Copper and Zinc Sulphates Lotion has been used as a wet dressing in eczema, impetigo, and intertrigo. Solutions of 0.25 to 0.5% of copper sulphate have been employed locally as astringents in eye infections. Crystals of copper sulphate are occasionally applied as a caustic to excessive granulation in burns or ulcers.

Copper sulphate is used in a concentration of 0.5 to 1 ppm to prevent the growth of algae in reservoirs, ponds, and swimming pools; 5 ppm will kill the fresh-water snails that act as intermediate hosts in the life-cycle of the parasites causing schistosomiasis and fascioliasis.

Reagents containing copper sulphate are used in tests for reducing sugars.

Deficiency. For reference to the administration of copper sulphate in copper-deficiency states, see under Copper (above).

Emesis in acute poisoning. Copper sulphate had no valid place as an emetic, because of the dangers of toxicity.— *Br. med. J.*, 1977, *2*, 977.

Herpes simplex keratitis. Copper sulphate iontophoresis (0.125% solution at 1 mA for 2 minutes) was used to treat 20 eyes of patients with either dendritic (epithelial and stromal) or disciform keratitis.— S. I. Brown *et al.*, *Archs Ophthal., N.Y.*, 1962, *67*, 453, per *J. Am. med. Ass.*, 1962, *180* (Apr. 28), A173.

Impetigo. For the use of copper and zinc sulphates lotion in the treatment of impetigo, see H. C. W. Stringer, *Drugs*, 1973, *6*, 413.

Molluscicidal action. A review of the use and toxicity of copper compounds as molluscicides.— T. C. Cheng and J. T. Sullivan, in *Molluscicides in Schistosomiasis Control*, T.C. Cheng (Ed.), London, Academic Press, 1974, p. 89. See also E. Paulini, *ibid.*, p. 155; E. A. Malek, *ibid.*, p. 171.

Other references: K. Y. Chu *et al.*, *Bull. Wld Hlth Org.* 1968, *39*, 320; L. S. Ritchie and L. A. Berríos-Durán, *ibid.*, 1969, *40*, 471.

Preparations

Lotions

Copper and Zinc Sulphates Lotion *(B.P.C. 1973)*. Copper and Zinc Lotion; Dalibour Water; Lotio Cupro-Zincica. Copper sulphate 1 g, zinc sulphate 1.5 g, concentrated camphor water 2.5 ml, water to 100 ml.

Similar preparations are included in some pharmacopoeias, with the synonym Dalibour or Alibour Water.

Sweitzer's Solution *(Rochester Methodist Hosp.)*. Copper sulphate 1 g, zinc sulphate 2 g, camphor water to 100 ml. To be diluted 1 to 16 or 1 to 32 with distilled water. Used as a wet dressing. Antibacterial and antifungal. Shelf-life 2 years.

Solutions

Copper Reagent. Benedict's Qualitative Reagent. Dissolve with the aid of heat sodium citrate 15 g, anhydrous sodium carbonate 13 g, and sodium bicarbonate 1 g in about 65 ml of water, cool, add a solution of copper sulphate 1.6 g in 15 ml of water, dilute to 100 ml and filter.

Potassium Cupri-tartrate Solution. Fehling's Solution. Solution No. 1: copper sulphate 3.464 g, sulphuric acid 0.05 ml, water to 50 ml. Solution No. 2: sodium potassium tartrate 17.6 g, sodium hydroxide 7.7 g, water to 50 ml. Mix equal volumes of Solution No. 1 and Solution No. 2 immediately before use.

Solution-tablets

Diagnostic Solution-tablets of Copper *(D.T.F.)*. Each contains anhydrous copper sulphate 18.75 mg, citric acid 300 mg, sodium hydroxide 250 mg, and anhydrous sodium carbonate 62.5 mg.

For a proprietary preparation of diagnostic solution-tablets containing copper sulphate, see Clinitest Reagent Tablets, p.527.

Proprietary Names of Copper Sulphate

Métacuprol *(Lemoine, Fr.)*.

Proprietary Copper-containing Intra-uterine Devices

Gravigard *(Searle, UK)*. An intra-uterine contraceptive device composed of copper-wound plastic. **Mini-Gravigard.** A smaller version of Gravigard. Both devices are stated to carry approximately 200 mm^2 of copper. (Also available as Gravigard in *Neth.*).

Multiload Cu250 *(Organon, UK)*. An intra-uterine contraceptive device composed of copper-wound plastic; stated to carry 250 mm^2 of copper.

Ortho Gyne-T *(Ortho-Cilag, UK)*. An intra-uterine contraceptive device composed of copper-wound plastic. The device is stated to carry 200 mm^2 of copper. (Also available as Gyne-T in *Fr., Neth.*).

Other Proprietary Names of Copper-containing Intra-uterine Devices

Copper-T 200 *(Neth.)*; D.I.U. ML Cu 250 *(Fr.)*; Gravigarde *(Fr.)*; Multiload ^{cu}250 *(Neth.)*; Stérilet T Au Cuivre 200, Sterlys *(both Fr.)*.

5286-z

Copper Acetate.
$(C_2H_3O_2)_2Cu,H_2O$=199.7.

CAS — 142-71-2 (anhydrous).

Pharmacopoeias. In *Span.*

Blue-green crystals or powder with a faint odour of acetic acid. **Soluble** in water.

Copper acetate has been used as an astringent and fungicide.

5287-c

Copper Aceto-Arsenite. Imperial, Paris, Parrot, Schweinfurth, or Vienna Green; CI Pigment Green 21; Colour Index No. 77410.
$Cu(C_2H_3O_2)_2,3Cu(AsO_2)_2$=1013.8.

CAS — 12002-03-8.

A brilliant bluish-green or deep green fine powder. Practically **insoluble** in water.

Copper aceto-arsenite was used for the control of the Colorado beetle, as a poison bait for caterpillars and grasshoppers, as a larvicide for the control of mosquitoes, and as a preservative for wood. The adverse effects of copper aceto-arsenite and their treatment are as for Arsenic Trioxide.

5288-k

Copper Chloride. Cupric Chloride.
$CuCl_2,2H_2O$=170.5.

CAS — 7447-39-4 (anhydrous); 10125-13-0 (dihydrate).

Greenish-blue deliquescent crystals. Freely **soluble** in water and alcohol.

Copper chloride has been used for its astringent and fungicidal properties as a substitute for copper sulphate.

5289-a

Copper Citrate *(B.P.C. 1949)*. Cupri Citras; Cupric Citrate.
$C_6H_4Cu_2O_7,2H_2O$=351.2.

CAS — 866-82-0 (anhydrous).

A green or bluish-green, odourless, crystalline powder. Slightly **soluble** in water; somewhat more soluble in alkali citrate solutions; soluble with decomposition in dilute ammonia solution and in mineral acids. **Store** in airtight containers.

Copper citrate was formerly used in trachoma as a 5% ointment for ulceration and granulation of the eyelids.

5290-e

Copper Naphthenate. The copper salt of naphthenic acids, a range of carboxylic acids, mostly derivatives of cyclopentane, obtained from petroleum.

CAS — 1338-02-9.

Copper naphthenate is used in veterinary practice for the treatment of ringworm and foot rot.
Zinc naphthenate is an ingredient of Tineafax Ointment (see p.732).

5291-l

Copper Subacetate *(B.P.C. 1934)*. Basic Copper Acetate; Copper Oxyacetate; Verdigris; Aerugo; Verdete. A basic copper acetate approximating to the formula $(C_2H_3O_2)_2Cu,Cu(OH)_2,5H_2O$.

CAS — 52503-64-7 (anhydrous).

Pharmacopoeias. In *Port.*

A greenish-blue powder or masses. Partly **soluble** in water with decomposition; soluble in ammonium carbonate solution; practically insoluble in alcohol.

Copper subacetate was formerly employed externally as an astringent, escharotic, and fungicide.

5292-y

Gold.
Au=196.9665.

CAS — 7440-57-5.

A bright-yellow, malleable, and ductile metal; the finely divided powder may be black, ruby, or purple.

Adverse Effects. Allergy to metallic gold is rare. For the systemic effects of gold salts, see under Sodium Aurothiomalate (below).

Allergy. A woman developed persistent, papular, eczematous lesions on both earlobes following ear piercing and wearing of gold ear-rings and subsequently developed a hypersensitivity to gold. The lesions were slow to respond to triamcinolone injections and were excised.— H. Petros and A. L. MacMillan, *Br. J. Derm.*, 1973, *88*, 505.

Necrotising vasculitis in a jeweller was induced by prolonged external contact with gold.— H. R. Roenigk and D. Handel, *Archs Derm.*, 1974, *109*, 253, per *J. Am. med. Ass.*, 1974, *227*, 959.

Further references: S. Comaish, *Archs Derm.*, 1969, *99*, 720 (dermatitis); E. Young, *Dermatologica*, 1974, *149*, 294 (dermatitis).

Radioactivity. A married couple both developed chronic skin lesions on their wedding-ring fingers. Their wedding rings were found to contain radioactive decay products with half-lives of over 20 years. Gold to be processed for dental use and jewellery should be routinely screened for radioactivity.— N. Simon and J. Harley, *J. Am. med. Ass.*, 1967, *200*, 254.

Uses. Gold, as a thin foil, has been applied to skin ulcers to promote healing. For the uses of radioactive gold, see Gold-198 under Radiopharmaceuticals, p.1390.

Topical application. In 13 patients, 22 ischaemic skin ulcers which had proved resistant to therapy with other agents were treated with gold leaf. After cleansing and debridement, the ulcers were wetted with alcohol and then covered with 4 to 8 layers of gold leaf and protective dressings. This procedure was repeated every 48 hours. The average decrease in area of 19 decubitus ulcers was 62%, whereas 3 control ulcers showed an average increase of 96%.— M. Wolf *et al.*, *J. Am. med. Ass.*, 1966, *196*, 693. A study in 44 patients with 64 skin ulcers of various types showed that treatment with gold leaf was no better than treatment with a simple dressing.— K. W. Smith *et al.*, *Archs Derm.*, 1967, *96*, 703, per *J. Am. med. Ass.*, 1967, *202*, (Dec. 11), A160.

5293-j

Auranofin. SKF D-39162. (1-Thio-β-D-glucopyranosato)(triethylphosphine)gold 2,3,4,6-tetra-acetate.
$C_{20}H_{34}AuO_9PS$=678.5.

CAS — 34031-32-8.

Auranofin has a gold content of about 29%.

It has been used similarly to sodium aurothiomalate (see p.934) in the treatment of rheumatoid arthritis. Favourable results have followed the use of 3-mg doses by mouth, twice daily.

References: A. E. Finkelstein *et al.*, *Ann. rheum. Dis.*, 1976, *35*, 251; F. -E. Berglöf *et al.*, *Arthritis Rheum.*, 1977, *20*, 108.

Manufacturers
Smith Kline & French, USA.

5294-z

Aurothioglucose *(U.S.P.)*. Gold Thioglucose; (D-Glucosylthio)gold; 1-Aurothio-D-glucopyranose. (1-Thio-D-glucopyranosato)gold.
$C_6H_{11}AuO_5S$=392.2.

CAS — 12192-57-3.

Pharmacopoeias. In *U.S.*

A yellow odourless or almost odourless powder. It contains a small amount of sodium acetate as a stabiliser and has a gold content of about 50%. Freely **soluble** in water; practically insoluble in alcohol, acetone, chloroform, and ether. A solution in water is dextrorotatory. A 1% solution in water has a pH of about 6.3. Aqueous solutions slowly decompose on standing. **Store** in airtight containers. Protect from light.

Adverse Effects, Treatment, and Precautions. As for Sodium Aurothiomalate, p.933.

Uses. Aurothioglucose has the same actions and uses as sodium aurothiomalate. It is administered intramuscularly as a suspension in oil in a weekly dose of 10 mg increasing gradually to 50 mg. Children, 6 to 12 years, may be given one-quarter the usual dose.

For reports suggesting that post-injection exacerbation of rheumatic symptoms and some other adverse reactions might be reduced by substituting aurothioglucose for sodium aurothiomalate or by substituting oily for aqueous injections of either salt, see Sodium Aurothiomalate, p.933.

Preparations

Sterile Aurothioglucose Suspension *(U.S.P.)*. Aurothioglucose Injection. A sterile suspension of aurothioglucose in a suitable vegetable oil. It may contain suitable thickening agents. Protect from light.

Proprietary Names
Aureotan *(Byk Gulden, Ger.)*; Auromyose *(Nourypharma, Neth.)*; Solganal *(Schering, USA)*.

5295-c

Aurothioglycanide. α-Auromercaptoacetanilide. 2-Aurothio-*N*-phenylacetamide.
C_8H_8AuNOS=363.2.

A greyish-yellow powder. Practically **insoluble** in water, chloroform, and ether. It has a gold content of about 54%.

Adverse Effects, Treatment, and Precautions. As for Sodium Aurothiomalate, p.933.

Uses. Aurothioglycanide has the same actions and uses as sodium aurothiomalate. It is more slowly absorbed than the water-soluble gold compounds.

5296-k

Sodium Aurothiomalate *(B.P.)*. Sod. Aurothiomal.; Gold Sodium Thiomalate *(U.S.P.)*; Sodium Aurothiosuccinate.

CAS — 12244-57-4 (xNa, anhydrous); 39377-38-3 (2 Na monohydrate).

Pharmacopoeias. In *Br.* and *U.S.*

Sodium aurothiomalate *B.P.* is a fine, pale yellow, hygroscopic powder with a slight odour. It consists mainly of the disodium salt of (aurothio)succinic acid ($C_4H_3AuNa_2O_4S$ = 390.1), loses not more than 2% of its weight on drying, and has a gold content of 44.5 to 46% calculated on the dried material; a 10% solution in water has a pH of 6 to 7.
Gold sodium thiomalate *U.S.P.* is a white to yellowish-white, odourless or almost odourless solid. It consists of a mixture of the monosodium and disodium salts of (aurothio)succinic acid ($C_4H_4AuNaO_4S$ = 368.1 and $C_4H_3AuNa_2O_4S$ = 390.1), loses not more than 8% of its weight on drying, and has a gold content of 44.8 to 49.6%, and 49 to 52.5% calculated on the

dried glycerol-free material; a 10% solution in water has a pH of 5.8 to 6.5.

Soluble 1 in less than 1 of water; practically insoluble in alcohol, ether, fixed oils, and most organic solvents. Solutions are **sterilised** by maintaining at 98° to 100° for 30 minutes with a bactericide or by filtration. **Store** in airtight containers. Protect from light.

Adverse Effects. Toxic reactions occur in up to about 40% of patients undergoing gold therapy, and over half affect the skin; in up to some 5% of patients reactions may be severe and, occasionally, even fatal; toxicity may be associated with eosinophilia and immunogenic changes indicative of hypersensitivity.

Toxic reactions commonly include stomatitis (often with a metallic taste) and pruritus (an early sign of intolerance); other reactions affecting the skin and mucous membranes include erythema, maculopapular eruptions, erythema multiforme, urticaria, eczema, seborrhoeic dermatitis, lichenoid eruptions sometimes leading to alopecia, exfoliative dermatitis, glossitis, pharyngitis, gastritis and colitis, vaginitis, and photosensitivity reactions, sometimes associated with dose-related pigmentation (chrysiasis).

Toxic effects on the blood include thrombocytopenia, leucopenia, agranulocytosis, and aplastic anaemia; fatal blood disorders may occur suddenly.

Effects on the kidneys include mild transient proteinuria which may lead to heavy proteinuria, haematuria, and nephrosis.

Other effects reported include pulmonary fibrosis, toxic hepatitis, peripheral neuritis, encephalitis, psychoses, peptic ulcer, and fever. Nitritoid reactions, with weakness, flushing, palpitations, and dyspnoea, may occur following injection of gold salts; local irritation may also follow injection, and sometimes there is initial exacerbation of the arthritic condition. Gold deposits occur in the eyes, occasionally causing keratitis and corneal ulceration.

Of 100 unselected patients undergoing gold therapy, mainly with sodium aurothiomalate, 13 suffered exacerbation of their rheumatic symptoms following the injections, and a further 2 reported increased fatigue and malaise. In 6 of the patients substitution of aurothioglucose for sodium aurothiomalate alleviated their symptoms suggesting that the reaction might be associated with the bioavailability of the gold salt. In general the post-injection reaction was mild and its major significance was its tendency to cause premature abandonment of gold therapy.— J. T. Halla *et al.*, *Arthritis Rheum.*, 1977, *20,* 1188.

In a study involving 98 patients with early rheumatoid arthritis, receiving sodium aurothiomalate injections, and studied over a period of a year, 30 (31%) suffered side-effects: proteinuria occurred in 6, allergic symptoms of the skin or mucous membranes with or without eosinophilia occurred in 23, and thrombocytopenia occurred in 1. Although the serum concentration of IgM was higher in those with side-effects, it remained within normal limits and the finding may have been coincidental; none of 32 other parameters studied showed any significant difference between those with or without side-effects. Earlier findings that gold nephropathy was commoner in seronegative patients could not be confirmed since 3 of the 6 patients with proteinuria were seropositive.— S. Jalava *et al.*, *Scand. J. Rheumatol.*, 1977, *6,* 206. IgA deficiency in 1 patient with rheumatoid arthritis being treated with sodium aurothiomalate.— D. R. Stanworth *et al.* (letter), *Lancet*, 1977, *1,* 1001.

Confirmation of earlier findings by G.S. Panayi *et al.* (*Br. med. J.*, 1978, *2,* 1326) of an association between the presence of HLA-DRw2 and DRw3 antigens and the toxicity of sodium aurothiomalate and penicillamine during treatment for rheumatoid arthritis. in a study of 91 patients with rheumatoid arthritis, 71 had toxic reactions to sodium aurothiomalate, penicillamine, or both. There was a highly significant association between the presence of antigens and the development of proteinuria during therapy with aurothiomalate and a similar trend in patients given penicillamine.— P. H. Wooley *et al.*, *New Engl. J. Med.*, 1980, *303,* 300.

Reviews of the side-effects of gold salts.— H. G. Petering, *Pharmac. Ther.*, 1976, *1,* 119; J. C. Renier and M. Boasson, *Thérapie*, 1976, *31,* 365.

Allergy. Ten of 11 patients who developed side-effects during gold therapy for rheumatoid arthritis had raised concentrations of immunoglobulin IgE, which reverted to normal within 2 months when treatment ceased. This suggested a hypersensitivity reaction.— P. Davis *et al.* (preliminary communication), *Br. med. J.*, 1973, *3,* 676. Gold salts had been suspected of causing polyarteritis and systemic lupus erythematosus.— P. D. B. Davies, *Br. J. Dis. Chest*, 1969, *63,* 57.

A patient who had developed contact dermatitis to gold one year earlier at the onset of her rheumatoid disease had pruritus, swelling, and pustulation of the affected areas when given a single test dose of sodium aurothiomalate 10 mg.— J. A. N. Rennie, *Br. med. J.*, 1976, *2,* 1294. Scepticism.— D. Dick (letter), *ibid.*, 1977, *1,* 51. A reply.— J. A. N. Rennie (letter), *ibid.*, 446.

Cardiovascular effects. Two patients developed nitritoid or vasomotor reactions while receiving sodium aurothiomalate for rheumatoid arthritis. Symptoms included facial flushing and vertigo. In 1 patient the reactions lasted for up to 3 hours and in the other patient they did not completely disappear until 30 hours later.— W. R. Austad (letter), *J. Am. med. Ass.*, 1970, *211,* 2158. Although vasomotor symptoms following sodium aurothiomalate injections in 2 patients were relieved within minutes of resting in a recumbent position, one patient developed a myocardial infarction. Aurothioglucose, which rarely produces vasomotor reactions might be preferable to sodium aurothiomalate in elderly patients with atherosclerosis or in patients with a history of cardiovascular disease.— N. L. Gottlieb and H. E. Brown, *Arthritis Rheum.*, 1977, *20,* 1026.

Effects on the blood. Although all of 4 patients with severe rheumatoid arthritis had marked leucopenia before the start of therapy, white-cell counts increased after successful treatment with sodium aurothiomalate.— J. D. C. Gowans and M. Salami, *New Engl. J. Med.*, 1973, *288,* 1007. See also E. R. Hurd and D. E. Cheatum, *J. Am. med. Ass.*, 1976, *235,* 2215.

There were 102 reports of adverse reactions to gold reported to the Committee on Safety of Medicines between June 1964 and September 1974. These included 41 reports of blood disorders including thrombocytopenia (11; 4 fatal), aplastic anaemia (16; 10 fatal), and agranulocytosis, pancytopenia, or leucopenia (9; 7 fatal), and gastro-intestinal haemorrhage (11; 2 fatal).— M. F. Cuthbert, *Curr. med. Res. Opinion*, 1974, *2,* 600. Deaths from blood dyscrasias had been reported between 1965 and 1971 to the Committee on the Safety of Medicines in 17 patients receiving gold for the treatment of rheumatoid arthritis. Studies in 55 similar patients treated during this period showed that abnormalities in blood count occurred in from 3 to 104 weeks in 47 patients receiving sodium aurothiomalate 50 mg weekly. Pancytopenia, fatal in 15 patients developed in 20 patients. Of 32 patients who developed thrombocytopenia, 6 received less than 200 mg of sodium aurothiomalate and 26 between 280 and 2050 mg; neutropenia developed in 3 other patients on the lower total dose.— A. G. L. Kay, *Br. med. J.*, 1976, *1,* 1266. See also *idem*, *Ann. rheum. Dis.*, 1973, *32,* 277. Pure red cell aplasia in a 20-year-old woman appeared to be due to sodium aurothiomalate; she had received a total of 120 mg.— G. Reid and A. C. Patterson, *Br. med. J.*, 1977, *2,* 1457.

A clinical and immunogenetic study of gold-induced thrombocytopenia.— J. S. Coblyn *et al.*, *Ann. intern. Med.*, 1981, *95,* 178.

Effects on the eyes. A 53-year-old woman who had received gold therapy for rheumatoid arthritis developed inflammation and ulcers of the eye and was found to have corneal deposits of metallic gold. Keratitis was an indication for stopping therapy, but the corneal deposits which often occurred in patients who had received 500 mg of gold were reversible and were not an indication for stopping therapy.— J. H. Rodenhäuser and T. Behrend, *Dt. med. Wschr.*, 1969, *94,* 2389, per *J. Am. med. Ass.*, 1969, *210,* 1944.

Effects on the kidneys. A clinical and pathological study of gold nephropathy. Of 75 patients receiving gold salts 5 developed proteinuria and in 2, criteria for the nephrotic syndrome were fulfilled.— D. S. Silverberg *et al.*, *Arthritis Rheum.*, 1970, *13,* 812. See also P. W. Vanace, *Arthritis Rheum.*, 1977, *20,* 548 (study in children). Other reports.— D. Hándlová, *Vnitř. Lék.*, 1968, *14,* 115; R. Wilkinson and D. W. Eccleston, *Br. med. J.*, 1970, *2,* 772; A. Katz and A. H. Little, *Archs Path.*, 1973, *96,* 133.

In 8 patients with probable gold-induced immune-complex nephropathy IgM-rheumatoid factor was absent, suggesting that the presence of IgM-rheumatoid factor might prevent gold-induced nephropathy.— B. V. Skrifvars *et al.*, *Ann. rheum. dis.*, 1977, *36,* 549.

Other studies on the causes of gold-induced nephropathy.— R. R. Tubbs *et al.* (letter), *New Engl. J. Med.*, 1977, *296,* 1413; G. W. Viol *et al.*, *Archs Path.*, 1977, *101,* 635.

Effects on the liver. Cholestatic jaundice occurred in 3 patients with rheumatoid arthritis who received total doses of sodium aurothiomalate of 37.5, 60, and 110 mg. All the patients recovered spontaneously.— M. Favreau *et al.*, *Ann. intern. Med.*, 1977, *87,* 717.

Effects on the lungs. Pulmonary fibrosis was reported in 1 patient after she had received a total dose of sodium aurothiomalate of 655 mg for the treatment of rheumatoid arthritis. Improvement followed during 1 year after stopping treatment with gold, but lung function deteriorated when treatment was restarted.— D. M. Geddes and J. Brostoff, *Br. med. J.*, 1976, *1,* 1444. Reversible gold-induced lung damage in a 41-year-old woman resembled adenocarcinoma; she recovered following withdrawal of gold and administration of prednisolone, although she was left with a pronounced restrictive lung disorder.— D. W. James *et al.*, *ibid.*, 1978, *1,* 1523.

Other reports.— R. H. Winterbauer *et al.*, *New Engl. J. Med.*, 1976, *294,* 919; S. Miyachi (letter), *ibid.*, *295,* 506; D. Geddes and J. Brostoff (letter), *ibid.*; G. S. Alarcón and E. Gotuzzo (letter), *ibid.*, 507.

Effects on the skin. A review of cutaneous reactions to gold salts.— J. Almeyda and H. Baker, *Br. J. Derm.*, 1970, *83,* 707.

In 10 patients with rheumatoid arthritis treated with gold, skin thickness decreased by a mean of 8.05%. There was no significant alteration in skin elasticity.— W. Harvey *et al.*, *Postgrad. med. J.*, 1974, *50, Suppl.* 2, 33.

Erythema nodosum. A woman with pemphigus vulgaris developed erythema nodosum after sodium aurothiomalate injections.— R. L. Stone *et al.*, *Archs Derm.*, 1973, *107,* 602.

Lichen planus and pityriasis rosea. In 37 patients who suffered skin eruptions during chrysotherapy, the most frequent clinical eruptions resembled non-specific dermatitis, lichen planus, and pityriasis rosea.— N. S. Penneys *et al.*, *Archs Derm.*, 1974, *109,* 372.

Toxic epidermal necrolysis. Toxic epidermal necrolysis which appeared in a woman with arthropathy had been blamed on gold, but might really have been idiopathic.— A. Lyell, *Br. J. Derm.*, 1967, *79,* 662.

Neurological effects. Despite low concentrations of gold in the urine and the CSF, encephalopathy in a 42-year-old man was associated with weekly injections of sodium aurothiomalate 10 to 15 mg to a total of 130 mg. Gold was withdrawn and prednisolone 30 mg daily and penicillamine 1 g daily administered; a month later he was well.— D. L. F. McAuley, *J. Neurol. Neurosurg. Psychiat.*, 1977, *40,* 1021.

Amyotrophic lateral sclerosis syndrome. A syndrome resembling amyotrophic lateral sclerosis with diffuse fasciculations and symmetrical weakness of arms and legs without sensory deficit, was believed to be associated with weekly administration of sodium aurothiomalate 150 mg. The symptoms slowly disappeared in the 2 months after stopping gold therapy.— D. E. Furst *et al.*, *Arthritis Rheum.*, 1977, *20,* 1473.

Guillain-Barré syndrome. Guillain-Barré syndrome in 2 patients associated with gold injections.— D. Bontoux *et al.*, *Revue Rhum. Mal. ostéo-artic.*, 1974, *41,* 48.

Treatment of Adverse Effects. Most of the toxic effects arising from gold therapy may be effectively treated with injections of dimercaprol (see p.383). Penicillamine (see p.387) may be given by mouth.

Skin disorders may require topical or systemic corticosteroid therapy; iodine solutions have been advocated for pigmentation.

Lung, kidney, and blood disorders may call for intensive supportive therapy involving corticosteroids and other immunosuppressive agents; blood transfusions may be required.

A review of the recognition and management of gold toxicity in 43 patients treated over a period of 5 years.— S. L. Burnstein *et al.*, *J. Am. osteop. Ass.*, 1977, *77,* 29.

The peripheral blood count of 2 patients with bone-marrow damage associated with gold therapy improved within 3 days of administration of acetylcysteine.— A. Lorber *et al.*, *J. clin. Pharmac.*, 1973, *13,* 332.

For the use of dimercaprol in the treatment of gold-induced thrombocytopenia, see Dimercaprol, p.383.

Precautions. Gold therapy is contra-indicated in renal or hepatic disease, severe anaemia, haemorrhagic conditions, diabetes, marked hypertension, heart failure, urticaria, eczema, and colitis. It is also contra-indicated in patients with a history of blood disorders or exfoliative dermatitis and in those recently subjected to irradiation.

As gold crosses the placental barrier and has caused foetal damage in *animals* it should not be given during pregnancy.

Gold salts are contra-indicated for the treatment of systemic lupus erythematosus; they should preferably be avoided in the elderly.

Concurrent administration of gold salts with other drugs capable of inducing blood disorders, such as phenylbutazone, oxyphenbutazone, antimalarials, and antineoplastic immunosuppressants should be undertaken with caution if at all. Penicillamine which also antagonises the action of gold should not be used concurrently.

Patients should be warned to report the appearance of sore throat or tongue, metallic taste, pruritus, rash, buccal ulceration, easy bruising, purpura, bleeding, pyrexia, indigestion, diarrhoea, or unexplained malaise.

The urine should be tested for albumin before each injection and the blood should be examined for signs of depressed haemopoiesis. Annual chest X-rays should be carried out.

While there are undoubtedly cases of acute idiosyncrasy to gold, deaths from gold toxicity are more commonly a result of the improper and incautious use of gold. The physician should see the patient at each injection to ask concerning the occurrence of metallic taste, sore throat, glossitis, skin eruption, diarrhoea, purpura or other unusual symptoms. During the first 4 weeks of a course a full blood count (including a numerical platelet estimation) should be carried out with each injection; the blood count and platelet estimation should be made before every second injection for the rest of the course; during maintenance treatment a full blood count should be made every 3 months. Urine should be tested for protein before each injection.— S. Kalowski, *May and Baker* (letter), *Med. J. Aust.*, 1976, *1*, 975. As a general rule blood should be taken each time a patient has an injection of gold and the subsequent dose should not be given unless the result of the blood count, including platelets, is known to be satisfactory; if there is a downward trend of platelets or granulocytes the count should be repeated and if the trend persists the next dose of gold not be given. Although patients on a low dose, such as sodium aurothiomalate 10 mg weekly, may not need such rigorous supervision, nevertheless blood counts should be done at least monthly.— A. Kay (letter), *Br. med. J.*, 1976, *1*, 1534 (Arthritis and Rheumatism Council Epidemiology Research Unit).

Administration in renal failure. Sodium aurothiomalate was reported to be 95% bound to plasma proteins. Its use should be avoided in patients with a glomerular filtration-rate of less than 50 ml per minute.— W. M. Bennett *et al.*, *Ann. intern. Med.*, 1980, *93*, 286.

Drug interactions. *Aspirin.* For a suggestion that concurrent gold administration might exacerbate aspirin-induced hepatic dysfunction, see Aspirin, p.239.

Indomethacin. Fatal aplastic anaemia occurred in a 70-year-old woman with rheumatoid arthritis who had completed a 10-month course of sodium aurothiomalate. She became ill 6 weeks later, 3 days after starting treatment with indomethacin 25 mg thrice daily.— E. Menkes and G. J. Kutas (letter), *Can. med. Ass. J.*, 1977, *117*, 118. Comment, with emphasis on the difficulties involved in determining whether indomethacin or gold caused aplastic anaemia.— C. A. Shearer (letter), *ibid.*, 1978, *118*, 18.

Phenylbutazone. Over the years many people had been given gold in association with phenylbutazone without ill-effects.— A. Kay, *Ann. rheum. Dis.*, 1973, *32*, 277. Concurrent administration of gold with pyrazolone-derived drugs such as phenylbutazone or oxyphenbutazone was contra-indicated.— R. G. Gray and N. L. Gottlieb (letter), *New Engl. J. Med.*, 1976, *295*, 506.

Effects on diagnostic tests. Gold could interfere technically with chemical estimations for PBI to produce erroneous lowered results.— *Drug & Ther. Bull.*, 1972, *10*, 69.

Sjögren's syndrome. Of 60 patients with rheumatoid arthritis 30% developed gold reactions compared with an incidence of only 17.7% in 41 patients also suffering from Sjögren's syndrome. Despite statements in the literature gold therapy was not contra-indicated in patients with Sjögren's syndrome.— M. H. Gordon *et al.*, *Ann. intern. Med.*, 1975, *82*, 47.

Absorption and Fate. Most gold compounds are poorly and irregularly absorbed from the gastro-intestinal tract. The water-soluble salts, such as sodium aurothiomalate, are absorbed readily after intramuscular injection and become bound to plasma proteins. Sodium aurothiomalate accumulates in the body and high concentrations occur in the kidney, liver, and spleen; providing the correct dosage balance is achieved, however, accumulation need not occur despite years of therapy. It is mainly excreted in the urine, with smaller amounts in the faeces. The serum half-life of gold clearance is about 5 or 6 days but after a course of treatment, gold may be found in the urine for up to 1 year owing to its presence in deep body compartments.

Following intramuscular injection of aqueous solution of sodium aurothiomalate 10 mg to 10 hospital in-patients with rheumatoid arthritis the average urinary excretion of gold in the first 24 hours was 270 µg and in the second 24 hours was 145 µg but this difference was not significant; faecal excretion in 5 patients ranged from 0 to 17 µg in the first 24 hours and 10 to 156 µg in the second 24 hours. Peak plasma concentrations were reached after 4 hours, declined rapidly between 4 and 36 hours, and then more slowly between 36 and 168 hours; the initial sharp decline was probably due to tissue absorption and the slower decline to urinary excretion. No correlation was found with faecal excretion although this was a large part of the total excretion.— M. Harth, *Clin. Pharmac. Ther.*, 1974, *15*, 354. See also R. C. Gerber *et al.*, *J. Lab. clin. Med.*, 1974, *83*, 778; B. R. Mascarenhas *et al.*, *Arthritis Rheum.*, 1972, *15*, 391; H. M. Rubinstein and A. A. Dietz, *Ann. rheum. Dis.*, 1973, *32*, 128; N. L. Gottlieb *et al.*, *Arthritis Rheum.*, 1974, *17*, 171.

A detailed review of the rational approach to gold administration on the basis of gold kinetic data. Although differences in excretion-rates of gold had been noted between subjects, undue sensitivity or resistance to therapy did not necessarily correlate with very slow or very rapid excretion.— A. Lorber, *Clin. Pharmacokinet.*, 1977, *2*, 127.

Pregnancy and the neonate. Gold was detected in the liver and kidney of an aborted foetus; the mother had been receiving sodium aurothiomalate at conception and it was for this reason that the pregnancy was terminated. Gold was also detected in the placenta.— I. Rocker and W. J. Henderson (letter), *Lancet*, 1976, *2*, 1246. The need for abortion in this patient was criticised.— A. J. Richards (letter), *ibid.*, 1977, *1*, 99. Reply.— I. Rocker (letter), *ibid.*

Analysis of the milk of a 35-year-old woman who was receiving sodium aurothiomalate and of the urine of her 15-month-old breast-fed daughter demonstrated that gold is secreted in the milk of mothers receiving gold salts and that small but significant amounts are absorbed into the infant's circulation.— R. A. F. Bell and I. M. Dale, *Arthritis Rheum.*, 1976, *19*, 1374.

Uses. Sodium aurothiomalate is used mainly for its anti-inflammatory effect in the treatment of rheumatoid arthritis. It is most effective in active progressive rheumatoid arthritis and of little or no value in the presence of extensive deformities. It is ineffective against other forms of arthritis.

Sodium aurothiomalate therapy should only be undertaken where facilities are available to carry out the tests specified under Precautions (above).

It is preferably given by deep intramuscular injection; an aqueous solution is usually employed but a suspension in oil has been used. Weekly doses of 1, 5, then 10 mg are given to test the patient's tolerance to the drug and these are usually followed by doses of up to 50 mg at weekly intervals to a total of about 1 g; maintenance therapy may be instituted consisting of 20 to 50 mg every 2 to 4 weeks.

For an initial 6 months children may be given maximum weekly doses of 10 mg for those weighing less than 25 kg, 20 mg for those weighing 25 to 50 kg, and 30 mg for those weighing over 50 kg. If an improvement is obtained maintenance therapy may then be continued with the same dosage at fortnightly or monthly intervals for 1 to 5 years.

An injection may produce an exacerbation of the symptoms and this may necessitate a reduction in the dosage.

Sodium aurothiomalate has been used in the treatment of chronic discoid lupus erythematosus unresponsive to other therapies; it has also been tried in the treatment of pemphigus and of bronchial asthma.

A review of the possible mode of action of gold compounds.— P. Bresloff, *Adv. Drug Res.*, 1977, *11*, 1. The localisation of gold in the synovial membrane in rheumatoid arthritis treated with sodium aurothiomalate.— H. Nakamura and M. Igarashi, *Ann. rheum. Dis.*, 1977, *36*, 209.

Asthma. In a double-blind study involving 79 patients with bronchial asthma a beneficial effect compared with control patients was noted in those receiving sodium aurothiomalate injections initially 10 mg weekly gradually increased to 100 mg weekly and subsequently given as 100 mg monthly.— M. Muranaka *et al.*, *Ann. Allergy*, 1978, *40*, 132.

Pemphigus. Gold injections appeared to be associated with a beneficial effect in 4 patients with pemphigus. Another 2 patients withdrew owing to the development of skin rashes.— H. Rotstein, *Aust. J. Derm.*, 1977, *18*, 119. See also N. S. Penneys *et al.*, *Archs Derm.*, 1973, *108*, 56.

Rheumatoid arthritis. Initial results of the Empire Rheumatism Council study (*Ann. rheum. Dis.*, 1960, *19*, 95) indicated that administration of sodium aurothiomalate 50 mg weekly for 20 doses had a beneficial effect on rheumatoid arthritis in 90 patients compared with 95 control patients, but follow-up of 159 of these patients (*Ann. rheum. Dis.*, 1961, *20*, 315) revealed that after about 24 months the benefit was lost. A. Lorber *et al.* (*Ann. rheum. Dis.*, 1973, *32*, 133) demonstrated that gold cumulation could be avoided by maintaining serum concentrations between 3 and 4 µg per ml, and subsequently J.W. Sigler *et al.* (*Ann. intern. Med.*, 1974, *80*, 21) reported encouraging results with a long-term maintenance regimen of 50 mg monthly for a period of 2 years. A. Lorber *et al.* (*Ann. rheum. Dis.*, 1973, *32*, 133) also proposed that maintenance of serum-gold concentrations above 3 µg per ml might confer significant clinical benefit but, possibly owing to the complex pharmacokinetics of gold, the issue has remained controversial, and R.C. Gerber *et al.* (*Ann. rheum. Dis.*, 1972, *31*, 308), N.L. Gottlieb *et al.* (*Arthritis Rheum.*, 1974, *17*, 171) and others have found no correlation between serum concentrations and response. J.M.M. McKenzie (*Rheumatol. Rehabil.*, 1977, *16*, 78) has, moreover, obtained an initial clinical response to weekly doses of 10 or 50 mg, the serum concentrations of gold again showing no correlation with clinical improvement. In addition, D.E. Furst *et al.* (*Arthritis Rheum.*, 1977, *20*, 1473), in a comparison of high-dose maintenance therapy of 150 mg weekly with conventional 50-mg weekly maintenance therapy, while decisively rejecting the high-dose therapy on the grounds of unacceptable toxicity, found no correlation between this toxicity and serum concentrations. In terms of duration of administration, however, in a long-term study covering 5 to 6 years R. Luukkainen *et al.* (*Scand. J. Rheumatol.*, 1977, *6*, 123) found significantly less progression of joint erosion in patients who received a total mean dose of 1858 mg compared with those who were obliged to stop therapy after a total mean dose of 254 mg.

Other studies.— Co-operating Clinics CommitteeAmerican Rheumatism Association, *Arthritis Rheum.*, 1973, *16*, 353; J. T. Sharp *et al.*, *Arthritis Rheum.*, 1977, *20*, 1179.

Comparison of aqueous and oily gold preparations. In a series of rheumatic patients oily injections of gold were found to be less toxic than aqueous injections, regardless of whether the salt used was sodium aurothiomalate or aurothioglucose.— J. S. Lawrence, *Ann. rheum. Dis.*, 1976, *35*, 171.

See also Adverse Effects abstracts (above).

Juvenile rheumatoid arthritis. Dosage of sodium aurothiomalate in children with juvenile rheumatoid arthritis (Still's disease) given at weekly intervals for 6 months, was: up to 20 kg body-weight, 5 mg; 20 to 30 kg, 10 mg; 30 to 50 kg, 20 mg; above 50 kg, 50 mg. If this was successful, the same doses were continued at fortnightly or monthly intervals.— B. M. Ansell, *Practitioner*, 1972, *208*, 91.

At least two-thirds of 22 patients with juvenile rheumatoid arthritis showed a good to excellent response to sodium aurothiomalate in a dose of 1 mg per kg body-weight at intervals of 1, 2, 3, or 4 weeks. In future studies of the treatment of juvenile rheumatoid arthritis with gold salts, 1 mg per kg body-weight weekly should be considered the basic dose, subsequently modified by determination of blood concentrations together with standard laboratory tests.— V. Hanson, *Arthritis Rheum.*, 1977, *20*, 548.

Reviews. For reviews of the use of sodium aurothiomalate and other gold salts in the treatment of progressive rheumatoid arthritis, see *J. Am. med. Ass.*, 1973, *224, Suppl.*, 662–805; G. E. Ehrlich, *J. Am. med. Ass.*, 1974, *228*, 94; *Lancet*, 1974, *1*, 789; *Br. med. J.*, 1975, *2*, 156.

Preparations

Gold Sodium Thiomalate Injection *(U.S.P.)*. A sterile solution of gold sodium thiomalate *U.S.P.* in Water for Injections. pH 5.8 to 6.5. Protect from light.

Sodium Aurothiomalate Injection *(B.P.)*. Sod. Aurothiomalate Inj. A sterile solution of sodium aurothiomalate in Water for Injections. Sterilised by maintaining at 98° to 100° with a bactericide, or by filtration. Protect from light.

Myocrisin *(May & Baker, UK)*. A brand of Sodium Aurothiomalate Injection, in ampoules of 1, 5, 10, 20, and 50 mg. (Also available as Myocrisin in *Austral., Denm., Norw., S.Afr., Swed.*).

Other Proprietary Names

Myochrysine *(Canad., USA)*; Tauredon *(Ger., Switz.)*.

5297-a

Sodium Aurothiosulphate *(B.P.C. 1949)*. Gold Sodium Thiosulphate.

$Na_3Au(S_2O_3)_2,2H_2O = 526.2$.

CAS — 10233-88-2 (anhydrous); 10210-36-3 (dihydrate).

Pharmacopoeias. In *Arg.*

White odourless glistening crystals with a sweet taste. **Soluble** 1 in 2 of water; practically insoluble in alcohol and most organic solvents. Solutions for injections are prepared by dissolving, immediately before use, the sterile contents of a sealed container in Water for Injections. **Protect** from light in sealed ampoules.

Adverse Effects, Treatment, and Precautions. As for Sodium Aurothiomalate, p.933.

Uses. Sodium aurothiosulphate has the same actions and uses as sodium aurothiomalate by which it has been largely superseded. It was administered intravenously (intramuscular injections were painful) and the dosage scheme was similar to that of the aurothiomalate.

Proprietary Names

Sanocrysin *(Ferrosan, Denm.)*.

5298-t

Lead.

Pb = 207.2.

CAS — 7439-92-1.

A grey, malleable and ductile metal.

Adverse Effects. Acute lead poisoning usually results from the accidental swallowing of soluble lead salts. The fatal dose of absorbed lead has been estimated as 500 mg; death of an adult has been reported following ingestion of 10 g of a lead salt; inevitable fatalities are reported to be associated with doses of 40 to 50 g. The symptoms are intense thirst, an astringent and metallic taste in the mouth, a burning abdominal pain, vomiting (sometimes with milky vomitus), diarrhoea or occasionally constipation, black stools, haemolysis and renal damage with oliguria, shock and coma.

Chronic poisoning is usually due to the accumulation of small quantities of lead in the body by inhalation, ingestion, or skin absorption. Most of these cases occur in young children from sucking lead paint or lead toys, though it is also an industrial hazard. Early symptoms are anorexia, constipation, headache, weakness, the development of a black or blue lead line on the gums (not seen in edentulous persons), and anaemia which is only sometimes characterised by large numbers of erythrocytes with basophilic stippling. There may be vomiting, irritability, incoordination, and painless peripheral neuritis with paralysis (wrist and foot drop) in more advanced cases and possibly renal damage. Encephalopathy with visual disturbance, persistent vomiting, ataxia, delirium, convulsions, and coma may develop especially in children. Lead also causes severe abdominal pain ('lead colic') and tonic contraction of the uterus which may result in abortion in pregnant women.

Organic lead compounds such as tetraethyl lead have a specific action on the nervous tissues. mental disturbances predominate, and convulsions may occur after severe exposure.

Maximum permissible atmospheric concentration of lead 150 µg per m^3; 100 µg per m^3 when derived from tetraethyl lead.

The Second International Workshop on Permissible Levels for Occupational Exposure to Inorganic Lead, 1976, recommended that individual blood-lead concentrations should not exceed 600 ng per ml for men. Taking into account the effects on the haematopoietic system at concentrations above 450 to 500 ng per ml and on nerve conduction velocity at concentrations between 500 and 600 ng per ml, it was, however, desirable to reduce individual exposure below this level. A health-based permissible concentration could not be agreed. Because of the theoretical risk of foetal damage, women of childbearing age should not be employed in situations where blood-lead concentrations might regularly exceed 400 ng per ml. The blood concentrations of both male and female workers should be known before employment.— R. L. Zielhuis, *Int. Archs occup. environ. Hlth*, 1977, *39*, 59.

Maximum tolerable weekly intake of lead for adults only: 3 mg per person or 50 µg per kg body-weight.— Twenty-second Report of Joint FAO/WHO Expert Committee on Food Additives, *Tech. Rep. Ser. Wld Hlth Org. No. 631*, 1978.

Action and environmental distribution. A detailed review of the pharmacology and toxicology of lead, including an account of its distribution in the environment.— R. A. Kehoe, *Pharmac. Ther.*, 1976, *1*, 161–88.

An extensive review of the exposure of humans to lead, including an account of the relative uptake from air as against absorption from the gastro-intestinal tract, mention of the cutaneous absorption of organic lead compounds, a description of the disposition of lead in the body and the effects of chelating agents, details of toxic effects on the blood and kidneys, and reference to nervous system toxicity.— P. B. Hammond, *A. Rev. Pharmac. & Toxic.*, 1977, *17*, 197–214.

Some other studies, reviews, and reports on the toxicology of lead and lead compounds.— Report of a WHO Expert Group on Trace Elements in Human Nutrition, *Tech. Rep. Ser. Wld Hlth Org. No. 532*, 1973, 46; J. S. Lin-Fu, *New Engl. J. Med.*, 1973, *289*, 1229 and 1289. A Report of an Inter-Departmental Working Group on Heavy Metals, Pollution Paper No. 2, London, HM Stationery Office, 1974; *Postgrad. med. J.*, 1975, *51*, 747–811; Food Additives and Contaminants Committee, *Review of the Lead in Food Regulations 1961*, FAC/REP/21, London, HM Stationery Office, 1975; Working Party on the Monitoring of Foodstuffs for Heavy Metals, *Survey of Lead in Food: First Supplementary Report*, London, HM Stationery Office, 1975; K. R. Mahaffey, *Pediatrics*, 1977, *59*, 448; *Environmental Health Criteria 3. Lead*, Geneva, Wld Hlth Org., 1977, per *Abstr. Hyg.*, 1977, *52*, 1153; *Lead and Health:* Report by the DHSS working party on lead in the environment, London, HM Stationery Office, 1980; *Lead in the Human Environment*, National Academy of Sciences, Washington DC, 1980.

Lead naphthenate. A study on the toxicity of lead naphthenate.— T. Van Peteghem and H. De Vos, *Br. J. ind. Med.*, 1974, *31*, 233.

Sources of poisoning. An account of the sources of lead and the effects of exposure.— *New Engl. J. Med.*, 1977, *297*, 943.

Some reports of lead poisoning and its sources.— W. Turner *et al.*, *Br. med. J.*, 1967, *3*, 56; M. J. Catton *et al.*, *ibid.*, 1970, *2*, 80 (burning battery cases); M. A. Warley *et al.* (letter), *ibid.*, 1968, *1*, 117 (eye cosmetic containing lead sulphide); P. C. Srivastava and S. Varadi (letter), *ibid.*, 578 (lipstick containing lead carbonate); B. Livesley and C. E. Sissons (letter), *ibid.*, 1968, *4*, 387 (torch-cutting lead-painted steel); A. D. F. Walls, *ibid.*, 1969, *1*, 98 (home-brewed cider); J. G. P. Power *et al.*, *ibid.*, 1969, *3*, 336 (lead chromate in chilli powder); M. Klein *et al.*, *New Engl. J. Med.*, 1970, *283*, 669 (apple juice stored in earthenware jar); F. W. Alexander and H. T. Delves, *Archs Dis. Childh.*, 1972, *47*, 446 (lead-containing paints and an eye cosmetic, /Surma/); C. L. Whitfield *et al.*, *Am. J. Med.*, 1972, *52*, 289 (moonshine liquor); M. K. Williams (letter), *Lancet*, 1972, *2*, 480 (barley-water in earthenware jars); K. G. A. Clark (letter), *ibid.*, 662 (cider in earthenware jars); G. J. A. I. Snodgrass *et al.* (letter), *Br. med. J.*, 1973, *4*, 230 (Indian lead-containing eye cosmetics); A. D. Beattie *et al.*, *Q. J. Med.*, 1975, *44*, 275 (abuse by self-injection of lead and opium pills); P. J. Landrigan *et al.*, *J. Am. med. Ass.*, 1975, *234*, 394; K. E. Anderson *et al.*, *Am. J. Med.*, 1977, *63*, 306 (indoor pistol ranges); Y. Yamamuta *et al.*, *Jap. J. ind. Hlth.*, 1975, *17*, 223 (tetraethyl lead in aviation fuel); *Lancet*, 1976, *2*, 1148 (Bal Jivan Chamco baby tonic); K. C. Perkins and F. A. Oski, *Pediatrics*, 1976, *57*, 426 (burning of newsprint); D. M. Switz *et al.*, *Archs intern. Med.*, 1976, *136*, 939 (bullet); E. L. Baker *et al.*, *New Engl. J. Med.*, 1977, *296*, 260 (contaminated clothing of lead workers); F. Beretta *et al.*, *Medna Lav.*, 1977, *68*, 340 (microwelding); R. L. Boeckx *et al.*, *Pediatrics*, 1977, *60*, 140; F. J. Coodin and R. Boeckx (letter), *New Engl. J. Med.*, 1978, *298*, 347 (both abuse, by inhalation, of lead-containing petrol); H. Chan *et al.*, *Clin. Toxicol.*, 1977, *10*, 273 (Chinese herbal medicines from Hong Kong); J. Clausen and S. C. Rastogi, *Br. J. ind. Med.*, 1977, *34*, 208 (lead naphthenate in high-pressure-resistant diesel engine lubricants); R. G. Feldman *et al.* (letter), *Lancet*, 1977, *1*, 89 (lead oxide fumes); J. Lightfoote *et al.*, *J. Am. med. Ass.*, 1977, *238*, 1539; *ibid.*, 1978, *239*, 1037 (both Chinese herbal remedy from Hong Kong); M. Lob and M. Berode, *Schweiz. med. Wschr.*, 1977, *107*, 1667 (glazed pottery); A. Canberk *et al.*, *Toxic. appl. Pharmac.*, 1978, *44*, 257 (print-shop workers); C. E. Searle and D. G. Harnden (letter), *Lancet*, 1979, *2*, 1070; H. A. Waldron (letter), *ibid* (hair-dye preparations, including Morgan's perfumed pomade); A. A. Attenburrow *et al.* (letter), *ibid.*, 1980, *1*, 323; M. Aslam *et al.* (letter), *ibid.*, 658 (differing findings on the hazards of Surma intoxication); A. Acra *et al.*, *ibid.*, 1981, *1*, 433 (lead-glazed pottery); *ibid.*, 1008 (lead in petrol); R. R. Jones (letter), *ibid.*, 1160 (lead in petrol); P. S. I. Barry (letter), *ibid.*, 1264 (the British Government's decision to reduce lead in petrol from 400 mg per litre to 150 mg per litre).

Water. For reports of toxicity following ingestion of lead in drinking water and for limits of lead in water, see Potable Water, in the section on Water, p.1669.

Diagnosis of lead poisoning. Of 85 children with blood-lead concentrations greater than 600 ng per ml, only 11% satisfied laboratory criteria of anaemia, coproporphyrinuria, lead lines, lead shadow in abdominal X-ray films, and stippling of erythrocytes.— O. M. Rennert *et al.*, *Clin. Pediat.* 1970, *9*, 9,, per *Clin. Med.*, 1970, *77* (Nov.), 39. Results of laboratory tests and assessment of questions concerning abdominal ache, constipation, and fatigue, and inspection for hand tremor in 489 factory workers exposed to lead, indicated that blood-lead measurement is the most meaningful way of monitoring workers exposed to lead. The toxic effect of lead did not appear to be associated with its action on the porphyrin metabolic pathway.— L. M. Irwig *et al.*, *Lancet*, 1978, *2*, 4.

Carboxyhaemoglobin concentrations were elevated in non-smoking workers occupationally exposed to lead; this might form the basis for a screening test.— W. R. Lee and H. Dhanapala (letter), *Br. med. J.*, 1977, *1*, 445.

Other references.— H. Sakurai *et al.*, *Archs environ. Hlth*, 1974, *29*, 157; J. J. Smulewicz, *Am. J. med. Sci.*, 1974, *267*, 49.

Effects on body systems. From a study in over 7000 lead workers, their life expectancy was calculated to be approximately the same as that of all USA males.— W. C. Cooper and W. R. Gaffey, *J. occup. Med.*, 1975, *17*, 100, per *Abstr. Hyg.*, 1975, *50*, 588.

Cardiovascular. A report of prolonged hypertension and blunted beta-adrenoceptor-mediated functions in a 65-year-old man after the inhalation of lead dust.— O. Bertel *et al.*, *Br. med. J.*, 1978, *1*, 551.

Cytogenetic. In a study of 150 men exposed to lead and who suffered from lead poisoning or demonstrated various degrees of absorption there was a decrease in fertility in those with lead poisoning or with moderate lead absorption. This was probably due to a direct effect on the gonads.— I. Lancranjan *et al.*, *Archs environ. Hlth*, 1975, *30*, 396, per *J. Am. med. Ass.*, 1975, *233*, 474. See also R. L. Zielhuis, *Int. Archs occup. environ. Hlth*, 1977, *39*, 59.

A study of 105 workers with varying degrees of lead exposure did not show a significant correlation between blood-lead concentrations and chromosome damage.—

G. Schwanitz *et al.*, *Dt. med. Wschr.*, 1975, *100*, 1007, per *J. Am. med. Ass.*, 1975, *233*, 571. See also M. Bauchinger *et al.*, *Mutat. Res.*, 1977, *56*, 75.

Nervous. In patients with motor neurone disease, 17% had a history of known contact with lead, long before the occurrence of the disease.— A. M. G. Campbell and E. R. Williams (letter), *Br. med. J.*, 1968, *4*, 582. See also A. M. G. Campbell *et al.*, *J. Neurol. Neurosurg. Psychiat.*, 1970, *33*, 877.

A study of 22 patients with multiple sclerosis compared with 22 controls indicated that blood concentrations of lead were similar in the 2 groups, and a single dose of penicillamine did not increase the urinary concentration of lead in these patients.— *J. R. Coll. gen. Pract.*, 1976, *26*, 622 (Report of the Birmingham Research Unit of the Royal College of General Practitioners and the Department of Social Medicine, University of Birmingham).

Renal. A discussion on acute renal failure in lead poisoning.— *Lancet*, 1978, *2*, 140.

Evidence for a role of lead in gout nephropathy.— V. Batuman *et al.*, *New Engl. J. Med.*, 1981, *304*, 520; M. C. Reif *et al.*, *ibid.*, 535. Further references: B. C. Campbell *et al.*, *Br. med. J.*, 1978, *2*, 1403.

Effects on children. Comments on evidence for and against the suggested association between subclinical lead poisoning and mental handicap in children. Findings remained difficult to evaluate.— *Lancet*, 1978, *1*, 365. See also *Br. med. J.*, 1977, *1*, 255.

In a study involving 2335 children considered not to have symptoms of lead intoxication, those with high concentrations of lead in the dentine of shed teeth performed neuropsychological tests less well than those with low lead concentrations. Disordered classroom behaviour could be correlated with increasing lead concentrations.— H. L. Needleman *et al.*, *New Engl. J. Med.*, 1979, *300*, 689. Comment.— J. S. Lin-Fu, *ibid.*, 731. Further comments and criticisms: M. S. Kramer (letter), *ibid.*, *301*, 161; D. M. Hall (letter), *ibid.*; J. F. Cole (letter), *ibid.*; A. Goldberg and M. R. Moore (letter), *ibid.*, 162; J. Coplan (letter), *ibid.*; D. R. Lynam (letter), *ibid.* Reply.— H. L. Needleman (letter), *ibid.*, 163. See also B. E. Clayton *et al.* (letter), *Lancet*, 1979, *1*, 324; H. L. Needleman (letter), *ibid.*, 1024; P. Graham (letter), *ibid.*; M. Barr *et al.* (letter), *ibid.*, 1289; H. L. Needleman and A. Leviton (letter), *ibid.*, *2*, 104.

See also Potable Water, in the section on Water, p.1669.

Lead in Food. In Great Britain, the amount of lead in food is controlled by the Lead in Food Regulations, 1979 (SI 1979: No. 1254) and Lead in Food (Scotland) Regulations, 1979 [SI 1979: No. 1641(S.139)]. These regulations restrict the amount of lead in food to a maximum of 1 ppm with the exception of foods specially prepared for infants and children, where a limit of 0.2 ppm is specified, and certain foods and drinks tabulated in the regulations for which limits ranging from 0.2 to 10 ppm are specified.

Provisional tolerable weekly intake of lead for adults only: 3 mg per person or 50 µg per kg body-weight.— Sixteenth Report of FAO/WHO Expert Committee on Food Additives, *Tech. Rep. Ser. Wld Hlth Org. No. 505*, 1972. See also *Fd Add. Ser. Wld Hlth Org. No. 4*, 1972.

The average lead content of the national diet of the UK in 1972–4 was 0.09 ppm, providing about 1 mg from food and 200 µg from beverages. Concentrations had fallen since an earlier report in 1972. Only 0.2% of nearly 11 000 water samples had lead concentrations higher than the WHO limit of 100 µg per litre (0.1 ppm).— Working Party on the Monitoring of Foodstuffs for Heavy Metals, *Survey of Lead in Food: First Supplementary Report*, London, HM Stationery Office, 1975.

Treatment of Adverse Effects. In acute poisoning following ingestion of soluble lead compounds the stomach should be emptied by aspiration and lavage, and a purgative such as sodium sulphate 30 g in 250 ml of water should be given.

Sodium calciumedetate (see p.391), in conjunction with dimercaprol (see p.383), should be given initially. Follow-up treatment with penicillamine (see p.387) may be continued for several months. Asymptomatic patients may be treated similarly or given penicillamine alone.

Abdominal colic may be relieved by administration of calcium salts by mouth or by intravenous injection. Atropine sulphate 1 mg may be given by subcutaneous injection, but cautious administration of morphine may be necessary.

In acute encephalopathy convulsions should be treated with the intravenous injection of diazepam and barbiturates, if necessary; an osmotic diuretic such as mannitol may be of value for the control of cerebral oedema. Intravenous administration of fluids should be limited to specific requirements in order to prevent exacerbation of cerebral oedema. Urine flow must be maintained; if there is significant renal impairment, peritoneal dialysis or haemodialysis must be undertaken in association with the chelating therapy.

Further exposure to lead should be prevented.

In 22 children who had suffered coma and/or convulsions from lead poisoning for 24 hours or more, 18 had been symptomatically treated for 4 to 30 days before diagnosis of lead poisoning. Cerebral symptoms had been precipitated by intravenous fluids and further damage was prevented by controlled fluid intake.— R. Coffin *et al.*, *J. Pediat.*, 1966, *69*, 198, per *Bull. Hyg.*, *Lond.*, 1967, *42*, 6.

For discussions on the treatment of lead poisoning, see *Med. Lett.*, 1972, *14*, 5; *Ann. intern. Med.*, 1972, *76*, 779..

For reports on the treatment of lead poisoning, see Dimercaprol, p.383, Disodium Edetate, p.384, Penicillamine, p.388, and Sodium Calciumedetate, p.391.

Precautions. Corticosteroids should not be given in lead poisoning as severe symptoms may be precipitated. Morphine may exacerbate cerebral symptoms.

The control of exposure of workers to lead in Great Britain is enforced by the Control of Lead at Work Regulations, 1980 (SI 1980: No. 1248).

Practical guidance with respect to the Control of Lead at Work Regulations, 1980.— Approved Code of Practice, Control of Lead at Work, Health and Safety Commission, London, HM Stationery Office, 1981.

Pregnancy and the neonate. A brief review of the potential foetal toxicity of maternal lead poisoning. Administration of a 7-day course of sodium calciumedetate, at her eighth month of pregnancy, to a woman with lead poisoning, appeared to have no adverse effects on the infant. Since foetal toxicity probably occurs in less than 25% of cases of lead poisoning in the last trimester it was not known whether the absence of any adverse effects of lead on the infant had been influenced by administration of sodium calciumedetate.— C. R. Angle and M. S. McIntire, *Am. J. Dis. Child.*, 1964, *108*, 436.

The use of lead nipple shields or lead acetate ointment by lactating mothers could produce sufficient quantities of lead in the milk to cause encephalitis in the suckling infant.— J. J. Rowan (letter), *Pharm. J.*, 1976, *2*, 184. See also Lead Acetate, p.936.

In an area of high atmospheric lead contamination the mean lead concentrations in maternal and foetal cord blood in 122 women were 412 and 379 ng per ml respectively compared with 147 and 118 ng per ml in 31 controls; birth weight and red cell values of the infants were not adversely affected.— A. R. L. Clark, *Postgrad. med. J.*, 1977, *53*, 674. See also D. G. Wibberley *et al.*, *J. med. Genet.*, 1977, *14*, 339.

Reports of prenatal lead intoxication: N. Singh *et al.*, *J. Pediat.*, 1978, *93*, 1019; A. E. Timpo *et al.*, *ibid.*, 1979, *94*, 765.

Absorption and Fate. Under normal circumstances about 5 to 10% of lead ingested in food is absorbed from the gastro-intestinal tract, mainly in the small intestine; some of the lead absorbed undergoes enterohepatic recycling. Lead is also absorbed by the lungs from dust particles. Inorganic lead is not absorbed through intact skin, but organic compounds such as lead naphthenate and tetraethyl lead may be absorbed rapidly.

Lead is distributed in the soft tissues, with higher concentrations in the liver and kidneys. In the blood it is associated with the erythrocytes. Over a period of time lead accumulates in the body and is deposited in calcified bone, hair, and teeth. Lead crosses the placental barrier. It is excreted in the urine, in sweat, and in milk.

The biological half-life of lead was 70 days.— W. A. Ritschel, *Drug Intell. & clin. Pharm.*, 1970, *4*, 332.

Uses of Lead Salts. Lead salts have an astringent action which is due to the formation of lead proteinate. They were formerly employed as soothing astringent applications, but the medicinal use of preparations containing lead is no longer recommended.

5299-x

Lead Acetate *(B.P.C. 1973).* Plumbi Acetas; Sugar of Lead; Azúcar de Plomo; Sal de Saturno; Bleiazetat; Acetato de Chumbo.

$(CH_3.CO_2)_2Pb,3H_2O=379.3$.

CAS — 301-04-2 (anhydrous).

Pharmacopoeias. In *Arg.*, *Aust.*, *Belg.*, *Cz.*, *Fr.*, *Ind.*, *It.*, *Neth.*, *Pol.*, *Port.*, and *Swiss.*

Small white transparent crystals or heavy crystalline masses with an acetous odour and a sweet astringent taste. It effloresces in warm air and absorbs carbon dioxide. It becomes anhydrous when dried at 40° and basic when heated.

Soluble 1 in 2 of water, usually forming an opalescent solution, 1 in 63 of alcohol, and 1 in 2 of glycerol. A solution in water is slightly alkaline to litmus. **Incompatible** with benzoates, carbonates, chlorides, ichthammol, iodides, phosphates, salicylates, sulphates, tannates, tannic acid, and acacia mucilage. **Store** in airtight containers.

Adverse Effects and Treatment. As for Lead (pp.935-6).

Application of lead acetate ointment to the breast had resulted in an infant ingesting sufficient quantities of lead to produce encephalitis.— J. A. Knowles, *J. Pediat.*, 1965, *66*, 1068.

Uses. Lead acetate has been used in a variety of preparations for external applications.

The use of lead acetate in cosmetics and toiletries is restricted in Great Britain under the Cosmetic Products Regulations 1978 (SI 1978: No. 1354).

Preparations

For details of lead lotions and other preparations containing lead acetate, see Martindale 27th Edn., p. 901.

5300-x

Lead Carbonate *(B.P.C. 1949).* White Lead; Cerussa; Lead Subcarbonate; Alvaiade. A basic lead carbonate corresponding approximately to

$2PbCO_3,Pb(OH)_2=715.6$.

CAS — 1344-36-1.

Pharmacopoeias. In *Aust.*, *Port.*, and *Span.*

A heavy, white, odourless, tasteless, amorphous powder or easily pulverisable masses. Practically **insoluble** in water and alcohol.

Adverse Effects, Treatment, and Precautions. As for Lead, pp.935-6.

Uses. Lead carbonate has been used as a 10% ointment.

5301-r

Lead Monoxide *(B.P.C. 1973).* Plumbi Monoxidum; Litharge; Plumbum Oxydatum Flavum; Plumbum Oxydatum Fusum; Massicot; Bleioxyd; Bleiglätte; Oxido Amarillo de Plomo; Oxido de Chumbo.

$PbO=223.2$.

CAS — 1317-36-8.

Pharmacopoeias. In *Aust.*, *Belg.*, *Cz.*, *Fr.*, *Hung.*, *Ind.*, *Jap.*, *Neth.*, *Pol.*, *Port.*, *Roum.*, *Rus.*, *Span.*, and *Swiss.*

Yellow, pale orange, or pale brick-red, odourless or almost odourless, heavy scales or powder. Very slightly **soluble** in water; practically insoluble in alcohol. **Store** in airtight containers.

Adverse Effects and Treatment. As for Lead (pp.935-6).

Uses. Lead monoxide is used in the preparation of lead plaster-mass.

5302-f

Lead Plaster-mass *(B.P.C. 1954).* Emp. Plumb. in Mass.; Diachylon Plaster-mass; Diachylon; Lead Plaster.

Pharmacopoeias. A similar preparation is included in several pharmacopoeias.

Crude lead oleate, prepared by heating lead monoxide and arachis or olive oil in water. It contains the equivalent of 31 to 34% of PbO.

The spread plaster has been used as a protective to corns, bunions, and abraded surfaces. The plaster-mass may be used in the preparation of adhesive bandages for the treatment of chronic leg ulcers in ambulant patients and of varicose veins. It is also used for plasters in cases where self-adhesive plaster-masses produce skin reactions.

Preparations

Diachylon Elastic Adhesive Bandage *(B.P.C. 1973).* Elastic Diachylon Bandage. Elastic cloth spread evenly with a diachylon mass. It should be warmed before application to the skin.

Ventilated Diachylon Elastic Adhesive Bandage *(B.P.C. 1973).* Ventilated Elastic Diachylon Bandage. Elastic cloth spread evenly with a diachylon mass so as to leave along its length strips of unspread fabric. The area of the unspread portions, excluding any margins, does not exceed 50% of the total area. It should be warmed before application to the skin.

NOTE. The diachylon mass for the above bandages, consists of lead soaps of the higher fatty acids to which suitable adhesives are added, and contains not less than 26.5% of Pb, calculated as PbO, with reference to the mass dried for 3 hours at 105°.

Lestreflex *(Seton, UK: Bateman-Jackson, UK).* A brand of Diachylon Elastic Adhesive Bandage and of Ventilated Diachylon Elastic Adhesive Bandage.

5303-d

Manganese.

Mn = 54.938.

CAS — 7439-96-5.

A greyish- or reddish-white, hard and brittle, metal. Although manganese deficiency has not been proved to cause disease in man, traces of manganese are considered to be essential to life. The daily human requirement is probably 2 to 3 mg.

Adverse Effects. Acute poisoning due to ingestion is rare owing to poor absorption. Symptoms of chronic poisoning include lethargy, oedema, and extrapyramidal effects, and have been associated with manganese-contaminated drinking water.

Chronic poisoning from inhalation of manganese dusts is an industrial hazard. Irritation and infections of the respiratory tract, headache, sleep disturbances, dermatitis, irritability, and liver enlargement occur, followed by a progressive deterioration in the central nervous system similar to the parkinsonian syndrome. Symptoms include weakness in the legs, increased muscle tone, hand tremor, slurred speech, muscular cramps, spastic gait, fixed facial expression, and mental deterioration.

There have also been reports of sialorrhoea, excessive perspiration, sexual disturbances, and blood changes. Very rarely hypothyroidism may occur.

Maximum permissible atmospheric concentration 5 mg per m^3. Maximum permissible atmospheric concentration of fumes 1 mg per m^3.

For a brief review of manganese deficiency and toxic effects see Report of a WHO Expert Group on Trace Elements in Human Nutrition, *Tech. Rep. Ser. Wld Hlth Org. No. 532,* 1973, 34.

For reports of industrial poisoning by manganese, see P. Schuler *et al., Ind. Med. Surg.,* 1957, *26,* 167; M. Wasserman and G. Mihail, *Acta Med. leg. soc.,* 1964, *17,* 61; S. Abd El Naby and M. Hassanein, *J. Neurol. Neurosurg. Psychiat.,* 1965, *28,* 282; K. A. Eiso, *Gig. Truda prof. Zabol.,* 1966, *10,* 39, per *Bull. Hyg., Lond.,* 1966, *41,* 1078; L. S. Khybyn, *Gig. Truda prof. Zabol.,* 1967, *11,* 51, per *Abstr. Wld Med.,* 1968, *42,* 327; M. L. Rawal, *Indian J. ind. Med.,* 1968, *14,* 41, per *Abstr. Hyg.,* 1969, *44,* 991; G. C. Cotzias *et al., Neurology, Minneap.,* 1968, *18,* 376; G. C. Cotzias, *ibid.,* 1155; S. V. Chandra *et al., Environ. Res.,* 1974, *7,* 374, per *Abstr. Hyg.,* 1975, *50,* 728.

Treatment of Adverse Effects. There is no specific therapy for manganese poisoning. Sodium calciumedetate has been used in the treatment of manganese poisoning but has been reported to be ineffective. Levodopa has been used to counter the neurological signs and symptoms of manganese poisoning (see p.886); amantadine (p.891) and hydroxytryptophan (p.1718) have also been given.

Sodium calciumedetate 2 g intravenously was given daily for 5 days to 6 men with manganese poisoning and repeated if necessary. Symptoms were relieved but not abolished and patients remained unfit for routine work.— F. Lautier, *Presse méd.,* 1963, *71,* 661, per *Pharmacy Dig.,* 1963, *27,* 508.

A man working in an atmosphere of manganese fumes developed an extrapyramidal disease and an extensor plantar response. The urine contained 4.58 µg of manganese per litre. A fellow worker, with a slightly higher concentration of manganese in the urine, had less severe symptoms. Both patients improved after treatment with disodium edetate, when concentrations of manganese in the urine increased to about 145 and 169 µg per litre respectively.— Whitlock C.M. *et al., Am. ind. Hyg. Ass. J.,* 1966, *27,* 454, per *Bull. Hyg., Lond.,* 1967, *42,* 614.

Uses. Manganese salts are occasionally used for their supposed effect in increasing the haematinic action of iron in the treatment of microcytic anaemia.

A review of the actions of manganese as a trace element covering the effects of deficiency, its pharmacokinetics, and its toxicity.— R. E. Burch *et al., Clin. Chem.,* 1975, *21,* 501.

Anaemia. For a report on the use of manganese in anaemia, see V. A. Bojko, *Terap. Arkh.,* 1964, *36,* 104, per *Abstr. Wld Med.,* 1965, *37,* 185.

Deficiency. After receiving a dietary regimen deficient in vitamin K, a volunteer was found to have an inadequate blood-clotting response to subsequent administration of vitamin K and was assumed to have a secondary deficiency, which on retrospective analysis appeared to be that of manganese. Other symptoms during the presumed deficiency included mild evanescent dermatitis, reddening of hair and beard, slowed growth of hair, nails and beard, occasional nausea and vomiting, coincident decrease of serum concentrations of phospholipids and triglycerides, and moderate weight loss; overall protein synthesis was not disturbed.— E. A. Doisy, in *Proceedings of the University of Missouri's Sixth Annual Conference on Trace Substances in Environmental Health,* D.D. Hemphill (Ed.), Columbia, University of Missouri, 1973, p. 193.

Some forms of convulsive disorders in children might be linked with manganese deficiency of the mother during pregnancy. The effects of the administration of manganese to children with convulsive disorders and low blood-manganese concentrations were being studied.— Y. Tanaka *et al., J. Am. med. Ass.,* 1977, *238,* 1805.

Further references: A. S. Prasad, *Trace Elements and Iron in Human Metabolism,* Chichester, John Wiley, 1978.

Parenteral nutrition. Manganese deficiency in total parenteral nutrition has not been explored, but in patients with liver disease, blood-manganese concentrations may rise to unacceptable levels, especially if solutions high in manganese are used.— K. N. Jeejeebhoy, in *Current Concepts in Parenteral Nutrition,* J.M. Greep *et al.* (Ed.), The Hague, Martinus Mijhoff, 1977, 351.

Parkinsonism. Of 15 patients with tardive and withdrawal dyskinesia who were treated with manganese chelate, 7 were cured completely within a day, 3 were much improved, 4 improved, and only 1 did not obtain any noticeable benefit.— R. A. Kunin (letter), *Am. J. Psychiat.,* 1976, *133,* 105.

5304-n

Manganese Sulphate *(B.P., B.P. Vet.).* Mang. Sulph. Manganese (II) sulphate tetrahydrate.

$MnSO_4,4H_2O = 223.1.$

CAS — 7785-87-7 (anhydrous); 10101-68-5 (tetrahydrate).

Pharmacopoeias. In *Br.*

Pale pink odourless or almost odourless crystals or crystalline powder with a somewhat saline acid taste. **Soluble** 1 in 1 of water; practically insoluble in alcohol. A 5% solution in water has a pH of not less than 5. Solutions are **sterilised** by autoclaving or by filtration.

Adverse Effects and Treatment. As for Manganese (above).

Uses. Manganese sulphate is an ingredient of Compound Ferrous Sulphate Tablets *B.P.C. 1973.* Doses of 0.5 to 2.5 mg have been given. It is also used in veterinary practice to prevent or treat manganese deficiency.

5306-m

Mercury *(B.P.C. 1963).*

Hydrargyrum; Hydrarg.; Hydrargyrum Depuratum; Quicksilver; Mercure; Quecksilber; Mercurio.

Hg = 200.59.

CAS — 7439-97-6.

Pharmacopoeias. In *Aust., Belg., Hung., Ind., It., Mex., Pol., Port., Span.,* and *Swiss.*

A shining, silvery white, very mobile liquid, easily divisible into globules, which readily volatilises on heating. Wt per ml about 13.55 g.

Practically **insoluble** in water, alcohol, and hydrochloric acid; soluble in nitric acid and in boiling sulphuric acid, forming solutions of mercuric and mercurous salts. **Incompatible** with aluminium.

Adverse Effects. Acute mercurial poisoning is generally caused by ingestion of soluble mercury compounds. The immediate symptoms include a metallic taste, thirst, severe abdominal pain, vomiting, ashy discoloration of the mouth and pharynx, and bloody diarrhoea. Recovery may follow treatment of early symptoms, but the local intestinal reaction may be severe enough to cause profound shock and death from circulatory failure. Stomatitis develops after about 24 hours and acute nephritis, anuria, and death may occur within 1 to 2 weeks. Colitis with prolonged diarrhoea and haemorrhage may also occur.

Stomatitis, salivation, metallic taste, diarrhoea, pneumonitis, and other respiratory symptoms, and renal damage with anuria, may follow inhalation of a high concentration of mercury vapour.

Chronic mercury poisoning may result from inhalation of mercury vapour, skin contact with mercury or mercury compounds, or ingestion of poorly soluble mercury salts over prolonged periods. It is characterised by tremor, motor and sensory disturbances, gastro-intestinal symptoms, dermatitis, liver and kidney damage, anaemia, mercurialentis, nephritis, and mental deterioration. Excessive salivation and loosening of teeth are signs of advanced poisoning. A blue line may be present on the gums.

Organic mercurial compounds such as methylmercury produce similar toxic effects, but they have a more selective action on the central nervous system and cause permanent damage.

Hypersensitivity and allergy to mercury and mercurial compounds has been reported.

Mercurialentis has been reported in patients treated with eye-drops containing an organomercurial preservative.

The use of mercury or mercurial salts in aperients or in dusting-powders and ointments in infants is the aetiological factor in acrodynia (pink disease).

The maximum permissible atmospheric concentrations of mercury are 50 µg per m^3 (all forms except alkyl) and 10 µg per m^3 (alkyl compounds).

Action and environmental distribution. A detailed review of the pharmacology and toxicology of mercury, including an account of its distribution in the environment.— H. G. Petering and L. B. Tepper, *Pharmac. Ther.,* 1976, *1,* 131.

Some other studies, reviews, and reports on the toxicology of mercury and mercury compounds.— T. W. Clarkson, *A. Rev. Pharmac.*, 1972, *12*, 375; M. M. Joselow *et al.*, *Ann. intern. Med.*, 1972, *76*, 119; *ibid.*, 779; *Environmental Health Criteria 1. Mercury*, Geneva, Wld Hlth Org., 1976, per *Abstr. Hyg.*, 1977, *52*, 614; A Report of an Inter-Departmental Working Group on Heavy Metals, *Pollution Paper No. 10*, London, HM Stationery Office, 1976; L. W. Chang, *Environ. Res.*, 1977, *14*, 329; I. M. Trachtenberg, *Z. ges. Hyg.*, 1977, *23*, 437; *Br. med. J.*, 1978, *1*, 599.

Sources of poisoning. A 23-year-old woman committed suicide by injecting 1 to 2 ml of metallic mercury into her forearm. She died 31 days after the injection. Mercury was detected in the blood, urine, kidneys, liver, lungs, spleen, heart, bile, colon, spinal cord, and brain on postmortem examination.— H. R. M. Johnson and O. Koumides, *Br. med. J.*, 1967, *1*, 340.

A 21-year-old woman injected 20 to 40 g of metallic mercury subcutaneously into her thighs. Maximum mercury concentrations of 180 μg per kg of blood and of 270 μg per litre of urine were found and both fell to normal after excision of the mercury deposits in the thighs. She was given 2 courses of dimercaprol, 6 mg per kg body-weight daily, each for 1 week. No clinical features of acute or chronic mercury poisoning developed.— D. M. Hill, *Br. med. J.*, 1967, *1*, 342.

A 48-year-old man died after the rupture within the nasopharynx of a bag containing 10 ml of mercury. About 4.5 ml of mercury was immediately recovered and the remainder was distributed in the lungs, stomach, and duodenum; a total of 8.2 ml was eventually recovered. The patient developed symptoms compatible with acute mercury poisoning and died from severe bronchial haemorrhage.— J. E. Zimmerman, *J. Am. med. Ass.*, 1969, *208*, 2158.

A 21-year-old boxer developed mercury granuloma with systemic absorption after injecting mercury into his arm in the mistaken belief that quicksilver would make his punches quicker.— F. B. Kern *et al.* (letter), *J. Am. med. Ass.*, 1972, *222*, 88. A 14-year-old boxer was admitted to hospital with general malaise, pleuritic chest pain, and shortness of breath of 24 hours' duration; he had received an intravenous injection of mercury 20 ml two days previously in the mistaken belief that it would strengthen his muscles. Treatment included nasal oxygen, analgesics, and intravenous fluids. X-ray examination revealed metallic densities in the lungs, the abdomen, and right ventricle. He showed gradual clinical improvement over 2 weeks and despite the massive dose showed no evidence of renal or hepatic damage. Eleven months later metallic densities were still seen in both lung fields. The patient had previously received intramuscular injections of mercury.— B. Celli and M. A. Khan, *New Engl. J. Med.*, 1976, *295*, 883.

Some other reports of mercury poisoning and its sources: J. F. Copplestone and D. A. McArthur, *Br. J. ind. Med.*, 1967, *24*, 77 (jewellery manufacture); H. B. Devlin and M. Sudlow, *Br. med. J.*, 1967, *1*, 347 (embolism from a syringe); V. Parameshvara, *Br. J. ind. Med.*, 1967, *24*, 73 (electric display sign); P. E. Pierce *et al.*, *J. Am. med. Ass.*, 1972, *220*, 1439 (contaminated pork); L. Wallach, *New Engl. J. Med.*, 1972, *287*, 178 (aspiration); M. E. Efrusy and W. O. Dobbins, *Am. J. dig. Dis.*, 1974, *19*, 373 (ruptured Cantor tube); H. Wüstner and C. E. Orfanos, *Dt. med. Wschr.*, 1975, *100*, 1694 (hair bleaches); V. J. Dzau *et al.*, *J. Am. med. Ass.*, 1977, *238*, 1531 (aspiration); W. K. Stewart *et al.*, *Br. J. ind. Med.*, 1977, *34*, 26 (laboratory use); J. E. Cummins and B. E. Nesbitt (letter), *Nature*, 1978, *273*, 96 (nucleic acid electrophoresis).

Spillage. A discussion of the problems of dealing with mercury spillage.— *Lancet*, 1975, *1*, 1021.

Allergy. Mercury-induced dermatitis in a 27-year-old woman caused by amalgam dental fillings.— J. Thomson and J. A. Russell, *Br. J. Derm.*, 1970, *82*, 292.

Other reports of hypersensitivity associated with mercury: J. D. Forbes and L. J. Miedler, *J. occup. Med.*, 1967, *9*, 368; J. K. Morgan, *Br. J. clin. Pract.*, 1968, *22*, 261; L. J. Miedler and J. D. Forbes, *Archs environ. Hlth*, 1968, *17*, 960.

Dentistry. Recommendations by the Commission on Dental Materials, Instruments, Equipment and Therapeutics on dental mercury hygiene.— *Br. dent. J.*, 1978, *144*, 87.

Reports and studies on the hazards of mercury exposure in dentistry: J. M. A. Lenihan *et al.*, *Br. dent. J.*, 1973, *135*, 365; J. T. Stevens *et al.*, *Milit. Med.*, 1975, *140*, 114; D. P. Merfield *et al.*, *Br. dent. J.*, 1976, *141*, 179; R. R. White and R. L. Brandt, *J. Am. dent. Ass.*, 1976, *92*, 1204; R. Wronski and F. Hartmann, *Dt. med. Wschr.*, 1977, *102*, 323; J. D. Cross *et al.* (letter), *Lancet*, 1978, *2*, 312.

Root fillings. There was no evidence of any danger from the mercury amalgam in dental root fillings.— *Br. med. J.*, 1973, *3*, 402. But see above under Allergy.

Diagnosis of mercury poisoning. Mercurialentis was considered a useful diagnostic aid to poisoning with mercury vapour.— V. Parameshvara, *Br. J. ind. Med.*, 1967, *24*, 73.

Effects on body systems. Detectable biological changes have been reported in workers exposed to less than 50 μg of mercury vapour per m³.— R. R. Lauwerys and J. P. Buchet, *Archs environ. Hlth*, 1973, *27*, 65, per *J. Am. med. Ass.*, 1973, *225*, 770.

Cytogenetic. Findings of increased chromosome aberrations in workers exposed to different compounds of mercury.— L. Verschaeve *et al.*, *Environ. Res.*, 1976, *12*, 306, per *J. Am. med. Ass.*, 1977, *237*, 1882.

Haematopoietic. A 59-year-old man employed filling thermometers with mercury developed aplastic anaemia and died. His urine contained 1.01 mg of mercury per litre.— D. R. Ryrie *et al.* (letter), *Br. med. J.*, 1970, *1*, 499. A similar report.— D. R. Wilson (letter), *ibid.*, 1966, *2*, 1534.

Nervous. A neuromuscular disorder responsive to neostigmine was discovered during electrophysiological testing of Iraqi patients poisoned by methylmercury. Neostigmine therapy resulted in considerable clinical improvement.— H. Rustam *et al.*, *Archs environ. Hlth*, 1975, *30*, 190, per *J. Am. med. Ass.*, 1975, *232*, 90.

Effects on children. The syndrome of acrodynia (pink disease), with symptoms of sweat rash, oedema of the extremities, photophobia, wasting, weakness, tachycardia, and diminished reflexes which affected young children was shown in the 1950's to be related to the administration of mercury in teething powders or to the absorption of mercury from dusting-powders and ointments. Many fatalities occurred. The prescribing of mercury for its purgative effects, as Mercury with Chalk or as mercurous chloride, and the administration of mercury in teething remedies was deprecated and the Council of the Pharmaceutical Society of Great Britain advised pharmacists to warn their customers of the dangers of preparations containing mercury and to use great discretion in the supply of such preparations.

Two instances of acrodynia in children were apparently due to ingestion of mercury. One child was given a total of 180 mg of mercury in the form of 'chocolate worm cake' and the other was given 180 mg of mercury in the form of mercury with chalk powders, and 3 Steedmans powders probably containing mercury. Both children recovered.— C. C. Forsyth and D. C. L. Savage (letter), *Br. med. J.*, 1968, *1*, 767.

Mercury poisoning occurred in 2 children, one of whom had the classical symptoms of acrodynia, after treatment of their eczema with folk-cures consisting of a belt of damp lint containing metallic mercury worn by one, and a yellow ointment containing metallic mercury 2% applied liberally to the skin of the other.— E. A. Magill, *Ulster med. J.*, 1975, *44*, 166.

Of 40 children with symptoms of mercury poisoning after the ingestion of mercury-treated grain in Iraq in 1971–2, follow-up 2 years later showed recovery of 6 of 6 with mild poisoning, 7 of 10 with moderate poisoning, 1 of 13 with severe poisoning, and none of 11 with very severe poisoning.— L. Amin-Zaki *et al.*, *Br. med. J.*, 1978, *1*, 613.

Other reports of mercury poisoning in children: J. B. P. Stephenson (letter), *Br. med. J.*, 1966, *1*, 1110; B. Egan and B. McNicholl (letter), *ibid.*, 1482.

For other reports of acrodynia, see Ammoniated Mercury, p.497 and Mercurous Chloride, p.940. See also Thiomersal, p.576.

Mercury in Food. Mercury is widely distributed in nature and is concentrated by some plants, by plankton, and by fish.

A review of alkylmercury contamination of foods. The estimated fatal dose of alkylmercury was approximately 1 mg daily, over a period of probably several weeks. The estimated acceptable daily intake was approximately 100 μg daily.— *J. Am. med. Ass.*, 1971, *215*, 287.

In certain countries foods were contaminated with mercury to an extent likely to cause intoxication. Fish and shellfish were foods likely to be affected; fish and shellfish from contaminated areas might contain more than 1 ppm compared with less than 0.1 ppm for fish from uncontaminated areas.— Fourteenth Report of FAO/WHO Expert Committee on Food Additives, *Tech. Rep. Ser. Wld Hlth Org. No. 462*, 1971.

Provisional tolerable weekly intake of mercury for man: up to 300 μg per person or 5 μg per kg body-weight. Not more than 200 μg per person or 3.3 μg per kg should be present as methylmercury expressed as mercury.— Sixteenth Report of FAO/WHO Expert Committee on Food Additives, *Tech. Rep. Ser. Wld Hlth Org. No. 505*, 1972. See also *Fd Add. Ser. Wld Hlth Org. No. 4*, 1972; Twenty-second Report of Joint FAO/WHO Expert Committee on Food Additives, *Tech. Rep. Ser. Wld Hlth Org. No. 631*, 1978.

Analysis of foodstuffs showed that in the UK the average mercury concentration in the diet was about 5 μg per kg which provided an estimated daily intake of 5 to 10 μg per person.— *Survey of Mercury in Food*, Minist. Agric. Fish. Fd, London, HM Stationery Office, 1971 and 1973.

A discussion of mercury in fish.— T. H. Jukes, *J. Am. med. Ass.*, 1975, *233*, 1001.

Reports on the Conference held in Baghdad, Iraq, 9–13 September 1974, on intoxication caused by alkylmercury-treated seed.— *Bull. Wld Hlth Org.*, 1976, *53*, *Suppl.*, 1–138. A summary of the main findings and recommendations of the Conference.— S. B. Skerfving and J. F. Copplestone, *ibid.*, *54*, 101.

Treatment of Adverse Effects. Acute poisoning due to the ingestion of soluble mercury compounds should be treated by immediate gastric aspiration and lavage preferably using 250 ml of a 5% solution of sodium formaldehyde sulphoxylate and leaving a further 100 or 200 ml in the stomach; alternatively a lavage solution of raw egg white may be used. Large quantities of milk or charcoal may also be given. Dimercaprol (see p.383) therapy should be started immediately. Penicillamine (see p.387) is an alternative form of chelation therapy but its role in acute mercury poisoning is less well established.

Water and electrolytes lost by vomiting and diarrhoea should be replaced, and adequate kidney function should be maintained; in the event of renal failure peritoneal dialysis or haemodialysis may be required.

A purgative such as sodium sulphate 30 g in 250 ml of water has also been advocated, and analgesics may be required.

Mercurials on the skin should be removed by copious washing with soap and water.

Response to the treatment of chronic mercurial poisoning is slow, and chelation therapy may promote the excretion of mercury without benefiting the clinical symptoms; administration of acetylpenicillamine (see p.380) has been reported to be more effective than dimercaprol and less toxic than penicillamine.

For reports on the treatment of mercury poisoning, see Dimercaprol, p.383, Succimer, p.393, and Penicillamine, p.388.

Dialysis. Haemodialysis could be life-saving in acute mercurial poisoning.— L. Sanchez-Sicilia *et al.*, *Ann. intern. Med.*, 1963, *59*, 692. Haemodialysis was considered to have contributed little to the recovery of a 14-year-old boy who had ingested mercuric cyanide.— E. P. Leumann and H. Brandenberg, *Clin. Toxicol.*, 1977, *11*, 301.

Resin. Studies in *mice* indicated that addition of a synthetic polythiol resin to food considerably increased the rate of excretion of mercury following administration of methylmercury and considerably reduced the absorption of methylmercury. It was considered that the enhanced excretion was caused by interruption of enterohepatic recycling.— T. W. Clarkson *et al.*, *Archs environ. Hlth*, 1973, *26*, 173. See also *idem*, *Fedn Proc.*, 1971, *30*, 543.

Precautions. Mercury and mercurials should not be given to infants or applied to their skin as they may cause acrodynia (pink disease). Maternal ingestion of mercury can cause damage to the foetus.

Mercurial compounds have interfered with protein-bound iodine estimations of thyroid function.— *Adverse Drug React. Bull.*, 1972, June, 104.

Mercury compounds could cause tar-coloured discoloration of the faeces.— R. B. Baran and B. Rowles, *J. Am. pharm. Ass.*, 1973, *NS13*, 139.

Pregnancy and the neonate. Some reports on adverse effects on the infants of mothers exposed to mercurials during pregnancy: R. D. Snyder, *New Engl. J. Med.*, 1971, *284*, 1014; *idem*, *Archs Neurol., Chicago*, 1972, *26*, 379; L. Amin-Zaki *et al.*, *Pediatrics*, 1974, *54*, 587; L. W. Chang *et al.*, *Environ. Res.*, 1977, *13*, 171; *idem*, *14*, 414.

Mercury is reported to be excreted in breast milk and can have adverse effects on the suckling infant.— T. E. O'Brien, *Am. J. Hosp. Pharm.*, 1974, *31*, 844.

A discussion on the possible danger to the foetus of maternal exposure to mercury.— *J. Am. med. Ass.*, 1975, *232*, 1105.

Absorption and Fate. There is little evidence to show that significant amounts of mercury are absorbed from globules in the gastro-intestinal tract but some absorption may follow mercury ingested in a finely divided form. Finely divided mercury is also absorbed through the skin and from the lungs and mercury vapour is also absorbed from the lungs. Mercury accumulates in the body and may be deposited in bone.

Soluble inorganic salts of mercury are readily absorbed from the gastro-intestinal tract and can also be absorbed through the skin. The mercury is distributed throughout the soft tissues with high concentrations in the kidneys; it is mainly excreted in the urine and through the colon, but traces are found in most body secretions. Most of the absorbed mercury is excreted within a week but traces may continue to be eliminated for many months.

Alkyl mercury compounds are also readily absorbed from both the gastro-intestinal and the respiratory tracts. They are distributed throughout the soft tissues with initial very high concentrations in the liver and kidneys and subsequent marked uptake by the nervous system. The half-life of methylmercury has been estimated to be 70 to 100 days, most being excreted in the faeces with extensive enterohepatic recycling.

Mercury diffuses across the placenta and is excreted in breast milk.

For details of the absorption, excretion, and distribution of elemental mercury, inorganic mercury, and organic mercury, see H. G. Petering and L. B. Tepper, *Pharmac. Ther.*, 1976, *1*, 131.

Ocular penetration of mercury (in thiomersal) from ophthalmic preservatives.— A. F. Winder *et al.*, *Lancet*, 1980, *2*, 237.

Uses. The hazards associated with mercury generally outweigh any therapeutic benefit and its clinical use has largely been abandoned. Mercurial diuretics such as Mersalyl (see p.607) are still occasionally employed but their use has generally been superseded by more modern diuretics, such as the thiazides. Ointments containing mercurials, such as Ammoniated Mercury (see p.497) have been used for some resistant skin disorders.

The ionisable mercury salts and certain organic compounds of mercury have been used as disinfectants, and some mercury salts are effective parasiticides and fungicides. The organic mercurials are also used as preservatives in eye-drops and injection solutions and for sterilisation of such solutions by heating with a bactericide.

A nitrated oxide of mercury, prepared by precipitation with ammonium hydroxide from a solution of mercury in nitric acid (Mercurius Solubilis; Merc. Sol.) is used in homoeopathic medicine.

It was considered unwise to use seed dressings of mercurial fungicides, especially alkylmercury compounds which accumulated in the nervous system causing irreversible damage.— Report of the 1972 Joint FAO/WHO Meeting on Pesticide Residues in Food, *Tech. Rep. Ser. Wld Hlth Org. No. 525*, 1973.

Transferable plasmid-mediated mercury resistance was detected in *Escherichia coli* isolated in Japan.— H. Nakahara *et al.*, *Antimicrob. Ag. Chemother.*, 1977, *11*, 999.

5307-b

Mercuric Chloride *(B.P.C. 1973, Eur. P.).* Mercuric Chlor.; Hydrargyri Perchloridum; Hydrarg. Perchlor.; Corrosive Sublimate; Mercury Bichloride; Mercury Perchloride; Hydrargyrum Bichloratum; Mercurique (Chlorure); Quecksilberchlorid; Bicloruro de Mercurio; Cloreto Mercúrico.

$HgCl_2$=271.5.

CAS — 7487-94-7.

Pharmacopoeias. In *Arg., Aust., Belg., Braz., Cz., Eur., Fr., Ger., It., Jap., Jug., Mex., Neth., Nord., Pol., Port., Rus., Span., Swiss,* and *Turk.*

A heavy, colourless or white, odourless, crystalline powder or crystalline masses. M.p. about 280°; it volatilises above 300°. **Soluble** 1 in 15 of water, 1 in 3 of alcohol, 1 in 25 of ether, and 1 in 15 of glycerol. A solution in water is acid to litmus. **Incompatible** with alkalis, alkaloids (especially if iodides are present), lead acetate, silver nitrate, proteins, and vegetable astringents. Solutions made with tap water may yield a slight deposit on standing. **Protect** from light.

For precautions to be taken in preparing and storing antiseptic solutions, see under Phenol, p.570.

NOTE. Solutions of mercuric chloride for external use should be coloured with indigo carmine as a safety precaution. When dispensing mercuric chloride, steel instruments such as spatulas must not be used, and surgical instruments must not be put into solutions of mercuric chloride. Solutions of mercuric chloride and other mercurials should not be allowed to come into contact with aluminium, for instance in screw caps or collapsible tubes.

Colouring of solutions. Mercuric chloride solution (0.1%) could be coloured by the addition of 0.1 ml of a 0.5% solution of methylene blue to 10 ml of solution, but a precipitate was formed when stronger solutions of mercuric chloride were used; 0.1 ml of indigo carmine solution (0.5%) or of trypan blue solution (0.343%) imparted a suitable colour to 10 ml of mercuric chloride solution, and no precipitation occurred in mercuric chloride solutions up to 2.5%.— K. J. Steel and W. R. L. Brown, *Pharm. J.*, 1957, *1*, 60.

Incompatibility. A 1% solution yielded a precipitate with phenol 0.5% or thiomersal 0.005%, a turbidity with benzalkonium chloride 0.02%, and a slight turbidity with phenethyl alcohol 0.5%.— S. W. Goldstein, *J. Am. pharm. Ass., pract. Pharm. Edn*, 1953, *14*, 498.

Adverse Effects, Treatment, Precautions, and Absorption and Fate. As for Mercury, pp.937-8. Mercuric chloride is readily absorbed from the gastro-intestinal tract and its effects are usually evident within 10 to 15 minutes.

Allergy. Of 877 persons with dermatitis or eczema submitted to patch testing with 0.1% aqueous solution of mercuric chloride, 4.5% gave a positive reaction.— E. Rudzki and D. Kleiniewska, *Br. J. Derm.*, 1970, *83*, 543. See also J. Hartung, *Berufsdermatosen*, 1965, *13*, 116; A. M. Kligman, *J. invest. Derm.*, 1966, *47*, 393.

Cancer implantations, prophylaxis. No signs of mercurialism occurred in 6 patients following the use of about 1 litre of a 0.2% solution of mercuric chloride to wash out the rectal stump and a further 300 ml to mop out the lumen of the colon and other tissues (these being dried up before the abdomen was closed) to prevent implantation of cancer cells during surgery for adenocarcinoma of the rectum. In 1 patient a maximum urinary concentration of 232 µg of mercury per litre followed the treatment.— H. B. Devlin (letter), *Br. med. J.*, 1967, *3*, 679. Because of the danger of renal tubular damage, illustrated by a case report, it was recommended that mercuric chloride solution should not be used as an irrigating agent in the peritoneal cavity.— J. C. Gingell *et al.* (letter), *ibid.*, 867. A patient sustained a superficial chemical burn due to interaction between mercuric chloride solution (used to reduce exfoliated malignant cells during rectal surgery) and an aluminium diathermy plate electrode beneath the patient.— A. G. Nash (letter), *ibid.*, 1973, *4*, 783.

Uses. The mercuric ion forms insoluble complexes with proteins and, by reason of this action on the proteins of bacterial cells, mercuric chloride is an antibacterial substance. To some extent its effect can be reversed by sulphydryl compounds. Its use is limited by its toxicity, its precipitating action on proteins, its irritant action on raw surfaces, its corrosive action on metals, and by the fact that its activity is greatly reduced in the presence of excreta or body fluids.

A 0.1% solution was formerly used as a disinfectant for the skin; its action was increased if alcohol (70%) was used as the vehicle.

Solutions of 0.001 to 0.025% were formerly used for irrigation or cleansing of wounds and 0.001% solutions for vaginal irrigation. Stronger concentrations should not be applied to raw surfaces or mucous membranes because mercuric chloride is rapidly absorbed and may cause acute toxicity. Salicylic Acid and Mercuric Chloride Lotion *B.P.C. 1973* has been used for the treatment of follicular infections.

Preparations

Harrington's Solution. Mercuric chloride 80 mg, alcohol (90%) 64 ml, hydrochloric acid 6 ml, and water 30 ml. Formerly used for pre-operative skin disinfection.

Mercuric Chloride Solution *(B.P. 1953).* Liq. Hydrarg. Perchlor.; Van Swieten's Solution. Mercuric chloride 0.1% in water. Protect from light.

5308-v

Mercuric Cyanide *(B.P.C. 1949).* Hydrargyri Cyanidum; Hydrarg. Cyanid.; Mercury Cyanide; Cyanuretum Hydrargyri; Hydrargyrum Cyanatum; Mercurique (Cyanure); Quecksilberzyanid; Cianeto de Mercúrio.

$Hg(CN)_2$=252.6.

CAS — 592-04-1.

Pharmacopoeias. In *Belg., Fr., Port.,* and *Span.*

Colourless or white, odourless, prismatic crystals. **Soluble** 1 in 13 of water, 1 in 3 of boiling water, 1 in 20 of alcohol, and 1 in 4 of glycerol; slightly soluble in ether. It is not decomposed by alkalis but it is decomposed by dilute hydrochloric acid with the evolution of hydrogen cyanide. **Protect** from light.

Adverse Effects, Treatment, and Precautions. As for Mercury pp.937-8.

Uses. Mercuric cyanide has the general properties of mercuric salts and was formerly used by local application for its disinfectant actions. It is not so irritating to the tissues as mercuric chloride but it is doubtful whether its disinfectant effect is as great. Solutions of 0.025 to 0.05% were formerly used as eye lotions.

5309-g

Red Mercuric Iodide *(B.P.C. 1954).* Hydrargyri Iodidum Rubrum; Hydrarg. Iod. Rub.; Mercuric Iodide; Hydrargyri Iodidum Praecipitatum; Hydrargyrum Biiodatum; Iodure Mercurique; Quecksilberjodid; Biyoduro de Mercurio.

HgI_2=454.4.

CAS — 7774-29-0.

Pharmacopoeias. In *Arg., Belg., Hung., It., Mex., Nord., Port., Span.,* and *Swiss.*

A scarlet-red odourless powder. Practically **insoluble** in water and chloroform; soluble 1 in 300 of alcohol (90%), 1 in 50 of castor oil, 1 in 150 of ether, and 1 in 230 of olive oil; readily soluble in solutions of iodides. **Protect** from light.

For a note on the incompatibility of mercurials with metals, see under Mercuric Chloride, p.939.

Adverse Effects, Treatment, and Precautions. As for Mercury, pp.937-8.

Uses. Red mercuric iodide resembles mercuric chloride in its actions and uses. Because of its sparing solubility, solutions in water or alcohol are obtained by the addition of a nearly equal weight of potassium iodide to form the soluble complex salt, mercuric potassium iodide, K_2HgI_4=786.4.

Solutions containing 0.02 to 0.05% were formerly used for applications to wounds and strengths of 0.01 to 0.02% were used as vaginal douches; alcoholic solutions containing 0.05 to 0.2% were used for skin disinfection. Ointments containing 1 or 2% were used in the treatment of ringworm and lupus; stronger ointments are irritant. It was also formerly given by mouth as an adjunct in the treatment of syphilis.

A preparation containing red mercuric iodide was formerly marketed in Great Britain under the proprietary name Neko (*Parke, Davis*).

5310-f

Red Mercuric Oxide *(B.P.C. 1949).* Hydrargyri Oxidum Rubrum; Hydrarg. Oxid. Rub.; Red Precipitate; Oxyde Mercurique Rouge; Rotes Quecksilberoxyd; Oxido Rojo de Mercurio.

HgO=216.6.

Pharmacopoeias. In *Arg., Chin., Port.,* and *Span.*

Odourless, orange-red scales or red powder, chemically identical with yellow mercuric oxide. **Protect** from light.

Adverse Effects, Treatment, and Precautions. As for Mercury, pp.937-8. Ointments of mercuric oxide should not be used while iodides are being given internally.

Uses. Red mercuric oxide has properties similar to those of the yellow oxide. A 10% ointment was formerly used in seborrhoea and as a parasiticide. It was not used ophthalmically because it was too irritant.

5311-d

Yellow Mercuric Oxide *(B.P.C. 1973).* Hydrargyri Oxydum Flavum; Hydrargyri Oxidum Flavum; Yellow Precipitate; Mercurique (Oxyde) Jaune; Gelbes Quecksilberoxyd; Oxido Amarillo de Mercurio.
HgO=216.6.

CAS — 21908-53-2.

Pharmacopoeias. In *Arg., Aust., Belg., Chin., Cz., Fr., Hung., Ind., Int., It., Jug., Mex., Pol., Port., Roum., Rus.,* and *Span.*

An orange-yellow odourless amorphous powder. Practically **insoluble** in water and alcohol; soluble in hydrochloric and nitric acids. A 20% suspension is neutral to litmus. **Incompatible** with bromides, iodides, sulphides, and cocaine hydrochloride. **Sterilise** by maintaining at 150° for 1 hour. **Protect** from light.

Adverse Effects, Treatment, and Precautions. As for Mercury, pp.937-8. Ointments of mercuric oxide should not be used while iodides are being given internally.

Uses. Yellow mercuric oxide has antibacterial properties and has been used in eye ointments for the treatment of blepharitis and conjunctivitis. Such ointments should not be used for prolonged periods as mercury may be absorbed by the eye.

Preparations

Mercuric Oxide Eye Ointment *(B.P.C. 1973).* Oculentum Hydrargyri Oxidi. A sterile eye ointment containing yellow mercuric oxide in Eye Ointment Basis. Prolonged use may be injurious to the eyes. **Golden Eye Ointment** is a similar preparation.

Pagenstecher's Ointment. Yellow mercuric oxide 4% in yellow soft paraffin has usually been supplied for this ointment in Great Britain. It has been used as an eye ointment.

Proprietary Names

Gul-øjenslave *(DAK, Denm.)*; Ophtosept *(Winzer, Ger.)*; Poenhidrargil *(Poen, Arg.)*.

5312-n

Mercuric Oxycyanide *(B.P.C. 1968).* Hydrargyri Oxycyanidum; Hydrarg. Oxycyanid.; Hydrargyrum Oxycyanatum; Oxycyanure Mercurique; Quecksilberoxyzyanid; Cianuro Básico de Mercurio.

CAS — 1335-31-5.

Pharmacopoeias. In *Aust., Belg., Cz., Int., Nord., Pol., Port., Roum., Rus., Span.,* and *Swiss,* the specified limits of HgO and $Hg(CN)_2$ varying slightly from those of the *B.P.C. 1968.*

A white odourless crystalline powder containing 14.5 to 16.5% of HgO and 83.5 to 85.5% of $Hg(CN)_2$. Almost completely **soluble** 1 in 35 of water; completely soluble 1 in 200 of water; sparingly soluble in alcohol; practically insoluble in chloroform and ether. A solution in water is alkaline to litmus; a 0.5% solution is no more than slightly hazy. Solutions are **sterilised** by filtration or prepared by an aseptic technique. **Store** in airtight containers. Protect from light.
For precautions to be taken in preparing and storing antiseptic solutions, see under Phenol, p.570.
For a note on the incompatibility of mercurials with metals, see under Mercuric Chloride, p.939.

Preservative for eye-drops. Benzalkonium chloride 0.01%, phenylmercuric borate 0.005%, or chlorhexidine gluconate 0.02% were suitable preservatives for mercuric oxycyanide eye-drops sterilised by filtration.— M. Van Ooteghem, *Pharm. Tijdschr. Belg.,* 1968, *45,* 69.

Adverse Effects, Treatment, and Precautions. As for Mercury, pp.937-8, but cyanide poisoning may also be present owing to the liberation of hydrocyanic acid in the stomach.

Uses. Mercuric oxycyanide is a mercurial disinfectant which has the advantage over mercuric chloride that it is less irritating and does not precipitate proteins. It was formerly used to treat conjunctivitis, in concentrations of 0.01 to 0.02%. Solutions should be freshly prepared without the aid of heat.

Proprietary Names

Kviksølv *(DAK, Denm.)*; Ocal *(Sopar, Belg.)*.

5313-h

Red Mercuric Sulphide *(B.P.C. 1934).* Hydrarg. Sulphid. Rub.; Mercuric Sulphide; Chinese Red; Cinnabar; Vermilion; Sulfure Mercurique; Rotes Quecksilbersulfid.
HgS=232.7.

CAS — 1344-48-5.

Pharmacopoeias. In *Chin., Cz., Hung.,* and *Swiss.*

A brilliant scarlet-red, odourless, heavy powder which is very soft to the touch. Practically **insoluble** in water and alcohol. **Protect** from light.

Red mercuric sulphide was formerly used in the form of an ointment (1 or 2%) as an antiseptic in chronic skin diseases.

Ethiops Mineral (black mercuric sulphide), an impure mercuric sulphide containing much free mercury and sulphur, is used as a pigment for rubber and plastics.

5314-m

Mercurous Chloride *(B.P.C. 1959).* Hydrargyri Subchloridum; Hydrarg. Subchlor.; Calomel; Calomelanos; Mercury Monochloride; Mercury Subchloride; Mild Mercurous Chloride; Hydrargyrosi Chloridum; Hydrargyrum Chloratum (Mite); Mercurius Dulcis; Mercureux (Chlorure); Quecksilberchlorür; Protocloruro de Mercurio; Cloreto Mercuroso.
HgCl=236.0.

CAS — 7546-30-7 (HgCl); 10112-91-1 (Hg_2Cl_2).

Pharmacopoeias. In *Arg., Aust., Belg., Fr., Hung., Ind., It., Mex., Nord., Pol., Port.,* and *Span.*
Several pharmacopoeias include also Precipitated Mercurous Chloride (Hydrargyri Subchloridum Praecipitatum), a white amorphous powder, to which the synonym 'White Precipitate' (Praecipitatum Album) is given by some pharmacopoeias (cf. Ammoniated Mercury).

An odourless, heavy, dull white powder which becomes yellow when triturated or compressed. It gradually darkens when exposed to light. Practically **insoluble** in water, alcohol, ether, and cold dilute mineral acids. **Incompatible** with alkali halides and soaps, many oxidising and reducing substances, and some alkaloids including cocaine and pilocarpine. It is blackened by contact with alkalis due to the formation of mercurous oxide. It forms a cement-like substance with mucilages of acacia and tragacanth. **Protect** from light.

Adverse Effects, Treatment, and Precautions. As for Mercury, pp.937-8. Though mercurous chloride, being an insoluble salt, is relatively non-toxic, it may give rise to systemic mercury poisoning if purgation does not occur and it is retained in the intestinal tract. The administration of mercurous chloride to infants has resulted in acrodynia and numerous fatalities have been reported.

Mercurous chloride could cause yellowish-green discoloration of the faeces.— R. B. Baran and B. Rowles, *J. Am. pharm. Ass.,* 1973, *NS13,* 139.

Two patients who had taken a laxative preparation containing mercurous chloride daily for a number of years suffered dementia, erethism, colitis, renal failure, and death.— L. E. Davis *et al., Archs Neurol., Chicago,* 1974, *30,* 428, per *J. Am. med. Ass.,* 1974, *228,* 1446.

Effects on children. A fatal case of acrodynia was reported in a six-month-old baby who had received 9 out-of-date mercurial teething powders containing 26% of mercurous chloride. A survey showed that the incidence and mortality-rate of pink disease had fallen dramatically since teething powders containing mercury were withdrawn from the British market in 1954. These results were interpreted as conclusive evidence that this disease was caused by the ingestion of mercury.— J. G. Dathan and C. C. Harvey, *Br. med. J.,* 1965, *1,* 1181.
See also Mercury, p.938.

Absorption and Fate. When taken by mouth, mercurous chloride passes through the stomach unchanged but under the conditions in the small intestine a small proportion is converted to irritant mercurial compounds. The unchanged mercurous chloride is eliminated in the faeces but some of the compounds formed may be absorbed and are eliminated as described under Mercury, p.939.

Uses. Mercurous chloride was formerly used mainly as a purgative. It was also used as an ointment or dusting-powder. Like other mercury compounds, mercurous chloride has an antisyphilitic action and ointments containing 30 to 50% were formerly used as prophylactics against syphilis.

5315-b

Mercury Salicylate *(B.P.C. 1949).* Hydrargyri Salicylas; Hydrarg. Salicyl.; Acidum Hydrargyrosalicylicum.

CAS — 5970-32-1.

Pharmacopoeias. In *Port.* and *Span.*

A white or faintly pink, odourless, amorphous powder, containing about 57% of Hg.
Practically **insoluble** in water and organic solvents; soluble in solutions of alkali hydroxides and carbonates and in warm solutions of alkali halides, the cooled solution depositing double salts. **Incompatible** with potassium iodide. **Protect** from light.

Adverse Effects, Treatment, and Precautions. As for Mercury, pp.937-8.

Uses. Mercury salicylate was formerly employed in the treatment of syphilis.

5316-v

Silver.

Ag=107.868.

CAS — 7440-22-4.

A pure white, malleable and ductile metal.

Adverse Effects, Treatment, and Precautions. Although poisoning has been reported following the intravenous administration of colloidal silver suspensions, acute poisoning does not follow oral ingestion, because the poor solubility of most silver compounds and the propensity of silver to react with protein to form insoluble salts, limits its absorption. The acute toxicity of soluble silver salts is associated with their corrosive action (see under Silver Nitrate, below).
Chronic silver exposure causes argyria which is considered solely to be a cosmetic problem and consists of an irreversible slate-blue discoloration of the skin caused by deposition of granules of a silver compound and metallic silver in the connective tissues; early signs occur near the teeth (the silver line) and in the eyes. Chronic application of topical preparations of silver salts may lead to argyria.
Although silver gradually accumulates in the body, unlike lead and mercury there is no evidence that it is a cumulative poison. Dimercaprol does not have any role in the removal of excess silver from the body.
Maximum permissible atmospheric concentration of silver metal 100 µg per m^3 and of soluble silver compounds 10 µg per m^3.

Action and environmental distribution. A review of the chemistry, pharmacology, and biological effects of silver, including an account of its distribution in the environment.— H. G. Petering, *Pharmac. Ther.,* 1976, *1,* 127.
See also *Argyria, The Pharmacology of Silver,* W.R. Hill and D.M. Pillsbury, London, Baillière Tindall and Cox, 1939.

Photosensitivity. The administration of silver salts might cause photosensitivity.— J. Kalivas, *J. Am. med. Ass.,* 1969, *209,* 1706.

Absorption and Fate. Silver and its salts are poorly absorbed from the gastro-intestinal tract and from mucous membranes owing to silver's property of reacting with protein to form insoluble compounds. Any silver that is absorbed is widely distributed throughout the body with gradual accumulation over the years. Some silver is excreted in the faeces but only trace amounts have been found in the urine.

Uses. In the form of its salts silver is used topically for its antibacterial activity. Soluble salts of silver are also used topically as astringents and caustics.

5317-g

Colloidal Silver. Argentum Colloidale; Argent Colloïdal par Voie Chimique; Collargol; Kolloides Silber; Plata Coloidal; Prata Coloidal.

CAS — 9007-35-6.

Pharmacopoeias. In *Arg., Aust., Belg., Fr., Hung., Port., Roum., Span.,* and *Swiss.*

A preparation of silver in combination with protein, usually containing 70 to 80% of Ag.

Green or bluish-black plates with a metallic lustre and a bitter metallic taste. Slowly **soluble** in water, yielding a colloidal solution of silver; practically insoluble in most organic solvents. Aqueous solutions should be freshly made, and filtered. **Incompatible** with dilute mineral acids and concentrated salt solutions; in the latter case the precipitate dissolves on diluting with water. **Protect** from light.

Adverse Effects, Treatment, and Precautions. As for Silver (above).

Uses. Colloidal silver has been applied topically in the form of a solution or ointment, 1 to 15%.

Proprietary Names

Néo-Collargol *(Martinet, Fr.).*

5318-q

Methargen. Disilver(I) 3,3′-methylenebis(naphthalene-2-sulphonate).

$C_{21}H_{14}Ag_2O_6S_2$=642.2.

CAS — 53370-43-7.

Methargen is used as a disinfectant. It has been applied topically as a 1% solution, cream, or emulsion, or in the form of impregnated gauze.

An alternative to the use of paste bandaging in gravitational ulcers was a tulle impregnated with methargen (Viacutan) laid over the ulcer and held in place with a cotton elastic bandage. In 45 patients receiving this treatment, complete healing of ulcers was apparent in half the patients in less than 8 weeks, and in all patients within 20 weeks.— S. Allen, *Practitioner,* 1969, *202,* 278.

5319-p

Silver Acetate. Argenti Acetas.

CH_3COOAg=166.9.

CAS — 563-63-3.

Pharmacopoeias. In *Aust.* and *Hung.*

An odourless, white or slightly greyish, crystalline powder or lustrous acicular crystals. **Soluble** 1 in 100 of water and 1 in 35 of boiling water; freely soluble in dilute nitric acid. **Protect** from light.

Silver acetate has been used similarly to silver nitrate in creams, eye lotions, and eye-drops.

It has been used in antismoking tablets.

Argyria. Argyria due to the use of antismoking lozenges (Respaton).— D. MacIntyre *et al., Br. med. J.,* 1978, *2,* 1749. See also D. Shelton and R. Goulding (letter), *ibid.,* 1979, *1,* 267.

Burns. In 22 patients with burns, treatment with silver acetate cream 0.5% was as effective as treatment with 0.5% solutions of silver nitrate. Smaller supplements of salt were needed and methaemoglobinaemia did not occur with silver acetate.— H. R. Butcher *et al., J. Trauma,* 1969, *9,* 359, per *J. Am. med. Ass.,* 1969, *208,* 2539.

5320-n

Colloidal Silver Iodide. Argenti Iodidum Colloidale. Silver iodide rendered colloidally stable by the presence of gelatin.

CAS — 7783-96-2 (silver iodide).

A pale yellow granular solid with a faint odour, containing about 20% of AgI. Freely **dispersible** in water, forming a milky opalescent colloidal suspension; slowly dispersible in glycerol; insoluble in fixed oils. **Protect** from light. Solutions should be freshly prepared.

Adverse Effects, Treatment, and Precautions. As for Silver (above).

Uses. Solutions containing 5 to 40% of colloidal silver iodide have been employed in the treatment of infections of the mucous membranes. Ointments, usually containing 5%, have been used in inflammatory conditions of the eye, ear, and nose.

5321-h

Silver Nitrate *(B.P., Eur. P., U.S.P.).* Argenti Nitras; Nitrato de Plata; Nitrato de Prata.

$AgNO_3$=169.9.

CAS — 7761-88-8.

Pharmacopoeias. In all pharmacopoeias examined except *Braz.* and *Chin.*

Colourless odourless crystals or white crystalline powder with a bitter metallic taste. On exposure to air or light in the presence of organic matter, silver nitrate becomes grey or greyish-black.

Soluble 1 in 0.5 of water, 1 in 0.1 of boiling water, 1 in 27 to 30 of alcohol, and 1 in 6.5 of boiling alcohol; slightly soluble in ether and glycerol. A 4% solution in water has a pH of 5.4 to 6.4. A 2.74% solution in water is iso-osmotic with serum.

Incompatible with organic material, e.g. rose water, if used instead of water for preparing a lotion; also with tartaric acid, hydrocyanic acid, alkalis, halogen acids and their salts, phosphates, tannins, and astringent preparations. Solutions should be freshly prepared; they are **sterilised** by autoclaving or by filtration. **Store** in airtight non-metallic containers. Protect from light. Solutions should be stored in alkali-free bottles and protected from light.

Incompatibility. A 1% solution yielded a precipitate with thiomersal 0.005%.— S. W. Goldstein and E. F. Ryan, *Drug Stand.,* 1952, *20,* 133. A 1% solution yielded a precipitate with benzalkonium chloride 0.02%.— S. W. Goldstein, *J. Am. pharm. Ass., pract. Pharm. Edn,* 1953, *14,* 498.

Preservative for eye-drops. Phenylmercuric borate 0.005% was a suitable preservative for silver nitrate eye-drops sterilised by filtration.— M. Van Ooteghem, *Pharm. Tijdschr. Belg.,* 1968, *45,* 69.

Adverse Effects. Symptoms of poisoning stem from the corrosive action of silver nitrate and include pain in the mouth, sialorrhoea, diarrhoea, vomiting, coma, and convulsions. The tissues and vomit are black. About 2 to 10 g may be fatal.

Chronic application to mucous surfaces or open wounds leads to argyria, see under Silver (above).

Absorption of the nitrate and reduction to nitrite may cause methaemoglobinaemia. Reaction with chloride in the body may cause hypochloraemia with associated hyponatraemia.

Argyria. Extensive argyria, affecting the skin, nail-beds, and viscera, occurred in a 46-year-old woman following the excessive use, over 2.5 years, of silver nitrate sticks for bleeding gums.— J. P. Marshall and R. P. Schneider, *Archs Derm.,* 1977, *113,* 1077.

Conjunctivitis. Conjunctivitis had occurred in neonates given 1% silver nitrate topically for prophylaxis of gonococcal ophthalmia neonatorum. The use of old solutions of silver nitrate which have become more concentrated could lead to corneal ulceration and opacification.— *Adverse Drug React. Bull.,* 1972, Oct., 112. In a study involving 450 neonates the incidence of chemical conjunctivitis following instillation of a 1% solution of silver nitrate was significantly reduced by subsequent irrigation with sterile water (incidence of 21.3%) compared with sodium chloride solution (34.7%) or boric acid and sodium borate solution (31.8%). The prevalence of chemical conjunctivitis was noted to be higher in infants with a low birth-weight.— S. Yasunaga and E. H. Kean, *Am. J. Dis. Child.,* 1977, *131,* 159.

Silver nitrate from a stick containing 75% was applied to the eyes of a newborn infant instead of a 1% solution. After 1 hour there was a thick purulent secretion, the eyelids were red and oedematous, and the conjunctiva markedly injected. The corneas had a blue-grey bedewed appearance with areas of corneal opacification. After treatment by lavage and topical application of antibiotics and homatropine 2% there was a marked improvement and after 1 week topical application of corticosteroids was started. Residual damage was limited to slight corneal opacity.— A. Hornblass (letter), *J. Am. med. Ass.,* 1975, *231,* 245.

Methaemoglobinaemia. Following application of dressings saturated with a 0.5% solution of silver nitrate, a 2-year-old girl with extensive burns developed methaemoglobinaemia associated with a heavy growth of nitrate-reducing bacteria. She recovered following administration of methylene blue.— B. Strauch *et al., New Engl. J. Med.,* 1969, *281,* 257. See also J. L. Ternberg and E. Luce, *Surgery,* 1968, *63,* 328.

Treatment of Adverse Effects. As soon as possible after ingestion a 1% solution of sodium chloride (10 g per litre) should be given repeatedly to precipitate insoluble silver chloride, and to prevent systemic chloride depletion. The stomach should be emptied by aspiration and lavage and sodium sulphate 30 g in 250 ml of water given as a purgative; sodium acid phosphate has also been recommended. Demulcents, such as milk, white of egg, or liquid paraffin may be given, and if pain is severe, morphine or pethidine should be administered.

Precautions. Silver nitrate stains the skin black and prolonged use of solutions may cause permanent staining. Topical application of silver nitrate solutions to extensive burns may cause hypochloraemia with associated hyponatraemia. Methaemoglobinaemia may occur in the presence of nitrate-reducing bacteria.

Silver compounds have interfered with protein-bound iodine estimations of thyroid function.— *Adverse Drug React. Bull.,* 1972, June, 104.

Absorption and Fate. As for Silver (above). Reduction of nitrate to the nitrite may occur in the presence of some bacteria.

Uses. Silver nitrate is employed for its caustic, astringent, and disinfectant properties. It has been used as a caustic to destroy warts and other small skin growths. A 1% solution has been used as a paint in pruritus ani or pruritus vulvae and as an application in non-specific infections. Compresses soaked in a 0.5% solution of silver nitrate are applied to severe burns to reduce infection.

Aqueous solutions containing 0.2 to 0.6% of silver nitrate have been used as eye lotions, and 1% eye-drops have been employed for the prophylaxis of ophthalmia neonatorum. Dilute solutions have been used as mouth-washes for the prevention of smoking.

Silver nitrate (Argentum Nitricum; Argent. Nit.) is used in homoeopathic medicine.

Aphthous ulcers. Silver nitrate had a limited role in the treatment of aphthous ulcers; it was not practicable to apply it to multiple lesions and larger lesions might develop.— H. A. Brody, *Clin. Med.,* 1972, *79* (Mar.), 18.

Burns. For studies on the relative merits of silver nitrate and silver sulphadiazine in the topical treatment of burns, see under Silver Sulphadiazine, p.1469.

For earlier reports on the use of silver nitrate in burns, see Martindale 27th Edn, p. 908.

Cystitis. Daily instillations of dilute silver nitrate solutions, aimed at distending the bladder, were useful in the treatment of interstitial cystitis, but less so than prednisolone.— *Br. med. J.,* 1972, *1,* 644.

Dental caries. Silver nitrate, used locally, had no effect in reducing dental caries; on the contrary it was suspected of causing greater destruction of dentine.— S. Gelbier (letter), *Br. dent. J.,* 1966, *121,* 499.

Epidermal necrolysis. Based on the treatment of 10 cases, the following was suggested as treatment for toxic epidermal necrolysis: continuous moist compresses of silver nitrate solution 0.25 to 0.5%, with generous wrapping to prevent excessive cooling; daily electrolyte estimations; and daily debridement; after about the fourth day the compresses could be replaced by dexamethasone/neomycin spray followed by inunction of wool alcohols ointment. A penicillin should be given routinely and steroids if vasculitis was present.— P. J. Koblenzer, *Archs Derm.*, 1967, *95*, 608.

Herpes simplex. Silver nitrate 1% had little effect *in vitro* or *in vivo* against herpes simplex virus type 2.— V. R. Coleman *et al.*, *Antimicrob. Ag. Chemother.*, 1973, *4*, 259. A further study.— F. Shimizu *et al.*, *ibid.*, 1976, *10*, 57.

Hydatid cysts. Intrahepatic cysts of *Echinococcus granulosus* were treated with excellent results in 20 patients by freezing the operation area then administering silver nitrate 0.5% to destroy the scolices.— I. Nazarian and F. Saidi, *Z. Tropenmed. Parasit.*, 1971, *22*, 188, per *Trop. Dis. Bull.*, 1971, *68*, 1356.

Ophthalmia neonatorum. In a study of the incidence of ophthalmia neonatorum in 220 000 births, it was found that in 92 865 cases where preparations other than silver nitrate were used the frequency of gonococcal ophthalmia neonatorum was 0.07% whereas where silver nitrate was used the rate was 0.1%. Silver nitrate did not always suppress the development of the condition and seemed no more effective than other agents. While a drop of 1% silver nitrate solution did no harm, there was little evidence that it did any good.— *Lancet*, 1949, *1*, 313.

Of the 49 states of the USA which had made regulations requiring routine prophylactic treatment of the eyes of newborn infants, 22 had specified silver nitrate applications. No evidence had been found to contra-indicate 1% silver nitrate drops when properly packed, handled, and administered. The increasing incidence of gonorrhoea had rendered continued routine prophylaxis necessary.—P.C. Barsam, *New Engl. J. Med.*, 1966, *274*, 731. Fewer local reactions occurred with penicillin than with silver nitrate eye-drops. Penicillin for neonatal prophylaxis should not be abandoned, since it did not appear to sensitise infants.—G. Nathenson (letter), *ibid.*, *275*, 280. Eye-drops containing less than 2% of silver nitrate were considered to be ineffective. Treatment was effective if applied early and prophylaxis was advised only in infants whose mothers were known or suspected to be infected.— E. B. Shaw (letter), *ibid.*, 281. See also P. Kober, *Medsche Klin.*, 1967, *62*, 424.

To prevent gonorrhoeal ophthalmia neonatorum, a 1% solution of silver nitrate was instilled at birth. The chemical conjunctivitis caused by silver nitrate was of short duration.— P. Thygeson, *J. Am. med. Ass.*, 1967, *201*, 902.

For reports on the chemical conjunctivitis associated with instillation of silver nitrate eye-drops and recommendations for reduction of the incidence, see Adverse Effects (above).

Pneumothorax. Spontaneous pneumothorax was successfully treated in 132 patients by pleurodesis induced with silver nitrate; repeated pleurodesis was necessary in only 2 patients. It was suggested that this therapy should be used for patients with only small or no blebs visible on thoracoscopy, or with only mild pre-existing lung disease.— I. Anderson and H. Nissen, *Dis. Chest*, 1968, *54*, 230, per *J. Am. med. Ass.*, 1968, *206*, 681.

Wounds. Silver nitrate solution 0.5% was more effective against Gram-positive than Gram-negative bacteria in the treatment of nonthermal war wounds. The solution did not hinder wound healing or epithelialisation of split thickness skin grafts.— J. P. Connors *et al.*, *Archs Surg., Chicago*, 1969, *98*, 119, per *J. Am. med. Ass.*, 1969, *207*, 580.

Preparations

Mitigated Silver Nitrate *(B.P.C. 1968)*. Argenti Nitras Mitigatus; Mitigated Caustic; Argenti Nitras Dilutus. Silver nitrate 1 and potassium nitrate 2, fused together and suitably moulded for application as a caustic to warts and condylomas. Protect from light.

A similar preparation is included in several pharmacopoeias.

Silver Nitrate Stain Remover *(Univ. of Iowa)*. Thiourea ($NH_2.CS.NH_2$=76.12) 8 g, citric acid monohydrate 8 g, water to 100 ml. It should be freshly prepared.

Toughened Silver Nitrate *(B.P.)*. Argenti Nitras Induratus; Toughened Caustic; Fused Silver Nitrate; Lunar Caustic; Moulded Silver Nitrate; Stylus Argenti Nitrici. Silver nitrate 95 and potassium nitrate 5, fused together and suitably moulded.

White or greyish-white cylindrical rods or cones, which become grey or greyish-black on exposure to light. Freely soluble in water; sparingly soluble in alcohol. Protect from light.

A similar preparation is included in several pharmacopoeias.

Toughened Silver Nitrate *(U.S.P.)*. Contains not less than 94.5% of $AgNO_3$, the remainder consisting of silver chloride. Store in airtight containers. Protect from light.

Creams

Silver Nitrate Cream. Silver nitrate, 0.5 or 2%, Xalifin-15 20%, water to 100%. The cream was stable with only slight discoloration when stored for 4 weeks in the dark at room temperature; at 0° to 4° there was no discoloration.—Pharm. Soc. Lab. Rep. P/68/15, 1968.

Eye-drops

Oculoguttae Argenti Nitratis pro Neonatis *(Dan. Disp.)*. Silver nitrate 670 mg, potassium nitrate 1.2 g, and Water for Injections, 98.13 g.

A similar preparation is included in *F.N.Belg.*

Silver Nitrate Eye-drops *(B.P.C. 1954)*. Gutt. Argent. Nit. Silver nitrate 0.5% w/v, potassium nitrate 1.33% w/v, in Solution for Eye-drops.

Nord. P. has 1% w/w with potassium nitrate 1% w/w in Water for Injections.

Ointments

Unguentum Argenti Nitratis Compositum. Compound Silver Nitrate Ointment. An ointment with this title is included in several pharmacopoeias. It contains silver nitrate 1% and Peru balsam 5 to 10% usually in a basis of yellow soft paraffin or yellow soft paraffin and wool fat.

Ophthalmic Solutions

Silver Nitrate Ophthalmic Solution *(U.S.P.)*. A solution of silver nitrate 0.95 to 1.05% in an aqueous medium. pH 4.5 to 6. It may contain sodium acetate as a buffer. Store in single-dose containers. Protect from light.

Solutions

Ammoniacal Silver Nitrate Solution *(U.S.N.F. XII, 1965)*. Ammoniacal Silver Nitrate, Howe. A solution of diamminosilver nitrate was prepared from silver nitrate 704 g, water 245 ml, and strong ammonia solution to dissolve all but the last trace of precipitate (about 680 ml).It contains 28.5 to 30.5% w/w of Ag and 9 to 9.7% w/w of NH_3. Store in small glass-stoppered containers or in ampoules. Protect from light.

This solution has been employed in dental surgery to deposit silver in exposed dentine or to fill up small crevices in the teeth. After the solution had been applied to the tooth it was followed by a reducing agent such as a 10% formaldehyde solution or eugenol to cause a deposit of metallic silver. The solution has also been employed in the treatment of fungous infections of the nails.

Solutio Argenti Nitratis cum Tetracaino *(Nord. P.)*. Silver nitrate 200 mg, amethocaine nitrate 100 mg, and water 99.7 g.

Proprietary Names

Helvedstensstifter *(Braun, Denm.)*; Lapis *(DAK, Denm.)*; Mova Nitrat Pippette *(Lindopharm, Ger.)*.

5322-m

Silver Protein *(B.P.C. 1968)*. Argentoproteinum; Strong Protein Silver; Strong Protargin; Argentum Proteinicum; Albumosesilber; Protargolum; Proteinato de Plata; Proteinato de Prata.

CAS — 9015-51-4.

Pharmacopoeias. In *Arg., Aust., Belg., Cz., Fr., Hung., Ind., Int., It., Jap., Pol., Port., Roum., Span.,* and *Turk.*

A brown odourless hygroscopic powder containing 7.5 to 8.5% of Ag.

Slowly **soluble** 1 in 2 of water; very slightly soluble in alcohol, chloroform, and ether. A solution in water is neutral to litmus. Solutions may be prepared by shaking the powder over the surface of cold water and allowing it to dissolve slowly, or by triturating the powder to a cream with water and diluting. Solutions are transparent and not coagulated by heat, nor precipitated by the addition of alkali, alkali sulphides, alkali salts, or albumin; they are relatively non-staining. **Store** in airtight containers. Protect from light.

Adverse Effects. As for Silver (above).

Uses. Silver protein solutions have antibacterial properties, due to the presence of low concentrations of ionised silver, and are used as eye-drops in the treatment of conjunctivitis. Solutions are relatively non-irritant unless they contain more than 10% of silver protein.

Preparations

Silver Protein Eye-drops *(B.P.C. 1963)*. Gutt. Argentoprot. A solution of silver protein 5%, with phenylmercuric acetate or nitrate 0.002%, in water. Prepared by dissolving, aseptically, the silver protein in a sterile 0.002% solution of phenylmercuric acetate or nitrate and transferring to the final sterilised container. The eye-drops must be freshly prepared. They are adversely affected by alkali. Protect from light.

Proprietary Names

Stillargol *(Mayoly-Spindler, Fr.)*.

5323-b

Mild Silver Protein *(B.P.C. 1968)*. Argentoproteinum Mite; Argentum Vitellinicum; Mild Silver Proteinate; Silver Nucleinate; Silver Vitellin; Mild Protargin; Vitelinato de Plata; Vitelinato de Prata.

NOTE. The name Mild Silver Protein is given to this compound because it is less bactericidal and less irritant than Silver Protein, though it contains more silver.

Pharmacopoeias. In *Arg., Belg., Fr., Ind., Mex., Port., Roum., Span., Swiss,* and *Turk.*

A hydroscopic brown powder or nearly black scales or granules with a slight odour and taste, containing 19 to 23% of Ag.

Soluble slowly but completely in water; very slightly soluble in alcohol, chloroform, and ether. After exposure to light it is incompletely soluble in water. A 5.51% solution in water is iso-osmotic with serum. **Incompatible** with cocaine hydrochloride, but compatible with 1% atropine sulphate solution. Incompatible with mineral acids, alkalis, tannins, and oxidising agents. **Store** in airtight containers. Protect from light.

Preservative for eye-drops. Phenylmercuric borate 0.005% was a suitable preservative for mild silver protein eye-drops sterilised by heating at 98° to 100° for 30 minutes.— M. Van Ooteghem, *Pharm. Tijdschr. Belg.*, 1968, *45*, 69.

Adverse Effects, Treatment, and Precautions. As for Silver (above).

Argyria. Argyria developed in an elderly woman after prolonged use of mild silver protein 10% nasal drops.— W. A. Parker, *Am. J. Hosp. Pharm.*, 1977, *34*, 287.

Uses. Mild silver protein solutions have antibacterial properties similar to those of silver protein solutions but they contain even lower concentrations of ionised silver and are consequently less irritant to the tissues. Mild silver protein may be used, therefore, in higher concentrations than silver protein, particularly where it is important to avoid irritation of mucous membranes. Mild silver protein, usually 1 to 5%, is used with ephedrine as drops or as a spray in nasal infections. It has been applied as a 20% solution in conjunctivitis and for the prophylaxis of ophthalmia neonatorum and as a 50% solution to corneal ulcers.

Rhinitis. Mild silver protein (Argyrol) has been used for many years in children with chronic purulent rhinitis and has some value in encouraging nose blowing. Its main disadvantage is the irreversible staining of handkerchiefs and pillows.— D. F. N. Harrison, *Prescribers' J.*, 1976, *16*, 69.

Preparations

Mild Silver Protein Eye-drops *(B.P.C. 1963)*. Gutt. Argentoprot. Mit. A solution of mild silver protein 20%, with phenylmercuric acetate or nitrate 0.002% in water. Prepared by dissolving, aseptically, the mild silver protein in a sterile 0.002% solution of phenylmercuric acetate or nitrate and transferring to the final sterilised container. The eye-drops must be freshly prepared. They are adversely affected by alkali. Protect from light.

A.P.F. (Mild Silver Protein Eye-Drops) has mild silver protein 20% and phenylmercuric nitrate 0.002% in Water for Injections.

Silver Protein and Ephedrine Instillation *(A.P.F.)*. Silver Protein and Ephedrine Nasal Drops. Mild silver protein 5 g, ephedrine 500 mg, phenylmercuric nitrate 2 mg, freshly boiled and cooled water to 100 ml. This solution should be recently prepared. Protect from light.

Proprietary Preparations

Argotone *(Rona, UK)*. Contains mild silver protein 1% and ephedrine hydrochloride 0.9% in 0.5% sodium chloride solution, available as **Nasal Drops** and as **Ready-Spray** nasal spray in plastic atomisers.

Other Proprietary Names

Argincolor *(Fr.)*; Argirol *(Spain)*; Vitargénol *(Fr.)*.

5324-v

Tin.

$Sn = 118.69$.

CAS — 7440-31-5.

A bright white, malleable but not very ductile, metal.

5325-g

Tin Oxide *(B.P.C. 1949)*. Stanni Oxidum; Stannous Oxide.

$SnO = 134.7$.

CAS — 21651-19-4.

A dark grey or black, odourless, tasteless powder. Practically **insoluble** in water and alcohol.

5326-q

Tin Powder *(B.P.C. 1949)*. Stanni Pulvis; Stann. Pulv. Metallic tin in the form of an extremely fine powder.

An odourless, tasteless, glistening, silver-grey powder. Practically **insoluble** in water and alcohol.

Adverse Effects, Treatment, and Precautions. Owing to their low solubility tin and tin oxide are very poorly absorbed from the gastro-intestinal tract and are not toxic. Chronic inhalation causes a benign form of pneumoconiosis.

Organic compounds of tin are highly toxic and cause severe neurological damage associated with oedema of the white matter of the brain. Treatment has been symptomatic. Contamination of the skin with organic tin compounds can cause severe burning.

Maximum permissible atmospheric concentration: inorganic compounds, except tin hydride and stannic oxide, 2 mg per m^3; organic compounds 100 μg per m^3.

Action and environmental distribution. A detailed account of the toxicology of tin.— J. M. Barnes and H. B. Stoner, *Pharmac. Rev.*, 1959, *11*, 211.

An evaluation of the toxicological data on tin and some tin salts in *animals* and man.— *Fd Add. Ser. Wld Hlth Org. No. 1*, 1972. See also Twenty-second Report of Joint FAO/WHO Expert Committee on Food Additives, *Tech. Rep. Ser. Wld Hlth Org. No. 631*, 1978.

A review of tin deficiency and toxic effects.— Report of a WHO Expert Group on Trace Elements in Human Nutrition, *Tech. Rep. Ser. Wld Hlth Org., No. 532*, 1973, 38.

Other references.— C. J. Benoy *et al.*, *Food & Cosmet. Toxicol.*, 1971, *9*, 645; A. P. DeGroot *et al.*, *ibid.*, 1973, *11*, 19.

Culinary utensils. Improved technology had reduced the average daily intake of tin from canned foods to about 4 mg. Providing the daily intake does not exceed 130 mg tin does not accumulate in the tissues.— *J. Am. med. Ass.*, 1974, *227*, 1450.

Organic tin poisoning. Stalinon, a remedy against boils, was alleged to have killed 102 people and to have left at least 100 others permanently affected. The preparation was dispensed in capsules each containing 15 mg of diiododiethyl tin and 100 mg of isolinoleic acid esters. A number of people took the capsules without untoward effects. In those who were affected, severe headache started about 4 days after ingestion and was accompanied by severe vomiting, disordered equilibrium, and retention of urine; diplopia and colic also occurred. In severe cases there was clouding of consciousness, proceeding to coma, and in some there was residual paraplegia. Cerebral oedema was found at necropsy. It was established that the clinical trial of Stalinon, on which depended the government sanction to market the preparation, was carried out on capsules supposed to contain 50 mg of diododiethyl tin but which in fact contained only 3 mg.— *Br. med. J.*, 1958, *1*, 515. See also T. Alajouanine *et al.*, *Revue neurol.*, 1958, *98*, 85.

Pregnancy and the neonate. Congenital malformations in 3 infants were associated with the administration of preparations containing tin and tin oxide to the mothers during pregnancy.— A. Notter *et al.*, *Bull. Féd. Socs Gynéc. Obstét. Lang. fr.*, 1968, *20*, *Suppl.*, 319.

Absorption and Fate. Tin is poorly absorbed from the gastro-intestinal tract. It is widely distributed in the body in small amounts and is mainly excreted in the faeces with no more than traces occurring in the urine.

Uses. Although there was no evidence to suggest that they were of value, tin and tin oxide were formerly given in doses of 0.5 to 1 g in the treatment of boils, carbuncles, and acne. They have been used in the treatment of tapeworm infection.

Tapeworm. Beneficial results had been reported in continental Europe with the use of preparations containing tin, in association with the oxide and the chloride, in the treatment of taeniasis, but their popularity has diminished with the introduction of newer taeniacides.— A. Davis, *Drug Treatment in Intestinal Helminthiases*, Geneva, World Health Organization, 1973.

Proprietary Preparations

Stannoxyl *(Cox Continental, UK)*. Tablets each containing tin powder 106.25 mg and tin oxide 18.75 mg. For furunculosis and other staphylococcal disorders. *Dose.* 16 tablets on the first day, decreasing by 2 tablets daily to a maintenance dose of 6 tablets daily.

5327-p

Zinc.

$Zn = 65.38$.

CAS — 7440-66-6.

A white metal with a bluish tinge; it is not very malleable or ductile.

Zinc is an essential element in nutrition and traces are present in many foods. It is a constituent of many enzyme systems, including carbonic anhydrase, alcohol dehydrogenase, and alkaline phosphatases, and it is present with insulin in the pancreas. Normal concentrations of zinc in plasma and serum range from 0.7 to 1.5 mg per litre. However in liver disease, diabetes, and following accidental or surgical injury urinary-zinc concentrations are increased.

A daily intake of 15 to 20 mg of zinc has been recommended but this may not be achieved with diets high in carbohydrate or vegetable protein. Reported effects of human zinc deficiency include delayed puberty and hypogonadal dwarfism.

Adverse Effects and Treatment. Chronic zinc poisoning in man has not been identified with certainty; it has been associated with anaemia which has responded to withdrawal of zinc and symptomatic therapy. Metal fume fever, with nausea, dyspnoea, and chest pain follows inhalation of zinc-containing dust. The acute toxicity of soluble zinc salts is associated with their corrosive action (see under Zinc Chloride, below).

A 16-year-old boy ingested 12 g of elemental zinc in an attempt to promote wound healing. Lethargy occurred 3 days after ingestion, and blood-zinc concentrations were elevated. Treatment with dimercaprol, 2.3 mg per kg body-weight intramuscularly every 4 hours for 4 injections, then once daily for 6 days, resulted in clinical improvement and a fall in zinc concentrations.— J. V. Murphy, *J. Am. med. Ass.*, 1970, *212*, 2119.

Chronic anaemia unresponsive to iron in 3 children was attributed to zinc poisoning. The urine contained 1.8 to 3.65 mg of zinc per litre (average in health 0.3 to 0.5 mg). Each of the children chewed metal toys made of zinc-containing alloy. When the toys were withdrawn the anaemia responded to continued treatment with iron.— V. D. Chunn, *Clin. Med.*, 1973, *80* (Mar.), 7.

A patient who took zinc sulphate 660 mg daily for just over a year for coeliac disease presented with profound hypochromic macrocytic anaemia, associated cardiac failure, and copper deficiency. Treatment consisted of slow transfusion of packed cells, copper sulphate 4 mg daily, and the withdrawal of zinc sulphate. The blood picture was normal 4 weeks later.— K. G. Porter *et al.* (letter), *Lancet*, 1977, *2*, 774.

Culinary utensils. A report of 8 outbreaks of food poisoning due to zinc: the source of zinc in 7 of the outbreaks was the galvanised container in which fruit had been soaked, cooked, or stored after cooking. Symptoms were mainly vomiting and nausea, with rapid recovery; the interval from ingestion to onset was short. Galvanised iron containers should not be used for cooking or storing acid fruits.— R. E. Jones *et al.*, *Mon. Bull. Minist. Hlth*, 1957, *16*, 241. See also under Dialysis (below).

Further references.— M. A. Brown *et al.*, *Archs environ. Hlth*, 1964, *8*, 657.

Dialysis. A 32-year-old woman developed severe nausea, vomiting, and fever on 6 occasions after home dialysis using water which had been stored in a galvanised tank. The plasma-zinc concentration 36 hours after the sixth home dialysis was 7 mg per litre and fell slowly after six weeks' hospital dialysis to 1.58 mg per litre. The red cell-zinc concentrations were respectively 35 and 12.3 mg per litre (normal 10 to 14 mg per litre). No further episodes occurred when the home water was deionised before use.— E. D. M. Gallery *et al.*, *Br. med. J.*, 1972, *4*, 331.

Dialysis anaemia attributed to zinc occurred in 9 of 10 patients in a dialysis unit and in 2 patients on home dialysis.— J. J. B. Petrie and P. G. Row, *Lancet*, 1977, *1*, 1178.. Criticism. No adverse effects occurred in patients undergoing dialysis with similar zinc concentrations in the dialysate. Other factors for the dialysis anaemia could be involved.— W. K. Stewart *et al.* (letter), *ibid.*, 1977, *2*, 139.

For reference to zinc deficiency in patients undergoing dialysis, see under Growth and Sexual Function (below).

Drinking water. A zinc content of more than 15 ppm would markedly impair the potability of drinking water.— *International Standards for Drinking Water*, 2nd Edn, Geneva, Wld Hlth Org., 1963.

Precautions. It has been suggested that concurrent administration with a zinc salt might diminish the effect of penicillamine.

Interactions. It was inadvisable to give zinc sulphate and penicillamine together as the latter might be inactivated.— W. H. Lyle, *Dista* (letter), *Lancet*, 1976, *2*, 684.

For a report of zinc acetate used in conjunction with penicillamine in the treatment of zinc deficiency, see Penicillamine, p.387.

Absorption and Fate. Zinc and its salts are poorly absorbed from the gastro-intestinal tract; only a small proportion of dietary zinc is absorbed. Zinc is distributed widely throughout the body and is excreted in the faeces with only traces appearing in the urine since the kidneys have little or no role in regulating the content of zinc in the body.

A review of studies of human zinc metabolism.— H. Spencer *et al.*, Intake, Excretion, and Retention of Zinc in Man, *Trace Elements in Human Health and Disease*, Vol. 1, A.S. Prasad and D. Oberleas (Ed.), London, Academic Press, 1976, p. 345.

Dietary effects. A study of the effects of foodstuffs on the absorption of zinc sulphate.— A. Pécoud *et al.*, *Clin. Pharmac. Ther.*, 1975, *17*, 469. See also J. L. Schelling *et al.* (letter), *Lancet*, 1973, *2*, 968.

Pregnancy and the neonate. Studies suggesting that low serum-zinc concentrations during pregnancy might be a sign of zinc deficiency with associated risks to mother and child.— S. Jameson, *Acta med. scand.*, 1976, *Suppl.*, 593, per *Abstr. Hyg.*, 1976, *51*, 1250.

Other references to *animal* and human studies: L. S. Hurley and H. Swenerton, *Proc. Soc. exp. Biol. Med.*, 1966, *123*, 692; K. Bilek *et al.*, *Arch. Gynaek.*, 1967, *204*, 97; K. M. Hambidge *et al.* (letter), *Lancet*, 1975, *1*, 577; C. H. Chang *et al.*, *J. pharm. Sci.*, 1977, *66*, 1755.

Uses. Zinc supplements (usually administered in the form of the sulphate) have been given in deficiency states and to accelerate wound healing associated with deficiency states. Zinc salts are used topically as mild astringents.

Deficiency. The mean concentration of zinc in the plasma was 960 μg per litre for healthy adults and 890 μg per litre for healthy children. Abnormally low concentrations were found in patients with alcoholic cirrhosis, other types of liver disease, active tuberculosis, indolent ulcers, uraemia, before and after a single haemodialysis, cardiac infarct, pulmonary infection, Down's syndrome, cystic fibrosis with growth retardation, in pregnancy, in women taking oral contraceptives, and in growth-retarded Iranian villagers.— J. A. Halsted and J. C. Smith, *Lancet*, 1970, *1*, 322. See also *Chronicle Wld Hlth Org.*, 1973, *27*, 534. There was no evidence that zinc supplements are of any use in the dietary regimen of *healthy* people.— *Med. Lett.*, 1978, *20*, 57.

Loss of weight, decreased libido, skin scaling, lethargy, and anorexia, together with biochemical changes in the zinc content of their plasma, red and white blood cells, and urine, was reported in subjects fed a dietary regimen containing all known essential nutrients, except zinc.— *J. Am. med. Ass.*, 1976, *235*, 2810.

For a detailed account of the role of zinc see, A. S. Prasad, Deficiency of Zinc in Man and its Toxicity, in *Trace Elements in Human Health and Disease*, Vol. 1, A.S. Prasad and D. Oberleas (Ed.), London, Academic Press, 1976, p. 1; K. M. Hambidge and P. A. Walravens, Zinc Deficiency in Infants and Preadolescent Children, *ibid.*, , p. 21.

Other reviews, reports, and studies on zinc requirements and deficiency: *Drug & Ther. Bull.*, 1973, *11*, 45; *Lancet*, 1973, *1*, 299; Report of a WHO Expert Group on Trace Elements in Human Nutrition, *Tech. Rep. Ser. Wld Hlth Org. No. 532*, 1973; R. E. Burch *et al.*, *Clin. Chem.*, 1975, *21*, 501; K. M. Hambidge, *Pediat. Clins N. Am.*, 1977, *24*, 95; G. S. Fell and R. R. Burns, *Proc. R. Soc. Med.*, 1976, *69*, 474; D. D. Ulmer, *New Engl. J. Med.*, 1977, *297*, 318; A. S. Prasad, *Trace Elements and Iron in Human Metabolism*, Chichester, John Wiley, 1978; Committee on Nutrition, *Pediatrics*, 1978, *62*, 408.

Acne. In a double-blind study in 64 patients with acne, treatment with zinc sulphate, as effervescent tablets containing the equivalent of 45 mg of zinc thrice daily, with or without added vitamin A, the mean acne score was reduced from 100% to 35% in 4 weeks, compared with 70 and 75% for vitamin A and placebo respectively. Continued treatment, for a total of 12 weeks, with zinc led to a reduction in acne score to 13%. Vitamin A did not produce added benefit.— G. Michaëlsson *et al.*, *Archs Derm.*, 1977, *113*, 31. Young male patients with severe acne vulgaris had a mean serum-zinc concentration significantly below that in patients with mild acne or in healthy subjects in a control group. The same difference was not found among young female patients. All the 173 patients in the study were over 15 years of age.— *idem*, *Br. J. Derm.*, 1977, *96*, 283. No significant differences were found between systemic treatment for acne with either oxytetracycline or zinc sulphate during a 12-week double-blind study in 37 patients.— *idem*, *97*, 561. Comments and criticisms.— *Br. med. J.*, 1977, *1*, 1493; S. C. Glover and M. I. White (letter), *ibid.*, 1977, *2*, 640; J. C. Fitzherbert (letter), *Med. J. Aust.*, 1977, *2*, 685.

There was no significant difference in response to placebo or zinc sulphate, providing the equivalent of 45 mg of zinc thrice daily, in a study of 39 patients with acne treated for 4 to 12 weeks.— K. Weismann *et al.*, *Acta derm.-vener., Stockh.*, 1977, *57*, 357.

Acrodermatitis enteropathica. Acrodermatitis enteropathica was considered to be a zinc-deficiency disorder. Nine children treated with zinc sulphate were completely free from symptoms. A small daily dose—35 mg of zinc sulphate providing about 8 mg of zinc—might suffice but the optimum daily dose appeared to be 150 mg providing 34 mg of zinc daily.— E. J. Moynahan (letter), *Lancet*, 1974, *2*, 399.

A 22-year-old woman with acrodermatitis enteropathica, who had been maintained on di-iodohydroxyquinoline 650 mg 3 or 4 times daily, showed complete remission within 4 days of starting zinc sulphate 220 mg (equivalent to 50 mg of zinc) thrice daily. Plasma-zinc concentrations rose to high-normal values. Zinc sulphate was discontinued after 10 days and a remission of 5 weeks obtained. When restarted, di-iodohydroxyquinoline was less effective, requiring a longer time and higher dose to achieve incomplete remission. After a period without medication zinc sulphate 50 mg (equivalent to 11.4 mg of zinc) twice daily was given and the clinical response was excellent although slightly slower than with the higher dose.— K. H. Neldner and K. M. Hambidge, *New Engl. J. Med.*, 1975, *292*, 879.

Two successful pregnancies in a woman with acrodermatitis enteropathica treated by zinc supplement.— D. P. Brenton *et al.*, *Lancet*, 1981, *2*, 500.

Further reports and comments: B. Portnoy and M. Molokhia, *Br. J. Derm.*, 1974, *91*, 701; *idem* (letter), *Lancet*, 1974, *2*, 663; R. I. Henkin and R. L. Aamodt (letter), *ibid.*, 1975, *1*, 1379; E. Guiraldes *et al.*, *ibid.*, 1975, *2*, 710; I. Polanco *et al.* (letter), *ibid.*, 1976, *1*, 430; B. Portnoy and M. Molokhia, *Br. J. Derm.*, 1976, *94*, 112; H. Reich *et al.*, *Dt. med. Wschr.*, 1976, *101*, 1724; I. L. Rubin *et al.*, *S. Afr. med. J.*, 1978, *53*, 497; P. A. Walravens *et al.*, *J. Pediat.*, 1978, *93*, 71.

Aphthous ulcers. Twelve of 17 patients with recurrent aphthous ulcers improved when treated with 50 to 150 mg of zinc daily given as zinc sulphate; ulcers were completely eradicated in 5 patients. Improvement appeared to be associated with zinc treatment in those patients with initial serum-zinc concentrations below 1.1 µg per ml.— H. W. Merchant *et al.*, *Sth. med. J.*, 1977, *70*, 559.

Coeliac disease. Correction of severe zinc deficiency in 6 patients with unresponsive coeliac disease produced immediate and sustained improvement subsequently maintained by a gluten-free diet.— M. Elmes *et al.*, *Q.J. Med.*, 1976, *45*, 696.

Cystic fibrosis. A report of zinc deficiency associated with cystic fibrosis, growth retardation, and hypogonadism.— J. A. Dodge and J. G. Yassa, *Br. med. J.*, 1978, *1*, 411.

Dementia. In a double-blind study of 30 geriatric patients with senile dementia 16 received zinc sulphate capsules, 220 mg (equivalent to 50 mg of zinc) thrice daily for 24 weeks, while 14 received placebo. Although psychological testing and psychiatric rating did not demonstrate any advantage of zinc sulphate over placebo some behavioural tests indicated that the patients receiving zinc sulphate deteriorated less rapidly. Diarrhoea occurred with zinc sulphate therapy.— A. W. Czerwinski *et al.*, *Clin. Pharmac. Ther.*, 1974, *15*, 436. A possible role of zinc in the pathology of dementia.— F. M. Burnet, *Lancet*, 1981, *1*, 186.

Diagnostic skin tests. Findings in 10 malnourished children following cutaneous application of zinc sulphate 1% in emulsifying ointment compared with application of emulsifying ointment alone, indicated that depressed cutaneous responses might be caused by zinc deficiency in protein-energy malnutrition. Results of skin tests in malnourished children to diagnose diseases such as tuberculosis might be enhanced by prior application of zinc.— M. H. N. Golden *et al.*, *Lancet*, 1978, *1*, 1226.

Furunculosis. Reduced serum concentrations of zinc were found in 15 patients with recurrent furunculosis. Treatment with zinc sulphate providing 45 mg of zinc thrice daily for 3 to 7 months in 8 of the patients was associated with regression of active lesions and no recurrence. This was superior to treatment by incision and antibiotic therapy in the other 7 patients.— I. Brody (letter), *Lancet*, 1977, *2*, 1358.

Gastric ulcer. In a double-blind study in patients with benign gastric ulcers, 10 were given zinc sulphate 220 mg (equivalent to 50 mg of zinc) thrice daily by mouth and 8 placebo. After 3 weeks patients taking zinc sulphate had an ulcer healing rate three times that of patients taking placebo, and more patients in the zinc sulphate group achieved complete healing. There was no evidence of zinc deficiency in any of the patients.— D. J. Frommer, *Med. J. Aust.*, 1975, *2*, 793. Comment.— M. J. S. Langman, *Drugs*, 1977, *14*, 105.

Further references: K. B. Orr (letter), *Med. J. Aust.*, 1976, *1*, 244.

Growth and sexual function. In a review of the role of zinc deficiency in retarded growth and sexual development of children, treatment with zinc was not found to increase growth or sexual development; retardation was considered to be due to protein malnutrition.— J. E. Caughey (letter), *Lancet*, 1973, *1*, 993. Treatment with zinc 40 mg daily as carbonate for 1 year produced a significant increase in height, weight, and bone-age in 20 boys.— J. G. Reinhold and H. A. Ronaghy (letter), *ibid.*, *2*, 50. See also H. A. Ronaghy *et al.*, *Am. J. clin. Nutr.*, 1974, *27*, 112.

The thymus was reduced in size after malnourishment. Supplementation with zinc as zinc acetate increased the size of thymus in a study of 8 recently malnourished children.— M. H. N. Golden *et al.* (preliminary communication), *Lancet*, 1977, *2*, 1057.

Reversal of zinc deficiency in 4 men with impotence associated with uraemia improved sexual function although not to the predialysis level. There was no improvement in 4 control patients. Initially zinc replacement was with zinc sulphate given by mouth but as this was inefficient zinc chloride was added to the dialysis bath.— L. D. Antoniou *et al.*, *Lancet*, 1977, *2*, 895. A report of reduced serum-zinc concentrations in 6 of 10 infertile men. Zinc sulphate increased plasma-testosterone concentration in 9 and sperm count in 8 men. One wife became pregnant.— T. R. Hartoma *et al.* (letter), *ibid.*, 1125.

In a double-bind study 7 male patients on regular haemodialysis had zinc solution added to the dialysis fluid to attain a final concentration of 400 µg per litre (6.1 µmol per litre); 7 similar control patients had distilled water added. No beneficial effect was noted on any aspect of sexual function in those given supplementary zinc.— A. C. Brook *et al.*, *Lancet*, 1980, *2*, 618. The poor results may have been due to the associated antihypertensive therapy the men were taking.— L. D. Antoniou and R. J. Shalhoub (letter), *ibid.*, 1034.

Further references: J. A. Halsted *et al.*, *Am. J. Med.*, 1972, *53*, 277; J. C. Smith *et al.*, *Science*, 1973, *181*, 954; *J. Am. med. Ass.*, 1976, *235*, 2810.

Hyperthyroidism. In 24 thyrotoxic patients zinc clearance was significantly higher than in 10 hypothyroid patients or 10 controls; plasma-zinc concentrations were comparable in the 3 groups. Zinc clearance was also correlated with a scale assessing the acuteness and severity of metabolic response to thyrotoxicosis (heart-rate, weight loss, serum concentrations of cholesterol, thyroxine, and triiodothyronine). The increased zinc clearance was probably due to catabolism. No clinical consequences were observed, but it might be important in malabsorption, zinc deficiency, phenylketonuria, or prolonged parenteral nutrition.— W. F. Bremner and G. S. Fell, *Postgrad. med. J.*, 1977, *53*, 143.

Leg ulcers. Patients with stasis leg ulcers had reduced radioactive zinc retention suggesting a rationale for zinc sulphate treatment.— T. Hawkins and J. Marks (letter), *Lancet*, 1976, *2*, 319.

See also under Wound Healing (below).

Porphyria. Zinc sulphate 220 mg (equivalent to 50 mg of zinc) every 8 hours by mouth relieved abdominal pain in a patient with acute intermittent porphyria.— W. Roman *et al.*, *Med. J. Aust.*, 1969, *1*, 633. A similar report.— W. Roman *et al.* (letter), *Lancet*, 1967, *2*, 716.

Rheumatoid arthritis. In a preliminary double-blind study of 24 patients with chronic, active, refractory rheumatoid arthritis, the addition of zinc sulphate 220 mg (equivalent to 50 mg of zinc) thrice daily produced beneficial results when compared with placebo. After 12 weeks all patients were given zinc sulphate for a further 12 weeks; those who had already received zinc continued to improve while those who had been on placebo began to improve.— P. A. Simkin, *Lancet*, 1976, *2*, 539.

Sickle-cell anaemia. Zinc deficiency in sickle-cell disease.— A. S. Prasad *et al.*, *Clin. Chem.*, 1975, *21*, 582.

Pica was associated with zinc deficiency in a child with sickle-cell disease. Correction of his deficiency abolished the abnormal appetite.— G. Karayalcin and P. Lanzkowsky (letter), *Lancet*, 1976, *2*, 687.

Taste perception. In 103 patients with diminished or distorted taste perception (hypogeusia, dysgeusia) and diminished or distorted smell perception (hyposmia, dysosmia) serum-zinc concentrations were significantly lower than in controls; the symptoms were alleviated by zinc supplements given by mouth.— *J. Am. med. Ass.*, 1974, *228*, 1669.

Results of a double-blind crossover study in 53 men and 53 women with taste and smell dysfunction did not indicate any significant difference between administration of 100 mg of elemental zinc daily in 4 divided doses and placebo.— R. I. Henkin *et al.*, *Am. J. med. Sci.*, 1976, *272*, 285.

Ulcerative colitis. In a double-blind study 50 mg of zinc given thrice daily as zinc sulphate, was of no benefit in 51 patients as an adjuvant in the treatment of ulcerative colitis or proctitis.— M. W. Dronfield *et al.*, *Gut*, 1977, *18*, 33.

Wound healing. Zinc sulphate, 660 mg daily in 3 divided doses, equivalent to 150 mg of elemental zinc, was found to increase the rate of healing of granulating wounds in a controlled study in 20 young men. Treated and control groups had comparable diets and their wounds received the same postoperative treatment. On average, wounds took 45.8 days to heal in patients receiving zinc sulphate and 80.1 days for the controls. There was no evidence of toxicity from the administration of zinc sulphate in capsules.— W. J. Pories *et al.*, *Lancet*, 1967, *1*, 121; *idem*, *Ann. Surg.*, 1967, *165*, 432. Criticisms and comments.— G. G. Power (letter), *Lancet*, 1967, *1*, 440. See also R. Simpson-White (letter), *ibid.*, 278; B. Williams (letter), *ibid.*, 330; C. B. Heald (letter), *ibid.*

In a controlled study in 104 patients, zinc sulphate 220 mg (equivalent to 50 mg of zinc) thrice daily after meals produced healing of leg ulcers in an average of 32 days compared with 77 days for patients given placebos.— S. L. Husain, *Lancet*, 1969, *1*, 1069.

Thrice daily application of an ointment containing zinc sulphate 1% in emulsifying ointment to one side of the body accelerated the healing of open skin sores in 7 of 8 severely malnourished children with symmetrical open skin sores of the limbs, compared with application of the basis to the other side. Both sides healed rapidly and symmetrically in the eighth child who was found to have been given oral zinc supplementation. It was concluded that the low plasma-zinc concentrations in malnourished children with skin sores reflect actual zinc deficiency, and not a spurious association caused by a lowering of plasma-zinc binding sites or redistribution of zinc within the body. Oral zinc supplements (Zn^{++} 2 mg per kg body-weight daily) are now given routinely to all malnourished children with broken skin.— M. H. N. Golden *et al.* (letter), *Lancet*, 1980, *1*, 1256.

Further references: W. J. Pories and W. H. Strain, *Trace Element Metabolism in Animals*, Proceedings of International Symposium by World Association for Animal Production/International Biological Programme, Aberdeen, July 1969, Edinburgh, Livingstone, 1970, p. 75; A. J. M. Brodribb and C. R. Ricketts, *Injury*, 1971, *3*, 25; T. Hallböök and E. Lanner, *Lancet*, 1972, *2*, 780; M. M. Molokhia and B. Portnoy (letter), *ibid.*, 1973, *1*, 41; M. W. Greaves and F. A. Ive, *Br. J. Derm.*, 1972, *87*, 632; R. Carruthers, *Drugs*, 1973, *6*, 161; R. I. Henkin, *New Engl. J. Med.*, 1974, *291*, 675; P. W. R. Lee *et al.*, *Surgery Gynec. Obstet.*, 1976, *143*, 549.

Parenteral nutrition. Analysis of solutions used for total parenteral nutrition demonstrated that most intravenous solutions given to patients for total parenteral nutrition contain very low concentrations of copper and minute quantities of selenium, but substantial amounts of zinc (which might come from the rubber stoppers). Although in some cases the zinc concentration might be adequate this might not always be so, it was thus essential to know not only the trace-element composition of intravenous solutions but also the zinc status of the patient.— M. Van Caillie *et al.*, *Lancet*, 1978, *2*, 200.

For details of parenteral solutions containing zinc, see under Amino Acids and Nutritional Agents, p.48.

5328-s

Zinc Acetate *(U.S.P., B.P.C. 1949).*
$(CH_3.CO_2)_2Zn,2H_2O = 219.5$.

CAS — 557-34-6 (anhydrous); 5970-45-6 (dihydrate).

Pharmacopoeias. In *U.S.*

Colourless or white crystals or granules with a faint acetous odour and a sharp disagreeable astringent metallic taste. It effloresces slowly to form a basic salt. **Soluble** 1 in 2.5 of water, 4 in 1 of boiling water, 1 in 30 of alcohol, and 1 in 3 of boiling alcohol. A 5% solution in water has a pH of 6 to 8. **Incompatible** with solutions of soluble carbonate, phosphates, tannic acid, and sulphurated potash. **Store** in airtight containers.

Zinc acetate resembles zinc sulphate (see below) in its actions. Dilute solutions (0.25%) have been used as eye lotions or eye-drops in the treatment of conjunctivitis. Zinc acetate was formerly used as an emetic. It is used in zinc-eugenol dental cements to accelerate setting.

Preparations

Zinc Acetate Eye-drops. Zinc acetate 250 mg, glycerol 1.5 g, sodium chloride 900 mg, chlorhexidine acetate 5 mg, Water for Injections to 100 ml. Sterilised by autoclaving.—P.L. Jeffs, *Australas. J. Pharm.*, 1962, *43*, 1031.

Zinc and Adrenaline Eye-drops. Zinc acetate 250 mg, adrenaline solution 8.5 ml, sodium metabisulphite 100 mg, chlorhexidine acetate 5 mg, Water for Injections to 100 ml. Sterilised by autoclaving.—P.L. Jeffs, *Australas. J. Pharm.*, 1962, *43*, 1031. See also under Adrenaline, p.5.

Zinc and Boric Eye-drops. Zinc acetate 250 mg, boric acid 1 g, glycerol 1.5 g, chlorhexidine acetate 5 mg, Water for Injections to 100 ml. Sterilised by autoclaving.—P.L. Jeffs, *Australas. J. Pharm.*, 1962, *43*, 1031.

5329-w

Zinc Chloride *(B.P., Eur. P., U.S.P.).* Zinci Chloridum; Zincum Chloratum.

$ZnCl_2 = 136.3$.

CAS — 7646-85-7.

Pharmacopoeias. In *Arg., Aust., Br., Eur., Fr., Ger., Hung., Jap., Mex., Neth., Nord., Pol., Port., Roum., Span., Swiss,* and *U.S.*

A white or almost white, odourless, deliquescent, caustic, crystalline powder or granules or opaque white masses or sticks. M.p. about 260°.

Soluble 1 in 0.5 of water if free from oxychloride, 1 in 1.5 of alcohol, and 1 in 2 of glycerol; soluble in acetone and ether. An approximately 10% solution in water has a pH of 4.6 to 6. **Incompatible** with soluble carbonates, phosphates, tannic acid, sulphurated potash, and silver salts. **Store** in airtight containers.

Zinc chloride almost always contains some oxychloride which produces a slightly turbid aqueous solution. Turbid solutions, except when intended for ophthalmic use, may be cleared by adding gradually a small amount of dilute hydrochloric acid. Solutions of zinc chloride should be filtered through asbestos or sintered glass, since they dissolve paper and cotton wool.

Adverse Effects. The ingestion of a large quantity of zinc chloride is rapidly followed by nausea and vomiting. Symptoms of poisoning stem from the corrosive action and include a burning sensation in the oesophagus and stomach; it often renders the mucous membranes white. Colic and bloody diarrhoea may follow, with convulsions, hypotension, and coma. Death may occur after only a few grams although recovery has followed much larger amounts.

Metal fume fever has occurred in industrial workers exposed to fumes from zinc chloride, molten zinc, or zinc oxide (see under Zinc, above).

Maximum permissible atmospheric concentration (fume) 1 mg per m^3.

A soldier died following the inhalation, in a confined space, of zinc chloride smoke during a Civil Defence exercise. He had severe retrosternal pain and was slightly cyanosed. Some 24 hours later his condition worsened progressively and death occurred on the eleventh day. Autopsy showed widespread consolidation of the lungs, oedema, areas of haemorrhage, and extensive necrosis and numerous punctate cysts had formed. Such patients should be observed at rest for at least 48 hours and should have a chest X-ray before returning to duty.— M. B. Macaulay and A. K. Mant, *J. R. Army med. Cps*, 1964, *110*, 27.

Treatment of Adverse Effects. The stomach should be emptied by aspiration and lavage, and demulcents such as milk or white of egg should be given freely. Administration of sodium calciumedetate by mouth and intravenously has been suggested. Morphine or pethidine may be given to relieve pain, and fluid and electrolyte balance should be corrected. Contamination of the skin and eyes should be treated by flooding with water.

Injury due to splashes of zinc chloride in the eye should be treated by immediate irrigation with neutral disodium edetate solution 0.05M.— R. E. Houle and W. M. Grant, *Am. J. Ophthal.*, 1973, *75*, 992. See also M. A. Johnstone *et al.*, *Am. J. Ophthal.*, 1973, *76*, 137.

Absorption and Fate. Zinc chloride is partially absorbed from the gastro-intestinal tract. For further details, see under Zinc (above).

Uses. Zinc chloride is a powerful caustic and astringent. A solution of zinc chloride 1% and zinc sulphate 2% has been used as an astringent mouth-wash. A 1 to 2% solution had been used for application to foul-smelling wounds and ulcers. A 10% solution has been used as an obtundent in dentistry.

Tissue fixative. Zinc chloride applied in a paste as a tissue fixative was successful in the removal of a neoplasm of the breast in an elderly woman. Layers of dead tissue were excised after each application until normal tissue was reached. The paste contained zinc chloride saturated solution 34.5 ml, antimony trisulphide (stibnite; about 180 μm powder) 40 g and *Sanguinaria canadensis* (adhesive) 10 g.— J. Sonneland, *Am. J. Surg.*, 1972, *124*, 391.

5330-m

Zinc Sulphate *(B.P., Eur. P.).* Zinc Sulph.; Zinc Sulfate *(U.S.P.)*; Zinci Sulfas; Zincum Sulfuricum.

$ZnSO_4,7H_2O = 287.5$.

CAS — 7733-02-0 (anhydrous); 7446-20-0 (heptahydrate).

NOTE. 'White vitriol' or 'white copperas' is crude zinc sulphate.

Pharmacopoeias. In all pharmacopoeias examined except *Roum.*

Odourless, colourless, transparent, efflorescent crystals or white crystalline powder with an astringent metallic taste. Each g of zinc sulphate represents 3.5 mmol (7 mEq) of zinc. Zinc sulphate 220 mg is approximately equivalent to 50 mg of zinc. It is efflorescent in dry air and loses 5 molecules of water of crystallisation, or 31.2% of its weight, when slowly heated to 50°, and a further molecule at 100°.

Soluble 1 in less than 1 of water, 1 in 0.2 of boiling water, and 1 in 2.5 of glycerol; practically insoluble in alcohol. A 5% solution in water has a pH of 4.4 to 5.6. A 7.65% solution in water is iso-osmotic with serum. Solutions are **sterilised** by autoclaving or by filtration. **Incompatible** with lead, calcium, and strontium salts, borax, alkali carbonates and hydroxides, silver protein, and tannins. **Store** in airtight containers.

Preservative for eye-drops. Phenylmercuric borate 0.005% was a suitable preservative for zinc sulphate eye-drops sterilised by filtration or by heating at 98° to 100° for 30 minutes.— M. Van Ooteghem, *Pharm. Tijdschr. Belg.*, 1968, *45*, 69.

Adverse Effects. Low doses of zinc sulphate may cause mild gastro-intestinal disturbances. Doses of 0.6 to 2 g are emetic. In overdosage it has corrosive effects similar to those of Zinc Chloride (above). See also under Zinc (above).

A 72-year-old woman died 47 days after the inadvertent infusion of zinc sulphate 7.4 g over 60 hours. Initial symptoms included hypotension, pulmonary oedema, diarrhoea and vomiting, jaundice, and oliguria; other features were cardiac arrhythmias, hyperamylasaemia, anaemia, and thrombocytopenia. Treatment included sodium calciumedetate (discontinued because of poor renal function), intravenous fluids, frusemide, and haemodialysis.— A. Brocks *et al.*, *Br. med. J.*, 1977, *1*, 1390.

A 15-year-old girl experienced epigastric discomfort on each occasion after taking zinc sulphate 220 mg as capsules twice daily; after 7 days she developed melaena and anaemia; endoscopy showed a haemorrhagic gastric erosion.— R. Moore, *Br. med. J.*, 1978, *1*, 754.

Treatment of Adverse Effects. As for Zinc Chloride (above).

Precautions. As for Zinc (above).

Patients should always be instructed to take zinc after meals.— M. M. Molokhia and B. Portnoy (letter), *Br. med. J.*, 1978, *1*, 1145.

Absorption and Fate. Zinc sulphate is partially absorbed from the gastro-intestinal tract. For further details, see under Zinc (above).

Uses. Zinc sulphate has been given internally in doses of up to 220 mg thrice daily to assist wound healing and in the treatment of acrodermatitis enteropathica. It was formerly used as a reflex emetic.

Externally, zinc sulphate is used as an astringent lotion for indolent ulcers and to assist granulation. It is used in conjunction with zinc chloride as an astringent mouth-wash. Solutions usually containing 0.25% of zinc sulphate are applied locally to relieve chronic inflammation of the cornea in conjunctivitis.

For references to the use of zinc sulphate, see under Zinc (above).

Preparations

Baths

Zinc Sulphate Bath *(B.P.C. 1949).* Balneum Zinci Sulphatis. Zinc sulphate 120 g in water 150 litres.

Eye Lotions

Collyrium Zinci Luteum *(Aust. P.).* Zinc sulphate 0.5, ammonium chloride 0.2, camphor 0.2, saffron 0.1, alcohol (70%) 10, Water for Injections to 100, all by wt.

Collyrium Zinci Sulfurici *(Cz. P.).* Zinc Sulphate Eye Lotion. Zinc sulphate 0.25%, boric acid 1.62%, borax 0.3%, and phenylmercuric borate 0.001%, in sterilised water.

Compound Zinc Sulphate Eye Lotion *(B.P.C. 1963)*. Collyr. Zinc. Sulph. Co.; Zinc Compound Eye Lotion. Zinc sulphate 343 mg, boric acid 2.29 g, freshly boiled and cooled water to 100 ml. It should be diluted with an equal volume of warm water before use.

Eye-drops

Zinc and Adrenaline Eye Drops *(A.P.F.)*. —see under Adrenaline, p.5.

Zinc Sulfate Ophthalmic Solution *(U.S.P.)*. A sterile aqueous solution of zinc sulphate made iso-osmotic by the addition of suitable salts; pH 5.8 to 6.2 or, if it contains sodium citrate, 7.2 to 7.8. Store in airtight containers.

Zinc Sulphate and Adrenaline Eye-drops *(B.P.)*. —see under Adrenaline, p.5.

Zinc Sulphate Eye Drops *(A.P.F.)*. Gutt. Zinc. Sulph.; Zinc and Boric Acid Eye Drops. Zinc sulphate 250 mg, boric acid 1.5 g, chlorbutol 500 mg, glycerol 1 ml, Water for Injections to 100 ml. Sterilised by autoclaving.

Zinc Sulphate Eye Drops *(B.P.)*. Gutt. Zinc. Sulph.; ZSU. A sterile solution of zinc sulphate 0.22 to 0.28%, with phenylmercuric acetate or nitrate 0.002%, in water. Sterilised by autoclaving, by filtration, or by maintaining at 98° to 100° for 30 minutes. If intended for use on more than one occasion they should not be used more than one month after first opening the container.

Studies of the stability and compatibility of benzalkonium chloride and phenethyl alcohol as preservatives of zinc sulphate eye-drops and zinc sulphate and adrenaline eye-drops.— Pharm. Soc. Lab. Rep. P/74/9, P/74/10, P/74/11, 1974.

Irrigations

Zinc Sulphate Irrigation *(B.P.C. 1959)*. Irrig. Zinc. Sulph. Zinc sulphate 1.03% in warm water.

Amended Formula. Zinc sulphate 5 g, water to 1 pint.—*Compendium of Past Formulae 1933 to 1966*, London, The National Pharmaceutical Union, 1969.

Lotions

Zinc Sulphate Lotion *(B.P.)*. Lot. Zinc. Sulph.; Lotio Rubra. Zinc Sulphate 1 g, amaranth solution 1 ml, water to 100 ml.

Zinc Sulphate Lotion *(St. Mark's Hosp.)*. Zinc sulphate 500 mg, compound lavender tincture 1 ml, water to 100 ml.

Mouth-washes

Zinc Sulphate and Zinc Chloride Mouth-wash *(B.P.C. 1973)*. Zinc sulphate 2 g, zinc chloride 1 g, dilute hydrochloric acid 1 ml, compound tartrazine solution 1 ml, double-strength chloroform water 50 ml, water to 100 ml. It should be diluted with 20 times its volume of warm water before use (15 ml to a tumblerful of warm water).

Proprietary Preparations

Zincfrin *(Alcon, UK: Farillon, UK)*. Eye-drops containing zinc sulphate 0.25% and phenylephrine hydrochloride 0.12%. For mild conjunctivitis and other mild eye disorders.

Zincomed *(Medo Chemicals, UK)*. Zinc sulphate, available as capsules of 220 mg.

Other Proprietary Names

Medizinc, Orazinc (both *USA*); Solvezinc *(Austral.)*; Solvezink *(Denm., Norw., Swed.)*; Verazinc *(USA)*; Zincaps *(Austral.)*; Zinc-220 *(USA)*; Zinklet *(Denm.)*.

Proprietary Names of Some Other Zinc Compounds

Zn-Plus (protein complex) *(Miller, USA)*.

Methylcellulose and Stabilising and Suspending Agents

5400-n

The stabilising and suspending agents described in this section all have the property of increasing the viscosity of water when dissolved or dispersed. The rheological properties of the dispersions can vary widely from thin liquids to thick gels.

They are used in emulsions as stabilisers and in some cases as emulsifying agents. They are used in suspensions for their rheological properties and for controlling flocculation. They are also used in the preparation of gels. Those agents of natural origin vary widely in their purity, uniformity, stability and other properties; they are also subject to microbial contamination.

The choice of a suitable emulsifier or stabiliser depends on whether the preparation is for internal or external use and whether the preparation is to be made extemporaneously or manufactured on a large scale and stored for prolonged periods. Emulsifying and suspending agents suitable for use in extemporaneously prepared products for *internal* use include acacia, methylcellulose and other cellulose derivatives, sodium alginate, and tragacanth. Those suitable for *external* use include bentonite, methylcellulose and other cellulose derivatives, sodium alginate, and tragacanth.

Agents that require dispersion using high-shear equipment and are more suitable for use in manufactured products for *internal* and *external* use include aluminium magnesium silicate and carbomer. Emulsifying agents suitable for internal and external use are also described in the sections on Cetomacrogol and Nonionic Surfactants, p.370 and Soaps and Anionic Surfactants, p.1439.

For a list of emulsifying agents and stabilisers permitted in foods, see Emulsifiers and Stabilisers in Food, p.370.

Many of the agents in this section are also used in the manufacture of tablets as disintegrants, binding and granulating agents and for film or enteric coating.

Because they swell in contact with intestinal fluids, several of these suspending agents are used as bulk laxatives and in the management of various bowel disorders; they include agar, ispaghula, methylcellulose, psyllium, and sterculia.

For further information on natural and semisynthetic polysaccharide gums, see *Industrial Gums, Polysaccharides and their Derivatives*, 2nd Edn, R.L. Whistler and J.N. BeMiller (Eds), London, Academic Press, 1973.

Sources of gums and their use in food.— R. L. Urquidi, *Int. Flavours & Food Addit.*, 1978, *9*, 73, per *Int. pharm. Abstr.*, 1978, *15*, 1032.

Bulk laxatives. The 4 types of hydrophilic agents used to increase the bulk of the stools by absorbing water were the cellulose ethers, such as methylcellulose; mucilaginous gums, such as sterculia; mucilaginous seeds and seed coats, such as ispaghula and psyllium; and various forms of wheat bran. Although pharmacologically inert they relieved constipation, haemorrhoids, and anal fissure by producing softer and larger stools and modifying colonic transit time. They were also used in the treatment of the irritable bowel, diverticular disease, diarrhoea, and in the management of colostomy and ileostomy. Side-effects such as flatulence, discomfort, and bolus formation could be reduced by ensuring adequate fluid intake.— *Drug & Ther. Bull.*, 1973, *11*, 77.

A discussion of the use of hydrophilic bulking agents in the treatment of constipation and allied disorders.— E. W. Godding, *Pharm. J.*, 1975, *2*, 34.

A brief discussion of precautions and adverse effects for bulk laxatives.— M. Samer, *Practitioner*, 1976, *216*, 661.

5401-h

Methylcellulose.

Metilcelulosa. A methyl ether of cellulose containing up to about 33% of methoxyl ($-OCH_3$) groups, calculated on the dry substance. The *B.P.* specifies 26 to 32% and 4 specific grades. The *U.S.P.* specifies 27.5 to 31.5%.

CAS — 9004-67-5.

Pharmacopoeias. In *Arg., Aust., Br., Braz., Fr., Hung., It., Jap., Roum., Span., Swiss,* and *U.S.*

A white or creamy-white, odourless, tasteless, somewhat hygroscopic fibrous powder or granules. It loses not more than 5% (*U.S.P.*) or 10% (*B.P.*) of its weight on drying.

Slowly **soluble** in cold water, yielding a clear or opalescent viscous colloidal solution; practically insoluble in hot water but dissolves on cooling; practically insoluble in alcohol, chloroform, and ether; soluble in a mixture of equal volumes of alcohol and chloroform, and in glacial acetic acid. A 1% solution in water has a pH of 6 to 8. **Incompatibilities** have been reported with aminacrine hydrochloride, chlorocresol, mercuric chloride, phenol, resorcinol, tannic acid, and silver nitrate.

Large amounts of electrolytes increase the viscosity of methylcellulose mucilages owing to salting-out of the methylcellulose; in very high concentrations of electrolytes, the methylcellulose may be completely precipitated in the form of a discrete or continuous gel. **Store** in a cool place in airtight containers. Solutions are sterilised by autoclaving.

The name 'methylcellulose' is commonly followed by a number indicating the approximate viscosity of a 2% w/v solution at 20°. The *B.P.* specifies **Methylcellulose 20** containing 26 to 32% of methoxyl groups and having a viscosity of a 2% solution at 20° of 17 to 23 centistokes. **Methylcellulose 450** contains 26 to 32% of methoxyl groups and a 2% solution at 20° has a viscosity of 350 to 550 centistokes. **Methylcellulose 2500** contains 27 to 29% of methoxyl groups and a 2% solution at 20° has a viscosity of 2200 to 2800 centistokes. **Methylcellulose 4500** contains 27 to 29% of methoxyl groups and a 2% solution at 20° has a viscosity of 4000 to 5000 centistokes.

To prepare a solution, slowly add the methylcellulose to about one-third the required amount of boiling water and stir the mixture until the material is thoroughly wetted; if the methylcellulose is not thoroughly wetted, lumps may be formed which are very difficult to disperse. Add the remainder of the water, preferably in the form of ice, and dissolve the wetted material with constant stirring.

Methylcellulose forms colourless, odourless, tasteless, inert, neutral mucilages, which are stable in acid or alkaline solution (pH 2 to 12) and in the presence of small concentrations of most electrolytes. Stock solutions should contain a suitable antimicrobial preservative such as phenylmercuric nitrate (0.001%). Various methylcelluloses, graded according to the viscosity of their solutions, are available commercially; the viscosities decrease with increase in temperature, which if raised sufficiently may result in precipitation of the methylcellulose, though on cooling the methylcellulose redissolves and the viscosity increases again; prolonged heating causes a permanent loss in viscosity but, unlike the natural gums, the viscosities remain stable for many months at normal temperatures.

Incompatibility. Methylcellulose formed complexes in solution with *p*-hydroxybenzoic acid, methyl hydroxybenzoate, propyl hydroxybenzoate, butyl hydroxybenzoate, and aminobenzoic acid; no apparent interaction occurred with ethyl aminobenzoate.— W. J. Tillman and R. Kuramoto, *J. Am. pharm. Ass., scient. Edn*, 1957, *46*, 211.

Methyl and propyl hydroxybenzoate reacted with methylcellulose, macrogols, povidone, and gelatin; there was no evidence of interaction of these hydroxybenzoates with carmellose sodium or tragacanth.— G. M. Miyawaki *et al.*, *J. Am. pharm. Ass., scient. Edn*, 1959, *48*, 315.

Methylcellulose reacted significantly with cetylpyridinium chloride but not with benzalkonium chloride.— P. P. Deluca and H. B. Kostenbauder, *J. Am. pharm. Ass., scient. Edn*, 1960, *49*, 430.

The presence of 1% methylcellulose caused an increase in the minimum inhibitory concentration of chloroxylenol of 81% against *Bacillus subtilis* and 400% against *Pseudomonas aeruginosa*. Activity against *Aspergillus niger* was unaffected.— M. D. Ray *et al.*, *J. pharm. Sci.*, 1968, *57*, 609.

Stability. Irreversible viscosity decreases could occur on heating dispersions of methylcellulose, ethylmethylcellulose, and carmellose sodium; the extent of the decrease varied with the temperature and time of heating and with the viscosity grade and type of derivative. Decrease in viscosity caused by heat in the presence of acid was greater than in neutral or alkaline dispersions. Viscosity changes could also occur in unheated dispersions in the presence of acid or alkali.

Small concentrations of salts decreased the viscosity of carmellose sodium sols but had no effect on methylcellulose sols and ethylmethylcellulose sols. Larger amounts caused the viscosities of methylcellulose sols and ethylmethylcellulose sols to increase. Industrial methylated spirit, propylene glycol, and glycerol increased the viscosities of all dispersions. The effect of sodium lauryl sulphate on carmellose sodium sols was similar to that of salts, and cetrimide precipitated the derivative. Dispersions of methylcellulose and of ethylmethylcellulose increased and then decreased in viscosity with increasing concentrations of sodium lauryl sulphate; cetrimide increased the viscosity. All derivatives were degraded by micro-organisms.

The viscosity of preserved dispersions of methylcellulose and of ethylmethylcellulose altered little over a year. The greatest decreases occurred in the highest viscosity grade samples stored at the highest temperature (30°). All dispersions of carmellose sodium decreased in viscosity over the storage period, storage in light producing the most unstable sols. The pH change of any dispersion on storage was negligible.— R. E. M. Davies and J. M. Rowson, *J. Pharm. Pharmac.*, 1957, *9*, 672; *idem*, 1958, *10*, 30.

Adverse Effects. Large quantities of methylcellulose and other bulk laxatives may temporarily increase flatulence and distension and intestinal obstruction has been reported after their administration. Oesophageal obstruction has also occurred when these agents have been swallowed dry.

Studies indicating that diets containing large amounts of nonabsorbable polysaccharides, such as cellulose, might decrease absorption of calcium, magnesium, zinc and phosphorus.— J. G. Reinhold *et al.*, *J. Nutr.*, 1976, *106*, 493; F. Ismail-Beigi *et al.*, *ibid.*, 1977, *107*, 510.

Precautions. Methylcellulose and other bulk laxatives should not be given to patients with intestinal obstruction, and they may be contra-indicated in patients with spastic bowel conditions. They should be taken with fluid to prevent faecal impaction or oesophageal obstruction.

Bulk laxatives lower the transit time through the gut and could affect the absorption of other drugs. Some bulk-forming agents may reduce postprandial blood glucose concentrations and may thereby alter insulin demand in patients with diabetes.

Bulk-forming laxatives may be contra-indicated in some patients with ulcerative colitis or regional ileitis.— *Med. Lett.*, 1975, *17*, 93.

Uses. Low-viscosity grades of methylcellulose, such as methylcellulose 20, are used as emulsifying agents for liquid paraffin and other mineral oils, and for vegetable oils such as arachis oil and olive oil; they are less efficient for emulsifying cod-liver oil. Emulsions are prepared by mixing the oil with the methylcellulose mucilage, preferably using a mechanical stirrer.

High-viscosity grades, such as methylcellulose 2500 or 4500, are used as thickening agents for medicated jellies and creams, as dispersing and thickening agents in suspensions, and as binding and disintegrating agents in tablets. A 0.5 to 1% solution of a high-viscosity grade has been used as a vehicle for eye-drops but hypromellose (see p.956) is now generally preferred for this purpose.

Medium- or high-viscosity grades, such as methylcellulose 450, 2500 or 4500, are used as bulk laxatives since by taking up moisture they increase the volume of the faeces and promote peristalsis. They are usually given in the form of granules or tablets, in a dosage of 1 to 6 g daily in divided doses taken with plenty of fluid. The effect of bulk laxatives is usually apparent within 12 to 24 hours, but up to 3 days of medication may be required to achieve the full effect. They are also given with a minimum amount of water, for the control of diarrhoea and in the management of ostomies. The value of using methylcellulose to relieve hunger in the management of obesity appears to be doubtful.

Methylcellulose is widely employed in the food industry and is used as an adhesive in plaster of Paris bandages.

For the use of a 1 or 2% aqueous solution of methylcellulose in conjunction with barium enema in a double contrast technique for the detection of diverticulosis and diverticular disease, see V. K. Clifton and A. I. Robertson, *Med. J. Aust.*, 1968, *2*, 899.

Studies in 9 healthy subjects showed that the addition of 5% methylcellulose to a 0.5% suspension of nitrofurantoin in water delayed the excretion of nitrofurantoin in urine. The amount excreted over 6 hours was significantly reduced.— H. Seager (letter), *J. Pharm. Pharmac.*, 1968, *20*, 968.

Estimated acceptable daily intake: up to 25 mg per kg body-weight, as the sum of total modified celluloses. The figure may be exceeded for dietetic purposes.— Seventeenth Report of FAO/WHO Expert Committee on Food Additives, *Tech. Rep. Ser. Wld Hlth Org. No. 539*, 1974.

For background toxicological information, see *Fd Add. Ser. Wld Hlth Org. No. 5*, 1974.

Binding agent for tablets. A study of the effect of some binding agents, including methylcellulose, on the mechanical properties of granules and their compression characteristics.— E. Doelker and E. Shotton, *J. Pharm. Pharmac.*, 1977, *29*, 193.

A study of the effect of methylcellulose, hydroxyethylcellulose and hydroxypropylcellulose on the disintegration and dissolution rates of tablets with changing temperature, when used as a binding agent.— H. Delonca *et al.*, *J. Pharm. Belg.*, 1978, *33*, 171.

Diverticular disease. In 6 patients with diverticular disease, treatment for 6 months with methylcellulose tablets led to reduction in rectosigmoid pressure; all patients became free of symptoms.— J. Hodgson, *Br. med. J.*, 1972, *3*, 729.

Haemostatic. Methylcellulose had been suggested for use as a haemostatic agent for topical use, mainly to reduce capillary bleeding. It was capable of absorbing 8 times its weight of fluid and after use could be easily and painlessly removed. Absorption of fluid caused the methylcellulose to swell thereby compressing the bleeding capillaries.— M. Verstraete, *Haemostatic Drugs, A Critical Appraisal*, The Hague, Martinus Nijhoff, 1977.

Obesity. As a bulk producing agent methylcellulose was not considered to have any special merit in the treatment of obesity; apples, celery, raw carrots, or salads were more palatable and equally effective.— J. Mayer, *New Engl. J. Med.*, 1966, *274*, 722.

When methylcellulose 0.5 or 1 g was given with water 30 minutes before a meal, gastric emptying began at once and by the time the subject started eating almost all the dose had moved into the small intestine. There was therefore no effect of increasing bulk in the stomach to produce satiety. Neither was there any evidence that increasing the volume of a meal with methylcellulose decreased the rate of ingestion since no extra chewing would be required. Satiety could not be produced by altering gastro-intestinal transport since peristalsis was increased by methylcellulose.— E. J. Drenick (letter), *J. Am. med. Ass.*, 1975, *234*, 271.

Use in ophthalmic ointment. An ophthalmic ointment containing methylcellulose 4% for protection of the eyes during anaesthesia did not absorb halothane to the same extent as the fat based protective eye ointments normally used. Water loss from the surface of the methylcellulose ointment led to the development of a sticky layer which effectively kept the eyes closed and thus prevented dehydration of the eyes.— P. Bundgaard-Nielsen *et al.*, *Arch. Pharm. Chemi, scient. Edn*, 1978, *6*, 121.

Use in ophthalmic solutions. The addition of 1% of methylcellulose 4000 to homatropine hydrobromide eye-drops increased the effect of the drug on the eye, the viscous nature of the preparation increasing the time of contact with the cornea and decreasing reflex lachrymation.— W. H. Mueller and D. L. Deardoff, *J. Am. pharm. Ass., scient. Edn*, 1956, *45*, 334.

In a controlled crossover study, a 2% pilocarpine hydrochloride solution containing 0.5% methylcellulose produced significantly greater miosis and lowering of intra-ocular pressure than a pilocarpine solution without methylcellulose.— J. S. Haas and D. L. Merrill, *Am. J. Ophthal.*, 1962, *54*, 21.

Preparations

Methylcellulose Vehicle. Methylcellulose '20' 0.75, Nipasept 0.1, water to 60; dissolve, then add propylene glycol 2, DC Antifoam Emulsion 'M30' 0.05, syrup to 100. Sterilise by autoclaving. Used for preparing suspensions from crushed tablets.— B.A. Miller, *St. Bart's Hosp., J. Hosp. Pharm.*, 1975, *33*, 89.

Gels and Mucilages

Hydrogelum Methylcellulosi *(Hung. P.).* Methylcellulose '450' 5 g, glycerol 10 g, solutio conservans (*Hung. P.*) 1 g, water to 100 g.

Methylcellulose Mucilage *(A.P.F.).* Mucil. Methylcellulos. Methylcellulose '20' 2 g, freshly boiled and cooled water to 100 ml.

Granules

Methylcellulose Granules *(B.P.).* Methylcellulose '2500' or '4500' 64 g, vanillin 200 mg, saccharin sodium 100 mg, amaranth, food grade of commerce, 20 mg, acacia powder 4 g, lactose 31.68 g. Mix, add sufficient water to form a coherent mass suitable for granulation, and pass through a No. 6 sieve; place the granules on a No. 22 sieve, reject the powder which passes through, and dry the granules at a temperature not exceeding 60°. Store in airtight containers.

Mouthwashes

Methylcellulose Mouthwash *(Bristol Roy. Infirm.).* Methylcellulose '450' 1 g, citric acid monohydrate 4.5 g, saccharin solution 0.5 ml, concentrated chloroform water 2.5 ml, water to 100 ml. Shelf-life 3 months. 15 ml to be diluted with half a tumblerful of water before use. A sialagogue.

For other formulas for use as sialagogues or saliva replacements, see Saliva Replacement Solution under Carmellose Sodium (p.951), and Lemon Mouthwash under Citric Acid (p.785). See also under Hypromellose, p.956.

Ophthalmic Solutions

Contact Lens Wetting Solution. Methylcellulose 0.5%, benzalkonium chloride 0.025%, chlorhexidine 0.005%, water to 100%.—L. Jenkin and R. Tyler-Jones, *Theory and Practice of Contact Lens Fitting*, London, Hatton Press, 1964.

Methylcellulose Ophthalmic Solution *(U.S.P.).* A sterile solution of methylcellulose. It may contain suitable antimicrobial, buffering, and stabilising agents. pH 6 to 7.8. Store in airtight containers. Used as artificial tears or contact lens solution.

Solutions

Methylcellulose Oral Solution *(U.S.P.).* A flavoured solution of methylcellulose, with alcohol 3.5 to 6.5%. Store at a temperature not exceeding 40° in airtight containers; avoid freezing. Protect from light.

Tablets

Methylcellulose Tablets *(U.S.P.).* Tablets containing methylcellulose.

Proprietary Preparations

Celacol M *(British Celanese, UK).* A brand of methylcellulose, available in a number of grades of viscosity. **Celacol MM** grades are soluble in a variety of organic solvents.

Celevac *(WB Pharmaceuticals, UK: Boehringer Ingelheim, UK).* Methylcellulose 450, available as **Tablets** of 500 mg and as sweetened **Granules** containing 64%.

Cellucon *(Medo Chemicals, UK).* Tablets each containing methylcellulose '2500' 500 mg.

Cologel *(Lilly, UK).* A flavoured liquid containing methylcellulose 9% and alcohol 5% (suggested diluent, water). For constipation. *Dose.* 5 to 15 ml thrice daily with water; maintenance, 5 to 15 ml daily.

Methocel A *(Dow, USA: K & K-Greeff, UK).* A brand of methylcellulose, available in a number of grades of viscosity.

Nilstim *(Trentham, UK: De Witt, UK).* Tablets each containing methylcellulose '2500' 400 mg and microcrystalline cellulose 220 mg. For appetite control and colostomy management. *Dose.* 2 tablets, with a drink, 15 minutes before the 2 principal meals of the day.

Other Proprietary Names

Austral.—Cellulone; *Canad.*—BFL, Lacril; *Denm.*—Viscosae.

5402-m

Acacia *(B.P., Eur. P.).* Acac.; Acaciae Gummi; Gum Acacia; Gum Arabic; Gummi Africanum; Gummi Arabicum; Gummi Mimosae; Gomme Arabique; Gomme de Sénégal.

CAS — 9000-01-5.

Pharmacopoeias. In all pharmacopoeias examined, except *Braz.*, *Chin.*, *Rus.*, and *Turk.* Not in *U.S.* but in *U.S.N.F. Ind.* specifies Indian Gum (from *A. arabica*).

The air-dried gummy exudation from the stem and branches of *Acacia senegal* (Leguminosae) and other species of *Acacia* of African origin. It consists of a complex calcium, magnesium, and potassium salt of arabic acid, a high molecular weight polysaccharide composed of D-galactose, L-arabinose, L-rhamnose, and D-glucuronic acid residues.

Almost odourless, yellowish-white to pale amber, rounded or ovoid, brittle tears with a bland mucilaginous taste. The tears are opaque, frequently with a cracked surface, and are easily broken into angular fragments with glistening surfaces. It loses not more than 15% of its weight when dried. At relative humidities between 25 and 65%, the equilibrium moisture content of powdered acacia is about 8 to 13%, but at relative humidities above 70% it absorbs substantial amounts of moisture.

Very slowly **soluble** 1 in 2 of water leaving only a very small residue and forming a slightly acid mucilage; practically insoluble in alcohol, chloroform, ether, glycerol, and oils. A solution in water is laevorotatory. Solutions are **sterilised** by autoclaving. **Incompatible** with alcohol, adrenaline, amidopyrine, apomorphine, bismuth subnitrate, borax, cresol, eugenol, ferric salts, gallic acid, lead subacetate, mercurous chloride, morphine, phenol, physostigmine, tannins, thymol, vanillin, and with acids unless well diluted. Acacia contains an oxidising enzyme which may affect preparations containing easily oxidised substances; the enzyme may be inactivated by heating at 100° for a short time. **Store** in a cool dry place in airtight containers.

Stock solutions should contain a suitable preservative.

The *B.P.* also describes Powdered Acacia; the *U.S.N.F.* also describes flake, granular, powdered, and spray-dried acacia.

Effect of gamma-irradiation. The sterilisation of acacia by irradiation with 25 000 Gy caused a loss of 16% in intrinsic viscosity in solutions prepared from it.— A. W. Hartman *et al.*, *J. pharm. Sci.*, 1975, *64*, 802.

Adverse Effects. Hypersensitivity reactions have occurred rarely after inhalation or ingestion of acacia.

Three renal transplant recipients found to be hypersensitive to prednisone tablets had reacted to the tragacanth and acacia used in their manufacture. Their symptoms subsided when a formulation using methylcellulose was substituted.— D. Rubinger *et al.* (letter), *Lancet*, 1978, *2*, 689.

Uses. Acacia forms viscous but not gelled solutions in water and is used with tragacanth as a suspending agent for resinous tinctures and non-dispersible powders in mixtures. Powdered acacia is used as an emulsifying agent for emulsions to be taken by mouth; 1 part of acacia is mixed with 4 parts of fixed oil or liquid paraffin and with 2 parts of water to form a primary emulsion; volatile oils require twice the proportion of gum and water.

Acacia is used as a demulcent in lozenges and pastilles where it provides slow disintegration. It may also be used with gelatin in micro-encapsulation procedures. It has been used as a granulating and binding agent for tablets but it has a tendency to prolong the disintegration time.

It is used in the food industry to retard sugar crystallisation, and as a thickener and emulsifier.

For a review of the chemistry and properties of acacia and other gums, see *The Chemistry and Rheology of Water-soluble Gums and Colloids*, SCI Monograph No. 24, London, Society of Chemical Industry, 1966.

Sensitivity reactions occurred rarely after inhalation or ingestion of acacia. Its use in food was not limited but further information was required.— *Fd Add. Ser. Wld Hlth Org. No. 5*, 1974.

Preparations

Acacia and Tragacanth Powder *(B.P.C. 1949)*. Pulv. Acac. et Trag.; Compound Powder of Acacia. Acacia 1 and tragacanth 1. A pill excipient.

Acacia Mucilage *(B.P. 1953)*. Mucilago Acaciae. Acacia 4 by wt, rinsed to remove dust, and dissolved in chloroform water 6 by vol. This quantity measures about 8¾ vol. It should be recently prepared. For suspending resinous tinctures, it is used in the proportion of 1 in 16 to 1 in 8 of the finished mixture.

A.P.F. includes benzoic acid 0.1%. Some pharmacopoeias include acacia mucilages of varying strengths, usually including a preservative such as sodium benzoate or methyl hydroxybenzoate.

Acacia Syrup *(U.S.N.F.)*. Acacia 10 g, sodium benzoate 100 mg, vanilla tincture 0.5 ml, sucrose 80 g, water to 100 ml. Store at a temperature not exceeding 40° in airtight containers.

Similar syrups are included in *Arg.P.*, *Port.P.*, and *Span.P.*

Gummi Arabicum Desenzymatum *(Aust. P., Roum. P., Span. P., Swiss P.)*. Obtained by evaporating the mucilage and powdering the residue; oxidase is thus destroyed.

5403-b

Agar *(U.S.N.F., B.P.C. 1954)*. Agar-agar; Japanese Isinglass; Layor Carang; Gélose; Colle du Japon; Gelosa.

CAS — 9002-18-0.

Pharmacopoeias. In *Arg., Aust., Braz., Chin., Cz., Fr., Hung., Ind., It., Jap., Jug., Mex., Nord., Pol., Port., Span.*, and *Swiss*. Also in *U.S.N.F.*

The dried hydrophilic colloidal substance extracted from *Gelidium cartilagineum* (Gelidiaceae), *Gracilaria confervoides* (Sphaerococcaceae), and related algae belonging to the Rhodophyceae. It consists chiefly of the calcium salt of the sulphuric acid ester of a linear polygalactose composed of D-galactose and 3,6-anhydro-L-galactose units.

Odourless or almost odourless, thin, greyish-white, translucent strips or flakes, or yellowish flattened bands, granules, or powder with a mucilaginous taste. It loses not more than 20% of its weight on drying. **Soluble** in boiling water; practically insoluble in organic solvents. It swells to a gelatinous mass in cold water; a 1.5% solution forms a stiff jelly on cooling. Solutions are **sterilised** by autoclaving. **Store** in a dry place.

Agars from different sources have different gelling powers. New Zealand agar 0.7%, Australian agar 2%, or South African agar 1%, will usually yield gels equivalent in strength to that produced by 1% of Japanese agar.

So-called agars, known as 'British agar' and 'Galway agar', are prepared chiefly from *Chondrus crispus* and *Gigartina stellata* (Gigartinaceae). The ash content of the 'agars' is usually very high.

The strength of agar gels is increased by ceratonia, dextrose, and sucrose. Gelatin, isinglass, sodium alginate, starch, and sterculia tend to weaken agar gels.

Adverse Effects and Precautions. As for Methylcellulose, p.947.

Uses. Agar is not digested and passes through the intestine almost unchanged. It has been used as a bulk laxative, since by taking up moisture it increases the volume of the faeces and promotes peristalsis. For this purpose it was taken in doses of 4 to 16 g once or twice daily crushed into small pieces and sprinkled on a little moist food such as stewed fruit.

Emulsions containing agar with liquid paraffin, phenolphthalein, and magnesium hydroxide have also been used but the small amount of agar in these acts solely as an emulsion stabiliser.

Agar is also used as the basis of many culture media for micro-organisms, and as a thickening agent in the food industry.

The properties of Spanish agar.— W. W. Binns *et al.*, *Pharm. J.*, 1970, *1*, 7.

The use of agar in food was limited only by good manufacturing practice. For background toxicological information, see *Fd Add. Ser. Wld Hlth Org. No. 5*, 1974.

A study in 80 premature infants given agar as a supplement to feeds indicated that it was of no value in the management of hyperbilirubinaemia in low birth-weight newborn infants.— C. Romagnoli *et al.*, *Archs Dis. Childh.*, 1975, *50*, 202.

5404-v

Althaea *(B.P.C. 1949)*. Alth.; Marshmallow; Marshmallow Root; Racine de Guimauve; Eibischwurzel; Raiz de Altea; Alteia.

Pharmacopoeias. In *Aust., Belg., Cz., Fr., Ger., Hung., It., Jug., Mex., Pol., Port., Roum., Rus., Span.*, and *Swiss*.

Althaea Leaf is included in *Aust., Belg., Cz., Fr., Hung., Jug., Pol.*, and *Roum.*, and Althaea Flower in *Belg., Fr.*

The dried peeled root of *Althaea officinalis* (Malvaceae), collected in the autumn from plants at least 2 years old and containing not less than 20% of water-soluble extractive. It contains 25 to 35% of mucilage. **Store** in a dry place.

Uses. Althaea is demulcent and emollient and was formerly used, in the form of an infusion or syrup, for irritation and inflammation of the mucous membranes of the mouth and pharynx. The leaves were similarly used. The root, flowers and leaves have been used as a poultice.

Preparations

Althaea Syrup *(B.P.C. 1949)*. Syr. Alth.; Marshmallow Syrup. Macerate althaea 4 g with water 56 ml for 12 hours, strain, filter into a tared vessel, and dissolve sucrose 90 g in the filtrate, heating to boiling; then allow to cool, replace any of the water lost by evaporation, strain, add chloroform 0.25 ml and shake until dissolved. *Dose.* 2 to 8 ml. A similar syrup is included in some pharmacopoeias.

5405-g

Aluminium Magnesium Silicate *(B.P.)*.

Magnesium Aluminum Silicate *(U.S.N.F.)*; Magnesium Aluminium Silicate; Saponite.

CAS — 1327-43-1; 12511-31-8.

The name Almasilate is applied to artificial aluminium silicate hydrate, for use as an antacid.

Pharmacopoeias. In *Br.* Also in *U.S.N.F.*

A hydrated native colloidal saponite freed from gritty particles. It is an odourless or almost odourless, tasteless creamy-white powder or small flakes. Practically **insoluble** in water, but swells to form a colloidal dispersion; practically insoluble in organic solvents. A 4% to 5% dispersion in water has a pH of 9 to 10.

The *B.P.* specifies that it loses not more than 10% of its weight when dried and also specifies a viscosity of about 250 centipoises for a 5% dispersion.

The *U.S.N.F.* specifies that it loses not more than 8% of its weight when dried and also describes 6 types with varying ranges of aluminium:magnesium content and varying viscosity ranges for dispersions of approximately 5%.

In preparing suspensions, the aluminium magnesium silicate is slowly added to the water with stirring until smooth.

Uses. Aluminium magnesium silicate is used, usually at a concentration of 0.5 to 2.5%, as a suspending and thickening agent and as an emulsion stabiliser in pharmaceutical preparations for internal and external use. Dispersions in water are thixotropic, and a 10% suspension is a firm gel. This viscosity of the suspensions is increased by heating, by the addition of electrolytes, and, at higher concentrations, by ageing.

It may be used in reduced amounts with other suspending agents and gums. Some grades are used as binding and disintegrating agents in tablets and in toothpastes.

An evaluation of aluminium magnesium silicate as an alternative to tragacanth.— C. A. Farley and W. Lund, *Pharm. J.*, 1976, *1*, 562.

Proprietary Preparations

Veegum *(Vanderbilt, USA: K & K-Greeff, UK)*. A brand of aluminium magnesium silicate. Available grades include **Veegum F**, a microfine powder; **Veegum HV**, a high-viscosity grade in the form of flakes; **Veegum K**, a grade producing stable suspensions with minimum thickening and flocculation in acid formulations; and **Veegum WG**, a powder.

Other Proprietary Names

Dianeusine *(Fr.)*; Sicco-Gynaedron *(Ger.)*.

5406-q

Apricot Gum. Gummi Armeniacae.

CAS — 56093-73-3.

Pharmacopoeias. In *Rus.*

A dried gummy exudation from the trunk and branches of the apricot tree, *Armeniaca vulgaris* (= *Prunus armeniaca*) (Rosaceae).

Apricot gum has properties resembling those of acacia.

5407-p

Bentonite *(B.P., Eur. P.)*. Bentonitum; Mineral Soap; Soap Clay; Wilkinite.

CAS — 1302-78-9.

Pharmacopoeias. In *Arg., Aust., Br., Cz., Eur., Fr., Ger., Ind., It., Jap., Neth.*, and *Swiss*. Also in *U.S.N.F.*

Native colloidal hydrated aluminium silicate, freed from gritty particles, consisting mainly of montmorillonite, $Al_2O_3,4SiO_2,H_2O$, but usually containing some magnesium and iron, together with small amounts of calcium carbonate and other minerals.

An odourless, hygroscopic, very fine, homogeneous, greyish-white powder with a yellowish tint, or pale buff-coloured powder, with a slight earthy taste. It loses 5 to 12% of its weight when dried.

Practically **insoluble** in water and in aqueous solutions, but swells into a homogeneous mass occupying about 12 times the volume of the dry powder. Practically insoluble, and does not swell, in organic solvents. A 2% suspension in water has a pH of 9.5 to 10.5. **Sterilised** by maintaining at 150° for 1 hour after drying at 100°; aqueous suspensions are sterilised by autoclaving.

Incompatible with strong electrolytes, positively charged particles and solutions, sulphurated potash, and acriflavine hydrochloride. **Store** in airtight containers.

Incompatibility. Suspensions of bentonite 5% containing concentrations of disinfectants likely to be encountered in practice were prepared and investigated. Bacteriological investigations indicated that cationic antibacterial substances were inhibited or inactivated by bentonite in aqueous suspensions but anionic and nonionic types were not affected. This inactivation was due to removal from solution of the cationic substance by a cation-exchange mechanism.— W. A. Harris, *Australas. J. Pharm.*, 1961, *42*, 583.

Uses. Bentonite absorbs water readily to form sols or gels, depending on its concentration, a preparation containing about 7% of bentonite being just pourable. The sols are suitable for suspending powders in aqueous preparations such as Calamine Lotion, and the gels for ointment and cream bases. These preparations have a pH of about 9; the gelling property of bentonite is much reduced in the presence of acid and increased by the addition of such alkaline substances as magnesium oxide.

In aqueous sols and gels, bentonite particles are negatively charged and flocculation occurs when electrolytes or positively charged suspensions are added. Because of this property bentonite is sometimes used in clarifying turbid liquids.

Sols and gels may conveniently be prepared by sprinkling the bentonite on the surface of hot water and allowing to stand for about 24 hours, stirring occasionally when the bentonite has become thoroughly wetted. A dispersion in water can also be prepared by first triturating the bentonite with glycerol or by mixing it with insoluble powders such as zinc oxide.

For suspending powders in aqueous preparations and for preparing cream bases containing suitable proportions of oil-in-water emulsifying agents such as Emulsifying Wax and Self-Emulsifying Glyceryl Monostearate, 2% of bentonite is adequate. A preparation containing 10 to 20% of bentonite and 10% of glycerol is also suitable as a basis. A sol containing 5% is convenient for dispensing purposes.

Bentonite should be sterilised before it is used for preparations intended for application to open wounds since it is liable to contain bacterial spores, including those of tetanus.

A 7% aqueous suspension of bentonite has been used for the treatment of poisoning by paraquat. Bentonite has also been used in the form of a gel as a bulk laxative.

Preparations

Bentonite Magma *(U.S.N.F.)*. Bentonite 5% w/w in water. Store in airtight containers.

5408-s

Bladderwrack *(B.P.C. 1949)*. Fucus; Seawrack; Kelpware; Tang.

Pharmacopoeias. In *Ger.* and *Pol. Ger.* also allows *Ascophyllum nodosum*.

The dried plant, *Fucus vesiculosus* (Fucaceae). It contains the gelatinous substance, algin, and at least 0.05% iodine. **Store** in a dry place. Protect from light.

Bladderwrack was formerly used in the management of obesity.

Kelp is a preparation of dried seaweed of various species that may be used as a domestic source of iodine.

Elevated concentrations of arsenic in urine were observed in 2 adults who ingested health food supplements derived from kelp. Concentrations slowly fell after discontinuation of the kelp tablets. Significant amounts of arsenic were subsequently found in several commercially available kelp products.— O. Walkiw and D. E. Douglas, *Clin. Toxicol.*, 1975, *8*, 325, per *Int. pharm. Abstr.*, 1976, *13*, 930.

5409-w

Carbomer *(B.P., U.S.N.F.)*. Carboxypolymethylene; Carboxyvinyl Polymer.

CAS — 54182-57-9.

Pharmacopoeias. In *Br.* Also in *U.S.N.F.*

A synthetic high molecular weight polymer of acrylic acid cross-linked with allylsucrose and containing 56 to 68% of carboxylic acid groups.

A white, fluffy, acid, hygroscopic powder with a slight characteristic odour. A 1% dispersion in water has a pH of about 3. Neutralised with alkali hydroxides or amines, it is **soluble** in water, alcohol, and glycerol. The *U.S.N.F.* specifies that the viscosity of a 0.5% neutralised solution is 30 000 to 40 000 centipoises.

In preparing a gel, the powder should first be dispersed in water with the aid of a high-speed stirrer, care being taken to avoid the formation of indispersible lumps. The solution is then neutralised with sodium hydroxide solution; 400 mg of sodium hydroxide neutralises 1 g of carbomer. The mixture should be slowly agitated with a broad paddle-type stirrer and care should be taken to avoid introducing air bubbles into the gel.

For gels in alcohols, glycols, and other organic solvents, a base must be chosen which reacts with carbomer to form a salt which is soluble in the particular solvent; bases which may be suitable for some solvents include ammonia solution, triethanolamine, and di-isopropanolamine.

Neutralised aqueous gels of carbomer are most viscous between pH 6 and pH 11; the viscosity is considerably reduced if the pH is less than 3 or greater than 12. Viscosity is also reduced in the presence of strong electrolytes. Gels rapidly lose viscosity on exposure to sunlight but this reaction can be minimised by the addition of an antioxidant. Aqueous gels are **sterilised** by autoclaving. **Store** in airtight containers. Protect from light.

Mucilages of carbomer should contain a suitable antimicrobial preservative; chlorocresol 0.1% or thiomersal 0.01% is suitable.

Effect of gamma-irradiation. The gel structure of gels based on carbomer was completely lost after gamma-irradiation. Addition of alcohol (95%) at a concentration of 5 to 10% provided suitable protection.— I. Adams *et al.*, *J. Pharm. Pharmac.*, 1972, *24*, 178P.

Incompatibility. Carbopol 934 was found to be incompatible in gels with phenol and was discoloured by resorcinol.— P. M. Caver *et al.*, *Am. J. Pharm.*, 1957, *129*, 118.

When added to solutions of Carbopol 934 in the concentrations commonly used for preservative purposes, benzoic acid and sodium benzoate caused a significant change in viscosity or a precipitate. When present in higher concentrations, benzalkonium chloride, benzethonium chloride, and phenylmercuric acetate caused a decrease in viscosity and the formation of a precipitate; thiomersal caused a significant decrease in viscosity only if present in excessive concentrations.— T. W. Schwarz and G. Levy, *Drug Stand.*, 1957, *25*, 154.

When, in preparing a suspension, Carbopol 934 was mixed with calamine or zinc oxide before being neutralised, an unsightly granular product of low viscosity resulted.— J. A. Lee and W. L. Nobles, *J. Am. pharm. Ass., scient. Edn*, 1959, *48*, 92.

Uses. Carbomer is used in the form of a neutralised gel as a suspending agent in pharmaceutical preparations for internal and external use. Concentrations of 0.1 to 0.4% are used in suspensions. In a concentration of 0.5 to 5%, carbomer is used as an aqueous ointment or gel basis. It is also used as a binding agent in tablets and in the formulation of prolonged-action preparations.

Carbomer is employed as an emulsifying agent in the preparation of oil-in-water emulsions for external use; for this purpose, it is neutralised partly with sodium hydroxide and partly with a long-chain amine such as stearylamine.

Carbomer reacts with basic drugs, such as ephedrine, to form a derivative which can be incorporated in gels; derivatives of this nature have been suggested for use in prolonged-action preparations.

It is widely used in the manufacture of cosmetics and in various industrial suspensions and emulsions.

For the use of carbomer for the thickening and gelling of glycols and macrogols and their derivatives without neutralisation, see W. Lang, *Drug Cosmet. Ind.*, 1972, *110* (Apr.), 52.

Formulas of gels, easily prepared in a hospital pharmacy and based on the use of carbomer, including a lubricant gel, gel for ultrasonography, rifamycin gel, anaesthetic lubricant gel, and progesterone hydroalcoholic gel.— F. Mathot, *Pharmakon*, 1977, *29*, 59, per *Int. pharm. Abstr.*, 1977, *14*, 826.

Studies on the rheological properties of Carbopol gels.— B. W. Barry and M. C. Meyer, *Int. J. Pharmaceut.*, 1979, *2*, 1 and 27.

A Carbopol imparted resistance to virus infection in *mice* when given by intraperitoneal injection 1 or 4 days before challenge with vaccinia virus or herpes simplex virus. An interferon-like substance was detected in the blood.— E. De Clercq and M. Luczak, *Arch. Virol.*, 1976, *52*, 151, per *Abstr. Hyg.*, 1978, *53*, 259.

Ophthalmic preparations. For reference to the suitability of aqueous gels containing carbomer for use in ophthalmic preparations, see F. Bottari *et al.*, *Farmaco, Edn prat.*, 1978, *33*, 434.

Use of sterilised gel. Gels have been repeatedly autoclaved without loss of viscosity and maintained their consistency over a pH range of 5 to 11; the sterilised gels adjusted to the desired pH might be of value in controlling the excoriation around fistulas and surgical incisions.— W. Saski, *Drug Stand.*, 1960, *28*, 79.

Proprietary Preparations

Carbopol 934 *(Goodrich, UK)*. A brand of carbomer. Grades are available for use in pharmaceutical preparations for internal or external use; it is also used in cosmetic and industrial products. **Carbopol 940** forms very clear gels in aqueous and non-aqueous vehicles and is used in cosmetics. **Carbopol 941** is used in cosmetic and other preparations where stability at low viscosity is required.

5410-m

Carmellose Calcium. Carboxymethylcellulose Calcium *(U.S.N.F.)*; Calcium Carboxymethylcellulose.

CAS — 9050-04-8.

Pharmacopoeias. In *Jap.* Also in *U.S.N.F.*

A white to yellowish-white hygroscopic powder. It loses not more than 10% of its weight on drying. It swells in water to form a suspension; practically **insoluble** in acetone, alcohol, chloroform, and ether. A 1% suspension in water has a pH of 4.5 to 6. **Store** in airtight containers.

5411-b

Carmellose Sodium. Sodium Carboxymethylcellulose *(B.P.C. 1973)*; Carboxymethylcellulose Sodium *(U.S.P.)*; Cellulose Gum; CMC; SCMC; Sodium Cellulose Glycollate.

CAS — 9004-32-4.

Pharmacopoeias. In *Arg.*, *Aust.*, *Braz.*, *Cz.*, *Fr.*, *Hung.*, *Jap.*, *Nord.*, *Roum.*, *Swiss*, and *U.S. U.S.N.F.* includes Croscarmellose Sodium, previously known as Modified Cellulose Gum, a cross-linked polymer of carmellose sodium, for use as a tablet disintegrant.

The sodium salt of a polycarboxymethyl ether of cellulose. It may be represented by the formula $[C_6H_{10-x}O_5(CH_2.CO_2Na)_x]_n$ where x represents the degree of substitution and n the number of anhydroglucose units in the molecule. The degree of polymerisation, n, affects the viscosity of solution and different grades of material are available which yield aqueous solutions having various viscosities covering the range 6 to 4000 centipoises in 1% solution.

Carmellose sodium is a white to cream-coloured, odourless or almost odourless, hygroscopic powder or granules with a bland mucilaginous taste. It loses not more than 10% of its weight on drying.

Soluble in water at all temperatures, yielding a clear solution; practically insoluble in alcohol, ether, and most other organic solvents. A 1% solution in water has a pH of 6 to 8.5. Mucilages are more sensitive to changes in pH than are those of methylcellulose. The viscosity of a carmellose sodium mucilage is decreased markedly below pH 5 or above pH 10.

The dry powder can be **sterilised** by maintaining the whole of the powder at 160° for 1 hour, but this causes a substantial decrease in viscosity and some deterioration in the properties of solutions prepared from the sterilised material. The sterilisation of solutions by heating also causes some lowering of viscosity but this is much less marked. When a solution is heated in an autoclave at 125° for 15 minutes and allowed to cool, the viscosity may be expected to decrease by about 25% and allowance should be made for this when calculating the amount of carmellose sodium to be included in a preparation which is to be sterilised.

Stock solutions should contain a suitable antimicrobial preservative.

Incompatibilities have been reported with strongly acidic solutions, and heavy metal ions such as aluminium, zinc, mercury, silver, and iron, but these may depend on the criterion used (e.g. appearance of a turbidity, loss in viscosity, or adsorption of the added substance), the concentration of both the carmellose sodium and the added substance, and the grade of carmellose sodium. **Store** in airtight containers.

For comparison of the stability of mucilages of carmellose sodium and other cellulose derivatives, see Methylcellulose, p.947.

Effect of gamma-irradiation. Irradiation of solutions of carmellose sodium caused a severe drop in viscosity by reducing chain length and molecular weight of the polymer. As low a dose as 57 Gy reduced viscosity by 48 to 66%.— L. J. Rasero and D. M. Skauen, *J. pharm. Sci.*, 1967, *56*, 724.

Adverse Effects and Precautions. As for Methylcellulose, p.947.

Background toxicological information.— *Fd Add. Ser. Wld Hlth Org. No. 5*, 1974.

Uses. Carmellose sodium is used as a suspending agent for insoluble powders in aqueous preparations for oral and parenteral administration and external application. It can also be used for dispersing the precipitate formed when resinous tinctures are added to water. It is employed in alkaline eye-drops used as artificial tears. It is used as an emulsifying agent for oil-in-water emulsions but it is less efficient than methylcellulose. For these purposes, 0.25 to 1% of a medium-viscosity grade is usually sufficient.

Higher concentrations, such as 4 to 6%, of a medium-viscosity grade are used in the preparation of gels which can be employed as bases for applications and pastes; glycerol is usually included in these preparations to prevent drying-out. It is added in the proportions of about 1 part to 9 to microcrystalline cellulose to improve dispersion.

Medium- and high-viscosity grades of carmellose sodium are used as bulk laxatives. For this purpose 4 to 10 g is given daily in divided doses, as tablets, with plenty of water. Carmellose sodium is an ingredient of protective preparations used in the fitting of ileostomy and colostomy appliances.

Carmellose sodium is widely used in the food industry.

Carmellose calcium is also used in pharmaceutical processes.

Estimated acceptable daily intake: up to 25 mg per kg body-weight, as the sum of total modified celluloses. The figure may be exceeded for dietetic purposes.— Seventeenth Report of the FAO/WHO Expert Committee on Food Additives, *Tech. Rep. Ser. Wld Hlth Org. No. 539*, 1974.

An evaluation of different viscosity grades of carmellose sodium as tablet disintegrants.— K. A. Khan and C. T. Rhodes, *Pharm. Acta Helv.*, 1975, *50*, 99.

An evaluation of the use of carmellose sodium as an alternative to tragacanth in the preparation of chalk or sulphadimidine mixtures.— C. A. Farley and W. Lund, *Pharm. J.*, 1976, *1*, 562.

Barium enema. Visualisation of the colonic mucosa with barium enema was improved when 0.5 or 1% of carmellose was added to the enema. The amended preparation gave results comparable with those achieved with barium enemas containing tannic acid 0.5%.— C. A. Perez and M. J. Friedenberg, *Am. J. Roentg.*, 1967, *99*, 98, per *Abstr. Wld Med.*, 1967, *41*, 735.

Obesity. Bulk-producing tablets containing carmellose sodium 100 mg, alginic acid 200 mg, and sodium bicarbonate 70 mg (Pretts) reduced hunger in patients following a restricted-intake diet.— R. S. Shearer, *Curr. ther. Res.*, 1976, *19*, 433.

Preparations

Suspending Vehicle *(Gt Ormond St Child. Hosp.)*. Carmellose sodium 1.1, methyl hydroxybenzoate 0.1, glycerol 6, syrup 35, water to 100. It should be freshly prepared.

Creams

Cremor ad Explorationem *(Dan. Disp.)*. Carmellose sodium 3 g, methyl hydroxybenzoate 100 mg, glycerol 10 g, water to 100 g. Sterilised by autoclaving. Store in a cool place.

Jellies

Jelly Basis. Carmellose sodium (medium viscosity) 5, glycerol 15, alkyl hydroxybenzoates 0.17, water to 100. The carmellose sodium and glycerol were mixed to form a slurry, added to hot water in which the preservative had been dissolved, and stirred vigorously until a gel formed.—H.H. Hutchins and R.E. Singiser, *J. Am. pharm. Ass., pract. Pharm. Edn*, 1955, *16*, 226.

Lubricating Jelly. Carmellose sodium 1.5 g, propylene glycol 25 ml, methyl hydroxybenzoate 150 mg, water to 100 ml. The methyl hydroxybenzoate was dissolved in the propylene glycol, the carmellose sodium added, and mixed thoroughly; the distilled water was boiled, the propylene glycol mixture added with constant stirring, and stirred until cold. The viscosity could be varied by altering the carmellose sodium content.—*Bull. Am. Soc. Hosp. Pharm.*, 1953, *10*, 153.

Mucilages

Mucilago Carboximethylcellulosi *(Nord. P.)*. Carboxymethylcellulose Mucilage. Carmellose sodium 2 g, alcohol 15 g, and water 83 g.

Pastes

Carboxymethylcellulose Sodium Paste *(U.S.P.)*. A paste containing carmellose sodium 16 to 17%. Store at a temperature not exceeding 30°.

Solutions

Saliva Replacement Solution *(Roy. Marsden Hosp.)*. Carmellose sodium (low-viscosity grade) 1 g, potassium chloride 62.5 mg, sodium chloride 86.5 mg, magnesium chloride 5.9 mg, calcium chloride 16.6 mg, potassium phosphate 80 mg, monobasic potassium phosphate 32.5 mg, sodium methyl hydroxybenzoate 230 mg, sodium fluoride 442 µg, sorbitol solution 3.3 ml, amaranth solution 0.006 ml, Lemon Trutype (*Bush Boake Allen*) 0.05 ml, sterile distilled water to 100 ml. Prepared as a substitute for Va-OraLube, for use in patients receiving radiotherapy for neoplasms of head and neck.

Va-OraLube. A saliva substitute solution developed specifically for use in patients receiving radiotherapy for malignancy of the head and neck. It is stated to contain potassium phosphates, potassium chloride, sodium chloride, magnesium chloride, calcium chloride, sodium fluoride (2 ppm of F), sorbitol, 'binder' [probably carmellose], flavouring, dye, preservative, and water. Specific gravity 1.0054. pH is 7.0. The viscosity and electrolyte concentration are adjusted to approximate whole saliva. The solution was used 1 to 8 times a day by 30 patients with dry mouth who were taking neuroleptics or tricyclic antidepressants. Relief of symptoms of dryness was immediate and complete following rinsing of the mouth with a small volume. The lubricant effect generally lasted from 1 to 3 hours.—W.E. Fann and I.L. Shannon, *Am. J. Psychiat.*, 1978, *135*, 251.

An initial appraisal of the problems involved in the formulation of an artifical saliva.— Pharm. Soc. Lab. Rep. P/80/2, 1980.

For other formulas for use as sialagogues or saliva replacements see Methylcellulose Mouthwash, p.948, and Lemon Mouthwash, p.785. See also under Hypromellose, p.956.

Tablets

Carboxymethylcellulose Sodium Tablets *(U.S.P.)*. Tablets containing carmellose sodium. Store in airtight containers.

Proprietary Preparations

Blanose Cellulose Gum *(Hercules, UK)*. A brand of carmellose sodium available in a number of viscosity grades.

Cekol *(Billerud-Uddeholm, Swed.: Berol Kemi, UK)*. A brand of carmellose sodium available in a number of viscosity grades.

Cellosize CMC *(British Celanese, UK)*. A brand of carmellose sodium available in a number of viscosity grades.

Cellulose Gum *(Hercules, UK)*. A brand of carmellose sodium available in a number of viscosity grades.

Colobase *(Coloplast, UK)*. A paste containing carmellose sodium, liquid paraffin, guar gum, cetyl alcohol, and artificial gum and resin. A protecting and sealing preparation for use around ostomies.

Courlose *(British Celanese, UK)*. A brand of carmellose sodium available in several grades. **Courlose P** is suitable for pharmaceutical purposes and is available in a number of viscosity grades.

Orabase *(Squibb Surgicare, UK)*. An ointment containing carmellose sodium 16.58%, pectin 16.58%, and gelatin 16.58% in Plastibase (a liquid paraffin-polyethylene basis). For protection of lesions of the mouth and skin.

Orahesive *(Squibb Surgicare, UK)*. A powder with adherent properties consisting of equal parts of carmellose sodium, pectin, and gelatin. For protection of lesions of the mouth and skin.

Stomahesive *(Squibb Surgicare, UK)*. An adhesive plaster containing carmellose sodium 20%, gelatin 20%, pectin 20%, and polyisobutylene 40%, with a polyethylene backing. For peristomal protection.

Stomahesive applied to the donor site after the harvesting of split-skin grafts in the treatment of burns and after excision of skin lesions virtually eliminated pain at the donor site. Removal of the dressing after 6 days usually disclosed full healing.— J. W. Fisher and M. Neal (letter), *Med. J. Aust.*, 1978, *1*, 42.

Varihesive *(Squibb Surgicare, UK)*. A dressing for leg ulcers containing carmellose sodium 20%, gelatin 20%, pectin 20%, and polyisobutylene 40%.

Use of Varihesive produced healing in 36 of 43 chronic leg ulcers. Patients with painful ulcers reported relief of pain when the dressings were used.— G. D. Tracy *et al.*, *Med. J. Aust.*, 1977, *1*, 777. See also P. J. Ashurst, *Practitioner*, 1975, *215*, 353.

Other Proprietary Names

Orora *(Belg.)*; Solvacton *(Arg.)*.

Carmellose sodium was also formerly marketed in Great Britain under the proprietary name Edifas B (*ICI Organics*).

5412-v

Carrageenan. Carrageenin; Carraghénates; Chondrus Extract; Irish Moss Extract.

CAS — 9000-07-1 (carrageenan); 11114-20-8 (κ-carrageenan); 9064-57-7 (λ-carrageenan).

Pharmacopoeias. In *Fr.*

A dried aqueous extract from species of *Chondrus*, *Gigartina*, *Eucheuma*, or other members of the families Gigartinaceae and Solieriaceae. It is a variable mixture of the ammonium, calcium, potassium, and sodium salts of two polysaccharides, κ-carrageenan, which contains D-galactose, 3,6-anhydro-D-galactose, and ester sulphate groups, and non-gelling λ-carrageenan which contains mono- and disulphate esters of D-galactose; the carrageenans may be separated by the selective precipitation of κ-carrageenan with potassium ions. It should not be hydrolysed or otherwise chemically degraded.

A white to yellowish, coarse or fine, almost odourless powder with a mucilaginous taste. It loses not more than 12% of its weight on drying.

Soluble 1 in 100 of water at 85° forming a viscous clear or slightly opalescent solution. It disperses more readily if first mixed with alcohol, glycerol, or syrup. A 2% solution may vary in viscosity from 50 to 3000 centipoises at 40°. The viscosity is affected by the presence of cations; potassium, calcium, and ammonium ions promote gel formation.

Uses. Carrageenan is an anionic polysaccharide used in the food industry as an emulsifying, suspending, and gelling agent. Degraded carrageenan does not possess the viscosity or gelling properties of carrageenan; it was formerly used to treat ulcerative colitis and peptic ulceration.

Estimated acceptable daily intake of undegraded carrageenan: up to 75 mg per kg body-weight. Low-molecular-weight or degraded carrageenan should not be used in food.— Seventeenth Report of the FAO/WHO Expert Committee on Food Additives, *Tech. Rep. Ser. Wld Hlth Org. No. 539*, 1974.

For background toxicological data on carrageenan and degraded carrageenan, see *Fd Add. Ser. Wld Hlth Org. No. 5*, 1974.

A review of the biological properties of carrageenan, with particular reference to its use in the screening of anti-inflammatory agents.— M. Di Rosa, *J. Pharm. Pharmac.*, 1972, *24*, 89.

Four types of carrageenan studied produced precipitation of plasma proteins and induced aggregation of human platelets *in vitro*. The order of potency of inducing aggregation was iota, lambda, gelcarin and kappa and this correlated with their reported relative activity as inflammatory agents.— R. M. McMillan *et al.*, *J. Pharm. Pharmac.*, 1979, *31*, 148.

Degraded carrageenan. No additional colonic symptoms were observed in 200 patients with peptic ulcer treated with degraded carrageenan (Ebimar), 5 g daily, and no absorption of the compound from the colon, or ulceration, or mucosal bleeding, occurred in 10 patients with ulcerative colitis treated with degraded carrageenan, 10 g daily.— S. Bonfils (letter), *Lancet*, 1970, *2*, 414.

Ulceration of the caecum occurred in 4 of 12 female *rats* given 5% degraded carrageenan in their drinking water for the first 6 months of life and whose mothers had been given the same compound during pregnancy. No ulcers were detected in the 12 control *rats*. Colonic ulceration due to degraded carrageenan was not limited to herbivores.— R. Marcus and J. Watt (letter), *Lancet*, 1971, *2*, 765. Bronchiectatic lesions were observed in 5 of 12 *rats* given degraded carrageenan.— *idem*, 766. A further warning concerning the potential hazards of degraded or undegraded carrageenan with reference to colorectal lesions and cancer in *animals*.— *idem*, 1980, *1*, 602. Strong agreement that the continued use of carrageenan as a food stabiliser should be seriously reconsidered. Experimental work has demonstrated adverse immunological effects and liver damage.— A. W. Thomson *et al.*, *ibid.*, 1034. The concern must be viewed with reservation.— S. Gangolli *et al.*, *British Industrial Biological Research Association*, *ibid.*, *2*, 87. See also H. P. Sarett, *Mead Johnson, USA*, *ibid.*, 1981, *1*, 151.

Suspending agent. Use as a suspending agent.— C. A. Farley and W. Lund, *Pharm. J.*, 1976, *1*, 562.

Proprietary Names

Coréine *(Daniel-Brunet, Fr.)*.

5413-g

Cellacephate *(B.P.)*. CAP; Cellulose Acetate Phthalate *(Eur. P., U.S.N.F.)*; Cellulosi Acetas Phthalas; Cellulosi Acetas Phtalas; Cellulosum Acetylphthalicum; Celophthalum.

CAS — 9004-38-0.

Pharmacopoeias. In *Aust.*, *Br.*, *Braz.*, *Cz.*, *Eur.*, *Fr.*, *Ger.*, *Hung.*, *It.*, *Jap.*, *Neth.*, *Nord.*, and *Swiss*. Also in *U.S.N.F.*

Cellulose in which about one-half the hydroxyl groups are acetylated and about one-quarter are esterified with 1 of the 2 acid groups of phthalic acid.

A hygroscopic, tasteless, white, free-flowing powder or colourless flakes, odourless or with a slight odour of acetic acid. The *B.P.* specifies 17 to 23% of acetyl groups and 30 to 40% of phthalyl groups, both calculated with reference to the anhydrous acid-free substance, and not more than 3% of free acid calculated as phthalic acid. The *U.S.N.F.* specifies 19 to 23.5% of acetyl groups and 30 to 36% of phthalyl groups, and not more than 6% of free acid. The equilibrium moisture content is about 5% at 50% relative humidity and about 9% at 75% relative humidity. Cellacephate hydrolyses fairly rapidly at moisture contents above about 6%.

Practically **insoluble** in water, alcohols, and chlorinated and non-chlorinated hydrocarbons; soluble in diethylene glycol, dioxan, and in solutions of alkali hydroxides and carbonates; soluble 1 in 4 of acetone containing 0.4% v/v of water (the solution may be slightly turbid if less water is present) and 1 in 6 of a mixture of equal volumes of ethyl acetate and isopropyl alcohol. Very slightly soluble in ether. A 15% solution in acetone containing 0.4% of water has a viscosity, at 20°, of 50 to 90 centipoises. **Store** in a cool place in airtight containers.

Uses. Cellacephate is unaffected by immersion in acid media in the stomach but softens and swells in intestinal fluid. It is used as an enteric-coating material for tablets and capsules. About 5 to 30% of plasticisers, such as diethyl phthalate, castor oil, or triacetin, are normally added to make coatings less brittle; a fatty or waxy substance such as carnauba wax may be added to retard penetration of water in acid media.

Preparations

Enteric Varnish. Vernix Enterosolubilis *(Nord. P.)*. Cellacephate 10 g, castor oil 500 mg, acetone 89.5 g.

Manufacturers

Eastman, UK.

5415-p

Dispersible Cellulose *(B.P.)*. Microcrystalline Cellulose and Carboxymethylcellulose Sodium *(U.S.N.F.)*.

Pharmacopoeias. In *Br.* Also in *U.S.N.F.*

An odourless tasteless white to off-white coarse to fine powder consisting of a colloid-forming attrited mixture of microcrystalline cellulose and carmellose sodium. It loses not more than 8% of its weight on drying.

Dispersible in water, with swelling, to produce a white, opaque dispersion or gel; practically insoluble in organic solvents and dilute acids. A dispersion in water has a pH of 6 to 8. **Store** in a cool dry place in airtight containers.

Grades containing 8.5, 11, and 11% of carmellose sodium and having viscosities of 120 cP in 2.1% solution, 120 cP in 1.2% solution, and 65 cP in 1.2% solution respectively are available.

Dispersible cellulose is used as a suspending agent.

Proprietary Preparations

Avicel RC *(FMC Corp., USA: Honeywill & Stein, UK)*. A brand of dispersible cellulose, available in 4 grades.

5414-q

Microcrystalline Cellulose *(B.P.C. 1973)*. Cellulosa Microgranulare; Cellulose Gel; Crystalline Cellulose.

CAS — 9004-34-6.

Pharmacopoeias. In *It.* and *Jap.* Also in *U.S.N.F. Br.* includes the dispersible grade under the title Dispersible Cellulose.

A fine, white or almost white, odourless or almost odourless, crystalline powder consisting of partially depolymerised cellulose, prepared by hydrolysis of purified wood cellulose. Molecular weight about 36 000.

Two pharmaceutical grades are commercially available, a colloidal water-dispersible powder and a non-dispersible powder. The colloidal water-dispersible grade has a much smaller average particle size than the non-dispersible grade and may contain a small percentage of carmellose sodium to aid its dispersion.

Both grades are practically **insoluble** in water but the colloidal grade is dispersible, forming colloidal suspensions at low concentrations and thixotropic gels at higher concentrations. Both grades are partially soluble in dilute alkalis, with swelling; practically insoluble in acids and most organic solvents. A 12.5% dispersion in water has a pH of 5.5 to 7.

Microcrystalline Cellulose (*U.S.N.F.*) contains 97 to 102% of cellulose, calculated on the dried basis, and forms with water a white opaque dispersion which does not form a supernatant liquid on standing.

Adverse Effects.

An evaluation of the toxicity of microcrystalline cellulose. It was not absorbed or digested by man and daily doses of up to 30 g were tolerated. Adverse effects seen in long-term *animal* studies were considered to be due to deficiencies in a diet with a high concentration of indigestible matter.— *Fd Add. Ser. Wld Hlth Org. No. 1*, 1972. See also *ibid.*, *No. 5*, 1974.

Uses. The colloidal grade of microcrystalline cellulose is used either alone or in conjunction with other cellulose derivatives such as carmellose sodium and hypromellose as a suspending agent for pharmaceutical preparations. The non-dispersible grade is used as a binder, filler, disintegrant, and lubricant in tablets; water-soluble active ingredients can be adsorbed on the material before compression. It has also been used in bulk-forming preparations with methylcellulose in the management of colostomies. The mixture has also been tried as a dietary aid, the intention being to relieve hunger.

Suspending agent. Properties and uses as a suspending agent.— W. D. Walkling and R. F. Shangraw, *J. pharm. Sci.*, 1968, *57*, 1927. See also C. A. Farley and W. Lund, *Pharm. J.*, 1976, *1*, 562.

Use in tablet manufacture. Reviews and studies of the use of microcrystalline cellulose in tablet manufacture.— E. J. Mendell, *Mfg Chem.*, 1972, *43* (May), 43; *ibid* (June), 31; R. L. Lamberson and G. E. Raynor, *Mfg Chem.*, 1976, *47* (June), 55; D. Sixsmith, *Mfg Chem.*, 1976, *47* (Aug.), 27; R. P. Bhatia *et al.*, *Drug Cosmet. Ind.*, 1978, *122* (Apr.), 38.

Further references: W. Feinstein and A. J. Bartilucci, *J. pharm. Sci.*, 1966, *55*, 332; G. R. Reier and R. F. Shangraw, *ibid.*, 510; E. Jaminet and H. Hess, *Pharm. Acta Helv.*, 1966, *41*, 39; M. A. Shah and R. G. Wilson, *J. pharm. Sci.*, 1968, *57*, 181.

Proprietary Preparations

Avicel PH *(FMC Corp., USA: Honeywill & Stein, UK)*. A brand of microcrystalline cellulose, available in 4 grades.

5416-s

Powdered Cellulose *(U.S.N.F.)*.

Pharmacopoeias. In *Fr.* and *Ger.* Also in *U.S.N.F.*

A purified mechanically disintegrated cellulose prepared from wood (alpha) cellulose. It loses not more than 7% of its weight when dried. The supernatant liquid of a 10% dispersion in water has a pH of 5 to 7.5.

Grades of different densities and particle size ranges are available.

Powdered cellulose is used as a tablet diluent, an adsorbent, and as a suspending agent.

Proprietary Preparations

Elcema *(Degussa, UK)*. Microfined cellulose, available in 4 grades.

5417-w

Ceratonia *(B.P.C. 1949)*. Cerat.; Ceratonia Gum; Carob Bean Gum; Carob Gum; Gomme de Caroube; Locust Bean Gum.

CAS — 9000-40-2.

Pharmacopoeias. In *Fr.*

The endosperms separated from the seeds of the locust bean tree, *Ceratonia siliqua* (Leguminosae). It is a high molecular weight polysaccharide containing D-galactose and D-mannose units. Powdered ceratonia is sometimes known as Cheshire gum. It loses not more than 15% of its weight on drying. **Dispersible** in water. Practically insoluble in alcohol. A 1% suspension has a pH of 5.3. **Store** in airtight containers.

Uses. Ceratonia has been used as a substitute for tragacanth. A mucilage, which is slightly more viscous than tragacanth mucilage, may be prepared by boiling 1 to 1.5% of powdered ceratonia with water.

On the toxicological data provided it was not possible to estimate an acceptable daily intake of ceratonia.— *Fd Add. Ser. Wld Hlth Org. No. 5*, 1974.

Proprietary Preparations

Arobon *(Nestlé, UK)*. A powder containing ceratonia 80%, starch 15%, and cocoa 5%. For diarrhoea. (Also available as Arobon in *Switz.*).

Nestargel *(Nestlé, UK)*. A thickening powder containing ceratonia 96.5% and calcium lactate 3.5%. For some vomiting in infants.

A preparation containing ceratonia was also formerly marketed in Great Britain under the proprietary name Carobel (*Cow & Gate*).

5418-e

Chondrus *(B.P.C. 1959)*. Chond.; Carrageen; Carragheen; Irish Moss.

Pharmacopoeias. In *Aust., Belg., Neth., Port.,* and *Swiss,* all of which allow also *Gigartina mamillosa* (Gigartinaceae).

The dried seaweed *Chondrus crispus* (Gigartinaceae) in yellowish, translucent, horny masses consisting of slender thalli from 5 to 15 cm in length. A 3% solution in boiling water forms a thick jelly on cooling.

Uses. Chondrus has been used as an emulsifying agent for cod-liver and other oils and as a substitute for gelatin in the preparation of jellies for invalids. A decoction has been employed as a demulcent in the treatment of coughs. Extracts of chondrus are used in the food industry (see Carrageenan, p.951).

Preparations

Chondrus Decoction *(B.P.C. 1949)*. Dec. Chond.; Decoction of Irish Moss; Mucilage of Irish Moss; Chondrus Mucilage. Washed chondrus 2.5 g, boiled with water for 15 minutes, strained while hot, and adjusted with water to 100 ml. *Dose.* 30 to 120 ml or more.

5419-l

Cydonia *(B.P.C. 1949)*. Quince Seed; Cydoniae Semen; Quittenkern.

CAS — 9011-85-2 (cydonin).

Pharmacopoeias. In *Swiss.*

The seeds of *Cydonia oblonga* (=*C. vulgaris*) (Rosaceae), containing about 20% of mucilage (cydonin). **Store** in a dry place.

Cydonia is soothing and demulcent. It has been used in the form of a decoction as an ingredient of, or as a basis for lotions and creams. A mucilage of cydonia has been used as a suspending agent.

5420-v

Dextrates *(U.S.N.F.)*.

CAS — 39404-33-6.

Pharmacopoeias. In *U.S.N.F.*

A purified mixture of saccharides obtained by the controlled enzymatic hydrolysis of starch. It loses 7.8 to 9.2% of its weight when dried. It contains the equivalent of 93 to 99% of dextrose, calculated on the dried basis. A 20% solution has a pH of 3.8 to 5.8.

Dextrates is used as a tablet binding and diluent.

5421-g

Ethylcellulose *(U.S.N.F.)*. An ethyl ether of cellulose containing 44 to 51% of ethoxyl ($-OC_2H_5$) groups, calculated on the dried basis.

CAS — 9004-57-3.

Pharmacopoeias. In *U.S.N.F.*

A free-flowing white to light tan powder. Its aqueous suspensions are neutral to litmus. Practically **insoluble** in water, glycerol, and propylene glycol. Ethylcellulose containing less than 46.5% of ethoxyl groups is freely soluble in chloroform, cyclohexane, methyl acetate, and tetrahydrofuran, and in mixtures of aromatic hydrocarbons with alcohol; ethylcellulose containing not less than 46.5% of ethoxyl groups is freely soluble in alcohol, chloroform, ethyl acetate, methyl alcohol, and toluene.

Water-soluble grades of ethylcellulose which have a lower degree of substitution are also manufactured, and these grades have properties similar to those of methylcellulose.

Uses. Ethylcellulose is used as a binder in tablets and as a film-coating material for tablets. It is also used in the manufacture of plastics and lacquers.

Proprietary Preparations

Aquacoat *(FMC Corp., USA: Honeywill & Stein, UK)*. A stable dispersion of ethylcellulose for use in tablet coating.

Ethocel *(Dow, USA: K & K-Greeff, UK)*. A range of ethylcellulose products available as **Medium** (45 to 46.5% ethoxy content) in viscosity grades of 50, 70, and 100 cP and **Standard** (48 to 49.5% ethoxy content) in viscosity grades of 7, 10, 20, 45, and 100 cP.

5422-q

Ethylhydroxyethylcellulose. An ether of cellulose in which both ethyl and hydroxyethyl groups are attached to the anhydroglucose rings of cellulose by ether linkages.

CAS — 9004-58-4.

A white or off-white granular powder which is odourless and tasteless. It contains about 8% of water. It swells in water and **disperses** to form a clear to opalescent viscous colloidal solution; practically insoluble in dehydrated alcohol, chloroform, and ether.

Stock solutions should contain a suitable antimicrobial preservative.

Uses. Ethylhydroxyethylcellulose has properties and uses similar to those of methylcellulose (see p.947). The viscosity and solubility are dependent on the relative proportions of the ethyl and hydroxyethyl groups.

Ethylhydroxyethylcellulose had a foaming power and a foam stability superior to those of methylcellulose. It had been employed in hand lotions, brushless shaving creams, and barrier creams, in strengths of 25 to 40% of a 2% aqueous solution. A formula for a barrier cream is provided.— H. Dietrich, *Soap chem. Spec.*, 1964, *40* (Nov.), 165.

Proprietary Preparations

Bermocoll E *(Berol Kemi, UK)*. A brand of ethylhydroxyethylcellulose, available in 10 viscosity grades.

Other Proprietary Names

Etulos *(Swed.)*.

5423-p

Ethylmethylcellulose. Methylethylcellulose. An ether of cellulose containing 14.5 to 19% of ethoxyl ($-OC_2H_5$) groups and 3.5 to 6.5% of methoxyl ($-OCH_3$) groups.

CAS — 9004-59-5.

A white or pale cream-coloured, almost odourless, fibrous solid or powder. The fibrous form loses not more than 15% and the powder not more than 10% of its weight on drying.

Dispersible in cold water to form aqueous solutions of poor clarity which undergo a reversible transformation from sol to gel upon heating and cooling, respectively. A 2.5% solution in water at 20° has a viscosity of about 20 to 60 centipoises. **Store** in airtight containers.

Adverse Effects.

For background toxicological information, see *Fd Add. Ser. Wld Hlth Org. No. 5*, 1974.

Uses. Ethylmethylcellulose has properties and uses similar to those of methylcellulose (see p.947) but solutions have poor clarity. It is not widely used in pharmacy but is employed extensively in the food industry.

Estimated acceptable daily intake: up to 25 mg per kg body-weight, as the sum of total modified celluloses. The figure may be exceeded for dietetic purposes.— Seventeenth Report of FAO/WHO Expert Committee on Food Additives, *Tech. Rep. Ser. Wld Hlth Org. No. 539*, 1974.

For comparison of the stability of mucilages of ethylmethylcellulose and other cellulose derivatives, see Methylcellulose, p.947.

Proprietary Preparations

Edifas A *(ICI Organics, UK)*. A brand of ethylmethylcellulose. **Cellofas A** is the corresponding industrial grade.

5424-s

Furcellaran. Danish Agar.

CAS — 9000-21-9.

An extract obtained from the seaweed *Furcellaria fastigiata*, consisting of a mixture of polysaccharides similar in structure to carrageenan (see p.951). The commercial product is the potassium chloride-precipitated fraction. It has properties similar to those of κ-carrageenan.

An off-white powder. It loses not more than 13% of its weight on drying. Practically **insoluble** in cold water and alcohol; soluble in hot water, forming a gel on cooling.

Furcellaran has been used in the food industry.

Estimated acceptable daily intake: up to 75 mg per kg body-weight.— Seventeenth Report of the FAO/WHO Expert Committee on Food Additives, *Tech. Rep. Ser. Wld Hlth Org. No. 539*, 1974.

For background toxicological information, see *Fd Add. Ser. Wld Hlth Org. No. 5*, 1974.

5425-w

Gelatin *(B.P., U.S.P.)*. Gelat.; Gelatina Alba; Gelatina Medicinalis; Gelatinum.

CAS — 9000-70-8.

Pharmacopoeias. In all pharmacopoeias examined except *Eur., Fr., Int.,* and *Neth.*

Colourless or pale yellowish or amber-coloured translucent sheets, shreds, flakes, powder, or granules with a slight odour and taste. It is a protein obtained by partial hydrolysis of animal collagenous tissues, such as skins, tendons, ligaments, and bones, with boiling water. It loses not more than 16% of its weight on drying. The *B.P.* specifies not more than 200 ppm of sulphur dioxide. The *U.S.P.* specifies not more than 40 ppm of sulphur dioxide; if for the manufacture of capsules or the coating of tablets it may contain 1500 ppm of sulphur dioxide, a suitable concentration of sodium lauryl sulphate, suitable antimicrobial agents, and may be coloured.

Practically **insoluble** in cold water, but swells and softens when immersed in it, gradually absorbing 5 to 10 times its weight of water; soluble in hot water, forming a jelly on cooling; practically insoluble in alcohol, chloroform, ether, and fixed and volatile oils; soluble in a mixture of glycerol and water, solution being aided by heat, and in 6M acetic acid. **Sterilised** by dry heat. Prolonged heating of solutions reduces gel strength and melting-point. **Incompatible** with alcohol, formaldehyde, mercury and other metal salts, and tannic acid. **Store** in airtight containers. The moisture content of powdered or finely divided gelatin varies rapidly with the humidity of the atmosphere to which it is exposed. It is stable in air when dry, but putrefies rapidly when moist or in solution.

Gelatins vary widely in quality and are usually graded by jelly strength, expressed as 'Bloom strength' or 'Bloom rating', which is the weight in grams which when applied to a plunger, 12.7 mm in diameter, under controlled conditions will produce a depression exactly 4 mm deep in a jelly matured at 10° and containing 6.67% w/w of gelatin in water. Gelatins with jelly strengths up to about 230 grams Bloom are available. The *B.P.* specifies a jelly strength of not less than 150 grams Bloom (assessed by the Bloom gelometer or the Boucher electronic jelly tester) and this is suitable for most pharmaceutical purposes but higher jelly strengths are preferable for gelatin capsules and for biological culture media.

Two types of gelatin are available for pharmaceutical use: *Type A*—derived from an acid-treated precursor and having an isoelectric point between pH 7 and 9; it is cationic and is most effective at a pH of about 3.2. *Type B*—derived from an alkali-treated precursor and having an isoelectric point between pH 4.7 and 5.2; it is anionic and is most effective at a pH of 7 to 8. To avoid incompatibility when gelatin is used with a second gum such as tragacanth, acacia, or agar, *Type B* should be used at alkaline pH. The names Pharmagel A and B are sometimes used for these gelatins in the USA.

The average mol. wt of gelatin in a preparation containing gelatin 4%, sodium chloride 0.85%, potassium chloride 0.038%, and calcium chloride 0.02% was 36 400 when autoclaved for 20 mintues at 15 lb pressure and 30 000 when autoclaved for 1 hour. When glycine 1% was added to the solution, the average mol. wt was 40 000 after autoclaving for 20 minutes and 35 000 after autoclaving for 1 hour.— Y. Gabr and A. Michael, *Arzneimittel-Forsch.*, 1967, *17*, 1211.

The photostability of gelatin films and capsules to ultraviolet light.— Y. Matsuda *et al.*, *Yakugakuzasshi*, 1979, *99*, 907, per *Int. pharm. Abstr.*, 1980, *17*, 741.

Standard for gelatin. A British Standard Specification for methods of sampling and testing gelatin (BS 757:1975) is published by the British Standards Institution.

Adverse Effects. Allergic and anaphylactic reactions have occurred after the infusion of gelatin or its derivatives.

In a randomised study of 750 patients, histamine-like side-effects were observed in 21.3% (96 of 450) of patients who received infusions of gelatin derivatives as plasma substitutes compared with 3.7% (11 of 300) of patients who received infusions of a dextran or hetastarch.— B. Schöning and H. Koch, *Anaesthesist*, 1975, *24*, 507.

There were 4 anaphylactic reactions in 6028 infusions of modified fluid gelatin.— J. Ring and K. Messmer, *Lancet*, 1977, *1*, 466.

A discussion on the adverse reactions to plasma substitutes including gelatin and its derivatives.— A. Doenicke *et al.*, *Br. J. Anaesth.*, 1977, *49*, 681.

Further references: J. Ring and K. Messmer, *Anaesthesist*, 1977, *26*, 279.

Treatment of Adverse Effects. Infusions containing gelatin should be discontinued immediately if allergic reactions occur. Administration of adrenaline, corticosteroids and antihistamines may be necessary in addition to supportive measures in the treatment of severe anaphylactic reactions.

Precautions. Precautions that should be observed with plasma expanders are described under Dextran 70 Intravenous Infusion, p.512, and these should be considered when gelatin and gelatin derivatives are used for this purpose.

Uses. Gelatin is a protein and is used as a nutrient. It is deficient in certain of the essential amino acids, notably tryptophan, but it yields a high proportion of lysine, an essential amino acid in which cereals and some other foods are deficient.

The daily administration of gelatin by mouth has been advocated for the treatment of brittle finger-nails and other non-mycotic defects of the nails but proof of the efficacy of such treatment is lacking.

Gelatin is used in the preparation of pastes, pastilles, pessaries, bougies, and suppositories. Gelatin is the main ingredient in hard and flexible capsule shells. Solutions containing 0.5 to 0.7% of gelatin in an iso-osmotic vehicle are used as artificial tears; a suitable bactericide, such as chlorbutol 0.5%, is usually added to the solution. Gelatin is also used for the microencapsulation of drugs, flavours, perfumes, and other industrial materials.

A gelatin, specially prepared from refined beef-bone collagen, has been used as a sterile 4 to 6% solution in iso-osmotic sodium chloride solution as a plasma expander, or to emulsify fat in intravenous 'feeding emulsions'. A polymer preparation derived from gelatin and urea, polygeline (see p.958), is also used as a plasma expander.

A preparation known as Pitkin's menstruum, consisting of gelatin, dextrose, and acetic acid in water (see below), has been employed as a vehicle for the injection of certain drugs, such as heparin, to delay their action. A solution of hydrolysed gelatin is used as a vehicle for Corticotrophin Gelatin Injection (see p.488). It may be prepared by heating a 16% w/w solution of gelatin in Water for Injections for sufficient time to give a solution which is mobile at 25°.

Gelatin, in the form of a water-insoluble film or porous sponge-like material, is used as a haemostatic, see Absorbable Gelatin Sponge and Absorbable Gelatin Film, p.737. When preparations containing gelatin are to be applied to abraded surfaces, the material should be sterilised, but prolonged heating reduces the strength of the gel.

The pharmaceutical uses and properties of gelatin.— R. T. Jones, *Process Biochem.*, 1970, *5*, *Part* 12, 2; *idem*, 1971, *6*, *Part* 7, 7; A. Widmann and R. J. Croome, *Pharmazeut. Ind.*, 1975, *37*, 650. See also *The Science and Technology of Gelatin*, A.G. Ward and A. Courts (Ed.), London, Academic Press, 1977.

Plasma substitute. A review of the use of gelatin and its derivatives as plasma substitutes.— A. Doenicke *et al.*, *Br. J. Anaesth.*, 1977, *49*, 681.

The value of gelatin preparations as alternatives to dextrans depends on rapid and complete excretion from the body, lack of effect on coagulation, and the possibility of using large doses which is desirable in some clinical conditions. Owing to their low molecular weight compared with dextrans their maintenance time in circulation is shorter; plasma expansion exceeds the infused volume. The haemodynamic effects last about 3 hours.— W. J. Rudowski, *Br. J. Hosp. Med.*, 1980, *23*, 389.

Test for pancreatic proteolytic activity. Following a gelatin-free diet, gelatin, in a dose of 28 g for adults and 14 g for children, was given dissolved in hot water and suitably flavoured. Excretion of hydroxyproline in the urine was compared with the rate of excretion during the gelatin-free diet period. Excretion of hydroxyproline was increased by about 7.7 mg per hour in healthy persons, compared with less than 4 mg per hour in patients with pancreatic or intestinal disease.— G. B. Theil *et al.*, *Am. J. dig. Dis.*, 1963, *8*, 1008.

Further references: H. D. Bronstein *et al.*, *Gastroenterology*, 1966, *50*, 621.

Preparations

Lamellae. Small medicated disks, about 3 mm in diameter, intended to dissolve in the lachrymal secretion; they are prepared by dissolving the medicament in a suitable water-soluble non-irritant basis. They are soluble in water at 37°.

Pitkin's Menstruum. (For intramuscular or subcutaneous injection). Gelatin 15 to 30%, dextrose 5 to 12%, glacial acetic acid 0.5%, distilled water to 100%.

Proprietary Preparations

Crodyne *(Croda, UK)*. A brand of gelatin.

Gelofusine *(Consolidated Chemicals, UK)*. A blood-plasma substitute for intravenous infusion containing gelatin (partially hydrolysed until the average molecular weight is 30 000) 4%, sodium chloride 0.85%, and calcium chloride 0.05%; it provides 146 mmol of Na, 5 mmol of Ca, and 156 mmol of Cl per litre.

Other Proprietary Names of Gelatin and Gelatin Derivatives

Gel-Phan *(Fr.)*; Neo-Plasmagel, Physiogel *(both Ger.)*.

5426-e

Ghatti Gum. Indian Gum.

CAS — 9000-28-6.

A gummy exudation from the stem of *Anogeissus latifolia* (Combretaceae). It consists of the calcium-magnesium salt of a complex high molecular weight polysaccharide containing L-arabinose, D-galactose, D-mannose, D-xylose, and D-glucuronic acid.

An off-white to buff-coloured powder. It loses not more than 14% of its weight on drying. **Soluble** 1 in 5 of water forming a very viscous mucilage; practically insoluble in alcohol.

Ghatti gum was formerly used in the food industry.

5427-l

Guar Gum *(U.S.N.F.)*. Guar Flour; Jaguar Gum.

CAS — 9000-30-0.

Pharmacopoeias. In *Fr.* and *Ind.* Also in *U.S.N.F.*

A gum obtained from the ground endosperms of the seeds of *Cyamopsis psoraloides* (=*C. tetragonolobus*) (Leguminosae). It contains not less than 66% of a high molecular weight hydrocolloidal polysaccharide, a galactomannan, composed of galactan and mannan units combined through glycosidic linkages.

A white to yellowish-white almost odourless powder with a characteristic taste. It loses not more than 15% of its weight on drying. **Dispersible** in hot or cold water to form a colloidal solution; practically insoluble in alcohol. A 0.5% solution is neutral to litmus. A 1% mucilage is similar in viscosity to acacia mucilage and a 3% mucilage is similar to tragacanth mucilage. Mucilages can be preserved with 0.2% of benzoic acid. **Incompatible** with acetone, alcohol, tannins, and strong acids and alkalis.

Physical properties.— I. A. Schlakman and A. J. Bartilucci, *Drug Stand.*, 1957, *25*, 149; R. J. Chudzikowski, *J. Soc. cosmet. Chem.*, 1971, *22*, 43.

Adverse Effects and Precautions. As for Methylcellulose p.947. Due to its unpalatability, guar gum taken in large doses may cause nausea and vomiting.

For background toxicological information on guar gum in food, see *Fd Add. Ser. Wld Hlth Org. No. 5*, 1974.

A comment on the risk of bezoar formation in diabetic patients with neuropathy receiving a fibre-rich dietary regimen.— B. Canivet *et al.* (letter), *Lancet*, 1980, *2*, 862.

Uses. Guar gum is used as a thickening agent and emulsion stabiliser. The stability of emulsions prepared with acacia can be considerably improved by the addition of 1% of guar gum. It is a poor suspending agent for insoluble powders. A 1 to 1.5% mucilage has been used as a binding and disintegrating agent in tablets.

Guar gum is also used as a suspending and thickening agent in the manufacture of various foods and has been used as a dietary bulking agent.

Guar gum could be incorporated into dough to give a palatable guar bread. For the preparation of bread containing 8 to 8.5 g guar gum per 100 g, replace each kg of flour in the usual bread recipe with a mixture of 800 g of flour, 150 g of guar gum and 50 g of dried vital wheat gluten and use additional yeast and water. The resulting dough requires care in cooking as it is more sensitive to timing than normal dough. Guar bread is bland and although more chewy it is an acceptable alternative to ordinary bread.— E. C. Apling *et al.* (letter), *Lancet*, 1977, *2*, 975.

The colonic response to guar gum. Addition to the diet increased faecal bulk and weight and shortened transit time through the gut. The effect of guar gum was less than that of bran.— J. H. Cummings *et al.*, *Lancet*, 1978, *1*, 5.

Effect on blood-glucose. References to guar gum reducing blood-glucose concentrations or insulin requirements in diabetics: D. J. A. Jenkins *et al.*, *Lancet*, 1976, *2*, 172 (with pectin); *idem*, *Ann. intern. Med.*, 1977, *86*, 20 (with or without pectin; in healthy subjects); *idem*, *Lancet*, 1977, *2*, 779; *idem*, *Br. med. J.*, 1978, *2*, 1744; T. M. S. Wolever *et al.* (letter), *Lancet*, 1978, *2*, 1381. See also D. J. A. Jenkins, *Lancet*, 1979, *2*, 1287. Criticisms.— J. I. Mann and H. C. R. Simpson (letter), *ibid.*, 1980, *1*, 44; J. Yudkin (letter), *ibid.*

Guar crispbread with soya beans reduced blood-glucose concentrations in diabetics to a greater extent than did guar crispbread alone.— D. J. A. Jenkins *et al.*, *Br. med. J.*, 1980, *281*, 1248.

Absence of effect of guar gum on blood-glucose concentrations: D. R. R. Williams and W. P. T. James (letter), *Lancet*, 1979, *1*, 271; M. Cohen and F. I. R. Martin (letter), *Br. med. J.*, 1979, *1*, 616.

The effects of guar gum with pectin on glucose absorption could be due simply to delayed gastric emptying.— S. Holt *et al.*, *Lancet*, 1979, *1*, 636.

Effect on serum lipids. Guar gum given in a daily dose of 15 g for 2 weeks reduced the mean serum-cholesterol concentration in 10 patients with type II hyperlipidaemia by 370 μg per ml (10.6%). In 3 patients who had received cholestyramine for over 2 years a reduction of 18.7% was obtained. Guar gum had no effect on the cholesterol concentration of a patient who had already been treated successfully with clofibrate. There was no significant change in serum-triglyceride concentrations in the 2-week period. Further study of guar gum as a hypocholesterolaemic agent was merited.— D. J. A. Jenkins *et al.*, *Am. J. clin. Nutr.*, 1979, *32*, 16. See also *idem*, 1975, *1*, 1116; *idem* (letter), *Lancet*, 1976, *2*, 1351; D. J. A. Jenkins, *ibid.*, 1979, *2*, 1287.

Proprietary Names

Guar gum was formerly marketed in Great Britain under the proprietary name Decorpa (*Norgine*) (see also under Sterculia).

5428-y

Hectorite

CAS — 12173-47-6.

Hectorite is one of the montmorillonite group of minerals. It is structurally similar to bentonite but the aluminium is largely replaced by magnesium and it contains small proportions of lithium and fluorine. Dried hectorite is white in colour. The purified substance absorbs more water than the bentonites and in concentrations of 1 to 2% it forms a transparent gel.

Hectorite has been used as a gelling, suspending, and emulsifying agent in external preparations.

Proprietary Preparations

Laponite *(Laporte, UK)*. A range of synthetic hectorite products, some of which contain no fluoride.

For reports on the properties and uses of Laponite, see B. S. Neumann and K. G. Sansom, *J. Soc. cosmet. Chem.*, 1970, *21*, 237; J. E. Carless and J. R. Nixon, *ibid.*, 427.

An evaluation of Laponite as a toothpaste binder.— B. J. R. Mayes, *Int. J. cosmet. Sci.*, 1979, *1*, 329.

Proprietary Preparations of Related Montmorillonites

Bentone EW (formerly known as Ben-A-Gel EW) *(Steetley Minerals, UK)*. A processed magnesium montmorillonite (hydrous magnesium silicate) used as a gelling, suspending, and emulsifying agent for aqueous systems.

Bentones *(Steetley Minerals, UK)*. A range of organically substituted montmorillonites; they are used for thickening and gelling organic liquids.

Sepiolite *(Steetley Minerals, UK)*. A white clay consisting of minute needles or laths of hydrated magnesium silicate. It has suspending, adsorptive, and clarifying properties.

5429-j

Hydroxyethylcellulose

CAS — 9004-62-0.

An ether of cellulose in which hydroxyethyl groups are attached to the anhydroglucose rings of cellulose by ether linkages. The substitution is not so well defined as in ethylcellulose or methylcellulose since some polyoxyethylene side chains are also present in the molecule.

A white or off-white powder which is odourless and tasteless. It contains about 5% of water. **Soluble** in cold or hot water, yielding clear solutions; insoluble in most organic solvents. A 2% solution in water has a pH of 6.5 to 8.5.

A solution in water is prepared by slowly sprinkling the hydroxyethylcellulose into the vortex formed by a mechanical stirrer. When a solution is heated, the viscosity decreases; unlike a solution of methylcellulose, a solution of hydroxyethylcellulose does not gel.

Stock solutions should contain a suitable antimicrobial preservative.

Solubility in organic solvents. One per cent solutions could be obtained in dilutions of alcohol up to 82% w/w, acetone up to 55% w/w, glycerol up to 85% w/w, and propylene glycol up to 71% w/w, but at the concentrations indicated flocculation was starting.— A. M. Dry and K. Steiger-Trippi, *Pharm. Acta Helv.*, 1964, *39*, 43.

Steroid suspensions. Hydroxyethylcellulose could cause caking of suspensions of corticosteroids.— J. H. Chapman and E. L. Neustadter, *J. Pharm. Pharmac.*, 1965, *17*, *Suppl.*, S138.

Uses. Hydroxyethylcellulose is used for the same purposes as methylcellulose (see p.947) but gives clearer solutions. Since it does not gel on heating, it may be useful in preparations where gel formation is undesirable.

Proprietary Preparations

Cellobond HEC *(BP Chemicals, UK: Hythe, UK)*. A brand of hydroxyethylcellulose, available in a number of grades giving different viscosities in aqueous solution.

K-Y Lubricating Jelly *(Johnson & Johnson, UK)*. A sterile, non-greasy jelly containing hydroxyethylcellulose. For application to surgeons' hands or gloves and to instruments; also used in electrotherapy.

Vaginal lubrication with K-Y Lubricating Jelly is effective in alleviating dyspareunia or even apareunia caused by excessive dryness.— *Drug & Ther. Bull.*, 1980, *18*, 55.

Natrosol 250 *(Hercules, UK)*. A brand of hydroxyethylcellulose, available in a number of viscosity grades.

Other Proprietary Names

Optocrymal *(Canad.)*.

5430-q

Hydroxyethylmethylcellulose. HEMC; Hydroxyethyl Methylcellulose. An ether of cellulose containing methoxyl and a small proportion of hydroxyethoxyl groups.

CAS — 9032-42-2.

Hydroxyethylmethylcellulose has similar properties and uses to methylcellulose (see p.947) but the presence of hydroxyethyl groups makes it more readily soluble in water; its solutions are more tolerant of salts and have a higher coagulation temperature.

For studies of the flow properties and the effect of additives on hydroxyethylmethylcellulose solutions, see M. A. Kassem and A. G. Mattha, *Pharm. Acta Helv.*, 1970, *45*, 345 and 355.

5431-p

Hydroxypropylcellulose. Hydroxypropyl Cellulose *(U.S.N.F.)*. An ether of cellulose containing not more than 80.5% of hydroxypropoxyl ($-OC_3H_6OH$) groups, calculated on the dried material. It may contain up to 0.6% of silicon dioxide or other suitable anticaking agents.

CAS — 9004-64-2.

Pharmacopoeias. In *Jap.* which specifies 53.4 to 77.5% of hydroxypropoxyl groups. Also in *U.S.N.F.*

A white to cream-coloured almost odourless and tasteless granular solid or powder. It loses not more than 5% of its weight on drying. **Soluble** in water below 40°, alcohol, chloroform, and propylene glycol, forming colloidal solutions; practically insoluble in hot water. A 1% solution in water has a pH of 5 to 8. The viscosity of a 10% solution is not less than 145 centipoises.

Adverse Effects.

For background toxicological information, see *Fd Add. Ser. Wld Hlth Org. No. 5,* 1974.

Uses. Hydroxypropylcellulose is used in the film coating of tablets, as a tablet excipient, as a thickener in elixirs, and as a stabiliser in foams, ointments, and lotions. Grades are available for use in the food industry.

Estimated acceptable daily intake: up to 25 mg per kg body-weight, as the sum of total modified celluloses. The figure may be exceeded for dietetic purposes.— Seventeenth Report of FAO/WHO Expert Committee on Food Additives, *Tech. Rep. Ser. Wld Hlth Org. No. 539,* 1974.

A reference to the studies using hydroxypropylcellulose (Klucel) for the preparation of slow-release covalently bonded oestrone or testosterone compounds which would hydrolyse during use.— S. Yolles, *J. parent. Drug Ass.*, 1978, *32*, 188.

A study on the texture and physical properties of frusemide tablets prepared with hydroxypropylcellulose mucilage. Hydroxypropylcellulose was considered to be a good binding agent. The film burst on drying during storage but the mechanical strength of the tablets remained almost unchanged.— K. Pintye-Hodi *et al.*, *Pharmazie*, 1979, *34*, 51, per *Int. pharm. Abstr.*, 1979, *16*, 1229.

Proprietary Preparations

Klucel *(Hercules, UK)*. A brand of hydroxypropylcellulose, available in a number of viscosity grades.

5432-s

Hypromellose *(B.P.C. 1973)*.

Hydroxypropylmethylcellulose; Hydroxypropyl Methylcellulose; Methyl Hydroxypropyl Cellulose; Methylcellulose Propylene Glycol Ether.

CAS — 8063-82-9.

Pharmacopoeias. U.S. specifies a range of hydroxypropyl methylcellulose, see below.

A mixed ether of cellulose containing, on the dried basis, 27 to 30% of methoxyl ($—OCH_3$) groups and 4 to 7.5% of hydroxypropoxyl ($—OC_3H_6OH$) groups, attached to the anhydroglucose rings of cellulose by ether linkages. This corresponds to Hydroxypropyl Methylcellulose 2906 *(U.S.P.)*.

A white or creamy-white, odourless, tasteless, fibrous powder or granules. It loses not more than 10% of its weight on drying. **Soluble** in cold water, forming a viscous colloidal solution which undergoes a reversible transformation from sol to gel upon heating and cooling, respectively; practically insoluble in alcohol, chloroform, and ether, but soluble in mixtures of methyl alcohol and methylene chloride. Certain grades are soluble in aqueous acetone, mixtures of methylene chloride and isopropyl alcohol, and other organic solvents. Aqueous solutions are tolerant to salts. A 1% solution has a pH of 6 to 8. **Store** in a cool place in airtight containers.

Stock solutions should contain a suitable antimicrobial preservative such as benzalkonium chloride.

The name 'hypromellose' is followed by a number indicating the approximate viscosity of a 2% solution at 20°. Hypromelloses of the following viscosities are described in the *B.P.C. 1973:*

Hypromellose 20. Viscosity of a 2% solution, at 20°, 15 to 25 centistokes.

Hypromellose 50. Viscosity of a 2% solution, at 20°, 40 to 60 centistokes.

Hypromellose 125. Viscosity of a 2% solution, at 20°, 110 to 140 centistokes.

Hypromellose 450. Viscosity of a 2% solution, at 20°, 350 to 550 centistokes.

Hypromellose 1500. Viscosity of a 2% solution, at 20°, 1200 to 1800 centistokes.

Hypromellose 4500. Viscosity of a 2% solution, at 20°, 3750 to 5250 centistokes.
Hypromellose 15 000. Viscosity of a 2% solution, at 20°, 12 000 to 18 000 centistokes.

5433-w

Hydroxypropyl Methylcellulose 1828.
(U.S.P.).

A propylene glycol ether of methylcellulose containing 16.5 to 20% of methoxyl groups and 23 to 32% of hydroxypropoxyl groups, calculated on the dried basis. It loses not more than 5% of its weight on drying.

5434-e

Hydroxypropyl Methylcellulose 2208.
(U.S.P.).

A propylene glycol ether of methylcellulose containing 19 to 24% of methoxyl groups and 4 to 12% of hydroxypropoxyl groups, calculated on the dried basis. It loses not more than 5% of its weight on drying.

5435-l

Hydroxypropyl Methylcellulose 2906.
(U.S.P.).

A propylene glycol ether of methylcellulose containing 27 to 30% of methoxyl groups and 4 to 7.5% of hydroxypropoxyl groups, calculated on the dried basis. It loses not more than 5% of its weight on drying.

5436-y

Hydroxypropyl Methylcellulose 2910.
(U.S.P.).

A propylene glycol ether of methylcellulose containing 28 to 30% of methoxyl groups and 7 to 12% of hydroxypropoxyl groups, calculated on the dried basis. It loses not more than 5% of its weight on drying.

Interactions. The solubility of hypromellose was reduced by dyes used in tablet coatings, including erythrosine BS. Rates of disintegration and dissolution of tablets coated with hypromellose could be adversely affected.— E. B. Prillig, *J. pharm. Sci.*, 1969, *58*, 1245.

Hypromellose in solution at a concentration of 0.5% bound 7% of benzalkonium chloride 0.5%. The inhibitory effect of benzalkonium chloride 0.003% against *Pseudomonas aeruginosa* was reduced by 13% in the presence of hypromellose 0.5%. The effect of hypromellose on the activity of benzalkonium chloride 0.01%, with or without disodium edetate was considered to be small.— T. F. J. Tromp *et al.*, *Pharm. Weekbl. Ned.*, 1976, *111*, 561.

Preparation of mucilage. Methods for preparing a mucilage of hypromellose were similar to those used for methylcellulose, but there was less tendency to form lumps and clarity was better with hypromellose. A suitable preservative for external preparations was phenylmercuric acetate or nitrate 0.001%.— G. Smith and J. A. Yacomeni, *Pharm. J.*, 1966, *1*, 447.

Stability of antibiotics in hypromellose solutions. The stability of 10 antibiotics when they were added to 3 commercially available 0.5% hypromellose solutions (Lacril, Tearisol, and Isoptotears).— E. Osborn *et al.*, *Am. J. Ophthal.*, 1976, *82*, 775.

Adverse Effects.

For background toxicological information, see *Fd Add. Ser. Wld Hlth Org. No. 5*, 1974.

Uses. Hypromellose has properties and uses similar to those of methylcellulose (see p.947) but it has several advantages. Since mucilages of hypromellose have greater clarity and fewer undispersed fibres are usually present, it is preferred to methylcellulose in the preparation of ophthalmic solutions; it prolongs the action of medicated eye-drops and is employed in alkaline eye-drops used as artificial tears to prevent damage to the cornea in patients with keratoconjunctivitis sicca or keratitis or during gonioscopy procedures. It is also used to moisten hard contact lenses and to lubricate artificial eyes.

Hypromellose has a slightly higher gel-point than the corresponding viscosity grade of methylcellulose; for example, a 2% solution of hypromellose 4500 gels at about 65°, whereas a 2% solution of methylcellulose 4500 gels at about 50°. It may be used instead of methylcellulose as an adhesive in plaster of Paris bandages. Certain grades have increased solubility in a wide range of solvents and are used in the film-coating of tablets.

Grades of hypromellose having a gel-point of about 90° are also available; they are not recommended for use in ophthalmic solutions but may be useful in jellies and ointments.

Estimated acceptable daily intake: up to 25 mg per kg body-weight, as the sum of total modified celluloses. The figure may be exceeded for dietetic purposes.— Seventeenth Report of FAO/WHO Expert Committee on Food Additives, *Tech. Rep. Ser. Wld Hlth Org. No. 539*, 1974.

A solution of hypromellose, to the formula of Hypromellose Eye-drops and flavoured, was used as a rinse for dry mouth.— *Drug & Ther. Bull.*, 1975, *13*, 38. It is considered that the use of the eye-drops as a mouth-rinse intended to be swallowed is not desirable because of the unsuitability of the borax/boric acid buffer and the benzalkonium chloride for internal use.— Pharm. Soc. Lab. Rep. P/80/2, 1980.

For other formulas used as saliva replacements or sialagogues, see Saliva Replacement Solution in Carmellose Sodium (p.951), Methylcellulose Mouthwash in Methylcellulose (p.948), and Lemon Mouthwash in Citric Acid (p.785).

Use in ophthalmic solutions. Measurements were made of the time taken for various ophthalmic vehicles to appear in the nose after passage through the lachrymal excretory system. Water appeared in 60 seconds, and 0.25, 0.5, 1, and 2.5% solutions of hypromellose in 90, 140, 210, and 255 seconds respectively. The 2.5% solution was not well tolerated and the 1% solution appeared to be ideal to permit maximum ocular absorption of a medicament.— M. L. Linn and L. T. Jones, *Am. J. Ophthal.*, 1968, *65*, 76.

In a double-blind crossover study, hypromellose in artificial tear solutions was retained in the eye longer than polyvinyl alcohol.— F. C. Bach *et al.*, *Ann. Ophthal.*, 1972, *4*, 116, per *Int. pharm. Abstr.*, 1974, *11*, 98.

Further references: *Drug & Ther. Bull.*, 1974, *12*, 81.

Spermicidal activity. Aqueous solutions of hypromellose 1 to 3% caused immediate and permanent immobilisation of human spermatozoa *in vitro*. Solutions of povidone with corresponding viscosities had no influence on sperm motility. Neither storage for 2.5 years nor marked decreases in viscosity affected the potency of the hypromellose solutions. Preliminary experiments with air-dried films of hypromellose gave less clear-cut results although sperm motility was abolished in the immediate contact zone.— K. Loewit, *Contraception*, 1977, *15*, 233.

Preparations

BJ6 Eye-drops *(Moorfields Eye Hosp.)*. Hypromellose '4000' 250 mg, sodium chloride 600 mg, sodium bicarbonate 450 mg, chlorhexidine acetate 10 mg, Water for Injections to 100 ml. pH about 8.45. Sterilised by maintaining at 98° to 100° for 30 minutes.

Hydroxypropyl Methylcellulose Ophthalmic Solution *(U.S.P.)*. A sterile solution of hydroxypropyl methylcellulose of a grade containing 19 to 30% of methoxyl groups and 4 to 12% of hydroxypropoxyl groups. It may contain suitable antimicrobial, buffering, and stabilising agents. pH 6 to 7.8. Store in airtight containers.

Hypromellose Eye Drops *(A.P.F.)*. Artificial-tears Solution. Hypromellose '4500' 300 mg, sodium chloride 900 mg, benzalkonium chloride solution 0.02 ml, disodium edetate 50 mg, Water for Injections to 100 ml. Sterilised by autoclaving. Redisperse the hypromellose by shaking whilst cooling.

NOTE. The *A.P.F.* directs that when Methylcellulose Eye Drops are requested, Hypromellose Eye Drops should be supplied.

Hypromellose Eye-drops *(B.P.C. 1973)*. Alkaline Eye-drops; Artificial Tears; HPRM. Hypromellose '4000', '4500', or '5000' 300 mg, sodium chloride 450 mg, potassium chloride 370 mg, borax 190 mg, boric acid 190 mg, benzalkonium chloride solution 0.02 ml, water to 100 ml. Thoroughly hydrate the hypromellose in 15 ml of water at 80° to 90° and add 35 ml of water, as ice. When homogeneous, mix with a solution of the sodium chloride, potassium chloride, borax, boric acid, and benzalkonium chloride in 40 ml of water. Make to volume with water, mix, and stand overnight. Decant and filter the supernatant liquid. Sterilise in the sealed final containers by autoclaving or maintaining at 98° to 100° for 30 minutes. Redisperse the coagulated hypromellose by shaking when cool. pH 8.4 to 8.6. Used for the replacement of deficient lachrymal secretion; it is not intended as a vehicle for other drugs. When the solution is supplied for use in gonioscopy procedures, the concentration of hypromellose may be increased; a concentration of 0.7 to 1.5% may be suitable.

NOTE. The *B.P.C.1973* directs that when Methylcellulose Eye-drops are requested, Hypromellose Eye-drops should be supplied.

The eye-drop solution met many of the requirements for a soaking and wetting solution for contact lenses. It had a pH of 8.4 to 8.6 and a good buffer capacity but patients preferred a less viscous preparation containing 0.15% hypromellose. The addition of a wetting agent to promote rapid wetting of the surface of plastic lenses was being considered.— W. Lund, *Pharm. J.*, 1969, *2*, 741.

User comfort of Hypromellose Eye-drops was reported to be related to viscosity and it was suggested that the viscosity of the *B.P.C. 1973* preparation might be too low for optimum comfort since most patients preferred drops with a viscosity of 20 centistokes. Viscosity values for eye-drops using 0.3% hypromellose (the concentration in the *B.P.C. 1973* formulation) were 5.4 and 7.7 centistokes with the 4500 and 5000 grades respectively. Viscosity increased as the concentration of hypromellose increased and a concentration of 0.4 to 0.45% of hypromellose 5000 would produce eye-drops with a viscosity of 15 to 20 centistokes. However increasing the viscosity had been shown to reduce the activity of benzalkonium chloride and microbiological studies should be carried out.— Pharm. Soc. Lab. Rep. P/76/12, 1976.

Proprietary Preparations

Celacol HPM *(British Celanese, UK)*. A brand of hypromellose, available in a number of grades of viscosity.

Isopto Alkaline *(Alcon, UK: Farillon, UK)*. A sterile buffered iso-osmotic solution of hypromellose 1%. For tear deficiencies. (Also available as Isopto-Alkaline in *S.Afr.*).

Isopto Plain *(Alcon, UK: Farillon, UK)*. A sterile buffered iso-osmotic solution of hypromellose 0.5%. For use as artificial tears. (Also available as Isopto-Plain in *S.Afr., Swed.*).

Methocel 2% *(Dispersa, Switz.: Martindale Samoore, UK)*. A sterile solution containing hypromellose 2%. For bonding lenses to the eye during gonioscopy.

Methocel E, F, J and K *(Dow, USA: K & K-Greeff, UK)*. Brands of hypromellose of pharmaceutical grade available in a number of different viscosities.

Tears Naturale *(Alcon, UK: Farillon, UK)*. Eye-drops containing hypromellose 0.5%, dextran '70' 0.1%. For use as artificial tears. (Also available as Tears Naturale in *Austral.*).

Other Proprietary Names

Isopto Tears *(Austral., Belg., Canad.)*; Methopt *(Austral.)*; Ultra Tears *(Switz.)*.

5437-j

Iceland Moss *(B.P.C. 1934)*. Cetraria; Lichen Islandicus; Lichen d'Islande.

Pharmacopoeias. In *Aust., Cz., Port., Span.,* and *Swiss.*

The dried lichen *Cetraria islandica* (Parmeliaceae). It has a mucilaginous and bitter taste. A 5% decoction gelatinises on cooling.

Iceland moss has demulcent properties and was formerly used as a decoction or as pastilles. The bitterness (due to cetraric acid) may be removed by maceration with water or a dilute solution of potassium carbonate.

5438-z

Isinglass *(B.P.C. 1949)*. Ichthyocolla; Colle de Poisson; Colla Piscium; Gelatina de Peixe.

Pharmacopoeias. In *Port.*

The dried swimming bladder of the sturgeon, *Acipenser huso*, and other species of *Acipenser* (Acipenseridae)

containing about 80% of collagen.
Odourless, semi-transparent, iridescent, membranous, whitish, horny or pearly shreds or thin sheets. Almost entirely **soluble** in boiling water and in most dilute acids and alkalis; practically insoluble in alcohol. A solution of 1 in 50 of boiling water forms a jelly on cooling.

NOTE. A similar material may be prepared from the swimming bladders of a number of fish other than the sturgeon and much of the commercial isinglass is from such sources.

Isinglass has been used as an adhesive in the preparation of protective plasters. It is used for clarifying beers and wines.

5439-c

Ispaghula *(B.P.C. 1968)*. Ispagh.; Isafgul; Isapgol; Spogel Seeds; Blond Psyllium; Indian Plantago Seed; Psylla Seeds.

Pharmacopoeias. In *Ind*. Also in *U.S.P.* (Plantago Seed) which allows also the seeds of *Plantago indica* and *P. psyllium*—see also Psyllium, p.959.

The dried ripe seeds of *Plantago ovata* (Plantaginaceae), containing mucilage and swelling in contact with moisture.

5440-s

Ispaghula Husk *(B.P.)*. Isapgol Husk.

Pharmacopoeias. In *Br.* and *Ind.*

The epidermis and collapsed adjacent layers removed from the dried ripe seeds of *Plantago ovata* (Plantaginaceae), containing mucilage and hemicelluloses.
Small, pale buff, brittle flakes; it loses not more than 12% of its weight on drying. Ispaghula husk swells rapidly in water forming a stiff mucilage.

Adverse Effects and Precautions. See Methylcellulose, p.947.

Uses. Both ispaghula and ispaghula husk are used as bulk laxatives in the treatment of chronic constipation. They are also used for the treatment of diarrhoea, irritable bowel syndrome, diverticulitis and in the management of colostomies and when excessive straining at stool must be avoided following ano-rectal surgery or in the management of haemorrhoids.
The effect of bulk-forming laxatives is usually apparent within 12 to 24 hours, but 2 to 3 days of medication may be required to achieve the full effect.
Ispaghula has been administered after soaking for several hours or as a powder in doses of 3 to 15 g. The husk is given in smaller doses of 3 to 5 g.

Diverticular disease. The effects of bran, ispaghula, and lactulose on colonic function were compared in 31 patients with diverticular disease. Treatment continued for 4 weeks with coarse cereal bran 20 g daily (7 patients), ispaghula husk as Fybogel, 2 sachets daily (14), and lactulose 20 to 40 ml daily (10). All preparations increased stool weight but only ispaghula had a significant effect. Bran reduced transit time and generally reduced colonic motility before and after food. Ispaghula increased basal motility but, like lactulose, had no significant effect on food-stimulated motility. Although all of the preparations relieved symptoms, bran remained the treatment of choice since it added to stool weight and lowered intraluminal pressure.— M. A. Eastwood *et al.*, *Gut*, 1978, *19*, 1144.

In a double-blind 4-month crossover study in 58 patients with symptomatic diverticular disease treated with bran (Energen bran crispbread) or ispaghula (Fybogel), only constipation was significantly affected.— M. H. Ornstein *et al.*, *Br. med. J.*, 1981, *282*, 1353.

Ileostomy control. In a comparison of the effects of codeine phosphate, diphenoxylate (as Lomotil), and ispaghula husk (as Isogel), taken before meals, on ileostomy output in 18 patients only codeine produced a significant fall in output. This was achieved by a reduction of water and electrolyte output with consequent thickening of its consistency. With Isogel ileostomy output was more viscid but water and electrolyte output was increased and there was danger of exacerbating water and electrolyte depletion.— C. R. Newton, *Gut*, 1978, *19*, 377.

Irritable bowel syndrome. In a double-blind study in 96 patients with irritable bowel syndrome ispaghula husk (Fybogel) one sachet twice daily, lorazepam 1 mg twice daily, and hyoscine butylbromide 10 mg four times daily were each more effective than a placebo, ispaghula significantly so. Treatment with more than one agent at a time increased the benefit.— J. A. Ritchie and S. C. Truelove, *Br. med. J.*, 1979, *1*, 376. Criticisms, particularly of the use of hyoscine butylbromide.— A. Herxheimer and J. J. Misiewicz (letter), *ibid.*, 752; K. D. MacRae (letter), *ibid.*; D. Gibbons (letter), *ibid.*

Proprietary Preparations of Ispaghula and Ispaghula Husk

Agiolax *(Madaus, Ger.: Rorer, UK)*. Granules containing ispaghula 54.2% and senna fruit 12.4%. For constipation. *Dose*. 1 to 2 teaspoonfuls, with liquid, twice daily.

Fybogel *(Reckitt & Colman Pharmaceuticals, UK)*. Ispaghula husk, available as granules in sachets containing 3.5 g, with sodium bicarbonate (Na 6 mmol; 6 mEq) and anhydrous citric acid. For patients requiring extra dietary fibre. *Dose*. The contents of 1 sachet, stirred into a glass of water, twice daily.

Isogel *(Allen & Hanburys, UK)*. Dried granules containing ispaghula husk. For chronic constipation and colostomy control. *Dose*. Two 5-ml spoonfuls, stirred in water, once or twice daily; children, one 5-ml spoonful.

Metamucil *(Searle, UK)*. A hydrophilic mucilloid from ispaghula mixed with an equal quantity of anhydrous dextrose. For constipation. *Dose*. 5 ml once to thrice daily; the dose should be added to water or other liquid, stirred briskly, and drunk at once, followed, if desired, by another glass of liquid. (Also available as Metamucil in *Neth.*, *USA*).

Metamucil 6.4 g given thrice daily to 2 healthy subjects for 6 weeks in a 10-week study increased excretion of faecal bile acids about threefold and reduced serum-cholesterol concentrations by a mean of 17%.— D. T. Forman *et al.*, *Proc. Soc. exp. Biol. Med.*, 1968, *127*, 1060.

Loss of diabetic control in a 38-year-old woman owing to the dextrose content of a Metamucil preparation (Metamucil Instant Mix).— J. Catellani and R. J. Collins (letter), *Lancet*, 1978, *2*, 98.

Regulan *(Searle, UK)*. Sachets of 6.4 g, containing 3.6 g of a hydrophilic mucilloid derived from ispaghula husk, with lime/lemon flavouring. For constipation and for patients requiring extra dietary fibre. *Dose*. The contents of one sachet once to thrice daily; 150 ml of cool water should be slowly added to the powder and the suspension drunk immediately.

Vi-Siblin *(Parke, Davis, UK)*. Granules containing ispaghula husk 66%. For chronic constipation. *Dose*. Two 5-ml spoonfuls, with water, one or more times daily.

Other Proprietary Names of Ispaghula and Ispaghula Husk

Ispaghul, Spagulax (both *Fr.*); Konsyl, LA Formula (both *USA*); Lunelax (*Swed.*).

5441-w

Linseed *(B.P.C. 1954)*. Linum; Flaxseed; Lini Semina; Lin; Leinsamen; Semen Lini; Semilla de Lino; Linho.

Pharmacopoeias. In *Aust.*, *Belg.*, *Chin.*, *Ger.*, *Hung.*, *Ind.*, *It.*, *Neth.*, *Nord.*, *Pol.*, *Port.*, *Roum.*, *Span.*, and *Swiss*.

The dried ripe seeds of *Linum usitatissimum* (Linaceae). The seeds contain mucilage and 30 to 40% of fixed oil. **Store** in a cool dry place.

Preparations of linseed have been administered for their demulcent action in the treatment of cough, and a mucilage (1 in 8), prepared by pouring boiling water over linseed and straining, has been used as a demulcent drink. The seeds have been used as a bulk laxative.

Proprietary Names
Linusit *(Fink, Ger.)*.

5442-e

Crushed Linseed *(B.P.C. 1954)*. Linum Contusum; Linseed Meal; Powdered Linseed; Lini Farina; Lini Semina Contusa; Lini Placentae Farina; Placenta Seminis Lini.

Pharmacopoeias. In *Hung.* and *Ind.*

Coarsely powdered linseed, recently prepared, containing not less than 30% of fixed oil. **Store** in a cool dry place.
Powdered linseed cake, left after extraction of oil, is sometimes known as 'linseed meal'; it contains 6 to 8% of oil.

Crushed linseed has been used as a poultice (cataplasma lini) to apply warmth and moisture locally for the relief of superficial or deep-seated inflammation. The poultice mass may be prepared by gradually adding 100 g of crushed linseed to 250 g of boiling water.

5443-l

Magnesium Silicate *(U.S.N.F.)*.

CAS — 1343-88-0.

Pharmacopoeias. In *U.S.N.F.*

A compound of magnesium oxide and silicon dioxide. It loses not more than 15% of its weight on drying. It contains not less than 15% of MgO and not less than 67% of SiO_2 after ignition. A 10% suspension in water has a pH of 7 to 10.8.

Magnesium silicate is used as a tablet excipient.

5444-y

Mallow Flowers. Malvae Flores; Mauve Sauvage; Malvenblüten.

Pharmacopoeias. In *Aust.*, *Belg.*, *Hung.*, *Port.*, and *Swiss*.

The dried flowers of the common mallow, *Malva sylvestris* or *M. mauritiana* (Malvaceae).

Mallow flowers are demulcent and emollient, containing much mucilage. A decoction of the flowers (and also of the leaves) has long been used as a domestic cough remedy.

5445-j

Mallow Leaves. Malvae Folia.

Pharmacopoeias. In *Aust.*, *Cz.*, *Hung.*, *Port.*, and *Swiss*.

The dried leaves of the common mallow, *Malva sylvestris*, and of the dwarf mallow, *M. neglecta*.

Mallow leaves have been used similarly to Mallow flowers.

5446-z

Oxypolygelatin

CAS — 9005-91-8.

A derivative of gelatin prepared by treating purified gelatin with glyoxal, followed by oxidation with hydrogen peroxide. It has an average molecular weight of about 31 000.

Adverse Effects, Treatment, and Precautions. As for Gelatin, p.954.

There were 2 anaphylactic reactions in 810 infusions of oxypolygelatin.— J. Ring and K. Messmer, *Lancet*, 1977, *1*, 466. See also H. W. Löding and P. Lawin, *Z. Prakt. Anaesth.*, 1972, *7*, 283; B. Schöning and H. Koch, *Anaesthesist*, 1975, *24*, 507.

Uses. Oxypolygelatin has been used similarly to Gelatin p.954 as a plasma substitute.

References: A. Doenicke *et al.*, *Br. J. Anaesth.*, 1977, *49*, 681.

Proprietary Names
Gelifundol *(Biotest, Ger.)*.

5447-c

Pectin *(U.S.P.)*.

CAS — 9000-69-5.

Pharmacopoeias. In *Aust.*, *Ind.*, *Span.*, and *U.S.*

A purified carbohydrate product obtained from

the dilute acid extract of the inner portion of the rind of citrus fruits or from apple pomace; it consists mainly of partially methoxylated polygalacturonic acids; when standardised to 150-Grade it yields not less than 6.7% of methoxy groups and not less than 74% of galacturonic acid, calculated on the dried basis.

A coarse or fine, yellowish-white, almost odourless powder with a mucilaginous taste. It loses not more than 10% of its weight on drying.

Almost completely **soluble** 1 in 20 of water, forming a viscous, opalescent, colloidal solution which flows readily and is acid to litmus; practically insoluble in alcohol and other organic solvents. It dissolves more readily in water if first moistened with alcohol, glycerol, or syrup, or if mixed with 3 or more parts of sucrose. **Incompatible** with alkalis, heavy metals, salicyclic acid, tannic acid, and strong alcohol. **Store** in airtight containers.

Commercial liquid pectin is the concentrated solution obtained by concentrating the dilute acid extract of citrus fruit, apples, or sugar beet and may contain other plant constituents derived from the source material.

Commercial powdered pectin is obtainable in a highly refined form and standardised to a definite 'setting power' or 'jelly grade' by the addition of dextrose or other sugars. It may also contain sodium, potassium, or calcium carbonates, bicarbonates, citrates, lactates, phosphates, or tartrates. The standard strength usually employed is '100-Grade', 1 part of which will set 100 parts of sugar in solution to a jelly of standard strength and firmness containing 65% of sugar. For toilet purposes, a pectin of about '190-Grade' is employed. For medicinal purposes, pure pectin, containing no added sugars, is used. Pectin *U.S.P.* may be standardised to '150-Grade' by the addition of sugars, and may contain sodium citrate or other buffers.

Adverse Effects and Precautions. As for Methylcellulose, p.947.

Background toxicological data on pectins and amidated pectins. In *rats*, high doses of pectin caused diarrhoea.— *Fd Add. Ser. Wld Hlth Org. No. 5,* 1974.

Markedly reduced absorption of digoxin was noted in a study of 10 healthy subjects following concurrent administration of a preparation containing kaolin and pectin.— D. D. Brown and R. P. Juhl, *New Engl. J. Med.*, 1976, *295,* 1034.

Uses. Apart from its commercial uses pectin has been employed for various therapeutic purposes. Internally, it may be used in the treatment of diarrhoea and is sometimes used in mixtures with kaolin.

Pectin has been employed as a haemostatic for internal and external haemorrhage, being given by mouth or used as a compress.

It is no longer used as a plasma substitute since it may cause degenerative changes in the liver and kidneys.

Pectin is an efficient emulsifying and gelling agent in acid media and is used in the preparation of pharmaceutical and cosmetic products. Its use is, however, limited by the fact that it is decomposed in alkaline media.

Temporary estimated acceptable daily intake of amidated pectins: up to 25 mg per kg body-weight.— Nineteenth Report of the Joint FAO/WHO Expert Committee on Food Additives, *Tech. Rep. Ser. Wld Hlth Org. No. 576,* 1975.

Administration. The unpalatability of pectin was overcome by incorporating 15 g of citrus pectin into a fruit gel containing raspberries 75 g, orange juice 70 g, sucrose 15 g and water 50 g.— R. M. Kay (letter), *Lancet,* 1976, *2,* 799.

Diarrhoea. A study of 204 patients with acute non-specific diarrhoea indicated that treatment with kaolin and pectin, diphenoxylate and atropine, or charcoal was no more effective than a controlled diet in reducing the frequency or looseness of stools.— K. Alestig *et al.*, *Practitioner,* 1979, *222,* 859.

Effect on blood-glucose. References to pectin reducing blood-glucose concentrations or insulin requirements.— D. J. A. Jenkins *et al.*, *Lancet,* 1976, *2,* 172 (with guar gum; in diabetics); *idem, Ann. intern. Med.*, 1977, *86,* 20 (with or without guar gum; in healthy subjects); T. Poynard *et al.* (letter), *Lancet,* 1980, *1,* 158. See also D. J. A. Jenkins, *ibid.*, 1979, *2,* 1287. Criticisms.— J. I. Mann and H. C. R. Simpson (letter), *ibid.*, 1980, *1,* 44; J. Yudkin (letter), *ibid.*

Addition of pectin 14.5 g to an oral glucose load test prevented the occurrence of hypoglycaemic symptoms and raised blood-glucose concentrations above control values in 9 patients who had experienced postprandial hypoglycaemia as a complication of gastric surgery. The most severely affected patient had subsequently received pectin 5 g twice daily for 5 weeks without further hypoglycaemic attacks. Pectin and other unabsorbable gelling agents may be of use in the treatment of abnormal carbohydrate absorption after gastric surgery.— D. J. A. Jenkins *et al.*, *Gastroenterology,* 1977, *73,* 215.

The effects of guar gum with pectin on glucose absorption could be due simply to delayed gastric emptying.— S. Holt *et al.*, *Lancet,* 1979, *1,* 636.

Effect on serum lipids. A review of the effect of dietary fibre, including pectin, on hyperlipidaemia.— D. J. A. Jenkins, *Lancet,* 1979, *2,* 1287.

Pectin 36 g daily for 2 weeks reduced the serum-cholesterol concentration in healthy volunteers by about 290 µg per ml.— D. J. A. Jenkins *et al.*, *Lancet,* 1975, *1,* 1116.

Pectin in a daily dose of about 12 g given for 4 weeks to 12 healthy subjects reduced total serum-cholesterol concentrations by about 8%. This was mainly due to a reduction in serum concentrations of low-density lipoprotein cholesterol and apolipoprotein-B. There was also an increase in wet-stool weight.— P. N. Durrington *et al.*, *Lancet,* 1976, *2,* 394. See also A. R. Leeds and M. A. Gassull (letter), *ibid.*, 637.

Pectin 20 g per day increased to 40 to 50 g daily, given for 2 weeks to 9 normolipidaemic and hyperlipidaemic patients, reduced the mean total serum cholesterol concentration by 13%. The effect was greater in the older patients with hypercholesterolaemia than in the young normocholesterolaemic subjects. Serum triglyceride concentrations were unaffected in both types of patients. The reduction in serum cholesterol appeared to be produced by increased elimination of cholesterol in the faeces as bile acids. Two of the hypercholesterolaemic patients had subsequently received pectin 30 g daily for one year with a permanent cholesterol reduction of about 15%. During the study faecal mass and dry weight were not consistently increased, suggesting that pectin may not be an ideal fibre for increasing faecal bulk in functional colonic disorders.— T. A. Miettinen and S. Tarpila, *Clinica chim. Acta,* 1977, *79,* 471.

Proprietary Names

Arhémapectine *(Gallier, Fr.)*; Sango-Stop *(Endopharm, Ger.)*.

5448-k

Plantain Seed. The seed of *Plantago major* var. *asiatica* .

Pharmacopoeias. In *Jap.*

Plantain seed has been suggested as a substitute for ispaghula.

References: S. M. J. S. Qadry, *J. Pharm. Pharmac.*, 1963, *15,* 552.

5449-a

Polygeline.

A polymer prepared by cross-linking polypeptides derived from denatured gelatin with a di-isocyanate to form urea bridges and having an average molecular weight of 35 000.

CAS — 9015-56-9.

Adverse Effects, Treatment, and Precautions. As for Gelatin, p.954.

In a randomised controlled single blind study, no allergic reactions were observed in 25 healthy subjects who received dimethindene 100 µg per kg body-weight and cimetidine 10 mg per kg both intravenously before receiving an infusion of Haemaccel 500 ml to replace 440 ml of blood previously withdrawn. Nine allergic reactions were observed in a similar control group.— W. Lorenz *et al.*, *Anaesthesist,* 1977, *26,* 644.

There were 9 anaphylactic reactions in 6151 infusions of polygeline.— J. Ring and K. Messmer, *Lancet,* 1977, *1,* 466.

Some other reports of anaphylactic or allergic reactions in patients given polygeline: N. Lund (letter), *Br. J. Anaesth.*, 1973, *45,* 929; K. Wisborg (letter), *ibid.*, 1975, *47,* 1116; W. Lorenz *et al.*, *ibid.*, 1976, *48,* 151; A. Doenicke *et al.*, *ibid.*, 1977, *49,* 681; M. K. Freeman, *Anaesthesia,* 1979, *34,* 341.

Absorption and Fate. Following infusion about 45% of a dose of polygeline is excreted within 12 hours, mostly in the urine. About 74% is reported to be excreted within 4 days. Serum half-lives of 4 to 8 hours have been reported.

In a study in 52 patients with normal or impaired renal function given 500 ml of polygeline 3.5% about 50% of the dose was excreted in the urine within 48 hours, chiefly within 12 hours, in those with normal renal function. Excretion was not impaired in those with a glomerular filtration-rate (GFR) of 31 to 90 ml per minute, slightly reduced in those with a GFR of 11 to 30 ml, reduced to 27% in 48 hours in those with a GFR of 2 to 10 ml, and to 9.3% in 48 hours in those with GFR of 0.5 to 2 ml. The proportion of polygeline excreted after 12 hours was increased in those with a low GFR. The mean half-life of the elimination phase was 505 minutes in those with adequate renal function increasing to 985 minutes in those with end-stage renal failure. Polygeline 500 ml of 3.5% solution could be given twice weekly for 1 to 2 months even in patients with total anuria.— H. Köhler *et al.*, *Eur. J. clin. Pharmac.*, 1978, *14,* 405.

Further references: L. Havers *et al.*, *Dt. med. Wschr.*, 1962, *87,* 730; W. Schwartzkopff *et al.*, *Z. ges. exp. Med.*, 1968, *147,* 202.

Uses. Polygeline has similar actions to gelatin (see p.954). It is given as a sterile 3.5% colloidal solution with suitable electrolytes as a plasma expander in hypovolaemia. It is also used in patients undergoing extracorporeal circulation and as a perfusion fluid for isolated organs.

A 3.5% solution of polygeline was used successfully as a vitreous substitute in 15 patients with retinal detachment.— J. A. Oosterhuis, *Archs Ophthal., N.Y.*, 1966, *76,* 374, per *Int. pharm. Abstr.*, 1966, *3,* 1593.

A review of the use of polygeline as a plasma substitute.— A. Doenicke *et al.*, *Br. J. Anaesth.*, 1977, *49,* 681.

The successful use of polygeline as the sole replacement fluid in plasma exchange.— A. J. Stellon and P. J. Moorhead, *Br. med. J.*, 1981, *282,* 698.

For the use of polygeline to reduce the adsorption of insulin on to plastic or glass, see Insulin Injection, p.844.

Proprietary Preparations

Haemaccel *(Hoechst, UK).* Polygeline, available as a 3.5% colloidal infusion solution, with the following electrolytes in each litre: sodium 145 mmol, potassium 5.1 mmol, calcium 6.26 mmol, and chloride 145 mmol. (Also available as Haemaccel in *Aust., Austral., Belg., Denm., Fr., Ger., Neth., Norw., Pol., Swed., Switz.*).

5450-e

Povidone

(B.P., U.S.P.). Polyvidone-Excipient; Polyvidone; Polyvidonum; Polyvinylpyrrolidone; PVP; Vinylpyrrolidinone Polymer. A mixture of essentially linear synthetic polymers of 1-vinyl-2-pyrrolidone of different chain lengths and molecular weights.

$(C_6H_9NO)_n = 111.1 \times n.$

CAS — 9003-39-8.

Pharmacopoeias. In *Br., Fr., Hung., It., Roum.,* and *U.S.* The grades described are not suitable for parenteral use.

U.S.N.F. includes Crospovidone, a synthetic cross-linked homopolymer of povidone, for use as a tablet excipient.

Povidone is a pharmaceutical grade of polyvinylpyrrolidone suitable for use in oral preparations and topical applications. A grade of povidone suitable for parenteral administration would have to comply with requirements additional to those provided in the *B.P., U.S.P.,* or other pharmacopoeias.

A fine white or very slightly cream-coloured, odourless or almost odourless, tasteless powder. It is hygroscopic, and significant amounts of moisture are absorbed at low relative humidities. The equilibrium moisture contents at 30, 50, and 70% relative humidity are 10, 20, and 40% respectively.

Soluble in water, alcohol, chloroform, and isopropyl alcohol; practically insoluble in acetone and ether. A 5% solution in water has a pH of 3 to 7. The viscosities of aqueous solutions of up to 10% do not differ significantly from those of water. The *B.P.* and *U.S.P.* state that the viscosity in aqueous solution, relative to water, is expressed as a K-value, ranging from 10 to 95. Aqueous solutions of grades suitable for injection are **sterilised** by autoclaving. **Store** in airtight containers.

Other grades of povidone are commercially available, including a grade for parenteral administration.

Povidone is available commercially in a number of mixtures of polymers, each product having a particular mean molecular weight, which is in the range of 10 000 to 700 000; solubilities decrease with increasing molecular weight and viscosities of solutions increase.

Interactions. Povidone formed a complex with erythrosine. The stability of erythrosine in solution was improved but the colour was slightly changed.— J. C. Anderson and G. M. Boyce, *J. pharm. Sci.*, 1969, *58*, 1425.

The effect of heat, preservatives, and additives on the viscosity of povidone solutions.— M. A. Kassem and A. G. Mattha, *Pharm. Acta Helv.*, 1970, *45*, 18 and 28.

Tests with 14 different preservatives indicated that inactivation by povidone was unlikely to be a formulation problem.— T. J. McCarthy, *Pharm. Weekbl. Ned.*, 1973, *108*, 449.

Adverse Effects. Injection of povidone can lead to deposits in various tissues and there may be inflammatory papulous or granulomatous responses with swelling and pain. Inhalation of excessive amounts may also affect lung tissue and pulmonary changes may lead to respiratory insufficiency.

Shock-like reactions have been reported in infants receiving intravenous injections of povidone.

Reviews of the adverse effects of povidone.— F. Cabanne *et al.*, *Annls Anat. path., Paris*, 1969, *14*, 419; W. Wessel *et al.*, *Arzneimittel-Forsch.*, 1971, *21*, 1468.

For background toxicological data, see *Fd Add. Ser. Wld Hlth Org. No. 5*, 1974.

Carcinogenic effect. Evidence of carcinogenic effect in rats.— W. C. Hueper, *Proc. Am. Ass. Cancer Res.*, 1956, *2*, 120; *idem*, *Cancer*, 1957, *10*, 8; *idem*, *Archs Path.*, 1959, *67*, 589. See also L. M. Lusky and A. A. Nelson, *Fedn Proc.*, 1957, *16*, Part 1, 318. Contrary findings.— *idem*, *J. natn. Cancer Inst.*, 1961, *26*, 229.

Cutaneous and granulomatous reactions. Papular dermatosis after the prolonged use of injections containing povidone.— F. Cabanne *et al.*, *Annls. Anat. path., Paris*, 1966, *11*, 385.

For a histological study of cutaneous infiltration, in 2 patients, due to povidone in posterior pituitary injections, see J. Thivolet *et al.*, *Br. J. Derm.*, 1970, *83*, 661.

A 54-year-old woman developed large foreign body granulomas in the breast and epigastric area after repeated injections of a depot preparation containing povidone, self-administered into the left breast. Povidone was identified in granulomatous tissue.— J. Gille and H. Brandau, *Geburtsch. Frauenheilk.*, 1975, *35*, 799.

Pseudotumours in the limbs of 2 patients contained foreign material which was probably associated with subcutaneous injections of a preparation containing procaine with povidone.— S. Soumerai, *J. med. Soc. New Jers.*, 1978, *75*, 407.

Hepatosplenomegaly. A 54-year-old woman with diabetes insipidus received intramuscular injections of a depot preparation of posterior-pituitary lobe containing povidone for 13 years. During treatment abcesses and inflammatory reactions occurred at the site of injection with infiltrations and swellings developing in various muscle groups. Hepatomegaly and splenomegaly became predominant symptoms with pancytopenia and spontaneous fracture of several vertebrae also occurring.— J. M. Bert *et al.*, *Sem. Hôp. Paris*, 1972, *48*, 1809.

Precautions. Precautions that should be observed with plasma expanders are described under Dextran 70 Intravenous Infusion, p.512, and these should be considered when povidone is used for this purpose.

Absorption and Fate. Povidone does not appear to be absorbed from the gastro-intestinal tract and is not metabolised following injection. Povidone is mainly excreted in the urine, the rate being dependent upon the molecular weight. Following intravenous injection about 70 to 90% of povidone with a molecular weight of about 25 000 or less is excreted within 24 to 72 hours in the urine; small amounts are excreted in the faeces. A substantial amount of povidone, particularly if of high molecular weight, may be stored for prolonged periods in organs rich in reticuloendothelial tissue.

Uses. Povidone is used in pharmacy as a suspending and dispersing agent, usually in concentrations of up to 10%. It is also used as a tablet binding and granulating agent, usually in a concentration of 0.5 to 5%, but a higher proportion may be necessary for some granules. It is particularly useful in the preparation of effervescent tablets and other tablets which are highly sensitive to water since it can be incorporated as a solution in an organic solvent such as alcohol.

It is also useful in the preparation of heat-sensitive tablets since granules prepared with a solution of povidone in an organic solvent of low boiling point can be dried in air at ordinary temperatures. It is employed as a dispersing agent for dyes in coloured tablets and as a stabilising agent in vitamin, enzyme, and salicylate preparations.

A 1 to 2% solution in alcohol is used as an aid to the granulation of very light powders prior to filling into capsules.

Solutions of povidone (10 to 25%) have been used as vehicles for such drugs as penicillin, cortisone, procaine, insulin, and iodine (see Povidone-Iodine, p.867), to delay their absorption and thus prolong their action. Its property of forming hard adherent films has been utilised in the formulation of film-coating solutions for tablets and in the formulation of skin sprays and hair lacquers in which it may be used as a copolymer with less hydrophilic compounds such as vinyl acetate.

Povidone has been used to reduce the irritant effects of drugs in ophthalmic preparations.

Povidone solutions may be used as artificial tears and to make the wearing of contact lenses more comfortable. A grade of povidone suitable for parenteral administration has been used as a plasma expander but dextran infusions are preferred.

An insoluble cross-linked form of polyvinylpyrrolidone sometimes known as polyvinylpolypyrrolidone or crospovidone is used as a tablet disintegrant.

For a review of the actions and uses of povidone, see W. Wessel *et al.*, *Arzneimittel-Forsch.*, 1971, *21*, 1468. See also L. Blecher and L. W. Burnette, *Bull. parent. Drug Ass.*, 1969, *23*, 124.

An intravenous infusion of 500 ml of 6% povidone in sodium chloride injection given over 2 hours was shown to decrease platelet adhesiveness in 6 of 8 fasting adults.— S. S. Sanbar *et al.*, *Lancet*, 1967, *2*, 917.

Available data on the storage of povidone used as a food additive in intestinal lymph nodes were insufficient. Because of general concern on the effects of stored macromolecules, the previous conditional acceptable daily intake was withdrawn.— Seventeenth Report of the FAO/WHO Expert Committee on Food Additives, *Tech. Rep. Ser. Wld Hlth Org. No. 539*, 1974.

Binding agent for tablets. A study of the effect of some binding agents, including povidone, on the mechanical properties of granules and their compression characteristics.— E. Doelker and E. Shotton, *J. Pharm. Pharmac.*, 1977, *29*, 193.

Cryopreservation. Povidone had been used in addition to glycerol as a cryoprotectant in the preservation of bone marrow.— D. E. Pegg, *Practitioner*, 1978, *221*, 543.

Effect on serum lipids. There were prompt and significant falls of about 28% in serum concentrations of cholesterol and triglyceride in 8 patients with hyperlipidaemia who were given 2 daily intravenous infusions of 500 ml of 6% povidone in sodium chloride injection. The maximum effects occurred 5 days after the infusion. The hypolipidaemic effect of the povidone persisted beyond the period of plasma-volume expansion.— S. S. Sanbar and G. Smet, *Circulation*, 1968, *38*, 771, per *J. Am. med. Ass.*, 1968, *206*, 923.

Test media. A brief study on the use of povidone in media for testing bacteria for sensitivity to antibiotics.— R. Bayston (letter), *J. antimicrob. Chemother.*, 1978, *4*, 291.

Preparations

P.V.P. 0.5% Eye-drops *(Moorfields Eye Hosp.).* Povidone 500 mg, hydroxyethylcellulose 500 mg, disodium edetate 100 mg, sodium acid phosphate 420 mg, sodium phosphate 1.43 g, thiomersal 5 mg, water to 100 ml. pH 6.8 to 7.4. Shelf-life 2 years. For patients using hydrophilic contact lenses, or as artificial tears.

P.V.P. 0.5% Alkaline Eye-drops *(Moorfields Eye Hosp.).* Povidone 500 mg, hydroxyethylcellulose 500 mg, disodium edetate 100 mg, sodium bicarbonate 1 g, sodium chloride 600 mg, thiomersal 5 mg, water to 100 ml. pH 8.0 to 8.6. Shelf-life 2 years. For patients using hydrophilic contact lenses, or as artificial tears.

Proprietary Preparations

Kollidon *(BASF, Ger.: Blagden, UK).* A brand of povidone, available in various grades for use in injections, and in oral and topical preparations.

Plasdone *(GAF, UK).* A brand of povidone available in various grades including **Plasdone K** for oral and topical use, and **Plasdone C** for use in injections. **Polyplasdone XL.** A brand of crospovidone; for use as a tablet disintegrant.

Other Proprietary Names

Bolinan (crospovidone)*(Fr.)*; Periston-N-Toxobin, Plassint (both *Ital.*); Protagent *(Ger.)*.

5451-l

Propylene Carbonate *(U.S.N.F.).* 4-Methyl-1,3-dioxolan-2-one.

$C_4H_6O_3$=102.1.

CAS — 108-32-7.

Pharmacopoeias. In *U.S.N.F.*

A clear colourless mobile liquid. Specific gravity 1.203 to 1.210. Freely **soluble** in water; miscible with alcohol and chloroform; practically insoluble in light petroleum. A 10% solution in water has a pH of 6.5 to 7.5. **Store** in airtight containers.

Propylene carbonate is used as a gelling agent.

5452-y

Psyllium *(B.P.C. 1973).* Psyll.; Psyllii Semen; Flea Seed; French Psyllium Seed; Psyllium Seed; Spanish Psyllium Seed; Flohsame.

Pharmacopoeias. In *Int.*, *Nord.*, and *Swiss*. Also in *U.S.P.* (Plantago Seed) which allows also the seeds of *Plantago ovata*—see also Ispaghula.

The dried ripe seeds of *Plantago afra* (=*P. psyllium*) or *P. indica* (=*P. arenaria*) (Spanish or French Psyllium Seed) (Plantaginaceae).

One g of seeds swells in 20 ml of water to occupy at least 14 ml after 24 hours. *U.S.P.* specifies at least 14 ml for *P. psyllium*, at least 10 ml for *P. ovata*, and at least 8 ml for *P. indica*. **Protect** from moisture.

Adverse Effects and Precautions. See Methylcellulose, p.947.

Rhinitis and wheezing occurred in 3 men exposed to psyllium powder during bulk-laxative production. All had reaginic skin sensitivity and 2 had positive bronchial inhalation challenges with a psyllium extract.— W. W. Busse and W. F. Schoenwetter, *Ann. intern. Med.*, 1975, *83*, 361.

Further references: H. S. Bernton, *Med. Ann. Distr. Columbia*, 1970, *39*, 313; R. Gross (letter), *J. Am. med. Ass.*, 1979, *241*, 1573.

Uses. Psyllium has properties and uses similar to those of ispaghula husk (see p.957). It is given in doses of 5 to 15 g. On account of its content of mucilage it is also used as a demulcent.

Proprietary Names
Effersyllium *(Stuart Pharmaceuticals, USA)*; Hydrocil Instant *(Rowell, USA)*; Osmolax *(Seclo, Fr.)*; Siblin *(Parke, Davis, Canad.)*; Syllact *(Wallace, USA)*.

5453-j

PVM/MA. PVMA-119. A 1:1 alternating linear copolymer of methyl vinyl ether and maleic anhydride.
$(C_7H_8O_4)_n$=156.1×*n*.

CAS — 9011-16-9.

A white powder. **Soluble** in hot water, slowly hydrolysing to free acid with a pH of 2 to 3. Neutralisation with a suitable base to pH 6 to 7 produces clear viscous gels. Viscosity is reduced at high pH values.

PVM/MA is used as a suspending agent and gelling agent for aqueous and aqueous-alcoholic solutions for external use, generally in concentrations of 0.75 to 3%. It has also been suggested as a film-coating agent for tablets.

Proprietary Preparations
Gantrez AN *(GAF, UK)*. PVM/MA, available in 4 grades of viscosity.

5454-z

Salep. Saleb Tuber; Tubera Salep.

Pharmacopoeias. In *Aust.* and *Port.*

The dried tubers of various orchidaceous plants, particularly the Early Purple Orchis, *Orchis mascula*, and other species of *Orchis* (Orchidaceae). The tubers are immersed in boiling water on collection and dried.

Salep contains mucilage and has nutritive and demulcent properties.
Mucilage of salep (Mucilago Salep) is prepared by boiling the powdered drug (1%) with water; alcohol (1 to 2%) is sometimes used to assist dispersion of the particles.

5455-c

Silica Gel *(U.S.N.F.)*.
SiO_2,xH_2O=60.08.

CAS — 63231-67-4.

Pharmacopoeias. In *U.S.N.F.*

A fine, white, odourless, hygroscopic, amorphous powder in which the diameter of the average particles ranges from 2 to 10 μm. It loses not more than 4% of its weight on drying.
Practically **insoluble** in water, alcohol, and other organic solvents; soluble in hot solutions of alkali hydroxides. A 5% suspension in water has a pH of 4 to 8. **Store** in airtight containers.

Silica gel is used pharmaceutically as a suspending, disintegrating, and anticaking agent. In granular form it is also used as a desiccant.

5456-k

Purified Siliceous Earth *(U.S.N.F.)*. Diatomite *(B.P.C. 1949)*; Purified Kieselguhr; Purified Infusorial Earth; Diatomaceous Earth; Terra Silicea Purificada.

Pharmacopoeias. In *U.S.N.F.*

An amorphous form of almost pure silicon dioxide with lesser amounts of crystalline polymorphs such as quartz and cristobalite obtained from siliceous deposits, consisting chiefly of frustules and fragments of diatoms, unicellular organisms belonging to the Bacillariaceae. The crude material is crushed, incinerated, boiled with dilute hydrochloric acid, washed, and calcined. A colloidal form of silicon dioxide is described under Colloidal Silicon Dioxide, p.960.
A fine, white, light grey, or pale buff, gritty, odourless, tasteless powder which adheres to the skin when rubbed.
Practically **insoluble** in water, organic solvents, dilute solutions of alkali hydroxides and acids, except hydrofluoric acid. It absorbs about 4 times its weight of water without becoming fluid.

Adverse Effects. As for Colloidal Silicon Dioxide.
Silicosis had been reported in 6 workers after relatively short periods of exposure to purified siliceous earth.— R. Beskow, *Scand. J. resp. Dis.*, 1978, *59*, 216, per *Abstr. Hyg.*, 1978, *53*, 1296.

Uses. Purified siliceous earth is used as a filtering medium. It has also been used in the preparation of dusting powders and as a basis for disinfectant powders.

5457-a

Colloidal Silicon Dioxide *(U.S.N.F.)*. Acidum Silicicum Colloidale; Colloidal Silica; Silice Precipitata; Hochdisperses Silicumdioxid.
SiO_2=60.08.

CAS — 7631-86-9 (silicon dioxide).

Pharmacopoeias. In *Aust., Ger., Hung.,* and *It.* Also in *U.S.N.F. Jap.* includes Light Anhydrous Silicic Acid which contains not less than 98% SiO_2 calculated on the incinerated basis.

A submicroscopic fumed silica, prepared by the vapour-phase hydrolysis of a silicon compound. It is a light, white, odourless, tasteless, non-gritty powder; particle size about 15 nm.
Practically **insoluble** in water, organic solvents, and acids, except hydrofluoric acid; soluble in hot solutions of alkali hydroxides. A 4% dispersion has a pH of 3.5 to 4.4. **Store** in airtight containers.

Adverse Effects. Colloidal silicon dioxide does not appear to be associated with silicosis.
For background toxicological information, see *Fd Add. Ser. Wld Hlth Org. No. 5*, 1974.

Uses. Colloidal silicon dioxide is used as a suspending agent and thickener in suspensions, ointments, and suppositories, as a stabiliser in emulsions, and as a filler in tablet coatings. It may also be used as a granulating agent and lubricant in tablets. As it absorbs a large quantity of water without liquefying, it is used as an anticaking agent to prevent clogging of hygroscopic powders.
Silicon dioxide (Silicea) is used in homoeopathic medicine.

The properties and uses of colloidal silicon dioxide in liquid products as a gelling and thixotropic agent.— K. A. Loftman, *Soap chem. Spec.*, 1966, *42* (Sept.), 70.

The use of colloidal silicon dioxide as a disintegrant in experimental lactose tablets.— A. M. Sakr *et al.*, *Mfg Chem.*, 1973, *44* (Jan.), 37.

The acceptable daily intake for man of silicon dioxide was only limited by good manufacturing practice.— Seventeenth Report of FAO/WHO Expert Committee on Food Additives, *Tech. Rep. Ser. Wld Hlth Org. No. 539*, 1974.

Colloidal silicon dioxide was not a satisfactory suspending agent for chalk or sulphadimidine mixtures.— C. A. Farley and W. Lund, *Pharm. J.*, 1976, *1*, 562.

The effect of colloidal silicon dioxide on the properties of rectal suppository formulations.— A. Moës, *J. Pharm. Belg.*, 1976, *31*, 355.

Proprietary Preparations
Aerosil *(Degussa, UK)*. A brand of colloidal silicon dioxide.

Cab-O-Sil *(K & K-Greeff, UK)*. A range of colloidal silicon dioxide powders.

Other Proprietary Names
Dissolvurol *(Fr.)*; Entero-Teknosal *(Ger.)*.

5458-t

Slippery Elm *(B.P.C. 1949)*. Ulmus Fulva; Slippery Elm Bark; Elm Bark; Ulmus.

The dried inner bark of *Ulmus fulva* (=*U. rubra*) (Ulmaceae). **Store** in a dry place.

Slippery elm contains much mucilage and was formerly used as a demulcent. A 2% suspension in water forms a thick fawn-coloured jelly. Mixed with hot water, the powder was also used as a poultice in abscesses and whitlows.
It was recommended by the Food Additives and Contaminants Committee that slippery elm bark be prohibited for use in foods as a flavouring agent.— *Report on the Review of Flavourings in Food,* FAC/REP/22, Ministry of Agriculture, Fisheries and Food, London, HM Stationery Office, 1976.

5459-x

Sodium Alginate *(B.P.C. 1973, U.S.N.F.)*. Algin; Sodium Polymannuronate.

CAS — 9005-38-3.

Pharmacopoeias. In *Aust., Fr.,* and *It.* Also in *U.S.N.F.*

It consists chiefly of the sodium salt of alginic acid, a polyuronic acid composed of residues of D-mannuronic and L-guluronic acids, and is obtained chiefly from algae belonging to the Phaeophyceae, mainly species of *Laminaria*.
A white or buff powder which is odourless or almost odourless and tasteless. It loses not more than 22% of its weight on drying. The *U.S.N.F.* specifies not more than 15% loss on drying.
Slowly **soluble** in water, forming an off-white to yellowish-brown viscous colloidal solution; practically insoluble in alcohol, chloroform, and ether, and in aqueous solutions containing more than 30% of alcohol. Various grades of sodium alginate are available which yield aqueous solutions having varying viscosities covering the range 20 to 400 centipoises in 1% solution at 20°. Sodium alginate is **sterilised** by autoclaving; solutions are similarly sterilised, but some loss of viscosity occurs, depending on the presence of other substances.
Incompatible with acridine derivatives, crystal violet, phenylmercuric acetate and nitrate, calcium salts, alcohol in concentrations greater than 5%, and heavy metals. High concentrations of electrolytes cause an increase in viscosity until salting-out of sodium alginate occurs; salting-out occurs if more than 4% of sodium chloride is present. Solutions are most stable between pH 4 and 10; alginic acid is precipitated below pH 3. **Store** in airtight containers. Solutions should not be stored in metal containers. Preparations for external use may be preserved by the addition of chlorocresol (0.1%), chloroxylenol (0.1%), or esters of *p*-hydroxybenzoic acid or, if the medium is acid, benzoic acid may be used.
In making preparations of sodium alginate, dispersion is more easily effected if the alginate is first mixed with 2 to 4% of alcohol, glycerol, propylene glycol, sugar, or other suitable dispersing agent.

Incompatibility. Tests carried out on the bactericidal activity of 3 cationic antiseptics, aminacrine, cetrimide, and crystal violet showed that in each case a marked decrease in activity occurred in the presence of sodium alginate. There was no correlation between reduction in bactericidal properties and precipitation. In contrast, the bacteriostatic activity of aminacrine was not lost even in the ratio of 1000 to 1 of alginate to aminacrine. Loss of bacteriostatic activity did occur, however, with 133 to 1 of alginate to cetrimide. Cationic antiseptics were unsatisfactory in alginate gels, though certain cationics might exert some preservative action.— G. Richardson and R. Woodford, *Pharm. J.*, 1964, *1*, 527.

Viscosity. The effects of temperature, pH, alcohol, glycerol, and electrolytes on the viscosity of alginate solutions.— R. Bolliger and K. Münzel, *Pharm. Acta Helv.*, 1958, *33*, 141 and 225, per *J. Pharm. Pharmac.*, 1958, *10*, 523 and 714.

There was a marked increase in the viscosity of solutions of sodium alginate which had been frozen and thawed. The increase was due and proportional to the amount of residual calcium present. Highly refined sodium alginate did not show this property. Small amounts of added calcium had practically no effect on the viscosity before freezing but caused a considerable increase after freezing and thawing.— G. Levy and T. W. Schwarz, *J. Am. pharm. Ass., scient. Edn*, 1958, *47*, 455.

Sodium alginate could be sterilised by ethylene oxide without loss of viscosity.— D. Coates and G. Richardson, *Can. J. pharm. Sci.*, 1974, *9*, 60.

The sterilisation of sodium alginate by irradiation with 25 000 Gy caused a loss of 70% in intrinsic viscosity in solutions prepared from it.— A. W. Hartman *et al.*, *J. pharm. Sci.*, 1975, *64*, 802.

Adverse Effects.

For background toxicological information, see *Fd Add. Ser. Wld Hlth Org. No. 5*, 1974.

Uses. Sodium alginate has little surface activity and its emulsifying power is chiefly achieved by increasing the viscosity of the aqueous phase. It is therefore used chiefly as a suspending and thickening agent and in the preparation of water-miscible pastes, creams, and gels.

A 1% solution has suspending properties similar to those of tragacanth mucilage and is capable of emulsifying an equal volume of vegetable oil by simple agitation; mineral oil emulsions require the addition of acacia. It may be used as a stabiliser for oil-in-water emulsions.

According to the viscosity required, from 1 to 10% is used in the preparation of pastes and creams, the addition of a trace of a soluble calcium salt increasing the viscosity in inverse ratio to the pH.

Sodium alginate is used as a binding and disintegrating agent in tablets and as a binding agent and demulcent in lozenges.

It is employed in making dental impression compounds and for coating dental plaster moulds. Sodium alginate is used as a thickening agent in liquid anionic detergents. It is widely used in the food industry.

Because of its property of instantaneous precipitation when brought into contact with free calcium ions, yielding calcium alginate, sodium alginate is employed as a haemostatic (see also Calcium Alginate, p.735).

It is also an ingredient of some antacid preparations used for gastric reflux.

Estimated acceptable daily intake: up to 25 mg, as alginic acid, per kg body-weight.— Seventeenth Report of FAO/WHO Expert Committee on Food Additives, *Tech. Rep. Ser. Wld Hlth Org. No. 539*, 1974.

Cooling solution for hypothermia. Sodium alginate 10 g, glycerol 5 g, sodium benzoate 1.33 g, water to 100 g. The solution was kept deep-frozen in nylon envelopes which were applied as corsets to induce hypothermia.— H. T. John *et al.* (letter), *Lancet*, 1967, *2*, 1310.

Effect on strontium absorption. The effectiveness of sodium alginate in selectively blocking the absorption of strontium (but not calcium) appeared to depend on its composition. Varieties with a high ratio of guluronic to mannuronic acids (G/M ratio) were found to be more effective in this respect. Tests showed that when an alginate with a G/M ratio of 97% was added to the diet in milk containing radioactive strontium-87m, it produced an average reduction of strontium in the plasma and urine of 83% and 87% respectively.— A. Sutton (letter), *Nature*, 1967, *216*, 1005. Similar reports.— J. Harrison *et al.*, *Can. med. Ass. J.*, 1966, *95*, 532; J. T. Triffitt (letter), *Nature*, 1968, *217*, 457.

Partially degraded alginates were more active in preventing the absorption of radioactive strontium given by mouth than unchanged sodium alginate. The degraded alginates formed relatively non-viscous solutions and were more easily administered.— Y. Tanaka *et al.*, *Can. med. Ass. J.*, 1968, *98*, 1179.

Suspending agent. The suspending properties of Alginate YZ 1% were studied in several *B.P.C.* mixtures. It was an effective suspending agent for paediatric sulphonamide mixtures but was less effective in chalk mixtures.— C. A. Farley and W. Lund, *Pharm. J.*, 1976, *1*, 562.

Tablet disintegrant. A calcium sodium alginate product, Alginate YZ, was found to be an effective tablet disintegrant, superior to Alginate P872 and a useful alternative to alginic acid. Unlike starch and Alginate P872, its disintegrant action was unaffected by the ingredients of the tablets. Dissolution tests on tablets incorporating Alginate YZ were considered to show that biological availability of the active ingredients would be satisfactory. The disintegration times of the tablets were increased when the alginate or alginic acid was incorporated inside the granules.— K. A. Khan and C. T. Rhodes, *Pharm. Acta Helv.*, 1972, *47*, 41.

The use of sodium alginate as a tablet binder and disintegrant in lactose tablets.— A. M. Sakr *et al.*, *Mfg Chem.*, 1972, *43* (Nov.), 38; *idem*, 1973, *44* (Jan.), 37.

Proprietary Preparations of Alginates

Alginate YZ (Formerly Alginate F417) *(Alginate Industries, UK)*. A tablet disintegrant containing sodium alginate 50% and calcium alginate 50%.

Manucol *(Alginate Industries, UK)*. Sodium alginate, available in a number of pharmaceutical grades. Alginic acid and calcium alginate are also available and are used as tablet disintegrants.

Manucol Ester *(Alginate Industries, UK)*. Propylene glycol alginate, available in several grades; a thickening, suspending and stabilising agent.

Estimated acceptable daily intake: up to 25 mg per kg body-weight.— Seventeenth Report of FAO/WHO Expert Committee on Food Additives, *Tech. Rep. Ser. Wld Hlth Org. No. 539*, 1974.

An evaluation of the toxicity of propylene glycol alginate in *animals*. It was found that only the propylene glycol moiety was absorbed and metabolised.— *Fd Add. Ser. Wld Hlth Org. No. 5*, 1974.

Manugel *(Alginate Industries, UK)*. Sodium alginate, available in a number of pharmaceutical grades, standardised for gel strength.

Manutex *(Alginate Industries, UK)*. Sodium alginate, available in several technical grades; stated to be suitable for use in external pharmaceutical preparations and cosmetics.

Ultraplast *(Wallace, Cameron, UK)*. A range of haemostatic dressings containing sodium and calcium alginates, available as **Dressings** and **Dressing Strips**, and as **Styptic Gauze**.

Ultrastat *(Wallace, Cameron, UK)*. A haemostatic aerosol containing sodium alginate 7% and chlorhexidine hydrochloride 0.1%.

Other Proprietary Names of Alginates

Coalgan-Ouate, Stop Hemo, Trophiderm *(all calcium alginate)(all Fr.)*.

A range of dressings containing calcium and sodium alginates was formerly marketed in Great Britain under the proprietary name Calgitex (*Medical Alginates*, now *Roussel*). Triethanolamine alginate was formerly marketed in Great Britain under the proprietary name Collatex T/RE (*Alginate Industries*).

5460-y

Sodium Starch Glycollate *(B.P.)*. Sodium Starch Glycolate *(U.S.N.F.)*; Sodium Carboxymethyl Starch; Starch Sodium Glycollate.

CAS — 9063-38-1.

Pharmacopoeias. In *Br.* Also in *U.S.N.F.*

The sodium salt of a poly-α-glucopyranose in which some of the hydroxyl groups are in the form of the carboxymethyl ether. It contains 2.8 to 4.5% of sodium, calculated on the washed and dried material. It may contain not more than 10% of sodium chloride.

A very fine, odourless, tasteless, white or off-white, free-flowing powder. It loses not more than 10% of its weight on drying. A 2% **dispersion** in cold water settles, on standing, to give a highly hydrated layer; practically insoluble in alcohol and most organic solvents. A 2% dispersion in water has a pH of 5.5 to 7.5.

Sodium starch glycollate is used as a disintegrating agent in tablet manufacture, and has been suggested for use as a suspending agent for extemporaneous preparations.

An evaluation of sodium starch glycollate as a tablet disintegrant.— E. Mendell, *Pharm. Acta Helv.*, 1974, *49*, 248.

Sodium starch glycollate was evaluated as an alternative to tragacanth in the extemporaneous preparation of paediatric chalk and sulphadimidine mixtures. The sedimentation volumes, appearance, and ease of redispersibility after standing favoured sodium starch glycollate 1% over cellulose and various derivatives, aluminium magnesium silicate, tragacanth, alginates, colloidal silicon dioxide, and other modified starches.— Pharm. Soc. Lab. Rep. No. P/75/4, 1975. Except in aromatic chalk and opium mixture, sodium starch glycollate produced suspensions with better redispersibility than aluminium magnesium silicate and 2 pregelatinised starches (Instant Clearjel and Snowflake Speciality Starch), and all were better than tragacanth in *B.P.C.* mixtures.— *ibid.*, P/75/9, 1975.. See also *ibid.*, P/76/1, 1976.; *ibid.*, P/76/3, 1976.; C. A. Farley and W. Lund, *Pharm. J.*, 1976, *1*, 562. See also G. Smith and I. E. E. McIntosh (letter), *ibid.*, 1976, *2*, 42.

The rheological properties of dispersions of sodium starch glycollate 1%, tragacanth 0.2%, and compound tragacanth powder 1% were similar and the small changes in viscosity on storage were preferable to the large increases that occurred with aluminium magnesium silicate 2%.— Pharm. Soc. Lab. Rep. No. P/75/10, 1975.

In a study of water-sorption properties, sodium starch glycollate and a cation-exchange resin (Amberlite IRP88) were extremely efficient disintegrants in a variety of tablet systems when compared with starch and carmellose sodium.— K. A. Khan and C. T. Rhodes, *J. pharm. Sci.*, 1975, *64*, 447.

An evaluation of the disintegration and compressibility of tablets using sodium starch glycollate as a tablet excipient.— R. P. Bhatia *et al.*, *Drug Cosmet. Ind.*, 1978, *122* (Apr.), 38.

Proprietary Preparations

Explotab *(Mendell, USA: K & K-Greeff, UK)*. A brand of sodium starch glycollate.

5461-j

Sterculia *(B.P.)*. Sterculia Gum; Indian Tragacanth; Karaya; Karaya Gum; Goma Caraia.

CAS — 9000-36-6.

Pharmacopoeias. In *Br.* and *Fr.*

The gum obtained from *Sterculia urens* and other species of *Sterculia* (Sterculiaceae). It consists of a complex, high molecular weight, partially acetylated polysaccharide composed of D-galacturonic acid (about 43%), D-galactose, and L-rhamnose and containing not less than 14% of volatile acid, calculated as acetic acid.

Irregular or vermiform, greyish or pinkish pieces with an odour resembling that of acetic acid. **Powdered Sterculia** is a white or buff-coloured powder containing not less than 10% of volatile acid, as acetic acid. It loses not more than 20% of its weight on drying.

Sparingly **soluble** in water, in which it swells to a homogeneous, adhesive, gelatinous mass; practically insoluble in alcohol and chloroform. **Store** at a temperature not exceeding 25°; powdered sterculia should be stored in airtight containers.

In distilled water, iso-osmotic saline, sodium hydroxide solution, or dilute hydrochloric acid, 5 g of a preparation containing sterculia (Normacol Special granules) showed marked swelling compared with preparations of psyllium (Isogel granules) and methylcellulose (Celevac granules).— J. D. Ireson and G. B. Leslie, *Pharm. J.*, 1970, *2*, 540.

Adverse Effects and Precautions. As for Methylcellulose, p.947.

Severe oesophageal obstruction occurred in an 80-year-old woman who swallowed 2 large teaspoonfuls of Normacol Standard with a little water each night. Large quantities of Normacol were subsequently aspirated from the bronchus; the oesophagus was intensely inflamed and the lower two-thirds was completely obstructed by a very large plug of Normacol granules, not all of which could be removed. Instructions for the administration of hygroscopic laxatives should emphasise the importance of taking adequate quantities of water immediately with the preparation. It may be unwise to recommend taking such preparations before retiring, especially if the patient is elderly or debilitated.— D. R. Sandeman *et al.* (letter), *Lancet*, 1980, *1*, 364. A similar report.— O. Voinchet and A. Mouchet, *Nouv. Presse méd.*, 1974, *3*, 1223.

Uses. Sterculia is used as a bulk laxative, since by taking up moisture it increases the volume of the faeces and promotes peristalsis. It is also used for the control of diarrhoea. It has adhesive properties and is used in the fitting of ileostomy and colostomy appliances and in dental fixative powders. It has also been used similarly to tragacanth to prepare bases for medicated jellies but it is a less efficient suspending agent.

It is used in industry as a thickening and suspending agent in the manufacture of lotions and pastes.

The acceptable daily intake of sterculia in food could not be determined from the toxicological data available. Further information on viscosity range was also required.— Twenty-first Report of the Joint FAO/FAO Expert Committee on Food Additives, *Tech. Rep. Ser. Wld Hlth Org. No. 617*, 1978.

Constipation. In a blind study in 175 constipated nursing mothers, treatment with preparations containing sterculia (Normacol Special) and sterculia with frangula (Normacol Standard) gave better relief with a lower incidence of side-effects in both mothers and infants than preparations containing senna (Senokot) or docusate sodium with danthron (Normax). In a similar study in 175 antenatal patients no treatment was judged to be superior.— J. O. Greenhalf and H. S. D. Leonard, *Practitioner*, 1973, *210*, 259.

Diverticular disease. In a double-blind study 10 patients with diverticular disease who took a preparation containing sterculia with alverine citrate 0.5% obtained more effective relief of their symptoms than 10 patients who took a similar preparation containing sterculia alone. The preparation containing alverine citrate also compared more favourably with the effects of coarse bran and was suitable for the treatment of diverticular disease in patients unable to tolerate bran.— G. S. Srivastava *et al.*, *Br. med. J.*, 1976, *1*, 315.

Fitting of colostomy appliances. Sterculia was used as an adhesive for colostomy bags and had the advantage over adhesive plasters and cements of being soothing to the skin and less likely to produce soreness. Sterculia could harden if exposed to warmth or sunshine.— J. C. Goligher and M. Pollard, *The Care of Your Colostomy*, 2nd Edn, London, Baillière Tindall, 1973.

Fitting of ileostomy appliances. In the fitting of a one-piece ileostomy appliance with latex, sterculia powder could be used in preparing washers by 2 methods. A moist ring of lint completely dipped in sterculia powder could be fitted around the stoma after the powder had begun to form a gel, or alternatively sterculia paste could be built up in a thick layer for an area of 1.25 cm around the stoma and then allowed to set. After either method, latex would then be spread completely over the washer and right up the stoma. As an adhesive, sterculia powder could be used to apply the flange of an ileostomy bag by forming a gel on the flange and on the area to be covered by the flange, but the adhesion would not be adequate to support the bag without a suitable belt. Sterculia was used mainly to fill the space between stoma and flange when a two-piece appliance was fitted.— *A New Life for Those with a Permanent Ileostomy*, 2nd Edn, London, Ileostomy Association of Great Britain.. See also J. C. Goligher and M. A. Pollard, *The Care of your Ileostomy*, Leeds, University Dept. of Surgery, 1972.

Pressure sores. The application of powdered sterculia stimulated granulation and healing of resistant bed sores in 2 patients.— M. R. Sather *et al.*, *Drug Intell. & clin. Pharm.*, 1977, *11*, 162.

Proprietary Preparations

Inolaxine Granules *(Dales, UK: Farillon, UK)*. Contain sterculia 98%. (Also available as Inolaxine in *Fr.*).

Normacol Standard *(Norgine, UK)*. Granules containing sterculia 62% and frangula 8%. For constipation. **Normacol Standard Sugar Free Formula**. Contains the same active ingredients but is free from sugar. **Normacol Special**. Granules containing sterculia 62%. For constipation, diverticular disease, and for colostomy and ileostomy control. **Normacol Antispasmodic**. Granules containing sterculia 62% and alverine citrate 0.5%. For spastic and hypertonic constipation. **Normacol X**. A composite pack containing Normacol Special 40 g and 2 tablets of danthron 200 mg. For preparation for abdominal radiological examination. *Dose*. The usual dose of Normacol preparations is one or two 5-ml spoonfuls once or twice daily.

Prefil *(Norgine, UK)*. Granules containing sterculia 55% and guar gum 5%. For appetite suppression. *Dose*. Two 5-ml spoonfuls, placed on the tongue and swallowed with plenty of water, half to one hour before meals.

Saltair Karaya Gum Powder *(Salt, UK)*. A brand of powdered sterculia.

Tex *(Simpla, UK)*. A brand of powdered sterculia; for peristomal use in conjunction with Gel an aluminium oxide basis.

Other Proprietary Names

Decorpa *(*see also under Guar Gum*) (Belg., Fr., Ger.)*; Karagum *(Austral.)*; Normalax *(Swed.)*.

5462-z

Tamarind Polyose. A polysaccharide extracted from the seeds of the tamarind, *Tamarindus indica* (Leguminosae).

A pale yellow odourless powder. It is **dispersible** in hot water to form a colloidal solution.

Tamarind polyose has been used as a binding agent in tablets, as a suspending agent for insoluble powders, and as an emulsifying agent.

5463-c

Tragacanth *(B.P., Eur. P., U.S.N.F.)*. Trag.; Gum Dragon; Gum Tragacanth; Tragacantha; Gomme Adragante; Tragant; Tragacanto; Goma Alcatira.

CAS — 9000-65-1.

Pharmacopoeias. In *Arg., Aust., Belg., Br., Cz., Eur., Fr., Ger., Hung., It., Jap., Jug., Mex., Neth., Nord., Pol., Port., Roum., Span., Swiss*, and *Turk*. Also in *U.S.N.F.*

The dried gummy exudation flowing naturally or obtained by incision from the trunk and branches of *Astragalus gummifer* and some other Asiatic species of *Astragalus* (Leguminosae) containing a water soluble polysaccharide, tragacanthin, and an insoluble methylated polysaccharide, bassorin; it yields on hydrolysis D-galacturonic acid, D-galactose, L-fucose, D-xylose, and L-arabinose; it also contains about 15% of water, traces of starch and altered cell walls, and about 2 to 3% volatile acid as acetic acid.

It is known in commerce as Persian tragacanth and occurs as thin, flattened, irregularly oblong or more or less curved, ribbon-like, white or pale yellow, somewhat translucent, horny flakes which are odourless and almost tasteless. Some indication of its suspending properties may be obtained from the apparent viscosity of its mucilage; commercial samples vary considerably in this property. **Powdered Tragacanth** is a white or yellowish-white colourless powder.

Sparingly **soluble** in water, in which it swells to a homogeneous, adhesive, gelatinous mass; practically insoluble in alcohol. A 1% solution has a viscosity of not less than 250 centipoises. Tragacanth gels may be **sterilised** by autoclaving. **Store** in airtight containers.

It is liable to microbial contamination with *Enterobacter* spp. and stock solutions should contain a suitable antimicrobial preservative. The use of dry heat or irradiation to reduce contamination may seriously impair the suspending properties of tragacanth. A suitable quality may, however, be achieved by gassing with ethylene oxide or slurrying with alcohol-water mixtures under appropriate conditions.

Hog gum, from species of *Prunus*, and sterculia gum are used in industry as substitutes for tragacanth.

Some samples of tragacanth responded to the test for peroxidases in the *B.P.* monograph for acacia and had been rejected. It was shown that the activity of peroxidase in tragacanth roughly paralleled the amount of starch, and was inversely proportional to the apparent viscosity of mucilages. This might reflect the conversion, in the plant, of starch to gum, and would explain why the finest grades with high viscosity contained no peroxidase or starch.— J. W. Fairbairn (letter), *J. Pharm. Pharmac.*, 1967, *19*, 191.

The physical properties of powders and gels of tragacanth of Turkish origin.— A. S. Geçgil *et al.*, *Planta med.*, 1975, *27*, 284.

Preservation of tragacanth jellies. The antibacterial action of chlorbutol, benzalkonium chloride, phenol, phenylmercuric acetate, thiomersal, and alkyl hydroxybenzoates was reduced in the presence of tragacanth.— P. C. Eisman, *J. Am. pharm. Ass., scient. Edn*, 1957, *46*, 144.

The most effective preservative at pH 7 or below was a mixture of methyl hydroxybenzoate 0.2% and propyl hydroxybenzoate 0.05%. Benzoic acid was ineffective; chlorbutol was effective against bacteria but not against fungi.— A. Taub *et al.*, *J. Am. pharm. Ass., scient. Edn*, 1958, *47*, 235. Jars of tragacanth gel containing lignocaine hydrochloride and preserved with methyl hydroxybenzoate 0.2% were found to be heavily contaminated with *Pseudomonas aeruginosa* after use. The gel was satisfactorily dispensed in small single-dose tubes.— I. Phillips, *Lancet*, 1966, *1*, 903.

Sterilisation. Gamma-irradiated samples of tragacanth mucilages were free from microbial contamination due to salmonellae and *Escherichia coli* but a pronounced decrease in viscosity occurred. It was suggested that minimal doses (1000 Gy) may be used to reduce the microbial load particularly if the initial contamination is not excessive.— G. P. Jacobs and R. Simes, *J. Pharm. Pharmac.*, 1979, *31*, 333.

Adverse Effects. Allergic reactions, sometimes severe, have occurred rarely after the ingestion or inhalation of tragacanth. Contact dermatitis has been reported following the external use of tragacanth.

Contact dermatitis in a 4-year-old boy, at the sites of ECG electrodes, was due to tragacanth in the electrode jelly.— R. J. Coskey, *Archs Derm.*, 1977, *113*, 839.

Three renal transplant recipients found to be hypersensitive to prednisone tablets had reacted to the tragacanth and acacia used in their manufacture. Their symptoms subsided when a formulation using methylcellulose was substituted.— D. Rubinger *et al.* (letter), *Lancet*, 1978, *2*, 689.

An immediate life-threatening allergic reaction in a 35-year-old woman was attributed to the tragacanth which was present in the beefburger she was eating.— D. Danoff *et al.* (letter), *New Engl. J. Med.*, 1978, *298*, 1095.

Uses. Tragacanth forms viscous solutions or gels with water, depending on the concentration. In dispensing aqueous preparations of tragacanth, the powdered tragacanth is first dispersed in a distributing agent, such as alcohol, essential oil, or glycerol, to prevent agglomeration on the addition of water.

Tragacanth, in the form of Tragacanth Mucilage or Compound Tragacanth Powder, is widely used to suspend heavy insoluble powders and sometimes with acacia to suspend many resinous tinctures. In lotions for external use tragacanth is preferable to acacia as a suspending agent. Tragacanth is added to emulsions prepared with acacia, in order to retard creaming, and is used as a thickening agent in the manufacture of creams, jellies, and pastes.

Bassorin Paste (Linimentum Exsiccans) is prepared by shaking vigorously in a wide-mouthed bottle 5% of tragacanth powder, 10% of alcohol, and 70% of water, and then adding 2% of glycerol, and water to 100%; it dries on the skin as a transparent film, easily removed by washing. It has been used as a basis for medicaments such as ichthammol, salicylic acid, resorcinol, and sulphur. Tragacanth is also used as the basis of lubricants for catheters and surgical instruments but such preparations must be sterilised as microbial contamination of tragacanth is common. It is also used in powder form as an adhesive for dentures.

Tragacanth (up to 5%) has been used as a excipient for pills and tablets containing no binding ingredient and in lozenges for its demulcent properties. It has also been used as a bulk laxative.

An acceptable daily intake of tragacanth in food could not be determined although additional toxicological data was available. Tragacanth was reported to affect hepatic metabolism in the *rat*.— Twenty-first Report of the Joint FAO/WHO Expert Committee on Food Additives, *Tech. Rep. Ser. Wld Hlth Org. No. 617*, 1978.

Metabolic effects. For the effect of tragacanth on postprandial blood-glucose concentrations, see D. J. A. Jenkins, *Br. med. J.*, 1978, *1*, 1392.

Paraffin emulsions. The rate of creaming was used to compare the stability of emulsions and it was found that tragacanth did not improve the stability of liquid paraffin-acacia emulsions even though the viscosity of the emulsion was increased.— R. A. Anderson and M. J. Woollard, *Australas. J. Pharm.*, 1962, *43*, 213.

Suspending agents. An evaluation of alternative suspending agents to tragacanth in the preparation of *B.P.C.* mixtures.— C. A. Farley and W. Lund, *Pharm. J.*, 1976, *1*, 562.

Preparations

Compound Tragacanth Paste *(B.P.C. 1954)*. Past. Trag. Co.; Catheter Lubricant; Lubricating Jelly. Tragacanth 2.29 g, glycerol 20 ml, alcohol 2.5 ml, phenylmercuric nitrate 11.4 mg, water to 100 ml. It is sterilised by maintaining the whole of the paste at a temperature of 98° to 100° for 30 minutes.

Compound Tragacanth Powder *(B.P.)*. Co. Trag. Pdr.; Pulvis Tragacanthae Compositus; Pulv. Trag. Co.; Tragacanth Powder Compound *(A.P.F.)*. Tragacanth 15, acacia 20, starch 20, and sucrose 45. Store in airtight containers.

It is used as a suspending agent for insoluble powders.

Hydroxybenzoate Gel *(A.P.F.)*. Catheter Lubricant; Surgical Lubricant. Propyl hydroxybenzoate 30 mg, methyl hydroxybenzoate 70 mg, tragacanth 3 g, glycerol 25 ml, water to 100 g. Sterilised by autoclaving. Lignocaine hydrochloride 2% or cyclomethycaine sulphate 0.75% may be added if required.

Phenylmercuric Nitrate Gel *(A.P.F.)*. Phenylmercuric Nitrate Glycanth. Phenylmercuric nitrate 10 mg, tragacanth 2.5 g, glycerol 25 ml, water to 100 g. Sterilised by maintaining at 98° to 100° for 30 minutes.

Tragacanth Mucilage *(B.P.C. 1973)*. Trag. Mucil. Tragacanth 1.25 g, alcohol (90%) 2.5 ml, chloroform water to 100 ml.

A.P.F. has a similar preparation with benzoic acid 100 mg added.

Port. P. and *Span. P.* have 10% w/w in water. *Arg. P.* has 5% w/w in chloroform water. *Dan. Disp.* has 1% with methyl hydroxybenzoate 0.2% in water, both w/w.

The maximum viscosity of tragacanth mucilage was obtained at pH 5, and raising or lowering the pH resulted in reduction of viscosity, e.g. the addition of benzoic acid as a preservative lowered the viscosity through the reduction in pH bringing about a degradation of the gum. Citrates also reduced the viscosity, probably through the formation of a complex with the calcium naturally present in tragacanth.— T. W. Schwarz *et al.*, *J. Am. pharm. Ass., scient. Edn*, 1958, *47*, 695.

5464-k

Verbascum Flowers. Mullein Flowers; Bouillon Blanc; Wollblumen.

Pharmacopoeias. In *Aust.*, *Belg.*, *Cz.*, *Fr.*, *Hung.*, and *Swiss.*

The dried corollas with adhering stamens of *Verbascum thapsiforme*, *V. phlomoides*, or *V. thapsus* (Scrophulariaceae).

Verbascum flowers have been extensively used in Europe in pulmonary complaints, usually as an infusion, often in conjunction with other herbs. It is doubtful whether they have any therapeutic value other than that of a demulcent.

Verbascum leaves have been similarly employed, usually as a liquid extract.

5465-a

Xanthan Gum *(U.S.N.F.)*. Corn Sugar Gum; Polysaccharide B 1459; Xantham Gum.

CAS — 11138-66-2.

Pharmacopoeias. In *U.S.N.F.*

A gum produced by a pure-culture fermentation of a carbohydrate with *Xanthomonas campestris* and purified. It is the sodium, potassium, or calcium salt of a high molecular weight partially acetylated polysaccharide containing D-glucose, D-mannose, and D-glucuronic acid units. It also contains not less than 1.5% of pyruvic acid.

A cream-coloured powder. It loses not more than 15% of its weight on drying. **Soluble** in hot and cold water. A solution in water is neutral to litmus. A 1% solution has a viscosity, at 24°, of not less than 600 centipoises.

Adverse Effects.

For background toxicological information, see *Fd Add. Ser. Wld Hlth Org. No. 6*, 1975.

Uses. Xanthan gum is used as a stabiliser, thickener, and emulsifier in the cosmetic and food industry.

Estimated acceptable daily intake: up to 10 mg per kg body-weight.— Eighteenth Report of the Joint FAO/WHO Expert Committee on Food Additives, *Tech. Rep. Ser. Wld Hlth Org. No. 557*, 1974.

Paraffin emulsions. When used to prepare 40% liquid paraffin emulsions, the optimum concentration of xanthan gum was 0.4 to 0.5% and there was no creaming of the emulsions after 6 months' storage. The emulsions were not thixotropic but could be poured from a bottle when shaken. A non-tacky film was left when the emulsions were applied to the skin. Comparable acacia emulsions required at least 25% acacia to prevent creaming in 6 months' storage.— O. E. Araujo, *J. pharm. Sci.*, 1967, *56*, 1141.

Suspending agent. A mucilage of xanthan gum 0.5 or 0.75% was a better suspending agent than tragacanth mucilage in compound lobelia and stramonium mixture. Xanthan gum mucilage was more difficult to prepare extemporaneously.— Pharm. Soc. Lab. Rep. P/77/5, 1977.

Metoclopramide and some other Anti-emetics

6540-r

Included in this section are some miscellaneous compounds used to treat or prevent nausea and vomiting.

6541-f

Metoclopramide Hydrochloride *(B.P.)*.

AHR-3070-C; MK 745. 4-Amino-5-chloro-*N*-(2-diethylaminoethyl)-2-methoxybenzamide hydrochloride monohydrate.
$C_{14}H_{22}ClN_3O_2,HCl,H_2O=354.3$.

CAS — 364-62-5 (metoclopramide); 7232-21-5 (hydrochloride, anhydrous); 54143-57-6 (hydrochloride, monohydrate).

Pharmacopoeias. In *Br. Chin.* includes metoclopramide. *Roum.* includes anhydrous metoclopramide hydrochloride.

A white or almost white, odourless or almost odourless, crystalline powder. M.p. about 185°. **Soluble** 1 in 0.7 of water, 1 in 3 of alcohol, and 1 in 55 of chloroform; practically insoluble in ether. A 10% solution in water has a pH of 4.5 to 6.5. **Protect** from light.

Some early work on the visual compatibility of metoclopramide hydrochloride with a number of individual drugs normally used pre- or postoperatively. Chemical stability had not been studied.— W. A. Parker and C. A. Shearer (letter), *Can. J. Hosp. Pharm.*, 1979, *32*, 38.

Adverse Effects. Metoclopramide may cause extrapyramidal reactions, especially in young patients. Although these reactions may occur following single doses or at therapeutic doses it has been considered that the risk may be reduced by keeping the daily dose below 500 µg per kg body-weight daily.

Other adverse effects include bowel upsets, drowsiness and fatigue, dizziness, restlessness, and anxiety. Galactorrhoea and gynaecomastia have been reported.

Hypertensive crises have occurred in patients with phaeochromocytomas given metoclopramide.

In a literature survey of reports on 1023 patients and a general practitioner survey in 788 patients, the incidence of side-effects was: drowsiness or lassitude 4% and 9.8% respectively; bowel disturbance 1.2% and 1.1%; extrapyramidal effects 1% and nil; dizziness or faintness 0.8% in both; and other effects 4.3% and nil.— O. P. W. Robinson, *Postgrad. med. J.*, 1973, *49* (July), *Suppl.* 4, 77.

Galactorrhoea occurring in a 41-year-old woman who had taken metoclopramide for about 4 months, ceased within 7 days when the drug was withdrawn.— W. A. Finnis *et al.* (letter), *Can. med. Ass. J.*, 1976, *115*, 845.

Cardiovascular effects. A hypertensive crisis followed the administration of metoclopramide in a patient with phaeochromocytoma.— P. F. Plouin *et al.* (letter), *Lancet*, 1976, *2*, 1357. Metoclopramide 10 mg by intravenous injection produced a striking and rapid increase in blood pressure in 2 patients with phaeochromocytoma and was associated with an increase in plasma-catecholamine concentration. These changes were not observed in 1 healthy subject, in 1 patient with moderate essential hypertension, and in another patient with renovascular hypertension.— E. Agabiti-Rosei *et al.* (letter), *ibid.*, 1977, *1*, 600.

Hypotension occurred in 4 patients undergoing surgery for repair of a ruptured intracranial aneurysm following intravenous administration of metoclopramide as an anti-emetic.— G. R. Park (letter), *Br. J. Anaesth.*, 1978, *50*, 1268.

Further references: M. Shaklai *et al.* (letter), *Br. med. J.*, 1974, *2*, 385 (multifocal supraventricular extrasystoles); H. J. Schulze and J. W. Winkler, *Dte Gesundh-Wes.*, 1978, *33*, 131 (bradycardia), per *Int. pharm. Abstr.*, 1978, *15*, 1018.

Extrapyramidal effects. Seven children with dystonic reactions due to a variety of drugs including metoclopramide had a greatly reduced urinary excretion of D-glucaric acid.— C. Cassimos *et al.*, *J. Pediat.*, 1975, *87*, 981, per *Int. pharm. Abstr.*, 1977, *14*, 782.

Hypertonia and opisthotonos in 1 child and hypertonia and oculogyric crisis in a second after taking metoclopramide; in the first case the dose was only slightly in excess of that recommended.— J. A. Sills and E. J. Glass (letter), *Br. med. J.*, 1978, *2*, 431.

Dystonic reactions occurring in 2 related children following the administration of therapeutic doses of metoclopramide.— A. R. Gatrad and A. H. Gatrad, *Br. J. clin. Pract.*, 1979, *33*, 111.

Fever in 2 patients associated with dystonic reactions to metoclopramide.— I. Wandless *et al.* (letter), *Lancet*, 1980, *1*, 1255.

Ten children experienced dystonic reactions with metoclopramide; daily doses ranged from 0.9 to 1.9 mg per kg body-weight daily. Five children accidentally poisoned with 50 to 100 mg of metoclopramide, representing 3.3 to 8.3 mg per kg, are reported; one developed slight extrapyramidal signs.— L. C. K. Low and K. M. Goel, *Archs Dis. Childh.*, 1980, *55*, 310.

Further references: M. C. Daele *et al.*, *Archs Dis. Childh.*, 1970, *45*, 130; P. S. Venkateswaran and A. G. Otto (letter), *Br. med. J.*, 1972, *4*, 178; S. M. Carter (letter), *Br. med. J.*, 1973, *4*, 491; K. L. De Silva *et al.*, *Practitioner*, 1973, *211*, 316; D. L. Cochlin, *Br. J. clin. Pract.*, 1974, *28*, 201; S. Melmed and H. Bank (letter), *Br. med. J.*, 1975, *1*, 331; C. H. Walsh (letter), *ibid.*, 737; T. K. Daneshmend and A. P. Manning, *Br. J. clin. Pract.*, 1978, *32*, 334; P. G. Reasbeck and A. Hossenbocus, *ibid.*, 1979, *33*, 31; G. U. Corsini *et al.* (letter), *Lancet*, 1979, *1*, 1344.

Tardive dyskinesia. A middle-aged man who had taken metoclopramide 80 mg daily for 4 years developed severe persistent facial dyskinesia (identical to the syndrome of tardive dyskinesia) when treatment suddenly ceased; symptoms were largely relieved by metoclopramide 30 mg daily but recurred when metoclopramide was withdrawn.— S. Lavy *et al.*, *Br. med. J.*, 1978, *1*, 77.

Extrapyramidal effects and tardive dyskinesia developed in 3 patients receiving long-term metoclopramide therapy. The symptoms disappeared or improved on discontinuing metoclopramide.— M. Kataria *et al.* (letter), *Lancet*, 1978, *2*, 1254.

Porphyria. A report of porphyria induced by metoclopramide in a young girl.— M. Doss *et al.* (letter), *Lancet*, 1981, *2*, 91.

Treatment of Adverse Effects. The treatment of extrapyramidal reactions is discussed under Chlorpromazine, p.1511.

Precautions. Metoclopramide should not be used where gastro-intestinal conditions might be adversely affected as in intestinal obstruction or immediately after surgery. There have been reports of hypertensive crises in patients with phaeochromocytoma given metoclopramide, thus its use is not recommended in such patients.

Children and young patients should be treated with care.

Care should also be exercised when using metoclopramide in patients taking other drugs that can also cause extrapyramidal reactions, such as the phenothiazines. Anticholinergic agents antagonise the effects of metoclopramide; narcotic analgesics may act similarly. Metoclopramide may affect the absorption of other drugs either by diminishing absorption from the stomach or by enhancing absorption from the small intestine. The effects of CNS depressants may be enhanced.

Metoclopramide given by mouth, intramuscularly, or intravenously caused a threefold to eightfold increase in circulating concentrations of prolactin.— A. S. McNeilly *et al.* (letter), *Br. med. J.*, 1974, *2*, 729. It would be unwise to give metoclopramide to patients with breast cancer, since some of these tumours were prolactin-dependent.— H. W. C. Ward (letter), *ibid.*, 1974, *3*, 169. Contrary views.— R. G. Wilson (letter), *ibid.*, 413; P. K. Bondy and T. J. Powles (letter), *ibid.*, 1974, *4*, 228.

Metoclopramide should not be used for symptomatic acute vomiting of unknown origin in small children.— A. Bloch (letter), *Br. med. J.*, 1978, *2*, 1092. A comment that the use of antidopaminergic drugs should be avoided in adolescents.— M. L. P. Gross (letter), *Lancet*, 1980, *2*, 479.

Administration in renal failure. A patient with renal impairment had developed metoclopramide-induced parkinsonism. Her plasma half-life for metoclopramide was grossly prolonged. Metoclopramide should be used with caution in patients with renal failure.— D. N. Bateman and D. S. Davies (letter), *Lancet*, 1979, *1*, 166. Similar findings had been reported in 7 patients.— A. Caralps (letter), *ibid.*, 554.

See also under Uses.

Pregnancy and the neonate. There had been no reported teratogenic effect following the use of metoclopramide during pregnancy where follow-up had been possible.— O. P. W. Robinson, *Postgrad. med. J.*, 1973, *49* (July), *Suppl.* 4, 80.

Absorption and Fate. Metoclopramide is rapidly absorbed from the gastro-intestinal tract and has been reported to undergo a high degree of first-pass hepatic metabolism. It is excreted in the urine as free and as conjugated metoclopramide and as metabolites. It is excreted in breast milk.

Following administration of metoclopramide 10 mg by mouth to 2 healthy subjects, about 78% of the dose was excreted in the urine in the first 24 hours. Blood concentrations of metoclopramide for 6 subjects who had received 10 mg reached a peak of about 40 ng per ml within the first 2 hours and the half-life of the drug for the period between 3 and 8 hours following the dosage was 4 hours. Administration of a 20-mg dose to 2 subjects indicated that the blood concentration was proportional to the dosage.— L. Teng *et al.*, *J. pharm. Sci.*, 1977, *66*, 1615.

The mean elimination half-life of metoclopramide in 7 healthy male subjects given 10 mg intravenously was about 166 minutes; plasma clearance was about 11 ml per minute per kg body-weight. Free and conjugated metoclopramide excreted in the urine over 36 hours in 3 of the subjects amounted to about 43% of the dose. Less than 20% was excreted unchanged. Gastric emptying was increased by metoclopramide 10 mg intravenously for at least 3 hours after injection.— D. N. Bateman *et al.*, *Br. J. clin. Pharmac.*, 1978, *6*, 401.

Samples of blood and expressed breast milk were taken from 10 patients who were breast-feeding their infants 2 hours after a dose of metoclopramide 10 mg. The mean plasma concentration of metoclopramide was 68.5 ng per ml while the mean concentration in breast milk was 125.7 ng per ml.— P. J. Lewis *et al.* (letter), *Br. J. clin. Pharmac.*, 1980, *9*, 217.

Further references: D. Schuppan *et al.*, *Arzneimittel-Forsch.*, 1979, *29*, 151; C. Graffner *et al.*, *Br. J. clin. Pharmac.*, 1979, *8*, 469; D. N. Bateman *et al.*, *ibid.*, 1980, *9*, 371.

Uses. Metoclopramide hydrochloride has central and anti-emetic properties as well as a positive effect on gastro-intestinal motility which appears to depend on the pre-existing tone of the gut. Some of its actions may be explained by a blockade of dopamine receptors and an increase in prolactin secretion.

Gastric peristalsis is increased leading to an increase in the gastric-emptying rate. Duodenal peristalsis may be increased which increases intestinal transit. The resting tone of the gastro-oesophageal sphincter is also increased.

Metoclopramide hydrochloride is used as an anti-emetic in the treatment of some forms of nausea and vomiting and to increase the gastro-intestinal motility. It is of little benefit in the prevention or treatment of motion sickness or in the treatment of nausea and vertigo due to Ménière's disease or other labyrinth disturbances. Metoclopramide hydrochloride may ease intubation procedures and speed up radiographic examinations. Conflicting results have been achieved in gastro-oesophageal reflux. There may be some benefit in migraine. Lactation may be improved.

It is usually administered by mouth in a dose equivalent to 10 mg of anhydrous metoclopramide hydrochloride thrice daily but may also be given by intramuscular or slow intravenous injection in the same dosage. The total daily dosage should not usually exceed 500 µg per kg body-weight.

Reviews of the actions and uses of metoclopramide: J. J. Misiewicz, *Gut*, 1973, *14*, 243; *Postgrad. med. J.*, 1973, *49* (July), *Suppl.* 4, 9–107; R. M. Pinder *et al.*, *Drugs*, 1976, *12*, 81; *Drug & Ther. Bull.*, 1976, *14*, 82; W. S. Nimmo, *Prescribers' J.*, 1977, *17*, 90; K. Schulze-Delrieu, *Gastroenterology*, 1979, *77*, 768; M. A. Smith and F. J. Salter, *Drug Intell. & clin. Pharm.*, 1980, *14*, 169; K. Schulze-Delrieu, *New Engl. J. Med.*, 1981, *305*, 28.

A comment that metoclopramide is a D_2 receptor antagonist.— P. Jenner and C. D. Marsden (letter), *Lancet*, 1979, *2*, 900.

Adjunct to X-ray examination. Studies in 125 patients showed that the transit time of barium to pass through the small intestine was 55 minutes in patients given metoclopramide and 163 minutes in patients given placebo. Examinations of the small bowel could be made in a shorter time when metoclopramide was used.— F. H. Howarth *et al.*, *Gut*, 1967, *8*, 628. See also W. B. James and A. G. Melrose, *Clin. Radiol.*, 1969, *20*, 57, per *Abstr. Wld Med.*, 1969, *43*, 711.

Administration in renal failure. A study of the pharmacokinetics of metoclopramide 10 mg by mouth and intravenously in 6 patients with chronic renal failure, 2 of whom were anephric. In addition to the reduced or non-existent renal clearance, total body clearance was also found to be substantially reduced in comparison with 7 subjects with normal renal function, and the terminal half-life was prolonged to about 14 hours. This suggests that the dose of metoclopramide in patients with renal failure should be reduced by at least 60% of that normally prescribed.— D. N. Bateman and R. Gokal (letter), *Lancet*, 1980, *1*, 982.

Diabetes mellitus. Uncontrolled diabetes mellitus in one patient due to gastroparesis diabeticorum: successful treatment with metoclopramide 10 mg before meals.— E. E. Muls and G. F. Lamberigts, *Postgrad. med. J.*, 1981, *57*, 185. See also G. F. Longstreth *et al.* (letter), *Ann. intern. Med.*, 1977, *86*, 195.

Diagnosis of pituitary adenomas. In 14 infertile women with hyperprolactinaemia the impaired prolactin responses to stimulation with protirelin 200 µg intravenously or metoclopramide 10 mg intravenously were reliable and clinically useful aids to diagnosis. Suppression tests using levodopa or bromocriptine were less reliable.— E. A. Cowden *et al.*, *Lancet*, 1979, *1*, 1155.

Dyspepsia. In a double-blind crossover trial 42 patients with flatulent dyspepsia received either metoclopramide 10 mg thrice daily or a placebo, each for 2 weeks. Metoclopramide was given before or after meals according to the timing of the symptoms. Significantly more patients preferred metoclopramide to placebo, and all symptoms were equally affected when improvement occurred.— A. G. Johnson, *Br. med. J.*, 1971, *2*, 25. See also *idem*, *Gut*, 1971, *12*, 421.

In a multicentre study, Maxolon 10 mg given every 8 hours was more effective than Asilone gel given before meals and at bedtime or Magnesium Trisilicate Mixture given after meals and at bedtime in the treatment of 69 patients with recurrent dyspepsia; patients received each treatment for 4 weeks.— D. J. W. de Almeida *et al.*, *Practitioner*, 1980, *224*, 105.

Gastric and duodenal ulcers. Metoclopramide was considered to be similar to carbenoxolone sodium in the treatment of gastric ulcer.— E. O. L. Hoskins, *Postgrad. med. J.*, 1973, *49*, *Suppl.* 4, 95. No benefit in acute exacerbations of duodenal ulceration.— M. G. Moshal, *ibid.*, 100.

In a double-blind randomised study in 48 patients with gastric ulcers who received either metoclopramide 10 mg thrice daily and at night or placebo for 4 to 8 weeks there was no significant difference in the numbers of healed gastric ulcers or rate of healing between the 2 groups. Twenty-four patients derived from both of these groups whose ulcers had healed then received a single maintenance dose of metoclopramide or placebo at night for a further 45 weeks. Two patients of the 9 who received metoclopramide and 7 of 15 who received placebo had a recurrence of ulcers. It was considered that metoclopramide might reduce recurrence of gastric ulcer.— A. G. Johnson *et al.*, *Clin. Trials J.*, 1977, *14*, (1), 3.

Gastro-oesophageal reflux. In 40 patients with gastro-oesophageal reflux or hiatus hernia, the intravenous injection of metoclopramide 10 mg caused no reduction in the degree of reflux within 5 to 10 minutes. Metoclopramide was unlikely to benefit patients with reflux oesophagitis.— J. N. Glanville and W. D. Walls, *Gut*, 1972, *13*, 31.

No gastro-oesophageal reflux was noted in 6 of 16 patients given a bolus injection of metoclopramide, and the number of movements causing reflux was diminished in the remainder.— C. Stanciu and J. R. Bennett, *Gut*, 1973, *14*, 275.

In a double-blind controlled trial in 31 patients with gastro-oesophageal reflux, metoclopramide was no more effective than placebo.— A. Paull and A. K. Grant, *Med. J. Aust.*, 1974, *2*, 627.

Doses higher than 10 mg normally used might be required for treating symptomatic gastro-oesophageal reflux secondary to lower oesophageal sphincter incompetence.— S. Cohen *et al.*, *Gastroenterology*, 1976, *70*, 484, per *Int. pharm. Abstr.*, 1976, *13*, 1031.

In a double-blind crossover study involving 18 patients with symptomatic gastro-oesophageal reflux and a subsequent 13 who crossed over only in the absence of considerable improvement in the initial treatment period, metoclopramide 10 mg 15 minutes before meals and 30 minutes before bedtime gave significantly more symptomatic improvement than placebo. Five patients in the metoclopramide group obtained 90% or more reduction in symptoms compared with none in the placebo group although the mean antacid intake remained the same for both groups. Side-effects of metoclopramide included marked nervousness and anxiety in 1 patient requiring withdrawal of therapy, nervousness in 2 and lethargy in 1 requiring dosage reduction, and gynaecomastia in 1.— R. W. McCallum *et al.*, *New Engl. J. Med.*, 1977, *296*, 354. See also *idem*, *Gastroenterology*, 1975, *68*, 1114.

Hiccup. For details of a protocol for the control of hiccups which involves the use of metoclopramide, see Chlorpromazine Hydrochloride, p.1515.

Hypotension. Severe orthostatic hypotension associated with a dopamine excess improved in one patient given metoclopramide 10 mg thrice daily for 5 days.— O. Kuchel *et al.*, *Ann. intern. Med.*, 1980, *93*, 841. Hypotension following metoclopramide injection.— M. S. Pegg (letter), *Anaesthesia*, 1980, *35*, 615.

See also under Adverse Effects, above.

Intubation, duodenal. A dose of 10 mg of metoclopramide given by intramuscular or intravenous injection facilitated the passage of a tube into the duodenum; hormonal stimulation of pancreatic secretion was not affected.— A. Delcourt and P. Wettendorff, *Gut*, 1968, *9*, 252. See also T. D. Bolin, *Med. J. Aust.*, 1969, *1*, 1078.

Endoscopy could be carried out successfully in patients with gastro-intestinal haemorrhage by giving diazepam as premedication and metoclopramide 10 mg intravenously. Up to 30 mg of metoclopramide in three doses was sometimes necessary to empty the stomach.— E. Bader (letter), *Lancet*, 1973, *1*, 101.

Lactation. See below under Pregnancy and the Neonate.

Migraine. A double-blind study of 50 patients with classical migraine indicated that metoclopramide had a beneficial effect in the treatment of migraine.— S. G. F. Matts, *Practitioner*, 1974, *212*, 887. See also *idem*, *Br. J. clin. Pract.*, 1972, *26*, 361; J. B. Hughes (letter), *Med. J. Aust.*, 1977, *2*, 580.

Metoclopramide was used in migraine because of its anti-emetic action and its effect on increasing the absorption of some other drugs.— M. Wilkinson, *Prescribers' J.*, 1980, *20*, 57.

Criticism of the use of metoclopramide analgesic combinations for migraine. It is doubtful if 5 to 10 mg of metoclopramide by mouth would reverse the delayed gastric empyting and hence absorption that occurs in migraine. There could be some antinauseant effect in patients without gastric stasis.— *Drug & Ther. Bull.*, 1980, *18*, 95.

Nausea and vomiting. Metoclopramide, 150 and 300 µg per kg body-weight intramuscularly or 20 mg by mouth or rectally as a suppository, had a significant anti-emetic action against apomorphine-induced vomiting. Its effects lasted 12 hours or more and were equal to those of prochlorperazine and superior to those of trimethobenzamide in effectiveness and duration of action.— R. L. Klein *et al.*, *Anesth. Analg. curr. Res.*, 1968, *47*, 259, per *Abstr. Wld Med.*, 1969, *43*, 89.

In a double-blind trial in women undergoing gynaecological laparotomies, there was less nausea, retching, and vomiting in 95 treated postoperatively with metoclopramide 10 mg intramuscularly than in 93 treated with perphenazine 5 mg.— B. Lind and H. Brevik, *Br. J. Anaesth.*, 1970, *42*, 614. Similar results with perphenazine and metoclopramide.— A. J. Handley, *Br. J. clin. Pract.*, 1967, *21*, 460.

Metoclopramide might be used as an anti-emetic in patients with parkinsonism without deterioration in function.— D. N. Bateman *et al.*, *Clin. Pharmac. Ther.*, 1978, *24*, 459.

Patients suffering from nausea or vomiting induced by cancer chemotherapy obtain no relief from metoclopramide.— W. S. Nimmo, *Prescribers' J.*, 1977, *17*, 90.

Metoclopramide given in large doses of 2 mg per kg body-weight by intravenous infusion with cisplatin significantly reduced the episodes of vomiting associated with cisplatin and decreased the volume of vomitus when compared with a placebo or with prochlorperazine 10 mg given intramuscularly in a controlled study involving 41 patients. The total dose of metoclopramide was 10 mg per kg given in 5 doses, each dose being given in 50 ml of sodium chloride injection and infused over 15 minutes.— R. J. Gralla *et al.*, *New Engl. J. Med.*, 1981, *305*, 905.

See also below under Pregnancy and the Neonate, Premedication, and Radiation Sickness.

For reports of domperidone being more effective as an anti-emetic than metoclopramide, see p.967.

Pregnancy and the neonate. In a study in 25 women in labour, metoclopramide 10 mg intramuscularly significantly increased the rate of gastric emptying, compared with a placebo, after a 750-ml test meal. There was no adverse effect on the foetus. The routine use of metoclopramide before emergency anaesthesia could reduce morbidity due to the aspiration of vomitus.— F. A. Howard and D. S. Sharp, *Br. med. J.*, 1973, *1*, 446.

Metoclopramide in a dose of 200 µg per kg body-weight did not promote gastric emptying in 15 low-birthweight babies.— I. Blumenthal and C. Costalos, *Br. J. clin. Pharmac.*, 1977, *4*, 207.

Lactation. Metoclopramide in doses of 10 mg or 15 mg thrice daily increased serum-prolactin concentrations and the quantity of breast milk whereas a dose of 5 mg thrice daily did not. The study involved 37 women with inadequate lactation and was placebo-controlled. Nine of the 27 mothers taking the effective doses were able to stop supplementary infant feeding. One child of a mother taking 45 mg had some intestinal discomfort.— A. Kauppila *et al.*, *Lancet*, 1981, *1*, 1175.

Further references: P. L. R. Sousa (letter), *Br. med. J.*, 1975, *1*, 512; P. J. Lewis *et al.* (letter), *Br. J. clin. Pharmac.*, 1980, *9*, 217.

Premedication. Metoclopramide 10 or 20 mg given with pethidine or morphine pre-operatively reduced the incidence of postoperative nausea and vomiting. When metoclopramide was given postoperatively it reduced the emetic effects of pethidine but not morphine.— R. A. E. Assaf *et al.*, *Br. J. Anaesth.*, 1974, *46*, 514.

Metoclopramide 10 and 20 mg was administered intramuscularly to 100 patients for premedication. Apart from restlessness there were no troublesome effects, but diazepam 10 mg produced a better response.— J. W. Dundee *et al.*, *Br. J. Anaesth.*, 1974, *46*, 509.

Psychosis. A report of *animal* studies indicating that metoclopramide can induce behavioural and biochemical supersensitivity. In schizophrenic in-patients metoclopramide in very large doses of up to 1 g daily was an effective antipsychotic agent; in some of the patients it induced extrapyramidal side-effects similar to those typically noted with standard neuroleptics.— M. Stanley *et al.* (letter), *Lancet*, 1979, *2*, 1190.

Radiation sickness. In a double-blind study radiation sickness was relieved in 20 of 38 patients with established sickness by treatment with metoclopramide 10 mg thrice daily, and in 23 of 38 patients by treatment with prochlorperazine 10 mg thrice daily.— H. W. C. Ward (letter), *Br. med. J.*, 1973, *2*, 52.

Preparations

Metoclopramide Injection *(B.P.)*. A sterile solution of metoclopramide hydrochloride in Water for Injections free from dissolved air; it contains suitable stabilising and buffering agents. Sterilised by autoclaving. pH 3 to 5. Potency is expressed in terms of the equivalent amount of anhydrous metoclopramide hydrochloride. Protect from light.

Metoclopramide Tablets *(B.P.)*. Tablets containing metoclopramide hydrochloride. Potency is expressed in terms of the equivalent amount of anhydrous metoclopramide hydrochloride. Protect from light.

Proprietary Preparations

Maxolon *(Beecham Research, UK)*. Metoclopramide hydrochloride, available as 2-ml **Ampoules** of an injection containing the equivalent of 5 mg of anhydrous metoclopramide hydrochloride per ml; as **Paediatric Liquid** containing the equivalent of 1 mg of anhydrous metoclopramide hydrochloride in each ml (suggested diluent, water); as **Syrup** containing the equivalent of 5 mg of anhydrous metoclopramide hydrochloride in each 5 ml (suggested diluent, water); and as scored **Tablets** each containing the equivalent of 10 mg of anhydrous metoclopramide hydrochloride. (Also available as Maxolon in *Austral., S.Afr.*).

Primperan *(Berk Pharmaceuticals, UK)*. Metoclopramide hydrochloride, available as 2-ml **Ampoules** of an injection containing the equivalent of 5 mg of anhydrous metoclopramide hydrochloride per ml; as **Syrup** containing the equivalent of 5 mg of anhydrous metoclopramide hydrochloride in each 5 ml (suggested diluent, syrup); and as scored **Tablets** each containing the equivalent of 10 mg of anhydrous metoclopramide hydrochloride. (Also available as Primperan in *Austral., Belg., Denm., Fr. (also as dihydrochloride), Neth., Norw., S.Afr., Spain, Switz.)*.

Other Proprietary Names

Arg.— Imperan *(as dihydrochloride)*, Netaf, Plasil, Primperil *(as dihydrochloride)*, Reliveran; *Austral.*— Metamide; *Canad.*— Maxeran, Reglan; *Denm.*— Emperal; *Ger.*— Paspertin; *Ital.*— Ananda, Clodil-ion, Clopan, Digetres, Metocobil, Placitril, Plasil, Regastrol, Viscal *(as dihydrochloride) Jap.*— Donopon-GP, Metoclol, Moriperan, Peraprin, Pramiel; *Spain*— Metagliz *(as glycyrrhizinate)*, Ulcofar *(as acetylglycyrrhizinate)*; *Switz.*— Paspertin; *USA*— Reglan.

Proprietary preparations containing metoclopramide and paracetamol (Paramax) or aspirin (Migravess) are included under Paracetamol and Aspirin, respectively.

6542-d

Benzquinamide Hydrochloride. P 2647 *(benzquinamide)*. 3-Diethylcarbamoyl-1,3,4,6,7,11b-hexahydro-9,10-dimethoxy-2*H*-benzo[*a*]quinolizin-2-yl acetate hydrochloride.

$C_{22}H_{32}N_2O_5,HCl=441.0$.

CAS — 63-12-7 (benzquinamide); 113-69-9 (hydrochloride).

Adverse Effects. The most common side-effect associated with benzquinamide is drowsiness. Other side-effects reported include allergy, dry mouth, shivering, sweating, hiccups, flushing, salivation, blurred vision, hypertension and hypotension, cardiac arrhythmias, headache, nervousness, and insomnia. Acute dystonic reactions have occasionally occurred.

Extrapyramidal effects. An acute dystonic reaction occurred in a 30-year-old man after the intramuscular injection of a single dose of benzquinamide. He had previously reacted similarly to prochlorperazine 10 mg by intramuscular injection. On both occasions symptoms were relieved by diphenhydramine given intramuscularly.— T. E. Rose and S. D. Averbuch (letter), *Ann. intern. Med.*, 1975, *83*, 231. A similar reaction occurred in a 28-year-old man with Hodgkin's disease minutes after he was given an intramuscular injection of benzquinamide 50 mg. He had also shown a similar reaction to injections of prochlorperazine.— W. R. Grove *et al.*, *Drug Intell. & clin. Pharm.*, 1976, *10*, 638.

Delirium induced in one patient by benzquinamide 25 mg was controlled within 2 minutes by physostigmine 1 mg given intravenously over 1 minute.— J. W. Chapin and D. W. Wingard, *Anesthesiology*, 1977, *46*, 364. For adverse comments on the use of physostigmine for the reversal of drug-induced reactions, see Physostigmine, p.1043.

Precautions. As for Metoclopramide Hydrochloride, p.964. Because of its mild anticholinergic activity the cautions described under Diphenidol, p.966 should be considered. There is no evidence of use in patients with phaeochromocytoma.

Absorption and Fate. Following intramuscular injection benzquinamide is metabolised in the liver and excreted in the urine and bile. Some unchanged benzquinamide is excreted in the urine. It is fairly extensively bound to plasma protein. It is reported to be absorbed following oral or rectal administration.

References: D. C. Hobbs and A. G. Connolly, *J. Pharmacokinet. Biopharm.*, 1978, *6*, 477, per *Int. pharm. Abstr.*, 1979, *16*, 368.

Uses. Benzquinamide hydrochloride has anti-emetic, antihistaminic, weak anticholinergic, and sedative properties and is used by deep intramuscular injection in a dose equivalent to 50 mg of benzquinamide to control nausea and vomiting. It acts within about 15 minutes of injection and a second dose of 50 mg may be given 1 hour later if necessary; subsequent doses of 50 mg may be repeated every 3 or 4 hours as necessary. It may also be given by slow intravenous injection in a dose of 25 mg given over a period of at least 1 minute in selected patients.

Benzquinamide should be given in reduced dosage in elderly patients.

Nausea and vomiting. Benzquinamide hydrochloride 100 mg given by mouth was more effective than prochlorperazine maleate 10 mg also given by mouth in inhibiting vomiting induced by apomorphine but its duration of action was much shorter.— R. L. Klein *et al.*, *Clin. Pharmac. Ther.*, 1970, *11*, 530.

Benzquinamide 50 mg intramuscularly given to 117 patients was more effective than thiethylperazine 10 mg intramuscularly given to 111 patients in the prevention of postoperative vomiting. Both drugs reduced the frequency of vomiting compared with a group of 100 patients who did not receive an anti-emetic drug. Drowsiness occurred in 21 patients given benzquinamide and in 28 given thiethylperazine.— H. Lutz and H. Immich, *Curr. ther. Res.*, 1972, *14*, 178.

Further references: G. Coruzzi *et al.*, *Farmaco Edn prat.*, 1980, *35*, 466.

Proprietary Names

Emete-con *(Roerig, USA)*.

6543-n

Diphenidol Hydrochloride. Difenidol Hydrochloride; SKF 478. 1,1-Diphenyl-4-piperidinobutan-1-ol hydrochloride.

$C_{21}H_{27}NO,HCl=345.9$.

CAS — 972-02-1 (diphenidol); 3254-89-5 (hydrochloride).

A white crystalline powder with a bitter taste. M.p. 214° to 221° with decomposition. Sparingly **soluble** in water and chloroform; soluble in alcohol; very slightly soluble in acetone; practically insoluble in ether. **Store** in airtight containers. Protect from light.

Adverse Effects. Adverse effects of diphenidol hydrochloride include auditory and visual hallucinations, disorientation, and confusion. Drowsiness, over-stimulation, depression, sleep disturbances, dry mouth, gastro-intestinal disturbances (including nausea and heartburn), blurred vision, and skin rashes may occur. Slight dizziness, jaundice, transient hypotension, and headache have been reported.

Precautions. Due to the risk of confusional states diphenidol should only be given to patients under close supervision. It is contra-indicated in renal failure and because of weak anticholinergic activity it should be used cautiously in patients with glaucoma, obstructive lesions of the gastro-intestinal or genito-urinary tracts, or sinus tachycardia.

Absorption and Fate. Diphenidol is absorbed from the gastro-intestinal tract and peak blood concentrations are obtained in 1½ to 3 hours. It is excreted in the urine and faeces.

Uses. Diphenidol hydrochloride is an anti-emetic agent claimed to control vertigo by means of a specific effect on the vestibular apparatus; it also has a weak peripheral anticholinergic action.

It is used for the symptomatic treatment of vertigo, nausea and vomiting due to Ménière's disease and other labyrinthine disturbances, irradiation sickness, and postoperative vomiting.

The usual dose is the equivalent of 25 to 50 mg of diphenidol by mouth every 4 hours. Alternatively 20 to 40 mg may be given by deep intramuscular injection, then 20 mg 1 hour later, if needed, and 20 to 40 mg every 4 hours subsequently. For rapid control of acute symptoms 20 mg may be given intravenously and repeated an hour later if needed. A total daily dose of 300 mg should not normally be exceeded.

Proprietary Names

Avomol *(Landerlan, Spain)*; Vontril *(Smith Kline & French, Austral.)*; Vontrol *(Smith Kline & French, Arg.; Smith Kline & French, Canad.; Smith Kline & French, S.Afr.; Smith Kline & French, USA)*; Ansmin, Antiul, Cephadol, Cerrosa, Deanosarl, Difenidolin, Maniol, Mecalmin, Meniedolin, Meranom, Midnighton, Pineroro, Satanolon, Solnomin, Tenesdol, Verterge, Wansar, Yesdol, Yophadol *(all Jap.)*.

6544-h

Domperidone. R 33812. 5-Chloro-1-{1-[3-(2-oxobenzimidazolin-1-yl)propyl]-4-piperidyl}benzimidazolin-2-one. $C_{22}H_{24}ClN_5O_2=425.9$.

CAS — 57808-66-9.

Adverse Effects, Treatment, and Precautions. Domperidone can be expected to have similar effects to Metoclopramide Hydrochloride, p.964. Extrapyramidal reactions have been reported.

Extrapyramidal effects. A 4-month-old infant developed severe extrapyramidal symptoms following a second dose of domperidone prescribed for vomiting.— P. Sol *et al.* (letter), *Lancet*, 1980, *2*, 802. On 2 occasions a 27-year-old woman developed severe extrapyramidal symptoms after intramuscular injection of domperidone.— O. Debontridder (letter), *ibid.; ibid.*, 1259.

Porphyria. A study in *rats*indicated that domperidone would probably not elicit an acute attack in susceptible porphyric individuals.— G. H. Blekkenhorst *et al.* (letter), *Lancet*, 1980, *1*, 1367. Criticisms of extrapolating data obtained from *animal* experiments to the treatment of human disease.— M. J. Brodie (letter), *ibid.*, *2*, 86; A. Gorchein (letter), *ibid.*, 152.

Absorption and Fate. Domperidone is absorbed from the gastro-intestinal tract and metabolised in the liver. It is excreted via the bile mainly as inactive metabolites.

Uses. Domperidone is a dopamine antagonist used similarly to metoclopramide hydrochloride in nausea and vomiting and to increase gastro-intestinal motility. It has been administered by mouth in doses of 10 to 20 mg thrice daily. It may also be given rectally, intramuscularly, or intravenously.

In vitro domperidone appears to be a potent antagonist of dopamine receptors but *in vivo* it cannot reach brain dopamine receptors, probably because it does not cross the blood-brain barrier. Thus, in man, it has potent anti-emetic properties without psychotropic or neurological effects.— J. M. Van Nueten and P. A. Janssen, in *Gastrointestinal Motility in Health and Disease*, W.L. Duthie (Ed.), Lancaster, MTP, 1978, p. 173. This information was also provided in a short review of domperidone which was reported to produce low concentrations in the brain and higher concentrations in the digestive tract.— A. J. Reyntjens *et al.*, *Arzneimittel-Forsch.*, 1978, *28*, 1194. However, extrapyramidal reactions have been reported, see Adverse Effects.

The results from a comparative study involving 201 patients given a barium meal suggested that although both domperidone and metoclopramide activated gastric emptying, accelerated bowel transit, and improved motor function in the proximal part of the gastro-intestinal tract, domperidone synchronised gastro-intestinal motor function due to protractive activity whereas metoclopramide acted as a 'hurrying' agent. Metoclopramide had a very marked short-lasting effect on antral peristalsis whereas such an effect was rare with domperidone.— R. Baeyens *et al.*, *Arzneimittel-Forsch.*, 1978, *28*, 682.

In a double-blind trial 129 patients received domperidone 10, 20, or 50 mg, or metoclopramide 20 mg, or a placebo by mouth 30 minutes before ingestion of a barium meal. Antral peristalsis, gastric emptying, and small bowel transit time were all significantly enhanced by domperidone 20 or 50 mg or metoclopramide 20 mg compared to a placebo.— A. De Schepper *et al.*, *Arzneimittel-Forsch.*, 1978, *28*, 1196.

In a double-blind study 8 patients with parkinsonism received domperidone 20 mg thrice daily half-an-hour before bromocriptine administration, and 9 similar patients received their bromocriptine therapy with placebo. In those receiving domperidone, a mean daily dose of bromocriptine of 148 mg was achieved before side-effects intervened, and a reduction in total disability of 76% occurred. In those receiving placebo, the bromocriptine dose could only be raised to a mean of 92 mg daily, and the reduction in total disability was a non-significant 42%. Substitution of domperidone for placebo in 5 of these patients permitted an increase in the bromocriptine dose from 59 to 114 mg daily with an average 75% overall improvement. The use of domperidone to limit the peripheral side-effects of bromocriptine permitted higher dosage and greater therapeutic effect. These results require confirmation by a long-term study after the optimum ratio of domperidone to bromocriptine has been achieved.— Y. Agid *et al.*, *Lancet*, 1979, *1*, 570.

Diabetes mellitus. A 48-year-old woman with severe diabetic gastroparesis and massive colonic dilatation obtained a dramatic clinical response to domperidone. She was referred for incapacitating constipation and despite treatment with All Bran and Metamucil, during the next 3 weeks spontaneous bowel movements were noticed 3 times only, and severe abdominal discomfort developed; massive gastric stasis was found radiologically in the absence of mechnical obstruction. Twenty-four hours after starting domperidone 10 mg intravenously every 4 hours, gastric stasis had completely disappeared. After changing to oral medication with 10 mg every 4 hours 3 spontaneous bowel movements occurred within the next 7 days; overnight residual gastric volumes were compatible with normal gastric emptying. Six weeks after hospital discharge a 1-kg gain in weight was accompanied by striking subjective improvement without any abdominal discomfort, and by far better control of diabetes. Domperidone may be of benefit not only in diabetic gastroparesis but also in otherwise refractory constipation in diabetic subjects.— M. Heer *et al.* (letter), *Lancet*, 1980, *2*, 1145. Similar benefit in several patients. However, not all gastroparetic patients respond well to dopaminergic receptor antagonist therapy and the authors cannot predict on any clinical criteria which patients will improve on domperidone.— S. J. Gordon and R. E. Joseph (letter), *ibid.*, 1981, *1*, 390.

Dyspepsia. In a double-blind study of 41 patients with chronic postprandial dyspepsia, domperidone 10 mg thrice daily before meals was more effective than placebo in relieving symptoms.— K. Haarmann *et al.*, *Postgrad. med. J.*, 1979, *55, Suppl.* 1, 24. A similar report.— W. Englert and D. Schlich, *ibid.*, 28. A similar report in 40 patients with dyspepsia due to delayed gastric emptying.— A. Bekhti and L. Rutgeerts, *ibid.*, 30.

Further references: W. Van Ganse *et al.*, *Curr. ther. Res.*, 1977, *23*, 695; J. Lienard *et al.*, *ibid.*, 1978, *23*, 529; E. Arts *et al.*, *J. int. med. Res.*, 1979, *7*, 158; R. Platteborse *et al.*, *Postgrad. med. J.*, 1979, *55, Suppl.* 1, 15; R. Deberdt, *ibid.*, 48.

Gastro-oesophageal reflux. Studies in 36 healthy subjects showed that domperidone 114 to 228 µg per kg body-weight intravenously increased lower oesophageal sphincter pressure and gastro-duodenal motility, but had no effect on gastric acid secretion or gastrin release. Lower oesophageal sphincter pressure was also increased in 9 patients with gastro-oesophageal reflux following high doses by mouth.— T. R. Weihrauch *et al.*, *Postgrad. med. J.*, 1979, *55, Suppl.* 1, 7.

Results of a placebo-controlled study in 15 patients indicated that domperidone does not seem to prevent exacerbations of disease in patients with chronic reflux oesophagitis and proven gastric motor failure; nor does it seem to increase the mechanical clearance activity of the oesophagus and the stomach.— K. Schulze-Delrieu *et al.* (letter), *Lancet*, 1981, *1*, 159.

Nausea and vomiting. In a double-blind study of 60 children aged between 2 and 6 years domperidone 30-mg suppositories, repeated 3 times if necessary at intervals of at least 3 hours, were more effective than either metoclopramide 10-mg suppositories or placebo, in the 24 hours of observation, in reducing the severity of nausea or vomiting occurring as a complication of acute gastroenteritis.— M. Van Eygen *et al.*, *Postgrad. med. J.*, 1979, *55, Suppl.* 1, 36.

In a 2-week double-blind study of 47 infants and children aged between 3 weeks and 8 years domperidone was more effective than metoclopramide or placebo in controlling the symptoms of chronic vomiting after food. The dose of both drugs was 0.3 mg per kg body-weight thrice daily given before meals as drops of a solution containing 10 mg per ml.— I. De Loore *et al.*, *Postgrad. med. J.*, 1979, *55, Suppl.* 1, 40.

Preliminary studies in 42 patients indicated that a suitable dosage regimen of domperidone to control postoperative nausea and vomiting was 20 mg intravenously initially followed by four doses of 10 mg by intravenous infusion in the following 24 hours. In a subsequent double-blind study of 106 patients, nausea and vomiting occurred in 3 of 53 patients treated with this regimen of domperidone administration and in 16 of 53 patients treated with placebo.— M. Boulanger *et al.*, *Postgrad. med. J.*, 1979, *55, Suppl.* 1, 45.

In a randomised crossover study in 18 children the incidence of nausea and vomiting, after cytotoxic chemotherapy, was significantly reduced when the children were given domperidone up to 1 mg per kg body-weight intravenously immediately before chemotherapy, compared with metoclopramide 500 µg per kg.— I. L. Swann *et al.*, *Br. med. J.*, 1979, *2*, 1188.

Further references: F. Dhondt *et al.*, *Curr. ther. Res.*, 1978, *24*, 912; J. Nogarède *et al.*, *Arzneimittel-Forsch.*, 1978, *28*, 686; M. Van Outryve *et al.*, *Postgrad. med. J.*, 1979, *55, Suppl.* 1, 33; R. Clara *et al.*, *ibid.*, 43; A. Reyntjens, *ibid.*, 50; D. P. D'Souza *et al.*, *Curr. ther. Res.*, 1980, *27*, 384.

Proprietary Preparations

Motilium *(Janssen, UK).* Domperidone, available as **Injection** containing 5 mg per ml in ampoules of 2 ml and as **Tablets** of 10 mg. (Also available as Motilium in *Neth., S.Afr.*).

6545-m

Metopimazine. EXP 999; RP 9965. 1-[3-(2-Methylsulphonylphenothiazin-10-yl)propyl]piperidine-4-carboxamide.

$C_{22}H_{27}N_3O_3S_2$=445.6.

CAS — 14008-44-7.

Metopimazine is an anti-emetic usually given in doses of 5 to 15 mg daily, by mouth or by rectum; 10 to 20 mg has been given by intramuscular injection.

In doses of 5 to 15 mg metopimazine was not effective in suppressing motion sickness 1½ to 24 hours after administration in paid volunteers.— H. O. Barber *et al.*, *Can. med. Ass. J.*, 1967, *97*, 1460.

In a double-blind study metopimazine 10 mg thrice daily was as effective an anti-emetic as prochlorperazine 5 mg thrice daily and both were better than a placebo for 50 patients with neoplasms who were receiving treatment with fluorouracil. Metopimazine 45 mg daily was given to patients receiving radiation therapy and had a slight sedative effect, but less than that caused by prochlorperazine 30 mg daily.— C. G. Moertel and R. J. Reitemeier, *J. clin. Pharmac.*, 1973, *13*, 283.

Following 2 double-blind studies in 183 patients with cancer receiving multiple combination chemotherapy, a minimum dose of 45 mg metopimazine per day was recommended as an anti-emetic during drug treatment.— L. Israel and C. Rodary, *J. int. med. Res.*, 1978, *6*, 235.

Further references: J. Gaillot and A. Bieder, *Farmaco, Edn prat.*, 1980, *35*, 3.

Proprietary Names

Vogalen *(Rhodia, Spain)*; Vogalene *(Rhodia, Arg.*; *Theraplix, Belg.*; *Théraplix, Fr.*; *RBS Pharma, Ital.*; *Théraplix, Neth.).*

6546-b

Oxypendyl Hydrochloride. Oxipendyl Dihydrochloride; Oxypendyl Dihydrochloride; Perthipendyl Dihydrochloride. 2-{4-[3-(Pyrido[3,2-*b*][1,4]benzothiazin-10-yl)propyl]piperazin-1-yl}ethanol dihydrochloride.

$C_{20}H_{26}N_4OS,2HCl$=443.4.

CAS — 5585-93-3 (oxypendyl); 17297-82-4 (hydrochloride).

Oxypendyl hydrochloride is an anti-emetic. Doses of 25 mg have been given 3 or 4 times daily by mouth. Doses of 30 mg have been given rectally and doses of 25 to 50 mg intramuscularly.

Proprietary Names

Pervetral *(Homburg, Ger.).*

Metronidazole and some other Antiprotozoal Agents

4750-z

The drugs described in this section are those primarily used in the treatment of amoebiasis, trichomoniasis, and trypanosomiasis. Some are also active in giardiasis and leishmaniasis.

Drugs used in the treatment of malaria are described in the section on chloroquine (see p.394).

A review of the choice and dosage of drugs in parasitic infections.— *Med. Lett.*, 1979, *21,* 105.

Amoebiasis. Amoebiasis is an infection with *Entamoeba histolytica*. Infection occurs from the ingestion of cysts, usually in contaminated food and drink. The cysts release trophozoites in the gastro-intestinal tract; reproduction occurs by fission of the trophozoites. Further cysts develop (rare in amoebic dysentery), are excreted in the faeces, and lead to transmission of the disease. Other trophozoites multiply and may invade the gut wall causing ulceration and, possibly after a long latent period, migrate to other tissues, especially the liver, where they may cause abscess formation.

The drugs used in the treatment of amoebiasis which are described in this section include derivatives of acetamide such as diloxanide furoate, alkaloids such as dehydroemetine and emetine, arsenical compounds such as acetarsol and carbarsone, derivatives of iodoquinoline such as clioquinol and di-iodohydroxyquinoline, and metronidazole and tinidazole. Also used in the treatment of amoebiasis but described elsewhere are antibiotics, including paromomycin and the tetracyclines, and chloroquine and niridazole.

The relative effectiveness of an amoebicide at the common sites of infection is determined by its absorption and tissue distribution characteristics. Metronidazole, niridazole, and tinidazole are effective at all the common sites of infection, but it is common practice, particularly with amoebicides active at specific sites, to give 2 or more amoebicides concomitantly.

Reviews of the treatment of amoebiasis.— C. Wilcocks, *Abstr. Wld Med.*, 1967, *41,* 241; *Br. med. J.*, 1970, *2,* 36; D. R. Seaton, *Practitioner,* 1971, *206,* 16; E. Barrett-Connor, *Ann. intern. Med.*, 1972, *77,* 797; R. Knight *et al.*, *Gut,* 1973, *14,* 145; A. M. Geddes, *Adv. Med. Topics Ther.*, 1976, *2,* 1; M. J. Miller, *Prog. Drug Res.*, 1976, *20,* 433; D. J. Krogstad *et al.*, *Ann. intern. Med.*, 1978, *88,* 89; R. Knight and S. G. Wright, *Gut,* 1978, *19,* 940; R. Knight, *J. antimicrob. Chemother.*, 1980, *6,* 577.

Amoebicides could be classified as: *direct acting amoebicides acting principally in the bowel lumen* such as the quinoline derivatives, the arsenical derivatives (acetarsol, carbarsone, and difetarsone), and other drugs including chlorbetamide, diloxanide, and paromomycin; *indirect acting amoebicides acting in the bowel lumen and wall* such as the tetracyclines and other antibiotics with amoebicidal activity; *tissue amoebicides acting principally in the bowel wall and liver* such as emetine, emetine bismuth iodide, and dehydroemetine; *tissue amoebicides acting principally in the liver* such as chloroquine; and *amoebicides effective at all sites* such as metronidazole and niridazole. In the treatment of asymptomatic intestinal amoebiasis any of the drugs active in the bowel lumen could be used but none was completely reliable; drugs with activity at other sites, such as the tetracyclines, emetine preparations, and possibly metronidazole might be effective. Mild to moderate amoebic dysentery should be treated with a tetracycline, a luminal amoebicide, and chloroquine and severe cases with emetine or dehydroemetine, a tetracycline, and a luminal amoebicide. Metronidazole might be useful. Relapses should be treated with the alternative drugs available. Hepatic amoebiasis should be treated with either metronidazole or a regimen of chloroquine, a luminal amoebicide, and either emetine or dehydroemetine. If dysentery was present, the dose of metronidazole should be increased and the regimen supplemented by tetracycline. There was no evidence of natural or acquired resistance by *Entamoeba histolytica* to amoebicides. To reduce the endemicity of amoebiasis, mass treatment could be given with a direct acting amoebicide or possibly with metronidazole, and prophylactically di-iodohydroxyquinoline or bismuth glycollylarsanilate could be used.— Report of the WHO Expert Committee on Amoebiasis, *Tech. Rep. Ser. Wld Hlth Org. No. 421,* 1969.

Metronidazole was the best treatment for mild to moderate amoebic dysentery. Alternatively, chlortetracycline or oxytetracycline with diloxanide furoate and chloroquine could be used. In very severe amoebic dysentery, electrolyte and fluid disturbances and anaemia should be corrected and treatment with metronidazole, tetracyclines, and diloxanide furoate given. Emetine or dehydroemetine could be substituted for metronidazole or given as well in very severe infections. Diloxanide furoate was effective in the treatment of cyst-passers. Di-iodohydroxyquinoline and tetracycline could also be used.— R. G. Hendrickse, *Br. med. J.*, 1973, *1,* 669.

A discussion on the possible differentiation of pathogenic from non-pathogenic *Entamoeba histolytica*.— *Lancet,* 1979, *1,* 303.

Trichomoniasis. Trichomoniasis is caused by invasion of the genital tract with *Trichomonas vaginalis*. Transmission is primarily sexual and the incubation period is 1 to 3 weeks. In females it may cause vaginitis and a vaginal discharge and may lead to urinary-tract infection. In males it may cause a low-grade urethritis.

The principal drugs used in the treatment of trichomoniasis and described in this section are acetarsol, metronidazole, nifuratel, nimorazole, and tinidazole. Also used and described elsewhere are clotrimazole, hachimycin, and natamycin.

A brief review.— M. J. Miller, *Prog. Drug Res.*, 1976, *20,* 433. See also *Br. J. vener. Dis.*, 1978, *54,* 69.

Trypanosomiasis. African trypanosomiasis (sleeping sickness) is caused by *Trypanosoma gambiense*, transmitted by river-haunting tsetse flies (*Glossina palpalis* and *G. tachinoides*), and *T. rhodesiense*, transmitted by open woodland tsetse flies of the species *Glossina*. Trypanosomiasis due to *T. gambiense* develops slowly over 2 to 3 years and is characterised by infection of the blood stream and lymph nodes followed by infection of the central nervous system. In *T. rhodesiense* infections involvement of the central nervous system rapidly follows infection of the blood stream and death frequently occurs within a year if the disease is untreated.

The principal drugs used in the treatment of the haemolymphatic phase are pentamidine and suramin; for CNS involvement melarsoprol is generally used.

South American trypanosomiasis (Chagas' disease) is caused by *T. cruzi*, carried by reduviid bugs which feed on human blood. Contamination of the skin by faeces of biting bugs is followed by penetration of skin abrasions, mucous membranes, and conjunctiva. Few drugs are available for treatment; nifurtimox and benznidazole have been used.

A review of the prophylactic management of trypanosomiasis.— E. Barrett-Connor, *Ann. intern. Med.*, 1972, *77,* 797.

Reviews of the management of trypanosomiasis.— W. H. R. Lumsden, *Br. med. Bull.*, 1972, *28,* 34; M. J. Miller, *Prog. Drug Res.*, 1976, *20,* 433; P. F. L. Boreham, *Pharm. J.*, 1978, *1,* 155.

A discussion of the limited compounds available for the treatment of Chagas' disease.— W. E. Gutteridge, *Trop. Dis. Bull.*, 1976, *73,* 699.

A report of a symposium on African trypanosomiasis.— *Annls Soc. belge Méd. trop.*, 1977, *57,* 188, per *Trop. Dis. Bull.*, 1978, *75,* 640.

A 'malignant' form of *Trypanosoma rhodesiense* infection in tourists.— P. G. Janssens and A. De Muynck, *Annls Soc. belge Méd. trop.*, 1977, *57,* 589, per *Abstr. Hyg.*, 1978, *53,* 1155.

The choice of treatment of trypanosomiasis is governed by the presence or absence of indications that trypanosomes have reached the CSF. In trypanosomiasis due to *Trypanosoma gambiense, suramin* (5 to 7 intravenous injections of 20 mg per kg body-weight, up to a maximum single dose of 1 g, at intervals of 5 to 7 days) is effective in the early stages of infection; alternatively, *pentamidine* (3 to 4 mg per kg given daily or on alternate days for 7 to 10 injections) may be given, provided it has not been used locally for mass prophylaxis against *T. gambiense*. When there is CNS involvement, *melarsoprol* (usually 3 courses of 3 daily intravenous injections of up to 3.6 mg per kg, each course separated by an interval of at least one week) is the drug of choice; treatment should preferably be preceded by 2 or 3 injections of *suramin*. *Melarsonyl potassium* (4 mg per kg given intramuscularly or subcutaneously in a regimen similar to that for melarsoprol) is indicated only when the intravenous route cannot easily be used. In *T. rhodesiense* infections *suramin* is again the drug of choice in the early stages and where there is CNS involvement *melarsoprol* and *suramin* should be used. *Nitrofurazone* (500 mg three or four times daily for 5 to 7 days) is used as an alternative in melarsoprol-resistant infections but its toxicity makes it unsuitable for regular use. Chemoprophylaxis in *T. rhodesiense* areas is not recommended.— Report of a Joint WHO Expert Committee and FAO Expert Consultation, *Tech. Rep. Ser. Wld Hlth Org. No. 635,* 1979.

4751-c

Metronidazole *(B.P., B.P. Vet., U.S.P.)*. Metronidaz.; Bayer 5360; RP 8823; NSC-50364; SC 10295. 2-(2-Methyl-5-nitroimidazol-1-yl)ethanol. $C_6H_9N_3O_3 = 171.2$.

CAS — 443-48-1.

Pharmacopoeias. In *Br., Braz., Chin., Cz., Jug., Nord., Roum.*, and *U.S.*

A white to pale yellow crystalline powder or crystals, odourless or with a slight odour and a bitter slightly saline taste. M.p. 159° to 163°. It darkens on exposure to light.

Soluble 1 in 100 of water, 1 in 200 of alcohol, and 1 in 250 of chloroform; slightly soluble in ether. A saturated solution in water has a pH of about 6.5. **Protect** from light.

Adverse Effects. Side-effects of metronidazole include gastro-intestinal discomfort, anorexia, nausea, coated tongue, dry mouth and unpleasant taste, headache, pruritus, and skin rash, and, less frequently vomiting, diarrhoea, weakness, vertigo, ataxia, depression, insomnia, drowsiness, urethral discomfort, and darkening of the urine. Occasionally there may be temporary moderate leucopenia. Peripheral neuropathy has been reported in patients on prolonged therapy.

Depression associated with metronidazole in 1 patient.— A. J. Giannini (letter), *Am. J. Psychiat.*, 1977, *134,* 329. See also A. J. Voth (letter), *Can. med. Ass. J.*, 1969, *100,* 1012; F. A. Whitlock and L. E. J. Evans, *Drugs,* 1978, *15,* 53.

Two patients who received metronidazole 3 to 6 g per m^2 body-surface every other day over a period of 10 days and 1 patient who received metronidazole 1 g per m^2 thrice daily for 7 days for radiosensitisation experienced major motor seizures.— S. Frytak *et al.*, *Ann. intern. Med.*, 1978, *88,* 361.

Colitis. For reports of *Clostridium difficile*-associated colitis following the use of metronidazole, see under Uses.

Mutagenic effects. Metronidazole had mutagenic effects in some strains of bacteria. Doses of 2 g were sometimes used and could produce serum-metronidazole concentrations of 30 to 45 μg per ml. Such concentrations could potentially increase the mutation-rate by a factor of 5 to 10. As the incidence of lung tumours in *mice* was also increased by metronidazole, nitroimidazole compounds should be used with caution and their use reappraised.— C. E. Voogd *et al.*, *Mutat. Res.*, 1974, *26,* 483, per *Trop. Dis. Bull.*, 1975, *72,* 66.

Increased chromosome aberrations were noted in patients following prolonged treatment with high doses of metronidazole.— F. Mitelman *et al.* (letter), *Lancet,* 1976, *2,* 802. No evidence of cytogenetic effect of metronidazole was found in a controlled study involving metronidazole and sulphasalazine. Such an effect could not be ruled out for sulphasalazine. Some patients in the previous study had received sulphasalazine in addition to metronidazole.— *idem*, 1980, *1*, 1249.

Mutagenic activity was found in the urine of 9 patients taking metronidazole orally and 1 using metronidazole vaginally. The effect was associated with unchanged metronidazole and at least 4 metabolites.— W. T. Speck *et al.*, *J. natn. Cancer Inst.*, 1976, *56*, 283.

The FDA believed that the risk of carcinogenesis from the use of metronidazole was low. Revised labelling recommended that the duration of treatment for trichomoniasis should be 7 days. Vaginal inserts would no longer be marketed.— *FDA Drug Bull.*, 1976, *6*, 22.

Absence of chromosome-breaking activity in 12 patients given metronidazole 200 mg thrice daily for 7 days. For all practical purposes metronidazole could be regarded as a safe drug for short-term treatment.— B. Hartley-Asp, *Leo* (letter), *Lancet*, 1979, *1*, 275. Criticism.— J. R. Coulter (letter), *Lancet*, 1979, *2*, 609. A reply.— B. Hartley-Asp (letter), *Lancet*, 1979, *2*, 981.

There was no appreciable increase in the expected incidence of cancer in a retrospective study of 771 women who had received metronidazole for the treatment of vaginal trichomoniasis diagnosed between 1960 and 1969.— C. M. Beard *et al.*, *New Engl. J. Med.*, 1979, *301*, 519. Similar findings in 2460 patients who received metronidazole between July 1969 and August 1973.— G. D. Friedman (letter), *ibid.*, 1980, *302*, 519. A view that it was too soon for valid conclusions to be drawn about the risk of cancer.— F. E. Mirer and M. A. Silverstein (letter), *ibid.* Further criticisms. Major congenital abnormalities occurred in 25% of infants exposed to metronidazole in the first trimester of pregnancy.— J. F. Haas (letter), *ibid.*, 520. Reply.— C. M. Beard (letter), *ibid.*

Neurological disorders. Reports of neuropathy: I. D. Ramsey (letter), *Br. med. J.*, 1968, *4*, 706; A. Coxon and C. A. Pallis, *J. Neurol. Neurosurg. Psychiat.*, 1976, *39*, 403; H. Schipper *et al.* (letter), *New Engl. J. Med.*, 1976, *295*, 901; W. G. Bradley *et al.*, *Br. med. J.*, 1977, *2*, 610; S. Hishon and J. Pilling (letter), *ibid.*, 832; I. J. Karlson and A. N. Hamlyn (letter), *ibid.*, 832; R. K. Kusumi *et al.*, *Ann. intern. Med.*, 1980, *93*, 59.

Pregnancy and the neonate. A pregnant woman aged 16 swallowed 21 tablets of metronidazole 200 mg. No treatment was given yet apart from transient disorientation no ill-effects resulted in either mother or foetus.— J. L. Fluker, *Br. J. vener. Dis.*, 1961, *36*, 280.

In 61 women who received metronidazole 200 mg thrice daily for 7 days, at various times during pregnancy, 3 gave birth to premature stillborn infants and 1 to an infant who later died of white asphyxia. There were no congenital malformations attributable to the drug. Metronidazole was considered quite safe when given in the second and third trimesters of pregnancy, but more evidence was required concerning its use during the first trimester.— P. Rodin and G. Hass, *Br. J. vener. Dis.*, 1966, *42*, 210.

A survey of the literature provided no positive evidence of teratogenicity associated with metronidazole; there might be an increased incidence if it was taken during the first trimester.— D. Chang and G. C. Cupit, *Drug Intell. & clin. Pharm.*, 1978, *12*, 409.

Metronidazole is carcinogenic in some *animals* and the urine of patients receiving metronidazole has been shown to be mutagenic in bacteria. Its use during the first trimester of pregnancy was not advised and possibly it should not be used during pregnancy at all.— *Med. Lett.*, 1979, *21*, 89.

See also under Mutagenic Effects, above.

Skin reactions. An eruption simulating pityriasis rosacea occurred on 2 occasions in a woman taking metronidazole.— J. C. Maize and K. J. Tomecki (letter), *Archs Derm.*, 1977, *113*, 1457.

Prophylactic treatment with metronidazole against amoebiasis repeatedly caused irritation and reddening of a pigmented patch of skin on a 40-year-old man.— R. P. C. Naik and G. Singh, *Dermatologica*, 1977, *155*, 59.

Precautions. Metronidazole should not be used in patients with blood dyscrasias or with active disease of the central nervous system. It is suggested that its use should be avoided during pregnancy.

Some authorities consider that women taking metronidazole should not breast-feed their babies.

When given in conjunction with alcohol, metronidazole may provoke a disulfiram-like reaction in some individuals.

Metronidazole enhances the anticoagulant effect of warfarin.

Metronidazole used in the treatment of mixed infections including trichomoniasis might make the detection of syphilis difficult.— I. I. Il'in *et al.*, *Vest. Derm. Vener.*, 1971, *45*, 74.

Candidal vaginitis following metronidazole therapy appeared to be more difficult to eradicate.— A. Palmer, *Practitioner*, 1975, *214*, 666.

Abnormally low serum aspartate aminotransferase (SGOT) values obtained in 18 patients during treatment with metronidazole were considered to be due to interference by metronidazole in the serum assay.— J. P. Rissing *et al.*, *Antimicrob. Ag. Chemother.*, 1978, *14*, 636.

Metronidazole is carcinogenic in some *animals* and the urine of patients receiving metronidazole has been shown to be mutagenic in bacteria. It would be prudent to use metronidazole as seldom as possible, and then in the lowest effective dosage for the shortest possible time. Its use during the first trimester of pregnancy was not advised and possibly it should not be used during pregnancy at all.— *Med. Lett.*, 1979, *21*, 89. See also Mutagenic Effects under Adverse Effects.

Interactions. Four of 20 chronic alcoholic patients who were taking disulfiram 500 mg daily developed acute psychosis or a confusional state when metronidazole 750 mg daily was given concomitantly. The daily dose of metronidazole was reduced to 250 mg for the next 9 patients, but 2 suffered a similar reaction. Symptoms arose on the tenth to fourteenth day of combined therapy, persisted or even increased in intensity for 2 to 3 days, then waned. Recovery took 1 to 2 weeks.— E. Rothstein and D. D. Clancy, *New Engl. J. Med.*, 1969, *280*, 1006.

In a 66-year-old woman who was taking oxytetracycline 250 mg four times daily for bronchitis, no improvement in her trichomonal vaginitis occurred when she received metronidazole 200 mg thrice daily for a week. On discontinuing oxytetracycline and repeating the course of metronidazole the vaginitis cleared.— S. Szanto (letter), *Br. med. J.*, 1971, *2*, 467.

Prolongation of prothrombin time in a 31-year-old woman on warfarin after a 10-day course of metronidazole.— F. J. Kazmier, *Mayo Clin. Proc.*, 1976, *51*, 782. In 8 healthy subjects concomitant administration of metronidazole enhanced the anticoagulant effect of racemic warfarin. The interaction could be reduced or even avoided by using *R*(+)-warfarin.— R. A. O'Reilly, *New Engl. J. Med.*, 1976, *295*, 354.

Absorption and Fate. Metronidazole is readily absorbed from the gastro-intestinal tract and from the rectal mucosa and widely distributed in body tissues. Maximum concentrations occur in the serum after about 1 hour and traces are detected after 24 hours.

At least half the dose is excreted in the urine as metronidazole and its metabolites, including an acid oxidation product, a hydroxy derivative, and a glucuronide. Metronidazole diffuses across the placenta, and is found in breast milk of nursing mothers in concentrations equivalent to those in the serum.

For the isolation and identification of the urinary oxidative metabolites of metronidazole, see J. E. Stambaugh *et al.*, *J. Pharmac. exp. Ther.*, 1968, *161*, 373.

The biological half-life of metronidazole was 6.2 hours after administration of 200-mg doses to 7 volunteers. The maximum serum concentration was 7.07 µg per ml.— P. G. Welling and A. M. Monro, *Arzneimittel-Forsch.*, 1972, *22*, 2128.

Metronidazole was less than 5% bound to plasma proteins.— D. R. Sanvordeker *et al.*, *J. pharm. Sci.*, 1975, *64*, 1797.

The concentration of metronidazole in pus from cerebral abscesses in 3 patients given 400 to 600 mg eight-hourly was 34.4 to 45 µg per ml, compared with concomitant serum concentrations of 11.5 to 35.1 µg per ml.— H. R. Ingham *et al.*, *Br. med. J.*, 1977, *2*, 991.

In 4 healthy patients given metronidazole 2.4 g by mouth concentrations in the CSF 90 minutes later were 6 to 22.7 µg per ml and represented 43% of the simultaneous serum concentrations.— A. M. H. Jokipii *et al.*, *J. antimicrob. Chemother.*, 1977, *3*, 239.

In 10 healthy subjects given metronidazole 400 mg either fasting or with food, the peak serum concentrations were similar but absorption was apparently delayed by food. In 9 patients with Crohn's disease, absorption of metronidazole was reduced in those with lesions of the upper small intestine. It was suggested that the dose should be related to the body-weight in all subjects.— A. Melander *et al.*, *Eur. J. clin. Pharmac.*, 1977, *12*, 69.

In 3 patients who had undergone surgery for common duct stones and who had received metronidazole 2 g by mouth, concentrations of metronidazole in serum and hepatic bile were comparable. In 55 patients studied during operation, having received metronidazole 500 mg intravenously, concentrations in gall-bladder bile and common-duct bile were comparable with those in serum when the biliary tract was not obstructed; when the common duct was blocked by a stone concentrations in gall-bladder bile were greatly reduced. In 5 patients with jaundice due to common-duct obstruction concentrations of metronidazole in common-duct bile were 56 to 99% of those in serum.— M. L. Nielsen and T. Justesen, *Scand. J. Gastroenterol.*, 1977, *12*, 1003.

Significant concentrations of metronidazole (above 8.5 µg per ml) were found in ear discharges from 8 of 12 patients with mixed aerobic/anaerobic infection of the middle ear given metronidazole 2.4 g two to four hours earlier. Similar results were obtained in patients undergoing ear surgery and given metronidazole 2 to 13 hours earlier. Clinical effects were not studied. The results did not yet justify a change in the recommended antimicrobial treatment of otitis media.— L. Jokipii *et al.*, *Archs Otorhinolar.*, 1978, *220*, 167.

In patients given suppositories containing metronidazole 1 g before and after surgery, serum-metronidazole concentrations postoperatively were at least 6 µg per ml in 34 of 38 patients.— G. W. Houghton and R. Templeton, *J. antimicrob. Chemother.*, 1978, *4*, *Suppl.* C, 91. Peak plasma concentrations of metronidazole of 5.5, 9.5, and 14 µg per ml occurred in 10 healthy subjects 4 hours after administration of suppositories containing 0.5, 1, and 2 g of metronidazole respectively.— T. Bergan and E. Arnold, *Chemotherapy, Basle*, 1980, *26*, 231.

In 13 women single 0.25-g doses of metronidazole produced mean peak serum concentrations, measured polarographically, of 5.1 µg per ml; values of 19.6 and 40.6 µg per ml were achieved after single doses of 1 and 2 g in 10 and 4 women respectively. Respective half-lives were 5.92, 7.8, and 8.78 hours. Protein binding was 10 to 20%. About 30 to 35% of the dose was recovered in the urine in 12 hours and more than 50% in 24 hours. Trichomonacidal concentrations of metronidazole were present in blood for 12 hours, 24 to 36 hours, and 48 hours respectively after the 3 dose schedules.— I. Amon *et al.*, *Int. J. clin. Pharmac.*, 1978, *16*, 384.

The plasma concentrations of metronidazole and its hydroxy metabolite ranged from 7.2 to 44.8 µg per ml and from 1.6 to 15.2 µg per ml respectively in 10 patients with anaerobic infections who received metronidazole 13.6 mg per kg body-weight by intravenous infusion over one hour followed by 1.43 mg per kg every hour for up to 12 days; the plasma concentrations of the acid metabolite ranged from 0 to 1.4 µg per ml. The ratio of metronidazole to hydroxy metabolite was about 1 in a patient taking phenytoin compared with 0.03 to 0.3 in the other 9 patients.— L. A. Wheeler *et al.*, *Antimicrob. Ag. Chemother.*, 1978, *13*, 205.

There was no significant difference between the bioavailability of 400 mg of metronidazole when given by mouth either as a single 400-mg tablet or as two 200-mg tablets or when given by intravenous infusion to 10 healthy male subjects. Mean elimination half-lives for metronidazole following each dose were 8.2, 8.4, and 8.3 hours respectively.— G. W. Houghton *et al.* (letter), *J. antimicrob. Chemother.*, 1979, *5*, 621. See also *idem*, *Br. J. clin. Pharmac.*, 1979, *8*, 337.

Pregnancy and the neonate. In 8 women given suppositories of metronidazole 1 g 8-hourly for 7 doses following caesarean section the mean concentration of metronidazole in breast milk 30 minutes after completing treatment was 10 µg per ml (maximum 25 µg per ml). There was unlikely to be any adverse effect in the breast-fed neonate; this did not necessarily apply to older infants who would take larger quantities of milk.— B. Moore and J. Collier (letter), *Br. med. J.*, 1979, *2*, 211.

Uses. Metronidazole has antiprotozoal and antibacterial actions and is effective against *Trichomonas vaginalis* and other protozoa including *Entamoeba histolytica* and *Giardia lamblia*, and against anaerobic bacteria.

It is used in the treatment of trichomoniasis of the genito-urinary tract in males and females; it does not affect the normal acidophilic flora of the vagina and it has no effect on *Candida* species. Resistant strains of *T. vaginalis* have occasionally been reported. In amoebiasis it is effective at all sites of infection and is used in the treatment of amoebic dysentery and amoebic liver abscess as well as for the eradication of *E. histolytica* from patients passing cysts. Metronidazole is also used in the treatment of giardiasis and of Vincent's infection, and in the prevention and treatment of anaerobic infections.

In trichomoniasis, the usual dose for adults and children over 10 years is 200 to 250 mg thrice daily after food for 7 days. A second course of treatment may be given, if needed, after an interval of 4 to 6 weeks. An alternative dosage schedule consists of 800 mg in the morning and 1.2 g at night on 2 consecutive days. Single doses of 2 g have also been used. The concomitant treatment of sexual consorts is recommended. In elderly women hormone therapy may be necessary to clear up vaginitis. The usual dose for children is: up to 3 years of age 150 mg daily for 7 days; 3 to 7 years 200 mg; and 7 to 10 years 300 mg.

In the treatment of amoebic dysentery a typical dose is 750 to 800 mg thrice daily for 5 to 10 days. Doses of 2 g once daily for 2 days have been suggested. Cure is assessed by the elimination of trophozoites and cysts from the faeces one month after treatment and by the resolution of rectal ulceration.

For the elimination of cysts from patients with asymptomatic amoebiasis doses of 400 to 800 mg thrice daily for 5 to 10 days have been used. A luminal amoebicide such as di-iodohydroxyquinoline or diloxanide furoate may be given concomitantly.

For the treatment of hepatic and other extra-intestinal amoebiasis doses of 500 to 800 mg thrice daily have been used. Single doses of 2.4 g, or single doses of 2 g once daily for 2 days, have been suggested. Treatment commonly includes the aspiration of liver abscess.

A suggested dose for children with amoebiasis: up to 3 years of age, one-quarter; 3 to 7 years, one-third; 7 to 10 years, one-half of the adult dose.

In giardiasis, the usual dose is 2 g daily for 3 successive days. Dosage for children is proportional, as for amoebiasis (above). An alternative suggested adult schedule is 250 mg thrice daily for 10 days.

In Vincent's infection, a dosage of 200 mg thrice daily or 400 mg twice daily is given for 3 days.

Metronidazole is also administered as the benzoyl derivative (see p.973). The hydrochloride (SC-32642) and phosphate (U-54555) are also under study.

Use in Anaerobic Infections. Metronidazole is active against obligate anaerobic bacteria such as *Bacteroides* and *Fusobacterium* spp. and is used in the treatment of infections due to such bacteria and in the prevention of postoperative anaerobic infections. It is bactericidal.

In the treatment of anaerobic infections the usual dose is 400 mg thrice daily for 7 days; children may be given 7.5 mg per kg body-weight thrice daily. Metronidazole may also be given rectally; a suppository containing 1 g may be given 8-hourly for 3 days, then 12-hourly until oral administration can be instituted. The rectal dose for children under 1 year is one-eighth of the adult dose; 1 to 5 years, one-quarter; 5 to 12 years, one-half. In severe infections metronidazole may be given intravenously—100 ml of a 0.5% solution is given at a rate of 5 ml per minute every 8 hours, with oral administration substituted as soon as possible. A similar parenteral dose has been used for prophylaxis. For children each intravenous dose contains 7.5 mg per kg.

For the prevention of anaerobic infection in gynaecological surgery metronidazole is given by mouth; the first dose is 1 g, then 200 mg thrice daily until starvation, followed by 200 mg thrice daily postoperatively for up to 7 days.

The following schedule may be used for the prevention of anaerobic infections during gastro-intestinal surgery: metronidazole 1 g by mouth for the first dose, then 200 mg eight-hourly during the 24 hours before starvation; this is followed by 1 g rectally starting 2 hours before surgery and continuing 8-hourly for up to 3 days, until oral administration of 200 to 400 mg thrice daily can be given to complete a 7-day course. If rectal administration continues after the third postoperative day the dose frequency should be reduced to 12-hourly. Various regimens using metronidazole in association with other antibacterial agents including neomycin, kanamycin, cephalosporins, or phthalylsulphathiazole have also been advocated. Children have been given metronidazole 5 mg per kg (up to 100 mg) by mouth 8-hourly for 48 hours with neomycin 125 mg (up to 1 year), 250 mg (1 to 5 years), or 500 mg (5 to 12 years) by mouth 6-hourly for 3 days before surgery, followed by metronidazole 125 to 500 mg rectally 8-hourly for 48 hours postoperatively.

For the prevention of anaerobic infection during appendicectomy metronidazole 1 g may be given as a suppository 2 hours before surgery then 8-hourly for 3 days, then 12-hourly; oral administration of 200 to 400 mg thrice daily, to complete a 7-day course, should commence as soon as possible. Children (5 to 12 years) have been given 500-mg doses rectally until oral administration (3.75 to 7.5 mg per kg) is possible.

Other appropriate antibacterial agents may be given concomitantly.

Reviews and discussions of the use of metronidazole.— R. Knight and S. G. Wright, *Gut,* 1978, *19,* 940; S. J. Eykyn, *Topics Ther.,* 1978, *4,* 18; E. J. Baines, *J. antimicrob. Chemother.,* 1978, *4, Suppl.* C, 97; R. H. George, *Prescribers' J.,* 1979, *19,* 118; *Aust. J. Pharm.,* 1979, *60,* 404; *Med. Lett.,* 1979, *21,* 89; S. M. Finegold, *Ann. intern. Med.,* 1980, *93,* 585; P. Goldman, *New Engl. J. Med.,* 1980, *303,* 1212; *idem,* 1981, *304,* 547; *Lancet,* 1981, *1,* 818.

The use of metronidazole for the prevention and treatment of dental caries.— Z. Tornyos *et al., Gyógyszerészet,* 1976, *20,* 72, per *Int. pharm. Abstr.,* 1977, *14,* 284.

The effect of metronidazole on the composition of bile.— T. S. Low-Beer, *Lancet,* 1978, *2,* 1063.

A discussion on the mechanism of antimicrobial action of metronidazole.— D. I. Edwards, *J. antimicrob. Chemother.,* 1979, *5,* 499.

Response of 3 patients with pneumatosis coli to treatment with metronidazole.— B. W. Ellis, *Br. med. J.,* 1980, *280,* 763. More experience is needed to establish the effectiveness and safety of antibiotic regimens for pneumatosis coli; metronidazole should be used with caution, possibly being restricted to patients in whom oxygen therapy has failed or is contra-indicated.— J. Gillon *et al.* (letter), *ibid.,* 1087.

Adjunct to radiotherapy. A review of the use of hypoxic sensitisers such as metronidazole and misonidazole as adjuncts to radiotherapy in patients with cancer.— J. D. Chapman, *New Engl. J. Med.,* 1979, *301,* 1429.

Administration of metronidazole 6 g per m^2 four hours before radiotherapy thrice weekly for 3 weeks to 16 fasting patients with supratentorial glioblastomas appeared to make the hypoxic tumour cells less resistant to radiotherapy compared with 15 control patients who received radiotherapy alone. Nitroimidazole derivatives might be useful radiosensitisers in human solid tumours.— R. Urtasun *et al., New Engl. J. Med.,* 1976, *294,* 1364. It was not clear whether the enhancing effect of metronidazole was a result of direct cytotoxicity or of radiosensitisation.— I. Tannock (letter), *ibid., 295,* 901. Follow-up of 13 patients in the radiotherapy group and 16 in the group receiving radiotherapy together with metronidazole confirmed the superiority of survival in the group receiving metronidazole as an adjunct.— R. C. Urtasun *et al.* (letter), *ibid.,* 1977, *296,* 757.

An apparently enhanced tumour response to radiotherapy in some of 36 patients with advanced head and neck tumours and 12 with alimentary metastatic adenocarcinoma, given metronidazole, might represent radiosensitisation, precision radiotherapy, or a direct cytotoxic effect of metronidazole, or a combined effect. Metronidazole was given in doses of 2.5 g daily for 5 days a week, to a total of up to 94 g.— A. B. M. F. Karim, *Br. J. Cancer,* 1978, *37, Suppl.* 3, 299.

Further references: R. L. Willson (letter), *Lancet,* 1976, *1,* 304; *ibid.,* 1978, *2,* 617; A. B. M. F. Karim (letter), *ibid.,* 891.

See also under Adverse Effects.

Administration in renal failure. Metronidazole was reported to be 20% bound to plasma proteins. The normal half-life was 6 to 14 hours. The interval between doses for bacterial infections should be extended from 8 hours to 12 hours in patients with a glomerular filtration-rate of less than 10 ml per minute. Concentrations of metronidazole were affected by haemodialysis.— W. M. Bennett *et al., Ann. intern. Med.,* 1980, *93,* 62.

Amoebiasis. For reviews of metronidazole in the treatment of amoebiasis, see *Br. med. J.,* 1970, *2,* 36; *Med. Lett.,* 1972, *14,* 39; *ibid.,* 1974, *16,* 7; E. B. Adams and I. N. MacLeod, *Medicine, Baltimore,* 1977, *56,* 315.

During a 12-month study mass treatment with metronidazole for control of amoebiasis was given to the 399 inhabitants of an Indian reservation; 4 persons developed amoebic dysentery compared with an incidence of 27 and 28 yearly in the 2 previous years. Persons weighing 50 kg and over received 2 g and those less than 50 kg received 43 mg per kg body-weight monthly for 3 doses. After 3 months the basic adult dose was reduced to 1.5 g given on alternate months, and because of a high incidence of vomiting the dose in infants and young children was reduced to 125 mg. Of the 4 patients who developed amoebiasis 2 had missed treatment for 3 or 4 months and 1 had vomited a dose 2 months earlier.— M. J. Miller *et al., Am. J. trop. Med. Hyg.,* 1972, *21,* 400, per *Trop. Dis. Bull.,* 1973, *70,* 244.

Since metronidazole did not always cure amoebiasis it was recommended that di-iodohydroxyquinoline should also be given in a dose of 2 g for adults or 40 mg per kg body-weight for a child, daily for 3 weeks.— H. B. Shookhoff and M. Katz (letter), *Lancet,* 1973, *2,* 1091. It was considered that metronidazole should be given alone for 1 or 2 ten-day courses before giving di-iodohydroxyquinoline.— F. E. Pittman (letter), *ibid.,* 1325; *idem,* 1974, *1,* 29. See also D. M. Weber, *J. Am. med. Ass.,* 1971, *216,* 1339.

A 63% cure-rate in amoebic cyst-passers (*Entamoeba histolytica* and *E. hartmanii*) after treatment with metronidazole 750 mg thrice daily for 5 days possibly reflected good absorption and therefore a low concentration in the bowel lumen.— R. Spillmann *et al., Am. J. trop. Med. Hyg.,* 1976, *25,* 549, per *Trop. Dis. Bull.,* 1977, *74,* 228.

A cure-rate of 53.3% in 30 patients with symptomatic intestinal amoebiasis treated with metronidazole 2 g daily (as a single dose) for 3 days.— N. P. Misra and R. C. Gupta, *J. int. med. Res.,* 1977, *5,* 434.

Recovery of 135 of 140 patients with pleuropulmonary amoebiasis (12 with pleural effusion, 35 with amoebic empyema, 20 with added bacterial infection, and 73 with pulmonary lesions) after treatment with metronidazole 800 mg thrice daily for 5 or 7 days, 400 mg thrice daily for 10 or 14 days, or occasionally 2 courses, with other appropriate treatment. There was no recurrence of amoebiasis in 83 patients followed for up to 2 years.— E. W. J. Cameron, *Chest,* 1978, *73,* 647.

For comparisons of tinidazole and metronidazole in the treatment of amoebiasis, see Tinidazole, p.984.

For the concomitant use of metronidazole and diloxanide furoate, see Diloxanide Furoate, p.978.

Liver abscess. In a trial in 80 adults with amoebic liver abscess who received metronidazole or other nitroimidazole derivatives, 79 were cured. Nimorazole and tinidazole appeared to have no advantages over metronidazole. It was suggested that failure of metronidazole in intestinal infections was best overcome by addition of a reliable luminal amoebicide.— S. J. Powell and R. Elsdon-Dew, *Am. J. trop. Med. Hyg.,* 1972, *21,* 518, per *Trop. Dis. Bull.,* 1973, *70,* 346.

A patient with hepatic amoebic abscess did not respond to metronidazole 750 mg eight-hourly with antibiotic therapy and drainage but recovered after therapy with chloroquine phosphate 1 g daily for 2 days then 500 mg daily and emetine hydrochloride 32 mg by intramuscular injection every 12 hours.— A. E. Stillman *et al., J. Am. med. Ass.,* 1974, *229,* 71.

For other unfavourable reports of the use of metronidazole in the treatment of patients with amoebic liver abscesses, see R. M. Henn and D. B. Collin, *J. Am. med. Ass.,* 1973, *224,* 1394; F. M. Griffin, *New Engl. J. Med.,* 1973, *288,* 1397; H. Wilde (letter), *ibid., 289,* 378; L. S. Fisher *et al., Am. J. med. Sci.,* 1976, *271,* 65.

Nine patients with amoebic liver abscess were treated with 2 intravenous infusions of metronidazole 1 g in dextrose injection given 24 hours apart and followed up with an oral dose of 400 mg thrice daily for 10 days. Pain and fever improved within 2 days and at the end of treatment all patients were considered cured.— K. G. Nair *et al.* (letter), *Lancet,* 1974, *1,* 1238.

Metronidazole usually in doses of 800 mg thrice daily for 5 days was considered to have replaced emetine as the drug of choice for the treatment of patients with amoebic liver abscess in Rhodesia; aspiration was also used when abscesses were large.— A. C. Lamont and A. C. B. Wicks, *Trans. R. Soc. trop. Med. Hyg.,* 1976, *70,*

302.

For further references to the use of metronidazole in hepatic amoebiasis, see Tinidazole, p.984.

For the use of diloxanide furoate together with metronidazole in the treatment of amoebic liver abscess, see Diloxanide Furoate, p.978.

Bacterial infections. Reviews and discussions of the use of metronidazole in anaerobic infections.— J. M. T. Hamilton-Miller, *J. antimicrob. Chemother.*, 1975, *1*, 273; R. N. Brogden *et al.*, *Drugs*, 1978, *16*, 387; *Drug & Ther. Bull.*, 1978, *16*, 9; A. J. Willis, *Br. J. Hosp. Med.*, 1978, *20*, 579; *Med. Lett.*, 1981, *23*, 13.

Metronidazole was rapidly effective in the topical treatment of anaerobically infected pressure sores. The lotion consisted of a 1% solution in sodium chloride solution 0.6% and was sterilised by autoclaving at 121° for 20 minutes.— P. H. Jones *et al.* (letter), *Lancet*, 1978, *1*, 214. A report of beneficial results with metronidazole 400 mg thrice daily by mouth for 7 days in patients with foul-smelling pressure sores or venous ulcers.— P. G. Baker and G. Haig, *Practitioner*, 1981, *225*, 569. Criticism of the study.— *Drug & Ther. Bull.*, 1981, *20*, 9.

The smell of some fungating tumours is identical to that associated with anaerobic infection, suggesting that it may be caused by colonisation of the tumour with anaerobes. A 48-year-old teacher with an offensive ulcerated right axillary tumour secondary to a breast carcinoma was accordingly given metronidazole 200 mg thrice daily. Within a week the odour had almost entirely disappeared and she was able to continue working as a teacher, which would otherwise have been impossible.— R. F. U. Ashford *et al.* (letter), *Lancet*, 1980, *1*, 874. Nine patients with fungating breast carcinoma causing an offensive smell were treated with metronidazole 400 mg thrice daily. The smell was reduced considerably in all 9 patients and in 4 it disappeared completely. Two patients experienced nausea which disappeared when the dose was reduced to 200 mg thrice daily, without impairing the clinical response. The topical efficacy of metronidazole 1% in 0.6% saline applied twice daily is now being investigated.— G. Sparrow *et al.* (letter), *ibid.*, 1185. See also D. C. Doll and K. J. Doll (letter), *Ann. intern. Med.*, 1981, *94*, 139 (malodorous tumours); J. Dankert *et al.* (letter), *Lancet*, 1981, *2*, 1295 (tumours of the ovary and cervix).

Further references: D. A. McGowan *et al.*, *Br. dent. J.*, 1977, *142*, 221; D. J. Sharp *et al.*, *J. antimicrob. Chemother.*, 1977, *3*, 233; H. Giamarellou *et al.*, *ibid.*, 347; S. Rom *et al.*, *Archs Dis. Childh.*, 1977, *52*, 740; C. H. Webb (letter), *Lancet*, 1977, *2*, 511; F. J. C. Hood, *J. antimicrob. Chemother.*, 1978, *4*, *Suppl.* C, 71; E. Bäck *et al.*, *Scand. J. infect. Dis.*, 1978, *10*, 152; R. D. Leach *et al.*, *Br. med. J.*, 1979, *2*, 5; B. Christensson *et al.*, *Scand. J. infect. Dis.*, 1979, *11*, 69; C. V. Sanders *et al.*, *Am. Rev. resp. Dis.*, 1979, *120*, 337; M. R. Perera *et al.*, *Lancet*, 1980, *2*, 629; S. Reilly and A. T. Willis (letter), *ibid.*, 970; M. Perera *et al.*, *J. antimicrob. Chemother.*, 1980, *6*, 105.

See also under Colitis and Vaginitis.

Antibacterial activity. The following anaerobic bacteria were inhibited by 3.1 µg per ml of metronidazole and killed by 6.3 µg per ml: *Bacteroides fragilis* and *melaninogenicus*, *Clostridium perfringens* and other species of clostridia, *Eubacterium*, *Fusobacterium*, *Peptococcus*, *Peptostreptococcus*, and *Veillonella spp*. *Proprionibacterium acnes* was relatively resistant. The same figures were achieved with tinidazole and ornidazole.— J. Wüst, *Antimicrob. Ag. Chemother.*, 1977, *11*, 631.

The median minimum inhibitory concentration of metronidazole against 40 strains of *Bacteroides* spp. was 0.25 µg per ml.— R. Wise *et al.*, *Chemotherapy, Basle*, 1977, *23*, 19.

Metronidazole inhibited 27, 45, 64, 73, and 100% of 11 strains of *Campylobacter fetus in vitro* at concentrations of 0.2, 0.4, 3.1, 6.2, and 12.5 µg per ml respectively.— A. W. Chow *et al.*, *Antimicrob. Ag. Chemother.*, 1978, *13*, 416.

At concentrations of about 5 times their MICs, metronidazole and nitrofurantoin had a similar bactericidal effect against 2 strains of *Bacteroides fragilis* and 2 of *Clostridium perfringens in vitro*. A more rapid effect was obtained with increasing concentrations of each drug. When used together against *Bacteroides fragilis* metronidazole and nitrofurantoin had an additive effect.— E. D. Ralph, *J. antimicrob. Chemother.*, 1978, *4*, 177.

Although the presence of aerobic bacteria in mixed cultures with *Bacteroides fragilis* did not inhibit the bactericidal activity of metronidazole against the latter organism it was considered that, *in vivo*, aerobic bacteria capable of inactivating metronidazole might still be capable of inhibiting the activity of metronidazole against anaerobes in mixed infections.— E. D. Ralph and D. A. Clarke, *Antimicrob. Ag. Chemother.*, 1978, *14*, 377.

When neomycin and metronidazole were given together to healthy subjects there was a reduction in both aerobic and anaerobic bacteria in the colon. Metronidazole alone had had no effect on anaerobic faecal bacteria and neomycin had been effective only against sensitive aerobes.— Y. Arabi *et al.*, *J. antimicrob. Chemother.*, 1979, *5*, 531.

Studies *in vitro* indicated that several organisms commonly found in the vagina are capable of absorbing and inactivating significant amounts of metronidazole at drug concentrations which are readily achievable in vaginal fluid. The effect may extend to other nitroimidazole drugs.— D. I. Edwards *et al.* (letter), *J. antimicrob. Chemother.*, 1979, *5*, 315. Criticism.— H. R. Ingham *et al.* (letter), *ibid.*, 734. Reply.— D. I. Edwards and D. Shanson (letter), *ibid.*, 1980, *6*, 402.

When incubated in suitable anaerobic condititons in the presence of metronidazole, the count of *Escherichia coli* and other Gram-negative facultative anaerobes was greatly reduced in 24 hours. This might explain why facultative anaerobes did not produce appreciable sepsis when metronidazole was used.— H. R. Ingham *et al.* (letter), *Lancet*, 1979, *2*, 902.

Metronidazole at the therapeutically attainable concentration of 10 µg per ml exhibited considerable activity against many Gram-negative facultative anaerobes examined but only under conditions of extreme anaerobiosis. All the organisms which were sensitive to metronidazole were found to inactive the compound under anaerobic and aerobic growth conditions.— H. R. Ingham *et al.*, *J. antimicrob. Chemother.*, 1980, *6*, 343.

A discussion on whether the efficacy of metronidazole against mixed infections, despite its lack of activity *in vitro* against aerobes, supports the hypothesis of bacterial synergy in the development of wound sepsis.— *Lancet*, 1980, *1*, 405. Comments and criticisms: F. Namavar *et al.* (letter), *ibid.*, 659; H. R. Ingham *et al.* (letter), *ibid;* J. Dankert *et al.* (letter), *ibid.*, 714; G. R. Jones (letter), *ibid.*, 829.

In a study of the activity of metronidazole used with 6 antimicrobial agents, the greatest enhancement of activity *in vitro* against 25 strains of *Bacteroides fragilis* was obtained when metronidazole was used with nalidixic acid, clindamycin, or rifampicin. However the effect was obtained against less than 50% of the strains and was reduced with a larger inoculum.— E. D. Ralph and Y. E. Amatnieks, *Antimicrob. Ag. Chemother.*, 1980, *17*, 379.

Metronidazole at a concentration of 1 µg per ml inhibited *in vitro* 98% of 84 strains of *Clostridium difficile* isolated from the stools of patients with antibiotic-associated diarrhoea or colitis; 99% of the strains were inhibited by 2 µg per ml.— J. Dzink and J. G. Bartlett, *Antimicrob. Ag. Chemother.*, 1980, *17*, 695.

Reports and studies of metronidazole-resistant strains of *Bacteroides fragilis*.— H. R. Ingham *et al.* (letter), *Lancet*, 1978, *1*, 214; V. O. Rotimi *et al.* (letter), *ibid.*, 1979, *1*, 833; M. L. Britz and R. G. Wilkinson, *Antimicrob. Ag. Chemother.*, 1979, *16*, 19.

Brain abscess. In 9 patients with intracranial abscess secondary to chronic middle-ear infection, *Bacteroides* spp. (usually *B. fragilis*) were cultured from pus from all patients and aerobic bacteria from 5. All patients were treated initially with metronidazole 400 to 600 mg eight-hourly by mouth or intravenously, penicillin 600 mg or ampicillin 500 mg six-hourly, and gentamicin 80 mg eight-hourly, subsequent antibiotic treatment being modified according to the bacteriological results. All the patients survived; one, who was comatose for many weeks, had residual cerebellar ataxia; the others were free from neurological deficit.— H. R. Ingham *et al.*, *Br. med. J.*, 1977, *2*, 991. Another report on the same patients.— *idem*, *J. antimicrob. Chemother.*, 1978, *4*, *Suppl.* C, 63. A further case.— R. H. George and A. J. Bint, *J. antimicrob. Chemother.*, 1976, *2*, 101.

Endocarditis. The successful use of metronidazole and ampicillin to control *Fusobacterium* endocarditis in a 27-year-old man; valve replacement was later needed.— J. Seggie, *Br. med. J.*, 1978, *1*, 960.

Further references.— J. N. Galgiani *et al.*, *Am. J. Med.*, 1978, *65*, 284; *J. Am. med. Ass.*, 1978, *239*, 2103.

Meningitis. For reports of the use of metronidazole in meningitis due to *Bacteroides*, *Fusobacterium*, and *Peptostreptococcus* spp., see L. R. O'Grady and E. D. Ralph, *Am. J. Dis. Child.*, 1976, *130*, 871; W. E. Feldman, *ibid.*, 880; B. W. Berman *et al.*, *J. Pediat.*, 1978, *93*, 793, per *Abstr. Hyg.*, 1979, *54*, 659; D. I. Peterson *et al.*, *Ann. Neurol.*, 1979, *6*, 364; C. S. Bryan *et al.*, *Sth. med. J.*, 1979, *72*, 494; J. F. Warner *et al.*, *Archs intern. Med.*, 1979, *139*, 167.

Pneumonia. A favourable report on the concomitant use of cephalosporins, penicillin, and metronidazole in 80 patients with chronic destructive pneumonia.— E. W. J. Cameron, *S. Afr. med. J.*, 1978, *54*, 57. Comment.— *Lancet*, 1980, *2*, 350.

Prophylaxis in surgery. Reports of regimens for surgical infection prophylaxis with metronidazole and other antibacterial agents: *Lancet*, 1974, *2*, 1540 (gynaecological surgery; metronidazole); A. T. Willis *et al.*, *Br. med. J.*, 1976, *1*, 318 (appendicectomy; metronidazole); A. T. Willis *et al.*, *Br. med. J.*, 1977, *1*, 607 (colonic surgery; metronidazole); S. A. Taylor and H. M. Cawdery, *Proc. R. Soc. Med.*, 1977, *70*, 481 (metronidazole with phthalylsulphathiazole); E. C. Ashby *et al.*, *Br. med. J.*, 1978, *2*, 1263 (prostatic biopsy; metronidazole with ampicillin or co-trimoxazole); N. Pashby and W. M. Mee, *J. antimicrob. Chemother.*, 1978, *4*, *Suppl.* C, 25 (appendicectomy; metronidazole); G. Gillespie and W. McNaught, *J. antimicrob. Chemother.*, 1978, *4*, *Suppl.* C, 29 (colonic surgery; metronidazole and kanamycin by mouth); M. R. B. Keighley *et al.*, *Lancet*, 1979, *1*, 894 (colorectal surgery; parenteral metronidazole and kanamycin); S. J. Eykyn *et al.*, *Lancet*, 1979, *2*, 761 (colorectal surgery; metronidazole intravenously); D. J. Pinto and P. J. Sanderson, *Br. med. J.*, 1980, *280*, 275 (appendicectomy; metronidazole and metronidazole with cephazolin or an aminoglycoside); A. V. Pollock and M. Evans (letter), *New Engl. J. Med.*, 1980, *303*, 1066 (colorectal surgery; comparison of neomycin and metronidazole with neomycin and erythromycin); M. M. Hares *et al.* (letter), *Lancet*, 1980, *1*, 1028 (amputation; metronidazole with neomycin compared with phenoxymethylpenicillin).

Further references to metronidazole being used in abdominal, gynaecological, or rectal surgery: C. Brass *et al.*, *Am. J. Surg.*, 1978, *135*, 91; *Lancet*, 1978, *2*, 1132; P. C. Appelbaum *et al.*, *S. Afr. med. J.*, 1978, *54*, 703; J. Goulton and P. G. Baker, *J. int. med. Res.*, 1978, *6*, 471; J. Goulton *et al.*, *ibid.*, 1979, *7*, 100; P. Jackson *et al.*, *N.Z. med. J.*, 1979, *89*, 243; D. Heginbotham and A. M. Rutherford, *ibid.*, 246; J. Rodgers *et al.*, *Br. J. Surg.*, 1979, *66*, 425; M. J. Greenall *et al.*, *ibid.*, 428; R. J. Salem *et al.*, *ibid.*, 430; T. Bjerkeset and A. Digranes, *Surgery, St Louis*, 1980, *87*, 560; T. B. Hagen *et al.*, *Acta chir. scand.*, 1980, *146*, 71; W. T. Morris *et al.*, *Aust. N.Z. J. Surg.*, 1980, *50*, 429; T. Bjerkeset, *Scand. J. Gastroenterol.*, 1980, *15*, *Suppl.* 58, 110; T. Løtveit *et al.*, *ibid.*, 111; T. Bergan *et al.*, *ibid.*, 113; F. Gottrup, *ibid.*, 114; M. Roland *et al.*, *ibid.*, 115; R. V. Fiddian, *ibid.*, 116; G. E. Foster *et al.*, *Lancet*, 1981, *1*, 769.

Use in obstetrics. Metronidazole, 500 mg given intravenously immediately before caesarean section, followed by 2 g rectally on completion of surgery, failed to reduce the incidence of postoperative infection in 35 patients compared with 38 patients who received a placebo. The use of short-course metronidazole cannot be justified in patients undergoing caesarean section but a longer course continuing after delivery may be effective in reducing postoperative morbidity.— L. McCowan and P. Jackson, *N.Z. med. J.*, 1980, *92*, 153.

Balantidiasis. Metronidazole in doses recommended for the treatment of amoebiasis failed to eliminate *Balantidium coli* from the stools of 3 of 5 patients. It was considered that metronidazole was not effective therapy for human balantidiasis.— J. W. Beasley and P. D. Walzer (letter), *Trans. R. Soc. trop. Med. Hyg.*, 1972, *66*, 519.

Metronidazole 200 mg twice daily for 5 days was effective in the treatment of a girl with a mixed bowel infection, including *Balantidium coli*, which had not responded to chloroquine or to chloramphenicol.— A. J. Radford, *Med. J. Aust.*, 1973, *1*, 238.

Twenty patients with balantidiasis were effectively treated with metronidazole. A dose of 1 g daily for adults or 500 mg daily for children for 5 days was as effective as 1.25 g and 750 mg respectively daily for 10 days.— A. Garcia-Laverde and L. De Bonilla, *Am. J. trop. Med. Hyg.*, 1975, *24*, 781, per *Trop. Dis. Bull.*, 1976, *73*, 235.

Colitis. Metronidazole 1.5 g daily produced rapid improvement in a patient with ampicillin-induced colitis.— H. T. Dinh *et al.* (letter), *Lancet*, 1978, *1*, 338. A dramatic clinical response had been obtained in 3 patients with pseudomembranous colitis, on administration of metronidazole 1.5 g daily for 15 days.— C. Matuchansky *et al.* (letter), *Lancet*, 1978, *2*, 580. Metronidazole by mouth eliminated *Clostridium difficile* and its toxin from 2 patients who had colitis after taking clindamycin.— N. L. Pashby *et al.*, *Br. med. J.*, 1979, *1*, 1605. *Clostridium difficile*-associated colitis in a patient treated with neomycin responded to treatment with metronidazole.— R. P. Bolton, *Br. med. J.*, 1979, *2*, 1479.

Two cases of *Clostridium difficile* colitis unresponsive to metronidazole.— G. A. G. Mogg *et al.* (letter), *Br. med. J.*, 1979, *2*, 335.

Clostridium difficile-associated colitis developed in a 46-year-old woman given metronidazole 250 mg thrice daily for 10 days. The patient had received no other antimicrobial agents in the previous year. *Clostridium difficile* and a cytopathic toxin neutralised by *Clostridium sordellii* antitoxin were isolated from stools. The isolate was susceptible to metronidazole at a concentration of 0.25 µg per ml.— R. Saginur *et al.*, *J. infect. Dis.*, 1980, *141*, 772. A report of pseudomembranous colitis associated with the use of metronidazole alone. *Clostridium difficile* was not isolated and might not be the sole causative agent.— G. Thomson *et al.*, *Br. med. J.*, 1981, *282*, 864.

Pseudomembranous colitis in a 15-year-old girl previously given cephazolin sodium and metronidazole responded to treatment with vancomycin followed by metronidazole. *Clostridium difficile* could not be detected.— R. K. S. Phillips *et al.*, *Br. med. J.*, 1981, *283*, 823.

Differing views on whether metronidazole should be used as an alternative to vancomycin in the treatment of pseudomembranous colitis.— R. P. Bolton (letter), *Br. med. J.*, 1981, *283*, 311; C. R. Pennington (letter), *ibid.*, 558; J. R. D. Brown (letter), *ibid.*, 1334.

For a view that metronidazole is a suitable drug for the treatment of pseudomembranous colitis, see Vancomycin Hydrochloride, p.1230.

Crohn's disease. Of 19 patients (6 with small-bowel diverticulosis and 13 with Crohn's disease) treated with metronidazole 200 mg eight-hourly for 4 weeks, 8 were unable to tolerate the drug because of severe lethargy, anorexia, nausea, and a sore furred tongue. Concentrations in serum were in the range 8 to 16 µg per ml.— J. H. B. Scarpello (letter), *Br. med. J.*, 1977, *1*, 104.

In a double-blind crossover study 20 patients with Crohn's disease, usually taking sulphasalazine or prednisone, or both, were treated for 2-month periods with metronidazole 250 mg four times daily or placebo, in addition to their usual treatment. There was no overall significant difference in the clinical or laboratory signs, but 6 patients with colonic involvement only showed striking improvement in diarrhoea, abdominal pain, and feeling of well-being.— P. Blichfeldt *et al.*, *Scand. J. Gastroenterol.*, 1978, *13*, 923.

Metronidazole 20 mg per kg body-weight daily in divided doses produced a decrease in drainage, erythema, and induration in all of 21 patients treated for chronic unremitting Crohn's disease. Nineteen patients had been unsuccessfully treated with other agents and 12 were on medication to which metronidazole was added. Of 17 patients who were maintained on metronidazole for 5 to 21 months, 10 had complete healing and 5 had advanced healing. Dosage had to be reduced in 4 patients and discontinued in one because of peripheral neuropathy.— L. H. Bernstein *et al.*, *Gastroenterology*, 1980, *79*, 357. Comment.— D. B. Sachar, *ibid.*, 393.

Further references: B. Ursing, *Scand. J. Gastroenterol.*, 1980, *15*, *Suppl.* 58, 117; J. P. Blomhoff, *ibid.*, 118.

Fascioliasis. Successful treatment of fascioliasis in 4 patients with metronidazole 1.5 g daily for 13 to 28 days.— B. Nik-Akhtar and V. Tabibi, *J. trop. Med. Hyg.*, 1977, *80*, 179, per *Trop. Dis. Bull.*, 1978, *75*, 376.

Filariasis. Metronidazole 400 mg thrice daily for 10 days was successful in the treatment of a patient with microfilariae resistant to treatment with diethylcarbamazine by mouth and by injection, and to injections of sodium fluoride.— P. D. Anjaria *et al.*, *J. Ass. Physns India*, 1972, *20*, 55, per *Trop. Dis. Bull.*, 1972, *69*, 941.

Giardiasis. Metronidazole in doses of 250 mg thrice daily for 7 days did not appear to be as effective as mepacrine in the treatment of giardiasis. It was more successful in the treatment of combined amoebiasis and giardiasis at a dose of 500 to 750 mg thrice daily for 10 days followed by di-iodohydroxyquinoline 650 mg thrice daily for 20 days.— M. S. Wolfe, *J. Am. med. Ass.*, 1975, *233*, 1362.

An 86.9% cure-rate in giardiasis after treatment with metronidazole 250 mg twice daily for 7 days.— G. C. Levi *et al.*, *Am. J. trop. Med. Hyg.*, 1977, *26*, 564, per *Trop. Dis. Bull.*, 1978, *75*, 648.

A 91% cure-rate in giardiasis after treatment with metronidazole 2 g once daily for 3 days.— S. G. Wright *et al.*, *Gut*, 1977, *18*, 343.

Cure in 11 of 15 patients with giardiasis given metronidazole 200 mg thrice daily for 7 days; in 14 of 15 when the course was repeated after a week; in 9 of 15 after a single dose of 2.4 g; and in 12 of 15 after 2.4 g daily for 2 days.— L. Jokipii and A. M. M. Jokipii, *Infection*, 1978, *6*, 92.

A recommended dose of metronidazole for giardiasis in infants and children: 15 to 25 mg per kg body-weight daily for 5 days.— S. Kavousi, *Am. J. trop. Med. Hyg.*, 1979, *28*, 19.

Further references: L. Jokipii and A. M. M. Jokipii, *J. infect. Dis.*, 1979, *140*, 984.

Guinea-worm infection. Treatment with metronidazole 200 mg thrice daily for 7 days was effective in all but 3 of 116 patients treated and all experienced relief of clinical symptoms; excision of lesions and treatment with procaine penicillin was also necessary for those patients with cellulitis. Side-effects which did not interfere with treatment were reported in 62 patients.— J. A. Antani *et al.*, *Am. J. trop. Med. Hyg.*, 1972, *21*, 178, per *Trop. Dis. Bull.*, 1973, *70*, 475.

For an unfavourable report of the use of metronidazole 200 mg thrice daily for 7 days in the treatment of guinea-worm infection, see D. R. Kulkarni and S. J. Nagalotimath (letter), *Trans. R. Soc. trop. Med. Hyg.*, 1975, *69*, 169.

An 85% cure-rate in 20 days in a double-blind study in which 118 patients with guinea-worm infection were given metronidazole 400 mg twice daily for 10 days.— D. S. Pardanani *et al.*, *Ann. trop. Med. Parasit.*, 1977, *71*, 45, per *Trop. Dis. Bull.*, 1977, *74*, 532.

Further references: R. Muller, *Bull. Wld Hlth Org.*, 1979, *57*, 683.

Leishmaniasis. Metronidazole in doses of 250 mg thrice daily for two ten-day periods with an interval of 10 days was successful in the treatment of cutaneous leishmaniasis in a 24-year-old man.— P. I. Long, *J. Am. med. Ass.*, 1973, *223*, 1378.

Metronidazole was not effective in the treatment of American leishmaniasis, due to *Leishmania brasiliensis*, in 5 of 6 patients.— B. C. Walton *et al.*, *J. Am. med. Ass.*, 1974, *228*, 1256.

Metronidazole 500 mg thrice daily for 4 to 8 weeks caused no changes in the lesions of 5 patients with Ethiopian mucocutaneous leishmaniasis.— A. Belehu *et al.*, *Br. J. Derm.*, 1978, *99*, 421.

For a report of the use of co-trimoxazole with metronidazole in the treatment of visceral leishmaniasis, see under Co-trimoxazole, p.1465.

Mononucleosis. A favourable report of the use of metronidazole in 'anginose' mononucleosis.— S. Å. Hedström *et al.*, *Scand. J. infect. Dis.*, 1978, *10*, 7, per *Abstr. Hyg.*, 1978, *53*, 515.

Skin disorders. Ten of 15 patients with rosacea of varying severity not responsive to tetracycline showed a good response to treatment with metronidazole 200 mg twice daily for 6 weeks; 2 of 14 similar patients responded to a placebo. One patient in each group withdrew from treatment after 2 to 3 days because of headache.— R. J. Pye and J. L. Burton, *Lancet*, 1976, *1*, 1211. See also E. M. Saihan and J. L. Burton, *Br. J. Derm.*, 1980, *102*, 443.

Five patients with acne improved when given metronidazole and this improvement was greater than that previously achieved with tetracycline in 2 of the patients.— S. Carne (letter), *Lancet*, 1976, *2*, 367.

Resolution of long-standing prurigo nodularis while receiving metronidazole.— S. M. Wood *et al* (letter), *Br. med. J.*, 1979, *1*, 552.

Syphilis. Metronidazole 2 to 4 g daily for 5 to 9 days healed syphilitic lesions after 4 to 7 days in 6 patients with secondary syphilis. Healing was complete in 2 to 3 weeks. Serum concentrations of metronidazole varied from 15 to 72 µg per ml.— A. H. Davies, *Br. J. vener. Dis.*, 1967, *43*, 197, per *Abstr. Hyg.*, 1968, *43*, 152. There was no evidence of healing in a syphilitic lesion after a week's treatment with metronidazole by mouth.— A. E. Wilkinson *et al.*, *Br. J. vener. Dis.*, 1967, *43*, 201, per *Abstr. Hyg.*, 1968, *43*, 152.

Trichomoniasis. Of 63 patients with vaginal trichomoniasis all of 52 followed up were free of infection 2 weeks after taking metronidazole 500 mg twice daily for 3 days.— H. Nouira, *Practitioner*, 1978, *220*, 790.

Metronidazole 800 mg or nimorazole 750 mg given every 12 hours for 2 days to women with trichomonal vaginitis produced cure-rates of 97.6% and 98.8% respectively.— A. Saeed *et al.*, *Br. J. clin. Pract.*, 1980, *34*, 41.

Reports and discussions on the resistance of *Trichomonas vaginalis* to metronidazole.— J. Thurner and J. G. Meingassner (letter), *Lancet*, 1978, *2*, 738; A. Forsgren and L. Forssman, *Br. J. vener. Dis.*, 1979, *55*, 351; R. Heyworth *et al.* (letter), *Lancet*, 1980, *2*, 476; J. G. Lossick (letter), *New Engl. J. Med.*, 1981, *304*, 735; P. Goldman (letter), *ibid.*; S. A. Waitkins and D. J. Thomas (letter), *Lancet*, 1981, *2*, 590; J. Goulton and S. Squires (letter), *ibid.*, 1982, *1*, 42.

Single-dose treatment. Metronidazole given as a single dose of 2 g was slightly more effective in curing trichomonal vaginitis than when given as the usual dose of 200 mg thrice daily for 7 days.— R. A. Underhill and J. E. Peck, *Br. J. clin. Pract.*, 1974, *28*, 134.

Metronidazole as a single 2-g dose gave a success-rate of 93% in women with trichomonal vaginitis, compared with an 89% response with the same dose of nimorazole.— J. D. H. Mahony *et al.*, *Br. J. clin. Pract.*, 1975, *29*, 71. See also J. S. McCann *et al.*, *Br. J. vener. Dis.*, 1972, *48*, 387, per *Abstr. Hyg.*, 1973, *48*, 425.

In 19 patients a single dose of 1.5 g of metronidazole for patients and their consorts was usually effective.— J. R. Dykers (letter), *New Engl. J. Med.*, 1976, *295*, 395.

Trichomonal vaginitis in 243 women was treated by a single 2-g dose of metronidazole; male consorts were given similar treatment. Of 203 women who were re-examined 190 were cured, 3 were re-infected and these and 3 others were cured by a further 2-g dose; 1 was pregnant and was not re-treated; the remaining 6 were cured after receiving 500 mg twice daily for 5 days or 250 mg thrice daily for 10 days, one needing metronidazole vaginal suppositories presumably because of failure to absorb the drug when given by mouth.— F. J. Fleury *et al.*, *Am. J. Obstet. Gynec.*, 1977, *128*, 320.

Further studies with favourable results of the use of single 2-g doses of metronidazole in the treatment of trichomonal vaginitis: J. R. Dykers, *Am. J. Obstet. Gynec.*, 1978, *132*, 579; R. N. Thin *et al.*, *Br. J. vener. Dis.*, 1979, *55*, 354; V. D. Hager *et al.*, *J. Am. med. Ass.*, 1980, *244*, 1219.

Tropical eosinophilia. Metronidazole 1 g thrice daily for 2 days was no more effective than doses of 400 mg thrice daily for 5 days for the treatment of tropical pulmonary eosinophilia; the cure-rate in each group of 20 patients was about 40% and the eosinophil count fell slowly. No relapses were reported among any of these patients.— N. R. Rao and V. V. Reddy, *J. trop. Med. Hyg.*, 1973, *76*, 147, per *Trop. Dis. Bull.*, 1973, *70*, 1112.

Improvement in the clinical index, with less improvement in the eosinophil count, in 20 patients with tropical eosinophilia treated with metronidazole 400 mg thrice daily for 5 days.— A. B. Vaidya *et al.*, *Indian J. med. Sci.*, 1976, *30*, 309, per *Trop. Dis. Bull.*, 1978, *75*, 1044.

Vaginitis. *Gardnerella vaginalis* (*Haemophilus vaginalis*) was implicated as a cause of nonspecific vaginitis. Clinical improvement and eradication of *G. vaginalis* was achieved in 80 of 81 women given metronidazole 500 mg twice daily for 7 days compared with 8 of 27 given ampicillin 500 mg four times daily for 7 days, 2 of 15 given doxycycline 100 mg twice daily for 7 days, and 1 of 7 who used a sulphonamide vaginal cream (Sultrin) twice daily for 10 days.— T. A. Pheifer *et al.*, *New Engl. J. Med.*, 1978, *298*, 1429.

During a placebo-controlled study of treatment regimens for *Gardnerella vaginalis* (*Haemophilus vaginalis*) vaginitis in 30 patients, sensitivity tests *in vitro* demonstrated a comparative insensitivity to metronidazole. Of 47 of the strains isolated, 33 showed sensitivity, 5 at 10 µg [per ml], 13 at 25 µg, and 15 at 50 µg. Despite this, 15 of 17 infected women showed clinical and bacteriological cure after administration of metronidazole 400 mg twice daily for 7 days; one was clinically cured but *G. vaginalis* was isolated in moderate growth, and one who was clinically and bacteriologically negative on follow-up subsequently relapsed. The effectiveness of metronidazole was difficult to reconcile with the comparative insensitivity *in vitro* of the organism and merits further study.— M. J. Balsdon *et al.*, *Lancet*, 1980, *1*, 501. Criticism.— B. A. Evans (letter), *ibid.*, 1029. Reply.— M. J. Balsdon and R. Maskell (letter), *ibid.*, *2*, 151. Findings suggesting that the efficacy of metronidazole in the treatment of vaginitis associated with *G. vaginalis* may be due in part to the activity of the 2-hydroxymethyl metabolite.— M. J. Balsdon and D. Jackson (letter), *ibid.*, 1981, *1*, 1112.

See also Trichomoniasis, above.

Vincent's infection. Metronidazole 200 mg thrice daily for a week or standard doses of phenoxymethylpenicillin for a week were both effective treatments for the acute phase of Vincent's infection, but should be followed by the appropriate dental care and maintenance to eliminate the infection.— A. D. Macalister, *Drugs*, 1973, *5*, 453. Metronidazole was preferred to penicillin in the treatment of acute ulcerative gingivitis as it avoided the risk of hypersensitivity and the development of resistance.— R. Duckworth, *Br. dent. J.*, 1973, *135*, 168.

Preparations

Metronidazole Tablets *(B.P.).* Tablets containing metronidazole.

Metronidazole Tablets *(U.S.P.).* Tablets containing metronidazole. Protect from light.

Proprietary Preparations

Flagyl *(May & Baker, UK).* Metronidazole, available as **Suppositories** of 0.5 and 1 g and as scored **Tablets** of 200 and 400 mg. **Flagyl Compak.** Packs containing 21 tablets (200 mg) and 14 vaginal tablets each containing nystatin 100 000 units. For vaginal trichomoniasis and candidiasis. *Dose.* 1 tablet thrice daily and 1 vaginal tablet night and morning for 7 days. (Also available as Flagyl in *Arg., Austral., Belg., Canad., Denm., Fr., Ger., Ital., Neth., Norw., NZ, S.Afr., Spain, Swed., Switz., USA*).

Flagyl Injection *(May & Baker, UK).* Metronidazole, available as a solution for intravenous infusion containing 5 mg per ml, in ampoules of 20 ml and in bottles or plastic bags containing 100 ml.

See under Benzoyl Metronidazole (p.974) for an oral suspension (Flagyl-S).

Vaginyl *(DDSA Pharmaceuticals, UK).* Metronidazole, available as scored tablets of 200 mg.

Other Proprietary Names

Arg.—Debetrol, Nalox, Tranoxa, Tricofin Oral; *Austral.*—Trichozole; *Canad.*—Neo-Tric, Novonidazol, Trikacide; *Denm.*—Elyzol, Trichomal; *Ger.*—Clont, Fossyol, Kreucosan, Rathimed N, Sanatrichom, Trichos Cordes, Tricho-Gynaedron oral; *Hung.*—Klion (see also under Benzoyl Metronidazole); *Ital.*—Deflamon, Gineflavir, Tricocet, Trivazol, Vagilen; *Jap.*—Meronidal, Nida, Salandol, Trichocide; *Norw.*—Elyzol; *Pol.*—Entizol; *Spain*— Tricowas B; *Swed.*— Elyzol; *Switz.*—Metrolag.

4752-k

Acetarsol *(B.P.).*

Acetarsolum; Acetarsone; Acetphenarsinum; Osarsolum; Acetaminohydroxyphenylarsonsäure. 3-Acetamido-4-hydroxyphenylarsonic acid.
$C_8H_{10}AsNO_5$=275.1.

CAS — 97-44-9.

Pharmacopoeias. In *Aust., Br., Fr., Int., Nord., Pol., Port., Rus., Span.,* and *Turk.*

A white odourless crystalline powder with a faintly acid taste containing about 27% of As. M.p. about 240° with decomposition.

Practically **insoluble** in cold water, alcohol, and dilute acids; soluble in dilute alkalis; moderately soluble in boiling water. A saturated solution in water is acid to litmus.

Adverse Effects. Acetarsol taken by mouth gives rise to gastro-intestinal irritation and to cutaneous eruptions as for Arsenic Trioxide (see p.1680). The use of vaginal tablets may give rise to local irritation; dermatitis has been reported.

Acute and fatal arsenical poisoning occurred in a 28-year-old woman. In an attempt to deal with resistant trichomonal vaginitis, the vagina had been packed for 2 alternate days with a total of 30 acetarsol pessaries.— D. A. L. Bowen *et al., Br. med. J.,* 1961, *1,* 1282.

Treatment of Adverse Effects. Symptoms of arsenical poisoning may be treated with dimercaprol (see p.383).

Precautions. Acetarsol is contra-indicated in the presence of cardiovascular disease, impaired liver or kidney function, optic neuritis, fever, or recent haemorrhage.

Absorption and Fate. Acetarsol is readily absorbed from the gastro-intestinal tract and most of the dose is excreted in the urine. Small amounts are stored in the liver and other tissues. Concentrations have been reported in the cerebrospinal fluid.

Uses. Acetarsol acts principally in the bowel lumen and has been used in the treatment of intestinal amoebiasis, being given by mouth in a dose of up to 250 mg twice daily for a period of 10 days, often in conjunction with other amoebicides. It has been largely replaced by less toxic drugs.

Trichomonal vaginitis has been treated by local application of acetarsol, in the form of vaginal tablets. Suppositories of acetarsol, usually containing 250 mg, have been employed in the treatment of proctitis.

Preparations

Acetarsol Pessaries *(B.P.).* Acetarsol Vaginal Tablets. Each contains acetarsol 250 mg, anhydrous dextrose 320 mg, and starch 350 mg. They may be prepared with any other suitable basis, including an effervescent basis. To be inserted, without previously moistening, into the vagina. *A.P.F.* and *Nord. P.* include similar pessaries.

Acetarsol Suppositories *(Middlesex Hosp.).* Acetarsol 250 mg, Witepsol H15 to 2 g. Shelf-life 6 months. For proctitis.

Acetarsol Tablets *(B.P.C. 1973).* Acetarsone Tablets. Tablets containing acetarsol.

Proprietary Preparations

SVC (Acetarsol Vaginal Compound) *(May & Baker, UK).* Effervescent vaginal tablets each containing acetarsol 250 mg, with carbohydrate. (Also available as SVC in *S.Afr.*).

Other Proprietary Names

Gynoplix *(Ital.)*; Stovarsol *(Fr.)*; Vagoflor *(Switz.)*.

4753-a

Acetarsol Sodium. The pentahydrate of the sodium salt of 3-acetamido-4-hydroxyphenylarsonic acid.
$C_8H_9AsNNaO_5,5H_2O$=387.2.

CAS — 5892-48-8 (anhydrous).

Pharmacopoeias. In *Fr.* and *Span.*

White crystals or a white crystalline powder. **Soluble** 1 in 7 of water; practically insoluble in alcohol, chloroform, acetone, and ether. A saturated solution in water has a pH of about 5.8.

Uses. Acetarsol sodium has been used for the administration of acetarsol by injection, subcutaneously or intravenously.

4754-t

Acinitrazole *(B. Vet. C. 1965).* Aminitrozole; Nithiamide; CL 5279. *N*-(5-Nitrothiazol-2-yl)acetamide.
$C_5H_5N_3O_3S$=187.2.

CAS — 140-40-9.

Pharmacopoeias. In *Cz.*

A buff or yellowish-buff, almost tasteless powder with a slight odour. Very slightly **soluble** in water; soluble 1 in 300 of alcohol and 1 in 900 of chloroform; slightly soluble in ether.

Acinitrazole has been used in veterinary medicine in the prevention and treatment of blackhead (histomoniasis) in turkeys. Reference has also been made to its use in swine dysentery.

Proprietary Names

Tricomon *(IBE, Spain)*; Tricosil *(Panthox & Burck, Ital.)*; Trigamma *(IBP, Ital.)*.

4755-x

Arsthinol. Arsthinenol. 2′-Hydroxy-5′-(4-hydroxymethyl-1,3,2-dithiarsolan-2-yl)acetanilide.
$C_{11}H_{14}AsNO_3S_2$=347.3.

CAS — 119-96-0.

An odourless white microcrystalline powder. Very slightly **soluble** in water and ether; soluble 1 in 40 of alcohol.

Adverse Effects. As for Acetarsol, above.

Uses. Arsthinol has been used in the treatment of intestinal amoebiasis.

4756-r

Benznidazole. Benzonidazole; Ro 7-1051. *N*-Benzyl-2-(2-nitroimidazol-1-yl)acetamide.
$C_{12}H_{12}N_4O_3$=260.3.

CAS — 22994-85-0.

Adverse Effects. Nausea, vomiting, abdominal pain, peripheral neuritis, and skin rash have been reported.

Uses. Benznidazole is of value in the treatment of acute and chronic South American trypanosomiasis (Chagas' disease) due to infection with *Trypanosoma cruzi.* A dose of 5 mg per kg body-weight daily for 30 to 60 days appears to be necessary.

Studies *in vitro* showed the minimum inhibitory concentration of benznidazole against *Bacteroides fragilis* to be 4 μg per ml.— A. V. Reynolds, *J. Pharm. Pharmac.,* 1979, *31, Suppl.,* 29P.

Peak plasma concentrations of 2.22 to 2.81 (average 2.54) μg per ml of benznidazole were obtained in 6 healthy subjects 3 to 4 hours after administration of a single 100-mg dose of benznidazole. The half-life of elimination ranged from 10.5 to 13.6 (average 12) hours. Benznidazole was about 44% bound to plasma proteins.— J. Raaflaub and W. H. Ziegler, *Arzneimittel-Forsch.,* 1979, *29,* 1611.

Chagas' disease. Benznidazole was given to 76 patients with Chagas' disease in the acute phase. A mean initial daily dose of 3.01 mg per kg body-weight was increased to a mean of 7.37 mg per kg by the end of a 30-day course. Of 73 patients available for follow-up 65 were considered, by repeated xenodiagnosis, to be free of infection. Skin reactions occurred in 11 patients.— C. A. Barclay *et al., Current Chemotherapy, Vol. 1,* W. Siegenthaler and R. Luthy (Ed.), Washington, American Society of Microbiology, 1978, 158.

Cure, as assessed by xenodiagnosis, was considered to have been achieved in all of 11 patients with chronic Chagas' disease given benznidazole 7 to 10 mg per kg body-weight daily for 60 days, in 7 of 8 treated similarly for 30 days, and in 13 of 14 given 4 to 5 mg per kg daily for 30 days. Side-effects occurred in 6 patients given the higher dose and in 1 given the lower dose.— J. A. Cerisola *et al., Current Chemotherapy, Vol. 1,* W. Siegenthaler and R. Luthy (Ed.), Washington, American Society of Microbiology, 1978, 159.

Acute or chronic Chagas' disease in 214 patients was treated with benznidazole; 92 received 8 mg or more per kg body-weight daily and 122 received 7 mg or less per kg. Persistent clearance, assessed by xenodiagnosis, occurred in 74 and 78% of patients respectively; acute and chronic disease responded similarly. Side-effects (nausea, vomiting, abdominal pain, peripheral neuritis, and skin rash) were common. A dose schedule of 5 mg per kg daily for 30 or 60 days was suggested.— J. R. Coura *et al., Current Chemotherapy, Vol. 1,* W. Siegenthaler and R. Luthy (Ed.), Washington, American Society of Microbiology, 1978, 161.

Leishmaniasis. Of 6 patients with mucocutaneous leishmaniasis treated with benznidazole 3 or 5 mg per kg body-weight daily in divided doses for 45 days 3 showed complete and 3 almost complete healing of cutaneous lesions; mucosal lesions showed less improvement. Follow-up 30 days later showed recrudescence of cutaneous lesions in 3 patients and of mucosal lesions in 5. Further study with larger doses was suggested.— S. D. Fava *et al., Current Chemotherapy, Vol. 1,* W. Siegenthaler and R. Luthy (Ed.), Washington, American Society of Microbiology, 1978, 163.

Proprietary Names

Radanil *(Roche, Arg.; Roche, Switz.)*; Rochagan *(Roche, Braz.)*.

4757-f

Benzoyl Metronidazole. RP 9712. 2-(2-Methyl-5-nitroimidazol-1-yl)ethyl benzoate.
$C_{13}H_{13}N_3O_4$=275.3.

CAS — 13182-89-3.

Oral suspensions containing benzoyl metronidazole are used as an acceptable tasteless form in which metronidazole can be administered to children. They are usually given before food.

Benzoyl metronidazole 200 mg is approximately equivalent to 124 mg of metronidazole.

Benzoyl metronidazole given to patients with amoebic dysentery in doses equivalent to metronidazole 750 mg thrice daily for 5 days for adults, and 50 mg per kg body-weight daily in divided doses for 7 days to children, cured 9 of 10 adults and 16 of 18 children aged 8 months to 11 years. Smaller doses given to 20 other adults were less effective. Thirty patients with amoebic liver abscesses were treated with the equivalent of 500 or 750 mg of metronidazole thrice daily for 5 days. One patient given the higher dose required additional treatment and 5 of the 30 still passed cysts after treatment. No side-effects other than nausea in 1 adult were reported.— S. J. Powell *et al.*, *S. Afr. med. J.*, 1973, *47*, 507, per *Trop. Dis. Bull.*, 1973, *70*, 746.

Further references: R. F. Roos, *S. Afr. med. J.*, 1978, *54*, 869; K. Aleskig *et al.*, *Scand. J. infect. Dis.*, 1980, *12*, 149.

Proprietary Preparations

Flagyl-S *(May & Baker, UK)*. Benzoyl metronidazole, available as suspension containing 320 mg in each 5 ml, equivalent to metronidazole 200 mg in each 5 ml. (Also available as Flagyl Suspension Buvable in *Fr.*).

Other Proprietary Names

Klion (see also under Metronidazole) *(Hung.)*.

4758-d

Bialamicol Hydrochloride *(B.P.C. 1963)*. Biallylamicol Hydrochloride; Biethylamicol Hydrochloride; CT 871; PAA 701; SN 6771. 3,3′-Diallyl-5,5′-bis(diethylaminomethyl)biphenyl-4,4′-diol dihydrochloride.
$C_{28}H_{40}N_2O_2,2HCl=509.6$.

CAS — 493-75-4 (bialamicol); 3624-96-2 (hydrochloride).

A white or almost white, odourless, crystalline powder. M.p. about 210°. **Soluble** 1 in 5 of water, 1 in 40 of alcohol, and 1 in 150 of chloroform; slightly soluble in ether.

Adverse Effects. Nausea and vomiting sometimes occur; skin rashes have been reported.

Uses. Bialamicol hydrochloride has been used in the treatment of intestinal amoebiasis. The usual dosage is 250 to 500 mg thrice daily for a 5-day course which may be repeated if necessary after a 3-week interval.

Preparations

Bialamicol hydrochloride is marketed in certain countries under the proprietary name Camoform (*Parke, Davis*).

4759-n

Bismuth Glycollylarsanilate *(B.P.C. 1963)*.

Bism. Glycollylarsan.; Glycobiarsol (*U.S.P.*). (Hydrogen *N*-glycoloylarsanilato)oxobismuth; Bismuthyl 4-glycolamidophenylarsonic acid.
$C_8H_9AsBiNO_6=499.1$.

CAS — 116-49-4.

Pharmacopoeias. In *Ind.* and *U.S.*

An odourless, yellowish-white to flesh-coloured, amorphous powder containing about 15% of As and about 40% of Bi. It decomposes on heating. Very slightly **soluble** in water and alcohol; practically insoluble in chloroform and ether; soluble in dilute hydrochloric acid. **Store** in airtight containers. Protect from light.

Adverse Effects. Arsenical intoxication has been reported, see under Arsenic Trioxide, p.1680. Suppositories containing bismuth glycollylarsanilate can cause local irritation.

Precautions. As for Acetarsol, p.973.

Uses. Bismuth glycollylarsanilate acts principally in the bowel lumen and has been used as an amoebicide in the treatment of intestinal amoebiasis. It may be given in conjunction with tetracycline and chloroquine in the prophylaxis and treatment of amoebiasis. The usual dosage is 500 mg by mouth thrice daily for 7 to 10 days. A rest period of 10 to 14 days should precede a second course of treatment.

Preparations

Glycobiarsol Tablets *(U.S.P.)*. Tablets containing bismuth glycollylarsanilate. Protect from light.

Proprietary Names

Wintodon *(Winthrop, Arg.)*.

4760-k

Broxaldine. Brobenzoxaldine. 5,7-Dibromo-2-methyl-8-quinolyl benzoate.
$C_{17}H_{11}Br_2NO_2=421.1$.

CAS — 3684-46-6.

Broxaldine has been used in conjunction with broxyquinoline in the treatment of intestinal infections, see below.

4761-a

Broxyquinoline.

Broxichinolinum. 5,7-Dibromoquinolin-8-ol.
$C_9H_5Br_2NO=303.0$.

CAS — 521-74-4.

Adverse Effects and Precautions. As for Clioquinol, p.975.

Optic atrophy in a 12-year-old boy might have been caused by broxyquinoline.— B. Strandvik and R. Zetterström, *Lancet*, 1968, *1*, 922.

There was no evidence that the risk of adverse effects was less for broxyquinoline than for clioquinol.— O. Hansson (letter), *Lancet*, 1977, *1*, 1152.

Uses. Broxyquinoline and broxaldine are halogenated quinoline derivatives related to Clioquinol (see p.975). They have been used together in the treatment of intestinal infections including amoebiasis, giardiasis, and diarrhoea following antibiotic therapy. The usual dose is 200 to 500 mg of broxyquinoline with 40 to 100 mg of broxaldine, thrice daily for not more than 4 weeks.

Amoebiasis. In an institute for mental defectives, 51 patients with intestinal amoebiasis were given broxyquinoline 800 mg and broxaldine 160 mg thrice daily for 10 days. Control of infection was achieved slowly; relapses, probably re-infections, were common. The treatment was effective against *Entamoeba histolytica*, *Giardia lamblia*, and *Trichomonas hominis*.— D. F. Sandars and G. N. Bianchi, *Med. J. Aust.*, 1970, *1*, 261.

Leprosy. Broxyquinoline with broxaldine produced a beneficial response in 13 patients with leprosy.— C. S. G. Sharma (letter), *Lancet*, 1975, *1*, 405.

Although there was a slight improvement in 10 of 14 patients with leprosy who were treated with broxyquinoline and broxaldine, the overall results were disappointing.— S. K. Hazra *et al.*, *Lepr. India*, 1979, *51*, 505, per *Trop. Dis. Bull.*, 1980, *77*, 742.

Proprietary Preparations

Intestopan *(Sandoz, UK)*. (Available only in certain countries). **Capsules Forte** each containing broxyquinoline 500 mg and broxaldine 100 mg and **Tablets** each containing broxyquinoline 200 mg and broxaldine 40 mg.

Other Proprietary Names

Colipar *(Fr.)*; Diromo *(Spain)*.

4762-t

Carbarsone *(U.S.P., B.P.C. 1963)*.

Carbars.; Carbarsonum; Aminarsonum. 4-Ureidophenylarsonic acid.
$C_7H_9AsN_2O_4=260.1$.

CAS — 121-59-5.

Pharmacopoeias. In *Int.*, *It.*, *Jug.*, *Mex.*, *Rus.*, *Turk.*, and *U.S.*

A white or almost white, almost odourless powder with a slightly acid taste.
Soluble 1 in 330 of water and 1 in 400 of alcohol; very slightly soluble in chloroform and ether; soluble in solutions of alkali hydroxides and carbonates. A saturated solution in water is acid to litmus.

Adverse Effects, Treatment, and Precautions. As for Acetarsol, p.973.
In therapeutic doses carbarsone is less toxic than acetarsol but it sometimes produces skin rashes and urticaria. It may occasionally cause gastro-intestinal symptoms and hepatitis; rarely, cases of severe encephalitis have been reported.

Severe cerebral and hepatic reactions occurred in 2 patients with intestinal amoebiasis, each treated for 10 days with 250 mg of carbarsone 4 times daily. Toxicity was considered to be due to slightly excessive dosage.— H. J. Swartz and H. Donnenfeld (letter), *J. Am. med. Ass.*, 1965, *191*, 678.

Absorption and Fate. Carbarsone is readily absorbed from the gastro-intestinal tract and is slowly excreted in the urine. Arsenic is reported to be liberated slowly.

Uses. Carbarsone acts principally in the bowel lumen and has been used in the treatment of intestinal amoebiasis. Carbarsone is usually administered by mouth in a dose of 250 mg twice or thrice daily for a period of 10 days, the course being repeated if necessary after an interval of at least 4 days. It is usually given to supplement other amoebicides.

Preparations

Carbarsone Capsules *(U.S.P.)*. Capsules containing carbarsone.
Carbarsone was formerly marketed in certain countries under the proprietary name Leucarsone (*May & Baker*).

4763-x

Carnidazole. R 25,831; R 28,096 (hydrochloride). *O*-Methyl [2-(2-methyl-5-nitroimidazol-1-yl)ethyl]thiocarbamate.
$C_8H_{12}N_4O_3S=244.3$.

CAS — 42116-76-7.

Adverse Effects. Gastro-intestinal side-effects and dizziness have been reported.

Uses. Carnidazole is a nitroimidazole derivative structurally related to metronidazole. It has been used with some success in the treatment of vaginal trichomoniasis, usually as a single dose of 1.5 or 2 g, as enteric-coated tablets.

References: A. Notowicz *et al.*, *Br. J. vener. Dis.*, 1979, *53*, 129; P. Chaudhuri and A. C. Drogendijk, *Eur. J. Obstet. Gynec. reprod. Biol.*, 1980, *10*, 325.

4764-r

Cephaëline Hydrochloride. 7′,10,11-Trimethoxyemetan-6′-ol dihydrochloride.
$C_{28}H_{38}N_2O_4,2HCl=539.5$.

CAS — 483-17-0 (cephaëline); 5853-29-2 (hydrochloride).

The dihydrochloride of cephaëline, an alkaloid of ipecacuanha. It is converted to emetine by methylation. It occurs as white crystals or crystalline powder. **Soluble** in water, alcohol, acetone, and chloroform. **Protect** from light.

Cephaëline hydrochloride has actions similar to emetine, but it is a less active amoebicide and a more powerful emetic. It has been used as an emetic and expectorant.

4765-f

Chiniofon *(B.P. 1948)*. Chinoiodine; Iodoquinoline; Iodo-oxyquinolinesulphonic Acid with Sodium Bicarbonate; Kiniofon; Quiniofon.

CAS — 8002-90-2.

Pharmacopoeias. In *Arg.*, *Belg.*, *Mex.*, *Nord.*, *Rus.*, and *Swiss.* Several specify 3 parts of acid and 1 part of sodium bicarbonate.

A mixture of approximately 4 parts of 8-hydroxy-7-iodoquinoline-5-sulphonic acid ($C_9H_6INO_4S$=351.1) and 1 part of sodium bicarbonate, containing about 28.9% of I.

A light yellow, odourless powder with a taste at first bitter but subsequently sweetish. **Soluble** 1 in 30 of water, with effervescence; practically insoluble in alcohol, chloroform, and ether. Aqueous solutions are decomposed by boiling. **Incompatible** with acids, alkalis, oxidising agents, and salts of heavy metals. **Store** in airtight containers. Protect from light.

4766-d

Chiniofon Sodium *(B.P.C. 1963).* Chiniof. Sod. Sodium 8-hydroxy-7-iodoquinoline-5-sulphonate. $C_9H_5INNaO_4S$=373.1.

Pharmacopoeias. In *Ind.*

An almost white, pale cream, or pinkish-cream, odourless or almost odourless, crystalline powder with a taste at first bitter but afterwards sweetish. **Soluble** 1 in 30 of water; practically insoluble in alcohol, chloroform, and ether. A 1% solution in water has a pH of 5.5 to 7.5.

Chiniofon and chiniofon sodium have been used in the treatment of intestinal amoebiasis, but are no longer considered effective.

Preparations

Solublettae Chiniofoni *(Nord. P.).* Chiniofon Solution-tablets. Each contains chiniofon 250 mg and urea 220 mg, prepared with tartaric acid 5 mg in alcohol q.s. (about 100 mg) and talc 25 mg.

4767-n

Chlorbetamide. Win 5047. 2,2-Dichloro-*N*-(2,4-dichlorobenzyl)-*N*-(2-hydroxyethyl)acetamide.
$C_{11}H_{11}Cl_4NO_2$=331.0.

CAS — 97-27-8.

A white crystalline powder with a slightly bitter taste. Very slightly **soluble** in water; soluble 1 in 20 of alcohol.

Chlorbetamide has been used as an amoebicide acting principally in the bowel lumen. Doses of 0.25 to 1 g daily have been given.

4768-h

Clamoxyquin Hydrochloride. CI 433; CN-17,900-2B; PAA-3854; NSC-20246. 5-Chloro-7-(3-diethylaminopropylaminomethyl)quinolin-8-ol dihydrochloride.
$C_{17}H_{24}ClN_3O,2HCl$=394.8.

CAS — 2545-39-3 (clamoxyquin); 4724-59-8 (hydrochloride).

Clamoxyquin hydrochloride is an amoebicide which has been used in intestinal amoebiasis. Clamoxyquin has also been used as the embonate salt ($C_{17}H_{24}ClN_3O,C_{23}H_{16}O_6,½H_2O$=719.2).

References: E. F. Elslager and D. F. Worth, *J. med. Chem.*, 1967, *10*, 1971.

4769-m

Clefamide *(B.P.C. 1973).* Chlorophenoxamide. 2,2-Dichloro-*N*-(2-hydroxyethyl)-*N*-[4-(4-nitrophenoxy)benzyl]acetamide.
$C_{17}H_{16}Cl_2N_2O_5$=399.2.

CAS — 3576-64-5.

A lemon-yellow, odourless or almost odourless, tasteless, crystalline powder. M.p. 134° to 137°. Practically **insoluble** in water; soluble 1 in 100 of alcohol, 1 in 80 of chloroform, 1 in 40 of ethyl acetate, and in acetone.

Adverse Effects. Flatulence sometimes occurs with therapeutic doses. Mild nausea, abdominal pain, and diarrhoea have been reported.

Absorption and Fate. Clefamide is poorly absorbed from the gastro-intestinal tract.

Uses. Clefamide is active principally in the bowel lumen and has been used principally in the treatment of asymptomatic intestinal amoebiasis. The usual dose was 1.5 g daily in divided doses for 10 days, increased, if necessary, to 2.25 g daily for a further 5 to 10 days.

Preparations

Clefamide Tablets *(B.P.C. 1973).* Tablets containing clefamide.

4770-t

Clioquinol *(B.P.).* Chinoform; Chloroiodoquine; Cliochinolum; Iodochlorhydroxyquin *(U.S.P.)*; Iodochlorhydroxyquinoline; Quiniodochlor; Vioformo. 5-Chloro-7-iodoquinolin-8-ol.
C_9H_5ClINO=305.5.

CAS — 130-26-7.

Pharmacopoeias. In *Aust., Br., Hung., Ind., It., Jug., Mex., Port., Swiss,* and *U.S.*

A yellowish-white to brownish-yellow, tasteless, voluminous powder with a slight characteristic odour containing not less than 97% of total phenols; *U.S.P.* specifies not less than 93% of C_9H_5ClINO. M.p. about 180° with decomposition. It darkens on exposure to light.

Practically **insoluble** in water and alcohol; soluble 1 in 43 of boiling alcohol and 1 in about 120 of chloroform; very slightly soluble in ether; soluble in dimethylformamide, pyridine, and hot ethyl acetate and hot glacial acetic acid. A 5% suspension in water is acid to phenolphthalein. **Incompatible** with oxidising agents. **Store** in airtight containers. Protect from light.

Adverse Effects. Clioquinol may rarely cause iodism in sensitive patients. Local application of clioquinol in ointments or creams may occasionally cause severe irritation.

In Japan, the epidemic development of subacute myelo-optic neuropathy (SMON) in the 1960's was associated with the ingestion of normal or high doses of clioquinol for prolonged periods and the Japanese SMON Research Commission concluded that there was a causal relationship. Symptoms include abdominal discomfort and diarrhoea, paraesthesias in the legs progressing to paraplegia in a small proportion of patients, loss of visual acuity sometimes leading to irreversible blindness, sensory disturbances, and a characteristic green pigmentation of the tongue, faeces, and urine. Although many patients improve when clioquinol is withdrawn, others may have residual disablement.

A few similar cases of subacute myelo-optic neuropathy have been reported from several other countries, nearly always in association with clioquinol or related hydroxyquinoline derivatives, such as broxyquinoline or di-iodohydroxyquinoline. It has also been suggested that the epidemic in Japan was due to genetic susceptibility; this possibility cannot be excluded. A concomitant virus infection has also been suggested.

Allergy. Of 4000 patients subjected to patch testing in 5 European clinics 1.4% of males and 1.9% of females showed positive reactions to clioquinol 5% in soft paraffin.— H. Bandmann *et al.*, *Archs Derm.*, 1972, *106*, 335.. See also E. Rudzki and D. Kleniewska, *Br. J. Derm.*, 1970, *83*, 543.

Further references: M. Kero *et al.*, *Contact Dermatitis*, 1979, *5*, 115.

Neurological disorders. *Mental confusion.* A 24-year-old man developed acute cerebral symptoms with mental confusion, hallucinations, and precoma, followed by retrograde amnesia for 4 to 5 days, after taking about 30 tablets of clioquinol for diarrhoea.— H. E. Kaeser and G. Scollo-Lavizzari, *Dt. med. Wschr.*, 1970, *95*, 394, per *J. Am. med. Ass.*, 1970, *211*, 1880.

An acute encephalopathic reaction occurred about 12 hours after ingestion of 4 g of clioquinol in 1 patient and 1.5 g of clioquinol in a second patient. Both suffered from headache, drowsiness, disorientation, and loss of memory.— T. M. Ferrier and M. J. Eadie, *Med. J. Aust.*, 1973, *2*, 1008.

Further references: M. Mumenthaler *et al.*, *J. Neurol. Neurosurg. Psychiat.*, 1979, *42*, 1084 (acute amnesia and long-lasting retrograde amnesia).

Subacute myelo-optic neuropathy. Reviews and discussions of neurological disorders, including subacute myelo-optic neuropathy, occurring in patients given clioquinol or other halogenated hydroxyquinolines.— *Med. Lett.*, 1971, *13*, 51; E. Nelson, *Ann. intern. Med.*, 1972, *77*, 468; J. Thomas, *Aust. J. Pharm.*, 1972, *53*, 282; M. G. Schultz, *J. Am. med. Ass.*, 1972, *220*, 273; G. P. Oakley, *ibid.*, 1973, *225*, 395; *Med. Lett.*, 1975, *17*, 105; *Lancet*, 1977, *1*, 534; O. de S. Pinto and D. Burley, *Ciba-Geigy, Switz.* (letter), *ibid.*, 1256; J. A. H. Lee (letter), *ibid.*, 1978, *2*, 738 and 1006; I. Shigematsu and H. Yanagawa (letter), *ibid.*, 945; *ibid.*, 1979, *1*, 375; M. Asao (letter), *ibid.*, 446; *ibid.*, 1980, *1*, 857; O. Hansson and A. Herxheimer (letter), *ibid.*, 1253; *ibid.*, 1254.

A survey of 263 patients in Japan with diseases of the digestive organs who had received clioquinol 0.6 to 1.6 g daily showed that 44 had developed neurological symptoms; there were no patients with neurological symptoms in 706 similar patients not receiving clioquinol. A further survey showed that 166 of 171 patients with subacute myelo-optic neuropathy had taken clioquinol for digestive disorders before the onset of neurological symptoms. Since the Ministry of Health and Welfare in Japan prohibited the production and sale of clioquinol in September 1970 very few patients had developed subacute myelo-optic neuropathy.— T. Tsubaki *et al.* (letter), *Lancet*, 1971, *1*, 696. A reply.— , *Ciba*, *ibid.*, 697.

In a national survey in Japan of patients with subacute myelo-optic neuropathy, 1839 were analysed and 1381 (75.1%) were found to have had clioquinol in the 6 months before the neuropathy. In a subgroup of 1092 patients who were in hospital when symptoms first occurred 944 (86.4%) had received clioquinol. The average total dose before the onset of neuropathy, where dosage details were known in 1007 patients, was 40.1 g. Visual impairment, then greenish discoloration of the tongue, were significantly related to dosage.— K. Nakae *et al.*, *Lancet*, 1973, *1*, 171. See also K. Nakae, *Lancet*, 1971, *2*, 510.

Fatal renal failure and subacute myelo-optic neuropathy occurred in a 55-year-old woman who had taken clioquinol for a prolonged period for ulcerative colitis.— G. de Crousaz *et al.* (letter), *Lancet*, 1973, *1*, 378.

The Committee on Safety of Medicines found no evidence of subacute myelo-optic neuropathy following clioquinol use in the UK although there might have been a few cases of reversible neurotoxicity from long exposure.— *Pharm. J.*, 1973, *1*, 510.

Reports of the Japanese SMON Research Commission.— *Jap. J. med. Sci. Biol.*, 1975, *28*, *Suppl.*

A survey of reports of subacute myelo-optic neuropathy associated with clioquinol use outside Japan.— G. Baumgartner *et al.*, *J. Neurol. Neurosurg. Psychiat.*, 1979, *42*, 1073.

Precautions. Clioquinol is contra-indicated in patients with impaired kidney or liver function, hyperthyroidism, or iodine intolerance. Clioquinol by mouth may interfere with determinations of protein-bound iodine for up to 3 months in tests for thyroid function. Its use is best avoided in patients with neurological disorders.

Serum concentrations of protein-bound iodine in 8 healthy adults increased significantly after taking clioquinol 500 mg daily for 14 days; in 6 the immediate post-treatment concentrations were in excess of 1 μg per ml.— P. H. Sönksen *et al.*, *Lancet*, 1968, *2*, 425. Similar effects after topical use in 4 patients.— I. S. Hodgson-Jones, *Trans. a. Rep. St John's Hosp. derm. Soc., Lond.*, 1970, *56*, 51, per *Drugs*, 1971, *1*, 491.

Absorption and Fate. Much of a dose of clioquinol passes through the gastro-intestinal tract without being absorbed, but a variable degree of absorption does occur. Some of the absorbed clioquinol is quickly excreted in the urine in conjugated form, but the remainder is more slowly excreted.

A green chelate of clioquinol with ferric iron has been found on the tongue and in the urine and faeces of patients after prolonged dosage.

Following a 250-mg dose of clioquinol, 6 healthy men excreted a mean of 12.6% of the dose in the urine as glucuronide during the following 10 hours.— L. Berggren and O. Hansson, *Clin. Pharmac. Ther.*, 1968, *9*, 67.

Clioquinol was absorbed from the gastro-intestinal tract. Maximum plasma concentrations occurred about 4 hours after a single dose of clioquinol by mouth. The apparent half-life ranged from 11 to 14 hours. Approximately 25% of a 750-mg dose was excreted in the urine over 72 hours. In volunteers given 500 mg thrice daily for 7 days then 250 mg thrice daily for 7 days, equilibrium was achieved by the fifth day. No clioquinol was detectable in the plasma 3 days after the last dose.— D. B.

Jack and W. Riess, *J. pharm. Sci.*, 1973, *62*, 1929.

The protein binding of clioquinol.— N. Hobara and K. Taketa, *Biochem. Pharmac.*, 1976, *25*, 1601, per *Int. pharm. Abstr.*, 1976, *13*, 1252.

About 3 to 4% of clioquinol applied to the skin was estimated to be absorbed. Four patients with dermatitis were treated with 15 to 20 g of clioquinol ointment 3% applied twice daily to 40% of the body area. A serum concentration of 0.8 to 1.2 µg per ml was achieved within 4 hours and maintained during treatment. The daily excretion in one patient was 15 to 20 mg, more than 95% being as conjugated metabolites. Serum-clioquinol concentrations were undetectable 5 days after treatment was stopped.— T. Fischer and P. Hartvig (letter), *Lancet*, 1977, *1*, 603.

Uses. Clioquinol has been used in the treatment of intestinal amoebiasis, particularly in cyst-passers. The usual dose is 250 mg three to six times daily for 10 days with repetition of the course after 7 to 10 days. Higher doses or longer courses increase the risk of neurotoxic side-effects.

It has been used for the prophylaxis and treatment of traveller's diarrhoea and similar infections but its value for this purpose is doubtful and such use is deprecated.

Clioquinol has antibacterial and antifungal activity and is used in creams and ointments, usually containing 3%, in the treatment of skin infections such as impetigo, infected wounds, ulcers, and burns, infectious eczematoid dermatitis, and in eczema and psoriasis complicated by bacterial infection.

Vaginal insufflations usually containing 25% of clioquinol have been used in the treatment of trichomonal vaginitis.

Clioquinol stains clothing and linen yellow on contact. It may stain the skin and discolour fair hair.

Tests *in vitro* showed that 52 strains of *Vibrio cholerae*, almost equally divided between eltor and other varieties, were sensitive to clioquinol. Variable sensitivity was demonstrated with various strains of *Escherichia coli, Pseudomonas aeruginosa, Ps. pseudomallei, Salmonella typhi, Shigella boydii, Sh. dysenteriae, Sh. flexneri*, and *Sh. sonnei*.— R. A. Finkelstein and J. Raungthum, *Bull. Wld Hlth Org.*, 1968, *38*, 803.

Clioquinol was bactericidal for plaque cultures of *Streptococcus mutans, Str. sanguis, Actinomyces viscosus*, and *Actinomyces naeslundii in vitro* at concentrations of 0.1, 1, 0.05, and 2% respectively.— J. M. Tanzer *et al.*, *Antimicrob. Ag. Chemother.*, 1978, *13*, 1044.

Skin infections. In a double-blind study, in 4 centres, in 277 patients with bacterial and/or fungous infections of the skin, treatment consisted of clioquinol 3% with hydrocortisone 1%, clioquinol 3%, hydrocortisone 1%, or the cream basis, applied thrice daily for 7 to 10 days. The combined formula was more effective than either of its components or its basis.— C. L. Carpenter *et al.*, *Curr. ther. Res.*, 1973, *15*, 650. A similar report.— H. I. Maibach, *Archs Derm.*, 1978, *114*, 1773.

Preparations

Creams

Clioquinol Cream *(B.P.)*. Clioquinol in very fine powder 3 g, chlorocresol 100 mg, cetomacrogol emulsifying ointment 30 g, freshly boiled and cooled water 66.9 g. Store at a temperature not exceeding 25° in well-closed containers which minimise evaporation and contamination. Protect from light. Avoid contact with aluminium. This cream may be prepared with any other suitable basis. Clioquinol may stain clothing or discolour fair hair.

Clioquinol Cream Aqueous *(A.P.F.)*. Iodochlorhydroxyquin Cream Aqueous. Clioquinol 3 g, cetomacrogol cream aqueous to 100 g. Protect from light and avoid contact with metals.

Hydrocortisone Acetate and Clioquinol Cream *(B.P.)*. Hydrocort. Acet. and Clioquinol Cream; Hydrocortisone and Clioquinol Ointment. Hydrocortisone acetate in very fine powder and clioquinol in very fine powder in a suitable basis. Store at a temperature not exceeding 25° in well-closed containers which minimise evaporation and contamination. Protect from light.
Avoid contact with aluminium. Clioquinol may stain clothing or discolour fair hair.

Iodochlorhydroxyquin Cream *(U.S.P.)*. Clioquinol Cream. Clioquinol in a suitable cream basis. Store in airtight containers. Protect from light.

Ointments

Clioquinol and Hydrocortisone Ointment *(St. John's Hosp.)*. Clioquinol 1%, hydrocortisone 0.5%, white soft paraffin to 100%.

Hydrocortisone and Clioquinol Ointment *(B.P.)*. Hydrocortisone in very fine powder and clioquinol in very fine powder in a suitable basis. Store at a temperature not exceeding 25°. Protect from light.

Iodochlorhydroxyquin Ointment *(U.S.P.)*. Clioquinol Ointment. Clioquinol in a suitable ointment basis. Store in airtight containers. Protect from light.

Powders

Compound Iodochlorhydroxyquin Powder *(U.S.P.)*. Compound Clioquinol Powder. Clioquinol 25 g, lactic acid 2.5 g, zinc stearate 20 g, and lactose 52.5 g. Protect from light.

For topical use or intravaginal insufflation in trichomonal vaginitis.

Tablets

Iodochlorhydroxyquin Tablets *(U.S.P.)*. Clioquinol Tablets. Tablets containing clioquinol. Store in airtight containers. Protect from light.

Proprietary Preparations

Barquinol HC *(Fisons, UK)*. Cream containing clioquinol 3% and hydrocortisone acetate 0.5%.

Entero-Valodon *(Wallace Mfg Chem., UK: Farillon, UK)*. Clioquinol, available as tablets of 250 mg.

Oralcer *(Vitabiotics, UK)*. Sustained-release pellets each containing clioquinol 35 mg and ascorbic acid 6 mg. For mouth ulcers. *Dose.* 6 to 8 pellets, dissolved slowly near the affected area, at hourly intervals on the first day, then 4 to 6 pellets daily.

An adverse report.— *Drug & Ther. Bull.*, 1973, *11*, 48.

Vioform-Hydrocortisone *(Ciba, UK)*. Preparations containing clioquinol 3% and hydrocortisone 1% available as **Cream** in a vanishing cream basis, and as **Ointment**.

Other Proprietary Names

Budoform, Cremo-Quin (both *Austral.)*; Enteritan *(Switz.)*; Entero-Vioform *(Austral., Canad., Ger., Neth., S.Afr.)*; Entero-Vioformio *(Ital.)*; Entero-Vioformo *(Arg., Spain)*; Vioform *(Austral., Canad., Ger., S.Afr., Switz., USA)*.

Clioquinol was also formerly marketed in Great Britain under the proprietary names Entero-Vioform and Vioform *(Ciba)*.

4771-x

Cloquinate. Chloquinate; Clochinatum. Chloroquine bis(8-hydroxy-7-iodoquinoline-5-sulphonate).
$C_{18}H_{26}ClN_3,(C_9H_6INO_4S)_2$=1022.1.

CAS — 7270-12-4.

Cloquinate is a neutral salt combining 1 molecule of chloroquine with 2 molecules of chiniofon (acid).

It has been used in the treatment of intestinal amoebiasis and extra-intestinal amoebic infections.

4772-r

Conessine Hydrobromide. Conessine Bromide; Bromhydrate de Conessine. 3β-Dimethylaminocon-5-enine dihydrobromide.
$C_{24}H_{40}N_2,2HBr$=518.4.

CAS — 546-06-5 (conessine); 5913-82-6 (hydrobromide).

The hydrobromide of an alkaloid obtained from the seeds of *Holarrhena antidysenterica*. It occurs as white odourless acicular crystals or microcrystalline powder with a very bitter taste. **Soluble** 1 in 5 of water and 1 in 11 of alcohol (90%); very slightly soluble in ether; practically insoluble in light petroleum.

Conessine hydrobromide was formerly used in the treatment of amoebic dysentery.

4773-f

Dehydroemetine Hydrochloride.

BT 436; DHE; 2,3-Dehydroemetine Hydrochloride; Ro 1-9334. 2,3-Didehydro-6′,7′,10,11-tetramethoxyemetan dihydrochloride; 3-Ethyl-1,6,7,11b-tetrahydro-9,10-dimethoxy-2-(1,2,3,4-tetrahydro-6,7-dimethoxy-1-isoquinolylmethyl)-4*H*-benzo[*a*]quinolizine dihydrochloride.
$C_{29}H_{38}N_2O_4,2HCl$=551.6.

CAS — 4914-30-1 (dehydroemetine); 2228-39-9 (hydrochloride).

A white odourless crystalline powder with a bitter taste. **Soluble** 1 in 30 of water.

Adverse Effects and Precautions. As for Emetine Hydrochloride, p.978.

Adverse reactions are usually milder and less frequent than with emetine.

About one-quarter of 50 patients with amoebiasis treated with dehydroemetine, 40 mg daily by subcutaneous injection for 10 days, showed a significant fall in blood pressure, and an increase in heart-rate; ECG recordings in over one-third of the patients showed significant changes in the T-wave amplitude. The cardiovascular toxicity of emetine in 65 similar patients treated in the same hospital was greater than that of the dehydroemetine-treated group.— R. M. Kapadia, *J. Indian med. Ass.*, 1964, *43*, 461, per *Trop. Dis. Bull.*, 1965, *62*, 413.

Six days after completing a 10-day course of treatment with dehydroemetine, 65 mg daily by intramuscular injection, a 25-year-old woman had an epileptiform seizure with cardiac irregularity and hypotension. ECG recordings showed depression and inversion of the T-waves. She gradually improved.— G. D. Lister, *J. trop. Med. Hyg.*, 1968, *71*, 219, per *Trop. Dis. Bull.*, 1969, *66*, 196.

Dehydroemetine-induced depression in one patient.— S. Sharma, *Indian J. med. Sci.*, 1976, *30*, 239, per *Trop. Dis. Bull.*, 1977, *74*, 1132.

A rise in serum-aminotransferase concentrations might occur during treatment with dehydroemetine.— F. Clark, *Adverse Drug React. Bull.*, 1977, Oct., 232.

Absorption and Fate. As for Emetine Hydrochloride, p.978.

Dehydroemetine is reported to be more quickly eliminated from the body than emetine and the risk of cumulation is less.

Uses. Dehydroemetine is used similarly to emetine hydrochloride (p.978) in the treatment of amoebiasis. Because of its more rapid elimination from the body, it can be given in higher doses for longer periods and, in cases of relapse, a course can be repeated after a shorter interval. It should not be given sooner than 45 days after a course of emetine.

Some success with dehydroemetine in the treatment of favus, leishmaniasis, and schistosomiasis has also been reported.

Dehydroemetine hydrochloride is administered by deep subcutaneous or deep intramuscular injection. The usual dose is 60 mg, or 1 mg per kg body-weight, daily for 6 to 10 days. Higher initial doses, up to 180 mg, may be employed in severe cases or the course may be extended to 15 days. In cases of relapse, the course may be repeated after an interval of 14 days.

Doses of 1.5 mg per kg have been suggested for the treatment of schistosomiasis.

Dehydroemetine has also been administered by mouth in similar doses as the hydrochloride, in a slow-release resinate, and as a complex iodide with bismuth.

Dehydroemetine 2.5 mg per kg body-weight thrice daily on alternate days for 30 doses was given to 17 patients infected with the fluke *Opisthorchis* with ova in the faeces. Two patients withdrew due to side-effects and 3 of the remaining 15 were cured. There was an overall percentage egg reduction of 85%.— L. Muangmanee *et al.*, *S.E. Asian J. trop. med. publ. Hlth*, 1974, *5*, 581, per *Trop. Dis. Bull.*, 1975, *72*, 733.

Amoebiasis. Dehydroemetine and emetine, in doses of 65 mg daily for 10 days, were considered to be equally effective in treating 50 patients with amoebic liver abscess. All patients were given chloroquine; di-iodohydroxyquinoline was given for intestinal amoebiasis and tetracycline for active dysentery. Dehydroemetine was considered less toxic than emetine.— S. J. Powell *et al.*, *Ann. trop. Med. Parasit.*, 1967, *61*, 26, per *Abstr. Wld Med.*, 1967, *41*, 925.

Children very ill with amoebic abscess were treated with dehydroemetine, or emetine, 2 mg per kg body-weight daily, given by subcutaneous injection in addition to either metronidazole 50 mg per kg daily or niridazole 25 mg per kg daily, both drugs being given for 10 days.— J. N. Scragg and S. J. Powell, *Archs Dis. Childh.*, 1970, *45*, 193, per R. Knight *et al.*, *Gut*, 1973, *14*, 145.

Herpes zoster. Twenty elderly patients with herpes zoster did not experience postherpetic neuralgia, and in 14 pain completely disappeared after treatment with dehydroemetine 60 mg given intramuscularly every 24 hours for 3 to 9 doses. In the other 6 patients pain diminished or disappeared in 2 to 4 weeks. No patients had active vesicles at the end of the first week of treatment. Of 20 similar patients treated with triamcinolone by mouth, 8 experienced postherpetic neuralgia and pain persisted for more than 6 months in 4.— E. Hernandez-Perez, *Cutis*, 1980, *25*, 424.

Preparations

Dehydroemetine hydrochloride is marketed in certain countries under the proprietary names Dametine (*E. Merck*) and Dehydroemetine Roche.

4774-d

Diethylamine Acetarsol. Diethylamine Acetarsone; Ethylacétphénarsine. The dihydrate of the diethylamine salt of 3-acetamido-4-hydroxyphenylarsonic acid.
$C_8H_{10}AsNO_5,C_4H_{11}N,2H_2O$=384.3.

CAS — 534-33-8 (anhydrous).

Pharmacopoeias. In *Belg.*

Colourless crystals or a white crystalline odourless powder with a slightly bitter taste. **Soluble** 1 in 3.5 of water, 1 in 1 of boiling water, and 1 in 7 of alcohol; practically insoluble in chloroform and ether.

Diethylamine acetarsol was formerly used in the treatment of rat-bite fever, relapsing fever, tropical eosinophilia, and some dermatoses.

Preparations

Diethylamine acetarsol was formerly marketed in certain countries under the proprietary name Acetylarsan (*May & Baker*).

4775-n

Difetarsone Sodium. Diphetarsone; RP 4763. Disodium *NN'*-ethylenebis(4-aminophenylarsonate) decahydrate.
$C_{14}H_{16}As_2N_2Na_2O_6,10H_2O$=684.3.

CAS — 3639-19-8 (difetarsone); 515-76-4 (sodium salt, anhydrous).

Difetarsone sodium has been used in the treatment of intestinal amoebiasis, usually in conjunction with a broad-spectrum antibiotic, in divided doses of up to 2 g daily for 10 days repeated after 5 to 6 weeks, if necessary. It has also been used in the treatment of whipworm and threadworm infection. See also Difetarsone-Spiramycin (below).

References to the treatment of whipworm infection: D. M. Lynch *et al.*, *Br. med. J.*, 1972, *4*, 73; N. M. Lenczner (letter), *Trans. R. Soc. trop. Med. Hyg.*, 1972, *66*, 510; D. R. O'Holohan and J. Hugoe-Matthews, *S.E. Asian J. trop. med. publ. Hlth*, 1972, *3*, 576, per *Trop. Dis. Bull.*, 1973, *70*, 669; C. J. Rubidge *et al.*, *S. Afr. med. J.*, 1973, *47*, 991, per *Trop. Dis. Bull.*, 1973, *70*, 1097; P. M. Leary *et al.*, *Archs Dis. Childh.*, 1974, *49*, 486.

Proprietary Names
Bémarsal *(Specia, Fr.)*.

4776-h

Difetarsone-Spiramycin. Diphetarsone-Spiramycin; RP 6753. The spiramycin salt of difetarsone, containing 66.2% of spiramycin base and 33.8% of difetarsone.

Difetarsone-spiramycin has been used similarly to difetarsone sodium in the treatment of intestinal amoebiasis and in threadworm and whipworm infestation.

Proprietary Names
Rovamycine-Difétarsone *(Specia, Fr.)*.

4777-m

Di-iodohydroxyquinoline *(B.P. 1973)*. Iodoquinol *(U.S.P.)*; Diiodohydroxyquin; Diiodohydroxyquinolinum; Diodoxyquinoléine. 5,7-Di-iodoquinolin-8-ol.
$C_9H_5I_2NO$=397.0.

CAS — 83-73-8.

Pharmacopoeias. In *Chin.*, *Fr.*, *Ind.*, *Int.*, *It.*, and *U.S.*

A light yellowish to tan-coloured, tasteless, microcrystalline powder, not readily wetted in water, odourless or with a slight odour.
Practically **insoluble** in water; sparingly soluble in alcohol, acetone, and ether. **Protect** from light.

Adverse Effects. As for Clioquinol, p.975.
Effects occasionally occurring include abdominal discomfort, diarrhoea, skin rash, acne, headache, pruritus ani, and furunculosis. Slight enlargement of the thyroid gland often occurs during treatment.

Neurological disorders. Reports of visual disturbances in children given di-iodohydroxyquinoline.— J. E. Etheridge and G. T. Stewart (letter), *Lancet*, 1966, *1*, 261; F. E. Pittman and M. Westphal (letter), *Lancet*, 1973, *2*, 566; M. M. Behrens (letter), *J. Am. med. Ass.*, 1974, *228*, 693.

Precautions. As for Clioquinol, p.975.

Control of acrodermatitis enteropathica by di-iodohydroxyquinoline was lost in a patient when she started taking an oral contraceptive.— M. J. Jackson, *J. clin. Path.*, 1977, *30*, 284.

Absorption and Fate. Di-iodohydroxyquinoline is partly and irregularly absorbed from the small intestine.

Following a 300-mg dose of di-iodohydroxyquinoline, 6 healthy men excreted a mean of 4.6% of the dose in the urine as glucuronide during the following 10 hours.— L. Berggren and O. Hansson, *Clin. Pharmac. Ther.*, 1968, *9*, 67.

Uses. Di-iodohydroxyquinoline acts principally in the bowel lumen and is used alone or with metronidazole in the treatment of intestinal amoebiasis, chiefly for cyst-passers. It has been used to supplement emetine or with chloroquine and tetracycline in amoebic dysentery. It has also been used in balantidiasis and giardiasis and has been used locally against *Trichomonas vaginalis*. Di-iodohydroxyquinoline has been used in the treatment of acrodermatitis enteropathica; it is reported to act by altering zinc absorption.
The usual dosage in the treatment of amoebiasis is 600 mg thrice daily for 20 days; for children the usual dose is 10 mg per kg body-weight thrice daily. It can be employed in ambulatory patients and asymptomatic carriers.

Most of 55 patients with ocreiform atrophy and superimposed dermatitis of the anterior surface of the lower leg responded well to an ointment containing di-iodohydroxyquinoline 3% and salicylic acid 2% in Emulsifying Ointment.— A. R. H. B. Verhagen and J. W. Koten, *Br. J. Derm.*, 1968, *80*, 682.

Di-iodohydroxyquinoline should not be used for the treatment of non-specific diarrhoea or other self-limiting conditions.— *Med. Lett.*, 1974, *16*, 71.

Acrodermatitis. A 5-month-old girl with acrodermatitis enteropathica obtained remission from diarrhoea and dermatitis when treated with di-iodohydroxyquinoline 200 mg thrice daily. She relapsed and was then given a diet of fresh whole human milk; treatment with di-iodohydroxyquinoline was continued in the same dosage. On this regimen a complete remission was obtained enabling the child to be weaned to a normal diet and treatment with di-iodohydroxyquinoline to be discontinued.— R. R. Schulze and R. K. Winkelmann, *Mayo Clin. Proc.*, 1966, *41*, 334.

In acrodermatitis enteropathica di-iodohydroxyquinoline acted by increasing the gastro-intestinal absorption as well as the retention of zinc.— M. J. Jackson, *J. clin. Path.*, 1977, *30*, 284. See also P. J. Aggett *et al.*, *Archs Dis. Childh.*, 1978, *53*, 691.

Aspergillosis. Of 13 patients with clinical pulmonary aspergillosis all had specific precipitins in their sera and most had *Aspergillus fumigatus* in their sputum. After treatment for 20 days with di-iodohydroxyquinoline 1.5 to 1.8 g daily precipitin tests became negative in 12 and the sputum was cleared in all those previously affected. Some patients experienced clinical benefit.— K. Horsfield *et al.*, *Thorax*, 1977, *32*, 250, per *Abstr. Hyg.*, 1977, *52*, 1131.

Preparations

Di-iodohydroxyquinoline Pessaries *(B.P.C. 1973)*. Each pessary contains di-iodohydroxyquinoline 100 mg, boric acid 65 mg, phosphoric acid 17 mg, lactose 180 mg, and anhydrous dextrose 300 mg; prepared by moist granulation and compression. They should be moistened with water before insertion into the vagina. Protect from light. *A.P.F.* has a similar formula.

Di-iodohydroxyquinoline Tablets *(B.P. 1973)*. Di-iodohydroxyquin. Tab. Tablets containing di-iodohydroxyquinoline. Protect from light.

Iodoquinol Tablets *(U.S.P.)*. Tablets containing di-iodohydroxyquinoline.

Proprietary Preparations

Diodoquin *(Searle, UK)*. Di-iodohydroxyquinoline, available as tablets of 650 mg. (Also available as Diodoquin in many other countries).

Embequin *(May & Baker, UK)*. (Available only in certain countries.) Di-iodohydroxyquinoline, available as tablets of 300 mg.

Other Proprietary Names

Dioxiquin *(Spain)*; Direxiode *(Austral., Belg., Fr., Switz.)*; Drioquilen *(Arg.)*; Floraquin *(Arg., Austral., Belg.)*; Moebiquin *(USA)*; Searlequin *(Arg.)*; Yodoxin *(USA)*.

A preparation containing di-iodohydroxyquinoline was formerly marketed in Great Britain under the proprietary name Floraquin (*Searle Pharmaceuticals*).

4778-b

Diloxanide *(B.P.C. 1963)*. Diloxan; RD 3803. 2,2-Dichloro-4'-hydroxy-*N*-methylacetanilide.
$C_9H_9Cl_2NO_2$=234.1.

CAS — 579-38-4.

A white or almost white, odourless, tasteless, crystalline powder. Slightly **soluble** in water; soluble 1 in 8 of alcohol, 1 in 35 of chloroform, and 1 in 66 of ether. **Protect** from light.

The actions and uses of diloxanide are described under Diloxanide Furoate (below). It has been given in doses of 1.5 g daily in divided doses.

Diloxanide was formerly marketed in certain countries under the proprietary name Entamide (*Boots*).

4779-v

Diloxanide Furoate *(B.P.)*. 4-(*N*-Methyl-2,2-dichloroacetamido)phenyl 2-furoate.
$C_{14}H_{11}Cl_2NO_4$=328.2.

CAS — 3736-81-0.

Pharmacopoeias. In *Br.*

A white or almost white, odourless, tasteless, crystalline powder. M.p. 114° to 116°.
Very slightly **soluble** in water; soluble 1 in 100 of alcohol, 1 in 2.5 of chloroform, and 1 in 130 of ether. **Protect** from light.

Adverse Effects. Flatulence, vomiting, pruritus, and urticaria may occasionally occur. Transient albuminuria has been reported.

Absorption and Fate. Diloxanide is readily absorbed from the gastro-intestinal tract and excreted in the faeces and urine. Diloxanide furoate is hydrolysed before absorption.

Uses. Diloxanide acts principally in the bowel lumen and is used in the treatment of intestinal amoebiasis. It is less effective in amoebic dysentery than in asymptomatic infection, but the furoate gives higher intestinal concentrations and is possibly more effective than metronidazole in the treatment of cyst-passers.
Diloxanide furoate is used in conjunction with chloroquine and tetracycline in amoebic dysentery and is used in the treatment of hepatic amoebiasis in conjunction with chloroquine and

dehydroemetine or emetine.

Diloxanide furoate is administered in a dosage of 500 mg thrice daily for 10 days. The dosage for children is 20 mg per kg body-weight daily, in divided doses, for 10 days. The course of treatment may be repeated if necessary.

Diloxanide furoate is also used concomitantly with metronidazole.

Amoebiasis. Diloxanide furoate 375 mg, tetracycline hydrochloride 250 mg, and chloroquine phosphate 100 mg, 4 times daily for 5 days, were given in capsules to 50 of 100 patients with dysentery due to *Entamoeba histolytica* and sometimes other parasites also. The other 50 received the same regimen without chloroquine. Children younger than 10 years received half this adult dose. The overall cure-rate for *E. histolytica* was 83%, and the efficacy of the preparations was not significantly different. Other protozoa and helminths were apparently not affected.— D. Botero, *Trans. R. Soc. trop. Med. Hyg.*, 1967, *61*, 769, per *Abstr. Wld Med.*, 1968, *42*, 497.

Diloxanide furoate 375 mg, tetracycline hydrochloride 250 mg, and chloroquine phosphate 100 mg, given 4 times daily for 5 days to 50 Costa Rican schoolboys, eliminated multiple intestinal protozoal infections within 2 days of completing the course. The recurrence-rate of *Giardia intestinalis* was 25% within 30 days, but *Entamoeba histolytica* did not recur for 90 days.— M. M. Schapiro, *Am. J. trop. Med. Hyg.*, 1967, *16*, 704, per *Trop. Dis. Bull.*, 1968, *65*, 766. A similar report.— E. Nnochiri, *J. trop. Med. Hyg.*, 1967, *70*, 224, per *Trop. Dis. Bull.*, 1968, *65*, 129.

Diloxanide furoate administered in a dose of 500 mg thrice daily for 10 days was effective in the treatment of 12 patients who were asymptomatic cyst carriers and 52 of 65 patients with non-dysenteric symptomatic intestinal amoebiasis. Flatulence was the only significant side-effect.— M. S. Wolfe, *J. Am. med Ass.*, 1973, *224*, 1601.

Diloxanide furoate was considered to be more effective than metronidazole in the treatment of non-dysenteric intestinal amoebiasis, and to be the drug of choice for this form of the disease.— R. Knight *et al.*, *Gut*, 1973, *14*, 145.

Diloxanide furoate 500 mg given with metronidazole 400 mg thrice daily for 5 days cleared amoebic cysts from the intestine in 59 of 60 patients treated and was considered to have cured liver abscesses in 58 of them. No relapses were noted during 3 months following treatment.— S. J. Powell *et al.*, *Ann. trop. Med. Parasit.*, 1973, *67*, 367, per *Trop. Dis. Bull.*, 1974, *71*, 44.

The standard regimen for the treatment of amoebiasis in American Indians in Saskatchewan was metronidazole 500 mg and diloxanide furoate 500 mg twice daily for 5 days.— R. D. P. Eaton *et al.*, *Can. J. publ. Hlth*, 1973, *64, Suppl.*, 47, per *Trop. Dis. Bull.*, 1974, *71*, 360.

Of 38 Peace Corps workers with amoebiasis in Ethiopia 36 were considered free of infection 1 to 2 months after treatment with metronidazole 750 mg thrice daily for 10 days followed by diloxanide furoate 500 mg thrice daily for 10 days.— J. L. Ey, *Ethiop. med. J.*, 1977, *15*, 101, per *Trop. Dis. Bull.*, 1979, *76*, 80.

A report of the successful treatment of a patient with *Entamoeba polecki* infection using metronidazole and diloxanide furoate.— J. S. Salaki *et al.*, *Am. J. trop. Med. Hyg.*, 1979, *28*, 190, per *Trop. Dis. Bull.*, 1980, *77*, 51.

Preparations

Diloxanide Furoate Tablets *(B.P.)*. Tablets containing diloxanide furoate. Protect from light.

Furamide *(Boots, UK)*. Diloxanide furoate, available as tablets of 500 mg. (Also available as Furamide in *Austral)*.

4780-r

Diminazene Aceturate *(B. Vet. C. 1965)*. 1,3-Bis(4-amidinophenyl)triazene bis(*N*-acetylglycinate) tetrahydrate.
$C_{22}H_{29}N_9O_6,4H_2O=587.6$.

CAS — 536-71-0 (diminazene); 908-54-3 (aceturate, anhydrous).

A yellow odourless powder. **Soluble** 1 in 14 of water; slightly soluble in alcohol; very slightly soluble in chloroform and ether.

Uses. Diminazene aceturate has trypanocidal, babesicidal, and bactericidal properties and is used in veterinary medicine in the treatment of trypanosomiasis and babesiasis. It has also been tried in human infections.

Babesiasis. The routine clinical use of pentamidine or diminazene aceturate in infections due to *Babesia microti* was not recommended except in patients without spleens, since normally the infection was self-limiting.— L. H. Miller *et al.*, *Ann. intern. Med.*, 1978, *88*, 200.

A patient infected with *Babesia microti* who had failed to respond to chloroquine had a rapid clinical and parasitologic response after administration of diminazene. However the patient developed Guillain-Barré syndrome after treatment and it was suggested that pentamidine might be preferable to diminazene in severe cases of human babesiasis.— T. K. Ruebush and A. Spielman, *Ann. intern. Med.*, 1978, *88*, 263.

Trypanosomiasis. Reference to use in human trypanosomiasis.— M. P. Hutchinson and H. J. C. Watson, *Trans. R. Soc. trop. Med. Hyg.*, 1962, *56*, 227; S. E. Temu, *Trans. R. Soc. trop. Med. Hyg.*, 1975, *69*, 277; East African Trypanosomiasis Research Organisation, *Trans. R. Soc. trop. Med. Hyg.*, 1975, *69*, 278.

Proprietary Names

Berenil *(veterinary) (Hoechst, UK)*; Ganaseg.

4781-f

Emetine and Bismuth Iodide *(B.P. 1973)*. Emet. Bism. Iod.; EBI.

CAS — 8001-15-8.

A complex iodide of emetine and bismuth containing 25 to 30% of emetine and 18 to 22.5% of Bi. It is a reddish-orange odourless powder with a bitter acrid taste. Practically **insoluble** in water and alcohol; soluble in acetone and, with decomposition, in concentrated acids and in alkaline solutions; practically insoluble in but slightly decomposed by dilute acids. **Store** in airtight containers. Protect from light.

Adverse Effects and Precautions. As for Emetine Hydrochloride (below).

When given by mouth emetine and bismuth iodide may cause nausea, vomiting, and diarrhoea.

Absorption and Fate. When given by mouth, emetine and bismuth iodide undergoes little decomposition until it reaches the small intestine, where emetine is liberated and exerts a local and systemic effect.

Uses. Emetine and bismuth iodide has actions similar to those of emetine hydrochloride and has been used in the treatment of asymptomatic intestinal amoebiasis. When given by mouth it is only slightly decomposed before reaching the small intestine where the bulk of the emetine is then released to give a high concentration in the intestine. It has been used with tetracycline and a luminal amoebicide such as diloxanide furoate in the treatment of severe amoebic dysentery with much tissue invasion.

The frequency with which it gives rise to unpleasant side-effects makes it unsuitable for routine therapy; patients should be confined to bed.

Emetine and bismuth iodide is usually administered in enteric-coated tablets or capsules but such preparations must disintegrate very readily in the intestine or they are valueless; when in capsules, the drug should not be suspended in an oily basis. The usual dose was 200 mg daily for 12 consecutive days if tolerated by the patient.

Preparations

Emetine and Bismuth Iodide Tablets *(B.P. 1973)*. Emet. Bism. Iod. Tab. Tablets containing emetine and bismuth iodide. They are enteric-and sugar-coated. Store at a temperature not exceeding 25° in airtight containers.

4782-d

Emetine Hydrochloride *(B.P., U.S.P.)*. Emet. Hydrochlor.; Emetini Hydrochloridum; Emetini Chloridum; Emetine Dihydrochloride; Ipecine Hydrochloride; Methylcephaëline Hydrochloride; Cloridrato de Emetina. 6′,7′,10,11-Tetramethoxyemetan dihydrochloride heptahydrate; (2*S*,3*R*,11b*S*)-3-Ethyl-1,3,4,6,7,11b-hexahydro-9,10-dimethoxy-2-[(1*R*)-1,2,3,4-tetrahydro-6,7-dimethoxy-1-isoquinolylmethyl]-2*H*-benzo[*a*]quinolizine dihydrochloride heptahydrate.
$C_{29}H_{40}N_2O_4,2HCl,7H_2O=679.7$.

CAS — 483-18-1 (emetine); 316-42-7 (hydrochloride, anhydrous); 7083-71-8 (hydrochloride, hydrate).

Pharmacopoeias. In *Arg., Aust., Belg., Br., Braz., Cz., Ger., Ind., Int., It., Jug., Mex., Nord., Port., Roum., Rus., Span., Swiss, Turk.*, and *U.S.* Many specify a variable proportion of water of crystallisation.

A white or very slightly yellow odourless crystalline powder with a bitter taste; it becomes faintly yellow on exposure to light. M.p. 235° to 255° after drying.

Soluble 1 in 8 of water, 1 in 12 of alcohol (90%), and 1 in 4 of chloroform; practically insoluble in ether. A solution in water is dextrorotatory. A 2% solution in water has a pH of 4 to 6. Solutions are **sterilised** by maintaining at 98° to 100° for 30 minutes with a bactericide or by filtration. **Store** in airtight containers. Protect from light.

The stability of emetine hydrochloride in solution: C. Schuyt *et al.*, *Pharm. Weekbl. Ned.*, 1977, *112*, 1125; *idem*, 1979, *114*, 186.

Adverse Effects. Emetine causes pain on injection and there may be associated muscle stiffness; there may be necrosis and abscess formation. After injection nausea, vomiting, and diarrhoea are common; there may be dizziness, headache, muscle weakness, urticaria or purpuric skin rash and, more rarely, mild sensory disturbances.

Cardiovascular effects are considered serious and include precordial pain, dyspnoea, tachycardia, and hypotension. Changes in the ECG, particularly flattening or inversion of the T-wave and prolongation of the Q-T interval, occur in many patients. Large doses or prolonged administration may cause lesions of the heart, gastro-intestinal tract, kidneys, liver, and skeletal muscle. Severe acute degenerative myocarditis may occur and may give rise to sudden cardiac failure and death. In some patients cardiotoxic effects have appeared after the completion of treatment with therapeutic doses.

Four patients given emetine for amoebiasis developed muscular weakness or peripheral neuritis after total doses ranging from 180 to 720 mg.— B. K. Chew and D. S. Yeoh, *Singapore med. J.*, 1966, *7*, 156, per *Trop. Dis. Bull.*, 1968, *65*, 32.

Precautions. Emetine is contra-indicated in cardiac or renal disease. Its use should be avoided during pregnancy and it should not be given to children, except in severe amoebic dysentery unresponsive to other drugs. It should be used with great caution in old or debilitated patients. ECG monitoring is advisable during treatment.

Absorption and Fate. After injection emetine hydrochloride is concentrated in the liver. Appreciable concentration occurs also in kidney, lung, and spleen. Very little of a parenteral dose is secreted into the intestinal lumen. Excretion occurs mainly in the urine, and is slow. Detectable concentrations may persist in urine 40 to 60 days after treatment has been discontinued. Cumulation may occur.

Uses. Emetine, an alkaloid of ipecacuanha, is an amoebicide acting principally in the bowel wall and in the liver. It is given by subcutaneous or intramuscular injection. In intestinal amoebiasis the symptoms are rapidly cleared by the first course of emetine injections and motile amoebae and cysts disappear, but more than 50% of patients later show cysts in their faeces and hence become carriers. Further treatment with emetine hydrochloride in these cases is of little value.

In severe amoebic dysentery it may be given with tetracycline and an amoebicide acting within the intestinal lumen such as diloxanide furoate.

In hepatic amoebiasis emetine may be given with chloroquine and an amoebicide acting within the intestinal lumen, but treatment with metronidazole is generally preferred.

Doses of emetine hydrochloride should never be larger than 60 mg daily and courses should not be longer than 10 days or repeated at intervals of less than 6 weeks. Children may be given 500 µg per kg body-weight twice daily (up to maximum of 60 mg daily) subcutaneously for 4 to 6 days. It is advisable for the patient to remain in bed during the emetine treatment and a careful watch should be kept on cardiac function with ECG monitoring; strenuous exercise should be avoided for several weeks.

Emetine hydrochloride has expectorant, diaphoretic, and emetic actions but is seldom used for these effects.

Amoebiasis. In a controlled study of 60 patients with amoebic liver abscess 20 were treated with emetine hydrochloride 65 mg daily parenterally for 10 days together with chloroquine 250 mg twice daily for 20 days; there was one failure due to fatal rupture of the abscess. ECG changes occurred in 7 patients and hypotension in 2. Of 20 treated with niridazole 500 mg thrice daily 2 refused treatment, 4 failed to complete the course of 10 days, and 14 were cured. Of 20 treated with metronidazole 400 mg thrice daily for 10 days 13 were cured; the remainder were judged clinical failures.— D. V. Datta *et al.*, *Am. J. trop. Med. Hyg.*, 1974, *23*, 586, per *Trop. Dis. Bull.*, 1974, *71*, 1259.

Aspergillosis. Pulmonary aspergillosis in 3 patients and otomycosis in 1 responded to emetine hydrochloride, 40 to 60 mg intramuscularly once daily for 7 to 10 days.— M. Jesiotr, *Scand. J. resp. Dis.*, 1973, 54, 326, per *Br. med. J.*, 1974, *2*, 133.

The MIC of emetine for an isolate of *Aspergillus niger* was in excess of 750 µg per ml, and for 22 other isolates of *Aspergillus* spp. it was in excess of 1.5 mg per ml. These values were not attainable clinically.— L. J. R. Milne and G. K. Crompton (letter), *Br. med. J.*, 1974, *3*, 803.

Fascioliasis. In 44 patients with fascioliasis, treatment for 18 days with emetine hydrochloride 30 mg daily by intramuscular injection to adults or chloroquine phosphate 150 mg twice daily by mouth to children for 3 weeks, was usually effective.— E. W. Hardman *et al.*, *Br. med. J.*, 1970, *3*, 502.

Leishmaniasis. Cultures from the lesions of a patient with leishmaniasis recidivens became negative after receiving intralesional injections of emetine hydrochloride once a week for 2 months. The patient had previously failed to respond to treatment with corticosteroids and antimonials and later flucytosine and amphotericin.— H. A. Cohen and A. Wahaba, *Acta derm.-vener., Stockh.*, 1979, *59*, 549, per *Trop. Dis. Bull.*, 1980, *77*, 472.

Tapeworm. *(Hymenolepis nana).* A child, aged 2½ years, with amoebic dysentery, harboured *Giardia intestinalis, Hymenolepis nana,* and several ectoparasites. Two courses of mepacrine with diloxanide furoate failed to affect the *Hymenolepis*. Further treatment with di-iodohydroxyquinoline and male fern extract was also unsuccessful. Finally, emetine hydrochloride 7.5 mg was given twice daily for 7 days, together with diloxanide furoate 125 mg thrice daily and *Hymenolepis* ova ceased to be excreted by the sixth day.— R. D. P. Eaton (letter), *Trans. R. Soc. trop. Med. Hyg.*, 1969, *63*, 153.

Preparations

Emetine Hydrochloride Injection *(U.S.P.).* A sterile solution of emetine hydrochloride in Water for Injections. pH 3 to 5. Protect from light.

Emetine Injection *(B.P.).* Emet. Inj. A sterile solution of emetine hydrochloride in Water for Injections, the acidity of the solution being adjusted by the addition of dilute hydrochloric acid to pH 3 (limits: pH 2.7 to 4). Sterilised by heating at 98° to 100° for 30 minutes with a bactericide, or by filtration. Protect from light.

A similar injection is included in several pharmacopoeias.

Injectabile Emetini *(Nord. P.).* Emetine Injection. Emetine hydrochloride 5 g, disodium edetate 10 mg, sodium chloride 400 mg, 0.1 M hydrochloric acid 1 g, Water for Injections to 100 ml. Sterilised by autoclaving.

Proprietary Names

Hemometina *(Cusi, Spain).*

4783-n

Etofamide. K 430; Ethychlordiphene. 2,2-Dichloro-*N*-(2-ethoxyethyl)-*N*-[4-(4-nitrophenoxy)benzyl]acetamide.

$C_{19}H_{20}Cl_2N_2O_5$=427.3.

CAS — 25287-60-9.

Etofamide has been used in the treatment of amoebiasis. It does not appear to be absorbed from the gastro-intestinal tract and high concentrations are found in the faeces for 3 days after administration of a single dose of 200 mg.

In 19 children with intestinal amoebiasis due to *Entamoeba histolytica;* etofamide 20 mg per kg body-weight daily for 3 days resulted in a parasitological cure in 18 of 19 patients. The remaining patient was cured after an additional 3-day treatment.— F. Biagi *et al.*, *Trans. R. Soc. trop. Med. Hyg.*, 1974, *68*, 368. See also I. de Carneri *et al.*, *Farmaco, Edn prat.*, 1972, *27*, 585; G. C. Levi *et al.*, *Revta Soc. bras. Med. trop.*, 1973, *7*, 335, per *Trop. Dis. Bull.*, 1975, *72*, 439; I. de Carneri *et al.*, *G. Mal. infett. parassit.*, 1976, *28*, 299, per *Trop. Dis. Bull.*, 1976, *73*, 931.

Proprietary Names

Kitnos.

4784-h

Furazolidone *(B.P., B.P. Vet.).* Nifurazolidonum. 3-(5-Nitrofurfurylideneamino)-2-oxazolidone.

$C_8H_7N_3O_5$=225.2.

CAS — 67-45-8.

Pharmacopoeias. In *Br., Braz., Chin., Cz., It., Nord., Roum.,* and *Rus.*

A yellow odourless crystalline powder, tasteless at first, followed by a bitter after-taste. M.p. about 259° with decomposition. Very slightly **soluble** in water and alcohol; slightly soluble in chloroform; practically insoluble in ether. The filtrate from a 1% suspension in water has a pH of 4.5 to 7. **Protect** from light.

Adverse Effects. Mild toxic symptoms, including headache, nausea, and vomiting, may occur; vesicular or morbilliform rashes may occur. Agranulocytosis has been reported. Acute haemolytic anaemia may occur in patients with a genetic deficiency of glucose-6-phosphate dehydrogenase.

A disulfiram-like reaction has been reported in patients taking alcohol while on furazolidone therapy.

When used intravaginally, it may occasionally give rise to vulvar oedema and pruritus.

A 56-year-old man who received furazolidone for 5 days for the treatment of suspected gastro-intestinal infection developed rigors and breathlessness. X-ray examination revealed diffuse mottling of the lungs which cleared after 7 days.— J. V. Collins and A. L. Thomas, *Postgrad. med. J.*, 1973, *49*, 518.

Serum sickness associated with the use of furazolidone in 2 patients; tartrazine present in the tablets might have been involved.— M. S. Wolfe and A. L. Moede, *Am. J. trop. Med. Hyg.*, 1978, *27*, 762.

Haemolytic anaemia. Experimental evidence suggested that the administration of 400 mg of furazolidone might produce significant haemolysis in Negroes with a deficiency of glucose-6-phosphate dehydrogenase.— Standardization of Procedures for the Study of Glucose-6-Phosphate Dehydrogenase, *Tech. Rep. Ser. Wld Hlth Org. No. 366,* 1967.

Precautions. Furazolidone inhibits some enzymes including monoamine oxidase. It is less potent than phenelzine but may enhance the effects of indirect acting sympathomimetics (see p.362) and antidepressants (see Precautions for Phenelzine Sulphate, p.128). Foods with a high tyramine content and alcoholic beverages should be avoided during and for a short period after treatment with furazolidone.

Furazolidone had no monoamine oxidase inhibiting activity but was converted to an active metabolite in rats, possibly 2-hydroxyethylhydrazine.— I. J. Stern *et al.*, *J. Pharmac. exp. Ther.*, 1967, *156*, 492.

Monoamine oxidase inhibition by furazolidone slowly increased as a function of the total dose but there was little risk of hypertension if treatment was limited to 400 mg daily for 5 days.— W. A. Pettinger *et al.*, *Clin. Pharmac. Ther.*, 1968, *9*, 442.

For a report of a toxic psychosis developing during treatment with furazolidone and amitriptyline, see under Amitriptyline Hydrochloride, p.112.

Transferable bacterial resistance. Transferable resistance to furazolidone had been observed between *Salmonella typhimurium* and *Escherichia coli.*— S. A. Kabins and S. Cohen (letter), *New Engl. J. Med.*, 1966, *275*, 1077.

Absorption and Fate. Most of a dose of furazolidone passes through the intestinal tract without being absorbed and is metabolised and inactivated in the intestine; about 5% is excreted in the urine together with coloured metabolites.

Studies in 12 healthy women indicated that little or no furazolidone was absorbed from the vagina.— G. Marion-Landais *et al.*, *Eaton, Curr. ther. Res.*, 1975, *18*, 510.

Uses. Furazolidone has antibacterial and antiprotozoal actions. In the treatment of diarrhoea and gastro-enteritis of bacterial origin it is given by mouth as tablets or suspension in a dosage of 100 mg four times daily for 2 to 5 days. Half this dose is given for prophylaxis. A suggested therapeutic dose, given 4 times daily, for infants aged 2 to 12 months is 12.5 mg; for children aged 1 to 4 years, 25 mg; and for children of 5 or over, 50 mg. It has also been used in the treatment of giardiasis.

Furazolidone has been used locally in conjunction with nifuroxime in the treatment of vaginal trichomoniasis or candidiasis as a powder for insufflation or as vaginal pessaries.

Cholera. In Calcutta, tests *in vitro* of sensitivity of 145 strains of *Vibrio cholerae* to furazolidone showed that the minimum inhibitory concentration for 80 strains was 1 µg per ml, and that sensitivity of strains to furazolidone decreased over a period of 6 years.— L. M. Prescott *et al.*, *Bull. Wld Hlth Org.*, 1968, *39*, 967.

Furazolidone was as effective as tetracycline in reducing the duration and volume of cholera diarrhoea, but it was less effective in eliminating vibrios from the intestinal tract.— A. W. Karchmer *et al.*, *Bull. Wld Hlth Org.*, 1970, *43*, 373.

Bacteriologically furazolidone 100 mg six-hourly for 3 days appeared to be less effective than tetracycline or minocycline in the treatment of cholera but the carrier state was lower after furazolidone.— D. N. G. Mazumdar *et al.*, *Indian J. med. Res.*, 1977, *66*, 917, per *Trop. Dis. Bull.*, 1978, *75*, 511.

Further references.— R. N. Chandhuri, *Lancet*, 1968, *1*, 332; N. F. Pierce *et al.*, *Br. med. J.*, 1968, *3*, 277; F. O'Grady, *Bull. Wld Hlth Org.*, 1976, *54*, 181.

Giardiasis. References: M. M. Rojas and J. W. Torrealba, *G.E.N.*, 1966, *21*, 127, per *Trop. Dis. Bull.*, 1967, *64*, 628; R. D. Botero *et al.*, *Revta Invest. Salud. Publ.*, 1973, *33*, 127, per *Trop. Dis. Bull.*, 1974, *71*, 1260; M. S. Wolfe, *J. Am. med. Ass.*, 1975, *233*, 1362; G. C. Levi *et al.*, *Am. J. trop. Med. Hyg.*, 1977, *26*, 564, per *Trop. Dis. Bull.*, 1978, *75*, 648.

Shigellosis. Furazolidone was ineffective in reducing the numbers of *Shigella* per g of faeces in 19 infants and children with shigellosis who were given 8 mg per kg body-weight daily in 4 divided doses for 5 days with kaolin and pectin. The results were similar to the natural course of the disease and furazolidone could not be recommended for shigellosis.— K. Haltalin and J. D. Nelson, *Am. J. Dis. Child.*, 1972, *123*, 40, per *Abstr. Hyg.*, 1972, *47*, 599.

A woman with co-trimoxazole-resistant shigellosis was treated with furazolidone 500 mg daily for 12 days. A week after completion of therapy her symptoms resolved and a stool culture was free of *Shigella;* 3 subsequent stool cultures at weekly intervals were also free.— D. E. Taylor *et al.* (letter), *Lancet*, 1980, *1*, 426.

Typhoid fever. References: M. El-S. Omar and M. F. A. Wahab, *J. trop. Med. Hyg.*, 1967, *70*, 43, per *Bull. Hyg., Lond.*, 1967, *42*, 1381; S. A. Kamat (letter), *J. Am. med. Ass.*, 1968, *206*, 2745; K. V. Thiruvengadam *et al.*, *J. Ass. Physns India*, 1971, *19*, 885, per *Br. med. J.*, 1973, *1*, 612; M. K. Punjani and J. S. Anand, *Indian Paediat.*, 1978, *15*, 769; S. P. Gupta *et al.*, *J. Ass. Physns India*, 1978, *26*, 573, per *Trop. Dis. Bull.*, 1980, *77*, 537.

Preparations

Furazolidone Tablets *(B.P.C. 1968)*. Tablets containing furazolidone. Protect from light.

Furoxone *(Norwich-Eaton, UK)*. Furazolidone, available as scored **Tablets** of 100 mg and as **Suspension** containing 25 mg in each 5 ml with kaolin 700 mg and pectin 75 mg (suggested diluent, water). *Dose*. 20 ml four times daily; children 2 to 12 months, 2.5 ml; 1 to 4 years, 5 ml; 5 years and older, 10 ml. (Also available as Furoxone in *Austral., Belg., Ital., Neth., S.Afr., USA*).

Proprietary preparations of furazolidone with nifuroxime are marketed in USA under the name Tricofuron (*Eaton*); this name is also applied to preparations containing only furazolidone.

Other Proprietary Names

Dialidene, Enterar *(both Ital.)*; Furoxane *(Fr.)*; Furoxona, Giardil *(both Arg.)*; Intefuran *(Ital.)*; Sirben *(Arg.)*; Tricofuron *(Fr.)*; Trifurox *(Norw.)*.

4785-m

Halquinol *(B.P.)*. Chlorhydroxyquinoline; Chlorquinol; Halquinols; SQ 16401. A mixture of the chlorinated products of quinolin-8-ol containing 57 to 74% of 5,7-dichloroquinolin-8-ol (chloroxine), 23 to 40% of 5-chloroquinolin-8-ol, and not more than 4% of 7-chloroquinolin-8-ol.

CAS — 8067-69-4.

Pharmacopoeias. In *Br. Cz.* has Chlorchinolinolum, a mixture of 5-chloro-and 5,7-dichloroquinolin-8-ol.

A yellowish-white to yellowish-grey voluminous powder with a faint cresol-like odour. Practically **insoluble** in water; soluble 1 in 250 of alcohol, 1 in 50 of chloroform, and 1 in 130 of ether; soluble in acids. **Incompatible** with many metal ions. Stable when dry but gradually volatilising in the presence of moisture at temperatures above 60°. **Protect** from light and avoid contact with metal.

Adverse Effects. Repeated application of halquinol may produce skin sensitisation. Skin rashes and pruritus have followed administration by mouth. Nausea and vomiting, headache, dizziness, and dysuria have been reported.

Reports of skin sensitivity in 3 patients following the application of a preparation containing halquinol 0.75% and triamcinolone acetonide 0.025%. All patients had used a preparation containing clioquinol 6 months to 2 years previously. Patch testing showed positive reactions to halquinol, chlorquinaldol, clioquinol, and di-iodohydroxyquinoline.— C. F. Allenby, *Br. med. J.*, 1965, *2*, 208.

A brief discussion of neuropathy and optic atrophy associated with halquinol.— O. Hansson and A. Herxheimer, *Lancet*, 1981, *1*, 450.

Uses. Halquinol has anti-amoebic, antibacterial, and antifungal actions. It has been used in the treatment of amoebiasis and in some cases of bacillary dysentery; it is not advocated in fulminating bacillary dysentery.

In amoebic and bacillary dysentery 3 to 4 g daily for 5 days was given. There should be a period of one month between courses.

Topically, it has been used in the treatment of infected skin conditions.

Halquinol had MICs ranging from 0.24 to 1.92 µg per ml against 12 different species of mycoplasma.— R. F. Cosgrove and S. Baines, *Squibb, Antimicrob. Ag. Chemother.*, 1978, *13*, 540.

5,7-Dichloroquinolin-8-ol was bactericidal for plaque cultures of *Streptococcus mutans, Str. sanguis, Actinomyces viscosus,* and *Actinomyces naeslundii in vitro* at concentrations of 0.05, 1, 2, and 0.2% respectively.— J. M. Tanzer *et al.*, *Antimicrob. Ag. Chemother.*, 1978, *13*, 1044.

Amoebiasis. References: P. P. Chanco *et al.*, *J. Philipp. med. Ass.*, 1965, *41*, 845, per *Trop. Dis. Bull.*, 1967, *64*, 167; R. Binato, *Hospital, Rio de J.*, 1966, *70*, 209, per *Trop. Dis. Bull.*, 1967, *64*, 168; S. Kumar *et al.*, *J. Ass. Physns India*, 1972, *20*, 775, per *Trop. Dis. Bull.*, 1973, *70*, 647.

Proprietary Names

Capitrol *(chloroxine) (Westwood, USA)*; Quixalin *(Squibb, S.Afr.)*; Quixaline *(Squibb, Belg.; Squibb, Fr.)*.

Halquinol was formerly marketed in Great Britain under the proprietary name Quixalin (*Squibb*).

4786-b

Holarrhena *(B.P.C. 1949)*. Kurchi; Conessi Bark; Tellicherry Bark.

Pharmacopoeias. In *Ind.*

The dried bark from the stem and root (*B.P.C. 1949*) or the dried bark from the stem (*Ind. P.*) of *Holarrhena antidysenterica* (Apocynaceae). It contains not less than 2% of total alkaloids, the principal alkaloid being conessine. **Store** in airtight containers.

Holarrhena is used in the treatment of amoebiasis but is probably less active than emetine. It has been used in India as a substitute for emetine in the treatment of amoebiasis, either as the liquid extract or as kurchi bismuth iodide.

Preparations

Kurchi Bismuth Iodide *(Ind. P.)*. A combination of bismuth iodide with the total alkaloids of holarrhena. It contains 23 to 27% of total alkaloids and 18 to 24% of bismuth. It is a fine, reddish-orange to dark red, odourless powder with a bitter acrid taste. Store in airtight containers. *Dose*. 300 to 600 mg.

Kurchi Liquid Extract *(Ind. P.)*. Holarrhena Liquid Extract. Prepared by percolation with alcohol (60%) and adjusted to contain 1% of total alkaloids. *Dose*. 8 to 16 ml.

4787-v

Melarsonyl Potassium. Melarsenoxide Potassium Dimercaptosuccinate; Mel W; Pentylthiarsphenylmelamine; RP 9955. Dipotassium 2-[4-(4,6-diamino-1,3,5-triazin-2-ylamino)phenyl]-1,3,2-dithiarsolan-4,5-dicarboxylate.

$C_{13}H_{11}AsK_2N_6O_4S_2$=532.5.

CAS — 37526-80-0 (melarsonyl); 13355-00-5 (potassium salt).

A white powder. **Soluble** in water. Aqueous solutions deteriorate on storage and should be used immediately after preparation; solutions for injection are prepared aseptically.

Adverse Effects and Treatment. As for Melarsoprol, p.980.

References: H. Collomb *et al.*, *Bull. Soc. méd. Afr. noire Langue franç.*, 1963, *8*, 61, per *Trop. Dis. Bull.*, 1964, *61*, 23; H. Collomb *et al.*, *Bull. Soc. méd. Afr. noire Langue franç.*, 1964, *9*, 325, per *Trop. Dis. Bull.*, 1965, *62*, 281.

Uses. Melarsonyl potassium is a water-soluble derivative of melarsoprol and may be administered by subcutaneous or intramuscular injection. It has been used in the treatment of *Trypanosoma gambiense* infections as an alternative to melarsoprol but it is considered less effective than melarsoprol in *T. rhodesiense* infections. The usual dosage employed has been 2 mg per kg body-weight increasing to 4 mg per kg, with a maximum of 200 mg for an adult and 2 mg per kg for a child, given intramuscularly daily for 4 days; the 4-day course of 4 mg per kg daily may be repeated after an interval of 7 to 10 days.

Filaria. *Wuchereria bancrofti*. Available evidence indicated that melarsonyl potassium was active against either periodic or sub-periodic *W. bancrofti*. Its main effect was produced on the adult worms. However, several deaths, apparently due to encephalopathy, had been reported following the use of melarsonyl potassium and it was not considered that such a risk should be incurred in the treatment of filariasis which was normally a non-fatal disease. Where it was used the size of the dose should be strictly limited as a precaution to reduce the risks involved.— Second Report of the Expert Committee on Filariasis, *Tech. Rep. Ser. Wld Hlth Org. No. 359*, 1967.

Guinea-worm. Melarsonyl potassium, 5 mg per kg body-weight up to a maximum of 200 mg, was given as a single dose to 45 patients with dracunculosis. Promethazine was also given to suppress allergic reactions. After 20 days, treatment was considered successful in 41 patients with disappearance of symptoms in 18 and expulsion of the worms in 23. In 2 patients treatment was less effective and in 2 ineffective.— C. Macario, *Bull. Soc. Path. exot.*, 1965, *58*, 1089, per *Trop. Dis. Bull.*, 1967, *64*, 769. See also S. Besse and C. Macario, *Bull. Soc. Path. exot.*, 1965, *58*, 1086.

Onchocerciasis. In the treatment of onchocerciasis, melarsonyl potassium had been given by intramuscular injection in doses of 200 mg daily for 4 days, the course being repeated after 10 to 14 days, or in a single dose of 7.5 to 10 mg per kg body-weight up to a maximum of 500 mg. Such treatment killed or sterilised most adult worms but had no effect on microfilariae. Peripheral neuritis had been reported after the use of melarsonyl potassium.— Second Report of a WHO Expert Committee on Onchocerciasis, *Tech. Rep. Ser. Wld Hlth Org. No. 335*, 1966. See also B. O. L. Duke, *Bull. Wld Hlth Org.*, 1970, *42*, 115.

Trypanosomiasis. References: Report of a Joint WHO Expert Committee and FAO Expert Consultation, *Tech. Rep. Ser. Wld Hlth Org. No. 635*, 1979.

Proprietary Names

Trimélarsan *(Specia, Fr.)*.

4788-g

Melarsoprol *(B.P. 1968)*. Melarsen Oxide-BAL; Mel B; RP 3854. 2-[4-(4,6-Diamino-1,3,5-triazin-2-ylamino)phenyl]-1,3,2-dithiarsolan-4-ylmethanol.

$C_{12}H_{15}AsN_6OS_2$=398.3.

CAS — 494-79-1.

A slightly cream-coloured or greyish cream-coloured, odourless or almost odourless powder with a bitter taste and containing about 18.5% of As. M.p. about 217° with decomposition.

Practically **insoluble** in water, alcohol, and ether; slowly soluble in cold propylene glycol but more readily soluble on warming. Solutions of melarsoprol in propylene glycol are **sterilised** by autoclaving.

Adverse Effects. Side-effects are common during treatment with melarsoprol partly because of its arsenical nature and partly because of its capacity for causing hypersensitivity reactions.

Melarsoprol is very irritant should extravasation occur.Vomiting and abdominal colic may occur, particularly after too rapid injection. Hypersensitivity reactions, peripheral neuropathy, and albuminuria may occur. Other side-effects reported include diarrhoea, cardiac arrhythmias, dermatitis, and hepatic disturbances.

The greatest risk however is from reactive encephalopathy, occurring in about 10% of patients and possibly due to the release of antigen from the trypanosomes; symptoms are tremor, convulsions, and coma; fatalities often occur. Less commonly haemorrhagic encephalopathy may occur.

Some references to encephalopathy with melarsoprol: K. Adriaenssens, *Annls Soc. belge Méd. trop.*, 1960, *4*, 701, per *Trop. Dis. Bull.*, 1961, *58*, 424; D. H. H. Robertson, *Trans. R. Soc. trop. Med. Hyg.*, 1963, *57*, 122; G. Sina *et al.*, *Annls Soc. belge Méd. trop.*, 1977, *57*, 67, per *Trop. Dis. Bull.*, 1977, *74*, 913.

Treatment of Adverse Effects. It has been suggested that the severity and incidence of toxic effects may be diminished if each dose of melarsoprol is preceded by treatment with promethazine hydrochloride and a corticosteroid.

The toxic effects of arsenic may be treated as described under Arsenic Trioxide, p.1681. Dimercaprol should be given but it has been reported to be of little benefit in some patients.

Hypersensitivity reactions occurring after the first course of treatment can be reduced by recommencing treatment with smaller and gradually increasing doses of melarsoprol in order to desensitise the patient, but some authorities consider that the use of small doses may increase the risk of resistance.

Precautions. Melarsoprol should not be administered during epidemics of influenza. It is contra-indicated in patients with impaired kidney or liver function. Severe haemolytic reactions have been reported in patients with glucose-6-phosphate dehydrogenase deficiency. It may precipitate erythema nodosum when administered to patients with leprosy.
Patients should be in hospital when they are treated with melarsoprol.

Absorption and Fate. Melarsoprol is reported to be fairly well absorbed if given by mouth but is usually given by intravenous injection. A small amount penetrates to the CSF where it has local trypanocidal action. It is rapidly excreted so any prophylactic effect is short-lived.

Eleven patients were given melarsoprol in a dose equivalent to 33.8 mg of arsenic daily for 3 days by intravenous injection. The mean blood-arsenic concentration was 480 µg per litre 15 minutes after injection and 185 µg per litre after 2 hours. Most of the excretion occurred in the first 3 days. There appeared to be no significant accumulation in the tissues.— B. Cristau *et al.*, *Medna trop.*, 1975, *35*, 389, per *Trop. Dis. Bull.*, 1976, *73*, 414.

Uses. Melarsoprol is a trypanocide which is effective in the treatment of all stages of *Trypanosoma gambiense* and *T. rhodesiense* infections, but because of its toxicity its use is usually reserved for later stages of the disease involving the central nervous system; it is often effective against infections that are resistant to tryparsamide. Resistance has been reported to develop.
Patients undergoing therapy with melarsoprol should be treated in hospital. The usual dosage is up to 3.6 mg per kg body-weight for an adult (with a maximum of 200 mg), given intravenously daily for 3 or 4 days; this course should be repeated after an interval of 7 to 10 days. A third course may be given if required. Children have been given 1.8 mg per kg. The initial dosage should be based on an assessment of the patient's general condition. Febrile or underweight patients with advanced meningo-encephalitis may be given preliminary treatment with up to 4 doses of suramin 250 to 500 mg, given on alternate days. Some authorities recommend initial doses of about 1.44 to 2.16 mg per kg especially to patients in poor condition. The injection should be given slowly, care being taken to prevent leakage into the surrounding tissues, and the patient should remain supine and fasting for at least 5 hours after the injection.
If a relapse occurs after the course of treatment, the infection is usually resistant to other forms of chemotherapy, but nitrofurazone (see p.499) may be tried with some chance of success.

Trypanosomiasis. After assessing the results of the follow-up of 71 patients (64 with *T. rhodesiense* and 7 with *T. gambiense* infections) treated with melarsoprol, it was concluded that a period of 3 years' observation was advisable to eliminate the possibility of relapse. Most relapses after an initial treatment with melarsoprol were evident in 6 to 12 months; the period shortened after unsuccessful treatment with the development of resistance to the drug. Nevertheless, cure might follow a second treatment with melarsoprol. Thereafter, re-treatment was unlikely to be successful in view of the rapid development of resistance to melarsoprol.— D. H. H. Robertson, *Trans. R. Soc. trop. Med. Hyg.*, 1963, *57*, 176.

Melarsoprol gave better results against *T. gambiense* than tryparsamide and pentamidine and was considered to be slightly superior to melarsonyl potassium. Pretreatment with promethazine hydrochloride and corticosteroids prevented untoward reactions.— Report of a Joint FAO/WHO Expert Committee, *Tech. Rep. Ser. Wld Hlth Org. No. 434*, 1969. See also Report of a Joint WHO Expert Committee and FAO Expert Consultation, *Tech. Rep. Ser. Wld Hlth Org. No. 635*, 1979.

For a report of the treatment of trypanosomiasis in a pregnant woman, with suramin and melarsoprol, see Suramin, p.984.

Preparations

Melarsoprol Injection *(B.P.)*. A sterile solution of melarsoprol 3.4 to 3.8% in propylene glycol containing 5% of water. Sterilised by autoclaving.

Proprietary Names

Arsobal *(Rhône-Poulenc, Fr.)*.

4789-q

Nifuratel.

Methylmercadone. 5-Methylthiomethyl-3-(5-nitrofurfurylideneamino)-2-oxazolidone.
$C_{10}H_{11}N_3O_5S=285.3$.

CAS — 4936-47-4.

Pharmacopoeias. In *Nord.*

A yellow crystalline powder with a characteristic odour of sulphur. M.p. 186° to 188°. Practically **insoluble** in water; soluble 1 in 400 of chloroform; sparingly soluble in acetone; soluble in dimethylformamide. **Protect** from light.

Adverse Effects. Gastro-intestinal discomfort and skin rashes occasionally occur with nifuratel.

Precautions. Nausea and flushing of the skin may occur if large quantities of alcohol are taken during treatment with nifuratel.

Absorption and Fate. When taken by mouth nifuratel is absorbed from the gastro-intestinal tract. A metabolite, with activity against bacteria but not against trichomonads, is excreted in the urine.

Uses. Nifuratel has antibacterial and antiprotozoal actions and is effective against some fungi including *Candida albicans*. It has been used in the treatment of candidal and trichomonal infections of the genito-urinary tract.
The dose for women is 200 mg by mouth thrice daily for 7 days together with one 250-mg pessary nightly for 10 nights. Local treatment has been used in pregnancy, 1 pessary being inserted nightly for 20 nights.
The dose for men is 200 mg thrice daily for 7 days.

The antimicrobial activity of nifuratel was compared with nitrofurantoin against 49 clinical isolates and 24 reference strains of *Bacteroides* or *Fusobacterium* spp. *in vitro*. The mean MICs were 7.7 µg per ml for nitrofurantoin and 0.28 µg per ml or less for nifuratel. Nifuratel had also been shown to be more effective against aerobic bacteria.— W. Brumfitt *et al.* (letter), *Lancet*, 1975, *1*, 460.

Giardiasis. References: M. A. B. Silva, *Revta bras. Med.*, 1973, *30*, 730, per *Trop. Dis. Bull.*, 1974, *71*, 363.

Proprietary Names

Inimur *(Woelm, Ger.)*; Macmiror *(Beta, Arg.; Poli, Ital.; Poli, Neth.; Adcock Ingram, S.Afr.; Farma-Lepori, Spain; Poli, Switz.)*; Omnes *(Cochard, Belg.; Fumouze, Fr.)*; Polmiror *(Astra, Denm.; Astra, Swed.)*.

Nifuratel was formerly marketed in Great Britain under the proprietary name Magmilor (*Calmic*).

4790-d

Nifurtimox.

Bayer 2502. Tetrahydro-3-methyl-4-(5-nitrofurfurylideneamino)-1,4-thiazine 1,1-dioxide.
$C_{10}H_{13}N_3O_5S=287.3$.

CAS — 23256-30-6.

A yellow solid. M.p. 180° to 182°. **Soluble** in water, acetone, methyl alcohol, and in a mixture of equal parts of dimethylformamide and pyridine. Dilute solutions in organic solvents should be protected from light.

Adverse Effects. Adverse effects are common and include anorexia with loss of weight, abdominal pain, nausea, and vomiting. Restlessness, nervous excitement, insomnia, drowsiness, headache, dizziness, arthralgia, loss of balance, depression, disorientation, paraesthesia, skin reactions, and convulsions have been reported.

Uses. Nifurtimox is of value in the treatment of acute and chronic South American trypanosomiasis (Chagas' disease) due to infection by *Trypanosoma cruzi*. It is better tolerated by children than by adults.
It has been found possible to reduce the doses given in early trials without loss of efficacy. Recommended doses are: adults 8 to 10 mg per kg body-weight daily for 120 days; children up to 10 years, 15 to 20 mg per kg daily; up to 16 years, 12.5 to 15 mg per kg daily. A 90-day course is probably adequate for children.

Chagas' disease. Success-rates of 90% (xenodiagnosis) and 80% (immunological response) had been achieved in 550 patients with acute Chagas' disease treated with nifurtimox. Of 89 patients with chronic Chagas' disease treated with nifurtimox 8 to 10 mg per kg body-weight daily for short (30 to 60 days) or long (90 to 120 days) periods 76 were considered to be free of infection (xenodiagnosis) after follow-up for at least 11 months. Results from treatment for short or long periods were comparable. The cure-rate was about 92% in Argentina, Chile, and Southern Brazil, and about 53% in central Brazil.— J. A. Cerisola, in *Chagas' Disease*, Proceedings of an International Symposium, New York City, 27 June 1977, Washington, Pan American Health Organization, Scientific Publication No. 347,, p. 35.

Further references: A. Rassi and H. de O. Ferreira, *Revta Soc. bras. Med. trop.*, 1971, *5*, 235, per *Trop. Dis. Bull.*, 1972, *69*, 885; G. C. Levi and V. A. Neto, *Revta Inst. Med. trop. S Paulo*, 1971, *13*, 369, per *Trop. Dis. Bull.*, 1972, *69*, 378; *Arzneimittel-Forsch.*, 1972, *22*, 1563–1642; J. A. Cerisola *et al.*, *Trop. Dis. Bull.*, 1973, *70*, 1153; H. Schenone *et al.*, *Boln chil. Parasit.*, 1972, *27*, 11, per *Trop. Dis. Bull.*, 1973, *70*, 327; S. G. Andrade and V. Macêdo, *Revta Inst. Med. trop. S Paulo*, 1973, *15*, 421, per *Trop. Dis. Bull.*, 1974, *71*, 1233; N. N. Silva *et al.*, *Revta Soc. bras. Med. trop.*, 1974, *8*, 325, per *Trop. Dis. Bull.*, 1975, *72*, 807; J. R. Cançado *et al.*, *Revta Inst. Med. trop. S Paulo*, 1975, *17*, 111, per *Trop. Dis. Bull.*, 1975, *72*, 808; J. R. Cançado *et al.*, *Revta goiana Med.*, 1976, *22*, 203, per *Trop. Dis. Bull.*, 1978, *75*, 767; J. L. da S. Baldy *et al.*, *Revta Inst. Med. trop. S Paulo*, 1979, *21*, 155, per *Trop. Dis. Bull.*, 1979, *76*, 914.

Proprietary Names

Lampit *(Bayer, Arg.; Bayer, Ger.)*.

4791-n

Nimorazole.

Nitrimidazine. 4-[2-(5-Nitroimidazol-1-yl)ethyl]morpholine.
$C_9H_{14}N_4O_3=226.2$.

CAS — 6506-37-2.

A whitish crystalline powder. M.p. about 110°.

Adverse Effects and Precautions. As for Metronidazole, p.968.

Absorption and Fate. Nimorazole is readily absorbed from the gastro-intestinal tract. Peak blood concentrations are achieved within 2 hours, and high concentrations are reported to occur in salivary and vaginal secretions. It is also absorbed after local application to the vagina. It is excreted in the urine together with 2 active metabolites.

Uses. Nimorazole which is a nitroimidazole like metronidazole has antiprotozoal actions and is effective against *Trichomonas vaginalis* and other protozoa, including *Entamoeba histolytica* and *Giardia lamblia*.
In the treatment of trichomoniasis, the usual dose is 2 g as a single dose with a main meal. Alternative regimens have been used: 3 doses of 1 g at intervals of 12 hours or 250 mg twice daily for 6 days. Sexual partners should be treated concomitantly.
In the treatment of Vincent's infection, nimorazole 500 mg is given twice daily for 2 days.
A suggested dose for amoebiasis is 500 mg twice daily for 5 days.

The median minimum inhibitory concentration of nimorazole against *Bacteroides* spp. was 0.25 µg per ml.— R. Wise *et al.*, *Chemotherapy, Basle*, 1977, *23*, 19.

Amoebiasis. References: A. V. M. Arrubarrena *et al.*, *Revta Gastroent. Méx.*, 1971, *36*, 140, per *Trop. Dis. Bull.*, 1972, *69*, 631; D. Sutrisno *et al.*, *Paediatrica Indones.*, 1978, *18*, 217, per *Trop. Dis. Bull.*, 1979, *76*, 766.

Balantidiasis. Of 17 children aged 3 to 15 years with ***Balantidium coli*** infections, 12 improved after treatment with nimorazole 500 mg daily for 5 days. Dizziness occurred in 3 patients and vomiting in 1.— R. D. Botero (letter), *Trans. R. Soc. trop. Med. Hyg.*, 1973, *67*, 145.

Giardiasis. In 20 patients with giardiasis, treatment with nimorazole eradicated infection, as judged by stool examinations 15 and 30 days after treatment. The dosage for adults was 1 g daily for 6 days and for children 375 mg daily for 5 days.— D. Huggins, *Hospital, Rio de J.*, 1970, *77*, 2053, per *Trop. Dis. Bull.*, 1971, *68*, 319. See also V. R. Pai *et al.*, *J. Ass. Physns India*, 1974, *22*, 531, per *Trop. Dis. Bull.*, 1975, *72*, 149.

Giardiasis was eradicated in all 49 patients who received nimorazole 2 to 2.5 g in divided doses over 2 to 5 days; these doses were also effective in eradicating amoebiasis in 7 other patients. A total dose of 1.5 g of nimorazole cured only 9 of 20 patients with giardiasis who were similarly treated.— J. L. Z. Louzada *et al.*, *Trib. méd., Paris*, 1971, *14*, 49, per *Trop. Dis. Bull.*, 1972, *69*, 910.

A cure-rate of 90.9% in 66 children with giardiasis given nimorazole 20 mg per kg body-weight daily for 5 days.— H. Schenone *et al.*, *Boln chil. Parasit.*, 1976, *31*, 12, per *Trop. Dis. Bull.*, 1977, *74*, 321.

A cure-rate of 94.1% in patients with giardiasis given nimorazole 250 mg twice daily for 5 days.— G. C. Levi *et al.*, *Am. J. trop. Med. Hyg.*, 1977, *26*, 564, per *Trop. Dis. Bull.*, 1978, *75*, 648.

Trichomoniasis. In a controlled study in 114 patients, treatment with nimorazole 250 mg twice daily for 6 days was effective in 39 of 57 (68%) patients with vaginal trichomoniasis whereas metronidazole 200 mg thrice daily for 7 days was effective in 51 of 57 (89%) similar patients. Anorexia and nausea occurred in 1 patient in each group.— B. A. Evans and R. D. Catterall, *Br. med. J.*, 1971, *4*, 146. Nimorazole 1 g every 12 hours for 3 doses was as effective as metronidazole 200 mg thrice daily for 7 days in the treatment of trichomonal vaginitis.— A. S. Wigfield, *Br. J. vener. Dis.*, 1975, *51*, 54, per *Abstr. Hyg.*, 1975, *50*, 382.

Nimorazole in single doses of 2 g cured 92% of 88 women with vaginal trichomoniasis; the cure-rate was 96% among 58 women whose partners also received treatment.— S. M. Ross, *Br. J. vener. Dis.*, 1973, *49*, 310, per *Abstr. Hyg.*, 1973, *48*, 730.

Of 150 patients given nimorazole 2 g daily in 2 divided doses on 2 successive days, 87 were found to be cured when examined at least 4 weeks later; 48 patients defaulted.— J. S. McCann *et al.*, *Br. J. vener. Dis.*, 1974, *50*, 375, per *Abstr. Hyg.*, 1975, *50*, 258.

A cure-rate of 90.5% in 59 women with trichomoniasis treated with nimorazole 300 mg twice daily for 7 days.— G. Eriksson and L. Wanger, *Br. J. vener. Dis.*, 1976, *52*, 276, per *Abstr. Hyg.*, 1976, *51*, 1164.

For further studies comparing the efficacy of nimorazole and metronidazole in the treatment of vaginal trichomoniasis, see under Metronidazole, p.972.

Further references: M. Moffett *et al.*, *Br. J. vener. Dis.*, 1971, *47*, 173; L. Cohen, *ibid.*, 177; *Drug & Ther. Bull.*, 1971, *9*, 103; A. N. McClean, *Br. J. vener. Dis.*, 1972, *48*, 69, per *Abstr. Hyg.*, 1972, *47*, 588; *Drug & Ther. Bull.*, 1973, *11*, 23; A. E. Tinkler, *Practitioner*, 1974, *212*, 115; S. Chandramani, *Br. J. clin. Pract.*, 1975, *29*, 114; M. J. Hayward and R. B. Roy, *Br. J. vener. Dis.*, 1976, *52*, 63.

Vincent's infection. In a double-blind study with 53 patients, nimorazole 250 mg thrice daily for 2 days was found to be as effective in the treatment of acute ulcerative gingivitis as metronidazole 200 mg thrice daily for 2 days.— J. Lozdan *et al.*, *Br. dent. J.*, 1971, *130*, 294.

Proprietary Preparations

Naxogin 500 *(Farmitalia Carlo Erba, UK)*. Nimorazole, available as scored tablets of 500 mg. (Also available as Naxogin in *Arg., Belg., Ital., Neth., S.Afr., Spain*).

Other Proprietary Names

Acterol Forte, Esclama *(both Ger.)*; Naxogyn *(Fr.)*; Sirledi *(Ital.)*.

4792-h

Ornidazole.

Ro-7-0207. 1-Chloro-3-(2-methyl-5-nitroimidazol-1-yl)propan-2-ol.
$C_7H_{10}ClN_3O_3$=219.6.

CAS — 16773-42-5.

A pale yellow crystalline powder. M.p. 74° to 79°. **Soluble** 1 in about 25 of water. A 1% solution has a pH of about 6.6.

Adverse Effects and Precautions. Side-effects include gastro-intestinal effects, dizziness, headache, drowsiness, muscle weakness, and skin reactions. Adverse reactions are claimed not to occur with alcohol. It should not be given to patients with active disease of the central nervous system.

For neuropathy associated with the use of ornidazole as a radiosensitiser, see H. Schipper (letter), *New Engl. J. Med.*, 1976, *295*, 901; R. C. Urtasan (letter), *ibid.*

Absorption and Fate. Ornidazole is readily absorbed from the gastro-intestinal tract. It is reported to be absorbed from the vaginal mucosa.

In 5 healthy women given ornidazole 1.5 g mean peak plasma concentrations of 33.2 µg per ml were achieved within 2 hours; the mean plasma half-life was 13.8 hours. Protein binding of 13.4% had been reported. Trichomonacidal concentrations were maintained for about 48 hours.— I. Matheson *et al.*, *Br. J. vener. Dis.*, 1977, *53*, 236.

The metabolism of ornidazole.— D. E. Schwartz *et al.*, *Xenobiotica*, 1979, *9*, 571.

Uses. Ornidazole has actions and uses similar to those of metronidazole (see p.969).

In amoebiasis and giardiasis the usual dose is 500 mg twice daily for 5 to 10 days. Children under 1 year, 1 to 6 years, and 7 to 12 years may be given respectively one-quarter, one-half, and three-quarters of the above dose.

In trichomoniasis a single dose of 1.5 g by mouth or 1 g by mouth with 500 mg vaginally may be given; 5-day courses of 1 g daily with or without concomitant vaginal therapy are also used. Sexual partners should be treated concomitantly.

Ornidazole has been used, usually in doses of 1 g daily by mouth or by slow intravenous injection, in the treatment of anaerobic infections.

Toxicological and clinical evaluation.— R. Richle *et al.*, *Arzneimittel-Forsch.*, 1978, *28*, 612.

Amoebiasis. In a double-blind study 17 of 18 patients with amoebic liver abscess were cleared of infection, with no relapses at 6 months, after treatment for 5 days with ornidazole 1.5 g daily, with multiple aspirations. The results were similar to those achieved in a further 18 patients treated with metronidazole.— A. Ruas *et al.*, *Cent. Afr. J. Med.*, 1973, *19*, 128, per *Trop. Dis. Bull.*, 1973, *70*, 1075.

Of 115 patients with intestinal amoebiasis 59 were treated with metronidazole 500 mg twice daily for 10 days and 56 with ornidazole in similar dosage. Parasitological failures and relapses were 6 and 2 for metronidazole and 1 and 9 for ornidazole.— R. D. Botero, *Am. J. trop. Med. Hyg.*, 1974, *23*, 1000, per *Trop. Dis. Bull.*, 1975, *72*, 240.

Further references.— S. A. Naoemar and B. Rukmono, *S.E. Asian J. trop. med. publ. Hlth*, 1973, *4*, 417; O. G. Sandia *et al.*, *Revta Inst. Med. trop. S Paulo*, 1977, *19*, 52.

Bacterial infections. Mixed aerobic-anaerobic infections were cured in 15 of 16 patients given ornidazole 500 mg by intravenous infusion over 30 minutes every 12 hours after an initial dose of 1 g. Oral administration at the same dose was substituted when possible. Duration of treatment ranged from 5 to 60 days (mean 21 days).— H. Giamarellou *et al.*, *J. antimicrob. Chemother.*, 1981, *7*, 569.

Antimicrobial action. The following anaerobic bacteria were inhibited by 3.1 µg per ml of ornidazole and killed by 6.3 µg per ml: *Bacteroides fragilis* and *melaninogenicus*, *Clostridium perfringens* and other species of clostridia, *Eubacterium*, *Fusobacterium*, *Peptococcus*, *Peptostreptococcus*, and Veillonella spp. *Propionibacterium acnes* was relatively resistant. The same figures were achieved with metronidazole and tinidazole.— J. Wüst, *Antimicrob. Ag. Chemother.*, 1977, *11*, 631.

Ornidazole inhibited about 62% of 55 strains of *Bacteroides fragilis in vitro* at a concentration of 1 µg per ml and metronidazole inhibited about 44%; both drugs inhibited all of the strains at 16 µg per ml. The activity of ornidazole was also similar to that of metronidazole against a further 229 anaerobic bacteria and most strains were inhibited at concentrations of 16 µg or less per ml. Strains of ***Propionibacterium, Streptococcus,*** and ***Actinomyces*** were significantly resistant to both drugs.— E. J. C. Goldstein *et al.*, *Antimicrob. Ag. Chemother.*, 1978, *14*, 609.

Crohn's disease. Use in Crohn's disease.— R. W. Ammann, *Schweiz. med. Wschr.*, 1978, *108*, 1075.

Giardiasis. Administration of a single dose of ornidazole 25 to 30 mg per kg body-weight cleared symptomatic giardiasis in 21 of 25 children aged 13 months to 14 years of age; one further patient was cleared with a second dose when his asymptomatic brother was also treated. Side-effects occurred in 4 patients (dizziness, 2; vomiting, 1; headache, vomiting, and abdominal pain, 1) and were not correlated with the dose.— H. P. T. Werkman and J. H. E. T. Meuwissen (letter), *Lancet*, 1979, *2*, 1373.

Further references: N. Iyngkaran *et al.*, *Scand. J. infect. Dis.*, 1978, *10*, 243; A. Sabchareon *et al.*, *S.E. Asian J. trop. med. publ. Hlth*, 1980, *11*, 280, per *Trop. Dis. Bull.*, 1981, *78*, 161.

Trichomoniasis. In a double-blind study all of 45 women with vaginal trichomoniasis were cleared of infection after a single dose of ornidazole 1.5 g by mouth; of 45 given tinidazole 2 g as a single dose 43 were cleared. Sexual partners were treated concomitantly.— L. Hillström *et al.*, *Br. J. vener. Dis.*, 1977, *53*, 193.

A success-rate of 98.5% was achieved in 68 women with vaginal trichomoniasis after treatment with ornidazole 1 to 2 g by mouth in one day, or 1 g in one day with 500 mg vaginally. Side-effects, usually mild, occurred in about 14% of the patients.— S. O. Chung *et al.*, *S.E. Asian J. trop. med. publ. Hlth*, 1978, *9*, 74.

Further references: T. H. Lean and D. Vengadasalam, *Br. J. vener. Dis.*, 1973, *49*, 69; M. Goisis *et al.*, *G. Mal. infett. parassit.*, 1975, *27*, 13, per *Abstr. Hyg.*, 1976, *51*, 427; M. Sköld *et al.*, *Br. J. vener. Dis.*, 1977, *53*, 44.

Proprietary Names

Tiberal *(Roche, Arg.; Roche, Ger.; Roche, S.Afr.; Roche, Switz.)*.

4793-m

Pentamidine Isethionate *(B.P.)*.

Pentamid. Isethion.; Pentamidini Isethionas; M & B 800. 4,4′-(Pentamethylenedioxy)dibenzamidine bis(2-hydroxyethanesulphonate).
$C_{19}H_{24}N_4O_2,2C_2H_6O_4S$=592.7.

CAS — 100-33-4 (pentamidine); 140-64-7 (isethionate).

Pharmacopoeias. In *Br.*, *Int.*, and *Turk.*

White or almost white, odourless, hygroscopic crystals or powder with a very bitter taste. M.p. 188° to 192°. Pentamidine isethionate 1.74 mg is approximately equivalent to 1 mg of pentamidine. **Soluble** 1 in 10 of water; soluble in glycerol; slightly soluble in alcohol; practically insoluble in acetone, chloroform, ether, and liquid paraffin. A 5% solution in water has a pH of 4.5 to 6.5. Aqueous solutions deteriorate on storage and should be used immediately after preparation; solutions for injection are prepared aseptically. **Store** in airtight containers.

Adverse Effects. The intramuscular injection of pentamidine isethionate often causes pain at the site of injection but this route of administration is preferable to intravenous injection; abscess formation has been reported.

Hyperglycaemia, hypoglycaemia, and haematological disturbances have been reported after treatment with pentamidine; vomiting and kidney and liver dysfunction may also occur.

The intravenous injection of pentamidine, and other diamidines, produces sudden hypotension if administered too rapidly. This may cause dizziness, headache, breathlessness, tachycardia, and fainting; occasionally, rigors have occurred after large doses.

Major complications in an infant who was thought to have *Pneumocystis carinii* pneumonia and was given pentamidine 4 mg per kg body-weight daily were local reactions and reversible uraemia.— *J. Am. med. Ass.*, 1974, *230*, 13.

Fever, tachycardia, hypotension, and profound fatal acidosis developed suddenly in a 14-year-old boy, with acute myeloid leukaemia in relapse, 11 hours after he was given a single dose of pentamidine 70 mg for the treatment of pneumonia due to *Pneumocystis carinii*.— F. R. Stark *et al.* (letter), *Lancet*, 1976, *1*, 1193.

Pentamidine isethionate inhibited platelet adhesiveness, platelet aggregation, and clot retraction *in vitro* in a dose-dependent manner. The thrombin clotting time was prolonged at concentrations of pentamidine of 5 µg per ml and above and the prothrombin time at concentrations above 10 µg per ml.— S. J. Kempin *et al.*, *Antimicrob. Ag. Chemother.*, 1977, *12*, 451.

Absorption and Fate. Pentamidine isethionate is absorbed from intramuscular injection sites and deposited in the tissues; only a small proportion of the dose is found in the blood.

Average low plasma-pentamidine concentrations of 400 ng per ml at 0.5 hour, 500 ng per ml at 1 hour, and 300 ng per ml at 3, 6, and 24 hours were observed in 7 patients given pentamidine 4 mg per kg body-weight intramuscularly. Measurement in 5 patients showed that half to two-thirds of the urinary excretion took place in the first 6 hours and after treatment was stopped decreasing amounts were found in the urine up to 8 weeks later.— T. P. Waalkes *et al.*, *Clin. Pharmac. Ther.*, 1970, *11*, 505.

Uses. Pentamidine isethionate is used in the treatment of early stages of African trypanosomiasis, especially in *Trypanosoma gambiense* infections. It does not attain sufficient concentration in the cerebrospinal fluid to be of value in the treatment of advanced trypanosomiasis in which the central nervous system is involved and treatment must be changed to melarsoprol.

Considerable confusion exists in the literature regarding the dose of pentamidine; WHO and some other authorities clearly express the individual dose as 3 to 4 mg of the base per kg body-weight; some other authorities quote a similar dose of the isethionate; the *B.P.* which does not express the dose in terms of body-weight expresses a dose of 150 to 300 mg in terms of the isethionate, which is equivalent to 86 to 172 mg of the base; 1.74 mg of the isethionate is approximately equivalent to 1 mg of the base.

The usual dose in the treatment of early trypanosomiasis is 3 to 4 mg of pentamidine per kg body-weight, as a 10% solution daily or on alternate days for 7 to 10 intramuscular injections.

Pentamidine is also given as a prophylactic, particularly against *T. gambiense* infection, in endemic areas in a dose of 4 mg per kg intramuscularly every 6 months. Before pentamidine is used for prophylaxis in a community, a careful examination should be made to detect patients in whom the disease has advanced beyond the early stages and these must be given a full course of treatment with a drug, such as melarsoprol or tryparsamide, which penetrates the blood-brain barrier.

Pentamidine is also used in the treatment of leishmaniasis (kala-azar) and is especially valuable in patients who do not respond to treatment with antimonial drugs. A dose of 2 to 4 mg per kg is given daily by intramuscular injection until 12 to 15 doses have been given; a second course of treatment may be given 1 or 2 weeks later.

Pentamidine has also been given by intramuscular injection, or in severe cases by slow intravenous injection, in the treatment of pneumonia due to *Pneumocystis carinii* in a dose of 4 mg per kg body-weight daily for 12 to 14 days.

Pentamidine mesylate has also been used.

Pentamidine isethionate showed slight activity *in vitro* against *Acanthamoeba* spp.— R. J. Duma and R. Finley, *Antimicrob. Ag. Chemother.*, 1976, *10*, 370.

Administration in renal failure. The interval between doses of pentamidine in the treatment of *Pneumocystis carinii* should be extended from 24 hours to 24 to 36 hours in patients with a glomerular filtration-rate (GFR) of 10 to 50 ml per minute, and to 48 hours in those with a GFR of less than 10 ml per minute.— W. M. Bennett *et al.*, *Ann. intern. Med.*, 1980, *93*, 62.

Babesiasis. The routine clinical use of pentamidine or diminazene aceturate in infections due to *Babesia microti* was not recommended except in patients without spleens, since normally the infection was self-limiting.— L. H. Miller *et al.*, *Ann. intern. Med.*, 1978, *88*, 200.

Since the use of diminazene in a patient infected with *Babesia microti* might have produced Guillain-Barré syndrome, it was suggested that pentamidine rather than diminazene might be preferable in severe cases of human babesiasis.— T. K. Ruebush and A. Spielman, *Ann. intern. Med.*, 1978, *88*, 263.

Pneumonia. *(Pneumocystis carinii).* A study of the use of pentamidine in the treatment of 74 patients with pneumonia considered to be due to *Pn. carinii.* About 77% of the patients who were treated for 9 days or longer with 4 mg per kg body-weight daily were considered cured. Because of the toxicity of pentamidine, the diagnosis of *Pn. carinii* infection should be confirmed before use.— K. A. Western *et al.*, *Ann. intern. Med.*, 1970, *73*, 695, per *Trop. Dis. Bull.*, 1971, *68*, 892.

Of 404 patients with known or suspected pneumonia due to *Pn. carinii*, treated with pentamidine isethionate, 69 of the 163 (42%) with confirmed pneumonia recovered. In 93 of the 163 patients treated for 9 days or more 59 (63%) recovered. Adverse reactions occurred in 189 patients and included alterations in renal function, hepatotoxicity, hypoglycaemia, haematological disturbances, skin rash, hypocalcaemia, hypotension, and local reactions.— P. D. Walzer *et al.*, *Ann. intern. Med.*, 1974, *80*, 83. See also G. W. Geelhoed *et al.*, *Ann. thorac. Surg.*, 1972, *14*, 335, per *J. Am. med. Ass.*, 1972, *222*, 1576.

Co-trimoxazole was as effective as pentamidine in the treatment of pneumonia due to *Pneumocystis carinii.* Co-trimoxazole had the advantages of being safer and of being effective by mouth.— W. T. Hughes *et al.*, *J. Pediat.*, 1978, *92*, 285.

Further references: J. Ruskin and J. S. Remington (letter), *J. Am. med. Ass.*, 1968, *203*, 604; J. P. Lillehei *et al.*, *ibid.*, *206*, 596; V. T. DeVita *et al.*, *New Engl. J. Med.*, 1969, *280*, 287; A. Lipson *et al.*, *Archs Dis. Childh.*, 1977, *52*, 314.

Trypanosomiasis. References: Report of a Joint WHO Expert Committee and FAO Expert Consultation, *Tech. Rep. Ser. Wld Hlth Org. No. 635*, 1979.

Preparations

Pentamidine Injection *(B.P.).* Pentamidine Isethionate Injection. A sterile solution of pentamidine isethionate in Water for Injections, prepared by dissolving, immediately before use, the sterile contents of a sealed container (Pentamidine Isethionate for Injection) in the requisite amount of Water for Injections.

Pentamidine Isethionate *(May & Baker, UK).* Available as powder for preparing injections in ampoules of 200 mg.

4794-b

Pentamidine Mesylate. Pentamidine Methanesulphonate; Pentamidine Dimethylsulphonate; RP 2512. 4,4′-(Pentamethylenedioxy)dibenzamidine dimethanesulphonate.

$C_{19}H_{24}N_4O_2,2CH_3SO_3H$=532.6.

CAS — 6823-79-6.

Pharmacopoeias. In *Fr.*

A white or very faintly pink, almost odourless, granular powder. Pentamidine mesylate 1.56 mg is approximately equivalent to 1 mg of pentamidine. Slightly **soluble** in water and alcohol; practically insoluble in acetone, chloroform, ether, and ethyl acetate. A 5% solution in water has a pH of 4.5 to 6.5.

Pentamidine mesylate has the same actions and uses as pentamidine isethionate.

Leishmaniasis. Eight patients with American leishmaniasis, 5 with the mucocutaneous form and 3 with the cutaneous form, were treated with pentamidine mesylate by intramuscular injection. Dosage was 120 mg on alternate days for 10 injections and further doses were given after 10 days to a total of 15 to 30 injections. Excellent results followed treatment in 5 patients, good in 2, but only fair in 1.— T. A. Furtado *et al.*, *Hospital, Rio de J.*, 1969, *75*, 1217, per *Trop. Dis. Bull.*, 1969, *66*, 907. For a similar report, see C. F. Lopes and M. A. De Almeida, *Hospital, Rio de J.*, 1968, *73*, 223, per *Trop. Dis. Bull.*, 1968, *65*, 987.

In 31 cases of diffuse cutaneous leishmaniasis the parasite was sensitive to pentamidine mesylate 4 mg per kg body-weight intramuscularly, the dose frequency depending upon appearance of toxic effects. Side-effects included abnormalities of glucose tolerance.— A. D. M. Bryceson, *Trans. R. Soc. trop. Med. Hyg.*, 1970, *64*, 369.

Proprietary Names

Lomidine *(Specia, Fr.; Rhône-Poulenc, Ger.).*

4795-v

Phanquone *(B.P. 1963).* C 11925; Phanquinone. 4,7-Phenanthroline-5,6-dione.

$C_{12}H_6N_2O_2$=210.2.

CAS — 84-12-8.

An orange, odourless, almost tasteless, crystalline powder. Slightly **soluble** in water; practically insoluble in alcohol and chloroform. **Store** in airtight containers. Protect from light.

Adverse Effects. Nausea, vomiting, slight burning sensation in the stomach, and transient dizziness may occur but can usually be avoided by taking phanquone with meals.

Absorption and Fate. Phanquone is absorbed from the gastro-intestinal tract and excreted in an active form in the bile and urine.

Uses. Phanquone has anti-amoebic and antibacterial actions. It is used chiefly in intestinal amoebiasis. The usual dose is 50 to 100 mg thrice daily for 5 to 10 days, the course being repeated, if necessary, after an interval of not less than 2 weeks.

The excretion of dark-coloured urine is attributed to the presence of metabolites of phanquone.

Proprietary Preparations

Entobex *(Ciba, UK).* (Available only in certain countries.) Phanquone, available as enteric-coated tablets of 50 mg.

4796-g

Stilbamidine Isethionate. M & B 744. Stilbene-4,4′-dicarboxamidine bis(2-hydroxyethanesulphonate).

$C_{16}H_{16}N_4,2C_2H_6O_4S$=516.6.

CAS — 122-06-5 (stilbamidine); 140-59-0 (isethionate).

Stilbamidine isethionate has antiprotozoal and antifungal properties and was formerly used in the treatment of the early stages of trypanosomiasis and in kala-azar. It is neurotoxic.

4797-q

Suramin *(B.P.C. 1973).* Suramin Sodium; Suraminum Natricum; Germanin; Bayer 205; Fourneau 309; Naganinum; Naganol. The symmetrical 3″-urea of the sodium salt of 8-(3-benzamido-4-methylbenzamido)naphthalene-1,3,5-trisulphonic acid.

$C_{51}H_{34}N_6Na_6O_{23}S_6$=1429.2.

CAS — 145-63-1 (acid); 129-46-4 (sodium salt).

Pharmacopoeias. In *Fr.*, *Int.*, *It.*, and *Rus.*

A white, pinkish-white, or slightly cream-coloured, odourless or almost odourless, hygroscopic powder with a slightly bitter alkaline taste. It contains not more than 10% of water. **Soluble** 1 in less than 1 of water; slightly soluble in alcohol; practically insoluble in chloroform and ether. Solutions deteriorate on storage and should be used immediately after preparation; solutions for injection are prepared aseptically. **Store** in a cool place in airtight containers. Protect from light.

Storage. A batch of suramin which had been stored in Ibadan, Nigeria, for 3 to 4 months produced less frequent albuminuria than a new batch which also produced dizziness, urticarial wheals, malaise, and tiredness, and acute nephritis in 1 patient. This confirmed the suggestion by F.C. Rodger (*Trans. R. Soc. trop. Med. Hyg.*, 1958, *52*, 462) that different batches of suramin had differing toxicity. Storage in the tropics probably also affected the potency.— E. Nnochiri, *Trans. R. Soc. trop. Med. Hyg.*, 1964, *58*, 413.

Adverse Effects. Suramin may cause nausea, vomiting, abdominal pain, diarrhoea, urticaria, collapse, paraesthesia, hyperaesthesia of the hands and soles of the feet, peripheral neuritis, fever, skin rash, dermatitis, photophobia, lachrymation, amblyopia, and uveitis. A serious effect is albuminuria, with the passage of casts and blood cells. Agranulocytosis and haemolytic anaemia are rare.

When used in onchocerciasis some of the effects may represent an allergic reaction to the killed filariae.

References: Second Report of a WHO Expert Committee on Onchocerciasis, *Tech. Rep. Ser. Wld Hlth Org. No. 335*, 1966.

Pregnancy and the neonate. Suramin had teratogenic effects in *mice*.— H. Tuchmann-Duplessis and L. Mercier-Parot, *C.r. Séanc. Soc. Biol.*, 1973, *167*, 1717, per *Trop. Dis. Bull.*, 1974, *71*, 1107. A woman with advanced trypanosomiasis was successfully treated with suramin and melarsoprol, in addition to supportive therapy, from the 20th week of pregnancy; she gave birth to an apparently normal child.— M. N. Lowenthal, *Med. J. Zambia*, 1971, *5*, 175, per *Trop. Dis. Bull.*, 1972, *69*, 495.

Precautions. It should not be used in the presence of renal disease or adrenal insufficiency.

Absorption and Fate. Following intravenous injection, suramin becomes bound to plasma proteins and a low concentration in plasma is maintained for up to 3 months.

Uses. Suramin is used in the treatment of the early stages of African trypanosomiasis, especially *Trypanosoma rhodesiense* infections, but as it does not reach the cerebrospinal fluid it is ineffective in the advanced disease when the central nervous system is affected.

Suramin is administered by intravenous injection. To test the patient's tolerance, it is advisable to begin treatment with an injection of 200 mg followed, if well tolerated after 24 to 48 hours by a dose of 20 mg per kg body-weight (up to 1 g) on days 1, 3, 8, 15, and 22. The urine should be tested before each dose, and if protein is present the dose should be reduced or administration delayed.

Combined therapy with tryparsamide has been used, particularly for late *T. gambiense* infection; 12 injections can be given intravenously at intervals of 5 days, each containing suramin up to 10 mg per kg body-weight (max. of 500 mg) and tryparsamide up to 30 mg per kg (max. of 1.5 g), as a 20% solution prepared immediately before use. Two or 3 such courses have been given at intervals of 1 month. Suramin is more commonly used in conjunction with melarsoprol.

Suramin has also been used in the prophylaxis of trypanosomiasis, in a dose of 1 g to provide protection for up to 3 months, but it may mask latent infections. As with pentamidine, it is important to detect more advanced infections and to treat these with melarsoprol.

Suramin is also effective in clearing the adult filariae of onchocerciasis but has only a limited action on microfilariae. The usual dose is 1 g (after an initial test dose) weekly for 5 or 6 weeks. Diethylcarbamazine is active on the microfilariae and the 2 drugs are sometimes used in conjunction.

Onchocerciasis. Less ocular deterioration was observed in a group of patients with onchocerciasis who had been treated 14 to 15 years earlier with a single full course of suramin 4.2 g, than was seen in a similar untreated group.— F. H. Budden, *Trans. R. Soc. trop. Med. Hyg.*, 1976, *70*, 484. The incidence of optic atrophy increased from 1 in 25 to 5 in 25 three years after patients had been treated with suramin 5.2 g (total dose) for ocular onchocerciasis. There was no change in the incidence (1 in 23) in 23 patients not given suramin.— B. Thylefors and A. Rolland, *Bull. Wld Hlth Org.*, 1979, *57*, 479.

Brief discussions of the treatment of onchocerciasis.— *Br. J. Ophthal.*, 1978, *62*, 427; B. Thylefors, *Bull. Wld Hlth Org.*, 1978, *56*, 63.

Further references: B. O. L. Duke *et al.*, *Tropenmed. Parasit.*, 1976, *27*, 133; J. Anderson *et al.*, *Tropenmed. Parasit.*, 1976, *27*, 263; J. Anderson *et al.*, *Tropenmed. Parasit.*, 1976, *27*, 279.

Trypanosomiasis. See Report of a Joint WHO Expert Committee and FAO Expert Consultation, *Tech. Rep. Ser. Wld Hlth Org. No. 635*, 1979.

Preparations

Suramin Injection *(B.P.C. 1973)*. A sterile solution of suramin in Water for Injections, prepared by dissolving, immediately before use, the sterile contents of a sealed container in the requisite amount of Water for Injections. Store the sealed container in a cool place. Protect from light.

Proprietary Names

Germanin *(Bayer, Ger.)*; Moranyl *(Specia, Fr.)*.

4798-p

Teclozan. Win 13,146. *NN'-p*-Phenylenedimethylenebis[2,2-dichloro-*N*-(2-ethoxyethyl)acetamide].

$C_{20}H_{28}Cl_4N_2O_4$=502.3.

CAS — 5560-78-1.

White crystals. M.p. about 142°. Slightly **soluble** in water.

Adverse Effects. Headache, nausea, vomiting, diarrhoea, and constipation have been reported, but teclozan is generally well tolerated.

Uses. Teclozan is used in the treatment of intestinal amoebiasis. About 20% of a dose is stated to be absorbed and to be rapidly excreted. The usual dose is 100 mg thrice daily for 5 days, or 500 mg daily, in divided doses, for 3 days.

Of 51 patients with chronic intestinal amoebiasis given teclozan 750 mg daily in divided doses after meals for 2 days, 43 were reported to be cured; a further 5 patients responded to a second course of treatment with teclozan. The drug was well tolerated.— D. Huggins, *Anais Esc. nac. Saúde públ. Med. trop.*, 1971, *5*, 29, per *Trop. Dis. Bull.*, 1972, *69*, 399.

Of 30 patients with mild amoebiasis, 25 were reported cured after receiving teclozan 100 mg thrice daily for 5 days; 2 patients required a second course of treatment and 3 remained resistant to teclozan. Two patients developed diarrhoea during treatment which was otherwise well tolerated.— A. Arcilla-Latonio *et al.*, *J. Philipp. med. Ass.*, 1972, *48*, 137, per *Trop. Dis. Bull.*, 1973, *70*, 345.

A cure-rate of 92.8% (at 4 weeks) was achieved in 28 boys with chronic amoebiasis given teclozan 100 mg thrice daily for 5 days.— A. Z. El-Abdin *et al.*, *J. Egypt. med. Ass.*, 1973, *56*, 174, per *Trop. Dis. Bull.*, 1974, *71*, 1028.

Cure in 56 of 60 patients with intestinal amoebiasis after treatment with teclozan 1.5 g in 3 divided doses in 24 hours.— P. Fernandes *et al.*, *Folha med.*, 1974, *69*, 293.

Cure in 26 of 27 children, aged 1 to 5 years, with amoebiasis (usually chronic) after treatment with teclozan 750 mg in 3 divided doses in 24 hours.— H. F. Bezerra *et al.*, *Revta bras. Med.*, 1977, *34*, *Suppl.* (Aug.), 50.

Proprietary Names

Falmonox *(Winthrop, Arg.; Winthrop, USA)*.

4799-s

Tinidazole.

CP 12574. 1-[2-(Ethylsulphonyl)ethyl]-2-methyl-5-nitroimidazole.

$C_8H_{13}N_3O_4S$=247.3.

CAS — 19387-91-8.

Colourless crystals. M.p. about 127°.

Adverse Effects and Precautions. As for Metronidazole, p.968.

Absorption and Fate. Tinidazole is absorbed from the gastro-intestinal tract.

Pharmacokinetics of tinidazole and metronidazole in man and in *mice*.— J. A. Taylor *et al.*, *Antimicrob. Ag. Chemother.*, 1969, 267.

The biological half-life of tinidazole was 12.7 hours after administration of 150 mg as a single dose and when administered twice daily for 7 days to 7 volunteers. The maximum serum concentration was 8.91 µg per ml.— P. G. Welling and A. M. Monro, *Arzneimittel-Forsch.*, 1972, *22*, 2128. See also B. A. Wood and A. M. Monro, *Br. J. vener. Dis.*, 1975, *51*, 51, per *Abstr. Hyg.*, 1975, *50*, 382.

The peak serum concentrations of tinidazole in 4 volunteers 6 to 11 hours after a single dose of 2 g were between 20 and 40 µg per ml, and 48 hours after ingestion the serum concentration was still above the minimal trichomonacidal concentration for most of the 8 strains of *Trichomonas vaginalis* examined.— A. Forsgren and J. Wallin, *Br. J. vener. Dis.*, 1974, *50*, 146 and 148, per *Abstr. Hyg.*, 1974, *49*, 593.

In 6 gynaecological patients given a single dose of tinidazole 2 g peak serum concentrations were 32 to 52 µg per ml 3 to 6 hours after the dose, and 18 to 35 µg per ml 8.5 to 15 hours after the dose. Concentrations in saliva, vaginal secretions, peritoneal fluid, and various tissue homogenates were broadly comparable with those in serum. The plasma half-life was about 13 hours.— T. Ripa *et al.*, *Chemotherapy, Basle*, 1977, *23*, 227, per *Int. pharm. Abstr.*, 1977, *14*, 1084.

In 4 healthy subjects given tinidazole 2 g concentrations in the CSF 90 minutes later (17 to 39 µg per ml) were 88% of those in serum.— A. M. M. Jokipii *et al.*, *J. antimicrob. Chemother.*, 1977, *3*, 239.

Uses. Tinidazole which is a nitroimidazole like metronidazole has antiprotozoal activity and is effective against *Trichomonas vaginalis*, *Entamoeba histolytica*, and *Giardia lamblia*. It is also active against anaerobic bacteria.

In trichomoniasis it is given by mouth in a dose of 150 mg twice daily for 7 days or as a single dose of 2 g to both men and women. It has been given in similar doses in the treatment of giardiasis.

In amoebiasis doses of 2 g once daily for 3 days are commonly used.

A review of tinidazole in the treatment of trichomoniasis, amoebiasis, and giardiasis.— P. R. Sawyer *et al.*, *Drugs*, 1976, *11*, 423.

Proceedings of a symposium on the use of tinidazole in the treatment of amoebiasis, giardiasis, and trichomoniasis.— *Drugs*, 1978, *15*, *Suppl.* 1, 1–60.

The following anaerobic bacteria were inhibited by 3.1 µg per ml of tinidazole and killed by 6.3 µg per ml: *Bacteroides fragilis* and *melaninogenicus*, *Clostridium perfringens* and other species of clostridia, *Eubacterium*, *Fusobacterium*, *Peptococcus*, *Peptostreptococcus*, and *Veillonella* spp. *Propionibacterium acnes* was relatively resistant. The same figures were achieved with metronidazole and ornidazole.— J. Wüst, *Antimicrob. Ag. Chemother.*, 1977, *11*, 631.

The median minimum inhibitory concentration of tinidazole against *Bacteroides* spp. was 0.12 µg per ml, compared with 0.25 µg per ml for metronidazole or nimorazole.— R. Wise *et al.*, *Chemotherapy, Basle*, 1977, *23*, 19.

The activities of clindamycin, tinidazole, and doxycycline *in vitro* were compared against 376 anaerobic bacteria. Clindamycin and tinidazole had MICs of 0.5 and 3 µg per ml respectively against 90% of 200 strains of *Bacteroides fragilis*. Tinidazole had an MIC of 12 µg per ml against 72 strains of the *Clostridium* spp. but benzylpenicillin and ampicillin were more active. Tinidazole was generally less active than benzylpenicillin, ampicillin, cephalothin, carbenicillin, erythromycin, chloramphenicol, tetracycline, and doxycycline against 20 strains of *Bacteroides melaninogenicus*, 54 of the *Fusobacterium* spp., and 30 strains of anaerobic Gram-positive cocci.— J. Klastersky *et al.*, *Antimicrob. Ag. Chemother.*, 1977, *12*, 563.

Amoebiasis. In a series of controlled studies 436 patients with intestinal amoebiasis were treated with tinidazole 600 mg twice daily for 5 days or 2 g once daily for 3 days, or metronidazole 400 mg thrice daily for 5 days or 2 g once daily for 3 days. Cure-rates for tinidazole were 97.2% and 88.3% respectively in patients passing trophozoites and 81.2% and 93.4% in those passing cysts, compared with 87.5% and 73.3%, and 84.2% and 47.3% for metronidazole. A cure-rate of 96% was achieved in 50 patients with hepatic amoebiasis given tinidazole 2 g once daily for 2 days, compared with 75.5% in 49 given metronidazole. A cure-rate of 88.3% was achieved in 94 patients with giardiasis given tinidazole in a mean dose of 61.8 mg per kg as a single dose, compared with 46.7% in 92 given metronidazole 56 mg per kg.— J. S. Bakshi *et al.*, *Drugs*, 1978, *15*, *Suppl.* 1, 33.

In a multicentre study in 8 countries a cure-rate of 95% was achieved in 502 patients with amoebiasis given tinidazole 2 g once daily (50 mg per kg body-weight for children) for 2 or 3 days. An excellent response was achieved in 60, and a good response in 17, of 82 with hepatic amoebiasis. A cure-rate of 88% was achieved in 74 children with giardiasis given a single dose of about 50 mg per kg. A cure-rate of 95.2% was achieved in 859 patients with trichomonal vaginitis given a single dose of 2 g.— V. V. Apte and R. S. Packard, *Drugs*, 1978, *15*, *Suppl*. 1, 43.

Of 88 aboriginal children infected with *Giardia lamblia* or *Entamoeba histolytica* 23 received a single dose of tinidazole 1 to 1.5 g, 23 tinidazole 1 to 1.5 g daily for 3 days, 23 metronidazole 200 mg twice daily for 5 days, and 19 were left untreated. Both metronidazole and tinidazole successfully cleared the majority of *G. lamblia* infections but *E. histolytica* infections were more effectively treated with tinidazole. A single dose of tinidazole was as effective as the longer regimen. No adverse reactions occurred with either drug.— J. S. Welch *et al.*, *Med. J. Aust.*, 1978, *1*, 469.

Further references: N. Islam and M. Hasan, *Curr. ther. Res.*, 1975, *17*, 161; J. N. Scragg *et al.*, *Archs Dis. Childh.*, 1976, *51*, 385.

Liver abscess. Tinidazole 57 mg per kg body-weight daily for 5 days or 50 mg per kg daily for 3 days was effective in the treatment of amoebic liver abscess in 23 of 25 children aged 3 months to 6 years.— J. N. Scragg and E. M. Proctor, *Archs Dis. Childh.*, 1977, *52*, 408.

Of 16 patients with hepatic amoebiasis 15 were cured after treatment with tinidazole 2 g as a single dose daily for 3 to 6 days, compared with 12 of 15 given metronidazole in the same dosage regimen for 4 to 10 days.— N. Islam and K. Hasan, *Drugs*, 1978, *15*, *Suppl*. 1, 26.

Further references.— H. A. Meyer, *E. Afr. med. J.*, 1974, *51*, 923, per *Trop. Dis. Bull.*, 1975, *72*, 720; S. N. Mathur *et al.*, *J. int. med. Res.*, 1977, *5*, 429; M. A. Quaderi *et al.*, *J. trop. Med. Hyg.*, 1978, *81*, 16.

Giardiasis. Cure in 35 of 38 children with giardiasis after a single dose of tinidazole; 2 others were cured after a second dose. Doses were: under 1 year, 500 mg; 7 years, 1 g; 12 years, 1.5 g.— S. Danzig and W. L. F. Hatchuel (letter), *S. Afr. med. J.*, 1977, *52*, 708, per *Trop. Dis. Bull.*, 1978, *75*, 783.

A cure-rate of 96.7% in patients with giardiasis treated with tinidazole 150 mg twice daily for 7 days.— G. C. Levi *et al.*, *Am. J. trop. Med. Hyg.*, 1977, *26*, 564, per *Trop. Dis. Bull.*, 1978, *75*, 648. See also S. Y. Salih and R. E. Abdalla, *J. trop. Med. Hyg.*, 1977, *80*, 11, per *Trop. Dis. Bull.*, 1977, *74*, 731.

Cure of 53 of 55 patients with giardiasis given tinidazole 2 g as a single dose.— N. A. El Masry *et al.*, *Am. J. trop. Med. Hyg.*, 1978, *27*, 201, per *Trop. Dis. Bull.*, 1978, *75*, 544.

See also under Amoebiasis, above.

Further references: L. Jokipii and A. M. M. Jokipii, *J. infect. Dis.*, 1979, *140*, 984; M. B. Tadros, *J. Egypt. Soc. Parasit.*, 1979, *9*, 467, per *Trop. Dis. Bull.*, 1980, *77*, 125; A. Sabchareon *et al.*, *S.E. Asian J. trop. med. publ. Hlth*, 1980, *11*, 280, per *Trop. Dis. Bull.*, 1981, *78*, 161.

Prophylaxis in surgery. In a prospective, randomised, double-blind study of 6 months' duration involving 71 patients 2 g of tinidazole given before surgery prevented wound infection after elective colonic surgery in 37 of 40 patients in comparison with 28 of 31 patients treated with placebo.— P. S. Hunt *et al.*, *Med. J. Aust.*, 1979, *1*, 107.

Postoperative infections occurred in 6 of 50 patients who received 2 g of tinidazole 12 to 18 hours before undergoing elective abdominal hysterectomy and 2 g 48 hours postoperatively; infections occurred in 28 of 50 similar control patients.— P. C. Appelbaum *et al.*, *Chemotherapy, Basle*, 1980, *26*, 145.

Further references: J. Adno and R. Cassel, *S. Afr. med. J.*, 1979, *56*, 565 (gynaecological surgery); M. Karhunen *et al.*, *Br. J. Obstet. Gynaec.*, 1980, *87*, 70 (hysterectomy).

Trichomoniasis. Tinidazole 2 g as a single dose produced parasitological cure in 47 of 50 patients with trichomoniasis, compared with 32 of 50 given metronidazole.— R. Anjaneyulu *et al.*, *J. int. med. Res.*, 1977, *5*, 438.

Further reports of the successful use of 2-g doses of tinidazole in women.— H. T. M. Rao and D. R. Shenoy, *J. int. med. Res.*, 1978, *6*, 46; J. P. Ward, *Med. J. Aust.*, 1976, *2*, 651; R. Jones and P. Enders, *ibid.*, 1977, *2*, 679; M. Massa *et al.*, *Boln chil. Parasit.*, 1976, *31*, 46, per *Trop. Dis. Bull.*, 1977, *74*, 291.

Successful use in men of single 1-g doses of tinidazole.— N. Kawamura, *Br. J. vener. Dis.*, 1978, *54*, 81, per *Abstr. Hyg.*, 1978, *53*, 465.

See also under Amoebiasis, above.

Vaginitis. Administration of a single dose of tinidazole 2 g to 35 women with *Gardnerella vaginalis (Haemophilus vaginalis)* infection led to disappearance of the bacteria in 33; of the other 2 women the count was reduced in one and a repeat treatment was successful in the second. Two women relapsed after 15 to 20 days and repeat treatment was successful. All the patients' partners were given the same dose of tinidazole, and abstinence from sexual intercourse was recommended for at least 24 hours.— M. Bardi *et al.* (letter), *Lancet*, 1980, *1*, 1029.

See also under Trichomoniasis, above.

Proprietary Names

Fasigin *(Pfizer, Ital.)*; Fasigyn *(Pfizer, Arg.*; *Pfizer, Austral.*; *Roerig, Belg.*; *Pfizer, Denm.*; *Pfizer, Neth.*; *Pfizer, Norw.*; *Pfizer, S.Afr.*; *Pfizer, Swed.*; *Pfizer, Switz.)*; Fasigyne *(Pfizer, Fr.)*; Simplotan *(Pfizer, Ger.)*; Trichogin *(Chiesi, Ital.)*; Tricolam *(Pfizer, Spain)*.

6000-c

Tryparsamide *(B.P. 1968)*. Tryparsam.; Tryparsamidum; Glyphenarsine; Tryparsone. Sodium hydrogen 4-(carbamoylmethylamino)phenylarsonate hemihydrate. $C_8H_{10}AsN_2NaO_4,\frac{1}{2}H_2O=305.1$.

CAS — 554-72-3 (anhydrous); 6159-29-1 (hemihydrate).

Pharmacopoeias. In *Ind.*, *Int.*, *It.*, *Mex.*, and *Turk.*

A colourless, odourless, crystalline powder which is slowly affected by light.

Soluble 1 in 1.5 of water, forming a neutral solution; soluble 1 in 3500 of alcohol; practically insoluble in chloroform and ether. A 4.62% solution is iso-osmotic with serum. Aqueous solutions deteriorate on storage and should be used immediately after preparation; solutions for injection are prepared aseptically. **Store** in a cool place in small airtight containers. Protect from light.

Adverse Effects. Side-effects include dizziness, tinnitus, nausea, vomiting, headache, fever, exfoliative dermatitis, allergic reactions, and bradycardia immediately after an injection. Liver damage may also occur.

The most serious toxic effect is upon the optic nerve. Treatment should be discontinued immediately if visual defects appear; though blindness may occur suddenly, especially if optic injury is already present, visual defects may not become apparent until a few weeks after a course of treatment has been completed.

Uses. Tryparsamide is trypanocidal. Because it penetrates the cerebrospinal fluid it has been used in the treatment of African trypanosomiasis with central nervous system involvement particularly in *Trypanosoma gambiense* infections. It has been given in doses of 30 to 60 mg per kg body-weight (up to maximum of 2 g) intravenously each week for 12 to 14 weeks. The trypanosomes may become resistant to tryparsamide. Because of the risk of blindness, melarsoprol is now preferred.

For the use of tryparsamide in conjunction with suramin, see p.984.

Preparations

Tryparsamide Injection *(B.P. 1968)*. Tryparsam. Inj. A sterile solution in Water for Injections, prepared by dissolving, immediately before use, the sterile contents of a sealed container in the requisite amount of Water for Injections.

Muscle Relaxants

5700-y

The skeletal muscle relaxants included in this section are of 2 main types: those with an action on the central nervous system, principally used for relieving painful muscle spasms or spasticity occurring in musculoskeletal and neuromuscular disorders; and those affecting neuromuscular transmission which are used as adjuncts in anaesthesia, particularly to enable adequate muscle relaxation to be achieved with light anaesthesia.

The drugs used in the treatment of muscle spasm diminish skeletal muscle tone and involuntary movement by a selective action on the central nervous system. Mephenesin (p.992), mephenesin carbamate (p.992), carisoprodol (p.988), chlorphenesin carbamate (p.988), chlorzoxazone (p.988), and cyclobenzaprine hydrochloride (p.989) are typical of this group. Dantrolene sodium (p.989) has been reported to have a direct action on muscle fibres and baclofen (p.987) has been reported to have a predominantly spinal action.

The drugs used as adjuncts to anaesthesia are of 2 types—non-depolarising agents and depolarising agents.

The non-depolarising agents interrupt neuromuscular transmission by competing with acetylcholine for receptor sites on the motor end-plate, thus reducing the response of the end-plate to acetylcholine. These are also called competitive neuromuscular blocking agents and their action is usually reversed by anticholinesterases, such as neostigmine. Alcuronium chloride (p.986), fazadinium bromide (p.991), gallamine triethiodide (p.991), pancuronium bromide (p.994), and tubocurarine chloride (p.999) are typical of this group.

The depolarising agents block neuromuscular transmission by producing a sustained partial depolarisation of the motor end-plate which renders the tissues incapable of responding to the transmitter. Their action is not reversed by anticholinesterases. Suxamethonium chloride (p.995) and suxethonium bromide (p.998) are typical of this group.

Generally, the non-depolarising agents, with a prolonged action, are used in major operations, while the depolarising agents, with a much shorter effect, are used for minor operations or manipulations.

It is common practice to use a short-acting depolarising drug, such as suxamethonium, for intubation, followed by a longer-acting non-depolarising drug, such as tubocurarine, to maintain muscle relaxation throughout an operation. Sometimes a depolarising drug may be given to facilitate closure of the muscular tissue. In such instances neostigmine should not be given to reverse the action of tubocurarine until the effects of the depolarising drug have ceased; the procedure is accordingly not recommended for routine practice.

Dual Block. Repeated doses of depolarising muscle relaxants can cause a change in response of the motor end-plate so that a non-depolarising block follows the primary depolarising block. When such a dual block (also termed a desensitisation block) has been established, it is usually reversible by anticholinesterases and intensified by non-depolarising drugs.

Mixed Block. Depolarising and non-depolarising muscle relaxants injected simultaneously give a mixed block in which it has been suggested that elements of both types of block might be present in different muscle fibres.

Prolonged apnoea or respiratory depression may follow the use of non-depolarising or depolarising muscle relaxants. After a non-depolarising drug, prolonged apnoea, unresponsive to neostigmine, may develop due to metabolic acidosis. Metabolic acidosis is generally considered to have been a major factor in cases formerly described as *neostigmine-resistant curarisation.* After the continuous infusion of a depolarising drug the resulting dual block may give prolonged respiratory depression related to the prolonged muscular relaxation, but apnoea rarely develops. After a depolarising drug prolonged respiratory depression may also occur in patients with low serum-pseudocholinesterase concentrations or with atypical pseudocholinesterase.

For relaxants of smooth muscle, see p.1059.

Reviews and comments: J. S. Cookson and W. D. M. Paton, *Anaesthesia*, 1969, *24*, 395; J. Stovner and I. Lund, *Br. J. Anaesth.*, 1970, *42*, 235; B. A. Callingham, *Pharm. J.*, 1972, *2*, 98; A. R. Hunter and S. A. Feldman, *Br. J. Anaesth.*, 1976, *48*, 277; J. Norman, *ibid.*, 1979, *51*, 471; S. A. Feldman, *Muscle Relaxants*, 2nd Edn, London, Saunders, 1979; J. C. De Lee and C. A. Rockwood, *Curr. ther. Res.*, 1980, *27*, 64; A. N. Győry, *Drugs*, 1980, *20*, 309; C. Lee and R. L. Katz, *Br. J. Anaesth.*, 1980, *52*, 173; G. H. Bush *et al.* (letter), *ibid.*, 962; C. Lee and R. L. Katz (letter), *ibid.*, 963; M. A. Thompson, *Br. J. Hosp. Med.*, 1980, *23*, 153.

A brief discussion of the use of neuromuscular blocking agents in controlled hypotension.— A. P. Adams, *Br. J. Anaesth.*, 1975, *47*, 777.

The duration of action of suxamethonium was less in London patients than in a comparable group of New York patients, and the duration and magnitude of action of tubocurarine was less in the London than the New York patients.— R. L. Katz *et al.*, *Br. J. Anaesth.*, 1969, *41*, 1041. The response of Los Angeles patients to suxamethonium was similar to that of London patients and not New York patients.— G. Levy, *ibid.*, 1970, *42*, 979.

Anaesthesia was induced with thiopentone in 70 patients and followed by a single dose of a non-depolarising muscle relaxant. There was a small decrease in plasma-potassium concentration following pancuronium (20 patients) and a smaller decrease after gallamine (20). No significant change occurred after tubocurarine (20) or fazadinium bromide (10).— I. M. Bali *et al.*, *Br. J. Anaesth.*, 1975, *47*, 505.

Concern at the use of muscle relaxants in intensive therapy units, although they are not sedative or analgesic agents, and a reminder of the horrors of being awake and intubated. Muscle relaxants should only be used for controlled ventilation in intensive therapy units if sedation proves inadequate or if a sleeping patient is not synchronising with a ventilator. The only limitation to the dose of opiate (or other sedative) given, is an untoward reaction or an unsatisfactory haemodynamic state. Worries about addiction are unnecessary.— C. M. H. M. Jones (letter), *Lancet*, 1980, *1*, 312. Agreement. Moreover anaesthetists commonly administer a muscle relaxant, rather than a narcotic or an analgesic, when patients make spontaneous coordinated limb movements during general anaesthesia. Although it is not known whether such movements indicate inadequate depression of conscious level, it is known that awareness during general anaesthesia is common.— A. Gilston (letter), *ibid.*, 480. A view that muscle relaxants in the intensive care setting are useful adjuncts.— D. Green (letter), *ibid.*, 715. Further comments.— *ibid.*, 746; *ibid.*, 1981, *1*, 427.

Pregnancy and the neonate. The effect of muscle relaxants in the newborn.— D. R. Cook, *Drugs*, 1976, *12*, 212.

The use of muscle relaxants in neonatal surgery.— E. Vivori and G. H. Bush, *Br. J. Anaesth.*, 1977, *49*, 51.

Reactions with other drugs. Interactions between muscle relaxants and other drugs.— I. H. Stockley, *Pharm. J.*, 1973, *2*, 152; H. H. Ali and J. J. Savarese, *Anesthesiology*, 1976, *45*, 216; T. N. Calvey, *Prescribers' J.*, 1980, *20*, 14.

Relative potency of muscle relaxants. The doses of relaxants needed to completely paralyse the grip of a 70-kg man were: gallamine 35 mg, suxamethonium 15 mg, tubocurarine 8 mg, alcuronium 5 mg, and pancuronium 1.5 mg. Maximum relaxation occurred in 45 to 60 seconds for suxamethonium and in 3 minutes for the other relaxants, and 75% of grip strength returned in 3 minutes for suxamethonium, 15 minutes for gallamine, and 20 minutes for the other relaxants. About 3 times these doses were required for endotracheal intubation in normal lightly anaesthetised subjects, or 3.5 times the dose for tubocurarine.— J. Stovner and I. Lund, *Br. J. Anaesth.*, 1970, *42*, 235.

Further references: N. E. Williams *et al.*, *Br. J. Anaesth.*, 1980, *52*, 1111.

5701-j

Alcuronium Chloride. Allnortoxiferin Chloride; Diallylnortoxiferine Dichloride; Diallyltoxiferine Chloride. *NN'*-Diallylbisnortoxiferinium dichloride pentahydrate.

$C_{44}H_{50}Cl_2N_4O_2,5H_2O = 827.9$.

CAS — 23214-96-2 (alcuronium); 15180-03-7 (chloride).

An odourless colourless crystalline powder. **Soluble** in water and alcohol. **Incompatible** with solutions of thiopentone sodium.

Adverse Effects, Treatment, and Precautions. As for Tubocurarine Chloride, p.999.

Alcuronium chloride has a smaller histamine-releasing effect than tubocurarine chloride.

Apnoea followed the intraperitoneal administration of streptomycin in a patient given alcuronium chloride. The patient was also receiving streptomycin parenterally for the treatment of tuberculosis.— R. V. Trubuhovich (letter), *Br. J. Anaesth.*, 1966, *38*, 843.

A 51-year-old woman who had received thiopentone sodium and suxamethonium without untoward effects developed an erythematous rash within 4 minutes of receiving alcuronium. When this sequence of drugs was followed on a second occasion the patient showed a similar reaction to alcuronium 12 mg given over 3 minutes.— C. S. Chan and M. L. Yeung, *Br. J. Anaesth.*, 1972, *44*, 103.

Anaphylaxis associated with alcuronium in 5 patients.— M. M. Fisher *et al.*, *Anaesth. & intensive Care*, 1978, *6*, 125.

Further references: M. L. Yeung *et al.*, *Anaesth. & intensive Care*, 1979, *7*, 62.

Absorption and Fate. When given intravenously, alcuronium is widely distributed throughout the body tissues; it is excreted unchanged, mainly by the kidneys.

Up to 2 hours after an intravenous injection of alcuronium in man the plasma concentration fell rapidly due to redistribution of the drug from the central to the peripheral compartment. The plasma concentration then fell more slowly, the half-life being about 3.3 hours. Alcuronium was not metabolised and about 80 to 85% was eliminated by the kidneys. About 10 to 15% was secreted into the bile and eliminated in the faeces. The half-life of the drug in an anuric patient was 16 hours.— J. Raaflaub and P. Frey, *Arzneimittel-Forsch.*, 1972, *22*, 73.

Further references: J. Walker *et al.*, *Eur. J. clin. Pharmac.*, 1980, *17*, 449.

Pregnancy and the neonate. Alcuronium, in a dose of 10 to 15 mg, was administered intravenously to 19 patients undergoing caesarean section. In 12 patients the alcuronium was administered over a few seconds; alcuronium 200 to 400 ng per ml was detected in the cord plasma of 11 of 13 neonates. In 7 patients in whom the administration time ranged from 2 to 6 minutes, the same amounts were detected in the cord plasma of 2 of 7 neonates. Neonatal plasma concentrations of alcuronium appeared to be independent of the maternal plasma concentrations at delivery, but related to the rate of injection. No evidence of neuromuscular block was seen in the neonates.— J. Thomas *et al.*, *Br. J. Anaesth.*, 1969, *41*, 297.

Uses. Alcuronium chloride is a non-depolarising muscle relaxant with effects similar to those of tubocurarine chloride (see p.999).

Alcuronium is used mainly as an adjuvant to anaesthesia to obtain greater muscle relaxation in surgical operations. An initial dose of 200 to 250 µg per kg body-weight intravenously is usually adequate to achieve 95% neuromuscular blockade. Muscle relaxation is obtained within about 2 minutes and the effect lasts for about 20 to 30 minutes. An initial dose of 300 µg per kg intravenously is reported to provide muscle relaxation for about 40 minutes. Supplementary doses of one-sixth to one-quarter the initial dose are reported to provide relaxation for additional periods of similar duration to the first. Somewhat smaller doses are required in patients anaesthetised with halothane 1.5 to 2%. Children may be given an initial dose of 125 to 200 µg per kg body-weight.

Ocular surgery. A study in 20 healthy subjects indicated that alcuronium may be a reasonable alternative to pancuronium for routine surgery of the open eye, particularly in elderly patients with limited cardiac reserve.— R. George *et al.*, *Br. J. Anaesth.*, 1979, *51*, 789.

Tetanus. Alcuronium was effective in controlling the spasms of tetanus; the problem of residual curarisation did not arise.— M. A. K. Omar (letter), *Br. med. J.*, 1979, *2*, 274.

Proprietary Preparations

Alloferin *(Roche, UK).* Alcuronium chloride, available as an injection containing 5 mg per ml in ampoules of 2 ml. (Also available as Alloferin in *Arg.*, *Austral.*, *Denm.*, *Ger.*, *Neth.*, *Norw.*, *S.Afr.*, *Swed.*, *Switz.*).

Other Proprietary Names

Alloférine *(Fr.).*

5702-z

Baclofen.

Ba 34647; Aminomethyl Chlorohydrocinnamic Acid. β-Aminomethyl-*p*-chlorohydrocinnamic acid; 4-Amino-3-(4-chlorophenyl)butyric acid.

$C_{10}H_{12}ClNO_2$=213.7.

CAS — 1134-47-0.

A white to off-white crystalline solid. M.p. about 207°. Slightly **soluble** in water; poorly soluble in organic solvents. **Store** in a cool place.

Adverse Effects. Nausea, vomiting, drowsiness, confusion, fatigue, and hypotonia may occur. Other side-effects include giddiness, hypotension, euphoria, hallucinations, depression, headache, diarrhoea or constipation, tremors, insomnia, visual disturbances, allergic skin reactions, pruritus, urinary disturbances, and hepatic impairment.

Baclofen is teratogenic in *animals*.

A report of breathlessness in 1 patient on baclofen 5 mg daily and marked abdominal distension in another.— F. Rigby, *Postgrad. med. J.*, 1972, *48* (Oct.), *Suppl.*, 28.

Deterioration of the EEG was reported in 2 epileptic patients while receiving baclofen.— R. N. Brogden *et al.*, *Drugs*, 1974, *8*, 1.

Impotence in 1 patient and worsening of urinary incontinence in 2.— D. W. Hedley *et al.*, *Postgrad. med. J.*, 1975, *51*, 615.

Decreased taste sensitivity was associated with baclofen in 1 patient.— H. Rollin, *Ann. Otol. Rhinol. Lar.*, 1978, *87*, 37.

Treatment of Adverse Effects. The stomach should be emptied by aspiration and lavage and general supportive measures employed. A high urinary output should be maintained by means of increased fluid intake and, if necessary, administration of diuretics. Convulsions occur mainly in patients with a history of epilepsy and should be treated symptomatically. Assisted respiration may be needed.

Overdosage with between 0.5 and 1.2 g of baclofen, together with alcohol, made a patient unconscious with epileptiform fits for 14 hours, despite gastric lavage given within 20 minutes of ingestion. After assisted respiration the patient woke but his previously spastic limbs were markedly flaccid for 3 days following the incident.— V. Paeslack, *Postgrad. med. J.*, 1972, *48* (Oct.), *Suppl.*, 30.

Use of atropine in baclofen overdosage.— R. E. Ferner, *Postgrad. med. J.*, 1981, *57*, 580.

Further references: G. W. Paulson, *Neurology, Minneap.*, 1976, *25*, 1105; D. J. Lipscomb and T. J. Meredith, *Postgrad. med. J.*, 1980, *56*, 108.

Precautions. Baclofen is contra-indicated in patients with a history of epilepsy or convulsive disorders. It should be used with caution in patients with a history of gastric and duodenal ulcer, severe psychiatric disorders, or impaired cerebrovascular system, in pulmonary insufficiency, renal impairment, and in patients receiving antihypertensive therapy. Patients with stroke tolerate baclofen poorly.

Patients taking baclofen should not take charge of vehicles, other means of transport, or machinery where loss of attention may lead to accidents.

It is recommended that baclofen should be used with caution in patients in whom spasticity is used to maintain posture or to increase function. Withdrawal of baclofen should be gradual.

Baclofen in doses of 75 mg daily might precipitate psychotic reactions in elderly patients.— *Med. J. Aust.*, 1972, *2*, 348.

The abrupt withdrawal of baclofen in a patient being treated for parkinsonism resulted in distressing hallucinations. This effect might have been due to altered dopamine metabolism.— A. J. Lees *et al.* (letter), *Lancet*, 1977, *1*, 858. Similar reports: O. B. Skausig and S. Korsgaard (letter), *ibid.*, 1258; R. Stien (letter), *ibid.*, 1977, *2*, 44.

Absorption and Fate. Baclofen is rapidly absorbed from the gastro-intestinal tract and is excreted mainly unchanged in the urine.

Baclofen was rapidly absorbed from the gastro-intestinal tract. An oral dose of baclofen 40 mg produced a peak plasma concentration of 0.6 µg per ml 2 hours after ingestion. About 40% of the dose was excreted in the urine within 6 hours, about 85% being unchanged baclofen, with a small amount of deaminated metabolite. Complete elimination was reached through the urine and faeces within 3 days.— J. W. Faigle and H. Keberle, *Postgrad. med. J.*, 1972, *48* (Oct.), *Suppl.*, 9.

Uses. Baclofen is an analogue of aminobutyric acid (p.1678). Its mode of action is not fully understood. It inhibits monosynaptic and polysynaptic transmission at the spinal level, and also depresses the CNS.

It is used for the symptomatic relief of muscular spasm due to conditions such as multiple sclerosis, and lesions of the spinal cord.

The initial dose is 5 mg thrice daily increased by 15 mg daily every fourth day to 20 mg thrice daily or until the desired therapeutic effect has been obtained. Doses of more than 80 to 100 mg daily are not generally recommended.

Reviews.— O. de S. Pinto *et al.*, *Postgrad. med. J.*, 1972, *48*, (Oct.), *Suppl.*, 18; *Drug & Ther. Bull.*, 1973, *11*, 63; D. B. Calne, *Prescribers' J.*, 1974, *14*, 59; R. N. Brogden *et al.*, *Drugs*, 1974, *8*, 1; *Aust. J. Pharm.*, 1978, *59*, 285; *Med. Lett.*, 1978, *20*, 43.

Action. A study indicating that the antispasticity activity of baclofen results in part from the (−)-stereoisomer inhibiting the release of excitatory amino acid neurotransmitters.— G. A. R. Johnston *et al.*, *J. Pharm. Pharmac.*, 1980, *32*, 230.

Huntington's chorea. Baclofen given in increasing doses to 2 patients with Huntington's chorea produced slight improvement at a dose of 60 mg daily.— N. -E. Andén *et al.* (letter), *Lancet*, 1973, *2*, 93.

Myotonia. Experience of the use of baclofen in 6 patients with myotonia suggested that baclofen might be an effective treatment.— P. Karli and L. Bergström (letter), *Lancet*, 1974, *1*, 1285.

Parkinsonism. In a double-blind crossover study in 12 patients with parkinsonism taking levodopa and a decarboxylase inhibitor, baclofen in a mean dose of 45 mg daily aggravated rigidity and functional disability, but there was a reduction in pain and the severity of dystonia in 4 patients with morning ('off-period') dystonia. Adverse effects were common.— A. J. Lees *et al.*, *J. Neurol. Neurosurg. Psychiat.*, 1978, *41*, 707.

Schizophrenia. Beneficial results were achieved in 13 chronic schizophrenic patients treated with baclofen.— P. K. Frederiksen (letter), *Lancet*, 1975, *1*, 702.

Unfavourable reports: G. M. Simpson *et al.* (letter), *Lancet*, 1976, *1*, 966; K. L. Davis *et al.* (letter), *ibid.*, 1245; R. Kuhn, *Arzneimittel-Forsch.*, 1976, *26*, 1187; N. C. Gulman *et al.*, *Acta psychiat. scand.*, 1976, *54*, 287; L. B. Bigelow *et al.*, *Am. J. Psychiat.*, 1977, *134*, 318; J. Wålinder *et al.* (letter), *New Engl. J. Med.*, 1977, *296*, 452.

Spasticity. A review on the treatment of spasticity including the use of baclofen.— R. R. Young and P. J. Delwaide, *New Engl. J. Med.*, 1981, *304*, 28 and 96.

There was improvement in spasticity in 6 patients with spinal cord disease who were given baclofen, 25 mg by intravenous injection, followed by 10 mg by mouth thrice daily for 10 days. For 1 patient oral administration could not be tolerated for more than 2 days because of nausea and vomiting. A double-blind trial in 23 patients with spasticity in lower limbs associated with spinal cord disease showed that baclofen 10 mg thrice daily was more effective than a placebo in reducing spasticity.— P. Hudgson *et al.*, *Postgrad. med. J.*, 1972, *48* (Oct.), *Suppl.*, 37. See also P. Hudgson and D. Weightman, *Br. med. J.*, 1971, *4*, 15.

Baclofen had become the treatment of choice for spinal spasticity; it was of no benefit to patients with cerebral lesions. Experience suggested that up to 150 mg daily might be tolerated; 4 divided doses were recommended. Elderly patients and patients with multiple sclerosis might not tolerate high doses. Central side-effects included confusion, euphoria, and depression.— D. J. Burke, *Drugs*, 1975, *10*, 112.

In view of the range of adverse effects of baclofen and of their possible severity the Australian Drug Evaluation Committee recommended that its use be restricted to suppression of voluntary muscle spasm in multiple sclerosis and in spinal lesions causing skeletal hypertonus and bladder dysfunction.— *Med. J. Aust.*, 1976, *1*, 322.

Baclofen was used in the long-term management of spasticity and muscle spasm in 113 patients for up to 6 years, in doses ranging from 30 to 200 mg daily. Of 9 patients with spasticity of cerebral origin only 3 experienced any relief of symptoms. Of 79 patients with spasticity due to spinal lesions improvement was slight in 28 and good in 41. In 87 patients with spasms, 51 showed marked improvement and 25 some improvement. Only 5 of 16 patients with urinary retention showed improvement. Side-effects occurred in 23 patients and included drowsiness (8), dreams (4), hallucinations (3), paranoia, euphoria, depression, headache, blurred vision, nausea, and tremor (2 each), visual illusions, vagueness, an aphrodisiac effect, anxiety, perioral numbness, diplopia, sweating, and weakness (1 each). One patient, who attempted suicide, took more than 1 g; he became comatose and required supportive treatment.— R. F. Jones and J. W. Lance, *Med. J. Aust.*, 1976, *1*, 654.

In a study of 11 patients with lower-limb spasticity, plasma-baclofen concentrations of over 400 ng per ml suppressed the muscle response to passive movement by about 50% but had little effect on the response to voluntary movement.— D. L. McLellan, *J. Neurol. Neurosurg. Psychiat.*, 1977, *40*, 30. Since relief of spasticity alone was unlikely to produce significant functional improvement, baclofen was probably best used in the management of non-ambulant patients not requiring their spasticity for support. Its role in ambulant patients was questionable.— *Lancet*, 1977, *2*, 594.

Further references: V. Paeslack, *Postgrad. med. J.*, 1972, *48* (Oct.), *Suppl.*, 30; P. Castaigne *et al.*, *Nouv. Presse méd.*, 1973, *2*, 2341, per *Int. pharm. Abstr.*, 1975, *12*, 347; M. A. Tudor (letter), *Lancet*, 1974, *1*, 136.

Cerebral palsy. In a double-blind crossover study in 20 children with cerebral palsy, baclofen was significantly more effective than placebo in relieving spasticity. In some patients there were improvements in walking ability, response to active and passive limb movements, self-help, and manual dexterity, and a reduction in scissoring. A suggested dose for children aged 2 to 7 years was 5 to 10 mg daily in divided doses gradually increased to a maximum of 30 to 40 mg daily; older children could tolerate 60 mg daily.— P. J. Milla and A. D. M. Jackson, *J. int. med. Res.*, 1977, *5*, 398.

Multiple sclerosis. Baclofen 5 mg thrice daily, gradually increased to an effective tolerable dose, was given to 35 patients with multiple sclerosis. The optimum dose ranged from 15 to 40 mg daily in 12 patients but 4 tolerated 60 to 80 mg daily. A reduction of spasticity was confirmed in 10 patients and troublesome muscle spasm was relieved in 8 of 21 patients. Withdrawal of baclofen was necessary in 19 patients because of increased weakness (9) and side-effects, including dizziness, drowsiness, and nausea (10).— D. W. Hedley *et al.*, *Postgrad. med. J.*, 1975, *51*, 615.

In a double-blind study of 16 patients with multiple sclerosis, baclofen in an optimum daily dose of 61.2 mg was compared with diazepam in an optimum daily dose of 26.8 mg. Both drugs were considered to have significantly reduced spasticity but there was no significant difference between them despite a significant preference for baclofen by the investigator.— A. From and A. Heltberg, *Acta neurol. scand.*, 1975, *51*, 158.

In a double-blind multicentre study in 106 patients with

multiple sclerosis, baclofen, in doses gradually increased to 80 mg daily if necessary, reduced symptoms of spasticity, compared with placebo.— B. A. Sachais *et al., Archs Neurol., Chicago*, 1977, *34*, 422. See also *J. Am. med. Ass.*, 1978, *239*, 2420.

Further references: W. Cendrowski and W. Sobczyk, *Eur. Neurol.*, 1977, *16*, 257.

Tardive dyskinesia. In a double-blind study in 19 patients with tardive dyskinesia induced by neuroleptic agents, baclofen, in doses of up to 60 mg daily for 2 weeks, reduced symptoms of dyskinesia in 15, with complete disappearence in 5, while neuroleptic medication continued.— S. Korsgaard, *Acta psychiat. scand.*, 1976, *54*, 17.

In a double-blind study baclofen 20 to 120 mg daily generally reduced hyperkinesia in 18 patients with neuroleptic-induced tardive dyskinesia most of whom continued to take neuroleptics, but increased parkinsonian symptoms. Sedation and confusion occurred in about half the patients, particularly in the elderly.— J. Gerlach *et al., Psychopharmacology*, 1978, *56*, 145.

Further references: G. M. Simpson *et al., Psychopharm. Bull.*, 1978, *14*, 16; J. Amsterdam and J. Mendels, *Am. J. Psychiat.*, 1979, *136*, 1197.

Trigeminal neuralgia. Seven of 10 patients with refractory trigeminal neuralgia benefited from treatment with baclofen in doses increased to 60 to 80 mg daily; 4 became free of pain and 3 had only 1 or 2 brief paroxysms daily.— G. H. Fromm *et al., Neurology, Minneap.*, 1979, *29*, 550.

Urinary retention. In 15 paraplegic patients the mean volume of residual urine fell from 115 to 63 ml with an accompanying fall in sphincter resistance, after treatment for 2 days with baclofen 20 mg daily by intravenous injection. The incidence of adverse reactions was low. Treatment was considered useful for active bladder training. Oral medication was not effective.— H. J. Hachen and V. Krucker, *Eur. Urol.*, 1977, *3*, 237.

Proprietary Preparations

Lioresal *(Ciba, UK)*. Baclofen, available as scored tablets of 10 mg. (Also available as Lioresal in *Arg., Austral., Belg., Canad., Denm., Fr., Ger., Ital., Neth., Norw., S.Afr., Spain, Switz., USA*).

5703-c

Carbolonium Bromide. Hexacarbacholine Bromide; Hexcarbocholine Bromide. *NN'*-Hexamethylenebis[(2-carbamoyloxyethyl)trimethylammonium] dibromide.
$C_{18}H_{40}Br_2N_4O_4$=536.3.

CAS — 13309-41-6 (carbolonium); 306-41-2 (bromide).

Carbolonium bromide has been used as a muscle relaxant during surgical operations under general anaesthesia.

References: *Lancet*, 1959, *2*, 648; K. Wiemers and W. Overbeck, *Br. J. Anaesth.*, 1960, *32*, 607; R. Hofmann and H. W. Opderbecke, *Geburtsh. Frauenheilk.*, 1971, *31*, 30.

Proprietary Names

Imbretil *(Chemie-Linz, Aust.; Hormonchemie, Ger.; Österreichische Stickstoffwerke, Switz.)*.

5704-k

Carisoprodol.

N-Isopropylmeprobamate. 2-Methyl-2-propyltrimethylene carbamate isopropylcarbamate.
$C_{12}H_{24}N_2O_4$=260.3.

CAS — 78-44-4.

A white odourless crystalline powder with a bitter taste. M.p. 92° to 94°.
Soluble 1 in 3300 of water; soluble in most common organic solvents; practically insoluble in vegetable oils.

Adverse Effects, Treatment, and Precautions. As for Meprobamate, p.1546.

A 45-year-old woman taking carisoprodol in a dosage of 350 mg thrice daily developed a rash which could also be produced by a test dose of 400 mg of meprobamate.— W. M. Honeycutt and A. C. Curtis, *J. Am. med. Ass.*, 1962, *180*, 691.

Overdosage. The main toxic effects in 2 men who took respectively 8.4 and 9.45 g of carisoprodol were drowsiness, dizziness, headache, vertigo, impairment of muscular coordination, and amnesia; slight tachycardia occurred in 1 man.— D. Goldberg, *Milit. Med.*, 1969, *134*, 597.

Absorption and Fate. Carisoprodol is metabolised in the liver and excreted by the kidneys.

Pregnancy and the neonate. Carisoprodol was excreted in human milk and might be present in concentrations 2 to 4 times that in maternal plasma.— T. E. O'Brien, *Am. J. Hosp. Pharm.*, 1974, *31*, 844.

Uses. Carisoprodol is a centrally acting muscle relaxant with actions similar to those of mephenesin (p.992) and a duration of effect of about 4 to 6 hours. It is used for the symptomatic relief of muscular spasm. The usual dose is 350 mg four times daily.

For a review of the analgesic and toxic effects of carisoprodol, and comparisons with codeine, see N. B. Eddy *et al., Codeine and its Alternates for Pain and Cough Relief*, Geneva, World Health Organization, 1970. See also *Bull. Wld Hlth Org.*, 1969, *40*, 1.

Carisoprodol had not been found of value in the treatment of painful musculoskeletal conditions; it had sedative effects, but did not relax muscles directly.— *Med. Lett.*, 1975, *17*, 42.

Proprietary Preparations

Carisoma *(Pharmax, UK)*. Carisoprodol, available as tablets of 125 and 350 mg.

Carisoma Compound *(Pharmax, UK)*. Tablets each containing carisoprodol 175 mg and paracetamol 350 mg. For musculoskeletal conditions associated with pain. *Dose.* 1 to 2 tablets thrice daily.

Other Proprietary Names

Caprodat *(Swed.)*; Flexartal *(Fr.)*; Mioxom *(Ital.)*; Relaxo-Powel *(Spain)*; Rela *(USA)*; Sanoma *(Ger.)*; Soma *(Canad., Ital., USA)*; Somadril *(Denm., Norw., Swed.)*; Somalgit Simple *(Spain)*.

NOTE. The name Soma has also been applied to a hallucinogenic fungus.

5705-a

Chlorphenesin Carbamate. 3-(4-Chlorophenoxy)propane-1,2-diol 1-carbamate.
$C_{10}H_{12}ClNO_4$=245.7.

CAS — 104-29-0 (chlorphenesin); 886-74-8 (carbamate).

An odourless white to off-white powder. M.p. about 90°. Practically **insoluble** in water; soluble in alcohol, acetone, and chloroform.

Adverse Effects, Treatment, and Precautions. As for Mephenesin, p.992.

Excitement and nervousness have been reported and allergic reactions have occurred. It should be given with caution to patients with impaired hepatic function.

A 12-g dose of chlorphenesin carbamate taken with suicidal intent caused only nausea and drowsiness lasting 6 hours.— L. J. Cass and W. S. Frederick, *J. new Drugs*, 1962, *2*, 366.

Absorption and Fate. Chlorphenesin carbamate is readily absorbed from the gastro-intestinal tract; peak serum concentrations are obtained 1 or 2 hours after administration and the serum half-life is about 4 hours. About 85% is excreted in the urine as the glucuronide within 24 hours.

References: A. A. Forist and R. W. Judy, *J. pharm. Sci.*, 1971, *60*, 1686; D. G. Kaiser and S. R. Shaw, *ibid.*, 1974, *63*, 1094; R. G. Stoll *et al., J. clin. Pharmac.*, 1974, *14*, 520.

Uses. Chlorphenesin carbamate is a centrally acting muscle relaxant related to mephenesin. It is used for the symptomatic relief of muscular spasm. The usual initial dose is 800 mg thrice daily reduced to 400 mg four times daily or less.

Chlorphenesin is also used as an antifungal agent.

Trigeminal neuralgia. Chlorphenesin carbamate gave marked relief of pain in 4 patients with trigeminal neuralgia and to 2 further patients whose symptoms were only partially controlled with carbamazepine or phenytoin. The initial dosage of 400 mg morning and midday and 800 mg at bedtime was gradually reduced, after pain was controlled, to the lowest effective dose.— D. J. Dalessio, *J. Am. med. Ass.*, 1973, *225*, 1659.

Proprietary Names

Maolate *(Upjohn, USA)*; Rinlaxer *(Jap.)*.

5706-t

Chlorzoxazone. Chlorobenzoxazolinone. 5-Chlorobenzoxazol-2(3*H*)-one.
$C_7H_4ClNO_2$=169.6.

CAS — 95-25-0.

Pharmacopoeias. In *Jap.* and *Nord.*

Odourless colourless crystals or white or almost white crystalline powder with a bitter taste. M.p. 190° to 194°.
Slightly **soluble** in water; soluble 1 in 20 of alcohol, 1 in 250 of chloroform, and 1 in 60 of ether; soluble in acetone, dimethylformamide, methyl alcohol, and dilute ammonia solution and alkalis. A solution in water is almost neutral to litmus. **Protect** from light.

Adverse Effects. Side-effects include nausea, vomiting, heartburn, abdominal discomfort, constipation, drowsiness, dizziness, skin rash, and headache. Jaundice in which chlorzoxazone was the suspected cause has been reported.

After taking a preparation of chlorzoxazone 250 mg and paracetamol 300 mg for low-back pain, a 21-year-old man experienced headache, spatial disorientation and a dream-like state, with nausea, vomiting, peripheral paraesthesia, and amnesia.— P. C. Liederman and R. A. Boldus, *J. Am. med. Ass.*, 1967, *202*, 64.

Precautions. Chlorzoxazone should not be given to patients with impaired liver function and should be discontinued if skin rash, pruritus, or signs of liver damage appear.

Chlorzoxazone could cause orange or purplish-red discoloration of the urine.— R. B. Baran and B. Rowles, *J. Am. pharm. Ass.*, 1973, *NS13*, 139.

Absorption and Fate. Peak blood concentrations occur 3 to 4 hours after a dose. Chlorzoxazone is rapidly converted to 6-hydroxychlorzoxazone which is excreted in the urine mainly as the glucuronide. It has a biological half-life of about 170 minutes.

In a healthy subject a peak plasma concentration of about 2.5 µg per ml occurred 4 hours after the administration of chlorzoxazone 300 mg by mouth. Less than 0.1% of the administered dose was excreted unchanged in the urine during the 24 hours following administration.— J. T. Stewart and C. W. Chan, *J. pharm. Sci.*, 1979, *68*, 910.

Uses. Chlorzoxazone is a centrally acting muscle relaxant with uses similar to those of mephenesin. The usual initial dose is 500 mg three or four times daily, with 250-mg doses for maintenance. Up to 750 mg three or four times daily has been given.

Chlorzoxazone 750 mg was more effective than diazepam 5 mg (both given 4 times daily) for relieving skeletal muscle spasm in 53 patients with sprains and contusions.— J. J. Scheiner, *Curr. ther. Res.*, 1976, *19*, 51.

Further references: J. J. Scheiner, *Curr. ther. Res.*, 1972, *14*, 168; J. M. Walker, *ibid.*, 1973, *15*, 248.

Proprietary Names

Biomioran *(Bioindustria, Ital.)*; Escoflex *(Streuli, Switz.)*; Paraflex *(Cilag-Chemie, Belg.; Astra, Denm.; Cilag, Ger.; Cilag-Chemie, Ital.; Cilag-Chemie, Neth.; Astra, Norw.; Astra, Swed.; Cilag-Chemie, Switz.; McNeil, USA)*; Solaxin *(Jap.)*.

5707-x

Curare *(B.P.C. 1934)*. Curara; Ourari; Urari; Woorali; Wourara.

CAS — 8063-06-7.

Pharmacopoeias. In *Span.*

An unstandardised extract derived mainly from the bark of various species of *Strychnos* and *Chondodendron* and prepared by evaporation of an aqueous decoction or infusion. It varies considerably in appearance and composition.

The physiologically active principle, (+)-tubocurarine chloride, has been isolated as a crystalline substance and *Chondodendron tomentosum* is now the usual source of the alkaloid. Tubocurarine chloride, which is now used in preference, is standardised spectrophotometrically; it is sometimes still referred to as curare in anaesthetic literature.

5708-r

Cyclobenzaprine Hydrochloride *(U.S.P.)*.

Proheptatriene Hydrochloride; CBZ *(cyclobenzaprine)*; MK-130 *(cyclobenzaprine)*; 9715 RP *(cyclobenzaprine)*. 3-(5*H*-Dibenzo[*a,d*]cyclohepten-5-ylidene)-*NN*-dimethylpropylamine hydrochloride.
$C_{20}H_{21}N,HCl=311.9$.

CAS — 303-53-7 (cyclobenzaprine); 6202-23-9 (hydrochloride).

A white or off-white odourless crystalline powder. M.p. 215° to 219° with a range of not more than 2°. Freely **soluble** in water, alcohol, and methyl alcohol; sparingly soluble in isopropyl alcohol; slightly soluble in chloroform and methylene chloride; practically insoluble in hydrocarbons.

Adverse Effects. Because of the structural similarity between cyclobenzaprine and the tricyclic antidepressants it would be reasonable to expect any of the side-effects described under amitriptyline hydrochloride (see p.110). Many of those effects have been reported. Drowsiness may occur in up to 40% of patients; dyspnoea and unpleasant taste have been reported.

Treatment of Adverse Effects. As for Amitriptyline Hydrochloride, p.111.
Dialysis is unlikely to be effective.

Precautions. As for Amitriptyline Hydrochloride, p.112.

Absorption and Fate. Cyclobenzaprine hydrochloride is readily, though variably, absorbed from the gastro-intestinal tract. It is extensively bound to plasma proteins and has a half-life of 1 to 3 days. It is extensively metabolised, and excreted via the kidneys. It probably appears in breast milk.

Comparison of the plasma concentrations after administration of the same dose of cyclobenzaprine by mouth or intravenous injection suggested that it may be metabolised in the intestinal tract or undergo a 'first-pass' effect in the liver.— H. B. Hucher *et al.*, *J. clin. Pharmac.*, 1977, *17*, 719.

Further references: H. B. Stucker and S. C. Stauffer, *J. pharm. Sci.*, 1976, *65*, 1253.

Uses. Cyclobenzaprine hydrochloride is a centrally acting muscle relaxant, chemically related to the tricyclic antidepressants. It appears to act at brain stem, rather than at spinal cord, levels. It is used for the symptomatic relief of muscle spasm. The usual dose is 10 mg thrice daily; the daily dose should not exceed 60 mg. Treatment for more than 2 or 3 weeks is not recommended. It is not considered effective in cerebral or spinal cord disease, or in cerebral palsy.

Reviews: *Med. Lett.*, 1978, *20*, 12.

Parkinsonism. Comparison with benztropine mesylate.— A. R. Potvin *et al.*, *Clin. Pharmac. Ther.*, 1977, *21*, 114.

Spasticity. Muscle spasm. In a double-blind trial 54 patients with muscle spasm associated with osteoarthritis of the neck or back were given cyclobenzaprine 20 to 40 mg daily in divided doses or a placebo. After 2 weeks' treatment symptoms were slightly less in patients receiving cyclobenzaprine, but after a further week without treatment there was little significant difference between the two groups. Drowsiness and dizziness occurred more frequently with cyclobenzaprine.— N. A. Bercel, *Curr. ther. Res.*, 1977, *22*, 462.

A controlled double-blind study lasting 2 weeks in 49 patients with long-term intractable pain of cervical and lumbar origin indicated comparable effectiveness of cyclobenzaprine hydrochloride 10 mg and diazepam 5 mg, both thrice daily. Dry mouth and drowsiness occurred more often with cyclobenzaprine than with diazepam.— B. R. Brown and J. Womble, *J. Am. med. Ass.*, 1978, *240*, 1151.

Analysis of 20 double-blind studies showed that cyclobenzaprine in a mean dose of about 32 mg daily was significantly more effective than placebo in the relief of skeletal muscle spasm. In patients with moderately severe or severe spasm cyclobenzaprine was more effective, in some parameters, than diazepam.— D. W. Nibbelink *et al.*, *Clin. Ther.*, 1978, *1*, 409.

The effectiveness of cyclobenzaprine hydrochloride in the treatment of muscle spasm was assessed by means of a postmarketing surveillance programme. In 4657 patients assessed, an excellent or good response was reported in 70%. Side-effects reported in the 4749 patients treated were drowsiness in 14.9%, dry mouth in 6.9%, dizziness in 2.8%, nervousness in 1.1%, fatigue in 1.5%, confusion in 1.5%, and nausea in 1.3%. Other side-effects reported included taste disturbance, tachycardia, disorientation, and hallucinations (all less than 1%). Cyclobenzaprine was discontinued in 101 patients because of adverse reactions.— D. W. Nibbelink and S. C. Strickland, *Curr. ther. Res.*, 1979, *25*, 564.

Further references: F. J. Azoury, *Curr. ther. Res.*, 1979, *26*, 189.

Preparations

Cyclobenzaprine Hydrochloride Tablets *(U.S.P.)*. Tablets containing cyclobenzaprine hydrochloride. The *U.S.P.* requires 75% dissolution in 30 minutes.

Proprietary Names

Flexeril *(Merck Sharp & Dohme, Canad.; Merck Sharp & Dohme, USA)*.

5709-f

Dantrolene Sodium.

F-440; F-368 *(dantrolene)*. The hemiheptahydrate of the sodium salt of 1-[5-(4-nitrophenyl)furfurylideneamino]-imidazolidine-2,4-dione.
$C_{14}H_9N_4NaO_5,3\frac{1}{2}H_2O=399.3$.

CAS — 7261-97-4 (dantrolene); 14663-23-1 (sodium salt, anhydrous); 24868-20-0 (sodium salt, hemiheptahydrate).

An orange powder. Slightly **soluble** in water; its solubility increases in alkaline solution. **Protect** from light.

Adverse Effects. The most common side-effects of dantrolene sodium are drowsiness, dizziness, weakness, general malaise, fatigue, and diarrhoea. Other side-effects reported include gastro-intestinal, cardiovascular, respiratory, urinary, musculoskeletal, neurological, and psychiatric symptoms. Pruritus and skin rashes may occur. Changes in liver-function tests, jaundice, and hepatitis have been reported; fatalities have occurred.
Dantrolene sodium in high doses is carcinogenic in some *animals*.

Abdominal distension and intestinal obstruction developed in 3 patients who were taking 50 mg or more of dantrolene four times a day.— S. A. Shaivitz (letter), *J. Am. med. Ass.*, 1974, *229*, 1282.

Dantrolene 75 mg daily in divided doses was poorly tolerated by 6 patients with amyotrophic lateral sclerosis. Side-effects also developed in another receiving 25 mg every 6 hours. Four patients developed severe muscle weakness and 5 developed sialorrhoea and dysphagia. One patient with borderline respiratory function developed respiratory depression after a single dose of 100 mg.— V. M. Rivera *et al.* (letter), *J. Am. med. Ass.*, 1975, *233*, 863.

Fatal bowel atony and hepatotoxicity in a patient taking dantrolene.— C. R. Goodman *et al.*, *N.Y. St. J. Med.*, 1977, *77*, 1759.

Dantrolene was reported to be epileptogenic.— *Lancet*, 1977, *2*, 594.

A report of pleural effusion in 4 patients of whom one also developed acute pericarditis and another pericardial effusions after receiving dantrolene sodium for at least 2 months.— M. L. Petusevsky *et al.*, *J. Am. med. Ass.*, 1979, *242*, 2772.

A report of the development of lymphocytic lymphoma in a patient associated with prolonged dantrolene therapy for progressive spastic paraplegia.— H. H. Wan and J. S. Tucker, *Postgrad. med. J.*, 1980, *56*, 261.

Liver damage. A revised package insert indicated that fatal hepatitis had been reported in about 0.1 to 0.2% of patients who had taken dantrolene for 60 days or more; symptomatic hepatitis had been seen in about 0.35 to 0.5% of patients who had taken dantrolene for 60 days or more. Liver dysfunction, as shown by blood abnormalities, had been seen in about 0.7 to 1% of all patients taking dantrolene for varying periods. The risk of hepatic injury appeared to be greater in patients over 35 years of age and in females. If observable benefit was not seen after 45 days' treatment dantrolene should be withdrawn.— *FDA Drug Bull.*, 1975, *5*, 12. See also *Bull. Nat. Clearinghouse Poison Control Centers*, Nov.–Dec., 1975.

An analysis of all the known cases of liver injury associated with dantrolene reported to the manufacturer or to the FDA. Fifty cases had been reported, with jaundice in 22; there were 14 fatalities. All the fatalities occurred in patients over 30 years of age who had taken dantrolene for at least 2 months. Eleven of the fatalities were in females. No liver damage occurred in patients under the age of 10 or treated for less than 1 month. Most of the cases and fatalities were in patients who had taken 300 mg or more daily. Damage was mainly hepatocellular with no evidence of hypersensitivity.— R. Utili *et al.*, *Gastroenterology*, 1977, *72*, 610.

Reports of liver damage: R. M. Ogburn *et al.* (letter), *Ann. intern. Med.*, 1976, *84*, 53; R. Schneider and D. Mitchell, *J. Am. med. Ass.*, 1976, *235*, 1590; S. R. Lundin *et al.*, *Drug Intell. & clin. Pharm.*, 1977, *11*, 278; J. H. Donegan *et al.*, *Am. J. dig. Dis.*, 1978, *23*, *Suppl.* (May), 48S; S. P. Wilkinson *et al.*, *Gut*, 1979, *20*, 33.

Treatment of Adverse Effects. The stomach should be emptied by aspiration and lavage and general supportive measures employed.
Large volumes of fluids should be administered to avoid the theoretical possibility of crystalluria.

Precautions. It is recommended that dantrolene sodium should not be used where spasticity is used to maintain posture or function and in patients with active liver disease; liver-function tests should be performed before and during treatment; if values rise treatment should generally be discontinued. It should be used with caution in patients with cardiac or pulmonary disorders and its use should be avoided during pregnancy and lactation.
Patients should not take charge of vehicles or machinery where loss of attention could cause accidents.
The effects of dantrolene sodium may be enhanced by tranquillisers. Concomitant administration with oestrogens may possibly increase the risk of liver damage.

A significant reduction in the binding of dantrolene to human serum albumin occurred in the presence of the tightly bound drugs, warfarin and clofibrate, but tolbutamide, which would similarly have been expected to displace dantrolene, increased the binding.— J. J. Vallner *et al.*, *J. pharm. Sci.*, 1976, *65*, 873.

A study of the effects of dantrolene sodium on *guinea-pig* isolated skeletal, smooth, and cardiac muscle. Reflex sympathetic activity might be an important factor in maintaining cardiac output in patients chronically treated with dantrolene. Serious interaction might occur following concurrent administration of drugs that impaired the activity of the sympathetic nervous system, such as adrenergic neurone blocking agents and beta-adrenoceptor blocking agents, or agents that interfered with calcium ion flux across cardiac cell membranes, such as verapamil or nifedipine. Experimental studies were needed.— W. C. Bowman and H. H. Khan, *J. Pharm. Pharmac.*, 1977, *29*, 628.

Absorption and Fate. Dantrolene sodium is incompletely absorbed from the gastro-intestinal tract. It is hydroxylated and a proportion is reduced to an acetylated amine derivative. About 25% is excreted in the urine mainly as the metabolites with a small amount of unchanged dantrolene, and about 45 to 50% appears in the bile.

In adults and children peak blood concentrations of dantrolene were obtained 4 to 6 hours after a single dose by mouth. The mean half-life was 8.7 hours.— M. H. M. Dykes, *J. Am. med. Ass.*, 1975, *231*, 862.

Plasma concentrations of dantrolene were assayed in 6 patients receiving chronic dantrolene therapy. In 4 patients dantrolene concentrations were fairly stable and remained between about 30 and 90 ng per ml, while concentrations fluctuated between 30 and 212 ng per ml in the other 2 patients. Plasma concentrations of 5-

hydroxydantroleneranged from about 100 to 300 ng per ml.— J. J. Vallner *et al.*, *Curr. ther. Res.*, 1979, *25*, 79.

Further references: P. L. Cox *et al.*, *J. pharm. Sci.*, 1969, *58*, 987; P. S. Leitman *et al.*, *Archs phys. Med.*, 1974, *55*, 388; W. J. Meyler *et al.*, *Eur. J. clin. Pharmac.*, 1979, *16*, 203.

Uses. Dantrolene sodium is a muscle relaxant reported to act by blocking muscle contraction beyond the neuromuscular junction. It is used for the symptomatic relief of muscular spasm due to conditions such as stroke, multiple sclerosis, spinal cord injury, and cerebral palsy.

The initial dose is 25 mg daily increased gradually over about 7 weeks to 100 mg four times daily or until the desired therapeutic effect has been obtained; dosage in excess of 400 mg daily is not recommended. The dose should be the lowest at which the desired response is obtained. If no response is achieved in 45 days treatment should be discontinued.

Dantrolene sodium is also used intravenously in the treatment of malignant hyperthermia. The initial dose is 1 mg per kg body-weight intravenously given rapidly, repeated, if necessary, to a total dose of 10 mg per kg.

Reviews of dantrolene sodium: *Med. Lett.*, 1974, *16*, 61; M. H. M. Dykes, *J. Am. med. Ass.*, 1975, *231*, 862; M. H. Barto, *Drug Intell. & clin. Pharm.*, 1975, *9*, 42; *Drug & Ther. Bull.*, 1976, *14*, 61; R. M. Pinder *et al.*, *Drugs*, 1977, *13*, 3.

It was considered that dantrolene acted directly on skeletal muscle at a site beyond the neuromuscular junction.— K. O. Ellis *et al.*, *J. pharm. Sci.*, 1973, *62*, 948.

Studies on isolated mammalian skeletal muscle indicated that the mechanism of action of dantrolene was by inhibition of release of calcium ions involved in the excitation-concentration coupling mechanism.— R. F. W. Moulds, *Br. J. Pharmac.*, 1977, *59*, 129.

Chorea. Six young adults with a lifelong history of distal unilateral or bilateral chorea and mild hemiatrophy, had a dramatic response to dantrolene.— H. Feit, *Neurology, Minneap.*, 1979, *29*, 1631.

Hyperpyrexia. Reviews and comments on the use of dantrolene sodium in the treatment of malignant hyperthermia: *Med. Lett.*, 1980, *22*, 61; F. R. Ellis and P. J. Halsall, *Br. J. Hosp. Med.*, 1980, *24*, 318; G. M. Hall, *Br. J. Anaesth.*, 1980, *52*, 847.

During *in vitro* studies of muscle fibres from *pigs* susceptible to malignant hyperthermia, dantrolene sodium protected fibres against and also reversed existing halothane-induced contraction; it appeared to act by inhibiting calcium release from sarcoplasmic reticulum and might be of value for pre-operative use in patients susceptible to malignant hyperthermia.— I. L. Anderson and E. W. Jones, *Anesthesiology*, 1976, *44*, 57, per *Drugs*, 1976, *11*, 473.

Studies in *dogs* and *sheep* indicated that dantrolene sodium had no effect on the cardiovascular or respiratory systems that would preclude its intravenous use in acute conditions where relaxation of skeletal muscle was required, such as malignant hyperthermia.— K. O. Ellis *et al.*, *J. pharm. Sci.*, 1976, *65*, 1359.

Dantrolene 5 mg per kg body-weight given by mouth (in the absence of an intravenous preparation) protected susceptible *pigs* from malignant hyperpyrexia when challenged with halothane or halothane with suxamethonium. Its use was recommended in patients at risk.— G. G. Harrison, *Br. J. Anaesth.*, 1977, *49*, 315.

A dose of dantrolene 2 mg per kg body-weight had been suggested for patients susceptible to malignant hyperpyrexia. Vomiting in a 35-kg patient given 50 mg four hours before surgery suggested that a lower dose of 0.5 to 1 mg per kg initially, allowing 1 or 2 days to reach 2 mg per kg, might be appropriate, the last dose being given 4 hours before surgery.— C. W. Free and M. P. C. Jaimon, *N.Z. med. J.*, 1978, *88*, 493.

Dental surgery was performed without complications and was well tolerated in a woman with a family history of malignant hyperthermia following treatment with dantrolene sodium 200 mg by mouth on the evening preceding surgery and again on the morning of surgery.— S. L. Bronstein *et al.*, *J. oral Surg.*, 1979, *37*, 719.

Possible malignant hyperthermia occurring postoperatively in a 6-month-old child responded to treatment with dantrolene sodium 50 mg intravenously.— D. K. Faust *et al.*, *Anesth. Analg.*, 1979, *58*, 33.

Successful use of dantrolene sodium intravenously for the treatment of malignant hyperthermia during surgery in a 28-year-old man; a total of 250 mg was given.— C. M. Friesen *et al.*, *Can. anaesth. Soc. J.*, 1979, *26*, 319.

Further references: F. Liebenschütz *et al.*, *Br. J. Anaesth.*, 1979, *51*, 899.

Heat stroke. A beneficial response to dantrolene in heat stroke.— J. S. Lydiatt and G. E. Hill (letter), *J. Am. med. Ass.*, 1981, *246*, 41.

Spasticity. A review on the treatment of spasticity including the use of dantrolene.— R. R. Young and P. J. Delwaide, *New Engl. J. Med.*, 1981, *304*, 28 and 96.

In a double-blind study in 5 centres, completed by 61 patients with spasticity, dantrolene 100 mg four times daily reduced muscle tension, assessed by tendon tap, by 40% compared with 15% for diazepam 5 mg four times daily and by 43% compared with 8% when assessed by tibial nerve stimulation. Subjectively both dantrolene and diazepam reduced spasticity and clonus. Subjective weakness and fatigue was common. There was no appreciable additive effect when the 2 drugs were given concomitantly.— R. E. Keenan *et al.*, *Clin. Ther.*, 1977, *1*, 48.

Dantrolene sodium 25 mg daily controlled muscle spasms and resulting pain in a 65-year-old man with advanced adenocarcinoma of the rectum and pelvic area.— A. Myers (letter), *J. Am. med. Ass.*, 1977, *237*, 2378.

In a 9-week double-blind crossover study of 35 patients with chronic spinal cord disease, dantrolene sodium 25 mg gradually increased to 100 mg four times a day was generally more effective than placebo in improving spasticity, knee and ankle clonus, gait, and flexor spasms. Eight patients withdrew from the study, 5 because of muscle weakness (2 in the placebo group), and one because of a maculopapular rash; other side-effects included depression in 3 patients.— R. Weiser *et al.*, *Practitioner*, 1978, *221*, 123.

Further references: S. B. Chyatte and J. V. Basmajian, *Archs phys. Med.*, 1973, *54*, 311; R. H. A. Haslam *et al.*, *Archs phys. Med.*, 1974, *55*, 384; M. Chipman *et al.*, *Dis. nerv. Syst.*, 1974, *35*, 27; F. U. Steinberg and K. L. Ferguson, *J. Am. Geriat. Soc.*, 1975, *23*, 70.

Multiple sclerosis. In a double-blind trial in 23 patients with multiple sclerosis with moderate to severe spasticity in the lower extremities, 11 received placebo and 12 received dantrolene sodium 25 mg four times a day, increased by weekly increments of 100 mg, if tolerated, up to a maximum of 800 mg daily. Mild improvement occurred in 3 patients with placebo and 4 with dantrolene sodium. Marked improvement occurred in 1 patient receiving dantrolene. Side-effects of weakness (6), dizziness, vertigo, and gastro-intestinal disturbance were common in the dantrolene group and 2 patients withdrew because of the severity of side-effects.— E. S. Tolosa *et al.* (letter), *J. Am. med. Ass.*, 1975, *233*, 1046.

In a double-blind study in 42 patients with stable multiple sclerosis dantrolene or diazepam relieved spasticity, clonus, and hyperreflexia. The doses in patients who chose to continue treatment after the study were dantrolene 118 ± 54 mg daily and diazepam 10.1 ± 5.5 mg daily.— R. T. Schmidt *et al.*, *J. Neurol. Neurosurg. Psychiat.*, 1976, *39*, 350.

A report of the use of dantrolene sodium in 5 patients as part of a regimen for the management of multiple sclerosis. All patients had a reduction in spasticity and contracture of leg muscles while taking dantrolene sodium 75 to 125 mg four times daily and apart from transient weakness no other side-effects were observed.— R. L. Reyes *et al.*, *Curr. ther. Res.*, 1978, *23*, 673.

Proprietary Preparations

Dantrium *(Norwich-Eaton, UK)*. Dantrolene sodium, available as capsules of 25 and 100 mg. (Also available as Dantrium in *Austral., Belg., Canad., Fr., Neth., NZ, S.Afr., USA*).

Dantrium Intravenous *(Norwich-Eaton, UK)*. Dantrolene sodium, available as powder for preparing injections, in vials of 20 mg, with mannitol 3 g and sodium hydroxide. For malignant hyperthermia.

Other Proprietary Names

Dantamacrin *(Ger.)*.

5710-z

Decamethonium Bromide *(U.S.P.)*. *NN'*-Decamethylenebis(trimethylammonium) dibromide.
$C_{16}H_{38}Br_2N_2$=418.3.

CAS — 156-74-1 (decamethonium); 541-22-0 (bromide).

Pharmacopoeias. In *U.S.*

A white hygroscopic crystalline powder, odourless or with a faint characteristic odour. M.p. about 265° with decomposition. Freely **soluble** in water and alcohol; practically insoluble in ether and ethyl acetate. **Store** in airtight containers.

Adverse Effects, Treatment, and Precautions. As for Suxamethonium Chloride, p.995.

Uses. Decamethonium bromide is a depolarising muscle relaxant used to obtain muscular relaxation during surgical operations and electroconvulsive therapy. The usual dose is 2 to 2.5 mg by intravenous injection given at the rate of 1 mg per minute, supplemented if necessary with 0.5 to 1 mg at intervals of 10 to 30 minutes.

Preparations

Decamethonium Bromide Injection *(U.S.P.)*. A sterile solution in Water for Injections adjusted if necessary to pH 4 to 7 with hydrochloric acid.

Proprietary Names

Syncurine *(Wellcome, Austral.; Wellcome, Canad.; Wellcome, USA)*.

5711-c

Decamethonium Iodide *(B.P.C. 1959)*. Decameth. Iod.; C 10; Decamethonium Biiodatum. *NN'*-Decamethylenebis(trimethylammonium) di-iodide.
$C_{16}H_{38}I_2N_2$=512.3.

CAS — 1420-40-2.

Pharmacopoeias. In *Cz., It.*, and *Pol.*

A white odourless crystalline powder with a bitter saline taste. M.p. 246° to 248°. **Soluble** 1 in 10 of water and 1 in 50 of alcohol; practically insoluble in acetone, chloroform, and ether. A saturated solution in water has a pH of 6 to 7. Solutions are **sterilised** by autoclaving or by filtration. **Incompatible** with phenylmercuric nitrate.

Adverse Effects, Treatment, and Precautions. As for Suxamethonium Chloride, p.995.

Decamethonium iodide may produce allergic reactions in patients sensitive to iodine.

Uses. Decamethonium iodide is a depolarising muscle relaxant which has been used to obtain muscular relaxation during surgical operations and electroconvulsive therapy. The usual dose in surgery is 3 to 5 mg by intravenous injection. The effect of a single injection lasts for 15 to 25 minutes, and supplementary doses of 0.5 to 3 mg may be given if required up to a total of 10 mg.

5712-k

Diplacine Hydrochloride. Diplacinum Dichloratum; Diplastin Hydrochloride; Diplatsin Hydrochloride. 4,4'-[*m*-Phenylenebis(oxyethylene)]bis(perhydro-1-hydroxy-7-hydroxymethyl-1*H*-pyrrolizinium) dichloride.
$C_{26}H_{42}Cl_2N_2O_6$=549.5.

CAS — 19918-85-5.

Diplacine hydrochloride is a muscle-relaxing agent with actions and uses similar to those of tubocurarine chloride (see p.999).

In a dose of 10 to 15 mg by intravenous injection, diplacine prevented muscle pains associated with the use of suxamethonium.— I. S. Zhorov *et al.*, *Br. J. Anaesth.*, 1967, *39*, 948.

5713-a

Elatine. An alkaloid obtained from *Delphinium elatum* (Ranunculaceae).
$C_{38}H_{50}N_2O_{10}$=694.8.

CAS — 26000-16-8.

A white crystalline powder. **Soluble** in water and organic solvents. **Protect** from light.

Elatine is a muscle relaxant used in the USSR with actions and uses similar to those of tubocurarine (see p.999).

5714-t

Fazadinium Bromide. AH 8165D. 1,1′-Azobis(3-methyl-2-phenyl-1*H*-imidazo[1,2-*a*]pyridinium) dibromide.
$C_{28}H_{24}Br_2N_6$=604.3.

CAS — 36653-54-0 (fazadinium); 49564-56-9 (bromide).

A yellow solid. Fazadinium bromide 1.36 mg is approximately equivalent to 1 mg of fazadinium. **Soluble** in water. A 2% solution has a pH of about 4. **Incompatible** with alkaline solutions.

In a study in 36 patients there was no difference in effect between formulations of fazadinium containing or not containing monothioglycerol.— P. Buckley and D. B. Scott (letter), *Br. J. Anaesth.*, 1977, *49*, 191.

Adverse Effects. As for Tubocurarine Chloride, p.999.
Tachycardia may occur after the use of fazadinium bromide, even after doses of 0.5 mg per kg body-weight, and may persist longer than the neuromuscular blockade. Local irritation at the site of injection has occurred, especially in children. Bronchospasm or urticaria has occasionally occurred, but histamine release does not appear to be a problem.

Treatment of Adverse Effects. As for Tubocurarine Chloride, p.999.

Precautions. As for Tubocurarine Chloride, p.999.
It should be used with care in patients with impaired renal function, in the elderly, and in patients with a low cardiac output or hypertension.
The effects of fazadinium are enhanced by ether, halothane, cyclopropane, and alphaxalone with alphadolone acetate, and may be enhanced by some aminoglycoside or polypeptide antibiotics and by raised body temperature. Concomitant administration with ketamine may increase tachycardia.

Absorption and Fate. About 30% of a dose of fazadinium bromide is excreted in the urine in 4 hours and 60 to 80% in 48 hours. Placental transfer is considered to be clinically insignificant.

A study of the pharmacokinetics of fazadinium in 10 anaesthetised patients given a single intravenous dose of 1.5 mg per kg body-weight. The serum half-life of the elimination phase was about 76 minutes and the mean plasma clearance, 132 ml per minute. About 50% of the dose was excreted, essentially unchanged, in the urine within 24 hours. Trace amounts of metabolites accounted for no more than 3% of the injected dose.— P. Duvaldestin *et al.*, *Br. J. Anaesth.*, 1978, *50*, 773.

In 5 patients given fazadinium bromide 70 mg intravenously the mean plasma concentration was greater than 10 µg per ml after 2 minutes and was 2.2 µg per ml after 1 hour.— J. D'Souza *et al.*, *J. Pharm. Pharmac.*, 1979, *31*, 416.

Further references: C. E. Blogg *et al.*, *Br. J. Anaesth.*, 1973, *45*, 1233; P. Duvaldestin *et al.*, *Br. J. Anaesth.*, 1979, *51*, 943 (in renal failure); P. Duvaldestin *et al.*, *Br. J. Anaesth.*, 1980, *52*, 7 (in liver disease).

Uses. Fazadinium bromide is a non-depolarising muscle relaxant, with a dose-dependent rapid onset and prolonged duration of action. Relaxation is evident in half to one minute; the effect lasts for about 30 minutes after doses equivalent to 0.5 mg of fazadinium per kg body-weight and up to 60 minutes after doses equivalent to 1 mg per kg. It is considered to have a mild ganglion-blocking effect. It does not appear to increase intra-ocular pressure.
Fazadinium bromide is used to facilitate endotracheal intubation and to provide muscular relaxation during surgery. The usual initial dose is the equivalent of 0.75 to 1 mg of fazadinium per kg, given intravenously; a subsequent dose one-quarter of the initial dose may be expected to prolong the effect for a further 10 to 20 minutes. Fazadinium has no advantages over suxamethonium for electroconvulsive therapy, and is not recommended for bronchoscopy.

Reviews.— *Drug & Ther. Bull.*, 1978, *16*, 90.

Fazadinium bromide is a non-depolarising muscle relaxant; it produces a rapid block with minimal cardiovascular and respiratory changes, no significant change in plasma potassium, and no fasciculation. The duration of action is longer in man than expected from animal work. The onset of effect is quicker than with suxamethonium and its duration is estimated to be comparable with pancuronium.— B. R. Simpson *et al.* (preliminary communication), *Lancet*, 1972, *1*, 516.

In 9 patients the haemodynamic and neuromuscular effects of fazadinium bromide were not influenced by moderate changes in respiratory acid-base status.— A. J. Coleman *et al.*, *Br. J. Anaesth.*, 1975, *47*, 365.

Intubation. Fazadinium bromide in a dose of 1.25 mg per kg body-weight was inferior to suxamethonium 1 mg per kg in a study in 60 patients requiring muscle relaxation for intubation.— H. S. A. Young *et al.*, *Br. J. Anaesth.*, 1974, *46*, 317.

Fazadinium bromide 0.5 and 1 mg per kg body-weight was compared with pancuronium 100 µg per kg in 3 groups of 20 patients during induction of anaesthesia prior to cardiac surgery. Both doses of fazadinium caused significant tachycardia and the higher dose arterial hypotension. There was no significant alteration in heart-rate or arterial pressure after pancuronium. Fazadinium at 0.5 mg per kg was unsatisfactory for tracheal intubation but at 1 mg per kg was comparable with pancuronium 100 µg per kg.— S. M. Lyons *et al.*, *Br. J. Anaesth.*, 1975, *47*, 725.

In a study in a 100 patients fazadinium 1 mg per kg body-weight provided better conditions for intubation during the first minute than did pancuronium 100 µg per kg. Fazadinium 500 µg per kg did not provide better conditions than pancuronium 80 µg per kg.— I. M. Corall *et al.*, *Br. J. Anaesth.*, 1977, *49*, 615.

Experience with 500 patients suggested that fazadinium was a useful alternative to suxamethonium for tracheal intubation; the usual dose was 750 µg per kg body-weight with a maximum of 45 mg; subsequent doses of 15 mg were given as required. The only consistent side-effect was tachycardia. The study had now been extended to 1000 patients.— D. E. Rowlands and K. Fidler, *Br. J. Anaesth.*, 1978, *50*, 289.

Although fazadinium had a significantly faster onset of action than pancuronium and tubocurarine it could not replace suxamethonium when rapid tracheal intubation was required under light general anaesthesia.— C. L. Blackburn and M. Morgan, *Br. J. Anaesth.*, 1978, *50*, 361.

Proprietary Preparations

Fazadon *(Duncan, Flockhart, UK)*. Fazadinium bromide, available as an injection containing the equivalent of 15 mg of fazadinium per ml, with sodium chloride 0.6% and α-thioglycerol 0.3%, in ampoules of 5 ml.

5720-k

Gallamine Triethiodide *(B.P., Eur. P., U.S.P.)*. Gallamini Triethiodidum; Bencurine Iodide. 2,2′,2″-(Benzene-1,2,3-triyltrioxy)tris(tetraethylammonium) tri-iodide.
$C_{30}H_{60}I_3N_3O_3$=891.5.

CAS — 153-76-4 (gallamine); 65-29-2 (triethiodide).

Pharmacopoeias. In *Arg., Br., Braz., Cz., Eur., Fr., Ger., Ind., Int., It., Jug., Neth., Nord., Swiss, Turk.,* and *U.S.*

A white, or faintly cream-coloured, hygroscopic, odourless or almost odourless powder with a slightly bitter taste. M.p. about 235° with decomposition.
Soluble 1 in 0.6 of water, 1 in 115 of alcohol, and 1 in 1500 of chloroform; slightly soluble in acetone; practically insoluble in ether. A 2% solution in water has a pH of 5.3 to 7. Aqueous solutions are stable and **compatible** with solutions of thiopentone sodium, providing the gallamine triethiodide solution is added to the thiopentone solution; they are **incompatible** with solutions of pethidine hydrochloride. Solutions are **sterilised** by autoclaving or by filtration. **Store** in airtight containers. Protect from light.

Adverse Effects. As for Tubocurarine Chloride, p.999. Tachycardia sometimes develops and persists for longer than the relaxant effect of the drug. Blood pressure may be raised. It has a smaller histamine-releasing effect than tubocurarine chloride.

Accidental subarachnoid injection of gallamine in a 48-year-old man, who subsequently underwent general anaesthesia and surgery, was followed 2 hours later by violent muscle spasms, pyrexia, profuse sweating, and increasing arterial pressure and heart-rate. About 4 hours later 15 ml of cerebrospinal fluid was withdrawn and was found still to contain gallamine. Treatment included intravenous injection of diazepam, hydrocortisone, dexamethasone, and infusion fluids. The patient survived.— T. W. Goonewardene *et al.*, *Br. J. Anaesth.*, 1975, *47*, 889.

Allergy. Bronchospasm, probable cardiac arrest, and an erythematous rash occurred in a 19-year-old patient due to an anaphylactoid reaction to gallamine triethiodide.— W. Sniper, *Anaesthesia*, 1971, *26*, 527.

Further reports.— M. Fisher (letter), *Br. J. Anaesth.*, 1977, *49*, 87; M. M. Fisher, *Anesth. & intensive Care*, 1978, *6*, 62.

Treatment of Adverse Effects. As for Tubocurarine Chloride, p.999.

Two patients undergoing bilateral nephrectomy received gallamine triethiodide; neuromuscular blockade was prolonged; haemodialysis was successful in effecting its removal.— M. M. Singer *et al.*, *Br. J. Anaesth.*, 1971, *43*, 404.

Further reference to dialysis: S. A. Feldman and J. A. Levi, *Br. J. Anaesth.*, 1963, *35*, 804.

Precautions. As for Tubocurarine Chloride, p.999.
Gallamine triethiodide should not be used in patients with renal impairment and should be used with caution in patients with hypertension or cardiac insufficiency when tachycardia would be undesirable; it should preferably be avoided in obstetric surgery until after the delivery of the foetus. It may produce allergic reactions in patients hypersensitive to iodine.
If used with cyclopropane anaesthesia, gallamine triethiodide may provoke ventricular arrhythmias.

Gallamine produced an acceptable cardiovascular stability when used after induction of anaesthesia with thiopentone in 20 patients with cardiac disease.— S. M. Lyons and R. S. J. Clarke, *Br. J. Anaesth.*, 1972, *44*, 575. See also B. R. Kennedy and J. V. Farman, *Br. J. Anaesth.*, 1968, *40*, 773.

Administration in renal failure. Gallamine could be given in usual doses to patients with a glomerular filtration-rate (GFR) above 50 ml per minute; its use should be avoided in those with a GFR of less than 50 ml per minute; recurarisation might occur up to 24 hours after surgery. Concentrations of gallamine were affected by haemodialysis and peritoneal dialysis.— W. M. Bennett *et al.*, *Ann. intern. Med.*, 1980, *93*, 286.

Further references: M. I. Ramzan *et al.*, *Br. J. clin. Pharmac.*, 1981, *12*, 141 (slower recovery).

Interactions. Enhancement of effect. A patient undergoing surgery received gallamine. Its action was terminated by atropine and neostigmine but neuromuscular blockade with apnoea developed when 300 mg of quinidine was given intramuscularly.— W. L. Way *et al.*, *J. Am. med. Ass.*, 1967, *200*, 153.

The intensity and duration of the neuromuscular block induced by gallamine was profoundly enhanced when diazepam, 150 to 200 µg per kg body-weight, was administered intravenously. Preliminary studies suggested that diazepam acted at the presynaptic membrane.— S. A. Feldman and B. E. Crawley (preliminary communication), *Br. med. J.*, 1970, *2*, 336. Diazepam did not enhance the neuromuscular blockade produced by tubocurarine or gallamine; in *rat* phrenic-nerve diaphragm it caused an increased contraction by a direct action on the muscle.— G. Moudgil and B. J. Pleuvry (letter), *ibid.*, 734. There was no evidence in *cats* of any alteration in the depth or duration of neuromuscular blockade induced by tubocurarine or gallamine if diazepam 200 to 400 µg per kg body-weight was given intravenously 5 minutes prior to the blocking agent or at the point of maximum blockade. Slight enhancement of the rate of recovery after diazepam 1 mg per kg was due to the diazepam solvent.— S. N. Webb and E. G. Bradshaw (letter), *ibid.*, 1971, *3*, 640. Investigations in *dogs* showed that diazepam significantly reversed the neuromuscular blockade induced by non-depolarising agents such as gallamine but augmented that of depolarising agents such as suxamethonium.— K. K. Sharma and U. C. Sharma, *J. Pharm. Pharmac.*, 1978, *30*, 64.

Absorption and Fate. Gallamine triethiodide is excreted unchanged in the urine. It diffuses across the placenta.

Gallamine or an active metabolite was found in the CSF of 6 patients after an intravenous injection of 2 to 3.8 mg per kg body-weight.— P. S. R. K. Haranath *et al.*, *Br. J. Pharmac.*, 1973, *48*, 640.

The clinical pharmacokinetics of gallamine triethiodide.— L. B. Wingard and D. R. Cook, *Clin. Pharmacokinet.*, 1977, *2*, 330.

A preliminary investigation of the renal and hepatic excretion of gallamine in 15 patients undergoing surgery showed that it was primarily excreted unchanged in the urine with negligible amounts in the bile. Observations in 3 patients indicated that poor urinary excretion of gallamine did not invariably result in persistent high serum concentrations or prolonged duration of neuromuscular effects.— S. Agoston *et al.*, *Br. J. Anaesth.*, 1978, *50*, 345.

Pregnancy and the neonate. Gallamine triethiodide 80 mg was given to 13 pregnant women immediately before delivery. The drug was found in the cord serum in high concentrations (up to 3 μg per ml) which were unrelated to the dose given to the mother and the concentration in the maternal serum, but there were no clinical effects in the babies.— J. S. Crawford and J. E. Gardiner, *Br. J. Anaesth.*, 1956, *28*, 154.

Uses. Gallamine triethiodide is a non-depolarising muscle relaxant with effects similar to those of tubocurarine chloride (p.999). Muscle relaxation commences within about 1 to 2 minutes of administration and lasts for about 20 to 30 minutes.

Gallamine triethiodide is used mainly as an adjuvant to anaesthesia to obtain greater muscular relaxation in surgical operations. The initial dose is usually 80 to 120 mg by intravenous injection and if necessary further doses of 20 to 40 mg may be given; an initial dose of 40 to 60 mg may be used to augment light anaesthesia for minor operations, with supplementary doses of 20 mg as required. It has been used in doses of 25 μg per kg body-weight for the diagnosis of myasthenia gravis. Children may be given an initial dose of 1.5 mg per kg body-weight intravenously. Gallamine has been given intramuscularly with or without hyaluronidase.

A comparative study of the administration of gallamine, tubocurarine, pancuronium, and hexafluorenium for the prevention of muscle fasciculations due to suxamethonium was carried out in 158 subjects; gallamine 10 to 20 mg administered 3 minutes before suxamethonium 1.5 mg per kg body-weight was recommended for clinical use.— D. J. Cullen, *Anesthesiology*, 1971, *35*, 572.

In 40 patients gallamine, 300 μg per kg body-weight given 3 minutes before induction of anaesthesia, was more effective than atropine, 6 μg per kg in 40 patients, in preventing slowing of the heart-rate after a second injection of suxamethonium—the incidence was 1 in 39 compared with 14 of 40. Both gallamine and atropine prevented junctional rhythm. Visible muscle fasciculations after the first dose of suxamethonium occurred in 1 of 40 patients after gallamine and in 33 of 40 after atropine.— R. K. Stoelting, *Anesth. Analg. curr. Res.*, 1977, *56*, 493.

Preparations

Gallamine Injection *(B.P.)*. A sterile solution of gallamine triethiodide in Water for Injections containing the equivalent of 0.1% of sulphur dioxide. Sterilised by autoclaving. pH 5.5 to 7.5. Protect from light.

Gallamine Triethiodide Injection *(U.S.P.)*. A sterile solution in Water for Injections. pH 6.5 to 7.5. Protect from light.

Flaxedil *(May & Baker, UK)*. Gallamine triethiodide, available as a 4% solution in ampoules of 2 ml. (Also available as Flaxedil in *Arg., Austral., Belg., Canad., Ger., Neth., S.Afr., Spain*).

Other Proprietary Names

Miowas G *(Spain)*; Relaxan *(Denm.)*.

5721-a

Hexafluorenium Bromide *(U.S.P.)*. Hexafluronium Bromide. *NN'*-Hexamethylenebis(fluoren-9-yldimethylammonium) dibromide.
$C_{36}H_{42}Br_2N_2$=662.5.

CAS — 4844-10-4 (hexafluorenium); 317-52-2 (bromide).

Pharmacopoeias. In *U.S.*

A white crystalline powder. Sparingly **soluble** in water; soluble in alcohol; practically insoluble in chloroform and ether. **Protect** from light.

Uses. Hexafluorenium bromide has been used to prolong the relaxant effects of suxamethonium chloride (see p.998); it is claimed to diminish suxamethonium-induced muscular fasciculations. The usual dose is 400 μg per kg body-weight 2 or 3 minutes before injection of suxamethonium; subsequent doses are 100 to 200 μg per kg as required.

The simultaneous administration of hexafluorenium bromide and suxamethonium should be avoided. Intermittent intravenous injection of 1.5 to 10 ml of a solution containing 2.5 mg of hexafluorenium bromide and 10 mg of suxamethonium per ml produced, in all of 6 patients, bronchospasm which persisted until the effect of the relaxants had worn off. One case terminated fatally.— B. Selvin and W. S. Howland, *Anesth. Analg. curr. Res.*, 1959, *38*, 332, per *Abstr. Wld Med.*, 1960, *27*, 506.

The use of hexafluorenium and suxamethonium in 93 patients undergoing abdominal surgery.— F. N. Campbell and M. Swerdlow, *Br. J. Anaesth.*, 1969, *41*, 962.

Hexafluorenium with suxamethonium was the technique of choice for patients with renal failure. Hexafluorenium 5 mg followed after 3 minutes by suxamethonium 10 mg produced relaxation for 20 to 30 minutes; a further dose of suxamethonium extended relaxation for a further 20 minutes, and could be repeated. For relaxation beyond 60 to 80 minutes the initial doses of each agent were repeated.— J. W. Kleine and A. Moesker (letter), *Br. J. Anaesth.*, 1976, *48*, 713.

Use of hexafluorenium with suxamethonium during anaesthesia might eliminate the undesirable effects of suxamethonium such as fasciculation, increased intraocular pressure, and the increases in serum-potassium concentration. The technique might be safe for anephric patients and for those in chronic renal failure.— P. A. Radnay *et al.*, *Br. J. Anaesth.*, 1979, *51*, 447.

For a comparative study of the effect of hexafluorenium bromide and other muscle relaxants for the prevention of muscle fasciculations due to suxamethonium, see Gallamine Triethiodide, above.

Preparations

Hexafluorenium Bromide Injection *(U.S.P.)*. A sterile solution in an aqueous solution of macrogols. When diluted with 4 volumes of water, the injection has a pH of 4 to 7.

Proprietary Names

Mylaxen *(Wallace, USA)*.

5722-t

Mephenesin *(B.P.C. 1973)*. Mephenes.; Cresoxydiol; Glykresin. 3-(*o*-Tolyloxy)propane-1,2-diol.
$C_{10}H_{14}O_3$=182.2.

CAS — 59-47-2.

Pharmacopoeias. In *Braz.*, *Ind.*, and *It.*

White, odourless or almost odourless, crystals or crystalline aggregates with a slightly bitter numbing taste. M.p. 70° to 73°.

Soluble 1 in 100 of water, 1 in 8 of alcohol, 1 in 12 of chloroform, and 1 in 7 of propylene glycol; soluble in ether. Solutions are **sterilised** by autoclaving or by filtration. **Store** at room temperature and avoid excessive heat.

Adverse Effects. Given by mouth, mephenesin may produce lassitude, anorexia, nausea, and vomiting. Leucopenia has been reported. Allergic reactions may occur. Overdosage may produce nystagmus, diplopia, weakness, and ataxia. Gross overdosage may produce respiratory paralysis, a fall in blood pressure, and heart block.

Unless well diluted, intravenous administration of alcoholic solutions of mephenesin may cause intravascular haemolysis and haemoglobinuria; fatalities due to renal anoxia and anuria have been reported. Local thrombosis may also occur at the site of injection.

In 4 women and 2 men, the colour of the hair changed from brunette to blonde during the first 3 to 4 months of treatment with mephenesin up to 10 to 12 g daily. Normal hair colour was restored about 3 months after withdrawal of the drug.— J. D. Spillane, *Br. med. J.*, 1963, *1*, 997.

Pulmonary eosinophilia had been reported following administration of mephenesin.— P. D. B. Davies, *Br. J. Dis. Chest*, 1969, *63*, 57.

Mephenesin could cause a rash similar to macular purpura and could cross-react with carbromal.— P. W. M. Copeman, *Br. J. Hosp. Med.*, 1972, *7*, 339.

Treatment of Adverse Effects. The stomach should be emptied by aspiration and lavage; general supportive measures are recommended.

Precautions. Mephenesin may enhance the effects of barbiturates and narcotics.

Mephenesin could interfere technically with laboratory estimations for 5-hydroxyindole-acetic acid and vanilmandelic acid in the urine to produce erroneous raised results.— *Drug & Ther. Bull.*, 1972, *10*, 69.

Absorption and Fate. Mephenesin is readily absorbed from the gastro-intestinal tract and distributed throughout most tissues of the body. After intravenous injection, mephenesin disappears from the plasma within 60 to 90 minutes. It is mainly metabolised in the liver; less than 2% is excreted unchanged in the urine, and about 50% is converted to inactive metabolites.

Uses. Mephenesin is a centrally acting muscle relaxant. It relaxes hypertonic muscles, lowers response to sensory stimuli, and depresses superficial reflexes.

Mephenesin is used for the symptomatic relief of muscular spasm and of spastic, hypertonic, and hyperkinetic conditions, such as parkinsonism, chorea, and athetosis.

Mephenesin has a duration of action of about 3 hours and is usually given by mouth after meals in a dose of 0.5 or 1 g one to six times daily according to the patient's requirements.

Mephenesin was formerly used in the treatment of anxiety and tension states, insomnia, alcoholism, arthritis, to obtain muscular relaxation for surgical operations, and in the treatment of tetanus.

It has been given intramuscularly as a 10% solution, or as a 1 or 2% solution by slow intravenous injection, or in an intravenous infusion.

Preparations

Mephenesin Injection *(B.P.C. 1968, Ind. P.)*. Mephenesin 10 g, propylene glycol 15 ml, alcohol 25 ml, Water for Injections to 100 ml. Store at room temperature. Solid matter may separate during storage and must be redissolved by warming before use. *Dose.* 1 to 10 ml by intramuscular injection or, well diluted, by intravenous infusion.

Proprietary Names

Decontractyl *(Robert & Carriere, Belg.*; *Robert et Carrière, Fr.*; *Robert et Carrière, Switz.)*; Relaxar *(Bouty, Ital.)*; Rhex *(Hobein, Ger.)*.

Mephenesin was formerly marketed in Great Britain under the proprietary name Myanesin *(Duncan, Flockhart)*.

5723-x

Mephenesin Carbamate. 3-(*o*-Tolyloxy)propane-1,2-diol 1-carbamate.
$C_{11}H_{15}NO_4$=225.2.

CAS — 533-06-2.

White crystals. M.p. 93°. Slightly **soluble** in water; very soluble in alcohol; soluble 1 in 50 of chloroform.

Uses. Mephenesin carbamate has actions and uses similar to those of mephenesin but has a longer duration of effect. It has been given in doses of 1 to 3 g three to five times daily after meals.

5724-r

Metaxalone. 5-(3,5-Xylyloxymethyl)oxazolidin-2-one. $C_{12}H_{15}NO_3$=221.3.

CAS — 1665-48-1.

A white odourless crystalline powder with a bitter taste. M.p. about 123°. Very slightly **soluble** in water; soluble in alcohol, acetone, chloroform, and propylene glycol.

Adverse Effects and Precautions. As for Chlorzoxazone, p.988.

Leucopenia, haemolytic anaemia, and jaundice have been reported.

Patients taking metaxalone excrete in the urine a metabolite which gives a false positive reaction for glycosuria.

Uses. The mode of action of metaxalone is not established. It is used for the relief of pain associated with acute muscular spasm. The usual dose is 800 mg three or four times daily.

In view of the adverse reactions and potential toxic effects reported for metaxalone, there seemed little reason for using it in preference to other available, less toxic drugs of this class.—Council on Drugs of AMA, *J. Am. med. Ass.*, 1964, *187*, 291.

Spasticity. Metaxalone was no better than a placebo in relieving skeletal muscle spasm in a double-blind study with 100 patients.— S. Diamond, *J. Am. med. Ass.*, 1966, *195*, 479.

In a multicentre double-blind trial, 228 patients with acute skeletal muscle spasm received metaxalone 800 mg four times daily or a placebo for 7 to 9 days. Improvement was significantly greater with metaxalone after 48 hours and at the end of the trial.— R. W. Dent and D. K. Ervin, *Curr. ther. Res.*, 1975, *18*, 433.

Proprietary Names

Skelaxin *(Robins, Canad.; Robins, USA).*

5725-f

Methocarbamol *(U.S.P.).*

Guaiphenesin Carbamate. 2-Hydroxy-3-(2-methoxyphenoxy)propyl carbamate.

$C_{11}H_{15}NO_5$=241.2.

CAS — 532-03-6.

Pharmacopoeias. In *Port.* and *U.S.*

A white powder, odourless or with a slight characteristic odour. M.p. about 94° or, if previously ground to a fine powder, about 90°. **Soluble** 1 in 40 of water; sparingly soluble in chloroform; soluble in alcohol only with heating; soluble in propylene glycol; practically insoluble in *n*-hexane. **Store** in airtight containers.

Adverse Effects. Side-effects reported include nausea, lightheadedness, dizziness, drowsiness, and allergic reactions.

After intravenous injection the patients may experience flushing, and a metallic taste; hypotension, bradycardia, and anaphylaxis have been reported.

A 48-year-old man who had received up to 10 g of methocarbamol for severe muscle spasm experienced paralytic ileus which was relieved by neostigmine. Abdominal symptoms first developed when he had received 7 g.— J. J. Kozma, *Clin. Med.*, 1964, *71*, 527.

In a study of 10 healthy subjects methocarbamol 1 g daily by intravenous injection on 3 successive days and 1 g every 30 minutes for 3 doses by intravenous injection on 3 successive days caused haemolysis of a relatively low order which did not exceed that occurring normally under certain physiological conditions such as exercise.— R. B. Scott *et al.*, *Clin. Pharmac. Ther.*, 1977, *21*, 208.

Treatment of Adverse Effects. As for Mephenesin, above.

Precautions. Preparations for injection may contain, as a solvent, a macrogol which could increase existing acidosis and urea retention in patients with renal impairment; such preparations should not be used in patients with known or suspected renal disease.

A 50-year-old woman with myasthenia gravis, controlled with pyridostigmine, experienced severe weakness after taking methocarbamol.— A. Podrizki (letter), *J. Am. med. Ass.*, 1968, *205*, 938.

Methocarbamol could cause discoloration of the urine, which became brown to black or green on standing.— R. B. Baran and B. Rowles, *J. Am. pharm. Ass.*, 1973, *NS13*, 139.

Absorption and Fate. Methocarbamol is absorbed from the gastro-intestinal tract and produces peak plasma concentrations after about 1 to 3 hours. Its activity derives from the intact molecule and only a small proportion is converted to guaiphenesin.

When methocarbamol was given to 2 subjects by mouth in doses of 0.2 and 1 g respectively it was rapidly absorbed, peak concentrations in the blood being reached in about 30 minutes. About 98% of the dose was excreted unchanged and as conjugated metabolites in the urine in 72 hours, most of it within 8 hours.— R. B. Bruce *et al.*, *J. pharm. Sci.*, 1971, *60*, 104.

Following the administration of methocarbamol 2 g to 7 volunteers, peak serum concentrations occurred at 1 hour in 4 subjects, at 2 hours in 2, and at 3 hours in 1. The mean biological half-life was 1.2 hours.— A. A. Forist and R. W. Judy, *J. pharm. Sci.*, 1971, *60*, 1686.

Uses. The mode of action of methocarbamol is not established. It is used for the symptomatic relief of muscular spasm. The usual initial dose is 1.5 g four times daily later reduced to a maintenance dose of about 4 g daily. If necessary it may be given by injection; up to 5 ml of a 10% solution may be given intramuscularly into each gluteal region; it may also be given intravenously at a rate of not more than 3 ml per minute, or by infusion in sodium chloride or dextrose injection. The parenteral dose should not exceed 3 g daily for 3 days. Extravasation should be avoided.

Methocarbamol has been given by intravenous injection as an adjunct in the treatment of tetanus in doses of up to 3 g every 6 hours until therapy by mouth is possible.

Children have been given 15 mg per kg bodyweight every 6 hours.

In a double-blind controlled trial in 9 patients with spastic multiple sclerosis, methocarbamol 2 g intravenously gave a decrease in spasticity ranging from 65% immediately after injection to 39% after 30 minutes. By comparision, placebo treatment produced a slight initial increase and a decrease of less than 30% in most patients. Methocarbamol was well tolerated and the reduction in muscle hypertonia lasted for at least 24 hours.— I. M. Levine *et al.*, *Neurology, Minneap.*, 1968, *18*, 69, per *Abstr. Wld Med.*, 1968, *42*, 639.

Further references: D. S. O'Doherty and C. D. Shields, *J. Am. med. Ass.*, 1958, *167*, 160; H. F. Forsyth, *ibid.*, 163; H. W. Park, *ibid.*, 168; J. L. Poppen and M. E. Flanagan, *ibid.*, 1959, *171*, 298; S. A. Tisdale and D. K. Ervin, *Curr. ther. Res.*, 1975, *17*, 525.

Spider bite (arachnidism). Methocarbamol was used in latrodectism to produce muscle relaxation and to relieve pain, nausea, and respiratory distress.— W. P. Horen, *Clin. Med.*, 1966, *73* (Aug.), 41.

Tetanus. Eleven patients in Nigeria suffering from tetanus of varying severity were treated with diazepam 20 mg and methocarbamol 1 g every 8 hours by intravenous infusion, supplementary intramuscular doses of diazepam being given as required. All the patients survived and the combined use of the 2 drugs was recommended, especially when intensive care units were not available. Penicillin and tetanus antitoxin were also given.— C. O. Anah, *Am. J. trop. Med. Hyg.*, 1974, *23*, 930.

Preparations

Methocarbamol Injection *(U.S.P.).* A sterile solution of methocarbamol in an aqueous solution of macrogol 300. pH 3.5 to 6.

Methocarbamol Tablets *(U.S.P.).* Tablets containing methocarbamol. Store in airtight containers.

Proprietary Preparations

Robaxin Injectable *(Robins, UK).* Contains methocarbamol 100 mg per ml in a 50% aqueous solution of macrogol 300, with sodium metabisulphite 0.1% in ampoules of 10 ml. **Robaxin-750.** Methocarbamol, available as scored tablets of 750 mg. (Also available as Robaxin in *Arg., Austral., Canad., Denm., Neth., Norw., S.Afr., Spain, Swed., Switz., USA*).

Robaxisal-Forte *(Robins, UK).* Scored tablets each containing methocarbamol 400 mg and aspirin 325 mg. For pain due to skeletal muscle spasm. *Dose.* 2 tablets 4 times daily.

Other Proprietary Names

Delaxin *(USA)*; Lumirelax *(Fr.)*; Methocabal *(Jap.)*; Miowas *(Ital., Spain)*; Robamol *(USA)*; Traumacut *(Ger.)*; Tresortil *(Denm.)*.

5726-d

Metocurine Iodide *(U.S.P.).*

Dimethyl Tubocurarine Iodide; Dimethyltubocurarine Iodide. (+)-6,6′,7′,12′-Tetramethoxy-2,2,2′,2′-tetramethyltubocuraranium di-iodide.

$C_{40}H_{48}I_2N_2O_6$=906.6.

CAS — 5152-30-7 (metocurine); 7601-55-0 (iodide).

NOTE. The name dimethyltubocurarine iodide was based on the old empirical formula for tubocurarine (see p.999).

Pharmacopoeias. In *U.S.*

A white to pale yellow odourless crystalline powder. **Soluble** 1 in 400 of water; slightly soluble in dilute acids and alkalis; very slightly soluble in alcohol; practically insoluble in chloroform and ether. **Incompatible** with sodium salts of barbiturates. **Store** in airtight containers.

Adverse Effects, Treatment, Precautions, and Absorption and Fate. As for Tubocurarine Chloride, p.999.

Metocurine iodide has been reported to have a smaller histamine-releasing effect than tubocurarine chloride but may produce allergic reactions in patients sensitive to iodine.

Pregnancy and the neonate. In 18 women undergoing caesarean section the concentration of metocurine in the umbilical vein compared with that in the maternal vein was 4, 7, 12, and 12% when metocurine was given, 2, 4, 6, and 10 minutes before delivery. It might be wise to avoid metocurine if the foetus was at risk.— I. Kivalo and S. Saarikoski, *Br. J. Anaesth.*, 1976, *48*, 239.

Uses. Metocurine iodide is a non-depolarising muscle relaxant with actions and uses similar to those of tubocurarine chloride (see p.999) but is between 2 and 3 times as potent. It has a longer duration of action, muscle relaxation being maintained for 25 to 90 minutes following a single dose.

The initial dose of metocurine iodide is usually 1.5 to 8 mg by intravenous injection over 1 minute, and further doses of 0.5 to 1 mg may be given as required.

In 15 patients undergoing surgery a dose of metocurine 300 µg per kg body-weight was necessary for consistent and adequate surgical relaxation. The effect was prolonged, more than 3 hours being needed for 50% recovery. Heart-rate and blood pressure were unchanged.— R. Hughes *et al.*, *Br. J. Anaesth.*, 1976, *48*, 969.

Metocurine had less effect on the myocardial tension-time index than pancuronium and was considered to be especially useful in patients with reduced cardiac reserve in whom increases in heart-rate and in blood pressure should be avoided.— J. W. Basta and M. Lightiger, *Anesthesiology*, 1977, *46*, 366.

The clinical pharmacology of metocurine.— J. J. Savarese *et al.*, *Anesthesiology*, 1977, *47*, 277.

Preparations

Metocurine Iodide Injection *(U.S.P.).* A sterile solution of metocurine iodide in iso-osmotic sodium chloride solution. Phenol 0.5%, or some other suitable bacteriostatic substance, is added to the injection in multidose containers.

Proprietary Names

Metubine Iodide *(Lilly, Canad.; Lilly, USA).*

5727-n

Pancuronium Bromide *(B.P.)*. Poncuronium Bromide; NA-97. 1,1′-(3α,17β-Diacetoxy-5α-androstan-2β,16β-ylene)bis(1-methylpiperidinium) dibromide.

$C_{35}H_{60}Br_2N_2O_4$=732.7.

CAS — 15500-66-0.

Pharmacopoeias. In *Br.*

White or almost white, odourless, hygroscopic crystals or crystalline powder with a bitter taste. It contains 5 to 8% of water. M.p. 215° with decomposition. **Soluble** 1 in 1 of water, 1 in 5 of alcohol and chloroform, 1 in 4 of dichloromethane, and 1 in 1 of methyl alcohol; practically insoluble in ether. A solution in water is dextrorotatory. Solutions are **sterilised** by filtration. **Store** at 2° to 8° in airtight containers.

Pancuronium bromide injection did not produce a visible precipitate when mixed in a syringe with thiopentone, methohexitone, propanidid, suxamethonium, pethidine, papaveretum, neostigmine, gallamine, tubocurarine, alcuronium, hydrocortisone, or promethazine.— D. Komesaroff and J. E. Field, *Med. J. Aust.*, 1969, *1*, 908.

Adverse Effects. As for Tubocurarine Chloride, p.999.

Pancuronium has relatively little cardiovascular activity although tachycardia has been reported. It has smaller histamine-releasing effect than tubocurarine chloride.

Following administration of pancuronium bromide 100 or 150 µg per kg body-weight intravenously to 100 infants, side-effects included excessive oral, pharyngeal, and tracheal secretions within 2 minutes of administration, and severe sweating in some patients.— E. J. Bennett *et al.*, *Anesth. Analg. curr. Res.*, 1971, *50*, 798.

Apnoea. Neuromuscular blockade persisted for about 4 hours after injection of pancuronium 6 mg followed by two 1-mg doses. Neostigmine and atropine failed to reverse the blockade. The patient was young and healthy.— M. A. Belafsky and H. L. Klawans, *Anesthesiology*, 1974, *40*, 295.

Bronchospasm. Symptoms of bronchospasm, probably due to histamine release, were associated with pancuronium in a patient undergoing anaesthesia for diagnostic procedures.— R. W. Buckland and A. F. Avery, *Br. J. Anaesth.*, 1973, *45*, 518. See also D. G. Tweedie and P. M. Ordish (letter), *ibid.*, 1974, *46*, 244.

Bronchospasm, pulmonary oedema, hypotension, cyanosis, and hypoxaemia occurred in a 57-year-old man given thiopentone and pancuronium bromide and recurred after a second injection of pancuronium several hours later. He had received pancuronium 6 weeks previously and a skin test was positive.— F. S. Brauer and C. R. Ananthanarayan, *Anesthesiology*, 1978, *49*, 434.

Cardiovascular effects. Following administration of pancuronium 40 µg per kg body-weight to 11 lightly anaesthetised individuals moderate elevation of pulse-rate was the only significant circulatory change.— F. F. Foldes *et al.*, *Anesthesiology*, 1971, *35*, 496, per *J. Am. med. Ass.*, 1972, *219*, 239.

Pancuronium bromide 4 mg increased the heart-rate in a 7-year-old boy with status asthmaticus and respiratory failure. Doses of 2 mg were required hourly for 19 hours followed by 1 mg, but the patient recovered without complication after 55 hours of controlled respiration.— L. R. Beam (letter), *J. Am. med. Ass.*, 1973, *223*, 1044. A similar report.— F. K. Orkin and J. R. P. Pegg (letter), *ibid.*, *224*, 630. The doses of pancuronium bromide which caused tachycardia were unnecessarily large for the production of muscular relaxation.— F. F. Foldes (letter), *ibid.*, *225*, 418.

Hypertension and tachycardia occurred in a patient with coronary artery disease given pancuronium bromide after induction of anaesthesia with morphine and nitrous oxide.— E. Grossman and A. M. Jacobi, *Anesthesiology*, 1974, *40*, 299.

Severe hypertension and tachycardia in a patient, with a history of obstructive lung disease, mild hypertension, and steroid-dependent asthma, given pancuronium. The effect was prevented by the prior administration of diazepam.— D. S. Fraley *et al.*, *Anesth. Analg. curr. Res.*, 1978, *57*, 265.

Pancuronium 20 to 80 µg per kg body-weight induced tachycardia in patients receiving balanced anaesthesia. Tachycardia was more pronounced when droperidol was also given.— P. Parmentier and P. Dagnelie, *Br. J. Anaesth.*, 1979, *51*, 157.

Further references: R. D. Miller *et al.*, *Anesthesiology*, 1975, *42*, 352, per *Int. pharm. Abstr.*, 1977, *14*, 491.

Hyperpyrexia. Pancuronium bromide caused muscular rigidity with hyperthermia within 40 to 60 seconds in 2 *pigs* who were also receiving halothane, nitrous oxide, and oxygen anaesthesia.— L. J. Chalstrey and G. B. Edwards, *Br. J. Anaesth.*, 1972, *44*, 91.

Treatment of Adverse Effects. As for Tubocurarine Chloride, p.999.

The use of haemodialysis to reverse pancuronium-induced muscular blockade unresponsive to edrophonium.— R. E. Abrams and T. F. Hornbein, *Anesthesiology*, 1975, *42*, 362, per *Int. pharm. Abstr.*, 1977, *14*, 469.

For the use of pyridostigmine bromide to reverse neuromuscular blockade induced by pancuronium bromide, see Pyridostigmine Bromide, p.1046.

Precautions. As for Tubocurarine Chloride, p.999.

There was a complete absence of cardiovascular side-effects when pancuronium bromide was used with halothane in 6 patients.— W. L. M. Baird and A. M. Reid, *Br. J. Anaesth.*, 1967, *39*, 775.

Three patients with liver dysfunction were resistant to pancuronium but several other patients responded normally.— W. L. M. Baird, *Proc. R. Soc. Med.*, 1970, *63*, 697.

Interactions. In 54 healthy patients undergoing minor surgery the frequency of bradycardia during antagonism of neuromuscular blockade with neostigmine was greater in patients given pancuronium than in those who had received alcuronium. There was no significant difference in patients given tubocurarine or pancuronium.— J. Heinonen and O. Takkunen, *Br. J. Anaesth.*, 1977, *49*, 1109.

While tubocurarine antagonised the onset and duration of suxamethonium block, pancuronium antagonised its onset but prolonged its duration.— A. D. Ivankovich *et al.*, *Can. Anaesth. Soc. J.*, 1977, *24*, 228.

Ventricular tachycardia occurred in 2 patients given pancuronium bromide while taking tricyclic anti-depressants. The effect was reproduced experimentally in 4 of 10 dogs.— M. F. Roizen and T. W. Feeley, *Ann. intern. Med.*, 1978, *88*, 64.

Diminished effect. Partial recovery from neuromuscular blockade after corticosteroids.— E. F. Meyers, *Anesthesiology*, 1977, *46*, 148; M. J. Laflin, *Anesthesiology*, 1977, *47*, 471.

Enhanced effect. Possible enhancement of pancuronium by thiotepa.— E. J. Bennett *et al.*, *Anesthesiology*, 1977, *46*, 220, per *Int. pharm. Abstr.*, 1977, *14*, 940.

Prolonged neuromuscular blockade had been reported in a patient given pancuronium bromide while taking lithium carbonate, and had been confirmed in *dogs*.— J. W. Jefferson (letter), *Ann. intern. Med.*, 1978, *88*, 577.

Potentiation of the effect of pancuronium by gentamicin sulphate in 1 patient.— *Med. J. Aust.*, 1979, *2*, 608.

Pregnancy and the neonate. Following administration of pancuronium 40 µg per kg body-weight to induce paralysis, 4 infants developed an alarming fall in transcutaneous oxygen tension, although ventilatory support had been adequate beforehand. Patients undergoing paralysis to improve oxygenation might experience significant and potentially injurious hypoxaemia.— J. B. Philips *et al.* (letter), *Lancet*, 1979, *1*, 877.

Absorption and Fate. Following intravenous injection pancuronium rapidly disappears from the blood. Small amounts cross the placenta.

The pharmacokinetics of pancuronium were studied in 9 patients who underwent surgery for total biliary obstruction. Plasma clearance was significantly reduced to less than half that in normal patients and the mean terminal plasma half-life of about 270 minutes was double the normal value. These changes were associated with prolonged neuromuscular blockade and could result in overdosage. Urinary excretion appeared to be unaffected by biliary obstruction. A mean of 40.6% of the dose was excreted unchanged in 24 hours with means of 9.6% excreted as the two monoacetyl metabolites and 2.1% as the dihydroxy metabolite.— A. A. Somogyi *et al.*, *Br. J. Anaesth.*, 1977, *49*, 1103.

The clinical pharmacokinetics of pancuronium bromide.— L. B. Wingard and D. R. Cook, *Clin. Pharmacokinet.*, 1977, *2*, 330.

A pharmacodynamic model for pancuronium.— C. J. Hull *et al.*, *Br. J. Anaesth.*, 1978, *50*, 1113.

Pregnancy and the neonate. The presence of pancuronium in the urine produced during the first 24 hours of life by 11 out of 20 male infants delivered by caesarean section from mothers who had received pancuronium showed that the drug could be transferred through the placenta within 5 minutes of administration. None of the infants showed evidence of neuromuscular blockade.— I. Speirs and A. W. Sim, *Br. J. Anaesth.*, 1972, *44*, 370.

In 15 patients undergoing caesarean section given pancuronium bromide 100 µg per kg body-weight intravenously with other agents, mean maternal arterial and umbilical venous serum concentrations of pancuronium bromide and metabolites were 520 and 120 ng per ml respectively at delivery (mean of 13 minutes after injection).— L. B. Wingard, *J. pharm. Sci.*, 1979, *68*, 914.

Further references: G. A. H. Heaney, *Br. J. Anaesth.*, 1974, *46*, 282; P. N. Booth *et al.*, *Anaesthesia*, 1977, *32*, 320; E. Abouleish *et al.*, *Br. J. Anaesth.*, 1980, *52*, 531.

Uses. Pancuronium bromide is a non-depolarising muscle relaxant with effects similar to those of tubocurarine chloride (p.999). Muscle relaxation commences within about 1 to 3 minutes of administration and lasts for about 45 minutes.

Pancuronium bromide is used mainly as an adjuvant to anaesthesia to obtain greater muscular relaxation in surgical operations. The initial dose is usually 40 to 100 µg per kg body-weight by intravenous injection, with supplementary doses of 10 to 40 µg per kg. Children may be given up to 80 µg per kg initially with supplementary doses of 10 to 20 µg per kg, and newborn infants 30 to 40 µg per kg initially with supplementary doses of up to 20 µg per kg. Patients under intensive care including those with intractable status asthmaticus or tetanus may be given 60 µg per kg intravenously every 1 to 1½ hours or 30 to 60 µg per kg intramuscularly every 1 to 2 hours.

Reviews of pancuronium bromide: T. M. Speight and G. S. Avery, *Drugs*, 1972, *4*, 163; M. F. Roizen and T. W. Feeley, *Ann. intern. Med.*, 1978, *88*, 64.

A study *in vitro* of serum from 14 subjects, aged 4 to 60 years, with normal reactions to suxamethonium demonstrated that pancuronium caused a powerful and highly selective inhibition of serum cholinesterase. The inhibition was reversible and competitive. Serum-cholinesterase activity decreased by about 60% three minutes after injection of pancuronium 100 µg per kg body-weight in 4 subjects. There was still a 40% depression 45 minutes after injection.— J. Stovner *et al.*, *Br. J. Anaesth.*, 1975, *47*, 949.

The peak neuromuscular blocking effect from pancuronium 50, 80, and 100 µg per kg body-weight given intravenously in a study of 9 patients occurred at 7, 2.5, and 2 minutes and lasted for 20, 40, and 60 minutes respectively. There was a correlation between serum-pancuronium concentrations and neuromuscular blockade.— S. Agoston *et al.*, *Anesthesiology*, 1977, *47*, 509.

Administration. An intravenous bolus injection and concomitant infusion of pancuronium was proposed for use in prolonged anaesthesia. Doses were calculated using pharmacokinetic principles to achieve a plasma concentration of 200 ng per ml which it was considered would provide adequate relaxation. Pancuronium, at an initial intravenous bolus dose of about 62.5 µg per kg body-weight was given to 16 surgical patients with constant infusion at about 350 ng per kg per minute as a solution containing 5 mg in 100 ml of sodium chloride injection. The regimen generally produced and maintained a predictable plasma concentration of pancuronium but monitoring of neuromuscular transmission was necessary to detect the excessive or inadequate dosage which might occur in some patients.— A. A. Somogyi *et al.*, *Br. J. Anaesth.*, 1978, *50*, 575.

In the elderly. Following an investigation in 75 elderly patients pancuronium bromide was considered to be a desirable drug for use in poor risk, elderly patients.— P. H. Lorhan and M. Lippmann, *Anesth. Analg. curr. Res.*, 1972, *51*, 914, per *Int. pharm. Abstr.*, 1974, *11*, 224. See also K. McLeod *et al.*, *Br. J. Anaesth.*, 1979, *51*, 435.

In liver disease. A study in 32 patients with chronic liver disease who underwent surgery concluded that pancuronium bromide could be substituted safely for tubocurarine. All patients exhibited pancuronium 'resistance' and required a mean total dose of 14.9 mg. Reversal effect was difficult in 2 patients with severe obstructive jaundice.— M. E. Ward *et al.*, *Br. J. Anaesth.*, 1975, *47*, 1199.

Serum and urinary concentrations of pancuronium were compared in 14 patients with cirrhosis of the liver and

12 patients without liver disease, all of whom underwent abdominal surgery and were given single doses of pancuronium ranging from 100 to 250 µg per kg body-weight. Mean distribution and elimination half-lives of about 24 and 208 minutes respectively in patients with cirrhosis were significantly prolonged when compared with values of 11 and 114 minutes respectively in the normal group. Elimination-rate constant and plasma clearance were decreased and distribution volume increased in the cirrhotic patients. There was a small increase in urinary excretion of pancuronium and its metabolites in the first 24 hours in patients with cirrhosis but not during the first 12 hours. Small amounts (about 5% of the dose) of the 3-hydroxy metabolite were present in only 3 of 11 cirrhotic patients. A prolonged duration of action of pancuronium could be expected in patients with cirrhosis of the liver and the increased distribution volume in these patients might necessitate a higher initial dose although the rate of disappearance of pancuronium from plasma would be slower than in patients without liver disease.— P. Duvaldestin *et al.*, *Br. J. Anaesth.*, 1978, *50*, 1131.

In renal failure. Pancuronium was a satisfactory muscle relaxant for 5 patients suffering from renal insufficiency.— S. Kamvyssi-Dea *et al.*, *Br. J. Anaesth.*, 1972, *44*, 1217.

Mean plasma-pancuronium concentrations 5 minutes after a dose of 4 mg were 600 and 460 ng per ml respectively in 6 patients with normal renal function and 7 patients with severe renal failure; after 4 hours the values were 67 and 180 ng per ml.— K. McLeod *et al.*, *Br. J. Anaesth.*, 1976, *48*, 341. See also W. Buzello and J. Ruthven-Murray, *Anaesthetist*, 1976, *25*, 440.

Studies in 10 anephric patients indicated that the plasma clearance of pancuronium was significantly reduced and the plasma half-life was increased, leading to prolonged neuromuscular blockade and slower rate of recovery.— A. A. Somogyi *et al.*, *Eur. J. clin. Pharmac.*, 1977, *12*, 23.

Pancuronium could be given in usual doses to patients with a glomerular filtration-rate (GFR) above 10 ml per minute; its use should be avoided in those with a GFR of less than 10 ml per minute; recurarisation might occur up to 24 hours after surgery and active metabolites may accumulate in end-stage renal disease.— W. M. Bennett *et al.*, *Ann. intern. Med.*, 1980, *93*, 286.

With suxamethonium. Pretreatment with pancuronium was less satisfactory than gallamine for preventing muscle fasciculations due to suxamethonium.— D. J. Cullen, *Anesthesiology*, 1971, *35*, 572. See also E. J. Bennett *et al.*, *Anesth. Analg. curr. Res.*, 1973, *52*, 892, per *J. Am. med. Ass.*, 1974, *227*, 813.

Pancuronium 500 µg per 70 kg body-weight was as effective as tubocurarine 3 mg per 70 kg in preventing gross fasciculations after suxamethonium, but was less effective in controlling fine fasciculations.— A. M. Domaoal *et al.*, *Anesth. Analg. curr. Res.*, 1975, *54*, 71, per *J. Am. med. Ass.*, 1975, *232*, 1412.

Asthma. Pancuronium bromide was a useful neuromuscular blocking agent in the treatment of medically irreversible status asthmaticus.— N. Levin and J. B. Dillon, *J. Am. med. Ass.*, 1972, *222*, 1265.

Hyperpyrexia. Halothane-induced contracture of muscle strips from patients susceptible to malignant hyperpyrexia was inhibited by methylprednisolone and pancuronium in concentrations equivalent to doses of 495 and 990 mg and 6 and 12 mg respectively. It was considered that pancuronium could be used cautiously in susceptible patients.— P. A. Cain and F. R. Ellis, *Br. J. Anaesth.*, 1977, *49*, 941. But see under Adverse Effects.

Pregnancy and the neonate. No evidence of adverse foetal effects was seen in a comparison of tubocurarine and pancuronium in patients undergoing caesarean section. Although no clear superiority of pancuronium over tubocurarine was demonstrated, blood pressure was better maintained in the pancuronium group.— J. B. Neeld *et al.*, *Anesth. Analg. curr. Res.*, 1974, *53*, 7, per *J. Am. med. Ass.*, 1974, *228*, 412.

Pancuronium bromide was a safe and well-tolerated muscle relaxant for anaesthesia in 25 neonates. It was 9 times as potent as tubocurarine at birth and 6 times as potent at 1 month old. Recommended intravenous doses of pancuronium were 30 µg per kg body-weight up to 1 week old, 60 µg per kg at 1 to 2 weeks, and 90 µg per kg at 2 to 4 weeks. Doses were reduced in prematurity, acidosis, hypothermia, and during antibiotic therapy, especially with kanamycin and gentamicin, when increased sensitivity was observed. Neuromuscular block was reversed with atropine 18 µg per kg body-weight and neostigmine 80 µg per kg intravenously.— E. J. Bennett *et al.*, *Br. J. Anaesth.*, 1975, *47*, 75.

Respiratory distress syndrome. The use of pancuronium to facilitate assisted respiration in 6 adults with respiratory distress syndrome.— R. W. Light *et al.*, *Anesth. Analg. curr. Res.*, 1975, *54*, 219, per *J. Am. med. Ass.*, 1975, *233*, 473.

The use of pancuronium bromide in infants with the respiratory distress syndrome.— M. J. Pollitzer *et al.*, *Lancet*, 1981, *1*, 346.

Preparations

Pancuronium Injection *(B.P.)*. A sterile solution of pancuronium bromide in sodium chloride injection; it contains a suitable stabilising agent and may contain an antimicrobial preservative. Sterilised by filtration. pH 3.8 to 4.2. Store at 2° to 8°, when it may be expected to retain its potency for not less than 2 years.

Pavulon *(Organon Teknika, UK)*. Pancuronium bromide, available as an injection containing 2 mg per ml, in ampoules of 2 ml, with sodium chloride, an acetate buffer, and benzyl alcohol 1%. (Also available as Pavulon in *Arg., Austral., Canad., Denm., Fr., Ital., Neth., Norw., S.Afr., Spain, Switz., USA*).

5728-h

Pridinol Hydrochloride. 1,1-Diphenyl-3-piperidinopropan-1-ol hydrochloride.
$C_{20}H_{25}NO,HCl=331.9$.

CAS — 511-45-5 (pridinol); 968-58-1 (hydrochloride).

Pridinol hydrochloride is used in the treatment of parkinsonism in a dose of 5 to 15 mg daily.

Proprietary Names
Parks 12 *(Hommel, Ger.; Hommel, Switz.)*.

5729-m

Pridinol Mesylate. 1,1-Diphenyl-3-piperidinopropan-1-ol methanesulphonate.
$C_{20}H_{25}NO,CH_3SO_3H=391.5$.

Pridinol mesylate is a muscle relaxant used in the symptomatic treatment of muscle spasm in doses of 2 to 8 mg thrice daily. It has also been given intramuscularly.

Proprietary Names
Lyseen *(Exa, Arg.; Hommel, Belg.; Hommel, Ger.; Bonomelli-Hommel, Ital.)*; Hikicenon, Loxeen, Mitanoline, Nonpressin, Tirashizin, Trilax *(all Jap.)*.

5730-t

Styramate. β-Hydroxyphenethyl carbamate.
$C_9H_{11}NO_3=181.2$.

CAS — 94-35-9.

An odourless crystalline powder. M.p. 108° to 110°. Sparingly **soluble** in water; soluble in alcohol, chloroform, and ether.

Adverse Effects. Gastric disturbances, drowsiness, dizziness, headache, and urticaria may occasionally occur.

Uses. Styramate is a centrally acting muscle relaxant with actions similar to those of mephenesin (see p.992). The usual dose is 200 to 400 mg four times daily.

Proprietary Names
Sinaxar *(Fawns & McAllan, Austral.; Christiaens, Belg.; Armour, Denm.; Armour, S.Afr.)*.

Styramate was formerly marketed in Great Britain under the proprietary name Sinaxar (*Armour*).

5731-x

Suxamethonium Bromide *(B.P.)*.

Suxameth. Brom.; Choline Bromide Succinate; Succinylcholine Bromide. 2,2′-Succinyldioxybis(ethyltrimethylammonium) dibromide dihydrate.
$C_{14}H_{30}Br_2N_2O_4,2H_2O=486.2$.

CAS — 306-40-1 (suxamethonium); 55-94-7 (bromide).

Pharmacopoeias. In *Br.*

A white or creamy-white almost odourless powder with a slightly saline taste. M.p. about 225°. Suxamethonium 1 mg (1 mg cation) is equivalent to 1.67 mg of suxamethonium bromide dihydrate and to 1.55 mg of anhydrous suxamethonium bromide.

Soluble 1 in 0.3 of water and 1 in 5 of alcohol; practically insoluble in chloroform and ether. A 1% solution in water has a pH of 4 to 5. Solutions deteriorate on storage and should be used immediately after preparation. It is rapidly hydrolysed by alkalis and therefore should not be mixed with thiopentone sodium. **Protect** from light.

Uses. Suxamethonium bromide has the same actions and is used for the same purposes as suxamethonium chloride and is administered by intravenous injection in similar doses of the cation.

Preparations

Suxamethonium Bromide Injection *(B.P.)*. Succinylcholine Bromide Injection. A sterile solution of suxamethonium bromide in Water for Injections, prepared by dissolving, immediately before use, the sterile contents of a sealed container (Suxamethonium Bromide for Injection) in the requisite amount of Water for Injections.

Brevidil M *(May & Baker, UK)*. Suxamethonium bromide, available as powder for preparing injections in ampoules of 67 mg (equivalent to 40 mg cation). (Also available as Brevidil M in *Austral., S.Afr.*).

5732-r

Suxamethonium Chloride *(B.P., Eur. P.)*.

Suxameth. Chlor.; Choline Chloride Succinate; Suxamethonii Chloridum; Succinylcholine Chloride *(U.S.P.)*; Succicurarium Chloride; Suxametonklorid. 2,2′-Succinyldioxybis(ethyltrimethylammonium) dichloride dihydrate.
$C_{14}H_{30}Cl_2N_2O_4,2H_2O=397.3$.

CAS — 71-27-2 (anhydrous); 6101-15-1 (dihydrate).

Pharmacopoeias. In *Aust., Br., Braz., Chin., Eur., Fr., Ger., Int., It., Jap., Jug., Neth., Nord., Pol., Roum., Swiss, Turk.,* and *U.S. Braz.* has the dihydrate or anhydrous salt; *Arg.* has the anhydrous salt.

A white or almost white, odourless or almost odourless, hygroscopic, crystalline powder with a saline taste. M.p. about 160°. Suxamethonium 1 mg (1 mg cation) is equivalent to 1.37 mg of suxamethonium chloride dihydrate and to 1.24 mg of anhydrous suxamethonium chloride.

Soluble 1 in 1 of water and 1 in 350 of alcohol; soluble in methyl alcohol and glacial acetic acid; very slightly soluble in acetic anhydride; practically insoluble in chloroform and ether. A 0.5% solution in water has a pH of 4 to 5. A 4.48% solution is iso-osmotic with serum. Solutions are **sterilised** by maintaining at 98° to 100° for 30 minutes with a bactericide or by filtration. It is rapidly destroyed by alkalis and therefore should not be mixed with thiopentone sodium. **Store** in airtight containers. Protect from light.

An aqueous solution of suxamethonium chloride iso-osmotic with serum (4.48%) caused 85% haemolysis of erythrocytes cultured in it for 45 minutes. The erythrocytes turned black.— E. R. Hammarlund and K. Pedersen-Bjergaard, *J. pharm. Sci.*, 1961, *50*, 24.

Storage. A solution of suxamethonium chloride 0.1 or 0.2% in dextrose injection or sodium chloride injection was stable for 1 week at 25° or for 4 weeks at 5°.— B. E. Kirschenbaum and C. J. Latiolais, *Am. J. Hosp. Pharm.*, 1976, *33*, 767.

Adverse Effects. Prolonged apnoea occurs in patients with low serum concentrations of pseudocholinesterase and in those with an atypical pseudocholinesterase. It has also been reported after high or repeated doses when a dual block (see p.986) has occurred. The administration of suxamethonium may be followed by bradycardia, often associated with cardiac arrhythmia; cardiac arrest has been reported. Sinus tachycardia and a rise in blood pressure has occurred after the continuous infusion of suxamethonium.

Malignant hyperpyrexia is a rare, often fatal, complication in patients anaesthetised with general anaesthetic agents and has been increasingly associated with concomitant administration of suxamethonium; it occurs in apparently healthy individuals genetically predisposed to this syndrome. The symptoms are increasing hyperthermia, muscular hypertonicity, with or without rigidity, acidosis, hyperkalaemia, and myoglobinuria. Ominous late developments include left heart failure, haemolysis, and signs of decerebration. Disseminated intravascular coagulation has been reported.

Hypersensitivity reactions to suxamethonium have been reported and bronchospasm has occasionally occurred.

Muscular pain similar to that following strenuous exercise may occur in the immediate postoperative period, particularly in patients who are ambulant in the early postoperative period but it is not related to dosage or the degree of fasciculation.

Myoglobinuria has been reported, either alone or associated with malignant hyperpyrexia.

Suxamethonium also causes a transient rise in intra-ocular pressure, and salivary gland enlargement. There may be some increase in bowel movements and in gastric and salivary secretions due to the muscarinic action of suxamethonium.

In a 49-year-old man, massive bilateral enlargement of the parotid, submaxillary, and sublingual salivary glands, with profuse production of watery saliva, occurred 5 minutes after intubation during anaesthesia which included an infusion of suxamethonium chloride. While the effect could not specifically be attributed to suxamethonium chloride, 6 similar cases had been reported.— L. I. Bonchek, *J. Am. med. Ass.*, 1969, *209*, 1716.

In a study in 36 adult males undergoing elective surgery, suxamethonium was administered intravenously at 6 rates, from 0.25 mg per second to 20 mg per second. The time to the first muscle fasciculation and the total fasciculation score were related to the rate of infusion, with the slowest rate having the lowest fasciculation score and the longest latency time. Infusion rates below 2 mg per second appear to offer a clinical method of reducing fasciculations and might diminish some of the deleterious sequelae of the administration of suxamethonium.— A. Feingold and J. L. Velazquez, *Br. J. Anaesth.*, 1979, *51*, 241.

Evidence to suggest that administration of suxamethonium in divided doses reduces muscle fasciculation but does not reduce postoperative muscle pain.— D. B. Wilson and J. W. Dundee, *Anesthesiology*, 1980, *52*, 273.

Allergy. Reports of allergy and hypersensitivity.— G. Jerums *et al.*, *Br. J. Anaesth.*, 1967, *39*, 73; A. M. Katz and P. G. Mulligan, *Br. J. Anaesth.*, 1972, *44*, 1097; J. M. Mandappa *et al.*, *Br. J. Anaesth.*, 1975, *47*, 523; M. Fisher (letter), *Br. J. Anaesth.*, 1977, *49*, 87; M. D. Matthews *et al.*, *Anaesth. & intensive Care*, 1977, *5*, 235; D. Royston and R. G. Wilkes, *Br. J. Anaesth.*, 1978, *50*, 611.

Apnoea. Reports and discussions of apnoea.— H. Lehmann and P. H. Simmons, *Lancet*, 1958, *2*, 981; H. M. Rubenstein *et al.*, *New Engl. J. Med.*, 1960, *262*, 1107; A. R. Hunter, *Anaesthesia*, 1966, *21*, 325 and 337; G. Pohlmann, *J. Am. med. Ass.*, 1966, *196*, 181; J. Horne *et al.*, *Anesthesiology*, 1973, *39*, 545; *Lancet*, 1973, *2*, 246; H. W. Bauld *et al.*, *Br. J. Anaesth.*, 1974, *46*, 273; C. S. Chan *et al.*, *Anaesth. & intensive Care*, 1977, *5*, 260; J. Viby-Mogensen and H. K. Hanel, *Acta Anaesth. scand.*, 1978, *22*, 371.

Cardiac arrhythmias. Of 96 fasting unpremedicated patients undergoing elective cardiac surgery who received suxamethonium 1 mg per kg body-weight intravenously, 73 showed ventricular arrhythmias.— W. F. M. List, *Anesth. Analg. curr. Res.*, 1971, *50*, 361, per *Int. pharm. Abstr.*, 1972, *9*, 545. Ventricular arrhythmia in 4 patients with polyneuropathy when they were given suxamethonium.— R. J. Fergusson *et al.*, *Br. med. J.*, 1981, *282*, 298.

Asystole in 2 patients given suxamethonium (with prior tubocurarine) and mention of 15 earlier cases.— C. H. McLeskey *et al.*, *Anesthesiology*, 1978, *49*, 208. See also A. L. Greenfield and H. Rosenberg, *ibid.*, 1980, *52*, 378.

Hyperkalaemia. In 6 patients, 2 of whom died, intravenous injection of suxamethonium was followed by circulatory arrest and/or severe hyperkalaemia. Increases in serum-potassium concentrations of up to 3.6 mmol per litre occurred within a few minutes of injection. Three of the patients had severe tetanus and 2 had uraemia. It was suggested that uraemia, with increased serum-potassium concentrations, and tetanus were contra-indications for the use of suxamethonium.— F. Roth and H. Wüthrich, *Br. J. Anaesth.*, 1969, *41*, 311.

The administration of suxamethonium to patients with burns, neurological disorders, muscular disease, tetanus, or massive trauma could produce acute hyperkalaemia resulting in serious or fatal cardiac arrhythmias.— H. Desmeules, *Can. med. Ass. J.*, 1973, *108*, 1527.

The effect of different anaesthetics on suxamethonium-induced hyperkalaemia was studied in 101 patients. Maximum increases in serum-potassium concentrations were: trichloroethylene 21.4%, chloroform 17.2%, halothane 15.1%, thiopentone 19.7%, and nitrous oxide controls 4.4%. Ten patients given tubocurarine 3 mg before induction with thiopentone and suxamethonium had a reduced maximum increase in serum potassium of 10.6%. It was concluded that hyperkalaemia was a combined effect of suxamethonium and the anaesthetic used.— V. J. Dhanaraj *et al.*, *Br. J. Anaesth.*, 1975, *47*, 516.

Evidence that muscle damage was the cause of increased plasma-potassium concentrations following administration of suxamethonium.— J. W. Dundee and I. M. Bali, *Br. J. clin. Pharmac.*, 1975, *2*, 376P.

Fifty-four patients undergoing surgery and 21 patients with chronic renal disease were given suxamethonium or suxethonium. Plasma-potassium concentrations rose in those given suxamethonium but not in those given suxethonium.— S. Day, *Br. J. Anaesth.*, 1976, *48*, 1011.

Further references: H. D. Weintraub *et al.*, *Br. J. Anaesth.*, 1969, *41*, 1048; A. A. Birch *et al.*, *J. Am. med. Ass.*, 1969, *210*, 490; *ibid.*, 549; L. H. Cooperman, *ibid.*, 1970, *213*, 1867; D. B. Cowgill *et al.*, *Anesthesiology*, 1974, *40*, 409.

Hyperpyrexia. A 13-year-old girl developed a fatal muscular rigidity with hyperthermia 50 minutes after receiving thiopentone, tubocurarine, and suxamethonium followed by anaesthesia with nitrous oxide, oxygen, and methoxyflurane.— D. G. Larard *et al.*, *Br. J. Anaesth.*, 1972, *44*, 93.

In 79 children undergoing ophthalmic operations who were given one of 5 anaesthetic sequences, it was found that significant increases in the serum-creatine phosphokinase concentration occurred among children who had received suxamethonium. Elevated concentrations of creatine phosphokinase had been reported in association with malignant hyperpyrexia.— R. K. R. Innes and J. H. Strømme, *Br. J. Anaesth.*, 1973, *45*, 185..

Metabolic, haemodynamic, and neuro-endocrine responses to suxamethonium in normal *pigs*, and in *pigs* susceptible to malignant hyperpyrexia.— G. A. Gronert and R. A. Theye, *Br. J. Anaesth.*, 1976, *48*, 513.

Further references: I. E. Purkis *et al.*, *Can. Anaesth. Soc. J.*, 1967, *14*, 183; M. A. Denborough *et al.*, *Lancet*, 1970, *1*, 1137; W. Kalow, *Fedn Proc.*, 1972, *31*, 1270; B. Peltz and J. Carstens, *Anaesthesia*, 1975, *30*, 346; M. A. Denborough, *Med. J. Aust.*, 1977, *2*, 757; D. E. Lees *et al.*, *Anesth. Analg. curr. Res.*, 1980, *59*, 514.

For a report of suxamethonium and atropine being associated with a high incidence of rigidity in patients who developed malignant hyperthermia, see Atropine, p.290.

Hypertonicity. Spasm of the masseter muscles preventing intubation and increased serum-creatine phosphokinase concentrations were attributed to suxamethonium in a 25-year-old woman being anaesthetised for tubal ligation.— P. K. Barnes, *Br. J. Anaesth.*, 1973, *45*, 759. See also D. D. Davies (letter), *ibid.*, 1970, *42*, 656; N. G. Caseby, *ibid.*, 1975, *47*, 1101.

Intra-ocular pressure. When suxamethonium chloride was used to facilitate endotracheal intubation prior to surgery, a transient rise in intra-ocular pressure was observed within 1 minute of injection in 20 of 29 patients. The raised pressure fell to or below pre-anaesthetic levels in all patients, including 10 with glaucoma, before surgery.— T. H. Taylor *et al.*, *Br. J. Anaesth.*, 1968, *40*, 113. See also K. Pandey *et al.*, *ibid.*, 1972, *44*, 191.

Failure of pancuronium to inhibit suxamethonium-induced increase in intra-ocular pressure.— D. J. Bowen *et al.*, *Br. J. Anaesth.*, 1976, *48*, 1201. Failure of non-depolarising muscle relaxants to inhibit suxamethonium-induced increase in intra-ocular pressure.— E. F. Myers *et al.*, *Anesthesiology*, 1978, *48*, 149.

Myoglobinuria. Two definite and 5 probable instances of myoglobinuria occurred in 24 ophthalmic patients who received repeated doses of suxamethonium during halothane anaesthesia.— M. M. Airaksinen and T. Tammisto, *Clin. Pharmac. Ther.*, 1966, *7*, 583. See also K. Jensen *et al.*, *Br. J. Anaesth.*, 1968, *40*, 329; C. A. B. McLaren, *ibid.*, 901.

Massive myoglobinuria precipitated by halothane and suxamethonium in a member of a family with elevation of serum creatine phosphokinase.— W. E. Moore *et al.*, *Anesth. Analg. curr. Res.*, 1976, *55*, 680.

A report of acute rhabdomyolysis, without pyrexia, associated with intra-operative cardiac arrest precipitated by suxamethonium and halothane.— H. Schaer *et al.*, *Br. J. Anaesth.*, 1977, *49*, 495.

Rhabdomyolysis associated with suxamethonium in a patient with Duchenne muscular dystrophy.— E. D. Miller *et al.*, *Anesthesiology*, 1978, *48*, 146, per *Int. pharm. Abstr.*, 1978, *15*, 408.

Further references: J. M. Gibbs, *Anaesth. & intensive Care*, 1978, *6*, 141.

Postoperative muscle pain. Of 289 patients given suxamethonium for bronchoscopy, 23.6% had muscle pains the following day.— C. A. Foster, *Br. med. J.*, 1960, *2*, 24.

A brief discussion of suxamethonium-induced muscle pain.— J. E. Riding, *Br. J. Anaesth.*, 1975, *47*, 91.

The incidence of postoperative muscle pain, due to suxamethonium, in 100 women undergoing tubal ligation in the lithotomy position was 42% compared with 20% in 50 pregnant women undergoing tubal ligation and first-trimester abortion in the same position; the incidence of intense fasciculation was 68% for the non-pregnant and 28% for the pregnant women.— S. Datta *et al.*, *Br. J. Anaesth.*, 1977, *49*, 625.

Of 52 children given suxamethonium 23 had electromyographic evidence of muscle action potential frequencies in excess of 50 Hz but only 2 of these had suxamethonium-induced pain. The frequency of 50 Hz, associated with pain in adults, was not applicable to children.— J. R. Fozard *et al.*, *Br. J. Anaesth.*, 1977, *49*, 1057.

Pseudocholinesterase (atypical). The occurrence of atypical pseudocholinesterase was estimated to occur unassociated with typical pseudocholinesterase in 1 in 3000 persons and followed a familial pattern.— D. H. Bush, *Br. J. Anaesth.*, 1961, *33*, 454.

Further references: F. M. M. Dewar and G. Wakefield, *Br. J. Anaesth.*, 1976, *48*, 707; D. R. Stanski *et al.*, *Anesthesiology*, 1977, *46*, 298; A. F. Kopman *et al.*, *Anesthesiology*, 1978, *49*, 142.

Tachyphylaxis. It was considered that tachyphylaxis and the change in the nature of the block caused by suxamethonium took place simultaneously and might be part of the same phenomenon.— N. Sugai *et al.*, *Br. J. clin. Pharmac.*, 1975, *2*, 487.

Further references: R. Hughes, *Br. J. Pharmac.*, 1973, *49*, 151P; C. Lee *et al.*, *Br. J. Anaesth.*, 1976, *48*, 91; C. Lee, *Br. J. Anaesth.*, 1976, *48*, 1097; C. Lee *et al.*, *Br. J. Anaesth.*, 1978, *50*, 189; M. J. Spurgeon, *Anesth. Analg. curr. Res.*, 1979, *58*, 57.

Treatment of Adverse Effects. Prolonged apnoea should be treated by assisted respiration with nitrous oxide and oxygen until spontaneous respiration is fully restored. Transfusion of fresh whole blood, frozen plasma, or other source of pseudocholinesterase will help the destruction of the suxamethonium. Neostigmine should not be used.

Sometimes, though not always, when the action of suxamethonium is prolonged, the neuromuscular block ceases to be depolarising in type and acquires some features of the paralysis produced by tubocurarine, i.e. dual block (see p.986). In these cases, assisted respiration should be continued until spontaneous respiration begins to return. A short-acting anticholinesterase such as edrophonium 10 mg may then be given intravenously. If an obvious improvement is maintained for several minutes, neostigmine, 1 to 2 mg, may be given. The immediate use of neostigmine is not advisable owing to the difficulty of determining the nature of the block.

The use of propanidid and lignocaine to reduce muscle fasciculations following the injection of suxamethonium.— E. N. S. Fry, *Br. J. Anaesth.*, 1975, *47*, 723. The technique appeared to depress the increase in serum-potassium concentration seen after the injection of suxamethonium.— *idem*, 1978, *50*, 841.

In a double-blind study in 53 patients undergoing bronchoscopy ascorbic acid 2 g daily for 2.5 days before and after examination had no effect on suxamethonium-induced pain.— J. B. Wood *et al.*, *Anaesthesia*, 1977,

32, 21.

Failure of tubocurarine or gallamine to prevent suxamethonium-induced increase in intra-ocular pressure.— E. F. Meyers *et al.*, *Anesthesiology*, 1978, *48*, 149, per *Int. pharm. Abstr.*, 1978, *15*, 422.

A study indicating that pretreatment with diazepam prevented suxamethonium-induced muscle fasciculations, hyperkalaemia, increased CPK concentrations, increased heart-rate and arterial pressure, and postoperative myalgia.— N. R. Fahmy *et al.*, *Clin. Pharmac. Ther.*, 1979, *26*, 395.

Results suggesting that thiopentone protects against suxamethonium-induced bradycardia during halothane anaesthesia.— J. Viby-Mogensen *et al.*, *Br. J. Anaesth.*, 1980, *52*, 1137.

Apnoea. The administration of about 200 ml of frozen serum was successful in ending apnoea, of 3 hours duration, due to suxamethonium. Fresh-frozen serum was found to have an average serum-pseudocholinesterase content of 120 units per ml, and compared favourably with the 30 units per ml found in whole blood.— J. Levin (letter), *Lancet*, 1966, *1*, 667. The findings of Levin with frozen serum were confirmed. A study had been made of the cholinesterase content of dried plasma which showed it to be within normal limits even after storage for 3 years at room temperature; the use of triple-strength reconstituted dried plasma was therefore considered likely to be equally as effective in apnoea as fresh blood or frozen plasma.— J. Ives *et al.* (letter), *Lancet*, 1966, *1*, 879.

Hyperkalaemia. Elevations of serum-potassium concentrations after the use of suxamethonium were reduced by the administration, 3 minutes earlier, of pancuronium 20 µg per kg body-weight.— H. N. Konchigeri and C. H. Tay, *Anesth. Analg. curr. Res.*, 1976, *55*, 474, per *J. Am. med. Ass.*, 1976, *236*, 2003.

Hyperpyrexia. In *pigs* the hyperthermic response was associated with a fall in the serum free thyroxine index and led to acidosis, pyrexia, rigor, and death. It was relieved by the cautious intravenous injection of successive small doses of liothyronine monitored by changes in temperature and in blood pH and pCO_2. An undue rise in serum free thyroxine index could be reversed by injection of magnesium sulphate or chloride or, if refractory, by the infusion of edetate. Six *pigs* treated with this regimen had survived.— D. Lister, *Br. med. J.*, 1973, *1*, 208.

For the recommended use of dantrolene for protection against malignant hyperpyrexia, see Dantrolene Sodium, p.990.

For the use of procaine in the treatment of malignant hyperpyrexia, see Procaine Hydrochloride, p.922.

Postoperative muscle pain. Frequency and severity of muscle pain developing in patients after injections of suxamethonium given during anaesthesia for bronchoscopy were reduced by an intramuscular dose of 500 to 750 µg of neostigmine given after bronchoscopy or by an intravenous injection of 3 to 5 mg of tubocurarine or 10 to 15 mg of diplacine given prior to the suxamethonium injection.— I. S. Zhorov *et al.*, *Br. J. Anaesth.*, 1967, *39*, 948.

Postoperative muscle pain induced by suxamethonium was significantly reduced in frequency, intensity, and duration by the prior intravenous injection of a single dose of lignocaine. Lignocaine prevented muscle fasciculation and slightly increased the duration of apnoea.— J. E. Usubiaga *et al.*, *Anesth. Analg. curr. Res.*, 1967, *46*, 225, per *Abstr. Wld Med.*, 1968, *42*, 255.

Diazepam 10 mg intravenously, given 5 minutes before suxamethonium, reduced the incidence, severity and duration of suxamethonium-induced muscle pain, compared with control, in a study in 50 patients.— R. S. Verma *et al.*, *Anesth. Analg. curr. Res.*, 1978, *57*, 295.

A view that efforts to reduce the frequency of suxamethonium-induced muscle pains in patients having major abdominal operations are not justified.— J. B. Brodsky and J. Ehrenwerth, *Br. J. Anaesth.*, 1980, *52*, 215.

For reports of the prevention of fasciculation due to suxamethonium, see under Gallamine Triethiodide, p.992, Pancuronium Bromide, p.995, and Tubocurarine Chloride, p.1000.

Precautions. Suxamethonium chloride is contra-indicated in patients who are burnt, exhibiting myotonia and muscular rigidity, or known to have atypical pseudocholinesterase. Suxamethonium chloride is also contra-indicated in patients with penetrating wounds of the eye or while the globe is open, or in massively traumatised patients. Its use is inadvisable in patients with low serum-pseudocholinesterase concentrations such as may occur in liver disease, malnutrition, severe anaemia, and in persons exposed to organophosphorus insecticides or weedkillers. Its use is also inadvisable in patients with advanced myasthenia gravis, neurological defects, or phaeochromocytoma.

It is not generally recommended in uraemic patients especially those with high serum-potassium concentrations. It should be used with caution in patients with cardiac disease. Atropine should be given before administration of suxamethonium chloride to prevent excessive bradycardia, bronchial secretion, or other muscarinic effects.

Administration of suxamethonium before or after the use of a non-depolarising relaxant such as tubocurarine may cause a mixed block (see p.986), but small doses of tubocurarine are sometimes given prior to suxamethonium to reduce muscle fasciculations and hyperkalaemia.

The effects of suxamethonium may be enhanced by some aminoglycoside or polypeptide antibiotics, narcotic analgesics, propanidid, quinidine, and by a decreased body temperature. The depolarising effects of suxamethonium may also be enhanced by neostigmine and other anticholinesterases; it has been recommended that eye-drops containing a long-acting anticholinesterase such as ecothiopate should be discontinued at least 2 weeks before the administration of suxamethonium.

Bradycardia due to suxamethonium may be enhanced by halothane or cyclopropane but diminished or prevented by thiopentone. The effects of digitalis may be enhanced by suxamethonium, leading to cardiac arrhythmias.

Injection of suxamethonium and other depolarising drugs led to an arousal response in the EEG which was accompanied by increases in heart-rate and blood pressure in patients anaesthetised with halothane. Administration of the non-depolarising drugs gallamine or alcuronium blocked any arousal response due to subsequent injection of suxamethonium.— K. Mori *et al.*, *Br. J. Anaesth.*, 1973, *45*, 604. See also N. Sugai *et al.*, *Br. J. clin. Pharmac.*, 1975, *2*, 391.

Plasma-cholinesterase concentrations were significantly reduced in 9 patients who underwent plasmaphaeresis. Suxamethonium should be used with caution in such patients.— G. J. Wood and G. M. Hall, *Br. J. Anaesth.*, 1978, *50*, 945. See also J. Lumley, *ibid.*, 1980, *52*, 1149.

A study in 15 patients undergoing surgery for duodenal ulcer and 14 patients with a normal gastro-intestinal tract concluded that there was no increased tendency to regurgitate during fasciculations induced by suxamethonium. This conclusion was not valid when there was an abnormality such as hiatus hernia in the gastro-oesophageal region.— G. Smith *et al.*, *Br. J. Anaesth.*, 1978, *50*, 1137.

A 56-year-old woman with Crohn's disease had prolonged apnoea following suxamethonium administration. Pseudocholinesterase values in this patient and in 2 others with Crohn's disease were subsequently found to be low. The low concentration of pseudocholinesterase found in Crohn's disease may be due to the disease itself, malnutrition, low serum albumin, or liver involvement. The frequency is not known, but anaesthetists should consider asking for measurement of pseudocholinesterase activity in Crohn's disease patients for whom surgery is planned.— S. N. Khalil *et al.* (letter), *Lancet*, 1980, *2*, 267.

For a report of bronchospasm in all of 6 patients who received suxamethonium and hexafluorenium bromide concomitantly, see Hexafluorenium Bromide, p.992.

Serum-cholinesterase concentrations were similar in 52 patients with chronic renal failure, 39 similar patients undergoing peritoneal dialysis, and 64 undergoing haemodialysis. Suxamethonium 50 to 100 mg was used in 81 of 90 patients undergoing renal transplantation. Although 26 had reduced cholinesterase values no problems were encountered except in 1 patient who experienced prolonged apnoea and who was found to have atypical cholinesterase inheritance.— D. W. Ryan, *Br. J. Anaesth.*, 1977, *49*, 945.

Interactions. Diminished effect. The duration of paralysis produced by 25 mg of suxamethonium was reduced by 20% following the intravenous administration of diazepam, 150 µg per kg body-weight, and the 25 to 75% recovery time shortened by 15%.— S. A. Feldman and B. E. Crawley (preliminary communication), *Br. med. J.*, 1970, *2*, 336. See also *idem* (letter), 1970, *1*, 691. Investigations in *dogs* showed that diazepam significantly reversed the neuromuscular blockade induced by non-depolarising agents such as gallamine but augmented that of depolarising agents such as suxamethonium.— K. K. Sharma and U. C. Sharma, *J. Pharm. Pharmac.*, 1978, *30*, 64.

Enhanced effect. When suxamethonium and oxytocin were employed simultaneously, suxamethonium produced a non-depolarising block, slower in onset, less intensive, and more prolonged than that normally associated with suxamethonium, and reversible by anticholinesterases.— R. J. H. Hodges (letter), *Br. med. J.*, 1958, *1*, 1416; R. J. H. Hodges *et al.*, *ibid.*, 1959, *1*, 413.

The neuromuscular blocking action of suxamethonium was enhanced by quinidine and by procainamide.— M. F. Cuthbert, *Br. J. Anaesth.*, 1966, *38*, 775.

The effects of suxamethonium were enhanced by procaine and lignocaine.— J. E. Usubiaga *et al.*, *Anesth. Analg. curr. Res.*, 1967, *46*, 39.

Sudden apnoea immediately followed intravenous injection of promazine hydrochloride 25 mg in a patient who had undergone a prolonged operative procedure during which a total of 550 mg of suxamethonium was used as a relaxant.— A. G. Regan and J. A. Aldrete, *Anesth. Analg. curr. Res.*, 1967, *46*, 315.

In 31 patients the period of apnoea following suxamethonium was on average 224 seconds longer when propanidid was given immediately prior to the injection of suxamethonium. The difference was ascribed to enzymic inhibition.— A. Doenicke *et al.*, *Br. J. Anaesth.*, 1968, *40*, 415.

A study in *cats* indicated that propranolol prevented fasciculations but enhanced neuromuscular blockade due to suxamethonium.— J. E. Usubiaga, *Anesthesiology*, 1968, *29*, 484.

Low serum-pseudocholinesterase concentrations were observed in 4 patients receiving phenelzine; 1 remained apnoeic for 1 hour following modified ECT.— P. O. Bodley *et al.* (preliminary communication), *Br. med. J.*, 1969, *3*, 510.

Despite warnings in the literature based on 1 report of an interaction, in a study of 6 surgical patients dexpanthenol was not found to enhance the effect of suxamethonium.— R. M. Smith *et al.*, *Anesth. Analg. curr. Res.*, 1969, *48*, 205.

Some cytotoxic drugs and whole body irradiation increased sensitivity to suxamethonium.— J. Stovner and I. Lund, *Br. J. Anaesth.*, 1970, *42*, 235.

Investigations in *rats* confirmed speculations (following 2 clinical cases) that magnesium enhanced neuromuscular blockade produced by tubocurarine, decamethonium, or suxamethonium.— M. M. Ghoneim and J. P. Long, *Anesthesiology*, 1970, *32*, 23.

The muscle relaxant properties of suxamethonium chloride were enhanced in *rats* treated with frusemide daily for a week.— E. Reyes and G. D. Appelt, *J. pharm. Sci.*, 1972, *61*, 562.

Ventricular fibrillation followed repeated doses of suxamethonium in a digitalised patient with hypercalcaemia.— R. B. Smith and J. Petruscak, *Anesth. Analg. curr. Res.*, 1972, *51*, 202, per *Int. pharm. Abstr.*, 1973, *10*, 20.

Neuromuscular blocking effects were enhanced by amphotericin.— *Med. Lett.*, 1973, *15*, 79.

Meturedepa might depress concentrations of pseudocholinesterase and so enhance the action of suxamethonium.— Horton J.A.G., *Adverse Drug React. Bull.*, 1975, Feb., 168.

Prolongation of suxamethonium-induced neuromuscular blockade in a woman taking lithium carbonate. This interaction was confirmed in *dogs*.— G. E. Hill *et al.*, *Anesthesiology*, 1976, *44*, 439.

Prolonged apnoea, after suxamethonium prior to ECT, in an 18-year-old woman with impaired liver function who had been treated with clindamycin; the pseudocholinesterase value was depressed.— D. Avery and R. Finn, *Dis. nerv. Syst.*, 1977, *38*, 473.

In 10 patients with typical plasma cholinesterase activity, neostigmine enhanced the block producd by suxamethonium whether it was of the depolarising or desensitisation type. In 5 patients with atypical cholinesterase, neostigmine enhanced the depolarising phase and antagonised the desensitising phase of the block.— A. Baraka, *Br. J. Anaesth.*, 1977, *49*, 479.

Prolongation of suxamethonium-induced neuromuscular blockade after prior administration of physostigmine.— A. F. Kopman *et al.*, *Anesthesiology*, 1978, *49*, 142.

Hyperkalaemia. Suxamethonium and decamethonium in normal doses increased serum concentrations of potassium. It was considered that depolarising muscle relaxants were contra-indicated in patients with abnormally high serum-potassium concentrations such as those with burns, severe trauma, or muscle denervation.— N. R. Fahmy *et al.*, *Anesthesiology*, 1975, *42*, 692.

Nine patients with severe intra-abdominal infection underwent repeat surgery with the use of suxamethonium; in 4, whose infection was of at least 14 days' duration, hyperkalaemia occurred with a rise of up to 2.95 mmol per litre; no significant rise occurred in the 5 with infection of not more than 9 days' duration. Those with severe intra-abdominal or systemic infection lasting longer than 1 week should be added to categories at risk from suxamethonium which should be avoided or, if essential, preceded by a non-depolarising muscle relaxant.— B. Kohlschütter *et al.*, *Br. J. Anaesth.*, 1976, *48*, 557.

Further references: G. A. Gronert and R. A. Theye, *Anesthesiology*, 1975, *43*, 89, per *Int. pharm. Abstr.*, 1977, *14*, 473; T. L. K. Rao and M. Shanmugam, *Anesth. Analg. curr. Res.*, 1979, *58*, 61.

Pregnancy and the neonate. Newborn infants had low levels of pseudocholinesterase and could therefore react adversely to suxamethonium chloride.— W. L. Nyhan, *J. Pediat.*, 1961, *59*, 1. See also E. K. Zsigmond and J. R. Downs, *Can. Anaesth. Soc. J.*, 1971, *18*, 278.

Prolonged apnoea occurred in both mother and neonate following caesarean section for which the mother received suxamethonium 100 mg. Both the mother and infant were atypical homozygotes deficient in pseudocholinesterase. Another atypical homozygotic mother also suffered prolonged apnoea following suxamethonium for caesarean section but the infant who was heterozygotic was not seriously affected.— A. Baraka *et al.*, *Anesthesiology*, 1975, *43*, 115, per *Drugs*, 1976, *11*, 76.

The distribution of suxamethonium in neonates.— M. Finster and G. F. Marx, *Anesthesiology*, 1976, *44*, 89.

Absorption and Fate. After injection, suxamethonium is hydrolysed by pseudocholinesterases in plasma and body tissues. One molecule of choline is split off rapidly to form succinylmonocholine which is then slowly hydrolysed to succinic acid and choline. Only a small proportion of suxamethonium is excreted unchanged in the urine. Succinylmonocholine has weak muscle-relaxant properties mainly of a non-depolarising nature.

Suxamethonium does not readily cross the placenta.

Studies of the enzymic inactivation of suxamethonium.— A. Doenicke *et al.*, *Br. J. Anaesth.*, 1968, *40*, 834.

Variant forms of serum cholinesterase and their effect on the metabolism of suxamethonium chloride.— B. La Du, *Ann. N.Y. Acad. Sci.*, 1971, *179*, 684. The pseudocholinesterase phenotypes of 182 patients with apnoea after suxamethonium and variations of the incidence of those phenotypes from those expected.— H. W. Goedde and K. Altland, *ibid.*, 695.

The pharmacokinetics of suxamethonium in infants, children, and adults.— D. R. Cook *et al.*, *Clin. Pharmac. Ther.*, 1976, *20*, 493.

The clinical pharmacokinetics of suxamethonium chloride.— L. B. Wingard and D. R. Cook, *Clin. Pharmacokinet.*, 1977, *2*, 330.

In 3 groups, each of 10 patients, the duration of suxamethonium-induced block in an occluded arm after occlusion for 1, 2, or 3 minutes was 68, 48, and 19% respectively of that in a non-occluded arm. It was considered that hydrolysis *in vivo* was slower than that recorded *in vitro*.— H. Holst-Larsen, *Br. J. Anaesth.*, 1976, *48*, 887. A similar report.— J. Wilson *et al.* (letter), *ibid.*, 1977, *49*, 90.

Pregnancy and the neonate. Small amounts of suxamethonium chloride had been detected in umbilical vein blood after intravenous administration to the mother of doses of 300 mg. The infant did not seem to be affected. — F. Moya and V. Thorndike, *Clin. Pharmac. Ther.*, 1963, *4*, 628. See also under Precautions.

Transient decreased respiration and tonus in an infant born to a woman who had received 140 mg of suxamethonium chloride during caesarean section.— W. D. Owens and G. L. Zeitlin, *Anesth. Analg. curr. Res.*, 1975, *54*, 38, per *Drug Intell. & clin. Pharm.*, 1975, *9*, 214.

Uses. Suxamethonium is a depolarising muscle relaxant. It acts in about 30 seconds following intravenous injection and has a duration of action averaging 3 to 5 minutes. It is used in surgical, anaesthetic, and other procedures in which a brief period of muscle relaxation is called for, as in intubation, endoscopies, and electroconvulsive therapy.

As the onset of relaxation is often preceded by a short period of painful muscle fasciculation, an intravenous anaesthetic, such as thiopentone sodium, should be given before suxamethonium is injected. Assisted respiration is necessary.

The usual single dose of suxamethonium chloride for an adult is 20 to 100 mg intravenously. Doses may be repeated if necessary with little danger of cumulative effect. A suggested dose for children is 1 to 2 mg per kg intravenously.

When a suitable vein is inaccessible suxamethonium may occasionally be given intramuscularly. A suggested intramuscular dose for adults and children is up to 2.5 mg per kg body-weight to a maximum total of 150 mg; the effect may be prolonged after intramuscular injection.

For prolonged procedures, as an alternative to repeated intravenous injections, sustained relaxation may be obtained by continuous intravenous infusion of a 0.1 to 0.2% solution, the rate of flow being adjusted as necessary. High doses may give rise to prolonged apnoea.

The duration of effect of suxamethonium has been increased by concomitantly administering hexafluorenium (see p.992).

The effect of dosage and rate of infusion on the duration of effect of suxamethonium.— M. D. Sokoll and R. D. Bastron, *Anesth. Analg. curr. Res.*, 1967, *46*, 682, per *J. Am. med. Ass.*, 1968, *203* (Jan. 22), A165.

A study of the neuromuscular effects of suxamethonium following single, intermittent, and continuous intravenous dosage in anaesthetised patients showed considerable variations in patient response. The initial neuromuscular block was depolarising, but became desensitising with increasing dosage and time. Recovery times of less than 30 minutes followed single intravenous doses of up to 3 mg per kg, continuous intravenous infusion for up to 1 hour, or intermittent infusion for several hours. Suxamethonium should be used only when intermittent muscle relaxation was required; when continuous prolonged relaxation was required, tubocurarine was to be preferred.— R. L. Katz and J. F. Ryan, *Br. J. Anaesth.*, 1969, *41*, 381.

The use of graded doses of suxamethonium and decamethonium in a patient with atypical cholinesterase.— S. Lee-Son *et al.*, *Anesthesiology*, 1975, *43*, 493, per *Int. pharm. Abstr.*, 1977, *14*, 431.

The effects of suxamethonium in 23 patients with traumatic nerve injuries.— A. Baraka, *Br. J. Anaesth.*, 1978, *50*, 195. Criticism.— W. Schreiber and J. Plötz (letter), *ibid.*, 1980, *52*, 842.

Electroconvulsive therapy. In a systematic dosage trial of suxamethonium for ECT, 500 µg per kg body-weight was found to give adequate blockade without increased frequency of cardiac arrhythmia or apnoea. This dose, with atropine and methohexitone, was recommended for starting a series of ECT sessions.— F. N. Pitts *et al.*, *Archs gen. Psychiat.*, 1968, *19*, 595, per *J. Am. med. Ass.*, 1968, *206*, 2138.

Tetanus. A patient with tetanus received suxamethonium, 1.5 to 3 mg per minute for 5½ days, with additional larger doses when required; a total of 22.5 g was given without toxic side-effects.— A. T. T. Forrester, *Br. med. J.*, 1954, *2*, 342.

In a patient with severe tetanus, suxamethonium 1 g intramuscularly produced relaxation of all muscles in 3 to 4 minutes. Twitching appeared in about 1½ hours, but did not become severe and opisthotonos did not recur until after 6 hours. Suxamethonium increased salivation but did not significantly increase bronchial secretion.— F. J. Curran *et al.*, *Anesth. Analg. curr. Res.*, 1968, *47*, 218, per *Int. pharm. Abstr.*, 1968, *5*, 1167.

Preparations

Sterile Succinylcholine Chloride *(U.S.P.)*. Sterile suxamethonium chloride suitable for parenteral use.

Succinylcholine Chloride Injection *(U.S.P.)*. A sterile solution of suxamethonium chloride in Water for Injections. pH 3 to 4.5. Potency is expressed in terms of anhydrous material. Store at 2° to 8°.

Suxamethonium Chloride Injection *(B.P.)*. Succinylcholine Chloride Injection. A sterile solution in Water for Injections. pH 3 to 5. Store at as low a temperature as possible above its freezing point and not exceeding 4°. Under these conditions it should retain its potency for at least 2 years.

Proprietary Preparations

Anectine *(Calmic, UK)*. Suxamethonium chloride, available as an injection containing 50 mg per ml in ampoules of 2 ml. (Also available as Anectine in *Austral.*, *Canad.*, *USA*).

Scoline *(Duncan, Flockhart, UK)*. Suxamethonium chloride, available as an injection containing 50 mg per ml, in ampoules of 2 ml and vials of 10 ml. (Also available as Scoline in *Austral.*, *Ital.*, *S.Afr.*).

Other Proprietary Names

Arg.—Paranoval; *Belg.*—Myoplegine; *Ger.*— Lysthenon, Pantolax, Succinyl-Asta; *Ital.*—Celocurin, Midarine, Myotenlis; *Neth.*—Curalest, Muscuryl, Succinyl; *Norw.*—Curacit (see also under Suxamethonium Iodide); *Swed.*—Celocurin-klorid; *Switz.*—Celocurin-Chlorid, Lysthenon, Midarine, Succinolin, Succinyl-Asta; *USA*—Quelicin, Sucostrin, Sux-Cert.

5733-f

Suxamethonium Iodide. Dithylinum; Suxamethonium Iodatum. 2,2′-Succinyldioxybis(ethyltrimethylammonium) di-iodide.

$C_{14}H_{30}I_2N_2O_4$=544.2.

CAS — 541-19-5.

Pharmacopoeias. In *Cz.*, *Pol.*, and *Rus.*

A white, odourless, slightly hygroscopic, crystalline powder. M.p. about 250°. Freely **soluble** in water; very slightly soluble in alcohol; practically insoluble in ether. A 1% solution in water has a pH of about 5. **Incompatible** with solutions of alkaline salts. **Store** in airtight containers. Protect from light.

Suxamethonium iodide has the same actions and is used for the same purposes as suxamethonium chloride.

Proprietary Names

Célocurine *(Kabivitrum, Fr.)*; Curacit (see also under Suxamethonium Chloride) *(GEA, Denm.)*.

5734-d

Suxethonium Bromide.

2,2′-Succinyldioxybis(diethyldimethylammonium) dibromide.

$C_{16}H_{34}Br_2N_2O_4$=478.3.

CAS — 111-00-2.

A slightly hygroscopic, white or slightly cream, crystalline powder. 1 mg Suxethonium (1 mg cation) is equivalent to 1.5 mg of suxethonium bromide.

Readily **soluble** in water, yielding weakly acidic solutions. Solutions for injection are prepared by dissolving immediately before use, the sterile contents of a sealed container in Water for Injections. It is rapidly hydrolysed by alkalis and therefore should not be mixed with solutions of thiopentone sodium. **Protect** from light.

Uses. Suxethonium bromide is a depolarising muscle relaxant with the same actions and uses as suxamethonium chloride (see p.995) but it has only about half the potency and a rather shorter duration of action, namely, 2 to 4 minutes. It is administered by intravenous injection, the dose being calculated on the basis of 1 to 1.25 mg cation (1.5 to 1.875 mg salt) per kg body-weight.

The absence of hyperkalaemia after suxethonium.— S. Day, *Br. J. Anaesth.*, 1976, *48*, 1011.

Proprietary Preparations

Brevidil E *(May & Baker, UK)*. Suxethonium bromide, available as powder for preparing injections in ampoules of 150 mg (equivalent to 100 mg cation). (Also available as Brevidil-E in *Austral.*, *S.Afr.*).

5735-n

Tolperisone Hydrochloride. 2,4'-Dimethyl-3-piperidinopropiophenone hydrochloride.
$C_{16}H_{23}NO,HCl = 281.8$.

CAS — 728-88-1 (tolperisone); 3644-61-9 (hydrochloride).

Adverse Effects. As for Chlorzoxazone, p.988. Diarrhoea has been reported.

Uses. Tolperisone hydrochloride is used for the symptomatic relief of muscle spasm in doses of 150 mg thrice daily.

Proprietary Names
Miodom *(Dominguez, Arg.)*; Mio-Relax *(LEFA, Spain)*; Mydocalm *(Richter, Denm.*; *Choay, Fr.*; *Gedeon Richter, Hung.*; *Katwijk, Neth.*; *Labatec-Pharma, Switz.)*; Abbsa, Arantoick, Atmosgen, Besnoline, Colmaite, Isocalm, Kineorl, Lasmon, Magnine, Menopatol, Metosomin, Minacalm, Muscalm, Naismeritin, Nichiperizone, Renbert, Rencarl, Roystajin, Sagereal, Sinorum, Tolisartine *(all Jap.)*.

5736-h

Tubocurarine Chloride *(B.P., Eur. P., U.S.P.)*.

Tubocurar. Chlor.; Tubocurarinii Chloridum; Tubocurarini Chloridum; *d*-Tubocurarine Chloride. (+)-7',12'-Dihydroxy-6,6'-dimethoxy-2,2',2'-trimethyltubocuraranium dichloride pentahydrate.
$C_{37}H_{42}Cl_2N_2O_6,5H_2O = 771.7$ (The empirical formula of tubocurarine chloride was formerly considered to be $C_{38}H_{44}Cl_2N_2O_6,5H_2O$).

CAS — 57-95-4 (tubocurarine); 57-94-3 (chloride, anhydrous); 6989-98-6 (chloride, pentahydrate).

Pharmacopoeias. In *Arg., Br., Braz., Cz., Eur., Fr., Ger., Ind., Int., It., Jap., Jug., Mex., Neth., Span., Swiss, Turk.*, and *U.S.*

The chloride of (+)-tubocurarine. It may be obtained from extracts of the stems of *Chondodendron tomentosum* (Menispermaceae). It is a white or slightly yellowish-white or greyish-white, odourless crystalline powder. M.p. about 270° with decomposition.

Soluble 1 in 20 of water and 1 in about 30 of alcohol; soluble in solutions of alkali hydroxides; practically insoluble in acetone, chloroform and ether. A 1% solution in water has a pH of 4 to 6. It is precipitated from aqueous solutions by sodium bicarbonate. Solutions are **sterilised** by distributing into ampoules, replacing the air with nitrogen or other suitable gas, sealing, and autoclaving. **Store** in airtight containers.

Incompatibility. Tubocurarine hydrochloride solution, 15 mg per ml, could usually be mixed with thiopentone sodium 2.5% solution in the proportion 1:19. If the pH of the resultant solution fell below 9.7, thiopentone was precipitated; above pH 9.7 the shelf-life of the mixture was limited to 48 hours.— C. Riffkin, *Am. J. Hosp. Pharm.*, 1963, *20*, 19.

A haze developed over 3 hours when tubocurarine chloride 60 mg per litre was mixed with trimetaphan camsylate 1 g per litre in dextrose injection.— B. B. Riley, *J. Hosp. Pharm.*, 1970, *28*, 228.

A haze developed in 15 minutes when methohexitone sodium 100 mg in 10 ml was mixed with tubocurarine chloride 12 mg in 4 ml.

Adverse Effects. In the doses commonly employed during anaesthesia, tubocurarine produces few side-effects providing efficient respiratory exchange is maintained. A fall in blood pressure and a slight increase in heart-rate usually occur. Occasionally, postoperative apnoea which is resistant to the action of neostigmine occurs (see p.986).

Rarely tubocurarine may cause bronchospasm due to histamine release.

Overdosage causes respiratory failure by paralysing the intercostal muscles and the diaphragm, and regurgitation of the stomach contents due to relaxation of the oesophageal muscle and sphincters.

Allergy. Reports of hypersensitivity.— V. Brandus *et al.*, *Br. J. Anaesth.*, 1973, *45*, 108; R. C. Rogoff *et al.*, *Anesthesiology*, 1974, *41*, 397; M. Fisher (letter), *Br. J. Anaesth.*, 1977, *49*, 87; A. C. Baldwin and M. D. Churcher, *Anaesthesia*, 1979, *34*, 339; B. C. Farmer and M. Sivarajan, *Anesthesiology*, 1979, *51*, 358.

Hyperpyrexia. Two cases of malignant hyperthermia where curare was probably the triggering drug. Each episode developed in a member of a known malignant hyperthermia family and developed despite preventive measures such as prophylactic cooling, and avoidance of potent inhalational anaesthetic agents and depolarising muscle relaxants.— B. A. Britt *et al.*, *Can. Anaesth. Soc. J.*, 1974, *21*, 371, per *J. Am. med. Ass.*, 1974, *230*, 771.

Muscle damage. An increase in serum-creatine phosphokinase concentration might result from muscle damage induced by injection of tubocurarine.— L. C. Cohen, *J. Am. med. Ass.*, 1972, *219*, 625.

Treatment of Adverse Effects. In respiratory failure following tubocurarine, respiration should be assisted and neostigmine methylsulphate should be given intravenously in a dose of 2 to 3 mg over 60 seconds with 0.6 to 1.2 mg of atropine sulphate. Additional neostigmine may be given but a total dose of 5 mg should not be exceeded.

In 3 patients with renal failure given tubocurarine, recurring dyspnoea or apnoea after neuromuscular blockade had apparently been reversed by neostigmine probably represented recurarisation. Pyridostigmine, with its longer action, might be preferable in such patients.— R. D. Miller and D. J. Cullen, *Br. J. Anaesth.*, 1976, *48*, 253.

Precautions. Tubocurarine chloride is contra-indicated, except as a diagnostic agent, in patients with myasthenia gravis and in some patients with respiratory insufficiency or pulmonary disease. It should be avoided or used with caution in patients with allergic disorders.

Care is necessary if tubocurarine chloride has to be given to a patient on 2 occasions within 24 hours, or in the presence of renal impairment. Patients with hepatic impairment may be relatively resistant to the effects of tubocurarine. Administration of tubocurarine either with or before a depolarising relaxant such as suxamethonium, may cause a muscle relaxation which is irreversible by neostigmine (see p.986).

The effects of tubocurarine are enhanced by ether and to a lesser extent by other inhalation anaesthetics; the hypotension produced by halothane anaesthesia is increased by tubocurarine. The effects of tubocurarine may be enhanced by some aminoglycoside or polypeptide antibiotics. The effects may also be enhanced by acidosis, hypokalaemia, raised body temperature, and by narcotic analgesics and quinidine.

Interactions. *Diminished effect.* For a review of the antagonism by adrenaline of the curare-induced neuromuscular block in *animals*, see W. C. Bowman and M. W. Nott, *Pharmac. Rev.*, 1969, *21*, 27.

In a study of the effect of alkalosis on tubocurarine requirements in 6 healthy subjects a 17% increase in the requirements was noted during hypocarbic anaesthesia (hypocapnic hyperventilation).— J. O. Bell and G. D. Blenkarn, *Anesth. Analg. curr. Res.*, 1972, *51*, 371, per *Int. pharm. Abstr.*, 1973, *10*, 375.

In *rats*, the muscle relaxation produced by tubocurarine chloride appeared to be antagonised by frusemide. This might have been the result of the formation of a complex between the 2 drugs.— E. Reyes and G. D. Appelt, *J. pharm. Sci.*, 1972, *61*, 562.

For a report of the reduction of the potency of non-depolarising muscle relaxants by immunosuppressants and guanethidine, see Azathioprine, p.190.

Enhanced effect. Parenteral administration of quinidine following the use of tubocurarine resulted in the recurarisation of a surgical patient.— W. L. Way *et al.*, *J. Am. med. Ass.*, 1967, *200*, 153.

In 43 patients undergoing surgery, halothane 1 to 2% increased the magnitude and duration of action of tubocurarine and decreased the activity of the abdominal muscles.— R. L. Katz and A. J. Gissen, *Anesthesiology*, 1967, *28*, 564, per *J. Am. med. Ass.*, 1967, *201* (July 24), A163.

A study in *cats* indicated that propranolol enhanced neuromuscular blockade due to tubocurarine.— J. E. Usubiaga, *Anesthesiology*, 1968, *29*, 484.

Prolonged curarisation in a patient with acute pancreatitis who received tubocurarine 20 mg was possibly due to hypocalcaemia and other factors associated with the pancreatitis.— B. D. McKie, *Br. J. Anaesth.*, 1969, *41*, 1091.

Procaine and lignocaine enhanced the effect of tubocurarine.— R. L. Katz and A. J. Gissen, *Acta anaesth. scand.*, 1969, *Suppl.* 36, 103.

Apparent enhancement of curarisation, with resistance to neostigmine, occurred in a 45-year-old patient given curare 12 mg over a 90-minute period for a surgical procedure after receiving a total of 11 g of colistin sulphomethate prior to surgery.— D. Gebbie, *Anesth. Analg. curr. Res.*, 1971, *50*, 109, per *Int. pharm. Abstr.*, 1971, *8*, 384.

Curariform effects were enhanced by amphotericin.— *Med. Lett.*, 1973, *15*, 79.

The prolongation of neuromuscular blockade in a patient was probably due to the enhancement of tubocurarine by magnesium sulphate.— A. J. C. de Silva, *Br. J. Anaesth.*, 1973, *45*, 1228. See also M. M. Ghoneim and J. P. Long, *Anesthesiology*, 1970, *32*, 23.

The effect of tubocurarine was enhanced by ketamine; pancuronium and suxamethonium were not affected.— R. R. Johnston *et al.*, *Anesth. Analg. curr. Res.*, 1974, *53*, 496, per *J. Am. med. Ass.*, 1974, *230*, 920.

Enhancement of the effect of tubocurarine by frusemide and possibly mannitol in 3 patients undergoing renal transplantation.— R. D. Miller *et al.*, *Anesthesiology*, 1976, *45*, 442.

Prolonged neuromuscular blockade in a patient given tubocurarine and trimetaphan (4.5 g in 90 minutes) for controlled hypotension.— S. L. Wilson *et al.*, *Anesth. Analg. curr. Res.*, 1976, *55*, 353.

Enhancement of the effect of tubocurarine by tobramycin.— P. M. Waterman and R. B. Smith, *Anesth. Analg. curr. Res.*, 1977, *56*, 587.

For reports of the effects of diazepam on non-depolarising neuromuscular blocking agents, see Gallamine Triethiodide, p.991.

Absorption and Fate. When given intravenously, tubocurarine is widely distributed throughout the body tissues and is concentrated at the neuromuscular junctions. It is slowly and irregularly absorbed following intramuscular injection. Tubocurarine, given in the usual dose range, does not pass the placental or blood-brain barrier in significant quantities. About 50% is excreted unchanged in the urine over several hours and the remainder is metabolised in the body.

The pharmacodynamics of tubocurarine.— L. B. Wingard and D. R. Cook, *Br. J. Anaesth.*, 1976, *48*, 839.

The clinical pharmacokinetics of tubocurarine chloride.— L. B. Wingard and D. R. Cook, *Clin. Pharmacokinet.*, 1977, *2*, 330.

In 4 subjects with normal renal function 38% of a dose of tubocurarine was excreted in 24 hours compared with 13% in 4 with renal failure who had just received renal transplants.— R. D. Miller *et al.*, *J. Pharmac. exp. Ther.*, 1977, *202*, 1.

Further references: M. I. Ramzan *et al.*, *Br. J. Anaesth.*, 1980, *52*, 893.

Blood-brain barrier. Samples of CSF collected from 6 patients after intravenous injection of tubocurarine 30 mg had detectable curare-like activity.— G. Devasankaraiah *et al.*, *Br. J. Pharmac.*, 1973, *47*, 787.

In 9 patients given single doses of tubocurarine (300 μg per kg body-weight) and 6 patients given 3 doses, concentrations in the CSF (up to 24.9 ng per ml) were considered unlikely to have a pharmacologic effect.— R. S. Matteo *et al.*, *Anesthesiology*, 1977, *46*, 396.

Pregnancy and the neonate. A young woman, about 28 weeks pregnant, with status epilepticus was given 15- to 30-mg doses of tubocurarine as needed, then every 2 hours, to control the fits. The total dose of tubocurarine was 245 mg. Premature labour occurred and after delivery the infant's heart beat was normal but there was no spontaneous activity or effort to breathe. Edrophonium 200 μg was injected through an umbilical catheter and within a few seconds the baby showed vigorous movements and began to breathe normally although it died 5½ hours after birth.— P. O. Older and J. M. Harris, *Br. J. Anaesth.*, 1968, *40*, 459.

Further references: J. B. E. Baker, *Pharmac. Rev.*, 1960, *12*, 37; F. Moya and V. Thorndike, *Clin. Pharmac. Ther.*, 1963, *4*, 628.

Uses. Tubocurarine is a non-depolarising muscle relaxant and when given by injection produces paralysis of voluntary muscle by blocking impulses at the neuromuscular junction. The action is rapid, effects beginning to appear within a minute or so after intravenous injection and lasting for 20 to 40 minutes; the maximum effect is attained within 3 to 5 minutes; with overdoses, respiratory paralysis usually occurs within 7 to 10 minutes.

In the dosage used clinically, tubocurarine chloride has no central stimulant, depressant, or analgesic action. It has histamine-releasing properties, and in doses probably larger than those used clinically, it blocks the action of acetylcholine at the autonomic ganglia.

Tubocurarine is used as an adjuvant to anaesthesia to obtain greater muscular relaxation in surgical operations and in orthopaedic manipulations. As the response is variable, it has been recommended that dosage should be based on an initial intravenous dose of 10 to 15 mg; undue susceptibility may be determined by giving a 5-mg dose prior to anaesthesia. Additional doses of 5 mg at intervals of about 25 minutes, up to a total of 40 mg, may be given if required. For children, the dose is 400 µg per kg body-weight intravenously; as premature and newborn infants may be more sensitive to tubocurarine, a dose of 200 to 250 µg per kg is suggested.

These doses apply to tubocurarine chloride used in conjunction with most of the usual anaesthetics. As ether has muscle-relaxant properties the dose of tubocurarine chloride required with it is only one-third to one-half of that usually recommended; lower doses should also be used with halothane to avoid hypotension. Patients must be provided with an effective airway and kept supplied with oxygen by means of a closed-circuit apparatus.

In most patients who have had large doses of tubocurarine over a long period, there will be some residual effect which will require reversal with neostigmine; the use of an additional dose of 5 to 10 mg of tubocurarine chloride to facilitate closure of the abdominal wall does not materially affect the ease with which this reversal can be accomplished. It is important that the patient should be breathing deeply and regularly before leaving the theatre.

Tubocurarine chloride is also used to control the muscle spasms and convulsions of tetanus, the usual initial dose being 75 to 150 µg per kg body-weight, intravenously, with subsequent doses as required. Tubocurarine chloride has also been given intramuscularly, sometimes with hyaluronidase to facilitate absorption.

The trauma in electroconvulsive therapy may be minimised by the administration, 5 minutes before induction of the shock, of tubocurarine chloride intravenously in a dose of up to 300 µg per kg body-weight, with atropine sulphate 0.6 to 1.2 mg, narcosis first being induced by thiopentone sodium 300 mg intravenously.

Tubocurarine chloride may be used as a diagnostic agent for myasthenia gravis but the procedure should only be used if other tests are indecisive. Patients suffering from this disease show exaggeration of the symptoms within 2 minutes after an intravenous injection of 15 µg per kg body-weight. As soon as a positive reaction is obtained 1.5 mg of neostigmine methylsulphate and 600 µg of atropine sulphate should be injected. Facilities for controlled respiration should be available.

Investigation of the serum protein pattern of 52 patients undergoing upper abdominal surgery showed a significant correlation between the immunoglobulin concentration in serum and the dose of tubocurarine required to maintain adequate muscular relaxation. This was attributed to the ability of immunoglobulin to bind tubocurarine.— A. Baraka and F. Gabali, *Br. J. Anaesth.*, 1968, *40*, 89. No correlation could be found between tubocurarine requirements and plasma protein fractions in 50 neonates.— E. Vivori *et al.*, *Br. J. Anaesth.*, 1974, *46*, 93.

Pretreatment with tubocurarine 3 mg abolished the fasciculations produced by suxamethonium without impairment of relaxation of hand, jaw, and respiratory muscles although 70 to 75% more suxamethonium was required for the same degree of block. Conditions for endotracheal intubation were excellent.— A. L. Pauca *et al.*, *Br. J. Anaesth.*, 1975, *47*, 1067.

Administration. In infants and children. Based on studies in 50 neonates recommended single initial doses of tubocurarine were: up to 1 week of age 250 µg per kg body-weight; 1 to 2 weeks 400 µg per kg; 2 to 4 weeks 500 µg per kg. Incremental dose of one-fifth or one-sixth of these doses were given as required. Initial doses were reduced in prematurity, acidosis, or hypothermia, and in the presence of antibiotics which might affect neurotransmission as well as of potent anaesthetics.— E. J. Bennett *et al.*, *Br. J. Anaesth.*, 1976, *48*, 687. See also N. G. Goudsouzian *et al.*, *Anesthesiology*, 1975, *43*, 416.

In renal failure. The action of tubocurarine was not unduly prolonged in patients with renal failure and increased transportation probably took place in the liver.— J. Stovner and I. Lund, *Br. J. Anaesth.*, 1970, *42*, 235.

Tubocurarine could be given in usual doses to patients with renal failure; the duration of action of each dose might be prolonged in patients with a glomerular filtration-rate of less than 10 ml per minute.— W. M. Bennett *et al.*, *Ann. intern. Med.*, 1980, *93*, 286.

Further references: K. B. Slawson, *Br. J. Anaesth.*, 1972, *44*, 277; D. K. F. Meijer *et al.*, *Anesthesiology*, 1979, *51*, 402.

Diagnosis of myasthenia gravis. The diagnosis of generalised myasthenia gravis, based on the administration of tubocurarine chloride 200 µg by regional intravenous injection into an arm. This resulted, 7 minutes later, in a mean reduction in grip-strength of about 68% in patients with generalised myasthenia, compared with about 10% in normal subjects and in patients with ocular myasthenia. The test gave unequivocally positive results in cases of myasthenia gravis which had not been confirmed by edrophonium.— F. F. Foldes *et al.*, *J. Am. med. Ass.*, 1968, *203*, 649.

Ocular surgery. Reduction of intra-ocular pressure by tubocurarine.— M. H. Al-Abrak and J. R. Samuel, *Br. J. Ophthal.*, 1974, *58*, 806.

Tetanus. In the treatment of severe tetanus tubocurarine was given intramuscularly in doses sufficient to give freedom from spasm for 2 hours at a time.— J. Macrae, *Br. med. J.*, 1973, *1*, 730. See also G. Clough and J. R. W. Dykes, *Br. J. Anaesth.*, 1973, *45*, 617.

Preparations

Tubocurarine Chloride Injection *(U.S.P.)*. A sterile solution in Water for Injections. pH 2.5 to 5.

Tubocurarine Injection *(B.P.)*. Tubocurar. Inj. A sterile 1% solution of tubocurarine chloride in Water for Injections free from dissolved air. Each ml contains 10 mg of tubocurarine chloride. pH 4 to 6.

Proprietary Preparations

Jexin *(Duncan, Flockhart, UK)*. Tubocurarine chloride, available as an injection containing 10 mg per ml, in ampoules of 1.5 ml.

Tubarine *(Calmic, UK)*. Tubocurarine chloride, available as an injection containing 10 mg per ml, in ampoules of 1.5 ml. (Also available as Tubarine in *Arg.*, *Austral.*, *Canad.*, *Ital.*, *S.Afr.*).

Other Proprietary Names

Curarin *(Ger., Ital.)*; Curarine *(Neth.)*; Intocostrin-T *(Ital.)*; Intocostrine-T *(Belg.)*; Tubarine Miscible *(Switz.)*; Tubocuran *(Denm.)*.

Narcotic Analgesics

6200-n

Narcotic analgesics, probably better described as opioid analgesics, are mainly used for the relief of moderate to severe pain. Non-narcotic or non-opioid analgesics, which often possess antipyretic and anti-inflammatory properties, are used for the relief of less severe pain; they are described under Aspirin and similar Analgesic and Anti-inflammatory Agents (p.234).

Narcotic analgesics are liable to produce dependence. Dependence of the morphine type and its treatment are described under Morphine (see p.1018).

The main narcotic analgesic is morphine (p.1018); it is also present in opium (p.1022) and papaveretum (p.1022). Diamorphine hydrochloride (p.1008), hydromorphone hydrochloride (p.1014), and oxymorphone hydrochloride (p.1022) are closely related morphine derivatives. Codeine (p.1004), dihydrocodeine tartrate (p.1010), and hydrocodone tartrate (p.1014) are much less liable to produce dependence and are used for the relief of less severe pain, often in conjunction with non-narcotic analgesics, and for suppression of cough. For drugs primarily used for the suppression of cough see under Pholcodine and some other Cough Suppressants (p.1260).

The principal synthetic drugs with morphine-like actions are pethidine hydrochloride (p.1026), anileridine (p.1002), dextromoramide tartrate (p.1005), dextropropoxyphene hydrochloride (p.1006), dipipanone hydrochloride (p.1011), and levorphanol tartrate (p.1015). Methadone hydrochloride (p.1015) and levomethadyl acetate (p.1014) are long-acting synthetic morphine-like drugs which have been used in the treatment of dependence.

Fentanyl citrate (p.1012) and phenoperidine hydrochloride (p.1028) are used with a major tranquilliser or neuroleptic agent, such as droperidol, to produce neuroleptanalgesia. This is a state of calm mental detachment with mild sedation accompanied by a high degree of analgesia that enables surgical operations and painful manipulative procedures to be undertaken with the cooperation of the patient.

Narcotic antagonists have been produced which reverse the actions of morphine-like drugs. Many of these antagonists retain some morphine-like actions. Drugs with both agonist and antagonist properties have been developed in an attempt to produce strong analgesics with a low dependence liability. Drugs with mixed agonist-antagonist properties which are used mainly as analgesics include buprenorphine hydrochloride (p.1002) and pentazocine (p.1024). Other antagonists are described under Narcotic Antagonists (p.1031).

A review of the pharmacology of synthetic opiate analgesics.— R. E. S. Bullingham, *Br. J. Hosp. Med.*, 1981, *25*, 59.

Analgesia. Reviews on the use of narcotic analgesics.— R. G. Twycross, *Postgrad. med. J.*, 1973, *49*, 732; J. M. Gibbs, *Drugs*, 1975, *9*, 373; *Med. Lett.*, 1975, *17* (Jan.), *Suppl.*, 48. A historical survey on the use of opioids in the management of pain, including their mode of action.— J. W. Lewis and M. J. Rance, *Pharm. J.*, 1978, *2*, 395; *idem*, 1979, *1*, 61; *Br. med. J.*, 1981, *282*, 1095.

The pharmacology and use of narcotic agonist and antagonist analgesics.— *Br. J. clin. Pharmac.*, 1979, *7*, *Suppl.* 3, 269S–326S.

The limitations of narcotics for sedation and analgesia for minor painful procedures.— *Med. Lett.*, 1977, *19*, 26.

A discussion on the advantages of patient-controlled analgesia.— *Lancet*, 1980, *1*, 289. Although intravenous patient-controlled analgesia may be suitable for relief of the pains of labour, it is of less use for the relief of continuous pain. Continuous intramuscular infusion via a portable syringe driver is suitable for the relief of postoperative pain and is safer and cheaper.— H. T. Davenport and B. M. Wright (letter), *ibid.*, 543.

In cancer and terminal pain. R. G. Twycross, *Br. med. J.*, 1975, *4*, 212 and 356; *idem*, *Pain*, 1977, *3*, 93; *Lancet*, 1978, *1*, 698; *Br. med. J.*, 1978, *1*, 459; D. W. Vere, *Topics Ther.*, 1978, *4*, 75; R. G. Twycross, *ibid.*, 94; R. C. Lamerton, *Practitioner*, 1979, *223*, 813; D. S. Shimm *et al.*, *J. Am. med. Ass.*, 1979, *241*, 2408; W. T. Beaver, *ibid.*, 1980, *244*, 2653.

In labour. A review of the use of analgesia in labour.— M. Rosen, *Br. J. Anaesth.*, 1979, *51*, *Suppl.* 1, 11S. See also D. B. Scott, *ibid.*, 1977, *49*, 11.

See also references to patient-controlled analgesia, above.

Postoperative. Discussions of the treatment of postoperative pain.— *Br. med. J.*, 1976, *2*, 664; *ibid.*, 1978, *2*, 517; C. L. Knight and M. Mehta, *Br. J. Hosp. Med.*, 1978, *19*, 462.

Neuroleptanalgesia. A review of the pharmacology of the analgesic drugs used in neuroleptanalgesia.— J. Edmonds-Seal and C. Prys-Roberts, *Br. J. Anaesth.*, 1970, *42*, 207.

6201-h

Enkephalins and Endorphins

Morphine and other narcotic analgesics are considered to produce many of their effects by actions at specific opiate receptors in the central nervous system. Endogenous peptides have been identified which possess opiate agonist activity. These include the enkephalins, met- and leu-enkephalin, and the endorphins, particularly beta-endorphin.

Enkephalins appear to be associated with neuronal systems in the brain and gastro-intestinal tract and to have a neurotransmitter role in these organs while beta-endorphin might have a hormonal role either within the pituitary or as a blood-borne hormone. In addition, beta-endorphin might have a more limited neurotransmitter role in the brain.

Beta-endorphin has analgesic activity if given into the CNS. A number of enkephalin or endorphin analogues are being or have been investigated including FK-33-824 [DAMME; (D-Ala^2, MePhe^4, Met (O)-ol)enkephalin], (D-Met^2, Pro^5)-enkephalinamide, metkephamid acetate (LY 127623), and (Des-Tyr)-γ-endorphin.

The identification of endogenous opioid pentapeptides.— J. Hughes *et al.*, *Nature*, 1975, *258*, 577.

An account of opiate receptors in the brain.— S. H. Snyder, *New Engl. J. Med.*, 1977, *296*, 266.

The distribution of endogenous opioid peptides in neurones of the human brain.— A. C. Cuello, *Lancet*, 1978, *2*, 291.

Dermorphins, potent opioid peptides from amphibian skin.— M. Broccardo *et al.*, *Br. J. Pharmac.*, 1981, *73*, 625.

Reviews. Some reviews on enkephalins and endorphins.— *Br. J. Anaesth.*, 1977, *49*, 523; R. Guillemin, *New Engl. J. Med.*, 1977, *296*, 226; J. Hughes and H. W. Kosterlitz, *Br. med. Bull.*, 1977, *33*, 157; *Br. med. J.*, 1978, *2*, 155; *Lancet*, 1978, *2*, 819; R. Guillemin, *Science*, 1978, *202*, 390; D. G. Smyth, *Pharm. J.*, 1979, *2*, 355; G. Metcalf, *Pharm. J.*, 1979, *2*, 356; W. E. Bunney *et al.*, *Ann. intern. Med.*, 1979, *91*, 239; *Br. med. J.*, 1980, *280*, 741; M. Schachter, *Br. J. Hosp. Med.*, 1981, *25*, 128.

Further references.— *Centrally Acting Peptides*, J. Hughes (Ed.), London, Macmillan, 1978; *Endorphins in Mental Health Research*, E. Usdin *et al.* (Ed.), London, Macmillan, 1979.

A discussion on endorphins and acupuncture.— *Lancet*, 1981, *1*, 480.

Increased met-enkephalin concentrations in the CSF of patients undergoing acupuncture.— V. Clement-Jones *et al.*, *Lancet*, 1980, *2*, 946. See also *idem*, 1979, *2*, 380.

Placebo effect. The possible involvement of endogenous morphine-like compounds in the placebo analgesic effect.— J. D. Levine *et al.*, *Nature*, 1978, *272*, 826; J. D. Levine *et al.*, *Lancet*, 1978, *2*, 654; P. Skrabanek (letter), *ibid.*, 791; A. D. Korczyn (letter), *ibid.*, 1304; A. Goldstein and P. Grevert (letter), *ibid.*, 1385.

Psychosis. Discussions on the possible role of endogenous opiate peptides in schizophrenia, mania, and psychosis.— A. Comfort, *Lancet*, 1977, *2*, 448; A. Dupont *et al.* (letter), *Lancet*, 1978, *2*, 1107; D. Janowsky *et al.* (letter), *Lancet*, 1978, *2*, 320; W. Domschke *et al.* (letter), *Lancet*, 1979, *1*, 1024; J. J. Hoo *et al.* (letter), *New Engl. J. Med.*, 1979, *301*, 946; F. D. Jones (letter), *ibid.*, 947.

Studies on endorphins in schizophrenia: J. M. van Ree *et al.* (letter), *Lancet*, 1980, *2*, 1363; B. Pethö *et al.* (letter), *ibid.*, 1981, *1*, 212.

6202-m

Alletorphine. *N*-Allylnoretorphine; R & S 218-M. (6*R*,7*R*,14*R*)-17-Allyl-7,8-dihydro-7-[(1*R*)-1-hydroxy-1-methylbutyl]-6-*O*-methyl-6,14-etheno-17-normorphine; (2*R*)-2-[(−)-(5*R*,6*R*,7*R*,14*R*)-9a-Allyl-4,5-epoxy-3-hydroxy-6-methoxy-6,14-ethenomorphinan-7-yl]pentan-2-ol.

$C_{27}H_{35}NO_4$=437.6.

CAS — 23758-80-7.

Crystals. M.p. 126°.

Alletorphine is a narcotic analgesic.

In a double-blind study in 142 patients who underwent abdominal surgery the analgesic effects on postoperative pain of alletorphine 560 µg per 70 kg body-weight and 350 µg per 70 kg were compared with morphine sulphate 10.5 mg per 70 kg, all intramuscularly. The higher dose of alletorphine was comparable with the morphine and cardiovascular and respiratory effects were not significantly different.— J. T. Macbeath and B. A. Moore, *Br. J. Anaesth.*, 1976, *48*, 97.

Manufacturers

Reckitt & Colman Pharmaceuticals, UK.

6203-b

Alphaprodine Hydrochloride *(U.S.P.)*. Nu 1196. (±)-*cis*-1,3-Dimethyl-4-phenyl-4-piperidyl propionate hydrochloride.

$C_{16}H_{23}NO_2$,HCl=297.8.

CAS — 77-20-3 (alphaprodine); 15867-21-7 (alphaprodine, ±); 561-78-4 (hydrochloride, ±).

Pharmacopoeias. In *U.S.*

A white crystalline powder with a slight odour and a bitter taste. M.p. 218° to 220°.

Soluble 1 in 2 of water, 1 in 7 of alcohol, 1 in 47 of acetone, and 1 in 3 of chloroform; very slightly soluble in ether. A 1% solution in water has a pH of 4.5 to 5.2. A 4.98% solution in water is iso-osmotic with serum.

An aqueous solution of alphaprodine hydrochloride iso-osmotic with serum (4.98%) caused 100% haemolysis of erythrocytes cultured in it for 45 minutes.— C. Sapp *et al.*, *J. pharm. Sci.*, 1975, *64*, 1884.

Dependence. The prolonged use of alphaprodine is liable to produce dependence of the morphine type (see p.1018).

Adverse Effects, Treatment, and Precautions. As for Morphine, p.1019.

Death of a child following use of alphaprodine in dental surgery.— C. H. Hine and A. Pasi, *Clin. Toxicol.*, 1972, *5*, 307.

Uses. Alphaprodine hydrochloride is an analgesic chemically related to and with an action resembling that of pethidine, but more rapid in onset and of shorter duration. Its main use is in obstetrics and as pre-operative medication in surgery and for minor surgical procedures.

Alphaprodine hydrochloride is administered by subcutaneous injection in a dose of 20 to 60 mg; the dose may be repeated at 2-hourly intervals to a maximum of 240 mg in 24 hours. This dose produces analgesia within 5 to 10 minutes, lasting for about 2 hours. In obstetrics, the initial dose is given after the cervix has begun to dilate, the last dose being given at least 2 hours prior to delivery to avoid depression of foetal respiration. Alphaprodine may also be given intravenously, a dose of 10 to 30 mg injected over a period of 3 to 4 minutes producing analgesia in 1 to 2 minutes, lasting for 30 to 60 minutes.

A comparison of diazepam and alphaprodine in cystoscopy.— C. E. Blackard *et al., Minn. Med.*, 1970, *53*, 11.

Preparations

Alphaprodine Hydrochloride Injection *(U.S.P.)*. A sterile solution of alphaprodine hydrochloride in Water for Injections pH 4 to 6.

Proprietary Names

Nisentil *(Roche, Canad.; Roche, USA)*.

6204-v

Anileridine *(U.S.P.)*.

Ethyl 1-(4-aminophenethyl)-4-phenylpiperidine-4-carboxylate.
$C_{22}H_{28}N_2O_2$=352.5.

CAS — 144-14-9.

Pharmacopoeias. In *U.S.*

A white to yellowish-white, odourless or almost odourless, crystalline powder. When exposed to light and air it oxidises and darkens in colour. There are 2 crystalline forms, melting at about 80° and about 89° respectively.

Very slightly **soluble** in water; soluble 1 in 2 of alcohol and 1 in 1 of chloroform; soluble in ether but solutions may be turbid. **Store** in airtight containers. Protect from light.

Incompatibility. For a report of incompatibilities of anileridine in intravenous solutions, see Codeine Phosphate, p.1004.

6205-g

Anileridine Hydrochloride *(U.S.P.)*.

$C_{22}H_{28}N_2O_2,2HCl$=425.4.

CAS — 126-12-5.

Pharmacopoeias. In *U.S.*

A white or almost white odourless crystalline powder. M.p. about 270° with decomposition. Anileridine hydrochloride 30 mg is approximately equivalent to 25 mg of anileridine. **Soluble** 1 in 5 of water and 1 in 80 of alcohol; practically insoluble in chloroform and ether. A 5% solution in water has a pH of 2.5 to 3. A 5.13% solution in water is iso-osmotic with serum. **Store** in airtight containers. Protect from light.

An aqueous solution of anileridine hydrochloride iso-osmotic with serum (5.13%) caused 12% haemolysis of erythrocytes cultured in it for 45 minutes.— C. Sapp *et al., J. pharm. Sci.*, 1975, *64*, 1884.

6206-q

Anileridine Phosphate.

$C_{22}H_{28}N_2O_2,H_3PO_4$=450.5.

CAS — 4268-37-5.

A white crystalline powder with a bitter taste. Anileridine phosphate 32 mg is approximately equivalent to 25 mg of anileridine. Very **soluble** in water. A solution in water has a pH of 3 to 4.

Dependence. Use of anileridine is liable to produce dependence of the morphine type (see p.1018).

Adverse Effects, Treatment, and Precautions. As for Morphine, p.1019.

Absorption and Fate. Anileridine and its salts are readily absorbed from the gastro-intestinal tract. It is broken down in the body and the metabolites are excreted in the urine together with about 5% of unchanged anileridine.

References: C. C. Porter, *J. Pharmac. exp. Ther.*, 1957, *120*, 447.

Uses. Anileridine is an analgesic chemically related to and with an action resembling that of pethidine (see p.1027). The usual dose as the hydrochloride by mouth is 25 mg every 6 hours. The usual subcutaneous or intramuscular dose for pain is 25 to 50 mg as the phosphate, every 4 to 6 hours, though for severe pain single doses of 75 mg have been given.

To support anaesthesia, 50 to 100 mg of anileridine, as the phosphate, is added to 500 ml of dextrose injection and the equivalent of 5 to 10 mg of anileridine is given by slow intravenous infusion followed by slow intravenous infusion of the solution at the rate of about 600 µg of anileridine per minute.

Preparations of Anileridine and its Salts

Anileridine Hydrochloride Tablets *(U.S.P.)*. Tablets containing anileridine hydrochloride. Potency is expressed in terms of the equivalent amount of anileridine. Store in airtight containers. Protect from light.

Anileridine Injection *(U.S.P.)*. A sterile solution of anileridine, prepared with the aid of phosphoric acid, in Water for Injections. Potency is expressed in terms of the equivalent amount of anileridine base. pH 4.5 to 5. Protect from light.

Proprietary Names of Anileridine and its Salts

Leritine *(Frosst, Canad.)*.

6207-p

Azidomorphine. 6-Deoxy-6-azidodihydroisomorphine. (6*R*)-6-Azido-6-deoxy-7,8-dihydromorphine; (5*R*,6*R*)-6-Azido-4,5-epoxy-9a-methylmorphinan-3-ol.
$C_{17}H_{20}N_4O_2$=312.4.

CAS — 22952-87-0.

Azidomorphine is reported to be a potent morphine-like agent.

References.— J. Knoll *et al., J. Pharm. Pharmac.*, 1973, *25*, 929; S. C. Clark *et al., Clin. Pharmac. Ther.*, 1976, *19*, 295; A. V. Karamanian *et al., Drug & Alcohol Depend.*, 1976, *1*, 319, per *Int. pharm. Abstr.*, 1977, *14*, 172.

6208-s

Bezitramide. R 4845. 4-[4-(2,3-Dihydro-2-oxo-3-propionyl-1*H*-benzimidazol-1-yl)piperidino]-2,2-diphenylbutyronitrile.
$C_{31}H_{32}N_4O_2$=492.6.

CAS — 15301-48-1.

A white amorphous or crystalline powder. Practically **insoluble** in water and dilute acids; soluble in acetone and chloroform; very slightly soluble in ether.

Bezitramide is a narcotic analgesic which has been used in doses of 5 mg in the treatment of severe pain. It has a slow onset of action which lasts for about 8 hours.

Significant reduction in pain was achieved with bezitramide 10 mg although this was less than that achieved with dextromoramide 10 mg in a study covering 47 patients. The study was ended prematurely because of the unacceptable level of side-effects with bezitramide which induced nausea, vomiting, drowsiness, dizziness, and sweating.— B. Kay, *Br. J. Anaesth.*, 1973, *45*, 623.

Further references: Sixteenth Report of the WHO Expert Committee on Drug Dependence, *Tech. Rep. Ser. Wld Hlth Org. No. 407*, 1969; H. Knape, *Br. J. Anaesth.*, 1970, *42*, 325; *idem*, 1971, *43*, 76; P. A. J. Janssen *et al., Arzneimittel-Forsch.*, 1971, *21*, 862; W. K. P. Amery *et al., ibid.*, 868; P. V. Admiraal *et al., Br. J. Anaesth.*, 1972, *44*, 1191.

Proprietary Names

Burgodin *(Janssen, Belg.; Janssen, Neth.)*.

6209-w

Buprenorphine Hydrochloride.

CL 112302; NIH 8805; UM 952; RX 6029-M *(buprenorphine)*. (6*R*,7*R*,14*S*)-17-Cyclopropylmethyl-7,8-dihydro-7-[(1*S*)-1-hydroxy-1,2,2-trimethylpropyl]-6-*O*-methyl-6,14-ethano-17-normorphine hydrochloride; (2*S*)-2-[(−)-(5*R*,6*R*,7*R*,14*S*)-9a-Cyclopropylmethyl-4,5-epoxy-3-hydroxy-6-methoxy-6,14-ethanomorphinan-7-yl]-3,3-dimethylbutan-2-ol hydrochloride.
$C_{29}H_{41}NO_4,HCl$=504.1.

CAS — 52485-79-7 (buprenorphine); 53152-21-9 (hydrochloride).

A white crystalline powder.

Dependence. Buprenorphine may have lower potential for producing dependence than morphine.

Adverse Effects. Buprenorphine appears to have similar adverse effects to morphine, with the possible exception of constipation. The most frequent side-effects of buprenorphine are drowsiness, nausea, vomiting, sweating, and dizziness. Respiratory depression, euphoria, miosis, and dry mouth may also occur.

Over 12 months 8187 patients were monitored for efficacy and untoward effects following administration of buprenorphine. Adverse effects reported were, nausea (8.8%), vomiting (7.4%), drowsiness (4.3%), sleeping (1.9%), dizziness (1.2%), sweating (0.98%), headache (0.55%), confusion (0.53%), lightheadedness (0.38%), blurred vision (0.28%), euphoria (0.27%), dry mouth (0.11%), depression (0.09%), and hallucinations (0.09%). Other adverse effects reported included amnesia, bloating, cough, cramp, diarrhoea, diplopia, and flatulence.— A. W. Harcus *et al., Br. med. J.*, 1979, *2*, 163.

A depressed patient who had been taking buprenorphine for more than 9 months claimed to have taken 35 to 40 buprenorphine tablets of 400 µg by dissolving the tablets in his mouth. He was conscious but drowsy and his temperature, respiration, blood pressure, and pulse-rate were normal. He vomited twice but suffered no further adverse effects. He discontinued buprenorphine and experienced no withdrawal symptoms.— C. D. Banks *et al., N.Z. med. J.*, 1979, *89*, 255.

Buprenorphine was given sublingually in doses of 150 to 800 µg to 141 patients with cancer pain. Of 94 patients who discontinued buprenorphine in less than 1 week, 50 did so because of side-effects and 29 because their previous analgesic was preferred. The remaining 47 patients continued taking buprenorphine for an average of 12 weeks. The main side-effects were dizziness, nausea, vomiting, drowsiness, dry mouth, and lightheadedness. Constipation was not reported and dependence and withdrawal did not occur in any patient.— D. S. Robbie, *Br. J. clin. Pharmac.*, 1979, *7, Suppl.* 3, 315S.

Treatment of Adverse Effects. Treatment is similar to that of morphine (see p.1019), *but* nalorphine and levallorphan are not antagonists. Naloxone (see p.1032) may be of benefit.

Precautions. As for Morphine, p.1019.

Buprenorphine has narcotic antagonist actions and may precipitate withdrawal symptoms if given to patients who have recently used other narcotic analgesics.

Buprenorphine should be used with caution in women during labour since the foetus is at risk from the absence of a dependable antagonist.

Absorption and Fate. Following intramuscular injection, buprenorphine rapidly produces peak plasma concentrations. It is metabolised chiefly in the liver and is excreted predominantly in the bile. Absorption also takes place through the buccal mucosa following sublingual administration.

Animal experiments indicate that buprenorphine is subject to considerable first-pass metabolism following administration by mouth, and that it crosses the blood-brain barrier and the placenta.

References: R. E. S. Bullingham *et al., Clin. Pharmac. Ther.*, 1980, *28*, 667.

Uses. Buprenorphine hydrochloride is an analgesic with actions and uses similar to those of morphine (see p.1020). In addition, it has weak narcotic antagonist properties. Following intramuscular injection analgesia is apparent within 30 to 60 minutes and lasts 6 to 8 hours. A similar response appears to be achieved following sublingual administration.

The dose by intramuscular or slow intravenous injection for moderate to severe pain is the equivalent of 300 to 600 µg of buprenorphine repeated every 6 to 8 hours as required. Doses of 400 µg are given sublingually every 6 to 8 hours.

Reviews of the actions and uses of buprenorphine.— *Drug & Ther. Bull.*, 1979, *17*, 17; R. C. Heel *et al.*, *Drugs*, 1979, *17*, 81.

For reviews of the pharmacology and clinical uses of narcotic analgesics including buprenorphine which are partial agonists and antagonists, see *Br. J. clin. Pharmac.*, 1979, *7*, *Suppl.* 3.

Anaesthesia. *Premedication.* In a study of 120 adults who received either buprenorphine 300 µg or morphine 10 mg as a premedicant before elective surgery, the frequency of nausea, vomiting, and giddiness was greater in the buprenorphine group.— J. W. Sear *et al.* (letter), *Br. J. Anaesth.*, 1979, *51*, 71.

Further references: B. Kay, *Br. J. Anaesth.*, 1980, *52*, 453 (comparison with fentanyl in analgesic supplemented anaesthesia); H. J. McQuay *et al.*, *ibid.*, 1013 (clinical effects during and after operation).

Analgesia. *Postoperative.* In a double-blind study in 172 patients buprenorphine 4 and 8 µg per kg body-weight were significantly more effective for the relief of postoperative pain than 2 µg per kg; for pain at rest buprenorphine 4 µg per kg was superior to pethidine 1 mg per kg, and 8 µg per kg was superior to pentazocine 600 µg per kg; for pain on movement buprenorphine 8 µg per kg was superior to pethidine. All drugs were given by intramuscular injection. Sedation was common and 2 patients taking buprenorphine 8 µg per kg had reduced respiratory frequency which did not cause clinical concern.— B. C. Hovell, *Br. J. Anaesth.*, 1977, *49*, 913.

Buprenorphine 5 µg per kg body-weight or pethidine 1 mg per kg were given by slow intravenous injection to 60 women immediately after lower abdominal surgery. Pain relief was similar with both drugs; it was at its greatest 1 hour after administration but was about 4 times as long with buprenorphine having a mean duration of about 10 hours. Side-effects were similar but dizziness, drowsiness, and vomiting were less frequent with buprenorphine. Marked miosis occurred within 10 minutes of injection of buprenorphine.— M. M. Kamel and I. C. Geddes, *Br. J. Anaesth.*, 1978, *50*, 599. See also B. Kay, *Br. J. Anaesth.*, 1978, *50*, 605; J. W. Downing *et al.*, *S. Afr. med. J.*, 1979, *55*, 1023.

In a double-blind study 29 patients were given buprenorphine or pethidine intravenously, by a patient-controlled demand machine, for postoperative pain. The relative potency of buprenorphine was considered to be 600 times that of pethidine. Mean total doses in the first 24 hours (and ranges) were: buprenorphine 15.3 µg per kg body-weight (range 4.2 to 57 µg per kg); pethidine 9.05 mg per kg (range 2.9 to 23 mg per kg).— K. Chakravarty *et al.*, *Br. med. J.*, 1979, *2*, 895.

Further references: G. Rolly and L. Versichelen, *Acta anaesth. belg.*, 1976, *27*, *Suppl.*, 134; *idem*, *27*, 183; J. W. Downing *et al.*, *Br. J. Anaesth.*, 1977, *49*, 251; A. B. Dobkin, *Can. Anaesth. Soc. J.*, 1977, *24*, 186; *idem*, 195; B. C. Hovell and A. E. Ward, *J. int. med. Res.*, 1977, *5*, 417; J. M. Gibbs and H. Johnson, *N.Z. med. J.*, 1978, *88*, 363; E. N. S. Fry, *Anaesthesia*, 1979, *34*, 549.

See also Anaesthesia, Premedication, above.

Cardiovascular disorders. Measurement of the haemodynamic effects of buprenorphine, 5 µg per kg body-weight given intravenously over 30 seconds, in 11 patients after open-heart surgery suggested that it was a suitable analgesic for patients with an unstable circulation.— F. L. Rosenfeldt *et al.*, *Br. med. J.*, 1978, *2*, 1602. See also F. L. Rosenfeldt *et al.*, *Br. J. clin. Pharmac.*, 1978, *5*, 362P. Comments.— D. W. Bethune (letter), *Br. med. J.*, 1979, *1*, 345; D. J. Coltart *et al.* (letter), *ibid.*; D. J. Coltart and A. D. Malcolm, *Br. J. clin. Pharmac.*, 1979, *7*, *Suppl.* 3, 309S.

Myocardial infarction. In 10 patients with myocardial infarction buprenorphine 300 µg intravenously caused a fall in systolic blood pressure which was not considered significant. In 43 further patients the effect of buprenorphine 400 µg sublingually was delayed compared with that of 300 µg intravenously. In a double-blind study in 118 patients the effect of buprenorphine 300 µg intravenously was significantly less, at 5 minutes, than that of diamorphine 5 mg intravenously, but at 15 minutes the effects were comparable. Buprenorphine was considered suitable for the relief of pain in myocardial infarction.— M. J. Hayes *et al.*, *Br. med. J.*, 1979, *2*, 300.

Sublingual buprenorphine might be useful in preventing recurrence of pain following myocardial infarction in patients treated at home.— H. C. R. Simpson (letter), *Br. med. J.*, 1979, *2*, 551.

Preparations

Temgesic (known in some countries as Buprex) *(Reckitt & Colman Pharmaceuticals, UK)*. Buprenorphine hydrochloride, available as an **Injection** containing the equivalent of buprenorphine 300 µg per ml, with dextrose 50 mg per ml, in ampoules of 1 and 2 ml and as **Sublingual Tablets** each containing the equivalent of 200 µg of buprenorphine. (Also available as Temgesic in *Eire*, *Norw.*).

6210-m

Butorphanol Tartrate *(U.S.P.)*. Levo-BC-2627 Tartrate. (−)-9a-Cyclobutylmethylmorphinan-3,14-diol hydrogen tartrate.

$C_{21}H_{29}NO_2,C_4H_6O_6$=477.6.

CAS — 42408-82-2 (butorphanol); 58786-99-5 (tartrate).

Pharmacopoeias. In *U.S.*

A white crystalline powder. M.p. 217° to 219° with decomposition. Sparingly **soluble** in water; slightly soluble in methyl alcohol; practically insoluble in alcohol, chloroform, ether, ethyl acetate, and hexane; soluble in dilute acids. A solution in water is slightly acidic. A solution in methyl alcohol is laevorotatory. **Store** in airtight containers.

Dependence. Butorphanol tartrate may have a lower potential for producing dependence than morphine.

Adverse Effects. As for Morphine, p.1019.

Results suggesting a ceiling effect to the respiratory depression induced by butorphanol.— H. Nagashima *et al.*, *Clin. Pharmac. Ther.*, 1976, *19*, 738; T. Kallos and F. Caruso, *ibid.*, 1977, *21*, 107.

Treatment of Adverse Effects. Treatment is similar to that for Morphine (see p.1019), *but* nalorphine and levallorphan are not suitable antagonists. However naloxone may be of benefit.

Precautions. As for Morphine, p.1019.

Butorphanol has narcotic antagonist actions and may precipitate withdrawal symptoms if given to patients who have recently used other narcotic analgesics.

Absorption and Fate. Butorphanol is absorbed from the gastro-intestinal tract but it undergoes extensive first-pass metabolism. Peak plasma concentrations occur 0.5 to 1 hour after intramuscular and 1 to 1.5 hours after oral administration. It is extensively metabolised through hydroxylation, *O*-dealkylation, and conjugation, less than 5% being excreted unchanged. Butorphanol and its metabolites are excreted mainly in the urine; about 11 to 14% of a parenteral dose is excreted in the bile. It crosses the placenta.

Uses. Butorphanol tartrate is an analgesic with actions and uses similar to those of morphine (see p.1020). In addition, it has weak narcotic antagonist properties. Analgesia is usually apparent within 30 minutes of intramuscular injection and may last for 3 to 4 hours.

For the relief of moderate to severe pain, butorphanol tartrate is given in doses of 1 to 4 mg every 3 to 4 hours by intramuscular injection. It may also be given in doses of 0.5 to 2 mg by intravenous injection.

Butorphanol tartrate has also been given by mouth in doses of 4 to 16 mg.

Reviews of the actions and uses of butorphanol.— R. C. Heel *et al.*, *Drugs*, 1978, *16*, 473; *Med. Lett.*, 1978, *20*, 111; B. Ameer and F. J. Salter, *Am. J. Hosp. Pharm.*, 1979, *36*, 1683; L. D. Vandam, *New Engl. J. Med.*, 1980, *302*, 381; J. R. Lewis, *J. Am. med. Ass.*, 1980, *243*, 1465.

Anaesthesia. *Premedication.* Intramuscular injections of butorphanol 1 or 2 mg with promethazine 25 or 50 mg and atropine 0.5 mg were used successfully as premedication in 109 patients being prepared for major surgery. Satisfactory sedation was obtained in 97% of the patients, with a mean onset time of 8 minutes.— M. Lippmann *et al.*, *J. int. med. Res.*, 1978, *6*, 455.

Further references: A. Delpizzo, *Curr. ther. Res.*, 1976, *20*, 763; L. C. Stehling and H. L. Zauder, *J. int. med. Res.*, 1978, *6*, 384.

Analgesia. In a double-blind study in 93 patients, butorphanol tartrate 8 mg was more effective in relieving musculoskeletal pain than codeine phosphate 60 mg. Both drugs were given by mouth four times daily for 3 days.— M. M. Gilbert *et al.*, *J. int. med. Res.*, 1978, *6*, 14.

See also below under Analgesia, Postoperative.

In labour. In a double-blind study in 200 women butorphanol 1 or 2 mg was as effective as pethidine 40 or 80 mg in relieving moderate to severe pain during the first stage of labour. Both drugs were given intravenously. The incidence of side-effects was less in patients receiving butorphanol.— R. Hodgkinson *et al.*, *J. int. med. Res.*, 1979, *7*, 224.

Further references: A. L. Maduska and M. Hajghassemali, *Can. Anaesth. Soc. J.*, 1978, *25*, 398.

Postoperative. Significant analgesia developed 1 minute after butorphanol 2 mg by intravenous injection in postoperative patients, with a peak after 4 to 5 minutes and duration of at least 60 minutes.— M. Lippmann *et al.*, *Curr. ther. Res.*, 1977, *22*, 276.

In a study of 41 patients with moderate to severe postoperative pain, significant analgesia occurred 30 minutes after administration of butorphanol tartrate 4 mg intramuscularly; the effect was greatest after 1 hour and persisted for up to 4 hours. The most common side-effect was sedation.— J. F. Zeedick, *Curr. ther. Res.*, 1977, *22*, 707.

Butorphanol 1 or 2 mg was as effective as pethidine 40 or 80 mg, each given by intramuscular injection in a double-blind study of 299 patients with moderate or severe postoperative pain. The incidence of side-effects was less in the group receiving butorphanol.— L. C. Stehling and H. L. Zauder, *J. int. med. Res.*, 1978, *6*, 306.

In a double-blind study in 127 women with episiotomy pain, butorphanol tartrate 8 or 16 mg was more effective in relieving pain and had a longer duration of action than codeine phosphate 60 mg. Both drugs were given by mouth four times daily.— H. M. Levin *et al.*, *J. int. med. Res.*, 1978, *6*, 24. Butorphanol tartrate and codeine phosphate produced similar effects in a double-blind study of 54 patients with postoperative pain.— J. F. Zeedick, *Curr. med. Res. Opinion*, 1979, *6*, 178.

Butorphanol tartrate 4 mg by mouth and paracetamol 650 mg each provided analgesia in a study of 120 patients with moderate to severe postoperative pain. A combination of the 2 analgesics provided greater analgesia for a longer period.— M. Lippmann *et al.*, *Clin. Pharmac. Ther.*, 1980, *27*, 267.

Further references: A. B. Dobkin *et al.*, *Clin. Pharmac. Ther.*, 1975, *18*, 547; A. Delpizzo, *Curr. ther. Res.*, 1976, *20*, 221; M. S. Gilbert *et al.*, *Clin. Pharmac. Ther.*, 1976, *20*, 359; M. Lippmann *et al.*, *Curr. ther. Res.*, 1977, *21*, 427; F. M. Galloway *et al.*, *Can. Anaesth. Soc. J.*, 1977, *24*, 90; W. C. North and D. R. Tielens, *Clin. Pharmac. Ther.*, 1977, *21*, 112; R. E. S. Young, *J. int. med. Res.*, 1977, *5*, 422; M. Lippmann *et al.*, *Curr. ther. Res.*, 1979, *26*, 181.

Preparations

Butorphanol Tartrate Injection *(U.S.P.)*. A sterile solution of butorphanol tartrate in Water for Injections. It may contain a suitable preservative and buffer. pH 3 to 5.5. Protect from light.

Proprietary Preparations

Stadol *(Bristol-Myers Pharmaceuticals, UK)*. Butorphanol tartrate, available as an injection containing 2 mg per ml, in vials of 1 and 2 ml. (Also available as Stadol in *Canad.*, *USA*).

6211-b

Codeine *(B.P., Eur. P., U.S.P.).* Codein.; Codeinum; Morphine Methyl Ether; Metilmorfina.

3-*O*-Methylmorphine monohydrate.

$C_{18}H_{21}NO_3,H_2O$=317.4.

CAS — 76-57-3 (anhydrous); 6059-47-8 (monohydrate).

Pharmacopoeias. In *Arg., Belg., Br., Eur., Fr., Ger., Int., It., Mex., Neth., Pol., Port., Roum., Rus., Span., Swiss, Turk.*, and *U.S.*

Codeine is obtained from opium or made by methylating morphine. It occurs as odourless colourless crystals or white crystalline powder with a bitter taste. M.p. 154° to 158° with a range of not more than 2°. It effloresces slowly in dry air and is affected by light.

Soluble 1 in 120 of water, 1 in 15 of boiling water, 1 in 2 of alcohol, 1 in 0.5 of chloroform, and 1 in 50 of ether; soluble in amyl alcohol, carbon disulphide, methyl alcohol, and in excess of aqueous ammonia; very soluble in dilute acids; slightly soluble in light petroleum; practically insoluble in excess of potassium hydroxide solution. A solution in water is laevorotatory. A 0.5% solution in water has a pH of more than 9. Solutions of codeine salts are **sterilised** by autoclaving or by filtration. **Incompatible** with bromides, iodides, and salts of heavy metals. **Store** in airtight containers. Protect from light.

Incompatibility. In the presence of moisture at 60°, aspirin acetylated codeine to 6-acetylcodeine. There was no reaction at room temperature at low moisture levels. The apparent activity and toxicity should not be altered by the acetylation according to the work of W.R. Buckett and others (*J. Pharm. Pharmac.*, 1964, *16*, 174).— A. L. Jacobs *et al.*, *J. pharm. Sci.*, 1966, *55*, 893. See also R. N. Galante *et al.*, *ibid.*, 1979, *68*, 1494.

6212-v

Codeine Hydrochloride.

$C_{18}H_{21}NO_3,HCl,2H_2O$=371.9.

CAS — 1422-07-7 (anhydrous).

Pharmacopoeias. In *Aust., Hung., Roum.*, and *Swiss.*

A white odourless crystalline powder with a bitter taste. **Soluble** 1 in 30 of water, 1 in 100 of alcohol (90%), and 1 in 800 of chloroform. **Protect** from light.

6213-g

Codeine Phosphate *(B.P., Eur. P., U.S.P.).*

Codeinii Phosphas; Codeini Phosphas; Methylmorphine Phosphate.

$C_{18}H_{21}NO_3,H_3PO_4,\frac{1}{2}H_2O$=406.4.

CAS — 52-28-8 (anhydrous); 41444-62-6 (hemihydrate); 5913-76-8 (sesquihydrate).

Pharmacopoeias. In all pharmacopoeias examined. All specify $1\frac{1}{2}H_2O$ or $\frac{1}{2}H_2O$.

Small odourless colourless crystals or white crystalline powder with a bitter taste.

Soluble 1 in 4 of water, 1 in 450 of alcohol, and 1 in 125 of boiling alcohol; practically insoluble in chloroform and ether. A solution in water is laevorotatory. A 4% solution in water has a pH of 4.2 to 5. A 7.29% solution is iso-osmotic with serum.**Sterilisation, incompatibilities** and **storage** as for Codeine, p.1004.

Incompatibility. Codeine phosphate was incompatible with phenobarbitone sodium, forming a codeine-phenobarbitone complex, and with potassium iodide, forming crystals of codeine periodide.— V. H. Bruin and W. H. Oliver, *Australas. J. Pharm.*, 1957, *38*, 226.

There was loss of clarity when intravenous solutions of codeine phosphate, anileridine hydrochloride, levorphanol tartrate, or methadone hydrochloride were mixed with those of aminophylline, ammonium chloride, amylobarbitone sodium, chlorothiazide sodium, heparin sodium, methicillin sodium, nitrofurantoin sodium, novobiocin sodium, pentobarbitone sodium, phenobarbitone sodium, phenytoin sodium, quinalbarbitone sodium, sodium bicarbonate, sodium iodide, sulphadiazine sodium, sulphafurazole sodium, or thiopentone sodium.— J. A. Patel and G. L. Phillips, *Am. J. Hosp. Pharm.*, 1966, *23*, 409.

6214-q

Codeine Sulphate. Codeine Sulfate *(U.S.P.).*

$(C_{18}H_{21}NO_3)_2,H_2SO_4,3H_2O$=750.9.

CAS — 1420-53-7 (anhydrous); 6854-40-6 (trihydrate).

Pharmacopoeias. In *U.S.*

White crystals or crystalline powder. **Soluble** 1 in 30 of water and 1 in 1300 of alcohol; practically insoluble in chloroform and ether. A solution in water is laevorotatory. **Store** in airtight containers. Protect from light.

Dependence. Prolonged use of high doses of codeine has produced dependence of the morphine type (see p.1018) in a very small proportion of users. Codeine produces less euphoria and sedation than morphine and is not a completely satisfactory substitute for morphine in morphine addicts. Withdrawal symptoms develop more slowly than with morphine and are milder.

A report on the use of codeine and glutethimide in combination by addicts.— J. N. DiGiacomo and C. L. King, *Int. J. Addict.*, 1970, *5*, 279.

For an extensive review of the incidence of codeine dependence, tolerance, withdrawal symptoms, and risk of abuse, indicating a low risk to public health from the common use of codeine and its preparations, see N. B. Eddy *et al.*, *Codeine and its Alternates for Pain and Cough Relief*, Geneva, World Health Organization, 1970. See also *Bull. Wld Hlth Org.*, 1968, *38*, 673.

Pregnancy and the neonate. Neonatal withdrawal symptoms associated with maternal use of codeine.— G. Van Leeuwen *et al.*, *Pediatrics*, 1965, *36*, 635.

Tolerance. Though the miosis that followed a single dose of codeine in healthy subjects was not reversed by nalorphine, when codeine was given in increasingly high doses as rapidly as the development of tolerance would allow (up to 240 mg by mouth 4 times daily) most subjects were found to react positively (with dilatation of the pupil) to the nalorphine test by the third day. When codeine was given intravenously by continuous infusion at a rate of 30 mg hourly to induce acute tolerance, after 8 hours 3 of 4 volunteers gave distinct positive reactions to nalorphine eye tests.— H. W. Elliott *et al.*, *Clin. Pharmac. Ther.*, 1967, *8*, 78.

Adverse Effects. As for Morphine, p.1019.

In therapeutic doses codeine is much less liable than morphine to produce adverse effects. Following large doses of codeine, excitement and, in children, convulsions may also occur.

Increases in intrabiliary pressure were observed after administration of 10 to 20 mg of codeine hydrochloride to 12 patients after cholecystectomy.— B. Jacobsson *et al.*, *Acta chir. scand.*, 1961, *122*, 407.

Allergy. For reports of allergic reactions to codeine, see under Morphine.

Overdosage. A report of acute codeine overdosage in 1 patient.— D. H. Huffman and R. L. Ferguson, *Johns Hopkins med. J.*, 1975, *136*, 183.

Blood concentrations of codeine ranged from 1.4 to 5.6 µg per ml in 8 adults whose deaths were attributed primarily to codeine overdosage. Pulmonary oedema was the main drug-related finding at autopsy.— J. A. Wright *et al.*, *Clin. Toxicol.*, 1975, *8*, 457. A report of pulmonary oedema occurring as a result of codeine overdosage.— J. Sklar and R. M. Timms, *Chest*, 1977, *72*, 230.

An evaluation of codeine intoxication in 430 children. Symptoms in decreasing order of frequency included sedation, rash, miosis, vomiting, itching, ataxia, and swelling of the skin. Respiratory failure occurred in 8 children and 2 died. All 8 had taken 5 mg or more per kg body-weight. In spite of this it was considered that a single overdose of 5 to 15 mg per kg would generally be tolerated by small children producing symptoms of overdosage without fatality. Treatment should include attention to respiration, emesis or gastric lavage, naloxone and, in all cases, charcoal and purgatives.— K. E. von Mühlendahl *et al.*, *Lancet*, 1976, *2*, 303.

The serum-concentration of codeine in a 3-month-old infant treated with a cough mixture containing codeine phosphate 10 mg per 5 ml was 12 µg per ml 3 days after the last dose. The infant subsequently died.— H. H. Ivey and J. Kattwinkel, *Pediatrics*, 1976, *57*, 164. A 3-month-old infant who had been born prematurely developed near fatal apnoea after two 5-ml doses of Actifed Compound Linctus [each 5 ml contains 10 mg of codeine phosphate]. Even if the recommended dose of 2.5 ml thrice daily for a 3-month-old infant had been given the codeine intake would have been dangerously high; there is clearly an urgent need to revise the dose recommendations for this product as they apply to young infants. Moreover, when prescribing for infants, prematurity should be taken into account.— T. C. R. Wilkes *et al.* (letter), *Lancet*, 1981, *1*, 1166.

Pregnancy and the neonate. Of 50 282 children born to mothers monitored by the Collaborative Perinatal Project, 1564 were found to have been exposed to narcotic analgesics, and possibly other drugs, at some time during the first 4 months of the pregnancy. Although there was little evidence of association between malformations and narcotic analgesic exposure in general a possible association between respiratory malformations and codeine (563 exposures) was noted.— O. P. Heinonen *et al.*, *Birth Defects and Drugs in Pregnancy*, Littleton MA, Publishing Sciences Group, 1977, p. 286.

Treatment of Adverse Effects and Precautions. As for Morphine, p.1019.

Codeine phosphate 50 mg alone and in combination with alcohol 0.5 g per kg body-weight had a deleterious effect on driving skills in both normal and emergency situations in a simulated driving test.— M. Linnoila and S. Häkkinen, *Clin. Pharmac. Ther.*, 1974, *15*, 368.

Severe narcosis occurred in a patient with hypocalcaemia from hypoparathyroidism when given codeine phosphate 30 mg every six hours. Naloxone reversed the narcosis.— D. F. Levine, *Postgrad. med. J.*, 1980, *56*, 736.

For a report questioning the use of codeine in antibiotic-induced diarrhoea, see Diphenoxylate Hydrochloride, p.1010.

Interactions. Codeine phosphate was adsorbed by light kaolin *in vitro*.— S. K. S. Yu *et al.*, *Aust. J. Pharm.*, 1976, *57*, 468.

Absorption and Fate. Codeine and its salts are absorbed from the gastro-intestinal tract. Ingestion of codeine phosphate produces peak plasma-codeine concentrations in about one hour. Codeine is metabolised by *O*-and *N*-demethylation in the liver to morphine and norcodeine. Codeine and its metabolites are excreted almost entirely by the kidney, mainly as conjugates with glucuronic acid.

The plasma half-life has been reported to be between 3 and 4 hours after administration by mouth or intramuscular injection.

After the administration of codeine phosphate 10 or 20 mg to 5 volunteers, normorphine was detected in the urine, in addition to other known metabolites. The quantities of each were total codeine 70%, total morphine 10%, total norcodeine 9%, and normorphine less than 4%.— W. O. R. Ebbighausen *et al.*, *J. pharm. Sci.*, 1973, *62*, 146.

The maximal rate of codeine metabolism appeared to be 30 mg per hour.— N. Nomof *et al.*, *Clin. Pharmac. Ther.*, 1974, *15*, 215.

A crossover study in 6 healthy subjects comparing oral administration of codeine phosphate 65 mg in analgesic tablets also containing aspirin, phenacetin, and caffeine, with intramuscular injection of codeine phosphate 65 mg. Following oral administration absorption of codeine phosphate was rapid with peak plasma-codeine concentrations of 102 to 140 ng per ml appearing after 0.75 to 1 hour; following intramuscular administration peak concentrations of 195 to 340 ng per ml appeared after 0.25 to 1 hour. The plasma half-life was between 3 and 4 hours following either route and the calculated bioavailability of the codeine in the tablets was a mean of 53% (range 42 to 71%) compared with the intramuscular preparation, presumably due to first-pass metabolism in the intestine and liver; this contrasted with the very low bioavailability of morphine following administration by mouth, presumably owing to more effective first-pass metabolism of morphine.— J. W. A. Findlay *et al.*, *Clin. Pharmac. Ther.*, 1977, *22*, 439.

In 6 healthy male subjects given radioactive codeine phosphate 30 mg by mouth peak plasma radioactivity occurred about 1 hour after administration and fell with a half-life of 3.1 hours. Within 4 hours a mean of 55.2% of the administered dose had been excreted in the urine with 95.1% being eliminated after 2 days. Similar results were obtained when the subjects were given 2 doses of 25 mg in solution 4 hours apart.— W. D. Bechtel and K. Sinterhauf, *Arzneimittel-Forsch.*, 1978,

28, 308.

Following the administration of codeine 30 mg by mouth to 2 healthy subjects hydrocodone, norhydrocodone, 6α-hydrocodol, and 6β-hydrocodol in addition to known metabolites were detected in the urine.— E. J. Cone *et al.*, *J. Pharm. Pharmac.*, 1979, *31*, 314.

Further references: D. P. Vaughan and A. H. Beckett, *J. Pharm. Pharmac.*, 1973, *25*, 104P (bioavailability); M. D. Solomon, *Clin. Toxicol.*, 1974, *7*, 255 (metabolism); J. W. A. Findlay *et al.*, *Clin. Pharmac. Ther.*, 1978, *24*, 60 (plasma concentrations of codeine and metabolites).

Protein binding. Codeine was about 25% bound to human serum proteins.— J. Judis, *J. pharm. Sci.*, 1977, *66*, 803.

Uses. Codeine is an analgesic with uses similar to those of morphine (see p.1020) but it is much less potent as an analgesic and has only mild sedative effects.

It is administered by mouth as the phosphate or sulphate in the form of linctuses for the relief of cough and as tablets for the relief of mild to moderate pain. The hydrochloride has also been given by mouth. The phosphate is also given by injection for the relief of pain.

Codeine and its salts are given in doses of 15 to 60 mg up to 6 times a day for the relief of pain. If these doses fail to relieve pain, larger doses rarely succeed and may give rise to restlessness and excitement. Children may be given 500 μg per kg body-weight 4 to 6 times daily.

Codeine and its salts are used to allay unproductive cough, usually in doses of 10 to 20 mg every 4 to 6 hours, to a maximum total of 120 mg in 24 hours. Children may be given up to 250 μg per kg every 4 to 6 hours. It is less constipating than morphine but it is used as tablets or in mixtures for the relief of diarrhoea.

Codeine, usually as the phosphate, is often administered by mouth with aspirin or paracetamol. Codeine camsylate and codeine hydrobromide are also used.

A comprehensive review of codeine as an analgesic and antitussive in relation to its dependence-producing potential and adverse effects compared with similar drugs. For mild to moderate pain codeine was effective in relatively non-toxic doses but the side-effects of high doses made it less useful than alternative drugs for severe pain. For cough suppression, alternatives were available with a lower dependence-producing liability and less side-effects but none of them had yet been proved to be therapeutically superior to codeine.— N. B. Eddy *et al.*, *Codeine and its Alternates for Pain and Cough Relief*, Geneva, World Health Organization, 1970; *idem*, *Bull. Wld Hlth Org.*, 1968, *38*, 673; *idem*, 1969, *40*, 1, 425, 639, and 721.

A study which suggests that codeine might facilitate acquisition, retention, and recall of simple learning.— R. Liljequist and M. J. Mattila, *Br. J. clin. Pharmac.*, 1977, *4*, 654P.

Administration. In children. On the basis of available data, codeine and other opiate cough suppressants should rarely be administered to children less than 6 to 12 months old. They should not be given in productive cough. When indicated for the treatment of nonproductive cough which interferes with sleep or school attendance, either codeine or dextromethorphan should be recommended in the form of single-ingredient preparations.— S. Segal *et al.*, *Pediatrics*, 1978, *62*, 118.

Administration in haemophilia. For the use of codeine in haemophiliacs, see Choline Salicylate, p.249.

Administration in renal failure. Codeine could be given in usual doses to patients with renal failure.— W. M. Bennett *et al.*, *Ann. intern. Med.*, 1980, *93*, 62.

Analgesia. Postpartum. In a double-blind study involving 5 groups of 46 postepisiotomy patients codeine sulphate 30 or 60 mg or dextropropoxyphene napsylate 50 or 100 mg, repeated after 4 hours, produced a significant increase in analgesia when compared to single doses or placebo. Adverse reactions were similar for all 5 treatments.— C. M. Gruber, *J. Am. med. Ass.*, 1977, *237*, 2734.

During a study of analgesics in postpartum uterine pain it was noted that codeine sulphate 60 mg was no more effective than placebo in this type of pain.— S. S. Bloomfield *et al.*, *Clin. Pharmac. Ther.*, 1977, *21*, 414.

Gastro-intestinal disorders. For a comparison of the effect of Lomotil tablets and codeine phosphate tablets on diarrhoea, see Diphenoxylate Hydrochloride, p.1011.

In a comparison of the effects of codeine phosphate, diphenoxylate (as Lomotil), and ispaghula (as Isogel), taken before meals, on ileostomy output in 18 patients only codeine produced a significant fall in output. This was achieved by a reduction of water and electrolyte output with consequent thickening of its consistency. With Isogel, ileostomy output was more viscid but water and electrolyte output was increased and there was danger of exacerbating water and electrolyte depletion.— C. R. Newton, *Gut*, 1978, *19*, 377.

In a double-blind study in 11 patients with chronic diarrhoea, loperamide 2 mg, diphenoxylate 5 mg with atropine, and codeine phosphate 30 mg had comparable antidiarrhoeal activity.— C. D. Shee and R. E. Pounder, *Br. med. J.*, 1980, *280*, 524.

For a report questioning the use of codeine in antibiotic-induced diarrhoea, see Diphenoxylate Hydrochloride, p.1010.

Narcolepsy. A 57-year-old man who had suffered from Gelineau's syndrome (rapid eye movement narcolepsy) for nearly 30 years noted disappearance of his narcolepsy, cataplexy, sleep paralysis, and hypnagogic hallucinations on receiving tablets of codeine phosphate 30 mg up to 8 times daily for Crohn's disease. Three years later he had an attack of cataplexy on the fifth day of a week when he was unable to obtain codeine phosphate. Both his bowel and his narcoleptic problems have subsequently been completely controlled with pentazocine tablets.— J. M. Harper (letter), *Lancet*, 1981, *1*, 92.

Preparations of Codeine and its Salts

For some other preparations containing codeine phosphate, see under Aspirin, p.243..

Injections

Codeine Phosphate Injection *(U.S.P.)*. A sterile solution of codeine phosphate in Water for Injections. pH 3 to 6. Protect from light. It should not be used if it is more than slightly discoloured or contains a precipitate.

Linctuses

Codeine Linctus *(A.P.F.)*. Linct. Codein. Codeine phosphate 25 mg, water 0.5 ml, glycerol 1 ml, squill oxymel 2 ml, concentrated chloroform water 0.1 ml, syrup to 5 ml. *Dose.* 5 ml.

Codeine Linctus *(B.P.)*. Linct. Codein. Codeine phosphate 15 mg, lemon syrup 1 ml, benzoic acid solution, chloroform spirit, and water of each 0.1 ml, compound tartrazine solution 0.05 ml, syrup to 5 ml. Protect from light. When a dose less than or not a multiple of 5 ml is prescribed the linctus should be diluted to 5 ml, or a multiple, with syrup. Such dilutions must be freshly prepared and not used more than 2 weeks after issue.
Dose. 5 ml.

Diabetic Codeine Linctus *(B.P.C. 1973)*. Codeine phosphate 15 mg, lemon spirit 0.005 ml, citric acid monohydrate 25 mg, benzoic acid solution 0.1 ml, chloroform spirit 0.1 ml, water 0.1 ml, compound tartrazine solution 0.05 ml, non-crystallising sorbitol solution to 5 ml. Protect from light. *Dose.* 5 ml. Each 5 ml contains about 4.2 g of carbohydrate providing about 67 kJ (16 kcal).

Diabetic Codeine Linctus *(Roy. Melb. Hosp.)*. Codeine phosphate 20 mg, glycerol 2 ml, concentrated chloroform water 0.125 ml, water to 5 ml.

Paediatric Codeine Linctus *(B.P.C. 1973)*. Paediatric Codeine Mixture; Codeine Linctus Paediatric. Codeine linctus 1 ml, syrup to 5 ml. It contains 3 mg of codeine phosphate in 5 ml. Protect from light. *Dose.* Children, up to 1 year, 5 ml; 1 to 5 years, 10 ml.

Syrups

Codeine Phosphate Syrup *(B.P.C. 1973)*. Syr. Codein. Phos. Codeine phosphate 25 mg, chloroform spirit 0.125 ml, freshly boiled and cooled water 0.075 ml, syrup to 5 ml. Protect from light. *Dose.* 2.5 to 10 ml.
Codeine Syrup *(A.P.F.)* has a similar formula containing concentrated chloroform water 0.075 ml instead of chloroform spirit.

Sirupus Codeinae *(Span. P.)*. Codeine 200 mg, alcohol (60%) 5 g, syrup to 100 g.
Arg. P., *Belg. P.*, *Port. P.*, and *Roum. P.* include similar preparations.

Syrupus Codeini *(Nord. P.)*. Codeine phosphate 250 mg, alcohol 250 mg, water 2 g, and black currant syrup 97.5 g.

Tablets

Codeine Phosphate Tablets *(B.P., U.S.P.)*. Codeine Phos. Tab.; Compressi Codeini Phosphatis. Tablets containing codeine phosphate. Protect from light.
Store in airtight containers.

Codeine Sulfate Tablets *(U.S.P.)*. Tablets containing codeine sulphate.

Proprietary Preparations of Codeine Salts

For some other proprietary preparations containing codeine phosphate, see under Aspirin, p.243, and Paracetamol, p.270..

Bepro *(Wallace Mfg Chem., UK: Farillon, UK)*. Syrup containing in each 5 ml codeine sulphate 6.25 mg, papaverine hydrochloride 625 μg, calcium iodide 50 mg, and glycerol 250 mg. For cough. *Dose.* 10 ml every 4 hours; children, 1.25 to 5 ml.

Diarrest *(Galen, UK)*. Liquid containing in each 5 ml codeine phosphate 5 mg, dicyclomine hydrochloride 2.5 mg, sodium chloride 50 mg, potassium chloride 40 mg, and sodium citrate 50 mg. For non-specific diarrhoea. *Dose.* 20 ml four times daily with water; children, 4 to 5 years, 5 ml; 6 to 9 years, 10 ml; 10 to 13 years, 15 ml.

A reminder that the essential consequence of acute diarrhoea is dehydration, and the fundamental treatment is rehydration.— W. A. M. Cutting and W. C. Marshall (letter), *Lancet*, 1979, *2*, 1022.

Kaodene *(Crookes Products, UK)*. Suspension containing in each 10 ml codeine phosphate 10 mg and light kaolin 3 g. For diarrhoea. *Dose.* 20 ml three or four times daily; children, 5 to 12 years, 10 ml.

A reminder that the essential consequence of acute diarrhoea is dehydration, and the fundamental treatment is rehydration.— W. A. M. Cutting and W. C. Marshall (letter), *Lancet*, 1979, *2*, 1022.

Tercolix *(Vestric, UK)*. An elixir containing in each 5 ml codeine phosphate 15 mg, terpin hydrate 30 mg, menthol 10 mg, pumilio pine oil 0.003 ml, cineole 0.004 ml, and glycerol 2 g (suggested diluent, glycerol and syrup: equal parts). For cough. *Dose.* 5 to 10 ml in a little warm water.

Other Proprietary Names of Codeine and its Salts

Codeine.—Codicept, Codipertussin *(resin complex) (both Ger.)*; Codeine Phosphate.—Codeinfos, Codeisan *(both Spain)*; Codlin *(Austral.)*; Paveral *(Canad.)*; Solcodein *(Spain)*; Tricodein *(Ger.)*.

6215-p

Dextromoramide.

Dextrodiphenopyrine; *d*-Moramid; Pyrrolamidol. (+)-1-(3-Methyl-4-morpholino-2,2-diphenylbutyryl)pyrrolidine.
$C_{25}H_{32}N_2O_2$=392.5.

CAS — 357-56-2.

A white, odourless, amorphous or microcrystalline powder with a bitter taste. M.p. 184°. Practically **insoluble** in water and light petroleum; soluble 1 in 50 of alcohol, 1 in 3 of chloroform, 1 in 30 of isopropyl alcohol, and 1 in 45 of methyl alcohol; slightly soluble in ether.

6216-s

Dextromoramide Tartrate *(B.P.)*.

Dextromoramide Acid Tartrate; Bitartrate de Dextromoramide.
$C_{25}H_{32}N_2O_2,C_4H_6O_6$=542.6.

CAS — 2922-44-3.

Pharmacopoeias. In *Br.*

A white odourless crystalline or amorphous powder with a bitter taste. M.p. about 190° with slight decomposition. Dextromoramide tartrate 6.9 mg is approximately equivalent to 5 mg of dextromoramide.

Soluble 1 in 25 of water, 1 in 85 of alcohol, 1 in 100 of acetone, and 1 in 40 of methyl alcohol; slightly soluble in chloroform and isopropyl alcohol; very slightly soluble in ether; practically insoluble in solutions of alkali hydroxides. A solution in 0.1M hydrochloric acid is dextrorotatory. A 1% solution in water has a pH of 3 to 4. Solutions may be **sterilised** by autoclaving or by filtration.

Dependence. The use of dextromoramide, especially for chronic conditions, may produce dependence of the morphine type (see p.1018).

In a case of marked dependence on dextromoramide a 68-year-old man with severe pain had 4400 tablets during 10½ months. Substitution with dihydrocodeine was unsuccessful but levorphanol 1.5 mg four times daily in conjunction with dihydrocodeine, chlorpromazine, and amitriptyline appeared to control the pain.— J. Cormack (letter), *Br. med. J.*, 1967, *1*, 362. Another similar report.— B. A. Juby (letter), *ibid.*

Gross abuse of dextromoramide in Australia.— D. B. Newgreen, *Aust. J. Pharm.*, 1980, *61*, 641.

Adverse Effects, Treatment, and Precautions. As for Morphine, p.1019.

From results of the use of dextromoramide intramuscularly in 107 patients in labour, it was not considered to be a useful or safe analgesic because of the incidence of severe and dangerous side-effects, including severe respiratory depression and deep narcosis. Nausea and vomiting occurred frequently and there was a threefold increase in the incidence of lethargy in babies. These effects usually occurred with doses of 10 mg or more.— W. P. Black, *Practitioner*, 1966, *197*, 348.

Unpleasant hallucinations occurred in 2 patients given dextromoramide 10 mg and chlorpromazine 25 mg.— D. P. Mason (letter), *Br. med. J.*, 1968, *1*, 55.

Uses. Dextromoramide tartrate is an analgesic related to methadone used in the treatment of moderate or severe pain. It is not recommended for use in obstetric analgesia. It is given by mouth, by rectum, or by subcutaneous or intramuscular injection, and similar analgesic effects are claimed for the same dose whether given by mouth or by injection. The analgesic effect begins after about 10 minutes and its duration of action is about 4 hours.

The usual dose is the equivalent of dextromoramide 5 mg by mouth or by injection increased if necessary up to 20 mg by mouth or 15 mg by injection.

Dextromoramide is also given rectally as suppositories containing the equivalent of 10 mg.

An initial dose equivalent to 88 µg per kg body-weight has been suggested for use in children.

Manufacturer's comments mainly on the analgesic effects of dextromoramide.— A. J. Grace (letter), *Br. med. J.*, 1980, *281*, 1285. Criticism. Dextromoramide was considered less suitable as an analgesic than morphine, diamorphine, or phenazocine for the control of pain in terminal illness.— A. T. Judd *et al.* (letter), *ibid.*, 1981, *282*, 75.

Preparations

Dextromoramide Injection *(B.P.C. 1973)*. Dextromoramide Tartrate Injection. A sterile solution of dextromoramide tartrate with sodium chloride in Water for Injections. Potency is expressed in terms of the equivalent amount of dextromoramide.

Dextromoramide Tablets *(B.P.)*. Tablets containing dextromoramide tartrate. Potency is expressed in terms of the equivalent amount of dextromoramide.

Palfium *(MCP Pharmaceuticals, UK)*. Dextromoramide tartrate, available as **Ampoules** each containing the equivalent of 5 or 10 mg of dextromoramide; as **Suppositories** each containing the equivalent of 10 mg of dextromoramide; and as scored **Tablets** each containing the equivalent of 5 or 10 mg of dextromoramide. (Also available as Palfium in *Austral., Belg., Denm., Fr., Ger., Neth., Switz., S.Afr.*).

Other Proprietary Names

Jetrium *(Ger.)*; Narcolo *(Ital.)*.

6217-w

Dextropropoxyphene Hydrochloride.

(B.P.). Propoxyphene Hydrochloride *(U.S.P.)*. (+)-(1*S*,2*R*)-1-Benzyl-3-dimethylamino-2-methyl-1-phenylpropyl propionate hydrochloride.

$C_{22}H_{29}NO_2,HCl=375.9$.

CAS — 469-62-5 (dextropropoxyphene); 1639-60-7 (hydrochloride).

Pharmacopoeias. In *Br.*, *Braz.*, and *U.S.*

A white or slightly yellow odourless powder with a bitter taste. M.p. 163.5° to 168.5° with a range of not more than 3°.

Soluble 1 in 0.3 of water, 1 in 1.5 of alcohol, and 1 in 0.6 of chloroform; soluble in acetone; practically insoluble in ether. A solution in water is dextrorotatory. Solutions for injection are **sterilised** by filtration. **Store** in airtight containers.

6218-e

Dextropropoxyphene Napsylate *(B.P.)*.

Propoxyphene Napsylate *(U.S.P.)*. Dextropropoxyphene naphthalene-2-sulphonate monohydrate.

$C_{22}H_{29}NO_2,C_{10}H_8O_3S,H_2O=565.7$.

CAS — 17140-78-2 (anhydrous); 26570-10-5 (monohydrate).

Pharmacopoeias. In *Br.* and *U.S.*

An odourless white powder with a bitter taste. M.p. 158° to 165° with a range of not more than 4°. Dextropropoxyphene napsylate 100 mg is approximately equivalent to 66 mg of dextropropoxyphene hydrochloride. Practically **insoluble** in water; soluble 1 in 13 to 15 of alcohol and 1 in 3 of chloroform; soluble in acetone and methyl alcohol. A solution in alcohol or chloroform is dextrorotatory. **Store** in airtight containers.

The napsylate is more stable than the hydrochloride in formulations containing aspirin.

Dependence. Prolonged use of dextropropoxyphene hydrochloride may lead to dependence of the morphine type (see p.1018).

During an epidemic of dextropropoxyphene abuse among American soldiers 13 died, pulmonary oedema being the primary finding at post mortem. Respiratory arrest, psychotic reactions, and dependence also occurred. In 7 patients who became dependent on the intravenous use of dextropropoxyphene, abscesses, cellulitis, thrombophlebitis, or sclerosis of the veins developed within 6 to 12 weeks despite the use of sterile vehicles and techniques. Withdrawal symptoms were mild.— F. S. Tennant, *Archs intern. Med.*, 1973, *132*, 191.

For further reports of dependence, see J. L. Claghorn and J. C. Schooler, *J. Am. med. Ass.*, 1966, *196*, 1089; R. C. Wolfe *et al.*, *Ann. intern. Med.*, 1969, *70*, 773; C. H. Salguero *et al.* (letter), *J. Am. med. Ass.*, 1969, *210*, 135; F. J. Kane and J. L. Norton (letter), *J. Am. med. Ass.*, 1970, *211*, 300; J. R. Lewis, *ibid.*, 1974, *228*, 1155; R. M. Whittington (letter), *Lancet*, 1979, *2*, 743.

Pregnancy and the neonate. Withdrawal symptoms occurred in an infant born to a woman who had taken dextropropoxyphene during pregnancy, the last dose being taken 11 hours before delivery.— W. W. Quillian and C. A. Dunn, *J. Am. med. Ass.*, 1976, *235*, 2128. See also H. K. Tyson, *J. Pediat.*, 1974, *85*, 684.

Treatment of dependence. Treatment of dextropropoxyphene dependence in a 41-year-old woman who had a history of multiple drug abuse consisted of withdrawing dextropropoxyphene and giving methadone on a reducing scale for 10 days.— R. Wall *et al.*, *Br. med. J.*, 1980, *280*, 1213. Comments.— N. Mellor (letter), *ibid.*, *281*, 617. Reply.— R. Wall (letter), *ibid.*

Adverse Effects. As for Morphine, p.1019, although in the recommended dosage the adverse effects of dextropropoxyphene are less marked. Gastro-intestinal effects are the most common. Liver impairment has been reported.

There are a disturbing number of fatalities from either accidental or intentional overdosage with dextropropoxyphene. Many reports emphasize the rapidity with which death ensues; death within an hour of overdosage is considered by some not to be uncommon. Overdosage is often complicated by patients also taking alcohol and using mixed preparations such as dextropropoxyphene with paracetamol or aspirin.

Symptoms of overdosage are similar to those of morphine poisoning (see p.1019). In addition patients may experience convulsions and psychotic reactions. There may be pulmonary oedema and cardiac arrhythmias.

Dextropropoxyphene injections are painful and have a very destructive effect on soft tissues and veins.

A discussion of the hazards of dextropropoxyphene.— *Br. med. J.*, 1977, *1*, 668.

Necrotising colitis, requiring surgery, in a 27-year-old woman who had taken about 75 Distalgesic tablets (dextropropoxyphene with paracetamol) was attributed to drug-induced hypotension.— R. S. J. Briggs *et al.* (letter), *Br. med. J.*, 1977, *2*, 1478.

Effects on liver. Reports of jaundice in patients taking dextropropoxyphene without paracetamol.— G. K. Daikos and J. C. Kosmidis, *J. Am. med. Ass.*, 1975, *232*, 835; T. H. Lee and P. J. Rees, *Br. med. J.*, 1977, *2*, 296; M. J. Ford *et al.*, *ibid.*, 674; *Med. J. Aust.*, 1979, *2*, 494.

Overdosage. A report on 30 fatalities due to dextropropoxyphene poisoning. All the victims were considered to have taken Distalgesic but paracetamol was considered to be of secondary importance. The mortality-rate from dextropropoxyphene poisoning might be much higher than 15% previously reported.— D. J. L. Carson and E. D. Carson, *Lancet*, 1977, *1*, 894. The cerebral depressant effect of dextropropoxyphene was often exacerbated by alcohol.— D. J. L. Carson and E. D. Carson (letter), *Br. med. J.*, 1976, *2*, 105.

A discussion of Distalgesic overdosage with mention of 33 fatalities and 60 cases of overdosage. Death was often rapid probably due to respiratory depression. Alcohol was often taken concomitantly and would have an additive effect.— R. M. Whittington, *Br. med. J.*, 1977, *2*, 172. See also F. G. Hails and R. M. Whittington (letter), *ibid.*, 1978, *2*, 1569.

Blood and liver concentrations of dextropropoxyphene following overdosage.— T. A. Rejent *et al.*, *Clin. Toxicol.*, 1977, *11*, 43.

A report on 82 cases of Distalgesic poisoning seen in 10 years. There was a high risk of death if 20 tablets were taken with a CNS depressant.— R. J. Young and A. A. H. Lawson, *Br. med. J.*, 1980, *280*, 1045. Comment.— P. S. Dwyer and I. F. Jones (letter), *ibid.*, *281*, 60.

Neonatal Distalgesic poisoning.— J. O. Beattie *et al.* (letter), *Lancet*, 1981, *2*, 49.

Further references: D. J. Young, *Archs intern. Med.*, 1972, *129*, 62; W. Q. Sturner and J. C. Garriott, *J. Am. med. Ass.*, 1973, *223*, 1125; J. Critchley *et al.* (letter), *Br. med. J.*, 1979, *1*, 342.

Pregnancy and the neonate. A report of congenital malformations in an infant born to a woman who had taken 20 to 36 capsules of dextropropoxyphene 65 mg daily during pregnancy and for several years before. The patient also took anti-emetics and phenytoin, mainly in the 2nd trimester. It was not possible to ascertain whether the causative agent was dextropropoxyphene.— M. V. Barrow and D. E. Souder (letter), *J. Am. med. Ass.*, 1971, *217*, 1551. See also C. A. D. Ringrose (letter), *Can. med. Ass. J.*, 1972, *106*, 1058.

Treatment of Adverse Effects. As for Morphine, p.1019.

Rapid treatment of overdosage with naloxone and assisted respiration is essential. Administration of activated charcoal may be of value but dialysis is of little value.

Convulsions may be controlled with diazepam 5 to 10 mg intravenously. Stimulants should not be used because of the risk of inducing convulsions.

Patients taking overdoses of dextropropoxyphene with paracetamol will also require treatment for paracetamol poisoning, and this is described on p.269.

Mixtures of dextropropoxyphene and aspirin may be involved; the treatment of aspirin poisoning is described on p.238.

Dextropropoxyphene poisoning required intensive supportive care including airways clearance, prevention of aspiration, and artificial ventilation. Naloxone should be given to all patients with serious toxicity as well as in less severe cases where drowsiness might be the only symptom as sudden deterioration could occur at a later stage. After waking the patient should be carefully observed for at least 24 hours as naloxone has a shorter duration of action than dextropropoxyphene and further doses might be required every 4 hours. Naloxone could be used as a diagnostic test of dextropropoxyphene poisoning, no response to up to three doses of 400 µg indicating that the condition was probably due to some other sedative drug, alcohol, or cerebral anoxia. If dextropropoxyphene was taken as Distalgesic, liver damage due to paracetamol might occur. Plasma-paracetamol concentrations should be estimated and, if high, specific treatment should be started.— *Lancet*, 1977, *2*, 542. For details of the management of paracetamol overdosage, see under Paracetamol, Treatment of Adverse Effects, p.269.

For comment on the *in vitro* adsorption of dextropropoxyphene by activated charcoal, see p.79.

Precautions. As for Morphine, p.1019.

It has been suggested that severely depressed

patients should be prescribed alternative analgesics. Alcohol and other central depressants may contribute to the hazards of dextropropoxyphene. The convulsant action of high doses of dextropropoxyphene may be enhanced by central nervous system stimulants.

Effects on diagnostic tests. Ingestion of dextropropoxyphene 65 mg thrice daily by a healthy subject was associated with significant depression of the urinary 17-hydroxycorticosteroids and 17-ketosteroids.— P. E. Cryer and J. Sode, *Ann. intern. Med.*, 1971, *75*, 697, per *Int. pharm. Abstr.*, 1972, *9*, 620.

Interactions. *Carbamazepine.* For the effect of dextropropoxyphene on carbamazepine, see Carbamazepine, p.1246.

Orphenadrine. A definite drug interaction between orphenadrine and dextropropoxyphene appeared to be unlikely.— R. E. Pearson and F. J. Salter, *New Engl. J. Med.*, 1970, *282*, 1215. No interaction occurred in 5 patients given the 2 drugs.— W. H. Puckett and J. A. Visconti, *ibid.*, *283*, 544. A 34-year-old man who had been receiving dextropropoxyphene for several days without ill effects developed marked mental confusion, anxiety, and tremors simulating stroke on the second day of receiving concomitant orphenadrine therapy.— W. Renforth, *ibid.*, 998.

Phenytoin. For the effect of dextropropoxyphene in increasing blood concentrations of phenytoin, see Phenytoin Sodium, p.1240.

Tobacco smoking. In a study of 835 patients who were arranged according to their cigarette smoking habits, dextropropoxyphene was ineffective in 10% of the non-smokers, in 15% of those who smoked up to 20 cigarettes a day, and in 20.3% of heavy smokers. This might be due to the smoking stimulating liver enzymes so increasing the metabolism of dextropropoxyphene.— Boston Collaborative Drug Surveillance Program, *Clin. Pharmac. Ther.*, 1973, *14*, 259.

Warfarin. For a report of dextropropoxyphene enhancing the anticoagulant effects of warfarin, see Warfarin Sodium, p.779.

Absorption and Fate. Dextropropoxyphene is readily absorbed from the gastro-intestinal tract, but it is subject to considerable first-pass metabolism. It is rapidly distributed and concentrated in the liver, lungs, and kidneys. Peak plasma concentrations occur about 1 to 2 hours after ingestion.

Dextropropoxyphene is *N*-demethylated to nordextropropoxyphene in the liver. It is excreted in the urine mainly as metabolites.

In patients who took lethal doses of dextropropoxyphene, concentrations found in the liver and lungs were 10 to 20 times higher than in the blood. It appeared that there might be an upper limit of dextropropoxyphene saturation in the blood of about 10 µg per ml after ingestion by mouth although the liver, lungs, and kidneys could accumulate much more. The average blood concentration in patients who took lethal doses was 4.72 µg per ml, suggesting an average absorbed quantity of 5.12 g. The drug was strongly bound to plasma proteins.— W. Q. Sturner and J. C. Garriott, *J. Am. med. Ass.*, 1973, *223*, 1125.

An oral dose of dextropropoxyphene 130 mg was given to normal subjects. The peak plasma concentration of dextropropoxyphene occurred after 1 to 2 hours followed by rapid elimination with an apparent half-life of 1.6 to 4.1 hours. The plasma concentration of the major metabolite, nordextropropoxyphene, reached a peak after 4 hours and thereafter slowly decayed with an apparent half-life of 11.5 to 28.8 hours. Individual differences in absorption and biotransformation might be responsible for the substantial variation in plasma dextropropoxyphene concentrations.— K. Verebely and C. E. Inturrisi, *Clin. Pharmac. Ther.*, 1974, *15*, 302.

Plasma concentrations in 4 subjects determined for up to 240 hours after single equivalent doses of dextropropoxyphene napsylate and dextropropoxyphene hydrochloride given at 6-week intervals in a crossover study indicated that the overall half-life of dextropropoxyphene was nearly 12 hours and norpropoxyphene nearly 37 hours.— R. L. Wolen *et al.*, *Clin. Pharmac. Ther.*, 1975, *17*, 15.

A study in 6 healthy subjects confirmed that although fatty, high-protein, or high-carbohydrate meals delayed dextropropoxyphene hydrochloride absorption, overall efficacy of absorption was not affected and appeared to be enhanced by the high-carbohydrate meal. Concurrent intake of large fluid volumes tended to reduce bioavailability from capsules.— P. G. Welling *et al.*, *Clin. Pharmac. Ther.*, 1976, *19*, 559. The peak plasma concentration of dextropropoxyphene occurred 2 hours after administration on an empty stomach; it was delayed by 1 hour after a meal of fat and carbohydrate, and by 2 hours after protein. However, carbohydrate and protein meals increased absorption.— M. N. Musa and L. L. Lyons, *Curr. ther. Res.*, 1976, *19*, 669.

Plasma-protein binding of dextropropoxyphene was not reduced in anephric patients.— K. M. Giacomini *et al.*, *J. clin. Pharmac.*, 1978, *18*, 106. Increased plasma concentrations of dextropropoxyphene in 7 anephric patients given dextropropoxyphene hydrochloride 130 mg.— T. P. Gibson *et al.*, *Clin. Pharmac. Ther.*, 1980, *27*, 665. See also *idem*, 1977, *21*, 103; K. M. Giacomini *et al.*, *ibid.*, 1980, *27*, 508.

Increased plasma concentrations of dextropropoxyphene and decreased plasma concentrations of nordextropropoxyphene in 4 cirrhotic patients and 4 patients with portacaval shunts given dextropropoxyphene hydrochloride 130 mg.— K. M. Giacomini *et al.*, *Clin. Pharmac. Ther.*, 1980, *28*, 417.

Further references: R. E. McMahon *et al.*, *Toxic. appl. Pharmac.*, 1971, *19*, 427; R. L. Wolen *et al.*, *Toxic. appl. Pharmac.*, 1971, *19*, 480; D. Perrier and M. Gibaldi, *J. clin. Pharmac.*, 1972, *12*, 449; J. F. Nash *et al.*, *J. pharm. Sci.*, 1975, *64*, 429; R. I. Poust *et al.*, *J. Am. pharm. Ass.*, 1976, *NS16*, 97; J. T. Wilson *et al.*, *Clin. Pharmac. Ther.*, 1976, *19*, 264; L. F. Gram *et al.*, *Clin. Pharmac. Ther.*, 1979, *26*, 473.

Uses. Dextropropoxyphene is an analgesic related to methadone. It is administered by mouth as the hydrochloride or napsylate to alleviate mild to moderate pain. It has little antitussive activity.

Dextropropoxyphene is mainly used in conjunction with other analgesics with anti-inflammatory and antipyretic effects, such as aspirin and paracetamol. The usual dose is 65 mg of dextropropoxyphene hydrochloride or 100 mg of the napsylate three or four times daily.

An extensive review of the actions and uses of dextropropoxyphene hydrochloride, with comparisons of its analgesic effect relative to codeine. Dextropropoxyphene was somewhat less potent than codeine.— N. B. Eddy *et al.*, *Codeine and its Alternates for Pain and Cough Relief*, Geneva, World Health Organization, 1970. See also *Bull. Wld Hlth Org.*, 1969, *40*, 1.

Other reviews: L. Lasagna, *Ann. intern. Med.*, 1976, *85*, 619; R. R. Miller, *Am. J. Hosp. Pharm.*, 1977, *34*, 413; *Drug & Ther. Bull.*, 1978, *16*, 71.

Administration in hepatic disease. See under Absorption and Fate.

Administration in renal failure. The normal dosage interval of 4 hours for dextropropoxyphene should be extended to 50 hours in patients with a glomerular filtration rate of less than 10 ml per minute. Concentrations of dextropropoxyphene are unaffected by haemodialysis or peritoneal dialysis.— W. M. Bennett *et al.*, *Ann. intern. Med.*, 1980, *93*, 62.

Increased plasma concentrations of dextropropoxyphene in anephric patients indicated that dextropropoxyphene should be used cautiously and in reduced dosage in patients with renal failure.— T. P. Gibson *et al.*, *Clin. Pharmac. Ther.*, 1980, *27*, 665.

Analgesia. A critical review of 20 double-blind clinical studies of dextropropoxyphene showed that it was no more effective than codeine or aspirin in analgesic effect, and might even be inferior to these analgesics.— R. R. Miller *et al.*, *J. Am. med. Ass.*, 1970, *213*, 996.

Dextropropoxyphene 65 mg was equivalent in analgesic potency to about 30 to 45 mg of codeine. In controlled trials, dextropropoxyphene 32 mg had been only inconsistently better than a placebo. When equal analgesic doses were used the side-effects of dextropropoxyphene and codeine were about the same.— *Med. Lett.*, 1970, *12*, 5 (National Academy of Sciences—National Research Council Panel on Drugs for Relief of Pain).

An assessment of Distalgesic concluded that the combination of dextropropoxyphene and paracetamol had few advantages, but a number of disadvantages, over paracetamol alone and that it should not be used unless paracetamol had failed to control pain.— *Drug & Ther. Bull.*, 1978, *16*, 71.

Treatment of dependence. Dextropropoxyphene hydrochloride 600 mg had produced miosis and subjective effects similar to those produced by morphine sulphate 20 mg subcutaneously. In 2 patients dependent on morphine 60 mg daily, dextropropoxyphene napsylate 1.2 g daily permitted withdrawal of morphine but mild abstinence persisted. When dextropropoxyphene was withdrawn a mild abstinence syndrome was precipitated. The usefulness of dextropropoxyphene in treating narcotic addiction was limited by its toxicity.— D. R. Jasinski *et al.*, *Archs gen. Psychiat.*, 1977, *34*, 227.

Further references: F. S. Tennant *et al.*, *J. Am. med. Ass.*, 1975, *232*, 1019; G. Udkow and M. Weintraub, *J. Pediat.*, 1978, *92*, 829.

Preparations of Dextropropoxyphene Salts

Dextropropoxyphene Capsules *(B.P.)*. Propoxyphene Capsules. Capsules containing dextropropoxyphene napsylate. Potency is expressed in terms of the equivalent amount of dextropropoxyphene.

Propoxyphene Hydrochloride and Acetaminophen Tablets *(U.S.P.)*. Tablets containing dextropropoxyphene hydrochloride and paracetamol. The *U.S.P.* requires 75% dissolution of dextropropoxyphene hydrochloride in 30 minutes. Store in airtight containers.

Propoxyphene Hydrochloride and APC Capsules *(U.S.P.)*. The *U.S.P.* requires that the amount of dextropropoxyphene hydrochloride in each capsule be specified; unless otherwise specified the capsules each contain aspirin 227 mg, phenacetin 162 mg, and caffeine 32.4 mg. The *U.S.P.* requires 85% dissolution of dextropropoxyphene hydrochloride and 75% dissolution of aspirin in 60 minutes. Store at 15° to 30° in airtight containers.

Propoxyphene Hydrochloride Capsules *(U.S.P.)*. Capsules containing dextropropoxyphene hydrochloride. The *U.S.P.* requires 85% dissolution in 60 minutes. Store in airtight containers.

Propoxyphene Napsylate and Acetaminophen Tablets *(U.S.P.)*. Tablets containing dextropropoxyphene napsylate and paracetamol. The *U.S.P.* requires 75% dissolution of dextropropoxyphene napsylate in 60 minutes. Store at 15° to 30° in airtight containers.

Propoxyphene Napsylate and Aspirin Tablets *(U.S.P.)*. Tablets containing dextropropoxyphene napsylate and aspirin. The *U.S.P.* requires 75% dissolution of dextropropoxyphene napsylate in 60 minutes. Store at 15° to 30° in airtight containers.

Propoxyphene Napsylate Oral Suspension *(U.S.P.)*. A suspension containing dextropropoxyphene napsylate with alcohol 0.5 to 1.5%. Store in airtight containers. Avoid freezing. Protect from light.

Propoxyphene Napsylate Tablets *(U.S.P.)*. Tablets containing dextropropoxyphene napsylate. The *U.S.P.* requires 75% dissolution in 60 minutes. Store in airtight containers.

Proprietary Preparations of Dextropropoxyphene Salts

Cosalgesic *(Cox Continental, UK)*. Tablets each containing dextropropoxyphene hydrochloride 32.5 mg and paracetamol 325 mg. Analgesic. *Dose.* 2 tablets 3 or 4 times daily.

Dextrogesic *(Unimed, UK)*. Tablets each containing dextropropoxyphene hydrochloride 32.5 mg and paracetamol 325 mg.

Distalgesic *(Dista, UK)*. Tablets each containing dextropropoxyphene hydrochloride 32.5 mg and paracetamol 325 mg. Analgesic. **Distalgesic Soluble.** Tablets each containing dextropropoxyphene napsylate 50 mg and paracetamol 325 mg. *Dose.* 2 tablets 3 or 4 times daily (the soluble tablets should be dissolved in water).

Dolasan *(Lilly, UK)*. Tablets each containing dextropropoxyphene napsylate 100 mg and aspirin 325 mg. Analgesic. *Dose.* 1 tablet 3 or 4 times daily.

Doloxene *(Lilly, UK)*. Capsules each containing dextropropoxyphene napsylate 100 mg equivalent to 65 mg of the hydrochloride. **Doloxene Compound.** Capsules each containing dextropropoxyphene napsylate 100 mg, aspirin 375 mg, and caffeine 30 mg. Analgesic. *Dose.* 1 capsule 3 or 4 times daily. (Also available as Doloxene in *Austral.*, *Denm.*, *Norw.*, *S.Afr.*, *Swed.*).

Napsalgesic Tablets *(Dista, UK)*. Each contains dextropropoxyphene napsylate 50 mg and aspirin 500 mg. Analgesic. *Dose.* 4 to 6 tablets daily in divided doses.

Other Proprietary Names of Dextropropoxyphene Hydrochloride

Arg.—Algafan; *Austral.*—Algaphan; *Belg.*—Algaphan, Dépronal; *Canad.*—Algodex, Depronal SA, Novopropoxyn, Pro-65, 642 Tablets; *Denm.*—Abalgin; *Fr.*—Antalvic, Dépronal; *Ger.*—Develin, Erantin; *Ital.*—Lenigesial (theobromine acetate derivative), Liberen, Tilene; *Neth.*—Depronal, Dolorphen; *S. Afr.*—Depronal-SA; *Spain*—Deprancol; *Swed.*—Dolotard; *Switz.*— Depronal Retard; *USA*—Daraphen, Darvon, Dolene, Dolocap, Mardon, Proxagesic, SK-65.

Dextropropoxyphene hydrochloride was also formerly marketed in Great Britain under the proprietary names Depronal SA (*Warner*) and SK-65 *(Smith Kline & French)*. A preparation containing dextropropoxyphene hydrochloride was also formerly marketed in Great Britain under the proprietary name Doloxytal *(Lilly)*.

Other Proprietary Names of Dextropropoxyphene Napsylate
Darvon-N *(Canad., USA)*.

6219-l

Diamorphine Hydrochloride *(B.P.)*.

Diamorph. Hydrochlor.; Diacetylmorphine Hydrochloride; Heroin Hydrochloride. 3,6-*O*-Diacetylmorphine hydrochloride monohydrate.
$C_{21}H_{23}NO_5,HCl,H_2O = 423.9$.

CAS — 561-27-3 (diamorphine); 1502-95-0 (hydrochloride, anhydrous).

Pharmacopoeias. In *Br.* and *Port.*

An almost white crystalline powder with a bitter taste, odourless when freshly prepared but develops an odour of acetic acid on storage. M.p. 229° to 233°.

Soluble 1 in 1.6 of water, 1 in 12 of alcohol, and 1 in 1.6 of chloroform; practically insoluble in ether. Solutions for injection are prepared by dissolving, immediately before use, the sterile contents of a sealed container in Water for Injections.

Incompatible with mineral acids and alkalis. Sodium chloride may precipitate diamorphine from concentrated solutions at a pH above 5.5.

Store in airtight containers. Protect from light. Diamorphine hydrolyses in aqueous solution to 3-*O*- and 6-*O*-acetylmorphine and morphine to a significant extent at room temperature; the rate of decomposition is at a minimum at about pH 4.

Degradation of diamorphine in solution.— E. A. Davey and J. B. Murray, *Pharm. J.*, 1969, *2*, 737.

Stability of diamorphine in chloroform water.— H. Cooper *et al.*, *Pharm. J.*, 1981, *1*, 682. Comment, including a reminder that the degradation product of diamorphine, monoacetyl morphine, is as potent as morphine, so that the 'efficacy half-life' is far longer than the more strictly interpreted pharmaceutical half-life.— R. G. Twycross (letter), *ibid.*, *2*, 218; I. M. Beaumont (letter), *ibid.*, 41.

Dependence. Use of diamorphine is liable to produce dependence of the morphine type (see p.1018).

Diamorphine and morphine were found to have essentially similar properties except for potency and absorption rate, and short-term addiction studies did not support the statement that tolerance develops more rapidly to diamorphine than to morphine.— W. R. Martin and H. F. Fraser, *J. Pharmac. exp. Ther.*, 1961, *133*, 388.

Pregnancy and the neonate. Thirteen infants born to mothers addicted to diamorphine had withdrawal symptoms evident 10 minutes to 48 hours after delivery; 6 had Apgar scores of 6 or less at 1 minute. Sedation was necessary in 9 of the 13 for periods of 3 to 67 days. Symptoms tended to recur when the infants were discharged from hospital and persisted for up to 6 months. Minor malformations were present in 2 infants.— M. M. Desmond *et al.*, *J. Pediat.*, 1972, *80*, 190.

Growth and development of 30 infants born to diamorphine addicts were related to the maternal pattern of diamorphine use and the severity of neonatal withdrawal symptoms. Withdrawal symptoms occurred in 80% of the infants, with subacute withdrawal symptoms lasting 3 to 6 months in 60%. Of 14 children followed for 1 year or longer, 7 demonstrated behavioural disturbances and 4 of these had associated growth impairment; 2 children had minor neurological abnormalities.— G. S. Wilson *et al.*, *Am. J. Dis. Child.*, 1973, *126*, 457. Development of preschool children of diamorphine-addicted mothers.— G. S. Wilson *et al.*, *Pediatrics*, 1979, *63*, 135, per *Int. pharm. Abstr.*, 1979, *16*, 455.

Of 149 children born to diamorphine addicts, 37% were of low birth-weight and 24% were born at less than 37 weeks gestation. Tobacco and alcohol abuse and poor maternal nutrition probably contributed to the growth retardation. The neonatal mortality rate was 6.7% and the stillbirth rate was 4%. Withdrawal symptoms were observed in 68% of the infants but no deaths were attributed directly to narcotic withdrawal.— H. S. Fricker and S. Segal, *Am. J. Dis. Child.*, 1978, *132*, 360.

Further references: A. M. Reddy *et al.*, *Pediatrics*, 1971, *48*, 353; R. L. Naeye *et al.*, *J. Pediat.*, 1973, *83*, 1055.

See also under Morphine, p.1018 and Methadone Hydrochloride, p.1015.

Tolerance. Cross-tolerance between methadone and diamorphine.— J. Volavka *et al.*, *J. nerv. ment. Dis.*, 1978, *166*, 104.

A study in healthy subjects and diamorphine-dependent patients indicated that tolerance developed to the miotic effects of repeated administration of diamorphine. The slope of the plot of pupil diameter against plasma concentration of morphine correlated with the daily dose of diamorphine and hence the effect of a test dose on pupil diameter could be used to predict the daily dose of diamorphine a patient was accustomed to.— K. H. Tress *et al.*, *Br. J. clin. Pharmac.*, 1978, *5*, 299. The duration of action was shorter in diamorphine-dependent subjects.— K. H. Tress and A. A. El-Sobky, *Br. J. clin. Pharmac.*, 1979, *7*, 213.

Adverse Effects and Treatment. As for Morphine, p.1019.

Pulmonary oedema after overdosage is a common cause of fatalities among diamorphine addicts. Nausea and vomiting are claimed to be less common than with morphine.

There are many reports of adverse effects associated with the abuse of diamorphine, usually obtained illicitly in an adulterated form.

Anisocoria (unevenly sized pupils) was frequently noted during withdrawal of subjects from diamorphine.— T. M. Cosgriff, *Archs Neurol., Chicago*, 1973, *29*, 200.

Oedema of the face, abdomen, and extremities, arthritis, and arthralgia were noted in patients maintained on methadone while secretly using heroin concurrently. These patients were identified by their puffy-faced appearance.— R. Tarail and W. D. Dorn (letter), *J. Am. med. Ass.*, 1974, *228*, 286.

A report of 8 deaths due to adulterated diamorphine. Lack of dosage standardisation was considered to be a major risk factor.— D. H. Huber *et al.*, *J. Am. med. Ass.*, 1974, *228*, 319.

The effect of diamorphine on reaction times, EEG, and other physiological parameters.— J. Volavka *et al.*, *Archs gen. Psychiat.*, 1974, *30*, 677.

There were very high serum concentrations of growth hormone in 24 diamorphine addicts; concentrations were still high in 11 after 6 months' abstinence from diamorphine.— A. H. Ghodse (letter), *Br. med. J.*, 1977, *1*, 1160.

For a report of medical complications associated with the self-administration of opiates, see Morphine, p.1018.

Effects on blood. A report in 5 male heroin users of a syndrome resembling acute thrombocytopenic purpura which was considered possibly to be a drug related immunologic response. All 5 patients had recently used 'brown heroin' before admission to hospital.— W. H. Adams *et al.*, *Ann. intern. Med.*, 1978, *89*, 207.

Further reports of thrombocytopenia in diamorphine users: D. H. Ryan (letter), *Ann. intern. Med.*, 1979, *90*, 852; R. A. Moss and D. B. Okun, *Archs intern. Med.*, 1979, *139*, 752.

Effects on cardiovascular system. Sudden death is not uncommon after parenteral administration of diamorphine.— S. M. Deglin *et al.*, *Drugs*, 1977, *14*, 29.

ECG abnormalities in acute diamorphine overdosage.— F. L. Glauser *et al.*, *Bull. Narcot.*, 1977, *29*, (Jan.–Mar.), 85.

Cerebral arteritis in a 20-year-old man occurred after the self-administration of diamorphine intravenously.— J. King *et al.*, *Med. J. Aust.*, 1978, *2*, 444.

Effects on kidneys. Studies in 8 patients with the nephrotic syndrome and who were also diamorphine addicts suggested an association between the diamorphine, its diluent, or its contamination and the renal disorder.— M. M. Kilcoyne *et al.*, *Lancet*, 1972, *1*, 17. See also T. K. S. Rao *et al.*, *New Engl. J. Med.*, 1974, *290*, 19. A study in 145 asymptomatic male diamorphine addicts did not support this suggestion.— J. A. L. Arruda *et al.*, *Archs intern. Med.*, 1975, *135*, 535.

Renal plasma flow and glomerular filtration-rate were reduced in patients who had taken an overdose of diamorphine.— F. L. Glauser *et al.*, *Am. J. med. Sci.*, 1976, *272*, 147, per *Int. pharm. Abstr.*, 1977, *14*, 1180.

Severe renal amyloidosis and nephrotic syndrome in 4 patients who had been diamorphine addicts for 14 to 27 years.— J. Scholes *et al.*, *Ann. intern. Med.*, 1979, *91*, 26.

Effects on liver. Abnormalities of liver function were seen in 35 of 46 patients dependent on diamorphine. High alcohol consumption was noted in 85% of these patients, indicating that this factor might be an important cause of chronic liver disease in drug addicts.— B. Stimmel *et al.*, *J. Am. med. Ass.*, 1972, *222*, 811. See also H. J. C. Ireton *et al.*, *Aust. N.Z. J. Med.*, 1974, *4*, 444.

Effects on muscle. A syndrome of acute rhabdomyolysis with myoglobinuria in 4 men followed intravenous injection of adulterated diamorphine. Acute renal failure occurred in 2 patients, 1 of whom survived, and was probably associated with the myoglobinuric state. Three patients survived and regained a major portion of their muscular function.— R. W. Richter *et al.*, *J. Am. med. Ass.*, 1971, *216*, 1172. See also R. J. Greenwood, *Postgrad. med. J.*, 1974, *50*, 772.

A study of 102 diamorphine addicts revealed antibodies to smooth muscle in 46% and lymphocytotoxic antibodies in 30%. In former addicts these antibodies were found in 10% and 15% respectively and in 5% and 2.5% of normal controls. Significant elevation of IgM was recorded in diamorphine addicts.— G. Husby, *Ann. intern. Med.*, 1975, *83*, 801.

Fever, paraspinal myalgias and periarthralgias occurred in 16 patients who had administered heroin intravenously. The underlying cause was unknown but may have been due to the heroin itself, described by a number of patients as brown heroin, or to an adulterant. The musculoskeletal complications were self-limited in those patients who were in hospital and received no heroin.— R. S. Pastan *et al.*, *Ann. intern. Med.*, 1977, *87*, 22.

Hyperkalaemia. A 25-year-old man, who was admitted to hospital in deep coma after injecting himself with an unknown quantity of 'street' heroin about 8 hours earlier, had severe hyperkalaemia with corresponding ECG abnormalities. His hyperkalaemia was considered to be the result of ischaemic injury to muscle during the period of unconsciousness and prolonged immobility following the overdose, with leakage of potassium ions from the muscles into the extracellular fluid.— C. J. Pearce and J. G. C. Cox (letter), *Lancet*, 1980, *2*, 923. Fatal hyperkalaemia in a 31-year-old man who had taken an overdose of diamorphine.— P. N. Trewby *et al.* (letter), *ibid.*, 1981, *1*, 327. A similar finding of hyperkalaemia in a 20-year-old man initially treated for diamorphine overdosage and shortly after readmitted with methadone overdosage. Injury to muscle together with moderately severe acidosis and renal insufficiency might have accounted for the severe hyperkalaemia.— L. G. Thijs *et al.* (letter), *ibid.*, 1245.

Effects on nervous system. Four cases of transverse myelitis were reported in Negro men taking adulterated diamorphine intravenously. In 3 of the men paralysis and sensory loss occurred within a few hours of injection. The thoracic spinal cord was involved in each case; a large necrotic lesion was found post mortem in 1 man at the level of the 9th to 11th thoracic vertebrae. A second man died but no autopsy was performed. Mild paralysis persisted in 1 man, and severe paralysis in the other.— R. W. Richter and R. N. Rosenberg, *J. Am. med. Ass.*, 1968, *206*, 1255.

Brachial and lumbosacral plexitis followed intravenous injection of adulterated diamorphine in 13 addicts. The component responsible for this effect was not identified.— Y. B. Challenor *et al.*, *J. Am. med. Ass.*, 1973, *225*, 958.

Two cases of acute polyneuritis (Guillain-Barré syndrome) occurred following intravenous administration of diamorphine. One patient had regularly used diamorphine intravenously for 1 year and the other had used amphetamine and barbiturates by mouth and diamorphine intravenously for about 8 months on an irregular basis.— W. R. Smith and A. F. Wilson, *J. Am. med. Ass.*, 1975, *231*, 1367.

Effect on sexual function. In a study of the effects of diamorphine use and subsequent abstinence in 31 male addicts it was noted that diamorphine alone or in association with methadone significantly suppressed plasma-testosterone concentrations. Recovery to normal concentrations occurred after about a month of abstinence. Significant suppression continued in a 15-year-old boy who had started to use diamorphine at the age of 12; this suggested that chronic diamorphine administration at a critical age might cause long-lasting sexual impairment.— J. H. Mendelson and N. K. Mello, *Clin. Pharmac. Ther.*, 1975, *17*, 529.

Immunological disorders. Hyperimmunoglobulinaemia appeared to be associated with parenteral administration of diamorphine in addicts.— P. Cushman, *Am. J. Epidem.*, 1974, *99*, 218.

In 38 diamorphine addicts there was a high incidence of immunological abnormalities: hypergammaglobulinaemia IgM 87%, IgG 63%, false positive test for syphilis 23%, and positive latex fixation test 21%. There was no consistent pattern in 10 addicts on methadone maintenance.— S. M. Brown *et al.*, *Archs intern. Med.*, 1974, *134*, 1001. In a study of immune function in 82 diamorphine addicts, slight abnormalities of humoral immunity were demonstrated with circulating immuno-complexes and increased concentrations of IgM. Contrary to the findings of S.M. Brown *et al.* cellular immunity was normal.— L. Ortona *et al.* (letter), *New Engl. J. Med.*, 1979, *300*, 45.

Overdosage. See under Effects on Cardiovascular System; Effects on Kidneys; Effects on Muscle, Hyperkalaemia; Pulmonary Oedema; Raised Intracranial Pressure.

Pulmonary oedema. The chronic use of diamorphine was associated with pulmonary abnormalities such as decrease in vital capacity. Extensive pulmonary oedema could occur following diamorphine overdose. The cause of this pulmonary oedema was not clear although several mechanisms had been proposed.— U. I. Frand *et al.*, *Ann. intern. Med.*, 1972, *77*, 29.

Further references: A. D. Steinberg and J. S. Karliner, *Archs intern. Med.*, 1968, *122*, 122; J. S. Karliner *et al.*, *Archs intern. Med.*, 1969, *124*, 350; W. J. Morrison *et al.*, *Radiology*, 1970, *97*, 347; K. Master (letter), *Ann. intern. Med.*, 1972, *77*, 817; E. C. Rosenow, *Ann. intern. Med.*, 1972, *77*, 977; M. L. Warnock *et al.*, *J. Am. med. Ass.*, 1972, *219*, 1051; E. M. Spiritus *et al.*, *Am. Rev. resp. Dis.*, 1973, *108*, 994.

Raised intracranial pressure. Raised intracranial pressure was noted in 12 of 42 patients suffering from an overdose of illicit diamorphine.— R. W. Richter *et al.*, *Bull. N.Y. Acad. Med.*, 1973, *49*, 3.

Precautions. As for Morphine, p.1019.

Serum creatine kinase values rose significantly in 3 of 10 patients given diamorphine 10 mg intramuscularly; this could cause confusion when these values were used for the assessment of cardiac infarction.— B. B. Scott *et al.*, *Br. med. J.*, 1974, *4*, 691.

Effects on blood glucose. In 12 diamorphine addicts, fasting blood sugar concentrations were normal but the response to a 50-g oral glucose-tolerance test was lower and delayed compared with controls, resting insulin concentrations were higher and the response to glucose was delayed, and resting growth hormone concentrations were higher and were not suppressed in response to glucose.— J. L. Reed and A. H. Ghodse, *Br. med. J.*, 1973, *2*, 582.

Interactions. After receiving cyamemazine 1.8 g and sulpiride 4.8 g intravenously over 48 hours for detoxification, a 25-year-old diamorphine addict developed hypertonia and malignant hyperthermia and died.— G. Bleichner *et al.* (letter), *Lancet*, 1981, *1*, 386.

Phaeochromocytoma. A 50-year-old man whose hypertension was increased and who developed tachycardia on several occasions after therapeutic doses of diamorphine was found to have a phaeochromocytoma. It was considered that diamorphine had liberated endogenous histamine and stimulated the release of catecholamines. Opiates were contra-indicated in patients with a phaeochromocytoma.— N. C. Chaturvedi *et al.*, *Br. med. J.*, 1974, *2*, 538.

Pregnancy and the neonate. Chromosomal aberrations were found in about 10% of 27 907 cells taken from 99 pregnant women dependent on diamorphine or methadone.— A. P. Amarose and M. J. Norusis, *Am. J. Obstet. Gynec.*, 1976, *124*, 635.

See also under Dependence, above.

Absorption and Fate. Diamorphine hydrochloride is well absorbed from the gastro-intestinal tract and following subcutaneous or intramuscular injection. It is rapidly converted to 6-*O*-monoacetylmorphine in the blood and then to morphine. Both diamorphine and monoacetylmorphine readily cross the blood-brain barrier. Morphine and morphine glucuronide are the main excretion products in the urine.

A review of the metabolism of diamorphine and morphine in man.— U. Boerner *et al.*, *Drug Metab. Rev.*, 1975, *4*, 39.

Metabolites of diamorphine excreted in the urine after intravenous administration were 6-monoacetylmorphine, morphine, and normorphine.— S. Y. Yeh and R. L. McQuinn, *J. pharm. Sci.*, 1975, *64*, 1237.

Following administration of diamorphine 10 mg per 70 kg body-weight intravenously to healthy, post-addict subjects the metabolites identified in urine were morphine, 6-acetylmorphine, normorphine, morphine 3-glucuronide, 6-acetylmorphine 3-glucuronide, and normorphine glucuronide. Morphine 3-glucuronide accounted for about 50% and morphine about 7% of the dose of diacetylmorphine.— S. Y. Yeh *et al.*, *J. pharm. Sci.*, 1977, *66*, 201.

Protein binding. Diamorphine was not significantly bound to human plasma protein in an *in vitro* system.— G. L. Cohn *et al.*, *Proc. Soc. exp. Biol. Med.*, 1974, *147*, 664.

Uses. Diamorphine hydrochloride resembles morphine in its action (see p.1020). It is a more potent analgesic than morphine but it has a shorter duration of action, its effect lasting only about 3 hours.

It is used for the relief of severe pain especially in terminal illnesses. It may be given by mouth or by subcutaneous or intramuscular injection in doses of 5 to 10 mg. Doses of 5 mg have been given intravenously to patients with a myocardial infarction. Diamorphine may also be used preoperatively and postoperatively.

The value of giving cocaine or a phenothiazine with morphine or diamorphine in severe pain is being questioned (see under Morphine, p.1020), as indeed is the practice of 'on-demand analgesia' versus that of continuous analgesia.

It is effective for the relief of cough and is used in doses of 1.5 to 6 mg, usually administered as a linctus. Because of its addictive properties, it should be used with discrimination and only when other less dangerous cough suppressants have proved inadequate.

In equianalgesic doses diamorphine had a shorter onset and duration of action and was more sedative than morphine but there was little difference between them in ability to relieve apprehension or cause euphoria. Both caused dizziness but diamorphine was less emetic than morphine.— J. W. Dundee *et al.*, *Lancet*, 1967, *2*, 221.

Administration, continuous subcutaneous. Excellent results with continuous subcutaneous analgesics and antiemetics in terminal care.— H. T. Hutchinson *et al.* (letter), *Lancet*, 1981, *2*, 1279.

Administration, epidural and intrathecal. A study in patients with low back pain indicated that epidural injection of fentanyl gave relief of pain lasting 90 minutes, whereas epidural injection of diamorphine gave pain relief lasting over 9 hours. Severe pruritus, which usually began about 30 minutes after the onset of analgesia, may limit the use of some epidural opiates; it was only weakly relieved by chlorpheniramine.— H. J. McQuay *et al.* (letter), *Lancet*, 1980, *1*, 768.

Experience with intrathecal diamorphine.— L. Kaufman (letter), *Lancet*, 1981, *2*, 1341.

Analgesia. *In labour.* Various treatments providing effective analgesia during labour were assessed in 150 births. Diamorphine in a dose of 10 mg was the most effective analgesic during the first stage of labour and relieved pain for up to 4 hours. Unlike morphine and pethidine, diamorphine seldom caused vomiting or other side-effects.— J. M. Beazley *et al.*, *Lancet*, 1967, *1*, 1033.

Terminal pain. In studies in 116 terminal carcinoma patients, morphine was substituted under double-blind conditions for diamorphine in a diamorphine and cocaine elixir in the ratio 2 for 1. Analysis of effective analgesic doses showed that diamorphine 1 part was equianalgesic with morphine 1.5 parts.— R. G. Twycross, *Br. J. Pharmac.*, 1972, *46*, 554P. See also R. G. Twycross *et al.*, *Br. J. clin. Pharmac.*, 1974, *1*, 491.

Of 500 consecutive patients admitted to hospital with terminal cancer more than 60% were maintained free of pain on a regular 4-hourly dose of 10 mg or less of diamorphine. Oral medication was adequate until the last 12 to 24 hours of life in 85%. There was no evidence that the patients became psychologically dependent or that diamorphine reduced mental alertness. Most patients also received other medication.— R. G. Twycross, *J. med. Ethics*, 1975, *1*, 10.

A double-blind comparative study of the efficacy of methadone or diamorphine with cocaine as analgesics in 46 patients with terminal cancer suggested that although methadone was a satisfactory substitute for diamorphine in some patients diamorphine should be used in very ill patients since it did not accumulate in the body to the same extent as methadone, thereby making dosage adjustment easier.— R. G. Twycross (letter), *Br. J. clin. Pharmac.*, 1977, *4*, 691. A criticism.— A. S. E. Fowle and E. Letley, *Wellcome* (letter), *Br. J. clin. Pharmac.*, 1978, *5*, 527. Reply.— R. G. Twycross (letter), *ibid.*, 528.

An account of the terminal care of a dying child. Diamorphine was prescribed unequivocally every 4 hours by mouth to control pain, and not, it is emphasised, only when required.— J. A. Chapman and J. Goodall, *Lancet*, 1980, *1*, 753.

A comparative study with morphine suggesting that diamorphine has no apparent unique advantages or disadvantages for the relief of postoperative pain in cancer patients.— R. F. Kaiko *et al.*, *New Engl. J. Med.*, 1981, *304*, 1501.

Further references: R. G. Twycross, *Int. J. clin. Pharmac.*, 1974, *9*, 184; R. G. Twycross, *Pain*, 1977, *3*, 93; B. M. Mount (letter), *Can. med. Ass. J.*, 1979, *120*, 405; M. Korcok (letter), *ibid.*, 406.

Cardiovascular disorders. *Myocardial infarction.* Diamorphine was the analgesic of choice for patients with acute myocardial infarction because its circulatory effects were few.— *Lancet*, 1976, *2*, 888.

Preparations

Elixirs

Diamorphine and Cocaine Elixir *(B.P.C. 1973).* Diamorphine hydrochloride 5 mg, cocaine hydrochloride 5 mg, syrup 1.25 ml, alcohol (90%) 0.625 ml, chloroform water to 5 ml. When specified by the prescriber, the proportion of diamorphine may be varied. It should be freshly prepared. *Dose.* Determined by the physician according to the patient's needs.

Stability testing on diamorphine and cocaine elixir differing from the *B.P.C.* formula only in cocaine indicated that, at 22°, 10% of the diamorphine hydrolysed in 8 weeks; storage at 4° halved the rate of hydrolysis, which was accelerated at 30° or 37°. There was no difference in stability between samples stored in the dark or in diffuse light. The use of honey or an aldose sugar instead of sucrose increased the rate of hydrolysis. Stability was increased by higher concentrations of alcohol and reduced by lower concentrations. The addition of chlorpromazine or prochlorperazine reduced the life (to 10% hydrolysis) to 2 weeks. In simulated gastric juice more than 75% of diamorphine was not hydrolysed after 4 hours at 37°.— R. G. Twycross and R. A. Gilhooley (letter), *Br. med. J.*, 1973, *4*, 552.

Further references on stability: G. K. Poochikian and J. C. Cradock, *J. pharm. Sci.*, 1980, *69*, 637.

Diamorphine, Cocaine, and Chlorpromazine Elixir *(B.P.C. 1973).* Diamorphine hydrochloride 5 mg, cocaine hydrochloride 5 mg, chlorpromazine elixir 1.25 ml (containing chlorpromazine hydrochloride 6.25 mg), alcohol (90%) 0.625 ml, chloroform water to 5 ml. When specified by the prescriber, the proportion of diamorphine may be varied. It should be freshly prepared. Protect from light. *Dose.* Determined by the physician according to the patient's needs.

NOTE. The administration of cocaine with diamorphine or morphine has been reported to be of no apparent benefit, see under Morphine.

Injections

Diamorphine Injection *(B.P.).* Diamorph. Inj. A sterile solution of diamorphine hydrochloride in Water for Injections prepared by dissolving, immediately before use, the sterile contents of a sealed container (Diamorphine Hydrochloride for Injection) in the requisite amount of Water for Injections.

Sodium chloride is unsuitable for adjusting the osmolarity of this injection as it precipitates diamorphine from solution. Protect from light.

Linctuses

Diamorphine Linctus *(B.P.C. 1973).* Diamorphine hydrochloride 3 mg, oxymel 1.25 ml, glycerol 1.25 ml, compound tartrazine solution 0.06 ml, syrup to 5 ml. It should be recently prepared. When a dose less than, or not a multiple of, 5 ml is prescribed the linctus should be diluted to 5 ml, or a multiple, with syrup. Such dilutions must be freshly prepared and not used more than 2 weeks after issue. *Dose.* 2.5 to 10 ml.

Proprietary Preparations

Diamorphine Tablets *(Roche, UK).* Diamorphine hydrochloride, available as tablets of 10 mg.

6220-v

Difenoxin Hydrochloride. R 15403; Difenoxylic Acid Hydrochloride. 1-(3-Cyano-3,3-diphenylpropyl)-4-phenylpiperidine-4-carboxylic acid hydrochloride.
$C_{28}H_{28}N_2O_2,HCl = 461.0$.

CAS — 28782-42-5 (difenoxin); 35607-36-4 (hydrochloride).

A white amorphous powder. M.p. 290°. Very slightly **soluble** in water; sparingly soluble in chloroform and solutions of sodium hydroxide; freely soluble in dimethyl sulphoxide.

Difenoxin is the principal metabolite of diphenoxylate and is used similarly (see p.1010). It has antidiarrhoeal activity about 5 times that of diphenoxylate.

References: I. van Wijngaarden and W. Soudijn, *Arzneimittel-Forsch.*, 1972, *22*, 513; C. J. E. Niemegeers *et al.*, *ibid.*, 516; R. Rubens *et al.*, *ibid.*, 526; J. Heykants, *ibid.*, 529; H. Schenker, *Schweiz. med. Wschr.*, 1976, *106*, 1650; N. Thurnherr and P. Spring, *Arzneimittel-Forsch.*, 1979, *29*, 559; R. Steffen, *ibid.*, 685; H. Pece, *ibid.*, 849.

Proprietary Names

(with atropine sulphate) Lyspafen (*Protea, Austral.*; *Fisons, S.Afr.*; *Cilag-Chemie, Switz.*); Motofen (*McNeil, USA*).

6221-g

Dihydrocodeine Phosphate. Hydrocodeine Phosphate.
$C_{18}H_{23}NO_3,H_3PO_4=399.4$.

CAS — 24204-13-5.

Pharmacopoeias. In *Jap.*

A white to yellowish-white odourless crystalline powder with a bitter taste. **Soluble** 1 in 3 of water; slightly soluble in alcohol. **Store** in airtight containers. Protect from light.

6222-q

Dihydrocodeine Tartrate *(B.P.)*.

Dihydrocodeine Acid Tartrate; Dihydrocodeine Bitartrate; Hydrocodeine Bitartrate. 7,8-Dihydro-3-*O*-methylmorphine hydrogen tartrate.
$C_{18}H_{23}NO_3,C_4H_6O_6=451.5$.

CAS — 125-28-0 (dihydrocodeine); 5965-13-9 (tartrate).

Pharmacopoeias. In *Aust.*, *Br.*, *Ger.*, and *Hung. Pol.* has the monohydrate.

Odourless colourless crystals or white crystalline powder with a bitter taste. M.p. 190° to 194°. **Soluble** 1 in 4.5 of water; sparingly soluble in alcohol; practically insoluble in ether. A solution in water is laevorotatory. A 10% solution in water has a pH of 3.2 to 4.2. Solutions for injection are **sterilised** by autoclaving or by filtration. **Protect** from light.

Dependence. Prolonged use of high doses of dihydrocodeine may produce dependence of the morphine type (see p.1018). Liability to abuse is about the same as for codeine.

Withdrawal symptoms occurred in a 6-week-old infant, who had received dihydrocodeine 2.5 mg per kg body-weight daily for 2 weeks, after abrupt withdrawal of the drug.— H. J. Hiller and E. Gladtke, *Dt. med. Wschr.*, 1974, *99*, 1502.

Case reports of 5 patients who had morphine-like side-effects when taking dihydrocodeine or withdrawal symptoms when medication ceased; doses were generally 60 to 90 mg four times daily.— P. Marks *et al.*, *Br. med. J.*, 1978, *1*, 1594.

Adverse Effects, Treatment, and Precautions. As for Morphine, p.1019, though side-effects from dihydrocodeine are less pronounced.

Five of 112 medical or surgical patients taking dihydrocodeine in usual doses had hallucinations and a further 4 had vivid dreams: 2 of 93 controls had hallucinations and 4 of 190 had vivid dreams.— M. Taylor *et al.*, *Br. med. J.*, 1978, *2*, 1198.

Toxicological investigations in 6 deaths associated with codeine or dihydrocodeine overdosage.— M. A. Peat and A. Sengupta, *Forensic Sci.*, 1977, *9*, 21.

Pregnancy and the neonate. Clinical depression of the newborn had been observed after use of dihydrocodeine during labour.— F. Moya and V. Thorndike, *Clin. Pharmac. Ther.*, 1963, *4*, 628.

Uses. Dihydrocodeine tartrate is used for the relief of mild to moderate pain. It has also been used as a cough suppressant. The usual dose by mouth is 30 mg after food every 4 to 6 hours, but up to 60 mg may be given if necessary.

Dihydrocodeine tartrate may also be given by deep subcutaneous or intramuscular injection in similar doses.

Dihydrocodeine phosphate has also been used as an analgesic.

For a review of the uses and side-effects of dihydrocodeine as an analgesic and cough suppressant in comparison with codeine, see N. B. Eddy, *Codeine and its Alternates for Pain and Cough Relief*, Geneva, World Health Organization, 1970; *idem*, *Bull. Wld Hlth Org.*, 1969, *40*, 1 and 639.

A preliminary study with dihydrocodeine suggesting that opiates may be of value in selected patients for the treatment of breathlessness.— A. A. Woodcock *et al.*, *New Engl. J. Med.*, 1981, *305*, 1611.

Preparations

Dihydrocodeine Injection *(B.P.)*. A sterile solution of dihydrocodeine tartrate in Water for Injections containing the equivalent of not more than 0.1% of sulphur dioxide. The solution is sterilised by autoclaving. pH 3 to 4.5. Protect from light.

Dihydrocodeine Tablets *(B.P.)*. Tablets containing dihydrocodeine tartrate. Protect from light.

Proprietary Preparations of Dihydrocodeine Tartrate

DF 118 *(Duncan, Flockhart, UK)*. Dihydrocodeine tartrate, available as **Elixir** containing 10 mg in each 5 ml as **Injection** containing 50 mg per ml, in ampoules of 1 ml; and as **Tablets** of 30 mg. (Also available as DF 118 in *Austral.*, *S.Afr.*).

Onadox-118 *(Duncan, Flockhart, UK)*. Tablets each containing dihydrocodeine tartrate 10 mg and soluble aspirin equivalent to aspirin 300 mg. Analgesic. *Dose.* 1 to 3 tablets, in water, 3 or 4 times daily after meals.

Paramol-118 *(Duncan, Flockhart, UK)*. Tablets each containing dihydrocodeine tartrate 10 mg and paracetamol 500 mg. Analgesic. *Dose.* 1 tablet every 4 hours to 2 tablets 4 times daily.

Other Proprietary Names of Dihydrocodeine Tartrate

Bicodein *(Spain)*; Fortuss *(Austral.)*; Paracodin (tartrate or hydrorhodanide) *(Austral., Ger., S.Afr., Switz.)*; Paracodina *(Spain)*; Remedacen (base-resin complex) *(Ger.)*; Rikodeine, Tuscodin (both *Austral.*).

6223-p

Diphenoxylate Hydrochloride *(B.P., U.S.P.)*.

Ethyl 1-(3-cyano-3,3-diphenylpropyl)-4-phenylpiperidine-4-carboxylate hydrochloride.
$C_{30}H_{32}N_2O_2,HCl=489.1$.

CAS — 915-30-0 (diphenoxylate); 3810-80-8 (hydrochloride).

Pharmacopoeias. In *Br.*, *Braz.*, and *U.S.*

A white or almost white odourless crystalline powder. M.p. 220° to 226°. Sparingly **soluble** in water and acetone; soluble 1 in 50 of alcohol, 1 in 40 of acetone, and 1 in 2.5 of chloroform; soluble in methyl alcohol; practically insoluble in ether and light petroleum; slightly soluble in isopropyl alcohol. A saturated solution in water has a pH of about 3.3.

Dependence. Prolonged use of diphenoxylate may produce dependence of the morphine type (see p.1018) but short-term administration in the recommended dosage with atropine sulphate carries a negligible risk of dependence. A dose of 40 to 60 mg of diphenoxylate hydrochloride may be followed by euphoria.

Adverse Effects. Reported side-effects include anorexia, nausea and vomiting, swelling of the gums, abdominal distention, paralytic ileus, toxic megacolon, headache, drowsiness, insomnia, dizziness, restlessness, euphoria, depression, numbness of the extremities, skin rash, and allergic skin reactions.

After overdosage, symptoms are similar to those of morphine poisoning (see p.1019).

Young children are particularly susceptible to overdosage. The presence of subclinical doses of atropine sulphate in preparations containing diphenoxylate may give rise to the side-effects of atropine in susceptible individuals or in overdosage—see Atropine, p.289.

For a report of intoxication with diphenoxylate simulating intestinal obstruction, see L. S. Figiel and S. J. Figiel, *Am. J. Gastroent., N.Y.*, 1973, *59*, 267.

Overdosage. A discussion of the toxic effects, particularly respiratory depression, of large doses of diphenoxylate. Surveillance of children in whom ingestion of Lomotil was suspected was obligatory for 48 to 72 hours in view of the slow absorption and long duration of action of diphenoxylate; late onset of respiratory depression should be anticipated.— *Br. med. J.*, 1973, *2*, 678. See also *J. Am. med. Ass.*, 1974, *230*, 14.

Further references to toxic effects of Lomotil overdosage in children.— W. Henderson and A. Psaila (letter), *Lancet*, 1969, *1*, 307; R. Wheeldon and H. J. Heggarty, *Archs Dis. Childh.*, 1971, *46*, 562; C. M. Ginsburg, *Am. J. Dis. Child.*, 1973, *125*, 241; B. H. Rumack and A. R. Temple, *Pediatrics*, 1974, *53*, 495; *Med. Lett.*, 1975, *17*, 104; S. M. Block *et al.*, *S. Afr. med. J.*, 1977, *51*, 553; J. A. Curtis and K. M. Goel, *Archs Dis. Childh.*, 1979, *54*, 222; E. A. Cutler *et al.*, *Pediatrics*, 1980, *65*, 157.

Treatment of Adverse Effects. As for Morphine, p.1019.

Patients should be observed for at least 24 hours after overdosage.

A survey of poisoning with diphenoxylate and atropine (Lomotil) showed that young children might develop pronounced symptoms after ingesting 1 to 5 tablets. In suspected poisoning the patient should be admitted to hospital and observed for at least 24 hours, as the atropine might delay the onset of symptoms. The patient should receive intensive supportive treatment and a narcotic antagonist such as naloxone if needed.— D. Penfold and G. N. Volans, *Br. med. J.*, 1977, *2*, 1401.

Further references: R. Wheeldon and H. J. Heggarty, *Archs Dis. Childh.*, 1971, *46*, 562; B. H. Rumack and A. R. Temple, *Pediatrics*, 1974, *53*, 495; A. W. Craft and J. R. Sibert, *Br. J. Hosp. Med.*, 1977, *17*, 469; M. L. Smith and T. L. Chambers (letter), *Br. med. J.*, 1978, *1*, 176; M. McGuigan and F. H. Lovejoy (letter), *Br. med. J.*, 1978, *1*, 990.

Precautions. As for Morphine, p.1019.

In certain countries diphenoxylate is contra-indicated in children less than 2 years of age.

Diphenoxylate is contra-indicated in the treatment of diarrhoea associated with pseudomembranous enterocolitis which may follow treatment with antibiotics such as clindamycin or lincomycin. It should be used with caution in patients with ulcerative colitis or obstructive bowel disorders.

In the presence of severe dehydration or electrolyte imbalance diphenoxylate should not be given before appropriate corrective therapy.

Diphenoxylate is structurally related to pethidine hydrochloride but has no analgesic effect and is unsuitable for parenteral administration.

The use of diphenoxylate hydrochloride 2.5 mg with atropine sulphate 25 µg (Lomotil) was contra-indicated in children under 2 years of age due to numerous poisoning reports.— G. Rosenstein *et al.*, *Pediatrics*, 1973, *51*, 132. The use of diphenoxylate 2.5 mg with atropine 25 µg (Lomotil) in children was difficult to justify.— J. A. Curtis and K. M. Goel, *Archs Dis. Childh.*, 1979, *54*, 222. Comments on diphenoxylate with atropine being used in the treatment of children in the tropics with diarrhoea.— S. Karan (letter), *ibid.*, 984; A. S. Limaye, *ibid.*; K. M. Goel, *ibid.*; A. J. R. Waterston, *ibid.*, 1980, *55*, 577; K. M. Goel, *ibid.*, 578; S. Karan, *ibid.*

The use of diphenoxylate with atropine (Lomotil) or codeine in the treatment of lincomycin-induced diarrhoea was questioned since, in a controlled study involving 200 healthy subjects, the highest incidence of diarrhoea was seen in those given either of these antidiarrhoeal treatments concomitantly with lincomycin given intramuscularly.— E. Novak *et al.*, *J. Am. med. Ass.*, 1976, *235*, 1451.

Absorption and Fate. Diphenoxylate is well absorbed from the gastro-intestinal tract and extensively metabolised in the liver to diphenoxylic acid (difenoxin) and hydroxydiphenoxylic acid. It is excreted mainly as metabolites in the urine and bile; it may also be excreted in breast milk. Absorption may be delayed in the presence of atropine sulphate.

The mean urinary and faecal excretion over 96 hours of total radioactivity from ^{14}C-diphenoxylate 5 mg given in alcohol to 3 subjects was 13.65% and 49.2% respectively. The major metabolites in the urine and faeces were diphenoxylic acid (difenoxin) and hydroxydiphenoxylic acid. Only a small percentage of diphenoxylate remained unchanged. Analysis of plasma radioactivity showed that diphenoxylic acid accounted for most of the activity. Plasma-diphenoxylate concentrations of 9.5 ng per ml occurred at 2 hours as did the peak of plasma diphenoxylic acid (40.1 ng per ml); the half-lives were 2.5 hours and 4.38 hours respectively.— A. Karim *et al.*, *Clin. Pharmac. Ther.*, 1972, *13*, 407.

See also under Difenoxin Hydrochloride.

Uses. Diphenoxylate hydrochloride is a derivative of pethidine but has no analgesic activity. It reduces intestinal motility and is used in the symptomatic treatment of acute and chronic diarrhoea. It is also used to reduce the frequency and fluidity of the stools in patients with colostomies or ileostomies. The usual initial dose is 5 mg four times daily, later reduced when the diarrhoea is controlled.

A suggested dose for children is: 2 to 5 years of age, 2.5 mg twice daily; 6 to 8 years, 2.5 mg thrice daily; 9 to 12 years, 2.5 mg four times daily; over 12 years, 5 mg thrice daily.

Preparations of diphenoxylate usually contain subclinical amounts of atropine sulphate in an attempt to prevent abuse by deliberate overdosage.

Diarrhoea. In a double-blind controlled trial, 23 patients with diarrhoea following vagotomy were given 3 treatments, each for 1 month; tablets containing diphenoxylate hydrochloride 5 mg and atropine sulphate 50 µg or codeine phosphate 15 mg or a placebo. The diphenoxylate and atropine preparation had a satisfactory constipating effect but did not appear to have any significant advantage over codeine phosphate. It appeared to be of little value in the prophylaxis of sudden episodic attacks or in the treatment of more continuous post-vagotomy diarrhoea.— C. D. Collins, *Br. med. J.*, 1966, *2*, 560.

Tablets each containing diphenoxylate hydrochloride 5 mg and atropine sulphate 50 µg were effective in controlling episodic diarrhoea following vagotomy in 8 out of 10 patients; a reduction in the sense of urgency was the benefit most appreciated. The usual dose was 2 tablets taken as a single dose at the onset of the attack.— A. G. Cox and F. C. Y. Cheng, *Br. J. clin. Pract.*, 1968, *22*, 211.

A study of 204 patients with acute non-specific diarrhoea indicated that treatment with kaolin and pectin, diphenoxylate and atropine, or charcoal was no more effective than a controlled diet in reducing the frequency or looseness of stools.— K. Alestig *et al.*, *Practitioner*, 1979, *222*, 859.

In a double-blind study in 11 patients with chronic diarrhoea loperamide 2 mg, diphenoxylate 5 mg with atropine, and codeine phosphate 30 mg had comparable antidiarrhoeal activity.— C. D. Shee and R. E. Pounder, *Br. med. J.*, 1980, *280*, 524.

For a report questioning the use of diphenoxylate in antibiotic-induced diarrhoea, see under Precautions.

Treatment of dependence. During a period of 7 years diphenoxylate 2.5 mg and atropine 25 µg (Lomotil), 1 to 2 tablets 4-hourly, in conjunction with chlormethiazole, 1 to 2 g four-hourly, was effective in treating the withdrawal phase in diamorphine and other narcotic drug dependence in 100 patients. This treatment was usually discontinued after 4 to 7 days following a gradual reduction in dosage.— M. M. Glatt, *Br. med. J.*, 1971, *3*, 105. See also M. M. Glatt *et al.*, *Br. J. Addict.*, 1970, *65*, 237.

Diphenoxylate hydrochloride plus atropine (Lomotil) suppressed the minor withdrawal symptoms which usually accompany methadone withdrawal and facilitated complete withdrawal following a period of methadone maintenance in 38 patients. Lomotil was given initially in a dose of 2 tablets thrice daily when withdrawal symptoms became troublesome. Lomotil was discontinued without incident in all patients.— M. H. Kleinman and D. Arnon, *Br. J. Addict.*, 1977, *72*, 167.

Preparations

Diphenoxylate Hydrochloride and Atropine Sulfate Oral Solution *(U.S.P.)*. Diphenoxylate Hydrochloride and Atropine Sulfate Solution. A solution of diphenoxylate hydrochloride and atropine sulphate. pH of a 50% dilution 3 to 3.7. It contains 13.5 to 16.5% of alcohol. Store in airtight containers. Protect from light.

Diphenoxylate Hydrochloride and Atropine Sulfate Tablets *(U.S.P.)*. Tablets containing diphenoxylate hydrochloride and atropine sulphate. Protect from light.

Proprietary Preparations

Lomotil *(Searle, UK)*. **Tablets** each containing diphenoxylate hydrochloride 2.5 mg and atropine sulphate 25 µg, and **Liquid** containing the equivalent of 1 tablet in each 5 ml. For the symptomatic relief of diarrhoea. *Dose.* Adults, 4 tablets or 20 ml of liquid initially then 2 tablets or 10 ml every 6 hours. (Also available as Lomotil in *Austral.*, *Canad.*, *S.Afr.*, *USA*).

A reminder that the essential consequence of acute diarrhoea is dehydration, and the fundamental treatment is rehydration.— W. A. M. Cutting and W. C. Marshall (letter), *Lancet*, 1979, *2*, 1022.

Lomotil with Neomycin *(Searle, UK)*. Scored **Tablets** each containing diphenoxylate hydrochloride 2.5 mg, atropine sulphate 25 µg, and neomycin sulphate 250 mg, and **Liquid** (suggested diluent, glycerol) containing the equivalent of 1 tablet in each 5 ml. For diarrhoea of bacterial origin. *Dose.* Adults, 4 tablets or 20 ml of liquid initially, followed by 2 tablets or 10 ml every 6 hours.

A reminder that the essential consequence of acute diarrhoea is dehydration, and the fundamental treatment is rehydration.— W. A. M. Cutting and W. C. Marshall (letter), *Lancet*, 1979, *2*, 1022.

Other Proprietary Names

(with atropine sulphate) Diarsed *(Fr.)*; Reasec *(Ital., Switz.)*; Retardin *(Denm., Norw., Swed.)*.

A preparation containing diphenoxylate hydrochloride and atropine sulphate was also formerly marketed in Great Britain under the proprietary name Reasec *(Janssen)*.

6224-s

Dipipanone Hydrochloride *(B.P.)*.

Dipipan. Hydrochlor.; Phenylpiperone Hydrochlorde; Piperidyl Methadone Hydrochloride; Piperidylamidone Hydrochloride. (±)-4,4-Diphenyl-6-piperidinoheptan-3-one hydrochloride monohydrate.
$C_{24}H_{31}NO,HCl,H_2O = 404.0$.

CAS — 467-83-4 (dipipanone).

Pharmacopoeias. In *Br.*

An almost odourless, white, crystalline powder with a bitter numbing and burning taste. M.p. 124° to 127°.

Soluble 1 in 40 of water, 1 in 1.5 of alcohol, and 1 in 6 of acetone; practically insoluble in ether. A 2.5% solution in water has a pH of 4 to 6. Solutions are **sterilised** by autoclaving or by filtration.

Dependence. Prolonged use of dipipanone may produce dependence of the morphine type (see p.1018).

References: I. P. James *et al.* (letter), *Br. med. J.*, 1976, *2*, 1448; D. H. Marjot (letter), *Br. med. J.*, 1978, *1*, 1214; *ibid.*, 1980, *281*, 290.

Adverse Effects, Treatment, and Precautions. As for Morphine, p.1019.

Intravenous injection may cause an alarming fall in blood pressure, and is not recommended. Dipipanone hydrochloride is often given with cyclizine hydrochloride to reduce the incidence of nausea and vomiting.

Ischaemic colitis requiring partial bowel resection occurred in a 25-year-old man after the intravenous injection of 3 Diconal tablets (each containing dipipanone hydrochloride 10 mg and cyclizine hydrochloride 30 mg) dissolved in tap water and the consumption of a large quantity of beer. The ischaemia was possibly caused by drug-induced hypotension.— A. R. Turnbull and P. Isaacson, *Br. med. J.*, 1977, *2*, 1000.

Absorption and Fate. Dipipanone hydrochloride is absorbed from the gastro-intestinal tract. It is metabolised in the liver and is excreted in the faeces and urine.

Uses. Dipipanone hydrochloride is an analgesic related to methadone. It is used in the treatment of moderate or severe pain. Following intramuscular injection the analgesic effect begins after about 15 minutes and lasts about 4 to 6 hours; following administration by mouth the effect begins within an hour and lasts about 6 hours.

It is usually given by mouth in a dose of 10 mg with cyclizine hydrochloride repeated every 6 hours. The dose may be increased if necessary in increments of 5 mg; it is seldom necessary to exceed a dose of 30 mg. It has also been given by subcutaneous or intramuscular injection in a dose of 12.5 to 25 mg repeated every 6 hours if necessary.

Preparations

Dipipanone Injection *(B.P.)*. A sterile solution of dipipanone hydrochloride in Water for Injections. The acidity is adjusted to pH 4.5 by the addition of hydrochloric acid (limits: 4 to 5.6). Sterilised by autoclaving. Protect from light.

Diconal (known in some countries as Wellconal) *(Calmic, UK)*. Scored tablets each containing dipipanone hydrochloride 10 mg and cyclizine hydrochloride 30 mg. For pain. *Dose.* 1 tablet, repeated if necessary every 6 hours. If this dosage is inadequate it may be increased by increments of half a tablet.

6225-w

Ethoheptazine Citrate.

Wy 401. Ethyl 1-methyl-4-phenylperhydroazepine-4-carboxylate dihydrogen citrate.
$C_{16}H_{23}NO_2,C_6H_8O_7 = 453.5$.

CAS — 77-15-6 (ethoheptazine); 6700-56-7 (citrate); 2085-42-9 (citrate, ±).

A white or almost white, almost odourless powder. M.p. about 140°. **Soluble** in water and alcohol; practically insoluble in ether. A 1% solution in water has a pH of 3.5 to 4.5. **Store** in airtight containers.

Adverse Effects. Nausea, vomiting, drowsiness, dizziness, epigastric distress, and pruritus may occur following administration of ethoheptazine citrate. Stimulation of the central nervous system has been reported following administration of large doses.

Ethoheptazine in doses of 2.1, 4.2, or 8.5 mg per kg body-weight intravenously caused visual and auditory hallucinations in 5 patients. The largest dose, given over a period of 4 minutes, caused epileptiform changes in the EEG.— R. O. Bauer *et al.*, *Pharmacologist*, 1965, *7*, 163.

Absorption and Fate. Ethoheptazine is readily absorbed from the gastro-intestinal tract and peak blood concentrations are reached in an hour. It is extensively metabolised in the liver and excreted in the urine.

Uses. Ethoheptazine citrate is structurally related to pethidine. It is employed as an analgesic in the treatment of mild to moderate pain, usually in conjunction with other analgesics such as aspirin or paracetamol. The usual dose is 75 to 150 mg three or four times daily.

Analgesia. Review: N. B. Eddy *et al.*, *Codeine and its Alternates for Pain and Cough Relief*, Geneva, World Health Organization, 1970. See also *idem*, *Bull. Wld Hlth Org.*, 1969, *40*, 1.

Proprietary Preparations

Equagesic (known in some countries as Ecuagesico) *(Wyeth, UK)*. Tablets each containing ethoheptazine citrate 75 mg, meprobamate 150 mg, and aspirin 250 mg. For pain, especially when accompanied by apprehension and anxiety. *Dose.* 2 tablets 3 or 4 times daily.

Zactipar (known in some countries as Zactane) *(Wyeth, UK)*. Tablets each containing ethoheptazine citrate 75 mg and paracetamol 400 mg. Analgesic. *Dose.* 1 or 2 tablets twice or thrice daily.

NOTE. The name Zactane is also applied to preparations containing only ethoheptazine citrate.

Zactirin (known in some countries as Zactrin and Zamintol) *(Wyeth, UK)*. Tablets each containing ethoheptazine citrate 75 mg, aspirin 325 mg, and calcium carbonate 97 mg. For pain. *Dose.* 1 or 2 tablets 2 to 4 times daily.

Other Proprietary Names

Panalgin *(Ital.)*.

6226-e

Ethylmorphine Hydrochloride *(B.P., Eur. P.)*.

Aethylmorphinae Hydrochloridum; Aethylmorphini Hydrochloridum; Ethylmorphini Hydrochloridum; Ethylmorphinium Chloride; Chlorhydrate de Codéthyline. 3-*O*-Ethylmorphine hydrochloride dihydrate.
$C_{19}H_{23}NO_3,HCl,2H_2O=385.9$.

CAS — 76-58-4 (ethylmorphine); 125-30-4 (hydrochloride, anhydrous).

Pharmacopoeias. In all pharmacopoeias examined except *Braz., Int., Turk.*, and *U.S.*

A white odourless crystalline powder with a bitter taste. M.p. about 123°, with decomposition. **Soluble** 1 in 12 of water, 1 in 25 of alcohol, 1 in 1 of warm alcohol, and 1 in 250 of chloroform; practically insoluble in ether. A 2% solution in water is laevorotatory and has a pH of 4 to 5.4. A 6.18% solution is iso-osmotic with serum. **Sterilisation** and **incompatibilities** as for Morphine, p.1018. **Protect** from light.

An aqueous solution of ethylmorphine hydrochloride iso-osmotic with serum (6.18%) caused 38% haemolysis of erythrocytes cultured in it for 45 minutes.— E. R. Hammarlund and K. Pedersen-Bjergaard, *J. pharm. Sci.*, 1961, *50*, 24.

Preservatives for eye-drops. Benzalkonium chloride 0.01% or phenylmercuric nitrate 0.002% were suitable preservatives for ethylmorphine hydrochloride eye-drops sterilised by filtration or heating at 98° to 100° for 30 minutes.— Pharm. Soc. Lab. Rep. P/65/5, 1965.

Benzalkonium chloride 0.01% or chlorhexidine gluconate 0.02% were suitable preservatives for ethylmorphine hydrochloride eye-drops sterilised by filtration.— M. Van Ooteghem, *Pharm. Tijdschr. Belg.*, 1968, *45*, 69.

Dependence. Prolonged use may lead to dependence of the morphine type (see p.1018).

Adverse Effects, Treatment, and Precautions. As for Morphine, p.1019.

Absorption and Fate. Ethylmorphine hydrochloride is absorbed from the gastro-intestinal tract.

Study of the metabolism of ethylmorphine in the foetal liver.— A. Rane and E. Ackermann, *Clin. Pharmac. Ther.*, 1972, *13*, 663.

Uses. Ethylmorphine hydrochloride has been used similarly to codeine as an analgesic and cough suppressant.

Ethylmorphine hydrochloride has been used as eye-drops containing 1 to 5% as a lymphagogue in the treatment of corneal ulcers, iritis, and glaucoma; it increases the blood supply to the tissues and may provoke a sharp burning sensation and some oedema of the conjunctiva, but this soon subsides.

Proprietary Names

Diosan Comp. *(Abello, Spain)*; Trachyl *(ethylmorphine methiodide) (Beytout, Fr.)*.

Ethylmorphine hydrochloride was formerly marketed in Great Britain under the proprietary name Renotin (*Lane & Stedman*).

6227-l

Etorphine Hydrochloride *(B.P. Vet.)*.

M 99; 19-Propylorvinol Hydrochloride. (6*R*, 7*R*, 14*R*)-7,8-Dihydro-7-(1-hydroxy-1-methylbutyl)-6-*O*-methyl-6,14-ethenomorphine hydrochloride; 2-[(−)-(5*R*, 6*R*, 7*R*, 14*R*)-4,5-Epoxy-3-hydroxy-6-methoxy-9a-methyl-6,14-ethenomorphinan-7-yl]pentan-2-ol hydrochloride.
$C_{25}H_{33}NO_4,HCl=448.0$.

CAS — 14521-96-1 (etorphine); 13764-49-3 (hydrochloride).

A white or almost white microcrystalline powder. **Soluble** 1 in 40 of water, 1 in 30 of alcohol, and 1 in 2200 of chloroform; practically insoluble in ether. A 2% solution in water has a pH of 4 to 5.5. **Protect** from light.

Dependence. Prolonged use of etorphine may lead to dependence of the morphine type (see p.1018).

References: D. R. Jasinski *et al.*, *Clin. Pharmac. Ther.*, 1975, *17*, 267.

Adverse Effects and Treatment. As for Morphine, p.1019. Spillage on the skin or splashes in the eyes or mouth should be treated immediately by lavage with copious quantities of water.

The accidental injection of some or all of the contents of a 2-ml syringe containing etorphine 2.45 mg and acepromazine 10 mg per ml (Immobilon, *Reckitt & Colman*, for use in large animals) in a healthy 41-year-old man produced dizziness, nausea, and coma. Two doses of nalorphine 10 mg with supportive measures were required to reverse the coma, and metoclopramide 10 mg was given intravenously to treat the nausea. The patient was out of danger in 6 hours.— S. Firn (letter), *Lancet*, 1973, *2*, 95. It was found later that the syringe contained 1 ml both before and after the accident. The effects were due to solution present on the needle.— *idem*, 1974, *1*, 577.

Further reports of etorphine (Immobilon) poisoning in man.— *Vet. Rec.*, 1976, *98*, 513; P. G. E. Goodrich (letter), *Vet. Rec.*, 1977, *100*, 458; C. M. Orr (letter), *Vet. Rec.*, 1977, *100*, 574.

Further references: G. N. Volans and B. A. Whittle (letter), *Br. med. J.*, 1976, *2*, 472; *Lancet*, 1977, *2*, 178.

Uses. A highly potent analgesic and narcotic. It is used with acepromazine maleate as a sedative to assist in the control of large animals and with methotrimeprazine for small animals. The duration of action of etorphine is 1 to 2 hours in animals but it may be longer in man, especially if the large animal preparation is involved.

Use of etorphine in veterinary surgical procedures.— J. L. Crooks *et al.*, *Vet. Rec.*, 1970, *87*, 498.

Further references: G. F. Blane *et al.*, *Br. J. Pharmac. Chemother.*, 1967, *30*, 11.

Preparations

Etorphine and Acepromazine Injection *(B.P. Vet.)*. A sterile solution containing in each ml etorphine hydrochloride 2.45 mg and acepromazine maleate 10 mg in Water for Injections containing a suitable preservative. pH 3.5 to 4.5. Sterilised by autoclaving or by filtration. Protect from light.

Etorphine and Methotrimeprazine Injection *(B.P. Vet.)*. A sterile solution containing in each ml etorphine hydrochloride 74 µg and methotrimeprazine 18 mg in Water for Injections containing suitable stabilising agents. pH 3.5 to 4.5 Sterilised by autoclaving or by filtration. Protect from light.

6228-y

Fentanyl Citrate *(B.P., B.P. Vet., U.S.P.)*.

Phentanyl Citrate; R 4263. *N*-(1-Phenethyl-4-piperidyl)propionanilide dihydrogen citrate.
$C_{22}H_{28}N_2O,C_6H_8O_7=528.6$.

CAS — 437-38-7 (fentanyl); 990-73-8 (citrate).

Pharmacopoeias. In *Br., Braz.*, and *U.S.*

White granules or a white glistening crystalline powder, odourless, with a bitter taste. M.p. 147° to 152°. **Soluble** 1 in 40 of water, 1 in 140 of alcohol, 1 in 350 of chloroform, 1 in 10 of methyl alcohol; slightly soluble in ether. Solutions are **sterilised** by autoclaving or by filtration. **Incompatible** with thiopentone, propanidid, and methohexitone. **Store** in airtight containers. Protect from light.

CAUTION. *Avoid contact with skin and the inhalation of particles of fentanyl citrate.*

Stability. Fentanyl was hydrolysed in acid solution by the cleavage of propionic acid but was unchanged in alkaline solution.— C. A. Janicki *et al.*, *J. pharm. Sci.*, 1968, *57*, 451.

Dependence. Prolonged use of fentanyl may lead to dependence of the morphine type (see p.1018).

Adverse Effects and Treatment. As for Morphine, p.1019. Atropine may be used to block the vagal effects of fentanyl such as bradycardia. Muscle rigidity may occur and has been reported to be alleviated by muscle relaxants.

Effects on muscle. A report of muscle rigidity occurring with fentanyl.— M. Rosenberg, *Anesth. Prog.*, 1977, *24*, 50. See also A. A. Bechtoldt and W. J. Murray, *Anesth. Analg. curr. Res.*, 1968, *47*, 395.

Effects on respiratory function. For reports on the effect of fentanyl in reducing the ventilatory response to carbon dioxide, see A. A. Bechtoldt and W. J. Murray, *Anesth. Analg. curr. Res.*, 1968, *47*, 395; L. D. Becker *et al.*, *Anesthesiology*, 1976, *44*, 291; M. F. Mulroy *et al.*, *Anesth. Analg. curr. Res.*, 1977, *56*, 826.

In 3 patients respiratory depression occurred 30 minutes to 4 hours after apparent recovery from the effects of fentanyl.— A. P. Adams and D. A. Pybus, *Br. med. J.*, 1978, *1*, 278. The patients were below average in weight and had also received other narcotic analgesics.— C. J. Wright (letter), *ibid.*, 441. The effects of the narcotic analgesics were enhanced by fentanyl.— J. H. Williams (letter), *ibid.*

Histamine release. A report of a significant histamine response occurring with fentanyl.— J. Hayden and E. Scott, *Anesth. Prog.*, 1974, *21*, 84.

Treatment of adverse effects. Physostigmine reversed the somnolence and disorientation that followed use of large doses of fentanyl and droperidol.— A. V. Bidwai *et al.*, *Anesthesiology*, 1976, *44*, 249.

Precautions. As for Morphine, p.1019. Care should be taken when fentanyl citrate is given to patients with myasthenia gravis. Care should be taken to avoid inhaling particles of fentanyl citrate or exposing the skin to it.

While using fentanyl citrate and droperidol for hypotensive anaesthesia it was noted in 22 patients that after an initial rapid fall, the systolic blood pressure could not be reduced below 90 to 100 mmHg, even by using concentrations of up to 6% of halothane.— P. J. Thompson (letter), *Br. med. J.*, 1969, *3*, 300.

In 8 patients undergoing neuroleptanalgesia with droperidol, diazepam, and fentanyl prior to carotid angiography, laryngeal reflex closure was repressed permitting aspiration of a test contrast medium. Neuroleptanalgesia should not be used without safeguarding the airway in patients liable to regurgitation and aspiration of gastric contents.— J. G. Brock-Utne *et al.*, *Br. J. Anaesth.*, 1976, *48*, 699. See also C. J. Kopriva *et al.*, *Anesthesiology*, 1974, *40*, 596; V. M. F. Hey and A. H. M. Z. Mollah (letter), *Lancet*, 1979, *1*, 552; L. Strunin and I. M. Corall (letter), *ibid.*, 673.

Unexpectedly high plasma-fentanyl concentrations occurred in a patient following epidural administration.— R. E. S. Bullingham *et al.* (letter), *Lancet*, 1980, *1*, 1361.

Effect on intracranial pressure. Fentanyl and droperidol given by injection reduced the CSF pressure of 8 of 9 patients with space-occupying intracranial lesions and in patients with normal CSF pathways. The CSF pressure was unaffected by phenoperidine and droperidol.— W. Fitch *et al.*, *Br. J. Anaesth.*, 1969, *41*, 800.

In 8 anaesthetised normocapnic patients with space-occupying intracranial lesions droperidol 7.5 to 12.5 mg caused an increase of intracranial pressure (ICP) in 4; a decrease in mean arterial pressure (MAP) (for the 8) from 99.9 to 85 mmHg resulted in a significant decrease from 79.9 to 57.8 mmHg in cerebral perfusion pressure (CPP). When fentanyl 200 to 300 µg was added there were minimal changes in ICP but a further decrease in MAP to 71.1 mmHg resulted in a further reduction in CPP to 47.8 mmHg. Neuroleptanalgesics should be used in patients with intracranial hypertension only if hypocapnia was established and if arterial pressure was near normal.— B. B. Misfeldt *et al.*, *Br. J. Anaesth.*, 1976, *48*, 963.

Fentanyl 200 µg was given intravenously to 10 anaesthetised patients, 9 of whom were hypocapnic, with space-occupying intracranial lesions. Increases or decreases in intracranial pressure occurred but were small and not significant. Mean arterial pressure and cerebral perfusion pressure were significantly reduced by fentanyl, although the changes were small unless the patient was already hypotensive. Fentanyl should not be given to such patients but otherwise it was a valuable adjunct to anaesthesia.— E. Moss *et al.*, *Br. J. Anaesth.*, 1978, *50*, 779.

Porphyria. A study in *rats* indicated that fentanyl should be regarded as potentially hazardous for patients with a hereditary hepatic porphyria.— G. H. Blekkenhorst *et al.* (letter), *Lancet*, 1980, *1*, 1367. Criticisms of extrapolating data obtained from *animal* experiments to the treatment of human disease.— M. J. Brodie (letter), *ibid.*, *2*, 86; A. Gorchein (letter), *ibid.*, 152.

Absorption and Fate. Fentanyl citrate is absorbed from the gastro-intestinal tract. After parenteral administration it has a rapid onset and short duration of action. It is rapidly metabolised, probably by oxidative *N*-dealkylation, and excreted mainly in the urine. The short duration of action is probably due to redistribution rather than metabolism and excretion. Up to 70% has been reported to be bound to plasma proteins.

A brief review of the pharmacokinetics of fentanyl during neuroleptanalgesia.— M. M. Ghoneim and K. Korttila, *Clin. Pharmacokinet.*, 1977, *2*, 344.

Following the intravenous administration of fentanyl citrate 0.1, 0.5, and 1 mg per m^2 body-surface to 14 patients during surgery serum-fentanyl concentrations decreased rapidly during the first 5 minutes to about 20% of the peak value, had stabilised at 1, 5, and 8 ng per ml respectively after about 2 hours, and thereafter continued to decrease very slowly. In 4 patients investigated, peak concentrations in CSF were below 4 ng per ml and occurred 10 to 40 minutes after administration. In 3 patients cumulative urinary fentanyl excretion was 14, 16, and 21% of the administered dose after 50 hours.— R. Schleimer *et al.*, *Clin. Pharmac. Ther.*, 1978, *23*, 188.

Comment by the manufacturer on the analgesic activity of fentanyl not being related to plasma concentrations.— R. F. Cookson (letter), *Br. J. Anaesth.*, 1980, *52*, 959.

Further references: S. Bower *et al.*, *Br. J. Anaesth.*, 1976, *48*, 1121; H. J. McQuay *et al.*, *ibid.*, 1979, *51*, 543; H. Stoeckel *et al.*, *ibid.*, 1979, *51*, 741; J. G. Bovill and P. S. Sebel, *ibid.*, 1980, *52*, 795; D. A. McClain and C. C. Hug, *Clin. Pharmac. Ther.*, 1980, *28*, 106; A. J. Koska *et al.*, *ibid.*, 1981, *29*, 100.

Uses. Fentanyl citrate is a potent analgesic, chemically related to pethidine, with actions similar to those of morphine (see p.1020) and pethidine (see p.1027).

Following intravenous injection the effect begins almost immediately, although maximum analgesia and respiratory depression may not occur for several minutes, and the average duration of action is 30 to 60 minutes; following intramuscular injection the effect begins in about 7 minutes and lasts 1 to 2 hours.

Fentanyl produces surgical analgesia and when a major tranquilliser or neuroleptic agent such as droperidol is added the patient can be maintained in a state of neuroleptanalgesia in which he is calm and indifferent to his surroundings and is able to cooperate with the surgeon. Nitrous oxide and oxygen may be given to produce light anaesthesia.

In anaesthesia where spontaneous respiration is maintained, an initial intravenous dose of the equivalent of 50 to 200 μg of fentanyl is given, with supplementary doses of 50 μg. In anaesthesia with controlled respiration, the initial dose is 300 to 3500 μg with supplementary doses of 100 to 200 μg. The initial doses in children are 3 to 5 μg per kg body-weight where spontaneous respiration is maintained or 10 to 15 μg per kg in anaesthesia with controlled respiration.

Doses of 50 to 100 μg of fentanyl may be given intramuscularly for the relief of postoperative pain, and repeated in 1 to 2 hours if necessary.

The pharmacology and pharmacokinetics of fentanyl.— W. Soudijn, in *Stress-free Anaesthesia*, C. Wood (Ed.), London, The Royal Society of Medicine, 1978, p. 3.

The effects of morphine sulphate and fentanyl citrate on tracheal smooth muscle.— I. Yasuda *et al.*, *Anesthesiology*, 1978, *49*, 117.

For reports of the reduction of side-effects of ketamine by droperidol and fentanyl citrate, see Ketamine Hydrochloride, p.751.

Administration. The duration of action of fentanyl was less than an hour while the effects of droperidol could last 6 to 7 hours. Therefore if repeated increments of the combined preparation were given droperidol overdosage might occur. The dosage of each should be estimated and then administered separately with increments of fentanyl being given as required for analgesia.— J. Adriani and M. Naraghi, *Conn. Med.*, 1976, *40*, 745.

Administration, epidural. A report on the use of epidural fentanyl (without preservative) for postoperative analgesia following elective caesarean section. Fentanyl 100 μg diluted with 8 ml of sodium chloride injection is given through an epidural catheter with the patient supine. Very satisfactory analgesia was obtained in 20 consecutive patients with no significant alteration in heart-rate, blood pressure, respiratory-rate, or level of consciousness. Onset of analgesia occurred in 4 to 10 minutes, reached a peak within 20 minutes, and lasted 200 to 400 minutes.— M. J. Wolfe and A. D. G. Nicholas (letter), *Lancet*, 1979, *2*, 150.

A study in patients with low back pain indicated that epidural injection of fentanyl gave relief of pain lasting 90 minutes, whereas epidural injection of diamorphine gave pain relief lasting over 9 hours. Severe pruritus, which usually began about 30 minutes after the onset of analgesia, may limit the use of some epidural opiates; it was only weakly relieved by chlorpheniramine.— H. J. McQuay *et al.* (letter), *Lancet*, 1980, *1*, 768.

Excellent results with epidural fentanyl citrate in a woman suffering intolerable pain as a result of widely disseminated skeletal metastases from carcinoma of the breast, together with fractures after a fall. The pain did not respond to frequent intramuscular injections of papaveretum 20 mg, and was unsatisfactorily managed by epidural bupivacaine which produced anaesthesia of the skin and faecal incontinence. It was found that fentanyl 50 μg diluted with 5 ml of physiological saline given hourly as a continuous infusion through a syringe pump produced complete analgesia. She recovered normal skin sensation and regained control of defaecation. Fentanyl citrate was given as Sublimaze, stated to be free from preservative.— R. M. B. Wright and T. Goroszeniuk (letter), *Lancet*, 1980, *2*, 1033.

For a report of disappointing results with epidural pethidine, phenoperidine, and fentanyl in labour, see Pethidine Hydrochloride, p.1027.

See also under Precautions, above.

Administration in renal failure. Fentanyl 75 μg administered to 6 patients with chronic renal failure and to 7 general surgical patients had no effect on cardiac output, arterial blood pressure, or heart-rate, but the drug increased the work of the heart.— J. W. Mostert *et al.*, *Br. J. Anaesth.*, 1970, *42*, 501.

Anaesthesia. The use of fentanyl, 25 μg per kg body-weight intravenously, together with alcuronium, nitrous oxide, and oxygen, following premedication with fentanyl and droperidol, was described for 52 patients aged 65 to 92 years who were undergoing orthopaedic surgery. Sequential injections of fentanyl 125 μg were given to maintain analgesia, and pentazocine 1 mg per kg was given postoperatively, to enable patients to recover consciousness. Freedom from pain continued for at least 5 hours.— K. Rifat, *Br. J. Anaesth.*, 1972, *44*, 175. A similar study in neonates and infants.— B. Kay, *Anesth. Analg. curr. Res.*, 1973, *52*, 970.

With experience of neuroleptanaesthesia in 500 patients most of whom were given droperidol with fentanyl along with nitrous oxide and muscle relaxants; the technique was considered suitable for elderly and poor-risk patients.— M. Morgan *et al.*, *Br. J. Anaesth.*, 1974, *46*, 288.

Anaesthesia with continuous infusion of fentanyl.— A. G. H. Cole *et al.*, *Br. J. Anaesth.*, 1980, *52*, 229P.

Further references to the use of fentanyl in neuroleptanaesthesia.— H. J. Wüst *et al.*, in *Stress-free Anaesthesia*, C. Wood (Ed.), London, The Royal Society of Medicine, 1978, p. 39.

Dental. In a randomised study in 100 patients undergoing dental surgery, cardiac arrhythmias were reduced by a regimen of fentanyl 1 μg per kg body-weight intravenously, tubocurarine 30 mg, thiopentone 5 to 6 mg per kg, nitrous oxide 67% in oxygen, and intermittent positive-pressure ventilation when compared with those given thiopentone, suxamethonium, halothane, nitrous oxide 62.5% in oxygen, with spontaneous ventilation. Immediate recovery was more rapid but the overall recovery time was similar. There was no significant difference in the incidence of nausea, vomiting, and postoperative pain.— V. J. E. Thomas *et al.*, *Br. J. Anaesth.*, 1976, *48*, 919.

High-dose fentanyl. A report of the regular use for more than a year of fentanyl for major vascular surgery—induction doses of 15 to 25 μg per kg body-weight were supplemented by regular increments of 250 to 500 μg. Hypercapnia, though present, appeared to be of little clinical importance. Opiate premedication should be avoided.— A. M. Florence (letter), *Br. med. J.*, 1978, *1*, 650. Comments.— *Lancet*, 1979, *1*, 81. Comments and corrections.— G. M. Hall and A. Holdcroft (letter), *ibid.*, 268; A. M. Florence (letter), *ibid.*. Criticism.— M. Johnstone (letter), *ibid.*, 378.

The effects of high doses of fentanyl on stress and metabolic response during major surgery.— G. M. Hall, in *Stress-free Anaesthesia*, C. Wood (Ed.), London, The Royal Society of Medicine, 1978, p. 19; A. Florence, *ibid.*, p. 23.

Fentanyl in doses up to 50 μg per kg body-weight was used as an anaesthetic for patients undergoing cardiac surgery. Complete anaesthesia was obtained with minimal cardiovascular effects in patients with mitral valve disease.— T. H. Stanley and L. R. Webster, in *Stress-free Anaesthesia*, C. Wood (Ed.), London, The Royal Society of Medicine, 1978, p. 27.

Discussion of the possibility that high doses of fentanyl (at least 50 μg per kg body-weight) might be of benefit in modifying the metabolic response to surgery.— G. M. Hall, *Br. J. Anaesth.*, 1980, *52*, 561.

Premedication. In a double-blind comparison on 100 patients, pethidine was more effective than fentanyl in producing total amnesia for pre-operative procedures and inhibiting muscular responses to surgical incision during nitrous oxide anaesthesia. Cardiovascular, respiratory, and metabolic functions remained more stable with fentanyl. In addition, there was no histamine reaction at the site of injection in comparison with pethidine.— J. W. Mostert *et al.*, *J. clin. Pharmac.*, 1968, *8*, 382.

A single-blind study involving 52 patients undergoing fibreoptic bronchoscopy indicating that a combination of fentanyl, diazepam, and atropine appears to be better premedication than papaveretum and hyoscine.— T. Goroszeniuk *et al.*, *Br. med. J.*, 1980, *281*, 486.

Further reports of the use of fentanyl citrate and droperidol as premedication for general anaesthesia.— S. J. Martin *et al.*, *Anesthesiology*, 1967, *28*, 458; J. G. Goodbody (letter), *Br. med. J.*, 1969, *4*, 368; M. Morgan, *ibid.*; F. S. Keddie (letter), *Br. med. J.*, 1969, *4*, 51; A. B. Dobkin *et al.*, *Anesth. Analg. curr. Res.*, 1970, *49*, 261.

Analgesia. *Postoperative.* To investigate the analgesic potency and respiratory depressant activity of fentanyl citrate, 75 patients were given intramuscular injections of 200 μg of fentanyl citrate or 10 mg of morphine sulphate postoperatively. The analgesics were comparable in relieving pain, and fentanyl had no advantage over morphine in speed of onset or duration of effects. Fentanyl depressed respiration more than morphine in the doses used and caused severe pain at the site of injection.— J. S. Finch and T. J. DeKornfeld, *J. clin. Pharmac.*, 1967, *7*, 46.

The use of fentanyl infusion, administered by a demand analgesia computer, for the relief of pain after peripheral vascular surgery. A basic dose of 30 μg per hour could be increased on demand up to a total of 150 μg per hour, and was as effective as epidural analgesia using bupivacaine.— W. D. White *et al.*, *Br. med. J.*, 1979, *2*, 166.

Further references: T. M. Hunt *et al.*, *Br. J. Anaesth.*, 1979, *51*, 785.

See also under Administration, Epidural.

Neuroleptanalgesia. A brief report on the use of neuroleptanalgesia, with fentanyl and droperidol, during the changing of burn dressings.— H. J. Birkhan (letter), *Lancet*, 1969, *2*, 111.

In 250 patients, fentanyl citrate and droperidol with diazepam produced satisfactory analgesia and sedation for peroral endoscopic examination.— H. I. Le Brun, *Gut*, 1976, *17*, 655.

See also under Anaesthesia, above.

Preparations

Fentanyl Citrate Injection *(U.S.P.)*. A sterile solution of fentanyl citrate in Water for Injections. pH 4 to 7.5. Potency is expressed in terms of the equivalent amount of fentanyl. Protect from light.

Sublimaze *(Janssen, UK)*. Fentanyl citrate, available as an injection containing the equivalent of 50 μg of fentanyl per ml, in ampoules of 2 and 10 ml. (Also available as Sublimaze in *Austral.*, *Canad.*, *S.Afr.*, *USA*).

Thalamonal Injection (known in *USA* as Innovar) *(Janssen, UK)*. A solution containing fentanyl citrate equivalent to fentanyl 50 μg and droperidol 2.5 mg per ml, in ampoules of 2 ml.

Other Proprietary Names

Fentanest *(Ital.)*; Haldid *(Denm.)*; Leptanal *(Norw., Swed.)*.

6229-j

Hydrocodone Hydrochloride. Dihydrocodeinone Hydrochloride.
$C_{18}H_{21}NO_3,HCl,2\frac{1}{2}H_2O=380.9$.

CAS — 25968-91-6 (anhydrous).

A white crystalline powder. **Soluble** 1 in 2 of water; soluble in alcohol. **Protect** from light.

6230-q

Hydrocodone Phosphate.
$C_{18}H_{21}NO_3,1\frac{1}{2}H_3PO_4=446.4$.

CAS — 34366-67-1.

Pharmacopoeias. In *Rus.*

A white or yellowish-white odourless crystalline powder with a bitter taste. **Soluble** in water; practically insoluble in alcohol, chloroform, and ether. **Protect** from light.

6231-p

Hydrocodone Tartrate.

Hydrocodone Acid Tartrate; Hydrocodone Bitartrate *(U.S.P.)*; Hydrocodoni Bitartras; Hydrocone Bitartrate; Dihydrocodeinone Acid Tartrate. 6-Deoxy-3-*O*-methyl-6-oxomorphine hydrogen tartrate hemipentahydrate; (−)-(5*R*)-4,5-Epoxy-3-methoxy-9a-methylmorphinan-6-one hydrogen tartrate hemipentahydrate.
$C_{18}H_{21}NO_3,C_4H_6O_6,2\frac{1}{2}H_2O=494.5$.

CAS — 125-29-1 (hydrocodone); 143-71-5 (tartrate, anhydrous); 34195-34-1 (tartrate, hemipentahydrate).

Pharmacopoeias. In *Aust., Belg., Cz., Ger., Hung., Int., Nord., Port., Swiss,* and *U.S. Turk.* has anhydrous.

White odourless crystals or crystalline powder with a slightly acid, bitter, saline taste.
Soluble 1 in 10 of water and 1 in 150 of alcohol; practically insoluble in chloroform and ether. A 2% solution in water is laevorotatory and has a pH of 3.2 to 3.8. Solutions containing 0.1% of sodium metabisulphite may be **sterilised** by autoclaving. **Incompatible** with alkalis, iodides, and tannic acid. **Store** in airtight containers. Protect from light.

Dependence. Prolonged use of hydrocodone may lead to dependence of the morphine type (see p.1018). It is more likely than codeine to produce dependence.

Abuse. Hydrocodone with phenyltoloxamine as cation exchange resin complexes (Tussionex) was being abused; its psychotropic effects lasted for about 8 hours.— Y. J. Berry (letter), *New Engl. J. Med.*, 1976, *295*, 286.

Adverse Effects, Treatment, and Precautions. As for Morphine, p.1019.

Overdose. Three deaths from pulmonary oedema associated with high concentrations of hydrocodone and phenyltoloxamine in body fluids following ingestion of a slow-release liquid preparation.— D. Vivian, *Drug Intell. & clin. Pharm.*, 1979, *13*, 445.

Uses. Hydrocodone tartrate has actions similar to those of codeine (see p.1005) but is more potent on a weight for weight basis. It is used chiefly for the relief of irritant cough, though it has no particular advantage over codeine. It is also used for the relief of moderate pain. Hydrocodone tartrate is taken by mouth in doses of 5 to 10 mg three or four times daily. It has been given by subcutaneous injection in doses of 5 to 15 mg, with a maximum of 45 mg daily.
The hydrochloride and the phosphate have also been used in similar doses.

Preparations

Hydrocodone Bitartrate Tablets *(U.S.P.)*. Tablets containing hydrocodone tartrate. Store in airtight containers. Protect from light.

Proprietary Names of Hydrocodone Hydrochloride

Dicodid (see also below) *(Knoll, Ger.; Knoll, Switz.)*.

Proprietary Names of Hydrocodone Tartrate

Biocodone *(Bios-Coutelier, Belg.)*; Broncodid *(Wolfs, Belg.)*; Codinovo *(Nourypharma, Neth.)*; Codone *(Lemmon, USA)*; Corutol DH *(Dow, Canad.)*; Dicodid (see also above)*(Knoll, Austral.; Knoll, Belg.; Knoll, Ger.; Knoll, Switz.; Knoll, USA)*; Hycodan *(Endo, Canad.; Endo, USA)*; Hycon *(Endo, Austral.)*; Nyodid *(Nyco, Norw.)*; Robidone *(Robins, Canad.)*.

Hydrocodone tartrate was formerly marketed in Great Britain under the proprietary name Dicodid (*Knoll, Ger.*).

6232-s

Hydromorphone. 7,8-Dihydromorphinone. 6-Deoxy-7,8-dihydro-6-oxomorphine; (−)-(5*R*)-4,5-Epoxy-3-hydroxy-9a-methylmorphinan-6-one.
$C_{17}H_{19}NO_3=285.3$.

CAS — 466-99-9.

A fine white or practically white odourless crystalline powder. M.p. about 260° with decomposition. Slightly **soluble** in water; freely soluble in alcohol; very soluble in chloroform. **Store** in airtight containers. Protect from light.

6233-w

Hydromorphone Hydrochloride *(U.S.P.)*.

Hydromorphoni Hydrochloridum; Dihydromorphinone Hydrochloride.
$C_{17}H_{19}NO_3,HCl=321.8$.

CAS — 71-68-1.

Pharmacopoeias. In *Arg., Aust., Braz., Ger., Int., Nord., Roum., Span., Swiss,* and *U.S.*

A white or almost white odourless crystalline powder with a bitter taste. **Soluble** 1 in 3 of water and 1 in 100 of alcohol (90%); practically insoluble in chloroform and ether. A solution in water is laevorotatory. Solutions are **sterilised** by autoclaving or by filtration. **Incompatibilities** as for Morphine, p.1018. **Store** in airtight containers. Protect from light.

Incompatibility. There was loss of clarity when intravenous solutions of hydromorphone hydrochloride were mixed with those of sodium bicarbonate or thiopentone sodium.— J. A. Patel and G. L. Phillips, *Am. J. Hosp. Pharm.*, 1966, *23*, 409.

Dependence. The use of hydromorphone may lead to dependence of the morphine type (see p.1018). As hydromorphone is more potent and has a shorter analgesic action than morphine, withdrawal symptoms occur sooner and are of greater intensity than for morphine.

Adverse Effects, Treatment, and Precautions. As for Morphine, p.1019.
Pain may occur at the injection site and local tissue irritation and induration may follow subcutaneous injection.

For a double-blind comparison of the respiratory depressant effects of hydromorphone and morphine, see C. R. Brown *et al.*, *Clin. Pharmac. Ther.*, 1973, *14*, 331.

Absorption and Fate. Hydromorphone is absorbed from the gastro-intestinal tract. It is metabolised and excreted in the urine mainly as conjugated hydromorphone.

Following administration of hydromorphone hydrochloride by mouth to 5 healthy former narcotic addicts, conjugated hydromorphone, hydromorphone, dihydroisomorphine, and dihydromorphine were identified in the urine. Conjugated hydromorphone was the major metabolite identified and was present in amounts ranging from 22 to 51% of the administered dose.— E. J. Cone *et al.*, *J. pharm. Sci.*, 1977, *66*, 1709.

Uses. Hydromorphone hydrochloride has a greater analgesic potency than morphine (see p.1020); following injection the analgesic effect usually occurs within 15 minutes and lasts about 5 hours.
It may be used for the relief of moderate and severe pain and is usually administered by subcutaneous or intramuscular injection in doses of 2 mg every 4 to 6 hours as necessary. It may be given by intravenous injection or by mouth in similar doses, or rectally in doses of 3 mg. In severe pain up to 4 mg every 4 to 6 hours may be required.
It has also been given, as a syrup, in doses of 1 mg repeated every 3 to 4 hours for the relief of non-productive cough.

Administration, epidural. Studies with epidural hydromorphone hydrochloride in healthy subjects, indicated that spinal opiate analgesia confined to the upper thoracic segments may modulate the afferent pathways of the Valsalva sympathetic response.— J. Leslie *et al.* (letter), *Lancet*, 1979, *2*, 151.

Preparations

Hydromorphone Hydrochloride Injection *(U.S.P.)*. A sterile solution in Water for Injections. pH 4 to 5.5. Protect from light.

Hydromorphone Hydrochloride Tablets *(U.S.P.)*. Tablets containing hydromorphone hydrochloride. Store in airtight containers. Protect from light.

Proprietary Names

Dilaudid *(Knoll, Austral.; Knoll, Ger.; Knoll, Switz.; Knoll, USA; Pentagone, Canad.)*.

6234-e

Ketobemidone. Cetobemidone. 1-(4-*m*-Hydroxyphenyl-1-methyl-4-piperidyl)propan-1-one.
$C_{15}H_{21}NO_2=247.3$.

CAS — 469-79-4.

Ketobemidone is a narcotic analgesic with actions and uses similar to those of morphine (see p.1018). The usual dose is 5 to 10 mg.

Obstetric analgesia with ketobemidone.— C. Carlsson *et al.*, *Br. J. Anaesth.*, 1980, *52*, 827.

Proprietary Names

Cliradon *(Ciba, Ger.; Ciba, Switz.)*.

6235-l

Levomethadyl Acetate.

LAAM; LAM; Levacetylmethadol; *l*-Acetylmethadol. (−)-4-Dimethylamino-1-ethyl-2,2-diphenylpentyl acetate.
$C_{23}H_{31}NO_2=353.5$.

CAS — 1477-40-3 (levomethadyl); 34433-66-4 (acetate).

The laevo isomer of methadyl acetate. M.p. about 70°.

Dependence, Adverse Effects, Treatment, and Precautions. As for Morphine, p.1018.

Effects on memory. The performance of tasks involving memory was not significantly different in 31 patients taking levomethadyl acetate 20 to 75 (mean 54) mg daily for 1 month or 15 to 100 (mean 60) mg at the end of 3 months, compared with a control group.— P. Grevert *et al.*, *Archs gen. Psychiat.*, 1977, *34*, 849.

Effects on sexual function. Measurement of plasma-testosterone concentrations in 13 men maintained on levomethadyl acetate indicated depression of plasma-testosterone concentrations in some instances to below the normal range for adult males.— J. H. Mendelson *et al.*, *Clin. Pharmac. Ther.*, 1976, *19*, 371.

Interactions. Both levomethadyl acetate and methadone might compete for plasma protein or tissue-binding sites. Differences in the attainment of a steady state after administration of levomethadyl acetate or more rapid excretion of methadone could lead to symptoms of withdrawal during a period of transfer from methadone to levomethadyl acetate maintenance therapy.— G. L. Henderson *et al.*, *Clin. Pharmac. Ther.*, 1977, *21*, 16.

Absorption and Fate. Levomethadyl acetate is absorbed from the gastro-intestinal tract. It has a slow onset and long duration of action, a single dose having a duration of action up to 72 hours. It is metabolised to compounds which have morphine-like activity and a long half-life. The metabolites *l*-α-noracetylmethadol and *l*-α-dinoracetylmethadol have been identified in plasma while methadol and normethadol have been identified in urine.

A study of the disposition of methadyl acetate in relation to pharmacological action.— R. F. Kaiko and C. E.

Inturrisi, *Clin. Pharmac. Ther.*, 1975, *18*, 96.

In a study of acute and chronic administration of levomethadyl acetate to replace oral methadone in 5 subjects and diamorphine in a further 5 subjects, the plasma decay curve was biexponential with an initial half-life of about 6 hours and a further half-life of about 50 hours. During chronic administration plasma concentrations of the metabolites noracetylmethadol acetate and dinoracetylmethadol acetate increased 5 and 13 times respectively and their half-lives were about 30 and more than 100 hours respectively; there appeared, however, to be little accumulation of levomethadyl acetate, no change occurring in the plasma decay curve. The findings suggested that the biological distribution of levomethadyl acetate was complex and its long duration of pharmacological action might be associated with at least 3 factors: *in vivo* generation of active metabolites, drug-tissue binding, and possibly enterohepatic recycling.— G. L. Henderson *et al.*, *Clin. Pharmac. Ther.*, 1977, *21*, 16.

Uses. Levomethadyl acetate is a long-acting narcotic analgesic which has been used in the management of chronic opiate dependence. It has been given in doses of up to 80 mg three times a week.

Methadyl acetate has been tried similarly.

High concentrations of levomethadyl acetate and its major metabolites had a negative chronotropic effect on isolated right atria of *guinea-pigs*. Prior administration of naloxone did not block this effect; levomethadyl acetate also diminished the positive chronotropic effect of noradrenaline.— J. L. Stickney, *Toxic. appl. Pharmac.*, 1977, *40*, 23.

Treatment of dependence. A comparative study in 193 heroin addicts indicated that levomethadyl acetate was as effective as methadone in the treatment of heroin addiction. Levomethadyl acetate induction was more difficult than methadone induction. Levomethadyl acetate was given on 3 days per week. There was a higher incidence of gastro-intestinal complaints in the levomethadyl acetate group while in the methadone group aching bones and joints, runny nose, and insomnia occurred more often.— E. C. Senay *et al.*, *J. Am. med. Ass.*, 1977, *237*, 138.

A comparative 40-week clinical study in 636 diamorphine addicts demonstrated that levomethadyl acetate was as effective as methadone for maintenance treatment of addicts. Side-effects were similar for both drugs. Levomethadyl acetate was given according to need in doses not exceeding 100 mg three days a week.— W. Ling *et al.*, *Archs gen. Psychiat.*, 1978, *35*, 345.

Further references: A. Zaks *et al.*, *J. Am. med. Ass.*, 1972, *220*, 811; S. K. Sim, *Can. med. Ass. J.*, 1973, *109*, 615; R. Levine *et al.*, *J. Am. med. Ass.*, 1973, *226*, 316; W. Ling *et al.*, *Archs gen. Psychiat.*, 1976, *33*, 709; J. Panell *et al.*, *Med. J. Aust.*, 1977, *2*, 150.

6236-y

Levorphanol Tartrate *(B.P., U.S.P.)*.

Levorphan Tartrate; Levorphanol Bitartrate; Methorphinan Tartrate. (−)-9a-Methylmorphinan-3-ol hydrogen tartrate dihydrate.

$C_{17}H_{23}NO,C_4H_6O_6,2H_2O=443.5$.

CAS — 77-07-6 (levorphanol); 125-72-4 (tartrate, anhydrous); 5985-38-6 (tartrate, dihydrate).

Pharmacopoeias. In *Br.*, *It.*, and *U.S.*

A white or almost white odourless crystalline powder with a bitter taste. M.p. 114° to 117°. **Soluble** 1 in 45 to 50 of water and 1 in 110 to 120 of alcohol; practically insoluble in chloroform. A solution in water is laevorotatory. A 0.2% solution in water has a pH of 3.4 to 4. Solutions are **sterilised** by autoclaving or by filtration. **Incompatible** with alkalis and thiopentone sodium. **Store** in airtight containers.

For a report of incompatibilities in intravenous solutions, see Codeine Phosphate, p.1004.

Dependence, Adverse Effects, Treatment, and Precautions. As for Morphine, p.1018.

Pregnancy and the neonate. Clinical depression of the newborn had been observed after use of levorphanol during labour.— F. Moya and V. Thorndike, *Clin. Pharmac. Ther.*, 1963, *4*, 628.

Absorption and Fate. Levorphanol is absorbed almost as well from the gastro-intestinal tract as when given by injection. It is probably conjugated and excreted in the urine as the glucuronide.

Uses. Levorphanol tartrate is an analgesic with effects similar to those of morphine (see p.1020), differing mainly in that it is almost as effective by mouth as by injection. The analgesic effect usually begins after about 10 to 30 minutes and lasts about 6 to 8 hours.

For severe pain, a dose of 1.5 to 4.5 mg may be given by mouth once or twice daily; the usual single dose by subcutaneous or intramuscular injection is 2 to 4 mg; it has been given by slow intravenous injection in a dose of 1 to 2 mg. It may also be used for supplementing nitrous oxide and oxygen anaesthesia in a dose of 250 or 500 µg intravenously, repeated as required.

Anaesthesia. For a report on the use of levorphanol as a supplement to nitrous oxide/oxygen anaesthesia, see J. W. Dundee *et al.*, *Anaesthesia*, 1969, *24*, 52. See also S. A. McDowell and J. W. Dundee, *Can. Anaesth. Soc. J.*, 1971, *18*, 541.

Effect on biliary tract. For an account of the comparative effects of a number of analgesics, including levorphanol tartrate, on the biliary tract, see Phenazocine Hydrobromide, p.1028.

Preparations

Levorphanol Injection *(B.P.)*. A sterile solution of levorphanol tartrate in Water for Injections, adjusted to pH 5.5 (range 5 to 6). Sterilised by autoclaving. Protect from light.

Levorphanol Tablets *(B.P.)*. Tablets containing levorphanol tartrate.

Levorphanol Tartrate Injection *(U.S.P.)*. A sterile solution in Water for Injections, pH 4.1 to 4.5.

Levorphanol Tartrate Tablets *(U.S.P.)*. Tablets containing levorphanol tartrate.

Proprietary Preparations

Dromoran (known in *Canad.* and *USA* as Levo-Dromoran and in some countries as Dalmadorm, Dalmate, or Dormador) *(Roche, UK)*. Levorphanol tartrate, available as 1-ml **Ampoules** of an injection containing 2 mg per ml and as **Tablets** of 1.5 mg. (Also available as Dromoran in *Austral.*, *Ger.*).

6237-j

Methadone Hydrochloride *(B.P., Eur. P., U.S.P.)*.

Methadone Hydrochlor.; Methadoni Hydrochloridum; Amidone Hydrochloride; Phenadone. (±)-6-Dimethylamino-4,4-diphenylheptan-3-one hydrochloride.

$C_{21}H_{27}NO,HCl=345.9$.

CAS — 76-99-3 (methadone); 297-88-1 (methadone, ±); 1095-90-5 (hydrochloride); 125-56-4 (hydrochloride, ±).

Pharmacopoeias. In *Arg.*, *Aust.*, *Belg.*, *Br.*, *Braz.*, *Cz.*, *Eur.*, *Ger.*, *Hung.*, *Ind.*, *Int.*, *It.*, *Jug.*, *Neth.*, *Nord.*, *Port.*, *Rus.*, *Swiss*, *Turk.*, and *U.S.*

Odourless colourless crystals or white crystalline powder with a bitter taste. M.p. 233° to 236°. **Soluble** 1 in 12 of water, 1 in 7 of alcohol, 1 in 350 of acetone, and 1 in 3 of chloroform; practically insoluble in ether and glycerol. A 1% solution in water has a pH of 4.5 to 6.5. An 8.59% solution is iso-osmotic with serum. Solutions are **sterilised** by autoclaving or by filtration and distributed in ampoules; chlorocresol should not be used as a bacteriostatic.

Incompatible with alkalis, chlorocresol, oxidising agents, iodides, mercury salts, saccharin sodium, and with a number of dyes, including amaranth and bordeaux B. **Store** in airtight containers. Protect from light.

An aqueous solution of methadone hydrochloride iso-osmotic with serum (8.59%) caused 100% haemolysis of erythrocytes cultured in it for 45 minutes. The solution turned dark brown.— E. R. Hammarlund and K. Pedersen-Bjergaard, *J. pharm. Sci.*, 1961, *50*, 24.

Incompatibility. For a report of incompatibilities in intravenous solutions, see Codeine Phosphate, p.1004.

Dependence. Prolonged use of methadone may lead to dependence of the morphine type (see p.1018). The withdrawal symptoms are less intense but more prolonged than those produced by morphine or diamorphine. They develop more slowly and do not usually appear until 24 to 48 hours after the last dose. Methadone is used for substitution therapy in those dependent on diamorphine and morphine (see under Uses).

Methadone hydrochloride produced subjective changes similar to those produced by diamorphine. It was about as potent as morphine by subcutaneous injection and half as potent by mouth. Chronic administration produced sedation, lethargic apathy, haemodilution, oedema, and reduced sexual interest and activity. Patients receiving and tolerant to methadone 100 mg daily still exhibited drug-seeking behaviour. At a dosage of 100 mg daily physical dependence and an abstinence syndrome developed similar to that produced by morphine except that the onset of the syndrome was slower. As in morphine-dependent subjects the acute syndrome was followed by a protracted syndrome.— W. R. Martin *et al.*, *Archs gen. Psychiat.*, 1973, *28*, 286.

Pregnancy and the neonate. In a comparison of 15 infants born to mothers receiving methadone maintenance and 38 born to untreated diamorphine addicts, withdrawal symptoms in the methadone group were more severe and more prolonged (6 to 16 days as against 2 to 8 days). It was considered that this might be due to greater placental passage and delayed renal excretion of methadone. Hypoglycaemia was present in 3 full-term infants in the methadone group.— B. K. Rajegowda *et al.*, *J. Pediat.*, 1972, *81*, 532.

In 105 pregnancies in patients dependent on methadone, mortality, complications of pregnancy, and neonatal growth and development were normal; one-third of the infants were premature, and most showed some signs of withdrawal symptoms.— G. Blinick *et al.*, *J. Am. med. Ass.*, 1973, *225*, 477.

Five cases of intra-uterine foetal death had been reported during methadone detoxification in the late mid-trimester or last trimester of pregnancy. Such detoxification should not be undertaken during pregnancy unless facilities were available for monitoring the concentrations of sympathomimetic amines in amniotic fluid.— F. P. Zuspan *et al.*, *Am. J. Obstet. Gynec.*, 1975, *122*, 43.

Withdrawal symptoms appeared in all except 1 of the infants born to 22 women taking methadone. The severity of withdrawal symptoms was related to the total dose of methadone ingested over the last 12 weeks of pregnancy, to the daily maternal dose at delivery, and to the maternal serum-methadone concentration at parturition. Concentrations in cord blood were lower than those in maternal serum. Concentrations in neonatal urine were 10 to 60 times those in cord blood. Infants were of lower birth weight than controls; a higher incidence of smoking might have been a contributory factor.— R. G. Harper *et al.*, *Am. J. Obstet. Gynec.*, 1977, *129*, 417.

Methadone withdrawal symptoms did not occur until the end of the first week of life in 2 infants whose mothers had been weaned from diamorphine to methadone during pregnancy. Infants born to such mothers should be watched for at least 7 days after birth.— R. E. Challis and J. W. Scopes (letter), *Lancet*, 1977, *2*, 1230. See also S. R. Kandall and L. M. Gartner, *Am. J. Dis. Child.*, 1974, *127*, 58.

For further reports on the neonatal withdrawal syndrome, see under Morphine.

Treatment of neonatal dependence. For reports on the treatment of neonatal narcotic dependence, see under Morphine.

Tolerance. A study of cross-tolerance between methadone and diamorphine in man.— J. Volavka *et al.*, *J. nerv. ment. Dis.*, 1978, *166*, 104.

Treatment of dependence. For a report on the use of diphenoxylate to facilitate methadone withdrawal, see under Diphenoxylate Hydrochloride.

Adverse Effects and Treatment. As for Morphine, p.1019.

Methadone has a relatively greater respiratory depressant effect than morphine. After gross overdosage symptoms are similar to those of morphine poisoning. Pulmonary oedema after overdosage is a common cause of fatalities among addicts.

Methadone causes pain at injection sites; subcutaneous injection causes local tissue irritation and induration.

A review of the side-effects which occurred in patients dependent on diamorphine when receiving maintenance treatment with methadone.— M. J. Kreek, *J. Am. med. Ass.*, 1973, *223*, 665.

Massive oedema and weight gain occurred in 3 patients during methadone maintenance.— B. Longwell *et al.*, *Int. J. Addict.*, 1979, *14*, 329.

For a comparison between isomers of methadone with regard to adverse effects, see under Uses.

Effects on sexual function. In 29 men receiving methadone maintenance therapy sexual function was markedly impaired. The ejaculate volume and seminal vesicular and prostatic secretions were reduced by over 50% in subjects receiving methadone compared with 16 diamorphine addicts and 43 control subjects. Serum-testosterone concentrations were about 43% lower in subjects receiving methadone than in diamorphine users or controls. The sperm count of subjects receiving methadone was over twice that of the controls reflecting a lack of sperm dilution by secondary-sex-organ secretions and the motility was markedly lower than normal.— T. J. Cicero *et al.*, *New Engl. J. Med.*, 1975, *292*, 882.

Further reports on the effect of methadone on sexual function.— F. Azizi *et al.*, *Steroids*, 1973, *22*, 467; J. Mintz *et al.*, *Archs gen. Psychiat.*, 1974, *31*, 700; R. Hanbury *et al.*, *Am. J. Drug Alcohol Abuse*, 1977, *4*, 13.

Gynaecomastia. Gynaecomastia had been noted in male subjects taking methadone.— B. L. Thomas (letter), *New Engl. J. Med.*, 1976, *294*, 169.

Histamine release. When methadone was injected intravenously into the arm below a sphygmomanometer cuff exerting a pressure just above the diastolic blood pressure, an immediate flare appeared when the cuff was released and wheals appeared within 30 seconds. The reaction spread down the arm and intense itching occurred; it cleared in 2½ hours.— D. I. Vollum, *Br. med. J.*, 1970, *2*, 647.

Overdosage. A 3-year-old child who took about 16 mg of methadone became deeply unconscious and cyanosed with shallow respirations, tachycardia, and a low blood pressure. He was treated with nalorphine intravenously and metaraminol intravenously and intramuscularly. An ECG showed a partial right bundle-branch block which later became complete. For several weeks the child remained drowsy with a striking insensitivity to pinprick, and was unable to see.— S. G. Ratcliffe, *Br. med. J.*, 1963, *1*, 1069.

Accidental methadone ingestion resulted in the deaths of 3 children aged between 1 and 3 years. Two of the children had methadone-blood concentrations of 1.1 μg per ml and one had a concentration of 90 μg of methadone per 100 g of liver.— J. E. Smialek *et al.*, *J. Am. med. Ass.*, 1977, *238*, 2516.

Pulmonary oedema. Pulmonary oedema developed in a 19-year-old girl 6 hours after she had ingested 80 mg of methadone hydrochloride. The patient recovered after treatment with nalorphine, sodium bicarbonate, frusemide, and respiratory assistance.— J. M. Kjeldgaard *et al.*, *J. Am. med. Ass.*, 1971, *218*, 882.

Precautions. As for Morphine, p.1019.

Methadone is not recommended for use in labour because its prolonged duration of action increases the risk of neonatal depression.

There is some evidence of accumulation.

Factors which changed the pH of the urine might upset the steady state of established methadone dose regimens.— R. C. Baselt and L. J. Casarett, *Clin. Pharmac. Ther.*, 1972, *13*, 64.

An 81-year-old woman with bony metastases from carcinoma of the breast was given methadone 5 mg thrice daily for 2 days; she became deeply unconscious but awoke immediately when given naloxone 400 μg intravenously.— P. Symonds (letter), *Br. med. J.*, 1977, *1*, 512. A further report of an enhanced effect of methadone in 3 patients with cancer.— D. S. Ettinger *et al.*, *Cancer Treat. Rep.*, 1979, *63*, 457.

Effects on diagnostic tests. *Direct Coombs' test.* No positive direct Coombs' tests (antiglobulin tests) were noted in long-term methadone maintenance therapy.— G. K. Sherwood *et al.*, *Blood*, 1972, *40*, 902.

Pregnancy tests. Contrary reports of methadone interfering or not with pregnancy tests.— C. A. Horwitz *et al.*, *J. Reprod. fert.*, 1973, *33*, 489; M. Dietrich *et al.* (letter), *Canad. med. Ass. J.*, 1974, *111*, 213.

Interactions. For reference to the possibility of methadone-withdrawal symptoms occurring during transfer to levomethadyl acetate maintenance therapy, see Levomethadyl Acetate, p.1014.

Antibiotics. Methadone had no antagonistic effect on the activities of nafcillin, carbenicillin, rifampicin, or gentamicin *in vitro* against *Staphylococcus aureus*, *Pseudomonas aeruginosa*, and *Serratia marcescens*. It was considered unlikely that methadone would interfere with antibiotic therapy of bacterial infections.— J. N. Sheagren *et al.*, *Antimicrob. Ag. Chemother.*, 1977, *12*, 748.

See also under Rifampicin, below.

Disulfiram. There were no contra-indications to the combined use of disulfiram and methadone.— C. V. Charuvastra *et al.*, *Archs gen. Psychiat.*, 1976, *33*, 391. Agreement, although disulfiram was found to enhance the demethylation of methadone and in some patients to alter its pharmacokinetics.— T. G. Tong *et al.*, *J. clin. Pharmac.*, 1980, *20*, 506.

Monoamine oxidase inhibitors. A report of the successful use of tranylcypromine in a patient receiving methadone maintenance therapy. No adverse interaction was observed.— G. Mendelson (letter), *Med. J. Aust.*, 1979, *1*, 400.

Phenytoin. A patient's usual dose of methadone failed to prevent withdrawal symptoms when he was also given phenytoin.— P. F. Finelli (letter), *New Engl. J. Med.*, 1976, *294*, 227. See also T. G. Tong *et al.*, *Ann. intern. Med.*, 1981, *94*, 349.

Rifampicin. Of 30 patients receiving methadone maintenance, 21 developed withdrawal symptoms following concurrent administration of rifampicin. In a study of 6 whose symptoms were severe, rifampicin was noted to lower plasma-methadone concentrations and to increase urinary excretion of the major metabolite.— M. J. Kreek *et al.*, *New Engl. J. Med.*, 1976, *294*, 1104.

Rifampicin 450 mg daily given as part of an antituberculous regimen involving streptomycin and isoniazid produced symptoms of methadone withdrawal in a patient receiving methadone maintenance at 40 mg daily. Withdrawal effects were abolished by increasing the methadone dose from 40 to 60 mg daily.— M. R. Bending and P. O. Skacel (letter), *Lancet*, 1977, *1*, 1211.

Pituitary-adrenal function. Plasma-cortisol concentrations were increased in 5 subjects when exposed to cold 21 hours after having taken their regular dose of methadone 50 or 80 mg. No increase was seen following cold exposure one hour after the dose or in healthy subjects at 1 or 21 hours.— P. F. Renault *et al.*, *Clin. Pharmac. Ther.*, 1972, *13*, 269.

Porphyria. Methadone probably did not precipitate acute porphyria.— *Drug & Ther. Bull.*, 1976, *14*, 55.

Pregnancy and the neonate. Clinical depression of the newborn had been observed after the use of methadone during labour. No correlation had been found between the clinical condition of the infants and the amount of methadone excreted in the urine during the first few days of life.— F. Moya and V. Thorndike, *Clin. Pharmac. Ther.*, 1963, *4*, 628.

Chromosomal aberrations were found in about 10% of 27 907 cells taken from 99 pregnant women dependent on diamorphine or methadone.— A. P. Amarose and M. J. Norusis, *Am. J. Obstet. Gynec.*, 1976, *124*, 635.

The death of a 5-week-old infant might have been the result of methadone ingestion in breast milk from the mother who received maintenance doses of methadone. The methadone-blood concentration of the infant at autopsy was 400 ng per ml.— J. E. Smialek *et al.*, *J. Am. med. Ass.*, 1977, *238*, 2516.

The amount of methadone in breast milk was unlikely to have any pharmacologic effect on the infant.— *Med. Lett.*, 1979, *21*, 52.

Absorption and Fate. Methadone is readily absorbed from the gastro-intestinal tract. It is widely distributed in the tissues and diffuses across the placenta. It is metabolised in the liver, mainly by *N*-demethylation and cyclisation, and the metabolites are excreted in the bile and urine. A variable amount of the dose appears in the urine unchanged. There is some evidence of accumulation.

A review of the relationship of the pharmacokinetics of morphine, methadone, and naloxone to pharmacological activity.— B. A. Berkowitz, *Clin. Pharmacokinet.*, 1976, *1*, 219.

A report of the concentrations of methadone and its metabolite 1,5-dimethyl-3,3-diphenyl-2-ethylidenepyrrolidine in various tissues in 11 subjects post mortem. Concentrations of 0.22 to 3.04 μg per ml, 1.56 to 42.5 μg per ml, and 0.52 to 132 μg per ml of methadone were present in the blood, bile, and urine respectively. The metabolite was present in large concentrations in the bile and urine.— A. E. Robinson and F. M. Williams, *J. Pharm. Pharmac.*, 1971, *23*, 353.

In a study of 50 patients being treated for diamorphine dependence with methadone the urinary excretion of methadone and its metabolite was found to be dose-dependent with nearly all of a dose of 160 mg being excreted in the urine, 60% as unchanged methadone. The ratio of metabolite to methadone excretion was found to be higher at high urine pH values and in women.— R. C. Baselt and L. J. Casarett, *Clin. Pharmac. Ther.*, 1972, *13*, 64.

The mean peak plasma-methadone concentration of 74 ng per ml in 5 subjects given 15 mg by mouth occurred at 4 hours. Over the first 24 hours 25% of the dose was excreted in the urine as almost equal parts of methadone and 1 of the 2 metabolites detected and during the next 72 hours an additional 25% of the dose was recovered. The renal clearance was found to be pH-dependent, the lower the pH the greater the clearance.— C. E. Inturrisi and K. Verebely, *Clin. Pharmac. Ther.*, 1972, *13*, 923. The mean apparent plasma half-life of methadone was calculated as 25 hours (range 13 to 47 hours).— *idem*, 633.

In a study of 17 patients receiving methadone maintenance therapy plasma concentrations fluctuated widely from day to day and week to week in individual patients. There was only rarely any relationship between symptom complaints and plasma-methadone concentrations so that determination of methadone concentrations was unlikely to be of any benefit.— W. H. Horns *et al.*, *Clin. Pharmac. Ther.*, 1975, *17*, 636.

Confirmation in 12 subjects receiving methadone-maintenance therapy that the most significant factor related to renal clearance in most patients was urinary pH.— G. D. Bellward *et al.*, *Clin. Pharmac. Ther.*, 1977, *22*, 92.

Further references on the metabolism and excretion of methadone.— E. Änggård *et al.*, *Clin. Pharmac. Ther.*, 1975, *17*, 258; L. W. Masten *et al.* (letter), *Nature*, 1975, *253*, 200; K. Verebely *et al.*, *Clin. Pharmac. Ther.*, 1975, *18*, 180; E. Änggård *et al.*, *Eur. J. clin. Pharmac.*, 1979, *16*, 53.

Accumulation. Studies in 3 patients given a 10 mg sustained-release tablet of methadone hydrochloride repeated after 12 hours and again after a further 13 hours indicated a satisfactory blood concentration 3 hours after the first dose and a peak 2 hours after the third dose—evidence of accumulation and a long half-life. The project of making a sustained release tablet was discontinued.— S. T. Leslie *et al.* (letter), *Br. med. J.*, 1977, *1*, 375. Comment: D. M. Rutherford and K. Raymond, *ibid.*, 774. Further evidence of accumulation.— R. G. Twycross (letter), *Br. J. clin. Pharmac.*, 1977, *4*, 691.

Since the antidiuretic and respiratory depressant effects of methadone were considerably longer than the analgesic effect studies were required to determine whether these were cumulative under clinical conditions.— G. D. Olsen *et al.*, *Clin. Pharmac. Ther.*, 1977, *21*, 147.

See also under Precautions, above.

Protein binding. Methadone was 8 to 44% bound to plasma albumin *in vitro;* binding was dependent on albumin concentration.— G. D. Olsen, *Science*, 1972, *176*, 525. Binding of methadone to human plasma proteins *in vitro* ranged from 71.7 to 87.5% over a range of methadone concentrations. The percent bound decreased as methadone concentrations increased.— G. D. Olsen, *Clin. Pharmac. Ther.*, 1973, *14*, 338.

Uses. Methadone hydrochloride is a potent analgesic with actions and uses similar to those of morphine (see p.1020) but having a less marked sedative action. The analgesic effect begins about 15 minutes after subcutaneous injection and about 45 minutes after administration by mouth, the effect usually lasting 3 to 4 hours. Accumulation may occur following repeated doses.

The fact that it gives less sedation makes it inferior to morphine for pre-operative medication. Administered in initial doses of 5 to 10 mg every 4 hours by mouth it is of value in the treatment of severe pain; doses of 30 mg have been given for very severe pain. For rapid action, methadone hydrochloride may be given by subcutaneous or intramuscular injection, usually in doses of 5 to 10 mg. It should not be given intravenously.

Methadone hydrochloride also has a depressant action on the cough centre and is given to control non-productive coughing of intractable disorders, such as lung cancer. For this purpose it is usually given in the form of a linctus in a dose of 2 mg every 4 hours. It has been suggested that children under 10 years of age may be given 250 µg, and older children 500 µg but children are very susceptible to the depressant effects of methadone and this use in children is not recommended.

Methadone hydrochloride is used as part of the treatment of dependence on narcotic drugs. Psychiatric support and rehabilitation are necessary during and after withdrawal (see also under Dependence, p.1015). Methadone has a longer duration of action than diamorphine and morphine and is usually administered once or twice daily. In the treatment of opiate withdrawal, or detoxification, methadone is given initially in doses sufficient to suppress withdrawal symptoms. A dose of 15 to 20 mg by mouth is usually sufficient, although higher doses may be required in some patients. After stabilisation the dose of methadone is gradually decreased until total withdrawal is achieved. Usually 1 mg of methadone can substitute for 30 mg of codeine, 2 mg of diamorphine, 4 mg of morphine, or 20 mg of pethidine. In some patients methadone is continued (methadone maintenance) as part of an overall treatment of the patient's dependence on other opiates; such patients are dependent on methadone. Methadone therapy of this nature in tolerant individuals does not act as a tranquilliser and symptoms of anxiety should not be treated by increased doses.

Results of a single-blind pilot study indicated that, although contributing no narcotic effects, some of the side-effects of methadone-maintenance therapy were caused by (+)-methadone. Results of a double-blind study of 66 patients comparing (−)-methadone with (±)-methadone did not, however, confirm this impression.— B. A. Judson *et al.*, *Clin. Pharmac. Ther.*, 1976, *20*, 445. In a study of the clinical effects and pharmacokinetics of racemic methadone compared with its isomers in 30 male subjects the half-life of (±)-methadone in blood was an average of about 22 hours compared with 24 hours for (−)-methadone and 25 hours for (+)-methadone. Further studies on the subjects in groups of 6 indicated that the effects of (+)-methadone 7.5 mg on respiration were not significantly different from a placebo response whereas (−)-methadone 7.5 mg and (±)-methadone 15 mg produced intense respiratory depression with a peak response after an average of about 4 hours and a return to control values at 72 hours for racemic methadone and a peak after an average of about 12 hours and a return to control values after an average of about 75 hours (variation 30 to 118 hours) in the case of (−)-methadone; 2 subjects given (+)-methadone 50 and 100 mg respectively both had small net depressions. The effects of (+)-methadone on pupillary constriction were again not significantly different from placebo but (±)- and (−)-methadone induced marked constriction with a peak effect at 2 hours and a duration lasting an average of 72 hours for racemic methadone and an average of 86 hours for (−)-methadone. Potency ratios for (−)- to (±)-methadone from blood concentration data were 3 for respiratory depression and 2.7 for miosis. The antidiuretic effect of racemic methadone was also more prolonged than the analgesic effect.— G. D. Olsen *et al.*, *Clin. Pharmac. Ther.*, 1977, *21*, 147.

Methadone 40 mg given to 7 volunteers produced a significant increase in serum-prolactin concentration when compared with placebo given to 7 control subjects. An antipsychotic effect was suggested.— M. S. Gold *et al.* (letter), *Lancet*, 1977, *2*, 398.

Administration. *In children.* An account of the terminal care of a dying child. The theoretical usefulness of methadone in controlling pain without inducing drowsiness was counteracted by its cumulative effect, and its use in children needs clarification.— J. A. Chapman and J. Goodall, *Lancet*, 1980, *1*, 753.

Administration in hepatic failure. A study of methadone disposition in patients with stable chronic liver disease suggesting that maintenance methadone dosage need not be changed.— D. M. Novick *et al.*, *Clin. Pharmac. Ther.*, 1981, *30*, 353.

Administration in renal failure. The interval between doses should be 6 hours in patients with a glomerular filtration-rate (GFR) of more than 50 ml per minute, 8 hours in those with a GFR of 10 to 50 ml per minute, and 8 to 12 hours in those with a GFR of less than 10 ml per minute. Concentrations of methadone were not affected by haemodialysis or peritoneal dialysis. Excretion was increased in acid urine.— W. M. Bennett *et al.*, *Ann. intern. Med.*, 1980, *93*, 62.

Methadone maintenance in a patient on chronic haemodialysis.— W. M. Glazer and G. L. Cohn, *Am. J. Psychiat.*, 1977, *134*, 931.

Analgesia. *Terminal pain.* A double-blind comparative study of the efficacy of methadone or diamorphine with cocaine as analgesics in 46 patients with terminal cancer suggested that although methadone was a satisfactory substitute for diamorphine in some patients, diamorphine should be used in very ill patients since it did not accumulate in the body to the same extent as methadone, thereby making dosage adjustment easier. The dangers of accumulation of methadone were stressed particularly in the elderly or debilitated.— R. G. Twycross (letter), *Br. J. clin. Pharmac.*, 1977, *4*, 691.

The use of methadone, on patient demand, for the relief of chronic cancer pain; by the 6th day the dose was 10 to 40 mg daily.— J. Säwe *et al.*, *Br. med. J.*, 1981, *282*, 771.

Cardiovascular disorders. For a comparison of methadone, diamorphine, morphine, and pentazocine in the relief of pain in myocardial infarction, see Pentazocine, p.1025.

Treatment of dependence. Some reviews and discussions of methadone maintenance treatment of narcotic addicts: V. P. Dole and M. E. Nyswander, *J. Am. med. Ass.*, 1976, *235*, 2117; N. E. Zinberg, *New Engl. J. Med.*, 1977, *296*, 1000. A critical review concluding that the value of methadone maintenance programmes in the treatment of narcotic addiction remains unproven.— M. Gossop, *Lancet*, 1978, *1*, 812.

The problems of *US* methadone maintenance regimens and the need to improve, rather than close, disorderly clinics.— V. P. Dole *et al.*, *New Engl. J. Med.*, 1982, *306*, 169.

In 900 patients dependent upon diamorphine, treatment with methadone appeared to result in a reduction in their convictions for crime. Of 723 male patients, 60% were usefully employed and about a further 30% were socially acceptable. Treatment consisted of initial doses of 10 mg of methadone twice daily, gradually increased over 4 to 6 weeks to a maintenance dose of 80 to 120 mg daily which was continued indefinitely. Patients did not experience euphoria or withdrawal symptoms with diamorphine but some patients continued on diamorphine intermittently.— V. P. Dole *et al.*, *J. Am. med. Ass.*, 1968, *206*, 2708. Comment by the AMA Methadone Maintenance Evaluation Committee.— *ibid.*, 2712. See also V. P. Dole, *J. Am. med. Ass.*, 1971, *215*, 1131.

Between 1972 and 1975 in Hong Kong one hundred diamorphine addicts were admitted to hospital for 2 weeks and stabilised on methadone 60 mg daily. Under double-blind conditions, after discharge from hospital, 50 then continued to be maintained on methadone 30 to 130 mg daily, and the other 50 were weaned off at a rate of 1 mg daily and subsequently maintained on placebo. After 32 weeks only 5 of the 50 control patients were still in the study compared with 38 of those receiving methadone-maintenance therapy. After 3 years only one control patient was still in the study compared with 28 on methadone therapy. Thirty-one of the control patients were removed from the study because of persistent use of diamorphine and 15 failed to attend for follow-up. By contrast, only 8 in the methadone-maintenance group were removed because of diamorphine use or because of persistent absence from the clinic. The rate of convictions per man-month of enrolment was more than twice as great for controls as for the treatment subjects. Fifty-two of the subjects who dropped out of the study were subsequently admitted to a methadone-maintenance programme and the retention rate was the same as for the original treatment group.— R. G. Newman and W. B. Whitehill, *Lancet*, 1979, *2*, 485.

Further references: A. D. Moffett *et al.*, *Clin. Med.*, 1971, *78* (Mar.), 29; J. M. Fultz and E. C. Senay, *Ann. intern. Med.*, 1975, *82*, 815; C. E. Riordan *et al.*, *J. Am. med. Ass.*, 1976, *235*, 2604; R. Smart *et al.*, *Can. J. publ. Hlth*, 1977, *68*, 55; J. Holmstrand *et al.*, *Clin. Pharmac. Ther.*, 1978, *23*, 175; M. S. Dalton and D. W. Duncan, *Med. J. Aust.*, 1979, *1*, 153.

For a comparison of methadone with levomethadyl acetate in the treatment of opiate dependence, see Levomethadyl Acetate, p.1015. For a comparison with clonidine, see p.141.

For reference to the use of naloxone mixed with methadone for methadone maintenance programmes, see Naloxone Hydrochloride, p.1033.

Withdrawal. An attempt was made to withdraw methadone from patients on methadone maintenance programmes; the mean dose of methadone was 31 mg daily. When withdrawal was attempted at the rate of 10% per week only 5 of 33 patients completed the schedule without interruption compared with 16 of 30 in whom withdrawal was attempted at the rate of about 3% per week; 6 and 10 patients respectively were considered abstinent at follow-up 1 month later. Withdrawal should not be attempted at a rate exceeding about 3% per week.— E. C. Senay *et al.*, *Archs gen. Psychiat.*, 1977, *34*, 361.

For reference to the control of methadone-withdrawal symptoms by administration of clonidine, see Clonidine, p.141.

For a report on the use of diphenoxylate during withdrawal from methadone maintenance, see Diphenoxylate Hydrochloride, p.1011.

Preparations

Injections

Methadone Hydrochloride Injection *(U.S.P.).* A sterile solution of methadone hydrochloride, 9.5 to 10.5 mg per ml, in Water for Injections. pH 3 to 6.5. Protect from light.

Methadone Injection *(B.P.).* Amidone Hydrochloride Injection. A sterile solution of methadone hydrochloride in Water for Injections. It is distributed in ampoules and sterilised by autoclaving.

Linctuses

Methadone Linctus *(B.P.).* Linct. Methadon.; Amidone Linctus. Methadone hydrochloride 2 mg, water 0.6 ml, compound tartrazine solution 0.04 ml, glycerol 1.25 ml, tolu syrup to 5 ml. When a dose less than or not a multiple of 5 ml is prescribed the linctus should be diluted to 5 ml, or a multiple, with syrup. Such dilutions must be freshly prepared and not used more than 2 weeks after issue.

For a report of incompatibility when Methadone Linctus was prepared with or diluted with syrup preserved with hydroxybenzoates, see under Sucrose, p.61.

Mixtures

Methadone Mixture 1 mg/1 ml *(D.T.F.).* Methadone hydrochloride 5 mg, syrup 2.5 ml, green S and tartrazine solution 0.01 ml, compound tartrazine solution 0.04 ml, double-strength chloroform water to 5 ml.

This preparation is intended only for drug-dependent persons and is 2.5 times the strength of Methadone Linctus (*B.P.*).

Solutions

Methadone Hydrochloride Oral Solution *(U.S.P.).* Contains methadone hydrochloride 9 to 11 mg in each ml, with a suitable preservative; it may contain suitable colouring and flavouring agents and surfactants. pH 3 to 6. To be diluted with water before being taken. Store at 15° to 30° in airtight containers. Protect from light.

Tablets

Methadone Hydrochloride Tablets *(U.S.P.).* Tablets containing methadone hydrochloride.

Methadone Tablets *(B.P.).* Amidone Hydrochloride Tablets. Tablets containing methadone hydrochloride.

Proprietary Preparations

Physeptone *(Wellcome, UK).* Methadone hydrochloride, available as **Injection** containing 10 mg per ml in ampoules of 1 ml; as **Linctus** containing 2 mg in each 5 ml (suggested diluent, syrup); and as scored **Tablets** of 5 mg. (Also available as Physeptone in *Austral.*, *Ital.*, *S.Afr.*).

Other Proprietary Names

Dolophine Hydrochloride *(USA)*; Eptadone *(Ital.)*; Heptanal *(Switz.)*; Ketalgin *(Switz.)*; Mephenon *(Belg., Ital.)*; L-Polamidon (laevo-isomer)*(Ger.)*; Symoron *(Neth.)*; Tussol *(Belg.)*.

6238-z

Metofoline Hydrochloride. Methopholine Hydrochloride; Methofoline Hydrochloride; Ro 4-1778. 1-(4-Chlorophenethyl)-1,2,3,4-tetrahydro-6,7-dimethoxy-2-methylisoquinoline hydrochloride.

$C_{20}H_{24}ClNO_2,HCl=382.3$.

CAS — 2154-02-1 (metofoline); 7558-47-6 (hydrochloride).

Metofoline hydrochloride is an analgesic with actions similar to those of codeine (see p.1004). It has been used for pre-operative medication and for the relief of mild to moderate acute and chronic pain in doses of 30 to 60 mg up to 4 times daily.

For a review comparing the analgesic effects of metofoline and codeine, see N. B. Eddy *et al.*, *Codeine and its Alternates for Pain and Cough Relief*, Geneva, World Health Organization, 1970. See also *idem*, *Bull. Wld Hlth Org.*, 1969, *40*, 1.

6239-c

Morphine *(B.P.C. 1934).* Morph.
(4a*R*,5*S*,7a*R*,8*R*,9c*S*)-4a,5,7a,8,9,9c-Hexahydro-12-methyl-8,9c-iminoethanophenanthro[4,5-*bcd*]furan-3,5-diol monohydrate.
$C_{17}H_{19}NO_3,H_2O$=303.4.

CAS — 57-27-2 (anhydrous); 6009-81-0 (monohydrate).

The principal alkaloid of opium. It occurs as an odourless white crystalline powder or colourless or white acicular crystals with a bitter taste. A solution in water is alkaline to litmus.

Soluble 1 in 5000 of water, 1 in 400 of boiling water, 1 in 250 of alcohol, 1 in 1500 of chloroform, 1 in 125 of glycerol, and 1 in 10 of oleic acid; practically insoluble in ether. **Protect** from light.

6240-s

Morphine Acetate *(B.P.C. 1934).* Morph. Acet.
$C_{17}H_{19}NO_3,C_2H_4O_2,3H_2O$=399.4.

CAS — 596-15-6 (anhydrous); 5974-11-8 (trihydrate).

A white amorphous or crystalline powder with a faintly acetous odour. **Soluble** 1 in 2.5 of water, 1 in 100 of alcohol, and 1 in 5 of glycerol; practically insoluble in ether. **Sterilisation** and **incompatibilities** are described under Morphine Hydrochloride, p.1018. **Store** in airtight containers. Protect from light.

Freeze-dried morphine acetate was stable and because of its solubility could be used to produce intramuscular injections providing up to 200 mg in a suitable volume.— G. K. Poochikian *et al.* (letter), *J. Am. med. Ass.*, 1980, *244*, 1434.

6241-w

Morphine Hydrochloride *(B.P., Eur. P.).*

Morph. Hydrochlor.; Morphini Hydrochloridum; Morphinii Chloridum; Morphinum Chloratum.
$C_{17}H_{19}NO_3,HCl,3H_2O$=375.8.

CAS — 52-26-6 (anhydrous); 6055-06-7 (trihydrate).

Pharmacopoeias. In all pharmacopoeias examined except *U.S.*

Odourless, colourless, silky crystals or crystalline powder or cubical white masses, with a bitter taste.

Soluble 1 in 24 of water, 1 in 100 of alcohol, and 1 in 10 of glycerol; practically insoluble in chloroform and ether. A solution in water is laevorotatory. Solutions in water have a pH of about 5. Solutions of morphine salts are **sterilised** by maintaining at 98° to 100° for 30 minutes with a bactericide or by filtration.

Morphine salts are **incompatible** with alkalis, bromides, iodides, potassium permanganate, tannic acid, and vegetable astringents; and with salts of iron, lead, manganese, silver, copper, and zinc; the alkalinity of glass bottles may precipitate some of the morphine from a solution of a salt. **Store** in airtight containers. Protect from light.

6242-e

Morphine Sulphate *(B.P.).*

Morph. Sulph.; Morphine Sulfate *(U.S.P.)*; Morphini Sulfas.
$(C_{17}H_{19}NO_3)_2,H_2SO_4,5H_2O$=758.8.

CAS — 64-31-3 (anhydrous); 6211-15-0 (pentahydrate).

Pharmacopoeias. In *Br.*, *Ind.*, *Int.*, *Mex.*, *Port.*, *Turk.*, and *U.S.*

Odourless, white, acicular crystals, cubical masses, or crystalline powder with a bitter taste. When exposed to air it gradually loses water of crystallisation. It darkens on prolonged exposure to light.

Soluble 1 in 21 of water and 1 in 1000 of alcohol; practically insoluble in chloroform and ether. A 2% solution is laevorotatory and is acid to methyl red. **Sterilisation** and **incompatibilities** are described under Morphine Hydrochloride, p.1018. **Store** in airtight containers. Protect from light.

Effect of gamma-irradiation. Gamma-irradiation at 250 000 Gy changed the colour of morphine sulphate powder from white to bright mustard yellow. Aqueous solutions remained clear and showed no change in pH, but they became coloured. There was some decrease in the content of anhydrous morphine and an increase in the amount of other alkaloids. Morphine Sulphate Injection became yellow and there was a decrease in the optical rotation but no loss of potency or change in pH.— *The Use of Gamma Radiation Sources for the Sterilisation of Pharmaceutical Products*, London, ABPI, 1960.

An aqueous solution of morphine 1% irradiated to 25 000 Gy showed a slight decrease in pH value but no change in morphine content could be measured.— E. L. Pandula *et al.*, *Radiosterilization of Medical Products*, Vienna, International Atomic Energy Agency, 1967, p. 83.

Incompatibility. There was loss of clarity when intravenous solutions of morphine sulphate were mixed with those of aminophylline, amylobarbitone sodium, chlorothiazide sodium, heparin sodium, methicillin sodium, nitrofurantoin sodium, novobiocin sodium, pethidine hydrochloride, phenobarbitone sodium, phenytoin sodium, sodium bicarbonate, sodium iodide, sulphadiazine sodium, sulphafurazole diethanolamine, or thiopentone sodium.— J. A. Patel and G. L. Phillips, *Am. J. Hosp. Pharm.*, 1966, *23*, 409.

Cloudiness developed when promethazine hydrochloride 12.5 mg was drawn up into a syringe containing morphine sulphate 8 mg.— N. M. Fleischer (letter), *Am. J. Hosp. Pharm.*, 1973, *30*, 665.

Morphine sulphate injection containing chlorocresol 0.2% was incompatible with chlorpromazine hydrochloride injection. Morphine injection without chlorocresol should be compatible.— J. B. Crapper, *Br. med. J.*, 1975, *1*, 33.

Stability. Stability of morphine in Kaolin and Morphine Mixture *B.P.*— K. Helliwell and P. Game, *Pharm. J.*, 1981, *2*, 128.

6243-l

Morphine Tartrate *(B.P.C. 1959).* Morph. Tart.
$(C_{17}H_{19}NO_3)_2,C_4H_6O_6,3H_2O$=774.8.

CAS — 302-31-8 (anhydrous); 6032-59-3 (trihydrate).

Minute, odourless, colourless, acicular, efflorescent crystals with a bitter taste. **Soluble** 1 in 10 of water and 1 in 1000 of alcohol; practically insoluble in chloroform and ether. **Sterilisation** and **incompatibilities** are described under Morphine Hydrochloride, p.1018. **Store** in airtight containers. Protect from light.

Dependence of the Morphine Type. Drug dependence of the morphine type is a state arising from repeated administration of morphine or a drug with morphine-like effects; it is characterised by an overwhelming need to continue taking the drug or one with similar properties, by a tendency to increase the dose owing to the development of tolerance, and by psychic or psychological and physical dependence on the drug.

Dependence on morphine may occur after treatment for 1 or 2 weeks with therapeutic doses; some physical dependence can be shown after only 2 or 3 days. Tolerance to many of the actions of morphine usually develops over 2 to 3 weeks on moderate therapeutic doses but develops more quickly with larger doses. On discontinuing morphine, tolerance declines over 2 weeks.

Abrupt withdrawal of opiates from persons physically dependent on them precipitates a withdrawal syndrome, the severity of which depends on the individual, the drug used, the size and frequency of the dose, and the duration of drug use. *Withdrawal symptoms* usually begin within a few hours, reach a peak within 36 to 72 hours, and then gradually subside. Withdrawal symptoms develop more slowly with methadone. Symptoms include yawning, mydriasis, lachrymation, rhinorrhoea, sneezing, muscle tremor, headache, weakness, sweating, anxiety, irritability, disturbed sleep or insomnia, restlessness, orgasm, anorexia, nausea, vomiting, loss of weight, diarrhoea, dehydration, leucocytosis, bone pain, abdominal and muscle cramps, increases in heart-rate, respiratory-rate, and blood pressure, rise in temperature, and gooseflesh and vasomotor disturbances.

Withdrawal symptoms may be terminated by a suitable dose of morphine or related drug.

Some physiological values may not return to normal for several months following the acute withdrawal syndrome.

Withdrawal therapy requires sustained surveillance and the patient should be persuaded to enter hospital or be referred to a treatment centre. Withdrawal may be effected slowly or rapidly. The usual method is to replace the drug of dependence by methadone (see p.1016), preferably as methadone mixture or linctus. Initially, 1 mg of methadone is substituted for each 4 mg of morphine. The methadone may then be slowly withdrawn over a period of about 3 weeks, treating withdrawal symptoms with sedatives if necessary. Cyclazocine (see p.1031) has also been used.

Psychotherapy and social rehabilitation are also needed. Relapses are frequent. For reports of the use of methadone in the treatment of drug dependence, see Methadone Hydrochloride, p.1017.

In many countries there are restrictions on the prescribing of narcotic drugs for addicts.

Major medical complications resulting from self-injection of opiates are overdose, pulmonary oedema and other pulmonary complications, hepatitis and liver disease, renal disease, and infections such as bacterial endocarditis, bacteraemia, osteomyelitis, malaria, tuberculosis, and abscesses. Unsterile injections, shared needles, and the presence of adulterants and particulate matter in injected material are probably responsible for many of these complications.— R. H. McDonald, in *Toxicology Annual 1974*, C.L. Winek (Ed.), New York, Marcel Dekker, 1975, pp. 91–127. Severe tetanus may also occur in narcotic addicts.— C. E. Cherubin, *Archs intern. Med.*, 1968, *121*, 156.

Epidemiology of hepatitis in drug addicts.— G. Raimondo *et al.*, *Lancet*, 1982, *1*, 249.

A discussion on the mechanisms involved in opiate addiction.— S. H. Snyder, *New Engl. J. Med.*, 1979, *300*, 465. See also L. Terenius, *Lakartidningen*, 1977, *74*, 4302; W. E. Bunney *et al.*, *Ann. intern. Med.*, 1979, *91*, 239.

Pregnancy and the neonate. Infants born to mothers dependent on diamorphine usually show signs of withdrawal 24 to 48 hours after birth. The most common symptoms of withdrawal are general hyperactivity, tremor, and irritability. Feeding difficulty and sleep disturbance may also be present. Convulsions have been reported but are uncommon with diamorphine. Withdrawal symptoms in infants dependent on methadone may be more severe, occur later, and require treatment for a longer period of time. Convulsions are more common during methadone withdrawal.— S. Pierog, in *Drug Abuse in Pregnancy and Neonatal Effects*, J.L. Rementería (Ed.), Saint Louis, C.V. Mosby, 1977, p. 95.

Further references: *Perinatal Addiction*, R.D. Harbison (Ed.), London, Spectrum Publications, 1975.

Treatment of neonatal dependence. Symptoms of diamorphine withdrawal occurred in 259 of 384 infants born to diamorphine-dependent mothers. Of these, 178 required treatment. All signs of withdrawal were effectively relieved by administration of chlorpromazine in a daily dose of 2.2 mg per kg body-weight in divided doses at 6-hourly intervals by mouth or by injection. The dose of chlorpromazine was gradually reduced over 10 to 40 days.— C. Zelson *et al.*, *Pediatrics*, 1971, *48*, 178.

Of 110 infants born to mothers, almost all of whom were taking methadone, diamorphine, or both, sometimes with other agents, 103 showed withdrawal symptoms; 51 needed treatment. There were no significant differences between those treated with methadone 250 µg six-hourly, increased to 500 µg six-hourly, phenobarbitone 5 to 8 mg per kg body-weight daily in 3 divided doses, or diazepam 0.5 to 2 mg eight-hourly. Withdrawal symptoms were less common in those whose mothers were taking less than 20 mg of methadone daily.— J. D. Madden *et al.*, *Am. J. Obstet. Gynec.*, 1977, *127*, 199.

The management of the neonatal narcotic withdrawal syndrome includes general supportive therapy as well as specific drug therapy. A quiet darkened environment may help calm the infant while adequate fluid and nutrient intake must be ensured. Camphorated opium tincture (Paregoric *U.S.P.*) has been widely used to treat withdrawal symptoms. An initial dose of 0.2 ml every 3 hours has been used. It is rarely necessary to exceed 0.7 ml per dose. After stabilisation the dose is gradually reduced over 25 to 45 days. The main adverse effects are constipation and lethargy. Diazepam has also been used in doses of 1 to 2 mg intramuscularly every 8 hours. Withdrawal can usually be accomplished within a week. Chlorpromazine has been given in doses of 2 to 3 mg per kg body-weight daily in divided doses by mouth or intramuscularly. Chlorpromazine can usually be withdrawn after 2 to 3 weeks. Phenobarbitone has been given to control symptoms of insomnia and irritability but it does not control gastro-intestinal disorders.— R. G. Harper and G. B. Edwards, in *Drug Abuse in Pregnancy and Neonatal Effects*, J.L. Rementería (Ed.), Saint Louis, C.V. Mosby, 1977, p. 103.

Treatment of dependence. Reviews. AMA Council on Mental Health, *J. Am. med. Ass.*, 1972, *219*, 1611; 1973, EURO 5423 IV (Copenhagen), (WHO Working Group Report), per *Abstr. Hyg.*, 1974, *49*, 558; M. M. Glatt, *A Guide to Addiction and its Treatment*, Lancaster, Medical and Technical Publishing, 1974.; *Br. med. J.*, 1979, *1*, 911; *Med. Lett.*, 1980, *22*, 73.

A discussion on the treatment of opiate-withdrawal symptoms with special reference to the use of clonidine.— *Lancet*, 1980, *2*, 349.

See also under Clonidine Hydrochloride, p.141.

See also under Pregnancy and the Neonate, above.

Adverse Effects. In normal doses the commonest side-effects of morphine and other narcotic analgesics are nausea, vomiting, constipation, drowsiness, and confusion. Micturition may be difficult and there may be ureteric or biliary spasm; there is also an antidiuretic effect. Dry mouth, sweating, facial flushing, vertigo, bradycardia, palpitations, orthostatic hypotension, hypothermia, restlessness, changes of mood, and miosis also occur. These effects occur more commonly in ambulant patients than in those at rest in bed. Raised intracranial pressure occurs in some patients.

Larger doses produce respiratory depression and hypotension, with circulatory failure and deepening coma. Convulsions may occur in infants and children. Death may occur from respiratory failure. Toxic doses vary considerably with the individual and addicts may tolerate large doses.

Due to the histamine-releasing effect, reactions such as urticaria and pruritus, occur in some individuals. Contact dermatitis has been reported and pain and irritation may occur on injection.

Anaphylactic reactions following intravenous injection of morphine and codeine have been reported.

For reviews of the toxic effects of narcotic analgesics, see R. E. Lister, *J. Pharm. Pharmac.*, 1966, *18*, 364; *Br. med. J.*, 1970, *2*, 587; W. E. Thornton and B. P. Thornton, *Am. J. Psychiat.*, 1974, *131*, 867.

Experience with epidural morphine (chloride) (2 mg in 10 ml physiological saline) for postoperative pain relief in 1200 patients, the first 242 of whom received a commercial preparation containing preservatives, and the remainder of whom were treated with preservative-free filtered solution. Side-effects regarded as related to epidural morphine were: nausea or vomiting (204 patients; 17%), blood pressure drop of 20 mmHg or more (24 patients; 2%), itching in the first 242 patients (36 patients; 15%), itching in the rest (9 patients; 1%), urinary retention (181 patients; 15%), and respiratory depression (1 patient). The 17% incidence of nausea and vomiting was considerably less than in a control group given morphine chloride 2 mg in physiological saline intravenously (57% incidence), as was the fall in blood pressure (2% against 14% in the controls). Itching was not affected by antihistamines and was probably caused by the preservatives; urinary retention might be a local anaesthetic effect; its frequency did not decrease with preservative-free solution. Although the incidence of respiratory depression is low following epidural morphine, it may still occur long after epidural infusion and patients must be closely monitored.— S. Reiz and M. Westberg (letter), *Lancet*, 1980, *2*, 203. Hallucinations may be a warning of impending intoxication when morphine is given epidurally.— A. Engquist *et al.* (letter), *ibid.*, 984. Late respiratory depression after concomitant use of morphine epidurally and parenterally.— L. L. Gustafsson *et al.* (letter), *ibid.*, 1981, *1*, 892. Shrinking pupils as a warning of respiratory depression after spinal morphine.— M. Bahar *et al.* (letter), *ibid.*, 893.

Allergy. Allergic reactions to cough syrups in patients sensitised to codeine and morphine.— R. Voorhorst and S. Sparreboom, *Ned. Tijdschr. Geneesk.*, 1977, *121*, 737.

Effects on liver. Serum concentrations of amylase and hydroxybutyric acid dehydrogenase may be raised after administration of opiates due to spasm of the sphincter of Oddi. The reason for the rise in serum-aspartate aminotransferase (SGOT) and serum-alanine aminotransferase (SGPT) concentrations following treatment with opiates or cholinergic agents was uncertain. It had also been reported that opiates could induce an increase in serum-lactic dehydrogenase concentration of hepatic origin by increasing intrabiliary pressure.— F. Clark, *Adverse Drug React. Bull.*, 1977, Oct., 232.

Effects on respiratory function. Morphine sulphate 7.5 mg by subcutaneous injection produced parallel decreases in hypoxic and hypercapnic ventilatory drives. It was possible that a decreased sensitivity to chemical stimuli to breathing might contribute to the respiratory depression.— J. V. Weil *et al.*, *New Engl. J. Med.*, 1975, *292*, 1103. See also R. F. Bedford and H. Wollman, *Anesthesiology*, 1975, *43*, 1.

The central nervous respiratory depressant action of narcotic analgesics.— H. L. Borison, *Pharmac. Ther.*, 1977, *3*, 227.

A study in 17 healthy subjects of the relationship between the plasma concentration of morphine and morphine-induced changes in ventilation and the ventilatory response to carbon dioxide. No relationship was demonstrated between the plasma concentration of morphine and the magnitude of the ventilatory effects of morphine between the subjects although both varied widely among the patients studied.— J. R. A. Rigg, *Br. J. Anaesth.*, 1978, *50*, 759 and 767.

Effects on sexual function. For the effects of narcotic analgesics on sexual function, see under Diamorphine Hydrochloride, p.1008, and Methadone Hydrochloride, p.1016.

Treatment of Adverse Effects. If the drug has been ingested, the stomach should be emptied by aspiration and lavage; a 0.02% aqueous solution of potassium permanganate (very pale pink) may be employed. A purgative such as sodium sulphate 30 g in 250 ml of water may be given to aid peristalsis.

Intensive supportive therapy may be necessary in order to correct respiratory failure and shock. In addition, the specific antagonist naloxone hydrochloride is used to counteract very rapidly the severe respiratory depression and coma produced by excessive doses of narcotic analgesics. A dose of 400 µg is given intravenously, repeated at intervals of 2 to 3 minutes if necessary. In children, a dose of 5 to 10 µg per kg body-weight may be given, while in neonates a dose of 10 µg per kg may be given. Naloxone may also be given by subcutaneous or intramuscular injection. The effect of naloxone may be of shorter duration than that of the narcotic analgesic and additional doses may be required to prevent relapses.

Nalorphine hydrobromide (p.1032) and levallorphan tartrate (p.1031) have also been used to antagonise the adverse effects of narcotic analgesics.

The use of narcotic antagonists such as naloxone, nalorphine, and levallorphan in persons physically dependent on morphine or related drugs may induce withdrawal symptoms.

Treatment of acute intoxication due to narcotic analgesics.— *Med. Lett.*, 1977, *19*, 13; E. J. Khantzian and G. J. McKenna, *Ann. intern. Med.*, 1979, *90*, 361.

Methods used *by addicts* to treat opiate overdose included intravenous administration of salt water, milk and vinegar, epsom salts, or sugar dissolved in water or milk. These methods were most dangerous as solutions were often very hyperosmotic and usually prepared with tap water and no sterilising precautions. Amphetamines, cocaine, adrenaline, and pentazocine administered intravenously were used less often and there was no clearly defined dose. This would be important in the use of cocaine which had a narrow margin between its stimulant and depressant effects. Other methods used were external stimulation with ice packs and the administration of emetics such as vinegar and salt water by mouth.— R. E. Kaufman and S. B. Levy, *J. Am. med. Ass.*, 1974, *227*, 411.

Precautions. Morphine is not usually given pre-operatively to children under 1 year of age, and it should be given with extreme care to newborn or premature infants for other conditions. The dosage should be reduced in elderly and debilitated patients.

Morphine is generally contra-indicated in respiratory depression, especially in the presence of cyanosis and excessive bronchial secretion, and after operations on the biliary tract. It is also contra-indicated in the presence of acute alcoholism, head injuries, and conditions in which intracranial pressure is raised. It should not be given during an attack of bronchial asthma or in heart failure secondary to chronic lung disease. It should be given with caution or in reduced doses to patients with hypothyroidism, adrenocortical insufficiency, impaired liver function, prostatic hypertrophy, or shock. It should be used with caution in patients with inflammatory or obstructive bowel disorders.

As serious and sometimes fatal reactions have occurred following administration of pethidine to patients receiving monoamine oxidase inhibitors, pethidine and related drugs are contra-indicated in patients taking monoamine oxidase inhibitors or within 14 days of stopping such treatment; morphine and other narcotic analgesics should be given with extreme caution. The depressant effects of morphine are enhanced by depressants of the central nervous system such as alcohol, anaesthetics, hypnotics and sedatives, and phenothiazines.

The administration of narcotic analgesics during labour may cause respiratory depression in the newborn infant.

Administration in liver disease. Care should be taken in administering drugs with high first-pass metabolism, such as narcotic analgesics, to cirrhotic patients as there is increased bioavailability and decreased clearance in these patients. Doses should be reduced significantly with these agents to avoid potential drug toxicity.— E. A. Neal *et al.*, *Gastroenterology*, 1979, *77*, 96.

Administration in renal failure. See under Uses.

Diabetes mellitus. Morphine could exacerbate diabetes mellitus.— *Drug & Ther. Bull.*, 1973, *11*, 5.

Interactions. Morphine and diamorphine were effective microsomal enzyme depletors.— L. W. Masten *et al.* (letter), *Nature*, 1975, *253*, 200.

Studies and discussions on the interactions of narcotic analgesics and of narcotic antagonists.— *Ann. N.Y. Acad. Sci.*, 1976, *281*, 244–371.

Cimetidine. Confusion and severe respiratory depression in a haemodialysis patient given both cimetidine and morphine.— A. Fine and D. N. Churchill (letter), *Can. med. Ass. J.*, 1981, *124*, 1434.

Dexamphetamine. For reference to the enhancement of morphine-induced analgesia by dexamphetamine, see Uses.

Phenothiazines. In a study in 6 healthy men morphine-induced respiratory depression was enhanced by prochlorperazine.— T. D. Mull and T. C. Smith, *Anesthesiology*, 1974, *40*, 581, per *Int. pharm. Abstr.*, 1975, *12*, 312.

Phaeochromocytoma. Opiates were contra-indicated in patients with a phaeochromocytoma as such drugs could liberate endogenous histamine and stimulate the release of catecholamines.— N. C. Chaturvedi *et al.*, *Br. med. J.*, 1974, *2*, 538.

Porphyria. Morphine probably did not precipitate acute porphyria.— *Drug & Ther. Bull.*, 1976, *14*, 55.

Pregnancy and the neonate. The effects of narcotic analgesics on maternal and foetal acid-base status.— A. Chang *et al.*, *Br. J. Obstet. Gynaec.*, 1976, *83*, 56.

A report of 32 pregnancies in 29 patients dependent on drugs; 24 pregnancies came to term and there were 23 surviving infants. There were no signs of narcotic withdrawal in the infants of 4 mothers dependent on 'soft drugs' (amphetamines, barbiturates, or methaqualone with diphenhydramine), of 1 mother who took pethidine, and of 4 mothers who had stopped taking diamorphine or methadone at least 3 weeks before delivery. The narcotic withdrawal syndrome occurred in 13 of 14 babies born to mothers taking diamorphine and/or methadone and required treatment for 14 to 58 days. It was recommended that in pregnant patients dependent on narcotics, methadone by mouth should be substituted for diamorphine, screening should be done for hepatitis-associated antigen, and during labour possible hepatotoxic anaesthetics should be avoided. Complete withdrawal of the drug of dependence should be avoided because of the risk of foetal distress or death. All neonates should be carefully observed for the first week of life. Chlorpromazine was given once symptoms developed.— A. C. Fraser, *Lancet*, 1976, *2*, 896.

Of 50 282 children born to mothers monitored by the Collaborative Perinatal Project 1564 were found to have been exposed to narcotic analgesics, and possibly other drugs, at some time during the first 4 months of the pregnancy. Although there was little evidence of association between malformations and narcotic analgesic exposure in general, a possible association between respiratory malformations and codeine (563 exposures) was noted.— O. P. Heinonen *et al.*, *Birth Defects and Drugs in Pregnancy*, Littleton MA, Publishing Sciences Group, 1977, p. 286.

Narcotic dependence did not appear to affect fertility in women, although multiple births might occur at a slightly higher frequency than in control populations. The incidence of congenital abnormalities among infants of drug-dependent mothers appears to be comparable with that of the general population but the infants appeared to be at risk from intra-uterine infection. Foetal withdrawal could result in foetal death. Growth retardation, a shorter gestational period, and premature birth were more common in infants exposed to diamorphine during pregnancy. Induction of some enzyme systems, including liver glucuronyl transferase and lung surfactant, also occured as a result of diamorphine use during pregnancy.— J. L. Rementería and L. Lotongkhum, in *Drug Abuse in Pregnancy and Neonatal Effects*, J.L. Rementería (Ed.), Saint Louis, C.V. Mosby, 1977, p. 3.

See also under Dependence, p.1018.

Ulcerative colitis. Opiates should be avoided in juvenile ulcerative colitis since they might induce spasm of the already narrowed colonic lumen.— M. Davidson, *New Engl. J. Med.*, 1967, *277*, 1408.

A retrospective study of 18 patients who had developed toxic megacolon revealed that 17 of the 18 had had opiate therapy either initiated or increased in dosage shortly before the development of toxic dilatation of the colon. In a further study in 14 patients with mild to moderately severe ulcerative colitis, small single doses of opium tincture were found to produce marked hypermotility of the pelvic colon.— J. M. Garrett *et al.*, *Gastroenterology*, 1967, *53*, 93.

Absorption and Fate. Morphine salts are absorbed from the gastro-intestinal tract but their effects by this route are not entirely predictable; after subcutaneous or intramuscular injection morphine is readily absorbed into the blood. It undergoes significant first-pass metabolism in the liver. Morphine is distributed throughout the body but mainly in the kidneys, liver, lungs, and spleen, with lower concentrations in the brain and muscles. Morphine diffuses across the placenta and traces also appear in milk and sweat.

Conjugation to morphine 3- and 6-glucuronides occurs in the liver and small proportions are metabolised by *N*-demethylation and *O*-methylation. About 10% of a dose of morphine is excreted through the bile into the faeces and the remainder is excreted in the urine, mainly as conjugates. About 90% of total morphine is excreted in 24 hours with traces up to 48 hours.

Urinary excretion patterns of morphine and codeine following consumption of morphine, codeine, diamorphine, and opium.— L. H. Yong and N. T. Lik, *Bull. Narcot.*, 1977, *29* (Jul.–Sept.), 45.

Pharmacokinetic studies of high-dose morphine sulphate in patients undergoing cardiac surgery indicated it was rapidly distributed throughout the body with an apparent elimination half-life (mean 137 minutes) similar to those reported after smaller doses. Hepatic clearance averaged about 25% of hepatic blood flow indicating that first-pass metabolism might be important following administration by mouth.— D. R. Stanski *et al.*, *Clin. Pharmac. Ther.*, 1976, *19*, 752.

There was a wide variation in the disposition of morphine 150 µg per kg body-weight given intramuscularly before anaesthesia to 36 patients and postoperatively to a further 5. No significant differences were found between the 2 groups. Peak plasma concentrations of morphine in the pre-anaesthetic group ranged from 30 to 160 ng per ml (mean 75.3 ng per ml) from 4 to 60 minutes (mean 27.8 minutes) after injection. In this group there was a significant difference between the mean elimination-rate constants for males and females and the half-life for males was longer than that in females. In the 5 patients given morphine postoperatively, peak plasma concentrations ranged from 30 to 130 ng per ml (mean 58.0 ng per ml) from 15 to 60 minutes (mean 37.0 minutes) after injection. The intravenous route is preferred to intramuscular injection for a more precise effect and it is considered that a continuous infusion technique should be developed for analgesia on a continuing basis.— J. R. A. Rigg *et al.*, *Br. J. Anaesth.*, 1978, *50*, 1125.

Further references: D. R. Stanski *et al.*, *Clin. Pharmac. Ther.*, 1978, *24*, 52 (kinetics of morphine given intramuscularly or intravenously); B. Dahlström *et al.*, *ibid.*, 1979, *26*, 354 (kinetics in children); J. Säwe *et al.*, *Clin. Pharmac. Ther.*, 1981, *30*, 629 (morphine kinetics in cancer patients).

Metabolism. A review of the metabolism of morphine and diamorphine.— U. Boerner *et al.*, *Drug Metab. Rev.*, 1975, *4*, 39.

The following metabolites were identified in morphine-dependent subjects receiving morphine sulphate 240 mg daily: morphine 3- and 6-glucuronides, morphine 3,6-diglucuronide, morphine 3-ethereal sulphate, normorphine, normorphine 6-glucuronide and possibly normorphine 3-glucuronide.— S. Y. Yeh *et al.*, *J. pharm. Sci.*, 1977, *66*, 1288.

Protein binding. Morphine was about 35% bound to human plasma protein, mainly to albumin. Binding was independent of morphine concentration but dependent on protein concentration.— G. D. Olsen, *Clin. Pharmac. Ther.*, 1975, *17*, 31. A study of morphine and phenytoin binding to plasma proteins in renal and hepatic failure.— G. D. Olsen *et al.*, *ibid.*, 677.

Further references: J. Judis, *J. pharm. Sci.*, 1977, *66*, 802; B. Fichtl and H. Kurz, *Eur. J. clin. Pharmac.*, 1978, *14*, 335.

Uses. Morphine is a narcotic analgesic obtained from opium. It acts mainly on the central nervous system and smooth muscle. Although morphine is predominantly a central nervous system depressant it has some central stimulant actions which result in nausea and vomiting and miosis. Morphine generally increases smooth muscle tone, especially the sphincters of the gastro-intestinal tract.

Morphine and related analgesics may produce both physical and psychological dependence and should therefore be used with discrimination (see p.1018). Tolerance may also develop.

Morphine is an analgesic used for the symptomatic relief of moderate to severe pain, especially that associated with neoplastic disease and for postoperative pain. When pain is likely to be of short duration, a short-acting analgesic is usually preferred. In acute conditions in which pain may be an important aid to diagnosis, analgesics may be withheld until diagnosis is made. In addition to relieving pain, morphine also alleviates the anxiety associated with severe pain. It is useful as a hypnotic where sleeplessness is due to pain, and may also relieve the pain of biliary or renal colic, although an antispasmodic may also be required since morphine may increase smooth muscle tone.

Morphine reduces intestinal motility and is used in the symptomatic treatment of diarrhoea. It also relieves the dyspnoea of left ventricular failure and of pulmonary oedema. It is effective for the suppression of cough, but codeine is usually preferred as there is less risk of dependence. Morphine has been used pre-operatively as an adjunct to anaesthesia for pain relief and to allay anxiety. It has also been used in high doses as a general anaesthetic in specialised procedures.

The value of giving cocaine or a phenothiazine with morphine or diamorphine in severe pain is being questioned, as indeed is the practice of 'on demand analgesia' versus that of continuous analgesia.

For the relief of pain, morphine sulphate is given in doses of 5 to 20 mg, usually by intramuscular or subcutaneous injection, every 4 hours. Children may be given 100 to 200 µg per kg body-weight up to a maximum of 15 mg. Morphine sulphate or hydrochloride may be given by mouth in doses of 10 to 20 mg. Morphine tartrate has also been given by injection. There are reports of epidural administration of morphine as the hydrochloride providing effective analgesia generally in chronic pain; doses of 2 mg have been employed.

A review of the non-analgesic effects of morphine.— B. A. Callingham, *Pharm. J.*, 1974, *2*, 84.

A review of the relationship of the pharmacokinetics of morphine, methadone, and naloxone to pharmacological activity.— B. A. Berkowitz, *Clin. Pharmacokinet.*, 1976, *1*, 219.

In 10 patients with normal heart function recovering from multiple trauma the injection of morphine 10 mg per 70 kg body-weight via a right atrial catheter significantly reduced mean arterial pressure and heart-rate, probably by means of peripheral vasodilatation. A reduction in the respiratory-rate and an increase in tidal volume were not considered to have contributed to the haemodynamic changes.— I. O. Samuel *et al.*, *Br. J. Anaesth.*, 1977, *49*, 927. In 10 similar patients morphine 10 mg per 70 kg, similarly given, increased forearm blood flow and reduced forearm vascular resistance; there was possibly a compensatory vasconstriction in some other part of the body.— *idem*, 935. See also R. Zelis *et al.*, *J. clin. Invest.*, 1974, *54*, 1247.

The effects of morphine sulphate on coronary blood flow.— D. M. Leaman *et al.*, *Am. J. Cardiol.*, 1978, *41*, 324.

The effects of morphine-nitrous oxide anaesthesia on cerebral blood flow and cerebral metabolism.— D. R. Jobes *et al.*, *Anesthesiology*, 1977, *47*, 16.

Administration. In a study in 45 patients relief from pain in the 72 hours following major surgery was significantly better in those given morphine by a constant infusion by infusion pump than in those given regular intramuscular doses or those given intramuscular doses as required. The respective mean total doses were 36 mg, 110 mg, and 140 mg.— P. C. Rutter *et al.*, *Br. med. J.*, 1980, *280*, 12. See also I. A. Orr *et al.*, *Br. med. J.*, 1981, *283*, 945 (continuous intravenous infusion).

Administration with cocaine. In a study in 400 terminal patients given morphine or diamorphine the addition of cocaine 10 mg per dose produced a small increase in alertness but stopping cocaine had no detectable effect. Cocaine was no longer used routinely. The inclusion of chlorpromazine was likely to antagonise any stimulant effect of the cocaine.— R. Twycross (letter), *Br. med. J.*, 1977, *2*, 1348. See also *Lancet*, 1979, *1*, 1220.

In a double-blind crossover study involving 27 patients with intractable pain a simple flavoured aqueous morphine solution was reported to be as effective for pain control as a standard Brompton Mixture containing a variable amount of morphine, cocaine 10 mg, alcohol (98%) 2.5 ml, syrup 5 ml and sufficient chloroform water to give a total volume of 20 ml. The morphine solution required some alcohol as a preservative.— R. Melzack *et al.*, *Can. med. Ass. J.*, 1979, *120* 435. A criticism of the degree of pain relief obtained from morphine given as the Brompton Mixture in terminally ill patients, advocating the use of intravenous morphine.— M. Keeri-Szanto (letter), *ibid.*, *121*, 17. A reply.— B. M. Mount, *ibid.*, 18.

Administration, epidural and intrathecal. Epidural administration of morphine 2 mg in 10 ml of dextrose injection or sodium chloride injection gave total relief of pain to 3 of 6 patients with chronic intractable pain, and more than 50% relief to the others. A further 4 patients with acute pain associated with surgery or trauma, obtained over 50% relief of pain. All patients obtained considerable analgesic effect within 2 to 3 minutes of injection, which seemed to reach a maximum after 10 to 15 minutes, and lasted 6 to 24 hours. Two of 3 patients who received placebo epidural saline injections obtained slight relief of pain that was less than the effect of subsequent morphine injections. Epidural bupivacaine gave effective relief but was less acceptable than the morphine owing to concomitant muscle weakness. The epidural morphine caused no signs of sympathetic block, such as postural hypotension, and wider clinical trials were considered justified.— M. Bahar *et al.*, *Lancet*, 1979, *1*, 527. Further observations from the same group. Morphine hydrochloride was given extradurally to 98 patients suffering from severe pain of differing origin and duration, including pain in malignancy, in labour, after surgery or trauma, and low-back pain. Complete or marked pain relief lasting at least 4 hours occurred in 55 patients and a further 23 achieved some relief. Thirty patients received single or repeated doses via an extradural needle, while 68 were given doses via an indwelling catheter once or twice daily for up to 8 days. Each dose of 2 to 3 mg consisted of 2 to 3 ml of a 0.1% solution of morphine hydrochloride in dextrose injection 10% diluted with 8 ml of sodium chloride injection. No preservatives were employed.— F. Magora *et al.*, *Br. J. Anaesth.*, 1980, *52*, 247.

Ten patients with severe pain were given morphine intrathecally as a hypertonic solution (morphine 1% and dextrose 15%) and immediately positioned in a 40° head-up position. Analgesia appeared after about 26 minutes, reached a peak after about an hour and lasted about 27 hours. No changes were noted in fine sensation, motor function, heart-rate, arterial pressure, and respiratory frequency; sedation was moderate or absent.— K. Samii *et al.* (letter), *Lancet*, 1979, *1*, 1142.

Morphine 2 mg given epidurally in 10 ml saline has been found to give inadequate analgesia in the immediate postoperative period but it usually gives good results on the day following surgery.— D. B. Scott and J. McClure (letter), *Lancet*, 1979, *1*, 1410. Disappointing results with epidural morphine in labour.— R. P. Husemeyer *et al.*, *ibid.*, *2*, 583. Disappointing results were obtained with epidural morphine in doses of 5 mg or 2 mg in a double-blind placebo-controlled study in 30 women on the day after abdominal hysterectomy. Acute pain may be more resistant to the method than chronic pain.— J. H. McClure *et al.*, *ibid.*, 1980, *1*, 975.

A study of the use of intrathecal morphine sulphate 1.5 mg as the sole analgesic during labour in 12 women. The injection abolished pain during the first stage of labour in all patients and the pain of the second stage was abolished in 4 and reduced in another 3. No loss of the 'pushing reflex' occurred so that full maternal co-operation in the second stage was achieved. Side-effects including itching of the face, mouth, eyes, and nose, and nausea and vomiting occurred but these were generally mild and easily treated.— P. V. Scott *et al.*, *Br. med. J.*, 1980, *281*, 351. This technique was not considered suitable for pain in labour in view of the high incidence of side-effects.— J. A. T. Duncan (letter), *ibid.*, 515; B. W. Perriss and A. F. Malins, *ibid.*

Continuous epidural analgesia through an implanted reservoir infusion pump.— D. W. Coombs *et al.* (letter), *Lancet*, 1981, *2*, 425.

Further references: J. Leslie *et al.* (letter), *Lancet*, 1979, *2*, 151 (action); E. T. Mathews and L. D. Abrams, *ibid* (open heart surgery); M. J. Cousins *et al.* (letter), *ibid.*, 584 (action); A. R. Bapat *et al.*, *ibid* (more effective in chronic than in acute pain); M. Zenz *et al.*, *ibid.*, 1981, *1*, 91 (beneficial long-term use in terminal cancer); D. J. Layfield *et al.*, *Br. med. J.*, 1981, *282*, 697 (ischaemic rest pain).

For the preparation of a suitable injection of morphine for epidural administration, see under Preparations, below.

Administration in liver disease. See under Precautions.

Administration in renal failure. Data for predicting removal of morphine by conventional haemodialysis.— T. P. Gibson and H. A. Nelson, *Clin. Pharmacokinet.*, 1977, *2*, 403.

Because of decreased plasma protein binding in uraemia, morphine should be given with caution to uraemic patients, particularly those with low serum albumin concentrations or liver disease.— W. M. Bennett, *Drugs*, 1979, *17*, 111. No dosage adjustment was recommended for patients with renal failure.— W. M. Bennett *et al.*, *Ann. intern. Med.*, 1980, *93*, 62.

Anaesthesia. *High-dose morphine.* Morphine administered at a maximum rate of 10 mg every 2 minutes until consciousness was lost or until a maximum total dose of 2 mg per kg body-weight was reached was compared with halothane as a primary anaesthetic agent in 128 patients undergoing open-heart surgery. Nitrous oxide and oxygen were used for induction. Hypertension was more frequent and greater with morphine. Overall mortality rates and durations of stay in the intensive care unit and in hospital were comparable in both groups of patients.— T. J. Conahan *et al.*, *Anesthesiology*, 1973, *38*, 528.

Up to 3 mg of morphine per kg body-weight was compared with 8 to 11 mg per kg during open-heart surgery. Oliguria, hypotension, and pooling occurred with the larger doses and doses above 3 mg per kg body-weight had little to recommend them.— T. H. Stanley *et al.*, *Anesthesiology*, 1973, *38*, 536.

In 10 healthy subjects the cardiovascular effects were studied of morphine 2 mg per kg body-weight administered intravenously at the rate of 10 mg per minute in association with oxygen followed by 70% nitrous oxide in oxygen. Total peripheral resistance increased and cardiac index and heart-rate decreased on addition of the nitrous oxide 70% suggesting that the combination might not be suitable for critically ill patients.— K. C. Wong *et al.*, *Anesthesiology*, 1973, *38*, 542.

A study of the kinetics of intravenous administration of high doses of morphine for anaesthesia in cardiac surgery patients.— D. R. Stanski *et al.*, *Clin. Pharmac. Ther.*, 1976, *19*, 752.

For a report on the use of high-dose morphine anaesthesia in the treatment of tetanus, see below under Tetanus.

Analgesia. *Postoperative.* In a double-blind single-dose study of 450 selected postoperative patients concurrent administration of dexamphetamine 10 mg intramuscularly doubled the analgesic potency of morphine sulphate; administration of 5 mg enhanced the analgesic potency by about 50%. Effects on blood pressure, pulse, and respiration rate were slight; sleepiness decreased slightly with increased doses of dexamphetamine; sweating increased significantly; dizziness and nausea increased slightly; also noted were other CNS effects, visual disturbances, flushing, and tremors. Increased side-effects were considered to be offset by the benefit of increased analgesia without increased sedation.— W. H. Forrest *et al.*, *New Engl. J. Med.*, 1977, *296*, 712. Criticism.— L. D. Vandam, *ibid.*, 750.

See also under Administration, above.

Cardiovascular disorders. *Myocardial infarction.* A study on the haemodynamic effects of intravenous morphine in 10 patients with acute myocardial infarction complicated by severe left ventricular failure suggested that the useful action of morphine in relieving distressing cardiac dyspnoea is not adequately explained by systemic venous pooling but rather that the effects of morphine on the central nervous system are more important.— A. D. Timmis *et al.*, *Br. med. J.*, 1980, *280*, 980.

For a comparison of morphine, diamorphine, methadone, and pentazocine in the relief of pain in cardiac infarction, see Pentazocine, p.1025.

Gastro-intestinal disorders. Opiates had no part to play in the treatment of infantile gastro-enteritis.— M. D. Holdaway, *Drugs*, 1977, *14*, 383.

Respiratory disorders. Use as an adjunct in the treatment of status asthmaticus.— P. Marchand and H. van Hasselt, *Lancet*, 1966, *1*, 227.

The effectiveness of morphine in pulmonary oedema was mainly due to its vasodilator action which led to increased peripheral pooling of blood.— *Lancet*, 1978, *1*, 972.

Tetanus. Morphine 1 to 2 mg per kg body-weight to a total of 3.1 g over 22 days was used to control autonomic hyperactivity in a patient who had developed generalised tetanus following injury. Dosage was reduced to 60 mg per day on the 23rd day and then discontinued.— M. A. Rie and R. S. Wilson, *Ann. intern. Med.*, 1978, *88*, 653.

Morphine 5 mg intravenously every 6 hours significantly reduced spontaneous sympathetic overactivity but had little effect on spasms induced by handling in 9 adults with tetanus.— N. Buchanan *et al.*, *Intensive Care Med.*, 1979, *5*, 65.

Preparations of Morphine and its Salts

Injections

Morphine and Atropine Injection *(B.P.).* Morph. and Atrop. Inj. A sterile solution of morphine sulphate 1 g, atropine sulphate 60 mg, sodium metabisulphite 100 mg, sodium chloride 690 mg, in Water for Injections to 100 ml. Sterilised by filtration. Protect from light.
Dose. 0.5 to 1 ml subcutaneously.

Morphine and Hyoscine Injection *(B.P.C. 1968).* Morphine and Scopolamine Injection. A sterile solution of morphine sulphate 1 g, hyoscine hydrobromide 40 mg, sodium metabisulphite 100 mg, sodium chloride 690 mg, in Water for Injections to 100 ml. Protect from light.
Dose. 0.5 to 1 ml subcutaneously.

Morphine Hydrochloride Injection *(Jap. P.).* A sterile solution of morphine hydrochloride in Water for Injections. Similar injections are described in other pharmacopoeias.

Morphine Sulfate Injection *(U.S.P.).* A sterile solution of morphine sulphate in Water for Injections. It may contain suitable antimicrobial agents. pH 2.5 to 6. Protect from light.

Morphine Sulphate Epidural Injection. An injection of morphine sulphate suitable for epidural administration without preservative or antioxidant could be prepared by packing 10 ml of a solution of morphine sulphate 2 mg in sodium chloride injection into 10 ml ampoules. Filtered oxygen-free nitrogen is bubbled through the solution for 5 seconds immediately before sealing the ampoule which is then autoclaved at 115° for 30 minutes. No breakdown of morphine has been detected in such ampoules after storage at room temperature for 4 months.— R.J. Bunn and R.M. Hobbs (letter), *Pharm. J.*, 1980, *1*, 334. Operating-theatre procedure demanded that the outside of the ampoule be sterile and to this end ampoules were being re-autoclaved in theatre with subsequent breakdown of the morphine. This problem was solved by suitably wrapping the ampoules in the pharmacy before the initial and sole autoclaving.— S. Turner and S. Potter, *ibid.*,*2*, 108.

Morphine Sulphate Injection *(B.P.).* Morph. Sulph. Inj.; Morphine Injection. A sterile solution of morphine sulphate in Water for Injections containing the equivalent of not more than 0.1% of sulphur dioxide. Sterilised by heating at 98° to 100° for 30 minutes with a bactericide, or by filtration. Protect from light.

Mixtures and Elixirs

Haustus MP *(Brompton Hosp.).* Morphine hydrochloride in the dose required, prochlorperazine mesylate 5 mg (as Stemetil Syrup), chloroform water to 10 ml.

NOTE. *Brompton Hosp.*, in common with some other hospitals, previously used a preparation containing cocaine hydrochloride as well as morphine hydrochloride, and known as Haustus E. Such formulations have largely fallen into disuse: see above under Administration with Cocaine, p.1020.

Various other names have been applied to mixtures containing morphine, diamorphine, and cocaine, including Mist. Euphoriens, Saunders' Mixture, Brompton Cocktail, and Brompton Mixture. The name Brompton Mixture was also applied to Mist. Tuss. Hydrocyan. (*N.F. 1939*) (*see Martindale, 27th Edn*, p. 973).

Morphine and Cocaine Elixir *(B.P.C. 1973).* Morphine hydrochloride 5 mg, cocaine hydrochloride 5 mg, syrup 1.25 ml, alcohol (90%) 0.625 ml, chloroform water to 5 ml. When specified by the prescriber, the proportion of morphine may be varied. It should be recently prepared. *Dose.* Determined by the physician according to the patient's needs.

Morphine, Cocaine, and Chlorpromazine Elixir *(B.P.C. 1973).* Morphine hydrochloride 5 mg, cocaine hydrochloride 5 mg, chlorpromazine elixir 1.25 ml, alcohol (90%) 0.625 ml, chloroform water to 5 ml. When specified by the prescriber, the proportion of morphine may be varied. It should be recently prepared. Protect from light. *Dose.* Determined by the physician according to the patient's needs.

NOTE. The administration of cocaine with diamorphine or morphine has been reported to be of no apparent benefit, see above.

Solutions

Morphine Hydrochloride Solution *(B.P.C. 1973).* Liq. Morph. Hydrochlor. Morphine hydrochloride 1 g, dilute hydrochloric acid 2 ml, alcohol (90%) 25 ml, freshly boiled and cooled water to 100 ml. Protect from light.
Dose. 0.5 to 2 ml.

Suppositories

Morphine Suppositories *(B.P.C. 1973).* Suppositories containing morphine hydrochloride or sulphate in theobroma oil or other suitable fatty basis. About 1.5 g of morphine hydrochloride or sulphate displaces 1 g of theobroma oil. Store in a cool place.

Tablets

Morphine Sulphate Tablets *(B.P.).* Morph. Sulph. Tab.; Tab. Morph. Sulph. Tablets containing morphine sulphate. Protect from light.

Proprietary Preparations of Morphine and its Salts

Cyclimorph 10 *(Calmic, UK).* An injection containing in each ml morphine tartrate 10 mg and cyclizine tartrate 50 mg, in ampoules of 1 ml. **Cyclimorph 15** contains in each ml morphine tartrate 15 mg and cyclizine tartrate 50 mg, in ampoules of 1 ml. For the relief of pain without causing nausea and vomiting.

Duromorph *(Laboratories for Applied Biology, UK).* Morphine in a long-acting microcrystalline form in aqueous suspension containing 64 mg in 1 ml for subcutaneous or intramuscular injection, available in ampoules of 1 ml.

MST-Continus *(Napp, UK).* Morphine sulphate, available as sustained-release tablets of 10 and 30 mg.
The 10-mg tablets were formerly known as MST-1.

Poor results with sustained-release tablets of morphine (MST-1) in the relief of postoperative dental pain, and re-emphasis that, whatever the formulation, morphine by mouth is not suitable for the treatment of acute pain. MST-1 may have a place in the treatment of chronic cancer pain, but further clinical and pharmacokinetic data are needed.— G. W. Hanks *et al.* (letter), *Lancet*, 1981, *1*, 732. MST-1 could be of benefit in some patients with cancer pain but the 10-mg strength means that some patients would have to take an absurdly large number of tablets.— R. G. Twycross (letter), *ibid.*, 892. See also J. K. Dewhurst (letter), *ibid.*; G. W. Hanks *et al.* (letter), *ibid.*, 1104; *Drug & Ther. Bull.*, 1981, *19*, 44.

Comment on the supply problem of Controlled Drugs from the general practice pharmacy, including mention of sustained-release tablets of morphine 30 mg and 60 mg (MST-3 Continus and MST-6 Continus, *Napp*).— S. Tempest (letter), *Pharm. J.*, 1981, *2*, 160.

Nepenthe Injection *(Evans Medical, UK).* Contains anhydrous morphine 0.84% (0.05% from papaveretum and 0.79% from morphine hydrochloride). **Nepenthe Oral Solution.** Contains anhydrous morphine 0.84% (0.05% from opium tincture and 0.79% morphine). *Dose.* 1 to 2 ml of Nepenthe Injection subcutaneously or intramuscularly repeated if required not more often than every four hours. Children 1 to 5 years of age may be given a maximum single dose of 0.25 to 0.5 ml and children 6 to 12 years of age a maximum single dose of 0.5 to 1 ml by subcutaneous or intramuscular injection. Nepenthe Oral Solution is given in similar doses by mouth. (Also available as Nepenthe in *Austral.*).

CAUTION. *Nepenthe Oral Solution may become concentrated through evaporation of the solvent. It should be stored in a cool place in airtight containers. If evaporation occurs during storage the solution should not be used because of risk of overdosage.*

A preparation containing morphine acetate was formerly marketed in Great Britain under the proprietary name Syrup Tussi Hydrobrom. *(Philip Harris).*

6244-y

Nalbuphine Hydrochloride. EN2234A. 17-Cyclobutylmethyl-7,8-dihydro-14-hydroxy-17-normorphine hydrochloride; (−)-(5*R*,6*S*,14*S*)-9a-Cyclobutylmethyl-4,5-epoxymorphinan-3,6,14-triol hydrochloride.
$C_{21}H_{27}NO_4,HCl = 393.9$.

CAS — 20594-83-6 (nalbuphine); 23277-43-2 (hydrochloride).

Dependence. Nalbuphine hydrochloride may produce dependence of the morphine type (p.1018). It is liable to abuse.

Adverse Effects, Treatment, and Precautions. As for Morphine, p.1019.

Uses. Nalbuphine hydrochloride has narcotic agonist and antagonist properties. It is used for the relief of moderate to severe pain. It is considered to produce similar analgesia to morphine and is given subcutaneously, intramuscularly, or intravenously in doses of 10 mg every 3 to 6 hours. Nalbuphine is reported to act within 15 minutes of subcutaneous or intramuscular injection or within 2 to 3 minutes of intravenous injection.

References: D. R. Jasinski and P. A. Mansky, *Clin. Pharmac. Ther.*, 1972, *13*, 78; S. Archer and W. F. Michne, *Prog. Drug Res.*, 1976, *20*, 45; *Med. Lett.*, 1979, *21*, 83; J. R. Lewis, *J. Am. med. Ass.*, 1980, *243*, 1465; A. Romagnoli and A. S. Keats, *Clin. Pharmac.*

Ther., 1980, *27*, 478; W. T. Beaver *et al.*, *ibid.*, 1981, *29*, 174; J. E. Stambaugh, *ibid.*, 284.

Proprietary Names
Nubain *(Endo, USA)*.

6245-j

Norpipanone Hydrochloride. Hoechst 10495. 4,4-Diphenyl-6-piperidinohexan-3-one hydrochloride.
$C_{23}H_{29}NO,HCl=371.9$.

CAS — 561-48-8 (norpipanone).

Crystals. M.p. 181° to 182°. **Soluble** in water and alcohol.

Norpipanone hydrochloride is a narcotic analgesic used to relieve pain in smooth muscle spasm and migraine. A dose of 6 mg three times daily has been used.

References: Thirteenth Report of a WHO Expert Committee on Addiction Producing Drugs, *Tech. Rep. Ser. Wld Hlth Org. No. 273*, 1964.

6246-z

Opium *(B.P.)*. Gum Opium; Raw Opium.

Pharmacopoeias. In all pharmacopoeias examined except *Braz., Eur., Fr., Jap.*, and *Rus.* The specified minimum content of anhydrous morphine varies slightly but is usually 9.5 or 10% or, alternatively, 12% calculated on the drug dried at 60°.

The dried or partly dried latex obtained by incision from the unripe capsules of *Papaver somniferum* (Papaveraceae). It has a strong characteristic odour and a bitter taste and contains not less than 9.5% of anhydrous morphine. **Incompatible** with vegetable astringents, alkaline carbonates, and salts of mercury, iron, lead, and zinc. The exuded latex is dried, by spontaneous evaporation or by artifical heat, and is manipulated to form cakes of uniform composition, variously shaped according to the country of origin, and known in commerce as Turkish, Indian, or European opium. The *B.P.* specifies Indian opium.

Opium contains a variable mixture of about 25 alkaloids, including morphine 9 to 17%, noscapine 2 to 9%, codeine 0.3 to 4%, and smaller proportions of thebaine, narceine, papaverine, and hydrocotarnine.

NOTE. The *B.P.* directs that when Opium is prescribed, Powdered Opium shall be dispensed.

6247-c

Powdered Opium *(B.P.)*. Pdrd. Opium; Standardised Opium Powder; Opii Pulvis Standardisatus; Opium Pulveratum; Opium Titratum; Pulvis Opii.

Pharmacopoeias. In all pharmacopoeias examined except *Braz., Eur.*, and *Fr. Mex.* and *U.S.* specify 10 to 10.5% of anhydrous morphine. *Swiss* specifies at least 10.5% of anhydrous morphine. *Jap.* also includes a diluted opium powder containing 1% of anhydrous morphine.

Opium, dried, powdered, and adjusted to contain 9.5 to 10.5% of anhydrous morphine; about 20 mg in 200 mg. **Store** in airtight containers.

Dependence. Prolonged use of opium may lead to dependence of the morphine type (see p.1018).

Adverse Effects and Treatment. As for Morphine, p.1019.

Adulteration of opium with arsenic in India, the intention being to provide stimulant or aphrodisiac properties. The concentration might be very low.— D. V. Datta and M. K. Kaul, *Bull. Narcot.*, 1977, *29* (July–Sept.), 41.

Further references: D. V. Datta (letter), *Lancet*, 1977, *1*, 484 and 903; R. D. P. Eaton (letter), *ibid.*, 903.

Carcinogenicity. The high incidence of oesophageal cancer in the Transkei and north-east Iran was shown by bacterial mutagenicity tests to be associated with ingestion of the pyrolysis products, tobacco pipe residues and opium dross, respectively.— T. Hewer *et al.*, *Lancet*, 1978, *2*, 494. Opium taking, including the eating of 'sukhte' (scrapings from opium pipes), was prevalent throughout Iran and could not be blamed for the high incidence of oesophageal cancer in particular population groups.— J. Kmet (letter), *ibid.*, 1371. Reply.— T. F. Hewer (letter), *ibid.*, 1979, *1*, 45.

Precautions. As for Morphine, p.1019.

Uses. Opium has analgesic and narcotic actions which are due mainly to its content of morphine (see p.1020).

It acts less rapidly than morphine since opium appears to be more slowly absorbed; the relaxing action of the papaverine and noscapine on intestinal muscle makes it more constipating than morphine.

Camphorated Opium Tincture (Paregoric) is given with expectorants for coughs. For its intestinal action opium is given as Aromatic Chalk with Opium Mixture.

Opium has been employed externally in liniments or lotions but there is no evidence of local analgesic action.

Treatment of neonatal narcotic dependence. Paregoric *(U.S.P.)* was usually given in initial doses of 0.2 ml by mouth every 3 hours for neonatal narcotic dependence, with increases of 0.05 ml every 3 hours until a controlling dose was reached. It was rarely necessary to exceed 0.7 ml per dose. The dose was maintained for about a week; mild tremulousness during the withdrawal period should not prevent further lowering of the dose but withdrawal from paregoric could take a long time since an over-rapid rate might lead to a recurrence of symptoms *Med. Lett.*, 1973, *15*, 47.

Further references: M. C. F. Semoff, *Ariz. Med.*, 1967, *24*, 933.

For further reports on the treatment of neonatal narcotic dependence, see p.1018.

Preparations

Extracts

Opium Dry Extract *(B.P.C. 1954)*. Ext. Opii Sicc.; Opium Extract; Extractum Opii Aquosum. A dry aqueous extract adjusted with calcium phosphate to contain 20% of anhydrous morphine. *Dose.* 15 to 60 mg. A similar extract is included in several pharmacopoeias.

Opium Liquid Extract *(B.P.C. 1954)*. Ext. Opii Liq. Opium dry extract 3.75 g, alcohol (90%) 20 ml, water to 100 ml. It contains 0.75% w/v of anhydrous morphine. *Dose.* 0.3 to 2 ml.

Linctuses

Opiate Squill Linctus *(B.P.)*. Linctus Scillae Opiatus; Compound Squill Linctus; Gee's Linctus; Squill Opiate Linctus. Equal volumes of camphorated opium tincture, squill oxymel, and tolu syrup; it may also contain 0.056% of powdered tragacanth or 0.011% of xanthan gum. It contains about 800 µg of anhydrous morphine in 5 ml. *Dose.* 5 ml. When a dose less than or not a multiple of 5 ml is prescribed, the linctus should be diluted to 5 ml, or a multiple, with syrup. Such dilutions must be freshly prepared and not used more than 2 weeks after issue.

NOTE. Clarification of this linctus can usually be accomplished by the addition of cetomacrogol (see p.373), though some batches of honey yield a preparation which cannot be clarified by this method. Clarified solutions do not, however, conform to the *B.P.* description of this linctus.

Paediatric Opiate Squill Linctus *(B.P.)*. Linctus Scillae Opiatus pro Infantibus; Squill Opiate Linctus Paediatric; Opiate Linctus for Infants. Camphorated opium tincture 0.3 ml, squill oxymel 0.3 ml, tolu syrup 0.3 ml, glycerol 1 ml, syrup to 5 ml. It contains about 150 µg of anhydrous morphine in 5 ml. *Dose.* Children, 5 to 10 ml. When a dose less than or not a multiple of 5 ml is prescribed, the linctus should be diluted to 5 ml, or a multiple, with syrup. Such dilutions must be freshly prepared and not used more than 2 weeks after issue.

For a report of incompatibility when Paediatric Opiate Squill Linctus was prepared with or diluted with syrup preserved with hydroxybenzoates, see under Sucrose, p.61.

Mixtures

Compound Camphorated Opium Mixture *(B.P.C. 1973)*. Mist. Opii Camph. Co.; Mist. Camph. Co. Camphorated opium tincture 1 ml, ammonium bicarbonate 100 mg, strong ammonium acetate solution 1 ml, water to 10 ml. It should be recently prepared. It contains about 500 µg of anhydrous morphine in 10 ml. *Dose.* 10 to 20 ml.

Pastilles

Opiate Squill Pastilles *(B.P.)*. Pastilli Scillae Opiati; Pastil. Scill. Opiat.; Gee's Linctus Pastilles; Gee's Pastilles. Each contains concentrated camphorated opium tincture 0.075 ml, squill liquid extract 0.03 ml, benzoic acid 600 µg, cinnamic acid 250 µg, glacial acetic acid 0.02 ml, and purified honey 0.2 ml in pastille basis. Each pastille contains about 300 µg of anhydrous morphine.

Tinctures

Camphorated Opium Tincture *(B.P.)*. Camph. Opium Tinct.; Tinct. Opii Camph.; Paregoric; Tinct. Camph. Co. Opium tincture 5 ml, benzoic acid 500 mg, camphor 300 mg, anise oil 0.3 ml, alcohol (60%) to 100 ml. It contains 0.045 to 0.055% w/v of anhydrous morphine; about 5 mg in 10 ml.
Dose. 2 to 10 ml.

Paregoric *(U.S.P.)* is similar and contains 0.035 to 0.045% of anhydrous morphine. Most other pharmacopoeias have a similar preparation containing 0.05% of anhydrous morphine.

Concentrated Camphorated Opium Tincture *(B.P.)*. Concentrated Camph. Opium Tinct.; Tinct. Opii Camph. Conc.; Liquor Opii Camphoratus Concentratus. Opium tincture 40 ml, benzoic acid 4 g, camphor 2.4 g, anise oil 2.4 ml, alcohol 40 ml, water to 100 ml. It is about 8 times as strong as Camphorated Opium Tincture *(B.P.)*.
Dose. 0.25 to 1.25 ml.

Opium Tincture *(B.P.)*. Laudanum. Prepared by maceration with water (boiling) and with alcohol and adjusted to contain 0.95 to 1.05% w/v of anhydrous morphine; about 20 mg in 2 ml.
Dose. 0.25 to 2 ml.

Most pharmacopoeias, including *U.S.P.* include a tincture of the same strength or 1% w/w.

Opium Tincture with Saffron *(B.P.C. 1934)*. Tincture Opii Crocata; Sydenham's Laudanum. A tincture prepared from opium, cinnamon, clove, and saffron, and adjusted to contain 1% w/v of anhydrous morphine.
Dose. 0.25 to 2 ml.

Several pharmacopoeias contain a similar preparation.

6248-k

Oxycodone Hydrochloride. Oxycodoni Hydrochloridum; Dihydrone Hydrochloride; Oxycone Hydrochloride; Thecodine; 7,8-Dihydro-14-hydroxycodeinone hydrochloride. 6-Deoxy-7,8-dihydro-14-hydroxy-3-*O*-methyl-6-oxomorphine hydrochloride trihydrate; (−)-(5*R*,14*S*)-4,5-Epoxy-14-hydroxy-3-methoxy-9a-methylmorphinan-6-one hydrochloride trihydrate.

$C_{18}H_{21}NO_4,HCl,3H_2O=405.9$.

CAS — 76-42-6 (oxycodone); 124-90-3 (hydrochloride, anhydrous).

Pharmacopoeias. In *Aust., Belg., Cz., Ger., Int., Jap., Jug., Nord., Port., Rus., Swiss*, and *Turk.* (mostly as trihydrate).

A white odourless crystalline powder with a bitter saline taste. M.p. about 275°. **Soluble** 1 in 6 of water, 1 in 60 of alcohol, and 1 in 600 of chloroform; practically insoluble in ether. A solution in water is neutral to litmus. **Incompatible** with alkalis, iodides, and tannic acid.

Dependence, Adverse Effects, Treatment, and Precautions. As for Morphine, p.1018.

Dyskinesia developed in a patient when she stopped taking a mixed analgesic preparation containing oxycodone. The condition was controlled by diphenhydramine.— G. Gardos (letter), *Lancet*, 1977, *1*, 759.

Absorption and Fate. Oxycodone is absorbed from the gastro-intestinal tract. It is metabolised to noroxycodone and both metabolite and unchanged drug are excreted in urine.

In 6 healthy subjects given a proprietary tablet containing oxycodone 4.5 mg with oxycodone terephthalate 380 µg, a mean plasma-oxycodone concentration of 18.4 ng per ml occurred 1 hour after administration.— N. L. Renzi and J. N. Tam, *J. pharm. Sci.*, 1979, *68*, 43.

Noroxycodone was the major metabolite of oxycodone.— S. H. Weinstein and J. C. Gaylord, *J. pharm. Sci.*, 1979, *68*, 527.

Uses. Oxycodone is used similarly to morphine (see p.1020) for the relief of pain. Oxycodone hydrochloride may be given by mouth or by subcutaneous injection in doses of 5 to 20 mg.

Oxycodone is also used as oxycodone pectinate which is given by intramuscular injection in doses of 10 to 20 mg. Its effects are of longer duration than those of the hydrochloride; a dose is effective for approximately 6 to 8 hours. The pectinate is also given rectally as suppositories.

Oxycodone terephthalate has also been given by mouth.

References: *Drug & Ther. Bull.*, 1979, *17*, 21.

Preparations

Injectabile Oxiconi 1% *(Nord. P.).* Oxycodone Hydrochloride Injection. Oxycodone hydrochloride 1 g, sodium metabisulphite 100 mg, sodium chloride 650 mg, 0.1 M hydrochloric acid 1 g, Water for Injections to 100 ml. Sterilised by autoclaving. Cresol 0.3% is a suitable preservative; *Dan. Disp.* specifies 0.1% methyl hydroxybenzoate.

Injectio Oxycodoni Composita *(Jap. P.).* A sterile solution of oxycodone hydrochloride 0.8% and hydrocotarnine hydrochloride 0.2% in Water for Injections.
Injectio Oxycodoni et Atropini Composita *(Jap. P.).* Contains in addition atropine sulphate 0.03%.

Solutio Thecodini 1% aut 2% pro Injectionibus *(Rus. P.).* Oxycodone Hydrochloride Injection. Oxycodone hydrochloride 1 g or 2 g, 0.1N hydrochloric acid 2 ml, Water for Injections to 100 ml; in ampoules of 1 ml. pH 2.8 to 4.

Proprietary Preparations of Oxycodone Pectinate

Oxycodone Suppositories (formerly known as Proladone) *(Boots, UK).* Oxycodone pectinate, available as suppositories each containing the equivalent of 30 mg of oxycodone (supplied only to special order). (Also available as Proladone in *Austral.*).

Other Proprietary Names of Oxycodone Salts

Hydrochloride: Endone *(Austral.)*; Eubine *(Fr.)*; Eukodal *(Ger.)*; Supeudol *(Canad.)*; Pectinate: Pancodone Retard *(Fr.)*.

6249-a

Oxymorphone Hydrochloride *(U.S.P.).*

Oximorphone Hydrochloride; 7,8-Dihydro-14-hydroxymorphinone hydrochloride. 6-Deoxy-7,8-dihydro-14-hydroxy-6-oxomorphine hydrochloride; (−)-(5*R*,14*S*)-4,5-Epoxy-3,14-dihydroxy-9a-methylmorphinan-6-one hydrochloride.
$C_{17}H_{19}NO_4,HCl = 337.8$.

CAS — 76-41-5 (oxymorphone); 357-07-3 (hydrochloride).

Pharmacopoeias. In *U.S.*

A white or slightly off-white odourless powder, darkening on exposure to light. It loses not more than 8% of its weight on drying. **Soluble** 1 in 4 of water, 1 in 100 of alcohol, and 1 in 25 of methyl alcohol; very slightly soluble in chloroform and ether. A solution in water is laevorotatory. Solutions in water are slightly acid. Solutions are **sterilised** by filtration. **Store** in airtight containers. Protect from light.

Dependence. Prolonged use of oxymorphone may lead to dependence of the morphine type (see p.1018).

Adverse Effects, Treatment, and Precautions. As for Morphine, p.1019.

Absorption and Fate. Oxymorphone hydrochloride is absorbed from the gastro-intestinal tract. It diffuses across the placenta.

Uses. Oxymorphone hydrochloride is an analgesic with uses similar to those of morphine (see p.1020). It is usually administered by subcutaneous or intramuscular injection in the treatment of moderate and severe pain, and by intravenous injection as an adjunct to anaesthesia. Oxymorphone is given in doses of 1 to 1.5 mg every 4 to 6 hours by intramuscular or subcutaneous injection; 500 µg may be given by intravenous injection.

Oxymorphone has also been administered by mouth in doses of 5 to 10 mg and is given rectally in a suppository in doses of 2 to 5 mg every 4 to 6 hours.

Unlike morphine, oxymorphone has little antitussive action.

Analgesia. In a double-blind crossover study in cancer patients, a single dose of oxymorphone given by mouth was considered to have one-sixth the potency of the same dose given by intramuscular injection. In a further study, oxymorphone had about 9 times the analgesic potency of morphine given by intramuscular injection.— W. T. Beaver *et al.*, *J. clin. Pharmac.*, 1977, *17*, 186.

Oxymorphone administered as a suppository was estimated to have one-tenth the analgesic effect of the same dose given by intramuscular injection.— W. T. Beaver and G. A. Feise, *J. clin. Pharmac.*, 1977, *17*, 276.

Reports on the use of oxymorphone in labour.— S. Ransom, *Anaesthesia*, 1966, *21*, 464; G. M. Eames and K. R. S. Pool, *Br. med. J.*, 1964, *2*, 353.

Preparations

Oxymorphone Hydrochloride Injection *(U.S.P.).* A sterile solution in Water for Injections. pH 2.7 to 4.5. Protect from light.

Oxymorphone Hydrochloride Suppositories *(U.S.P.).* Suppositories containing oxymorphone hydrochloride. Store at 2° to 8°.

Proprietary Names

Numorphan *(Endo, Canad.; Endo, S.Afr.; Endo, USA).*

6250-e

Papaveretum *(B.P.C. 1973).*

Opium Concentratum; Extractum Concentratum Opii; Alkaloidorum Opii Hydrochloridum; Omnoponum; Opialum. The hydrochlorides of alkaloids of opium, containing the equivalent of anhydrous morphine 47.5 to 52.5%, anhydrous codeine 2.5 to 5%, noscapine 16 to 22%, and papaverine 2.5 to 7%.

CAS — 8002-76-4.

Pharmacopoeias. Similar preparations of mixed opium alkaloids are included in *Jap., Pol., Roum.*, and *Rus.*

A white, light-brown, or brownish-grey powder. **Soluble** 1 in 15 of water; less soluble in alcohol. Solutions are **sterilised** by maintaining at 98° to 100° for 30 minutes with a bactericide or by filtration; chlorocresol should not be used as the bactericide. **Protect** from light.

Dependence, Adverse Effects, Treatment, and Precautions. As for Morphine, p.1018.

A well-built 14-year-old boy about to undergo operation was given, intramuscularly, papaveretum 20 mg with hyoscine hydrobromide 400 µg (adult dose). Ninety minutes later he had an intense itching at the back of the shoulder and then a single major epileptiform convulsion lasting about a minute followed by postictal stupor for 30 minutes.— R. P. Holmes (letter), *Br. J. Anaesth.*, 1968, *40*, 633.

Pregnancy and the neonate. Clinical depression of the newborn had been observed after the use of papaveretum during labour.— F. Moya and V. Thorndike, *Clin. Pharmac. Ther.*, 1963, *4*, 628.

Uses. Papaveretum has the analgesic and narcotic properties of morphine (see p.1020); 20 mg is equivalent clinically to 10 to 15 mg of morphine.

In adults it is generally administered by subcutaneous or intramuscular injection in doses of 10 to 20 mg. Infants aged up to 1 month may be given 150 µg per kg body-weight and infants aged up to 1 year, 200 µg per kg. Children aged 1 to 5 years may be given 2.5 to 5 mg and children aged 6 to 12 years, 5 to 10 mg. It is employed in conjunction with hyoscine for pre-operative medication and has been given with hyoscine and atropine to produce partial anaesthesia and 'twilight sleep'.

Papaveretum may also be given by mouth in doses of 10 to 20 mg.

Analgesia. *Postoperative.* A technique for providing postoperative pain relief is being developed. When analgesia is first required papaveretum is injected intravenously in boluses of 2 mg each minute until adequate analgesia is achieved as confirmed by the patient's comfort and ability to cough without pain. An hour later 4 mg is injected over 12 hours. After the first 24 hours the 4-mg dose may be reduced by 1 mg every 12-hour period.— E. N. S. Fry (letter), *Br. med. J.*, 1976, *2*, 817.

In 17 men given papaveretum intravenously in titrated doses for postoperative pain the dose range was 9 to 30 mg, and 6 to 25 mg in 44 women. The dose correlated poorly with age and body-weight. The dose should be titrated intravenously and 3 repeat doses could then be given intramuscularly with intervals of 4, 6, and 8 hours.— E. N. S. Fry and S. Deshpande, *Br. med. J.*, 1977, *2*, 870.

A study comparing 2 methods of administration of papaveretum for the relief of postoperative pain in patients who had undergone cholecystectomy. In 11 patients a loading dose of 1 mg per minute of papaveretum was given by continuous intravenous infusion until the patient would breathe deeply and cough effectively without undue pain followed by eight times this loading dose given by continuous intravenous infusion over 48 hours and a further 11 patients were given papaveretum 250 µg per kg body-weight intramuscularly every four hours as necessary. Significantly greater relief of pain was experienced in the group who received the intravenous regimen, which may have reflected the larger dose of papaveretum given to this group, but was associated with a greater degree of respiratory depression and potentially life-threatening changes in the respiratory pattern which included apnoea with consequent hypoxia. These findings suggest that the fear that large doses of analgesics will cause respiratory complications, which often accounts for inadequate postoperative pain relief, is well founded.— J. A. Catling *et al.*, *Br. med. J.*, 1980, *281*, 478. This technique of the intravenous infusion of papaveretum originally described by the author (*Br. med. J.*, 1976, *2*, 817, see above) was no longer used by him. Buprenorphine and fentanyl are given pre-operatively and papaveretum 10 to 20 mg is given intramuscularly as soon as the patient gains consciousness but before severe pain is felt.— E. N. S. Fry (letter), *ibid.*, 807.

Preparations

Papaveretum Injection *(B.P.C. 1973).* A sterile solution of papaveretum 2% w/v and glycerol 1.4% w/v in Water for Injections. It may contain a bactericide; phenylmercuric nitrate 0.002% is suitable. It is supplied in single-dose containers. Protect from light. It contains the equivalent of about 10 mg of anhydrous morphine in 1 ml. *Dose.* Adults subcutaneously or intramuscularly, 0.5 to 1 ml; children, intramuscularly, up to 1 month, 0.0075 ml per kg body-weight; 1 to 12 months, 0.01 ml per kg body-weight; 1 to 5 years, 0.125 to 0.25 ml; 6 to 12 years, 0.25 to 0.5 ml.

Sterilisation. Some samples of papaveretum gave a precipitate when heated in the presence of phenylmercuric nitrate.— *Pharm. J.*, 1956, *2*, 345 (Pharm. Soc. Lab. Rep.).

Papaveretum Tablets *(B.P.C. 1973).* Tablets containing papaveretum.

Solutio Omnoponi 1% aut 2% pro Injectionibus *(Rus. P.).* Morphine hydrochloride 670 mg or 1.34 g, noscapine 270 mg or 540 mg, papaverine hydrochloride 36 mg or 72 mg, codeine 72 mg or 144 mg, thebaine 5 mg or 10 mg, 1N hydrochloric acid 0.97 to 0.98 ml or 1.94 to 1.96 ml, Water for Injections to 100 ml; in ampoules of 1 ml. pH 2.5 to 3.5.

Proprietary Preparations

Omnopon *(Roche, UK).* Papaveretum, available as 1-ml **Ampoules** of an injection containing 20 mg per ml and as **Tablets** of 10 mg. (Also available as Omnopon in *Austral., S.Afr.*).

Omnopon-Scopolamine *(Roche, UK).* An injection containing papaveretum 20 mg and hyoscine hydrobromide 400 µg per ml, in ampoules of 1 ml.

Pantopon *(Roche, UK).* Tubunic ampoule syringes of 1 ml each containing soluble hydrochlorides of alkaloids of opium equivalent to anhydrous morphine 10 mg, anhydrous codeine 1.8 mg, noscapine 2.2 mg, and papaverine 2 mg. (Also available as Pantopon in *Belg., Ger., USA*).

Other Proprietary Names

Escopon *(Switz.).*

6251-l

Pentazocine *(B.P., U.S.P.).* NIH 7958; Win 20 228. ($2R^*$,$6R^*$,$11R^*$)-1,2,3,4,5,6-Hexahydro-6,11-dimethyl-3-(3-methylbut-2-enyl)-2,6-methano-3-benzazocin-8-ol.
$C_{19}H_{27}NO$=285.4.

CAS — 359-83-1.

Pharmacopoeias. In *Br.*, *Nord.*, and *U.S.*

A white or pale tan-coloured odourless or almost odourless powder. M.p. 147° to 158°. Pentazocine 100 mg is approximately equivalent to 112.8 of pentazocine hydrochloride or 131.6 mg of pentazocine lactate. Practically **insoluble** in water; soluble 1 in 11 to 15 of alcohol, 1 in 2 of chloroform, 1 in 33 of ether; soluble in acetone; sparingly soluble in ethyl acetate. **Store** in airtight containers. Protect from light.

6252-y

Pentazocine Hydrochloride *(B.P., U.S.P.).*
$C_{19}H_{27}NO,HCl$=321.9.

CAS — 2276-52-0; 64024-15-3.

Pharmacopoeias. In *Br.*, *Nord.*, and *U.S.*

A white to pale cream-coloured odourless crystalline powder. There are 2 forms, melting at about 218° and about 254° respectively. **Soluble** 1 in 30 of water, 1 in 16 of alcohol, 1 in 4 of chloroform; very slightly soluble in acetone; practically insoluble in ether. A 1% solution in water has a pH of 4 to 6. **Store** in airtight containers. Protect from light.

6253-j

Pentazocine Lactate. Pentazocini Lactas.
$C_{19}H_{27}NO,C_3H_6O_3$=375.5.

CAS — 17146-95-1.

Pharmacopoeias. In *Nord.*

A white to cream-coloured odourless or almost odourless powder. **Soluble** 1 in 25 of water, 1 in 12 of alcohol, 1 in 25 of chloroform, 1 in 1500 of ether. Solutions for injection are **sterilised** by autoclaving or by filtration. **Incompatible** in solution with diazepam and chlordiazepoxide and with alkaline substances such as aminophylline and soluble barbiturates. **Protect** from light.

Dependence. Prolonged use of high doses of pentazocine may produce dependence. It is subject to abuse.

Abuse. Pentazocine abuse was widespread among 'street addicts'. It was often used in combination with tripelennamine, commonly referred to as 'T's and Blues'; the crushed tablets were dissolved in water and usually injected intravenously.— C. V. Showalter and L. Moore (letter), *J. Am. med. Ass.*, 1978, *239*, 1610. See also *FDA Drug Bull.*, 1978, *8*, 34; W. J. Bailey (letter), *J. Am. med. Ass.*, 1979, *242*, 2392; C. V. Showalter, *ibid.*, 1980, *244*, 1224.

Dependence. Pentazocine was capable of producing mild physical and somewhat greater psychic dependence.— Seventeenth Report of the WHO Expert Committee on Drug Dependence, *Tech. Rep. Ser. Wld Hlth Org. No. 437*, 1970.

Four women received pentazocine 135 to 960 mg daily by intramuscular injection for about a year. When cessation of pentazocine was attempted they suffered severe withdrawal symptoms 12 hours after the last dose. Tremor, sweating, severe chills, and leg muscle cramps were followed by abdominal cramps, nausea, vomiting, itching, and rhinorrhoea. The most lasting symptoms were abdominal cramps, nausea, and feeling cold. Methadone was used successfully to counteract these withdrawal symptoms.— J. C. Schoolar *et al.* (letter), *Lancet*, 1969, *1*, 1263. Comments and criticism.— J. M. Mungavin (letter), *ibid.*, 1969, *2*, 56.

A 20-year-old woman had been taking pentazocine for 2 years and was unable to stop taking the drug because of severe withdrawal effects. At presentation she was taking 300 to 400 mg daily intravenously. Withdrawal symptoms lasted 2 weeks and included backache, nausea, vomiting, anorexia, sweating, agitation, and severe cramps, abdominal pain, and depression unresponsive to tricyclic antidepressants. She had been successfully rehabilitated. Five similar patients had been treated; all had withdrawal symptoms and all had relapsed. The possibility of stricter statutory control was suggested.— A. King and T. A. Betts, *Br. med. J.*, 1978, *2*, 21. Comment.— C. G. Nicol, *Winthrop* (letter), *ibid.*, 357.

Further references: R. G. Sandoval and R. I. H. Wang, *New Engl. J. Med.*, 1969, *280*, 1391; R. D. Alarcon *et al.*, *Johns Hopkins med. J.*, 1971, *129*, 311; J. A. Inciardi and C. D. Chambers, *N.Y. St. J. Med.*, 1971, *71*, 1727.

Pregnancy and the neonate. Withdrawal symptoms developed, 10 hours after delivery, in an infant whose mother had taken pentazocine 50 mg thrice daily during the last 6 weeks of pregnancy.— O. Preis *et al.*, *Am. J. Obstet. Gynec.*, 1977, *127*, 205.

Further references to neonatal withdrawal symptoms R. L. Goetz and R. V. Bain, *J. Pediat.*, 1974, *84*, 887; J. W. Scanlon, *J. Pediat.*, 1974, *85*, 735; T. O. Reeds, *J. Pediat.*, 1975, *87*, 324.

Adverse Effects. The most frequent side-effects of pentazocine are light- headedness, dizziness, nausea and vomiting, sedation, and sweating. It may also cause headache, dry mouth, constipation, flushing of the skin, respiratory depression, tachycardia, hypotension, raised intracranial pressure, transient hypertension, mood changes, nightmares, paraesthesia, pruritus, biliary tract spasm, and urinary retention. Changed uterine contractions, muscle tremor, insomnia, disorientation, hallucinations, disturbances of vision, transient eosinophilia, chills, and allergic reactions have also occurred. After large intravenous doses grand mal convulsions have been noted.

Pentazocine injections may be painful. Local tissue damage at injection sites has been reported, particularly after subcutaneous injection or multiple doses.

Effects on the blood. Agranulocytosis associated in one patient with pentazocine.— A. Marks and N. Abramson (letter), *Ann. intern. Med.*, 1980, *92*, 433.

Effects on mental state. A review of the psychotomimetic side-effects of pentazocine.— C. E. Coursey, *Drug Intell. & clin. Pharm.*, 1978, *12*, 341.

Sixteen of 202 patients taking pentazocine in normal doses by mouth or intramuscular injection developed perceptual changes including visual and auditory hallucinations.— A. J. J. Wood *et al.*, *Br. med. J.*, 1974, *1*, 305.

Of 65 patients given pentazocine 40 to 50 mg intramuscularly (repeated as required), for postoperative pain, 24 had hallucinations in the 24 hours following surgery, compared with 7 of 49 patients given morphine in 10-mg doses.— J. I. Alexander and A. A. Spence (letter), *Br. med. J.*, 1974, *2*, 224. See also *Br. med. J.*, 1974, *1*, 297.

Ten of 105 medical or surgical patients taking pentazocine in usual doses had hallucinations and a further 10 had vivid dreams.— M. Taylor *et al.*, *Br. med. J.*, 1978, *2*, 1198.

Effects on muscle and skin. Of 51 patients given pentazocine, 25 to 100 mg by mouth 4 times daily for 3 days, treatment was discontinued in 1 after 24 hours because of cramp in the legs.— S. Lipton, *Br. J. Anaesth.*, 1972, *44*, 869.

Toxic epidermal necrolysis in a 62-year-old man was attributed to pentazocine; he had taken 50 to 75 mg every 4 hours for 8 days. He was severely dehydrated and had a blood-urea concentration of 4.3 mg per ml, but recovered after fluid replacement and other intensive treatment.— J. A. A. Hunter and A. M. Davison, *Br. J. Derm.*, 1973, *88*, 287.

Six patients who had been given pentazocine intramuscularly for less than 3 months suffered severe induration of soft tissues at pentazocine injection sites. In 1 patient induration was severe and produced ankylosis of the knee joints and limited the range of motion in the hips and shoulders. Four patients had not exceeded the recommended doses.— T. F. Beckner (letter), *J. Am. med. Ass.*, 1974, *227*, 1383.

Fibrous myopathy occurred in 3 patients who had been self-administering pentazocine intramuscularly in daily dosages up to 360 mg for years. Fibrotic induration of quadriceps and deltoid muscles, muscle weakness, and limitation of motion due to fibrotic muscle contracture were the main symptoms.— S. J. Oh *et al.*, *J. Am. med. Ass.*, 1975, *231*, 271. Similar reports of fibrous myopathy following repeated injections of pentazocine.— J. C. Steiner *et al.*, *Archs Neurol., Chicago*, 1973, *28*, 408; D. Fleiss (letter), *J. Am. med. Ass.*, 1975, *232*, 1126; B. E. Levin and W. K. Engel, *J. Am. med. Ass.*, 1975, *234*, 621.

Woody sclerosis of the skin at subcutaneous injection sites in one patient was attributed to repeated injections of pentazocine lactate over a prolonged period.— B. L. Schiff and A. B. Kern, *J. Am. med. Ass.*, 1977, *238*, 1542. Similar reports: J. B. Winfield and K. Greer (letter), *ibid.*, 1973, *226*, 189; B. Cosman *et al.*, *Plastic reconstr. Surg.*, 1977, *59*, 255.

Pulmonary oedema. Pulmonary oedema occurred immediately after the intravenous injection of pentazocine 30 mg in 1 patient with a recent myocardial infarction.— M. Murtadha (letter), *Lancet*, 1977, *1*, 373.

Treatment of Adverse Effects. Treatment is similar to that for morphine (see p.1019), *but* nalorphine and levallorphan are not antagonists and may add to the depressant effects of pentazocine. Naloxone hydrochloride 400 µg by subcutaneous, intramuscular, or intravenous injection is a specific antidote; this dose may be repeated at intervals of 2 to 3 minutes.

For a reference to the successful use of naloxone in pentazocine intoxication, see Naloxone Hydrochloride, p.1033.

Precautions. As for Morphine, p.1019.

Pentazocine has weak narcotic antagonist actions and may precipitate withdrawal symptoms if given to patients who have recently used other narcotic analgesics.

Pentazocine should be given with caution to patients prone to seizures.

When frequent injections are needed, pentazocine should be given intramuscularly and the injection sites should be varied.

It has been suggested that because of its cardiovascular effects, pentazocine might not be suitable for patients suffering myocardial infarctions.

Enhanced bioavailability and decreased clearance of pentazocine in patients with cirrhosis.— E. A. Neal *et al.*, *Gastroenterology*, 1979, *77*, 96.

Antagonist effects. Not only was pentazocine an antagonist to morphine but to some extent it was also an antagonist to itself. If an initial dose was followed too closely by a second dose some loss of pain relief could occur. Pentazocine should be used only when it was clear that no other analgesic would be needed in the immediate future or had been administered in the immediate past.— A. R. Hunter, *Practitioner*, 1973, *211*, 476.

Effects on diagnostic tests. Serum creatine kinase values rose significantly in 3 of 15 patients given pentazocine 30 mg intramuscularly; this could cause confusion when these values were used for the assessment of cardiac infarction.— B. B. Scott *et al.*, *Br. med. J.*, 1974, *4*, 691.

Interactions. *Doxapram.* In healthy subjects doxapram 60 mg intramuscularly given with pentazocine 30 mg reduced the amount of respiratory depression produced by the narcotic; the effect was considered to be simply additive.— J. C. Gasser (letter), *Br. J. Anaesth.*, 1977, *49*, 952. See also J. C. Gasser and J. W. Bellville, *Anaesthesist*, 1975, *24*, 526.

Hydroxyzine. Enhanced respiratory depression with hydroxyzine and pentazocine.— J. C. Gasser and J. W. Bellville, *Anesthesiology*, 1975, *43*, 599.

Monoamine oxidase inhibitors. For a report of *animal* studies suggesting that the effect of pentazocine was enhanced by monoamine oxidase inhibitors, see K. J. Rogers and J. A. Thornton, *Br. J. Anaesth.*, 1968, *40*, 146.

Promethazine. An investigation in 36 women following elective caesarean section indicated that the average initial dose requirement of pentazocine was not affected by concurrent administration of promethazine but the average maintenance dose was reduced by one-third.— M. Keeri-Szanto and B. Remington, *Clin. Pharmac. Ther.*, 1972, *13*, 143.

Tobacco smoking. Higher maintenance doses of pentazocine were required by patients who were smokers and/or city-dwellers than by those who were non-smokers and/or lived in the countryside.— M. Keeri-Szanto and J. R. Pomeroy, *Lancet*, 1971, *1*, 947. A study in 70 urban subjects indicated that smokers metabolised about 40% more pentazocine than non-smokers, although there was large inter-subject variation. It was suggested that tobacco smoking induces liver enzymes responsible for drug oxidation.— D. P. Vaughan *et al.*, *Br. J. clin. Pharmac.*, 1976, *3*, 279.

Porphyria. From studies in *rats* of the porphyrinogenic effect of various drugs used in anaesthesia it is suggested that pentazocine should not be given to patients with porphyria.— R. K. Parikh and M. R. Moore, *Br. J. Anaesth.*, 1978, *50*, 1099.

Absorption and Fate. Pentazocine is absorbed from the gastro-intestinal tract; following administration by mouth, peak plasma concentrations are reached in 1 to 3 hours. After intramuscular injection, peak plasma concentrations are reached in 15 minutes to 1 hour. Pentazocine is metabolised in the liver and only a small proportion of the dose administered appears unchanged in the urine. It diffuses across the placenta.

In 4 healthy subjects, the amount of unchanged pentazocine excreted in acid urine 32 hours after intravenous and oral administration was 8 to 24% and 3 to 15% respectively of the dose administered. After 48 hours, 0.1 to 2% of the unchanged drug was recovered in the faeces regardless of the route of administration.— A. H. Beckett *et al.*, *J. Pharm. Pharmac.*, 1970, *22*, 123. In 5 of 7 subjects given pentazocine by mouth the proportion excreted as free pentazocine in the urine within 24 hours was between 2 and 4.5%; in the other 2 subjects the proportions were 10.6 and 12.4% respectively and in these 7 subjects the amount of pentazocine excreted as glucuronide was consistently greater than the amount of free pentazocine. In 2 subjects given 30 mg per 70 kg body-weight intramuscularly the 24-hour urinary excretion of free pentazocine was 1.3 and 9.6% respectively.— B. Berkowitz, *Ann. N.Y. Acad. Sci.*, 1971, *179*, 269.

The range of pentazocine binding to plasma protein in the blood from 20 healthy subjects was 56 to 66% whereas in 22 patients the range extended to 48 to 75%. *In vitro* studies on the blood of healthy subjects indicated that 48% of the total amount of pentazocine in whole blood was in the red blood-cells, 33% was bound to the plasma proteins, and 19% was in the plasma water. In subjects with abnormally high or low red blood-cell counts, response to pentazocine might therefore be altered.— M. Ehrnebo *et al.*, *Clin. Pharmac. Ther.*, 1974, *16*, 424.

Measurements of the mean plasma concentration of pentazocine in 5 healthy subjects, made for up to 6 hours after administration indicated that the bioavailability of the dose given by mouth was 18.4% (range 11.1 to 31.6%) of the administered dose. Plasma half-lives of the intravenously and orally administered doses were 203 and 177 minutes respectively.— M. Ehrnebo *et al.*, *Clin. Pharmac. Ther.*, 1977, *22*, 888.

Further references: B. A. Berkowitz *et al.*, *Clin. Pharmac. Ther.*, 1969, *10*, 320; L. Paalzow and A. Arbin, *J. Pharm. Pharmac.*, 1972, *24*, 552; S. Agurell *et al.*, *ibid.*, 1974, *26*, 1.

Pregnancy and the neonate. Pentazocine had not been detected in the milk of lactating mothers.— B. E. Takyi, *J. Hosp. Pharm.*, 1970, *28*, 317.

Uses. Pentazocine is an analgesic with actions and uses similar to those of morphine (see p.1020). In addition, it has weak narcotic antagonist actions. For the relief of moderate to severe pain, 30 mg of pentazocine intramuscularly is reported to be equivalent to about 10 mg of morphine subcutaneously or intramuscularly. The analgesic effect declines more rapidly than that of morphine.

Pentazocine is administered by mouth as capsules or tablets of the hydrochloride. The usual dose is the equivalent of 25 to 100 mg of pentazocine every 3 to 4 hours; it should not be necessary to exceed 600 mg daily. Children aged 6 to 12 may be given 25 mg every 3 to 4 hours.

Pentazocine is administered by subcutaneous, intramuscular, and intravenous injection as the lactate for the relief of moderate to severe pain. The usual dose is the equivalent of pentazocine 30 to 60 mg intramuscularly or subcutaneously every 3 to 4 hours; it should not be necessary to exceed 360 mg daily. Intravenous doses of 30 mg are also used. For children, the maximum single dose subcutaneously or intramuscularly should not exceed 1 mg per kg body-weight, or 500 µg per kg intravenously.

Pentazocine is also given rectally as the lactate in suppositories usually in a dose of the equivalent of pentazocine 50 mg up to 4 times daily.

Reviews of pentazocine: R. N. Brogden *et al.*, *Drugs*, 1973, *5*, 6; W. H. Forrest, *Ann. intern. Med.*, 1974, *81*, 644; *Med. Lett.*, 1976, *18*, 46.

The laevo isomer of pentazocine was a potent respiratory depressant, 13 mg having about the same effect as morphine 10 mg, whereas the dextro isomer, in doses of 30 and 60 mg, had no more effect on respiration than a placebo, according to a crossover study with 6 volunteers. Laevo-pentazocine appeared to give rise more frequently to lightheaded, dreamy, relaxed, and euphoric states, and dextro-pentazocine to mild depression and anxiety.— J. W. Bellville and W. H. Forrest, *Clin. Pharmac. Ther.*, 1968, *9*, 142.

Pentazocine, administered in 5 sequential intravenous injections of 600 µg per kg body-weight, raised the systolic blood pressure by about 30%, the diastolic pressure by about 10%, and the heart-rate by about 13% in 5 conscious patients. In 5 anaesthetised patients, a fall in blood pressure of about 25% occurred, with some fluctuations, and the heart-rate was reduced by about 20 to 25%.— T. Tammisto *et al.*, *Br. J. Anaesth.*, 1970, *42*, 317.

A report of the clinical effects of pentazocine given by mouth in 616 hospitalised medical patients and parenterally in 816.— R. R. Miller, *J. clin. Pharmac.*, 1975, *15*, 198. Criticism.— G. W. McCarl, *Winthrop* (letter), *ibid.*, 718. Reply.— R. R. Miller (letter), *ibid.*, 719.

Administration in renal failure. Pentazocine could be given in usual doses to patients with renal failure.— W. M. Bennett *et al.*, *Ann. intern. Med.*, 1980, *93*, 62.

Administration in haemophilia. For the use of pentazocine in haemophiliacs, see Choline Salicylate, p.249.

Anaesthesia. Dental anaesthesia was achieved by giving pentazocine 30 mg intravenously with diazepam at the rate of 2.5 mg intravenously per 30 seconds till sedation was evident. Complicated dental surgery was possible if local anaesthesia was added.— P. Sykes (letter), *Br. med. J.*, 1977, *2*, 832.

Good operating conditions were achieved in 45 of 100 patients undergoing cystoscopy and related procedures by premedication with diazepam 10 mg by mouth 2 hours before surgery and induction of anaesthesia with pentazocine 1 mg per kg body-weight and diazepam 20 to 40 mg intravenously; 34 patients required supplements of nitrous oxide, and 21 required nitrous oxide and alphadolone with alphaxalone.— T. G. C. Smith *et al.*, *Br. J. Anaesth.*, 1977, *49*, 509.

Premedication. In a double-blind study in patients about to undergo minor gynaecological operations, 50 were given 10 mg of morphine intramuscularly and 50 others 20 mg of pentazocine about 1 hour pre-operatively. Results in the 2 groups showed that sedation or relief from anxiety was very similar.— W. Norris and A. B. M. Telfer, *Br. J. Anaesth.*, 1968, *40*, 341.

Pentazocine 50 mg, taken by 50 healthy gynaecological patients, had a slight sedative effect but was no more effective than a placebo in reducing anxiety in a further 50 patients.— W. Norris and A. B. M. Telfer, *Br. J. Anaesth.*, 1970, *42*, 151.

Cardiovascular disorders. *Myocardial infarction.* Pentazocine 60 mg intravenously appeared to be a suitable analgesic for patients with a recent myocardial infarction. Studies in 10 patients showed that, unlike morphine, its use was not generally followed by hypotension, an increase in the respiratory dead-space/tidal volume ratio, or an increase in the difference between alveolar and arterial oxygen tensions. Because such changes were associated with a bad prognosis in myocardial infarction, it was suggested that pentazocine should be used in preference to morphine as an analgesic in patients with myocardial infarction. Morphine and pentazocine caused respiratory depression, but pentazocine could be expected not to have serious adverse effects on arterial oxygen tension.— S. Lal *et al.*, *Lancet*, 1969, *1*, 379 and 381.

Diamorphine 5 mg, methadone 10 mg, morphine 10 mg, and pentazocine 30 mg, given intravenously, gave complete relief of pain due to suspected myocardial infarction in 47, 32, 17, and 19% of 118 patients respectively after 10 minutes and in 34, 50, 52, and 33% after 120 minutes. Each drug allayed anxiety, caused drowsiness in most patients, nausea and vomiting in some, and reduced the mean respiratory-rate. In contrast to the other drugs, pentazocine produced a rise in systolic blood pressure when this was below 120 mmHg; when the blood pressure exceeded 120 mmHg, the incidence of a fall in blood pressure was less with pentazocine than for the other treatments. The results suggested that diamorphine might be considered to be the analgesic of choice in a situation where rapid relief of pain was essential, but pentazocine with its low addiction potential and lower incidence of blood pressure reduction might be the most suitable treatment for pain in patients with a suspected cardiac infarction.— M. E. Scott and R. Orr, *Lancet*, 1969, *1*, 1065.

Discussion on the haemodynamic changes associated with pentazocine in patients with myocardial infarction. The effect on the ischaemic myocardium is not clear. Diamorphine is preferred.— *Lancet*, 1976, *2*, 888. *Animal* studies had demonstrated that pentazocine had a positive inotropic action on the heart and should therefore be used with caution in cardiac infarction.— T. N. Appleyard and J. A. Thornton (letter), *ibid.*, 1025. See also G. Lee *et al.*, *Am. J. Med.*, 1976, *60*, 949.

Effect on biliary tract. The rise in biliary pressure in 31 patients was less with pentazocine than with pethidine or phenazocine and much less than with morphine.— G. Economou and J. N. Ward-McQuaid, *Gut*, 1971, *12*, 218.

Effect on colon. In 5 healthy men, 5 patients with the irritable bowel syndrome, and 5 with diverticular disease, colonic motor activity was significantly reduced after they were given pentazocine 300 µg per kg body-weight intravenously or 500 µg per kg intramuscularly. Pentazocine was useful for the treatment of such disorders.— C. Stanciu and J. R. Bennett, *Br. med. J.*, 1974, *1*, 312.

Hiccup. Pentazocine 30 mg intravenously was effective in the relief of hiccup.— E. N. S. Fry (letter), *Br. med. J.*, 1977, *2*, 704.

Narcolepsy. For a report of pentazocine controlling the symptoms of narcolepsy, see Codeine Phosphate, p.1005.

Neuroleptanalgesia. Pentazocine and phenoperidine were equally satisfactory as analgesics for neuroleptanalgesia in 55 patients. Phenoperidine caused more marked cardiovascular changes and increases in arterial carbon-dioxide tension. Pentazocine was a suitable alternative to phenoperidine in conjunction with droperidol in neuroleptanalgesia.— B. Kay *et al.*, *Br. J. Anaesth.*, 1970, *42*, 329.

Preparations of Pentazocine Salts

Pentazocine Hydrochloride and Aspirin Tablets *(U.S.P.)*. Tablets containing pentazocine hydrochloride and aspirin. Potency is expressed in terms of the equivalent amount of pentazocine. The *U.S.P.* requires 80% dissolution of pentazocine and 70% dissolution of aspirin in 30 minutes. Store in airtight containers. Protect from light.

Pentazocine Hydrochloride Tablets *(U.S.P.)*. Tablets containing pentazocine hydrochloride. Potency is expressed in terms of the equivalent amount of pentazocine. Store in airtight containers. Protect from light.

Pentazocine Lactate Injection *(B.P.)*. Pentazocine Injection. A sterile solution in Water for Injections prepared from pentazocine and lactic acid. Sterilised by autoclaving. Potency is expressed in terms of the equivalent amount of pentazocine. pH 4 to 5. Protect from light.

Pentazocine Lactate Injection *(U.S.P.)*. A sterile solution of pentazocine lactate in Water for Injections prepared from pentazocine and lactic acid. Potency is expressed in terms of the equivalent amount of pentazocine. pH 4 to 5.

Pentazocine Tablets *(B.P.)*. Tablets containing pentazocine hydrochloride. They may be film-coated.

Proprietary Preparations of Pentazocine Salts

Fortagesic *(Winthrop, UK)*. Tablets each containing pentazocine hydrochloride equivalent to pentazocine 15 mg and paracetamol 500 mg. For muscular and articular pain. *Dose.* Adults, 2 tablets 3 or 4 times daily; not recommended for children under 7 years.

Fortral *(Winthrop, UK)*. Pentazocine hydrochloride, available as **Capsules** of 50 mg and **Tablets** of 25 mg. **Fortral Injection.** Contains pentazocine lactate equivalent to 30 mg pentazocine per ml, in ampoules of 1 and 2 ml. **Fortral Suppositories.** Each contains pentazocine lactate equivalent to pentazocine 50 mg. (Also available as Fortral in *Aust.*, *Austral.*, *Belg.*, *Denm.*, *Fr.*, *Ger.*, *Iceland*, *Neth.*).

Other Proprietary Names of Pentazocine Hydrochloride and Pentazocine Lactate

Algopent *(Ital.)*; Fortalgesic *(Swed., Switz.)*; Fortralin *(Fin., Norw.)*; Fortwin *(Ind.)*; Liticon, Pentafen, Pentalgina (all *Ital.*); Sosegon *(Arg., S.Afr., Spain)*; Talwin *(Canad., Ital., USA)*.

6254-z

Pethidine Hydrochloride *(B.P., B.P. Vet.)*.

Pethidinae Hydrochloridum; Pethidini Hydrochloridum; Meperidine Hydrochloride *(U.S.P.)*. Ethyl 1-methyl-4-phenylpiperidine-4-carboxylate hydrochloride.

$C_{15}H_{21}NO_2,HCl=283.8$.

CAS — 57-42-1 (pethidine); 50-13-5 (hydrochloride).

Pharmacopoeias. In *Arg., Aust., Belg., Br., Braz., Chin., Cz., Eur., Fr., Ger., Hung., Ind., Int., It., Jap., Jug., Mex., Neth., Nord., Port., Roum., Swiss, Turk.*, and *U.S.*

A white odourless crystalline powder, with a slightly acid bitter taste. M.p. 186° to 190°.

Very **soluble** in water; soluble 1 in 20 of alcohol; soluble in chloroform; practically insoluble in ether. A 2% solution in water has a pH of 4.5 to 5.5. A 4.8% solution is iso-osmotic with serum. Solutions are **sterilised** by autoclaving or by filtration. **Incompatible** with alkalis, iodine, iodides, and thiopentone sodium. **Protect** from light.

An aqueous solution of pethidine hydrochloride iso-osmotic with serum (4.8%) caused 98% haemolysis of erythrocytes cultured in it for 45 minutes.— E. R. Hammarlund and K. Pedersen-Bjergaard, *J. pharm. Sci.*, 1961, *50*, 24.

Incompatibility. There was loss of clarity when intravenous solutions of pethidine hydrochloride were mixed with those of aminophylline, amylobarbitone sodium, heparin sodium, methicillin sodium, morphine sulphate, nitrofurantoin sodium, pentobarbitone sodium, phenobarbitone sodium, phenytoin sodium, sodium bicarbonate, sodium iodide, sulphadiazine sodium, sulphafurazole diethanolamine, or thiopentone sodium.— J. A. Patel and G. L. Phillips, *Am. J. Hosp. Pharm.*, 1966, *23*, 409.

Stability. Pethidine hydrochloride was stable for at least 24 hours at room temperature in dextrose 5% and 4% and in sodium chloride injection and sodium chloride injection diluted 1 in 5.— L. Rudd and P. Simpson (letter), *Med. J. Aust.*, 1978, *2*, 34.

Dependence. Prolonged use of pethidine may lead to dependence of the morphine type (see p.1018). Doses as large as 3 or 4 g daily may be taken by addicts. As tolerance to the central nervous system stimulant and anticholinergic effects is not complete with these very large doses, muscle twitching, tremor, mental confusion, hallucinations, and sometimes convulsions may be present. Withdrawal symptoms appear more rapidly than with morphine and are of shorter duration.

Adverse Effects. As for Morphine, p.1019.

Constipation and urinary retention occur less frequently than with morphine. Intravenous injection may produce vasodilatation and hypotension. After overdosage, symptoms are generally similar to those of morphine poisoning, however stimulation of the central nervous system and convulsions may also occur, especially in tolerant individuals or following toxic doses by mouth. Local reactions often follow injection of pethidine; general hypersensitivity reactions occur rarely.

Three cases of toxic epidermal necrolysis have been reported to be associated with the use of pethidine.— E. D. Lowney *et al.*, *Archs Derm.*, 1967, *95*, 359.

Of 26 294 consecutive patients monitored in the Boston Collaborative Drug Surveillance Program, 366 received pethidine by mouth and adverse reactions were reported in 16, mainly involving the gastro-intestinal tract. A further 3268 patients received pethidine by injection, and adverse effects were reported in 102, involving the central nervous system in 38.— R. R. Miller and H. Jick, *J. clin. Pharmac.*, 1978, *18*, 180.

Effects on vision. Visual disturbances occurred after intravenous injection of pethidine hydrochloride 50 mg in 4 normal subjects and were sometimes noted after the intramuscular injection of 100 mg.— L. E. Mather *et al.*, *Br. J. Anaesth.*, 1975, *47*, 1269.

Effects on respiratory function. In 3 healthy subjects pethidine 50 mg daily, by mouth, for 2 days had a bronchoconstrictor effect.— R. B. Douglas *et al.* (letter), *Br. med. J.*, 1976, *2*, 880.

Respiratory arrest occurred postoperatively in a woman after a usual dose of pethidine.— R. K. Stoelting, *Anesth. Analg. curr. Res.*, 1977, *56*, 727.

Treatment of Adverse Effects. As for Morphine, p.1019.

Diazepam or thiopentone sodium may be required to control convulsions.

In 26 newborn infants whose mothers had received pethidine within 4 hours prior to delivery, naloxone 35 or 70 µg was injected into the umbilical vein to treat respiratory depression. Since only a slight and delayed pethidine antagonist action was observed following doses of 35 µg, it was suggested that a 70-µg dose might be more suitable. No excitatory effects were noted. Another 16 newborn infants similarly received nalorphine 500 or 700 µg. Restoration of respiration function was obtained, but there was a pronounced and undesirable excitatory action.— J. E. H. Brice *et al.*, *Archs Dis. Child.*, 1979, *54*, 356.

Precautions. As for Morphine, p.1019.

It should be given cautiously to patients with supraventricular tachycardia.

Very severe reactions, including cerebral excitement, confusion, convulsions, hyperpyrexia, hypertension, severe respiratory depression, cyanosis, coma and occasionally death have followed administration of pethidine to patients receiving monoamine oxidase inhibitors. Concurrent administration of pethidine and phenothiazines has produced severe hypotensive episodes and prolonged the respiratory depression due to pethidine.

The metabolism of pethidine was reduced in neonates, during pregnancy, and in women taking some oral contraceptives.— J. S. Crawford and S. Rudofsky, *Br. J. Anaesth.*, 1966, *38*, 446. A study in women who had not taken an oral contraceptive for at least 1 year, women currently taking a 'combined' oral contraceptive, and in men showed no differences in serum concentrations, metabolism, or excretion patterns of pethidine between the 3 groups.— J. E. Stambaugh and I. W. Wainer, *J. clin. Pharmac.*, 1975, *15*, 46.

A weight-related dose of pethidine given with an anaesthetic produced significantly higher plasma concentrations in elderly subjects than in younger subjects.— K. Chan *et al.*, *Br. J. clin. Pharmac.*, 1975, *2*, 297.

The prolongation of the half-life of pethidine in patients with viral hepatitis.— T. S. McHorse *et al.*, *Gastroenterology*, 1975, *68*, 775.

For the effect of pethidine when given to patients undergoing anaesthesia with trichloroethylene, see Trichloroethylene, p.761.

Effects on driving. Studies in healthy subjects indicated that patients should not drive or operate machinery for 24 hours after receiving pethidine 75 mg intramuscularly.— K. Korttila and M. Linnoila, *Anesthesiology*, 1975, *42*, 685.

Interactions. *Bupivacaine.* Pethidine increased the amount of unbound bupivacaine in plasma *in vitro*.— M. M. Ghoneim and H. Pandya, *Br. J. Anaesth.*, 1974, *46*, 435.

Debrisoquine. Administration of pethidine to *rabbits* pretreated with debrisoquine provoked a toxic reaction characterised by motor restlessness, shivering-like tremor, hyperexcitability, tachypnoea, dilated pupils, and hyperpyrexia; the symptoms persisted for nearly 3 hours. The mode of action was unclear but debrisoquine has monoamine oxidase inhibiting properties, enhances serotonin, and inhibits hepatic *N*-demethylation of pethidine.— O. H. Osman and I. B. Eltayeb, *J. Pharm. Pharmac.*, 1977, *29*, 143.

Diazepam. In healthy adults the respiratory depression produced by pethidine 1.5 mg per kg body-weight intravenously was not increased by the simultaneous administration of diazepam 150 µg per kg intravenously.— E. K. Zsigmond *et. al.*, *J. clin. Pharmac.*, 1974, *14*, 377.

Monoamine oxidase inhibitors. Two patients, treated with iproniazid for angina of effort, were precipitated into coma by intramuscular injections of pethidine. Prednisolone caused prompt reversal of the conditions.— J. C. Shee, *Br. med. J.*, 1960, *2*, 507.

A man of 63, who had taken phenelzine sulphate for several months, was given an intramuscular injection of 100 mg of pethidine as an analgesic after an operation. His respiration became stertorous and suddenly ceased and his pulse became hardly palpable. From a state of cyanosis, rigidity, and coma, he was partially restored in a few minutes by artificial respiration but he remained unconscious for an hour.— D. C. Taylor (letter), *Lancet*, 1962, *2*, 401. See also D. P. Cocks and A. Passmore-Rowe (letter), *Br. med. J.*, 1962, *2*, 1545.

A man with hypertension, who was taking pargyline 100 mg and hydrochlorothiazide 50 mg daily, was premedicated with pethidine 100 mg and hyoscine hydrobromide. Within minutes he became rigid and comatose with generalised tonic spasm but slowly recovered when treated with oxygen and an intravenous dextrose solution.— I. M. Vigran, *J. Am. med. Ass.*, 1964, *187*, 953.

A 73-year-old man, who was taking mebanazine, was given pethidine as part of his premedication for a routine bladder examination. He died from shock and pulmonary haemorrhage.— *Pharm. J.*, 1965, *2*, 341.

Inhibition of *N*-demethylation of pethidine might be involved in the interaction between pethidine and monamine oxidase inhibitors.— N. R. Eade and K. W. Renton, *J. Pharmac. exp. Ther.*, 1970, *173*, 31. See also B. Clark *et al.*, *Br. J. Pharmac.*, 1972, *44*, 89. For the effect of monoamine oxidase inhibitors on *N*-demethylation and hydrolysis of pethidine, see N. R. Eade and K. W. Renton, *Biochem. Pharmac.*, 1970, *19*, 2243.

Phenobarbitone. Prolonged sedation occurred in a patient receiving phenobarbitone and given pethidine. Investigation in another 4 patients and 1 healthy subject indicated that phenobarbitone induced *N*-demethylation of pethidine with increased production of norpethidine which accounted for the CNS toxicity.— J. E. Stambaugh *et al.*, *Lancet*, 1977, *1*, 398.

Phenytoin. Reduced half-life of pethidine on concomitant administration of phenytoin.— S. M. Pond and K. M. Kretschzmar, *Clin. Pharmac. Ther.*, 1981, *30*, 680.

Prochlorperazine. A study in 6 healthy subjects demonstrated that concurrent administration of prochlorperazine with pethidine prolonged the respiratory depression due to pethidine.— S. M. Steen and M. Yates, *Clin. Pharmac. Ther.*, 1972, *13*, 153.

Promazine. A primigravida aged 22 was given intravenous premedication consisting of pethidine 100 mg with promazine 50 mg in 20 ml of saline. Five minutes after the injection the membranes were ruptured and 15 minutes after the injection the foetal heart-rate was 72; the patient appeared pale and shocked with a thready pulse of 120 and systolic blood pressure of 70 mmHg. About an hour after the original injection a baby was delivered by caesarean section. The child was flaccid and asphyxiated at birth and died 40 hours after delivery. Previous experience with pethidine-promazine mixtures intramuscularly and intravenously had been entirely without mishap.— A. G. Amias and D. Fairbairn, *Br. med. J.*, 1963, *2*, 432. Reasons for doubting that the death was caused by the use of pethidine and promazine.— D. O'Sullivan (letter), *ibid.*, 748. Two years previously, a temporary severe drop in blood pressure with slowing of the foetal heart occurred in 6 patients given the same mixture. No subsequent cases had occurred.— D. J. P. O'Meara (letter), *ibid.*, 749.

An obstetric patient aged 17 years was admitted at term and received pethidine 100 mg with promazine 50 mg, intramuscularly, prior to vaginal examination. She collapsed shortly afterwards and became cyanosed. Her limbs were spastic and her pulse was imperceptible. She recovered with symptomatic treatment.— I. A. Donaldson (letter), *Br. med. J.*, 1963, *2*, 1592.

Phaeochromocytoma. Pethidine provoked episodes of hypertension on 5 occasions when given postoperatively to a patient with non-resectable phaeochromocytoma. The effect was suppressed when labetalol was being given.— C. A. Lawrence, *Br. med. J.*, 1978, *1*, 149.

Porphyria. Pethidine probably did not precipitate acute porphyria.— *Drug & Ther. Bull.*, 1976, *14*, 55.

Pregnancy and the neonate. Signs of foetal depression were not apparent when delivery occurred within 1 hour of pethidine administration. Depression was present in 6 of 24 infants delivered 1 to 3 hours after injection, and in all of 5 infants delivered 3 to 6 hours after injection.— J. C. Morrison *et al.*, *Am. J. Obstet. Gynec.*, 1973, *115*, 1132. See also F. Moya and V. Thorndike, *Clin. Pharmac. Ther.*, 1963, *4*, 628; R. M. Rothberg *et al.*, *Biol. Neonate*, 1978, *33*, 80.

The pO_2 fell immediately after the administration of pethidine 50 mg in 4 of 9 women in late pregnancy or labour, and in 13 of 19 similar women after the administration of 100 mg with levallorphan 1.25 mg. Abnormal heart-rate patterns were recorded in 8 foetuses.— A. Huch *et al.*, *J. Obstet. Gynaec. Br. Commonw.*, 1974, *81*, 608.

Maternally administered pethidine reduced neonatal serum-bilirubin concentrations, although the magnitude of the effect was small.— J. H. Drew and W. H. Kitchen, *J. Pediat.*, 1976, *89*, 657.

The effects of analgesia during labour were assessed in

920 neonates on the first and second days of life. In infants whose mothers had received pethidine, responses were depressed on both days; the depression was greatest with the highest dose of pethidine (75 to 150 mg within 4 hours of delivery). Depression produced by pethidine and anaesthetic agents was additive. Babies delivered under chloroprocaine epidural anaesthesia suffered least depression.— R. Hodgkinson *et al.*, *Can. Anaesth. Soc. J.*, 1978, *25*, 405.

A study was conducted in 145 women who received either pethidine or epidural bupivacaine or no analgesic during labour. Apgar scores of 7 or less at 1 minute occurred in 10 infants in the pethidine group, in 2 infants in the bupivacaine group and no infants in the control group. There was no significant difference in Apgar scores at 5 minutes. The elimination half-lives of pethidine and bupivacaine in infants were 22.4 hours and 14 hours respectively. There were no significant behavioural differences in infants during the first 6 weeks of life.— B. A. Lieberman *et al.*, *Br. J. Obstet. Gynaec.*, 1979, *86*, 598.

Comment on behavioural studies on the effect on the infant of pethidine analgesia in labour.— *Lancet*, 1981, *2*, 291.

See also under Interactions, Promazine, above.

Absorption and Fate. Pethidine hydrochloride is readily absorbed from the gastro-intestinal tract, and is partly bound to plasma proteins. It is metabolised in the liver by hydrolysis to pethidinic acid or demethylation to norpethidine and hydrolysis to norpethidinic acid, followed by conjugation with glucuronic acid. At the usual values of urinary pH or if the urine is alkaline, excretion of unchanged pethidine is negligible; urinary excretion of pethidine and norpethidine is enhanced by acidification of the urine. Pethidine crosses the placenta and appears in milk.

A review of the clinical pharmacokinetics of pethidine.— L. E. Mather and P. J. Meffin, *Clin. Pharmacokinet.*, 1978, *3*, 352.

Investigations in 8 healthy subjects and 10 patients with cirrhosis of the liver who were given single rapid intravenous injections of pethidine 800 µg per kg body-weight indicated that the elimination of pethidine was prolonged in cirrhosis, probably due to impairment of the drug-metabolising activity in the liver. The terminal pethidine-plasma half-life was an average of about 3 hours in the healthy subjects and 7 hours in the patients.— U. Klotz *et al.*, *Clin. Pharmac. Ther.*, 1974, *16*, 667. See also E. A. Neal *et al.*, *Gastroenterology*, 1979, *77*, 96; S. M. Pond *et al.*, *Clin. Pharmac. Ther.*, 1981, *30*, 183.

Following administration of pethidine hydrochloride 100 mg by mouth to 4 healthy subjects systemic availability, calculated from drug clearance following intravenous injection of 50 mg in the same subjects, was 47 to 71%. Double absorption peaks were possibly associated with the action of pethidine on the gut, or a recycling process.— L. E. Mather and G. T. Tucker, *Clin. Pharmac. Ther.*, 1976, *20*, 535. A study in 6 healthy subjects indicated that fluctuations in the plasma concentrations of pethidine were unlikely to be explained by enterogastric or enterohepatic recycling.— R. Dunkerley *et al.*, *Clin. Pharmac. Ther.*, 1976, *20*, 546.

In 5 healthy subjects given pethidine 36 mg per m^2 body-surface intramuscularly 9 to 27.8% and 4.4 to 13% of the administered dose was excreted in the urine within 24 hours as pethidinic acid and norpethidinic acid respectively.— I. W. Wainer and J. E. Stambaugh, *J. pharm. Sci.*, 1978, *67*, 116.

See also K. Chan, *J. Pharm. Pharmac.*, 1979, *31*, 672 (influence of urinary pH).

Pethidine clearance during continuous intravenous infusions in postoperative patients.— K. L. Austin *et al.*, *Br. J. clin. Pharmac.*, 1981, *1*, 25.

Further references to the pharmacokinetics of pethidine.— L. E. Mather *et al.*, *Clin. Pharmac. Ther.*, 1975, *17*, 21; J. E. Stambaugh *et al.*, *J. clin. Pharmac.*, 1976, *16*, 245.

Pregnancy and the neonate. Studies in 15 women in labour suggested that blood concentrations of pethidine in the newborn were greater than in the mother, but the reverse for pentazocine. Pethidine was perhaps transferred across the placenta more rapidly than pentazocine.— A. H. Beckett and J. F. Taylor, *J. Pharm. Pharmac.*, 1967, *19*, *Suppl.*, 50S. See also S. E. F. O'Donoghue (letter), *Nature*, 1971, *229*, 124.

Twelve women in labour were given one dose of pethidine 150 mg intramuscularly 1 to 4 hours before delivery and most of the infants at birth had plasma concentrations of 500 ng per ml or less. When pethidine was given within 1 hour of delivery, infant plasma concentrations were much higher as they also were when 3 mothers were given 2 doses of pethidine within 8 hours of delivery. The ratio of cord to maternal plasma concentrations for all 19 was 0.74. All babies eliminated pethidine from the blood within 148 hours.— L. V. Cooper *et al.*, *Archs Dis. Childh.*, 1977, *52*, 638.

A study of the excretion of pethidine and norpethidine by 7 neonates, whose mothers had received pethidine intramuscularly or intravenously, showed that the amounts excreted increased significantly with the dose-delivery interval up to 5 hours. Most of the placentally-transferred pethidine should be excreted by the 3rd day.— M. I. J. Hogg *et al.*, *Br. J. Anaesth.*, 1977, *49*, 891.

Protein binding of pethidine was measured in 9 pairs of plasma samples obtained at delivery from mothers and neonates. Protein binding in the mothers was 63.3% while in the neonates it was 51.7%.— R. L. Nation, *Clin. Pharmac. Ther.*, 1981, *29*, 472.

Further references: J. C. Morrison *et al.*, *Am. J. Obstet. Gynec.*, 1976, *126*, 997; J. Caldwell *et al.*, *Br. J. clin. Pharmac.*, 1977, *4*, 715P; D. Morgan *et al.*, *Clin. Pharmac. Ther.*, 1978, *23*, 288; J. Caldwell *et al.*, *Life Sci.*, 1978, *22*, 589; J. Caldwell *et al.*, *Br. J. clin. Pharmac.*, 1978, *5*, 362P; T. A. Moreland *et al.*, *Archs Dis. Childh.*, 1980, *55*, 78; B. R. Kuhnert *et al.*, *Clin. Pharmac. Ther.*, 1980, *27*, 486; R. L. Nation, *Clin. Pharmacokinet.*, 1980, *5*, 340; P. L. Morselli *et al.*, *ibid.*, 485.

Uses. Pethidine hydrochloride is an analgesic which has the actions and uses of morphine (p.1020) and can be used for the relief of most types of moderate to severe pain including postoperative pain and the pain of labour. It is also used as pre-operative medication and as an adjunct to anaesthesia. It has little effect on cough or on diarrhoea. Pethidine also has local anaesthetic and slight atropine-like actions.

A dose of 60 to 100 mg of pethidine is approximately equivalent in analgesic effect to 10 mg of morphine. The analgesic effect of pethidine hydrochloride is shorter than for morphine and usually lasts for 2 to 4 hours.

For the relief of pain, pethidine hydrochloride is given in doses of 50 to 100 mg by mouth or by intramuscular injection. These doses may be repeated every 3 to 4 hours if necessary. Up to 150 mg may be required for the relief of severe pain. Pethidine may also be given in the same dosage by subcutaneous injection and, in reduced doses, by intravenous injection. The usual dose for pre-operative medication is 50 to 100 mg by subcutaneous or intramuscular injection. In children, doses of 1 to 1.5 mg per kg body-weight may be given by mouth or by intramuscular or subcutaneous injection.

In obstetric analgesia 50 to 100 mg may be given by intramuscular or subcutaneous injection as soon as contractions occur at regular intervals. This dose may be repeated after 1 to 3 hours if necessary. Pethidine does not diminish the force of uterine contraction but it may prolong labour and may produce respiratory depression in the newborn (see under Precautions).

Pethidine has also been used in conjunction with chlorpromazine or promethazine to produce special types of basal narcosis known as 'potentiated anaesthesia' and 'artificial hibernation'.

An injection of pethidine hydrochloride and levallorphan tartrate is claimed to have the same analgesic potency as pethidine alone but to reduce the risk of respiratory depression.

In a controlled study in 40 convalescent patients, pethidine 1 mg per kg body-weight intravenously over 3 minutes increased blood flow by up to 100% in the forearm and leg while venous and arterial resistance decreased. In 6 patients with heart failure, blood flow was only increased by up to 50% though venous tone and heart-rate were increased.— M. Nadasdi and T. T. Zsotér, *Clin. Pharmac. Ther.*, 1969, *10*, 239. See also J. W. Mostert *et al.*, *Br. J. Anaesth.*, 1970, *42*, 501; C. E. Reier and R. E. Johnstone, *Anesth. Analg. curr. Res.*, 1970, *49*, 119; B. E. Strauer, *Klin. Wschr.*, 1973, *51*, 1105.

Administration. *In the elderly.* Lower initial doses should be used in the elderly and doses titrated to the needs of the patient.— D. E. Wallace and A. S. Watanabe, *Drug Intell. & clin. Pharm.*, 1977, *11*, 597.

See also under Absorption and Fate.

Administration, epidural. To obviate the need for repeated subarachnoid injections to obtain analgesia in severe intractable pain, pethidine was injected through an indwelling epidural catheter. In 7 patients with severe postoperative pain, preservative-free pethidine hydrochloride in physiological saline 100 mg in 10 ml, provided onset of pain relief at 5 minutes which corresponded to high CSF-pethidine concentrations of 0.5 to 2 µg per ml. Complete pain relief occurred in all patients in 12 to 20 minutes and corresponded to CSF-pethidine concentrations of 10 to 20 µg per ml. Typical peak blood-pethidine concentrations occurred after approximately 40 minutes with a mean absorption half-life of 25 minutes. Over periods of 2 to 4 days pethidine given as required provided analgesia lasting 4.5 to 20 hours (mean 6 hours). In 6 patients with chronic intractable cancer pain, complete relief was obtained after pethidine hydrochloride 30 mg in 6 ml; blood-pethidine concentrations were less than those previously determined by intravenous infusion to be analgesic in these patients, and analgesia lasted 4.5 to 18 hours (mean 8 hours). Absence of increased analgesia when analgesic concentrations in the blood were eventually reached following the 100-mg injections and reversal only of concomitant transitory mild sedation by intravenous injection of naloxone, strongly suggested that the initial analgesic effect of the high doses of epidural pethidine was due to a spinal action. No changes in sensory, sympathetic, or motor function were detected, indicating that this form of analgesia may have considerable advantages for relief of severe pain.— M. J. Cousins *et al.* (letter), *Lancet*, 1979, *1*, 1141. A note of caution regarding the high dose of pethidine used. A frail 76-year-old woman given pethidine 50 mg in 10 ml epidurally developed virtual apnoea, and a heavy 42-year-old woman given 100 mg developed very slow respiration.— D. B. Scott and J. McClure (letter), *ibid.*, 1410.

Disappointing results have been obtained using epidural opiates in labour. In 10 patients given pethidine 25 to 50 mg in 10 ml saline, good analgesia was often produced within 10 minutes and lasted about an hour, but the response was very variable; some patients obtained no relief, and tolerance might begin after the third or fourth injection. Phenoperidine 1 mg in 10 to 12 ml saline, and fentanyl 100 µg in 10 to 12 ml saline, increased the response little or not at all.— B. W. Perriss (letter), *Lancet*, 1979, *2*, 422.

Administration in hepatic disease. For a report of increased half-life of pethidine in patients with cirrhosis, see under Absorption and Fate.

Administration in renal failure. Norpethidine accumulated more rapidly in patients in renal failure than in cancer patients with normal renal function following administration of pethidine. CNS excitation in 2 patients receiving multiple doses of pethidine was associated with high concentrations of norpethidine. Therefore pethidine should be given with caution to patients in renal failure, especially when repeated doses are given.— H. H. Szeto *et al.*, *Ann. intern. Med.*, 1977, *86*, 738. See also M. M. Reidenberg, *Hosp. Pharm.*, 1978, *13*, 339. Pethidine could be given in usual doses to patients with renal failure.— W. M. Bennett *et al.*, *Ann. intern. Med.*, 1980, *93*, 62.

Data for predicting removal of pethidine by conventional haemodialysis.— T. P. Gibson and H. A. Nelson, *Clin. Pharmacokinet.*, 1977, *2*, 403.

Anaesthesia. *Premedication.* Pethidine 1 mg per kg body-weight, diazepam 250 µg per kg, and flunitrazepam 20 µg per kg intramuscularly were compared as premedicants in a double-blind study in 145 children, aged 0 to 15 years, undergoing otolaryngological surgery. All drugs were anxiolytic in the children 5 years and older, but diazepam was less effective in children under 5 years.— L. Lindgren *et al.*, *Br. J. Anaesth.*, 1979, *51*, 321.

Analgesia. *In labour.* A review of the use of systemic and inhalational analgesia in labour.— M. Rosen, *Br. J. Anaesth.*, 1979, *51*, *Suppl.* 1, 11S.

Of 152 women in whom the foetus was considered to be at risk of hypoxia, all were given pethidine during the first stage of labour; 51 needed no further analgesic; 51 were given trichloroethylene during the late first stage and during the second stage of labour; and 50 were similarly given nitrous oxide 50% with oxygen 50%. The pH of foetal scalp blood 35 to 55 minutes later had fallen by a mean of 0.015, 0.04, and 0.009 respectively in the 3 groups; pCO_2 rose by 2 and 6.4 mmHg and fell by 2 mmHg respectively; and pO_2 fell by 3.4 and 5.4 mmHg and rose by 0.9 mmHg respectively. Apgar scores at 1 minute were 6.7, 6.17, and 7.42, and at 5 minutes 8.85, 8.43, and 9.2 respectively. Not only was nitrous oxide/oxygen safer than trichloroethylene; it had positive benefits.— T. J. Phillips and R. R. Macdonald, *Br. med. J.*, 1971, *3*, 558.

In a study in 663 women in labour more than 75% of those who received pethidine during the first stage stated that they obtained little or no relief of pain. Nearly 50% of those who received nitrous oxide 50% in oxygen obtained satisfactory relief which was not improved when pethidine was given concomitantly.— A. Holdcroft and M. Morgan, *J. Obstet. Gynaec. Br. Commonw.*, 1974, *81*, 603.

A sequential study in 121 patients in labour, given pethidine 100 mg intravenously or pethidine 100 mg plus naloxone 400 µg, showed that naloxone reduced the analgesic effect of pethidine without reducing the incidence of nausea and vomiting; naloxone slightly reduced the incidence of dizziness.— C. B. Girvan *et al.*, *Br. J. Anaesth.*, 1976, *48*, 563.

For further reports on the use of pethidine in labour, see C. H. de Boer and S. S. Chau (letter), *Lancet*, 1967, *2*, 1256; Y. Sica-Blanco *et al.*, *Am. J. Obstet. Gynec.*, 1967, *97*, 1096; G. D. Malkasian *et al.*, *Obstet. Gynec.*, 1967, *30*, 568; J. S. Crawford, *Practitioner*, 1974, *212*, 677.

See also under Precautions and Absorption and Fate.

Postoperative. In a small trial in patients who had had upper abdominal surgery the demand for pethidine, from a patient demand apparatus, fell quickly over the first 24 hours. No patient made a demand near the maximum. The average dose was 8.1 mg per kg body-weight in 24 hours with a range of 2.9 to 23 mg per kg.— M. Rosen and M. D. Vickers (letter), *Br. med. J.*, 1979, *1*, 1278.

A favourable report of the continuous intravenous infusion of pethidine for postoperative pain; the usual dose was 300 µg per kg body-weight per hour.— J. J. Church, *Br. med. J.*, 1979, *1*, 977.

Further reports on the use of pethidine by intravenous infusion for postoperative analgesia.— J. V. Stapleton *et al.* (letter), *Br. med. J.*, 1978, *2*, 1499; H. T. Davenport and B. M. Wright (letter), *Br. med. J.*, 1979, *1*, 1561; J. V. Stapleton *et al.*, *Anaesth. & intensive Care*, 1979, *7*, 25.

Further reports on the use of pethidine for postoperative analgesia.— M. Keeri-Szanto and S. Heaman, *Surgery Gynec. Obstet.*, 1972, *134*, 647; F. M. Galloway *et al.*, *Can. Anaesth. Soc. J.*, 1977, *24*, 90; A. E. Pflug and J. J. Bonica, *Archs Surg., Chicago*, 1977, *112*, 773.

Cardiovascular disorders. *Myocardial infarction.* Pethidine hydrochloride, in a dose of 100 mg by intravenous injection, given to patients with myocardial infarction caused a transient rise in systemic arterial pressure and systemic vascular resistance and increased the heart-rate. Ten to 15 minutes after the injection, these cardiovascular effects had fallen to below the pretreatment levels. Because of these effects pethidine could not be recommended for the relief of pain in myocardial infarction.— H. A. Rees *et al.*, *Lancet*, 1967, *2*, 863.

In order to reduce the neural and humoral consequences of anxiety and pain in myocardial infarction pethidine hydrochloride 50 to 100 mg was mixed with promethazine hydrochloride 25 mg and injected intravenously over a period of 4 to 5 minutes until the patient became pleasantly drowsy.— P. Nixon (letter), *Br. med. J.*, 1975, *2*, 87. See also P. G. F. Nixon *et al.*, *Lancet*, 1968, *1*, 726.

Effect on biliary tract. For reports of the comparative effects of a number of analgesics, including pethidine hydrochloride, on the biliary tract, see Pentazocine Hydrochloride, p.1025, and Phenazocine Hydrobromide, p.1028.

Hiccup. Pethidine 50 mg intravenously relieved hiccup of long duration, or during anaesthesia, within 2 minutes. If 50 mg was not enough an extra 25 mg could be given. The initial dose of 50 mg might be repeated within 1 hour if the hiccup returned but it should not be repeated a second time for at least 3 hours.— N. L. Wulfsohn (letter), *Lancet*, 1954, *2*, 289.

Preparations

Compound Injection of Pethidine *(Gt Ormond St Child. Hosp.).* Dr. Cope's Injection. Pethidine hydrochloride 2.5 g, chlorpromazine hydrochloride 625 mg, promethazine hydrochloride 625 mg, sodium sulphite 40 mg, sodium metabisulphite 80 mg, hydroquinone 20 mg, Water for Injections to 100 ml. Sterilised by autoclaving in ampoules of alkali-free glass. Protect from light; the solution should not be used if it has turned pink. Shelf-life 1 year. *Dose.* For premedication of children, 1 ml per 10 kg body-weight intramuscularly ½ to ¾ hour before operating. Max. dose 1.5 ml. It is intended for children under 15 kg.

Meperidine Hydrochloride Injection *(U.S.P.).* A sterile solution of pethidine hydrochloride in Water for Injections. pH 3.5 to 6.

Meperidine Hydrochloride Syrup *(U.S.P.).* A syrup containing pethidine hydrochloride. pH 3.5 to 3.9. Store in airtight containers. Protect from light.

Meperidine Hydrochloride Tablets *(U.S.P.).* Tablets containing pethidine hydrochloride. Protect from light.

Pethidine Injection *(B.P.).* Pethidine Hydrochloride Injection. A sterile solution of pethidine hydrochloride in Water for Injections. Sterilised by autoclaving.

Pethidine Tablets *(B.P.).* Pethidine Hydrochloride Tablets. Tablets containing pethidine hydrochloride.

Proprietary Preparations

Pethidine Roche *(Roche, UK).* Pethidine hydrochloride, available as **Injection** containing 50 mg per ml, in ampoules of 1 and 2 ml, and as **Tablets** of 25 and 50 mg.

Pethilorfan *(Roche, UK).* An injection containing in each ml pethidine hydrochloride 50 mg and levallorphan tartrate 625 µg, in ampoules of 1 and 2 ml.

Other Proprietary Names

Centralgin *(Switz.)*; Demer-Idine *(Canad.)*; Demerol *(Arg., Canad., USA)*; Dolantin *(Ger., Switz.)*; Dolantine *(Belg.)*; Doloneurin *(Neth.)*; Dolosal *(Belg., Fr.)*; Pethoid *(Austral.)*.

A preparation containing pethidine hydrochloride and promethazine hydrochloride was formerly marketed in Great Britain under the proprietary name Pamergan P100. A preparation containing in addition atropine sulphate was formerly marketed under the proprietary name Pamergan AP100/25 (*May & Baker*).

6255-c

Phenadoxone Hydrochloride. B.P. 1953; 6-Morpholino-4,4-diphenylheptan-3-one hydrochloride.
$C_{23}H_{29}NO_2,HCl=387.9$.

CAS — 467-84-5 (phenadoxone); 545-91-5 (hydrochloride).

A white odourless crystalline powder with a slightly bitter taste. **Soluble** 1 in 25 of water and 1 in 10 of alcohol; very soluble in chloroform. A 5% solution in water has a pH of 3.5 to 5.

Adverse Effects, Treatment, and Precautions. As for Morphine, p.1019.

Uses. It is an analgesic with a short duration of effect which was formerly used for the relief of pain, in doses of 25 to 50 mg by mouth and 5 to 15 mg subcutaneously or intramuscularly.

6256-k

Phenazocine Hydrobromide *(B.P. 1973).*

1,2,3,4,5,6-Hexahydro-6,11-dimethyl-3-phenethyl-2,6-methano-3-benzazocin-8-ol hydrobromide hemihydrate.
$C_{22}H_{27}NO,HBr,½H_2O=411.4$.

CAS — 127-35-5 (phenazocine); 1239-04-9 (hydrobromide, anhydrous).

A white odourless microcrystalline powder with a bitter taste. **Soluble** 1 in 350 of water, 1 in 45 of alcohol, and 1 in 140 of chloroform; practically insoluble in ether. A 0.2% solution in water has a pH of 5 to 7. Solutions for injection are **sterilised** by autoclaving. **Protect** from light.

Dependence. Prolonged use of phenazocine may lead to dependence of the morphine type (see p.1018).

Adverse Effects, Treatment, and Precautions. As for Morphine, p.1019.

Phenazocine has less sedative effects and is less likely to cause constipation than is morphine but it is more likely to cause respiratory depression.

Pregnancy and the neonate. Clinical depression of the newborn had been observed after the use of phenazocine during labour.— F. Moya and V. Thorndike, *Clin. Pharmac. Ther.*, 1963, *4*, 628.

Absorption and Fate. Phenazocine is absorbed from the gastro-intestinal tract. It is metabolised in the liver.

Uses. Phenazocine hydrobromide is an analgesic with actions and uses similar to those of morphine (see p.1020).

Phenazocine acts within 20 minutes after administration by mouth, intramuscularly, or sublingually; the analgesic effect lasts up to 6 hours. For pre-operative medication, a dose of 1 to 2 mg is given intramuscularly 45 to 60 minutes before operation. As an adjunct to anaesthesia, 0.5 to 1 mg has been given intravenously. The usual dose as an analgesic is 1 to 3 mg intramuscularly every 4 to 6 hours if necessary.

The usual dose by mouth is 5 mg every 4 to 6 hours, though single doses of 20 mg may be given.

Effect on biliary tract. Because morphine and pethidine were known to cause spasm of the common bile-duct sphincter and to increase the pressure in the bile-duct, they were not considered suitable analgesics for use in patients with biliary tract disease. The effects of 5 alternative analgesics on bile-duct pressure were therefore compared. Phenazocine in a dose of 2 mg by intramuscular injection caused no rise in bile-duct pressure on 4 occasions and a slight rise on 2 occasions. Dextropropoxyphene hydrochloride in a dose of 100 mg by intramuscular injection [provided specially by the manufacturer] caused no increase in pressure on 3 occasions and no increase occurred when it was given by mouth. Phenoperidine, in a dose of 2 mg by intramuscular injection and 1 mg by intravenous injection, was given on 11 occasions; slight increases in bile-duct pressure occurred on 3 occasions, including both occasions when the drug was given by intravenous injection. Marked or moderate rises in pressure followed intramuscular injections of levorphanol and dextromoramide. Because dextropropoxyphene had only a comparatively weak analgesic effect and because phenoperidine was a short-acting analgesic, phenazocine was considered to be the most suitable analgesic for biliary pain.— D. S. Hopton and H. B. Torrance, *Gut*, 1967, *8*, 296.

For a comparative study of the effect of morphine, pethidine, pentazocine, and phenazocine on biliary pressure, see Pentazocine, p.1025.

Preparations

Phenazocine Injection *(B.P. 1973).* A sterile solution of phenazocine hydrobromide in Water for Injections containing 1.5% of propylene glycol and suitable buffering agents. pH 2.8 to 3.6. Protect from light.

Phenazocine Tablets *(B.P. 1973).* Tablets containing phenazocine hydrobromide. Protect from light.

Narphen *(Smith & Nephew Pharmaceuticals, UK).* Phenazocine hydrobromide, available as scored tablets of 5 mg.

6257-a

Phenoperidine Hydrochloride. R 1406.

Ethyl 1-(3-hydroxy-3-phenylpropyl)-4-phenylpiperidine-4-carboxylate hydrochloride.
$C_{23}H_{29}NO_3,HCl=403.9$.

CAS — 562-26-5 (phenoperidine); 3627-49-4 (hydrochloride).

A white odourless crystalline powder with a bitter, slightly numbing taste. **Soluble** 1 in 50 of water, 1 in 10 of alcohol (90%), and 1 in 3 of chloroform; slightly soluble in acetone; practically insoluble in ether. Solutions are **sterilised** by autoclaving or by filtration. **Incompatible** with propanidid and solutions of methohexitone sodium and thiopentone sodium.

Dependence, Adverse Effects, and Treatment. As for Morphine, p.1018.

Atropine may be used to block the vagal effects of phenoperidine such as bradycardia.

Phenoperidine hydrochloride and morphine sulphate intravenously in doses of 1.5 mg and 10 mg per 70 kg body-weight respectively had comparable respiratory depressant effects. The effects of phenoperidine were of longer duration than those of morphine.— S. Jennett *et al.*, *Br. J. Anaesth.*, 1968, *40*, 864.

Precautions. As for Morphine, p.1019.
Muscular rigidity may occur; this has been reported to be alleviated by muscle relaxants.

It had been reported that phenoperidine could be given without ill effects to patients on monoamine oxidase inhibitors. However, since it was partially metabolised to pethidine, it was advisable to use alternative methods of anaesthesia in patients taking monoamine oxidase inhibitors.— H. Schnieden, *Prescribers' J.*, 1966, *6*, 82.

Prior beta-blockade with propranolol probably contributed to severe hypotension in a patient with tetanus given phenoperidine; earlier doses of phenoperidine had not caused hypotension.— K. L. Woods (letter), *Br. med. J.*, 1978, *2*, 1164.

Absorption and Fate. Phenoperidine is absorbed from the gastro-intestinal tract. About one-half of an injected dose is excreted unchanged in the urine; the remainder is metabolised in the liver to pethidine and pethidinic acid, which are mainly excreted in the urine.

Five anaesthetised patients were given phenoperidine 2 mg intravenously. The distribution half-life (in 4 patients) ranged from 3.19 to 14.23 minutes while the elimination half-life ranged from 47.31 to 162.30 minutes. Chromatographic studies identified phenoperidine, pethidine, and norpethidine in the urine.— L. Milne *et al.*, *Br. J. Anaesth.*, 1980, *52*, 537.

Uses. Phenoperidine hydrochloride is a potent analgesic, chemically related to pethidine, with similar actions to morphine (see p.1020). By injection its effects last for up to 1 hour.
Phenoperidine hydrochloride produces surgical analgesia and when a major tranquilliser or neuroleptic agent such as droperidol is added, the patient can be maintained in a state of neuroleptanalgesia in which he is calm and indifferent to his surroundings and is able to cooperate with the surgeon. Nitrous oxide and oxygen may be given to produce light anaesthesia.
In anaesthesia where spontaneous respiration is maintained, an average initial intravenous dose of phenoperidine hydrochloride is up to 1 mg; supplements of 500 µg may be given approximately every 40 to 60 minutes. In similar conditions children have been given 30 to 50 µg per kg body-weight. In anaesthesia with controlled respiration, the initial dose is 2 to 5 mg with supplementary doses of 1 mg; children have been given 100 to 150 µg per kg.
Intramuscular injections may be given for analgesia.
Phenoperidine has also been used to depress respiration in long-term assisted ventilation.

Anaesthesia. In 25 patients whose anaesthesia included phenoperidine 2 mg with supplements of 0.5 to 1 mg, postoperative pain was less at 1 and 2 hours than in 25 patients whose anaesthesia included halothane 0.5%, but the number of doses of narcotic analgesics in the first 24 hours was not reduced and the pain scores over the first 3 days were not significantly different. Phenoperidine might have a cumulative effect after narcotic premedication or a sedative effect.— J. J. Henderson and G. D. Parbrook, *Br. J. Anaesth.*, 1976, *48*, 587.

Phaeochromocytoma. Experience of surgery in 102 patients with phaeochromocytoma suggested that droperidol and phenoperidine was the anaesthetic procedure of choice; it had been used in 38 patients with a decrease in the incidence of arrhythmia and a greater stability of blood pressure. Maintenance of blood pressure after removal of the tumour by maintenance of blood volume was superior to the use of noradrenaline.— J. M. Desmonts *et al.*, *Br. J. Anaesth.*, 1977, *49*, 991.

Proprietary Preparations

Operidine *(Janssen, UK)*. Phenoperidine hydrochloride, available as an injection containing 1 mg per ml, in ampoules of 2 ml. (Also available as Operidine in *Austral.*).

NOTE: Operidine is used as a synonym for pethidine hydrochloride in *Jap. P.*

Other Proprietary Names

Lealgin *(Swed.)*; R.1406 *(Fr.)*.

6258-t

Piminodine Esylate. Piminodine Ethanesulphonate. Ethyl 1-(3-anilinopropyl)-4-phenylpiperidine-4-carboxylate ethanesulphonate.
$C_{23}H_{30}N_2O_2,C_2H_6O_3S=476.6$.

CAS — 13495-09-5 (piminodine); 7081-52-9 (esylate).

A colourless crystalline powder with a slightly bitter taste. M.p. 128° to 135°. Slightly **soluble** in water and ether; soluble 1 in 6 of alcohol and 1 in 2 of chloroform. A 0.8% solution in water has a pH of about 4.8. **Store** in airtight containers. Protect from light.

Dependence, Adverse Effects, Treatment, and Precautions. As for Morphine, p.1018.

Uses. Piminodine esylate is an analgesic related chemically and pharmacologically to pethidine with uses similar to those of morphine (see p.1020).
It has been given in doses of 25 to 50 mg by mouth, every 4 to 6 hours and 10 to 20 mg by subcutaneous or intramuscular injection, every 4 hours if necessary.

6259-x

Piritramide.

R 3365; Pirinitramide. 1-(3-Cyano-3,3-diphenylpropyl)-4-piperidinopiperidine-4-carboxamide.
$C_{27}H_{34}N_4O=430.6$.

CAS — 302-41-0.

A crystalline powder. M.p. 149° to 150°.

Dependence, Adverse Effects, Treatment, and Precautions. As for Morphine, p.1018.

Absorption and Fate. Piritramide has been reported to be metabolised in the liver and excreted in the faeces.

Uses. Piritramide is a narcotic analgesic with actions similar to those of morphine (see p.1020). It has a duration of action of about 6 hours after intramuscular injection. It is given in the treatment of postoperative pain in a dose of 20 mg by intramuscular injection, repeated every 6 hours if necessary to a max. of 4 doses.
Piritramide may also be administered as the hydrogen tartrate.

In a double-blind study of 240 patients with postoperative pain piritramide 20 mg intramuscularly appeared to be equal in analgesic effect to morphine 15 mg intramuscularly. At this strength the hypnotic effect of piritramide was greater but there was a smaller incidence of other side-effects.— B. Kay, *Br. J. Anaesth.*, 1971, *43*, 1167.

Proprietary Preparations

Dipidolor *(Janssen, UK)*. Piritramide, available as 2-ml ampoules of an injection containing 10 mg per ml. (Also available as Dipidolor in *Belg., Ger., Neth.*).

Other Proprietary Names

Piridolan *(Norw., Swed.)*.

6260-y

Poppy Capsule *(B.P.C., 1949)*. Papav. Cap.; Poppy Heads; Fruit du Pavot; Mohnfrucht; Fruto de Adormidera; Dormideiras.

Pharmacopoeias. In *Belg., Chin., Port.,* and *Span.*

The dried fruits of *Papaver somniferum* (Papaveraceae), collected before dehiscence has occurred, containing about 0.1 to 0.3% of morphine with traces of other opium alkaloids; the seeds are devoid of alkaloid but contain about 50% of oil.

A brief discussion of experimental poppy culture.— J. L. Jones, *Pharm. J.*, 1973, *1*, 471.

Poppy capsule is mildly sedative and has been used as a liquid extract or syrup in cough mixtures.

Dependence. A report of 9 Asians dependent on poppy capsules, seen at a Birmingham hospital.— S. M. Smith and I. Burnside, *Br. med. J.*, 1972, *1*, 480. See also M. M. Glatt and M. M. Hossain, *ibid.*, 1963, *2*, 102.

6261-j

Thebacon Hydrochloride. Acethydrocodone Hydrochloride; Acetyldihydrocodeinone Hydrochloride; Dihydrocodeinone Enol Acetate Hydrochloride. 6-*O*-Acetyl-7,8-dihydro-3-*O*-methyl-6,7-didehydromorphine hydrochloride; (−)-(5*R*)-4,5-Epoxy-3-methoxy-9a-methylmorphin-6-en-6-yl acetate hydrochloride.
$C_{20}H_{23}NO_4,HCl=377.9$.

CAS — 466-90-0 (thebacon).

Thebacon hydrochloride is a narcotic analgesic used for the relief of pain and as a cough suppressant in doses of 2.5 to 5 mg.

Proprietary Names

Acedicon *(Boehringer Ingelheim, Ger.; Boehringer Ingelheim, Ital.)*; Acedicone *(Boehringer Ingelheim, Belg.)*; Thebacetyl *(Bios-Coutelier, Belg.)*.

6262-z

Tilidate Hydrochloride. Tilidine Hydrochloride; Gö 1261 C; W 5759A. (±)-Ethyl *trans*-2-dimethylamino-1-phenylcyclohex-3-ene-1-carboxylate hydrochloride hemihydrate.
$C_{17}H_{23}NO_2,HCl,\frac{1}{2}H_2O=318.8$.

CAS — 20380-58-9 (tilidate); 27107-79-5 (hydrochloride, anhydrous).

A white crystalline powder with a bitter taste. M.p. 162°. **Soluble** in water.

Dependence, Adverse Effects, Treatment, and Precautions. As for Morphine, p.1018. Tilidate hydrochloride is subject to abuse.

Dependence. Study of tilidate abuse and dependence.— H. Beil and A. Trojan, *Münch. med. Wschr.*, 1976, *118*, 634.

Effects on respiratory function. A crossover study of the comparative respiratory depression of tilidate and morphine in 6 healthy subjects. The respiratory depression of both drugs was effectively antagonised by naloxone.— A. Romagnoli and A. S. Keats, *Clin. Pharmac. Ther.*, 1975, *17*, 523.

Absorption and Fate. Tilidate is absorbed from the gastro-intestinal tract. It is metabolised and excreted in the urine mainly as metabolites.

Following administration of radioactive tilidate 50 mg by mouth to a healthy subject 93.6% of the radioactivity had been eliminated in the urine within 48 hours with a half-life of 8 hours. Less than 0.2% of the urinary radioactivity corresponded to unchanged tilidate and 2 and 3% respectively to nortilidate and bisnortilidate.— K. -O. Vollmer and A. v. Hodenberg, *Arzneimittel-Forsch.*, 1977, *27*, 1706.

Further references: K. -O. Vollmer and H. Achenbach, *Arzneimittel-Forsch.*, 1974, *24*, 1237; H. Hengy *et al.*, *J. pharm. Sci.*, 1978, *67*, 1765.

Uses. Tilidate hydrochloride is a narcotic analgesic used in the control of moderate to severe pain. A dose, in terms of the anhydrous hydrochloride, of 50 to 100 mg up to 4 times daily has been suggested.
Tilidate hydrochloride has sometimes been given with naloxone in an attempt to prevent abuse.

Early studies.— *Arzneimittel-Forsch.*, 1970, *20*, 977–998.

A comparison of the effects of tilidate 50 mg, pethidine 100 mg, and placebo in the relief of postoperative pain.— A. L. Mauro and M. Shapiro, *Curr. ther. Res.*, 1974, *16*, 725.

Further references: G. Navarro *et al.*, *Clin. Pharmac. Ther.*, 1974, *15*, 215; T. Tammisto and I. Tigerstedt, *Acta anaesth. scand.*, 1975, *19*, 296; N. Maranetra and M. C. F. Pain, *Med. J. Aust.*, 1976, *1*, 397.

Proprietary Names

Kitadol *(Larma, Spain)*; Lak *(Bernabó, Arg.)*; Tilitrate *(Substancia, Spain)*; Tilsa *(Ferrer, Spain)*; Valoron *(Substantia, Belg.; Warner, S.Afr.; Gödecke, Switz.)*.

6263-c

Tramadol Hydrochloride. CG 315E; U 26225A. (±)-*trans*-2-Dimethylaminomethyl-1-(3-methoxyphenyl)cyclohexanol hydrochloride.
$C_{16}H_{25}NO_2,HCl=299.8$.

CAS — 27203-92-5 (tramadol); 36282-47-0 (hydrochloride).

A white, odourless, crystalline powder with a bitter taste. M.p. 179° to 180°.
Readily **soluble** in water. A 1% solution in water has a pH of 5.4.

Tramadol hydrochloride is a narcotic analgesic given by intramuscular or intravenous injection in doses of 50 to 100 mg or as suppository in doses of 100 mg.

References: *Arzneimittel-Forsch.*, 1978, *28*, 97–217.

Proprietary Names
Crispin *(Jap.)*; Tramal *(Grünenthal, Ger.)*.

6264-k

Trimeperidine Hydrochloride. Promedolum. 1,2,5-Trimethyl-4-phenyl-4-piperidyl propionate hydrochloride. $C_{17}H_{25}NO_2,HCl=311.9$.

CAS — 64-39-1 (trimeperidine); 125-80-4 (hydrochloride).

Pharmacopoeias. In *Rus.*

A white odourless or almost odourless crystalline powder with a bitter taste. Freely **soluble** in water and chloroform; soluble in alcohol; practically insoluble in ether.

Trimeperidine hydrochloride is a narcotic analgesic with actions and uses similar to those of pethidine hydrochloride (see p.1026).
It is administered by mouth in doses of 50 mg or subcutaneously in doses of 40 mg.

Narcotic Antagonists

7300-y

Included in this section are drugs that reverse the actions of morphine and related narcotics. Some of these narcotic antagonists such as nalorphine, levallorphan, and cyclazocine may also possess some agonist activity. Naloxone has no agonist activity and is considered to be a pure narcotic antagonist.

Narcotic antagonists with agonist activity that are used as analgesics are included in the section on narcotic analgesics, p.1001.

Reviews of narcotic antagonists.— S. Archer and W. F. Michne, *Prog. Drug Res.*, 1976, *20*, 45–100; R. B. Resnick, *Int. J. Addict.*, 1977, *12*, 863; H. D. Kleber, *Int. J. Addict.*, 1977, *12*, 857.

For discussion on the pharmacology and use of narcotic agonist and antagonist analgesic drugs, see *Br. J. clin. Pharmac.*, 1979, *7*, *Suppl.* 3, 269S–326S.

7301-j

Cyclazocine. Win 20 740. 3-Cyclopropylmethyl-1,2,3,4,5,6-hexahydro-6,11-dimethyl-2,6-methano-3-benzazocin-8-ol.

$C_{18}H_{25}NO=271.4$.

CAS — 3572-80-3.

Dependence. As for Nalorphine Hydrobromide, p.1031.

Adverse Effects and Precautions. As for Nalorphine Hydrobromide, p.1031.

Agitation, anxiety, and insomnia have been reported.

The irritability and insomnia that occurred when the dose of cyclazocine was rapidly increased in detoxified narcotic addicts could be antagonised by naloxone 0.5 to 1 g daily by mouth. It was only necessary in a few patients.— M. Fink *et al.*, *Am. J. Nurs.*, 1971, *71*, 1359.

Uses. Cyclazocine is a narcotic antagonist with properties similar to those of nalorphine hydrobromide (see p.1032). It also has analgesic properties but because of its psychotomimetic side-effects it is unsuitable for this purpose. It has a longer duration of action than morphine and is effective when given by mouth.

Cyclazocine has been used in the treatment of narcotic dependence; following withdrawal of narcotic analgesics, a small dose of cyclazocine given by mouth blocks the euphoric and other effects of narcotic drugs for up to 24 hours. The dose of cyclazocine is then increased to about 4 mg daily and maintained at this level until abstinent behaviour has been achieved. Doses of 10 mg have been used to extend the duration of diamorphine blockade to 48 hours.

Cyclazocine was found to be effective by mouth and to have an extended action. Tolerance developed to the subjective effects of cyclazocine but not to its morphine-antagonising action when given chronically to 6 subjects in doses of 2 mg per 70 kg of body-weight twice daily. The toxic and euphoriant actions of even very large doses of morphine and diamorphine were abolished, as was the development of physical dependence.— W. R. Martin *et al.*, *Clin. Pharmac. Ther.*, 1966, *7*, 455.

Treatment of narcotic dependence. References: Fifteenth Report of WHO Expert Committee on Dependence-Producing Drugs, *Tech. Rep. Ser. Wld Hlth Org. No. 343*, 1966; A. M. Freedman *et al.*, *J. Am. med. Ass.*, 1967, *202*, 191; R. Resnick, *Am. J. Psychiat.*, 1974, *131*, 595; H. Kleber *et al.*, *Archs gen. Psychiat.*, 1974, *30*, 37.

7302-z

Diprenorphine Hydrochloride *(B.P. Vet.).* M5050. (6*R*,7*R*,14*S*)-17-Cyclopropylmethyl-7,8-dihydro-7-(1-hydroxy-1-methylethyl)-6-*O*-methyl-6,14-ethano-17-normorphine hydrochloride; 2-[(−)-(5*R*,6*R*,7*R*,14*S*)-9a-Cyclopropylmethyl-4,5-epoxy-3-hydroxy-6-methoxy-6,14-ethanomorphinan-7-yl]propan-2-ol hydrochloride.

$C_{26}H_{35}NO_4,HCl=462.0$.

CAS — 14357-78-9 (diprenorphine); 16808-86-9 (hydrochloride).

A white or almost white crystalline powder. **Soluble** 1 in 30 of water, 1 in 160 of alcohol, and 1 in 2500 of chloroform; practically insoluble in ether. A 2% solution in water has a pH of 4.5 to 6. **Protect** from light.

Diprenorphine hydrochloride is a narcotic antagonist which is used in veterinary medicine to reverse the effects of etorphine hydrochloride.

References: G. F. Blane, *J. Pharm. Pharmac.*, 1967, *19*, 367; G. F. Blane and D. Dugdall, *ibid.*, 1968, *20*, 547; J. L. Crooks *et al.*, *Vet. Rec.*, 1970, *87*, 498.

Preparations

Diprenorphine Injection *(B.P. Vet.).* A sterile solution of diprenorphine hydrochloride in Water for Injections containing chlorocresol and methylene blue. pH 3.5 to 4.5. Sterilise by autoclaving or by filtration. Protect from light. Potency is expressed in terms of diprenorphine.

7303-c

Levallorphan Tartrate *(B.P., U.S.P.).* (−)-9a-Allylmorphinan-3-ol hydrogen tartrate.

$C_{19}H_{25}NO,C_4H_6O_6=433.5$.

CAS — 152-02-3 (levallorphan); 71-82-9 (tartrate).

Pharmacopoeias. In *Br.*, *Swiss*, *Turk.*, and *U.S.*

A white or almost white odourless crystalline powder with an intensely bitter taste. M.p. 174° to 177°.

Soluble 1 in about 20 of water and 1 in 100 of alcohol; 1 in 5000 of ether, 1 in 3300 of chloroform, 1 in 13 of methyl alcohol, and 1 in 665 of isopropyl alcohol; practically insoluble in light petroleum. A solution in water is laevorotatory. A 0.2% solution in water has a pH of 3.2 to 4. A 9.4% solution in water is iso-osmotic with serum. Solutions are **sterilised** by autoclaving or by filtration. **Store** in airtight containers. Protect from light.

An aqueous solution of levallorphan tartrate iso-osmotic with serum (9.4%) caused 59% haemolysis of erythrocytes cultured in it for 45 minutes. The solution and cells turned brown.— C. Sapp *et al.*, *J. pharm. Sci.*, 1975, *64*, 1884.

Incompatibility. Particulate matter was observed within 2 hours when 1 ml of commercial levallorphan tartrate injection was mixed with 5 ml of sterile water and 1 ml of commercial injection solutions of methicillin sodium, or sulphafurazole diethanolamine.— R. Misgen, *Am. J. Hosp. Pharm.*, 1965, *22*, 92.

Adverse Effects and Precautions. As for Nalorphine Hydrobromide, p.1031.

Absorption and Fate. Levallorphan tartrate acts within a few minutes of intravenous injection and its effects have been reported to last for up to 4 hours. It crosses the placenta.

Uses. Levallorphan has actions similar to those of nalorphine (p.1032). Small doses of levallorphan antagonise the respiratory depression of narcotic drugs but larger doses also antagonise their analgesic actions.

In the treatment of narcotic overdosage, an initial dose of 1 mg of levallorphan tartrate may be given intravenously followed by 1 or 2 doses of 0.5 mg at intervals of 5 to 10 minutes, if necessary. In children, 20 µg per kg body-weight may be given.

For respiratory depression of the newborn, a dose of 1 mg may be given intravenously to the mother 5 to 10 minutes before delivery, or 50 to 250 µg may be injected into the umbilical vein of the newborn infant. If this vein cannot be used, the injection may be given subcutaneously or intramuscularly.

Reference: W. U. Reidt *et al.*, *Am. Rev. resp. Dis.*, 1961, *83*, 481.

Preparations

Levallorphan Injection *(B.P.).* A sterile solution of levallorphan tartrate in Water for Injections, adjusted to pH 4.5 (range: pH 4 to 5). Sterilised by autoclaving. Protect from light.

Levallorphan Tartrate Injection *(U.S.P.).* A sterile solution of levallorphan tartrate in Water for Injections. pH 4 to 4.5.

Lorfan *(Roche, UK).* Levallorphan tartrate, available as an injection containing 1 mg per ml, in ampoules of 1 ml. (Also available as Lorfan in *Austral.*, *Canad.*, *Ger.*, *Switz.*, *USA*).

7304-k

Nalorphine Hydrobromide *(B.P., B.P. Vet.).* Nalorph. Hydrobrom. 17-Allyl-17-normorphine hydrobromide; (−)-(5*R*,6*S*)-9a-Allyl-4,5-epoxymorphin-7-en-3,6-diol hydrobromide.

$C_{19}H_{21}NO_3,HBr=392.3$.

CAS — 62-67-9 (nalorphine); 1041-90-3 (hydrobromide).

Pharmacopoeias. In *Br.*, *Braz.*, *Chin.*, *Hung.*, and *It.*

A white to creamy-white odourless crystalline powder. M.p. about 260° with decomposition. **Soluble** 1 in 24 of water and 1 in 35 of alcohol. A solution in methyl alcohol is laevorotatory. A 2% solution in water is acid to methyl red. Aqueous solutions may deposit crystals of the dihydrate; the dihydrate is readily soluble in dehydrated alcohol but the solution rapidly yields a deposit of the anhydrous salt. Solutions are **sterilised** by autoclaving or by filtration. **Store** in airtight containers. Protect from light.

7305-a

Nalorphine Hydrochloride *(U.S.P.).* Nalorphini Hydrochloridum; Nalorphinium Chloride.

$C_{19}H_{21}NO_3,HCl=347.8$.

CAS — 57-29-4.

Pharmacopoeias. In *Arg.*, *Fr.*, *Ind.*, *Int.*, *Jug.*, *Nord.*, *Turk.*, and *U.S.*

A white or almost white odourless crystalline powder with a bitter taste; it slowly darkens on exposure to air and light. M.p. 260° to 263°. **Soluble** 1 in 8 of water and 1 in 35 of alcohol; practically insoluble in chloroform and ether; soluble in dilute solutions of alkali hydroxides. A solution in water is laevorotatory. Solutions in water have a pH of about 5; a 6.36% solution is iso-osmotic with serum. Solutions are **sterilised** by autoclaving or by filtration and kept in alkali-free containers. **Store** in airtight containers. Protect from light.

Dependence. Mild withdrawal effects have been reported following the prolonged administration of nalorphine, but it has little liability to abuse.

Healthy subjects given progressively larger doses of nalorphine became tolerant to its effects and were cross-tolerant to the effects of cyclazocine. On withdrawal, an abstinence syndrome developed which was milder than that for morphine but similar to that of cyclazocine.— W. R. Martin and C. W. Gorodetzky, *J. Pharmac. exp. Ther.*, 1965, *150*, 437. A study of the dependence-producing potential of cyclazocine.— W. R. Martin *et al.*, *ibid.*, 426.

Adverse Effects and Precautions. Nalorphine may give rise to drowsiness, irritability, miosis, pallor, bradycardia, hypotension, and sweating. Occasionally, nausea and a feeling of drunkenness may occur. Nalorphine may also cause respiratory depression and disturbing psychotic effects. In those dependent on narcotic drugs, the administration of nalorphine may be followed by a typical withdrawal syndrome.

Nalorphine must only be used to treat respiratory depression due to narcotic analgesics.

In a study in 6 healthy persons, the respiratory depressant effect of 13.5 mg of nalorphine was about equivalent to 10 mg of morphine. When both drugs were given together, intramuscularly, in various dosages, the resulting effects on the respiration were complex: with 5 mg of morphine, increasing the dose of nalorphine produced greater depression than increasing it with 10 mg of morphine. The interaction of the 2 drugs was regarded as an example of 'competitive dualism'. The antagonism by nalorphine of the respiratory depression produced by morphine was primarily related to differences in the intrinsic action of each drug, and not simply due to mutually competitive affinities for certain receptor sites.— J. W. Bellville and G. Fleischli, *Clin. Pharmac. Ther.*, 1968, *9*, 152.

In patients given narcotic antagonists who have apparently recovered from their narcotic overdose, observation must be continued for up to 48 hours as the half-life of the antagonist was generally shorter than that of the narcotic.— R. Tarala and L. E. J. Evans (letter), *Lancet*, 1973, *2*, 1201.

Further references: R. E. Lister, *J. Pharm. Pharmac.*, 1966, *18*, 364; J. R. Lawrence and R. Lee, *Lancet*, 1975, *2*, 717.

Pregnancy and the neonate. In studies on pregnant women before the onset of labour, nalorphine was found to cause mild respiratory acidosis in the mother and metabolic acidosis in the foetus. Naloxone did not cause acidosis in mother or foetus.— A. Chang *et al.*, *Med. J. Aust.*, 1976, *1*, 263.

See also under Uses.

Absorption and Fate. Nalorphine is poorly absorbed when given by mouth. When administered by injection, it readily passes into the brain and across the placenta.

It is largely metabolised in the liver and excreted in the urine. About 2 to 6% of the dose is excreted unchanged in the urine.

Uses. Nalorphine is a narcotic antagonist with some agonist properties that reduces or abolishes the depressant actions of morphine and other narcotic substances but not those of the barbiturates or other non-narcotic depressants. Nalorphine has analgesic properties but is unsuitable for use as an analgesic because of its unpleasant side-effects. It is used to reverse narcotic-induced respiratory depression when it will exert an effect within 1 or 2 minutes of intravenous injection. In general naloxone is preferred as a narcotic antagonist.

Nalorphine hydrobromide is usually given by intravenous injection in a dose of 5 to 10 mg, repeated in 10 to 15 minutes if necessary. Some authorities recommend that a total dosage of 40 mg should not be exceeded but considerably larger amounts have been given in severe poisoning; single doses of 40 mg have occasionally been given; it acts within about 1 minute after intravenous injection. It may also be given intramuscularly or subcutaneously. The usual supportive measures should also be employed in cases of severe narcotic poisoning.

Nalorphine hydrobromide has also been used to reverse neonatal respiratory depression following administration of narcotic analgesics to the mother. For this purpose an intravenous injection of 10 mg has been given to the mother about 10 minutes before the expected time of delivery, alternatively 0.25 to 1 mg injected directly into the umbilical vein of the newborn infant.

Nalorphine hydrochloride is used similarly.

There was no maximum dose of nalorphine; each patient should be given the dose required to cope with his condition. Doses of up to 105 mg have been given in 1 hour without respiratory depression. Continuous intravenous infusions might have to be given following single bolus injections.— J. A. H. Forrest and H. Mathew (letter), *Lancet*, 1973, *2*, 211.

Further references: *Narcotic Antagonists, Advances in Biochemical Psychopharmacology*, Vol. VIII, M.C. Braude *et al.* (Ed.), New York, Raven Press, 1973.

Nalorphine pupil test. The value of the nalorphine pupil test for diagnosing the use of narcotic analgesics was confirmed in 79 male addicts; 67 physically dependent on diamorphine and 12 opium addicts. In all of them, the subcutaneous injection of nalorphine hydrobromide 3 mg consistently reversed the drug-induced miosis and produced a mean increase in pupil size of at least 0.375 mm, at some time between 1 and 16 hours after the last dose of narcotic. The most responsive period (95% of positive reactions) was between 1 and 4 hours. Correlation between the pupil response and urine tests for morphine was positive in all but 1 addict (98.7%) on the first day of narcotic withdrawal.— E. L. Way *et al.*, *Clin. Pharmac. Ther.*, 1966, *7*, 300. See also K. D. Parker *et al.*, *J. forens. Sci.*, 1966, *11*, 152.

Pregnancy and the neonate. Although nalorphine had a more prolonged effect than naloxone in reversing pethidine-induced neonatal respiratory depression, it was associated with irritability, excessive crying, and reduced sucking reflex.— J. E. H. Brice *et al.*, *Archs Dis. Childh.*, 1978, *53*, 837. A similar report.— J. E. H. Brice *et al.*, *Archs Dis. Childh.*, 1979, *54*, 356.

Preparations of Nalorphine Hydrobromide and Hydrochloride

Nalorphine Injection *(B.P.).* Nalorphine Hydrobromide Injection. A sterile solution of nalorphine hydrobromide in Water for Injections. The acidity is adjusted to pH 3 (limits: pH 2.7 to 3.3) by the addition of hydrobromic acid. Sterilised by autoclaving. Protect from light.

Nalorphine Hydrochloride Injection *(U.S.P.).* A suitably buffered sterile solution in Water for Injections. pH 6 to 7.5.

Proprietary Names of Nalorphine Hydrobromide and Hydrochloride

Lethidrone *(Wellcome, Austral.; Wellcome, S.Afr.; Wellcome, Switz.)*; Norfin *(Lusofarmaco, Ital.)*.

Nalorphine hydrobromide was formerly marketed in Great Britain under the proprietary name Lethidrone *(Wellcome)*.

7306-t

Naloxone Hydrochloride *(U.S.P.).* EN 1530;

Allylnoroxymorphone Hydrochloride. 17-Allyl-6-deoxy-7,8-dihydro-14-hydroxy-6-oxo-17-normorphine hydrochloride; (−)-(5*R*,14*S*)-9a-Allyl-4,5-epoxy-3,14-dihydroxymorphinan-6-one hydrochloride.

$C_{19}H_{21}NO_4,HCl=363.8$.

CAS — 465-65-6 (naloxone); 357-08-4 (hydrochloride, anhydrous); 51481-60-8 (hydrochloride, dihydrate).

Pharmacopoeias. In *Braz.* and *U.S.* (anhydrous or dihydrate).

A white to slightly off-white powder. **Soluble** in water, dilute acids, and strong alkalis; slightly soluble in alcohol; practically insoluble in chloroform and ether. A solution in water is laevorotatory. Aqueous solutions are acidic. A 8.07% solution in water is iso-osmotic with serum. **Store** in airtight containers. Protect from light.

An aqueous solution of naloxone hydrochloride iso-osmotic with serum (8.07%) caused 35% haemolysis of erythrocytes cultured in it for 45 minutes.— C. Sapp *et al.*, *J. pharm. Sci.*, 1975, *64*, 1884.

Dependence. Prolonged administration of naloxone does not lead to tolerance or dependence. It has no abuse potential.

Adverse Effects and Precautions. Unlike nalorphine hydrobromide, naloxone appears to be almost devoid of side-effects in patients who are not dependent on narcotic analgesics. Nausea and vomiting have been reported, and sedation may occur in patients who have not taken narcotics.

In those dependent on narcotic drugs, the administration of naloxone may be followed by a typical withdrawal syndrome.

When naloxone was used postoperatively to reverse respiratory depression due to morphine, 19 of 21 patients had transient nausea and vomiting, usually within 5 minutes.— D. E. Longnecker *et al.*, *Anesth. Analg. curr. Res.*, 1973, *52*, 447.

Ventricular tachycardia and fibrillation occurred on 2 occasions following the use of naloxone to reverse the effects of morphine in cardiac surgery.— L. L. Michaelis *et al.*, *Ann. thorac. Surg.*, 1974, *18*, 608.

Acute pulmonary oedema followed the use of naloxone in one patient to reverse morphine anaesthesia.— J. W. Flacke *et al.*, *Anesthesiology*, 1977, *47*, 376.

Interactions. Studies and discussions on the interactions of narcotic analgesics and of narcotic antagonists.— *Ann. N.Y. Acad. Sci.*, 1976, *281*, 244–371.

Absorption and Fate. Naloxone is absorbed from the gastro-intestinal tract but it is subject to considerable first-pass metabolism. It is largely metabolised in the liver and is excreted in conjugated form in the urine. It has a short plasma half-life.

A review of the relationship of the pharmacokinetics of morphine, methadone, and naloxone to pharmacological activity.— B. A. Berkowitz, *Clin. Pharmacokinet.*, 1976, *1*, 219.

Naloxone was metabolised by *N*-dealkylation and reduction of the 6-keto group, and the glucuronides of these 2 metabolites, with the glucuronide of unchanged naloxone, were excreted in the urine.— S. H. Weinstein *et al.*, *J. pharm. Sci.*, 1971, *60*, 1567.

After administration by mouth to a healthy subject naloxone hydrochloride was rapidly absorbed into the blood stream and reached a plasma concentration comparable to that obtained following intravenous administration. The material in the plasma, however, was not free naloxone, but a metabolite which did not have the same biological potency. The plasma half-life of naloxone was calculated to be 90 minutes in a healthy subject, 100 minutes in an opiate-dependent patient while receiving diamorphine, or 70 minutes when free from opiates.— J. Fishman *et al.*, *J. Pharmac. exp. Ther.*, 1973, *187*, 575. The half-time of recovery in the case of ventilatory response was estimated to be about 15 to 20 minutes for naloxone.— J. M. Evans *et al.*, *Br. med. J.*, 1974, *2*, 589.

Pregnancy and the neonate. Peak plasma concentrations of 4.0 to 5.4 ng per ml and 9.2 to 20.2 ng per ml were achieved 40 minutes after the injection of 35 or 70 µg respectively of naloxone hydrochloride into the umbilical vein in a study of 12 newborn infants. The concentrations then declined exponentially at similar rates in both groups; mean half-lives were 3.5 hours for those receiving 35 µg and 2.6 hours for those receiving 70 µg. A dose of 200 µg was given intramuscularly to 20 neonates and peak plasma concentrations of 11.3 to 34.7 ng per ml were detected at 0.5 to 2 hours. Plasma concentrations declined rapidly between 1 and 6 hours then more slowly between 6 and 36 hours.— J. E. H. Brice *et al.*, *Br. J. clin. Pharmac.*, 1979, *8*, 412P. Further details. At 24 to 36 hours plasma concentrations following the intramuscular injection were as high as those recorded 4 hours after intravenous injection of 35 µg. This may explain the prolonged duration of action of naloxone when given intramuscularly.— T. A. Moreland *et al.*, *ibid.*, 1980, *9*, 609.

Uses. Naloxone is a specific narcotic antagonist which, unlike nalorphine, has no morphine-like actions. It is also an effective antagonist for mixed agonist-antagonist analgesics such as pentazocine. It can also reverse some of the adverse effects of narcotic antagonists with agonist properties. Because naloxone has no respiratory depressant activity it may be given to patients merely suspected of narcotic overdosage without risk of enhancing respiratory depression. It reverses narcotic analgesia and has no analgesic properties of its own. Naloxone acts within 2 minutes of intravenous injection and usually within 2 or 3 minutes of subcutaneous or intramuscular injection. Very much higher doses are required by mouth.

In the treatment of known or suspected narcotic overdose, an initial dose of 400 µg of naloxone hydrochloride may be given subcutaneously, intramuscularly, or intravenously and repeated at intervals of 2 or 3 minutes. If significant improvement has not been obtained after 2 or 3 doses the condition of the patient may be due to other causes. In children 5 to 10 µg per kg body-weight may be given, similarly repeated at intervals of 2 or 3 minutes. Further injections may be required after 45 minutes or less. Patients should always be closely observed since duration of action of the narcotic may exceed that of naloxone.

Naloxone hydrochloride may be used postoperatively in intravenous doses of 1.5 to 3 µg per kg body-weight to counteract narcotic-induced respiratory depression.

Neonatal respiratory depression resulting from administration of narcotic analgesics during labour may be reversed by naloxone hydrochloride. The usual dose is 10 µg per kg body-weight given by intravenous, intramuscular, or subcutaneous injection to the infant, repeated if necessary. Alternatively a single dose of 200 µg (60µg per kg) intramuscularly at birth has been suggested.

Naloxone hydrochloride has been used to produce narcotic blockade for the maintenance of addicts after narcotic withdrawal. Doses of up to 3 g by mouth have been used to provide blockade for 24 hours. It has also been used cautiously in small doses to diagnose narcotic dependence by precipitating the withdrawal syndrome.

Reviews of the uses of naloxone: *Lancet*, 1975, *1*, 734; W. R. Martin, *Ann. intern. Med.*, 1976, *85*, 765; *Drug & Ther. Bull.*, 1981, *19*, 83.

Naloxone reversed narcotic-induced biliary spasm.— R. L. McCammon *et al.*, *Anesthesiology*, 1978, *48*, 437.

In 4 healthy subjects naloxone 1.2 mg intravenously largely reversed pentazocine-induced delay in gastric emptying and delayed absorption of paracetamol. Naloxone might be useful to reverse narcotic effects on gastric emptying before the induction of anaesthesia during labour or in recurrent vomiting.— W. S. Nimmo *et al.*, *Br. med. J.*, 1979, *2*, 1189.

A suggestion that naloxone could be used to suppress raised serum-prolactin concentrations in patients with prolactin-secreting pituitary tumours.— B. A. Schainker and T. J. Cicero (letter), *New Engl. J. Med.*, 1979, *300*, 563. Available data suggested that opiate-receptor blockade would probably not replace bromocriptine for the medical management of hyperprolactinaemia.— N. G. Baranetsky *et al.* (letter), *New Engl. J. Med.*, 1979, *301*, 164.

Naloxone reversed morphine-induced peripheral vasodilatation.— R. A. Cohen and J. D. Coffman, *Clin. Pharmac. Ther.*, 1980, *28*, 541.

Naloxone reversal of ischaemic neurological deficits.— D. S. Baskin and Y. Hosobuchi, *Lancet*, 1981, *2*, 272. Criticism.— P. A. J. Hardy (letter), *ibid.*, 1052.

Naloxone reversal of urinary retention after epidural morphine.— N. Rawal *et al.* (letter), *Lancet*, 1981, *2*, 1411.

Further references on the effects of naloxone: J. Vardi *et al.*, *Curr. ther. Res.*, 1979, *26*, 1015 (parkinsonism); J. A. Summerfield (letter), *Br. J. clin. Pharmac.*, 1980, *10*, 180 (itching); M. Kyriakides *et al.* (letter), *Lancet*, 1980, *1*, 876; S. N. Sullivan, *ibid.*, 1140 (both obesity); N. J. Brandt *et al.*, *New Engl. J. Med.*, 1980, *303*, 914; S. H. Snyder, *ibid.*, 934 (both encephalomyelopathy); D. B. Dunger *et al.*, *Lancet*, 1980, *1*, 1277 (hypothalamic syndrome).

Administration in renal failure. Naloxone could be given in usual doses to patients with renal failure.— W. M. Bennett *et al.*, *Ann. intern. Med.*, 1980, *93*, 62.

Diagnosis of narcotic dependence. Naloxone could be used as a diagnostic agent to determine physical dependence on opiates. The heart-rate, blood pressure, temperature, pupil size, presence of gooseflesh on the thorax, presence of sweating, lachrymation, yawning, or rhinorrhoea were noted before and after the administration of naloxone 160 µg intramuscularly. If no gooseflesh was present after 20 to 30 minutes the drug was administered intravenously in a dose of 240 µg and the observations repeated. The intensity of symptoms such as gooseflesh indicated the degree of dependence.— P. H. Blachly, *J. Am. med. Ass.*, 1973, *224*, 334. See also *idem* (letter), *New Engl. J. Med.*, 1972, *286*, 951.

Further references: R. I. H. Wang *et al.*, *Clin. Pharmac. Ther.*, 1974, *16*, 653; B. A. Judson *et al.*, *Clin. Pharmac. Ther.*, 1980, *27*, 492.

Pain insensitivity. A patient with congenital insensitivity to pain had an increased threshold of nociceptive flexion reflex when compared with healthy subjects. Naloxone reduced this threshold and indicated that congenital insensitivity to pain could be related to a tonic hyperactivity of a morphine-like pain-inhibitory system antagonised by naloxone.— H. Dehen *et al.* (letter), *Lancet*, 1977, *2*, 293.

Tests in a 29-year-old woman with congenital insensitivity to pain indicated that naloxone might be a possible means of treatment.— H. Yanagida (letter), *Lancet*, 1978, *2*, 520. Comment.— J. C. Willer *et al.* (letter), *ibid.*, 739.

Pregnancy and the neonate. In a double-blind study naloxone 40 µg was injected within 1 minute of birth into the umbilical vein of 10 infants born to mothers who had received pethidine during labour; the alveolar PCO_2 was significantly lower, 30 minutes later, than in 18 controls and alveolar ventilation was significantly increased; these changes were no longer significant at 4 to 48 hours; there was no difference between the groups in respect of feeding behaviour or response to an auditory stimulus. In a further study the alveolar PCO_2 was significantly lower and alveolar ventilation significantly increased for 48 hours in 15 infants given naloxone 200 µg intramuscularly within 1 minute of birth, when compared with 15 controls; milk consumption was increased and the time to stop reacting to a repeated auditory stimulus was reduced.— P. C. Weiner *et al.*, *Br. med. J.*, 1977, *2*, 228; *idem*, 229. Follow-up of 19 children showed that naloxone did not significantly affect development.— P. C. Wiener and S. Wallace (letter), *Br. med. J.*, 1980, *280*, 252.

Further references: J. M. Evans *et al.*, *Lancet*, 1975, *1*, 734; J. M. Evans *et al.*, *Br. med. J.*, 1976, *2*, 1098; T. Gerhardt *et al.*, *J. Pediat.*, 1977, *90*, 1009; J. E. H. Brice *et al.*, *Archs Dis. Childh.*, 1978, *53*, 837; J. E. H. Brice *et al.*, *Archs Dis. Childh.*, 1979, *54*, 356.

For a comparison of the effects of naloxone and nalorphine on maternal and foetal blood pH, see Nalorphine, p.1032.

Psychiatric disorders. *Mania.* In a double-blind placebo-controlled crossover study, small but significant decreases in ratings for mania were noted following infusions of naloxone in 12 manic or hypomanic patients. Contrary to reported findings of a decrease in *rats*, a non-significant rise in growth hormone concentrations was noted. These preliminary findings support a role for endorphins in the regulation of manic symptoms. The role of concurrent administration of psychotropic drugs, which many of the patients were receiving, needs further study.— D. Janowsky *et al.* (letter), *Lancet*, 1978, *2*, 320. Naloxone was not found to have any effect on serum-prolactin concentrations in 8 healthy subjects or in 16 psychiatric patients (8 of whom were receiving antipsychotic medication), although the symptoms of 12 of the patients with manic symptoms appeared to decrease after naloxone infusion.— *idem*, 637.

Schizophrenia. Naloxone 10 mg given by intravenous infusion to 9 patients with chronic schizophrenia, in a double-blind study, was associated with reduction of hallucinations in 6 patients, slight improvement in 1 patient, and no improvement in the other 2; the effect lasted for from 3 hours in 2 patients up to 48 hours in 1 patient. Results were considered suggestive of involvement of endogenous opioids in some schizophrenic symptoms.— S. J. Watson *et al.*, *Science*, 1978, *201*, 73.

Auditory hallucinations in a 28-year-old woman were relieved by opiates and by naloxone 400 µg which might be a useful emergency treatment; endorphins and opiate receptors might be involved in the pathogenesis of auditory hallucinations.— M. Orr and C. Oppenheimer, *Br. med. J.*, 1978, *1*, 481.

During a random double-blind study in 14 schizophrenic patients and 5 with affective disorders, the intravenous administration of naloxone 400 µg and of doses up to 10 mg did not produce any marked improvement in most of the ratings of behaviour studied.— G. C. Davis *et al.*, *Science*, 1977, *197*, 74.

Intravenous injections of naloxone 400 µg were no better than a placebo for reducing the incidence of hallucinations during a study in 7 patients with chronic schizophrenia.— J. Volavka *et al.*, *Science*, 1977, *196*, 1227. A report of another study which failed to demonstrate any effect of naloxone on schizophrenia.— J. Lipinski *et al.* (letter), *Lancet*, 1979, *1*, 1292.

Further references: P. A. Berger *et al.*, *Am. J. Psychiat.*, 1981, *138*, 913.

Respiratory-tract disorders. A study of naloxone in patients with chronic obstructive pulmonary disease.— T. V. Santiago *et al.*, *New Engl. J. Med.*, 1981, *304*, 1190.

Shock. Intravenous administration of naloxone 10 µg per kg body-weight immediately raised the blood pressure and reduced the heart-rate of an 8-year-old child with apparently irreversible septic shock associated with meningococcal infection. The child subsequently received 2 subcutaneous injections of naloxone 200 µg, and after about an hour the cardiovascular indices stabilised. Naloxone might be tried in septic and other shock which has not responded to traditional intensive therapy and seems irreversible.— M. Tiengo (letter), *Lancet*, 1980, *2*, 690.

Although both patients subsequently died, intravenous administration of naloxone was associated with significant improvement in circulatory indices in one patient with cardiogenic shock and one with septic shock. Both patients had been unresponsive to conventional therapy, including dopamine, but it was considered that both the naloxone and conventional treatment probably contributed to the improvement.— R. Dirksen *et al.* (letter), *Lancet*, 1980, *2*, 1360. Naloxone reversed septic shock unresponsive to dopamine in a woman with terminal carcinoma. She did not respond to a dose of 10 µg per kg body-weight but immediately improved after receiving 100 µg per kg.— D. J. M. Wright *et al.* (letter), *ibid.*, 1361.

Use by continuous intravenous infusion in septic shock.— W. R. Swinburn and P. Phelan (letter), *Lancet*, 1982, *1*, 167.

Concern that anecdotal evidence may encourage unrestrained use of opiate antagonists in shock.— J. W. Holaday and A. I. Faden (letter), *Lancet*, 1981, *2*, 201.

Further references: W. P. Peters *et al.*, *Lancet*, 1981, *1*, 529; R. Dirksen *et al.* (letter), *ibid.*, 607; K. Lenz *et al.*, *ibid.*, 834; J. Burnie, *ibid.*, 942.

Treatment of alcohol overdosage. A report of a study in 100 patients with suspected alcohol-induced coma, confirming that naloxone in doses of up to 1.2 mg can reverse alcohol-induced coma in some cases. This re-emphasises the value of using naloxone both diagnostically and therapeutically in the unconscious patient, although it must be recognised that a response can no longer be used as specific evidence of opiate poisoning.— D. B. Jefferys *et al.* (letter), *Lancet*, 1980, *1*, 308. See also A. I. Mackenzie, *ibid.*, 1979, *1*, 733. Evidence that naloxone is not an effective antagonist of alcohol.— M. J. Mattila *et al.*, *ibid.*, 1981, *1*, 775. Failure of naloxone to reverse alcohol intoxication.— D. M. Catley *et al.* (letter), *ibid.*, 1263.

Treatment of diazepam overdosage. For a report on the successful use of naloxone in the treatment of diazepam overdosage, see E. F. Bell, *J. Pediat.*, 1975, *87*, 803. See also C. Jordan *et al.*, *Br. J. Anaesth.*, 1979, *51*, 570P.

Treatment of narcotic dependence. When given by mouth as a single dose, as much as 3 g of naloxone hydrochloride was required to provide satisfactory blockade to 50 mg of diamorphine for 24 hours.— A. Zaks *et al.*, *J. Am. med. Ass.*, 1971, *215*, 2108.

Naloxone was about 50 times less potent by mouth than parenterally and it was possible to formulate a mixture containing methadone hydrochloride and naloxone hydrochloride which was indistinguishable from methadone alone by mouth, but which had significantly less miotic, behavioural, and subjective effects than methadone alone when abused parenterally, because of the naloxone. Such a mixture had a reduced parenteral abuse potential in both opiate-dependent and non-dependent subjects. There was, however, a risk in opiate-dependent subjects that illicit parenteral administration of the mixtures could precipitate a dangerous abstinence syndrome.— J. G. Nutt and D. R. Jasinski, *Clin. Pharmac. Ther.*, 1974, *15*, 156.

A preliminary study in 33 addicted subjects, of a method of inducing narcotic withdrawal with naloxone so that naltrexone-maintenance therapy could be introduced without precipitating the abstinence syndrome. The procedure involved repeated injections of naloxone and took 1 or 2 days according to the severity of addiction; naloxone was also given by mouth to identify subjects liable to severe and prolonged gastro-intestinal symptoms. Less severely addicted patients were able to make the transition from opiate dependence to naltrexone maintenance within 48 hours after their last opiate dose.— R. B. Resnick *et al.*, *Clin. Pharmac. Ther.*, 1977, *21*, 409.

Treatment of narcotic overdosage. All of 9 patients who were unconscious due to narcotic intoxication with dipipanone, pethidine, diamorphine, pentazocine, or dihydrocodeine recovered consciousness within 1 to 2 minutes of naloxone 0.4 to 1.2 mg being given by intravenous injection, and their respiratory rate and volume increased. Additional doses of 0.4 to 1.2 mg were necessary depending on the state of consciousness and respiration. There was no response in 13 patients suffering from an overdose of non-narcotic CNS depressants when given naloxone but neither was there any deterioration. Tremor and hyperventilation were associated with the abrupt return to consciousness in some patients.— L. E. J. Evans *et al.*, *Lancet*, 1973, *1*, 452. See also L. E. J. Evans (letter), *Br. med. J.*, 1973, *2*, 717.

For the use of naloxone in the treatment of apomorphine-induced emesis, see Apomorphine Hydrochloride, p.892.

Preparations

Naloxone Hydrochloride Injection *(U.S.P.)*. A sterile iso-osmotic solution in Water for Injections. It may contain suitable preservatives. Potency is expressed in terms of anhydrous naloxone hydrochloride. pH 3 to 4.5. Protect from light.

Narcan *(Du Pont Pharmaceuticals, UK)*. Naloxone hydrochloride, available as an injection containing 400 µg per ml, in ampoules of 1 ml. **Narcan Neonatal.** Naloxone hydrochloride, available as an injection containing 20 µg per ml, in ampoules of 2 ml. (Also available as Narcan in *Aust., Austral., Belg., Canad., Fr., Ital., Neth., S.Afr., Switz., USA*).

Other Proprietary Names

Nalonee *(Denm., Fin., Iceland, Norw., Swed.)*; Narcanti *(Ger.)*.

7307-x

Naltrexone Hydrochloride. EN-1639A.

17-Cyclopropylmethyl-6-deoxy-7,8-dihydro-14-hydroxy-6-oxo-17-normorphine hydrochloride; (−)-(5*R*,14*S*)-9a-Cyclopropylmethyl-4,5-epoxy-3,14-dihydroxymorphinan-6-one hydrochloride. $C_{20}H_{23}NO_4,HCl=377.9$.

CAS — 16590-41-3 (naltrexone); 16676-29-2 (hydrochloride).

Adverse Effects and Precautions. As for Naloxone, p.1032.

Nausea, abdominal pain, headache, and skin rash have been reported.

No withdrawal effects were reported in patients for whom treatment with naltrexone in daily doses of 30 mg or 50 mg was stopped abruptly.— S. Archer and W. F. Michne, *Prog. Drug Res.*, 1976, *20,* 45.

A double-blind study in 40 patients showed naltrexone to have fewer induction side-effects than cyclazocine.— L. S. Brahen *et al.*, *Archs gen. Psychiat.*, 1977, *34,* 1181.

Absorption and Fate. Naltrexone is well absorbed from the gastro-intestinal tract. It has a long duration of action.

Following administration of naltrexone as initial doses of 100 mg and as chronic doses of 100 mg daily to 4 ex-addict subjects, it was rapidly absorbed and steady-state equilibrium readily achieved without accumulation of naltrexone or its metabolite β-naltrexol. Absorption was complete (less than 0.5% of free naltrexone being recovered in the 24-hour faeces) but plasma concentrations varied substantially especially in the first few hours (peak concentrations ranging from 15.2 to 64.2 ng per ml occurring, usually, after 1 hour in the acute study) this variation narrowing (to 2.1 to 3.0 ng per ml) by 24 hours, suggesting that absorption and distribution were the greatest variables. Recovery of the daily dose was double that of the initial dose with an average of about 70% in the 24-hour urine, 3.5% in the faeces, and the missing 27% might be unidentified metabolites; this 2-fold recovery on chronic administration suggested saturation of the binding sites. Peak concentrations of β-naltrexol occurred after 1 or (usually) 2 hours in both studies and concentrations of the metabolite were 1.5 to 10 times higher than those of naltrexone, this proportion not changing between the acute and the chronic phase of the study, suggesting that naltrexone did not induce its own metabolism. Plasma concentrations of naltrexone declined biexponentially with an average estimated secondary half-life of about 10.3 hours in the acute study, and 9.7 hours in the chronic study; there was a third extremely low phase with an estimated half-life of 96 hours. Although naltrexone is considered a nearly pure antagonist, a slight agonist effect was noted on the pupil, this being signifcantly greater in the chronic phase of the study; the metabolite responsible for this was not known.— K. Verebey *et al.*, *Clin. Pharmac. Ther.*, 1976, *20,* 315.

Further references: K. Verebey *et al.*, *Res. Commun. chem. Path. Pharmac.*, 1975, *12,* 67; E. J. Cone *et al.*, *J. pharm. Sci.*, 1975, *64,* 618; E. J. Cone *et al.*, *Res. Commun. chem. Path. Pharmac.*, 1978, *20,* 413.

Protein binding. The *in vitro* binding of naltrexone in human plasma was about 20%.— T. M. Ludden *et al.*, *J. pharm. Sci.*, 1976, *65,* 712.

Uses. Naltrexone hydrochloride is a narcotic antagonist that can be given by mouth. It has a much longer duration of action than naloxone. Naltrexone hydrochloride has been given to former diamorphine addicts to prevent relapse in doses of 50 mg daily. Alternate-day therapy has been tried.

Naltrexone was about 17 times as potent as nalorphine and did not cause dysphoria. Its duration of action was longer than that of naloxone and shorter than that of cyclazocine. A daily dose of 50 mg by mouth caused blockade of the effects of morphine and diamorphine comparable with that caused by cyclazocine 4 mg daily.— W. R. Martin *et al.*, *Archs gen. Psychiat.*, 1973, *28,* 784.

Studies in the effect of single doses of naltrexone 20 to 160 mg in 8 ex-addict subjects.— E. R. Gritz *et al.*, *Clin. Pharmac. Ther.*, 1976, *19,* 773.

Further references: P. F. Renault, *Bull. Narcot.*, 1978, *30* (Apr.–June), 21; *Archs gen. Psychiat.*, 1978, *35,* 335.

Manufacturers

Endo, USA.

Neostigmine and other Parasympathomimetics

4500-x

Parasympathomimetic agents may be classified into 2 distinct pharmacological groups:
The true *parasympathomimetics* or cholinomimetics, typified by the choline esters and pilocarpine, which produce the effects of parasympathetic nerve stimulation. They possess the muscarinic rather than the nicotinic effects of acetylcholine (see p.1037). They include: bethanechol, p.1037, carbachol, p.1038, methacholine, p.1042, and pilocarpine, p.1044.
Anticholinesterases, which inhibit the enzymic hydrolysis of acetylcholine by cholinesterases. Consequently acetylcholine accumulates and its actions are prolonged and intensified. Some anticholinesterases react *'reversibly'* with cholinesterases; such drugs include: ambenonium, p.1037, galantamine, p.1041, neostigmine, p.1035, physostigmine, p.1042, and pyridostigmine, p.1045. Other anticholinesterases react *'irreversibly'* with cholinesterases; such drugs include: demecarium, p.1039, dyflos, p.1039, ecothiopate, p.1040, and pyrophos, p.1046.

4501-r

Neostigmine Bromide *(B.P., Eur. P., U.S.P.).*

Neostig. Brom.; Neostigmini Bromidum; Neostigminii Bromidum; Neostigminum Bromatum; Synstigmine Bromide. 3-(Dimethylcarbamoyloxy)-*NNN*-trimethylanilinium bromide.
$C_{12}H_{19}BrN_2O_2$=303.2.

CAS — 59-99-4 (neostigmine); 114-80-7 (bromide).

Pharmacopoeias. In *Aust., Br., Braz., Chin., Cz., Eur., Fr., Ger., Hung., Ind., Int., It., Jug., Mex., Neth., Nord., Roum., Swiss, Turk.,* and *U.S.*

Odourless colourless crystals or a white crystalline, slightly hygroscopic powder with a bitter taste. M.p. 171° to 176° with decomposition.
Soluble 1 in 0.5 of water, 1 in 8 of alcohol, and 1 in 5 of chloroform; practically insoluble in ether. A solution in water is neutral to litmus. Solutions are **sterilised** by autoclaving (adjusted to pH 4 to 6) or by filtration. **Incompatible** with alkalis and iodine. **Store** in airtight containers. Protect from light.

Neostigmine ointment 5% was effectively sterilised by irradiation at 45 000 Gy; the content of neostigmine bromide was slightly reduced but no degradation products could be detected by thin-layer chromatography.— B. P. Jacob and K. Leupin, *Pharm. Acta Helv.*, 1974, *49*, 12.

Adverse Effects, Treatment, and Precautions. As for Neostigmine Methylsulphate, below.

A fatality in a 9-year-old child who received 15 mg of neostigmine daily for megacolon was considered due to a period of constipation which allowed the normal daily dose to remain in the gastro-intestinal tract. When normal gastro-intestinal motility was achieved, absorption of a lethal dose occurred. It was recommended that neostigmine doses be withheld if megacolon patients became constipated for longer than 2 or 3 days.— J. C. Briggs *et al.*, *Br. med. J.*, 1969, *4*, 344.

Absorption and Fate. See Neostigmine Methylsulphate, below.

In 3 fasting myasthenic patients given a single dose of neostigmine 30 mg, peak plasma concentrations (range 4 to 9 ng per ml) occurred 1 to 2 hours after administration and the mean plasma half-life was 0.87 hours (range 0.71 to 1.00 hours). Comparison of these data with those obtained from 4 non-myasthenic patients given neostigmine intravenously indicated a bioavailability of 1 to 2% for neostigmine administered orally. In a further 4 myasthenic patients the plasma-neostigmine concentration 4 hours after the first dose of the day was about 3 ng per ml in 3 patients receiving repeated doses of neostigmine 15 mg with pyridostigmine 60 mg and was about 10 times higher (20 to 40 ng per ml) in the fourth patient who received repeated doses of neostigmine 150 mg with pyridostigmine 60 mg.— S. -M. Aquilonius *et al.*, *Eur. J. clin. Pharmac.*, 1979, *15*, 367.

Uses. Neostigmine bromide has the actions and uses of neostigmine (see Neostigmine Methylsulphate). Neostigmine bromide 15 mg by mouth is reported to be approximately equivalent to neostigmine methylsulphate 0.5 to 1 mg subcutaneously or intramuscularly.
It is given by mouth in the treatment of myasthenia gravis usually in daily doses of 75 to 300 mg although more may be required; the dose should be divided throughout the day and, if necessary, the night according to the response of the patient and larger portions of the total daily dose may be given at times of greater fatigue. Atropine sulphate 500 µg thrice daily, or another anticholinergic, may be given thrice daily to afford relief from side-effects; these may also be minimised by taking neostigmine bromide with meals to slow absorption although in severe cases neostigmine may be required before meals to permit swallowing of an adequate amount of food.
The action of neostigmine on myasthenia gravis may be enhanced by concomitant administration of ephedrine hydrochloride.

Both myasthenia gravis and schizophrenia in a 12-year-old boy were successfully treated with neostigmine bromide 15 mg four times daily.— R. C. Schnackenberg and G. Holmes, *Am. J. Psychiat.*, 1977, *134*, 1025.

Pregnancy and the neonate. Reports of the use of neostigmine bromide in the treatment of heartburn of pregnancy.— M. Dumont and P. Bourbon, *Presse méd.*, 1950, *58*, 646; D. Bower, *J. Obstet. Gynaec. Br. Commonw.*, 1960, *68*, 846.

Preparations

Injectabile Neostigmini *(Nord. P.).* Neostigmine Injection. A sterile aqueous solution of neostigmine bromide 0.05%, sodium chloride 0.9%, and 0.1M hydrochloric acid 0.1%. *Dan. Disp.* specifies 1% w/v benzyl alcohol as preservative.
A similar preparation is included in the *Swiss. P.*

Neostigmine Bromide Tablets *(U.S.P.).* Tablets containing neostigmine bromide. Store in airtight containers.

Neostigmine Tablets *(B.P.).* Neostig. Tab. Tablets containing neostigmine bromide. Protect from light.

Proprietary Preparations

Prostigmin Tablets *(Roche, UK).* Scored tablets each containing neostigmine bromide 15 mg. (Also available as Prostigmin in *Austral., Canad., Denm., Ger., Neth., Norw., S.Afr., Swed., Switz., USA*).

Other Proprietary Names

Juvastigmin *(Austral., Switz.)*; Prostigmina *(Ital.)*; Prostigmine *(Belg., Fr.)*.

See also under Neostigmine Methylsulphate.

4502-f

Neostigmine Methylsulphate *(B.P.).*

Neostig. Methylsulph.; Neostigmine Methylsulfate *(U.S.P.)*; Neostigmini Methylsulfas; Proserinum.
$C_{13}H_{22}N_2O_6S$=334.4.

CAS — 51-60-5.

Pharmacopoeias. In *Arg., Aust., Br., Braz., Chin., Ger., Hung., Ind., Int., It., Jap., Jug., Mex., Pol., Port., Rus., Turk.,* and *U.S.*

Odourless colourless crystals or a white crystalline powder with a bitter taste. M.p. 144° to 149°.
Soluble 1 in 0.5 of water and 1 in 6 of alcohol. A solution in water is neutral to litmus. A 5.22% solution is iso-osmotic with serum. Solutions are **sterilised** by autoclaving or by filtration. **Store** in airtight containers. Protect from light.

Adverse Effects. Side-effects include salivation, anorexia, nausea and vomiting, abdominal cramps and diarrhoea. Symptoms of overdosage include sweating, lachrymation, watery nasal discharge, eructation, involuntary defaecation and urination, flushing, miosis, conjunctival congestion, ciliary spasm, brow ache, nystagmus, restlessness, agitation, fear, excessive dreaming, increased bronchial secretion combined with bronchoconstriction, bradycardia and hypotension, muscle cramps, scattered fasciculations and eventually severe weakness and paralysis, convulsions, and coma.
It has also been stated that paradoxical effects could occur due to interaction between nicotinic and muscarinic actions; a consequence of this could be some evidence of an acceleration of pulse-rate and elevation of blood pressure. Death may follow due to cardiac arrest or central respiratory paralysis and pulmonary oedema. The major symptom of overdosage in myasthenia gravis is increased muscular weakness.

Treatment of Adverse Effects. If neostigmine has been taken by mouth the stomach should be emptied by aspiration and lavage. Give atropine sulphate 1 to 2 mg intravenously, intramuscularly, or subcutaneously to control the muscarinic effects. This dose may be repeated every 2 to 4 hours as necessary. Supportive treatment includes intravenous administration of diazepam 5 to 10 mg; muscle twitching may be controlled with small doses of tubocurarine (together with assisted respiration); oxygen may be required.

Precautions. Neostigmine methylsulphate is contra-indicated in mechanical intestinal or urinary obstruction. When it is given by injection, atropine should always be available to counteract any reactions in patients excessively susceptible to the action of neostigmine.
Neostigmine methylsulphate should be used with caution in patients with bradycardia, bronchial asthma, cardiac disease, epilepsy, hypotension, parkinsonism, or peptic ulceration. It should not be used in conjunction with depolarising muscle relaxants such as suxamethonium. It should not be used during cyclopropane or halothane anaesthesia although it may be used after withdrawal of these agents.
Neostigmine methylsulphate should be used with caution in patients with myasthenia gravis to avoid provoking a cholinergic crisis with increased muscular weakness.
Parasympathomimetics should not be given by injection to patients with diabetes or gangrene.

In 83 patients with chronic ulcerative colitis, postoperative leakage from ileorectal anastomoses occurred in 12 out of 33 who received neostigmine during the anaesthetic to reverse the muscle relaxant compared with 2 leakages out of 50 who did not receive neostigmine.— C. M. A. Bell and C. B. Lewis, *Br. med. J.*, 1968, *3*, 587.

An intravenous injection of 2 to 2.5 mg of neostigmine with, or preceded by 0.6 to 1.2 mg of atropine, greatly increased bowel activity in unanaesthetised patients and in 38% of patients anaesthetised with anaesthetics other than halothane. In the patients anaesthetised with 1 to 2% of halothane, bowel activity was reduced. It was suggested that recently constructed ileorectal anastomoses were particularly at risk when neostigmine was used to reverse muscle relaxation; atropine did not reduce the risk.— J. L. Wilkins *et al.*, *Br. med. J.*, 1970, *1*, 793.

Interactions. Severe bradycardia occurred after simultaneous administration of atropine and neostigmine, to reverse pancuronium-induced neuromuscular blockade, in a patient on long-term propranolol therapy.— D. H. Sprague, *Anesthesiology*, 1975, *42*, 208.

The modification of glucocorticoid action in patients with myasthenia gravis by anticholinesterase.— W. Jubiz and A. W. Meikle, *Drugs*, 1979, *18*, 113.

Reversal of neuromuscular blockade. The neuromuscular block induced by tubocurarine, metocurine, or gallamine, during halothane anaesthesia was antagonised by a single dose of neostigmine preceded by atropine but was potentiated by a second dose given 2 to 3 minutes later. A possible explanation was that the tetanus had fully recovered after the first dose and that the second dose was acting on normal unblocked muscle. It was suggested that neostigmine in doses used clinically may produce an acetylcholine-induced block which could be a potential hazard in clinical anaesthesia.— R. Hughes *et al.*, *Br. J. Anaesth.*, 1979, *51*, 568P. See also R. Hughes and J. P. Payne, *Br. J. Anaesth.*, 1977, *49*, 1172; J. P. Payne *et al.*, *ibid.*, 1980, *52*, 69.

Absorption and Fate. Neostigmine is poorly absorbed from the gastro-intestinal tract. It is metabolised partly by hydrolysis of the ester linkage.

When neostigmine was given by mouth to 2 patients with myasthenia gravis less then 5% was found unchanged in the urine; after intramuscular injection up to 67% was found unchanged in the urine.— P. T. Nowell *et al.*, *Br. J. Pharmac. Chemother.*, 1962, *18*, 617.

Neostigmine was rapidly eliminated from the plasma of 5 patients to whom 5 mg of the methylsulphate had been given to antagonise residual neuromuscular block. The plasma concentration of neostigmine declined to about 8% of its initial value after 5 minutes with a distribution half-life of less than one minute. Elimination half-life ranged from about 15 to 30 minutes. Trace amounts of neostigmine could be detected in the plasma after one hour.— N. E. Williams *et al.*, *Br. J. Anaesth.*, 1978, *50*, 1065.

In 4 non-myasthenic patients given neostigmine 2.5 or 3 mg intravenously to antagonise the neuromuscular block after general surgery the mean plasma half-life of neostigmine was 0.89 hours (range 0.79 to 1.01 hours).— S. -M. Aquilonius *et al.*, *Eur. J. clin. Pharmac.*, 1979, *15*, 367.

In patients with myasthenia gravis given a single dose of neostigmine methylsulphate intramuscularly the mean plasma half-life was 71.9 minutes. Approximately 50% of the dose was eliminated unchanged in the urine within 24 hours with 15% appearing as 3-hydroxyphenyltrimethylammonium and about 15% as other metabolites. It was suggested that metabolism and biliary excretion may play significant roles in the elimination of neostigmine.— S. M. Somani *et al.*, *Clin. Pharmac. Ther.*, 1980, *28*, 64.

Further references.— T. N. Calvey *et al.*, *Br. J. clin. Pharmac.*, 1979, *7*, 149; R. Cronnelly *et al.*, *Anesthesiology*, 1979, *51*, 222.

Uses. Neostigmine inhibits cholinesterase activity and prolongs and intensifies the muscarinic and nicotinic effects of acetylcholine (see p.1037). It probably also has direct effects on skeletal muscle fibres. The anticholinesterase actions of neostigmine are reversible. It is used mainly for its action on skeletal muscle, and less frequently to increase the activity of smooth muscle.

Neostigmine methylsulphate is used in the treatment of myasthenia gravis in usual doses of 1 to 2.5 mg daily given in divided doses by subcutaneous, intramuscular, or intravenous injection according to the severity of the condition. Larger doses may sometimes be required. Whenever possible treatment should be by mouth with neostigmine bromide (see p.1035). It has also been used intramuscularly with atropine sulphate in the diagnosis of myasthenia gravis. If the muscarinic effects of neostigmine are troublesome, they can be controlled by prior administration of atropine by mouth or by injection. Neostigmine methylsulphate is also used to curtail the muscular relaxation produced by non-depolarising muscle relaxants such as tubocurarine and gallamine; for adults the usual dose is 2 to 3 mg given concomitantly with 0.6 to 1.2 mg of atropine sulphate by slow intravenous injection over a period of 60 seconds. Additional neostigmine may be given until the muscle power is normal but a total of 5 mg should not be exceeded. The recommended ratio of atropine to neostigmine given varies from 1:2 to 1:3. A suggested dose for children is 50 µg per kg body-weight. Lower doses of neostigmine are used in the USA.

It is also used in the treatment of paralytic ileus and postoperative urinary retention, in doses of 0.5 to 1 mg. For expelling intestinal flatus prior to radiography of the gall-bladder, kidneys, or ureters, a single dose of 500 µg has sometimes been used.

A solution containing from 3 to 5% has been instilled to lower intra-ocular pressure in the treatment of glaucoma.

Adjunct to bowel X-ray. In 77% of 96 adults and 1 child given neostigmine methylsulphate 500 to 750 µg by subcutaneous or intramuscular injection immediately after radiological examination of the stomach and duodenum, filling of the terminal ileum and caecum with contrast agent occurred within 1 hour. Increasing the dose to 1 mg did not significantly improve the effect. Changes of the mucous membranes were not observed.— J. H. A. Müller, *Dte GesundhWes.*, 1968, *23*, 391.

Administration in renal failure. Studies during anaesthesia indicated that the mean serum elimination half-life of neostigmine was 79.8 minutes in 8 patients with normal renal function but was prolonged to a mean of 181.1 minutes in 4 anephric patients.— R. Cronnelly *et al.*, *Anesthesiology*, 1979, *51*, 222.

The interval between doses of neostigmine should be extended from 6 hours to 12 to 18 hours in patients with a glomerular filtration-rate of less than 10 ml per minute.— W. M. Bennett *et al.*, *Ann. intern. Med.*, 1980, *93*, 286.

Diagnosis of neuromuscular disorders. Neostigmine 1 mg intramuscularly, with atropine 600 µg to lessen side-reactions, was used in the differential diagnosis of neuromuscular disease by observing the occurrence of muscle fasciculations at 30-minute intervals for 2 hours. Fasciculations occurred in 51 of 66 patients with neurogenic atrophy, none of 52 with myopathy, and 7 of 104 control subjects.— A. N. Patel and R. K. Swami, *New Engl. J. Med.*, 1969, *281*, 523.

Myasthenia gravis. A detailed account of the nature of myasthenia gravis and its management.— D. B. Drachman, *New Engl. J. Med.*, 1978, *298*, 136 and 186.

Further reviews, studies, and comments on the treatment of myasthenia gravis using anticholinesterases.— W. Flacke, *New Engl. J. Med.*, 1973, *288*, 27; C. W. H. Havard, *Br. med. J.*, 1973, *3*, 437; J. C. Walsh, *Med. J. Aust.*, 1974, *1*, 997; A. B. Loach *et al.*, *Br. med. J.*, 1975, *1*, 309; C. W. H. Havard, *ibid.*, 1975, *4*, 152; D. Grob, *A. Rev. Pharmac. & Toxic.*, 1976, *16*, 215; *Drug & Ther. Bull.*, 1977, *15*, 29; C. W. H. Havard, *Br. med. J.*, 1977, *2*, 1008.

An infant born to a woman suffering from myasthenia gravis was diagnosed as suffering from neonatal myasthenia gravis. The child responded to neostigmine methylsulphate intramuscularly. After 2 weeks sucking pressures before and after edrophonium chloride were the same and electromyelographic recording confirmed the absence of muscle weakness. Neostigmine therapy was discontinued without ill-effect.— A. A. Hutchison *et al.*, *Br. med. J.*, 1975, *4*, 623.

The management of myasthenia gravis in a 6-month-old child with neostigmine and pyridostigmine.— F. Oberklaid and I. J. Hopkins, *Archs Dis. Childh.*, 1976, *51*, 719.

The continuous subcutaneous injection of neostigmine, in doses of up to 50 mg daily, was helpful in the control of severe myasthenia gravis in a 27-year-old woman.— J. P. Bingle *et al.*, *Br. med. J.*, 1979, *1*, 1050.

With plasmaphaeresis. Reports and comments on the treatment of myasthenia gravis with anticholinesterases in association with plasmaphaeresis.— P. C. Dau *et al.*, *New Engl. J. Med.*, 1977, *297*, 1134; J. Newsom-Davis *et al.* (letter), *ibid.*, 1978, *298*, 456; P. C. Dau *et al.* (letter), *ibid.*, 457; J. Keesey (letter), *ibid.*, 1029; J. Newsom-Davis *et al.*, *Lancet*, 1979, *1*, 464; P. O. Behan *et al.*, *ibid.*, 1979, *2*, 438; P. Kornfeld *et al.* (letter), *ibid.*, 629.

Pregnancy and the neonate. A report of the use of neostigmine in the treatment of heartburn of pregnancy.— C. L. Sullivan, *Am. J. Obstet. Gynec.*, 1950, *60*, 205.

See also under Myasthenia Gravis, above.

Reversal of neuromuscular blockade. When reversal of curarisation in 31 patients was undertaken using simultaneous intravenous injections of atropine 20 µg per kg body-weight and neostigmine 50 µg per kg, no serious cardiac hazards were encountered if hyperventilation was maintained throughout the recovery period.— A. Baraka, *Br. J. Anaesth.*, 1968, *40*, 30. See also *idem.*, 27.

Simultaneous injection of atropine with neostigmine intravenously over 60 seconds appeared to be the most suitable method for the reversal of neuromuscular blockade.— V. Rosner *et al.*, *Br. J. Anaesth.*, 1971, *43*, 1066.

No undesirable haemodynamic side-effects occurred in 20 children in whom tubocurarine-induced neuromuscular blockade was reversed with neostigmine 50 µg per kg body-weight and atropine 20 µg per kg.— M. R. Salem *et al.*, *Br. J. Anaesth.*, 1977, *49*, 901.

For references to the use of glycopyrronium bromide with neostigmine for reversing neuromuscular block, see Glycopyrronium Bromide, p.301.

See also under Precautions (above).

Snake bite. Neostigmine 500 µg intravenously, repeated on 2 occasions, was successfully used in the treatment of snake bite [probably cobra] in a 10-year-old child; it was considered to have reversed respiratory paralysis caused by the neurotoxin component of the venom.— R. W. Naphade and R. N. Shetti, *Br. J. Anaesth.*, 1977, *49*, 1065. Neostigmine would be of no value in the treatment of bites from snakes of which the venom has neurotoxins which act presynaptically, including the Asian krait, the Australian tiger snake, and the taipan.— T. Brophy and S. K. Sutherland (letter), *Br. J. Anaesth.*, 1979, *51*, 264.

Use in paraplegics. A discussion of the intrathecal use of neostigmine methylsulphate in a test of impotence in paraplegics.— L. Guttmann and J. J. Walsh, *Paraplegia*, 1971, *9*, 39.

Preparations

Neostigmine Injection *(B.P.)*. Neostig. Inj. A sterile solution of neostigmine methylsulphate in Water for Injections. Sterilised by autoclaving. pH 4.5 to 6.5. Protect from light.

Neostigmine Methylsulfate Injection *(U.S.P.)*. A sterile solution of neostigmine methylsulphate in Water for Injections. pH 5 to 6.5. Protect from light.

Prostigmin Injection *(Roche, UK)*. Contains neostigmine methylsulphate 0.5 or 2.5 mg per ml, in ampoules of 1 ml. (Also available as Prostigmin in *Austral.*, *Canad.*, *Denm.*, *Ger.*, *Neth.*, *Norw.*, *S.Afr.*, *Swed.*, *Switz.*, *USA*).

Other Proprietary Names

Intrastigmina *(Ital.)*; Juvastigmin *(Austral., Switz.)*; Prostigmina *(Ital.)*; Prostigmine *(Belg., Fr.)*.

See also under Neostigmine Bromide.

4503-d

Aceclidine Hydrochloride. 3-Acetoxyquinuclidine hydrochloride; 3-Quinuclidinyl acetate hydrochloride. $C_9H_{15}NO_2,HCl = 205.7$.

CAS — 827-61-2 (aceclidine); 6109-70-2 (hydrochloride).

Adverse Effects, Treatment, and Precautions. As for Neostigmine Methylsulphate, p.1035.

A study indicating that usual therapeutic doses of aceclidine strongly interfere with colour vision.— J. Laroche and C. Laroche, *Annls pharm. Fr.*, 1977, *35*, 173.

Uses. Aceclidine hydrochloride is a parasympathomimetic agent with little if any anticholinesterase activity. It is used to lower intra-ocular pressure in patients with open-angle glaucoma.

Aceclidine could be used in the treatment of open-angle glaucoma if pilocarpine was not tolerated or became ineffective.— J. H. Romano, *Br. J. Ophthal.*, 1970, *54*, 510.

Eye-drops containing aceclidine 4% had an effect on intra-ocular pressure similar to that of pilocarpine 2%. Eye-drops containing aceclidine 0.5 to 4% all had a duration of action of at least 7 hours.— S. M. Drance *et al.*, *Archs Ophthal., N.Y.*, 1972, *88*, 394.

Further references.— T. W. Lieberman and I. H. Leopold, *Am. J. Ophthal.*, 1967, *64*, 405; M. D. Mashkovsky and C. A. Zaitseva, *Arzneimittel-Forsch.*, 1968, *18*, 320; P. Bastide *et al.*, *ibid.*, 1968, *18*, 322.

Proprietary Names

Glaucostat *(Chibret, Belg.; Merck Sharp & Dohme-Chibret, Fr.; Bournonville, Neth.)*.

4504-n

Aceclidine Salicylate. Aceclidinum. 3-Acetoxyquinuclidine salicylate. $C_9H_{15}NO_2,C_7H_6O_3 = 307.3$.

CAS — 6821-59-6.

Pharmacopoeias. In *Rus.*

A white crystalline powder. M.p. 137° to 141°. Freely

soluble in water; soluble in alcohol; practically insoluble in ether. A 5% solution in water has a pH of 5.2 to 6.2. Solutions in water may be **sterilised** by filtration. **Store** in airtight containers. Protect from light.

Adverse Effects, Treatment, and Precautions. As for Neostigmine Methylsulphate, p.1035.

Uses. Aceclidine salicylate is a parasympathomimetic agent used to lower intra-ocular pressure in patients with open-angle glaucoma. In the USSR it is also used to enhance the tone of smooth muscles of the intestine, bladder, and uterus.

4505-h

Acetylcholine Bromide. Acetylcholini Bromidum. $C_7H_{16}BrNO_2$=226.1.

CAS — 66-23-9.

Deliquescent colourless crystals or white crystalline powder with an unpleasant smell and a saline taste. Freely **soluble** in water; soluble in alcohol; practically insoluble in ether. Decomposed by hot water and alkalis. **Store** in airtight containers. Protect from light.

Acetylcholine bromide has actions and uses similar to those of Acetylcholine Chloride.

4506-m

Acetylcholine Chloride.

Acetylcholinum Chloratum; Acetylcholinii Chloridum; Cloreto de Acetil-colina. (2-Acetoxyethyl)trimethylammonium chloride. $C_7H_{16}ClNO_2$=181.7.

CAS — 51-84-3 (acetylcholine); 60-31-1 (chloride).

Pharmacopoeias. In *Aust., Belg., Cz., Fr., Jug., Mex., Span., Swiss,* and *Turk. Jap.* includes Acetylcholine Chloride for Injection.

A white, very hygroscopic, crystalline powder with a faint amine-like odour and a sharply saline taste. M.p. about 150°.

Very **soluble** in water yielding unstable solutions; very soluble in alcohol and propylene glycol; freely soluble in chloroform and acetic acid; practically insoluble in ether. A 10% solution in water has a pH of about 5. Solutions for injection are prepared by dissolving the sterile contents of a sealed ampoule in Water for Injections immediately before use. **Incompatible** with alkalis and acids. **Store** in containers sealed by fusion of the glass. Protect from light.

Adverse Effects, Treatment, and Precautions. As for Methacholine Chloride, p.1042.

Hypotension and bradycardia developed in a 65-year-old woman immediately after the injection of acetylcholine chloride 20 mg into the anterior chamber of the eye following cataract extraction.— M. Babinski *et al., Archs Ophthal., N.Y.*, 1976, *94*, 675.

Uses. Acetylcholine is a chemical transmitter with a very wide range of actions in the body; it is a powerful quaternary ammonium parasympathomimetic agent but its action is transient as it is rapidly destroyed by cholinesterase. It is released from post-ganglionic parasympathetic nerves and also from some post-ganglionic sympathetic nerves to produce peripheral actions which correspond to those of muscarine. It is accordingly a vasodilator and cardiac depressant, its vasodilator action being most marked in the peripheral vascular areas. It is a stimulant of the vagus and parasympathetic nervous system and has a tonic action on smooth muscle; it also increases the lachrymal, salivary, and other secretions. All the muscarinic actions of acetylcholine are abolished by atropine.

Acetylcholine also has actions which correspond to those of nicotine and is accordingly a stimulant of skeletal muscle, the autonomic ganglia, and the adrenal medulla. The nicotinic actions of acetylcholine on skeletal muscle are blocked by tubocurarine; they are also inhibited by massive administration or discharge of acetylcholine itself which has clinical application in relation to the mode of action of depolarising muscle relaxants such as suxamethonium (see Muscle Relaxants, p.986).

Acetylcholine chloride is instilled as a freshly prepared 1% solution as a miotic in cataract surgery to constrict the pupil in seconds; it may also be used in penetrating keratoplasty and in simple iridectomy for glaucoma.

It has also been used in a wide variety of conditions such as Raynaud's disease, intermittent claudication, trophic ulcers, gangrene, postoperative distension and paralytic ileus, paroxysmal tachycardia, and (by subconjunctival injection) in spasm of the retinal arteries and chronic glaucoma, but with variable results, probably owing to its transient action.

Adjunct to eye surgery. The use of acetylcholine as a miotic agent was considered to be a valuable adjunct in corneal crafting from the results obtained in a study with 106 patients. Irrigated into the anterior chamber after cataract extraction, acetylcholine induced prompt and effective miosis which protected the vitreous face and facilitated the placement of corneal sutures. Solutions of 0.5 and 1% strength were considered the most effective. The miotic action was fairly short and required augmentation with a longer-acting agent such as pilocarpine.— R. D. Harley and J. E. Mishler, *Br. J. Ophthal.*, 1966, *50*, 429.

Acetylcholine chloride 1% in a solution of mannitol (Miochol) was injected into the anterior chamber of the eye as a miotic after the removal of cataractous lenses from 9 patients. It was found to induce regular, round constriction of the pupil without producing irritation or iritis, immediate or delayed. On average, a reduction in pupil size of 2.2 mm was achieved in 76.6 seconds.— G. V. Catford and E. Millis, *Br. J. Ophthal.*, 1967, *51*, 183. See also A. B. Rizzuti, *Am. J. Ophthal.*, 1967, *63*, 484.

Cardiac arrhythmias. Mention of the use of acetylcholine in the treatment of supraventricular tachycardia.— R. J. T. Woodland (letter), *Br. med. J.*, 1979, *2*, 1514.

Intermittent claudication. A report of beneficial results with acetylcholine and lignocaine in 6 patients with intermittent claudication and 3 patients with early gangrene of the toes.— R. J. T. Woodland (letter), *Br. med. J.*, 1969, *1*, 253.

Proprietary Preparations

Miochol *(CooperVision, UK).* An ophthalmic solution containing acetylcholine chloride 1% and mannitol 3%. It is prepared immediately before use by mixing the contents of 2 compartments of a Univial (a 2-chambered vial); 1 compartment contains acetylcholine chloride 20 mg and mannitol 60 mg, and the other contains 2 ml of Water for Injections. Any solution not used should be discarded. (Also available as Miochol in *Canad., Swed.*).

Other Proprietary Names

Covochol *(S.Afr.).*

4507-b

Ambenonium Chloride *(U.S.P.).*

Ambestigmini Chloridum; Win 8077. *NN'*-[Oxalylbis(iminoethylene)]bis[(2-chlorobenzyl)diethylammonium] dichloride. $C_{28}H_{42}Cl_4N_4O_2$=608.5.

CAS — 7648-98-8 (ambenonium); 115-79-7 (chloride, anhydrous); 52022-31-8 (chloride, tetrahydrate).

Pharmacopoeias. In *U.S. Rus. P.* includes the ethanolate under the title Oxazylum.

An equilibrium mixture of anhydrous material and the tetrahydrate. A white odourless powder. It loses not more than 11.5% of its weight on drying. M.p. about 200°. **Soluble** 1 in 5 of water and 1 in 20 of alcohol; slightly soluble in chloroform; practically insoluble in acetone and ether. Solutions are **sterilised** by autoclaving or by filtration. **Store** in airtight containers.

Adverse Effects, Treatment, and Precautions. As for Neostigmine Methylsulphate, see p.1035.

As there is only slight warning of overdosage routine administration of atropine with ambenonium is contra-indicated because the muscarinic symptoms of overdosage may be suppressed leaving only the more serious nicotinic effects (fasciculation and paralysis of voluntary muscle).

Acute cholinergic crises developed in 2 patients given ambenonium chloride for chronic cystitis and bladder distension. The first patient took 5 mg four times daily for about 19 days, and the second 3 doses of 10 mg over about 20 hours. Treatment consisted in the withdrawal of ambenonium and the intravenous administration of up to 1 mg of atropine. It was emphasised that neither of these patients had myasthenia nor was taking a ganglion-blocking drug.— D. B. Sachar, *New Engl. J. Med.*, 1964, *271*, 1260.

Uses. Ambenonium is an inhibitor of cholinesterase activity with actions similar to those of neostigmine (see Neostigmine Methylsulphate, p.1036), but of longer duration. Ambenonium chloride is given by mouth in the treatment of myasthenia gravis and may be of value in patients who cannot tolerate neostigmine. It is administered 3 to 4 times daily, usually in doses of 5 to 25 mg. Patients receiving a daily dosage in excess of 200 mg require careful observation for untoward effects.

Myasthenia gravis. In 33 patients with myasthenia gravis treated with ambenonium chloride 37.5 to 300 mg daily, 13 patients obtained as good or better relief with fewer side-effects than after previous anticholinesterase therapy. Two patients required atropine to treat gastro-intestinal symptoms, 1 suffered dizziness with doses of 200 to 300 mg daily, and another had abdominal pain after about 300 mg daily.— M. R. Westerberg, *Archs Neurol. Psychiat.*, 1956, *56*, 91.

Further references.— F. Nicholas, *Clin. Med.*, 1964, *71*, 1727.

Urinary retention and constipation. Twenty patients with atony of the bladder or bowel were given doses of ambenonium chloride varying from 5 mg four times daily to 25 mg thrice daily and all derived benefit.— G. M. Mahoney *et al., New Engl. J. Med.*, 1959, *260*, 1065.

Preparations

Ambenonium Chloride Tablets *(U.S.P.).* Tablets containing ambenonium chloride. Potency is expressed in terms of the anhydrous material. The *U.S.P.* requires 80% dissolution in 15 minutes. Store in airtight containers.

Mytelase *(Sterling Research, UK).* Scored tablets each containing ambenonium chloride 10 mg. (Also available as Mytelase in *Austral., Belg., Denm., Fin., Fr., Ger., Ital., Neth., Swed., Switz., USA*).

4508-v

Benzpyrinium Bromide. Benzopyrinium Bromide; Benzstigmini Bromidum. 1-Benzyl-3-dimethylcarbamoyloxypyridinium bromide. $C_{15}H_{17}BrN_2O_2$=337.2.

CAS — 587-46-2.

Benzpyrinium is an inhibitor of cholinesterase activity with actions similar to those of neostigmine (see Neostigmine Methylsulphate, p.1035) but it is slightly less potent.

It was formerly used for the treatment of postoperative intestinal atony, postoperative urinary retention, and simple delayed menstruation in doses of 2 mg intramuscularly.

4509-g

Bethanechol Chloride *(U.S.P.).*

Carbamylmethylcholine Chloride; Bethanecholi Chloridum. (2-Carbamoyloxypropyl)trimethylammonium chloride.

$C_7H_{17}ClN_2O_2$=196.7.

CAS — 674-38-4 (bethanechol); 590-63-6 (chloride).

Pharmacopoeias. In *Jap., Turk.*, and *U.S.*

Colourless or white hygroscopic crystals or white crystalline powder usually having a slight amine-like odour. There are two crystalline forms one melts at about 211° and the other at about 219°.

Soluble 1 in 1 of water and 1 in 10 of alcohol; less soluble in dehydrated alcohol; practically insoluble in chloroform and ether. A 1% solution in water has a pH of 5.5 to 6.5. A 3.05% solution is iso-osmotic with serum. **Store** in airtight containers.

Adverse Effects. As for Methacholine Chloride, p.1042. Untoward effects related to the cardiovascular system are less liable to occur.

Miliaria crystallina occurred as a complication to treatment with bethanechol in a diabetic patient. The reaction was limited to the extremities.— P. G. Rochmis and B. S. Koplon, *Archs Derm.*, 1967, *95*, 499.

Treatment of Adverse Effects. As for Neostigmine Methylsulphate, p.1035.

Precautions. As for Methacholine Chloride, p.1042. Bethanechol chloride should not be given during pregnancy. It should not be used after a gastro-intestinal anastomosis until healing has taken place, or in the presence of peritonitis or mechanical intestinal or urinary obstruction.

Uses. Bethanechol chloride is a quaternary ammonium parasympathomimetic agent with the muscarinic actions of acetylcholine (see p.1037). It is not readily inactivated by cholinesterases so that its actions are more prolonged than those of acetylcholine.

Because it has little if any nicotinic actions, bethanechol may be preferred to carbachol for the treatment of gastric retention following vagotomy, in postoperative abdominal distension, and in some forms of urinary retention, including that following surgery. It is given subcutaneously or by mouth, a dose of 5 mg subcutaneously producing a rapid but transitory increase in the tone and motility of the stomach, intestine, and urinary bladder; this amount may be repeated after 15 to 30 minutes if necessary. It should not be given by intramuscular or intravenous injection.

Doses by mouth range from 5 to 50 mg up to 4 times daily. It should be taken on an empty stomach. The beneficial effect usually occurs within 30 to 90 minutes and lasts about an hour.

Of 12 patients with chronic Chagas' disease and megacolon who showed no abnormalities after oesophageal manometric studies, 9 showed a marked increase in spontaneous activity in the lower body of the oesophagus after a subcutaneous injection of bethanechol 2.5 mg. The procedure might be of diagnostic value.— P. Heitman and J. Espinoza, *Gut*, 1969, *10*, 848.

In a controlled crossover study of 20 patients with chronic heartburn which was not effectively controlled by antacids, bethanechol 25 mg four times daily for 2 months was significantly superior to placebo in improving symptoms and decreasing the use of antacids.— R. L. Farrell *et al.*, *Ann. intern. Med.*, 1974, *80*, 573.

Treatment of reflux oesophagitis with bethanechol.— K. D. Thanik *et al.*, *Ann. intern. Med.*, 1980, *93*, 805.

Malakoplakia. Administration of bethanechol chloride 40 mg daily corrected the decreased bactericidal activity of mononuclear cells of a patient with malakoplakia and monocyte functional defects. Following surgery the patient had developed infections which had responded poorly to drainage, antibiotic therapy, and plasma, whereas during 11 months of bethanechol therapy he had suffered no fever or evidence of infection, his cutaneous sinuses and internal fistulas closed promptly, and he gained 15 kg in weight. *In vitro* the cell defect was corrected by carbachol as well as bethanechol. Although the association between malakoplakia and monocyte functional defects was not fully understood it was clear that cholinergic agonists could be helpful in the therapy of malakoplakia.— N. I. Abdou *et al.*, *New Engl. J. Med.*, 1977, *297*, 1413.

Reversal of anticholinergic action. A report of the beneficial use of bethanechol chloride to alleviate side-effects due to tricyclic antidepressant therapy in 20 patients.— H. C. Everett, *Am. J. Psychiat.*, 1975, *132*, 1202.

Blurred vision experienced by a patient receiving fluphenazine and benztropine was alleviated by the addition of bethanechol chloride 25 mg thrice daily to his therapy.— D. S. P. Schubert, *Am. J. Psychiat.*, 1979, *136*, 110.

Preparations

Bethanechol Chloride Injection *(U.S.P.)*. A sterile solution in Water for Injections. pH 5.5 to 7.5.

Bethanechol Chloride Tablets *(U.S.P.)*. Tablets containing bethanechol chloride. Store in airtight containers.

Proprietary Preparations

Mechothane *(Macarthys, UK)*. Bethanechol chloride, available as ampoules of 5 mg.

Myotonine Chloride *(Glenwood, UK)*. Bethanechol chloride, available as scored tablets of 10 and 25 mg.

Other Proprietary Names

Austral.—Urecholine, Urocarb; *Belg.*—Muscaran; *Canad.*—Duvoid, Urecholine; *Ital.*— Urecholine; *Jap.*—Besacolin; *Switz.*—Myocholine, Urecholine; *USA*—Duvoid, Myotonachol, Urecholine, Vesicholine.

4510-f

Calabar Bean *(B.P.C. 1934)*. Physostigma; Ordeal Bean; Chopnut; Fève de Calabar.

The ripe seeds of *Physostigma venenosum* (Leguminosae).

The poisonous properties of calabar bean are due chiefly to the presence, in the cotyledons only, of 0.04 to 0.3% of physostigmine. It is used only as the source of physostigmine.

4511-d

Carbachol *(U.S.P., B.P. 1973)*.

Carbach.; Carbacholum; Carbacholum Chloratum; Carbacholine; Choline Chloride Carbamate; Carbamoylcholine Chloride; Carbamylcholine Chloride. *O*-Carbamoylcholine chloride; (2-Carbamoyloxyethyl)trimethylammonium chloride.

$C_6H_{15}ClN_2O_2$=182.6.

CAS — 51-83-2.

Pharmacopoeias. In *Arg., Aust., Braz., Cz., Ind., Int., It., Mex., Nord., Rus., Swiss, Turk.*, and *U.S.*

White or faintly yellow hygroscopic crystals or crystalline powder, odourless or with a faint amine-like odour. M.p. 200° to 204° with decomposition.

Soluble 1 in 1 of water and 1 in 50 of alcohol; very slightly soluble in dehydrated alcohol, more readily soluble on boiling; practically insoluble in acetone, chloroform, and ether. Solutions in water are neutral to litmus. Solutions are **sterilised** by autoclaving or by filtration. Aqueous solutions are most stable to autoclaving when buffered to pH 3.5. Up to 5% decomposition may occur when unbuffered solutions are heated in an autoclave, and the decomposition increases the pH of the solutions; such autoclaved solutions should not be stored for more than a year. **Incompatible** with alkalis, iodine, and silver salts. **Store** in airtight containers. Protect from light.

Incompatibility. Chlorocresol (0.025 to 0.1%) and chlorbutol (0.5%) were both found to be incompatible with a solution of carbachol (0.8%) and sodium chloride (0.69%), very slight precipitates forming on heating and increasing on standing.— Pharm. Soc. Lab. Rep. No. 911, 1962.

Stability in solution. Reports of stability tests.— P. Lundgren, *Acta pharm. suec.*, 1969, *6*, 799; R. Puckett and R. D. Poe, *J. pharm. Sci.*, 1969, *58*, 602.

Adverse Effects. As for Methacholine Chloride, p.1042. Untoward effects related to the cardiovascular system are less liable to occur.

A 58-year-old man developed oesophageal rupture 2 hours after a subcutaneous injection of carbachol to relieve urinary retention. There was some delay in diagnosis and the patient died on the 24th day.— P. Cochrane, *Br. med. J.*, 1973, *1*, 463.

A report of life-threatening attacks of profuse sweating, intestinal cramps, explosive defaecation, hypothermia, hypotension, and bradycardia in a 36-year-old man due to carbachol intoxication. A 10-year-old boy had died following similar attacks associated with repeated carbachol ingestion.— B. Sangster *et al.*, *Neth. J. Med.*, 1979, *22*, 27.

Treatment of Adverse Effects. As for Neostigmine Methylsulphate, p.1035.

Precautions. As for Methacholine Chloride, p.1042.

It is recommended that carbachol should not be used as eye-drops in patients with a corneal abrasion as there may be excessive absorption.

The sensitivity of asthmatic patients to carbachol bronchoconstriction was increased when inhalation of carbachol was preceded by maximum respiratory manoeuvres. Lung-function tests involving respiratory manoeuvres probably overestimated bronchial sensitivity.— J. Orehek *et al.*, *Br. med. J.*, 1975, *1*, 123.

Uses. Carbachol is a quaternary ammonium parasympathomimetic agent with the muscarinic and nicotinic actions of acetylcholine (see p.1037). It is not readily inactivated by cholinesterases so that its actions are more prolonged than those of acetylcholine. It is given by subcutaneous injection or by mouth. It should not be given by intramuscular or intravenous injection.

Carbachol has been used in the treatment of postoperative intestinal atony and postoperative retention of urine, for which it has been given by subcutaneous injection in a dose of 250 µg repeated twice at 30-minute intervals when necessary or in doses of up to 4 mg by mouth. It has also been used to stop supraventricular paroxysmal tachycardia when all other measures have failed.

Carbachol has a miotic action and eye-drops containing 0.75 to 3% have been used to lower intra-ocular pressure in glaucoma, sometimes in conjunction with other miotics such as physostigmine.

Carbachol has also been used by intra-ocular irrigation, 0.4 to 0.5 ml of a 0.01% solution being instilled into the anterior chamber of the eye, to produce miosis after cataract surgery.

Carbachol was not considered suitable in the treatment of accommodative esotropia because of its irregular onset and short duration of action.— H. P. Williams, *Br. J. Ophthal.*, 1974, *58*, 668.

Adjunct to eye surgery. Carbachol solution 0.01% was considered to be effective and non-irritating when used as a miotic after the lens was removed in cataract surgery. In 40 patients complete miosis occurred in about 85 seconds and pupils were reduced in size from a diameter of about 6 mm to about 2.8 mm five minutes after injection.— H. Beasley *et al.*, *Archs Ophthal., N.Y.*, 1968, *80*, 39.

Effect on bowel function. An injection of carbachol increased coordinated propulsion in the bowel fourfold in healthy persons and more than tenfold in diarrhoeic or constipated patients. In patients with abnormal bowel function, big increases in multihaustral propulsion and peristalsis occurred in the colon after carbachol and haustral propulsion was diminished. Haustral propulsion was increased in healthy persons.— J. A. Ritchie, *Gut*, 1968, *9*, 502.

Truncal vagotomy in patients with chronic duodenal ulcer brought about a drop in gastric acid and pepsin production, but the stimulatory effect of a submaximal dose of carbachol, 2 µg per kg body-weight given by subcutaneous injection, was not greater after the operation than before, and its administration could not be used as the basis of a test for the completeness of vagotomy.— D. J. Cowley, *Gut*, 1972, *13*, 99.

Glaucoma. In the treatment of simple glaucoma, carbachol was considered to be a useful alternative to pilocarpine and to other miotics where resistance or intolerance had developed. Solutions of 0.75, 1.5, and 3% could be used every 4 to 8 hours.— J. J. Kanski, *Br. J. Ophthal.*, 1968, *52*, 936.

Sun-blindness. Even in comparatively late cases of sun-blindness the symptoms could in many instances be alleviated immediately by retrobulbar injections of carbachol 250 µg.— S. Gebertt, *Br. med. J.*, 1956, *1*, 95.

Preparations

Eye-drops

Carbachol Eye-drops *(B.P.C. 1973).* CAR. A sterile solution containing up to 3% of carbachol, with 0.02% of benzalkonium chloride solution, in water. Sterilised by autoclaving or by filtration or by maintaining at 98° to 100° for 30 minutes. This solution is adversely affected by alkali.

A.P.F. has carbachol 750 mg, sodium chloride 700 mg, benzalkonium chloride solution 0.02 ml, disodium edetate 50 mg, Water for Injections to 100 ml; sterilised by autoclaving.

Another formula: carbachol 800 mg, anhydrous dextrose 5 g, chlorhexidine acetate 5 mg, Water for Injections to 100 ml; sterilised by autoclaving.—P.L. Jeffs, *Australas. J. Pharm.*,1962, *43*, 1031.

Injections

Carbachol Injection *(B.P. 1973).* A sterile solution in Water for Injections, with the addition of 5% of anhydrous dextrose.

Injectabile Carbacholini *(Nord. P.).* Carbachol Injection. Carbachol 250 µg, sodium chloride 9 mg, Water for Injections to 1 ml. Sterilised by autoclaving. A suitable preservative is 0.001% phenylmercuric nitrate. *Dan. Disp.* specifies 1% w/v benzyl alcohol.

Solutions

Carbachol Intraocular Solution *(U.S.P.).* A sterile solution of carbachol in an aqueous vehicle. It contains no preservatives or antimicrobial agents. pH 5 to 7.5. Any unused portion remaining after first opening the container should be discarded. Store at 15° to 30° in airtight containers and avoid freezing.

Carbachol Ophthalmic Solution *(U.S.P.).* A sterile solution of carbachol in an iso-osmotic aqueous vehicle; it may contain suitable preservatives and antimicrobial agents. pH 5 to 7. Store in airtight containers.

Tablets

Tablettae Carbacholini *(Nord. P.).* Carbachol Tablets. Each contains carbachol 2 mg.

Proprietary Preparations

Isopto Carbachol *(Alcon, UK: Farillon, UK).* Eye-drops containing carbachol 3%, with hypromellose 1%. (Also available as Isopto Carbachol in *Austral.*, *Canad.*, *Neth.*, *Switz.* Also available as Isopto-Carbachol in *Norw.*, *S.Afr.*).

Other Proprietary Names

Denm.— Karbakolin Isopto; *Ger.*—Doryl; *Ital.*—Carbyl; *Neth.*—Doryl; *Norw.*— Miostat Carbachol; *Swed.*—Isopto-Karbakolin; *Switz.*—Doryl, Spersacarbachol.

4512-n

Demecarium Bromide *(U.S.P.).* BC 48.

3,3′-[*NN*′-Decamethylenebis(methylcarbamoyloxy)]bis(*NNN*-trimethylanilinium) dibromide.

$C_{32}H_{52}Br_2N_4O_4$=716.6.

CAS — 56-94-0.

Pharmacopoeias. In *U.S.*

A white or slightly yellow, slightly hygroscopic, crystalline powder. M.p. 163° to 168° with decomposition. Freely **soluble** in water and alcohol; soluble in ether; sparingly soluble in acetone. A 1% solution in water has a pH of 5 to 7. Solutions may be **sterilised** by autoclaving or by filtration. **Store** in airtight containers. Protect from light.

Adverse Effects. As for Neostigmine Methylsulphate, p.1035. Demecarium is an 'irreversible' cholinesterase inhibitor and the toxic effects may be prolonged.

Treatment of Adverse Effects. As for Organophosphorus Insecticides, p.833. Pralidoxime has been reported to be more active in counteracting the effects of dyflos and ecothiopate than of demecarium.

Precautions. As for Dyflos, p.1039.

Uses. Demecarium is an inhibitor of cholinesterase with actions similar to those of dyflos (see p.1040). Its miotic action begins within about 20 minutes of its application and may persist for a week or more. It causes a reduction in intra-ocular pressure which is maximal in 24 hours and may persist for 9 days or more. It may be administered in aqueous solution.

Demecarium bromide is used in the treatment of open-angle glaucoma by local instillation into the affected eye. The dosage varies from 1 to 2 drops of a 0.25% solution twice weekly, preferably at bedtime, to 1 or 2 drops twice daily. It may be used alone or in conjunction with other topical agents or with a systemically administered carbonic anhydrase inhibitor.

Demecarium bromide has also been used in the management of accommodative convergent strabismus (esotropia).

Glaucoma. Demecarium bromide in 0.1, 0.25, and 0.5% solution was used to treat 106 eyes of 59 patients, the frequency being from twice weekly to twice daily. Intra-ocular pressure was controlled in most cases where other treatment had failed. The trial showed that the lower concentrations should be used and the frequency adapted to the individual but never more than twice daily.— N. Krishna and I. H. Leopold, *Am. J. Ophthal.*, 1960, *49*, 554.

Preparations

Demecarium Bromide Ophthalmic Solution *(U.S.P.).* A sterile aqueous solution of demecarium bromide with a suitable antimicrobial agent. pH 5 to 7.5. Store in airtight containers. Protect from light.

Tosmilen *(Sinclair, UK).* Demecarium bromide, available as eye-drops containing 0.25 and 0.5% in aqueous solution. (Also available as Tosmilen in *Austral.*, *Denm.*, *Ger.*, *Neth.*, *Switz.*).

Other Proprietary Names

Humorsol *(USA)*; Tonilen *(Spain)*; Tosmilène *(Fr.)*; Visumiotic *(Arg.)*.

4513-h

Distigmine Bromide. BC 51; Hexamarium Bromide; Bispyridostigmine Bromide. 1,1′-Dimethyl-3,3′-[*NN*′-hexamethylenebis(methylcarbamoyloxy)]dipyridinium dibromide.

$C_{22}H_{32}Br_2N_4O_4$=576.3.

CAS — 15876-67-2.

A crystalline powder. Freely **soluble** in water. Solutions are **sterilised** by autoclaving.

Adverse Effects, Treatment, and Precautions. As for Neostigmine Methylsulphate, p.1035.

A faecal fistula developed in a patient who was treated with distigmine bromide on the thirteenth day after extra-peritoneal anterior resection. He suddenly passed bright blood per rectum and developed left suprapubic pain with evidence of an anastomotic leak.— E. G. Muir, *Proc. R. Soc. Med.*, 1968, *61*, 401.

Absorption and Fate. Distigmine is poorly absorbed from the gastro-intestinal tract. It has been stated that 1 to 2% of a dose by mouth is excreted in the urine in 24 hours compared with 50% of a dose given intramuscularly.

Uses. Distigmine is an inhibitor of cholinesterase with actions similar to those of neostigmine (see Neostigmine Methylsulphate, p.1036) but of longer duration. Maximum inhibition of plasma cholinesterase occurs 9 hours after a single intramuscular dose, and persists for about 24 hours. It is used in the prevention and treatment of postoperative intestinal atony and urinary retention; 500 µg of distigmine bromide may be injected intramuscularly about 12 hours after surgery and may be repeated every 24 hours until normal function is restored. Distigmine bromide may also be given by mouth in a dose of 5 mg daily thirty minutes before breakfast.

Distigmine bromide in conjunction with short-acting parasympathomimetics has been given for the treatment of myasthenia gravis, but should only be given by mouth. Doses of up to 20 mg daily for adults and 10 mg daily for children have been used.

In 36 adult males with neurogenic bladders (upper motor neurone type), distigmine bromide 500 µg intramuscularly produced a significant reduction in bladder size within 25 minutes in 15. Of the remaining patients 10 had demonstrable urinary-tract obstruction. In 7 patients with lower motor neurone type neurogenic bladders, a significant response occurred in 1 patient.— J. Yeo *et al.*, *Med. J. Aust.*, 1974, *2*, 201. See also *idem*, 1973, *1*, 116.

Myasthenia gravis. Twelve of 17 patients with myasthenia gravis benefited from treatment with distigmine bromide 5 to 15 mg daily usually given in conjunction with short-acting supplementary drugs.— E. Hokkanen, *Nord. Med.*, 1966, *76*, 937.

Proprietary Preparations

Ubretid *(Berk Pharmaceuticals, UK).* Distigmine bromide, available in 1-ml **Ampoules** of an injection containing 500 µg per ml and as scored **Tablets** of 5 mg. (Also available as Ubretid in *Austral.*, *Ger.*, *Neth.*, *S.Afr.*, *Switz.*).

4514-m

Dyflos *(B.P.C. 1968).* Isoflurophate *(U.S.P.)*; DFP; Di-isopropyl Flurophosphate; Di-isopropylfluorophosphonate; Fluostigmin. Di-isopropyl phosphorofluoridate.

$C_6H_{14}FO_3P$=184.1.

CAS — 55-91-4.

Pharmacopoeias. In *Arg.* and *U.S.*

A clear, colourless, or faintly yellow, almost odourless, mobile liquid. Relative density about 1.05. **Soluble** 1 in 65 of water; soluble in alcohol, chloroform, ether, and vegetable oils. Solutions in water are unstable and are hydrolysed, with the evolution of hydrogen fluoride, to the extent of 50% in 16 hours. **Store** at 8° to 15° in sealed containers.

CAUTION. *The vapour of dyflos is very toxic and only solutions in arachis oil should be used therapeutically. Contaminated material should be immersed in a 2% aqueous solution of sodium hydroxide for several hours. Dyflos can be removed from the skin by washing with soap and water.*

Adverse Effects. As for Neostigmine Methylsulphate, p.1035.

Dyflos is an 'irreversible' cholinesterase inhibitor and the toxic effects may be prolonged.

Systemic toxicity occurs after inhalation of the vapour.

A review and discussion on the use of miotics and the incidence of retinal detachment.— J. J. Alpar, *Ann. Ophthal.*, 1979, *11*, 395. See also H. Beasley and F. T. Fraunfelder, *Ophthalmology*, 1979, *86*, 95.

Treatment of Adverse Effects. As for Organophosphorus Insecticides, p.833.

Precautions. Pain, headache, and dimness of vision may occur during the first few days of treatment. Dyflos and other 'irreversible' anticholinesterases should be used with caution in acutely ill and allergic patients. It should not be used simultaneously with acetylcholine and should not be used in patients with bronchial asthma, cardiac disease, parkinsonism, peptic ulceration, epilepsy, bradycardia, intestinal or urinary-tract obstruction, or hypotension.

Dyflos is also contra-indicated in acute closed-angle glaucoma since a further rise in intra-ocular pressure is more likely to occur. It should not be used when there is retinal damage. Treatment with dyflos carries a high risk of the development of cataracts. Iris cysts occur fairly frequently in children and may be prevented by the concurrent administration of adrenaline or phenylephrine eye-drops.

Dyflos reduces serum cholinesterase activity and enhances the effects of depolarising muscle relaxants such as suxamethonium; cyclopropane or halothane anaesthesia should not be used until the effects have worn off. There is a risk of hyphaemia if ophthalmic surgery is carried out on treated patients. The effects of 'irreversible' anticholinesterases may be antagonised by the prior administration of physostigmine or neostigmine.

Absorption and Fate. Dyflos is readily absorbed from the gastro-intestinal tract, from skin and mucous membranes, and from the lungs. Dyflos interacts with cholinesterases producing stable phosphonylated and phosphorylated derivatives which are then hydrolysed by phosphorylphosphatases. These products of hydrolysis are excreted mainly in the urine with less than 5% appearing in the faeces; phosphorus-containing metabolites persist in the body for more than 10 days.

Uses. Dyflos is an inhibitor of cholinesterase with actions similar to those of neostigmine (see Neostigmine Methylsulphate, p.1036) but much more prolonged. Unlike neostigmine it combines irreversibly with cholinesterases. Dyflos has a more powerful miotic action which begins within 5 to 10 minutes and may persist for 2 to 4 weeks; it causes a reduction in intra-ocular pressure which is maximal in 24 hours and may persist for a week.

Dyflos has been used mainly in the treatment of glaucoma, particularly in simple glaucoma and glaucoma following cataract extraction. It has usually been employed as a 0.1% solution in arachis oil, 1 drop having been instilled into the conjunctival sac once or twice daily. Where a single daily instillation is sufficient, the inconvenience of ciliary spasm may be avoided by using the drops at night before retiring.

Dyflos has also been used, usually as a 0.025% ointment, in the management of accommodative convergent strabismus (esotropia).

Dyflos was formerly administered intramuscularly in the treatment of myasthenia gravis and paralytic ileus but has been superseded by cholinesterase inhibitors with a less prolonged action.

Preparations

Dyflos Eye Drops *(A.P.F.)*. DFP Eye Drops. Strong dyflos eye-drops 25 ml, arachis oil, freed from moisture by heating at 120° and sterilised by maintaining at 160° for 2 hours, to 100 ml. Prepared aseptically. Protect from moisture.

Dyflos Eye Drops Strong *(A.P.F.)*. Strong DFP Eye Drops. Dyflos 0.1% in arachis oil, freed from moisture by heating at 120° and sterilised by maintaining at 160° for 2 hours. Prepared aseptically. Protect from moisture.

Isoflurophate Ophthalmic Ointment *(U.S.P.)*. A sterile eye ointment containing dyflos 0.0225 to 0.0275% in a suitable anhydrous basis.

Proprietary Names

DFP-Oel *(Winzer, Ger.)*; Diflupyl *(Labaz, Fr.; Labaz, Neth.)*; Floropryl *(Merck Sharp & Dohme, USA)*.

4515-b

Ecothiopate Iodide *(B.P.)*.

Echothiophate Iodide *(U.S.P.)*; Echothiopate Iodide; Ecostigmine Iodide; MI 217. (2-Diethoxyphosphinylthioethyl)trimethylammonium iodide.

$C_9H_{23}INO_3PS$=383.2.

CAS — 6736-03-4 (ecothiopate); 513-10-0 (iodide).

Pharmacopoeias. In *Br.* and *U.S.*

A white crystalline hygroscopic powder with an alliaceous odour. M.p. about 119° with decomposition. **Soluble** 1 in 1 of water, 1 in 25 of alcohol, and 1 in 3 of methyl alcohol; practically insoluble in other organic solvents. A solution in water has a pH of about 4. **Store** at 2° to 8° in airtight containers. Protect from light.

Stability in solution. Degradation of ecothiopate iodide was at a minimum below pH 5 and had a first-order reaction-rate. Below pH 5 degradation products included ethanol and above pH 9 (2-mercaptoethyl)trimethylammonium iodide.— A. Hussain *et al., J. pharm. Sci.*, 1968, *57*, 411.

Adverse Effects. As for Neostigmine Methylsulphate, p.1035.

Ecothiopate is an 'irreversible' cholinesterase inhibitor and the toxic effects may be prolonged. Plasma and erythrocyte cholinesterases may be diminished by treatment with ecothiopate eye-drops. Acute iritis or precipitation of acute glaucoma may occasionally follow treatment with ecothiopate.

Cholinergic crisis. A 57-year-old man with glaucoma who had been using ecothiopate eye-drops in both eyes for at least 9 months developed an acute cholinergic crisis which responded to treatment with atropine 2 mg intravenously and intramuscularly and pralidoxime chloride 2 g intravenously. It was not certain whether intoxication had occurred through topical therapy or whether the man had taken ecothiopate orally.— M. Hallett and R. F. Cullen, *J. Am. med. Ass.*, 1972, *222*, 1414.

Effects on cholinesterase. Systemic side-effects occurred in 3 of 10 patients being treated with eye-drops containing 0.06% ecothiopate, in 5 of 22 with 0.125% eye-drops, and 2 of 7 with 0.25% eye-drops. Investigations showed that cholinesterases in plasma and red blood-cells were depressed within 6 weeks by ecothiopate administered as eye-drops, and recovery took at least 8 weeks when treatment was stopped.— P. E. A. Hiscox and C. McCulloch, *Can. J. Ophthal.*, 1966, *1*, 274.

The use of 1 drop of ecothiopate iodide eye-drops 0.06% daily for 8 to 12 weeks in 21 children resulted in a reduction of blood-cholinesterase concentrations to a mean of 48% of pretreatment values. The reduction commenced within 2 weeks of initiation of treatment and reached a maximum within 5 to 7 weeks.— P. P. Ellis and M. Esterdahl, *Archs Ophthal., N.Y.*, 1967, *77*, 598.

Further references.— T. E. Eilderton *et al., Can. Anaesth. Soc. J.*, 1968, *15*, 291.

Effects on the eyes. *Glaucoma.* A 7-year-old boy who had been treated for several weeks with ecothiopate iodide eye-drops 0.125% for accommodative esotropia, developed bilateral closed-angle glaucoma. A striking feature was the marked decrease in depth of the anterior chamber of each eye, possibly due to severe ciliary spasm. Treatment with atropine eye ointment 1% was rapidly effective.— D. E. P. Jones and D. M. Watson, *Br. J. Ophthal.*, 1967, *51*, 783.

Lenticular opacities. In a survey of patients with chronic simple glaucoma who had been treated with ecothiopate iodide, 19 were found to have developed cataracts, characterised by anterior subcapsular lens opacities; 15 of these had clear lenses prior to ecothiopate treatment.— A. de Roelth, *J. Am. med. Ass.*, 1966, *195*, 664.

Further references.— R. N. Shaffer and J. Hetherington, *Am. J. Ophthal.*, 1966, *62*, 613; U. Axelsson, *Acta Ophthalmol.*, 1968, *46*, 83; R. A. Thoft, *Archs Ophthal., N.Y.*, 1968, *80*, 317.

Retinal detachment. A review and discussion on the use of miotics and the incidence of retinal detachment.— J. J. Alpar, *Ann. Ophthal.*, 1979, *11*, 395. See also H. Beasley and F. T. Fraunfelder, *Ophthalmology*, 1979, *86*, 95.

Effects on respiratory function. Bronchospasm which did not respond to standard treatment occurred in a 60-year-old woman and she did not improve until the use of ecothiopate eye-drops was discontinued.— C. Fratto, *Ann. intern. Med.*, 1978, *88*, 362.

Treatment of Adverse Effects. As for Organophosphorus Insecticides, p.833.

Precautions. As for Dyflos, p.1039.

It should be used with great care in patients with a history of retinal detachment or iodine hypersensitivity.

Treatment with ecothiopate eye-drops should be stopped if persistent diarrhoea, urinary incontinence, sweating, cardiotoxicity, or muscle weakness occurs.

Because of the incidence of cataract in patients on anticholinesterase therapy such as demecarium, dyflos, or ecothiopate, these drugs should not be used if glaucoma could be controlled by pilocarpine in conjunction with adrenaline and, if necessary, the use of carbonic anhydrase inhibitors.— R. N. Shaffer and J. Hetherington, *Am. J. Ophthal.*, 1966, *62*, 613.

Examination of 100 drainage operations (Scheie's) showed that ecothiopate iodide had an adverse effect on the outcome of the operations.— W. H. G. Douglas and T. G. Ramsell, *Br. J. Ophthal.*, 1969, *53*, 472.

Interactions. Normal caudal epidural anaesthesia using chloroprocaine was observed in a 75-year-old woman with low plasma cholinesterase activity secondary to chronic treatment with ecothiopate iodide eye-drops. Although chloroprocaine is metabolised by plasma cholinesterase it was believed that redistribution from the site of action and not alternative metabolic pathways accounted for the normal action. It was suggested that chloroprocaine was probably safe to use in patients with reduced cholinesterase activity resulting from the use of anticholinesterases such as ecothiopate.— J. B. Brodsky and F. A. Campos, *Anesthesiology*, 1978, *48*, 288.

Pregnancy and the neonate. A 22-year-old West Indian, without apparent genetic abnormality, was treated with ecothiopate iodide eye-drops 0.125% for glaucoma for several months during pregnancy. Her serum-pseudocholinesterase activity at delivery, 2 months after withdrawal of ecothiopate treatment, was lower than would have been expected, but returned to normal within a month. The infant's pseudocholinesterase activity was elevated and rose sharply over the first 3 months of life, possibly due to transplacental diffusion, causing depression of pseudocholinesterase during foetal life with a subsequent rise after birth.— D. A. Birks *et al., Archs Ophthal., N.Y.*, 1968, *79*, 283.

Uses. Ecothiopate is an inhibitor of cholinesterase with actions similar to those of dyflos. Its miotic action begins within 10 to 45 minutes of its application and may persist for 1 to 4 weeks; it causes a reduction in intra-ocular pressure which is maximal after 24 hours and may persist for 4 days. It may be administered in aqueous solution.

Ecothiopate iodide is used mainly in the treatment of open-angle glaucoma by local instillation into the affected eye. The strength of solution is adjusted according to the patient's needs from 0.03% to 0.25% and drops are instilled once or twice daily. Whenever possible treatment should be at bedtime. Pilocarpine eye-drops should be administered for at least 2 months before starting high strengths of ecothiopate eye-drops. It may be used alone or in conjunction with other topical agents or with a systemically administered carbonic anhydrase inhibitor.

Ecothiopate iodide has also been used in the management of accommodative convergent strabismus (esotropia).

The use of ecothiopate in the management of errors of refraction.— S. W. Cohen, *Am. J. Ophthal.*, 1966, *62*, 303.

Glaucoma. Control of ocular tension at night was always satisfactory with ecothiopate 0.06%, but was not satisfactory in a large proportion of patients treated with pilocarpine 2%.— P. C. Barsam and H. P. Vogel, *Am. J. Ophthal.*, 1964, *57*, 241.

Satisfactory control occurred with ecothiopate iodide in 14 of 17 eyes with chronic closed-angle glaucoma which was previously not controlled with pilocarpine and acetazolamide.— J. D. Sussman, *Am. J. Ophthal.*, 1965, *59*, 308.

Tonographic study showed that the addition of adrenaline to ecothiopate eye-drops made a substantial contribution to the normalisation of resistance to outflow in patients with ocular hypertension.— P. C. Kronfeld, *Archs Ophthal., N.Y.*, 1967, *78*, 140.

In the majority of 44 patients with open-angle glaucoma ecothiopate was as effective alone as when given with pilocarpine.— M. M. Kini *et al., Archs Ophthal., N.Y.*, 1973, *89*, 190.

Myasthenia gravis. Ecothiopate was used to treat 12 myasthenic patients, poorly controlled on short-acting anticholinesterases, and gave good results initially in 10. Subsequent control could not be maintained in 5 patients and in these the drug was discontinued. Of the remainder, 2 had remissions, 1 died of lung cancer, and the other 4 were successfully maintained on ecothiopate for over 6 years (2 of these required additional small supplements of pyridostigmine before meals to relieve bulbar symptoms). The 2 patients receiving ecothiopate alone required about 10.5 and 7 mg daily in divided doses for control.— F. F. Foldes *et al., Clin. Pharmac. Ther.*, 1966, *7*, 620.

Preparations

Echothiophate Iodide for Ophthalmic Solution *(U.S.P.)*. Sterile Ecothiopate Iodide. It may contain mannitol or other suitable diluent. Store at a temperature not exceeding 8° in airtight containers.

Phospholine Iodide *(Ayerst, UK).* Ecothiopate iodide, supplied as powder for the preparation of eye-drops containing 0.03, 0.06, 0.125, and 0.25%, with potassium acetate 40 mg, and 5-ml ampoules of diluent containing chlorbutol 0.5%, mannitol 1.2%, boric acid, and anhydrous sodium phosphate. (Also available as Phospholine Iodide in *Austral., Belg., Canad., Denm., Fr., Ital., Norw., S.Afr., Switz., USA*).

Other Proprietary Names

Echodide *(USA)*; Ecofilina *(Venez.)*; Iodeto de fosfolina *(Braz.)*; Phospholinjodid *(Ger.)*; Yoduro de fosfolina *(Mex.)*.

4516-v

Edrophonium Chloride *(B.P., U.S.P.)*.

Edrophonii Chloridum. Ethyl(3-hydroxyphenyl)dimethylammonium chloride.

$C_{10}H_{16}ClNO = 201.7$.

CAS — 312-48-1 (edrophonium); 116-38-1 (chloride).

Pharmacopoeias. In *Br., Int.,* and *U.S.*

A white odourless crystalline powder with a bitter saline taste. M.p. 165° to 170° with decomposition.

Soluble 1 in 0.5 of water and 1 in 5 of alcohol; practically insoluble in chloroform and ether. A 10% solution in water has a pH of 4 to 5. A 3.36% solution is iso-osmotic with serum. Solutions are **sterilised** by autoclaving or by filtration. **Store** in airtight containers. Protect from light.

Adverse Effects, Treatment, and Precautions. As for Neostigmine Methylsulphate, p.1035.

Diagnosis of myasthenia gravis. A warning against the use of 10 mg of edrophonium intravenously as a test for myasthenia gravis; it might cause failure of respiratory and bulbar muscles and excessive secretion of saliva and bronchial secretions.— D. L. McLellan (letter), *Br. med. J.*, 1973, *3*, 634.

Effects on the heart. A 66-year-old woman given edrophonium chloride 10 mg by rapid intravenous injection developed sinus bradycardia with ventricular asystole requiring cardiac massage and atropine for return to normal sinus rhythm.— R. M. Rossen *et al., J. Am. med. Ass.*, 1976, *235*, 1041.

Further references.— G. H. Mayor and P. W. Willis, *Sth. med. J.*, 1976, *69*, 1437; J. A. Youngberg, *Anesthesiology*, 1979, *50*, 234.

Absorption and Fate. Following intravenous injection the action of edrophonium is rapid in onset and of short duration.

A study in 5 surgical patients on the plasma elimination half-lives of edrophonium chloride after intravenous injection indicated that an initial rapid phase of elimination (range 0.54 to 1.92 minutes) was followed by a much slower decline (range 24.23 to 45.00 minutes). It was suggested that the rapid fall in the plasma concentration of edrophonium was not primarily due to metabolism and excretion but to the rapid uptake of the drug by other tissues.— T. N. Calvey *et al., Clin. Pharmac. Ther.*, 1976, *19*, 813.

Uses. Edrophonium has actions similar to those of neostigmine (see Neostigmine Methylsulphate, p.1036) but its effect on skeletal muscle is claimed to be particularly prominent. Its action is rapid in onset and of short duration.

Edrophonium chloride is of particular value in the diagnosis of myasthenia gravis. It is given by intravenous injection in doses of 2 to 10 mg; the usual procedure is to inject 2 mg and, if no adverse reaction occurs within 30 seconds, to continue with the injection of a further 8 mg. The dose of edrophonium chloride for a child is 200 µg per kg body-weight by intravenous injection; one-fifth of this dose should be given initially and if no adverse reaction occurs the rest may be given; 2 mg may be given by intramuscular injection when intravenous injection is difficult. Atropine should always be available when the test is carried out.

In patients with myasthenia gravis, there is immediate subjective improvement and muscle strength increases. This effect usually lasts only for about 5 minutes, after which time the typical signs and symptoms return; because of its brief action the drug is not suitable for the routine treatment of myasthenia gravis.

Lower doses of edrophonium chloride are used to determine whether or not a patient with severe symptoms of myasthenia gravis and respiratory failure is suffering from the effects of inadequate or excessive treatment with anticholinesterase drugs. If treatment has been inadequate, edrophonium chloride will produce an immediate amelioration of symptoms, whereas in cholinergic crises due to over-treatment the symptoms will be aggravated.

Edrophonium chloride was originally introduced for the reversal of the effects of tubocurarine and other non-depolarising muscle relaxants. A dose of 5 to 10 mg was given by intravenous injection and repeated every 5 to 10 minutes up to 40 mg if necessary. The briefness of its action limits its usefulness and neostigmine is preferred. Where prolonged apnoea occurs in a patient treated with a depolarising muscle relaxant, such as suxamethonium, edrophonium 10 mg may be given intravenously to determine the presence of a dual block.

Doses of 10 to 20 mg have been given intravenously in the treatment of paroxysmal tachycardia.

Cardiac arrhythmias. Edrophonium was considered to be a safe and useful agent for the differentiation of supraventricular arrhythmias and in the conversion of paroxysmal atrial tachycardia to normal sinus rhythm.— A. J. Moss and L. M. Aledort, *Am. J. Cardiol.*, 1966, *17*, 58.

A single rapid intravenous infusion of edrophonium 5 mg, repeated if no slowing occurred within 2 minutes, was used successfully to treat 14 patients with supraventricular arrhythmias, 12 of whom had received digitalis to the limit of safety. When ventricular slowing occurred a continuous infusion of edrophonium in dextrose injection was given at a rate of 0.25 to 2 mg per minute for 30 minutes to 30 hours. To avoid serious bradycardia or ventricular tachycardia, however, an initial dose of edrophonium 2 mg was recommended with increments of 2 mg per minute until 10 mg had been infused; the continuous infusion should start at 250 µg per minute.— J. Frieden *et al., Am. J. Cardiol.*, 1971, *27*, 294.

Edrophonium, 10 mg was given by rapid intravenous injection on 103 occasions to 84 patients and was a useful vagotonic drug in the differentiation of cardiac arrhythmias. Poor results were obtained in the conversion of atrial tachycardia to normal sinus rhythm. In view of the risk of producing alarming atrioventricular block it was recommended that edrophonium should not be given to patients with atrial flutter or tachycardia who were receiving digitalis. Other side-effects included premature ventricular beats, abdominal cramps, salivation, nausea, blurring of vision, lachrymation, and leg cramps; paradoxical transient cardiac speeding occurred in 1 patient in sinus rhythm.— R. C. V. Reddy *et al., Am. Heart J.*, 1971, *82*, 742.

Further references.— J. D. Cantwell *et al., Archs intern. Med.*, 1972, *130*, 221; R. R. Miller *et al., Am. Heart J.*, 1977, *93*, 222.

Diagnosis of myasthenia gravis. Re-evaluation of edrophonium tonography in 22 myasthenic patients and 28 control cases confirmed that it was a valuable and reliable test in the diagnosis of myasthenia gravis. Positive results were also obtained in 6 control patients who had other defects of neuromuscular transmission.— S. H. Wray and D. Pavan-Langston, *Neurology, Minneap.*, 1971, *21*, 586.

Diagnosis of visual defects in myasthenia gravis. The rapid improvement in uni-ocular accommodation in 8 of 9 patients (6 of whom had generalised myasthenia gravis and 3 had ocular myasthenia), following a single intravenous injection of 10 mg of edrophonium chloride brought to light defects of visual accommodation, suggesting that, in myasthenia, effects were not limited to disturbance of the external ocular and other skeletal muscles.— N. Manson and G. Stern, *Lancet*, 1965, *1*, 935.

Further references.— J. A. Retzlaff *et al., Am. J. Ophthal.*, 1969, *67*, 13, per *Mayo Clin. Proc.*, 1969, *44*, 210; J. R. Keane and W. F. Hoyt, *J. Am. med. Ass.*, 1970, *212*, 1209.

Preparations

Edrophonium Chloride Injection *(U.S.P.).* A sterile solution of edrophonium chloride in Water for Injections. pH 5 to 5.8.

Edrophonium Injection *(B.P.).* A sterile solution of edrophonium chloride in Water for Injections. Sterilised by autoclaving. pH 5 to 6. Protect from light.

Tensilon *(Roche, UK).* Edrophonium chloride, available as an injection containing 10 mg per ml, in ampoules of 1 ml. (Also available as Tensilon in *Canad., USA*).

4517-g

Galantamine Hydrobromide.

Galanthamini Hydrobromidum; Galanthamine Hydrobromide.

$C_{17}H_{21}NO_3,HBr = 368.3$.

CAS — 357-70-0 (galantamine); 1953-04-4 (hydrobromide).

Pharmacopoeias. In *Chin.* and *Rus.*

The hydrobromide of galantamine, an alkaloid obtained in the USSR from the bulbs of the Caucasian snowdrop (Voronov's snowdrop), *Galanthus woronowii* (Amaryllidaceae); it is also present in other closely related species.

Galantamine hydrobromide occurs as a fine white crystalline powder with a bitter taste. Sparingly **soluble** in water; practically insoluble in alcohol, chloroform, and ether. Solutions may be **sterilised** by maintaining at 98° to 100° for 30 minutes with a bactericide or by filtration.

Adverse Effects, Treatment, and Precautions. As for Neostigmine Methylsulphate, p.1035.

Uses. Galantamine hydrobromide is an inhibitor of cholinesterase activity, with actions similar to those of neostigmine (see Neostigmine Methylsulphate, p.1036). It is used in the USSR in myasthenia, myopathy, and motor and sensory impairment arising from diseases and traumatic injuries of the nervous system. It may also be used to curtail the muscle relaxation produced by non-depolarising muscle relaxants such as tubocurarine and gallamine.

A review of the sources, structure, characterisation, extraction, toxicity, and action of galantamine.— J. R. Boissier *et al., Ann. pharm. franç.*, 1960, *18*, 888.

Reversal of anticholinergic action. Galantamine hydrobromide 500 µg per kg body-weight, given intravenously, rapidly reversed the central anticholinergic syndrome produced by injection of hyoscine hydrobromide 2 mg intravenously. Ten healthy subjects became alert within 5 to 10 minutes and were completely awake after 30 minutes.— A. Baraka and S. Harik, *J. Am. med. Ass.*, 1977, *238*, 2293. Comments. A brief discussion of the pharmacology and potential use of galantamine hydrobromide in poisoning by anticholinergic drugs.— D. A. Cozanitis and E. Toivakka (letter), *ibid.*, 1978, *240*, 108.

Reversal of neuromuscular blockade. Galantamine had a wide therapeutic margin, was well tolerated, and had a consistent effect which was no longer lasting than other antagonists of non-depolarising muscle relaxants. Up to 20 to 25 mg in divided doses of 5 to 10 mg, equivalent to 0.5 to 1 mg of neostigmine, were recommended for complete muscle relaxation. It had mild central stimulant properties and because of a slight muscarinic action, it was not always necessary for atropine to be given before galantamine therapy. Galantamine, 5 to 10 mg twice daily by intramuscular injection, had also been used to stimulate postoperative peristalsis.— O. Mayrhofer, *Bull. schweiz. Akad. med. Wiss.*, 1967, *23*, 48.

Neostigmine 2.5 mg was superior to galantamine 25 mg in reversing neuromuscular blockade due to tubocurarine.— J. De Angelis and L. F. Walts, *Anesth. Analg. curr. Res.*, 1972, *51*, 196.

Further references.— H. Foitzik and P. Lawin, *Z. prakt. Anaesth. Wiederbeleb.*, 1972, *7*, 203; H. Foitzik *et al., ibid.*, 1973, *8*, 18.

Preparations

Solutio Galanthamini Hydrobromidi pro Injectionibus *(Rus. P.).* Galantamine Hydrobromide Injection. A solution of galantamine hydrobromide in Water for Injections; in ampoules of 1 ml. pH 5 to 7. Sterilised in steam at 100° for 30 minutes.

Proprietary Names

Nivalina *(UCB, Ital.)*.

4518-q

Jaborandi *(B.P.C. 1949).* Jaborandi Leaves; Pilocarpus.

Pharmacopoeias. In *Fr.* and *Port.* from *P. microphyllus;* in *Braz.* from *P. microphyllus, P. jaborandi* (Pernambuco jaborandi), and *P. pennatifolius* (Paraguay jaborandi); and in *Span.* and *Swiss* from *P. jaborandi.*

The dried leaflets of Maranham jaborandi, *Pilocarpus microphyllus* (Rutaceae), containing not less than 0.4% of alkaloids, calculated as pilocarpine. **Store** in airtight containers. Protect from light.

Adverse Effects, Treatment, and Precautions. As for Neostigmine Methylsulphate, p.1035.

Uses. The actions of jaborandi are mainly those of its principal alkaloid, pilocarpine. Jaborandi was formerly added to hair lotions for its supposed effect in stimulating hair growth but the use of *P. jaborandi* and its galenical preparations in cosmetic products is now prohibited in Great Britain and some other countries.

Preparations

Jaborandi Liquid Extract *(B.P.C. 1949).* Ext. Jaborand. Liq. Prepared by percolation with alcohol (45%) and standardised to contain 0.5% w/v of alkaloids calculated as pilocarpine.

Jaborandi Tincture *(B.P.C. 1949).* Tinct. Jaborand. Jaborandi liquid extract 1 in 5, in alcohol (45%). *Dose.* 0.6 to 2 ml.

4519-p

Methacholine Bromide. Methacholini Bromidum.
$C_8H_{18}BrNO_2$=240.1.

CAS — 333-31-3.

Pharmacopoeias. In *Nord.*

A white, crystalline, very hygroscopic powder with a faint amine-like odour. M.p. about 148°. **Soluble** 1 in 0.3 of water, 1 in 0.8 of alcohol (90%), and 3 in 4 of chloroform; practically insoluble in ether. A freshly prepared 5% solution in water has a pH of about 5. A 3.77% solution is iso-osmotic with serum. **Store** in airtight containers.

Methacholine bromide has actions and uses similar to those of methacholine chloride but, being less hygroscopic, it is more suitable for administration in tablet form. It has been given in doses of 200 to 600 mg daily.

4520-n

Methacholine Chloride *(B.P.C. 1973, U.S.P.).*

Acetyl-β-methylcholine Chloride; Methacholinium Chloratum. (2-Acetoxypropyl)trimethylammonium chloride.
$C_8H_{18}ClNO_2$=195.7.

CAS — 55-92-5 (methacholine); 62-51-1 (chloride).

Pharmacopoeias. In *Braz., Ind., It., Mex., Swiss,* and *U.S.*

Colourless, very hygroscopic crystals, or a white crystalline powder, odourless or with a slight odour. M.p. 170° to 173°. **Soluble** 1 in 0.4 of water, 1 in 1.2 of alcohol, and 1 in 2.1 of chloroform. A 2% solution in water has a pH of 4.5 to 5.5. A 3.21% solution is iso-osmotic with serum. Solutions are **sterilised** by filtration. **Store** in airtight containers.

Adverse Effects. Toxic symptoms include nausea and vomiting, flushing, sweating, salivation, lachrymation, eructation, involuntary defaecation and urination, transient dyspnoea, palpitations, bradycardia and peripheral vasodilatation leading to hypotension, transient heart block, and a feeling of constriction under the sternum. When given by injection, methacholine may cause a terrifying sensation of choking.

Treatment of Adverse Effects. As for Neostigmine Methylsulphate, p.1035.

Precautions. Methacholine chloride should not be given to patients suffering from allergic conditions, especially asthma, or to patients with Addison's disease, intestinal or urinary obstruction, coronary occlusion, hyperthyroidism, or peptic ulcer. It should be used with caution in elderly patients.

It should not be administered concurrently with neostigmine, physostigmine, or other anticholinesterases, unless a prolonged effect is required, when doses should be reduced. It should not be used in patients with hypertension as it may cause a precipitous fall in blood pressure.

Atropine should be available to counteract any reactions in patients excessively susceptible to the action of methacholine.

Serious untoward reactions occurring in 3 patients given methacholine in conjunction with neostigmine for paroxysmal supraventricular tachycardia were relieved in 2 patients by atropine intravenously but the third patient died.— R. H. Furman and A. J. Geiger, *J. Am. med. Ass.,* 1952, *149,* 269.

Uses. Methacholine is a quaternary ammonium parasympathomimetic agent with the muscarinic actions of acetylcholine (see p.1037). It is not readily inactivated by cholinesterases so that its actions are more prolonged than those of acetylcholine.

Methacholine chloride has been used to terminate attacks of supraventricular paroxysmal tachycardia, the usual dose being 10 to 25 mg subcutaneously; this may be repeated in 30 minutes if necessary. It should not be given by intravenous or intramuscular injection.

Methacholine has been used by mouth and subcutaneously in the treatment of Raynaud's syndrome, scleroderma, and other vasospastic conditions of the extremities. It has also been administered locally by iontophoresis.

Eye-drops containing 2.5% of methacholine chloride are used in the diagnosis of Adie's pupil; miosis occurs in the affected pupil within 30 minutes, whereas the normal pupil is unaffected. Eye-drops (10 to 20%) have also been used in the treatment of simple glaucoma but other miotics are generally preferred.

Preparations

Amechol (Methacholine) Eye-drops *(Moorfields Eye Hosp.).* Methacholine chloride 2.5%, phenylmercuric nitrate 0.002%, water to 100%. Store in a refrigerator. Shelf-life 3 months.

4521-h

Physostigmine *(B.P.C. 1973, U.S.P.).*

Physostigmina; Eserine. (3a*S*,8a*R*)-1,2,3,3a,8,8a-Hexahydro-1,3a,8-trimethylpyrrolo[2,3-*b*]indol-5-yl methylcarbamate.
$C_{15}H_{21}N_3O_2$=275.3.

CAS — 57-47-6.

An alkaloid obtained from the calabar bean, the seed of *Physostigma venenosum* (Leguminosae). It occurs as colourless or almost colourless, odourless or almost odourless, crystals or a white microcrystalline powder which become pink on exposure to heat, light, air, or contact with traces of metals, owing to the formation of rubreserine. M.p. not lower than 103°.

Soluble 1 in 75 of water, 1 in 10 of alcohol, 1 in 1 of chloroform, 1 in 30 of ether, and 1 in 180 of soft paraffin; soluble, on warming, 1 in 100 of castor oil; very soluble in dichloromethane; soluble in fixed oils. A solution in benzene is laevorotatory. Sterile oily solutions are prepared aseptically. **Store** in airtight containers. Protect from light.

Physostigmine has the actions and uses described under Physostigmine Salicylate. It is used for the preparation of oily eye-drops.

Preparations

Physostigmine Oily Eye-drops *(B.P.C. 1963).* Gutt. Physostig. Oleos.; Eserine Oily Eye-drops. A sterile solution containing 1% w/v of physostigmine in sterilised castor oil. Protect from light. *A.P.F.* (Physostigmine Eye Drops Oily) has 0.25, 0.5, and 1% solutions.

4522-m

Physostigmine Aminoxide Salicylate. Physostigmine *N*-Oxide Salicylate; Eserine Aminoxide Salicylate.
$C_{15}H_{21}N_3O_3,C_7H_6O_3$=429.5.

Crystals which become red on exposure to heat, light, and air. M.p. 90°.

Physostigmine aminoxide salicylate is an inhibitor of cholinesterase activity that has been given in doses of 3 mg thrice daily before meals for the relief of constipation. It has also been advocated for the treatment of some skin disorders.

Proprietary Names

Génésérine 3 *(Amido, Fr.).*

4523-b

Physostigmine Salicylate *(B.P., Eur. P., U.S.P.).*

Physostig. Sal.; Physostigminii Salicylas; Physostigmini Salicylas; Eserinii Salicylas; Eserine Salicylate; Fisostigmina Salicilato.
$C_{15}H_{21}N_3O_2,C_7H_6O_3$=413.5.

CAS — 57-64-7.

Pharmacopoeias. In all pharmacopoeias examined except *Braz., Chin.,* and *Span.*

Colourless or white odourless crystals or white powder with a slightly bitter taste. M.p. 184° to 186°. The crystals and their aqueous solution become red on exposure to heat, light, air, and contact with traces of metals, owing to the formation of rubreserine; the change is less rapid in faintly acid solution.

Soluble 1 in 75 to 90 of water, 1 in 25 of alcohol, 1 in 6 of chloroform, and 1 in 250 of ether. A solution in water is laevorotatory. Solutions are **sterilised** by maintaining at 98° to 100° for 30 minutes with a bactericide or by filtration; the pH should be kept below 4 and an antoxidant should be included. **Incompatible** with acids, alkalis, iodine, and salts of iron and silver. **Store** in airtight containers. Protect from light.

Solutions should be freshly prepared or, if kept, stored in hermetically sealed containers. It has been reported that storage in plastic syringes in the light renders physostigmine ineffective.

Preservative for eye-drops. Phenylmercuric borate 0.005% was a suitable preservative for physostigmine salicylate eye-drops sterilised by filtration.— M. Van Ooteghem, *Pharm. Tijdschr. Belg.,* 1968, *45,* 69.

Stability of solutions of physostigmine salts. Ascorbic acid (0.1%) in solutions containing 1% of physostigmine hydrobromide prevented oxidation for 6 months under normal storage conditions. A pale brown colour developed owing to oxidation of the ascorbic acid. Sodium metabisulphite (0.1%) was less effective.— W. Swallow, *Pharm. J.,* 1951, *1,* 11.

Eye-drops containing physostigmine salicylate 1% and sodium chloride 0.75% lost 1% of their physostigmine content in 3 months at 20°; at 30°, 3% was lost. Heating at 100° for 15 minutes resulted in a loss of 1 to 4% and the development of a red colour. Discoloration was prevented by the addition of 0.1% of sodium metabisulphite but this resulted in the solution becoming too acid on storage. The inclusion of 2% of sodium acid citrate was sufficient to buffer the solution to pH 5 and such solutions showed a loss of 1 to 2% with no discoloration or pH change on heating at 100° for 15 minutes; the loss on storage at 20° for 6 months was 10%. The addition of disodium edetate did not prevent discoloration.— J. Mørch, *Dansk Tidsskr. Farm.,* 1958, *32,* 93.

The degradation products of physostigmine which might be formed after heat sterilisation of eye-drops were eseroline, rubreserine, eserine blue, and eserine brown. The anticholinesterase activity *in vitro* of eseroline and rubreserine was 1000 to 5000 times less than that of physostigmine. Eserine blue was the most potent degradation product and was 100 to 500 times less active than physostigmine.— B. A. Hemsworth and G.

B. West (letter), *J. Pharm. Pharmac.*, 1968, *20*, 406; *idem*, *J. pharm. Sci.*, 1970, *59*, 118.

The effect of pH and sodium metabisulphite on the stability of physostigmine solutions to heat and gamma irradiation showed that maximum stability at 90° occurred between pH 2.2 and 3; sodium metabisulphite 0.5% w/v improved stability towards irradiation but not to degradation by heat.— G. Fletcher and D. J. G. Davies, *J. Pharm. Pharmac.*, 1968, *20*, *Suppl.*, 108S.

Physostigmine salicylate was most stable in aqueous solution at about pH 3.6 at 25°, with a time for 10% decomposition of about 90 years.— I. Christenson, *Acta pharm. suec.*, 1969, *6*, 287.

Physostigmine eye-drops 0.25, 0.5, or 1%, prepared to the *B.P.C. 1973* formula (pH 3.6 to 3.8) and sterilised by heating or by filtration retained more than 99% of their activity after storage at 25° for 1 year. A faint pink colour occurred after sterilisation by heat, and in all samples after storage for 1 year.— A. R. Rogers and G. Smith, *Pharm. J.*, 1973, *2*, 353.

A report of possible degradation of physostigmine in solutions also containing sodium bisulfite.— A. Hussain *et al.*, *J. pharm. Sci.*, 1978, *67*, 742. See also A. Hussain and K. Iga, *J. parent. Drug Ass.*, 1979, *33*, 32.

Adverse Effects. As for Neostigmine Methylsulphate, p.1035.

Toxic effects are usually more severe than those occurring with neostigmine.

Effects on the eyes. A review and discussion on the use of miotics and the incidence of retinal detachment.— J. J. Alpar, *Ann. Ophthal.*, 1979, *11*, 395. See also H. Beasley and F. T. Fraunfelder, *Ophthalmology*, 1979, *86*, 95.

Treatment of Adverse Effects. As for Neostigmine Methylsulphate, p.1035.

A 22-year-old student who took 1 g of physostigmine salicylate developed nausea, abdominal pain, and terrifying hallucinations. Seventy-five minutes later gastric lavage was performed with dilute potassium permanganate solution (using a total of 1 g in 8 litres of water), forced alkaline diuresis was started, and small doses of atropine sulphate were given by intravenous injection. When 1.05 mg of atropine had been given his heart-rate rose to 200 per minute and multifocal ventricular ectopic beats developed. Treatment with atropine was stopped. He later became cyanosed and large quantities of watery fluid were aspirated from the airways. Mechanical ventilation was started. Because of convulsions, at first controlled with calcium gluconate, and generalised muscular twitching he was paralysed with tubocurarine. Later, diazepam was given in addition. Two doses of pralidoxime mesylate 500 mg at 5-minute intervals improved muscular tone. He made a successful recovery.— G. Cumming *et al.*, *Lancet*, 1968, *2*, 147. A slow intravenous injection of 5 mg of propranolol might reduce the heart-rate and avert the danger of ventricular fibrillation in physostigmine poisoning. Propranolol in conjunction with atropine had been found a safe procedure, slowing the heart-rate to its low intrinsic level.— A. Valero (letter), *ibid.*, 459.

Precautions. As for Neostigmine Methylsulphate, p.1035.

A prolonged response to suxamethonium occurred in a 25-year-old woman undergoing caesarean section who had, about 15 minutes earlier, received physostigmine salicylate 2 mg intravenously followed by 2 mg intramuscularly to control the adverse effects of the premedication.— A. F. Kopman *et al.*, *Anesthesiology*, 1978, *49*, 142.

Absorption and Fate. Physostigmine salicylate is readily absorbed from the gastro-intestinal tract, subcutaneous tissues, and mucous membranes. It is largely destroyed in the body by hydrolysis of the ester linkage by cholinesterases; a 1-mg dose injected subcutaneously has been claimed to be destroyed in 2 hours. Little is excreted in the urine.

Uses. Physostigmine is an inhibitor of cholinesterase activity with actions similar to those of neostigmine (see Neostigmine Methylsulphate, p.1036).

Physostigmine is used mainly as a miotic. The pupils begin to constrict within 10 minutes of application and the effect lasts for about 12 hours. It may be used to counteract the dilatation of the pupil caused by atropine, homatropine, or cocaine; in these circumstances it may, however, produce considerable irritation and pain due to spasm. Physostigmine is also used to decrease intra-ocular pressure in glaucoma.

Unlike neostigmine, physostigmine crosses the blood-brain barrier and can reverse the central as well as the peripheral effects of anticholinergic agents such as atropine. Physostigmine, 0.5 to 2 mg subcutaneously, intramuscularly, or intravenously, repeated every 1 or 2 hours as necessary, has been advocated for the reversal of anticholinergic poisoning associated with overdosage of anticholinergic agents and tricyclic antidepressants. In general, however, such treatment is not recommended (see Anticholinergic Poisoning, below).

Physostigmine was considered to cause a rapid miosis which was maximal in 30 minutes and lasted 24 to 72 hours. In concentrations of 0.25 to 1% it could be used twice or thrice daily for simple glaucoma, for closed-angle glaucoma, and to counter mydriasis, except in retrobulbar anaesthesia.— J. J. Kanski, *Br. J. Ophthal.*, 1968, *52*, 936.

Studies into the action of physostigmine on memory.— B. H. Peters and H. S. Levin, *Archs Neurol., Chicago*, 1977, *34*, 215; *J. Am. med. Ass.*, 1978, *239*, 2419; K. L. Davis *et al.*, *Science*, 1978, *201*, 272; K. L. Davis *et al.* (letter), *New Engl. J. Med.*, 1979, *301*, 946.

Alzheimer's disease. Improvement in memory.— B. H. Peters and H. S. Levin, *Ann. Neurol.*, 1979, *6*, 219. See also C. M. Smith and M. Swash (letter), *Lancet*, 1979, *1*, 42.

Further references: O. Muramoto *et al.*, *Archs Neurol., Chicago*, 1979, *36*, 501.

Anaesthesia. Physostigmine administered intramuscularly in a dose of 50 µg per kg body-weight to children after hyoscine premedication prevented the delirium which often occurred.— D. S. Nelson, *J. Am. med. Ass.*, 1973, *223*, 132.

Studies on physostigmine for the reversal of postanaesthetic effects.— J. Brebner and L. Hadley, *Can. Anaesth. Soc. J.*, 1976, *23*, 574; A. V. Bidwai *et al.*, *Anesthesiology*, 1976, *44*, 249; D. B. Smith *et al.*, *Anesth. Analg. curr. Res.*, 1976, *55*, 478; G. E. Hill *et al.*, *Can. Anaesth. Soc. J.*, 1977, *24*, 707.

Anticholinergic poisoning. Although physostigmine can reverse effects of anticholinergic and tricyclic antidepressant poisoning, most reviewers agree that in general such a use is inappropriate and hazardous. R.W. Newton (*J. Am. med. Ass.*, 1975, *231*, 941) concluded from a study of 21 patients suffering from tricyclic overdosage that in the routine management of tricyclic poisoning the hazards of the cholinergic properties of physostigmine, in particular the risk of inducing respiratory difficulty, outweigh any benefits of an early return to consciousness. In order to counteract the peripheral cholinergic actions of physostigmine, yet benefit from its central cholinergic properties, S.-M. Aquilonius and U. Hedstrand (*Acta anaesth. scand.*, 1978, *22*, 40) administered propantheline bromide to 10 patients with tricyclic poisoning before giving physostigmine; as anticipated successful reversal of central effects of the tricyclics was achieved without significant peripheral cholinergic toxicity, but the beneficial effect of physostigmine on consciousness lasted less than 1 hour and one patient suffered grand mal seizures. They concluded that the use of physostigmine had not been shown to affect the mortality-rate in tricyclic poisoning and might exacerbate the risk of grand mal seizures. Nevertheless some (see H. Pall *et al.*, *Acta pharmac. tox.*, 1977, *41*, *Suppl.* 2, 171 who have employed continuous intravenous infusion) do consider that seriously poisoned patients may benefit from physostigmine administration and that not only does it have a beneficial effect on the central aspects of anticholinergic poisoning but that some of the adverse cardiac effects of tricyclics may be also reversed. However, as a serious complication of physostigmine administration, they pointed out that 2 patients, both known chronic alcoholics developed acute pancreatitis. Physostigmine has a shorter duration of action than most anticholinergic agents, and a considerably shorter duration of action than most tricyclics, therefore reports of the successful use of physostigmine have highlighted the need for repeated doses over periods of hours or days (see R.H. Brier (letter), *Ann. intern. Med.*, 1978, *89*, 579). Briefly discussing the difficulties in the diagnosis and treatment of anticholinergic poisoning E.D. Caine (*New Engl. J. Med.*, 1979, *300*, 1278) suggested that although physostigmine can be beneficial when absolutely necessary to maintain the patient's safety, its use could lead to severe cardiac and respiratory effects, and that in uncomplicated cases of overdosage, to await the spontaneous remission of toxicity could be the safest treatment of all.

Individual reports of the use of physostigmine in poisoning with anticholinergic agents, antihistamines, antipsychotic agents, and tricyclic antidepressants.— K. Leczyka and K. Trembla, *Pol. med. J.*, 1969, *8*, 381 (atropine; reversal of coma); K. C. Ullman *et al.* (letter), *Lancet*, 1970, *1*, 252 (hyoscine hydrobromide; improvement in psychiatric symptoms); S. E. Young *et al.*, *Am. J. Ophthal.*, 1971, *72*, 1136 (hyoscine eye-drops; control of central and peripheral toxicity); M. K. El-Yousef *et al.* (letter), *J. Am. med. Ass.*, 1972, *220*, 125 (benztropine mesylate in association with antipsychotics or tricyclic antidepressants; reversal of psychoses); B. H. Rumack, *Pediatrics*, 1973, *52*, 449 (anticholinergic agents); J. S. Burks *et al.*, *J. Am. med. Ass.*, 1974, *230*, 1405 (amitriptyline and imipramine); J. S. Gillick, *Br. J. Anaesth.*, 1974, *46*, 793 (atropine); B. D. Snyder *et al.*, *J. Am. med. Ass.*, 1974, *230*, 1433 (amitriptyline); J. H. Lee *et al.*, *Anesthesiology*, 1975, *43*, 683 (diphenhydramine and promethazine; reversal of depression and excitement); P. C. Holinger and H. L. Klawans, *Am. J. Psychiat.*, 1976, *133*, 1018 (amitriptyline; reversal of coma); B. D. Snyder *et al.* (letter), *New Engl. J. Med.*, 1976, *295*, 1435 (orphenadrine citrate; reversal of agitated delirium); S. P. Wright, *Clin. Pediat.*, 1976, *15*, 1123 (imipramine; beneficial effect on cardiac arrhythmia); J. W. Chapin and D. W. Wingard, *Anesthesiology*, 1977, *46*, 364 (benzquinamide; control of delirium); P. A. Janson *et al.*, *J. Am. med. Ass.*, 1977, *237*, 2632 (doxepin hydrochloride); P. Schuster *et al.*, *Clin. Toxicol.*, 1977, *10*, 437 (clozapine; reversal of delirium); S. F. Wang and C. L. Marlowe, *Pediatrics*, 1977, *59*, 301 (chlorpromazine; reversal of coma); D. Weisdorf *et al.*, *Clin. Pharmac. Ther.*, 1978, *24*, 663 (phenothiazines; reversal of central anticholinergic syndrome and cardiac abnormalities); C. D. Berkowitz, *J. Pediat.*, 1979, *95*, 144 (amantadine); P. J. Cowen, *Postgrad. med. J.*, 1979, *55*, 556 (promethazine; control of psychosis); G. Cleghorn and G. Bourke (letter), *Lancet*, 1980, *2*, 368 (promethazine and imipramine).

Further reviews, comments, and studies.— R. A. Munoz, *Am. J. Psychiat.*, 1976, *133*, 1085; J. K. Van De Ree *et al.*, *Neth. J. Med.*, 1977, *20*, 149; J. T. Biggs, *Hosp. Pract.*, 1978, *13*, 79; P. J. Perry *et al.*, *Am. J. Hosp. Pharm.*, 1978, *35*, 725; S. Nattel *et al.*, *Clin. Pharmac. Ther.*, 1979, *25*, 96; *Med. Lett.*, 1980, *22*, 55; M. V. Rudorfer (letter), *Lancet*, 1980, *2*, 589.

Ataxia. A report of the beneficial effect of physostigmine in patients with familial ataxias.— R. A. P. Kark *et al.*, *Neurology, Minneap.*, 1977, *27*, 70.

Gilles de la Tourette's syndrome. The reduction of tics after treatment with physostigmine in patients with the Tourette syndrome appears to be due to an increase in central cholinergic activity. Six patients with frequent and relatively constant motor tics given a peripheral anticholinergic agent, propantheline 90 µg per kg body-weight intravenously, followed by physostigmine 50 µg per kg infused intravenously over one hour had a significant decrease in tic frequency with the greatest effect 30 minutes after the infusion.— S. M. Stahl and P. A. Berger (letter), *New Engl. J. Med.*, 1980, *302*, 1311. See also *idem*, 298.

Mania. Three patients with mania given infusions of physostigmine were calmed but their thought processes were not changed.— B. J. Carroll *et al.* (letter), *Lancet*, 1973, *1*, 427.

In 8 patients with mania the slow intravenous infusion of physostigmine salicylate changed thought content and mood from mania towards depression.— K. L. Davis *et al.*, *Archs gen. Psychiat.*, 1978, *35*, 119.

Further references.— D. S. Janowsky *et al.* (letter), *Lancet*, 1972, *1*, 1236; *idem*, *Archs gen. Psychiat.*, 1973, *28*, 542.

Pediculosis. In patients with *Phthirus pubis* infection, the parasites had been removed from the eyelashes by application of a 0.25% physostigmine ophthalmic ointment by means of a cotton-tipped applicator.— A. B. Ackerman, *New Engl. J. Med.*, 1968, *278*, 950.

Tardive dyskinesia. Results of a double-blind placebo-controlled study involving 12 patients with tardive dyskinesia indicated that physostigmine reduced dyskinetic movements, but the mechanism by which this was achieved, whether by sedation or specific cholinergic activity, needed further evaluation.— C. A. Tamminga *et al.*, *Am. J. Psychiat.*, 1977, *134*, 769.

Preparations

Physostigmine Eye Ointment *(B.P.C. 1963).* Eserine Eye Ointment. Physostigmine salicylate in eye ointment basis. Store below 15°.

Physostigmine Injection *(Ind. P.).* Physostigmine salicylate in Water for Injections containing sodium metabisulphite 0.05%.

Physostigmine Salicylate Injection *(U.S.P.)*. A sterile solution of physostigmine salicylate in Water for Injections; it may contain an antimicrobial agent and an antioxidant. pH 4 to 6. Protect from light. Do not use if more than slightly discoloured.

Physostigmine Salicylate Ophthalmic Solution *(U.S.P.)*. A sterile aqueous solution of physostigmine salicylate. It may contain suitable antimicrobial agents, buffers, stabilisers, and suitable additives to increase its viscosity. pH 2 to 4. Store in airtight containers. Protect from light.

Proprietary Names

Antilirium *(O'Neal, Canad.; O'Neal, USA)*; Fisostin *(Tubi Lux, Ital.)*; Isopto-Eserine *(Alcon, USA)*.

4524-v

Physostigmine Sulphate *(B.P., B.P. Vet.)*.

Physostig. Sulph.; Physostigmine Sulfate *(U.S.P.)*; Eserine Sulphate.

$(C_{15}H_{21}N_3O_2)_2,H_2SO_4$=648.8.

CAS — 64-47-1.

Pharmacopoeias. In *Br., Braz., Jap., Port., Span.,* and *U.S.*

A white or almost white, deliquescent, odourless or almost odourless, microcrystalline powder with a slightly bitter taste. M.p. 143° to 147°. The powder and its aqueous solution become red on exposure to heat, light, air, and contact with traces of metals, owing to the formation of rubreserine; the change is less rapid in acid solution.

Soluble 1 in less than 1 of water and of alcohol; soluble in chloroform; very lightly soluble in ether. A 1% solution is laevorotatory and has a pH of 3 to 4. Solutions are **sterilised** by maintaining at 98° to 100° for 30 minutes with a bactericide or by filtration. **Store** in airtight containers. Protect from light.

Stability of solutions of physostigmine salts. For reports on the stability of solutions of physostigmine salts, see under Physostigmine Salicylate, p.1042.

Physostigmine sulphate has the actions and uses described under Physostigmine Salicylate. As it is more soluble than the salicylate and is compatible with a wider range of preservatives it is usually preferred for the preparation of eye-drops.

Preparations

Physostigmine and Pilocarpine Eye-drops *(B.P.C. 1973)*. Eserine and Pilocarpine Eye-drops. A sterile solution containing up to 0.5% of physostigmine sulphate and up to 4% of pilocarpine hydrochloride, with 0.2% of sodium metabisulphite and 0.02% v/v of benzalkonium chloride solution in water. Sterilised by filtration or by maintaining at 98° to 100° for 30 minutes. The solution is adversely affected by alkalis. Protect from light.

Physostigmine Eye Drops *(A.P.F.)*. Eserine Eye-drops. Physostigmine sulphate 500 mg, sodium metabisulphite 100 mg, sodium chloride 800 mg, benzalkonium chloride solution 0.02 ml, disodium edetate 50 mg, Water for Injections to 100 ml. Sterilised by maintaining at 98° to 100° for 30 minutes. Protect from light.

Physostigmine Eye Drops *(B.P.)*. Eserine Eye Drops; Physostigmine Sulphate Eye Drops; ESR. A sterile solution of physostigmine sulphate in water containing not more than 0.2% of sulphur dioxide. When intended for use on more than one occasion they also contain benzalkonium chloride 0.01% and should not be used more than one month after first opening the container.

Physostigmine Sulfate Ophthalmic Ointment *(U.S.P.)*. A sterile eye ointment containing physostigmine sulphate.

4525-g

Pilocarpine *(U.S.P.)*. (3*S*,4*R*)-3-Ethyldihydro-4-[(1-methyl-1*H*-imidazol-5-yl)methyl]-furan-2(3*H*)-one.

$C_{11}H_{16}N_2O_2$=208.3.

CAS — 92-13-7.

Pharmacopoeias. In *U.S.*

An alkaloid obtained from the leaflets of *Pilocarpus microphyllus* (Rutaceae) and other species of *Pilocarpus*. A viscous, hygroscopic, colourless, oily liquid or crystals. M.p. about 34°. **Soluble** in water, alcohol, chloroform; sparingly soluble in ether; practically insoluble in light petroleum; soluble 1 in 350 of sesame oil. A solution in phosphate buffer is dextrorotatory. **Store** at a temperature not exceeding 8° in airtight containers. Protect from light.

Pilocarpine has actions and uses similar to those described under Pilocarpine Hydrochloride. It is used in the management of glaucoma. A reservoir containing pilocarpine may be placed in the conjunctival sac to provide a continuous dose.

A discussion on the use of pilocarpine Ocuserts in the treatment of chronic glaucoma.— *Drug & Ther. Bull.*, 1978, *16*, 45.

Further references.— K. L. Macoul and D. Pavan-Langston, *Archs Ophthal., N.Y.*, 1975, *93*, 587; *Med. Lett.*, 1975, *17*, 27.

Preparations

Pilocarpine Ocular System *(U.S.P.)*. A sterile device containing pilocarpine intended to permit the gradual release of pilocarpine. The *U.S.P.* requires the release of not less than 80% and not more than 120% of the labelled content in one week. Store at a temperature not exceeding 8°.

Ocusert Pilo-20 *(May & Baker, UK)*. An ocular therapeutic system for placement in the conjunctival sac consisting of a reservoir containing pilocarpine 5 mg, and delivering pilocarpine at an average rate of 20 µg per hour for 1 week. **Ocusert Pilo-40** contains pilocarpine 11 mg, and delivers 40 µg per hour. Store at 2° to 8°. (Also available as Ocusert Pilo-20 and Pilo-40 in *Austral., Canad., USA*).

Other Proprietary Names

Ocusert P20/P40 *(Ger., Ital., Neth.)*; Pilomann-Öl *(Ger.)*; Pilosyst 20/40 Ocusert *(Switz.)*; Thilo-Carpin (borate) *(Ger.)*.

4526-q

Pilocarpine Hydrochloride *(B.P., B.P. Vet., U.S.P.)*.

Pilocarp. Hydrochlor.; Pilocarpini Hydrochloridum; Pilocarpini Chloridum; Pilocarpinium Chloratum.

$C_{11}H_{16}N_2O_2,HCl$=244.7.

CAS — 54-71-7.

Pharmacopoeias. In *Arg., Aust., Br., Braz., Cz., Ger., Hung., It., Jap., Jug., Mex., Nord., Pol., Port., Roum., Rus., Span., Swiss,* and *U.S.*

Odourless or almost odourless hygroscopic colourless crystals or white crystalline powder with a slightly bitter taste. M.p. 199° to 205°.

Soluble 1 in less than 1 of water, 1 in 3 of alcohol, and 1 in 360 of chloroform; practically insoluble in ether. A solution in water is dextrorotatory. A 0.5% solution in water has a pH of 3.8 to 5.2. A 4.08% solution is iso-osmotic with serum. Solutions are **sterilised** by autoclaving or by filtration. **Incompatible** with alkalis, chlorhexidine acetate, iodine, silver salts, phenylmercuric salts, and mercurous chloride. **Store** in airtight containers. Protect from light.

Preservative for eye-drops. Benzalkonium chloride 0.01% or chlorhexidine gluconate 0.02% were suitable preservatives for pilocarpine hydrochloride eye-drops sterilised by filtration. Benzalkonium chloride 0.01% was also a suitable preservative for the eye-drops when sterilised by heating at 98° to 100° for 30 minutes.— M. Van Ooteghem, *Pharm. Tijdschr. Belg.*, 1968, *45*, 69.

Stability of solutions of pilocarpine salts. Ophthalmic solutions of pilocarpine hydrochloride were apparently more stable in the presence of methylcellulose but less stable in the presence of phosphate buffer, pH 6.2 during storage for 5 months.— I. R. Brown *et al.*, *Can. J. pharm. Sci.*, 1966, *1*, 22.

Aqueous solutions of pilocarpine hydrochloride or nitrate were stable, but because of their acidic reaction (about pH 4) might cause pain on instillation into the eye. Solutions adjusted to pH 7 with sodium bicarbonate retained 97% of activity after heating at 100° for 30 minutes, and 90% of activity after subsequent storage at 25° for 3 weeks, or 5° for 12 weeks. Solutions adjusted to pH 6.5 with borax or sodium hydroxide retained 98% of activity after heating at 100° for 30 minutes and 90% of activity after subsequent storage at 25° for 5 weeks or 5° for 20 weeks.— R. A. Anderson and S. D. Fitzgerald, *Australas. J. Pharm.*, 1967, *48*, S108.

Simple aqueous solutions of pilocarpine salts had a pH of about 4 and were relatively stable, but in a phosphate buffer of pH 6.8 the stability was reduced due to formation of isopilocarpine, according to S. Riegelman and D.G. Vaughan (*J. Am. pharm. Ass., pract. Pharm. Edn*, 1958, *19*, 537). That other changes also occurred was shown by colour reactions and fall in pH on storage. In a phosphate-free buffer in the range pH 5.6 to 6.7 there was a first-order reaction-rate between protonated pilocarpine and hydroxyl ions.— R. A. Anderson, *Can. J. pharm. Sci.*, 1967, *2*, 25.

Pilocarpine solutions at pH 6.5 were found to have a greater ocular hypotensive effect in patients with glaucoma than solutions at pH 4, although they had to be renewed more frequently since they were less stable.— R. A. Anderson and J. B. Cowle, *Br. J. Ophthal.*, 1968, *52*, 607.

The hydrolysis and epimerisation of pilocarpine nitrate in aqueous solution.— M. A. Nunes and E. Brochmann-Hanssen, *J. pharm. Sci.*, 1974, *63*, 716.

Further references: R. Fagerström, *J. Pharm. Pharmac.*, 1963, *15*, 479; K. Baeschlin and J. C. Etter, *Pharm. Acta Helv.*, 1969, *44*, 348; P. -H. Chung *et al.*, *J. pharm. Sci.*, 1970, *59*, 1300; S. S. Larsen, *Dansk. Tidsskr. Farm.*, 1971, *45*, 317; I. S. Gibbs and M. M. Tuckerman, *J. pharm. Sci.*, 1974, *63*, 276.

Adverse Effects, Treatment, and Precautions. As for Neostigmine Methylsulphate, p.1035.

Effects on the blood. An aqueous solution of pilocarpine hydrochloride iso-osmotic with serum (4.08%) caused 89% haemolysis of erythrocytes cultured in it for 45 minutes.— E. R. Hammarlund and K. Pedersen-Bjergaard, *J. pharm. Sci.*, 1961, *50*, 24.

Effects on the ears. In a 76-year-old woman with glaucoma, use of pilocarpine 4% eye-drops, 2 drops 6 times daily, resulted in disturbances in the middle ear and Eustachian tube. After reducing the dose to 1 drop and compressing the lachrymal sac for 5 minutes after each instillation ear symptoms disappeared within a few days.— R. M. Moose (letter), *J. Am. med. Ass.*, 1974, *230*, 1255.

Effects on the eyes. A review and discussion on the use of miotics and the incidence of retinal detachment.— J. J. Alpar, *Ann. Ophthal.*, 1979, *11*, 395. See also H. Beasley and F. T. Fraunfelder, *Ophthalmology*, 1979, *86*, 95.

A central macular hole developed in 1 eye of a patient following the bilateral use of pilocarpine 2% eye-drops.— R. S. Garlikov and R. G. Chenoweth, *Ann. Ophthal.*, 1975, *7*, 1313.

A study indicating that usual therapeutic doses of pilocarpine strongly interfere with colour vision.— J. Laroche and C. Laroche, *Annls pharm. Fr.*, 1977, *35*, 173.

A paradoxical increase in intra-ocular pressure occurred in a patient with unilateral angle-recession glaucoma given pilocarpine eye-drops.— B. S. Bleiman and A. L. Schwartz, *Archs Ophthal., N.Y.*, 1979, *97*, 1305.

Effects on the gastro-intestinal tract. Gastro-intestinal spasm and nausea associated with the use of pilocarpine eye-drops.— R. S. Sando, *Pa Med.*, 1980, *83* (Apr.), 24.

Uses. Pilocarpine is a parasympathomimetic agent with the muscarinic effects of acetylcholine (see p.1037).

Pilocarpine hydrochloride is used in solutions of 1 to 5% as a miotic to constrict the pupil and decrease the intra-ocular pressure in glaucoma and detachment of the retina. It is also used to antagonise the effects of short-acting mydriatics on the eye. As a miotic, it is only about half as active as physostigmine and its action is less complete and of shorter duration but it also causes less irritation; a slight increase of intra-ocular pressure may occur at first. With the 1% solution the pupils begin to constrict about 10 minutes after application and the effect lasts about 6 hours.

Pilocarpine 2.5 to 5 mg has been given by mouth to counteract some of the common side-effects of ganglion-blocking agents, such as dryness of the mouth, constipation, and impaired vision.

Pilocarpine 1% counteracted the mydriatic effects of sympathomimetic agents, such as phenylephrine and hydroxyamphetamine in concentrations usually used in ophthalmology, within 30 minutes. After mydriasis with parasympathomimetic agents, such as tropicamide and homatropine, pilocarpine did not cause effective miosis.— L. M. Anastasi *et al.*, *Archs Ophthal., N.Y.*, 1968, *79*, 710.

Administration. The use of pilocarpine alginate in the form of lamellae could prolong the miotic effect of pilocarpine to about 7 to 8 hours.— S. P. Loucas and H. M. Haddad (letter), *J. pharm. Sci.*, 1972, *61*, 985.

The management of 22 patients with acute closed-angle glaucoma by means of a hydrophilic contact lens presoaked in 1% pilocarpine.— J. S. Hillman, *Br. J. Ophthal.*, 1974, *58*, 674.

A study in 13 healthy subjects suggested that pilocarpine 2% administered in castor oil solution might have a greater degree and duration of action than administration in aqueous solution.— S. A. Smith *et al.*, *Br. J. Ophthal.*, 1978, *62*, 314.

The use of pilocarpine gel in patients with increased intraocular pressure.— I. Goldberg *et al.*, *Am. J. Ophthal.*, 1979, *88*, 843.

Further references.— M. Ruben and R. Watkins, *Br. J. Ophthal.*, 1975, *59*, 455; A. T. Birmingham, *Br. J. Ophthal.*, 1976, *60*, 568; R. R. File and T. F. Patton, *Archs Ophthal., N.Y.*, 1980, *98*, 112.

Glaucoma. Pilocarpine was used in concentrations up to 3% for the pre-operative or medical treatment of closed-angle glaucoma, but up to 6% for use up to 6 times daily for patients with open-angle glaucoma. It was relatively free from local and systemic side-effects and could be used synergistically with physostigmine 0.125 to 0.5%.— V. J. Marmion, *Prescribers' J.*, 1966, *6*, 68.

Pilocarpine produced in 10 to 15 minutes a miosis which lasted for 6 to 8 hours. It had marked vasodilatory effects. Solutions of 0.5 to 4% should be used at least 3 times a day for simple glaucoma though in acute closed-angle glaucoma it could be administered as often as once a minute.— J. J. Kanski, *Br. J. Ophthal.*, 1968, *52*, 936.

A comparison was made of various regimens using pilocarpine in the initial treatment of primary closed-angle glaucoma in 20 patients. It was concluded that 1 drop of pilocarpine eye-drops 2% instilled 3 to 4 hours after an intravenous injection of acetazolamide 500 mg was sufficient to terminate an acute attack.— F. Ganias and R. Mapstone, *Br. J. Ophthal.*, 1975, *59*, 205.

Pilocarpine was used in provocative tests to determine which eyes at risk were likely to develop closed-angle glaucoma.— R. Mapstone, *Br. J. Ophthal.*, 1976, *60*, 115.

Ocular hypertension. Tonographic study in patients with ocular hypertension showed no additive ocular hypotensive effect when physostigmine 1% was added to pilocarpine 4% eye-drops, but true additive effect was seen after the addition of adrenaline to pilocarpine eye-drops.— P. C. Kronfeld, *Archs Ophthal., N.Y.*, 1967, *78*, 140.

The maximal pressure reduction in 12 patients with ocular hypertension occurred 2 hours after instillation of one dose of pilocarpine eye-drops 1, 2, 4, or 8% into one eye. All strengths produced an increase in intra-ocular pressure during the first hour.— S. M. Drance and P. A. Nash, *Can. J. Ophthal.*, 1971, *6*, 9.

Reversal of anticholinergic action. In 12 patients with blurred vision as a consequence of antipsychotic therapy administration of pilocarpine 2% eye-drops produced improvement in vision in all.— J. G. Carter *et al.* (letter), *Am. J. Psychiat.*, 1977, *134*, 941.

Preparations

Oculoguttae Pilocarpini 2% *(Nord. P.).* Pilocarpine Hydrochloride Eye-drops. Pilocarpine hydrochloride 2 g, sodium chloride 450 mg, Water for Injections to 100 g. Sterilised by autoclaving. Phenylmercuric nitrate 0.001% may be added as a preservative.

Pilocarpine Eye Drops *(A.P.F.).* Pilocarpine hydrochloride 0.5, 1, 2, or 4%, benzalkonium chloride solution 0.02% v/v, disodium edetate 0.05%, sodium chloride 0.8, 0.7, 0.4, and 0% respectively, Water for Injections to 100%. Sterilise by autoclaving.

Pilocarpine Eye Drops *(B.P.).* Pilocarpine Hydrochloride Eye Drops; PIL. A sterile solution of pilocarpine hydrochloride in water. When intended for use on more than one occasion they contain benzalkonium chloride 0.01%, and should not be used more than one month after first opening the container.

Pilocarpine Eye Drops Buffered *(A.P.F.).* Pilocarpine hydrochloride 0.5, 1, 2, or 4%, borax 0.1, 0.2, 0.4, and 0.8% respectively or a sufficient quantity to adjust to a pH of 6.5, benzalkonium chloride solution 0.02% v/v, disodium edetate 0.05%, sodium chloride 0.7, 0.5, 0.2, and 0% respectively, Water for Injections to 100%. Sterilised by maintaining at 98° to 100° for 30 minutes. They should be freshly prepared. Store below 25° and use within 2 months.

Pilocarpine Hydrochloride Ophthalmic Solution *(U.S.P.).* A sterile, buffered, aqueous solution. It may contain suitable antimicrobial agents, stabilisers, and additives to increase its viscosity. pH 3.5 to 5.5. Store in airtight containers.

Proprietary Preparations

Isopto Carpine *(Alcon, UK: Farillon, UK).* Eye-drops containing pilocarpine hydrochloride 0.5, 1, 2, 3, or 4%, with hypromellose 0.5%. (Also available as Isopto Carpine in *Austral., Canad., Neth., Switz.* Also available as Isopto-Carpine in *Norw., S.Afr.*).

Sno pilo *(Smith & Nephew Pharmaceuticals, UK).* Eye-drops containing pilocarpine hydrochloride 0.5, 1, 2, 3, or 4%, with polyvinyl alcohol.

Other Proprietary Names

Arg.—Isopto Carpina; *Austral.*—Neutracarpine, Pilopt, PV Carpine; *Canad.*—Adsorbocarpine; *Denm.*— Pilokarpin Isopto, Spersacarpine; *Fr.*—Isopto Pilocarpine; *Ger.*— Pilocar, Pilomann, Spersacarpin; *Ital.*—Liocarpina, Pilotonina; *Norw.*—Spersakarpin; *S.Afr.*—Pilocar; *Spain*—Faring-S, Isopto Carpina, Veriscarpina; *Swed.*—Isopto-Pilokarpin, Spersacarpine; *Switz.*—Spersacarpine; *USA*—Adsorbocarpine, Mi-Pilo, Pilocar.

4527-p

Pilocarpine Nitrate *(B.P., Eur. P., U.S.P.).*

Pilocarp. Nit.; Pilocarpinii Nitras; Pilocarpini Nitras; Pilocarpinium Nitricum.

$C_{11}H_{16}N_2O_2,HNO_3=271.3$.

CAS — 148-72-1.

Pharmacopoeias. In *Arg., Belg., Br., Braz., Eur., Fr., Ger., Ind., Int., It., Mex., Neth., Port., Roum., Span., Swiss, Turk.*, and *U.S.*

Odourless colourless crystals or white crystalline powder with a faintly bitter taste. M.p. 171° to 179° with decomposition.

Soluble 1 in 8 of water and 1 in 160 of alcohol; practically insoluble in chloroform and ether. A solution in water is dextrorotatory. A solution in water is acid to litmus. Solutions are **sterilised** by autoclaving or by filtration. **Incompatible** with alkalis, iodine, and chlorhexidine acetate; solutions containing more than 1% are incompatible with benzalkonium chloride. **Store** in airtight containers. Protect from light.

Preservative for eye-drops. Phenylmercuric borate 0.005% or chlorhexidine gluconate 0.02% were suitable preservatives for pilocarpine nitrate eye-drops sterilised by filtration. Phenylmercuric borate 0.005% was also a suitable preservative for the eye-drops sterilised by heating at 98° to 100° for 30 minutes.— M. Van Ooteghem, *Pharm. Tijdschr. Belg.*, 1968, *45*, 69.

Stability of solutions of pilocarpine salts. For reports on the stability of solutions of pilocarpine salts, see under Pilocarpine Hydrochloride, p.1044.

Pilocarpine nitrate has the actions and uses of pilocarpine as described under Pilocarpine Hydrochloride, p.1044.

The use of pilocarpine nitrate intradermally to assess the therapeutic efficacy of dapsone in patients with maculoanaesthetic leprosy.— P. B. Joshi, *Lepr. India*, 1976, *48*, 55.

Preparations

Pilocarpine Nitrate Ophthalmic Solution *(U.S.P.).* A sterile, buffered, aqueous solution. It may contain suitable antimicrobial agents, stabilisers, and additives to increase its viscosity. pH 4 to 5.5. Store in airtight containers. Protect from light.

Minims Pilocarpine Nitrate *(Smith & Nephew Pharmaceuticals, UK).* Sterile eye-drops containing pilocarpine nitrate 1, 2, or 4% in single-use disposable applicators.

Other Proprietary Names

Arg.—Piloplos; *Canad.*—PV Carpine; *Fr.*—Chibro-Pilocarpine, Dulcicarpine, Marticarpine, Pilo; *Ger.*—Miopos, Pilopos, Vistacarpin; *S.Afr.*—PV-Carpine; *Swed.*—Licarpin; *Switz.*—Chibro-Pilocarpine.

4528-s

Pyridostigmine Bromide *(B.P., U.S.P.).*

Pyridostig. Brom.; Pyridostigmini Bromidum.

3-Dimethylcarbamoyloxy-1-methylpyridinium bromide.

$C_9H_{13}BrN_2O_2=261.1$.

CAS — 155-97-5 (pyridostigmine); 101-26-8 (bromide).

Pharmacopoeias. In *Br., Int., Nord.*, and *U.S.*

A white or almost white deliquescent crystalline powder with an agreeable characteristic odour and a bitter taste. M.p. 153° to 157°.

Soluble 1 in less than 1 of water, 1 in less than 1 of alcohol, and 1 in 1 of chloroform; slightly soluble in light petroleum; practically insoluble in ether. A 4.13% solution in water is iso-osmotic with serum. Solutions are **sterilised** by autoclaving or by filtration. **Store** in airtight containers. Protect from light.

Adverse Effects, Treatment, and Precautions. As for Neostigmine Methylsulphate, p.1035.

Alopecia. Toxic alopecia associated with pyridostigmine therapy.— L. M. Field (letter), *Archs Derm.*, 1980, *116*, 1103.

Pregnancy and the neonate. A mother with myasthenia who excreted pyridostigmine more slowly than other myasthenic patients was overtreated with the drug during pregnancy. She gave birth to a child who showed clinical signs of myasthenia at 24 hours. Neuromuscular transmission improved after an intravenous injection of 100 µg of neostigmine, which was maintained in progressively decreasing dosage for 12 days.— G. A. Buckley *et al.*, *Br. J. Pharmac.*, 1968, *34*, 203P.

Reversal of neuromuscular blockade. A prolonged response to suxamethonium following the reversal of pancuronium-induced neuromuscular blockade occurred in an 82-year-old man who had been given a total dose of pyridostigmine 30 mg over 15 minutes together with atropine.— E. W. Bentz and R. K. Stoelting, *Anesthesiology*, 1976, *44*, 258.

Absorption and Fate. Pyridostigmine is poorly absorbed from the gastro-intestinal tract; it is excreted mainly in the urine.

During prolonged administration of pyridostigmine by mouth 2 to 16% was excreted unchanged in the urine. Pyridostigmine was found in the urine up to 2 days after discontinuation of the drug.— P. T. Nowell *et al.*, *Br. J. Pharmac. Chemother.*, 1962, *18*, 617.

Pyridostigmine and three metabolites were isolated from the urine of 3 patients with myasthenia gravis given pyridostigmine. One metabolite was found to be 3-hydroxy-*N*-methylpyridinium; the other two were not identified.— S. M. Somani *et al.*, *Clin. Pharmac. Ther.*, 1972, *13*, 393.

A report of poor control of myasthenia gravis in 4 patients due to malabsorption of pyridostigmine given by mouth.— S. L. Cohan *et al.*, *Neurology, Minneap.*, 1977, *27*, 299.

In 4 patients with myasthenia gravis affecting the adductor pollicis muscle a positive correlation between plasma-pyridostigmine concentration required to restore normal transmission (range 27.8 to 125.7 ng per ml) and a significant effect on neuromuscular transmission was observed in 2 patients. In a fifth patient with myasthenia gravis and suffering from ptosis but with no involvement of the adductor pollicis muscle a significant increase in the diameter of the eyelid fissure occurred with a plasma-pyridostigmine concentration of about 10 ng per ml.— K. Chan and T. N. Calvey, *Clin. Pharmac. Ther.*, 1977, *22*, 596. See also T. N. Calvey and K. Chan, *ibid.*, *21*, 187; K. Chan and T. N. Calvey, *Eur. Neurol.*, 1977, *16*, 69.

Uses. Pyridostigmine bromide is an inhibitor of cholinesterase activity with actions similar to those of neostigmine (see Neostigmine Methylsulphate, p.1036), but is slower in onset and of longer duration; it is only about one-fourth as active as neostigmine.

Pyridostigmine bromide is mainly used in the treatment of myasthenia gravis, usually in daily doses of 0.3 to 1.2 g although more may be required; the dose should be divided throughout the day and, if necessary, the night according to the response of the patient and larger portions of the total daily dose may be given at times of greater fatigue. It may also be given by subcutaneous or intramuscular injection. In severe cases it can also be given by very slow intravenous injection. It does not always relieve the symptoms of myasthenia gravis as completely as neostigmine but it may produce fewer gastro-intestinal disturbances, and its prolonged effect often provides more sustained relief and it is particularly suitable for treatment at night. A suggested dose for children is 7 mg per kg body-weight daily in 6 divided doses.

In paralytic ileus or postoperative urinary retention, a dose of 1 to 2 mg may be given intramuscularly. To curtail the muscular relaxation produced by non-depolarising muscle relaxants, such as tubocurarine and gallamine, an initial dose of 2 to 5 mg may be given intravenously and repeated to a total of 10 mg but it is less satisfactory than neostigmine.

Administration in renal failure. A 58-year-old woman with myasthenia gravis who had received pyridostigmine 420 to 660 mg daily for 14 years had to have the dose frequently reduced, finally to 60 mg daily, after developing visceral lupus erythematosus with rapidly progressive renal failure which required chronic dialysis. In spite of this dose reduction 2 severe cholinergic crises developed, the second ending fatally. It was suggested that an accumulation of pyridostigmine, normally excreted by the kidney, had occurred during dialysis.— R. Korz *et al., Dt. med. Wschr.*, 1978, *103*, 1485.

In patients receiving pyridostigmine for the reversal of non-depolarising muscular blockade following anaesthesia pyridostigmine kinetics were not significantly different in 5 following renal transplantation from those in 5 with normal renal function but in 4 anephric patients the elimination half-life was significantly increased and the plasma clearance significantly decreased. It appeared that approximately 75% of the plasma clearance of pyridostigmine depended on renal function.— R. Cronnelly *et al., Clin. Pharmac. Ther.*, 1980, *28*, 78.

Myasthenia gravis. The management of myasthenia gravis in a 6-month-old child with neostigmine and pyridostigmine. Good control was achieved with a pyridostigmine dose of 50 mg every 4 hours, but this had to be increased to 80 mg then 100 mg 5 times daily. The child died several months later following inhalation of vomitus.— F. Oberklaid and I. J. Hopkins, *Archs Dis. Childh.*, 1976, *51*, 719.

Reversal of neuromuscular blockade. Investigations in 100 surgical patients indicated that pyridostigmine bromide 10 to 20 mg effectively antagonised pancuronium and appeared to be a safe alternative to neostigmine for the reversal of neuromuscular blockade due to pancuronium bromide.— M. Lippmann and R. C. Rogoff, *Anesth. Analg. curr. Res.*, 1974, *53*, 20.

Further references.— P. G. McNall *et al., Anesth. Analg. curr. Res.*, 1969, *48*, 1026; A. W. Gotta and C. A. Sullivan, *Can. Anaesth. Soc. J.*, 1970, *17*, 527.

For a reference to the use of glycopyrronium bromide with pyridostigmine for reversing neuromuscular blockade, see Glycopyrronium Bromide, p.301.

See also under Precautions (above).

Preparations

Pyridostigmine Bromide Injection *(U.S.P.)*. A sterile solution of pyridostigmine bromide in a suitable vehicle. pH 4.5 to 5.5. Protect from light.

Pyridostigmine Bromide Syrup *(U.S.P.)*. A syrup containing 1.08 to 1.32 g of pyridostigmine bromide in each 100 ml. Store in airtight containers. Protect from light.

Pyridostigmine Bromide Tablets *(U.S.P.)*. Tablets containing pyridostigmine bromide. Store in airtight containers.

Pyridostigmine Injection *(B.P.)*. Pyridostig. Inj.; Pyridostigmine Bromide Injection. A sterile solution of pyridostigmine bromide in Water for Injections. Sterilised by autoclaving. pH 5.7 to 6.3. Protect from light.

Pyridostigmine Tablets *(B.P.)*. Pyridostig. Tab. Tablets containing pyridostigmine bromide. Protect from light.

Proprietary Preparations

Mestinon *(Roche, UK)*. Pyridostigmine bromide, available as 1-ml **Ampoules** of an injection containing 1 mg per ml and as scored **Tablets** of 60 mg. (Also available as Mestinon in *Austral., Belg., Canad., Denm., Fr., Ger., Ital., Neth., Norw., S.Afr., Spain, Switz., USA*).

Other Proprietary Names

Regonol *(Canad., USA)*.

4529-w

Pyrophos. Tetraethyl monothiopyrophosphate.
$C_8H_{20}O_6P_2S$=306.2.

CAS — 645-78-3.

A pale yellow oily liquid with a characteristic odour. **Soluble** 1 in 1000 of water; soluble in organic solvents. Oily solutions are stable but aqueous solutions are unstable due to hydrolysis. **Protect** from light.

Pyrophos is an inhibitor of cholinesterase with actions similar to those of dyflos (see p.1039). Its miotic action begins within about 10 minutes of its application and may persist for as long as 12 days. It has been used in the USSR in the treatment of certain types of glaucoma by instillation into the conjunctival sac, usually as a 0.01% solution in liquid paraffin or persic oil.

Nitrofurantoin and some other Urinary Antimicrobial Agents

5650-t

The urinary antimicrobial agents described in this section are used in the treatment and prophylaxis of infections of the lower urinary tract. In general antibiotics or sulphonamides are preferred in the treatment of infections of the urinary tract.

Urinary-tract infection, or significant bacteriuria, is said to be present if culture of a midstream specimen of urine (MSU) indicates that there are more than 100 000 organisms per ml. Infections may be differentiated into those of the upper tract, involving the renal parenchyma, and those of the lower tract or bladder and urethra.

The choice of antimicrobial agent is largely determined by the sensitivity of the infecting organism. The majority of acute infections are caused by *Escherichia coli* and, to a lesser extent, *Proteus* spp. The range of organisms isolated is much wider in hospital than in domiciliary practice. Other bacteria include *Klebsiella* spp., *Streptococcus faecalis, Staphylococcus epidermidis,* and *Pseudomonas aeruginosa.* In chronic infections more than one kind of organism is often present.

Relief from some acute infections of the lower urinary tract may be hastened by promoting diuresis without unduly affecting antimicrobial activity in the urine and a high fluid intake is beneficial. Dysuria is generally relieved, but infection not eradicated, following the administration of potassium or sodium citrate. Acidification of the urine may inhibit bacterial growth and is essential when hexamine is given. Organic acids such as mandelic acid have a greater antibacterial effect than can be accounted for by changes in urinary pH alone. The effects of sulphonamides and some antibiotics are enhanced by alkalinisation of the urine. Ascorbic acid or sodium bicarbonate may be given to adjust pH but such agents should not be used in patients with renal failure.

Antimicrobial agents which are eliminated in an active form through the kidneys may be used to treat infection of the urinary tract. In some instances antibacterial concentrations may be obtained in the urine by administering doses too small to achieve effective concentrations in the blood, thereby diminishing the systemic toxicity of the treatment. However, while such treatment may produce amelioration of bacteriuria, an effective antibacterial concentration in the tissues as well as in the urine may be necessary for the eradication of infection.

In acute infections treatment is given for at least 7 to 10 days; in chronic or recurrent infections, both intermittent and continuous courses of treatment have been advocated. Chronic infection is generally associated with some abnormality of the urinary tract and the infection is not likely to be eradicated by drug treatment alone.

Nitrofurantoin, a nitrofuran derivative, and also hexamine mandelate and hippurate are used prophylactically. Nitrofurantoin or nalidixic acid may be of value in controlling infections resistant to other agents.

The urine should be examined bacteriologically 1 week and 4 to 6 weeks after antimicrobial treatment and then at increasing intervals for 12 to 18 months to detect symptomatic recurrences.

Urinary-tract infections. A 3-year study of 63 girls with covert (or asymptomatic) bacteriuria demonstrated that treatment had no significant effect and was not considered essential.— D. C. L. Savage *et al., Lancet,* 1975, *1,* 358.

A follow-up study over 9 to 18 years of the long-term effects of bacteriuria detected in 60 schoolgirls indicated that they had considerably more recurrent infections and urological abnormalities and were at high risk of bacteriuria during pregnancy when compared with 38 matched controls. Bacteriuria also occurred in 7 of the 65 children of the study subjects compared with none of the 24 children born to control subjects. Only one of the 60 subjects developed substantially reduced renal function but even so, the study demonstrates that screening for bacteriuria in schoolgirls detects those at risk of considerable morbidity from recurrent infection and a small number with major urological abnormalities. Since all episodes of bacteriuria were treated with short courses of chemotherapy some renal damage may have been prevented.— J. Y. Gillenwater *et al., New Engl. J. Med.,* 1979, *301,* 396.

Recommended terminology of urinary-tract infection.— *Br. med. J.,* 1979, *2,* 717 (Report by the MRC Bacteriuria Committee). Comments.— N. B. Eastwood (letter), *ibid.,* 938; H. G. Hanley (letter), *ibid.*

Discussions on the treatment of urinary-tract infections.— R. S. Nanra, *Drugs,* 1976, *11,* 441; R. R. Bailey, *ibid.,* 1977, *13,* 137; A. W. Asscher, *Br. med. J.,* 1978, *1,* 1531; *ibid.,* 1649.

Further references.— A. J. Wing, *Br. med. J.,* 1970, *3,* 753; P. E. Gower, *Prescribers' J.,* 1971, *11,* 78; *Drug & Ther. Bull.,* 1972, *10,* 41; P. J. Little, *Drugs,* 1972, *3,* 414; *ibid., 4,* 132; K. F. Fairley, *ibid.,* 1973, *6,* 417; R. R. Bailey, *ibid.,* 1974, *8,* 54; A. P. Ball *et al., ibid.,* 1975, *10,* 1.

In pregnancy. The treatment of urinary-tract infection in pregnancy.— P. J. Little, *Drugs,* 1977, *14,* 390.

Prophylaxis. In a prospective study of prophylactic therapy in 249 men with urinary-tract infection, treated initially with antibiotics, 165 completed 25 months of continuous treatment with sulphamethizole, nitrofurantoin, hexamine mandelate, or placebo. Follow-up was continued for up to 10 years after the start of therapy in 65 patients. Continuous therapy, especially with nitrofurantoin and hexamine mandelate, reduced the recurrence-rate of bacteriuria and acute exacerbations during the first year, but thereafter control of bacteriuria gradually diminished. Side-effects developed in 8 of the 249 during 25 months of treatment and these were—nitrofurantoin: skin eruptions (2), repetitive asthma (1), peripheral neuropathy (1); hexamine mandelate: skin eruptions (1), dyspnoea and dysuria (1), severe diarrhoea (1); and sulphamethizole: hepatotoxicity (1). One patient developed reversible interstitial pneumonia after taking nitrofurantoin for 37 months. Continuous therapy was not necessary in all patients with bacteriuria since a 'cure' was achieved in 25% of patients who received a single short course of antibiotic therapy.— R. B. Freeman *et al., Ann. intern. Med.,* 1975, *83,* 133. See also C. M. Kunin, *ibid.,* 273.

In 14 patients with chronic or recurrent urinary-tract infection nitrofurantoin, nalidixic acid, cephalexin, benzylpenicillin, or sulphonamides taken as a single prophylactic dose, after sexual intercourse, significantly reduced the incidence of infections.— K. L. Vosti, *J. Am. med. Ass.,* 1975, *231* 934.

5651-x

Nitrofurantoin *(B.P.).* Nitrofurant.; Nitrofurantoinum; Furadoninum. 1-(5-Nitrofurfurylideneamino)hydantoin; 1-(5-Nitrofurfurylideneamino)imidazolidine-2,4-dione.

$C_8H_6N_4O_5$=238.2.

CAS — 67-20-9 (anhydrous); 17140-81-7 (monohydrate).

Pharmacopoeias. In *Br., Chin., Cz., Int., It., Jug., Nord., Pol., Roum., Swiss,* and *Turk. Rus.* specifies the monohydrate; *Braz.* and *U.S.* specify anhydrous or monohydrate.

Yellow odourless or almost odourless crystals or fine powder with a bitter taste. It is discoloured by alkalis and by exposure to light.

Soluble 1 in 5000 of water, 1 in 2000 of alcohol, 1 in 200 of acetone, 1 in 16 of dimethylformamide, and 1 in 70 of macrogol 300. **Store** at a temperature not exceeding 25° in airtight containers and avoid contact with metals other than stainless steel or aluminium. Protect from light.

5652-r

Nitrofurantoin Sodium.

$C_8H_5N_4NaO_5$=260.1.

CAS — 54-87-5.

A yellow to orange-coloured powder.

Crystal size. Nitrofurantoin in 'macrocrystals' of 75 to 180 µm produced ample urinary concentration with satisfactory total urinary excretion.— H. E. Paul *et al., J. pharm. Sci.,* 1967, *56,* 882.

In a study in 399 patients with a history of nitrofurantoin intolerance, capsules of nitrofurantoin in coarse particule size produced gastro-intestinal intolerance much less frequently than commercial nitrofurantoin tablets.— F. J. Hailey and H. W. Glascock, *Curr. ther. Res.,* 1967, *9,* 600.

In 10 healthy men, microcrystalline nitrofurantoin in tablets was excreted in the urine more readily than macrocrystalline nitrofurantoin in gelatin capsules. It was considered that macrocrystals in a capsule were absorbed more slowly than microcrystals in a tablet form.— J. D. Conklin; F. J. Hailey, *Clin. Pharmac. Ther.,* 1969, *10,* 534.

Further references: J. D. Conklin *et al., J. pharm. Sci.,* 1969, *58,* 1365.

Incompatibility. Nitrofurantoin 36 mg was 'physically incompatible' with tetracycline 50 mg in 100 ml of dextrose injection.— R. D. Dunworth and F. R. Kenna, *Am. J. Hosp. Pharm.,* 1965, *22,* 190.

There was loss of clarity when intravenous solutions of nitrofurantoin sodium were mixed with insulin, narcotic salts, noradrenaline acid tartrate, procaine hydrochloride, prochlorperazine maleate, promethazine hydrochloride, protein hydrolysate, streptomycin sulphate, tetracycline hydrochloride (in dextrose injection), vancomycin hydrochloride, ammonium chloride injection, or lactated Ringer's injection.— J. A. Patel and G. L. Phillips, *Am. J. Hosp. Pharm.,* 1966, *23,* 409.

A haze or precipitate was observed within an hour when an average dose of nitrofurantoin sodium was mixed in dextrose injection with polymyxin B sulphate. Nitrofurantoin was also reported to be incompatible with amphotericin and kanamycin sulphate, and with tetracycline hydrochloride in dextrose but not sodium chloride solution.— J. M. Meisler and M. W. Skolaut, *Am. J. Hosp. Pharm.,* 1966, *23,* 557.

Nitrofurantoin sodium in dextrose injection was incompatible with metaraminol tartrate; the pH fell to 7.2 and a brown precipitate was formed.— M. Edward, *Am. J. Hosp. Pharm.,* 1967, *24,* 440.

Nitrofurantoin sodium was incompatible with amikacin sulphate in a variety of diluents.— B. C. Nunning and A. P. Granatek, *Curr. ther. Res.,* 1976, *20,* 417.

Solubility. The dissolution-rate of a molar 1:5 nitrofurantoin and deoxycholic acid co-precipitate was 6 times faster than that of the drug alone or in a physical mixture with deoxycholic acid. The absorption from the co-precipitate in 4 subjects was also greater than that of nitrofurantoin alone, 50 to 80% more unchanged nitrofurantoin being excreted in 24 hours.— R. G. Stoll *et al., J. pharm. Sci.,* 1973, *62,* 65.

The effect of pH on the dissolution of nitrofurantoin.— T. R. Bates *et al., J. pharm. Sci.,* 1974, *63,* 643. See also— L. -K. Chen *et al., ibid.,* 1976, *65,* 868.

Low concentrations of urea increased the solubility of nitrofurantoin in aqueous solution but, at a concentration above about 2% at 30° and 2.35% at 37°, solubility was markedly decreased. Urea concentration in the urine was usually about 2%.— D. E. Cadwallader *et al.* (letter), *J. pharm. Sci.,* 1975, *64,* 886. Creatinine, either alone or in the presence of urea, increased the solubility of nitrofurantoin. These effects might explain the absence of crystalluria with high doses of nitrofurantoin.— L. -K. Chen *et al., ibid.,* 1976, *65,* 868.

The dissolution rate of nitrofurantoin was increased by preparing a solid dispersion in macrogol 6000.— A. S. Geneidi *et al., J. pharm. Sci.,* 1978, *67,* 114.

Adverse Effects. Nitrofurantoin may cause nausea, vomiting, drowsiness, and headache. Polyneuritis, usually related to high blood concentrations, has occurred in patients with impaired renal function or after prolonged administration or the administration of large doses. Nystagmus and alopecia have occurred.

Allergic reactions such as skin rashes and fever may occur and, more rarely, serious acute pulmonary sensitivity reactions including symptoms of asthma and oedema. Chronic pulmonary symptoms may develop insidiously in patients on long-term therapy and these are not always reversible.

Other adverse effects include megaloblastic anaemia, agranulocytosis, haemolytic anaemia in persons with a genetic deficiency of glucose-6-phosphate dehydrogenase, and liver damage.

In a study of 757 courses of treatment with nitrofurantoin side-effects sufficiently severe to require treatment, reduction, or discontinuation of dosage, or avoidance of further exposure occurred on 70 occasions (31 allergic) and included gastro-intestinal, dermatological, haematological, and other effects. The side-effects were significantly dose-dependent, occurring in 1.6% of patients receiving less than 4 mg per kg body-weight and in 23.6% of those receiving more than 7 mg per kg. Reactions were more frequent in females and the risk of reactions increased with increased exposure to the drug.— J. Koch-Weser *et al.*, *Archs intern. Med.*, 1971, *128*, 399. See also R. A. Delaney *et al.*, *Am. J. Pharm.*, 1977, *149*, 26; L. Holmberg *et al.*, *Am. J. Med.*, 1980, *69*, 733.

In a controlled study of 24 patients with chronic pyelonephritis who had previously stopped taking nitrofurantoin because of toxicity, 2 of 12 patients given nitrofurantoin 100 mg in conjunction with deglycyrrhizinated liquorice 250 mg thrice daily experienced side-effects attributed to nitrofurantoin compared with 10 of 12 given nitrofurantoin alone.— R. Gromotka *et al.*, *Arzneimittel-Forsch.*, 1972, *22*, 627.

Three elderly patients with indwelling catheters developed crystalluria after treatment with prophylactic doses of nitrofurantoin.— J. B. MacDonald and E. T. MacDonald, *Br. med. J.*, 1976, *2*, 1044.

Allergy. A review of the pulmonary reactions to nitrofurantoin.— E. C. Rosenow, *Ann. intern. Med.*, 1972, *77*, 977.

Reports of pulmonary reactions following long-term treatment with nitrofurantoin.— O. Bäck *et al.* (letter), *lancet*, 1974, *1*, 930; I. Strandberg *et al.*, *Acta med. scand.*, 1974, *196*, 483; S. J. Simonian *et al.*, *Ann. thorac. Surg.*, 1977, *24*, 284; H. Rantala *et al.* (letter), *Lancet* 1979, *2*, 799; N. S. Jayasundera *et al.*, *J. Am. med. Ass.*, 1980, *243*, 769.

A report of a lupus-like syndrome occurring in 3 subjects after treatment with nitrofurantoin.— O. Selroos and J. Edgren, *Acta med. scand.*, 1975, *197*, 125.

In a study of 76 women and 5 men with hypersensitivity reactions to nitrofurantoin, 66 had pulmonary reactions. A preparation containing nitrofurantoin with ascorbic acid appeared to cause significantly fewer hypersensitivity reactions than those containing only nitrofurantoin.— A. R. A. Sovijärvi *et al.*, *Scand. J. resp. Dis.*, 1977, *58*, 41.

Blood disorders. A 41-year-old woman with chronic pyelitis was given nitrofurantoin 100 mg 4 times daily for 3 days. She developed haemolytic anaemia which was associated with erythrocyte enolase deficiency.— M. Stefanini, *Am. J. clin. Path.*, 1972, *58*, 408.

An analysis of blood dyscrasias reported to the Swedish Adverse Drug Reaction Committee for the 5-year period 1966–70 showed that thrombocytopenia attributable to nitrofurantoin had been reported on 3 occasions. It was estimated that reported figures represented one-third of the true frequency.— L. E. Böttiger and B. Westerholm, *Br. med. J.*, 1973, *3*, 339.

Gastro-intestinal side-effects. For reports relating the incidence of gastro-intestinal side-effects to the crystal size of nitrofurantoin, see under Crystal Size (p.1047) and Urinary-tract Infections (p.1049).

Hepatitis. Reports of hepatitis associated with nitrofurantoin: D. E. Hatoff *et al.*, *Am. J. Med.*, 1979, *67*, 117; J. R. Sharp *et al.*, *Ann. intern. Med.*, 1980, *92*, 14; M. Black *et al.*, *ibid.*, 62; K. G. Tolman, *ibid.*, 119.

Intracranial hypertension. Bulging of the anterior fontanelle, with a poor response to stimuli, developed in a 10-month-old child after treatment for 7 days with nitrofurantoin 25 mg thrice daily; the likely diagnosis was benign intracranial hypertension, possibly due to nitrofurantoin.— D. B. Sharma and A. James (letter), *Br. med. J.*, 1974, *4*, 771.

A report of benign intracranial hypertension developing in a 23-year-old woman during a 10-day course of nitrofurantoin 200 mg daily.— G. R. Mushet (letter), *Archs Neurol., Chicago*, 1977, *34*, 257.

Polyneuropathy. Polyneuropathies developed in 5 patients after treatment with nitrofurantoin for urinary infection. Four patients had urinary-tract obstruction or chronic renal infection. Dosage in most cases varied from 200 to 400 mg daily for 10 days to 7 months, but 1 patient had had 300 to 600 mg daily intermittently for several years. Paraesthesia in the extremities was followed by muscle weakness and sensory impairment. Recovery was complete only if the drug was withdrawn before marked muscle weakness had occurred.— C. J. Rubenstein, *J. Am. med. Ass.*, 1964, *187*, 647.

In a review of 137 cases, symptoms of neuropathy usually occurred within 45 days of starting nitrofurantoin therapy. The degree of recovery depended on the severity of the symptoms but had no apparent relationship to dosage.— J. F. Toole and M. L. Parrish, *Neurology, Minneap.*, 1973, *23*, 554.

A 73-year-old man developed progressive peripheral neuropathy and cerebellar dysfunction during therapy with nitrofurantoin 400 mg daily for 15 weeks.— R. W. Graebner and A. Herskowitz, *Archs Neurol., Chicago*, 1973, *29*, 195.

Precautions. Nitrofurantoin should not be given to patients with impaired renal function since antibacterial concentrations in the urine may not be attained and toxic concentrations in the plasma can occur. It is also contra-indicated in patients known to be hypersensitive, in those with a deficiency of glucose-6-phosphate dehydrogenase, and in infants less than one month old. Nitrofurantoin should be avoided during the first trimester of pregnancy.

Patients should be warned to report early signs of polyneuritis such as paraesthesia. It might be advisable to check patients undergoing prolonged therapy for changes in pulmonary function.

Nitrofurantoin and nalidixic acid are antagonistic *in vitro* and should not be used together. Nitrofurantoin has also been reported to antagonise the effects of oxolinic acid *in vitro* against some organisms. It has been suggested that alcohol and nitrofurantoin could produce a disulfiram-like reaction.

Nitrofurantoin could cause rust-yellow or brownish discoloration of the urine.— R. B. Baran and B. Rowles, *J. Am. pharm. Ass.*, 1973, *NS13*, 139.

Nitrofurantoin induced haemolytic anaemia in subjects with glucose-6-phosphate dehydrogenase deficiency; this abnormality was common in West African, Mediterranean, Middle Eastern, and southern Chinese people.— *Drug & Ther. Bull.*, 1974, *12*, 69.

Reduced rate and extent of absorption of nitrofurantoin following administration with magnesium trisilicate.— V. F. Naggar and S. A. Khalil, *Clin. Pharmac. Ther.*, 1979, *25*, 857.

Antimicrobial Action. Nitrofurantoin is bactericidal *in vitro* to most Gram-positive and Gram-negative urinary-tract pathogens and minimum inhibitory concentrations have been reported to range from 4 to 100 µg per ml. *Pseudomonas aeruginosa* is usually resistant and most strains of *Proteus* spp. are moderately resistant. It is most active in acid urine, and if the pH exceeds 8 most of the antibacterial activity is lost. Resistance rarely develops during nitrofurantoin treatment.

Antagonism between nitrofurantoin and nalidixic acid and nitrofurantoin and oxolinic acid has been demonstrated *in vitro*.

Nitrofurantoin is considered to act by interfering with bacterial enzymes involved in carbohydrate metabolism.

Studies *in vitro* showed the minimum inhibitory concentration of nitrofurantoin against *Bacteroides fragilis* to be 7.65 µg per ml.— Reynolds A.V., *J. Pharm. Pharmac.*, 1979, *31*, *Suppl.*, 29P.

For a report of the effect of nitrofurantoin with metronidazole against *Bacteroides fragilis*, see Metronidazole, p.971.

For reports of nitrofurantoin inhibiting the antimicrobial actions of nalidixic acid and oxolinic acid, see Nalidixic Acid, p.1052 and Oxolinic Acid, p.1053 respectively.

Bacterial resistance. Fifty-six of 301 strains of *Escherichia coli*, 15 of 25 strains of *Klebsiella*, and 14 of 20 strains of *Proteus* isolated from out-patients in Stockholm during 1971/72 were resistant to nitrofurantoin. In one case resistance to nitrofurantoin was transferred.— M. Jonsson, *Scand. J. infect. Dis.*, 1973, *5*, 41.

Transferable bacterial resistance. There was no evidence that resistance to nitrofurantoin had been transferred among the enterobacteriaceae by a resistance-transfer factor.— H. W. Glascock (letter), *New Engl. J. Med.*, 1966, *275*, 1077. See also P. Chadwick and M. Niell, *Can. med. Ass. J.*, 1973, *109*, 691.

Transfer of resistance to nitrofurantoin was found in only 3 of 42 strains of Gram-negative bacteria.— M. Jonsson *et al.*, *Scand. J. infect. Dis.*, 1972, *4*, 133. Eleven of 20 strains of *Salmonella* isolated in a hospital were resistant to nitrofurantoin. In 1 strain resistance could be transferred, but transferability was lost from the first to subsequent isolates.— *idem*, 209.

Absorption and Fate. Nitrofurantoin is readily absorbed from the gastro-intestinal tract and 25 to 60% is bound to plasma proteins. The plasma half-life is about 20 minutes. Nitrofurantoin diffuses across the placenta; low concentrations appear in the foetal circulation and have been detected in milk. About 40% of a dose is excreted rapidly in the urine as nitrofurantoin. Average doses give a concentration of 50 to 200 µg per ml in the urine in patients with normal renal function.

The absorption of nitrofurantoin is dependent on crystal size. The macrocrystalline form has slower dissolution and absorption rates, produces lower serum concentrations than the microcrystalline form, and takes longer to achieve peak concentrations in the urine.

Nitrofurantoin disposition.— B. Hoener and S. E. Patterson, *Clin. Pharmac. Ther.*, 1981, *29*, 808.

Bioavailability. A study of the bioavailability of nitrofurantoin.— M. C. Meyer *et al.*, *J. pharm. Sci.*, 1974, *63*, 1693. See also D. E. Cadwallader *et al.*, *J. Am. pharm. Ass.*, 1975, *NS15*, 409.

Urinary concentrations of nitrofurantoin were increased when it was given after food. Increases of up to 40% occurred in dosage forms with the poorest dissolution characteristics.— H. A. Rosenberg and T. R. Bates, *Clin. Pharmac. Ther.*, 1976, *20*, 227.

Excretion. The rate of excretion of nitrofurantoin in the urine of 10 healthy persons and of 16 patients who had undergone gastric resection was greater after the administration of enteric-coated tablets than after plain uncoated tablets.— G. Stoffels *et al.*, *Arzneimittel-Forsch.*, 1968, *18*, 360.

The total excretion of nitrofurantoin within 12 hours of its administration was almost doubled by the concomitant administration of pyridoxine.— I. Amon *et al.*, *Dte GesundhWes.*, 1973, *28*, 1153, per *Int. pharm. Abstr.*, 1974, *11*, 200. A similar report.— A. Mattheus and H. Heise, *Dte GesundhWes.*, 1973, *28*, 716, per *Int. pharm. Abstr.*, 1973, *10*, 899.

A crossover study in 6 healthy fasted subjects compared urinary excretion of macrocrystalline nitrofurantoin 100 mg given alone with that when propantheline 30 mg was taken 45 minutes previously. Prior administration of propantheline produced a significant increase in nitrofurantoin excretion, probably due to delayed gastric emptying. The administration of nitrofurantoin with food might have a similar effect.— J. M. Jaffe (letter), *J. pharm. Sci.*, 1975, *64*, 1730.

Uses. Nitrofurantoin is used in the treatment of urinary-tract infections although sulphonamides or antibiotics are generally the agents of choice. Antimicrobial concentrations are not reached in the blood but nitrofurantoin is concentrated in the urine and bactericidal concentrations are achieved. It is widely used prophylactically and for long-term suppressive therapy.

It is given by mouth usually in a dose of 100 mg four times daily, during or immediately after meals, and at bedtime with food or cold milk. Treatment is usually continued for up to 14 days. A usual prophylactic dose is 50 to 100 mg at bedtime.

Infants over 1 month of age and older children may be given 1.25 to 1.75 mg per kg body-weight 4 times daily by mouth. The dosage should be reduced if continued beyond 10 to 14 days or if used for prophylaxis.

Nitrofurantoin sodium has been given parenterally to patients unable to take the drug by mouth; the usual dose is the equivalent of 180 mg of nitrofurantoin twice daily intramuscularly in diluent free from hydroxybenzoates, cresol, or phenol or by intravenous infusion in at least 500 ml of diluent.

At certain concentrations *in vitro* nitrofurantoin sodium caused immobilisation of sperm. Irrigation of the vas during vasectomy produced postoperative sterility in 14 of 16 men. The procedure might reduce the need for sperm analysis and might be of value if follow-up was difficult.— P. S. Albert *et al., J. Urol.*, 1975, *113*, 69.

Dysentery. Nitrofurantoin had been reported to be effective in shigella infections.— G. T. Keusch and G. F. Grady (letter), *New Engl. J. Med.*, 1972, *286*, 107.

Ureterovesical reflux. For a report on the use of nitrofurantoin, 50 to 100 mg four times a day, for ureterovesical reflux, see P. G. Klotz, *Can. med. Ass. J.*, 1969, *100*, 4.

Urinary-tract infections. A review of the use of nitrofurantoin in the treatment of urinary-tract infections.— *Med. Lett.*, 1971, *13*, 99. See also *ibid.*, 1980, *22*, 36.

In a double-blind study of patients with urinary-tract infections macrocrystalline nitrofurantoin and standard crystalline nitrofurantoin had similar cure-rates but only 8 of 46 in the macrocrystalline group experienced nausea and vomiting compared with 19 of 44 in the crystalline group. Side-effects in 7 patients in the latter group were severe enough to stop treatment.— S. Kalowski *et al., New Engl. J. Med.*, 1974, *290*, 385. See also *Drug & Ther. Bull.*, 1974, *12*, 47.

The use of nitrofurantoin should be restricted to the treatment of lower urinary-tract infections in patients with normal renal function.— *Br. med. J.*, 1976, *1*, 4.

From a study of the relative incidences of urinary infections in 147 males and 664 females during the first 3 months of 1976 it was considered that nitrofurantoin, which was ineffective against *Proteus* spp. *in vivo*, was not the drug of choice for treating boys.— J. Crump *et al.* (letter), *Lancet*, 1976, *1*, 1184.

Prophylaxis. In an initial study of 52 women with a history of recurrent urinary-tract infection, treatment with nitrofurantoin 50 to 100 mg taken at bedtime after emptying the bladder prevented infection in 46 over a period ranging from 10 to 260 weeks. Of the 6 who had bacteriuria 5 had some abnormality of the urinary tract. Side-effects of nausea and skin reaction occurred in 5 patients, 3 of whom withdrew from the study. In a second double-blind study 3 of 25 women given nitrofurantoin 50 mg each night became infected compared with 15 of 25 given placebo.— R. R. Bailey *et al., Lancet*, 1971, *2*, 1112.

Nitrofurantoin prophylaxis was adequate for the simpler problems of re-infection but where bacteriuria persisted co-trimoxazole was indicated.— T. A. Stamey *et al., New Engl. J. Med.*, 1977, *296*, 780.

Nitrofurantoin in a daily dose of 25 mg for girls weighing less than 20 kg and 50 mg for heavier girls was significantly more effective than placebo in preventing reccurrences of urinary-tract infection in a double-blind crossover study of 18 girls aged between 3 and 13 years. There were 35 episodes of bacteriuria during the placebo period and 2 during the treatment period; both periods lasted for 6 months.— J. A. Lohr *et al., Pediatrics* 1977, *59*, 562.

For reference to the beneficial use of low-dose nitrofurantoin prophylaxis following urinary-tract infections, see Co-trimoxazole, p.1466.

Preparations

Nitrofurantoin Mixture *(B.P.)*. Nitrofurantoin Suspension. A homogeneous suspension of nitrofurantoin in a suitable flavoured vehicle. Store at a temperature not exceeding 25°. Protect from light. The mixture should not be diluted.

Nitrofurantoin Oral Suspension *(U.S.P.)*. A suspension of nitrofurantoin 0.46 to 0.54% w/v in a suitable aqueous basis. pH 4.5 to 6.5. Store in airtight containers. Protect from light.

Nitrofurantoin Tablets *(B.P.)*. Tablets containing nitrofurantoin. Store at a temperature not exceeding 25°. Protect from light.

Nitrofurantoin Tablets *(U.S.P.)*. Tablets containing nitrofurantoin. Potency is expressed in terms of anhydrous nitrofurantoin. The *U.S.P.* requires 25% dissolution in 60 minutes. Store in airtight containers. Protect from light.

Proprietary Preparations

Berkfurin *(Berk Pharmaceuticals, UK)*. Nitrofurantoin, available as scored tablets of 50 and 100 mg.

Ceduran *(Tillotts, UK)*. Scored tablets each containing nitrofurantoin 100 mg and deglycyrrhizinised liquorice (containing not more than 3% glycyrrhizinic acid) 250 mg. For urinary-tract infections. *Dose.* Acute infections, 3 or 4 tablets daily; chronic infections, 1 or 2 tablets daily.

Furadantin *(Norwich-Eaton, UK)*. Nitrofurantoin, available as **Suspension** containing 25 mg in each 5 ml (dilution not recommended) and as scored **Tablets** of 50 and 100 mg. (Also available as Furadantin in *Austral., Ger., Ital., Norw., S.Afr., Switz., USA*).

Furan *(Chelsea Drug & Chemical, UK)*. Nitrofurantoin, available as scored tablets of 50 and 100 mg.

Macrodantin *(Norwich-Eaton, UK)*. Nitrofurantoin macrocrystals, available as capsules of 50 and 100 mg. The crystal size is designed to control absorption and reduce nausea. (Also available as Macrodantin in *Austral., Canad., S.Afr., USA*).

Urantoin *(DDSA Pharmaceuticals, UK)*. Nitrofurantoin, available as tablets of 50 and 100 mg.

Other Proprietary Names

Arg.—Furadantina; *Belg.*—Furadantine, Ituran; *Canad.*—Furatine, Nephronex, Nifuran, Novofuran; *Fr.*—Furadantine, Furadöine; *Ger.*—Cystit, Fua-Med, Ituran, Nierofu, Phenurin, Urolong, Uro-Tablinen; *Ital.*— Chemiofuran, Cistofuran, Furil, Nitrofurin G.W., Urolisa; *Jap.*—Urefuran, Uretoin, Urosagen; *Neth.*—Furadantine; *Spain*—Furantoina, Furobactina, Micturol Simple; *Switz.*—Urodin, Urolong, Uvamin retard; *USA*—Cyantin, Ivadantin, Nitrex, Trantoin.

5653-f

Ammonium Mandelate.

$C_8H_7O_3NH_4$=169.2.

CAS — 530-31-4.

A white, very hygroscopic, almost odourless, crystalline powder with an unpleasant acrid taste. It discolours on exposure to light.

Very **soluble** in water; sparingly soluble in alcohol. Solutions in water are slightly acid to litmus. **Store** in airtight containers. Protect from light.

Ammonium mandelate has actions similar to those of mandelic acid (see p.1051) and was formerly used, in the form of a mixture, as a urinary antiseptic. It has been given in doses of 3 g four times daily.

5654-d

Calcium Mandelate *(B.P.C. 1954)*. Calcium Amygdalate.

$(C_8H_7O_3)_2Ca$=342.4.

CAS — 134-95-2.

Pharmacopoeias. In *Arg., Ind., Nord., Span.*, and *Swiss.*

A white crystalline powder with a slight aromatic odour and a slightly saline taste. **Soluble** 1 in 100 of water and 1 in 4500 of alcohol (90%). Solutions in water are neutral or faintly acid to litmus. **Incompatible** with oxidising and reducing agents and with carbonates, phosphates, and sulphates. Calcium mandelate is not easily wetted with water and wetting agents are usually added to its pharmaceutical preparations.

Calcium mandelate has actions similar to those of mandelic acid (see p.1051), the acid being liberated in the stomach. It has been administered as granules or as a flavoured powder suspended in water in the treatment of urinary-tract infections in doses of 2 to 4 g.

5655-n

Cinoxacin. Azolinic Acid; 64716. 1-Ethyl-1,4-dihydro-4-oxo-1,3-dioxolo[4,5-*g*]cinnoline-3-carboxylic acid.

$C_{12}H_{10}N_2O_5$=262.2.

CAS — 28657-80-9.

White crystals. M.p. about 265°. Practically **insoluble** in water.

Cinoxacin is an antimicrobial agent with properties similar to those of nalidixic acid (see p.1051). In the treatment of urinary-tract infections the usual dose is 500 mg twice daily for 7 to 14 days; for prophylaxis a single dose of 500 mg daily at bedtime may be given.

Absorption and fate. Pharmacokinetic studies with cinoxacin.— R. L. Wolen *et al., Clin. Pharmac. Ther.*, 1976, *19*, 119; S. Colleen *et al., J. antimicrob. Chemother.*, 1977, *3*, 579; R. A. P. Burt *et al., Br. J. Urol.*, 1977, *49*, 147; H. R. Black *et al., Antimicrob. Ag. Chemother.*, 1979, *15*, 165; N. Rodriguez *et al., ibid.*, 465.

Administration in renal failure. A study suggesting that for patients with a creatinine clearance rate of less than 30 ml per minute, one-half to one-quarter of the normal dose of cinoxacin should be given.— J. J. Szwed *et al., J. antimicrob. Chemother.*, 1978, *4*, 451.

Further references: S. Maigaard *et al., Antimicrob. Ag. Chemother.*, 1979, *16*, 411; M. B. Affrime *et al., Clin. Pharmac. Ther.*, 1980, *27*, 243.

Antimicrobial action. References indicating that the antibacterial spectrum of cinoxacin is similar to that of nalidixic acid.— R. M. Lumish and C. W. Norden, *Antimicrob. Ag. Chemother.*, 1975, *7*, 159; R. N. Jones and P. C. Fuchs, *ibid.*, 1976, *10*, 146; R. C. Gordon *et al., ibid.*, 918; E. Rubinstein and B. Shainberg, *ibid.*, 1977, *11*, 577; P. A. Mårdh *et al., J. antimicrob. Chemother.*, 1977, *3*, 411.

Urinary-tract infections. A discussion of the actions and uses of cinoxacin in urinary-tract infections.— *Drug & Ther. Bull.*, 1980, *18*, 47.

Of 20 patients with urinary-tract infection treated for 10 days with cinoxacin 250 mg every 6 hours 19 were cleared of their infection during or immediately after treatment.— A. P. Panwalker *et al., Antimicrob. Ag. Chemother.*, 1976, *9*, 502.

Further references: S. N. Rous, *J. Urol.*, 1978, *120*, 196 (treatment); R. R. Landes, *ibid.*, 1980, *123*, 47 (prophylaxis).

Proprietary Preparations

Cinobac *(Lilly, UK)*. Cinoxacin, available as capsules of 500 mg.

5656-h

Dihydroxymethylfuratrizine. *N*-[6-(5-Nitrofurfurylidenemethyl)-1,2,4-triazin-3-yl]iminodimethanol.

$C_{11}H_{11}N_5O_5$=293.2.

CAS — 794-93-4.

A yellow crystalline powder. M.p. about 157° with decomposition. Practically **insoluble** in water and most organic solvents; soluble in dimethylformamide.

Dihydroxymethylfuratrizine is a nitrofuran antibacterial agent which was formerly used in the treatment of urinary-tract infections.

5657-m

Hexamine *(B.P.C. 1959)*. Methenamine

(U.S.P.); Aminoform; Formine; Hexamethylenamine; Urotropine; Esametilentetrammina; Esammina; Metenamina. Hexamethylenetetramine; 1,3,5,7-Tetraazatricyclo[3.3.1.1^{3,7}]decane.

$C_6H_{12}N_4$=140.2.

CAS — 100-97-0.

Pharmacopoeias. In *Arg., Aust., Belg., Braz., Chin., Cz., Fr., Ger., Hung., Ind., It., Mex., Neth., Pol., Port., Roum., Rus., Span., Swiss* and *U.S.*

Almost odourless, colourless, lustrous crystals or white crystalline powder with a bitter-sweet taste. It sublimes at about 260° without melting.

Soluble 1 in 1.5 of water, 1 in 8 of alcohol (90%), 1 in 12 of chloroform, and 1 in 320 of ether. A 10% solution in water has a pH of between 8 and 8.8. A 3.68% solution is iso-osmotic with serum. **Incompatible** with tannins and oxidising agents; it is decomposed by acids and acid salts. **Store** in airtight containers.

An aqueous solution of hexamine iso-osmotic with serum (3.68%) caused 100% haemolysis of erythrocytes cultured in it for 45 minutes.— E. R. Hammarlund and K. Pedersen-Bjergaard, *J. pharm. Sci.*, 1961, *50*, 24.

Adverse Effects. Comparatively large amounts of formaldehyde are formed during prolonged administration or when large doses are used, and may give rise to gastro-intestinal upsets, painful and frequent micturition, cystitis, haematuria, proteinuria, and renal and bladder lesions. The effect of the formaldehyde may be diluted by administering sodium bicarbonate or large quantities of water but it is then less effective. Skin rashes have occasionally been reported.

A detailed toxicological evaluation of hexamine in *animals*. There did not appear to be any confirmation of a carcinogenic hazard in *rats* or their offspring.— *Fd Add. Ser. Wld Hlth Org. No. 1,* 1972.

For background toxicological information, see *Fd Add. Ser. Wld Hlth Org. No. 5,* 1974.

Antimicrobial Action. The antimicrobial action of hexamine is due to formaldehyde which is liberated during acid hydrolysis. All micro-organisms are susceptible to formaldehyde and hexamine is effective *in vitro* against a range of Gram-negative and Gram-positive organisms.

It is less effective than either hexamine hippurate or hexamine mandelate. Minimum inhibitory concentrations have been reported to range from 1.25 to more than 20 mg per ml.

For reports on the antibacterial action of hexamine and its salts, see H. Seneca *et al., J. Urol.,* 1967, *97,* 1094.

Absorption and Fate. Hexamine is readily absorbed from the gastro-intestinal tract and is rapidly eliminated unchanged in the urine. In acid urine, hexamine is slowly hydrolysed with the liberation of formaldehyde; the same reaction occurs in the acid gastric secretion and may account for a loss of 10 to 30% of the administered dose.

Uses. Hexamine is used, usually as the hippurate or mandelate, in the treatment of urinary-tract infections.

Topically, hexamine has been used in deodorant preparations, since in the presence of acidic decomposition products on the skin it liberates formaldehyde.

Hexamine is a permitted preservative for use in Provolone cheese and marinated herrings and mackerel.

Estimated acceptable daily intake: up to 150 µg per kg body-weight. The toxic effects were due to liberated formaldehyde and formic acid. Because of possible nitrosamine formation it should not be used with nitrites.— Seventeenth Report of FAO/WHO Expert Committee on Food Additives, *Tech. Rep. Ser. Wld Hlth Org. No. 539,* 1974.

A favourable report of the use of hexamine topically in hyperhidrosis.— S. I. Cullen, *Archs Derm.,* 1975, *111,* 1158.

Preparations

Methenamine and Sodium Biphosphate Tablets *(U.S.P.).* Tablets containing hexamine and sodium acid phosphate. Store in airtight containers.

Methenamine Elixir *(U.S.P.).* Contains hexamine, with 19 to 21% of alcohol. Store in airtight containers.

Methenamine Tablets *(U.S.P.).* **Hexamine Tablets** *(B.P.C. 1954).* Tablets containing hexamine. The tablets should be dissolved in water before administration.

Proprietary Names

Aci-steril (as orthophosphate) *(Heyl, Ger.)*; Antihydral *(Robugen, Ger.)*; Jodoibs (as ethyliodide) *(Benvegna, Ital.)*; Uromandelin *(Lazar, Arg.)*; Urotropina *(Schering, Arg.; Schering, Ital.)*.

5658-b

Hexamine Anhydromethylenecitrate. Hexacitraminum; Hexamethylentetraminum Anhydromethylencitricum; Esammina citrica. Hexamethylenetetramine, compound with 5-oxo-1,3-dioxolane-4,4-diacetic acid.
$C_6H_{12}N_4,C_7H_8O_7=344.3$.

CAS — 6190-43-8.

Pharmacopoeias. In *It.*

A white, odourless, crystalline powder with an acid taste. **Soluble** in water.

Hexamine anhydromethylenecitrate has been given similarly to other hexamine compounds for urinary-tract infections in doses of 0.5 to 1 g three or four times daily.

Proprietary Names

Elmitolo *(Bayer, Ital.)*.

5659-v

Hexamine Camphorate. Hexacamphaminum.
$(C_6H_{12}N_4)_2,C_{10}H_{16}O_4=480.6$.

CAS — 630-55-7.

Pharmacopoeias. In *Swiss.*

A white powder with a faint odour of camphor, and an acid, slightly bitter, taste. **Soluble** in water, alcohol, and chloroform.

Hexamine camphorate has been given similarly to other hexamine compounds for urinary-tract infections in doses of 1.5 to 4.5 g daily.

5660-r

Hexamine Hippurate.

Methenamine Hippurate. Hexamethylenetetramine hippurate.
$C_6H_{12}N_4,C_9H_9NO_3=319.4$.

CAS — 5714-73-8.

A white crystalline powder. M.p. 105° to 110°. **Soluble** in water and alcohol.

Adverse Effects. As for Hexamine, p.1050.

Side-effects in 5 of 18 patients given hexamine hippurate 4 g daily were nausea and vomiting (3), erythematous rash (1), and pruritus (1).— A. R. Gerstein *et al., J. Urol.,* 1968, *100,* 767.

In 29 patients given hexamine hippurate 1 g twice daily severe nausea developed in 2 and stomatitis in 1.— G. R. Gibson, *Med. J. Aust.,* 1970, *1,* 167.

Precautions. Hexamine hippurate is contra-indicated in patients with hepatic insufficiency, severe renal failure, severe dehydration, or metabolic acidosis.

It should not be used to treat acute parenchymal infections of the kidney.

Hexamine hippurate should not be given concomitantly with sulphonamides, as crystalluria may occur, or with alkalising agents such as potassium citrate.

Administration in renal failure. Hexamine hippurate was not recommended for urinary-tract infections if the creatinine clearance was less than 20 ml per minute.— J. S. Cheigh, *Am. J. Med.,* 1977, *62,* 555.

Pregnancy and the neonate. In 5 pregnant women given hexamine hippurate, urine concentrations of oestriol promptly fell to below normal values. Treatment continued to delivery and the infants were not adversely affected.— S. Kivinen and R. Tuimala, *Br. med. J.,* 1977, *2,* 682.

Antimicrobial Action. Hexamine hippurate has the antimicrobial action of hexamine (see p.1050); hippuric acid, a bacteriostat, may also contribute to its action. It is effective *in vitro* against *Escherichia coli, Pseudomonas aeruginosa, Klebsiella pneumoniae,* and some *Staphylococcus* and *Streptococcus* spp.

Minimum inhibitory concentrations are reported to range from 0.625 to 2.5 mg per ml; concentrations of up to 10 mg per ml are required to inhibit the growth of *Klebsiella aerogenes* and some strains of *Proteus vulgaris.*

Antimicrobial resistance does not appear to occur.

A correlation of antibacterial activity with urinary hexamine hippurate, and free formaldehyde concentrations, pH, and volume.— H. Miller and E. Phillips, *Invest. Urol.,* 1970, *8,* 21.

Absorption and Fate. As for Hexamine, above.

More than 90% of the hexamine moiety is claimed to be excreted in the urine; about 13% is converted to formaldehyde.

Antibacterial activity is demonstrated in the urine within 30 minutes of a dose.

Uses. Hexamine hippurate is used in the treatment of infections of the urinary tract. It is only active in acid urine, when formaldehyde is released, and this acidity is generally maintained by the presence of hippuric acid.

Acute urinary infections should be treated with antibiotics or sulphonamides but hexamine hippurate may be used in the treatment of chronic or recurrent infections and asymptomatic bacteriuria. It is of value in long-term therapy because acquired resistance does not appear to develop.

The usual dose is 1 g twice daily. Children aged 1 to 5 years may be given one-quarter the adult dose and children 6 to 12 years may be given half the adult dose.

Urinary-tract infections. A comparative crossover study of hexamine hippurate (Hiprex) 1 g twice daily and hexamine mandelate (Mandelamine) 1 g four times daily in 73 patients demonstrated that while both treatments were satisfactory for the prevention of lower urinary-tract infection, the incidence of side-effects, particularly gastro-intestinal, was significantly lower with hexamine hippurate.— J. G. Gow, *Practitioner,* 1974, *213,* 97.

In a study in geriatric patients with indwelling catheters, hexamine hippurate 2 g thrice daily reduced the complications associated with an indwelling catheter.— B. Norberg *et al., Eur. J. clin. Pharmac.,* 1979, *15,* 357.

Further references: H. Seneca *et al., J. Urol.,* 1967, *97* 1094; A. R. Gerstein *et al., ibid.,* 1968, *100,* 767; G. R. Gibson, *Med. J. Aust.,* 1970, *1,* 167.

In pregnancy. Reduction of the number of premature births among Chicago babies was claimed after treatment with hexamine hippurate of prepartum mothers who had confirmed bacteriuria. Of 3000 pregnant women screened, 305 had significant infection which was cleared in 255 patients after treatment for 2 weeks; the incidence of premature births was 10.6%. In the 20 000 prepartum patients seen in clinics, the incidence was 14%. Of 7000 patients screened later, bacteriuria was found in some 653 and cleared in about 70% with hexamine treatment; the incidence of premature births was 6.1%. In a simultaneous study, the incidence of premature births was 18% among 73 women with untreated bacteriuria. The most common infecting organism was *Escherichia coli.*— *J. Am. med. Ass.,* 1967, *201* (July 3), A27.

Proprietary Preparations

Hiprex *(Carnegie, UK).* Hexamine hippurate, available as scored tablets of 1 g. (Also available as Hiprex in *Austral., Belg., Ger., Norw., Swed., Switz., USA*).

Other Proprietary Names

Haiprex *(Denm.)*; Hipeksal *(Norw.)*; Hippramine *(S.Afr.)*; Hip-Rex *(Canad.)*; Urex *(USA)*.

5661-f

Hexamine Mandelate.

Methenamine Mandelate *(U.S.P.)*; Mandelato de Metenamina. Hexamethylenetetramine mandelate.
$C_6H_{12}N_4,C_8H_8O_3=292.3$.

CAS — 587-23-5.

Pharmacopoeias. In *Braz.* and *U.S.*

A white crystalline almost odourless powder with a sour taste, containing not less than 95.5% of $C_6H_{12}N_4,C_8H_8O_3$ and not less than 50% of mandelic acid ($C_8H_8O_3$). M.p. about 127° with decomposition.

Very **soluble** in water; soluble 1 in 10 of alcohol, 1 in 20 of chloroform, and 1 in 350 of ether. Solutions in water have a pH of about 4.

Adverse Effects. As for Hexamine, p.1050.

Giddiness and tinnitus have been reported to occur with mandelic acid.

A 2½-year-old child who accidentally ingested at least 8 g of hexamine mandelate developed haemorrhagic cystitis, mild transient uraemia, and acidosis. He recovered without specific treatment.— R. P. Ross and G. F. Conway, *Am. J. Dis. Child.*, 1970, *119*, 86.

Precautions. As for Hexamine Hippurate, p.1050.

Two senile patients with dysphagia developed lipoid pneumonia after therapy with hexamine mandelate oral suspension the principal vehicle of which was sesame oil. Both recovered when the medication was withdrawn.— R. J. Timmerman and J. A. Schroer, *J. Am. med. Ass.*, 1973, *225*, 1524.

Administration in renal failure. Hexamine mandelate was not recommended for urinary-tract infections if the creatinine clearance was less than 20 ml per minute.— J. S. Cheigh, *Am. J. Med.*, 1977, *62*, 555.

Dosage of hexamine mandelate could be unchanged in mild or moderate renal failure; it should be avoided if the glomerular filtration-rate was less than 10 ml per minute.— W. M. Bennett *et al.*, *Ann. intern. Med.*, 1980, *93*, 62.

Crystalluria. Administration of hexamine mandelate with sulphamethizole produced marked turbidity in the urine of 9 of 23 patients, the turbidity increasing with a fall of pH. Sulphamethizole was found to constitute 63% of the precipitate. Tests *in vitro* showed that hexamine and formaldehyde produced a precipitate with sulphamethizole at pH 5 to 6.— J. H. Lipton, *New Engl. J. Med.*, 1963, *268*, 92.

Laboratory estimations. Patients taking hexamine mandelate might show an apparent elevation of urinary excretion of 17-hydroxycorticosteroids if a colorimetric method using phenylhydrazine was performed.— L. E. Braverman *et al.*, *Clin. Chem.*, 1968, *14*, 374.

Hexamine mandelate could cause interference in laboratory tests for catecholamines.— *Med. Lett.*, 1971, *13*, 82.

Artificially high concentrations of urinary oestrogens could be recorded in patients taking hexamine mandelate.— *Adverse Drug React. Bull.*, 1972, June, 104.

Antimicrobial Action. Hexamine mandelate has the antimicrobial actions of both hexamine (see p.1050) and mandelic acid (see below). It is effective *in vitro* against *Escherichia coli, Pseudomonas aeruginosa, Proteus vulgaris,* and some *Klebsiella, Staphylococcus,* and *Streptococcus* spp.

Minimum inhibitory concentrations are reported to range from 2.5 to 5 mg per ml.

Antimicrobial resistance does not appear to occur.

Absorption and Fate. As for Hexamine, p.1050.

Uses. Hexamine mandelate is used in the treatment of infections of the urinary tract. It is only active in acid urine (pH below 5.5), when formaldehyde is released, and acidification of the urine by administration of ammonium chloride or ascorbic acid may be necessary. If urea-splitting bacteria such as *Proteus* or *Pseudomonas* spp. are present in the urine they may produce so much ammonia that the urine cannot be acidified.

Acute urinary infections should be treated with antibiotics or sulphonamides but hexamine mandelate may be useful in chronic or recurrent urinary infections. It is suitable for long-term use because acquired resistance does not appear to develop.

The usual dose in adults is 1 g four times daily, after meals and at bedtime. A suggested dose for children is 50 mg per kg body-weight daily in 4 divided doses, with an initial dose of 100 mg per kg in the first 24 hours for children over 6 years.

Urinary-tract infections. Treatment with hexamine mandelate and ascorbic acid both 1 g every 6 hours was considered to be ineffective in the suppression of, or as prophylactic treatment against, chronic urinary infections in a study of para- or quadriplegic patients who had indwelling urinary catheters or who had received intermittent catheterisation.— B. Vainrub and D. M. Musher, *Antimicrob. Ag. Chemother.*, 1977, *12*, 625.

For a comparative study of hexamine hippurate and hexamine mandelate, see Hexamine Hippurate, above.

Preparations

Methenamine Mandelate Oral Suspension *(U.S.P.)*. A suspension of hexamine mandelate in a vegetable oil. Store in airtight containers.

Methenamine Mandelate Tablets *(U.S.P.)*. Tablets containing hexamine mandelate.

Proprietary Preparations

G-500 Tablets *(Cox, UK)*. Enteric-coated tablets each containing hexamine mandelate 250 mg and racemethionine 250 mg. For chronic urinary-tract infections.

Mandelamine *(Warner, UK)*. Hexamine mandelate, available as enteric-coated tablets of 250 and 500 mg. (Also available as Mandelamine in *Austral., Belg., Ger., S.Afr., Switz., USA*).

Other Proprietary Names

Cedulamin *(Switz.)*; Hexydal *(Norw.)*; Lemandine *(Spain)*; Mandaze *(Austral.)*; Metenamin *(Denm.)*; Methandine *(Canad.)*; Reflux *(Neth.)*; Renelate *(USA)*; Sterine *(Canad.)*; Urocedulamin *(Neth.)*.

5662-d

Mandelic Acid *(B.P.C. 1959)*. Amygdalic Acid; Phenylglycollic Acid; Racemic Mandelic Acid. 2-Hydroxy-2-phenylacetic acid.

$C_8H_8O_3$=152.1.

CAS — 90-64-2; 17199-29-0 (+); 611-72-3 (±); 611-71-2 (−).

Pharmacopoeias. In *Arg., Aust.,* and *Neth.*

White, almost odourless crystals with an acid saline taste, turning yellow on exposure to light. M.p. 119° to 121°. **Soluble** 1 in 6 of water, 1 in 1 of alcohol, 1 in 45 of chloroform, and 1 in 6 of ether. **Incompatible** with calcium salts. **Store** in airtight containers. Protect from light.

Mandelic acid has bacteriostatic properties and has been used in the treatment of urinary-tract infections, usually as the ammonium or calcium salt.

It is excreted unchanged in the urine and has been effective against infections due to *Escherichia coli* and *Streptococcus faecalis* provided that the pH is maintained below 5.5. It has been given in doses of 2 to 4 g. See also Hexamine Mandelate, p.1051.

5663-n

Nalidixic Acid *(B.P., U.S.P.)*. Nalidixinic Acid; Win 18 320. 1-Ethyl-1,4-dihydro-7-methyl-4-oxo-1,8-naphthyridine-3-carboxylic acid.

$C_{12}H_{12}N_2O_3$=232.2.

CAS — 389-08-2.

Pharmacopoeias. In *Br., Braz., Chin., Cz., It., Jap.,* and *U.S.*

An almost white or very pale yellow odourless or almost odourless crystalline powder. M.p. 225° to 231°.

Practically **insoluble** in water; soluble 1 in 910 of alcohol, 1 in 350 of acetone, and 1 in 35 of chloroform; very slightly soluble in ether; soluble in solutions of alkali hydroxides and carbonates. Solutions are **sterilised** by autoclaving. **Store** in airtight containers. Protect from light.

Adverse Effects. Common side-effects include nausea and vomiting. Diarrhoea, gastro-intestinal bleeding, muscular weakness, myalgia, phototoxicity, and allergic reactions have occurred.

Effects on the central nervous system include visual disturbances , headache, dizziness, and drowsiness; acute psychoses have been reported. Convulsions have occurred after high doses or in patients with predisposing factors such as cerebrovascular insufficiency, parkinsonism, and epilepsy. There have been reports of intracranial hypertension in infants and young children.

Rarely, cholestatic jaundice, thrombocytopenia and leucopenia have occurred as has haemolytic anaemia in patients who may or may not be deficient in glucose-6-phosphate dehydrogenase.

The Committee on Safety of Drugs had received 518 reports of reactions to nalidixic acid during the period 1964 to 1969. These included reports of visual disturbances (219) and skin reactions (148). Nalidixic acid was believed to be the only drug involved in 97 of the skin reactions; of these 25 were phototoxic, 24 urticarial, 17 'drug rash' erythema, and 15 maculopapular.— S. Alexander and L. Forman, *Br. J. Derm.*, 1971, *84*, 429.

Severe metabolic acidosis with serum concentrations of nalidixic acid 297 µg per ml was reported in a previously healthy 18-year-old man who had taken an overdose of nalidixic acid together with probenecid and other drugs. The mean serum concentration of nalidixic acid 8 hours after dosage was increased 3-fold when the dose followed probenecid 500 mg in 2 subjects.— H. Dash and J. Mills (letter), *Ann. intern. Med.*, 1976, *84*, 570.

Arthralgia. A 22-year-old woman with acute pyelonephritis, who was known to experience visual disturbances when treated with nalidixic acid, developed severe arthralgia after receiving 4 doses each of 500 mg at 6-hourly intervals. Treatment was discontinued and the patient recovered gradually without disability.— R. R. Bailey *et al.*, *Can. med. Ass. J.*, 1972, *107*, 604, per *letter*

Haemolytic anaemia. Reports of haemolytic anaemia occurring in infants and adults, some of whom were deficient in glucose-6-phosphate dehydrogenase.— E. M. Belton and R. V. Jones (letter), *Lancet*, 1965, *2*, 691; L. P. Vargas and C. S. González (letter), *ibid.*, 1967, *2*, 97; B. K. Mandal and J. Stevenson (letter), *ibid.*, 1970, *1*, 614. Australian Drug Evaluation Committee, *Med. J. Aust.*, 1972, *1*, 435; L. Alessio and G. Morselli (letter), *Br. med. J.*, 1972, *4*, 110; C. Gilbertson and D. R. Jones (letter), *ibid.*, 493.

Hyperglycaemia. A girl aged 14 took 6.5 g of nalidixic acid and developed convulsions, hyperglycaemia, and glycosuria. She was not treated with insulin because the plasma-acetone test was negative. She recovered slowly over about 4 days.— M. A. Islam and T. Sreedharan, *J. Am. med. Ass.*, 1965, *192*, 1100.

Hyperglycaemia (1.95 mg per ml) and convulsions developed in a 31-year-old woman who had taken nalidixic acid 1 g four times daily for 2 days.— A. G. Fraser and A. D. B. Harrower, *Br. med. J.*, 1977, *2*, 1518.

Intracranial hypertension. Reports of intracranial hypertension occurring in infants and children given nalidixic acid.— L. O. Boréus and B. Sundström, *Br. med. J.*, 1967, *2*, 744; E. E. Anderson *et al.*, *J. Am. med. Ass.*, 1971, *216*, 1023; T. Deonna and J. P. Guignard, *Archs Dis. Childh.*, 1974, *49*, 743.

Lupus erythematosus. A lupus erythematosus-like disease was associated with treatment with nalidixic acid in a 70-year-old woman who developed a rash on the 28th day of treatment. Laboratory tests revealed a positive antinuclear factor and lupus erythematosus (LE) cells. When the patient inadvertently took nalidixic acid 6 months later she developed a severe itching rash, diffuse myalgia, and arthralgia accompanied by the reappearance of antinuclear factor and LE cells.— A. Rubinstein (letter), *New Engl. J. Med.*, 1979, *301*, 1288.

Precautions. Nalidixic acid should be given with care to patients with damage of the central nervous system, to patients subject to convulsions, and to those with impaired renal or hepatic function.

Its use should be avoided in babies less than 3 months old or during the first trimester of pregnancy.

Exposure to strong sunlight should be avoided during treatment.

Nitrofurantoin and nalidixic acid are antagonistic *in vitro* and should not be used together.

Nalidixic acid may cause false positive reactions in urine tests for glucose using copper reduction methods.

Interactions. Nalidixic acid was highly bound to albumin and displaced warfarin from its binding sites *in vitro*. J. Koch-Weser and E. M. Sellers, *New Engl. J. Med.*, 1971, *285*, 547.

For a report of the prolongation of the prothrombin time in a patient taking warfarin and nalidixic acid, see Warfarin Sodium, p.779.

For the effect of nalidixic acid on nicoumalone, see Nicoumalone, p.772.

Laboratory estimations. False elevations of urinary 17-ketosteroid concentrations were observed in 2 patients who were taking nalidixic acid. A similar elevation was seen in 2 volunteers who received trial doses. No effect was observed on 17-hydroxycorticosteroid determinations. The addition of nalidixic acid to normal urine samples gave misleading results in the Zimmerman reaction for urinary steroids.— O. Llerena and O. H. Pearson, *New Engl. J. Med.*, 1968, *279*, 983.

Nalidixic acid interfered with the estimation of plasma concentrations of 11-hydroxycorticosteroids.— *Adverse*

Drug React. Bull., 1972, June, 104.

Nalidixic acid could interfere technically with laboratory estimations for vanilmandelic acid in the urine (Pisano method) to produce erroneous raised results— *Drug & Ther. Bull.*, 1972, *10*, 69.

Nalidixic acid could interfere with the Autoanalyser I method of measuring glucose by reducing the reagent, alkaline ferricyanide.— J. Millhouse, *Adverse Drug React. Bull.*, 1974, Dec., 164.

Antimicrobial Action. Nalidixic acid is bactericidal and inhibits Gram-negative micro-organisms including *Escherichia coli, Klebsiella aerogenes, Kleb. pneumoniae, Salmonella* spp., *Shigella* spp., and *Proteus* spp. *Brucella* spp. may be sensitive. Minimum inhibitory concentrations are reported to range from about 5 to 75 µg per ml. Many organisms are inhibited by 10 µg per ml or less. *Pseudomonas aeruginosa* is usually resistant. Bacterial resistance may develop rapidly, sometimes within a few days and cross-resistance with oxolinic acid occurs.

Unlike nitrofurantoin, Gram-positive urinary-tract pathogens are relatively resistant also the antibacterial activity of nalidixic acid is not significantly affected by differences in urinary pH. Antagonism between nitrofurantoin and nalidixic acid has been demonstrated *in vitro.*

Nalidixic acid is considered to act by inhibiting the replication of bacterial DNA.

For a study of the activity of nalidixic acid with various antibiotics on 95 strains of Enterobacteriaceae, see J. Michel *et al., Antimicrob. Ag. Chemother.*, 1973, *4*, 201.

Nitrofurantoin had been reported to inhibit the antimicrobial activity of nalidixic acid *in vitro.*— G. P. C. Westwood and W. L. Hooper (letter), *Lancet*, 1975, *1*, 460.

Nalidixic acid altered the protein patterns in sensitive but not resistant *E. coli.*— L. Chao, *Antimicrob. Ag. Chemother.*, 1977, *11*, 167.

Rifampicin and nalidixic acid enhanced the activity of each other when used together *in vitro* against various Gram-negative bacteria and suppressed the emergence of resistant bacteria that occurred when each drug was used alone.— D. Greenwood and J. Andrew, *J. antimicrob. Chemother.*, 1978, *4*, 533.

For a report that the bactericidal effect of nalidixic acid decreased as the concentration increased see below under Dosage.

For a report that oxolinic acid was more effective *in vitro* than nalidixic acid or cinoxacin against 138 strains of *Shigella sonnei* and *Sh. flexneri*, see Oxolinic Acid, p.1053.

Bacterial resistance. A study *in vitro* of the emergence of resistance to nalidixic acid in *E. coli* suggested that whereas uncomplicated urinary-tract infections might respond to minimal therapy with nalidixic acid, more complicated infections would require prolonged and high-dose therapy to reduce the emergence of organisms resistant to nalidixic acid.— D. Greenwood and F. O'Grady, *Antimicrob. Ag. Chemother.*, 1977, *12*, 678.

Absorption and Fate. Nalidixic acid is readily absorbed from the gastro-intestinal tract. The plasma half-life is about 90 minutes and peak plasma concentrations of 20 to 50 µg per ml have been reported 2 hours after the administration of 1 g by mouth. About 90% of the drug is bound to plasma proteins.

It is rapidly metabolised, mainly to hydroxynalidixic acid which also has antibacterial activity and accounts for about 30% of active drug in the blood. About 80% of a dose appears in the urine within 8 hours, most of the nalidixic acid and its active metabolite having been conjugated in the liver to inactive glucuronides but urinary concentrations of free drug and active metabolite ranging from 25 to 250 µg per ml are achieved after a single 1-g dose. Hydroxynalidixic acid accounts for about 85% of this activity.

Only traces of nalidixic acid appear in milk and cerebrospinal fluid. About 4% of a dose is excreted in the faeces.

The peak urine concentrations of total nalidixic acid bound and free were 2.2 mg per ml and occurred about 3 hours after administration of 1 g by mouth to 5 patients with normal kidney function.— P. Brühl *et al., Arzneimittel-Forsch.*, 1973, *23*, 1311. See also P. T. Mannisto, *Clin. Pharmac. Ther.*, 1976, *19*, 37.

Further references: N. Ferry *et al., Clin. Pharmac. Ther.*, 1981, *29*, 695.

Uses. Nalidixic acid is used in the treatment of urinary-tract infections due to Gram-negative micro-organisms other than *Pseudomonas* spp., which are usually not susceptible. It has been used in acute and chronic infections and may be effective in urinary infections which have not responded to treatment with antibiotics or sulphonamides. Its antibacterial activity does not appear to be influenced by urinary pH although the concomitant administration of sodium bicarbonate or sodium citrate does increase the concentration of active drug in the urine. It has also been used in the treatment of bacterial dysentery. Although *Brucella* spp. may be sensitive brucellosis tends to be treated with other antimicrobial compounds.

The usual adult dose is 4 g daily in 4 divided doses for at least 7 days in acute infections. If therapy continues for longer than 2 weeks, for instance in the treatment of chronic or persistent infections, the dose should usually be halved. Children may be given 50 mg per kg body-weight daily in 2 to 4 divided doses.

A suggested dose of nalidixic acid, in conjunction with sodium citrate, is 660 mg thrice daily for 3 days.

The sodium salt of nalidixic acid has been given by intravenous infusion.

Dosage. Blood concentrations were enhanced when nalidixic acid was taken at least 1 hour before meals instead of after meals. Dosage should be adjusted to body-weight, the initial adult dosage being about 15 to 16 mg per kg body-weight 4 times daily.— E. W. McChesney *et al., J. pharm. Sci.*, 1967, *56*, 594.

Although nalidixic acid was bactericidal against various Gram-negative bacteria in concentrations of 50 to 200 µg per ml, as the concentration increased the bactericidal effect decreased and it was bacteriostatic at 400 µg per ml. As normal doses gave a urine concentration of 200 to 350 µg per ml within 4 to 6 hours this was above the most lethal concentration and it was suggested that decreased doses be used.— G. C. Crumplin and J. T. Smith, *Antimicrob. Ag. Chemother.*, 1975, *8*, 251. The induction rate of bacterial resistance during treatment with nalidixic acid 1 g four times daily for 10 days was only about 7% in 27 consecutive patients. Reports of excessive resistance could be attributed to the use of lower doses.— T. A. Stamey and J. Bragonje, *J. Am. med. Ass.*, 1976, *236*, 1857. Reducing the dose of nalidixic acid in urinary-tract infections from 4 g to 1.5 g daily could reduce adverse reactions and was not associated with an increase in the incidence of bacterial resistance.— R. R. Bailey (letter), *ibid.*, 1977, *237*, 2720. See also T. A. Stamey (letter), *ibid.*

Dosage in renal failure. Nalidixic acid was not recommended for urinary-tract infections if the creatinine clearance was less than 20 ml per minute.— J. S. Cheigh, *Am. J. Med.*, 1977, *62*, 555.

The dosage interval of nalidixic acid was not affected in renal failure.— P. Sharpstone, *Br. med. J.*, 1977, *2*, 36.

The half-life of nalidixic acid was increased from 1.5 to 21 hours in end-stage renal failure. It could be given in usual doses in mild or moderate renal failure; it should be avoided if the glomerular filtration-rate was less than 10 ml per minute because metabolites accumulated.— W. M. Bennett *et al., Ann. intern. Med.*, 1980, *93*, 62.

Dysentery. Infants and children with shigellosis were given either nalidixic acid 13.75 mg per kg body-weight or ampicillin 25 mg per kg every 6 hours for 5 days. Clearance of shigella occurred more slowly and relapses were more frequent with nalidixic acid.— K. C. Haltalin *et al., Archs Dis. Childh.*, 1973, *48*, 305.

Urinary-tract infections. From a study of the relative incidences of urinary infections in 147 males and 664 females during the first 3 months of 1976 it was considered that nalidixic and oxolinic acids, having little activity against Gram-positive organisms, should be avoided for the treatment of young women.— J. Crump *et al.* (letter), *Lancet*, 1976, *1*, 1184.

Reports of the use of nalidixic acid with sodium citrate in the treatment of urinary-tract infections: T. A. McAllister, *Practitioner* 1981, *225*, 575; J. G. Winwick and S. J. Savage, *J. int. med. Res.*, 1981, *9*, 58.

Preparations

Nalidixic Acid Mixture *(B.P.)*. A suspension of nalidixic acid in a suitable flavoured vehicle, which may be coloured. It may contain suitable antimicrobial preservatives. When a dose less than, or not a multiple of, 5 ml is prescribed, the mixture should be diluted to 5 ml, or a multiple, with syrup. Such dilutions must be freshly prepared and should not be used later than 2 weeks after issue.

Nalidixic Acid Oral Suspension *(U.S.P.)*. A suspension containing nalidixic acid in a suitable aqueous vehicle. Store in airtight containers.

Nalidixic Acid Tablets *(B.P.)*. Tablets containing nalidixic acid. Protect from light.

Nalidixic Acid Tablets *(U.S.P.)*. Tablets containing nalidixic acid. The *U.S.P.* requires 80% dissolution in 30 minutes. Store in airtight containers.

Proprietary Preparations

Mictral *(Winthrop, UK)*. Granules containing in each 7-g sachet nalidixic acid 660 mg, sodium citrate 3.75 g, anhydrous citric acid 250 mg, and sodium bicarbonate 250 mg. For lower urinary-tract infections. *Dose.* The contents of one sachet in water thrice daily for 3 days.

Negram *(Sterling Research, UK)*. Nalidixic acid, available as **Suspension** containing 60 mg per ml (suggested diluent, syrup), and as scored **Tablets** of 500 mg. (Also available as Negram in *Aust., Austral., Belg., Denm., Fin., Fr., Iceland, Neth., Norw., Swed., Switz.*).

Other Proprietary Names

Arg.—Wintomylon; *Canad.*—NegGram; *Ger.*—Nogram; *Ind.*—Gramoneg; *Ital.*—Chemiurin, Dixiben, Dixilina, Dixinal, Dixurol, Enexina, Eucistin, Faril, Nalicidin, Nalidixin, Naligen, Naligram, Nalissina, Nalix, Naluran (sodium salt), Naxuril, Negabatt, Neg-Gram, Pielos, Specifin, Uralgin, Uretrene, Uriclar, Uri-Flor, Urisco, Uristeril, Urodixin, Urogram, Urolex, Uromina, Uronax, Uroneg, Uropan, Valuren; *Jap.*—Entolon, Innoxalon, Jicsron, Kusnarin, Nalidicron, Nalitucson, Narigix, Nicelate, Oxoranil, Poleon, Sicmylon, Unaserus, Uroman, Wintomylon, Wintron; *S.Afr.*—Wintomylon; *Spain*—Nalidixin, Nalidixol, Nogermin, Notricel, Wintomylon; *USA*—NegGram.

5664-h

Nitroxoline. 5-Nitroquinolin-8-ol.
$C_9H_6N_2O_3$=190.2.

CAS — 4008-48-4.

A yellow crystalline powder. M.p. 179° to 182°. Sparingly **soluble** in alcohol and ether; freely soluble in alkali and hot hydrochloric acid.

Nitroxoline is a urinary antiseptic and has been given in doses of 300 to 500 mg daily.

The treatment of chronic urinary-tract infections with nitroxoline.— B. von Rütte and I. Delnon, *Schweiz. med. Wschr.*, 1968, *98*, 1864.

The inhibitory effect of nitroxoline on *Mycobacterium* spp.— H. O. K. Tanzil *et al., Am. Rev. resp. Dis.*, 1973, *108*, 147, per *Abstr. Hyg.*, 1974, *49*, 235.

Proprietary Names

Nibiol *(Debat, Belg.; Debat, Fr.; Debat, Neth.; Roussel-Amor Gil, Spain; Debat, Switz.)*; Uro-Coli *(Roussel Maestretti, Ital.)*.

5665-m

Oxolinic Acid. W 4565. 5-Ethyl-5,8-dihydro-8-oxo-1,3-dioxolo[4,5-*g*]quinoline-7-carboxylic acid.
$C_{13}H_{11}NO_5$=261.2.

CAS — 14698-29-4.

Crystals. M.p. 313° to 314°. **Soluble** in alkaline solutions.

Adverse Effects. Side-effects appear to be similar to those seen with nalidixic acid (see p.1051) and include nausea and vomiting, visual disturbances, dizziness, restlessness, insomnia, and irritability. Drowsiness has been reported. Stimulant effects on the central nervous system are more common than with nalidixic acid.

Side-effects occurred in 23 of 44 patients given 51 courses of oxolinic acid 1 g daily usually for 14 days. Most of the side-effects were mild. Fifteen of 20 patients with gastro-intestinal disturbances experienced nausea. Symptoms were systemic in 8, cardiopulmonary in 5, and neurological in 5.— D. J. D'Alessio *et al.*, *Antimicrob. Ag. Chemother.*, 1967, 490.

Precautions. Oxolinic acid should be used with caution in patients with severely impaired renal function or with convulsive disorders. Its use should be avoided during the first trimester of pregnancy and during lactation. Its use is also probably best avoided in infants. The stimulant effect on the central nervous system may be increased in elderly patients.

Nitrofurantoin has been reported to antagonise the activity of oxolinic acid against some organisms *in vitro*.

Oxolinic acid may give false positive reactions in urine tests for glucose using copper reduction methods.

Antimicrobial Action. Oxolinic acid is bactericidal and has a similar antibacterial spectrum to nalidixic acid and inhibits Gram-negative organisms including *Escherichia coli*, *Proteus* spp., and *Klebsiella* spp. Minimum inhibitory concentrations below 5 µg per ml are reported. *Pseudomonas aeruginosa* is usually resistant.

Gram-positive bacteria are relatively resistant although activity against *Staphylococcus aureus* has been demonstrated.

Bacterial resistance may develop rapidly and cross-resistance with nalidixic acid occurs. Also, nitrofurantoin may antagonise the activity of oxolinic acid against some organisms.

Oxolinic acid probably acts by inhibiting the synthesis of bacterial DNA.

Oxolinic acid was active *in vitro* against Gram-negative bacteria with the exception of *Pseudomonas* spp. Minimum inhibitory concentrations ranged from 0.19 to 1.56 µg per ml. It was also active against *Staph. aureus*, but inactive against most other Gram-positive bacteria. Oxolinic acid was effective *in vivo* against *Pr. vulgaris*, *Pr. mirabilis*, *E. coli*, *Kleb. pneumoniae*, and *Staph. aureus*.— F. J. Turner *et al.*, *Antimicrob. Ag. Chemother.*, 1967, 475. Further references: D. J. D'Alessio *et al.*, *ibid.*, 490; H. Neussel and G. Linzenmeier, *Chemotherapy, Basle*, 1973, *18*, 253.

Nitrofurantoin inhibited the antimicrobial action of oxolinic acid against *Pr. mirabilis* and other nonlactose-fermenting organisms *in vitro*.— G. P. C. Westwood and W. L. Hooper (letter), *Lancet*, 1975, *1*, 460.

Oxolinic acid was more active *in vitro* than nalidixic acid or cinoxacin against 138 strains of *Shigella sonnei* and *Sh. flexneri* with an MIC of 1.56 µg per ml compared with 6.25 µg per ml for the other two.— R. C. Gordon *et al.*, *Antimicrob. Ag. Chemother.*, 1976, *10*, 918.

Studies *in vitro* indicated that oxolinic acid had greater inhibitory activity than ampicillin against *Salmonella typhi* from chronic typhoid carriers.— C. M. Nolan and J. Rosenfeld, *Curr. ther. Res.*, 1977, *21*, 736.

Bacterial resistance. Oxolinic acid was effective against all Gram-negative organisms tested except *Ps. aeruginosa;* resistance developed in 4.8% of patients.— K. N. Ghatikar, *Curr. ther. Res.*, 1974, *16*, 130.

Of 475 strains of various organisms resistant to nalidixic acid, only 1 strain of *Pr. mirabilis* and 1 of *Staph. aureus* were fully sensitive to oxolinic acid and another 34 strains were moderately sensitive.— R. N. Grüneberg (letter), *Lancet*, 1974, *2*, 1088.

Absorption and Fate. Oxolinic acid is absorbed from the gastro-intestinal tract. A plasma half-life of 6 to 7 hours has been reported. It is extensively metabolised and conjugated and excreted in the urine. Some metabolites are active.

Excretion in milk and faeces is also stated to occur.

The administration of 750 mg of oxolinic acid every 12 hours in 8 patients resulted in average serum concentrations of 1.9 µg per ml after 7 days, with a peak 2 hours after a dose. In 20 patients with impaired renal function, the average concentration was 6.1 µg per ml 2 hours after a dose. The average urinary concentrations were 44 to 96 µg per ml in patients with normal renal function and 35 to 76 µg per ml in those with impaired function. The excretion of oxolinic acid was very variable, with an average of about 6.5% in each group.— P. O. Madsen and P. R. Rhodes, *J. Urol.*, 1971, *105*, 870.

Between 80 and 85% of oxolinic acid was bound to serum protein.— R. C. Gordon *et al.*, *Antimicrob. Ag. Chemother.*, 1976, *10*, 918.

Further references: D. J. D'Alessio *et al.*, *Antimicrob. Ag. Chemother.*, 1967, 490; F. J. DiCarlo *et al.*, *Archs int. Pharmacodyn. Thér.*, 1968, *174*, 413; P. T. Mannisto, *Clin. Pharmac. Ther.*, 1976, *19*, 37.

Uses. Oxolinic acid has actions and uses similar to those of nalidixic acid (see p.1052). It is used in the treatment of urinary-tract infections due to Gram-negative organisms other than *Pseudomonas* spp. The adult dose is 750 mg every 12 hours for 7 to 14 days, preferably after food.

Dysentery. In 25 subjects with induced shigellosis, a negative stool count was achieved after 5 days' treatment in 4 of 6 patients who received oxolinic acid, 1 of 6 who received oxolinic acid and diphenoxylate plus atropine (Lomotil), and none of the patients who received either diphenoxylate or placebo. Fever was prolonged in 2 men who received diphenoxylate.— H. L. DuPont and R. B. Hornick, *J. Am. med. Ass.*, 1973, *226*, 1525.

Urinary-tract infections. When used in the treatment of chronic bacteriuria, oxolinic acid 2 g daily was associated with less bacterial resistance than nalidixic acid 4 g daily, but relapse often occurred upon withdrawal of the drug.— E. Atlas *et al.*, *Ann. intern. Med.*, 1969, *70*, 713.

Of 290 patients with urinary-tract infections treated with oxolinic acid for 10 to 15 days, 83% were clinically cured and 80% bacteriologically cured—a few relapsed. Resistant strains developed in 4.8%. The dose was 750 mg once or twice daily with lower doses for children. Side-effects, chiefly nausea and vomiting, occurred in 29 patients.— K. N. Ghatikar, *Curr. ther. Res.*, 1974, *16*, 130.

In a clinical study 106 patients with urinary-tract infection due to Gram-negative organisms, mainly *E. coli*, received oxolinic acid 750 mg twice daily for 7 days. Of these 86 were treated successfully. In a further 32, Gram-negative organisms isolated were not sensitive to oxolinic acid. Side-effects occurred in 16 of 138 patients treated and included nausea or vomiting (6), restlessness (4), insomnia (5), chest pain and pounding (1), and a feeling of doom (1).— B. S. Pearson, *Med. J. Aust.*, 1975, *1*, 140.

An unfavourable review of the use of oxolinic acid for the treatment of urinary tract infections.— *Med. Lett.*, 1976, *18*, 2 and 20. See also *Drug & Ther. Bull.*, 1975, *13*, 70.

From a study of the relative incidences of urinary infections in 147 males and 664 females during the first 3 months of 1976 it was considered that nalidixic and oxolinic acids, having little activity against Gram-positive organisms, should be avoided for the treatment of young women.— J. Crump *et al.* (letter), *Lancet*, 1976, *1*, 1184.

Oxolinic acid 15 to 20 mg per kg body-weight daily in 2 divided doses was given for 14 to 21 days to children aged 1½ to 16 years with urinary-tract infections. The infecting organism was eradicated in 26 of 30 children including 11 of 13 with an underlying structural or functional abnormality. Bacterial resistance had developed in the 4 who did not respond. There was no bacteriological relapse in 19 children 6 weeks after treatment. Mild side-effects occurred in 17. The results indicated that if the urine was not sterile after 5 days of treatment bacterial resistance was likely to have developed.— R. M. Shapera and J. M. Matsen, *Am. J. Dis. Child.*, 1977, *131*, 34.

Proprietary Names

Decme *(Poli, Ital.)*; Emyrenil *(Emyfar, Spain)*; Gramurin *(Chinoin, Hung.)*; Nefroclar *(Hosbon, Spain)*; Nidantin *(Sasse, Ger.)*; Ossian *(Bioindustria, Ital.)*; Oxobid *(Warner, NZ)*; Oxoboi *(Boi, Spain)*; Oxoinex *(Inexfa, Spain)*; Oxol *(Casen-Roncales, Spain)*; Oxalin *(Prodes, Spain)*; Oxolina *(Armour, Ital.)*; Pietil *(Argentia, Arg.)*; Prodoxol *(Warner, S.Afr.)*; Tilvis *(Scharper, Ital.)*; Tiurasin *(Bouty, Ital.)*; Tropodil *(Elea, Arg.)*; Urinox *(Warner, Arg.)*; Uristatic *(Frumtost, Spain)*; Uritrate *(Parke, Davis, Ital.; Substancia, Spain)*; Uro-Alvar *(Alvarez Gómez, Spain)*; Uropax *(LEFA, Spain)*; Urotrate *(Substantia, Fr.)*; Uroxol *(Ausonia, Ital.)*; Utibid *(Warner, Austral.; Parke, Davis, USA)*.

Oxolinic acid was formerly marketed in Great Britain under the proprietary name Prodoxol (*Warner*).

5666-b

Pipemidic Acid. 1489 RB; Piperamic Acid. 8-Ethyl-5,8-dihydro-5-oxo-2-(piperazin-1-yl)pyrido[2,3-*d*]pyrimidine-6-carboxylic acid.

$C_{14}H_{17}N_5O_3$=303.3.

CAS — 51940-44-4.

A yellowish-white powder with a bitter taste. M.p. about 260°. Slightly **soluble** in water and organic solvents. Soluble in acid and alkaline solutions.

Pipemidic acid is an antimicrobial agent with properties similar to those of nalidixic acid (see p.1051) and is given in the treatment of urinary-tract infections in doses of 400 mg morning and night. It is stated to be effective against some organisms resistant to piromidic acid (see below) and nalidixic acid.

A clinical study in children.— Y. Kotani *et al.*, *Chemotherapy, Tokyo*, 1975, *23*, 2893.

Studies in obstetrics and gynaecology indicated that the amount of pipemidic acid diffusing across the placenta was very small.— M. Kanao *et al.*, *Chemotherapy, Tokyo*, 1975, *23*, 2939. Antimicrobial activity.— M. Shimizu *et al.*, *Antimicrob. Ag. Chemother.*, 1975, *8*, 132.

The inhibition of R-plasmid transfer by pipemidic acid.— S. Nakamura *et al.*, *Antimicrob. Ag. Chemother*, 1976, *10*, 779.

An average peak serum concentration of 2.7 µg per ml (range 2 to 3.3 µg) was obtained 2 hours after administration of pipemidic acid 400 mg to 5 subjects with normal renal function.— G. Montay *et al.*, *Thérapie*, 1977, *32*, 553.. Further references.— M. Shimizu *et al.*, *Antimicrob. Ag. Chemother.*, 1975, *7*, 441.

Epidermal necrolysis. A 25-year-old woman developed toxic epidermal necrolysis (Lyell's syndrome) about 2 weeks after she had started treatment with pipemidic acid 800 mg daily.— F. Vachon *et al.*, *Nouv. Presse méd.*, 1977, *6*, 1239.

Proprietary Names

Deblaston *(Madaus, Ger.)*; Pipemid *(Gentili, Ital.)*; Pipram *(Bellon, Fr.; RBS Pharma, Ital.)*; Urotractin *(Zambeletti, Ital.)*.

5667-v

Piromidic Acid. PD-93. 8-Ethyl-5,8-dihydro-5-oxo-2-(pyrrolidin-1-yl)pyrido[2,3-*d*]pyrimidine-6-carboxylic acid.

$C_{14}H_{16}N_4O_3$=288.3.

CAS — 19562-30-2.

A yellowish-white or pale yellow powder, almost odourless and tasteless. Practically **insoluble** in water and alcohol; slightly soluble in chloroform; soluble in solutions of sodium hydroxide.

Piromidic acid is an antimicrobial agent with properties similar to those of nalidixic acid (see p.1051) but it is less active. Organisms resistant to nalidixic acid are also resistant to piromidic acid. Its use has been suggested in the treatment of infections of the urinary, gastro-intestinal, and biliary tracts in a dose of 2 g daily in divided doses.

Comparison with nalidixic acid.— M. Shimizu *et al.*, *Antimicrob. Ag. Chemother.*, 1970, 117.

Metabolism.— M. Shimizu *et al.*, *Antimicrob. Ag. Chemother.*, 1970, 123; Y. Sekine *et al.*, *Xenobiotica*, 1976, *6*, 185.

Renal failure in 2 patients possibly associated with the administration of piromidic acid.— *Japan med. Gaz.*, 1978, *15* (Apr. 20), 10.

Proprietary Names

Bactamyl *(Carrion, Fr.)*; Coltix *(Gramon, Arg.)*; Panerco *(Erco, Denm.)*; Pirodal *(ISF, Ital.)*; Septural *(Grünenthal, Ger.)*; Uriclor *(Almirall, Spain)*; Actrun C, Panacid *(both Jap.)*.

Oxygen and some other Gases

5200-c

This section includes monographs on oxygen, carbon dioxide, helium and nitrogen. Some compressed and liquefied gases are used as refrigerants and aerosol propellents and some of these are included.

5201-k

Oxygen *(B.P., Eur. P., U.S.P.)*. Oxygenium; Ossigeno; Sauerstoff.
O_2=31.9988.

CAS — 7782-44-7.

Pharmacopoeias. In all pharmacopoeias examined except *Rus.*

A colourless odourless tasteless gas. It contains not less than 99% v/v of O_2, the residue consisting either of argon with a trace of nitrogen or of hydrogen. Oxygen intended for aviation or mountain rescue must have a sufficiently low moisture content to avoid blocking of valves by freezing.

Soluble 1 in 32 of water by volume and 1 in 7 of alcohol by volume at normal temperature and pressure. **Store** under compression in metal cylinders.

In the UK cylinders of oxygen are painted black with a white shoulder. Cylinders of oxygen mixed with carbon dioxide are painted black with grey and white quarterings on neck and shoulder. Cylinders of oxygen mixed with helium are painted black with brown and white quarterings on neck and shoulder. The name or chemical symbol of the gas or gases should be stencilled in paint on the shoulder of the cylinder and clearly and indelibly stamped on the cylinder valve.

For identification colours for medical gas cylinders, see British Standards Specification BS 1319C: 1976.

Adverse Effects. Prolonged administration of high concentrations of oxygen (greater than about 40%) may damage the pulmonary epithelium leading to pulmonary oedema and generalised atelectasis. Retrolental fibroplasia has occurred in premature infants treated with concentrations of more than 50% of oxygen.

Hyperbaric oxygen at pressures over 2 atmospheres has led to convulsions.

A review of oxygen toxicity.— L. Frank and D. Massaro, *Am. J. Med.*, 1980, *69*, 117.

Short-term memory was impaired in 12 men performing a step tracking task whilst breathing oxygen from a demand-type mask compared with breathing air from a mask.— E. C. Poulton, *Aerospace Med.*, 1974, *45*, 482, per *J. Am. med. Ass.*, 1974, *229*, 348.

Effect on eyes. For a review of retrolental fibroplasia caused by oxygen in infants, see P. J. Evans, *Practitioner*, 1970, *205*, 468.

A 32-year-old man with myasthenia gravis had been given air containing 80% oxygen for 150 days when he complained of darkness of central vision in both eyes. On examination atrophy of the retinal arteries was found. The cause was considered to be exposure to high oxygen concentrations.— T. Kobayashi and S. Murakami, *J. Am. med. Ass.*, 1972, *219*, 741.

Effect on lungs. An extensive review, with 540 references, of the pulmonary toxicity of oxygen.— J. M. Clark and C. J. Lambertsen, *Pharmac. Rev.*, 1971, *23*, 37.

Normobaric oxygen toxicity of the lung.— S. M. Deneke and B. L. Fanburg, *New Engl. J. Med.*, 1980, *303*, 76.

Examination of the lungs of 70 patients who died after prolonged artificial ventilation with a high concentration of oxygen revealed in many of them a beefy oedematous appearance. The changes in lung structure were not related to the duration of artificial ventilation alone, but followed the prolonged delivery of a high concentration of oxygen, though no definite cause-and-effect relationship could be established. High concentrations of oxygen necessary to maintain the arterial oxygen tension should be reduced as soon as was consistent with the patient's safety.— G. Nash *et al.*, *New Engl. J. Med.*, 1967, *276*, 368.

Oxygen had been given from birth during part of the first 6 hours, or continuously, to 49 of 60 infants, mostly premature, who were found at post mortem to have had lung haemorrhage. No similar evidence of haemorrhage was found in 23 further infants who had not received oxygen or had received none during the first 6 hours.— D. R. Shanklin and S. L. Wolfson, *New Engl. J. Med.*, 1967, *277*, 833. In a 10-year review of pulmonary haemorrhage, no systematic differences were found in its incidence in the years when the use of oxygen was curtailed compared with its greater use in later years.— M. E. Avery and R. A. deLemos (letter), *ibid.*, 1968, *278*, 338. Comment on the role of oxygen and other factors in the incidence of bronchopulmonary dysplasia in preterm infants.— *Lancet*, 1980, *1*, 690.

Lung changes (hyaline membranes or proliferative pneumonitis) in 21 patients who died after oxygen therapy for injury or exposure to smoke indicated that pneumonitis was associated with breathing 60 to 100% oxygen for at least 2 days. The threshold value for damage appeared to be 40% oxygen. Those respiring 25 to 40% oxygen for days developed only subclinical focal lung lesions or had no changes.— S. Sevitt, *J. clin. Path.*, 1974, *27*, 21. Despite the high concentrations of oxygen given to 7 miners who were victims of a pit explosion only one had any evidence of pulmonary fibrosis and this was focal.— P. S. Hasleton *et al.*, *J. clin. Path.*, 1981, *34*, 1147.

Heart block. In 3 of 5 patients treated with hyperbaric oxygen at 5 to 30 lb per in^2, bundle branch block occurred within a few minutes of commencing treatment. ECG recordings were normal 30 to 60 minutes after leaving the chamber. In 2 of the patients no such effect was seen when their toxic infection and fever had subsided.— H. D. Jones (letter), *Lancet*, 1968, *1*, 822.

Precautions. Any fire or spark is highly dangerous in the presence of increased oxygen concentrations especially when oxygen is used under pressure.

Growth of surface cultures of bacteria was found to be inhibited in atmospheres in which the partial pressure of oxygen exceeded 600 mmHg, the degree of inhibition being proportional to the partial pressure of oxygen. In deep cultures incubated in 3 atmospheres of oxygen, growth was more rapid and heavier than in cultures incubated in air at normal atmospheric pressure. The results suggested caution was necessary in treating patients with deep-seated aerobic infections with hyperbaric oxygen.— C. A. Pennock, *Lancet*, 1966, *1*, 1348. See also J. M. Stark and J. S. Orr (letter), *ibid.*, 1966, *2*, 108.

Coronary vasoconstriction could occur, particularly in patients with diseased arteries, following the inhalation of 100% oxygen.— M. G. Bourassa *et al.*, *Am. J. Cardiol.*, 1969, *24*, 172, per *Abstr. Wld Med.*, 1970, *44*, 120.

Uses. Oxygen is given by inhalation to correct hypoxaemia in conditions causing under-ventilation of the lungs, such as exacerbations of chronic bronchitis, pneumonia, or pulmonary oedema, in extensive fibrosing alveolitis, and in conditions where the oxygen content of the air breathed is inadequate as at high altitudes; it is also used in circulatory failure associated with conditions such as myocardial infarction or after cardiac arrest. Oxygen is of value in the treatment of carbon monoxide poisoning and in providing enhanced oxygenation in severe anaemia or in the treatment of respiratory depression until more specific treatments are started. It may be useful in the management of abdominal distension and in removing accumulated nitrogen from other cavities. Oxygen is also given by inhalation to subjects working in pressurised spaces and to divers to reduce the concentration of nitrogen inhaled. It is used as a diluent of volatile and gaseous anaesthetics.

The addition of 5 or 7% of carbon dioxide to inhaled oxygen stimulates the respiratory centre and causes deeper breathing, except in patients who have stopped breathing; this effect may be diminished by depressants.

In obstructive airway disease, in conditions such as bronchitis and emphysema, oxygen is usually administered to give an inspired concentration of about 30%. High concentrations are to be avoided as they may enhance carbon-dioxide retention and narcosis.

In conditions not usually associated with retention of carbon dioxide, such as pneumonia, pulmonary oedema, fibrosing alveolitis, or circulatory failure, oxygen may be administered in concentrations of up to 100%. The concentration should be reduced as soon as possible. In crush injuries of the chest or in respiratory depression due to poisoning, oxygen may be administered in conjunction with assisted respiration. High concentrations of oxygen may be administered in carbon monoxide poisoning, but in severe cases treatment with hyperbaric oxygen at 2 atmospheres absolute may be preferred.

Oxygen concentrations of up to 35% may be employed in asphyxia in the newborn and in conditions associated with respiratory distress in infants; higher concentrations should only be used for short periods under carefully controlled conditions.

Oxygen may be administered by means of a nasal catheter, face mask, or oxygen tent. Face masks are commonly employed for domiciliary oxygen therapy when flow-rates are 2 or 4 litres per minute and oxygen concentrations usually 28%.

Metal cylinders containing oxygen should be fitted with a reducing valve by which the rate of flow can be controlled. It is important that the reducing valve should be free from all traces of oil or grease, as otherwise a violent explosion may occur. Also, if the reducing valve is of the rubber-bellows type, the tap of the reducer should always be opened before opening the main oxygen tap on the cylinder; opening the main tap with the reducing valve tap closed has been known to cause spontaneous fire.

Oxygen under pressure, i.e. hyperbaric oxygen, is administered by enclosing the patient in a special high-pressure chamber. It is used to correct hypoxaemia in conditions such as arterial disease, asphyxia in the newborn, congenital heart disease, and poisoning by carbon monoxide. It is also used to enhance the effectiveness of irradiation in the treatment of malignant disease, and as an adjunct in the treatment of severe anaerobic infections.

A discussion on acute oxygen therapy.— *Lancet*, 1981, *1*, 980. Comments on the use of humidifiers.— J. B. Wood and C. Frith (letter), *ibid.*, 1426; G. Lazlo (letter), *ibid.*, *2*, 104.

Comment on the use of oxygen insufflation of the peritoneum for the detection of inguinal hernia in children.— *Br. med. J.*, 1974, *3*, 540.

Abdominal distension. The intestinal gas-filled cysts resolved in 2 patients with pneumatosis cystoides intestinalis following treatment with oxygen by inhalation. However in both cases this was only temporary. One patient underwent further treatment with consequent improvement but the other patient refused more oxygen and 13 months after her colon had become apparently normal following the oxygen her cysts were as widespread as before treatment.— W. van der Linden (letter), *Lancet*, 1974, *2*, 1388. See also R. H. L. Down and W. M. Castleden, *Br. med. J.*, 1975, *1*, 493.

Four patients with pneumatosis cystoides intestinalis were successfully treated with oxygen therapy. The disease recurred in 1 patient after 6 months.— N. M. Simon *et al.*, *J. Am. med. Ass.*, 1975, *231*, 1354.

For further references, see A. E. Mackinnon *et al.*, *Archs Dis. Childh.*, 1977, *52*, 956; R. Güller *et al.*, *Dt. med. Wschr.*, 1977, *102*, 1869; S. Holt *et al.*, *Gut*, 1979, *20*, 493.

See also Paralytic Ileus under Hyperbaric Oxygen Therapy, below.

Administration. References to various methods of administering oxygen.— M. Catterall *et al.*, *Lancet*, 1967, *1*, 415; C. J. Woods (letter), *ibid.*, 617; J. M. Collis and D. W. Bethune (letter), *ibid.*, 787; G. S. Robertson, *ibid.*, 1969, *1*, 801; J. M. Leigh (letter), *Br. med. J.*, 1970, *4*, 620; S. A. Friedman *et al.*, *J. Am. med. Ass.*, 1974, *228*, 474; E. J. M. Campbell and K. B. Minty, *Lancet*, 1976, *1*, 1199; M. G. Harries, *Practitioner*, 1978, *221*, 616; M. K. Benson, *Prescribers' J.*, 1979, *19*, 9.

Cardiovascular disorders. Administration of oxygen before or during the slow injection of an intravenous anaesthetic was considered to be highly desirable for patients with severe heart disease.— S. M. Lyons and R. S. J. Clark, *Br. J. Anaesth.*, 1972, *44*, 575.

Cor pulmonale. In a study in 26 patients with chronic hypoxic cor pulmonale with pulmonary hypertension the breathing of 30% oxygen during exercise reduced hypoxia and increased exercise tolerance (walking distance) but the gain in exercise tolerance was nullified when they had to carry their liquid oxygen supply (weight 4.5 kg).— R. J. E. Leggett and D. C. Flenley, *Br. med. J.*, 1977, *2*, 84.

See also under Respiratory Disorders, below.

Myocardial infarction. A review of the use of oxygen in acute myocardial infarction.— *Lancet*, 1969, *2*, 525. See also A. J. Moss, *Ann. intern. Med.*, 1975, *83*, 897; *Br. med. J.*, 1976, *1*, 731.

In a double-blind study of 157 patients with uncomplicated myocardial infarction the administration of oxygen did not cause greater benefits than the administration of compressed air. Arterial pO_2 values and serum aspartate aminotransferase (SGOT) concentrations were higher among the 80 patients given oxygen.— J. M. Rawles and A. C. F. Kenmure, *Br. med. J.*, 1976, *1*, 1121.

See also under Hyperbaric Oxygen Therapy, below.

Patent ductus arteriosus. The successful use of oxygen in 3 infants, each at least 35 weeks (gestational plus postnatal) of age, to close patent ductus arteriosus.— P. M. Dunn and B. D. Speidel (letter), *Lancet*, 1973, *2*, 333.

Decompression sickness. For a report on nitrogen-oxygen mixtures in the treatment of divers with decompression sickness, see Nitrogen, p.1057.

Diagnostic test. Continuous positive airway pressure with oxygen 100% could be used as an adjunct to differentiate cardiac and pulmonary disease in neonates. In neonates with pulmonary disease the arterial oxygen pressure tended to show a significant increase, but in congenital heart disease or persistent foetal circulation there was little or no change.— P. S. Rao *et al.*, *Archs Dis. Childh.*, 1978, *53*, 456.

Effect on exercise. An unfavourable review of the use of oxygen before, during, or after exercise to improve athletic performance.— *Med. Lett.*, 1978, *20*, 28.

Headache. The author achieved relief of cluster headaches by inhaling oxygen.— J. F. Janks (letter), *J. Am. med. Ass.*, 1978, *239*, 191.

Hyperbaric oxygen therapy. Reviews.— *Lancet*, 1968, *2*, 336; *Med. Lett.*, 1978, *20*, 51.

The use of oxygen at a pressure of 2 or 3 atmospheres rapidly relieved anoxia, enhanced the action of ionising radiations on tissue, and preserved viability in tissues and organs stored at low temperatures. Prolonged exposure to hyperbaric oxygen had adversely affected renal function and vision, but heart muscle, which could readily take up oxygen, had been relatively immune from toxicity. Hyperbaric oxygen had not materially improved the clinical prognosis after myocardial infarction. It had inhibited α-toxin production by *Clostridium welchii* without killing the organism. Topical application of oxygen at 3 atmospheres was better than at 2 atmospheres in the treatment of open wounds infected with clostridia, but the clinical advantage of hyperbaric oxygen in tetanus had not been established. Wounds exposed to hyperbaric oxygen tended to remain dry and systemic infection-rates were reduced; this application might be useful in the badly burnt patient. In poisoning by carbon monoxide, cyanide, or chlorinated hydrocarbons, tissue hypoxia could be reversed by exposure of the patient to hyperbaric oxygen.— A. R. Behnke and H. A. Saltzman, *New Engl. J. Med.*, 1967, *276*, 1423 and 1478. See also *J. Am. med. Ass.*, 1978, *239*, 1011 (burns); R. A. Neubauer (letter), *ibid.*, 1393 (leg ulcers). See also under Precautions.

Improvement in cognition in elderly men given hyperbaric oxygen.— E. A. Jacobs *et al.*, *New Engl. J. Med.*, 1968, *281*, 753. See also *J. Am. med. Ass.*, 1975, *231*, 238. No improvement.— A. Raskin *et al.*, *Archs gen. Psychiat.*, 1978, *35*, 50.

Nine patients with air embolism sustained during haemodialysis were treated with hyperbaric oxygen within 10 minutes to 3 hours of diagnosis. There had been only slight improvement in their condition after conventional treatment but all cardiopulmonary and neurological abnormalities were greatly improved in 7 patients after 10 minutes at 6 atmospheres absolute. One patient improved at a lower pressure but the ninth required prolonged compression before improvement. On discharge from the chamber no patient had symptoms of air embolism.— S. E. Baskin and R. F. Wozniak, *New Engl. J. Med.*, 1975, *293*, 184.

Anaemia. Hyperbaric oxygen was used successfully in the treatment of a woman with hypoxia due to idiopathic auto-immune haemolytic anaemia. After 5 days' treatment the haemoglobin concentration had risen from 3 g per 100 ml to 5 g per 100 ml.— O. Myking and A. Schreiner, *J. Am. med. Ass.*, 1974, *227*, 1161.

The use of hyperbaric oxygen in patients with blood loss anaemia who refused transfusion.— G. B. Hart, *J. Am. med. Ass.*, 1974, *228*, 1028.

Carbon monoxide poisoning. Reports on the use of hyperbaric oxygen in the treatment of carbon monoxide poisoning: G. Smith *et al.*, *Lancet*, 1962, *1*, 816; M. E. Sluyter and I. Boerema, *Ned. Tijdschr. Geneesk.*, 1962, *106*, 826; J. Thurston (letters), *Br. med. J.*, 1968, *4*, 386 and 772; *idem*, 1969, *1*, 446.

Cardiovascular disorders. Myocardial infarction. Studies in 10 patients being treated for myocardial infarction with high pressure oxygen showed that blood pressure, systemic vascular resistance, and arterial pO_2 rose progressively. Reduction in cardiac output and stroke-volume were also noted. High pressure oxygen was considered to be of value to patients with severe hypoxia, hypotension, and metabolic acidosis; it could limit the extent of infarction. No evidence of oxygen toxicity was noted.— A. J. V. Cameron *et al.*, *Lancet*, 1966, *2*, 833.

Of forty patients with cardiac infarction thirty-seven were successfully treated by intermittent exposure to oxygen at a maximum pressure of 2 atmospheres. Severe chest pain was quickly relieved in 23 patients and dyspnoea in 14; pulmonary oedema was not relieved for several hours.— R. Ashfield and C. J. Gavey, *Postgrad. med. J.*, 1969, *45*, 648, per *Abstr. Wld Med.*, 1970, *44*, 285.

See also above.

Gas gangrene. A brief review of the role of hyperbaric oxygen in the treatment of gas gangrene.— *Br. med. J.*, 1972, *3*, 715. See also J. C. Davis *et al.*, *J. Am. med. Ass.*, 1973, *224*, 205.

For reports of the use of hyperbaric oxygen in the treatment of gas gangrene, see S. C. Karz *et al.*, *J. Am. med. Ass.*, 1971, *217*, 962; B. Roding *et al.*, *Surgery Gynec. Obstet.*, 1972, *134*, 579; A. J. Keogh (letter), *Br. med. J.*, 1972, *4*, 175; D. L. Fowler *et al.*, *J. Am. med. Ass.*, 1977, *238*, 882; H. Nier *et al.*, *Dt. med. Wschr.*, 1978, *103*, 1958; H. U. Cameron and M. Ford, *Can. med. Ass. J.*, 1978, *119*, 1207.

Malignant neoplasms. Reviews of hyperbaric oxygen with radiation in the treatment of malignant neoplasms: H. A. S. van den Brenk, *J. Am. med. Ass.*, 1971, *217*, 948 (head and neck); J. R. Glassburn *et al.*, *Cancer*, 1977, *39*, 751.

Results were disappointing following 2363 treatments with hyperbaric oxygen in conjunction with radiotherapy for carcinoma of the bronchus and bladder. It was suggested that hyperbaric oxygenation might increase the growth of metastases.— I. S. Cade and J. B. McEwen, *Cancer*, 1967, *20*, 817, per *J. Am. med. Ass.*, 1967, *200* (June 12), A227.

Results of radiotherapy treatment under hyperbaric oxygen were assessed in 1669 cancer patients registered for study between 1963 and 1976. Hyperbaric oxygen was found significantly to improve the results of radiotherapy, both in terms of survival and local tumour control, for tumours in the head and neck, and in the uterine cervix. Although some improvement in survival appeared to occur in carcinoma of the bronchus the results were not statistically significant; no improvement was noted in carcinoma of the bladder. Side-effects included occasional oxygen convulsions and refusal of therapy owing to claustrophobia.—Report of a Medical Research Council Working Party, *Lancet*, 1978, *2*, 881.

Osteomyelitis. A favourable report of the use of hyperbaric oxygen to treat intractable mandibular osteomyelitis in 1 patient.— E. G. Mainous *et al.*, *Milit. Med.*, 1975, *140*, 196.

Paralytic ileus. Hyperbaric oxygen had been used successfully in 12 patients with paralytic ileus unresponsive to conventional treatment. It was given at 2½ atmospheres for 1 hour twice daily for a total of 4 to 10 hours. Recovery was often rapid.— R. E. Loder, *Br. med. J.*, 1977, *1*, 1448.

Spinal cord injuries. Favourable reports of the use of hyperbaric oxygen therapy in patients with spinal cord injuries.— J. D. Yeo *et al.*, *Med. J. Aust.*, 1978, *2*, 572; R. F. Jones *et al.*, *ibid.*, 573. See also G. Bedbrook, *ibid.*, 618.

Vertigo. All 7 patients with vertigo achieved a good response when exposed to hyperbaric oxygen at 2 atmospheres absolute for 2 hours for total periods of 6 to 30 hours. Vertigo and nausea and vomiting disappeared in 4 patients and was greatly reduced in 2.— S. Nair *et al.* (preliminary communication), *Lancet*, 1973, *1*, 184.

Respiratory disorders. In 8 patients with acute exacerbations of respiratory failure due to chronic bronchitis the mean arterial pO_2 was 44.8 mmHg and the mean arterial pCO_2 was 60.4 mmHg. After the administration of 30% oxygen these values were 68 and 65.8 mmHg respectively. The mean venous pO_2 was 27.9 mmHg before oxygenation and 36.1 mmHg after. In 8 patients with pulmonary oedema (consequent on myocardial infarction in 6) mean arterial pO_2 and pCO_2 values were 55.5 and 31.8 mmHg and were raised to 288.4 and 35.7 mmHg respectively after oxygenation with 60 to 90% oxygen; venous pO_2 rose from 26.3 to 35.7 mmHg. An adequate venous pO_2 was necessary to ensure capillary oxygenation. In patients with bronchitis and a raised pCO_2, 30% oxygen was unlikely to lead to ventilatory depression. In patients with pulmonary oedema and a low or normal pCO_2, high concentrations of oxygen were not only necessary but safe.— D. C. Flenley *et al.*, *Br. med. J.*, 1973, *1*, 78. See also P. M. Warren *et al.*, *Lancet*, 1980, *1*, 467.

A discussion of postoperative hypoxaemia and the administration of oxygen.— J. M. Leigh, *Br. J. Anaesth.*, 1975, *47*, 108. See also G. B. Drummond and D. Wright, *Br. J. Anaesth.*, 1976, *48*, 270.

Discussions of the postanaesthetic use of oxygen.— *Br. med. J.*, 1978, *2*, 1452; P. S. Parfrey *et al.* (letter), *Br. med. J.*, 1978, *2*, 1713.

In a long-term comparative study of patients with hypoxaemic chronic obstructive lung disease continuous oxygen therapy was associated with a lower mortality than 12-hour nocturnal oxygen therapy.— Nocturnal Oxygen Therapy Trial Group, *Ann. intern. Med.*, 1980, *93*, 391. Comment.— S. D. Roberts, *ibid.*, 499. A multicentre controlled study in patients with chronic bronchitis and emphysema complicated by hypoxic cor pulmonale indicated that long-term oxygen therapy could reduce mortality over 3 years in both men and women but the effect only became evident in men after 500 days had elapsed. Patients received oxygen for 15 hours each day at a flow-rate of 2 litres per minute or no oxygen.—Report of the Medical Research Council Working Party, *Lancet*, 1981, *1*, 681. Comments on long-term oxygen therapy at home in patients with advanced chronic bronchitis and other chronic obstructive lung diseases.— *Lancet*, 1981, *1*, 701; *Br. med. J.*, 1981, *282*, 1909; *Lancet*, 1981, *2*, 670.

Breathlessness and exercise tolerance were improved in 'pink and puffing' patients with fixed airways obstruction when they breathed oxygen, regardless of whether the cylinder was carried by the patient or an assistant.— A. A. Woodcock *et al.*, *Lancet*, 1981, *1*, 907.

A study on nocturnal hypoxaemia and ECG changes in patients with chronic obstructive airways disease.— V. G. Tirlapur *et al.*, *New Engl. J. Med.*, 1982, *306*, 125. Comment on oxygen therapy.— A. J. Block, *ibid.*, 166.

References to the use of oxygen in respiratory failure: L. W. Faulks *et al.*, *Med. J. Aust.*, 1975, *1*, 69; J. E. Hodgkin *et al.*, *J. Am. med. Ass.*, 1975, *232*, 1243; R. A. L. Brewis, *Br. med. J.*, 1978, *1*, 898; T. L. Petty *et al.*, *Archs intern. Med.*, 1979, *139*, 28; *Lancet*, 1979, *1*, 1172; D. M. Davies (letter), *ibid.*, 1290; L. Gattinoni *et al.*, *Lancet*, 1980, *2*, 292.

Asphyxia in the newborn. The arterial oxygen tension in premature babies should be maintained in the range 60 to 90 mmHg. Too high a concentration in inspired air could cause eye and lung damage but too low a concentration could cause permanent brain damage.— *Drug & Ther. Bull.*, 1974, *12*, 45.

See also under Respiratory Distress Syndrome, below.

Asthma. Recommendations on the use of oxygen in the treatment of acute asthma.— M. C. F. Pain, *Drugs*, 1976, *12*, 231.

Pneumonia. Oxygen in the treatment of pneumonia.— C. M. Ogilvie, *Br. med. J.*, 1978, *1*, 771.

Respiratory distress syndrome. The management of hyaline membrane disease in infants, with special reference to the use of oxygen.— E. O. R. Reynolds, *Br. med. Bull.*, 1975, *31*, 18.

A review of the management of idiopathic respiratory distress syndrome in the newborn (hyaline membrane disease); conservative treatment alone was unsuitable for all but mild cases. The arterial pO_2 should ideally be maintained at 70 to 90 mmHg. If ambient oxygen concentrations greater than 30% were required, monitoring of the pO_2 was mandatory; continuous measurement of the ambient oxygen concentration was equally important. An arterial pO_2 above 120 mmHg might cause retrolental fibrosis. Maintenance of the rectal temperature at 37.5° kept oxygen consumption to a minimum, and the oxygen and air mixture should be warmed to 35° and humidified to 90 to 100% relative humidity.— *Drug & Ther. Bull.*, 1976, *14*, 37.

See also under Diagnostic Test, above.

Preparations

Carboxygenum *(Nord. P.)*. A mixture of oxygen 96% v/v and carbon dioxide 4% v/v.

Carbogen. A name given to mixtures of carbon dioxide and oxygen in various proportions.

5202-a

Carbon Dioxide *(B.P., Eur. P., U.S.P.)*.

Carbon Diox.; Carbonei Dioxydum; Carbonei Dioxidum; Carbonic Anhydride; Carbonic Acid Gas.

CO_2=44.01.

CAS — 124-38-9.

Pharmacopoeias. In *Arg., Belg., Br., Braz., Chin., Cz., Eur., Fr., Ger., Hung., Ind., Int., It., Jap., Jug., Neth., Pol., Swiss, Turk.*, and *U.S.*

A colourless odourless gas which does not support combustion. It is about 1½ times as heavy as air. A solution in water has weakly acid properties. Carbon dioxide can be liquefied by pressure at 31° or lower; at 31° a pressure of 72 atmospheres is required.

Soluble 1 in about 1 of water by volume at normal temperature and pressure. **Store** under compression in metal cylinders, at a temperature not exceeding 31°.

In the UK cylinders of carbon dioxide are painted grey. The name of the gas or the chemical symbol 'CO_2' should be stencilled in paint on the shoulder of the cylinder and clearly and indelibly stamped on the cylinder valve.

Liquid carbon dioxide and solid carbon dioxide are described below.

Adverse Effects. Above a concentration of 6%, carbon dioxide gives rise to headache, dizziness, mental confusion, palpitations, hypertension, and dyspnoea, and depression of the central nervous system. However concentrations of about 30% have a stimulating effect and may produce convulsions. Higher concentrations are depressant; inhalation of 50% carbon dioxide is reported to produce central effects similar to anaesthetics. The inhalation of high concentrations may produce respiratory acidosis.

Abrupt withdrawal of carbon dioxide after prolonged inhalation commonly produces pallor, hypotension, dizziness, severe headache, and nausea or vomiting.

Maximum permissible atmospheric concentration 5000 ppm.

The accidental exposure of a patient for about 8 minutes to a nitrous oxide-oxygen-carbon dioxide mixture estimated to contain about 60% of carbon dioxide and 7% of oxygen resulted in severe cyanosis, 'tracheal tug', reduced depth of respiration, rapid gasping 'frog-like' respiratory efforts, full and bounding pulse, and dilated pupils. There were no muscle twitchings or convulsions. The patient recovered uneventfully after artificial respiration with oxygen.— O. P. Dinnick (letter), *Br. J. Anaesth.*, 1968, *40*, 36.

Toxicity during use in laparoscopy. Hazardous increases in blood concentrations of carbon dioxide following the use of carbon dioxide for inflation of the abdomen during laparoscopy in 100 patients; 17 experienced cardiac arrhythmias, compared with 2 of 45 patients for whom nitrous oxide was used.— D. B. Scott and D. G. Julian, *Br. med. J.*, 1972, *1*, 411. Criticisms and comments on anaesthetic and technique.— J. E. Utting (letter), *ibid.*, 566; T. Sayer (letter), *ibid;* N. L. M. Gordon *et al.* (letter), *ibid.*, 625; P. Steptoe and F. M. Campbell (letter), *ibid.*

Hypotension in 1 patient and transient cardiac arrest in another, both undergoing laparoscopy after termination of pregnancy, were probably due to gas embolism from the carbon dioxide used for insufflation.— M. B. Barnett and D. T. Y. Liu (letter), *Br. med. J.*, 1974, *1*, 328.

Precautions. Carbon dioxide should be used with caution in respiratory obstruction and in pulmonary oedema, because the carbon dioxide tension in the blood is already increased and the enhanced respiratory effort may cause or increase pulmonary oedema.

The ability of the respiration to respond to carbon dioxide is diminished in patients with respiratory depression or those who have been given morphine or other depressants and in the anaesthetised or narcotised patient coma may follow inhalation of concentrations of carbon dioxide as low as 5% in oxygen.

Uses. Carbon dioxide is important for regulating the acid-base balance of the blood and tissues. Increased metabolic activity results in a corresponding increase in the proportion of carbon dioxide in the tissues and a decrease in the proportion of oxygen.

Although carbon dioxide stimulates respiration, it is seldom used for this purpose. Treatment of carbon monoxide poisoning with carbon dioxide is discouraged.

Carbon dioxide, when given by mouth in solution or as carbonates or bicarbonates, promotes the absorption of liquids by the mucous membranes. For this reason aerated waters rapidly relieve thirst, hasten the action of alcohol, and soon cause diuresis. Some carbonates in the stomach increase the secretion of gastric acid, and this effect should be borne in mind when they are prescribed to relieve hyperacidity. Effervescing waters are useful for masking the unpleasant taste of saline aperients.

Carbon dioxide gas is sometimes used as an inert gas to replace air in containers holding oxidisable substances when the pH is suitable.

Laboratory studies indicated that high concentrations of carbon dioxide in the presence of some serum components stimulated erythropoiesis in bone-marrow cultures.— H. J. Morton, *Nature*, 1967, *215*, 1166.

The ventilatory response to carbon dioxide in 21 Nigerian patients with homozygous sickle-cell disease was not different from that in healthy patients.— O. O. Elegbeleye *et al.*, *Br. J. Anaesth.*, 1976, *48*, 249.

The respiratory response to inhalation of carbon dioxide was significantly lower in 13 patients with endogenous depression than in 32 patients with reactive depression and 18 healthy subjects.— J. Damas-Mora *et al.* (letter), *Lancet*, 1978, *1*, 616.

Cerebral fat embolism. A man of 33 with cerebral fat embolism who was deeply comatose and had decerebrate rigidity recovered after treatment with 20% carbon dioxide in oxygen for 5½ hours. Carbon dioxide was chosen as it was the most potent of the agents known to increase cerebral blood flow.— B. Broom, *Lancet*, 1961, *1*, 1324.

Diagnosis of cardiac disease. For a report of carbon dioxide cineangiocardiography in the diagnosis of pericardial disease, see A. F. Turner *et al.*, *Am. J. Roentg.*, 1966, *97*, 342.

Liquid Carbon Dioxide is a limpid colourless liquid which is immiscible with water but readily dissolves in alcohol, ether, and volatile oils; at atmospheric pressure it boils at about −78°.

Use in food. The Food Additives and Contaminants Committee recommended that carbon dioxide be permitted for use as a solvent in food provided that the maximum concentration for oil in the carbon dioxide was 2 ppm.— *Report on the Review of Solvents in Food*, FAC/REP/25, Ministry of Agriculture, Fisheries and Food, London, HM Stationery Office, 1978.

Carbon dioxide is permitted for use in food under The Miscellaneous Additives in Food Regulations 1974 (SI 1974: No. 1121) for England and Wales and The Miscellaneous Additives in Food (Scotland) Regulations 1974 [SI 1974: No. 1338 (S. 116)].

Solid Carbon Dioxide, or 'dry ice', is obtainable commercially and is widely used in refrigeration; owing to its low thermal conductivity it is more stable than liquid carbon dioxide. A less compact form known as 'carbon dioxide snow' is formed as the compressed gas evaporates from a storage cyclinder. The carbon dioxide immediately freezes on issuing from the nozzle, and by collecting the 'snow' in a suitable receptacle it can be formed into a stick or crayon like an ordinary candle, or it may be compressed into a mould and cut to any shape with a knife. The cylinders used for this purpose are fitted with an internal tube. The 'snow' evaporates slowly—a crayon 12.5 cm by 2.5 cm will last about 1 to 2 hours. As many as 30 applications can be made with this size.

Solid carbon dioxide, which has a temperature of −80°, has a destructive action on tissues and is used to destroy warts and naevi by being applied with a light pressure for 5 to 6 seconds. The application is almost painless, but the solid should be shaped to suit the part to be treated. The surrounding tissue should be covered with soft paraffin. A wheal is afterwards formed, followed by a vesicle, but very little scarring occurs. If a second application is necessary, the inflammation from the first must be allowed to subside.

The use of solid carbon dioxide as an aerosol propellent.— L. W. Haase, *Mfg Chem.*, 1970, *41* (Feb.), 69.

Warts. References: K. D. Crow and O. L. S. Scott, *Lancet*, 1954, *2*, 312 and 660; M. H. Bunney, *Drugs*, 1977, *13*, 445.

5203-t

Helium *(B.P., U.S.P.)*.

He=4.0026.

CAS — 7440-59-7.

Pharmacopoeias. In *Br., Int.*, and *U.S.*

A colourless odourless tasteless gas which is not combustible and does not support combustion; it has a relative density not greater than 0.16. The *B.P.* specifies not less than 98% v/v of He and the *U.S.P.* not less than 99%. It is supplied in metal cylinders.

Soluble 1 in 72.5 of water by volume at normal temperature and pressure. **Store** under compression in metal cylinders.

In the UK cylinders of helium are painted brown; cylinders of oxygen and helium mixture are painted black with brown and white quarterings on neck and shoulder. The name or chemical symbol of the gas or gases should be stencilled in paint on the shoulder of the cylinder and clearly and indelibly stamped on the cylinder valve.

Uses. As helium is less dense than nitrogen the breathing of a mixture of 80% helium and 20% oxygen requires less effort than breathing air. Such mixtures have been used in patients with acute obstructions of the upper respiratory tract. Mixtures of helium and oxygen are used by divers or others working under high pressure to prevent the development of caisson disease; they are preferred to compressed air since they do not cause nitrogen narcosis.

Breathing helium speeds up the vocal pattern and increases vocal pitch.

Metabolism in hyperbaric helium atmospheres.— L. W. Raymond *et al.*, *J. appl. Physiol.*, 1968, *24*, 678.

Helium was considered to be about 8.5 times less narcotic than nitrogen when used together with oxygen by divers.— C. Edmonds and R. L. Thomas, *Med. J. Aust.*, 1972, *2*, 1416.

Contradictory comments on the value of helium-oxygen mixtures in inhalation therapy.— T. L. Petty, *J. Am. med. Ass.*, 1977, *238*, 1957; D. F. Egan, *ibid.*, 1958.

Helium and oxygen mixtures in decompression sickness.— C. H. Brookings and N. K. I. McIver (letter), *Lancet*, 1978, *2*, 468; P. B. James *et al.* (letter), *ibid.*, 469.

5204-x

Nitrogen *(U.S.N.F.)*. Nitrogenium; Azote.

N_2=28.0134.

CAS — 7727-37-9.

Pharmacopoeias. In *Aust., Cz., Fr., Hung., Jap., Jug., Nord.,* and *Swiss.* Also in *U.S.N.F.*

A colourless odourless tasteless gas which is non-inflammable and does not support combustion.

Soluble 1 in 65 of water by volume and 1 in 9 of alcohol by volume, at normal temperature and pressure. **Store** under compression in metal cylinders.

In the UK cylinders of nitrogen are painted grey with black neck and shoulder. The name of the gas or the chemical symbol 'N_2' should be stencilled in paint on the shoulder of the cylinder and clearly and indelibly stamped on the cylinder valve.

Adverse Effects. Nitrogen narcosis has been reported from nitrogen breathed at high pressure as in deep-water diving.

A report of onychodystrophies in 2 patients after liquid nitrogen therapy for verruca vulgaris.— C. M. Caravati *et al., Archs Derm.*, 1969, *100*, 441.

Syncope occurred in 2 patients during the application of liquid nitrogen for the removal of warts.— A. M. Epstein and J. L. Shupack (letter), *Archs Derm.*, 1977, *113*, 847.

A tingling sensation persisting for 2 days in the last 2 fingers of the hand followed the application of liquid nitrogen to a wart on the elbow of a 21-year-old man; numbness of the hand followed and ulnar neuropathy was apparent 6 months later.— P. F. Finelli, *Archs Derm.*, 1975, *111*, 1340.

Uses. Nitrogen is used as a diluent for pure oxygen or other active gases and as an inert gas to replace air in containers holding oxidisable substances. Liquid nitrogen is used as a cryotherapeutic agent for the removal of warts and malignant growths.

The use of nitrogen probes in cryosurgery in the treatment of second- and third-degree haemorrhoids.— K. L. Williams *et al., Br. med. J.*, 1973, *1*, 666.

Decompression therapy. Three divers with refractory decompression sickness requiring exposure to compressed air for durations leading to pulmonary oxygen toxicity were satisfactorily treated with nitrogen-oxygen. The use of nitrogen-oxygen mixtures with an inspired pO_2 of 0.5 bar or less allows a potentially indefinite duration of recompression at raised environmental pressure.— J. N. Miller *et al., Lancet*, 1978, *2*, 169. Criticisms.— C. H. Brookings and N. K. I. McIver (letter), *ibid.*, 468; P. B. James *et al.* (letter), *ibid.*, 469. Reply.— T. G. Shields and D. H. Elliott (letter), *ibid.*, 782. Further comment.— J. N. Miller and L. Fagraeus (letter), *ibid.*

Malignant neoplasms. References: A. A. Gage, *J. Am. med. Ass.*, 1968, *204*, 565; *J. Am. med. Ass.*, 1968, *205* (Aug. 26), A25; J. H. Beggs, *J. Am. med. Ass.*, 1968, *206*, 1570; R. C. Marcove and T. R. Miller, *J. Am. med. Ass.*, 1969, *207*, 1890.

Warts. A brief note on the use of liquid nitrogen in the treatment of warts.— M. H. Bunney, *Drugs*, 1977, *13*, 445.

5205-r

Refrigerants and Aerosol Propellents

A number of compressed and liquefied gases are used as refrigerants and as aerosol propellents; these include nitrogen, nitrous oxide, carbon dioxide, propane, and the butanes. Halogenated hydrocarbons, sometimes called fluorocarbons, were widely used but because of environmental hazards their use has been severely restricted; they are still used in pharmacy.

Reviews: A. E. M. Mclean, *Br. J. clin. Pharmac.*, 1977, *4*, 663; *Mfg Chem.*, 1979, *50* (April), 43.

The use of ethylene oxide mixed with an aerosol propellent (Freon) for the surface sterilisation of heat- and/or moisture-sensitive materials.— J. H. Robertson *et al., Bull. parent. Drug Ass.*, 1977, *31*, 265. See also S. B. Benyamin *et al., J. Pharm. Belg.*, 1976, *31*, 436.

Adverse Effects. The toxicity to humans of gases used as refrigerants and aerosol propellents appears to be slight if they are not abused. There may be some CNS depression; asphyxia may be the main problem. Direct inhalation of halogenated hydrocarbons by asthmatics receiving routine inhalational therapy is considered safe although abuse may cause cardiac arrhythmias.

A review of the toxicity in *animals* of 15 hydrocarbon propellents used in aerosols. Trichlorofluoromethane, dichlorofluoromethane, trichlorotrifluoroethane, and trichloroethane were classified as low-pressure propellents of high toxicity; dichlorotetrafluoroethane as a low-pressure propellent of intermediate toxicity; dichlorodifluoromethane as a high-pressure propellent of intermediate toxicity; and chloropentafluoroethane and difluoroethane as high-pressure propellents of low toxicity.— D. M. Aviado, *Toxicity of Propellants*, Progress in Drug Research Vol. 18, E. Jucker (Ed.), Basle, Birkhäuser Verlag, 1974, p. 365.

A comprehensive review of the toxicity of aerosols.— D. M. Aviado, *J. clin. Pharmac.*, 1975, *15*, 86. See also *Lancet*, 1975, *1*, 1073.

A review of the toxicology of halogenated hydrocarbons.— K. C. Back and E. W. Van Stee, *A. Rev. Pharmac. & Toxic.*, 1977, *17*, 83.

Skin sensitivity to trichlorofluoromethane, as shown by patch tests, in 3 patients, one of whom was also sensitive to dichlorodifluoromethane.— W. G. van Ketel, *Contact Dermatitis*, 1976, *2*, 115.

High concentrations of halogenated hydrocarbons in air may induce narcosis.— *Br. med. J.*, 1979, *2*, 322.

Abuse. Deaths following abuse of aerosols: M. Bass, *J. Am. med. Ass.*, 1970, *212*, 2075; *Pharm. J.*, 1973, *2*, 146. See also *ibid.*, 171; *Med. J. Aust.*, 1975, *2*, 202.

Effect on heart and lungs. A study involving 8 asthmatic patients using aerosols propelled by trichlorofluoromethane and dichlorodifluoromethane indicated that except with grossly excessive use of an aerosol inhaler in a short period of time, predicted myocardial concentrations of fluorocarbon in man were much less than the concentrations shown to sensitise the heart of conscious *dogs* to adrenaline.— C. T. Dollery *et al., Clin. Pharmac. Ther.*, 1974, *15*, 59.

Monochlorodifluoromethane aerosol, used by pathology students to accelerate the freezing of specimens for section, was associated with a 3.6 times greater risk of palpitations compared with similar workers not exposed to the propellent.— F. E. Speizer *et al., New Engl. J. Med.*, 1975, *292*, 624.

The death of a 4-year-old boy was believed to have been caused by his spraying the contents of an aerosol deodorant in his bath, thus displacing the air and leading to toxic fluorocarbon concentrations.— I. G. Jefferson (letter), *Lancet*, 1978, *1*, 779.

An increase in respiratory resistance occurred in 25 patients with asthma and 3 laryngectomised patients after aerosol propellents had been sprayed into the buccal or nasal cavity. It was suggested that this bronchoconstrictor reflex was elicited by the local low-temperature stimulus produced by the propellent.— D. Nolte *et al., Dt. med. Wschr.*, 1979, *104*, 172.

Comment on the surge in asthma fatalities that occurred in the 1960s and the growing realisation that pressurised aerosols were probably not the main culprit.— *Lancet*, 1979, *2*, 337.

Absorption and Fate. There appears to be little absorption following inhalation of aerosol propellents or refrigerants.

In 2 patients studied about 0.1% of a dose of radioactive dichlorodifluoromethane or of trichlorofluoromethane inhaled was metabolised and excreted as carbon dioxide; up to 0.1% was also found in the urine within 72 hours.— G. W. Mergner *et al., Anesthesiology*, 1975, *42*, 345.

Proprietary Refrigerants and Aerosol Propellents

Arcton Propellents *(ICI Mond, UK)*. A range of halogen derivatives of hydrocarbons used as aerosol propellents and refrigerants.

Arklone *(ICI Mond, UK)*. A brand of trichlorotrifluoroethane for dry-cleaning and industrial purposes.

Calor Aerosol Propellants *(Calor, UK)*. A range of propellents based upon low-boiling-point hydrocarbons, available in 5 grades.

Isceon Propellents *(ISC Chemicals, UK)*. A range of halogen derivatives of hydrocarbons used as aerosol propellents, refrigerants, and solvents.

PR Spray *(Boots, UK)*. A refrigerant skin spray containing dichlorodifluoromethane 15% and trichlorofluoromethane 85%.

Skefron *(Smith Kline & French, UK)*. A refrigerant skin spray, containing dichlorodifluoromethane 15% and trichlorofluoromethane 85%.

Other Proprietary Names

Austral.—Dermamist, Frezan, Forane; *Belg.*—Cryofluorane; *Canad.*—Freeze-O-Derm; *Fr.*—Cryofluorane, Flugene, Forane; *Ger.*—Frigen, Kaltron, Provotest; *Spain*—Forane; *USA*—Freon, Genetron, Isotron, Ucon.

NOTE. Forane is also a proprietary name for Isoflurane.

A preparation containing dichlorodifluoromethane and trichlorofluoromethane was also formerly marketed in Great Britain under the proprietary name Coolspray (*Bengué*).

5206-f

Dichlorodifluoromethane *(B.P., U.S.N.F.)*. Difluorodichloromethane; Propellent 12; Refrigerant 12.

CCl_2F_2=120.9.

CAS — 75-71-8.

Pharmacopoeias. In *Br.* Also in *U.S.N.F.*

A colourless non-inflammable gas with a faint ethereal odour which, when liquefied by compression, forms a clear colourless liquid. It is supplied compressed in metal containers. Wt per ml about 1.5 g at −35° and about 1.35 g at 15°. B.p. about −29.8°. In the liquid state it is practically **immiscible** with water but miscible with dehydrated alcohol. **Store** in a cool place free from materials of an inflammable nature, in suitable metal containers.

Dichlorodifluoromethane is used as a refrigerant and as an aerosol propellent, see above. A spray is used as a local anaesthetic, the intense cold produced by the rapid evaporation of the spray making the tissues insensitive.

Maximum permissible atmospheric concentration 1000 ppm.

Estimated acceptable daily intake up to 1.5 mg per kg body-weight.— Nineteenth Report of the Joint FAO/WHO Expert Committee on Food Additives, *Tech. Rep. Ser. Wld Hlth Org. No. 576*, 1975.

A placebo-controlled study of the bronchoconstriction induced in 9 healthy non-smokers following use of 6 hair sprays containing trichlorofluoromethane, dichlorodifluoromethane, alcohol, and perfume in varying proportions. It was considered that the alcohol content might contribute to the decreases in lung function.— E. Zuskin *et al.* (letter), *Lancet*, 1978, *2*, 1203.

Cryosurgery. The use of dichlorodifluoromethane for the removal of cataracts by cryosurgery.— D. M. Worthen and R. F. Brubaker, *Archs Ophthal.*, 1967, *78*, 451; J. M. Stewart *et al., Med. J. Aust.*, 1967, *2*, 643.

A report of the use of a halogenated hydrocarbon (monochlorodifluoromethane) for tonsillectomy by cryosurgery in 64 patients.— R. Rabkin, *Archs Otolar.*, 1968, *88*, 547.

Use in food. The use of dichlorodifluoromethane is permitted in frozen food under The Miscellaneous Additives in Food Regulations 1980 (SI 1980: No. 1834) for England and Wales and The Miscellaneous Additives in Food (Scotland) Regulations 1980 [SI 1980: No. 1889 (S.176)]. See also *Report on the Review of Solvents in Food*, FAC/REP/25, Ministry of Agriculture, Fisheries and Food, London, HM Stationery Office, 1978..

See also estimated acceptable daily intake, above.

5207-d

Dichlorotetrafluoroethane *(B.P., U.S.N.F.)*. Tetrafluorodichloroethane; Propellent 114; Refrigerant 114. 1,2-Dichloro-1,1,2,2-tetrafluoroethane.

$CClF_2.CClF_2$=170.9.

CAS — 76-14-2.

Pharmacopoeias. In *Br.* Also in *U.S.N.F.*

A colourless non-inflammable gas with a faint ethereal odour which, when liquefied by compression, forms a clear colourless liquid. It is supplied compressed in metal containers. Wt per ml about 1.63 g at −35° and about 1.49 g at 15°. B.p about 3.5°. In the liquid state it is practically **immiscible** with water, but miscible with dehydrated alcohol. **Store** in a cool place free from material of an inflammable nature, in suitable metal containers.

A refrigerant and aerosol propellent, see above.
Maximum permissible atmospheric concentration 1000 ppm.

5208-n

Trichlorofluoromethane *(B.P.)*. Fluorotrichloromethane; Trichloromonofluoromethane *(U.S.N.F.)*; Propellent 11; Refrigerant 11.
CCl_3F=137.4.

CAS — 75-69-4.

Pharmacopoeias. In *Br.* Also in *U.S.N.F.*

A clear, colourless, non-inflammable, volatile liquid with a faint ethereal odour. It is supplied compressed in metal containers. Wt per ml 1.61 g at −35° and about 1.5 g at 15°. B.p. about 23.7°. In the liquid state it is practically **immiscible** with water but miscible with dehydrated alcohol. **Store** in a cool place, free from materials of an inflammable nature, in suitable metal containers.

Stability. At low oxygen concentrations, trichlorofluoromethane reacted with alcohol to form acetaldehyde, hydrochloric acid, and dichlorofluoromethane. Higher oxygen concentrations depressed free radical chain reactions by formation of peroxides but promoted electrochemical corrosion. Nitromethane was an effective stabiliser. Trichlorofluoromethane also reacted with water or aqueous alcohol to form acids.— P. A. Sanders, *Soap chem. Spec.*, 1966, *42* (July), 74.

Methyl isocyanide was identified as the foul-smelling compound produced when trichlorofluoromethane stabilised with nitromethane was stored in iron or steel containers. Nitromethane was reduced to methylamine, and in the presence of oxygen and water methyl isocyanide was formed.— S. Temple and R. G. Hirsch, *du Pont de Nemours, USA, J. Soc. cosmet. Chem.*, 1977, *28*, 765.

A refrigerant and aerosol propellent, see above. Maximum permissible atmospheric concentration 1000 ppm.

Adverse effects. A deodorant aerosol containing a mixture of dichlorodifluoromethane and trichlorofluoromethane as propellent produced a hallucinogenic effect when deliberately abused, but one containing dichlorodifluoromethane alone did not.— R. A. Kramer and P. Pierpaoli, *Pediatrics*, 1971, *48*, 322.

In a comparative study of the cardiopulmonary toxicity of 9 propellents and halothane in *dogs*, the most toxic was trichlorofluoromethane, which depressed respiratory minute volume, reduced mean blood pressure, and accelerated heart-rate. Trichlorofluoromethane was one of the most widely used aerosol propellents.— M. A. Belej and D. M. Aviado, *J. clin. Pharmac.*, 1975, *15*, 105.

Distribution. Fluorocarbons, especially the less volatile trichlorofluoromethane, occurred in the arterial and venous blood in peak concentrations of 1.7 µg per ml after the use of inhalers. Volunteers who inhaled 1 dose every 10 minutes for 6 hours did not have a progressive rise in the blood concentration.— C. T. Dollery *et al.* (preliminary communication), *Lancet*, 1970, *2*, 1164.

Blood concentrations of trichlorofluoromethane reached 0.13 to 2.6 µg per ml after 2 inhalations of an aerosol in 9 asthmatics and controls. The half-life in blood was 0.3 to 1.5 minutes. These concentrations were not considered to be high enough to sensitise the heart to adrenergic compounds.— J. W. Paterson *et al.*, *Lancet*, 1971, *2*, 565.

Papaverine and some other Smooth Muscle Relaxants

5220-x

This section includes a miscellaneous group of compounds used as antispasmodics in a variety of conditions affecting the vascular system and the gastro-intestinal and genito-urinary tracts. Anticholinergic smooth muscle relaxants are described in the section on Atropine and other Anticholinergic Agents, p.289. Skeletal muscle relaxants are described in the section on Muscle Relaxants (see p.986). Vasodilators are described on p.1614.

5221-r

Papaverine *(B.P.C. 1949)*. 6,7-Dimethoxy-1-(3,4-dimethoxybenzyl)isoquinoline.

$C_{20}H_{21}NO_4$=339.4.

CAS — 58-74-2.

Pharmacopoeias. In *Ind.*

An alkaloid obtained from opium or prepared synthetically. Odourless tasteless crystals or white crystalline powder. Practically **insoluble** in water; sparingly soluble in alcohol and ether. **Store** in airtight containers. Protect from light.

5222-f

Papaverine Cromesilate. Papaverine 6,7-dihydroxycoumarin-4-methanesulphonate.

$C_{20}H_{21}NO_4,C_9H_6O_7S$=597.6.

CAS — 63817-84-5.

5223-d

Papaverine Hydrochloride *(B.P., Eur. P., U.S.P.)*. Papaver. Hydrochlor.; Papaverini Hydrochloridum; Papaverinii Chloridum; Papaverinium Chloride.

$C_{20}H_{21}NO_4,HCl$=375.9.

CAS — 61-25-6.

Pharmacopoeias. In all pharmacopoeias examined.

Odourless white or almost white crystals or crystalline powder with a slightly bitter taste. M.p. about 220° with decomposition.

Soluble 1 in 30 to 40 of water, 1 in 120 of alcohol, and 1 in 10 of chloroform; practically insoluble in ether. A 2% solution in water has a pH of 3 to 4.5. Solutions are **sterilised** by autoclaving or by filtration. **Incompatible** with bromides, iodine and iodides, alkalis, and tannins. Precipitation may occur when Papaverine Hydrochloride Injection is added to Lactated Ringer's Injection. **Store** in airtight containers. Protect from light.

Bioavailability. A review of the bioavailability of papaverine hydrochloride.— H. B. Kostenbauder *et al.*, *J. Am. pharm. Ass.*, 1977, *NS17*, 303.

Further references: M. C. Meyer *et al.*, *J. clin. Pharmac.*, 1979, *19*, 435.

Discoloration and stability in solutions. Papaverine hydrochloride injection which had changed from colourless to yellow on storage was found, by paper chromatography, to contain papaveraldine, papaverinol, and 8 unidentified compounds.— E. Pawelczyk and T. Hermann, *Dissnes pharm. Pharmac.*, 1966, *17*, 569, per *Pharm. J.*, 1974, *1*, 587.

Papaverine hydrochloride solutions, sterilised by autoclaving or filtration, developed a pale yellow colour on storage for a year at 25° or a month at 37°, but there was no loss of potency after 4 years at 25° or 18 months at 37°. The addition of 0.005% disodium edetate inhibited colour formation at pH 3 to 4 for at least 2 years, probably by the chelation of iron. Light and air increased discoloration.— D. E. Griffith, *J. pharm. Sci.*, 1967, *56*, 1197.

5224-n

Papaverine Sulphate *(B.P.C. 1963)*. Papaver. Sulph.

$(C_{20}H_{21}NO_4)_2,H_2SO_4,5H_2O$=866.9.

CAS — 32808-09-6 (anhydrous).

Pharmacopoeias. In *Nord.*

Odourless white crystals or white or almost white crystalline powder with a slightly bitter taste. **Soluble** 1 in 2 of water, 1 in 20 of alcohol, and 1 in 5000 of ether; slightly soluble in chloroform. A 2% solution in water has a pH of about 3. Solutions are **sterilised** by autoclaving or by filtration. **Store** in airtight containers. Protect from light.

Adverse Effects and Precautions. Side-effects of papaverine include gastro-intestinal disturbance, flushing of the face, headache, drowsiness, skin rash, sweating, and vertigo. Jaundice and eosinophilia occur and may be due to hypersensitivity. Papaverine should be used with caution intravenously since it can cause cardiac arrhythmias; a slow rate of injection is recommended. Intravenous injection is contra-indicated in patients with complete atrioventricular block. Papaverine should be used with caution in patients with glaucoma.

For a report of papaverine decreasing the effectiveness of levodopa, see Levodopa, p.885.

Liver dysfunction. Reports of hypersensitivity reactions.— V. Rønnov-Jessen and A. Tjernlund, *New Engl. J. Med.*, 1969, *281*, 1333; H. W. Kiaer *et al.*, *Archs Path.*, 1974, *98*, 292; G. B. Snider and S. A. Gogate, *Ohio St. med. J.*, 1978, *74*, 571.

Reversible hepatitis in a 62-year-old woman was associated with papaverine given for about 3 years.— R. Poupon *et al.*, *Gastroenterol. clin. biol.*, 1978, *2*, 305.

Six of 14 elderly patients receiving papaverine 600 mg daily developed biochemical evidence of altered hepatic function.— M. S. Pathy and A. J. Reynolds, *Postgrad. med. J.*, 1980, *56*, 488.

Absorption and Fate. Papaverine is readily absorbed when given by mouth. Its biological half-life is reported to be between one and two hours.

Most of a dose is metabolised in the liver and excreted in the urine, almost entirely as demethylated glucuronide-conjugated phenolic metabolites, mostly the 4′-hydroxypapaverine glucuronide.

Uses. Papaverine relaxes smooth muscle directly. It has been given to relieve ischaemia and is present in some cough preparations. However, there is little evidence to justify its clinical use.

Papaverine has usually been given as the hydrochloride in doses of up to 600 mg daily. Sustained-release preparations have been used. It has also been given by injection using the intra-arterial, intramuscular, or intravenous routes (but see Adverse Effects and Precautions). The cromesilate, hydrobromide, phenylglycolate, sulphate, and teprosilate have also been used.

In a double-blind study involving 57 elderly patients with mental impairment due, it was believed, to cerebral arteriosclerosis, those treated with papaverine hydrochloride 300 mg twice daily as a sustained-release preparation showed significantly greater improvement in many parameters than those treated with placebo; memory was not improved. Two patients experienced mild drowsiness and vertigo respectively.— R. M. Ritter *et al.*, *Clin. Med.*, 1971, *78* (Apr.), 18. See also L. M. McQuillan *et al.*, *Curr. ther. Res.*, 1974, *16*, 49.

Mean regional cerebral blood flow increased by 10.7% in 5 patients with cerebral ischaemia given papaverine 60 mg intravenously.— H. Herrschaft, *Arzneimittel-Forsch.*, 1976, *26*, 1240.

The use of papaverine infusions in the management of acute mesenteric ischaemia.— S. J. Boley *et al.*, *Curr. Probl. Surg.*, 1978, *15*, (Apr.), 12.

A review of the use of vasodilators, including papaverine, in the treatment of senile dementias.— J. A. Yesavage *et al.*, *Archs gen. Psychiat.*, 1979, *36*, 220.

Migraine. Papaverine 150 mg twice daily was given to 20 patients with migraine attacks occurring more than once a week and 18 reported freedom from attacks. None of the patients had previously been adequately controlled with other drugs.— C. M. Poser (letter), *Lancet*, 1974, *1*, 1290.

Further references: N. Vijayan, *Headache*, 1977, *17*, 159.

Psoriasis. In a double-blind study involving 45 patients with psoriasis significant improvement was obtained with papaverine cream 1%. The clinical potency appeared to be approximately equivalent to that of hydrocortisone cream 0.5 to 1%.— J. J. Voorhees *et al.*, *Clin. Pharmac. Ther.*, 1974, *16*, 919. The efficacy of papaverine for the topical treatment of psoriatic skin lesions could be due to its action as a potent inhibitor of phosphodiesterase; a threefold increase in cyclic adenosine phosphate phosphodiesterase activity had been reported in such lesions.— M. A. Stawiski *et al.*, *J. invest. Derm.*, 1975, *64*, 124, per B. Weiss and W. N. Hait, *A. Rev. Pharmac. & Toxic.*, 1977, *17*, 454.

Preparations of Papaverine Salts

Papaverine Hydrochloride Injection *(U.S.P.)*. A sterile solution in Water for Injections. pH not below 3.

Papaverine Hydrochloride Tablets *(U.S.P.)*. Tablets containing papaverine hydrochloride. The *U.S.P.* requires 80% dissolution in 30 minutes. Store in airtight containers.

Proprietary Names of Papaverine Hydrochloride

Artegodan *(Artesan, Ger.)*; Cerebid *(Saron, USA)*; Cerespan *(USV Pharmaceutical Corp., USA)*; Dilaspan *(Parkdale, USA)*; Dipav *(Lemmon, USA)*; Dylate *(Elder, USA)*; Kavrin *(Hyrex, USA)*; Myobid *(Laser, USA)*; P-200 *(Boots, USA)*; Pameion *(Simes, Ital.)*; Panergon *(Mack, Illert., Ger.*; *Mack, Switz.)*; Papaverlumin Fuerte *(Pidefé, Spain)*; Pavabid *(Marion Laboratories, USA)*; Pava-2 Caps *(General Pharm. Prods, USA)*; Pavacap *(Reid-Provident, USA)*; Pavacen *(Central Pharmacal, USA)*; Pavakey *(Key, USA)*; Pavased *(Mallard, USA)*; Pavatran *(Mayrand, USA)*; Pava-Wol *(Wolins, USA)*; Paveron *(Karlspharma, Ger.)*; Pavine TD *(Lexalabs, USA)*; Qua-Bid *(Quaker, USA)*; Sustaverine *(ICN, USA)*; Therapav *(Berlex, USA)*; Vasal *(Tutag, USA)*; Vasocap *(Keene, USA)*; Vaso-Pav *(UAD, USA)*; Vasospan *(Ulmer, USA)*.

Proprietary Names of Other Papaverine Salts

Albatran (codecarboxylase derivative) *(Beaufour, Fr.)*; Kaldil (teprosilate) *(Bruneau, Fr.)*; Maspaver (sulphate) *(Juste, Spain)*; Permavérine (cromesilate) *(Armstrong, Arg.*; *Robert et Carrière, Fr.)*.

5225-h

Alverine. Dipropyline; Phenpropamine. *N*-Ethyl-3,3′-diphenyldipropylamine.

$C_{20}H_{27}N$=281.4.

CAS — 150-59-4.

5226-m

Alverine Citrate.

$C_{20}H_{27}N,C_6H_8O_7$=473.6.

CAS — 5560-59-8.

A white to off-white powder with a sweet odour and a slightly bitter taste. M.p. 100° to 103°. Slightly **soluble** in water and chloroform; sparingly soluble in alcohol; very slightly soluble in ether. A 0.5% solution in water has a pH of 3.5 to 4.5. **Store** in airtight containers. Protect from light.

Adverse Effects. Hypotension, drowsiness, dizziness, weakness, headache, and dry mouth may occur. A feeling of inebriation has been reported following the intravenous administration of alverine.

Uses. Alverine is used as an antispasmodic in disorders of the gastro-intestinal and genito-urinary tracts. It is given by mouth as the citrate in doses of 60 to 120 mg (approximately equivalent to 40 to 80 mg of alverine), by suppository as alverine in doses of 80 mg, and by intramuscular or slow intravenous injection as the tartrate in doses equivalent to 40 mg of alverine.

Proprietary Preparations

Spasmonal *(Norgine, UK)*. Alverine citrate, available as tablets of 60 mg.

Other Proprietary Names

Profenil Faible *(Canad.)*; Spasmavérine (also as tartrate)*(Fr., Switz.)*.

5227-b

Ambucetamide. A 16. 2-Dibutylamino-2-(4-methoxyphenyl)acetamide.
$C_{17}H_{28}N_2O_2$=292.4.

CAS — 519-88-0.

Uses. Ambucetamide 100 mg has been given with paracetamol for the relief of dysmenorrhoea.

Proprietary Preparations

Femerital *(MCP Pharmaceuticals, UK)*. Scored tablets each containing ambucetamide 100 mg and paracetamol 250 mg. For primary dysmenorrhoea. *Dose.* 1 to 2 tablets thrice daily.

5228-v

Amprotropine Phosphate. 3-Diethylamino-2,2-dimethylpropyl (±)-tropate dihydrogen phosphate.
$C_{18}H_{29}NO_3,H_3PO_4$=405.4.

CAS — 148-32-3 (amprotropine); 134-53-2 (phosphate).

A white crystalline powder with a faint odour and a bitter taste. Freely **soluble** in water. **Incompatible** with alkalis.

Uses. Amprotropine phosphate, which has been reported to have a direct action on smooth muscle, has been used as an antispasmodic in doses of 50 to 100 mg three or four times daily.

5229-g

Bietamiverine Hydrochloride. Dietamiverine Dihydrochloride. 2-Diethylaminoethyl 2-phenyl-2-piperidinoacetate dihydrochloride.
$C_{19}H_{30}N_2O_2,2HCl$=391.4.

CAS — 479-81-2 (bietamiverine); 2691-46-5 (hydrochloride).

A white crystalline powder. M.p. 194° to 195°.

Uses. Bietamiverine hydrochloride has been used in the treatment of dysmenorrhoea and intestinal and urinary muscle spasms in doses of up to 300 mg daily.

Proprietary Names

Fine-Dol *(Isola-Ibi, Ital.)*; Novosparol *(Prophin, Ital.)*; Spasmisolvina *(Dessy, Ital.)*.

5230-f

Camylofin Hydrochloride. Acamylophenine Hydrochloride; Camylofin Dihydrochloride. Isopentyl 2-(2-diethylaminoethylamino)-2-phenylacetate dihydrochloride.
$C_{19}H_{32}N_2O_2,2HCl$=393.4.

CAS — 54-30-8 (camylofin); 5892-41-1 (hydrochloride).

Crystals. M.p. 172° to 178°. **Soluble** in water.

Uses. Camylofin hydrochloride is given as an antispasmodic in functional disorders of the gastro-intestinal tract in doses of 50 to 100 mg twice to thrice daily. It has also been used as camylofin bis(noramidopyrine mesylate).

Proprietary Names

Avacan *(Asta, Denm.; Asta, Ger.; Schering, Ital.; Asta, Neth.; Noristan, S.Afr.)*.

5231-d

Dimoxyline Phosphate. LO 8146; Dioxyline Phosphate. 1-(4-Ethoxy-3-methoxybenzyl)-6,7-dimethoxy-3-methylisoquinoline dihydrogen phosphate.
$C_{22}H_{25}NO_4,H_3PO_4$=465.4.

CAS — 147-27-3 (dimoxyline); 5667-46-9 (phosphate).

A white crystalline powder. M.p. about 198° with decomposition. **Soluble** 1 in 25 of water and 1 in 320 of alcohol.

Adverse Effects. Side-effects include nausea, vomiting, dizziness, sweating, flushing of the skin, sedation, and abdominal cramp.

Absorption and Fate. Dimoxyline phosphate is absorbed from the gastro-intestinal tract. It is reported to be metabolised in the liver and excreted via the kidneys.

Uses. Dimoxyline is a synthetic analogue of papaverine (see p.1059). It has been tried in conditions in which there is reflex spasm of blood vessels in limbs or lungs, and in other conditions involving spasm of smooth muscle. Doses of 100 to 400 mg of the phosphate have been given three or four times daily.

Proprietary Names

Paveril Phosphate *(Lilly, USA)*; Paverona *(Lilly, Ital.)*.

5232-n

Ethaverine Hydrochloride. 1-(3,4-Diethoxybenzyl)-6,7-diethoxyisoquinoline hydrochloride.
$C_{24}H_{29}NO_4,HCl$=432.0.

CAS — 486-47-5 (ethaverine); 985-13-7 (hydrochloride).

The tetraethoxy analogue of papaverine (see p.1059); ethaverine hydrochloride has been used similarly in doses of 100 or 200 mg thrice daily by mouth.

References.— W. J. Oswald and D. H. Baeder, *Sth. med. J.*, 1975, *68*, 1481; G. R. Asby *et al.*, *Curr. ther. Res.*, 1974, *16*, 1096.

Proprietary Names

Cardiostron *(Solco, Ger.)*; Cebral *(Kenwood, USA)*; Circubid *(Merchant, USA)*; Eta-Lent *(Roger, USA)*; Ethaquin *(Ascher, USA)*; Ethatab *(Glaxo, USA)*; Ethavex *(Econo Med, USA)*; Isovex *(Medics, USA)*; Laverin *(Lemmon, USA)*; Pavaspan *(Jamieson-McKames, USA)*; Plaquivérine *(Monal, Fr.)*.

5233-h

Flavoxate Hydrochloride.

DW 61; Rec 7-0040. 2-Piperidinoethyl 3-methyl-4-oxo-2-phenyl-4*H*-chromene-8-carboxylate hydrochloride.
$C_{24}H_{25}NO_4,HCl$=427.9.

CAS — 15301-69-6 (flavoxate); 3717-88-2 (hydrochloride).

Adverse Effects. Flavoxate hydrochloride causes adverse anticholinergic effects including increased intra-ocular pressure. There may be gastro-intestinal disturbances and hypersensitivity reactions. Other adverse effects include headache, sedation, vertigo, and confusion. Leucopenia has been reported rarely.

Precautions. Flavoxate hydrochloride should not generally be used in patients with obstructive conditions of the intestinal or urinary tracts. It should be used with care in patients with glaucoma.

Absorption and Fate. Flavoxate is absorbed from the gastro-intestinal tract. Part of the dose is metabolised, mainly to 3-methylflavone-8-carboxylic acid. There is some urinary excretion.

References: C. Benvenuti *et al.*, *Farmaco, Edn prat.*, 1977, *32*, 99; *Aust. J. Pharm.*, 1979, *60*, 400.

Uses. Flavoxate hydrochloride is an antispasmodic with some structural similarity to propantheline. It is used in the management of some disorders of the lower urinary tract in doses of 100 or 200 mg three or four times daily.

In 24 patients with bladder spasm associated with a variety of urological disorders, treatment (under double-blind conditions) with flavoxate 200 mg four times daily resulted in moderate improvement or complete relief of frequency in 15 of 21 patients, of urgency in 16 of 20 patients, of suprapubic pain in 11 of 19 patients, of dysuria in 9 of 16 patients, and of nocturia in 10 of 15 patients. Flavoxate appeared to be a little more effective than propantheline, 30 mg four times daily, given to 22 similar patients. Dryness of the mouth occurred in 1 patient given flavoxate, abdominal pains in one, and headache in one; 2 of these patients discontinued treatment.— D. V. Bradley and R. J. Cazort, *J. clin. Pharmac.*, 1970, *10*, 65.

A brief discussion of functional abnormalities of the bladder and appropriate drug therapy.— S. L. Stanton, *Br. med. J.*, 1978, *1*, 1607.

Further references: P. F. Kohler and P. A. Morales, *J. Urol.*, 1968, *100*, 729; *Med. Lett.*, 1971, *13*, 107; *Drug & Ther. Bull.*, 1972, *10*, 11; A. Cova and I. Setnikar, *Arzneimittel-Forsch.*, 1975, *25*, 1707; V. J. Gururaj *et al.*, *Clin. Med.*, 1975, *82*, (June), 25; E. Pedersen, *Urol. int.*, 1977, *32*, 202.

Proprietary Preparations

Urispas *(Syntex, UK)*. Flavoxate hydrochloride, available as tablets of 100 mg. (Also available as Urispas in *Austral., Neth., S.Afr., Switz., USA*).

Other Proprietary Names

Bradalone *(Jap.)*; Genurin *(Ital., Spain)*; Spasuret *(Ger.)*; Urispadol *(Denm.)*.

5234-m

Flopropione. Fluropropiofenone; Phloropropiophenone; RP 13907. 2′,4′,6′-Trihydroxypropiophenone.
$C_9H_{10}O_4$=182.2.

CAS — 2295-58-1.

Flopropione is reported to have antispasmodic properties and to be an antagonist of serotonin.

Proprietary Names

Labrodax *(Rhodia, Arg.; Specia, Belg.)*; Bilup, Compacsul, Cospanon, Cospuron, Ecapron, Ephtanon, Flopion, Floveton, Gallepronin, Gasstenon, Mirulevatin, Nichipanon, Padeskin, Pasmus, Pellegal, Sartiron, Spasmoril, Supanate, Toriphenon, Trytalon, Tuflit (all *Jap.*).

5235-b

Loperamide Hydrochloride *(U.S.P.)*.

R 18553. 4-(4-*p*-Chlorophenyl-4-hydroxypiperidino)-*NN*-dimethyl-2,2-diphenylbutyramide hydrochloride.
$C_{29}H_{33}ClN_2O_2,HCl$=513.5.

CAS — 53179-11-6 (loperamide); 34552-83-5 (hydrochloride).

Pharmacopoeias. In *U.S.*

A white or yellowish-white amorphous or micro-crystalline powder. M.p. about 225° with some decomposition. Slightly **soluble** in water and dilute acids; freely soluble in chloroform, isopropyl alcohol, and methyl alcohol.

Adverse Effects and Treatment. Abdominal pain and other gastro-intestinal disturbances, dry mouth, dizziness, and fatigue have occurred. Skin rash has also been reported. Depression of the CNS may be seen in overdosage, and naloxone (see p.1032) has been recommended in addition to gastric lavage in the management of poisoning.

Toxic megacolon developed in a patient with ulcerative colitis within 3 weeks of beginning treatment with loperamide.— J. W. Brown, *J. Am. med. Ass.*, 1979, *241*, 501.

Precautions. Loperamide is probably best avoided in the treatment of acute infective diarrhoea until more is known of its safety and efficacy (see Uses). It should not be used to treat young children.

Patients with inflammatory bowel disease receiving loperamide should be carefully observed for signs of toxic megacolon.

Absorption and Fate. Loperamide is incompletely absorbed from the gastro-intestinal tract. Its elimination half-life is reported to range from 7 to 15 hours. It is mainly excreted in the faeces.

Loperamide probably accumulates in the wall of the small intestine and is released extremely slowly.— M. Wüster and A. Herz, *Archs Pharmac.*, 1978, *301*, 187.

References to the pharmacokinetics of loperamide: J. Heykants *et al.*, *Arzneimittel-Forsch.*, 1974, *24*, 1649; M. Michiels *et al.*, *Life Sci.*, 1977, *21*, 451; H. S. Weintraub *et al.*, *Curr. ther. Res.*, 1977, *21*, 867; J. M. Killinger *et al.*, *J. clin. Pharmac.*, 1979, *19*, 211.

Uses. Loperamide inhibits peristalsis and is used in the treatment of some diarrhoeas. Studies remain to be done to show the value of loperamide in acute infective diarrhoea. It should not be used to treat young children.

Loperamide is also used in ileostomy management to control the volume of discharge.

The usual initial dose of loperamide hydrochloride is 4 mg, followed by 2 mg after each loose stool, up to a total of 16 mg daily.

Reviews of loperamide: *Med. Lett.*, 1977, *19*, 73; *Drug & Ther. Bull.*, 1977, *15*, 61; R. C. Heel *et al.*, *Drugs*, 1978, *15*, 33.

Diarrhoea. Loperamide has been reported to control acute and chronic diarrhoea and some of the studies have involved comparisons with diphenoxylate (H. Verhaegen *et al.*, *Arzneimittel-Forsch.*, 1974, *24*, 1657; J. Dom *et al.*, *ibid.*, 1660; W. Amery *et al.*, *Curr. ther. Res.*, 1975, *17*, 263; W. Pelemans and G. Vantrappen, *Gastroenterology*, 1976, *70*, 1030; P. Mainguet and R. Fiasse, *Gut*, 1977, *18*, 575; C.D. Shee and R.E. Pounder, *Br. med. J.*, 1980, *280*, 524). Following a report by B. Sandhu *et al.* (*Lancet*, 1979, *2*, 689) that loperamide might possess antisecretory properties, W.A.M. Cutting and W.C. Marshall (*Lancet*, 1979, *2*, 1022) pointed out that this property should not obscure the fact that rehydration was the most important therapy for acute diarrhoea. J. Heap of *Janssen* (*Lancet*, 1979, *2*, 1299) agreed with this although he did not agree with Cutting and Marshall's doubts about loperamide being recommended for the symptomatic control of acute and chronic diarrhoea of any aetiology especially in children. However, B. Sandhu *et al.* in further correspondence (*Lancet*, 1980, *1*, 483) stated that loperamide should not be used in acute infective diarrhoea in childhood since colonisation might be facilitated and prolonged. This use was also criticised by K.E. von Mühlendahl *et al.* (*Lancet*, 1980, *1*, 209); in addition they pointed to doubtful evidence of paralytic ileus occurring in 4 children given loperamide. The manufacturers in the UK agreed that the efficacy and safety of loperamide in acute infective diarrhoea had not been proved although clinical studies were under way. Subsequently 3 children were reported by H. Marcovitch (*Lancet*, 1980, *1*, 1413) to have suffered drowsiness, irritability, and unacceptable behaviour and personality changes within 3 to 5 days of starting treatment with loperamide.

Ileostomy. In a double-blind trial 20 patients with ileostomy were given, after a 3-day drug-free period, loperamide 4 mg twice daily for 4 days adjusted up to 12 mg daily for the next 3 days if needed, followed by placebo, or vice versa. Median faecal output was 645, 500, and 600 g daily respectively for the drug-free, loperamide, and placebo regimens. Loperamide was useful for controlling excessive ileostomy loss. Several patients noticed increased urine losses; one suffered pain due to increased faecal consistence.— G. N. Tytgat and K. Huibregtse, *Br. med. J.*, 1975, *2*, 667. See also G. N. Tytgat (letter), *ibid.*, 1975, *3*, 489; G. N. Tytgat *et al.*, *Am. J. dig. Dis.*, 1977, *22*, 669.

Preparations

Loperamide Hydrochloride Capsules *(U.S.P.)*. Capsules containing loperamide hydrochloride.

Imodium *(Janssen, UK)*. Loperamide hydrochloride, available as **Capsules** of 2 mg and as **Syrup** containing 1 mg in each 5 ml. (Also available as Imodium in *Aust., Austral., Belg., Canad., Denm., Fr., Ger., Ital., Neth., S.Afr., Switz., USA*).

A reminder that the essential consequence of acute diarrhoea is dehydration, and the fundamental treatment is rehydration.— W. A. M. Cutting and W. C. Marshall (letter), *Lancet*, 1979, *2*, 1022.

Other Proprietary Names

AMI-29, Blox *(both Ital.)*; Colifilm *(Arg.)*; Dissenten *(Ital.)*; Elcoman *(Arg.)*; Fortasec *(Spain)*; Lopemid *(Ital.)*; Regulane, Suprasec *(both Arg.)*.

5236-v

Mebeverine Hydrochloride. CSAG 144.

4-[Ethyl(4-methoxy-α-methylphenethyl)amino]-butyl veratrate hydrochloride.

$C_{25}H_{35}NO_5,HCl = 466.0$.

CAS — 3625-06-7 (mebeverine); 2753-45-9 (hydrochloride).

A white crystalline powder.

Uses. Mebeverine hydrochloride is given as an antispasmodic in gastro-intestinal disorders in doses of 135 mg thrice daily before meals.

References: A. M. Connell, *Br. med. J.*, 1965, *2*, 848; P. S. Gupta *et al.*, *Br. J. clin. Pract.*, 1972, *26*, 35; *ibid.*, 215; C. Tasman-Jones, *N.Z. med. J.*, 1973, *77*, 232.

Proprietary Preparations

Colofac *(Duphar, UK)*. Mebeverine hydrochloride, available as tablets of 135 mg. (Also available as Colofac in *Austral.*).

Other Proprietary Names

Duspatal *(Ger., Ital., Neth.)*; Duspatalin *(Belg., Denm., Fr., S.Afr., Spain, Switz.)*.

5237-g

Moxaverine Hydrochloride. Meteverinum Hydrochloride. 1-Benzyl-3-ethyl-6,7-dimethoxyisoquinoline hydrochloride.

$C_{20}H_{21}NO_2,HCl = 343.9$.

CAS — 10539-19-2 (moxaverine); 1163-37-7 (hydrochloride).

Crystals. M.p. 208° to 214° with decomposition. Very sparingly **soluble** in cold water; more soluble in hot water; soluble in hot alcohol.

Uses. Moxaverine hydrochloride has a similar structure to papaverine (see p.1059) and has been used as an antispasmodic and in vascular disorders. The base has also been used.

Mean regional cerebral blood flow increased by 13.5 and 11.8% in 5 and 10 patients with cerebral ischaemia given moxaverine 150 mg and 150 mg with procaine hydrochloride respectively by intravenous injection.— H. Herrschaft, *Arzneimittel-Forsch.*, 1976, *26*, 1240.

Proprietary Names

Eupaverin *(E. Merck, Ger.; E. Merck, Neth.; E. Merck, Swed.)*; Eupaverina *(Bracco, Ital.; Igoda, Spain)*; Kollateral-forte *(Permicutan, Ger.)*.

5238-q

Octamylamine Hydrochloride. Octisamyl Hydrochloride. *N*-Isopentyl-1,5-dimethylhexylamine hydrochloride.

$C_{13}H_{29}N,HCl = 235.8$.

CAS — 502-59-0 (octamylamine); 5964-56-7 (hydrochloride).

White crystals. M.p. 121°. **Soluble** in water, alcohol, and ether.

Uses. Octamylamine hydrochloride has actions similar to papaverine (see p.1059) and is used as an antispasmodic in a dose of 100 to 200 mg.

Proprietary Names

Octometine *(Veride, Belg.; Biosédra, Fr.)*.

5239-p

Phenetamine. UCB 1545; Phenecyclamine. 2-(α-Cyclohexylbenzyl)-*NNN′N′*-tetraethylpropane-1,3-diamine. Feclemine.

$C_{24}H_{42}N_2 = 358.6$.

CAS — 3590-16-7.

Phenetamine has been used as an antispasmodic in functional disorders of the uterus and colon.

Proprietary Names

Fenetamin *(also as embonate) (Isola-Ibi, Ital.)*.

5240-n

Pipoxolan Hydrochloride. 5,5-Diphenyl-2-(2-piperidinoethyl)-1,3-dioxolan-4-one hydrochloride.

$C_{22}H_{25}NO_3,HCl = 387.9$.

CAS — 23744-24-3 (pipoxolan); 18174-58-8 (hydrochloride).

A white odourless crystalline powder. **Soluble** in water.

Uses. Pipoxolan hydrochloride has been used as an antispasmodic agent in doses of 10 to 30 mg twice or thrice daily by mouth or by rectum.

Proprietary Names

Paraespas *(Ima, Arg.)*; Rocofin *(Alter, Spain)*; Rowapraxin *(Sanico, Belg.; Rowa-Wagner, Ger.; Rowa, S.Afr.)*.

5241-h

Pitofenone Hydrochloride. Methyl 2-[4-(2-piperidinoethoxy)benzoyl]benzoate hydrochloride.

$C_{22}H_{25}NO_4,HCl = 403.9$.

CAS — 54063-52-4 (pitofenone).

Uses. Pitofenone hydrochloride has been used as an antispasmodic in doses of up to 30 mg daily, by mouth, rectally, or by intramuscular or slow intravenous injection.

5242-m

Pramiverine Hydrochloride. HSP 2986. *N*-Isopropyl-4,4-diphenylcyclohexylamine hydrochloride.

$C_{21}H_{27}N,HCl = 329.9$.

CAS — 14334-40-8 (pramiverine); 14334-41-9 (hydrochloride).

Uses. Pramiverine hydrochloride has been used as an antispasmodic in functional disorders of the gastro-intestinal tract in doses of up to 8 mg daily by mouth. It has also been given rectally and by intramuscular or intravenous injection.

References: *Arzneimittel-Forsch.*, 1976, *26*, 686–752.

Proprietary Names

Raptalgin *(Merck, Arg.)*; Sistalgin *(Cascan, Ger.; Bracco, Ital.)*.

5243-b

Proxazole Citrate. AF-634; PZ-17105. *NN*-Diethyl-2-[3-(α-ethylbenzyl)-1,2,4-oxadiazol-5-yl]ethylamine dihydrogen citrate.

$C_{17}H_{25}N_3O,C_6H_8O_7 = 479.5$.

CAS — 5696-09-3 (proxazole); 132-35-4 (citrate).

Uses. Proxazole citrate has actions similar to papaverine (see p.1059). It has been given as an antispasmodic in doses of 100 to 200 mg thrice daily by mouth. It has also been given rectally and by intramuscular or intravenous injection.

Proxazole administered parenterally increased the regional cerebral blood flow in 23 patients with cerebrovascular disease.— W. -D. Heiss *et al.*, *Arzneimittel-Forsch.*, 1973, *23*, 772. No significant change in mean regional cerebral blood flow was observed in 10 patients with cerebral ischaemia given proxazole 40 mg intravenously.— H. Herrschaft, *Arzneimittel-Forsch.*, 1976, *26*, 1240.

In a controlled trial in 330 patients proxazole 400 mg daily for 30 days significantly reduced the psychic and neurological manifestations of cerebrovascular insufficiency compared with a control group.— G. Esposito and M. De Gregorio, *Arzneimittel-Forsch.*, 1974, *24*, 1692.

Proprietary Names

Recidol *(Lampugnani, Ital.)*; Solacil *(Finadiet, Arg.)*; Toness *(Angelini, Ital.; Alter, Spain)*.

5244-v

Racefemine Fumarate. 3697 CB. (±)-α-Methyl-*N*-(1-methyl-2-phenoxyethyl)phenethylamine hydrogen fumarate.
$C_{18}H_{23}NO,C_4H_4O_4$=385.5.

CAS — 22232-57-1 (racefemine); 1590-35-8 (fumarate).

Uses. Racefemine fumarate has been used as a uterine relaxant in doses of up to 200 mg daily, by mouth. The dextrorotatory isomer, dextrofemine, is used intravenously in doses of up to 50 mg.

Proprietary Names
Dysmalgine *(Clin-Comar-Byla, Fr.)*.

5245-g

Trimethyldiphenylpropylamine Hydrochloride. *N,N*,1-Trimethyl-3,3-diphenylpropylamine hydrochloride.
$C_{18}H_{23}N,HCl$=289.8.

CAS — 13957-55-6 (trimethyldiphenylpropylamine); 22173-83-7 (hydrochloride).

Trimethyldiphenylpropylamine hydrochloride has been used as an antispasmodic.

Proprietary Names
Recipavrin *(Recip, Swed.)*.

5246-q

Trospium Chloride. 3α-Benziloyloxynortropane-8-spiro-1′-pyrrolidinium chloride.
$C_{25}H_{30}ClNO_3$=428.0.

CAS — 10405-02-4.

Uses. Trospium chloride is used for the relief of spasm of smooth muscle, chiefly of the gastro-intestinal and genital tracts. It is given in doses of 2 to 4 mg thrice daily, and 200 micrograms by intramuscular or slow intravenous injection as a single dose. It is also used as suppositories.

Proprietary Names
Spasmex *(Pfleger, Ger.)*.

Paraffins and similar Bases

6400-s

This section includes a number of substances used mainly as bases for the preparation of creams, emulsions, ointments, and suppositories. They are used either as inert carriers for drugs or for their various emulsifying and emollient properties. Some are also used to improve the texture, stability or water repellent properties of the final preparation. Other substances used in the preparation of bases can be found in the sections on Cetomacrogol and Nonionic Surfactants p.370, Glycerol, Glycols and Macrogols p.706, and Soaps and other Anionic Surfactants p.1439.

For a survey of formulation requirements for topical preparations, including ointments and emulsion bases, see R. L. Goldemburg, *Drug Devel. Comm.*, 1976, *2*, 43.

6401-w

Hard Paraffin *(B.P.)*. Paraffinum Durum; Paraff. Dur.; Paraffin *(U.S.N.F.)*; Paraffin Wax; Paraffinum Solidum; Hartparaffin.

CAS — 8002-74-2.

NOTE. Paraffinum Solidum (*Jug. P.*, *Span. P.*, and *Swiss P.*) is ceresin.

Pharmacopoeias. In *Aust.*, *Belg.*, *Br.*, *Chin.*, *Ger.*, *Hung.*, *Ind.*, *It.*, *Jap.*, *Neth.*, *Nord.*, *Pol.*, and *Port.* Also in *U.S.N.F.* Various melting-points are specified.

A mixture of solid hydrocarbons consisting mainly of *n*-paraffins and, to a lesser extent, of their isomers, obtained by distillation from petroleum or from the oil produced in the destructive distillation of shale.

It is a colourless or white, odourless, tasteless, translucent, wax-like solid, frequently showing a crystalline structure, and is slightly greasy to the touch. The *B.P.* specifies m.p. 50° to 57°; the *U.S.N.F.* specifies 47° to 65°. When melted, the liquid is free from fluorescence by daylight. It burns with a luminous flame and is characterised by its stability to most chemical reagents. Hard paraffins of other melting-points are available.

Practically **insoluble** in water and alcohol; soluble in chloroform, ether, light petroleum, volatile oils, and most warm fixed oils; freely soluble in carbon disulphide; practically insoluble in acetone. An alcoholic extract is neutral to litmus. It is **sterilised** by maintaining at 150° for 1 hour. **Store** at a temperature not exceeding 40°. Protect from light.

Adverse Effects. Injection of paraffins into tissues may cause a granulomatous reaction which may be considerably delayed in onset.

Maximum permissible atmospheric concentration of paraffin wax fumes 2 mg per m^3.

Uses. Hard paraffin is employed principally as a stiffening ingredient in ointment bases.

A variety of hard paraffin with a melting-point of 43° to 46° is employed in physiotherapy for the relief of pain in inflamed joints and sprains. For this purpose it is used in the form of paraffin-wax baths, the limb being repeatedly immersed in the melted wax until 5 or 6 coats of wax have been applied. The part is then wrapped in jaconet and cotton wool for about half an hour and then the wax peeled off, leaving an erythema of the skin. When the affected part cannot be immersed in the wax, several coats of wax may be applied by means of a brush or spray.

The lower-melting hard paraffin was formerly used in plastic surgery, but granulomatous reactions have occurred following its injection into tissues.

Preparations

Paraffin No. 7. Mix hard paraffin 67, soft paraffin 25, and olive oil 5, and add resorcinol 1 (dissolved in alcohol) and eucalyptus oil 2. Formerly used as a protective covering for burns and wounds; it has a m.p. of about 48°.

Proprietary Preparations of Similar Waxes

Glokem *(ABM Chemicals, UK)*. A range of diamide (D series) or ester amide (E series) waxes based chiefly on long-chain alkyl acids. For use in the preparation of ointment bases and to raise the softening-point of ointment bases in tropical conditions.

6402-e

Liquid Paraffin *(B.P., B.P. Vet.)*. Liquid Petrolatum; Mineral Oil *(U.S.P.)*; Heavy Liquid Petrolatum; White Mineral Oil; Oleum Petrolei; Oleum Vaselini; Paraffinum Liquidum; Paraffinum Subliquidum; Vaselinum Liquidum; Huile de Vaseline Épaisse; Dickflüssiges Paraffin; Vaselinöl.

CAS — 8012-95-1.

Pharmacopoeias. In all pharmacopoeias examined except *Eur.* and *Int.* Various viscosities and specific gravities are specified. See also Light Liquid Paraffin.

Liquid paraffin is a mixture of liquid hydrocarbons, varying in composition according to the source of the petroleum from which it is obtained; the *B.P.* permits up to 10 ppm of tocopherol or butylated hydroxytoluene as a stabiliser; the *U.S.P.* permits a suitable stabiliser.

It is a transparent, colourless, almost odourless and tasteless, oily liquid, free from fluorescence by daylight. The *B.P.* specifies wt per ml 0.83 to 0.89 g and kinematic viscosity at 37.8° not less than 64 centistokes. The *U.S.P.* specifies specific gravity 0.845 to 0.905 and kinematic viscosity at 40° not less than 34.5 centistokes.

Practically **insoluble** in water and alcohol; soluble in acetone, chloroform, and ether; miscible with carbon disulphide, light petroleum, fixed oils (except castor oil), and volatile oils. It is **sterilised** by maintaining at 150° for 1 hour. **Store** in airtight containers. Protect from light.

NOTE. In *B.P. 1968* and earlier editions the specified wt per ml was 0.87 to 0.89 g and a lighter grade was described as light liquid paraffin (see p.1064).

Effect of gamma-irradiation. Liquid paraffin, in completely-filled soft plastic tubes, showed bubbles of gas after irradiation, the bubbles being larger at the higher level of irradiation (250 000 Gy). The iodine value was increased after irradiation at both high and low (25 000 Gy) levels of irradiation.— *The Use of Gamma Radiation Sources for the Sterilisation of Pharmaceutical Products*, London, ABPI, 1960.

Mineral Hydrocarbons in Food. The Mineral Hydrocarbons in Food Regulations, 1966, and The Mineral Hydrocarbons in Food (Scotland) Regulations, 1966, prohibit, subject to certain exemptions, the use in Great Britain of any mineral hydrocarbon in the composition or preparation of food. The exemptions are dried fruit (0.5%), citrus fruit (0.1%), sugar confectionery (0.2%), any chewing compound (60% of solid mineral hydrocarbon), the rind of any whole pressed cheese, and eggs through dipping or spraying for preserving; in all these exemptions the mineral hydrocarbons permitted must comply with specifications laid down in a schedule to the Regulations.

Adverse Effects. Excessive dosage may result in anal seepage and irritation. Liquid paraffin is absorbed to a slight extent, especially if emulsified, and may give rise to granulomatous reactions. Similar reactions follow the injection of liquid paraffin and may be considerably delayed in onset. Lipoid pneumonia has been reported following the use of liquid paraffin nasal drops or spray solutions or following inhalation of oil taken by mouth.

Prolonged use should be avoided.

The carcinogenic action of mineral oils; a chemical and biological study.— *Report of the MRC Carcinogenic Action of Mineral Oils Committee, Special Report Series No. 306*, London, HM Stationery Office, 1968.

For reports of chronic toxicity from mineral oils in industry, see W. J. Lloyd (letter), *Br. med. J.*, 1968, *4*, 830; M. Sutton (letter), *ibid.*, 1969, *1*, 116; *ibid.*, 1973, *3*, 44.

For background toxicological information on food grade mineral oil, see *Fd Add. Ser. Wld Hlth Org. No. 5*, 1974.

Granuloma. Subcutaneous paraffinomas occurred in the scalp, neck and scrotum of a patient following the dubious practice of injecting liquid paraffin into these sites for pain relief. This led to soft tissue infection and osteomyelitis 28 years later. Marked calcification was seen in radiographs after 35 years.— E. L. Lame *et al.*, *Milit. Med.*, 1974, *139*, 818.

A 49-year-old Asian woman developed paraffinoma of the face with painful swelling and redness of the skin 7 months after receiving injections of liquid paraffin in both cheeks and around the eyes for cosmetic purposes. Although her condition improved after surgery and maintenance on prednisone, surgical removal of all affected tissue appeared to be the only effective treatment for this condition.— J. J. Bloem and I. van der Waal, *Oral Surg.*, 1974, *38*, 675.

Florid chronic inflammatory local reactions with cyst formation and calcification occurred in one patient more than 60 years after intramammary injection of liquid paraffin.— C. Thiels and K. Dumke, *Fortschr. Röntgenstr.*, 1977, *126*, 173.

Lipoid pneumonia. Lipoid pneumonia with lipoid granulomata occurred in a 75-year-old man who had applied a mentholated petroleum preparation intranasally daily for 12 years.— B. Varkey and A. V. P. Kutty (letter), *Ann. intern. Med.*, 1976, *84*, 176. See also *New Engl. J. Med.*, 1977, *296*, 1105.

Skin reaction. In investigating an irritant reaction to a cosmetic preparation, a mineral oil produced no effect when applied alone, but did so when used in conjunction with sodium alkyl sulphate. No further irritant reactions occurred when the mineral oil was changed.— M. M. Rieger and G. W. Battista, *J. Soc. cosmet. Chem.*, 1964, *15*, 161.

Precautions. Prolonged ingestion of liquid paraffin may interfere with the absorption of fat-soluble vitamins and should be avoided. It should not be used when abdominal pain, nausea, or vomiting is present.

Absorption and Fate. Liquid paraffin may be absorbed to a slight extent from the gastro-intestinal tract, especially if emulsified.

Uses. Taken internally, liquid paraffin acts as a lubricant and, since it keeps the stools soft, it has been widely employed in chronic constipation, especially in the presence of haemorrhoids or other painful conditions of the anus and rectum. For this purpose, 10 to 30 ml has been given daily, either in divided doses or at bedtime.

Externally, liquid paraffin may be used as an ingredient of ointment bases, as an emollient to the skin in irritant conditions, and to remove crusts. Sterilised liquid paraffin is used as an aseptic dressing and as a lubricant for catheters and surgical instruments.

For a range of cosmetic formulations incorporating liquid paraffin, including hair creams and hand cleansers, see G. A. Parnassum, *Soap Perfum. Cosm.*, 1968, *41*, 35 and 97.

Sterile liquid paraffin was introduced into the bladders of 20 patients to replace a similar volume of infected residual urine which could not be voided, so that as the supernatant layer it would be expelled last. Patients returned periodically for replacement of retained urine. There was a reduction in infections and symptoms in about 50% of the patients.— J. E. Dees, *J. Urol.*, 1970, *103*, 152.

Peritonitis due to talc or starch was relieved in 50% of *animals* given liquid paraffin by intraperitoneal infusion within 72 hours of the powder. Symptoms subsided in 1 patient with peritonitis due to starch who was given 25 ml of sterile liquid paraffin intraperitoneally.— L. Katsilabros (letter), *Lancet*, 1973, *1*, 397. Paraffinomas were a hazard to the use of paraffin in the peritoneum.— J. S. Campbell and I. W. D. Henderson (letter), *ibid.*, 775; I. Penn (letter), *ibid.*, 776.

Preparations

Emulsions

Liquid Paraffin and Magnesium Hydroxide Emulsion *(B.P.)*. Emuls. Paraff. Liq. et Mag. Hydrox.; Liquid Paraffin and Magnesium Hydroxide Mixture; Mixture of Magnesium Hydroxide and Liquid Paraffin; Mist. Mag. Hydrox. et Paraff. Liq. Liquid paraffin 2.5 ml, chloroform spirit 0.15 ml, and magnesium hydroxide mixture 7.35 ml. Store at a temperature not exceeding 20° and avoid freezing. *Dose.* 5 to 20 ml.

Liquid Paraffin and Phenolphthalein Emulsion *(B.P.)*. Liquid Paraffin and Phenolphthalein Mixture; Compound Liquid Paraffin Emulsion. Phenolphthalein, micro-crystalline, 30 mg, liquid paraffin emulsion to 10 ml. Store at a temperature not exceeding 20° and avoid freezing.

A.P.F. has phenolphthalein 30 mg, liquid paraffin emulsion (*A.P.F.*) to 10 ml. Dose 5 to 20 ml.

Liquid Paraffin Emulsion *(A.P.F.)*. Emuls. Paraff. Liq. Liquid paraffin 50 ml, acacia 12.5 g, saccharin sodium 5 mg, benzoic acid solution 2.5 ml, vanillin 50 mg, chloroform 0.25 ml, water to 100 ml. Suitable alternative emulsifying agents may replace the acacia. *Dose.* 10 to 30 ml.

Liquid Paraffin Emulsion *(B.P.)*. Liquid Paraffin Mixture; Emulsio Paraffini Liquidi; Emuls. Paraff. Liq. Liquid paraffin 5 ml, methylcellulose '20' 200 mg, chloroform 0.025 ml, benzoic acid solution 0.2 ml, vanillin 5 mg, saccharin sodium 500 µg, water to 10 ml. Mix the methylcellulose with 1.2 ml of boiling water and, when the powder is thoroughly hydrated add sufficient water in the form of ice to produce 3.5 ml, and stir until homogeneous; add the other ingredients (except the liquid paraffin), the saccharin sodium being first dissolved in water, adjust to 5 ml with water, and mix; add the liquid paraffin with constant stirring and pass through a homogeniser. Store at a temperature not exceeding 20° and avoid freezing. *Dose.* 10 to 30 ml.

NOTE. Incompatibilities, due to the 'salting-out' of the methylcellulose, may occur if this preparation is dispensed with electrolytes, such as magnesium sulphate, in moderately high concentrations.

Liquid Paraffin Emulsion *(B.P. 1958, Ind. P.)*. Liquid paraffin 5 ml, acacia 1.25 g, tragacanth 50 mg, glycerol 1.25 ml, sodium benzoate 50 mg, vanillin 5 mg, chloroform 0.025 ml, water to 10 ml. *Dose.* 8 to 30 ml.

Liquid Paraffin Emulsion with Magnesium Sulphate. Difficulty encountered in dispensing a stable mixture containing magnesium sulphate and liquid paraffin emulsion could be overcome by using liquid paraffin emulsion *B.P. 1958*, which contained acacia and tragacanth, in place of methylcellulose.—G. Smith and J.A. Yacomeni, *Pharm. J.*, 1966, *1*, 447.

Liquid Paraffin Emulsion with Cascara *(B.P.C. 1973)*. Liquid Paraffin and Cascara Mixture. Cascara elixir 0.625 ml, liquid paraffin emulsion to 10 ml. *Dose.* 10 to 30 ml.

A.P.F. has the same formula with liquid paraffin emulsion (*A.P.F.*).

Mineral Oil Emulsion *(U.S.P.)*. Liquid paraffin 50 ml, acacia 12.5 g, syrup 10 ml, vanillin 4 mg, alcohol 6 ml, water to 100 ml. The vanillin may be replaced by not more than 1% of other official flavouring substances; sweet orange-peel tincture 6 ml or benzoic acid 200 mg may replace the alcohol as a preservative. Store in airtight containers.

Enemas

Mineral Oil Enema *(U.S.P.)*. Consists of liquid paraffin.

Lotions

Massage Lotion *(Hadassah Univ. Hosp.)*. Liquid paraffin 5 g, white soft paraffin 12.6 g, emulsifying wax 3.15 g, alcohol (95%) 25 ml, lavender oil 0.1 ml, water to 100 g. Used for bedsores.

Ointments

Ointment Basis. Dissolve, with the aid of heat, Polythene (mol. wt 21 000) 5 g in liquid paraffin 95 g and cool the solution at 10° per second from just above its cloud point to just below its gel point. A soft ointment basis was formed which varied little in consistency over the temperature range −15° to +60°. A proprietary preparation of similar composition was available in USA under the name Plastibase (*Squibb*).— M.N. Mutimer *et al.*, *J. Am. pharm. Ass., scient. Edn*, 1956, *45*, 101.

Proprietary Preparations

Agarol *(Warner, UK)*. An emulsion containing liquid paraffin 31.9% and phenolphthalein 1.32% with agar 0.2%. *Dose.* 5 to 15 ml, according to age, at night, and repeated 2 hours after breakfast if necessary.

Oilatum Emollient *(Stiefel, UK)*. Contains liquid paraffin 63.7% and acetylated wool alcohols 5%. For ichthyosis and related dry skin conditions.

Petrolagar Emulsion (Blue Label) *(Wyeth, UK)*. Contains liquid paraffin 7% and light liquid paraffin 18%. **(Red Label)** contains, in addition, phenolphthalein 0.35%. *Dose.* 10 ml night and morning.

Other Proprietary Names

Fr.—Lansoÿl, Nujol, Parlax; *Ger.*—Granugenol, Obstinol mild, Sanato-Lax; *Ital.*—Granugenolo; *Spain*—Ventricol.

6403-l

Light Liquid Paraffin. Paraffinum Liquidum Leve; Paraff. Liq. Lev.; Light Liquid Petrolatum; Light Mineral Oil *(U.S.P.)*; Light White Mineral Oil; Spray Paraffin; Paraffinum Liquidum Tenue; Paraffinum Perliquidum; Huile de Vaseline Fluide; Dünnflüssiges Paraffin; Vaselina Liquida.

NOTE. The name Parolein has been applied to light liquid paraffin, particularly when used as eye-drops.

Pharmacopoeias. In *Arg., Fr., Ger., Ind., Jap., Neth., Port., Span., Swiss,* and *U.S.*

A variety of liquid paraffin of specific gravity 0.818 to 0.880 and lower kinematic viscosity (not greater than 33.5 centistokes at 40°) than the oil for internal administration. **Store** in airtight containers. Protect from light.

Adverse Effects and Precautions. As for Liquid Paraffin, p.1063.

Uses. Light liquid paraffin has been used to cleanse dry and inflamed skin and to facilitate the removal of dermatological preparations. It was formerly used as a vehicle for nasal spray solutions but its use for this purpose is not recommended since it inhibits ciliary action and may also give rise to lipoid pneumonia.

Proprietary Preparations

Astrolene *(Astor, UK)*. A range of light liquid paraffins of kinematic viscosity 4 to 18 cS at 37.8°.

Other Proprietary Names

Salus-öl *(Ger.)*.

6404-y

White Soft Paraffin *(B.P.)*.

Paraffinum Molle Album; Paraff. Moll. Alb.; White Petrolatum *(U.S.P.)*; White Petroleum Jelly; Vaseline Officinale.

Pharmacopoeias. In all pharmacopoeias examined except *Braz., Eur., Fr., Int.,* and *Rus. Chin. P.* does not differentiate between white and yellow soft paraffin. Many pharmacopoeias use the title Vaselinum Album; in Great Britain the name 'Vaseline' is a trade-mark.

White soft paraffin is bleached yellow soft paraffin.

Protect from light.

A study of the rheological variation between 6 grades of white soft paraffin *B.P.*— B. W. Barry and A. J. Grace, *J. Pharm. Pharmac.*, 1970, *22*, *Suppl.*, 147S.

6405-j

Yellow Soft Paraffin *(B.P.)*.

Paraffinum Molle Flavum; Paraff. Moll. Flav.; Petrolatum *(U.S.P.)*; Petroleum Jelly; Yellow Petrolatum; Yellow Petroleum Jelly.

Pharmacopoeias. In *Aust., Br., Chin., Cz., Hung., Ind., Jap., Jug., Mex., Neth., Nord., Pol., Swiss,* and *U.S.*
U.S. permits a suitable stabiliser. *Chin. P.* does not differentiate between white and yellow soft paraffin. Many pharmacopoeias use the title Vaselinum Flavum; in Great Britain the name 'Vaseline' is a trade-mark.

A purified semi-solid mixture of hydrocarbons obtained from petroleum. It is a pale yellow to light amber-coloured, translucent, soft, unctuous mass, not more than slightly fluorescent by daylight even when melted, odourless when rubbed on the skin, and almost tasteless. The *B.P.* specifies m.p. 38° to 56°. The *U.S.P.* specifies 38° to 60°.

Practically **insoluble** in water, alcohol, and acetone; soluble in carbon disulphide, chloroform, ether, light petroleum, and most fixed and volatile oils, the solutions sometimes showing a slight opalescence. An alcoholic extract is neutral to litmus. It is **sterilised** by maintaining at 150° for 1 hour.

Effect of gamma-irradiation. Tin tubes completely filled with white soft paraffin became distended and the fold partially unrolled after irradiation (25 000 Gy). Two of 3 tubes only about 80% filled were unchanged, but the third was distended. Irradiation at a higher level (250 000 Gy) burst open tubes which were completely filled and partially unrolled those incompletely filled. Soft plastic tubes filled so as not to leave an air space showed no apparent change after irradiation.— *The Use of Gamma Radiation Sources for the Sterilisation of Pharmaceutical Products*, London, ABPI, 1960.

Adverse Effects. As for Hard Paraffin, p.1063.

Bilateral granulomas of the breasts in a young woman resulted from multiple injections of warm molten soft paraffin into each breast to increase their size. The granulomas were successfully removed by surgery.— R. B. Crosbie and H. D. Kaufman, *Br. med. J.*, 1967, *3*, 840.

Myospherulosis. Myospherulotic lesions, which appeared to be composed of shrunken distorted erythrocytes, were associated with the packing of cavities, following ENT surgery, with soft paraffin-based ointments containing tetracyclines.— *Lancet*, 1978, *2*, 358.

Uses. Soft paraffin is not readily absorbed by the skin. It is used as an emollient and protective ointment basis for surface action. Sterilised dressings containing yellow soft paraffin or its preparations are often used for wound dressings as they are easily removed. Crude yellow soft paraffin is also used as a sunscreening agent.

Observations of the nature, structure, and properties of soft paraffins.— P. Mannheim, *Soap Perfum. Cosm.*, 1966, *39*, 313. See also A. J. Franks, *ibid.*, 316.

In 14 experiments, white soft paraffin completely suppressed transepidermal water loss in 9, and partially suppressed it in 5. When 5% propylene glycol was added, suppression was complete in 3 of 5 experiments and partial in 1; no suppression was demonstrated in 1 experiment.— *Chemist Drugg.*, 1968, *190*, 534.

The use of soft paraffin as a moisturiser in cosmetics.— F. Tranner, *Cosmet. Toilet.*, 1978, *93*, (Mar.), 81.

Ointment bases. Paraffin Ointment, Simple Ointment, and Wool Alcohols Ointment as ointment bases which were largely composed of paraffins were criticised on the following grounds: (a) they did not rub into the skin, (b) they were unpleasant to use and easily rubbed on to clothing, (c) they tended to reduce the action of active ingredients, and (d) they created an unpleasant feeling of warmth. It was stated that the bases could be improved by the inclusion of 15 to 20% of fatty acid esters such as isopropyl myristate or of acetoglycerides in place of an equivalent amount of soft paraffin.— G. M. Howard, *Perfum. essent. Oil Rec.*, 1960, *51*, 613.

Preparations

Paraffin Gauze Dressing *(B.P.)*. Tulle Gras Dressing. A cotton, cotton and viscose, or viscose gauze, impregnated with yellow or white soft paraffin, sealed in suitable containers, and sterilised by a suitable sterilisation process. The degree of loading with paraffins may be 'light' or 'normal'. The soft paraffin may be replaced by a mixture of soft paraffin and hard paraffin when the dressing is required for use in tropical countries.

It is used in the treatment of wounds, such as burns and scalds, and for skin grafts.

Petrolatum Gauze *(U.S.P.)*. Sterilised absorbent cotton or cotton and viscose gauze saturated with sterilised white soft paraffin; it contains 70 to 80% by weight of soft paraffin.

Eye Ointments

Simple Eye Ointment *(B.P.)*. Eye Ointment Basis; Eye Ointment Base *(A.P.F.)*; Oculentum Base. Liquid paraffin 10, wool fat 10, yellow soft paraffin 80. Sterilised by maintaining at 150° for 1 hour; *A.P.F.* specifies 150° to 160° for not less than 2 hours.

In *B.P.C. 1973* eye ointments intended for use in tropical or subtropical climates the proportion of paraffins may be varied or hard paraffin may be included when prevailing high temperatures would otherwise make the ointment too soft.

The *B.P.C. 1973* states that when Non-medicated Eye Ointment is ordered or prescribed, this ointment is supplied.

Nord. P. (Oculentum Simplex) has liquid paraffin 20 and yellow soft paraffin 80, sterilised by maintaining at 140° for 3 hours.

Ointments

Hydrophilic Ointment *(U.S.P.)*. White soft paraffin 25 g, stearyl alcohol 25 g, propylene glycol 12 g, sodium lauryl sulphate 1 g, methyl hydroxybenzoate 25 mg, propyl hydroxybenzoate 15 mg, and water 37 g. Store in airtight containers.
Jap. P. includes a similar ointment.

Hydrophilic Petrolatum *(U.S.P.)*. Cholesterol 3, stearyl alcohol 3, white beeswax 8, white soft paraffin 86.
Jap. P. (Vaselinum Hydrophilicum) permits cetyl alcohol or stearyl alcohol.

Paraffin Ointment *(B.P.)*. Unguentum Paraffini. Hard paraffin 3, white beeswax 2, cetostearyl alcohol 5, and white soft paraffin 90. Store at a temperature not exceeding 25°.

Parenol *(B.P.C. 1949)*. Solid Parenol. White or yellow soft paraffin 65 g, wool fat 15 g, and water 20 g.

Simple Ointment *(B.P., Ind. P.)*. Unguentum Simplex; Ung. Simp. Wool fat 5, hard paraffin 5, cetostearyl alcohol 5, and white or yellow soft paraffin 85. Unless otherwise directed, when simple ointment is used in a white ointment it should be prepared with white soft paraffin and when used in a coloured ointment it should be prepared with yellow soft paraffin. Store at a temperature not exceeding 25°.
A.P.F. (Simple Ointment White) has the same formula made only with white soft paraffin.

Unguentum Molle *(Nord. P.)*. Wool fat 20 and yellow soft paraffin 80.

Unguentum Simplex *(Belg. P.)*. Onguent Simple. Equal parts of wool fat and white soft paraffin.

White Ointment *(U.S.P.)*. White beeswax 5, white soft paraffin 95. *Jap. P.* has hydrous wool fat 5, white beeswax 5, and white soft paraffin 90.

Yellow Ointment *(U.S.P.)*. Yellow beeswax 5 and yellow soft paraffin 95.

Proprietary Preparations

Jelonet *(Smith & Nephew, UK)*. A brand of Paraffin Gauze Dressing. (Also available as Jelonet in *Austral., S.Afr.*).

Peritex *(Southon-Horton, UK)*. A tulle dressing impregnated with soft paraffin, for use on burns and wounds.

Ultrabase *(Schering, UK)*. An emollient cream containing white soft paraffin, liquid paraffin, and stearyl alcohol.

Unguentum Merck *(E. Merck, UK)*. Contains white soft paraffin 32%, liquid paraffin 3%, cetostearyl alcohol 9%, polysorbate '40' 6%, glyceryl monostearate 3%, propylene glycol 5%, Miglyol '812' 2%, silicic acid 0.1%, and sorbic acid 0.2%. For use as an emollient and as a diluent for dermatological preparations.

Erythematous deterioration of psoriasis lesions in a 31-year-old woman receiving treatment was found to be due to sorbic acid present in Unguentum Merck used as a diluent of the steroid ointment prescribed.— E. M. Saihan and R. R. M. Harman, *Br. J. Derm.*, 1978, *99*, 583.

Other Proprietary Names

Dermosa Cusi Lubricante *(Spain)*; Red Veterinary Petrolatum, RVP *(bothUSA)*; Unitulle *(Austral.)*.

6406-z

Barrier Creams

The term 'barrier creams' is used to describe ointments, creams, or lotions that are applied to prevent damage to the skin. Barrier creams vary widely in composition. They should be easy to apply, easily washed off with soap and water, bacteriostatic, non-hygroscopic, non-transferable, non-sticky, and stable (to avoid the necessity of frequent application), and they must not act as heat insulators

Barrier creams are used to prevent damage to the skin by mechanical, chemical, or bacteriological action. The bases are usually slightly absorbed by the skin and fill the hair follicles with inert material. The preparation may contain suitable powders such as zinc oxide, kaolin, Fuller's earth, and talc to protect against mechanical irritants. Silicones may be included for their water-repellent and protective properties. As these creams are in daily use over long periods, they must not contain substances that are deleterious to the skin.

Some types of barrier cream form a flexible film when allowed to dry on the skin, and intrusion of contaminants is prevented for some hours. The film swells on washing the hands with soap and water and is removed together with superimposed dirt.

Barrier creams should not remove the natural grease, weaken the horny skin layer, or have a drying, oxidising, or reducing action. The pH should be from 5.5 to 6.5.

The choice of a suitable preparation depends on the specific type of contamination against which protection is desired. Contaminants may be divided into 2 main groups, water-miscible and water-immiscible substances, the first group including acid and neutral irritants, alkalis and soaps, explosives, and photographic chemicals, and the second including such substances as paraffin oils, paints, dusts, and tars.

Numerous proprietary barrier creams are marketed and many of these are issued with precise details of the contaminants against which they are effective.

A short review of barrier creams, with typical formulas.— P. Alexander, *Mfg Chem.*, 1968, *39* (Nov.), 33.

For other formulas for barrier creams, see under Silicones, p.1069.

Proprietary Preparations

HEB Waterproof *(Waterhouse, UK)*. A barrier cream containing cetostearyl alcohol, emulsifying wax, liquid paraffin, soft paraffin, wood fat, preservatives, and water.

Kerodex *(Sterling Industrial, UK)*. A range of water-resistant and water-soluble barrier creams for protection against a wide range of irritants. **Kerodex 77**. A gel formulation containing no silicones.

Rozalex *(Sterling Industrial, UK)*. A range of water-resistant and oil-resistant barrier creams for protection against a wide range of irritants. Skin cleansers and reconditioning creams are also available.

6407-c

White Beeswax *(B.P.)*. Cera Alba; White Wax *(U.S.N.F.)*; Cire Blanche; Gebleichtes Wachs; Cera Blanca; Cêra Branca.

CAS — 8012-89-3.

Pharmacopoeias. In *Arg., Aust., Belg., Br., Cz., Fr., Ger., Hung., Ind., It., Jap., Jug., Mex., Neth., Nord., Pol., Port., Roum., Span.,* and *Swiss.* Also in *U.S.N.F.*

Bleached yellow beeswax. A white or yellowish-white solid, translucent in thin layers, with a faint characteristic odour. Relative density about 0.96. M.p. 61° to 65°.

6408-k

Yellow Beeswax *(B.P.)*. Cera Flava; Yellow Wax *(U.S.N.F.)*; Cire Jaune; Gelbes Wachs; Cera Amarilla; Cêra Amarela.

CAS — 8012-89-3.

Pharmacopoeias. In *Arg., Aust., Belg., Br., Chin., Ger., Ind., Jap., Mex., Neth., Nord., Pol., Port., Roum., Span.,* and *Swiss.* Also in *U.S.N.F.*

The wax obtained by melting with hot water the walls of the honeycomb of the bee, *Apis mellifera* (Apidae), and removing the foreign matter. It contains about 70% of esters, chiefly myricyl palmitate. It is a yellow or light brown solid with an agreeable honey-like odour, brittle when cold, plastic when warmed in the hand. Relative density about 0.96. M.p. 61° to 65°.

Practically **insoluble** in water; sparingly soluble in alcohol; soluble in chloroform, ether, fixed and volatile oils, and warm carbon disulphide.

Adverse Effects. Hypersensitivity reactions to beeswax have been reported.

Occupational dermatitis in a 65-year-old beekeeper was found to be due to poplar resins in the beeswax.— H. W. Rothenborg, *Archs Derm.*, 1967, *95*, 381, per *J. Am. med. Ass.*, 1967, *200* (Apr. 24), A190.

Uses. Yellow beeswax is used as an ingredient of ointments and enables water to be incorporated to produce water-in-oil emulsions. White beeswax is similarly employed; it is occasionally used to adjust the melting-point of suppositories.

Preparations

Aseptic Surgical Wax *(B.P.C. 1949)*. Cera Aseptica Chirurgicalis; Horsley's Wax; Bone Wax. A sterile mixture of yellow beeswax 7 and olive oil 2 with phenol 1, all by wt. Cover with a 0.2% w/v solution of mercuric chloride and protect from light in sterile bottles in a cool place. When required for use the containers should be heated to 100° for 5 minutes and the contents poured into a 0.2% w/v solution of mercuric chloride warmed to 40°. It has been used for preventing haemorrhage in cranial surgery.

This preparation should not be confused with a proprietary preparation of yellow beeswax known as Bonewax.

Cera Styptica *(Jap. P.)*. Styptic Wax. Yellow beeswax 73 g, fixed oil 22 g, and phenol 5 g.

Cerato *(Arg. P.)*. White beeswax 25 g, olive oil 75 g.

Cold Cream *(A.P.F.)*. Ceratum Hydrosum; Crem. Refrig. Oleos.; Ung. Refrig. White beeswax 17 g, liquid paraffin 45 g, borax 1 g, and freshly boiled and cooled water 37 ml.

Galen's Wax. Cérat de Galien *(F.N. Fr.)*. White beeswax 130 g, almond oil 535 g, distilled rose water 330 g, and borax 5 g.

Simple Ointment *(Jap. P.)*. Yellow beeswax 33 g, vegetable oil to 100 g.

Proprietary Preparations

Bonewax *(Ethicon, UK)*. Consists of refined white beeswax 90% and isopropyl palmitate 10%, available as 2.5-g sticks, individually wrapped and sterilised.

This preparation should not be confused with Aseptic Surgical Wax which is also known as Bone Wax.

Gelucire 62/05 *(Alfa, UK)*. A beeswax derivative with controlled hydrophilic properties; an excipient for encapsulation of liquids into hard gelatin capsules.

6409-a

Ceresin. Cerasin; Mineral Wax; Purified Ozokerite.

CAS — 8001-75-0.

Pharmacopoeias. In *Jug., Span.,* and *Swiss*, with the title Paraffinum Solidum.

A mixture of solid hydrocarbons obtained by the purification of ozokerite, a naturally occurring solid paraffin. It is a colourless, odourless, waxy, microcrystalline solid resembling white beeswax. M.p. 50° to 75°.

Practically **insoluble** in water; soluble 1 in 30 of dehydrated alcohol; soluble in chloroform, ether, fixed and volatile oils, and light petroleum. **Sterilised** by heating for 1½ hours at 160° or 4 hours at 140°.

See also Microcrystalline Wax, p.1067.

Except in certain Eastern European countries, the terms ozokerite and ceresin were applied also to waxes obtained from mineral oil fractions with special characteristics. The waxes were microcrystalline hydrocarbons with complex molecular structures including side chains and ring formations. They were practically oil-free, with a solidification point between 65° and 75°, good paste-forming capacity with paraffin wax, and high solvent-retention value—the property of slowing down the evaporation of volatile liquids with which they were mixed; these features were valuable in stabilising polishing pastes.— *Soap chem. Spec.*, 1964, *40*, 111.

Uses. Ceresin is used as a substitute for beeswax or hard paraffin.

6410-e

Cetostearyl Alcohol *(B.P.)*. Cetostearyl Alc.; Cetylstearylalkohol; Alcohol Cetylicus et Stearylicus.

CAS — 8005-44-5.

Pharmacopoeias. In *Aust., Belg., Br., Cz., Ger., Jug.,* and *Roum.* Also in *U.S.N.F.*

A mixture of solid aliphatic alcohols, mainly stearyl and cetyl alcohols, obtained by the reduction of the appropriate fatty acids, or from sperm oils. It usually consists of about 50 to 70% of stearyl alcohol and 20 to 35% of cetyl alcohol. *U.S.N.F.* specifies not less than 90% of stearyl and cetyl alcohols and not less than 40% of stearyl alcohol. M.p. 43° to 53°.

A white or cream-coloured unctuous mass, or almost white flakes or granules, with a faint characteristic odour and a bland taste. It melts to a clear colourless or pale yellow liquid, free from cloudiness or suspended matter. Solidifying-point 45° to 53°.

Practically **insoluble** in water; soluble in ether; less soluble in alcohol and light petroleum.

The composition of cetostearyl alcohol.— A. W. Mace, *J. Pharm. Pharmac.*, 1975, *27*, 209.

Cetostearyl alcohol has similar properties to cetyl alcohol. In conjunction with suitable hydrophilic substances, such as sulphated fatty alcohols as in Emulsifying Wax (see p.1441) and cetomacrogol as in Cetomacrogol Emulsifying Wax (see p.374), it produces oil-in-water emulsions which are stable over a wide pH range.

It increases the viscosity of water-in-oil emulsions, thereby improving their stability, and improves the emollient properties of paraffin ointments.

See also Higher Fatty Alcohols, p.1066.

Cetostearyl alcohol sometimes causes contact allergy.— M. Hannuksela, *Int. J. cosmet. Sci.*, 1979, *1*, 257.

Proprietary Preparations

Laurex CS *(Albright & Wilson, Marchon Division, UK).* A brand of cetostearyl alcohol.

6411-l

Cetyl Alcohol *(U.S.N.F.).* 1-Hexadecanol; Hexadecyl Alcohol; Cetanol; Álcool Cetílico.

CAS — 36653-82-4.

Pharmacopoeias. In *Aust., Cz., Fr., Jap., Jug., Neth., Nord., Port., Span.,* and *Swiss.* Also in *U.S.N.F.*

A mixture of solid aliphatic alcohols consisting chiefly of cetyl alcohol, $C_{16}H_{33}OH$. Cetyl alcohol of commerce usually contains 60 to 70% cetyl alcohol and 20 to 30% stearyl alcohol. Pure cetyl alcohol is also available. *U.S.N.F.* specifies not less than 90% of cetyl alcohol, the remainder consisting chiefly of related alcohols.

It occurs as white unctuous flakes, cubes, or granules, with a faint characteristic odour and bland taste. M.p. 45° to 50°. It is non-irritating, does not become rancid, and is stable to light and air.

Practically **insoluble** in water; soluble 1 in 10 of alcohol, 1 in 3 of chloroform and ether; soluble in carbon disulphide and light petroleum; miscible when melted with fixed oils and fats, liquid paraffin, and hard paraffin. **Store** in a cool place.

Cetyl alcohol is used as a constituent of ointments and creams, especially those in which it is desired to incorporate water or an aqueous solution.

A mixture of 19 parts of soft paraffin and 1 part of cetyl alcohol will absorb from 40 to 50% of its weight of water; if 10% of wool fat is added to the mixture, the proportion of water can be further increased. When a large proportion of water is present in cetyl alcohol creams, the addition of a preservative is desirable. A mixture of 1 part of cetyl alcohol and 15 parts of arachis oil may be used as a basis for suppositories. See also Higher Fatty Alcohols p.1066.

Cetyl alcohol was claimed to provide greater emolliency than isopropyl myristate. It had lubricating properties and, because of its compatibility with aluminium chlorhydroxide-propylene glycol complex, was used in antiperspirant aerosols as well as in hand and skin creams and lotions.— *Mfg Chem.*, 1972, *43* (Jan.), 70.

Cetyl alcohol sometimes causes contact allergy.— M. Hannuksela, *Int. J. cosmet. Sci.*, 1979, *1*, 257.

Preparations

Unguentum Cetylicum *(Belg. P., Cz. P., Span. P., Swiss P.).* Cetylic Ointment. Cetyl alcohol 4, wool fat 10, and white soft paraffin 86.

Unguentum Cetylicum cum Aqua *(Swiss P.).* Unguentum Cetylicum Hydrosum *(Cz. P.).* Cetylic ointment 6 and water 4.

Belg. P. has cetylic ointment 7 and water 3.

Unguentum Hydrophilicum I *(Swiss P.).* Pommade Hydrophile Non Ionogène. Cetyl alcohol 10 g, hydrogenated arachis oil 20 g, polysorbate '60' 5 g, propylene glycol 10 g, methyl hydroxybenzoate 70 mg, propyl hydroxybenzoate 30 mg, and water to 100 g. **Unguentum Hydrophilicum II** (*Swiss P.*). Pommade Hydrophile Aniono-active. A similar formula to Unguentum Hydrophilicum I with polysorbate '60' replaced by sodium lauryl sulphate 1 g.

Proprietary Preparations

Laurex 16 *(Albright & Wilson, Marchon Division, UK).* A brand of cetyl alcohol.

6412-y

Cholesterol *(U.S.P.).* Cholesterin. Cholest-5-en-3β-ol.

$C_{27}H_{46}O$=386.7.

CAS — 57-88-5.

Pharmacopoeias. In *Aust., Braz., Cz., Jap., Pol., Roum., Span.,* and *U.S.*

White or faintly yellow, almost odourless, pearly leaflets, needles, powder, or granules. M.p. 147° to 150°. It acquires a yellow to pale tan colour on prolonged exposure to light. It is a constituent of all animal cells and occurs in most foods; Wool Alcohols (see p.1071) contains not less than 30% of cholesterol.

Practically **insoluble** in water; slowly soluble 1 in 100 of alcohol and 1 in 50 of dehydrated alcohol; soluble in acetone, chloroform, dioxan, ether, ethyl acetate, light petroleum, and vegetable oils. Clear aqueous solutions may be prepared with the aid of cetomacrogol or macrogol fatty esters. **Store** in airtight containers in a cool place. Protect from light.

Solubility. The solubility of cholesterol in various fats and oils.— D. Kritchevsky and S. A. Tepper, *Proc. Soc. exp. Biol. Med.*, 1964, *116*, 104.

Pectin 0.5% and acacia 0.5% markedly increased the aqueous solubility of cholesterol. Its solubility was also increased by 6 and 10% dextran.— D. K. Madan and D. E. Cadwallader (letter), *J. pharm. Sci.*, 1970, *59*, 1362.

Uses. Cholesterol imparts water-absorbing power to ointments and is used as an emulsifying agent. Cholesterol is employed as an anti-irritant in spirituous 'hair tonics' in concentrations of up to 2% and it is incorporated in many cosmetic ointments.

Cholesterol has a physiological role.

6413-j

Coconut Oil *(B.P.).* Oleum Cocois; Coconut Butter; Oleum Cocos Raffinatum; Oleum Cocosis; Aceite de Coco.

CAS — 8001-31-8.

Pharmacopoeias. In *Br.* and *Jap.*

A white or pearl-white unctuous mass; odourless or with an odour of coconut and a bland taste, obtained by expression from the dried solid part of the endosperm of the coconut, the fruit of *Cocos nucifera* (Palmae). M.p. 23° to 26°.

Practically **insoluble** in water; soluble 1 in 2 of alcohol (at 60°); freely soluble in chloroform, ether, carbon disulphide, and light petroleum. It readily becomes rancid on exposure to air. **Store** at a temperature not exceeding 25° in well-filled airtight containers. Protect from light.

NOTE. Fractionated coconut oil is described in the section on Fixed Oils, p.696.

Uses. Coconut oil forms a readily absorbable ointment basis and is used particularly in preparations applied to the scalp. It is used commercially in the preparations of 'marine' or sea-water soaps, as coconut-oil soaps are not easily precipitated by sodium chloride.

Preparations

Coconut Oil Compound Ointment. See under Coal Tar, p.506.

Coconut Oil Soap Solution *(B.P.C. 1934).* Liq. Sap. Ol. Cocois. Prepared from coconut oil 18.31 g, potassium hydroxide 1.97 g, sodium hydroxide 1.97 g, water to 100 ml and saturated with thymol. Used as a shampoo and skin cleanser.

Acidum Cocos *(Nord. P.).* A mixture of fatty acids, chiefly lauric acid, $C_{11}H_{23}.CO_2H$, and myristic acid, $C_{13}H_{27}.CO_2H$, prepared by the hydrolysis of coconut oil and distillation of the isolated fatty acids. A yellowish greasy solid with an odour of coconut and a bland taste. M.p 21 to 29°. Very slightly soluble in water; very soluble in alcohol, chloroform, and ether. Store in a cool place.

Cobee *(PVO International, USA: Alfa, UK).* A range of natural and hydrogenated coconut oils. For use as emollients and bases for pharmaceutical preparations.

6414-z

Higher Fatty Alcohols

Higher fatty alcohols is a general term for the higher members of the series of the saturated aliphatic monohydric alcohols. They are found in waxes or in the wax-like unsaponifiable constituents of some fats. As these sources, with few exceptions, are severely limited, the higher fatty alcohols are prepared by the catalytic hydrogenation of the higher fatty acids.

The main sources of these acids are fixed oils and fats which, on hydrolysis, give mixtures of acids. As these mixtures are not separated in commerce but are hydrogenated directly, the higher aliphatic alcohols consist of mixtures of alcohols, the composition of which depends upon the source of the fixed oil or fat used to obtain the acids.

The higher fatty alcohols are solid white crystalline substances, melting without decomposition. They are stable to alkalis and acids, and after boiling with alcoholic potassium hydroxide they are precipitated unchanged when the solution is diluted with water. The alcohols dissolve in concentrated sulphuric acid in the cold to form alkyl sulphates, the sodium salts of which are known commercially as sulphated fatty alcohols—see p.1439.

Two higher fatty alcohols, cetyl alcohol (see p.1066) and stearyl alcohol (see p.1070), as well as the mixed alcohols, cetostearyl alcohol (see p.1065), are used in cosmetic and pharmaceutical products. They possess good emollient properties without being greasy and they increase the viscosity, improve the texture, and aid the stability of water-in-oil emulsions. Moreover, the pure substances do not turn rancid. They possess some emulsifying powers which, in formulas for water-in-oil emulsions, allow a reduction of the amounts of other emulsifying agents used; they are also readily absorbed by the skin, thus increasing the efficacy of the preparations containing them.

Proprietary Preparations

Lanbritol Wax N21 *(Ronsheim & Moore, UK).* A nonionic self-emulsifying wax prepared from higher fatty alcohols. It forms oil-in-water emulsions which are stable in the presence of anionic and cationic medicaments, and inorganic salts of monovalent and polyvalent metals.

Stearal *(Amerchol, USA: Anstead, UK).* A straight-chain fatty alcohol; used to increase the viscosity of emulsions.

6415-c

Hard Fat *(B.P., Eur. P.).* Adeps Solidus; Adeps Neutralis; Massa Estearínica; Glycérides Semi-synthétiques Solides; Hartfett; Neutralfett.

Pharmacopoeias. In *Aust., Belg., Br., Eur., Fr., Ger., Hung., It., Neth., Nord.,* and *Port.*

A mixture of mono-, di-, and triglycerides of the saturated fatty acids $C_9H_{19}COOH$ to $C_{17}H_{35}COOH$.
A white brittle, solid which is unctuous to the touch, almost odourless and tasteless and free from rancid odour. M.p. 33° to 36°. The melted substance is colourless or slightly yellowish and forms a stable emulsion when shaken with an equal amount of hot water.
Practically **insoluble** in water; slightly soluble in alcohol; freely soluble in ether, soluble in acetone and chloroform; miscible with theobroma oil and other oils. **Incompatible** with alkaline substances. **Store** in airtight containers. Protect from light.

Uses. The name Hard Fat is applied to a range of bases with varying degrees of hardness and differing melting ranges. These bases are used for the preparation of suppositories in place of theobroma oil over which they have certain advantages.
They are less liable to rancidity than theobroma oil, the narrower interval between their melting and setting points reduces the tendency to sedimentation of solid medicaments, and their solidifying points are not affected by over-heating. They have water-absorbent and emulsifying properties and the melted mass sets quickly on cooling to provide suppositories with a clean polished appearance.
Bases with appropriate melting-points can be selected for counteracting the lowering of melting-point caused by certain medicaments and for providing bases suitable for use in different climates.

Some Proprietary Suppository Bases

Coberine *(Loders & Nucoline, UK).* A substitute for theobroma oil, prepared by solvent fractionation of vegetable oils and selective blending of the glyceride fractions.

Massa Estarinum *(Dynamit Nobel, UK).* A range of suppository bases consisting of mixtures of mono-, di-, and triglycerides of saturated fatty acids.

Massuppol *(Croklaan, Neth.: Loders & Nucoline, UK).* A suppository basis consisting of glyceryl esters, mainly of lauric acid, to which a very small amount of glyceryl monostearate has been added to improve its water-absorbing capacity. The basis is very hard and completely melts below body-temperature; it is not affected by overheating and, on cooling, sets rapidly. **Massuppol 15.** A grade designed for cold moulding.

Suppocire *(Alfa, UK).* A range of suppository bases consisting of mixtures of mono-, di-, and triglycerides of vegetable oils and of polyoxyethylene glycerides.

Witepsol Suppository Bases *(Dynamit Nobel, UK).* A range of suppository bases consisting of triglycerides of saturated vegetable fatty acids.

For information on other suppository bases, see under Glycerol (p.707), Macrogols (p.711), Fractionated Palm Kernel Oil (p.1068), and Theobroma Oil (p.1071).

6416-k

Isopropyl Myristate *(B.P.C. 1973, U.S.N.F.).* Isopropyl Myrist.

$(CH_3)_2CH.O.CO.(CH_2)_{12}.CH_3=270.5$.

CAS — 110-27-0.

Pharmacopoeias. In *Aust.* Also in *U.S.N.F.* which specifies esters of isopropyl alcohol and saturated high molecular weight fatty acids, principally myristic acid; it contains not less than 90% of $C_{17}H_{34}O_2$.

A clear colourless or almost colourless, almost odourless, mobile oily liquid with a bland taste. Wt per ml 0.85 to 0.855 g. F.p. about 5°.
Practically **insoluble** in water, glycerol, and propylene glycol; soluble 1 in 3 of alcohol; miscible with chloroform, ether, liquid hydrocarbons, and fixed oils. **Incompatible** with hard paraffin, producing a granular mixture. **Store** in airtight containers. Protect from light.

Uses. Isopropyl myristate is resistant to oxidation and hydrolysis and does not become rancid; it is free from irritant and sensitising properties and is absorbed fairly readily by the skin.
It may be used in external preparations in place of vegetable oils, and in emollient ointments and creams, yielding products which are relatively free from greasiness.
It is a solvent for many substances applied externally and is of value as a vehicle when direct contact and penetration of the medicament are required.
Other isopropyl fatty acid esters, including di-isopropyl adipate, isopropyl laurate, isopropyl linoleate, and isopropyl palmitate (p.1067) have similar properties and are used for similar purposes to those of isopropyl myristate.

Use in food. The Food Additives and Contaminants Committee were unable to recommend the use of isopropyl myristate as a solvent in food at a concentration of use in food as consumed above 5 ppm. Further toxicity studies were required.— *Report on the Review of Solvents in Food,* FAC/REP/25, Ministry of Agriculture, Fisheries and Food, London, HM Stationery Office, 1978.

Proprietary Preparations

Ceraphyls *(Van Dyk, USA: Black, UK).* A range of emollient substances, some imparting water-repellent films without greasiness or tackiness. **Ceraphyl 230** is di-isopropyl adipate and **Ceraphyl IPL** is isopropyl linoleate.

Crodamols *(Croda, UK).* A range of emollient substances, including **Crodamol DA** (di-isopropyl adipate), **Crodamol IPL** (isopropyl laurate), and **Crodamol IPM** (isopropyl myristate).

Emulsiderm *(Dermal Laboratories, UK).* Emulsion containing isopropyl myristate 25%, liquid paraffin 25%, and benzalkonium chloride 0.5%. For skin application or as a bath additive in dry skin conditions.

Promyr *(Amerchol, USA: Anstead, UK).* A brand of isopropyl myristate. **Propal.** A material with similar properties but a higher melting point.

6417-a

Isopropyl Palmitate *(U.S.N.F.).*
$(CH_3)_2CH.O.CO.(CH_2)_{14}.CH_3=298.5$.

CAS — 142-91-6.

Pharmacopoeias. In *U.S.N.F.*

Esters of isopropyl alcohol and saturated high molecular weight fatty acids; it contains not less than 90% of $C_{19}H_{38}O_2$. Specific gravity 0.850 to 0.855. **Store** in airtight containers. Protect from light.

Isopropyl palmitate has similar properties and uses to those of isopropyl myristate (p.1067).

Proprietary Preparations

Crodamol IPP *(Croda, UK).* A brand of isopropyl palmitate.

6418-t

Japan Wax. Cera Rhois.

CAS — 8001-39-6.

A white to yellowish fat obtained by warm compression from the fruit rind of *Rhus succedanea* (Anacardiaceae) and bleached by sunlight. It consists chiefly of palmitin and palmitic acid.

Japan wax is used in the manufacture of polishes.

6419-x

Kokum Butter. Oleum Garciniae; Goa Butter; Mangosteen Oil.

Pharmacopoeias. In *Ind.*

The solid fat expressed from the seeds of *Garcinia indica* (Guttiferae) and purified. It is a white or greyish-white fat which is almost odourless and tasteless. M.p. 39° to 42°.

Kokum butter has been used as a suppository basis.

6420-y

Lard *(B.P.C. 1963).* Adeps; Prepared Lard; Adeps Suillus (Depuratus); Adeps Lotus; Axungia; Axonge; Schweineschmalz; Grasa de Cerdo; Manteca de Cerdo; Banha.

Pharmacopoeias. In *Aust., Cz., Ger., Jap., Mex., Pol., Port., Roum.,* and *Span.*

The purified fat of the hog, *Sus scrofa* (Suidae), prepared from the 'flare' or omentum. **Store** in a cool place in airtight containers. Protect from light.

Uses. Lard has been used as an ointment basis but it has been superseded by more stable vehicles. It is readily absorbed by the skin but is unpleasantly greasy and it is liable to become rancid on exposure to light and air, which makes it offensive in use and unsatisfactory for application to sensitive tissues.

6421-j

Benzoinated Lard *(B.P.C. 1954).* Adeps Benz.; Axonge Benzoinée; Benzoeschmalz; Grasa de Cerdo Benzoinada; Manteca Benzoinada; Banha Benzoinada.

Pharmacopoeias. In *Cz., Mex., Port.,* and *Span.* From 1 to 3% of Siam benzoin is used and some include 5 to 6% of anhydrous sodium sulphate.

Prepared by heating lard with 2% Siam benzoin at about 65° for 1 hour, straining, and stirring until cold. Substances extracted from the Siam benzoin help to prevent rancidity due to the growth of micro-organisms. **Store** in airtight containers. Protect from light.

Benzoinated lard should not be used as a basis for eye ointments or in the preparation of ointments containing alkaloidal bases.

6422-z

Microcrystalline Wax *(U.S.N.F.).*

Pharmacopoeias. In *U.S.N.F.*

A mixture of straight-chain, branched-chain, and cyclic hydrocarbons, obtained by solvent fractionation of the still bottom fraction of petroleum by suitable dewaxing or de-oiling means.
A white or cream-coloured odourless waxy solid. M.p. 54° to 102°. Practically **insoluble** in water; sparingly soluble in dehydrated alcohol; soluble in chloroform, ether, volatile oils, and in most warm fixed oils. **Store** in airtight containers.
See also Ceresin, p.1065.

Microcrystalline wax is a stiffening agent and tablet-coating agent.

6423-c

Oleyl Alcohol *(U.S.N.F.).*

CAS — 143-28-2.

Pharmacopoeias. In *U.S.N.F.*

A mixture of unsaturated and saturated high molecular weight fatty alcohols consisting chiefly of oleyl alcohol, $C_{18}H_{36}O = 268.5$.
A clear colourless to light yellow oily liquid with a faint characteristic odour and a bland taste. M.p. 13° to 19°. Practically **insoluble** in water; soluble in alcohol, ether, isopropyl alcohol, and light liquid paraffin. **Store** at 15° to 30° in well-filled airtight containers.

Oleyl alcohol has been used as an emulsion stabiliser and as a skin emollient.

Oleyl alcohol and sorbitan mono-oleate might diminish the activity of chlorpromazine.— A. Mériaux-Brochu and J. Paiement, *Can. J. pharm. Sci.*, 1977, *12*, 97.

Proprietary Preparations

Novol *(Croda, UK)*. A brand of oleyl alcohol.

6424-k

Palm Kernel Oil *(B.P.C. 1949)*. Oleum Palmae Nuclei; Palm-nut Oil.

CAS — 8023-79-8.

A fat expressed from the kernels of the fruit of the palm tree, *Elaeis guineensis* (Palmae).

Palm kernel oil has been used as an ointment basis. It is similar to coconut oil (see p.1066) in its properties and it has been used in the manufacture of soaps and margarine.

6425-a

Fractionated Palm Kernel Oil *(B.P.)*.

Pharmacopoeias. In *Br.* The standards of the *B.P.* monograph encompass several different suppository bases.

A white, solid, odourless, tasteless, brittle fat, obtained by selective solvent fractionation and hydrogenation of the natural oil expressed from the kernels of *Elaeis guineensis* (Palmae). M.p. 31° to 36°.

Practically **insoluble** in water and alcohol; soluble in chloroform, ether, and light petroleum. **Store** at a temperature not exceeding 25°.

Fractionated palm kernel oil is used instead of theobroma oil as a fatty basis for suppositories. It has also been used in chocolate.

Proprietary Preparations

Extracoa *(Loders & Nucoline, UK)*. A brand of fractionated palm kernel oil. M.p. 31 to 32°.

Supercoa *(Loders & Nucoline, UK)*. A brand of fractionated palm kernel oil. M.p. 33.5 to 35.5°.

6426-t

Silicones

Silicones are polymers with a structure consisting of alternate atoms of silicon and oxygen, organic groups such as methyl or phenyl being attached to the silicon atoms.

The dimethicones, or dimethyl polysiloxane fluids, are the most important; they are fluid polymers with the general formula $CH_3.[Si(CH_3)_2.O]_n.Si(CH_3)_3$.

The viscosity of silicone polymers rises with increase in molecular weight and fluids are available throughout the range of 0.65 to 3 million centistokes. The various grades are distinguished by numbers, each number approximately corresponding to the viscosity of the particular grade. Higher polymers take the form of greases, waxes, and resins. Silicone rubbers can be prepared and are widely used in medicine and pharmacy on account of their chemical inertness and resistance to heat treatment. They may be permeable to moisture when used as closures.

The silicone fluids are colourless, odourless, and tasteless. They are stable to heat and resistant to most chemicals, apart from some concentrated acids and strong alkali solutions. Solubility in organic solvents decreases with increase in the molecular weight of the silicone.

Grades of methylphenyl silicones are available which have greater compatibility with organic solvents and are soluble in aqueous alcohol and in liquid paraffin.

Silicones are **sterilised** by maintaining at 150° for 1 hour.

6427-x

Dimethicones *(B.P.)*.

Dimethylpolysiloxane; Dimethyl Silicone Fluid; Dimethylsiloxane; Dimeticone; Methyl Polysiloxane; Huile de Silicone; Siliconum Liquidum; Permethylpolysiloxane. Poly(dimethylsiloxane). $CH_3.[Si(CH_3)_2.O]_nSi(CH_3)_3$.

CAS — 9006-65-9.

Pharmacopoeias. In *Br., Chin.,* and *Fr.*

Dimethicone may be prepared by hydrolysing a mixture of dichlorodimethylsilane, $(CH_3)_2SiCl_2$, and chlorotrimethylsilane, $(CH_3)_3SiCl$. The products of hydrolysis contain active silanol groups (SiOH) through which condensation polymerisation proceeds. By varying the proportion of chlorotrimethylsilane, which acts as a chain terminator, silicones of varying molecular weight may be prepared.

As the molecular weight increases, the products become more viscous, and fluids are available throughout the viscosity range of 0.65 centistokes to 3 million centistokes. The various grades are distinguished by numbers, each number approximately corresponding to the viscosity in centistokes.

Clear colourless or pale yellow, odourless or almost odourless liquids, practically **immiscible** with water, alcohol, acetone, and methyl alcohol, and miscible with chlorinated hydrocarbons, ether, solvent naphtha, and xylene; dimethicones 20, 200, 350, and 500 are also miscible with amyl acetate, cyclohexane, kerosene, and petroleum spirit. Their viscosities, in centistokes, at 25° are:dimethicone '20'—17 to 23; dimethicone '200'—190 to 210; dimethicone '350'—330 to 370; dimethicone '500'—475 to 525. Dimethicone 20 has a wt per ml of 0.94 to 0.965 g. Dimethicone 200, 350, 500, and 1000, all have a wt per ml of 0.965 to 0.98 g.

6428-r

Activated Dimethicone.

Simethicone *(U.S.P.)*; Activated Polymethylsiloxane.

CAS — 8050-81-5.

Pharmacopoeias. In *U.S.*

A mixture of liquid dimethicones containing finely divided silicon dioxide to enhance the defoaming properties of the silicone. It is a grey, translucent, almost odourless, tasteless fluid, containing 4 to 7% w/w of silicon dioxide. The viscosity of the supernatant liquid, after separation of the silicon dioxide, is not less than 300 centistokes.

Practically **insoluble** in water and dehydrated alcohol; soluble 1 in 10 of chloroform and ether leaving a residue of silicon dioxide. **Store** in airtight containers.

Adsorption by antacids. The defoaming activity of activated dimethicone was reduced in conjunction with some common antacids and decreased further on storage. These antacids, particularly aluminium hydroxide and magnesium carbonate, adsorbed the silicone.— M. Rezak, *J. pharm. Sci.*, 1966, *55*, 538.

Adverse Effects of Silicones. Injection of silicones into tissues may cause a granulomatous reaction.

Physiologically, the silicones were extremely inert and application of silicone fluids to the skin and ordinary handling over a period of years by laboratory workers of various methyl and phenyl silicone polymers caused no skin disorders or sensitisation, nor was absorption observed. The organic silicon compounds were not toxic in themselves, with the exception of those containing unhydrolysed chlorine atoms which released hydrochloric acid in the presence of water.— *Chem. Prod.*, 1963, *26* (Aug.), 22.

A few isolated and incompletely documented deaths had been reported following the injection of liquid silicones into tissues for cosmetic purposes. The fate of some 15% of silicone liquid injected into laboratory *animals* had not been traced.— J. E. Murray and R. M. Goldwyn (letter), *New Engl. J. Med.*, 1966, *275*, 336.

Repeated injections of silicone fluid into the breasts in 2 women were followed by extensive bilateral granulomatous mastitis.— W. St. C. Symmers, *Br. med. J.*, 1968, *3*, 19. See also J. S. Nosanchuk, *Archs Surg., Chicago*, 1968, *97*, 583.

White plugs which contained fat, dimethicone, and silica were found in the retinal vessels of 2 patients who underwent open-heart surgery. A defoaming agent containing dimethicone fluid and silica gel (Antifoam A, *Dow Corning*) had been used in the perfusion.— I. M. Williams, *Br. J. Ophthal.*, 1975, *59*, 81.

Migration of silicone and granulomatous hepatitis occurred in 2 patients who had received silicone injections to the breasts, malar areas, and trochanters. Another developed rock-hard red breasts with skin changes and an enlarged liver after injections of silicone to the breasts. A fourth patient died shortly after receiving silicone injections to the breasts; death appeared to result from severe bilateral pulmonary oedema.— R. Ellenbogen *et al.*, *J. Am. med. Ass.*, 1975, *234*, 308.

An estimate that at least 12 000 women in the Las Vegas area had received 'bootleg silicone injections' (using a nonmedical-grade silicone) mostly in the breast area for cosmetic purposes, at least 1% of them developed complications each year. Infections which had occurred after the injections usually developed within a short time but had been reported up to 5 years later. Some infections responded to antibiotic therapy while others resulted in necrosis and sloughing of the skin and involved tissue. Migration of the injected material had occasionally occurred. Cyst formation was probably the most frequent complication occurring either shortly after injection or years later. Granuloma formation was less common but was considered to be a more formidable problem and was sometimes accompanied by skin changes including pigment changes, lymphoedema, silicoma of the skin, vesicle formation, and ulceration. Complications occurred irrespective of the site and had developed up to 9 years later. Medical-grade silicone was probably little safer than other types of silicone.— E. H. Kopf *et al.*, *Rocky Mtn med. J.*, 1976, *73*, 77. See also *J. Am. med. Ass.*, 1976, *236*, 959.

In a woman with silicone elastomer finger-joint prostheses, fracture of the prostheses resulted in synovitis due to the presence of silicone particles in the synovium. A second woman with intact silicone elastomer finger-joint prostheses had lymphadenopathy with silicone particles in the axillary lymph node.— A. J. Christie *et al.*, *J. Am. med. Ass.*, 1977, *237*, 1463.

Over a period of 10 years 92 patients received injections of medical-grade silicone. Granulomas subsequently developed in 13 injection sites, usually within 1 year but some took a few years to develop and one appeared after 7 years.— T. F. Wilkie, *Plastic reconstr. Surg.*, 1977, *60*, 179.

A 55-year-old woman developed severe swelling, marked tenderness and erythema at the sites of injection and periorbital oedema after receiving injections of silicone in the facial area. A scratch test proved positive for allergy to silicone. The patient responded well to steroid therapy, but later her symptoms recurred without further exposure to silicone preparations. Recurrence may have been due to the use of cosmetics containing silicates.— M. J. Fellner and D. Rudikoff, *Int. J. Derm.*, 1979, *18*, 375.

Refractile particles in the livers of haemodialysis patients. Silicone used in the dialysis equipment might have been the cause.— A. S. -Y. Leong *et al.* (letter), *Lancet*, 1981, *1*, 889. Silicone-induced splenomegaly in a dialysis patient. The dialysis equipment contained silicone and histologic examination showed foreign-body inclusions in the spleen.— J. Bommer *et al.*, *New Engl. J. Med.*, 1981, *305*, 1077. Malignant lymphoma with intranodal refractile particles after insertion of silicone prostheses.— J. M. Digby and A. L. Wells (letter), *Lancet*, 1981, *2*, 580.

For a report of a dimethicone additive used in cooking oil being associated with a diminished effect of warfarin and phenindione, see Warfarin Sodium, p.777.

Uses of Silicones. Silicones are water-repellent and have a low surface tension. They are used in barrier creams for protecting the skin against water-soluble irritants. Creams, lotions, and ointments containing 10 to 30% of a dimethicone are employed for the prevention of bedsores and napkin rash and to protect the skin against trauma due to incontinence or colostomy discharge.

Silicone preparations should not be applied where free drainage is necessary or to inflamed or abraded skin; they may be irritant to the eyes, but a special grade has been suggested as a lubricant for artificial eyes.

Silicones are used as antifoaming agents, and the addition of 4 to 8% of finely divided silicon dioxide increases the antifoaming activity of dimethicones. Dimethicones activated with silicon dioxide act by changing the surface tension of gas bubbles, thereby causing them to coalesce. They are used in the treatment of flatulence and meteorism, for the elimination of gas, air, or foam from the gastro-intestinal tract prior to radiography, and for the relief of abdominal distension and dyspepsia. Doses of up to 2 g daily have been used, often in conjunction with antacids such as aluminium hydroxide. Silicones are also used topically as wound dressings.

Silicones are used as lubricants for hypodermic syringes; a methylphenyl silicone is often preferred because of its better lubricating properties and greater stability at high temperatures. Ampoules, vials, and other glassware may be coated with a thin film of silicone; solutions and suspensions may be drained completely from containers which have been so treated. An advantage in coating measures with silicones is that the meniscus of aqueous liquids in such measures is almost flat.

Blood may take longer to coagulate when collected in silicone-treated glassware.

Silicone Treatment of Glassware. A typical method is to rinse clean dry vials with a 2% solution of dimethicone '1000' in xylene or carbon tetrachloride, drain off the excess solution and dry the vials at 110°; they are then heated at 250° to 275° for 3 hours to bond the silicone to the glass. A grade of silicone (MS 1107) is available which is used in the same way but can be 'cured' in 1 to 2 hours at 100° or 20 minutes at 150°. In this case ethyl acetate or *n*-hexane is used as the solvent.

If the article cannot be heat-treated it may be made water-repellent by the use of dimethyldichlorosilane. The article is rinsed with a solution of the chlorosilane and allowed to dry. There is usually sufficient absorbed water on the surface to hydrolyse the chlorosilane to a silicone. The apparatus should be washed before use with water to remove traces of hydrochloric acid. This process is not suitable for articles subject to corrosion by hydrochloric acid.

Tentative estimated acceptable daily intake of dimethicones with a relative molecular mass in the range of 200 to 300: up to 1.5 mg per kg body-weight.— Twenty-third Report of the Joint FAO/WHO Expert Committee on Food Additives, *Tech. Rep. Ser. Wld Hlth Org. No. 648*, 1980. For background toxicological information on dimethicones and activated dimethicone, see *Fd Add. Ser. Wld Hlth Org. No. 6*, 1975.

The use of silicones on vials and closures for parenteral products.— C. Riffkin, *Bull. parent. Drug Ass.*, 1968, *22*, 66.

Silicones in cosmetics and toiletries.— F. C. Saunders, *Mfg Chem.*, 1969, *40* (Oct.), 27.

The use of silicone foam sponge as a wound dressing.— R. A. B. Wood and L. E. Hughes, *Br. med. J.*, 1975, *4*, 131. See also J. Macfie and J. McMahon, *Br. J. Surg.*, 1980, *67*, 85; R. H. P. Williams *et al.*, *Br. med. J.*, 1981, *282*, 21.

Abdominal discomfort. In a study of 1092 patients who had undergone abdominal hysterectomy or caesarean section, 655 were given activated dimethicone 80 mg every 4 hours for 14 doses. There was a reduction in nausea, abdominal distension, severity of gas pain, and the amount of narcotic analgesic required compared with the untreated group. Similar results were obtained in a double-blind study of a further 200 patients.— A. Gibstein *et al.*, *Obstet. Gynec.*, 1971, *38*, 386.

It was recommended that dimethicone be taken before meals.— *Drug & Ther. Bull.*, 1972, *10*, 9.

Of 41 patients with functional upper gastro-intestinal disorders who were given 50-mg tablets of activated dimethicone or a placebo, the 20 patients receiving activated dimethicone were improved and there was little change in the group receiving placebo.— J. E. Bernstein and A. M. Kasich, *J. clin. Pharmac.*, 1974, *14*, 617.

A study in 15 healthy subjects indicated that activated dimethicone accelerated the passage of gas through the intestine. It did not affect the total volume of gas expelled.— I. E. Danhof and J. J. Stavola, *Obstet. Gynec.*, 1974, *44*, 148, per *Int. pharm. Abstr.*, 1978, *15*, 931.

Activated dimethicone was considered to be of no value in the treatment of flatulence associated with gastro-intestinal disorders.— *Med. Lett.*, 1975, *17*, 80.

Antifoaming activity. Froth tests showed that the defoaming properties of dimethicone in antacid preparations were due to the presence of free dimethicone. Omission of silica had little effect on the defoaming action. It was suggested that the aluminium hydroxide and talc components were responsible for dispersing the dimethicone, and silica was not necessary for 'activation'.— J. E. Carless *et al.*, *J. Pharm. Pharmac.*, 1973, *25*, 849.

Bedsores. Controlled studies had shown that silicone emulsions or creams must contain 20% of silicone to be effective.— G. W. Roberts (letter), *Lancet*, 1960, *1*, 283.

A bedsore in an 86-year-old man healed completely in 4.5 months when a cream containing 20% dimethicone (Vasogen) was applied twice daily. Within 2 days of the treatment starting the serous secretion ceased and the surface of the ulcer began to heal.— P. McEwan (letter), *Lancet*, 1968, *1*, 45.

An assessment of preparations for bedsores, including silicones.— *Drug & Ther. Bull.*, 1977, *15*, 69.

Burns. For a report of the use of silicone-soaked mittens in the treatment of burnt hands, see *J. Am. med. Ass.*, 1968, *206*, 2641.

Immersion of burnt hands in gloves soaked in liquid silicone led to early debridement and removal of the eschar. There was lack of pain during treatment and control of infection was good.— J. W. Batdorf *et al.*, *Archs Surg., Chicago*, 1969, *98*, 469.

See also Use in Physiotherapy, below.

Immersion foot. A condition described as 'immersion foot' developed in the feet of US soldiers from constant exposure to warm water in the lowlands of Vietnam. Protection was afforded by a preparation made from methylsilicone, fluorosilicone, and silica as an aerosol, liquid, and grease. It was applied freshly each day to the feet and/or socks.— L. J. Buckels *et al.*, *J. Am. med. Ass.*, 1967, *200*, 681.

Rheumatic disorders. Reports of benefit from intra-articular injections of dimethicone in osteoarthritis and rheumatoid arthritis: B. Helal and B. S. Karadi, *Ann. phys. Med.*, 1968, *9*, 334; B. Helal *et al.*, *Int. Surg.*, 1970, *54*, 317. See also B. Helal (letter), *Br. med. J.*, 1970, *2*, 50.

A study indicating that dimethicone 200 is less effective than hydrocortisone acetate in normal saline when given by intra-articular injection to increase the range of knee-joint movement in patients with osteoarthritis or rheumatoid arthritis.— M. Corbett *et al.*, *Br. med. J.*, 1970, *1*, 24.

In a controlled study in 40 osteoarthritic knees intra-articular injection of saline appeared more beneficial than dimethicone 300 in reducing pain, although the effect was not noticeable a month later. Stiffness was not affected by either injection. Synovial reactions to silicone, severe in 1 patient, occurred in 3 patients.— V. Wright *et al.*, *Br. med. J.*, 1971, *2*, 370.

Silicones were of unproven value in the treatment of osteoarthritis.— F. D. Hart, *Practitioner*, 1974, *212*, 244.

Ultrasonography. The quality of sound transmission in the abdomen of patients undergoing ultrasonography was improved by prior administration of activated dimethicone 80 mg four times a day for 1 or 2 days.— G. Sommer *et al.*, *Radiology*, 1977, *125*, 219, per *Int. pharm. Abstr.*, 1978, *15*, 776.

Use in ophthalmology. M. F. Armaly, *J. Am. med. Ass.*, 1966, *198*, 214; R.C. Watzke, *Archs Ophthal., N.Y.*, 1967, *77*, 185.

Use in physiotherapy. Dimethicone 20 was used in the treatment of hands damaged by trauma or operation. The hands were immersed and exercised in the oil for 20 minutes up to 3 times daily, often starting the day after injury. The treatment facilitated movement of the hands and debridement of dead tissue and hastened the formation of granulation tissue.— D. Gifford, *Physiotherapy, Lond.*, 1974, *60*, 350.

See also Burns above.

Preparations Containing Silicones

Creams and Ointments

Dimethicone Cream *(B.P.C. 1973)*. Cremor Dimethiconi; Crem. Dimethic.; Dimethicone Cream Aqueous *(A.P.F.)*; Silicone Cream. Dimethicone '350' 10 g, chlorocresol 100 mg, cetrimide 500 mg, cetostearyl alcohol 5 g, liquid paraffin 40 g, and freshly boiled and cooled water 44.4 g. Store in a cool place in well-closed containers which prevent evaporation and contamination.

Silicone-Hydrocortisone Barrier Cream *(Roy. Victoria Infirm.)*. Dimethicone '400' 10, hydrocortisone 1, liquid paraffin 37, cetostearyl alcohol 3, Polawax 5, chlorocresol 0.1, water to 100. Shelf-life 1 month. Store at 4° to 8°.

Mixtures

Simethicone Oral Suspension *(U.S.P.)*. A suspension containing activated dimethicone. pH 4.4 to 4.6. Store in airtight containers. Protect from light.

Tablets

Simethicone Tablets *(U.S.P.)*. Tablets containing activated dimethicone.

Proprietary Preparations of Silicones

Andursil *(Geigy, UK)*. **Suspension** containing in each 5 ml activated dimethicone 150 mg, aluminium hydroxide equivalent to Al_2O_3 200 mg, magnesium hydroxide 200 mg, and aluminium hydroxide-magnesium carbonate co-dried gel 200 mg and **Tablets** each containing activated dimethicone 250 mg and aluminium hydroxide-magnesium carbonate co-dried gel 750 mg. For gastric disorders. *Dose.* 5 to 10 ml of suspension or 1 or 2 tablets 3 or 4 times daily and at bedtime, or as required.

Antasil *(Stuart, UK)*. **Liquid** containing in each 5 ml activated dimethicone 150 mg, dried aluminium hydroxide 400 mg, and magnesium hydroxide 400 mg and **Tablets** each containing activated dimethicone 250 mg, dried aluminium hydroxide 400 mg, and magnesium hydroxide 400 mg. For gastric hyperacidity and flatulence. *Dose.* 5 to 30 ml of liquid, or 1 or 2 tablets, between meals and at bedtime.

Asilone *(Berk Pharmaceuticals, UK)*. **Gel** and **Suspension** containing in each 5 ml activated dimethicone 135 mg, dried aluminium hydroxide 420 mg, and light magnesium oxide 70 mg and **Tablets** each containing activated dimethicone 270 mg and dried aluminium hydroxide 500 mg. For dyspepsia, flatulence, and associated disorders. *Dose.* 5 to 10 ml or 1 or 2 tablets before meals and at bedtime.

Asilone for Infants *(Berk Pharmaceuticals, UK)*. Suspension containing in each 5 ml activated dimethicone 27 mg, dried aluminium hydroxide 84 mg, and light magnesium oxide 14 mg. *Dose.* Infants 1 to 3 months, 2.5 ml three or four times daily before or during feeds; older children, 5 ml three or four times daily before or during feeds.

Diloran *(Rona, UK)*. **Suspension** containing in each 10 ml activated dimethicone 25 mg, magnesium oxide 320 mg, and aluminium hydroxide-magnesium carbonate co-dried gel 80 mg and **Tablets** each containing activated dimethicone 25 mg, magnesium oxide 340 mg, and aluminium hydroxide-magnesium carbonate co-dried gel 85 mg. For gastric hyperacidity and flatulence. *Dose.* 10 to 20 ml of suspension or 1 or 2 tablets, sucked or chewed, thrice daily between meals and at bedtime.

Diovol *(Pharmax, UK)*. **Suspension** containing in each 5 ml dimethicone 25 mg, aluminium hydroxide 200 mg, and magnesium hydroxide 200 mg. **Tablets** each containing dimethicone 25 mg, aluminium hydroxide-magnesium carbonate co-dried gel 300 mg, and magnesium hydroxide 100 mg. For gastric hyperacidity and flatulence. *Dose.* 10 to 20 ml of suspension thrice daily, or 1 or 2 tablets, chewed or sucked, as required; children, 6 to 12 years, half the adult dose.

Dow Corning 360 Medical Fluid *(Dow Corning, UK)*. A brand of dimethicone, available in 8 viscosity grades ranging from 20 to 12 500 centistokes. For use as a lubricant and for protection of the skin.

Dow Corning Antifoam M Compound *(Dow Corning, UK)*. A pharmaceutical grade of dimethicone blended with silicon dioxide, with a viscosity of 2500 to 3500 cP. **Dow Corning Antifoam M 30 Emulsion** contains 30% of Dow Corning Antifoam M Compound.

Dow Corning Silastic Foam Dressing *(Dow Corning, UK)*. A liquid silicone preparation containing stannous octoate as a curing agent, forming in use a spongy elastomer. For the management of open granulating wounds.

Phazyme *(Stafford-Miller, UK)*. Tablets each containing, in an outer layer, activated dimethicone 20 mg and, in a coated core for release in the duodenum, activated dimethicone 40 mg and pancreatin containing 480 *B.P.*

units of amylase activity, 240 *B.P.* units of lipase activity, and 50 *B.P.* units of protease activity. For discomfort due to gastro-intestinal gas. *Dose.* 1 or 2 tablets with meals and at night.

Polyalk *(Galen, UK).* **Gel** and **Suspension** both containing in each 5 ml activated dimethicone 125 mg, dried aluminium hydroxide 440 mg and light magnesium oxide 70 mg and **Tablets** each containing activated dimethicone 250 mg and dried aluminium hydroxide 500 mg. Antacid and antiflatulent. *Dose.* 5 to 10 ml of suspension or 1 or 2 tablets, sucked or chewed, before meals and at bedtime if required.

Polycrol *(Nicholas, UK).* **Gel** containing in each 5 ml activated dimethicone 25 mg, aluminium hydroxide mixture 4.75 ml, and magnesium hydroxide 100 mg. **Forte Gel** containing in each 5 ml activated dimethicone 125 mg, aluminium hydroxide mixture 4.75 ml, and magnesium hydroxide 100 mg. **Tablets** each containing activated dimethicone 25 mg, aluminium hydroxide-magnesium carbonate co-dried gel 275 mg, and magnesium hydroxide 100 mg. **Forte Tablets** each containing activated dimethicone 250 mg, aluminium hydroxide-magnesium carbonate co-dried gel 275 mg, and magnesium hydroxide 100 mg. For gastro-intestinal disorders. *Dose.* 5 to 10 ml of gel or 1 or 2 tablets, chewed or sucked, thrice daily after meals.

Repelcote *(Hopkin & Williams, UK).* A 2% solution of dimethyldichlorosilane in trichloroethane. For the silicone treatment of glassware; no baking is required.

Rikospray Silicone *(Riker, UK).* An aerosol containing aldioxa 0.5% and cetylpyridinium chloride 0.02%, in a basis of dimethicone '1000'. For bedsores and napkin rash and for colostomy hygiene.

Silastic 382 Medical Grade Elastomer *(Dow Corning, UK).* An elastomer base composed of dimethicone and silicon dioxide with a curing agent containing stannous octoate. For the fabrication of surgical implants and prostheses. **Silastic Medical Adhesive Silicone Type A** bonds silicone elastomer to itself and to other materials. **Dow Corning Medical Adhesive B Spray** bonds ostomy appliances, prostheses, and dressings to the skin. **Dow Corning 355 Medical Adhesive.** A liquid form of Medical Adhesive B for use with a brush. **Dow Corning Remover** removes Dow Corning Medical Adhesive B from the skin and other materials.

Silicone Fluids F 111 *(ICI Organics, UK).* A brand of dimethicone available in 11 viscosity grades ranging from 20 to 100 000 centistokes.

Siloxyl *(Concept Pharmaceuticals, UK).* **Tablets** each containing activated dimethicone 250 mg and dried aluminium hydroxide 500 mg. **Suspension.** Contains in each 5 ml activated dimethicone 125 mg, dried aluminium hydroxide 420 mg, and light magnesium oxide 70 mg. Antacid and antiflatulent. *Dose.* 5 to 10 ml of suspension or 1 to 2 tablets, sucked or chewed, between meals and at bedtime; children, 5 ml of suspension.

Siopel Cream *(ICI Pharmaceuticals, UK).* An oil-in-water cream containing dimethicone 10%, with cetrimide 0.3%. For protection of the skin in occupational dermatoses and incontinence, and in colostomy and similar conditions. (Also available as Siopel in *S.Afr.*).

Sprilon (known in some countries as Evalgan or Silon) *(Pharmacia, UK: Farillon, UK).* A pressurised spray containing dimethicone 1.2 g, zinc oxide 14.4 g, and ointment basis to 60 g. For eczema and leg ulcers, the prevention of bedsores, and protection of the skin in incontinence.

Stuart Silicone Protective *(Stuart, UK).* A pressurised spray containing castor oil 1%, terpineol 1%, and dimethicone, with propellent. For bedsores.

Sylopal *(Norton, UK: Vestric, UK).* Suspension containing dimethicone 125 mg, light magnesium oxide 70 mg, and aluminium hydroxide mixture to 5 ml. For gastric hyperacidity and flatulence. *Dose.* 5 to 10 ml before food and at bedtime.

Translet Skin Cream (formerly known as Ostomy Plus Three) *(Franklin Medical, UK).* Contains dimethicone 2.5%, stearic acid 18.5%, liquid paraffin 3.2%, glyceryl monostearate 0.5%, propylene glycol alginate 0.5%, and glycerol 2.1%. For protection of the skin in colostomy and similar conditions.

Unigest *(Unigreg, UK: Vestric, UK).* Capsules each containing dimethicone '500' 250 mg, aluminium hydroxide 50 mg, magnesium carbonate 50 mg, and magnesium hydroxide 100 mg. For flatulence and dyspepsia. *Dose.* 1 or 2 capsules, swallowed whole, after meals and at bedtime.

Vasogen *(Pharmax, UK).* Cream containing dimethicone 20%, zinc oxide 7.5%, and calamine 1.5% in an oil-in-water emulsion. For bedsores, napkin rash, and dermatoses.

Other Proprietary Names of Silicones

Arg.—Carbogasol Liquido, Factor A-G Comprimidos; *Austral.*—Dermafilm, Infacol, Mylicon, Skin Repair; *Belg.*—Polysilon Gel; *Canad.*—Barriere, Ovol; *Denm.*—Aeropax, Ceolat, Heydogen, Mylicon, Silan; *Fr.*—Polysilane, Siligaz; *Ger.*—Bicolon, Ceolat, Endo-Paractol, Lefax, Sab Simplex; *Ital.*—Kestomatine, Mylicon, Silican; *Jap.*—Dipoxane; *Neth.*—Aeropax, Ceolat, Disflatyl, Meteorex; *Norw.*—Ceolat, Minifom, Siloxan; *Spain*—Aero-Red, Aerosilane, Enterosilicona, Kestomal Infantil, Nogasilan; *Swed.*—Minifom; *Switz.*—Aeropax, Ceolat, Heydogen; *USA*—Mylicon, Silain.

Dimethicone or activated dimethicone were also formerly marketed in Great Britain under the proprietary names Lancepol Paediatric (*Lancet Pharmaceuticals*, now *Kirby-Warrick*) and Polycrol S (*Nicholas*).

Preparations containing silicones were also formerly marketed in Great Britain under the proprietary names Mylanta (*Parke, Davis*), Silicone 555 (*Aerosol Marketing & Chemical Co.*), Silocalm (*Concept Pharmaceuticals*), Simeco (*Wyeth*), and Syl (*Reckitt & Colman Pharmaceuticals*).

6429-f

Spermaceti *(B.P.C. 1968).* Cetaceum; Blanc de Baleine; Cire de Cachalot; Walrat; Esperma de Ballena; Espermacete.

CAS — 8002-23-1.

Pharmacopoeias. In *Arg., Aust., Belg., Cz., Fr., Ger., Hung., It., Jug., Nord., Pol., Port., Roum., Span., Swiss,* and *Turk.*

A solid wax obtained from the mixed oils from the head, blubber, and carcase of the sperm whale, *Physeter catodon* (=*P. macrocephalus*) (Physeteridae), and the bottle-nosed whale, *Hyperoödon rostratus* (Ziphiidae).

Translucent, crystalline, pearly-white, unctuous masses with little odour and taste. It consists mainly of cetyl palmitate and cetyl myristate; at least 70% of the alcohols present are cetyl alcohol and not more than 10% of the fatty acids are stearic and higher acids. M.p. 44° to 52°. Sp. gr. about 0.94. It is readily inflammable and burns with a bright, somewhat sooty flame.

Practically **insoluble** in water and cold alcohol; soluble 1 in 20 of boiling alcohol, 1 in 2.5 of chloroform, and 1 in 7 of ether; soluble in carbon disulphide and in fixed and volatile oils; slightly soluble in cold light petroleum.

Composition. An accurate description of the composition of spermaceti, based on thin-layer and gas chromatography, would be a mixture of hexadecyl (cetyl) esters of fatty acids between C_{26} and C_{38} with cetyl laurate, cetyl myristate, cetyl palmitate, and cetyl stearate comprising at least 85% of the total esters.— P. J. Holloway, *J. Pharm. Pharmac.*, 1968, *20*, 775.

6430-z

Cetyl Esters Wax *(U.S.N.F.).* Synthetic Spermaceti.

Pharmacopoeias. In *U.S.N.F.*

A mixture consisting primarily of esters of saturated fatty alcohols (C_{14} to C_{18}) and saturated fatty acids (C_{14} to C_{18}). White to off-white translucent flakes with a crystalline structure and a pearly lustre when caked; it has a faint odour and a bland taste. M.p. 43° to 47°. Practically **insoluble** in water and cold alcohol; soluble in chloroform, ether, fixed and volatile oils, and boiling alcohol. **Store** in a dry place at a temperature not exceeding 40°.

Uses. Spermaceti has been used as an ingredient of some cold creams; a synthetic version is now used.

Preparations

Cold Cream *(U.S.P.).* Cetyl esters wax 12.5 g, white beeswax 12 g, liquid paraffin 56 g, borax 500 mg, water 19 ml. For other formulas for cold creams, see Beeswax (p.1065) and Rose Oil (p.682).

Proprietary Preparations

Crodamol SS *(Croda, UK).* A brand of cetyl esters wax.

Cyclol SPS *(Witco, UK).* A brand of cetyl esters wax.

6431-c

Squalane *(U.S.N.F.).* Cosbiol; Dodecahydrosqualene; Perhydrosqualène; Spinacane. 2,6,10,15,19,23-Hexamethyltetracosane. $C_{30}H_{62}$=422.8.

CAS — 111-01-3.

Pharmacopoeias. In *Fr.* Also in *U.S.N.F.*

A saturated hydrocarbon obtained by hydrogenation of squalene, an aliphatic dihydrotriterpene occurring in certain fish oils, particularly shark-liver oil from which a commercial grade of squalane is obtained by direct hydrogenation.

It is a colourless, almost odourless and tasteless, inert, transparent, oily liquid, non-drying and not liable to rancidity. Specific gravity 0.807 to 0.810.

Practically **insoluble** in water; very slightly soluble in dehydrated alcohol; soluble in chloroform, ether, light petroleum, and oils; slightly soluble in acetone, glacial acetic acid, and methyl alcohol.

Uses. Squalane is miscible with human sebum of which it may possibly be a constituent. It is used as an ingredient of ointment bases to which it imparts increased skin permeability.

A comparison of the properties and toxicity of squalane and a synthetic substitute, hydrogenated polyisobutene (Polysynlane).— T. R. Davis, *Cosmet. Toilet.*, 1976, *91* (Jan.), 33.

Proprietary Preparations

Dermalex Skin Lotion *(Dermalex, UK).* Contains squalane 3%, hexachlorophane 0.5%, and allantoin 0.25%. For prevention of bedsores and for incontinence rash.

For a double-blind study of the use of Dermalex Skin Lotion in the prevention of pressure sores, see M. F. Green *et al.*, *Mod. Geriat.*, 1974, *4*, 376.

Natuderm *(Burgess, UK).* An emollient cream with a lipid component stated to be similar in composition to human sebum.

Initial experience with Natuderm, a new skin film emulsion analogue cream.— A. R. Maisley and J. H. R. Brook, *Br. J. clin. Pract.*, 1980, *34*, 178.

Robane *(Robeco Chemicals, USA: Anstead, UK).* A brand of purified squalane.

6432-k

Stearyl Alcohol *(U.S.N.F.).* Octadecyl Alcohol; Alcool Stéarylique.

CAS — 112-92-5.

Pharmacopoeias. In *Fr. It.,* and *Jap.* Also in *U.S.N.F.*

A mixture of solid aliphatic alcohols. The *U.S.N.F.* specifies not less than 90% of stearyl alcohol $C_{18}H_{37}OH$, the remainder consisting chiefly of related alcohols.

White unctuous flakes or granules with a faint characteristic odour and a bland taste. M.p. 55° to 60°. Practically **insoluble** in water; soluble in alcohol, chloroform, ether, and vegetable oils. **Store** in a cool place.

Adverse Effects. Stearyl alcohol may occasionally cause contact dermatitis.

Reports of contact dermatitis.— *Drug Cosmet. Ind.*, 1974, *114* (May), 116; I. Pevny and M. Uhlich, *Hautarzt*, 1975, *26*, 252.

Uses. Stearyl alcohol has similar properties to and is used for the same purposes as cetyl alcohol (see p.1066), but it produces somewhat firmer preparations.

See also Higher Fatty Alcohols, p.1066.

Proprietary Preparations

Laurex 18 *(Albright & Wilson, Marchon Division, UK).* A brand of stearyl alcohol.

6433-a

Suet *(B.P.C. 1949).* Sevum; Prepared Suet; Mutton Suet; Sebum; Sebum Ovillum Depuratum; Suif de Mouton Purifié; Hammeltalg; Sebo.

CAS — 8022-87-5.

The purified internal fat of the abdomen of the sheep, *Ovis aries* (Bovidae). A firm, white, nearly odourless, unctuous fat with a bland taste.

Practically **insoluble** in water and cold alcohol; soluble 1 in 45 of boiling alcohol and 1 in 60 of ether. M.p. 45° to 50°. Becomes rancid and unfit for use on prolonged exposure to air.

6434-t

Beef Suet. Sebum Bovinum; Sevum Bovinum; Beef Tallow.

Pharmacopoeias. In *Jap.*

The purified internal fat of the ox, *Bos taurus* var. *domesticus* (Bovidae).

Uses. Suet and beef suet have been used in some countries in place of lard and benzoinated lard.

6435-x

Theobroma Oil *(B.P.).* Oleum Theobromatis; Ol. Theobrom.; Cacao Butter; Cocoa Butter *(U.S.N.F.)*; Oleum Cacao; Butyrum Cacao; Beurre de Cacao; Burro di Cacao; Manteca de Cacao; Manteiga de Cacau; Kakaobutter.

CAS — 8002-31-1.

Pharmacopoeias. In *Arg., Aust., Belg., Br., Cz., Ger., Hung., It., Jap., Jug., Mex., Neth., Nord., Pol., Port., Roum., Rus., Span., Swiss,* and *Turk.* Also in *U.S.N.F.*

A solid fat expressed from the roasted seeds of *Theobroma cacao* (Sterculiaceae). It is a yellowish-white, somewhat brittle solid, becoming white on keeping with a slight odour of cocoa and a bland characteristic taste. It is sometimes deodorised. M.p. 31° to 34°. It contains about 55% of oleopalmitostearin and up to 2% of theobromine.

Slightly **soluble** in alcohol; freely soluble in chloroform, ether, and light petroleum; soluble in boiling dehydrated alcohol. **Store** in a cool place and protect from light.

Uses. Theobroma oil is employed as a basis for suppositories, pessaries, and bougies. Theobroma oil exhibits polymorphism and if the basis is heated to more than 36° during preparation the solidification point will be appreciably lowered due to the formation of metastable states, leading to subsequent difficulty in setting.

Certain medicaments, such as phenol, chloral hydrate, and resorcinol, cause an appreciable lowering of the melting-point of theobroma oil when warmed with it. In preparing suppositories containing these, the melting-point may be brought back to normal by incorporating a little white beeswax. This addition may be avoided, except in the case of suppositories containing volatile oils, by using the minimum amount of heat.

In hot climates, it is customary to incorporate 5 to 15% of white beeswax according to the prevailing temperature.

Theobroma oil is sometimes an ingredient of emollient ointments and it is also used as a lubricant in massage.

It is a major ingredient of chocolate.

For information on other suppository bases, see under Hard Fat (p.1067), Glycerol (p.707), Macrogols (p.711), and Fractionated Palm Kernel Oil (p.1068).

6436-r

Wool Alcohols *(B.P.).* Wool Wax Alcohols; Lanolin Alcohols *(U.S.N.F.)*; Alcoholia Lanae; Alcolanum; Lanalcolum; Wollwachsalkohole.

CAS — 8027-33-6.

Pharmacopoeias. In *Aust., Br., Cz., Ger., Hung., Ind., Jug., Roum.,* and *Swiss.* Also in *U.S.N.F.*

A golden-brown solid, somewhat brittle when cold but plastic when warm, with a faint characteristic odour. The *B.P.* specifies m.p. not below 58°; the *U.S.N.F.* specifies not below 56°. It consists of the alcoholic fraction of the product obtained by saponification of the wool grease of the sheep, and contains not less than 30% of cholesterol. The *B.P.* specifies 500 to 1000 ppm of butylated hydroxyanisole or butylated hydroxytoluene as an antoxidant; the *U.S.N.F.* permits up to 1000 ppm of a suitable antoxidant. It also contains 10 to 13% of isocholesterol with other steroid and triterpene alcohols.

Practically **insoluble** in water; moderately soluble in alcohol; completely soluble 1 in 25 of boiling dehydrated alcohol; freely soluble in chloroform, ether, and light petroleum. **Store** at a temperature not exceeding 25° in airtight containers. Protect from light.

Adverse Effects. Wool alcohols sometimes has a slightly irritant action. Hypersensitivity may occur.

Of 4000 patients subjected to patch testing in 5 European clinics 2% of males and 3.1% of females showed positive reactions to wool alcohols 30% in soft paraffin.— H. Bandmann *et al., Archs Derm.,* 1972, *106,* 335.

Positive reactions to wool alcohols 30% in soft paraffin occurred in 31 (1.2%) of 2538 patients with eczema and suspected of having contact sensitivities.— M. Hannuksela *et al., Contact Dermatitis,* 1976, *2,* 105.

Uses. Wool alcohols is used in the preparation of Wool Alcohols Ointment and other ointments and is a good emulsifying agent for water-in-oil emulsions, since emulsions so made do not darken on the surface or acquire an objectionable odour in hot weather.

The addition of 5% of wool alcohols permits a threefold increase in the amount of water which can be incorporated in soft paraffin and such emulsions are not 'cracked' by the addition of weak acids; they may be improved and made more stable by the addition of cetostearyl alcohol. Proportions of wool alcohols up to 2.5% may also be added to oil-in-water emulsions to improve the texture, stability, and emollient properties.

A review of distilled wool alcohols.— E. W. Clark, *Drug Cosmet. Ind.,* 1968, *103* (Sept.), 46; *idem,* (Oct.), 74.

In 11 experiments, wool alcohols ointment did not suppress transepidermal water loss.— *Chemist Drugg.,* 1968, *190,* 534.

Preparations

Hydrous Ointment *(B.P.).* Oily Cream *(A.P.F.)*; Unguentum Aquosum; Ung. Aquos.; Wool Alcohols Cream. Wool alcohols ointment 50 g, phenoxyethanol 1 g, dried magnesium sulphate 500 mg, water 48.5 g.

Store at a temperature not exceeding 25° in non-absorbent containers. Any aqueous liquid which separates may be reincorporated by stirring. When hydrous ointment is used in a white ointment it should be prepared from wool alcohols ointment made with white soft paraffin and when used in a coloured ointment it should be prepared from wool alcohols ointment made with yellow soft paraffin.

A.P.F. has wool alcohols ointment (*A.P.F.*) 50% with freshly boiled and cooled water.

Addition of magnesium sulphate 0.5% enhanced the stability and appearance of Hydrous Ointment. Wool alcohols from different sources exerted only negligible effects on the stabilised creams. Further studies on the optimum concentration of magnesium sulphate and on suitable preservative systems were necessary.— Pharm. Soc. Lab. Rep. P/74/7, 1974.

Incompatibility. Hydrous ointment was incompatible with phenol 1%, ichthammol 5%, and coal tar solution 10%. Compatible with salicylic acid 10%, benzoic acid 10%, crude coal tar 15%, and ammoniated mercury 10%. Separation in 2 weeks occurred with ichthammol 1% and resorcinol 5 to 10%.— J. Ashley, *Australas. J. Pharm.,* 1955, *36,* 989.

Wool Alcohols Ointment *(B.P., Ind. P.).* Ung. Alcoh. Lan. Wool Alcohols 6%, with hard paraffin, white soft paraffin or yellow soft paraffin, and liquid paraffin. The proportions of the paraffins may be varied to produce an ointment having suitable properties. When wool alcohols ointment is used in a white ointment it should be prepared with white soft paraffin and when used in a coloured ointment it should be prepared with yellow soft paraffin. Store at a temperature not exceeding 25°.

A.P.F. has wool alcohols 6 g, hard paraffin 17 g, white soft paraffin 17 g, liquid paraffin 60 g.

Wool Alcohols Ointment *(Ger. P.).* Lanae Alcoholum Unguentum. Wool alcohols 6, cetostearyl alcohol 0.5, white soft paraffin 93.5.

Proprietary Preparations

See under Wool Fat.

6437-f

Wool Fat *(B.P.).* Adeps Lanae; Anhydrous Lanolin *(U.S.P.)*; Purified Lanolin; Refined Wool Fat; Cera Lanae; Lanoléine; Graisse de Suint Purifiée; Wollfett; Lanolina; Suarda; Wollwachs.

CAS — 8006-54-0.

Pharmacopoeias. In all pharmacopoeias examined except *Eur., Fr.,* and *Int.*

A pale yellow, tenacious, unctuous substance with a faint characteristic odour. It is the purified anhydrous waxy substance obtained from the wool of the sheep, *Ovis aries* (Bovidae). It consists mainly of fatty acid esters of cholesterol, lanosterol, and fatty alcohols. M.p. 36° to 44°. The *B.P.* permits not more than 200 ppm of butylated hydroxytoluene. 10 g absorbs not less than 20 ml of water.

Practically **insoluble** in water; sparingly soluble in cold alcohol; soluble 1 in about 75 of boiling alcohol; soluble in chloroform, ether, acetone, and carbon disulphide. It is **sterilised** by maintaining at 150° for 1 hour. **Store** at a temperature not exceeding 25°.

Technical Anhydrous Lanolin. A British Standard for technical anhydrous lanolin has been published (BS 3488: 1962).

Detergents in wool fat. Wool grease was normally recovered from wool by centrifuging woolscouring liquors. At one time soap was used and could be removed during refining, but it had been replaced by nonoxinol detergents which contaminated the grease and might remain in the lanolin after refining. Twenty commercial samples of wool grease contained from 0.55 to 2.4% of detergent, and this could affect their emulsifying properties.— C. A. Anderson *et al., J. Pharm. Pharmac.,* 1966, *18,* 809.

Adverse Effects. Wool fat may produce skin sensitisation.

A review of allergy to hydrous wool fat and wool alcohols.— R. Breit and H. -J. Bandmann, *Br. J. Derm.,* 1973, *88,* 414. See also *Br. med. J.,* 1973, *2,* 379.

Patch tests on 270 consecutive eczematous patients (130 females and 140 males) gave positive reactions to wool fat and/or wool alcohols in 14 (10.8%) of the females and 6 (4.3%) of the males.— K. Wereide, *Acta derm.-vener., Stockh.,* 1965, *45,* 15.

The incidence of specific allergy to hydrous wool fat in the general population was calculated to be no more than 9.7 per million.— E. W. Clark, *J. Soc. Cosmet. Chem.,* 1975, *26,* 323.

Positive reactions to hydrous wool fat occurred in 14 (0.6%) of 2538 patients with eczema and suspected of having contact sensitivities.— M. Hannuksela *et al., Contact Dermatitis,* 1976, *2,* 105.

Further references: E. Cronin, *Br. J. Derm.,* 1966, *78,* 167; A. A. Fisher *et al., Archs Derm.,* 1971, *104,* 286.

The allergens of wool fat appeared to be in the content of natural free fatty alcohols rather than in the total alcohols. The incidence of allergy was increased by the presence of detergent. A method is described for the removal of free fatty alcohols and detergent from wool fat.— E. W. Clark *et al.*, *Contact Dermatitis*, 1977, *3*, 69.

Uses. Wool fat resembles the sebaceous secretion of the human skin. By itself it is not readily absorbed, but when mixed with a suitable vegetable oil or with soft paraffin it gives emollient creams which penetrate the skin and thus facilitate the absorption of drugs. It does not readily become rancid.

Wool fat can absorb about 30% of water and is of value in the preparation of water-in-oil emulsions. Thus, by the addition of a small quantity of wool fat, soft or liquid paraffin can be formed into stable emulsions with water.

A number of derivatives and modifications of wool fat are available possessing properties similar to those of wool fat with certain advantages.

Liquid lanolin is a viscous liquid consisting of liquid esters derived by fractionation from wool fat; it blends well with both mineral and vegetable oils and is used as an emulsifying agent and emollient in skin creams and lotions. It is absorbed by the skin without the tackiness of wool fat.

Water-soluble lanolins are produced by reacting wool fat with ethylene oxide yielding polyoxyethylene derivatives, both liquid and solid. They give clear or slightly opalescent solutions in water and are used in cosmetic creams as emulsifying agents and emollients.

Hydrogenated wool fat is also available. It is a white odourless product free from stickiness but otherwise having similar properties to wool fat with water-absorbing capacity increased by about 50%.

In 4 experiments, wool fat did not suppress transepidermal water loss.— *Chemist Drugg.*, 1968, *190*, 534.

Proprietary Preparations of Wool Fat or Wool Fat Derivatives

Abracol VPX *(Bush Boake Allen, UK)*. An emulsifying agent based on a mixture of cholesterols and paraffins. It is used for producing water-in-oil emulsions and creams, the heat stability of which increases with the water content and with the addition of a small proportion of glycerol.

Acetadeps *(Westbrook, UK)*. A wax obtained by acetylation of wool fat. It is used as an oil-soluble emollient.

Acetulan *(Amerchol, USA: Anstead, UK)*. A liquid fraction of acetylated wool alcohols. It is an odourless, neutral, pale yellow liquid of low viscosity, soluble in alcohol, liquid paraffin, and vegetable oils, and is used for reducing greasiness and for improving spread and texture in emulsified and anhydrous systems.

Acylan *(Croda, UK)*. A brand of acetylated wool fat. It is a yellow unctuous solid with protective and emollient properties.

Albalan *(Westbrook, UK)*. A wax obtained from wool fat by the removal of the liquid components; it is used for producing heat-stable water-in-oil emulsions.

Amerchols *(Amerchol, USA: Anstead, UK)*. A range of surface-active emulsifying agents based on wool fat. **Amerchol C** is a semi-solid preparation used to assist release of active ingredients from ointment bases. **Amerchol CAB** is a solid preparation containing free sterols and higher alcohols; it is used as an emulsifying agent and as a component of anhydrous bases. **Amerchol H-9** is a soft solid preparation containing free sterols and higher alcohols; it is used as an emollient and emulsifying agent, particularly in burn ointments. **Amerchol L-101** is a liquid preparation containing free sterols and higher alcohols; it is used as a secondary emulsifying agent, stabiliser, and emollient in oil-in-water emulsions, and as a primary emulsifying agent for water-in-oil emulsions.

Amerlate LFA *(Amerchol, USA: Anstead, UK)*. A waxy solid consisting of lanolin acids; it is used as a wetting and dispersing agent for powders.

Amerlate P *(Amerchol, USA: Anstead, UK)*. The isopropyl esters of wool fat fatty acids. It is a soft butter-like solid with the properties of a pigment-dispersing agent, lubricant, conditioner, and moisturiser, and may be used as a supplementary water-in-oil emulsifying agent. **Amerlate W** is a similar product.

Aqualose *(Westbrook, UK)*. A range of water-soluble derivatives of wool fat, including ethoxylated wool fat (**Aqualose L30** and **L75**), alkoxylated liquid lanolin (**Aqualose LL100**), ethoxylated wool alcohols (**Aqualose W20**), and solubilised unmodified wool fat (**Aqualose SLW** and **SLT**). **Aqualose L75/50** and **Aqualose W20/50** are 50% aqueous solutions of the anhydrous derivatives.

Argobase *(Westbrook, UK)*. A range of absorption bases consisting of wool fat or wool alcohols blended with inert hydrocarbons. They are good emollient emulsifying agents, and are available in the following grades: **L1**, a liquid basis; **S1**, a solid basis with m.p. of 31 to 38°; and **EU**, a brand of Wool Alcohols Ointment. **Argobase 125.** A solution of wool alcohols in light liquid paraffin.

Argonol *(Westbrook, UK)*. A range of liquid lanolins in the following grades: **Argonol 40** is a partially modified liquid fraction of wool fat; **Argonol 60** and **Argonol 50 Super** are liquid fractions of wool fat; **Argonol ACE 2**and **Argonol ACE 5** consist principally of acetylated wool alcohols; **Argonol ISO** is a blend of wool fat, wool alcohols, and isopropyl esters; **Argonol RIC-2** is a blend of wool fat, and esters of ricinoleic acid, with some free alcohols of high mol. wt. All are oil-soluble emollients.

Argowax *(Westbrook, UK)*. Brands of wool alcohols.

Corona and Coronet *(Croda, UK)*. Brands of wool fat.

Cremba *(Croda, UK)*. An absorption base consisting of a mixture of cholesterol-rich extracts of hydrous wool fat and inert hydrocarbon bases. It is an emollient emulsifying agent producing water-in-oil emulsions.

Crestalan *(Croda, UK)*. A range of greaseless emollients derived from fractionated liquid lanolin and isopropyl esters. They are pale yellow liquids with a faint odour.

Crodalan AWS *(Croda, UK)*. A surface-active emollient based on acetylated ethoxylated wool alcohols; it is used as an oil-in-water emulsifying agent. **Crodalan LA.** A brand of acetylated wool alcohols. It is a clear yellow liquid, free from stickiness, with emollient properties.

Crodalan IPL *(Croda, UK)*. An emollient consisting of isopropyl esters of fractionated wool fat acids; available as a yellow liquid or a soft yellow paste.

Fluicol *(Croda, UK)*. A nonionic liquid containing segregation products of wool alcohols; for the preparation of water-in-oil emulsions and as a stabiliser or emollient in oil-in-water emulsions.

Fluilan *(Croda, UK)*. A brand of liquid lanolin. Soluble in mineral and vegetable oils and used for preparing water-in-oil emulsions and as a stabiliser in oil-in-water emulsions. **Fluilanol** is a brand of nonionic self-emulsifying liquid lanolin.

Golden Fleece *(Westbrook, UK)*. A range of wool fats.

Hartolan and Super Hartolan *(Croda, UK)*. Brands of wool alcohols. Super Hartolan has a m.p. between 60° and 70°.

Hartolite *(Croda, UK)*. A blend of wool alcohols and liquid paraffin. It is used as a water-in-oil emulsifying agent for making heat-stable emulsions.

Isocreme Absorption Base *(Croda, UK)*. A product of similar composition and with similar uses to Cremba.

Iscolan *(Croda, UK)*. An emollient based on isostearyl alcohol and wool fat acids. It is a pale yellow liquid.

Lanesta *(Westbrook, UK)*. A range of isopropyl esters of wool fat acids. **Lanesta L** is a pale yellow liquid, soluble in oils and alcohol; **Lanesta P** is a yellow butter-like solid with a faint odour; **Lanesta S** is a pale yellow, almost odourless, soft paste, tending to separate slightly. All have high emollient, penetrative, and moisturising properties.

Lanexol AWS *(Croda, UK)*. A brand of alkoxylated liquid lanolin. It is a viscous amber liquid soluble in alcohol and water.

Lanocerin *(Amerchol, USA: Anstead, UK)*. A wax obtained from wool fat; it is used as an emulsion stabiliser.

Lanogels *(Amerchol, USA: Anstead, UK)*. A range of nonionic surfactants derived from wool fat.

Lanogene (sometimes described as lanolin oil) *(Amerchol, USA: Anstead, UK)*. A wax-free oil-soluble fraction of wool fat. **Isopropylan 33** is a mixture of Lanogene and isopropyl esters of lanolin acids.

Lanolin Deodorized AAA Anhydrous *(Amerchol, USA: Anstead, UK)*. A soft grade of lanolin.

Liquid Base 3896 *(Croda, UK)*. A similar product to Fluicol.

Modulan *(Amerchol, USA: Anstead, UK)*. A brand of acetylated wool fat consisting of a pale yellow, almost odourless, unctuous solid melting at 30° to 40°, approximating human skin fats. It is soluble in oils and is used as a hypoallergenic hydrophobic emollient and superfatting agent in aerosols, soaps, and oil-in-water emulsions.

OHlan *(Amerchol, USA: Anstead, UK)*. A waxy solid obtained by hydroxylation of wool fat. It is used as an emulsifying agent and stabiliser in water-in-oil emulsions.

Polychols *(Croda, UK)*. A range of water-dispersible or water-soluble ethoxylated wool alcohols; used as oil-in-water emulsifying agents and as solubilising, gelling, and dispersing agents.

Polylan *(Amerchol, USA: Anstead, UK)*. An oily liquid consisting of polyunsaturated esters of wool alcohols and linoleic acid; it is used as an emollient and lubricant.

Satulan *(Croda, UK)*. Hydrogenated wool fat. It is a white odourless fatty substance, free from stickiness, with emollient and emulsifying properties similar to wool fat.

Sebase *(Westbrook, UK)*. An anhydrous self-emulsifying cream basis consisting of ethoxylated wool fat derivatives with emulsifiers, emollients, lubricants, and stabilisers. It is a soft, pale yellow, almost odourless, waxy solid; it melts to a clear liquid, and forms stable oil-in-water emulsions (pH about 5) with all proportions of water.

Solan E *(Croda, UK)*. A polyoxyethylene derivative of wool fat giving clear solutions with water.

Solulans *(Amerchol, USA: Anstead, UK)*. A range of polyoxyethylene derivatives of wool fat or wool alcohols, some wholly or partially acetylated. They are non-greasy clear liquids or waxy solids, soluble in water, alcohol, and some oils, and are used for their emollient properties in external preparations. **Solulans PB.** A range of propylene oxide derivatives of wool alcohols, with emollient properties.

White Swan *(Croda, UK)*. A brand of wool fat.

Yeoman *(Croda, UK)*. A brand of wool fat.

Other Proprietary Names of Wool Fat or Wool Fat Derivatives

Eucerin *(Austral.)*.

Wool fat derivatives were also formerly marketed in Great Britain under the proprietary names Alcolose W2, Argonol LIN (both *Westbrook*), and Lanex (*Croda*).

6438-d

Hydrous Wool Fat *(B.P.)*. Adeps Lanae Hydrosus; Lanolin *(U.S.P.)*; Hydrous Lanolin; Cera Lanae cum Aqua; Lanoléine Hydratée; Graisse de Suint Hydratée; Lanolina Hidratada.

Pharmacopoeias. In *Br., Braz., Cz., Ind., It., Jap., Neth., Nord., Pol., Roum., Rus.*, and *U.S.* Various water contents are specified.
Aust. has wool fat 70, liquid paraffin 10, and water 20. *Ger.* has wool fat 65, liquid paraffin 15, and water 20. *Span.* has wool fat 65, olive oil 15, and water 20. *Swiss* has wool fat 70, olive oil 10, and water 20

A yellowish-white ointment basis prepared from wool fat 7 and water 3.

Practically **insoluble** in water; chloroform and ether dissolve only the fats it contains. More water, up to about equal weights of fat and water, may be incorporated in hydrous wool fat without affecting its consistency. **Store** at a temperature not exceeding 25° in airtight containers.

Adverse Effects. See under Wool Fat.

Uses. Hydrous wool fat is used as a component of ointment bases.

Preparations

Hydrous Wool Fat Ointment *(B.P.C. 1973)*. Unguentum Adipis Lanae Hydrosi. Equal parts of hydrous wool fat and yellow soft paraffin. It should be kept in containers which prevent evaporation.

Proprietary preparations of wool fats are described under Wool Fat, p.1072.

Parathyroid and Calcitonin

8050-t

Parathyroid hormone is a single-chain polypeptide isolated from the parathyroid glands. It contains 84 amino acids and in man the first 34 appear to be responsible for the hormonal activity. The amino-acid sequence varies according to the source.
Parathyroid hormone has a hypercalcaemic effect while calcitonin has a hypocalcaemic effect.

8051-x

Parathyroid Injection *(U.S.P.)*. Inj. Parathyroid; Parathyroid Extract; Parathyroid Solution; Parathyreoidinum pro Injectionibus.

CAS — 9002-64-6 (parathyroid hormone).

Pharmacopoeias. In *Mex.*, *Span.*, and *U.S.*

A sterile solution in Water for Injections of the water-soluble hormone from the parathyroid glands of mammals, which has the property of increasing the calcium content of the blood. pH 2.5 to 3.5. It possesses a potency per ml of not less than 100 *U.S.P.* parathyroid units, each unit representing one-hundredth of the amount required to raise the calcium content of 100 ml of the blood serum of normal dogs 1 mg within 16 to 18 hours after administration.
Parathyroid injection may be diluted with dextrose injection 2.5 to 5%. Sodium chloride solutions should not be used as they often cause precipitation. **Store** at 2° to 15° and avoid freezing.

Unit. 200 units of parathyroid hormone, bovine, for bioassay are contained in approximately 0.6 mg of freeze-dried trichloroacetic acid extract of bovine parathyroid glands, with lactose 5 mg in one ampoule of the first International Reference Preparation (1974).
2 units of parathyroid hormone, bovine, for immunoassay are contained in approximately 1 μg of freeze-dried purified isohormone I from bovine parathyroids, with albumin 200 μg and lactose 1 mg in one ampoule of the first International Reference Preparation (1974).
MRC and *U.S.P.* units are approximately equivalent to international units.

The preparation established as the first International Reference Preparation of parathyroid hormone, bovine, for bioassay had been widely used with an assigned potency approximately numerically equivalent to that of a pharmacopoeial preparation from one country and had been acceptable; it was defined on this basis. A more highly purified preparation, calibrated in terms of the International Reference Preparation, should be used in some assays to avoid anomalous results. In the absence of purified human parathyroid hormone a preparation of purified bovine parathyroid hormone which had proved useful for immunoassays was established as the reference preparation; it could be used only in suitable assay systems.— Twenty-sixth Report of the WHO Expert Committee on Biological Standardization, *Tech. Rep. Ser. Wld Hlth Org. No. 565*, 1975.

Adverse Effects. Overdosage with parathyroid causes an abnormally high concentration of calcium in the blood, the symptoms of which are weakness, anorexia, vomiting and diarrhoea; if treatment is maintained despite these signs, mobilised calcium may be deposited in soft tissues such as in the kidney, or further toxic effects of calcium excess may occur, possibly progressing to coma and death. Hypersensitivity reactions may occur.
See also under Calcium, Adverse Effects, p.619.

An immediate-type generalised reaction, consistent with anaphylaxis, occurred in one patient after the intravenous administration of bovine parathyroid hormone.— J. N. O'Rourke *et al.*, *J. Allergy & clin. Immunol.*, 1973, *52*, 56, per *J. Am. med. Ass.*, 1973, *226*, 492.

A report suggesting a relationship between high blood concentrations of parathyroid hormone and uraemic neuropathy.— M. M. Avram *et al.*, *New Engl. J. Med.*, 1978, *298*, 1000. Criticisms of the suggestion.— H. P. Sauerwein and R. T. Krediet (letter), *ibid.*, *299*, 362; A. I. Arieff and R. W. Schmidt (letter), *ibid.* Reply.— M. M. Avram *et al.* (letter), *ibid.*, 363.

Precautions. Parathyroid should be used with caution in patients with renal or cardiac disease. Skin tests for sensitisation should be carried out prior to intravenous administration.

Absorption and Fate. As parathyroid hormone is destroyed by proteolytic enzymes it is given by injection. Cleavage to peptide fragments occurs after administration, probably in the liver and kidney, and these fragments may still retain antigen activity although they are probably inactive as hormones. Less than 1% of the parathyroid hormone is excreted in the urine.
Although the half-life of parathyroid hormone has been reported to be only a few minutes, the onset of action is slow. It has been stated that the response may last up to 36 hours.

The clearance of bovine parathyroid hormone in normal subjects, anephric patients, and patients with chronic renal failure.— S. E. Papapoulos *et al.*, *Clin. Endocr.*, 1977, *7*, 211.

A discussion on the peripheral metabolism of parathyroid hormone.— K. J. Martin *et al.*, *New Engl. J. Med.*, 1979, *301*, 1092.

Uses. Parathyroid hormone is involved in the plasma-calcium balance. It also has actions on bone, kidney, and the gastro-intestinal tract. It increases bone resorption and stimulates production of 1,25-dihydroxycholecalciferol in the kidney. Renal excretion of inorganic phosphate is increased but overall that of calcium is decreased. It acts on the wall of the gut to increase absorption of calcium and phosphate and this is probably an indirect result of stimulating 1,25-dihydroxycholecalciferol production.
Parathyroid hormone has been used to raise the plasma-calcium concentration in acute hypoparathyroidism with tetany. It has no place in long-term treatment, which is carried out with vitamins of the D group (see p.1658). Tetany resulting from disturbances in metabolism unrelated to abnormal parathyroid function should not be treated with parathyroid preparations.
It has also been used as a diagnostic agent in the differential diagnosis of hypoparathyroidism and pseudo-hypoparathyroidism.
Parathyroid injection is usually given subcutaneously or intramuscularly, but in emergencies it may be given intravenously. The intramuscular route may be preferable.
In the acute tetany of hypoparathyroidism, a usual adult dose is 20 to 40 units every 12 hours. Its onset of action is slow, so that intravenous injection of calcium is necessary for immediate relief.
Parathyroid therapy must be used with caution to avoid excess of calcium in the blood and it is important that treatment should be controlled by frequent analyses of the serum calcium which should not be allowed to rise above 3.0 mmol per litre (120 μg per ml). Treatment should be discontinued as soon as symptoms of overdosage appear.

A review of the parathyroid glands: physiology, hypoparathyroidism, and hyperparathyroidism.— S. Tomlinson and J. L. H. O'Riordan, *Br. J. Hosp. Med.*, 1978, *19*, 40.

Resistance, demonstrated by the presence of antibodies, occurred in a woman who was hypoparathyroid following subtotal thyroidectomy and who was treated on several occasions with parathyroid extract.— R. A. Melick *et al.*, *New Engl. J. Med.*, 1967, *276*, 144.

Differential diagnosis of hypoparathyroidism. The differing effects of parathyroid extract, given as a single intravenous infusion, on urinary cyclic adenosine monophosphate excretion and on serum concentration of 1,25-dihydroxycholecalciferol, provided a clear distinction between 2 patients, one with surgical hypoparathyroidism and the other with pseudohypoparathyroidism.— R. S. Mason *et al.* (letter), *Ann. intern. Med.*, 1980, *92*, 260.

The effect of parathyroid extract, given as a single intravenous infusion, on the plasma concentration of 1,25-dihydroxycholecalciferol in 3 children; one had osteoporosis, the second suspected hypoparathyroidism, and the third hypophosphataemic rickets. The response may be useful as an investigational tool.— D. Aarskog and L. Aksnes (letter), *Lancet*, 1980, *1*, 362.

Osteoporosis. In 20 patients with severe vertebral crush fractures and 1 patient with a history of fractures of the long bones given synthetic human parathyroid hormone fragment (PTH 1-34) as once-daily subcutaneous injections for 6 to 24 months calcium and phosphate balances improved in some patients but there was no significant improvement overall. There were, however, substantial increases in iliac trabecular bone volume and this new bone was histologically normal. It was suggested that as vertebrae are normally more than 75% composed of trabecular bone this hormone fragment might usefully increase the strength of the vertebrae in patients with axial osteoporosis.— J. Reeve *et al.*, *Br. med. J.*, 1980, *280*, 1340; *ibid.*, *281*, 198. See also J. Reeve *et al.*, *Lancet*, 1976, *1*, 1035.

Synthetic fragments of human parathyroid hormone probably do not duplicate the biological effects of the intact hormone *in vivo*. Results in the treatment of involutional osteoporosis with human parathyroid hormone fragment (1-34) have been somewhat disappointing.— B. Frame and S. D. Rao, *Ann. intern. Med.*, 1980, *93*, 928.

Proprietary Names
Parathorm *(Hormonchemie, Ger.)*; Para-Thor-Mone *(Lilly, Austral.)*.

Parathyroid injection was formerly marketed in Great Britain under the proprietary name Para-Thor-Mone *(Lilly)*.

8052-r

Calcitonin. Thyrocalcitonin.

CAS — 9007-12-9.

A hormone, formed in the mammalian thyroid parafollicular cells and the ultimobranchial bodies in non-mammalian vertebrates, or obtained by synthesis, which has the property of lowering the calcium content of blood. It is a polypeptide containing 32 amino acids. The amino-acid sequence varies greatly from species to species.

8053-f

Calcitonin (Pork) *(B.P.)*. A polypeptide hormone of ultimobranchial origin extractable from pork thyroid. It has a molecular weight of about 3600. It contains not less than 60 units per mg calculated with reference to the dried material.

CAS — 12321-44-7.

Pharmacopoeias. In *Br.*

A white or almost white powder. It loses not more than 6% of its weight on drying. **Soluble** in water and in solutions of alkali hydroxides; practically insoluble in acetone, alcohol, chloroform, and ether; sparingly soluble in solutions of mineral acids. **Store** at a temperature not exceeding 25°. Protect from light. Under these conditions it may be expected to retain its potency for not less than 2 years. Solutions for injection should be used within 24 hours of preparation or, if stored at 2° to 10°, within 7 days.

8054-d

Salcatonin *(B.P.)*. Calcitonin (Salmon). A polypeptide having the structure of salmon calcitonin I. It contains not less than 4000 units per mg calculated with reference to the peptide con-

tent.

CAS — 47931-85-1.

Pharmacopoeias. In *Br.*

A white fluffy powder containing not less than 80% of peptide, not more than 15% of acetic acid, and not more than 10% of water, and not more than 20% of acetic acid and water. **Soluble** at least 1 in 5 of water (pH 4 to 6); very slightly soluble in alcohol; soluble 1 in 10 of methyl alcohol; soluble in glacial acetic acid. A 1% solution has a pH of 4 to 6.

Store at 2° to 8°. Protect from light. Under these conditions it may be expected to retain its potency for not less than 2 years.

Units. One unit of calcitonin, porcine, for bioassay is contained in approximately 10 µg of freeze-dried purified porcine calcitonin, with mannitol 5 mg in one ampoule of the first International Reference Preparation (1974).

80 units of calcitonin, salmon, for bioassay are contained in approximately 20 µg of freeze-dried synthetic salmon calcitonin, with mannitol 2 mg in one ampoule of the first International Reference Preparation (1974).

One unit of calcitonin, human, for bioassay is contained in approximately 8.5 µg of freeze-dried synthetic human calcitonin peptide with mannitol 10 mg in one ampoule of the first International Reference Preparation (1978).

Potency is estimated by comparing the hypocalcaemic effect, in *rats*, with that of the standard preparation, and is expressed in international or MRC units which are considered to be equivalent. Calcitonin activity has also been expressed in terms of the Hammersmith unit (1 international unit is approx. equivalent to 1000 Hammersmith units) and the Hirsch unit (1 international unit is approx. equivalent to 100 Hirsch units).

Adverse Effects, Treatment, and Precautions. Calcitonin (pork) or salcatonin may cause tingling or flushing of the face or extremities; gastro-intestinal disturbances may also occur. These side-effects usually settle as treatment progresses. An unpleasant taste, inflammatory reactions at the injection site, skin rash, and disturbances of glucose metabolism have been reported. Circulating antibodies may develop but resistance to treatment does not necessarily follow. Synthetic human calcitonin may be effective in overcoming resistance to other calcitonins.

In patients with a history of allergy a skin test with a 1:100 dilution should be performed before administration.

Calcitonin should be used with caution during pregnancy. It is better avoided during lactation.

Troublesome side-effects may be reduced by administration at bed-time or by prior administration of an anti-emetic.

Hypomagnesaemia in 2 children with osteogenesis imperfecta during treatment with salcatonin. In one child the side-effect appeared to be dose-related. The second child had other electrolyte imbalances, but also intercurrent infection and vomiting.— G. P. August *et al., J. Pediat.*, 1977, *91*, 1001.

Antibodies developed within 3 to 18 months in 11 of 16 patients with Paget's disease of bone treated for a mean of 29 months with salcatonin, but antibody titres later fell in 9 of the 11. The development of antibodies was only rarely the cause of clinical resistance.— N. J. Y. Woodhouse *et al., Br. med. J.*, 1977, *2*, 927.

Formation of antibodies to synthetic human calcitonin during treatment of Paget's disease.— F. M. Dietrich *et al., Acta endocr., Copenh.*, 1979, *92*, 468. Human calcitonin produced a hypocalcaemic response in 5 patients with Paget's disease of bone who had serum antibodies to salcatonin.— S. Rojanasathit *et al., Lancet*, 1974, *2*, 1412.

Pizotifen to prevent side-effects of calcitonin.— A. J. Crisp (letter), *Lancet*, 1981, *1*, 775.

Effect on glucose metabolism. Blood-sugar concentrations were increased by salcatonin in 9 patients.— A. Gattereau *et al.* (letter), *Lancet*, 1977, *2*, 1076. It was very unlikely that calcitonin would cause diabetes mellitus.— I. M. A. Evans *et al.* (letter), *ibid.*, 1978, *1*, 280.

A report of marked deterioration in control in a previously well controlled diabetic during treatment with porcine calcitonin.— D. W. Thomas *et al.* (letter), *Med. J. Aust.*, 1979, *2*, 699.

Further references.— J. Blahos *et al., Endokrinologie*, 1976, *68*, 226.

Interactions. In 7 healthy men the diuresis and natriuresis induced by calcitonin were significantly reduced when indomethacin 25 mg four times daily was given for a week.— D. B. Barnett *et al., Br. med. J.*, 1975, *3*, 686.

The addition of salcatonin to hydrochlorothiazide treatment for idiopathic hypercalciuria reduced serum potassium concentrations and these were not increased to usual values when potassium supplements were given by mouth. Serum potassium should be monitored regularly in such patients.— W. C. Sturtridge *et al., Can. med. Ass. J.*, 1977, *117*, 1031.

Absorption and Fate. Degradation of calcitonin occurs mainly in the kidneys. A small proportion of any injected dose is excreted in the urine. Calcitonin is reported not to cross the placenta.

The distribution and clearance of calcitonin in *animals* and man.— H. P. J. Bennett and C. McMartin, *Pharmac. Rev.*, 1978, *30*, 247.

The metabolic clearance-rate of synthetic human calcitonin was studied in 13 normal patients and 13 uraemic patients. The plasma clearance of calcitonin appeared to involve 3 exponential functions with calculated half-lives of 2.8, 11.5, and 317.8 minutes. In uraemic patients the calculated half-lives of these 3 components were 4.5, 22.5, and 1564.3 minutes.— R. Ardaillou *et al., J. clin. Invest.*, 1970, *49*, 2345.

Maximum plasma concentrations occurred about 30 minutes after subcutaneous administration of synthetic human calcitonin 100 units to patients with osteitis deformans.— J. C. Stevenson and I. M. A. Evans, *Drugs*, 1981, *21*, 257.

Uses. Calcitonin has a hypocalcaemic action due to inhibition of bone resorption. Naturally-occurring porcine calcitonin and synthetic salmon calcitonin (salcatonin) are in clinical use and salcatonin is the more potent. Synthetic human calcitonin is also being used and would be expected to have a lower antigenicity than the other two forms.

Calcitonins are used in the treatment of selected patients with diseases characterised by bone resorption and re-formation, such as osteitis deformans (Paget's disease of bone). They are also used for hypercalcaemia from a variety of causes including vitamin D intoxication, neoplastic disease, thyrotoxicosis, and hyperparathyroidism.

Biochemical improvement may be monitored by measurement of serum-alkaline phosphatase and urinary-hydroxyproline excretion values; dosage may be reduced as these values fall.

In osteitis deformans the usual dose range for calcitonin (pork) by subcutaneous or intramuscular injection is 80 units thrice weekly to 160 units daily. For salcatonin given by similar routes the range is 50 units thrice weekly to 100 units daily.

In the treatment of hypercalcaemia calcitonin (pork) up to 4 units per kg body-weight may be given by intramuscular or subcutaneous injection according to the patient's needs. It has also been given intravenously in doses of 50 to 100 units. Plasma-calcium concentrations should be monitored during treatment. Salcatonin has been given in doses of up to 400 units every 6 to 8 hours by subcutaneous or intramuscular injection; another suggested regimen is 4 units per kg body-weight given every 12 hours, increased if necessary to a maximum of 8 units per kg every 6 hours. Doses greater than 8 units per kg are considered to have no additional benefit.

Other calcitonin analogues or derivatives have also been prepared for investigation.

A review of calcitonin.— L. A. Austin and H. Heath, *New Engl. J. Med.*, 1981, *304*, 269. See also L. J. Deftos and B. P. First, *Ann. intern. Med.*, 1981, *95*, 192.

Some relief of bone-pain was observed during long-term administration of calcitonin (pork) to patients suffering from neoplastic osteolysis.— T. Barreca *et al., Curr. ther. Res.*, 1979, *26*, 644..

Salcatonin 60 to 120 µg daily had a beneficial influence on the clinical course of 51 patients with acute pancreatitis compared to 52 similar patients used as controls.— F. Paul *et al., Dt. med. Wschr.*, 1979, *104*, 615.

Action. For the role of calcitonin in the control of blood calcium, see K. J. Catt, *Lancet*, 1970, *2*, 255.

Reports and comments on the physiological role of calcitonin and the influence of sex, race, and age upon it.— C. J. Hillyard *et al., Lancet*, 1978, *1*, 961 (lower plasma concentrations in women than in men); I. Holló (letter), *ibid.*, 1362; H. Heath (letter), *ibid.*; I. MacIntyre *et al.* (letter), *ibid.*, 1978, *2*, 158; T. Cundy *et al.* (letter), *ibid.*, 159; J. C. Stevenson and C. J. Hillyard (letter), *Lancet*, 1979, *2*, 694; L. J. Deftos *et al., New Engl. J. Med.*, 1980, *302*, 1351 (influence of age and sex); A. J. Padilla (letter), *ibid.*, *303*, 821; L. J. Deftos (letter), *ibid.*, 822.

Studies and comments on the possible physiological role of calcitonin in pregnancy.— J. C. Stevenson *et al., Lancet*, 1979, *2*, 769; R. Kumar *et al., New Engl. J. Med.*, 1980, *302*, 1143; J. Kovarik *et al.* (letter), *Lancet*, 1980, *1*, 199.

A study of histological and biochemical indexes of bone turnover in 27 nephrectomised patients receiving haemodialysis; evidence that endogenous calcitonin might have a possible role in renal osteodystrophy.— J. A. Kanis *et al., New Engl. J. Med.*, 1977, *296*, 1073. Comment.— J. F. Habener and A. L. Schiller, *ibid.*, 1112. Further comments.— H. S. Grunstein *et al.* (letter), *ibid.*, *297*, 401; F. Quarto di Palo (letter), *ibid.*, 402. Reply.— J. A. Kanis *et al.* (letter), *ibid.* See also K. L. Becker *et al.* (letter), *ibid.*, 403.

Hypercalcaemia. Control of hypercalcaemia in multiple myeloma using calcitonin injections in association with administration of inorganic phosphate solution by mouth.— N. Brautbar and R. Luboshitzky, *Archs intern. Med.*, 1977, *137*, 914.

The effect of synthetic human calcitonin 2 mg six-hourly by continuous intravenous infusion for 48 hours on hypercalcaemia in 10 patients with metastatic breast cancer. A sustained fall in serum-calcium concentrations was seen in 8 of the 10 who had bony metastases, and this reduction continued in 4 when changed to other treatment.— T. D. Koelmeyer *et al., N.Z. med. J.*, 1978, *87*, 434.

Calcitonin produces a rapid fall in serum-calcium concentrations and an early indication of a likely response can be obtained from the fall in the 6 hours after the first injection. However, about one fifth of patients are reported not to respond and reductions of more than 0.7 mmol of calcium per litre are considered unusual even in severe hypercalcaemia. Alternative treatment should be tried early in the seriously ill patient if there is no response to calcitonin.— *Br. med. J.*, 1980, *280*, 204.

Further references to the use of calcitonins in hypercalcaemia.— O. L. Silva and K. L. Becker, *Archs intern. Med.*, 1973, *132*, 337; C. R. Paterson, *Postgrad. med. J.*, 1974, *50*, 158; A. R. Behn and T. E. T. West, *Br. med. J.*, 1977, *1*, 755 (multiple myeloma); L. A. Wisneski *et al., Clin. Pharmac. Ther.*, 1978, *24*, 219; M. L. Binstock and G. R. Mundy, *Ann. intern. Med.*, 1980, *93*, 269 (malignant disease: given with prednisone).

Mental disorders. Salcatonin controlled 2 episodes of psychotic agitation with hyperthermia in one patient with malignant catatonia. The patient's condition might have been associated with increased concentrations of calcium.— J. S. Carmen and R. J. Wyatt (letter), *Lancet*, 1977, *2*, 1124.

Salcatonin administered to patients with primary psychotic disorders tended to worsen depression but to reduce agitation during the succeeding 24 hours.— J. S. Carman and R. J. Wyatt, *Archs gen. Psychiat.*, 1979, *36*, 72.

Osteitis deformans. The incidence, symptoms, and treatment of Paget's disease of bone.— R. Smith, *Br. med. J.*, 1977, *1*, 365. See also *Lancet*, 1978, *1*, 914.

Paget's disease of bone and its treatment, including a discussion of therapeutic aims, patient selection, and the choice of drug.— H. K. Ibbertson *et al., Drugs*, 1979, *18*, 33.

Reviews of calcitonins in the treatment of osteitis deformans.— *J. Am. med. Ass.*, 1975, *232*, 1156; *Br. med. J.*, 1975, *3*, 505; A. Avramides, *Clin. Orthop.*, 1977, *127*, 78; I. M. A. Evans, *Lancet*, 1979, *2*, 1232; J. C. Stevenson and I. M. A. Evans, *Drugs*, 1981, *21*, 257; D. J. Hosking, *Br. med. J.*, 1981, *283*, 686.

A metabolic study of 4 patients with osteitis deformans

showed that during treatment with salcatonin for periods of up to 19 months, calcium, phosphorus, and magnesium balances were not affected while bone turnover decreased.— D. G. Oreopoulos *et al.*, *Can. med. Ass. J.*, 1977, *116*, 851. See also W. C. Sturtridge *et al.*, *ibid.*, *117*, 1031.

Reports, studies, and discussions on calcitonins in the treatment of osteitis deformans and its complications.— J. DeRose *et al.*, *Am. J. Med.*, 1974, *56*, 858 (long-term subcutaneous self-administration); R. A. Melick *et al.*, *Br. med. J.*, 1976, *1*, 627 (improvement in a patient with spinal column involvement); A. Avramides *et al.*, *J. clin. Endocr. Metab.*, 1976, *42*, 459; T. J. Martin *et al.*, *Aust. N.Z. J. Med.*, 1977, *7*, 36 (porcine calcitonin); M. -H. Nicolle *et al.*, *Thérapie*, 1977, *32*, 603 (marked improvement in paraplegic symptoms with relapse on stopping porcine calcitonin); W. C. Sturtridge *et al.*, *Can. med. Ass. J.*, 1977, *117*, 1031 (sustained improvement in 40% to 50% of patients receiving salcatonin); W. E. Plehwe *et al.*, *Med. J. Aust.*, 1977, *1*, 577 (decrease in serum-alkaline phosphatase unrelated to clinical improvement); C. P. Williams *et al.*, *J. clin. Path.*, 1978, *31*, 1212 (histological and biochemical changes during treatment); *Med. Lett.*, 1978, *20*, 78 (disadvantages of salcatonin compared with disodium etidronate).

Administration. Although it was generally accepted that the treatment of Paget's disease [of bone] required large doses of calcitonin, 1 unit of calcitonin (pork) thrice weekly for 3 months followed by a gap of 2 months gives therapeutic results which compare favourably with published reports on large doses of calcitonin. Moreover side-effects do not occur with low dosage which has the further advantage of having practically no antigenicity.— G. Milhaud (letter), *Lancet*, 1978, *1*, 1153. Criticism.— I. M. A. Evans and I. MacIntyre (letter), *ibid.*, 213.

Combination therapy. Treatment of osteitis deformans with disodium etidronate and calcitonin.— D. J. Hosking *et al.*, *Lancet*, 1976, *1*, 615; I. MacIntyre *et al.* (letter), *ibid.*, 757; D. J. Hosking and O. L. M. Bijovet (letter), *ibid.*, 970.

Treatment of osteitis deformans with mithramycin and calcitonin.— A. G. Hadjipavlou *et al.*, *J. Bone Jt Surg.*, 1977, *59A*, 1045.

Deafness. In 10 patients with Paget's disease of bone treated with calcitonin (pork) or salcatonin progression of hearing loss was less than in 7 untreated patients.— L. R. Solomon *et al.*, *Br. med. J.*, 1977, *2*, 485. In a study of 13 patients with Pagetoid deafness treatment for 3 years with calcitonin was of no benefit.— G. S. Walker *et al.*, *Br. med. J.*, 1979, *2*, 364. See also P. M. G. B. Grimaldi *et al.*, *Br. med. J.*, 1975, *2*, 726.

Human calcitonin. A review of human calcitonin in osteitis deformans.— F. R. Singer, *Clin. Orthop.*, 1977, *127*, 86.

Calcitonin has a place in the treatment of the juvenile condition, hereditary bone dysplasia with hyperphosphatasaemia, which resembles adult Paget's disease. It is essential to use the non-antigenic human hormone, since treatment may be lifelong.— I. M. Evans, *Lancet*, 1979, *2*, 1232. See also F. H. Doyle *et al.*, *Br. J. Radiol.*, 1974, *47*, 9; V. Dunn *et al.*, *Am. J. Roentg.*, 1979, *132*, 541.

Further references.— N. J. Y. Woodhouse *et al.*, *Lancet*, 1971, *1*, 1139; *idem*, 1972, *2*, 992; F. H. Doyle *et al.*, *Br. J. Radiol.*, 1974, *47*, 1; P. B. Greenberg *et al.*, *Am. J. Med.*, 1974, *56*, 867.

Sarcoma. Porcine calcitonin was effective in controlling bone pain but appeared to have no effect on the progression of a sarcoma complicating Paget's disease in a 68-year-old man.— P. C. Bartley *et al.*, *Med. J. Aust.*, 1979, *1*, 99. A similar report.— I. G. Walton and J. A. Strong (letter), *Lancet*, 1973, *1*, 887.

Osteogenesis imperfecta. A discussion of the clinical presentation of osteogenesis imperfecta.— R. Smith, *Br. med. J.*, 1977, *1*, 365.

Fifty patients, 48 of them children from 6 months to 15 years of age, received salcatonin 2 units per kg bodyweight thrice weekly subcutaneously for periods up to 48 months together with calcium supplements. Half of them had osteogenesis imperfecta tarda and half osteogenesis imperfecta congenita. The annual fracture-rate was reduced in children, and densitometric studies indicated that bone mineral loss might be reduced, at least in children below 5 years. Some patients had objective evidence of increased strength and mobility, and these also experienced subjective improvement; others reported aching bone pain during treatment. Stress fractures were occasionally found. The optimal dose and duration of treatment, and whether or not salcatonin can be used prophylactically, remain to be determined. Selection of patients is necessary.— S. Castells *et al.*, *J. Pediat.*, 1979, *95*, 807.

Further references.— S. Castells, *Curr. ther. Res.*, 1974, *16*, 1; G. P. August *et al.*, *J. Pediat.*, 1977, *91*, 1001 (hypomagnesaemia during calcitonin therapy); E. Rosenberg *et al.*, *J. clin. Endocr. Metab.*, 1977, *44*, 346.

Osteoporosis. In 12 of 25 patients with osteoporosis, salcatonin and calcium supplements for 10 to 29 months produced a small increase in total body calcium; 75% of patients had a decrease in back pain, which eventually disappeared in 50%. X-rays showed no skeletal improvement.— S. Wallach *et al.*, *Curr. ther. Res.*, 1977, *22*, 556.

A study in 19 healthy men, 30 healthy women, 18 women taking an oestrogen with progestogen oral contraceptive preparation, and 13 women in the third trimester of pregnancy, indicated that plasma-calcitonin concentrations of women are lower than those of men but, during pregnancy or oral contraceptive administration, exceed those of men. These findings lent support to the implication of a study by P. Lewis *et al.*(*J. Endocr.*, 1971, *49*, 9) that calcitonin might be partly a hormone of skeletal maintenance. Studies directed at finding whether reduced plasma-calcitonin concentrations might be associated with post menopausal osteoporosis are required.— C. J. Hillyard *et al.*, *Lancet*, 1978, *1*, 961. Plasma-calcitonin concentrations rose sharply during administration of oestrogens to healthy postmenopausal women. Oestrogen lack may have a lowering effect on calcitonin secretion which may in turn lead to postmenopausal bone loss. Thus calcitonin may be of value in the prevention of postmenopausal osteoporosis as well as in its treatment.— J. C. Stevenson *et al.*, *Lancet*, 1981, *1*, 693.

A very brief discussion on the use of calcitonin in the treatment of postmenopausal osteoporosis. Calcitonin alone does not appear to be effective; combined with calcium and vitamin D it may help to retard bone loss.— *Med. Lett.*, 1980, *22*, 45.

Sudeck's atrophy. Calcitonin is as effective as corticosteroids in treating the burning pain and oedema of Sudeck's atrophy of the foot, provided it is given early enough; it also has fewer side-effects.— *Br. med. J.*, 1979, *2*, 26.

For the unsuccessful use of salcatonin in a patient with reflex sympathetic dystrophy syndrome (Sudeck's atrophy), see N. N. S. Kay *et al.*, *Br. med. J.*, 1977, *1*, 1575.

In 10 patients with Sudeck's syndrome given calcitonin (pork) 160 units daily intramuscularly for 1 week then 480 units weekly for 3 to 5 weeks, treatment was effective only in patients with first stage or in the transition from first to second stage disease. Salcatonin was now the drug of choice in Sudeck's syndrome.— K. J. Münzenberg, *Dt. med. Wschr.*, 1978, *103*, 26.

Preparations

Calcitonin (Pork) Injection *(B.P.)*. A sterile solution of calcitonin (pork) in a suitable solvent. pH 3.5 to 5.5. It is prepared by dissolving the contents of a sealed container [Calcitonin (Pork) for Injection] in the solvent. The container may contain added inert substances and the solvent contains a suitable antimicrobial preservative. The sealed container should be stored at a temperature not exceeding 25°. Protect from light. Under these conditions the contents may be expected to retain their potency for not less than 2 years. After reconstitution the solution should be used within 24 hours or within a week if stored at 2° to 8°.

Salcatonin Injection *(B.P.)*. A sterile solution of salcatonin in Water for Injections; it may contain suitable buffering and stabilising agents. Sterilised by filtration. pH 3.9 to 4.5. Store at 2° to 8°. Protect from light. Under these conditions it may be expected to retain its potency for not less than 2 years.

Calcitare *(Armour, UK)*. Calcitonin (pork), available in vials of 160 units, supplied with gelatin diluent, for intramuscular or subcutaneous injection. (Also available as Calcitare in *Austral., Belg., Denm., Neth., Norw., S.Afr.*).

Calsynar *(Armour, UK)*. Synthetic salcatonin, available in vials containing 400 units in 2 ml of saline/acetate diluent, for intramuscular or subcutaneous injection. (Also available as Calsynar in *Austral., Neth., S.Afr.*).

Other Proprietary Names

Calcimar (salcatonin) *(Canad., USA)*; Calcitar (pork) *(Fr., Ital., Jap.)*; Calcitonina (salcatonin) *(Ital.)*; Calsyn (salcatonin) *(Fr.)*; Cibacalcin (human) *(Neth., NZ)*; Cibacalcin DC (human) *(Neth.)*; Miacalcic (salcatonin) *(Austral., Norw., NZ, Swed.)*; Staporos (pork) *(Fr.)*.

Synthetic salcatonin was also formerly marketed in Great Britain under the proprietary name Miacalcic (*Sandoz*).

Penicillins and other Antibiotics

1-z

Antibiotics are substances, produced in substrates during the growth of micro-organisms, which in low concentrations destroy or inhibit the growth of other species of micro-organisms. The term is somewhat outdated since it has been extended to include chemically related and derived substances which are produced wholly or partly by chemical synthesis. The elucidation of the chemical structure of the antibiotics produced by fermentation has permitted the synthesis of related antibiotic substances which possess additional, different, or therapeutically more effective antimicrobial properties.

Though antibiotics are generally considered as antimicrobial in their activity, there are many compounds classified as antibiotics which have little or no activity against micro-organisms; some with marked activity against the growth of neoplasms are described in the section on Antineoplastic Agents (p.171).

Antibiotics and other agents which are mainly used for their action against mycobacteria are described in the sections on Tuberculostatics and Tuberculocides (p.1564) and Sulphones and other Antileprotic Agents (p.1487).

There are many substances with anti-infective activity, other than antibiotics, which are used to combat infective diseases whether they are caused by viruses, bacteria, fungi, protozoa, worms, or flukes. Agents with activity against viruses are described under Idoxuridine and some other Antiviral Agents (p.820). Antibacterial agents other than antibiotics are described in the sections on Nitrofurantoin and some other Urinary Antimicrobial Agents (p.1047) and Sulphonamides and Trimethoprim (p.1457). Griseofulvin and other Antifungal Agents (p.714) includes antibiotics and other substances active against fungi. For antiprotozoal substances see the sections on Chloroquine and other Antimalarials (p.394) and Metronidazole and some other Antiprotozoal Agents (p.968); metronidazole is also used in the treatment of anaerobic bacterial infections. Agents used in the treatment of worm and fluke infestations are described under Anthelmintics and Schistosomicides (p.86).

In addition, Disinfectants and Antiseptics (p.547) are used to kill or inhibit the growth of micro-organisms. Vaccines (p.1586) and preparations of immunoglobulin (see p.329) are used to protect against infection.

Antimicrobial Action. The distinction between *bacteriostatic* antibiotics which reversibly inhibit the growth of susceptible micro-organisms and *bactericidal* antibiotics which kill the organisms is based on determinations of their effects *in vitro* on certain strains of micro-organisms. Provided the results are obtained with concentrations of antibiotics attainable in serum and tissues by the administration of therapeutic doses, the distinction remains clinically valid. Given in high therapeutic doses, the aminoglycosides, cephalosporins, penicillins, and polymyxins may be bactericidal by this criterion, whereas chloramphenicol, erythromycin, and the tetracyclines are usually bacteriostatic. An antibiotic which is bactericidal in a certain concentration may become bacteriostatic at lower concentrations. The maintenance of a bactericidal effect depends upon adequate dosage and tissue penetration.

As a guide to the sensitivity of any specific micro-organism to an antibiotic, the *minimum inhibitory concentration* (MIC) is utilised. This is the lowest concentration of antibiotic which will inhibit the growth of a given strain of micro-organism under controlled conditions, and is usually expressed in terms of μg of antibiotic per ml of medium. Similarly, the *minimum bactericidal concentration* (MBC) may also be used. The MIC of a bactericidal antibiotic is usually within one or two dilutions of its MBC.

For brief reviews of the different modes of action of antibiotics, see *Lancet*, 1966, *2*, 484; *ibid.*, 1967, *1*, 321; J. T. Smith, *Pharm. J.*, 1968, *1*, 7; F. W. O'Grady, *Proc. R. Soc. Med.*, 1971, *64*, 529.

A study on subinhibitory concentrations of antibiotics. The minimum antibiotic concentration (MAC) has been defined as the minimum concentration affecting the morphology of bacteria or the rate of growth, expressed as a fraction of the MIC or MBC.— U. Zanon (letter), *J. antimicrob. Chemother.*, 1977, *3*, 106. A discussion on the inhibitory effects of antibiotics at concentrations below their MICs.— G. N. Rolinson, *J. antimicrob. Chemother.*, 1977, *3*, 111.

Testing Bacteria for Sensitivity to Antibiotic Action. Two principal methods are available for testing bacteria for sensitivity to antibiotic action. The dilution method is reasonably precise but time consuming and one test determines only the action of one antibiotic on a given bacterial strain. It is used mainly for research purposes although it is sometimes used in practice where the dose has to be calculated on activity as in endocarditis or where slowly growing organisms such as *Mycobacterium tuberculosis* or *Actinomyces israelii* are to be tested. The impregnated filter paper disk method is less exact, but is able to test simultaneously the effect of several antibiotics on a given strain; it is mainly used for routine diagnostic procedures.

In the tube dilution method doubling dilutions of a given antibiotic are made and inoculated with an overnight broth culture of the bacterial strain under investigation. After overnight incubation, the highest dilution at which no bacterial growth occurs is taken as the end-point of the titration. This is the minimum inhibitory concentration (MIC). A similar method may be used for determining the minimum bactericidal concentration (MBC); any tubes with no growth are subcultured and those which show no growth on antibiotic-free medium demonstrate bactericidal activity. An agar dilution method is also available.

In the disk diffusion method the whole surface of a culture plate is inoculated with the strain of organism under investigation and filter paper disks containing specified concentrations of various antibiotics are laid on the surface of the plate. After overnight incubation the zone of inhibition of growth surrounding each disk is measured. Disks of low or high potency are used according to the clinical conditions and special features of each individual case.

A review of laboratory tests used to guide antimicrobial therapy.— J. E. Rosenblatt, *Mayo Clin. Proc.*, 1977, *52*, 611.

Computer analysis of the sensitivity of micro-organisms in detecting subgroups with varying sensitivities, variation in sensitivity with time or source, and multiple resistance.— T. F. O'Brien *et al.*, *J. Am. med. Ass.*, 1969, *210*, 84.

The isolation and sensitivity of uncommon *Pseudomonas* spp.— G. L. Gilardi, *Ann. intern. Med.*, 1972, *77*, 211.

A method for antibiotic sensitivity testing which combined the simplicity of the disk method with the quantitative result from serial dilution was based on the observation that, when a thin layer of agar was covered with paper impregnated with antibiotic, diffusion of the antibiotic was rapid and uniform distribution in the agar was achieved after only a few hours. Known concentrations of antibiotic could be obtained in agar rapidly and after inoculation and incubation, growth or inhibition of the test organism could be observed.— G. N. Rolinson and E. J. Russell, *Lancet*, 1971, *2*, 745.

The interpretation of antibiotic sensitivity tests.— *Med. Lett.*, 1972, *14* (Jan. 21), 24. See also.— M. J. Marshall and C. A. Field, *J. antimicrob. Chemother.*, 1975, *1*, *Suppl.* (Sept.), 13; *Med. Lett.*, 1980, *22*, 22; C. Krasemann and G. Hildenbrand, *J. antimicrob. Chemother.*, 1980, *6*, 181 (agar diffusion tests).

Criticisms of the MIC as a measure of sensitivity to antibiotics.— I. Phillips *et al.*, *J. antimicrob. Chemother.*, 1976, *2*, 31; S. Selwyn (letter), *J. antimicrob. Chemother.*, 1976, *2*, 221. Greater reliance on MBCs was unlikely to be the answer.— D. Greenwood (letter), *J. antimicrob. Chemother.*, 1976, *2*, 312.

A method for determining the sensitivity of *Chlamydia trachomatis*, using a simple doubling dilution technique in a cell culture system.— G. L. Ridgway *et al.*, *J. antimicrob. Chemother.*, 1976, *2*, 71.

A method for the determination of the sensitivity *in vitro* of *Nocardia* and *Actinomadura* spp.— G. F. Carroll *et al.*, *Am. J. clin. Path.*, 1977, *68*, 279.

A comparative study of 4 disk diffusion tests.— D. F. J. Brown and D. Kothari, *J. antimicrob. Chemother.*, 1978, *4*, 19. See also *idem*, 27.

A suggestion for the standardisation of inoculum numbers in MIC determinations.— D. B. Wheldon and M. P. E. Slack (letter), *J. antimicrob. Chemother.*, 1978, *4*, 578.

Determinations of MBC should be carried out using at least 2 media and treatment started with the antibiotic having the lowest MBC in all media used.— L. R. Peterson *et al.*, *Antimicrob. Ag. Chemother.*, 1978, *13*, 665.

An assay utilising the reduction of nitrates to nitrites by *Haemophilus influenzae* was in good agreement with a standard micro-broth-dilution assay but was considered to be more sensitive in detecting viable bacteria.— W. Fleming and J. Fierer, *Antimicrob. Ag. Chemother.*, 1978, *13*, 791.

Susceptibility testing with the Bauer-Kirby disk was unsuitable for the differentiation of partially resistant from fully sensitive strains of *Neisseria gonorrhoeae*.— R. M. Robins-Browne *et al.*, *J. antimicrob. Chemother.*, 1979, *5*, 67.

A comparison of anaerobic bacteria susceptibility to 7 antimicrobial agents using different tests. The greatest number of discrepancies between methods were seen with tetracycline.— J. E. Rosenblatt *et al.*, *Antimicrob. Ag. Chemother.*, 1979, *15*, 351.

An evaluation of Autobac I *(Pfizer, USA)*, a semi-automated method for rapid antibiotic susceptibility testing.— G. R. Funnell and M. D. G. Guinness, *Antimicrob. Ag. Chemother.*, 1979, *16*, 255.

Chlorhexidine may interfere with microbiological antibiotic assays and should not be used before such a procedure.— P. Larsson and M. Rylander (letter), *J. antimicrob. Chemother.*, 1980, *6*, 682.

Resistance. Resistance of a micro-organism to an antibiotic may be natural or acquired. The emergence of antibiotic-resistant bacteria is closely linked to the extent that antibiotics are used in man and in items of his diet; resistant strains may appear rapidly or slowly depending on the organism, the amount and type of antibiotic used, and the way in which it is used.

Resistance may develop by *selection* of resistant strains during the use of an antibiotic. It may be acquired by random *mutation* which can occur rapidly as a single step or more gradually in a step-wise manner. Earlier evidence that resistance can be acquired by *adaptation* to the environment does not appear to have been substantiated. Resistance may also be transferred from one organism to another and this is discussed in more detail below.

Several mechanisms may be responsible for the resistance of organisms to antibiotics. The *intrinsic resistance* of Gram-negative bacilli to benzylpenicillin is due to the impermeability of the cell wall to the antibiotic and the same may apply to methicillin-resistant strains of staphylococci. *Inactivating enzymes* produced by bacteria are also responsible for resistance. Beta-lactamases such as penicillinase are a group of enzymes which hydrolyse the beta-lactam ring of penicillins and cephalosporins; they are produced by many bacteria including *Staph. aureus*, *Bacillus* and *Clostridium* spp., and all Gram-negative organisms. Chloramphenicol and the aminoglycosides are also inactivated by enzymes. The *inhibition of uptake* of antibiotic is responsible for the resistance of bacteria to tetracycline. The phenomenon of *tolerance* to penicillin in strains of *Staph. aureus* has been described by L.D. Sabath *et al.* (*Lancet*, 1977, *1*, 443). Tolerant strains can be detected by measuring minimum inhibitory concentrations and minimum bactericidal concentrations since in such organisms the antibiotic concerned is inhibitory but, contrary to its usual activity, not bactericidal. More recently tolerance has been reported with other antibiotics and other bacteria.

Organisms resistant to one antibiotic may become resistant to another and this is termed *cross-resistance*. There is often complete cross-resistance between structurally related antibiotics such as the tetracyclines.

Resistance may be acquired by the *transfer* of genetic material from one organism to another. This may be achieved by *transduction* which involves the transfer by bacteriophage of DNA carrying a gene for resistance, or by *conjugation*, when genetic material in the form of extrachromosomal circular particles of DNA (known as plasmids or episomes) is passed from one bacterium to another while they are in contact. These transferable resistance plasmids, termed *R-plasmids* or *R-factors*, consist of 2 parts, one coding for drug resistance and the other for transfer. The 2 parts may be linked to form a single unit which transfers intact to the recipient bacterium. The intestinal tract is an important site for the transfer of bacterial resistance and R-plasmids are the major source of acquired antibiotic resistance in enterobacteria. Some transference has been observed in burns and in peritoneal dialysis fluid. Transfer also appears to occur outside the body,probably in sewage and other very contaminated surface water.

Resistance to several antibiotics is termed multiple or multiply resistance and may be transferred from one bacterial species to another. Plasmids may confer resistance by specifying the production of enzymes such as the beta-lactamases or by bringing about permeability changes in the bacterial cell wall. Fortunately, it appears that if the antibiotics involved are witheld, transferable resistance can be lost spontaneously within weeks or months of its appearance.

The proceedings of a symposium on bacterial resistance.— *J. antimicrob. Chemother.*, 1977, *3*, *Suppl.* C, 1-84.

Reviews of the resistance of bacteria to antibiotics.— L. P. Garrod, *Br. med. J.*, 1976, *2*, 933; J. D. Williams, *Prescribers' J.*, 1977, *17*, 102; W. C. Noble and J. Naidoo, *Br. J. Derm.*, 1978, *98*, 481; F. J. Buckwold and A. R. Ronald, *J. antimicrob. Chemother.*, 1979, *5*, 129.

Reports and discussions on the mechanisms of resistance to antibiotics.— J. W. Costerton and K. -J. Cheng, *J. antimicrob. Chemother.*, 1975, *1*, 363; B. W. Holloway and L. V. Asche, *Drugs*, 1977, *14*, 283; M. A. Chan and M. Goldner, *J. antimicrob. Chemother.*, 1978, *4*, 39; C. Watanakunakorn, *ibid.*, 561; S. G. B. Amyes, *ibid.*, 1980, *6*, 303; S. M. Bell *et al.* (letter), *Lancet*, 1981, *1*, 846; R. W. Lacey and V. L. Lord (letter), *ibid.*, 1049 (new type of beta-lactamase resistance in *Staph. aureus*).

Discussions on the beta-lactamases produced by Gram-negative bacteria.— R. B. Sykes and M. Matthew, *J. antimicrob. Chemother.*, 1976, *2*, 115; D. Greenwood, *ibid.*, 1977, *3*, 7; M. Matthew, *ibid.*, 1979, *5*, 349.

Reports on the incidence of resistance to antibiotics.— G. A. J. Ayliffe *et al.*, *J. clin. Path.*, 1977, *30*, 40; Y. Miyamoto *et al.*, *Antimicrob. Ag. Chemother.*, 1978, *13*, 399; G. A. J. Ayliffe *et al.*, *Lancet*, 1979, *1*, 538.

Report of a WHO Meeting on Surveillance for the Prevention and Control of Health Hazards due to Antibiotic-resistant Enterobacteria.— *Tech. Rep. Ser. Wld Hlth Org. No. 624*, 1978.

Transferable resistance. For a detailed review of resistance to antibiotics by enteric bacteria in *animals* and the transmission of the resistance to other micro-organisms, with a consideration of the hazards to public health, see *Report of the Joint Committee on the Use of Antibiotics in Animal Husbandry and Veterinary Medicine*, London, HM Stationery Office, 1969.

The demonstration in urine of R-factor-mediated resistance by *Serratia marcescens* to ampicillin, carbenicillin, chloramphenicol, kanamycin, streptomycin, and tetracycline.— D. R. Schaberg *et al.*, *Antimicrob. Ag. Chemother.*, 1977, *11*, 449.

A discussion on the spread of R-factors in organisms other than the Enterobacteriaceae.— J. D. Williams, *J. antimicrob. Chemother.*, 1978, *4*, 6.

An *in vitro* study indicated that strains of *Streptococcus faecalis* could transfer erythromycin-resistance to group A, B, and D streptococci. Large scale use of macrolide antibiotics and virginiamycin for growth promotion in animal husbandry could lead to a reservoir of macrolide-resistant group-D streptococci indigenous in animals which could transfer resistance to the virulent group A and group B streptococci.— J. D. A. van Embden *et al.* (letter), *Lancet*, 1978, *1*, 655.

A report of *Salmonella typhimurium* type 204 resistant to chloramphenicol, streptomycin, sulphonamides, and tetracyclines, and of type 193 resistant to ampicillin, chloramphenicol, neomycin/kanamycin, streptomycin, sulphonamides, and tetracyclines. Prudence was needed in the use of antibiotics in veterinary practice to prevent the emergence of resistant strains for the treatment of which the clinician's choice would be extremely limited.— E. J. Threlfall *et al.*, *Br. med. J.*, 1978, *2*, 997.

Reports of transferable multiple resistance.— V. M. Olexy *et al.*, *Antimicrob. Ag. Chemother.*, 1979, *15*, 93; D. N. Gerding *et al.*, *ibid.*, 608; P. L. Sadowski *et al.*, *ibid.*, 616; E. J. Threlfall *et al.* (letter), *Lancet*, 1980, *1*, 1247 (*Vibrio cholerae* El Tor); C. S. Heymann *et al.* (letter), *Lancet*, 1981, *1*, 553; P. C. Applebaum (letter), *ibid* (*Haemophilus influenzae*).

Absorption and Fate. Antibiotics which are well absorbed from the alimentary tract may be given by mouth. However, the instability of many other antibiotics to acid makes their parenteral administration necessary. For patients with a severe, life-threatening infection, parenteral administration is the most effective and rapid means of producing an antimicrobial concentration of antibiotic in the blood and other tissues. Intramuscular injection is the commonest route, but some antibiotics which are painful and irritant when injected into muscle are usually administered intravenously. Alternatively, antibiotics such as the penicillins may be given intramuscularly with a local anaesthetic to reduce pain.

The efficacy with which an orally administered antibiotic is absorbed is not necessarily reflected in its plasma concentration since some compounds are rapidly removed from circulation by the liver and appear in relatively high concentration in the bile. Reabsorption of an antibiotic which has been preferentially concentrated in bile may prolong its therapeutic activity. Chelation of the tetracycline antibiotics with aluminium, calcium, magnesium, and possibly other cations may delay or prevent their absorption after administration by mouth in conjunction with antacid preparations given to reduce gastric upset.

The absorption of many antibiotics given by mouth is affected by food and it is common practice to give many of them before meals.

Binding to plasma proteins decreases the concentration of free antibiotic available but also delays excretion of the antibiotic by the kidney tubules, so prolonging its presence in the circulation. However, there is controversy over the significance of the effect of protein binding on activity.

Penetration of an antibiotic into infected tissue depends on local vascularity. Diffusion into abscesses or exudates in body cavities may be slow and severely limited.

Chloramphenicol is one of the few antibiotics that can enter the cerebrospinal fluid when the meninges are normal although with many antibiotics penetration is facilitated when the meninges are inflamed. In infections of the CNS, adequate concentrations of antibiotics such as gentamicin may only be achieved by intrathecal injection.

General reviews.— C. M. Kunin, *Clin. Pharmac. Ther.*, 1974, *16*, 251; M. S. S. Chow and R. A. Ronfeld, *J. clin. Pharmac.*, 1975, *15*, 405.

A brief review of comparisons of the absorption and excretion of antibiotics by young and elderly patients.— D. P. Richey and A. D. Bender, *A. Rev. Pharmac. & Toxic.*, 1977, *17*, 49.

A review of the pharmacokinetics of antimicrobial agents with respect to the liver and hepatotoxicity.— S. P. Barrett and P. J. Watt, *J. antimicrob. Chemother.*, 1979, *5*, 337. See also D. E. Rollins and C. D. Klaassen, *Clin. Pharmacokinet.*, 1979, *4*, 368 (biliary excretion).

The serum concentration of an antibiotic administered by continuous intravenous infusion could be calculated in µg per ml by multiplying a tenth of the antibiotic's half-life expressed in minutes by the dose in mg infused per minute. This formula could be modified for patients with renal impairment by assessing the prolongation of half-life from the reduced creatinine clearance.— F. O'Grady *et al.* (letter), *Lancet*, 1971, *2*, 209.

A discussion on the absorption and fate of antibiotics after administration by extra-vascular injection.— D. S. Reeves, *J. antimicrob. Chemother.*, 1975, *1*, 350.

Although sex-linked differences in drug kinetics exist for some antibiotics such as cephradine, chloramphenicol, gentamicin, kanamycin, penicillin, rifampicin, and tetracycline, in general they do not call for dosage modification.— J. F. Giudicelli and J. P. Tillement, *Clin. Pharmacokinet.*, 1977, *2*, 157.

Absorption and fate in infants and children. The pharmacokinetics of penicillins when given by mouth to newborn infants (in the first 48 hours of life) were examined. After the first dose peak serum concentrations were reached at 2 hours with flucloxacillin (7 infants), between 4 and 9 hours with amoxycillin (7 infants), at 9 hours with ampicillin (9 infants), and at 15 hours with ampicillin when given in combination with flucloxacillin (4 infants). There was considerable individual variation. Because of the delay in achieving peak concentrations the first dose should be given by intramuscular injection and treatment by mouth started at the same time and continued 6-hourly. Amoxycillin was not better absorbed than ampicillin. Less than 30% of the antibiotics was excreted in the urine during the first 24 hours.— M. D. Cohen *et al.*, *Archs Dis. Childh.*, 1975, *50*, 230.

A study on the effect of food on the absorption of antibiotics in infants and children.— G. H. McCracken *et al.*, *Pediatrics*, 1978, *62*, 738.

Further references: M. Gavend and G. Bessard, *Archs fr. Pédiat.*, 1976, *33*, 809; P. L. Morselli *et al.*, *Clin. Pharmacokinet.*, 1980, *5*, 485 (neonates and infants).

Diffusion. Proceedings of a symposium on the tissue penetration of antibiotics.— *Scand. J. infect. Dis.*, 1978, *Suppl.* 14, 1-315.

Ascitic fluid. Ampicillin, benzylpenicillin, cephalothin, cephazolin, chloramphenicol, clindamycin, gentamicin, and tobramycin, each diffused into ascitic fluid in a study of 20 patients with ascites and peritonitis following intravenous or intramuscular administration. Antibiotic concentration in ascitic fluid exceeded 50% of serum concentrations in 16 patients and about half the ascitic-fluid concentrations exceeded 90% of the serum concentrations. Intraperitoneal instillation of antibiotics was not considered to be necessary except for critically ill patients.— D. N. Gerding *et al.*, *Ann. intern. Med.*, 1977, *86*, 706.

Bone. Antibiotic concentrations in pus and bone of children with osteomyelitis.— T. R. Tetzlaff *et al.*, *J. Pediat.*, 1978, *92*, 135.

Further references: R. L. Parsons, *J. antimicrob. Chemother.*, 1976, *2*, 228.

Cerebrospinal fluid. A review of the penetration of antibiotics into the cerebrospinal fluid and brain tissue.— R. W. A. Barling and J. B. Selkon, *J. antimicrob. Chemother.*, 1978, *4*, 203.

Pleural fluid. A discussion on the penetration of antibiotics into the pleural fluid and its clinical implications.— H. Lode, *J. antimicrob. Chemother.*, 1979, *5*, 122.

Sputum. In patients with cystic fibrosis and respiratory infections, the sputum antibiotic concentrations were not directly related to those of the serum.— B. A. Saggers and D. Lawson, *Archs Dis. Childh.*, 1968, *43*, 404.

Synovial fluid. Antibiotic concentrations in suppurative synovial fluid.— J. D. Nelson *et al.*, *J. Pediat.*, 1978, *92*, 131.

Wound fluid. Antibiotic concentrations in wound fluid after intravenous administration.— D. H. Bagley *et al.*, *Ann. Surg.*, 1978, *188*, 202.

Plasma concentrations. Discussions on the relevance of measuring blood concentrations of antibiotics.— W. L. Hewitt and M. C. Z. McHenry, *Med. Clins N. Am.*, 1978, *62*, 1119; G. W. Rylance and T. A. Moreland, *Archs Dis. Childh.*, 1980, *55*, 89.

Pregnancy and the neonate. A review of the pharmacokinetics of antibiotics in pregnancy and labour.— A.

Philipson, *Clin. Pharmacokinet.*, 1979, *4*, 297.

A brief review of the excretion of antibiotics in breast milk.— J. T. Wilson *et al.*, *Clin. Pharmacokinet.*, 1980, *5*, 1.

The pharmacokinetics of antibiotics given to mothers during childbirth.— R. L. Nation, *Clin. Pharmacokinet.*, 1980, *5*, 340.

Following maternal administration, bacteriostatic concentrations of all antibiotics could be found in foetal blood. Penicillin and tetracycline concentrations in the foetus were from 25 to 75% of the maternal concentration and streptomycin about 50%. Erythromycin crossed the placenta when more than 800 mg was taken, but the foetal concentration was only about 25% of the maternal concentration. Effective concentrations of chloramphenicol crossed the placenta.— M. C. Dentkos, *Am. J. Hosp. Pharm.*, 1966, *23*, 139.

See also under Absorption and Fate in Infants and Children (above).

Protein binding. Protein binding was considered in general to reduce the activity of antibiotics and although there might be occasions when the slow release from the bound state might be desirable it was considered that it was unlikely to be so with the beta-lactam antibiotics. The disadvantages of protein binding could be intensified by any metabolic inactivation as with cephalothin.— S. Selwyn, *Lancet*, 1976, *2*, 616.

A review of the protein binding of antimicrobial agents with the clinical pharmacokinetic and therapeutic implications. Both protein binding and membrane penetration correlated well with lipid solubility so that extensive drug protein binding was often counteracted by greater intrinsic antimicrobial activity.— W. A. Craig and P. G. Welling, *Clin. Pharmacokinet.*, 1977, *2*, 252. See also G. N. Rolinson, *J. antimicrob. Chemother.*, 1980, *6*, 311.

A conclusion that the penetration of antibiotic into tissue fluid is independent of the fraction of free drug in the blood.— A. P. Gillett and R. Wise, *Lancet*, 1978, *1*, 962. Contrary findings in *animal* studies.— L. R. Peterson and D. N. Gerding (letter), *ibid.*, *2*, 376. See also S. Selwyn (letter), *Lancet*, 1978, *1*, 1104; R. Wise and A. P. Gillett (letter), *ibid.*; R. Wise *et al.* (letter), *ibid.*, *2*, 431.

Further references: N. Buchanan, *S. Afr. med. J.*, 1977, *52*, 733.

Choice of Antibiotic. Before choosing an antibiotic it is advisable to consider whether such treatment is essential and whether a single antibiotic,several antibiotics, or antibiotic therapy in conjunction with surgery should be used. Consideration should also be given to the length of the course of treatment, particularly if a response does not occur as expected, and alternative treatments must be considered for any patient who does not respond.

Ideally, the choice of antibiotic is made on the results of sensitivity tests which should be carried out on specimens from every patient. Results should be interpreted with reference to the response achieved with the indicated treatment in similar conditions. When it is necessary to treat patients before sensitivity tests have been carried out, the known local patterns of bacterial resistance should be taken into account before deciding initial antibiotic treatment. Sensitivity tests should still be done, as results can confirm the choice or indicate a change.

The severity and type of infection and the state of the patient influence the choice of an antibiotic, its route of administration, and whether a bactericidal or bacteriostatic effect is indicated. Severe infections usually require treatment with bactericidal agents. The parenteral route of administration is the most reliable in such patients and intravenous or more direct routes produce peak antibiotic concentrations rapidly. Oral administration is convenient but should only be used when reliable absorption and a rapid effect are not essential. A few antibiotics are administered topically; it is advisable that those that are so used should preferably not be those given systemically.

The chosen antibiotic must be as safe as possible and a balance has to be achieved between toxicity, effectiveness, and duration of treatment.

A review of the use of antibiotics in elderly patients.— J. Modai and Y. Coquin, *Thérapie*, 1975, *30*, 359.

For general reviews of the actions and uses of the penicillins, see M. Barza, *Am. J. Hosp. Pharm.*, 1977, *34*, 57; C. J. Wilkowske, *Mayo Clin. Proc.*, 1977, *52*, 616; R. Wise, *Br. med. J.*, 1978, *1*, 1679; W. E. Farrar, *J. antimicrob. Chemother.*, 1980, *6*, 573.

The Rational Choice of Antibacterial Agents, R.P. Mouton *et al.* (Ed.), London, Kluwer Harrap, 1977.

The choice of antibiotics.— *Prescribers' J.*, 1977, *17*, 124; P. E. Hermans, *Mayo Clin. Proc.*, 1977, *52*, 603; R. Wise, *Practitioner*, 1977, *219*, 449; R. A. V. Benn, *Drugs*, 1977, *13*, 297; A. J. Bint and D. S. Reeves, *Br. J. Hosp. Med.*, 1978, *19*, 335; A. P. Gillett *et al.*, *Br. med. J.*, 1978, *2*, 335; R. A. Gleckman and A. L. Eposito, *Sth. med. J.*, 1979, *72*, 721; M. Shapiro *et al.*, *J. infect. Dis.*, 1979, *139*, 698; A. M. Geddes, *Prescribers' J.*, 1979, *19*, 72; P. Noone, *Practitioner*, 1979, *223*, 450; *Med. Lett.*, 1980, *22*, 5.

Guidelines for the management of accidents involving micro-organisms, including the use of antibiotics.— *Bull. Wld Hlth Org.*, 1980, *58*, 245.

Abscess, brain. Recommendations for the treatment of brain abscesses according to their site of origin. Abscesses of *sinusitic origin* are frequently caused by *Streptococcus milleri*—benzylpenicillin 9.6 to 14.4 g daily must be included in the regimen; abscesses of *otitic origin* are caused by a wide range of aerobic and anaerobic bacteria—benzylpenicillin and chloramphenicol, with or without metronidazole, ampicillin, or co-trimoxazole should be used; abscesses of *metastatic or cryptogenic origin* may be streptococcal or due to a mixture of bacteria—multiple broad-spectrum treatment, including penicillin, should be used until bacteriological results are available; *spinal and post-traumatic intracranial abscesses* are usually due to *Staphylococcus aureus* and fusidic acid is probably the treatment of choice.— J. de Louvois, *J. antimicrob. Chemother.*, 1978, *4*, 395. See also J. de Louvois *et al.*, *Br. med. J.*, 1977, *2*, 985. A review of the choice of treatment for brain abscesses including criticism of the recommendations of de Louvois. Metronidazole should be included in the treatment of abscesses of *sinusitic origin* and probably also those of otitic origin. For abscesses due to *Staph. aureus*, fusidic acid should be used with another antibiotic to prevent the emergence of resistance.— *Lancet*, 1978, *2*, 1081.

Abscess, liver. A review of the presentation, diagnosis, and management of pyogenic liver abscess seen in 16 patients over a period of 9 years. Appropriate high-dose bactericidal chemotherapy together with aspiration under ultrasonographic guidance seems to be the best treatment, and to reduce greatly the need for surgery. Closed aspiration was done in 7 patients together with the following antimicrobial chemotherapy for 2 to 10 weeks: metronidazole in association with gentamicin, cephradine, or ampicillin (5 patients), ampicillin alone in one, and penicillin alone in one. Two patients had poor clinical and bacteriological response to oral chloramphenicol to which the isolates were sensitive *in vitro*.— M. R. Perera *et al.*, *Lancet*, 1980, *2*, 629.

Anaerobic infections. Reviews.— A. T. Willis, *Br. J. Hosp. Med.*, 1978, *20*, 579; M. S. Sprott and H. R. Ingham, *Drugs*, 1979, *18*, 137.

Arthritis, bacterial. A short discussion on the treatment of acute bacterial arthritis.— L. J. Strausbaugh and T. El Hadidi, *Practitioner*, 1979, *222*, 395.

Cystic fibrosis. Discussions on the use of antibiotics in the management of cystic fibrosis.— R. Dinwiddie, *Practitioner*, 1980, *224*, 291; M. Mearns, *Prescribers' J.*, 1980, *20*, 45.

Diarrhoea. A review of the incidence of carriers of enteropathogenic *Escherichia coli*, criticising the use of antibiotics for the treatment of diarrhoea. Control measures centering on fluid and electrolyte replacement were advocated.— U. Bollag, *Trans. R. Soc. trop. Med. Hyg.*, 1978, *72*, 588.

A review of the prophylaxis and treatment of traveller's diarrhoea.— *Med. Lett.*, 1979, *21*, 41. See also A. G. Higginson, *Practitioner*, 1979, *223*, 529.

See also under Enteric Infections, below.

Dosage in infants and children. Reviews of the use of antibiotics in neonatal infections, with recommended doses.— P. A. Davies, *Br. med. J.*, 1978, *2*, 676; H. C. Spratt, *Drugs*, 1978, *16*, 226.

Reviews of antimicrobial agents and their use in infants and children.— H. F. Eichenwald and G. H. McCracken, *J. Pediat.*, 1978, *93*, 337; G. H. McCracken and H. F. Eichenwald, *J. Pediat.*, 1978, *93*, 357.

See also Neonatal Infections (below).

Dosage in renal failure. References and reviews: *Drug & Ther. Bull.*, 1969, *7*, 53; G. D. Chisholm, *Med. J. Aust.*, 1970, *1*, *Suppl.* (June 13), 25; A. J. Wing, *Br. med. J.*, 1970, *4*, 35; F. O'Grady, *Br. med. Bull.*, 1971, *27*, 142; C. M. Kunin, *Hosp. Pract.*, 1972, *7*, 141; E. A. Jackson and D. C. McLeod, *Am. J. Hosp. Pharm.*, 1974, *31*, 36 and 137; G. E. Mawer, *Adverse Drug React. Bull.*, 1975, June, 176; G. B. Appel and H. C. Neu, *New Engl. J. Med.*, 1977, *296*, 663 and 722; W. M. Bennett, *Drugs*, 1979, *17*, 111; J. Fabre *et al.*, *Clin. Pharmacokinet.*, 1980, *5*, 441.

Endocarditis. A review of infective endocarditis and its treatment. In patients with medical endocarditis suggested antibiotic treatment after taking blood for cultures but before receiving the laboratory results is: benzylpenicillin 6 g in association with gentamicin 160 to 240 mg in 24 hours, both drugs being given in intermittent bolus dosage. If staphylococcal infection is likely, sodium fusidate 500 mg thrice daily should be added.— C. M. Oakley, *Br. J. Hosp. Med.*, 1980, *24*, 232.

Further reviews of the treatment of endocarditis.— B. Watt, *J. antimicrob. Chemother.*, 1978, *4*, 107; A. P. Ball and A. M. Geddes (letter), *ibid.*, 381; P. D. Welsby, *Postgrad. med. J.*, 1978, *54*, 321; *Br. med. J.*, 1979, *2*, 4; A. E. Dormer, *Practitioner*, 1980, *224*, 255; J. A. Lowes *et al.*, *Lancet*, 1980, *1*, 133; C. M. Oakley and J. H. Darrell, *Prescribers' J.*, 1980, *20*, 98; D. Kaye, *Am. J. Med.*, 1980, *69*, 650; M. A. Sande and W. M. Scheld, *Ann. intern. Med.*, 1980, *92*, 390.

Studies *in vitro* indicated that the synergistic activity of nafcillin or oxacillin when used together with gentamicin against strains of enterococci was reduced in the presence of serum. Methicillin used together with gentamicin in broth or serum was synergistic against none of the strains. It was recommended that the semisynthetic penicillinase-resistant penicillins should not be used as primary agents in treatment of patients with enterococcal endocarditis. In such patients, benyzlpenicillin plus an aminoglycoside should be used as initial treatment.— R. H. Glew and R. C. Moellering, *Antimicrob. Ag. Chemother.*, 1979, *15*, 87.

Further references: B. Abrams *et al.*, *Ann. intern. Med.*, 1979, *90*, 789; A. W. Karchmer *et al.*, *J. Am. med. Ass.*, 1979, *241*, 1801; P. J. Geiseler (letter), *Lancet*, 1981, *1*, 659; P. A. Oill *et al.* (letter), *New Engl. J. Med.*, 1981, *305*, 101.

Enteric infections. In a statement prepared by R.W. Townley for the Australian Paediatric Association, the inclusion of antibiotics in preparations used for the treatment of acute enteritis was considered to be therapeutically useless, unnecessarily expensive, and an environmental hazard. As from August 1975 these preparations were not available under the Australian health service.— *Aust. J. Pharm.*, 1975, *56*, 317.

A brief discussion on the antibiotic treatment of typhoid fever.— A. M. Geddes, *J. antimicrob. Chemother.*, 1977, *3*, 382.

A review of enteric infections and their treatment in infants and children.— M. I. Marks, *Drugs*, 1978, *16*, 219.

Further references: U. Kindler *et al.*, *Dt. med. Wschr.*, 1977, *102*, 1720; U. Clibon and S. L. Barriere, *J. Am. pharm. Ass.*, 1977, *NS17*, 80.

See also under Diarrhoea, above.

Eye infections. General reviews: P. Trevor-Roper, *Prescribers' J.*, 1976, *16*, 124; D. W. Sabiston, *Drugs*, 1977, *14*, 207; J. L. Baum, *New Engl. J. Med.*, 1978, *299*, 28; D. L. Easty, *Practitioner*, 1980, *224*, 593.

The use of antibiotics for bacterial conjunctivitis.— *Med. Lett.*, 1976, *18*, 70.

Gonorrhoea. Reviews: *Med. Lett.*, 1979, *21*, 66; R. D. Catterall, *Prescribers' J.*, 1980, *20*, 86.

Despite an overall trend towards the constant or increasing resistance of *Neisseria gonorrhoeae* and the emergence of beta-lactamase-producing strains, a single dose of penicillin was still the drug of choice for the initial treatment of gonorrhoea. There was, however, an urgent need for new antibiotics active against beta-lactamase-producing and -nonproducing gonococci. The following regimens for the treatment of gonorrhoea should be considered. Single-dose regimens: penicillins; benzylpenicillin 3 g or procaine penicillin 4.8 g intramuscularly, or ampicillin 3.5 g by mouth all given with probenecid 1 or 2 g; aminoglycosides; spectinomycin 2 g or kanamycin 2 g intramuscularly. Multiple-dose regimens: tetracycline 500 mg four times daily for 4.5 days or co-trimoxazole 6 tablets once daily for 3 days.— *Neisseria gonorrhoeae and gonococcal infections*, Report of a WHO Scientific Group, *Tech. Rep. Ser. Wld Hlth Org. No. 616*, 1978.

Recommendations from the US Public Health Service for the treatment of gonorrhoea.— *Morb. Mortal.*, 1979, *28*, 13. See also *Ann. intern. Med.*, 1979, *90*, 809;

W. M. McCormack, *Ann. intern. Med.*, 1979, *90*, 845.

For details of recommended doses, see under Amoxycillin, p.1090, Ampicillin, p.1095, Erythromycin, p.1159, Procaine Penicillin, p.1206, Spectinomycin Hydrochloride, p.1212, and Tetracycline Hydrochloride, p.1220. See also Cefoxitin Sodium, p.1121 and Cefuroxime Sodium, p.1122.

Comment on the emergence of penicillinase-producing strains of *Neisseria gonorrhoeae* with cross-resistance to antibiotics other than penicillin.— *Lancet*, 1981, *1*, 816.

Legionnaires' disease. Proceedings of a symposium on legionnaires' disease.— *Ann. intern. Med.*, 1979, *90*, 489-703.

The most effective antimicrobial agents against legionnaires' disease bacterium in a study in embryonated eggs from *hens* were in descending order: rifampicin, gentamicin, streptomycin, erythromycin, sulphadiazine, and chloramphenicol.— V. J. Lewis *et al.*, *Antimicrob. Ag. Chemother.*, 1978, *13*, 419.

See also under Erythromycin, p.1160.

Meningitis. Although the value of intrathecal administration of antibiotics in meningitis remained unclear it still seemed wise to continue with this technique in severe infections.— *Lancet*, 1976, *2*, 1068. See also C. Y. Yeung, *Archs Dis. Childh.*, 1976, *51*, 686.

Antibiotic treatment before referral to hospital in 31 of 104 patients with bacterial meningitis did not affect the bacterial diagnosis or prognosis.— F. K. Rømer, *Lancet*, 1977, *2*, 345.

A discussion on neonatal meningitis and suggested doses for its treatment. *E. coli* was still one of the commonest causes of the disease in the UK.— P. A. Davies, *Br. J. Hosp. Med.*, 1977, *18*, 425. See also H. P. Lambert, *J. antimicrob. Chemother.*, 1977, *3*, 381.

From 1973 to 1976 group B streptococci accounted for 52% of 70 cases of neonatal meningitis, *E. coli* for 14% and *Listeria monocytogenes* for 6%. Beyond the neonatal period *Haemophilus influenzae* type b was the principal cause in the USA. Initial treatment with ampicillin 100 to 200 mg per kg body-weight daily intravenously and gentamicin 5 to 7.5 mg per kg daily intramuscularly was recommended for neonatal meningitis of unknown aetiology. In older infants ampicillin 200 to 300 mg per kg daily and chloramphenicol 100 mg per kg daily, both intravenously, should be used. Benzylpenicillin 90 to 150 mg per kg daily intravenously was preferred for group B streptococcal, pneumococcal, or meningococcal meningitis.— G. H. McCracken and H. F. Eichenwald, *J. Pediat.*, 1978, *93*, 357. See also G. A. Ahronheim, *Drugs*, 1978, *16*, 136.

Neisseria meningitidis, Streptococcus pneumoniae, and *H. influenzae* accounted for most cases of pyogenic meningitis. Meningococcal and pneumococcal meningitis were treated with benzylpenicillin 1.2 to 1.8 g intravenously every 4 hours. Meningitis caused by *H. influenzae*mainly affected children below school age and good results were achieved with ampicillin and chloramphenicol although with the emergence of ampicillin-resistant strains chloramphenicol may become the antibiotic of first choice.— H. P. Lambert, *Br. med. J.*, 1978, *2*, 259.

A discussion on the treatment of bacterial meningitis.— G. D. Overturf and P. F. Wehrle, *Drugs*, 1979, *18*, 65.

For the treatment of Gram-negative bacterial meningitis and ventriculitis, see Gentamicin Sulphate, p.1172.

Otitis media. The choice of antibiotic for acute otitis media.— *Br. med. J.*, 1976, *2*, 1407; N. Roydhouse, *Drugs*, 1978, *15*, 393; S. H. Sell *et al.*, *Sth. med. J.*, 1978, *71*, 1493; J. F. Neil, *Prescribers' J.*, 1980, *20*, 39; *ibid.*, June (correction).

Peritonitis. Peritoneal lavage in the treatment of peritonitis.— M. Stephen and J. Loewenthal, *Surgery, St Louis*, 1979, *85*, 603.

Pertussis. The role of antibiotics in the treatment of pertussis.— *Br. med. J.*, 1978, *1*, 1007. See also R. B. Elliott, *Drugs*, 1977, *14*, 220; H. Lambert, *J. antimicrob. Chemother.*, 1979, *5*, 329.

Pregnancy and the neonate. Reviews of the chemotherapy of infections in pregnancy.— W. Mosimann, *Schweiz. med. Wschr.*, 1975, *105*, 257; P. J. Little, *Drugs*, 1977, *14*, 390; A. J. Weinstein, *Drugs*, 1979, *17*, 56.

Neonatal infections. The proceedings of a symposium on perinatal and neonatal infections.— R. Hurley *et al.* (Ed.), *J. antimicrob. Chemother.*, 1979, *5*, *Suppl.* A, 1–89.

Reviews and discussions on the treatment of neonatal infections.— *Br. med. J.*, 1979, *2*, 1385; H. B. Valman, *ibid.*, 1980, *280*, 772; *Drug & Ther. Bull.*, 1981, *19*, 13; J. D. Siegel and G. H. McCracken, *New Engl. J. Med.*, 1981, *304*, 642; *Lancet*, 1981, *2*, 181 (group B streptococci).

See also Dosage in Infants and Children and Meningitis (above) and Respiratory Distress Syndrome (below).

Respiratory distress syndrome. A policy of immediate antibiotic therapy in infants with respiratory distress.— T. J. French *et al.* (letter), *Lancet*, 1978, *2*, 997. Not all neonates with group B streptococcal infection show early warning signs but a review of experience indicated that the deaths attributable to such infection were confined to infants who were either preterm or of low birth-weight. All such infants are now given penicillin which is stopped if cultures are negative after 2 days and there are no signs suggestive of infection.— M. A. Hall *et al.* (letter), *ibid.*, 1254. The view that antibiotics have no place in the treatment of the respiratory distress syndrome, although some infants may need antibiotics since the group B streptococcus may produce symptoms similar to those of severe respiratory distress syndrome.— H. B. Valman, *Br. med. J.*, 1979, *2*, 1483.

Respiratory infections. A discussion on the choice of antibiotic for the treatment of bronchitis and pneumonia.— G. K. Crompton, *Prescribers' J.*, 1978, *18*, 14 and 74. See also R. G. Petersdorf and H. Featherstone, *Am. Rev. resp. Dis.*, 1978, *117*, 1; H. B. Valman, *Br. med. J.*, 1980, *280*, 1438 (older infants).

Bronchitis. The treatment of bronchitis.— A. E. Tattersfield, *Br. med. J.*, 1978, *1*, 1123; M. W. Burns, *Drugs*, 1979, *18*, 58; D. T. D. Hughes and D. W. Empey, *Practitioner*, 1979, *223*, 771; *Med. Lett.*, 1980, *22*, 68.

Pneumonia. The treatment of pneumonia.— C. M. Ogilvie, *Br. med. J.*, 1978, *1*, 771; R. B. Cole, *Practitioner*, 1979, *223*, 765.

The choice of antibiotics for the treatment of staphylococcal pneumonia.— R. Bagg, *J. antimicrob. Chemother.*, 1978, *4*, 297.

Comment on the treatment of pneumonia in acute leukaemia.— *Br. med. J.*, 1980, *281*, 1235.

Episodes of acute bacterial pneumonia, due to a Gram-negative weakly acid-fast bacterium designated Pittsburgh Pneumonia Agent (PPA), occurred in 8 immunosuppressed patients within 3 weeks of starting high daily doses of corticosteroids. All of the patients were given broad-spectrum antibiotics but only 3 survived and no pattern of antibiotic efficacy emerged. Susceptibility studies *in vitro* indicated that erythromycin, rifampicin, and co-trimoxazole had activity against PPA.— R. L. Myerowitz *et al.*, *New Engl. J. Med.*, 1979, *301*, 953. A further report of an unidentified acid-fast bacterium causing pulmonary infections in 5 similar patients. The organism could not be cultured.— B. H. Rogers *et al.*, *ibid.*, 959. Comment.— M. N. Swartz, *ibid.*, 995. See also A. M. Ackley (letter), *Lancet*, 1981, *1*, 221.

Septicaemia. Discussions on the use of antibiotics in septicaemia.— A. M. Geddes, *Br. med. J.*, 1978, *2*, 181. See also P. G. Reasbeck (letter), *Br. med. J.*, 1978, *2*, 566; P. Noone *et al.*, *J. antimicrob. Chemother.*, 1978, *4*, *Suppl.* C, 83; *Br. med. J.*, 1980, *280*, 1240.

Skeletal infections. A discussion of the choice of antibiotic for osteomyelitis.— *Lancet*, 1975, *1*, 153. See also F. A. Waldvogel and H. Vasey, *New Engl. J. Med.*, 1980, *303*, 360.

Bacterial infections of the skeletal system and their treatment in infants and children.— G. A. Ahronheim, *Drugs*, 1978, *16*, 210. See also T. R. Tetzlaff *et al.*, *J. Pediat.*, 1978, *92*, 485.

Skin disorders. General reviews.— D. A. Bremner, *Drugs*, 1977, *13*, 52; M. I. Marks, *Drugs*, 1978, *16*, 202 (infants and children).

Recommendations for the topical use of antibiotics in infants and children.— S. Segal *et al.*, *Pediatrics*, 1977, *59*, 1041.

A description of prickly heat. Topically applied antibacterial agents consistently prevent anhidrosis induced by polyethylene occlusion.— *Lancet*, 1979, *1*, 305.

Acne. The American Ad Hoc Committee on the Use of Antibiotics in Dermatology reported that erythromycin, clomocycline, and co-trimoxazole were roughly as effective as tetracycline for the treatment of acne vulgaris. The use of an antibiotic effective against the strain of *Corynebacterium acne* in the individual patient and dispensed in a suitable basis to enhance the penetration from a topical preparation might provide the best management of severe acne.— *Br. med. J.*, 1976, *1*, 1423. See also *J. Am. med. Ass.*, 1975, *234*, 1058.

Further references: W. J. Cunliffe, *Br. J. Hosp. Med.*, 1978, *20*, 24.

Storage of aortic valves. A solution used for the sterilisation and storage of aortic valves for transplantation: Hank's balanced salt solution [volume not stated] with the addition of penicillin 50 units, streptomycin 1 mg, kanamycin 1 mg, and amphotericin 25 units.— B. G. Barratt-Boyes *et al.*, *Circulation*, 1977, *55*, 353.

Syphilis. For a review of the use and toxic effects of antibiotics other than penicillin for the treatment of syphilis, see O. Idsøe *et al.*, *Bull. Wld Hlth Org.*, 1972, *47*, *Suppl.*, 44 and 51. See also W. M. Platts, *Drugs*, 1973, *5*, 144.

For tests used in the detection of syphilis, see Laboratory Diagnosis of Venereal Disease, *Public Health Laboratory Service Monograph Series No. 1*, London, HM Stationery Office, 1972.

The American Public Health Service's treatment schedules for syphilis.— *Obstet. Gynec.*, 1976, *48*, 727. See also *Med. Lett.*, 1977, *19*, 105.

A discussion on the treatment of neurosyphilis with reference to recent doubts about the effectiveness of benzathine penicillin.— R. D. Catterall, *Br. J. Hosp. Med.*, 1977, *17*, 585.

Urinary-tract infections. General reviews of the choice of treatment of urinary-tract infections.— R. S. Nanra, *Drugs*, 1976, *11*, 441; *Med. Lett.*, 1977, *19*, 87; A. W. Asscher, *Br. med. J.*, 1978, *1*, 1531; *Drug & Ther. Bull.*, 1979, *17*, 81.

Reviews of the treatment of urinary-tract infections in infants and children.— J. M. Stansfeld, *Practitioner*, 1977, *218*, 59; M. H. Winterborn, *Br. J. Hosp. Med.*, 1977, *17*, 453; M. I. Marks, *Drugs*, 1978, *16*, 147.

The use of single-dose antibiotic therapy in the management of urinary-tract infection.— K. F. Fairley *et al.*, *Med. J. Aust.*, 1978, *2*, 75; R. R. Bailey, *Drugs*, 1979, *17*, 219; J. D. Anderson, *J. antimicrob. Chemother.*, 1980, *6*, 170; *Lancet*, 1981, *1*, 26.

The value of the determination of antibiotic concentrations in tissue and in urine in the treatment of urinary-tract infections.— P. Naumann, *J. antimicrob. Chemother.*, 1978, *4*, 9.

Of 43 women shown by the absence of antibody coating on the infecting bacteria to have amoxycillin-susceptible urinary-tract infections limited to the bladder, all responded to amoxycillin therapy; of 18 shown to have antibody-coated bacteria 9 relapsed within a week of completion of therapy and 3 relapsed again following treatment with other agents. The presence of antibody coating indicates upper urinary-tract infection while the absence of coating indicates lower urinary-tract infection.— L. S. T. Fang *et al.*, *New Engl. J. Med.*, 1978, *298*, 413.

Asymptomatic bacteriuria. A 3-year study of 63 girls with covert (or asymptomatic) bacteriuria demonstrated that treatment had no significant effect and was not considered essential.— D. C. L. Savage *et al.*, *Lancet*, 1975, *1*, 358.

Although treatment of asymptomatic bacteriuria reduced the infection in 110 schoolgirls compared with 98 controls followed-up for a mean period of 4 years, there was no significant difference in clinical outcome. Kidney scars that were associated with infection appeared to develop before the age of 5 years. It might be more beneficial to study these younger girls.— Cardiff-Oxford Bacteriuria Study Group, *Lancet*, 1978, *1*, 889. Comment.— J. M. Smellie and I. C. S. Normand (letter), *ibid.*, 1199. Corrections.— R. Mayon-White and A. W. Asscher (letter), *ibid.*, 1200. Criticism of statement that 'screening for occult bacteriuria cannot......be recommended in schoolgirls'. Results of a similar programme had indicated that this conclusion was unjustified.— G. Turner *et al.* (letter), *ibid.*, 1978, *2*, 1147.

A follow-up study over 9 to 18 years of the long-term effects of bacteriuria detected in 60 schoolgirls indicated that they had considerably more recurrent infections and urological abnormalities and were at high risk of bacteriuria during pregnancy when compared with 38 matched controls. Bacteriuria also occurred in 7 of the 65 children of the study subjects compared with none of the 24 children born to control subjects. Only one of the 60 subjects developed substantially reduced renal function but even so, the study demonstrates that screening for bacteriuria in schoolgirls detects those at risk of considerable morbidity from recurrent infection and a small number with major urological abnormalities. Since all episodes of bacteriuria were treated with short courses of chemotherapy some renal damage may have been prevented.— J. Y. Gillenwater *et al.*, *New Engl. J. Med.*, 1979, *301*, 396.

Findings that bacteriuria in old age is associated with a reduction in survival.— A. S. Dontas *et al.*, *New Engl. J. Med.*, 1981, *304*, 939..

Vaginitis. A study demonstrating that *Gardnerella vaginalis* (*Haemophilus vaginalis*) was generally the predominant organism in vaginal fluid from women with non-specific vaginitis although concentrations of anaerobic *Bacteroides* and *Peptococcus* spp. were also significantly increased. The relative pathogenic roles of anaerobes and of *G. vaginalis* in nonspecific vaginitis remain unclear.— C. A. Spiegel *et al.*, *New Engl. J. Med.*, 1980, *303*, 601. Comment.— R. H. Kaufman, *ibid.*, 637.

Combined Antibiotic Action. The concurrent administration of 2 or more antibiotics or other antimicrobial agents has been widely employed but the only clear indications for combined therapy are: the treatment of mixed infections, brain abscess and intra-abdominal or pelvic infections are very likely to be in this category; the production of synergism; the prevention of the emergence of resistant organisms; and the initial treatment of unidentified life-threatening infections. The use of fixed-dose combined preparations is generally not recommended.

Synergism occurs between penicillin and streptomycin or gentamicin in enterococcal endocarditis and has been reported between tetracycline and streptomycin in brucellosis. Enhanced activity against *Pseudomonas aeruginosa* has been demonstrated with carbenicillin and gentamicin and similarly with ticarcillin and tobramycin. Synergism between penicillins and/or cephalosporins has been demonstrated against Gram-negative organisms in which beta-lactamase production is responsible for resistance to one agent alone. In such an instance, methicillin or cloxacillin has increased the combined activity of the antibiotics by inhibiting enzymic degradation of the more susceptible antibiotic. However, antagonism between combinations of penicillins and cephalosporins has been demonstrated by J.F. Acar *et al.* (*J. clin. Invest.*, 1975, *55*, 446) and may be due to competition for, or alteration of, cellular binding sites. Recently, the beta-lactamase inhibitor clavulanic acid has been used with penicillinase-sensitive antibiotics in an attempt to extend their range of activity.

In the treatment of tuberculosis, several antimicrobial agents are always used together in order to delay the emergence of resistant strains of mycobacteria.

Care is necessary in prescribing combined therapy, since some antibiotics may interfere with the activity of others. In general, it has been predicted that interference will occur between the respective activities of a bactericidal and a bacteriostatic antibiotic given concurrently, but not between 2 bactericidal antibiotics although this interference may not necessarily be significant *in vivo*.

The combined use of antibiotics with similar adverse effects may be a problem; for example, the aminoglycosides and some cephalosporins are potentially nephrotoxic. Supra-infection may result because of the broad spectrum of activity of combined antibiotic treatment.

Reviews of the combined use of antibiotics.— A. J. Weinstein, *Med. J. Aust.*, 1977, *2*, *Suppl.* 3, 19; J. J. Rahal, *Medicine*, 1978, *57*, 179; *Lancet*, 1978, *2*, 80. See also T. Matthews (letter), *ibid.*, 376.

It was suggested that caution be exercised in the simultaneous clinical use of antibiotics such as chloramphenicol, lincomycin and the macrolides, acting on the 50S subunit of bacterial ribosomes.— B. Weisblum (letter), *Lancet*, 1967, *1*, 843.

A report of incompatibilities and interactions between penicillins and aminoglycoside antibiotics in concentrated solutions for intramuscular injection.— B. Lynn and A. Jones, *Beecham Research*, *Advances in Antimicrobial and Antineoplastic Chemotherapy*, Vol. I, pt 1, Urban and Schwarzenberg, 1972, 701.

Combinations of bacteriostatic and bactericidal antibiotics were not necessarily antagonistic; cephalothin or penicillin with rolitetracycline showed some enhanced activity *in vitro* against *Staphylococcus aureus* and *Escherichia coli*.— F. D. Daschner, *Antimicrob. Ag. Chemother.*, 1976, *10*, 802.

When erythromycin and benzylpenicillin were used together against isolates of *Staph. aureus* that were inducibly resistant to both antibiotics alone, the isolates were susceptible because of inhibition of penicillinase induction by erythromycin; this effect was not seen when resistance to erythromycin was constitutive.— N. E. Allen and J. K. Epp, *Lilly, USA*, *Antimicrob. Ag. Chemother.*, 1978, *13*, 849.

Further references: *Clinical Use of Combinations of Antibiotics*, J. Klastersky (Ed.), London, Hodder and Stoughton, 1975; N. A. Simmons, *J. antimicrob. Chemother.*, 1975, *1*, 257; C. Watanakunakorn and C. Glotzbecker, *Antimicrob. Ag. Chemother.*, 1977, *11*, 88; L. J. Lincoln *et al.*, *Antimicrob. Ag. Chemother.*, 1977, *12*, 484; E. T. Anderson *et al.*, *Chemotherapy, Basle*, 1978, *24*, 45.

Prophylactic Use of Antibiotics. There are few occasions when the prophylactic use of antibiotics is justifiable. Patients at risk of developing endocarditis, including those with valvular heart disease or other cardiac abnormalities and those with a history of endocarditis or rheumatic fever, should be given antibiotics prophylactically when about to undergo dental operations, tonsillectomy, or other procedure liable to lead to bacteraemia. The antibiotic should be administered so that the peak plasma concentration coincides with the operation. Benzylpenicillin and procaine penicillin, with or without an aminoglycoside, may be given before the procedure and antibiotic cover continued for 48 hours.

Patients who have had rheumatic fever may require prolonged prophylaxis against recurrent streptococcal infection. Phenoxymethylpenicillin 125 mg twice daily by mouth or a monthly intramuscular injection of benzathine penicillin 1.125 g may provide reliable prophylaxis.

Antibiotics have been administered prophylactically to patients with chronic bronchitis.

Antibiotics, mainly the aminoglycosides, are sometimes given to suppress the intestinal flora in patients receiving chemotherapy for leukaemia, who are at special risk of acquiring infection.

The prophylactic use of antibiotics in surgery is controversial but their systemic use has been recommended in patients undergoing gastro-intestinal operations and in other types of surgery including cardiovascular, gynaecological, and orthopaedic operations. Antibiotics frequently used include cephalosporins, penicillins, and aminoglycosides. They should be injected immediately before, and if necessary, during the operation so that adequate concentrations are present. To reduce the risk of supra-infection, prophylaxis should generally not continue for longer than 24 to 48 hours. When anaerobic organisms are likely to be a problem, metronidazole (see p.969) may be used.

Antibiotics have occasionally been administered to patients with viral infections to lessen the risk of secondary infection.

Reviews of the prophylactic use of antibiotics.— W. Brumfitt and J. M. T. Hamilton-Miller, *J. antimicrob. Chemother.*, 1975, *1*, 163; *J. Am. med. Ass.*, 1977, *237*, 1134; I. Jacoby *et al.*, *Med. Clins N. Am.*, 1978, *62*, 1083; H. C. Neu, *J. antimicrob. Chemother.*, 1979, *5*, 331.

A discussion on the prevention of infection in minor accidental wounds.— G. D. Chisholm (letter), *J. antimicrob. Chemother.*, 1976, *2*, 109.

The use of antibiotics and other antimicrobial agents to eliminate most pathogenic organisms from patients undergoing bone-marrow transplantation.— H. F. L. Guiot and R. van Furth, *Br. med. J.*, 1977, *1*, 800.

Bronchitis prophylaxis. A review of chemoprophylaxis in chronic bronchitis.— D. Hughes, *J. antimicrob. Chemother.*, 1976, *2*, 320.

Long-term prophylaxis with antibiotics during the winter had generally been abandoned. The only current place for prophylaxis was in providing cover during general anaesthesia.— *Lancet*, 1975, *1*, 505.

Cholera prophylaxis. Mass chemoprophylaxis against cholera had not been shown to be of value. The elimination of intestinal flora could predispose to cholera by upsetting defence mechanisms.— W. H. Barker and E. J. Gangarosa (letter), *Lancet*, 1973, *2*, 1265.

Endocarditis prophylaxis. As protection against the development of subacute bacterial endocarditis, patients with rheumatic heart disease should be given an intramuscular injection of procaine penicillin 600 mg and crystalline benzylpenicillin 360 mg in a single injection together with 1 g of streptomycin 1 or 2 hours before any surgical operation. Subsequently, procaine penicillin 600 mg and streptomycin 1 g should be given intramuscularly daily for 2 days. Because of the possible presence of penicillin-resistant organisms during penicillin prophylaxis, other combinatios of drugs including erythromycin, streptomycin, vancomycin, and cephaloridine had been recommended. Patients sensitive to penicillin should be given erythromycin 250 mg four times daily for 3 days, starting 8 hours before the operation.— Report of a WHO Expert Committee on Prevention of Rheumatic Fever, *Tech. Rep. Ser. Wld Hlth Org. No. 342*, 1966.

Recommended prophylactic antibiotic regimens for use in patients at risk of developing bacterial endocarditis.— *Circulation*, 1977, *56*, 139A (Report of the Committee on Prevention of Rheumatic Fever and Bacterial Endocarditis of the American Heart Association). See also *Med. Lett.*, 1979, *21*, 73. Critical comments on the report.— *Br. med. J.*, 1977, *2*, 1564; D. C. Shanson, *J. antimicrob. Chemother.*, 1978, *4*, 2; R. G. Petersdorf, *Am. J. Med.*, 1978, *65*, 220; *Br. med. J.*, 1979, *1*, 290; P. A. Oill *et al.* (letter), *New Engl. J. Med.*, 1981, *305*, 101.

There was no indication for routine antibiotic cover at childbirth in women at risk of endocarditis. Appropriate antibiotic therapy would be used if sepsis were present or suspected.— H. A. Fleming (letter), *Lancet*, 1977, *1*, 144. A contrary view.— M. de Swiet, *Prescribers' J.*, 1979, *19*, 59. See also D. Sugrue *et al.*, *Br. Heart J.*, 1980, *44*, 499.

Further references: C. Ward *et al.*, *Postgrad. med. J.*, 1977, *53*, 353; L. Weinstein, *J. Am. med. Ass.*, 1978, *240*, 2485; *Br. med. J.*, 1979, *1*, 1004; *Br. med. J.*, 1979, *2*, 785; G. A. Pankey, *Am. Heart J.*, 1979, *98*, 102; C. Oakley and W. Somerville, *Br. Heart J.*, 1981, *45*, 233; O. Scott, *Archs Dis. Childh.*, 1981, *56*, 581.

Dental procedures. Patients with heart disease might require the administration of antibiotics before and up to 48 hours after tooth extraction to counteract the consequent transient bacteraemia.— Standing Dental Advisory Committee, *Emergencies in Dental Practice*, London, HM Stationery Office, 1967.

Discussions on the use of antibiotics for prophylaxis in dentistry.— *Br. dent. J.*, 1978, *144*, 236; A. D. Wright, *ibid.*, 351. See also D. Barrett (letter), *ibid.*, *145*, 36; B. Hemphill (letter), *ibid.*, 91; D. A. McGowan, *J. antimicrob. Chemother.*, 1978, *4*, 486.

Further references: I. Phillips *et al.*, *J. med. Microbiol.*, 1976, *9*, 393.

Leukaemia. The prevention of infections in acute leukaemia.— *Lancet*, 1978, *2*, 769.

A report of the beneficial effects of a protected environment and prophylactic antibiotics, given orally or intravenously, in patients undergoing chemotherapy for acute leukaemia. Such patients had a lower risk of fatal infection, higher complete remission-rate, and longer survival than patients treated similarly in a conventional hospital room.— V. Rodriguez *et al.*, *Medicine, Baltimore*, 1978, *57*, 253.

Further references: A. S. Levine *et al.*, *New Engl. J. Med.*, 1973, *288*, 477; *Lancet*, 1974, *2*, 764; P. F. M. Wrigley, *Adv. Med. Topics Ther.*, 1976, *2*, 78; F. A. Gill *et al.*, *Cancer*, 1977, *39*, 1704; L. Balducci *et al.*, *Sth. med. J.*, 1979, *72*, 889; *Lancet*, 1980, *1*, 25; *Med. Lett.*, 1981, *23*, 55.

Meningitis prophylaxis. Infant contacts of patients with influenzal meningitis should be closely supervised and treated, if signs of infection occurred, with ampicillin trihydrate, 50 mg per kg body-weight daily, or with chloramphenicol, 100 mg per kg daily, for 4 days. In cases of meningococcal meningitis, intimate contacts, both children and adults, should be treated prophylactically with sulphadiazine or, in the case of resistant organisms, with penicillin, for 2 to 4 days. Antibiotic prophylaxis was unnecessary for contacts of other types of purulent meningitis.— L. L. Coriell, per *J. Am. med. Ass.*, 1967, *201*, 281. See also M. S. Artenstein, *ibid.*, 1975, *231*, 1035; W. A. Littlejohns, *J. antimicrob. Chemother.*, 1977, *3*, 9.

Rheumatic fever prophylaxis. To prevent first attacks of rheumatic fever during streptococcal infections or to prevent recurrence of infection in patients who had had rheumatic fever, suggested treatment was benzylpenicillin 1.2 g intramuscularly followed by phenoxymethylpenicillin 250 mg or benzylpenicillin 300 mg thrice daily by mouth for 10 days. Continuous prophylaxis in patients who had had rheumatic fever was provided by benzylpenicillin 120 mg or phenoxymethylpenicillin 125 mg given by mouth twice daily. Alternatively, a monthly injection of 1.125 g of benzathine penicillin was suitable. To reduce the risk of endocarditis in patients with rheumatic heart disease about to undergo dental extraction or other similar operations, 180 mg of benzylpenicillin or 300 mg of procaine penicillin should be given intramuscularly 1 hour before the operation and 300 mg of procaine penicillin 6 to 12 hours after surgery. If necessary phenoxymethylpenicillin 250 mg every 6 hours should be given for 2 days.— *Prevention of Initial Attacks and Recurrences of Rheumatic Fever*, London, Ministry of Health, 1965. For a similar report, see Report of a WHO Expert Committee on Prevention of Rheumatic Fever, *Tech. Rep. Ser. Wld Hlth Org. No. 342,* 1966.

After a primary attack of rheumatic fever, penicillin should be given for 5 years, or until the patient left school, as a protection against further streptococcal infection. Oral phenoxymethylpenicillin 250 mg daily, or monthly intramuscular injections of benzathine penicillin (usual dose 1.125 g) were the treatments recommended, though the latter was considered more likely to be effective. Neither treatment would influence progressive fibrosis in patients who had already sustained cardiac damage.— Report of a Sub-Committee of the Standing Medical Advisory Committee, *Rheumatic Fever in Scotland*, London, HM Stationery Office, 1967. The recommendation that treatment should be continued for 5 years could be criticised. It had been shown by R. Leonard and N.K. Wenger (*Am. J. Dis. Child.*, 1966, *111*, 533) that recurrences could follow up to 20 years after the first episode of rheumatic carditis and it seemed wise therefore to continue treatment until the age of 17 or 18 in children and for at least 5 years when the first episode occurred at or above the age of 13 years.— *Lancet*, 1967, *2*, 29.

Penicillin is the drug of choice in the treatment of streptococcal upper respiratory-tract infections to prevent primary attacks of rheumatic fever. A single intramuscular dose of benzathine penicillin 900 mg or 450 mg for patients under about 30 kg body-weight is recommended. Alternatively a 10-day course of oral benzylpenicillin 120 to 150 mg thrice or 4 times daily may be given. Patients allergic to penicillin can be given erythromycin; tetracycline should not be used because of the very high prevalence of resistant strains. Prevention of recurrent rheumatic fever depended on continuous prophylaxis and is recommended for all patients with a history of rheumatic fever, those with rheumatic heart disease, or those with Sydenham's chorea. Benzathine penicillin 900 mg intramuscularly every 4 weeks is the most effective treatment. Oral prophylaxis with benzylpenicillin 120 to 150 mg twice daily or sulphadiazine 1 g daily may be used in patients at lower risk of recurrence. Firm guidelines regarding duration of prophylaxis cannot yet be given.— *Circulation*, 1977, *55*, Jan (Report of the Committee on Rheumatic Fever and Bacterial Endocarditis of the American Heart Association). Comment on the report. Phenoxymethylpenicillin is preferable to benzylpenicillin when oral treatment is required; the use of sulphadiazine is also questioned.— *Br. med. J.*, 1977, *2*, 1564. See also *Bull. Wld Hlth Org.*, 1978, *56*, 887 (WHO Memorandum).

It was recommended that under streptococcal pharyngitis epidemic situations all nonallergic patients with pharyngitis should be given penicillin therapy.— R. K. Tompkins *et al.*, *Ann. intern. Med.*, 1977, *86*, 481. See also A. L. Bisno, *ibid.*, 494; R. H. Pantell, *ibid.*, 497; *Lancet*, 1981, *1*, 311.

In the control of rheumatic heart disease in developing countries, pharyngitis should be treated with one injection of benzathine penicillin (900 mg in adults and 450 mg in children); sulphadiazine and tetracycline should not be used. In the secondary prevention of rheumatic fever the schedule recommended in 1966 (*Tech. Rep. Ser. Wld Hlth Org. No. 342*) is still valid but injections of benzathine penicillin every 3 weeks rather than monthly are preferable. The length of prophylaxis is still disputed.— *Chronicle Wld Hlth Org.*, 1980, *34*, 389.

Further references: N. S. Blackman and L. Kuskin, *Clin. Pediat.*, 1972, *11*, 15; G. Peter and A. L. Smith, *New Engl. J. Med.*, 1977, *297*, 311 and 365; J. E. Parrillo *et al.*, *New Engl. J. Med.*, 1979, *300*, 296.

Surgical infection prophylaxis. Reviews and discussions of antibiotics in surgical infection prophylaxis.— A. D. Roy, *J. antimicrob. Chemother.*, 1976, *2*, 233; *J. Am. med. Ass.*, 1977, *237*, 1003; *Lancet*, 1977, *1*, 1351; *Br. med. J.*, 1977, *2*, 1500; G. W. Chodak and M. E. Plaut, *Obstet. Gynec.*, 1978, *51*, 123; B. A. Cunha *et al.* (letter), *Lancet*, 1978, *1*, 207; S. A. Berger *et al.*, *Surgery Gynec. Obstet.*, 1978, *146*, 469; H. Ellis, *Postgrad. med. J.*, 1978, *54*, 367; S. W. B. Newsom, *J. antimicrob. Chemother.*, 1978, *4*, 389; *Med. Lett.*, 1979, *21*, 73; A. M. Clarke, *J. antimicrob. Chemother.*, 1979, *5*, 493; *Br. med. J.*, 1980, *280*, 1241; M. R. B. Keighley, *Br. J. Hosp. Med.*, 1980, *23*, 465; *Br. med. J.*, 1980, *280*, 882; *ibid.*, 1063; *Drug & Ther. Bull.*, 1981, *19*, 45.

Treatment with antibiotics and chemotherapeutic agents prior to colonic surgery was generally considered justifiable, but staphylococcal enterocolitis might occur because of the resistance of the organism. Systemic chemotherapy for the prevention of wound infection after general surgery had been disappointing.— *Lancet*, 1968, *1*, 831. See also F. P. Herter and C. A. Slanetz, *Am. J. Surg.*, 1967, *113*, 165.

For reports of the ineffectiveness of antibiotic prophylaxis in patients undergoing various surgical procedures, see H. Clark, *Am. Heart J.*, 1969, *77*, 767; T. K. Day, *Lancet*, 1975, *2*, 1174; R. Truesdale *et al.*, *J. Am. med. Ass.*, 1979, *241*, 1254; H. -J. Peters, *Dt. med. Wschr.*, 1979, *104*, 347.

In a study of 830 patients who underwent appendicectomy, postoperative infections occurred in 123 of 553 patients who did not receive prophylactic antibiotic treatment. *Bacteroides fragilis* was the commonest organism isolated from all patients. It was considered that the use of clindamycin, lincomycin, or metronidazole for prophylaxis in patients undergoing appendicectomy was more appropriate than other antibiotics because of their higher antimicrobial activity against anaerobic bacteria.— D. A. Leigh, *J. antimicrob. Chemother.*, 1978, *4*, *Suppl.* C, 15. A survey of the use of antibacterial agents for prophylaxis of infection in appendicectomy.— W. B. Campbell, *Br. med. J.*, 1980, *281*, 1597. Antibiotic lavage to prevent wound sepsis after appendicectomy.— Z. H. Krukowski and N. A. Matheson (letter), *Lancet*, 1981, *1*, 948.

Continuous prophylaxis with antibiotics should be used after splenectomy up to the age of 5 years.— A. J. Ammann and L. K. Diamond (letter), *New Engl. J. Med.*, 1978, *299*, 778.

Recipients of kidney transplants undergoing any operation were given a single intravenous bolus injection of antibiotics on induction of anaesthesia. The regimen included ampicillin 2 g, oxacillin 2 g, and gentamicin 1.5 mg per kg body-weight. Clindamycin 400 mg was substituted for the penicillins in allergic patients.— N. L. Tilney *et al.*, *New Engl. J. Med.*, 1978, *299*, 1321.

Further references: C. R. Whitney *et al.*, *Archs Ophthal., N.Y.*, 1972, *87*, 155; G. A. Kune and J. G. W. Burdon, *Med. J. Aust.*, 1975, *2*, 627; J. H. Grossman and R. L. Adams, *Obstet. Gynec.*, 1979, *53*, 23.

Urinary-tract infection prophylaxis. There was a lower incidence of recurrence of pyelonephritis requiring rehospitalisation in women maintained on antibiotics following an acute episode of antepartum pyelonephritis than in those who had treatment withdrawn after management of the acute episode.— R. E. Harris and L. C. Gilstrap, *Obstet. Gynec.*, 1974, *44*, 637.

Antibiotic prophylaxis using 9 doses of cephazolin sodium 500 mg every 8 hours was no better than placebo against catheter-associated bacteriuria in a study of 196 patients undergoing elective surgery. Prophylaxis was not recommended in patients with non-severe underlying conditions and undergoing short-term bladder catheterisation.— M. R. Britt *et al.*, *Antimicrob. Ag. Chemother.*, 1977, *11*, 240.

Venereal disease prophylaxis. The administration of benzathine penicillin 1.8 g was an adequate prophylactic treatment against infection with syphilis; tetracycline or erythromycin could be used if the patient was allergic to penicillin. Prophylaxis against gonorrhoea in male subjects consisted of 2.4 g of procaine penicillin, with twice this dose for female subjects. Oxytetracycline 1.5 g as a single dose could be used for patients allergic to penicillin.— W. J. Brown, *J. Am. med. Ass.*, 1968, *205*, 653.

Antibiotic Policies. In hospitals, various policies have been advocated with the object of conserving the usefulness of antibiotics as long as possible. Restriction of antibiotics to patients for whom no alternative treatment is available, combined therapy to achieve quicker and more complete elimination of the micro-organisms and thus reduce the emergence of resistant strains, changing from an antibiotic to which resistance has appeared to another to which the organism is susceptible in the hope that resistance to the first antibiotic will diminish, the use of many different antibiotics, none of them used widely enough to permit a significant resistance to arise, and the holding of some antibiotics in reserve, are among the control measures advocated. The induction of resistance should be reduced by employing adequate doses of antibiotics and by avoiding the use of antibiotics for trivial infection and unnecessary prophylaxis.

A discussion on antibiotic policies.— G. A. J. Ayliffe, *J. antimicrob. Chemother.*, 1975, *1*, 255.

Six antibiotics—ampicillin, cephradine, cloxacillin, erythromycin, oxytetracycline, and penicillin (benzylpenicillin and phenoxymethylpenicillin) covered 98% of requirements over a 2-year period. There was widespread resistance to ampicillin in *Staph. aureus*, Enterobacteriaceae, and *Bacteroides*; otherwise resistance was not a problem.— R. W. Lacey, *Br. med. J.*, 1979, *1*, 1389.

Hazards of Antibiotic Therapy. Most antibiotics given by mouth in large enough doses may cause gastro-intestinal irritation. Severe and sometimes fatal pseudomembranous colitis has occurred, especially with clindamycin and lincomycin. Antibiotics may also interfere with the absorption of essential food factors such as vitamins of the B group by provoking diarrhoea or by reducing the numbers of micro-organisms synthesising vitamins in the intestines.

Supra-infection is usually attributable to the suppression of antibiotic-susceptible micro-organisms which normally provide natural competition to prevent the unlimited multiplication of antibiotic-resistant micro-organisms. The administration of broad-spectrum antibiotics, especially by mouth, may result in supra-infection with *Candida* and other yeasts, filamentous fungi, coliform organisms, *Proteus*, or *Pseudomonas* species, affecting the mouth, gastro-intestinal tract, or upper respiratory tract. A more serious infection is staphylococcal enterocolitis which follows the overgrowth of antibiotic-resistant staphylococci. If supra-infection occurs the antibiotic should be withdrawn and other measures to which the supra-infection responds should be substituted.

Compounds may cause pain when given by intramuscular injection and thrombophlebitis when given intravenously.

Allergy and hypersensitivity reactions to antibiotics are particularly troublesome with the penicillins and streptomycin. The topical application of neomycin and other antibiotics increases the risk of inducing sensitisation and allergic reactions in a previously sensitised person may be severe and life-threatening. They often take the form of an urticarial rash and angioneurotic oedema, and may involve bronchospasm and cardiovascular failure. Adrenaline, antihistamines, and corticosteroids are used to treat severe or persistent toxic symptoms. Allergic contact dermatitis has been reported in persons who regularly handle antibiotics. The topical use of antibiotics is also associated with an increased incidence of bacterial resistance.

Tetracycline has a tendency to be concentrated in developing teeth and bones and to cause liver dysfunction when unusually high serum concentrations are reached. The aminoglycosides, polymyxins, tetracyclines, and lincomycins are liable to cause apnoea by blocking neuromuscular transmission if given in large doses, especially if introduced into the peritoneal cavity. Many antibiotics cause damage to the kidneys; a few may damage the eighth cranial nerve or the bone marrow, especially if abnormally high serum concentrations result from impaired excretion. Antibiotics which readily diffuse across the placenta, such as tetracyclines, may be toxic to the foetus if given during pregnancy. The inability of premature and newborn infants to conjugate some antibiotics in the liver may be a factor in toxicity.

The untoward effects of antibiotic therapy on the gastro-intestinal tract, with recommendations for their management.— C. M. Kunin, *Clin. Pharmac. Ther.*, 1967, *8*, 495; E. R. Smith and S. J. M. Goulston, *Drugs*, 1975, *10*, 329; *Br. med. J.*, 1975, *4*, 243.

For comments on the dangers of using antibiotics in eye diseases, see J. S. Cant, *Practitioner*, 1969, *202*, 787.

Skin colonisation with Gram-negative organisms was a hazard of antibiotic therapy in patients with hepatic failure given extracorporeal liver perfusions.— R. V. Mummery *et al.*, *Lancet*, 1971, *2*, 60.

The adverse effects of antibiotics on the immune response.— A. Tarnawski and B. Batko (letter), *Lancet*,

1973, *1*, 674; Y. H. Thong (letter), *Med. J. Aust.*, 1978, *1*, 444.

The toxicity of antibiotics.— G. E. Mawer, *Prescribers' J.*, 1977, *17*, 116.

A discussion of the hazards of topical antibiotics.— *Br. med. J.*, 1977, *1*, 1494.

A warning of the consequences, possibly fatal, attributed to the release of endotoxin following the too rapid destruction of Gram-negative organisms *in vivo* by antibiotics. Fatalities had occurred with gentamicin, tetracycline, and with chloramphenicol.— D. A. B. Hopkin (letter), *Lancet*, 1977, *2*, 603.

Blood disorders. A study in neutropenic patients indicated that antimicrobials have a leading role in drug-induced neutropenia.— S. A. Weitzman *et al.*, *Lancet*, 1978, *1*, 1068.

Effect on EEG. In a study of 95 patients, it was found that intravenous injections of polymyxin B, erythromycin, colistin, lincomycin, or ampicillin accelerated basic EEG rhythms, while intravenous injections of oleandomycin, chloramphenicol, novobiocin, tetracycline, oxytetracycline, oxacillin, methicillin, or cephaloridine retarded them. Polymyxin B produced the greatest degree of acceleration, and cephaloridine the greatest degree of deceleration.— S. Doutlik *et al.*, *Arzneimittel-Forsch.*, 1967, *17*, 1177.

Hepatotoxicity. A short discussion on antimicrobial agents and hepatotoxicity.— *Br. med. J.*, 1980, *280*, 1486.

Interactions. Reviews of the interactions of antibiotics: J. Koch-Weser and E. M. Sellers, *New Engl. J. Med.*, 1971, *285*, 547; S. A. Kabins, *J. Am. med. Ass.*, 1972, *219*, 206; I. H. Stockley, *Pharm. J.*, 1973, *1*, 36; A. M. Geddes, *Prescribers' J.*, 1976, *16*, 9; A. J. Bint and I. Burtt, *Drugs*, 1980, *20*, 57.

Oral contraceptives. A brief discussion on the effect of antimicrobial agents on the efficacy of oral contraceptives.— M. L'E. Orme and D. J. Back, *J. antimicrob. Chemother.*, 1979, *5*, 124.

Nephrotoxicity. A review of the nephrotoxicity of antimicrobial agents.— G. B. Appel and H. C. Neu, *New Engl. J. Med.*, 1977, *296*, 663, 722, and 784. See also S. K. Agarwal (letter), *New Engl. J. Med.*, 1977, *297*, 224; M. L. Graber and D. S. Gluckin (letter), *ibid.*; R. D. Meyer (letter), *ibid.*, 225; G. B. Appel and H. C. Neu (letter), *ibid.*

Antibiotic damage to damaged kidneys.— *Lancet*, 1978, *2*, 558.

Pregnancy and the neonate. Sixty of 836 mothers of congenitally malformed infants had used antibiotics during the first trimester of pregnancy, compared with 42 in 836 controls. The case : control incidence ratio of 1.43 was not significant.— G. Greenberg *et al.*, *Br. med. J.*, 1977, *2*, 853.

Pseudomembranous colitis. Reports leading to the identification of a toxin produced by *Clostridium difficile* as a cause of antibiotic-associated pseudomembranous colitis.— H. E. Larson *et al.*, *Br. med. J.*, 1977, *1*, 1246; G. D. Rifkin *et al.*, *Lancet*, 1977, *2*, 1103; H. E. Larson and A. B. Price, *Lancet*, 1977, *2*, 1312; J. G. Bartlett *et al.*, *New Engl. J. Med.*, 1978, *298*, 531; A. Kappas *et al.*, *Br. med. J.*, 1978, *1*, 675; R. H. George *et al.*, *Br. med. J.*, 1978, *1*, 695; W. L. George *et al.*, *Lancet*, 1978, *1*, 802; H. E. Larson *et al.*, *Lancet*, 1978, *1*, 1063; *Lancet*, 1978, *1*, 1080.

A review of antibiotic-associated pseudomembranous colitis. The disorder has now been associated with many antimicrobial agents including amoxycillin, ampicillin, cefuroxime, cephazolin, clindamycin, co-trimoxazole, lincomycin, and tetracycline, as well as combinations of drugs, particularly aminoglycosides with metronidazole, and usually occurs in postoperative patients. Diagnosis is dependent on the demonstration of a neutralisable toxin in the stool and elimination of toxin-producing strains of *Clostridium difficile* from the colon is achieved with vancomycin, oral doses of 125 mg being given four times a day for 5 days.— M. R. B. Keighley, *Drugs*, 1980, *20*, 49. Clindamycin and lincomycin have accounted for 80% of the reports of antibiotic-associated colitis submitted to the Committee on Safety of Medicines from 1964 to 1978.— *Br. med. J.*, 1981, *282*, 1913.

Results of a Boston Collaborative Drug Surveillance Program indicated that of 26 294 hospital in-patients monitored from 1966 to 1975, 8948 received at least one antibiotic or antibacterial agent, but none developed drug-induced colitis while in hospital. Of the 8948, a total of 3988 received ampicillin, 437 received chloramphenicol, 90 received lincomycin, 163 received clindamycin, and 1517 received tetracycline. All 7 who were admitted with antibiotic-induced colitis were female; 6 had been taking lincomycin (5 from New Zealand) and 1 (also from New Zealand) had been taking ampicillin. None of another 24 783 patients interviewed in 1972 had a diagnosis of drug-induced colitis. Antibiotic-induced colitis, in general, appeared to be rare, although it might be more common in New Zealand. Unlike the findings of F.J. Tedesco *et al.* (*Ann. intern. Med.*, 1974, *81*, 429) these data also appeared to indicate that serious clindamycin-induced colitis is an uncommon reaction, but agreed with those of F.J. Tedesco (*Am. J. dig. Dis.*, 1975, *20*, 295) that ampicillin-associated colitis is rare.— R. R. Miller and H. Jick, *Clin. Pharmac. Ther.*, 1977, *22*, 1.

Following gastro-intestinal operations diarrhoea developed in 46 (39%) of 119 patients who received antibiotic therapy and in only 12 (10%) of 122 who did not. Nine of the patients with diarrhoea had a neutralisable faecal toxin characteristic of pseudomembranous colitis, and all of these patients had toxigenic strains of *Cl. difficile* identified in their stools, although sigmoidoscopy revealed a membrane in only 3 cases, and biopsy in only 5. If pseudomembranous colitis is defined by the presence of a neutralised faecal toxin, results of diagnosis using the conventional methods of sigmoidoscopy and rectal biopsy are often unreliable.— M. R. B. Keighley *et al.*, *Lancet*, 1978, *2*, 1165.

Comment on the difficulty of defining pseudomembranous colitis.— A. B. Price and H. E. Larson (letter), *Lancet*, 1979, *1*, 443.

Further references to pseudomembranous colitis: A. Wald *et al.*, *Ann. intern. Med.*, 1980, *92*, 798 (not associated with antibiotics); P. R. Mills *et al.* (letter), *Lancet*, 1981, *1*, 552 (evidence that pseudomembranous colitis can be infectious).

Antibiotics in Food

The use of antibiotics for the treatment of bovine mastitis or other infections in animals, the feeding of antibiotics to young farm stock to accelerate growth, or the employment of antibiotics in various ways as food preservatives or to control diseases of plants may result in possible hazards to human health due to traces of antibiotics being present in food. These hazards may include direct toxic effects, hypersensitivity reactions, and the production of antibiotic resistance in pathogenic organisms transmissible to man.

For a discussion of the uses of antibiotics in animal husbandry with a consideration of the hazards to public health, see *Report of the Joint Committee on the Use of Antibiotics in Animal Husbandry and Veterinary Medicine*, London, HM Stationery Office, 1969.

ANTIBIOTICS IN VETERINARY MEDICINE

The use of antibiotics either by mouth or by injection for the treatment of animal diseases did not normally result in an accumulation of the antibiotics in the tissues. Analytical data and clinical experience indicated that the antibiotics were rapidly eliminated. Nevertheless, in order to ensure that there were no antibiotic residues in human food derived from treated animals, a WHO Expert Committee (*Tech. Rep. Ser. Wld Hlth Org. No. 260*, 1963) recommended that an interval should be allowed between the last treatment and the time of slaughter. Usually 48 hours was sufficient for the elimination of the antibiotic but this might not be so and manufacturers should state on the label the interval that was required. The Committee recommended that eggs from poultry receiving therapeutic amounts of antibiotics should not be sold for human consumption.

ANTIBIOTIC RESIDUES IN MILK

When antibiotics are administered parenterally in full therapeutic doses some excretion occurs in the milk. A much more important cause of the presence of antibiotics in cows' milk is intramammary injection via the teat canal for the treatment of mastitis. Antibiotics used for this purpose include procaine penicillin, cloxacillin, cephalonium, cephoxazole, dihydrostreptomycin, erythromycin, neomycin, spiramycin, and the tetracyclines. It is recommended that milk from treated animals should not be used as long as antibiotic residues can be detected in it.

For comments on the hazards of antibiotics in milk, see Report of Expert Committee on the Public Health Aspects of the Use of Antibiotics in Food and Feedstuffs, *Tech. Rep. Ser. Wld Hlth Org. No. 260*, 1963.

Manufacturers of antibiotic preparations for injecting into the teat canal should be asked to formulate them so that they were eliminated within 48 hours and to label them with instructions to withhold milk from the market for a specified time after their use. Dyes included with the medication as 'markers' by which the presence of antibiotic could be easily detected were unsatisfactory but the search for a suitable marker—not necessarily a dye—should be continued.— *Report of the Milk Hygiene Subcommittee of the Milk and Milk Products Technical Advisory Committee*, London, HM Stationery Office, 1963.

In 2 surveys, each for periods of 7 months, 3.9 and 3.8% respectively of milk samples were found to contain 0.05 units or more per ml of penicillin.— A. H. Parry *et al.*, *Mon. Bull. Minist. Hlth*, 1966, *25*, 92.

Following the intramammary injection of oxytetracycline, residues from treated quarters persisted as long as 5.5 days. Residues in the milk from untreated quarters appeared to be due to transfer via the circulation.— S. E. Katz *et al.*, *J. Ass. off. anal. Chem.*, 1973, *56*, 706.

ANTIBIOTIC SUPPLEMENTS FOR ANIMAL FEEDS

Small quantities of certain antibiotics are added to the feed of young animals with the object of stimulating the rate of growth.

In the European Economic Community the use of antibiotics in feeding stuffs is controlled by Directive 70/524/EEC of 23 November 1970; this Directive has been subject to many amendments. Antibiotics, permitted or provisionally permitted (subject to specified conditions) are avoparcin, bacitracin zinc, bambermycin, lincomycin, mocimycin, monensin sodium, nosiheptide, spiramycin, tylosin, and virginiamycin. Carbadox, nitrovin, and olaquindox are also used as growth promoters.

The EEC Directive also covers coccidiostats and other medicinal substances, together with vitamins, minerals, and pharmaceutical adjuvants.

In the UK implementation of the Directive in respect of antibiotics and medicinal substances is by control of the relevant product licences under the provisions of The Medicines Act 1968. Implementation of the Directive in Great Britain in respect of non-medicinal substances is by means of The Fertilisers and Feeding Stuffs Regulations 1973 (SI 1973: No. 1521) as amended (SI 1976: No. 840 and SI 1977: No. 115). The Directive is not considered to prohibit the addition in Great Britain of other antibiotics or medicinal substances to feeding stuffs for medicinal use under veterinary direction.

The administration of antibiotics to farm livestock at subtherapeutic concentrations posed certain hazards to human and animal health. There was evidence to show that enteric bacteria of animal origin were commonly ingested by man and an infection by an organism with multiple drug resistance could endanger the life of the patient. Further, transfer of resistance from nonpathogenic to pathogenic organisms could occur. It was recommended that the use without prescription of antibiotics in animal feeding stuffs should be restricted to those antibiotics which had little or no application as therapeutic agents in man or animals and which would not impair the efficacy of a prescribed therapeutic drug through the development of resistant strains of organisms.— *Report of the Joint Committee on the Use of Antibiotics in Animal Husbandry and Veterinary Medicine* [Swann Report], London, HM Stationery Office, 1969. Comments on the effects of legislation passed in Great Britain as a result of the Swann report and the emergence of multiple drug resistance in *Salmonella typhimurium* in bovines.— *Br. med. J.*, 1980, *280*, 1195; H. W. Smith (letter), *ibid.*, 1537; M. Richmond (letter), *ibid.*, 1615.

The amounts of antibiotics added to animal feeds should not be greater than were required to produce the desired effect and any increase above approved levels should only follow thorough investigations into the necessity for such an increase and any possible consequences. Similarly adequate study of the effects that could arise from using mixtures should be carried out before 2 or more antibiotics were added to a feed. No antibiotic should be used if there was any risk to the animal or any effect on the wholesomeness of foods of animal origin. Nor should antibiotics be used that gave rise to residues in eggs or milk. Should the use of antibiotics be unavoidable in lactating animals then the milk should be discarded until the residue could no longer be detected.— Twelfth Report of the Joint FAO/WHO

Expert Committee on Food Additives, *Tech. Rep. Ser. Wld Hlth Org. No. 430,* 1969. See also Report of Expert Committee on the Public Health Aspects of the Use of Antibiotics in Food and Feedstuffs, *Tech. Rep. Ser. Wld Hlth Org. No. 260,* 1963.

The deposition of chloramphenicol in egg albumen and yolk after ingestion by poultry.— C. S. Sisodia and R. H. Dunlop, *Can. vet. J.,* 1972, *13,* 279, per *Int. pharm. Abstr.,* 1974, *11,* 402.

Residues of oxytetracycline were determined in the eggs and tissues of poultry given oxytetracycline supplements in a concentration of 25 to 200 g per ton. Cooking destroyed all residues in muscle but livers retained 50% of uncooked concentrations.— S. E. Katz *et al., J. Ass. off. anal. Chem.,* 1973, *56,* 77, per *Int. pharm. Abstr.,* 1973, *10,* 838. Similar studies with chlortetracycline.— *idem, J. Ass. off. anal. Chem.,* 1972, *55,* 128 and 134.

A discussion of the use of antibiotics as supplements in animal feeding and the emergence of resistant strains.— *Br. med. J.,* 1974, *2,* 235. See also T. H. Jukes, *J. Am. med. Ass.,* 1975, *232,* 292; P. Pohl, *J. antimicrob. Chemother.,* 1977, *3, Suppl.* C, 67.

Calves and swine fed with a diet containing subtherapeutic concentrations of oxytetracycline for 28 days and inoculated with *Salmonella typhimurium* showed a decrease in the shedding of *S. typhimurium* in time compared with unmedicated inoculated controls. In chickens there was a slight sporadic increase in resistant colonies. It was considered that there was no evidence that continuous low-level feeding of oxytetracycline to animals was associated with an increased incidence of salmonellosis in animals or humans.— D. G. Evangelisti *et al., Antimicrob. Ag. Chemother.,* 1975, *8,* 664.

The use of neomycin and oxytetracycline in feeds for poultry, pigs, and calves was not considered to affect the quantity, prevalence, and shedding of *S. typhimurium.*— A. E. Girard *et al., Pfizer, USA, Antimicrob. Ag. Chemother.,* 1976, *10,* 89.

Although chlortetracycline 110 mg added to each kg of feed reduced the quantity, duration, and prevalence of faecal shedding of *S. typhimurium* from swine when the infecting strains were susceptible to chlortetracycline, all these factors were increased when the strains were resistant and the transmission of *Salmonella* between animals was enhanced.— R. D. Williams *et al., Antimicrob. Ag. Chemother.,* 1978, *14,* 710.

Further references: J. D. A. van Embden *et al.* (letter), *Lancet,* 1978, *1,* 655; J. I. Rood *et al., Antimicrob. Ag. Chemother.,* 1978, *13,* 871; S. B. Levy, *J. infect. Dis.,* 1978, *137,* 689.

ANTIBIOTICS AS FOOD PRESERVATIVES

Certain antibiotics have been shown to increase the shelf or storage life of several kinds of processed and fresh foods. The antibiotics used in food preservation in certain countries have included chlortetracycline, oxytetracycline, nisin, and nystatin.

In Great Britain the use of antibiotics as food preservatives is limited by the Preservatives in Food Regulations, 1979 (SI 1979: No. 752) and the Preservatives in Food (Scotland) Regulations, 1979 [SI 1979: No. 1073 (S.96)]. Under these regulations, cheese, clotted cream, or any canned food may have nisin in it or on it.

Generally, antibiotics should only be considered for use as direct food additives if they did not affect microbial spoilage of food so as to result in danger to the consumer, were not of therapeutic importance, and did not give rise to cross-resistance or affect the clinical use of other antibiotics. Information should be obtained on the effects on the normal body flora of an antibiotic suggested for use as an intentional food additive. The usual standards of food hygiene should not be permitted to diminish because of the use of an antibiotic as a food additive.— Twelfth Report of the Joint FAO/WHO Expert Committee on Food Additives, *Tech. Rep. Ser. Wld Hlth Org. No. 430,* 1969.

ANTIBIOTICS IN PLANT DISEASE CONTROL

Antibiotics are used in the treatment of some bacterial and mycotic diseases of plants. In Great Britain the use of antibiotics for horticultural purposes is limited by the Pesticides Safety Precautions Scheme and the Medicines (Prohibition of Non-medicinal Antimicrobial Substances) Order 1977 (SI 1977: No. 2131). Under this order preparations for horticultural use as fungicides may contain streptomycin provided they have been rendered unfit for any medicinal purpose, and unpalatable to such a degree as to prevent their consumption by human beings, by the addition of a sufficient quantity of a suitable substance. Oxytetracycline and cycloheximide have also been used in plant disease control.

Antibiotic Groups. Although antibiotics are a very diverse class of compounds they are often classified and discussed in groups. They may be classified according to their mode of action or spectrum of antimicrobial activity but generally antibiotics with similar chemical structures are grouped together.

The Aminoglycosides

The aminoglycosides are a closely-related group of bactericidal antibiotics derived from bacteria of the order Actinomycetales or, more specifically, the genus *Streptomyces* (framycetin, kanamycin, neomycin, paromomycin, streptomycin, and tobramycin) and the genus *Micromonospora* (gentamicin and sissomicin). They are polycationic compounds which are generally used as the sulphate and contain 2-deoxystreptamine (or streptose in streptomycin) with cyclic amino-sugars attached by glycosidic linkages. They have also been termed aminoglycosidic aminocyclitols.

The aminoglycosides have broadly similar toxicological features. Ototoxicity is a major limitation to their use; streptomycin and gentamicin are generally considered to be more toxic to the vestibular branch of the eighth cranial nerve and neomycin and kanamycin to be more toxic to the auditory branch. Other adverse effects common to the group include nephrotoxicity, neuromuscular blocking activity, and allergy, including cross-reactivity.

The pharmacokinetics of the aminoglycosides are very similar. Little is absorbed from the gastro-intestinal tract but they are generally well-distributed in the body after parenteral administration although penetration into the cerebrospinal fluid is poor. They are excreted unchanged in the urine by glomerular filtration.

The aminoglycosides have a similar antimicrobial spectrum and are thought to act by interfering with bacterial protein synthesis, possibly by binding irreversibly to the 30S portion of the bacterial ribosome. They are most active against Gram-negative rods. *Staphylococcus aureus* is susceptible to the aminoglycosides but otherwise most Gram-positive bacteria, and also anaerobic bacteria, are naturally resistant. They show enhanced activity with penicillin against some streptococci. Bacterial resistance to streptomycin may occur by mutation whereas with the other aminoglycosides it is usually associated with the plasmid-mediated production of inactivating enzymes which are capable of phosphorylation, acetylation, or adenylation. As many as 9 enzymes have been identified.

Streptomycin was the first aminoglycoside to become available commercially and was isolated from a strain of *Streptomyces griseus* in 1944. Its use is now restricted mainly to the treatment of tuberculosis when it is always adminstered in association with other drugs such as rifampicin, isoniazid, and ethambutol because of the rapid development of resistance. *Dihydrostreptomycin,* a reduction product of streptomycin, is no longer used because of its toxicity. The *neomycin* complex of antibiotics were the next to be isolated; neomycin itself is mainly a mixture of the B and C isomers and neomycin B is considered to be identical with *framycetin.* Because of their toxicity they are not given systemically. The same applies to *paromomycin* which is used in the treatment of intestinal amoebiasis. *Kanamycin* is less toxic than neomycin and can be used systemically. However, it is not active against *Pseudomonas aeruginosa* and has generally been replaced by gentamicin, although it has been used in penicillin-resistant gonorrhoea and streptomycin-resistant tuberculosis.

Gentamicin was isolated from *Micromonospora purpurea* in 1963 and, being active against *Ps. aeruginosa* and *Serratia marcescens,* is widely used in the treatment of life-threatening infections. *Tobramycin* is closely related to kanamycin but has an antimicrobial spectrum very similar to that of gentamicin and is reported to be more active against *Ps. aeruginosa.* Although there is cross-resistance between gentamicin and tobramycin, tobramycin may be inactivated by fewer bacterial enzymes. *Amikacin,* a semi-synthetic derivative of kanamycin, has a side-chain rendering it less susceptible to inactivating enzymes. It has a spectrum of activity like that of gentamicin but Gram-negative bacteria resistant to gentamicin, tobramycin, and kanamycin are often sensitive. Two more recent additions to the aminoglycoside group of antibiotics include *sissomicin* which is structurally related to gentamicin, the two antibiotics exhibiting cross-resistance, and *netilmicin,* the *N*-ethyl derivative of sissomicin, which may be active against some gentamicin-resistant strains.

Because of their potential toxicity and antimicrobial spectrum, aminoglycoside antibiotics should in general only be used for the treatment of serious infections. Doses must be carefully regulated to maintain plasma concentrations within the therapeutic range but avoiding accumulation, especially in patients with renal impairment. Neomycin and framycetin, which are considered too toxic to be given parenterally, have been given by mouth to suppress the intestinal flora. The topical use of neomycin and gentamicin has been associated with allergic reactions and the emergence of resistant bacteria. Gentamicin or tobramycin are the antibiotics of choice in the treatment of life-threatening infections due to aminoglycoside-sensitive organisms and are often used in association with carbenicillin or ticarcillin. With the continuing emergence of resistant strains, amikacin and netilmicin should be reserved for severe infections resistant to gentamicin and the other aminoglycosides.

The Cephalosporins

The cephalosporins are semi-synthetic antibiotics derived from cephalosporin C a natural antibiotic produced by the mould *Cephalosporium acremonium.* The active nucleus, 7-aminocephalosporanic acid, is very closely related to the penicillin nucleus, 6-aminopenicillanic acid, and consists of a beta-lactam ring fused with a 6-membered dihydrothiazine ring and having an acetoxymethyl group at position 3. Cephalosporin C has a side-chain at position 7 derived from D-α-aminoadipic acid and is significantly less active than benzylpenicillin against susceptible Gram-positive and Gram-negative bacteria. Chemical modification of positions 3 and 7 has resulted in a series of antibiotics with different characteristics. Substitution at the 7-amino group tends to affect antibacterial action whereas at position 3 it may have more of an effect on pharmacokinetic properties.

The cephalosporins are bactericidal and, similarly to the penicillins, they act by inhibiting synthesis of the bacterial cell wall. They are active against a wide range of Gram-positive and Gram-negative bacteria, including penicillinase-producing staphylococci, but not against enterococci. Newer cephalosporins show activity against *Pseudomonas* spp. Methicillin-resistant strains of *Staphylococcus aureus* are usually resistant to the cephalosporins. Susceptible Gram-positive cocci are more sensitive to the penicillins.

Cephalothin was the first cephalosporin to become available and has been widely used, especially in the USA; like *cephacetrile* and *cefapirin* it retains the 3-acetoxy group of the parent compound, cephalosporin C. All 3 antibiotics are relatively unstable in the body and despite different substituents at the 7-position have similar antibacterial activity. The first cephalosporin to be used in the UK was *cephaloridine.* It has the same group at position 7 as cephalothin but the pyridinium group at position 3 has rendered it metabolically stable. *Cephazolin* has different groups at positions 3 and 7 and is also stable with very similar activity to that of cephaloridine although, like cephalothin, intramuscular injections are painful whereas cephaloridine is said to be virtually painless.

Cephaloglycin was the first of this group of antibiotics to be active by mouth although absorption is poor and, having a 3-acetoxy group, it is metabolically unstable. *Cephalexin*, with the same group at position 7 as cephaloglycin but a methyl group at 3, has a structure analogous to that of ampicillin; it is stable and almost completely absorbed from the gastro-intestinal tract, as is *cephradine* which has a similar structure and properties to those of cephalexin. Both cephalexin and cephradine are less potent than cephalothin or cephaloridine.

The cephalosporins mentioned so far have very similar antibacterial spectra and although differing in their potency are usually more active against Gram-positive than Gram-negative bacteria; *Enterobacter* and indole-positive *Proteus* spp. are generally resistant. The newer cephalosporins are resistant to many Gram-negative beta-lactamases and are relatively more active against Gram-negative bacteria and less active against Gram-positive bacteria. *Cephamandole* was one of the first of the so-called beta-lactamase-resistant cephalosporins to become available and has a broader spectrum of activity than cephalothin or cephaloridine. It is more active against many Enterobacteriaceae and against *Haemophilus influenzae*; Gram-positive cocci tend to be less sensitive. Similarly, *cefuroxime* is resistant to most Gram-negative beta-lactamases and is very active against *H. influenzae* and *Neisseria spp. Cefotaxime* is the first cephalosporin reported to be active against *Pseudomonas aeruginosa* and other Gram-negative bacteria are also more sensitive to it than to cefuroxime, including *H. influenzae*.

Cefaclor, like cephalexin and cephradine, can be taken by mouth, but it is more active against Gram-negative bacteria and may be less resistant to staphylococcal penicillinase.

Like the penicillins, the cephalosporins are generally well-tolerated apart from hypersensitivity reactions. Some cross-reactivity between the two groups of antibiotics has been reported and patients known to be allergic to penicillins should be treated with care. Nephrotoxicity may be a problem with cephaloridine and some consider that for this reason it should be withdrawn from use.

The established cephalosporins have not been regarded as antibiotics of first choice in the treatment of infections. They may be of value in some patients who are sensitive to penicillin and against certain bacteria such as *Klebsiella* spp. and penicillin-resistant staphylococci. The newer cephalosporins have a broader spectrum of activity and their place in antibiotic therapy remains to be determined.

The Cephamycins

The cephamycins are a family of beta-lactam antibiotics derived from actinomycetes. Cephamycin C is produced naturally by *Streptomyces lactamdurans* and is related structurally to cephalosporin C. *Cefoxitin*, as a semi-synthetic derivative of cephamycin C, has a carbamoyl group at position 3 and, like the other cephamycins, a 7-α-methoxy group in addition to the D-α-aminoadipic acid chain. Resistance to beta-lactamases is thought to result from steric hindrance by this methoxy group. Cefoxitin has similar antimicrobial activity to that of cephamandole and cefuroxime but, unlike the cephalosporins, is active against *Bacteroides fragilis*.

The Chloramphenicols

Chloramphenicol is an antibiotic which was first isolated from cultures of *Streptomyces venezuelae* in 1947 but is now produced synthetically. It has a relatively simple structure and is a derivative of dichloroacetic acid with a nitrobenzene moiety. Chloramphenicol was the first broad-spectrum antibiotic to be discovered; it acts by interfering with bacterial protein synthesis and is mainly bacteriostatic. Its range of activity is similar to that of tetracycline and includes Gram-positive and Gram-negative bacteria, rickettsias, and chlamydias. The sensitivity of *Salmonella typhi, Haemophilus influenzae*, and *Bacteroides fragilis* to chloramphenicol provides the principal indications for its use.

After one or two years' use chloramphenicol was found to have a serious and sometimes fatal depressant effect on the bone marrow. The 'grey syndrome', another potentially fatal adverse effect, was reported later in newborn infants. As a result of this toxicity the use of chloramphenicol has been restricted in many countries; it should only be given when there is no suitable alternative and never for minor infections.

Chloramphenicol is active when given by mouth and, unlike most other antibiotics, it diffuses into the cerebrospinal fluid even when the meninges are not inflamed. The majority of a dose is inactivated in the liver, only a small proportion appearing unchanged in the urine.

Chloramphenicol is still the treatment of choice for typhoid fever in many countries although resistance is sometimes a problem. Ampicillin became the preferred antibiotic for *Haemophilus influenzae* infections, especially meningitis, but the emergence of ampicillin-resistant strains has led to a reappraisal of the use of chloramphenicol. Many workers now consider that ampicillin and chloramphenicol should both be given to patients with meningitis until the sensitivity of the infecting organisms is known. Chloramphenicol is also effective against many anaerobic bacteria and may be valuable in such conditions as cerebral abscess where anaerobes such as *Bacteroides fragilis* are often involved.

Chloramphenicol sodium succinate is used parenterally and the palmitate, which is almost tasteless, is given in oral suspensions. Ophthalmic preparations of chloramphenicol are used widely for a variety of infections.

Thiamphenicol is a semisynthetic derivative of chloramphenicol in which the nitro group on the benzene ring has been replaced by a methylsulphonyl group, resulting, in general, in a loss of activity *in vitro*. It has been claimed that thiamphenicol is less toxic than chloramphenicol and there have been fewer reports of aplastic anaemia but reversible bone-marrow depression may occur more frequently. Unlike chloramphenicol, thiamphenicol is not metabolised in the liver to any extent and is excreted largely unchanged in the urine. It has been used similarly to chloramphenicol in some countries.

Azidamfenicol is another analogue of chloramphenicol which has been used topically in the treatment of eye infections.

Fusidic Acid

Fusidic acid is an antibiotic which is derived from strains of the fungus *Fusidium coccineum*. It has a steroid structure and is related to cephalosporin P, an antibiotic produced by *Cephalosporium acremonium* which also produces cephalosporin C from which the cephalosporin antibiotics are derived. Fusidic acid has a narrow spectrum of antibacterial activity but is very active against *Staphylococcus aureus*, including penicillinase-producing strains. Unfortunately resistance to fusidic acid is readily acquired and it is often given in conjunction with other antibiotics; the topical use of fusidic acid in a hospital environment has been associated with an increased incidence of resistance.

It penetrates well into most body tissues and fluids, apart from the cerebrospinal fluid, a property of value in infectious conditions such as abscesses and osteomyelitis. Fusidic acid is used in the treatment of staphylococcal infections, especially those resistant to other antibiotics. The sodium salt, sodium fusidate, is given by mouth and is also used in topical preparations; fusidic acid itself is available as a suspension for oral use and as a gel. For severe staphylococcal infections the antibiotic is given intravenously as diethanolamine fusidate.

The Lincomycins

Lincomycin is an antibiotic produced by a strain of *Streptomyces lincolnensis* and was first described in 1962; *clindamycin* is the 7-chloro-7-deoxy derivative of lincomycin.

Although not related structurally to erythromycin and the other macrolide antibiotics, lincomycin has similar antimicrobial activity and acts at the same site on the bacterial ribosome to suppress protein synthesis. Chloramphenicol also acts at this site and these 3 antibiotics are potentially antagonistic.

Lincomycin is bacteriostatic or bactericidal depending on the concentration and is active mainly against Gram-positive bacteria, including penicillin-resistant strains of *Staphylococcus aureus*, and against *Bacteroides* spp; clindamycin is qualitatively similar but more active than lincomycin *in vitro*. Cross-resistance occurs between lincomycin, clindamycin, and erythromycin.

The lincomycins have been used, like erythromycin, as an alternative to penicillin but reports of the occurrence of severe and sometimes fatal pseudomembranous colitis in association with lincomycin and clindamycin have led to the recommendation that they should only be used in severe infections when there is no suitable alternative.

Both lincomycin and clindamycin can be given orally and parenterally but clindamycin is much better absorbed from the gastro-intestinal tract and less affected by the presence of food in the stomach. They both penetrate well into bone and have been used successfully in osteomyelitis. They have also been used topically in the treatment of severe acne vulgaris.

The main indication for the use of lincomycin or clindamycin is now in the treatment of severe anaerobic infections although metronidazole (see p.969) may be a more suitable choice in such infections.

The Macrolides

The macrolides are a large group of antibiotics mainly derived from *Streptomyces* spp. and having a common macrocyclic lactone ring to which one or more sugars are attached. They are all weak bases and only slightly soluble in water. Their properties are very similar and in general they have low toxicity and the same spectrum of antimicrobial activity with cross-resistance between individual members of the group. The macrolide antibiotics are bacteriostatic or bactericidal, depending on the concentration and the type of micro-organism, and are thought to interfere with bacterial protein synthesis. Their antimicrobial spectrum is similar to that of benzylpenicillin but they are also active against such organisms as *Mycoplasma pneumoniae* and some rickettsias and chlamydias.

Erythromycin was discovered in 1952 and is the only macrolide antibiotic to be used widely. It is destroyed by gastric acid and must therefore be given as enteric-coated tablets or as one of its more stable salts or esters such as the stearate or ethylsuccinate. The estolate has been associated with hepatotoxicity and some authorities feel that its use is no longer justified. Erythromycin lactobionate or gluceptate may be given intravenously and the ethylsuccinate intramuscularly. Erythromycin is used as an alternative to penicillin, especially in patients who are allergic to penicillin, and, similarly to tetracycline, in the treatment of infections due to *Mycoplasma pneumo-*

niae and *Chlamydia trachomatis*, and in acne vulgaris.

The other macrolide antibiotics include *spiramycin* which has been used extensively in Europe and has been claimed to be effective in the treatment of toxoplasmosis. High tissue concentrations are achieved and maintained for longer than with the other macrolides.

Oleandomycin has been used orally and parenterally as the phosphate. Its ester, *triacetyloleandomycin*, is better absorbed from the gastro-intestinal tract but, like erythromycin estolate, has proved hepatotoxic. *Kitasamycin* has been used in Japan and *midecamycin* in France.

Two more recent macrolide antibiotics, *josamycin* and *rosaramicin*, also appear to have similar properties to erythromycin. Josamycin may be more active *in vitro* than erythromycin against some anaerobic bacteria and rosaramicin is generally more active against Gram-negative bacteria. Rosaramicin, unlike the other macrolides mentioned, is obtained from a *Micromonospora* spp.

Pristinamycin, not strictly a macrolide antibiotic, is a cyclic peptide derived from *Streptomyces pristinaspiralis* and has been described as a depsipeptide. It has been used in France, especially in the treatment of staphylococcal infections.

The Penicillins

Penicillin was the first antibiotic to be used therapeutically and was originally obtained, as a mixture of penicillins known as F, G, X, and K, from the mould *Penicillium notatum*. Better yields were achieved using *P. chrysogenum* and benzylpenicillin (penicillin G) was selectively produced by adding the precursor phenylacetic acid to the fermentation medium. The term 'penicillin' is now used generically for the entire group of natural and semisynthetic penicillins. Penicillins are still the most widely used antibiotics; they are generally well tolerated, apart from hypersensitivity reactions, and are bactericidal by virtue of their inhibitory action on the synthesis of the bacterial cell wall.

They all have the same ring structure and are monobasic acids which readily form salts and esters; 6-aminopenicillanic acid, the penicillin nucleus, consists of a fused thiazolidine ring and a beta-lactam ring with an amino group at the 6-position.

The earlier or so-called 'natural' penicillins were produced by adding different side-chain precursors to fermentations of the *Penicillium* mould; *benzylpenicillin*, with a phenylacetamido side-chain at the 6-position, and *phenoxymethylpenicillin* (penicillin V), with a phenoxyacetamido side-chain, were 2 of the first and are still widely used. Benzylpenicillin can be considered the parent compound of the penicillins and is active mainly against Gram-positive bacteria and *Neisseria*spp. It is inactivated by penicillinase-producing bacteria and because of its instability in gastric acid it is usually injected. Long-acting preparations include *procaine penicillin* and *benzathine penicillin* which slowly release benzylpenicillin after injection. Phenoxymethylpenicillin is acid-stable and therefore given by mouth but it is also inactivated by penicillinase. It is generally used for relatively mild infections.

When no side-chain precursor is added to the fermentation medium 6-aminopenicillanic acid itself is obtained. It may be produced in large amounts from benzylpenicillin or phenoxymethylpenicillin by the use of amidases. A range of penicillins has been synthesised from 6-aminopenicillanic acid by substitution at the 6-amino position in an effort to improve on the instability of benzylpenicillin to gastric acid and penicillinases, to widen its antimicrobial spectrum, and to reduce its rapid rate of renal excretion. Two phenoxypenicillins in which the side-chain is α-phenoxypropionamido (*phenethicillin*) or α-phenoxybutyramido (*propicillin*) are more stable to acid than benzylpenicillin but offer no advantage over phenoxymethylpenicillin.

Methicillin has a 2,6-dimethoxybenzamido group at the 6-position and was the first penicillin found to be resistant to destruction by staphylococcal penicillinase. However, it is not acid-resistant and has to be injected. The isoxazolyl penicillins, *cloxacillin, dicloxacillin, flucloxacillin*, and *oxacillin*, are resistant to penicillinase and gastric acid. They have very similar chemical structures and differ mainly in their absorption characteristics. *Nafcillin* is a similar penicillinase-resistant antibiotic but is irregularly absorbed when taken by mouth.

Ampicillin has a D(−)-α-aminophenylacetamido side-chain and a broader spectrum of activity than benzylpenicillin; although generally less active against Gram-positive bacteria, some Gram-negative organisms including *Escherichia coli, Haemophilus influenzae*, and *Salmonella* spp. are sensitive although resistance is being reported increasingly. *Pseudomonas* spp. are not sensitive. Ampicillin is acid-stable and can be given by mouth but is destroyed by penicillinase.

Amoxycillin, with a D(−)-α-aminohydroxyphenylacetamido side-chain, only differs from ampicillin by the addition of a hydroxyl group, but is better absorbed from the gastro-intestinal tract. A number of pro-drugs including *bacampicillin, hetacillin, metampicillin, pivampicillin*, and *talampicillin* are also said to be better absorbed and are hydrolysed to ampicillin *in vivo*.

Carbenicillin, with an α-carboxyphenylacetamido side-chain, has marked activity against *Pseudomonas aeruginosa* and some *Proteus* spp. but otherwise is generally less active than ampicillin. It has to be given by injection and large doses are required. *Carfecillin* and *carindacillin* are the phenyl and indanyl esters of carbenicillin respectively and are hydrolysed to carbenicillin *in vivo* when taken by mouth. *Sulbenicillin* has an α-phenylsulphoacetamido side-chain and ticarcillin an α-carboxythienylacetamido side-chain and both have similar activity to carbenicillin; *ticarcillin* appears to be more active against *Ps. aeruginosa*. *Azlocillin* and *mezlocillin* are 2 closely-related ureido-penicillins reported to be more active than carbenicillin against *Ps. aeruginosa* and to have a wider range of activity.

Recently *mecillinam*, a penicillanic acid derivative with a substituted amidino group in the 6-position, has been introduced. Unlike the 6-aminopenicillanic acid derivatives it is active mainly against Gram-negative bacteria including ampicillin-resistant strains of *E. coli*, although *Ps. aeruginosa, H. influenzae*, and *Bacteroides* spp. are considered resistant. Mecillinam is not active orally and is given by mouth as *pivmecillinam* which is hydrolysed to mecillinam on absorption.

The beta-lactamase inhibitor *clavulanic acid* may be of value in extending the antimicrobial range of the penicillin and cephalosporin antibiotics.

The Polymyxins

The polymyxins are water-soluble basic antibiotics produced by the growth of different strains of *Bacillus polymyxa* (=*B. aerosporus*). They are cyclic polypeptides, have a molecular weight of about 1000, and readily form salts with acids.

Two similar antibacterial substances were originally isolated independently in 1947 in Great Britain and USA, the British material being named 'aerosporin' and the American, 'polymyxin'. At least 3 other antibacterial substances were subsequently isolated from different strains of *B. polymyxa* and it was agreed that the generic name 'polymyxin' should be applied to this group of antibiotics, aerosporin becoming polymyxin A and the other original polymyxin becoming polymyxin D; the 3 later-discovered related substances were named polymyxin B, C, and E, respectively. 'Aerosporin' is now a proprietary name for polymyxin B sulphate and the name colistin is used for polymyxin E.

Only *polymyxin B* and *colistin* are used clinically. They have similar bactericidal activity against Gram-negative bacteria, especially *Pseudomonas*, but are potentially nephrotoxic and neurotoxic and have largely been replaced by other less toxic antibiotics such as gentamicin, carbenicillin, or the cephalosporins. Polymyxin B and colistin are not absorbed when taken by mouth and the sulphates have been used in gastro-intestinal infections. Polymyxin B sulphate or colistin sulphomethate sodium may be administered parenterally for the treatment of pseudomonal infections resistant to other antibiotics; *sulphomyxin sodium*, a sulphomethylated form of polymyxin B was formerly available for intramuscular injection. Both polymyxin B and colistin are used topically.

The Rifamycins

The rifamycins also known as ansamycins or rifomycins are a group of antibiotics isolated from a strain of *Streptomyces mediterranei*.

The two rifamycins, *rifamide* and *rifamycin sodium*, described in this section are mainly of historical interest since more effective treatment can usually be provided with other antibiotics. They are active against Gram-positive organisms, some Gram-negative organisms, and *Mycobacterium tuberculosis*. Neither is absorbed following administration by mouth; both give high biliary concentrations following parenteral administration.

The main rifamycin is *rifampicin*, a derivative of rifamycin SV that can be given by mouth. It is described in the section on Tuberculostatics and Tuberculocides, p.1577.

The Tetracyclines

The tetracyclines are a group of antibiotics, originally derived from certain *Streptomyces* spp., having the same tetracyclic nucleus, naphthacene, and similar properties. Unlike the penicillins and aminoglycosides they are bacteriostatic at the concentrations usually achieved in the body but act similarly to the aminoglycosides by interfering with protein synthesis in susceptible organisms.

Tetracyclines all have a broad spectrum of activity which includes Gram-positive and Gram-negative bacteria, chlamydias, rickettsias, and mycoplasma, but the emergence of resistant strains and the development of other antimicrobial agents has reduced their value. Adverse effects have also restricted their usefulness. Gastro-intestinal disturbances are common and other important toxic effects include anti-anabolic effects, especially in patients with renal impairment; fatty changes in the liver, associated with the intravenous administration of tetracycline; deposition in bones and teeth, precluding their use in late pregnancy and young children; and photosensitivity, especially with demeclocycline. Allergic reactions are relatively uncommon. Intramuscular injections are painful and tetracyclines are preferably given by mouth. Because of these adverse effects tetracyclines should be avoided in pregnant women, children, and, apart from doxycycline, patients with renal failure.

The first tetracycline to be introduced was *chlortetracycline* in 1948 and, like chloramphenicol which was discovered about the same time, it was found to have a broad spectrum of activity and to be active by mouth unlike benzylpenicillin or streptomycin the only other antibiotics then in use. The discovery of chlortetracycline was followed closely by that of *oxytetracycline* and then *tetracycline*, a reduction product of chlortetracycline which may be produced semisynthetically. All 3 have very similar properties although oxytetracycline may cause less staining of teeth. *Demeclocycline*, demethylated chlortetracycline, is reportedly more active *in vitro* than tetracycline against certain species, is more readily absorbed, and has a longer half-life; recommended doses have sometimes been given twice daily. However, phototoxic reactions have been reported most frequently with demeclocycline and it probably causes the most marked discoloration of teeth. It has been used with some success in patients with the syndrome of inappropriate secretion of antidiuretic hormone.

The 4 tetracyclines mentioned so far (chlortetracycline, oxytetracycline, tetracycline, and demeclocycline) are all natural products that have been isolated from *Streptomyces* spp. The more recent tetracyclines, clomocycline, methacycline, doxycycline, and minocycline are semisynthetic derivatives. *Lymecycline* and *rolitetracycline* are more water-soluble tetracyclines and have been used parenterally. *Methacycline*, like demeclocycline, has a longer half-life than tetracycline and has been given twice daily. *Doxycycline* and *minocycline*, 2 more recent semisynthetic tetracycline derivatives, are both more active *in vitro* than tetracycline against many species. More importantly, minocycline is active against some tetracycline-resistant strains of staphylococci, streptococci, *Escherichia coli*, and *Haemophilus influenzae*. Both antibiotics are well absorbed and, unlike the other tetracyclines, absorption is not significantly affected by the presence of food. They can be given in lower doses than the older members of the group and, having long half-lives, doxycycline is usually given once daily and minocycline twice daily. Doxycycline appears to have no anti-anabolic effect and can be given to patients with renal impairment; some workers also consider that minocycline can be used in such patients. Both doxycycline and minocycline are more lipid-soluble than the other tetracyclines and they penetrate well into tissues.

Because of the emergence of resistant organisms and the discovery of agents with narrower antimicrobial spectra, tetracyclines are not generally the antibiotics of choice in Gram-positive or Gram-negative infections. However they have a place in the treatment of chlamydial infections such as trachoma, rickettsial infections such as typhus, mycoplasmal infections such as atypical pneumonia, and in acute exacerbations of chronic bronchitis, non-specific urethritis, brucellosis, plague, and cholera; low doses are used in the long-term treatment of severe acne. The tetracyclines have also been useful in the treatment of penicillin-allergic patients suffering from venereal diseases, anthrax, or actinomycosis.

Tetracycline and oxytetracycline are still widely used despite their irregular absorption; doxycycline and minocycline are given in smaller doses and may be preferable in patients prone to diarrhoea.

Miscellaneous Antibiotics

There are a number of antibiotics which do not belong to any of the groups already mentioned. They include *fosfomycin*, an antibiotic which appears to be unrelated to other antimicrobial agents. It is active against a range of Gram-positive and Gram-negative organisms and has been given by mouth and by injection. *Spectinomycin* is an aminocyclitol antibiotic with some similarities to streptomycin; it is not an aminoglycoside. Spectinomycin is active against a wide range of bacteria but its clinical use is restricted to the treatment of gonorrhoea. *Vancomycin* has a glycopeptide structure and is very active against Gram-positive cocci. Unfortunately it has proved rather toxic and for systemic use can only be given intravenously. Vancomycin is reserved for the treatment of severe staphylococcal infections and in the treatment and prophylaxis of endocarditis when other antibiotics cannot be used either because of patient sensitivity or bacterial resistance. Vancomycin is poorly absorbed when taken by mouth; it has been used in the treatment of pseudomembranous colitis. *Virginiamycin* belongs to a large group of naturally-occurring substances which have a cyclic peptide structure. It has been used in the treatment of infections due to Gram-positive cocci and is an additive for animal feeding stuffs.

2-c

Adicillin. Aminocarboxybutylpenicillin; Cephalosporin N; Penicillin N; Synnematin B. (6*R*)-6-(D-5-Amino-5-carboxyvaleramido)penicillanic acid.
$C_{14}H_{21}N_3O_6S$=359.4.

CAS — 525-94-0.

A penicillin obtained from the mould *Emericellopsis salmosynnematum* (*Cephalosporium salmosynnematum*).

Soluble in water; practically insoluble in alcohol, acetone, and ether. Unstable in acid solution. **Store** in a cool place in airtight containers.

Adicillin was reported to be less active than benzylpenicillin against Gram-positive micro-organisms but more active against Gram-negative species, especially the *Salmonella* and *Proteus* groups. It is inactivated by penicillinase.

Adicillin was formerly given by intramuscular injection in the treatment of typhoid fever and of gonorrhoea.

184-z

Amikacin *(U.S.P.)*. 6-*O*-(3-Amino-3-deoxy-α-D-glucopyranosyl)-4-*O*-(6-amino-6-deoxy-α-D-glucopyranosyl)-1-*N*-[(2*S*)-4-amino-2-hydroxybutyryl]-2-deoxy-D-streptamine.

$C_{22}H_{43}N_5O_{13}$=585.6.

CAS — 37517-28-5.

A semisynthetic derivative of kanamycin A. A white crystalline powder containing not less than 900 μg of amikacin per mg, calculated on the anhydrous basis. Sparingly **soluble** in water. A solution in water is dextrorotatory. A 1% solution in water has a pH of 9.5 to 11.5. **Store** in airtight containers.

3-k

Amikacin Sulphate. Amikacin Sulfate; BB-K8.

$C_{22}H_{43}N_5O_{13}, 2H_2SO_4$=781.8.

CAS — 39831-55-5.

Freely **soluble** in water. A solution for injection is adjusted to pH 4.5 with sulphuric acid and is stable for 3 years when **stored** at up to 25°; it may darken from colourless to pale yellow.

Amikacin sulphate is **incompatible** with amphotericin, ampicillin sodium, cefapirin sodium, cephalothin sodium, chlorothiazide sodium, erythromycin gluceptate, heparin, nitrofurantoin sodium, novobiocin sodium, phenytoin sodium, sulphadiazine sodium, thiopentone sodium, and warfarin sodium, and, in concentrated solutions, with carbenicillin sodium. Occasional incompatibilities have occurred, depending on the composition and strength of the vehicle, with chlortetracycline hydrochloride, oxytetracycline hydrochloride, tetracycline hydrochloride, and vitamins of the B group with vitamin C; with cephazolin sodium turbidity has developed after 8 hours; loss of potency has occurred with potassium chloride in a vehicle of dextran 75 injection and sodium chloride injection.

Amikacin sulphate 1.3 g is approximately equivalent to 1 g of amikacin (1 million units).

Amikacin *base* is a white crystalline substance; m.p. 201° to 204° with decomposition; soluble in water; a 1% solution in water has a pH of 9.5 to 11.5. The 'equilibrium solubility' at 25° is approximately 185 mg per ml. When a solution containing about 185 mg per ml was autoclaved for 30 minutes at 120° there was no loss of potency but a light yellow or amber colour developed. A 30% v/v solution of the 250 mg-per-ml commercial solution (sulphate) is isotonic with sodium chloride injection 0.9%.— M. A. Kaplan *et al.*, *Curr. ther. Res.*, 1976, *20*, 352.

References to compatibility studies.— B. C. Nunning and A. P. Granatek, *Curr. ther. Res.*, 1976, *20*, 359; B. C. Nunning *et al.*, *Curr. ther. Res.*, 1976, *20*, 369; B. C. Nunning and A. P. Granatek, *ibid.*, 417.

For the effect of ticarcillin on amikacin, see Gentamicin Sulphate, p.1166.

Adverse Effects, Treatment, and Precautions. As for Gentamicin Sulphate, p.1166. The ototoxicity of amikacin appears to be similar to that of Kanamycin Sulphate, p.1175.

High frequency hearing loss was found in 71 (4.6%) of 1548 patients who had received amikacin and increased serum-creatinine concentrations were measured in 135.— A. Z. Lane *et al.*, *Bristol Laboratories, USA*, *Am. J. Med.*, 1977, *62*, 911.

Four of 26 patients treated with gentamicin developed nephrotoxicity compared with none of 27 given amikacin. Ototoxicity developed in 2 patients from each treatment group.— S. A. Lerner *et al.*, *Am. J. Med.*, 1977, *62*, 919. For a report suggesting that amikacin was no more nephrotoxic or ototoxic than gentamicin, see Uses below.

Amikacin had an unusually short half-life in 5 patients with burns. Serum concentrations should be monitored and the dosage adjusted accordingly to achieve therapeutic concentrations of 20 to 30 μg per ml.— D. E. Zaske *et al.*, *Surgery*, 1978, *84*, 603.

See under Absorption and Fate (below) for a report of the serum half-life of amikacin being significantly prolonged in infants with hypoxia and in premature infants.

For reports of other compounds affecting the antimicrobial activity of amikacin, see below under Antimicrobial Action.

For comparative studies of the toxicity of amikacin and netilmicin, see Netilmicin Sulphate, p.1192.

Nephrotoxicity. In healthy subjects the urinary excretion of alanine aminopeptidase, an enzyme in the proximal tubule, was determined as an index of kidney damage caused by aminoglycoside antibiotics. After 3 days' treatment, the greatest loss of alanine aminopeptidase was associated with amikacin, suggesting the greatest potential for kidney damage, and least with tobramycin, with intermediate values for gentamicin, netilmicin and sissomicin.— A. W. Mondorf *et al.*, *Eur. J. clin. Pharmac.*, 1978, *13*, 133.

In a prospective study, nephrotoxicity occurred in 6 of 60 patients given amikacin and 7 of 56 given gentamicin an average of 10 days after treatment was started, and serum-creatinine concentrations continued to rise for as long as 9 days after it was stopped. This toxicity was associated with plasma concentrations of more than 38.5 μg per ml and 10 μg per ml for amikacin and gentamicin, respectively, and trough concentrations of amikacin above 10 μg per ml.— C. R. Smith *et al.*, *Johns Hopkins med. J.*, 1978, *142*, 85.

Neuromuscular blockade. For reference to the possible prolongation of neuromuscular blockade by amikacin, see Y. Hashimoto *et al.*, *Anesthesiology*, 1978, *49*, 219.

Ototoxicity. Perceptive hearing loss occurred in 13 of 44 patients undergoing 55 courses of treatment with amikacin, generally in a dose of 20 to 25 mg per kg body-weight daily to a maximum of 1.5 g daily. The hearing loss was permanent in 10 of the 13 patients but did not progress when amikacin was withdrawn. Factors associated with ototoxicity included a duration of therapy of 10 days or more with more than 15 g, previous treatment with aminoglycosides, and peak and trough blood concentrations of 32 and 10 μg per ml respectively. It was recommended that serial audiograms be carried out if amikacin therapy is prolonged with a dose greater than 15 g or if the patient has previously been treated with an aminoglycoside. Ototoxicity might also be controlled by monitoring blood concentrations.— R. E. Black *et al.*, *Antimicrob. Ag. Chemother.*, 1976, *9*, 956.

Overdosage. There was no evidence of nephrotoxicity or ototoxicity in a 60-year-old woman following the accidental administration of amikacin 9 g by intravenous infusion over 6 hours. Haemodialysis started 12 hours after administration of amikacin did not influence amikacin clearance.— P. W. L. Ho *et al.*, *Ann. intern. Med.*, 1979, *91*, 227. See also J. P. Flandrois *et al.*, *Infection*, 1979, *7*, 190.

Antimicrobial Action. Amikacin is bactericidal and has a mode of action and antimicrobial spectrum similar to that of gentamicin (see p.1168). It is reported to be degraded by only one of the

9 aminoglycoside-inactivating enzymes known to be produced by bacteria and is active against some strains of Gram-negative bacteria which are resistant to gentamicin, tobramycin, and kanamycin, including *Pseudomonas aeruginosa* and *Serratia marcescens*. Minimum inhibitory concentrations ranging from 0.5 to 16 µg per ml have been reported for Gram-negative bacteria.

Of 152 strains of 9 species of organisms that had developed resistance to the aminoglycosides 86.2, 67.1, 60.5, and 8.6% respectively were resistant to kanamycin, gentamicin, tobramycin, and amikacin.— K. E. Price *et al.*, *Antimicrob. Ag. Chemother.*, 1974, *5*, 143.

A comparison of the antimicrobial activity *in vitro* of amikacin, gentamicin, kanamycin, and tobramycin. Gentamicin and tobramycin generally showed the highest activity but amikacin was the most active against sensitive organisms that had developed resistance to the other aminoglycosides.— A. V. Reynolds *et al.*, *Br. med. J.*, 1974, *3*, 778.

A crossover comparison was made of amikacin 5 mg per kg body-weight intramuscularly and gentamicin 1.5 mg per kg intramuscularly using the disk method, the inocular-replicating method, and a tube dilution technique, in 5 patients with malignant tumours but no signs of impaired renal or hepatic function. Amikacin was found to be less active on a weight basis against *Escherichia coli*, *Proteus* spp., and *Klebsiella* spp. Amikacin and gentamicin were found to be equally active against *Ps. aeruginosa*. Amikacin was found to be active against gentamicin-resistant strains, especially *Klebsiella* strains.— J. Klastersky *et al.*, *Clin. Pharmac. Ther.*, 1975, *17*, 348.

A report of the antibacterial activity of amikacin related to its resistance to bacterial enzymes.— K. E. Price *et al.*, *J. infect. Dis.*, 1976, *134*, *Suppl.* (Nov.), S249.

The activity of 9 aminoglycosides and spectinomycin was tested *in vitro* against 351 strains of Enterobacteriaceae, 34 of *Ps. aeruginosa*, 38 gentamicin-sensitive and 42 gentamicin-resistant strains of the *Pseudomonas* spp., 20 of the *Acinetobacter* spp., 17 of *Haemophilus influenzae*, and 41 strains of *Neisseria gonorrhoeae;* amikacin inhibited 99, 79, 97, 21, 100, 100, and 46% of the strains respectively at a concentration of 16 µg per ml. Resistance to kanamycin was more common than resistance to gentamicin or to amikacin and resistance to all 3 antibiotics occurred in 40 Gram-negative organisms.— I. Phillips *et al.*, *J. antimicrob. Chemother.*, 1977, *3*, 403.

Amikacin *in vitro* in concentrations of 1.6 µg per ml inhibited 69 of 100 cultures of *Mycobacterium tuberculosis;* 3.2 µg per ml inhibited 30 of the remaining cultures, and 6.4 µg per ml inhibited the final culture.— P. R. J. Gangadharam and E. R. Candler, *Tubercle*, 1977, *58*, 35. See also J. A. G. Rodriguez *et al.* (letter), *J. antimicrob. Chemother.*, 1978, *4*, 293.

Amikacin had an MIC of 3.1 µg or less per ml against 5 of 10 strains of organisms in the *Mycobacterium fortuitum* complex. At a similar concentration, streptomycin, gentamicin, and sissomicin inhibited 1, 2, and 1 strain respectively.— W. E. Sanders *et al.*, *Antimicrob. Ag. Chemother.*, 1977, *12*, 295. See also J. A. Garcia-Rodriguez and F. Martin-Luengo, *Tubercle*, 1978, *59*, 277; D. F. Welch and M. T. Kelly, *Antimicrob. Ag. Chemother.*, 1979, *15*, 754.

Amikacin *in vitro* inhibited 44% of 27 strains of *Nocardia asteroides* at concentrations less than 0.25 µg per ml and inhibited all 27 strains at 1 µg per ml.— J. R. Dalovisio and G. A. Pankey, *Antimicrob. Ag. Chemother.*, 1978, *13*, 128. Amikacin was the most effective of 7 aminoglycosides tested *in vitro* against *Nocardia asteroides*.— J. A. Garcia-Rodriguez *et al.* (letter), *J. antimicrob. Chemother.*, 1979, *5*, 610.

Excessively high rates of false resistance to amikacin obtained using the 10-µg disk in diffusion susceptibility tests were best resolved by using a 30-µg disk.— J. A. Washington *et al.*, *Antimicrob. Ag. Chemother.*, 1979, *15*, 400.

Further references: J. B. Howard and G. H. McCracken, *Antimicrob. Ag. Chemother.*, 1975, *8*, 86; M. I. Marks, *J. clin. Pharmac.*, 1975, *15*, 246; T. T. Yoshikawa *et al.*, *Antimicrob. Ag. Chemother.*, 1978, *13*, 177; C. Watanakunakorn and C. A. Kauffman, *Infection*, 1978, *6*, 111.

For a comparative study of the activities of tobramycin, amikacin, sissomicin, and gentamicin against 408 strains of Gram-negative rods, in which amikacin was the most active against gentamicin-resistant organisms, see Gentamicin, p.1168.

For a comparison of the activities *in vitro* of amikacin, netilmicin, and gentamicin against isolates of *Serratia marcescens*, see Netilmicin, p.1192.

For the activity of amikacin against gentamicin-resistant *Ps. aeruginosa*, see Tobramycin, p.1226.

Diminished activity. A report of colistin diminishing the activity *in vitro* of amikacin against gentamicin-resistant strains of *Ps. aeruginosa*.— Y. Kobayashi, *Keio J. Med.*, 1976, *25*, 151.

For a study indicating that daunorubicin or cytarabine reduced the activity of amikacin *in vitro* against some Gram-negative organisms, see Gentamicin, p.1168.

Enhanced activity. Enhanced activity was demonstrated *in vitro* for a combination of amikacin and trimethoprim against several strains of *Klebsiella pneumoniae*, *Serratia marcescens* and *E. coli*. No enhanced effect was observed against *Pseudomonas aeruginosa*.— T. L. Parsley *et al.*, *Antimicrob. Ag. Chemother.*, 1977, *12*, 349.

A study showing enhanced activity for amikacin and cephazolin against *Klebsiella* spp.— J. Klastersky *et al.*, *J. infect. Dis.*, 1976, *134*, 271.

For reports of ticarcillin and amikacin showing enhanced activity *in vitro* against *Ps. aeruginosa*, see Ticarcillin, p.1225.

Resistance. Amikacin-resistant strains of Gram-negative bacteria have been reported; cross-resistance with other aminoglycoside antibiotics may occur.

A report of the emergence of strains of *Providencia stuartii* resistant to amikacin.— G. D. Overturf *et al.*, *Surgery, St Louis*, 1976, *79*, 224.

Resistance to amikacin developed in *Ps. aeruginosa* in a patient treated with amikacin for 4 days. The organism remained sensitive to tobramycin.— I. D. Amirak *et al.* (letter), *Lancet*, 1977, *1*, 537.

Further references: J. Davies and P. Courvalin, *Am. J. Med.*, 1977, *62*, 868; M. H. Perlin and S. A. Lerner, *Antimicrob. Ag. Chemother.*, 1979, *16*, 598.

Absorption and Fate. As for Kanamycin Sulphate, p.1176.

Amikacin is rapidly absorbed after intramuscular injection and peak plasma concentrations of about 20 µg per ml are achieved one hour after a 500-mg dose, reducing to about 2 µg per ml 10 hours after injection. A plasma concentration of 38 µg per ml has been reported after the intravenous infusion of 500 mg over 30 minutes, reduced to 18 µg per ml one hour later. Amikacin has been detected in body tissues and fluids after injection; it crosses the placenta but does not readily penetrate into the cerebrospinal fluid.

A plasma half-life of about 2 hours has been reported in patients with normal renal function. Most of a dose is excreted by glomerular filtration in the urine within 24 hours. It is removed by haemodialysis; peritoneal dialysis is not so efficient.

A comparative study of the pharmacokinetics of amikacin and kanamycin.— J. T. Clarke *et al.*, *Clin. Pharmac. Ther.*, 1974, *15*, 610.

The mean serum half-life of amikacin after an intramuscular injection of 7.5 mg per kg body-weight was 1.74 hours in 10 healthy subjects, 7.45 hours in 5 patients with a creatinine-clearance rate [CCR] of 20 to 80 ml per minute, 23.31 hours in 5 patients with a CCR of 5 to 20 ml per minute, and about 58 hours in 1 patient with a CCR of less than 5 ml per minute. The corresponding percentages of the dose recovered in the urine within 24 hours were about 80, 59, 28, and 7.5% respectively. The mean serum half-life was 5.71 hours in 5 patients during an 8-hour haemodialysis session.— A. Leroy *et al.*, *J. antimicrob. Chemother.*, 1976, *2*, 373. See also under Dosage in Renal Failure in Uses.

The mean peak serum concentrations of amikacin in 6 healthy subjects were 7.8 and 20.2 µg per ml after intramuscular injections of 125 and 500 mg respectively and occurred after 1.0 and 1.8 hours; the mean plasma half-lives were 4.66 and 2.79 hours respectively. The same doses given intravenously produced mean plasma half-lives of 2.8 and 3.37 hours respectively. The proportion of the dose recovered in the urine appeared to be less after the higher dose irrespective of the route of administration.— R. A. Yates *et al.*, *J. antimicrob. Chemother.*, 1978, *4*, 335.

Further references: G. P. Bodey *et al.*, *Antimicrob. Ag. Chemother.*, 1974, *5*, 508; V. L. Yu, *J. Am. med. Ass.*, 1977, *238*, 943; M. J. Kendall *et al.*, *J. antimicrob. Chemother.*, 1978, *4*, 459; J. M. Walker *et al.*, *J. antimicrob. Chemother.*, 1979, *5*, 95; J. -C. Pechere and R. Dugal, *Clin. Pharmacokinet.*, 1979, *4*, 170.

Absorption and fate in infants and children. The pharmacokinetics of amikacin in the newborn were comparable with those of kanamycin and mean serum-amikacin concentrations of 17 to 20 µg per ml had been recorded 30 minutes after 7.5 mg per kg body-weight given intramuscularly. Measurements made after several days' administration to 11 infants showed a mean peak serum-amikacin concentration of 21.1 µg per ml after intramuscular injection. Reduced concentrations were measured in 5 of the 11 after several intravenous injections and were associated with a birth-weight of 1.92 kg or less. Amikacin diffused into the CSF in concentrations ranging from 0.8 to 9.2 µg per ml 1 to 12 hours after 7.5 mg per kg given intramuscularly (mean 4.4 µg per ml). When 45 children with various bacterial infections were treated with amikacin 36 had a satisfactory clinical response, a bacteriological response occurring within 72 hours in 21 and after 72 hours in 14.— J. B. Howard *et al.*, *Antimicrob. Ag. Chemother.*, 1976, *10*, 205.

In a study of the serum pharmacokinetics of amikacin given by intravenous and intramuscular injection to 36 neonates, the serum half-life was significantly prolonged in infants with hypoxia and in premature infants. The mean half-life for 11 hypoxaemic infants was 7.3 hours compared with 4.8 hours for the 25 nonhypoxaemic infants. The 12 nonhypoxaemic infants who were premature had a mean serum half-life of 5.7 hours compared with 4 hours for the 13 who were full-term. A loading dose was not considered necessary for neonates and it was recommended that serum concentrations of amikacin should be monitored in newborn infants.— M. G. Myers *et al.*, *Antimicrob. Ag. Chemother.*, 1977, *11*, 1027.

Amikacin 7.5 mg per kg body-weight was given by intramuscular injection to 41 children. Peak concentrations of amikacin occurred at the same time (1.5 hours) in muscle, fat, and serum, mean values being 2.2, 1.9, and 14.9 µg per ml respectively.— F. Daschner *et al.*, *Antimicrob. Ag. Chemother.*, 1977, *11*, 1081.

A pharmacokinetic study of amikacin in 20 children aged from 4 to 16 years.— B. Vogelstein *et al.*, *J. Pediat.*, 1977, *91*, 333.

Studies on the pharmacokinetics of amikacin in children with cancer.— T. G. Cleary *et al.*, *Antimicrob. Ag. Chemother.*, 1979, *16*, 829; W. G. Kramer *et al.*, *Clin. Pharmac. Ther.*, 1979, *26*, 635.

Diffusion. Amikacin diffused into interstitial fluid. This diffusion was related to the amount of protein binding.— J. S. Tan and S. J. Salstrom, *Antimicrob. Ag. Chemother.*, 1977, *11*, 698.

Bronchial secretions. Studies on the concentrations of amikacin achieved in bronchial secretions.— W. L. Dull *et al.*, *Antimicrob. Ag. Chemother.*, 1979, *16*, 767; G. Mombelli *et al.*, *ibid.*, 1981, *19*, 72.

Cerebrospinal fluid. Concentrations of amikacin in cerebrospinal fluid were undetectable in 18 of 24 healthy subjects 1 to 8.5 hours after an intramuscular injection of amikacin 7.5 mg per kg body-weight, and were less than 500 ng per ml in the other 6. Mean serum concentrations of amikacin at 1, 2, and 4 hours after administration were 19.7, 17.2, and 12.0 µg per ml respectively.— D. J. Briedis and H. G. Robson, *Antimicrob. Ag. Chemother.*, 1978, *13*, 1042.

Peritoneal fluid. Peritoneal diffusion was more effective with amikacin than gentamicin or benzylpenicillin in a *rabbit* sterile peritonitis model. The peritoneal fluid concentration of each antibiotic as a percentage of the respective peak serum concentration was 71% for amikacin, 37% for gentamicin and 23% for benzylpenicillin.— R. R. MacGregor, *Antimicrob. Ag. Chemother.*, 1977, *11*, 110.

Renal cortex. Renal cortical concentrations of amikacin ranged from 365 to 1030 µg per g and medullary concentrations from 270 to 718 µg per g in postmortem tissue from 5 patients who had received amikacin 0.25 to 8 hours before death.— C. Q. Edwards *et al.*, *Antimicrob. Ag. Chemother.*, 1976, *9*, 925.

Pregnancy and the neonate. Amikacin 7.5 mg per kg body-weight given intramuscularly to 11 women in the terminal stage of labour 1 hour before the expected time of incision of the amnion during caesarean section produced maternal blood and urine concentrations of amikacin of 24.2 and 99.8 µg per ml respectively while foetal blood and urine concentrations were 4.3 and 1.2 µg per ml respectively.— F. Flores-Mercado *et al.*, *J. int. med. Res.*, 1977, *5*, 292. See also B. Bernard *et al.*, *J. infect. Dis.*, 1977, *135*, 925.

See also Absorption and Fate in Infants and Children, above.

Uses. Amikacin is a semisynthetic aminoglycoside antibiotic derived from kanamycin and is used similarly to gentamicin (see p.1170) in the treatment of severe Gram-negative infections. It is given as the sulphate, and is generally reserved for the treatment of severe infections caused by susceptible bacteria which are resistant to gentamicin and tobramycin. As with gentamicin, amikacin may be used with carbenicillin or other penicillins, and with cephalosporins; the injections should be given separately.

A suggested dose for adults and children is the equivalent of 15 mg of amikacin per kg body-weight daily in equally divided doses every 8 or 12 hours by intramuscular injection, up to a maximum of 1.5 g daily in adults. The same doses may be given by slow intravenous injection over 2 to 3 minutes or by intravenous infusion. In adults, 500 mg in 200 ml of diluent has been infused over 30 to 60 minutes; for infants, infusions over 1 to 2 hours have been suggested. To reduce the risk of ototoxicity treatment should preferably not continue for longer than 7 to 10 days, the total dose given to adults should not exceed 15 g, and peak plasma concentrations greater than 30 μg per ml or trough plasma concentrations greater than 10 μg per ml should be avoided. In patients with impaired renal function doses should be reduced or the intervals between them prolonged.

Amikacin has been given by intrathecal injection in conjunction with systemic administration. A 0.25% solution has been instilled into body cavities in adults.

Reviews of the actions and uses of amikacin.— *Lancet*, 1975, *2*, 804; *Med. Lett.*, 1976, *18*, 97; *Drug & Ther. Bull.*, 1977, *15*, 63; *Lancet*, 1977, *1*, 891; D. O. Schiffman, *J. Am. med. Ass.*, 1977, *238*, 1547; D. Andrews, *Can. J. Hosp. Pharm.*, 1977, *30*, 146; *Aust. J. Pharm.*, 1978, *59*, 677; R. D. Meyer, *Ann. intern. Med.*, 1981, *95*, 328.

See also under Gentamicin Sulphate, p.1171, for general reviews of the aminoglycoside antibiotics.

The proceedings of symposiums on the actions and uses of amikacin.— *J. infect. Dis.*, 1976, *134*, *Suppl.* (Nov.), S235-S460; *Am. J. Med.*, 1977, *62*, 863-966.

For reports on the use of amikacin with other antibiotics in neutropenic patients, see D. M. Hahn *et al.*, *Antimicrob. Ag. Chemother.*, 1977, *12*, 618 (cephalothin); W. K. Lau *et al.*, *Am. J. Med.*, 1977, *62*, 959 (carbenicillin); J. Klastersky *et al.*, *Cancer Treat. Rep.*, 1977, *61*, 1433 (carbenicillin and cephazolin).

Dosage. The use of lean body mass to calculate amikacin dosage.— T. H. Hallynck *et al.* (letter), *J. antimicrob. Chemother.*, 1980, *6*, 286.

Dosage in infants and children. Of 30 children aged 2 months to 13 years with various Gram-negative infections and treated with amikacin intramuscularly 24 responded satisfactorily after 5 to 14 days' treatment. Three dosage schedules were used: 3.75 mg per kg body-weight every 12 hours, 7.5 mg per kg every 12 hours and 7.5 mg per kg every 24 hours. The lowest dose was considered suitable for most Gram-negative infections.— J. I. Ramirez *et al.*, *J. int. med. Res.*, 1976, *4*, 1.

A study of the kinetics and dosage calculations for amikacin in neonates.— H. Sardemann *et al.*, *Clin. Pharmac. Ther.*, 1976, *20*, 59.

From a study in 20 children aged from 4 to 16 years it was concluded that doses of amikacin should be based on body-surface rather than body-weight because renal clearance is higher in children than in adults.— B. Vogelstein *et al.*, *J. Pediat.*, 1977, *91*, 333.

A suggested dose of amikacin for infants of more than 37 weeks' gestation is 7.5 mg per kg body-weight given intramuscularly or by very slow bolus intravenous injection every 12 hours for the first 48 hours of life and then every 8 hours. For immature infants (those of less than 37 weeks' gestation) this dose should be given every 12 hours for the first week of life and then every 8 hours.— P. A. Davies, *Br. med. J.*, 1978, *2*, 676. See also H. C. Spratt, *Drugs*, 1978, *16*, 226. From the results of a study in premature infants (gestational age 26 to 34 weeks) who were treated with amikacin in a dose of 7.5 mg per kg body-weight every 12 hours by intramuscular injection, it was recommended that an initial loading dose of 10 mg per kg should be given in severe infections.— S. V. Want *et al.*, *J. antimicrob. Chemother.*, 1979, *5*, 527.

Amikacin 7.5 to 20 mg per kg body-weight daily given intramuscularly every 12 hours for 5 to 21 days cured 92 of 93 children (aged 1 month to 12 years) with septicaemia or infections of the gastro-intestinal tract, urinary tract, or upper or lower respiratory tract.— A. E. Cedrato *et al.*, *Curr. ther. Res.*, 1978, *24*, 123.

Further references: G. H. McCracken, *J. Pediat.*, 1977, *91*, 358.

See also under Absorption and Fate.

Dosage in renal failure. Absorption studies of amikacin in 9 patients with varying degrees of renal impairment and in 4 patients with normally functioning kidneys indicated that the serum half-life could be estimated by multiplying the serum-creatinine concentration in mg per 100 ml by a factor of 3.— J. Levy and J. Klastersky, *J. clin. Pharmac.*, 1975, *15*, 705.

The calculated half-life of amikacin in 6 patients with end-stage renal failure was 28 hours; on haemodialysis the serum half-life was 3.75 hours but clearance over 4 hours ranged from 29 to 81%. Peritoneal dialysis did not reduce the half-life in 3 patients; about 20% of the dose was recovered in the first 12 hours and 57% in 48 hours. Serum concentrations should be monitored.— T. Madhavan *et al.*, *Antimicrob. Ag. Chemother.*, 1976, *10*, 464.

Amikacin was reported not to be bound to plasma proteins. The normal half-life of 2 to 2.5 hours was increased to 30 hours in end-stage renal failure. The interval between doses should be extended from 8 to 12 hours to 12 to 18 hours in patients with a glomerular filtration-rate (GFR) above 50 ml per minute, to 24 to 36 hours in those with a GFR of 10 to 50 ml per minute, and to 36 to 48 hours in those with a GFR of less than 10 ml per minute. Concentrations of amikacin were affected by haemodialysis and peritoneal dialysis.— W. M. Bennett *et al.*, *Ann. intern. Med.*, 1977, *86*, 754. See also *idem*, 1980, *93*, 62.

Data for predicting removal of amikacin by conventional haemodialysis.— T. P. Gibson and H. A. Nelson, *Clin. Pharmacokinet.*, 1977, *2*, 403.

The mean elimination half-life of amikacin was 86.5 hours in 6 anephric patients, decreasing to 5.6 hours during haemodialysis and 44.3 hours in 4 patients with minimal residual kidney function, decreasing to 17.9 hours during peritoneal dialysis. For anephric patients on weekly dialysis a dose of 5 to 7 mg per kg body-weight intravenously immediately after dialysis will suffice. Patients with a creatinine clearance-rate between 2 and 5 ml per minute might need an extra dose after 4 days.— L. Regeur *et al.*, *Antimicrob. Ag. Chemother.*, 1977, *11*, 214. See also R. D. Meyer *et al.*, *Chemotherapy, Basle*, 1978, *24*, 172.

Further references: A. Leroy *et al.*, *J. antimicrob. Chemother.*, 1976, *2*, 373; M. C. McHenry *et al.*, *J. infect. Dis.*, 1976, *134*, *Suppl.* (Nov.), S343; G. B. Appel and H. C. Neu, *New Engl. J. Med.*, 1977, *296*, 663; R. D. Meyer (letter), *ibid.*, *297*, 225; G. B. Appel and H. C. Neu (letter), *ibid.*

Gram-negative infections, miscellaneous. Amikacin 7.5 mg per kg body-weight every 12 hours by intramuscular or intravenous injection was given to 35 patients with 36 serious Gram-negative infections, 13 of which were gentamicin-resistant. Treatment was continued for 6 to 50 days. A cure was achieved in 17 infections and improvement or cure with clinical superinfection in a further 12. Gentamicin-resistant infections were cured in 6 of 13 infections with complete failure in only one. Minor ototoxicity occurred in 6 patients who were treated for more than 2 weeks or had received previous aminoglycoside therapy. Possible nephrotoxicity was found in 6 patients.— R. D. Meyer *et al.*, *Ann. intern. Med.*, 1975, *83*, 790.

Amikacin was effective in about 70% of 49 cases of infection mainly due to Gram-negative organisms in 39 cancer patients with neutropenia. Best results were achieved when serum-amikacin concentrations were maintained at about 15 μg per ml by continuous intravenous infusion but uraemia and deafness were associated with high doses, uraemia being significantly more common with serum concentrations greater than 15 μg per ml and with repeated courses. There was one fatality possibly due to the accidental rapid infusion of amikacin through a subclavian catheter.— M. Valdivieso *et al.*, *Am. J. med. Sci.*, 1975, *270*, 453. In a similar study, amikacin was effective in 13 of 24 infections caused by Gram-negative bacteria resistant to gentamicin.— M. Valdivieso and G. P. Bodey, *Am. J. med. Sci.*, 1977, *273*, 177.

For discussions on infections caused by *Serratia marcescens* and amikacin as the possible treatment of choice, see A. P. Ball, *J. antimicrob. Chemother.*, 1976, *2*, 317; *Lancet*, 1977, *1*, 636.

In a comparative study of amikacin and gentamicin, amikacin was found to be effective therapy for severe Gram-negative infections its overall efficacy being similar to that of gentamicin; it was no more nephrotoxic or ototoxic than gentamicin. Of 39 patients who received amikacin 8 mg per kg body-weight by intravenous injection over 30 minutes initially, subsequently adjusted to maintain plasma concentrations of 20 to 40 μg per ml 1 hour after infusion, it was effective in 10 of 12 bacteraemias, 21 of 24 urinary-tract infections, 2 of 5 pneumonias, and 4 of 6 other serious infections; of 32 who similarly received gentamicin 2 mg per kg subsequently adjusted to maintain plasma concentrations of 5 to 10 μg per ml 1 hour after infusion, it was effective in 12 of 15 bacteraemias, 15 of 18 urinary-tract infections, 2 of 4 pneumonias, and 3 of 3 other serious infections. Of patients evaluated for nephrotoxicity 11% of 62 who received amikacin and 8% of 62 who received gentamicin developed definite symptoms. Of patients evaluated for auditory toxicity 6% of 34 who received amikacin and 10% of 30 who received gentamicin developed symptoms; a further 2 in the amikacin group developed transitory tinnitus.— C. R. Smith *et al.*, *New Engl. J. Med.*, 1977, *296*, 349.

Amikacin 0.5 to 1.5 g daily given, by intramuscular or slow intravenous injection (over 2 to 3 minutes), for 3 to 12 days to 12 patients produced a cure or clinical improvement in 12 of 13 infections produced by *Klebsiella aerogenes* resistant to gentamicin, kanamycin, tobramycin, ampicillin, and several other antibiotics *in vitro*. Results were similar in a further 15 patients who received 18 courses of treatment. Renal function deteriorated in several patients during treatment but it may not have always been due to amikacin.— D. C. E. Speller *et al.*, *J. antimicrob. Chemother.*, 1977, *3*, 483.

Amikacin eradicated *Ps. aeruginosa* from the sputum of 2 of 18 patients with cystic fibrosis and respiratory infections undergoing 22 courses of therapy. However, there was clinical improvement in 19 of the courses. Carbenicillin was also given in 8 of the courses.— W. K. Lau *et al.*, *Pediatrics*, 1977, *60*, 372.

Further references: A. A. Pollock *et al.*, *J. Am. med. Ass.*, 1977, *237*, 562; V. L. Yu *et al.*, *J. Am. med. Ass.*, 1977, *238*, 943; F. P. Tally and S. L. Gorbach, *Am. J. Med.*, 1977, *62*, 940; R. Feld *et al.*, *J. infect. Dis.*, 1977, *135*, 61; J. Klastersky *et al.*, *Am. J. med. Sci.*, 1977, *273*, 157.

Meningitis. The intrathecal administration of amikacin 20 mg daily in the treatment of meningitis due to *Kleb. pneumoniae* in one patient. Some deafness occurred but could not be proved to be due to amikacin.— C. S. Block *et al.* (letter), *Lancet*, 1977, *1*, 1371.

Further references: B. Hamory *et al.*, *J. Am. med. Ass.*, 1976, *236*, 1973; A. R. Sklaver *et al.*, *Archs intern. Med.*, 1978, *138*, 713; P. F. Wright *et al.*, *J. infect. Dis.*, 1981, *143*, 141.

Urinary-tract infections. Amikacin given intramuscularly usually in a dose of 500 mg every 12 hours was effective in treating 12 episodes of urinary-tract infections in 11 patients. In each case the infection was due to strains of *Proteus rettgeri* resistant to gentamicin and kanamycin.— P. M. Sharp *et al.*, *Antimicrob. Ag. Chemother.*, 1974, *5*, 435.

Of 29 children with acute or chronic pyelonephritis and 1 child with a urinary-tract infection, all aged between 2 months and 11 years, 23 were cured after treatment with amikacin 5 mg per kg body-weight administered intramuscularly as a single dose or in 2 divided doses daily for 10 days. All the treatment failures occurred in children with chronic pyelonephritis. Of 30 adult patients with acute or chronic pyelonephritis who received amikacin 500 mg every day similarly, 29 were cured. There was no evidence of nephrotoxicity or ototoxicity during therapy.— I. Mimica *et al.*, *Curr. ther. Res.*, 1978, *23*, 555.

In a randomised double-blind study in 50 patients with urinary-tract infection amikacin 375 mg thrice daily intramuscularly was more effective than gentamicin 80 mg thrice daily. Decreased doses were used in patients with impaired renal function.— D. Höffler, *Dt. med. Wschr.*, 1978, *103*, 2071.

Further references: A. J. Khan *et al.*, *Pediatrics*, 1976, *58*, 873; S. Maigaard *et al.*, *Antimicrob. Ag. Chemother.*, 1978, *14*, 544.

Preparations

Amikacin Sulfate Injection *(U.S.P.)*. A sterile solution of amikacin sulphate in Water for Injections, with suitable buffers and preservatives. pH 3.5 to 5.5. It contains the equivalent of 50 or 250 mg of amikacin per ml.

Amikin Injection *(Bristol-Myers Pharmaceuticals, UK)*. Contains amikacin sulphate, equivalent to amikacin 250 mg per ml, in vials of 2 ml, with methyl and propyl hydroxybenzoates. (Also available as Amikin in *Austral., Canad., Eire, S.Afr., Switz., USA*).

Amikin Paediatric Injection *(Bristol-Myers Pharmaceuticals, UK)*. Contains amikacin sulphate equivalent to amikacin 50 mg per ml, in ampoules of 2 ml (free from preservatives).

Other Proprietary Names

Amiklin *(Fr.)*; Amukin *(Belg., Neth.)*; BB-K8 *(Ital., Mex.)*; Biclin *(Spain)*; Biklin *(Arg., Denm., Ger., Jap., Swed.)*; Pierami *(Ital.)*.

4-a

Amoxycillin. Amoxicillin; Amoxicilline; BRL 2333; D(−)-α-Amino-*p*-hydroxybenzylpenicillin. (6*R*)-6-[α-D-(4-Hydroxyphenyl)glycylamino]penicillanic acid.

$C_{16}H_{19}N_3O_5S$=365.4.

CAS — 26787-78-0.

5-t

Amoxycillin Sodium. The sodium salt of amoxycillin.

$C_{16}H_{18}N_3NaO_5S$=387.4.

CAS — 34642-77-8.

A white or off-white powder. Each g represents about 2.6 mmol (2.6 mEq) of sodium. Amoxycillin sodium 1.06 g is approximately equivalent to 1 g of amoxycillin. **Soluble** 1 in less than 1 of water. A 10% solution in water has a pH of 8 to 10. A 5% solution is approximately iso-osmotic with serum.

The **stability** of aqueous solutions decreases markedly as the concentration increases. At concentrations up to 5% amoxycillin sodium is stable for 6 hours in Sodium Chloride Intravenous Infusion, for 3 hours in sodium lactate solutions, and for 1 hour in solutions containing 4 to 5% dextrose.

Polymerisation. A study of polymeric impurities in samples of amoxycillin sodium.— M. G. De Angeli *et al.*, *Farmaco, Edn prat.*, 1980, *35*, 100.

Stability in solution. Optimum storage conditions for aqueous solutions of amoxycillin were considered to be in the pH range of 5.8 to 6.5 using a citrate buffer. There was maximum stability at pH 5.77.— H. Zia *et al.*, *Can. J. pharm. Sci.*, 1977, *12*, 80.

6-x

Amoxycillin Trihydrate *(B.P.)*. Amoxicillin *(U.S.P.)*. The trihydrate of amoxycillin.

$C_{16}H_{19}N_3O_5S,3H_2O$=419.4.

CAS — 61336-70-7.

Pharmacopoeias. In *Br.* and *U.S.*

A white or almost white odourless or almost odourless crystalline powder. Amoxycillin trihydrate 1.15 g is approximately equivalent to 1 g of amoxycillin. **Soluble** 1 in 400 of water, 1 in 1000 of alcohol, 1 in 200 of methyl alcohol; practically insoluble in chloroform, ether, carbon tetrachloride, and fixed oils. A 0.2% solution in water has a pH of 3.5 to 5.5. **Store** below 25° in airtight containers.

Adverse Effects and Treatment. As for Ampicillin, p.1092.

In 2 girls with infectious mononucleosis the administration of amoxycillin led to the development of a rash similar to that seen in such patients after ampicillin.— R. Mulroy (letter), *Br. med. J.*, 1973, *1*, 554. A similar report.— P. W. M. Copeman and R. Scrivener (letter), *ibid.*, 1977, *1*, 1354.

Pseudomembranous colitis, associated with the administration of amoxycillin 250 mg thrice daily for 5 days, occurred in a 10-year-old boy.— S. Similä *et al.* (letter), *Lancet*, 1976, *2*, 317.

Precautions. As for Ampicillin, p.1093.

Amoxycillin like ampicillin should not be given in infectious mononucleosis.— J. D. Williams and A. M. Geddes (letter), *Br. med. J.*, 1973, *2*, 116. Ampicillin caused skin rashes in 90% of patients with infectious mononucleosis whereas 2 of 7 patients with this disease and given amoxycillin developed a rash.— E. T. Knudsen (letter), *ibid.*, 240.

In the opinion of the Australian Adverse Drug Reactions Advisory Committee, amoxycillin was contra-indicated in infectious mononucleosis and was not suitable for the treatment of acute pharyngitis where the infecting organism was unknown.— *Aust. J. Pharm.*, 1978, *59*, 91.

For a reference to impaired absorption in patients with coeliac disease, see below under Absorption and Fate.

Antimicrobial Action. Amoxycillin is bactericidal, is effective against the same range of organisms as ampicillin (see p.1093), and has a similar mode of action. It has been reported that amoxycillin predominantly inhibits side-wall synthesis in susceptible bacteria while ampicillin mainly inhibits cross-wall synthesis. Amoxycillin has been reported to be slightly more active than ampicillin against some streptococci and *Salmonella* spp. but less active against *Shigella* spp. It is inactivated by penicillinase and complete cross-resistance has been reported between amoxycillin and ampicillin.

Minimum inhibitory concentrations ranging from 0.01 to 5 μg per ml have been reported.

The minimum inhibitory concentration of amoxycillin against *Streptococcus pyogenes, Streptococcus pneumoniae,* and penicillin-susceptible strains of *Staphylococcus aureus* was less than 0.1 μg per ml. The MIC for most strains of *Escherichia coli, Proteus mirabilis,* and *Salmonella* was less than 10 μg per ml, and 0.5 μg per ml for *Haemophilus* strains and *Neisseria gonorrhoeae*. Amoxycillin inhibited 65% of enterococci at a concentration of 1 μg per ml. The strains of *Klebsiella, Enterobacter, Serratia,* and *Pseudomonas* tested were resistant to 250 μg or more per ml of amoxycillin. The antibacterial activity of amoxycillin was almost identical with that of ampicillin and it was equally bound to proteins.— H. C. Neu and E. B. Winshell, *Antimicrob. Ag. Chemother.*, 1970, 407.

At the concentrations mentioned, amoxycillin inhibited the growth of the following organisms: 0.02 μg per ml, *Str. pneumoniae* and *N. gonorrhoeae*; 0.1 μg per ml, *Staph. aureus*; 0.25 μg per ml, *Haemophilus influenzae*; 0.5 μg per ml, *Str. faecalis*; 1.25 μg per ml, *Salmonella* spp.; 2.5 μg per ml, *Pr. mirabilis* and *Shigella sonnei*; 5 μg per ml, *E. coli*.— R. Sutherland *et al.*, *Br. med. J.*, 1972, *3*, 13. See also R. Sutherland and G. N. Rolinson, *Antimicrob. Ag. Chemother.*, 1970, 411.

Of 68 strains of *H. influenzae,* 7 were inhibited by amoxycillin at a concentration of 0.12 μg per ml, 59 at 0.25 μg per ml, and 2 at 0.5 μg per ml. Amoxycillin was always slightly less active than ampicillin but the MICs were always well within peak plasma concentrations.— J. D. Williams and J. Andrews, *Br. med. J.*, 1974, *1*, 134.

Amoxycillin inhibited the majority of 262 strains of anaerobic bacteria at 16 μg or less per ml, including about 22 of 42 strains of *Bacteroides fragilis*.— V. L. Sutter and S. M. Finegold, *Antimicrob. Ag. Chemother.*, 1976, *10*, 736.

A study in *mice* showed that the greater therapeutic activity of amoxycillin in infected *animals* compared with ampicillin was due to its greater bacteriolytic activity *in vivo*.— K. R. Comber *et al.*, *Beecham Research, Antimicrob. Ag. Chemother.*, 1977, *12*, 736.

Amoxycillin inhibited 25, 42, 52, 80, and all of 92 strains of *Neisseria gonorrhoeae in vitro* at an MIC of 30, 60, 125, 250, and 500 ng per ml respectively.— B. A. Watts *et al.*, *J. antimicrob. Chemother.*, 1977, *3*, 331.

Enhanced activity. The bactericidal activity of amoxycillin was generally enhanced *in vitro* against strains of *Streptococcus faecalis* over the first 6 hours when used with a sub-inhibitory concentration of an aminoglycoside antibiotic to which the strain was sensitive. A similar effect was obtained against 1 strain of each of *Str. salivarius* and *Str. bovis* when amoxycillin was used with gentamicin sulphate.— M. J. Basker and R. Sutherland, *J. antimicrob. Chemother.*, 1977, *3*, 273.

Further references: M. Matsuura *et al.*, *Antimicrob. Ag. Chemother.*, 1980, *17*, 908 (enhanced activity with amoxycillin and clavulanic acid against beta-lactamase-producing bacteria).

Absorption and Fate. Amoxycillin trihydrate is rapidly absorbed when given by mouth; it is not converted to ampicillin. It is widely distributed and is reported to produce peak antibiotic plasma concentrations that are up to twice as high as those from the same dose of ampicillin. Peak plasma-amoxycillin concentrations of about 5 μg per ml have been observed 2 hours after a dose of 250 mg, with detectable amounts present for up to 8 hours. Doubling the dose can produce double the concentration. The presence of food in the stomach does not appear to diminish absorption significantly.

Amoxycillin is given by injection as the sodium salt and a peak plasma concentration of about 14 μg of amoxycillin per ml has been reported to occur one hour after the intramuscular injection of a dose equivalent to 500 mg of amoxycillin. However, in general, similar concentrations are achieved with intramuscular and oral administration.

Up to 20% is bound to plasma proteins in the circulation and plasma half-lives of about one hour have been reported. Amoxycillin diffuses across the placenta; little appears to be excreted in breast milk. It penetrates well into purulent and mucoid sputum and low concentrations have been found in ocular fluid. Concentrations of the antibiotic have been detected in the CSF of patients with inflamed meninges given amoxycillin intravenously.

About 60% of an oral dose of amoxycillin is excreted unchanged in the urine in 6 hours by glomerular filtration and tubular secretion. Urinary concentrations range from about 0.3 to 1.3 mg per ml after a dose of 250 mg. Up to 75% of a parenteral dose has been reported to be excreted unchanged in the urine within 6 hours. Probenecid retards renal excretion. High concentrations have been reported in bile.

In a crossover study with healthy volunteers the mean peak serum concentration of amoxycillin was 5.2 μg per ml 1 hour after a 250-mg dose compared with 4 μg per ml for ampicillin 2 hours after a 500-mg dose. The ingestion of food with amoxycillin had no effect on its absorption. Probenecid increased the serum concentration of amoxycillin and delayed its excretion. After a 250-mg dose of amoxycillin the urine concentrations ranged from 0.31 to 9 mg per ml. From 65 to 95% of a dose was excreted in 6 hours.— H. C. Neu and E. B. Winshell, *Antimicrob. Ag. Chemother.*, 1970, 423.

The mean peak serum concentrations of amoxycillin 2 hours after a dose by mouth to fasting subjects were: 125 mg, 2.7 μg per ml; 250 mg, 5.1 μg per ml; 500 mg, 10.8 μg per ml; and 1 g, 20.6 μg per ml. For the 250-mg and 500-mg doses, these values were twice those obtained after the same doses of ampicillin. Peak levels in non-fasting subjects were only slightly lower than in fasting subjects. Only unchanged amoxycillin was detected in the urine, 58 to 68% of a dose being excreted in 6 hours.— R. Sutherland *et al.*, *Br. med. J.*, 1972, *3*, 13.

The mean peak serum concentration of amoxycillin was 7.6 μg per ml after a 500-mg dose, compared with 3.2 μg per ml for the same dose of ampicillin. Urinary recovery for amoxycillin at 8 hours was 60% and for ampicillin 34%. Serum half-lives were similar, 61.3 minutes for amoxycillin and 60.3 minutes for ampicillin.— R. C. Gordon *et al.*, *Antimicrob. Ag. Chemother.*, 1972, *1*, 504.

In 4 healthy subjects given amoxycillin 250 mg after a meal, peak concentrations of 5 to 7.2 μg per ml occurred 2 hours after the dose, but fell to less than 1 μg per ml within 6 hours. Similar values were obtained in 3 patients with pernicious anaemia. The half-life was 77.5 minutes after single doses and 92.2 minutes after 8 days' treatment. Concentrations in the urine 2 hours after a dose were 344 μg per ml; a mean of 64% of a dose was recovered in the urine in 6 hours. In patients with renal failure peak serum concentrations of 10.1 μg per ml were reached 3 to 4 hours after a single dose. The half-life was prolonged (128 to 911 minutes) in patients with a creatinine clearance of less than 50 ml per minute. Concentrations in urine were lower and a mean of 38% of a dose was recovered in 6 hours. The half-life was markedly prolonged in 3 patients on regular dialysis.— D. H. Lawson *et al.*, *Postgrad. med. J.*, 1974, *50*, 500.

The absorption of amoxycillin was impaired in patients with coeliac disease.— R. L. Parsons *et al.*, *J. antimicrob. Chemother.*, 1975, *1*, 39.

The pharmacokinetics of amoxycillin.— D. A. Spyker *et al.*, *Antimicrob. Ag. Chemother.*, 1977, *11*, 132.

In a double-blind crossover study in 16 healthy subjects who received a single 500-mg dose of amoxycillin or ampicillin, food had no significant effect on the absorption of amoxycillin but the absorption of ampicillin was significantly reduced when taken after a meal.— F. N. Eshelman and D. A. Spyker, *Beecham, USA, Antimicrob. Ag. Chemother.*, 1978, *14*, 539. A similar study in 6 healthy subjects demonstrated that the absorption of both antibiotics was reduced when single doses were given after food.— P. G. Welling *et al.*, *J. pharm. Sci.*, 1977, *66*, 549.

Further references: D. Zarowny *et al.*, *Clin. Pharmac. Ther.*, 1974, *16*, 1045; P. J. Little and B. A. Peddie, *Med. J. Aust.*, 1974, *2*, 598; R. N. Brogden *et al.*, *Drugs*, 1975, *9*, 88; P. Ball *et al.* (letter), *J. antimicrob. Chemother.*, 1978, *4*, 385 (elderly patients); C. M. Ginsburg *et al.*, *Pediatrics*, 1979, *64*, 627 (comparison with ampicillin in infants and children); T. L. Lee *et al.*, *J. pharm. Sci.*, 1979, *68*, 454 (urinary excretion); R. C. Rudoy, *Antimicrob. Ag. Chemother.*, 1979, *15*, 628 (paediatric patients; intravenous use).

Diffusion into body fluids. Amoxycillin was given in a dose of 500 mg four times daily to 22 patients with pneumonia or acute exacerbations of chronic bronchitis. The mean sputum concentrations at 2 to 3 and 6 hours after a dose were 0.52 and 0.53 μg per ml respectively. Corresponding serum concentrations were 11 and 3.5 μg per ml. The mean concentration in saliva at 2 hours was 0.32 μg per ml. Clinical response occurred more rapidly when the sputum concentration exceeded 0.25 μg per ml but elimination of the organism was related to the pathogen rather than the concentration of amoxycillin.— S. M. Stewart *et al.*, *Thorax*, 1974, *29*, 110. In patients with acute exacerbations of chronic bronchitis sputum concentrations of amoxycillin increased proportionally with dose. Results in 30 patients with chronic bronchitis indicated that amoxycillin penetrated best into sputum containing about 50% pus.— A. Ingold, *Br. J. Dis. Chest*, 1975, *69*, 211.

In a study of 22 children with chronic otitis media, mean concentrations of 6.2 and 1.48 μg per ml of antibiotic were achieved in the middle-ear fluid 1 to 2 hours after 1-g oral doses of amoxycillin and ampicillin respectively. Serum concentrations were not significantly different.— J. J. Klimek *et al.*, *J. infect. Dis.*, 1977, *135*, 999.

Mean CSF concentrations of amoxycillin in 12 healthy subjects given 33 mg per kg body-weight by intravenous infusion were 350 and 360 ng per ml, ½ and 3½ hours respectively after administration. Higher concentrations were achieved with the same dose of ampicillin given to a further 9 healthy subjects.— N. Clumeck *et al.*, *Antimicrob. Ag. Chemother.*, 1978, *14*, 531. In the presence of meningeal inflammation in 13 patients with tuberculous meningitis, concentrations of amoxycillin in the CSF ranged from 0.1 to 1.5 μg per ml 2 hours after administration of 1 g by mouth and represented about 1 to 21% of the concurrent serum concentrations. Following administration of 2 g intravenously, as the sodium salt, concentrations in the CSF ranged from 2.9 to 40 μg per ml at 1.5 hours and from 2.6 to 27 μg per ml at 4 hours and represented about 8 to 93% and 47 to 475% respectively of the concurrent serum concentrations.— L. J. Strausbaugh *et al.*, *Antimicrob. Ag. Chemother.*, 1978, *14*, 899. See also J. C. Craft *et al.*, *Antimicrob. Ag. Chemother.*, 1979, *16*, 346 (the effect of probenecid on amoxycillin concentrations in the CSF in bacterial meningitis).

Further references to the diffusion of amoxycillin: M. Onsrud *et al.*, *Acta obstet. gynec. scand.*, 1979, *58*, 401 (peritoneal fluid); L. Weingartner *et al.*, *Int. J. clin. Pharmac. Ther. Toxic.*, 1980, *18*, 185 (bronchial secretions).

Metabolism. About 24% of a dose of amoxycillin 250 mg was metabolised and about 33% of a 500-mg dose. After 6 hours, 63% of a 250-mg dose, given to 10 healthy subjects, was recovered unchanged in the urine and 20% was excreted as penicilloic acid.— M. Cole *et al.*, *Antimicrob. Ag. Chemother.*, 1973, *3*, 463.

There was no evidence of active metabolites of amoxycillin in the urine of healthy subjects following administration of amoxycillin trihydrate.— M. C. Cole and B. Ridley (letter), *J. antimicrob. Chemother.*, 1978, *4*, 580.

Uses. Amoxycillin is the 4-hydroxy analogue of ampicillin (see p.1091) and has similar actions and uses. It is given by mouth, as the trihydrate, in lower doses than ampicillin to treat infections due to susceptible Gram-positive and Gram-negative organisms; it is less effective in the treatment of shigellosis. The usual dose is the equivalent of 250 mg of amoxycillin thrice daily; 500 mg thrice daily may be required in some severe infections and higher doses are used in salmonellal infections. Children up to 10 years of age may be given the equivalent of 125 to 250 mg thrice daily; under 20 kg body-weight a dose of 20 to 40 mg per kg daily has been suggested.

Amoxycillin is given as a single dose of 3 g, often with probenecid 1 g, in the treatment of gonorrhoea. For uncomplicated acute urinary-tract infections two 3-g doses of amoxycillin may be given with 10 to 12 hours between doses. A single 3-g dose may be given for the prophylaxis of endocarditis in susceptible patients about 1 hour before procedures such as dental extractions; children may be given half the adult dose.

Amoxycillin is administered by injection as amoxycillin sodium and in moderate infections the equivalent of 500 mg of amoxycillin may be given intramuscularly every 8 hours. If pain is experienced the injection can be prepared using a 0.5% solution of procaine hydrochloride or a 1% solution of lignocaine hydrochloride. In severe infections the equivalent of 1 g of amoxycillin may be given every 6 hours by slow intravenous injection over 3 to 4 minutes or by infusion over 30 to 60 minutes. Children up to 10 years of age may be given the equivalent of 50 to 100 mg per kg body-weight daily by injection in divided doses.

Reports and reviews of amoxycillin.— *Chemotherapy, Basle*, 1973, *18, Suppl.*, 1; R. N. Brogden *et al.*, *Drugs*, 1974, *7*, 326; *idem*, 1975, *9*, 88; H. C. Neu, *ibid.*, 81; R. N. Brogden *et al.*, *ibid.*, 1979, *18*, 169; H. C. Neu, *Ann. intern. Med.*, 1979, *90*, 356.

A study of the absorption, excretion, and effectiveness of amoxycillin in 69 patients with various infections. Maximum serum concentrations of amoxycillin were achieved after 2 hours and averaged 4.52 μg per ml after a 250-mg dose, and 10.45 μg per ml after a 500-mg dose. The total amount of amoxycillin recovered from urine ranged from 43.8 to 52.6% of the administered dose. The MIC of amoxycillin for 20 haemophilus strains was 0.1 to 1 μg per ml. Fifty-six of the 69 patients were successfully treated. Amoxycillin seemed better absorbed than equivalent doses of ampicillin but had similar antibacterial activity against enterobacteria and less activity against *Haemophilus influenzae*. Three patients developed maculopapular skin rashes, 2 dyspepsia, 1 pruritus vulvae, 1 nausea, and 1 vomiting.— J. Kosmidis *et al.*, *Br. J. clin. Pract.*, 1972, *26*, 341.

Bronchitis. In a study of 100 patients with acute purulent exacerbations of bronchitis, amoxycillin 500 mg thrice daily for 10 days given to 50 patients was as effective as co-trimoxazole 2.88 g daily, given to men, or 1.92 g daily, given to women, also for 10 days. Amoxycillin was more effective in preventing relapse.— A. Pines *et al.*, *Chemotherapy, Basle*, 1977, *23*, 58.

Further references: A. L. Molla, *Practitioner*, 1974, *212*, 123; G. A. Bell *et al.*, *Br. J. clin. Pract.*, 1974, *28*, 89.

Dosage in infants and children. A study of the pharmacokinetics of amoxycillin in neonates and premature infants. Therapeutic concentrations were achieved, without accumulation, when 50 mg per kg body-weight was given by mouth every 12 hours. In severe infection this dose could be given 8-hourly.— L. Weingärtner *et al.*, *Int. J. clin. Pharmac. Biopharm.*, 1977, *15*, 184. A suggested dose of amoxycillin for older infants was 50 mg per kg body-weight daily in 3 divided doses.— *Br. med. J.*, 1980, *280*, 703.

Dosage in renal failure. For patients undergoing haemodialysis 1 g of amoxycillin could be injected at the end of the dialysis session and repeated every 12 to 36 hours.— G. Humbert *et al.*, *Antimicrob. Ag. Chemother.*, 1979, *15*, 28. See also E. L. Francke *et al.*, *Clin. Pharmac. Ther.*, 1979, *26*, 31.

The normal half-life for amoxycillin of 0.9 to 2.3 hours was increased to 5 to 20 hours in end-stage renal failure. The interval between doses should be extended from 8 hours to up to 12 hours in patients with a glomerular filtration-rate (GFR) of 10 to 50 ml per minute, and to up to 16 hours in those with a GFR of less than 10 ml per minute, though normal doses were necessary for urinary-tract infections. Concentrations of amoxycillin were affected by haemodialysis but not by peritoneal dialysis.— W. M. Bennett *et al.*, *Ann. intern. Med.*, 1980, *93*, 62.

Further references: J. Sabto *et al.*, *Med. J. Aust.*, 1973, *2*, 537 (dialysis); G. B. Appel and H. C. Neu, *New Engl. J. Med.*, 1977, *296*, 663; R. H. Jones, *J. Infect.*, 1979, *1*, 235 (peritoneal dialysis).

Endocarditis prophylaxis. Amoxycillin was considered to be preferable to phenoxymethylpenicillin for prophylaxis of endocarditis since it provided higher serum concentrations during the 6 to 8 hours following dental extraction.— D. C. Shanson *et al.*, *J. antimicrob. Chemother.*, 1978, *4*, 431.

Studies in subjects given 3 or 4 g of amoxycillin as a single dose suggested that a 3-g dose would provide adequate prophylaxis against endocarditis; the dose should be taken one hour before dental surgery and possibly repeated 8 to 9 hours after surgery. It was not suitable for patients undergoing general anaesthesia or for those with prosthetic heart valves.— D. C. Shanson *et al.*, *Br. med. J.*, 1980, *280*, 446.

Gonorrhoea. Amoxycillin 2 g initially then 1 g five hours later was used to treat 100 men with acute gonorrhoea. Of the 81 followed up 2 had not responded. Blood concentrations were well above the MICs of test strains of gonococci.— R. R. Wilcox, *Br. J. vener. Dis.*, 1974, *50*, 120. See also *idem*, 1972, *48*, 504; C. D. Alergant, *ibid.*, 1973, *49*, 274.

In a comparison of amoxycillin 3 g alone with ampicillin 3.5 g with probenecid 1 g in 58 men and 56 women with gonorrhoea the failure-rate in anogenital gonorrhoea was 4.2 and 1.7% respectively and the difference was not significant. All 4 patients with oropharyngeal gonorrhoea failed to respond to ampicillin as did 1 of 3 given amoxycillin.— W. W. Karney *et al.*, *Antimicrob. Ag. Chemother.*, 1974, *5*, 114.

A single dose of amoxycillin 3 g with probenecid 1 g by mouth was effective in 86 of 87 male patients with urethral gonorrhoea.— A. M. Z. Walker and J. W. Tapsall (letter), *Med. J. Aust.*, 1977, *2*, 785.

In a double-blind study of 104 patients with anogenital gonorrhoea cure-rates achieved with amoxycillin 1 g and probenecid 1 g or amoxycillin 3 g and probenecid 1 g were 86% and 94.4% respectively; the difference was not significant.— R. N. Thin *et al.*, *Br. J. vener. Dis.*, 1977, *53*, 118.

The US Public Health Service recommended ampicillin 3.5 g or amoxycillin 3 g, either with probenecid 1 g by mouth as one regimen for the treatment of uncomplicated gonorrhoea in men and women. However, this treatment was considered to be slightly less effective than that with procaine penicillin or tetracycline. Ampicillin or amoxycillin could be used in other gonococcal infections.— *Morb. Mortal.*, 1979, *28*, 13.

Further references: R. W. Mitchell and H. G. Robson, *Can. med. Ass. J.*, 1974, *111*, 1198; U. Nwokolo, *Med. J. Zambia*, 1975, *9*, 102; J. D. Price and J. L. Fluker, *Br. J. vener. Dis.*, 1975, *51*, 398.

Leptospirosis. Amoxycillin 2 g or ampicillin 3 g daily for 6 days was successfully used for the treatment of leptospirosis in 27 patients.— D. Münnich and M. Lakatos, *Chemotherapy, Basle*, 1976, *22*, 372.

Meningitis. A study in 21 children indicated that amoxycillin sodium is as effective as ampicillin sodium in the treatment of bacterial meningitis due to *H. influenzae*. Amoxycillin sodium 50 mg per kg body-weight was given every 6 hours intravenously over 15 minutes for 14 days.— C. M. Nolan *et al.*, *Antimicrob. Ag. Chemother.*, 1979, *16*, 171.

Further references to amoxycillin in meningitis: J. C. Craft *et al.*, *Antimicrob. Ag. Chemother.*, 1979, *16*, 346 (with probenecid).

Otitis media. In a double-blind study of 383 infants and children with acute otitis media, amoxycillin 30 mg per kg body-weight daily was more effective in promoting an initial response in pneumococcal infection (31% of infections) than phenoxymethylpenicillin, erythromycin estolate, or erythromycin with triple sulphonamides. For haemophilus infections (22%), cure-rates with amoxycillin and the erythromycin-sulphonamide combination were significantly better than with the other 2 regimens.— J. E. Howard *et al.*, *Am. J. Dis. Child.*, 1976, *130*, 965. See also *Br. med. J.*, 1976, *2*, 1407.

Salmonellal infections. Seven patients with enteric fever became symptom-free and afebrile after treatment with amoxycillin 500 mg every 8 hours and in 6 the *S. typhi* or *S. paratyphi A* was eradicated. One patient with acute brucellosis improved when treated with amoxycillin but relapsed.— Z. Farid *et al.* (letter), *Lancet*, 1974, *1*, 350.

Amoxycillin was a suitable alternative to chloramphenicol in the treatment of typhoid fever and had fewer side-effects. Amoxycillin 1 g was given every 6 hours for 14 days to 61 patients and chloramphenicol 1 g every 8 hours to 63 patients until fever subsided then 500 mg every 8 hours for 1 week and 250 mg every 6 hours to a total treatment period of at least 14 days and a total dose of not more than 30 g. Patients in both groups showed striking improvement within 72 to 96 hours. Further investigation was indicated, especially into the long-term carrier state.— N. Pillay *et al.*, *Lancet*, 1975, *2*, 333.

In a study in 155 children with typhoid fever clinical, bacteriological, and temperature response were better in those treated with amoxycillin 100 mg per kg body-weight daily for 21 days than in those given chloramphenicol 50 mg per kg daily.— J. N. Scragg, *Br. med. J.*, 1976, *2*, 1031. See also J. N. Scragg and O. P. W. Robinson (letter), *J. antimicrob. Chemother.*, 1980, *6*, 156.

Experience in 30 patients with glucose 6-phosphate dehydrogenase deficiency or haematological complications after chloramphenicol suggested that amoxycillin 1 g six-hourly for 12 to 16 days was suitable for patients with typhoid fever.— A. M. Afifi *et al.*, *Br. med. J.*, 1976, *2*, 1033.

Amoxycillin 2 g (as the trihydrate) thrice daily for 28 days eradicated *Salmonella typhi* in 9 of 10 enteric carriers. Of 5 other carriers who received a reduced dose of 1 g thrice daily because of gastro-intestinal side-effects 2 were cured. The mean serum-amoxycillin concentrations were about 10.4 and 3 μg per ml in 5 cured and 4 failed patients respectively.— C. M. Nolan and P. C. White, *J. Am. med. Ass.*, 1978, *239*, 2352.

Further references: R. H. Gilman *et al.*, *J. infect. Dis.*, 1975, *132*, 630.

Urinary-tract infections. Bacteriological success-rates in 135 patients with urinary-tract infections who were treated with amoxycillin 250 mg thrice daily were 81% after the first week and 83% after the second week. The clinical success-rate was 96% on both occasions. Diarrhoea, the most common side-effect, necessitated withdrawal of treatment in 1 patient.— J. D. Price and J. W. Harding, *Br. J. clin. Pract.*, 1973, *27*, 165.

A general-practice study in 110 patients with urinary-tract infection suggested that a 3-day course of amoxycillin 500 mg thrice daily was as effective as a 10-day course.— C. A. C. Charlton *et al.*, *Br. med. J.*, 1976, *1*, 124.

Of 19 women with lower urinary-tract bacteriological infections 15 were infected with amoxycillin-sensitive organisms and 11 were considered cured at 6 weeks following 7 days' treatment with amoxycillin 250 mg thrice daily. Upper urinary-tract bacteriological infections occurred in 4 men and 19 women and of the 16 patients who were available to follow-up and whose infections were susceptible to amoxycillin, 8 were considered cured at 6 weeks following amoxycillin 500 mg thrice daily for 14 days. Peri-urethral supra-infection occurred in 19 of 28 women in whom swabs were taken before and after treatment.— A. R. Ronald *et al.*, *Antimicrob. Ag. Chemother.*, 1977, *11*, 780.

Further references: P. Tan *et al.*, *Chemotherapy, Basle*, 1973, *18, Suppl.*, 69; P. R. Grob *et al.*, *Practitioner*, 1977, *219*, 258.

For the use of amoxycillin in association with clavulanic acid in the treatment of urinary-tract infections, see Clavulanic Acid, p.1144.

Single-dose therapy. Of 22 women shown by the antibody-coated bacteria technique (a non-invasive technique) to have amoxycillin-susceptible urinary-tract infections limited to the lower urinary tract, all responded to amoxycillin 3 g given as a single dose and were free of symptoms within 24 to 48 hours of treatment; identical results were obtained with 21 similar women given a conventional course of amoxycillin 250 mg four times daily for 10 days. Side-effects in the single-dose group included mild gastro-intestinal disturbances in 3 women and worsening of rash in 1 woman with infective mononucleosis; in the conventional therapy group mild gastro-intestinal disturbances occurred in 8 women and symptomatic candidal vulvovaginitis in 9.— L. S. T. Fang *et al.*, *New Engl. J. Med.*, 1978, *298*, 413. In a comparative study in 74 patients with urinary-tract infections the cure-rate of 67% in those given a single 3-g dose of amoxycillin was significantly lower than the 80% cure-rate achieved in those who took 250 mg thrice daily for 10 days. In the single-dose group there was a high incidence of diarrhoea (17.5%), which in some cases was explosive and incapacitating.— D. A. Leigh *et al.* (letter), *J. antimicrob. Chemother.*, 1980, *6*, 403.

Criticism of treatment regimens for cystitis involving one or two 3-g doses of amoxycillin. Since amoxycillin is excreted very rapidly, frequent small doses would be more appropriate.— D. Greenwood *et al.* (letter), *Lancet*, 1980, *1*, 197.

Further references to single-dose therapy with amoxycillin: R. R. Bailey, *Drugs*, 1977, *13*, 137; R. R. Bailey and G. D. Abbott, *Nephron*, 1977, *18*, 316; P. M. Rogers, *Br. J. clin. Pract.*, 1980, *34*, 327; R. H. Rubin *et al.*, *J. Am. med. Ass.*, 1980, *244*, 561; W. E. Stamm, *ibid.*, 591.

Preparations

Amoxicillin Capsules *(U.S.P.)*. Capsules containing amoxycillin trihydrate equivalent to 250 or 500 mg of amoxycillin. Store at 15° to 30° in airtight containers.

Amoxicillin for Oral Suspension *(U.S.P.)*. Contains amoxycillin trihydrate with one or more suitable buffers, colouring and flavouring agents, preservatives, stabilisers, sweeteners, and suspending agents. Store at 15° to 30° in airtight containers. When reconstituted it contains the equivalent of 25 or 50 mg of amoxycillin per ml. pH 5 to 7.5.

Amoxycillin Capsules *(B.P.)*. Capsules containing amoxycillin trihydrate. Potency is expressed in terms of anhydrous amoxycillin. Store at a temperature not exceeding 30°.

Proprietary Preparations

Amoxil *(Bencard, UK)*. Amoxycillin trihydrate, available as **Capsules** containing the equivalent of 250 or 500 mg of amoxycillin; as **Dispersible Tablets** containing the equivalent of 500 mg; as **Paediatric Suspension** (supplied as powder for preparation with water before use) containing the equivalent of 125 mg in 1.25 ml; as **Sachets** (containing powder for preparation with water before use) containing the equivalent of 3 g; and as **Syrup** (supplied as powder for preparation with water before use) containing the equivalent of 125 or 250 mg in each 5 ml (suggested diluent, syrup). **Amoxil Injection**. Amoxycillin sodium (supplied as powder for solution before use), in vials containing the equivalent of 0.25, 0.5, or 1 g of amoxycillin. (Also available as Amoxil in *Austral.*, *S.Afr.*, *USA*).

Amoxycillin trihydrate is also an ingredient of Augmentin preparations (see Clavulanic Acid, p.1144).

Other Proprietary Names of Amoxycillin, Amoxycillin Sodium, and Amoxycillin Trihydrate

Arg.—Amoxidal, Amoxipenil, Fullcilina, Larocilin, Penamox; *Austral.*—Moxacin; *Belg.*—Clamoxyl, Hiconcil, Moxaline, Novabritine; *Canad.*—Amoxican, Moxilean, Novamoxin, Penamox, Polymox; *Denm.*—Draximox, Imacillin; *Fin.*—Clamox; *Fr.*—Clamoxyl, Hiconcil; *Ger.*—Amoxypen, Clamoxyl; *Ital.*—Alfamox, AM 73, Amox, Amoxibiotic, Amoxillin, Amoxipen, Amplimox, Aspenil, Ibiamox, Isimoxin, Majorpen, Mopen, Moxal, Overal Ilfi, Pamocil, Paradroxil, Piramox, Simoxil, Simplamox, Sintoplus, Velamox, Zimox (lactate); *Jap.*—Amolin, Clamoxyl, Delacillin, Efpenix, Hiconcil, Himino Max, Pasetocin, Sawacillin, Widecillin; *Neth.*—Clamoxyl, Flemoxin; *Norw.*—Imacillin; *Spain*—Actimoxi, Agerpen, Alfida, Amo-Flamisan, Amox, Amoxaren, Ardine, Bioxidona, Clamoxyl, Co-Amoxin, Dacala, Damoxicil, Eupen, Hosboral, Kapoxi, Morgenxil, Olmopen, Precopen, Raylina, Reloxyl, Sintedix, Superpeni, Tolodina; *Swed.*—Bristamox, Imacillin; *Switz.*—Clamoxyl; *USA*—Larotid, Polymox, Robamox, Sumox, Trimox, Utimox, Wymox.

7-r

Amphomycin. Amfomycin. An antimicrobial substance produced by the growth of *Streptomyces canus*.

CAS — 1402-82-0.

It is an amphoteric acidic polypeptide with surfactant properties in slightly acid or neutral solutions. **Soluble** in water and alcohol.

The calcium salt of amphomycin is soluble 1 in 200 of water and 1 in 80 of methyl alcohol. Aqueous solutions at pH 7 retain their activity for at least a month at room temperature.

Amphomycin has an antibacterial action against Gram-positive bacteria, especially cocci, and was formerly used mainly as the calcium salt in ointments with neomycin and hydrocortisone in the treatment of impetigo and infected dermatitis.

Amphomycin was formerly marketed in Great Britain under the proprietary name Ecomytrin (*Warner*), known in USA as Amphocortin..

8-f

Ampicillin *(B.P., B.P. Vet.)*. Ampicillinum; Anhydrous Ampicillin; Aminobenzylpenicillin. (6*R*)-6-(α-D-Phenylglycylamino)penicillanic acid. $C_{16}H_{19}N_3O_4S$=349.4.

CAS — 69-53-4.

Pharmacopoeias. In *Br.*, *Braz.*, *Int.*, *It.*, *Jap.*, and *Turk.* *U.S.* permits anhydrous or the trihydrate.

A white almost odourless crystalline powder with a bitter taste. It absorbs insignificant amounts of moisture at 25° at relative humidities up to about 80%, but under damper conditions it absorbs significant amounts.

Soluble 1 in 170 of water; practically insoluble in alcohol, acetone, chloroform, ether, carbon tetrachloride, and fixed oils. A 0.25% solution in water has a pH of 3.5 to 5.5. It is more **stable** than phenoxymethylpenicillin in acid solution. **Store** at a temperature not exceeding 25° in airtight containers.

The solubilities of ampicillin and ampicillin trihydrate in water were determined at different temperatures. Ampicillin decreased in solubility with increases in temperature, but the reverse occurred with the trihydrate. One part of ampicillin was soluble in the following parts of water: at 7.5°, 65.8; 20°, 74.6; 30°, 83.3; 40°, 87; and 50°, 90.9. Comparable solubilities for the trihydrate were: at 7.5°, 182; 20°, 167; 30°, 125; 40°, 100; and 50°, 71.4. The transition temperature was 42°. There was no interconversion of anhydrous ampicillin to the trihydrate except by seeding with trihydrate crystals. The thermodynamic activity of the anhydrous form was greater and so ought to produce greater physiological activity. Since the anhydrous form was not converted to trihydrate at room and body temperature, the differing activity was retained clinically.— J. W. Poole and C. K. Bahal, *J. pharm. Sci.*, 1968, *57*, 1945.

Stability. In a study of the effect of polymers on the stability of ampicillin tablets prepared by direct compression, PVM/MA copolymer gave the best results.— S. Niazi *et al.*, *Drug Devel. Comm.*, 1976, *2*, 241.

9-d

Ampicillin Sodium *(B.P., B.P. Vet.)*. Ampicillin Sod.; Ampicillinum Natricum; Sodium Ampicillin; Ampicillinnatrium. The sodium salt of ampicillin . $C_{16}H_{18}N_3NaO_4S$=371.4.

CAS — 69-52-3.

Pharmacopoeias. In *Br.*, *Braz.*, *Int.*, *It.*, *Jap.*, *Jug.*, *Nord.*, *Roum.*, and *Turk.*
U.S.P. has Sterile Ampicillin Sodium.

A white to off-white, odourless or almost odourless, crystalline or amorphous powder with a bitter taste, containing not less than 87% of ampicillin. It is hygroscopic and absorbs substantial amounts of moisture, even at low relative humidities. Each g represents about 2.7 mmol (2.7 mEq) of sodium. Ampicillin sodium 1.06 g is approximately equivalent to 1 g of ampicillin.

Soluble 1 in 2 of water and 1 in 50 of acetone; slightly soluble in chloroform; practically insoluble in ether, liquid paraffin, and fixed oils. With alcohol, ampicillin sodium forms a colloidal dispersion which gels on standing. A 10% solution in water has a pH of 8 to 10.

Store at a temperature not exceeding 25° in airtight containers; if it is intended for injection, the containers should be sterile and sealed to exclude micro-organisms.

Stability. The stability of solutions of ampicillin sodium is dependent on the concentration, the nature of the vehicle, and temperature.

Stability decreases as the concentration of ampicillin sodium increases; at 5° solutions containing 1% and 5% should retain 90% of their potency for 7 days and 24 hours respectively; solutions containing 10% and 25% may retain 80% of their potency for 24 hours and 6 hours respectively.

Stability decreases in the presence of dextrose, laevulose, and lactate. Sodium Chloride Intravenous Infusion is a suitable vehicle. If solutions containing dextrose or invert sugar are required the concentration of ampicillin should not exceed 0.2% and they should be given within 4 hours, preferably less; solutions in Sodium Lactate Intravenous Infusion should not exceed 3% and should be given within 4 hours.

Stability decreases as the temperature increases

but reports of the effect of freezing are conflicting.

Incompatible with amikacin sulphate, chlorpromazine hydrochloride, clindamycin phosphate, colistin sulphomethate sodium, dopamine hydrochloride, erythromycin ethylsuccinate and lactobionate, hydralazine hydrochloride, kanamycin sulphate, lincomycin hydrochloride, protein hydrolysate, and prochlorperazine mesylate; loss of potency has occurred with polysaccharides such as dextran 40 and with hydrocortisone sodium succinate; occasional incompatibility, depending generally on the pH and the vehicle, has occurred with gentamicin sulphate, lignocaine hydrochloride, oxytetracycline hydrochloride, polymyxin B sulphate, streptomycin sulphate, and tetracycline hydrochloride.

Incompatibility. Ampicillin was incompatible in solution with *adrenaline, chloramphenicol sodium succinate, chlortetracycline, noradrenaline, novobiocin, pentobarbitone, phenobarbitone, polymyxin B, protein hydrolysate, sulphafurazole, suxamethonium,* and *thiopentone sodium*.— *Med. Lett.*, 1972, *14* (Jan.), *Suppl.*, 32.

Ampicillin was reported to be incompatible with *atropine sulphate, calcium chloride, calcium gluconate, metaraminol tartrate,* and *vitamins of the B group with vitamin C* in an infusion fluid.— B. Flouvat and P. Lechat, *Thérapie*, 1974, *29*, 337.

Ampicillin sodium formed unacceptable levels of particulate matter when mixed with a total parenteral nutrient solution containing *amino acids* 4.25% and *dextrose* 25%.— N. Athanikar *et al., Am. J. Hosp. Pharm.*, 1979, *36*, 511.

Further references: B. Lynn, *Chemist Drugg.*, 1967, *187*, 157; *idem, J. Hosp. Pharm.*, 1970, *28*, 71; B. B. Riley, *ibid.*, 228; B. Lynn, *ibid.*, 1971, *29*, 183.

Polymerisation. A study of the polymerisation of ampicillin in aqueous solution.— E. J. Kuchinskas and G. N. Levy, *J. pharm. Sci.*, 1972, *61*, 727.

Dimerisation and hydrolysis reactions, followed by polymerisation, were responsible for most of the degradation of ampicillin in solution.— H. Bundgaard, *Acta pharm. suec.*, 1976, *13*, 9.

Studies on the rate of formation of polymers in injections of ampicillin sodium 20% during storage for up to 24 hours.— E. Cavatorta *et al., Farmaco, Edn prat.*, 1980, *35*, 273.

Stability. Ultraviolet irradiation for 2 hours had a destructive effect on ampicillin sodium.— A. A. Kassem and E. H. Girgis, *Bull. Fac. Pharm., Cairo*, 1970, *9*, 157.

Stability in solution. In a study of the kinetics and mechanism of degradation of ampicillin in solution, minimum hydrolysis occurred at pH 5.85, while in citrate buffer maximum stability occurred at pH 4.85.— J. P. Hou and J. W. Poole, *J. pharm. Sci.*, 1969, *58*, 447.

Accelerated degradation of benzylpenicillin sodium, ampicillin sodium, carbenicillin sodium, and phenoxymethylpenicillin potassium in neutral and alkaline sucrose solutions was due to a nucleophilic displacement reaction with the formation of sucrose penicilloate esters. These esters might be antigenic and their presence should be avoided by maintaining the pH of solutions of penicillins and sucrose at 6 to 6.5.— H. Bundgaard and C. Larsen, *Int. J. Pharmaceut.*, 1978, *1*, 95.

There was a linear relationship between the degradation-rate of benzylpenicillin and ampicillin and the concentration (up to 10%) of aqueous solutions of glucose, laevulose, sucrose, dextran, sorbitol, mannitol, and glycerol to which they were added. The rate-accelerating effect was directly proportional to hydroxide ion concentration up to pH about 10.5 and it proceeded through a nucleophilic pathway with the intermediate formation of penicilloyl esters. These esters might contribute to the allergic reactions which occurred with penicillin and their formation could be reduced or avoided by adjusting the pH of these penicillin-containing solutions to between 6 and 6.5.— H. Bundgaard and C. Larsen, *Arch. Pharm. Chemi, scient. Edn*, 1978, *6*, 184.

Further references on the stability of solutions.— B. Lynn, *Pharm. J.*, 1966, *1*, 115; J. F. Gallelli, *Am. J. Hosp. Pharm.*, 1967, *24*, 425; B. Lynn, *J. Hosp. Pharm.*, 1970, *28*, 71; J. Jacobs *et al., Drug Intell. & clin. Pharm.*, 1970, *4*, 204; D. R. Savello and R. F. Shangraw, *Am. J. Hosp. Pharm.*, 1971, *28*, 754; B. Lynn, *J. Hosp. Pharm.*, 1971, *29*, 183; J. Jacobs *et al., J. clin. Path.*, 1973, *26*, 742; J. Ashwin and B. Lynn, *Pharm. J.*, 1975, *1*, 487; B. E. Kirschenbaum and C. J. Latiolais, *Am. J. Hosp. Pharm.*, 1976, *33*, 767; G. Stjernström *et al., Acta pharm. suec.*, 1978, *15*, 33.

10-c

Ampicillin Trihydrate *(B.P., B.P. Vet.)*.

Ampicillin; Ampicillinum Trihydratum. The trihydrate of ampicillin.

$C_{16}H_{19}N_3O_4S,3H_2O$=403.4.

CAS — 7177-48-2.

Pharmacopoeias. In *Br., Braz., Cz., Int., It., Jug., Nord.,* and *Roum.* In *Jap.* and *U.S.* under the title Ampicillin.

A white practically odourless crystalline powder with a bitter taste. A 0.25% solution in water has a pH of 3.5 to 5.5. Ampicillin trihydrate 1.15 g is approximately equivalent to 1 g of ampicillin. **Soluble** 1 in 150 of water; practically insoluble in alcohol, acetone, chloroform, ether, carbon tetrachloride, and fixed oils. It absorbs insignificant amounts of moisture at 25° at relative humidities up to about 80%; under damper conditions it absorbs significant amounts. **Store** at a temperature not exceeding 25° in airtight containers.

Trace amounts of 2-hydroxy-3-phenylpyrazine, a fluorophore, had been detected in some commercially available products of ampicillin trihydrate.— M. J. Lebelle *et al., J. Pharm. Pharmac.*, 1979, *31*, 441.

Incompatibility. A study of the effect of the antibiotic and preservative on each other's binding to pharmaceutical adjuvants in mixtures containing chlorocresol or benzalkonium chloride and ampicillin trihydrate.— M. A. El-Nakeeb and M. H. Ali, *Mfg Chem.*, 1976, *47* (Mar.), 37.

Stability in solution. The half-life of a 0.1% solution of ampicillin trihydrate in 50% aqueous alcohol at pH 1.3 and 35° was 660 minutes.— B. Lynn, *Chemist Drugg.*, 1967, *187*, 134.

A suspension containing ampicillin trihydrate 67 mg per ml was stable for 18 months at 5°. During this period the pH fell from 6.1 to 5.6.— C. Bergwitz-Larsen and Å. G. Pilbrant, *Acta pharm. suec.*, 1973, *10*, 317.

A solution of ampicillin trihydrate 1.28 mg per ml in dextrose solution 5% showed a significant decrease in concentration after 48 hours at room temperature.— J. W. Munson *et al., J. pharm. Sci.*, 1979, *68*, 1333.

Adverse Effects. As for Benzylpenicillin, p.1103. Allergic reactions occur in sensitised persons. Skin rashes are the most common side-effect and are either urticarial or maculopapular; the urticarial reactions are typical of penicillin hypersensitivity while the maculopapular eruptions are characteristic of ampicillin and often appear about 5 days after treatment has finished. Removal of allergenic foreign material from ampicillin has been reported to reduce the incidence of maculopapular eruptions. Most patients with infectious mononucleosis develop a skin rash when treated with ampicillin.

Diarrhoea, nausea, and vomiting have occurred and raised serum aminotransferase concentrations have occasionally been reported. Severe pseudomembranous colitis has recently been reported in some patients. Supra-infections with *Pseudomonas* and *Candida* have also occurred.

Crystalluria occurred in 4 patients with meningitis within 24 hours of starting treatment with ampicillin, given intravenously.— J. L. Potter *et al., Pediatrics*, 1971, *48*, 636. Another similar report in one patient.— H. M. Jones and W. A. Schrader (letter), *Am. J. clin. Path.*, 1972, *58*, 220.

Non-allergic fever was observed on the 3rd to 8th day of treatment in 11 of 110 patients with scarlet fever treated with ampicillin.— J. Ström (letter), *Br. med. J.*, 1973, *1*, 419.

In an uncontrolled study of the side-effects of ampicillin given to 400 children in doses of 50 to 200 mg per kg body-weight daily, vomiting and severe diarrhoea were rare but moderate diarrhoea was common. Erythematous maculopapular skin rashes occurred in 3 to 7% and urticarial rashes in 1%. Perineal candidiasis occurred in some infants, usually with mild diarrhoea, and, unlike the other side-effects, was dose-related.— J. W. Bass *et al., J. Pediat.*, 1973, *83*, 106.

Non-specific abdominal pain had been reported on 6 occasions in women aged 33 to 58 years given ampicillin by mouth.— G. K. Davies *et al.* (letter), *Lancet*, 1974, *2*, 167.

Raised amino-acid excretion occurred in 2 infants given ampicillin and 1 was initially diagnosed as having maple-syrup-urine disease before the role of ampicillin was discovered.— S. F. Cahalane and C. Mullins (letter), *Lancet*, 1975, *1*, 812.

Allergy. A rash was reported in 9.5% of 422 patients treated with ampicillin, in 4.5% of 622 patients treated with other penicillins, and in 1.8% of 2941 patients not receiving these drugs. The risk of a rash occurring after ampicillin and other penicillins was 7.7 and 2.7% respectively. The occurrence of a rash after ampicillin was unaffected by the route of administration, but with other penicillins a rash appeared more frequently after an injection than after administration by mouth.— S. Shapiro *et al., Lancet*, 1969, *2*, 969. There was no association between the mean daily dose of ampicillin and the frequency of drug rash, nor was rash associated with duration of treatment.— *idem* (letter), 1970, *1*, 194.

When purified ampicillin and standard ampicillin were given by mouth to 1068 and 1077 patients respectively, 15 patients (1.4%) in the first group and 33 patients (3.1%) in the second group developed skin rashes, usually within 3 days of starting treatment.— E. T. Knudsen *et al., Br. med. J.*, 1970, *1*, 469. Criticism.— O. B. Fardig *et al.* (letter), *ibid.*, *2*, 735.

Reactions to ampicillin occurred not only in patients with infectious mononucleosis and lymphatic leukaemia, but also in those with cytomegalovirus mononucleosis.— H. P. Lambert *et al.* (letter), *Br. med. J.*, 1972, *1*, 688.

Of 50 patients with adverse reactions to ampicillin therapy, 34 developed maculopapular rash and 16 had urticaria. There were no reactions to skin tests in the first group, but in the second, 6 of the 16 had a positive reaction. Of these 6, 4 developed urticaria again when challenged with a further dose of ampicillin. It was concluded that maculopapular rashes were probably not of allergic origin but that about 25% of patients with urticaria manifested true allergic reactions to ampicillin.— C. W. Bierman *et al., J. Am. med. Ass.*, 1972, *220*, 1098.

The incidence and characteristics of skin rashes were studied in 933 patients treated with ampicillin; those with infectious mononucleosis or a history of allergy to penicillin were excluded. The overall incidence of rashes was 7.3% (males 3.7%, females 13.4%). Those given ampicillin initially by injection appeared more likely to develop rash than those given treatment by mouth. The median time of onset of rash was 9 days after commencing treatment and the median duration was 6 days; in some patients the rash faded during continued treatment. The incidence of rashes was somewhat lower (5.8%) in those given ampicillin of low protein content than in those given material of higher protein content (incidence 8.5%). The rash was macular or maculopapular in most patients and was not considered allergic. Future treatment with ampicillin or other penicillin was not therefore contra-indicated. The incidence of rashes was significantly higher in patients with viral infections than in those with other infections; a higher incidence had previously been reported in infectious mononucleosis, in cytomegalovirus mononucleosis, and in lymphatic leukaemia.— *Br. med. J.*, 1973, *1*, 7 (Report of a Collaborative Study Group).

Only 1 of 10 patients with lymphoproliferative disease with infective complications developed a skin rash, found to be non-specific, following treatment with a specially prepared polymer-free ampicillin. Three of the patients were sensitive to a high-dose ampicillin polymer during skin tests.— A. C. Parker and J. Richmond, *Br. med. J.*, 1976, *1*, 998.

Occurrence of the non-allergic maculopapular rash that often accompanies the use of ampicillin was not a contra-indication to its subsequent use and such patients should not automatically be labelled penicillin-allergic.— B. Sokoloff (letter), *Pediatrics*, 1977, *59*, 637. Distinguishing between maculopapular rashes, which had not been conclusively proved to be non-allergic, and allergic urticarial rashes was not easy and the 2 types often occurred together. Skin-testing for hypersensitivity to penicillin should be used.— A. B. Campbell and L. F. Soyka (letter), *ibid.*, 638.

Further reports of allergic reactions associated with ampicillin: R. H. Poe *et al., Chest*, 1980, *77*, 449 (adult respiratory distress syndrome).

Arthritis. A 23-year-old woman developed arthritis in the right knee in association with ampicillin-induced colitis.— B. M. Rothschild *et al., Archs intern. Med.*, 1977, *137*, 1605.

Blood disorders. One patient with jaundice developed thrombocytopenia associated with ampicillin.— A. P. Brooks (letter), *Lancet*, 1974, *2*, 723.

A haemorrhagic diathesis has been seen following ampicillin.— K. Andrassy *et al.* (letter), *New Engl. J. Med.*, 1975, *292*, 109.

Agranulocytosis. Agranulocytosis occurred in an elderly patient with nephrolithiasis and urinary-tract infection after administration of ampicillin but resolved on withdrawal of the drug.— M. Graf and A. Tarlov, *Ann. intern. Med.*, 1968, *69*, 91.

Colitis. A self-limiting pseudomembranous colitis was reported in a 3-year-old girl who had faecal retention 4 days after completing 5 days' treatment with ampicillin 60 mg per kg body-weight daily, for acute otitis media; diarrhoea and fever occurred after a further 9 days.— D. L. Christie and M. E. Ament, *J. Pediat.*, 1975, *87*, 657.

A 73-year-old woman undergoing condylar arthroplasty of the knee was given ampicillin and cloxacillin prophylactically. Diarrhoea and vomiting occurred on the tenth postoperative day and diarrhoea persisted when the antibiotics were given intramuscularly for a further 13 days. Pseudomembranous enterocolitis was diagnosed 7 days later; the condition did not respond to codeine phosphate; hypoproteinaemia and oedema developed and the patient died.— L. Read and J. R. Cove-Smith, *Postgrad. med. J.*, 1977, *53*, 324.

Of 3988 hospital in-patients in a Boston Collaborative Drug Surveillance Program who received ampicillin none developed colitis. Of 26 294 hospital in-patients monitored only 1 had been admitted with ampicillin-associated colitis. Of a further 24 783 interviewed none had ampicillin-associated colitis. These data confirmed the findings of F.J. Tedesco (*Am. J. dig. Dis.*, 1975, *20*, 295) that ampicillin-associated colitis is rare.— R. R. Miller and H. Jick, *Clin. Pharmac. Ther.*, 1977, *22*, 1.

Findings in 4 of 5 patients with pseudomembranous colitis compared with healthy subjects suggested that a faecal toxin associated with pseudomembranous colitis is produced by *Clostridium difficile* and that this is the likely cause of pseudomembranous colitis. Antibiotic treatment might alter the conditions that limit the replication and persistence of *Cl. difficile* so that a susceptible individual exposed to *Cl. difficile* develops colitis.— H. E. Larson *et al.*, *Lancet*, 1978, *1*, 1063. Comment.— *ibid.*, 1080. The possible association of *Cl. perfringens* with pseudomembranous colitis following a course of ampicillin.— J. N. Schwartz *et al.*, *J. Pediat.*, 1980, *97*, 661.

A report of 5 patients who suffered acute bloody diarrhoea associated with administration of ampicillin, amoxycillin, or phenoxymethylpenicillin. Pseudomembranous colitis was excluded and it was believed that the diarrhoea was allergic in origin.— R. B. Toffler *et al.*, *Lancet*, 1978, *2*, 707.

Pseudomembranous colitis in an acutely ill 27-month-old boy who died after a month of intractable diarrhoea was associated with the administration of ampicillin.— W. A. Auritt *et al.*, *J. Pediat.*, 1978, *93*, 882.

Further reports of pseudomembranous colitis associated with ampicillin.— J. P. Keating *et al.*, *Am. J. Dis. Child.*, 1974, *128*, 369; D. Berkowitz *et al.*, *Am. J. Gastroent., N.Y.*, 1976, *66*, 362; W. R. Bartle and F. G. Saibil, *Can. med. Ass. J.*, 1977, *116*, 162; J. -P. Buts *et al.*, *Gastroenterology*, 1977, *73*, 823.

For further references to pseudomembranous colitis associated with antibiotic therapy, see Clindamycin Hydrochloride, p.1144.

Effect on serum aminotransferase. For a report of elevated serum aspartate aminotransferase (SGOT) values following the intramuscular administration of ampicillin, see Carbenicillin, p.1111.

Intracranial hypertension. Reversible increased intracranial pressure with bulging of the anterior fontanelle and increased cerebrospinal fluid pressure was associated in 6 infants with ampicillin.— D. Ehrlich *et al.*, *Harefuah*, 1973, *85*, 112.

Nephrotoxicity. Interstitial nephritis occurred in a 43-year-old woman given ampicillin in a dose of 200 mg per kg body-weight over 24 hours. After treatment she recovered completely.— D. Maxwell *et al.*, *J. Am. med. Ass.*, 1974, *230*, 586. See also E. J. Ruley and L. M. Lisi, *J. Pediat.*, 1974, *84*, 878; A. J. Woodroffe, *Med. J. Aust.*, 1975, *1*, 65; H. G. Rennke *et al.* (letter), *New Engl. J. Med.*, 1980, *302*, 691; A. L. Linton *et al.*, *Ann. intern. Med.*, 1980, *93*, 735.

Ototoxicity. Ototoxicity was not confirmed in a follow-up study of 37 children who had been treated with ampicillin, usually in daily doses of 400 mg per kg body-weight intravenously, for *Haemophilus influenzae* meningitis.— H. Dahnsjö *et al.*, *Acta paediat. scand.*, 1976, *65*, 733.

Of 47 children treated for *Haemophilus influenzae* meningitis, 3 showed some sensorineural loss of hearing. They included 1 of 27 given ampicillin only, 1 of 12 given chloramphenicol only, and 1 of 8 given both antibiotics. Two of the 3 children with loss of hearing had received ampicillin intravenously 300 mg per kg body-weight and 460 mg per kg daily respectively. Doses in most of the other children given ampicillin did not exceed 250 mg per kg daily. Ampicillin may be ototoxic when given intravenously in very high doses.— F. E. Jones and D. R. Hanson, *Develop. Med. Child Neurology*, 1977, *19*, 593.

A further report of ototoxicity associated with ampicillin.— M. Koskiniemi *et al.*, *Acta paediat. scand.*, 1978, *67*, 17.

Skin reactions. Of the 39 946 medical in-patients monitored by the Boston Collaborative Drug Surveillance Program, 5311 received ampicillin and 1040 received amoxycillin. Of the ampicillin recipients 289 (5.4%) had a rash within 14 days of the first dose; of the amoxycillin recipients 70 (6.7%) had a rash during the same period. It is concluded that the rate of rash attributable to the 2 drugs is similar.— J. Porter and H. Jick (letter), *Lancet*, 1980, *1*, 1037.

See also under Allergy (above).

Treatment of Adverse Effects. When cutaneous reactions to ampicillin occur they may subside spontaneously within a few hours or days. Control of the reactions may be attempted by the administration of antihistamines.

At the first sign of an immediate allergic reaction 0.3 to 1 ml of Adrenaline Injection should be given intramuscularly (or in severe cases 0.2 ml well diluted intravenously) followed by a further dose if no improvement occurs. Urticaria may be treated with corticosteroids by mouth.

See also under Benzylpenicillin, p.1105.

Metronidazole 1.5 g daily produced rapid improvement in a patient with ampicillin-induced colitis.— H. T. Dinh *et al.* (letter), *Lancet*, 1978, *1*, 338.

Precautions. Ampicillin is contra-indicated in patients known to be sensitive to penicillin and it should be used with caution in patients with known histories of allergy. Reduced doses may be required in patients with impaired renal function. It should preferably not be given to patients with infectious mononucleosis since they are especially susceptible to ampicillin-induced skin rashes.

See also under Benzylpenicillin, p.1105.

The incidence of side-effects in patients with renal disease who were treated with ampicillin 500 mg six-hourly was greater than in patients with normal renal function (56% compared with 6.1%); mean blood concentrations were 32 µg per ml compared with 1.9 µg per ml. Reactions in patients with impaired renal function occurred in a mean of 8.3 days. Permanent reduction in renal function occurred in 3 patients after reactions. Adequate blood concentrations of 2.7 µg per ml were obtained by a reduced dose of 100 mg eight-hourly.— H. A. Lee and L. F. Hill, *Br. J. clin. Pract.*, 1968, *22*, 354.

Ampicillin should be avoided in infectious mononucleosis, cytomegalovirus infection, and lymphocytic leukaemias because of the increased risk of rash.— T. F. Murphy (letter), *Ann. intern. Med.*, 1979, *91*, 324.

Biliary obstruction. Bile-duct obstruction caused impaired absorption of ampicillin.— *Drug & Ther. Bull.*, 1976, *14*, 57.

Effect on urine estimations. Ampicillin could interfere with paper chromatographic estimations of urinary amino acids by producing drug spots.— *Drug & Ther. Bull.*, 1972, *10*, 69.

Interactions. *Allopurinol.* In a study of 1324 patients who were receiving ampicillin 15 of 67 patients (22.4%) who were also receiving allopurinol developed a skin rash compared with 94 of the remainder (7.5%). Either allopurinol or the hyperuricaemia was considered to be responsible for the increased incidence of skin rash.— *New Engl. J. Med.*, 1972, *286*, 505 (Boston Collaborative Drug Surveillance Program).

Beta-blockers. For a report of ampicillin reducing the elimination half-life of practolol given by mouth but not by intravenous injection, see Practolol, p.1349.

Chloramphenicol. Eight of 11 children treated for *Haemophilus influenzae* meningitis with ampicillin and chloramphenicol had long-term sequelae compared with 4 of 32 given ampicillin alone and 4 of 22 given chloramphenicol alone. An increased risk was suggested for this combination.— J. Lindberg *et al.*, *Pediatrics*, 1977, *60*, 1. Further references: T. Matthews (letter), *Lancet*, 1978, *2*, 376.

See also under Antimicrobial Action (below).

Oral contraceptives. A suggestion that ampicillin might diminish the effectiveness of oral contraceptives.— D. J. Back and M. L'E. Orme, *Prescribers' J.*, 1977, *17*, 137. Contrary results.— C. I. Friedman *et al.*, *Obstet. Gynec.*, 1980, *55*, 33.

Pregnancy and the neonate. In 3 women in late pregnancy ampicillin 2 g daily for 3 days reduced the mean plasma concentrations of total oestriol conjugates, oestriol 16α-glucuronide, oestrone conjugates, and oestradiol conjugates. It had little effect on unconjugated oestrogen concentrations and no effect on progesterone. Ampicillin probably inhibited steroid conjugate hydrolysis in the gut H. Adlercreutz *et al.*, *Am. J. Obstet. Gynec.*, 1977, *128*, 266. A similar report.— M. J. Tikkanen *et al.* (letter), *Br. med. J.*, 1973, *2*, 369.

In a study in pregnant women, plasma concentrations of ampicillin and pivampicillin were shown to be significantly lower than expected. It was necessary to double the dose in pregnant women to achieve plasma concentrations comparable to those in non-pregnant women.— A. Philipson, *Am. J. Obstet. Gynec.*, 1978, *130*, 674.

Antimicrobial Action. Ampicillin is bactericidal and has a similar mode of action to that of benzylpenicillin. It resembles benzylpenicillin in its action against Gram-positive organisms, including *Streptococcus faecalis*, *Str. pneumoniae*, and haemolytic streptococci but, apart perhaps from *Str. faecalis*, it is less potent than benzylpenicillin. *Listeria monocytogenes* is also highly sensitive. Its action is similar to that of the tetracyclines and chloramphenicol against Gram-negative organisms, particularly *Haemophilus influenzae*, salmonellae, and most strains of *Escherichia coli*; highly resistant strains of *H. influenzae* have been reported. *Neisseria gonorrhoeae*, *N. meningitidis*, *Bordetella pertussis*, *Proteus mirabilis*, and *Brucella* spp. are also sensitive. Ampicillin is effective against some shigellae but strains can acquire resistance rapidly.

Minimum inhibitory concentrations for Gram-positive organisms have been reported to range from 0.02 to 5 µg per ml and for Gram-negative organisms from 0.02 to 8 µg per ml. It is inactive against most strains of *Pseudomonas aeruginosa*.

Phospholipids had a greater affinity for benzylpenicillin than for ampicillin. The higher concentrations of lipids in the cell walls of Gram-negative organisms, preventing benzylpenicillin reaching the cell membrane, were considered to be the cause of the bacterial resistance of these organisms to penicillin and of their sensitivity to ampicillin.— J. M. Padfield and I. W. Kellaway, *J. Pharm. Pharmac.*, 1973, *25*, 285.

Of 68 strains of *H. influenzae*, 67 were inhibited by ampicillin at a concentration of 0.12 µg per ml, and 1 at 0.25 µg per ml. These concentrations were well within the peak blood concentrations of ampicillin.— J. D. Williams and J. Andrews, *Br. med. J.*, 1974, *1*, 134. Of 104 strains of *H. influenzae* isolated from children, 30 produced beta-lactamase and required 2 µg or more of ampicillin per ml for inhibition; 5 strains were not inhibited by 128 µg per ml. MICs for strains not producing beta-lactamase ranged from 0.06 to 1 µg per ml.— E. O. Mason *et al.*, *Antimicrob. Ag. Chemother.*, 1980, *17*, 470. See also Resistance, below.

Ampicillin inhibited the majority of 222 strains of anaerobic bacteria at 16 µg or less per ml, including 19 of 34 strains of *Bacteroides fragilis*.— V. L. Sutter and S. M. Finegold, *Antimicrob. Ag. Chemother.*, 1976, *10*, 736. In a further study the majority of 265 strains of anaerobic bacteria, including 19 of 41 strains of *Bacteroides fragilis*, were inhibited by ampicillin 8 µg per ml.— P. C. Appelbaum and S. A. Chatterton, *ibid.*, 1978, *14*, 371.

Ampicillin inhibited 33, 49, 59, 87, and all of 92 strains of *N. gonorrhoeae in vitro* at an MIC of 30, 60, 125, 250, and 500 ng per ml respectively.— B. A. Watts *et al.*, *J. antimicrob. Chemother.*, 1977, *3*, 331.

MBCs of ampicillin greatly exceeded MICs against 40 strains of *Lactobacilli in vitro*.— A. S. Bayer *et al.*, *Antimicrob. Ag. Chemother.*, 1978, *14*, 720.

Activity of ampicillin with chloramphenicol. Mutual antagonism did not occur when ampicillin and chloramphenicol were used together *in vitro* against ampicillin-resistant or ampicillin-sensitive strains of *H. influenzae* type b. However, ampicillin and chloramphenicol had an indifferent effect on each other's activity against the majority of strains.— F. S. Cole *et al.*, *Antimicrob. Ag.*

Chemother., 1979, *15*, 415. The effects of ampicillin with chloramphenicol *in vitro* against *H. influenzae* were variable and appeared to depend mainly on the concentration of chloramphenicol. No apparent antagonism occurred with high concentrations of chloramphenicol (5 to 10 μg per ml) but low concentrations (1 to 2 μg per ml) were antagonistic to the bactericidal activity of ampicillin. Ampicillin did not antagonise the effect of chloramphenicol.— A. M. R. Mackenzie, *J. antimicrob. Chemother.*, 1979, *5*, 693.

When ampicillin and chloramphenicol were used together *in vitro* against 21 strains of *N. meningitidis* their activities were antagonistic against 13 strains, additive against 5, and synergistic against 3. Against 21 strains of *Str. pneumoniae* their activities were antagonistic for 1 strain, additive for 14, and synergistic for 6.— W. E. Feldman and T. Zweighaft, *Antimicrob. Ag. Chemother.*, 1979, *15*, 240.

Diminished activity. The antibacterial action of ampicillin against *Staphylococcus aureus* was inhibited *in vitro* by clindamycin.— P. D. Meers (letter), *Lancet*, 1973, *2*, 573.

Mecillinam had an antagonistic effect on the activity *in vitro* of ampicillin against 3 of 29 strains of *Bacteroides* spp.— I. Trestman *et al.*, *Antimicrob. Ag. Chemother.*, 1979, *16*, 283.

Enhanced activity. The bactericidal activity of ampicillin against *E. coli*, *Pr. mirabilis*, and *Enterobacter* spp. was enhanced *in vitro* by kanamycin.— R. J. Bulger and U. Roosen-Runge, *Am. J. med. Sci.*, 1969, *258*, 7.

A more rapid bactericidal effect *in vitro* was achieved against group B streptococci when gentamicin was used with ampicillin instead of ampicillin alone.— V. Schauf *et al.*, *J. Pediat.*, 1976, *89*, 194.

The activity of ampicillin *in vitro* against *E. coli* was enhanced when used with human serum.— B. S. Dutcher *et al.*, *Antimicrob. Ag. Chemother.*, 1978, *13*, 820.

Up to 64 μg per ml of ampicillin or amoxycillin was required to inhibit 15 beta-lactamase-producing strains of *N. gonorrhoeae in vitro*, but less than 4 μg per ml when either antibiotic was used together with clavulanic acid in the ratio of 2 to 1.— P. Piot *et al.*, *Antimicrob. Ag. Chemother.*, 1979, *15*, 535.

Further reports of enhanced activity *in vitro* with ampicillin and other antibiotics: E. Grunberg and R. Cleeland, *J. antimicrob. Chemother.*, 1977, *3*, *Suppl.* B, 59 (with mecillinam); C. Watanakunakorn and C. Glotzbecker, *J. antimicrob. Chemother.*, 1978, *4*, 539 (with sissomicin or netilmicin against enterococci); M. D. Cooper *et al.*, *Antimicrob. Ag. Chemother.*, 1979, *15*, 484 (with aminoglycosides against aminoglycoside-resistant group B streptococci); J. Garau and S. A. Kabins, *J. antimicrob. Chemother.*, 1979, *5*, 31 (with oxacillin against enterococci); J. Mizoguchi *et al.*, *Antimicrob. Ag. Chemother.*, 1979, *16*, 439 (with dicloxacillin against beta-lactamase-producing *Citrobacter freundii*); W. M. Scheld *et al.*, *Antimicrob. Ag. Chemother.*, 1979, *16*, 271 (with mecillinam against *E. coli* and *Kleb. pneumoniae*); A. S. Bayer *et al.*, *Antimicrob. Ag. Chemother.*, 1980, *17*, 359 (with aminoglycosides against antibiotic-tolerant lactobacilli); R. Hone and M. Foley (letter), *J. antimicrob. Chemother.*, 1980, *6*, 410 (with mecillinam against *Proteus* spp.); R. Yogev *et al.*, *Antimicrob. Ag. Chemother.*, 1980, *17*, 461 (with nafcillin against ampicillin-resistant *H. influenzae*).

For a study of the synergistic activity of ampicillin and fosfomycin against strains of shigellae and salmonellae, see Fosfomycin, p.1165.

Resistance. Ampicillin is inactivated by penicillinase and penicillinase-producing strains of *Staphylococcus aureus*, *Proteus* spp., *E. coli*, and *Klebsiella* spp. are resistant. In Gram-negative organisms resistance factors can occur causing resistance to ampicillin and other antibiotics. Resistance has been reported in other strains of *E. coli*, in *Bacteroides* spp., shigellae, and *Salmonella* spp.

Type b strains of *Haemophilus influenzae*, highly resistant to ampicillin, are frequently reported and the incidence of resistance appears to be increasing.

Resistance of bacteroides. Of 60 strains of *Bacteroides fragilis* 56 were resistant to ampicillin.— O. A. Okubadejo *et al.*, *Br. med. J.*, 1973, *2*, 212.

Resistance of haemophilus. When sensitivity tests of strains of *H. influenzae* were read macroscopically results were influenced by the inoculum size. Microscopic examination revealed that the turbidity in heavily inoculated broth was due to L-forms which gave the impression of resistance. This could be avoided by reducing the inoculum to 10^5 organisms per ml, reading the doubling dilution technique microscopically, and expressing the MIC as the lowest concentration of antibiotic that contains no coccobacillary forms.— D. E. Roberts (letter), *Lancet*, 1974, *2*, 157.

The resistance of 5 isolates of *H. influenzae* to ampicillin was due to beta-lactamases similar to those mediated by R-factors. Studies with *H. influenzae* and *E. coli* suggested that both bacteria inhibited the entry of ampicillin to the bacteria but that this inhibition was much less with *H. influenzae*. This might account for the difficulty in detecting *H. influenzae* resistance with low concentrations of ampicillin.— A. A. Medeiros and T. F. O'Brien, *Lancet*, 1975, *1*, 716.

Plasmid-mediated R-factors, the same as those from the Enterobacteriaceae, had been detected in strains of *H. influenzae* producing resistance to ampicillin and tetracycline. There had also been a few reports of chloramphenicol-resistant *H. influenzae*.— R. Laufs *et al.*, *Dt. med. Wschr.*, 1978, *103*, 658.

Resistance to ampicillin was present in 13 of 168 (7.7%) strains of *H. influenzae*, 148 of 334 (44.3%) *H. parainfluenzae*, 2 of 4 (50%) *H. haemolyticus*, 20 of 68 (29.4%) *H. parahaemolyticus*, and 3 of 14 (21.4%) strains of other spp. of *Haemophilus* (X-dependent).— A. P. Gillett *et al.* (letter), *Br. med. J.*, 1978, *2*, 278.

Confirmation of a second mechanism of ampicillin resistance in *H. influenzae*, not associated with beta-lactamase production.— S. M. Bell and D. Plowman, *Lancet*, 1980, *1*, 279. Failure to demonstrate the presence of beta-lactamase in over 50% of the strains was probably due to overestimation of the incidence of ampicillin resistance. Of 31 ampicillin-resistant strains of *H. influenzae* studied over 2 years only 1 lacked evidence of beta-lactamase. Moreover, the Center for Disease Control, in Atlanta, is aware of fewer than 10 *H. influenzae* isolates in the US in the past 4 years that were ampicillin resistant but beta-lactamase negative.— R. Yogev (letter), *ibid.*, 934. Comments.— A. J. Howard and C. J. Hince (letter), *ibid.*, 1359; S. M. Bell and D. E. Plowman (letter), *ibid.*; D. B. Wheldon and M. P. E. Slack (letter), *ibid.*, *2*, 149; A. Griffiths (letter), *ibid.*, 150; S. M. Bell and D. E. Plowman (letter), *ibid.*, 422.

Further reports of ampicillin-resistant *Haemophilus*: W. J. Thomas *et al.* (letter), *Lancet*, 1974, *1*, 313 (*H. influenzae*); V. Syriopoulou *et al.*, *J. Pediat.*, 1976, *89*, 839 (incidence of resistant *H. influenzae*); A. J. Howard *et al.*, *Br. med. J.*, 1978, *2*, 1657 (*H. influenzae*); R. Schwartz *et al.*, *J. Am. med. Ass.*, 1978, *239*, 320 (incidence of resistant *H. influenzae*); J. I. Ward *et al.*, *J. infect. Dis.*, 1978, *138*, 421 (prevalence of resistant *H. influenzae*); J. L. Brunton *et al.*, *Antimicrob. Ag. Chemother.*, 1979, *15*, 294 (*H. ducreyi*); D. P. Jubelirer and A. S. Yeager, *J. Pediat.*, 1979, *95*, 415 (simultaneous recovery of ampicillin-sensitive and ampicillin-resistant *H. influenzae* type b in meningitis); I. Braveny and K. Machka (letter), *Lancet*, 1980, *2*, 752 (*H. influenzae* and *H. parainfluenzae*); L. Jokipii and A. M. M. Jokipii, *J. antimicrob. Chemother.*, 1980, *6*, 623 (prevalence of resistant *H. influenzae*); S. M. Markowitz, *Antimicrob. Ag. Chemother.*, 1980, *17*, 80 (ampicillin-resistant non-beta-lactamase-producing *H. influenzae*); J. D. Nelson (letter), *J. Am. med. Ass.*, 1980, *244*, 239 (prevalence of resistant *H. influenzae*); S. Simasathien *et al.*, *Lancet*, 1980, *2*, 1214 (*H. influenzae*).

Resistance of nocardia. Results of a study *in vitro* of the susceptibility of isolates of the *Nocardia* spp. to beta-lactam antibiotics suggested that factors other than, or in addition to, beta-lactamase production were responsible for resistance to ampicillin or carbenicillin.— R. J. Wallace *et al.*, *Antimicrob. Ag. Chemother.*, 1978, *14*, 704.

Resistance of salmonellae. Ampicillin resistance among *S. typhimurium* was reversed when ampicillin was used with appropriate anti-plasmid compounds such as mepacrine or tilorone.— F. E. Hahn and Ciak. J., *Antimicrob. Ag. Chemother.*, 1977, *11*, 176.

Resistance of shigellae. During a 4½-year period 503 strains of *Shigella* spp. were isolated and the incidence of ampicillin resistance rose from 8% in the first year to 95% at the end of the study.— S. Ross *et al.*, *J. Am. med. Ass.*, 1972, *221*, 45. See also R. C. Tilton *et al.* (letter), *ibid.*, *222*, 487.

Both transferable and non-transferable types of resistance to ampicillin were detected in strains of *Shigella sonnei*. Different beta-lactamases were involved for each type with the non-transferable form being considered to be of a low level and the transferable form due to an R-factor to be of a high level.— J. T. Smith *et al.*, *Antimicrob. Ag. Chemother.*, 1974, *6*, 418.

Further references: C. F. Peng, *Chin. J. Microbiol.*, 1975, *8*, 12; M. M. Rahaman *et al.* (letter), *Lancet*, 1974, *1*, 406.

Resistance of streptococci. Strains of *Str. pneumoniae* from 5 children were partially resistant to ampicillin.— P. C. Appelbaum *et al.*, *Lancet*, 1977, *2*, 995.

A report of the increasing resistance of oral α-haemolytic streptococci to ampicillin in Northern Ireland.— R. H. Elliott and J. M. Dunbar, *Br. dent. J.*, 1977, *142*, 283.

A report of *Str. faecalis* in a 75-year-old man with endocarditis, that exhibited tolerance to ampicillin with an MIC of 1.6 μg per ml and an MBC of over 100 μg per ml.— M. McDonald *et al.* (letter), *Lancet*, 1980, *2*, 321.

Absorption and Fate. Ampicillin is relatively stable in the acid gastric secretion and is well absorbed from the gastro-intestinal tract after oral administration. Food can interfere with the absorption of ampicillin so doses should be taken 30 minutes to an hour before meals. Peak concentrations in plasma are obtained in about 2 hours and following a dose of 500 mg by mouth are reported to range from 2 to 6 μg per ml. Doubling the dose can produce double the concentration. Ampicillin is given by injection as the sodium salt and following the intramuscular administration of 500 mg peak plasma concentrations occur at about 1 hour and are reported to range from 7 to 14 μg per ml.

About 20% is bound to plasma proteins in the circulation and plasma half-lives of about 1 to 2 hours have been reported. It diffuses across the placenta into the foetal circulation and concentrations can persist in amniotic fluid. Concentrations can be detected in the milk of nursing mothers. There is little diffusion into the cerebrospinal fluid except when the meninges are infected, when high concentrations are achieved. Concentrations of ampicillin are found in ascitic, pleural, joint, and ocular fluids.

Renal clearance of ampicillin is slower than that of benzylpenicillin and occurs partly by glomerular filtration and partly by tubular secretion. About 30% of an orally administered dose is excreted unchanged in the urine in 6 hours; urinary concentrations range from 0.25 to 1 mg per ml following a dose of 500 mg. After 500 mg is given parenterally 70 to 75% is excreted in the urine within 6 hours. A high concentration is reached in bile and some is excreted in the faeces. Renal elimination is retarded by the concomitant use of probenecid.

A review of the pharmacokinetics of the penicillins.— M. Barza and L. Weinstein, *Clin. Pharmacokinet.*, 1976, *1*, 297.

The degree of binding of penicillins to serum proteins was least with methicillin and ampicillin, intermediate with benzylpenicillin and phenoxymethylpenicillin, and high (90% or more) with oxacillin, cloxacillin, nafcillin, and dicloxacillin. Dicloxacillin gave the highest serum concentration of total antibiotic after a single oral dose, followed in decreasing order by cloxacillin, oxacillin, nafcillin, and ampicillin. The concentration of free antibiotic in serum was highest with ampicillin, followed by cloxacillin. There was no significant difference between the remaining beta-lactamase-resistant compounds. After injection, nafcillin produced much lower serum concentrations of total antibiotic than the others, but the amount of free compound available did not significantly differ from that of oxacillin, and exceeded that of dicloxacillin. Free methicillin exceeded more than tenfold the concentration of other penicillins resistant to beta-lactamase. The urinary recovery of antibiotics suggested that nafcillin and oxacillin were absorbed equally well from the alimentary canal, despite the difference in their serum concentration, and that the absorption of dicloxacillin was not complete. Larger amounts of methicillin than of other antibiotics appeared in the urine.— C. M. Kunin, *Clin. Pharmac. Ther.*, 1966, *7*, 166.

Peak serum concentrations were higher and occurred earlier after the administration of anhydrous ampicillin than after the trihydrate form. These results corresponded with solubility and dissolution-rate data.— J. W. Poole *et al.*, *Curr. ther. Res.*, 1968, *10*, 292.

The biological half-life of ampicillin was 0.75 to 2 hours in adults (4 to 6 hours in renal failure), 2.2 to 3.4 hours (according to age) in infants born at term, and 1.9 to 3.6 hours (according to age) in premature infants.— W. A. Ritschel, *Drug Intell. & clin. Pharm.*, 1970, *4*, 332.

In infants the serum half-life was 1.2 hours at 1 month but 4 hours at 1 week, due to immature kidney function.— J. M. Rosenberg and K. Mann, *ibid.*, 1973, *7*, 346.

In a study with healthy volunteers the mean serum concentration of ampicillin sodium was 6.79 µg per ml 1 hour after a 500-mg dose given intramuscularly. Serum concentrations were 1.84, 2.75, and 4.84 µg per ml 2 hours after the intramuscular administration of 250, 500, and 1000 mg respectively of ampicillin trihydrate. The absorption of ampicillin trihydrate was slower than its elimination.— J. T. Doluisio *et al.*, *J. pharm. Sci.*, 1971, *60*, 715.

After an intravenous injection of ampicillin 1 g the mean serum half-life was 74 minutes. Probenecid increased this time to 137 minutes. Probenecid also increased the biliary concentration of ampicillin.— J. Kampmann *et al.*, *Br. J. Pharmac.*, 1973, *47*, 782.

Although there was little impairment in absorption of ampicillin in 14 patients with gastric achlorhydria and 22 patients with partial gastrectomy compared with 21 healthy subjects, absorption appeared to be impaired in 18 patients with obstructive jaundice.— J. A. Davies and J. M. Holt, *J. antimicrob. Chemother.*, 1975, *1*, *Suppl.* (Sept.), 69.

A study of the biliary excretion of ampicillin.— J. M. Brogard *et al.*, *Chemotheraphy, Basle*, 1977, *23*, 213.

A study on the pharmacokinetics of ampicillin and its prodrugs bacampicillin and pivampicillin in 5 subjects.— M. Ehrnebo *et al.*, *J. Pharmacokinet. Biopharm.*, 1979, *7*, 429.

In 24 patients with spontaneous bacterial meningitis treated with a constant-rate intravenous infusion of ampicillin in a dose of 150 mg per kg body-weight daily, large differences in serum-ampicillin concentrations (9.4 to 92 µg per ml) were noted when measured on day 5.— E. Bouvet *et al.*, *Br. med. J.*, 1980, *280*, 1164.

Bioavailability. A review of the bioavailability of various ampicillin preparations.— W. J. Jusko *et al.*, *J. Am. pharm. Ass.*, 1975, *NS15*, 591.

A comparative study on the bioavailability of 4 different brands of ampicillin and a preparation of talampicillin.— J. M. T. Hamilton-Miller and W. Brumfitt, *J. antimicrob. Chemother.*, 1979, *5*, 699.

Diffusion into body fluids and tissues. Ten young children with acute exudative otitis media received an intramuscular injection of ampicillin, in a dose of 250 mg for those weighing less than 11.2 kg and 500 mg for the other children. Ampicillin concentrations in the exudate ranged from 1.6 to 19 µg per ml which exceeded the MIC against the usual organisms causing otitis media. Blood concentrations of ampicillin ranged from 6.3 to 46 µg per ml.— J. D. Coffey, *J. Pediat.*, 1968, *72*, 693.

The average concentration of ampicillin in the synovial fluid of 19 patients about 2 hours after being given 500 mg every 6 hours for 2 days was 1.8 µg per ml compared to a serum-ampicillin concentration of 2.9 µg per ml. Samples withdrawn from 4 patients 3½ to 7 hours after the dose showed an average synovial concentration of 0.68 µg per ml and an average serum concentration of 0.75 µg per ml which did not indicate any accumulation. Higher concentrations were found in the lighter patients and in women.— E. A. Baciocco and R. L. Iles, *Clin. Pharmac. Ther.*, 1971, *12*, 858.

Both ampicillin and cloxacillin diffused into the synovial fluid of patients with osteoarthritis or rheumatoid arthritis and the concentrations were related to the degree of protein binding. For ampicillin, where 86 to 87% of the quantity in the serum was free, 70% of the serum concentration was achieved in the synovial fluid, mostly in the free state, and for cloxacillin, which was highly bound to serum-protein, the mean peak concentration in synovial fluid was 22% of that in the serum.— A. Howell *et al.*, *Clin. Pharmac. Ther.*, 1972, *13*, 724. In a study involving 21 infants and children with suppurative arthritis, adequate concentrations of ampicillin were achieved after 50 mg per kg body-weight was given by mouth. Similar peak serum and joint fluid concentrations occurred 2 hours after a dose. Further results with cephalexin, cloxacillin, dicloxacillin, and benzylpenicillin suggested that the degree of binding to plasma protein did not influence the diffusion of antibiotics into joint fluid.— J. D. Nelson *et al.*, *J. Pediat.*, 1978, *92*, 131.

Mean CSF concentrations of ampicillin in 9 healthy subjects given 33 mg per kg body-weight by intravenous infusion were 460 and 700 ng per ml, ½ and 3½ hours respectively after administration. Higher concentrations were achieved than with the same dose of amoxycillin given to 12 further healthy subjects.— N. Clumeck *et al.*, *Antimicrob. Ag. Chemother.*, 1978, *14*, 531.

Tissue concentrations in human tonsils of benzylpenicillin, ampicillin, and lincomycin given intravenously before tonsillectomy.— J. Gabka and W. Platz, *Arzneimittel-Forsch.*, 1978, *28*, 87.

Metabolism. About 21% of a dose of ampicillin 250 or 500 mg was metabolised. After 12 hours about 26% of a 500-mg dose, taken by 6 healthy subjects, was recovered unchanged in the urine and 7% was excreted as penicilloic acid. When ampicillin 250 mg was taken by 10 subjects about 43% was excreted unchanged within 6 hours and 11% as penicilloic acid.— M. Cole *et al.*, *Antimicrob. Ag. Chemother.*, 1973, *3*, 463. See also H. Knothe *et al.*, *Arzneimittel-Forsch.*, 1974, *24*, 951.

A comparison of the metabolism of ampicillin in 9 patients with chronic cirrhosis and in 8 healthy subjects.— G. P. Lewis and W. J. Jusko, *Clin. Pharmac. Ther.*, 1975, *18*, 475.

There was no evidence of active metabolites of ampicillin in the urine of healthy subjects following administration of ampicillin trihydrate.— M. Cole and B. Ridley (letter), *J. antimicrob. Chemother.*, 1978, *4*, 580.

Pregnancy and the neonate. The concentrations of ampicillin in maternal and cord sera and in the amniotic fluid were measured in 42 women who had been given ampicillin, 500 mg six-hourly by mouth. At the time of amniotomy or amniocentesis, the concentration in the amniotic fluid varied between 0.42 and 5.1 µg per ml and at the time of delivery the concentration in the cord sera ranged between 0.24 and 2 µg per ml. It was concluded that the concentrations in amniotic fluid and maternal serum were probably sufficiently high to be effective against a high proportion of the bacteria likely to be encountered in intrapartum infections, but the concentrations in the cord serum would probably be ineffective against a significant proportion of them.— T. E. Blecher *et al.*, *Br. med. J.*, 1966, *1*, 137. In a study of 25 pregnant women given ampicillin intravenously before undergoing an abortion it was found that plasma concentrations in the mother and the foetus were equal at 90 minutes but that transplacental diffusion appeared to be slower than diffusion to maternal tissues.— L. -O. Boréus, *Acta pharmac. tox.*, 1971, *29*, *Suppl.* 3, 250.

Two hours after the administration of ampicillin 500 mg to a nursing mother the concentration in a milk sample was 70 µg per ml; the amount likely to be taken by a suckling infant was well below the normal paediatric dose.— B. E. Takyi, *J. Hosp. Pharm.*, 1970, *28*, 317.

In 42 newborn infants given a single dose of ampicillin, 50 mg per kg body-weight by intragastric tube, mean serum concentrations (assessed in some of the infants at each time point) at 30 minutes were 2.71 µg per ml, rising to 20.15 µg per ml at 4 hours, and then gradually falling with values at 12 hours still higher than those at 30 minutes.— A. Sabra *et al.*, *Curr. ther. Res.*, 1973, *15*, 866. For the pharmacokinetics of ampicillin in neonates, see also J. M. Kaplan *et al.*, *J. Pediat.*, 1974, *84*, 571; O. M. J. Driessen *et al.*, *Eur. J. clin. Pharmac.*, 1978, *13*, 449; O. M. J. Driessen *et al.*, *Eur. J. clin. Pharmac.*, 1979, *15*, 133.

Further references to the pharmacokinetics of ampicillin in pregnancy: A. Philipson, *J. infect. Dis.*, 1977, *136*, 370.

Uses. Ampicillin is used in the treatment of infections of the respiratory tract such as pneumonia and bronchitis and is especially effective where *Haemophilus influenzae* is the causative organism although the incidence of resistant strains is increasing. It is ineffective in mycoplasmal pneumonia and in infections due to penicillinase-producing organisms. Ampicillin is also employed in the treatment of infections of the urinary tract due to *Escherichia coli, Proteus mirabilis,* and *Streptococcus faecalis.*

Ampicillin is used in the treatment of gonorrhoea and when given with probenecid 1 g, single doses of 2 to 3.5 g are generally effective. Ampicillin is given in haemophilus meningitis; high parenteral doses of 150 to 300 mg per kg body-weight daily in divided doses are required and should be given for at least 10 days. Increasing resistance is a problem. Meningitis caused by *Listeria monocytogenes* has responded successfully to similar doses of ampicillin.

Because it is excreted in high concentration in the bile it has been used in the treatment of infections of the biliary and intestinal tracts caused by *E. coli,* salmonellae, and shigellae although resistance may be a problem.

Ampicillin is given by mouth as the anhydrous form or as the trihydrate. The potassium salt has also been given by mouth. The usual dose for adults in the treatment of infections due to Gram-positive organisms and those due to *H. influenzae* is 250 to 500 mg of ampicillin every 6 hours and for infections of the gastro-intestinal tract and of the urinary tract due to Gram-negative organisms, 500 to 750 mg every 6 to 8 hours. For enteric infections 1 or 2 g is given four times daily for 2 weeks in the acute condition or for 4 to 12 weeks in the carrier state. It is recommended that ampicillin be taken ½ to 1 hour before food. Children may be given half the adult dose.

Ampicillin is administered by injection as ampicillin sodium. It is normally given intramuscularly in doses of up to the equivalent of 3 g of ampicillin daily or it may be given by slow intravenous injection over 3 to 4 minutes or by infusion. Solutions of ampicillin sodium given by infusion should be administered within one hour of preparation. If intramuscular injections are painful they may be prepared using a procaine hydrochloride solution. Doses equivalent to 500 mg daily have been administered by intraperitoneal and intrapleural injection. The equivalent of 500 mg, dissolved if necessary in a 0.5% solution of procaine hydrochloride, has also been given daily by intra-articular injection.

In meningitis, systemic treatment may be supplemented with intrathecal injections of ampicillin. The usual daily intrathecal dose is the equivalent of 5 mg for infants from birth up to 2 years of age, 10 mg for children up to 12 years of age, and 20 mg for adults. The dose should be dissolved in sodium chloride injection 0.9% immediately before use to give a solution containing 10 mg per ml.

A short comparative review of ampicillin and other aminopenicillins.— H. C. Neu, *Drugs*, 1975, *9*, 81.

In most clinical situations there was no evidence that amoxycillin or talampicillin had any advantages over ampicillin.— *Drug & Ther. Bull.*, 1977, *15*, 65; J. M. T. Hamilton-Miller, *J. antimicrob. Chemother.*, 1978, *4*, 193.

The proceedings of a symposium on ampicillin and other aminopenicillins.— *Infection*, 1979, *7*, *Suppl.* 5, S423–S512.

Bronchitis. In 6 patients with chronic haemophilus bronchial infections, treatment with ampicillin, 1 g every 6 hours for at least 10 days, failed to affect sputum purulence. The presence of large numbers of enterobacteria suggested that they might produce enough penicillinase to reduce concentrations of ampicillin in sputum to less than those required to control *H. influenzae.* When cloxacillin, generally 1 g six-hourly, was given to prevent inactivation of ampicillin given 1 hour later, sputum purulence was reduced in all except 1 patient within 6 days.— J. L. Maddocks and J. R. May, *Lancet*, 1969, *1*, 793.

Ampicillin 2 g daily was as effective as tetracycline 2 g daily in the treatment of acute exacerbations in 79 patients with chronic bronchitis. Although *H. influenzae* and *Streptococcus pneumoniae* were eradicated from the sputum 60% of the time clinical improvement was not specifically linked to clearance of these organisms. Neither ampicillin nor tetracycline could be shown to be more effective than a placebo as a prophylactic agent against acute attacks of bronchitis.— H. H. Hahn *et al.*, *Antimicrob. Ag. Chemother.*, 1972, *2*, 45.

Cephalexin or ampicillin 500 mg taken four times a day for 10 days were considered to be equally effective in the treatment of 111 patients with acute bronchitis or acute exacerbations of chronic bronchitis.— D. M. Cooke and R. T. Garrett, *Glaxo*, *J. antimicrob. Chemother.*, 1975, *1*, *Suppl.* (Sept.), 99.

Crohn's disease. A review of the aetiology and treatment of Crohn's disease including the use of ampicillin and tetracycline.— P. Brown, *Med. J. Aust.*, 1974, *1*, 269.

Dosage in infants and children. In children requiring ampicillin for prophylaxis during surgery the recommended daily dose by mouth was 50 to 200 mg per kg body-weight in 4 doses and by injection 100 to 300 mg per kg in 4 doses.— W. L. Buntain *et al.*, *Mayo Clin. Proc.*, 1972, *47*, 654.

A dose of 50 to 150 mg per kg body-weight daily by mouth or 150 to 400 mg per kg by injection was recommended for children requiring treatment with ampicillin. Neonates should receive 100 mg per kg in 3 divided doses for the first 2 weeks of life then in 4 to 6 divided doses.— M. I. Marks *et al.*, *Can. med. Ass. J.*, 1973, *109*, 213.

Doses of ampicillin in excess of 300 mg per kg body-weight daily were generally not justified in infants and children.— H. F. Eichenwald and G. H. McCracken, *J. Pediat.*, 1978, *93*, 337. See also G. H. McCracken and H. F. Eichenwald, *ibid.*, 357.

The suggested dose of ampicillin for infants of more than 37 weeks' gestation was 50 mg per kg body-weight given intramuscularly or intravenously, by very slow bolus injection, every 12 hours for the first 48 hours of life, every 8 hours from the 3rd day to 2 weeks, then every 6 hours. For immature infants (those of less than 37 weeks' gestation) this dose should be given every 12 hours for the first week of life, every 8 hours from then to 4 weeks of age, and every 6 hours thereafter.— P. A. Davies, *Br. med. J.*, 1978, *2*, 676. See also H. C. Spratt, *Drugs*, 1978, *16*, 226; H. B. Valman, *Br. med. J.*, 1980, *280*, 457.

Dosage in renal failure. A review of the use of antibiotics, including ampicillin, in the treatment of patients with renal and hepatic insufficiency.— D. L. Giusti, *Drug Intell. & clin. Pharm.*, 1973, *7*, 62.

Seven patients undergoing intermittent peritoneal dialysis for acute or chronic renal failure, who were also receiving ampicillin, oxacillin, or tetracycline parenterally, were studied to determine antibiotic concentrations in serum and peritoneal fluid. Renal impairment maintained the serum concentrations of ampicillin and tetracycline longer so that their dosage should be lowered, but oxacillin was unaffected and should be given in normal doses. Peritoneal dialysis did not affect dosage requirements. Four patients who received ampicillin or tetracycline for local prophylaxis in their intraperitoneal infusions were studied. Ampicillin was absorbed and inadequate concentrations were maintained for local prophylaxis. Forty per cent of the tetracycline was inactivated by calcium and magnesium in the dialysing fluid and a large proportion of the remainder was absorbed, producing blood concentrations which were inadequate for systemic therapy but were high enough to cause adverse reactions.— J. Ruedy, *Can. med. Ass. J.*, 1966, *94*, 257.

When ampicillin 250 mg was added to each litre of peritoneal dialysis fluid, blood concentrations of up to 53.6 μg per ml were obtained. The high concentrations were well tolerated but adequate therapeutic concentrations were obtained by the addition of 50 mg per litre. Satisfactory response of renal infection in patients with low urinary ampicillin concentrations suggested adequate parenchymal penetration.— H. A. Lee and L. F. Hill, *Br. J. clin. Pract.*, 1968, *22*, 354. See also J. S. Cheigh, *Am. J. Med.*, 1977, *62*, 555.

The pharmacokinetics of ampicillin and hetacillin, which was found to be equivalent to ampicillin, were studied following intravenous administration in healthy subjects and in 6 anephric patients. About 92% of a dose was excreted by the kidney in the healthy subjects but there was considerable retention in the anephric patients and about 40% was dialysed in 7.5 hours. Maintenance doses were calculated and it was recommended that anephric patients be given 3.5% of the normal maintenance dose, anephric patients on dialysis 12%, patients with glomerular filtration-rates of up to 25 ml per minute 11%, of 25 to 50 ml per minute 24%, 50 to 75 ml per minute 36%, and [75] to 100 ml per minute 49%.— W. J. Jusko *et al.*, *Clin. Pharmac. Ther.*, 1973, *14*, 90.

Data for predicting removal of ampicillin by conventional haemodialysis.— T. P. Gibson and H. A. Nelson, *Clin. Pharmacokinet.*, 1977, *2*, 403.

The normal half-life for ampicillin of 1.5 hours was increased to 7 to 20 hours in end-stage renal failure. The interval between doses should be from 6 to 12 hours in patients with a glomerular filtration-rate (GFR) of 10 to 50 ml per minute, and from 12 to 16 hours in those with a GFR of less than 10 ml per minute, though normal doses were necessary for urinary-tract infections. Concentrations of ampicillin were affected by haemodialysis but not by peritoneal dialysis.— W. M. Bennett *et al.*, *Ann. intern. Med.*, 1980, *93*, 62. See also P. Sharpstone, *Br. med. J.*, 1977, *2*, 36; G. B. Appel and H. C. Neu, *New Engl. J. Med.*, 1977, *296*, 663.

See also under Precautions (above).

Encephalopathy. Ampicillin reduced gastric ammonia concentrations significantly in uraemic and non-uraemic patients with hepatic encephalopathy and was considered to be superior to neomycin.— S. Meyers and C. S. Lieber, *Gastroenterology*, 1976, *70*, 244.

Endocarditis. Ampicillin, 200 mg per kg body-weight daily in divided doses at 4-hourly intervals by rapid intravenous infusion, was recommended to treat children who developed postoperative endocarditis due to *Escherichia coli*. Higher doses were necessary where the organism had developed some resistance. Kanamycin, 15 mg per kg daily by intramuscular injection at 8- to 12-hour intervals, could be added if the response to ampicillin alone was inadequate. Auditory and renal function should be monitored if kanamycin injections were given. The duration of therapy should be at least 4 weeks.— R. E. Stanton *et al.*, *New Engl. J. Med.*, 1968, *279*, 737.

In the treatment of endocarditis due to group D streptococci, benzylpenicillin or ampicillin had a synergistic effect with kanamycin or gentamicin.— C. J. Wilkowske *et al.*, *Antimicrob. Ag. Chemother.*, 1970, 195. The association of ampicillin or benzylpenicillin with gentamicin appeared to be synergistic in 7 patients with enterococcal endocarditis.— P. Serra *et al.*, *Archs intern. Med.*, 1977, *137*, 1562.

Prophylaxis. For patients at risk of developing bacterial endocarditis ampicillin 1 g intramuscularly or intravenously with gentamicin 1.5 mg per kg body-weight, up to a maximum of 80 mg, intramuscularly or intravenously, or streptomycin 1 g intramuscularly can be given 30 to 60 minutes before operations or procedures involving the gastro-intestinal and genito-urinary tracts. Suitable doses for children are: ampicillin 50 mg per kg, gentamicin 2 mg per kg, and streptomycin 20 mg per kg. Additional doses might be necessary during prolonged procedures.— *Circulation*, 1977, *56*, 139A (Report of the Committee on Prevention of Rheumatic Fever and Bacterial Endocarditis of the American Heart Association). A recommended oral dose of ampicillin for such patients is 3.5 g with probenecid 1 g taken one to two hours before the procedure, then 15 mg per kg every six hours for 4 doses. In addition, streptomycin 1 g is given intramuscularly one hour before the procedure and a further dose 12 hours later.— *Med. Lett.*, 1977, *19*, 40.

See also under Prophylactic Use of Antibiotics, p.1080.

Enteritis. Ampicillin 100 to 200 mg per kg body-weight daily could be given orally or parenterally to infants and children with salmonellal gastro-enteritis, enteric fever, or shigellosis, although *Shigella sonnei* and *flexneri* are becoming increasingly resistant.— M. I. Marks, *Drugs*, 1978, *16*, 219.

Further references: K. C. Haltalin *et al.*, *Am. J. Dis. Child.*, 1972, *124*, 554; R. H. Gilman *et al.*, *Antimicrob. Ag. Chemother.*, 1980, *17*, 402, (*Shigella dysenteriae* and *S. flexneri*); F. A. Barada and R. L. Guerrant, *Antimicrob. Ag. Chemother.*, 1980, *17*, 961 (co-trimoxazole as the treatment of choice in adults where ampicillin resistance among *Shigella* is common).

Epiglottitis. A child with epiglottitis rapidly improved on intubation and the intravenous administration of ampicillin. The strain of *Haemophilus influenzae* type b was, however, relatively resistant to ampicillin, and some strains are much more resistant. It is therefore suggested that chemotherapy in epiglottitis and haemophilus meningitis should begin with ampicillin in association with chloramphenicol.— D. Hansman (letter), *Lancet*, 1979, *1*, 1354. See also H. S. Faden, *Pediatrics*, 1979, *63*, 402.

Eye infections. Ampicillin 100 mg in 0.5 ml could be given daily for 7 to 10 days by slow subconjunctival injection in the treatment of susceptible corneal infections.— F. P. Furgiuele, *Drugs*, 1978, *15*, 310.

Gonorrhoea. In a study involving 5117 patients with uncomplicated gonorrhoea, treatment with ampicillin 3.5 g and probenecid 1 g was less effective than an intramuscular injection of procaine penicillin 4.8 g after probenecid 1 g.— R. E. Kaufman *et al.*, *New Engl. J. Med.*, 1976, *294*, 1.

A single oral dose of ampicillin 3.5 g with probenecid 1 g was a recommended treatment for gonorrhoea. In Europe ampicillin 2 g with probenecid had proved adequate. While this treatment was marginally less effective than that with procaine penicillin, administration was simpler with costs still being reasonable when the savings in syringes and needles were considered.— *Neisseria gonorrhoeae and gonococcal infections*, Report of a WHO Scientific Group, *Tech. Rep. Ser. Wld Hlth Org. No. 616*, 1978. The US Public Health Service recommended ampicillin 3.5 g or amoxycillin 3 g, each with probenecid 1 g by mouth as one regimen for the treatment of uncomplicated gonorrhoea in men and women. However, this treatment was considered to be slightly less effective than that with procaine penicillin or tetracycline. Ampicillin or amoxycillin could be used in other gonococcal infections.— *Morb. Mortal.*, 1979, *28*, 13.

Further references: A. Bro-Jørgensen and T. Jensen, *Br. J. vener. Dis.*, 1971, *47*, 443; J. John and F. J. G. Jefferiss, *ibid.*, 1973, *49*, 362; R. B. Roy and S. M. Laird, *ibid.*, 1974, *50*, 117.

See also under Choice of an Antibiotic, p.1078.

Granuloma inguinale. Granuloma inguinale in 4 patients responded to treatment with ampicillin; lesions disappeared and there was no recurrence 4 to 6 months later. The dose was 250 mg four times daily for 3½ to 11 weeks in 3 patients; the fourth patient, who had relapsed after earlier treatment with tetracycline, received 500 mg four times daily for 12 weeks.— M. A. Thew *et al.*, *J. Am. med. Ass.*, 1969, *210*, 866. Ampicillin 500 mg every 6 hours for 14 days has been found effective.— *Br. med. J.*, 1981, *282*, 461.

Haemophilus infections. A study of 34 children at a day-care centre in the USA showed that vaccination with *Haemophilus influenzae* type b polysaccharide vaccine did not reduce the carrier rate of *H. influenzae* type b disease, nor did it prevent the acquisition of organisms by non-carriers. One child who had been identified as a carrier developed meningitis 4 months after vaccination. Of 6 children who were asymptomatic carriers, and who were treated with ampicillin trihydrate 100 mg per kg body-weight daily for 10 days, 3 still had positive cultures 1 and 7 days after treatment. Although ampicillin did not appear effective in reducing the carrier-rate it was still considered the safest and most acceptable control measure available.— C. M. Ginsburg *et al.*, *J. Am. med. Ass.*, 1977, *238*, 604.

Soft-tissue infections and bacteraemia caused by ampicillin-resistant *H. influenzae* type b were treated successfully with high doses of ampicillin intravenously (200 to 400 mg per kg body-weight daily) in 6 children.— D. Murphy and J. Todd, *J. Pediat.*, 1979, *94*, 983.

Further references P. A. Oill *et al.*, *Archs intern. Med.*, 1979, *139*, 985 (adult bacteraemic *H. parainfluenzae* infections).

See also under Bronchitis and Epiglottitis (both above) and Meningitis (below).

Leptospirosis. Ampicillin 3 g or amoxycillin 2 g daily for 6 days were successfully used for the treatment of leptospirosis in 27 patients.— D. Münnich and M. Lakatos, *Chemotherapy, Basle*, 1976, *22*, 372.

Listeriosis. Ampicillin 125 to 250 mg by intramuscular injection every 12 hours for 1 week followed by 125 mg twice or thrice daily by mouth for a further 2 weeks, was found to be more effective in the treatment of neonatal listeriosis than tetracycline, chloramphenicol, or benzylpenicillin.— L. Weingärtner and S. Ortel, *Dt. med. Wschr.*, 1967, *92*, 1098. See also A. M. Visintine *et al.*, *Am. J. Dis. Child.*, 1977, *131*, 393.

A comment on the incidence of perinatal listeriosis. For both the pregnant woman and the newborn infant the treatment of choice is ampicillin in association with either kanamycin or gentamicin, though where meningitis is present chloramphenicol should be used with ampicillin instead. Some workers now favour 2 or 3 weeks' treatment and although dosage is not often reported it should probably start with intravenous ampicillin 200 to 400 mg per kg body-weight.— *Lancet*, 1980, *1*, 911. Criticism.— S. N. Cohen (letter), *ibid.*, *2*, 32. Reply.— *ibid.*

Further references: M. H. Robertson *et al.*, *Archs Dis. Childh.*, 1979, *54*, 549 (ampicillin and gentamicin).

Meningitis. Ampicillin 400 mg per kg body-weight was given daily in the treatment of meningitis to produce adequate CSF concentrations and was continued for 5 days after the patient was afebrile to ensure that the focus of infection was cleared. Treatment usually lasted 10 to 14 days in infants. Since the blood-brain barrier became increasingly impermeable to ampicillin as the patient improved it was imperative that the dose should not be reduced at the end of treatment.— A. L. Smith, *Pediatrics*, 1973, *52*, 597. A study in 202 patients with bacterial meningitis who received ampicillin in a dose of either 150 or 400 mg per kg body-weight daily suggested that the high-dosage regimen offers no significant benefit over the low-dosage regimen and that ampicillin remains the treatment of choice for most cases of bacterial meningitis including those due to *H. influenzae*.— G. R. Greene *et al.*, *Antimicrob. Ag. Chemother.*, 1979, *16*, 198.

A brief discussion of the initial treatment of meningitis in children and consideration of the American Academy of Pediatrics' advice (*Pediatrics*, 1975, *55*, 145) that in areas where resistant strains of *H. influenzae* had been recognised and where this organism was suspected to be the pathogen initial treatment of meningitis should include benzylpenicillin or ampicillin plus chloramphenicol 100 mg per kg body-weight daily. It was considered that resistance was so widespread in the USA that treatment of children aged more than 2 years with bacterial meningitis should automatically include chloramphenicol 100 mg per kg daily.— *Med. Lett.*, 1975, *17*,

15. Two strains of *H. influenzae* type b, one sensitive to ampicillin, the other resistant, were isolated during the treatment of meningitis originally attributed to sensitive strains. Ampicillin resistance should be borne in mind before discontinuing chloramphenicol in severe *H. influenzae* infection, even if the initial cultures suggest sensitivity to ampicillin.— P. Mac Mahon and P. Ramberan (letter), *Lancet*, 1980, *1*, 1080.

Ampicillin sodium 200 mg per kg body-weight daily for 10 days was used to treat 62 children with *Haemophilus* meningitis. Half the children were treated intravenously for 10 days and the other half intravenously for 5 days then intramuscularly for 5 days; the response was similar in both groups. Positive cultures were still present in 14 patients on day 2 but all organisms were sensitive and all CSF cultures were negative by 48 hours. Neurological sequelae occurred in 78% of the patients with delayed eradication of infection compared with 13% of those with prompt responses.— H. D. Wilson and K. C. Haltalin, *Am. J. Dis. Child.*, 1975, *129*, 208.

A discussion on the use of ampicillin and chloramphenicol in the treatment of *H. influenzae* meningitis.— R. J. Fallon, *J. antimicrob. Chemother.*, 1976, *2*, 3. See also R. C. Gehrz *et al.*, *Am. J. Dis. Child.*, 1976, *130*, 877; R. D. Feigin *et al.*, *J. Pediat.*, 1976, *88*, 542.

A 3-week-old infant with *Salmonella typhi* meningitis was successfully treated with ampicillin sodium 400 mg per kg body-weight daily and gentamicin 7.5 mg per kg daily, both given intravenously.— B. K. Burton *et al.*, *Am. J. Dis. Child.*, 1977, *131*, 1031.

Ampicillin and carbenicillin were equally effective in the treatment of purulent meningitis due to susceptible organisms in a study of 86 patients. All patients were given an initial loading dose of 65 mg of antibiotic per kg body-weight intravenously followed by 200 or 400 mg per kg daily in 6 divided doses generally to a maximum of 28 days.— G. D. Overturf *et al.*, *Antimicrob. Ag. Chemother.*, 1977, *11*, 420.

In a retrospective comparison of the treatment of *H. influenzae* meningitis with parenteral ampicillin, usually 200 mg per kg body-weight daily, or triple therapy with chloramphenicol, a sulphonamide, and a penicillin, there was no significant difference in final outcome. However there were 6 cases of defective vestibular function and 3 children became deaf in the group given ampicillin; no cases were found in those given chloramphenicol. Although these differences between groups were not statistically significant the use of ampicillin needed re-evaluating.— M. Koskiniemi *et al.*, *Acta paediat. scand.*, 1978, *67*, 17.

Ampicillin 12 to 20 g daily by intermittent intravenous infusion for about 17 days was used successfully in 5 patients with meningitis produced by *Listeria monocytogenes*. On the third to fifth day of treatment serum concentrations of ampicillin in 4 of the patients ranged from 110 to 250 µg per ml, 30 minutes after an infusion of 50 to 60 mg per kg body-weight and concentrations in cerebrospinal fluid ranged from 5 to 8 µg per ml 40 minutes after administration. In the remaining patient, who had severe renal impairment, serum and CSF concentrations on the fourth day of treatment were 150 and 60 µg per ml respectively.— S. Iwarson *et al.*, *J. antimicrob. Chemother.*, 1978, *4*, 229.

For further references to the use of ampicillin and chloramphenicol in the treatment of *H. influenzae* meningitis, see Chloramphenicol, p.1140.

For reports on the use of ampicillin in association with gentamicin in the treatment of Gram-negative bacterial meningitis and ventriculitis, see Gentamicin Sulphate, p.1172.

See also under Choice of an Antibiotic, p.1079.

Mononucleosis. Most patients with infectious mononucleosis developed hypersensitivity reactions to ampicillin. No rash or other evidence of hypersensitivity developed in 10 patients given graduated doses up to a full therapeutic dose some months after their initial reaction.— I. J. Nazareth (letter), *Br. med. J.*, 1971, *3*, 48. A 6-year-old child was given ampicillin without untoward reaction 16 weeks after a hypersensitivity reaction when treated for infectious mononucleosis.— S. A. Haider, *ibid.*, 1971, *4*, 364.

See also under Adverse Effects.

Nocardiosis. Ampicillin and a preparation of trisulfapyrimidines together reduced to ¼ or less the MIC of ampicillin or trisulfapyrimidines alone against 3 of 4 isolates of *Nocardia asteroides*. The isolates were from 4 patients with renal transplants 3 of whom were successfully treated for nocardial infections with the above combined therapy.— M. G. Orfanakis *et al.*, *Antimicrob. Ag. Chemother.*, 1972, *1*, 215.

Otitis media. Ampicillin was considered the antibiotic of choice for acute otitis media, especially in children under 3 years when the infecting organism was commonly *Haemophilus influenzae*.— J. A. Bosso and J. R. Jackman, *Drug Intell. & clin. Pharm.*, 1977, *11*, 665. See also *Br. med. J.*, 1976, *2*, 1407.

A report of a fatal case of otitis media, and a reminder to the clinician of the need to treat otitis media with early, appropriate chemotherapy, which is usually ampicillin or amoxycillin.— N. A. Cooper *et al.* (letter), *Lancet*, 1980, *1*, 418.

Further references to the treatment of otitis media: O. E. Laxdal *et al.*, *Can. med. Ass. J.*, 1970, *102*, 263; R. D. Bland, *Pediatrics*, 1972, *49*, 187; P. A. Shurin *et al.*, *J. Pediat.*, 1980, *96*, 1081.

Pelvic inflammatory disease. For a report of the successful use of ampicillin with an initial dose of procaine penicillin in the treatment of women with acute pelvic inflammatory disease, see Tetracycline Hydrochloride, p.1221.

Pertussis. A heavy growth of *Bordetella pertussis* was eradicated from the sputum of an adult after 36 hours of treatment with ampicillin.— C. D. Ribeiro (letter), *Lancet*, 1981, *1*, 951.

Pneumonia. Patients with pneumonia (excluding those critically ill and in whom death was considered possible within 24 hours) were treated in a controlled study with ampicillin 1 g daily (43 patients), ampicillin 1 g plus prednisolone 20 mg daily (20 patients), ampicillin 2 g daily (43 patients), or ampicillin 2 g plus prednisolone 20 mg daily (20 patients). Ampicillin was given for 7 or 14 days and prednisolone for 7 days. Patients taking ampicillin 1 g responded more rapidly (as judged by resolution of fever) than those taking 2 g and the difference was significant at day 6. Patients taking prednisolone responded more rapidly (though the difference was not significant) than those taking ampicillin alone. There was no difference in the rate of clearance of pathogens or of improvement in radiological appearance. Skin rash appeared only in those taking ampicillin 2 g and was not suppressed by prednisolone.— V. U. McHardy and M. E. Schonell, *Br. med. J.*, 1972, *4*, 569. The greater improvement (as regards fever) in those taking ampicillin 1 g daily than in those taking 2 g daily might have been due to ampicillin causing non-allergic fever.— J. Ström (letter), *ibid.*, 1973, *1*, 419.

Salmonellal infections. Salmonellae were excreted in faeces for longer after convalescence from *Salmonella typhimurium* food poisoning when ampicillin 1 g or chloramphenicol 1 g was given daily for 3 days. Of 185 patients given an antibiotic, salmonellae were excreted for 12 days after exposure by 65.4% and for 31 days by 27%. For 87 patients who were not treated the corresponding figures were 42.5 and 11.5% respectively. In 9.7% of those given an antibiotic, salmonellal strains initially sensitive to several antibiotics acquired resistance to 1 or more. This effect was not seen in untreated patients.— B. Aserkoff and J. V. Bennett, *New Engl. J. Med.*, 1969, *281*, 636.

Paratyphoid fever. In a study of 41 patients with paratyphoid fever treated with ampicillin, chloramphenicol, or both, there was a 21% failure-rate with ampicillin and an 8% failure-rate with chloramphenicol. Therapy with both antibiotics concomitantly was effective in all patients.— M. F. A. Wahab *et al.*, *Ann. intern. Med.*, 1969, *70*, 913.

Typhoid fever. Ampicillin 4 g daily given for 90 days to 10 patients who were typhoid carriers eliminated *Salmonella typhi* organisms from the stools of 9. These patients had consistently negative stool cultures over an 18-month follow-up period.— W. E. Phillips, *J. Am. med. Ass.*, 1971, *217*, 913.

In 50 patients with typhoid fever treated with chloramphenicol 2 g daily in 4 doses for 15 days together with ampicillin 1 g intramuscularly every 6 hours until 2 days after defervescence or for at least 7 days, the mean duration of fever was significantly reduced to 3.9 days compared with 5.4 days in 50 similar patients treated with chloramphenicol alone. Two patients treated with chloramphenicol alone relapsed; none of those treated with both drugs relapsed.— F. De Ritis *et al.*, *Br. med. J.*, 1972, *4*, 17.

Neither ampicillin nor co-trimoxazole should be considered suitable alternatives to chloramphenicol in the treatment of typhoid fever in most countries. Ampicillin might be used to start treatment in a widespread epidemic of typhoid caused by individual chloramphenicol-resistant strains of *Salmonella typhi* or in hyperendemic typhoid due to an assortment of chloramphenicol-resistant strains until the sensitivity of the infecting strain could be determined.— E. S. Anderson (letter), *Lancet*, 1973, *2*, 1494.

Ampicillin or co-trimoxazole were recommended in the treatment of typhoid fever due to *S. typhi* resistant to chloramphenicol, streptomycin, sulphonamide, and tetracycline. Chloramphenicol was still recommended for susceptible infections.— T. Butler *et al.*, *Antimicrob. Ag. Chemother.*, 1977, *11*, 645.

High doses of ampicillin given by mouth were considered to be no better than lower doses or than chloramphenicol for the treatment of typhoid fever in a study of 24 children aged 3 to 16 years; they were given ampicillin 150 or 300 mg per kg body-weight daily by mouth, ampicillin (discontinued because of urticaria) followed by chloramphenicol 25 to 50 mg per kg daily, or chloramphenicol 50 to 100 mg per kg daily alone and reduced by half after 2 to 5 days. Fever subsided in up to 5 days among children given chloramphenicol and in 3 to 20 days among those given ampicillin. Relapses 8 to 22 days after treatment occurred in 1 of 13 children given ampicillin alone, in 2 of 5 given both drugs, and in 3 of 6 given chloramphenicol. These children and 9 others (5 treated with ampicillin, 2 treated with both drugs, and 2 given chloramphenicol alone) were found to be asymptomatic excretors of *S. typhi* and were treated again until their stools were negative. Further treatment was with ampicillin given by mouth or by injection, or with co-trimoxazole 0.32 to 1.6 g daily for up to 14 days.— G. Hardy *et al.*, *Can. med. Ass. J.*, 1977, *116*, 761.

See also under Chloramphenicol, p.1140.

Shigellosis. Co-trimoxazole was considered to be more effective than ampicillin in a study of 19 children with shigellosis. There was a marked decrease in the sensitivity of *Shigella* spp. to ampicillin.— M. J. Chang *et al.*, *Pediatrics*, 1977, *59*, 726.

Silicosis. *Branhamella* (*Neisseria*) *catarrhalis*, isolated from 11 retired coalminers with anthracosilicosis, generally responded to treatment with ampicillin, a beta-lactamase-positive strain, resistant to ampicillin, responded to cefuroxime.— G. Ninane *et al.*, *Br. med. J.*, 1978, *1*, 276.

Streptococcal infections. ***Prophylaxis in neonates.*** Ampicillin sodium 500 mg intravenously every 6 hours during labour prevented the transmission of early-onset group B streptococcus disease to 34 neonates, whose mothers had been colonised with group B streptococci. Early-onset group B streptococcus disease developed in 14 of 24 infants whose mothers were not treated with ampicillin during labour.— M. D. Yow *et al.*, *J. Am. med. Ass.*, 1979, *241*, 1245.

See also under Benzylpenicillin, p.1109.

Surgical infection prophylaxis. Antibiotic treatment with ampicillin 500 mg or tetracycline 500 mg (or 200 mg if given by intramuscular injection) every 6 hours reduced the duration of fever in patients who had undergone appendicectomy for perforated appendix and did not undergo intraperitoneal drainage, but had no effect on patients who required appendicectomy for other reasons.— C. J. Magarey *et al.*, *Lancet*, 1971, *2*, 179.

Of 59 patients who received 1 g of ampicillin topically into the wound after closure of the peritoneum in surgery of the alimentary or biliary tract, 4 developed wound sepsis. Of 53 patients who received 600 mg of benzylpenicillin and 2 g of sulphadiazine topically, 11 became infected.— T. A. M. Stoker and H. Ellis, *Br. J. Surg.*, 1972, *59*, 184.

A double-blind study in 267 patients showed no statistical difference in the incidence of wound sepsis following abdominal surgery whether the wound was treated with ampicillin 1 g, ampicillin 500 mg and cloxacillin 500 mg, or no antibiotic.— M. J. Jensen *et al.*, *Br. J. clin. Pract.*, 1975, *29*, 115.

Ampicillin, given prophylactically to 100 patients undergoing vaginal hysterectomy, significantly reduced postoperative pelvic infection and duration of hospital stay when compared with 100 control patients. Two doses of 500 mg were taken 12 and 6 hours before surgery and 500 mg was given intravenously at surgery and for 4 repeated doses.— M. W. Glover and J. R. van Nagell, *Am. J. Obstet. Gynec.*, 1976, *126*, 385. See also M. E. Boyd and R. Garceau, *ibid.*, *125*, 581.

In a study in 423 surgical patients 1 g of cephaloridine or ampicillin in 2 ml of sterile water was instilled into the wound before closure. In patients at high risk (obesity or colorectal surgery) the primary sepsis-rate with cephaloridine was 14.1% and with ampicillin, 36.1%. In the remaining patients similar rates of 6.5 and 4.4% were achieved with cephaloridine and ampicillin respectively.— A. V. Pollock *et al.*, *Br. J. Surg.*, 1977, *64*, 322.

The prophylactic use of intravenous ampicillin and flucloxacillin in patients undergoing total hip replacement.— R. L. Parsons *et al.*, *Br. J. clin. Pharmac.*, 1978, *6*, 135.

For the use of ampicillin as prophylaxis against bacteraemia after transrectal biopsy, see Metronidazole, p.971.

Urinary-tract infections. A controlled study of the comparative effect of ampicillin, nitrofurantoin, and trisulfapyrimidines on acute urinary-tract infections in 119 children did not show any difference in therapeutic effectiveness.— E. C. Burke and G. B. Stickler, *Mayo Clin. Proc.*, 1969, *44*, 318.

Treatment with ampicillin, erythromycin, and sodium bicarbonate with a high fluid intake for 10 days was as effective as sulphafurazole or nitrofurantoin for 3 weeks in a study involving 24 children with malformations or neurological disturbances of the urinary tract and infections with L-phase organisms. All children were given low maintenance doses of sulphafurazole or nitrofurantoin. Relapse-rates were 22% for the antibiotic group and 62% for the other group.— H. Gnarpe, *Scand. J. infect. Dis.*, 1974, *6*, 75.

Ampicillin and co-trimoxazole were equally effective against susceptible acute urinary-tract infections in a study of 34 children.— N. S. Ellerstein *et al.*, *Pediatrics*, 1977, *60*, 245.

Cephradine and ampicillin eradicated acute urinary-tract infections with equal success in a study of 63 women.— B. I. Davies, *J. antimicrob. Chemother.*, 1977, *3*, 219.

Of 18 patients with urinary-tract infections and significant bacteruria given ampicillin 300 mg with dicloxacillin 200 mg six-hourly for 7 to 10 days, 12 were cured compared with only 7 of 18 patients given ampicillin 500 mg six-hourly alone.— G. F. Abbate *et al.*, *Arzneimittel-Forsch.*, 1978, *28*, 1008.

For a comparison of ampicillin, cephalexin, co-trimoxazole, and trimethoprim alone in the treatment of urinary-tract infections, see Co-trimoxazole, p.1466.

Vaginitis. For a report of the failure of ampicillin to eradicate *Gardnerella vaginalis* (*Haemophilus vaginalis*) from 19 of 27 patients with non-specific vaginitis, see Metronidazole, p.972.

Preparations

Capsules

Ampicillin Capsules *(B.P.).* Capsules containing ampicillin or ampicillin trihydrate. Potency is expressed in terms of anhydrous ampicillin. Store at a temperature not exceeding 30°.

Ampicillin Capsules *(U.S.P.).* Capsules containing 125, 250, or 500 mg of anhydrous ampicillin or ampicillin trihydrate equivalent to 250 or 500 mg of anhydrous ampicillin. Store in airtight containers.

Eye Ointments

Ampicillin Eye Ointment. Ampicillin or ampicillin sodium 2, liquid paraffin 25, white soft paraffin to 100. If stored in a moisture-proof container there would be little loss of potency in 1 year's storage at room temperature.— B. Lynn, *Chemist Drugg.*, 1967, *187*, 157.

Eye-drops

Ampicillin Eye-drops. Ampicillin sodium 1, phenylmercuric nitrate 0.002, Water for Injections to 100. Sterilised by filtration. This solution might be expected to lose approximately 8% of its potency in 7 days at refrigerator temperature or more than 20% in 3 days at 23°. It could also be used for ear-drops.— B. Lynn, *Chemist Drugg.*, 1967, *187*, 157.

Injections

Ampicillin Injection *(B.P.).* Ampicillin Sodium Injection. A sterile solution of ampicillin sodium in Water for Injections prepared by dissolving, immediately before use, the sterile contents of a sealed container (Ampicillin Sodium for Injection) in the requisite amount of Water for Injections. The amount of ampicillin sodium in a sealed container is expressed in terms of the equivalent amount of anhydrous ampicillin. *U.S.P.* includes Sterile Ampicillin Sodium.

Sterile Ampicillin for Suspension *(U.S.P.).* A dry mixture of ampicillin trihydrate and one or more suitable buffers, preservatives, stabilisers, and suspending agents. pH after reconstitution 5 to 7.

Mixtures and Suspensions

Ampicillin for Oral Suspension *(U.S.P.).* Ampicillin, anhydrous or trihydrate, containing one or more suitable colours, flavours, buffers, preservatives, and sweeteners. Store in airtight containers. When reconstituted it contains 25, 50, or 100 mg of ampicillin per ml. pH after reconstitution 5 to 7.5.

A recommended formula for a suspension of ampicillin prepared extemporaneously from the contents of capsules and buffered to a pH of between 4.5 and 6. If stored at room temperature the shelf-life was only 4 to 5 days but if stored in a cool place the shelf-life was at least 2 weeks.— G. C. Brown and J. B. Kayes, *J. clin. Pharm.*, 1976, *1*, 29.

Ampicillin Mixture *(B.P.C. 1973).* Ampicillin Syrup. A suspension of ampicillin or ampicillin trihydrate in a suitable flavoured vehicle; it is prepared freshly by dispersing a powder of the dry mixed ingredients in the specified volume of water. pH 4.5 to 6.5. The mixture loses not more than 10% potency when stored for a week at 15°. When Strong Ampicillin Mixture or Strong Ampicillin Syrup is prescribed, a suspension containing 250 mg of ampicillin, or the equivalent amount of the trihydrate, in 5 ml is supplied. When a dose less than 5 ml is prescribed, the mixture should be diluted to 5 ml with syrup. Such dilutions must be freshly prepared. The mixture and diluted mixture should be stored in a cool place and used within 1 week of preparation.

Pessaries and Suppositories

Ampicillin Pessaries and Suppositories. Pessaries and suppositories containing 100 mg and 500 mg respectively of ampicillin sodium in theobroma oil were suggested. The free acid did not diffuse from the base so well. The density of ampicillin sodium compared with theobroma oil was 1.42.— B. Lynn, *Chemist Drugg.*, 1967, *187*, 157.

Tablets

Ampicillin Tablets *(U.S.P.).* Tablets containing 250 or 500 mg of anhydrous ampicillin or (chewable tablets) ampicillin or ampicillin trihydrate equivalent to 125 or 250 mg of anhydrous ampicillin. Store in airtight containers.

Paediatric Ampicillin Tablets *(B.P.C. 1973).* Tablets containing ampicillin or ampicillin trihydrate. Store in a cool place in airtight containers.

Proprietary Preparations

Amfipen *(Brocades, UK).* Ampicillin, available as **Capsules** of 250 and 500 mg; as **Syrup** (supplied as powder for preparation with water before use) containing 125 mg in each 5 ml; and as **Syrup Forte** (supplied as powder for preparation with water before use) containing 250 mg in each 5 ml. **Amfipen Injection.** Ampicillin sodium (supplied as powder for solution before use), in vials containing the equivalent of 250 or 500 mg of ampicillin. (Also available as Amfipen in *Neth., Switz.*).

Ampiclox Injection *(Beecham Research, UK).* Vials each containing ampicillin sodium equivalent to ampicillin 250 mg and cloxacillin sodium equivalent to cloxacillin 250 mg, for the preparation of injections. *Dose.* The contents of 1 or 2 vials every 4 to 6 hours.

Ampiclox Neonatal *(Beecham Research, UK).* **Injection** (supplied as powder for solution before use) in vials each containing ampicillin sodium equivalent to ampicillin 50 mg and cloxacillin sodium equivalent to cloxacillin 25 mg, and **Oral Suspension** (supplied as sugar-free powder for preparation with water before use) containing in each dose of 0.6 ml ampicillin trihydrate equivalent to ampicillin 60 mg and cloxacillin sodium equivalent to cloxacillin 30 mg. *Dose.* The contents of 1 vial by intramuscular or intravenous injection thrice daily; or 0.6 ml of drops every 4 hours.

Britcin *(DDSA Pharmaceuticals, UK).* Ampicillin trihydrate, available as capsules each containing the equivalent of ampicillin 250 and 500 mg.

Magnapen *(Beecham Research, UK).* **Capsules** each containing ampicillin trihydrate equivalent to ampicillin 250 mg and flucloxacillin sodium equivalent to flucloxacillin 250 mg; **Injection** (supplied as powder for solution before use) in 500-mg vials each containing ampicillin sodium equivalent to ampicillin 250 mg and flucloxacillin sodium equivalent to flucloxacillin 250 mg or 1-g vials each containing double those quantities; and **Syrup** (supplied as powder for preparation with water before use) containing in each 5 ml ampicillin trihydrate equivalent to ampicillin 125 mg and flucloxacillin sodium equivalent to flucloxacillin 125 mg (suggested diluent, syrup). *Dose.* 1 capsule, 10 ml of syrup, or 500 mg by injection 4 times daily; children 2 to 10 years, half the above dose.

Penbritin *(Beecham Research, UK).* Ampicillin trihydrate, available as **Capsules** containing the equivalent of 250 and 500 mg of ampicillin; as **Paediatric Suspension** (supplied as powder for preparation with water before use) containing the equivalent of 125 mg in each 1.25 ml (suggested diluent, syrup); as scored **Paediatric Tablets** containing the equivalent of 125 mg; as **Syrup** (supplied as powder for preparation with water before use) containing the equivalent of 125 mg in each 5 ml (suggested diluent, syrup); and as **Syrup Forte** (supplied as powder for preparation with water before use) containing the equivalent of 250 mg in each 5 ml (suggested diluent, syrup). **Penbritin Injection** (supplied as powder of ampicillin sodium for solution before use), available in vials containing the equivalent of 250 and 500 mg of ampicillin. (Also available as Penbritin in *Arg., Austral., Belg., Canad., Neth., S.Afr., Switz., USA*).

Pentrexyl *(Bristol-Myers Pharmaceuticals, UK).* Ampicillin trihydrate, available as capsules containing the equivalent of 250 or 500 mg of ampicillin. (Also available as Pentrexyl in *Belg., Spain.* Available as Pentrexyl containing ampicillin sodium in *Denm., Norw., Spain*).

Vidopen *(Berk Pharmaceuticals, UK).* Ampicillin trihydrate, available as **Capsules** each containing the equivalent of 250 or 500 mg of ampicillin; as **Syrup** (supplied as powder for preparation with water before use) containing the equivalent of 125 mg in each 5 ml (suggested diluent, syrup); and as **Syrup Forte** (supplied as powder for preparation with water before use) containing the equivalent of 250 mg in each 5 ml (suggested diluent, syrup).

Other Proprietary Names of Ampicillin, Ampicillin Sodium, and Ampicillin Trihydrate

Arg.—Aletmicina, Dotirol, Grampenil, Hostes, Orbecilina *(ampicillin sodium with ampicillin benzathine)*, Pentrexyl-K *(potassium)*, Poenbiotico, Principen, Tolimal, Trifacilina, Viacilina-A; *Austral.*—Austrapen, Bristin; *Belg.*—Ampibel, Fortapen; *Canad.*—Amcill, Ampicin, Ampilean, Biosan; *Fr.*—Ampicil, Penbritine, Pénicline, Totapen, Ukapen; *Ger.*—Amblosin, Ampi-Tablinen, Binotal, Cuxacillin, Cymbi, Deripen, DuraAmpicillin, Pen-Bristol, Penbrock, Suractin *(potassium)*; *Hung.*—Semicillin; *Ind.*—Roscillin; *Ital.*—Ampen, Ampibiotic, Ampibronc Capsules, Ampicil, Ampicina, Ampifen, Ampilan, Ampilisa, Ampilux, Ampisint, Ampitex, Ampivax, Ampi-Zoja, Amplibios, Amplicid, Amplipen, Amplipenyl, Ampliscocil, Amplital, Amplizer, Anidropen, Anticyl, Argocillina, Binotal, Bio-ampi, Biocellina, Citicil, Eurocillin, Farmampil, Germicillina, Geycillina, Gramcillina, Lampocillina, Napicil, Overcillina, Pen Ampil, Penberin, Penisint BG, Pentrexil, Platocillina, Principen, Radiocillina, Saicil, Sernabiotic, Sesquicillina, Sintopenyl, Tauglicolcillina *(ampicillin sulphoguaiacolate)*, Totaciclina; *Jap.*—Adobacillin, Ampipenix, Bionacillin, Bonapicillin, Domicillin, Iwacillin, Marisilan, NC Cilin, Penimic, Pharcillin, Racenacillin, Synpenin, Tokiocillin, Totacillin; *S.Afr.*—Ampil, Famicillin, Pentrex, Petercillin, Synthecillin; *Spain*—Amblosin, Ampi-Biopharma, Ampicil, Ampiciman, Ampi-Framan, Ampikel, Ampiland, Ampinebiot, Ampinova, Ampinoxi, Ampi-Oral, Ampiorus, Ampi-Vial 500, Amplimedix Inyec., Bemicina *(ampicillin arginine)*, Benusel Oral, Binotal, Britapen, Cilleral, Espectrosira, Espimin-Cilina Caps, Fidesbiotic, Fuerpen, Gobemicina, Guicitrina, Lifeampil, Morepen, Novoexpectro, Nuvapen, Nuvapen Retard *(ampicillin sodium with ampicillin benzathine)*, Penimaster, Peninovel, Penorsin, Plumericin, Prestacilina, Quimetam, Resan, Sumipanto, Togram, Trafarbiot, Ultrabion Oral, Urebion Ampicillina; *Swed.*—Doktacillin; *Switz.*—Ampilag, Cimexillin, Helvecillin, Penbristol, Rivocillin; *USA*—A-Cillin, Alpen, Alpen-N, Amcill, Amcill-S, Amperil, D-Amp, Omnipen, Omnipen-N, Pen A, Pen A/N, Penbritin-S, Pensyn, Pensyn-N, Polycillin, Polycillin-N, Principen, Principen/N, Robamox, SK-Ampicillin, SK-Ampicillin-N, Supen, Totacillin, Totacillin-N.

A preparation containing ampicillin trihydrate, sulphadimidine, and light kaolin was formerly marketed in Great Britain under the proprietary name Penbritin KS (*Beecham Research*).

11-k

Avoparcin. Compound 254. A glycopeptide antibiotic produced by *Streptomyces candidus* or by any other means.

CAS — 37332-99-3.

It is used as a food additive in veterinary practice to promote growth.

References: *Drugs Today*, 1978, *14*, 41.

12-a

Azidamfenicol. Bayer 52910; Azidamphenicol; Azidoamphenicol. 2-Azido-*N*-[(*αR,βR*)-*β*-hydroxy-*α*-hydroxymethyl-4-nitrophenethyl]acetamide.
$C_{11}H_{13}N_5O_5$=295.3.

CAS — 13838-08-9.

Crystals. M.p. 107°. **Soluble** 1 in 50 of water.

Azidamfenicol is an antibiotic which is related structurally to chloramphenicol (see p.1136) and has been given as eye-drops.

A report of the antimicrobial activity *in vitro* of a preparation containing azidamfenicol, clotrimazole, and dexamethasone.— C. Poitschek *et al., Arzneimittel-Forsch.*, 1978, *28*, 232.

Proprietary Names

Leucomycin-N *(Bayer, Ger.)*; Thilocanfol *(Thilo, Ger.)*.

13-t

Azidocillin. Azidobenzylpenicillin; BRL 2534; SPC 297D. (6*R*)-6-(D-2-Azido-2-phenylacetamido)penicillanic acid.
$C_{16}H_{17}N_5O_4S$=375.4.

CAS — 17243-38-8.

Azidocillin has actions and uses similar to those of benzylpenicillin (see p.1102). It is acid-stable and absorbed from the gastro-intestinal tract. Azidocillin diffuses across the placenta and about 50 to 75% is excreted in the urine. It has been given sometimes as the sodium or potassium salt in doses of 750 mg twice daily.

The absorption of azidocillin.— E. Hansson *et al., Antimicrob. Ag. Chemother.*, 1967, 568.

In a study in 16 children azidocillin 500 mg produced similar free serum-antibiotic concentrations to 250 mg of ampicillin. The half-life of azidocillin was 0.54 hours compared with 1.39 hours for ampicillin while plasma binding was 84 and 18% for azidocillin and ampicillin respectively. Both had MICs of 0.02 µg per ml for *Streptococcus pneumoniae* and 0.5 µg per ml for *Haemophilus influenzae*.— M. F. Michel *et al., Chemotherapy, Basle*, 1973, *18*, 77.

In 10 healthy adults given azidocillin 750 mg by mouth mean peak serum concentrations of 6.1, 0.5, and 0.045 µg per ml occurred 1.5, 4, and 6 hours respectively after administration. After 9 hours about 58% of the administered dose was recovered in the urine.— C. Simon *et al., Arzneimittel-Forsch.*, 1976, *26*, 424.

Further references to pharmacokinetic studies: O. Wasz-Höckert *et al., Scand. J. infect. Dis.*, 1970, *2*, 125 (transplacental diffusion); T. Brusis *et al., Infection*, 1977, *5*, 26.

Antimicrobial action. See B. Sjoberg *et al., Antimicrob. Ag. Chemother.*, 1967, 560; U. Forsgren, *ibid.*, 1968, 449; B. A. Watts *et al., J. antimicrob. Chemother.*, 1977, *3*, 331.

Bronchitis. Comparisons of twice daily and thrice daily administration of azidocillin in acute attacks of chronic bronchitis.— O. Wieser and H. Weuta, *Br. J. clin. Pract.*, 1980, *34*, 101.

Pertussis. Azidocillin 60 mg per kg body-weight daily by mouth for 5 days eliminated *Bordetella pertussis* from the nasal swabs of 12 children with whooping cough.— C. Simon *et al., Arzneimittel-Forsch.*, 1976, *26*, 424.

Proprietary Names of Azidocillin and its Salts

Astracilina *(Astra, Arg.)*; Globacillin *(sodium) (Astra, Denm.; Astra, Norw.; Astra, Swed.)*; Nalpen *(potassium) (Beecham-Wülfing, Ger.; Bencard, Neth.)*; Syncillin *(sodium) (Tropon, Ger.)*.

14-x

Azlocillin Sodium. BAY e 6905. Sodium (6*R*)-6-[D-2-(2-oxoimidazolidine-1-carboxamido)-2-phenylacetamido]penicillanate.
$C_{20}H_{22}N_5NaO_6S$=483.5.

CAS — 37091-66-0 (azlocillin); 37091-65-9 (sodium salt).

A white to pale yellow almost odourless crystalline powder. Each g represents about 2.1 mmol (2.1 mEq) of sodium.

Adverse Effects, Treatment, and Precautions. As for Benzylpenicillin, p.1103.

Antimicrobial Action. Azlocillin has a range of antimicrobial activity similar to, but wider than, that of carbenicillin (p.1111) and is reported to be more active than carbenicillin *in vitro*, especially against *Pseudomonas aeruginosa*.

The activity *in vitro* of azlocillin against 578 clinical isolates, 479 of which were Gram-negative bacilli and 99 Gram-positive cocci. Susceptible organisms included *Pseudomonas aeruginosa* and indole-positive and -negative *Proteus* spp. *E. coli* and *Serratia* spp. showed moderate sensitivity while *Klebsiella* and *Enterobacter* spp. were less sensitive. Among the streptococci, *Str. pyogenes* was susceptible, but sensitivity varied among strains of *Str. pneumoniae*. Penicillin-sensitive, though not penicillin-resistant, strains of *Staph. aureus* were also sensitive. In a comparative study of azlocillin, carbenicillin, ticarcillin, BL-P 1654, and mezlocillin, mezlocillin was the most effective antibacterial agent except against *Ps. aeruginosa* where azlocillin and BL-P 1654 were most effective.— D. Stewart and G. P. Bodey, *Antimicrob. Ag. Chemother.*, 1977, *11*, 865.

In a comparison *in vitro*, azlocillin was more active than mezlocillin against *Ps. aeruginosa* and was 8 times more active than carbenicillin against susceptible strains.— R. Wise *et al., Antimicrob. Ag. Chemother.*, 1978, *13*, 559.

Azlocillin inhibited all of 20 strains of *Ps. aeruginosa in vitro* at a concentration of 31.2 µg per ml and was more active than mezlocillin or ticarcillin.— L. Coppens and J. Klastersky, *Antimicrob. Ag. Chemother.*, 1979, *15*, 396. A comparison of the effects of azlocillin and ticarcillin against *Ps. aeruginosa* demonstrated differing bactericidal effects which appeared to be related primarily to dose-related differences in the inhibition of cell-wall synthesis and also to the instability of azlocillin to pseudomonal beta-lactamases. A greater inoculum effect was seen with azlocillin and, unlike ticarcillin, azlocillin failed to cause any significant lysis. During bactericidal tests, azlocillin was inactivated whereas there was no loss of ticarcillin activity.— A. R. White *et al., Beecham Research, Antimicrob. Ag. Chemother.*, 1980, *18*, 182.

Further references: G. P. Bodey *et al., Antimicrob. Ag. Chemother.*, 1978, *13*, 14; G. P. Bodey and B. Le Blanc, *ibid.*, *14*, 78; B. Chattopadhyay and I. Hall (letter), *Lancet*, 1979, *1*, 391; C. N. Baker *et al., Antimicrob. Ag. Chemother.*, 1980, *17*, 757.

For comparisons of the activity *in vitro* of azlocillin, mezlocillin, and other antibiotics, see Mezlocillin Sodium, p.1184.

Absorption and Fate. Azlocillin is poorly absorbed from the gastro-intestinal tract.

The mean serum half-life of azlocillin was 47.6 minutes in 10 healthy subjects and 293.3 minutes in 8 patients with a glomerular filtration-rate of less than 10 ml per minute, after an intravenous injection of 2 g. In 12 subjects with normal renal function about 52% of the dose appeared in the urine in the first 2 hours after administration and about 65% within 24 hours. About 28% of azlocillin was bound to plasma proteins in 5 healthy subjects and 25% in 4 patients on haemodialysis.— P. Fiegel and K. Becker, *Antimicrob. Ag. Chemother.*, 1978, *14*, 288.

The mean serum concentration of azlocillin in 10 healthy subjects was 236.5 µg per ml 1 hour after an infusion of 5 g given over 15 minutes and had fallen to 44.3 µg per ml at 6 hours. Serum concentrations of azlocillin were significantly higher than those produced by the same doses of mezlocillin or ticarcillin up to 6 hours after administration.— L. Coppens and J. Klastersky, *Antimicrob. Ag. Chemother.*, 1979, *15*, 396.

Further references to pharmacokinetic studies with azlocillin: H. Lode *et al., Infection*, 1977, *5*, 163; J. M. Aletta *et al., Clin. Pharmac. Ther.*, 1980, *27*, 563 (haemodialysis); A. Leroy *et al., Antimicrob. Ag. Chemother.*, 1980, *17*, 344 (impaired renal function); U. Sitka *et al., Chemotherapy, Basle*, 1980, *26*, 171 (neonates).

Uses. Azlocillin sodium is a ureido-penicillin, closely related to mezlocillin sodium (p.1184), and is used in the treatment of pseudomonal infections. It is given in doses equivalent to 2 to 5 g of azlocillin every 8 hours by intravenous injection or infusion. In patients with a creatinine clearance of less than 30 ml per minute doses should be given every 12 hours. Azlocillin is removed by dialysis.

Doses of 2 g or less may be administered by bolus injection as a 10% solution in Water for Injections; higher doses should be infused over 20 to 30 minutes.

Suggested doses of azlocillin for children, to be given every 8 hours, are: 1 to 2 years (10 to 13 kg body-weight), 500 mg; 2 to 6 years (13 to 20 kg), 0.5 to 1 g; over 6 years (over 20 kg), 1 to 3 g. A dose of 50 mg per kg body-weight every 8 hours has been recommended for infants over 3 kg and a similar dose every 12 hours for those below 3 kg and for premature infants.

A brief review of azlocillin.— *Drug & Ther. Bull.*, 1981, *19*, 65.

In 28 severely ill patients including 9 with renal insufficiency, *Ps. aeruginosa*, which was causing septicaemia or respiratory, urinary, or wound infections, was eliminated in 18 by azlocillin 4 to 6 g daily intravenously for 6 to 28 days. Necrotising otitis externa in a further 2 patients was cured after 57 and 116 days of therapy. No serious side-effects occurred.— E. B. Helm *et al., Dt. med. Wschr.*, 1977, *102*, 1211.

The successful use of azlocillin 5 g intravenously 6-hourly for 10 days in the treatment of pseudomonal meningitis. The concentration in the CSF after 7 days of treatment was 5 µg per ml, 5 times the MIC.— C. J. Ellis and P. H. Walter, *Br. med. J.*, 1979, *2*, 767.

See also under Mezlocillin Sodium, p.1185.

Proprietary Preparations

Securopen *(Bayer, UK)*. Azlocillin sodium, available as powder for preparing injections, in vials containing the equivalent of azlocillin 0.5, 1, and 2 g and infusion vials containing the equivalent of 5 g. (Also available as Securopen in *Ger., Neth.*).

15-r

Bacampicillin Hydrochloride. Carampicillin; EPC 272. 1-(Ethoxycarbonyloxy)ethyl (6*R*)-6-(*α*-D-phenylglycylamino)penicillanate hydrochloride.
$C_{21}H_{27}N_3O_7S$, HCl=502.0.

CAS — 50972-17-3 (bacampicillin); 37661-08-8 (hydrochloride).

A white crystalline powder. Bacampicillin hydrochloride 1.44 g is approximately equivalent to 1 g of ampicillin. **Soluble** 1 in 15 of water, 1 in 7 of alcohol, and 1 in 10 of chloroform. Practically insoluble in ether.

Bacampicillin hydrochloride has the actions and uses of ampicillin (see p.1091) to which it is rapidly hydrolysed after absorption. It is given in doses of 400 or 800 mg twice or thrice daily. Peak plasma-ampicillin concentrations of up to 8 and 14 µg per ml have been reported about one hour after 400- and 800-mg doses of bacampicillin hydrochloride, with about 70% of a dose excreted in the urine. A serum half-life for bacampicillin of 50 to 112 minutes has been reported.

A brief review of bacampicillin.— *Med. Lett.*, 1981, *23*, 49.

A study of the antibacterial activity and pharmacokinetics of bacampicillin and ampicillin. A much sharper and higher peak serum concentration was reached after administration of bacampicillin, indicating bioavailability about 40% greater than after an equimolar dose of ampicillin.— M. Rozencweig *et al., Clin. Pharmac. Ther.*, 1976, *19*, 592.

In a randomised crossover study 11 healthy subjects were given single oral doses of bacampicillin 400 mg and equimolar doses of ampicillin (278 mg), pivampicillin (398 mg), and amoxycillin (291 mg). Mean peak serum concentrations were: bacampicillin 8.27 µg per ml, ampicillin 3.70 µg per ml, pivampicillin 7.14 µg per ml, and amoxycillin 7.68 µg per ml with a significant difference between ampicillin and the other 3 drugs. Serum half-lives were 0.75, 1.09, 0.96, and 0.95 hours respectively. Ampicillin had about two-thirds of the bioavailability of bacampicillin and pivampicillin.— J. Sjövall *et al., Antimicrob. Ag. Chemother.*, 1978, *13*, 90.

In a crossover study in 10 healthy subjects, serum concentrations of ampicillin were similar after single equimolar doses of bacampicillin by mouth and ampicillin by intramuscular injection. Absorption-rates were also similar and bacampicillin had a mean bioavailability of 87% compared with 71% for ampicillin.— T. Bergan, *Antimicrob. Ag. Chemother.*, 1978, *13*, 971.

In 9 infants (aged 2 to 9 months) given bacampicillin 10 mg per kg body-weight, the mean peak serum concentration of ampicillin was about 6 µg per ml and was estimated to occur about 0.4 hours after administration. The mean serum half-life was 0.8 hours.— T. Bergan *et al., J. antimicrob. Chemother.*, 1978, *4*, 79.

Further pharmacokinetic studies with bacampicillin: F. P. V. Maesen *et al., J. antimicrob. Chemother.*, 1976, *2*,

279 (concentrations of ampicillin in serum and sputum); P. T. Männistö *et al.* (letter), *ibid.*, 1979, *5*, 236 (concentrations of ampicillin in serum and bronchial mucosa); J. S. Tan and S. -J. Salstrom, *Antimicrob. Ag. Chemother.*, 1979, *15*, 510 (concentrations of ampicillin in serum and interstitial fluid).

References to the clinical use of bacampicillin: B. I. Davies *et al.*, *Scand. J. resp. Dis.*, 1978, *59*, 249 (bronchitis); S. Bengtsson *et al.*, *J. antimicrob. Chemother.*, 1979, *5*, 211 (gonorrhoea); P. J. Spengler and L. D. Edwards, *Br. J. vener. Dis.*, 1980, *56*, 151 (gonorrhoea).

Proprietary Preparations

Ambaxin *(Upjohn, UK)*. Bacampicillin hydrochloride, available as scored tablets of 400 mg.

Other Proprietary Names

Bacacil *(Arg., Switz.)*; Penglobe *(Arg., Belg., Denm., Fr., Ger., Neth., Swed.)*; Spectrobid *(USA)*.

16-f

Bacitracin *(U.S.P., B.P. 1968)*. Bacitracinum.

CAS — 1405-87-4.

Pharmacopoeias. In *Arg., Belg., Braz., Cz., Ind., Int., It., Jug., Mex., Nord., Port., Swiss, Turk.*, and *U.S.*, which also includes Sterile Bacitracin.

Bacitracin is a polypeptide produced by the growth of an organism of the *licheniformis* group of *Bacillus subtilis*.

It is a white to pale buff hygroscopic powder, odourless or with a slight odour, with a bitter taste. It contains not less than 40 units per mg.

Freely **soluble** in water; soluble in alcohol, methyl alcohol, and glacial acetic acid, the solution in the organic solvents usually showing some insoluble residue; practically insoluble in acetone, chloroform, and ether. A solution containing 10 000 units per ml has a pH of 5.5 to 7.5.

Bacitracin is precipitated from solutions and inactivated by salts of many of the heavy metals; it is also inactivated by benzoates, salicylates, and tannates. Solutions in water deteriorate at room temperature, but if stored at 2° to 8° they may be expected to retain their potency for 1 week; when stored at 25°, solutions should be used within 48 hours. The dry powder is relatively stable at room temperature but deteriorates on heating. **Store** in a cool place in airtight containers. Protect from light.

Stability in ointments. Bacitracin was stable in anhydrous bases such as paraffins, white wax, or wool fat. It was not affected by the addition of hydroquinone, ascorbyl palmitate, cetyl alcohol, calamine, zinc oxide, or benzocaine. It was slowly inactivated in bases containing steryl alcohol, cholesterol, polyoxyethylene derivatives, and sodium lauryl sulphate. It was rapidly inactivated in bases containing water, macrogols, propylene glycol, glycerol, cetylpyridinium chloride, benzalkonium chloride, ichthammol, phenol, and tannic acid.— J. M. Plaxco and W. J. Husa, *J. Am. pharm. Ass., scient. Edn*, 1956, *45*, 141.

Stability in solution. The deterioration which occurred was probably a process of oxidation initiated by light. Solutions in which the air had been replaced by nitrogen showed a loss in activity not greater than 10% after 3 months' storage in diffused light.— V. Würtzen, *Dansk Tidsskr. Farm.*, 1954, *28*, 34.

There was no significant loss of potency when bacitracin powder was added to 3 commercially available 0.5% hypromellose solutions in plastic squeezy bottles (Lacril, pH 5.9; Tearisol, pH 7.3; Isoptotears, pH 7.4) and the resulting solutions of bacitracin 9600 units per ml kept at 25° for 7 days.— E. Osborn *et al.*, *Am. J. Ophthal.*, 1976, *82*, 775.

Units. One unit of bacitracin is contained in 0.01351 mg of the second International Standard Preparation (1964) of bacitracin zinc which contains 74 units per mg.

Adverse Effects. When administered by intramuscular injection, bacitracin can be nephrotoxic. Nephrotoxicity may also occur after local application over the site of abdominal operations or after instillation into infected cavities. Local application of bacitracin has been associated with severe allergic disorders.

Allergy. A 50-year-old woman suffered an anaphylactic allergic reaction after the application of an ointment containing bacitracin to a skin-graft donor site.— M. A. Vale *et al.* (letter), *Archs Derm.*, 1978, *114*, 800.

Further references: G. Roupe and Ö. Strannegård, *Archs Derm.*, 1969, *100*, 450.

Antimicrobial Action. Bacitracin interferes with bacterial cell wall synthesis and is active against many Gram-positive bacteria including staphylococci, streptococci, clostridia and *Corynebacterium diphtheriae*; it is also active against *Treponema pallidum* and some Gram-negative cocci.

Absorption and Fate. Bacitracin is not appreciably absorbed from the gastro-intestinal tract. When administered by intramuscular injection it is rapidly absorbed; doses of 200 to 300 units per kg body-weight every 6 hours produce plasma concentrations of up to 2 units per ml. About 30% of a single injected dose is excreted in the urine within 24 hours. Bacitracin readily diffuses into the pleural and ascitic fluids but little passes into the cerebrospinal fluid.

The half-life of bacitracin in serum was 1.5 hours and 9 to 31% was excreted in the urine.— C. M. Kunin, *Ann. intern. Med.*, 1967, *67*, 151.

Uses. Bacitracin is mainly used as an external application to the skin or the eye, in the treatment of infections due to susceptible organisms. It is usually given with other antibiotics such as neomycin. Bacitracin zinc (see below) is used similarly.

Bacitracin is no longer considered suitable for intramuscular use.

Bacitracin has been instilled into the peritoneal cavity or sprayed over operation wounds although absorption may occur. It was formerly given by mouth to reduce the gastro-intestinal flora. Bacitracin methylene disalicylate has been used as a feed supplement for pigs.

The bacitracin-inhibition test for the identification of beta-haemolytic streptococci of the Lancefield group A.— D. J. Coleman *et al.*, *J. clin. Path.*, 1977, *30*, 421.

Colitis. Reports of the use of bacitracin by mouth in the treatment of pseudomembranous colitis.— T. -W. Chang *et al.*, *Gastroenterology*, 1980, *78*, 1584; F. J. Tedesco, *Dig. Dis. Scis*, 1980, *25*, 783.

Skin disorders. A study in newborn infants showed that bacitracin ointment appeared to be as efficient as 3% hexachlorophane emulsions in reducing staphylococcal sepsis.— J. D. Johnson *et al.*, *Pediatrics*, 1976, *58*, 354.

For reports of the use of neomycin with bacitracin in the treatment of skin infections, see Neomycin Sulphate, p.1190.

Preparations

Bacitracin Ophthalmic Ointment *(U.S.P.)*. A sterile preparation of bacitracin 500 units per g in an anhydrous ointment basis.

Bacitracin Ointment *(U.S.P.)*. Bacitracin 500 units per g in an anhydrous ointment basis. It may contain a suitable anaesthetic.

Other preparations containing bacitracin are described under Neomycin Sulphate, p.1191..

For a proprietary preparation of bacitracin, see under Polymyxin B Sulphate, p.1206..

Other Proprietary Names

Baciguent *(Canad., USA)*; Bacitin *(Canad.)*.

17-d

Bacitracin Zinc *(B.P., U.S.P.)*. Zinc Bacitracin; Bacitracins Zinc Complex.

CAS — 1405-89-6.

Pharmacopoeias. In *Br.* and *U.S.*

A zinc salt or salts of bacitracin, containing not less than 55 units per mg of bacitracin and 4 to 6% of zinc, calculated on the dried material. The *U.S.P.* specifies not less than 40 units per mg and not less than 10% of zinc.

A white or pale buff or tan hygroscopic powder, odourless or with a slight odour and with a bitter taste.

Soluble 1 in 900 of water and 1 in 500 of alcohol; very slightly soluble in ether; practically insoluble in chloroform. A saturated solution in water has a pH of 6 to 7.5. **Store** in a cool place in airtight containers; if intended for parenteral administration as a spray in body cavities the containers should be sterile and sealed to exclude micro-organisms.

Effect of gamma-irradiation. Bacitracin zinc powder was unchanged in colour at 25 000 Gy and slightly deeper in colour at 250 000 Gy. The potency of 65.6 units per mg fell to 60.9 units per mg at 25 000 Gy and to 48.1 at 250 000 Gy.— *The Use of Gamma Radiation Sources for the Sterilisation of Pharmaceutical Products*, London, ABPI, 1960.

Stability. Bacitracin zinc was more stable than bacitracin and could be stored for 18 months at temperatures up to 40° without appreciable loss. Lozenges of bacitracin zinc and ointments and tablets containing bacitracin zinc with neomycin were more stable than the corresponding bacitracin preparations. Bacitracin zinc was less bitter than bacitracin and the taste was more readily disguised.— H. M. Gross *et al.*, *Drug Cosmet. Ind.*, 1954, *75*, 612.

Bacitracin zinc has the actions described under bacitracin; it is used in lozenges, ointments, dusting-powders, aerosol sprays and solutions for bladder irrigation, often in conjunction with other antibiotics such as neomycin and polymyxin B, or with hydrocortisone, for topical application. Absorption from open wounds and from the bladder may lead to adverse effects.

Bacitracin zinc is used as an additive for animal feeding stuffs.

Preparations containing bacitracin zinc are described under Neomycin Sulphate, p.1191..

For proprietary preparations of bacitracin zinc, see under Hydrocortisone, p.474, Neomycin Sulphate, p.1191, and Polymyxin B Sulphate, p.1206..

18-n

Bekanamycin Sulphate. Bekanamycini Sulfas; Aminodeoxykanamycin Sulfate; Kanamycin B Sulphate; KDM; NK 1006. 6-*O*-(3-Amino-3-deoxy-α-D-glucopyranosyl)-2-deoxy-4-*O*-(2,6-diamino-2,6-dideoxy-α-D-glucopyranosyl)-D-streptamine sulphate.

$C_{18}H_{37}N_5O_{10}, 2.5H_2SO_4$=728.7.

CAS — 4696-76-8 (bekanamycin); 70550-99-1 (sulphate).

Pharmacopoeias. In *Jap.*

An aminoglycoside antibiotic obtained from a mutant strain of *Streptomyces kanamyceticus*. An odourless or almost odourless white amorphous powder with a slightly bitter taste. Bekanamycin sulphate 1.5 g is approximately equivalent to 1 g of bekanamycin. Freely **soluble** in water; practically insoluble in most organic solvents.

It has actions similar to those of kanamycin sulphate (see p.1175). It has been used in the treatment of infections due to susceptible organisms in doses equivalent to 400 to 600 mg of bekanamycin daily by intramuscular injection in 2 or 3 divided doses.

In the treatment of gonorrhoea, a single intramuscular injection of bekanamycin 1.2 g produced a cure-rate of 93%—equivalent to the cure-rate following kanamycin 2 g. Pain at the injection site occurred in some patients.— A. Guerrieri *et al.*, *Clin. Med.*, 1975, *82* (Jan.), 25.

Bekanamycin was more active than kanamycin but less active than amikacin, gentamicin, dibekacin, or sissomicin *in vitro* against 200 strains of *Pseudomonas aeruginosa*, and inhibited 2, 37 and 155 strains at concentrations of 0.156, 1.25, and 10 μg per ml respectively.— A. G. Paradelis *et al.*, *Antimicrob. Ag. Chemother.*, 1978, *14*, 514.

Proprietary Names

Coltericin *(Argentia, Arg.)*; Kanendomicina *(LEFA, Spain)*; Kanendomycin *(Jap.)*; Stereocidin *(Crinos, Ital.)*.

19-h

Benethamine Penicillin *(B.P.C. 1973).*
Beneth. Penicil. Benzyl(phenethyl)ammonium (6*R*)-6-(2-phenylacetamido)penicillanate.
$C_{15}H_{17}N,C_{16}H_{18}N_2O_4S=545.7$.
CAS — 751-84-8.

A white or almost white, odourless or almost odourless, crystalline powder; it is almost tasteless but causes a local sensation of numbness. Benethamine penicillin 1 g is approximately equivalent to 600 mg of benzylpenicillin (1 million units).
Soluble 1 in 1500 of water, 1 in 100 of acetone (50%), 1 in 50 of chloroform, and 1 in 50 of methyl alcohol (75%). A 1.5% suspension in water has a pH of 5.5 to 7. **Store** in a cool place in airtight containers; if intended for injection, the containers should be sterile and sealed to exclude micro-organisms.

Benethamine penicillin is a poorly soluble derivative of benzylpenicillin (see p.1102) with similar properties and is given intramuscularly in doses of 300 to 600 mg every 3 or 4 days. It is not recommended for chronic, severe, or deep-seated infections such as subacute bacterial endocarditis or meningitis. After intramuscular injection it is slowly absorbed and releases benzylpenicillin into the circulation for 4 to 5 days. Benethamine penicillin is usually given in conjunction with benzylpenicillin and procaine penicillin to produce both an immediate and a prolonged effect.

Gonorrhoea. Of 103 men with gonorrhoea given a single dose of 1.25 million units of Triplopen, 9 relapsed within 14 days; of 103 given twice the dose of Triplopen, 7 relapsed similarly; of 104 given 1.25 million units of Triplopen plus 2.88 g of co-trimoxazole as a single dose, 3 relapsed; of 25 given a single dose of 2.88 g of co-trimoxazole, 7 relapsed.— A. S. Wigfield *et al.*, *Br. J. vener. Dis.*, 1973, *49*, 277.

Preparations

Fortified Benethamine Penicillin Injection *(B.P.C. 1973).* Penicillin Triple Injection; Benethamine Penicillin with Benzylpenicillin Sodium and Procaine Penicillin Injection; Triple Penicillin Injection. A sterile suspension of benethamine penicillin and procaine penicillin, with appropriate pharmaceutical adjuvants, in a solution of benzylpenicillin sodium in Water for Injections. Usual strength: benethamine penicillin 500 000 units, benzylpenicillin sodium 500 000 units, procaine penicillin 250 000 units. It contains no bactericide and is prepared aseptically by adding Water for Injections to the contents of a sealed container shortly before use. Store in a cool place and use within 7 days, or within 14 days when stored at 2° to 10°; if stored at temperatures approaching 20°, it should be used within 4 days. *Dose.* 1.2 million units, intramuscularly as a single dose, repeated if necessary every 3 or 4 days.

Triplopen *(Glaxo, UK).* A brand of Fortified Benethamine Penicillin Injection. *Dose.* The contents of 2 vials as a single dose or of 1 vial daily or every 2 or 3 days.

Other Proprietary Names
Benapen *(S.Afr.).*

20-a

Benzathine Penicillin *(B.P., B.P. Vet.).* Penicillin G Benzathine *(U.S.P.)*; Benzathini Benzylpenicillinum; Benzylpenicillinum Benzathinum; Benzathine Penicillin G; Benzathine Benzylpenicillin; Benzethacil; Benzilpenicilina Benzatinica; Dibenzylamine Penicillin G; Dibenzyl Penicillin; Penzaethinum G. *NN'*-Dibenzylethylenediammonium bis[(6*R*)-6-(2-phenylacetamido)penicillanate].
$C_{16}H_{20}N_2(C_{16}H_{18}N_2O_4S)_2=909.1$.
CAS — 1538-09-6 (anhydrous); 5928-83-6 (monohydrate); 41372-02-5 (tetrahydrate).

Pharmacopoeias. In *Arg., Aust., Br., Braz., Cz., Eur., Fr., Ger., Ind., Int., It., Jap., Jug., Neth., Pol., Port., Turk.*, and *U.S.*, most of which specify the tetrahydrate and contain not less than 1000 to 1200 units per mg. *Br.* specifies 5 to 8% w/w water of crystallisation.

A white, odourless, almost tasteless, hygroscopic powder. Benzathine penicillin 900 mg is approximately equivalent to 720 mg of benzylpenicillin (1.2 million units).
Soluble 1 in 6000 of water, 1 in 65 of alcohol, 1 in 10 of formamide, and 1 in 7 of dimethylformamide; practically insoluble in chloroform and ether. A saturated solution in water has a pH of 5 to 7.5. Aqueous suspensions are most stable when buffered to pH 6 to 7 and stored at low temperatures; such suspensions containing 25 to 50 mg per ml may be expected to retain 90% of their potency for 2 years if stored below 25°. **Store** at a temperature not exceeding 30° in airtight containers. Protect from light. If intended for injection the containers should be sterile and sealed to exclude micro-organisms.

Effect of gamma-irradiation. Benzathine penicillin powder became off-white at 25 000 Gy and pale cream-coloured at 250 000 Gy. The initial potency of 1180 units per mg fell to 1164 at 25 000 Gy and to 1146 at 250 000 Gy. An aqueous suspension became off-white at 25 000 Gy and cream-coloured at 250 000 Gy. The initial potency of 282 080 units per ml changed to 284 150 at 25 000 Gy and to 279 000 at 250 000 Gy.— *The Use of Gamma Radiation Sources for the Sterilisation of Pharmaceutical Products,* London, ABPI, 1960.

Adverse Effects, Treatment, and Precautions. As for Benzylpenicillin, p.1103.
Benzathine penicillin should not be used in the initial treatment of severe acute infections.

Ischaemia. Two children, aged 3 years or less, developed regional ischaemia with shock after an intramuscular injection of benzathine penicillin, 1 after a second dose of 450 mg, the other after a third dose of 900 mg. Acute pain was followed by ischaemia of the buttock, abdominal wall, perineum, and legs. Recovery was not complete for several days.— J. Gerbeaux *et al.*, *Presse méd.*, 1966, *74*, 229. See also C. P. Darby *et al.*, *Clin. Pediat.*, 1973, *12*, 485.

A report of the accidental intra-arterial injection of benzathine penicillin in 2 infants causing arteriolar obstruction followed by gangrene of the affected limb.— J. M. Wynne, *Archs Dis. Childh.*, 1978, *53*, 396. See also H. Schanzer *et al.*, *J. Am. med. Ass.*, 1979, *242*, 1289.

Skin reactions. Skin rashes were not an adequate indication of sensitivity to penicillin. Of 208 children with group A streptococcal infection and a history of penicillin sensitivity, 1 developed a skin rash and 1 urticaria when they were given either benzathine penicillin 450 mg and procaine penicillin 600 mg, or benzathine penicillin 900 mg. Children who received the mixture recovered from their infection more rapidly than those who received benzathine penicillin.— *J. Am. med. Ass.*, 1969, *210*, 1181.

Absorption and Fate. When benzathine penicillin is given by intramuscular injection, it forms a depot from which benzylpenicillin is slowly released; a single dose of 900 mg is reported to give an effective concentration of penicillin in the blood for up to 4 weeks.
Benzathine penicillin is stable in the presence of gastric juice and its absorption from the gastro-intestinal tract is not appreciably affected by the presence of food. However, the amounts that are absorbed are smaller than those from the same dose of a soluble penicillin though children may absorb more than adults. When benzathine penicillin is given by mouth in adequate doses, the maximum concentration of penicillin in the blood is produced less rapidly than after a corresponding dose of a soluble salt of penicillin but effective blood concentrations persist for a longer time—up to 6 hours.

After a single intramuscular dose of an aqueous injection containing 900 mg of benzathine penicillin, 600 mg of procaine penicillin, and 360 mg of benzylpenicillin potassium, mean daily serum concentrations 3, 4, 5, 6, and 7 days later were 60, 44, 42, 36, and 34 ng per ml respectively. When the dose was halved the mean serum concentrations fell by about one-half.— A. E. Tinkler and R. Shannon, *Bull. Wld Hlth Org.*, 1966, *35*, 857.

Benzathine penicillin 37.5 mg per kg body-weight given intramuscularly to 125 neonates produced peak serum concentrations of 1.23 µg per ml at 13 to 24 hours and concentrations decreased to 0.65 µg per ml by the fourth day. More than 100 µg per ml of penicillin was present in the urine of some infants throughout the first week of life. Antibacterial activity in serum was higher in neonates than in children and adults.— J. O. Klein *et al.*, *J. Pediat.*, 1973, *82*, 1065.

Diffusion into body fluids and tissues. A single intramuscular injection of benzathine penicillin 75 mg per kg of body-weight was given to 59 infants born to mothers with syphilis. A mean peak serum concentration of 2.54 µg per ml occurred at 24 hours after the dose and at least 0.42 µg per ml of penicillin was found at 120 hours. Peak concentrations of penicillin in the CSF, noted between 12 and 24 hours, only ranged from 0.012 and 0.21 µg per ml and were not adequate for neonates with possible neurosyphilis.— M. E. Speer *et al.*, *J. Pediat.*, 1977, *91*, 996.

Uses. Benzathine penicillin is used for the treatment of infections due to micro-organisms highly susceptible to benzylpenicillin (see p.1105). In acute infections, and when bacteraemia is present, the initial treatment should be with benzylpenicillin by injection.
Benzathine penicillin is given by deep intramuscular injection in a usual dose of 900 mg for the treatment of streptococcal infections and for the prophylaxis of secondary infections before tonsillectomy or dental extractions. Children may be given intramuscular doses of 225 to 675 mg according to body-weight. To prevent recurrences of acute rheumatic fever 900 mg may be given intramuscularly every 4 weeks; doses of 450 mg or 900 mg have been recommended for children.
Benzathine penicillin may be used in the treatment of syphilis, usually in a single dose of 1.8 g intramuscularly. However, since inadequate penetration into the cerebrospinal fluid has been reported in patients with neurosyphilis, procaine penicillin is often preferred. Benzathine penicillin should not be used in the treatment of gonorrhoea.
For mild infections in adults, benzathine penicillin has been given by mouth in a dose of 450 mg every 6 to 8 hours although phenoxymethylpenicillin is usually preferred. Children have been given half the adult dose.

A review of the use and side-effects of intramuscular injections of benzathine penicillin and of benzathine penicillin with procaine penicillin.— *Med. Lett.*, 1974, *16*, 87.

Diphtheria. Benzathine penicillin given as a single intramuscular dose was as effective in treating carriers as erythromycin during a diphtheria epidemic.— R. V. McCloskey *et al.*, *Ann. intern. Med.*, 1971, *75*, 495.

Rheumatic fever prophylaxis. When studied under controlled conditions for 4 years, a monthly prophylactic injection of 900 mg of benzathine penicillin reduced the incidence of streptococcal infections in patients aged 5 to 17, who had had rheumatic fever, to 6.6 per 100 patient-years, and the incidence of rheumatic recurrences to 0.6 per 100 patient-years. The comparable figures were 22.7 and 4.8 when patients were given a monthly regimen of benzylpenicillin potassium 240 mg thrice daily for 10 days followed by 240 mg daily. From a review of prophylactic trials, injections of benzathine penicillin were the treatment of choice.— A. R. Feinstein *et al.*, *J. Am. med. Ass.*, 1968, *206*, 565.

Of 129 children in Barbados who had had rheumatic fever, 115 were considered to have received adequate prophylaxis against recurrence. The regimen was 900 mg of benzathine penicillin monthly (*Br. med.J.*, 1972, *3*, 387). In the 115 children 97% adherence to the regimen was achieved; 2 relapsed. Three of 14 who had received inadequate prophylaxis (69% adherence to schedule) relapsed.— T. A. Hassell and K. L. Stuart, *Br. med. J.*, 1974, *2*, 39.

See also under Prophylactic Use of Antibiotics, p.1080.

Streptococcal infections, other. In the control of epidemics of streptococcal infections, benzathine penicillin 900 mg by intramuscular injection for the total population was the best method of treatment. Administration of penicillin by mouth for 10 days or more was also effective. Once the epidemic was under control, it was possible to prevent infection building up again by giving new members of the community a single injection of combined short- and long-acting penicillins.— Report of a WHO Expert Committee on Prevention of Rheumatic Fever, *Tech. Rep. Ser. Wld Hlth Org. No. 342*, 1966.

See also P. Ferrieri *et al.*, *J. infect. Dis.*, 1974, *129*, 429.

A report of failure of penicillin to eradicate group A streptococci during an outbreak of pharyngitis in a semi-closed population of over 300 adults and children despite the sensitivity of strains *in vitro*. The antibiotics given were either benzathine penicillin intramuscularly or phenoxymethylpenicillin by mouth (or erythromycin by mouth for allergic subjects). Findings suggested that many of the treatment failures were streptococcal carriers and not acutely infected individuals. An unusual aspect was the high rate of treatment failure after intramuscular benzathine penicillin therapy.— A. S. Gastanaduy *et al.*, *Lancet*, 1980, *2*, 498.

Syphilis. Benzathine penicillin was given in a single dose of 37.5 mg per kg body-weight to 4 infants with congenital syphilis but since penicillin activity in the CSF was detected in only 1 infant treatment was considered to be inadequate.— J. M. Kaplan and G. H. McCracken, *J. Pediat.*, 1973, *82*, 1069.

Benzathine penicillin 1.8 g followed 3 to 5 days later with 1.8 g and again 3 to 5 days later with 900 mg was effective in the treatment of 40 patients with secondary syphilis, producing seroconversion in them all.— R. D. Durst *et al.*, *Archs Derm.*, 1973, *108*, 663.

In 1976 the US Public Health Service recommended a single dose of benzathine penicillin 1.8 g intramuscularly as an alternative to procaine penicillin in primary, secondary, and latent syphilis of less than one year's duration. In late syphilis the same dose should be given weekly for 3 successive weeks.— *Obstet. Gynec.*, 1976, *48*, 727. See also *Med. Lett.*, 1977, *19*, 105.

Twelve of 13 patients with syphilis given benzathine penicillin 2.7 g weekly by intramuscular injection for 4 weeks had no penicillin detectable in the CSF after treatment.— J. A. Mohr *et al.*, *J. Am. med. Ass.*, 1976, *236*, 2208.

Yaws. Active yaws was found in 294 of 3422 children examined in the West Indies. Benzathine penicillin was given intramuscularly to infected children in a dose based on age, up to 900 mg, while the remainder received a smaller dose. Only 3 notifications of yaws were made in the district during the next 2 years.— R. E. M. Lees and G. H. K. Gentle, *W. Indian med. J.*, 1967, *16*, 228. See also R. E. M. Lees, *Can. J. publ. Hlth*, 1973, *64*, *Suppl.*, 52.

Preparations

Benzathine Penicillin Tablets *(B.P. 1958)*. Benzathine Penicillin G Tablets. Tablets containing benzathine penicillin.

Fortified Benzathine Penicillin Injection *(B.P.C. 1973)*. Benzathine Penicillin with Benzylpenicillin Potassium and Procaine Penicillin Injection. A sterile suspension of benzathine penicillin and procaine penicillin, with appropriate pharmaceutical adjuvants, in a solution of benzylpenicillin potassium in Water for Injections. It contains no bactericide and is prepared aseptically by adding Water for Injections to the contents of a sealed container shortly before use. The injection should be used immediately after preparation, or, if stored at 2° to 4°, within 7 days. *Dose.* 0.9 to 1.2 million units by deep intramuscular injection as a single dose, repeated if necessary every 2 or 3 days.

Penicillin G Benzathine Oral Suspension *(U.S.P.)*. Benzathine penicillin with one or more suitable buffers, colouring, flavouring and dispersing agents, and preservatives. pH 6 to 7. It contains the equivalent of 30 000 or 60 000 units of benzylpenicillin per ml. Store in airtight containers.

Penicillin G Benzathine Tablets *(U.S.P.)*. Tablets containing benzathine penicillin equivalent to 200 000 units of benzylpenicillin. Store in airtight containers.

Sterile Penicillin G Benzathine Suspension *(U.S.P.)*. A sterile suspension of benzathine penicillin in Water for Injections with one or more suitable dispersing agents, buffers, preservatives, and suspending agents. pH 5 to 7.5. It contains the equivalent of 300 000 units of benzylpenicillin per ml or per container. Store at 2° to 8°.

Proprietary Preparations

Penidural *(Wyeth, UK)*. Benzathine penicillin, available as **Oral Suspension** containing 229 mg in each 5 ml (suggested diluent, syrup) and as **Oral Drops** containing 115 mg per ml in bottles of 10 ml. **Penidural-LA** (Penidural Long-Acting Injection). An aqueous suspension of benzathine penicillin containing 229 mg per ml in vials of 10 ml; for deep intramuscular injection. (Also available as Penidural in *Austral.*, *Neth.*, *NZ*).

Other Proprietary Names

Arg.—Benzetacil L-A, Pen-di-Ben; *Austral.*—Bicillin, LPG; *Belg.*—Penadur LA; *Canad.*—Bicillin; *Fr.*—Extencilline; *Ger.*—Tardocillin; *Ital.*—Diaminocillina, Wycillina AP; *S.Afr.*—Penilente-LA; *Spain*—Benzetacil Simple, Brevicilina Simple, Cepacilina, Pipercilina, Tardopenil; *Switz.*—Penadur; *USA*—Bicillin, Bicillin L-A, Permapen.

NOTE. The name Bicillin is used in Great Britain as a proprietary name for a preparation containing procaine penicillin and benzylpenicillin sodium (see p.1207).

21-t

Benzathine Phenoxymethylpenicillin.

Penicillin V Benzathine *(U.S.P.)*; Phenoxymethylpenicillini Dibenzylaethylendiaminum. *NN'*-Dibenzylethylenediammonium bis[(6*R*)-6-(2-phenoxyacetamido)penicillanate].

$(C_{16}H_{18}N_2O_5S)_2,C_{16}H_{20}N_2=941.1$.

CAS — 5928-84-7 (anhydrous); 63690-57-3 (tetrahydrate).

Pharmacopoeias. In *Aust.* and *U.S.*

An almost white powder with a characteristic odour. Benzathine phenoxymethylpenicillin 1.3 g is approximately equivalent to 1 g of phenoxymethylpenicillin. **Soluble** 1 in 3200 of water, 1 in 330 of alcohol, 1 in 42 of chloroform, 1 in 910 of ether, and 1 in 37 of acetone. A saturated solution in water has a pH of 4 to 6.5. **Store** in airtight containers.

Benzathine phenoxymethylpenicillin has the actions and uses of phenoxymethylpenicillin. It has been given in doses of 250 mg.

Preparations

Penicillin V Benzathine Oral Suspension *(U.S.P.)*. A suspension of benzathine phenoxymethylpenicillin with one or more suitable buffers, colouring, dispersing, and flavouring agents, and preservatives. It contains the equivalent of 17.7 or 35.4 mg of phenoxymethylpenicillin per ml. pH 6 to 7. Store at 2° to 8° in airtight containers.

Proprietary Names

Benoral (see also under Benorylate) *(Galepharma, Spain)*; Cilicaine V *(Sigma, Austral.)*; Falcopen-V *(Faulding, Austral.)*; Kelacilline *(Kela, Belg.)*; Meropenin *(Astra, Swed.)*; Minervacil *(Byk, Neth.)*; Monocillin (see also under Phenoxymethylpenicillin) *(Chassot, Switz.)*; Oracilline (see also under Phenoxymethylpenicillin) *(Theraplix, Belg.*; *Théraplix, Fr.)*; Ospen (see also under Phenoxymethylpenicillin) *(Sandoz, Ger.*; *Sandoz, Switz.)*; Penorline *(Allard, Fr.)*; Phenocillin *(Streuli, Switz.)*; PVF *(Frosst, Canad.)*; Stabicilline (see also under Phenoxymethylpenicillin) *(Vifor, Switz.)*; Vicalin *(Malco, Austral.)*; Vicin *(Knoll, Austral.)*.

181-l

Benzylpenicillin.

Crystalline Penicillin G; Penicillin; Penicillin G. (2*S*,5*R*,6*R*)-3,3-Dimethyl-7-oxo-6-phenylacetamido-4-thia-1-azabicyclo[3.2.0]heptane-2-carboxylic acid; (6*R*)-6-(2-Phenylacetamido)penicillanic acid.

$C_{16}H_{18}N_2O_4S=334.4$.

CAS — 61-33-6.

The name benzylpenicillin is commonly used to describe either benzylpenicillin potassium or benzylpenicillin sodium as these are the forms in which benzylpenicillin is used.

In *Martindale*, benzylpenicillin means either the potassium or sodium salt.

182-y

Benzylpenicillin Potassium *(B.P., Eur. P.)*.

Benzylpenicillin; Penicillin; Crystalline Penicillin G; Penicillin G; Penicillin G Potassium. Potassium (6*R*)-6-(2-phenylacetamido)penicillanate.

$C_{16}H_{17}KN_2O_4S=372.5$.

CAS — 113-98-4.

Pharmacopoeias. In all pharmacopoeias examined except *Braz.*, *Nord.*, and *U.S.*; *U.S.* includes Sterile Penicillin G Potassium. *B.P. Vet.* includes Benzylpenicillin which may be either the potassium or sodium salt.

The potassium salt of 6-phenylacetamidopenicillanic acid, an antimicrobial acid produced by growing certain strains of *Penicillium notatum* or related moulds under appropriate conditions in a suitable culture medium, or produced by any other means. It contains not less than 96% of total penicillins. Each g represents about 2.7 mmol (2.7 mEq) of potassium. Benzylpenicillin potassium 600 mg has generally been considered to be approximately equivalent to 1 million units (1 mega unit).

A white finely crystalline powder with a faint characteristic odour. At relative humidities up to 55% it absorbs insignificant amounts of moisture at 25°; between 55 and 80% it absorbs larger but still small amounts of moisture, but under damper conditions it absorbs substantial amounts. Very **soluble** in water; soluble in alcohol and glycerol; practically insoluble in chloroform, ether, fixed oils, and liquid paraffin. Its solutions are dextrorotatory. A 10% solution in water has a pH of 5.5 to 7.5. A 5.48% solution is iso-osmotic with serum. **Store** at a temperature not exceeding 30° in airtight containers. If it is intended for injection, the containers should be sterile and sealed to exclude micro-organisms.

Stability and **incompatibility**. As for Benzylpenicillin Sodium (below).

Stability in solution. The stability of citrate-buffered benzylpenicillin potassium, when added to dextrose injection in a strength of 540 µg per ml, depended on the pH of the dextrose. At pH 4.5 over 10% potency was lost in 4 hours after mixing. Solutions in the range pH 4.5 to 5.5 should be administered immediately. A pH above 8 led to a rapid loss of penicillin potency. Mixtures of penicillin-dextrose with *aminophylline* 500 mg per litre, *pentobarbitone sodium* 500 mg per litre, *metaraminol tartrate* 100 mg per litre, and *vitamin-B complex with vitamin C* (pH 3.9) lost potency rapidly.— E. A. Parker *et al.*, *Abbott, Bull. parent. Drug Ass.*, 1967, *21*, 197.

Solutions of benzylpenicillin potassium in water, alcohol 40%, alcohol 70%, and benzyl alcohol 0.5% retained 85.1, 84.1, 85, and 82% potency respectively after storage for 10 days at room temperature.— A. B. Segelman and N. R. Farnsworth (letter), *J. pharm. Sci.*, 1970, *59*, 726.

Solutions of benzylpenicillin potassium in either sucrose 10% or dextrose 5% at 37° were inactivated and the pH fell from 9 to 8.5. After storage for 24 hours the activity of the solutions was negligible.— M. S. Simberkoff *et al.*, *New Engl. J. Med.*, 1970, *283*, 116.

22-x

Benzylpenicillin Sodium *(B.P., Eur. P.)*.

Benzylpenicillin; Benzylpenicillinum Natricum; Penicillin; Crystalline Penicillin G; Penicillin G; Penicillin G Sodium. Sodium (6*R*)-6-(2-phenylacetamido)penicillanate.

$C_{16}H_{17}N_2NaO_4S=356.4$.

CAS — 69-57-8.

Pharmacopoeias. In all pharmacopoeias examined except *Cz.* and *U.S.*; *U.S.* includes Sterile Penicillin G Sodium. *B.P. Vet.* includes Benzylpenicillin which may be either the potassium or sodium salt.

The sodium salt of 6-phenylacetamidopenicillanic acid, an antimicrobial acid produced by growing certain strains of *Penicillium notatum* or related moulds under appropriate conditions in a suitable culture medium, or produced by any other means. It contains not less than 96% of total penicillins. Each g represents about 2.8 mmol (2.8 mEq) of sodium. Benzylpenicillin sodium 600 mg has generally been considered to be approximately equivalent to 1 million units (1 mega unit).

A white to slightly yellow finely crystalline powder with a faint characteristic odour. At relative humidities up to 55% it absorbs insignificant amounts of moisture at 25°; between 55 and 70% it absorbs significant amounts of moisture and under damper conditions it absorbs substantial amounts.

Very **soluble** in water; soluble in alcohol and glycerol; practically insoluble in chloroform, ether, fixed oils, and liquid paraffin. Its solutions are dextrorotatory. A 10% solution in water has a pH of 5.5 to 7.5. **Store** in a cool place at a temperature not exceeding 30° in airtight containers. If it is intended for injection, the containers should be sterile and sealed to exclude micro-organisms.

Benzylpenicillin sodium or potassium, provided it contains less than 0.5% moisture and is stored in airtight containers, is relatively **stable** at room temperature for 2 to 3 years. Loss of potency occurs more rapidly at higher temperatures. Benzylpenicillin sodium or potassium is hydrolysed in aqueous solutions by degradation of the β-lactam ring and hydrolysis is accelerated by increased temperature. Degradation products include biologically inactive penicillic and penicilloic acids which lower the pH and cause a progressive increase in the rate of deterioration. By buffering solutions to pH 6 to 7 (optimum 6.8) deterioration is retarded. Dilute solutions are more stable than concentrated ones.

Injections of benzylpenicillin sodium or potassium stored at 2° to 10° should be used within 7 days of preparation if unbuffered or within 14 days if buffered. At temperatures approaching 20°, unbuffered injection solutions should be used within 24 hours and buffered solutions within 4 days.

Benzylpenicillin sodium or potassium is **incompatible** with metal ions, especially those of copper, zinc, and mercury, which attack the thiazolidine ring, and the use of zinc compounds in the processing of rubber may be responsible for the inactivation of penicillin solutions by rubber tubing and vial caps.

Benzylpenicillin sodium or potassium is also inactivated by oxidising and reducing agents, alcohols, glycerol, macrogols, and other hydroxy compounds. However, impurities may be responsible for the inactivation. In slightly alkaline solutions it is rapidly inactivated by cysteine and other aminothiol compounds. It is incompatible with sympathomimetic amines, the degree of incompatibility being dependent on concentrations, pH of vehicles, and time.

The acidity of autoclaved dextrose solutions destroys the activity of benzylpenicillin sodium or potassium which should not be given in dextrose injection although either salt may be injected into the tubing of the giving set after being well diluted with sodium chloride injection. Care should also be taken when benzylpenicillin sodium or potassium is added to solutions containing tetracycline hydrochloride and some other antibiotics as incompatibilities may occur.

A large number of micro-organisms are insensitive to penicillin and may produce the enzyme, penicillinase, which is capable of destroying penicillin. The addition of a bacteriostat inhibits the production of penicillinase by micro-organisms and assists in maintaining the potency of solutions.

A macromolecular component, which may be associated with allergenicity, has been reported by F.R. Batchelor *et al.* (*Lancet*, 1967, *1*, 1175) and G.T. Stewart (*ibid.*, 1177) (see under Adverse Effects) to be formed by polymerisation in solutions of benzylpenicillin sodium or potassium, and it is suggested that solutions of penicillins and cephalosporins should be prepared immediately before injection.

Effect of gamma-irradiation. Benzylpenicillin sodium powder became off-white at 25 000 Gy and buff-coloured at 250 000 Gy. Solutions remained colourless at 25 000 Gy but became pale brown at 250 000 Gy. The initial potency of 1660 units per mg fell to 1650 at 25 000 Gy and to 1611 at 250 000 Gy.— *The Use of Gamma Radiation Sources for the Sterilisation of Pharmaceutical Products*, London, ABPI, 1960.

Incompatibility. *Wool alcohols, hard paraffin, macrogols, cetostearyl alcohol, self-emulsifying stearyl alcohol, cocoa butter, emulsifying wax, lanolin, crude cholinesterinated bases*, and many ionic and nonionic *surfactants* had an adverse effect on the stability of penicillin.— W. A. Woodard, *J. Pharm. Pharmac.*, 1952, *4*, 1009.

The following types of compound were reported to be incompatible with benzylpenicillin: *alcohols, glycerol, glycol, sugars, acids, amines, aminacrine hydrochloride, ephedrine, procaine, heavy metals, rubber tubing, thiamine hydrochloride, zinc oxide, oxidising agents, oxidised cellulose, iodine, iodides, thiols, thiomersal, chlorocresol*, and *resorcinol*. A review, with bibliography, of the pharmaceutics of penicillin.— M. A. Schwartz and F. H. Buckwalter, *J. pharm. Sci.*, 1962, *51*, 1119.

Surfactants, preservatives, and *thickening agents* reduced the stability of benzylpenicillin sodium, phenoxyethylpenicillin potassium, phenoxymethylpenicillin potassium, and dimethoxyphenylpenicillin sodium in aqueous buffered solution. Stability was not influenced by the degree of polymerisation of macrogols and cellulose ethers. Micellar surfactants increased the hydrolytic decomposition of the β-lactam ring.— K. Thoma *et al.*, *Acta pharm. hung.*, 1965, *35*, 1.

There was loss of clarity when intravenous solutions of benzylpenicillin were mixed with those of *cephalothin sodium, hydroxyzine hydrochloride, lincomycin hydrochloride, metaraminol tartrate, noradrenaline acid tartrate, phenytoin sodium, prochlorperazine maleate, promethazine hydrochloride, tetracycline hydrochloride, vancomycin hydrochloride*, or (in dextrose injection) *promazine hydrochloride* or *thiopentone sodium*.— J. A. Patel and G. L. Phillips, *Am. J. Hosp. Pharm.*, 1966, *23*, 409. *Cephalothin* 1 g per litre was physically compatible with a buffered solution of benzylpenicillin.— E. A. Parker, *ibid.*, 1969, *26*, 543. A similar report.— *idem*, 1970, *27*, 492.

Benzylpenicillin sodium 600 mg was incompatible with *tetracycline hydrochloride* 100 mg in 2 ml of water below pH 2.5, with *oxytetracycline hydrochloride* 100 mg in 2.1 ml of water at pH 2, and with *erythromycin ethylsuccinate* 100 mg in 2 ml of aqueous basis at pH 6.— B. Lynn, *J. Hosp. Pharm.*, 1970, *28*, 71.

A haze developed over 3 hours when benzylpenicillin 6 g per litre was mixed with *amphotericin* 200 mg per litre in Dextrose Intravenous Infusion 5%, and with *chlorpromazine hydrochloride* 200 mg per litre and *prochlorperazine mesylate* 100 mg per litre in Sodium Chloride Intravenous Infusion.— B. B. Riley, *J. Hosp. Pharm.*, 1970, *28*, 228.

There was an immediate loss of benzylpenicillin potency when intramuscular injections of benzylpenicillin and *gentamicin, kanamycin* or *streptomycin* were mixed.— B. Lynn and A. Jones, *Advances in Antimicrobial and Antineoplastic Chemotherapy*, Vol. I, pt 1, Munich, Urban and Schwarzenberg, 1972, p. 701.

Benzylpenicillin was incompatible with *vitamins of the B group with vitamin C* in an infusion fluid.— B. Flouvat and P. Lechat, *Thérapie*, 1974, *29*, 337.

Benzylpenicillin was compatible with Ascorbic Acid Injection *U.S.P.* (sodium ascorbate). Reports of incompatibility were a function of pH rather than a characteristic of the ascorbate ion.— H. J. Pfeifer and J. W. Webb, *Am. J. Hosp. Pharm.*, 1976, *33*, 448.

Preservation in solution. Phenylmercuric borate 0.005% was a suitable preservative for benzylpenicillin eye-drops sterilised by filtration.— M. Van Ooteghem, *Pharm. Tijdschr. Belg.*, 1968, *45*, 69.

Stability. Ultraviolet irradiation for 2 hours had a destructive effect on benzylpenicillin sodium.— A. A. Kassem and E. H. Girgis, *Bull. Fac. Pharm., Cairo*, 1970, *9*, 157.

Benzylpenicillin was unstable in oleaginous preparations containing colloidal silica.— H. Zia *et al.*, *Can. J. pharm. Sci.*, 1974, *9*, 117.

Stability in solution. Benzylpenicillin 600 mg per litre was stable for 6 hours at room temperature in Water for Injections (pH 5.8), or sodium chloride injection (pH 5.7) but lost 10 to 12% potency after 24 hours. Injections with a pH further removed from the optimum range of 6 to 7 were only stable for 6 to 7 hours.— E. A. Parker, *Am. J. Hosp. Pharm.*, 1967, *24*, 434.

A report of the effect of pH, electrolytes, bicarbonates, lactate and phosphate buffers, some carbohydrates, and alcohol on the stability of benzylpenicillin in infusion fluids.— P. Lundgren and L. Landersjö, *Acta pharm. suec.*, 1970, *7*, 509, per *Pharm. J.*, 1971, *2*, 32.

Solutions of benzylpenicillin sodium in water, sodium chloride 0.9% solution, and citrate buffer (pH 6.5) were stable for 12 weeks at −25°.— S. S. Larsen, *Dansk Tidsskr. Farm.*, 1971, *45*, 307.

Solutions of benzylpenicillin sodium 12 500 units per ml in normal saline maintained their potency for 6 hours at 20° to 25° and lost about 10% of their potency after 24 hours. Similar solutions in normal saline containing 20% of Alevaire lost about 10% of the potency in 6 hours and about 30% in 24 hours.— B. Lynn, *Pharm. J.*, 1973, *1*, 19.

Benzylpenicillin, phenoxymethylpenicillin, and dicloxacillin formed complexes in solution with *sucrose* and their degradation rates were increased. Ampicillin was only slightly affected by sucrose.— S. L. Hem *et al.*, *J. pharm. Sci.*, 1973, *62*, 267. Accelerated degradation of benzylpenicillin sodium, ampicillin sodium, carbenicillin sodium, and phenoxymethylpenicillin potassium in neutral and alkaline sucrose solutions was due to a nucleophilic displacement reaction with the formation of sucrose penicilloate esters. These esters might be antigenic and their presence should be avoided by maintaining the pH of solutions of penicillins and sucrose at 6 to 6.5.— H. Bundgaard and C. Larsen, *Int. J. Pharmaceut.*, 1978, *1*, 95.

Solutions of benzylpenicillin 333 000 units per ml were prepared by adding powder for injection to each of 3 commercially available 0.5% hypromellose solutions in plastic squeezy bottles (Lacril, pH 5.9; Tearisol, pH 7.3; Isoptotears, pH 7.4). The solutions had relative antibiotic potencies of 74% after 3 days and only 25% after 7 days when stored at 25°.— E. Osborn *et al.*, *Am. J. Ophthal.*, 1976, *82*, 775.

The presence of carbohydrate was a determining factor for the stability of benzylpenicillin in alkaline solution. Above pH 8, for example when *aminophylline, sodium bicarbonate*, or *trometamol* were added to dextrose or fructose solutions, the degradation of benzylpenicillin was so rapid that its addition to such mixtures should be avoided. Trace amounts of iron accelerated this degradation.— L. Landersjö *et al.*, *Acta pharm. suec.*, 1977, *14*, 293.

Glucose and fructose accelerated the degradation of benzylpenicillin in weakly alkaline solutions (pH 8.5 to 9.25) due to a nucleophilic reaction involving the formation of penicilloyl carbohydrate esters which were hydrolysed to penicilloic acid. Ferrous ions catalysed the degradation of benzylpenicillin in a 10% fructose solution by accelerating ester formation.— C. Larsen and H. Bundgaard, *Arch. Pharm. Chemi, scient. Edn*, 1978, *6*, 33.

There was a linear relationship between the degradation-rate of benzylpenicillin and ampicillin and the concentration (up to 10%) of aqueous solutions of glucose, fructose, sucrose, dextran, sorbitol, mannitol, and glycerol to which they were added. The rate-accelerating effect was directly proportional to hydroxide ion concentration up to pH about 10.5 and it proceeded through a nucleophilic pathway with the intermediate formation of penicilloyl esters. These esters might contribute to the allergic reactions which occurred with penicillin and their formation could be reduced or avoided by adjusting the pH of these penicillin-containing solutions to between 6 and 6.5.— H. Bundgaard and C. Larsen, *Arch. Pharm. Chemi, scient. Edn*, 1978, *6*, 184.

It was suggested that penicillamine, which was detected in benzylpenicillin solutions of neutral pH, was formed from the degradation of benzylpenicillenic acid, an isomer of benzylpenicillin.— M. Jemal *et al.*, *J. pharm. Sci.*, 1978, *67*, 302.

Further references: L. Landersjö *et al.*, *Acta pharm. suec.*, 1978, *15*, 161; H. Bundgaard, *Arch. Pharm. Chemi, scient. Edn*, 1980, *8*, 161.

Sterilisation. Penicillin could be sterilised by exposing the dry powder to ethylene oxide vapour or by adding this chemical to a solution of the antibiotic. No loss in potency or increase in acute toxicity resulted from such treatments. Extreme desiccation must be avoided.— S. Kaye *et al.*, *J. Lab. clin. Med.*, 1952, *40*, 67.

Units. One unit of penicillin was contained in 0.0005988 mg of the second International Standard Preparation (1952) of benzylpenicillin sodium which contained 1670 units per mg. The International Standard was discontinued in 1968 since penicillin can now be characterised completely by chemical tests.

Adverse Effects. When benzylpenicillin is administered to a hypersensitive patient, anaphylactic shock with collapse and sometimes death may occur within minutes. A generalised sensitivity reaction can occur within 1 to 3 weeks with urticaria, fever, eosinophilia, joint pains, angioneurotic oedema, erythema multiforme, and exfoliative dermatitis, although an accelerated urticarial reaction can develop within hours.

Since the topical application or inhalation of

penicillin was condemned as a major cause of sensitisation, this effect is now initiated mainly through the therapeutic use of parenteral and oral preparations. Sensitisation also occurs in industrial and hospital workers exposed to penicillin and may result from the ingestion of food, such as milk and meat products, containing penicillin residues.

Intravenous doses over 6 g have been associated with haemolytic anaemia in patients with circulating IgG antibody. Prolongation of bleeding time and defective platelet function has also been observed with high doses of benzylpenicillin.

Protein contaminants have been partly responsible for the sensitivity reactions to penicillins but so too has a protein residue isolated from commercial 6-aminopenicillanic acid so that patients who are allergic to benzylpenicillin are allergic to the 6-aminopenicillanic acid nucleus found in all penicillins. Sensitised patients may also react to the cephalosporins.

Glossitis, angular and aphthous stomatitis, and darkening of the tongue are liable to follow the use of penicillin as lozenges and occasionally by injection.

Convulsions and other signs of toxicity to the central nervous system may occur with very high doses of benzylpenicillin, particularly when administered intravenously to infants and the elderly, to patients with renal failure, or when administered intrathecally in doses above 12 mg. Nephrotoxicity has occurred in some patients with diminished renal function given large doses of benzylpenicillin. Acute interstitial nephritis, a hypersensitivity reaction, has also been reported.

Disturbances of blood electrolytes may follow the administration of large doses of the potassium and sodium salts of benzylpenicillin.

Some patients in the early stages of syphilis may experience a Herxheimer reaction shortly after starting treatment with penicillin. It is possibly due to the release of endotoxins from the killed treponemes and symptoms include fever, sweating, headache, malaise, and reactions at the site of the lesions. The reaction can be dangerous in cardiovascular syphilis or where there is a serious risk of increased local damage such as primary optic atrophy or nerve deafness.

Administration of penicillin by mouth is liable to produce transient diarrhoea and, sometimes, nausea, heartburn, and pruritus ani.

A report of abdominal pain following the intravenous administration of benzylpenicillin.— P. C. Robinson *et al.*, *Aust. N.Z. J. Med.*, 1979, *9*, 69.

Allergy. An impurity of high molecular weight which gave strong passive cutaneous anaphylactic reactions in *animals* was isolated from solutions of the sodium salt of 6-aminopenicillanic acid; a similar impurity was isolated from commercial benzylpenicillin solutions. The impurity was of protein origin and immunological studies showed it to have penicilloyl specificity. Another antigen, with penicilloyl specificity, derived from the penicillin molecule presumably by polymerisation, was found to form on storage in solutions of benzylpenicillin and of the sodium salt of 6-aminopenicillanic acid from which the high-molecular-weight impurity had been removed.— F. R. Batchelor *et al.*, *Lancet*, 1967, *1*, 1175. See also H. Bundgaard, *J. clin. Hosp. Pharm.*, 1980, *5*, 73 (polymerisation and reactions with carbohydrates).

Intradermal or scratch tests with solutions containing 1 µg or less of the protein residues obtained from the sodium salt of 6-aminopenicillanic acid produced strong reactions in 6 patients with proven hypersensitivity to penicillins. Two of the patients reacted to test doses of 10 µg of commercial batches of the sodium salt of 6-aminopenicillanic acid but only 1 reacted to a solution which had been dialysed to remove the protein residue. Doses of 10 ng of the protein residue from commercial benzylpenicillin produced a similar response in 2 hypersensitive patients, but dialysed benzylpenicillin was given without untoward effect to 2 hypersensitive patients. Dialysed solutions of benzylpenicillin, when stored at 25° to 37°, were found to form 30 mg of sulphurous polymer in 1 hour and 440 mg in 24 hours per 100 g of starting material; the polymer might act as a carrier of the allergen and it was suggested that penicillins and cephalosporins should be injected immediately after being dissolved.— G. T. Stewart, *Lancet*, 1967, *1*, 1177. The macromolecular residues contained a polymer and had been found to be proteinaceous.— *idem* (letter), *Lancet* 1968, *1*, 1088. See also E. T. Knudsen *et al.*, *ibid.*, 1967, *1*, 1184.

Allergic reactions to penicillin had been reported to vary from 0.7 to 10% and sudden reactions, resembling anaphylactic reactions in *animals*, had occurred in about 0.015 to 0.04% of patients treated. The fatality-rate was 0.0015 to 0.002%. A review of 151 deaths after penicillin treatment showed that almost 70% had received penicillin previously and about a third had shown some evidence of allergy. Where death occurred, adverse effects generally appeared either immediately on administering the dose or within 15 minutes.— O. Idsøe *et al.*, *Bull. Wld Hlth Org.*, 1968, *38*, 159.

The Boston Collaborative Drug Surveillance Program monitored consecutively 32 812 medical inpatients. Drug-induced anaphylaxis occurred in 1 of 2150 patients given benzylpenicillin.— J. Porter and H. Jick, *Lancet*, 1977, *1*, 587.

A brief review of penicillin allergy.— *Drug & Ther. Bull.*, 1975, *13*, 9. See also C. H. Dash, *J. antimicrob. Chemother.*, 1975, *1*, *Suppl.* (Sept.), 107.

For other references to hypersensitivity, see Martindale 27th Edn, p. 1083.

Blood disorders. A 12-year-old boy developed pancytopenia after treatment for 23 days with benzylpenicillin to a total of about 276 g. The condition reappeared 17 days later after a challenge dose of about 600 mg. It was believed that benzylpenicillin blocked the release of mature cells from the bone marrow.— B. Joorabchi and E. Kohout, *Br. med. J.*, 1973, *2*, 26.

A report of leucopenia during treatment with benzylpenicillin.— B. Colvin *et al.*, *Br. Heart J.*, 1974, *36*, 216.

Coagulation disorder. A haemorrhagic diathesis occurred in one patient with renal failure given benzylpenicillin 6 g daily. Five other patients undergoing heart surgery had prolonged bleeding times with related changes in the blood picture associated with doses of 18 and 24 g of benzylpenicillin daily. High doses of benzylpenicillin were considered to cause a latent coagulation disorder that might become clinically apparent in the presence of pre-existing haemostatic defects, as in uraemia or after surgery.— K. Andrassy *et al.*, *Lancet*, 1976, *2*, 1039. See also P. L. Roberts (letter), *Ann. intern. Med.*, 1974, *81*, 267; M. J. Lacombe *et al.*, *Nouv. Presse méd.*, 1974, *3*, 1435; C. H. Brown *et al.*, *Blood*, 1976, *47*, 949.

Haemolytic anaemia. Haemolytic anaemia could occur following large doses of penicillin, usually benzylpenicillin, particularly in patients who had received large doses of the drug in the past and who were given penicillin again in doses of about 6 g or more daily. This effect should be considered in patients with diseases such as subacute bacterial endocarditis and septicaemia which were commonly associated with anaemia, since haemolysis due to the antibiotic might be unrecognised.— *Br. med. J.*, 1968, *3*, 4.

Further reports of haemolytic anaemia.— P. Spath *et al.*, *Schweiz. med. Wschr.*, 1973, *103*, 383; J. P. Cazenave, *Sem. Hôp. Paris*, 1973, *49*, 307; C. A. Ries *et al.*, *J. Am. med. Ass.*, 1975, *233*, 432; A. F. Dove *et al.*, *Br. med. J.*, 1975, *3*, 684; G. W. G. Bird *et al.* (letter), *Lancet*, 1975, *2*, 462; F. N. Jackson and J. P. Jaffe, *J. Am. med. Ass.*, 1979, *242*, 2286; T. R. Spitzer (letter), *Lancet*, 1981, *1*, 1361.

Positive Coombs' test. Positive direct Coombs' tests, sometimes associated with haemolysis, had been found in patients treated with penicillin. Specific antibodies had been detected in some cases, but the effect did not appear to be dose-related. Haemolysis abated when penicillin was withdrawn and corticosteroids given; Coombs' tests remained positive, however, for at least 2 weeks after stopping penicillin treatment.— *J. Am. med. Ass.*, 1967, *202* (Oct. 16), A38.

Electrolyte disturbances. Studies in 8 healthy persons and 8 patients with renal lesions showed that benzylpenicillin sodium 18 g and benzylpenicillin potassium 6 g increased the urinary excretion of sodium and decreased the urinary excretion of chloride to a greater degree than did sodium and potassium chloride. Kaliuresis was increased by benzylpenicillin sodium in the patients. It was suggested that not more than 6 g of benzylpenicillin potassium should be given in an hour, and that it should be alternated with the sodium salt.— M. Hohenegger and K. H. Spitzy, *Arzneimittel-Forsch.*, 1966, *16*, 1345.

Five of 6 patients with subacute bacterial endocarditis developed hypokalaemia and metabolic alkalosis within 3 to 6 days of treatment with 60 g of benzylpenicillin sodium daily. Urinary potassium excretion was an important factor in causing hypokalaemia, and it was considered that penicillin could promote urinary potassium excretion by acting as a non-reabsorbable anion. The use of benzylpenicillin potassium or concomitant administration of potassium-sparing diuretics might prevent potassium depletion when massive doses of penicillin were necessary.— F. P. Brunner and P. G. Frick, *Br. med. J.*, 1968, *4*, 550. Infusions of penicillin 60 g daily had been performed in patients for up to 3 months without evidence of electrolyte imbalance, neurotoxicity, marked changes in serum osmolality, or haemolysis. A continuous infusion with three 500-ml volumes of sodium chloride solution 0.18% to which had been added benzylpenicillin in quantities of 18, 24, and 18 g respectively had been given, each dose being composed of approximately equal parts of the sodium and potassium salts. Alternatively, sodium and potassium concentrations in serum could be altered by adjusting this ratio.— H. Smith and S. E. J. Young (letter), *ibid.*, 1969, *1*, 53.

Granuloma. A 36-year-old man who had bilateral subareolar injections of a penicillin preparation developed bilateral breast enlargement with induration and discoloration. The condition persisted for 6 years and was diagnosed as granuloma. The reaction was attributed to an unknown adjuvant in the injections.— R. M. Schmidt and J. W. C. Hagstrom (letter), *J. Am. med. Ass.*, 1969, *209*, 1088.

Lupus erythematosus. Penicillin had been implicated in the causation of systemic lupus erythematosus.— D. Alarcón-Segovia, *Mayo Clin. Proc.*, 1969, *44*, 664.

Nephrotoxicity. Clinical features of an allergic reaction were associated with renal failure in 7 patients during prolonged treatment with large doses of benzylpenicillin or methicillin. Renal disease subsided in 6 patients when the antibiotic was discontinued. Three patients had received methicillin in doses of 6 to 24 g daily, 3 had received benzylpenicillin 7.2 to 36 g daily, and 1 had received methicillin 4 to 6 g daily in conjunction with benzylpenicillin 12 g daily. Renal biopsy in 4 patients showed tubular damage and interstitial accumulation of mononuclear cells and eosinophils.— D. S. Baldwin *et al.*, *New Engl. J. Med.*, 1968, *279*, 1245.

A report of interstitial nephritis and pneumonitis occurring in a 64-year-old man who became dyspnoeic, confused, and oliguric, within about one month of starting a course of benzylpenicillin 30 g daily intravenously. Haemodialysis was necessary and skin rash, eosinophilia, fever, and confusion persisted until vancomycin was given in place of penicillin. Interstitial pulmonary infiltrates resolved slowly.— M. Geller *et al.*, *Ann. Allergy*, 1976, *37*, 183.

Further references: R. W. Schrier *et al.*, *Ann. intern. Med.*, 1966, *64*, 116; R. B. Colvin *et al.* (letter), *ibid.*, 1974, *81*, 404.

Neurotoxicity. Reviews on the neurotoxicity of penicillin: B. Fossieck and R. H. Parker, *J. clin. Pharmac.*, 1974, *14*, 504; P. J. Nicholls, *J. antimicrob. Chemother.*, 1980, *6*, 161.

Four patients with renal failure who were given benzylpenicillin potassium by intravenous injection in doses ranging from 15 to 24 g daily developed encephalopathy characterised by impaired sensorium, myoclonus, and seizures. In 3 of the patients, the encephalopathy was considered to have contributed to their subsequent death. The frequency of this complication demanded the need for caution when large doses of penicillin were administered to uraemic patients.— H. A. Bloomer *et al.*, *J. Am. med. Ass.*, 1967, *200*, 121.

Signs of neurotoxicity, including myoclonic jerks, seizures, and coma, in 8 of 15 patients were possibly caused by excessive concentrations of penicillin in cerebrospinal fluid. Doses of either benzylpenicillin potassium or sodium, ranged from 300 mg every 2 hours to 12 g every 4 hours, administered intravenously. Seizures decreased in frequency within 12 to 24 hours of treatment being stopped.— H. Smith *et al.*, *Archs intern. Med.*, 1967, *120*, 47.

A 3-year-old boy had convulsions and died after 600 mg of penicillin was injected into the spinal cavity.— *Br. med. J.*, 1970, *3*, 412.

A patient with pneumonia who was given a total of 13.2 g of benzylpenicillin in 40 hours, after previous treatment with gentamicin, ampicillin, and tetracycline, developed generalised seizures and died of Gram-negative bronchopneumonia. His kidney function was not significantly impaired and the seizures were considered to be due to a cerebral abscess found at post mortem. It was suggested that penicillin neurotoxicity should not be suspected in patients with normal or only slightly abnormal kidney function unless the dosage was higher than 48 g daily.— D. W. Love and F. J. Salter, *Am. J. Hosp. Pharm.*, 1972, *29*, 424.

The Boston Collaborative Drug Surveillance Program monitored consecutively 32 812 medical inpatients. Drug-induced convulsions occurred in 5 of 3901 patients given penicillins. Four were given benzylpenicillin intravenously and 1 was given oxacillin intravenously.— J. Porter and H. Jick, *Lancet*, 1977, *1*, 587.

A report of sciatic neuritis associated with a penicillin injection.— E. W. Massey and A. B. Pleet, *Anesth. Analg. curr. Res.*, 1979, *58*, 63.

Skin reactions. Fifteen cases of toxic epidermal necrolysis had been reported associated with the use of penicillin or its derivatives.— E. D. Lowney *et al.*, *Archs Derm.*, 1967, *95*, 359.

Reference to the Stevens-Johnson syndrome being associated with the administration of penicillin.— J. R. Caldwell and L. E. Cluff, *J. Am. med. Ass.*, 1974, *230*, 77.

See also Allergy (above).

Treatment of Adverse Effects. When cutaneous reactions occur they may subside spontaneously within a few hours or days or when penicillin is withdrawn. Control of the reactions may be attempted by the administration of antihistamines or, should there be no response, of corticosteroids. Desensitisation has been attempted when treatment with penicillin has been considered essential.

At the first sign of an immediate reaction to penicillin treatment, 0.3 to 1 ml of Adrenaline Injection should be given intramuscularly (or in severe cases 0.2 ml well diluted intravenously) followed by a further dose if no improvement occurs. This should be followed by an antihistamine, such as diphenhydramine or chlorpheniramine, given parenterally and a corticosteroid given intravenously. If bronchospasm is severe aminophylline (250 mg in 10 ml) may be given intravenously. Assisted respiration is necessary if there is upper airways obstruction and plasma or suitable electrolyte solutions should be given intravenously if circulatory failure occurs.

Urticaria and joint pains, if severe, may be treated with corticosteroids by mouth.

Penicillinase (see p.654) was formerly advocated for the early treatment of allergic shock caused by penicillin but it may itself be responsible for allergic reactions and its use is no longer recommended.

For discussions on the treatment of allergic reactions to penicillin and desensitisation using graded doses, see B. B. Levine, *New Engl. J. Med.*, 1966, *275*, 1115; G. Westerman *et al.*, *J. Am. med. Ass.*, 1966, *198*, 173.

Four of 9 patients who developed skin rashes during penicillin therapy for bacterial endocarditis were given systemic steroids and their penicillin therapy was continued as recommended by A.J. Raper and V.E. Kemp (*New Engl. J. Med.*, 1965, *273*, 297).— J. A. Lowes *et al.*, *Lancet*, 1980, *1*, 133.

A 60-year-old woman with analgesic nephropathy receiving regular haemodialysis developed penicillin intoxication with severe central nervous system symptoms following treatment with intravenous benzylpenicillin for suspected septicaemia. Plasma-penicillin concentrations were reduced considerably following the addition of charcoal haemoperfusion to the haemodialysis and the patient recovered without residual neurological abnormalities. It appeared that standard haemodialysis was insufficient to prevent an accumulation of penicillin following the administration of large doses and it was suggested that charcoal haemoperfusion is far more efficient than dialysis in removing penicillin and should be the treatment of choice for penicillin intoxication.— C. J. Wickerts *et al.*, *Br. med. J.*, 1980, *280*, 1254.

Further references: J. Pedersen-Bjergaard, *Acta allerg.*, 1969, *24*, 333; J. S. Staffurth, *Prescribers' J.*, 1972, *12*, 76; V. Gotz, *Drug Intell. & clin. Pharm.*, 1976, *10*, 333; *Med. Lett.*, 1978, *20*, 14; *J. Am. med. Ass.*, 1980, *243*, 1704.

Overdosage. The recovery of a woman who was accidentally given benzylpenicillin 1.2 g intrathecally in mistake for 12 mg. Intravenous phenytoin and diazepam did not control the seizures which developed 45 minutes later, therefore she was paralysed, intubated, ventilated, and given thiopentone sodium by infusion. A neurosurgeon drained off 50 ml of CSF and replaced it with 40 ml of physiological saline. A further 40 ml of CSF was drained off 12 hours later, and 30 hours after the overdose the thiopentone infusion was stopped. Despite infusion of dopamine the patient remained severely hypotensive for a further 4 days; 36 hours after the thiopentone withdrawal several focal seizures and one grand mal seizure were controlled with intravenous clonazepam and sodium valproate by mouth. She remained unresponsive for 10 days; at 2 weeks she was speaking a little and beginning to feed herself; at 3 weeks she was walking unaided and her performance on simple verbal and arithmetic tests was better than on admission, but her short-term memory was poorer.— C. Marks and B. H. Cummins (letter), *Lancet*, 1981, *1*, 658.

For a suggested method of treating intrathecal overdosage with benzylpenicillin, see Sodium Diatrizoate, p.436.

Precautions. Penicillin should not be given for trivial infections. If a patient is known to be hypersensitive to penicillin, an antibiotic of another class should be given. However, sensitised patients may react to the cephalosporins. Penicillin should be given with caution to patients with a history of allergy, especially to other drugs. Care is necessary if large doses of the potassium or sodium salts are given to patients with impaired renal function or congestive heart failure or if large doses are given intrathecally. Because of the Herxheimer reaction care is also necessary when treating some patients with syphilis (see under Adverse Effects).

Contact with penicillin should be avoided since skin sensitisation may occur.

One of the dangers of penicillin therapy is the emergence of **supra-infection** by resistant species such as *Proteus, Pseudomonas,* and *Candida* (p.1081) which do not respond to further penicillin therapy, and may ultimately lead to death. One of the most serious of these is staphylococcal enterocolitis due to penicillin-resistant strains. If this occurs, another antibiotic to which the organism is sensitive should be substituted immediately. Systemic mycotic infections may sometimes occur.

Antibiotics such as penicillin should be avoided during treatment for urticaria.— P. W. M. Copeman, *Br. J. Hosp. Med.*, 1972, *7*, 339.

Prophylaxis with benzylpenicillin 120 mg administered twice daily by mouth to 277 children with rheumatism masked streptococcal infections with an antistreptolysin O response, giving throat cultures that were falsely negative. Of 244 siblings with clinical infections not receiving prophylaxis, only 4.1% had negative cultures compared with 34.4% of 61 clinical infections in rheumatic children.— B. F. Massell and L. H. Honikman, *J. Am. med. Ass.*, 1972, *221*, 1123.

Penicillin was unlikely to occur in blue cheeses made in the traditional manner so that patients sensitive to penicillin could eat such cheeses.— *Br. med. J.*, 1973, *3*, 44. See also *ibid.*, 585.

Effect on blood estimations. Pseudobisalbuminaemia could confuse blood estimations for albumin by electrophoresis in patients taking penicillin.— *Drug & Ther. Bull.*, 1972, *10*, 69.

Effect on urine estimations. The administration of penicillin could interfere with measurements of urinary 17-hydroxycorticosteroids.— J. M. Rosenberg and I. S. Kampa, *Drug Intell. & clin. Pharm.*, 1973, *7*, 33.

False-positive reactions for proteinuria had been noted in patients taking derivatives of penicillin.— K. Andrassy *et al.* (letter), *Lancet*, 1978, *2*, 154.

Interactions. *Aspirin, sulphamethoxypyridazine,* and *sulphaethidole* inhibited the serum-binding of benzylpenicillin *in vitro* and *in vivo*.— C. M. Kunin, *Clin. Pharmac. Ther.*, 1966, *7*, 180.

Probenecid, phenylbutazone, sulphinpyrazone, aspirin, sulphaphenazole, and *indomethacin* all prolonged the plasma half-life of benzylpenicillin.— J. Kampmann *et al.*, *Clin. Pharmac. Ther.*, 1972, *13*, 516.

In 1 of 5 subjects the absorption and elimination of oral benzylpenicillin was increased while taking *cimetidine*, probably because of transient achlorhydria.— A. J. Fairfax *et al.*, *Br. med. J.*, 1978, *1*, 820.

A report of enhanced action of *warfarin* in 1 patient receiving benzylpenicillin.— M. A. Brown *et al.*, *Can. J. Hosp. Pharm.*, 1979, *32*, 18. See also S. M. Wallace and M. A. Brown, *ibid.*, 78.

Reports on the antimicrobial activity of benzylpenicillin being diminished and enhanced are given in the section on Antimicrobial Action.

Interference with blood grouping. Penicillin in doses greater than 12 g daily might interfere with blood grouping and compatibility tests.— M. A. M. Ali, *Prescribers' J.*, 1970, *10*, 60.

Tests for Hypersensitivity. Skin tests with penicillin are of limited value; scratch tests followed, if negative, by intradermal tests have been used but negative results are unreliable and severe reactions have sometimes been provoked in sensitised persons even by dilute solutions. Skin tests with penicillin combined with a polypeptide (see Penicilloyl-polylysine, p.522) have been carried out, but may give unreliable results. A minor determinant mixture of benzylpenicillin and its degradation products has been used alone or with penicilloyl-polylysine and negative results appear to be more reliable.

A number of *in vitro* laboratory tests, including the basophil degranulation test, the histamine release test, and the lymphocyte transformation test, have been developed for the detection of hypersensitivity to penicillin. None of them has proved entirely dependable so far.

The following tests for hypersensitivity to penicillin were studied in 10 healthy subjects and 15 persons with a past history of penicillin reactions: (a) the skin test with penicilloyl-polylysine, (b) the direct basophil test, (c) the basophil degranulation test, and (d) the fluorometric histamine release test. No test proved as sensitive as the patients' histories of previous reactions.— S. S. Resnik and W. B. Shelley, *J. invest. Derm.*, 1965, *45*, 269.

Penicillin was necessary in the treatment of 29 patients who gave a history of previous penicillin reactions but who had negative skin tests with hapten antigens. No patients suffered anaphylactic or immediate urticarial reactions and only 5 had delayed maculopapular eruptions. It was considered that the results of skin testing were more reliable than the patients' histories.— M. J. Fellner *et al.*, *Archs Derm.*, 1971, *103*, 371.

A report of the successful use of skin testing for penicillin hypersensitivity with penicilloyl-polylysine and a minor determinant mixture of benzylpenicillin and its derivatives.— N. F. Adkinson *et al.*, *New Engl. J. Med.*, 1971, *285*, 22. See also B. B. Levine, *ibid.*, 1972, *286*, 42; C. W. Parker, *ibid.*, 1975, *292*, 957; G. R. Green *et al.*, *J. Allergy & clin. Immunol.*, 1977, *60*, 339; *Med. Lett.*, 1978, *20*, 14.

For earlier reports of various hypersensitivity tests, see Martindale 27th Edn, p.1084.

Antimicrobial Action. Benzylpenicillin has bacteriostatic and bactericidal actions, depending on its concentration, against most Gram-positive bacteria and Gram-negative cocci, and against some spirochaetes and actinomycetes. It is considered to act by inhibiting transpeptidase, the enzyme responsible for cross-linking of peptidoglycan during the final stage of synthesis of the bacterial cell wall, and so exerts its effect against dividing bacteria. Its action is inhibited by the enzyme penicillinase, produced during the growth of certain micro-organisms, but not by serum, pus, or the products of the autolysis of tissue.

The following pathogenic organisms are usually sensitive to benzylpenicillin in the concentrations commonly achieved in the body during treatment: *Actinomyces israelii, Bacillus anthracis, Clostridium* spp., *Corynebacterium diphtheriae, Erysipelothrix rhusiopathiae, Leptospira* spp., *Listeria monocytogenes, Neisseria* spp., *Spirillum minus, Streptobacillus moniliformis, Treponema* spp., and some staphylococci, streptococci, and a few of the larger viruses. Some strains of *Haemophilus* spp. are relatively susceptible. The minimum inhibitory concentrations of benzylpenicillin for these organisms have been reported to range from 0.006 to 2 μg per ml.

Among pathogenic micro-organisms naturally insensitive to benzylpenicillin are *Brucella, Mycobacterium, Pasteurella* (except *P. multocida*), *Proteus* (apart from some strains of *Pr. mirabilis*), *Pseudomonas, Vibrio, Klebsiella*, the *Escherichia coli* group, some of the *Streptococcus viridans* group, fungi (though not *Actinomyces*), mycoplasmas, rickettsias, and most viruses.

The sensitivity of bacteria to benzylpenicillin varies widely even among the genera which are normally susceptible. Gonococci (*Neisseria gonorrhoeae*), though Gram-negative, have been among the most sensitive although the overall trend in various parts of the world has been towards constant or increasing resistance. Streptococci are very sensitive followed closely by meningococci (*Neisseria meningitidis*) and by non-penicillinase-producing staphylococci.

See also p.1085 for a brief discussion on the penicillin group of antibiotics.

Reviews on the mode of action of the penicillins: *Lancet*, 1972, *2*, 468; A. Tomasz, *Ann. Rev. Microbiol.*, 1979, *33*, 113. See also *Lancet*, 1978, *2*, 1083.

In a study of 23 antibiotics, benzylpenicillin and phenoxymethylpenicillin were the most active against 78 strains of *Streptococcus pneumoniae*.— L. D. Sabath *et al.*, *Antimicrob. Ag. Chemother.*, 1970, 53.

Using a standardised disk-diffusion technique 98% of 140 isolates of beta-haemolytic streptococci were shown to be sensitive to benzylpenicillin in a concentration of 2 μg and using an agar-dilution technique 100% of 133 streptococcal isolates were shown to be sensitive to benzylpenicillin in a concentration of 100 ng per ml. The disk-diffusion technique was considered to be suitable for *in vitro* testing.— M. I. Marks *et al.*, *Can. med. Ass. J.*, 1973, *108*, 1274.

In a study *in vitro* of the susceptibility of *Staph. aureus* and *Staph. epidermidis* to 65 antimicrobial agents with antistaphylococcal activity, rifampicin was the most active overall. Amongst the 16 penicillins, benzylpenicillin or phenoxymethylpenicillin was the most active but only against penicillin-sensitive strains; for all strains dicloxacillin, cloxacillin, and nafcillin were the most active.— L. D. Sabath *et al.*, *Antimicrob. Ag. Chemother.*, 1976, *9*, 962.

Benzylpenicillin was active against the majority of 486 strains of anaerobic bacteria at 32 μg or less per ml. About 55 of 76 strains of *Bacteroides fragilis* were inhibited at this concentration, which was considered attainable with high parenteral doses.— V. L. Sutter and S. M. Finegold, *Antimicrob. Ag. Chemother.*, 1976, *10*, 736. In a further study the majority of 265 strains of anaerobic bacteria, including 25 of 41 strains of *Bacteroides fragilis*, were inhibited by benzylpenicillin 8 μg per ml.— P. C. Appelbaum and S. A. Chatterton, *ibid.*, 1978, *14*, 371.

Sensitivity tests with 20 antibiotics on 57 strains of *Clostridium perfringens* showed that benzylpenicillin and amoxycillin were the most effective, each inhibiting all strains with 0.12 μg per ml. The semisynthetic penicillins, the cephalosporins, chloramphenicol, and clindamycin were also effective. Infections should be treated with benzylpenicillin. If there was penicillin-hypersensitivity a cephalosporin could be used; chloramphenicol or clindamycin might be alternatives. Neither erythromycin nor tetracycline should generally be considered.— J. D. Schwartzman *et al.*, *Antimicrob. Ag. Chemother.*, 1977, *11*, 695.

Benzylpenicillin inhibited 11, 39, 43, 47, 58, 72, 88 and all of 92 strains of *Neisseria gonorrhoeae in vitro* at an MIC of 8, 16, 30, 60, 125, 250, 500, and 1000 ng per ml respectively.— B. A. Watts *et al.*, *J. antimicrob. Chemother.*, 1977, *3*, 331. See also J. R. Dillon *et al.* (letter), *ibid.*, 1978, *4*, 477; W. H. Hall *et al.*, *Antimicrob. Ag. Chemother.*, 1979, *15*, 562; M. Gedebou and A. Tassew, *Bull. Wld Hlth Org.*, 1980, *58*, 67 and 73.

MBCs of benzylpenicillin greatly exceeded MICs against 40 strains of *Lactobacilli in vitro*.— A. S. Bayer *et al.*, *Antimicrob. Ag. Chemother.*, 1978, *14*, 720. See also Enhanced Activity (below).

Diminished activity. The bactericidal activity of benzylpenicillin on *Vibrio cholerae* was suppressed by the addition of chloramphenicol, chlortetracycline, demeclocycline, erythromycin, kanamycin, neomycin, oleandomycin, oxytetracycline, paromomycin, streptomycin, or tetracycline. Bacitracin, cephalothin, colistin, cycloserine, polymyxin, and vancomycin did not affect the bactericidal properties of benzylpenicillin.— T. Chang and L. Weinstein (letter), *Nature*, 1966, *211*, 763.

There was no evidence of clinical antagonism between benzylpenicillin and chloramphenicol in 65 of 66 patients given both antibiotics for bronchitis or bronchopneumonia.— P. Ardalan, *Prax. Pneumol.*, 1969, *23*, 772.

Studies of the antibacterial action of chloramphenicol together with benzylpenicillin against *Neisseria meningitidis* showed that if chloramphenicol was present only in low concentrations (0.1 to 5 μg per ml) it antagonised the action of benzylpenicillin. However, chloramphenicol 10 μg per ml together with benzylpenicillin 0.6 μg per ml had the same rate of action as either drug alone.— E. Yourassowsky and R. Monsieur, *Arzneimittel-Forsch.*, 1971, *21*, 1385.

Chloroquine phosphate decreased the antibacterial effect *in vitro* of benzylpenicillin and phenoxymethylpenicillin against *Staph. aureus*.— M. A. Toama *et al.*, *J. pharm. Sci.*, 1978, *67*, 23.

Polymyxin B protected *Proteus mirabilis in vitro* against usually bactericidal concentrations of benzylpenicillin.— I. J. Sud and D. S. Feingold, *Antimicrob. Ag. Chemother.*, 1978, *14*, 916.

Enhanced activity. Benzylpenicillin had a greater enhanced activity *in vitro* when used with netilmicin or sissomicin than when used with streptomycin or kanamycin, against the majority of 14 streptomycin-susceptible strains of enterococci and against 6 strains that were resistant to streptomycin. The rate of killing was dependent on the concentration of the aminoglycoside used.— C. C. Sanders, *Antimicrob. Ag. Chemother.*, 1977, *12*, 195. The activities of benzylpenicillin and netilmicin were enhanced *in vitro* against 28 strains of *Streptococcus faecalis* when used together.— O. M. Korzeniowski *et al.*, *ibid.*, 1978, *13*, 430. See also J. Carrizosa and D. Kaye, *ibid.*, 505 (benzylpenicillin and netilmicin); F. Soriano and D. Greenwood, *J. clin. Path.*, 1979, *32*, 1174 (benzylpenicillin and gentamicin).

The MICs of benzylpenicillin or cephalothin *in vitro* against 55 penicillin-resistant strains of the *Bacteroides* spp. were reduced when used with clavulanic acid 1 or 5 μg per ml, but the MICs against resistant strains of *Clostridium clostridiiforme* and *Clostridium ramosum* were unaffected.— J. Wüst and T. D. Wilkins, *Antimicrob. Ag. Chemother.*, 1978, *13*, 130.

Benzylpenicillin or ampicillin in association with either streptomycin or gentamicin demonstrated enhanced bactericidal activity *in vitro* against 17 isolates of lactobacilli tolerant to benzylpenicillin and ampicillin. Combinations of benzylpenicillin with streptomycin or gentamicin were equally bactericidal and the activity of benzylpenicillin with streptomycin was statistically greater than that of ampicillin with streptomycin.— A. S. Bayer *et al.*, *Antimicrob. Ag. Chemother.*, 1980, *17*, 359.

Resistance. Resistance of micro-organisms to benzylpenicillin is usually natural and is associated with insensitive organisms and those which produce penicillinase, the enzyme which destroys the antibiotic. Resistance among staphylococci is common and the replacement of susceptible staphylococci by penicillinase-producing staphylococci has been responsible for the emergence of resistance in this organism, especially in hospitals.

Recently, two new mechanisms of resistance to penicillin have been reported, one where tolerance develops (L.D. Sabath *et al.*,*Lancet*, 1977, *1*, 443) and the other where penicillin is thought to be destroyed by an enzyme produced by the host cells (P. Barnes and P.M. Waterworth, *Br. med. J.*, 1977, *1*, 991; J. de Louvois and R. Hurley, *ibid.*, 998).

Penicillin-resistant strains of *Streptococcus pyogenes* and *Neisseria meningitidis* are rare, but reports of resistant *Str. pneumoniae* are increasing.

Some strains of *N. gonorrhoeae* have become less sensitive to penicillin and in 1976 the existence of a penicillinase-producing gonococcus was reported for the first time.

A 46-year-old man with a pleural effusion due to haemolytic group B streptococci sensitive to penicillin by the disk test failed to respond to vigorous treatment with benzylpenicillin. Aspirated pus contained no penicillin and was able to inactivate penicillin, 4 other penicillins, and 7 cephalosporins. It was considered that failure of treatment was due to an enzyme (not a β-lactamase) probably from the cell wall of the patient's leucocytes.— P. Barnes and P. M. Waterworth, *Br. med. J.*, 1977, *1*, 991. Four of 22 samples of human pus inactivated up to 95% of added penicillin within 1 hour *in vitro*; a similar effect, in 3 samples tested, occurred with cephaloridine and ampicillin, but not with streptomycin or fusidic acid. It was considered due to an enzyme in the pus, possibly an amidase; beta-lactamase was not detected.— J. de Louvois and R. Hurley, *ibid.*, 998. See also *ibid.*, 986.

For a possible association between the lipid content of the cell walls of Gram-negative organisms and their resistance to benzylpenicillin, see Ampicillin, p.1093.

Resistance of Bacteroides. Of 60 strains of *Bacteroides fragilis* 59 were resistant to benzylpenicillin.— O. A. Okubadejo *et al.*, *Br. med. J.*, 1973, *2*, 212.

Beta-lactamase-producing strains of *Bacteroides* spp. and *Staph. aureus* were present in the tonsils of 23 and 24 of 50 children with chronic recurrent tonsillitis, respectively. It was considered that these beta-lactamase-producing organisms might protect penicillin-susceptible group A β-haemolytic streptococci resulting in the failure of penicillin treatment.— I. Brook *et al.* (letter), *Lancet*, 1981, *1*, 332.

Resistance of gonococci. Discussions on the emergence of *Neisseria gonorrhoeae* resistant to penicillin: *Br. med. J.*, 1976, *2*, 963; *ibid.*, 1977, *1*, 1618; J. R. Saunders, *Nature*, 1977, *266*, 586; A. E. Wilkinson, *J. antimicrob. Chemother.*, 1977, *3*, 197; R. S. Morton, *Med. J. Aust.*, 1978, *2*, 95; *Lancet*, 1981, *1*, 816.

A report on the susceptibility patterns of 2 strains of *N. gonorrhoeae* which, although non-beta-lactamase producing, were unusually resistant to penicillin.— R. Shtibel (letter), *Lancet*, 1980, *2*, 39. Comments.— J. H. Darrell and R. S. Mitchison (letter), *ibid.*, 202; E. G. Dowsett (letter), *ibid.*; A. D. Seth and N. A. Johnston (letter), *ibid.*, 531.

A survey of beta-lactamase-producing gonococcal isolates reported in Great Britain. Epidemiological data suggest that there are 2 separate endemic zones of infection—one in South-east Asia and the other in West Africa. The penicillinase-producing *N. gonorrhoeae* (PPNG) from these 2 areas differ in auxotyping and in the molecular mass of the R plasmid. Epidemics caused by PPNG have been reported in a number of countries including Great Britain, the majority originating from the Far East and West Africa. The number of cases of PPNG infections reported in Great Britain since 1977 are: 1977, 15 cases; 1978, 31; 1979, 104; and 1980 (to October), 170. This compares with a total number of new cases of gonorrhoea reported annually of about 61 000. The majority of these PPNG infections were contracted overseas but in 1979, 41 patients (39%) reported contracting their infections in Great Britain. Although the current incidence of PPNG in Great Britain was low compared with that in Singapore and the Philippines, continued epidemiological assessment is essential.— N. A. Johnston *et al.*, *Lancet*, 1981, *1*, 263.

Further reports of beta-lactamase-producing penicillin-resistant gonococci.— I. Phillips, *Lancet*, 1976, *2*, 656; W. A. Ashford *et al.*, *ibid.*, 657; A. Percival *et al.*, *ibid.*, 1379; M. Lindon and G. Handke (letter), *Med. J. Aust.*, 1976, *2*, 660; K. S. Thompson (letter), *ibid.*, 1977, *1*, 676; A. F. Hallett *et al.* (letter), *Lancet*, 1977, *1*, 1205; L. P. Elwell *et al.*, *Antimicrob. Ag. Chemother.*, 1977, *11*, 528; G. Muller and N. Sonnichsen, *Dte GesundhWes.*, 1978, *33*, 1249, per *Int. pharm. Abstr.*, 1979, *16*, 31; R. N. Thin, *Br. J. vener. Dis.*, 1980, *56*, 193; H. Bijkerk, *ibid.*, 243; J. D. A. van Embden *et al.* (letter), *Lancet*, 1981, *1*, 938 (penicillinase-producing gonococci in the Netherlands carrying 'Africa' plasmid in association with transfer plasmid).

Resistance of meningococci. Over a 2-year period 8 patients with meningitis failed to respond to benzylpenicillin and culture of the isolated organism demonstrated penicillin-resistant *N. meningitidis*.— P. Contoyiannis and D. A. Adamopoulos (letter), *Lancet*, 1974, *1*, 462.

Resistance of staphylococci. Seven strains of *Staph. aureus* displayed a form of resistance to penicillins termed *tolerance* where the minimum inhibitory concentration was low but the minimum bactericidal concentration high.— L. D. Sabath *et al.*, *Lancet*, 1977, *1*, 443. Using a method that tests the entire bacterial population of the original blood culture, all of 34 bacteraemic strains of *Staph. aureus* were found to contain tolerant organisms, suggesting that all such strains contain tolerant bacteria.— H. E. Bradley *et al.* (letter), *ibid.*, 1979, *1*, 150. See also E. V. Haldane and S. Affias (letter), *ibid.*, 1977, *2*, 39; *Drugs*, 1977, *14*, 396. Comment on penicillin-tolerant bacteria and the view that laboratories should be prepared to measure MICs and MBCs of isolates from serious infections where delayed or poor response to therapy is unexplained. Disk sensitivity tests alone may be misleading.— *Lancet*, 1980, *1*, 856.

A beta-lactamase-producing strain of *Staph. aureus* was susceptible to benzylpenicillin; production of this enzyme did not necessarily afford resistance to the penicillins.— S. Sachithanandam *et al.*, *Antimicrob. Ag. Chemother.*, 1978, *13*, 289.

Of 200 strains of *Staph. aureus* 163 were resistant to penicillin, but patients were still responsive, probably because the strains produced only small amounts of penicillinase.— Z. A. Hassam *et al.*, *Br. med. J.*, 1978, *2*, 536.

See also under Resistance of Bacteroides (above).

Resistance of streptococci. The increasing resistance of pneumococci.— *Lancet*, 1977, *2*, 803. Of 866 strains of

Str. pneumoniae one had a reduced sensitivity to penicillin.— A. J. Howard *et al., Br. med. J.*, 1978, *1*, 1657. None of 74 recently isolated strains of *Str. pneumoniae* were highly resistant to benzylpenicillin and all but 5 had MICs of 0.062 µg or less per ml. The highest MIC was 0.5 µg per ml for one strain.— C. Watanakunakorn and C. Glotzbecker, *J. antimicrob. Chemother.*, 1980, *6*, 83.

Relative resistances to benzylpenicillin of 6 strains of *Str. pneumoniae* isolated in 1977 could be detected by a microdilution method but not by the standard disk diffusion test.— M. Tarpay, *Antimicrob. Ag. Chemother.*, 1978, *14*, 628.

After the isolation from a 3-year-old boy of a pneumococcus resistant to benzylpenicillin, erythromycin, clindamycin, tetracycline, chloramphenicol, and co-trimoxazole, screening of patients and staff in 2 hospitals in Johannesburg during August 1977 revealed that 160 of 543 patients and 8 of 434 staff were carriers of penicillin-resistant pneumococci although beta-lactamase activity could not be demonstrated. The majority were multi-resistant strains and were mainly carried by children under 3 years old who had received multiple antibiotics. The elimination of resistant pneumococci was attempted in all carriers and they were treated with rifampicin and fusidic acid, rifampicin and erythromycin, or minocycline. Resistance to rifampicin occurred during treatment in some strains. The empirical use of penicillin in the treatment of pneumococcal infection was no longer justified. Worldwide surveillance was necessary to assess the prevalence of resistant strains and if these spread, prophylaxis with pneumococcal vaccine might be useful, although the protection afforded to children under 2 years old was uncertain.— M. R. Jacobs *et al., New Engl. J. Med.*, 1978, *299*, 735. See also M. Finland, *ibid.*, 770; M. R. Jacobs and H. J. Koornhof, *J. antimicrob. Chemother.*, 1978, *4*, 481; H. J. Koornhof *et al., Morb. Mortal.*, 1978, *27*, 1; J. R. Armstrong and S. L. Narasimhan (letter), *New Engl. J. Med.*, 1979, *300*, 499; D. Hansman (letter), *ibid.*; M. R. Jacobs *et al.* (letter), *ibid.*; S. David (letter), *ibid.*, 500; M. Finland (letter), *ibid.*

Findings of a high prevalence of penicillin-insensitive pneumococci in Port Moresby, Papua New Guinea. Among resistant strains MICs of benzylpenicillin ranged from 0.1 to 1.0 µg per ml. Hence they are unlikely to cause therapeutic problems in the treatment of pneumonia since high plasma concentrations of benzylpenicillin are readily obtained. The situation is different in meningitis, however, since even when the meninges are inflamed peak concentrations of benzylpenicillin in the CSF are only about 1 µg per ml. All the strains encountered in the present study were sensitive to chloramphenicol and also to erythromycin, lincomycin, and tetracycline. Therefore, chloramphenicol can be used as an alternative to penicillin in the treatment of pneumococcal meningitis in Papua New Guinea.— M. Gratten *et al., Lancet*, 1980, *2*, 192. Comment.— M. A. Knowles and G. C. Turner (letter), *ibid.*, 478.

Further reports of penicillin-resistant pneumococci.— D. Hansman and M. M. Bullen (letter), *Lancet*, 1967, *2*, 264; L. Devitt *et al., Med. J. Aust.*, 1977, *1*, 586; P. C. Appelbaum *et al., Lancet*, 1977, *2*, 995; J. M. S. Dixon *et al., Can. med. Ass. J.*, 1977, *117*, 1159; R. C. Cooksey *et al., Antimicrob. Ag. Chemother.*, 1978, *13*, 645; D. Hansman, *Med. J. Aust.*, 1978, *2*, 295; G. A. Ahronheim *et al., Am. J. Dis. Child.*, 1979, *133*, 187; H. F. Pabst and J. Nigrin (letter), *Lancet*, 1979, *2*, 359; D. C. Shanson *et al.* (letter), *ibid.*, 956; A. J. Saah *et al., J. Am. med. Ass.*, 1980, *243*, 1824.

Reports of penicillin-tolerant streptococci: J. T. Noble *et al.* (letter), *Lancet*, 1980, *2*, 982 (group G streptococci); D. Portnoy *et al., Can. med. Ass. J.*, 1980, *122*, 69 (bacterial endocarditis due to a penicillin-tolerant group C streptococcus). See also *Lancet*, 1980, *1*, 856.

Absorption and Fate. Benzylpenicillin rapidly appears in the blood following intramuscular injection of water-soluble salts, and maximum concentrations are usually reached in 15 to 30 minutes; peak plasma concentrations of about 12 µg per ml have been reported after doses of 600 mg with therapeutic plasma concentrations for most susceptible organisms detectable for about 5 hours.

Though plasma-penicillin concentrations do not necessarily indicate those that can be expected to prevail in the tissues, they are a useful guide to dosage. The minimum inhibitory concentration of benzylpenicillin ranges from 0.006 to 2 µg per ml and optimum bactericidal concentrations are considered to be 5 to 10 times greater. Higher concentrations are required for less sensitive organisms.

When given by mouth, benzylpenicillin is inactivated fairly rapidly by the acid gastric secretions and only about 30% is absorbed, albeit rapidly, mainly from the duodenum. Buffers have been given simultaneously in an attempt to reduce the destruction by gastric secretions but excess of alkalis must be avoided since they also destroy the antibiotic.

Absorption is somewhat slower after oral than after intramuscular administration and the maximum plasma-penicillin concentration may not be attained for about an hour. In order to attain plasma-penicillin concentrations after oral administration comparable to those following intramuscular injection, up to 5 times as much benzylpenicillin may be necessary. Absorption varies greatly in different individuals and is better in patients suffering from gastric hypoacidity; in infants, whose acidity is low, absorption is almost complete. Absorption may also be increased in elderly patients as their gastric acidity decreases.

Food reduces the absorption of benzylpenicillin and oral doses are best given no later than half an hour before and no earlier than 2 to 3 hours after a meal.

Some of the less soluble penicillins, such as phenoxymethylpenicillin and benzathine penicillin, are more resistant to inactivation by gastric secretions and are better absorbed from the gastro-intestinal tract.

Benzylpenicillin is widely distributed at varying concentrations in body tissues and fluids. It appears in pleural, pericardial, peritoneal, and synovial fluids but diffuses less readily into the eye and only to a small extent into abscess cavities and avascular areas. Inflamed tissue is more readily penetrated.

Benzylpenicillin diffuses across the placenta into the foetal circulation, and small amounts appear in the milk of nursing mothers, but very little passes into the CSF, unless the meninges are inflamed.

The plasma half-life is about 30 minutes although it may be longer in infants and the elderly because of incomplete renal function. Approximately 45 to 65% is reported to be bound to plasma protein.

It is rapidly excreted by the renal tubules, causing a steep decline in plasma-penicillin concentrations and about 20% of a dose given by mouth appears in the urine. About 60 to 90% of a dose of aqueous benzylpenicillin given intramuscularly appears in the urine, usually in the first hour. Significant concentrations are achieved in bile. However, in patients with normal renal function only small amounts are excreted via the bile and as penicillin is destroyed by penicillinase-producing micro-organisms in the lower gastro-intestinal tract, little or none appears in the faeces.

Tubular excretion is inhibited by probenecid (see p.420), which is sometimes given to increase plasma-penicillin concentrations.

A discussion on the metabolism of benzylpenicillin in premature and full-term infants.— H. D. Riley, *J. clin. Pharmac.*, 1967, *7*, 312. Absorption in full-term infants.— G. H. McCracken *et al., J. Pediat.*, 1973, *82*, 692.

The biological half-life of benzylpenicillin was 0.5 to 1 hour; in renal failure this might be increased to 7 to 10 hours.— W. A. Ritschel, *Drug Intell. & clin. Pharm.*, 1970, *4*, 332.

The half-life of benzylpenicillin when infused in doses to achieve a continuous serum concentration of 0.56 µg per ml was increased by probenecid. However, when given in doses to achieve a concentration of 6 µg per ml, the half-life was not significantly increased. Phenoxymethylpenicillin by mouth had a similar effect to probenecid and was considered preferable due to its own antibiotic properties.— K. H. Spitzy *et al., Advances in Antimicrobial and Antineoplastic Chemotherapy*, Vol. I, pt 1, Munich, Urban and Schwarzenberg, 1972, p. 47.

Studies in 61 patients aged 20 to 91 years showed an inverse relationship between serum-benzylpenicillin half-life which varied from 16 to 164 minutes and endogenous creatinine clearance which varied from 168 to 9 ml per minute. The older the patient the lower the creatinine clearance and the longer the serum half-life. Aspirin, indomethacin, phenylbutazone, probenecid, sulphinpyrazone, and sulphaphenazole prolonged benzylpenicillin half-life.— J. Kampmann *et al., Clin. Pharmac. Ther.*, 1972, *13*, 516.

A mean of 19% of a 300 mg intramuscular dose of benzylpenicillin was recovered as penicilloic acid from the urine of 6 healthy subjects.— M. Cole *et al., Antimicrob. Ag. Chemother.*, 1973, *3*, 463.

A review of the pharmacokinetics of the penicillins.— M. Barza and L. Weinstein, *Clin. Pharmacokinet.*, 1976, *1*, 297.

There were sex-linked differences in the kinetics of benzylpenicillin and other antibiotics but dosage modification was not required.— J. F. Giudicelli and J. P. Tillement, *Clin. Pharmacokinet.*, 1977, *2*, 157.

Diffusion into body fluids and tissues. Benzylpenicillin was found in fluid from the middle ear of patients with secretory or acute suppurative otitis media who had been given intramuscular injections 1 to 3 hours previously. When oxytetracycline was used concentrations were only found in those patients with acute suppurative otitis media.— H. Silverstein *et al., Pediatrics*, 1966, *38*, 33.

In 3 patients given a dose of 600 mg of benzylpenicillin intramuscularly, concentrations of 0.5 to 2.6 µg per ml were found in bile 1 hour later and peak concentrations of 10 to 20 µg per ml were reached 2 to 4 hours after the injection.— G. Acocella *et al., Gut*, 1968, *9*, 536.

Benzylpenicillin, 1.92 g given intravenously when the meninges were not inflamed, produced concentrations in most specimens of brain tissue sufficient to inhibit sensitive Gram-positive cocci.— P. W. Kramer *et al., J. Neurosurg.*, 1969, *31*, 295.

Benzylpenicillin, 14.5 mg to 40 mg per kg body-weight intramuscularly or intravenously or 75 mg per kg daily by continuous infusion, was administered to 4 children with septic joint disease. Synovial fluid withdrawn 0.25 to 6 hours after a dose contained 0.08 to 5.4 µg per ml of penicillin; the concentrations were generally 50% or more of the serum concentrations.— J. D. Nelson, *New Engl. J. Med.*, 1971, *284*, 349.

Benzylpenicillin in high concentrations killed gonococci within phagocytes. Low concentrations only killed the extracellular organisms.— D. R. Veale *et al., Lancet*, 1975, *1*, 306.

Tissue concentrations in human tonsils of benzylpenicillin, ampicillin, and lincomycin given intravenously before tonsillectomy.— J. Gabka and W. Platz, *Arzneimittel-Forsch.*, 1978, *28*, 87.

A study of penicillin concentrations in serum and CSF of patients receiving different preparations of penicillin to treat late-acquired or congenital syphilis.— E. M. C. Dunlop *et al., J. Am. med. Ass.*, 1979, *241*, 2538.

Elimination in renal failure. The penicillin half-life in serum was prolonged in 10 uraemic patients who were given 3 g of benzylpenicillin intravenously when compared with 10 normal subjects given the same dose. A logarithmic relationship was established between rising half-life of serum penicillin, falling rate of glomerular filtration, and effective renal plasma flow.— M. E. Plaut *et al., J. Lab. clin. Med.*, 1969, *74*, 12.

Protein binding. A study of protein binding of penicillins to human serum albumin.— H. Zia *et al., Can. J. pharm. Sci.*, 1980, *15*, 14.

Uses. Benzylpenicillin is used in the treatment of a variety of infections due to susceptible organisms, including wound infections, abscesses, boils, diphtheria, acute tonsillitis, actinomycosis, anthrax, gas gangrene, tetanus, erysipelas, pneumococcal pneumonia, scarlet fever, rheumatic fever, some types of subacute bacterial endocarditis, acute osteomyelitis, otitis media, mastoiditis, meningococcal infections, Vincent's infection, gonorrhoea, syphilis, rat-bite fever, leptospirosis, yaws, and pinta.

Benzylpenicillin is also used prophylactically before dental and surgical procedures in patients at risk of developing endocarditis and to prevent a recurrence of rheumatic fever. Whenever possible, cultural identification of the infecting organism and sensitivity tests should be carried out, but treatment should be started immediately in severe infections that are suspected to be caused by organisms normally sensitive to benzylpenicillin. When the results of the sensitivity tests are known the dosage and frequency of administration can be adjusted or another antibiotic used if necessary.

The dose of benzylpenicillin should be sufficient to achieve an optimum bactericidal concentration in the blood as rapidly as possible, and for many of the infections listed above doses of 300 to 600 mg two to four times daily, by intramuscular or intravenous injection, are adequate. Infants and children from 1 month to 12 years may be given 10 to 20 mg per kg body-weight daily in divided doses, neonates may be given 30 mg per kg daily.

In subacute bacterial endocarditis prolonged treatment is required and, depending on the organism responsible, 3 to 18 g daily by intermittent intravenous injection or by continuous infusion, sometimes together with an aminoglycoside such as streptomycin, may be necessary to clear all bacteria from the vegetations. Doses of at least 24 g daily may be needed when the organism is relatively resistant. Treatment should continue for 4 to 6 weeks.

A continuous serum-penicillin concentration of just above 0.018 µg per ml is effective in the treatment of syphilis when maintained for at least 7 to 10 days, but in practice the concentration is often maintained for at least 15 to 20 days. Treatment with parenteral penicillin is therefore more easily carried out using slow-release preparations such as benzathine penicillin (see p.1101) or procaine penicillin (see p.1206).

Despite the changing sensitivity pattern of *Neisseria gonorrhoeae* and the emergence of penicillinase-producing strains, penicillin is still the treatment of first choice for gonorrhoea in many parts of the world. The usual dose is 3 g intramuscularly given with probenecid, usually 1 g. Procaine penicillin is also used, and is often preferred.

In the treatment of meningeal infections, doses of 600 mg to 1.8 g are given, usually intravenously, every 2 to 4 hours for about 2 weeks. Intrathecal injections are not often used but where they are felt to be necessary in severely ill patients then 6 to 12 mg is given daily. The dose administered intrathecally should never exceed 12 mg. Children may be treated with daily intravenous doses of 40 to 240 mg per kg body-weight; in some instances intrathecal injections of 1.5 to 3 mg have been used.

For intramuscular administration, doses up to 300 mg should be dissolved in 1 ml of Water for Injections and larger doses in 2 ml. All except very weak solutions are hyperosmotic and sodium chloride injection should not be used as the solvent. For intrathecal injection, benzylpenicillin 6 mg is usually dissolved in 10 ml of sodium chloride injection or cerebrospinal fluid and injected slowly.

In some severe infections, such as subacute bacterial endocarditis, meningitis, and peritonitis, doses of at least 24 g daily may be necessary and can be given by intermittent intravenous injection or continuous infusion. It has been recommended that intravenous doses of benzypenicillin above 1.2 g should be administered slowly at not more than 300 mg per minute to avoid irritation of the central nervous system.

For subconjunctival injection, 300 mg of benzylpenicillin may be dissolved in 0.5 ml of lignocaine and adrenaline injection, or other suitable solvent. Benzylpenicillin has been given by mouth in a dose ranging from 0.5 to 3 g daily in the treatment of infections of moderate severity but one of the acid-resistant penicillins, such as phenoxymethylpenicillin, is preferred.

Actinomycosis. High doses of 6 to 12 g of benzylpenicillin daily for 6 to 8 weeks were recommended in the treatment of abdominal actinomycosis since various bacteria, apart from *Actinomyces israelii*, had been isolated from the abscess.— H. J. Klasen, *Ned. Tijdschr. Geneesk.*, 1971, *115*, 1212.

Treatment of actinomycosis consisted of benzylpenicillin 1.2 g every 8 hours for 6 weeks followed by a 6-week course of procaine penicillin 600 mg once or twice daily, together with an oral penicillin. Streptomycin, tetracycline, or a sulphonamide might be added if indicated by sensitivity tests.— A. Sakula, *Practitioner*, 1974, *212*, 335.

Further references: M. Fradis *et al.*, *Archs Otolar.*, 1976, *102*, 87.

Amanita poisoning. The technique of using large doses of penicillin to treat amanita poisoning was based on displacing the toxins from serum albumin. However, equilibrium dialysis failed to reveal any binding, thus if penicillin was effective then another mechanism was involved.— L. Fiume *et al.* (letter), *Lancet*, 1977, *1*, 1111.

The intravenous infusion of benzylpenicillin sodium had a beneficial effect in *dogs* given sublethal doses of *Amanita phalloides* and the effect of combined treatment with silymarin required further investigation.— G. L. Floersheim *et al.*, *Toxic. appl. Pharmac.*, 1978, *46*, 455.

Anthrax. Two men developed cutaneous anthrax after contact with infected bone meal. One patient, who also had a *Staphylococcus epidermidis* infection, recovered after treatment with benzylpenicillin, 600 mg six-hourly for 12 days, but the second patient showed little improvement after 24 hours following treatment with benzylpenicillin 600 mg every 4 hours and streptomycin by parenteral injection was added for 5 days. A hypersensitivity reaction after 7 days led to replacement of penicillin with tetracycline, 250 mg six-hourly, for a further 10 days. In both patients, oedema subsided after a week's treatment, with resolution of scabs 4 weeks and 3 months later respectively.— A. H. Knight *et al.*, *Br. med. J.*, 1969, *1*, 416.

A further reference: H. A. Ronaghy *et al.*, *Curr. ther. Res.*, 1972, *14*, 721.

Arthritis, gonococcal. The recommended treatment for gonococcal arthritis was 300 mg of benzylpenicillin by injection 4-hourly until the acute joint inflammation subsided, usually within 3 to 7 days, followed by either 2 g of phenoxymethylpenicillin by mouth daily, or aqueous procaine penicillin 360 mg intramuscularly every 12 hours, for 2 weeks. Intra-articular injections of penicillin were not advised.— H. Keiser *et al.*, *New Engl. J. Med.*, 1968, *279*, 234.

Benzylpenicillin, 720 mg given every 12 hours by intramuscular injection together with probenecid, 500 mg four times daily to 1 patient, or as intravenous injections of benzylpenicillin, 6 g daily for 10 days, to another was successfully used in the treatment of 2 women with gonococcal arthritis.— A. Fam *et al.*, *Can. med. Ass. J.*, 1973, *108*, 319.

Cataract extraction. Postoperative subconjunctival injections of benzylpenicillin 120 mg in conjunction with either streptomycin 20 000 units or colistin sulphomethate sodium 20 mg were effective in preventing endophthalmitis following cataract extraction in 1212 patients; the injections were well tolerated even in patients hypersensitive to penicillin.— J. R. Cassidy, *Am. J. Ophthal.*, 1967, *64*, 1081.

Dental prophylaxis. For references to the prophylactic use of benzylpenicillin before dental procedures in patients at special risk, see under Endocarditis (below) and Prophylactic Use of Antibiotics, p.1080.

Dosage in infants and children. By intramuscular injection the total daily dose of benzylpenicillin in children should be 12 to 30 mg per kg body-weight and by intravenous injection 12 to 300 mg per kg daily. Neonates should receive 30 mg per kg daily in 2 or 3 doses.— M. I. Marks *et al.*, *Can. med. Ass. J.*, 1973, *109*, 309.

The suggested dose of benzylpenicillin for infants of more than 37 weeks' gestation was 30 mg per kg body-weight given intramuscularly or intravenously, by very slow bolus injection, every 12 hours for the first 48 hours of life, every 8 hours from the 3rd day to 2 weeks, then every 6 hours. For immature infants (those of less than 37 weeks' gestation) this dose should be given every 12 hours for the first week of life, every 8 hours from then to 4 weeks of age, and every 6 hours thereafter.— P. A. Davies, *Br. med. J.*, 1978, *2*, 676.

Further references: H. C. Spratt, *Drugs*, 1978, *16*, 226; G. H. McCracken and H. F. Eichenwald, *J. Pediat.*, 1978, *93*, 357; H. B. Valman, *Br. med. J.*, 1980, *280*, 457.

Dosage in renal failure. A method for achieving optimal serum-benzylpenicillin concentrations in patients with renal failure. Daily maintenance dose of benzylpenicillin in units = total plasma clearance of benzylpenicillin (ml per min) multiplied by the desired mean serum-benzylpenicillin concentration (µg per ml) and by 2300.— C. S. Bryan and W. J. Stone, *Ann. intern. Med.*, 1975, *82*, 189.

Data for predicting removal of benzylpenicillin by conventional haemodialysis.— T. P. Gibson and H. A. Nelson, *Clin. Pharmacokinet.*, 1977, *2*, 403.

The normal half-life for benzylpenicillin of 0.5 hour was increased to 6 to 20 hours in end-stage renal failure. The interval between doses should be extended from 8 hours to 8 to 12 hours in patients with a glomerular filtration-rate (GFR) between 10 and 50 ml per minute and to 12 to 18 hours when the GFR is less than 10 ml per minute. Alternatively, doses could be reduced to 75% of the standard dose when the GFR is between 10 and 50 ml per minute and to 25 to 50% in patients with a GFR below 10 ml per minute. Concentrations of benzylpenicillin were affected by haemodialysis but not by peritoneal dialysis.— W. M. Bennett *et al.*, *Ann. intern. Med.*, 1980, *93*, 62. Further references: C. M. Kunin, *Ann intern. Med.*, 1967, *67*, 151; D. L. Giusti, *Drug Intell. & clin. Pharm.*, 1973, *7*, 62; P. Sharpstone, *Br. med. J.*, 1977, *2*, 36; G. B. Appel and H. C. Neu, *New Engl. J. Med.*, 1977, *296*, 663.

Endocarditis. Reviews of the recommended treatment for bacterial endocarditis.— R. Benn, *Drugs*, 1976, *12*, 374; C. Oakley, *Br. med. J.*, 1978, *2*, 489 and 804.

In patients with undiagnosed bacterial endocarditis, penicillin 24 g intravenously and streptomycin 1 g daily, were the basis of treatment. Penicillin was administered in intermittent high doses; massive doses were effective even with organisms of low sensitivity. Methicillin replaced penicillin if no response occurred in 72 hours. In patients allergic to penicillin, cephalothin was used.— *Med. J. Aust.*, 1970, *1*, 1132.

In the treatment of endocarditis due to group D streptococci benzylpenicillin or ampicillin had a synergistic effect with kanamycin or gentamicin.— C. J. Wilkowske *et al.*, *Antimicrob. Ag. Chemother.*, 1970, 195. There was no additional benefit when gentamicin was added to treatment with benzylpenicillin, methicillin, or nafcillin in 40 patients with endocarditis due to *Staph. aureus*.— C. Watanakunakorn and I. Baird, *Am. J. med. Sci.*, 1977, *273*, 133.

Four patients with enterococcal endocarditis and 2 with enterococcal meningitis were successfully treated with benzylpenicillin and gentamicin. Doses of gentamicin ranged from 60 to 100 mg every 8 hours and for penicillin were 12 to 18 g every 24 hours; treatment lasted 11 to 42 days.— A. J. Weinstein and R. C. Moellering, *J. Am. med. Ass.*, 1973, *223*, 1030. Criticism of the use of gentamicin with benzylpenicillin in the early stages of the treatment of enterococcal endocarditis because of the possibility of nephrotoxicity. The use of streptomycin with benzylpenicillin was recommended.— D. Kaye *et al.* (letter), *ibid.*, *224*, 1426.

There was enhanced antibacterial activity when penicillin and streptomycin were tested together against *Streptococcus viridans*. The mixture was used successfully in the treatment of 35 patients with endocarditis due to penicillin-sensitive *Str. viridans*.— J. C. Wolfe and W. D. Johnson, *Ann. intern. Med.*, 1974, *81*, 178.

A report of endocarditis associated with *Cardiobacterium hominis* in 4 patients. Treatment with benzylpenicillin or ampicillin 12 g daily for 3 weeks was suggested when the presence of a Gram-negative, facultatively anaerobic organism was demonstrated in patients with endocarditis in natural heart valves.— J. E. Geraci *et al.*, *Mayo Clin. Proc.*, 1978, *53*, 49.

A favourable report of the use of benzylpenicillin with gentamicin in infective endocarditis due to *Actinobacillus actinomycetemcomitans*.— G. Lalonde and R. Hand, *Can. med. Ass. J.*, 1980, *122*, 316.

See also under Choice of An Antibiotic (p.1078).

Prophylaxis. To reduce the risk of endocarditis in persons with rheumatic heart diseases who were to undergo dental extraction or operation such as tonsillectomy, the following bactericidal regimen, to be commenced an hour beforehand, was advocated: benzylpenicillin 180 mg and procaine penicillin 300 mg given intramuscularly; followed, 6 to 12 hours after operation, by a further 300 mg of procaine penicillin. This could be followed, in cases of doubt, by oral treatment with phenoxymethylpenicillin 250 mg or benzylpenicillin 300 mg given every 6 hours for 2 days. In patients already receiving penicillin prophylactically, where there was a risk of infection by penicillin-resistant organisms, alternative protection with tetracycline, erythromycin, or vancomycin should be considered.— *Prevention of Initial Attacks and Recurrences of Rheumatic Fever*, London, Ministry of Health, 1965.

Despite antibiotic cover with total doses of 2.4 g of benzylpenicillin and 4.5 g of cloxacillin for a dental operation, a patient developed endocarditis caused by penicillin-sensitive streptococci.— D. T. Durack and W. A. Littler (letter), *Lancet*, 1974, *2*, 846.

A study of the efficacy of penicillin prophylaxis in children with cardiac disease known to be at risk for bacterial endocarditis indicated that testing of the MBC is the only reliable method of determining penicillin resistance in viridans streptococci and endurance and tolerance should be considered when penicillin prophylaxis for bacterial endocarditis fails.— Y. Holloway *et al.* (letter), *Lancet*, 1980, *1*, 589. See also L. Pulliam *et al.* (letter), *Lancet*, 1979, *2*, 957 (further reference to penicillin tolerance).

See also under Prophylactic Use of Antibiotics, p.1080.

Eye infections. Four cases of gonorrhoeal ophthalmia, 2 in infants and 2 in young adults, responded rapidly to local treatment with eye-drops, which contained benzylpenicillin 6 mg per ml, instilled initially every 15 minutes. Penicillin was also given intramuscularly.— T. Hansen *et al.* (letter), *J. Am. med. Ass.*, 1966, *195*, 1156. This was still the recommended treatment.— J. L. Baum, *New Engl. J. Med.*, 1978, *299*, 28.

Propylaxis. Gonococcal ophthalmia could be prevented in the newborn infant by instilling 1 or 2 drops of penicillin eye-drops containing 6 mg per ml or by applying a penicillin eye ointment containing 0.6 or 60 mg per g. Intramuscular injections of 30 to 60 mg could also be used.— *Med. Lett.*, 1970, *12*, 38. The preferred method of prophylaxis against *Neisseria gonorrhoeae* in neonates was still the use of silver nitrate 1% eye-drops.— J. L. Baum, *New Engl. J. Med.*, 1978, *299*, 28.

Gonorrhoea. Probenecid 1 g by mouth together with benzylpenicillin sodium 3 g administered in 8 ml of 0.5% lignocaine solution intramuscularly was effective in the treatment of 99% of 832 patients with gonorrhoea. There was a marked improvement in the sensitivity *in vitro* of *Neisseria gonorrhoeae* during the period of the study.— G. A. Olsen and G. Lomholt, *Br. J. vener. Dis.*, 1969, *45*, 144. See also R. C. F. Gray *et al.*, *ibid.*, 1970, *46*, 401.

From a comparison of various treatment regimens in 98 patients with the gonococcal arthritis-dermatitis syndrome the following were recommended in uncomplicated infection: benzylpenicillin, at least 6 g daily, intravenously for about 3 days followed by ampicillin 2 g daily by mouth to complete at least 10 days of treatment, or a loading dose of ampicillin 3.5 g with probenecid 1 g followed by ampicillin 2 g daily for 7 to 14 days.— H. H. Handsfield *et al.*, *Ann. intern. Med.*, 1976, *84*, 661. See also R. M. Blankenship *et al.*, *New Engl. J. Med.*, 1974, *290*, 267.

Benzylpenicillin 3 g intramuscularly given with probenecid 1 or 2 g by mouth was a recommended single-dose regimen for the treatment of gonorrhoea.— *Neisseria gonorrhoeae and gonococcal infections*, Report of a WHO Scientific Group, *Tech. Rep. Ser. Wld Hlth Org. No. 616*, 1978.

See also under Choice of an Antibiotic, p.1078.

Intrathecal administration. The usual intrathecal dose of benzylpenicillin was 6 mg dissolved in 10 ml of sodium chloride injection and injected slowly once daily. For infants and children 100 µg per kg body-weight, diluted appropriately, was recommended.— F. C. Wood and C. Dash, *Glaxo* (letter), *Br. med. J.*, 1978, *2*, 1090. A view that penicillin should not be administered intrathecally to children since it had no therapeutic value and dosage errors were often made, with fatal results.— H. B. Valman, *Br. med. J.*, 1980, *280*, 1588.

Leptospirosis. Penicillin 1.44 g daily had been recommended for the treatment of leptospirosis if treatment was started before the fourth day of illness. The initial dose should be 3.6 to 6 g if treatment was started on the fourth day or later and treatment continued for 6 days with a daily dose of 1.44 g. In very ill patients, up to 24 g of penicillin should be given on the first day in intravenous fluids. Leptospirosis could also be treated with tetracycline, 2 g daily for 7 days. Of patients with leptospirosis given 360 mg of penicillin 4-hourly for the first 24 hours, then 6-hourly, 83% suffered Herxheimer reactions.— L. H. Turner, *Br. med. J.*, 1969, *1*, 231. See also Report of a WHO Expert Group on Current Problems in Leptospirosis Research, *Tech. Rep. Ser. Wld Hlth Org. No. 380*, 1967; A. Sakula and W. Moore, *Br. med. J.*, 1969, *1*, 226.

Penicillin was not considered to have any value in the treatment of leptospirosis even when given in the early stages.— R. D. Lockhart (letter), *Br. med. J.*, 1973, *3*, 173.

In 8 patients with leptospirosis treated in the early stages with penicillin, the cell count of the CSF in the second week was significantly lower than in 18 patients not given penicillin. Penicillin given in the early stages appeared to be of some benefit.— J. H. Lawson (letter), *Br. med. J.*, 1973, *4*, 109.

Lyme disease. A report of the beneficial effect of benzylpenicillin in the treatment of Lyme disease (erythema chronicum migrans).— A. C. Steere *et al.*, *Ann. intern. Med.*, 1980, *93*, 1.

Meningitis. A prospective study of the pharmacokinetics of benzylpenicillin in 24 children aged 2 weeks to 11 years with pneumococcal, group A streptococcal, or meningococcal meningitis. Therapy was initiated with chloramphenicol 100 mg per kg body-weight daily intraveneously in 4 divided doses (discontinued as soon as the organism had been identified), together with benzylpenicillin 150 mg per kg daily in 6 divided doses infused intravenously over a 15-minute period. The mean CSF-penicillin concentration was 800 ng per ml throughout the 4-hour dosage interval on the first day, declining to 700 ng per ml on the fifth day, and 300 ng per ml on the tenth;expressing this as a percentage of the simultaneous serum concentration the mean of all values regardless of time was 18.4% on the first day declining to 9.9% and 4.9% on the fifth and tenth days respectively; this pattern correlated with return of the CSF protein pattern to normal. All CSF cultures obtained 18 to 24 hours after the onset of therapy were sterile and a mean peak concentration of penicillin in CSF of 960 ng per ml was obtained at least transiently on all 3 study days half to 1 hour after infusion, suggesting that the treatment regimen was adequate. Higher dosages might, however, be necessary for organisms with an unusually high MIC to penicillin; in view of wide variations from the mean found in this and other studies, monitoring of CSF-penicillin concentrations might also be indicated for such cases.— J. P. Hieber and J. D. Nelson, *New Engl. J. Med.*, 1977, *297*, 410.

Further references: V. Vic-Dupont *et al.*, *Presse méd.*, 1969, *77*, 155.

See also Choice of an Antibiotic, p.1079.

For a comparison of benzylpenicillin and chloramphenicol in the treatment of group A meningococcal meningitis, see Chloramphenicol, p.1140.

Meningococcal infections. A discussion on meningococcal septicaemia; the antibiotic of choice is benzylpenicillin given by intramuscular or intravenous injection.— *Br. med. J.*, 1979, *2*, 953.

See also Meningitis, above.

Prophylaxis. A recommendation that a mouth-to-mouth resuscitation contact of a patient with meningococcal infection should be admitted to hospital and started on 7.2 g of benzylpenicillin intravenously over 24 hours, after blood has been drawn for culture. The patients are discharged 2 days later if they remain free of symptoms and if blood cultures are sterile.— M. R. Achong (letter), *Lancet*, 1979, *2*, 1025. Experience over the past 22 years has indicated that the risk is negligible.— S. S. Cutler (letter), *ibid.*, 1074.

Paresis. New neurological signs were found in 25 of 64 patients who had been treated for paresis with penicillin. The proportion of patients with new neurological signs was 3 times greater in patients who had been given penicillin and malaria treatment than in those treated with penicillin alone. Courses of penicillin treatment ranged from 1.8 to 18 g; there was no correlation between size of dose and the likelihood of developing new symptoms.— E. Wilner and J. A. Brody, *Lancet*, 1968, *2*, 1370.

Pelvic inflammatory disease. Reference to the use of benzylpenicillin in pelvic inflammatory disease: G. Schnider *et al.*, *Obstet. Gynec.*, 1979, *54*, 554; C. J. Van Gelderen, *S.Afr. med. J.*, 1980, *58*, 246.

Pneumococcal infection prophylaxis. Prophylactic penicillin 125 mg twice daily indefinitely was recommended after splenectomy in patients with thalassaemia.— B. Modell, *Archs Dis. Childh.*, 1977, *52*, 489.

Pneumococcal vaccine (Pneumovax) failed to protect 2 children with sickle-cell anaemia from penumococcal infection. Apart from the problem of penicillin-resistant pneumococci, the usefulness of long-term prophylaxis with penicillin in such patients has been limited by poor patient compliance. However, since the calculated protective effect of the vaccine is only about 50%, patients homozygous for sickle-cell disease should receive penicillin prophylaxis starting at 6-months-old and pneumococcal vaccination when they are at least 2-years-old.— V. I. Ahonkhai *et al.*, *New Engl. J. Med.*, 1979, *301*, 26.

Rheumatic fever. A recommended treatment for acute rheumatism in children was benzylpenicillin 300 mg twice daily by intramuscular injection for at least 10 days, followed by phenoxymethylpenicillin 250 mg twice daily by mouth.— R. G. Mitchell, *Practitioner*, 1972, *208*, 86.

Prophylaxis. For the use of benzylpenicillin in the prophylaxis of rheumatic fever, see Prophylactic Use of Antibiotics, p.1080.

Skin infections. An outbreak of idiopathic erysipelas in a psychiatric hospital, unresponsive to ampicillin, was successfully controlled by benzylpenicillin. The organism was identified as group A streptococcus M-type 1.— E. G. Dowsett, *Br. med. J.*, 1975, *1*, 500.

Streptococcal infections, other. A brief discussion on the treatment of infections produced by Lancefield group B streptococci.— R. G. Finch, *J. antimicrob. Chemother.*, 1978, *4*, 198.

Prophylaxis in neonates. A discussion on the prevention of group B streptococcal infections in neonates.— *Lancet*, 1978, *2*, 1240. Comment.— I. Blumenthal (letter), *ibid.*, 1383.

During a review period from January 1969 to May 1974, of 1208 infants with a gestational age less than 35 weeks, 11 had early-onset group B streptococcal septicaemia and 10 died. Benzylpenicillin 30 to 60 mg per kg body-weight intravenously or intramuscularly daily was then administered within 2 hours of birth to all infants with a gestational age less than 35 weeks (or subsequently weighing less than 2500 g). Of 983 infants given penicillin only one developed group B streptococcal septicaemia and none died.— D. J. Lloyd *et al.*, *Lancet*, 1979, *1*, 713. Findings at variance.— R. S. Ramamurthy *et al.* (letter), *ibid.*, *2*, 246. Rearrangement by D.J. Lloyd *et al.* (*Lancet*, 1979, *1*, 713) of their data into weight groups, and into infants who did and did not receive penicillin might improve the case for the efficacy of penicillin prophylaxis. The wisdom of the proposal of A.J. Steigman *et al.* (*Pediatrics*, 1978, *62*, 842) for controlled studies seems more compelling than ever.— B. F. Anthony (letter), *ibid.*, 751. A controlled study over 25 months in 18 738 newborn infants to determine the effect of a single intramuscular dose of benzylpenicillin, given within one hour of delivery, on the incidence of neonatal group B streptococcal infections. Although the suppressive effect of prophylactic benzylpenicillin on colonisation and disease rates due to penicillin-susceptible organisms was encouraging, routine administration at birth cannot be recommended until the effect on the incidence of disease caused by penicillin-resistant pathogens has been fully defined.— J. D. Siegel, *New Engl. J. Med.*, 1980, *303*, 769. Further comments.— S. P. Gotoff and K. M. Boyer (letter), *ibid.*, 1981, *304*, 484; A. M. Walker and K. J. Rothman (letter), *ibid.*, 485; J. D. Siegel *et al.* (letter), *ibid.*

Surgical infection prophylaxis. A study of 85 cases of clostridial infection, including 56 of gas gangrene, where most of the serious infections followed amputations of the leg, suggested that penicillin prophylactically was necessary for patients at high risk from gas-gangrene organisms emanating from the bowel. Treatment should commence at operation and continue at 300 mg every 6 hours for 1 week.— M. T. Parker, *Br. med. J.*, 1969, *3*, 671.

For further references to surgical infection prophylaxis, see Prophylactic Use of Antibiotics, p.1081.

Syphilis. A detailed review of penicillin in the treatment of syphilis.— O. Idsøe *et al.*, *Bull. Wld Hlth Org.*, 1972, *47*, *Suppl.*, 5. See also *Obstet. Gynec.*, 1976, *48*, 727; R. D. Catterall, *Br. J. Hosp. Med.*, 1977, *17*, 585; *Med. Lett.*, 1977, *19*, 105.

In a survey of 460 patients treated, during 6 years in Sydney, for primary syphilis with 5 doses, and for secondary syphilis with 7 doses of a preparation containing benzylpenicillin, benzathine penicillin, and procaine penicillin (Bi-Cillin All-Purpose), it was considered that this treatment was not adequate for secondary syphilis and that the sensitivity of *Treponema pallidum* to penicillin might have decreased.— G. Hatos, *Med. J. Aust.*, 1972, *2*, 415.

Conventional doses of benzylpenicillin were not effective in the treatment of neurosyphilis, but 16 patients responded satisfactorily to very high doses given by intravenous infusion over 3 to 5 days.— G. Ritter *et al.*, *Münch. med. Wschr.*, 1975, *117*, 1383.

Tetanus. A report on the management of tetanus in neonates, including the use of benzylpenicillin.— J. M. Adams *et al.*, *Pediatrics*, 1979, *64*, 472.

Urinary-tract infections. In a study of 242 patients with urinary-tract infections due to Gram-negative organisms, 94 were treated with benzylpenicillin potassium 500 mg every 6 hours for 14 days and were compared with the other patients who were treated with ampicillin, nalidixic acid, nitrofurantoin, tetracycline, or sulphamethoxazole. At 3 weeks 56.2% of the 242 patients and 60% of those given benzylpenicillin potassium were bacteriologically free of infection. At 7 weeks 23.2% of 108 patients had relapsed including 27% of the benzylpenicillin group. None of the patients treated with sulphamethoxazole or nalidixic acid relapsed.— J. Hulbert, *Lancet*,

1972, *2*, 1216.

Whipple's disease. The treatment of choice in Whipple's disease was penicillin 600 mg four times a day for 2 weeks, followed by phenoxymethylpenicillin 250 mg four times a day by mouth for 3 months. This should be satisfactory in producing long-term remission.— *Med. J. Aust.*, 1974, *1*, 646. Experience in a patient with Whipple's disease, who had been treated with procaine penicillin and then maintained on benzylpenicillin by mouth, suggests that current guidelines for treatment may need modifying. Symptoms were resolved although penicillin apparently suppressed but did not prevent CNS disease—subtle neurological changes occurred and there was abrupt onset of meningitis, ataxia, and encephalopathy when penicillin was withdrawn after 2 years. The patient was subsequently maintained indefinitely on chloramphenicol.— M. Feldman *et al.*, *Ann. intern. Med.*, 1980, *93*, 709.

Wound infection. Benzylpenicillin was administered intravenously in doses of 600 mg to 1.8 g hourly in the treatment of patients with clostridial gas gangrene. Two patients in renal failure received 600 mg every 4 hours, and 1 patient who received 1.8 g hourly for 2 weeks developed haemolytic anaemia. Of 20 patients treated, 16 survived.— I. P. Unsworth, *Med. J. Aust.*, 1973, *1*, 1077.

Preparations

Capsules

Penicillin G Potassium Capsules *(U.S.P.)*. Capsules containing benzylpenicillin potassium equivalent to 250 000 or 400 000 units of benzylpenicillin. Store in airtight containers.

Eye Ointments

Penicillin Eye Ointment *(B.P.C. 1959)*. Oculent. Penicil. Benzylpenicillin q.s., liquid paraffin 5 g, and white soft paraffin 95 g. Melt together the liquid paraffin and the white soft paraffin, filter while hot through coarse filter-paper in a heated funnel, sterilise the filtrate by maintaining at 150° for 1 hour, and allow to cool; using aseptic precautions, incorporate the benzylpenicillin in the basis. Store in a cool dry place.

Eye-drops

Penicillin Eye-drops *(B.P.C. 1959)*. Benzylpenicillin Eye-drops; Gutt. Penicil. Benzylpenicillin with 0.5% w/v of sodium citrate in Solution For Eye-drops. Store in a cool place and use within 4 days.

A suitable formula for benzylpenicillin eye-drops: benzylpenicillin 15 mg, sodium citrate 50 mg, and phenylmercuric nitrate 0.002% in 10 ml of Water for Injections. Prepared aseptically.— D. O. Crompton, *Drugs*, 1973, *6*, 267.

Injections

Benzylpenicillin Injection *(B.P.)*. Penicillin Injection. A sterile solution of benzylpenicillin potassium or benzylpenicillin sodium in Water for Injections, prepared by dissolving the sterile contents of a sealed container in the requisite amount of Water for Injections. It may contain a suitable buffering agent. Store at a temperature between 2° and 8° and use within 7 days of preparation or within 14 days if a buffering agent is present. If stored at temperatures approaching 20°, it should be used within 24 hours of preparation or within 4 days if a buffering agent is present.

U.S.P. has Penicillin G Potassium for Injection and Penicillin G Sodium for Injection. Both are suitably buffered.

Lozenges

Penicillin Lozenges *(B.P.C. 1973)*. Benzylpenicillin Lozenges. Lozenges containing benzylpenicillin. Each lozenge weighs about 1 g. Store and supply in airtight containers and keep in a cool dry place.

Solutions

Penicillin G Potassium for Oral Solution *(U.S.P.)*. A dry mixture of benzylpenicillin potassium and one or more suitable buffers, colouring and flavouring agents, diluents, and preservatives. Store in airtight containers. When reconstituted it contains the equivalent of 20 000, 25 000, 40 000, 50 000, 80 000, or 100 000 units of benzylpenicillin per ml. pH 5.5 to 7.5.

Solution-tablets

Buffered Benzylpenicillin Solution-tablets *(B.P.C. 1968)*. Buffered Penicillin Solution-tablets; Penicillin and Sodium Citrate Solution-tablets; Solvellae Penicillini et Sodii Citratis. Each contains benzylpenicillin 9 mg (15 000 units) and sodium citrate 30 mg. They are intended for use in dispensing preparations for external use. They should not be used for dispensing eye-drops unless sterile and they are not suitable for preparing injections. Store in a cool place in airtight containers.

Penicillin G Potassium Tablets for Oral Solution *(U.S.P.)*. Tablets containing benzylpenicillin potassium equivalent to 100 000, 200 000, or 250 000 units of benzylpenicillin. Store in airtight containers.

Tablets

Benzylpenicillin Tablets *(B.P.)*. Penicillin Tablets; Penicillin G Tablets. Tablets containing benzylpenicillin potassium or benzylpenicillin sodium. Potency is expressed in terms of the equivalent amount of benzylpenicillin. They may be coated. Store at a temperature not exceeding 30°.

Penicillin G Potassium Tablets *(U.S.P.)*. Tablets containing benzylpenicillin potassium equivalent to 100 000, 200 000, 250 000, 400 000, 500 000, 800 000, or 1 million units of benzylpenicillin. Store in airtight containers.

Proprietary Preparations

Crystapen G *(Glaxo, UK)*. Benzylpenicillin potassium, available as **Syrup** (supplied as granules for preparation with water before use) containing 125 and 250 mg in each 5 ml (suggested diluent, syrup) and as **Tablets** of 250 mg. (Also available as Crystapen G in *Austral.*).

Crystapen Injection *(Glaxo, UK)*. Benzylpenicillin sodium, available as powder for preparing injections, in vials of 300 and 600 mg (unbuffered), and in vials of 3 and 6 g (buffered with sodium citrate 4.5%). (Also available as Crystapen in *Austral.*, *Canad.*, *NZ*, *S.Afr.*).

Crystapen Intrathecal *(Glaxo, UK)*. Benzylpenicillin sodium, available as unbuffered powder for preparing intrathecal injections, in ampoules of 12 mg.

Other Proprietary Names of Benzylpenicillin Potassium

Arg.— Cristapen; *Austral.*— Abbocillin-G; *Canad.*— Falapen, Megacillin *(see also under Clemizole Penicillin, Phenoxymethylpenicillin, and Procaine Penicillin)*, Novopen *(see also under Benzylpenicillin Sodium)*, P-50; *Spain*— Cidan-Cilina *(see also under Benzylpenicillin Sodium)*, Lasacilina, Penifasa '450' Simple, Unicilina Potasica; *USA*— Hyasorb, M-Cillin B, Paclin G, Pentids, Pfizerpen G, Sugracillin.

Benzylpenicillin potassium was also formerly marketed in Great Britain under the proprietary name Tabillin (*Boots*).

Other Proprietary Names of Benzylpenicillin Sodium

Fr.— Spécilline G; *NZ*— Gonopen; *S.Afr.*— Novopen *(see also under Benzylpenicillin Potassium)*; *Spain*— Cidan-Cilina *(see also under Benzylpenicillin Potassium)*, Cilipen, Crisocilin-G, Dermosa Cusi Penicilina, Natricilin, Penilevel, Penimiluy, Sanciline, Sodipen, Unicilina, Unicilina Sodica.

A preparation containing benzylpenicillin sodium and streptomycin sulphate was formerly marketed in Great Britain under the proprietary name Crystamycin (*Glaxo*).

Proprietary Names of some other Benzylpenicillin Salts

Canad.— P.G.A. *(benzylpenicillin ammonium)*.

23-r

BL-P 1654. (6*R*)-6-[D-2-(3-Amidinoureido)-2-phenylacetamido]penicillanic acid.
$C_{18}H_{22}N_6O_5S$=434.5.

CAS — 28889-87-4.

BL-P 1654 is a ureido-penicillin with activity broadly similar to that of carbenicillin (see p.1111). Against *Pseudomonas aeruginosa*, the minimum bactericidal concentration is much higher than the minimum inhibitory concentration. Nephrotoxicity has been demonstrated in *animals* and clinical use appears unlikely.

From the MIC values BL-P 1654 appeared to be 8 to 16 times as active as carbenicillin against 89 isolates of *Ps. aeruginosa*. However the minimum bactericidal concentration was 16 to 64 times higher than the MIC for all strains. Resistance rapidly developed *in vitro*.— E. R. Wald *et al.*, *Antimicrob. Ag. Chemother.*, 1975, *7*, 336.

BL-P 1654 was generally slightly less active than ticarcillin and carbenicillin except against *Staph. epidermidis* and enterococci. There was a marked inoculum effect when BL-P 1654 was tested against *Ps. aeruginosa* and there was a discrepancy between minimum inhibitory and bactericidal concentrations.— T. C. Eickhoff and J. M. Ehret, *Antimicrob. Ag. Chemother.*, 1976, *10*, 241. See also C. C. Sanders and W. E. Sanders, *ibid.*, 1975, *7*, 435.

Further references to the antimicrobial action of BL-P 1654: R. E. Van Scoy *et al.*, *Antimicrob. Ag. Chemother.*, 1970, 12; K. E. Price *et al.*, *ibid.*, 17; L. J. Adler *et al.*, *ibid.*, 63; G. P. Bodey and D. Stewart, *Appl. Microbiol.*, 1971, *21*, 710; S. G. Sackel *et al.*, *Antimicrob. Ag. Chemother.*, 1977, *12*, 31.

Pharmacokinetic studies with BL-P 1654: G. P. Bodey *et al.*, *Antimicrob. Ag. Chemother.*, 1974, *5*, 366; J. T. Clarke *et al.*, *ibid.*, *6*, 729.

Manufacturers
Bristol, USA.

24-f

Carbenicillin Sodium *(B.P.)*.
Carbenicillin Disodium; Carbenicillinnatrium; BRL 2064; CP 15639-2; α-Carboxybenzylpenicillin Sodium. The disodium salt of (6*R*)-6-(2-carboxy-2-phenylacetamido)penicillanic acid.
$C_{17}H_{16}N_2Na_2O_6S$=422.4.

CAS — 4697-36-3 (acid); 4800-94-6 (disodium salt).

Pharmacopoeias. In *Br.*, *Braz.*, *Jap.*, and *Nord.* *Nord.* and *U.S.* include an injection grade.

A white or almost white, odourless, hygroscopic, crystalline powder with a bitter taste. It contains not less than 89% of $C_{17}H_{16}N_2Na_2O_6S$, calculated on the anhydrous substance. Each g represents about 4.7 mmol (4.7 mEq) of sodium. Carbenicillin sodium 1.1 g is approximately equivalent to 1 g of carbenicillin. **Soluble** 1 in 1.2 of water and 1 in 25 of alcohol; practically insoluble in chloroform and ether. A 10% solution in water has a pH of 6 to 8. A 4.4% solution in water is iso-osmotic with serum. **Store** at a temperature not exceeding 5° in airtight containers which should be sterile and sealed to exclude micro-organisms. Protect from light.

Incompatible with amphotericin, chloramphenicol sodium succinate, erythromycin ethylsuccinate, kanamycin sulphate, oxytetracycline hydrochloride, streptomycin sulphate, tetracycline hydrochloride, vitamins of the B group with vitamin C, and, in concentrated solutions, with amikacin sulphate. Incompatibility with gentamicin has been reported.

Incompatibility. For a list of incompatibilities including *phenytoin* and sympathomimetic agents, see *Med. Lett.*, 1972, *14* (Jan.), *Suppl.*, 32.

A white precipitate was formed when carbenicillin and *promethazine* were mixed in an intravenous solution.— G. E. Otterman and D. W. Samuelson (letter), *Am. J. Hosp. Pharm.*, 1979, *36*, 1156.

Further references: B. Lynn, *J. Hosp. Pharm.*, 1970, *28*, 71; B. B. Riley, *ibid.*, 228; B. Lynn (letter), *Lancet*, 1971, *1*, 654; B. Lynn and A. Jones, *Beecham Research, Advances in Antimicrobial and Antineoplastic Chemotherapy*, Vol. 1, pt 1, Munich, Urban and Schwarzenberg, 1972, p. 701; B. Flouvat and P. Lechat, *Thérapie*, 1974, *29*, 337.

For the inactivation of gentamicin by carbenicillin, see Gentamicin Sulphate, p.1166.

For a report of incompatibility with tobramycin, see Tobramycin, p.1226.

Stability in solution. A 10% loss of potency was noted in 6 hours in a solution of carbenicillin sodium 5 g per 500 ml of sodium lactate injection. A solution containing 15 g per 500 ml was stable for 6 hours in Aminosol Vitrum and for 24 hours in Aminosol-Glucose and Aminosol-Fructose-Ethanol at 23°. A solution containing 1 g per litre in a peritoneal dialysis solution (Dialaflex 62) was stable for up to 3 hours at 37°. An intramuscular solution containing 1 g of carbenicillin sodium in 2 ml of water lost 20% potency in 3 days at 23° and less than 5% in 6 days at 5°. Because concentrated solutions might form polymers, injections should be freshly prepared.— B. Lynn, *J. Hosp. Pharm.*, 1970, *28*, 71 .

After the addition of 5 g of carbenicillin sodium to 500 ml of 5 infusion solutions the percentage potencies at 4, 8, 12, and 24 hours were—dextrose injection: 100, 95.6, 97, and 116.1; sodium chloride and dextrose injection: 100, 84.2, 96.5, and 94.7; sodium lactate injection: 87.8, 82.9, 85.4, and 69.5; modified compound sodium lactate injection: 100, 94.3, 103.7, and 88.6; sodium chloride injection: 85.2, 86.9, 94.3, and 70.5. Loss of potency was generally associated with a progressive fall in pH.— J. Jacobs *et al.*, *Drug Intell. & clin. Pharm.*, 1970, *4*, 204.

Carbenicillin 0.2% in a 20% solution of tyloxapol 0.125%, sodium bicarbonate 2%, and glycerol 5% (Alevaire) in sodium chloride injection lost 4% potency after 6 hours and 26% after 24 hours when stored at 20°.— B. Lynn, *J. Hosp. Pharm.*, 1971, *29*, 183.

Carbenicillin sodium was only moderately stable in acid media, with a half-life at 25° and pH 2 of 140 minutes and at 37° and pH 2.9 of about 30 minutes. It was most stable at pH 6 to 9. Carbenicillin sodium 1 g per litre was stable and compatible for 24 hours in dextrose injection, sodium chloride injection, maintenance electrolytes in dextrose injection, and in mixtures in dextrose injection with potassium chloride, sodium bicarbonate, hydrocortisone sodium succinate, gentamicin sulphate, and ampicillin sodium (all within the range pH 5.2 to 8.3). In vitamin-B complex with ascorbic acid injection in dextrose injection (pH 3.6), carbenicillin was stable for 24 hours at 5° but lost nearly 50% of its potency at 25°.— E. D. Zost and V. A. Yanchick, *Am. J. Hosp. Pharm.*, 1972, *29*, 135.

The degradation of carbenicillin sodium was at a minimum at pH 6.5.— H. Zia *et al.*, *Can. J. pharm. Sci.*, 1974, *9*, 112.

There was no significant loss of potency when carbenicillin for injection was dissolved in water, added to 3 commercially available 0.5% hypromellose solutions in plastic squeezy bottles (Lacril, pH 5.9; Tearisol, pH 7.3; Isoptotears, pH 7.4), and the resulting solutions, containing carbenicillin 6.2 mg per ml, kept at 25° for 7 days.— E. Osborn *et al.*, *Am. J. Ophthal.*, 1976, *82*, 775.

Accelerated degradation of benzylpenicillin sodium, ampicillin sodium, carbenicillin sodium, and phenoxymethylpenicillin potassium in neutral and alkaline sucrose solutions was due to a nucleophilic displacement reaction with the formation of sucrose penicilloate esters. These esters might be antigenic and their presence should be avoided by maintaining the pH of solutions of penicillins and sucrose at 6 to 6.5.— H. Bundgaard and C. Larsen, *Int. J. Pharmaceut.*, 1978, *1*, 95.

Further references: B. E. Kirschenbaum and C. J. Latiolais, *Am. J. Hosp. Pharm.*, 1976, *33*, 767; H. Colding and G. E. Andersen, *Antimicrob. Ag. Chemother.*, 1978, *13*, 555.

Adverse Effects and Treatment. As for Benzylpenicillin, p.1103.

Purpura and haemorrhage have been reported. Convulsions have occurred in patients with renal impairment given high doses. Electrolyte disturbances may follow the administration of large doses of carbenicillin sodium.

Allergy. The Boston Collaborative Drug Surveillance Program monitored consecutively 32 812 medical inpatients. Drug-induced anaphylaxis occurred in 1 of 113 patients given carbenicillin.— J. Porter and H. Jick, *Lancet*, 1977, *1*, 587.

Blood disorders. Two patients developed reversible granulocytopenia when treated with carbenicillin. One had 4 episodes after amounts varying from 510 to 720 g and the other had an episode after 96 g given over 16 days.— M. P. Reyes *et al.*, *Am. J. Med.*, 1973, *54*, 413.

Coagulation disorder. Of 30 patients who received carbenicillin sodium in doses of 500 to 750 mg per kg body-weight daily, purpura and bleeding from mucous membranes occurred in 6. The bleeding appeared within 12 hours of starting therapy and took from 3 to 7 days to disappear after discontinuation of the drug.— P. D. McClure *et al.* (letter), *Lancet*, 1970, *2*, 1307. See also A. Lurie *et al.* (letter), *ibid.*, 1970, *1*, 1114.

Platelet function was affected in 17 subjects receiving 20 to 40 g of carbenicillin daily and in 5 patients receiving 20 to 30 g daily. In some cases bleeding times, plasma prothrombin times, and clot retraction were disturbed for up to 12 days after the carbenicillin was stopped. This suggested an effect not only on circulating platelets but also on megakaryocytes. The increase in bleeding time appeared to be dose-dependent.— C. H. Brown *et al.*, *New Engl. J. Med.*, 1974, *291*, 265. Bleeding had also been seen after ampicillin, benzylpenicillin, methicillin, and ticarcillin but not after cephalothin, dicloxacillin, or flucloxacillin.— K. Andrassy *et al.* (letter), *ibid.*, 1975, *292*, 109.

Further references: B. A. Waisbren *et al.* (letter), *J. Am. med. Ass.*, 1971, *217*, 1243; M. Yudis *et al.* (letter), *Lancet*, 1972, *2*, 599; D. A. Lederer *et al.*, *J. Pharm. Pharmac.*, 1973, *25*, 876.

See also Haemorrhagic Cystitis, (below).

Electrolyte disturbances. Reports of hypokalaemia associated with carbenicillin sodium.— B. I. Hoffbrand and J. D. M. Stewart (letter), *Br. med. J.*, 1970, *4*, 746; J. Klastersky *et al.* (letter), *Ann. intern. Med.*, 1973, *78*, 774; S. V. Cabizuca and K. B. Desser, *J. Am. med. Ass.*, 1976, *236*, 956; F. B. Stapleton *et al.*, *Am. J. Dis. Child.*, 1976, *130*, 1104.

Haemorrhagic cystitis. Erythrocyturia with painful, frequent voiding, sterile urine, and moderate leucocyturia was noted in 7 children with cystic fibrosis during and after intravenous administration of carbenicillin 500 mg per kg body-weight daily. The symptoms started on the third to the eighth day and continued up to 2 weeks after stopping carbenicillin. An eighth child suffered painless haematuria during carbenicillin therapy. Subsequent administration of the same dose to 2 of the children caused the symptoms to recur after 3 days despite prophylactic administration of antihistamines to one. During such therapy the urine should be monitored daily and treatment withdrawn as soon as microscopic erythrocyturia is found. Dosage reduction had not been tried; tobramycin was given instead.— N. E. Møller (letter), *Lancet*, 1978, *2*, 946.

Hepatotoxicity. The intramuscular injection of carbenicillin or ampicillin had resulted in a rise of serum aspartate aminotransferase (SGOT) values, whereas the same dose by intravenous injection had not. This indicated that muscle damage and not liver damage was responsible for the effect.— A. K. Knirsch and E. J. Gralla, *New Engl. J. Med.*, 1970, *282*, 1081. Rises in SGOT values had also occurred after the intravenous administration of carbenicillin.— D. W. Gump (letter), *ibid.*, 1489.

In 4 patients carbenicillin sodium was associated with mild, reversible, anicteric hepatitis on 8 occasions.— F. M. Wilson *et al.*, *J. Am. med. Ass.*, 1975, *232*, 818.

Nephrotoxicity. Acute interstitial nephritis developed in a 66-year-old man given carbenicillin sodium 24 g daily for more than 3 weeks; he also received gentamicin and small intermittent doses of frusemide but the penicillin was considered responsible.— G. B. Appel *et al.*, *Archs intern. Med.*, 1978, *138*, 1265. See also G. A. Roselle *et al.*, *Sth. med. J.*, 1978, *71*, 84.

Neurotoxicity. A 48-year-old woman developed seizures following treatment with 50 g of carbenicillin administered intravenously over 2 days. The convulsive episodes abated when carbenicillin was discontinued, but severe neuromyal irritability and hyperreflexia developed when carbenicillin was started again and disappeared when the dose was reduced.— N. A. Kurtzman *et al.*, *J. Am. med. Ass.*, 1970, *214*, 1320.

A 36-year-old woman with chronic active pyelonephritis who was treated with carbenicillin 5 g every 6 hours developed acute metabolic acidosis and grand mal seizures on the 13th day of treatment. Excessively high blood concentrations of carbenicillin were noted in the presence of renal impairment.— A. Whelton *et al.*, *J. Am. med. Ass.*, 1971, *218*, 1942.

Precautions. Carbenicillin sodium is contra-indicated in patients known to be sensitive to penicillin and it should be given with caution to patients with known histories of allergy or with impaired renal function. Because of its sodium content, it should be given cautiously to patients on a restricted sodium diet.

Carbenicillin sodium and gentamicin have been shown to be incompatible *in vitro* and should be administered separately when both are required. For comments on the use of these two antibiotics see Gentamicin Sulphate, p.1168.

The high specific gravity of a patient's urine was attributed to his carbenicillin treatment for burns. His daily dose was 30 g which could have produced a daily excretion of 24 g in his urine. A similar situation could occur with benzylpenicillin. As burned patients might have their fluid management monitored by the specific gravity of their urine, care should be taken not to misinterpret any measurements.— C. Deziel *et al.* (letter), *Lancet*, 1977, *2*, 980. A similar report of hypersthenuria in 2 patients.— L. A. Zwelling and J. E. Balow, *Ann. intern. Med.*, 1978, *89*, 225.

For the effect of other agents on the antimicrobial activity of carbenicillin, see below under Antimicrobial Action.

Antimicrobial Action. Carbenicillin has a mode of action similar to that of benzylpenicillin and is bactericidal *in vitro* against many strains of *Escherichia coli, Salmonella, Shigella, Haemophilus influenzae,* and *Neisseria* and is comparable with ampicillin though it is less active. Its activity against Gram-positive micro-organisms is less than that of benzylpenicillin. *Klebsiella* spp. are usually insensitive. It is active against most strains of indole-positive *Proteus* spp. including *Pr. morganii, Pr. rettgeri,* and *Pr. vulgaris,* but not against penicillinase-producing strains of *Pr. mirabilis.* The most important feature of carbenicillin is its activity against *Pseudomonas aeruginosa*, but some strains have shown resistance to carbenicillin and are not inhibited by concentrations of 200 μg per ml. The antimicrobial action of carbenicillin can be enhanced by gentamicin (see p.1168).

Carbenicillin in a concentration of 12.5 μg per ml inhibited the growth of 89% of *Proteus* spp. and 44% of *E. coli* which were tested. Only 13% of *Ps. aeruginosa* strains were inhibited by concentrations of 50 μg per ml but 81% were inhibited by 100 μg per ml. The strains of *Str. faecalis* tested were sensitive to concentrations of between 12.5 and 50 μg per ml. *Klebsiella* spp. tested were resistant. Minimum inhibitory concentrations with a large inoculum were usually one- or two-fold greater than with a small inoculum and for all organisms tested the concentration of carbenicillin required to kill more than 99% of an inoculum was between 2 and 4 times greater than the inhibitory concentration.— W. Brumfitt *et al.*, *Lancet*, 1967, *1*, 1289.

For 99 of 143 strains of *Pseudomonas* spp. the MIC of carbenicillin was 200 to 300 μg per ml. Most strains of *E. coli* and *Proteus* spp. were inhibited by 25 μg per ml or less. Strains of *Klebsiella* spp. were resistant to carbenicillin.— G. P. Bodey and L. M. Terrell, *J. Bact.*, 1968, *95*, 1587.

An additive or slightly antagonistic effect against *Ps. aeruginosa* was found *in vitro* for carbenicillin with polymyxin B sulphate as well as the synergism between carbenicillin and gentamicin.— T. C. Eickhoff, *Appl. Microbiol.*, 1969, *18*, 469.

In a study *in vitro* of the susceptibility of Gram-negative bacilli to carbenicillin, most strains of *Enterobacteriaceae* (except *Kleb. pneumoniae* and *Pr. vulgaris*) and strains of *Ps. aeruginosa, Ps. stutzeri, Acinetobacter lwoffii* and *Acinetobacter anitratus* were susceptible to carbenicillin in concentrations of 100 μg per ml.— J. A. Washington, *Mayo Clin. Proc.*, 1972, *47*, 332.

In a study of the activities of penicillins and cephalosporins *in vitro* against 5 beta-lactamase-producing and 5 non-producing strains of *H. influenzae*, ampicillin and benzylpenicillin were significantly less active against the β-lactamase-producing strains but carbenicillin was highly active against all of the strains and relatively resistant to hydrolysis. Although cephamandole was hydrolysed its activity was similar to that of carbenicillin.— S. Kattan *et al.*, *J. antimicrob. Chemother.*, 1975, *1*, 79.

Carbenicillin inhibited the majority of 486 strains of anaerobic bacteria at 128 μg per ml, including 72 of 76 strains of *Bacteroides fragilis*.— V. L. Sutter and S. M. Finegold, *Antimicrob. Ag. Chemother.*, 1976, *10*, 736. Similar results were achieved in a further study.— P. C. Appelbaum and S. A. Chatterton, *ibid.*, 1978, *14*, 371.

Carbenicillin inhibited 4, 32, 42, 44, 61, 70, 90, and all of 92 strains of *Neisseria gonorrhoeae* at an MIC of 8, 16, 30, 60, 250, 500, 1000, and 2000 ng per ml respectively.— B. A. Watts *et al.*, *J. antimicrob. Chemother.*, 1977, *3*, 331.

Carbenicillin had an MIC of 16 μg per ml against 100 strains of *Staph. aureus* but the MBC for the majority of strains was much higher. Twenty-five of the strains gave a positive carbenicillinase test but there was no correlation between carbenicillinase production and values for the MIC or MBC.— C. Watanakunakorn and C. Glotzbecker, *J. antimicrob. Chemother.*, 1979, *5*, 151.

An inoculum effect was found *in vitro* with carbenicillin or cephamandole against isolates of *H. influenzae* type b, especially ampicillin-resistant strains.— V. P. Syriopoulou *et al.*, *Antimicrob. Ag. Chemother.*, 1979, *16*, 510.

Further references: J. D. King *et al.*, *J. clin. Path.*, 1980, *33*, 297 (*Ps. aeruginosa*); D. Greenwood and A. Eley (letter), *J. antimicrob. Chemother.*, 1980, *6*, 672 (*Ps. aeruginosa*).

For comparative studies of carbenicillin and ticarcillin see, Ticarcillin Sodium, p.1224.

For a report of piperacillin being more active than carbenicillin or ticarcillin against 612 isolates of aerobic bacteria, see Piperacillin, p.1202.

Diminished activity. Antagonism occurred against some strains of *Staph. aureus* when the activity of carbenicillin was tested *in vitro* with mithramycin.— J. Y. Jacobs *et al.*, *Antimicrob. Ag. Chemother.*, 1979, *15*,

580.

For the antagonistic effect of colistin and carbenicillin against *Pseudomonas*, see Colistin Sulphate, p.1150.

Enhanced activity. Acetylcysteine and carbenicillin or ticarcillin had additive or enhanced inhibitory activity *in vitro* against strains of *Ps. aeruginosa*.— M. F. Parry and H. C. Neu, *J. clin. Microbiol.*, 1977, *5*, 58.

Enhanced activity against isolates of *Ps. aeruginosa* was demonstrated *in vitro* when piperacillin, ticarcillin, or carbenicillin were used with gentamicin, tobramycin, or amikacin.— P. Chanbusarakum and P. R. Murray, *Antimicrob. Ag. Chemother.*, 1978, *14*, 505.

The activities of gentamicin, tobramycin, or amikacin were determined *in vitro* against 138 strains of gentamicin-resistant Gram-negative bacteria when used with carbenicillin, azlocillin, or mezlocillin. Potentially useful synergy was considered to occur between gentamicin and carbenicillin, azlocillin, or mezlocillin against *Ps. aeruginosa* and between gentamicin and carbenicillin against *Proteus*, *Providencia*, *Acinetobacter*, and *Alcaligenes* spp. There appeared to be no relationship between the hydrolysis of the penicillin by beta-lactamases and the synergistic action of the penicillin and gentamicin.— W. Farrell *et al.*, *J. antimicrob. Chemother.*, 1979, *5*, 23.

Carbenicillin was synergistic when used *in vitro* with amikacin, gentamicin, or tobramycin against the majority of 20 strains of *Serratia marcescens* that were relatively resistant to carbenicillin or aminoglycoside antibiotics alone.— M. Y. C. Lin *et al.*, *J. antimicrob. Chemother.*, 1979, *5*, 37.

Further reports of enhanced activity *in vitro* with carbenicillin and other agents: B. Light and H. G. Riggs, *Antimicrob. Ag. Chemother.*, 1978, *13*, 979 (with triethylenetetramine dihydrochloride against *Ps. aeruginosa*); J. Y. Jacobs *et al.*, *ibid.*, 1979, *15*, 580 (with mitomycin against *Staph. aureus*); I. Trestman *et al.*, *ibid.*, *16*, 283, (with mecillinam against *Bacteroides* spp.); C. Watanakunakorn and C. Glotzbecker, *J. antimicrob. Chemother.*, 1979, *5*, 151 (with aminoglycosides against *Staph. aureus*); G. F. Gerberick and P. A. Castric, *Antimicrob. Ag. Chemother.*, 1980, *17*, 732 (with glycine or edetic acid against *Ps. aeruginosa*); G. Masuda *et al.*, *ibid.*, 334 (with gentamicin against *Ps. aeruginosa*).

Resistance. Carbenicillin is inactivated by penicillinase. Resistance to carbenicillin has developed in *Pseudomonas aeruginosa* following treatment with carbenicillin. This resistance may arise by genetic mutation or by the transfer of resistance factors (R-factors) to and from certain strains of Enterobacteriaceae. Some strains of *Ps. aeruginosa* produce a specific β-lactamase, carbenicillinase, and transferable resistance appears to be associated with this production.

Carbenicillin resistance, acquired *in vitro* by *E. coli* strain K12 from a resistant strain of *Ps. aeruginosa* found in a human burn, was transferred from the *E. coli* strain to a sensitive strain of *Ps. aeruginosa* found in mixed infection on *mouse* burns. Some strains of *Klebsiella* or *Proteus* spp. isolated from burns were found to transfer the same pattern of resistance to a sensitive *E. coli* or *Ps. aeruginosa* strain. Carbenicillin resistance was often associated with resistance to tetracycline, kanamycin, ampicillin, and cephaloridine, thus greatly decreasing the effectiveness of multiple antibiotic therapy.— E. Roe *et al.*, *Lancet*, 1971, *1*, 149.

After a ban on the use of carbenicillin in a burns unit, strains of Gram-negative organisms were still found for some time which possessed the R-factor although none was found in the staff's faeces. Severe restriction on the use of tetracycline, kanamycin, ampicillin and cephaloridine which were associated with the R-factor was instituted and could have had a part to play in maintaining the absence of organisms carrying the R-factor. Tests carried out during this period of control showed some return of sensitivity.— E. J. L. Lowbury *et al.*, *Lancet*, 1972, *2*, 941. See also *ibid.*, 961.

There was cross-resistance between ampicillin and carbenicillin for strains of *Shigella sonnei*. Over approximately 2.5 years the incidence of carbenicillin-resistant strains increased from virtually zero to 55%.— S. Ross *et al.*, *J. Am. med. Ass.*, 1972, *221*, 45.

Mucoid strains of *Ps. aeruginosa* isolated from the sputum of 2 patients with cystic fibrosis were more resistant to carbenicillin than non-mucoid strains from the same sputum samples.— J. R. W. Govan (letter), *J. antimicrob. Chemother.*, 1976, *2*, 215.

A report of *Ps. aeruginosa* resistant to gentamicin with carbenicillin.— I. M. Baird *et al.*, *Antimicrob. Ag. Chemother.*, 1976, *10*, 626.

Further references: R. B. Sykes and M. H. Richmond, *Lancet*, 1971, *2*, 342; A. E. Jephcott *et al.* (letter), *ibid.*, 1973, *1*, 272.

For a report of R-factors determining multiple resistance to gentamicin and carbenicillin among strains of *Ps. aeruginosa*, see Gentamicin Sulphate, p.1169.

For a report of a strain of *Ps. aeruginosa* resistant to polymyxin showing cross-resistance to carbenicillin, see Polymyxin B Sulphate, p.1205.

Absorption and Fate. Carbenicillin is not absorbed from the gastro-intestinal tract. The intramuscular injection of 1 g produces a plasma concentration of about 30 µg per ml after 1 hour, 20 µg per ml after 2 hours, and more than 10 µg per ml for a further 2 hours. Doubling the dose can double the concentration. Approximately 50% is reported to be bound to plasma proteins. The average biological half-life is reported to be 1 hour. Renal clearance of carbenicillin is similar to but slower than that of ampicillin. About 80% of the dose appears unchanged in the urine, in concentrations of 2 to 4 mg per ml, within 6 hours.

An intravenous injection of 1 g produces a peak plasma concentration of about 140 µg per ml after 15 minutes, falling to about 30 µg per ml after 2 hours, and falling rapidly during the next 2 hours. Urinary concentrations of 5 to 10 mg per ml follow the intravenous injection of 1 g. After 5 g by intravenous injection, plasma concentrations of more than 300 µg per ml are achieved in 15 minutes, falling to about 125 µg per ml after 2 hours. The continuous intravenous infusion of 12 to 30 g of carbenicillin sodium, with probenecid by mouth to delay excretion, produces plasma concentrations of 50 to 400 µg per ml. Distribution of carbenicillin in the body is similar to that of other penicillins. Small amounts have been detected in human milk. There is little diffusion into the cerebrospinal fluid except when the meninges are inflamed. Relatively high concentrations have been reported in bile.

One hour after a 1-g intramuscular dose of carbenicillin serum concentrations ranged from 10 to 40 µg per ml and 6 hours after the dose they ranged from 2 to 11 µg per ml. Urinary concentrations were usually between 0.7 and 2 mg per ml and about 65% of the injected dose was excreted within the first 6 hours. In patients with impaired renal function much higher serum concentrations were attained and only about 20% of the injected dose appeared in the urine within 6 hours.— W. Brumfitt *et al.*, *Lancet*, 1967, *1*, 1289.

In a study of subjects given carbenicillin 2 g intravenously the mean serum concentration in 5 normal subjects was about 103 µg per ml and the mean serum half-life was about 1 hour. The mean serum half-life was increased in 9 patients with liver disease, in 11 with oliguric renal failure, and in 5 patients with oliguria and liver disease to 1.9, 15.7, and 23.2 hours respectively. Significant amounts of carbenicillin were removed by haemodialysis and half-lives could be reduced by 53 to 70%.— T. A. Hoffman *et al.*, *Ann. intern. Med.*, 1970, *73*, 173.

In a study of 27 neonates given carbenicillin peak serum concentrations of 147 µg per ml were achieved in babies of normal birth-weight and 174 µg per ml in those of low birth-weight after doses of 100 mg per kg body-weight intramuscularly. The average 12-hourly excretion was 36% in those of low birth-weight and 61% in those of normal weight and excretion correlated with creatinine clearance. Serum half-life was 2.7 hours in neonates of normal weight and 4 hours in those of low weight.— C. D. Morehead *et al.*, *Antimicrob. Ag. Chemother.*, 1972, *2*, 267. See also H. Neussel and H. Olbing, *Int. Z. klin. Pharmak.*, 1972, *5*, 444.

The serum-carbenicillin half-life in an anephric patient was 29.5 hours, a concentration of 204 µg per ml being attained after the ½-hour infusion of 100 mg per kg body-weight. Serum concentrations estimated from a graph of the regression of carbenicillin against time were within 5 to 10 µg per ml of the actual figure. Haemodialysis for 6 hours reduced serum carbenicillin by about 50 µg per ml.— J. D. Nelson and E. W. Reimold (letter), *Lancet*, 1973, *1*, 486.

Five patients with kidney disease were given carbenicillin 5 g by intravenous infusion 2 hours before nephrectomy. The mean serum-carbenicillin concentration at the time of nephrectomy was 277 µg per ml and kidney concentrations were 173, 173, and 181 µg per g of cortex, medulla, and papilla respectively. Dehydrated *dogs* given carbenicillin were found to have increased renal medullary, papillary, and urine concentrations of carbenicillin when compared to results from hydrated *dogs*.— A. Whelton *et al.*, *Ann. intern. Med.*, 1973, *78*, 659.

Mean peak serum-carbenicillin concentrations of about 500 µg per ml were obtained at the end of an infusion of carbenicillin 5 g given over 30 minutes to healthy subjects and concentrations remained above 100 µg per ml for 3 hours. Probenecid did not enhance the peak concentration. When the same dose was given over 4 hours peak concentrations of 170 µg per ml were achieved at the end of the infusion. Concentrations above 100 µg per ml were obtained between 2 and 5 hours when probenecid was given and the peak concentration was 230 µg per ml.— B. Lynn, *Eur. J. Cancer*, 1973, *9*, 425.

A comparative study of the pharmacokinetics of carbenicillin, piperacillin, and ticarcillin.— B. R. Meyers *et al.*, *Antimicrob. Ag. Chemother.*, 1980, *17*, 608.

Further references: G. P. Bodey *et al.*, *Am. J. med. Sci.*, 1969, *257*, 185; H. C. Standiford *et al.*, *J. infect. Dis.*, 1970, *122*, *Suppl.*, 9; J. D. Nelson and G. H. McCracken, *Pediatrics*, 1973, *52*, 801; D. Höffler *et al.*, *Dt. med. Wschr.*, 1974, *99*, 399; J. M. Brogard *et al.*, *J. int. med. Res.*, 1974, *2*, 142.

Diffusion into body fluids and tissues. Carbenicillin sodium administered by subconjunctival injection penetrated the normal non-inflamed eye.— G. L. Boyle *et al.*, *Am. J. Ophthal.*, 1972, *73*, 754.

In a study of the diffusion of 7 different antibiotics into bone, carbenicillin, clindamycin, and methicillin diffused there with the greatest frequency.— J. D. Smilack *et al.*, *Antimicrob. Ag. Chemother.*, 1976, *9*, 169.

Carbenicillin diffused into interstitial fluid. This diffusion was related to the amount of protein binding.— J. S. Tan and S. J. Salstrom, *Antimicrob. Ag. Chemother.*, 1977, *11*, 698.

Metabolism. Only about 2% of a 500 mg intramuscular dose of carbenicillin, given to 6 healthy subjects, was metabolised and recovered in the urine as penicilloic acid within 12 hours. About 82% of the dose was excreted unchanged.— M. Cole *et al.*, *Antimicrob. Ag. Chemother.*, 1973, *3*, 463.

Uses. Carbenicillin is used in the treatment of infections due to *Pseudomonas aeruginosa*, when large doses are given intravenously. It has also been administered intramuscularly or intravenously in the treatment of serious infections due to non-penicillinase producing strains of *Proteus* spp. and to some strains of *Escherichia coli*.

Carbenicillin is often used with gentamicin (see p.1170) since the 2 antibiotics have been shown to be synergistic, and though some inactivation has been reported the mixture appears to be clinically useful; it is advisable to administer the injections separately and the monitoring of serum-gentamicin concentrations is recommended. The emergence of *Pseudomonas* resistance may also be inhibited when patients are treated with the 2 antibiotics.

For severe systemic infections the usual adult dose is the equivalent of 20 to 30 g of carbenicillin daily in divided doses by intravenous infusion or injection, usually every 4 to 6 hours. Carbenicillin should be injected slowly over 3 to 4 minutes and infusions should be given rapidly over 30 to 40 minutes since infusion over longer periods may not produce therapeutic concentrations. The concomitant administration of probenecid 1 g thrice daily by mouth may lead to higher and more prolonged serum concentrations of carbenicillin but is not recommended in patients with impaired renal function. Doses of carbenicillin may need to be reduced in renal failure.

For meningitis, intravenous therapy is reinforced by a daily intrathecal injection of the equivalent of 20 to 40 mg of carbenicillin; infants from birth up to about 2 years may be given 5 to 10 mg and older children 10 to 20 mg. In each case the higher dose should be used for infections due to *Ps. aeruginosa*. Doses are dissolved in sodium chloride injection immediately before use to give a solution containing 10 mg per ml; if the required dose is higher than 20 mg a more concentrated solution may be prepared so that a 2-ml dose volume is not exceeded.

In the treatment of urinary infections the usual dose is the equivalent of 4 to 8 g daily in divided doses by intramuscular injection. Probenecid should not be used.

The usual recommended dose for children is the equivalent of 50 to 100 mg per kg body-weight daily intramuscularly and 250 to 500 mg per kg daily intravenously, according to the severity of the infection.

If the pain following intramuscular injection is troublesome carbenicillin can be administered in a 0.5% solution of lignocaine hydrochloride.

As an adjunct to systemic use, carbenicillin may be given by intra-articular injection in doses of 500 mg to 1 g and by intrapleural injection in doses of 1 g daily; a 25% solution in lignocaine and adrenaline injection has been recommended for subconjunctival use. The equivalent of carbenicillin 250 to 500 mg dissolved in 3 to 5 ml of water may be nebulised and inhaled 4 times daily. A 0.2% solution of carbenicillin has been suggested for local irrigation.

Reviews of carbenicillin.— W. L. Hewitt and R. E. Winters, *J. infect. Dis.*, 1973, *127, Suppl.*, S120; *J. Am. med. Ass.*, 1977, *237*, 1366 and 1367; C. D. Peterson *et al.*, *Drug Intell. & clin. Pharm.*, 1977, *11*, 482.

A study of carbenicillin given to 74 patients with serious infections caused by *Ps. aeruginosa, Proteus* spp., and *E. coli*. In peritoneal infections, carbenicillin was added to the peritoneal dialysis fluid in a concentration of 100 µg per ml, in some cases in addition to intramuscular treatment.— W. Brumfitt *et al.*, *Lancet*, 1967, *1*, 1289.

References to the use of carbenicillin, with cephalosporins or aminoglycosides, for the treatment of infections in neutropenic patients with neoplastic disease.— H. Gaya, *Br. J. Hosp. Med.*, 1975, *13*, 124; P. J. Burke *et al.*, *Johns Hopkins med. J.*, 1976, *139*, 1; W. K. Lau *et al.*, *Am. J. Med.*, 1977, *62*, 959 (with amikacin or gentamicin); G. P. Bodey *et al.*, *Am. J. med. Sci.*, 1977, *273*, 309 (with cephalothin or cephazolin); S. C. Schimpff *et al.*, *J. infect. Dis.*, 1978, *137*, 14; G. P. Bodey *et al.*, *ibid.*, *Suppl.*, S139 (with cephamandole); G. P. Bodey *et al.*, *Am. J. Med.*, 1979, *67*, 608 (with cephamandole or tobramycin); B. F. Issell *et al.*, *Am. J. med. Sci.*, 1979, *277*, 311 (with tobramycin).

Abscess. Two patients with lung abscess infected with *Ps. aeruginosa* were successfully treated by instillation into the lung of carbenicillin and colistin in one and carbenicillin and gentamicin in the other.— S. W. B. Newsom *et al.* (letter), *Lancet*, 1974, *2*, 530.

Anaerobic infections. The beneficial response of severe anaerobic infections, especially those due to *Bacteroides fragilis*, to treatment with carbenicillin.— R. M. Swenson and B. Lorber, *Antimicrob. Ag. Chemother.*, 1976, *9*, 1025. See also H. Thadepalli and J. T. Huang, *Curr. ther. Res.*, 1977, *22*, 549; E. L. Westerman *et al.*, *Am. J. med. Sci.*, 1978, *276*, 159; I. Brook, *Infection*, 1979, *7*, 247; *idem*, *Laryngoscope, St Louis*, 1979, *89*, 1129.

Carbenicillin or ticarcillin are not antibiotics of first choice in the treatment of anaerobic infections and in general should be reserved for *Ps. aeruginosa* infection.— D. G. Maki *et al.*, *J. infect. Dis.*, 1978, *138*, 859.

Bronchitis. The efficacy of carbenicillin, colistin, and gentamicin was compared in 81 patients with severe bronchial infection due to *Ps. aeruginosa*. Colistin caused little or no clinical improvement. Carbenicillin, 4 to 8 g intramuscularly and 4 g in 20 ml of saline by inhalation daily, with probenecid, 4 g by mouth daily, led to a slight or pronounced clinical improvement in 12 of 15 patients. The regimen of carbenicillin with gentamicin, 100 mg thrice daily by intramuscular injection and 40 mg four times a day by inhalation, gave better results than carbenicillin alone. Carbenicillin 18 g daily administered by slow intravenous infusion to 7 very seriously ill patients followed by intramuscular therapy led to slight or marked improvement in 6 patients, though in 6 initial carbenicillin resistance had been present.— A. Pines *et al.*, *Br. med. J.*, 1970, *1*, 663.

Burns. Strains of *Ps. aeruginosa* highly resistant to carbenicillin had been isolated from burns. Treatment of patients with severe infections caused by strains of *Pseudomonas* still sensitive to carbenicillin should consist of carbenicillin in conjunction with gentamicin or polymyxin. The combined treatment was indicated because both of the latter retained their activity against the carbenicillin-resistant strains, and a synergism has been noted between carbenicillin and gentamicin.— E. J. L. Lowbury *et al.*, *Lancet*, 1969, *2*, 448.

For earlier references to the use of carbenicillin in patients with burns and pseudomonal infections, see Martindale 27th Edn, p. 1092.

Dosage in infants and children. The recommended daily dose of carbenicillin for children was 300 to 600 mg per kg body-weight given intravenously in divided doses every 2 to 4 hours for systemic infections or 100 to 200 mg per kg intramuscularly or intravenously for urinary-tract infections due to *Proteus* or *Pseudomonas* spp. In neonates the recommended dose was 100 mg per kg every 6 hours by intravenous injection.— M. I. Marks *et al.*, *Can. med. Ass. J.*, 1973, *109*, 49.

The suggested dose of carbenicillin for infants of more than 37 weeks' gestation was 100 mg per kg body-weight given intramuscularly or intravenously, by very slow bolus injection, every 12 hours for the first 48 hours of life, every 8 hours from the 3rd day to 2 weeks, then every 6 hours. For immature infants (those of less than 37 weeks' gestation) this dose should be given every 12 hours for the 1st week of life, every 8 hours from then to 4 weeks of age, and every 6 hours thereafter.— P. A. Davies, *Br. med. J.*, 1978, *2*, 676.

Further references: J. D. Nelson and G. H. McCracken, *Pediatrics*, 1973, *52*, 801; H. C. Spratt, *Drugs*, 1978, *16*, 226; G. H. McCracken and H. F. Eichenwald, *J. Pediat.*, 1978, *93*, 357.

Dosage in renal failure. From an investigation in 8 patients with severe renal failure a dosage schedule of carbenicillin, 2 g intravenously every 8 hours, was recommended for such patients to maintain serum concentrations of about 100 µg per ml. The mean serum half-life of carbenicillin was 12.5 hours. During haemodialysis or peritoneal dialysis the half-life of carbenicillin was reduced and the dosage should be repeated every 4 or 6 hours respectively. Peritoneal clearance was poor.— J. B. Eastwood and J. R. Curtis, *Br. med. J.*, 1968, *1*, 486.

For patients with urinary, respiratory, or wound infections together with renal failure, 2 g of carbenicillin followed by 1 g intramuscularly every 6 hours was considered necessary. A dose of 2 g would be required every 6 hours with return of reasonable renal function, and during peritoneal dialysis and haemodialysis. In pseudomonal septicaemia with renal failure, 4 g of carbenicillin should be given initially by intravenous injection followed by 2 to 4 g six-hourly by slow injection or continuous infusion. Additional doses would be required during dialysis.— M. Johny *et al.*, *Med. J. Aust.*, 1969, *2*, 681.

Data for predicting removal of carbenicillin by conventional haemodialysis.— T. P. Gibson and H. A. Nelson, *Clin. Pharmacokinet.*, 1977, *2*, 403.

After a loading dose of 4 to 6 g carbenicillin could be given in a dose of 4 to 5 g every 4 hours to patients with a creatinine clearance (CC) of 40 to 80 ml per minute, 2 to 4 g every 6 to 12 hours to those with a CC of 20 to 30 ml per minute, and 2 g every 12 hours to those with a CC of 5 to 10 ml per minute. In haemodialysis 2 g could be given every 12 to 24 hours and 2 g after dialysis; in peritoneal dialysis, 2 g could be given every 6 to 12 hours. Doses of 100 to 200 mg were used in each 2 litres of dialysate.— J. S. Cheigh, *Am. J. Med.*, 1977, *62*, 555.

The normal half-life for carbenicillin of 1.5 hours was increased to 10 to 20 hours in end-stage renal failure. The interval between doses should be extended from 4 hours to 8 to 12 hours in those with a glomerular filtration-rate (GFR) of more than 50 ml per minute, to 12 to 24 hours in those with a GFR of 10 to 50 ml per minute, and to 24 to 48 hours in those with a GFR of less than 10 ml per minute. Alternatively doses could be reduced to 75%, 50%, and 25% in those with a GFR of more than 50 ml per minute, 10 to 50 ml per minute, or less than 10 ml per minute respectively. Concentrations of carbenicillin were affected by haemodialysis or peritoneal dialysis.— W. M. Bennett *et al.*, *Ann. intern. Med.*, 1980, *93*, 62.

Further references: P. Sharpstone, *Br. med. J.*, 1977, *2*, 36; G. B. Appel and H. C. Neu, *New Engl. J. Med.*, 1977, *296*, 663.

Gonorrhoea. A comparison of carbenicillin with procaine penicillin in the treatment of uncomplicated gonorrhoea.— M. Nelson, *Sth. med. J., Nashville*, 1973, *66*, 921.

Meningitis. Intravenous therapy with carbenicillin was supplemented with intrathecal or intraventricular doses in 2 women with meningitis. The first, with *Ps. aeruginosa* meningitis, received 40 mg daily intrathecally and 30 mg daily intraventricularly as well as 6 to 20 g daily intravenously with probenecid 2 g daily by mouth. The second, with paracolon meningitis, received 25 mg into each brain ventricle 8-hourly as well as 24 g daily by intravenous infusion and probenecid 3 g daily by mouth. In each patient the infection was rapidly controlled.— A. E. Richardson *et al.*, *Postgrad. med. J.*, 1968, *44*, 844.

Four infants with meningitis due to *Pr. mirabilis* or *Pr. morganii* were successfully treated with carbenicillin given intravenously in doses of 300 to 800 mg per kg body-weight daily for 22 to 42 days. Two children experienced reversible alterations in liver function.— S. Ross *et al.*, *J. infect. Dis.*, 1970, *122, Suppl.*, S62.

Ampicillin and carbenicillin were equally effective in the treatment of purulent meningitis due to susceptible organisms in a study of 86 patients. All patients were given an initial loading dose of 65 mg of antibiotic per kg body-weight intravenously followed by 200 or 400 mg per kg daily in 6 divided doses generally to a maximum of 28 days.— G. D. Overturf *et al.*, *Antimicrob. Ag. Chemother.*, 1977, *11*, 420. Carbenicillin offers no advantage over ampicillin for the treatment of children with meningitis caused by ampicillin-sensitive *H. influenzae* type b; chloramphenicol should be used against ampicillin-resistant strains.— *Med. Lett.*, 1979, *21*, 45.

Pneumonia. Carbenicillin alone or with gentamicin was used successfully to treat 42 children with aspiration pneumonia. Infecting organisms included Gram-positive cocci, *Bacteroides fragilis, B. melaninogenicus, Klebsiella pneumoniae,* and *Ps. aeruginosa*.— I. Brook, *Curr. ther. Res.*, 1978, *23*, 136.

Pseudomonal infections. Of 17 patients with pseudomonal infections and 3 with other Gram-negative bacillary infections treated with carbenicillin, 6 were cured. Five patients relapsed between 12 and 23 days later due to re-infection with *Ps. aeruginosa* with marked resistance to the drug. Seizures occurred in 2 severely uraemic patients given 4 g, and pulmonary oedema in 1 given 24 g daily.— T. A. Hoffman and W. E. Bullock, *Ann. intern. Med.*, 1970, *73*, 165.

Carbenicillin when administered in a daily dose of 30 g by intravenous infusion to adults and 20 g per m^2 body-surface to children under 15 years was effective in the treatment of 44 of 59 episodes of pseudomonal infections.— G. P. Bodey *et al.*, *J. Am. med. Ass.*, 1971, *218*, 62.

Carbenicillin 15 g per m^2 body-surface and colistin sulphomethate sodium 100 to 600 mg per m^2 daily were administered intravenously every 6 or 12 hours for the treatment of severe pseudomonal infections in 9 children with leukaemia. Two with cellulitis and septicaemia and 1 with septicaemia were cured of the infection and improvement was seen in a further 2 with cellulitis and septicaemia and 1 with septicaemia. No side-effects attributable to antibiotic therapy were seen.— C. B. Pratt and D. L. Dugger, *Curr. ther. Res.*, 1971, *13*, 182.

Carbenicillin and tobramycin produced a favourable response in 9 of 10 children with cystic fibrosis suffering from *Ps. aeruginosa* infections.— P. Déry, *J. Am. med. Ass.*, 1977, *237*, 1415. A retrospective study of 160 patients with cystic fibrosis, 80 of whom had persistent colonisation of the respiratory tract with *Ps. aeruginosa*, showed that treatment with antibiotics, including carbenicillin and aminoglycosides did not eradicate *Ps. aeruginosa* and their continued use seemed to contribute to the persistence of infection and to the appearance of mucoid strains.— L. L. Kulczycki *et al.*, *J. Am. med. Ass.*, 1978, *240*, 30. See also P. H. Beaudry *et al.*, *J. Pediat.*, 1980, *97*, 144.

Use with gentamicin. For reports on the use of carbenicillin in conjunction with Gentamicin Sulphate, see p.1173.

Preparations

Carbenicillin Injection *(B.P.)*. A sterile solution of carbenicillin sodium in Water for Injections prepared, immediately before use, by dissolving the sterile contents of a sealed container in the requisite amount of Water for Injections. Potency is expressed in terms of the equivalent amount of carbenicillin. It should be used immediately. *U.S.P.* includes Sterile Carbenicillin Disodium.

Pyopen *(Beecham Research, UK)*. Carbenicillin sodium, available as powder for preparing injections in vials each containing the equivalent of 1 and 5 g of carbenicillin, and in infusion bottles containing the equivalent of 5 g. (Also available as Pyopen in *Arg., Austral., Belg., Canad., Fr., Ital., Jap., Neth., S.Afr., Spain, Switz., USA*).

Other Proprietary Names

Anabactyl *(Ger.)*; Carbapen *(Austral.)*; Fugacillin *(Denm., Norw., Swed.)*; Geopen (see also under Carindacillin Sodium) *(Ital., USA)*: Microcillin *(Ger.)*; Pyocianil *(Ital.)*; Rexcilina *(Spain)*.

25-d

Carfecillin Sodium. BRL 3475; Carbenicillin Phenyl Sodium. Sodium (6*R*)-6-(2-phenoxycarbonyl-2-phenylacetamido)penicillanate.
$C_{23}H_{21}N_2NaO_6S$=476.5.

CAS — 27025-49-6 (acid); 21649-57-0 (sodium salt).

Each g represents about 2.1 mmol (2.1 mEq) of sodium. Carfecillin sodium 1.3 g is approximately equivalent to 1 g of carbenicillin.

Adverse Effects, Treatment, and Precautions. As for Carbenicillin Sodium, p.1111. Nausea and diarrhoea have been reported in about 5% of patients given carfecillin sodium.

Antimicrobial Action. As for Carbenicillin Sodium, p.1111.

Absorption and Fate. Carfecillin sodium is absorbed from the gastro-intestinal tract and is rapidly hydrolysed in the gastric mucosa and the liver to carbenicillin and phenol. Following a dose of 1 g of carfecillin sodium plasma concentrations of 5 to 10 µg per ml of carbenicillin and urine concentrations of 0.3 to 1 mg per ml of carbenicillin may be achieved.

In 4 healthy volunteers given carfecillin 500 mg as a single dose, mean peak serum concentrations of about 3 µg per ml were achieved about 90 minutes after the dose; in 6 given 1 g peak concentrations of about 5 µg per ml were achieved about 100 minutes after the dose; these concentrations were inadequate to treat systemic infection with *Pseudomonas aeruginosa*. Mean urine concentrations in the first 4 hours after the 500-mg and 1-g doses were respectively 112 µg per ml (range 54 to 180) and 434 µg per ml (range 52 to 1120). Of 35 patients with urinary-tract infection 21 were cleared of infection after treatment for 7 days with 1 g eight-hourly; failures included 4 of 12 with infection due to *Ps. aeruginosa*, 6 of 9 due to *Escherichia coli*, 1 due to *Proteus mirabilis*, and 1 due to *Staphylococcus aureus*.— P. J. Wilkinson *et al.*, *Br. med. J.*, 1975, *2*, 250.

A mean peak serum-carbenicillin concentration of only 1.38 µg per ml was achieved in 11 fasting subjects 2 hours after a 500-mg dose of carfecillin. A mean peak urine concentration of 830 µg per ml occurred between 2 and 4 hours but, as with serum concentrations, there was considerable individual variation. About 27% of the dose was recovered from the urine, as carbenicillin, over 6 hours.— D. A. Leigh and K. Simmons, *J. antimicrob. Chemother.*, 1976, *2*, 293.

Further references: Z. Modr *et al.*, *Int. J. clin. Pharmac. Biopharm.*, 1977, *15*, 81; H. Graber *et al.*, *ibid.*, 1978, *16*, 59.

Uses. Carfecillin sodium is given by mouth in doses of 0.5 to 1 g thrice daily for the treatment of urinary-tract infections due to *Pseudomonas* spp. and other sensitive bacteria including *Escherichia coli* and *Proteus* spp. Children from 2 to 10 years may be given half the adult dose; a recommended dose range is 30 to 60 mg per kg body-weight daily. It is not used for the treatment of systemic infections since attainable plasma-carbenicillin concentrations are too low to be effective.

A review of carfecillin.— *Drug & Ther. Bull.*, 1975, *13*, 35. See also E. T. Knudsen (letter), *Br. med. J.*, 1974, *4*, 530; R. Wise, *J. antimicrob. Chemother.*, 1975, *1*, 4.

Urinary-tract infections. Clinical improvement was seen in 180 of 203 patients with urinary-tract infections given carfecillin sodium 500 mg thrice daily for 7 days.— L. J. Lees and J. W. Harding, *Br. J. clin. Pract.*, 1974, *28*, 349.

Carfecillin 500 mg thrice daily for 7 days cured 44 of 58 patients with urinary-tract infections caused mainly by *E. coli* or *Ps. aeruginosa*, but 12 patients became re-infected. Resistant strains of *Klebsiella* spp. were responsible for re-infection in 9 who had previously had pseudomonal infections.— D. A. Leigh and K. Simmons, *J. antimicrob. Chemother.*, 1976, *2*, 293. See also J. Borowski *et al.*, *ibid.*, 175.

Proprietary Preparations

Uticillin *(Beecham Research, UK)*. Carfecillin sodium, available as tablets of 500 mg. (Also available as Uticillin in *Jap.,S.Afr.*).

NOTE

Uticillin VK is a proprietary name for Phenoxymethylpenicillin Potassium p.1201.

Other Proprietary Names

Gripenin-O *(Jap.)*; Pencina *(Switz.)*.

26-n

Carindacillin Sodium. Carbenicillin Indanyl Sodium *(U.S.P.)*; CP-15464-2. Sodium (6*R*)-6-[2-(indan-5-yloxycarbonyl)-2-phenylacetamido]-penicillanate.
$C_{26}H_{25}N_2NaO_6S$=516.5.

CAS — 35531-88-5 (acid); 26605-69-6 (sodium salt).

Pharmacopoeias. In *U.S.*

A white to off-white crystalline powder with a bitter taste. **Soluble** in water and alcohol. A 10% solution in water has a pH of 5 to 8. Each g represents about 1.9 mmol (1.9 mEq) of sodium. Carindacillin sodium 1.4 g is approximately equivalent to 1 g of carbenicillin.

Adverse Effects, Treatment, and Precautions. As for Carbenicillin Sodium, p.1111.
Side-effects that have been reported with carindacillin sodium include bitter taste, nausea, vomiting, diarrhoea, skin rashes and dizziness

Colitis. Reports of pseudomembranous colitis associated with carindacillin sodium T. F. O'Meara and R. A. Simmons (letter), *Ann. intern. Med.*, 1980, *92*, 440; H. A. Saadah (letter), *ibid.*, *93*, 645.

Antimicrobial Action. As for Carbenicillin Sodium, p.1111.
Carindacillin has a lower MIC for Gram-positive organisms and *Klebsiella pneumoniae* than carbenicillin *in vitro* but due to the rapid metabolism of the ester this is not observed *in vivo*.

Absorption and Fate. Carindacillin sodium is administered by mouth and is hydrolysed releasing carbenicillin. Peak plasma-carbenicillin concentrations of at least 10 µg per ml occur about 1.5 hours after a dose of 1 g of carindacillin sodium. Low concentrations of carindacillin can be detected in the plasma; these are highest at 30 minutes and negligible at 1.5 hours. Carindacillin is reported to be 98% bound to plasma proteins. A dose of 1 g maintains a urine-carbenicillin concentration of 1 mg per ml for about 3 hours. The indanol moiety is excreted in the urine as conjugates.

Following a dose of 1 g of carindacillin in 6 healthy subjects, peak serum concentrations of carbenicillin of at least 6.3 µg per ml were achieved in 2 hours. In 5 of the subjects probenecid 500 mg given 1 and 8 hours before carindacillin 1 g increased the fasting mean peak serum concentration of carbenicillin from 10.4 to 23.7 µg per ml. Concentrations of at least 640 µg per ml of carbenicillin were detected in urine collected over 6 hours when probenecid was not given and 312 µg per ml when probenecid was given.— J. L. Bran *et al.*, *Clin. Pharmac. Ther.*, 1971, *12*, 525.

Following oral administration, carindacillin sodium was rapidly absorbed and hydrolysed to yield carbenicillin, the indanol fraction being excreted in the urine as glucuronide and sulphate ester conjugates. Peak serum concentrations of carbenicillin occurred 1 to 2 hours after administration in 24 normal volunteers and reached near zero levels in 6 hours. Peak serum levels and serum half-life were increased in patients with renal failure but urine concentrations in these patients were sufficient to inhibit most organisms causing urinary-tract infections.— R. B. Bailey *et al.*, *Postgrad. med. J.*, 1972, *48*, 422.

Further references: K. Butler *et al.*, *J. infect. Dis.*, 1973, *127*, *Suppl.*, S97; A. K. Knirsch *et al.*, *ibid.*, S105; Z. Modr *et al.*, *Int. J. clin. Pharmac. Biopharm.*, 1977, *15*, 81.

Uses. Carindacillin sodium is given by mouth usually in doses equivalent to 382 to 764 mg of carbenicillin four times daily for the treatment of urinary-tract infections due to *Pseudomonas* spp., *E. coli*, and sensitive *Proteus* spp. It is not used for the treatment of systemic infections since attainable plasma-carbenicillin concentrations are too low to be effective.

A review of carindacillin.— *Med. Lett.*, 1973, *15*, 29.

Dosage in renal failure. In a study of 20 patients with chronic renal disease and varying degrees of renal impairment a dose of 1 g of carindacillin sodium produced urine concentrations that were considered adequate to treat susceptible urinary-tract infections in patients with mild or moderate renal insufficiency (creatinine clearances of 33 to 84 and 17 to 22 ml per minute respectively).— C. E. Cox, *J. infect. Dis.*, 1973, *127*, *Suppl.*, S157.

In a study of patients with reduced kidney function, 3 of 4 patients with a creatinine clearance of less than 30 ml per minute achieved urine concentrations of carbenicillin considered to exceed only transiently the MICs for *E. coli*, *Klebsiella*, and *Enterobacter* spp. when given carindacillin sodium 1 g.— H. Nakano *et al.*, *Chemotherapy, Basle*, 1977, *23*, 299.

Gonorrhoea. Carindacillin sodium 1.5 g with probenecid 1 g was used to treat 50 men with gonorrhoea. Follow-up of 42 showed that 37 were cured; 3 had been re-infected and 2 failed to respond.— V. S. Rajan and J. E. H. Sng, *Singapore med. J.*, 1974, *15*, 37.

Prostatitis. A report of the successful use of carindacillin sodium 1 g four times a day in patients with acute or chronic prostatitis.— R. A. Oliveri *et al.*, *Curr. ther. Res.*, 1979, *25*, 415.

Urinary-tract infections. Carindacillin 2 or 4 g daily by mouth was given for 14 days to 26 patients with genito-urinary infection. There was bacteriological cure in 13 of 15 with *E. coli*, 3 of 15 with *Proteus* spp., and 3 of 5 with *Ps. aeruginosa*, but one patient with *Klebsiella* failed to respond. About a third of a dose was excreted in the urine within 6 hours, giving urine concentrations of 0.274 to 2.16 mg per ml.— J. F. Wallace *et al.*, *Antimicrob. Ag. Chemother.*, 1970, 223.

Carindacillin in a dose of 1 g four times daily usually for 2 weeks given to 28 patients with urinary-tract infections due to *E. coli*, *Pr. mirabilis*, *Ps. aeruginosa*, *Enterobacter aerogenes*, enterococci, and *Citrobacter* cleared all symptoms within 72 hours and eliminated the infecting organism in all patients. Four weeks later 16 patients were still free of infection, 4 had relapsed, and 8 were infected with a new organism. Most patients complained of the taste and smell of carindacillin; pruritus causing withdrawal of treatment occurred in 2, nausea in 2, and diarrhoea in 1. Laboratory studies after treatment demonstrated mild eosinophilia in 2 and elevation of serum aminotransferases in 2.— J. L. Bran *et al.*, *Clin. Pharmac. Ther.*, 1971, *12*, 525.

There were no significant differences in response to carindacillin 1 g, ampicillin 0.5 or 1 g, or cephaloglycin 500 mg given four times daily to 56 patients with urinary-tract infections due to Gram-negative organisms.— K. M. Ries *et al.*, *J. infect. Dis.*, 1973, *127*, *Suppl.*, S148.

Further references: M. Turck, *J. infect. Dis.*, 1973, *127*, *Suppl.*, S133; D. A. Baker and V. T. Andriole, *ibid.*, S136; W. J. Holloway and W. A. Taylor, *ibid.*, S143; M. Westenfelder and P. O. Madsen, *ibid.*, S154; *Br. med. J.*, 1973, *3*, 555; H. G. E. Michiels *et al.*, *Curr. med. Res. Opinion*, 1978, *5*, 394; H. Seneca, *J. Am. Geriat. Soc.*, 1979, *27*, 222.

Preparations

Carbenicillin Indanyl Sodium Tablets *(U.S.P.)*. Carindacillin Sodium Tablets. Tablets containing carindacillin sodium equivalent to carbenicillin 382 mg. Store in airtight containers.

Proprietary Names

Carindapen *(Pfizer, Ger.)*; Geocillin *(Roerig, USA)*; Geopen *(see also under Carbenicillin Sodium) (Pfizer, Austral.; Pfizer, Denm.; Pfizer, Ital.; Pfizer, Switz.)*; Geopen-U *(Jap.)*; G.U.-Pen *(Pfizer, Belg.; Pfizer, Neth.)*; Unipen 500 *(Pfizer, Spain)*.

27-h

Cefaclor *(U.S.P.)*. 99638. (7*R*)-3-Chloro-7-(α-D-phenylglycylamino)-3-cephem-4-carboxylic acid monohydrate.
$C_{15}H_{14}ClN_3O_4S,H_2O$=385.8.

CAS — 53994-73-3 (anhydrous); 70356-03-5 (monohydrate).

Pharmacopoeias. In *U.S.*

A white to off-white crystalline powder. It has a

potency of not less than 860 μg per mg. **Soluble** 1 in 100 of water; very slightly soluble in chloroform, ether, and methyl alcohol. A 2.5% aqueous suspension has a pH of 3 to 4.5. **Store** in airtight containers.

Stability in solution. Buffered solutions of cefaclor at pH 2.5, 4.5, 6, 7, and 8 stored for 72 hours at 4° contained 95, 93, 71, 46, and 34% of their initial activity respectively; stored at 25° for 72 hours the solutions contained 95, 69, 16, 5, and 3%, and at 37°, solutions at pH 2.5, 4.5, and 6 contained 80, 15, and 5%. After 24 hours solutions at pH 7 or 8 contained only 3% of the initial activity. Freshly prepared human serum or plasma containing cefaclor lost 8 and 51% of its cefaclor activity respectively when incubated for 6 hours at 4° and 25° and lost 48% when incubated for 2 hours at 37°. The rate of loss of the activity of cefaclor when added to commercially prepared pooled human serum was about 15, 45, and 68% per hour at 4, 25, and 37°.— M. A. Foglesong *et al.*, *Antimicrob. Ag. Chemother.*, 1978, *13*, 49.

Adverse Effects and Precautions. As for Cephalexin, p.1123.

Allergy. A cluster of hypersensitivity reactions occurred in 8 children receiving cefaclor for the treatment of persistent otitis media; 6 were taking cefaclor for the second time. A generalised pruritic rash and arthritis appeared from 5 to 19 days after the initiation of treatment with cefaclor and generally disappeared within 4 to 5 days of discontinuation. Signs of erythema multiforme developed in 6 of the children and purpura in 4.— D. L. Murray *et al.* (letter), *New Engl. J. Med.*, 1980, *303*, 1003.

Antimicrobial Action. Cefaclor is bactericidal and has antimicrobial activity similar to that of cephalexin (see p.1123) but is reported to be more active against Gram-negative bacteria such as *Escherichia coli, Klebsiella pneumoniae,* and *Proteus mirabilis*, and especially against *Haemophilus influenzae*, including ampicillin-resistant strains, and against *Neisseria gonorrhoeae.* It may be less resistant to staphylococcal penicillinase than cephalexin or cephradine and a marked inoculum effect has occurred *in vitro.*

Cefaclor had a similar antimicrobial spectrum to cephalexin and cephradine but in general was substantially more active; cephradine was the least active. With an inoculum size of 10^4 colony-forming units (CFU) per ml, MICs for cefaclor, cephalexin, and cephradine against *H. influenzae* were 2, 8, and 16 μg per ml respectively and 2, 32, and 64 μg per ml for beta-lactamase-producing strains; there was a marked inoculum effect when it was increased to 10^6 CFU per ml, especially with cefaclor. The inoculum effect with *Staph. aureus* was very variable, but cephalexin was the least affected by penicillinase-producing strains and cefaclor was the most affected by such strains.— N. J. Bill and J. A. Washington, *Antimicrob. Ag. Chemother.*, 1977, *11*, 470. See also M. S. Silver *et al.*, *ibid.*, *12*, 591; S. Mirrett and L. B. Reller, *Curr. ther. Res.*, 1979, *26*, 145; R. Wise *et al.*, *J. antimicrob. Chemother.*, 1979, *5*, 601.

In an *in vitro* study of 261 clinical isolates, cefaclor and cephalexin were less active than cephalothin against *Staph. aureus*. Cefaclor was generally the most active against *E. coli, Kleb. pneumoniae*, and *Pr. mirabilis*, although the inoculum effect was greater than with cephalothin.— J. Santoro and M. E. Levison, *Antimicrob. Ag. Chemother.*, 1977, *12*, 442.

Cefaclor and cefatrizine had similar activity to cephalexin and cephradine against staphylococci, streptococci, and anaerobes but greater activity against *E. coli, Klebsiella* spp., *Pr. mirabilis*, and *H. influenzae*.— R. J. Fass and R. B. Prior, *Curr. ther. Res.*, 1978, *24*, 352.

Cefaclor had a similar activity to cephamandole, and was more active than cephazolin, cephalothin, or cephalexin *in vitro* against 67 strains of *Salmonella typhi* and 54 strains of *S. paratyphi A.* Cefaclor had an MIC of 0.39, 0.78, and 1.56 μg per ml respectively against 55, 97, and 100% of the strains of *S. typhi* and an MIC of 0.78, 1.56, and 3.12 μg per ml respectively against 9, 87, and 100% of the strains of *S. paratyphi A.*— L. J. Strausbaugh *et al.*, *Antimicrob. Ag. Chemother.*, 1978, *13*, 134.

Cefaclor was generally less effective *in vitro* than cephamandole or cephazolin against 331 aerobes and less effective than cephamandole, cephazolin, cephalothin, or cephradine against 271 anaerobes. At 16 μg per ml cefaclor inhibited 68% of all aerobes tested and nearly 80% of 211 enteropathogenic organisms isolated from cases of infantile diarrhoea, including *E. coli, Salmonella,* and *Shigella.* The activities of benzylpenicillin and cefaclor were not enhanced when used together.— V. T. Bach *et al.*, *Antimicrob. Ag. Chemother.*, 1978, *13*, 210.

A test using a standardised diffusion disk containing cephalothin 30 μg was fairly reliable for predicting susceptibility of isolates of pyogenic Gram-positive cocci and of *E. coli* to cefaclor but was unreliable for isolates of enterococci and the *Enterobacter* spp. Clinical studies should be accompanied by laboratory studies with a candidate cefaclor disk.— S. Shadomy and M. Carver, *Antimicrob. Ag. Chemother.*, 1978, *13*, 228.

Cefaclor had a similar activity to cephalexin *in vitro* against Gram-positive bacteria but was more active against *Haemophilus influenzae* including beta-lactamase-producing isolates. All of 10 strains of *H. influenzae* were inhibited by 12.5 μg per ml of cefaclor compared with 50 μg per ml of cephalexin. Cefaclor was also generally more active than cephalexin against other Gram-negative bacteria but less resistant to beta-lactamases.— H. C. Neu and K. P. Fu, *Antimicrob. Ag. Chemother.*, 1978, *13*, 584. See also W. M. Scheld *et al.*, *ibid.*, 1977, *12*, 290; C. C. Sanders, *ibid.*, 490. At 6.25 μg per ml, 100, 11, and 3% of 33 beta-lactamase-negative and 31 beta-lactamase-positive isolates of *H. influenzae* were inhibited by cefaclor, cephalexin, and cephradine, respectively. The actions of cefaclor, trimethoprim, or erythromycin were considered to be synergistic when used with sulphamethoxazole.— R. Sinai *et al.*, *Antimicrob. Ag. Chemother.*, 1978, *13*, 861.

Cefaclor had an MIC of 8 μg or less per ml against 181 of 201 strains of *Staph. aureus in vitro* while cephalothin had an MIC of 1 μg or less per ml against 195.— B. M. Gray *et al.*, *Antimicrob. Ag. Chemother.*, 1978, *13*, 988.

Cefaclor appeared to be 10 times more active than cephalexin or cephradine against 15 strains of *Neisseria gonorrhoeae*, although there was an inoculum effect with one of 2 beta-lactamase-producers tested.— R. Wise (letter), *J. antimicrob. Chemother.*, 1978, *4*, 578.

Cefaclor was more active than cephalexin against strains of *Staph. aureus*, streptococci, and anaerobic bacteria *in vitro* but was less active than benzylpenicillin. Cefaclor was also more active than cephalexin or benzylpenicillin against facultative Gram-negative bacteria but none of the antibiotics was very active against strains of *Pseudomonas* or indole-positive *Proteus*, *Providencia*, or other Enterobacteriaceae. Cefaclor was highly active against *Pasteurella multocida*. Neither of the cephalosporins was active against *Bacteroides fragilis*.— F. P. Tally *et al.*, *J. antimicrob. Chemother.*, 1979, *5*, 159.

Further references: B. R. Meyers and S. Z. Hirschman, *J. clin. Pharmac.*, 1978, *18*, 85.

For further comparisons *in vitro* of cefaclor with other cephalosporins active by mouth, see Cefatrizine, p.1117.

Absorption and Fate. Cefaclor is absorbed from the gastro-intestinal tract but plasma concentrations are slightly lower than those achieved with cephalexin or cephradine. Doses of 250 and 500 mg by mouth produce peak plasma concentrations of about 6 and 13 μg per ml respectively at 1 hour; absorption is delayed by the presence of food. Half-lives ranging from 30 minutes to 1 hour have been reported.

Cefaclor appears to be widely distributed in the body and is rapidly excreted by the kidneys, at least 50% of a dose appearing in the urine within 6 hours. Probenecid delays excretion.

An oral dose of 250 mg given to healthy subjects produced a mean peak serum concentration of 6.01 μg per ml for cefaclor compared with 9.43 μg per ml for cephalexin; half-lives were 0.58 and 0.8 hours respectively.— O. M. Korzeniowski *et al.*, *Antimicrob. Ag. Chemother.*, 1977, *12*, 157.

Mean peak plasma concentrations of cefaclor were 12.4 or 5 μg per ml in 5 healthy fasting subjects after taking 500 or 250 mg of cefaclor respectively. About half of a dose was excreted in the urine within 4 hours of administration. Ingestion of food significantly reduced the absorption of cefaclor. The mean plasma half-life of cefaclor was 0.8 hours after the 500 mg dose and this was increased to 1.3 hours when taken with 1 g of probenecid. The peak plasma concentration of cefaclor ranged from 12.1 to 23.2 μg per ml in 7 fasting patients with impaired renal function after the 500 mg dose and was 19.7 μg per ml in 4 anephric patients. Plasma half-lives ranged from 1.5 to 3.5 hours in the patients with impaired renal function and were 2.8 and 2.1 hours after and during dialysis respectively in the anephric patients.— J. Santoro *et al.*, *Antimicrob. Ag. Chemother.*, 1978, *13*, 951.

The pharmacokinetics of cefaclor were studied in 17 patients with end-stage renal disease (creatinine clearance of less than 5 ml per minute). A mean peak plasma concentration of 48.3 μg per ml was obtained in 6 fasting patients after a 1-g dose and occurred within 4 hours of administration; the mean plasma half-life was 2.3 hours. A haemodialysis session of 5.5 hours starting 2 hours after the same dose reduced the mean half-life to 1.6 hours and about 35% of the dose was recovered in the dialysate. There was no evidence of drug accumulation in 5 patients who received cefaclor 500 mg every 6 hours for 36 hours and plasma concentrations were maintained between 10.6 and 16 μg per ml.— S. J. Berman *et al.*, *Antimicrob. Ag. Chemother.*, 1978, *14*, 281. See also D. A. Spyker *et al.*, *ibid.*, 172. The peak serum concentration of cefaclor in 5 patients with mild to moderate renal impairment ranged from 23 to 11.9 μg per ml from 1 to 4 hours after administration of a single 500-mg dose and remained above 5 μg per ml at 4 hours. The serum half-life ranged from about 1.4 to 2.7 hours. Urinary concentrations during the first 24 hours were considered to be high enough to inhibit many common urinary pathogens. It was suggested that a 500-mg dose of cefaclor could be given every 8 to 12 hours to these patients but in patients undergoing haemodialysis, monitoring of serum concentrations was required. Haemodialysis was effective in clearing cefaclor.— G. Gartenberg *et al.*, *J. antimicrob. Chemother.*, 1979, *5*, 465. Criticism and comments.— J. P. Fillastre *et al.* (letter), *ibid.*, 1980, *6*, 155. See also Dosage in Renal Failure in Uses (below).

Mean peak plasma concentrations of cefaclor in 10 healthy subjects were 6.31, 15.22, and 25.44 μg per ml one hour after administration of doses of 0.25, 0.5, and 1 g respectively; mean plasma half-lives were 0.49, 1.0, and 0.76 hours and urinary concentrations were about 273, 799, and 2000 μg per ml respectively during the 6 hours after administration. About 47 to 51% of a dose was excreted in the urine.— G. R. Hodges *et al.*, *Antimicrob. Ag. Chemother.*, 1978, *14*, 454.

Average peak serum concentrations of cefaclor of 2.44, 3.73, 5.10, and 10.19 μg per ml occurred 1 hour after administration of 100, 150, 250, and 500 mg respectively in a study involving 50 fasting healthy subjects. The mean plasma half-life was about 40 minutes and 71 to 75% of a dose was recovered in the urine in the first 6 hours after administration; over half of each dose was recovered in the first 2 hours. In 6 subjects who received cefaclor after food, absorption was reduced, producing lower and sometimes delayed mean peak serum concentrations, but urinary recovery was similar to that in fasting subjects.— A. Glynne *et al.*, *J. antimicrob. Chemother.*, 1978, *4*, 343.

The pharmacokinetics of cefaclor were studied in 28 children aged 4 to 63 months who were treated for impetigo, pharyngitis or otitis media. The mean serum concentrations of cefaclor 30 minutes after administration of cefaclor 10 mg per kg body-weight were 10.8 μg per ml in fasting children and 6.7 μg per ml in those who received the antibiotic and milk concomitantly; corresponding concentrations after 15 mg per kg were 13.1 and 10.9 μg per ml respectively. Although peak serum concentrations of cefaclor were smaller in non-fasting children the overall absorption of cefaclor was similar for both groups. Serum half-lives of cefaclor ranged from 36 to 46 minutes after 15 mg per kg and from 55 to 60 minutes after 10 mg per kg. Mean concentrations of cefaclor in saliva up to 6 hours after administration of 15 mg per kg were similar to the corresponding serum concentrations.— G. H. McCracken *et al.*, *J. antimicrob. Chemother.*, 1978, *4*, 515.

Cefaclor was about 50% bound to plasma proteins *in vitro*.— F. P. Tally *et al.*, *J. antimicrob. Chemother.*, 1979, *5*, 159.

Further references to pharmacokinetic studies of cefaclor: B. R. Meyers *et al.*, *J. clin. Pharmac.*, 1978, *18*, 174; H. Lode *et al.*, *Antimicrob. Ag. Chemother.*, 1979, *16*, 1; P. G. Welling *et al.*, *Int. J. clin. Pharmac. Biopharm.*, 1979, *17*, 397.

Uses. Cefaclor, a cephalosporin antibiotic, is administered by mouth in the treatment of susceptible infections including those of the respiratory and urinary tracts. The usual dose is 250 mg every 8 hours although up to 4 g daily has been given. A suggested dose for children is 20 mg per kg body-weight daily increased if necessary to 40 mg per kg daily but not exceeding a total daily dose of 1 g.

Reviews of cefaclor.— *Drug & Ther. Bull.*, 1979, *17*, 69; *Med. Lett.*, 1979, *21*, 85; *Postgrad. med. J.*, 1979, *55*, *Suppl.* 4, 1–101; H. D. Bergman, *Drug Intell. & clin. Pharm.*, 1980, *14*, 11.

Of 73 children aged 1 to 13 years with staphylococcal bullous impetigo who were evaluated after receiving cefaclor 30 mg per kg body-weight daily in 3 or 4 divided doses for 5 to 10 days, 66 were cleared of lesions and of 5 who were considered to have improved 3 were cleared after a further 4 days of therapy. One child developed diarrhoea and treatment was discontinued after 5 days, when his lesions had healed.— B. M. Gray *et al.*, *Antimicrob. Ag. Chemother.*, 1978, *13*, 988.

In a study of 95 infants with acute otitis media, cefaclor in a dose of 60 mg per kg body-weight daily was more effective than 40 mg per kg daily and results were comparable with those previously achieved using amoxycillin.— J. D. Nelson *et al.*, *Am. J. Dis. Child.*, 1978, *132*, 992.

Further references: L. J. Baraff *et al.*, *Curr. ther. Res.*, 1977, *22*, 536; C. M. Ginsberg and G. H. McCracken, *J. Pediat.*, 1980, *96*, 340.

Dosage in renal failure. The half-life of cefaclor after a 250 mg dose was 0.4 to 1.1 hours in 6 healthy subjects [creatinine clearance rate (CCR): 93 to 125 ml per minute], 0.6 to 1.1 hours in 3 elderly patients (CCR:81 to 87 ml per minute), 0.8 to 3.5 hours in 11 patients with renal disease of long duration (CCR: 6 to 59 ml per minute), and 2.5 to 3.04 hours in 5 patients requiring haemodialysis. About 50 to 70% of the dose was recovered in the urine of the healthy subjects within 8 hours. From a nomogram constructed from the results it was recommended that patients with severely impaired renal function should receive one-quarter of the usual 24-hour maintenance dose in a 24-hour period, those with a CCR of less than 40 ml per minute, half of the dose, and that modification of the dose for patients with a CCR greater than 40 ml per minute was unnecessary.— R. Bloch *et al.*, *Antimicrob. Ag. Chemother.*, 1977, *12*, 730.

The normal half-life for cefaclor of 0.75 hour was increased to 2.8 hours in end-stage renal failure. In patients with a glomerular filtration-rate (GFR) of 10 to 50 ml per minute 50 to 100% of the normal dose could be given and in those with a GFR of less than 10 ml per minute the dose should be reduced to 33%. Concentrations of cefaclor were not affected by haemodialysis.— W. M. Bennett *et al.*, *Ann. intern. Med.*, 1980, *93*, 62.

See also above under Absorption and Fate.

Preparations

Cefaclor Capsules *(U.S.P.)*. Capsules containing cefaclor. Potency is expressed in terms of the equivalent amount of anhydrous cefaclor. Store in airtight containers.

Cefaclor for Oral Suspension *(U.S.P.)*. A dry mixture of cefaclor and one or more suitable buffers, colours, diluents, and flavours. Potency is expressed in terms of the equivalent amount of anhydrous cefaclor. pH of the reconstituted suspension 2.5 to 4.5. Store in airtight containers.

Distaclor *(Dista, UK)*. Cefaclor, available as **Capsules** of 250 mg and as **Suspension** (supplied as granules for preparation with water before use) containing 125 or 250 mg in each 5 ml (suggested diluents, syrup or water).

Other Proprietary Names

Ceclor *(USA)*; Panoral *(Ger.)*.

28-m

Cefadroxil *(U.S.P.)*. BL-S578; MJF 11567-3. (7*R*)-7-(α-D-4-Hydroxyphenylglycylamino)-3-methyl-3-cephem-4-carboxylic acid monohydrate.

$C_{16}H_{17}N_3O_5S, H_2O$=381.4.

CAS — 50370-12-2 (anhydrous); 66592-87-8 (monohydrate).

Pharmacopoeias. In *U.S.*

A white crystalline powder containing the equivalent of 900 to 1050 µg of cefadroxil monohydrate per mg, calculated on the anhydrous basis. **Soluble** in water. A 5% solution in water has a pH of 4 to 6. **Store** in airtight containers.

Adverse Effects and Precautions. As for Cephalexin, p.1123.

Antimicrobial Action. Cefadroxil is an analogue of cephalexin (p.1123) and has similar antimicrobial activity *in vitro.*

Cefadroxil had similar inhibitory activity to that of cephalexin and cephradine against 602 clinical isolates of Gram-positive and Gram-negative bacteria.— R. E. Buck and K. E. Price, *Antimicrob. Ag. Chemother.*, 1977, *11*, 324.

Absorption and Fate. Cefadroxil is well-absorbed from the gastro-intestinal tract and concentrations in the plasma and urine are more sustained than with cephalexin.

In a comparative study in healthy fasted subjects, cephalexin and cephradine were more rapidly absorbed than cefadroxil. Mean peak plasma concentrations after a 500-mg dose by mouth were about 16 µg per ml for cefadroxil, 21 µg per ml for cephalexin, and 18 µg per ml for cephradine but concentrations were sustained for longer with cefadroxil and 4 hours after a dose were about 5, 1, and 1 µg per ml respectively; corresponding half-lives were 1.27, 0.57, and 0.61 hours. Cefadroxil was 20% bound to plasma proteins compared with 17% for cephalexin. The presence of food had no significant effect on the absorption of cefadroxil or cephalexin. Mean urinary concentrations 0 to 3, 3 to 6, and 6 to 12 hours after a 500-mg dose were 1211, 1113, and 167 µg per ml for cefadroxil, 1783, 607, and 78 µg per ml for cephalexin, and 2136, 582, and 61 µg per ml for cephradine. About 88% of a dose of cefadroxil or cephalexin was excreted in the urine.— M. Pfeffer *et al.*, *Antimicrob. Ag. Chemother.*, 1977, *11*, 331. See also A. I. Hartstein *et al.*, *ibid.*, *12*, 93.

Mean peak serum concentrations of cefadroxil in healthy subjects after 0.5- and 1-g doses were 15.04 and 26.32 µg per ml respectively 2 hours after administration and 33.88 µg per ml 3 hours after a 1.5-g dose. There was little evidence of drug accumulation in serum after repeated dosage. The mean serum half-lives of cefadroxil after the 0.5-, 1-, and 1.5-g doses were 1.18, 1.51, and 1.99 hours respectively. In a placebo-controlled double-blind study in a further 29 healthy subjects cefadroxil produced significantly greater and more sustained serum concentrations than cephalexin after equal doses. Serum half-lives for cefadroxil and cephalexin were 1.66 and 0.91 hours respectively after a dose of 1.5 g four times daily.— E. R. Jolly *et al.*, *Curr. ther. Res.*, 1977, *22*, 727.

The pharmacokinetics of cefadroxil were studied in 30 children aged 13 months to 12 years. The mean peak serum concentrations of cefadroxil were 10.1 µg per ml in 10 fasting children and 7.4 µg per ml in 11 children who were given milk with cefadroxil 10 mg per kg body-weight and occurred 1 hour after administration; mean peak serum concentrations in 16 fasting children and in 17 children who were given milk with a dose of 15 mg per kg were 13.7 and 11.0 µg per ml respectively. Cefadroxil was detected in the serum at least 6 hours after administration and the serum half-life of cefadroxil ranged from 1.3 to 1.5 hours. Mean urinary concentrations of cefadroxil were 1.70 and 2.62 mg per ml, 0 to 2 and 2 to 4 hours after administration of the dose of 15 mg per kg respectively and 2.98 and 0.99 mg per ml, 0 to 3 and 3 to 6 hours after the dose of 10 mg per kg respectively.— C. M. Ginsburg *et al.*, *Antimicrob. Ag. Chemother.*, 1978, *13*, 845.

The pharmacokinetics of cefadroxil in patients with renal insufficiency.— R. E. Cutler *et al.*, *Clin. Pharmac. Ther.*, 1979, *25*, 514; G. Humbert *et al.*, *Chemotherapy, Basle*, 1979, *25*, 189.

Further references to pharmacokinetic studies of cefadroxil: D. M. Henness *et al.*, *Clin. Ther.*, 1978, *1*, 263; H. Lode *et al.*, *Antimicrob. Ag. Chemother.*, 1979, *16*, 1.

Uses. Cefadroxil, a cephalosporin antibiotic, is administered by mouth in the treatment of susceptible infections including those of the respiratory and urinary tracts. The usual daily dose is 1 or 2 g, given as a single dose or in 2 divided doses.

Reviews of cefadroxil.— P. J. Santella *et al.*, *J. int. med. Res.*, 1978, *6*, 441; *Med. Lett.*, 1979, *21*, 85.

Cefadroxil 1 g twice daily or cephalexin 500 mg four times daily both for 10 days produced a cure 5 to 9 days after treatment in 263 of 282 and 267 of 292 patients respectively who had acute urinary-tract infections. Relapse or re-infection occurred in 50 patients who had taken cefadroxil and in 36 who had taken cephalexin. Nausea and vomiting were more common in patients taking cefadroxil but the incidence was reduced when the medication was taken with meals. Monilial vaginitis, yeast infections, burning, itching, or other vaginitis occurred in 14 patients taking cefadroxil and in 27 taking cephalexin.— D. M. Henness and D. Richards, *Curr. ther. Res.*, 1978, *23*, 547.

Cefadroxil was used to treat 363 patients with respiratory-tract infections due to Gram-positive or Gram-negative organisms. Doses were usually 1 to 2 g daily in adults and 40 to 50 mg per kg body-weight daily for children. Duration of treatment ranged from 3 to 30 days. The overall clinical success-rate was 97.5%. Side-effects occurred in 28 (7.7%) patients, the majority being gastro-intestinal disturbances.— P. J. Santella and B. Tanrisever, *Curr. ther. Res.*, 1979, *25*, 210.

Further references to the use of cefadroxil: F. F. Mercado *et al.*, *J. int. med. Res.*, 1978, *6*, 271; P. J. Santella and E. Berman, *Curr. ther. Res.*, 1978, *23*, 148; C. M. Ginsburg and G. H. McCracken, *J. Pediat.*, 1980, *96*, 340; D. M. Henness and W. Woodhams, *Curr. ther. Res.*, 1980, *27*, 263.

Dosage in renal failure. The normal half-life for cefadroxil of 1.4 hours was increased to 20 to 25 hours in end-stage renal failure. The interval between doses should be extended from 8 hours to 12 to 24 hours in patients with a glomerular filtration-rate (GFR) of 10 to 50 ml per minute and to 24 to 48 hours in patients with a GFR of less than 10 ml per minute. Concentrations of cefadroxil were affected by haemodialysis.— W. M. Bennett *et al.*, *Ann. intern. Med.*, 1980, *93*, 62. The view that the normal dosage interval should be 12 or 24 hours and that a 12-hour dosage interval may still be used even in patients with a creatinine clearance-rate as low as 25 ml per minute.— G. R. McKinney, *Mead Johnson, USA* (letter), *ibid.*, 784. Reply.— R. A. Parker and W. M. Bennett (letter), *ibid.*

Preparations

Cefadroxil Capsules *(U.S.P.)*. Capsules containing the equivalent of 500 mg of anhydrous cefadroxil. Store in airtight containers.

Cefadroxil for Oral Suspension *(U.S.P.)*. A dry mixture of cefadroxil and one or more suitable buffers, colours, diluents, and flavours. Potency is expressed in terms of the equivalent amount of anhydrous cefadroxil. pH of the reconstituted suspension 4.5 to 6. Store in airtight containers.

Proprietary Names

Duracef *(Mead Johnson, Belg.)*; Duricef *(Mead Johnson, USA)*; Oracefal *(Bristol, Fr.)*; Ultracef *(Bristol, USA)*.

29-b

Cefapirin Sodium. BL-P1322; Cephapirin Sodium. Sodium (7*R*)-7-[2-(4-pyridylthio)acetamido]cephalosporanate; Sodium (7*R*)-3-acetoxymethyl-7-[2-(4-pyridylthio)acetamido]-3-cephem-4-carboxylate.

$C_{17}H_{16}N_3NaO_6S_2$=445.4.

CAS — 21593-23-7 (cefapirin); 24356-60-3 (sodium salt).

Pharmacopoeias. In *U.S.* as Sterile Cephapirin Sodium.

A white to off-white crystalline powder, odourless or with a slight odour. Each g represents about 2.3 mmol (2.3 mEq) of sodium. Cefapirin sodium 1.05 g is approximately equivalent to 1 g of cefapirin. **Soluble** 1 in less than 2 of water, 1 in 400 of dehydrated alcohol, and 1 in 2000 of acetone, chloroform, and ether. A 1% solution in water has a pH of 6.5 to 8.5.

Incompatible with amikacin sulphate, oxytetracycline hydrochloride, phenytoin sodium, polymyxin B sulphate, sulphadiazine sodium, tetracycline hydrochloride, thiopentone sodium, and, dependent on the vehicle, with aminophylline, chlortetracycline hydrochloride, and kanamycin sulphate.

Effect of gamma-irradiation. The potency of cefapirin sodium powder was reduced by 3.4% after a radiation dose of 50 000 Gy and by 1.3% after 25 000 Gy (the commonly employed sterilisation dose). Radiolysis was negligible when the dose was reduced to 10 000 Gy.— G. P. Jacobs, *Int. J. appl. Radiat. Isotopes*, 1980, *31*, 91.

Incompatibility. References: V. K. Prasad *et al.*, *Curr. ther. Res.*, 1974, *16*, 505 and 540.

Stability in solution. No significant changes occurred in solutions of cefapirin in Water for Injections, dextrose injection 5%, or sodium chloride injection 0.9% stored for at least 60 days in the frozen state.— M. A. Kaplan and A. P. Granatek, *Curr. ther. Res.*, 1974, *16*, 573.

The physical and chemical stability of cefapirin sodium solutions.— V. K. Prasad *et al.*, *Curr. ther. Res.*, 1974, *16*, 1214.

Solutions containing cefapirin sodium 50 to 400 mg per ml in Water for Injections are stable for 12 hours at 25° or 10 days at 4°. Solutions containing 20 to 100 mg per ml in dextrose injection 5% or sodium chloride injection 0.9% are stable for 24 hours at 25° or 10 days at 4°.— B. E. Kirschenbaum and C. J. Latiolais, *Am. J.*

Hosp. Pharm., 1976, *33*, 767. See also C. J. Latiolais (letter), *ibid.*, 1120.

Adverse Effects and Precautions. As for Cephalothin Sodium, p.1128.

It is recommended that cefapirin should be given with care in reduced dosage to patients with renal impairment.

For the report of an illness resembling serum sickness in 30 subjects receiving high doses of cephalothin and cefapirin over a prolonged period, see Cephalothin Sodium, p.1128.

Blood disorders. A report of neutropenia in 1 patient associated with cefapirin therapy for 6 days. The neutrophil count returned to normal when cefapirin was discontinued.— M. E. Levison *et al.*, *Antimicrob. Ag. Chemother.*, 1972, *1*, 174.

Thrombophlebitis. Only 2 instances of mild phlebitis were noted in 10 healthy volunteers receiving cefapirin by intravenous infusion whereas there were 8 including one thrombophlebitis in 10 volunteers receiving cephalothin. The strengths of the solutions used were 0.5 g in 250 ml every 6 hours for the first 24 hours, then 1 g in 250 ml every 6 hours for 4 days.— A. Z. Lane *et al.*, *Antimicrob. Ag. Chemother.*, 1972, *2*, 234.

See also under Cephalothin Sodium, p.1129.

Antimicrobial Action. The antibacterial activity of cefapirin is almost identical to that of cephalothin (see p.1129).

All 30 isolates of *Staph. aureus* were killed by 5 µg or less per ml of cefapirin. A concentration of 7.5 µg per ml killed 30 isolates of *E. coli*, *Pr. mirabilis*, and 80% of 30 isolates of *Klebsiella*. Other *Proteus* spp., *Enterobacter*, and *Pseudomonas* spp. were resistant. Increasing the size of the inoculum decreased the susceptibility of the sensitive bacteria.— P. Weisner *et al.*, *Antimicrob. Ag. Chemother.*, 1972, *1*, 303.

Further references: S. J. Bodner and M. G. Koenig, *Am. J. med. Sci.*, 1972, *263*, 43; J. L. Brown *et al.*, *Antimicrob. Ag. Chemother.*, 1972, *1*, 35.

Absorption and Fate. Cefapirin is poorly absorbed from the gastro-intestinal tract and is given by intramuscular or intravenous injection as the sodium salt. Plasma concentrations of 16 to 24 µg per ml have been reported 30 minutes after a dose of 1 g given intramuscularly. Up to 50% of a dose is bound to plasma proteins and the plasma half-life is about 36 minutes.

Similarly to cephalothin, high concentrations are excreted in the urine and about 40% of a dose appears as the less active deacetylated metabolite. About 1% may be excreted in bile.

A review.— C. H. Nightingale *et al.*, *J. pharm. Sci.*, 1975, *64*, 1899.

Cefapirin sodium in doses of 12.5 and 20 mg per kg body-weight given to 10 children aged 8.5 months to 12 years by intramuscular injection produced peak serum concentrations of 7.6 and 14.5 µg per ml respectively within about 30 minutes. Serum concentrations were insignificant after 4 hours. Similar doses given by rapid intravenous injection to 1 boy produced peak concentrations of 44 and 54 µg per ml respectively within 15 minutes. One child excreted about 53% of a dose given intramuscularly within 4 hours.— R. C. Gordon *et al.*, *Curr. ther. Res.*, 1971, *13*, 398.

In a study of 5 healthy volunteers given 1 g of cefapirin sodium intravenously, the average serum-cefapirin concentration was 73 µg per ml 15 minutes after injection and fell to zero at 6 hours; the serum half-life was 21 minutes. During the first 6 hours 72% of the dose was excreted in the urine in an average concentration of 2.6 mg per ml. Negligible amounts were excreted in the next 6 hours. Another 5 volunteers given 1 g intramuscularly achieved serum concentrations of 24 µg per ml after 30 minutes falling to 0.2 µg per ml at 6 hours; the serum half-life was 47 minutes. About 53% was excreted in the urine within 6 hours in an average concentration of 1.3 mg per ml. A further 6% was excreted in the next 6 hours. All subjects complained of moderate pain after intramuscular injection.— J. Axelrod *et al.*, *J. clin. Pharmac.*, 1972, *12*, 84.

Cefapirin was metabolised to desacetylcefapirin in healthy subjects. Although plasma concentrations of the metabolite ranged from 0.3 to 2.5 µg per ml compared with cefapirin concentrations of 1.7 to 63.6 µg per ml over the same period following 1 g intravenously about 45% of the dose was excreted in the urine as desacetylcefapirin over 6 hours and about 49% as cefapirin. It was considered that cefapirin underwent renal metabolism. The plasma half-life of cefapirin was about 0.5 hours and that of desacetylcefapirin 0.43 hours. The metabolite had 54% of the activity of the parent compound against *Sarcina lutea*.— B. E. Cabana *et al.*, *Bristol Laboratories, USA*, *Antimicrob. Ag. Chemother.*, 1976, *10*, 307.

For a comparison of the pharmacokinetics of cefapirin, cephamandole, and cephalothin, see M. Barza *et al.*, *Antimicrob. Ag. Chemother.*, 1976, *10*, 421.

An investigation of the renal excretion of cefapirin suggested that active tubular reabsorption of the drug occurs as well as tubular secretion.— A. Arvidsson *et al.*, *Clin. Pharmac. Ther.*, 1979, *25*, 870.

Further references to pharmacokinetic studies of cefapirin: A. G. Paradelis *et al.*, *Arzneimittel-Forsch.*, 1977, *27*, 2167.

Diffusion. Studies in orthopaedic patients indicated good penetration of cefapirin into bone. Following therapeutic doses, concentrations of 2 to 28 µg per g were achieved in bone, and 5.75 to 42 µg per ml in synovial fluid.— D. J. Schurman *et al.*, *Curr. ther. Res.*, 1976, *20*, 194.

Similar concentrations of cephalothin and cefapirin were obtained in the plasma and interstitial fluid of 12 healthy subjects in a crossover study following 1-g doses given by intravenous infusion.— J. S. Tan and S. -J. Salstrom, *Antimicrob. Ag. Chemother.*, 1979, *15*, 510.

Uses. Cefapirin sodium is a cephalosporin antibiotic with actions and uses similar to those of cephalothin (see p.1128).

The equivalent of 2 to 6 g of cefapirin is given daily in 4 to 6 divided doses by intramuscular injection or intravenously by slow injection over 3 to 5 minutes or by intermittent infusion. In severe infections up to 12 g daily may be given. A suggested dose for children is 40 to 80 mg per kg body-weight daily in 4 divided doses.

Reduced doses may be necessary in patients with impaired renal function.

In a study of 27 patients with various infections 25 responded to treatment with cefapirin sodium 2 to 8 g daily by intravenous or intramuscular injection. All the patients given intramuscular injections complained of pain but neither pain nor phlebitis was a problem following intravenous injections. Three patients had increased serum aspartate aminotransferase (SGOT) values, 3 had eosinophilia, and 1 developed anaemia, leucopenia, and neutropenia.— J. L. Bran *et al.*, *Antimicrob. Ag. Chemother.*, 1972, *1*, 35.

Further references: S. J. Bodner and M. G. Koenig, *Am. J. med. Sci.*, 1972, *263*, 43; J. Inagaki and G. P. Bodey, *Curr. ther. Res.*, 1973, *15*, 37; *Med. Lett.*, 1974, *16*, 53.

Dosage in infants and children. Cefapirin sodium was administered parenterally to 19 children aged 2 months to 12 years of age in doses of 50 to 80 mg per kg body-weight daily in the treatment of infections and was effective in 17. One child developed raised BUN values and anaemia but had recently been given kanamycin. Eosinophilia developed in 8 of the 16 patients who showed no eosinophilia at the start of treatment.— R. C. Gordon *et al.*, *Curr. ther. Res.*, 1971, *13*, 398. See also A. J. Khan and C. V. Pryles, *ibid.*, 1973, *15*, 198.

Dosage in renal failure. The plasma half-life of cefapirin was about 105 to 108 minutes in patients undergoing haemodialysis and 96 minutes in non-dialysed patients with chronic renal failure. To maintain the MIC for most Gram-positive and Gram-negative organisms in the blood and urine non-dialysed patients with renal failure should receive 15 to 18 mg per kg body-weight every 12 hours and dialysed patients the same dose just before dialysis and then every 12 hours.— R. V. McCloskey *et al.*, *Antimicrob. Ag. Chemother.*, 1972, *1*, 90.

The normal half-life for cefapirin of 0.6 hours was increased to 2.4 hours in end-stage renal failure. The interval between doses should be extended from 6 hours to 12 hours in patients with a glomerular filtration-rate of less than 10 ml per minute. Concentrations of cefapirin were affected by haemodialysis.— W. M. Bennett *et al.*, *Ann. intern. Med.*, 1977, *86*, 754. See also *idem*, 1980, *93*, 62.

The mean plasma concentration of cefapirin was 216 µg per ml, 30 minutes after the end of a 30-minute intravenous infusion of cefapirin 40 mg per kg body-weight, and had fallen to 33 µg per ml at the end of a 5.5-hour haemodialysis session in 9 patients with end-stage renal disease. The mean half-life of cefapirin was 2.8 hours. There was no evidence of drug accumulation in a further 5 patients who received 50 mg per kg in 75 ml of sodium chloride injection during the initial and final 30 minutes of five consecutive haemodialysis sessions each lasting 5.5 hours. The mean serum concentrations of cefapirin between sessions varied from 297 to 5 µg per ml. A similar infusion was used successfully to treat 9 patients with infections due to *Escherichia coli* or *Staphylococcus aureus*.— S. J. Berman *et al.*, *Antimicrob. Ag. Chemother.*, 1978, *13*, 4.

Pneumonia. Of 50 infants with bronchial pneumonia given a twice-daily dose of cefapirin sodium for up to 19 days, 40 were cured and 6 improved. The daily dose was 60 to 150 mg per kg body-weight, producing an average peak serum level of about 13.7 µg per ml.— A. Cedrato and A. Larguia, *Clin. Med.*, 1973, *80* (Oct.), 27.

Cefapirin was effective in the treatment of 30 children with pneumonia and empyema caused by various organisms which were eliminated from pleural pus within 48 hours. Concentrations of 23 to 37 µg per ml were achieved in pleural pus within 2 hours.— H. Trujillo *et al.*, *J. int. med. Res.*, 1974, *2*, 125.

Preparations

Sterile Cephapirin Sodium *(U.S.P.)*. A grade of cefapirin sodium for injection. Potency is expressed in terms of the equivalent amount of cefapirin.

Proprietary Names

Ambrocef *(Lusofarmaco, Ital.)*; Ambrotina *(Lusofarmaco, Ital.)*; Brisfirina *(Bristol-Myers, Spain)*; Brisporin *(Bristol Italiana Sud, Ital.)*; Bristocef *(Bristol, Ger.)*; Cefadyl *(Bristol, Canad.; Bristol, USA)*; Céfaloject *(Bristol, Fr.)*; Cefatrexil *(Mead Johnson, Arg.)*; Cefatrexyl *(Bristol, Austral.; Mead Johnson, Belg.; Jap.; Bristol, NZ; Bristol, Switz.)*.

30-x

Cefatrizine. BL-S640; SKF 60771; S-640P. (7*R*)-7-(α-D-4-Hydroxyphenylglycylamino)-3-(1*H*-1,2,3-triazol-4-ylthiomethyl)-3-cephem-4-carboxylic acid.

$C_{18}H_{18}N_6O_5S_2$=462.5.

CAS — 51627-14-6.

Cefatrizine is a cephalosporin antibiotic with actions and uses similar to those of cephalexin (see p.1123). It is active by mouth and has been given in doses of up to 2 g daily.

Antimicrobial action. The antimicrobial activity of cefatrizine was comparable *in vitro* with that of cephalexin, except that it appeared to be more effective against strains of *Enterobacter*, *Haemophilus*, and *Proteus*. It was not inactivated by beta-lactamases from 14 strains of *Salmonella typhimurium* and it was active against ampicillin-resistant *H. influenzae*. No enhanced effect was observed with cefatrizine and gentamicin, carbenicillin, kanamycin, or polymyxin.— C. C. Blackwell *et al.*, *Antimicrob. Ag. Chemother.*, 1976, *10*, 288. For similar activity to ampicillin against *H. influenzae* as well as activity against 4 ampicillin-resistant strains, see T. Brotherton *et al.*, *ibid.*, 322.

Cefatrizine had MICs of 1.06, 0.10, 0.22, 2.30, 2.52, and 4.24 µg per ml respectively against 25 strains of *Staphylococcus aureus*, 20 of *Streptococcus pyogenes*, 16 of *Streptococcus pneumoniae*, 25 of *Escherichia coli*, 21 of *Klebsiella pneumoniae*, and 24 of *Proteus mirabilis*, and had a similar or superior activity *in vitro* to cefaclor, cephalexin, cephaloglycin, or cephradine against these organisms. Cefatrizine was also active against several indole-positive *Proteus* species. None of the cephalosporins was very active against enterococci *Enterobacter cloacae*, or *Enterobacter aerogenes*.— S. Shadomy *et al.*, *Antimicrob. Ag. Chemother.*, 1977, *12*, 609.

The activity of cefatrizine against 400 clinical isolates of Gram-positive and Gram-negative bacteria compared with cephalexin, cephalothin, cephamandole, and cefoxitin.— H. C. Neu and K. P. Fu, *Antimicrob. Ag. Chemother.*, 1979, *15*, 209.

Further references: F. Leitner *et al.*, *Antimicrob. Ag. Chemother.*, 1975, *7*, 298; C. Watanakunakorn *et al.*, *ibid.*, 381; G. D. Overturf *et al.*, *ibid.*, *8*, 305.

Absorption and fate. A single oral dose of cefatrizine 1 g was given to 22 pregnant patients up to 23 hours prior to surgical abortion. Mean maternal-serum concentrations of cefatrizine 1, 2, 4, and 8 hours after administration were 3.7, 7.9, 6.5, and 1.6 µg per ml respectively. Maternal-serum half-life was estimated at 2.4 hours compared with 4.4 hours for placental serum. Cefatrizine concentrations in foetal serum, kidney, lung, amniotic fluid, bile, and urine reached 1.66, 2.76, 2.46, 1.02, 1.56, and 2.75 µg per ml or g respectively. No cefatrizine was detected in the foetuses from 11 women whose abortion was achieved with a dinoprost infusion. All women had been given cefatrizine 1 g.— B. Bernard *et al.*, *Antimicrob. Ag. Chemother.*, 1977, *12*, 231.

Uses. All of 20 children with tonsillitis, otitis media, or impetigo were free of symptoms after treatment with cefatrizine 13 to 47 mg per kg body-weight (mean 29 mg per kg) daily for 5 days. One child developed diarrhoea and a second had moderate eosinophilia.— L. J. Baraff *et al.*, *Curr. ther. Res.*, 1977, *21*, 187.

Cefatrizine 500 mg taken every 12 hours produced a clinical and bacteriological cure in 20 of 24 patients with skin and soft-tissue infections and cephalexin 500 mg taken every 6 hours produced a cure in 21 of 24 similar patients. Most patients received a 10-day course but some patients were given up to 20 days' treatment with cefatrizine and up to 40 days with cephalexin. Treatment failures occurred in both groups with infections produced by *Streptococcus epidermidis* and *Peptococcus* J. R. Dalovisio *et al.*, *Curr. ther. Res.*, 1978, *23*, 417.

Cefatrizine 0.75 to 2 g given daily for up to 10 days to 34 patients with genito-urinary tract infections, 56 with respiratory tract infections and 11 with soft-tissue infections produced a clinical cure in 25, 52, and 11 patients respectively. No new strains of bacteria resistant to cefatrizine appeared during therapy and all relapses were produced by sensitive bacteria. Side-effects which were experienced by 19 patients included diarrhoea, headache, nausea and vomiting, rashes, elevations of liver enzyme values, and eosinophilia and were responsible for 4 patients discontinuing treatment.— B. S. Ribner *et al.*, *Curr. ther. Res.*, 1978, *24*, 614.

Further references: R. Del Busto *et al.*, *Antimicrob. Ag. Chemother.*, 1976, *9*, 397.

Manufacturers
Bristol, USA.

31-r

Cefazaflur Sodium. SKF 59962. Sodium (7*R*)-3-(1-methyl-1*H*-tetrazol-5-ylthiomethyl)-7-(2-trifluoromethylthioacetamido)-3-cephem-4-carboxylate.
$C_{13}H_{12}F_3N_6NaO_4S_3$=492.4.

CAS — 58665-96-6 (cefazaflur); 52123-49-6 (sodium salt).

Cefazaflur sodium is a cephalosporin antibiotic with similar antibacterial activity to that of Cephalothin Sodium, p.1129.

Antimicrobial action of cefazaflur.— G. W. Counts *et al.*, *Antimicrob. Ag. Chemother.*, 1977, *11*, 708; N. Aswapokee and H. C. Neu, *ibid.*, 1979, *15*, 444.

In 7 healthy subjects given cefazaflur 1 g by intramuscular injection, the mean peak serum concentration was about 25 µg per ml after 30 minutes.The apparent serum half-life was about 50 minutes. Cefazaflur was not strongly bound to plasma proteins and so was rapidly eliminated in the urine; about 90% of the dose was recovered after 6 hours and about 93% after 24 hours. Side-effects included slight local pain (1 subject), discomfort after injection (3), and eosinophilia (1). It was suggested that cefazaflur might be useful for the treatment of Gram-negative urinary-tract infections.— C. Harvengt *et al.*, *J. clin. Pharmac.*, 1977, *17*, 128.

Manufacturers
Smith Kline & French, USA.

187-a

Cefoperazone Sodium. T-1551; CP-52640-2. Sodium (7*R*)-7-[(*R*)-2-(4-ethyl-2,3-dioxopiperazin-1-ylcarboxamido)-2-(4-hydroxyphenyl)acetamido]-3-[(1-methyl-1*H*-tetrazol-5-yl)thiomethyl]-3-cephem-4-carboxylate.
$C_{25}H_{26}N_9NaO_8S_2$=667.6.

CAS — 62893-19-0 (cefoperazone); 62893-20-3 (sodium salt).

Cefoperazone is a cephalosporin antibiotic with a wide spectrum of activity similar to that of cefotaxime (p.1118). It is administered parenterally as the sodium salt.

International symposium on cefoperazone sodium.— *Drugs*, 1981, *22*, *Suppl.* 1, 1-124.

A review of cefoperazone.— *Drugs*, 1981, *22*, 423.

Studies on the antimicrobial activity *in vitro* of cefoperazone: H. C. Neu *et al.*, *Antimicrob. Ag. Chemother.*, 1979, *16*, 150; N. Matsubara *et al.*, *ibid.*, 731; M. V. Borobio *et al.*, *ibid.*, 1980, *17*, 129; W. H. Hall *et al.*, *ibid.*, 273; R. R. Bulger and J. A. Washington, *ibid.*, 393; A. M. Hinkle *et al.*, *ibid.*, 423; S. D. R. Lang *et al.*, *ibid.*, 488; K. Sato *et al.*, *ibid.*, 736; R. N. Jones *et al.*, *ibid.*, 743; C. N. Baker *et al.*, *ibid.*, 757; D. Kaye *et al.*, *ibid.*, 957; B. Van Klingeren *et al.* (letter), *J. antimicrob. Chemother.*, 1980, *6*, 674.

Cefoperazone had some activity *in vitro* against enterococci.— T. M. File and J. S. Tan (letter), *Lancet*, 1981, *2*, 477.

A pharmacokinetic study of cefoperazone.— A. -F. Allaz *et al.*, *Schweitz. med. Wschr.*, 1979, *109*, 1999.

Beneficial results were achieved with cefoperazone in 30 elderly patients with urinary-tract infections. A dose of 2 g was dissolved in 6 ml of a 0.5% lignocaine solution and given by intramuscular injection every 12 hours for 7 days.— R. Vryens *et al.*, *Curr. ther. Res.*, 1980, *27*, 757.

Diarrhoea and some nausea associated with cefoperazone.— R. Norrby and K. Alestig (letter), *Lancet*, 1981, *2*, 1417.

Interactions. *Alcohol.* In 3 of 4 healthy subjects who took alcoholic beverages 36 hours after a dose of cefoperazone, alcohol intolerance occurred. In one subject the syndrome developed on 3 separate occasions.— D. S. Reeves and A. J. Davies (letter), *Lancet*, 1980, *2*, 540. See also F. G. McMahon (letter), *J. Am. med. Ass.*, 1980, *243*, 2397.

Proprietary Names
Cefobid *(Pfizer, Hong Kong)*; Cefobine *(Pfizer, Fr.)*; Cefobis *(Pfizer, Ger.*; *Pfizer, Switz.)*.

32-f

Cefotaxime Sodium. HR 756; RU 24756. Sodium (7*R*)-7-[(*Z*)-2-(2-aminothiazol-4-yl)-2-(methoxyimino)acetamido]cephalosporanate; Sodium (7*R*)-3-acetoxymethyl-7-[(*Z*)-2-(2-aminothiazol-4-yl)-2-(methoxyimino)acetamido]-3-cephem-4-carboxylate.
$C_{16}H_{16}N_5NaO_7S_2$=477.4.

CAS — 63527-52-6 (cefotaxime); 64485-93-4 (sodium salt).

An odourless, white to slightly cream-coloured powder. Each g represents 2.09 mmol (2.09 mEq) of sodium. Cefotaxime sodium 1.05 g is approximately equivalent to 1 g of cefotaxime.

Freely **soluble** in water; practically insoluble in organic solvents. A 10% solution has a pH of about 5.5.

Adverse Effects and Precautions. As for Cephalothin Sodium, p.1128.

Nephrotoxicity. A study in 3 patients demonstrated no evidence for direct tubular toxicity of cefotaxime.— G. Ninane (letter), *Lancet*, 1979, *1*, 332. A study in healthy subjects indicating that cefotaxime is not nephrotoxic.— A. W. Mondorf (letter), *ibid.*, *2*, 799.

In 6 patients with renal failure given cefotaxime 0.5 to 1.5 g daily, renal function remained stable during treatment; renal function also remained stable in 9 further patients without renal failure.— N. Clumeck *et al.* (letter), *Lancet*, 1979, *1*, 835.

Antimicrobial Action. Cefotaxime has a wider antibacterial spectrum than that of cefuroxime (see p.1121). It is active *in vitro* against *Pseudomonas aeruginosa* at relatively high concentrations and is reported to be more potent than cefuroxime against many Gram-negative bacteria including *Haemophilus influenzae.*

Cefotaxime was generally more active *in vitro* than carbenicillin or cephazolin against strains of *Ps. aeruginosa, Serratia marcescens, Providencia stuartii*, and the Enterobacteriaceae and was highly active against strains of *Salmonella typhi*. Cephazolin and cefotaxime had a similar activity against penicillin-susceptible and penicillin-resistant strains of *Staphylococcus aureus*. Cefotaxime was more active than ampicillin against strains of *H. influenzae* and more active than benzylpenicillin against *Neisseria gonorrhoeae.*— R. Wise *et al.*, *Antimicrob. Ag. Chemother.*, 1978, *14*, 807.

In a study of 431 bacterial isolates cefotaxime was about 100 times more active than cefuroxime or cefoxitin against *Escherichia coli, Klebsiella aerogenes*, and *Proteus mirabilis* and 40 times more active against *Salmonella typhimurium*. Against species usually reported to be cephalosporin-resistant cefotaxime was about 1000 times more active against *Proteus morganii* and *Providencia stuartii* and 100 to 300 times more active against *Pr. vulgaris, Pr. rettgeri*, and *Serratia marcescens*; it was much more active than cefuroxime against *Enterobacter* spp. Against *Ps. aeruginosa* cefotaxime was 4 times more active than carbenicillin and against *H. influenzae* it was 30 times more active than cefuroxime. Differences in activity against *Bacteroides fragilis* and Gram-positive cocci were less marked. Mean MICs for cefotaxime included 0.027 µg per ml for *H. influenzae*, 0.048 µg per ml for indole-positive *Proteus* spp., 0.066 µg per ml for *E. coli*, 0.14 µg per ml for *Serratia marcescens*, and 13.69 µg per ml for *Ps. aeruginosa*.— J. M. T. Hamilton-Miller *et al.*, *J. antimicrob. Chemother.*, 1978, *4*, 437.

Cefotaxime was more active *in vitro* than cephamandole, cefuroxime, cefoxitin, cephaloridine, or cephazolin against 160 strains of *H. influenzae* (including 15 beta-lactamase-producing strains), over 90% of isolates being inhibited by 0.03 µg or less per ml. Against 194 gentamicin-resistant Gram-negative rods, cefotaxime was generally more active than cephamandole, cefuroxime, or cefoxitin especially against *Ps. aeruginosa* and *Klebsiella, Providencia*, and *Enterobacter* spp. Cefoxitin was the most active against 54 strains of *Bacteroides fragilis* and although 8 ampicillin-sensitive strains were also sensitive to 8 µg or less per ml of cefotaxime and the other cephalosporins tested, strains less sensitive to ampicillin were also less susceptible to the cephalosporins.— F. A. Drasar *et al.*, *J. antimicrob. Chemother.*, 1978, *4*, 445.

In a comparative study of cefotaxime and a number of cephalosporins and penicillins against 659 isolates, cefotaxime was found to have a wide spectrum of activity. It was the most active beta-lactam antibiotic against Enterobacteriaceae and MICs against *Neisseria gonorrhoeae* and *H. influenzae* were similar to those with ampicillin. Cefotaxime was more active than carbenicillin against *Ps. aeruginosa* but less active than piperacillin or gentamicin. It was more active than carbenicillin against *Bacteroides fragilis* but less active than cefoxitin. Synergy was exhibited with gentamicin against some strains of indole-positive *Proteus* and *Ps. aeruginosa*. Cefotaxime was less active than cephalothin or cephamandole against *Staph. aureus*.— H. C. Neu *et al.*, *Antimicrob. Ag. Chemother.*, 1979, *15*, 273.

Cefotaxime was more active *in vitro* than benzylpenicillin, cephamandole, cefoxitin, or tetracycline against 192 isolates of *Neisseria gonorrhoeae in vitro* including 23 strains resistant to less than 0.5 µg per ml of penicillin, and inhibited 175 strains at a concentration of 0.008 µg per ml and 191 at 0.03 µg per ml. Cefotaxime was also the most active against 3 beta-lactamase-producing isolates of *N. gonorrhoeae*.— P. R. Murray *et al.*, *Antimicrob. Ag. Chemother.*, 1979, *15*, 452. See also P. Piot *et al.*, *ibid.*, 535; C. N. Baker *et al.*, *ibid.*, 1980, *17*, 757.

All but one of 150 strains of *N. meningitidis* were inhibited by cefotaxime 0.008 µg per ml. These concentrations are much lower than those for cefuroxime, cefoxitin, or benzylpenicillin. When account is taken of the concentrations of 0.3 to 15 µg per ml of cefotaxime found in CSF, and the MICs for *H. influenzae* of up to 0.06 µg per ml and for *Streptococcus pneumoniae* of up to 0.016 µg per ml, cefotaxime may be the drug of first choice in the treatment of bacterial meningitis outside, and possibly in, the neonatal period.— W. M. Brown and R. J. Fallon (letter), *Lancet*, 1979, *1*, 1246.

Cefotaxime was the only cephalosporin of 7 tested (including cefuroxime) that was more active than ampicillin against 21 non-beta-lactamase-producing strains of *Haemophilus* and the most active antibiotic against 18 beta-lactamase-producing strains.— H. W. Van Landuyt and M. Pyckavet, *Antimicrob. Ag. Chemother.*, 1979, *16*, 109. Cefotaxime and moxalactam were highly active against all isolates of *H. influenzae* tested, irrespective of beta-lactamase production.— J. H. Jorgensen *et al.*, *ibid.*, 1980, *17*, 516. See also I. Braveny and K. Machka (letter), *Lancet*, 1980, *2*, 752.

A study *in vitro* indicated that hydrolysis by beta-lactamases was a major mechanism in the resistance of *Bacteroides fragilis* to cefotaxime. There was an increase in susceptibility of the strains to cefotaxime in the presence of clavulanic acid 500 ng per ml.— R. Wise (letter), *J. antimicrob. Chemother.*, 1979, *5*, 115.

Diffusion disk susceptibility testing with cefotaxime indicated that a 30-µg disk provided data for the susceptibility of *Ps. aeruginosa*, but produced very large zones of inhibition against Enterobacteriaceae. A 5-µg disk appeared to provide the most useful susceptibility data for *Staph. aureus* and Enterobacteriaceae.— N. Aswapokee *et al.*, *Antimicrob. Ag. Chemother.*, 1979, *16*, 164. A further study on disk susceptibility testing of cefotaxime.— P. C. Fuchs *et al.*, *ibid.*, 1980, *18*, 88.

Of 53 clinical isolates of *Ps. aeruginosa*, 96% and 78% were susceptible to moxalactam and cefotaxime, respectively, at concentrations of 62.5 µg per ml.— V. L. Yu *et al.*, *Antimicrob. Ag. Chemother.*, 1980, *17*, 96.. In a comparative study *in vitro* of 4 cephalosporins with anti-pseudomonal activity, MICs against carbenicillin-sensitive strains of *Ps. aeruginosa* were: ceftazidime, about 1 μg per ml; cefoperazone, 2 to 4 μg per ml; moxalactam, 4 to 8 μg per ml; and cefotaxime, 8 to 16 μg per ml.— B. Van Klingeren *et al.* (letter), *J. antimicrob. Chemother.*, 1980, *6*, 674.

The desacetyl metabolite of cefotaxime had about one-tenth the activity of cefotaxime *in vitro* against the common Enterobacteriaceae but was somewhat more active than cephazolin, cefuroxime, or cefoxitin. The metabolite had no useful activity against *Ps. aeruginosa* and was less active than cefotaxime or cefoxitin against *Staph. aureus* or *Bacteroides fragilis*.— R. Wise *et al.*, *Antimicrob. Ag. chemother.*, 1980, *17*, 84.

Further comparisons of the antibacterial activity of cefotaxime and other cephalosporin antibiotics: G. W. Counts and M. Turck, *Antimicrob. Ag. Chemother.*, 1979, *16*, 64; R. P. Mouton *et al.*, *ibid.*, 757; M. V. Borobio *et al.*, *ibid.*, 1980, *17*, 129; W. H. Hall *et al.*, *ibid.*, 273; D. Greenwood *et al.*, *ibid.*, 397; S. D. R. Lang *et al.*, *ibid.*, 488; J. H. Jorgensen *et al.*, *ibid.*, 937; S. Masuyoshi *et al.*, *ibid.*, *18*, 1; P. C. Appelbaum *et al.* (letter), *Lancet*, 1981, *2*, 472.

Diminished activity. For the effect of cefoxitin on cefotaxime and cefuroxime *in vitro*, see Cefuroxime Sodium, p.1121.

Absorption and Fate. Cefotaxime is administered by injection as the sodium salt. It is rapidly absorbed after intramuscular injection and mean peak serum concentrations of 11.9 and 25.3 μg per ml have been reported about 30 minutes after the equivalent of 0.5 and 1 g of cefotaxime respectively. Immediately after the intravenous injection of 0.5, 1 or 2 g of cefotaxime mean peak serum concentrations of 38, 102, and 215 μg per ml, respectively, have been achieved with concentrations ranging from 1 to 3.27 μg per ml after 4 hours. Concentrations have been detected in serum 8 hours after injection by either route. About 40% is reported to be bound to plasma proteins; the elimination half-life of cefotaxime is about 1.2 hours. It is widely distributed in body tissues and fluids; therapeutic concentrations have been achieved in the cerebrospinal fluid when the meninges are inflamed. It diffuses across the placenta and is excreted in breast milk.

Cefotaxime is partially metabolised to desacetyl cefotaxime, which has some activity, and to inactive metabolites. Cefotaxime is eliminated mainly by the kidneys and about 60% of a dose has been recovered unchanged in the urine within 24 hours; a further 20% is excreted as the desacetyl metabolite. Tubular secretion is blocked by probenecid. Cefotaxime is also excreted in bile.

Pharmacokinetic studies of cefotaxime: R. Lüthy *et al.*, *Antimicrob. Ag. Chemother.*, 1979, *16*, 127; K. P. Fu *et al.*, *ibid.*, 592; F. Esmieu *et al.*, *J. antimicrob. Chemother.*, 1980, *6*, *Suppl.* A, 83; H. C. Neu *et al.*, *Clin. Pharmac. Ther.*, 1980, *27*, 677.

Uses. Cefotaxime is a cephalosporin antibiotic and is given as the sodium salt by intramuscular or intravenous injection in the treatment of susceptible infections. In moderate infections the equivalent of 1 g of cefotaxime is administered 12-hourly. In severe infections up to 12 g may be given daily in 3 or 4 divided doses; pseudomonal infections usually require more than 6 g daily. Children may be given the equivalent of 100 to 150 mg of cefotaxime per kg body-weight (50 mg per kg for neonates) daily in 2 to 4 divided doses, increased to 200 mg per kg daily if necessary. Doses of cefotaxime should be reduced in severe renal failure.

In the treatment of gonorrhoea a single 1-g dose of cefotaxime by intramuscular or intravenous injection has been suggested.

Cefotaxime sodium may also be given by intravenous infusion. The equivalent of 1 to 2 g of cefotaxime is dissolved in 40 to 100 ml of Water for Injections, sodium chloride injection, dextrose injection, or other suitable fluid, and administered over 20 to 60 minutes.

A brief review of cefotaxime.— *Med. Lett.*, 1981, *23*, 61.

The proceedings of a symposium on cefotaxime.— *J. antimicrob. Chemother.*, 1980, *6*, *Suppl.* A, 1—303.

Dosage in renal failure. A recommendation that the dose of cefotaxime be reduced from 1 g twice daily to 500 mg twice daily in the severely compromised patient with renal failure, when the creatinine clearance is less than 5 ml per minute.— R. Wise and N. Wright (letter), *Lancet*, 1981, *1*, 1106. See also R. Wise *et al.*, *Antimicrob. Ag. Chemother.*, 1981, *19*, 526.

Gonorrhoea. A report of the successful use of cefotaxime to treat a 22-year-old woman with acute gonorrhoea caused by a beta-lactamase-producing strain of *Neisseria gonorrhoeae*. She was given 2 g of cefotaxime (as 1 g in 1% lignocaine given intramuscularly into each buttock).— R. C. B. Slack *et al.* (letter), *Lancet*, 1980, *1*, 431.

The suggestion that uncomplicated gonorrhoea caused by beta-lactamase-producing strains of *N. gonorrhoeae* should be treated with cefotaxime 500 mg by intramuscular injection.— A. J. Boakes *et al.* (letter), *Lancet*, 1981, *2*, 96.

Further references to cefotaxime in gonorrhoea: V. S. Rajan *et al.*, *Br. J. vener. Dis.*, 1980, *56*, 255; M. L. Simpson *et al.*, *Antimicrob. Ag. Chemother.*, 1981, *19*, 798.

Haemophilus infections. The successful use of cefotaxime for ampicillin-resistant haemophilus infections.— S. W. B. Newsom *et al.* (letter), *Lancet*, 1981, *1*, 667.

See also Meningitis (below).

Meningitis. Intravenous administration of cefotaxime to 13 children with bacterial meningitis, due to *Haemophilus influenzae*, β-haemolytic streptococcus group B, *Streptococcus pneumoniae*, *Staphylococcus epidermidis*, *Neisseria meningitidis*, *Escherichia coli*, or *Pseudomonas aeruginosa*, most of whom had not responded to other antibiotics, indicated that cefotaxime penetrates into the CSF in sufficient amounts to give therapeutic concentrations resulting in cure. Ten of the 13 patients were cured; one relapsed with a new infecting organism but was again cured with cefotaxime, and a further child with *E. coli* meningitis who also received cefotaxime 100 μg intraventricularly was also cured. Laboratory results in one hospital where the children were treated intravenously, indicated that CSF concentrations were high as early as one hour after intravenous injection of 50 mg per kg body-weight and remained high for at least 7 hours after injection, being considerably higher than serum concentrations 4 hours after injection. In a second hospital the highest CSF concentrations were found 2 hours after intravenous injection of 25 mg per kg and seemed to depend on the day of meningitis (treatment), and the number of cells in the CSF; the considerably lower CSF concentrations found may have been related to the assay method used, but still exceeded the MICs for the causative organisms.— B. H. Belohradsky *et al.*, *Lancet*, 1980, *1*, 61. Experience with cefotaxime in treating cerebral infections has been encouraging but controlled clinical studies are necessary before it can be recommended as the drug of choice.— P. M. Shah (letter), *ibid.*, 490.

Proprietary Preparations

Claforan *(Roussel, UK)*. Cefotaxime sodium, available as powder for preparing injections, in vials containing the equivalent of cefotaxime 0.5, 1, and 2 g. Protect from light. (Also available as Claforan in *Eire, Ger., Hong Kong, Ital.*).

33-d

Cefoxitin Sodium. MK-306; L-620,388.

Sodium (7*S*)-3-carbamoyloxymethyl-7-methoxy-7-[2-(2-thienyl)acetamido]-3-cephem-4-carboxylate.

$C_{16}H_{16}N_3NaO_7S_2$=449.4.

CAS — 35607-66-0 (cefoxitin); 33564-30-6 (sodium salt).

Pharmacopoeias. U.S. includes Sterile Cefoxitin Sodium.

Cefoxitin is a semisynthetic cephamycin antibiotic derived from cephamycin C which is produced naturally by *Streptomyces lactamdurans*.

The sodium salt is a white to off-white, somewhat hygroscopic powder with a slight characteristic odour. *U.S.P.* specifies the equivalent of 850 to 1000 μg of cefoxitin per mg. Each g represents 2.23 mmol (2.23 mEq) of sodium. Cefoxitin sodium 1.05 g is approximately equivalent to 1 g of cefoxitin. Very **soluble** in water; sparingly soluble in alcohol and dimethylformamide; slightly soluble in acetone; soluble in methyl alcohol; practically insoluble in chloroform and ether. A 10% solution in water has a pH of 4.2 to 7.

Store in airtight containers. Injections containing 1 g in 10 ml should be used within 24 hours of preparation if stored at 25° and within 96 hours if stored between 2° and 10°. Cefoxitin sodium tends to darken on storage.

Crystalline cefoxitin sodium was both chemically and physically more stable than the amorphous form.— E. R. Oberholtzer and G. S. Brenner, *J. pharm. Sci.*, 1979, *68*, 863.

Cefoxitin sodium in solution was compatible with and stable in a wide variety of frequently used intravenous infusion fluids for at least 24 hours at room temperature.— M. J. O'Brien *et al.*, *Am. J. Hosp. Pharm.*, 1979, *36*, 33.

Adverse Effects. As for Cephalothin Sodium, p.1128.

About 8% of 1924 patients from 108 studies experienced drug-related adverse effects after receiving cefoxitin. After intravenous infusion, thrombophlebitis was reported in 89 of 1678 patients (5.3%) and occurred more frequently when indwelling polyethylene catheters were used rather than butterfly needles. Skin rashes occurred in 2.2% of patients. Reported changes in laboratory estimations after intravenous cefoxitin included eosinophilia (2.9% of patients tested), positive direct Coombs' tests (2.4%, haemolysis was not reported), increased serum aminotransferases (about 3%), and increased serum creatinine (0.7%). Intramuscular injections prepared with 0.5 or 1% lignocaine solutions were well-tolerated by 159 of 175 patients.— C. van Winzum, *J. antimicrob. Chemother.*, 1978, *4*, *Suppl.* B, 91. See also R. Norrby *et al.*, *Merck Sharp & Dohme, USA*, *J. Infect.*, 1979, *1*, *Suppl.* 1, 57.

Blood disorders. A report of cefoxitin-induced acute leucopenia.— M. Shansky and C. W. Greenlaw (letter), *Ann. intern. Med.*, 1980, *92*, 874.

Precautions. As for Cephaloridine, p.1126.

There is some evidence of cross-allergenicity between cephamycins and other beta-lactam antibiotics. Cefoxitin should not be given to patients who are known to be allergic to cephalosporins and should be given with great care to those who are allergic to penicillin or have known histories of allergy, especially to drugs.

It is recommended that cefoxitin should be given in reduced dosage to patients with impaired renal function.

Interactions. The serum half-life of cefoxitin is not affected to a measurable extent by concomitant administration with moderate doses of frusemide.— B. Trolløfors and R. Norrby (letter), *J. antimicrob. Chemother.*, 1980, *6*, 405.

Interference with laboratory estimations. Serum-creatinine estimations should be delayed until at least 2 and preferably 4 hours after cefoxitin administration, and, as the creatinine clearance may be falsely high, such estimations should not be relied on clinically.— S. R. Durham *et al.*, *J. clin. Path.*, 1979, *32*, 1148.

Antimicrobial Action. Cefoxitin is a cephamycin antibiotic which differs structurally from the cephalosporins by the addition of a 7α-methoxy group to the 7β-aminocephalosporanic acid nucleus. Like the other beta-lactam antibiotics it is bactericidal and is considered to act through the inhibition of bacterial cell wall synthesis.

Cefoxitin is resistant to most beta-lactamases. It has a broad spectrum of activity against Gram-positive and Gram-negative bacteria, similar to that of cephamandole and cefuroxime, but is generally more active against indole-positive *Proteus* spp. and less active against *Haemophilus influenzae*, *Staphylococcus aureus*, and *Enterobacter* spp. *Pseudomonas* spp. and most enterococci are resistant.

Cefoxitin is active against *Bacteroides fragilis*.

Both cefoxitin and cephamandole were active *in vitro* against cephalothin- and gentamicin-susceptible strains of *Klebsiella pneumoniae*, however, only cefoxitin inhibited resistant isolates (17 of 20 isolates being inhibited by 12.5 μg or less per ml of cefoxitin). Resistance was mediated by beta-lactamase activity; cefoxitin was not susceptible to degradation whereas cephamandole was.— R. T. Jackson *et al., Antimicrob. Ag. Chemother.*, 1977, *11*, 84. Preliminary findings from 51 isolates of *Kleb. aerogenes* resistant to gentamicin showed that while all strains were fully sensitive to cefoxitin, some strains had resistance to cefuroxime.— C. J. Noble *et al.* (letter), *Lancet*, 1979, *1*, 832.

Cephamandole was more active *in vitro* than cefoxitin against 18 isolates of *Proteus mirabilis*, 15 of *Enterobacter aerogenes* and 17 of *Enterobacter cloacae* but less active against 21 of *E. coli* and 19 of *Kleb. pneumoniae*.— S. Shadomy *et al., Antimicrob. Ag. Chemother.*, 1978, *13*, 412.

The majority of 48 isolates of penicillin-sensitive gonococci were inhibited by 0.25 μg per ml of cefoxitin compared with 0.03 μg per ml of benzylpenicillin. Against inocula of beta-lactamase producing gonococci of increasing size, MICs for cefoxitin were 1 μg per ml compared with 0.03 to 0.12 μg per ml for cefuroxime which did show a slight inoculum effect. Although there was no inoculum effect with cefoxitin, cefuroxime was still more active weight for weight.— I. Phillips, *J. antimicrob. Chemother.*, 1978, *4, Suppl.* B, 61.

For further comparisons of cefoxitin with the cephalosporins, see W. H. Hall *et al., Curr. ther. Res.*, 1977, *21*, 374; T. Une and S. Mitsuhashi, *Arzneimittel-Forsch.*, 1977, *27*, 89; W. L. George *et al., Antimicrob. Ag. Chemother.*, 1978, *13*, 484; H. C. Neu and K. P. Fu, *ibid.*, 584; J. H. Jorgensen *et al., Curr. ther. Res.*, 1979, *25*, 74; A. Vuye *et al., J. antimicrob. Chemother.*, 1979, *5*, 293; R. R. Bulger and J. A. Washington, *Antimicrob. Ag. Chemother.*, 1980, *17*, 393.

Further references: H. Wallick and D. Hendlin, *Antimicrob. Ag. Chemother.*, 1974, *5*, 25; A. K. Miller *et al., ibid.*, 33; R. C. Moellering *et al., ibid.*, *6*, 320; F. P. Tally *et al., ibid.*, 1975, *7*, 128; *J. antimicrob. Chemother.*, 1978, *4, Suppl.* B, 1-68; R. N. Brogden *et al., Drugs*, 1979, *17*, 1; J. A. Garcia-Rodriguez *et al.* (letter), *J. antimicrob. Chemother.*, 1979, *5*, 616.

For comparative studies of the antimicrobial activity of cefoxitin with other cephalosporins, see Cephamandole, p.1131 and Cefuroxime, p.1121.

Activity against anaerobic bacteria. Cefoxitin was more effective than cephalothin or benzylpenicillin against *Bacteroides fragilis* but benzylpenicillin was more active against the other anaerobic bacteria tested.— D. K. Henderson *et al., Antimicrob. Ag. Chemother.*, 1977, *11*, 679.

The activities of cefaclor, cephalexin, cephalothin, cephazolin, cephamandole, and cefoxitin were compared *in vitro* against 408 clinical isolates of anaerobic bacteria. Apart from *Lactobacillus* spp. and *Bacteroides fragilis*, the majority of Gram-positive and -negative bacteria were inhibited by 16 μg per ml of each antibiotic. Cephazolin was the most active against 11 isolates of *Lactobacillus* whereas cefoxitin, cephalexin, and cefaclor were relatively inactive. Cefoxitin was the only antibiotic with signficant activity against *Bacteroides fragilis* and 70% of 51 isolates were inhibited by 16 μg per ml.— A. W. Chow and D. Bednorz, *Antimicrob. Ag. Chemother.*, 1978, *14*, 668. See also V. T. Bach *et al., ibid.*, 1977, *11*, 912.

Of 10 cephalosporin antibiotics, clindamycin, benzylpenicillin, and dicloxacillin, cefoxitin and benzylpenicillin were the most active *in vitro* against 24 strains of *Eikenella corrodens*.— E. J. C. Goldstein *et al., Antimicrob. Ag. Chemother.*, 1978, *14*, 639.

Diminished activity. Antagonism occurred between cefoxitin and cefuroxime when tested *in vitro* against *Enterobacter cloacae*.— B. Chattopadhyay and I. Hall (letter), *J. antimicrob. Chemother.*, 1979, *5*, 490. See also Cefuroxime Sodium, p.1121.

Enhanced activity. Studies *in vitro* indicating synergism between cefoxitin and benzylpenicillin or carbenicillin against *Bacteroides fragilis, E. coli*, and enterococci.— V. T. Bach and H. Thadepalli, *Curr. ther. Res.*, 1977, *21*, 537.

There was little if any synergy *in vitro* between mezlocillin and cefoxitin against beta-lactamase-producing strains of Enterobacteriaceae, *Pseudomonas*, and *Enterobacter*, but some synergy against *Bacteroides fragilis*.— R. Wise *et al., J. antimicrob. Chemother.*, 1979, *5*, 301.

Resistance. Only cefoxitin and cephalothin appeared resistant to inactivation by beta-lactamase-producing *Staph. aureus* in a study of 8 cephalosporins.— I. W. Fong *et al., Antimicrob. Ag. Chemother.*, 1976, *9*, 939.

In a study of the beta-lactamase activities of 64 strains of *Bacteroides fragilis*, 7 cephalosporins showed variable susceptibility to hydrolysis but cefoxitin was not hydrolysed by any of the subspecies.— T. Leung and J. D. Williams, *J. antimicrob. Chemother.*, 1978, *4, Suppl.* B, 47. Resistance to cephamycins by cefoxitin-resistant strains of *Bacteroides fragilis* could not be correlated with the production of beta-lactamase.— K. Dornbusch *et al., ibid.*, 1980, *6*, 207.

There was little correlation between beta-lactamase production and decreased susceptibility of strains of Enterobacteriaceae to cephamandole or cefoxitin. It was suggested that other characteristics might be responsible for resistance.— J. L. Ott *et al., Antimicrob. Ag. Chemother.*, 1979, *15*, 14.

Further references: H. R. Onishi *et al., Antimicrob. Ag. Chemother.*, 1974, *5*, 38; H. C. Neu, *ibid.*, 1974, *6*, 170; A. D. Russell *et al., J. antimicrob. Chemother.*, 1978, *4, Suppl.* B, 33.

Absorption and Fate. Cefoxitin is not absorbed from the gastro-intestinal tract; it is given parenterally as the sodium salt. After 1 g by intramuscular injection a peak plasma concentration of 22.5 μg per ml at 20 minutes has been reported whereas concentrations of 124, 74, and 27 μg per ml have been achieved after the intravenous injection of 1 g over 3, 30, and 120 minutes respectively. Similarly to cephalothin, cefoxitin is about 70% bound to plasma proteins; it has a half-life of 45 to 60 minutes. Cefoxitin is widely distributed in the body but there is normally little penetration into the cerebrospinal fluid. It diffuses across the placenta and has been detected in the milk of nursing mothers.

The majority of a dose is excreted unchanged by the kidneys, about 2% being metabolised to descarbamylcefoxitin which is virtually inactive. High concentrations of cefoxitin are achieved in the urine by glomerular filtration and tubular secretion and 77 to 99% of a dose is recovered within 12 hours; probenecid slows this excretion. Small amounts of cefoxitin appear in bile.

For reviews of the absorption and fate of cefoxitin, see J. J. Schrogie *et al., Merck Sharp & Dohme, USA, J. antimicrob. Chemother.*, 1978, *4, Suppl.* B, 69; R. N. Brogden *et al., Drugs*, 1979, *17*, 1.

In an evaulation of cefoxitin in 38 patients with miscellaneous infections the mean serum-cefoxitin concentrations 30 minutes after an infusion of 1 g given as a 1% solution over 20 to 40 minutes was 32 μg per ml in the patients with normal renal function. Six hours after the infusion the mean concentration was less than 3 μg per ml. Concentrations in ascitic fluid exceeded those in the serum when measured in 3 patients, 2 of whom had renal impairment. There was no evidence of diffusion into the cerebrospinal fluid in 2 patients, one with no meningeal inflammation and the other with pleocytosis.— P. N. R. Heseltine *et al., Antimicrob. Ag. Chemother.*, 1977, *11*, 427.

Use of lignocaine hydrochloride 0.5 or 1% solution as a solvent for cefoxitin sodium reduced the pain of intramuscular injection without apparently affecting the pharmacokinetics of cefoxitin.— P. F. Sonneville *et al., Eur. J. clin. Pharmac.*, 1977, *12*, 273.

After the intravenous infusion of cefoxitin 30 mg per kg body-weight over 30 minutes the serum half-life which was 0.78 hours in 5 healthy subjects was prolonged up to about 22 hours, in 20 uraemic patients according to the degree of renal impairment. About 86% of the initial serum concentration was removed by haemodialysis in 5 patients.— J. P. Fillastre *et al., J. antimicrob. Chemother.*, 1978, *4, Suppl.* B, 79.

Further references to the pharmacokinetics of cefoxitin: J. Kosmidis *et al., Br. med. J.*, 1973, *4*, 653; W. Brumfitt *et al., Antimicrob. Ag. Chemother.*, 1974, *6*, 290; C. S. Goodwin *et al., ibid.*, 338; P. F. Sonneville *et al., Eur. J. clin. Pharmac.*, 1976, *9*, 397; C. Simon *et al., Arzneimittel-Forsch.*, 1978, *28*, 1541; M. J. Garcia *et al., Eur. J. clin. Pharmac.*, 1979, *16*, 119; R. Wise *et al., J. Infect.*, 1979, *1, Suppl.* 1, 49; N. Buchanan *et al.* (letter), *Br. J. clin. Pharmac.*, 1980, *9*, 623; W. E. Feldman *et al., Antimicrob. Ag. Chemother.*, 1980, *17*, 669.

Diffusion. Studies on cefoxitin concentrations in the cerebrospinal fluid of patients with meningitis.— P. A. A. Galvao *et al., Antimicrob. Ag. Chemother.*, 1980, *17*, 526; G. Humbert *et al., ibid.*, 675.

Uses. Cefoxitin sodium, a cephamycin antibiotic, is given intravenously by slow injection over 3 to 5 minutes or by infusion in the treatment of susceptible infections. Intramuscular injections are painful but may be prepared using 2 ml of a 0.5 or 1% solution of lignocaine hydrochloride.

The usual dose of cefoxitin is 1 or 2 g every 8 hours although it may be given more frequently (every 4 or 6 hours) and in severe infections up to 12 g daily has been recommended. A suggested dose for children of 2 years and older is 80 to 160 mg per kg body-weight daily in divided doses, increased to 200 mg per kg daily in severe infections.

In renal insufficiency, dosage should be reduced according to the creatinine-clearance rate, after an initial loading dose of 1 to 2 g. Suggested maintenance doses are: 1 to 2 g every 8 to 12 hours with a clearance of 30 to 50 ml per minute, 1 to 2 g every 12 to 24 hours with a clearance of 10 to 29 ml per minute, 0.5 to 1 g every 12 to 24 hours with a clearance of 5 to 9 ml per minute, and 0.5 to 1 g every 24 to 48 hours when the clearance is below 5 ml per minute.

Reviews of the actions and uses of cefoxitin.— *J. antimicrob. Chemother.*, 1978, *4, Suppl.* B, 1-256; *Chemotherapy, Tokyo*, 1978, *26, Suppl.* 1;; *Drug & Ther. Bull.*, 1979, *17*, 35; *Med. Lett.*, 1979, *21*, 13; R. N. Brogden *et al., Drugs*, 1979, *17*, 1; H. C. Neu, *ibid.*, 153.

Cefoxitin 1 or 2 g was infused as a 1 or 2% solution in sodium chloride or dextrose injection over 20 to 40 minutes every 4 or 6 hours in 38 patients with a variety of infections. Bacteriological confirmation of infection was obtained in 33 patients and 18 achieved a bacteriological and 26 a clinical cure. The infections included pneumonia, peritonitis, and soft tissue and urinary-tract infections, caused by a range of bacteria. *Pseudomonas aeruginosa* and *Enterobacter* spp. were resistant to cefoxitin and both aerobic and anaerobic Gram-positive organisms were less sensitive to cefoxitin than to cephalothin; however, Gram-negative aerobes were more sensitive to cefoxitin. Side-effects included burning on infusion in 2 patients and phlebitis in 12. Renal function deteriorated in 4 although in 2 this was not unexpected. Eosinophilia was noted in 6 and a false-positive Coombs' test in 2 patients.— P. N. R. Heseltine *et al., Antimicrob. Ag. Chemother.*, 1977, *11*, 427.

Cefoxitin given by intravenous infusion over a period of 20 to 30 minutes in a usual dose of 6 to 12 g daily in the form of the sodium salt was used successfully to treat 37 of 42 patients with various aerobic and anaerobic infections. Of the 5 treatment failures 2 were due to infections produced by *Serratia marcescens*. One patient developed a severe clinical superinfection with *Pseudomonas aeruginosa*.— S. R. Nair and C. E. Cherubin, *Antimicrob. Ag. Chemother.*, 1978, *14*, 866.

Abdominal sepsis was cured in 30 of 34 patients after the intravenous injection of cefoxitin every 8 hours for 5 to 7 days. The individual doses used were: 2 g for adults, 1.5 g for older children, and 1 g for younger children. A 15-month-old baby was given 0.5 g every 8 hours. A cefoxitin-resistant strain of *Bacteroides fragilis* was isolated from a septicaemic patient who failed to respond.— A. M. Geddes and R. M. L. Wilcox, *J. antimicrob. Chemother.*, 1978, *4, Suppl.* B, 151.

Cefoxitin 150 mg per kg body-weight daily in divided doses every 6 hours was given by intravenous or intramuscular injection to 32 infants and children aged from 3 to 151 months (mean, 26 months) and 17 of 19 patients with proven infections were clinically and bacteriologically cured. However, *Streptococcus pneumoniae* was isolated from the CSF of one patient with facial cellulitis before and during treatment with cefoxitin and *Haemophilus influenzae* from the CSF of a patient with septic arthritis after 10 days of treatment. The risk of inadequately treated bacterial meningitis might limit the use of cefoxitin as initial treatment in infants and children.— W. E. Feldman *et al., Antimicrob. Ag. Chemother.*, 1980, *17*, 669.

Further references: R. V. McCloskey, *Antimicrob. Ag. Chemother.*, 1977, *12*, 636; M. Gurwith *et al., ibid.*, 1978, *13*, 255; N. Christophidis *et al., Med. J. Aust.*, 1978, *1*, 512; S. Alvarez and W. J. Mogabgab, *Curr. ther. Res.*, 1978, *24*, 327; A. M. Geddes *et al., Scand. J. infect. Dis.*, 1978, *13, Suppl.*, 78; P. J. Little and B. A. Peddie, *N.Z. med. J.*, 1978, *88*, 46; F. P. Tally *et al., J. antimicrob. Chemother.*, 1979, *5*, 101; J. A. Jacobson *et al., Antimicrob. Ag. Chemother.*, 1979, *16*, 183.

Dosage in renal failure. The normal half-life for cefoxitin of 0.7 hour was increased to 13 to 22 hours in patients with end-stage renal failure. The normal dose interval of 6 to 8 hours should be increased to 8 to 12 hours in patients with a glomerular filtration-rate (GFR) of 10 to 50 ml per minute and to 24 hours in those with a GFR of less than 10 ml per minute. Concentrations of cefoxitin were affected by haemodialysis.— W. M. Bennett *et al., Ann. intern. Med.*, 1980,

93, 62.

Gonorrhoea. Cefoxitin was as effective as procaine penicillin in curing penicillin-sensitive gonorrhoea and significantly more effective in treating gonorrhoea due to penicillin-resistant strains of *N. gonorrhoeae*. Single doses of cefoxitin 2 g in 4 ml of a 0.5% lignocaine solution were given intramuscularly to patients with gonococcal urethritis. Each patient also took probenecid 1 g by mouth. All of 54 men given cefoxitin were cured including 21 with penicillinase-producing gonococci. Cefoxitin appears to be an effective alternative to spectinomycin in the single-dose treatment of penicillin-resistant gonococcal urethritis.— S. W. Berg *et al.*, *New Engl. J. Med.*, 1979, *301*, 509.

Patients infected with a beta-lactamase-producing strain of *N. gonorrhoeae*, also resistant to spectinomycin, could be treated with cefoxitin 2 g by intramuscular injection, preceded by 1 g of probenecid by mouth.— *Lancet*, 1981, *1*, 1221.

Preparations

Sterile Cefoxitin Sodium *(U.S.P.)*. Cefoxitin sodium suitable for parenteral use.

Mefoxin *(Merck Sharp & Dohme, UK)*. Cefoxitin sodium, available as powder for preparing injections, in vials each containing the equivalent of cefoxitin 1 or 2 g. (Also available as Mefoxin in *Austral., Canad., Fr., Ital., Lux., Neth., NZ, USA*).

Other Proprietary Names

Mefoxitin *(Denm., Ger., Swed., Switz.)*.

34-n

Ceftezole Sodium. Sodium (7*R*-7-[2-(1*H*-tetrazol-1-yl)acetamido]-3-(1,3,4-thiadiazol-2-ylthiomethyl)-3-cephem-4-carboxylate.

$C_{13}H_{11}N_8NaO_4S_3$=462.4.

CAS — 26973-24-0 (ceftezole); 41136-22-5 (sodium salt).

Ceftezole sodium is a cephalosporin antibiotic with similar properties to those of cephazolin (see p.1133). It has been given by intramuscular or intravenous injection in doses equivalent to 0.5 to 4 g of ceftezole daily.

For studies of the actions and uses of ceftezole, see *Chemotherapy, Tokyo*, 1976, *24*, 573-1252.

Absorption and fate.— M. Nishida *et al.*, *Antimicrob. Ag. Chemother.*, 1976, *10*, 1.

Proprietary Names

Celoslin *(Fujisawa, Jap.)*; Falomesin *(Chugai, Jap.)*.

35-h

Cefuroxime Sodium.

640/359. Sodium (7*R*)-3-carbamoyloxymethyl-7-[(2*Z*)-2-(2-furyl)-2-methoxyiminoacetamido]-3-cephem-4-carboxylate.

$C_{16}H_{15}N_4NaO_8S$=446.4.

CAS — 55268-75-2 (cefuroxime); 56238-63-2 (sodium salt).

A white to faintly yellow powder. Each g represents 2.24 mmol (2.24 mEq) of sodium. Cefuroxime sodium 1.05 g is approximately equivalent to 1 g of cefuroxime. Freely **soluble** in water, slightly soluble in alcohol, and sparingly soluble in methyl alcohol. A 10% solution in water has a pH of about 7. **Store** below 25°; protect from light.

Suspensions of cefuroxime sodium for intramuscular injection and solutions for direct intravenous injection should be used within 5 hours of preparation if stored below 25° or within 48 hours if stored between 2° and 10°. Darkening of the solution may occur on storage. Solutions for intravenous infusion in sodium chloride injection 0.9%, dextrose injection 5%, and injections of sodium chloride and dextrose or of compound sodium lactate may be expected to retain their potency for up to 24 hours at 25°.

Stability. Cefuroxime sodium was stable in 0.5 or 1% lignocaine hydrochloride solutions and such solutions could be used for the preparation of intramuscular injections. Mixtures of cefuroxime sodium and aminoglycosides might be physically incompatible. There was a loss of potency of about 15% when cefuroxime sodium 5 mg per ml in a 2.74% sodium bicarbonate solution was stored for 24 hours at 25°, significant yellowing of the solution also occurred.— M. J. Hartley *et al.*, *Pharm. J.*, 1978, *2*, 288.

Adverse Effects and Precautions. As for Cephalothin Sodium, p.1128.

Cefuroxime may cause false-negative reactions in the ferricyanide test for glucose.

It is recommended that cefuroxime should be given with care in reduced dosage to patients with renal impairment.

There were no signs of nephrotoxicity in 19 of 20 patients with pre-existing renal impairment when they were treated with cefuroxime, with or without frusemide, for 2 weeks. Decreased renal function occurred in one patient who had received an overdose of cefuroxime.— B. Trollfors *et al.*, *J. antimicrob. Chemother.*, 1980, *6*, 665.

Antimicrobial Action. Cefuroxime, like the other cephalosporins, is bactericidal and it has a broad spectrum of activity similar to that of cephamandole. It penetrates well through bacterial cell walls and is resistant to most beta-lactamases produced by Gram-negative bacteria. It is generally more active than cephalothin against Gram-negative bacteria including Enterobacteriaceae such as *Escherichia coli*, *Proteus mirabilis*, and *Klebsiella* and *Enterobacter* spp. Cefuroxime is very active against *Haemophilus influenzae*, including beta-lactamase-producing strains, and the *Neisseria* spp., including penicillin-resistant gonococci. It generally has similar or less activity against Gram-positive cocci than the older cephalosporins. *Pseudomonas* spp. are resistant.

In a study of the activity of 8 cephalosporins and benzylpenicillin *in vitro* against *Neisseria gonorrhoeae*, cefuroxime was the most active of the cephalosporins and was as active as benzylpenicillin against strains sensitive to penicillin. The order of effectiveness of the other cephalosporins was cephamandole, cefoxitin, cephalothin, cephazolin, cephradine, cephalexin, and cephaloridine. Cefuroxime and cefoxitin were equally active against penicillin-resistant strains of *N. gonorrhoeae* but the remaining cephalosporins were less active and were in order of effectiveness; cephazolin, cephamandole, cephalothin, cephaloridine, cephalexin, and cephradine.— I. Phillips *et al*, *J. antimicrob. Chemother.*, 1976, *2*, 31. Against inocula of beta-lactamase producing gonococci of increasing size, MICs for cefoxitin were 1 µg per ml compared with 0.03 to 0.12 µg per ml for cefuroxime which did show a slight inoculum effect. Although there was no inoculum effect with cefoxitin, cefuroxime was still more active weight for weight.— *idem*, 1978, *4*, *Suppl.* B, 61.

Cefuroxime had an MIC of up to 0.25 µg per ml against penicillinase-producing gonococci and showed no appreciable inoculum effect. It was 10 times more active than cephalexin.— A. Percival *et al.*, *Lancet*, 1976, *2*, 1379.

Cefuroxime was as effective as ampicillin against *H. influenzae* except for beta-lactamase producing strains which were more sensitive to cefuroxime.— R. B. Sykes *et al.*, *Glaxo*, *Antimicrob. Ag. Chemother.*, 1977, *11*, 599.

The antimicrobial action of cefuroxime was compared *in vitro* with that of cephalothin against 5887 clinical bacterial isolates. Cefuroxime was generally more effective against the Enterobacteriaceae, *H. influenzae* and other *Haemophilus* species, and *Streptococcus pneumoniae*. *Neisseria meningitidis* was considered to be especially sensitive to cefuroxime, 72% of isolates being inhibited at 0.06 µg per ml. Cefuroxime was less effective than cephalothin against *Staphylococcus aureus* and showed weak activity against *Bacteroides fragilis* although other anaerobic organisms were more sensitive with MICs usually of 2 to 8 µg per ml.— R. N. Jones *et al.*, *Antimicrob. Ag. Chemother.*, 1977, *12*, 47.

An *in vitro* comparison of the activity of cefuroxime with that of cephamandole, cephazolin, cefoxitin, cephaloridine, cephradine, and cephalothin against 397 bacterial isolates.— A. L. Barry *et al.*, *Proc. R. Soc. Med.*, 1977, *70*, *Suppl.* 9, 63.

Cefuroxime appeared to be one of the most resistant cephalosporins to each of 2 beta-lactamases from *Staph. aureus*. Hydrolysis of cefuroxime was not detected whereas cephalothin, cephaloridine, and cephazolin were all hydrolysed in increasing amounts in the order listed.— M. Laverdiere *et al.*, *Proc. R. Soc. Med.*, 1977, *70*, *Suppl.* 9, 72.

Cefuroxime had a similar or greater activity *in vitro* compared with cephamandole against 168 isolates of cephalothin-resistant Enterobacteriaceae but was less active against 12 isolates of indole-positive *Proteus* spp. The activity of cefoxitin was also similar to or greater than cefuroxime or cephamandole against all the isolates except those of the *Enterobacter* spp.— W. L. George *et al.*, *Antimicrob. Ag. Chemother.*, 1978, *13*, 484.

In a study *in vitro* of the activity of cefuroxime against 604 bacterial isolates, streptococci other than *Str. faecalis* were inhibited by 0.4 µg per ml or less and staphylococci by 0.2 µg per ml or less. MICs for beta-lactamase-containing staphylococci were 0.8 to 6.2 µg per ml; methicillin-resistant *Staph. aureus* and *Staph. epidermidis* were inhibited by 1.6 to 6.2 µg per ml. All of 30 strains of *N. gonorrhoeae*, *N. meningitidis*, and *H. influenzae* were inhibited by 1.6 µg per ml or less of cefuroxime. At a concentration of 12.5 µg per ml, 83% of strains of *E. coli*, 100% of *Salmonella*, 58% of *Shigella*, 95% of *Citrobacter*, 100% of *Kleb. pneumoniae*, 56% of *Enterobacter*, 90% of *Pr. mirabilis*, 72% of *Pr. rettgeri*, and 57% of *Providencia* were inhibited but only 16% of *Serratia marcescens*, 37% of *Pr. morganii*, and 43% of *Acinetobacter* strains were inhibited by 12.5 µg per ml. *Pseudomonas* spp. were resistant and only 24% of 17 strains of *Bacteroides fragilis* were inhibited at 50 µg per ml. Minimum bactericidal concentrations were the same or twice the minimum inhibitory concentrations for the majority of Enterobacteriaceae except with the *Enterobacter* spp., some of which had an MBC 64 times greater than the MIC. Against Gram-positive cocci cefuroxime had similar activity to cephalothin and cephamandole but was much less active against *Str. faecalis*. Against Enterobacteriaceae cefuroxime was more active than cephalothin and similar to cephamandole but is demonstrated greater resistance to beta-lactamase hydrolysis.— H. C. Neu and K. P. Fu, *Antimicrob. Ag. Chemother.*, 1978, *13*, 657.

In a preliminary study cefuroxime was more active *in vitro* against *Treponema pallidum* than cephazolin or cephacetrile. The minimum immobilising concentration for cefuroxime was 0.0125 µg per ml compared with 0.0016 µg per ml for benzylpenicillin.— L. Xerri and P. Orsolini (letter), *J. antimicrob. Chemother.*, 1978, *4*, 189.

Preliminary findings from 51 isolates of *Klebsiella aerogenes* resistant to gentamicin showed that while all strains were fully sensitive to cefoxitin, some strains had resistance to cefuroxime.— C. J. Noble *et al.* (letter), *Lancet*, 1979, *1*, 832.

MICs for cefuroxime against some strains of indole-positive *Proteus* were lower when tested on agar than in broth. A similar effect was obtained against *Streptococcus faecalis*.— M. Rylander *et al.*, *Antimicrob. Ag. Chemother.*, 1979, *15*, 572.

Further references: C. H. O'Callaghan *et al.*, *J. Antibiot., Tokyo*, 1976, *29*, 29; R. Norrby *et al.*, *Antimicrob. Ag. Chemother.*, 1976, *9*, 506; C. H. O'Callaghan *et al.*, *ibid.*, 511; D. M. Ryan *et al.*, *ibid.*, 520; S. Eykyn *et al.*, *ibid.*, 690; D. Greenwood *et al.*, *J. antimicrob. Chemother.*, 1976, *2*, 337; S. Goto, *Proc. R. Soc. Med.*, 1977, *70*, *Suppl.* 9, 56; M. H. Richmond, *ibid.*, 77; R. N. Brogden *et al.*, *Drugs*, 1979, *17*, 233; J. H. Jorgensen *et al.*, *Curr. ther. Res.*, 1979, *25*, 74; L. O. Potaschmacher *et al.*, *J. clin. Path.*, 1979, *32*, 944; M. V. Borobio *et al.*, *Antimicrob. Ag. Chemother.*, 1980, *17*, 129; W. Brown and R. J. Fallon, *J. antimicrob. Chemother.*, 1980, *6*, 91.

Diminished activity. Zones of inhibition for *Enterobacter* normally susceptible to cefuroxime or cefotaxime and resistant to cefoxitin were reduced when cefotaxime or cefuroxime were tested on agar plates in the presence of cefoxitin. On retesting the strains were found to be susceptible. However, when cultures were grown in broth in the presence of cefuroxime or cefotaxime with cefoxitin, resistant strains were isolated which inactivated several other cephalosporins and penicillins. Cultures rapidly reverted to susceptible when cefoxitin was removed from the media.— P. M. Waterworth and A. M. Emmerson, *Antimicrob. Ag. Chemother.*, 1979, *15*, 497.

Enhanced activity. Synergy or an additive effect against *E. coli*, *Klebsiella*, and *Serratia* spp. was demonstrated *in vitro* between aminoglycosides, especially amikacin, and cefuroxime.— H. Gaya *et al.*, *Proc. R. Soc. Med.*, 1977, *70*, *Suppl.* 9, 51.

Absorption and Fate. Cefuroxime is poorly absorbed from the gastro-intestinal tract and is given by intramuscular or intravenous injection as the sodium salt. Peak plasma concentrations of 26 to 34 µg per ml have been achieved 0.5 to 1 hour after an intramuscular dose of 750 mg with measurable amounts present 8 hours after a dose; after 750 mg given intravenously concentrations from 50 to 70 μg per ml have been reported. About 33% is bound to plasma proteins; the plasma half-life is about 70 minutes.

Cefuroxime is widely distributed in the body and has been found in pleural fluid, sputum, bone, synovial fluid, and aqueous humour. It diffuses across the placenta but only achieves therapeutic concentrations in the CSF when the meninges are inflamed.

At least 85% of a dose is excreted, mainly unchanged, by glomerular filtration and renal tubular secretion within 6 hours; high concentrations are achieved in the urine. Probenecid blocks some renal excretion. Small amounts of cefuroxime are excreted in bile.

Mean peak serum concentrations of 14.8, 25.7, 34.6, or 40 μg per ml were achieved 29 to 45 minutes after cefuroxime 0.25, 0.5, 0.75, or 1 g was given intramuscularly to 33 healthy subjects. Measurable concentrations were present 8 hours after the injection of 0.5 g or more. After intravenous doses of cefuroxime 0.25, 0.5, or 1 g given over 3 minutes to 9 healthy subjects, mean concentrations of 39, 66, or 99 μg per ml were obtained. Cefuroxime had an ultimate serum half-life of about 70 minutes and in 5 subjects given 1 g intramuscularly about 33% was bound to plasma proteins. More than 95% of a dose was excreted unchanged in the urine in 24 hours; high urinary concentrations were achieved 1 to 2 hours after injection and ranged from 0.5 to 7 mg per ml. From 43 to 54% of a dose was calculated as being secreted through the kidney tubules.— R. D. Foord, *Antimicrob. Ag. Chemother.*, 1976, *9*, 741.

The mean serum concentrations of cefuroxime in 7 healthy subjects reached a peak of 37.8 μg per ml at the end of a 30 minute intravenous infusion of cefuroxime 500 mg given in 90 ml of sodium chloride injection and remained above 10 μg per ml for at least 1.5 hours after the start of the infusion; after a similar 750-mg dose the mean serum concentration reached a peak of 51 μg per ml and remained above 10 μg per ml for at least 2.5 hours. After the 500 and 750-mg doses 97.8 and 95.7% of the doses respectively were recovered in the urine within 24 hours of administration and the estimated serum half-lives of cefuroxime were 111 and 126 minutes respectively.— C. S. Goodwin *et al.*, *J. antimicrob. Chemother.*, 1977, *3*, 253.

The mean serum half-life of cefuroxime ranged from 1.15 to 1.7 hours and the mean urinary excretion of cefuroxime up to 8 hours after administration was 84% of the dose. Mean serum concentrations of cefuroxime 30 minutes after the end of an intermittent infusion were 44, 73, and 145 μg per ml after a dose of 1, 1.5, and 2 g respectively.— R. Norrby *et al.*, *J. antimicrob. Chemother.*, 1977, *3*, 355.

Mean peak serum concentrations of cefuroxime after 0.5, 0.75, and 1 g given intramuscularly were 24.8, 27, and 33 μg per ml respectively and serum half-lives were 63.7, 88.2, and 115 minutes; the mean percentages of the dose of cefuroxime recovered in the urine within 8 hours of administration were about 69, 82, and 83% respectively but 97% was recovered after an intravenous dose of 1 g. There was no evidence of accumulation of cefuroxime in serum.— G. K. Daikos *et al.*, *J. antimicrob. Chemother.*, 1977, *3*, 555.

A study of the factors affecting the intramuscular absorption of cefuroxime.— S. M. Harding *et al.*, *J. antimicrob. Chemother.*, 1979, *5*, 87.

A study on concentrations of cefuroxime in the serum, bile, muscle, and skin after intravenous administration in patients undergoing cholecystectomy.— M. Severn and S. J. A. Powis, *J. antimicrob. Chemother.*, 1979, *5*, 183.

The pharmacokinetics of cefuroxime in patients with renal insufficiency.— R. van Dalen *et al.*, *J. antimicrob. Chemother.*, 1979, *5*, 281.

Further references to the pharmacokinetics of cefuroxime:— P. E. Gower and C. H. Dash, *Eur. J. clin. Pharmac.*, 1977, *12*, 221; *Proc. R. Soc. Med.*, 1977, *70*, *Suppl.* 9, 19-50; R. N. Brogden *et al.*, *Drugs*, 1979, *17*, 233.

Diffusion. Reports on the penetration of cefuroxime into the cerebrospinal fluid.— L. Corbeel *et al.* (letter), *Archs Dis. Childh.*, 1979, *54*, 729; H. Friedrich *et al.*, *Chemotherapy, Basle*, 1980, *26*, 91; C. Müller *et al.*, *J. antimicrob. Chemother.*, 1980, *6*, 279; J. Modai (letter), *ibid.*, 680.

Pregnancy and the neonate. Studies on the transplacental diffusion of cefuroxime.— I. Craft *et al.*, *Br. J. Obstet. Gynaec.*, 1981, *88*, 141 (intramuscular); P. Bousfield *et al.*, *ibid.*, 146 (intravenous).

Uses. Cefuroxime is a cephalosporin antibiotic and is given as the sodium salt by intramuscular or intravenous injection in the treatment of susceptible infections. A usual dose is the equivalent of 750 mg of cefuroxime every 8 hours but in more severe infections up to 1.5 g may be given 6-hourly; a dose of 1.5 g in 50 ml of Water for Injections may be infused over 30 minutes. Infants and children can be given 30 to 60 mg per kg body-weight daily increased to 100 mg per kg daily if necessary. Doses should be reduced in impaired renal function.

In the treatment of penicillin-resistant gonorrhoea a single dose of 1.5 g by intramuscular injection has been suggested.

For reports and reviews of the actions and uses of cefuroxime, see *Proc. R. Soc. Med.*, 1977, *70*, *Suppl.* 9, 1-214; H. C. Neu, *Ann. intern. Med.*, 1978, *89*, 719; R. N. Brogden *et al.*, *Drugs*, 1979, *17*, 233; *Drug & Ther. Bull.*, 1979, *17*, 35.

Further references to the use of cefuroxime: A. M. Geddes *et al.*, *Scand. J. infect. Dis.*, 1978, *13*, *Suppl.*, 78; N. J. Mitchell *et al.*, *J. antimicrob. Chemother.*, 1980, *6*, 393; P. Guérisse (letter), *Lancet*, 1981, *2*, 96.

Dosage in renal failure. Recommendations for the adjustment of dosage intervals of cefuroxime in patients with renal insufficiency. Concentrations were affected by haemodialysis.— R. van Dalen *et al.*, *J. antimicrob. Chemother.*, 1979, *5*, 281.

Gonorrhoea. In a study of the treatment of acute uncomplicated gonorrhoea 17 of 18 men given a single intramuscular dose of cefuroxime 1 g were cured and 60 of 62 given 1.5 g. The patients also received probenecid 1 g.— J. D. Price and J. L. Fluker, *Br. J. vener. Dis.*, 1978, *54*, 165.

Cure-rates of 94.8 to 99.6% were achieved with cefuroxime in 1196 patients with uncomplicated gonorrhoea. Cefuroxime was given intramuscularly in doses of 1 or 1.5 g or 0.75 g was given in association with probenecid 1 g by mouth.— W. Fowler *et al.*, *Br. J. vener. Dis.*, 1978, *54*, 400.

Ophthalmia neonatorum caused by beta-lactamase-producing gonococci in premature identical twins was successfully treated with sulphacetamide 30% eye-drops every 6 hours and erythromycin by drip feed replaced after 24 hours by cefuroxime 100 mg per kg body-weight daily intramuscularly in 3 divided doses for 7 days. Recovery of gonococci from sites other than the eye pointed to the need for systemic antigonococcal treatment in such babies.— E. M. C. Dunlop *et al.*, *Br. med. J.*, 1980, *281*, 483.

Meningitis. Seven children with meningitis due to *Neisseria meningitidis* or *Haemophilus influenzae* were successfully treated with cefuroxime 25 mg per kg body-weight infused over 20 minutes every 4 hours generally in addition to ampicillin, chloramphenicol, and sulphadimidine. CSF concentrations of cefuroxime (measured in 3 children) were between 1.5 and 9 μg per ml and exceeded the MICs for the infecting organisms.— J. A. Kuzemko and S. R. Walker, *Archs Dis. Childh.*, 1979, *54*, 235.

Further references: Swedish Study Group, *Lancet*, 1982, *1*, 295.

Proprietary Preparations

Zinacef *(Glaxo, UK)*. Cefuroxime sodium, available as powder for preparing injections, in vials containing the equivalent of 0.25, 0.75, or 1.5 g of cefuroxime. Protect from light. (Also available as Zinacef in *Ger.*, *Neth.*, *S.Afr.*, *Swed.*).

Other Proprietary Names

Curoxim, Itorex, Ultroxim *(all Ital.)*.

36-m

Cephacetrile Sodium.
B 73-56; Ba 36278A; Cefacetrile Sodium. Sodium (7*R*)-7-(2-cyanoacetamido)cephalosporanate; Sodium (7*R*)-3-acetoxymethyl-7-(2-cyanoacetamido)-3-cephem-4-carboxylate.

$C_{13}H_{12}N_3NaO_6S = 361.3$.

CAS — 10206-21-0 (cephacetrile); 23239-41-0 (sodium salt).

A crystalline powder. Each g represents about 2.8 mmol (2.8 mEq) of sodium. Cephacetrile sodium 1.07 g is approximately equivalent to 1 g of cephacetrile. Readily **soluble** in water.

Adverse Effects and Precautions. As for Cephalothin Sodium, p.1128.

It is recommended that cephacetrile should be given with care in reduced dosage to patients with renal impairment.

After an infusion of cephacetrile 8 g over 30 minutes, 9 of 15 healthy subjects had temporary proximal renal tubule damage, shown by increased excretion of alanine-aminopeptidase (a brush-border enzyme).— A. W. Mondorf *et al.*, *Eur. J. clin. Pharmac.*, 1978, *13*, 357.

Antimicrobial Action. Cephacetrile is bactericidal and has an antibacterial activity similar to that of cephalothin. It is reported to be less susceptible to inactivation by beta-lactamases than either cephaloridine or cephalothin.

The minimum inhibitory concentrations of cephacetrile *in vitro* were 0.1 to 0.4 μg per ml for susceptible Gram-positive strains and 3 to 15 μg per ml for Gram-negative strains F. Knüsel *et al.*, *Antimicrob. Ag. Chemother.*, 1970, 140.

Cephacetrile was more resistant to hydrolysis by beta-lactamase enzymes of several Gram-negative organisms than either cephaloridine or cephalothin.— H. C. Neu and E. B. Winshell, *J. Antibiot., Tokyo*, 1972, *25*, 400.

Further references: F. Kradolfer *et al.*, *Antimicrob. Ag. Chemother.*, 1970, 150; *Lancet*, 1973, *2*, 364; J. Gelzer and P. N. Maurice (letter), *ibid.*, 855; J. D. Williams and J. Andrews, *Br. med. J.*, 1974, *1*, 134; S. Eykyn and I. Phillips (letter), *ibid.*, 1974, *2*, 59.

Absorption and Fate. Cephacetrile is poorly absorbed from the gastro-intestinal tract and is given by intramuscular or intravenous injection. Following a dose of 1 g given intramuscularly peak plasma concentrations ranging from 13 to 23 μg per ml have been achieved within one hour. From 30 to 40% of cephacetrile may be bound to plasma proteins and reported values for plasma half-lives range from 0.5 to 1.5 hours. Cephacetrile diffuses into bone and the cerebrospinal fluid and also across the placenta into the foetal circulation.

It is excreted in the urine mainly by glomerular filtration but with some renal tubular secretion; up to 25% may appear as the desacetyl metabolite. About 70% of an intramuscular dose is excreted within 6 hours; urine concentrations of at least 3 mg per ml have been reported. Biliary excretion is low in patients with normal renal function.

A review.— C. H. Nightingale *et al.*, *J. pharm. Sci.*, 1975, *64*, 1899.

The mean serum concentration of cephacetrile 15 minutes after intravenous injection of 500 mg to 5 healthy male subjects was 30.7 μg per ml. Antibacterial activity of the serum had a mean half-life of 33.2 minutes; 33 to 36% was bound to serum. Urinary excretion accounted for a mean of 84.3% activity over 10 hours, maximum excretion occurring in the first 2 hours.— D. K. Luscombe *et al.*, *Antimicrob. Ag. Chemother.*, 1973, *3*, 677.

In a study of 23 patients with varying degrees of renal function about 97% of a dose of cephacetrile was excreted in the urine of those with normal kidney function when the biological half-life was about 1 hour. In anuric patients the half-life was about 30 hours; in patients with chronic stable renal disease the half-lives could be estimated by multiplying the serum-creatinine concentrations by 1.5 or dividing the urea concentration by 14.— P. Spring *et al.*, *Schweiz. med. Wschr.*, 1973, *103*, 783.

Cephacetrile was administered in a dose of 1 g in a 2% lignocaine solution to 10 subjects on 2 occasions, once into the anterolateral aspect of the thigh and once into the upper outer quadrant of the buttock. Significantly higher serum-cephacetrile concentrations were obtained at 30 minutes after injection into the thigh than into the buttock. There was a similar trend with gentamicin but this was not significant.— D. S. Reeves *et al.*, *Lancet*, 1974, *2*, 1421.

Further references: A. R. Nissenson *et al.*, *Clin. Pharmac. Ther.*, 1972, *13*, 887; L. Dettli *et al.*, *Advances in Antimicrobial and Antineoplastic Chemotherapy*, Vol. I, pt 1, Munich, Urban and Schwarzenberg, 1972, 57; F. Reutter and P. N. Maurice, *ibid.*, 59; P. N. Maurice *et al.*, *Schweiz. med. Wschr.*, 1973, *103*, 718; J. M. Brogard *et al.*, *Antimicrob. Ag. Chemother.*, 1973, *3*, 19; A. Dominguez-Gil *et al.*, *Eur. J. clin. Pharmac.*, 1979, *16*, 49.

Diffusion. Into *bone*: H. Stuflesser *et al.* (letter), *J. antimicrob. Chemother.*, 1978, *4*, 188. *cerebrospinal fluid*: L. Dettli (letter), *Br. med. J.*, 1976, *2*, 110; A. Windorfer and U. Gasteiger, *Infection*, 1977, *5*, 242.

Uses. Cephacetrile sodium is a cephalosporin antibiotic with the actions and uses of Cephaloridine, p.1127.

Cephacetrile 2 to 6 g daily is given by intramuscular or slow intravenous injection in 4 divided doses; in severe infections up to 12 g daily may be given, if necessary by infusion. A suggested dose for children is 50 to 100 mg per kg body-weight daily.

Reduced doses should be used in patients with impaired renal function.

For reports of the actions and uses of cephacetrile, see F. Kradolfer *et al.*, *Schweiz. med. Wschr.*, 1973, *103*, 711; G. R. Hodges *et al.*, *Antimicrob. Ag. Chemother.*, 1973, *3*, 228; G. G. Jackson *et al.*, *ibid.*, 1974, *5*, 247; *Arzneimittel-Forsch.*, 1974, *24*, 1446-1533; A. L. Kaplan and A. A. Acosta, *Curr. ther. Res.*, 1975, *18*, 793 (salpingitis); J. L. Zehnder *et al.*, *Obstet. Gynec.*, 1976, *47*, 423 (pelvic inflammatory disease).

Proceedings of a symposium on cephacetrile.— *Infection*, 1976, *4*, *Suppl.* 3, S171-S282.

Meningitis. From studies of serum and CSF concentrations, cephacetrile could be recommended in the treatment of neonatal meningitis caused by *Klebsiella pneumoniae*. The following intravenous regimens were suggested: in neonates over 2 kg at birth, an initial daily dose of 150 mg per kg body-weight in 2 equal doses reduced to 80 mg per kg on day 2; in neonates up to 2 kg, an initial daily dose of 100 mg per kg in 2 doses reduced to 60 mg per kg on day 2.— A. Windorfer and U. Gasteiger, *Infection*, 1977, *5*, 242.

Urinary-tract infections. Cephacetrile 1 g in 2 ml of a 2% lignocaine solution was given intramuscularly every 12 hours for 5 days to 21 patients with urinary-tract infections and 15 were bacteriologically cured.— R. Wise *et al.*, *Chemotherapy, Basle*, 1974, *20*, 177. See also C. Panticelli *et al.*, *Eur. J. clin. Pharmac.*, 1974, *7*, 331.

Proprietary Names

Celospor *(Ciba, Fr.; Ciba, Ger.; Grünenthal, Ger.; Chinoin, Hung.; Ciba, Ital.; Jap.; Ciba, Spain; Ciba-Geigy, Switz.)*; Celtol *(Jap.)*.

37-b

Cephalexin *(B.P., U.S.P.)*. 66873; Cefalexin.

(7*R*)-3-Methyl-7-(α-D-phenylglycylamino)-3-cephem-4-carboxylic acid monohydrate.

$C_{16}H_{17}N_3O_4S,H_2O$=365.4.

CAS — 15686-71-2(anhydrous); 23325-78-2(monohydrate).

Pharmacopoeias. In *Br.*, *Braz.*, *Jap.*, and *U.S.*

A white to cream-coloured, slightly hygroscopic, crystalline powder with a characteristic odour. The *B.P.* specifies 95 to 103% of cephalexin and *U.S.P.* not less than 900 μg per mg, both calculated on the anhydrous basis. **Soluble** 1 in 100 of water and 1 in 30 of 0.2% hydrochloric acid; slightly soluble in dioxan, dimethylacetamide, and dimethylformamide; very slightly soluble in acetone; practically insoluble in alcohol, chloroform, and ether; soluble in solutions of dilute alkalis. A 0.5% solution has a pH of 3.5 to 5.5. Aqueous solutions and suspensions decompose on storage but have optimum stability at pH 4.5. **Store** at a temperature not exceeding 30° in airtight containers. Protect from light.

For a discussion of the physical properties and a consideration of the problems in the formulation of cephalexin, see C. M. Bond *et al.*, *Pharm. J.*, 1970, *2*, 210. Cephalexin could be formulated as a sustained-release tablet.— H. Schneider *et al.*, *J. pharm. Sci.*, 1978, *67*, 1620.

Cephalexin, crystallised from water at room temperature, separated from solution as the dihydrate but converted to the monohydrate at relative humidities below 70% R. R. Pfeiffer *et al.*, *J. pharm. Sci.*, 1970, *59*, 1809.

Apparent pKa values determined for cephalexin at 35° were 2.56 and 6.88.— T. Yamana and A. Tsuji, *J. pharm. Sci.*, 1976, *65*, 1563.

Effect of gamma-irradiation. Tests indicated that cephalexin powder may be irradiated safely at the commonly employed sterilisation dose of 25 000 Gy.— G. P. Jacobs, *Int. J. appl. Radiat. Isotopes*, 1980, *31*, 91.

Stability. Cephalexin in horse serum was stable for at least 30 days when stored at −10°. Repeated thawing and freezing did not affect its stability. After 30 days at 4° cephalexin retained 56% activity.— M. A. Foglesong, *Antimicrob. Ag. Chemother.*, 1977, *11*, 174.

Stability in solution. Studies on the degradation of cephalexin in aqueous solution.— H. Bundgaard, *Arch. Pharm. Chemi, scient. Edn*, 1976, *4*, 25; *idem*, 1977, *5*, 149.

Adverse Effects. Side-effects of cephalexin include nausea, vomiting, diarrhoea, and abdominal discomfort. Skin rashes occur in about 1% of patients treated with cephalexin and rises in serum aminotransferases have been noted. Eosinophilia and neutropenia have occurred in a few patients. Supra-infection with resistant micro-organisms, particularly *Candida*, may follow treatment.

Hypokalaemia occurred in 9 of 11 patients with leukaemia after being given courses of gentamicin 80 mg intravenously every 8 hours with cephalexin 1 g every 6 hours. Most of the patients were also receiving anti-neoplastic therapy.— G. P. Young *et al.* (letter), *Lancet*, 1973, *2*, 855.

A 70-year-old white man with diabetes was treated with cephalexin 500 mg every 6 hours for urinary-tract infection. He developed nephrohepatotoxicity which was reversed when the drug was withdrawn.— C. G. Fung-Herrera and W. P. Mulvaney, *J. Am. med. Ass.*, 1974, *229*, 318.

Blood disorders. An acute haemolysis was observed in a haemophilic patient who, having received blood transfusions and a high potency human antihaemophilic globulin preparation after crush injury, was treated with ampicillin 1 g daily for 9 days, followed by cephalexin 2 g daily for 13 days. The haemolytic episode commenced on the 9th day of treatment with cephalexin and ceased when the drug was withdrawn.— C. D. Forbes *et al.*, *Postgrad. med. J.*, 1972, *48*, 186.

A report of acute reversible agranulocytosis associated with the administration of cephalexin.— M. Le Porrier *et al.*, *Ann. Méd. interne*, 1976, *127*, 461.

Colitis. An 83-year-old man developed pseudomembranous colitis after receiving courses of cephalexin, cephalothin sodium, and cephazolin sodium.— J. F. Tures *et al.*, *J. Am. med. Ass.*, 1976, *236*, 948.

Nephrotoxicity. Reports of nephrotoxicity associated with cephalexin.— C. G. Fung-Herrera and W. P. Mulvaney, *J. Am. med. Ass.*, 1974, *229*, 318; S. Verma and E. Kieff, *ibid.*, 1975, *234*, 618; A. L. Linton *et al.*, *Ann. intern. Med.*, 1980, *93*, 735.

Neurotoxicity. A 46-year-old woman with uraemia who was treated with cephalexin for suspected bacterial endocarditis developed convulsions and a toxic psychosis which were attributed to raised serum levels of cephalexin, as high as 120 μg per ml. The patient returned to normal 11 days after cessation of treatment with cephalexin.— B. M. Saker *et al.*, *Med. J. Aust.*, 1973, *1*, 497.

Precautions. Patients who are known or suspected to be allergic to other cephalosporins should not be treated with cephalexin and care is necessary in treating patients known to be hypersensitive to penicillin or with known histories of allergy. Reduced dosage is recommended in patients with impaired kidney function.

The urine of patients taking cephalexin may give a false positive reaction for glucose with copper-reduction reagents.

Positive results to the Coombs' test have been reported with cephalexin.

Mean peak plasma concentrations of cephalexin were reduced in healthy subjects when they also took cholestyramine.— R. L. Parsons and G. M. Paddock, *J. antimicrob. Chemother.*, 1975, *1*, *Suppl.* (Sept.), 59.

See also Absorption and Fate.

Antimicrobial Action. Cephalexin is bactericidal and has antimicrobial activity similar to that of cephaloridine or cephalothin against both Gram-positive and Gram-negative organisms, though it is generally less potent. Some strains of Gram-negative organisms may be inhibited only by concentrations that can usually be achieved only in the urinary tract. *Haemophilus influenzae* shows varying sensitivity to cephalexin. Enterococci, *Bacteroides*, *Enterobacter*, *Proteus* apart from *Pr. mirabilis*, and *Pseudomonas* spp. are resistant to cephalexin. It is reported to be more active in alkaline than in acid media.

Beta-lactamases inhibit cephalexin but it is more resistant to staphylococcal penicillinase than cephazolin or cephaloridine. Methicillin-resistant strains of staphylococci are usually resistant to cephalexin.

MICs of cephalexin for the majority of group A streptococci were 0.78 μg or less per ml; for pneumococci 0.19 to 3.13 μg per ml; for all except 2 resistant strains of coagulase-positive staphylococci 0.95 to 3.9 μg per ml. The minimum bactericidal concentration differed little from these figures, except for penicillin-resistant coagulase-positive staphylococci for which it was higher. MICs for *Escherichia coli* and *Proteus mirabilis* were 7.8 to 15.6 μg per ml; for *Salmonella* spp. 3.9 to 7.8 μg per ml. Some *Klebsiella-Aerobacter* spp. had an MIC of 3.9 to 31.3 μg per ml, while others, in addition to enterococci and *Pseudomonas* spp., were resistant.— R. L. Perkins *et al.*, *Am. J. med. Sci.*, 1968, *256*, 122.

Of 68 strains of *Haemophilus influenzae* 5 were inhibited by cephalexin at a concentration of 1 μg per ml, 16 at 2 μg per ml, 15 at 4 μg per ml, 26 at 8 μg per ml, and 6 at 16 μg per ml.— J. D. Williams and J. Andrews, *Br. med. J.*, 1974, *1*, 134. Of 36 strains, 2 had an MIC of cephalexin of 0.39 μg per ml; 2 of 0.78 μg per ml; 4 of 1.56 μg per ml; 8 of 3.12 μg per ml; 11 of 6.25 μg per ml; 7 of 12.5 μg per ml; and 2 of 25 μg per ml.— S. Eykyn and I. Phillips (letter), *ibid.*, 1974, *2*, 59.

Cephalexin had an MIC of 3.12 and 6.25 μg per ml respectively against 73 and 100% of 67 strains of *Salmonella typhi* and an MIC of 6.25 and 12.5 μg per ml against 31 and 98% of 54 strains of *S. paratyphi A*.— L. J. Strausbaugh *et al.*, *Antimicrob. Ag. Chemother.*, 1978, *13*, 134.

For comparisons of the activities of cephalexin, cephradine, cefaclor, and cefatrizine see Cefaclor, p.1115.

Absorption and Fate. Cephalexin is almost completely absorbed from the gastro-intestinal tract and produces peak plasma concentrations about 1 hour after administration. A dose of 500 mg produces a mean peak plasma concentration of about 18 μg per ml, about the same as the concentration produced by an equal dose of cephaloridine given intramuscularly and greater than that produced by cephalothin. If cephalexin is taken with food there is delayed and slightly reduced absorption and there may be delayed elimination from the plasma. About 10 to 15% of a dose is bound to plasma proteins.

The biological half-life has been reported to range from 0.6 to at least 1.2 hours and this increases with reduced renal function. About 80% or more of a dose is excreted unchanged in the urine in the first 6 hours by glomerular filtration and tubular secretion; urinary concentrations greater than 1 mg per ml have been achieved after a dose of 500 mg. Probenecid delays urinary excretion and has been reported to increase biliary excretion. Cephalexin is widely distributed in the body but does not enter the cerebrospinal fluid in significant quantities unless the meninges are inflamed. It diffuses across the placenta and small quantities are found in the milk of nursing mothers. Therapeutically effective concentrations may be found in the bile.

A short review.— C. H. Nightingale *et al.*, *J. pharm. Sci.*, 1975, *64*, 1899.

After single doses of 0.25, 0.5, and 1 g of cephalexin given by mouth to healthy persons, peak serum concentrations at 1 hour averaged 6.8, 17.6, and 25 μg per ml respectively. After 4 hours, serum concentrations were 0.6, 1.5, and 3.1 μg per ml respectively. The percentages of the dose recovered in urine during the first 6 hours were 96, 93, and 85 respectively.— R. L. Perkins *et al.*, *Am. J. med. Sci.*, 1968, *256*, 122. A similar report.— P. E. Gower and C. H. Dash, *Br. J. Pharmac.*, 1969, *37*, 738.

The absorption of cephalexin administered by injection.— J. B. de Maine and W. M. M. Kirby, *Antimicrob. Ag. Chemother.*, 1970, 190; J. A. Davies and J. M. Holt, *J. clin. Path.*, 1972, *25*, 518; P. E. Gower *et al.*, *J. Pharm. Pharmac.*, 1973, *25*, 376; P. Nicholas *et al.*, *J. clin. Pharmac.*, 1973, *13*, 463.

A crossover study in 9 healthy subjects given 5 doses of cephalexin or cephradine 1 g every six hours in differing formulations indicated that the two drugs were pharmacokinetically equivalent.— E. Finkelstein *et al.*, *J. pharm. Sci.*, 1978, *67*, 1447. See also M. Chow *et al.*, *J. clin. Pharmac.*, 1979, *19*, 185.

A report of the use of a sustained-release preparation of cephalexin in children.— M. Hori *et al.*, *Jap. J. Antibiot.*, 1978, *31*, 59.

A study in 15 children indicated that there was no substantial effect on absorption when cephalexin was taken with meals.— T. R. Tetzlaff *et al.*, *J. Pediat.*, 1978, *92*, 292.

Absorption and fate in disease states. The absorption and urinary excretion of cephalexin were increased in patients with coeliac disease or small bowel diverticulosis but absorption was reduced and delayed in patients with Crohn's disease or fibrocystic disease. Cephalexin appeared to be more suitable than co-trimoxazole in the treatment of infections in patients with malabsorption syndromes.— R. L. Parsons and G. M. Paddock, *J. antimicrob. Chemother.*, 1975, *1*, *Suppl.* (Sept.), 59.

There was little impairment in absorption of cephalexin in 18 patients with obstructive jaundice, 14 with gastric achlorhydria, 22 with partial gastrectomy and 6 patients with congestive cardiac failure compared with 21 healthy subjects. Although absorption was not impaired in 9 elderly subjects (mean age 78 years) serum concentrations of cephalexin were sustained compared with those in 12 younger subjects (mean age 29 years).— J. A. Davies and J. M. Holt, *J. antimicrob. Chemother.*, 1975, *1*, *Suppl.* (Sept.), 69.

Absorption and fate in renal impairment. Cephalexin was given in a dose of 500 mg to 18 healthy persons and 9 patients with renal failure. The biological half-life was 1.4 hours in healthy persons compared with 14.4 hours in patients with renal failure and there was a substantial change in distribution indicated by the smaller apparent volume of distribution in patients with renal failure compared with that in healthy persons.— M. Gibaldi and D. Perrier, *J. clin. Pharmac.*, 1972, *12*, 201. See also C. M. Kunin and Z. Finkelberg, *Ann. intern. Med.*, 1970, *72*, 349; D. A. Spyker *et al.*, *Antimicrob. Ag. Chemother.*, 1978, *14*, 172.

Serum concentrations of cephalexin 4 hours after a single 250-mg dose were in general related to the serum-creatinine concentration.— R. H. Butcher *et al.*, *Med. J. Aust.*, 1972, *2*, 1282.

Diffusion. For reports on the diffusion of cephalexin into body fluids, see G. L. Boyle *et al.*, *Am. J. Ophthal.*, 1970, *69*, 868 (aqueous humour); J. E. L. Sales *et al.*, *Br. med. J.*, 1972, *3*, 441 (bile); G. M. Halprin and S. M. McMahon, *Antimicrob. Ag. Chemother.*, 1973, *3*, 703; A. Kohonen *et al.*, *Ann. clin. Res.*, 1975, *7*, 50; F. Daschner, *Münch. med. Wschr.*, 1977, *119*, 339 (sputum).

Studies suggesting that the degree of binding to plasma proteins does not influence the diffusion of antibiotics, including cephalexin, into body fluids.— A. P. Gillett and R. Wise, *Lancet*, 1978, *1*, 962 (tissue fluid); J. D. Nelson *et al.*, *J. Pediat.*, 1978, *92*, 131 (synovial fluid).

Pregnancy and the neonate. Cephalexin 500 mg was given at induction of labour to 20 women and repeated every 6 hours until delivery; bacteriostatic concentrations of cephalexin (against *Staphylococcus aureus*) were rapidly achieved in all mothers. Lower bacteriostatic concentrations were achieved in the cord blood of 10 of the infants at delivery. Neither maternal blood nor cord blood had bacteriostatic concentrations if delivery was delayed more than 18 hours, possibly because pylorospasm reduced absorption. This effect was not overcome by doubling the dose in a further 20 women.— M. L. Paterson *et al.*, *Clin. Med.*, 1972, *79* (Mar.), 22.

Newborn infants up to the age of 3 days absorbed 50 to 60% of cephalexin given as a syrup. The high plasma concentrations seen 8 to 12 hours after the dose were attributed to the reduced renal function of infants.— R. Boothman *et al.*, *Archs Dis. Childh.*, 1973, *48*, 147.

A mean peak serum concentration of about 4.5 µg per ml was obtained in 13 neonates 6 hours after administration of cephalexin 15 mg per kg body-weight 2 hours after a feed; the half-life for cephalexin was 63 hours.— J. A. Raeburn *et al.*, *J. antimicrob. Chemother.*, 1975, *1*, *Suppl.* (Sept.), 53.

Uses. Cephalexin, a cephalosporin antibiotic, is administered by mouth for the treatment of infections of the respiratory and urinary tracts and other infections due to sensitive organisms. For severe infections treatment with parenteral cephalosporins is to be preferred. It is not destroyed by gastric acid but absorption may be delayed by food in the stomach or small intestine. It is more resistant to staphylococcal penicillinase than is cephaloridine or cephazolin.

The usual dose is 250 to 500 mg every 6 hours; in severe or deep-seated infections the dose can be increased to 3 to 6 g daily but when high doses are required the use of a parenteral cephalosporin should be considered. Infants and children may be given 25 to 100 mg per kg body-weight daily in divided doses to a maximum of 4 g daily. In patients with impaired kidney function smaller doses should be employed.

Cephalexin sodium has occasionally been administered by intravenous or intramuscular injection.

Reviews of cephalexin.— R. S. Griffith and H. R. Black, *Med. Clins N. Amer.*, 1970, *54*, 1229; S. Eykyn, *J. clin. Path.*, 1971, *24*, 419; *Med. Lett.*, 1971, *13*, 25; T. M. Speight *et al.*, *Drugs*, 1972, *3*, 9; M. Finland, *ibid.*, 1.

Of 21 patients with soft tissue infections good clinical response to cephalexin 500 mg every 6 to 8 hours occurred in 15 patients. Good response was also shown in 3 of 9 patients with urinary-tract infections and in 4 of 8 with respiratory infections. Of 37 patients treated with cephalexin, infections were controlled in 24. Organisms which responded to cephalexin were *Clostridium welchii, Staph. aureus, Staph. albus, Proteus mirabilis, Klebsiella* spp., and *E. coli*.— L. N. Roberts, *J. clin. Pharmac.*, 1973, *13*, 276.

Cephalexin sodium given intravenously or intramuscularly in a dose of 1 g four times daily for 7 to 10 days was effective in treating infection following surgery in 14 of 20 patients. Two of 12 patients given the same dose of cephalexin sodium prophylactically after transvesical prostatectomy developed an infection, compared with 10 of 15 patients in a control group not receiving antibiotic therapy.— S. P. F. Hughes *et al.*, *Br. J. clin. Pract.*, 1974, *28*, 51. See also R. Svensson and S. Seeberg, *Scand. J. infect. Dis.*, 1974, *6*, 279.

For the proceedings of a conference on cephalexin and cephaloridine, see *J. antimicrob. Chemother.*, 1975, *1*, *Suppl.* (Sept.), 1-139.

Dosage in renal failure. Cephalexin 500 mg was given to 12 patients 1 hour before starting maintenance haemodialysis. The mean serum half-life was reduced to 4.6 hours and the mean serum concentration 15 hours after administration at the end of dialysis was 3.3 µg per ml which compares with 21.8 hours and 14.7 µg per ml respectively in patients given the same dose between dialyses. The recommended dose for patients on intermittent haemodialysis was 500 mg daily plus 500 mg at the end of each dialysis.— R. R. Bailey *et al.*, *Postgrad. med. J.*, 1970, *46*, *Suppl.*, 60.

After a loading dose of 500 mg cephalexin could be given in a dose of 500 mg every 4 to 6 hours to patients with a creatinine clearance of 40 to 80 ml per minute, 500 mg every 8 to 12 hours to those with a clearance of 20 to 30 ml per minute, 250 mg every 12 hours to those with a clearance of 10 ml per minute, and 250 mg every 12 to 24 hours to those with a clearance of 5 ml per minute. In haemodialysis 250 mg could be given every 12 to 24 hours and 500 mg after dialysis.— J. S. Cheigh, *Am. J. Med.*, 1977, *62*, 555. Similar reports.— J. A. Linquist *et al.*, *New Engl. J. Med.*, 1970, *283*, 720; S. A. Kabins *et al.*, *Am. J. med. Sci.*, 1970, *259*, 133.

Blood-cephalexin concentrations could be altered by haemodialysis and peritoneal dialysis.— P. Sharpstone, *Br. med. J.*, 1977, *2*, 36.

Data for predicting removal of cephalexin by conventional haemodialysis.— T. P. Gibson and H. A. Nelson, *Clin. Pharmacokinet.*, 1977, *2*, 403.

Further references: D. L. Giusti, *Drug Intell. & clin. Pharm.*, 1973, *7*, 252; G. B. Appel and H. C. Neu, *New Engl. J. Med.*, 1977, *296*, 663; W. M. Bennett *et al.*, *Ann. intern. Med.*, 1980, *93*, 62.

See also under Absorption and Fate.

Gonorrhoea. Cephalexin was given in doses of 2 to 6 g daily for 2 to 4 days in the treatment of proven gonorrhoea in 21 men and 5 women. The organisms were eliminated in 14 patients after 1 course of treatment, but in 3 others there were relapses, even at increased dosage and in a further 4, organisms resistant to cephalexin were found.— C. F. D. Ackman *et al.*, *Can. med. Ass. J.*, 1972, *106*, 350.

Of 50 women with gonorrhoea 48 were considered cured and of 103 men 99 were considered cured after a single dose of ten 500-mg tablets of cephalexin and four 500-mg tablets of probenecid, administered over about 30 minutes.— R. R. Landes *et al.*, *Clin. Med.*, 1972, *79* (June), 23.

Further references to cephalexin in gonorrhoea: J. A. Aluoch and Odhiambo-Olel, *E. Afr. med. J.*, 1978, *55*, 519.

Otitis media. Cephalexin was used in the treatment of 97 children with otitis media. The usual dosage was 100 mg per kg body-weight daily by mouth for 10 to 12 days. Therapy failed in 7 children; *Haemophilus influenzae* was responsible for 5 failures and *Streptococcus pneumoniae* for 2.— S. E. McLinn *et al.*, *J. Am. med. Ass.*, 1975, *234*, 171.

Cephalexin should not be used to treat otitis media due to *Haemophilus influenzae*.— B. W. Stechenberg *et al.*, *Pediatrics*, 1976, *58*, 532.

Pharyngitis. Reports of the use of cephalexin in the treatment of pharyngitis in children.— M. Stillerman *et al.*, *Am. J. Dis. Child.*, 1972, *123*, 457; W. M. Gooch *et al.*, *Clin. Med.*, 1972, *79* (Dec.), 11; J. M. Matsen *et al.*, *Antimicrob. Ag. Chemother.*, 1974, *6*, 501.

Respiratory infections, other. A report of cephalexin in the treatment of *pneumonia*.— I. M. Rosenthal *et al.*, *Postgrad. med. J.*, 1971, *47*, *Suppl.*, 51.

Reports of the use of cephalexin in *bronchitis*.— A. Pines, *Br. J. clin. Pract.*, 1972, *26*, 209; *Practitioner*, 1972, *208*, 421 (Report No. 167 of the General Practitioner Research Group,); D. M. Cooke and R. T. Garrett, *J. antimicrob. Chemother.*, 1975, *1*, *Suppl.* (Sept.), 99 (comparison with ampicillin); J. Cooper and F. B. McGillion, *Practitioner*, 1978, *221*, 428 (comparison with co-trimoxazole).

Cephalexin in the management of patients with pulmonary disease due to *cystic fibrosis*.— V. A. Loening-Baucke *et al.*, *J. Pediat.*, 1979, *95*, 630.

Shigellosis. From a study of children and infants with diarrhoea, in which *Shigella* was present in 42%, it was considered that cephalexin was not suitable for the treatment of shigellosis due to ampicillin-resistant organisms.— J. D. Nelson and K. C. Haltalin, *Antimicrob. Ag. Chemother.*, 1975, *7*, 415.

Syphilis. The use of cephalexin in the treatment of syphilis. A regimen giving a total dose of 30 g was as effective as erythromycin or tetracycline but 15 g was not. Penicillin was still the treatment of choice where possible.— W. C. Duncan and J. M. Knox, *Archs Derm.*, 1974, *110*, 77.

Urinary-tract infections. Cephalexin 0.5 or 1 g four times a day for 14 days was given to 18 patients with urinary-tract infections. From 29 to 89% of the daily ingested dose was excreted in the urine in 24 hours. Urinary concentrations of 920 to 4700 µg per ml were obtained. Peak blood concentrations occurred 30 minutes to 2 hours after ingestion of cephalexin. Seven of 12 patients became faecal carriers of *Pseudomonas aeruginosa* and 4 of 12 carriers of *Proteus*, significantly more than in a control group receiving no antibiotics. Cephalexin eliminated the infecting organism in 75% of the patients.— H. Gaya *et al.*, *Br. med. J.*, 1970, *3*, 624. Comments.— J. C. Gould and A. J. Keay (letter), *ibid.*, 1970, *4*, 56; C. N. Brown and G. E. Mallett, *Lilly* (letter), *ibid.*, 116; C. H. Dash and P. E. Gower (letter), *ibid.*, 181.

Similar results were obtained with cephalexin and ampicillin in the treatment of urinary-tract infections in 62 patients.— J. A. Davies *et al.*, *Br. med. J.*, 1971, *3*, 215.

In 22 patients with frequent symptomatic urinary infection, treatment for 6 months with cephalexin 500 mg by mouth daily was successful in 17, partially successful in 1, and a failure in 4. Radiological abnormalities were present in 14 patients including the 4 failures. Cephalexin was withdrawn in 1 patient due to sensitivity reaction.— K. F. Fairley *et al.*, *Med. J. Aust.*, 1974, *1*, 318.

Recurrence of infection occurred in 1 of 25 women with a history of recurrent urinary-tract infections within 6 months of starting prphylaxis with cephalexin 125 mg taken at night, compared with 13 of 25 who received a placebo. No further relapses occurred in 20 patients receiving cephalexin and in 10 receiving placebo who were followed up for 12 months from the start of the study.— P. E. Gower, *J. antimicrob. Chemother.*, 1975, *1*, *Suppl.* (Sept.), 93.

A recommendation that cephalexin be used to treat ampicillin-resistant urinary-tract infections in pregnancy.— *Br. med. J.*, 1977, *2*, 690.

For a comparison of ampicillin, cephalexin, co-trimoxazole, and trimethoprim alone in the treatment of urinary-tract infections, see Co-trimoxazole, p.1466.

Preparations

Cephalexin Capsules *(B.P.)*. Capsules containing cephalexin. Store at a temperature not exceeding 30°. Protect from light.

Cephalexin Capsules *(U.S.P.)*. Capsules containing the equivalent of 125, 250, or 500 mg of anhydrous cephalexin. Store in airtight containers.

Cephalexin for Oral Suspension *(U.S.P.)*. A dry mixture of cephalexin with one or more suitable diluents, buffers, colours, and flavours. Store in airtight containers. The suspension is prepared by the addition of diluent before issue. When reconstituted it contains the equivalent of 25, 50, or 100 mg of anhydrous cephalexin per ml. pH 3 to 6.

Cephalexin Mixture *(B.P.C. 1973)*. A suspension of cephalexin in a suitable flavoured vehicle; it is freshly prepared by dispersing granules of the dry mixed ingredients in the specified vol. of water. pH 3 to 6. Store in a cool place.

Cephalexin Tablets *(B.P.)*. Tablets containing cephalexin. They may be film-coated. Store at a temperature not exceeding 30°.

Cephalexin Tablets *(U.S.P.)*. Tablets containing the equivalent of 0.5 or 1 g of anhydrous cephalexin. Store in airtight containers.

Proprietary Preparations

Ceporex *(Glaxo, UK)*. Cephalexin, available as **Capsules** and **Tablets** of 250 and 500 mg; as **Paediatric Drops** (supplied as granules for preparation with water before use) containing 125 mg in each 1.25 ml; as **Suspension** containing 125 or 250 mg in each 5 ml in a vehicle containing vegetable oil (dilution not recommended); and as **Syrup** (supplied as granules for preparation with water before use) containing 125, 250, or 500 mg in each 5 ml (suggested diluent, water). (Also available as Ceporex in *Austral., Belg., Canad., Ital., Neth., S.Afr., Spain, Switz.*).

Keflex *(Lilly, UK)*. Cephalexin, available as **Capsules** containing 250 and 500 mg; as **Suspension** (supplied as granules for preparation with water before use) containing 125 and 250 mg in each 5 ml (suggested diluent, syrup); as **Tablets** containing 250 and 500 mg. (Also available as Keflex in *Austral., Canad., Denm., Jap., Norw., S.Afr., Switz., USA*).

Other Proprietary Names

Arg.—Ceporexin, Keforal, Septilisin; *Aust.*—Cepexin; *Belg.*—Keforal; *Fin.*—Ceporexina; *Fr.*—Céporexine, Keforal; *Ger.*—Ceporexin, Oracef; *Hung.*—Pyassan; *Ital.*—Alfaspoven *(cephalexin sodium)*, Ausocef, Bor-cef, Cefadros, Cefaxin, Ceflor, Cepoven *(cephalexin sodium)*, Chemosporal, Domucef, Farexin, Ibilex, Keforal, Latoral, Lorexina, Sasperos; *Jap.*—Cephalomax, Cephazal, Cepol, CEX, Cipomin, Derantel, Derantel-D, Garasin, Iwalexin, Larixin, Madlexin, Mepilacin-DS, Ohlexin, Oracocin, Oroxin, Rinesal, Segoramin, Sencephalin, Syncel, Taicelexin, Tokiolexin, Tokiolexin-DS, Xahl; *Neth.*—Keforal; *Norw.*—Ceporexine; *Spain*—Acaxina, Acinipan, Amplicefal, Ampligram *(see also under Cephaloridine)*, Basporin, Bilatox, Bioporina Oral *(see also under Cephaloridine)*, Brisoral, Cefa-Iskia, Cefa-Reder, Cefabiot Oral *(see also under Cephaloridine)*, Cefadina, Cefaleh Ina, Cefalekey, Cefalepir, Cefalescord, Cefalival, Cefalogobens Oral *(see also under Cephaloridine)*, Cefaloticum, Cefaloto, Ceferran, Cefexin, Cefibacter, Cefipan Oral *(see also under Cephaloridine)*, Cilicef Oral *(see also under Cephaloridine)*, Cusisporina Cefalexina *(see also under Cephaloridine)*, Efalexin, Erifalecin, Falecina, Fergon *(see also under Ferrous Gluconate)*, Grafalex, Henina Oral *(see also under Cephaloridine)*, Huberlexina Oral *(see also under Cephaloridine)*, Janocilin, Kefloridina, Kelfison Oral *(see also under Cephaloridine)*, Laquisporin, Lefosporina, Lerporina, Lexibiotico *(see also under Cephaloridine)*, Libesporal, Llenas Biotic Oral *(see also under Cephaloridine)*, Llonexina, Mecilex, Neolexina, Nilexina, Ortisporina, Porinabis, Pracefal, Prindex, Rogeridina *(see also under Cephaloridine)*, Sartosona, Sayra, Septosporina, Sporal, Talinsul Oral *(see also under Cephaloridine)*, Testaxina, Torlasporin, Ultralexin *(cephalexin lysinate)*, Vapocilin; *Swed.*—Ceporexine, Oralexine; *Switz.*—Palitrex.

38-v

Cephaloglycin *(U.S.P.)*. Cefaloglycin. (7*R*)-7-(α-D-Phenylglycylamino)cephalosporanic acid dihydrate; (7*R*)-3-Acetoxymethyl-7-(α-D-phenylglycylamino)-3-cephem-4-carboxylic acid dihydrate.

$C_{18}H_{19}N_3O_6S,2H_2O=441.5$.

CAS — 3577-01-3 (anhydrous); 22202-75-1 (dihydrate).

Pharmacopoeias. In *U.S.*

A white to off-white crystalline powder. It contains not less than 900 µg of cephaloglycin per mg, calculated on the anhydrous basis. Slightly **soluble** in water; practically insoluble in most organic solvents. A 5% suspension in water has a pH of 3 to 5.5. *Store* in airtight containers.

Stability. Cephaloglycin in horse serum lost more than 50% of the initial activity when stored for 30 days at −10° or at 4°.— M. A. Foglesong, *Antimicrob. Ag. Chemother.*, 1977, *11*, 174.

Stability in solution. A study on the degradation of cephaloglycin in aqueous solution.— H. Bundgaard, *Arch. Pharm. Chemi, scient. Edn*, 1976, *4*, 25.

Adverse Effects and Precautions. As for Cephalexin, p.1123, although gastro-intestinal side-effects are generally more severe with cephaloglycin. Diarrhoea occurs in about 5% of patients and it may be severe and persistent enough to cause the treatment to be withdrawn. Nausea and vomiting also occur and abdominal pain, gastro-intestinal bleeding, and severe enterocolitis have occasionally been reported.

Antimicrobial Action. Cephaloglycin is bactericidal and has a spectrum of activity similar to that of cephalexin (p.1123) but is slightly more active against Gram-positive organisms. It is most active against streptococci at pH values below 7, but its maximum activity against *E. coli* occurs at pH 6.5 to 8.

References: C. M. Kunin and D. Brandt, *Am. J. med. Sci.*, 1968, *255*, 196; W. D. Johnson *et al.*, *J. Am. med. Ass.*, 1968, *206*, 2698; W. E. Wick *et al.*, *Appl. Microbiol.*, 1971, *21*, 426.

Absorption and Fate. Cephaloglycin is only partly absorbed from the gastro-intestinal tract and produces low plasma concentrations; peak values of 0.5 to 2 µg per ml are obtained with doses of 0.5 to 1 g. About 25% of a dose is reported to be excreted in the urine by glomerular filtration and tubular secretion, mainly as active desacetylcephaloglycin. Doses of 250 and 500 mg produce over 8 hours mean urine concentrations of 200 and 350 µg per ml respectively. Peak urine concentrations may exceed 1.3 mg per ml after a 500 -mg dose. There is little binding to plasma proteins.

A brief review of cephaloglycin.— C. H. Nightingale *et al.*, *J. pharm. Sci.*, 1975, *64*, 1899.

In subjects with normal renal function, cephaloglycin 0.5 and 1 g by mouth gave mean peak serum concentrations of 0.22 µg per ml at 2 hours and 0.46 µg per ml at 1 hour respectively, and mean urine concentrations ranging from 18 to 255 and 57 to 200 µg per ml respectively after 2 to 4 hours. After anhydrous cephaloglycin 0.5 and 1 g, the mean peak serum concentrations were 0.8 µg per ml at 4 hours and 0.84 µg per ml at 2 hours respectively, and urinary concentrations ranging from 60 to 282, and 58 to 1100 µg per ml respectively after 2 to 4 hours.— R. L. Perkins *et al.*, *Clin. Pharmac. Ther.*, 1969, *10*, 244.

Uses. Cephaloglycin is a cephalosporin antibiotic and has been used in the treatment of infections of the urinary tract due to sensitive organisms. It does not produce sufficiently high serum concentrations to be useful in the treatment of systemic infections. The usual dose is the equivalent of 250 to 500 mg of anhydrous cephaloglycin by mouth four times daily; children have been given 25 to 50 mg per kg body-weight daily in divided doses.

Preparations

Cephaloglycin Capsules *(U.S.P.)*. Capsules containing cephaloglycin equivalent to 250 mg of anhydrous cephaloglycin. Store in airtight containers.

Proprietary Names

Kafocin *(Lilly, USA)*.

39-g

Cephalonium. 87/90; Carbamoylcefaloridine. (7*R*)-3-(4-Carbamoyl-1-pyridiniomethyl)-7-[2-(2-thienyl)acetamido]-3-cephem-4-carboxylate.

$C_{20}H_{18}N_4O_5S_2=458.5$.

CAS — 5575-21-3.

A cephalosporin antibiotic used in veterinary practice.

Manufacturers

Glaxo, UK.

40-f

Cephaloridine *(B.P., Eur. P.)*. Cefaloridine; Cefaloridinum; Ceph. 87/4. (7*R*)-3-(1-Pyridiniomethyl)-7-[2-(2-thienyl)acetamido]-3-cephem-4-carboxylate.

$C_{19}H_{17}N_3O_4S_2=415.5$.

CAS — 50-59-9.

Pharmacopoeias. In *Br., Eur., Fr., Ger., It., Jap.,* and *Neth. U.S.P.* includes Sterile Cephaloridine.

A white or almost white crystalline powder, with a slight odour of pyridine, and a bitter taste. The *B.P.* specifies not less than 95% of cephaloridine calculated on the anhydrous basis; *U.S.P.* specifies not less than 900 µg per mg. The α-form contains not more than 0.5% of water and the δ-form not more than 3%.

Soluble 1 in 5 of water, 1 in 1000 of alcohol; practically insoluble in chloroform, ether, and most other organic solvents. A 10% solution in water has a pH of 4 to 6. A 12.2% solution in water is approximately iso-osmotic with serum. **Store** in a cool dry place in sterile containers sealed to exclude micro-organisms and as far as possible moisture. Protect from light.

Injections of cephaloridine are prepared aseptically and should be used within 24 hours when stored at a temperature not exceeding 20°, or within 4 days when stored at a temperature between 2° and 8°. Refrigerated solutions should be gently warmed before administration to dissolve crystals.

Cephaloridine is unstable in solutions which contain both dextrose and sodium bicarbonate and its addition to solutions below pH 4 or above pH 7.5 is not advised. Cephaloridine is **incompatible** with high molecular weight compounds and alkaline earth metals.

The polymorphism of cephaloridine crystals.— J. H. Chapman *et al.*, *J. pharm. Pharmac.*, 1968, *20*, 418.

Effect of gamma-irradiation. Cephaloridine powder was apparently unaffected by radiation doses of up to 50 000 Gy, indicating that it may be safely irradiated at the commonly employed sterilisation dose of 25 000 Gy.— G. P. Jacobs, *Int. J. appl. Radiat. Isotopes*, 1980, *31*, 91.

Incompatibility. Cephaloridine was incompatible in solution with *amylobarbitone, benzylpenicillin, calcium chloride, calcium gluceptate, calcium gluconate, chlorpromazine, chlortetracycline, colistin sulphomethate sodium, diphenhydramine, erythromycin gluceptate* and *lactobionate, gentamicin, hydrocortisone,* the *hydroxybenzoates, hydroxyzine, kanamycin, lincomycin, magnesium salts, methylphenidate, oxytetracycline, pentobarbitone, phenobarbitone, phenytoin, polymyxin B, prochlorperazine, protein hydrolysate, tetracycline, thiopentone sodium,* and *vitamin-B complex.*— *Med. Lett.*, 1972, *14* (Jan.), *Suppl.*, 32.

A precipitate was observed when cephaloridine 2 g per litre was added to dextrose injection 5% or sodium chloride injection 0.9% containing *heparin sodium* 20 000 units per litre.— J. Jacobs *et al.*, *J. clin. Path.*, 1973, *26*, 742.

Cephaloridine lost about 11 to 18% of its antimicrobial activity *in vitro* in the presence of a number of vitamins including *thiamine, riboflavine, pyridoxine, nicotinamide, ascorbic acid,* or *aminobenzoic acid.*— M. A. El-Nakeeb *et al., Can, J. pharm. Sci.,* 1976, *11,* 85.

Stability. Cephaloridine in horse serum lost 29% of its initial activity when stored for 30 days at −10°. Its stability was also affected by repeated thawing and freezing. After 30 days at 4° it possessed less than 50% of its initial activity.— M. A. Foglesong, *Antimicrob. Ag. Chemother.,* 1977, *11,* 174.

Stability in solution. There was no loss in activity over a period of 24 hours when cephaloridine was dissolved in calcium gluconate or dextran solution or added to an infusion containing thiopentone sodium. Colistin sulphomethate sodium could be added to infusion fluid containing cephaloridine without loss of activity for a period of 24 hours.— C. L. J. Coles and K. A. Lees (letter), *Pharm. J.,* 1971, *1,* 153.

Cephaloridine 1 g per 100 ml retained 92.5% activity in dextrose injection 5% at 5° after 14 days and 97.1% activity at 25° after 24 hours. In sodium chloride injection 0.9% the comparable figures were 95.4% and 100% respectively.— J. M. Mann *et al., Am. J. Hosp. Pharm.,* 1971, *28,* 760.

Cephaloridine 20 g per 100 ml in aqueous solution retained 96.5% activity for 7 days and 99.5% for 42 days when stored at −20° immediately after reconstitution. Occasional precipitation occurred on thawing when sodium chloride injection 0.9% or dextrose injection 5% was used as solvent.— J. C. Boylan *et al., Am. J. Hosp. Pharm.,* 1972, *29,* 687.

Solutions of cephaloridine 32 mg per ml were prepared by adding powder for injection to each of 3 commercially available 0.5% hypromellose solutions in plastic squeezy bottles (Lacril, pH 5.9; Tearisol, pH 7.3; Isoptotears, pH 7.4). Cephaloridine was insoluble in Lacril and Isoptotears and had to be dissolved in saline first. The solutions had relative antibiotic potencies of 94% after 3 days and 64% after 7 days when stored at 25°.— E. Osborn *et al., Am. J. Opthal.,* 1976, *82,* 775.

Adverse Effects. Allergic reactions, including pruritus, urticaria, and skin rashes, may occur especially in patients hypersensitive to penicillin. Rarely, there may be mild transient neutropenia, elevated serum aspartate aminotransferase (SGOT) values, and an increased prothrombin time. Neurological disturbances have occurred occasionally. Supra-infection by resistant organisms such as *Candida* and *Pseudomonas* has been reported. The most serious adverse effect is acute and potentially fatal renal failure. This is probably due to proximal tubular necrosis and appears to be dose-related as it occurs more frequently when the total daily dose exceeds 4 to 6 g. Patients with existing renal impairment are at special risk.

Two anephric patients on haemodialysis shed finger-nails and, later, toe-nails after treatment with large doses of cephaloridine (up to 8 g daily) and cloxacillin (up to 10 g daily). None of 34 other patients in the haemodialysis unit had any abnormality of the nails. The 2 affected patients were the only 2 given large doses of the antibiotics.— J. B. Eastwood *et al., Br. J. Derm.,* 1969, *81,* 750.

A report of convulsions in an infant following the intrathecal administration of cephaloridine 50 mg.— H. Yoshioka *et al., Infection,* 1975, *3,* 123.

Allergy. An 18-year-old woman suffered a severe anaphylactic reaction following intravenous administration of 1 g of cephaloridine.— Y. Saleh and E. Tischler, *Med. J. Aust.,* 1974, *2,* 490.

Cephaloridine had been shown to produce a histamine-like reaction as well as an allergic reaction.— G. M. Halpern (letter), *Med. J. Aust.,* 1975, *1,* 366.

See also under Precautions.

Colitis. Fatal pseudomembranous colitis occurred in a woman who had received cephaloridine for 3 days and cephalothin for about 3 further days.— J. Tan *et al., J. Am. med. Ass.,* 1979, *242,* 749.

Nephrotoxicity. For reviews of the nephrotoxicity of cephalosporins, see G. B. Appel and H. C. Neu, *New Engl. J. Med.,* 1977, *296,* 663; M. Barza, *J. infect. Dis.,* 1978, *137, Suppl.* (May), S60; *Lancet,* 1979, *1,* 962.

No laboratory evidence of nephrotoxicity was found in 10 patients given cephaloridine 2 to 4 g daily by intramuscular injection for 8 days to treat urinary-tract infections. Nephrotoxicity was felt to be unlikely if the serum concentration of cephaloridine was kept below 100 μg per ml.— J. F. Winchester and A. C. Kennedy, *Lancet,* 1972, *2,* 514. Of 13 patients with renal failure attributed to cephaloridine, 6 had been given daily doses of 4 g or less.— D. Kleinknecht *et al.* (letter), *Ann intern. Med.,* 1974, *80,* 421.

Common factors in 96 instances of possible cephaloridine nephrotoxicity included a dosage of more than 6 g daily, patients with doubtful or impaired renal function sometimes treated without reduction of dosage, patients usually aged over 50 years, a primary diagnosis of bacterial endocarditis, lung infection or septicaemia, reductions in renal clearance produced by surgical trauma, hypersensitivity reactions to penicillin or cephaloridine, concomitant use of other potentially nephrotoxic antibiotics, and the use of diuretics.— R. D. Foord, *Glaxo, J. antimicrob. Chemother.,* 1975, *1, Suppl.* (Sept.), 119.

Precautions. Patients who are hypersensitive to penicillins may be able to tolerate therapeutic doses of cephaloridine but instances of an immunological cross-reaction to both antibiotics have been reported and sudden, severe, and sometimes fatal reactions have occurred. Patients who are known to be allergic to penicillins should therefore be treated with great care with cephaloridine. Care is also necessary when cephaloridine is given to patients with known histories of allergy.

Since increased prothrombin times have been reported it may be advisable to give cephaloridine with care to patients taking anticoagulants. The concomitant use of diuretics such as frusemide and other nephrotoxic antibiotics such as gentamicin increases the risk of kidney damage.

Cephaloridine should be given with caution and in reduced doses to patients with renal impairment.

Positive results to the direct Coombs' test have been found during treatment with cephaloridine and these can interfere with blood cross-matching. The Coombs' test employs a diagnostic antiglobulin reaction to detect the antibody on the surface of the red blood cell. The direct test uses the patient's own red blood cells.

The urine of patients being treated with cephaloridine may give false positive reactions for glucose with copper-reduction reagents.

The majority of patients with a history of allergy to penicillin appeared not to have reacted to a cephalosporin.— C. H. Dash, *Glaxo, J. antimicrob. Chemother.,* 1975, *1, Suppl.* (Sept.), 107. Allergic reactions have been reported to occur in 2 to 5% of all persons receiving cephalosporins and in 5 to 16% of patients with a history of penicillin allergy (B.E. Murray and R.C. Moellering, *Clin. Ther.,* 1979, *2,* 155). Most authorities consider that it is safer to avoid giving any of the cephalosporins or cephamycins to patients with a history of anaphylaxis or immediate-type hypersensitivity reaction to the penicillins although it is not unreasonable to consider their cautious use when indicated in patients with a history of less severe reactions to the penicillins, such as eosinophilia, morbilliform rash, or drug fever.— R. C. Moellering, *J. Am. med. Ass.,* 1980, *244,* 2562.

A review of immunological cross-reactivity between penicillins and cephalosporins.— L. D. Petz, *J. infect. Dis.,* 1978, *137, Suppl.* (May), S74.

Interactions. When urine of patients treated with cephaloridine was tested for protein with 20% of sulphosalicylic acid, a heavy white precipitate developed if cephaloridine concentrations were 40 mg per ml or more. This precipitate was indistinguishable from that seen in proteinuria due to renal damage and awareness of this false positive reaction was important in the treatment of the patients.— M. Levy and M. Eliakim (letter), *J. Am. med. Ass.,* 1972, *219,* 908.

Concurrent administration of frusemide and cephaloridine in healthy subjects could reduce renal clearance of cephaloridine with consequent increase in plasma concentrations; in some instances cephaloridine-plasma concentrations were doubled.— W. J. Tilstone *et al., Clin. Pharmac. Ther.,* 1977, *22,* 389.

For the effect of other drugs on the antimicrobial activity of cephaloridine, see below under Antimicrobial Action.

Antimicrobial Action. Cephaloridine is bactericidal and acts similarly to the penicillins by inhibiting synthesis of the bacterial cell wall. It is active against a wide range of Gram-positive and Gram-negative organisms. Both penicillinase and non-penicillinase-producing staphylococci are sensitive but cephaloridine is inhibited by the enzyme more than most other cephalosporins; methicillin-resistant *Staphylococcus aureus* is usually resistant to this group of antibiotics. Other susceptible Gram-positive bacteria include streptococci, but not *Streptococcus faecalis, Bacillus anthracis, Clostridium* spp., *Corynebacterium diphtheriae,* and *Listeria monocytogenes.* The cephalosporins are generally not very active against enterococci. Among the Gram-negative organisms, it is active against *Neisseria, Salmonella,* and *Shigella* spp., *Bordetella pertussis, Klebsiella pneumoniae, Proteus mirabilis,* and some strains of *Escherichia coli* and *Haemophilus influenzae.* Cephaloridine is inactive against *Bacteroides fragilis, Enterobacter aerogenes, Pseudomonas* spp., mycobacteria, mycoplasmas, and fungi.

The minimum inhibitory concentrations of cephaloridine for susceptible Gram-positive organisms range from about 0.01 to 1 μg per ml; for most susceptible Gram-negative organisms concentrations of at least 1 μg per ml are required for inhibition.

For a brief discussion on the cephalosporin group of antibiotics, see p.1083.

A discussion of the antibacterial activity of cephalosporins *in vitro.*— J. A. Washington, *Mayo Clin. Proc.,* 1976, *51,* 237.

The Quality-control Committee of the Public Health Laboratory Service recommended that disk diffusion methods should not be employed for the sensitivity testing of *Staph. aureus* to the cephalosporins since they produced misleading results.— R. Blowers *et al.* (letter), *Br. med. J.,* 1973, *3,* 46.

Cephamandole was the most active of 8 cephalosporins *in vitro* against 100 isolates of *H. influenzae* and had an MIC of 0.78 μg or less per ml against 97; the order of decreasing activity of the other cephalosporins was cefapirin, cephalothin, cefoxitin, cephaloridine, cephazolin, cephradine, and cephalexin. The most active cephalosporins against 100 strains of *Str. pneumoniae* were, in order, cephaloridine, cefapirin, cephamandole, cephazolin, and cephalothin and all inhibited 90 strains at a concentration of 0.19 μg per ml; cefoxitin, cephradine, and cephalexin were less active and required 3.12 μg per ml for similar inhibition.— E. Yourassowsky *et al., J. antimicrob. Chemother.,* 1976, *2,* 55. For earlier reports of the activity of cephaloridine and other cephalosporins against *H. influenzae,* see J. D. Williams and J. Andrews, *Br. med. J.,* 1974, *1,* 134; S. Eykyn and I. Phillips (letter), *ibid.,* 1974, *2,* 59.

Cephazolin and then cephaloridine underwent the greatest inactivation by beta-lactamase-producing *Staph. aureus* in a study of 8 cephalosporins. Some inactivation occurred in decreasing order of severity in cephalexin, cephradine, cefapirin, and cephamandole. Cephalothin and cefoxitin appeared to be resistant to inactivation. It was considered that cephalothin was generally the best cephalosporin to use in severe staphylococcal infections.— I. W. Fong *et al., Antimicrob. Ag. Chemother.,* 1976, *9,* 939. In a study *in vitro* of the susceptibility of *Staph. aureus* and *Staph. epidermidis* to 65 antimicrobial agents with antistaphylococcal activity, rifampicin was the most active overall. Amongst 12 cephalosporins, cephaloridine and nitrocefin sodium [$C_{21}H_{15}N_4NaO_8S_2$=538.5] were the most active with cephaloglycin, cephradine, cephalexin, and cefoxitin being the least active.— L. D. Sabath *et al., Antimicrob. Ag. Chemother.,* 1976, *9,* 962. The activity of 19 cephalosporin antibiotics was measured *in vitro* against 105 isolates of *Staph. aureus* and *Staph. epidermidis.* Most of the antibiotics showed an inoculum effect against some of the strains but this was greatest with cephaloridine or nitrocefin. Of those drugs normally given intravenously, cefapirin, cephalothin, or cefazaflur were generally most active against 66 strains of methicillin-susceptible staphylococci and overall cephalosporins given parenterally were more active than those given by mouth except for cefaclor. The activity of both types of cephalosporin was generally poor against 39 methicillin-resistant strains.— M. Laverdiere *et al., Antimicrob. Ag. Chemother.,* 1978, *13,* 669.

Cephaloridine was the most active of 5 parenteral cephalosporins *in vitro* against 43 lactobacilli with cephazolin and cephamandole being next most active.— A. S. Bayer *et al., Antimicrob. Ag. Chemother.,* 1979, *16,* 112.

Diminished activity. Antagonism occurred against some strains of *Staph. aureus* when the activity of cephaloridine was tested *in vitro* with actinomycin D or mithramycin.— J. Y. Jacobs *et al., Antimicrob. Ag. Chemother.*, 1979, *15*, 580.

Enhanced activity. Synergism usually occurred against strains of *Staph. aureus* when cephaloridine was tested *in vitro* with mitomycin.— J. Y. Jacobs *et al., Antimicrob. Ag. Chemother.*, 1979, *15*, 580.

Resistance. Gram-positive cocci have not been shown to develop resistance readily to cephaloridine. There is some cross-resistance between cephaloridine and the penicillins. Cephaloridine may be inactivated by penicillinase. It is also inactivated by beta-lactamases (cephalosporinases) produced by certain Gram-negative organisms. Cloxacillin or methicillin may inhibit the action of the enzyme on cephaloridine.

Cephaloridine was less resistant to staphylococcal penicillinase than cephazolin, cephalothin, and cephalexin. Cephalexin was most resistant. Cephaloridine was not considered suitable for staphylococcal infections.— R. W. Lacey and A. Stokes, *J. clin. Path.*, 1977, *30*, 35.

Whereas beta-lactamase production was a major factor in the resistance of *Ps. aeruginosa* to benzylpenicillin, ampicillin, or cephaloridine, a permeability barrier was mainly responsible for the organism's resistance to methicillin, cephalothin, cephazolin, or cephalexin.— H. Ohmori *et al., Antimicrob. Ag. Chemother.*, 1977, *12*, 537.

Absorption and Fate. Cephaloridine is poorly absorbed from the gastro-intestinal tract and must be given by injection. It is widely distributed in body tissues and fluids except the brain and cerebrospinal fluid although it diffuses into the CSF when the meninges are inflamed. Cephaloridine diffuses across the placenta into the foetal circulation and it is excreted in the milk of nursing mothers. Only about 20% of a dose is bound to plasma proteins. The biological half-life of cephaloridine has been reported to be about 1 to 1.5 hours.

Peak plasma concentrations of 15 to 20 µg per ml are achieved ½ to 1 hour after the intramuscular injection of 500 mg and 30 to 35 µg per ml after a 1-g dose; detectable amounts are reported to be present at least 8 hours after a dose.

Cephaloridine is rapidly excreted unchanged in urine mainly by glomerular filtration and about 80% is eliminated within 24 hours. High urine concentrations of 0.4 to 1 mg per ml have been reported following normal dosage. A small amount is excreted in bile.

A review of the pharmacokinetics and uses of the cephalosporins.— C. H. Nightingale *et al., J. pharm. Sci.*, 1975, *64*, 1899.

Cephaloridine was bound to a negligible extent to serum proteins. The half-life in serum was 1.5 hours and 70% was excreted in urine.— C. M. Kunin, *Ann. intern. Med.*, 1967, *67*, 151.

Variations in urine-cephaloridine concentrations were found between 4 of 17 early-stream, midstream and terminal-stream urine samples from 8 subjects. It was suggested that the urine in the bladder was not homogeneous.— D. S. Reeves *et al., Lancet*, 1974, *1*, 1258. Significantly greater urine concentrations of cephaloridine were achieved following the administration of doses of 500 mg in 2 ml of sodium chloride injection into the anterolateral aspect of the thigh than into the upper outer quadrant of the buttock in a study of 10 subjects. There was no significant difference in serum concentrations.— *idem*, *2*, 1421.

Cephaloridine 1 g was given as an intravenous bolus injection in 20 ml of sodium chloride injection to 10 healthy subjects after anaesthetic induction for surgery. Mean serum concentrations of cephaloridine fell rapidly reaching about one-quarter the initial concentration after 2 hours and then more slowly over the following 4 hours. The ultimate mean half-life of cephaloridine was about 123 minutes.— D. D. Mathews, *J. antimicrob. Chemother.*, 1975, *1*, *Suppl.* (Sept.), 37.

Findings of a study *in vitro* suggested that for cephalosporin antibiotics, a longer half-life might be more useful than obtaining initial higher peak serum concentrations.— S. Grasso *et al., Antimicrob. Ag. Chemother.*, 1978, *13*, 570.

An investigation of the renal excretion of cephaloridine suggested that active tubular reabsorption of the drug occurs as well as tubular secretion.— A. Arvidsson *et al., Clin. Pharmac. Ther.*, 1979, *25*, 870.

Further references: J. W. Kislak *et al., Am. J. med. Sci.*, 1966, *251*, 433; P. De Schepper *et al., J. clin. Pharmac.*, 1973, *13*, 83; A. G. Paradelis *et al., Arzneimittel-Forsch.*, 1977, *27*, 2167.

Diffusion. Cephaloridine 2 g, given intravenously when the meninges were not inflamed, produced concentrations in most specimens of brain tissue sufficient to inhibit sensitive Gram-positive cocci.— P. W. Kramer *et al., J. Neurosurg.*, 1969, *31*, 295.

High concentrations of cephaloridine, lasting at least 8 hours, were found, after a 1 g intravenous dose, in the secondary aqueous humour of patients in whom the primary humour of the anterior eye had been aspirated.— R. E. Records, *Archs Ophthal., N.Y.*, 1969, *81*, 331.

After an intramuscular injection of 30 mg per kg body-weight therapeutic concentrations of cephaloridine were found in the aqueous humour.— A. B. Richards *et al., Br. J. Ophthal.*, 1972, *56*, 531.

In 21 patients, given a single intramuscular injection of cephaloridine 1 g prior to surgery for retinal detachment, the serum concentrations varied from 8.9 to 23.8 µg per ml and the subretinal fluid concentrations varied from 0.7 to 3.7 µg per ml, after 1.25 to 2.5 hours.— A. H. Chignell, *Br. J. Ophthal.*, 1973, *57*, 421.

Cephaloridine 100 mg per kg body-weight daily was given intravenously for 14 to 21 days to 8 children with osteomyelitis. Concentrations in pus of up to 12.3 µg per ml and in bone of up to 6.6 µg per g were achieved. Mean values generally exceeded the minimum bactericidal concentration for *Staphylococcus aureus*. Two children treated intramuscularly also achieved concentrations in pus and bone.— T. R. Tetzlaff *et al., J. Pediat.*, 1978, *92*, 135.

Further references: W. Barr and R. M. Graham, *J. Obstet. Gynaec. Br. Commonw.*, 1967, *74*, 739 (transplacental diffusion); G. Acocella *et al., Gut*, 1968, *9*, 536 (bile).

Uses. Cephaloridine is a cephalosporin antibiotic. It may be used in the treatment of infections of the respiratory and urinary tracts and other infections due to susceptible organisms including those caused by penicillin-resistant staphylococci. Nephrotoxicity limits its use. Its activity may be reduced by high concentrations of penicillinase; it is inactivated by cephalosporinase.

A usual dose is 0.5 to 1 g two or three times daily by intramuscular injection. It can also be given intravenously. Children may be given 20 to 40 mg per kg body-weight daily in divided doses. Larger doses are indicated in severe infections and in those due to Gram-negative micro-organisms; a daily dosage of 6 g for adults and 4 g for children should not normally be exceeded. A maximum daily dose of 4 g is recommended for patients over the age of 50 years and in any patient who has undergone surgery within 48 hours.

In pneumococcal meningitis, high total daily doses of 70 to 100 mg per kg have been supplemented by the intrathecal administration of up to 50 mg in 2 to 10 ml of sodium chloride injection or the patient's cerebrospinal fluid each day. A suggested daily intrathecal dose for children is 500 µg per kg; total daily doses of up to 12.5 mg in infants and 25 mg in children have also been recommended. The use of larger doses can cause meningism.

Cephaloridine should preferably not be given to patients with impaired renal function because of its nephrotoxicity. If administration is essential smaller doses should be employed; with creatinine clearances of less than 10 ml per minute the daily dose should not exceed 500 mg and with clearances of 10 to 20 and 20 to 40 ml per minute the daily dose should not exceed 1 and 2 g respectively.

In the treatment of corneal infections systemic treatment may be supplemented by the subconjunctival injection of cephaloridine 50 to 100 mg.

For reviews and clinical evaluations of cephaloridine and the other cephalosporins, see *J. antimicrob. Chemother.*, 1975, *1*, *Suppl.* (Sept.), 1-139; R. C. Moellering and M. N. Swartz, *New Engl. J. Med.*, 1976, *294*, 24; *Med. Lett.*, 1976, *18*, 33; *J. Am. med. Ass.*, 1977, *237*, 1243; M. Barza and P. V. W. Miao, *Am. J. Hosp. Pharm.*, 1977, *34*, 621; R. L. Thompson, *Mayo Clin. Proc.*, 1977, *52*, 625; *Lancet*, 1978, *1*, 863; J. D. Williams, *J. antimicrob. Chemother.*, 1978, *4*, 109; R. Wise, *Br. med. J.*, 1978, *2*, 40; S. Selwyn (letter), *ibid.*, 277; R. W. Lacey (letter), *ibid.*; R. C. Moellering, *J. infect. Dis.*, 1978, *137*, *Suppl.* (May), S2; R. G. Petersdorf and H. Featherstone, *Am. Rev. resp. Dis.*, 1978, *117*, 1; B. E. Murray and R. C. Moellering, *Clin. Ther.*, 1979, *2*, 155; C. H. O'Callaghan, *J. antimicrob. Chemother.*, 1979, *5*, 635; S. Selwyn (letter), *ibid.*, 1980, *6*, 401; A. J. Weinstein, *Drugs*, 1980, *20*, 137.

For a report of the successful use of cephaloridine with chloramphenicol in the treatment of infections due to highly resistant strains of Enterobacteriaceae, see Chloramphenicol, p.1139.

Bronchitis. Reports of the use of cephaloridine in the treatment of bronchitis.— A. Pines *et al., Br. J. Dis. Chest*, 1967, *61*, 101; K. M. Citron *et al., Lancet*, 1968, *2*, 592; A. Pines *et al., Br. J. Dis. Chest*, 1971, *65*, 91.

Dosage in infants and children. The suggested dose of cephaloridine for infants of more than 37 weeks' gestation was 15 mg per kg body-weight given intramuscularly every 12 hours in the first 48 hours of life, otherwise every 8 hours. For immature infants (those of less than 37 weeks' gestation) 15 mg per kg could be given every 12 hours for the first week of life and every 8 hours thereafter.— P. A. Davies, *Br. J. Hosp. Med.*, 1972, *8*, 13.

Dosage in renal failure. Reviews of the use of cephaloridine in patients with impaired renal function: L. D. Bechtol, *Curr. ther. Res.*, 1972, *14*, 790; L. Giusti, *Drug Intell. & clin. Pharm.*, 1973, *7*, 252.

In patients with oliguria, intervals between doses of cephaloridine should be increased to every 24 hours.— C. M. Kunin, *Ann. intern. Med.*, 1967, *67*, 151.

The dosage interval of cephaloridine should be increased from 6 hours in normal patients to 12 hours in those with mild renal failure; it should be avoided in moderate and severe renal failure. Blood-cephaloridine concentrations could be altered by haemodialysis and peritoneal dialysis.— P. Sharpstone, *Br. med. J.*, 1977, *2*, 36.

Data for predicting removal of cephaloridine by conventional haemodialysis.— T. P. Gibson and H. A. Nelson, *Clin. Pharmacokinet.*, 1977, *2*, 403.

Meningitis. High systemic doses of cephaloridine failed to arrest clinical deterioration or to eliminate the micro-organism in 3 infants with *Haemophilus influenzae* meningitis, despite the achievement of inhibitory serum and cerebrospinal fluid concentrations.— S. H. Walker and C. C. Collins, *Am. J. Dis. Child.*, 1968, *116*, 285.

In a review of 106 patients with meningitis reported to have been treated with cephaloridine or cephalothin it was considered that the antibiotics were unreliable without additional intrathecal medication.— L. S. Fisher *et al., Ann. intern. Med.*, 1975, *82*, 689. See also S. A. Kabins (letter), *ibid.*, *83*, 428.

Surgical infection prophylaxis. After cephaloridine was administered parenterally in 3 doses to patients with 376 surgical wounds, 34 (9.1%) became infected compared with 57 (14.7%) of 386 wounds in patients not receiving cephaloridine.— C. Evans and A. V. Pollock, *Br. J. Surg.*, 1973, *60*, 434. An analysis of results obtained in a number of studies.— A. V. Pollock and M. Evans, *Br. med. J.*, 1977, *1*, 20. See also *idem*, *2*, 124.

There were fewer postoperative pelvic infections and there was less postoperative morbidity in 50 women given cephaloridine 3 g on the day of vaginal hysterectomy than in 50 similar women given placebo.— W. J. Ledger *et al., Am. J. Obstet. Gynec.*, 1973, *115*, 766.

In a study involving 246 patients who underwent appendicectomy, cephaloridine 1 g given by intramuscular injection pre-operatively and thereafter every 6 hours for 3 days (a 500-mg dose was used in children under 11 years), significantly reduced the overall incidence of wound infection as did extraperitoneal wound drainage. When both procedures were used the infection-rate was further reduced.— N. W. Everson *et al., Br. J. Surg.*, 1977, *64*, 236. See also L. E. Ivarsson, *Acta chir. scand.*, 1977, *143*, 469; P. D. Foster and R. D. O'Toole, *J. Am. med. Ass.*, 1978, *239*, 1411.

Two cases of deep infection developed within 6 months after 146 operations for total hip replacement when the patients were given cephaloridine prophylactically, and 2 after 157 operations in patients given flucloxacillin. The low incidence was comparable with that achieved in ultra-clean-air environments. The regimens were: cephaloridine 1 g intraveneously on induction of anaesthesia followed by 1 g intramuscularly 6 and 12 hours later; flucloxacillin 500 mg intramuscularly one hour before surgery then 4 times daily for 14 days, intramuscularly for one day then by mouth. The simplicity of the cephaloridine regimen was an advantage.— J. P. Pollard *et al., Br. med. J.*, 1979, *1*, 707. See also S. P. F. Hughes *et al., J. antimicrob. Chemother.*, 1975, *1*,

Suppl. (Sept.), 41; G. Wewalka and M. Endler, *Arzneimittel-Forsch.*, 1978, *28*, 72.

Local use of cephaloridine. In a group of 401 patients undergoing surgery a topical solution of cephaloridine 1 g in 2 ml was applied to the wounds of 188 patients, the rest acting as controls. The rate of infection of clean wounds was not significantly different in the 2 groups but infection of contaminated wounds was reduced from 38.7% in the controls to 12.8% in the treated patients. However in infected wounds of treated patients the percentage of organisms resistant was double that of infected controls.— C. Evans *et al.*, *Br. J. Surg.*, 1974, *61*, 133.

Cephaloridine was applied topically to over 1200 patients over a period of 4 years for the prophylaxis of wound sepsis. In 1971 the resistance-rate for cephaloridine was 20.4% and in 1974 it was 20.5%.— A. V. Pollock and M. Evans (letter), *Br. med. J.*, 1975, *3*, 436.

Cephaloridine 1 g in 2 ml by intra-incisional instillation was significantly more effective in preventing wound infection than Polybactrin sprayed into the wound at laparotomy. Of 148 laparotomy patients given cephaloridine, 16 developed wound infection compared with 33 of 152 given Polybactrin. The difference was more pronounced in primary rather than secondary wound infection.— N. Menzies-Gow *et al.* (letter), *Lancet*, 1977, *2*, 196. Criticism. Cephaloridine was considered unsuitable for use in laparotomies because of the resistance of *Bacteroides* spp., probably the main pathogenic hazard in colorectal surgery, and the variability in the sensitivity of coliforms.— R. B. Galland *et al.* (letter), *ibid.*, 304.

Further reports of the instillation of cephaloridine into surgical wounds: I. L. Rosenberg and A. V. Pollock (letter), *Br. med. J.*, 1974, *2*, 558 (compared with gentamicin); A. V. Pollock and M. Evans, *J. antimicrob. Chemother.*, 1975, *1*, *Suppl.* (Sept.), 71 (compared with framycetin); A. V. Pollock *et al.*, *Br. J. Surg.*, 1977, *64*, 322 (compared with ampicillin).

Syphilis. Twenty-three patients with early syphilis were treated successfully with cephaloridine 500 mg intramuscularly each day for 10 days, excluding Saturday and Sunday. None of the 5 patients known to be hypersensitive to penicillin suffered any side-effects. A further 15 patients were treated, with apparent success, but were not available for follow-up.— J. M. Glicksman *et al.*, *Archs intern. Med.*, 1968, *121*, 342.

Preparations

Cephaloridine Injection *(B.P.)*. A sterile solution in Water for Injections, prepared by dissolving the sterile contents of a sealed container (Cephaloridine for Injection) in the requisite amount of Water for Injections. pH 4 to 6. Store at a temperature not exceeding 20° and use within 24 hours, or at 2° to 8° and use within 4 days.

Ceporin *(Glaxo, UK)*. Cephaloridine, available as powder for preparing injections, in vials of 250 mg, 500 mg, and 1 g as the δ form. (Also available as Ceporin in *Ital.*, *Switz.*).

Other Proprietary Names

Arg.—Ceflorin; *Aust.*—Glaxoridin; *Austral.*—Ceporan, Loridine; *Belg.*—Cepalorin, Keflodin; *Canad.*—Ceporan; *Denm.*—Ceporan; *Fr.*—Céporine, Keflodin; *Ger.*—Cepaloridin; *Ital.*—Dinasint, Faredina, Keflodin, Latorex, Lauridin, Sasperin, Sintoridyn; *Jap.*—CER; *Neth.*—Cepalorin, Keflodin; *Norw.*—Keflodin; *S.Afr.*—Ceporan; *Spain*—Acaporina, Aliporina, Amplicerina, Ampligram Inyec. *(see* also under Cephalexin*)*, Bioporina *(see* also under Cephalexin*)*, Cefabena, Cefabiot inyectable *(see* also under Cephalexin*)*, Cefalisan, Cefalobiotic, Cefalogobens Inyectable *(see* also under Cephalexin*)*, Cefalomiso, Cefamusel, Cefaresan, Cefipan *(see* also under Cephalexin*)*, Ceporan, Cilicef Inyec. *(see* also under Cephalexin*)*, Cilifor, Cobalcina, Cusisporina Inyec. *(see* also under Cephalexin*)*, Eldia, Endosporol, Enebiotico, Filoklin, Gencefal, Henina Inyectable *(see* also under Cephalexin*)*, Huberlexina Inyectable *(see* also under Cephalexin*)*, Intrasporin, Janosina, Keflodin, Kelfison Inyec. *(see* also under Cephalexin*)*, Lexibiotico Inyec. *(see* also under Cephalexin*)*, Libesporina, Liexina, Llenas Biotic Inyec. *(see* also under Cephalexin*)*, Lloncefal, Poricefal, Prinderin, Rogeridina Inyec. *(see* also under Cephalexin*)*, Sporanicum, Talinsul Inyec. *(see* also under Cephalexin*)*, Tapiola, Testadina, Totalmicina; *Swed.*—Ceporan; *USA*—Loridine.

41-d

Cephalothin Sodium *(B.P., U.S.P.)*. Sodium Cephalothin; Cefalotin Sodium. Sodium (7*R*)-7-[2-(2-thienyl)acetamido)cephalosporanate; Sodium (7*R*)-3-acetoxymethyl-7-[2-(2-thienyl)acetamido]-3-cephem-4-carboxylate. $C_{16}H_{15}N_2NaO_6S_2$=418.4.

CAS — 153-61-7 (cephalothin); 58-71-9 (sodium salt).

Pharmacopoeias. In *Br.*, *Braz.*, *Jap.*, and *U.S.*

A white to off-white, almost odourless, crystalline powder with a bitter taste. Each g represents 2.39 mmol (2.39 mEq) of sodium. Cephalothin sodium 1.06 g is approximately equivalent to 1 g of cephalothin.

Soluble 1 in 3.5 of water and 1 in 700 of alcohol; practically insoluble in chloroform, ether, and most other organic solvents. A 10% solution in water has a pH of 4.5 to 7. A sterile mixture of cephalothin sodium and sodium bicarbonate produces a solution with a pH of 6 to 8.5 when reconstituted with Water for Injections. **Store** at a temperature not exceeding 25° in airtight containers. If it is intended for parenteral administration, the containers should be sterile and sealed to exclude micro-organisms. Protect from light.

Injections of cephalothin sodium should be used within 6 hours when stored at room temperature, or within 48 hours when stored at a temperature between 2° and 10°. Refrigerated solutions should be gently warmed before administration to dissolve any crystals. Discoloration occurs on storage of concentrated solutions.

Incompatible with amikacin sulphate, aminophylline, soluble barbiturates, calcium chloride, calcium gluceptate, calcium gluconate, chlortetracycline hydrochloride, colistin sulphomethate sodium, diphenhydramine hydrochloride, erythromycin gluceptate, erythromycin lactobionate, gentamicin sulphate, kanamycin sulphate, neomycin sulphate, oxytetracycline hydrochloride, polymyxin B sulphate, sulphafurazole diethanolamine, tetracycline hydrochloride, and tobramycin sulphate. Occasional incompatibilities have occurred with benzylpenicillin, hydrocortisone sodium succinate, methylprednisolone sodium succinate, methicillin sodium, phenytoin sodium, prochlorperazine, and vitamins of the B group with vitamin C.

Effect of gamma-irradiation. The potency of cephalothin sodium powder was reduced by 3.1% after a radiation dose of 50 000 Gy and by 2.1% after 25 000 Gy (the commonly employed sterilisation dose). Radiolysis was negligible when the dose was reduced to 10 000 Gy.— G. P. Jacobs, *Int. J. appl. Radiat. Isotopes*, 1980, *31*, 91.

Incompatibility. In addition to the drugs mentioned above, cephalothin was incompatible in solution with *chlorpromazine, hydroxyzine, lincomycin, magnesium salts, methylphenidate*, and *protein hydrolysate*.— *Med. Lett.*, 1972, *14* (Jan.), *Suppl.*, 32.

Cephalothin was incompatible with *antihistamines, canrenoate potassium, lignocaine, metaraminol tartrate, noradrenaline acid tartrate*, and *suxamethonium* in an infusion fluid.— B. Flouvat and P. Lechat, *Thérapie*, 1974, *29*, 337.

Further references: J. A. Patel and G. L. Phillips, *Am. J. Hosp. Pharm.*, 1966, *23*, 409; J. M. Meisler and M. W. Skolaut, *ibid.*, 557; M. Edward, *ibid.*, 1967, *24*, 440; E. A. Parker, *ibid.*, 1970, *27*, 492.

Stability. There was a mean loss in activity of about 36% when cephalothin was incubated for 5 hours in human serum at 37° in the presence of air. Cephazolin lost about 4% activity under the same conditions.— D. Pitkin *et al.*, *Antimicrob. Ag. Chemother.*, 1977, *12*, 284. See also M. A. Foglesong, *ibid.*, *11*, 174.

Stability in solution. Cephalothin sodium was stable in dextrose injection 5% in the pH range 3.6 to 7.6 for 6 hours but a significant loss in activity occurred after 24 hours.— E. A. Parker, *Am. J. Hosp. Pharm.*, 1970, *27*, 492.

Cephalothin sodium 1 g per 100 ml retained 90.6% activity in dextrose injection 5% at 5° after 14 days, and 89.6% at 25° after 24 hours. In sodium chloride injection 0.9%, the comparable figures were 89.4% and 90.1% activity respectively.— J. M. Mann *et al.*, *Am. J. Hosp. Pharm.*, 1971, *28*, 760.

Cephalothin sodium 23 g per 100 ml and 10 g per 100 ml in aqueous solution retained 98.6% and 96% activity respectively for 42 days when stored at −20° immediately after reconstitution. Occasional precipitation occurred on thawing when sodium chloride injection 0.9% or dextrose injection 5% was used as solvent.— J. C. Boylan *et al.*, *Am. J. Hosp. Pharm.*, 1972, *29*, 687.

Solutions of cephalothin 65 mg per ml were prepared by adding powder for injection to each of 3 commercially available 0.5% hypromellose solutions in plastic squeezy bottles (Lacril, pH 5.9; Tearisol, pH 7.3; Isoptotears, pH 7.4). The solutions had relative antibiotic potencies of 89% after 3 days and 75% after 7 days when stored at 25°.— E. Osborn *et al.*, *Am. J. Ophthal.*, 1976, *82*, 775.

Units. One unit of cephalothin is contained in 0.0010661 mg of the first International Reference Preparation (1965) of cephalothin sodium which contains 938 units per mg.

Adverse Effects. Cephalothin has side-effects similar to those of cephaloridine (p.1126) except that there is reported to be less risk of nephrotoxicity with cephalothin and that there is greater pain following the intramuscular injection of cephalothin. Thrombophlebitis has occurred usually after infusion for at least 3 days of more than 6 g daily.

Other effects include urticaria, skin reactions, eosinophilia, neutropenia, and an auto-immune type of haemolytic anaemia. Thrombocytopenia and elevated serum aspartate aminotransferase (SGOT) values have been reported.

A 59-year-old man received cephalothin sodium 500 mg intramuscularly every 6 hours following aortic valve replacement. Shortly afterwards he developed tachycardia with haemolysis and hyperpyrexia. When cephalothin waa discontinued his condition improved rapidly.— G. M. Lemole *et al.*, *J. Am. med. Ass.*, 1972, *221*, 593.

Two patients with myelogenous leukaemia and fever developed supraventricular tachycardia during the slow intravenous infusion of cephalothin sodium.— R. A. Kaslow (letter), *J. Am. med. Ass.*, 1972, *222*, 833.

Meningitis which developed in 5 patients who were receiving cephalothin was considered to be a hazard in patients with bacteraemia who were being treated with antibiotics which were not easily absorbed into the cerebrospinal fluid.— R. J. Mangi *et al.*, *Ann. intern. Med.*, 1973, *78*, 347. Comment.— *Br. med. J.*, 1973, *3*, 366; W. I. H. Shedden, *Lilly* (letter), *ibid.*, 638.

Allergy. Of 54 patients who received cephalothin, 7 had an allergic reaction; 2 had anaphylaxis, 2 urticaria, and 3 maculopapular rashes. Five of these 7 patients had a history of penicillin allergy and 6 of the 11 patients with a history of penicillin allergy had a positive skin test with penicilloyl-polylysine. Allergic reactions to cephalothin appeared to occur more frequently in Negro women than in Negro men or white persons.— R. Thoburn *et al.*, *J. Am. med. Ass.*, 1966, *198*, 345.

In a study of 174 patients who were given intravenous injections of benzylpenicillin or cephalothin sodium, cross-allergy between the antibiotics was demonstrated. Patients who had received no cephalothin developed anticephalothin antibodies after treatment with penicillin and the titres of antipenicillin antibodies were increased by treatment with cephalothin.— G. N. Abraham *et al.*, *Clin. exp. Immun.*, 1968, *3*, 343.

An illness resembling serum sickness without consistent oedema and neurological abnormalities occurred in 30 subjects receiving intravenous doses of cephalothin and cefapirin 2 g four times daily. Symptoms, first noted in 4 patients on the 11th day of administration and in all by the 28th day, disappeared within a few days of stopping the antibiotic and were considered to be due to a hypersensitivity reaction either to the cephalosporin or a degradation product. The high incidence might have been due to the rapid rate of infusion or the high doses.— W. E. Sanders *et al.*, *New Engl. J. Med.*, 1974, *290*, 424.

A report of 2 cases in which administration of cephalothin sodium during surgery resulted in anaphylaxis and death. One patient had a history of allergy to penicillin.— F. G. Spruill *et al.*, *J. Am. med. Ass.*, 1974, *229*, 440.

The Boston Collaborative Drugs Surveillance Program monitored consecutively 32 812 medical inpatients. Drug-induced anaphylaxis occurred in 1 of 1273 patients given cephalothin sodium.— J. Porter and H. Jick, *Lancet*, 1977, *1*, 587.

Antibodies to cephalothin were present in the serum of 2 patients who had received whole blood from donor blood which was found to have plasma-cephalothin antibodies. One of the patients experienced a mild allergic reaction when treated with cephalothin.— D. R. Branch and H. Gifford, *J. Am. med. Ass.*, 1979, *241*, 495.

Blood disorders. Thrombocytopenia occurred in 2 patients treated with cephalothin; it might be due to a specific anticephalothin antibody.— H. R. Gralnick *et al.*, *Ann. intern. Med.*, 1972, *77*, 401.

Red-cell aplasia in a 67-year-old man was considered to be due to cephalothin.— D. MacCulloch *et al.* (letter), *Br. med. J.*, 1974, *4*, 163.

In 1974 the incidence of cephalothin-induced granulocytopenia in one hospital was 4 of about 3800 patients who had received the drug. There were 2 further instances of granulocytopenia in the first half of 1975.— M. -A. DiCato and L. Ellman (letter), *Ann. intern. Med.*, 1975, *83*, 671.

A report of 4 cases of agranulocytosis occurring during treatment with cephalothin.— P. Galanaud *et al.*, *Ann. Méd. interne*, 1976, *127*, 579.

Haemolytic anaemia. Of 25 penicillin-sensitive patients, 13 developed haemolytic anaemia when treated with cephalothin sodium. Severe allergic reactions also occurred. Of 118 students who had been exposed to penicillin but not to cephalothin sodium, 43 had antibodies which reacted with cephalothin-coated cells.— *J. Am. med. Ass.*, 1968, *206*, 1701. Two patients developed haemolytic anaemia after treatment with cephalothin sodium. Erythrocytes from both patients were positive in the direct Coombs' test and the patients had antibodies which reacted with cephalothin-coated cells.— H. R. Gralnick *et al.*, *ibid.*, 1971, *217*, 1193. A further case.— R. N. Rubin and E. R. Burka (letter), *Ann. intern. Med.*, 1977, *86*, 64.

Colitis. An 83-year-old man developed pseudomembranous colitis after receiving courses of cephalexin, cephalothin sodium, and cephazolin sodium.— J. F. Tures *et al.*, *J. Am. med. Ass.*, 1976, *236*, 948. Further reports.— D. F. Hutcheon *et al.*, *Am. J. dig. Dis.*, 1978, *23*, 321; J. Tan *et al.*, *J. Am. med. Ass.*, 1979, *242*, 749; J. G. Bartlett *et al.*, *ibid.*, 2683; S. T. Donta *et al.*, *Archs intern. Med.*, 1980, *140*, 574.

The intraperitoneal administration of cephalothin appeared to be the cause of diarrhoea, mediated by *Clostridium difficile* toxin, in a 62-year-old man. He was treated successfully with vancomycin.— D. L. Coleman *et al.* (letter), *Lancet*, 1981, *1*, 1004.

Nephrotoxicity. Acute renal failure occurred in 5 patients during cephalothin sodium therapy. Rash occurred in 2 patients and eosinophilia in 2. Renal function deteriorated 3 to 10 days after cephalothin therapy was begun and spontaneously improved within 1 to 11 days after it was withdrawn.— J. R. Burton *et al.*, *J. Am. med. Ass.*, 1974, *229*, 679. See also S. Müller *et al.*, *Schweiz. med. Wschr.*, 1973, *103*, 889.

Common factors in 63 instances of possible cephalothin nephrotoxicity included a dosage of more than 12 g daily, patients with doubtful or impaired renal function sometimes treated without reduction of dosage, patients usually aged over 50 years, a primary diagnosis of bacterial endocarditis, lung infection, or septicaemia, reductions in renal clearance produced by surgical trauma, hypersensitivity reactions to penicillin or cephalothin, concomitant use of other potentially nephrotoxic antibiotics or of diuretics.— R. D. Foord, *Glaxo*, *J. antimicrob. Chemother.*, 1975, *1*, *Suppl.* (Sept.), 119.

For reports of nephrotoxicity in patients given colistin sulphomethate and cephalothin concomitantly, see Colistin Sulphomethate Sodium, p.1150.

With aminoglycosides. Review of data from the Boston Collaborative Drug Surveillance Program revealed no enhanced renal toxicity arising from the use of gentamicin with cephalothin. Increases in blood urea nitrogen values were found in 22 of 334 patients given gentamicin, 10 of 492 given cephalothin, and 23 of 247 given both antibiotics.— W. L. Fanning *et al.*, *Antimicrob. Ag. Chemother.*, 1976, *10*, 80.

In a prospective double-blind study of 90 patients with suspected sepsis 12 of 47 (25.5%) who received cephalothin plus an aminoglycoside antibiotic (gentamicin or tobramycin) developed definite nephrotoxicity compared with only 3 of 43 (7%) who received methicillin plus gentamicin or tobramycin; possible or definite nephrotoxicity developed in 17 of the 47 and 7 of the 43 respectively. Both differences were statistically significant. No significant difference was found between gentamicin and tobramycin in relation to nephrotoxicity.— J. C. Wade *et al.*, *Lancet*, 1978, *2*, 604. When the antibiotics were given for longer than 10 days methicillin with gentamicin was strongly nephrotoxic.— L. Yver (letter), *ibid.*, 1314.

A study in *rats* indicated that cephalothin or carbenicillin exerted a protective effect against the nephrotoxicity of gentamicin. Carbenicillin produced this effect at a lower dose than cephalothin.— R. Bloch *et al.*, *Antimicrob. Ag. Chemother.*, 1979, *15*, 46.

For other reports of nephrotoxicity in patients given cephalothin in association with gentamicin, see J. P. Fillastre *et al.*, *Br. med. J.*, 1973, *2*, 396; P. Noone *et al.* (letter), *ibid.*, 776; E. L. Gurwich *et al.*, *Am. J. Hosp. Pharm.*, 1978, *35*, 1402; J. H. Schwartz and P. Schein, *Cancer*, 1978, *41*, 769.

For further reports of nephrotoxicity in patients being treated with gentamicin and cephalothin, see Gentamicin Sulphate, p.1167.

Psychosis. A report of a toxic paranoid reaction precipitated in 1 patient by cephalothin.— G. Murray (letter), *Drug Intell. & clin. Pharm.*, 1974, *8*, 71.

Thrombophlebitis. Of 94 patients being treated with cephalothin 19 (20%) developed severe phlebitis associated with drug administration compared with 11 of 120 (9%) who received cefapirin. When intravenous infusion sites were evaluated 100 of 276 (36%) veins receiving cephalothin and 103 of 355 (29%) veins receiving cefapirin developed phlebitis and severe phlebitis occurred in 25 (9%) and 14 (4%) veins respectively. The efficacy of both drugs in the treatment of infections was similar.— J. Inagaki and G. P. Bodey, *Curr. ther. Res.*, 1973, *15*, 37. In a single-blind study of 120 patients there was no difference between cephalothin and cefapirin in the incidence and severity of phlebitis.— A. S. Cross and E. C. Tramont, *Antimicrob. Ag. Chemother.*, 1976, *9*, 722. See also A. P. Sorrentino *et al.*, *Am. J. Hosp. Pharm.*, 1976, *33*, 642.

There was no difference in the incidence of phlebitis produced by buffered and unbuffered infusions of cephalothin in doses of 2 g given over 5 to 15 minutes every 6 hours for 48 hours.— J. Carrizosa *et al.*, *Antimicrob. Ag. Chemother.*, 1974, *5*, 192. The incidence of phlebitis was significantly lower with a buffered infusion compared with an unbuffered one when 1 g was given over 15 minutes every 2 hours for 4 days.— M. G. Bergeron *et al.*, *ibid.*, 1976, *9*, 646.

A comparison of the incidence of phlebitis caused by infusions of cephalothin, cefapirin, and cephamandole. The incidence of moderate phlebitis was lowest with cephalothin and highest with cephamandole. More doses of cefapirin were required to produce moderate phlebitis than of the other 2.— S. Berger *et al.*, *Antimicrob. Ag. Chemother.*, 1976, *9*, 575. The incidence of thrombophlebitis was no greater with intravenous infusions of these 3 cephalosporins when compared with water, all given in dextrose injection with sodium chloride injection 0.2%, in a study of 16 subjects. However, the thrombophlebitis caused by cephalothin was more severe.— W. T. Siebert *et al.*, *ibid.*, *10*, 467.

See also under Cefapirin Sodium, p.1117.

Precautions. As for Cephaloridine, p.1126.

The concomitant use of cephalothin and gentamicin or other nephrotoxic antibiotics appears to increase the risk of kidney damage. It is recommended that cephalothin be given with care in reduced dosage to patients with renal impairment. Since it is metabolised in the liver it should be given with caution to patients with hepatic failure.

A report of severe encephalopathy occurring in a man with renal failure who received a total of 22 g of cephalothin over 5 days. Very high cephalothin concentrations in the CSF (9.6 µg per ml) and serum (170 µg per ml) were recorded.— M. -J. Wu *et al.* (letter), *Ann. intern. Med.*, 1978, *89*, 429.

Interactions. The rate of urinary excretion of cephalothin was not affected by the administration of frusemide, mercaptomerin, or mannitol in 5 healthy persons.— A. D. Tice *et al.*, *Antimicrob. Ag. Chemother.*, 1975, *7*, 168.

See also under Antimicrobial Action, below.

Interference with laboratory estimations. Cephalothin sodium could interfere with the glucose test (Benedict's) to produce erroneous raised results.— M. Lubrau, *Med. Clins N. Am.*, 1969, *53*, 211.

When urine of patients treated with cephalothin was tested for protein with 20% sulphosalicylic acid, a heavy white precipitate developed if cephalothin concentrations were 10 mg per ml or more. This precipitate was indistinguishable from that seen in proteinuria due to renal damage and awareness of this false positive reaction is important in the treatment of the patients.— M. Levy and M. Eliakim (letter), *J. Am. med. Ass.*, 1972, *219*, 908.

Cephalothin interfered with the determination of creatinine concentrations in plasma and urine using the Jaffé method and might produce falsely high values. This effect should be borne in mind when monitoring renal function.— L. I. Rankin *et al.*, *Antimicrob. Ag. Chemother.*, 1979, *15*, 666.

Cephalosporins with a 3-acetoxymethyl group, including cephalothin, cephaloglycin, cephacetrile, cefapirin, and cefotaxime, are deacetylated by lysed whole blood and this should be taken into account when assays must be run in whole blood or on tissues containing whole blood.— W. E. Wright and J. A. Frogge, *Antimicrob. Ag. Chemother.*, 1980, *17*, 99.

Antimicrobial Action. Cephalothin is bactericidal and has the same mode of action and spectrum of activity as cephaloridine (see p.1126). However, it is less active than cephaloridine against Gram-positive organisms. Cephalothin is inhibited by staphylococcal penicillinase to a lesser extent than is cephaloridine.

The minimum inhibitory concentration for most Gram-positive organisms ranges from 0.06 to 1 µg per ml; for most Gram-negative organisms concentrations of at least 1 µg per ml are required to inhibit growth.

At a concentration of 10 µg per ml of serum, which was usually attainable with 500 mg of cephalothin intramuscularly, there was inhibition of 82% of strains of *Proteus mirabilis*, 10% of *Klebsiella* spp., 58% of *E. coli*, 54% of paracolon types, but of only 8% of indole-positive *Proteus* strains. Cephalothin was not active against *Ps. aeruginosa*.— M. Turck *et al.*, *Ann. intern. Med.*, 1965, *63*, 199.

For reports of the activity of cephalothin and other cephalosporins against *Haemophilus influenzae*, see J. D. Williams and J. Andrews, *Br. med. J.*, 1974, *1*, 134; S. Eykyn and I. Phillips (letter), *ibid.*, 1974, *2*, 59.

Only cefoxitin and cephalothin appeared resistant to inactivation by beta-lactamase-producing *Staph. aureus* in a study of 8 cephalosporins. It was considered that cephalothin was generally the best cephalosporin to use in severe staphylococcal infections.— I. W. Fong *et al.*, *Antimicrob. Ag. Chemother.*, 1976, *9*, 939.

Ten antibiotics were tested for their activity *in vitro* against 50 strains of *Haemophilus parainfluenzae*. All strains were sensitive to carbenicillin, cephalothin, chloramphenicol, colistin, gentamicin, and kanamycin and showed variable susceptibilities to erythromycin and tetracycline. Three strains were resistant to ampicillin and penicillin.— J. B. Mayo and L. R. McCarthy, *Antimicrob. Ag. Chemother.*, 1977, *11*, 844.

Cephalothin had an MIC of 0.78, 1.56, 3.12, 6.25, and 12.5 µg per ml respectively against 48, 89, 97, 98 and 100% of 67 strains of *Salmonella typhi* and an MIC of 3.12, 6.25, and 12.5 µg per ml respectively against 22, 94, and 96% of 54 strains of *S. paratyphi A*.— L. J. Strausbaugh *et al.*, *Antimicrob. Ag. Chemother.*, 1978, *13*, 134.

A report of the activities of 6 cephalosporins, including cephalothin, against 408 clinical isolates of anaerobic bacteria.— A. W. Chow and D. Bednorz, *Antimicrob. Ag. Chemother.*, 1978, *14*, 668. See also V. L. Sutter and S. M. Finegold, *ibid.*, 1976, *10*, 736.

A study of the accuracy of diffusion susceptibility tests with disks containing 30 µg of cephamandole or cephalothin indicated that although the same interpretive zone standards could be applied to tests with either disk the two drugs could not be tested interchangeably.— A. L. Barry *et al.*, *Antimicrob. Ag. Chemother.*, 1979, *15*, 140.

Diminished activity. When cephalothin was used with gentamicin or vancomycin in *mice* infected with methicillin-resistant *Staph. epidermidis*, there was an increased death-rate compared with the use of any of the drugs alone. The antagonism was not due to drug-drug inactivation.— F. D. Lowy *et al.*, *Antimicrob. Ag. Chemother.*, 1979, *16*, 314.

Enhanced activity. The MICs of benzylpenicillin or cephalothin *in vitro* against 55 penicillin-resistant strains of the *Bacteroides* spp. were reduced when used with clavulanic acid 1 or 5 µg per ml, but the MICs against resistant strains of *Clostridium clostridiiforme* and *Clostridium ramosum* were unaffected.— J. Wüst and T. D. Wilkins, *Antimicrob. Ag. Chemother.*, 1978, *13*, 130.

Sera containing cephalothin and gentamicin had a greater bactericidal activity against *Kleb. pneumoniae* than that containing ticarcillin and gentamicin and sera containing ticarcillin and cephalothin was the least active.— J. Murillo *et al.*, *Antimicrob. Ag. Chemother.*, 1978, *13*, 992.

A report of enhanced activity *in vitro* with cephalothin and rifampicin or vancomycin against methicillin-resistant *Staph. epidermidis*.— M. E. Ein *et al.*, *Antimicrob. Ag. Chemother.*, 1979, *16*, 655. See also Diminished Activity (above).

For a report of sodium clavulanate enhancing the effect of cephalothin *in vitro* against cephalothin-resistant strains of *Klebsiella pneumoniae*, see p.1143.

For reports of synergy between gentamicin and cephalothin, see Gentamicin Sulphate, p.1169.

Resistance. As for Cephaloridine, p.1127.
Cephalothin is less susceptible than cephaloridine to inhibition by penicillinase.

Of 400 strains of *Salmonella* isolated from patients in USA during 1967, 8% were resistant to cephalothin; 24.5% of *S. typhimurium* strains were resistant. Assessment of resistance was based upon a zone of inhibition of 11 mm or less using disks containing 30 µg of cephalothin sodium.— S. A. Schroeder *et al.*, *J. Am. med. Ass.*, 1968, *205*, 903.

Strains of *Str. pneumoniae* isolated from 5 children were partially resistant to cephalothin.— P. C. Appelbaum *et al.*, *Lancet*, 1977, *2*, 995.

A clinical isolate of *E. coli*, normally susceptible to cephalothin, was capable of degrading cephalothin after prolonged incubation in broth containing the drug at a greater concentration than its MIC. Studies suggested the presence of an acylesterase.— T. Nishiura *et al.*, *Antimicrob. Ag. Chemother.*, 1978, *13*, 1036.

Methicillin-resistant coagulase-negative staphylococci showed nearly total cross-resistance to 8 cephalosporins tested *in vitro*, including cephalothin. Beta-lactamases produced by the staphylococci had little hydrolytic effect on the cephalosporins and there was no correlation between anti-staphylococcal activity and resistance to beta-lactamases.— J. F. John and W. F. McNeill, *Antimicrob. Ag. Chemother.*, 1980, *17*, 179.

Tolerance. Of 7 strains of *Staph. aureus* displaying a form of resistance to penicillins termed tolerance, 5 were cross-tolerant to the bactericidal effect of cephalothin.— L. D. Sabath *et al.*, *Lancet*, 1977, *1*, 443. Of 30 isolates of *Staph. aureus*, 19 were tolerant to the bactericidal effect of oxacillin or cephalothin but none were tolerant to gentamicin. Tolerance was unrelated to phage type.— J. J. Bradley *et al.*, *Antimicrob. Ag. Chemother.*, 1978, *13*, 1052.

MBCs of cephalothin greatly exceeded MICs against 40 strains of *Lactobacilli in vitro*.— A. S. Bayer *et al.*, *Antimicrob. Ag. Chemother.*, 1978, *14*, 720.

A report of tolerance to cephalothin by Lancefield group G streptococci.— J. T. Noble *et al.* (letter), *Lancet*, 1980, *2*, 982.

Absorption and Fate. Cephalothin is poorly absorbed from the gastro-intestinal tract. About 65% of cephalothin in the circulation following parenteral administration is bound to plasma proteins compared with about 20% for cephaloridine. It is widely distributed in body tissues and fluids except the brain and cerebrospinal fluid. When the meninges are inflamed lower CSF concentrations are achieved with cephalothin than cephaloridine. It readily diffuses across the placenta into the foetal circulation and has been detected in breast milk. The biological half-life varies from about 30 to 50 minutes, and is shorter than that of cephaloridine.
After intramuscular injection peak plasma concentrations of about 10 and 20 µg per ml are achieved within 30 minutes of doses of 0.5 and 1 g respectively but rapidly decline within 4 hours. Concentrations of 30 to 60 µg per ml have been reported 15 minutes after the intravenous injection of a 1-g dose; a range of 14 to 20 µg per ml has been achieved by the continuous intravenous infusion of 500 mg per hour.
Unlike cephaloridine about 20 to 30% of cephalothin is rapidly deacetylated in the liver and about 60% of a dose is excreted in the urine by the renal tubules within 6 hours as cephalothin and the relatively inactive metabolite. High urine concentrations of 0.8 and 2.5 mg per ml have been observed following doses of 0.5 and 1 g. Probenecid blocks the renal excretion of cephalothin. A small amount is excreted in bile.

A review of the pharmacokinetics and clinical use of cephalosporin antibiotics including cephalothin.— C. H. Nightingale *et al.*, *J. pharm. Sci.*, 1975, *64*, 1899.

A study of the reversibility of the plasma-protein binding of cephalothin *in vitro*.— M. Barza *et al.*, *Antimicrob. Ag. Chemother.*, 1972, *1*, 427.

Following administration of cephalothin intravenously to 5 adults (5 to 37.5 mg per kg body-weight) and 5 children (10 to 25 mg per kg) the mean elimination half-life from serum was 13.5 and 18.6 minutes respectively. The rapid clearance suggested that clinical regimens using a 4- to 6-hour dosing schedule might result in concentrations below the minimum inhibitory concentration of most susceptible organisms for approximately 50% of each treatment period.— T. F. Rolewicz *et al.*, *Clin. Pharmac. Ther.*, 1977, *22*, 928.

Further references to pharmacokinetic studies of cephalothin: A. G. Paradelis *et al.*, *Arzneimittel-Forsch.*, 1977, *27*, 2167; K. W. Miller *et al.*, *Clin. Pharmac. Ther.*, 1979, *26*, 54 (in cardiopulmonary bypass surgery).

Diffusion. Cephalothin 1 g was given intravenously or intraperitoneally to 11 patients with cirrhosis and ascites. Intraperitoneal administration was more effective in maintaining high concentrations of cephalothin in the ascitic fluid, effective concentrations remaining 11 hours after administration.— D. E. Wilson *et al.*, *Am. J. med. Sci.*, 1967, *253*, 449.

Cephalothin 2 to 4 g every 4 to 6 hours was infused intravenously over 15 to 30 minutes in 14 patients, and produced serum concentrations of 0.6 to 218.3 µg per ml. No cephalothin could be found in the cerebrospinal fluid of 5 patients. In patients with a raised CSF protein content or cell content, concentrations of less than 1 µg per ml were usually found in the CSF. In 1 patient with inflamed meninges the CSF contained cephalothin 5 µg per ml.— P. I. Lerner, *Am. J. med. Sci.*, 1969, *257*, 125.

Cephalothin 2 g, given intravenously when the meninges were not inflamed, produced concentrations in brain tissue sufficient to inhibit sensitive Gram-positive cocci.— P. W. Kramer *et al.*, *J. Neurosurg.*, 1969, *31*, 295.

Cephalothin diffused into interstitial fluid. This diffusion was related to the amount of protein binding.— J. S. Tan and S. J. Salstrom, *Antimicrob. Ag. Chemother.*, 1977, *11*, 698. See also *idem*, 1979, *15*, 510.

For further reports of diffusion, see M. A. MacAulay and D. Charles, *Am. J. Obstet. Gynec.*, 1968, *100*, 940 (transplacental diffusion); J. D. Nelson, *New Engl. J. Med.*, 1971, *284*, 349 (synovial fluid); J. M. Brogard *et al.*, *Chemotherapy, Basle*, 1973, *18*, 212; J. Mendelson *et al.*, *Antimicrob. Ag. Chemother.*, 1974, *6*, 659 (bile); R. H. Fitzgerald *et al.*, *ibid.*, 1978, *14*, 723 (bone and synovial tissue).

Uses. Cephalothin sodium is a cephalosporin antibiotic with a bactericidal action and is used similarly to cephaloridine (see p.1127), in the treatment of soft tissue infections and infections of the respiratory and urinary tracts. It is less susceptible to penicillinase than cephaloridine and may be more effective in infections caused by penicillin-resistant staphylococci. It is probably less likely to cause renal damage.
Cephalothin sodium is given by slow intravenous injection over 2 to 5 minutes or by intermittent or continuous infusion. It may be given intramuscularly but this route is painful. The usual dose is the equivalent of 0.5 to 1 g of cephalothin every 4 to 6 hours; doses of 12 g daily may be given in severe infections. Because of its shorter half-life cephalothin needs to be given more often than cephaloridine. Children may be given 80 to 160 mg per kg body-weight daily in divided doses. Higher doses of up to 270 mg per kg daily have been employed.
Reduced doses are recommended for patients with impaired renal function; patients with anuria may be given maintenance doses of 1.5 or occasionally 3 g daily in divided doses. With creatinine clearances below 10, 25, 50, or 80 ml per minute doses of 0.5, 1, 1.5, or 2 g respectively may be given every 6 hours.

Cephalothin was given to 65 patients in daily doses ranging from 2 to 12 g, with a mean of 4.3 g. Total doses ranged from 8 to 608 g, with a mean of 88 g, and duration of therapy from 2 to 82 days, with a mean of 16.8 days. Cure or improvement occurred in 78%. Seven patients of the 65 developed clinically significant supra-infection due to *Klebsiella-Aerobacter*, *Pseudomonas aeruginosa*, or *Candida albicans*, and all 7 died. There were 25 untoward reactions in 23 patients. In addition, 4 patients developed phlebitis and 1 an abscess at the injection site. Among 22 penicillin-allergic patients there were 9 probable hypersensitivity reactions to cephalothin, compared with 5 such reactions among 43 patients with no history of penicillin allergy; the commonest manifestation was eosinophilia.— S. L. Merrill *et al.*, *Ann. intern. Med.*, 1966, *64*, 1.

Tobramycin 4 mg per kg body-weight and cephalothin 100 mg per kg were given daily by intramuscular or intravenous injection for 6 to 18 days to 35 patients with serious bacterial infections and severe blood diseases. A favourable response to treatment was obtained in 7 of 11 patients with septicaemia, 17 of 20 with urinary-tract infections, and 3 of 4 patients with bronchopneumonia. Most patients who did not respond had acute leukaemia.— A. G. Papayannis *et al.*, *J. antimicrob. Chemother.*, 1977, *3*, 311. For further reports of the use of cephalothin with other antibiotics in neutropenic patients, see D. M. Hahn *et al.* (letter), *Antimicrob. Ag. Chemother.*, 1977, *12*, 618 (amikacin); G. P. Bodey *et al.*, *Am. J. med. Sci.*, 1977, *273*, 309 (carbenicillin).

For reviews of the cephalosporins, see Cephaloridine, p.1127.

Administration, intraperitoneal. Intraperitoneal irrigations with cephalothin were carried out in 94 surgical operations in 92 patients but there was no difference in wound infection, sepsis, or deaths between these patients and a control group given sodium chloride injection.— W. M. Rambo, *Am. J. Surg.*, 1972, *123*, 192.

There was no significant difference in the development of peritonitis in a double-blind study of 36 patients undergoing peritoneal dialysis given either placebo or cephalothin sodium in the dialysis fluid. However, there was a significantly greater incidence of positive cultures in the patients given placebo.— J. Axelrod *et al.*, *Archs. intern. Med.*, 1973, *132*, 368.

In 14 patients with generalised peritonitis, prolonged peritoneal lavage, with a dialysis solution containing kanamycin 40 µg per ml and cephalothin 100 µg per ml, was performed continuously for 2 to 10 days. The antibiotics were changed if organisms proved resistant to either drug. Additional antibiotics were given systemically to 10 patients. Of 11 patients in whom the causative lesion was repaired, 1 patient died from gastro-intestinal haemorrhage and chest infection 5 weeks after lavage ceased. Three patients in whom the causative lesion was not repaired died.— R. C. Atkins *et al.*, *Med. J. Aust.*, 1976, *1*, 954.

Dosage in renal failure. In patients with oliguria, intervals between doses of cephalothin should be increased to every 24 hours.— C. M. Kunin, *Ann. intern. Med.*, 1967, *67*, 151.

Six patients on a regular haemodialysis programme were given 1 g of cephalothin intravenously 60 hours before and again just before dialysis. The average serum concentration 15 minutes after the 2nd injection was 107 µg per ml and this fell during dialysis to a mean of 13 µg per ml at 10 hours, the mean half-life during dialysis being 3.3 hours. It was considered that a 1-g dose given just before haemodialysis would provide an adequate concentration during the dialysis and that 1 g given between dialyses would provide only adequate concentrations for 48 to 72 hours. Cephalothin should not be used to treat Gram-negative infections in patients undergoing dialysis.— R. C. Venuto and M. E. Plaut, *Antimicrob. Ag. Chemother.*, 1970, 50.

A review of the clinical use of cephalothin in patients with renal and hepatic insufficiency.— D. L. Giusti, *Drug Intell. & clin. Pharm.*, 1973, *7*, 252. Comment.— S. L. Barriere (letter), *ibid.*, 526. A reply.— D. L. Giusti (letter), *ibid.*

The normal half-life for cephalothin of 0.5 to 0.9 hours was increased to 3 to 18 hours in end-stage renal failure. The interval between doses should be extended from 6 hours to 8 to 12 hours in patients with a glomerular filtration-rate of less than 10 ml per minute. Concentrations of cephalothin were affected by haemodialysis and peritoneal dialysis.— W. M. Bennett *et al.*, *Ann. intern. Med.*, 1977, *86*, 754. See also *idem*, 1980, *93*, 62.

The dosage interval should be increased from 6 to 8 hours in patients with moderate renal failure, and to 12 to 24 hours in those with severe renal failure.— P. Sharpstone, *Br. med. J.*, 1977, *2*, 36.

After a loading dose of 1 to 3 g cephalothin could be given in a dose of 1 to 2 g every 4 to 6 hours to patients with a creatinine clearance (CC) of 40 to 80 ml per minute, every 6 to 8 hours to those with a CC of 10 to 30 ml per minute, and every 8 to 12 hours to those with a CC of 5 ml per minute. In haemodialysis 1 to 2 g could be given every 8 to 12 hours and 1 to 2 g after dialysis.— J. S. Cheigh, *Am. J. Med.*, 1977, *62*, 555.

Data for predicting removal of cephalothin by conventional haemodialysis.— T. P. Gibson and H. A. Nelson, *Clin. Pharmacokinet.*, 1977, *2*, 403.

Meningitis. For a review of the use of cephalothin and cephaloridine in the treatment of bacterial meningitis, see Cephaloridine, p.1127.

Open-heart surgery. A total of 28 g of cephalothin sodium was given intravenously to each of 100 patients over the 48 hours during and immediately following open-heart surgery. Despite the relatively high dosage and the simultaneous use of frusemide, no nephrotoxic effects were found and cephalothin sodium was considered to be safe and effective. Infections produced by organisms resistant to cephalothin were due to *Pseudomonas aeruginosa* (1), *Escherichia coli* (5), and *Staphylococcus aureus* (1).— W. H. Bain *et al.*, *J. antimicrob. Chemother.*, 1977, *3*, 339. Criticism.— A. Herxheimer (letter), *ibid.*, 621. See also S. W. B. Newsom, *J. antimicrob. Chemother.*, 1978, *4*, 389.

A regimen consisting of cephalothin sodium, cephalexin, and gentamicin was considered to have provided effective prophylaxis against local and systemic bacterial infection in 101 patients who had undergone open-heart surgery.— C. H. Anyanwu and M. H. Yacoub, *Curr. ther. Res.*, 1978, *23*, 1.

Further references: L. Gonzalez-Lavin *et al.*, *Clin. Med.*, 1970, *77* (Dec.), 31; J. E. Conte *et al.*, *Ann. intern. Med.*, 1972, *76*, 943.

For a report of the prophylactic use of cephalothin and cephamandole during cardiac surgery, see Cephamandole, p.1133.

Osteomyelitis. Cephalothin was used to provide antibiotic cover in 14 patients with *Staph. aureus* osteomyelitis undergoing amputation of the toe or part of the foot; 1 g was given intravenously 4-hourly for 2 weeks commencing 2 or 3 days before surgery, followed by cephalexin 6 g daily by mouth for 4 weeks.— M. D. Kerstein, *Curr. ther. Res.*, 1974, *16*, 306.

Staphylococcal infections. For a report suggesting treatment of infections due to methicillin-resistant *Staph. aureus* with cephalothin in conjunction with kanamycin, see Kanamycin Sulphate, p.1177.

Surgical infection prophylaxis. In a study over 3.5 years involving 930 vaginal hysterectomies, the morbidity-rate and incidence of bacteriuria was about 10% in 333 patients who received cephalothin 1 g intramuscularly one hour before operation, 1 g intravenously during operation, and 1 g intramuscularly or intravenously every 6 hours for the next 72 hours; occasionally an oral cephalosporin was used postoperatively. In the remainder, to whom cephalothin was only given if it was required therapeutically after hysterectomy, morbidity and bacteriuria occurred in about 30% of patients.— L. F. Peterson *et al.*, *Curr. ther. Res.*, 1977, *22*, 792. See also J. L. Allen *et al.*, *Obstet. Gynec.*, 1972, *39*, 218.

Gas gangrene developed in 4 patients with open fractures treated with surgical debridement and prophylactic cephalothin sodium by intravenous injection. Five of 11 human isolates of *Clostridium* species tested demonstrated resistance to cephalothin.— J. A. Mohr *et al.*, *J. Am. med.Ass.*, 1978, *239*, 847.

A report indicating that, unlike cephaloridine and cephazolin, cephalothin may not be effective in the prophylaxis of surgical wound infection.— H. C. Polk *et al.*, *J. Am. med. Ass.*, 1980, *244*, 1353.

Further references: N. G. Waterman *et al.*, *Archs Surg., Chicago*, 1968, *97*, 365; K. Kjellgren and H. Sellström, *Acta chir. scand.*, 1977, *143*, 473; K. A. Hamod *et al.*, *Am. J. Obstet. Gynec.*, 1980, *136*, 976 (single dose).

See also under Intraperitoneal Administration and Open-heart Surgery (above).

Syphilis. Cephalothin 1 g was given intramuscularly every 12 hours to 25 men (including 4 who were sensitive to penicillin) for 20 days for those with primary and for 25 days for those with secondary syphilis. There was rapid resolution of the lesions and all positive blood tests became negative within 3 months. None of the patients with a history of penicillin reactions suffered reactions with cephalothin. The duration of follow-up was 6 months to 2 years and no recurrences were noted.— G. Nicolis and A. Loucopoulos, *Br. J. vener. Dis.*, 1974, *50*, 270.

Preparations

Cephalothin Injection *(B.P.)*. A sterile solution of cephalothin sodium in Water for Injections. It is prepared by dissolving the sterile contents of a sealed container (Cephalothin Sodium for Injection) in the requisite amount of Water for Injections. pH 4.5 to 7. Store at 2° to 8° and use within 48 hours of preparation.

Cephalothin Sodium for Injection *(U.S.P.)*. A sterile mixture of cephalothin sodium and one or more suitable buffers. Potency is expressed in terms of the equivalent amount of cephalothin. The injection is prepared by the addition of diluent before use. pH 6 to 8.5.

Keflin *(Lilly, UK)*. Cephalothin sodium, available as powder for preparing injections, in vials each containing the equivalent of 1 or 4 g of cephalothin. (Also available as Keflin in *Arg., Belg., Canad., Denm., Fr., Ital., Neth., Norw., Spain, USA*).

Other Proprietary Names

Averon *(Spain)*; Cephation *(Jap.)*; Ceporacin *(Austral., Belg., Canad., Neth., Spain)*; Cepovenin *(Ger.)*; CET, Coaxin *(both Jap.)*; Keflin N *(Switz.)*; Keflin Neutral *(Austral., S.Afr.)*; Seffin *(Arg.)*; Synclotin, Toricelocin *(both Jap.)*.

42-n

Cephamandole.

Cefamandole; 83405. (7*R*)-7-D-Mandelamido-3-(1-methyl-1*H*-tetrazol-5-ylthiomethyl)-3-cephem-4-carboxylic acid.
$C_{18}H_{18}N_6O_5S_2$=462.5.

CAS — 34444-01-4.

Stability. Cephamandole in horse serum was stable for at least 30 days when stored at −10°. Repeated thawing and freezing did not affect its stability. After 30 days at 4° cephamandole retained 70% activity.— M. A. Foglesong, *Antimicrob. Ag. Chemother.*, 1977, *11*, 174.

43-h

Cephamandole Nafate.

Cefamandole Nafate *(U.S.P.)*; 106223. Sodium (7*R*)-7-[(2*R*)-2-formyloxy-2-phenylacetamido]-3-(1-methyl-1*H*-tetrazol-5-ylthiomethyl)-3-cephem-4-carboxylate.
$C_{19}H_{17}N_6NaO_6S_2$=512.5.

CAS — 42540-40-9.

Pharmacopoeias. In *U.S.*

A crystalline powder containing the equivalent of 810 to 1000 μg of cephamandole per mg, calculated on the anhydrous basis. 1.11 g of cephamandole nafate approximately equivalent to 1 g of cephamandole activity represents 2.2 mmol (2.2 mEq) of sodium. Proprietary preparations (Kefadol and Mandol) contain sodium carbonate and the total sodium content of these preparations is approximately 3.3 mmol (3.3 mEq) per g of cephamandole activity.

Freely **soluble** in water; practically insoluble in most organic solvents. A 10% solution has a pH of 3.5 to 7.

Formulations of cephamandole nafate available for injection contain sodium carbonate and are **incompatible** with solutions containing calcium or magnesium salts. When reconstituted with water the sodium carbonate rapidly hydrolyses about 30% of the ester to cephamandole; during storage of the reconstituted solution at room temperature carbon dioxide is produced. Solutions for injection should be used within 96 hours if stored at 5° or within 24 hours if kept at 25°. **Store** in airtight containers.

Adverse Effects and Precautions. As for Cephalothin Sodium, p.1128. Cephamandole should be given with care in reduced dosage to patients with renal impairment.

Blood disorders. During a study of parenteral cephamandole sodium in the management of peritoneal and soft-tissue sepsis, cephamandole appeared to induce prolonged prothrombin time in 3 patients, all of whom suffered major gastro-intestinal bleeds, one of which was fatal. All 3 patients had been maintained without food or drink by mouth for at least 7 days, and it is considered that sufficient antibiotic was excreted through the bile into the gut lumen to alter the bacterial intestinal flora and suppress synthesis of vitamin K; renal failure, in the patient who died, may also have been important. Timely injections of vitamin K may be warranted in patients on antibiotics where oral intake of nutrients is restricted.— C. A. Hooper *et al.* (letter), *Lancet*, 1980, *1*, 39.

Interactions. Alcohol. A report of a disulfiram-like reaction to alcohol in a man receiving cephamandole.— H. Portier *et al.* (letter), *Lancet*, 1980, *2*, 263. A further report.— S. Drummer *et al.* (letter), *New Engl. J. Med.*, 1980, *303*, 1417.

See also under Cefoperazone, p.1118 and Latamoxef, p.1177.

Skin reactions. A report of toxic epidermal necrolysis associated with the administration of cephamandole.— R. N. Greenberg *et al.*, *Antimicrob. Ag. Chemother.*, 1979, *15*, 337.

Thrombophlebitis. For comparative studies of thrombophlebitis arising from cephamandole infusions, see Cephalothin Sodium p.1129.

Antimicrobial Action. Cephamandole is bactericidal and has a broader spectrum of activity than the older cephalosporins, including cephaloridine and cephalothin. It generally has similar or less activity against Gram-positive cocci but is resistant to some beta-lactamases produced by Gram-negative bacteria and is more active against many of the Enterobacteriaceae including *Escherichia coli* and *Klebsiella* spp. and especially *Enterobacter* and indole-positive *Proteus* spp. Like cefuroxime, cephamandole is very active *in vitro* against *Haemophilus influenzae* although an inoculum effect has been reported. *Pseudomonas* spp. are resistant.

Cephamandole was the most active of 7 cephalosporins against *E. coli* but it was not resistant to all 4 of the beta-lactamases tested. Cefoxitin and to a lesser extent cefuroxime were resistant to the beta-lactamases and only slightly less active than cephamandole against *E. coli*.— M. H. Richmond and S. Wotton, *Antimicrob. Ag. Chemother.*, 1976, *10*, 219.

The activities of cephamandole, cefoxitin, cephalexin, and cephalothin were compared *in vitro* in broth and agar dilutions against 645 strains of bacteria from clinical sources. Cephamandole and cephalothin were the most effective against Gram-positive organisms while cephamandole and cefoxitin were most effective against Gram-negative organisms. Cephamandole was more active than cefoxitin against *Pr. mirabilis, Pr. rettgeri,* and *Enterobacter* spp. as well as *N. meningitidis, N. gonorrhoeae*, and *H. influenzae*. An inoculum effect was demonstrated for cephamandole when testing *H. influenzae*.— T. C. Eickhoff and J. M. Ehret, *Antimicrob. Ag. Chemother.*, 1976, *9*, 994. Another study of the activity *in vitro* of cefoxitin and cephamandole showed diminished activity of cephamandole in broth compared with agar medium; this was not the case with cefoxitin. The main advantage of cephamandole over cefoxitin was in its action against *Enterobacter* spp.— H. G. Adams *et al.*, *ibid.*, 1019. Discrepancies in the sensitivity of *Enterobacter* spp. to cephamandole measured by agar and broth dilutions appeared to be due to a relatively high mutation-rate to resistance.— C. M. Findell and J. C. Sherris, *ibid.*, 970.

Depending on the test used, cephamandole nafate had about one-tenth the antibacterial activity *in vitro* of cephamandole but since cephamandole nafate was rapidly hydrolysed to cephamandole the activities *in vivo* were virtually identical.— J. R. Turner *et al.*, *Lilly, USA*, *Antimicrob. Ag. Chemother.*, 1977, *12*, 67. Since cephamandole nafate did not have the equivalent antibiotic activity of cephamandole *in vitro*, it was recommended that before microbiological assay the nafate should be hydrolysed. It might be advisable to use either the sodium or lithium salts of cephamandole in microbiological studies.— C. L. Winely *et al.*, *Antimicrob. Ag. Chemother.*, 1979, *16*, 424.

A report of penicillinase-producing gonococci being sensitive to cephamandole.— A. F. Hallett *et al.* (letter), *Lancet*, 1977, *1*, 1205.

The *in vitro* activity of cephamandole against Gram-negative organisms did not correlate well with its stability to beta-lactamases.— K. P. Fu and H. C. Neu, *J. infect. Dis.*, 1978, *137*, *Suppl.* (May), S38.

The activities of ampicillin, cephamandole, cefoxitin, cefaclor, and cefatrizine were compared *in vitro* against 100 isolates of *Haemophilus influenzae.* Of 68 isolates which did not produce beta-lactamase all were inhibited by ampicillin 1 μg or less per ml, 99% by cephamandole 2 μg per ml or cefoxitin 8 μg per ml, and more than 95% by cefaclor or cefatrizine 16 μg per ml. Cephamandole had an MIC of 2 μg per ml against 84% of 32 isolates which were resistant to ampicillin, 31 of which produced a beta-lactamase, while cefoxitin had an MIC of 8 μg per ml against 82% and 16 μg per ml against 98%; cefaclor or cefatrizine 16 μg per ml inhibited about 85 to 90% of the isolates.— J. H. Jorgensen and

G. A. Alexander, *Antimicrob. Ag. Chemother.*, 1978, *13*, 342. See also S. Kattan *et al.*, *J. antimicrob. Chemother.*, 1975, *1*, 79; W. H. Hall *et al.*, *Curr. ther. Res.*, 1977, *21*, 374; P. H. Azimi, *Antimicrob. Ag. Chemother.*, 1978, *13*, 955; E. Yourassowsky *et al.*, *ibid.*, 1979, *15*, 325; C. Watanakunakorn and C. Glotzbecker, *ibid.*, 836; V. P. Syriopoulou *et al.*, *ibid.*, *16*, 510 (inoculum effect).

Cephamandole had a similar activity to cefaclor, and was more active than cephazolin, cephalothin or cephalexin *in vitro* against 67 strains of *Salmonella typhi* and 54 strains of *S. paratyphi A*. Cephamandole had an MIC of 0.39, 0.78, and 3.12 µg per ml respectively against 92, 98 and 100% of the strains of *S. typhi* and an MIC of 1.56 and 3.12 µg per ml respectively against 94 and 100% of the strains of *S. paratyphi A*.— L. J. Strausbaugh *et al.*, *Antimicrob. Ag. Chemother.*, 1978, *13*, 134.

A study of the accuracy of diffusion susceptibility tests with disks containing 30 µg of cephamandole or cephalothin indicated that although the same interpretive zone standards could be applied to tests with either disk the two drugs could not be tested interchangeably.— A. L. Barry *et al.*, *Antimicrob. Ag. Chemother.*, 1979, *15*, 140.

For further comparisons of cephamandole with other cephalosporins, see L. Verbist, *Antimicrob. Ag. Chemother.*, 1976, *10*, 657; D. C. Blair *et al.*, *Curr. ther. Res.*, 1977, *22*, 861; C. Watanakunakorn and C. Glotzbecker, *ibid.*, 1978, *24*, 149; W. L. George *et al.*, *Antimicrob. Ag. Chemother.*, 1978, *13*, 484; H. C. Neu and K. P. Fu, *ibid.*, 584; V. C. Simon *et al.*, *J. antimicrob. Chemother.*, 1978, *4*, 85; J. H. Jorgensen *et al.*, *Curr. ther. Res.*, 1979, *25*, 74; C. Thornsberry *et al.*, *J. antimicrob. Chemother.*, 1979, *5*, 137; W. H. Hall *et al.*, *Antimicrob. Ag. Chemother.*, 1980, *17*, 273.

Enhanced activity. The antibacterial activity *in vitro* of cephamandole against strains of *Bacteroides fragilis* was increased on average more than 100-fold by erythromycin. An optimum effect was achieved with concentrations of 200 ng per ml for erythromycin and 400 ng per ml for cephamandole.— R. S. Griffith *et al.*, *Antimicrob. Ag. Chemother.*, 1977, *11*, 813.

Synergy was demonstrated *in vitro* in 12 to 46% of 63 strains of *Enterobacter*, *E. coli*, and *Klebsiella* when cephamandole was used with gentamicin or amikacin. For *Enterobacter* and *Klebsiella* synergy was most likely with isolates resistant to cephamandole.— K. P. Fu and H. C. Neu, *J. infect. Dis.*, 1978, *137*, *Suppl.* (May), S38.

Resistance. Strains of *Str. pneumoniae* isolated from 5 children were partially resistant to cephamandole.— P. C. Appelbaum *et al.*, *Lancet*, 1977, *2*, 995.

There was little correlation between beta-lactamase production and decreased susceptibility of strains of Enterobacteriaceae to cephamandole or cefoxitin. It was suggested that other characteristics might be responsible for resistance.— J. L. Ott *et al.*, *Antimicrob. Ag. Chemother.*, 1979, *15*, 14. Studies *in vitro* indicated the presence of cefoxitin-inducible beta-lactamases among many strains of cephalothin-resistant, cephamandole-susceptible Enterobacteriaceae. The enzymes were highly active against cephamandole but less so against cefoxitin.— C. C. Sanders and W. E. Sanders, *ibid.*, 792.

Absorption and Fate. Cephamandole is poorly absorbed from the gastro-intestinal tract. It is given by intramuscular or intravenous injection as the nafate which is rapidly hydrolysed to release cephamandole *in vivo*. Similarly to cephalothin, peak plasma concentrations for cephamandole of at least 12 and 20 µg per ml have been achieved up to 1 hour after intramuscular doses of 0.5 and 1 g respectively; concentrations are very low after 6 hours. Immediately after the intravenous infusion of 1 g over 30 minutes an average plasma concentration of 85 µg per ml has been reported. About 70% is bound to plasma proteins. Plasma half-lives vary from about 0.7 to 1.2 hours depending on the route of injection.

Cephamandole diffuses into the CSF when the meninges are inflamed and penetrates into bone and joint fluid. It is rapidly excreted unchanged by glomerular filtration and renal tubular secretion; about 80% of a dose is excreted within 6 hours and high urinary concentrations are achieved. Probenecid blocks some renal excretion. A small amount of cephamandole is excreted in bile.

Two doses of probenecid 500 mg given 6 hours apart nearly doubled the peak serum concentrations of cephamandole, given in a dose of 1 g intramuscularly, from 20.4 to 37 µg per ml. The half-life of cephamandole was extended from 1.1 to 2 hours with reduction in the rate of urinary excretion.— R. S. Griffith *et al.*, *Antimicrob. Ag. Chemother.*, 1977, *11*, 809.

Blood concentrations and urinary excretion of cephamandole in 30 children and infants (3 months to 13 years) were similar to those previously reported by B.R. Meyers *et al.* (*Antimicrob. Ag. Chemother.*, 1976, *9*, 140) in healthy adults. The half-life for cephamandole following intramuscular administration was about 66 minutes in children under 1 year and 88 minutes in children 1 year or over; half-lives following intravenous injection were about 46 and 48 minutes respectively.— C. T. Chang *et al.*, *Antimicrob. Ag. Chemother.*, 1978, *14*, 838.

In a study of 10 healthy subjects serum concentrations of cephamandole were about 5 times higher than those of cephalothin 0.5 to 1 hour after an intravenous injection of 1 g of cephamandole or cephalothin. The mean serum concentration of cephamandole 3 hours after administration was 2.2 µg per ml compared with less than 0.1 µg per ml for cephalothin.— V. C. Simon *et al.*, *J. antimicrob. Chemother.*, 1978, *4*, 85.

A comparison of the pharmacokinetics of cephamandole and other cephalosporins.— H. C. Neu, *J. infect. Dis.*, 1978, *137*, *Suppl.* (May), S80. See also W. E. Grose *et al.*, *Clin. Pharmac. Ther.*, 1976, *20*, 579; I. W. Fong *et al.*, *Antimicrob. Ag. Chemother.*, 1976, *9*, 65; M. Barza *et al.*, *ibid.*, *10*, 421; R. S. Griffith *et al.*, *Lilly, USA*, *ibid.*, 814.

Cephamandole nafate 1 g was administered intramuscularly to 22 patients with varying degrees of renal function. Mean peak plasma concentrations which occurred 1 to 2 hours after administration ranged from 17 µg per ml in patients with normal renal function to 42 µg per ml in anephric patients. Mean plasma half-lives were 1.49 hours in patients with normal renal function, 2.42 hours in patients with a creatinine clearance rate (CCR) of 39 to 50 ml per minute, 6.03 hours in patients with a CCR of 7 to 20 ml per minute, and 11.48 hours in anephric patients. Haemodialysis resulted in increased elimination of cephamandole. Whereas patients with a CCR of 39 ml or more per minute excreted about 48% of a dose in the urine within 8 hours, patients with a CCR of less than 20 ml per minute excreted only about 17%. Since there was significant variance in calculated plasma half-lives in patients with a CCR of less than 20 ml per minute it was recommended that in these patients doses should be adjusted according to serum-cephamandole concentrations.— A. W. Czerwinski and J. A. Pederson, *Antimicrob. Ag. Chemother.*, 1979, *15*, 161. See also B. R. Meyers and S. Z. Hirschman, *ibid.*, 1977, *11*, 248; H.-E. Mellin *et al.*, *ibid.*, 262; D. Höffler *et al.*, *Dt. med. Wschr.*, 1978, *103*, 1334; J. M. Brogard *et al.*, *J. clin. Pharmac.*, 1979, *19*, 366.

A study on the pharmacokinetics of cephamandole in patients undergoing haemodialysis.— J. G. Gambertoglio *et al.*, *Clin. Pharmac. Ther.*, 1979, *26*, 592. See also R. L. Nielsen *et al.*, *Antimicrob. Ag. Chemother.*, 1979, *16*, 683.

Diffusion. Cephamandole diffused into interstitial fluid. This diffusion was related to the amount of protein binding.— J. S. Tan and S. J. Salstrom, *Antimicrob. Ag. Chemother.*, 1977, *11*, 698.

Cephamandole 37 mg per kg body-weight given intravenously every 6 hours was used successfully to treat 62 children with various infections. Concentrations in the cerebrospinal fluid of 11 children ranged from 0.25 to 2.4 µg per ml; serum concentrations ranged from 0.86 to 30.2 µg per ml. CSF concentrations were 4% of the mean serum concentration in children without active meningitis and 23% of the mean serum concentration in children with active meningitis.— S. H. Walker and V. P. Gahol, *Antimicrob. Ag. Chemother.*, 1978, *14*, 315. See also E. A. Steinberg *et al.*, *ibid.*, 1977, *11*, 933.

The mean peak concentrations of cephamandole, cephazolin, and cephalothin in bile were 352, 46, and 12 µg per ml respectively in 8 patients 30 minutes after receiving 1 g of each antibiotic intravenously on separate occasions; the mean peak serum concentrations were 55.0, 92.8, and 32.4 µg per ml. The amount of cephamandole, cephazolin, and cephalothin excreted in the bile up to 6 hours after administration was 4.12, 1.2, and 0.25 mg respectively.— K. R. Ratzan *et al.*, *Antimicrob. Ag. Chemother.*, 1978, *13*, 985.

Concentrations of cephamandole were achieved in aqueous humour after intravenous injection.— J. L. Axelrod and R. S. Kochman, *Am. J. Ophthal.*, 1978, *85*, 342.

Uses. Cephamandole is a cephalosporin antibiotic and is given, as the nafate, by intramuscular injection, by slow intravenous injection over 3 to 5 minutes, or by intermittent or continuous infusion in the treatment of susceptible infections. The equivalent of 0.5 up to 2 g of cephamandole may be given every 4 to 8 hours depending on the severity of the infection. Children can be given 50 to 150 mg per kg body-weight daily but the maximum adult dose must not be exceeded. Doses should be reduced in impaired renal function.

If necessary, intramuscular injections may be prepared using a 0.5% solution of lignocaine hydrochloride.

Cephamandole lithium is available for use in sensitivity tests *in vitro*.

Proceedings of a symposium on cephamandole.— *J. infect. Dis.*, 1978, *137*, *Suppl.* (May), S1-S194.

For brief reviews of cephamandole, see *Drug & Ther. Bull.*, 1979, *17*, 35; *Med. Lett.*, 1979, *21*, 13.

In a study involving 88 febrile patients with cancer, 36 of 60 infectious episodes responded to treatment with carbenicillin and cephamandole. Carbenicillin 30 g was given daily by intermittent infusion and in addition cephamandole 3 g in 50 ml of dextrose injection was given intravenously over 30 minutes every 6 hours or 3 g was given over 30 minutes followed immediately by the continuous infusion of 3 g in 200 ml of dextrose injection every 6 hours. Response-rates were substantially better in severely neutropenic patients when cephamandole was given by continuous infusion, otherwise there was no significant difference between the 2 regimens.— G. P. Bodey *et al.*, *J. infect. Dis.*, 1978, *137*, *Suppl.* (May), S139. See also *idem*, *Am. J. Med.*, 1979, *67*, 608.

Cephamandole was successfully used in association with gentamicin or tobramycin to treat severe Gram-negative infections in 31 patients. Creatinine clearance values remained within the normal range.— L. O. Gentry, *J. infect. Dis.*, 1978, *137*, *Suppl.* (May), S144.

Further references: W. Rosett *et al.*, *Am. J. med. Sci.*, 1977, *274*, 153.

Anaerobic infections. Cephamandole 2 g was given every 3 to 4 hours by intravenous infusion over 10 to 20 minutes (dosage adjusted in renal failure) to 31 patients with anaerobic infections. Some patients also received tobramycin. Of 27 patients evaluated after 5 days of therapy 26 had a satisfactory response but a significant number of adverse effects was encountered at this high dose. Adverse effects included a positive Coombs' test (6), transient liver function abnormalities (6), phlebitis (6), reversible neutropenia (3), fever (1), eosinophilia (2), and toxic epidermal necrolysis (1).— R. N. Greenberg *et al.*, *Antimicrob. Ag. Chemother.*, 1979, *15*, 337.

Dosage in infants and children. Cephamandole 100 mg per kg body-weight daily was given intravenously in divided doses every 6 hours for 5 to 17 days to 47 children (4 months to 17 years) who had infections which included bacteraemia, ethmoiditis and periorbital cellulitis, soft tissue infection, pneumonia, and lymphadenitis. The clinical response was prompt in all but 2 patients who developed a generalised erythematous and/or pruritic rash and were withdrawn from treatment. Eosinophilia occurred in 18 patients.— P. H. Azimi, *Antimicrob. Ag. Chemother.*, 1978, *13*, 955. A further report of the use of cephamandole in infants and children.— W. J. Rodriguez *et al.*, *J. infect. Dis.*, 1978, *137*, *Suppl.* (May), S150.

Cephamandole 33 mg per kg body-weight given intramuscularly every 8 hours for 6 to 9 days was successful in the treatment of 23 neonates with pustular skin infections produced by *Staph. aureus*. Serum concentrations of cephamandole were similar when given intramuscularly or intravenously producing higher serum concentrations and longer half-lives than those observed in older infants and children.— M. M. Agbayani *et al.*, *Antimicrob. Ag. Chemother.*, 1979, *15*, 674.

Dosage in renal failure. Although cephamandole nafate given intramuscularly to 11 patients with chronic renal failure was not significantly removed from the serum during haemodialysis or peritoneal dialysis, it was considered that an initial loading dose calculated as 186 mg per m^2 body-surface should be used during dialysis followed by half this dose every half-life (7.2 hours during peritoneal dialysis and 6.6 hours during haemodialysis).— M. J. Ahern *et al.*, *Antimicrob. Ag. Chemother.*, 1976, *10*, 457. In a similar study involving 15 patients with stable chronic renal failure and given cephamandole nafate 1 g by intravenous injection, the half-life of 7.7 hours for cephamandole was reduced to about 6 hours by haemodialysis. It was considered that intravenous doses should be given 24 hours apart to patients with severe renal failure and that this would also apply in those undergoing haemodialysis; as long as a patient had received a dose just before haemodialysis an additional dose would not be required at the end of dialysis.— G. B. Appel *et al.*, *ibid.*, 623.

The normal half-life for cephamandole of 1 hour was increased to 11 hours in end-stage renal failure. The interval between doses should be extended from 4 to 6 hours to 6 hours in patients with a glomerular filtration-rate (GFR) above 50 ml per minute, to 6 to 9 hours in those with a GFR of 10 to 50 ml per minute, and to 9 hours in those with a GFR of less than 10 ml per minute. Alternatively, doses could be reduced to 25 to 50% and 25% in those with a GFR of 10 to 50 ml and less than 10 ml per minute respectively. Concentrations of cephamandole were affected by haemodialysis.— W. M. Bennett *et al.*, *Ann. intern. Med.*, 1980, *93*, 62.

See also under Absorption and Fate (above).

Haemophilus infections. The view that cephamandole should not be used for the treatment of serious, invasive *Haemophilus* infections. *H. influenzae* meningitis has been reported to occur during therapy and cephamandole has been found relatively inefficient in the treatment of such meningitis.— M. I. Marks, *J. Pediat.*, 1981, *98*, 910. See also P. H. Azimi and P. A. Chase, *ibid.*, 995; S. A. Chartrand *et al.*, *ibid.*, 1003.

See also under Meningitis (below).

Meningitis. Of 26 patients with purulent meningitis (16 due to *N. meningitidis*, 3 to *H. influenzae*, 1 to *Str. pneumoniae*, and 6 unclassified) 24 recovered, including the 3 infected with *H. influenzae*, after treatment with cephamandole 175 to 200 mg per kg body-weight daily given intravenously in 6 divided doses.— O. M. Korzeniowski *et al.*, *J. infect. Dis.*, 1978, *137*, *Suppl.* (May), S169. Treatment with cephamandole 200 mg per kg body-weight daily intravenously failed to eradicate the infection in 3 children with *H. influenzae* type b meningitis, despite susceptibility *in vitro* and evidence of penetration into the CSF.— E. A. Steinberg *et al.*, *ibid.*, S180. Cephamandole was not recommended for the treatment of ampicillin-resistant *H. influenzae* meningitis because of the inoculum effect noted *in vitro*.— V. P. Syriopoulou *et al.*, *Antimicrob. Ag. Chemother.*, 1979, *16*, 510.

See also Haemophilus Infections (above).

Open-heart surgery. No infections occurred in 30 patients up to 6 months after undergoing prosthetic cardiac valve insertion after they received an intramuscular injection of 20 mg per kg body-weight of cephamandole or cephalothin before surgery. Plasma concentrations 30 minutes after injection ranged from 25 to 66 μg per ml for cephamandole and from 20 to 40 μg per ml for cephalothin and remained above 6 μg per ml for both antibiotics during the period of cardiopulmonary bypass. Although cephamandole was found in atrial muscle and valve tissue in all of 15 patients who received cephamandole, concentrations of cephalothin were undetectable in similar samples in the majority of patients who received cephalothin.— G. L. Archer *et al.*, *Antimicrob. Ag. Chemother.*, 1978, *13*, 924.

In 16 patients undergoing cardiopulmonary bypass surgery lasting up to 220 minutes and given cephamandole 20 mg per kg body-weight by intravenous infusion over 15 minutes at the time of anaesthesia induction, the mean half-life of cephamandole during bypass (113.2 minutes) was significantly increased compared to the mean terminal half-life (52 minutes) in 5 healthy subjects. Throughout the procedure plasma-cephamandole concentrations were maintained above the minimum inhibitory concentration for those organisms most likely to cause postoperative infection. It was concluded that if a dose of 20 mg per kg is given within an hour of the start of cardiovascular surgery a supplemental dose is not needed until the patient has been on cardiopulmonary bypass for at least 4 hours.— R. E. Polk *et al.*, *Clin. Pharmac. Ther.*, 1978, *23*, 473.

Pneumonia. In a randomised double-blind study there was no significant difference in the response or cure-rate of 96 patients with clinical and radiographic evidence of pneumonia who received cephamandole 1 g or benzylpenicillin 360 mg intravenously every 6 hours. Of the 49 patients with pneumonia due to *Str. pneumoniae* alone, all 24 treated with cephamandole and all 25 treated with benzylpenicillin responded to therapy. There was no significant difference in the number of side-effects reported by 93 of the patients evaluated who received benzylpenicillin or cephamandole, although 1 patient receiving cephamandole developed a positive direct Coombs' test.— B. G. Petty *et al.*, *Antimicrob. Ag. Chemother.*, 1978, *14*, 13.

Further references: C. A. Perlino and M. E. Plaut, *Curr. ther. Res.*, 1977, *22*, 807; I. V. Hoverman and L. O. Gentry, *ibid.*, 1978, *24*, 622; M. E. Plaut and C. A. Perlino, *J. infect. Dis.*, 1978, *137*, *Suppl.* (May), S133.

Salmonellal infections. The successful management of *S. typhi* bacteraemia in 1 patient with cephamandole 2 g intravenously every 6 hours for 14 days.— S. Z. Hirschman *et al.*, *Antimicrob. Ag. Chemother.*, 1977, *11*, 369.

Urinary-tract infections. Eleven of 26 patients with pyelonephritis and 3 of 5 with cystitis were re-infected with the same or different organisms within 10 days of completing at least 5 days of therapy with cephamandole 1.5 to 8 g given daily by intravenous or intramuscular injection in divided doses. The number of re-infections produced by *Pseudomonas aeruginosa* suggested that the use of cephamandole could lead to secondary infections by such resistant organisms. One patient developed a maculopapular rash and 3 patients who received intramuscular therapy complained of pain at the site of injection.— H. D. Short *et al.*, *J. antimicrob. Chemother.*, 1976, *2*, 345.

Cephamandole or cephazolin 500 mg given intramuscularly every 8 hours for 7 days were equally effective in the treatment of complicated urinary-tract infections in 65 elderly men.— U. Hoyme and P. O. Madsen, *J. infect. Dis.*, 1978, *137*, *Suppl.* (May), S100.

Preparations

Cefamandole Nafate for Injection *(U.S.P.)*. A sterile mixture of cephamandole nafate and one or more suitable buffers. Potency is expressed in terms of the equivalent amount of cephamandole. pH of a 10% solution 6 to 8.

Kefadol *(Lilly, UK)*. Cephamandole nafate, available as powder for preparing injections, in vials each containing the equivalent of 0.5, 1, or 2 g of cephamandole, with anhydrous sodium carbonate equivalent to about 1.2 mmol (1.2 mEq) of sodium per g of cephamandole.

Continued production of carbon dioxide after the repackaging of reconstituted solutions of Mandol (cephamandole nafate) into syringes led to an explosive-like reaction in which the rubber closure was forced out of the syringe body.— M. A. Palmer and C. C. Fraterrigo (letter), *Am. J. Hosp. Pharm.*, 1979, *36*, 596; *idem*, 1025. When intended for intramuscular or direct intravenous injection Mandol solution should be left in the original containers and withdrawn into syringes immediately before use.— P. R. Klink and C. W. McKeehan, *Lilly, USA* (letter), *ibid.*, 597.

Other Proprietary Names of Cephamandole Nafate

Mandokef *(Denm., Ger., S.Afr., Spain, Switz.)*; Mandol *(Austral., Canad., Neth., NZ, USA)*.

44-m

Cephazolin Sodium.

46083; SKF 41558; Cefazolin Sodium. Sodium (7*R*)-3-(5-methyl-1,3,4-thiadiazol-2-ylthiomethyl)-7-[2-(1*H*-tetrazol-1-yl)acetamido]-3-cephem-4-carboxylate.
$C_{14}H_{13}N_8NaO_4S_3$=476.5.

CAS — 25953-19-9 (cephazolin); 27164-46-1 (sodium salt).

Pharmacopoeias. U.S.P. includes Sterile Cefazolin Sodium.

A white to off-white almost odourless crystalline powder with a bitter taste. Each g represents about 2.1 mmol (2.1 mEq) of sodium. Cephazolin sodium 1.05 g is approximately equivalent to 1 g of cephazolin.

Freely **soluble** in water; slightly soluble in methyl alcohol; very slightly soluble in alcohol; practically insoluble in acetone, ether, and chloroform. A 10% solution in water has a pH of 4.5 to 6.

Injections of cephazolin sodium should be used within 24 hours when stored at room temperature, or within 96 hours when stored at a temperature between 2° and 10°. Refrigerated solutions should be warmed gently before administration to dissolve any crystals.

Cephazolin sodium is stated to be **incompatible** with amylobarbitone sodium, calcium gluceptate, calcium gluconate, chlortetracycline hydrochloride, colistin sulphomethate sodium, erythromycin gluceptate, kanamycin sulphate, oxytetracycline hydrochloride, pentobarbitone sodium, polymyxin B sulphate, and tetracycline hydrochloride. With amikacin sulphate turbidity is reported to develop after 8 hours.

The initial pH of a 0.5 to a 33% solution of cephazolin sodium in Water for Injections ranged from 5.37 to 5.60.— M. Bornstein *et al.*, *Am. J. Hosp. Pharm.*, 1974, *31*, 296.

Cephazolin sodium when added to either sodium chloride 0.9% or dextrose 5% in water to give concentrations of 10 mg per ml for intermittent infusion, may be filtered through a Millipore membrane filter without adversely affecting the concentration of active drug.— D. J. Stennett *et al.*, *Am. J. Hosp. Pharm.*, 1979, *36*, 657.

Stability. There was a mean loss in activity of about 36% when cephalothin was incubated for 5 hours in human serum at 37° in the presence of air. Cephazolin lost about 4% activity under the same conditions.— D. Pitkin *et al.*, *Antimicrob. Ag. Chemother.*, 1977, *12*, 284. See also M. A. Foglesong, *ibid.*, *11*, 174.

Stability in solution. Cephazolin sodium 500 mg in 100 ml was stable at 5° or 25° in Water for Injections, sodium chloride injection 0.9%, dextrose injection 5%, or lactated ringer's injection.— M. Bornstein *et al.*, *Am. J. Hosp. Pharm.*, 1974, *31*, 296.

Adverse Effects. Side-effects are similar to those of cephalothin sodium (p.1128) but phlebitis after the intravenous administration of cephazolin sodium and pain after intramuscular injection appear to be less frequent.

A 31-year-old man given cephazolin intramuscularly for infection due to *Listeria monocytogenes* developed meningitis. Cephazolin did not reliably penetrate the CSF. It should not be used in bacterial meningitis and only with caution in infections that might result in meningitis.— B. Lorber *et al.* (letter), *Ann. intern. Med.*, 1975, *82*, 226. See also B. Ribner *et al.* (letter), *ibid.*, *83*, 37.

Blood disorders. In 20 patients treated with cephazolin 1.5 to 4 g daily for 7 to 70 days, mainly for respiratory or urinary-tract infections, haematologic side-effects were transient and included leucopenia in 1 patient, eosinophilia in 2, slight thrombocytopenia in 2, and positive conversion of direct Coombs' test in 4. Anaemia present in 8 patients prior to therapy worsened slightly in 2, and 5 patients became anaemic during treatment.— M. Nakamura *et al.*, *Arzneimittel-Forsch.*, 1973, *23*, 1260.

Increased thrombin, prothrombin, and partial thromboplastin times were noted in a patient 12 days after the start of cephazolin therapy 0.5 g every 8 hours. These returned to normal 48 hours after stopping cephazolin but abnormalities recurred within 10 days of starting a second course.— P. I. Lerner and A. Lubin (letter), *New Engl. J. Med.*, 1974, *290*, 1324.

Colitis. For reports of pseudomembranous colitis associated with cephazolin, see H. J. Fee *et al.*, *Am. J. Surg.*, 1977, *133*, 247; J. F. Tures *et al.*, *J. Am. med. Ass.*, 1976, *236*, 948.

Neurotoxicity. Convulsions in a 52-year-old man with renal failure were associated with treatment with cephazolin 12 g daily later reduced to 2 g daily.— M. E. Gardner *et al.*, *Drug Intell. & clin. Pharm.*, 1978, *12*, 268. See also R. L. Yost *et al.*, *Am. Surg.*, 1977, *43*, 417.

Precautions. As for Cephaloridine, p.1126.

It is recommended that cephazolin should be given with care and in reduced dosage to patients with renal impairment.

The serum-protein binding of cephazolin fell from an average of 72.5 down to an average of 22.4% in 12 uraemic patients who underwent dialysis.— D. S. Greene and A. D. Tice, *J. pharm. Sci.*, 1977, *66*, 1508.

Antimicrobial Action. As for Cephaloridine, p.1126. It is more active against *Escherichia coli*. Cephazolin is considered to be more susceptible to beta-lactamases than other cephalosporins.

Apart from a few strains of *E. coli* most Gram-negative organisms resistant to cephalothin were also resistant to cephazolin.— J. P. Phair *et al.*, *Antimicrob. Ag. Chemother.*, 1972, *2*, 329.

The antibacterial activity of cephazolin was compared with that of cephalexin, cephaloridine, and cephalothin against various Gram-negative organisms. Cephazolin was the most active against *E. coli* and *Shigella* spp. Against *Salmonella* spp. its activity was equivalent to cephalexin and cephaloridine and greater than cephalothin. Against *Klebsiella* cephazolin was more active than cephaloridine or cephalexin but less active than cephalothin.— C. Campello *et al.*, *G. Mal. infett. parassit.*, 1973, *25*, 407, per *Abstr. Hyg.*, 1974, *49*, 143.

Cephazolin was active *in vitro* against ampicillin-susceptible and resistant strains of *E. coli* in lower concentrations than other cephalosporins.— D. Greenwood *et al.*, *Antimicrob. Ag. Chemother.*, 1975, *7*, 191.

Cephazolin and then cephaloridine underwent the greatest inactivation by beta-lactamase-producing *Staph. aureus* in a study of 8 cephalosporins.— I. W. Fong *et al.*, *Antimicrob. Ag. Chemother.*, 1976, *9*, 939. See also C. Regamey *et al.*, *J. infect. Dis.*, 1975, *131*, 291.

Tests *in vitro* showed that 63% of 38 strains of *Enterobacter* and 50% of 252 strains of *Klebsiella* were resistant to cephazolin.— C. Krasemann and C. Peckelsen, *Dt. med. Wschr.*, 1977, *102*, 87.

Enhanced activity. For reports of cephazolin with other antibiotics showing enhanced activity against enterococci *in vitro*, see M. Bourque *et al.*, *Antimicrob. Ag. Chemother.*, 1976, *10*, 157 (gentamicin); J. Klastersky *et al.*, *J. infect. Dis.*, 1976, *134*, 271 (amikacin); H. C. Neu and K. P. Fu, *Antimicrob. Ag. Chemother.*, 1978, *13*, 813 (azlocillin).

Enhanced activity *in vitro* with cephazolin and amikacin against 7 of 9 oxacillin-resistant strains of *Staph. aureus*.— J. Levy and J. Klastersky, *J. antimicrob. Chemother.*, 1979, *5*, 365.

Absorption and Fate. Cephazolin sodium is poorly absorbed from the gastro-intestinal tract and is given by intramuscular or intravenous injection. Following a dose of 500 mg given intramuscularly, peak plasma concentrations of 30 µg or more per ml are obtained within 1 hour and measurable amounts are present at least 8 hours after a dose; these concentrations are higher than those achieved with equivalent doses of cephaloridine and cephalothin. Up to 90% of cephazolin may be bound loosely to plasma proteins and the plasma half-life in patients with normal renal function is about 1.8 hours. Cephazolin diffuses into bone and ascitic, pleural, and synovial fluid but not appreciably into the cerebrospinal fluid. It diffuses across the placenta into the foetal circulation and low concentrations are excreted in the milk of nursing mothers.

Cephazolin is excreted unchanged in the urine, mainly by glomerular filtration with some renal tubular secretion, at least 80% of a dose given intramuscularly being excreted within 24 hours. Urine concentrations of more than 1 and 4 mg per ml have been reported after intramuscular doses of 0.5 and 1 g respectively. High biliary concentrations have been reported.

A review.— C. H. Nightingale *et al.*, *J. pharm. Sci.*, 1975, *64*, 1899.

After an intramuscular injection of 500 mg of cephazolin in 3 healthy subjects, the peak serum concentrations and urine concentrations were 34.1 µg per ml and 4 mg per ml respectively after 1 hour and 6.2 µg per ml and 20.6 µg per ml respectively after 6 hours. An average of 62.6% of the drug was excreted in the urine within 6 hours.— S. Ishiyama *et al.*, *Antimicrob. Ag. Chemother.*, 1970, 476.

Cephazolin, given by intramuscular injection in an average dose of 14.9 mg per kg body-weight to 10 volunteers produced a peak serum concentration of 52.2 µg per ml 2 hours later, with a mean serum half-life of 153 minutes. Over 80% of the dose was excreted in the urine within 8 hours. These injections prepared in sodium chloride injection caused pain lasting up to 4 hours. Similar doses given intravenously in 100 ml of dextrose injection over 30 minutes to 10 other volunteers produced a mean peak serum concentration of 143.6 µg per ml within 30 minutes, with a serum half-life of 69 minutes. Over 90% of the dose was excreted within 8 hours.— P. Nicholas *et al.*, *J. clin. Pharmac.*, 1973, *13*, 325. See also P. De Schepper *et al.*, *ibid.*, 83.

Comparisons of the pharmacokinetics of cephazolin with those of other cephalosporins.— W. M. M. Kirby and C. Regamey, *J. infect. Dis.*, 1973, *128*, *Suppl.*, S341; T. Bergan, *Chemotherapy, Basle*, 1977, *23*, 389.

The biliary excretion of cephazolin.— K. R. Ratzan *et al.*, *Antimicrob. Ag. Chemother.*, 1974, *6*, 426; J. M. Brogard *et al.*, *J. infect. Dis.*, 1975, *131*, 625; A. R. McLeish *et al.*, *Surgery, St Louis*, 1977, *81*, 426.

In 10 healthy subjects given cephazolin 500 mg intramuscularly the mean half-life was about 2.2 hours. About 48% of the dose was recovered from the urine within 6 hours. In 10 patients on dialysis administration of the same dose of cephazolin between treatments produced a mean peak serum concentration of 73.2 µg per ml, falling to 43.1 µg per ml at 12 hours, and 34.2 µg per ml at 24 hours, with an average half-life of 25.7 hours. When cephazolin was administered at the beginning of dialysis the mean peak concentration was similar, but decreased more rapidly to 24.9 µg per ml at 6 hours, with a half-life of 3.3 hours.— J. M. Brogard *et al.*, *J. clin. Pharmac.*, 1977, *17*, 225. For further studies in patients with renal impairment, see also A. Leroy *et al.*, *Curr. ther. Res.*, 1974, *16*, 878; C. P. Craig and S. I. Rifkin, *Clin. Pharmac. Ther.*, 1976, *19*, 825; L. B. Hiner *et al.*, *J. Pediat.*, 1980, *96*, 335.

Further references to pharmacokinetic studies of cephazolin: A. G. Paradelis *et al.*, *Arzneimittel-Forsch.*, 1977, *27*, 2167; R. D. Smyth *et al.*, *Antimicrob. Ag. Chemother.*, 1979, *16*, 615 (high doses); K. W. Miller *et al.*, *Clin. Pharmac. Ther.*, 1980, *27*, 550 (effect of cardiopulmonary bypass).

Diffusion. Cephazolin given intravenously diffused poorly into the interstitial fluid and this was a reflection of its high degree of protein binding.— J. S. Tan and S. J. Salstrom, *Antimicrob. Ag. Chemother.*, 1977, *11*, 698. Contrary results following intramuscular injection were found in *rabbits*.— C. Carbon *et al.*, *ibid.*, 594.

Cephazolin penetrated the pleural fluid to achieve effective therapeutic concentrations in spite of a high degree of protein-binding. Mean concentrations at 30, 60, and 120 minutes were 37, 15, and 12 µg per ml in patients from a group of 9 given 1 g intravenously. A dose of 0.5 g given intramuscularly to another 9 produced mean concentrations of 9, 15, and 53 µg per ml at 60, 120, and 240 minutes.— D. R. Cole and J. Pung, *Antimicrob. Ag. Chemother.*, 1977, *11*, 1033.

Cephazolin 50 mg per kg body-weight daily was given intravenously for 14 to 21 days to 4 children with osteomyelitis. Concentrations in pus ranged from 5.5 to 13.3 µg per ml and in bone from 3.2 to 5.5 µg per g. In 4 similar children given cephazolin intramuscularly, concentrations in pus ranged from 8.7 to 9.8 µg per ml; concentrations of 3.1 and 3.2 µg per g were achieved in 2 of 3 bone specimens available but antimicrobial activity was not detected in the third specimen. Mean values generally exceeded the minimum bactericidal concentration for *Staphylococcus aureus*. The penetration of cephazolin in pus was 15% and in bone 7% of the peak serum concentration.— T. R. Tetzlaff *et al.*, *J. Pediat.*, 1978, *92*, 135.

Satisfactory concentrations of cephazolin were achieved in bone, hip capsule, and plasma when 4 g was given intravenously to 7 patients before hip joint replacement.— R. L. Parsons *et al.*, *Br. J. clin. Pharmac.*, 1978, *5*, 331. See also *idem*, *J. antimicrob. Chemother.*, 1976, *2*, 228.

Further references to the diffusion of cephazolin: C. H. Nightingale *et al.*, *Antimicrob. Ag. Chemother.*, 1980, *17*, 595 (atrial appendage and pericardial fluids); J. H. Saunders and S. D. McPherson, *Am. J. Ophthal.*, 1980, *89*, 564 (ocular penetration after subconjunctival injection); N. Yamada *et al.*, *Am. J. Obstet. Gynec.*, 1980, *136*, 1036 (uterine tissue).

Pregnancy and the neonate. Reports of the transplacental diffusion of cephazolin.— B. Bernard *et al.*, *J. infect. Dis.*, 1977, *136*, 377; A. Dekel *et al.*, *Harefuah*, 1977, *93*, 133.

The transfer of cephazolin into breast milk.— H. Yoshioka *et al.*, *J. Pediat.*, 1979, *94*, 151.

Uses. Cephazolin sodium is a cephalosporin antibiotic with the actions and uses of Cephaloridine, p.1127.

The usual adult dose is the equivalent of 500 mg of cephazolin every 12 hours by intramuscular or slow intravenous injection over 3 to 5 minutes or by infusion, increased if necessary to 0.5 to 1 g every 6 hours; 6 g daily has been given in severe infections. Children over 1 month may be given 25 to 50 mg per kg body-weight daily in divided doses increased in severe infections to a maximum of 100 mg per kg daily.

Reduced doses should be employed in patients with impaired renal function. After a loading dose of 500 mg patients with anuria may be given up to 200 mg every 24 hours; with a creatinine clearance below 20 ml per minute maintenance doses of 75 to 400 mg may be given every 24 hours and with clearances below 40 and 70 ml per minute doses of 125 to 600 mg and 0.25 to 1.25 g respectively may be given every 12 hours.

Reports and reviews of cephazolin.— *J. infect. Dis.*, 1973, *128*, *Suppl.* (Oct.), S307-S424; *Med. Lett.*, 1974, *16*, 1; *Drug & Ther. Bull.*, 1974, *12*, 95; R. Quintiliani and C. H. Nightingale, *Ann. intern. Med.*, 1978, *89*, 650.

All of 13 children with pneumonia due to various organisms and 7 of 9 with urinary-tract infection chiefly due to *E. coli* responded satisfactorily to treatment with cephazolin 25 to 50 (mean 28.5) mg per kg body-weight daily in 4 doses by intramuscular injection. Two children with urinary-tract infection developed supra-infection due to *Pseudomonas*. Mean peak serum concentrations in 10 children who received 6.26 mg per kg were 33.6 µg per ml at 30 minutes falling to 5.9 µg per ml at 4 hours; about 75% of the dose was recovered in the urine. Three children developed a mild eosinophilia, 1 a rash possibly due to cephazolin, and 1 minor changes in liver-function tests.— A. J. Khan, *Curr. ther. Res.*, 1973, *15*, 727.

For a report of the similar efficacy of cephazolin and cephradine when given intravenously to 180 patients, see Cephradine, p.1136.

Administration, intraperitoneal. From results of a study in 9 patients undergoing peritoneal dialysis it appeared that a suitable intraperitoneal dose for cephazolin would be 150 mg added to each litre of dialysis fluid with an additional initial dose of 250 to 500 mg given parenterally. Intraperitoneal administration of cephazolin was generally well tolerated but one patient developed abdominal pain.— D. Kaye *et al.*, *Antimicrob. Ag. Chemother.*, 1978, *14*, 318.

Dosage in renal failure. Haemodialysis over 4 hours removed about 46% of cephazolin and patients undergoing haemodialysis should receive a further half dose after haemodialysis. Peritoneal dialysis did not affect the half-life of cephazolin.— T. Madhavan *et al.*, *Antimicrob. Ag. Chemother.*, 1975, *8*, 63.

The normal half-life for cephazolin of 1.4 to 2.2 hours was increased to 18 to 36 hours in end-stage renal failure. The interval between doses should be extended from 8 hours to 12 hours in those with a glomerular filtration-rate (GFR) of 10 to 50 ml per minute, and to 24 to 48 hours in those with a GFR of less than 10 ml per minute. Alternatively, doses could be reduced to 50% and 25% in those with a GFR of 10 to 50 and less than 10 ml per minute respectively. Concentrations of cephazolin were affected by haemodialysis but not by peritoneal dialysis.— W. M. Bennett *et al.*, *Ann. intern. Med.*, 1977, *86*, 754. See also *idem*, 1980, *93*, 62; C. P. Craig and S. I. Rifkin, *Clin. Pharmac. Ther.*, 1976, *19*, 825; P. Sharpstone, *Br. med. J.*, 1977, *2*, 36.

After a loading dose of 500 mg cephazolin could be given in the usual dose to patients with a creatinine clearance of 60 to 80 ml per minute, 250 mg every 6 hours to those with a clearance of 30 to 50 ml per minute, 250 mg every 6 to 12 hours to those with a clearance of 10 to 20 ml per minute, and 250 mg every 48 hours to those with a clearance of 5 ml per minute. In haemodialysis 250 mg could be given every 48 hours and 250 mg after dialysis.— J. S. Cheigh, *Am. J. Med.*, 1977, *62*, 555.

Although the rate of absorption was not appreciably influenced by renal function, elimination of cephazolin was prolonged in patients with impairment. It was recommended that for a 500-mg dose given intramuscularly the interval between doses should be 8, 12, 24, and 36 hours for patients with creatinine clearances of 60, 30 to 60, 15 to 30, and 15 ml per minute respectively.— T. Bergan *et al.*, *J. antimicrob. Chemother.*, 1977, *3*, 435.

Data for predicting removal of cephazolin by conventional haemodialysis.— T. P. Gibson and H. A. Nelson, *Clin. Pharmacokinet.*, 1977, *2*, 403.

Further references: A. Leroy *et al.*, *Curr. ther. Res.*, 1974, *16*, 878; J. M. Brogard *et al.*, *J. clin. Pharmac.*, 1977, *17*, 225.

Endocarditis. A report of 2 patients with staphylococcal endocarditis treated unsuccessfully with cephazolin.— R. E. Bryant and R. H. Alford, *J. Am. med. Ass.*, 1977, *237*, 569. Cephazolin was considered to be of value in endocarditis due to *Staph. aureus*.— D. Kaye *et al.* (letter), *ibid.*, 2601. See also R. E. Bryant and R. H. Alford (letter), *ibid.*, 1978, *239*, 1130; D. Kaye *et al.* (letter), *ibid.*

Osteomyelitis. Cephazolin 4 to 8 g given intravenously or intramuscularly daily for 10 to 90 days cured 15 of 16 episodes of severe osteomyelitis or septic arthritis or both in 15 patients. Eight patients subsequently received cephalexin 1 to 4 g daily and one received ampicillin 2 g daily, all by mouth. Peak concentrations of cephazolin in serum ranged from 25 to 216 µg per ml in 11 patients and peak concentrations in bone from 5 patients ranged from less than 0.6 to 10.6 µg per g. Infecting organisms included *Staphylococcus aureus*, Streptococci, *E. coli, Klebsiella pneumoniae, Proteus mirabilis, Neisseria gonorrhoeae*, and *Salmonella enteritidis*.— R. J. Fass, *Antimicrob. Ag. Chemother.*, 1978, *13*, 405.

Respiratory infections. For reports on the use of cephazolin in the treatment of respiratory-tract infections, see A. Pines *et al.*, *Chemotherapy, Basle*, 1977, *23*, 114 (bronchitis); M. J. Raff *et al.*, *Int. J. clin. Pharmac. Biopharm.*, 1978, *16*, 78 (pneumonia); S. G. Jenkinson *et al.*, *J. Am. med. Ass.*, 1979, *241*, 2815 (pneumococcal pneumonia); G. R. Plotkin (letter), *ibid.*, *242*, 1848 (criticism); S. G. Jenkinson (letter), *ibid* (reply).

Salmonellal infections. Nine patients with acute enteric fever due in 7 to *Salmonella typhi* and in 2 to *S. paratyphi* B were effectively treated with cephazolin 3 to 6 g by intravenous or intramuscular injection daily in divided doses for 11 to 16 days. One patient relapsed during a follow-up period of 5 to 8 weeks. Intravenous administration was associated with frequent and severe phlebitis.— M. Uwaydah, *Antimicrob. Ag. Chemother.*, 1976, *10*, 52.

Surgical infection prophylaxis. The incidence of wound sepsis was 16.9% in 65 patients after cholecystectomy, 3.2% in 63 similar patients given cephazolin sodium 1 g intramuscularly 1 hour before surgery, and 5.5% in 73 patients given 1 g before surgery and 500 mg every 8 hours for 5 days postoperatively.— C. J. L. Strachan *et al.*, *Br. med. J.*, 1977, *1*, 1254.

In a randomised clinical study 250 women undergoing abdominal or vaginal hysterectomy received peri-operative cephazolin while 265 similar women received placebo. In both the vaginal and the abdominal hysterectomy groups patients receiving cephazolin had significantly lower rates of standard febrile morbidity, received fewer therapeutic courses of antibiotics, and had shorter hospital stays. There was no increase in side-effects in the cephazolin group. Cephazolin was given intramuscularly in a dose of 1 g one to two hours before surgery, followed by second and third doses 6 and 12 hours after the first.— B. F. Polk *et al.*, *Lancet*, 1980, *1*, 437.

In a placebo-controlled study of prophylactic cephazolin in total hip replacement, benefit was restricted to patients undergoing surgery in conventional rather than 'hypersterile' operating theatres. Cephazolin was given in doses of 1 g every 6 hours, starting at induction of anaesthesia.— C. Hill *et al.*, *Lancet*, 1981, *1*, 795.

Further references to surgical infection prophylaxis with cephazolin: H. H. Stone *et al.*, *Ann. Surg.*, 1976, *184*, 443 (gastric, biliary, or colonic surgery); G. Wewalka and M. Endler, *Arzneimittel-Forsch.*, 1978, *28*, 72 (orthopaedic surgery); R. Wong *et al.*, *Obstet. Gynec.*, 1978, *51*, 407 (caesarean section); J. P. Phelan and S. C. Pruyn, *Am. J. Obstet. Gynec.*, 1979, *133*, 474 (caesarean section); R. C. Kester *et al.*, *Curr. med. Res. Opinion.*, 1979, *6*, 44 (peripheral vascular reconstruction or amputation).

Urinary-tract infections. For a report that cephazolin and cephamandole were equally effective in the treatment of urinary-tract infections, see Cephamandole, p.1133.

For the failure of cephazolin sodium to prevent catheter-associated bacteriuria, see Prophylactic Use of Antibiotics, p.1081.

Preparations

Sterile Cefazolin Sodium *(U.S.P.)*. A grade of cephazolin sodium for injection. Potency is expressed in terms of the equivalent amount of cephazolin.

Kefzol *(Lilly, UK)*. Cephazolin sodium, available as powder for preparing injections, in vials each containing the equivalent of 0.5 or 1 g of cephazolin. (Also available as Kefzol in *Austral., Belg., Canad., Denm., Fr., Neth., S.Afr., Switz., USA*).

Other Proprietary Names

Arg.—Cefalomicina; *Belg.*—Cefacidal; *Canad.*—Ancef; *Denm.*—Cefacidal; *Fr.*—Céfacidal; *Ger.*—Elzogram, Gramaxin, Zolicef; *Ital.*—Acef, Atirin, Cefamezin, Cefazina, Cromezin, Kezolin, Recef, Totacef, Zolin, Zolisint; *Neth.*—Cefacidal; *Spain*—Areuzolin, Brizolina, Caricef, Cefamezin, Fidesporin, Kefol, Lifezolina, Novaporin; *Swed.*—Celmetin; *USA*—Ancef.

180-e

Cephoxazole Sodium. Cefoxazole Sodium; 291/1 (acid). Sodium (7*R*)-7-[3-(2-chlorophenyl)-5-methylisoxazole-4-carboxamido]cephalosporanate; Sodium (7*R*)-3-acetoxymethyl-7-[3-(2-chlorophenyl)-5-methylisoxazole-4-carboxamido]ceph-3-em-4-carboxylate. $C_{21}H_{17}ClN_3NaO_7S$=513.9.

CAS — 36920-48-6 (cephoxazole).

Cephoxazole sodium is a cephalosporin antibiotic used in veterinary practice.

Manufacturers
Glaxo, UK.

45-b

Cephradine *(B.P., U.S.P.)*. SQ 11436; Cefradine. (7*R*)-7-(α-D-Cyclohexa-1,4-dienylglycylamino)-3-methyl-3-cephem-4-carboxylic acid. $C_{16}H_{19}N_3O_4S$=349.4.

CAS — 38821-53-3.

Pharmacopoeias. In *Br.* and *U.S.* which also includes Sterile Cephradine

A white to cream-coloured crystalline powder with a characteristic odour. *B.P.* specifies not less than 95% of cephradine and *U.S.P.* not less than 900 μg per mg, both calculated on the anhydrous basis. **Soluble** 1 in about 50 of water at pH 6; less soluble at acid or neutral pH; soluble 1 in 70 of methyl alcohol; freely soluble in propylene glycol; sparingly soluble in acetone; practically insoluble in alcohol, chloroform, and ether. A 1% solution in water has a pH of 3.5 to 6. **Store** at a temperature not exceeding 30°. Protect from light.

Injections of cephradine should be used within 2 hours when stored at room temperature or within 24 hours if stored at 5°. Some injections contain sodium carbonate and are **incompatible** with solutions such as compound sodium lactate injection which contain calcium salts.

The addition of 2% procaine hydrochloride to intramuscular injections of cephradine in 16 subjects did not significantly alter the bioavailability of cephradine compared with similar injections reconstituted with sterile water.— R. A. Vukovich *et al.*, *Curr. ther. Res.*, 1975, *18*, 711.

Stability in solution. The stability of cephradine in various infusion fluids.— D. Adam, *Münch. med. Wschr.*, 1974, *116*, 1945.

Adverse Effects and Precautions. As for Cephalexin, p.1123.. Intramuscular injections of cephradine can be painful and thrombophlebitis has occurred following intravenous injection. Reduced dosage is necessary in patients with impaired renal function.

Colitis. A report of pseudomembranous colitis leading to death in a 67-year-old woman given cephradine 500 mg four times daily.— R. J. Newman and C. M. McCollum, *Br. J. clin. Pract.*, 1979, *33*, 32.

Antimicrobial Action. Cephradine has an antimicrobial action similar to that of cephalexin (see p.1123).

The antibacterial activities of cephradine and cephalexin were almost identical against *Staphylococcus aureus, Staph. pyogenes*, and various Gram-negative organisms.— J. D. Williams and A. M. Geddes (letter), *Br. med. J.*, 1973, *2*, 613.

Reports of the varying activity of cephradine against strains of *Haemophilus influenzae*.— S. Selwyn (letter), *Br. med. J.*, 1974, *1*, 388; S. Eykyn and I. Phillips (letter), *ibid.*, 1974, *2*, 59; R. Sinai *et al.*, *Antimicrob. Ag. Chemother.*, 1978, *13*, 861.

In a study of the susceptibility of the cephalosporins to penicillinase of *Staph. aureus*, cephradine was the most resistant, then in decreasing order of stability cephalexin, cephalothin, cephazolin and least resistant cephaloridine.— R. W. Lacey and A. Stokes, *J. clin. Path.*, 1977, *30*, 35.

Strains of *Salmonella typhi* resistant to chloramphenicol and relatively resistant to ampicillin had been found susceptible to cephradine.— A. G. Paradelis *et al.* (letter), *J. antimicrob. Chemother.*, 1977, *3*, 627. Multi-resistant strains of *Salmonella wien* and *S. heidelberg* were reported to be very sensitive to cephradine with MICs ranging from 0.156 to 0.312 μg per ml.— *idem*, 1978, *4*, 386.

Activity of cephradine against anaerobes.— W. Brumfitt *et al.*, *Lancet*, 1982, *1*, 394.

For comparisons *in vitro* of the activities of cephradine, cephalexin, cefaclor, and cefatrizine, see Cefaclor, p.1115.

Enhanced activity. A report of enhanced activity *in vitro* with cephradine and mecillinam against 18 of 36 multi-resistant strains of Gram-negative bacilli.— B. Chattopadhyay and I. Hall, *J. antimicrob. Chemother.*, 1979, *5*, 549.

Absorption and Fate. Cephradine is rapidly absorbed from the gastro-intestinal tract. Doses of 250 and 500 mg given by mouth produce peak plasma concentrations ranging from 6 to 9 and 11 to 18 μg per ml respectively at 1 hour and are similar to those achieved with cephalexin. A more rapid absorption with a higher peak plasma concentration may be achieved if the same dose is given as a syrup. Absorption is delayed by the presence of food. About 6 to 20% is reported to be bound to plasma proteins. A plasma half-life of about 50 minutes has been reported. It diffuses across the placenta into the foetal circulation and is excreted in small amounts in the milk of nursing mothers.

Cephradine is excreted unchanged in the urine by glomerular filtration and tubular secretion, almost all of a dose being recovered within 6 hours. Urinary concentrations greater than 1 mg per ml have been achieved after a 500-mg dose by mouth.

Probenecid delays excretion.

Following intramuscular injection peak plasma concentrations of about 6 μg per ml are achieved within 1 to 2 hours of a dose of 500 mg and about 10 μg per ml within 2 hours of 1 g. About 60% is excreted in the urine within 6 hours and about 92% within 24 hours.

A short review.— C. H. Nightingale *et al.*, *J. pharm. Sci.*, 1975, *64*, 1899.

Twelve subjects, 6 fasting and 6 not, received a single dose of cephradine 500 mg by mouth. A peak serum concentration of 18.3 μg per ml was reached at 1 hour in fasting volunteers and in non-fasting ones a peak of 19.2 μg per ml was reached. The average recovery of cephradine from urine in 6 hours was 87 and 93.6% in fasting and non-fasting persons respectively. Similar values were obtained when the same volunteers were given cephalexin 500 mg. Absorption and excretion of both drugs was more rapid in fasting volunteers.— C. Harvengt *et al.*, *J. clin. Pharmac.*, 1973, *13*, 36. See also T. W. Mischler *et al.*, *ibid.*, 1974, *14*, 604.

Absorption of cephradine after intramuscular injection was lower in 6 healthy women than in 6 healthy men, especially after injection into the gluteus maximus.— R. A. Vukovich *et al.*, *Clin. Pharmac. Ther.*, 1975, *18*, 215.

A crossover study in 9 healthy subjects given 5 doses of cephalexin or cephradine 1 g every six hours by mouth in differing formulations indicated that the two drugs were pharmacokinetically equivalent.— E. Finkelstein *et al.*, *J. pharm. Sci.*, 1978, *67*, 1447.

Further references to the pharmacokinetics of cephradine: J. Klastersky *et al.*, *Chemotherapy, Basle*, 1973, *18*, 191; A. Zaki *et al.*, *J. clin. Pharmac.*, 1974, *14*, 118; A. G. Paradelis *et al.*, *Arzneimittel-Forsch.*, 1977, *27*, 2167.

Diffusion. Following the intramuscular injection of cephradine 500 mg in 15 patients undergoing thoracic surgery, mean plasma concentrations and mean lung-tissue concentrations were 7.6 μg and 3.1 μg at 30 minutes and 6.5 μg and 2.6 μg at 60 minutes respectively. Lung-tissue concentrations were about 40% of plasma concentrations from 30 to 120 minutes following administration. It was suggested that cephradine could be of use in thoracic infection and doses larger than 500 mg would be required to provide therapeutically effective concentrations in both plasma and lung tissue.— I. J. Kiss *et al.*, *Br. J. clin. Pharmac.*, 1976, *3*, 891.

Pregnancy and the neonate. Cephradine concentrations of 1 to 3 μg per ml were achieved in the amniotic fluid of women given 500-mg doses of cephradine by mouth. An average concentration of 0.6 μg per ml was achieved in the milk of 6 nursing mothers who took 500 mg every 6 hours for 2 days.— T. W. Mischler *et al.*, *Clin.*

Pharmac. Ther., 1974, *15*, 214. See also T. W. Mischler *et al.*, *J. reprod. Med.*, 1978, *21*, 130.

Further references to transplacental diffusion of cephradine: I. Craft and T. C. Forster, *Antimicrob. Ag. Chemother.*, 1978, *14*, 924.

Uses. Cephradine, a cephalosporin antibiotic, is administered by mouth similarly to cephalexin (see p.1124) and by intramuscular or intravenous injection similarly to cephaloridine (see p.1127) in the treatment of susceptible infections.

Cephradine is given by mouth or injection in doses of 250 or 500 mg four times daily. In severe infections up to 4 g daily may be given. The usual daily dose by mouth for children is 25 to 50 mg per kg body-weight; by injection 50 to 100 mg per kg increasing to 300 mg per kg daily in severe infections.

Reduced dosage is recommended in patients with impaired renal function.

For reports and reviews of the actions and uses of cephradine, see *J.Ir. med. Ass.*, 1973, *66* (Mar. 24), *Suppl.*, 1-37; *Drug & Ther. Bull.*, 1973, *11*, 47; *Med. Lett.*, 1974, *16*, 99.

Cephradine was recommended for the eradication of penicillinase-producing staphylococci despite the fact that the MIC was substantially higher than concentrations achieved by the recommended doses.— J. D. Williams and A. M. Geddes (letter), *Br. med. J.*, 1973, *2*, 116.

Cephradine was chosen as the cephalosporin of choice for the Westminster Hospital Group following an *in vitro* and *in vivo* comparison of 5 cephalosporins (cephaloridine, cephalothin, cephalexin, cephradine, and cephazolin). Seven representative penicillins were also evaluated in parallel. The main organisms studied were *Staph. aureus* and *Pr. mirabilis*. Cephradine and cephalexin were the least affected by protein binding and increases in MIC and MBC (minimal bactericidal concentration) in serum were less with these two cephalosporins. Cephradine showed the greatest resistance to beta-lactamases. It was as resistant to metabolism as cephaloridine, cephalexin, and cephazolin. Its therapeutic ratio was greater, its renal safety was as good as cephalexin and better than the other three, and it was better distributed. Also cephradine could be given by more routes than the others.— S. Selwyn, *Lancet*, 1976, *2*, 616. Criticisms.— I. Phillips and S. Eykyn (letter), *ibid.*, 900; D. S. Reeves (letter), *ibid.*; W. Brumfitt and J. Hamilton-Miller (letter), *ibid.* A reply.— S. Selwyn (letter), *ibid.*, 901.

Cephradine and cephazolin given by intravenous injection were of similar efficacy in the treatment of 180 patients with urinary-tract infections, pneumonia, septicaemia, skin and soft tissue infections, or multiple infections. Side-effects were similar in both groups and included phlebitis or thrombophlebitis at the injection site, diarrhoea, and eosinophilia.— D. L. Caloza *et al.*, *Squibb, USA*, *Antimicrob. Ag. Chemother.*, 1979, *15*, 119.

Further references to the use of cephradine: A. B. Brosof and T. Q. Spitzer, *Curr. ther. Res.*, 1979, *26*, 317 (bone infections due to *Staph. aureus*); S. E. McLinn, *J. int. med. Res.*, 1979, *7*, 546 (otitis media); J. Mendelson *et al.*, *Obstet. Gynec.*, 1979, *53*, 31 (surgical infection prophylaxis).

Dosage in infants and children. After ingestion of cephradine 15 mg per kg body-weight by 16 children aged 13 months to 8.25 years, mean peak serum concentrations of 21.3 and 9.9 µg per ml were attained at 30 minutes in fasting and non-fasting children respectively; at 6 hours, 64% and 87% of the children had measurable antimicrobial activity in serum. Serum half-lives were 0.8 and 1 hour. A dose of 15 mg per kg given every 12 hours for children older than 9 months might be insufficient and a dose of 60 mg per kg given daily in 4 divided doses about every 6 hours was recommended.— C. M. Ginsburg and G. H. McCracken, *Antimicrob. Ag. Chemother.*, 1979, *16*, 74.

Dosage in renal failure. A dosage schedule for cephradine in patients with varying degrees of renal impairment: those with creatinine clearances of up to 5, from 5 to 20, and above 20 ml per minute could be given 250 mg every 12 hours, 250 mg every 6 hours, and 500 mg every 6 hours respectively. Patients on long-term intermittent haemodialysis could be given 250 mg at the beginning of dialysis, 250 mg after 12 hours, and 250 mg 42 hours after the beginning of dialysis. A dose of 250 mg could be given at the beginning of the next dialysis procedure provided this was 30 hours or more after the previous dose.— A. E. Solomon *et al.*, *Br. J. clin. Pharmac.*, 1975, *2*, 443.

The normal half-life for cephradine of 1.3 hours was increased to 8 to 15 hours in end-stage renal failure. Doses should be reduced to 50% in patients with a glomerular filtration-rate (GFR) of 10 to 50 ml per minute, and to 25% in those with a GFR of less than 10 ml per minute. Concentrations of cephradine were affected by haemodialysis and peritoneal dialysis.— W. M. Bennett *et al.*, *Ann. intern. Med.*, 1977, *86*, 754. See also *idem*, 1980, *93*, 62.

The dosage interval of cephradine should be increased from 6 hours in normal patients to 12 hours in those with mild renal failure, 24 hours in those with moderate renal failure, and 48 hours in those with severe renal failure.— P. Sharpstone, *Br. med. J.*, 1977, *2*, 36.

Endocarditis. Cephradine 500 mg every 3 hours by intravenous injection was ineffective in the treatment of endocarditis in 1 patient despite an MIC of 0.312 µg per ml against *Str. viridans* which was the causative organism. Benzylpenicillin 12 g intravenously daily in divided doses with an antihistamine to control a sensitivity rash was effective.— P. R. Daggett and A. W. Nathan (letter), *Lancet*, 1975, *2*, 877.

Gonorrhoea. Cephradine 2 g by intramuscular injection and a further 2-g dose 8 hours later was given to 58 men with acute gonorrhoea. Only 1 patient required a further 1-g dose on examination 24 hours later and all were considered cured during follow-up for 30 days.— A. Theodoridis *et al.*, *Curr. ther. Res.*, 1976, *19*, 20.

Syphilis. A report on the successful use of cephradine, 1 g intramuscularly every 12 hours for 15 days, in the treatment of infectious syphilis.— A. Theodoridis *et al.*, *Curr. ther. Res.*, 1976, *20*, 254.

Urinary-tract infections. In 53 infections in 51 patients with recurrent urinary-tract infection, cephradine 500 mg by mouth 4 times a day for 7 to 10 days was successful in 19 of 20 patients with bladder infections, 18 of 30 with kidney infections, and 2 of 3 others. Side-effects included development of vaginal *Candida albicans* infection in 6 patients, depression in 1, transient rise in liver enzymes in 3, and abdominal pain in 2, necessitating withdrawal of the drug in 1 patient.— J. A. Whitworth *et al.*, *Med. J. Aust.*, 1973, *2*, 742.

Similar beneficial results were obtained when ampicillin or cephradine 500 mg four times daily for one week was taken by 63 women with acute urinary-tract infections.— B. I. Davies, *J. antimicrob. Chemother.*, 1977, *3*, 219.

Further references to cephradine in urinary-tract infections: G. H. B. Wurth and T. K. Clarke, *Curr. med. Res. Opinion*, 1976, *4*, 139; J. H. Lipton, *Curr. ther. Res.*, 1977, *22*, 253; J. Cooper *et al.*, *J. antimicrob. Chemother.*, 1980, *6*, 231; C. M. Evans *et al.*, *Curr. med. Res. Opinion*, 1980, *6*, 386.

Preparations

Cephradine Capsules *(B.P.)*. Capsules containing cephradine.
U.S.P. specifies 250 or 500 mg. Store at a temperature not exceeding 30° in airtight containers.

Cephradine for Injection *(U.S.P.)*. A dry mixture of cephradine and one or more suitable buffers and solubilising agents. The injection is prepared by the addition of diluent before use. pH of a 1% solution 8 to 9.6.

Cephradine for Oral Suspension *(U.S.P.)*. A dry mixture of cephradine and one or more suitable buffers, diluents, and colouring and flavouring agents. Store in airtight containers. The suspension is prepared by the addition of diluent before issue and contains 25 or 50 mg per ml. pH 3.5 to 6.

Cephradine Tablets *(U.S.P.)*. Tablets containing cephradine. Store in airtight containers.

Sterile Cephradine *(U.S.P.)*. Cephradine suitable for parenteral use. pH of a 1% solution 3.5 to 6.

Proprietary Preparations

Velosef *(Squibb, UK)*. Cephradine, available as **Capsules** of 250 and 500 mg and as **Syrup** (supplied as powder for preparation with water before use) containing 125 and 250 mg in each 5 ml (suggested diluent, syrup). (Also available as Velosef in *Austral., Belg., Canad., Denm., Fr., Neth., USA*).

Velosef for Injection *(Squibb, UK)*. Cephradine, blended with arginine, available as powder for preparing injections, in vials containing cephradine 0.5, 1, and 2 g.

Other Proprietary Names

Anspor *(USA)*; Cefamid, Cefradex *(both Ital.)*; Cefradina *(Spain)*; Cefril *(S.Afr.)*; Cefro *(Jap.)*; Cefrum, Citicef *(both Ital.)*; Dicefalin *(Jap.)*; Eskacef *(Austral., Belg., Fr., Ger., Ital., Spain)*; Eskefrin *(Arg.)*; Lisacef *(Ital.)*; Maxisporin *(Belg., Neth.)*; Medicef *(Ital.)*; Megacef *(Fr.)*; Noblitina *(Spain)*; Protocef *(Ital.)*; Sefril *(Ger., Spain, Switz.)*; Velocef *(Arg., Ital., Spain)*.

Cephradine was also formerly marketed in Great Britain under the proprietary name Eskacef (*Smith Kline & French*).

46-v

Chloramphenicol *(B.P., B.P. Vet., Eur. P., U.S.P.)*.

Chloramphen.; Chloramphenicolum; Laevomycetinum; Chloranfenicol; Cloranfenicol; Kloramfenikol. 2,2-Dichloro-*N*-[(*αR*,*βR*)-*β*-hydroxy-*α*-hydroxymethyl-4-nitrophenethyl]acetamide.

$C_{11}H_{12}Cl_2N_2O_5$=323.1.

CAS — *56-75-7*.

Pharmacopoeias. In all pharmacopoeias examined except *Braz.* and *Chin.*
Rus. also includes chloramphenicol stearate.

An antimicrobial substance produced by the growth of certain strains of *Streptomyces venezuelae*, but now mainly prepared synthetically.

Fine, white to greyish-white or yellowish-white, odourless crystals, needles, or elongated plates, with a very bitter taste. M.p. 149° to 153°. *U.S.P.* specifies not less than 900 µg per mg.

Soluble 1 in 400 of water, 1 in 2.5 of alcohol, and 1 in 7 of propylene glycol; freely soluble in acetone and ethyl acetate; slightly soluble in acids, alkalis, chloroform, and ether; practically insoluble in light petroleum and vegetable oils. A solution in dehydrated alcohol is dextrorotatory and a solution in ethyl acetate is laevorotatory. A 0.5% suspension in water has a pH of 4.5 to 7.5. Solutions are **sterilised** by filtration. **Store** in airtight containers. Protect from light.

NOTE. Propylene glycol must not be used as a solvent for chloramphenicol in eye-drops or nasal drops since it causes a marked burning sensation.

A study on the 3 polymorphic forms of chloramphenicol stearate.— R. Cameroni *et al.*, *Farmaco, Edn prat.*, 1978, *33*, 141.

Bilirubin could interfere with the colorimetric assay of chloramphenicol. A method using activated charcoal was devised to overcome the problem.— E. O. Mason *et al.*, *Antimicrob. Ag. Chemother.*, 1979, *15*, 544.

Incompatibility. An immediate precipitate was formed when chloramphenicol 500 mg and erythromycin 250 mg or tetracycline hydrochloride 500 mg were mixed in 1 litre of 5% dextrose solution.— H. R. Grant, *Hosp. Pharmst*, 1962, *15*, 67.

A haze developed over 3 hours when chloramphenicol 4 g per litre was mixed with chlorpromazine hydrochloride 200 mg per litre or prochlorperazine mesylate 100 mg per litre in sodium chloride injection, but an immediate precipitate was formed when chlorpromazine hydrochloride was added in dextrose injection.— B. B. Riley, *J. Hosp. Pharm.*, 1970, *28*, 228.

Loss of activity. Chloramphenicol was less active against *Staphylococcus aureus* in the presence of carmellose sodium, methylcellulose, tragacanth, sodium alginate, bentonite, and polysorbate 80.— M. A. El-Nakeeb and R. T. Yousef, *Acta pharm. suec.*, 1968, *5*, 1.

A study on the adsorption of chloramphenicol *in vitro* on various antacids.— S. A. Khalil *et al.*, *Pharmazie*, 1976, *31*, 105.

A study of the effect of the antibiotic and preservative on each other's binding to pharmaceutical adjuvants in mixtures containing benzalkonium chloride or chlorocresol and chloramphenicol.— M. A. El-Nakeeb and M. H. Ali, *Mfg Chem.*, 1976, *47* (Mar.), 37..

Release from suppositories. Sodium lauryl sulphate 1% or polysorbates '61' or '65' 5% increased the rate of release of chloramphenicol from suppositories made with macrogol 1500. Compound bases, except those containing macrogol 1500 with added sodium lauryl sulphate, did not enhance activity. Stability was adequate for 6 months.— L. Adám *et al.*, *Revtă med., Turgu Mures*, 1967, *13*, 356, per *Int. pharm. Abstr.*, 1968, *5*, 690. See also M. A. Ghafoor and C. L. Huyck, *Am. J. Pharm.*, 1962, *134*, 63.

Solubility. Urea increased the solubility of chloramphenicol in water. A solid solution of chloramphenicol in urea had a dissolution-rate up to 4 times that of chloramphenicol alone.— A. H. Goldberg *et al.*, *J. pharm. Sci.*, 1966, *55*, 581.

The solubility of chloramphenicol in water was increased

by the addition of benzalkonium chloride. The 2 substances had a synergistic action *in vitro* against *Pseudomonas aeruginosa*.— R. T. Yousef and A. A. Ghobashy, *Acta pharm. suec.*, 1968, *5*, 385.

Stability in solution. Chloramphenicol in aqueous solution was very stable over a wide pH range. Hydrolysis did not occur at ordinary temperatures at pH 2 to 7. Decomposition was catalysed by mono-hydrogen phosphate and mono- and di-hydrogen citrate ions and undissociated acetic acid, and it was recommended that only weakly buffered solutions should be dispensed.— T. Higuchi *et al.*, *J. Am. pharm. Ass., scient. Edn*, 1954, *43*, 129.

Aqueous solutions lost about half their chloramphenicol content by hydrolysis on storage for 290 days at 20° to 22°; under the same conditions, solutions buffered (with borax) at pH 7.4 lost about 14%. The loss on heating the solutions at 100° for 15 minutes was about 3%.— A. Brunzell, *Svensk farm. Tidskr.*, 1957, *6*, 129.

Chloramphenicol was degraded by light in 0.25% aqueous solution and the solution became yellow and acid. The major degradation products were formed by oxidation, reduction, and subsequent condensation.— I. K. Shih, *J. pharm. Sci.*, 1971, *60*, 1889.

Stability of preparations. Chloramphenicol ointment and eye ointment were stable for 2 years at 20° to 25°. Chloramphenicol ear-drops and eye-drops (*B.P.C.*) and chloramphenicol cream (*D.T.F.*) retained more than 90% of their potencies after 2 years, 3 to 4 months, and 5 months respectively. After heating the eye-drops at 115° to 116° for 30 minutes, 15% hydrolysis occurred, and after heating with a bactericide at 100° for 30 minutes, 3 to 4% hydrolysis occurred.— K. C. James and R. H. Leach, *J. Pharm. Pharmac.*, 1970, *22*, 607.

Sterilisation of solutions. Chloramphenicol in aqueous solution could be heated at 100° for 30 minutes, with a predicted loss of only 3.66% potency. A loss of 10% potency would occur in 29 minutes at 115°. Heating at 98° to 100° for 30 minutes would be an acceptable method of sterilisation for chloramphenicol eye-drops and the drops would not lose more than 10% potency in 4 months' storage at 20° or 2 years at 4°.— M. Heward *et al.*, *Pharm. J.*, 1970, *1* 386. Comments.— K. C. James and R. H. Leach, *ibid.*, 477.

Adverse Effects. The most serious adverse effect of chloramphenicol is its depression of the bone marrow, which can take 2 different forms. The first is a dose-related reversible depression occurring usually when plasma-chloramphenicol concentrations reach 25 to 35 µg per ml and is characterised by morphological changes in the bone marrow, decreased iron utilisation, mild anaemia, leucopenia, and thrombocytopenia. This effect may be due to inhibition of protein synthesis in the mitochondria of bone marrow cells.

The second and apparently unrelated form of bone-marrow toxicity is severe irreversible aplastic anaemia which is reported to have an estimated incidence of 1 in 4000 to 1 in 100 000. The aplasia usually develops after a latent period of weeks or even months and it is considered that victims may have some biochemical predisposition. Unfortunately there is no way of identifying susceptible patients and because the 2 forms of toxicity are distinct blood counts are of no value. It is estimated that up to 80% of these patients may die. Survival is most likely in those with early onset aplasia but they may subsequently develop myeloblastic leukaemia.

Haemolytic anaemia has occurred in some persons with a genetic deficiency of glucose-6-phosphate dehydrogenase activity.

A toxic manifestation—'the grey syndrome'—characterised by vomiting, abdominal distension, ashen colour, hypothermia, irregular respiration, progressive pallid cynanosis, and shock, followed by death in a few hours or days, has occurred in premature and other newborn infants receiving large doses of chloramphenicol. In most cases, the dose of chloramphenicol has been more than 25 mg per kg body-weight daily. A similar syndrome has been reported in adults and older children given very high doses.

Prolonged oral administration of chloramphenicol may induce bleeding, either by bone-marrow depression or by reducing the intestinal flora with consequent inhibition of vitamin K synthesis and greatly increased prothrombin time.

Peripheral as well as optic neuritis has been reported in patients receiving chloramphenicol, usually over prolonged periods. Although ocular symptoms are often reversible if treatment is withdrawn early, optic atrophy with blindness has occurred.

Local hypersensitivity reactions may occur and erythema multiforme (Stevens-Johnson syndrome) has occasionally been reported. Gastro-intestinal symptoms including nausea, vomiting, and diarrhoea can follow oral administration but are less common than with the tetracyclines. Disturbances of the oral and intestinal flora may cause stomatitis, glossitis, and rectal or vaginal irritation.

Chloramphenicol intoxication in premature infants was due to a deficiency of glucuronyl transferase activity.— J. M. Lord, *Hosp. Top.*, 1968, *46*, 83, per *Int. pharm. Abstr.*, 1968, *5*, 502.

Allergy. Of 620 persons with dermatitis or eczema submitted to patch testing with chloramphenicol 50% in yellow soft paraffin, 1.7% gave a positive reaction.— E. Rudzki and D. Kleniewska, *Br. J. Derm.*, 1970, *83*, 543.

Alopecia. Reversible alopecia and bone-marrow depression occurred in a 3-year-old child, with cystic fibrosis, who was given chloramphenicol 70 mg per kg body-weight daily for about 10 weeks.— J. P. Kapp *et al.*, *Clin. Pediat.*, 1977, *16*, 64.

Blood disorders. Reviews.— B. C. P. Polak *et al.*, *Acta med. scand.*, 1972, *192*, 409; A. A. Yunis, in *Blood Disorders due to Drugs and Other Agents*, R.H. Girdwood (Ed.), Amsterdam, Excerpta Medica, 1973, 107-26.

Single courses of 10 g of chloramphenicol could cause fatal aplasia.— A. A. Sharp, *Br. med. J.*, 1963, *1*, 735.

Granulocytopenia, thrombocytopenia, and moderate anaemia followed the use of 0.5% aqueous chloramphenicol eye-drops for 2 out of every 3 days for 23 months in a man aged 36 with a family history of hypersensitivity to chloramphenicol.— R. L. Rosenthal and A. Blackman, *J. Am. med. Ass.*, 1965, *191*, 136. A report of aplastic anaemia in a patient eventually found to have been using eye-drops containing chloramphenicol.— G. Carpenter (letter), *Lancet*, 1975, *2*, 326. Fatal aplastic anaemia following the use of chloramphenicol eye ointment.— S. M. Abrams *et al.*, *Archs intern. Med.*, 1980, *140*, 576. Comment.— *Med. Lett.*, 1980, *22*, 96.

Five patients developed hepatitis then fatal aplastic anaemia following the administration of chloramphenicol.— R. Hodgkinson, *Med. J. Aust.*, 1973, *1*, 939.

An analysis of blood dyscrasias reported to the Swedish Adverse Drug Reaction Committee for the 5-year period 1966-70 showed that aplastic anaemia attributable to chloramphenicol had been reported on 5 occasions (4 fatal). It is estimated that reported figures represented one-third of the true frequency.— L. E. Böttiger and B. Westerholm, *Br. med. J.*, 1973, *3*, 339.

In a study of 76 infants and children aged 2 months to 15 years who received chloramphenicol in doses of 31 to 133 mg per kg body-weight daily for 10 to 76 days for infections, hyperferraemia occurred in 36 and haemopoietic toxicity in 21. Hyperferraemia was more common in children above 6 years and at dosage levels above 75 mg per kg body-weight daily. In 15 patients with haemopoietic toxicity chloramphenicol was continued and 10 received additional phenylalanine or riboflavine; recovery was variable. However therapy should be discontinued if neutropenia or thrombocytopenia develop.— D. W. O'G. Hughes, *Med. J. Aust.*, 1973, *2*, 1142.

Both chloramphenicol and thiamphenicol inhibited colony formation by normal bone marrow *in vitro* at concentrations considered to be close to those achieved therapeutically. However, bone marrow from 2 patients, one with chloramphenicol-induced aplastic anaemia and the other with a history of such anaemia did not react to chloramphenicol.— A. Howell *et al.*, *Lancet*, 1975, *1*, 65. Bone-marrow precursors from patients with chloramphenicol-induced aplastic anaemia were not necessarily resistant to chloramphenicol *in vitro*.— P. Kern *et al.* (letter), *ibid.*, 1190.

Despite features of dose-related reversible bone-marrow depression in a 23-year-old man given benzylpenicillin and chloramphenicol intravenously, the condition progressed to fatal aplastic anaemia 12 days after chloramphenicol had been withdrawn.— R. S. Daum *et al.*, *J. Pediat.*, 1979, *94*, 403.

Fatal bone-marrow hypoplasia in a shepherd using chloramphenicol spray.— G. S. Del Giacco *et al.* (letter), *Lancet*, 1981, *1*, 945.

Further references: T. Nagao and A. M. Mauer, *New Engl. J. Med.*, 1969, *281*, 7; B. Modan *et al.*, *Am. J. med. Sci.*, 1975, *270*, 441; R. S. Pekarek *et al.*, *Clin. Chem.*, 1975, *21*, 528.

Haemolytic anaemia. Chloramphenicol 1 to 2 g daily had been reported to cause haemolytic anaemia in certain individuals with a deficiency of glucose-6-phosphate dehydrogenase in conjunction with factors such as infection.— E. Beutler, *Pharmac. Rev.*, 1969, *21*, 73.

Chloramphenicol also caused haemolytic anaemia in patients with a deficiency of erythrocyte glutathione peroxidase.— M. Steinberg and T. Necheles, *Am. J. Med.*, 1971, *50*, 542, per M. Swanson, *Drug Intell. & clin. Pharm.*, 1973, *7*, 6.

Chloramphenicol did not cause haemolysis in Chinese patients with glucose-6-phosphate dehydrogenase deficiency.— T. K. Chan *et al.*, *Br. med. J.*, 1976, *2*, 1227.

Leukaemia. See below.

Colitis. Not one of 437 hospital in-patients in a Boston Collaborative Drug Surveillance Program who received chloramphenicol developed colitis.— R. R. Miller and H. Jick, *Clin. Pharmac. Ther.*, 1977, *22*, 1.

Encephalitis. Reversible symptoms of encephalopathy developed in 3 patients treated with chloramphenicol.— P. H. Levine *et al.*, *Clin. Pharmac. Ther.*, 1970, *11*, 194.

Leukaemia. Three patients treated with chloramphenicol developed pancytopenia leading to myeloblastic leukaemia. The continued widespread administration of chloramphenicol, often for trivial complaints, was considered to be a possible cause of some forms of leukaemia, particularly those of the relatively indolent hypoplastic type.— M. J. Brauer and W. Dameshek, *New Engl. J. Med.*, 1967, *267*, 1003.

Three further cases of acute leukaemia had occurred in patients previously treated with chloramphenicol. This took the total reported in the literature up to 27.— P. Lechat *et al.*, *Thérapie*, 1976, *31*, 129.

Further references: T. Cohen and W. P. Creger, *Am. J. Med.*, 1967, *43*, 762.

Optic neuritis. Reports of optic neuritis associated with chloramphenicol.— N. N. Huang *et al.*, *J. Pediat.*, 1966, *68*, 32; S. Charache *et al.*, *Johns Hopkins med. J.*, 1977, *140*, 121; L. Rothkoff *et al.*, *Ann. Ophthal.*, 1979, *11*, 105 (optic atrophy after irrigation of the lachrymal ducts); V. Godel *et al.*, *Archs Ophthal.*, *N.Y.*, 1980, *98*, 1417.

Ototoxicity. Chloramphenicol sodium succinate 5% in Ringer's solution and propylene glycol 10% both caused irreversible deafness when instilled into the middle ear cavity in *guinea-pigs*. It was recommended that propylene glycol should not be used as a solvent for chloramphenicol ear drops, and that higher concentrations of chloramphenicol should not be used in the middle-ear cavity.— T. Morizono and B. M. Johnstone, *Med. J. Aust.*, 1975, *2*, 634.

Of 47 children treated for *Haemophilus influenzae* meningitis, 3 showed some loss of hearing. They included 1 of 27 given ampicillin only, 1 of 12 given chloramphenicol only, and 1 of 8 given both antibiotics.— F. E. Jones and D. R. Hanson, *Develop. Med. Child Neurology*, 1977, *19*, 593.

Treatment of Adverse Effects. Chloramphenicol should be discontinued immediately on the appearance of toxic symptoms. Blood transfusions are of little avail when aplastic anaemia has developed; treatment with androgens such as oxymetholone and corticosteroids has been reported to be of benefit in some patients.

Allergic skin rashes may be treated with antihistamines by mouth. Vitamins of the B group have been given in the treatment of the optic neuritis induced by chloramphenicol. Phytomenadione may be tried to prevent gastro-intestinal haemorrhage due to lowered prothrombin values during prolonged treatment with chloramphenicol.

Early toxic changes occurring in the bone marrow of children, following treatment with chloramphenicol, were reversed, generally within 2 to 4 days, by a daily dose of 100 mg per kg body-weight of L-phenylalanine.— D. Ingall *et al.*, *New Engl. J. Med.*, 1965, *272*, 180.

In patients with impaired renal function, chloramphenicol could be removed from the body by dialysis. Clearance was about one-third that of creatinine.— C. M. Kunin, *Ann. intern. Med.*, 1967, *67*, 151. See also Dosage in Renal Failure, below under Uses.

Reports on the treatment of accidental chloramphenicol overdosage in infants.— S. M. Mauer *et al.*, *J. Pediat.*, 1980, *96*, 136 (charcoal haemoperfusion); D. L. Kessler *et al.*, *ibid.*, 140 (exchange transfusion).

Precautions. Chloramphenicol is contra-indicated in patients with a history of hypersensitivity or toxic reactions. It should never be given for minor infections or for prophylaxis. Repeated courses and prolonged treatment should be avoided.

Reduced doses should be given to patients with impaired liver function. Uraemic patients may be more susceptible to the depressant effect of chloramphenicol on bone marrow but reducing the dose may result in inadequate plasma concentrations. Routine periodic blood examinations are advisable in all patients including infants; these examinations will not warn of aplastic anaemia.

Because of the risk of the 'grey syndrome' newborn infants should never be given chloramphenicol, unless it may be life-saving and there is no alternative treatment. The use of chloramphenicol is probably best avoided during pregnancy; nursing infants should be observed with care since chloramphenicol given to the mother is excreted in the milk.

Concomitant administration of chloramphenicol with other drugs liable to depress bone-marrow function should be avoided.

Chloramphenicol may interfere with the development of immunity and it should not be given during active immunisation.

Chloramphenicol enhances the effects of coumarin anticoagulants (see under Dicoumarol, p.771, and Warfarin Sodium, p.776), some hypoglycaemic agents (see under Chlorpropamide, p.852, and Tolbutamide, p.860), and phenytoin (see p.1238).

A study indicating that usual therapeutic doses of chloramphenicol interfere with colour vision.— J. Laroche and C. Laroche, *Annls pharm. fr.*, 1972, *30*, 433.

A report of HL-A antigen changes in patients treated with chloramphenicol.— A. Ben-David *et al.*, *Tissue Antigens*, 1973, *3*, 378, per P. Lechat *et al.*, *Thérapie*, 1976, *31*, 129.

For a report of the effect of malnutrition on the metabolism of chloramphenicol, see below under Absorption and Fate.

Interactions. *Alcohol.* Mention of a potential disulfiram-like reaction with alcohol and chloramphenicol.— *FDA Drug Bull.*, 1979, *9*, 10.

Antibiotics. Eight of 11 children treated for *Haemophilus influenzae* meningitis with ampicillin and chloramphenicol had long-term sequelae compared with 4 of 32 given ampicillin alone and 4 of 22 given chloramphenicol alone. An increased risk was suggested for this combination.— J. Lindberg *et al.*, *Pediatrics*, 1977, *60*, 1. See also T. Matthews (letter), *Lancet*, 1978, *2*, 376.

For reports of the effects of other antibiotics on the antimicrobial activity of chloramphenicol, see below under Antimicrobial Action.

Anticonvulsants. In a newborn infant with *Escherichia coli* meningitis unresponsive to ampicillin and gentamicin, chloramphenicol was given intravenously for 3 weeks and blood concentrations measured after each injection. The dose had to be increased gradually from 20 to 95 mg per kg body-weight daily in order to maintain the blood concentration in the therapeutic range of 10 to 20 μg per ml. The concomitant use of phenobarbitone and phenytoin might have stimulated the metabolism of chloramphenicol.— S. B. Black *et al.*, *J. Pediat.*, 1978, *92*, 235.

Phenobarbitone reduced the blood-choramphenicol concentration in 2 children being treated with the antibiotic for meningitis due to *H. influenzae*.— R. A. Bloxham *et al.*, *Archs Dis. Childh.*, 1979, *54*, 76.

For the effect of chloramphenicol on serum concentrations of *phenobarbitone*, see Phenobarbitone, p.813.

Cyclophosphamide. The biotransformation of cyclophosphamide into its active metabolites was retarded by chloramphenicol.— O. K. Faber *et al.*, *Br. J. clin. Pharmac.*, 1975, *2*, 281.

Diuretics. The urinary excretion of chloramphenicol in healthy subjects was decreased by frusemide but the excretion of its metabolites as aryl amines and total nitro compounds was increased.— O. Schück *et al.*, *Experientia*, 1975, *31*, 1434. The urinary excretion of chloramphenicol and its metabolites was increased in healthy subjects when ethacrynic acid, hydrochlorothiazide, or clopamide were taken with a 1-g dose of chloramphenicol. There were no significant changes in serum concentrations of chloramphenicol and its metabolites.— O. Schück *et al.*, *Int. J. clin. Pharmac. Biopharm.*, 1978, *16*, 217.

Paracetamol. In 6 patients given chloramphenicol 1 g intravenously the mean half-life of 3.25 hours (assessed from blood samples taken 0.5, 1, 1.5, and 2 hours after the dose) was increased to 15 hours after paracetamol 100 mg was given intravenously 2 hours after the chloramphenicol.— N. Buchanan and G. P. Moodley, *Br. med. J.*, 1979, *2*, 307.

Antimicrobial Action. Chloramphenicol is a broad-spectrum antibiotic (see p.1084) which acts by interfering with bacterial protein synthesis. It is usually bacteriostatic and is effective against a wide range of Gram-negative and Gram-positive organisms. *Salmonella typhi, Haemophilus influenzae, Neisseria meningitidis,* and *Bordetella pertussis* are particularly susceptible, and most strains are inhibited by concentrations of less than 2 μg per ml. Chloramphenicol is active against anaerobic bacteria and an MIC of 8 μg or less per ml has been reported for most strains of *Bacteroides fragilis*. It has antirickettsial activity, and is also active against chlamydias of the psittacosis-lymphogranuloma group, and against *Vibrio* spp. *Pseudomonas aeruginosa* is usually resistant. It has some activity against *Mycoplasma pneumoniae*.

Gentamicin did not affect the activity of chloramphenicol against *Bacteroides fragilis*. However, chloramphenicol inhibited the bactericidal activity of gentamicin against *E. coli*.— J. Klastersky and M. Husson, *Antimicrob. Ag. Chemother.*, 1977, *12*, 135.

Chloramphenicol was bactericidal *in vitro* against most isolates of meningeal pathogens such as *H. influenzae, Streptococcus pneumoniae*, and *N. meningitidis* at clinically achievable concentrations but was only bacteriostatic against the Enterobacteriaceae and *Staphylococcus aureus*.— J. J. Rahal and M. S. Simberkoff, *Antimicrob. Ag. Chemother.*, 1979, *16*, 13.

Reports of the activity *in vitro* of chloramphenicol against: *Campylobacter fetus*.— A. W. Chow *et al.*, *Antimicrob. Ag. Chemother.*, 1978, *13*, 416. *Haemophilus* spp.— J. D. Williams and J. Andrews, *Br. med. J.*, 1974, *1*, 134; J. B. Mayo and L. R. McCarthy, *Antimicrob. Ag. Chemother.*, 1977, *11*, 844; G. W. Hammond *et al.*, *Antimicrob. Ag. Chemother.*, 1978, *13*, 608; E. O. Mason *et al.*, *Antimicrob. Ag. Chemother.*, 1980, *17*, 470. *Legionella pneumophila*.— C. Thornsberry *et al.*, *Antimicrob. Ag. Chemother.*, 1978, *13*, 78. *Listeria monocytogenes*.— G. L. Wiggins *et al.*, *Antimicrob. Ag. Chemother.*, 1978, *13*, 854. *Neisseria gonorrhoeae*.— P. D. Duck *et al.*, *Antimicrob. Ag. Chemother.*, 1978, *14*, 788. *Shigella sonnei*.— G. I. Barrow and C. Ellis, *Mon. Bull. Minist. Hlth*, 1967, *26*, 250. *Vibrio* spp.— L. M. Prescott *et al.*, *Bull. Wld Hlth Org.*, 1968, *39*, 967; F. O'Grady *et al.*, *Bull. Wld Hlth Org.*, 1976, *54*, 181; S. W. Joseph *et al.*, *Antimicrob. Ag. Chemother.*, 1978, *13*, 244. *Yersinia enterocolitica*.— M. Raevuori *et al.*, *Antimicrob. Ag. Chemother.*, 1978, *13*, 888.

For details of the antagonism of the antibacterial action of benzylpenicillin against *N. meningitidis* by low concentrations of chloramphenicol and for a report that benzylpenicillin and chloramphenicol were not considered to be antagonistic, see Benzylpenicillin, p.1106.

Activity against anaerobic bacteria. A study *in vitro* of the activity of 10 antimicrobial agents against 124 strains of *Bacteroides fragilis* and 57 strains of other anaerobic bacteria indicated that clindamycin, metronidazole, and chloramphenicol were the most effective agents against *B. fragilis*.— J. Dubois *et al.*, *J. antimicrob. Chemother.*, 1978, *4*, 329.

Activity of ampicillin with chloramphenicol. See under Ampicillin, p.1093.

Diminished activity. Antagonism between chloramphenicol and aminoglycoside antibiotics has been reported *in vitro* and has been confirmed *in vivo* in *animals*.— P. J. Sanderson (letter), *Lancet*, 1978, *2*, 210.

Antagonism occurred against some strains of *Staph. aureus* when the activity of chloramphenicol was tested *in vitro* with bleomycin.— J. Y. Jacobs *et al.*, *Antimicrob. Ag. Chemother.*, 1979, *15*, 580.

For a report of various compounds decreasing the activity of chloramphenicol, see above under Incompatibility.

Enhanced activity. Synergism usually occurred when chloramphenicol was tested *in vitro* with actinomycin D or mitomycin against *Staph. aureus*. The effect of mitomycin was obtained at concentrations below those usually obtainable in serum.— J. Y. Jacobs *et al.*, *Antimicrob. Ag. Chemother.*, 1979, *15*, 580.

For a study of the enhanced activity of chloramphenicol and fosfomycin against strains of *Shigella* and *Salmonella*, see Fosfomycin, p.1165.

For a report of enhanced activity with chloramphenicol and benzalkonium chloride, see above under Solubility.

Resistance. The incidence of resistance to chloramphenicol has increased slowly and resistant strains of the majority of sensitive species have been reported. Resistance is plasmid-mediated and may be transferable. There is evidence of weak cross-resistance between chloramphenicol and erythromycin and chloramphenicol and tetracyclines. Cross-resistance with thiamphenicol also occurs.

Acetylation of chloramphenicol was considered to be the primary biochemical mechanism in bacterial resistance mediated by the R-factor.— W. V. Shaw and J. Unowsky, *J. Bact.*, 1968, *95*, 1976. Similar findings in *Streptococcus pneumoniae*.— A. Dang-Van *et al.*, *Antimicrob. Ag. Chemother.*, 1978, *13*, 577.

R-plasmid mediated resistance to chloramphenicol in strains of *Escherichia coli* might involve more than acetyltransferase activity.— T. Yokota *et al.*, *Antimicrob. Ag. Chemother.*, 1977, *11*, 952.

Resistance of Bacteroides. Severe anaerobic infections, mainly due to *Bacteroides fragilis*, in 10 patients who failed to respond to chloramphenicol but were later successfully treated with clindamycin.— H. Thadepalli *et al.*, *Curr. ther. Res.*, 1977, *22*, 421.

A report of strains of *B. fragilis* moderately resistant (MIC 12.5 μg per ml) to chloramphenicol due to production of chloramphenicol acetyltransferase.— M. L. Britz and R. G. Wilkinson, *Antimicrob. Ag. Chemother.*, 1978, *14*, 105.

The identification in a strain of *Bacteroides ochraceus* of a conjugative plasmid which specifies resistance to chloramphenicol, tetracycline, kanamycin, and streptomycin and which could be transferred by conjugation to *E. coli*.— D. G. Guiney and C. E. Davis, *Nature*, 1978, *274*, 181. See also J. R. Saunders, *ibid.*, 113.

Resistance of Haemophilus. Plasmid-mediated resistance to chloramphenicol and tetracycline in *Haemophilus influenzae*.— B. Van Klingeren *et al.*, *Antimicrob. Ag. Chemother.*, 1977, *11*, 383.

Meningitis due to chloramphenicol-resistant *H. influenzae* type b.— A. -L. Kinmonth *et al.*, *Br. med. J.*, 1978, *1*, 694.

A clinical isolate of *H. influenzae* resistant to chloramphenicol, ampicillin, and tetracycline; resistance was shown to be transferable.— L. E. Bryan, *Antimicrob. Ag. Chemother.*, 1978, *14*, 154.

The sensitivity of 523 clinical isolates of *H. influenzae* and *H. parainfluenzae* was investigated in a multicentre study in 8 cities in West Germany. Of 7 chloramphenicol-resistant strains (MIC more than 4 μg per ml), one was resistant to chloramphenicol only, 3 to chloramphenicol and tetracycline, 2 to chloramphenicol, tetracycline, and ampicillin, and 1 to chloramphenicol, tetracycline, and co-trimoxazole.— I. Braveny and K. Machka (letter), *Lancet*, 1980, *2*, 752.

Further references: P. Cavanagh *et al.* (letter), *Lancet*, 1975, *1*, 696; A. Manten *et al.* (letter), *ibid.*, 1976, *1*, 702; R. Laufs *et al.*, *Dt. med. Wschr.*, 1978, *103*, 658; A. J. Howard *et al.*, *Br. med. J.*, 1978, *1*, 1657; S. Simasathien *et al.*, *Lancet*, 1980, *2*, 1214.

Resistance of Salmonellae. Of 8 isolates of *Salmonella typhi* from Vietnamese patients, 4 were resistant to chloramphenicol, tetracycline, sulphadiazine, and streptomycin and transferable resistance was demonstrated in 3 of the strains. These results could not be applied to the patients and chloramphenicol was given as standard treatment; those with resistant organisms had prolonged febrile courses and 1 died. Ampicillin or co-trimoxazole was recommended for the treatment of enteric fever in Vietnam.— T. Butler *et al.*, *Lancet*, 1973, *2*, 983. Comment.— *ibid.*, 1008. Transferable resistance to chloramphenicol would occur in *S. typhi* only where typhoid was a common disease and where the antibiotic was used indiscriminantly. Chloramphenicol remained the drug of choice for typhoid in most countries; where there were epidemics associated with resistant *S. typhi* treatment could be started with ampicillin until results of sensitivity tests were available. During 1972 the Enteric Reference Laboratory received 119 cultures of *S. typhi*, 31 from Great Britain and 88 from 23 other countries. Two cultures, both from Mexico, were resistant.— E. S. Anderson (letter), *ibid.*, 1494.

A study of multiple-drug resistance in isolates of *Salmonella* in India over the period 1972–8 indicated that since 1975 appreciable numbers of serotypes from human and non-human sources had emerged with multiple resistance to between 2 to 6 antimicrobial agents. Isolates of *S. typhi* uniformly resistant to chloramphenicol, streptomycin, sulphafurazole and tetracycline had been obtained. All the isolates studied were sensitive *in vitro* to co-trimoxazole.— K. B. Sharma *et al.*, *J. antimicrob. Chemother.*, 1979, *5*, 15.

S. typhi, in a patient with enteric fever, acquired resistance to both chloramphenicol and co-trimoxazole during treatment.— N. Datta *et al.*, *Lancet*, 1981, *1*, 1181.

Further references: C. K. J. Paniker and K. N. Vimala (letter), *Nature*, 1972, *239*, 109; G. Overturf *et al.*, *New Engl. J. Med.*, 1973, *289*, 463; *Br. med. J.*, 1975, *2*, 582; J. D. Brown *et al.*, *J. Am. med. Ass.*, 1975, *231*, 162; W. R. Sanborn *et al.* (letter), *Lancet*, 1975, *2*, 408; C. E. Cherubin *et al.*, *J. infect. Dis.*, 1977, *135*, 807; R. Virgilio and A. M. Cordano, *Revta lat.-am. Microbiol.*, 1978, *19*, 67, per *Trop. Dis. Bull.*, 1979, *76*, 148.

Resistance of streptococci. Of 1176 strains of group A streptococci isolated in Japan in the period 1972 to 1974, 241 were resistant to tetracycline, 234 to tetracycline and chloramphenicol, 427 to tetracycline, chloramphenicol, erythromycin, oleandomycin, josamycin, mydecamycin, and lincomycin, and 19 to chloramphenicol alone. Seven of 83 strains of group B streptococci were resistant to tetracycline and chloramphenicol and 26 to tetracycline alone. It was considered that because resistance to a single macrolide antibiotic was rare and that acquisition of resistance to tetracycline and/or chloramphenicol appeared to be a prerequisite for resistance to macrolide antibiotics, restriction of the use of tetracycline and chloramphenicol would lead to a decline in the frequency of macrolide-antibiotic resistance.— Y. Miyamoto *et al.*, *Antimicrob. Ag. Chemother.*, 1978, *13*, 399.

Chloramphenicol-resistant pneumococci in West Africa.— D. Hansman (letter), *Lancet*, 1978, *1*, 1102.

Three of 866 strains of *Str. pneumoniae* were resistant to chloramphenicol.— A. J. Howard *et al.*, *Br. med. J.*, 1978, *1*, 1657. See also J. Garau *et al.* (letter), *Lancet*, 1981, *2*, 147.

Further references: M. Nakae *et al.*, *Antimicrob. Ag. Chemother.*, 1977, *12*, 427.

Absorption and Fate. Chloramphenicol is readily absorbed when given by mouth. Blood concentrations of about 10 µg per ml may be reached 2 hours after a single dose of 1 g; a dose of 500 mg every 6 hours usually maintains blood concentrations above 4 µg per ml. Higher blood concentrations are not achieved by parenteral administration of similar doses.

Chloramphenicol is widely distributed in body tissues and fluids; it enters the cerebrospinal fluid, even in the absence of meningitis, giving concentrations of about 30 to 50% of those existing in the blood; it diffuses across the placenta into the foetal circulation, into breast milk, and into the aqueous and vitreous humours of the eye. Up to about 60% in the circulation is bound to plasma protein.

Chloramphenicol is excreted mainly in the urine but only 5 to 10% of a dose appears unchanged; the remainder is inactivated in the liver, mostly by conjugation with glucuronic acid; reduction to aryl amines has also been reported. About 3% is excreted in the bile. However, most is reabsorbed and only about 1%, mainly in the inactive form, is excreted in the faeces.

Although peritoneal dialysis did not remove significant amounts of chloramphenicol there was significant absorption from the peritoneal cavity.— P. A. Greenberg and J. P. Sanford, *Ann. intern. Med.*, 1967, *66*, 465.

Some 24% of chloramphenicol was bound in the body to serum proteins. The biological half-life in serum was 1.6 to 3.3 hours and 5 to 15% was excreted in urine.— C. M. Kunin, *Ann. intern. Med.*, 1967, *67*, 151. The biological half-life of chloramphenicol was 3.5 to 5 hours.— W. A. Ritschel, *Drug Intell. & clin. Pharm.*, 1970, *4*, 332.

In a study of 170 men and 142 women given various antibiotics, blood concentrations following chloramphenicol 500 mg were 34 and 33% higher in the females at 1 and 2 hours.— R. Scotti, *Chemotherapy, Basle*, 1973, *18*, 205.

In a study of 21 patients there was a significant correlation between serum trough concentrations of chloramphenicol and dose in patients with normal liver function but no such correlation in patients with impaired liver function. Mean serum protein binding of chloramphenicol was 53% in 10 patients with normal liver function, 42% in 15 patients with cirrhosis, and 32% in 20 premature infants. Reduced binding in neonates suggests that a lower therapeutic range of total chloramphenicol concentration of 3.5 to 13.9 µg per ml might be required compared with the usual adult range of 5 to 20 µg per ml. Half of the patients with impaired liver function had serum concentrations of above 25 µg per ml after usual doses of chloramphenicol. The degree of intrapatient variation suggests that frequent monitoring of serum concentrations is necessary with empirical adjustment of dosage when indicated.— J. R. Koup *et al.*, *Antimicrob. Ag. Chemother.*, 1979, *15*, 651.

There was no detectable systemic absorption of chloramphenicol after instillation of chloramphenicol eye-drops 2-hourly for 5 to 7 days.— G. E. Trope *et al.*, *Br. J. Ophthal.*, 1979, *63*, 690.

Absorption and fate in disease states. In a study of the metabolism of chloramphenicol in malnourished children only 35 to 55% of an oral dose, given as the palmitate, appeared in the conjugated form compared with 75 to 80% in normal children.— S. Mehta *et al.*, *Am. J. clin. Nutr.*, 1975, *28*, 977.

Absorption and fate in infants and children. See A. Windorfer and W. Pringsheim, *Eur. J. Pediat.*, 1977, *124*, 129; S. B. Black *et al.*, *J. Pediat.*, 1978, *92*, 235; C. A. Friedman *et al.*, *ibid.*, 1979, *95*, 1071; L. K. Pickering *et al.*, *ibid.*, 1980, *96*, 757; J. P. Glazer *et al.*, *Pediatrics*, 1980, *66*, 573; C. M. Sack *et al.*, *ibid.*, 579; J. R. Koup *et al.*, *Clin. Pharmacokinet.*, 1981, *6*, 83. See also above.

Bioavailability. Bioavailability studies on 5 commercial sugar-coated chloramphenicol tablets.— H. Ogata *et al.*, *J. pharm. Sci.*, 1979, *68*, 712.

The absorption-rates as shown by urinary excretion were similar for chloramphenicol and its cationic acrylic resin coprecipitate; the anionic coprecipitate studied was absorbed more slowly, but the extent of absorption was equal for all the preparations examined.— A. Ghanem *et al.*, *Can. J. pharm. Sci.*, 1980, *15*, 17.

Diffusion. *Ascitic fluid.* D. N. Gerding *et al.*, *Ann. intern. Med.*, 1977, *86*, 708.

Brain. Of 5 antibiotics, including ampicillin and chloramphenicol, given in usual doses to patients with non-inflamed meninges, only chloramphenicol achieved concentrations in brain tissue sufficient to inhibit Gram-negative pathogens. The administration of dexamethasone had no effect on this diffusion.— P. W. Kramer *et al.*, *J. Neurosurg.*, 1969, *31*, 295.

Peak serum concentrations of chloramphenicol and concentrations in cerebrospinal fluid ranged from 14.1 to 54.4 µg per ml and from 13.0 to 36.6 µg per ml respectively in 3 premature infants with intracranial sepsis who received chloramphenicol 25 to 35 mg per kg body-weight daily in 2 divided intravenous infusions of one hour each.— L. M. Dunkle, *Antimicrob. Ag. Chemother.*, 1978, *13*, 427.

Following doses of chloramphenicol of 25 mg per kg body-weight given to 2 infants with hydrocephalus and ventriculitis peak serum and peak ventricular fluid concentrations occurred after 30 minutes and 3 hours respectively. The peak ventricular fluid concentration was 57.5% of the peak serum concentration in one patient and only 22.5% in the other.— R. Yogev and T. Williams, *Antimicrob. Ag. Chemother.*, 1979, *16*, 7.

Eye. The penetration of chloramphenicol from eye-drops or ointment was assessed in 183 patients. The concentration of chloramphenicol in tears fell below 1 µg per ml within about 5 minutes of a single application of a 0.5% solution to the eye and repeated instillation during several hours was necessary to achieve a concentration in aqueous humour of 1 µg per ml. A single application of chloramphenicol 1% ointment produced concentrations in aqueous humour of about 2 µg per ml at 2 hours, falling to 1 µg per ml at 4 hours; repeated applications of the ointment every 15 minutes gave a concentration of up to 77 µg per ml.— C. Hanna *et al.*, *Archs Ophthal., N.Y.*, 1978, *96*, 1258.

Saliva. Studies in 20 patients being treated with chloramphenicol indicated that serum and saliva concentrations were significantly but variably related and therefore saliva concentrations could not be relied upon as a guide to therapy.— J. R. Koup *et al.*, *Antimicrob. Ag. Chemother.*, 1979, *15*, 658.

Uses. The liability of chloramphenicol to provoke life-threatening adverse effects, particularly bone-marrow aplasia, severely limits its clinical usefulness. It should never be given for minor infections and regular blood estimations should be made during treatment of all patients. Typhoid fever and similar salmonellal infections are the prime indications for the use of chloramphenicol, though it will not eliminate the carrier state.

It is used in serious infections due to *Haemophilus influenzae*, including meningitis attributed to ampicillin-resistant strains, but if children are to be treated the 'grey syndrome' should be taken into consideration; it has been incorporated into cystic fibrosis regimens. Chloramphenicol has also been used to eradicate vibrios from patients with cholera, to treat severe anaerobic infections due to *Bacteroides fragilis* especially those involving the central nervous system, and rickettsial infections such as typhus and Rocky Mountain spotted fever when tetracyclines are not indicated. Chloramphenicol is applied topically for a variety of eye infections due to sensitive organisms and has also been used in skin infections.

Chloramphenicol is usually administered by mouth in capsules or as a suspension of chloramphenicol palmitate (see p.1141). For adults the usual dose is 500 mg every 6 hours or 50 mg per kg body-weight daily. In the treatment of typhoid fever a higher initial dose should not be given because of the release of endotoxins from the infecting organisms. Treatment should be continued for 2 or 3 days after the patient's temperature has returned to normal so as to minimise the risk of relapse, but it is inadvisable to employ prolonged courses and for this reason a maximum total dose of 26 g has been recommended although in severe infections higher doses have been given.

For children, the usual daily dose is 25 to 50 mg per kg body-weight, given in divided doses at intervals of 6 hours. Doses of up to 100 mg per kg daily have occasionally been given.

In cases of severe infection, premature and full-term infants may be given daily doses of up to 25 mg per kg body-weight and full-term infants over the age of 2 weeks may be given up to 50 mg per kg. However, chloramphenicol should only be used when there is no other suitable treatment for the severe infection and when blood concentrations can be monitored.

Chloramphenicol may be administered by injection as the water-soluble Chloramphenicol Sodium Succinate (p.1142).

Reviews of chloramphenicol.— H. C. Meissner and A. L. Smith, *Pediatrics*, 1979, *64*, 348; A. Kucers, *J. antimicrob. Chemother.*, 1980, *6*, 1.

The proceedings of a 1973 symposium on the metabolism, pharmacokinetics, toxicity, actions including immunosuppressant effects, and uses of chloramphenicol and thiamphenicol.— *Postgrad. med. J.*, 1974, *50* (Oct.), *Suppl.*, 5.

Chloramphenicol reduced the white cell and blast count in a patient with chronic myeloid leukaemia.— M. A. Schwarz and B. G. Firkin, *Med. J. Aust.*, 1976, *1*, 687. See also B. Klein *et al.*, *Acta haemat.*, 1980, *64*, 246.

Cephaloridine 1 g with chloramphenicol 2 g given daily for 3 weeks was used successfully to treat a patient with an infection produced by a strain of *Proteus rettgeri* highly resistant to several antibiotics including cephaloridine. A second patient with an infection produced by a strain of *Serratia liquefaciens* similarly resistant was successfully treated with cephaloridine 3 g and chloramphenicol 3 g daily for 10 days. It was stressed that this combination should only be used when resistance was due to beta-lactamase production and when high concentrations of the antibiotics could be achieved.— T. Sacks *et al.* (letter), *J. antimicrob. Chemother.*, 1977, *3*, 525.

Treatment aimed at eradicating a possible reservoir of infection due to a Gram-positive bacterium in the bone marrow consisted in one patient of chloramphenicol 6 g daily given intravenously for 10 days then 1 g daily by mouth for one month; this was then replaced by cephalexin given for a further 10 months. Since then the patient has remained well for a year.— G. L. Archer *et al.*, *New Engl. J. Med.*, 1979, *301*, 897.

Dosage. To minimise the risk of death from aplastic anaemia, chloramphenicol should not be given in doses exceeding 30 mg per kg body-weight daily, nor in courses of more than 7 days, and the dose should be kept low if it has to be given to patients with defective renal function.— P. H. Willcox (letter), *Br. med. J.*, 1967, *2*, 443.

For a method of predicting individual daily dosage requirements of chloramphenicol from a single serum assay following an initial dose, see J. R. Koup *et al.*, *Clin. Pharmacokinet.*, 1979, *4*, 460.

Dosage in hepatic failure. For a report of reduced protein binding and elevated serum concentrations of chloramphenicol in patients with impaired liver function, see above under Absorption and Fate.

Dosage in infants and children. For references to the use of chloramphenicol in infants and children, see P. A. Davies, *Br. J. Hosp. Med.*, 1972, *8*, 13; P. A. Davies, *Br. med. J.*, 1978, *2*, 676; H. C. Spratt, *Drugs*, 1978, *16*, 226; G. H. McCracken and H. F. Eichenwald, *J. Pediat.*, 1978, *93*, 357.

For reference to the reduced protein binding of chloramphenicol in premature infants, see above under Absorption and Fate.

Dosage in renal failure. Chloramphenicol should be avoided in moderate or severe renal failure.— P. Sharpstone, *Br. med. J.*, 1977, *2*, 36.

The dose of chloramphenicol should be reduced by 10% in uraemic patients.— G. B. Appel and H. C. Neu, *New Engl. J. Med.*, 1977, *296*, 663.

Data for predicting removal of chloramphenicol by conventional haemodialysis.— T. P. Gibson and H. A. Nelson, *Clin. Pharmacokinet.*, 1977, *2*, 403.

Chloramphenicol was reported to be 60% bound to plasma proteins; binding might be slightly decreased in end-stage renal disease and cirrhosis. The normal half-life of 2.5 hours was increased to 3 to 7 hours in end-stage renal failure; the half-life might be markedly prolonged in the joint presence of renal and hepatic impairment. Chloramphenicol could be given in usual doses to patients with renal failure. Concentrations of chloramphenicol were affected by haemodialysis, but not by peritoneal dialysis.— W. M. Bennett *et al.*, *Ann. intern. Med.*, 1980, *93*, 62.

Further references: H. G. Wolters and D. Hoffler, *Dt. med. Wschr.*, 1970, *95*, 2019; J. S. Cheigh, *Am. J. Med.*, 1977, *62*, 555.

Effect on leucocyte migration. Chloramphenicol inhibited leucocyte migration (leucotaxis) *in vitro*.— A. Forsgren and D. Schmeling, *Antimicrob. Ag. Chemother.*, 1977, *11*, 580.

Eye infections. Reports of the successful use of chloramphenicol eye-drops in the treatment of conjunctivitis due to *Neisseria meningitidis*.— D. Hansman (letter), *Br. med. J.*, 1972, *1*, 748. *Yersinia enterocolitica* (chloramphenicol and penicillin were also given systemically).— E. P. Crichton (letter), *Can. med. Ass. J.*, 1978, *118*, 22. See also *ibid.*, 490 and 901.

The incidence of eye infections following 20 000 cataract operations was 0.11%. When chloramphenicol 0.4% was used topically with polymyxin B and erythromycin for prophylaxis the incidence of infections fell to 0.02% in 15 000 operations compared with an incidence of 0.6% when neomycin was substituted for chloramphenicol.— H. F. Allen and A. B. Mangiaracine, *Archs Ophthal., N.Y.*, 1974, *91*, 3.

Late complications of chemical burns of the eye included adhesions of the globe to the lid; liberal and frequent application of chloramphenicol eye ointment or eye-drops was desirable. Chloramphenicol should also be used after the removal of a foreign body from the eye.— P. A. Gardiner, *Br. med. J.*, 1978, *2*, 1347.

Chloramphenicol 1 mg by subconjunctival injection or 1 to 2 mg by intravitreal injection could be given daily for 7 to 10 days in the treatment of corneal infections.— F. P. Furgiule, *Drugs*, 1978, *15*, 310.

Haemophilus infections. Chloramphenicol was considered the antibiotic of choice for life-threatening haemophilus infections, including epiglottitis, because of the emergence of beta-lactamase-producing strains of *Haemophilus influenzae* type b.— D. C. Turk (letter), *Br. med. J.*, 1976, *2*, 1385.

A suggestion that chemotherapy in epiglottitis and haemophilus meningitis should begin with ampicillin in association with chloramphenicol.— D. Hansman (letter), *Lancet*, 1979, *1*, 1354.

Further references: M. G. Addy *et al.*, *Br. med. J.*, 1972, *1*, 40; B. Wolman *et al.* (letter), *ibid.*, 246; G. Delage *et al.* (letter), *J. Pediat.*, 1977, *90*, 319; A. M. Gellady *et al.*, *Pediatrics*, 1978, *61*, 272; N. F. R. Williams *et al.*, *Can. med. Ass. J.*, 1978, *118*, 63.

See also under Meningitis.

Leprosy. Chloramphenicol 1 g thrice daily by mouth or intramuscular injection was used to treat 30 African patients with erythema nodosum leprosum and 1 with acute peripheral neuritis. All patients with severe forms of the disease improved but not those with few persistent moderate lesions. Relapse occurred in 30% of patients after 15 days to 4 months.— P. Saint-André *et al.*, *Afr. Med.*, 1973, *12*, 871, per *Trop. Dis. Bull.*, 1975, *72*, 41.

Melioidosis. Experience in Vietnam indicated that chloramphenicol 12 g, kanamycin sulphate 4 g, and novobiocin sodium 6 g, daily, might be required to control a serious infection. Further antibiotic dosage would depend on clinical responses. Minimum duration of therapy advised was not less than 4 weeks.— E. B. Cooper, *J. Am. med. Ass.*, 1967, *200*, 452. See also M. C. Patterson *et al.*, *ibid.*, 447.

Meningitis. The US Public Health Service recommended that chloramphenicol might be used in penicillin-sensitive patients with gonococcal meningitis.— *Morb. Mortal.*, 1979, *28*, 13.

Meningitis caused by *Campylobacter fetus* subspp. *jejuni* in a 34-year-old man was successfully treated with chloramphenicol. The organism was resistant to ampicillin but was sensitive also to metronidazole.— R. Norrby *et al.*, *Br. med. J.*, 1980, *280*, 1164.

Further references: L. R. O'Grady and E. D. Ralph, *Am. J. Dis. Child.*, 1976, *130*, 871; W. E. Feldman, *Am. J. Dis. Child.*, 1976, *130*, 880 (anaerobic meningitis).

For a report of penicillin-insensitive pneumococci in Papua New Guinea, and the recommendation that chloramphenicol can be used as an alternative in the treatment of pneumococcal meningitis there, see Benzylpenicillin, p.1107.

See also under Choice of an Antibiotic, p.1079.

Haemophilus influenzae meningitis. A retrospective comparative study of the therapy of *H. influenzae* meningitis with chloramphenicol and ampicillin in 116 and 136 children respectively showed that ampicillin-treated patients had a higher degree of fever and remained febrile longer than those treated with chloramphenicol. Also, 6 of those who received ampicillin suffered bacteriological relapse whereas there was no relapse in the chloramphenicol-treated patients.— P. G. Shackelford *et al.*, *New Engl. J. Med.*, 1972, *287*, 634. See also *ibid.*, 664.

Because of ampicillin-resistant *H. influenzae* it was considered reasonable to include chloramphenicol 100 mg per kg body-weight daily by intravenous injection in the initial treatment of bacterial meningitis in children aged more than 2 months in North America. The American Academy of Pediatrics recommended in 1975 that in areas where resistance had occurred and when *H. influenzae* type b was suspected to be the pathogen the initial treatment of meningitis should include benzylpenicillin or ampicillin with chloramphenicol 100 mg per kg daily.— *Med. Lett.*, 1975, *17*, 15.

A discussion on the use of ampicillin and chloramphenicol in the treatment of *H. influenzae* meningitis.— R. J. Fallon, *J. antimicrob. Chemother.*, 1976, *2*, 3. See also R. D. Feigin *et al.*, *J. Pediat.*, 1976, *88*, 542; W. E. Feldman, *Pediatrics*, 1978, *61*, 406.

See also under Chloramphenicol Sodium Succinate, p.1142 for reference to the incompatibility of chloramphenicol with ampicillin.

Comment on the treatment of *H. influenzae* meningitis in children and results indicating that treatment with chloramphenicol by mouth was as effective and safe as intravenous therapy with chloramphenicol.— *J. Am. med. Ass.*, 1980, *244*, 1883.

For a warning that initial chloramphenicol therapy should not be discontinued too soon in severe *H. influenzae* infection, see Ampicillin, p.1096.

For a comparison of the treatment of *H. influenzae* meningitis with ampicillin or triple therapy with chloramphenicol, a sulphonamide, and a penicillin, see Ampicillin, p.1097.

Meningococcal meningitis. In a study in Nigeria, where 30% of group A meningococci were resistant to sulphonamides, 123 patients with group A meningococcal meningitis were treated with either chloramphenicol or benzylpenicillin; the results were considered comparable but chloramphenicol was cheaper. Of 65 and 68 treated respectively with chloramphenicol and benzylpenicillin 9 and 10 respectively were considered treatment failures. Of 5 treated with chloramphenicol and who had severe neurological signs at 5 days, 4 improved remarkably before follow-up, as did 5 of 8 similar patients who had been treated with benzylpenicillin.— H. C. Whittle *et al.*, *Br. med. J.*, 1973, *3*, 379.

Meningococcal meningitis was cured in 35 of 49 children over 1-year-old by a single injection of chloramphenicol given intramuscularly as an oily suspension. Only 4 of 17 children with pneumococcal meningitis were cured. The dose ranged from 1 to 3 g according to age.— P. Saliou *et al.*, *Méd. trop. Marseille*, 1977, *37*, 189. See also S. S. Wali *et al.*, *Trans. R. Soc. trop. Med. Hyg.*, 1979, *73*, 698.

Pneumonia. Chloramphenicol 500 mg six-hourly for 7 days was successful in the treatment of a patient with pneumonia due to *Flavobacterium meningosepticum*.— D. Teres, *J. Am. med. Ass.*, 1974, *228*, 732.

Rocky Mountain spotted fever. Of 13 patients with Rocky Mountain spotted fever, all of 10 patients given chloramphenicol survived and one given tetracycline made a slow recovery.— G. W. Hazard *et al.*, *New Engl. J. Med.*, 1969, *280*, 57.

Salmonellal infections. In 144 patients with salmonellal enteric fever the mean time taken to abolish fever was 5.1 days when chloramphenicol, 50 mg per kg body-weight daily, was administered. Ampicillin, 100 mg per kg daily, abolished fever in 6.5 days, and a combination of both antibiotics in 4.9 days. Treatment was continued for 7 days after the patients had become afebrile. In the ampicillin group the failures (23%) subsequently responded to chloramphenicol, and no failure occurred in the other 2 groups. A similar response occurred in 121 patients with non-specific enteric fever. Temporary carriers occurred only in the chloramphenicol-treated group. It was concluded that chloramphenicol was the most effective treatment, with ampicillin as an effective alternative.— R. P. Robertson *et al.*, *New Engl. J. Med.*, 1968, *278*, 171.

Chloramphenicol by mouth or intramuscular injection was compared with ampicillin and co-trimoxazole in the treatment of 89 patients with bacteriologically confirmed typhoid fever. Chloramphenicol 50 mg per kg body-weight given by mouth daily in divided doses for 12 days provided the best treatment. Chloramphenicol given by mouth produced higher blood concentrations than the same dose given intramuscularly. However, in a second smaller study just involving these 2 routes of administration of chloramphenicol the response from the oral route was no better than that from the intramuscular route.— M. J. Snyder *et al.*, *Lancet*, 1976, *2*, 1155.

In a comparative study of chloramphenicol and co-trimoxazole in patients with typhoid and paratyphoid fever, treatment with chloramphenicol was more successful initially but gave rise to a greater number of carriers.— S. Ramachandran *et al.*, *J. trop. Med. Hyg.*, 1978, *81*, 36.

A favourable report of surgery with peritoneal irrigation, using a solution of dextran in which chloramphenicol 4 g per litre together with aprotinin 1 million units had been dissolved, in the treatment of typhoid perforation.— O. A. Badejo and A. O. Arigbabu, *Gut*, 1980, *21*, 141.

Further references: K. P. Mokhobo, *S.Afr. med. J.*, 1975, *49*, 55; M. Uwaydah, *J. antimicrob. Chemother.*, 1975, *1*, 135; J. Brodie, *J. Hyg., Camb.*, 1976, *76*, 191; S. K. Samantray *et al.*, *Practitioner*, 1977, *218*, 400; D. Portnoy and S. Seah, *Can. med. Ass. J.*, 1979, *120*, 1264.

For a study showing amoxycillin to be superior to chloramphenicol in typhoid fever, see Amoxycillin, p.1091.

See also under Ampicillin, p.1097.

See also under Resistance, p.1138.

Skin disorders. A report of similar beneficial results with topical preparations of chloramphenicol (Actinac) or benzoyl peroxide (PanOxyl 5 Acne Gel) in the treatment of acne.— W. J. Cunliffe *et al.*, *Practitioner*, 1980, *224*, 952.

Trachoma. For the use of chloramphenicol in conjunction with sulphonamides in the treatment of trachoma, see M. H. Bhimani, *Dar es Salaam med. J.*, 1969, *1*, 65, per *Trop. Dis. Bull.*, 1970, *67*, 1044.

Typhus. For a comparison of doxycycline, chloramphenicol, and co-trimoxazole in the treatment of typhus, see Doxycycline Hydrochloride, p.1157.

Preparations

Capsules

Chloramphenicol Capsules *(B.P.)*. Capsules containing chloramphenicol. Store at a temperature not exceeding 30°.

U.S.P. specifies 50, 100, or 250 mg. Store in airtight containers.

Creams

Chloramphenicol Cream *(D.T.F.)*. Chloramphenicol 1 g, propylene glycol 50 g, macrogol '4000' 49 g.

Ear-drops

Chloramphenicol Ear Drops *(B.P., A.P.F.).* Auristillae Chloramphenicolis. Chloramphenicol in propylene glycol. Protect from light. Small amounts of water reduce the solubility of chloramphenicol in propylene glycol.

For a report of ototoxicity in *guinea-pigs*, see p.1137.

Eye Ointments

Chloramphenicol Eye Ointment *(B.P.).* Oculentum Chloramphenicolis; Chloramphenicol Ophthalmic Ointment. A sterile eye ointment containing chloramphenicol in Simple Eye Ointment or other suitable basis.

Nord. P. and *U.S.P.* (Chloramphenicol Ophthalmic Ointment) include a similar ointment.

Chloramphenicol Eye Ointment *(A.P.F.).* Chloramphenicol 1% in Eye Ointment Base (*A.P.F.*). Prepared using an aseptic technique.

Eye-drops

Chloramphenicol Eye Drops *(B.P.).* Guttae Chloramphenicolis; CPL. A sterile solution of chloramphenicol in water containing suitable buffers and 0.002% of phenylmercuric acetate or nitrate. pH 7 to 7.5. Store at 2° to 8° when they may be expected to retain their potency for 18 months, or at a temperature not exceeding 25° when they may be expected to retain their potency for 4 months. Protect from light. Eye-drops intended for use on more than one occasion should not be used later than one month after first opening the container.

Chloramphenicol Eye Drops *(A.P.F.).* Chloramphenicol 500 mg, boric acid 1.5 g, borax 300 mg, phenylmercuric nitrate 2 mg, and Water for Injections to 100 ml.

Chloramphenicol for Ophthalmic Solution *(U.S.P.).* A sterile dry mixture of chloramphenicol with or without one or more suitable buffers, diluents, and preservatives. Store in airtight containers. The solution is prepared by the addition of diluent before use and contains not less than 1 mg of chloramphenicol per ml. It may contain cortisone or hydrocortisone or a suitable ester of either. pH 7.1 to 7.5.

Chloramphenicol Ophthalmic Solution *(U.S.P.).* A sterile buffered solution of chloramphenicol. pH 7 to 7.5. Store in airtight containers.

Preservative for eye-drops. Benzalkonium chloride 0.01% or phenylmercuric borate 0.005% were suitable preservatives for chloramphenicol eye-drops sterilised by filtration.— M. Van Ooteghem, *Pharm. Tijdschr. Belg.*, 1968, *45*, 69.

Injections

Chloramphenicol Injection *(U.S.P.).* A sterile solution of chloramphenicol 250 mg per ml in one or more suitable solvents. It may contain suitable buffers. pH 4.7 to 5.

Solutions

Chloramphenicol Solution for Burns. Chloramphenicol 100 mg, polymyxin B sulphate 100 000 units, neomycin [sulphate] 50 mg, sodium chloride 0.9% solution to 100 ml. Chloramphenicol sodium succinate should not be used as it was inactive when applied topically.—R.J. Kellogg and T.A. Stolee (letter), *Am.J. Hosp. Pharm.*,1972, *29*, 386.

Proprietary Preparations

Actinac *(Roussel, UK).* Powder containing in each g chloramphenicol 40 mg, hydrocortisone acetate 40 mg, butoxyethyl nicotinate ($C_{12}H_{17}NO_3$=223.3) 24 mg, allantoin 24 mg, and precipitated sulphur 320 mg, supplied with bottles of aqueous diluent for preparing a lotion. For acne.

Alcon Opulets Chloramphenicol 0.5% *(Alcon, UK: Farillon, UK).* Sterile eye-drops containing chloramphenicol 0.5%, in single-use disposable applicators. Store at 5°; protect from light.

Chloromycetin *(Parke, Davis, UK).* Chloramphenicol, available as **Capsules** of 250 mg; as **Ear-drops Topical 10%** containing 10% in propylene glycol; as **Ophthalmic Ointment** containing 1%; as **Chloromycetin Redidrops (Ophthalmic)** containing 0.5% in aqueous solution with boric acid, borax, and phenylmercuric acetate; and as **Chloromycetin Pure**, chloramphenicol in powder form. (Also available as Chloromycetin in *Arg., Austral., Belg., Canad., Denm., Ital., Norw., S.Afr., Swed., Switz., USA*).

Chloromycetin-Hydrocortisone Ophthalmic Ointment *(Parke, Davis, UK).* Contains chloramphenicol 1% and hydrocortisone acetate 0.5%.

Kemicetine *(Farmitalia Carlo Erba, UK).* Chloramphenicol, available as sterile powder in vials of 1 g. (Also available as Kemicetine in *S.Afr.*).

Minims Chloramphenicol *(Smith & Nephew Pharmaceuticals, UK).* Sterile eye-drops containing chloramphenicol 0.5% in single-use disposable applicators. Store at 5°.

Sno phenicol *(Smith & Nephew Pharmaceuticals, UK).* Eye-drops containing chloramphenicol 0.5% with polyvinyl alcohol. Store at 5°.

Other Proprietary Names

Arg.—Bioticaps *(see also Chloramphenicol Sodium Succinate)*, Cloroptic, Farmicetina *(see also Chloramphenicol Cinnamate)*, Iprobiot, Pantofenicol *(pantothenate) (see also Chloramphenicol Palmitate)*, Quemicetina *(also stearate) (see also Chloramphenicol Sodium Succinate)*, Sintomicetina *(see also Chloramphenicol Palmitate)*; *Austral.*—Chlomin, Chloramol *(see also Chloramphenicol Sodium Succinate)*, Chloroptic, Chlorsig, Opclor; *Belg.*—Fenicol, Globenicol *(see also Chloramphenicol Palmitate and Chloramphenicol Sodium Succinate)*, Kemicetina, Synthomycetine *(see also Chloramphenicol Sodium Succinate)*; *Canad.*—Chloroptic, Fenicol, Isopto Fenicol, Novochlorocap, Pentamycetin, Sopamycetin; *Fr.*—Cébénicol, Ophtaphénicol, Tifomycine; *Ger.*—Aquamycetin *(see also Chloramphenicol Sodium Succinate)*, Chloroptic, Kamaver *(see also Chloramphenicol Palmitate)*, Leukomycin, Oleomycetin, Pantovernil, Paraxin; *Ind.*—Ranphenicol *(see also Chloramphenicol Palmitate and Chloramphenicol Sodium Succinate)*; *Ital.*—Cafenolo, Chemicetina *(also stearate) (see also Chloramphenicol Sodium Succinate)*, Chemyzin, Cloramfen, Levomicetina, Lomecitina, Micoclorina *(also glycinate sulphate)*, Micodry *(chloramphenicol palmitoylglycolate)*, Mycetin, Sificetina; *Neth.*—Globenicol *(see also Chloramphenicol Palmitate and Chloramphenicol Sodium Succinate)*; *Norw.*—Oftalent; *S.Afr.*—Chloramex, Chlorcol, Chloroptic, Lennacol, Troymycetin; *Spain*—Chemicetina, Cloramplast, Clorbiotina *(also glycinate sulphate)*, Cloromicetin, Cloromoin, Cloromycetin *(see also Chloramphenicol Palmitate and Chloramphenicol Sodium Succinate)*, Plastodermo; *Switz.*—Cutispray No. 4, Doctamicina, Isopto Fenicol, Labamicol, Rivomycine, Septicol *(see also Chloramphenicol Palmitate and Chloramphenicol Sodium Succinate)*, Spersanicol; *USA*—Amphicol, Antibiopto, Econochlor, Mychel, Ophthoclor.

Preparations containing chloramphenicol were also formerly marketed in Great Britain under the proprietary names Ginetris (*Montedison* now *Farmitalia Carlo Erba*) and Otopred Ear Drops (*Loveridge*).

47-g

Chloramphenicol Cinnamate *(B.P.C. 1968).* (2*R*,3*R*)-2-(2,2-Dichloroacetamido)-3-hydroxy-3-(4-nitrophenyl)propyl cinnamate.

$C_{20}H_{18}Cl_2N_2O_6$=453.3.

CAS — 14399-14-5.

A white or yellowish-white, odourless, crystalline powder; it is tasteless or almost tasteless. M.p. about 119°.

Very slightly **soluble** in water; soluble, at 20°, 1 in 25 of alcohol, 1 in 50 of chloroform, and 1 in 500 of ether. A 10% suspension in water is neutral to litmus. **Protect** from light.

Chloramphenicol cinnamate has the actions and uses of chloramphenicol (see p.1136) and was administered by mouth as a flavoured aqueous suspension.

Proprietary Names

Farmicetina *(Montedison, Arg.) (see also Chloramphenicol)*.

48-q

Chloramphenicol Palmitate *(B.P., U.S.P.).*

Chloramphen. Palm.; Chloramphenicol α-Palmitate; Palmitylchloramphenicol. (2*R*, 3*R*)-2-(2,2-Dichloroacetamido)-3-hydroxy-3-(4-nitrophenyl)propyl palmitate.

$C_{27}H_{42}Cl_2N_2O_6$=561.5.

CAS — 530-43-8.

Pharmacopoeias. In *Br., Braz., Cz., Fr., Hung., It., Jap., Jug., Nord., Swiss, Turk.*, and *U.S.*

A fine, white, unctuous, crystalline powder with a faint odour and a bland mild taste. M.p. 87° to 95°. Chloramphenicol palmitate 174 mg is approximately equivalent to 100 mg of chloramphenicol.

Practically **insoluble** in water; soluble 1 in 45 of alcohol, 1 in 6 of chloroform, and 1 in 14 of ether; freely soluble in acetone; soluble in ethyl acetate; very slightly soluble in light petroleum. A solution in dehydrated alcohol is dextrorotatory. **Store** in airtight containers. Protect from light.

Chloramphenicol palmitate occurs in several polymorphic forms. Although any polymorph may be used in making preparations the final product must contain the desired polymorph B. The *B.P.* specifies a limit for polymorph A in Chloramphenicol Palmitate Mixture.

Absorption. Three polymorphic forms of the palmitate were demonstrated, of which polymorph B was the best absorbed. Peak blood concentrations were up to 8 times higher for polymorph B than Polymorph A, both of about 5 μm particle size. Increasing the mean diameter of form B to 25 μm did not reduce blood concentrations.— A. J. Aguiar *et al.*, *J. pharm. Sci.*, 1967, *56*, 847.

Suspensions containing the equivalent of 250 mg of chloramphenicol as the polymorph A or amorphous forms of chloramphenicol palmitate with 2% of polysorbate 80 were administered to up to 10 children aged 5 to 7 years. Serum concentrations of chloramphenicol after 2 and 4 hours were less after administration of suspensions containing polymorph A compared with the amorphous form. After 6 hours, the blood concentration was higher with the polymorph A suspension and at 8 hours there was little difference between the two.— S. Banerjee *et al.*, *J. pharm. Sci.*, 1971, *60*, 153.

The hydrolysis of chloramphenicol palmitate polymorphs A and B by pancreatin.— H. Andersgaard *et al.*, *Acta pharm. suec.*, 1974, *11*, 239.

Stability. The formulation of a stable chloramphenicol palmitate suspension.— A. Moës, *Pharm. Acta Helv.*, 1968, *43*, 290.

The polymorph B (α-form) of chloramphenicol palmitate was stable at room and higher temperatures; aqueous suspensions were also stable, with and without wetting agents. Polymorph C was less stable and rapidly converted to polymorph A (β-form) at elevated temperatures.— L. Borka, *Acta pharm. suec.*, 1971, *8*, 365.

Chloramphenicol palmitate suspension in a syrup basis became curdled and discoloured after storage in a rigid amber polyvinyl chloride bottle for 2 years, but kept well when stored in amber glass bottles for the same period.— R. C. Shah *et al.*, *Pharm. J.*, 1978, *2*, 58.

Chloramphenicol palmitate has the actions and uses of chloramphenicol (see p.1136) and is administered by mouth in equivalent doses as a flavoured aqueous suspension. It is hydrolysed to chloramphenicol in the gastro-intestinal tract.

Sequential measurement of CSF-chloramphenicol concentrations over a 6-hour dosage interval in a patient with an indwelling lumbar subarachnoid catheter. Therapeutic concentrations (5 μg or more per ml) were achieved during the entire dosage interval after oral administration of chloramphenicol palmitate suspension 12.5 mg per kg body-weight every 6 hours.— E. R. Rensimer *et al.* (letter), *Lancet*, 1981, *1*, 165.

Preparations

Chloramphenicol Palmitate Mixture *(B.P.).* Chloramphenicol Mixture; Chloramphenicol Palmitate Suspension. A suspension of chloramphenicol palmitate in very fine particles in a suitably flavoured vehicle. Potency is expressed in terms of the equivalent amount of chloramphenicol. When a dose less than or not a multiple of 5 ml is prescribed, the mixture should be diluted to 5 ml, or a multiple, with syrup. Such dilutions must be freshly prepared and not used more than 2 weeks after issue. Protect from light.

Chloramphenicol Palmitate Oral Suspension *(U.S.P.).* A suspension containing chloramphenicol palmitate with one or more suitable buffers, preservatives, colouring, flavouring, and suspending agents. It contains the equivalent of 31.25 mg of chloramphenicol per ml. pH 4.5 to 7. Store in airtight containers. Protect from light.

Chloramphenicol Palmitate Suspension *(F.N. Belg.).* A suspension containing chloramphenicol palmitate 350 mg in each 5 ml.

Proprietary Preparations

Chloromycetin Palmitate Suspension *(Parke, Davis, UK).* A suspension containing in each 5 ml chloramphenicol palmitate equivalent to 125 mg of chloramphenicol (suggested diluent, syrup). (Also available as Chloromycetin Palmitate Suspension in *Arg., Austral., Belg., Canad., Ital., S.Afr., Switz., USA*).

Other Proprietary Names

Arg.—Pantofenicol, Sintomicetina *(both also under*

Chloramphenicol); *Denm.*—Chloramex; *Ger.*—Kamaver (see also Chloramphenicol); *Ind.*—Ranphenicol (see also Chloramphenicol and Chloramphenicol Sodium Succinate); *Ital.*—Paidomicetina; *Neth.*—Globenicol (see also Chloramphenicol and Chloramphenicol Sodium Succinate); *Spain*—Cloromisol, Cloromycetin (see also Chloramphenicol and Chloramphenicol Sodium Succinate); *Switz.*—Septicol (see also Chloramphenicol and Chloramphenicol Sodium Succinate).

49-p

Chloramphenicol Sodium Succinate *(B.P., B.P. Vet.).*

Chloramphen. Sod. Succ.; Chloramphenicol α-Sodium Succinate. Sodium (2*R*,3*R*)-2-(2,2-dichloroacetamido)-3-hydroxy-3-(4-nitrophenyl)propyl succinate.

$C_{15}H_{15}Cl_2N_2NaO_8$=445.2.

CAS — 982-57-0.

Pharmacopoeias. In *Br., Cz.,* and *Jap. U.S.* includes Sterile Chloramphenicol Sodium Succinate.

A white or yellowish-white hygroscopic, odourless or almost odourless powder with a bitter saline taste. Chloramphenicol sodium succinate 140 mg is approximately equivalent to 100 mg of chloramphenicol.

Soluble 1 in less than 1 of water, 1 in 1 of alcohol; practically insoluble in chloroform and ether. A 25% solution in water has a pH of 6 to 7. A 6.8% solution in water is iso-osmotic with serum. **Store** in airtight containers. Protect from light. If intended for injection the containers should be sterile and sealed to exclude micro-organisms.

Sterile solutions are stable for 30 days at room temperature. A slight change of colour is not indicative of loss of potency, but cloudy solutions should not be employed.

Incompatibility. There was loss of clarity when intravenous solutions of chloramphenicol sodium succinate were mixed with those of *benzyl alcohol, erythromycin gluceptate, hydroxyzine hydrochloride, novobiocin sodium, oxytetracycline hydrochloride, phenytoin sodium, prochlorperazine maleate, promethazine hydrochloride, tetracycline hydrochloride, tripelennamine hydrochloride,* or *vancomycin hydrochloride.*— J. A. Patel and G. L. Phillips, *Am. J. Hosp. Pharm.*, 1966, *23*, 409. A similar report.— R. Misgen, *Am. J. Hosp. Pharm.*, 1965, *22*, 92.

A haze or precipitate was observed within an hour when an average dose of chloramphenicol sodium succinate was mixed in dextrose injection with *polymyxin B sulphate, tetracycline hydrochloride,* or certain strengths of *erythromycin lactobionate.* A precipitate occurred with *hydrocortisone sodium succinate* on standing.— J. M. Meisler and M. W. Skolaut, *Am. J. Hosp. Pharm.*, 1966, *23*, 557.

Diluents containing benzyl alcohol were satisfactory for the preparation of chloramphenicol sodium succinate solutions.— E. A. Parker, *Abbott* (letter), *Am. J. Hosp. Pharm.*, 1969, *26*, 197.

Chloramphenicol sodium succinate was incompatible with *aminophylline, benzyl alcohol, calcium chloride, suxamethonium,* or *vitamins of the B group with vitamin C,* in an infusion fluid.— B. Flouvat and P. Lechat, *Thérapie*, 1974, *29*, 337. For a further list of incompatibilities including *ampicillin, ascorbic acid, carbenicillin, chlorpromazine, chlortetracycline, gentamicin, heparin, methylprednisolone, phenothiazines, procaine, promazine, protein hydrolysate, sulphadiazine,* and *vitamin-B complex,* see *Med. Lett.*, 1972, *14* (Jan.), *Suppl.*, 32.

For conflicting reports of incompatibility between methicillin sodium and chloramphenicol sodium succinate, see Methicillin Sodium, p.1182.

Adverse Effects, Treatment, and Precautions. As for Chloramphenicol, p.1137.

Patients experience a bitter taste 15 to 20 seconds after an intravenous injection of chloramphenicol sodium succinate and the taste persists for 2 to 3 minutes.

For a report of ototoxicity in *guinea-pigs*, see p.1137.

Absorption and Fate. Chloramphenicol is rapidly liberated from chloramphenicol sodium succinate after parenteral administration. It is reported that about one-half of the chloramphenicol present in blood is in the active form and plasma concentrations are lower than those achieved with a comparable dose of chloramphenicol given by mouth. Higher concentrations are achieved after intravenous injection than after intramuscular injection.

Unchanged chloramphenicol sodium succinate, free chloramphenicol, and metabolites are excreted in the urine.

The biological half-life of chloramphenicol succinate was 3.5 to 5 hours in adults, 4 hours in children, and 8 to 22 hours (according to age) in premature infants.— W. A. Ritschel, *Drug Intell. & clin. Pharm.*, 1970, *4*, 332.

Further references: R. L. Slaughter *et al.*, *Clin. Pharmac. Ther.*, 1980, *28*, 69 (pharmacokinetics in critically ill patients); R. E. Kauffman *et al.*, *J. Pediat.*, 1981, *98*, 315.

Uses. Chloramphenicol sodium succinate has the antimicrobial action and uses of chloramphenicol (see p.1138). Because of its solubility in water, chloramphenicol sodium succinate is suitable for parenteral administration in aqueous solution. It is given usually by intravenous injection when oral administration of chloramphenicol is not feasible. However, patients should be changed to oral therapy as soon as possible.

A solution containing the equivalent of 10% of chloramphenicol in Water for Injections or other suitable diluent is given intravenously over at least one minute; chloramphenicol as the sodium succinate may also be given by slow intravenous infusion. Solutions containing the equivalent of 10% of chloramphenicol have been given subcutaneously and solutions containing the equivalent of 25 to 40% have been given by deep intramuscular injection.

The dose must be adjusted according to the severity of the infection. Adults may be given the equivalent of 1 g of chloramphenicol every 6 or 8 hours or 50 to 100 mg per kg body-weight daily; children may be given the equivalent of 50 or in some severe infections 100 mg per kg daily in divided doses. The doses for infants are the same as those for chloramphenicol given by mouth, see p.1139.

Chloramphenicol arginine succinate has also been given by intramuscular injection.

Preparations

Chloramphenicol Sodium Succinate Injection *(B.P.).* Chloramphen. Sod. Succ. Inj. A sterile solution of chloramphenicol sodium succinate in Water for Injections, prepared by dissolving the sterile contents of a sealed container (Chloramphenicol Sodium Succinate for Injection) in the requisite amount of Water for Injections. Potency is expressed in terms of the equivalent amount of chloramphenicol. Protect from light and use within 24 hours of preparation.

Sterile Chloramphenicol Sodium Succinate *(U.S.P.).* A grade of chloramphenicol sodium succinate for injection. Potency is expressed in terms of the equivalent amount of chloramphenicol.

Proprietary Preparations

Chloromycetin Succinate *(Parke, Davis, UK).* Chloramphenicol sodium succinate, available as powder for preparing injections, in vials each containing the equivalent of chloramphenicol 0.3 and 1.2 g. (Also available as Chloromycetin Succinate in *Arg., Austral., Belg., Canad., Denm., Norw., S.Afr., Swed., Switz., USA*).

Kemicetine Succinate *(Farmitalia Carlo Erba, UK).* Chloramphenicol sodium succinate, available as powder for preparing injections in vials each containing the equivalent of 1 g of chloramphenicol.

Other Proprietary Names

Arg.—Bioticaps, Quemicetina (both also under Chloramphenicol); *Austral.*—Chloramol (see also Chloramphenicol); *Belg.*—Globenicol (see also under Chloramphenicol and Chloramphenicol Palmitate), Synthomycetine (see also Chloramphenicol); *Fr.*—Solnicol Ercé; *Ger.*—Aquamycetin (hydrogen succinate) (see also Chloramphenicol), Nevimycin; *Ind.*—Ranphenicol (see also Chloramphenicol and Chloramphenicol Palmitate); *Ital.*—Biomicin, Chemicetina (see also Chloramphenicol), Succicaf; *Jap.*—Paraxin Succinat A (arginine succinate); *Neth.*—Globenicol (hydrogen succinate) (see also Chloramphenicol and Chloramphenicol Palmitate); *Spain*—Cloromycetin (see also Chloramphenicol and Chloramphenicol Palmitate); *Switz.*—Septicol (see also Chloramphenicol and Chloramphenicol Palmitate), Solu-Paraxin; *USA*—Mychel-S.

50-n

Chlortetracycline.

7-Chlorotetracycline.

$C_{22}H_{23}ClN_2O_8$=478.9.

CAS — 57-62-5.

A yellow crystalline powder. Very slightly **soluble** in water; slightly soluble in alcohol, acetone, and ethyl acetate; practically insoluble in ether.

51-h

Chlortetracycline Calcium.

The calcium salt of chlortetracycline.

CAS — 5892-31-9.

A white powder. Practically **insoluble** in water.

52-m

Chlortetracycline Hydrochloride *(B.P., B.P. Vet., Eur. P., U.S.P.).*

Chlortetracyc. Hydrochlor.; Chlortetracyclini Hydrochloridum; Biomycin.

$C_{22}H_{23}ClN_2O_8$,HCl=515.3.

CAS — 64-72-2.

NOTE. Aureomycin and aureomycin hydrochloride were used as nonproprietary names for chlortetracycline hydrochloride; these names are now used in some countries as proprietary names.

Pharmacopoeias. In *Arg., Aust., Belg., Br., Braz., Cz., Eur., Fr., Ger., Ind., Int., It., Jug., Neth., Rus., Span., Swiss,* and *U.S.*

An antimicrobial substance produced by the growth of certain strains of *Streptomyces aureofaciens* or by any other means.

Yellow odourless crystals with a bitter taste, containing not less than 950 units per mg of dried substance. **Soluble** 1 in 75 to 110 of water and 1 in 250 to 560 of alcohol; soluble in solutions of alkali hydroxides and carbonates; practically insoluble in acetone, chloroform, dioxan, ether, light petroleum, and propylene glycol. A 1% solution in water has a pH of 2.3 to 3.3. Solutions in water at 37° lose about 50% of their activity in 24 hours; neutral and alkaline solutions are rapidly inactivated. **Store** in airtight containers. If it is intended for injection the containers should be sterile and sealed to exclude micro-organisms. Protect from light.

Chlortetracycline hydrochloride is **incompatible** with calcium chloride, cephaloridine, cephalothin sodium, cephazolin sodium, and lactated ringer's injection, and incompatibility has also been reported with amikacin sulphate, ammonium chloride, calcium gluconate, cefapirin sodium, colistin sulphomethate sodium, compound sodium lactate injection, dextrans, laevulose, polymyxin B sulphate, promazine hydrochloride, protein hydrolysate, riboflavine, Ringer's injection, and ristocetin.

Effect of gamma-irradiation. The chemical and biological activity of chlortetracycline and oxytetracycline was not changed significantly by irradiation to 50 000 Gy. In aqueous solutions, significant inactivation of both antibiotics occurred with a dose as low as 250 Gy.— J. Holland *et al.*, *Radiosterilization of Medical Products*, Vienna, International Atomic Energy Agency, 1967, 69.

Incompatibility. See— R. C. Bogash, *Bull. Am. Soc. Hosp. Pharm.*, 1955, *12*, 445; H. R. Grant, *Hosp. Pharmst*, 1962, *15*, 67; J. A. Patel and G. L. Phillips, *Am. J. Hosp. Pharm.*, 1966, *23*, 409; J. M. Meisler and M. W. Skolaut, *Am. J. Hosp. Pharm.*, 1966, *23*, 557.

Units. One unit of chlortetracycline is contained in 0.001 mg of the second International Standard Preparation (1969) of chlortetracycline hydrochloride which contains 1000 units per mg.

Adverse Effects and Precautions. As for Tetracycline Hydrochloride, p.1217. Chlortetracycline tends to produce a grey-brown discoloration of teeth.

Bleeding and eventually death occurred in 2 patients who received chortetracycline parenterally in doses of up to 3 g daily for several days postoperatively. Both patients had liver injuries and the coagulation defect could have been due to this cause.— W. D. Schwindt and W. Kisken, *Am. J. Surg.*, 1967, *113*, 837.

A study indicating that usual therapeutic doses of chlortetracycline interfere with colour vision.— J. Laroche and C. Laroche, *Annls pharm. fr.*, 1972, *30*, 433. See also *idem*, 1970, *28*, 333.

Absorption and Fate. As for Tetracycline Hydrochloride, p.1219.

Chlortetracycline, unlike the other tetracyclines, is reported to be rapidly inactivated in the body. It is largely eliminated by biliary excretion, only about 15% being excreted in the urine and although it is not recommended in patients with renal impairment accumulation would not be likely.

Some 47% of chlortetracycline was bound in the body to serum proteins. The half-life in serum was 5.6 hours and 18% was excreted in urine.— C. M. Kunin, *Ann. intern. Med.*, 1967, *67*, 151.

The biological half-life of chlortetracycline was variously reported as 2.3 to 5.6 hours; in renal failure this might be increased to 7 to 11 hours.— W. A. Ritschel, *Drug Intell. & clin. Pharm.*, 1970, *4*, 332.

Pregnancy and the neonate. The concentration of chlortetracycline in foetal blood was one-fourteenth that of the maternal blood.— P. Demers *et al.*, *Can. med. Ass. J.*, 1968, *99*, 849.

Uses. Chlortetracycline hydrochloride has the antimicrobial activity and uses described under Tetracycline Hydrochloride (see p.1218).

The usual dose is 250 to 500 mg four times daily by mouth, preferably one hour before, or 2 hours after, meals. Suggested doses for children have been 10 to 50 mg per kg body-weight daily but chlortetracycline should only be used after considering the effects on teeth.

The MIC of chlortetracycline *in vitro* against 17 strains of *Chlamydia trachomatis* ranged from 0.125 to 1.0 μg per ml.— H. J. Blackman *et al.*, *Antimicrob. Ag. Chemother.*, 1977, *12*, 673.

Trachoma. Chlamydial ophthalmia in infants should be treated with chlortetracycline cream 1% and erythromycin 30 mg per kg body-weight [daily] for 21 days; failures could occur with topical treatment only. Silver nitrate prophylaxis was ineffective against *Chlamydia trachomatis*.— G. L. Ridgway, *Archs Dis. Childh.*, 1978, *53*, 447. See also G. L. Ridgway and J. D. Oriel (letter), *New Engl. J. Med.*, 1977, *297*, 512.

For earlier reports of the use of chlortetracycline eye ointment in the treatment of trachoma, see Martindale 27th Edn, p. 1113.

Preparations

Capsules

Chlortetracycline Capsules *(B.P.)*. Caps. Chlortetracyc. Capsules containing chlortetracycline hydrochloride. The *B.P.* requires 70% dissolution in 45 minutes. Store at a temperature not exceeding 30°. *U.S.P.* (Chlortetracycline Hydrochloride Capsules) specifies 50, 100 or 250 mg. Store in airtight containers. Protect from light.

Eye Ointments

Chlortetracycline Eye Ointment *(A.P.F.)*. Chlortetracycline hydrochloride 1% in Eye Ointment Base (*A.P.F.*). Prepare using an aseptic technique.

Chlortetracycline Eye Ointment *(B.P.C. 1973)*. Contains sterile chlortetracycline hydrochloride in Eye Ointment Basis or any other suitable sterile basis. Protect from light.

Chlortetracycline Hydrochloride Ophthalmic Ointment *(U.S.P.)*. Contains chlortetracycline hydrochloride 1% in a suitable ointment basis.

Ointments

Chlortetracycline Ointment *(B.P.C. 1973)*. Contains chlortetracycline hydrochloride up to 3% in wool fat 10% and yellow soft paraffin to 100% or any other suitable basis. When a lower strength is prescribed the 3% ointment may be diluted with a basis of 10% wool fat in yellow soft paraffin.

A.P.F. has a similar formula.

Chlortetracycline Ointment 1% *(St. John's Hosp.)*. Chlortetracycline hydrochloride 1, wool fat 10, white soft paraffin to 100.

Proprietary Preparations

Aureomycin *(Lederle, UK)*. Chlortetracycline hydrochloride, available as **Capsules** of 250 mg; as **Cream** containing 3%; as **Ointment** containing 3%; as **Ophthalmic Ointment** containing 1%; and as **Powder**. (Also available as Aureomycin in *Austral., Belg., Canad., Denm., Ger., Neth., Norw., S.Afr., Swed., Switz., USA*).

Other Proprietary Names for Chlortetracycline Hydrochloride

Aureomicina *(Ital., Spain)*; Auréomycine *(Fr.)*; Aureum *(Ital.)*; Chlortet *(Austral.)*; Clorciclina *(Ital.)*.

63-g

Ciclacillin. Cyclacillin *(U.S.P.)*; Wy 4508. (6*R*)-6-(1-Aminocyclohexanecarboxamido)penicillanic acid.
$C_{15}H_{23}N_3O_4S$=341.4.

CAS — 3485-14-1.

Pharmacopoeias. In *U.S.*

A crystalline solid with a characteristic odour. **Soluble** 1 in 30 of water. It contains not less than 900 μg per mg. M.p. about 181°. A 1% solution has a pH of 4 to 6.5. **Store** in airtight containers.

Adverse Effects, Treatment, and Precautions. As for Ampicillin, p.1092.

Whereas side-effects were reported in 128 of 1286 patients (10%) treated with ciclacillin, side-effects developed in 202 of 1129 patients (18%) who received ampicillin. Diarrhoea and skin rash were the side-effects most often reported.— J. A. Gold *et al.*, *Antimicrob. Ag. Chemother.*, 1979, *15*, 55.

See also under Absorption and Fate (below).

Absorption and Fate. Ciclacillin is well-absorbed from the gastro-intestinal tract and peak serum concentrations of about 12 μg per ml have been reported after a single 500-mg dose. About 80% of a dose is excreted in the urine within 6 hours, mainly as ciclacillin.

Ciclacillin 250 mg produced blood concentrations that at 30 minutes were 5 times higher than the peak concentrations of ampicillin achieved 1 hour after a dose of 250 mg. Ciclacillin was rapidly excreted, about 80% of the dose appearing in the urine mostly within 6 hours.— C. G. Hertz, *Antimicrob. Ag. Chemother.*, 1973, *4*, 361.

Investigation in *rats* demonstrated that ciclacillin caused sex-related nephropathy. The nephrotoxic effect was noted only in male *rats* and in correlation with this a metabolite of ciclacillin, 1-aminocyclohexanecarboxylic acid accumulated to a greater extent in the male. Nephrotoxicity was not noted in *dogs, rhesus monkeys*, or man. In man ciclacillin was well absorbed by mouth yielding peak concentrations in serum within 30 minutes after dosing; most of it was cleared from the blood within 6 hours because of a high rate of renal excretion. The principal excretion product in man was unchanged ciclacillin (60 to 70% of the dose), about 15 to 20% was penicilloic acid, and about 1 to 2% was 1-aminocyclohexanecarboxylic acid, this amount being independent of the sex of the subjects.— W. E. Tucker *et al.*, *Toxic. appl. Pharmac.*, 1974, *29*, 1.

Further references to pharmacokinetic studies with ciclacillin: M. Stillerman and H. D. Isenberg, *Antimicrob. Ag. Chemother.*, 1970, 270; K. F. Wagner *et al.*, *Antimicrob. Ag. Chemother.*, 1980, *17*, 89.

Uses. Ciclacillin is an antibiotic closely related to ampicillin (p.1091) and has a similar antimicrobial spectrum but is less active *in vitro*, with MICs reported to range from 0.1 to 32 μg per ml. Ciclacillin is given in usual doses of 250 or 500 mg four times daily. Children may be given half the adult dose.

A brief review of ciclacillin.— *Med. Lett.*, 1980, *22*, 13.

Ciclacillin was of similar efficacy to ampicillin in the treatment of 1819 patients with infections of the genito-urinary or respiratory tract, infections of the skin and soft tissues, or otitis media.— J. A. Gold *et al.*, *Antimicrob. Ag. Chemother.*, 1979, *15*, 55.

Further references: B. Arend *et al.*, *Arzneimittel-Forsch.*, 1975, *25*, 1382; G. H. Warren, *Chemotherapy, Basle*, 1976, *22*, 154.

Preparations

Cyclacillin for Oral Suspension *(U.S.P.)*. A dry mixture of ciclacillin with one or more suitable buffers, colours, flavours, preservatives, sweeteners, and suspending agents. pH of the reconstituted suspension 4.5 to 6.5. Store in airtight containers.

Cyclacillin Tablets *(U.S.P.)*. Tablets containing ciclacillin. Store in airtight containers.

Calthor *(Ayerst, UK)*. Ciclacillin, available as **Suspension** (supplied as granules for preparation with water before use) containing 125 or 250 mg in each 5 ml and as scored **Tablets** of 250 or 500 mg.

Other Proprietary Names

Citocilina *(Spain)*; Citocillin *(S.Afr.)*; Citosarin *(Jap.)*; Cyclapen-W *(USA)*; Orfilina *(Spain)*; Ultracillin *(Ger., Switz.)*; Vastcillin, Vatracin *(both Jap.)*; Vipicil *(Arg.)*; Wyvital *(Jap.)*.

153-p

Clavulanic Acid. BRL 14151; MM 14151. (*Z*)-(2*R*,5*R*)-3-(2-Hydroxyethylidene)-7-oxo-4-oxa-1-azabicyclo[3.2.0]heptane-2-carboxylic acid.
$C_8H_9NO_5$=199.2.

CAS — 58001-44-8; 61177-45-5 (potassium salt); 57943-81-4 (sodium salt).

Clavulanic acid is produced by cultures of *Streptomyces clavuligerus*. It has a beta-lactam structure resembling that of the penicillin nucleus except that the fused thiazolidine ring of the penicillins is replaced by an oxazolidine ring. In general, clavulanic acid has only weak antibacterial activity but it is a potent progressive inhibitor of beta-lactamases produced by many bacteria including *Staphylococcus aureus*, the Enterobacteriaceae, *Haemophilus influenzae, Neisseria gonorrhoeae*, and *Bacteroides fragilis*, and consequently enhances the activity *in vitro* of penicillin and cephalosporin antibiotics against many resistant strains. The activity of cefoxitin, which is thought to be resistant to most beta-lactamases, does not appear to be enhanced.

Clavulanic acid is given by mouth, as potassium clavulanate, in association with amoxycillin in the treatment of various infections. The equivalent of 125 mg of clavulanic acid together with the equivalent of amoxycillin 250 mg may be given thrice daily; doses may be doubled in severe infections. Sodium clavulanate has also been used.

Reviews on clavulanate with amoxycillin: R. N. Brogden *et al.*, *Drugs*, 1981, *22*, 337; *Drug & Ther. Bull.*, 1982, *20*, 21.

Proceedings of a symposium on clavulanate-potentiated amoxycillin.— G. N. Rolinson and A. Watson (Ed.), Oxford, Excerpta Medica, 1980.

Antimicrobial action. A discussion on the inhibition of beta-lactamases.— J. M. T. Hamilton-Miller, *J. antimicrob. Chemother.*, 1977, *3*, 195.

In a study *in vitro* of *Escherichia coli*, sodium clavulanate produced rapid cell lysis at a concentration above 50 μg per ml and had the same mode of action as a beta-lactam antibiotic.— B. G. Spratt *et al.*, *Antimicrob. Ag. Chemother.*, 1977, *12*, 406.

The MIC of benzylpenicillin *in vitro* was reduced against *Bacteroides fragilis*, and against beta-lactamase-producing strains of *N. gonorrhoeae* and *Staph. aureus* when used with clavulanic acid. The activity of amoxycillin *in vitro* against beta-lactamase-producing strains of *E. coli, Klebsiella* spp., and indole-negative strains of *Proteus* spp. was also enhanced when used with clavulanic acid. However, 2 beta-lactamase-producing strains of *Pseudomonas aeruginosa* remained resistant to carbenicillin in the presence of clavulanic acid. Concentrations of clavulanic acid used were 1, 5, or 10 μg per ml.— R. Wise *et al.*, *Antimicrob. Ag. Chemother.*, 1978, *13*, 389.

Cephalothin had an MIC of 64 μg or more per ml against 10 strains of *Kleb. pneumoniae* resistant to cephalothin, and sodium clavulanate had a mean MIC of 28 μg per ml. When used with clavulanate 1 μg per ml all the isolates were inhibited by cephalothin 8 μg per ml or by cephalothin 4 μg per ml when used with clavulanate 5 or 10 μg per ml. However, the enhancing effect of sodium clavulanate on cephalothin was much less for 10 cephalothin-susceptible strains (MIC 16 μg per ml) than for resistant isolates which suggested that the major effect was due to beta-lactamase inhibition. Sodium clavulanate also failed to enhance the activity of cefoxitin.— R. T. Jackson *et al.*, *Antimicrob. Ag. Chemother.*, 1978, *14*, 118.

Clavulanic acid used alone *in vitro* had a low degree of antibacterial activity against strains of *Staph. aureus*, Enterobacteriaceae, *Pseudomonas aeruginosa, Bacteroides fragilis*, and *Haemophilus influenzae* but inhibited the majority of *N. gonorrhoeae* at a concentration of 0.1 μg per ml. Clavulanic acid enhanced the activity of ampicillin *in vitro* against beta-lactamase-producing strains of *N. gonorrhoeae, H. influenzae, E. coli, Salmonella typhi,* and *Shigella sonnei* over the concentration range of 1 part of clavulanic acid with 1 to 10 parts of ampicillin. Clavulanic acid also enhanced the activity of amoxycillin and cephalosporin antibiotics against strains of the Enterobacteriaceae and *Staph. aureus*.— H. C. Neu and K. P. Fu, *Antimicrob. Ag. Chemother.*, 1978, *14*, 650.

The MIC of sodium clavulanate *in vitro* against strains of *N. gonorrhoeae* ranged from 1 to 5 μg per ml. When used at subinhibitory concentrations sodium clavulanate reduced the MICs of benzylpenicillin, ampicillin, and amoxycillin against beta-lactamase-producing strains of *N. gonorrhoeae* more than 32-fold but had little effect on the MICs for non-beta-lactamase-producing strains. The effect of sodium clavulanate on the activity of cefoxitin was minimal against either type of strain.— J. M. Miller *et al., Antimicrob. Ag. Chemother.*, 1978, *14*, 794.

Further references: R. Wise (letter), *Lancet*, 1977, *2*, 145; C. Reading and M. Cole, *Antimicrob. Ag. Chemother.*, 1977, *11*, 852; J. Wüst and T. D. Wilkins, *ibid.*, 1978, *13*, 130; B. Van Klingeren and M. Dessens-Kroon (letter), *J. antimicrob. Chemother.*, 1979, *5*, 322; D. Greenwood *et al., ibid.*, 539; B. Olsson *et al., Antimicrob. Ag. Chemother.*, 1979, *15*, 263; P. Piot *et al., ibid.*, 535; K. P. Fu and H. C. Neu, *ibid.*, *16*, 561; M. Matsuura *et al., ibid.*, 1980, *17*, 908; R. Wise *et al., J. antimicrob. Chemother.*, 1980, *6*, 197.

For a report of the effect of clavulanic acid on the activity of ticarcillin, see Ticarcillin, p.1225.

Infections. A study of 3 dosage regimens of amoxycillin trihydrate with clavulanic acid in 60 patients with mainly amoxycillin-resistant urinary-tract infections. Administration of amoxycillin trihydrate 500 mg with potassium clavulanate 125 mg every 8 hours for 7 days, eradicated a high proportion of urinary-tract infections caused by amoxycillin-resistant organisms. Of the 2 other regimens, a dose of amoxycillin trihydrate 250 mg (with sodium clavulanate 125 mg) was too low, whereas a dose of potassium clavulanate 250 mg (with amoxycillin trihydrate 500 mg) was poorly tolerated and did not improve the rate of cure; clinical findings that the clavulanate dose of 250 mg was unnecessary were supported by bacteriological studies. Of 20 patients given the higher dose of clavulanate with amoxycillin, mild transient eosinophilia was noted in 4, and 8 complained of nausea (2 of whom were unable to complete the study because of vomiting). Administration with meals appeared to reduce the prevalence of nausea. Pharmacokinetic studies in healthy subjects indicated that clavulanic acid had no significant effect on the absorption, distribution, or excretion of amoxycillin. Both agents were rapidly absorbed from the gastro-intestinal tract, reaching peak serum concentrations about 60 minutes after administration; both had overall serum half-lives of 60 to 70 minutes; most of the amoxycillin was recovered in the urine within 6 hours, but less than 50% of clavulanic acid was; urinary concentrations of clavulanic acid in excess of those required to inhibit most plasmid-mediated beta-lactamases were present throughout the 6 hours following both the 125-mg and the 250-mg clavulanate dosage regimens.— A. P. Ball *et al., Lancet*, 1980, *1*, 620.

Further references to the use of clavulanic acid in association with amoxycillin: G. Ninane *et al.* (letter), *Lancet*, 1978, *2*, 257; D. A. Leigh *et al., J. antimicrob. Chemother.*, 1981, *7*, 229; P. Ball *et al., ibid.*, 441.

Proprietary Preparations

Augmentin *(Beecham Research, UK)*. **Tablets** and **Dispersible Tablets** each containing potassium clavulanate equivalent to clavulanic acid 125 mg and amoxycillin trihydrate equivalent to amoxycillin 250 mg.

53-b

Clemizole Penicillin. Penicillinclemizole. 1-[1-(4-Chlorobenzyl)benzimidazol-2-ylmethyl]pyrrolidinium (6*R*)-6-(2-phenylacetamido)penicillanate.
$C_{16}H_{18}N_2O_4S,C_{19}H_{20}ClN_3$=660.2.

CAS — 6011-39-8.

Clemizole penicillin is a long-acting preparation of benzylpenicillin (see p.1102) which has been used similarly to procaine penicillin. Clemizole penicillin 1.2 g contains about 600 mg (1 million units) of benzylpenicillin.

References: O. Delzant, *Revue int. Servs Santé Armées*, 1970, *43*, 233, per *Abstr. Hyg.*, 1970, *45*, 1384.

Proprietary Names

Megacillin *(Grünenthal, Ger.; Grünenthal, Switz.)*(see also under Benzylpenicillin, Phenoxymethylpenicillin, and Procaine Penicillin); Prevecillin *(Grünenthal, S.Afr.)*.

54-v

Clindamycin Hydrochloride *(B.P., U.S.P.)*.

Chlorodeoxylincomycin Hydrochloride; (7*S*)-Chloro-7-deoxylincomycin; U 21251. Methyl 6-amino-7-chloro-6,7,8-trideoxy-*N*-[(2*S*,4*R*)-1-methyl-4-propylprolyl]-1-thio-β-L-*threo*-D-*galacto*-octopyranoside hydrochloride monohydrate.
$C_{18}H_{33}ClN_2O_5S,HCl,H_2O$=479.5.

CAS — 18323-44-9 (clindamycin); 21462-39-5 (hydrochloride, anhydrous); 58207-19-5 (hydrochloride, monohydrate).

NOTE. The name Clinimycin was formerly used for Clindamycin. It has been used for a preparation of oxytetracycline (see p.1198).

Pharmacopoeias. In *Br., Braz.*, and *U.S.*

A white or almost white crystalline powder, odourless or with a faint mercaptan-like odour, and with a bitter taste. Clindamycin hydrochloride 1.09 g is approximately equivalent to 1 g of clindamycin. **Soluble** 1 in 2 of water, 1 in 200 of alcohol, and 1 in 4 of dimethylformamide; freely soluble in methyl alcohol; very slightly soluble in chloroform; practically insoluble in acetone. A solution in water is dextrorotatory. A 10% solution in water has a pH of 3 to 5.5. **Store** at a temperature not exceeding 30° in airtight containers.

In buffered aqueous solution, clindamycin showed maximum stability at pH 3 to 5; after storage for 2 years at 25° not more than 10% degradation would occur in the pH range 1 to 6.5. At pH 0.4 to 4 hydrolysis of clindamycin to 1-dethiomethyl-1-hydroxyclindamycin and methyl mercaptan occurred; at pH 5 to 10 lincomycin was formed.— T. O. Oesterling, *J. pharm. Sci.*, 1970, *59*, 63.

Units. One unit of clindamycin is contained in 0.0011947 mg of the first International Reference Preparation (1971) of clindamycin hydrochloride which contains 837 units per mg.

Adverse Effects. Clindamycin hydrochloride may cause diarrhoea, which can be severe and persistent, nausea, vomiting, abdominal cramps, and abnormality of taste. Severe pseudomembranous colitis has occurred in some patients and has occasionally been fatal. Colitis and diarrhoea have been reported during treatment and after its completion. Some reports suggest that the intestinal effects may be due to superinfection. Hypersensitivity reactions, including skin rashes and urticaria, may occur and transient leucopenia and eosinophilia, elevations of alkaline phosphatase and serum aminotransferases and jaundice have been reported. Agranulocytosis, thrombocytopenia, and erythema multiforme have been observed. Phlebitis may occur with large intravenous doses.

Few adverse reactions had occurred in about 22 000 casualty patients given lincomycin or clindamycin over 4 years. Three patients had a skin rash after clindamycin and an occasional patient complained of diarrhoea.— D. H. Wilson (letter), *Br. med. J.*, 1974, *4*, 288. Of 70 patients taking clindamycin 150 mg twice daily for acne, 12% developed mild diarrhoea within 2 or 3 weeks.— W. J. Cunliffe and S. G. Tan (letter), *ibid.*, 289.

Contact dermatitis developed in a patient who used a topical preparation containing clindamycin hydrochloride 1% for the treatment of pruritic acne lesions.— R. J. Coskey (letter), *Archs Derm.*, 1978, *114*, 446.

Colitis. Discussions on colitis associated with the administration of clindamycin, lincomycin, and other antibiotics.— F. E. Pittman, *Adverse Drug React. Bull.*, 1977, Apr., 220; N. D. Gallagher and S. J. M. Goulston, *Drugs*, 1978, *16*, 385; D. A. Leigh, *J. antimicrob. Chemother.*, 1978, *4*, 195; *Br. med. J.*, 1978, *1*, 669; *J. Am. med. Ass.*, 1978, *239*, 2101; *Br. med. J.*, 1979, *2*, 349; F. E. Pittman, *Adverse Drug React. Bull.*, 1979, Apr., 268.

Three patients who received clindamycin 600 mg daily for 5, 6, and 7 days respectively developed severe colitis of several weeks' duration.— L. E. Cohen *et al., J. Am. med. Ass.*, 1973, *223*, 1379.

In a prospective study of 200 patients treated with clindamycin by mouth or injection 42 (21%) developed diarrhoea and 20 (10%) had proctoscopic evidence of pseudomembranous colitis. The colitis was not dose-dependent but it was more common following administration by mouth than injection.— F. J. Tedesco *et al., Ann. intern. Med.*, 1974, *81*, 429. See also *idem*, 547.

Discussion of the role of Lomotil in antibiotic-associated colitis.— F. E. Pittman (letter), *Ann. intern. Med.*, 1975, *83*, 124; F. J. Tedesco and D. H. Alpers (letter), *ibid.*, 125.

Of 163 hospital in-patients in a Boston Collaborative Drug Surveillance Program who received clindamycin none developed colitis.— R. R. Miller and H. Jick, *Clin. Pharmac. Ther.*, 1977, *22*, 1. Although diarrhoea occurred in 46 of 145 patients given clindamycin, in 16 there was an established clinical cause and pseudomembranous colitis was not seen in any patient.— R. E. Condon and M. J. Anderson, *Archs Surg., Chicago*, 1978, *113*, 794. See also A. M. Geddes (letter), *Br. med. J.*, 1974, *4*, 591.

A report of pseudomembranous colitis in 5 children who had received either clindamycin, ampicillin, or benzylpenicillin.— J. -P. Buts *et al., Gastroenterology*, 1977, *73*, 823.

Diarrhoea occurred in 38 of 1484 children given 10-day courses of clindamycin. [Colitis was not seen].— M. F. Randolph and K. E. Morris, *Clin. Pediat.*, 1977, *16*, 722.

Diarrhoea associated with topical clindamycin therapy had been reported in 3 patients.— D. A. Voron (letter), *Archs Derm.*, 1978, *114*, 798.

Severe diarrhoea occurred in 25 of 160 patients who received clindamycin or lincomycin for bacterial infections, but it could not be related to a change in faecal flora. Diarrhoea occurred more frequently when clindamycin was given prophylactically and the incidence was higher in women (19%) than in men (13%) and in patients over 60 years of age. Clindamycin should be used cautiously in elderly patients.— D. A. Leigh and K. Simmons, *J. clin. Path.*, 1978, *31*, 439.

Between 1964 and 1978 the Committee on Safety of Medicines (according to Adverse Reaction Series No.17, 1979) had received 174 reports of colitis attributed to antibiotics; 116, including 27 deaths, were associated with clindamycin and 27, including 10 deaths, with lincomycin. All but 4 of the reports associated with clindamycin were received after 1974, when the condition known as pseudomembranous colitis was identified. Clindamycin and lincomycin should not be given for minor infections.— *Pharm. J.*, 1979, *1*, 518.

Further references: R. F. Wells *et al.* (letter), *Lancet*, 1974, *1*, 66; J. G. P. Sissons *et al.* (letter), *ibid.*, 172; J. R. Stroehlein *et al.* (letter), *ibid.*, 221; J. M. Temperley (letter), *ibid.*; S. P. Wilkinson (letter), *ibid.*, 415; F. J. Tedesco *et al., New Engl. J. Med.*, 1974, *290*, 841; J. R. Stroehlein *et al., Mayo Clin. Proc.*, 1974, *49*, 240; R. Wise *et al.* (letter), *Lancet*, 1974, *1*, 878; C. H. Ramirez-Ronda (letter), *Ann. intern. Med.*, 1974, *81*, 860; *Med. Lett.*, 1974, *16*, 73; M. S. Wolfe (letter), *J. Am. med. Ass.*, 1974, *229*, 266; *Br. med. J.*, 1974, *4*, 65; H. W. Steer (letter), *Lancet*, 1974, *1*, 1176; *idem* (letter), 1975, *1*, 411; J. J. Marr *et al., Gastroenterology*, 1975, *69*, 352; K. M. Das and W. F. Erber (letter), *Ann. intern. Med.*, 1975, *82*, 426; B. R. Miller and M. H. Wheeler (letter), *Br. med. J.*, 1975, *3*, 433; S. A. Kabins and T. J. Spira (letter), *Ann. intern. Med.*, 1975, *83*, 830; H. W. Steer, *Gut*, 1975, *16*, 695; J. L. Unger *et al., Am. J. dig. Dis.*, 1975, *20*, 214; L. J. Hoberman *et al., ibid.*, 1976, *21*, 1; F. J. Tedesco, *ibid.*, 26; *Lancet*, 1976, *1*, 405; J. F. Munk *et al., Med. J. Aust.*, 1976, *2*, 95; W. V. Bogomoletz, *Gut*, 1976, *17*, 483; E. C. Sweeney and J. P. Sheehan, *Br. med. J.*, 1979, *2*, 1188.

See also Hazards of Antibiotic Therapy, p.1082 and Lincomycin Hydrochloride, p.1178.

Erythema multiforme. A patient who had been taking clindamycin 150 mg four times daily for a dental infection developed erythema multiforme (the Stevens-Johnson syndrome) 14 days after the start of treatment. Her condition improved after she received prednisone 60 mg daily (decreasing after 6 days) for 3 weeks.— D. D. Fulghum and P. M. Catalano, *J. Am. med. Ass.*, 1973, *223*, 318.

Hepatotoxicity. Liver enzyme abnormalities occurred in a patient receiving clindamycin phosphate intravenously.

Biopsy demonstrated lobular disruption, pseudogranulomas, necrosis, eosinophilic bodies, and mononuclear cell infiltration. The liver enzymes returned to normal when clindamycin was withdrawn and biopsy taken 15 days later showed improvement.— M. Elmore *et al.*, *Am. J. Med.*, 1974, *57*, 627.

Oesophageal ulceration. A report of oesophageal ulceration due to the disintegration of a capsule of clindamycin in the oesophagus.— D. R. Sutton and J. K. Gosnold (letter), *Br. med. J.*, 1977, *1*, 1598.

Treatment of Adverse Effects. Clindamycin should be withdrawn if significant diarrhoea or colitis occurs. Vancomycin in doses of 125 to 500 mg by mouth every 6 hours has been used successfully in the treatment of antibiotic-associated pseudomembranous colitis.

In vitro studies indicated that cholestyramine and colestipol hydrochloride bind the *Clostridium difficile* toxin which is implicated in antibiotic-associated colitis.— T. W. Chang *et al.* (letter), *Lancet*, 1978, *2*, 258. These anionic-exchange resins would probably be beneficial *in vivo* but might interfere with the therapeutic action of vancomycin if used concomitantly.— R. H. George *et al.* (letter), *ibid.*, 624.

A report of the treatment of antibiotic-associated pseudomembranous colitis with cholestyramine.— E. W. Kreutzer and F. D. Milligan, *Johns Hopkins med. J.*, 1978, *143*, 67.

Metronidazole by mouth eliminated *Cl. difficile* and its toxin from 2 patients who had colitis after taking clindamycin.— N. L. Pashby *et al.*, *Br. med. J.*, 1979, *1*, 1605.

See also under Metronidazole, p.971, for both favourable and unfavourable reports of its use in colitis.

For reports of the successful use of vancomycin in the treatment of antibiotic-induced colitis, see Vancomycin Hydrochloride, p.1230.

Precautions. Clindamycin should not be given to patients known to be hypersensitive or who have experienced reactions with lincomycin. It should not be used in patients with diarrhoeal states and it should be used with caution in patients with impaired liver and renal function.

Since clindamycin is reported to possess neuromuscular blocking activity it should be used with care with other drugs with similar activity.

A report that diabetic patients tend to have lower plasma concentrations of clindamycin than other patients after intramuscular administration.— R. J. Fass and S. Saslaw, *Am. J. med. Sci.*, 1972, *263*, 369.

Clindamycin 300 mg was given intramuscularly to 6 healthy subjects, 9 patients with renal disease, and 10 with liver disease. The mean biological half-lives were 3 hours in the healthy subjects, 2.9 hours in those with kidney disorders, and 6.4 (2.6 to 14.2) hours in those with liver disease. Clindamycin should not be given to patients with severe liver disease.— R. Brandl *et al.*, *Dt. med. Wschr.*, 1972, *97*, 1057. See also G. R. Avant *et al.*, *Am. J. dig. Dis.*, 1975, *20*, 223. Five hours after the administration of clindamycin 600 mg by intravenous injection the mean serum concentration in patients with moderate to severe hepatic dysfunction was 24.3 µg per ml whereas in patients with normal function it was 8.3 µg per ml. It was suggested that the dose of clindamycin should be modified in patients with liver disease.— D. N. Williams *et al.*, *Antimicrob. Ag. Chemother.*, 1975, *7*, 153. Clindamycin 300 mg was given intravenously every 12 hours for 2 days to patients with cirrhosis or acute or chronic hepatitis or to controls. There was no deterioration in the liver disorder. Although there was a slight but significant delay in excretion between controls and patients with cirrhosis the half-lives in all groups were considered to be in normal ranges.— D. R. Hinthorn *et al.*, *ibid.*, 1976, *9*, 498.

Increased absorption of clindamycin occurred in Crohn's disease and coeliac disease.— *Drug & Ther. Bull.*, 1976, *14*, 57.

Interactions. In 16 healthy subjects given clindamycin alone and with a kaolin-pectin suspension it was found that the suspension had no effect on the extent of clindamycin absorption but did markedly reduce the absorption rate.— K. S. Albert *et al.*, *J. pharm. Sci.*, 1978, *67*, 1579.

For a report of antineoplastic antibiotics affecting the activity of clindamycin against *Staphylococcus aureus in vitro*, see under Antimicrobial Action.

Antimicrobial Action. Clindamycin has an antimicrobial spectrum similar to that of lincomycin (see p.1178) but its activity against sensitive organisms is greater.

Minimum inhibitory concentrations for sensitive Gram-positive cocci have been reported to range from about 0.002 to 0.8 µg per ml. Most strains of *Bacteroides* spp. have been found to be inhibited by 2 µg or less per ml of clindamycin.

Clindamycin possessed marked antiplasmodial activity.— C. Lewis, *J. Parasitol.*, 1968, *54*, 169.

A comparison was made of the activities *in vitro* of clindamycin, lincomycin, and erythromycin against several micro-organisms. Clindamycin was most active at high pH. Clindamycin was more active than lincomycin against all the organisms used except *Streptococcus faecalis*, against which both were ineffective. Clindamycin was equally or more effective than erythromycin against β-haemolytic streptococci, *Str. viridans*, *Str. pneumoniae*, and erythromycin-sensitive *Staphylococcus aureus*. It was usually more active than erythromycin against *Clostridium welchii*, and was active against erythromycin-resistant staphylococci. It was less active than erythromycin against *Haemophilus influenzae*, *Str. faecalis*, and *Neisseria gonorrhoeae*.— I. Phillips *et al.*, *Br. med. J.*, 1970, *2*, 89.

The MIC of clindamycin for 50 strains of *H. influenzae* was 0.12 to 4 µg per ml, and 42 strains were sensitive to 2 µg or less per ml. Peak serum concentrations were about 6 µg per ml and average concentrations about 3 µg per ml, so that clindamycin might be of use in bronchitis caused by *H. influenzae*.— K. Zinnemann and J. Frazer (letter), *Br. med. J.*, 1970, *2*, 481. Of 68 strains of *H. influenzae* 9 were inhibited by clindamycin at a concentration of 0.25 µg per ml, 30 at 0.5 µg per ml, 18 at 1 µg per ml, and 11 at 2 µg per ml. — J. D. Williams and J. Andrews, *ibid.*, 1974, *1*, 134.

Sensitivity tests showed that 475 of 500 strains of *Staph. aureus* and 78 of 100 strains of *H. influenzae* were sensitive to 2 µg per ml of clindamycin. Most strains of *Staph. aureus* were inhibited in concentrations of 0.2 µg or less per ml.— A. M. Geddes *et al.*, *Br. med. J.*, 1970, *2*, 703.

Erythromycin and clindamycin were the most active of 21 antimicrobial agents tested *in vitro* against 56 strains of *Gardnerella vaginalis* (*Haemophilus vaginalis*); all strains were inhibited by 0.06 µg or less per ml.— L. R. McCarthy *et al.*, *Antimicrob. Ag. Chemother.*, 1979, *16*, 186.

Further references: K. Williams *et al.*, *Med. Lab. Technol.*, 1972, *29*, 233; S. Feltham *et al.* (letter), *J. antimicrob. Chemother.*, 1979, *5*, 731.

For the effects of clindamycin on the antimicrobial activity of gentamicin and ampicillin, see Gentamicin Sulphate, p.1168 and Ampicillin, p.1094.

Activity against anaerobic bacteria. Clindamycin had an MIC of 0.5 µg per ml against 90% of 200 strains of *Bacteroides fragilis* and was more active than tinidazole, doxycycline, chloramphenicol, erythromycin, benzylpenicillin, tetracycline, ampicillin, carbenicillin, and cephalothin. Clindamycin and benzylpenicillin were the most active against 20 strains of *B. melaninogenicus* and doxycycline, clindamycin, and benzylpenicillin were the most active against *Fusobacterium* spp. Clindamycin was less active than benzylpenicillin or ampicillin against *Clostridia* spp. but it had an MIC of about 1.5 µg per ml against 30 strains of anaerobic Gram-positive cocci.— J. Klastersky *et al.*, *Antimicrob. Ag. Chemother.*, 1977, *12*, 563.

Clindamycin was more active than erythromycin against all of 265 strains of anaerobic bacteria. All of 41 strains of *Bacteroides fragilis* were inhibited by 2 µg or less per ml of clindamycin whereas only 29% of the strains were inhibited by 8 µg per ml of erythromycin.— P. C. Appelbaum and S. A. Chatterton, *Antimicrob. Ag. Chemother.*, 1978, *14*, 371. See also V. L. Sutter and S. M. Finegold, *Antimicrob. Ag. Chemother.*, 1976, *10*, 736.

A study *in vitro* indicated that clindamycin, metronidazole, and chloramphenicol were the most effective agents against *Bacteroides fragilis* and of the cephalosporins tested cefoxitin was the most active.— J. Dubois *et al.*, *J. antimicrob. Chemother.*, 1978, *4*, 329.

Further references: S. J. Bodner *et al.*, *Antimicrob. Ag. Chemother.*, 1972, *2*, 57; O. A. Okubadejo *et al.* (letter), *Lancet*, 1973, *1*, 147; *idem*, *Br. med. J.*, 1973, *2*, 212.

Enhanced activity. A report of the enhanced inhibitory activity of both clindamycin and metronidazole against 12 of 17 strains of *Bacteroides fragilis* when used together *in vitro*.— D. F. Busch *et al.*, *J. infect. Dis.*, 1976, *133*, 321. See also E. D. Ralph and Y. E. Amatnieks, *Antimicrob. Ag. Chemother.*, 1980, *17*, 379.

Diminished activity. Antagonism occurred against some strains of *Staph. aureus* when the activity of clindamycin was tested *in vitro* with actinomycin D, daunorubicin, doxorubicin, bleomycin, or mithramycin and synergism usually occurred when clindamycin was tested with mitomycin. The effect of mitomycin was obtained at concentrations below those usually obtainable in serum.— J. Y. Jacobs *et al.*, *Antimicrob. Ag. Chemother.*, 1979, *15*, 580.

Enhanced activity. There was enhanced activity *in vitro* against strains of *Escherichia coli* when clindamycin or erythromycin were tested with gentamicin or colistin.— B. Leng *et al.*, *Antimicrob. Ag. Chemother.*, 1975, *8*, 164. See also R. J. Fass *et al.*, *Antimicrob. Ag. Chemother.*, 1974, *6*, 582.

Resistance. As for Lincomycin Hydrochloride, p.1178.

Cross-resistance occurs between clindamycin, lincomycin, and erythromycin.

Resistance of group A streptococci to clindamycin occurred in patients with burns who received the standard dose recommended for moderate infections of 150 mg four times a day for 5 days.— J. Kohn and A. J. Evans (letter), *Br. med. J.*, 1970, *2*, 423.

Minimum bactericidal concentrations of clindamycin greatly exceeded MICs against 40 strains of *Lactobacilli*.— A. S. Bayer *et al.*, *Antimicrob. Ag. Chemother.*, 1978, *14*, 720.

Further reports of the isolation of clindamycin-resistant bacteria: *Corynebacterium xerosis*.— R. K. Porschen *et al.*, *Am. J. clin. Path.*, 1977, *68*, 290. *Staphylococcus aureus*.— C. Watanakunakorn, *Am. J. Med.*, 1976, *60*, 419; C. E. Cherubin and S. R. Nair, *J. Am. med. Ass.*, 1978, *239*, 626; Z. A. Hassam *et al.*, *Br. med. J.*, 1978, *2*, 536. *Streptococcus pneumoniae*.— L. A. A. Champion *et al.*, *J. Pediat.*, 1978, *92*, 505.

Resistance of Bacteroides. Clindamycin-resistant strains of *Bacteroides fragilis* were isolated from two patients in different institutions.— J. S. Salaki *et al.*, *Am. J. Med.*, 1976, *60*, 426.

For a report of some lincomycin-resistant strains of *B. fragilis* being inhibited by clindamycin, see Lincomycin Hydrochloride, p.1178.

For a report of anaerobic infections responding to clindamycin after showing resistance to chloramphenicol, see Chloramphenicol, p.1138.

Absorption and Fate. About 90% of a dose of clindamycin hydrochloride is absorbed from the gastro-intestinal tract and peak plasma concentrations are achieved more rapidly than with lincomycin (see p.1178); concentrations of about 2.5 µg per ml occur within 1 hour after a 150-mg dose of clindamycin, with average concentrations of about 0.7 µg per ml after 6 hours. After doses of 300 and 600 mg peak plasma concentrations of 4 and 8 µg per ml, respectively, have been reported. The biological half-life is about 2.5 hours. Absorption is not significantly diminished by food in the stomach but the rate of absorption may be reduced.

Clindamycin is widely distributed in body fluids and tissues including bone but it does not reach the CSF in significant concentrations. It diffuses across the placenta into the foetal circulation and has been reported to appear in breast milk. High concentrations occur in bile. About 10% of a dose is excreted in the urine as active clindamycin and about 4% in the faeces; the remainder is inactivated in the liver. Increased urinary recovery of clindamycin has been reported in patients with liver disease. It is not effectively removed from the blood by dialysis.

Clindamycin was bound to serum proteins to the extent of 93.6%.— R. C. Gordon *et al.*, *J. pharm. Sci.*, 1973, *62*, 1074.

In 18 patients with acne vulgaris who had applied an aqueous/alcoholic solution of clindamycin hydrochloride 1% twice to 4 times daily for 6 to 150 days there was no evidence of systemic absorption.— R. J. Algra *et al.*, *Archs Derm.*, 1977, *113*, 1390. Urinary concentrations of clindamycin of up to 0.7 µg per ml had been reported in 4 of 9 subjects who had received daily topical applications containing clindamycin 20 mg for 1 to 7 weeks.— D. A. Voron (letter), *Archs Derm.*, 1978, *114*, 798.

Further references: D. C. McLeod, *Clin. Drug Abstr.*, 1973, *16*, 142, per *Drug Intell. & clin. Pharm.*, 1973, *7*, 575.

For varying reports on the effects of renal impairment on the serum concentrations of clindamycin, see Dosage in Renal Failure, below.

Pregnancy and the neonate. Tests on aborted foetuses showed that both clindamycin and erythromycin given by mouth to the mothers crossed the placental barrier, although erythromycin was less predictable than clindamycin. Foetal tissues, especially liver, were able to concentrate the antibiotics.— A. Philipson *et al.*, *New Engl. J. Med.*, 1973, *288*, 1219.

Further references: A. J. Weinstein *et al.*, *Am. J. Obstet. Gynec.*, 1976, *124*, 688.

Uses. Clindamycin is a chlorinated derivative of the antibiotic lincomycin (see p.1178) and has similar properties although it is better absorbed from the gastro-intestinal tract and is more active. Clindamycin is used in the treatment of serious anaerobic infections especially those caused by *Bacteroides fragilis*. It has been recommended as an alternative to penicillin in some severe staphylococcal and streptococcal infections, including staphylococcal osteomyelitis. Because of its potential toxicity (see Adverse Effects) clindamycin should only be used when there is no suitable alternative.

Clindamycin is given by mouth as the hydrochloride in doses equivalent to 150 to 300 mg every 6 hours. In severe infections a dose of 450 mg may be given 6-hourly. The capsules should be taken with a glass of water. For children over the age of 1 month, the usual dose is 8 to 16 mg per kg body-weight daily in four divided doses or up to 20 mg per kg daily in divided doses in severe infections. (See also under Clindamycin Palmitate Hydrochloride, below.)

It may be given by injection as clindamycin phosphate (see below). Clindamycin palmitate hydrochloride (see below) is used in oral liquid preparations.

A guide to the use of clindamycin and lincomycin.— Veterans Administration Ad Hoc Interdisciplinary Advisory Committee on Antimicrobial Drug Usage, *J. Am. med. Ass.*, 1977, *237*, 1482. See also L. P. Rhodes (letter), *ibid.*, *238*, 852.

Clindamycin phosphate in a usual dose of 300 to 600 mg twice or thrice daily was given by intramuscular injection to 219 patients, the majority of whom had suspected or established infections of the gastro-intestinal or genital tracts after surgery. Many patients received additional antibiotics and in some the parenteral course of clindamycin was followed by clindamycin by mouth. Of 203 patients evaluated 186 had a favourable response to treatment and there was no significant difference between the cure-rates obtained with the various regimens. Gastro-intestinal side-effects due to antibiotic therapy occurred in 27 patients and treatment was discontinued in 7 patients because of diarrhoea. The incidence of diarrhoea was 3 times higher in patients who received antibiotics for prophylaxis compared with those who received treatment for proven infections.— D. A. Leigh *et al.*, *J. antimicrob. Chemother.*, 1977, *3*, 493.

An infection caused by *Pasteurella multocida* in a 3-year-old child was successfully treated with ampicillin and clindamycin.— I. Böhlck, *Dt. med. Wschr.*, 1978, *103*, 1143.

Further references to the use of clindamycin in various infections: A. M. Geddes *et al.*, *Br. med. J.*, 1970, *2*, 703; R. J. Fass and S. Saslaw, *Am. J. med. Sci.*, 1972, *263*, 369; M. D. Kerstein, *Curr. ther. Res.*, 1972, *14*, 107; K. W. Riebe and T. O. Oesterling, *Upjohn, Bull. parent. Drug Ass.*, 1972, *26*, 139; W. Schumer *et al.*, *Archs Surg., Chicago*, 1973, *106*, 578; W. G. L. Carr, *Curr. ther. Res.*, 1973, *15*, 630; A. W. Chow *et al.*, *Archs intern. Med.*, 1974, *134*, 78; R. G. Finch *et al.*, *J. antimicrob. Chemother.*, 1975, *1*, 297.

Actinomycosis. A 57-year-old man was successfully treated for actinomycosis with clindamycin 600 mg intravenously every 6 hours for 5 weeks. Clindamycin would be given by mouth for up to 1 year. He had previously developed an anaphylactoid reaction when treatment with benzylpenicillin was attempted.— H. D. Rose and M. W. Rytel (letter), *J. Am. med. Ass.*, 1972, *221*, 1052.

Anaerobic infections. Proceedings of a symposium on the role of clindamycin in anaerobic infections.— *J. infect. Dis.*, 1977, *135*, *Suppl.* Mar., S1-S136.

Of 19 patients with various severe infections due to anaerobic organisms and treated with clindamycin phosphate equivalent to 600 to 900 mg of clindamycin intravenously and/or intramuscularly to a total daily dose of 1.2 to 2.7 g for up to 52 days, 18 were assessed as bacteriologically and clinically cured. One patient received phenoxymethylpenicillin 2 g daily by mouth and 8 had clindamycin hydrochloride 0.9 to 1.2 g daily also by mouth after they had responded to clindamycin phosphate. Eosinophilia occurred in 3 patients, signs of altered liver function in 8, phlebitis in 1, and rashes in 2 which caused discontinuation of treatment. Two of the 5 patients who received clindamycin intramuscularly complained of local discomfort from 900-mg doses.— R. J. Fass *et al.*, *Ann. intern. Med.*, 1973, *78*, 853.

Clindamycin phosphate was given intravenously in doses of 300 to 450 mg every 6 to 8 hours to 42 patients with severe anaerobic infection. The mean serum concentration was always well in excess of the MIC. The mortality-rate in the 19 patients with bacteraemia was 21% compared with 27% in 48 similar patients treated with chloramphenicol. The infected sites healed in 21 of 23 non-bacteraemic patients and of 32 of the total group on whom follow-up cultures were done, 31 were cured bacteriologically. Treatment was well tolerated.— A. W. Chow *et al.*, *Archs intern. Med.*, 1974, *134*, 78. A similar report.— S. L. Gorbach and H. Thadepalli, *ibid.*, 87.

Of 18 patients with *Bacteroides fragilis* infection 14 responded to treatment with clindamycin. The response-rate (78%) was little higher than 93 (65%) in 142 patients given no antibiotics or antibiotics to which the organism was not sensitive.— D. A. Leigh, *Br. med. J.*, 1974, *3*, 225.

Further references: E. V. Haldane and C. E. van Rooyen, *Can. med. Ass. J.*, 1972, *107*, 1177; J. G. Bartlett *et al.*, *New Engl. J. Med.*, 1972, *287*, 1006; P. C. T. Dickinson and P. Saphyakhajon, *Can. med. Ass. J.*, 1975, *111*, 945; J. Klastersky *et al.*, *Antimicrob. Ag. Chemother.*, 1979, *16*, 366.

Use with aminoglycosides. The response to clindamycin given parenterally with kanamycin was similar in 21 women with severe obstetric-gynaecological infections to that with benzylpenicillin and kanamycin in 23 similar women. The penicillin regimen was ineffective in *B. fragilis* infection and the clindamycin regimen in enterococcal infection.— W. J. Ledger *et al.*, *Obstet. Gynec.*, 1974, *43*, 490.

Excellent results were obtained following concurrent administration of clindamycin and gentamicin to 38 patients with life-threatening infections, 29 of whom had failed to respond to prior antibiotic therapy. The good results were mainly attributed to the activity of clindamycin against anaerobic bacteria, particularly *B. fragilis*. Of the patients treated 30 recovered, 2 improved but required alternative therapy owing to the development of rashes, and 6 relapsed or failed to respond.— R. J. Fass *et al.*, *Archs intern. Med.*, 1977, *137*, 28.

Further references: A. W. Chow *et al.*, *Can. med. Ass. J.*, 1976, *115*, 1225; G. K. M. Harding *et al.*, *J. infect. Dis.*, 1980, *142*, 384.

For a report of the use of clindamycin with tobramycin in febrile leukaemic patients, see Tobramycin, p.1227.

Diphtheria. Clindamycin 150 mg four times a day for 7 days was as effective as benzathine penicillin or erythromycin in the treatment of diphtheria patients and carriers.— *J. Am. med. Ass.*, 1973, *226*, 1166. See also R. V. McCloskey *et al.*, *Ann. intern. Med.*, 1974, *81*, 788.

Dosage in renal failure. The mean half-life of clindamycin after a 150-mg dose was 2.15 hours in 4 healthy subjects, 1.58 hours in 5 patients with terminal renal failure, and 1.85 hours in 4 similar patients during dialysis. Clindamycin could be given in normal doses to patients on dialysis.— J. B. Eastwood and P. E. Gower, *Postgrad. med. J.*, 1974, *50*, 710.

Intravenous infusion of 300 mg of clindamycin in 7 patients in renal failure produced an average peak serum concentration of 12.8 μg per ml, which approximately corresponded to the serum concentration produced by a 900-mg dose in normal subjects. It was recommended that the dose of clindamycin phosphate intravenously for subjects in renal failure should be at least half the normal recommended dose.— A. M. Joshi and R. M. Stein, *J. clin. Pharmac.*, 1974, *14*, 140.

Peritoneal dialysis did not affect serum concentrations of clindamycin, but peak concentrations were twice as high in anephric patients as in normal subjects and so the normal dose should be halved for such patients.— R. F. Malacoff *et al.*, *Antimicrob. Ag. Chemother.*, 1975, *8*, 574.

The half-life for clindamycin was 2 to 2.5 hours in healthy persons and 1.5 to 3.5 hours in end-stage renal failure. Clindamycin could be given in usual doses to patients with impaired renal function. Concentrations of clindamycin were not affected by haemodialysis or peritoneal dialysis.— W. M. Bennett *et al.*, *Ann. intern. Med.*, 1977, *86*, 754. See also *idem*, 1980, *93*, 62.

A suggested dose for uraemic patients was clindamycin 300 mg every 8 hours.— G. B. Appel and H. C. Neu, *New Engl. J. Med.*, 1977, *296*, 663.

Further references: B. A. Peddie *et al.*, *Aust. N.Z. J. Med.*, 1975, *5*, 198; T. P. Gibson and H. A. Nelson, *Clin. Pharmacokinet.*, 1977, *2*, 403; J. S. Cheigh, *Am. J. Med.*, 1977, *62*, 555; A. P. Roberts *et al.*, *Eur. J. clin. Pharmac.*, 1978, *14*, 435.

Dry socket. Clindamycin was as effective as phenoxymethylpenicillin in controlling dry socket.— W. R. E. Laird *et al.*, *Br. dent. J.*, 1972, *133*, 106.

Endocarditis. Clindamycin 900 mg intravenously every 8 hours for 6 weeks was successful in the treatment of pneumococcal endocarditis in a patient with penicillin allergy.— J. T. Keane and H. D. Rose, *J. Am. med. Ass.*, 1973, *226*, 1120.

Further references: R. Freeman and D. W. Roberts, *Postgrad. med. J.*, 1976, *52*, 595.

Hidradenitis. Two patients with chronic suppurative hidradenitis obtained considerable benefit from clindamycin therapy. Although surgery and intensive local cleaning, debridement, and hydrotherapy remain the primary means of treatment in the chronic case, where anaerobes are recovered, antibiotics active against *Bacteroides* spp. might reduce the foul-smelling discharge and improve the chances of successful surgery.— D. E. Brenner and D. P. Lookingbill (letter), *Lancet*, 1980, *2*, 921. Comments.— A. S. Highet *et al.* (letter), *ibid.*, 1203; L. E. Hughes (letter), *ibid.*, 1981, *1*, 51.

Malaria. Of 12 patients with chloroquine-resistant falciparum malaria, 5 were cured after treatment with clindamycin 450 mg (for adults) 8-hourly for 3 days. Of 6 given clindamycin in the same dose plus quinine 540 mg (given as sulphate) every 8 hours for 3 days, 4 were cured but 5 had unacceptable side-effects. Of 8 given clindamycin plus quinine, each at approximately half dosage, 3 were cured and 5 had unacceptable side-effects. Quinine alone cleared 3 patients of parasitaemia, but with recrudescence.— A. P. Hall *et al.*, *Br. med. J.*, 1975, *2*, 12.

Further references: L. H. Miller *et al.*, *Am. J. trop. Med. Hyg.*, 1974, *23*, 565.

Osteomyelitis. In a retrospective study, 33 of 35 children aged 5 to 15 years with acute osteomyelitis were successfully treated with clindamycin 75 or 150 mg 4 times daily for 4 to 8 weeks. Therapy for 4 weeks was adequate.— M. R. Wharton and F. H. Beddow, *Postgrad. med. J.*, 1975, *51*, 166.

Clindamycin was used successfully in the treatment of acute and chronic osteomyelitis in 25 and 4 children respectively. The majority of patients were given the equivalent of 50 mg per kg body-weight daily by intravenous injection for 3 weeks followed by 25 mg per kg daily by mouth for 4 to 6 weeks. *Staphylococcus aureus* was isolated in 22 of the patients and nearly all isolates were penicillin-resistant.— W. Rodriguez *et al.*, *Am. J. Dis. Child.*, 1977, *131*, 1088.

The successful use of clindamycin in the treatment of bone and joint infections.— A. M. Geddes *et al.*, *J. antimicrob. Chemother.*, 1977, *3*, 501.

Otitis media. A report on the use of clindamycin in the treatment of chronic recurrent suppurative otitis media in children.— I. Brook, *J. Lar Otol.*, 1980, *94*, 607.

Pneumonia. Clindamycin had a beneficial effect in 9 patients with pulmonary infections due to *Mycoplasma pneumoniae*.— J. Axelrod *et al.*, *Antimicrob. Ag. Chemother.*, 1972, *2*, 499. It was no more effective than placebo in 9 further patients with *M. pneumoniae*.— J. D. Smilack *et al.*, *J. Am. med. Ass.*, 1974, *228*, 729.

All of 28 children with aspiration pneumonia due to aerobic and anaerobic bacteria responded to therapy with clindamycin phosphate 25 to 40 mg per kg body-weight given daily in 3 divided doses. Gentamicin 3 to 6 mg per kg given daily in 3 divided doses was added to the regimen when aerobic Gram-negative bacilli were predominant. The average length of treatment was about 14 days.— I. Brook, *Antimicrob. Ag. Chemother.*, 1979, *15*, 342.

Further references: J. R. Bongiorno *et al.*, *Curr. ther. Res.*, 1971, *13*, 667; P. Sen *et al.*, *Archs intern. Med.*, 1974, *134*, 73.

Skin infections. The beneficial effect of clindamycin hydrochloride 150 mg daily on severe acne vulgaris in 21 patients.— W. J. Cunliffe *et al.*, *Br. J. Derm.*, 1972, *87*, 37. See also W. J. Cunliffe and J. A. Cotterill, *Practitioner*, 1973, *210*, 698.

Clindamycin 150 mg thrice daily for one week then twice daily for 2 weeks was effective in the treatment of 16 of 18 patients with acne.— *Br. med. J.*, 1975, *1*,

399.

From a study of 142 patients with acne lasting from 4 to 7 years it was considered that clindamycin should not be denied to patients because of the side-effects but should be restricted to those with moderate to severe acne unresponsive to treatment with tetracycline, erythromycin, co-trimoxazole, or topical preparations.— S. G. Tan and W. J. Cunliffe, *Br. J. Derm.*, 1976, *94*, 313.

Topical use. A report of the successful topical treatment of acne vulgaris using clindamycin phosphate 1% in *N*-methyl-2-pyrrolidone.— W. Resh and R. B. Stoughton, *Archs Derm.*, 1976, *112*, 182.

A local survey of the formulations used in dispensing topical clindamycin preparations (usually 1%) from commercially-available clindamycin capsules or injections.— N. C. Lacina *et al.*, *Am. Pharm.*, 1978, *NS18* (Oct.), 30.

Guidelines for the extemporaneous compounding of clindamycin preparations for topical use in acne. A suitable procedure for preparing a clear clindamycin solution consisted of shaking the contents of clindamycin capsules with a vehicle of isopropyl alcohol or alcohol 70%, propylene glycol 10%, and water 20%. A 6- to 8-week shelf-life was considered reasonable for the solution.— R. J. Orr *et al.*, *Am. Pharm.*, 1978, *NS18* (Nov.), 23.

Topical 1% solutions of clindamycin phosphate or hydrochloride reduced inflammatory lesions by about 70% when used for at least 3 months in a study involving 15 patients with acne. The vehicle used for each solution was isopropyl alcohol (91%) 8 parts and one part each of water and propylene glycol, by volume.— J. D. Guin, *Int. J. Derm.*, 1979, *18*, 164.

Further references: R. B. Stoughton, *Archs Derm.*, 1979, *115*, 486; A. A. Fisher, *Cutis*, 1979, *23*, 406; *idem*, 1980, *25*, 474; R. B. Stoughton *et al.*, *ibid.*, *26*, 424.

For conflicting reports on the systemic absorption of clindamycin after its topical use, see under Absorption and Fate.

Surgical infection prophylaxis. Results of a placebo-controlled double-blind study involving 80 patients assessing the surgical treatment of acute abscesses with and without antibiotic cover (clindamycin injection before operation, or capsules after operation, or both) appeared to confirm that a single injection of an effective antibiotic before surgery is sufficient to protect the patient against bacteraemia and permit optimum healing.— P. W. H. Blick *et al.*, *Br. med. J.*, 1980, *281*, 111.

Preparations

Clindamycin Capsules *(B.P.)*. Capsules containing clindamycin hydrochloride. Potency is expressed in terms of the equivalent amount of clindamycin. Store at a temperature not exceeding 30°.

Clindamycin Hydrochloride Capsules *(U.S.P.)*. Capsules containing clindamycin hydrochloride. Potency is expressed in terms of the equivalent amount of clindamycin. Store in airtight containers.

Clindamycin Topical Solution *(Rochester Methodist Hosp.)*. Clindamycin (as hydrochloride) 1, isopropyl alcohol 56, propylene glycol 10, water 34. pH adjusted to 5. Shelf-life 9 months.

Proprietary Preparations

Dalacin C *(Upjohn, UK)*. Clindamycin hydrochloride, available as capsules each containing the equivalent of clindamycin 75 or 150 mg. (Also available as Dalacin C in *Arg.*, *Austral.*, *Belg.*, *Canad.*, *Ital.*, *Neth.*, *S.Afr.*, *Switz.*).

NOTE. The name Dalacin was formerly applied to streptovaricin..

Other Proprietary Names

Cleocin *(USA)*; Dalacin *(Denm., Norw., Spain)*; Dalacina *(Swed.)*; Dalacine *(Fr.)*; Sobelin *(Ger.)*.

The above proprietary names are also applied to preparations of clindamycin palmitate hydrochloride or clindamycin phosphate.

55-g

Clindamycin Palmitate Hydrochloride.

(U.S.P.). U 25179E. Clindamycin 2-palmitate hydrochloride.

$C_{34}H_{63}ClN_2O_6S,HCl$=699.9.

CAS — 36688-78-5 (clindamycin palmitate); 25507-04-4 (hydrochloride).

Pharmacopoeias. In *U.S.*

A white to off-white amorphous powder with a characteristic odour and taste. The *U.S.P.* specifies not less than the equivalent of 540 µg of clindamycin per mg. Clindamycin palmitate hydrochloride 1.6 g is approximately equivalent to 1 g of clindamycin. Freely **soluble** in water, alcohol, chloroform, and ether; very soluble in dimethylformamide and ethyl acetate. A 1% solution in water has a pH of 2.8 to 3.8. **Store** in airtight containers.

Adverse Effects, Treatment, and Precautions. As for Clindamycin Hydrochloride, p.1144.

Absorption and Fate. Clindamycin palmitate hydrochloride is rapidly hydrolysed following oral administration to provide free clindamycin. Plasma concentrations of about 2 to 4 µg per ml have been achieved in children given the equivalent of 2 to 4 mg of clindamycin per kg body-weight every 6 hours. A biological half-life of about 2 hours is reported in children.

Studies of 52 children aged 6 months to 14 years indicated that the equivalent of clindamycin 8 to 16 mg per kg body-weight daily in divided doses gave effective serum concentrations during a 17-dose course of clindamycin palmitate hydrochloride in flavoured granules. Tolerance was good and 75% of the children found the preparation palatable. There was no drug accumulation or increase in metabolism due to enzyme induction.— R. M. DeHaan and D. Schellenberg, *J. clin. Pharmac.*, 1972, *12*, 74.

In a crossover study of the absorption of clindamycin 12 men received clindamycin 300 mg as a suspension prepared from the palmitate hydrochloride, while fasting, immediately before food, or 1 hour after food. Serum concentrations of clindamycin were higher at the peak time of 1 hour when the drug was given immediately before food than when it was given to fasting patients. Serum concentrations were lower at 0.5 and 1 hour but higher at 3 and 4 hours when patients received the drug 1 hour after food than when they were given it immediately before food. With all drug regimens clindamycin appeared in the blood within half an hour.— R. M. DeHaan *et al.*, *J. clin. Pharmac.*, 1972, *12*, 205.

A comparison of the blood concentrations attained with doses of clindamycin as the hydrochloride, palmitate, and phosphate.— C. M. Metzler *et al.*, *J. pharm. Sci.*, 1973, *62*, 591.

Uses. Clindamycin palmitate hydrochloride has the actions and uses of Clindamycin Hydrochloride, p.1144. It is suitable for the preparation of flavoured syrups. Children may be given the equivalent of 8 to 25 mg of clindamycin per kg body-weight daily in divided doses. Children under one-year-old or weighing 10 kg or less should receive at least the equivalent of 37.5 mg of clindamycin thrice daily.

Preparations

Clindamycin Palmitate Hydrochloride for Oral Solution *(U.S.P.)*. A dry mixture with one or more suitable diluents, buffers, colouring and flavouring agents, and preservatives. Store in airtight containers. The solution is prepared by the addition of diluent before issue, and contains the equivalent of 15 mg of clindamycin per ml. pH 2.5 to 5.

Dalacin C Paediatric *(Upjohn, UK)*. Contains in each 5 ml clindamycin palmitate hydrochloride equivalent to clindamycin 75 mg (supplied as granules for preparation with water before use; suggested diluent, water). (Also available as Dalacin C in *Austral.*, *Belg.*, *Canad.*, *Ital.*, *Neth.*, *S.Afr.*, *Switz.*).

NOTE. The name Dalacin was formerly applied to streptovaricin..

Other Proprietary Names

Cleocin *(USA)*; Dalacin *(Denm., Norw., Spain)*; Dalacina *(Swed.)*; Dalacine *(Fr.)*; Sobelin *(Ger.)*.

The above proprietary names are also applied to preparations of clindamycin hydrochloride or clindamycin phosphate.

56-q

Clindamycin Phosphate *(U.S.P.)*. U 28 508.

Clindamycin 2-(dihydrogen phosphate).

$C_{18}H_{34}ClN_2O_8PS$=505.0.

CAS — 24729-96-2.

Pharmacopoeias. In *U.S.*

A white to off-white, odourless or almost odourless, hygroscopic, crystalline powder with a bitter taste. Clindamycin phosphate 1.2 g is approximately equivalent to 1 g of clindamycin. **Soluble** 1 in 2.5 of water; slightly soluble in dehydrated alcohol; very slightly soluble in acetone; practically insoluble in chloroform and ether. A 1% solution in water has a pH of 3 to 4.5. A 10.73% solution in water is iso-osmotic with serum. **Store** in airtight containers.

It is reported to be **incompatible** with aminophylline, ampicillin sodium, barbiturates, calcium gluconate, magnesium sulphate, phenytoin sodium, and vitamins of the B group. Solutions with tobramycin sulphate in dextrose injection are reported to be unstable.

Clindamycin phosphate was less bitter than clindamycin hydrochloride, and was most stable in solution at pH 3.5 to 6.5.— T. O. Oesterling and E. L. Rowe, *J. pharm. Sci.*, 1970, *59*, 175.

An aqueous solution of clindamycin phosphate iso-osmotic with serum (10.73%) caused 58% haemolysis of erythrocytes cultured in it for 45 minutes. The solution and cells turned brown.— C. Sapp *et al.*, *J. pharm. Sci.*, 1975, *64*, 1884.

Adverse Effects, Treatment, and Precautions. As for Clindamycin Hydrochloride, p.1144.

A report of an anaphylactic reaction to intravenous infusion of clindamycin.— A. J. Pomerance *et al.* (letter), *Drug Intell. & clin. Pharm.*, 1979, *13*, 348.

Absorption and Fate. Clindamycin phosphate is biologically inactive but is rapidly hydrolysed in the blood to clindamycin. When the equivalent of 300 mg of clindamycin is injected intramuscularly every 8 hours a mean peak plasma concentration of 6 µg per ml is achieved within 3 hours; 600 mg every 12 hours gives a peak concentration of 9 µg per ml. In children, peak concentrations may be reached within one hour. When the same doses are infused intravenously every 8 hours peak concentrations of 7 and 10 µg per ml are achieved by the end of infusion.

About 8% and 28% of intramuscular and intravenous doses of clindamycin, respectively, have been recovered from the urine within 8 hours.

A dose of clindamycin phosphate equivalent to 150 mg of clindamycin per m^2 body-surface given to 4 children intramuscularly produced adequate serum activity of 2.4 µg per ml at 8 hours, the half-life of serum activity being 3.4 hours. A dose of 117 mg per m^2 in 8 children produced an inadequate mean serum concentration of 1 µg per ml at 8 hours where the half-life was 2.4 hours.— R. E. Kauffman *et al.*, *Clin. Pharmac. Ther.*, 1972, *13*, 704.

In a study of 19 patients treated with clindamycin phosphate given parenterally, the equivalent of 900 mg of base was the usual dose which was given intravenously every 8 hours. After 30-minute infusions serum concentrations ranged from 11.1 to 39 µg per ml with a mean of 23.6 µg per ml. At 2 to 4 hours concentrations were 3.4 to 15 µg per ml (mean 9.6 µg per ml) and by 8 hours 0.9 to 10.7 µg per ml (mean 5.4 µg per ml). Maximum concentrations at 1 to 4 and at 8 hours in the 5 patients given 900 mg intramuscularly were similar to those after intravenous injection.— R. J. Fass *et al.*, *Ann. intern. Med.*, 1973, *78*, 853.

A comparison of the blood concentrations attained with doses of clindamycin as the hydrochloride, palmitate, and phosphate.— C. M. Metzler *et al.*, *J. pharm. Sci.*, 1973, *62*, 591.

Clindamycin phosphate given intravenously was rapidly hydrolysed to clindamycin which disappeared from serum within 2 hours. Doses up to 4.8 g daily produced no toxic effects. Activity in bile, due to a *N*-demethyl derivative, persisted for up to 18 hours. Following intramuscular injection a peak serum concentration of clindamycin was found within 2 to 3 hours, with some still present after 4 hours, and the salivary concentration reached a peak at about 90 to 120 minutes after administration. Activity in urine, due to metabolites, persisted for up to 4 days after a single dose of clindamycin phosphate. The minimum effective dose was considered to be 300 mg every 12 hours.— R. M. DeHaan *et al., J. clin. Pharmac.*, 1973, *13*, 190.

Clindamycin phosphate 600 mg was given intravenously to 14 patients about 1 hour before biliary tract surgery; 7 had total obstruction of the common bile duct and 7 had patent biliary tracts. Those with patent ducts had average serum concentrations of 19.2 and 14.5 μg per ml at 30 and 60 minutes respectively and achieved high concentrations of clindamycin in specimens of gall-bladder bile (33.9 μg per ml), common duct bile (41.7 μg per ml), gall-bladder wall (12.0 μg per g), and liver (33.9 μg per g) obtained during surgery. In those with obstructed ducts average serum concentrations were 15.4 and 11.3 μg per ml at 30 and 60 minutes respectively. They had no measurable drug in the common duct bile and a reduced concentration in the gall-bladder wall (4.6 μg per g). Concentrations in the liver were however slightly higher (41.5 μg per g) than in the other group and clindamycin could therefore be used for intrahepatic infections in patients with common bile duct obstruction.— R. E. Brown *et al., Ann. intern. Med.*, 1976, *84*, 168.

Further references: V. Balachandar *et al., Clin. Med.*, 1973, *80* (Apr.), 24.

Diffusion. The mean serum-clindamycin concentration in 30 patients undergoing hip replacement was 7.33 μg per ml at the time of operation, after 1 days' therapy with clindamycin phosphate 300 mg every 8 hours by intramuscular injection. Mean bone concentration was 2.63 μg per g and the mean ratio of bone: serum concentration was 0.40±0.30.— P. Nicholas *et al., Antimicrob. Ag. Chemother.*, 1975, *8*, 220. See also J. D. Smilack *et al., ibid.*, 1976, *9*, 169.

Mean concentrations of clindamycin in femoral bone from 8 patients given 300 mg four times daily by intravenous infusion ranged from 0.4 to 4.9 μg per g and from 0.4 to 6 μg per g when determined by an agar diffusion method or an electrophoretic method respectively; corresponding serum concentrations ranged from 1.7 to 24 μg per ml in 7 patients. Use of the electrophoretic method may have reduced the binding capacity of the bone.— K. Dornbusch *et al., J. antimicrob. Chemother.*, 1977, *3*, 153.

Concentrations of clindamycin exceeded 2.5 μg per g in 32 of 40 tissue samples (primarily skin and bone) taken from 29 patients undergoing excision of decubitus ulcers 30 to 90 minutes after an intravenous infusion of 600 mg as the phosphate given over 10 minutes, and were greater than simultaneous concentrations in serum in 16 of 32 samples.— S. A. Berger *et al., Antimicrob. Ag. Chemother.*, 1978, *14*, 498.

Further references: D. N. Gerding *et al., Ann. intern. Med.*, 1977, *86*, 708; S. A. Berger *et al., Archs Surg., Chicago*, 1978, *35*, 1094; P. Baird *et al., Postgrad. med. J.*, 1978, *54*, 65.

Uses. Clindamycin phosphate has the actions and uses of clindamycin hydrochloride (see p.1144). It is administered by intramuscular injection or slow intravenous infusion in doses equivalent to 0.6 to 2.7 g of clindamycin daily in divided doses. Higher doses have been given intravenously in very severe infections but no more than 1.2 g should be infused in 1 hour. Children over the age of 1 month may be given the equivalent of 15 to 40 mg per kg body-weight daily in divided doses; in severe infections they should receive a total dose of not less than 300 mg of clindamycin daily.

Preparations

Clindamycin Phosphate Injection *(U.S.P.).* A sterile solution in Water for Injections with one or more suitable preservatives and sequestering agents. pH 5.5 to 7. It contains the equivalent of 150 mg of clindamycin per ml.

Clindamycin Phosphate Topical Solution *(U.S.P.).* A solution containing clindamycin phosphate. Potency is expressed in terms of the equivalent amount of clindamycin. pH 4 to 7. Store in airtight containers.

Sterile Clindamycin Phosphate *(U.S.P.).* Clindamycin phosphate suitable for parenteral use.

Proprietary Preparations

Dalacin C Phosphate Sterile Solution *(Upjohn, UK).* Clindamycin phosphate, available as injection containing the equivalent of 150 mg of clindamycin per ml, in ampoules of 2 and 4 ml. (Also available as Dalacin C in *Arg., Austral., Belg., Canad., Neth., S.Afr., Switz.*).

NOTE. The name Dalacin was formerly applied to streptovaricin..

Other Proprietary Names

Cleocin *(USA)*; Dalacin *(Denm., Norw.)*; Dalacina *(Swed.)*; Sobelin *(Ger.)*.

The above proprietary names are also applied to preparations of clindamycin hydrochloride and clindamycin palmitate hydrochloride.

57-p

Clometocillin Potassium. Penicillin 356 *(clometocillin)*; 3,4-Dichloro-α-methoxybenzylpenicillin potassium. Potassium (6*R*)-6-[2-(3,4-dichlorophenyl)-2-methoxyacetamido]penicillanate.

$C_{17}H_{17}Cl_2KN_2O_5S = 471.4$.

CAS — 1926-49-4 (clometocillin); 15433-28-0 (potassium salt).

Clometocillin has actions and uses similar to those of benzylpenicillin (see p.1102) but is acid-stable and well-absorbed from the gastro-intestinal tract. It has been given in a dose of 500 mg twice daily.

Antibacterial activity of clometocillin.— P. J. Van Dijck *et al., Antibiotics Chemother.*, 1962, *12*, 192.

Proprietary Names

Rixapen *(RIT, Belg.; Smith Kline & French, Fr.)*.

58-s

Clomocycline Calcium.

An insoluble complex prepared from clomocycline sodium (see below) and a soluble calcium salt.

CAS — 1181-54-0 (clomocycline).

59-w

Clomocycline Sodium.

Chlormethylencycline Sodium; Methylolchlortetracycline Sodium; N^2-(Hydroxymethyl)chlortetracycline Sodium. The sodium salt of 7-chloro-N^2-(hydroxymethyl)tetracycline.

$C_{23}H_{24}ClN_2NaO_9 = 530.9$.

A yellow powder with a bitter taste. Very **soluble** in water. A 2% solution in water has a pH of about 8.4. Solutions in water lose most of their activity after 24 hours. **Store** in airtight containers. Protect from light.

Adverse Effects and Precautions. As for Tetracycline Hydrochloride, p.1217.

Pregnancy and the neonate. A report of the birth of an infant with multiple abnormalities to a woman who had taken clomocycline for the first 8 weeks of pregnancy. A causal relationship was not established but it was considered that prolonged tetracycline treatment for acne should not be given to women having unprotected intercourse and that is should be withdrawn as soon as possible in an unplanned pregnancy.— R. Corcoran and J. M. Castles, *Br. med. J.*, 1977, *2*, 807.

Absorption and Fate. As for Tetracycline Hydrochloride, p.1219.

Clomocycline sodium is absorbed from the gastro-intestinal tract and serum concentrations of about 1 μg per ml have been reported to follow 2 or 3 hours after a single 170-mg dose and concentrations of about 2 μg per ml after repeated doses. Its biological half-life is about 5.7 hours. About 30% of the administered dose is excreted in the urine.

Uses. Clomocycline sodium has the antimicrobial activity and uses described under Tetracycline Hydrochloride (see p.1218).

It is given by mouth in capsules, and has been used as a syrup containing clomocycline calcium. The usual adult dose is 170 mg four times daily but the dose may be doubled in severe infections. A suggested dose for children has been 12 mg per kg body-weight of clomocycline sodium daily in divided doses but the effects of tetracyclines on teeth should be considered.

Skin disorders. Clomocycline produced marked improvement in 10 of 24 patients with pustular or pustular and cystic acne and moderate improvement in a further 12. The patients had shown negligible improvement with previous local and antibiotic therapy. Dosage was usually 170 mg four times daily for 1 week, then 170 mg twice daily, and treatment lasted for 2 weeks to 11 months. One patient experienced heartburn and another an irritant erythematous macular rash.— J. L. Verbov, *Br. J. clin. Pract.*, 1968, *22*, 37. See also M. Ganpule, *Practitioner*, 1968, *201*, 479.

In a double-blind crossover study completed by 40 of 60 patients with persistent palmoplantar pustulosis, 15 responded to treatment with clomocycline 170 mg thrice daily for 2 weeks and then twice daily for 10 weeks, 1 responded to treatment and the placebo, and 2 patients responded only to the placebo. There was no response in 22 patients.— J. M. Ward *et al., Br. J. Derm.*, 1976, *95*, 317.

Proprietary Preparations

Megaclor *(Pharmax, UK).* Clomocycline sodium, available as capsules of 170 mg.

60-m

Cloxacillin Sodium *(B.P., B.P. Vet., U.S.P.).*

Cloxacillinum Natricum; Sodium Cloxacillin; BRL 1621; P 25. Sodium (6*R*)-6-[3-(2-chlorophenyl)-5-methylisoxazole-4-carboxamido]penicillanate monohydrate.

$C_{19}H_{17}ClN_3NaO_5S,H_2O = 475.9$.

CAS — 61-72-3 (cloxacillin); 642-78-4 (sodium salt, anhydrous); 7081-44-9 (sodium salt, monohydrate).

Pharmacopoeias. In *Br., Int., Jap., Jug., Nord., Roum.,* and *U.S.*

A white, odourless, hygroscopic, crystalline powder with an intensely bitter taste. Each g represents about 2.1 mmol (2.1 mEq) of sodium. Cloxacillin sodium 1.09 g is approximately equivalent to 1 g of anhydrous cloxacillin. The *B.P.* specifies not less than 95% of cloxacillin calculated as the anhydrous substance. *U.S.P.* specifies not less than 825 μg of cloxacillin per mg.

Soluble 1 in 2.5 of water, 1 in 30 of alcohol, and 1 in 500 of chloroform. A 10% solution in water has a pH of 5 to 7. Solutions containing 2.5 to 20% may be expected to lose about 5% of their activity when stored for 7 days in a refrigerator. At room temperature, losses of up to 15% may be expected over 4 days, but thereafter the rate of decomposition may be accelerated. The use of buffering agents is of little advantage.

Store at a temperature not exceeding 25° in airtight containers; if it is intended for injection, the containers should be sterile and sealed to exclude micro-organisms.

Incompatible with ascorbic acid, chlorpromazine hydrochloride, erythromycin ethylsuccinate, gentamicin sulphate, oxytetracycline hydrochloride, polymyxin B sulphate, and tetracycline hydrochloride. Some loss of potency has been reported with colistin sulphomethate sodium and kanamycin sulphate.

Incompatibility. Solutions of cloxacillin sodium equivalent to cloxacillin 1% with hydrocortisone sodium succinate 0.02% in sodium chloride injection 0.9%, dextrose injection 5%, or sodium chloride and dextrose injection at 25° were stable over 24 hours. Cloxacillin sodium 2 mg per ml in sodium chloride injection lost 11% potency over 6 hours and 52% over 24 hours when stored at 23° with a solution of tyloxapol 0.125%, sodium bicarbonate 2%, and glycerol 5% (Alevaire).— B. Lynn, *J. Hosp. Pharm.*, 1971, *29*, 183.

Further references: B. Lynn, *J. Hosp. Pharm.*, 1970, *28*, 71; B. B. Riley, *ibid.*, 228; B. Lynn and A. Jones, *Beecham Research, Advances in Antimicrobial and Antineoplastic Chemotherapy*, Vol. I, pt 1, Munich, Urban and Schwarzenberg, 1972, p. 701; B. Flouvat and P. Lechat, *Thérapie*, 1974, *29*, 337.

Stability in solution. The half-life of a 0.1% solution of cloxacillin sodium in 50% aqueous alcohol at pH 1.3 and 35° was 160 minutes.— B. Lynn, *Chemist Drugg.*, 1967, *187*, 134.

A 10% loss of potency in 8 hours was noted in solutions of cloxacillin sodium 5 g in 500 ml of sodium bicarbonate injection 1.4% but solutions in Aminosol Vitrum, Aminosol-Fructose-Ethanol, and Aminosol-Glucose were stable for 24 hours at 23°. A solution of cloxacillin sodium 500 mg per litre in a peritoneal dialysis solution (Dialaflex 62) retained 95% potency for up to 3 hours at 37°.— B. Lynn, *J. Hosp. Pharm.*, 1970, *28*, 71.

The activity of solutions of cloxacillin sodium in either sucrose 10% or dextrose 5% at 37° was negligible after 24 hours.— M. S. Simberkoff *et al.*, *New Engl. J. Med.*, 1970, *283*, 116.

In aqueous solutions of cloxacillin sodium, maximum stability occurred at pH 6.3.— H. Bundgaard and K. Ilver, *Dansk Tidsskr. Farm.*, 1970, *44*, 365.

Orbenin syrup suffered no loss of potency when diluted with syrup and stored at 20° for 5 days.— L. Gould and M. W. Brown (letter), *Pharm. J.*, 1974, *1*, 276.

Cloxacillin sodium should not be added to lactate solutions or, in concentrations less than 4 g per litre, to carbohydrate solutions with a pH below 4. Temperature affected the stability and an increase of 5° to 6° could double the degradation-rate. Acetic acid, acetate ions, bicarbonate, dihydrogen and monohydrogen phosphate ions, citric acid, and dihydrogen and monohydrogen citrate ions could catalyse the degradation of cloxacillin, while unprotonated citrate ion was non-catalytic.— L. Landersjö *et al.*, *Acta pharm. suec.*, 1974, *11*, 563.

Adverse Effects and Treatment. As for Benzylpenicillin, p.1103.

Febrile reactions were noted in 9 patients after the intravenous infusion of cloxacillin. Shaking chills and fever lasting 20 to 30 minutes occurred, in some patients after each dose and in others only intermittently.— J. Portnoy *et al.* (letter), *Can. med. Ass. J.*, 1975, *112*, 280.

Blood disorders. Agranulocytosis developed in a 42-year-old man about one month after starting treatment with cloxacillin 500 mg four times daily.— E. L. Westerman *et al.*, *Am. J. clin. Path.*, 1978, *69*, 559.

Hepatotoxity. Intrahepatic cholestatic jaundice which occurred in a woman receiving nitrofurantoin, ampicillin, and cloxacillin re-appeared when the patient was treated with cloxacillin 2 years later. A macrophage inhibition factor test confirmed that cloxacillin was the offending drug.— R. Enat *et al.*, *Br. med. J.*, 1980, *280*, 982.

Precautions. Cloxacillin sodium is contra-indicated in patients known to be sensitive to penicillin and it should be given with caution to patients with known histories of allergy. It should not be given by subconjunctival injection or used in eye-drops.

In a study in neonates given ampicillin, cloxacillin, flucloxacillin, or sulphafurazole, all except ampicillin reduced bilirubin-binding capacity. Sulphafurazole was already known to have precipitated kernicterus in preterm infants and it was suggested that cloxacillin and flucloxacillin should be used with caution in jaundiced neonates.— Friedman L.A. and P. J. Lewis, *Br. J. clin. Pharmac.*, 1977, *4*, 395P. See also *idem*, 1980, *9*, 61.

Interactions. Aspirin, sulphamethoxypyridazine, and sulphaethidole inhibited the serum-binding of cloxacillin *in vitro* and *in vivo*.— C. M. Kunin, *Clin. Pharmac. Ther.*, 1966, *7*, 180.

Cloxacillin affected the estimation of urinary 17-oxosteroids and 17-oxogenic steroids.— *Adverse Drug React. Bull.*, 1972, June, 104.

Antimicrobial Action. Cloxacillin sodium is bactericidal with a mode of action similar to that of benzylpenicillin. It has an antibacterial spectrum similar to that of methicillin and is active against most Gram-positive organisms and *Neisseria* spp. On the basis of minimum inhibitory concentrations, its activity against both penicillin-resistant and penicillin-sensitive staphylococci is 4 to 8 times that of methicillin sodium but against penicillin-sensitive staphylococci its activity is only about one-quarter that of benzylpenicillin or phenoxymethylpenicillin. A minimum inhibitory concentration against penicillin-resistant staphylococci of 0.25 to 0.5 µg per ml has been reported. Its activity against streptococci is less than that of benzylpenicillin but sufficient to be useful when these organisms are present with penicillin-resistant staphylococci.

In an *in vitro* study, flucloxacillin was bactericidal against 88% of 26 penicillin-resistant isolates of *Staphylococcus aureus* at 0.4 µg per ml and against all of them at 6.2 µg per ml; cloxacillin was bactericidal against 81% of the isolates at 0.8 µg per ml and against all at 12.5 µg per ml; and oxacillin was bactericidal against 88% of the isolates at 0.2 µg per ml and against all at 1.6 µg per ml.— M. G. Bergeron *et al.*, *Am. J. med. Sci.*, 1976, *271*, 13.

For a report of cloxacillin being one of the most active penicillins against *Staph. aureus* and *Staph. epidermidis*, see Benzylpenicillin, p.1106.

Resistance. As for Methicillin Sodium, p.1183.

Skin lesions in which *Corynebacterium diphtheriae* were present were found to be resistant to treatment with cloxacillin, and showed slow response to treatment with erythromycin and penicillin.— W. H. Cockcroft *et al.*, *Can. med. Ass. J.*, 1973, *108*, 329.

Absorption and Fate. Cloxacillin sodium is absorbed after oral administration but absorption is reduced by food in the stomach or small intestine. After an oral dose of 500 mg, a peak plasma concentration of 8 to 10 µg per ml is obtained in fasting subjects in 1 hour and a therapeutic concentration persists for up to about 4 hours. Absorption is more complete when given by intramuscular injection and peak plasma concentrations of about 15 µg per ml have been observed 30 minutes after a dose of 500 mg. Doubling the oral or intramuscular dose can double the plasma concentration. About 94% of cloxacillin in the circulation is bound to plasma proteins. Some 35% of an oral dose is excreted in the urine and up to 10% in the bile.

Cloxacillin diffuses across the placenta into the foetal circulation and it is excreted in the milk of nursing mothers. It does not penetrate well into normal cerebrospinal fluid but some antimicrobial activity has been observed in pleural and synovial fluids.

Serum concentrations are enhanced if probenecid is given concomitantly.

The biological half-life of cloxacillin was reported to be 1.5 hours.— F. O'Grady *et al.* (letter), *Lancet*, 1971, *2*, 209. A report of it being 0.5 hours.— W. M. Bennett *et al.*, *J. Am. med. Ass.*, 1973, *223*, 991.

The pharmacokinetics of cloxacillin in healthy subjects and patients on chronic intermittent haemodialysis.— E. H. Nauta and H. Mattie, *Br. J. clin. Pharmac.*, 1975, *2*, 111.

Cloxacillin was reported to be absorbed from the peritoneal cavity.— J. S. Cheigh, *Am. J. Med.*, 1977, *62*, 555.

Diffusion into body fluids. Cloxacillin 500 mg every 6 hours was given to a 10-year-old girl with septic arthritis and 2 hours 50 minutes after the last dose specimens of synovial fluid and serum were obtained. The concentration of cloxacillin in the serum was 7.7 µg per ml and in synovial fluid 3.8 µg per ml. Intra-articular treatment was considered unnecessary and undesirable.— J. H. Newman (letter), *Br. med. J.*, 1974, *3*, 472.

In a study of infants and children with suppurative arthritis, the concentration of cloxacillin achieved in joint fluid was about 65% of the serum concentration 2 hours after 25 mg per kg body-weight was given by mouth. When compared with other antibiotics, the degree of binding to plasma proteins did not appear to influence diffusion.— J. D. Nelson *et al.*, *J. Pediat.*, 1978, *92*, 131.

See also Ampicillin p.1095.

Metabolism. About 22% of a 500-mg dose of cloxacillin was metabolised. Within 12 hours of the dose being taken by 6 healthy subjects about 49% was recovered in the urine, 11% as penicilloic acid.— M. Cole *et al.*, *Antimicrob. Ag. Chemother.*, 1973, *3*, 463.

Oral and intravenous doses of cloxacillin showed similar patterns of plasma concentration and degradation, indicating little metabolism in the gastro-intestinal tract; metabolites probably include penicilloic and penilloic acids.— K. Hellström *et al.*, *Eur. J. clin. Pharmac.*, 1974, *7*, 125.

The metabolite of cloxacillin had similar antibacterial properties to the parent compound and accumulated in patients with renal impairment.— H. H. W. Thijssen and H. Mattie, *Antimicrob. Ag. Chemother.*, 1976, *10*, 441.

Plasma concentrations. Plasma concentrations of cloxacillin after 250 mg given intravenously per hour for 3 hours to normal subjects were about 15 and 0.6 µg per ml at the end of infusion and after 2 hours respectively. The urinary clearance-rate was 162.2 ml per minute and a total of 62% of the dose was excreted in the urine.— J. E. Rosenblatt *et al.*, *Archs intern. Med.*, 1968, *121*, 345.

When 7 fasting subjects were given cloxacillin 250 mg the mean peak serum-cloxacillin concentration was 4.8 µg per ml and when the same subjects were given a dose of 500 mg the mean peak serum concentration was 6.4 µg per ml.— G. P. Bodey *et al.*, *Clin. Pharmac. Ther.*, 1972, *13*, 512.

In 5 children (age 1 week to 2 years) with staphylococcal infection given oxacillin sodium 25 mg per kg body-weight intramuscularly peak serum concentrations, 30 minutes after administration, ranged from 45 to 86 µg per ml with a mean elimination half-life of 78 minutes. After 7 to 10 days, treatment was changed to cloxacillin 25 mg per kg by mouth four times daily with peak concentrations, 1 to 2 hours after administration, of 28 to 80 µg per ml and a mean elimination half-life of 71 minutes.— G. J. Burckart *et al.*, *Am. J. Hosp. Pharm.*, 1978, *35*, 1380.

Uses. Cloxacillin is used for the treatment of infections due to staphylococci resistant to benzylpenicillin; it is also used for mixed streptococcal and staphylococcal infections when the staphylococci are penicillin-resistant. It is slightly less resistant to staphylococcal penicillinase than methicillin. It is resistant to inactivation by the gastric juice and is suitable for administration by mouth. It should be given about 1 hour before meals as the presence of food in the stomach and small intestine reduces absorption.

Though cloxacillin is more active than methicillin against moderately active penicillinase-producing staphylococci, methicillin may be more effective in infections due to types that are highly active producers of penicillinase.

Cloxacillin is sometimes given with ampicillin in infections due to beta-lactamase-producing Gram-negative organisms since it may inhibit the destruction of ampicillin.

The usual dose of cloxacillin is the equivalent of 500 mg four times daily by mouth or 250 mg in 1.5 ml of Water for Injections, or if necessary 0.5% lignocaine hydrochloride solution, by intramuscular injection every 4 to 6 hours. The equivalent of 500 mg in 10 ml of Water for Injections may be given by slow intravenous injection over 3 to 4 minutes every 4 to 6 hours or by intravenous infusion. Cloxacillin has been administered by intra-articular injection, dissolved if necessary in a 0.5% solution of lignocaine hydrochloride, and by intrapleural injection in doses of 500 mg daily. Using powder for injection, up to 250 mg has been dissolved in 3 ml of sterile water and inhaled by nebuliser four times daily. Doses may be doubled in severe infections.

Children up to 2 years of age may be given one-quarter the adult dose and those aged 2 to 10 years, one-half the adult dose.

In staphylococcal meningitis systemic treatment has been supplemented with intrathecal injections of cloxacillin. The usual daily intrathecal dose is the equivalent of 5 mg for infants from birth up to 2 years of age, 10 mg for children up to 12 years of age, and 20 mg for adults. The dose should be dissolved in sodium chloride injection 0.9% immediately before use to give a solution containing 10 mg per ml.

A guide to the use of penicillinase-resistant penicillins.— Veterans Administration Ad Hoc Interdisciplinary Advisory Committee on Antimicrobial Drug Usage, *J. Am. med. Ass.*, 1977, *237*, 1605.

Bronchitis. For a report of cloxacillin being given to prevent the inactivation of ampicillin by penicillinase in patients with bronchial infections, see Ampicillin, p.1095.

Dosage in infants and children. The recommended dose of cloxacillin for children was 50 to 100 mg per kg body-weight daily given by mouth in divided doses every 6 hours before meals. The recommended dose by injection was 100 to 200 mg per kg daily.— M. I. Marks *et al.*, *Can. med. Ass. J.*, 1973, *109*, 309.

The suggested dose of cloxacillin for infants of more than 37 weeks' gestation was 25 mg per kg body-weight given intramuscularly or intravenously by very slow bolus injection, every 12 hours for the first 48 hours of life, every 8 hours from the 3rd day to 2 weeks, then every 6 hours. For immature infants (those of less than 37 weeks' gestation) this dose should be given every 12 hours for the 1st week of life, every 8 hours from then to 4 weeks of age, and every 6 hours thereafter.— P. A. Davies, *Br. med. J.*, 1978, *2*, 676. See also H. C. Spratt, *Drugs*, 1978, *16*, 226.

Further references: G. H. McCracken and H. F. Eichenwald, *J. Pediat.*, 1978, *93*, 357.

Dosage in renal failure. Anuric patients with a creatinine clearance of 10 ml or less per minute could be given cloxacillin 250 mg to 1 g by mouth every 6 hours.— D. L. Giusti, *Drug Intell. & clin. Pharm.*, 1973, *7*, 62.

The normal half-life for cloxacillin of 0.4 to 0.6 hour was increased to 0.8 hour in end-stage renal failure. It could be given in usual doses to patients with renal failure. Concentrations of cloxacillin were not affected by haemodialysis.— W. M. Bennett *et al.*, *Ann. intern. Med.*, 1980, *93*, 62. See also P. Sharpstone, *Br. med. J.*, 1977, *2*, 36.

Further references: T. P. Gibson and H. A. Nelson, *Clin. Pharmacokinet.*, 1977, *2*, 403.

Osteomyelitis. Of 19 patients with chronic staphylococcal osteomyelitis given cloxacillin (17) or phenoxymethylpenicillin (2) 5 g with probenecid 2 g daily for 2 to 18 months, 16 remained well and symptom-free 7 to 9 years later. Two patients had died from an unrelated disease and 1 was lost to follow-up. Maintenance antibiotic therapy was given to 8 patients.— S. M. Bell, *Med. J. Aust.*, 1976, *2*, 591.

A suggested dose for cloxacillin in the initial treatment of osteomyelitis in children was 150 to 200 mg per kg body-weight daily given intravenously in 4 to 6 divided doses.— G. A. Ahronheim, *Drugs*, 1978, *16*, 210.

Further references: J. H. Green, *Br. med. J.*, 1967, *2*, 414.

Staphylococcal infections. The administration of cloxacillin 500 mg four times daily by mouth to a total of 8 to 30 g was followed by a good clinical response and eradication of staphylococci in 11 of 15 infections of bone, urine, or sputum due to penicillinase-producing staphylococci. In only 3 of 17 skin and wound infections were similar results obtained. Gram-negative organisms were responsible for 16 to 17 persisting infections.— J. P. Anderson and B. L. Dodson, *Br. J. clin. Pract.*, 1966, *20*, 409.

Cloxacillin and sodium fusidate together with ampicillin were each considered suitable for the treatment of arterial or venous shunts that were suspected of being infected. The dose of cloxacillin and sodium fusidate was 500 mg initially, then 250 mg four times a day. Ampicillin was discontinued if bacterial investigation showed the presence of *Staph. aureus*.— R. Rao *et al.*, *Br. med. J.*, 1972, *3*, 618.

See also Osteomyelitis (above).

Preparations

Capsules

Cloxacillin Capsules *(B.P.)*. Capsules containing cloxacillin sodium. Potency is expressed in terms of the equivalent amount of cloxacillin. Store at a temperature not exceeding 30°.

Cloxacillin Sodium Capsules *(U.S.P.)*. Capsules containing cloxacillin sodium equivalent to 125, 250, or 500 mg of cloxacillin. Store in airtight containers.

Ear-drops

Cloxacillin Ear-drops. Cloxacillin sodium 1, phenylmercuric nitrate 0.002 or methyl hydroxybenzoate 0.1, sodium citrate 0.5, Water for Injections to 100. Sterilised by filtration. Addition of glycerol or propylene glycol would decrease the stability of the preparation. This solution might be expected to lose about 5% potency in 7 days at about 4°, or up to 15% in 4 days at room temperature.— B. Lynn, *Chemist Drugg.*, 1967, *187*, 157.

Elixirs and Solutions

Cloxacillin Elixir *(B.P.C. 1973)*. Cloxacillin Syrup. A solution of cloxacillin sodium in a suitable coloured flavoured vehicle. pH 5 to 6. It is prepared freshly by dissolving a powder consisting of the dry mixed ingredients in the specified volume of water. When a dose less than 5 ml is prescribed, the elixir should be diluted to 5 ml with syrup. Such dilutions must be freshly prepared. The elixir and diluted elixir should be stored in a cool place and used within 1 week of preparation.

Cloxacillin Sodium for Oral Solution *(U.S.P.)*. A dry mixture of cloxacillin sodium and one or more suitable buffers, colouring and flavouring agents, and preservatives. Store in airtight containers. It contains the equivalent of 25 or 50 mg of cloxacillin per ml when reconstituted. pH when reconstituted 5 to 7.5.

Injections

Cloxacillin Injection *(B.P.)*. A sterile solution of cloxacillin sodium in Water for Injections, prepared by dissolving the sterile contents of a sealed container in the requisite amount of Water for Injections. pH 5 to 7. The amount of cloxacillin sodium in a sealed container is expressed in terms of the equivalent amount of cloxacillin. The injection should be used within 30 minutes of preparation.

Proprietary Preparations

Orbenin *(Beecham Research, UK)*. Cloxacillin sodium, available as **Capsules** each containing the equivalent of 250 and 500 mg of cloxacillin; as **Injection** in vials each containing the equivalent of 0.25, 0.5, and 1 g of cloxacillin for solution before use; as **Syrup** (suggested diluent, syrup) containing in each 5 ml the equivalent of 125 mg of cloxacillin (supplied as a powder for preparation with water before use). (Also available as Orbenin in *Austral., Belg., Canad., Ital., Neth., S.Afr., Spain, Switz.*).

Other Proprietary Names

Austral.—Austrastaph; *Belg.*—Penstapho N; *Canad.*—Bactopen, Cloxapen, Cloxilean, Novocloxin, Tegopen; *Denm.*—Ekvacillin; *Fr.*—Cloxypen, Orbénine, Staphybiotic; *Ital.*—Cloxapen; *Jap.*—Clocillin; *Norw.*—Ekvacillin; *Swed.*—Ekvacillin; *USA*—Cloxapen, Tegopen.

61-b

Colistin Sulphate *(B.P.)*.

Colistin Sulfate *(U.S.P.)*; Polymyxin E Sulphate. The sulphate of a mixture of antimicrobial peptides produced by a strain of *Bacillus polymyxa* var. *colistinus*.

CAS — 1066-17-7 (colistin); 1264-72-8 (sulphate).

Pharmacopoeias. In *Br., Fr., Jap., Jug.,* and *U.S.*

A white to cream-coloured odourless hygroscopic powder with a bitter taste. The *B.P.* specifies not less than 19 000 units per mg; *U.S.P.* specifies not less than 500 μg of colistin per mg.

Soluble 1 in less than 2 of water and 1 in 300 of alcohol; slightly soluble in methyl alcohol; practically insoluble in acetone, chloroform, ether, and propylene glycol. A solution in water is laevorotatory. A 1% solution in water has a pH of 4 to 5.8. Aqueous solutions may be expected to retain their potency for 4 weeks when stored at room temperature or for 8 weeks when stored at 2° to 4°. **Store** in airtight containers. Protect from light.

The base is precipitated from aqueous solution above pH 7.5.

Colistin was incompatible with *soluble barbiturates* and *cyanocobalamin* in an infusion fluid.— B. Flouvat and P. Lechat, *Thérapie*, 1974, *29*, 337.

Units. One unit of colistin is contained in 0.00004878 mg of the first International Standard Preparation (1968) of colistin sulphate which contains 20 500 units per mg. See also under Uses.

Adverse Effects. Colistin sulphate is poorly absorbed from the gastro-intestinal tract and adverse effects do not normally follow its administration in the usual oral doses. Rashes and overgrowth of non-susceptible organisms, particularly *Proteus* spp., may occur.

Ototoxicity. A solution of colistin applied directly into the middle ear of *guinea pigs* caused substantial sensory cell damage in the cochlea.— H. Stupp *et al.*, *Audiology*, 1973, *12*, 350.

Antimicrobial Action. The antimicrobial spectrum and mode of action of colistin is similar to that of polymyxin B (see p.1205) but it is slightly less active. About 50% of its activity *in vitro* is lost in the presence of large amounts of serum.

The minimum inhibitory concentrations of colistin against sensitive organisms have been reported to range from 0.2 to 80 units per ml.

The use of disks of colistin sulphate in sensitivity tests.— P. N. Edmunds (letter), *Lancet*, 1974, *2*, 1526. A reply.— S. F. Sullman, *Pharmax* (letter), *ibid.*, 1975, *1*, 277.

A report of colistin diminishing the activity *in vitro* of amikacin against gentamicin-resistant strains of *Ps. aeruginosa*.— Y. Kobayashi, *Keio J. Med.*, 1976, *25*, 151.

The mean MIC of colistin against 6 isolates of the legionnaires' disease bacterium was 72 units per ml.— C. Thornsberry *et al.*, *Antimicrob. Ag. Chemother.*, 1978, *13*, 78.

Diminished activity. Physiological concentrations of calcium present in serum inhibited the *in vitro* antibacterial activity of colistin against *Ps. aeruginosa*.— S. D. Davis *et al.*, *J. infect. Dis.*, 1971, *124*, 610.

Colistin and sulphamethoxazole were antagonistic *in vitro* when tested against *Ps. aeruginosa*. There was also some indication that carbenicillin and colistin were antagonistic.— A. C. Dalton and M. E. Plaut, *Am. J. med. Sci.*, 1971, *261*, 335.

Enhanced activity. In 19 of 20 strains of *Ps. aeruginosa*, sulphamethoxazole and sulphamethizole enhanced the bactericidal effects of colistin.— N. A. Simmons and D. J. McGillicuddy, *Br. med. J.*, 1969, *3*, 693.

Resistance. Bacteria do not readily acquire resistance to colistin, but when resistance does occur there is complete cross-resistance between polymyxin B and colistin.

Absorption and Fate. Colistin sulphate is poorly absorbed from the gastro-intestinal tract.

Uses. Colistin is a polymyxin antibiotic and is given by mouth, as the sulphate, for the treatment of gastro-enteritis due to susceptible micro-organisms. It has been effective in intestinal infections due to *Escherichia coli*, but less satisfactory results have been obtained in *Shigella* and *Salmonella* infections.

An international standard preparation of colistin has been established by the WHO (see above) and based on this 50 mg of colistin sulphate is approximately equivalent to 1 million units of colistin. In the *USA* the potency of the national standard is expressed in terms of μg per mg but it is accepted for comparative purposes that each 'μg' of colistin is equivalent to 30 units.

The usual adult dose is 1.5 to 3 million units thrice daily; up to 18 million units has been given daily. Children weighing up to 15 kg body-weight may be given 250 000 to 500 000 units thrice daily and those weighing from 15 to 30 kg may be given 0.75 to 1.5 million units thrice daily.

Colistin sulphate has also been applied topically as an ointment, powder, or solution in a concentration of 1%.

Colistin sulphomethate sodium (see below) is administered parenterally.

A brief review of the polymyxins.— D. Andrews, *Can. J. Hosp. Pharm.*, 1978, *31*, 215.

For reports of a regimen including framycetin, colistin, and nystatin (FRACON) for sterilisation of the gastro-intestinal tract, see Framycetin Sulphate, p.1166.

For reference to the use of colistin sulphate as part of an oral non-absorbable antibiotic regimen for patients with acute non-lymphoblastic leukaemia, see Neomycin Sulphate, p.1190.

For reports on the use of colistin in the treatment of enteritis and eye infections, see Martindale 27th Edn, p. 1121.

Preparations

Colistin Sulfate for Oral Suspension *(U.S.P.)*. A dry mixture of colistin sulphate with one or more suitable buffers, diluents, colouring, flavouring, and dispersing agents. Store in airtight containers. Protect from light. The suspension is prepared by the addition of diluent before issue and contains the equivalent of 5 mg of colistin per ml. pH 5 to 6.

Colistin Tablets *(B.P.)*. Tablets containing colistin sulphate. Protect from light.

Colomycin *(Pharmax, UK)*. Colistin sulphate, available as sterile **Powder** for topical use; as **Syrup** (supplied as powder for preparation with water before use) containing 250 000 units in each 5 ml and as scored **Tablets** of 1.5 million units.

Other Proprietary Names

Belcomycine *(Neth.)*; Colimicina *(Ital.)* (see also Colistin Sulphomethate Sodium); Colimycine *(Belg., Fr., Switz.)* (see also Colistin Sulphomethate Sodium); Coly-Mycin S

(*USA*).

NOTE. Colimycin is the name given to a Russian antibiotic, of the neomycin group.

62-v

Colistin Sulphomethate Sodium (*B.P.*).

Colistimethate Sodium; Colistineméthanesulfonate Sodique; Sodium Colistimethate; Sodium Colistinmethanesulphonate. An antimicrobial substance prepared from colistin sulphate by the action of formaldehyde and sodium bisulphite, whereby amino groups are sulphomethylated.

CAS — 8068-28-8.

Pharmacopoeias. In *Br., Fr.,* and *Jap. U.S.* includes Sterile Colistimethate Sodium.

A white to cream-coloured odourless powder with a bitter taste. The *B.P.* specifies not less than 11 500 units per mg; *U.S.P.* specifies not less than 390 μg of colistin per mg.

Soluble 1 in less than 2 of water and 1 in 500 of alcohol; soluble in methyl alcohol; practically insoluble in acetone, chloroform, ether, and propylene glycol. A solution in water is laevorotatory. A 1% solution in water has a pH of 6.2 to 7.5. A 6.73% solution is iso-osmotic with serum.

Store in airtight containers. If intended for injection the containers should be sterile and sealed to exclude micro-organisms. Protect from light.

Incompatible with carbenicillin sodium, cephaloridine, cephalothin sodium, cephazolin sodium, and erythromycin lactobionate.

The diffusion and stability of colistin sulphomethate in 18 ointment and cream bases.— E. G. Beveridge, *Pharmax, Pharm. J.,* 1965, *1,* 319.

Incompatibility. A haze or precipitate was observed within an hour when an average dose of colistin sulphomethate sodium was mixed in dextrose injection with *cephalothin sodium, erythromycin lactobionate,* or *hydrocortisone sodium succinate,* and on standing with *chlortetracycline hydrochloride.*— J. M. Meisler and M. W. Skolaut, *Am. J. Hosp. Pharm.,* 1966, *23,* 557.

Colistin sulphomethate sodium was rapidly inactivated in the presence of *carbenicillin*; about 40% of the potency was lost in 3 minutes. Carbenicillin was not affected.— B. Lynn (letter), *Lancet,* 1971, *1,* 654.

Colistin sulphomethate sodium lost 30% of its activity 30 minutes after mixing with *methicillin sodium* at concentrations used for intramuscular administration.— B. Lynn, in *Clinical Use of Combinations of Antibiotics,* J. Klastersky (Ed.), London, Hodder and Stoughton, 1975, p.24.

For a further list of incompatibilities including *erythromycin gluceptate, hydroxyzine, kanamycin,* and *tetracycline,* see *Med. Lett.,* 1972, *14,* (Jan.), *Suppl.,* 32.

Stability in solution. Solutions of colistin salts were relatively stable at pH 2 to 6 but decreased in potency above pH 6.— B. S. Schwartz *et al., Antibiotics A.,* 1959-60, 41.

Colistin sulphomethate sodium was stable in the dry state for prolonged periods at room temperature, with insignificant losses after storage for 18 months. Aqueous solutions buffered with citrate over the pH range of 4 to 7 were stable for periods of up to 30 days. It was gradually hydrolysed in solutions above pH 9 with precipitation of colistin base. A mixture of colistin sulphomethate sodium, phosphate buffer, and cinchocaine hydrochloride, as dry powder for reconstitution, was found to be stable for periods of up to 12 months.— F. C. Ninger and B. S. Schwartz, *J. Am. pharm. Ass.,* 1962, *NS2,* 215.

Units. One unit of colistin sulphomethate is contained in 0.00007874 mg of the first International Reference Preparation (1966) of colistin sulphomethate which contains 12 700 units per mg. See also under Uses.

Adverse Effects and Precautions. As for Polymyxin B Sulphate, p.1204.

Adverse effects developed in 72 ot 288 patients (25.1%) given 317 courses of treatment with colistin sulphomethate intramuscularly; 205 patients were given a total dose of less than 1 g, 69 between 1 and 2 g, and 43 were given doses greater than 2 g. Nephrotoxicity occurred in 20.2% of courses; the incidence increased with the age of the patient and with the concomitant administration of cephalothin sodium. Neurotoxic reactions, mainly paraesthesias and respiratory depression with apnoea, were found in 7.3% and allergic reactions in 2.2% of courses. There was a higher reaction-rate for any given dose calculated on body-weight in heavy patients than in lighter patients.— J. Koch-Weser *et al., Ann. intern. Med.,* 1970, *72,* 857.

There was a lower incidence of side-effects following colistin sulphomethate sodium than polymyxin B given in therapeutically effective doses to 45 patients with urinary-tract infections.— M. F. Pedersen *et al., Investve Urol.,* 1971, *9,* 234.

Nephrotoxicity. Colistin 26 million units daily was given to 14 severely ill patients with refractory *Klebsiella* chest and/or urinary-tract infections. Acute renal failure, sometimes with acute tubular necrosis, was evident in all patients, and contributed to the final cause of death in some of the 8 patients who died.— D. J. E. Price and D. I. Graham, *Br. med. J.,* 1970, *4,* 525. Criticisms.— E. Sproston and M. P. McConnell, *Pharmax* (letter), *ibid.,* 748.

Acute renal failure occurred in 4 patients given colistin sulphomethate sodium. All the patients had reduced glomerular filtration-rates and had either received cephalothin before, or concomitantly with, colistin sulphomethate sodium. It was recommended that dosage should be calculated from a measure of the glomerular filtration-rate rather than from body-weight.— S. Adler and D. P. Segel, *Am. J. med. Sci.,* 1971, *261,* 109.

Neuromuscular blockade. Respiratory arrest occurred in a man with myasthenia gravis 2½ hours after he received an intramuscular injection of colistin sulphomethate sodium. Recovery of respiratory function took 11 days but other affected muscles improved after the intramuscular injection of neostigmine methylsulphate 2 mg and an intravenous injection of edrophonium chloride 10 mg.— D. A. Decker and R. W. Fincham, *Archs Neurol., Chicago,* 1971, *25,* 141.

A report of prolonged respiratory depression due to interaction of pancuronium bromide with colistin in one patient. A normal pattern of breathing was reinstated after 20 ml of a 10% solution of calcium gluconate was given in 2 divided doses.— M. M. Giala and A. G. Paradelis (letter), *J. antimicrob. Chemother.,* 1979, *5,* 234.

Neurotoxicity. A 26-year-old woman with diabetes and renal failure developed a severe polyneuropathy which coincided with high blood concentrations of colistin sulphomethate sodium following daily doses of 1 million units and which resolved when treatment was discontinued.— J. F. Bridgman and S. M. Rosen (letter), *Br. med. J.,* 1971, *2,* 527. See also G. Richet *et al., ibid.,* 1970, *2,* 394.

A patient developed myopathy with inflammatory signs and disturbances of the CNS following treatment with colistin sulphomethate sodium intramuscularly.— M. Vanhaeverbeek *et al., J. Neurol. Neurosurg. Psychiat.,* 1974, *37,* 1343.

Treatment of Adverse Effects. As for Polymyxin B Sulphate, p.1205.

There have been conflicting reports of the value of peritoneal dialysis or haemodialysis in the removal of excessive amounts of colistin from the blood.

A 10-month-old boy developed acute renal failure after the accidental administration of an overdose of colistin sulphomethate. Two exchange transfusions were used successfully to remove colistin after peritoneal dialysis had failed. Renal function appeared to return to normal and no neurotoxicity was seen.— J. M. Brown *et al., Med. J. Aust.,* 1970, *2,* 923.

See under Dosage in renal failure (below) for references to the effects of dialysis on blood concentrations of colistin.

Absorption and Fate. Colistin sulphomethate sodium is poorly absorbed from the gastro-intestinal tract. Peak plasma concentrations of 125 to 190 units per ml occur 2 hours after an intramuscular injection of 1.5 million units. Detectable concentrations persist for about 8 hours.

Colistin is mainly excreted by glomerular filtration and up to 80% of a parenteral dose of the sulphomethate sodium may be excreted in the urine within 8 hours. Excretion is more rapid in children than in adults; it is diminished in patients with impaired kidney function. Colistin diffuses across the placenta but diffusion into the cerebrospinal fluid is negligible except occasionally in infants. It has been detected in bile and in breast milk.

Colistin was only bound to a limited extent to serum proteins in the body. The half-life in serum was 1.6 to 2.7 hours and 40 to 80% was excreted in urine.— C. M. Kunin, *Ann. intern. Med.,* 1967, *67,* 151.

The methanesulphonate derivative of colistin was pharmacologically and clinically different from the base. Its renal excretion was much more rapid, and the resulting urinary concentration of antibiotic higher. A maximum dose of 5 mg per kg body-weight daily was recommended.— R. M. Gabrielson, *Warner-Chilcott Laboratories* (letter), *New Engl. J. Med.,* 1968, *279,* 1400.

The biological half-life of colistin sulphomethate sodium was variously reported as 9 hours in newborn infants falling to 2.6 hours 3 or 4 days later and 2.3 to 2.6 hours (according to age) in premature infants.— W. A. Ritschel, *Drug Intell. & clin. Pharm.,* 1970, *4,* 332.

Colistin sulphomethate was administered intramuscularly in a dose of 75 mg to 10 healthy persons and 8 patients with renal failure. The biological half-life was 4.8 hours in normal persons and 18 hours in patients with renal failure. A substantial change in drug distribution occurred as indicated by the smaller volume of distribution in the patients with renal failure.— M. Gibaldi and D. Perrier, *J. clin. Pharmac.,* 1972, *12,* 201.

Colistin sulphomethate sodium was absorbed from the peritoneal cavity.— J. S. Cheigh, *Am. J. Med.,* 1977, *62,* 555.

Colistin sulphomethate sodium was reported to be more than 75% bound to plasma proteins.— W. M. Bennett *et al., Ann. intern. Med.,* 1977, *86,* 754.

Diffusion. *Placenta.* M. A. MacAulay and D. Charles, *Clin. Pharmac. Ther.,* 1967, *8,* 578.

Uses. Colistin sulphomethate sodium has the antimicrobial action described under colistin sulphate. It is the form of colistin used for parenteral administration.

It may also be applied topically in a concentration of 1% or given as an aerosol for respiratory infections in doses similar to those given by injection, and supplemented by parenteral administration. In the treatment of eye infections 1% in lignocaine injection 0.5% has been given by subconjunctival injection.

An international reference preparation of colistin sulphomethate has been established by the WHO (see p.1150) and based on this 80 mg of colistin sulphomethate is approximately equivalent to 1 million units of colistin sulphomethate. In the *USA* the potency of the national standard is expressed in terms of μg per mg but it is accepted for comparative purposes that each 'μg' of colistin base is equivalent to 30 units.

The normal dose for adults is 6 million units daily in divided doses by intramuscular injection or intravenously by slow injection or infusion; up to 9 million units has been given. Children may be given 50 000 units per kg body-weight by intramuscular injection daily in 3 divided doses. Doses should be reduced in renal impairment.

Colistin sulphomethate sodium has been given intrathecally as a single daily injection of 500 to 1000 units per kg body-weight.

Colistin sulphomethate sodium given as an aerosol in doses of 50 or 100 mg thrice daily for 7 days eradicated or reduced the sputum colony counts in 18 of 20 patients with infections of the respiratory tract due mainly to *Pseudomonas aeruginosa, Klebsiella pneumoniae,* and *Kleb. aerogenes.* Supra-infection with *Proteus* and *Serratia* occurred in 3 patients. Recurrence of infection was noted in 6 patients.— H. D. Rose *et al., J. clin. Pharmac.,* 1970, *10,* 274.

Ps. aeruginosa was present in the sputum of 34 of 63 patients as a commensal. In 14 patients with chronic infections aerosol inhalations of colistin sulphomethate sodium or of gentamicin were of little value, but systemic antibiotic treatment achieved temporary suppression of the organism. In 10 patients (7 with chronic bronchitis) *Pseudomonas* appeared to interfere with antibiotic therapy directed at other organisms; when *Pseudomonas* was eliminated by aerosol therapy other organisms responded to antibiotics. In 5 patients with acute pseudomonas infections immediate systemic therapy was necessary.— M. W. Burns, *Br. med. J.,* 1973, *3,* 382.

Co-trimoxazole and colistin sulphomethate showed enhanced activity against multiple drug-resistant strains of *Serratia marcescens*. Four of 6 patients with serious *Serratia* infections responded to treatment with 1.92 g of co-trimoxazole and 2 to 5 mg per kg body-weight of colistin sulphomethate daily.— F. E. Thomas *et al.*, *Antimicrob. Ag. Chemother.*, 1976, *9*, 201.

Dosage in renal failure. From an investigation in 4 patients with severe renal failure a dosage schedule for colistin sulphomethate sodium of 2 to 3 mg per kg body-weight intravenously every 3 days was suggested and no modification was required when peritoneal dialysis was employed as peritoneal clearance was poor. The rate of disappearance of colistin was increased during haemodialysis and a dose of 2 to 3 mg per kg intravenously at the end of each dialysis was suggested.— J. R. Curtis and J. B. Eastwood, *Br. med. J.*, 1968, *1*, 484.

Recommended dosages of colistin sulphomethate sodium in patients with renal insufficiency: when endogenous creatinine clearance exceeded 20 ml per minute, 75 to 100% of the recommended daily dose divided into doses every 12 hours; when clearance was between 5 and 20 ml per minute, 50% of the usual daily dose divided into doses every 12 hours; when clearance was less than 5 ml per minute, 30 to 35% of the normally recommended dose divided into doses every 12 to 18 hours. If the patient was severely ill and essentially anuric, an initial dose of 75 mg could be given by intramuscular injection, after which the recommended dosage was advised. In essentially anuric patients, colistin blood concentrations fell by 75% after 24 hours and by 97% after 72 hours following a single injection of 2 mg per kg body-weight and would not maintain therapeutic blood concentrations until diuresis occurred. Concentrations were not significantly affected by haemodialysis and patients undergoing peritoneal dialysis only lost about 1 mg of colistin sulphomethate sodium per hour.— N. J. Goodwin and E. A. Friedman, *Ann. intern. Med.*, 1968, *68*, 984.

The dosage interval of colistin should be increased from 12 hours in normal patients to 24 hours in those with mild renal failure, 48 hours in those with moderate renal failure, and 72 hours in those with severe renal failure. Blood-colistin concentrations could be altered by haemodialysis and peritoneal dialysis; concentrations should be monitored in severe renal failure.— P. Sharpstone, *Br. med. J.*, 1977, *2*, 36. See also W. M. Bennett *et al.*, *Ann. intern. Med.*, 1980, *93*, 62.

Further references: H. M. Swick *et al.*, *J. Pediat.*, 1969, *74*, 976; G. B. Appel and H. C. Neu, *New Engl. J. Med.*, 1977, *296*, 663.

Preparations

Colistin Sulphomethate Injection *(B.P.)*. Colistin Sulphometh. Inj.; Colistin Injection. A sterile solution of colistin sulphomethate sodium, prepared by dissolving the sterile contents of a sealed container (Colistin Sulphomethate Sodium for Injection) in the requisite amount of Sodium Chloride Intravenous Infusion. Store at 2° to 8° and use within 48 hours.

For intravenous infusions, freshly prepared solutions should be used and the infusion completed within 6 hours.

Sterile Colistimethate Sodium *(U.S.P.)*. A grade of colistin sulphomethate sodium for injection.

Colomycin Injection *(Pharmax, UK)*. Colistin sulphomethate sodium, available as powder in vials of 0.5 and 1 million units.

Other Proprietary Names

Colimicina *(Ital., Spain)* (see also Colistin Sulphate); Colimycin *(Denm., Norw.)*; Colimycine *(Fr., Neth., Switz.)* (see also Colistin Sulphate); Coly-Mycin M *(Austral., Canad., USA)*.

NOTE. Colimycin is also the name given to a Russian antibiotic, of the neomycin group..

64-q

Cycloserine *(B.P., U.S.P.)*. Cycloserinum; D-Cycloserine. (+)-(*R*)-4-Aminoisoxazolidin-3-one.
$C_3H_6N_2O_2$=102.1.

CAS — 68-41-7.

Pharmacopoeias. In *Br., Cz., Int., Jap., Jug.*, and *U.S. Hung.* has the hydrogen tartrate.

An antimicrobial substance produced by the growth of certain strains of *Streptomyces orchidaceus* or *S. garyphalus*, or obtained by synthesis.

A white or pale yellow, hygroscopic, crystalline powder, odourless or with a slight odour, with a slightly bitter taste. Its activity diminishes on absorbing water. The *B.P.* specifies not less than 98%, calculated on the dried substance; *U.S.P.* specifies not less than 900 µg per mg.

Soluble 1 in 10 of water and 1 in 50 of alcohol; slightly soluble in chloroform and ether. A 10% solution in water has a pH of 5.7 to 6.3. **Store** at a temperature not exceeding 25° in airtight containers.

Stability in capsules and tablets. Investigations into the deterioration of cycloserine tablets and capsules indicated that humidity was a more important factor than temperature, and that deterioration occurred more rapidly with capsules than with tablets.— K. V. N. Rao *et al.*, *Bull. Wld Hlth Org.*, 1968, *39*, 781.

Stability in solution. Cycloserine was stable in solutions of pH 6 to 8.— P. -A. Jonsson and B. Turesson, *Svensk Farm. Tidskr.*, 1968, *72*, 963.

Adverse Effects. The side-effects of cycloserine appear to be dose-related; at therapeutic doses of 500 mg daily up to 30% of patients may experience side-effects. These are mainly neurological and include dizziness, headache, sedation, speech difficulties, confusion, tremor, convulsions, paresis, hyperreflexia, paraesthesias, coma, depression, and psychoses. Toxic reactions may be reduced by keeping plasma concentrations below 25 µg per ml.

Allergic skin reactions occur occasionally and serum aminotransferase values may be raised, especially in patients with a history of liver disease. Anaemias have been reported.

Treatment of Adverse Effects. Convulsions and other toxic effects on the central nervous system usually disappear when treatment is withdrawn, although specific treatment may be necessary. Pyridoxine has been employed to diminish side-effects during treatment but severe toxic effects are most effectively prevented by adjusting the dose so as to avoid high blood concentrations of cycloserine.

Overdosage may require gastric lavage and symptomatic treatment. Peritoneal dialysis has been tried as has forced diuresis.

Precautions. Cycloserine is contra-indicated in epileptics or mentally unstable patients. Great care is necessary in alcoholics and in patients with impaired renal function. Cycloserine should be given in reduced dosage to patients with impaired renal function and serum concentrations should be checked frequently.

Cycloserine appeared to enhance the toxic effects of alcohol on the CNS in 2 patients.— F. Glass *et al.*, *Arzneimittel-Forsch.*, 1965, *15*, 684.

Antimicrobial Action. Cycloserine interferes with bacterial cell-wall synthesis. It inhibits the growth of virulent strains of *Mycobacterium tuberculosis* and other mycobacteria; strains that have developed resistance to streptomycin, isoniazid, or aminosalicyclic acid may be susceptible to cycloserine. Minimum inhibitory concentrations range from 10 to 20 µg per ml. It has some activity against Gram-negative bacteria, including *Escherichia coli*, and against Gram-positive bacteria. The antimicrobial action of cycloserine is antagonised by D-alanine.

In a synthetic culture medium free from D-alanine, the minimum inhibitory concentration for 2 strains of *E. coli* and 1 of *Salmonella typhimurium* ranged from 2 to 5 µg per ml. In a concentration of 10 µg per ml cycloserine had a bactericidal effect comparable to that of ampicillin or cephaloridine. The bactericidal action was inhibited by chloramphenicol or tetracycline.— A. Manten *et al.*, *Chemother. Rev.*, 1968, *13*, 242, per *Abstr. Wld Med.*, 1969, *43*, 178.

The minimum inhibitory concentration of cycloserine for *M. tuberculosis*, strain H37Rv, was greatly diminished when an acridine, such as acriflavine, ethacridine, mepacrine, or proflavine was added in sub-bacteriostatic concentrations.— V. N. Soloviev and V. S. Zueva (letter), *Lancet*, 1968, *2*, 412.

Sodium salicylate antagonised the antimicrobial activity of cycloserine *in vitro*.— M. J. Mattila *et al.*, *Arzneimittel-Forsch.*, 1972, *22*, 1769.

Resistance. *Mycobacterium tuberculosis* develops resistance to cycloserine to a lesser extent than to streptomycin. Development of bacterial resistance is delayed when cycloserine is administered in conjunction with other antituberculous agents. Resistant strains of *Staph. aureus* and *E. coli* have occurred.

Absorption and Fate. Cycloserine is absorbed from the gastro-intestinal tract. Effective plasma concentrations are reached in 3 to 8 hours depending on the dose. Peak plasma concentrations averaging about 4 µg per ml have been achieved with a single dose of 250 mg, and of 15 µg per ml after 1 g. Repeated doses produce considerably higher plasma concentrations. The plasma half-life is estimated to be about 10 hours.

Cycloserine diffuses across the placenta and also diffuses into the cerebrospinal, pleural, and ascitic fluids. It also appears in the milk of nursing mothers. Up to 60% of a dose appears unchanged in the urine within 24 hours; a further 10% may be excreted over the next 48 hours. Little is found in the faeces.

Less than 20% of cycloserine was bound to serum proteins.— M. J. Mattila *et al.*, *Arzneimittel-Forsch.*, 1972, *22*, 1769.

Uses. Cycloserine is used in conjunction with other antituberculous agents in the treatment of pulmonary tuberculosis. It may also be given for urinary-tract infections due to sensitive micro-organisms, particularly *Escherichia* spp., if other treatments are of no avail.

Cycloserine has occasionally been used in the treatment of leprosy.

Cycloserine is administered by mouth in doses of 250 mg once or twice daily. This can be increased to 250 mg three or four times daily if necessary. However, the total daily dose should not exceed 1 g and plasma concentrations should be kept below 25 µg per ml. Children have been given up to 10 mg per kg body-weight daily in divided doses, adjusted according to the blood concentration.

References: J. M. Murdoch *et al.*, *Practitioner*, 1966, *196*, 800; C. V. Ramakrishnan *et al.*, *Tubercle*, 1967, *48*, 114; *Scand. J. resp. Dis.*, 1970, *Suppl.* No.71, 13-326.

Preparations

Cycloserine Capsules *(B.P., U.S.P.)*. Capsules containing cycloserine. Store at a temperature not exceeding 30°. *U.S.P.* specifies 250 mg. Store in airtight containers.

Cycloserine Tablets *(B.P.)*. Tablets containing cycloserine. Store at a temperature not exceeding 25°.

Proprietary Preparations

Cycloserine, Lilly *(Lilly, UK)*. Available as capsules of 125 and 250 mg.

Other Proprietary Names

Ciclovalidin *(Ital.)*; Closina *(Austral.)*; Farmiserina *(Spain)*; Micoserina *(Ital.)*; Seromycin *(USA)*; Setavax *(Spain)*.

65-p

Demeclocycline *(U.S.P.)*. Demethylchlortetracycline. 7-Chloro-6-demethyltetracycline.
$C_{21}H_{21}ClN_2O_8$=464.9.

CAS — 127-33-3.

Pharmacopoeias. In *U.S.*

A yellow odourless crystalline powder with a bitter taste, containing not less than the equivalent of 970 µg of demeclocycline hydrochloride per mg, calculated on the anhydrous basis. Sparingly **soluble** in water; soluble 1 in 200 of alcohol and 1 in 40 of methyl alcohol; soluble in dilute hydrochloric acid, and solutions of alkali hydroxides and carbonates. A 1% solution in water has a pH of 4 to 5.5. **Store** in airtight containers. Protect from light.

66-s

Demeclocycline Hydrochloride *(B.P., Eur. P., U.S.P.).*

Demeclocyclini Hydrochloridum; Demethylchlortetracycline Hydrochloride; Demethylchlortetracyclini Chloridum.

$C_{21}H_{21}ClN_2O_8$, HCl=501.3.

CAS — 64-73-3.

Pharmacopoeias. In *Br., Eur., Fr., Ger., It., Neth., Nord., Swiss,* and *U.S.*

An antimicrobial substance produced by the growth of *Streptomyces aureofaciens* or by any other means. It occurs as a yellow, odourless, amphoteric, crystalline powder with a bitter taste. The *B.P.* specifies not less than 950 units per mg and *U.S.P.* specifies not less than 900 µg per mg, both calculated on the anhydrous basis.

Soluble 1 in 30 to 60 of water, 1 in 45 to 200 of alcohol, 1 in 50 of methyl alcohol; practically insoluble in acetone, chloroform, and ether; soluble in aqueous solutions of alkali hydroxides and carbonates. A 1% solution in water has a pH of 2 to 3. **Store** in airtight containers. Protect from light.

Loss of activity. The sulphates of copper, nickel, ferrous iron, and magnesium all destroyed or reduced the activity of demeclocycline when added to a solution of the antibiotic. Tests *in vitro* showed enhancement of antibiotic activity in the presence of zinc sulphate.— M. E. Hamner, *Antibiotics Chemother.,* 1961, *11,* 498.

Storage. Demeclocycline showed no loss in potency after storage for 30 days at 37° and 100% relative humidity.— V. C. Walton *et al., J. pharm. Sci.,* 1970, *59,* 1160.

Accelerated degradation studies showed that there was no significant loss of potency of demeclocycline hydrochloride when stored in ampoules at 37° for 2 years.— J. W. Lightbown *et al., Bull. Wld Hlth Org.,* 1972, *47,* 343.

Units. One unit of demeclocycline is contained in 0.001 mg of the first International Reference Preparation (1962) which contains 1000 units per mg.

Adverse Effects. As for Tetracycline Hydrochloride, p.1217. Allergic reactions appear to be more common with demeclocycline and phototoxic reactions occur more frequently than with other tetracyclines. Demeclocycline probably produces the most marked tooth discoloration, turning affected teeth a strong yellow.

Reversible nephrogenic diabetes insipidus has been reported in patients treated with demeclocycline.

Nephrotoxicity. Reversible dose-dependent polyuria occurred in 8 of 24 patients given various doses of demeclocycline. This action appeared to be due to a blocking of the activity of antidiuretic hormone.— I. Singer and D. Rotenberg, *Ann. intern. Med.,* 1973, *79,* 679.

Nonoliguric acute renal failure occurred in a patient with cirrhosis given demeclocycline 300 mg thrice daily. Demeclocycline should be used with great caution in correcting impaired renal diluting ability especially in cirrhotic patients.— J. R. Oster and M. Epstein (letter), *Lancet,* 1977, *1,* 52.

Further references: H. Roth *et al., Archs intern. Med.,* 1967, *120,* 433; F. Carrilho *et al., Ann. intern. Med.,* 1977, *87,* 195; *Br. med. J.,* 1978, *2,* 1405; P. L. Padfield *et al., Postgrad. med. J.,* 1978, *54,* 623.

Photosensitivity. Three patients developed a lichenoid eruption about 14 days after a photosensitive reaction to demeclocycline.— H. E. Jones *et al., Archs Derm.,* 1972, *106,* 58.

A 64-year-old woman who developed photodermatitis one day after treatment with demeclocycline developed photo-onycholysis 5 weeks later.— H. J. N. Bethell, *Br. med. J.,* 1977, *2,* 96.

Further references: H. Blank *et al., Archs Derm.,* 1968, *97,* 1; P. Frost *et al., J. Am. med. Ass.,* 1971, *216,* 326.

Treatment. Recurrence of a photosensitive reaction to demeclocycline was considered to be due to inadequate treatment with prednisone which was given for only 3 days. It was recommended that corticosteroid treatment should be gradually withdrawn over 2 to 3 weeks.— G. Kahn and J. K. Legg, *Archs Derm.,* 1971, *103,* 94.

Precautions. As for Tetracycline Hydrochloride, p.1218.

A study indicating that usual therapeutic doses of demeclocycline interfere with colour vision.— J. Laroche and C. Laroche, *Annls pharm. fr.,* 1972, *30,* 433. See also *idem,* 1970, *28,* 333.

Interactions. Diuresis induced by amiloride and metolazone was enhanced in a patient when demeclocycline was given concomitantly.— R. R. Ghose and R. Bonser (letter), *Br. med. J.,* 1978, *1,* 1282.

Antimicrobial Action. Demeclocycline hydrochloride has a range and mode of antimicrobial action similar to that of tetracycline hydrochloride (see p.1218). It is more effective *in vitro* than tetracycline against some species such as *Streptococcus viridans* and *Haemophilus influenzae.*

Absorption and Fate. As for Tetracycline Hydrochloride, p.1219.

After oral administration, demeclocycline hydrochloride is absorbed more readily than tetracycline hydrochloride but is excreted much more slowly. Plasma concentrations of up to 2.4 µg per ml have been reported 3 to 4 hours after an oral dose of 300 mg and persist for longer than after a similar dose of tetracycline, only falling to about 1 µg per ml after 24 hours.

The renal clearance of demeclocycline is about half that of tetracycline.

Some 41 to 90% of demeclocycline was bound in the body to serum proteins. The half-life in serum was 12.3 hours and 42% was excreted in urine.— C. M. Kunin, *Ann. intern. Med.,* 1967, *67,* 151.

The administration of demeclocycline hydrochloride 300 mg every 12 hours to 9 healthy subjects resulted in mean serum concentrations of about 0.70 µg per ml after 2 hours, falling to 0.39 µg after 12 hours, rising and maintained between about 1 and 2.2 µg after the first 24 hours' treatment. About 38 mg of the drug was recovered from the urine during the first 24 hours.— L. P. Olon and D. N. Holvey, *Clin. Med.,* 1968, *75* (Jan.), 33.

Uses. Demeclocycline hydrochloride has uses similar to those of tetracycline hydrochloride (see p.1220). It is excreted more slowly and effective blood concentrations are maintained for a longer period. The base is used in oral liquid preparations.

The usual adult dosage is 600 mg of demeclocycline hydrochloride daily by mouth in 2 or 4 divided doses preferably one hour before or 2 hours after meals. Children have been given 6 to 12 mg per kg body-weight daily in divided doses (but see Adverse Effects).

In the treatment of mycoplasmal pneumonia the adult dose is 900 mg daily in divided doses. Up to 1.2 g daily has been given to adults in the treatment of chronic hyponatraemia associated with the inappropriate secretion of antidiuretic hormone, when water restriction has proved ineffective.

Ascites. Administration of demeclocycline 300 mg thrice daily for 10 days in addition to a maintenance regimen of diuretics with fluid and salt restriction, resolved all symptoms of hypovolaemia and postural changes in blood pressure and pulse in a 66-year-old woman with severe ascites. Within 2 weeks of discontinuing demeclocycline, symptoms of hypovolaemia returned. Mild renal insufficiency occurred during administration of demeclocycline.— R. Kirkpatrick (letter), *J. Am. med. Ass.,* 1978, *239,* 616.

Hyponatraemia. Demeclocycline hydrochloride 1.2 g daily for 7 to 10 days, reducing to 600 mg daily after 10 days, corrected hyponatraemia and induced production of hypotonic urine with beneficial clinical effects in 7 patients with lung cancer and inappropriate hypersecretion of antidiuretic hormone. Demeclocycline appears to be the drug of choice in the chronic form of this syndrome even though it moderately impairs renal function.— A. De Troyer, *J. Am. med. Ass.,* 1977, *237,* 2723.

In all of 10 patients with hyponatraemia owing to inappropriate secretion of antidiuretic hormone, administration of demeclocycline 600 to 1200 mg daily restored serum-sodium concentrations to a mean of about 139 µmol per litre within 5 to 14 days, permitting unrestricted water intake. Lithium carbonate 600 to 900 mg daily administered to 3 of the patients had been ineffective and had serious side-effects in 2; further study of it was abandoned. One patient with a 22-year history of hyponatraemia had an initial excellent response to demeclocycline which was lost on reduction of the dose to 600 mg daily but regained at 900 mg daily and still maintained 11 months later, indicating that response was very sensitive to dose.— J. N. Forrest *et al., New Engl. J. Med.,* 1978, *298,* 173. The patients had small-cell bronchogenic carcinoma. Antineoplastic chemotherapy effectively controls the secondary syndrome of inappropriate secretion of antidiuretic hormone in such patients and is the treatment of choice in previously untreated patients.— M. H. Cohen *et al.* (letter), *ibid.,* 1423. Four of the 10 patients had small-cell carcinoma of the lung which was unresponsive to radiotherapy and/or chemotherapy.— J. N. Forrest *et al.* (letter), *ibid.*

A study indicating that the nephrotoxicity of demeclocycline severely limits its usefulness in treating hyponatraemia in patients with cirrhosis.— P. D. Miller *et al., J. Am. med. Ass.,* 1980, *243,* 2513. Agreement that demeclocycline should not be used in patients with cirrhosis. Its use in patients with congestive heart failure should be equally suspect.— M. Geheb and M. Cox, *ibid.,* 2519.

Further references: A. De Troyer and J. -C. Demanet, *New Engl. J. Med.,* 1975, *293,* 915; A. De Troyer *et al.* (letter), *Ann. intern. Med.,* 1976, *85,* 336; W. H. Perks *et al.* (letter), *Lancet,* 1976, *2,* 1414; R. W. Schrier, *New Engl. J. Med.,* 1978, *298,* 214; A. Tanay *et al., Ann. intern. Med.,* 1979, *90,* 50.

Oedema. Five of 6 patients with oedema due to congestive heart failure, unresponsive to diuretics, responded to treatment with demeclocycline 1.2 g daily; there was progressive weight loss, increased diuresis and salt excretion, and decreased urine osmolality.— D. Z. de Beyl *et al., Br. med. J.,* 1978, *1,* 760.

Oedema in a patient with severe congestive heart failure responded well to demeclocycline 150 mg twice daily, together with diuretics.— R. S. A. Bonser and R. R. Ghose, *Postgrad. med. J.,* 1980, *56,* 121.

See also under Hyponatraemia (above).

Preparations

Demeclocycline Capsules *(B.P.).* Demethylchlortetracycline Capsules. Capsules containing demeclocycline hydrochloride. Store at a temperature not exceeding 30°. *U.S.P.* (Demeclocycline Hydrochloride Capsules) specifies 75, 150, or 300 mg. Store in airtight containers. Protect from light.

Demeclocycline Hydrochloride Tablets *(U.S.P.).* Tablets containing demeclocycline hydrochloride 75, 150, or 300 mg. Store in airtight containers. Protect from light.

Demeclocycline Oral Suspension *(U.S.P.).* Contains the equivalent of 15 mg of demeclocycline hydrochloride per ml; it may contain one or more suitable buffers, preservatives, stabilising, and suspending agents. pH 4 to 5.8. Store in airtight containers. Protect from light.

Proprietary Preparations

Ledermycin *(Lederle, UK).* **Capsules** each containing 150 mg of demeclocycline hydrochloride; **Drops** containing in each ml demeclocycline base equivalent to demeclocycline hydrochloride 60 mg; **Syrup** containing in each 5 ml demeclocycline base equivalent to demeclocycline hydrochloride 75 mg (dilution not recommended); and **Tablets** each containing 300 mg of demeclocycline hydrochloride. (Also available as Ledermycin in *Belg., Denm., Ger., Neth., Norw., S.Afr., Switz.*).

Other Proprietary Names for Demeclocycline and Demeclocycline Hydrochloride

Arg.— Ledermicina; *Canad.*— Declomycin; *Fr.*— Ledermycine; *Ital.*— Actaciclina, Bioterciclin, Clortetrin, Demeplus, Deme-Proter, Demetetra, Demetraciclina, Demetraclin, Detracin, Detravis, Dimeral, Diuciclin (also demeclocycline magnesium), Elkamicina, Fidocin, Isodemetil, Latomicina, Ledermicina, Magis-Ciclina, Mirciclina, Neo Cromaciclin, Tetradek, Tollerclin, Veraciclina; *Spain*— Benaciclin, Complecicilin, Ledermicina, Provimicina, Wolnerciclina; *USA*— Declomycin.

A preparation containing demeclocycline and nystatin was formerly marketed in Great Britain under the proprietary name Lederstatin (*Lederle*).

67-w

Dibekacin Sulphate. 3′,4′-Dideoxykanamycin B. 6-*O*-(3-Amino-3-deoxy-α-D-glucopyranosyl)-2-deoxy-4-*O*-(2,6-diamino-2,3,4,6-tetradeoxy-α-D-glucopyranosyl)-D-streptamine sulphate.

$C_{18}H_{37}N_5O_8,xH_2SO_4$=451.5 (dibekacin).

CAS — 34493-98-6 (dibekacin); 58580-55-5 (sulphate).

A white or yellowish-white odourless powder with a bitter taste. Very **soluble** in water; practically insoluble in acetone, alcohol, and other organic solvents.

Dibekacin is an aminoglycoside antibiotic derived from kanamycin with actions and uses similar to those of gentamicin (see p.1166). It has been given in a dose of 1 mg per kg body-weight by intramuscular injection or intravenous infusion over half an hour 2 to 3 times daily.

The pharmacokinetics of dibekacin in normal subjects and patients with renal impairment.— F. Yamasaku and T. Kabasawa, *Chemotherapy, Tokyo,* 1976, *24,* 1520; A. Leroy *et al., J. antimicrob. Chemother.,* 1980, *6,* 113.

Dibekacin at a concentration of 4 µg per ml inhibited 91% of 351 strains of Enterobacteriaceae, 88% of 34 strains of *Pseudomonas aeruginosa,* 75% of 20 strains of the *Acinetobacter* spp., 90% of 17 strains of *Haemophilus influenzae,* and none of 41 strains of *Neisseria gonorrhoeae.*— I. Phillips *et al., J. antimicrob. Chemother.,* 1977, *3,* 403.

Dibekacin had a similar activity to gentamicin sulphate against 218 strains of *Ps. aeruginosa in vitro*; the activities of both drugs were innoculum-dependent. The majority of 29 strains of *Ps. maltophilia* and 10 of *Ps. cepacia* were resistant to both drugs.— K. Tsuchiya and M. Kondo, *Takeda, Jap., Antimicrob. Ag. Chemother.,* 1978, *13,* 536.

Dibekacin was more active than amikacin, gentamicin, kanamycin, bekanamycin, or sissomicin *in vitro* against 200 strains of *Ps. aeruginosa* and inhibited 49, 160, 183, and all of the strains at concentrations of 0.156, 0.625, 1.25, and 5 µg per ml respectively. Several strains highly resistant to gentamicin were susceptible to dibekacin.— A. G. Paradelis *et al., Antimicrob. Ag. Chemother.,* 1978, *14,* 514.

Dibekacin was less active *in vitro* than gentamicin against strains of *Escherichia coli,* indole-positive strains of the *Proteus* spp., and *Serratia marcescens* and of similar activity against *Ps. aeruginosa* and *Klebsiella pneumoniae.*— F. Daschner and H. Langmaack (letter), *J. antimicrob. Chemother.,* 1978, *4,* 286.

Proprietary Names

Decabicin *(LEFA, Spain)*; Klobamicina *(Almirall, Spain)*; Orbicin *(Pfizer, Ger.; Mack, Illert., Ger.)*; Panimycin *(Jap.).*

68-e

Dicloxacillin Sodium *(U.S.P.).*

Sodium Dicloxacillin; BRL 1702; P 1011. Sodium (6*R*)-6-[3-(2,6-dichlorophenyl)-5-methylisoxazole-4-carboxamido]penicillanate monohydrate.

$C_{19}H_{16}Cl_2N_3NaO_5S,H_2O$=510.3.

CAS — 3116-76-5 (dicloxacillin); 343-55-5 (sodium salt, anhydrous); 13412-64-1 (sodium salt, monohydrate).

Pharmacopoeias. In *Braz., Jap.,* and *U.S. U.S.* also includes Sterile Dicloxacillin Sodium.

A white to off-white crystalline powder with a bitter taste. Each g represents approximately 2 mmol (2 mEq) of sodium. Dicloxacillin sodium 1.09 g is approximately equivalent to 1 g of anhydrous dicloxacillin. *U.S.P.* specifies not less than the equivalent of 850 µg of dicloxacillin per mg. Freely **soluble** in water; soluble in methyl alcohol; practically insoluble in ether. A 1% solution in water has a pH of 4.5 to 7.5. **Store** in airtight containers.

Incompatibility. Dicloxacillin sodium was incompatible with *stearic acid.* A dry mixture lost potency on storage.— H. Jacobson and G. Reier, *J. pharm. Sci.,* 1969, *58,* 631.

Stability in solution. The activity of solutions of dicloxacillin sodium in either sucrose 10% or dextrose 5% at 37° was negligible after 24 hours.— M. S. Simberkoff *et al., New Engl. J. Med.,* 1970, *283,* 116.

Adverse Effects and Treatment. As for Benzylpenicillin, p.1103.

Increased concentrations of serum aspartate aminotransferase (SGOT) have been reported with dicloxacillin.

Colitis. A report of abdominal cramps and bloody diarrhoea associated with the administration of dicloxacillin by mouth.— V. L. Fox, *Pediatrics,* 1979, *63,* 676.

The isolation of toxin-producing *Clostridium difficile* from 2 children with dicloxacillin- and oxacillin-associated diarrhoea, respectively.— I. Brook, *Pediatrics,* 1980, *65,* 1154.

Ischaemia. Ischaemia followed by gangrene requiring amputation occurred in the hand and lower arm of 2 patients each given dicloxacillin accidentally by intra-arterial injection.— H. Ehringer *et al., Wien. med. Wschr.,* 1971, *121,* 710.

Precautions. As for Cloxacillin Sodium, p.1149.

Dicloxacillin should be given cautiously to infants.

A report of enhanced renal excretion of dicloxacillin in patients with cystic fibrosis.— W. J. Jusko *et al., Pediatrics,* 1975, *56,* 1038.

Interactions. Aspirin, sulphamethoxypyridazine, and sulphaethidole inhibited the serum-binding of dicloxacillin *in vitro* and *in vivo.*— C. M. Kunin, *Clin. Pharmac. Ther.,* 1966, *7,* 180. See also K. A. DeSante *et al., J. clin. Pharmac.,* 1980, *20,* 534.

Studies of blood concentrations and excretion rates in 9 healthy persons indicated that the metabolism of ampicillin potassium and dicloxacillin sodium did not differ significantly when the drugs were given alone or in combination.— P. C. Gooding *et al., Curr. ther. Res.,* 1972, *14,* 43.

Antimicrobial Action. Dicloxacillin sodium has a range of antimicrobial activity similar to that of cloxacillin (see p.1149), but is generally reported to be more active.

For a report of dicloxacillin being one of the most active penicillins against *Staph. aureus* and *Staph. epidermidis,* see Benzylpenicillin, p.1106.

Resistance. As for Methicillin Sodium, p.1183.

Absorption and Fate. Dicloxacillin is readily absorbed when given by mouth but absorption is reduced by food in the stomach or small intestine. Absorption is greater with dicloxacillin than cloxacillin or oxacillin and plasma concentrations 1 hour after a 500-mg dose may range from 9.5 to 19.5 µg per ml and persist for about 4 hours. Doubling the dose can double the plasma concentration. However, protein-binding is greater with dicloxacillin, about 97% being bound to plasma proteins. Plasma-dicloxacillin concentrations tend to be more prolonged and this may be due to slower elimination as well as better absorption. About 70% of a dose given by mouth is excreted in the urine. Serum concentrations are enhanced if probenecid is given concomitantly. Dicloxacillin diffuses across the placenta.

Dicloxacillin given by mouth was better absorbed than either oxacillin or cloxacillin, and of doses given, 60, 21, and 40% respectively were eliminated in the urine within 8 hours. Dicloxacillin diffused into CSF in the absence of meningeal inflammation. Dicloxacillin should be given at not more than 6-hourly intervals, and doses of 500 mg should be adequate in staphylococcal infections.— T. Knott *et al., Arzneimittel-Forsch.,* 1965, *15,* 331.

The biological half-life of dicloxacillin was reported to be 0.5 hours.— W. M. Bennett *et al., J. Am. med. Ass.,* 1973, *223,* 991. The half-life was reported to be 0.71 hours.— W. A. Craig and P. G. Welling, *Clin. Pharmacokinet.,* 1977, *2,* 252.

A comparative study of the elimination, distribution, and absorption of dicloxacillin and cloxacillin in healthy subjects; higher serum concentrations of dicloxacillin were attributed to better absorption and slower renal elimination, no significant differences being found in the body distribution. Details of the kinetics of dicloxacillin were studied in patients undergoing haemodialysis; an elimination half-life of 129 minutes was found, compared with one of 42 minutes in the healthy subjects, and about 76% of an oral dose was absorbed which was greater than the amount absorbed by healthy subjects.— E. H. Nauta and H. Mattie, *Clin. Pharmac. Ther.,* 1976, *20,* 98.

Diffusion into body fluids and tissues. In a study of infants and children with suppurative arthritis, the concentration of dicloxacillin achieved in joint fluid was about 70% of the serum concentration 2 hours after 25 mg per kg body-weight was given by mouth. When compared with other antibiotics, the degree of binding to plasma proteins did not appear to influence diffusion.— J. D. Nelson *et al., J. Pediat.,* 1978, *92,* 131.

Dicloxacillin 50 mg per kg body-weight daily was given intramuscularly for 14 to 21 days to 8 children with osteomyelitis. Concentrations could only be detected in 4 of 8 specimens of pus and ranged from 1.4 to 71.0 µg per ml. In bone from 6 children concentrations ranged from 1.8 to 21.6 µg per g. Mean values in pus and bone exceeded the MBC for *Staph. aureus.*— T. R. Tetzlaff *et al., J. Pediat.,* 1978, *92,* 135.

Metabolism. About 10% of a 500-mg dose of dicloxacillin was metabolised. Within 12 hours of the dose being taken by 6 healthy subjects about 37% was recovered in the urine, 4% as penicilloic acid.— M. Cole *et al., Antimicrob. Ag. Chemother.,* 1973, *3,* 463.

Dicloxacillin was metabolised to a slightly less potent antibacterial compound that probably accumulated in patients with renal impairment.— H. H. W. Thijssen and H. Mattie, *Antimicrob. Ag. Chemother.,* 1976, *10,* 441.

Plasma concentrations. For reports of serum concentrations after the administration of dicloxacillin, see E. A. De Felice, *J. clin. Pharmac.,* 1967, *7,* 275; J. E. Rosenblatt *et al., Archs intern. Med.,* 1968, *121,* 345; J. T. Doluisio *et al., J. pharm. Sci.,* 1971, *60,* 715.

Pregnancy and the neonate. Dicloxacillin diffused across the placenta at term. The transfer from maternal to cord blood was similar to that which occurred with antibiotics that were not bound to serum proteins.— M. A. MacAulay *et al., Am. J. Obstet. Gynec.,* 1968, *102,* 1162.

Uses. Dicloxacillin sodium is used for the treatment of infections due to staphylococci resistant to benzylpenicillin. It is also used for the treatment of mixed streptococcal or pneumococcal and staphylococcal infections when the staphylococci are penicillin-resistant. Its resistance to inactivation by staphylococcal penicillinase is reported to be slightly greater than that of cloxacillin.

Dicloxacillin sodium is administered by mouth, about 1 hour before meals. The usual dose for adults is the equivalent of 0.25 to 1 g of dicloxacillin every 4 to 6 hours according to the severity of the infection. Children may be given the equivalent of 12 to 100 mg of dicloxacillin per kg body-weight daily in divided doses.

Dicloxacillin sodium has also been given intramuscularly in doses equivalent to 0.25 to 1 g of dicloxacillin every 6 hours.

A clinical evaluation of the parenteral use of dicloxacillin.— S. C. Deresinski and D. A. Stevens, *Curr. ther. Res.,* 1975, *18,* 151.

A guide to the use of penicillinase-resistant penicillins.— Veterans Administration Ad Hoc Interdisciplinary Advisory Committee on Antimicrobial Drug Usage, *J. Am. med. Ass.,* 1977, *237,* 1605.

Dosage in renal failure. In patients with anuria and a creatinine clearance of 10 ml or less per minute, the maximum recommended dose of dicloxacillin was 500 mg every 6 hours. Patients with renal and hepatic disease should receive lower doses.— D. L. Giusti, *Drug Intell. & clin. Pharm.,* 1973, *7,* 62.

Data for predicting removal of dicloxacillin by conventional haemodialysis.— T. P. Gibson and H. A. Nelson, *Clin. Pharmacokinet.,* 1977, *2,* 403.

The normal half-life for dicloxacillin of 0.5 to 0.9 hour was increased to 1 to 1.6 hours in end-stage renal failure. It could be given in usual doses to patients with renal failure. Concentrations of dicloxacillin were not affected by haemodialysis.— W. M. Bennett *et al., Ann. intern. Med.,* 1980, *93,* 62.

Further references showing that haemodialysis had no effect on dicloxacillin.— T. W. Williams *et al., Antimicrob. Ag. Chemother.,* 1967, 767; R. V. McCloskey and C. P. Hayes, *ibid.,* 770; G. B. Appel and H. C. Neu, *New Engl. J. Med.,* 1977, *296,* 663.

Osteomyelitis. A report on the use of high doses of dicloxacillin in the treatment of staphylococcal osteomyelitis in children.— Y. J. Bryson *et al., J. Pediat.,* 1979, *94,* 673.

Urinary-tract infections. Of 18 patients with urinary-tract infections and significant bacteriuria given ampicillin 300 mg with dicloxacillin 200 mg six-hourly for 7 to 10 days, 12 were cured, 3 improved, 1 failed to respond, and 2 later developed supra-infections. In a similar group of 18 patients given only ampicillin 500 mg six-hourly for the same period 7 were cured, 7 improved, and 4 failed to respond.— G. F. Abbate *et al.*, *Arzneimittel-Forsch.*, 1978, *28*, 1008.

Preparations

Dicloxacillin Sodium Capsules *(U.S.P.)*. Capsules containing dicloxacillin sodium equivalent to 62.5, 125, 250, or 500 mg of dicloxacillin. Store in airtight containers.

Dicloxacillin Sodium for Oral Suspension *(U.S.P.)*. A dry mixture of dicloxacillin sodium and one or more suitable buffers, colouring and flavouring agents, and preservatives. Store in airtight containers. The suspension is prepared by the addition of diluent before issue. pH 4.5 to 7.5.

Proprietary Names

Dichlor-Stapenor *(Bayer, Ger.)*; Diclo *(FIRMA, Ital.)*; Diclocil *(Bristol, Belg.*; *Bristol, Fr.*; *Bristol Italiana Sud, Ital.*; *Bristol, Neth.*; *Antibioticos, Spain*; *Bristol, Switz.)*; Diclocila *(Bristol, Swed.)*; Diclocillin *(Aristochimica, Ital.)*; Diclomax *(Pulitzer, Ital.)*; Dicloxapen *(Magis, Ital.)*; Diflor *(Coli, Ital.)*; Dycill *(Beecham, USA)*; Dynapen *(Bristol, Canad.*; *Bristol, USA)*; Maclicine *(Christiaens, Belg.)*; Novapen *(IBP, Ital.)*; Pathocil *(Wyeth, USA)*; Stafopenin *(Astra, Swed.)*; Veracillin *(Ayerst, USA)*.

69-l

Diethanolamine Fusidate *(B.P.C. 1968)*.

The diethanolamine salt of fusidic acid.

$C_{35}H_{59}NO_8=621.9$.

CAS — 16391-75-6.

A white or almost white, odourless or almost odourless, crystalline powder with a bitter taste. Diethanolamine fusidate 1.15 g is approximately equivalent to 1 g of sodium fusidate. **Soluble** 1 in 3 of water, 1 in 2.5 of alcohol, 1 in 70 of acetone, and 1 in 7 of chloroform; very slightly soluble in ether. A 3% solution in water has a pH of 7 to 8.5; a 10% solution is colourless or almost colourless. **Store** in airtight containers. Protect from light.

Diethanolamine fusidate has the actions and uses described under Sodium Fusidate, p.1210. It is administered by intravenous infusion.

Proprietary Preparations

Fucidin for Intravenous Infusion *(Leo, UK)*. Diethanolamine fusidate, available as powder for preparing solutions, in vials of 580 mg (equivalent to sodium fusidate 500 mg), supplied with 50-ml vials of phosphate-citrate buffered solvent. (Also available as Fucidin for Intravenous Infusion in *Denm.*, *Norw.*, *S.Afr.* Available as Fucidin Oral Suspension in *Austral.*).

Other Proprietary Names

Fucidine *(Ger.)* (see also under Sodium Fusidate).

71-g

Dihydrostreptomycin Sulphate *(B.P. 1958, B.P. Vet.)*.

4-*O*-[2-*O*-(2-Deoxy-2-methylamino-α-L-glucopyranosyl)-5-deoxy-3-*C*-hydroxymethyl-α-L-lyxofuranosyl]-*NN'*-diamidino-D-streptamine sulphate.

$(C_{21}H_{41}N_7O_{12})_2,3H_2SO_4=1461.4$.

CAS — 128-46-1 (dihydrostreptomycin); 5490-27-7 (sulphate).

Pharmacopoeias. In *Arg.*, *Aust.*, *Belg.*, *Fr.*, *Ind.*, *It.*, *Mex.*, *Nord.*, *Port.*, and *Swiss*.

Dihydrostreptomycin (*Span. P.*) is the hydrochloride or the sulphate.

A sterile white hygroscopic solid with a slightly bitter taste. *B.P.1958* specified not less than 700 units (microgram equivalents of dihydrostreptomycin base) per mg; *B.P. Vet.* specifies not less than 720 units per mg. Dihydrostreptomycin sulphate 1.25 g is approximately equivalent to 1 g of dihydrostreptomycin.

Very **soluble** in water; practically insoluble in alcohol, acetone, chloroform, and ether. A 25% solution in water has a pH of 4.5 to 7. A 19.4% solution is iso-osmotic with serum. Solutions for injection are prepared by dissolving the sterile contents of a sealed container in Water for Injections. The sulphate is **incompatible** with streptomycin calcium chloride and with acids and alkalis.

Store at a temperature not exceeding 30° in sterile containers.

Dihydrostreptomycin was incompatible with *soluble barbiturates, calcium gluconate, calcium gluceptate, heparin, noradrenaline acid tartrate*, and *sulphafurazole diethanolamine* in an infusion fluid.— B. Flouvat and P. Lechat, *Thérapie*, 1974, *29*, 337.

Units. One unit of dihydrostreptomycin is contained in 0.001219 mg of the second International Standard Preparation (1966) of dihydrostreptomycin sulphate which contains 820 units per mg.

Dihydrostreptomycin sulphate has actions and uses similar to those of Streptomycin Sulphate, p.1213. However, it is more ototoxic. It was given intramuscularly in doses equivalent to 0.5 to 1 g of dihydrostreptomycin.

Dihydrostreptomycin pantothenate was formerly available, in association with the sulphate, and was used similarly.

Dihydrostreptomycin sulphate is an ingredient of Guanimycin Suspension Forte, see under Sulphaguanidine, p.1478.

Proprietary Names

Abiocine *(Lepetit, Fr.)*; Diestreptopab *(Martin Santos, Spain)*; Dihidro-Cidan Sulfato *(Cidan, Spain)*; Enterastrept *(Heyl, Ger.)*; Estreptoluy *(Miluy, Spain)*; Sanestrepto *(Santos, Spain)*; Solvo-strept *(Heyl, Ger.)*.

72-q

Doxycycline *(U.S.P.)*.

Doxycycline Monohydrate. 6-Deoxy-5β-hydroxytetracycline monohydrate.

$C_{22}H_{24}N_2O_8,H_2O=462.5$.

CAS — 564-25-0 (anhydrous); 17086-28-1 (monohydrate).

Pharmacopoeias. In *U.S.*

A yellow crystalline powder. Very slightly **soluble** in water; sparingly soluble in alcohol; practically insoluble in chloroform and ether; freely soluble in dilute acids and alkali hydroxides. A 1% aqueous suspension has a pH of 5 to 6.5. **Store** in airtight containers. Protect from light.

73-p

Doxycycline Calcium.

A complex prepared from doxycycline hydrochloride and calcium chloride.

74-s

Doxycycline Hydrochloride *(B.P.)*.

Doxycycline Hyclate *(U.S.P.)*; Doxycyclini Chloridum; 6-Deoxy-5β-hydroxytetracycline Hydrochloride. Doxycycline hydrochloride hemiethanolate hemihydrate.

$C_{22}H_{24}N_2O_8,HCl,½C_2H_5OH,½H_2O=512.9$.

CAS — 10592-13-9 ($C_{22}H_{24}N_2O_8,HCl$); 24390-14-5 ($C_{22}H_{24}N_2O_8,HCl,½C_2H_5OH,½H_2O$).

Pharmacopoeias. In *Br.*, *Braz.*, *Cz.*, *Nord.*, and *U.S.*

A yellow crystalline powder with a slight ethanolic odour and a bitter taste containing not less than 822 units per mg. M.p. about 200° with decomposition. Doxycycline hydrochloride 115 mg is approximately equivalent to 100 mg of doxycycline. **Soluble** 1 in 3 of water, 1 in 60 of alcohol, and 1 in 4 of methyl alcohol; practically insoluble in chloroform and ether; soluble in solutions of alkali hydroxides and carbonates. A 1% solution in water has a pH of 2 to 3. **Store** in airtight containers. Protect from light.

Solutions in sodium chloride injection or dextrose injection should be used within 12 hours of preparation and protected from direct sunlight; they may be stored for up to 72 hours at a temperature between 2° and 8°.

Loss of activity. Riboflavine reduced the antimicrobial activity *in vitro* of doxycycline hydrochloride by 56.5%.— M. A. El-Nakeeb *et al.*, *Can. J. pharm. Sci.*, 1976, *11*, 85.

Units. One unit of doxycycline is contained in 0.0011494 mg of the first International Reference Preparation (1975) of doxycycline hydrochloride which contains 870 units per mg.

Adverse Effects. As for Tetracycline Hydrochloride, p.1217.

Doxycycline has a low affinity for binding with calcium and work in *animals* suggests that it may cause less tooth-staining than other tetracyclines.

Deposition in bones and teeth. Of 25 children who had been born prematurely and who had received doxycycline in total doses of from 9 to 37 mg soon after birth, only 1 was found to have a discoloration of the milk teeth. The upper incisors had a slight spotted discoloration.— G. Forti and C. Benincori (letter), *Lancet*, 1969, *1*, 782.

Effect on the gastro-intestinal tract. A report of oesophageal ulceration, in a patient with a normal oesophagus, following ingestion of a doxycycline capsule.— L. Bokey and T. B. Hugh, *Med. J. Aust.*, 1975, *1*, 236. Similar reports.— R. Schneider, *Am. J. dig. Dis.*, 1977, *22*, 805; E. Kobler *et al.*, *Dt. med. Wschr.*, 1978, *103*, 1035; M. Giger *et al.*, *ibid.*, 1038.

Precautions. As for Tetracycline Hydrochloride, p.1218.

Absorption of doxycycline appears to be less affected by milk or food than the other tetracyclines. Doxycycline may also be less likely to aggravate renal disease.

A study indicating that usual therapeutic doses of doxycycline interfere with colour vision.— J. Laroche and C. Laroche, *Annls pharm. fr.*, 1972, *30*, 433.

Renal function deteriorated acutely but reversibly in a patient with chronic renal failure given doxycycline for 14 days.— L. H. Orr *et al.*, *Archs intern. Med.*, 1978, *138*, 793.

Interactions. In 5 subjects the mean half-life of doxycycline after a 100-mg intravenous dose was significantly reduced from a mean of 15.3 hours to a mean of 11.1 hours after the administration for 10 days of phenobarbitone 50 mg thrice daily. In 5 further patients on long-term barbiturates the mean half-life was 7.7 hours. Phenytoin similarly reduced the half-life of doxycycline.— P. J. Neuvonen and O. Penttilä, *Br. med. J.*, 1974, *1*, 535.

The mean half-life of doxycycline after intravenous injection of 100 mg was 15.1 hours in 9 controls, but was 7.2 hours in 7 patients who had taken phenytoin for from 4 months to 10 years, 8.4 hours in 5 patients who had taken carbamazepine for from 4 months to 4 years, and 7.4 hours in 4 patients taking phenytoin and carbamazepine.— O. Penttilä *et al.*, *Br. med. J.*, 1974, *2*, 470.

Concurrent oral ferrous sulphate administration lowered the serum concentration of doxycycline administered by mouth, and shortened the serum half-life after a single intravenous injection. The interaction could not be avoided completely by leaving a 3-hour interval between doses of the two drugs.— P. J. Neuvonen and O. Penttilä, *Eur. J. clin. Pharmac.*, 1974, *7*, 361. The therapeutic effect of doxycycline was not considered to be at risk provided doxycycline and iron were given several hours apart.— V. M. K. Venho *et al.*, *Eur. J. clin. Pharmac.*, 1978, *14*, 277.

Antimicrobial Action. Doxycycline hydrochloride has a range of antimicrobial activity and mode of action similar to that of tetracycline hydrochloride (see p.1218). It is more effective than tetracycline against many species.

Doxycycline and clindamycin had MICs of less than 6 μg per ml against 54 strains of *Fusobacterium* spp.; benzylpenicillin had similar activity and ampicillin, cephalothin, carbenicillin, erythromycin, chloramphenicol, tetracycline, and tinidazole were less active. Against 322 strains of other anaerobic bacteria including *Bacteroides fragilis*, *B. melaninogenicus*, *Clostridium* spp., and Gram-positive cocci, doxycycline was slightly more active than tetracycline but generally much less active than clindamycin and many of the other antibiotics.— J. Klastersky *et al.*, *Antimicrob. Ag. Chemother.*, 1977, *12*, 563.

For comparative studies of the activities of doxycycline and minocycline and the sensitivity of tetracycline-resistant bacteria to doxycycline, see Minocycline Hydrochloride, p.1185.

Diminished activity. Riboflavine reduced the antimicrobial activity of doxycycline hydrochloride *in vitro* by 56.5%.— M. A. El-Nakeeb *et al.*, *Can. J. pharm. Sci.*, 1976, *11*, 85.

Absorption and Fate. As for Tetracycline Hydrochloride, p.1219.

Doxycycline hydrochloride is readily absorbed from the gastro-intestinal tract and 2 hours after a 200-mg dose plasma concentrations of 2.6 μg per ml, falling to 1.45 μg per ml at 24 hours, have been reported. Following repeated doses of 100 mg daily, concentrations of about 2 μg per ml are maintained. Similar values are reported after intravenous infusions.

Absorption is not significantly affected by the presence of food in the stomach or duodenum. Up to 90% of doxycycline in the circulation is reported to be bound to plasma proteins. Its biological half-life varies from about 15 hours after a single dose to 22 hours after repeated doses. Doxycycline is more lipid-soluble than tetracycline. It is widely distributed in body tissues and fluids but only low concentrations are achieved in cerebrospinal fluid. Doxycycline is slowly excreted, mainly in the urine. It is stated not to accumulate in patients with renal impairment although excretion in the urine is reduced; doxycycline may be excreted directly into the gastro-intestinal tract in these patients. Nevertheless there have been reports of some accumulation in renal failure. There is also some inactivation in the liver but up to 25% of a dose has been excreted in the faeces in an active form.

Doxycycline in a dose of 200 mg produced peak serum concentrations after 4 hours of 9 μg per ml in patients with impaired kidney function and 4.2 μg per ml in other patients. The urine concentration, 24 hours after administration, was 20.9 μg per ml in patients with normal kidney function, a value much greater than the MIC for most sensitive organisms. Urine measurements of patients with renal failure showed low doxycycline concentrations.— W. A. Mahon *et al.*, *Can. med. Ass. J.*, 1970, *103*, 1031. Doxycycline appears to accumulate to some extent in impaired renal function. After a 200-mg intravenous dose, the serum half-life was significantly prolonged from 13.8 to 20.6 hours in 8 patients with chronic stable renal failure (creatinine clearance less than 5 ml per minute) compared with 8 subjects with normal renal function. In those with renal failure only 2% of the dose was recovered in the urine over 72 hours compared with 57% in normal subjects.— D. Heaney and G. Eknoyan, *Clin. Pharmac. Ther.*, 1978, *24*, 233.

In 6 healthy subjects urinary excretion of doxycycline after a single 200-mg dose by mouth was 60.8% when urine pH was 7.4 to 8.0 and 37.1% at pH 5.3 to 6.3. The mean half-life in each case was 9 and 13.2 hours respectively. During a multiple dose regimen urinary excretion of doxycycline was 65% at pH 7.7 to 8.4 and 52.8% at pH 5.6 to 6.7. The mean half-lives under these conditions were 11.8 and 17 hours respectively.— J. M. Jaffe *et al.*, *J. pharm. Sci.*, 1974, *63*, 1256.

A mean peak serum concentration of 15.29 μg per ml was measured fluorimetrically 4 hours after a 500-mg dose of doxycycline was taken by 11 Nigerian subjects.— B. K. Adadevoh *et al.*, *Br. med. J.*, 1976, *1*, 880.

Evidence suggesting that doxycycline is probably not metabolised.— A. P. De Leenheer and H. J. C. F. Nelis, *J. pharm. Sci.*, 1979, *68*, 999.

Further references: J. Fabre *et al.*, *Schweiz. med. Wschr.*, 1967, *97*, 915; M. L. Nielsen *et al.*, *Acta pharmac. tox.*, 1971, *29*, 314; P. Lee *et al.*, *N.Z. med. J.*, 1972, *75*, 355; K. Alestig, *Scand. J. infect. Dis.*, 1973, *5*, 193; K. Alestig, *Scand. J. infect. Dis.*, 1974, *6*, 265; G. E. Marlin and S. Cheng, *Med. J. Aust.*, 1979, *1*, 575.

Diffusion. Lung and bronchial tissue. J. Gartmann, *Schweiz. med. Wschr.*, 1972, *102*, 1484; H. Thadepalli *et al.*, *Chest*, 1980, *78*, 304.

Seminal fluid. H. Gnarpe and J. Friberg, *Am. J. Obstet. Gynec.*, 1972, *114*, 963.

Sinus secretions. C. Lundberg *et al.* (letter), *Lancet*, 1968, *2*, 107.

Sputum. D. MacCulloch *et al.*, *N.Z. med. J.*, 1974, *80*, 300; R. W. Ruhen and M. K. Tandon, *Med. J. Aust.*, 1976, *1*, 151; B. J. S. Hartnett and G. E. Marlin, *Thorax*, 1976, *31*, 144; C. G. C. MacArthur *et al.*, *J. antimicrob. Chemother.*, 1978, *4*, 509.

Tonsils. A. Miniti *et al.*, *Revta Hosp. Clin. Fac. Med. Univ. S Paulo*, 1970, *25*, 371.

Transplacental diffusion. H. J. Wallner and A. Schmiedel, *Münch. med. Wschr.*, 1975, *117*, 349.

Uses. Doxycycline hydrochloride is used for the same purposes as tetracycline hydrochloride (see p.1220). It is readily absorbed and excreted more slowly than most other tetracyclines and effective blood concentrations are maintained for longer periods so that dosage once daily is usually adequate.

It may be given, with care, to patients with renal impairment but its low renal clearance could make it unsuitable for the treatment of urinary-tract infections.

Doxycycline is administered in capsules as the hydrochloride or in syrup or suspension as the calcium chelate or monohydrate. The hydrochloride may also be given by intravenous infusion. The usual dose is the equivalent of 200 mg of doxycycline initially, followed by 100 mg daily. Children weighing less than 45 kg may be given 4.4 mg per kg body-weight initially and thereafter 2.2 mg per kg daily but the effect of tetracyclines on teeth should be considered. In severe infections the initial dosage is maintained throughout the course of treatment. The equivalent of 300 or 600 mg has been given over one day in the treatment of gonorrhoea.

Doxycycline 200 mg daily intravenously was given to 56 patients with malignant diseases who were susceptible to infection. No impairment of kidney or liver function occurred. Blood concentrations of doxycycline ranged from 1 to 6 μg per ml and were sufficient to inhibit most Gram-positive cocci including tetracycline-resistant organisms. Infections due to Enterobacteriaceae, *Pseudomonas*, and enterococci were less effectively treated. Of 30 infectious episodes caused by these organisms only 12 responded to treatment. Overall, 37 of 56 patients were effectively treated. However, serious supra-infection occurred in 7 patients and was fatal in 1 of them.— J. Klastersky *et al.*, *Curr. ther. Res.*, 1972, *14*, 49. See also *idem*, *Int. J. clin. Pharmac. Biopharm.*, 1975, *11*, 19.

For the proceedings of symposiums on doxycycline, see *Chemotherapy, Basle*, 1975, *21*, *Suppl.* 1, 1-148; *Scand. J. infect. Dis.*, 1976, *Suppl.* 9, 1-113.

Anthrax. There was rapid systemic improvement in 33 patients with cutaneous anthrax given one dose of doxycycline 7 to 32 mg per kg body-weight. All lesions were free of infection within 4 days.— S. N. Saggar *et al.*, *E. Afr. med. J.*, 1974, *51*, 889.

Bronchitis. There was no significant difference in the rate or degree of conversion of sputum from purulent to mucoid in a double-blind study carried out by the Research Committee of the British Thoracic and Tuberculosis Association on 60 patients with acute exacerbations of bronchitis given doxycycline or oxytetracycline.— J. H. Angel, *B.T.T.A. Rev.*, 1972, *2*, 41. See also *Br. J. Dis. Chest*, 1973, *67*, 114.

A study using doxycycline and placebo indicating that in otherwise healthy patients with cough and purulent sputum the symptoms would usually get better without antibiotic treatment.— N. C. H. Stott and R. R. West, *Br. med. J.*, 1976, *2*, 556. Comment.— *ibid.*, 550.

Further references: H. Swarz, *Curr. med. Res. Opinion*, 1977, *5*, 234; G. J. Pandy, *Med. J. Aust.*, 1979, *1*, 264.

Chancroid. Doxycycline 300 mg was effective within 1 to 6 days in the treatment of 30 of 31 patients with chancroid.— T. J. Stamps, *J. trop. Med. Hyg.*, 1974, *77*, 55.

In a study of 62 patients with chancroid, treatment with a single 300-mg dose of doxycycline was compared with sulphafurazole 1 g given four times daily for 1 week. At follow-up after 1 week there was an inadequate response in 8 of 30 patients who received doxycycline and in 6 of 19 who received sulphafurazole. Rates of lesion-healing in the 2 groups were similar but it was considered that the advantage of compliance in the doxycycline group was offset by the side-effect of vomiting.— G. W. Hammond *et al.*, *J. antimicrob. Chemother.*, 1979, *5*, 261.

Cholera. Doxycycline 2 mg per kg body-weight initially, at 12 hours, then daily for 4 days or a total of 5 doses given to 17 patients with actively purging cholera was as effective as tetracycline 20 mg per kg daily given to 15 patients in divided 6-hourly doses for 4 days and more effective than placebo. However, vibrios were eradicated more rapidly with tetracycline (1.8 days) than with doxycycline (2.6 days). In spite of this and of a risk of incomplete absorption due to reduced transit time in cholera, the reduced number of doses of doxycycline and its safety in renal impairment offered advantages over tetracycline.— M. M. Rahaman *et al.*, *Antimicrob. Ag. Chemother.*, 1976, *10*, 610.

In a comparative study in cholera patients, doxycycline 300 mg as a single dose was almost as effective as tetracycline 500 mg every 6 hours for 48 hours.— S. De *et al.*, *Bull. Wld Hlth Org.*, 1976, *54*, 177.

In cholera patients, a single 200-mg dose of doxycycline was as effective as 100 mg, repeated after 12 hours and then given daily for 3 days. Tetracycline remained the treatment of choice.— D. A. Sack *et al.*, *Antimicrob. Ag. Chemother.*, 1978, *14*, 462.

Prophylaxis. From a study in 276 contacts of cholera patients, 137 of whom were given doxycycline, a single dose of doxycycline was considered an effective prophylactic agent. The dose was 300 mg for persons over 15 years of age and 6 mg per kg body-weight for younger persons.— P. G. Sen Gupta *et al.*, *Bull. Wld Hlth Org.*, 1978, *56*, 323.

Diarrhoea. Prophylaxis. In a double-blind study involving 18 Peace Corps volunteers who took doxycycline 200 mg on the flight out and 100 mg daily for their first 3 weeks in Kenya only 1 (6%) suffered travellers' diarrhoea whereas of 21 who took placebo capsules 9 (43%) suffered 1 or more episodes. The protective effect of doxycycline in travellers' diarrhoea was associated with the absence of detectable enterotoxigenic *Escherichia coli* and appeared to persist for a week after the antibiotic was discontinued.— D. A. Sack *et al.*, *New Engl. J. Med.*, 1978, *298*, 758. Daily administration of doxycycline should probably continue while the subject is at risk, although long-term prophylaxis is not recommended until more information is available.— J. B. Armstrong, *Pfizer* (letter), *Can. med. Ass. J.*, 1979, *120*, 794. Similar results were achieved among 50 volunteers in Morocco, but the indiscriminate use of doxycycline prophylaxis should be discouraged.— R. B. Sack *et al.*, *Gastroenterology*, 1979, *76*, 1368.

Concern about the potential hazards of giving doxycycline prophylactically to large numbers of travellers.— R. L. Guerrant and J. M. Hughes (letter), *New Engl. J. Med.*, 1978, *299*, 1412; M. H. Merson, *Gastroenterology*, 1979, *76*, 1485.

See also under Cholera (above).

Dosage in renal failure. A comparison of doxycycline with oxytetracycline in 9 patients with impaired renal function undergoing haemodialysis showed that production of urea was higher in the patients when they received 250 mg oxytetracycline every 6 or every 12 hours than when they received doxycycline 200 mg initially and 100 mg daily for 6 days. Three other patients were given doxycycline 200 mg daily. The mean urea production in these was higher than that of patients on the lower dose of doxycycline. The serum half-life of doxycycline was 17 hours and during dialysis 18 hours, while the half-life of oxytetracycline varied between 40 and 72 hours reduced to 14 to 20 hours during dialysis.— T. Morgan and N. Ribush, *Med. J. Aust.*, 1972, *1*, 55.

In 15 patients with renal failure given doxycycline, 200 mg on the first day and then 100 mg daily for 7 days, the mean serum-creatinine concentration rose from 375 to 500 μmol per litre, the mean serum-urea concentration from 21 to 23.3 μmol per litre, and the mean serum-uric acid concentration from 478 to 548 μmol per litre; these rises were not significant and there was no accumulation of doxycycline in the serum.— A. Kasanen *et al.*, *Curr. ther. Res.*, 1974, *16*, 243.

A recommended dosage of doxycycline in patients undergoing haemodialysis was 200 mg intravenously initially followed by 200 mg daily by mouth or intravenous injection.— J. F. Mahony and D. Lloyd-Jones, *Med. J. Aust.*, 1975, *2*, 673.

The normal half-life for doxycycline of 14 to 25 hours was increased to 15 to 36 hours in end-stage renal failure. The normal dosage interval of 12 hours should be increased up to 18 hours in patients with a glomerular filtration-rate (GFR) of 10 to 50 ml per minute and from 18 to 24 hours in patients with a GFR of less than 10 ml per minute. Concentrations of doxycycline were not affected by haemodialysis or peritoneal dialysis.— W. M. Bennett *et al.*, *Ann. intern. Med.*, 1980, *93*, 62.

Further references: Ø. Stenbaek *et al.*, *Scand, J. infect.*

Dis., 1973, *5*, 199; C. Simon *et al.*, *Schweiz. med. Wschr.*, 1975, *105*, 1615.

See also under Absorption and Fate (above).

Gonorrhoea. One dose of doxycycline 300 mg given to 40 patients with confirmed gonorrhoea was effective in 29 (72.5%) and was not considered adequate. One patient vomited after taking the dose on an empty stomach.— M. G. Mutchnick, *Br. J. vener. Dis.*, 1972, *48*, 381.

There were no failures among 100 women with gonorrhoea treated with 2 doses of doxycycline 300 mg given 8 hours apart and 2 failures among 50 given 1 dose of cephaloridine 2 g intramuscularly. These results were similar to those obtained with penicillin therapy.— J. Söltz-Szöts and E. Kokoschka, *Br. J. vener. Dis.*, 1973, *49*, 177.

In a study of 1124 patients with gonorrhoea treated with 2 doses of ampicillin 1 g given 5 hours apart or 1 dose of doxycycline 300 mg the failure-rates for men were 1.1% with ampicillin and 8.1% with doxycycline while those for women were 1.0% and 5.7% respectively. Side-effects were more common with doxycycline.— W. Enfors and G. Eriksson, *Br. J. vener. Dis.*, 1975, *51*, 99.

Legionnaires' disease. Experience suggesting that doxycycline is clinically effective in legionnaires' disease. Erythromycin remains the drug of choice, but if the diagnosis is uncertain and legionnaires' disease is only one of a number of diagnostic possibilities, empirical therapy with doxycycline is preferred.— B. A. Cunha and M. Jonas (letter), *Lancet*, 1981, *1*, 1107.

Mycoplasmal infections and infertility. T-strain mycoplasmas were isolated from 54 infertile couples. Both partners were treated with doxycycline 200 mg on day 7 of the menstrual cycle then 100 mg daily until the 16th day, monthly for 3 months and thereafter 200 mg daily for 10 days monthly. Pregnancy occurred in 15 of the couples.— J. Friberg and H. Gnarpe, *Am. J. Obstet. Gynec.*, 1973, *116*, 23.

In a study of the role of mycoplasmal infection in infertility 35 couples were given doxycycline 100 mg twice on the first day then once daily for 27 days; 25 had mycoplasmal infections of the genital tract before treatment and 2 were culture-positive 14 days after treatment. No association was found between infertility and infection with T-strain *Mycoplasma* or *Mycoplasma hominis*.— J. de Louvois *et al.*, *Lancet*, 1974, *1*, 1073.

Although doxycycline eradicated *Mycoplasma* spp. this was of no benefit in the treatment of infertility in a controlled study of 120 patients.— R. F. Harrison *et al.*, *Lancet*, 1975, *1*, 605.

Pneumonia. No difference was found in efficacy between doxycycline, tetracycline, and oxytetracycline in reducing morbidity in patients with pneumonia due to *Mycoplasma pneumoniae*.— W. M. Gooch and W. J. Mogabgab, *Antimicrob. Ag. Chemother.*, 1970, 291.

Further references: V. P. Nagpal and J. R. Harries, *E. Afr. med. J.*, 1974, *51*, 778; P. A. Abiose *et al.*, *Curr. ther. Res.*, 1977, *21*, 458.

See also under Legionnaires' Disease, above.

Relapsing fever, louse-borne. Doxycycline in a single dose of 100 mg was effective in the treatment of 26 patients with confirmed louse-borne relapsing fever who were followed up for 2 weeks. Each patient experienced a Herxheimer reaction and in 5 the cardiac failure with hypotension required treatment with digoxin 500 µg intravenously. Also 10 patients with serologically confirmed typhus were given doxycycline 100 mg and between 38 and 128 hours they became afebrile and symptom-free.— P. L. Perine *et al.*, *Lancet*, 1974, *2*, 742.

Skin disorders. For a report of the use of doxycycline in the treatment of acne, see Oxytetracycline Hydrochloride, p.1197.

Surgical infection prophylaxis. From a study of 20 patients who underwent surgery where intra-abdominal infection was suspected, treatment with doxycycline or doxycycline and gentamicin was associated with a high level of post-operative infections.— R. A. Klein *et al.*, *J. Am. med. Ass.*, 1977, *238*, 1933.

In a study involving 118 patients undergoing colorectal surgery doxycycline, 200 mg given 4 to 6 hours preoperatively and then 100 mg daily for 5 days, reduced the incidence of wound infections, septicaemia, and intra-abdominal complications from 45% to 12.1%.— H. Höjer and J. Wetterfors, *Ann. Surg.*, 1978, *187*, 362.

Experience involving 2950 women undergoing induced abortion indicated that a single prophylactic dose of doxycycline 500 mg by mouth considerably reduced the incidence of pelvic infection after abortion, compared with placebo.— C. Brewer, *Br. med. J.*, 1980, *281*, 780.

Further references: W. L. Hengeveld, *Curr. med. Res. Opinion*, 1977, *4*, 505.

Syphilis. Doxycycline 100 mg twice daily for 28 days, repeated every 3 to 4 months, was effective and well tolerated in 51 patients with syphilis at various stages.— Y. Onoda, *Br. J. vener. Dis.*, 1979, *55*, 110.

Trachoma. Doxycycline administered in single daily doses of 2.5 to 4 mg per kg body-weight on 5 days each week over 40 days to American Indian children with chronic trachoma was more effective than placebo. Serum concentration of the drug remained adequate through much of the treatment period but the drug concentration in tears fluctuated.— I. Hoshiwara *et al.*, *J. Am. med. Ass.*, 1973, *224*, 220.

A double-blind controlled study of topical oxytetracycline twice daily for 7 days each month or doxycycline 5 mg per kg body-weight once a month by mouth in hyperendemic trachoma. There was no marked difference between the two treatments.— S. Darougar *et al.*, *Br. J. Ophthal.*, 1980, *64*, 291.

Typhus. In a study in 65 patients with epidemic typhus the response (in terms of clinical improvement and speed of defervescence) in 26 given doxycycline 200 mg as a single dose was comparable with that in 21 given chloramphenicol 800 mg four times daily for about 8 days. There was little response in 18 patients given co-trimoxazole.— J. Huys *et al.*, *Trans. R. Soc. trop. Med. Hyg.*, 1973, *67*, 718.

A single dose of doxycycline 200 mg was as effective as a 7-day course of treatment with tetracycline for patients with scrub typhus.— G. W. Brown *et al.*, *Trans. R. Soc. trop. Med. Hyg.*, 1978, *72*, 412.

Further references: J. G. Olson *et al.*, *Am. J. trop. med. Hyg.*, 1980, *29*, 989.

Urinary-tract infections. While doxycycline might be a useful form of tetracycline for administration to patients with impaired renal function, its efficacy in urinary-tract infection was doubtful.— *Med. Lett.*, 1972, *14*, 3.

Doxycycline 300 mg was effective in about 93% of 213 patients with gonococcal or non-gonococcal urethritis. Gastro-intestinal effects were reduced by giving the dose with reconstituted dried milk.— G. Masterton and C. B. S. Schofield, *Br. J. vener. Dis.*, 1972, *48*, 121. In an attempt to reduce gastro-intestinal side-effects doxycycline was administered as a syrup rather than a capsule in a single dose of 300 mg to 266 male patients with urethritis and only 5 suffered side-effects. Of the 244 patients followed up, only 21 failed to respond and 13 were re-infected. When compared with the results in the above study the response was similar in gonorrhoea but poorer in non-gonococcal urethritis.— C. B. S. Schofield and G. Masterton, *Br. J. vener. Dis.*, 1974, *50*, 303.

In a study of 62 women with acute urethral syndrome, doxycycline was significantly more effective than placebo in eradicating urinary symptoms, pyuria, and the infecting micro-organisms, including coliforms, staphylococci, or *Chlamydia trachomatis*. Women without pyuria did not benefit from treatment with doxycycline.— W. E. Stamm *et al.*, *New Engl. J. Med.*, 1981, *304*, 956.

Further references: A. Lassus *et al.*, *Br. J. vener. Dis.*, 1971, *47*, 126; H. M. Perroud and J. F. Vulliemin, *Schweiz. med. Wschr.*, 1978, *108*, 412.

Preparations

Doxycycline Calcium Oral Suspension *(U.S.P.)*. It is prepared from doxycycline hydrochloride and contains one or more suitable buffers, diluents, preservatives, colouring agents, and flavouring agents. It contains the equivalent of 10 mg of doxycycline per ml. pH 6.5 to 8. Store in airtight containers. Protect from light.

Doxycycline Capsules *(B.P.)*. Capsules containing doxycycline hydrochloride. Potency is expressed in terms of the equivalent amount of doxycycline. Store at a temperature not exceeding 30°. *U.S.P.* (Doxycycline Hyclate Capsules) specifies the equivalent of 50 or 100 mg of doxycycline. Store in airtight containers. Protect from light.

Doxycycline for Oral Suspension *(U.S.P.)*. Doxycycline with one or more suitable suspending and dispersing agents. It may contain one or more suitable buffers, diluents, colouring agents, flavouring agents, and preservatives. Store in airtight containers. Protect from light. The suspension is prepared by the addition of diluent before issue and contains 5 mg per ml. pH 5 to 6.5.

Doxycycline Hyclate for Injection *(U.S.P.)*. A dry mixture of doxycycline hydrochloride and a suitable buffer. The injection is prepared by the addition of diluent before use. pH 1.8 to 3.3. Potency is expressed in terms of the equivalent amount of doxycycline.

Doxycycline Hyclate Tablets *(U.S.P.)*. Tablets containing doxycycline hydrochloride. Potency is expressed in terms of the equivalent amount of doxycycline. The *U.S.P.* requires 55% dissolution in 60 minutes and 85% dissolution in 90 minutes. Store in airtight containers. Protect from light.

Proprietary Preparations

Vibramycin *(Pfizer, UK)*. Doxycycline hydrochloride, available as capsules each containing the equivalent of 100 mg of doxycycline. **Vibramycin Syrup** contains the equivalent of 50 mg of doxycycline (as the calcium chelate) in each 5 ml (suggested diluent, syrup). (Also available as Vibramycin in *Austral.*, *Canad.*, *Denm.*, *Ger.*, *Jap.*, *Neth.*, *Norw.*, *S.Afr.*, *Switz.*, *USA*).

Vibramycin-D *(Pfizer, UK)*. Dispersible tablets each containing doxycycline 100 mg in a basis flavoured with black currant.

Other Proprietary Names for Doxycycline and Doxycycline Hydrochloride

Arg.—Vibramicina; *Austral.*—Doxin; *Belg.*—Vibramycine; *Fr.*—Vibramycine, Vibraveineuse; *Ger.*—Doxitard, Vibravenös; *Ind.*—Tetradox; *Ital.*—Amplidox, Bassado, Biostar, Cirenyl, Dossil, Doxacin, Doxi, Doxibiotic, Doxidima, Doxigram, Doxilen, Doxileo, Doxina, Doxivis, Ecodox, Ekaciclina, Emidox, Esaciclina, Esadoxi, Falorciclina, Farmodoxi, Furdox, Germiciclin, Ghimadox, Gibidox, Gram-Val, Icidox, Iclados, Isodox, Lampodox, Microciclina, Minidox, Miraclin, Monodoxin, Neociclina, Novaciclin, Philcociclina, Pocaciclina, Radox, Samecin, Saramicina, Semelciclina, Semelin, Severciclina, Sferamicina, Sincromicyn, Stamicina, Tecacin, Tecnomicina, Unacil, Uniciclina, Unidox, Vibradoxil, Vibralex, Vibramicina, Vip-Ciclina, Ximicina; *Jap.*—Hydramycin, Liomycin, Roximycin; *Neth.*—Doxymycin, Dumoxin; *Norw.*—Doxylin, Dumoxin, Idocyklin; *Spain*—Clisemina, Dosil, Dox-Life, Doxaclen, Doxiclat, Doxiclin, Doxinate, Doxitrecina, Farmacina, Fenoseptil (dodecylsulfamate), Fortaciclina, Geobiotico Depot (see also Oxytetracycline), Hiclamicina, Libeciclina, Liviatin, Nivocilin, Noveciclina, Peraseptum, Plenomicin (phosphate), Relociclina, Retens, Rodomicina, Solupen, Tetrasan, Unidoxi, Vibracina, Vibravenosa; *Swed.*—Idocyklin; *Switz.*—Vibravenös; *USA*—Doxychel, Vibra-Tabs.

NOTE. The name Solupen was formerly used for preparations containing benzylpenicillin.

75-w

Enramycin. Enduracidin.

CAS — 11115-82-5.

Enramycin is a polypeptide antibiotic derived from cultures of *Streptomyces fungicidicus* B5477 and active against Gram-positive bacteria. It was formerly given by intramuscular injection and has been used as an animal feed additive.

Manufacturers

Takeda, Jap.

76-e

Epicillin.

SQ 11302. (6*R*)-6-(α-D-Cyclohexa-1,4-dienylglycylamino)penicillanic acid.

$C_{16}H_{21}N_3O_4S = 351.4$.

CAS — 26774-90-3.

A crystalline powder. **Soluble** 1 in 250 of water.

At 25° epicillin trihydrate was about 4 times more soluble in water than the anhydrous form. Respective solubilities were 1 in 56 and 1 in 250.— J. P. Hou and A. Restivo (letter), *J. pharm. Sci.*, 1975, *64*, 710.

Adverse Effects, Treatment, and Precautions. As for Ampicillin, p.1092.

Gastro-intestinal effects are the most common side-effects with epicillin. Skin rashes and pruritus, drowsiness, dizziness, headache, and vaginitis have occurred.

Antimicrobial Action. Epicillin is bactericidal and has a spectrum of activity similar to that of ampicillin (see p.1093). It is reported to be more active against *Pseudomonas aeruginosa* than ampicillin but less active than carbenicillin. Most sensitive organisms are inhibited by 1 µg or less per ml. Epicillin is inactivated by penicillinase and there is cross-resistance with ampicillin.

The antimicrobial activity of epicillin was similar to that of ampicillin except that epicillin inhibited *Ps. aerugi-*

nosa at 9.4 μg per ml whereas ampicillin required 25 μg per ml. Epicillin was bactericidal at concentrations near the MIC.— H. Basch *et al.*, *Infect. & Immunity*, 1971, *4*, 44.

Absorption and Fate. Epicillin is readily absorbed from the gastro-intestinal tract. Peak plasma concentrations of 2 to 9 μg per ml have been reported 2 hours after a dose of 500 mg with a plasma half-life of about 60 minutes. From 10 to 30% may be bound to plasma proteins. Epicillin is excreted in the urine, about 30% of a dose being recovered, mainly unchanged, within 6 hours.

Pregnancy and the neonate. The diffusion of epicillin into amniotic fluid and breast milk.— T. W. Mischler *et al.*, *J. reprod. Med.*, 1978, *21*, 130.

Uses. Epicillin has actions and uses similar to those of ampicillin (see p.1091). It is administered by mouth in the treatment of susceptible infections in doses of 250 to 500 mg every 6 hours. Children weighing less than 20 kg may be given 25 to 100 mg per kg body-weight daily in divided doses. Epicillin sodium has been administered by intramuscular and intravenous injection.

A review of epicillin covering antibacterial activity, resistance, adverse effects, absorption and fate, and uses.— R. N. Brogden and G. S. Avery, *Drugs*, 1972, *3*, 314.

Good response to treatment with epicillin sodium 250 mg to 1 g every 6 hours by intravenous or intramuscular injection followed by epicillin by mouth in similar doses was observed in 47 of 50 patients with acute infective illnesses, including meningitis, typhoid fever, each in 1 patient, superficial infections in 4, respiratory-tract infections in 22, genito-urinary infections in 13 of 15, and gonorrhoea in 3 of 4. Total dosage was up to 56.5 g of epicillin. There was no evidence of undue pain due to injection. Phlebitis developed in 1 patient. A mild maculopapular rash occurred in 1 patient on the 2nd day and in another on the 10th day but the rashes cleared when epicillin was withdrawn. Slight nausea and looseness of stools were each reported in 1 patient.— B. M. Limson *et al.*, *Med. J. Aust.*, 1972, *2*, 1348. See also B. M. Limson *et al.*, *Clin. Med.*, 1974, *81* (June), 33.

Epicillin sodium was administered intramuscularly or intravenously to 34 patients with acute infections. Adults received 1 to 4 g daily and children 50 to 200 mg per kg body-weight. Good to excellent results were seen in 27. The only side-effect noted was pain at the site of injection in 1 patient.— B. D. Alora *et al.*, *Curr. ther. Res.*, 1972, *14*, 358.

In 62 children with bacteriologically-confirmed infections of the pharynx or middle ear, an excellent response was obtained in 55 and a good response in 7 after treatment with epicillin 250 mg four times daily for patients weighing 20 kg or more and 12.5 mg per kg body-weight four times daily for lighter patients, given for 5 to 9 days.— J. Alban, *Curr. ther. Res.*, 1974, *16*, 24.

Further references: J. E. Beck *et al.*, *Curr. ther. Res.*, 1971, *13*, 530; P. D. Reyes-Javier, *ibid.*, 602; D. W. Feeney *et al.*, *N.Z. med. J.*, 1972, *75*, 77.

Enteritis. Clinical and bacteriological cure was obtained in 29 of 33 patients with gastro-intestinal infections due to *Salmonella* or *Shigella* organisms which were treated with epicillin 500 mg thrice daily for 10 days. In 2 further patients *in vitro* tests showed organism resistance to epicillin, but 1 was cured on treatment. Side-effects were slight.— L. Landa, *Curr. ther. Res.*, 1971, *13*, 654.

Of 50 patients with acute enteric fever given epicillin 1 g every 6 hours by mouth, 43 responded well and were afebrile within 10 days. Treatment failure occurred in 6 and therapy was withdrawn in 1 due to the development of a severe urticarial rash.— A. Hassau *et al.*, *J. int. med. Res.*, 1977, *5*, 91.

Gonorrhoea. Epicillin 3.5 g with probenecid 1 g cured 114 of 117 patients with urogenital or rectal gonorrhoea. Unfortunately there was a high frequency of postgonococcal urethritis; it occurred in 31 of 68 men cured of urethral gonorrhoea.— E. Stolz *et al.*, *Dermatologica*, 1978, *157*, 254.

Further references: S. Öhman and J. Wallin, *Curr. ther. Res.*, 1975, *17*, 427.

Skin infections. Epicillin 500 mg every 12 hours for 5 to 14 days was given to 55 Egyptian patients aged 6 to 47 years with skin infections due to susceptible *Staphylococcus aureus* or *Streptococcus pyogenes*. There was a good to excellent response in 35 of 37 patients with impetigo, in 10 patients with ecthyma, and in 7 of 8 patients with folliculitis.— M. El-Zawahry *et al.*, *Br. J. Derm.*, 1976, *95*, 177.

Proprietary Names

Dexacilina (also as sodium salt) (*Squibb, Arg.*); Dexacillin (also as hydrochloride or sodium salt) (*Squibb, Austral.*; *Squibb, Belg.*; *Squibb, Ital.*); Dexacilline (*Squibb, Fr.*); Dex-Cillin (*Squibb, S.Afr.*); Florispec (also as sodium salt) (*Squibb, Neth.*); Omnisan (*SIFSA, Spain*); Spectacillin (also as sodium salt) (*Sandoz, Ger.*; *Sandoz, Switz.*).

77-1

Erythromycin *(B.P., B.P. Vet., Eur. P., U.S.P.).*

Erythromycinum; Eritromicina. Erythromycin A is (2*R*,3*S*,4*S*,5*R*,6*R*,8*R*,10*R*,11*R*,12*S*,13*R*) -3-(2,6-dideoxy-3-*C*,3-*O*-dimethyl-α-L-*ribo*-hexopyranosyloxy)-5-(3,4,6-trideoxy-3-dimethylamino-β-D-*xylo*-hexopyranosyloxy)-6,11,12-trihydroxy-2,4,6,8,10,12-hexamethyl-9-oxopentadecan-13-olide.

$C_{37}H_{67}NO_{13}$=733.9.

CAS — 114-07-8 (erythromycin A).

Pharmacopoeias. In *Belg.*, *Br.*, *Braz.*, *Cz.*, *Eur.*, *Fr.*, *Ger.*, *Ind.*, *Int.*, *It.*, *Jap.*, *Jug.*, *Neth.*, *Rus.*, *Swiss*, *Turk.*, and *U.S.*

Braz., *Ind.*, and *U.S.* specify not less than 85% of erythromycin, calculated with reference to the dried substance.

Erythromycin is an antimicrobial substance produced by the growth of certain strains of *Streptomyces erythreus* and is a mixture consisting largely of erythromycin A with lesser amounts of erythromycins B and C. It readily forms salts with inorganic and organic acids, and also forms esters.

It occurs as white or slightly yellow, odourless or almost odourless, slightly hygroscopic crystals or powder with a bitter taste, containing not more than 6.5% of water. The *B.P.* specifies not less than 920 units per mg and the *U.S.P.* not less than 850 μg per mg, both calculated on the anhydrous basis.

Soluble 1 in 1000 of water; less soluble at higher temperatures; soluble 1 in 5 of alcohol, 1 in 6 of chloroform, and 1 in 5 of ether; soluble in methyl alcohol and dilute hydrochloric acid. A solution in dehydrated alcohol is laevorotatory. A 0.067% solution in water has a pH of 8 to 10.5. It is stable in the dry state and solutions deteriorate only slowly at room temperature but more rapidly at 60° and above. **Store** below 30° in airtight containers. Protect from light.

The water solubility and bitterness of the salts of erythromycin were related to the size of the alkyl group attached to the acid used to prepare the salt. In addition, the bitterness was related to the stability of the salt. The stearyl sulphate salt was the least bitter.— P. H. Jones *et al.*, *J. pharm. Sci.*, 1969, *58*, 337.

Physical characterisation of erythromycin as anhydrate, monohydrate, and dihydrate crystalline solids. The anhydrate had the slowest dissolution rate and the dihydrate the fastest. Anhydrate crystals of erythromycin appeared to be the most stable form and their melting point of 190° to 193° was probably the true value for crystalline erythromycin base.— P. V. Allen *et al.*, *J. pharm. Sci.*, 1978, *67*, 1087.

Incompatibility. A precipitate was formed when erythromycin 250 mg was mixed with *chloramphenicol* 500 mg, *oxytetracycline hydrochloride* 250 mg, or *tetracycline hydrochloride* 500 mg in 1 litre of dextrose solution (5%).— H. R. Grant, *Hosp. Pharmst*, 1962, *15*, 67.

Erythromycin was very much less active against *Staphylococcus aureus* in the presence of *magnesium trisilicate*, *sodium alginate*, *pectin*, and *bentonite* and less active with *calamine*, *silica* (Aerosil), *methylcellulose*, *carmellose*, and *polysorbate 80*.— M. A. El-Nakeeb and R. T. Yousef, *Acta pharm. suec.*, 1968, *5*, 1.

Units. One unit of erythromycin is contained in 0.001087 mg of the second International Standard Preparation (1978) of erythromycin A base which contains 920 units per mg.

Adverse Effects. Gastro-intestinal disturbances are fairly common with erythromycin, especially with large doses, but serious side-effects are rare. Supra-infection following the oral administration of erythromycin is also rare, as is sensitisation to erythromycin; skin reactions have been reported. Reversible deafness has occurred after high doses of erythromycin.

Colitis. A report of pseudomembranous colitis associated with the administration of erythromycin ethylsuccinate.— N. M. Gantz *et al.*, *Ann. intern. Med.*, 1979, *91*, 866.

Hepatotoxicity. For reports of hepatotoxicity associated with erythromycin, see Erythromycin Estolate (p.1161), Erythromycin Ethylsuccinate (p.1162), and Erythromycin Propionate (p.1163).

Ototoxicity. Partial deafness developed in a woman after 4 days' therapy with erythromycin 4 g daily. When the dose was reduced to 2 g daily 3 days later her hearing returned to normal.— M. R. Eckman *et al.* (letter), *New Engl. J. Med.*, 1975, *292*, 649.

Reversible loss of hearing occurred in 2 patients, with uraemia and liver disease, given erythromycin 4 g daily by intravenous injection of the lactobionate; it was associated with very high blood concentrations of erythromycin.— G. V. Quinnan and W. R. McCabe (letter), *Lancet*, 1978, *1*, 1160. See also U. Mintz *et al.* (letter), *J. Am. med. Ass.*, 1973, *225*, 1122.

Administration of erythromycin stearate 500 mg four times daily to 2 patients on chronic intermittent dialysis caused reversible ototoxicity.— W. F. van Marion *et al.* (letter), *Lancet*, 1978, *2*, 214.

Further references to ototoxicity associated with the administration of erythromycin: W. Lornoy and J. Steyaert (letter), *Acta clin. belg.*, 1979, *34*, 111 (lactobionate); J. -P. Méry and A. Kanfer (letter), *New Engl. J. Med.*, 1979, *301*, 944; P. Thompson *et al.*, *J. Otolar.*, 1980, *9*, 60 (stearate).

Precautions. Erythromycin should not be used in patients with a known history of allergy to it and should be given with caution to patients with impaired liver function.

A study indicating that usual therapeutic doses of erythromycin interfere with colour vision.— J. Laroche and C. Laroche, *Annls pharm. fr.*, 1972, *30*, 433.

To avoid the ototoxicity of erythromycin in patients with renal failure it is suggested that the daily dosage should not exceed 1.5 g in patients with serum creatinine above 180 μmol per litre; hearing acuity should be tested before and during treatment, especially in the elderly; and erythromycin should not be given with other potentially ototoxic drugs.— J. -P. Méry and A. Kanfer (letter), *New Engl. J. Med.*, 1979, *301*, 944.

Interactions. Erythromycin might interfere with fluorimetric estimations of urinary catecholamines.— J. Millhouse, *Adverse Drug React. Bull.*, 1974, Dec 164.

For the effect of erythromycin on plasma-*theophylline* concentrations, see Aminophylline, p.343.

For the effect of erythromycin and other macrolide antibiotics on *carbamazepine*, see Carbamazepine, p.1246.

For a report of erythromycin enhancing the effect of *warfarin*, see Warfarin Sodium, p.779.

Antimicrobial Action. Erythromycin is a macrolide antibiotic which acts by interfering with bacterial protein synthesis and is bacteriostatic or bactericidal depending on its concentration and the type of organism. Activity increases with increases in pH up to about pH 8.5. Its range of antimicrobial action is similar to that of penicillin. It is active against most Gram-positive and some Gram-negative bacteria including *Neisseria* spp., *Haemophilus influenzae*, and *Bordetella pertussis*, against spirochaetes and some rickettsias and chlamydias. *Mycoplasma pneumoniae* is very sensitive to erythromycin; this is not so with *Mycoplasma hominis*. *Streptococcus pneumoniae* and haemolytic streptococci are highly sensitive but staphylococci (including those resistant to penicillin) are rather less sensitive. Although the Enterobacteriaceae are generally resistant to erythromycin, some strains of *Escherichia coli* and *Klebsiella* spp. have been reported to be sensitive at an alkaline pH. The Gram-negative bacterium responsible for legionnaires' disease and known as *Legionella pneumophila* is reported to be sensitive to erythromycin.

The minimum inhibitory concentrations of erythromycin for sensitive micro-organisms have been reported to range from less than 0.1 to about 2 μg per ml.

For a brief discussion on the macrolide group of antibiotics, see p.1084.

The susceptibility *in vitro* of 5 strains of *Mycoplasma pneumoniae* was tested to 21 antibiotics. Erythromycin was the most active followed by oleandomycin; streptomycin was also very active. The penicillins were inactive and cephaloridine, cephalothin sodium, and polymyxin B were effective only in concentrations which would preclude their clinical use. Demeclocycline hydrochloride and tetracycline were the most effective of the tetracyclines tested. Kanamycin and gentamicin were also effective. Only the efficacy of erythromycin was unaffected by inoculum size.— R. L. Jao and M. Finland, *Am. J. med. Sci.*, 1967, *253*, 639.

The sensitivity *in vitro* of 36 strains of *Bordetella pertussis* was tested to 9 antibiotics. Erythromycin was the most active. Lincomycin and cephalothin were least effective; ampicillin, chloramphenicol, kanamycin, and oxytetracycline had moderate activity; and benzylpenicillin and streptomycin were slightly less effective.— J. W. Bass *et al.*, *Am. J. Dis. Child.*, 1969, *117*, 276.

Claims that erythromycin and lincomycin were antagonistic were not confirmed when the two antibiotics were tested together against *E. coli*.— E. R. Garrett *et al.*, *J. pharm. Sci.*, 1970, *59*, 1448. A study on several interactions between erythromycin and lincomycin in *Streptococcus pyogenes*.— D. I. Annear, *J. med. Microbiol.*, 1978, *11*, 193.

Of 68 strains of *H. influenzae*, 34 were inhibited by erythromycin at a concentration of 0.06 μg per ml, 17 at 0.12 μg per ml, 13 at 0.25 μg per ml, and 4 at 0.5 μg per ml.— J. D. Williams and J. Andrews, *Br. med. J.*, 1974, *1*, 134. See also E. M. Ndawula and P. J. Sanderson (letter), *J. antimicrob. Chemother.*, 1980, *6*, 687.

Erythromycin was active *in vitro* against *Chlamydia trachomatis*,the MIC against 15 strains ranging from 0.1 to 0.5 μg per ml.— C. -C. Kuo *et al.*, *Antimicrob. Ag. Chemother.*, 1977, *12*, 80. See also H. J. Blackman *et al.*, *Antimicrob. Ag. Chemother.*, 1977, *12*, 673; C. K. Lee *et al.*, *Antimicrob. Ag. Chemother.*, 1978, *13*, 441.

Of 141 isolates of *Ureaplasma urealyticum* from patients with non-specific urethritis, 14 were resistant to oxytetracycline 600 ng per ml or minocycline 150 ng per ml. All the isolates were sensitive to erythromycin 80 ng per ml.— R. T. Evans and D. Taylor-Robinson, *J. antimicrob. Chemother.*, 1978, *4*, 57.

Erythromycin inhibited about 92, 98, and 100% of 517 of non-beta-lactamase-producing isolates of *Neisseria gonorrhoeae in vitro* at an MIC of 0.5, 1, and 2 μg per ml respectively. It inhibited about 39, 92, and 100% of 13 beta-lactamase-producing isolates at MICs of 0.5, 1, and 2 μg per ml.— J. R. Dillon *et al.* (letter), *J. antimicrob. Chemother.*, 1978, *4*, 477.

The causative organism in legionnaires' disease was reported to be sensitive to erythromycin.— J. S. Bennett (letter), *Can. med. Ass. J.*, 1978, *118*, 1031. The bacterium responsible for legionnaires' disease has been classified as a new species, *Legionella pneumophila*.— D. J. Brenner *et al.*, *Ann. intern. Med.*, 1979, *90*, 656. The mean MIC of erythromycin against 6 isolates of the legionnaires' disease bacterium was 0.18 μg per ml.— C. Thornsberry *et al.*, *Antimicrob. Ag. Chemother.*, 1978, *13*, 78.

Erythromycin and clindamycin were the most active of 21 antimicrobial agents tested *in vitro* against 56 strains of *Gardnerella vaginalis* (*Haemophilus vaginalis*); all strains were inhibited by 0.06 μg or less per ml.— L. R. McCarthy *et al.*, *Antimicrob. Ag. Chemother.*, 1979, *16*, 186.

For a report of the activity of cephamandole against strains of *Bacteroides fragilis* being increased more than 100-fold by erythromycin, see Cephamandole, p.1132.

For reports of clindamycin being more active than erythromycin against *Bacteroides fragilis*, see Clindamycin Hydrochloride, p.1145.

Diminished activity. For a report of various compounds decreasing the activity of erythromycin against *Staph. aureus*, see above under Incompatibility.

Enhanced activity. Synergism occurred against some strains of *Staphylococcus aureus* when the activity of erythromycin was tested *in vitro* with daunorubicin, mitomycin, or doxorubicin.— J. Y. Jacobs *et al.*, *Antimicrob. Ag. Chemother.*, 1979, *15*, 580.

For a report of the enhanced activity *in vitro* of erythromycin with gentamicin or colistin against strains of *Escherichia coli*, see Clindamycin Hydrochloride, p.1145.

Resistance. Though bacteria, especially staphylococci and streptococci, rapidly develop resistance to erythromycin *in vitro*, the development of resistant strains *in vivo* is not usually a serious clinical problem during successful short courses of treatment; during prolonged treatment of infections more difficult to eradicate, the development of resistant strains is common.

Cross-resistance occurs between erythromycin and the other macrolide antibiotics, lincomycin, and clindamycin. Week cross-resistance between erythromycin and chloramphenicol has been reported.

Resistance of campylobacter. A report from Sweden that about 10% of clinical isolates of *Campylobacter* spp. tested were highly resistant to erythromycin.— M. Walder and A. Forsgren (letter), *Lancet*, 1978, *2*, 1201. The incidence of resistance was much lower in Scotland (Edinburgh) W. A. T. Brunton *et al.* (letter), *ibid.*, 1385. Only 2 of 200 isolates of *Campylobacter jejuni* tested were resistant to erythromycin.— M. A. Karmali *et al.* (letter), *Can. med. Ass. J.*, 1980, *123*, 263.

Resistance of corynebacteria. Two strains of *Corynebacterium diphtheriae* isolated from skin lesions of 2 patients were resistant to erythromycin and lincomycin. The MICs were 1 and 2 mg per ml respectively.— C. H. Jellard and A. E. Lipinski (letter), *Lancet*, 1973, *1*, 156. See also M. B. Coyle *et al.*, *Antimicrob. Ag. Chemother.*, 1979, *16*, 525.

Resistance of pneumococci. Between January 1969 and September 1973, none of 4724 isolates of pneumococci were resistant to erythromycin whereas from October 1973 to December 1977, 64 of 8995 isolates were resistant. Of the 38 resistant strains isolated, 14 were also highly resistant to lincomycin and clindamycin.— J. M. S. Dixon and A. E. Lipinski, *Can. med. Ass. J.*, 1978, *119*, 1044. Of 866 strains of *Streptococcus pneumoniae* none was resistant to erythromycin.— A. J. Howard *et al.*, *Br. med. J.*, 1978, *1*, 1657.

Resistance of staphylococci. There was a decrease in the proportion of erythromycin-resistant *Staphylococcus aureus* isolated from burns in a hospital burns unit following the withdrawal of routine prophylaxis with erythromycin. Resistance to several other antibiotics also declined. Further use of erythromycin in the unit increased the numbers of resistant isolates which again fell when the use of erythromycin was discontinued.— H. A. Lilly and E. J. Lowbury, *J. antimicrob. Chemother.*, 1978, *4*, 545.

Further references: R. W. Lacey, *J. clin. Path.*, 1977, *30*, 602; J. O. Forfar, *Scott. med. J.*, 1977, *22*, 381.

Resistance of streptococci. Of 1176 strains of group A streptococci isolated in Japan in the period 1972 to 1974, 427 were resistant to tetracycline, chloramphenicol, erythromycin, oleandomycin, josamycin, midecamycin, and lincomycin. It was considered that because resistance to a single macrolide antibiotic was rare and that acquisition of resistance to tetracycline and/or chloramphenicol appeared to be a prerequisite for resistance to macrolide antibiotics, restriction of the use of tetracycline and chloramphenicol would lead to a decline in the frequency of macrolide-antibiotic resistance.— Y. Miyamoto *et al.*, *Antimicrob. Ag. Chemother.*, 1978, *13*, 399. See also M. Nakae *et al.*, *Antimicrob. Ag. Chemother.*, 1977, *12*, 427.

An *in vitro* study indicated that strains of *Str. faecalis* could transfer erythromycin-resistance to group A, B, and D streptococci. Large scale use of macrolide antibiotics and virginiamycin for growth promotion in animal husbandry could lead to a reservoir of macrolide-resistant group-D streptococci indigenous in animals which could transfer resistance to the virulent group A and group B streptococci.— J. D. A. van Embden *et al.* (letter), *Lancet*, 1978, *1*, 655.

Further references: K. Sprunt *et al.*, *Pediatrics*, 1970, *46*, 84; J. M. S. Dixon and A. E. Lipinski, *Antimicrob. Ag. Chemother.*, 1972, *1*, 333.

See also under Resistance of Pneumococci.

Absorption and Fate. Erythromycin is destroyed by gastric acid, and is usually administered either as base in enteric-coated tablets or as the more stable salts or esters. Food can interfere with the absorption of erythromycin so it is best taken 30 minutes or more before food. Plasma half-lives from 1.2 to 4 hours have been reported. A peak plasma-erythromycin concentration of about 0.5 μg per ml is achieved within 4 hours of a dose of 250 mg of the base. However, after 250 mg has been given every 6 hours for a few days, peak plasma concentrations of 1 to 2 μg per ml occur within 2 to 4 hours of a dose.

Erythromycin is widely distributed throughout body tissues and fluids with some retention in the liver and spleen. Diffusion into the aqueous, but not the vitreous humour of the eye has been reported to be good. Only low concentrations appear in cerebrospinal fluid unless the meninges are inflamed. Up to 20% of the maternal plasma concentration of erythromycin has been measured in the blood of the foetus; it appears in breast milk. Erythromycin is excreted in high concentrations in the bile and up to 5% of an oral dose appears in the urine; considerable amounts may also be inactivated in the body.

Intravenous administration causes higher but less sustained plasma concentrations and a greater degree of urinary excretion.

Some 18% of erythromycin in the circulation was bound to serum proteins. The half-life in serum was 1.4 hours and 15% was excreted in urine.— C. M. Kunin, *Ann. intern. Med.*, 1967, *67*, 151.

About 81% of erythromycin was bound to serum proteins when measured by ultrafiltration and about 84% when equilibrium dialysis was used.— R. G. Wiegand and A. H. C. Chun, *J. pharm. Sci.*, 1972, *61*, 425.

About 73% of erythromycin and 92.6% of erythromycin propionate was bound to serum proteins as measured by ultrafiltration with 100% serum and tube dilution. The low degree of protein-binding previously reported could have been due to measurements based only on tube dilution and not using whole serum.— R. C. Gordon *et al.*, *J. pharm. Sci.*, 1973, *62*, 1074.

Biliary excretion of erythromycin after parenteral administration.— P. Chelvan *et al.*, *Br. J. clin. Pharmac.*, 1979, *8*, 233.

Bioavailability. A review of the bioavailability of preparations of erythromycin base and the stearate.— C. H. Nightingale *et al.*, *J. Am. pharm. Ass.*, 1976, *NS16*, 203.

Diffusion. The antibiotic activity of erythromycin in synovial fluid was comparable with that in blood plasma.— *J. Am. med. Ass.*, 1968, *205*, (July 15), A34.

Uses. Erythromycin is used as an alternative to penicillin in the treatment of infections due to Gram-positive cocci, especially streptococci, in clostridial infections, and in those due to *Listeria monocytogenes*. In penicillin-sensitive patients it is given in place of penicillin in the prophylaxis of endocarditis and rheumatic fever and in the treatment of syphilis and gonorrhoea. *Haemophilus influenzae* is susceptible to erythromycin though in otitis media adequate inhibitory concentrations may not be achieved in the exudate.

Erythromycin is effective in the treatment of diphtheria and the carrier state and in the management of pertussis, when it may be used to render the patient non-infectious and is also given prophylactically to contacts. It is used in infections due to *Mycoplasma pneumoniae* and *Chlamydia trachomatis*, in legionnaires' disease, in intestinal amoebiasis, and, similarly to tetracycline, in the treatment of severe acne vulgaris.

An effective blood concentration for moderately severe infections in adults may be maintained by a dosage of 250 mg every 6 hours; for severe infections 2 to 4 g may be given daily. For children the dose is usually about 30 to 50 mg per kg body-weight daily although it may be doubled in severe infections. To avoid destruction by gastric juice, erythromycin is usually given as enteric-coated tablets, preferably on an empty stomach, as its absorption is delayed by the presence of food. It is also given as the estolate, ethylsuccinate, or stearate.

In the patient who is unable to take erythromycin by mouth and in severely ill patients in whom it is necessary to attain an immediate high blood concentration, erythromycin may be given intravenously in the form of one of its more soluble salts such as the lactobionate.

Erythromycin may also be given intramuscularly as a solution of erythromycin ethylsuccinate.

Reports and reviews on the actions and uses of erythromycin.— C. M. Ginsburg and H. F. Eichenwald, *J.*

Pediat., 1976, *89*, 872; R. W. Lacey, *Postgrad. med. J.*, 1977, *53*, 195; *Med. Lett.*, 1978, *20*, 94; *Curr. med. Res. Opinion*, 1978, *5*, *Suppl.* 2, 1–68; J. L. Straughan, *S. Afr. med. J.*, 1978, *53*, 527; M. W. McKendrick, *J. antimicrob. Chemother.*, 1979, *5*, 495; P. G. Welling, *ibid.*, 633; *Curr. med. Res. Opinion*, 1979, *6*, *Suppl.* 3, 1–66; *ibid.*, 1980, *6*, *Suppl.* 8, 1–109.

In a comparison of erythromycin salts in aqueous suspensions used for 10-day courses in the treatment of acute β-haemolytic streptococcal pharyngitis in 110 children, there were relapses within 21 days in 7 of 58 children treated with erythromycin stearate and in 1 of 52 children treated with erythromycin estolate in equivalent doses.— D. C. Ryan *et al.*, *Med. J. Aust.*, 1973, *1*, 20. The above study was considered lacking in fundamental safeguards since the rate of defaulting in the taking of doses was not known and no measures were taken to avoid re-infection of patients.— A. McLeay and P. Cooke (letter), *ibid.*, 213.

A report of 6 patients with infections due to *Corynebacterium bovis*, an organism mainly affecting *cows* and dairy produce. A wide range of antibiotics was effective in sensitivity tests. As some ampicillin resistance was observed, erythromycin was considered an appropriate antibiotic for the treatment of infections due to this organism.— J. A. Vale and G. W. Scott, *Lancet*, 1977, *2*, 682.

Erythromycin stearate was significantly more effective than rosaramicin in reducing carrier-rates in a study involving 87 nasal carriers of *Staphylococcus aureus* and both were more effective than a placebo when given in doses of 1 g daily for 7 days. Carrier-rates increased towards the original values in both antibiotic-treated groups once therapy was stopped.— S. Z. Wilson *et al.*, *Antimicrob. Ag. Chemother.*, 1979, *15*, 379.

Q fever in 5 patients (diagnosed retrospectively) responded promptly to treatment with erythromycin lactobionate intravenously.— L. J. D'Angelo and R. Hetherington, *Br. med. J.*, 1979, *2*, 305.

Administration, rectal. A report of the successful use of erythromycin suppositories in a patient who had undergone an almost total small bowel resection. Suppositories of erythromycin base in Witepsol H15 were prepared; a displacement value of 3.7 was calculated for erythromycin. Adequate serum concentrations were achieved by the insertion four times daily of two 4-g suppositories, each containing 1 g of erythromycin.— S. Hall and S. Potter (letter), *Pharm. J.*, 1981, *2*, 115.

Amoebiasis. *For reports of the use of erythromycin in the treatment of amoebiasis, see Martindale 27th Edn*, p.1134.

Anaerobic infections. Erythromycin was effective in 14 of 17 patients with anaerobic infections.— E. J. C. Goldstein *et al.*, *J. Am. med. Ass.*, 1979, *242*, 435.

Bronchitis. Erythromycin or ampicillin 500 mg four times daily were equally effective in the treatment of infective exacerbations of chronic bronchitis. Side-effects were less frequent with erythromycin.— R. F. Willey *et al.*, *Br. J. Dis. Chest*, 1978, *72*, 13.

Campylobacter infections. A premature infant born to a woman suffering from campylobacter diarrhoea was given gentamicin parenterally to prevent invasive infection. On the fifth postnatal day the infant's intestine was infected with campylobacter, and erythromycin stearate 20 mg every eight hours by mouth was started, the gentamicin being stopped the following day. Subsequent faecal specimens did not yield campylobacter, and the erythromycin was stopped after 5 days. It was considered that the parenteral gentamicin may have prevented the development of symptoms and possibly invasive infection while permitting intestinal multiplication. It was presumed that the rapid disappearance of the campylobacter after starting oral therapy was due to the erythromycin, which is accordingly recommended from birth in such situations.— S. L. Mawer and B. A. M. Smith (letter), *Lancet*, 1979, *1*, 1041.

Further references: M. B. Skirrow, *Br. med. J.*, 1977, *2*, 9; C. D. Ribeiro (letter), *Lancet*, 1978, *2*, 270; S. G. Boyd and J. M. Murdoch (letter), *J. antimicrob. Chemother.*, 1979, *5*, 728.

Chlamydial infections. Erythromycin was recommended instead of a tetracycline for the treatment of chlamydial infections in pregnant or lactating women or in young children.— *Drug & Ther. Bull.*, 1978, *16*, 37.

A report of a man with chronic non-bacterial prostatitis which could have been a manifestation of delayed hypersensitivity to *Chlamydia trachomatis*. He was treated with erythromycin stearate 500 mg every 6 hours for 5½ months; he experienced acute exacerbation of symptoms after 3 weeks, which subsided after 2 weeks, and subsequently his symptoms improved. His wife was given erythromycin for 3 weeks.— R. C. Ballard *et al.* (letter), *Lancet*, 1979, *2*, 1305.

For further reports and reviews, see also under Tetracycline Hydrochloride, p.1220.

See also under Trachoma, below.

Diphtheria. In a comparison in 294 subjects between a single injection of benzathine penicillin and a 7-day course of clindamycin or erythromycin by mouth, erythromycin was recommended as the drug of choice for the treatment of diphtheria carriers.— R. V. McCloskey *et al.*, *Ann. intern. Med.*, 1974, *81*, 788. Bacteriological follow-up should be carried out 2 weeks after completing treatment with erythromycin or penicillin.— L. W. Miller *et al.*, *Antimicrob. Ag. Chemother.*, 1974, *6*, 166.

The successful use of erythromycin with diphtheria antitoxin to treat a 10-week-old child with a toxigenic strain of *Corynebacterium diphtheriae mitis*. Carriers were also treated with erythromycin.— L. E. Simmons *et al.*, *Lancet*, 1980, *1*, 304.

Dosage in renal failure. The normal half-life for erythromycin of 1.2 to 2.6 hours was increased to 4 to 6 hours in end-stage renal failure. It could be given in usual doses to patients with renal failure.— W. M. Bennett *et al.*, *Ann. intern. Med.*, 1977, *86*, 754. See also *idem*, 1980, *93*, 62. Erythromycin was reported not to be dialysable.— J. S. Cheigh, *Am. J. Med.*, 1977, *62*, 555.

Data for predicting removal of erythromycin by conventional haemodialysis.— T. P. Gibson and H. A. Nelson, *Clin. Pharmacokinet.*, 1977, *2*, 403.

Further references: P. G. Welling and W. A. Craig, *J. pharm. Sci.*, 1978, *67*, 1057.

See also under Precautions (above).

Endocarditis prophylaxis. A warning that the oral flora of patients on short-term or long-term erythromycin therapy contains *Streptococcus viridans* resistant to serum concentrations of erythromycin attainable with the recommended bacterial endocarditis regimen [see p.1080].— K. Bromberg *et al.* (letter), *Ann. intern. Med.*, 1980, *93*, 931.

Gonorrhoea. Erythromycin was not considered to be an effective treatment alternative for pregnant women with gonorrhoea who were allergic to penicillin.— S. T. Brown *et al.*, *J. Am. med. Ass.*, 1977, *238*, 1371.

The US Public Health Service recommended erythromycin 500 mg four times daily for 7 days as one regimen for the treatment of disseminated gonococcal infection. In neonatal gonococcal ophthalmia, erythromycin eye ointment or eye-drops could be used prophylactically but for treatment penicillin must be given systemically.— *Morb. Mortal.*, 1979, *28*, 13.

Legionnaires' disease. A discussion of legionnaires' disease. Treatment with antibiotics, primarily erythromycin, is thought to be of value in most cases; it seems to have little effect on the early progressive and potentially fatal disease.— *Br. med. J.*, 1980, *280*, 591. See also A. C. Miller, *J. antimicrob. Chemother.*, 1981, *7*, 217.

Erythromycin was recommended for the treatment of legionnaires' disease at a suggested dose of 0.5 to 1 g every 6 hours for adults and 15 mg per kg body-weight every 6 hours for children other than neonates.— Center for Disease Control, *Ann. intern. Med.*, 1978, *88*, 363.

Two renal transplant patients who contracted legionnaires' disease, responded to a high dosage of erythromycin, starting with 1.2 g intravenously every 6 hours.— J. O'H. Tobin *et al.*, *Lancet*, 1980, *2*, 118.

A report of legionnaires' disease in a 6-month-old infant. She recovered rapidly on erythromycin 250 mg every 6 hours by mouth.— R. M. Simpson *et al.* (letter), *Lancet*, 1980, *2*, 740.

A description, based on 16 cases of distinctive neurological findings associated with legionnaires' disease. Erythromycin is the drug of choice but where response is poor the addition of rifampicin is recommended.— D. H. Kennedy *et al.* (letter), *Lancet*, 1981, *1*, 940.

Otitis media. In a study of 81 children with otitis media due to *Haemophilus influenzae*, erythromycin ethylsuccinate equivalent to erythromycin 50 mg per kg body-weight daily combined with trisulphapyrimidines [sulphadiazine, sulphamerazine, and sulphadimidine in equal parts] 150 mg per kg daily was significantly more effective than erythromycin used alone. However, there was no significant difference in the results obtained with ampicillin 50 to 60 mg per kg daily and those achieved with either the combined regimen or erythromycin alone.— S. H. Sell *et al.*, *Sth. med. J.*, 1978, *71*, 1493.

Pertussis. A discussion on the use of erythromycin and other antimicrobial agents in the treatment and prevention of pertussis.— H. Lambert, *J. antimicrob. Chemother.*, 1979, *5*, 329.

Prophylaxis. Erythromycin 1 to 1.5 g daily for 14 days was effective in the prophylaxis of pertussis in hospital staff; symptoms developed in only 1 of 8 patients who became infected after prophylaxis. Since chemoprophylaxis was considered to be a temporary measure pertussis vaccine was evaluated in other members of the staff.— C. C. Linnemann *et al.*, *Lancet*, 1975, *2*, 540.

Erythromycin 50 mg per kg body-weight was given intramuscularly each day for 5 days to 7 infants in contact with an index case infected with *Bordetella pertussis*. Two of the infants had positive cultures for the organism but showed no symptoms and 2 days after treatment started, cultures were negative. None of the other 5 babies developed symptoms or infection.— W. A. Altemeier and E. M. Ayoub, *Pediatrics*, 1977, *59*, 623.

Erythromycin, 25 mg per kg body-weight daily for 14 days, eliminated *Bordetella pertussis* from the respiratory tract. It could be given to unvaccinated children and infants to prevent transmission within a family.— A. G. Ironside (letter), *Br. med. J.*, 1979, *1*, 619.

Reports of the failure of prophylaxis with erythromycin for pertussis contacts in the community.— P. R. Grob (letter), *Lancet*, 1981, *1*, 772; M. Spencely and H. P. Lambert (letter), *ibid.*

Further references: S. Ware (letter), *Lancet*, 1977, *2*, 872; G. C. Arneil and T. A. McAllister, *Practitioner*, 1977, *219*, 855; *Br. med. J.*, 1978, *1*, 1007; L. J. Baraff *et al.*, *Pediatrics*, 1978, *61*, 224.

Relapsing fever, louse-borne. For a study concluding that the treatment of choice was a single 500-mg dose of tetracycline or erythromycin by mouth, see Tetracycline Hydrochloride, p.1222.

Skin disorders. Erythrasma, caused by *Corynebacterium minutissimum*, responded to treatment with erythromycin 250 mg four times a day for 14 days. Tetracyclines were also effective.— O. L. S. Scott and M. L. Johnson, *Practitioner*, 1969, *202*, 37.

In 72 patients with impetigo, *Staphylococcus aureus* was isolated from 87%. Forty-one patients with widespread impetigo or with lesions of the scalp or beard area were treated for 7 days systemically with erythromycin ethylsuccinate 250 mg six-hourly or 40 mg per kg body-weight daily for children. Of 39 seen 4 weeks later 7 had recurrences; of these, 5 had familial contacts with impetigo or the offending organism.— B. L. Connor, *Br. J. Derm.*, 1972, *87*, *Suppl.* 8, 48.

Erythromycin applied topically in a concentration of 2% was effective in reducing inflammatory lesions in 10 patients with acne. It was less effective in reducing comedones.— J. E. Fulton and G. Pablo, *Archs Derm.*, 1974, *110*, 83.

In a double-blind placebo-controlled study of 69 patients with grade II or III acne a 2% solution of erythromycin offered little therapeutic benefit.— R. A. Prince *et al.*, *Drug Intell. & clin. Pharm.*, 1981, *15*, 372.

Further references to the topical use of erythromycin: M. W. Greaves, *Practitioner*, 1976, *217*, 585; R. L. Dobson and B. S. Belknap, *J. Am. Acad. Derm.*, 1980, *3*, 478; C. L. Feucht *et al.*, *ibid.*, 483; A. A. Fisher, *Cutis*, 1980, *25*, 474; L. Rivkin and M. Rapaport, *ibid.*, 552.

References to the systemic use of erythromycin in the treatment of acne: *Archs Derm.*, 1975, *111*, 1630; R. Marks, *Practitioner*, 1977, *219*, 840; L. Hellgren and J. Vincent, *Dermatologica*, 1978, *156*, 105.

See also under Tetracycline Hydrochloride, p.1222.

Surgical infection prophylaxis. Reference to the prophylactic use of neomycin and erythromycin base before colonic surgery.— J. S. Clarke *et al.*, *Ann. Surg.*, 1977, *186*, 251. The wound infection rate was reduced from 25% to 5% when metronidazole were substituted for erythromycin.— C. Brass *et al.*, *Am. J. Surg.*, 1978, *135*, 91.

For a report of surgical infection prophylaxis with neomycin and erythromycin being less effective than prophylaxis with neomycin and metronidazole, see Neomycin Sulphate, p.1190.

Syphilis. Erythromycin in doses of 3 g daily for 10 days was more effective for the treatment of early syphilis than in doses of 2 g daily for 10 days, and as effective as tetracycline 3 g daily for 10 days, and benzathine penicillin 1.8 g as a single injection.— A. L. Schroeter *et al.*, *J. Am. med. Ass.*, 1972, *221*, 471.

The US Public Health Service recommended erythromycin 500 mg taken four times daily for 15 days as one regimen for the treatment of early syphilis in patients who were allergic to penicillin.— *Obstet. Gynec.*, 1976, *48*, 727.

Trachoma. Topical treatment of neonatal ocular chlamydial infection with topical antibiotics alone was inadequate. Since tetracyclines could not be used systemically in babies owing to possible damage to bones and teeth, erythromycin 30 mg per kg body-weight [daily] given for 21 days together with application of chlortetracycline eye-ointment had been very effective in over 20 cases.— G. L. Ridgway and J. D. Oriel (letter), *New Engl. J. Med.*, 1977, *297*, 512. See also G. L. Ridgway, *Archs Dis. Childh.*, 1978, *53*, 447.

The prophylactic application of 1% erythromycin eye ointment prevented chlamydial conjunctivitis in infants born to women infected with *Chlamydia trachomatis* but did not prevent respiratory infection.— M. R. Hammerschlag *et al.*, *J. Am. med. Ass.*, 1980, *244*, 2291.

Further references: M. L. Tarizzo and R. Nataf, *Revue int. Trachome*, 1969-70, *46*, 7.

Urinary-tract infections. Reports of inferior results with erythromycin when compared with tetracyclines in the treatment of non-gonococcal urethritis.— R. R. Willcox, *Br. J. vener. Dis.*, 1968, *44*, 157; G. W. Csonka and R. J. Spitzer, *Br. J. vener. Dis.*, 1969, *45*, 52.

Treatment with erythromycin estolate 500 mg or 1 g thrice daily for 14 days in conjunction with sodium bicarbonate 18 g daily to render the urine alkaline eliminated the infecting Gram-negative bacteria from the urine of 27 of the 37 patients with chronic bacteriuria. Five of the 10 patients who did not respond had taken the treatment irregularly. After 3 weeks 17 patients were culture-negative. At further follow-up 14 of 15 patients had negative urine cultures from 2 to 6 months later and of the 7 followed for 6 to 24 months 6 remained negative.— S. H. Zinner *et al.*, *Lancet*, 1971, *1*, 1267. See also J. Klastersky *et al.*, *Curr. ther. Res.*, 1971, *13*, 427.

Of 32 men with non-specific urethritis, ureaplasmas were isolated from 6 and chlamydias from 5 of 19 investigated for this organism. Two further patients had both ureaplasmas and chlamydias. After treatment with erythromycin stearate 500 mg four times daily for 14 days ureaplasmas had cleared in all 6 and chlamydias had cleared in 3 of the 5 previously positive patients. Of the 2 patients with a double infection 1 was completely cleared and 1 was still ureaplasma positive. All but 1 of the remaining patients with symptoms present but cultures negative had symptoms alleviated by erythromycin therapy.— C. Rana *et al.*, *Med. J. Aust.*, 1978, *1*, 409. Unless the presence of gonococci had been excluded, tetracycline and not erythromycin should be used for the treatment of non-specific urethritis.— L. Kowal (letter), *ibid.*, 1978, *2*, 30.

For a review of the treatment of nongonococcal urethritis, see Tetracycline Hydrochloride, p.1222.

Vaginitis. In a preliminary study erythromycin was not effective for the treatment of vaginitis associated with *Gardnerella vaginalis* (*Haemophilus vaginalis*).— M. A. Durfee *et al.*, *Antimicrob. Ag. Chemother.*, 1979, *16*, 635.

Preparations

Erythromycin Ointment *(U.S.P.)*. Erythromycin 10 mg per g in a suitable ointment basis.

Erythromycin Ophthalmic Ointment *(U.S.P.)*. A sterile eye ointment containing erythromycin 5 mg per g in a suitable basis.

Erythromycin Tablets *(B.P.)*. Tablets containing erythromycin. They are enteric-coated and either film- or sugar-coated.

Erythromycin Tablets *(U.S.P.)*. Tablets containing erythromycin 250 or 500 mg or, if enteric-coated, 100 or 250 mg.

Proprietary Preparations

Erycen *(Berk Pharmaceuticals, UK)*. Erythromycin, available as enteric-coated tablets of 250 mg.

Erythromid *(Abbott, UK)*. Erythromycin, available as enteric-coated tablets of 250 mg. (Also available as Erythromid in *Canad.*).

Ilotycin *(Lilly, UK)*. Erythromycin, available as tablets of 250 mg. (Also available as Ilotycin in *Canad.*, *Neth.*, *Switz.*, *USA*).

Retcin *(DDSA Pharmaceuticals, UK)*. Erythromycin,available as enteric-coated tablets of 250 mg.

Other Proprietary Names

Arg.— Emu-Ve, Oftalmolets, Pantomicina (see also Erythromycin Ethylsuccinate); *Austral.*— Bram-mycin, Emu-V, Eratrex, Eryc, Ilocap; *Belg.*— Emu-V; *Canad.*— E-Mycin (see also Erythromycin Stearate); *Fr.*— Abboticine (see also Erythromycin Ethylsuccinate and Erythromycin Stearate); *Ger.*— Erycinum (see also Erythromycin Gluceptate), Paediathrocin (see also Erythromycin Ethylsuccinate); *Ital.*— Iloticina, Proterytrin (see also Erythromycin Estolate, Erythromycin Ethylsuccinate, and Erythromycin Lactobionate); *S.Afr.*— Biorythrin, Emu-V; *Spain*— Endoeritrin, Orizina, Pantomicina; *USA*— E-Mycin (see also Erythromycin Stearate), Robimycin.

78-y

Erythromycin Estolate *(B.P., U.S.P.)*. Erythromycin Propionate Lauryl Sulphate; Propionyl Erythromycin Lauryl Sulphate. Erythromycin 2′-propionate dodecyl sulphate.

$C_{40}H_{71}NO_{14},C_{12}H_{26}O_4S = 1056.4$.

CAS — 3521-62-8.

Pharmacopoeias. In *Br.*, *Cz.*, *Jug.*, and *U.S.*

A white, odourless or almost odourless, almost tasteless, crystalline powder containing not less than 610 units per mg. Erythromycin estolate 1.44 g is approximately equivalent to 1 g of erythromycin. Practically **insoluble** in water; soluble 1 in 2 of alcohol, 1 in 10 of chloroform, and 1 in 15 of acetone; practically insoluble in dilute hydrochloric acid. A saturated solution in water has a pH of 4.5 to 7. **Store** in airtight containers. Protect from light.

A study indicating that erythromycin estolate could exist in both crystalline and amorphous states, as well as an intermediate phase.— J. Piccolo, *Can. J. pharm. Sci.*, 1979, *14*, 99.

Adverse Effects. As for Erythromycin, p.1158. Signs of liver damage consisting of upper abdominal pain, fever, liver enlargement, eosinophilia, raised serum bilirubin, and changes in other liver-function tests indicative of cholestasis, and jaundice (reversible on discontinuing treatment) have been reported in patients receiving erythromycin estolate for more than 10 days or immediately on starting a second course. These hepatotoxic effects appear to be limited almost entirely to adult patients.

In one year there were 6 cases of infantile hypertrophic pyloric stenosis out of an infant population of 963; 5 of these cases were attributed to erythromycin estolate given in a daily dose of 40 mg per kg body-weight. Vomiting began within 48 hours of starting erythromycin estolate in all 5 children and their condition deteriorated despite subsequent withdrawal of the antibiotic. Surgical treatment was required and a pyloric mass was confirmed in each of the 5 infants.— J. A. Sanfilippo, *J. pediat. Surg.*, 1976, *11*, 177.

Hepatotoxicity. The Committee on Safety of Medicines reported in Adverse Reaction Leaflet No. 10 that it had received 41 reports of jaundice associated with erythromycin, 40 of which related to erythromycin estolate. The jaundice usually lasted for 1 or 2 weeks and was reversible after the antibiotic was withdrawn. There were no fatalities. The Committee was not able to advise whether the risk of jaundice with erythromycin estolate was offset by greater efficacy.— *Pharm. J.*, 1973, *2*, 59.

Up to May 1973 the Australian Drug Evaluation Committee had received 113 reports of jaundice or cholestasis associated with erythromycin estolate; only 2 of these dealt with children under the age of 6 years. Since the Committee did not consider that the estolate was more effective than other forms of erythromycin, its use, apart from the low-dose paediatric formulations, should be restricted.— *Med. J. Aust.*, 1973, *2*, 192.

Studies with various substituted erythromycin preparations in a subject who had experienced a hepatotoxic reaction with erythromycin estolate demonstrated that the hepatotoxicity was associated with the propionyl group.— K. G. Tolman *et al.*, *Ann. intern. Med.*, 1974, *81*, 58.

A report of hepatotoxicity in a 7-year-old boy given erythromycin estolate.— J. D. Lloyd-Still *et al.*, *Am. J. Dis. Child.*, 1978, *132*, 320.

A report of complete biliary obstruction in a 6-week-old infant associated with the administration of erythromycin estolate.— D. Krowchuk and J. H. Seashore, *Pediatrics*, 1979, *64*, 956.

The FDA was beginning procedures for the removal from the market of solid dosage forms of erythromycin estolate because of a greater risk of hepatotoxicity than that associated with other forms of erythromycin.— *FDA Drug Bull.*, 1979, *9*, 26.

Further references: L. G. Cacace *et al.*, *Drug Intell. & clin. Pharm.*, 1977, *11*, 22; B. Young and W. R. Bartle, *Can. pharm. J.*, 1977, *110*, 423; B. G. Rowsell, *Can. pharm. J.*, 1978, *111*, 112; U. Gafter *et al.*, *N.Y. St. J. Med.*, 1979, *79*, 87.

Precautions. Erythromycin estolate should not be given to patients with impaired liver function or to patients who have developed jaundice or other symptoms of liver toxicity during previous treatment with erythromycin estolate. A second course of treatment with this ester should be given with caution.

It should not be used in patients with a known history of allergy to erythromycin.

Seven young men without evidence of jaundice or oedema were each given 1 g of erythromycin estolate 8-hourly for 4 doses, in each of 2 cycles of treatment 6 days apart. During 1 cycle they also took either sodium bicarbonate 18 g or acetazolamide 500 mg daily. All subjects apparently showed transient and sometimes marked elevations of serum aspartate aminotransferase (SGOT) values. The results were found to be due to a false positive colorimetric reaction, attributed to an unidentified trypsin-stable substance in the blood, possibly a metabolite of the antibiotic. Despite this finding, the authors stressed, any apparent rise in SGOT should not be disregarded during erythromycin estolate therapy, where real elevations of SGOT values had been demonstrated.— L. D. Sabath *et al.*, *New Engl. J. Med.*, 1968, *279*, 1137.

Pregnancy and the neonate. Of 298 pregnant women who took erythromycin estolate, clindamycin, or placebo for 3 weeks or longer, about 14, 4, and 3% respectively had abnormally high serum aspartate aminotransferase (SGOT) values. Erythromycin estolate should probably not be given to pregnant women.— W. M. McCormack *et al.*, *Antimicrob. Ag. Chemother.*, 1977, *12*, 630.

Absorption and Fate. Erythromycin estolate is more stable than the free base to the acid of gastric juice; following administration by mouth, it is rapidly absorbed, whether given in the fasting state or with food, and appears in the blood as erythromycin base or as erythromycin propionate which hydrolyses to erythromycin. It is not clear whether the circulating concentrations of active base produced by erythromycin estolate are higher than those from other preparations though it appears that this may be so.

A detailed study *in vitro* of the antibacterial activity of 2′-esters of erythromycin suggested that they were only active when hydrolysed to erythromycin.— P. L. Tardrew *et al.*, *Abbott, USA*, *Appl. Microbiol.*, 1969, *18*, 159.

Serum concentrations of erythromycin were very variable in 20 subjects given the estolate by mouth; mean concentrations 4 hours after a dose of 250 mg were 0.71 μg per ml in 8 men and 0.56 μg per ml in 12 women. The variability was attributed to the fact that erythromycin was distributed through total body-water and the amount absorbed appeared to be in direct proportion to body-weight.— B. Lake and S. M. Bell, *Med. J. Aust.*, 1969, *1*, 449.

A bioavailability study on preparations of erythromycin estolate.— R. Dugal *et al.*, *Can. J. pharm. Sci.*, 1976, *11*, 92.

In 28 children given single and multiple doses of erythromycin estolate or ethylsuccinate, higher concentrations of erythromycin were achieved in both serum and tonsils after the estolate.— C. M. Ginsburg *et al.*, *J. Pediat.*, 1976, *89*, 1011. See also L. D. Bechtol *et al.*, *Curr. ther. Res.*, 1976, *20*, 610; *idem*, 1981, *29*, 52; P. Patamasucon *et al.*, *Antimicrob. Ag. Chemother.*, 1981, *19*, 736.

In 10 healthy subjects higher plasma concentrations of total antibiotic were achieved with erythromycin estolate than with equivalent doses of the stearate but concentrations of free base were lower although more consistent. Increased absorption occurred with the estolate in the presence of food whereas the absorption of stearate was reduced.— P. G. Welling *et al.*, *J. pharm. Sci.*, 1979, *68*, 150. Single-dose studies in healthy subjects indicated that absorption of erythromycin estolate (as capsules) was enhanced after food compared to that after a 12-hour fast. Food had little effect on the bioavailability of erythromycin ethylsuccinate suspension or enteric-coated erythromycin tablets.— L. D. Bechtol *et al.*, *Curr. ther. Res.*, 1979, *25*, 618.

Further references to comparative bioavailability studies of erythromycin estolate and other erythromycin preparations: A. R. DiSanto *et al.*, *J. clin. Pharmac.*, 1980, *20*, 437 (estolate and erythromycin base); J. Henry *et al., Postgrad. med. J.*, 1980, *55*, 707 (estolate, propionate, and stearate); G. J. Yakatan *et al., J. clin. Pharmac.*, 1980, *20*, 625 (estolate, stearate, and erythromycin base).

For a comparison with erythromycin stearate, see Erythromycin Stearate, p.1163.

Uses. Erythromycin estolate has the actions and uses of erythromycin (see p.1158) and is administered by mouth in capsules or tablets or as an aqueous suspension in similar doses.

Preparations

Erythromycin Estolate Capsules *(B.P.)*. Capsules containing erythromycin estolate. Potency is expressed in terms of the equivalent amount of erythromycin. Store at a temperature not exceeding 30°.

Erythromycin Estolate Capsules *(U.S.P.)*. Capsules containing erythromycin estolate equivalent to 125 or 250 mg of erythromycin. Store in airtight containers.

Erythromycin Estolate for Oral Suspension *(U.S.P.)*. A dry mixture of erythromycin estolate with one or more suitable buffers, diluents, colouring, flavouring, and dispersing agents. Store in airtight containers. The suspension is prepared by the addition of diluent before issue and contains the equivalent of 25 mg of erythromycin per ml or (pediatric drops) 100 mg per ml. pH 5 to 7 or (pediatric drops) 5 to 5.5.

Erythromycin Estolate Oral Suspension *(U.S.P.)*. A suspension of erythromycin estolate with one or more suitable buffers, diluents, colouring, flavouring, and dispersing agents. It contains the equivalent of 25, 50 or 100 mg of erythromycin per ml. Store at a temperature not exceeding 8° in airtight containers. pH 3.5 to 6.5.

Erythromycin Estolate Tablets *(U.S.P.)*. Tablets containing erythromycin estolate equivalent to 125 or 250 mg (chewable tablets) or 500 mg of erythromycin. Store in airtight containers.

Proprietary Preparations

Ilosone *(Dista, UK)*. Erythromycin estolate, available as **Capsules** each containing the equivalent of 250 mg of erythromycin base; as **Suspension 125 mg** containing the equivalent of 125 mg of erythromycin in each 5 ml (suggested diluent, syrup); as **Suspension Forte** containing the equivalent of 250 mg of erythromycin in each 5 ml; and as **Tablets** each containing the equivalent of 500 mg of erythromycin. (Also available as Ilosone in *Austral., Belg., Canad., Ital., S.Afr., Switz., USA*).

Other Proprietary Names

Austral.—Eromycin; *Canad.*—Novorythro *(see also* Erythromycin Stearate*)*; *Fr.*—Propiocine Enfant; *Ger.*—Neo-Erycinum, Togiren; *Ital.*—Erimec, Eritrobios, Eritrobiotic, Eritroger, Estomicina, Manilina, Marocid, Mistral, Proterytrin *(see also* Erythromycin, Erythromycin Ethylsuccinate, and Erythromycin Lactobionate*)*, Roxochemil, Stellamicina *(see also* Erythromycin Lactobionate*)*; *Jap.*—Taimoxin; *S.Afr.*—Purmycin; *Spain*—Dreimicina, Eritro-Wolf, Eritrocin, Eritroveinte, Espimina, Neo-Iloticina; *Switz.*—Cimetrin.

79-j

Erythromycin Ethyl Carbonate *(B.P.C. 1968)*. Erythromycin Ethylcarbonate. Erythromycin 2′-(ethylcarbonate).

$C_{40}H_{71}NO_{15}$=806.0.

CAS — 7218-80-6.

A white, odourless, crystalline powder with a less bitter taste than erythromycin. It contains not less than 775 units per mg. Erythromycin ethyl carbonate 1.1 g is approximately equivalent to 1 g of erythromycin. Slightly **soluble** in water and cyclohexane; soluble 1 in 10 of alcohol, 1 in 8 of chloroform, and 1 in 35 of ether; freely soluble in acetone, dioxan, and methyl alcohol. A 20% suspension in water has a pH of 6.3 to 8.

Erythromycin ethyl carbonate has the actions and uses of erythromycin (see p.1158) and was formerly used for the preparation of flavoured suspensions for oral administration.

80-q

Erythromycin Ethylsuccinate *(U.S.P.)*.

Erythromycin 2′-(ethylsuccinate).

$C_{43}H_{75}NO_{16}$=862.1.

CAS — 1264-62-6.

Pharmacopoeias. In *Jap.* and *U.S.*

A white or slightly yellow, odourless or almost odourless, almost tasteless, crystalline powder. Erythromycin ethylsuccinate 1.17 g is approximately equivalent to 1 g of erythromycin. Very slightly **soluble** in water; freely soluble in alcohol, chloroform, and liquid macrogols. A 1% suspension in water has a pH of 6 to 8.5. **Incompatible** with ampicillin sodium and cloxacillin sodium. **Store** in airtight containers.

The effect of sodium carboxymethylcellulose, bentonite, and agar on bioavailability of erythromycin ethylsuccinate from mixtures.— P. Kahela *et al., Drug Dev. ind. Pharm.*, 1978, *4*, 261.

Erythromycin ethylsuccinate has the actions and uses of erythromycin (see p.1158) and is administered by mouth in tablets or as a suspension in similar doses. It is also given by deep intramuscular injection as a solution in a liquid macrogol with butyl aminobenzoate and benzyl alcohol; the addition of water to such solutions causes a precipitate to form, so that they cannot be administered by the intravenous or subcutaneous routes. Adults may be given the equivalent of 100 mg of erythromycin intramuscularly every 4 to 8 hours but in severe infections intravenous injection of the lactobionate is preferred. Intramuscular injections are not recommended for children.

In 18 children aged 6 to 23 months given erythromycin ethylsuccinate 40 to 50 mg per kg body-weight daily the mean serum concentration was about 3.05 µg per ml after 1½ hours when given with food and 1.51 µg per ml after 1 hour when fasting. Fasting serum concentrations were comparable to those found in adults receiving therapeutic doses.— T. C. Coyne *et al., J. clin. Pharmac.*, 1978, *18*, 194.

A bioavailability study of erythromycin ethylsuccinate from tablet and mixture forms and a comparison with equivalent doses of erythromycin stearate.— A. -S. Malmborg, *Curr. ther. Res.*, 1980, *27*, 733. See also J. P. Butzler *et al., Chemotherapy, Basle*, 1979, *25*, 367.

Colitis. See Adverse Effects of Erythromycin, p.1158.

Hepatotoxicity. Cholestatic jaundice occurred in a patient given erythromycin ethylsuccinate.— G. Klatskin, Toxic and Drug-Induced Hepatitis, in *Diseases of the Liver*, L. Schiff (Ed.) Philadelphia, Lipincott, 1975, 644.

Further reports of hepatotoxicity associated with erythromycin ethylsuccinate: J. H. Bena, *J. Kansas med. Soc.*, 1979, *80*, 418; A. L. Viteri *et al., Gastroenterology*, 1979, *76*, 1007; D. Sullivan *et al., J. Am. med. Ass.*, 1980, *243*, 1074.

Preparations

Erythromycin Ethylsuccinate and Sulfisoxazole Acetyl for Oral Suspension *(U.S.P.)*. A dry mixture of erythromycin ethylsuccinate and acetyl sulphafurazole with one or more suitable buffers, colours, flavours, surfactants, and suspending agents. Potency is expressed in terms of the equivalent amounts of erythromycin and sulphafurazole. When no strength is specified a suspension containing in each ml the equivalent of 40 mg of erythromycin and the equivalent of 120 mg of sulphafurazole is supplied. pH of the reconstituted suspension 5 to 7. Store in airtight containers.

Erythromycin Ethylsuccinate for Oral Suspension *(U.S.P.)*. A dry mixture of erythromycin ethylsuccinate with one or more suitable buffers, diluents, colouring, flavouring, and dispersing agents. Store in airtight containers. The suspension is prepared by the addition of diluent before issue and contains the equivalent of 40 mg of erythromycin per ml. pH 7 to 9.

Erythromycin Ethylsuccinate Injection *(U.S.P.)*. A sterile solution of erythromycin ethylsuccinate in macrogol 400 with butyl aminobenzoate 2% and a suitable preservative. It contains the equivalent of erythromycin 50 mg per ml. For intramuscular use only.

Erythromycin Ethylsuccinate Oral Suspension *(U.S.P.)*. A suspension of erythromycin ethylsuccinate with one or more suitable buffers, preservatives, colouring, flavouring, and dispersing agents. pH 6.5 to 8.5. It contains the equivalent of 40 or 80 mg of erythromycin per ml. Store at a temperature not exceeding 8° in airtight containers.

Erythromycin Ethylsuccinate Tablets *(U.S.P.)*. Tablets containing erythromycin ethylsuccinate equivalent to 400 mg or (chewable tablets) 200 mg of erythromycin. Store in airtight containers.

Proprietary Preparations

Erythroped *(Abbott, UK)*. Erythromycin ethylsuccinate, available as a suspension (supplied as granules for preparation with water before use) containing the equivalent of 250 mg of erythromycin in each 5 ml (suggested diluent, syrup). **Erythroped Forte**. Contains the equivalent of 500 mg of erythromycin in each 5 ml. **Erythroped PI.** Contains the equivalent of 125 mg of erythromycin in each 5 ml. (Also available as Erythroped in *S.Afr.*).

Other Proprietary Names

Arg.—Ambamida, Pantomicina *(see also* Erythromycin*)*; *Austral.*—EES 200, Erythrocin IM; *Belg.*—Abboticine *(see also* Erythromycin and Erythromycin Stearate*)*, Erythrocine *(see also* Erythromycin Lactobionate and Erythromycin Stearate*)*, Erythroforte 500; *Canad.*—EES 200, EES 400; *Denm.*—Abboticin *(see also* Erythromycin Lactobionate and Erythromycin Stearate*)*; *Fr.*—Abboticine *(see also* Erythromycin and Erythromycin Stearate*)*, Erythrocine *(see also* Erythromycin Lactobionate and Erythromycin Stearate*)*; *Ger.*—Anamycin, Eromerzin, Erythrocin IM, Paediathrocin *(see also* Erythromycin*)*; *Ital.*—Eritrocina *(see also* Erythromycin Stearate*)*, Proterytrin *(see also* Erythromycin, Erythromycin Estolate, and Erythromycin Lactobionate*)*; *Jap.*—Eryromycen, Erythro-ES, Erythromycin-ES, Esinol, Esmycin, Minotin, Refkas, Takasunon *(see also* Erythromycin Stearate*)*; *Neth.*—Abboticine *(see also* Erythromycin and Erythromycin Stearate*)*, Erythrocine *(see also* Erythromycin Lactobionate and Erythromycin Stearate*)*; *Norw.*—Abboticin *(see also* Erythromycin Lactobionate and Erythromycin Stearate*)*; *Switz.*—Erythrocine *(see also* Erythromycin Lactobionate and Erythromycin Stearate*)*; *USA*—EES, E-Mycin E, Erythrocin IM, Pediamycin, Wyamycin E.

Erythromycin ethylsuccinate for intramuscular injection was formerly marketed in Great Britain under the proprietary name Erythrocin IM (*Abbott*).

81-p

Erythromycin Gluceptate.

Erythromycin glucoheptonate.

$C_{37}H_{67}NO_{13},C_7H_{14}O_8$=960.1.

CAS — 23067-13-2.

Pharmacopoeias. U.S. includes Sterile Erythromycin Gluceptate.

A white, odourless or almost odourless, slightly hygroscopic powder. Erythromycin gluceptate 1.3 g is approximately equivalent to 1 g of erythromycin.

Freely **soluble** in water, alcohol, and methyl alcohol; slightly soluble in acetone and chloroform; practically insoluble in ether. A 5% solution in water is neutral or slightly acid. A 2.5% solution in water is stable at 2° to 4° for about 7 days. **Store** in airtight containers.

Incompatible with amikacin sulphate, cephaloridine, cephalothin sodium, and cephazolin sodium.

Incompatibility. Particulate matter was observed within 2 hours when 1 ml of commercial erythromycin gluceptate injection was mixed with 5 ml of sterile water and 1 ml of any of the following commercial injection solutions: *chloramphenicol sodium succinate, phenobarbitone sodium*, and *phenytoin sodium*. Though no precipitate occurred the manufacturer stated that erythromycin gluceptate was incompatible with *Prochlorperazine edisylate*.— R. Misgen, *Am. J. Hosp. Pharm.*, 1965, *22*, 92.

There was loss of clarity when intravenous solutions of erythromycin gluceptate were mixed with those of *chloramphenicol sodium succinate, heparin sodium, novobiocin sodium, pentobarbitone sodium, phenobarbitone sodium, phenytoin sodium, quinalbarbitone sodium, streptomycin sulphate*, or *tetracycline hydrochloride*.— J. A. Patel and G. L. Phillips, *Am. J. Hosp. Pharm.*, 1966, *23*, 409.

For a list of incompatibilities including *carbenicillin sodium, cephalothin sodium, colistin sulphomethate sodium, protein hydrolysate injection, thiopentone sodium*, and *vitamin-B complex*, see *Med. Lett.*, 1972, *14* (Jan.), *Suppl.*, 32.

Stability in solution. Erythromycin gluceptate solutions were stable only between pH 6 and 7.5, and lost 70 to 80% potency in 15 minutes at pH 4.5. Its addition to dextrose injection raised the pH by 0.95 to 1.7 units, so that unless the pH of the dextrose injection (limits 3.5 to 6.5) was above 5.05, stability could not be assured during administration. Aminophylline raised the pH to 8.3 and caused loss of potency.— M. Edward, *Am. J. Hosp. Pharm.*, 1967, *24*, 440.

Erythromycin gluceptate retained its potency almost unchanged for 24 hours in sodium chloride injection or dextrose injection buffered to pH 7 to 8.— R. F. Bergstrom and A. L. Fites (letter), *Am. J. Hosp. Pharm.*, 1975, *32*, 241.

Erythromycin gluceptate has the actions and uses of erythromycin (see p.1158).

It is suitable for the preparation of solutions for intravenous administration. Oral administration of erythromycin should replace parenteral administration as soon as practicable.

The usual dose for adults is the equivalent of 250 to 500 mg of erythromycin in 100 to 250 ml of dextrose injection or sodium chloride injection by slow intravenous infusion over 20 to 60 minutes every 6 hours or the equivalent of 1 to 2 g of erythromycin by slow intravenous infusion over 24 hours.

For the preparation of solutions of erythromycin gluceptate for injection, a primary solution should be prepared by dissolving erythromycin gluceptate, equivalent to 250 or 500 mg of erythromycin, in at least 10 ml of Water for Injections or the equivalent of 1 g in at least 20 ml. This solution may be diluted further with sodium chloride injection or dextrose injection. To avoid gel formation or slow and incomplete solution of the drug, sodium chloride injection should not be used in preparing the primary solution.

For a report of higher prostate concentrations being achieved with rosaramicin than with erythromycin gluceptate taken by mouth, see Rosaramicin, p.1209.

Preparations

Sterile Erythromycin Gluceptate *(U.S.P.)*. A grade of erythromycin gluceptate for injection in vials containing the equivalent of 0.25, 0.5, or 1 g of erythromycin. pH of a 2.5% solution 6 to 8.

Proprietary Names

Erycinum *(Schering, Ger.)* (see also Erythromycin); Ilotycin Gluceptate *(Lilly, Austral.; Lilly, Switz.; Dista, USA)*.

82-s

Erythromycin Lactobionate.

Erythromycin mono(4-*O*-β-D-galactopyranosyl-D-gluconate).

$C_{37}H_{67}NO_{13},C_{12}H_{22}O_{12}$=1092.2.

CAS — 3847-29-8.

Pharmacopoeias. In *Roum. U.S.P.* includes Erythromycin Lactobionate for Injection.

White or slightly yellow crystals or powder with a faint odour. Erythromycin lactobionate 1.5 g is approximately equivalent to 1 g of erythromycin. Freely **soluble** in water, alcohol, and methyl alcohol; slightly soluble in acetone and chloroform; practically insoluble in ether. A 5% solution in water has a pH of 6.5 to 7.5. A 5% solution in water is stable at 2° to 4° for about 14 days. In acidic solutions, erythromycin lactobionate is unstable and rapidly loses potency below pH 5.5. **Incompatible** with ampicillin sodium, cephalothin sodium, colistin sulphomethate sodium, heparin sodium, and acidic substances such as metaraminol tartrate, gentamicin sulphate, and tetracyclines.

Incompatibility. A haze or precipitate was observed within an hour when an average dose of erythromycin lactobionate was mixed in dextrose injection with *colistin sulphomethate sodium* or *heparin*, and on standing with *cephalothin sodium. Tetracycline hydrochloride* inactivated erythromycin because of its acidity and *hydrocortisone sodium succinate* was incompatible at certain concentrations.— J. M. Meisler and M. W. Skolaut, *Am. J. Hosp. Pharm.*, 1966, *23*, 557. A report of precipitation occurring when erythromycin lactobionate was mixed with *hydrocortisone sodium phosphate* in dextrose saline solution.— J. P. Richardson (letter), *Pharm. J.*, 1979, *2*, 29.

A precipitate was formed when a solution of erythromycin lactobionate was mixed with solutions of *ampicillin sodium* or *cloxacillin sodium*, but there was no precipitate when it was mixed with methicillin sodium.— B. Lynn, *Chemist Drugg.*, 1967, *187*, 157.

For a list of incompatibilities including *aminophylline, ascorbic acid, carbenicillin, chloramphenicol, metaraminol, protein hydrolysate injection, thiopentone sodium*, and *vitamin-B complex*, see *Med. Lett.*, 1972, *14* (Jan.), *Suppl.*, 32.

Stability. Dry powdered erythromycin lactobionate was stable for at least a year when stored in the dark at room temperature. It was inactivated by light and increase in temperature. Aqueous solutions could be stored for 1 to 2 weeks in a refrigerator without significant loss of activity. The lactobionate, both in the powdered form and in aqueous solution, was less stable to heat than erythromycin base.— H. W. Unterman *et al.*, *Farmacia, Buc.*, 1964, *12*, 625, per *Int. pharm. Abstr.*, 1965, *2*, 1042.

Stability in solution. Erythromycin lactobionate in dextrose injection at pH 6.38 lost 14% of its activity after 6 hours and 15% after 6 hours in 5% dextrose in sodium chloride injection at pH 5.39. There was no significant loss of potency after 24 hours in sodium chloride injection.— J. N. Bair and D. P. Carew, *Bull. parent. Drug Ass.*, 1965, *19*, 153. Other similar reports.— E. A. Parker, *Abbott, ibid.*, 1967, *21*, 197; *idem, Am. J. Hosp. Pharm.*, 1967, *24*, 434; *idem*, 1969, *26*, 412.

Erythromycin lactobionate 500 mg in 100 ml of dextrose injection or sodium chloride injection was stable for 21 days at 25°.— J. F. Gallelli *et al.*, *Am. J. Hosp. Pharm.*, 1969, *26*, 630.

Erythromycin lactobionate has the actions and uses of erythromycin (see p.1158). It is suitable for the preparation of solutions for intravenous injection to patients who are unable to tolerate oral medication or when it is necessary to produce a high blood concentration of erythromycin to control severe infections. Oral administration of erythromycin should replace parenteral administration as soon as practicable.

The usual dose for adults is the equivalent of 300 mg of erythromycin, by intravenous injection over a period of 5 minutes, every 6 hours, or the equivalent of 1 to 2 g of erythromycin daily by intermittent intravenous infusion over 20 to 60 minutes every 6 hours or by infusion over 24 hours. The equivalent of 4 g daily has been recommended for severe infections. Children may be given the equivalent of 30 to 50 mg per kg body-weight daily in divided doses.

For the preparation of solutions of erythromycin lactobionate for injection, a primary solution containing not more than 5% of erythromycin should be prepared with Water for Injections or dextrose injection. For intravenous injection it should be diluted at least 5 times with sodium chloride injection or other solution. For intravenous infusion it is further diluted. To avoid precipitation of the drug, sodium chloride injection or other inorganic salt solution should not be used in preparing the primary solution.

In 6 healthy subjects given erythromycin 2 g by infusion of the lactobionate over 12 hours, the mean peak plasma concentration of erythromycin at about 1 hour was 6.1 μg per ml with a second peak of 7.2 μg per ml at 4 hours. Effective concentrations were maintained at least 8 hours after the end of infusion.— R. L. Parsons *et al.*, *Postgrad. med. J.*, 1978, *54*, 68. See also M. A. Neaverson, *Curr. med. Res. Opinion*, 1976, *4*, 359.

Between 0.5 and 1 g of erythromycin lactobionate was administered by continuous infusion to 8 patients before undergoing hip surgery. Concentrations in cancellous bone ranged from 0.6 to 11.5 μg per g with a mean value about 30% of the corresponding serum concentrations.— V. T. Rosdahl *et al.*, *J. antimicrob. Chemother.*, 1979, *5*, 275.

Ototoxicity. For reports on the use of erythromycin lactobionate being associated with reversible loss of hearing, see under Adverse Effects in Erythromycin, p.1158.

Preparations

Erythromycin Lactobionate for Injection *(U.S.P.)*. A sterile salt prepared from erythromycin and lactobionic acid by freeze-drying; it contains a suitable preservative. pH of a 5% solution 6.5 to 7.5. It contains the equivalent of 0.3, 0.5, or 1 g per container.

Erythrocin I.V. Lactobionate *(Abbott, UK)*. Erythromycin lactobionate, available as powder for preparing intravenous injections in vials each containing the equivalent of 0.3 or 1 g of erythromycin. (Also available as Erythrocin IV in *Austral., Ger., USA*).

Other Proprietary Names

Denm.—Abboticin (see also Erythromycin Ethylsuccinate and Erythromycin Stearate); *Ital.*—Proterytrin (see also Erythromycin, Erythromycin Estolate, and Erythromycin Ethylsuccinate), Stellamicina (see also Erythromycin Estolate); *Neth.*—Erythrocine (see also Erythromycin Ethylsuccinate and Erythromycin Stearate); *Norw.*—Abboticin (see also Erythromycin Ethylsuccinate and Erythromycin Stearate); *Switz.*—Erythrocine Lactobionate.

83-w

Erythromycin Propionate. Erythromycin 2′-propionate.

$C_{40}H_{71}NO_{14}$=790.0.

CAS — 134-36-1.

Pharmacopoeias. In *Fr.* and *Roum.*

A white odourless powder with a slightly bitter taste. Erythromycin propionate 1.08 g is approximately equivalent to 1 g of erythromycin. Slightly **soluble** in water; freely soluble in alcohol, acetone, and chloroform.

Erythromycin propionate has the actions of erythromycin (see p.1158) and has been used similarly to the estolate, the lauryl sulphate salt of erythromycin propionate, in a dose equivalent to 1 to 2 g of erythromycin daily.

Hepatotoxicity. Severe abdominal pains, cholestatic jaundice, and eosinophilia occurred in a patient after erythromycin propionate was given.— D. Pessayre and J. P. Benhamou (letter), *Br. med. J.*, 1979, *1*, 1357.

For a report of the hepatotoxicity of erythromycin estolate being associated with the propionyl group, see Erythromycin Estolate, p.1161.

Proprietary Names

Éry 500 *(Bouchara, Fr.)*; Propiocine *(Roussel, Fr.)*.

84-e

Erythromycin Stearate *(B.P., U.S.P.)*.

The stearate of erythromycin with some uncombined stearic acid and sodium stearate.

$C_{37}H_{67}NO_{13},C_{18}H_{36}O_2$=1018.4.

CAS — 643-22-1.

Pharmacopoeias. In *Br., Fr.*, and *U.S.*

Colourless or slightly yellow crystals or a white or slightly yellow powder, odourless or with a slight earthy odour, with a slightly bitter taste. The *B.P.* specifies that it should contain not less than 77% of erythromycin stearate (equivalent to approximately 50% of erythromycin), 5 to 18.5% of free stearic acid, not more than 6% of sodium stearate, and not more than 4% of water. It contains not less than 550 units per mg.*U.S.P.* specifies a potency equivalent to not less than 550 μg of erythromycin per mg.

Practically **insoluble** in water and acetone; partly soluble in alcohol, chloroform, ether, isopropyl alcohol, and methyl alcohol. Solubility in some organic solvents appears to be dependent on the composition of the salt. A saturated solution in water is alkaline to litmus. **Store** in airtight containers.Protect from light.

Adverse Effects and Precautions. As for Erythromycin, p.1158.

Absorption and Fate. Erythromycin stearate is relatively stable in gastric acid and when given by mouth it releases active erythromycin in the duodenum.

Ten per cent of erythromycin administered as stearate was found to be unbound to serum proteins whereas only 1.5% of erythromycin estolate was free. Though the total serum concentration of erythromycin propionate was 3 times higher than that of erythromycin, this was considered to be less important for determining therapeutic efficacy. The half-lives in blood were 1.18 and about 1.6 hours respectively.— R. G. Wiegand and A. H. C. Chun, *J. pharm. Sci.*, 1972, *61*, 425.

In a study on the absorption of erythromycin stearate, all volunteers given 250 mg every six hours for 5 doses had therapeutically adequate serum concentrations after 24 hours. The serum half-life of erythromycin stearate was found to be 1.4 hours.— E. Triggs and M. A. Neaverson (letter), *Med. J. Aust.*, 1973, *2*, 344.

Bioavailability studies on different preparations of erythromycin stearate.— E. J. Triggs and J. J. Ashley, *Med. J. Aust.*, 1978, *2*, 121; R. Mäntylä *et al.*, *Ann. clin. Res.*, 1978, *10*, 258; N. Berend *et al.*, *Curr. med. Res. Opinion*, 1979, *6*, 118; G. J. Yakatan *et al.*, *J. Pharmacokinet. Biopharm.*, 1979, *7*, 355; C. W. Clarke *et al.*, *J. antimicrob. Chemother.*, 1980, *6*, 389.

A mean peak serum-erythromycin concentration of 2.65 μg per ml occurred 2 hours after administration of erythromycin stearate equivalent to erythromycin 500 mg by mouth, with 250 ml of water, to 6 healthy subjects in the fasting state. In the same subjects following a standard meal high in carbohydrate, fat, or protein, or in a fasting state with only 20 ml of water, peak serum concentrations were reduced by about 50%. It was suggested that erythromycin stearate should be administered on an empty stomach with an adequate amount of water.— P. G. Welling *et al.*, *J. pharm. Sci.*, 1978, *67*, 764.

Erythromycin was better absorbed when 15 healthy subjects took erythromycin stearate immediately before food rather than on an empty stomach. A mean peak plasma concentration of 2.8 μg per ml occurred one hour after a 500-mg dose was taken just before a standardised breakfast compared with only 1.3 μg per ml two hours after a similar dose was taken in the fasting state. Tablets of erythromycin stearate should be taken just before a meal and not as previously recommended.— A. -S. Malmborg, *Curr. med. Res. Opinion*, 1978, *5*, *Suppl.* 2, 15. See also *idem*, *J. antimicrob. Chemother.*, 1979, *5*, 591. Confirmation that preparations of erythromycin stearate should be given immediately before food for consistent and rapid absorption. In this study food did not affect the bioavailability of a preparation of erythromycin base.— J. Rutland *et al.*, *Br. J. clin. Pharmac.*, 1979, *8*, 343.

Uses. Erythromycin stearate has the actions and uses of erythromycin, (see p.1158) and is administered by mouth as tablets or as a flavoured suspension in similar doses.

Preparations

Erythromycin Mixture *(B.P.C. 1973)*. Erythromycin Suspension. A suspension of erythromycin stearate containing the equivalent of 2% of erythromycin in a suitable coloured flavoured vehicle.
The mixture and its dilutions with syrup should be stored in a cool place. When a dose less than 5 ml is prescribed, the mixture should be diluted to 5 ml with syrup. Such dilutions must be freshly prepared and not used more than 2 weeks after issue. *Dose.* Children, every 6 hours; up to 1 year, 2.5 ml; 1 to 5 years, 5 ml; 6 to 12 years, 10 ml.

Erythromycin Stearate for Oral Suspension *(U.S.P.)*. A dry mixture of erythromycin stearate with one or more suitable buffers, diluents, colouring, flavouring, and dispersing agents. Store in airtight containers. The suspension is prepared by the addition of diluent before issue and contains the equivalent of 25 or 50 mg of erythromycin per ml. pH 6 to 9.

Erythromycin Stearate Tablets *(B.P.)*. Erythromycin Stear. Tab. Tablets containing erythromycin stearate. Potency is expressed in terms of the equivalent amount of erythromycin. They are film-coated. Protect from light. *U.S.P.* specifies the equivalent of 75, 100, 125, 250, or 500 mg of erythromycin. Store in airtight containers.

Proprietary Preparations

Erythrocin *(Abbott, UK)*. Erythromycin stearate, available as **Filmtabs** (film-coated tablets) each containing the equivalent of 250 or 500 mg of erythromycin and **Oral Suspension** containing the equivalent of 100 mg of erythromycin in each 5 ml (suggested diluent, syrup without preservative). (Also available as Erythrocin in *Austral.*, *Canad.*, *Ger.*, *S.Afr.*, *USA*).

Other Proprietary Names

Arg.—Celtiacina; *Austral.*—E-Mycin *(see also* Erythromycin*)*, Erostin, Ethryn; *Belg.*—Erythrocine *(see also* Erythromycin Ethylsuccinate and Erythromycin Lactobionate*)*; *Canad.*—Novorythro *(see also* Erythromycin Estolate*)*; *Denm.*—Abboticin *(see also* Erythromycin Ethylsuccinate and Erythromycin Lactobionate*)*; *Fr.*—Abboticine *(see also* Erythromycin and Erythromycin Ethylsuccinate*)*; *Ger.*—DuraErythromycin; *Ital.*—Eritrocina *(see also* Erythromycin Ethylsuccinate*)*, Rossomicina; *Jap.*—Erythro-S, Takasunon *(see also* Erythromycin Ethylsuccinate*)*; *Neth.*—Erythrocine *(see also* Erythromycin Ethylsuccinate and Erythromycin Lactobionate*)*; *Norw.*—Abboticin *(see also* Erythromycin Ethylsuccinate and Erythromycin Lactobionate*)*; *S.Afr.*—Eromel, Rythrocaps; *Spain*—Torlamicina; *Swed.*—Abboticin *(see also* Erythromycin Ethylsuccinate and Erythromycin Lactobionate*)*, Bristamycin; *Switz.*—Eritrolag, Erythrocine *(see also* Erythromycin Ethylsuccinate and Erythromycin Lactobionate*)*; *USA*—Bristamycin, Dowmycin-E, Erypar, Ethril, Pfizer-E, SK-Erythromycin.

85-l

Flucloxacillin Sodium *(B.P.)*.

Floxacillin Sodium; BRL 2039 (for the acid). Sodium (6*R*)-6-[3-(2-chloro-6-fluorophenyl)-5-methylisoxazole-4-carboxamido]penicillanate monohydrate.

$C_{19}H_{16}ClFN_3NaO_5S,H_2O = 493.9$.

CAS — 5250-39-5 (flucloxacillin); 1847-24-1 (sodium salt, anhydrous); 34214-51-2 (sodium salt, monohydrate).

Pharmacopoeias. In *Br.*

A white or almost white hygroscopic crystalline powder with a characteristic bitter taste. Each g represents about 2 mmol (2 mEq) of sodium. Flucloxacillin sodium 1.09 g is approximately equivalent to 1 g of anhydrous flucloxacillin. **Soluble** 1 in 1 of water, 1 in 8 of alcohol, 1 in 8 of acetone, and 1 in 2 of methyl alcohol. A 10% solution in water has a pH of 5 to 7. The optimum pH for the stability of citrate-buffered solutions is 6.5 and aqueous 10% solutions at pH 6 to 7 may be expected to retain at least 90% potency for 7 days at 20° to 25°. Solutions containing 0.1% in injections of sodium chloride, dextrose, sodium chloride and dextrose, or sodium lactate may be expected to lose up to 6% of their activity at room temperature in 24 hours. **Store** at a temperature not exceeding 25° in airtight containers; if it is intended for injection, the containers should be sterile and sealed to exclude micro-organisms.

Incompatible with colistin sulphomethate sodium, gentamicin, kanamycin, and polymyxin B sulphate; loss of potency after mixing with streptomycin has also been reported.

Incompatibility. Flucloxacillin sodium equivalent to flucloxacillin 0.2% in a 20% solution of tyloxapol 0.125%, sodium bicarbonate 2%, and glycerol 5% (Alevaire) lost 11% potency over 6 hours and 66% over 24 hours when stored at 20°.— B. Lynn, *J. Hosp. Pharm.*, 1971, *29*, 183.

Further references: B. Lynn and A. Jones, *Beecham Research, Advances in Antimicrobial and Antineoplastic Chemotherapy*, Vol. I, pt 1, Munich, Urban and Schwarzenberg, 1972, 701.

Stability in solution. The stability of aqueous solutions of flucloxacillin sodium.— B. Lynn, *J. Hosp. Pharm.*, 1971, *29*, 183.

Adverse Effects and Treatment. As for Benzylpenicillin, p.1103.

Precautions. As for Cloxacillin Sodium, p.1149.

Antimicrobial Action. Flucloxacillin sodium has an antibacterial activity similar to that of cloxacillin sodium (see p.1149).

Flucloxacillin was active against a number of Gram-positive bacilli and against Gram-negative cocci, except *Streptococcus faecalis*. Gram-negative bacteria were relatively insensitive; Enterobacteriaceae required up to 500 μg or more per ml for inhibition of growth. Concentrations of 5 to 12.5 μg per ml inhibited the growth of *Haemophilus influenzae*, *Bordetella pertussis*, *Pasteurella septica*, and *Brucella abortus*. Gonococci, meningococci, and β-haemolytic streptococci were inhibited by 0.1 μg per ml of flucloxacillin. Penicillinase-producing staphylococci were usually inhibited by flucloxacillin in concentrations of 0.25 to 0.5 μg per ml.— R. Sutherland *et al.*, *Br. med. J.*, 1970, *4*, 455.

In an *in vitro* study, flucloxacillin was bactericidal against 88% of 26 penicillin-resistant isolates of *Staphylococcus aureus* at 0.4 μg per ml and against all of them at 6.2 μg per ml; cloxacillin was bactericidal against 81% of the isolates at 0.8 μg per ml and against all at 12.5 μg per ml; and oxacillin was bactericidal against 88% of the isolates at 0.2 μg per ml and against all at 1.6 μg per ml.— M. G. Bergeron *et al.*, *Am. J. med. Sci.*, 1976, *271*, 13.

Resistance. As for Methicillin Sodium, p.1183.

Flucloxacillin was less resistant to staphylococcal penicillinase than methicillin, cloxacillin, and nafcillin.— R. W. Lacey and A. Stokes, *J. clin. Path.*, 1977, *30*, 35.

Absorption and Fate. Flucloxacillin sodium, like dicloxacillin sodium, is better absorbed from the gastro-intestinal tract than cloxacillin sodium, but absorption is also reduced by food in the stomach or small intestine. After an oral dose of 250 to 500 mg, in fasting subjects, peak serum concentrations in about 1 hour may range from 3 to 27 μg per ml, with mean peak concentrations of about 11 to 15 μg per ml; a therapeutic concentration persists for about 4 hours. A similar pattern follows the intramuscular injection of flucloxacillin sodium but peak concentrations are achieved in about 30 minutes. Doubling the dose can double the plasma concentration. About 95% of flucloxacillin in the circulation is bound to plasma proteins. Some 50% of a dose by mouth and up to 90% of an intramuscular dose is excreted in the urine within 6 hours.

Serum concentrations are enhanced if probenecid is given concomitantly.

A comparison of the pharmacokinetics of flucloxacillin, cloxacillin, and oxacillin in 10 healthy subjects who took 500 mg four times daily for 8 days.— M. G. Bergeron *et al.*, *Am. J. med. Sci.* 1976, *271*, 13.

Further references: R. Sutherland *et al.*, *Br. med. J.*, 1970, *4*, 455; G. P. Bodey *et al.*, *Clin. Pharmac. Ther.*, 1972, *13*, 512; C. Kamme and B. Ursing, *Scand. J. infect. Dis.*, 1974, *6*, 273; E. H. Nauta and H. Mattie, *Br. J. clin. Pharmac.*, 1975, *2*, 111.

Diffusion into body tissues and fluids. Flucloxacillin 0.5 or 1 g was given intramuscularly to 10 patients about 2 hours before undergoing total hip replacement for osteoarthritis; bone and serum were sampled simultaneously at operation. The mean serum concentration of flucloxacillin was 8.9 (range 4.6 to 17) μg per ml in 10 patients while the mean concentration of flucloxacillin in washings from trabecular bone was 1.3 (range 0.3 to 2.2) μg per ml. From 0.3 to 2 (mean 0.9) μg per ml of flucloxacillin was present in the washings of compact bone of 9 patients, but was undetectable in the remaining patient. Marrow aspirate or supernatant from marrow aspirate of 4 patients contained from less than 0.8, 2.5, 5.9, and 13 μg per ml of flucloxacillin respectively. Contamination of bone washings with blood was estimated to account for no more than 26% of the flucloxacillin.— P. F. Unsworth *et al.*, *J. clin. Path.*, 1978, *31*, 705. See also J. P. Pollard *et al.*, *J. antimicrob. Chemother.*, 1979, *5*, 721 (concentrations of flucloxacillin in the femoral head and joint capsule).

Metabolism. About 10% of a 500-mg dose of flucloxacillin was metabolised. Within 12 hours of the dose being taken by 6 healthy subjects about 44% was recovered in the urine, 4% as penicilloic acid.— M. Cole *et al.*, *Antimicrob. Ag. Chemother.*, 1973, *3*, 463.

The metabolite of flucloxacillin had similar antibacterial properties to the parent compound and accumulated in patients with renal impairment.— H. H. W. Thijssen and H. Mattie, *Antimicrob. Ag. Chemother.*, 1976, *10*, 441.

Uses. Flucloxacillin sodium is used for the treatment of infections due to staphylococci resistant to benzylpenicillin; it is also used for mixed streptococcal and staphylococcal infections when the staphylococci are penicillin-resistant. It is suitable for administration by mouth and should be given about 1 hour before meals as the presence of food in the stomach reduces absorption.

Flucloxacillin sodium is administered 4 times daily in a dose equivalent to 250 mg of flucloxacillin, by mouth or by intramuscular injection in 1.5 ml of Water for Injections or 0.5% lignocaine hydrochloride solution, if necessary. Intravenously, the equivalent of 250 to 500 mg of flucloxacillin in 10 ml of Water for Injections may be given 4 times daily by slow injection over 3 to 4 minutes or by intravenous infusion. Doses may be doubled in severe infections.

Flucloxacillin 250 to 500 mg daily has also been administered by intra-articular injection, dissolved if necessary in a 0.5% solution of lignocaine hydrochloride, and by intrapleural injection in a dose of 250 mg daily. Using powder for injection, up to 250 mg has been dissolved in 3 ml of sterile water and inhaled by nebuliser 4 times daily.

Children up to 2 years of age may be given one-quarter the adult dose and those aged 2 to 10 years, one-half the adult dose.

In staphylococcal meningitis systemic treatment has been supplemented with intrathecal injections of flucloxacillin. The usual daily intrathecal dose is the equivalent of 5 mg for infants from birth up to 2 years of age, 10 mg for children up to 12 years of age, and 20 mg for adults. The dose should be dissolved in sodium chloride injection 0.9% immediately before use to give a solution containing 10 mg per ml.

Burns. Of 5302 isolates of *Staph. aureus* obtained from 34 burnt patients, 2476 were moderately sensitive to methicillin at 37° but resistant at 30°. Zones of inhibition with flucloxacillin disks were not greatly different at 30° or 37°. *Staph. aureus* was eliminated from 10 of 21 burns in 9 of 17 patients treated for 4 days with flucloxacillin 250 mg six-hourly but in none of 17 controls.— E. J. L. Lowbury *et al.*, *Br. med. J.*, 1977, *1*, 1054.

In a study of patients with burns infected with *Staph. aureus* all patients with methicillin-sensitive strains who received flucloxacillin 500 mg every 6 hours were cleared of or had a reduction in the number of bacteria after 4 days' treatment. Results obtained with the same dose (500 mg) against methicillin-resistant strains were similar to those obtained with 250 mg against methicillin-sensitive strains.— A. Kidson *et al.*, *J. antimicrob. Chemother.*, 1979, *5*, 359.

Dosage in infants and children. A suggested dose of flucloxacillin for older infants was 50 mg per kg body-weight daily, given by mouth in 3 divided doses.— *Br. med. J.*, 1980, *280*, 703.

Dosage in renal failure. Flucloxacillin could be given in usual doses to patients with renal failure.— G. B. Appel and H. C. Neu, *New Engl. J. Med.*, 1977, *296*, 663.

Surgical infection prophylaxis. Tissue and fluid concentrations of ampicillin and flucloxacillin were measured after the prophylactic intravenous bolus injection of the combined antibiotics (as Magnapen 4 g) immediately before the induction of anaesthesia in 7 patients undergoing total hip replacement. Despite considerable individual variation, concentrations of flucloxacillin in plasma, bone, hip capsule, and drain fluid generally exceeded its MIC against penicillinase-producing *Staph. aureus*. The MICs of both antibiotics were also exceeded for most other sensitive pathogens. Postoperatively patients were given flucloxacillin 1 g and ampicillin 1 g (as Magnapen) intramuscularly every 6 hours for up to 72 hours until the removal of drains from the wound.— R. L. Parsons *et al.*, *Br. J. clin. Pharmac.*, 1978, *6*, 135.

For a further report of the use of flucloxacillin in the prophylaxis of infection in total hip replacement, see Cephaloridine, p.1127.

Preparations

Flucloxacillin Capsules *(B.P.)*. Capsules containing flucloxacillin sodium. Potency is expressed in terms of the equivalent amount of flucloxacillin. Store at a temperature not exceeding 30°.

Flucloxacillin Injection *(B.P.)*. A sterile solution of flucloxacillin sodium prepared by dissolving, immediately before use, the sterile contents of a sealed container (Flucloxacillin Sodium for Injection) in the requisite amount of Water for Injections. The amount of flucloxacillin sodium in a sealed container is expressed in terms of the equivalent amount of flucloxacillin. The injection should be used within 30 minutes of preparation.

Proprietary Preparations

Floxapen *(Beecham Research, UK)*. Flucloxacillin sodium, available as **Capsules** each containing the equivalent of 250 or 500 mg of flucloxacillin; as **Syrup** (supplied as powder for preparation with water before use) containing the equivalent of 125 mg of flucloxacillin in each 5 ml (suggested diluent, syrup); and as **Injection** (supplied as powder for solution before use) in vials each containing the equivalent of 250 or 500 mg of flucloxacillin. (Also available as Floxapen in *Austral.*, *Belg.*, *Ital.*, *Neth.*, *NZ*, *S.Afr.*, *Switz.*).

Other Proprietary Names

Dumpikal *(Spain)*; Flopen *(Austral.)*; Flupen *(Ital.)*; Heracillin *(Denm., Swed.)*; Penplus *(Ital.)*; Staphylex *(Ger.)*.

179-a

Fosfomycin.
MK-955; Phosphonomycin.
(−)-(1*R*,2*S*)-(1,2-Epoxypropyl)phosphonic acid.
$C_3H_7O_4P = 138.1$.

CAS — 23155-02-4.

An antibiotic isolated from *Streptomyces fradiae*, *Streptomyces viridochromogenes*, and *Streptomyces wedmorensis* or produced synthetically.

Adverse Effects. Gastro-intestinal disturbances, transient increases in serum concentrations of aminotransferases, and skin rashes have been reported following the use of fosfomycin. Eosinophilia has also occurred.

Antimicrobial Action. Fosfomycin is a bactericidal antibiotic and is reported to interfere with the first step in the synthesis of bacterial cell walls. It is active *in vitro* against a range of Gram-positive and Gram-negative bacteria including *Staphylococcus aureus*, some streptococci, most Enterobacteriaceae, *Neisseria* spp., and some strains of *Pseudomonas aeruginosa*. *Bacteroides* spp. are not sensitive. MICs are very variable and depend on the type of test media used as well as inoculum size. Bacterial resistance to fosfomycin has been reported.

References.— R. Ansorg, *Infection*, 1978, *6*, 73.

Enhanced activity. The activity of fosfomycin was enhanced to some degree *in vitro* against various Gram-negative and Gram-positive bacteria when used with beta-lactam or aminoglycoside antibiotics, chloramphenicol, rifamycin, lincomycin, tetracycline, or erythromycin. *Mice* infected with *Ps. aeruginosa* had greater rates of survival when given fosfomycin with carbenicillin or gentamicin compared with rates when given each antibiotic alone.— T. Olay *et al.*, *J. antimicrob. Chemother.*, 1978, *4*, 569.

The activity of fosfomycin used alone or with chloramphenicol or ampicillin was studied *in vitro* against 90 strains of *Salmonella* and 50 strains of *Shigella*. Fosfomycin had an MIC of 4, 8, 16, 32, and 64 µg per ml respectively against 4.4, 40, 71.1, 81.1, and 92.2% of the *Salmonella* strains and 4, 8, 22, 46, and 60% of the *Shigella* strains. When used together, the activities of fosfomycin and ampicillin were enhanced against 74 and additive against 7 of the *Salmonella* strains and enhanced against 27 and additive against 9 of the *Shigella* strains. Chloramphenicol and fosfomycin enhanced each others activity against 56 strains of *Salmonella* and 29 strains of *Shigella* when used together and their activities were additive against 9 strains of *Salmonella* and 10 strains of *Shigella*. There was no antagonistic effect when fosfomycin was used with chloramphenicol or ampicillin.— E. J. Perea *et al.*, *Antimicrob. Ag. Chemother.*, 1978, *13*, 705.

Absorption and Fate. Fosfomycin is poorly absorbed from the gastro-intestinal tract. Peak plasma concentrations of about 3 and 5 µg per ml have been reported 2 hours after oral doses of 0.5 and 1 g respectively, compared with concentrations of about 17 and 28 µg per ml one hour after similar doses given intramuscularly; the plasma half-life varies from 1.5 to 2 hours. Fosfomycin does not appear to be bound to plasma proteins. It diffuses across the placenta and is widely distributed in body fluids including the cerebrospinal fluid; small amounts have been found in breast milk and bile. The majority of a parenteral dose is excreted unchanged in the urine, by glomerular filtration, within 24 hours.

Pharmacokinetics of fosfomycin after intravenous administration.— K. C. Kwan *et al.*, *J. pharm. Sci.*, 1971, *60*, 678.

Uses. Fosfomycin is an antibiotic which appears to be unrelated to other antimicrobial agents in current use. It has been given by mouth as the calcium salt and by intramuscular or intravenous injection as the sodium salt in the treatment of a variety of infections including those of the urinary, gastro-intestinal, and respiratory tracts. Usual adult doses have ranged from 2 to 4 g daily in divided doses, although up to 16 g daily has been administered intravenously in severe infections. Children have been given 100 to 200 mg per kg body-weight daily in divided doses.

Reports of studies on fosfomycin.— *Antimicrob. Ag. Chemother.*, 1969, 284-351; D. Hendlin *et al.*, *Science*, 1969, *166*, 122 and 123; *Chemotherapy, Tokyo*, 1975, *23*, 1649.

Fosfomycin calcium (a suspension containing 50 mg per ml fosfomycin) 100 to 200 mg per kg body-weight daily in divided doses was given for about 7 days to 42 premature infants and children, including 3 carriers, with gastro-enteritis due to *Escherichia coli*. After a second course of treatment in 11 cases (6 re-infections, 5 relapses) a 92% cure was achieved. Fosfomycin was partly absorbed, a mean blood concentration of 2.8 (100 mg per kg) to 4.6 µg per ml (200 mg per kg) being detected in 23 patients 1 hour after the first dose. The remainder was eliminated in the faeces. In 11 patients (200 mg per kg) a mean of 3.7 µg per g of faeces was measured on day 3 to 4 of treatment. Fosfomycin was well tolerated.— F. Baquero *et al.*, *Archs Dis. Childh.*, 1975, *50*, 367.

Proceedings of a symposium on the actions and uses of fosfomycin.— A. Gallego and J. M. Rubio (Ed.), *Chemotherapy, Basle*, 1977, *23*, *Suppl.* 1, 1-447.

Proprietary Names of Fosfomycin Calcium and Fosfomycin Sodium

Fosfocin *(Crinos, Ital.)*; Fosfocina *(CEPA, Spain)*; Fosfocine *(Midy, Fr.)*; Fosfotricina *(Italfarmaco, Ital.)*; Francital *(Francia Farm., Ital.)*; Lancetina *(Lancet, Ital.)*; Selemicina *(Italchemi, Ital.)*; Valemicina *(Farmochimica Italiana, Ital.)*; Veramina *(Roux-Ocefa, Arg.)*.

86-y

Framycetin Sulphate
(B.P., B.P. Vet.). The sulphate of neomycin B.
$C_{23}H_{46}N_6O_{13},3H_2SO_4 = 908.9$.

CAS — 119-04-0 (framycetin); 28002-70-2 (sulphate).

Pharmacopoeias. In *Br.* and *Fr. Fr. P.* specifies 2.5 H_2SO_4.

Framycetin is an antimicrobial substance produced by certain strains of *Streptomyces fradiae* or *Streptomyces decaris* or by any other means. It contains not more than 3% of neomycin C (see p.1188) and not more than 1% of neomycin A. A white or yellowish-white, odourless or almost odourless, tasteless, hygroscopic powder containing not less than 630 units per mg.

Soluble 1 in 1 of water; practically insoluble in alcohol, chloroform, and ether. A solution in water is dextrorotatory. A 1% solution in water has a pH of 6 to 7. Buffered aqueous solutions are stable at room temperature. **Store** at a temperature not exceeding 30° in airtight containers. If it is intended for injection, the containers should be sterile and sealed to exclude micro-organisms. Protect from light.

Units. One unit of framycetin is contained in 0.001492 mg of the first International Reference Preparation (1970) of framycetin sulphate which contains 670 units per mg.

Framycetin sulphate has actions and uses similar to those of neomycin sulphate (p.1188) and is administered topically in the treatment of infections of the skin, eye, and ear. Adults have been given doses of up to 2 or sometimes 4 g daily by mouth for enteric infections.

Framycetin has been given prophylactically with colistin and nystatin (FRACON) to reduce the intestinal flora in patients with leukaemia.

References to the subconjunctival injection of framycetin.— A. J. Bron *et al.*, *Br. J. Ophthal.*, 1970, *54*, 615; N. E. Christy and P. Lall, *Archs Ophthal., N.Y.*, 1973, *90*, 361.

Suppression of intestinal flora. In 38 patients with

acute leukaemia framycetin in a dose of 750 mg twice daily by mouth reduced the incidence of septicaemia arising from the bowel by 49% compared with a control group of 66 similar patients.— M. J. Keating and D. G. Penington, *Med. J. Aust.*, 1973, *2*, 213.

A schedule of antibiotics not absorbed from the gastro-intestinal tract and including framycetin, colistin, and nystatin with amphotericin lozenges and topical applications of chlorhexidine preparations was effective in preventing infection in a controlled study of 113 patients being treated for acute nonlymphoblastic leukaemia.— R. A. Storring *et al.*, *Lancet*, 1977, *2*, 837. Gastro-intestinal sterilisation with framycetin, colistin, and nystatin (FRACON) was associated with the healing of a high rectal fistula in a patient with aplastic anaemia.— A. J. Barrett *et al.* (letter), *ibid.*, 1229.

For reference to the replacement of framycetin sulphate as part of an oral non-absorbable antibiotic regimen by neomycin sulphate, see Neomycin Sulphate, p.1190.

Preparations

Framycetin Sulphate Gauze Dressing *(D.T.F.)*. Open mesh cotton gauze of leno weave impregnated with a white soft paraffin and wool fat basis containing framycetin sulphate 1%, sterilised. It is supplied in 10-cm squares as single pieces.

Proprietary Preparations

Framycort *(Fisons, UK)*. Preparations containing framycetin sulphate 0.5% and hydrocortisone acetate 0.5%, available as **Ear- and Eye-drops, Eye Ointment,** and **Ointment**.

Framygen *(Fisons, UK)*. Framycetin sulphate, available as **Cream** containing 0.5%; as **Ear-and Eye-drops** containing 0.5%; and as **Eye Ointment** containing 0.5%. (Also available as Framygen in *Austral.*).

Sofradex *(Roussel, UK)*. **Eye-Ear Drops** containing framycetin sulphate 0.5%, dexamethasone sodium *m*-sulphobenzoate equivalent to dexamethasone 0.05%, and gramicidin 0.005%; and **Eye-Ear Ointment** containing framycetin 0.5%, dexamethasone 0.05%, and gramicidin 0.005%.

Soframycin *(Roussel, UK)*. Framycetin sulphate, available as **Eye-drops** containing 0.5%; as **Eye Ointment** containing 0.5%; as **Sterile Powder** for the preparation of solutions for local and topical use and for intrathecal injection, in vials of 500 mg; and as scored **Tablets** of 250 mg. (Also available as Soframycin in *Austral., Canad., Denm., Neth., S.Afr., Switz.*).

Soframycin Skin Cream *(Roussel, UK)*. Contains framycetin sulphate 1.5% and gramicidin 0.005% in a water-miscible basis; **Soframycin Skin Ointment** contains framycetin sulphate 1.5% and gramicidin 0.005% in a basis containing soft paraffin and hydrous wool fat.

Soframycin Nebuliser *(Roussel, UK)*. Nasal spray containing framycetin sulphate 1.25%, gramicidin 0.005% and phenylephrine hydrochloride 0.25%.

Sofra-Tulle *(Roussel, UK)*. A sterile paraffin gauze dressing impregnated with framycetin sulphate 1%. (Also available as Sofra-Tulle in *Austral., Canad., Neth., Norw., S.Afr., Switz.*).

Other Proprietary Names

Isoframicol *(Fr.)*; Perframyl *(Arg.)*; Soframycine *(Belg., Fr.)*; Tuttomycin *(Ger.)*.

A preparation containing framycetin sulphate and light kaolin was formerly marketed in Great Britain under the proprietary name Enterfram (*Fisons*).

87-j

Fusafungine.

A depsipeptide antibiotic of *Fusarium lateritium*.

CAS — 1393-87-9.

Fusafungine occurs as a white or slightly yellowish crystalline powder with a slight odour and a very bitter taste. M.p. 122° to 128°. It contains at least 2 amino acids. Practically **insoluble** in water; very soluble in alcohol and methyl alcohol; soluble in chloroform, propylene glycol, and oils; slightly soluble in glycerol. Solutions in oil may be **sterilised** by maintaining at 150° for 1 hour. The dry substance and solutions in oil are stable.

Fusafungine is active against some Gram-positive and Gram-negative organisms and *Candida albicans*. It has also been stated to possess anti-inflammatory activity.

It is used in the form of an aerosol spray as an 0.25% solution in the treatment of infections of the upper respiratory tract.

References: D. Haler, *J. int. med. Res.*, 1977, *5*, 61; J. C. Vallé-Jones, *ibid.*, 65; M. F. Osman, *ibid.*, 139.

Proprietary Preparations

Locabiotal *(Servier, UK)*. An aerosol spray containing fusafungine 0.25% in solution in isopropyl myristate with a flavouring agent, delivering 125 µg in each metered dose, in a container fitted with nasal and oral nozzles. *Dose*. Nasal, 3 metered doses 5 times daily; oral, 5 doses 5 times daily. Children: nasal, 1 to 3 doses 5 times daily; oral, 2 to 4 doses thrice daily. (Also available as Locabiotal in *Arg., Belg., Fr., Ital., S.Afr., Switz.*).

Other Proprietary Names

Fusaloyos *(Spain)*; Locabiosol *(Ger.)*.

88-z

Fusidic Acid

(B.P.). SQ 16603. *ent*-16α-Acetoxy-3β,11β-dihydroxy-4β,8β,14α-trimethyl-18-nor-5β,10α-cholesta-(17*Z*)-17(20),24-dien-21-oic acid hemihydrate.

$C_{31}H_{48}O_6,\frac{1}{2}H_2O=525.7$.

CAS — 6990-06-3 (anhydrous).

An antimicrobial substance produced by the growth of certain strains of *Fusidium coccineum* (K. Tubaki).

A white odourless or almost odourless crystalline powder. M.p. about 193°. Practically **insoluble** in water; soluble 1 in 5 of alcohol, 1 in 4 of chloroform, and 1 in 60 of ether. **Store** in airtight containers. Protect from light.

Fusidic acid has the actions and uses of Sodium Fusidate, p.1210. It is used for the preparation of aqueous suspensions for administration by mouth and the following doses of fusidic acid have been recommended for children: up to 1 year, 50 mg per kg body-weight daily in 3 divided doses; 1 to 5 years, 250 mg thrice daily; and 5 to 12 years, 500 mg thrice daily (250 mg of fusidic acid is stated to be therapeutically equivalent to 175 mg of sodium fusidate).

Fusidic acid is also used in gels.

Preparations

Fusidic Acid Mixture *(B.P.C. 1973)*. Fusidic Acid Suspension. A suspension of fusidic acid in a suitable coloured flavoured aqueous basis. pH 4.8 to 5.2. The mixture should not be diluted; a dose of 2.5 ml may be measured in a 5-ml spoon, but smaller doses should be measured in a graduated pipette. Protect from light.

When Fusidate Mixture is prescribed, Fusidic Acid Mixture shall be supplied.

Proprietary Preparations

Fucidin Suspension *(Leo, UK)*. Contains fusidic acid 250 mg (stated to be therapeutically equivalent to sodium fusidate 175 mg) in each 5 ml (dilution not recommended). **Fucidin Cream.** Contains fusidic acid 2%. **Fucidin Gel.** Contains fusidic acid 2% in a water-miscible basis. **Fucidin H Gel.** Contains in addition, hydrocortisone acetate 1%. **Fucidin Caviject.** Sterile Fucidin Gel in single-dose applicators containing 7 g. (Also available as Fucidin in *Denm., Ital., Norw., Switz.*).

89-c

Gentamicin Sulphate

(B.P.). Gentamicin Sulfate *(U.S.P.)*. The sulphates of a mixture of antimicrobial substances produced by *Micromonospora purpurea*.

CAS — 1403-66-3 (gentamicin); 1405-41-0 (sulphate).

Pharmacopoeias. In *Br., Braz.,* and *U.S.*

Gentamicin sulphate is a complex mixture of the sulphates of gentamicin C_1, gentamicin C_{1A}, and gentamicin C_2. It contains when dried 31 to 34% of sulphate and not less than 590 units of gentamicin per mg; 80 000 units of gentamicin is approximately equivalent to 80 mg of gentamicin. A white to buff-coloured powder containing not more than 15% of water.

Soluble in water; practically insoluble in alcohol, chloroform, and ether. A solution in water is dextrorotatory. A 4% solution in water has a pH of 3.5 to 5.5. Solutions are **sterilised** by filtration. **Store** in airtight containers.

Incompatible with amphotericin, cephalosporins, erythromycin, heparin, penicillins, sodium bicarbonate, and sulphadiazine sodium. When gentamicin is given with carbenicillin or other penicillins, administration at different sites is recommended.

Aqueous solutions of gentamicin turned brown when autoclaved and this could be prevented by the addition of concentrations of sodium metabisulphite as low as 80 µg per ml. Potency was not affected by autoclaving.— *Pharm. J.*, 1976, *1*, 229.

Potency of gentamicin sulphate was lost in plastic disposable syringes and a brown precipitate formed. Storage in glass disposable syringes should not exceed 30 days.— B. Weiner *et al.*, *Am. J. Hosp. Pharm.*, 1976, *33*, 1254.

The preparation and properties of liposome-associated gentamicin.— J. R. Morgan and K. E. Williams, *Antimicrob. Ag. Chemother.*, 1980, *17*, 544.

For reports of interference with assays for aminoglycosides, see under Precautions.

Incompatibility. Gentamicin 10 µg per ml in serum (representing the peak serum concentration likely to be achieved after an intramuscular or intravenous injection) lost 50% of its activity in 36 hours at 37° when *carbenicillin* was added. *Ampicillin, benzylpenicillin, cloxacillin,* and *methicillin* caused a loss of 20% or more in gentamicin activity after 48 hours when added in concentrations of 200 µg per ml but no significant loss in concentrations of 50 µg per ml. No inactivation of gentamicin occurred with *cephaloridine* or *cephalothin*. Gentamicin 160 µg per ml was stable for 48 hours at room temperature in dextrose solution 5%, dextrose-saline solution, and saline solution. When *carbenicillin* was added a significant loss of potency occurred in 30 minutes and 50% was lost in 8 to 12 hours. With *ampicillin*, 50% loss of gentamicin activity occurred after 2 hours. Visible precipitates occurred with *cephalothin* and *cloxacillin*.— P. Noone and J. R. Pattison, *Lancet*, 1971, *2*, 575.

For a list of incompatibilities including *chloramphenicol sodium succinate* and *vitamin-B complex*, see *Med. Lett.*, 1972, *14* (Jan.), *Suppl.*, 32.

Stability tests *in vitro* indicated that ticarcillin caused significantly less inactivation of aminoglycoside antibiotics, particularly amikacin and netilmicin, than did carbenicillin.— L. K. Pickering and P. Gearhart, *Antimicrob. Ag. Chemother.*, 1979, *15*, 592.

Further references: B. B. Riley, *J. Hosp. Pharm.*, 1970, *28*, 228; J. Jacobs *et al.*, *J. clin. Path.*, 1973, *26*, 742.

For the effect of dopamine hydrochloride on gentamicin, see Dopamine Hydrochloride, p.9.

Stability. There was no significant loss of potency when gentamicin injection was added to commercially available gentamicin 0.3% eye-drops and the resulting solution of 14 mg per ml kept at 25° for 7 days.— E. Osborn *et al.*, *Am. J. Ophthal.*, 1976, *82*, 775.

Units. One unit of gentamicin is contained in 0.00156 mg of the first International Reference Preparation (1968) of gentamicin sulphate which contains 641 units per mg.

Adverse Effects. As for Neomycin Sulphate, p.1189.

Vestibular damage is more common than hearing loss which, when it occurs, is greatest in the high-tone range. Patients with renal impairment are especially susceptible to ototoxicity; high total doses of gentamicin and previous exposure to other ototoxic drugs are contributary factors. Ototoxicity has also been reported after the topical treatment of severe burns with gentamicin.

Reversible nephrotoxicity may occur and acute renal failure has been reported, often in association with the concurrent administration of a cephalosporin antibiotic.

Plasma concentrations above 10 to 12 µg per ml are associated with a high risk of toxicity although individual tolerance may vary. Trough plasma concentrations, that is those immediately before the next dose, may be the best guide to cumulation of gentamicin; a trough concentration of more than 2 µg per ml may be associated with toxicity.

Gentamicin has a neuromuscular blocking action

but is less potent than neomycin. Hypersensitivity reactions have occurred, especially after local use, and cross-sensitivity with neomycin and kanamycin may occur.

Infrequent effects reported include anaemia, purpura, convulsions, increased serum aminotransferase values, and increased serum-bilirubin concentrations.

A review of the toxicity of gentamicin.— W. L. Hewitt, *Postgrad. med. J.*, 1974, *50* (Nov.), *Suppl.* 7, 55.

An accidental overdose of 160 mg of gentamicin (2 mg per kg body-weight) instead of 2 mg was given intrathecally on two occasions to a patient; the only signs of toxicity were transient calf pain and weakness.— J. Smilack and R. V. McCloskey (letter), *Ann. intern. Med.*, 1972, *77*, 1002.

A report of Fanconi syndrome associated with the administration of gentamicin.— J. C. Russo and R. D. Adelman, *J. Pediat.*, 1980, *96*, 151.

Allergy. An anaphylactic reaction to gentamicin in one patient. Collapse with tachycardia, hypotension, and apnoea occurred within a minute of starting to inject 80 mg intravenously.— F. J. Hall (letter), *Lancet*, 1977, *2*, 455. A large or concentrated dose of an antibiotic could produce adverse effects due to the release of endotoxin in patients whose bloodstreams contained a heavy infection of Gram-negative bacteria. This should be considered as a cause of anaphylaxis. One patient had died in endotoxic shock 20 minutes after receiving gentamicin intravenously for a suspected heavy bacteraemia following surgical disturbance of a large pelvic abscess.— D. A. B. Hopkin (letter), *ibid.*, 603.

Alopecia. A 15-year-old boy complained of dizziness, tinnitus, and blurred vision during treatment with gentamicin, and there was progressive loss of hair and eyebrows. The blood concentration of gentamicin was 14 µg per ml. Hair began to grow again when treatment was discontinued.— H. Yoshioka and I. Matsuda (letter), *J. Am. med. Ass.*, 1970, *211*, 123.

Blood disorders. A report of granulocytopenia after gentamicin and diazepam.— R. Bussien, *Nouv. Presse méd.*, 1974, *3*, 1236. For a report of reversible agranulocytosis in 1 patient given gentamicin, see J. C. Chang and B. Reyes, *J. Am. med. Ass.*, 1975, *232*, 1154.

Amikacin, gentamicin, kanamycin, netilmicin, or tobramycin *in vitro* increased granulocyte adherence and slightly decreased migration, with no change in phagocytosis.— M. M. Seklecki *et al.*, *Antimicrob. Ag. Chemother.*, 1978, *13*, 552.

A report of thrombocytopenia associated with the administration of gentamicin.— J. -H. Chen *et al.*, *N. Y. St. J. Med.*, 1980, *80*, 1134.

Electrolyte disturbances. Two patients developed hypomagnesaemia, hypocalcaemia, and hypokalaemia as a result of renal wasting of magnesium and potassium shortly after receiving large doses of gentamicin (total doses of 1.32 and 10.99 g). Tetany developed in 1 patient and continuous intravenous infusion of calcium was necessary. Hypocalcaemia was associated with inappropriately low serum-immunoreactive parathyroid hormone concentrations. Serum calcium, magnesium, and potassium should be monitored in patients receiving large doses of gentamicin.— R. S. Bar *et al.*, *Ann. intern. Med.*, 1975, *82*, 646.

Hypocalcaemia, hypomagnesaemia, and hypokalaemia were associated with aminoglycoside therapy in 17 patients with malignant disease. Five developed progressive renal failure and there were 12 deaths. Antineoplastic agents and especially doxorubicin might have exacerbated this metabolic disturbance.— M. J. Keating *et al.*, *Cancer*, 1977, *39*, 1410.

Further references: A. M. Holmes *et al.*, *Q.J. Med.*, 1970, *39*, 299; G. P. Young *et al.* (letter), *Lancet*, 1973, *2*, 855; S. V. Cabizuca and K. B. Desser, *J. Am. med. Ass.*, 1976, *236*, 956; C. J. H. Kelnar *et al.*, *Archs Dis. Childh.*, 1978, *53*, 817.

Intracranial hypertension. Benign intracranial hypertension in a 26-year-old man with cystic fibrosis was attributed to gentamicin which had been given, 80 mg intramuscularly twice daily, for 5 days prior to his admission to hospital with headaches and transient blurring of vision. Gentamicin was discontinued on the second day in hospital and the headaches subsided.— R. Boe and C. S. Conner (letter), *J. Am. med. Ass.*, 1973, *226*, 567.

Nephrotoxicity. On 19 occasions when patients with renal allografts were given courses of gentamicin, urine-enzyme activity rose, indicative of renal damage. Serum-creatinine and urinary-protein concentrations generally rose. The damage was usually reversible. Increased urine-enzyme activity was not indicative of allograft rejection if the patient was receiving gentamicin.— J. M. Wellwood *et al.*, *Br. med. J.*, 1975, *3*, 278. Urine-enzyme activity in the assessment of renal disease.— *idem*, 408.

Acute renal failure appeared in 5 patients over 45 years of age 8 to 17 days after the start of treatment with gentamicin 1.7 to 2.88 g given over 12 to 18 days; oliguria was not seen. Recovery took an average of 42 days and was complete in 4 patients.— N. E. Gary *et al.*, *Archs intern. Med.*, 1976, *136*, 1101.

A study in 64 seriously ill patients, average age 65 years, who received standard doses of gentamicin sulphate for up to an average of 11 days indicated that tissue accumulation of gentamicin was greater in 17 of the patients who experienced nephrotoxic effects than in the 47 patients who had no apparent change in renal function.— J. J. Schentag *et al.*, *J. Am. med. Ass.*, 1978, *240*, 2067. In a study of 114 patients who received gentamicin, amikacin, or tobramycin, aminoglycoside nephrotoxicity was found to be dependent on tissue accumulation and not simply elevated serum concentrations. The antibiotic should be withdrawn if aminoglycoside nephrotoxicity occurs since renal function will continue to deteriorate despite a reduction in dosage.— J. J. Schentag *et al.*, *J. surg. Res.*, 1979, *26*, 270.

A report of interstitial nephritis attributed to gentamicin.— D. Saltissi *et al.*, *Br. med. J.*, 1979, *1*, 1182. See also C. T. Flynn (letter), *ibid.*, 1628.

A study of 127 patients who received gentamicin, tobramycin, or amikacin indicated that aminoglycoside-induced auditory toxicity and nephrotoxicity were independent events.— C. R. Smith *et al.*, *Antimicrob. Ag. Chemother.*, 1979, *15*, 780.

Daily urinary cast counts could be used to identify early renal tubular damage in patients receiving aminoglycosides.— J. J. Schentag *et al.*, *Antimicrob. Ag. Chemother.*, 1979, *16*, 468. A report of the measurement of lysozyme excretion in the urine to detect early gentamicin-induced nephrotoxicity before serum creatinine rises.— G. Nicot *et al.* (letter), *New Engl. J. Med.*, 1980, *303*, 48.

In a double-blind comparison of toxicity, in patients who had received at least 9 doses of antibiotic, tobramycin caused nephrotoxicity less frequently than gentamicin but there was no significant difference in the incidence of auditory toxicity. Nephrotoxicity, defined in terms of an increase in serum creatinine, occurred in 19 of 72 patients (26%) receiving gentamicin compared with 9 of 74 (12%) given tobramycin; the severity of nephrotoxicity was similar in both groups. Auditory toxicity developed in 5 of 47 patients given gentamicin and 5 of 44 given tobramycin.— C. R. Smith *et al.*, *New Engl. J. Med.*, 1980, *302*, 1106. See also M. E. Plaut *et al.* (letter), *Lancet*, 1979, *2*, 526; A. M. Emmerson *et al.* (letter), *ibid.*, 1980, *1*, 96; G. D. Kumin, *J. Am. med. Ass.*, 1980, *244*, 1808. A study demonstrating no significant difference between the nephrotoxicity of gentamicin and tobramycin.— I. W. Fong *et al.*, *J. antimicrob. Chemother.*, 1981, *7*, 81.

Further references: T. Kahn and R. M. Stein (letter), *Lancet*, 1972, *1*, 498; P. Jungers *et al.*, *Nouv. Presse méd.*, 1977, *6*, 923; *Lancet*, 1978, *2*, 558.

In association with cephalosporins. A 40-year-old man with malignant lymphoma who developed acute tubular necrosis after treatment with gentamicin sulphate 1 mg per kg body-weight and cephalothin sodium 2 g every 6 hours intravenously for 10 days died of renal failure and disseminated lymphosarcoma.— S. N. Bobrow *et al.*, *J. Am. med. Ass.*, 1972, *222*, 1546.

Three patients developed reversible acute renal failure when treated with gentamicin 4.4 to 6 mg per kg body-weight daily in conjunction with cephalothin 6 to 12 g daily.— D. Kleinknecht *et al.* (letter), *Lancet*, 1973, *1*, 1129.

Review of data from the Boston Collaborative Drug Surveillance Program revealed no enhanced renal toxicity arising from the use of gentamicin with cephalothin. Increases in blood urea nitrogen values were found in 22 of 334 patients given gentamicin, 10 of 492 given cephalothin, and 23 of 247 given both antibiotics.— W. L. Fanning *et al.*, *Antimicrob. Ag. Chemother.*, 1976, *10*, 80.

A discussion on whether cephalosporin antibiotics potentiate or antagonise the nephrotoxic effects of aminoglycoside antibiotics.— F. P. Marsh, *J. antimicrob. Chemother.*, 1978, *4*, 103. There is little justification for the use of a cephalosporin in association with an aminoglycoside.— P. Noone (letter), *ibid.*, 465. See also F. P. Marsh (letter), *ibid.*, 577.

See also Cephalothin Sodium, p.1129.

Neuromuscular blockade. Neuromuscular blockade and profound respiratory depression occurred in a 59-year-old man during treatment with gentamicin intramuscularly in a dose of 60 mg every 8 hours. Breathing improved following the intravenous administration of 1 g of calcium chloride and withdrawal of gentamicin. It was considered that renal impairment, cumulative effects of gentamicin, and lowered serum calcium might possibly have facilitated the neuromuscular blocking action of gentamicin.— W. A. Warner and E. Sanders, *J. Am. med. Ass.*, 1971, *215*, 1153.

A 64-year-old man with severe Parkinson's disease developed profound transitory muscular weakness due to neuromuscular blockade during 4 days of treatment with gentamicin 80 mg intramuscularly, reduced to 45 mg on day 2, every 8 hours.— J. L. Holtzman (letter), *Ann. intern. Med.*, 1976, *84*, 55.

Further references to aminoglycoside antibiotics and neuromuscular blockade: A. G. Paradelis (letter), *J. antimicrob. Chemother.*, 1979, *5*, 737.

Neurotoxicity. A woman with meningitis was treated with gentamicin sulphate and tobramycin sulphate intrathecally and intramuscularly. She developed evidence of arachnoiditis and symptoms of polyradiculitis. Neurological symptoms improved when therapy was withdrawn and recurred when intrathecal administration was started again.— J. W. Hollifield *et al.*, *J. Am. med. Ass.*, 1976, *236*, 1264.

Meningeal irritation following the intrathecal administration of gentamicin.— R. M. Buckley *et al.*, *Am. J. med. Sci.*, 1977, *274*, 207. See also I. Watanabe *et al.*, *Ann. Neurol.*, 1978, *4*, 564. The absence of any significant ill effects following the intrathecal injection of 160 mg of gentamicin.— J. Smilack and R. V. McCloskey (letter), *Ann. intern. Med.*, 1972, *77*, 1002.

A report of polyneuropathy and, in part, encephalopathy occurring in 4 patients following treatment with gentamicin.— A. Bischoff *et al.*, *Schweiz. med. Wschr.*, 1977, *107*, 3.

Ototoxicity. In a study carried out over a period of 7 years, 1327 patients were treated with gentamicin, 3 mg or more per kg body-weight daily. Of these, 31 (2.3%) developed significant ototoxicity which could be attributed to gentamicin.— G. M. Arcieri *et al.*, *Med. J. Aust.*, 1970, *1*, *Suppl.* (June 13), 30.

References to the incidence of ototoxicity in infants and children.— J. Elfving *et al.*, *Chemotherapy, Basle*, 1973, *18*, 141; P. Echeverria *et al.*, *ibid.*, 1978, *24*, 267; T. Finitzo-Hieber *et al.*, *Pediatrics*, 1979, *63*, 443.

Vestibular toxicity was evident in 12 of 22 patients with chronic renal failure treated with gentamicin for severe infections. Maintenance of balance was more badly disturbed than expected in 3 of these patients possibly due not only to vestibular loss but also to loss of proprioception secondary to polyneuropathy resulting from chronic renal failure. Four patients with extensive burns receiving gentamicin suffered both vestibular and cochlear toxicity with moderate to severe hearing loss. This higher incidence of cochlear toxicity could have been due to the additional use of topical gentamicin in these patients.— V. S. Dayal *et al.*, *Archs Otolar.*, 1974, *100*, 338.

The Boston Collaborative Drug Surveillance Program monitored consecutively 32 812 medical inpatients. Drug-induced deafness occurred in 4 of 1125 patients given gentamicin.— J. Porter and H. Jick, *Lancet*, 1977, *1*, 587.

Permanent deafness in one ear and partial deafness in the other occurred in a man with advanced renal failure given gentamicin. There were no vestibular symptoms.— D. A. Moffat and R. T. Ramsden, *J. Lar. Otol.*, 1977, *91*, 511.

Ototoxicity was considered to be more often associated with sustained plasma concentrations of aminoglycosides than with high peak concentrations. There was no conclusive evidence for more than marginal differences between the ototoxicity of commonly used aminoglycosides.— J. M. Symonds, *J. antimicrob. Chemother.*, 1979, *4*, 199.

Further references: G. G. Jackson and G. Arcieri, *J. infect. Dis.*, 1971, *124*, *Suppl.*, 130; V. S. Dayal *et al.*, *Ann. Otol. Rhinol. Lar.*, 1979, *88*, 36.

See also under Nephrotoxicity (above).

Psychosis. Visual hallucinations were reported in 3 patients who had each received a total of 880 mg, 780 mg, and 1200 mg of gentamicin respectively by intramuscular injection; normal mental states were recovered within 72 hours of withdrawal of gentamicin.— G. J. Byrd (letter), *Drug Ther.*, 1976, *6*, 11. See also G. J. Byrd, *J. Am. med. Ass.*, 1977, *238*, 53.

Treatment of Adverse Effects. Gentamicin may be removed by haemodialysis or peritoneal dialysis. Calcium salts given intravenously have been used to counter the neuromuscular blockade caused by gentamicin and the use of neostigmine has also been suggested.

Haemoperfusion through acrylic resin-coated charcoal together with haemodialysis removed about 70% of the gentamicin given, in excessive dosage, to an anuric patient.— N. Wright and A. Bhamjee, *Postgrad. med. J.*, 1980, *56*, 140.

Precautions. Gentamicin is contra-indicated in patients with a known history of allergy to it and probably to other aminoglycosides. If symptoms of ototoxicity occur gentamicin should be withdrawn immediately.

Gentamicin should be given with care and in reduced dosage to patients with impaired renal function. Plasma concentrations of gentamicin should be checked frequently in these patients and the dosage should be adjusted if the plasma concentration approaches 10 to 12 μg per ml or if the concentration immediately before the next dose exceeds 2 μg per ml.

Care should be exerted when gentamicin is given to patients receiving other drugs with a neuromuscular blocking activity or which are ototoxic or nephrotoxic. Anti-emetics may mask ototoxic symptoms.

Since gentamicin has been shown to be incompatible with carbenicillin sodium *in vitro* the two antibiotics should be administered separately when both are required. No antagonism has been shown *in vivo* except when the two antibiotics have been used together in patients with severe renal impairment, when the activity of gentamicin has been diminished.

Many workers consider that gentamicin should not be used topically because of the serious risk of developing bacterial resistance.

A report of serum-gentamicin concentrations being reduced in febrile subjects.— J. E. Pennington *et al.*, *J. infect. Dis.*, 1975, *132*, 270.

The potential hazard of gentamicin therapy in patients with ascites was demonstrated in a man with high predose concentrations of gentamicin. His ascitic fluid might have acted as a reservoir of gentamicin.— S. K. Seth and T. D. Moore (letter), *Ann. intern. Med.*, 1979, *91*, 134.

Interactions. High concentrations (18.75 mg per ml) of sulphacetamide increased the mean bactericidal concentration of gentamicin *in vitro* against 37 strains of *Pseudomonas aeruginosa*. As such concentrations are often reached the use of sulphacetamide with gentamicin in the treatment of eye infections was not recommended.— L. M. Burger *et al.*, *Am. J. Ophthal.*, 1973, *75*, 314.

Studies in *animals* demonstrating enhancement of ear and kidney damage resulting from concurrent administration of frusemide and aminoglycoside antibiotics.— I. Ohtani *et al.*, *Chemotherapy, Tokyo*, 1977, *25*, 2348. Concurrent administration of frusemide and gentamicin in healthy subjects reduced renal clearance of gentamicin with consequent increase in plasma concentrations; in some instances plasma-gentamicin concentrations had been increased by 70%.— W. J. Tilstone *et al.*, *Clin. Pharmac. Ther.*, 1977, *22*, 389.

A report of reduced ticarcillin and gentamicin concentrations in the serum of patients receiving the 2 antibiotics together when compared with each of the drugs given together with cephalothin.— J. Murillo *et al.*, *J. Am. med. Ass.*, 1979, *241*, 2401.

For reports on the effects of other drugs on the antimicrobial activity of gentamicin, see below.

Interference with aminoglycoside assays. The radionuclide gallium-67 was found to interfere with radio-enzymatic assays of aminoglycoside antibiotics. A method of overcoming this problem is described. Several other radionuclides tested did not affect the assay.— I. Bhattacharya *et al.*, *Antimicrob. Ag. Chemother.*, 1978, *14*, 448. See also K. Shannon *et al.* (letter), *J. antimicrob. Chemother.*, 1980, *6*, 285.

In the presence of zinc salts, assays for aminoglycosides could give falsely low concentrations.— R. H. George and D. E. Healing (letter), *J. antimicrob. Chemother.*, 1978, *4*, 186.

A study on the following factors which affect the measurements of serum-gentamicin concentrations by the luciferase method: sodium phosphate, glucose, and heparin.— L. Nilsson, *Antimicrob. Ag. Chemother.*, 1980, *17*, 918.

Pregnancy and the neonate. If given during pregnancy gentamicin sulphate might cause damage to the eighth cranial nerve of the foetus.— G. M. Stirrat, *Prescribers' J.*, 1973, *13*, 135.

Antimicrobial Action. Gentamicin is bactericidal with greater antibacterial activity than streptomycin, neomycin, or kanamycin although it acts similarly by inhibiting protein synthesis in susceptible bacteria. It is effective against many strains of Gram-negative bacteria including species of *Escherichia, Enterobacter, Klebsiella, Salmonella, Serratia, Shigella,* some *Proteus* and, unlike kanamycin and the earlier aminoglycosides, against *Pseudomonas aeruginosa.* Minimum inhibitory concentrations have been reported to range from 0.06 to 8 μg per ml.

Among the Gram-positive organisms *Staphylococcus aureus* is highly sensitive to gentamicin with minimum inhibitory concentrations being reported within the range of 0.125 to 1 μg per ml. Other Gram-positive cocci are less sensitive but *Bacillus, Clostridium,* and *Corynebacterium* spp. and *Listeria monocytogenes* may be inhibited by normal concentrations.

Gentamicin and carbenicillin have an enhanced antimicrobial action *in vivo* against *Pseudomonas* when given together. A similar activity has been reported for gentamicin and cephalothin against *Klebsiella* as well as for gentamicin and benzylpenicillin against *Streptococcus faecalis* and *Str. viridans.*

Gentamicin is active against some strains of *Mycobacterium tuberculosis* and mycoplasmas have been reported sensitive; yeasts and fungi are resistant.

It is more active in an alkaline medium.

For a brief discussion on the aminoglycoside group of antibiotics, see p.1083.

Sensitivity studies carried out on 20 strains of *Aeromonas hydrophila* demonstrated that all were inhibited by 3 μg per ml of gentamicin, 5 μg per ml of chloramphenicol, 10 μg per ml of nalidixic acid, and 50 μg per ml of nitrofurantoin.— J. A. Washington, *Ann. intern. Med.*, 1972, *76*, 611.

The activities of gentamicin, amikacin, tobramycin, and sissomicin were compared *in vitro* in a study of 196 gentamicin-resistant Gram-negative rods and 212 similar strains sensitive to gentamicin. Organisms with an MIC of gentamicin of 8 μg per ml or more were considered resistant. Gentamicin was the most active against all the sensitive organisms except for *Pseudomonas* spp. which were most sensitive to tobramycin. Amikacin was the most active against gentamicin-resistant organisms; sissomicin showed little activity against resistant organisms and MICs against the gentamicin-sensitive rods were generally higher than those of gentamicin.— F. A. Drasar *et al.*, *Br. med. J.*, 1976, *2*, 1284. See also I. Phillips *et al.*, *J. antimicrob. Chemother.*, 1977, *3*, 403.

The majority of 190 strains of *Yersinia enterocolitica* were inhibited *in vitro* by 1 μg per ml of gentamicin, netilmicin, or tobramycin, by 2 μg per ml of neomycin or amikacin, or by 8 μg per ml of kanamycin.— M. Raevuori *et al.*, *Antimicrob. Ag. Chemother.*, 1978, *13*, 888. See also S. Hammerberg *et al.*, *Antimicrob. Ag. Chemother.*, 1977, *11*, 566.

Although the majority of strains of *Vibrio parahaemolyticus* and *Vibrio alginolyticus* were susceptible to gentamicin by agar diffusion tests, susceptibility could not be measured by MIC methods because sodium chloride in the medium diminished the activity of gentamicin.— S. W. Joseph *et al.*, *Antimicrob. Ag. Chemother.*, 1978, *13*, 244.

Studies of the activity of gentamicin against *Ps. aeruginosa in vitro* and in *mice* suggested that current susceptibility criteria could lead to overestimated activity and hence underdosing with gentamicin.— T. I. Nicas and L. E. Bryan, *Antimicrob. Ag. Chemother.*, 1978, *13*, 796.

In a study of the activity *in vitro* of 29 antimicrobial agents against 95 strains of *Campylobacter fetus* subsp. *jejuni*, furazolidone and gentamicin were the most active. The penicillins and cephalosporins were generally inactive.— R. Vanhoof *et al.*, *Antimicrob. Ag. Chemother.*, 1978, *14*, 553. See also M. Walder, *ibid.*, 1979, *16*, 37.

Gentamicin was found to be more active than cephalothin, vancomycin, or rifampicin *in vitro* against methicillin-resistant isolates of *Staph. epidermidis* but caused the emergence of strain variants. When gentamicin was used with cephalothin, vancomycin, or rifampicin there was no improvement in bactericidal activity but no strain variants emerged. Gentamicin was also the most effective antibiotic in *mice* infected with *Staph. epidermidis*, but gentamicin with vancomycin was the most effective regimen. Rifampicin and vancomycin used together were generally as effective as gentamicin alone both *in vitro* and in *mice*. When cephalothin was used with gentamicin or vancomycin or when gentamicin was used with nafcillin in *mice* there was an increased death-rate compared with the use of any of the drugs alone. The antagonism was not due to drug-drug inactivation.— F. D. Lowy *et al.*, *Antimicrob. Ag. Chemother.*, 1979, *16*, 314.

A study of the reliability of some agar diffusion assays for aminoglycoside antibiotics.— G. Kahlmeter, *J. antimicrob. Chemother.*, 1980, *6*, 43.

Diminished activity. Magnesium and to a lesser extent calcium increased the MIC of gentamicin *in vitro* against *Ps. aeruginosa*.— D. N. Gilbert *et al.*, *J. infect. Dis.*, 1971, *124, Suppl.*, S37. The activity *in vitro* of gentamicin against *Ps. aeruginosa* was antagonised by physiological concentrations of calcium present in serum but to a lesser extent than the antagonism of colistin.— S. D. Davis and A. Iannetta, *Appl. Microbiol.*, 1972, *23*, 775.

The antibacterial activity of gentamicin was decreased by 9 to 14% in the presence of heparin concentrations up to 100 units per ml. Inhibition increased with concentration, reaching 56% with a concentration of heparin 1000 units per ml. Underestimation of gentamicin activity would be most likely when small quantities of blood were collected in capillary tubes containing relatively large amounts of heparin. Concentrations of heparin reached in the blood of patients receiving heparin were too low to affect gentamicin.— C. Regamey *et al.*, *Antimicrob. Ag. Chemother.*, 1972, *1*, 329.

Large concentrations of sulphacetamide significantly increased the mean bactericidal concentration of gentamicin *in vitro* against *Ps. aeruginosa*. High concentrations of sulphafurazole significantly decreased the MIC of gentamicin against *Ps. aeruginosa* but had no significant effect on the mean bactericidal concentration.— L. M. Burger *et al.*, *Am. J. Ophthal.*, 1973, *75*, 314.

The antimicrobial activity of gentamicin *in vitro* against *Staph. aureus, E. coli, Kleb. aerogenes,* and *Enterobacter* and *Proteus* spp. was reduced in anaerobic and hypercapnic conditions. Kanamycin, tobramycin, and amikacin were similarly affected.— A. V. Reynolds *et al.*, *Lancet*, 1976, *1*, 447.

The antibacterial activity *in vitro* of gentamicin or tobramycin against *Ps. aeruginosa* was antagonised by acetylcysteine.— M. F. Parry and H. C. Neu, *J. clin. Microbiol.*, 1977, *5*, 58.

When used at concentrations achievable in serum, daunorubicin or cytarabine reduced the activity of gentamicin or amikacin against some strains of *Kleb. pneumoniae* and *Ps. aeruginosa* but not against *E. coli*.— M. R. Moody *et al.*, *Antimicrob. Ag. Chemother.*, 1978, *14*, 737.

Chloramphenicol and gentamicin might be antagonistic.— P. J. Sanderson (letter), *Lancet*, 1978, *2*, 210.

Antagonism occurred against some strains of *Staph. aureus* when the activity of gentamicin was tested *in vitro* with actinomycin D or doxorubicin.— J. Y. Jacobs *et al.*, *Antimicrob. Ag. Chemother.*, 1979, *15*, 580.

Effect with clindamycin. Clindamycin inhibited the antistaphylococcal activity of gentamicin *in vitro*.— P. D. Meers (letter), *Lancet*, 1973, *2*, 573. Antagonism was demonstrated against strains of *Str. mutans*.— R. J. Snyder *et al.*, *Antimicrob. Ag. Chemother.*, 1975, *7*, 333.

Although clindamycin had been reported to inhibit *in vitro* the activity of gentamicin on *E. coli* and *Kleb. pneumoniae*, no confirmation was found in a *murine* model of *E. coli* infection involving gentamicin or amikacin with clindamycin.— E. Ekwo and G. Peter, *Antimicrob. Ag. Chemother.*, 1976, *10*, 893.

Gentamicin had no effect on the activity of clindamycin against *Bacteroides fragilis* and neither did clindamycin affect the activity of gentamicin against *E. coli*.— J. Klastersky and M. Husson, *Antimicrob. Ag. Chemother.*, 1977, *12*, 135.

Further references: D. J. H. Payne and O. A. Okubadejo (letter), *Lancet*, 1973, *2*, 845; O. A. Okubadejo and J. Allen, *J. antimicrob. Chemother.*, 1975, *1*, 403.

Enhanced activity. The MICs of carbenicillin and gentamicin against a clinical isolate of *Ps. aeruginosa in vitro* were substantially reduced when they were used with triethylenetetramine dihydrochloride.— B. Light and H. G. Riggs, *Antimicrob. Ag. Chemother.*, 1978, *13*, 979.

Synergism usually occurred when gentamicin was tested

in vitro with mitomycin against some strains of *Staph. aureus*. The effect of mitomycin was obtained at concentrations below those usually obtainable in serum.— J. Y. Jacobs *et al.*, *Antimicrob. Ag. Chemother.*, 1979, *15*, 580.

With cefotaxime. Enhanced activity *in vitro* against aminoglycoside-resistant *Ps. aeruginosa*.— P. R. Murray, *Antimicrob. Ag. Chemother.*, 1980, *17*, 474.

With cephalothin. For reports of enhanced activity *in vitro* against *Klebsiella* spp., see J. Klastersky *et al.*, *Am. J. med. Sci.*, 1971, *262*, 283; R. M. D'Alessandri *et al.*, *Antimicrob. Ag. Chemother.*, 1976, *10*, 889. Against staphylococci, see J. Klastersky, *Antimicrob. Ag. Chemother.*, 1972, *1*, 441; R. L. Marier *et al.*, *ibid.*, 1975, *8*, 571.

With cephazolin. Cephazolin with gentamicin showed enhanced activity against enterococci *in vitro*.— M. Bourque *et al.*, *Antimicrob. Ag. Chemother.*, 1976, *10*, 157.

With co-trimoxazole. Enhanced activity *in vitro* against *E. coli* and *Kleb. pneumoniae*.— J. W. Paisley and J. A. Washington, *Antimicrob. Ag. Chemother.*, 1978, *14*, 656.

With minocycline. Demonstration *in vitro* of enhanced antimicrobial activity with a combination of gentamicin and minocycline against the Enterobacteriaceae, especially *E. coli*.— R. J. Fass *et al.*, *Antimicrob. Ag. Chemother.*, 1976, *10*, 34.

With the penicillins. For reports of enhanced activity *in vitro* against *Str. faecalis*, see M. J. Basker and R. Sutherland, *J. antimicrob. Chemother.*, 1977, *3*, 273 (amoxycillin); S. A. Calderwood *et al.*, *Antimicrob. Ag. Chemother.*, 1977, *12*, 401. Against Enterobacteriaceae, see H. C. Neu and K. P. Fu, *Antimicrob. Ag. Chemother.*, 1978, *13*, 813 (azlocillin). Against *Listeria monocytogenes*, see G. L. Wiggins *et al.*, *Antimicrob. Ag. Chemother.*, 1978, *13*, 854 (ampicillin). Against *Staph. aureus*, see C. U. Tuazon *et al.*, *Curr. ther. Res.*, 1978, *23*, 760 (nafcillin); R. J. P. Hemmer *et al.*, *Antimicrob. Ag. Chemother.*, 1979, *15*, 34 (methicillin); C. Watanakunakorn and C. Glotzbecker, *J. antimicrob. Chemother.*, 1979, *5*, 151 (carbenicillin); J. H. Licht, *Archs intern. Med.*, 1979, *139*, 1094 (penicillinase-resistant penicillin). Against aminoglycoside-resistant group B streptococci, see M. D. Cooper *et al.*, *Antimicrob. Ag. Chemother.*, 1979, *15*, 484 (ampicillin). Against antibiotic-tolerant lactobacilli, see A. S. Bayer *et al.*, *Antimicrob. Ag. Chemother.*, 1980, *17*, 359 (benzylpenicillin or ampicillin).

For the enhancement of activity of gentamicin against *Ps. aeruginosa* and *Providencia* by carbenicillin or cephalothin, see Tobramycin, p.1226.

For details of the synergistic activity of gentamicin and carbenicillin, see Use with Carbenicillin, p.1173.

Resistance. An increase in the incidence of resistant staphylococci, *Pseudomonas aeruginosa*, and other Gram-negative bacteria has followed the increased parenteral and local use of gentamicin. Resistance may be transferable and result from the plasmid-mediated production of inactivating enzymes. There may be cross-resistance between gentamicin and other aminoglycosides including neomycin, kanamycin, and tobramycin.

From 1 to 2% of all Gram-negative rods isolated in a London hospital were resistant to gentamicin, a 2-fold increase over the previous 18 months. They included *Ps. aeruginosa* (about 5%), *Klebsiella* and *Enterobacter* spp. (7%), and *Acinetobacter* spp. (20%), compared with only about 0.1% of *Escherichia coli* and *Proteus mirabilis*. The use of gentamicin given parenterally had more than doubled over the previous 4 years.— F. A. Draser *et al.*, *Br. med. J.*, 1976, *2*, 1284.

Gentamicin resistance in Japan.— H. Nakahara *et al.* (letter), *Lancet*, 1977, *1*, 911.

It was considered that gentamicin 240 mg daily would be effective only against very susceptible bacteria with an MIC of up to 1 µg per ml.— R. Bickenbach *et al.*, *Arzneimittel-Forsch.*, 1977, *27*, 2023.

A study of resistance to aminoglycoside antibiotics among the Enterobacteriaceae and *Acinetobacter* spp. Of the 142 strains tested, 120 were resistant to streptomycin, 69 to kanamycin, 76 to gentamicin, 52 to tobramycin, and 12 to amikacin. Most gentamicin-resistant strains were resistant to the other antibiotics except dibekacin and tobramycin which were active against about half of the strains and amikacin which was active against about three quarters of the strains. The majority of gentamicin-resistant strains produced inactivating or modifying enzymes.— K. P. Shannon *et al.*, *J. antimicrob. Chemother.*, 1978, *4*, 131.

A discussion of resistance to antibiotics related to topical use.— *Br. med. J.*, 1978, *2*, 649.

Resistance of some clinical isolates of *Acinetobacter calcoaceticus* subsp. *anitratus* to high concentrations of kanamycin, tobramycin, and amikacin was associated with the production of an aminoglycoside-modifying acetyltransferase and resistance to kanamycin and neomycin was associated with a phosphotransferase. Strains resistant to lower concentrations of the antibiotics did not have this enzyme activity. Strains resistant to gentamicin could not be shown to produce resistance by enzymatic modification.— B. E. Murray and R. C. Moellering, *Antimicrob Ag. Chemother.*, 1979, *15*, 190.

Further references: D. Christol *et al.*, *Presse méd.*, 1971, *79*, 467; B. H. Minshew *et al.*, *Antimicrob. Ag. Chemother.*, 1977, *12*, 688; S. J. Seligman, *ibid.*, 1978, *13*, 70; L. E. Bryan *et al.*, *ibid.*, 1979, *15*, 7.

Resistance of Enterobacteriaceae. In 2 patients with meningitis due to *E. coli* originally sensitive to gentamicin, resistant strains appeared after a few days' treatment.— A. G. L. Whitelaw *et al.* (letter), *Br. med. J.*, 1974, *2*, 613.

Of 23 isolates of Gram-negative bacilli resistant to gentamicin, 5 strains of *Enterobacter cloacae* were also resistant to tobramycin, neomycin, kanamycin, paromomycin, spectinomycin, ampicillin, carbenicillin, streptomycin, sulphonamides, tetracycline, and cephalexin. Transferable resistance to *E. coli* was demonstrated for gentamicin and 7 of the other antibiotics. Other organisms resistant to gentamicin included *Providencia stuartii* (3) and *Ps. aeruginosa* (5).— S. M. Poston *et al.*, *J. antimicrob. Chemother.*, 1976, *2*, 189.

A report of the emergence of gentamicin-resistant *Klebsiella* after 7 years' use. In some strains this resistance was transferable. All resistant strains were susceptible to amikacin and netilmicin.— R. P. Rennie and I. B. R. Duncan, *Antimicrob. Ag. Chemother.*, 1977, *11*, 179.

Gentamicin-resistant *Kleb. aerogenes* was isolated from the urine of 17 of 237 male patients in a urological ward. Faecal samples from 25 of the men were examined and 2 had resistant *Klebsiella*. Resistance was plasmid-mediated but amikacin, tobramycin, and nalidixic acid remained active against the resistant epidemic strain.— M. W. Casewell *et al.*, *Lancet*, 1977, *2*, 444.

Exposure to gentamicin produced an increase in the resistance to tobramycin of a strain of *E. coli* which possessed an R-factor conferring resistance to gentamicin. The R-factor did not affect the intrinsic susceptibility of the organism to tobramycin. It was suggested that prior treatment of gentamicin-resistant organisms with gentamicin could affect their subsequent response to other aminoglycosides.— S. L. Mawer and D. Greenwood, *J. clin. Path.*, 1978, *31*, 12.

Further references: M. S. Shafi and N. Datta, *Lancet*, 1975, *1*, 1355; P. B. Iannini *et al.*, *Ann. intern. Med.*, 1976, *85*, 161; F. E. Thomas *et al.*, *Archs. intern. Med.*, 1977, *137*, 581; E. Rosenthal and U. Kohns, *Dt. med. Wschr.*, 1977, *102*, 1350; I. Forbes *et al.*, *Med. J. Aust.*, 1977, *1*, 14; N. J. Roberts and R. G. Douglas, *Antimicrob. Ag. Chemother.*, 1978, *13*, 214; L. Verbist *et al.*, *J. antimicrob. Chemother.*, 1978, *4*, 47.

Resistance of Pseudomonas. During an 18-month period none of 197 isolates of *Ps. aeruginosa* was resistant to gentamicin and 1 of 191 isolates was resistant to carbenicillin. In the next 9 months the incidence increased to 11 of 145 (7.6%) isolates, and 19 of 141 (13.5%) respectively and in the next 6 months to 20 of 142 (14%) isolates and 33 of 145 (23%) respectively. The oral use of gentamicin appeared to be associated with the induction of gentamicin resistance.— W. H. Greene *et al.*, *Ann. intern. Med.*, 1973, *79*, 684.

There was a high incidence of R-factors determining multiple resistance to antibiotics including gentamicin and carbenicillin among hospital isolates of *Ps. aeruginosa*. The factors were readily transferred to other strains of *Ps. aeruginosa* but not to *E. coli* or *Pr. mirabilis*.— T. R. Korfhagen *et al.*, *Antimicrob. Ag. Chemother.*, 1975, *7*, 64. See also T. R. Korfhagen and J. C. Loper, *ibid.*, 69; P. Kontomichalou *et al.*, *ibid.*, 1976, *9*, 866; I. M. Baird *et al.*, *ibid.*, *10*, 626.

Of 1162 isolates of *Ps. aeruginosa* and 394 of *Serratia marcescens*, 222 (19.1%) and 197 (50%) respectively were resistant to gentamicin. Amikacin was active against 79% and all respectively of the resistant strains. Tobramycin and sissomicin had little advantage over gentamicin.— R. D. Meyer *et al.*, *Lancet*, 1976, *1*, 580. A similar report.— C. A. Kauffman *et al.*, *Antimicrob. Ag. Chemother.*, 1978, *13*, 918. Of 84 strains of *Ps. aeruginosa* resistant to gentamicin (MIC of 40 µg or more per ml) 95, 14, and 7% were susceptible to amikacin, tobramycin, and sissomicin respectively. Netilmicin inhibited 35% of the strains at a concentration of 5 µg per ml and 50% of the strains at 10 µg per ml.— N. J. Legakis *et al.* (letter), *J. antimicrob. Chemother.*, 1979, *5*, 487.

Gentamicin-resistant strains of *Ps. aeruginosa* were isolated from 6 patients and one nurse was found to be a carrier. Plasmid-mediated resistance to kanamycin, sissomicin, tobramycin, sulphonamides, and mercuric chloride was detected. Aminoglycoside resistance was due to acetyltransferase activity.— F. R. Falkiner *et al.*, *J. clin. Path.*, 1977, *30*, 731.

The majority of 44 isolates of *Ps. aeruginosa* and 42 other strains of the *Pseudomonas* spp., that were resistant to gentamicin *in vitro* did not appear to produce inactivating enzymes that accounted for their resistance; resistance to kanamycin appeared to be due to the action of an enzyme.— I. Phillips *et al.*, *J. antimicrob. Chemother.*, 1978, *4*, 121.

Further references: P. Chadwick, *Can. med. Ass. J.*, 1973, *109*, 585; D. V. Seal and J. E. M. Strangeways (letter), *Lancet*, 1975, *1*, 48; M. Barnham *et al.* (letter), *ibid.*, 576; S. Eykyn and I. Phillips (letter), *ibid.*, 861; M. Haas *et al.*, *Antimicrob. Ag. Chemother.*, 1976, *9*, 945; S. Biddlecombe *et al.*, *ibid.*, 951; I. A. Holder (letter), *J. antimicrob. Chemother.*, 1976, *2*, 309; S. L. Mawer and D. Greenwood (letter), *Lancet*, 1977, *1*, 749; D. V. Seal and J. E. M. Strangeways (letter), *ibid.*, 856; F. L. Ruben *et al.*, *Am. J. med. Sci.*, 1978, *275*, 173; K. Bridges *et al.*, *Br. med. J.*, 1979, *1*, 446.

For a report of a strain of *Ps. aeruginosa* resistant to polymyxin showing cross-resistance to gentamicin, see Polymyxin B Sulphate, p.1205.

Resistance of staphylococci. An isolate of *Staphylococcus aureus* resistant to gentamicin, kanamycin, and tobramycin. Resistance was mediated by an inactivating enzyme.— A. Porthouse *et al.*, *Lancet*, 1976, *1*, 20. See also D. C. E. Speller *et al.*, *ibid.*, 464; R. E. Warren and S. O. B. Roberts (letter), *ibid.*, 543.

A report of the identification of phosphotransferase and acetyltransferase from a gentamicin-resistant strain of *Staph. aureus*. The enzymes were active against some other aminoglycoside antibiotics.— D. F. J. Brown *et al.* (letter), *Lancet*, 1976, *2*, 419. See also K. P. Shannon and I. Phillips (letter), *ibid.*, 580.

An outbreak of gentamicin-resistant strains of *Staph. aureus* involving 23 patients and 3 members of staff in the Dermatological Unit of a hospital appeared to be associated with the increased topical use of gentamicin.— T. D. Wyatt *et al.*, *J. antimicrob. Chemother.*, 1977, *3*, 213.

A strain of *Staph. aureus* resistant to gentamicin, kanamycin, tobramycin, or sissomicin but susceptible to amikacin, streptomycin, netilmicin, methicillin, tetracycline, or chloramphenicol was isolated from neonatal infants in the USA.— L. Vogel *et al.*, *Antimicrob. Ag. Chemother.*, 1978, *13*, 466.

A study *in vitro* indicated that although isolates of *Staph. aureus* contained acetyl-, adenylyl-, and phosphotransferase activity, the phosphotransferase reaction was most responsible for their resistance to gentamicin, amikacin, or netilmicin. The resistance was considered to be plasmid-mediated.— D. F. Scott *et al.*, *Antimicrob. Ag. Chemother.*, 1978, *13*, 641.

An epidemic of gentamicin-resistant *Staph. aureus* affected 24 adults and children in one hospital over a 10-week period. The gentamicin-resistant staphylococcal isolates showed 3 distinct phage susceptibility patterns in 2 distinct phage groups, which could most readily be explained by limited transfer of genetic information coding for antibiotic resistance between staphylococcal strains. It was considered that *in vivo* plasmid transfer was the most plausible explanation for the distinct difference in phage-typing patterns, although this could not be confirmed by laboratory testing.— G. P. Greenhood *et al.*, *Lancet*, 1979, *1*, 289.

During the period from June 1976 to December 1977, 90 hospitalised patients were found to be colonised or infected with gentamicin-resistant strains of *Staph. aureus*; 65 had acquired these strains during hospitalisation. Apart from those in 11 of 16 plastic surgery patients no common phage type was found amongst the strains. Cross-resistance to tobramycin occurred in most of the strains tested but 90% or over were susceptible to 8 µg per ml of amikacin or 4 µg per ml of netilmicin.— F. J. Buckwold *et al.*, *Antimicrob. Ag. Chemother.*, 1979, *15*, 152.

Further references: A. J. Bint *et al.*, *J. clin. Path.*, 1977, *30*, 165; J. E. Dowding, *Antimicrob. Ag. Chemother.*, 1977, *11*, 47; D. O. Wood *et al.*, *ibid.*, *12*, 513; C. Watanakunakorn, *J. antimicrob. Chemother.*, 1978, *4*, 561; W. C. Noble and J. Naidoo, *Br. J. Derm.*, 1978, *98*, 481; H. Faden *et al.*, *J. Am. med. Ass.*, 1979, *241*, 143; *Lancet*, 1981, *2*, 127.

Resistance of streptococci. The sensitivity to gentamicin of group B streptococci isolated from vaginal swabs prior to delivery was 53% in 1973 and 17% in 1974.— T. M. S. Reid, *Br. med. J.*, 1975, *2*, 533.

An investigation of aminoglycoside resistance occurring in strains of *Streptococcus faecalis*.— M. J. Basker *et al.*, *J. clin. Path.*, 1977, *30*, 375.

Absorption and Fate. Gentamicin is poorly absorbed from the gastro-intestinal tract but rapidly absorbed after intramuscular injection, peak plasma concentrations being reached in half to 1 hour, and effective concentrations being still present 4 hours after injection. A dose equivalent to 1 mg of gentamicin per kg body-weight produces average peak plasma concentrations of about 4 μg per ml although there may be considerable individual variation and higher concentrations in patients with renal impairment. After intramuscular injection, gentamicin appears in body fluids but there is little diffusion into the cerebrospinal fluid and even when the meninges are inflamed effective concentrations may not be achieved; diffusion into the eye is also poor. Gentamicin crosses the placenta but only small amounts have been reported in breast milk.

Systemic absorption has been reported after the topical application of gentamicin to patients with burns, especially from a cream rather than an ointment.

The biological half-life has been variously reported as 1 to 4 hours. Gentamicin is excreted in the urine by glomerular filtration and after the first day or two of administration at least 70% of a dose may be recovered in 24 hours. Small amounts have been detected in the bile.

A review of the clinical pharmacokinetics of aminoglycoside antibiotics.— J. -C. Pechere and R. Dugal, *Clin. Pharmacokinet.*, 1979, *4*, 170.

When 10 patients were given an intravenous infusion of gentamicin 40 mg as the sulphate per m^2 body-surface over 2 hours the mean peak serum concentration was 4.5 μg per ml at 2 hours. The serum half-life was 2 hours and serum concentrations greater than 1 μg per ml were maintained for 6 hours. Six patients were treated with 30 mg per m^2 administered in the same way every 6 hours and measurements on day 3 showed a mean peak serum concentration of 4.2 μg per ml and a serum half-life of approximately 2 hours. One of these patients had impaired renal function and maintained serum-gentamicin concentrations of at least 11 μg per ml with a peak measured on day 3 of 18 μg per ml. No further accumulation was noted on day 10. Only 1 of 4 patients studied had detectable gentamicin concentrations in their CSF. Eight of 38 patients treated with gentamicin usually in conjunction with carbenicillin had signs of nephrotoxicity and 11 of 25 treated patients had lowered creatinine clearances associated with gentamicin.— V. Rodriguez *et al.*, *Clin. Pharmac. Ther.*, 1970, *11*, 275.

A study in 3 volunteers showed that the renal clearance of gentamicin was not significantly affected by changes of urine pH.— C. Mariel *et al.* (letter), *Br. med. J.*, 1972, *2*, 406.

Intrathecal injections of gentamicin 4 mg given to 12 patients produced CSF concentrations of up to 45 μg per ml which were eliminated within 2 to 24 hours to residual concentrations of 0.3 μg per ml. At 14 hours the concentrations in all samples were 7.8 μg or less.— J. J. Rahal (letter), *Ann. intern. Med.*, 1972, *77*, 1003.

Gentamicin 80 mg given as a slow bolus intravenous injection produced a peak serum concentration of about 10 μg per ml in 5 healthy subjects. A dose of 1 mg per kg body-weight produced a marginally lower peak concentration which fell quicker than with the standard dose.— B. C. Stratford *et al.*, *Lancet*, 1974, *1*, 378. Toxic concentrations could have been achieved as gentamicin 1 mg per kg body-weight given to 5 healthy men in a rapid bolus intravenous injection over 10 seconds produced a mean peak serum concentration of 18.3 μg per ml at 2.5 minutes falling to 9.3 μg per ml at 10 minutes and 5.1 μg per ml at 1 hour.— R. R. Bailey and K. L. Lynn (letter), *ibid.*, 730.

Peak serum concentrations of gentamicin in 10 patients who received gentamicin 280 mg by intramuscular injection ranged from 9.9 to 15.8 (mean 12.71) μg per ml and occurred 0.5 to 2 hours after administration. The mean serum concentration was 2.54 μg per ml 6 hours after administration and the serum half-life was 2.15 hours. The percentages of the dose recovered in the urine within 2, 4 and 24 hours of administration were about 35, 60 and 86% respectively. There were no signs of ototoxicity or nephrotoxicity after injection.— C. Thuillier *et al.* (letter), *J. antimicrob. Chemother.*, 1977, *3*, 527.

Gentamicin 0.4 to 7 mg per kg body-weight (the lower doses being used in renal impairment) given intravenously to 47 patients daily for an average of 10 days was shown to persist in the body. Peak and trough serum concentrations rose gradually in most patients during treatment then declined in 2 phases after the last dose. The first phase was similar to that seen during each interval between doses and was mainly influenced by renal function. The second phase was slow with an average half-life of 112 hours. Kidney-cortex concentrations were at least 100 times those in serum and 40% of the total gentamicin in the body was present in the kidneys.— J. J. Schentag and W. J. Jusko (letter), *Lancet*, 1977, *1*, 486.

In a study of 16 patients with various infections who received from 1 to 11.6 g of gentamicin by intramuscular or intravenous injection over a period of 5 to 76 days, gentamicin could be detected several weeks later in serum and urine. The mean half-life of gentamicin for the terminal phase of elimination from serum was estimated to be 11.8 days and in urine the mean terminal half-life was 9.5 days. It was considered that gentamicin had an affinity for some human tissues and that the two-compartment open model used for describing the pharmacokinetics of gentamicin might be inadequate.— G. Kahlmeter *et al.*, *J. antimicrob. Chemother.*, 1978, *4*, 143.

The disposition of gentamicin C_1, C_{1a} and C_2.— R. L. Nation *et al.*, *Eur. J. clin. Pharmac.*, 1978, *13*, 459.

Gentamicin pharmacokinetics in kwashiorkor.— N. Buchanan *et al.*, *Br. J. clin. Pharmac.*, 1979, *8*, 451.

The pharmacokinetics of aminoglycoside antibiotics in burn patients.— R. J. Sawchuk and T. S. Rector, *Clin. Pharmacokinet.*, 1980, *5*, 548.

Further references: P. Naumann and W. Auwärter, *Arzneimittel-Forsch.*, 1968, *18*, 1119; B. R. Meyers and S. Z. Hirschman, *J. clin. Pharmac.*, 1972, *12*, 321; J. Mendelson *et al.*, *Antimicrob. Ag. Chemother.*, 1973, *4*, 538; T. W. Wilson *et al.*, *Clin. Pharmac. Ther.*, 1973, *14*, 815; D. Kaye *et al.*, *J. infect. Dis.*, 1974, *130*, 150; G. Kahlmeter and C. Kamme (letter), *Lancet*, 1975, *1*, 286.

For reference to sex-linked differences in gentamicin kinetics, see p.1077.

Absorption and fate in infants and children. In the newborn, the biological half-life of gentamicin was 144 minutes, in infants 85 minutes, and in older children 63 to 67 minutes.— H. -J. Rohwedder and U. Goll, *Dt. med. Wschr.*, 1970, *95*, 1171.

The pharmacokinetics of gentamicin given intravenously to neonates showed that this route was a suitable alternative to intramuscular injection.— G. H. McCracken *et al.*, *Pediatrics*, 1977, *60*, 463.

For reports of the pharmacokinetics of gentamicin in children given doses based on body-weight or body-surface, see G. R. Siber *et al.*, *J. Pediat.*, 1979, *94*, 135; W. E. Evans *et al.*, *ibid.*, 139.

Further references: D. B. Haughey *et al.*, *J. Pediat.*, 1980, *96*, 325 (premature neonates); R. M. Kliegman *et al.*, *ibid.*, 927 (exchange transfusion in neonates).

See also under Uses.

Absorption from wounds. References.— H. H. Stone *et al.*, *Am. Surg.*, 1968, *34*, 639.

Diffusion. Bile. Peak concentrations of gentamicin were found in the bile 2 to 3 hours after an injection of gentamicin 1 mg per kg body-weight in 16 patients and gentamicin was still present after 8 hours. Ten of the patients who had no cystic duct obstruction had a mean biliary concentration of 2 μg per ml.— H. A. Pitt *et al.*, *J. infect. Dis.*, 1973, *127*, 299.

Bronchial secretions. Following intramuscular injection of 2 mg per kg body-weight of gentamicin to 5 patients, a mean peak serum concentration of 6.75 μg per ml was reached after 1 hour; very low concentrations were detected in bronchial secretions (range 0.1 to 4.3 μg per ml). When the same dose of gentamicin was given endotracheally the mean concentration in bronchial secretions was 43.4 μg per ml after 4 hours, and 13.8 μg per ml after 6 hours; serum concentrations of gentamicin after endotracheal administration were very low.— W. Odio *et al.*, *J. clin. Pharmac.*, 1975, *15*, 518.

Cervical fluid, mucus, and menses. G. Creatsas *et al.*, *Int. J. clin. Pharmac. Biopharm.*, 1979, *17*, 225.

Eye. Gentamicin 40 mg given by subconjunctival injection to 21 patients generally produced an effective concentration in the aqueous humour.— M. B. R. Mathalone and A. Harden, *Br. J. Ophthal.*, 1972, *56*, 609. Gentamicin eye-drops did not produce an effective concentration in the aqueous humour.— J. S. Hillman *et al.*, *ibid.*, 1979, *63*, 794.

Peritoneal fluid. The diffusion of gentamicin into peritoneal fluid during spontaneous peritonitis was therapeutically adequate in 8 cirrhotic patients. In 3 further patients with cirrhotic ascites but without peritonitis, concentrations of gentamicin in the peritoneal fluid were lower in one and undetectable in 2.— G. D. Richey and C. J. Schleupner, *Antimicrob. Ag. Chemother.*, 1981, *19*, 312.

Renal cortex. Renal cortical concentrations of gentamicin ranged from 140 to 540 μg per g and medullary concentrations from 128 to 230 μg per g in postmortem tissue from 4 patients who had received gentamicin within 1 to 8 hours of death.— C. Q. Edwards *et al.*, *Antimicrob. Ag. Chemother.*, 1976, *9*, 925. An *in vitro* study on *rat* tissue indicated that the uptake of gentamicin by the renal cortex was an active process requiring aerobic phosphorylation.— C. H. Hsu, *ibid.*, 1977, *12*, 192.

Synovial fluid. The concentration of gentamicin in synovial fluid ranged from 54 to 147% of simultaneous serum concentrations in 5 patients with non-traumatic joint effusions 60 to 120 minutes after they received gentamicin 1 to 1.5 mg per kg body-weight intramuscularly.— T. H. Dee and F. Kozin, *Antimicrob. Ag. Chemother.*, 1977, *12*, 548. See also D. C. Marsh *et al.*, *J. Am. med. Ass.*, 1974, *228*, 607.

Pregnancy and the neonate. Gentamicin 40 mg given by intramuscular injection to 37 pregnant women just before delivery produced a mean peak serum concentration of 3.65 μg per ml within 30 minutes and a peak of 1.25 μg per ml in the cord serum within 1 to 2 hours.— H. Yoshioka *et al.*, *J. Pediat.*, 1972, *80*, 121.

The rate of elimination of gentamicin in postpartum women.— D. E. Zaske *et al.*, *Obstet. Gynec.*, 1980, *56*, 559.

See also under Absorption and Fate in Infants and Children.

Protein binding. Gentamicin did not exhibit any protein binding in studies *in vitro* of human serum under controlled physiological conditions using an ultrafiltration technique.— R. C. Gordon *et al.*, *Antimicrob. Ag. Chemother.*, 1972, *2*, 214.

Studies *in vitro* indicated that a mean of 27.3, 20.5, and 16.7% of gentamicin was bound to serum proteins in the presence of zero, physiologic, and elevated concentrations respectively of calcium and magnesium ions. Higher degrees of protein binding occurred in plasma and in serum containing heparin indicating that the apparent increase in plasma-protein binding was due to a direct binding of gentamicin to the heparin used as an anticoagulant. No difference in the binding capacity was found between sera obtained from healthy subjects and that from uraemic patients receiving chronic haemodialysis.— D. R. Myers *et al.*, *Clin. Pharmac. Ther.*, 1978, *23*, 356.

Uses. Gentamicin sulphate is an aminoglycoside antibiotic and is used to treat septicaemia, including neonatal sepsis, and other severe systemic infections due to sensitive Gram-negative organisms. To delay the development of resistance it is often given in conjunction with carbenicillin for the treatment of infections that are sensitive to both antibiotics, but they should be administered separately. There is also evidence for enhanced antimicrobial activity against *Pseudomonas* when both antibiotics are used. Gentamicin and benzylpenicillin show enhanced activity against *Streptococcus faecalis* and *Str. viridans* and they may be used in the treatment and prophylaxis of endocarditis caused by these organisms; again, the injections should be administered separately. In the treatment of urinary-tract infections with gentamicin, alkalis should be given concomitantly to raise the urinary pH above 7.

Gentamicin is also used topically in concentrations of 0.1 to 0.3% and, occasionally, systemically to treat staphylococcal infections but as topical use may lead to the emergence of resistance this method of administration is considered to be inadvisable.

Gentamicin sulphate is usually given intramuscularly every 8 hours; the total daily dose is the equivalent of 3 to 5 mg of gentamicin per kg body-weight. The same dose may be given to children but the equivalent of 5 to 7.5 mg of gentamicin per kg daily in divided doses is recommended for infants and neonates. The course of treatment should generally be limited to 7 to 10 days and plasma concentrations of gentamicin should not exceed 10 to 12 µg per ml. Dosage should be reduced in renal impairment.

Gentamicin has been given intravenously by bolus injection over 3 minutes or by dilution in up to 100 ml of fluid and infusion over 20 minutes. Doses for intravenous administration are the same as those used intramuscularly. It has sometimes been given by mouth for enteric infections and to suppress intestinal flora. In meningitis it has been administered intrathecally or, more usually, intraventricularly in doses of 1 mg or more daily in conjunction with intramuscular therapy. Doses of 10 to 40 mg have been given by subconjunctival injection.

A bone cement impregnated with gentamicin is used in orthopaedic surgery. Acrylic beads containing gentamicin and threaded on to surgical wire are implanted in the management of bone infections.

Reviews of the actions and uses of gentamicin and other aminoglycosides: M. Barza and R. T. Scheife, *Am. J. Hosp. Pharm.*, 1977, *34*, 723; G. B. Appel and H. C. Neu, *Ann. intern. Med.*, 1978, *89*, 528; P. Noone, *Br. med. J.*, 1978, *2*, 549 and 613; J. D. Williams and T. Leung, *Topics Ther.*, 1978, *4*, 36; I. P. Folb, *S. Afr. med. J.*, 1979, *55*, 807; *Med. Lett.*, 1980, *22*, 85; R. P. Mouton, *J. antimicrob. Chemother.*, 1980, *6*, 166.

Gentamicin was substituted for kanamycin to control an outbreak of infections due to R-factor-mediated kanamycin-resistant enteric bacteria in a nursery. Within a month the kanamycin-resistant organisms were virtually eliminated. Over 15 months there was a significant increase in resistant Gram-negative intestinal flora.— J. A. Franco *et al.*, *Am. J. Dis. Child.*, 1973, *126*, 318.

Gentamicin appeared to be the best treatment for *Bacillus cereus* infections.— P. C. B. Turnbull *et al.*, *Br. med. J.*, 1977, *1*, 1628.

The effective use of gentamicin in peritoneal infections due to sensitive organisms in 14 children undergoing peritoneal dialysis.— R. E. Day and R. H. R. White, *Archs Dis. Childh.*, 1977, *52*, 56.

Bronchitis and bronchiectasis. In 23 men with chronic purulent bronchitis or purulent bronchiectasis, which had not responded to intensive antibiotic therapy, treatment with gentamicin was successful on 7 of 36 occasions. *Pseudomonas aeruginosa* and *Klebsiella pneumoniae* were repeatedly isolated in profuse growth. Gentamicin was administered by intramuscular injection alone in doses of 200 to 360 mg daily, by aerosol inhalation alone in doses of 20 mg in 5 ml of normal saline 4 times daily, or by both routes in similar dosage.— A. Pines *et al.*, *Br. med. J.*, 1967, *2*, 543.

All of 7 patients with tracheobronchial infections improved when given gentamicin 240 mg daily through their endotracheal tubes. Five of the patients had concentrations of more than 20 µg per ml in the respiratory secretions. Of 8 similar patients given gentamicin intramuscularly, none had detectable concentrations in their respiratory secretions and only 2 patients improved.— J. Klastersky *et al.*, *Chest*, 1972, *61*, 117, per *J. Am. med. Ass.*, 1972, *220*, 440. See also M. Peromet *et al.*, *Chemotherapy, Basle*, 1973, *19*, 211; J. Klastersky *et al.*, *Int. J. clin. Pharmac. Ther. Toxic.*, 1973, *7*, 279.

Burns. Because of the development of resistance by *Pseudomonas*, only burns covering more than 20% of the body surface should be treated topically and systemically with gentamicin.— B. G. MacMillan, *J. infect. Dis.*, 1969, *119*, 492.

In a review of 192 burnt patients treated with topical gentamicin 0.1%, 66 with silver nitrate solution 0.5%, 56 with mafenide acetate cream 10%, and 40 with silver sulphadiazine, together with topical antibiotics, the overall mortality-rates were 12.5, 27, 18, and 17.5% respectively; the proportion of deaths due to sepsis (usually due to *Pseudomonas*) was lowest in those treated with mafenide (2 of 10) compared with 14 of 24, 11 of 18, and 4 of 7 in the gentamicin, silver nitrate, and silver sulphadiazine groups respectively. Gentamicin (especially as cream) and mafenide appeared to penetrate the wound, while silver nitrate had little penetrating ability.— R. P. Hummel *et al.*, *Ann. Surg.*, 1970, *172*, 370.

Further references: *Lancet*, 1969, *2*, 629; C. F. T. Snelling *et al.*, *Can. med. Ass. J.*, 1978, *119*, 466; I. A. Holder *et al.*, *J. antimicrob. Chemother.*, 1979, *5*, 455.

Campylobacteriosis. A review of campylobacter enteritis; in campylobacter septicaemia the treatment of choice is gentamicin.— *Lancet*, 1978, *2*, 135.

Dosage. Of 21 patients who had valley blood-gentamicin concentrations of 2 µg or more per ml 8 developed a rise in serum creatinine. In 86 patients studied it was established that to ensure an initial peak concentration of more than 4 µg per ml a loading dose of 2 mg per kg body-weight must be given.— J. G. Dahlgren *et al.*, *Antimicrob. Ag. Chemother.*, 1975, *8*, 58.

An assessment of bolus injection over 3 to 5 minutes versus slow infusion over 2 hours in 63 patients. Bolus administration was considered to be a safe technique.— J. Mendelson *et al.*, *Antimicrob. Ag. Chemother.*, 1976, *9*, 633. Gentamicin given by large-volume infusions resulted in subtherapeutic blood concentrations as the elimination half-life was reduced and the total clearance enhanced.— S. Kaumeier and P. Lücker, *Arzneimittel-Forsch.*, 1977, *27*, 1212.

A dosage chart for the calculation of gentamicin doses based on administration predominantly by the intravenous route and on the use of lean body-weight rather than total body-weight to calculate volume of distribution.— J. H. Hull and F. A. Sarubbi, *Ann. intern. Med.*, 1976, *85*, 183. See also J. S. Raichlen (letter), *Ann. intern. Med.*, 1976, *85*, 827; J. H. Hull and F. A. Sarubbi (letter), *Ann. intern. Med.*, 1976, *85*, 827. Confirmation of the value of this nomogram in predicting serum-gentamicin concentrations.— W. L. Russell *et al.*, *Am. J. Hosp. Pharm.*, 1978, *35*, 570. See also T. L. Yeh *et al.* (letter), *Am. J. Hosp. Pharm.*, 1978, *35*, 902; W. J. Sawyer (letter), *Am. J. Hosp. Pharm.*, 1978, *35*, 1343.

Discussions on the use of nomograms to calculate doses of gentamicin and other aminoglycoside antibiotics.— G. E. Mawer, *Adv. Med. Topics Ther.*, 1976, *2*, 36; D. S. Reeves, *J. antimicrob. Chemother.*, 1977, *3*, 533.

Treatment of febrile episodes in 50 patients with neutropenic blood disorders was more effective when the dose of gentamicin given with a fixed dose of clindamycin was adjusted according to a nomogram than when both drugs were given in a fixed dose.— P. M. Wilkinson *et al.*, *J. antimicrob. Chemother.*, 1977, *3*, 297.

A review of the relationship between serum concentrations of gentamicin and its efficacy or toxicity concluded that peak and trough concentrations should be measured in all patients receiving full therapeutic doses and in those in whom renal function or extracellular fluid volumes are abnormal. Peak serum concentrations of gentamicin should be in the range of 5 to 8 µg per ml.— M. Barza and M. Lauermann, *Clin. Pharmacokinet.*, 1978, *3*, 202.

The calculation of gentamicin and tobramycin doses in obese patients.— S. N. Schwartz *et al.*, *J. infect. Dis.*, 1978, *138*, 499.

Gentamicin dosage based on body-surface rather than body-weight produced predictable peak serum concentrations in a study of 58 patients aged from 8 months to 73 years and given doses of 60 mg per m^2 intravenously.— G. R. Siber *et al.*, *J. Pediat.*, 1979, *94*, 135. In 35 children, gentamicin dosage calculated by body-weight or body-surface was equally unpredictable; it should be based on the monitoring of serum concentrations.— W. E. Evans *et al.*, *J. Pediat.*, 1979, *94*, 139.

Dosage in infants and children. In infants an initial dose of 3 mg per kg body-weight followed by 2 mg per kg every 8 hours for 14 doses produced adequate serum-gentamicin concentrations which were not considered toxic. As high concentrations of gentamicin were found in kidney and lung tissue the volume of distribution was greater than the extracellular space.— R. D. G. Milner *et al.*, *Archs Dis. Childh.*, 1972, *47*, 927.

An intramuscular dose of 2.5 mg per kg body-weight produced adequate serum-gentamicin concentrations of 4 to 5 µg per ml in the neonate and young infant. This dose should be repeated every 12 hours for the first week of life and then every 8 hours. For intraventricular or intrathecal injection, a dose of 1 mg or possibly 2 mg once daily was recommended until cultures were sterile. For urinary-tract infections 1 mg per kg body-weight every 8 hours was considered suitable.— J. D. Nelson and G. H. McCracken, *Am. J. Dis. Child.*, 1972, *124*, 13. Although many neonates given gentamicin intramuscularly according to the above schedule failed to achieve optimum serum concentrations of 4 µg per ml some had pre-dose serum concentrations greater than 1 µg per ml, indicating possible accumulation. This occurred in 12 of 18 neonates of 25 to 30 weeks' gestation and in 11 of 40 preterm infants with a gestational age of 31 to 38 weeks. It was concluded that in preterm neonates of less than 31 weeks' gestation, the interval between doses should be greater than 12 hours. Small-for-dates neonates could require doses higher than 2.5 mg per kg body-weight, because of the larger volume of distribution.— B. M. Assael *et al.*, *Archs Dis. Childh.*, 1977, *52*, 883.

A suggested dose of gentamicin for infants of more than 37 weeks' gestation is 2.5 mg per kg body-weight given intramuscularly or by very slow bolus intravenous injection every 12 hours for the first 48 hours of life and then every 8 hours. For immature infants (those of less than 37 weeks' gestation) this dose should be given every 12 hours for the first week of life and then every 8 hours. A dose of 1 to 2 mg is recommended for intraventricular injection, the smaller dose for premature infants; larger doses may be necessary if there is hydrocephalus.— P. A. Davies, *Br. med. J.*, 1978, *2*, 676. See also H. C. Spratt, *Drugs*, 1978, *16*, 226.

Further references: T. A. McAllister and D. G. Young, *Archs Dis. Childh.*, 1974, *49*, 495; P. Echeverria *et al.*, *J. Pediat.*, 1975, *87*, 805; H. F. Eichenwald and G. H. McCracken, *J. Pediat.*, 1978, *93*, 337; G. H. McCracken and H. F. Eichenwald, *J. Pediat.*, 1978, *93*, 357; W. E. Evans *et al.*, *Clin. Pharmacokinet.*, 1980, *5*, 295; S. Sirinavin *et al.*, *J. Pediat.*, 1980, *96*, 331; H. B. Valman, *Br. med. J.*, 1980, *280*, 457.

See also under Dosage (above).

Dosage in renal failure. Gentamicin was given to 17 patients with renal failure and severe infections in a loading dose of 1.7 mg per kg body-weight intramuscularly followed by a dose every 8 hours calculated according to a dosage nomogram based on an elimination constant and creatinine clearance and designed to lead to safe inhibitory serum concentrations, usually of 3 to 8 µg per ml. There was no evidence of ototoxicity or nephrotoxicity in any of the 17 patients.— R. A. Chan *et al.*, *Ann. intern. Med.*, 1972, *76*, 773.

The plasma half-life could be estimated in patients with renal failure by quadrupling the creatinine clearance expressed in mg per 100 ml.— R. E. Cutler *et al.*, *J. Am. med. Ass.*, 1972, *219*, 1037.

An evaluation of a dosage nomogram for gentamicin in 36 patients with varying degrees of renal function.— G. E. Mawer *et al.*, *Br. J. clin. Pharmac.*, 1974, *1*, 45.

In a comparison of the 2 regimens for gentamicin administration recommended for patients with impaired renal function, one being prolonged intervals between doses, the other a loading dose followed at the usual intervals by reduced maintenance doses, there did not appear to be a difference in the risk of nephrotoxicity for the 20 patients studied. No comparison could be made of the efficacy.— E. L. Goodman *et al.*, *Antimicrob. Ag. Chemother.*, 1975, *8*, 434.

After a loading dose of 1 to 2 mg per kg body-weight gentamicin could be given in a dose of 1 to 1.5 mg per kg every 8 hours to patients with a creatinine clearance (CC) of 60 to 80 ml per minute, 0.5 to 0.8 mg per kg to those with a CC of 30 to 40 ml per minute, 0.3 mg per kg to those with a CC of 10 to 20 ml per minute, and 0.2 mg per kg to those with a CC of 5 ml per minute. An alternative dosage for those with a CC of 30 to 80 ml per minute was 0.5 mg per kg at a frequency (in hours) of 4 times the serum-creatinine concentration (in mg per 100 ml). In haemodialysis 0.25 mg per kg could be given every 12 hours, or 1 to 1.5 mg per kg after dialysis; in peritoneal dialysis 1 mg per kg could be given every 12 hours.— J. S. Cheigh, *Am. J. Med.*, 1977, *62*, 555.

Data for predicting removal of gentamicin by conventional haemodialysis.— T. P. Gibson and H. A. Nelson, *Clin. Pharmacokinet.*, 1977, *2*, 403.

In a study involving 10 patients with chronic renal failure, mean tissue concentrations of gentamicin in the renal cortex and medulla were only 1.2 and 0.7 µg per g, respectively, when they were given the doses recommended for their degree of renal failure. No gentamicin was detected in the cortex of one patient nor in the medulla of 3.— W. M. Bennett *et al.*, *J. Lab. clin. Med.*, 1977, *90*, 389.

Nomograms based on serum-creatinine concentrations were of little value in assessing aminoglycoside dosage in 20 patients after renal transplantation or on haemodialysis. In 2 patients concentrations of gentamicin were reduced when carbenicillin was given concomitantly. In 1 patient there were increased peak and trough concentrations of gentamicin when flucytosine was given while in a second patient a reduced dose of gentamicin was needed. Cephalexin and cephradine might have contributed to deteriorating renal function in 2 patients.— P. Noone *et al.*, *Br. med. J.*, 1978, *2*, 470.

In children with renal failure a suggested dosage schedule for gentamicin was 1 mg per kg body-weight by intramuscular injection at intervals of three times the serum half-life, which could be calculated from the creatinine clearance.— H. Yoshioka *et al.*, *Archs Dis. Childh.*, 1978, *53*, 334.

The normal half-life for gentamicin of 2 hours was

increased to 24 to 48 hours in end-stage renal failure. The interval between doses should be extended from 8 hours to 8 to 12 hours in patients with a glomerular filtration-rate (GFR) above 50 ml per minute, to 12 to 24 hours in those with a GFR of 10 to 50 ml per minute, and to 24 to 48 hours in those with a GFR of less than 10 ml per minute; alternatively doses should be reduced to 75 to 100%, 50 to 75%, and 25 to 50% of normal respectively. Concentrations of gentamicin were affected by haemodialysis or peritoneal dialysis; 4 to 5 mg could be added to each litre of peritoneal dialysate to obtain satisfactory serum concentrations.— W. M. Bennett *et al.*, *Ann. intern. Med.*, 1980, *93*, 62.

Further references: J. R. Curtis *et al.*, *Br. med. J.*, 1967, *2*, 537; G. E. Schumacher, *Am. J. Hosp. Pharm.*, 1975, *32*, 299; W. J. Jusko *et al.*, *Kidney Int.*, 1976, *9*, 430; P. Sharpstone, *Br. med. J.*, 1977, *2*, 36; G. B. Appel and H. C. Neu, *New Engl. J. Med.*, 1977, *296*, 663; L. Létourneau-Saheb *et al.*, *Int. J. clin. Pharmac. Biopharm.*, 1977, *15*, 116.

Ear infections. Of 49 patients with chronic ear discharge treated with ear-drops containing gentamicin sulphate equivalent to 0.3% gentamicin base and hydrocortisone acetate 1% (Gentisone HC) thrice daily, 36 showed a dry ear with no signs of infection, 7 showed reduced otorrhoea, and 5 showed persistent otorrhoea.— A. G. Kilcoyne, *Practitioner*, 1973, *211*, 91.

For comments on the possible ototoxicity of some antibiotic ear-drops including gentamicin, see *Lancet*, 1976, *1*, 896.

Endocarditis. Of 7 patients with enterococcal endocarditis 6 were successfully treated with ampicillin in association with gentamicin and 1 with benzylpenicillin with gentamicin. The association of ampicillin or benzylpenicillin with gentamicin appeared to be synergistic.— P. Serra *et al.*, *Archs intern. Med.*, 1977, *137*, 1562.

Recommendations that gentamicin should now replace streptomycin for use with penicillin in the treatment of enterococcal endocarditis.— *Lancet*, 1978, *2*, 80; C. Oakley, *Br. med. J.*, 1978, *2*, 489 and 804; B. Watt, *J. antimicrob. Chemother.*, 1978, *4*, 107.

Prophylaxis. The view that penicillin (or ampicillin) plus gentamicin should be used for prophylaxis against enterococcal endocarditis.— P. A. Oill *et al.* (letter), *New Engl. J. Med.*, 1981, *305*, 101.

Enteritis. Gentamicin, 12.5 mg per lb body-weight daily by mouth, alleviated symptoms of acute gastro-enteritis in 5 of 6 infants in a specialised ward, where cross-infection had occurred with a pathogenic strain of *E. coli* (0114) resistant to the other antibiotics tested.— H. B. Valman and M. J. Wilmers, *Lancet*, 1969, *1*, 1122. Comments.— T. P. Mann (letter), *ibid.*, 1311; R. T. D. Emond *et al.* (letter), *ibid.*, 1312. Reply.— M. J. Wilmers and H. B. Valman (letter), *ibid.*, 1969, *2*, 113.

Gentamicin was given by mouth in a dose of 4 mg per kg body-weight and intramuscularly in a dose of 2 mg per kg for 5 days to 90 infants with acute gastro-enteritis due to *E. coli.* There was a dramatic and rapid response in 83 (92%). One infant died.— M. Coetzee and P. M. Leary, *Archs Dis. Childh.*, 1971, *46*, 646.

Gentamicin was considered effective in preventing necrotising enterocolitis in babies at risk. None of 20 infants given 2.5 mg per kg body-weight by mouth every 6 hours for a week developed this condition compared with 4 of 22 similar control infants. Prophylaxis with gentamicin by mouth was recommended for all infants under 1.5 kg body-weight, all requiring umbilical catheters, all premature babies with a history of foetal distress, Apgar score less than 7 at one or five minutes, or any hypotension and/or hypoxia after birth.— L. Grylack and J. W. Scanlon (letter), *Lancet*, 1977, *2*, 506.

Eye infections. Thirty-six patients with bacterial conjunctivitis were treated with gentamicin eye-drops 0.3% four or five times daily and continued for at least 3 days after subsidence of symptoms. Symptomatic relief was obtained by 20 patients within 24 hours, by 7 patients within 48 hours, and by 5 patients within 72 hours; 4 patients showed a poor response. Gram-negative organisms responded most promptly. In addition, 2 patients with infected sockets reported absence of discharge within 3 to 4 days, and 2 patients with senile mature cataracts and positive eye cultures had negative cultures within 1 week. Transient stinging occurred in 15 patients.— A. H. Halasa, *Am. J. Ophthal.*, 1967, *63*, 1699.

The incidence of endophthalmitis was about 2.8% in 400 patients undergoing cataract extraction in eye camps in South India and treated with chloramphenicol topically and by mouth peri-operatively. The incidence was reduced to 0.37% in 1626 similar patients treated by a single injection of gentamicin 50 µg into the anterior chamber of the eye postoperatively and given no chloramphenicol or other antibiotic.— G. A. Peyman *et al.*, *Br. J. Ophthal.*, 1977, *61*, 260.

Further references: M. S. Tarakji and K. F. Tabbara, *Br. J. Ophthal.*, 1976, *60*, 750; F. T. Feaster *et al.*, *Am. J. Ophthal.*, 1978, *85*, 114; J. A. Smith, *ibid.*, 1980, *89*, 449.

Gonorrhoea. Although gentamicin 240 mg either as a single dose or 2 divided doses, on successive days, given to 85 men with gonorrhoea produced adequate serum concentrations to inhibit gonococci, the failure-rates were 15 and 10.5% respectively. Gentamicin was only considered suitable where patients might also have an early syphilitic lesion.— G. D. Morrison and D. S. Reeves, *Br. J. vener. Dis.*, 1973, *49*, 513. See also W. Bowie *et al.*, *Br. J. vener. Dis.*, 1974, *50*, 208.

Gram-negative infections, miscellaneous. A peak serum-gentamicin concentration of 5 µg per ml was achieved within 3 days in all 17 of 20 episodes of Gram-negative urinary-tract infection which responded to treatment with gentamicin. Similar concentrations were achieved in all of 15 episodes of wound infection, but 3 failed to respond. In 25 episodes of Gram-negative pneumonia, 18 achieved a concentration of 8 µg per ml and of these 16 were cured; only 3 of the 7 who failed to reach 8 µg per ml were cured. Of 15 episodes of septicaemia, including 11 in the above groups, 10 recovered after achieving concentrations of 5 µg per ml. Two patients given gentamicin and cephaloridine developed renal failure—fatal in 1. There was no evidence of hearing loss due to gentamicin. It was recommended that in severe infections dosage should aim at peak concentrations of at least 5 µg per ml and preferably 8 to 12 µg per ml, and should not be reduced unless concentrations exceeded 15 µg per ml. In renal failure or prolonged treatment 'trough' concentrations immediately before a dose should also be assayed.— P. Noone *et al.*, *Br. med. J.*, 1974, *1*, 477. See also P. Noone and B. T. Rogers, *J. clin. Path.*, 1976, *29*, 652.

References to the use of gentamicin in the treatment of infections caused by *Serratia marcescens*.— A. P. Ball, *J. antimicrob. Chemother.*, 1976, *2*, 317; *Lancet*, 1977, *1*, 636; *Br. med. J.*, 1977, *1*, 1177; J. Gray *et al.*, *J. antimicrob. Chemother.*, 1978, *4*, 551.

Systemic infection due to *Yersinia enterocolitica* in a 72-year-old woman responded to treatment with gentamicin; a blood culture was sterile within 48 hours of starting treatment.— S. L. Narasimhan *et al.*, *Can. med. Ass. J.*, 1978, *118*, 682. See also L. Mantse *et al.*, *Can. med. Ass. J.*, 1978, *119*, 922.

For a report of the successful treatment of severe Gram-negative infections using gentamicin or tobramycin in association with cephamandole, see Cephamandole, p.1132.

Listeriosis. For the use of gentamicin in association with ampicillin in the treatment of listeriosis, see Ampicillin, p.1096.

Melioidosis. A 28-year-old man developed multiple complications of wounds including fulminant *Pseudomonas pseudomallei* septicaemic melioidosis which was successfully treated with gentamicin sulphate. He received a total of 1.22 g of gentamicin intramuscularly over a period of 14 days. He was given an initial loading dose of 5 mg per kg body-weight, followed by 4 mg per kg every 48 hours for the first week then every 72 hours during the second week. At the end of 2 weeks there was marked improvement but chloramphenicol was given for 2 weeks because of a positive wound culture and to prevent relapses.— J. E. Zimmerman, *J. Am. med. Ass.*, 1970, *213*, 2266.

Meningitis and ventriculitis. Patients with meningitis due to Gram-negative organisms were given gentamicin 4 mg intrathecally once or twice daily for 3 to 10 days as well as 80 to 240 mg intramuscularly daily and in some cases other antibiotics. Concentrations of gentamicin in the cerebrospinal fluid in 11 of 14 samples were 19 to 46 µg per ml at 8 hours but at 20 hours two-thirds were less than 3 µg per ml. In order to maintain therapeutic concentrations in the cerebrospinal fluid a dose of 4 mg intrathecally repeated every 18 hours was suggested for adults, and systemic therapy with 5 mg per kg body-weight should be carried out.— J. J. Rahal *et al.*, *New Engl. J. Med.*, 1974, *290*, 1394.

Gentamicin 1 mg daily by lumbar intrathecal injection for a minimum of 3 days had no beneficial effect when it was given to 52 of 117 infants with Gram-negative enteric meningitis, all of whom were receiving ampicillin intravenously and gentamicin intramuscularly.— G. H. McCracken and S. G. Mize, *J. Pediat.*, 1976, *89*, 66 (Report of the Neonatal Meningitis Cooperative Study Group). If evidence of ventriculitis is found in such infants, treatment with gentamicin 2 to 3 mg daily by intraventricular injection should be started.— G. H. McCracken and H. F. Eichenwald, *J. Pediat.*, 1978, *93*, 357. Results of a multicentre study in the USA and Latin America involving 52 infants with both meningitis and ventriculitis, caused mainly by *Escherichia coli* in the USA and *Salmonella* spp. in Latin America. A more than threefold higher death-rate was unexpectedly found among those who received intraventricular gentamicin in addition to systemic ampicillin and gentamicin therapy, compared with those who received systemic ampicillin and gentamicin therapy alone, and the study was therefore terminated early. On the basis of data obtained from this study, intraventricular therapy cannot be recommended for the routine management of neonatal meningitis caused by Gram-negative enteric bacilli.— G. H. McCracken *et al.*, *Lancet*, 1980, *1*, 787 (Report of the Second Neonatal Meningitis Cooperative Study Group). Criticisms. It is considered that the study is inconclusive.— A. B. Kaiser *et al.* (letter), *ibid.*, *2*, 252. Similar criticisms.— R. E. Warren and N. R. C. Roberton (letter), *ibid.*; L. Corbeel *et al.* (letter), *ibid.*; W. Frederiksen and P. Schouenborg (letter), *ibid.*, 253. Reply.— G. H. McCracken and S. G. Mize (letter), *ibid.* A suggestion that intraventricular injection of gentamicin to children with ventriculitis who show a positive Gram-negative culture might release a fatal dose of endotoxin.— D. A. B. Hopkin (letter), *ibid.*, 799.

For discussions on the systemic and intraventricular use of gentamicin in the treatment of neonatal meningitis and the doubtful value of intrathecal injections of gentamicin, see P. A. Davies, *Br. J. Hosp. Med.*, 1977, *18*, 425; H. P. Lambert, *J. antimicrob. Chemother.*, 1977, *3*, 381; G. A. Ahronheim, *Drugs*, 1978, *16*, 136.

Gentamicin is the antibiotic most often used for the intralumbar or intraventricular treatment of Gram-negative bacterial meningitis. The manufacturer has recommended daily doses of 4 to 8 mg for adults and 1 to 3 mg for children.— *Med. Lett.*, 1977, *19*, 94. Intraventricular administration of aminoglycoside antibiotics should not be used routinely to treat neonates with meningitis caused by Gram-negative bacilli.— *ibid.*, 1979, *21*, 52.

A 3-week-old infant with *Salmonella typhi* meningitis was treated successfully with ampicillin 400 mg per kg body-weight daily and gentamicin 7.5 mg per kg daily, both given intravenously.— B. K. Burton *et al.*, *Am. J. Dis. Child.*, 1977, *131*, 1031.

Salmonellal infections. Gentamicin, 60 mg by intramuscular injection every 12 hours, and ampicillin, 1 g given intravenously every 6 hours, combined with drainage, were used to remove a liver abscess from a man with *Salmonella paratyphi B* infection which was resistant to ampicillin alone. Complete eradication of the organism followed treatment later with chloramphenicol, 2 g daily for 2 weeks.— M. Poon and M. G. Sanders, *Can. med. Ass. J.*, 1972, *107*, 529.

Skin infections. Gentamicin cream 0.1% was no more effective than a placebo cream in a double-blind study of the treatment of pyogenic infections of the skin. Where improvement was noted it was due to washing and removal of crusts.— S. T. Zaynoun *et al.*, *Br. J. Derm.*, 1974, *90*, 331.

For reports and comments on the topical use of antibiotics, see Neomycin Sulphate, p.1190.

Suppression of intestinal flora. A group of 19 patients with acute leukaemia received gentamicin 200 mg, vancomycin 500 mg, and nystatin 1 to 4 g every 6 hours for prophylactic suppression of intestinal flora. Therapy was discontinued in 1 patient who developed severe vomiting and diarrhoea. Bacterial growth was suppressed in 18 patients and fungal growth in 7 for the duration of treatment. Compared with a control group of 28 patients previously treated there was a reduction in infective episodes but no significant difference in remission rates.— J. A. Levi *et al.*, *Med. J. Aust.*, 1973, *1*, 1025.

Further references: A. S. Levine *et al.*, *Eur. J. Cancer*, 1975, *11*, *Suppl.*, 57; D. M. Hahn *et al.*, *Antimicrob. Ag. Chemother.*, 1978, *13*, 958.

Surgical infection prophylaxis. Gentamicin 80 mg intramuscularly or placebo was given pre-operatively to 80 patients undergoing colonic or rectal operations. There was no significant difference in the incidence of postoperative wound infection, intraperitoneal abscess formation, and faecal fistula between 41 patients who received gentamicin and 39 who received placebo. However mortality was lower in the gentamicin group.— R. C. Burton *et al.*, *Med. J. Aust.*, 1975, *2*, 597.

In a controlled study, 150 patients, some of whom were jaundiced and all of whom were undergoing surgery of the biliary tract, were given rifamide which achieved high biliary concentrations, gentamicin which achieved low concentrations, or no antibiotic. The incidence of wound infection and bacteraemia was reduced significantly only in the gentamicin group and adequate serum concentrations were considered more important than biliary concentrations in such patients. Postoperative infection was only reduced when the bile contained bacteria at operation.— M. R. B. Keighley *et al.*, *Gut*, 1976, *17*, 495.

Wound infection occurred postoperatively in 1 of 27 patients undergoing colorectal surgery and given antibiotic coverage for 5 days with gentamicin in conjunction with lincomycin or metronidazole. Extrinsic infection due to faecal contamination occurred in one other patient in this group. Of 25 control patients, 12 developed wound infection and 1 died of sepsis. Since 2 of 14 patients given lincomycin developed pseudomembranous colitis this antibiotic was exchanged for metronidazole 1 g every 8 hours as a suppository or 500 mg intravenously every 8 hours. The initial dose of gentamicin was 1.6 mg per kg body-weight by intravenous or intramuscular injection initially then adjusted to maintain a plasma-gentamicin concentration of between 3 and 10 µg per ml.— R. S. Feathers *et al.*, *Lancet*, 1977, *2*, 4.

Further references: N. Pashby and W. M. Mee, *J. antimicrob. Chemother.*, 1978, *4*, *Suppl.* C, 25.

For the use of a regimen containing gentamicin, cephalothin, and cephalexin as antibiotic prophylaxis in open-heart surgery, see Cephalothin Sodium, p.1131.

Urinary-tract infections. Results of a trial, in which 32 patients of all ages with varied infections of the urinary tract were treated with gentamicin sulphate, showed the usefulness of the antibiotic for short-term therapy particularly where it was unreasonable to delay treatment until the results of sensitivity tests were known. Dosage was between 1 and 1.3 mg per kg body-weight daily, though in 2 patients 2.2 mg per kg daily was given. The treatment removed *Escherichia coli* in 10 of 12 patients, *Pseudomonas aeruginosa* in 4 of 7, and *Proteus* spp. in 7 of 8. In 7 patients who showed re-infection 6 weeks later, the infecting organisms were different in 4 patients.— R. A. H. Mooney and C. H. L. Howells, *Br. J. clin. Pract.*, 1969, *23*, 19.

The use of a single daily dose schedule with 160 mg of gentamicin daily for 8 to 15 days in the treatment of urinary-tract infection. This schedule was successful in 10 of 11 patients compared with a thrice-daily schedule which was successful in 8 of 10 patients.— E. Labovitz *et al.*, *Antimicrob. Ag. Chemother.*, 1974, *6*, 465 . See also N. Principi *et al.*, *Helv. paediat. Acta*, 1977, *32*, 343; V. Prát *et al.*, *Infection*, 1978, *6*, 29.

Gentamicin C_1 (Sch 13706), one of the 3 components of gentamicin, was as effective as gentamicin in complicated urinary-tract infections. A slight impairment of renal function after repeated doses of gentamicin was not noted with gentamicin C_1.— A. Mosegaard *et al.*, *Antimicrob. Ag. Chemother.*, 1975, *7*, 328.

Use with Carbenicillin. In a study of 425 Enterobacteriaceae including 87 strains of *Pseudomonas*, 80% of all organisms and 87% of the *Pseudomonas* strains were inhibited by 3.1 µg per ml of gentamicin with 100 µg per ml of carbenicillin. The mixture was synergistic (defined as a 4-fold decrease in the MIC of both antibiotics) against 32% of the *Pseudomonas* strains.— J. Klastersky *et al.*, *Am. J. med. Sci.*, 1970, *260*, 373, per *Int. pharm. Abstr.*, 1971, *8*, 606.

In 2 patients, one with normal and the other with impaired renal function, a profound fall in gentamicin-serum concentrations occurred when carbenicillin was given concomitantly with gentamicin. The results were confirmed in *animals*. Studies *in vitro* of a solution of gentamicin 5 µg and carbenicillin 200 µg per ml demonstrated inactivation of gentamicin.— J. E. McLaughlin and D. S. Reeves, *Lancet*, 1971, *1*, 261. Though inactivation of gentamicin by carbenicillin might be important when renal excretion was grossly impaired, or when the drugs were given by slow infusion, experience of using the drugs together during 4 years had been satisfactory.— S. Eykyn *et al.* (letter), *ibid.*, 545. A further study on the inactivation of gentamicin by carbenicillin and by ticarcillin in patients with renal failure.— F. R. Ervin *et al.*, *Antimicrob. Ag. Chemother.*, 1976, *9*, 1004.

Gentamicin 80 mg intramuscularly or 60 mg intravenously every 6 hours and carbenicillin 5 g intravenously every 4 hours brought about prolonged improvement in 38 patients and temporary improvement in 3 when they were administered empirically to 75 acutely ill, febrile patients with cancer and granulocytopenia. Infection was confirmed in 48 patients and *Ps. aeruginosa* was isolated in 21. Prolonged improvement occurred in 14 of these 21 patients and temporary improvement was noted in another 3. The treatment was found to be less effective in other Gram-negative infections. Supra-infection occurred in 8 patients.— S. Schimpff *et al.*, *New Engl. J. Med.*, 1971, *284*, 1061. For similar reports, see P. J. Burke *et al.*, *Johns Hopkins med. J.*, 1976, *139*, 1; W. K. Lau *et al.*, *Am. J. Med.*, 1977, *62*, 959; M. Gurwith *et al.*, *Am. J. Med.*, 1978, *64*, 127.

A carbenicillin-gentamicin combination, in concentrations that could be achieved clinically in serum, inhibited 114 clinical isolates of *Ps. aeruginosa* at lower concentrations *in vitro* than those required with the individual antibiotics. In 16 isolates the combination had no advantage over the most effective antibiotic alone. In strains highly resistant to gentamicin the combination was no more effective than carbenicillin alone.— R. M. Kluge *et al.*, *Ann. intern. Med.*, 1974, *81*, 584. A report in neonates.— J. D. Nelson and G. H. McCracken, *Pediatrics*, 1973, *52*, 801.

A recommendation by the EORTC International Antimicrobial Therapy Project Group that gentamicin with carbenicillin or ticarcillin be used for the initial empirical treatment of infection in febrile granulocytopenic patients with cancer.— *J. infect. Dis.*, 1978, *137*, 14.

The activity of gentamicin was determined *in vitro* against 138 strains of gentamicin-resistant Gram-negative bacteria when used with carbenicillin, azlocillin, or mezlocillin. Potentially useful enhancement was considered to occur between gentamicin and carbenicillin, azlocillin, or mezlocillin against *Pseudomonas aeruginosa* and between gentamicin and carbenicillin against the *Proteus*, *Providencia*, *Acinetobacter*, and *Alcaligenes* spp. There appeared to be no relationship between the hydrolysis of the penicillin by beta-lactamases and the enhanced action of the penicillin and gentamicin.— W. Farrell *et al.*, *J. antimicrob. Chemother.*, 1979, *5*, 23. See also S. M. Pogwizd and S. A. Lerner, *Antimicrob. Ag. Chemother.*, 1976, *10*, 878; R. H. Glew *et al.*, *Antimicrob. Ag. Chemother.*, 1977, *11*, 1036; P. Chanbusarakum and P. R. Murray, *Antimicrob. Ag. Chemother.*, 1978, *14*, 505; M. Y. C. Lin *et al.*, *J. antimicrob. Chemother.*, 1979, *5*, 37.

For reports of incompatibilities of gentamicin with Penicillins, see p.1166.

Cystic fibrosis. Carbenicillin with gentamicin did not eliminate pulmonary infections in patients with cystic fibrosis but they did improve lung function.— B. Boxerbaum *et al.* (letter), *J. Pediat.*, 1972, *81*, 188.

Preparations

Creams

Gentamicin Cream *(B.P.)*. A viscous oil-in-water emulsion containing gentamicin sulphate in solution in the aqueous phase. Potency is expressed in terms of the equivalent amount of gentamicin. Store at a temperature not exceeding 25° in well-closed containers which minimise evaporation and contamination. *U.S.P.* (Gentamicin Sulfate Cream) specifies the equivalent of 0.1% of gentamicin. Store at a temperature not exceeding 40° in airtight containers.

Eye Ointments

Gentamicin Sulfate Ophthalmic Ointment *(U.S.P.)*. A sterile eye ointment containing gentamicin sulphate equivalent to 3 mg of gentamicin per g. Store at a temperature not exceeding 40°.

Eye-drops

Gentamicin Eye Drops *(B.P.)*. GNT. A sterile solution of gentamicin sulphate in water. Sterilised by filtration. Potency is expressed in terms of the equivalent amount of gentamicin. Eye-drops intended for use on more than one occasion should not be used later than one month after first opening the container.

Gentamicin Sulfate Ophthalmic Solution *(U.S.P.)*. A sterile buffered solution of gentamicin sulphate with preservatives containing the equivalent of 3 mg of gentamicin per ml. pH 6.5 to 7.5. Store at a temperature not exceeding 40° in airtight containers.

Injections

Gentamicin Injection *(B.P.)*. A sterile solution of gentamicin sulphate in Water for Injections containing suitable stabilising agents. Sterilised by filtration. pH 3 to 4.5.

Gentamicin Sulfate Injection *(U.S.P.)*. A sterile solution of gentamicin sulphate in Water for Injections. It may contain suitable buffers, preservatives, and sequestering agents unless intended for intrathecal use, when it contains only suitable agents to adjust tonicity. pH 3 to 5.5.

Ointments

Gentamicin Ointment *(B.P.)*. Gentamicin Sulphate Ointment. A dispersion of gentamicin sulphate in very fine particles in white soft paraffin or other anhydrous greasy basis. Potency is expressed in terms of the equivalent amount of gentamicin. Store at a temperature not exceeding 25°. *U.S.P.* (Gentamicin Sulfate Ointment) specifies the equivalent of 1 mg of gentamicin per g. Store at a temperature not exceeding 40° in airtight containers.

Proprietary Preparations

Alcomicin *(Alcon, UK: Farillon, UK)*. Gentamicin sulphate, available as eye-drops containing the equivalent of gentamicin 0.3%.

Cidomycin *(Roussel, UK)*. Gentamicin sulphate, available as **Cidomycin Injectable**, containing the equivalent of 40 mg (40 000 units) of gentamicin per ml with preservatives, in ampoules, disposable syringes, and vials of 2 ml, and the equivalent of 80 mg (80 000 units) per ml, in disposable syringes of 1.5 ml; as **Cidomycin Injectable Paediatric** containing the equivalent of 10 mg (10 000 units) per ml, in vials of 2 ml; as **Cidomycin Intrathecal Injectable** containing the equivalent of 5 mg (5000 units) per ml, in ampoules of 1 ml; as **Cidomycin Sterile Powder** for preparing subconjunctival injections, in bottles containing the equivalent of 1 g; and as **Cream** and **Ointment**, each containing the equivalent of 0.3% of gentamicin. (Also available as Cidomycin in *Austral.*, *Canad.*, *S.Afr.*).

Garamycin *(Kirby-Warrick, UK)*. Gentamicin sulphate, available as **Injection** containing in each ml the equivalent of 40 mg of gentamicin base, in ampoules and vials of 2 ml, and as **Paediatric Injection** containing in each ml the equivalent of 10 mg, in vials of 2 ml. (Also available as Garamycin in *Austral.*, *Canad.*, *Denm.*, *Neth.*, *Norw.*, *S.Afr.*, *Switz.*, *USA*).

Gentamicin BDH *(E. Merck, UK)*. Gentamicin sulphate, available as solutions for injection, containing the equivalent of gentamicin 5 mg per ml in ampoules of 2 ml, the equivalent of 40 mg per ml in ampoules of 2 ml, and the equivalent of 60 mg per ml in ampoules of 2 ml.

Gentamicin L-BDH *(E. Merck, UK)*. Gentamicin sulphate, available as solutions for intrathecal injection, containing the equivalent of gentamicin 500 µg per ml in ampoules of 2 ml and the equivalent of 2.5 mg per ml in ampoules of 2 ml.

Genticin *(Nicholas, UK)*. Gentamicin sulphate, available as **Injection** containing in each ml the equivalent of 40 mg (40 000units) of gentamicin base, with methyl hydroxybenzoate 1.8 mg, propylhydroxybenzoate 200 µg, and sodium metabisulphite 3.2 mg, in ampoules and vials of 2 ml; as **Paediatric Injection** containing in each ml the equivalent of 10 mg (10 000 units) of gentamicin, with methyl hydroxybenzoate 1.3 mg, propyl hydroxybenzoate 200 µg, and sodium metabisulphite 3.2 mg, in vials of 2 ml; as **Intrathecal Injection** containing in each ml the equivalent of 1 mg (1000 units) of gentamicin and sodium chloride 8.5 mg, in ampoules of 2 ml; as **Eye-Ear Drops** containing the equivalent of 0.3% of gentamicin; as **Pure Powder** for preparing injections in packs containing the equivalent of 1 and 10 g of gentamicin; and as **Cream** and **Ointment** each containing the equivalent of 0.3% of gentamicin. **Genticin HC Cream** and **Ointment** contain, in addition, hydrocortisone acetate 1%.

Gentigan *(E. Merck, UK)*. Gentamicin sulphate, available as injection containing the equivalent of gentamicin 40 mg per ml, in ampoules of 2 ml.

Gentisone HC *(Nicholas, UK)*. Ear-drops containing gentamicin sulphate equivalent to gentamicin 0.3% and hydrocortisone acetate 1%. For otitis externa and chronic otitis media.

Minims Gentamicin *(Smith & Nephew Pharmaceuticals, UK)*. Sterile eye-drops containing gentamicin sulphate equivalent to gentamicin 0.3%, in single-use disposable applicators.

Other Proprietary Names

Arg.—Gentamina, Glevomicina, Rovixida, Sintepul; *Aust.*—Refobacin; *Belg.*—Geomycine; *Fr.*—Gentalline; *Ger.*—Refobacin, Sulmycin; *Ital.*—Genalfa, Gentalyn, Gentibioptal, Genticol, Ribomicin; *Jap.*—Gentacin; *Spain*—Biogen, Espectrocina, Genta-Gobens, Gentadavur, Gentallenas, Gentamin, Gentamival, Gento, Gentoma, Nuclogen, Sulgemicin; *Swed.*—Garamycina; *USA*—Genoptic.

Preparations containing gentamicin sulphate and polymethylmethacrylate, intended for the management of bone infections, are described under Methylmethacrylate, p.1727.

90-s

Gramicidin *(U.S.P.)*. Gramicidin D; Gramicidin (Dubos).

CAS — 1405-97-6.

NOTE. The name gramicidin was formerly applied to tyrothricin. Gramicidin should also be distinguished from gramicidin S ('Soviet gramicidin').

Pharmacopoeias. In *U.S.*

An antimicrobial cyclic polypeptide produced by the growth of *Bacillus brevis* Dubos; it may be obtained from tyrothricin (see p.1228), of which it is one of the principal components, by extraction with a mixture of acetone and ether.

It occurs as a white or almost white, odourless, crystalline powder containing not less than 900 μg of gramicidin per mg. M.p. 229° or higher. Practically **insoluble** in water, chloroform, and ether; soluble in alcohol, acetic acid, and propylene glycol; slightly soluble in acetone and dioxan. **Store** in airtight containers.

Units. One unit of gramicidin is contained in 0.001 mg of the first International Reference Preparation (1966) which contains 1000 units per mg.

Adverse Effects and Precautions. As for Tyrothricin, p.1229.

Uses. Gramicidin has actions similar to those of tyrothricin (see p.1228) and is too toxic to be administered systemically. It has been used for the local treatment of susceptible infections.

Some proprietary compound preparations are available containing gramicidin with neomycin sulphate (see under Neomycin Sulphate, p.1191)..

Proprietary Names

Bafucin *(Ferrosan, Swed.)*.

91-w

Gramicidin S. Gramicidin C; Soviet Gramicidin.

$C_{60}H_{92}N_{12}O_{10}$=1141.5.

CAS — 113-73-5.

Pharmacopoeias. Rus. includes a sterile 2% alcoholic solution (Solutio Gramicidini S 2%); this solution is diluted with 100 volumes of water or of alcohol (70%) before use.

An antimicrobial cyclic polypeptide produced by the growth of *Bacillus brevis* Gause-Brazhnikova, or by synthesis. It is a white crystalline powder. Alcoholic solutions are stable when **stored** in a cool place and protected from light.

Units. One unit of gramicidin S was contained in 0.001002 mg of the first International Reference Preparation (1962) which contained 998 units per mg. The International Reference Preparation was discontinued in 1973.

Gramicidin S has actions and uses similar to those of gramicidin.

183-j

Hetacillin *(U.S.P.).* Hetacillinum; Isopropylidene-aminobenzylpenicillin; BL-P 804; BRL 804; Phenazacillin. (6*R*)-6-(2,2-Dimethyl-5-oxo-4-phenylimidazolidin-1-yl)penicillanic acid.

$C_{19}H_{23}N_3O_4S$=389.5.

CAS — 3511-16-8.

Pharmacopoeias. In *U.S.*

A white or off-white crystalline powder. *U.S.P.* specifies not less than the equivalent of 810 μg of ampicillin per mg. Practically **insoluble** in water and most organic solvents; soluble in methyl alcohol and in dilute solutions of sodium hydroxide. **Store** in airtight containers.

92-e

Hetacillin Potassium *(U.S.P.).* Hetacillinum Kalicum; Isopropylideneaminobenzylpenicillin Potassium. The potassium salt of hetacillin.

$C_{19}H_{22}KN_3O_4S$=427.6.

CAS — 5321-32-4.

Pharmacopoeias. In *Jap.* and *U.S.*

A white to light buff crystalline powder. Each g represents about 2.3 mmol (2.3 mEq) of potassium. Hetacillin potassium 1.1 g is approximately equivalent to 1 g of hetacillin and 900 mg of ampicillin. The *U.S.P.* specifies not less than the equivalent of 735 μg of ampicillin per mg. Freely **soluble** in water; soluble in alcohol. A 1% solution in water has a pH of 7 to 9. A 5.5% solution in water is iso-osmotic with serum. **Store** in airtight containers.

The stability of hetacillin in aqueous solution.— E. J. Kuchinskas and G. N. Levy, *J. pharm. Sci.*, 1972, *61*, 727.

Hetacillin in aqueous solution was hydrolysed to ampicillin and acetone. The half-life for the removal of the acetone moiety from hetacillin was nearly 8 hours.— G. N. Levy *et al.*, *J. pharm. Sci.*, 1974, *63*, 1197.

Hetacillin has the actions of ampicillin (see p.1091), to which it is rapidly converted after administration by mouth or by injection. It has been given in doses equivalent to 225 to 450 mg of ampicillin 4 times daily by mouth and has been given by injection.

The recommended doses of hetacillin were considered to be too low.— *Med. Lett.*, 1971, *13*, 49; *ibid.*, 1972, *14*, 38.

A study indicating that usual therapeutic doses of hetacillin strongly interfere with colour vision.— J. Laroche and C. Laroche, *Annls pharm. fr.*, 1977, *35*, 173.

Further references: D. Gotlieb *et al.*, *Clin. Med.*, 1970, *77* (Oct.), 21; M. C. Faria *et al.*, *ibid.*, 1971, *78*, (Nov.), 32; L. Mir *et al.*, *ibid.*, 1972, *79*, (July), 28; W. J. Jusko and G. P. Lewis, *J. pharm. Sci.*, 1973, *62*, 69.

Preparations

Hetacillin for Oral Suspension *(U.S.P.).* Hetacillin with one or more suitable colouring and flavouring agents, preservatives, sweeteners, and suspending agents. Store in airtight containers. The suspension is prepared by the addition of diluent before issue. pH 2 to 5. When reconstituted it contains the equivalent of 22.5, 45, or 112.5 mg of ampicillin per ml.

Hetacillin Potassium Capsules *(U.S.P.).* Capsules containing the equivalent of 112.5, 225, or 450 mg of ampicillin. Store in airtight containers.

Hetacillin Tablets *(U.S.P.).* Tablets containing the equivalent of 112.5 mg of ampicillin; they should be chewed then swallowed. Store in airtight containers.

Proprietary Names

Etaciland *(Landerlan, Spain)*; Etasepti *(Iskia, Spain)*; Hetancinato *(Miluy, Spain)*; Hystra *(Cidan, Spain)*; Versapen (also hydrochloride) *(Allard, Fr.*; *Bristol Italiana Sud, Ital.*; *Bristol-Myers, Spain*; *Bristol, USA)*; Versapen-K *(Bristol, USA)*; Viderbiotic *(Sintex, Spain)*.

93-l

Hydrabamine Phenoxymethylpenicillin.

Penicillin V Hydrabamine *(U.S.P.). NN'*-Bis-[(1,2,3,4,4a,9,10,10a-octahydro-7-isopropyl-1,4a-dimethylphenanthr-1-yl)methyl]ethylenediamine bis[(6*R*)-6-(2-phenoxyacetamido)penicillanate].

$(C_{16}H_{18}N_2O_5S)_2,C_{42}H_{64}N_2$=1297.8.

CAS — 6591-72-6.

Pharmacopoeias. In *U.S.*

An almost white powder with a characteristic odour. Hydrabamine phenoxymethylpenicillin 1.85 g is approximately equivalent to 1 g of phenoxymethylpenicillin. Very slightly **soluble** in water, alcohol, and ether; soluble 1 in 1.5 of chloroform. **Store** in airtight containers.

Hydrabamine phenoxymethylpenicillin has the actions and uses of phenoxymethylpenicillin (see p.1199). It has been given in doses of 250 mg. The hydrabamine portion of the molecule is not absorbed to any significant extent after oral administration.

Preparations

Penicillin V Hydrabamine Oral Suspension *(U.S.P.).* A suspension of hydrabamine phenoxymethylpenicillin with one or more suitable dispersing agents, buffers, preservatives, and colouring and flavouring agents. pH 4.5 to 6.5. It contains the equivalent of 36 mg of phenoxymethylpenicillin per ml. Store at a temperature not exceeding 25° in airtight containers. Protect from light.

Penicillin V Hydrabamine Tablets *(U.S.P.).* Tablets containing hydrabamine phenoxymethylpenicillin equivalent to 125 or 250 mg of phenoxymethylpenicillin; they should be chewed then swallowed. Store in airtight containers.

Proprietary Names

Abbocillin-V *(Abbott, Austral.)*; Compocillin *(Abbott, Austral.)*; Compocillin-V *(Abbott, Austral.*; *Abbott, NZ*; *Abbott, S.Afr.*; *Ross, USA)*; Flavopen *(G.P. Laboratories, Austral.)*; Pfipen V (see also Phenoxymethylpenicillin) *(Pfizer, Austral.)*.

94-y

Josamycin. EN-141. 3-Acetoxy-5-[3,6-dideoxy-4-*O*-(2,6-dideoxy-4-*O*-isovaleryl-3-*C*-methyl-α-L-*ribo*-hexopyranosyl)-3-dimethylamino-β-D-glucopyranosyloxy]-6-formylmethyl-9-hydroxy-4-methoxy-8-methylhexadecan-10,12-dien-15-olide.

$C_{42}H_{69}NO_{15}$=828.0.

CAS — 56689-45-3.

Pharmacopoeias. In *Jap.*

Josamycin is a macrolide antibiotic obtained from cultures of *Streptomyces narbonensis* var. *josamyceticus*, or by other means.

It is a white to yellowish-white odourless crystalline powder with a bitter taste. Very slightly **soluble** in water; very soluble in alcohol, chloroform, ether, and methyl alcohol; freely soluble in acetone; and very slightly soluble in light petroleum.

Josamycin has antibacterial activity similar to that of erythromycin (see p.1158) but may be more active *in vitro* against some anaerobic bacteria. It has been given by mouth in doses of 0.6 to 2 g daily in divided doses in the treatment of susceptible infections.

Absorption and fate. The pharmacokinetics of josamycin following administration by mouth were similar to those of erythromycin stearate in a study of 21 healthy subjects. Josamycin tended to accumulate over the first 48 hours of administration and the plasma half-life varied from 1.34 to 1.56 hours. The urinary excretion over 24 hours ranged from 4.4 to 17.5% as treatment progressed. Josamycin was also present in saliva, sweat, and tears and mean concentrations of 1.03, 0.95, and 2.62 μg per ml respectively were measured in 4 subjects given 1.5 g as a loading dose then 0.5 g every six hours for 10 days.— L. J. Strausbaugh *et al.*, *Antimicrob. Ag. Chemother.*, 1976, *10*, 450.

Antimicrobial action. In a comparative study *in vitro* josamycin showed similar activity to erythromycin and clindamycin against Gram-positive aerobic cocci. It was more active than erythromycin and ampicillin against anaerobes, 90% of isolates of *Bacteroides fragilis* being inhibited by 0.78 μg per ml, and comparable with clindamycin.— E. L. Westerman *et al.*, *Antimicrob. Ag. Chemother.*, 1976, *9*, 988. Against *Bacteroides fragilis*, josamycin had similar inhibitory activity but less bactericidal activity than metronidazole, rosaramicin, or clindamycin.— J. Santoro *et al.*, *Antimicrob. Ag. Chemother.*, 1976, *10*, 188.

Josamycin was as or more active than erythromycin *in vitro* against anaerobic Gram-positive organisms and against *Bacteroides* spp.; it was inactive against *Fusobacterium* spp. About 75% of anaerobic organisms tested were inhibited by 1.56 μg per ml of josamycin. At 3.12 μg per ml all strains of *Bacteroides fragilis* were inhibited and at this concentration josamycin was as active as clindamycin. As such a serum concentration was not achieved with oral therapy, the treatment of anaerobic infections with josamycin would have to await a parenteral form. A concentration of 1.56 μg per ml of josamycin inhibited 95 of 96 strains of Gram-positive aerobic organisms; this activity was less than that of erythromycin.— R. E. Reese *et al.*, *Antimicrob. Ag. Chemother.*, 1976, *10*, 253.

Josamycin and rosaramicin were considered comparable to erythromycin in their action *in vitro* against some aerobic Gram-positive cocci. They were inferior to clindamycin against anaerobes.— S. Shadomy *et al.*, *Antimicrob. Ag. Chemother.*, 1976, *10*, 773.

Josamycin was less active *in vitro* than erythromycin against *Staphylococcus aureus* and streptococci, and less active than clindamycin against *Bacteroides fragilis*. It had similar activity to erythromycin against isolates of *Clostridium* spp.— T. J. Cleary *et al.*, *Curr. ther. Res.*, 1978, *23*, 351.

Further references: E. Yourassowsky, *Arzneimittel-Forsch.*, 1972, *22*, 2005; D. Bock and W. Ritzerfeld, *Arzneimittel-Forsch.*, 1974, *24*, 140; W. L. Fanning *et al.*, *Curr. ther. Res.*, 1976, *20*, 99.

Infections. Josamycin 500 mg four times daily for 7 days was as effective as erythromycin in the same dose in mycoplasmal pneumonia in a double-blind study of 21 patients.— R. P. Wenzel *et al.*, *Antimicrob. Ag.*

Chemother., 1976, *10*, 899.

Josamycin 1.5 g daily was as effective as erythromycin stearate 1 g daily, both in divided doses, in reducing the nasal carriage of *Staph. aureus* in a controlled study of 75 subjects.— S. Z. Wilson *et al.*, *Antimicrob. Ag. Chemother.*, 1977, *11*, 407.

Proprietary Names
Jomybel *(Yamanouchi, Belg.)*; Josacine (also propionate) *(Spret-Mauchant, Fr.)*; Josamy *(Jap.*; *Endo, USA)*.

95-j

Kanamycin Acid Sulphate *(B.P.)*.

A form of kanamycin sulphate prepared by adding sulphuric acid to a solution of kanamycin sulphate and drying by a suitable method.
$C_{18}H_{36}N_4O_{11},1.7H_2SO_4=651.2$.

Pharmacopoeias. In *Br.* and *It. It.* specifies either the monosulphate or acid sulphate.

A white or almost white, odourless or almost odourless, hygroscopic powder containing not less than 670 units per mg and 23 to 26% of sulphate, calculated on the dried material. Kanamycin acid sulphate 1.34 g is approximately equivalent to 1 g of kanamycin.

Soluble 1 in 1 of water; practically insoluble in alcohol, acetone, chloroform, and ether. A solution in water is dextrorotatory. A 1% solution in water has a pH of 6 to 8.5. **Store** in airtight containers. If it is intended for injection the containers should be sterile and sealed to exclude micro-organisms. Protect from light.

96-z

Kanamycin Sulphate *(B.P.)*.

Kanamycin Sulfate *(U.S.P.)*; Kanamycin A Sulphate. 6-*O*-(3-Amino-3-deoxy-α-D-glucopyranosyl)-4-*O*-(6-amino-6-deoxy-α-D-glucopyranosyl)-2-deoxy-D-streptamine monosulphate.
$C_{18}H_{36}N_4O_{11},H_2SO_4=582.6$.

CAS — 59-01-8 (kanamycin); 25389-94-0 (sulphate).

Pharmacopoeias. In *Br.*, *It.*, *Jap.*, *Roum.*, *Rus.*, and *U.S.*
It. specifies either the monosulphate or acid sulphate; *Jap.* has xH_2SO_4.

The sulphate of an antimicrobial substance produced by the growth of *Streptomyces kanamyceticus* or by any other means.

A white or almost white, odourless, crystalline powder. It contains not less than 750 units per mg and 15.7 to 17.3% of sulphate, calculated on the dried material, and not more than 3% (*B.P.*) or 5% (*U.S.P.*) of kanamycin B (see p.1100). Kanamycin monosulphate 1.2 g is approximately equivalent to 1 g of kanamycin.

Soluble 1 in 8 of water; practically insoluble in alcohol, acetone, chloroform, ether, and ethyl acetate. A solution in water is dextrorotatory. A 1% solution in water has a pH of 6 to 8.5. **Store** in airtight containers. If it is intended for injection, the containers should be sterile and sealed to exclude micro-organisms. Protect from light.

INCOMPATIBILITY has been reported with amphotericin, ampicillin sodium, cefapirin sodium, cephalothin sodium, cephazolin sodium, chlorpheniramine maleate, colistin sulphomethate sodium, flucloxacillin sodium, heparin, hydrocortisone sodium succinate, lincomycin hydrochloride, methohexitone sodium, nitrofurantoin sodium, novobiocin sodium, phenobarbitone sodium, phenytoin sodium, prochlorperazine edisylate, sulphadiazine sodium, and sulphafurazole diethanolamine; loss of potency of both penicillin and kanamycin has been reported with carbenicillin sodium, cloxacillin sodium, and methicillin sodium.

Incompatibility. Kanamycin was incompatible with *aminophylline, canrenoate potassium, hydroxydione sodium succinate,* or *methylprednisolone sodium succinate* in an intravenous infusion fluid.— B. Flouvat and P. Lechat, *Thérapie*, 1974, *29*, 337.

For a list of further incompatibilities including *calcium gluconate, chlorpromazine, colistin sulphomethate sodium, novobiocin, pentobarbitone, polymyxin B, promazine, protein hydrolysate injection, quinalbarbitone sodium, sodium bicarbonate, thiopentone sodium,* and *vitamin-B complex,* see *Med. Lett.*, 1972, *14* (Jan.), *Suppl.*, 32.

Further references: R. Misgen, *Am. J. Hosp. Pharm.*, 1965, *22*, 92; J. M. Meisler and M. W. Skolaut, *ibid.*, 1966, *23*, 557; B. B. Riley, *J. Hosp. Pharm.*, 1970, *28*, 228; B. Lynn and A. Jones, *Beecham Research, Advances in Antimicrobial and Antineoplastic Chemotherapy*, Vol. 1, pt 1, Munich, Urban and Schwarzenberg 1972, p. 701.

Loss of activity. The antimicrobial activity of kanamycin sulphate was reduced in the presence of ascorbic acid.— M. A. El-Nakeeb *et al.*, *Can. J. pharm. Sci.*, 1976, *11*, 85.

Stability in solution. Solutions of kanamycin sulphate were stable in dextrose injection and sodium chloride injection.— *Med. Lett.*, 1972, *14* (Jan.), *Suppl.*, 32.

There was no significant loss of potency when kanamycin injection was added to 3 commercially available 0.5% hypromellose solutions in plastic squeezy bottles (Lacril, pH 5.9; Tearisol, pH 7.3; Isoptotears, pH 7.4) and the resulting solutions of kanamycin 30 mg per ml kept at 25° for 7 days.— E. Osborn *et al.*, *Am. J. Ophthal.*, 1976, *82*, 775.

Units. One unit of kanamycin is contained in 0.001232 mg of the first International Reference Preparation (1959) of kanamycin sulphate which contains 812 units per mg.

The dose of kanamycin is normally expressed in terms of the base; 1 g of kanamycin base is approximately equivalent to 1 million units.

Adverse Effects. As for Neomycin Sulphate, p.1189.

Nausea, vomiting, and diarrhoea have been reported following oral administration and staphylococcal enterocolitis may occur. A malabsorption syndrome may also occur although the risk is less with kanamycin than with neomycin.

Minor side-effects such as skin rash, fever, headache, and paraesthesia sometimes occur. Mild reversible renal disturbance is common.

The most serious toxic effect is damage to the eighth cranial nerve resulting in irreversible loss of hearing especially if the course of treatment is prolonged or if there is impaired kidney function. Vestibular damage is less common.

The occurrence of neurotoxic reactions is greatly reduced if the dose is adjusted so that the concentration of kanamycin in the plasma does not exceed 30 µg per ml and the total dose does not exceed about 15 g in 15 days. Neurotoxic reactions occur less frequently in well-hydrated patients under 40 years of age with normal renal function, if treatment is not prolonged. Neuromuscular blockade with respiratory depression has followed intraperitoneal applications of kanamycin in anaesthetised patients.

Hepatotoxicity. Kanamycin was the cause of hepatitis in 1 patient.— S. Imoto *et al.* (letter), *Ann. intern. Med.*, 1979, *91*, 129.

Neuromuscular blockade. A 51-year-old man with chronic renal disease became paralysed after treatment with kanamycin and colistin. His pupils were dilated and fixed but he could hear. The paralysis was due to a block in neuromuscular transmission. He was treated with calcium intravenously and neostigmine. Antibiotic concentrations were not high.— M. P. McQuillen *et al.*, *Archs Neurol., Chicago*, 1968, *18*, 402.

Ototoxicity. Of 17 patients treated for Gram-negative infections with kanamycin in a total dosage of between 1 and 9 g over 1½ to 9 days, 3 developed ototoxic lesions. Sudden and severe hearing loss occurred in 1 patient with renal failure and septicaemia who received only 1 g of kanamycin. Ototoxic symptoms developed in 7 patients and tinnitus in 6 of these patients often preceded or accompanied the onset of hearing impairment.— G. A. Toma and B. J. Main, *Postgrad. med. J.*, 1967, *Suppl.*, May, 46.

A report of intra-uterine and maternal ototoxicity following the administration of kanamycin and ethacrynic acid to a 20-year-old woman with chronic renal disease in the 7th month of pregnancy.— H. C. Jones, *J. natn. med. Ass.*, 1973, *65*, 201.

The Boston Collaborative Drug Surveillance Program monitored consecutively 32 812 medical in-patients. Drug-induced deafness occurred in 5 of 372 patients given kanamycin. One of these patients had previously developed deafness while receiving ethacrynic acid.— J. Porter and H. Jick, *Lancet*, 1977, *1*, 587.

Treatment of Adverse Effects. Kanamycin may be removed by haemodialysis or peritoneal dialysis. Calcium gluconate intravenously or neostigmine has been employed, not always successfully, to counter the neuromuscular blockade caused by kanamycin.

Calcium ions inhibited the antimicrobial activity *in vitro* of kanamycin against some organisms, so that prophylactic administration of calcium salts with kanamycin in an attempt to reduce antibiotic-induced neuromuscular blockade could be unwise.— K. Sakurai *et al.*, *Am. Surg.*, 1965, *31*, 165.

Precautions. Kanamycin is contra-indicated for intestinal disinfection when an obstruction is present and in patients with a history of allergy to it. It should not be given parenterally for trivial infections or to patients with impaired hearing; if tinnitus or dizziness occurs during treatment, kanamycin should be withdrawn immediately.

Kanamycin should be used with care and in reduced dosage in patients with impaired renal function. Elderly patients and patients receiving treatment for longer than 15 days should be carefully observed for signs of ototoxicity.

As with streptomycin (see p.1214) and the other aminoglycosides kanamycin should be used with caution in patients with myasthenia gravis or those receiving other drugs with neuromuscular blocking activity, anticoagulants, anti-emetics, and other ototoxic agents.

Like neomycin (p.1189), kanamycin by mouth might impair the absorption of other drugs.

For the effect of other drugs on the antimicrobial activity of kanamycin, see below under Antimicrobial Action.

Antimicrobial Action. Kanamycin sulphate is bactericidal and has a mode of action similar to that of streptomycin (p.1214) and the other aminoglycoside antibiotics. It is active against a range of Gram-negative organisms including *Escherichia coli, Enterobacter, Klebsiella, Proteus, Serratia, Salmonella* and *Shigella* spp. *Haemophilus influenzae, Brucella*, and *Neisseria* spp. are also sensitive but *Pseudomonas aeruginosa* and *Bacteroides* spp. are invariably resistant. Among Gram-positive organisms only *Staphylococcus aureus* and *epidermidis* are sensitive although *Streptococcus faecalis* may be inhibited by kanamycin in association with benzylpenicillin. Some strains of *Mycobacterium tuberculosis* are sensitive. Kanamycin is ineffective against *Treponema pallidum*, mycoplasmas, yeasts, and fungi.

The minimum inhibitory concentration of kanamycin for susceptible organisms ranges from 0.5 to 8 µg per ml.

It is most active in an alkaline medium.

For a report of the antimicrobial action of ampicillin being enhanced by kanamycin, see Ampicillin, p.1094.

Diminished activity. The antimicrobial activity of kanamycin sulphate was reduced in the presence of ascorbic acid.— M. A. El-Nakeeb *et al.*, *Can. J. pharm. Sci.*, 1976, *11*, 85.

For the effect of calcium on kanamycin, see Treatment of Adverse Effects, above.

Enhanced activity. Kanamycin killed 23 of 25 clinically isolated strains of *Klebsiella* in a concentration of 3.9 µg per ml. Synergism between kanamycin and cephalothin was demonstrated against 13 strains, and no instance of antagonism occurred. Twenty-three strains were inhibited by the presence of 2 µg per ml of each drug, and all 25 were inhibited by a concentration of 8 µg per ml, these concentrations being readily attained in therapy. There was evidence of the development of resistance.— R. J. Bulger, *Ann. intern. Med.*, 1967, *67*, 523.

The MIC of kanamycin for *M. tuberculosis*, strain H37Rv, was greatly diminished when an acridine, such as acriflavine, ethacridine, mepacrine, or proflavine was added in sub-bacteriostatic concentrations.— V. N. Soloviev and V. S. Zueva (letter), *Lancet*, 1968, *2*, 412.

There was enhanced activity against some strains of

Staph. aureus when kanamycin was tested *in vitro* with actinomycin D.— J. Y. Jacobs *et al., Antimicrob. Ag. Chemother.*, 1979, *15*, 580.

For a comparison of the effect of netilmicin, sissomicin, and kanamycin on the activity of benzylpenicillin on enterococci, see Benzylpenicillin, p.1106.

Resistance. Resistance has been observed in strains of most of the organisms reported to be sensitive to kanamycin and a trend towards increasing resistance has been reported.

There is cross-resistance between kanamycin, neomycin, and paromomycin and partial cross-resistance between kanamycin and streptomycin.

Absorption and Fate. Little kanamycin is absorbed after administration by mouth but accumulation in patients with renal failure may produce significant plasma concentrations. After intramuscular injection kanamycin is rapidly absorbed and distributed in tissue fluids. Peak plasma concentrations of about 20 and 30 μg per ml are attained in about 1 hour following doses of 0.5 and 1 g respectively but amounts are negligible after 12 hours. There is little evidence of kanamycin being bound to plasma proteins. A plasma half-life of about 3 hours has been reported but it may be longer in elderly patients and especially in premature and newborn infants.

Kanamycin is rapidly excreted by glomerular filtration and most of a parenteral dose appears in the urine within 6 hours, during which time concentrations in excess of 100 μg per ml may be produced. Only a small amount is excreted in the bile. Kanamycin does not diffuse into the cerebrospinal fluid if the meninges are not inflamed. It has been detected in cord blood and in breast milk. When kidney function is impaired the concentration of kanamycin in plasma progressively increases to a level at which neurotoxic effects may be produced.

Reports of biological half-lives for kanamycin: 3 hours.— C. M. Kunin, *Ann. intern. Med.*, 1967, *67*, 151. 2 to 4 hours in adults (4 to 5 days in renal failure) and 6 to 18 hours (according to age) in premature infants.— W. A. Ritschel, *Drug Intell. & clin. Pharm.*, 1970, *4*, 332. 5 hours.— F. O'Grady *et al.* (letter), *Lancet*, 1971, *2*, 209.

Kanamycin did not exhibit any protein binding in studies *in vitro* of human serum under controlled physiological conditions using an ultrafiltration technique.— R. C. Gordon *et al., Antimicrob. Ag. Chemother.*, 1972, *2*, 214.

The pharmacokinetics of kanamycin by intravenous infusion and intramuscular injection.— J. T. Clarke *et al., Clin. Pharmac. Ther.*, 1974, *15*, 610. See also J. -C. Pechere and R. Dugal, *Clin. Pharmacokinet.*, 1979, *4*, 170.

For reference to sex-linked differences in kanamycin kinetics, see p.1077.

Absorption and fate in infants and children. In 65 neonates treated with kanamycin 7.5 or 10 mg per kg body-weight by intramuscular injection every 12 hours, mean peak serum concentrations varied with dose, birth-weight, and postnatal age and were lower in infants weighing 2 kg or more at birth. Half-lives were correlated inversely with gestational and chronological age. In 21 infants with meningitis given kanamycin 7.5 mg per kg intramuscularly every 12 hours, peak concentrations detected in the CSF 3 to 4 hours after administration ranged from 2.4 to 12 μg per ml (mean of 5.6 μg per ml) compared with a mean peak serum concentration of 13 μg per ml. Penetration into the CSF roughly correlated with the degree of meningeal inflammation.— J. B. Howard and G. H. McCracken, *J. Pediat.*, 1975, *86*, 949.

Diffusion. The average serum and synovial fluid concentrations of kanamycin in samples taken from 7 patients within 2 hours of completing 2 days' treatment with 15 mg per kg body-weight daily given intramuscularly in 2 divided doses were 18 and 16 μg per ml respectively.— E. A. Baciocco and R. L. Iles, *Clin. Pharmac. Ther.*, 1971, *12*, 858.

Although a higher concentration of kanamycin was found in the CSF of neonates without meningitis after an intramuscular injection of 12.5 mg per kg body-weight than after 7.5 mg per kg the concentrations achieved were not in the desired therapeutic range.— L. L. McDonald and J. W. St. Geme, *Antimicrob. Ag. Chemother.*, 1972, *2*, 41. See also under Absorption and Fate in Infants and Children (above).

Uses. Kanamycin is an aminoglycoside antibiotic used in the short-term treatment of infections due to susceptible Gram-negative organisms, especially *Proteus* spp. It has been used to treat staphylococcal infections when other treatment is unsuitable and has sometimes been used as a secondary antituberculous agent, but other safer agents are usually preferred.

Kanamycin sulphate is usually given by intramuscular injection. To avoid loss of hearing it is advisable to restrict the total daily dose for adults to the equivalent of 15 mg per kg body-weight of kanamycin, to a maximum of 1.5 g given in 2 to 4 divided doses, and to limit the course of treatment to a maximum of 10 to 15 g. If there is no response within 3 to 4 days, treatment should be changed. Children can receive the same daily dose of 15 mg per kg.

In overwhelming infections, kanamycin may be given as a slow intravenous infusion of a 0.25% solution at the rate of 3 to 4 ml per minute to a total of 15 mg per kg body-weight daily in 2 or 3 divided doses; daily doses of up to 30 mg per kg have also been recommended. As an adjunct to systemic therapy a recommended daily intrathecal dose is the equivalent of 25 to 50 mg of kanamycin although up to 100 mg has been given over 24 hours. Children may be given 2.5 to 12.5 mg daily but higher doses have been used.

Kanamycin has been used similarly to neomycin as an intestinal antiseptic. In the treatment of intestinal infections the equivalent of 1 to 2 g of kanamycin has been given daily by mouth in 4 divided doses. For pre-operative use, the equivalent of 1 g of kanamycin may be given every hour for 4 hours, then 1 g every 6 hours for 36 to 72 hours. In the management of hepatic coma 8 to 12 g daily may be given. The increasingly frequent occurrence of resistant organisms in the bowel may diminish the effectiveness of kanamycin administered by mouth.

For the inhalation treatment of respiratory infections kanamycin has been administered 2 to 4 times daily as an aerosol containing 250 mg in 1 ml of water diluted with 3 ml of saline.

Doses of kanamycin should be reduced when there is renal impairment.

Kanamycin, given as a single intramuscular dose of 2 g, has been used in the treatment of penicillin-resistant gonorrhoea.

See Gentamicin Sulphate, p.1171 for general reviews of the aminoglycoside antibiotics.

Administration by aerosol. References M. I. Lifschitz and C. R. Denning, *Clin. Pharmac. Ther.*, 1971, *12*, 91; S. M. Ayres *et al., Curr. ther. Res.*, 1972, *14*, 153.

Administration, intraperitoneal. For the use of kanamycin and cephalothin in prolonged peritoneal lavage in generalised peritonitis, see Cephalothin, p.1130.

Dosage in infants and children. A dose of 5 mg per kg body-weight of kanamycin given intramuscularly to 16 children aged 2 months to 12 years produced a mean peak serum concentration of 10.9 μg per ml at 30 minutes compared with a peak of 17.6 μg per ml at 1 hour in 10 children given 10 mg per kg. As optimum peak therapeutic concentrations were considered to range from 15 to 25 μg per ml in spite of much lower MICs, the 5 mg per kg dose was probably too low. It was estimated that a dose of 10 mg per kg given intramuscularly every 8 hours would produce an average peak serum concentration of 18.4 μg per ml at steady state and as paediatric therapy usually ranged from 5 to 10 days the total dose need generally not exceed 300 mg per kg. The proposed dose of 10 mg per kg every 8 hours should be assessed.— J. P. Hieber and J. D. Nelson, *Antimicrob. Ag. Chemother.*, 1976, *9*, 899.

The suggested dose of kanamycin for infants of more than 37 weeks' gestation was 7.5 mg per kg body-weight intramuscularly or as a very slow bolus intravenous injection every 12 hours for the first 48 hours of life, then 10 mg per kg every 8 hours. For immature infants (those of less than 37 weeks' gestation) 7.5 mg per kg could be given every 12 hours for the first week of life then 10 mg per kg every 8 hours. A suggested intraventricular dose was 3 mg, or 2 mg for premature infants.— P. A. Davies, *Br. med. J.*, 1978, *2*, 676. See also H. C. Spratt, *Drugs*, 1978, *16*, 226.

Revised intramuscular doses of kanamycin for infants weighing less than 2 kg at birth were: 12-hourly doses of 7.5 mg per kg body-weight for those aged 7 days or less or 10 mg per kg for those over 7 days. For infants over 2 kg at birth body-weight: 10 mg per kg every 12 hours for those aged 7 days or less or every 8 hours for those over 7 days. If necessary, doses could be given by constant intravenous infusion over 20 minutes. Kanamycin was considered safe when given in these doses for not more than 12 days.— H. F. Eichenwald and G. H. McCracken, *J. Pediat.*, 1978, *93*, 337.

A dose of kanamycin in newborn infants of 7.5 mg per kg body-weight every 12 hours by intramuscular injection was recommended in order to achieve maximum plasma concentrations between 15 and 30 μg per ml.— O. M. J. Driessen *et al., Eur. J. clin. Pharmac.*, 1979, *15*, 133.

Results indicating that in older children kanamycin in a dose of 30 mg per kg body-weight daily intramuscularly or intravenously produced optimal peak serum concentrations without drug accumulation or toxicity. This dose, given in 3 divided doses, is recommended for children over 2 months of age, but must be reconsidered if therapy beyond 14 days is necessary.— J. P. Hieber *et al., J. Pediat.*, 1980, *96*, 1089.

Further references: H. J. Simon and S. G. Axline, *Ann. N.Y. Acad. Sci.*, 1966, *132*, 1020; M. Yow, *ibid.*, 1037; G. J. Yakatan *et al., Clin. Pharmac. Ther.*, 1978, *24*, 90.

Dosage in renal failure. In 10 patients with varying degrees of renal function, the serum concentrations of kanamycin and creatinine were measured after intramuscular injections of 500 mg of kanamycin sulphate. The half-life in hours of kanamycin was about 3.3 times the creatinine concentration in mg per 100 ml. In patients with normal renal function an intramuscular dose of 7 mg per kg body-weight every 12 hours (3 times the half-life of 3 to 5 hours in such patients) was usually appropriate. In patients with renal failure a similar dose every third half-life period would provide adequate blood concentrations. In anuric patients a similar initial dose would not need to be repeated. In patients treated with haemodialysis, the initial dose should be repeated after every other period of 6 to 8 hours of dialysis.— R. E. Cutler and B. M. Orme, *J. Am. med. Ass.*, 1969, *209*, 539.

Of 12 patients with renal failure given 3 injections of kanamycin 7.5 mg per kg body-weight at an interval in hours equal to 3 times the serum creatinine in mg per 100 ml, a satisfactory clinical response occurred in 9 patients. The observed half-life of kanamycin in hours was 5.2 times the creatinine concentration in mg per 100 ml.— R. V. McCloskey and G. G. Becker, *Antimicrob. Ag. Chemother.*, 1970, 161.

A computerised mathematical model for predicting the dosage and serum concentrations of kanamycin in patients with renal insufficiency using the patients' age, sex, body-weight, and serum creatinine as the minimum input data.— G. E. Mawer *et al., Lancet*, 1972, *1*, 12. The programme was extended to produce a dosage nomogram for kanamycin using the serum-creatinine concentration, weight, and age of the patient. This should produce serum-kanamycin concentrations of 10 to 30 μg per ml 2 hours after each dose.— *idem* (letter), 1972, *2*, 45.

After a loading dose of 7 mg per kg body-weight kanamycin could be given in a dose of 7 mg per kg every third half-life (half-life=3 times serum-creatinine concentration in mg per 100 ml) to patients with a creatinine clearance (CC) of 40 to 80 ml per minute, in a dose of 250 mg every 24 hours to those with a CC of 20 to 30 ml per minute, every 48 hours to those with a CC of 10 ml per minute, and 7 mg per kg every 5 to 7 days to those with a CC of 5 ml per minute. In haemodialysis 7 mg per kg could be given every other haemodialysis; in peritoneal dialysis 3.5 mg per kg, or 250 mg, could be given every 24 hours.— J. S. Cheigh, *Am. J. Med.*, 1977, *62*, 555.

Further references: C. M. Kunin, *Ann. N.Y. Acad. Sci.*, 1966, *132*, 811; *idem, Ann. intern. Med.*, 1967, *67*, 151; T. P. Gibson and H. A. Nelson, *Clin. Pharmacokinet.*, 1977, *2*, 403; P. Sharpstone, *Br. med. J.*, 1977, *2*, 36; W. M. Bennett *et al., Ann. intern. Med.*, 1980, *93*, 62.

Encephalopathy. Kanamycin given by mouth and then intramuscularly to 14 patients with cirrhosis of the liver reduced blood and urine ammonia and urine amino acid concentrations but had no effect on plasma amino acids. Ten of the patients had chronic hepatic encephalopathy and 6 improved when kanamycin was given intramuscularly.— F. Nealon *et al., Clin. Pharmac. Ther.*,

1971, *12*, 298.

Enterocolitis. Kanamycin given prophylactically prevented necrotising enterocolitis in infants under 1.5 kg body-weight at birth.— E. A. Egan *et al.*, *J. Pediat.*, 1976, *89*, 467. See also E. A. Egan *et al.* (letter), *J. Pediat.*, 1977, *90*, 331. Two of 9 infants under 2 kg body-weight given kanamycin 15 mg per kg daily for at least 6 days to prevent necrotising enterocolitis developed the condition. The enterocolitis was due to *Staphylococcus epidermidis* that was resistant to kanamycin, gentamicin, oxacillin and benzylpenicillin. Strains with a similar resistance pattern were isolated from 6 of the other infants and from a further child with meningitis. The organism was not recovered from children in the nursery 5 months after kanamycin prophylaxis was stopped.— M. M. Conroy *et al.* (letter), *Lancet*, 1978, *1*, 613.

Gonorrhoea. References G. W. Csonka, *Postgrad. med. J.*, 1967, (May), *Suppl.*, 63; T. F. Keys *et al.*, *J. Am. med. Ass.*, 1969, *210*, 857; J. L. Fluker and A. B. Hewitt, *Br. J. vener. Dis.*, 1970, *46*, 454; R. Pang *et al.*, *Br. med. J.*, 1979, *1*, 380.

Leprosy. Kanamycin 1 g daily for 90 days given to 10 patients with lepromatous leprosy produced results similar to those achieved with rifamycin and oxytetracycline, a response being obtained within 30 days. There was transient albuminuria in 6 and hearing impairment in 8 patients. It was recommended that treatment should not exceed 30 days.— D. V. A. Opromolla and S. C. Almeida, *Revta bras. Leprol.*, 1970, *37*, 17, per *Trop. Dis. Bull.*, 1972, *69*, 753.

Meningitis. Six infants were treated with intramuscular and with intrathecal or intraventricular injections of kanamycin for the treatment of meningitis and ventriculitis due to *Proteus*, *Klebsiella aerogenes*, and *Escherichia coli*. In 4 patients, the organisms became resistant to all drugs except kanamycin. The cerebrospinal fluid became sterile in 4 children, but only 2 of these survived.— J. Lorber, *Postgrad. med. J.*, 1967, (May), *Suppl.*, 52.

Plague. Kanamycin was effective in the treatment of 13 patients with bubonic plague although 1 who developed meningitis also required ampicillin. Four out of 5 patients with bubonic-septicaemic plague responded to kanamycin but 1 subsequently developed a fatal plague meningitis. The 5 strains of *Yersinia pestis* tested by the disk method were sensitive, with the MIC for 4 of the strains being less than 0.75 to 6.25 µg per ml.— J. R. Cantey, *Ann. intern. Med.*, 1972, *76*, 871.

Staphylococcal infections. Synergism between kanamycin and cephalothin at growth inhibiting concentrations was demonstrated in 7 of 9 strains of *Staphylococcus aureus* resistant to methicillin, but synergism at minimum bactericidal concentrations was evident in only 5. Synergism between kanamycin and methicillin occurred in 2 and 3 strains respectively. No antagonism between the antibiotics was noted. It was suggested that in selected cases of methicillin-resistant staphylococcal infection kanamycin with either cephalothin or methicillin could be given as initial treatment whilst awaiting the results of *in vitro* tests for synergism.— R. J. Bulger, *Lancet*, 1967, *1*, 17. A criticism and a reply.— S. J. Seligman and R. J. Bulger (letters), *ibid.*, 390 and 391. See also R. J. Bulger (letter), *Br. med. J.*, 1967, *4*, 805.

Surgical infection prophylaxis. Before undergoing elective excision of colorectal carcinoma, 47 patients received an oral antibiotic regimen of metronidazole 1.2 g daily by mouth for 2 days (the last dose given 36 hours before operation to avoid systemic blood concentrations), and kanamycin 3 g by mouth for 3 days (the last dose given 12 hours before operation). Forty-six similar patients received a regimen of 3 doses of metronidazole 500 mg by slow intravenous infusion and kanamycin 1 g intramuscularly or intravenously (these doses given in the anaesthetic room before operation, at 18.00 hours on the evening of operation, and at 6.00 hours the following morning). Abdominal wound sepsis occurred in only 3 patients (6.5%) in the systemic therapy group; in the oral therapy group it occurred in 17 (36%), and 15 of these 17 patients had resistant bacteria in the colon at operation which were the organisms isolated from the subsequent septic lesion. In 6 of the oral group patients, large numbers of kanamycin-resistant *Staphylococcus aureus* were recorded; antibiotic-associated pseudomembranous colitis occurred in 7 patients, 6 of them in the oral group.— M. R. B. Keighley *et al.*, *Lancet*, 1979, *1*, 894. Mention of results indicating that metronidazole with kanamycin had no advantage over metronidazole alone when given by mouth to patients undergoing colonic surgery.— G. Proud and J. Chamberlain (letter), *ibid.*, *2*, 1017.

Urinary-tract infections. A single intramuscular injection of kanamycin sulphate 500 mg was effective in eradicating bladder infections in 36 of 39 patients and upper-tract infections in 18 of 65 patients.— A. R. Ronald *et al.*, *J. Am. med. Ass.*, 1976, *235*, 1854.

Preparations

Kanamycin Injection *(B.P.)*. A sterile solution of kanamycin sulphate in Water for Injections containing sulphuric acid and suitable buffering and stabilising agents (pH 4 to 6), or a solution prepared by dissolving the contents of a sealed container of kanamycin acid sulphate (Kanamycin Acid Sulphate for Injection) in Water for Injections immediately before use (pH 6.5 to 7.5). Protect from light.

Kanamycin Sulfate Capsules *(U.S.P.)*. Capsules containing kanamycin sulphate equivalent to 500 mg of kanamycin. Store in airtight containers.

Kanamycin Sulfate Injection *(U.S.P.)*. A sterile solution of kanamycin sulphate with suitable buffers and preservatives. pH 3.5 to 5. It contains the equivalent of 37.5, 250, or 333.3 mg of kanamycin per ml.

Proprietary Preparations

Kannasyn *(Winthrop, UK)*. Kanamycin, available as **Powder** for preparing injections, in vials containing the equivalent of 1 g of kanamycin (as acid sulphate), and as **Solution** containing the equivalent of 250 mg of kanamycin (as sulphate) per ml with sodium metabisulphite and sodium citrate as stabilising agents and methyl and propyl hydroxybenzoates as preservatives, in vials of 4 ml.

Kantrex *(Bristol-Myers Pharmaceuticals, UK)*. Kanamycin sulphate, available as **Capsules** containing the equivalent of 250 mg of kanamycin and as **Injection** in single-use vials containing the equivalent of 1 g of kanamycin in 3 ml, with sodium citrate and preservative. (Also available as Kantrex in *Arg.*, *Austral.*, *Canad.*, *Denm.*, *Ital.*, *Norw.*, *S.Afr.*, *Spain*, *Switz.*, *USA*).

Other Proprietary Names

Arg.—Cristalomicina; *Austral.*—Kanasig; *Belg.*—Kamynex, Kanacyn, Kanamytrex; *Fr.*—Kamycine; *Ger.*—Kanamytrex; *Ital.*—Kanacet, Kanacetic, Kanapiam, Kanatrol, Keimicina; *Neth.*—Kamynex, Kanacyn; *Spain*—Kanabiot, Kanafluid, Kanahidro, Kanaqua, Kanescin; *USA*—Klebcil.

Preparations containing kanamycin sulphate were also formerly marketed in Great Britain under the proprietary names Kanfotrex (*Bristol*) and Kantrexil (*Bristol*).

97-c

Kitasamycin. Leucomycin.

CAS — 1392-21-8.

Pharmacopoeias. In *Jap.* which also includes Acetylkitasamycin.

An antimicrobial substance produced by *Streptomyces kitasatoensis*. A white to light yellowish-white odourless powder with a bitter taste. Sparingly **soluble** in water; very soluble in alcohol, acetone, chloroform, ether, and methyl alcohol; freely soluble in carbon tetrachloride; practically insoluble in light petroleum.

Kitasamycin is a macrolide antibiotic with similar actions and uses to Erythromycin, (p.1158), but weaker antimicrobial activity. It has been given by mouth in doses of 1 to 1.4 g daily or by slow intravenous injection in doses of 200 mg every 6 to 8 hours. The tartrate has also been used.

In 81 patients with acute respiratory infections, including 56 with mixed bacterial infections, kitasamycin 1.6 g daily for 5 days, resulted in bacteriological and clinical cure in 34 and clinical cure only in 25. In 10 patients with wound infections, all were considered cured clinically, but 1 was a bacteriological failure.— B. C. Stratford and S. Dixson, *Med. J. Aust.*, 1974, *1*, 1029.

Proprietary Names

Ayermicina *(Ayerst, Ital.)*.

186-k

Latamoxef Sodium. 6059-S; LY 127935; Moxalactam Disodium. (7*R*)-7-[2-Carboxy-2-(4-hydroxyphenyl)acetamido]-7-methoxy-3-(1-methyl-1*H*-tetrazol-5-ylthiomethyl)-1-oxa-3-cephem-4-carboxylic acid, disodium salt. $C_{20}H_{18}N_6Na_2O_9S$=564.4.

CAS — 64952-97-2 (latamoxef); 64953-12-4 (disodium salt).

Each g of latamoxef sodium represents 3.5 mmol (3.5 mEq) of sodium. Latamoxef sodium 1.08 g is approximately equivalent to 1 g of latamoxef.

Latamoxef is an antibiotic closely related to the cephalosporins and has a wide antibacterial spectrum of activity similar to that of cefotaxime (p.1118). It is administered parenterally as the sodium salt and has been given by intravenous injection in doses equivalent to 1 to 2 g of latamoxef every 8 hours.

A brief review of latamoxef sodium, a 1-oxacephalosporin antibiotic in which the sulphur atom of the beta-lactam nucleus is replaced by oxygen. Studies *in vitro* have demonstrated that latamoxef has a very broad spectrum of activity against most beta-lactamase-producing Gram-negative bacteria, including many resistant to aminoglycosides and other cephalosporins, and in general it is 8 to 32 times more active than cefoxitin, cefuroxime, or cephazolin, but less active than cefotaxime. Latamoxef is active against *Haemophilus influenzae* and some strains of *Bacteroides fragilis*, with activity against anaerobes comparable to that of cefoxitin and cefotaxime. It has moderate activity, similar to that of cefotaxime, against *Pseudomonas aeruginosa*. Against Gram-positive bacteria, latamoxef has only moderate activity and, like other cephalosporins, is inactive against enterococci.

Latamoxef has a long half-life and after intramuscular or intravenous injection peak serum concentrations are reported to be high with inhibitory activity persisting for 8 to 12 hours. Penetration into the cerebrospinal fluid is superior to that of other cephalosporins and limited clinical experience has suggested that latamoxef is safe and effective in meningitis and other severe infections caused by Gram-negative bacilli in infancy. It should not be used alone in neonatal meningitis until the pathogen has been identified because of its poor activity against group B streptococci and should not be used in adult meningitis because of its relatively low activity against pneumococci. Satisfactory responses to latamoxef have been reported in a variety of infections but not in pseudomonal infections of the urinary tract. Latamoxef may be of value in the management of coliform and *Haemophilus* meningitis and in infections caused by Gram-negative bacilli resistant to other antibiotics. Alcohol intolerance similar to the disulfiram reaction has been reported as has hypoprothrombinaemia with bleeding in some patients.— *Lancet*, 1981, *2*, 23. Another brief review mentions in addition to these adverse effects, thrombophlebitis, anaphylaxis and other hypersensitivity reactions, diarrhoea, pseudomembranous colitis, convulsions, and superinfections with enterococci, *Pseudomonas*, and *Candida*.— *Med. Lett.*, 1982, *24*, 13.

Studies on the antimicrobial activity *in vitro* of latamoxef: H. C. Neu *et al.*, *Antimicrob. Ag. Chemother.*, 1979, *16*, 141 and 528; M. Barza *et al.*, *ibid.*, 287; G. M. Trager *et al.*, *ibid.*, 297; R. Wise *et al.*, *ibid.*, 341; R. J. Fass, *ibid.*, 503; D. J. Flournoy and F. A. Perryman, *ibid.*, 641; T. P. Felegie *et al.*, *ibid.*, 833; D. G. Delgado *et al.*, *ibid.*, 864; S. S. Weaver *et al.*, *ibid.*, 1980, *17*, 92; V. L. Yu *et al.*, *ibid.*, 96; M. V. Borobio *et al.*, *ibid.*, 129; W. H. Hall *et al.*, *ibid.*, 273; T. Yoshida *et al.*, *ibid.*, 302; R. R. Bulger and J. A. Washington, *ibid.*, 393; L. G. Reimer *et al.*, *ibid.*, 412; E. O. Mason *et al.*, *ibid.*, 470; S. D. R. Lang *et al.*, *ibid.*, 488; J. H. Jorgensen *et al.*, *ibid.*, 516; K. Sato *et al.*, *ibid.*, 736; R. N. Jones *et al.*, *ibid.*, 750; C. N. Baker *et al.*, *ibid.*, 757; J. H. Jorgensen *et al.*, *ibid.*, 937; C. A. Warren *et al.*, *J. antimicrob. Chemother.*, 1980, *6*, 607; B. Van Klingeren *et al.* (letter), *ibid.*, 674; I. Brook (letter), *ibid.*, 676; C. Watanakunakorn and C. Glotzbecker, *Curr. ther. Res.*, 1980, *27*, 287; J. P. Maskell and M. Nasu (letter), *Lancet*, 1981, *1*, 733.

Pharmacokinetic studies of latamoxef: S. H. Landesman *et al.*, *Am. J. Med.*, 1980, *69*, 92 (CSF); J. N. Parsons *et al.*, *Antimicrob. Ag. Chemother.*, 1980, *17*, 226; R. Wise *et al.*, *J. antimicrob. Chemother.*, 1980, *6*, 319; U. B. Schaad *et al.*, *J. Pediat.*, 1981, *98*, 129.

Reports on the clinical use of latamoxef sodium: R. S. Gibbs *et al.*, *Antimicrob. Ag. Chemother.*, 1980, *17*, 1004; R. W. Tofte *et al.*, *ibid.*, 1981, *19*, 740; J. R. Lentino *et al.*, *ibid.*, 801; U. B. Schaad *et al.*, *J. Pediat.*, 1981, *98*, 129 (meningitis).

A report of enterococcal superinfection and colonisation in 9 patients, including bacteraemia in 2, after treatment with latamoxef sodium for serious infections due to other bacterial pathogens.— V. L. Yu, *Ann. intern. Med.*, 1981, *94*, 784.

Interactions. *Alcohol.* Two patients receiving latamoxef sodium developed a disulfiram-like reaction to alcohol.— H. C. Neu and A. S. Prince (letter), *Lancet*, 1980, *1*, 1422.

Proprietary Names
Moxam *(Lilly, USA).*

98-k

Lincomycin Hydrochloride *(B.P., B.P. Vet., U.S.P.).*

Methyl 6-amino-6,8-dideoxy-*N*-[(2*S*,4*R*)-1-methyl-4-propylprolyl]-1-thio-α-D-*erythro*-D-*galacto*-octopyranoside hydrochloride monohydrate.

$C_{18}H_{34}N_2O_6S,HCl,H_2O = 461.0$.

CAS — 154-21-2 (lincomycin); 859-18-7 (hydrochloride, anhydrous); 7179-49-9 (hydrochloride, monohydrate).

Pharmacopoeias. In *Br.*, *Jap.* and *U.S.*

A monobasic antibiotic produced by the growth of *Streptomyces lincolnensis* var. *lincolnensis* or by any other means.

A white or almost white crystalline powder, odourless or with a slight characteristic odour and a bitter taste. The *B.P.* specifies that it contains not less than 82.5% of lincomycin (calculated with reference to the anhydrous substance) of which not more than 5% is lincomycin B. The *U.S.P.* specifies not less than 790 µg of lincomycin per mg. Lincomycin hydrochloride 1.13 g is approximately equivalent to 1 g of lincomycin.

Soluble 1 in 1 of water, 1 in 40 of alcohol, and 1 in 20 of dimethylformamide; soluble in methyl alcohol; very slightly soluble in acetone; practically insoluble in chloroform and ether. A solution in water is dextrorotatory. A 10% solution of lincomycin hydrochloride in water has a pH of 3 to 5.5. Solutions are **sterilised** by filtration. **Store** at a temperature not exceeding 30° in airtight containers. If it is intended for parenteral administration, the containers should be sterile and sealed to exclude micro-organisms.

Lincomycin hydrochloride is stated to be **incompatible** with kanamycin sulphate and novobiocin sodium.

Incompatibility. There was loss of clarity when intravenous solutions of lincomycin hydrochloride were mixed with those of *benzylpenicillin* or *phenytoin sodium*.— J. A. Patel and G. L. Phillips, *Am. J. Hosp. Pharm.*, 1966, *23*, 409.

Lincomycin hydrochloride 600 mg in 2 ml was visually compatible for at least 1 hour when used as the solvent for *benzylpenicillin, cloxacillin sodium*, or *methicillin sodium*, and with *ampicillin sodium* or *carbenicillin sodium* when the penicillin was first dissolved in 2 ml of water.— B. Lynn, *J. Hosp. Pharm.*, 1970, *28*, 71.

A crystalline precipitate occurred when lincomyin hydrochloride 2.4 g per litre was mixed with *sulphadiazine sodium* 4 g per litre in dextrose injection or sodium chloride injection.— B. B. Riley, *J. Hosp. Pharm.*, 1970, *28*, 228.

Lincomycin was incompatible with *canrenoate potassium* in an intravenous infusion fluid.— B. Flouvat and P. Lechat, *Thérapie*, 1974, *29*, 337.

For a further list of incompatibilities including *carbenicillin, cephalothin, cloxacillin, hydrocortisone, novobiocin, streptomycin*, and *vitamin-B complex*, see *Med. Lett.*, 1972, *14* (Jan.), *Suppl.*, 32.

Stability in solution. Solutions of lincomycin were stable in sodium chloride injection and dextrose injection for 24 hours at room temperature.— *Med. Lett.*, 1972, *14* (Jan.), *Suppl.*, 32.

Units. One unit of lincomycin is contained in 0.0011351 mg of the first International Reference Preparation (1965) of lincomycin hydrochloride which contains 881 units per mg.

Adverse Effects. Severe and persistent diarrhoea has occurred and some patients have developed severe and sometimes fatal pseudomembranous colitis; both conditions have been reported during and after a course of lincomycin hydrochloride. Some reports suggest that the intestinal effects may be due to superinfection. Nausea, vomiting, abdominal cramps, pruritus ani, stomatitis, glossitis, and abnormality of taste may occur; hypersensitivity reactions are rare. Agranulocytosis, leucopenia, and thrombocytopenia have been reported, as have raised serum aspartate aminotransferase (SGOT) values. Phlebitis may occur when large doses of lincomycin hydrochloride are given intravenously. Hypotension and on rare occasions cardiac arrest have followed too rapid intravenous injections.

A patient given lincomycin 4 to 6 g daily by rapid intermittent intravenous infusion developed reversible glucose intolerance, hyperlipidaemia, and hypertriglyceridaemia.— C. J. O'Connell and M. E. Plaut, *Curr. ther. Res.*, 1969, *11*, 478.

Chest compliance decreased within 15 minutes of the inadvertent administration of a 12-g bolus intravenous injection of lincomycin instead of 1.2 g. Cardiac arrest immediately followed intubation. It was considered that cardiac arrest was not due to reflex bradycardia or hypoxia after intubation but to a cardiac depressant action.— J. L. Daubeck *et al.*, *Anesth. Analg. curr. Res.*, 1974, *53*, 563.

A 10-year-old girl with osteomyelitis erroneously received lincomycin 6 g intravenously on 2 occasions within 10 hours without signs of toxicity, apart from fatigue and unpleasant taste sensation.— K. Widhalm and G. Salzman, *Arzneimittel-Forsch.*, 1978, *28*, 1428.

Colitis. Of 25 patients who received lincomycin with other antibiotics as prophylaxis after undergoing surgery for the large bowel 6, with an average age of 68 years, developed pseudomembranous colitis; it did not occur in 33 similar patients who received lincomycin alone for 5 days.— C. E. Clark *et al.*, *J. antimicrob. Chemother.*, 1976, *2*, 167.

The incidence of diarrhoea in a group of patients treated with lincomycin or clindamycin was closely comparable with a similar group receiving ampicillin. Of 96 receiving lincomycin, only 1 developed pseudomembranous colitis after 2 prolonged courses.— M. B. Robertson *et al.*, *Med. J. Aust.*, 1977, *1*, 243. See also M. B. Robertson and K. J. Breen (letter), *ibid.*, 466.

Of 90 hospital in-patients in a Boston Collaborative Drug Surveillance Program who received lincomycin none developed colitis. Of 26 294 hospital in-patients monitored 6 had been admitted with lincomycin-associated colitis. All were female and had taken the antibiotic by mouth; 1 had also received 4 injections; 5 were from New Zealand which, with the cases reported by A.J.Scott *et al.* (*Lancet*, 1973, *2*, 1232) might point to a geographical distribution.— R. R. Miller and H. Jick, *Clin. Pharmac. Ther.*, 1977, *22*, 1.

Diarrhoea occurred in 11 of 30 subjects who took lincomycin 500 mg every 8 hours for 7 days but in none of a further 18 subjects who took gentamicin 80 mg every 8 hours in addition to lincomycin.— E. Fesce *et al.*, *Int. J. clin. Pharmac. Biopharm.*, 1978, *16*, 495.

Antibiotic-induced diarrhoea was seen in 43 (12%) of 368 patients given lincomycin or clindamycin but there were no cases of pseudomembranous colitis.— D. A. Leigh *et al.*, *J. antimicrob. Chemother.*, 1980, *6*, 639.

Further references: G. B. Manashil and J. A. Kern, *Am. J. Gastroent.*, 1973, *60*, 394; J. Sneddon (letter), *Lancet*, 1974, *1*, 221; W. P. Dyck *et al.* (letter), *ibid.*, 272; F. E. Pittman *et al.* (letter), *ibid.*, 451; *Br. med. J.*, 1974, *4*, 65; W. N. Hubbard, *Upjohn, USA* (letter), *Lancet*, 1974, *1*, 172; F. E. Pittman *et al.*, *Archs intern. Med.*, 1974, *134*, 368; J. F. Munk and K. J. Breen (letter), *Med. J. Aust.*, 1975, *1*, 839; J. F. Munk *et al.*, *Med. J. Aust.*, 1976, *2*, 95.

See also under Clindamycin Hydrochloride, p.1144.

Treatment of Adverse Effects. As for Clindamycin Hydrochloride, p.1145.

The development of watery diarrhoea in a 71-year-old woman during treatment with lincomycin was due to toxins from lincomycin-resistant *Clostridium sporogenes* and *C. difficile*, both of which were eradicated by treatment with vancomycin given in 2 courses each lasting 10 days.— T. J. Marrie *et al.*, *Can. med. Ass. J.*, 1978, *119*, 1058.

See also below under Precautions.

Precautions. Lincomycin should not be given to patients who are known to be hypersensitive or who have experienced reactions with clindamycin. It should not be used in patients with diarrhoeal states and it should be used with care in patients with impaired liver and renal function. Kaolin and cyclamates reduce the absorption of lincomycin from the gastro-intestinal tract.

Since lincomycin is reported to possess neuromuscular blocking activity it should be used carefully with other drugs with similar activity.

Large doses of lincomycin, given rapidly by intravenous injection, seemed to be associated with cardiopulmonary arrest; 4 such cases had been observed. The same doses, given slowly, were well tolerated. Doses of 4 g or more should be dissolved in at least 500 ml of fluid and infused at a rate of not more than 100 ml per hour.— B. A. Waisbren (letter), *J. Am. med. Ass.*, 1968, *206*, 2118.

The use of diphenoxylate with atropine (Lomotil) or codeine in the treatment of lincomycin-induced diarrhoea was questioned since, in a controlled study involving 200 healthy subjects, the highest incidence of diarrhoea was seen in those given either of these antidiarrhoeal treatments concomitantly with lincomycin given intramuscularly.— E. Novak *et al.*, *J. Am. med. Ass.*, 1976, *235*, 1451.

Pregnancy and the neonate. A study over 7 years of the children of mothers who received lincomycin in the 3 trimesters of pregnancy indicated that the incidence of abnormalities was no greater than in a normal population.— A. Mickal and J. D. Panzer, *Am. J. Obstet. Gynec.*, 1975, *121*, 1071.

Antimicrobial Action. Lincomycin is bacteriostatic or bactericidal depending on the concentration and has a range of antimicrobial activity and mode of action similar to that of erythromycin. It is active against *Streptococcus pyogenes, Str. pneumoniae, Str. viridans, Staphylococcus aureus, Corynebacterium diphtheriae, Bacillus anthracis*, and some *Clostridia* spp. However, *Neisseria gonorrhoea, N. meningitidis*, and *Haemophilus influenzae* are sensitive to erythromycin but relatively resistant to lincomycin and the mycoplasmas, apart from *Mycoplasma hominis*, are less sensitive. The enterobacteria and *Str. faecalis* are resistant. Most strains of *Bacteroides* spp. have been reported to be inhibited by about 6 µg or less per ml of lincomycin.

The minimum inhibitory concentrations of lincomycin have been reported to range from 0.02 to 3.1 µg per ml for many strains of *Str. pyogenes, Str. pneumoniae*, and *Staph. aureus*.

For a brief discussion on the lincomycin antibiotics, see p.1084.

Of 68 strains of *H. influenzae* 1 was inhibited by lincomycin at a concentration of 1 µg per ml, 16 at 2 µg per ml, 19 at 4 µg per ml, 23 at 8 µg per ml, and 9 at 16 µg per ml.— J. D. Williams and J. Andrews, *Br. med. J.*, 1974, *1*, 134.

For references to an interaction between lincomycin and erythromycin *in vitro*, see Erythromycin, p.1159.

Resistance. A varied incidence of staphylococcal resistance has been reported. Cross-resistance occurs between lincomycin, clindamycin, and erythromycin. Some erythromycin-resistant organisms may be sensitive to lincomycin but resistance may develop *in vivo*. Resistance to lincomycin has also been reported in pneumococci and haemolytic streptococci.

Of 1176 strains of group A streptococci isolated in Japan in the period 1972 to 1974, 241 were resistant to tetracycline, 234 to tetracycline and chloramphenicol, 427 to tetracycline, chloramphenicol, erythromycin, oleandomycin, josamycin, midecamycin, and lincomycin, and 19 to chloramphenicol alone.— Y. Miyamoto *et al.*, *Antimicrob. Ag. Chemother.*, 1978, *13*, 399. See also M. Nakae *et al.*, *Antimicrob. Ag. Chemother.*, 1977, *12*, 427.

Three strains of *Bacteroides fragilis* isolated in 3 successive weeks were all resistant to lincomycin. One strain was inhibited *in vitro* by clindamycin 45 µg per ml and the other 2 by clindamycin 2.5 µg per ml.— M. Rahman (letter), *J. antimicrob. Chemother.*, 1978, *4*, 381.

For reports of *Corynebacterium diphtheriae* and pneumococci resistant to lincomycin and erythromycin, see Erythromycin, p.1159.

Absorption and Fate. About 20 to 35% of a dose of lincomycin given by mouth is absorbed from the gastro-intestinal tract and following a 500-mg dose, peak plasma concentrations of 1 to 6 µg per ml are reached within 2 to 4 hours; detectable concentrations may persist for about 12 hours. Administration after meals reduces peak values by 50% or more. Lincomycin is widely distributed in the tissues including bone and body fluids but diffusion into the cerebrospinal fluid is poor unless the meninges are inflamed. It diffuses across the placenta and is excreted in the milk of nursing mothers.

The intramuscular injection of 600 mg produces peak plasma concentrations of 8 to 12 µg per ml within 1 to 2 hours decreasing to 1 µg at 24 hours; concentrations of 6 to 13 µg per ml have been maintained when this dose is given 8-hourly. The intravenous infusion of 300 and 600 mg over 2 hours gives peak concentrations of about 10 and 16 µg per ml respectively.

The biological half-life of lincomycin is about 5 hours. About 5 to 10% of a 500-mg dose given by mouth is excreted in the urine within 24 hours but 30% or more of a dose given parenterally may be excreted in the urine, most of it within 4 hours. It is not effectively removed from the blood by dialysis. High concentrations are achieved in the bile and about 40% of a dose given by mouth and up to 14% of a dose given by injection can be excreted in the faeces. It is considered that lincomycin not accounted for by urinary and faecal excretion is inactivated, probably in the liver.

Some 80 to 90% of lincomycin in the circulation was bound to serum proteins. The biological half-life in serum was 4.4 to 4.7 hours and 10 to 15% was excreted in urine.— C. M. Kunin, *Ann. intern. Med.*, 1967, *67*, 151. Using the ultrafiltration method 71.9% of lincomycin was bound to serum proteins.— R. C. Gordon *et al.*, *J. pharm. Sci.*, 1973, *62*, 1074.

Studies of serum concentrations of lincomycin after its administration rectally indicated that absorption was greater from an aqueous solution than from a suppository. Absorption from an aqueous solution administered rectally averaged from about one-half to approximately the same absorption attained following administration of the same dose by mouth, depending upon whether the subjects were fasting or had had enemas.— J. G. Wagner *et al.*, *J. clin. Pharmac.*, 1968, *8*, 154.

Daily infusions of lincomycin 4.8 to 8.4 g as the hydrochloride in divided doses over 2 hours for 7 days produced no toxic reactions in 16 healthy subjects when compared with 16 controls. The average peak serum concentration after 1.2 g was about 24 µg per ml with a nadir concentration of about 10 µg per ml. The CSF concentration measured in 1 subject was 1.9 µg per ml when his serum concentration was 25.49 µg per ml.— E. Novak *et al.*, *Clin. Pharmac. Ther.*, 1971, *12*, 793.

Diffusion. Lincomycin, 600 mg every 12 hours intramuscularly, starting the evening before thoracotomy, produced a mean serum concentration of 6.8 µg per ml and a pleural fluid concentration of 5.2 µg per ml 1 to 3 hours after operation in 34 patients. After administration of lincomycin thrice daily by mouth in doses of 0.5 to 1 g, the mean concentrations were 5.1 and 1.9 µg per ml respectively from 1 to 3 hours after operation.— P. A. Thomas and P. C. Jolly, *Am. Rev. resp. Dis.*, 1967, *96*, 1044.

Lincomycin, 600 mg intramuscularly every 8 hours, was given to 11 patients. The CSF concentration was 7 µg per ml in 1 patient with inflamed meninges and smaller concentrations were found in 3 patients 2 of whom had viral meningitis. Lincomycin was not detected in the CSF of the other 7 patients.— P. I. Lerner, *Am. J. med. Sci.*, 1969, *257*, 125.

Twelve patients undergoing total hip replacement received lincomycin 600 mg intramuscularly 6 hours before surgery, 600 mg by intravenous infusion during surgery, and 600 mg intramuscularly every 12 hours postoperatively until the drains were removed at 72 hours. The mean concentrations of lincomycin in ground bone, hip capsule, and synovial fluid from samples taken at operation were 20.1, 9.4, and 5.4 µg per g. Plasma concentrations in samples taken immediately postoperatively ranged from 0.98 to 21.20 µg per ml. Lincomycin was considered to provide adequate cover but, as 2 patients developed pseudomembranous colitis, toxicity restricted its use.— R. L. Parsons *et al.*, *Br. J. clin. Pharmac.*, 1977, *4*, 433. See also G. Linzenmeier *et al.*, *Arzneimittel-Forsch.*, 1968, *18*, 204; V. Vacek and M. Hejzlar, *ibid.*, 1457; K. Dornbusch *et al.*, *J. antimicrob. Chemother.*, 1977, *3*, 153.

Tissue concentrations in human tonsils of lincomycin given intravenously before tonsillectomy.— J. Gabka and W. Platz, *Arzneimittel-Forsch.*, 1978, *28*, 87.

Pregnancy and the neonate. In a study in 60 women given lincomycin 600 mg by intramuscular injection (usually a single dose) shortly before delivery, peak maternal blood concentrations occurred about 45 minutes after injection and peak cord blood concentrations occurred about 55 minutes after injection. Mean concentrations at 2 hours were 8.22 and 2.10 µg per ml respectively in 10 mothers and 5 babies respectively; both concentrations fell progressively, with mean values of 3.31 and 1.27 µg per ml at 8 hours. The passage of lincomycin into the amniotic fluid was slower and more variable and was also more persistent. Lincomycin was possibly implicated in persistent neuromuscular block, unresponsive to neostigmine, in 1 patient after caesarean section.— N. M. Duignan *et al.*, *Br. med. J.*, 1973, *3*, 75.

Uses. Lincomycin is an antibiotic which has been used effectively in the treatment of infections due to staphylococci, streptococci, and *Bacteroides fragilis* although its chlorinated derivative, clindamycin (see p.1144), is often preferred. However, because of their effects on the gastro-intestinal tract their use is best limited to severe infections where there is no other suitable alternative. Lincomycin, like clindamycin, penetrates bone and has been used successfully in the treatment of acute and chronic osteomyelitis.

Lincomycin hydrochloride is administered by mouth in doses equivalent to 500 mg of lincomycin before food 3 or 4 times daily; by intramuscular injection, 600 mg once or twice daily; by slow intravenous infusion over not less than one hour, 600 mg twice or thrice daily in 250 ml of Sodium Chloride Intravenous Infusion or Dextrose Intravenous Infusion 5%. Higher doses have been given in very severe infections. Children over the age of 1 month may be given 30 to 60 mg per kg body-weight daily in divided doses by mouth or 10 to 20 mg per kg daily in divided doses by intramuscular injection or intravenous infusion.

Lincomycin blocked the formation of lithocholic acid in *monkeys* given chenodeoxycholic acid and prevented the development of hepatic lesions.— G. Salen *et al.* (letter), *Lancet*, 1975, *1*, 1082.

Actinomycosis. For a report of the successful treatment of actinomycosis with lincomycin in 4 patients hypersensitive to penicillin, see J. A. Mohr *et al.*, *J. Am. med. Ass.*, 1970, *212*, 2260.

Dosage in hepatic failure. The mean serum half-life for lincomycin was 8.96 hours (range 6.11-11.8 hours) in 9 patients with hepatic insufficiency, but normal renal function, given 600 mg intramuscularly compared with 4.85 hours (range 4.45 to 5.67 hours) in 6 controls with normal hepatic and renal functions. Doses may need to be reduced in patients with liver disease.— H. M. Bellamy *et al.*, *Antimicrob. Ag. Chemother.*, 1966, 36.

Dosage in renal failure. In patients with oliguria, intervals between doses of lincomycin should be increased to every 12 hours.— C. M. Kunin, *Ann. intern. Med.*, 1967, *67*, 151.

The normal half-life for lincomcyin of 4 to 5 hours was increased to 10 hours in end-stage renal failure. The interval between doses should be extended from 6 hours to 12 hours in those with a glomerular filtration-rate (GFR) of 10 to 50 ml per minute, and to 24 hours in those with a GFR of less than 10 ml per minute. Concentrations of lincomycin were not affected by haemodialysis or peritoneal dialysis.— W. M. Bennett *et al.*, *Ann. intern. Med.*, 1977, *86*, 754. See also *idem*, 1980, *93*, 62.

Further references: T. P. Gibson and H. A. Nelson, *Clin. Pharmacokinet.*, 1977, *2*, 403; P. Sharpstone, *Br. med. J.*, 1977, *2*, 36; G. B. Appel and H. C. Neu, *New Engl. J. Med.*, 1977, *296*, 663.

Endocarditis. A 43-year-old woman with endocarditis due to *Coxiella burnetii* was successfully treated with lincomycin, 1.5 g six-hourly, with tetracycline, 2 g daily, added after 2 weeks. This therapy was maintained for more than 14 months with satisfactory improvement in her condition.— W. P. G. Turck and M. B. Matthews (letter), *Br. med. J.*, 1969, *1*, 185. Lincomycin, in association with tetracycline, seemed more effective than tetracycline alone in controlling Q fever endocarditis.— W. P. G. Turck (letter), *Br. med. J.*, 1978, *1*, 1052.

Meningitis. Intrathecal administration of lincomycin to 15 patients with meningitis gave good to excellent results in 13 patients. From previous studies in *dogs* the optimum intrathecal dose was determined as 1 to 2 mg daily.— Y. Miyazaki, *Arzneimittel-Forsch.*, 1973, *23*, 940.

Osteomyelitis. An excellent bacteriological and clinical response occurred in 25 patients with osteomyelitis who were treated for a prolonged period with lincomycin, 500 mg six-hourly.— N. L. McMillan *et al.*, *Practitioner*, 1967, *198*, 390. A similar report.— S. I. Hnatko, *Can. med. Ass. J.*, 1967, *97*, 580.

Skin infections. *Topical use.* Reference to the use of a 5% solution of lincomycin in isopropyl alcohol or alcohol for the topical treatment of acne.— B. W. Lee (letter), *Archs Derm.*, 1978, *114*, 1551.

Surgical infection prophylaxis. Although lincomycin has been used successfully for prophylaxis, sometimes with tobramycin (R.B. Galland *et al.*, *Lancet*, 1977, *2*, 1043), in patients undergoing colorectal surgery, fatal pseudomembranous colitis had been associated with such a regimen. Metronidazole with gentamicin might prove the most effective regimen for systemic prophylaxis in colorectal surgery.— Keighley M.R.B. *et al.*, *J. antimicrob. Chemother.*, 1978, *4*, *Suppl.* C, 33.

Preparations

Lincomycin Capsules *(B.P.)*. Capsules containing lincomycin hydrochloride. Potency is expressed in terms of the equivalent amount of lincomycin. Store at a temperature not exceeding 30°.

Lincomycin Hydrochloride Capsules *(U.S.P.)*. Capsules containing lincomycin hydrochloride equivalent to 250 or 500 mg of lincomycin. Store in airtight containers.

Lincomycin Hydrochloride Syrup *(U.S.P.)*. Contains lincomycin hydrochloride with one or more suitable preservatives, colouring, flavouring, and sweetening agents. pH 3 to 5.5. It contains the equivalent of 25 or 50 mg of lincomycin per ml. Store in airtight containers.

Lincomycin Injection *(B.P.)*. A sterile solution of lincomycin hydrochloride in Water for Injections. pH 3 to 5.5. Sterilised by filtration. Potency is expressed in terms of the equivalent amount of lincomycin. Store at a temperature not exceeding 30°. Protect from light. Under these conditions it may be expected to retain its potency for not less than 5 years. *U.S.P.* (Lincomycin Hydrochloride Injection) specifies the equivalent of 300 mg of lincomycin per ml, with benzyl alcohol as a preservative.

Proprietary Preparations

Lincocin *(Upjohn, UK)*. Lincomycin hydrochloride, available as 2-ml **Ampoules** of an injection containing the equivalent of 300 mg of lincomycin per ml; as **Capsules** each containing the equivalent of 500 mg of lincomycin; and as **Syrup** containing the equivalent of 250 mg of lincomycin in each 5 ml (suggested diluent, syrup). (Also available as Lincocin in *Austral., Belg., Canad., Denm., Ital., Neth., Norw., S.Afr., Spain, Switz., USA*).

Mycivin *(Boots, UK)*. Lincomycin hydrochloride, available as 2-ml ampoules of an injection containing the equivalent of 300 mg of lincomycin per ml.

Other Proprietary Names

Albiotic *(Ger., Ind.)*; Cillimicina *(Ital., Spain)*; Cillimycin *(Ger., Norw.)*; Frademicina *(Arg.)*; Lincocine *(Fr.)*.

99-a

Lividomycin. Lividomycin A. 4-*O*-(2-Amino-2,3-dideoxy-α-D-*ribo*-hexopyranosyl)-2-deoxy-5-*O*-[3-*O*-(4-*O*-α-D-mannopyranosyl-2,6-diamino-2,6-dideoxy-β-L-idopyranosyl)-β-D-ribofuranosyl]-D-streptamine.
$C_{29}H_{55}N_5O_{18}$=761.8.

CAS — 36441-41-5.

An antimicrobial substance produced by the growth of *Streptomyces lividus*.

A white amorphous odourless powder with a bitter taste. **Soluble** in water and methyl alcohol. Solutions are stable at neutral or alkaline pH.

Lividomycin is an aminoglycoside antibiotic with actions and uses similar to those of kanamycin (see p.1175), although it has some activity against *Pseudomonas aeruginosa*. It has been given, sometimes as the sulphate, in a dose of 1 g daily by intramuscular injection.

The activity of lividomycin against *Ps. aeruginosa* and its inactivation by phosphorylation induced by resistant strains.— F. Kobayashi *et al.*, *Antimicrob. Ag. Chemother.*, 1972, *1*, 17.

A report of transferable resistance of *Escherichia coli* to lividomycin.— M. Yamaguchi *et al.*, *Antimicrob. Ag. Chemother.*, 1972, *1*, 139. See also *idem*, *2*, 142.

Further references: C. Vitali *et al.*, *Annali Sclavo*, 1973, *15*, 329.

Absorption and fate. A mean peak serum concentration of 13.2 µg per ml was achieved one hour after the intramuscular injection of lividomycin 350 mg in 8 healthy subjects. The serum half-life was about 2 hours; 63% of the dose was excreted in the urine within 6 hours and

82% within 24 hours. The half-life was about 8 hours in 12 patients with a creatinine-clearance rate [CCR] of 20 to 80 ml per minute, 18 hours in 8 patients with a CCR of 5 to 20 ml per minute, and 40 hours in 20 patients with a CCR of less than 5 ml per minute. Corresponding percentages of the dose recovered in the urine within 24 hours were about 64, 36, and 0% respectively. The serum half-life was about 7 hours in 12 patients during an 8-hour haemodialysis session. It was suggested that for uraemic patients the normal dose should be given at intervals equal to 3 times the serum half-life or a normal dose should be given, followed every 12 hours by a sustaining dose related to the CCR.— A. Leroy *et al.*, *J. antimicrob. Chemother.*, 1976, *2*, 373. See also G. Humbert *et al.*, *Curr. ther. Res.*, 1974, *16*, 232.

Tuberculosis, pulmonary. A preliminary study of lividomycin given intramuscularly in a dose of 1 g thrice weekly with a daily regimen of aminosalicylic acid and isoniazid to 7 patients with untreated cavity pulmonary tuberculosis. All 7 became sputum-negative within 3 months.— M. Tsukamura, *Tubercle*, 1972, *53*, 43.

Urinary-tract infections. Lividomycin 1 g daily by intramuscular injection for 3 days, was as effective as kanamycin in acute cystitis, and when given for 7 days was as effective as kanamycin in acute pyelonephritis or urinary-tract infection following prostatectomy.— J. Kumazawa and S. Momose, *Curr. ther. Res.*, 1973, *15*, 873.

Proprietary Names

Livaline (sulphate) *(Bellon, Fr.)*.

100-a

Lymecycline *(B.P.)*.

Limeciclina; Tetracycline-L-methylenelysine. A water-soluble combination of tetracycline, lysine, and formaldehyde with a molecular weight of approximately 603.

CAS — 992-21-2.

Pharmacopoeias. In *Br.* and *It.*

A yellow very hygroscopic powder which darkens an exposure to light and air and contains not more than 5% w/w of water. It contains not less than 900 units per mg of anhydrous lymecycline. Lymecycline 204 mg is approximately equivalent to 150 mg of tetracycline and to 162 mg of tetracycline hydrochloride. **Soluble** 1 in less than 1 of water; slightly soluble in alcohol and methyl alcohol; practically insoluble in acetone, chloroform, and ether. A solution in water is laevorotatory. A 1% solution in water has a pH of 7.8 to 8.1. It is inactivated in solutions of pH less than 2 and is slowly destroyed at pH 7 or above. **Store** at a temperature not exceeding 25° in airtight containers. If it is intended for injection the containers should be sterile and sealed to exclude micro-organisms. **Protect** from light.

When stored in a cool place, capsules of lymecycline and lymecycline for the preparation of intramuscular injections may be expected to retain their potency for 18 and 16 months respectively.— H. L. Clarke, *Carlo Erba, Personal Communication*, 1971.

Accelerated degradation studies showed that the loss of potency of lymecycline powder stored in ampoules at −20° would be less than 1% over 10 years.— J. W. Lightbown *et al.*, *Bull. Wld Hlth Org.*, 1972, *47*, 343.

Units. One unit of lymecycline is contained in 0.0010548 mg of the second International Reference Preparation (1971) which contains 948 units per mg.

Adverse Effects and Precautions. As for Tetracycline Hydrochloride, p.1217.

Gastro-intestinal side-effects have been reported to be less with lymecycline than with tetracycline.

Absorption and Fate. As for Tetracycline Hydrochloride, p.1219.

Lymecycline is more readily absorbed from the gastro-intestinal tract than is tetracycline and similar blood concentrations are achieved with smaller doses. When the dose is doubled an almost correspondingly higher blood concentration has been reported to occur.

When lymecycline was given to 8 healthy subjects in a dose either of 150 mg four times daily or 300 mg twice daily, for 3 days, adequate blood concentrations were attained. Values ranged from 0.72 to 2.75 μg per ml, calculated as tetracycline, at various times from 2 to 50 hours after commencing treatment with the first regimen to 1.9 to 2.55 μg per ml for the second. Fasting did not greatly affect the blood concentrations.— L. Vitartali and A. Pisani-Ceretti (letter), *Lancet*, 1968, *1*, 923.

A mean concentration of 1.4 μg of lymecycline per ml was achieved in sinus secretions 3 to 5 hours after 300 mg was taken by 15 patients on twice-daily dosage.— K. Lundin and J. -E. Brorson (letter), *J. antimicrob. Chemother.*, 1978, *4*, 187.

Uses. Lymecycline has antimicrobial activity and uses similar to those of tetracycline hydrochloride (see p.1218). It is more completely absorbed than tetracycline hydrochloride when taken by mouth and smaller doses may be employed.

The usual adult dose is the equivalent of 600 mg of tetracycline base by mouth daily in 2 or 4 divided doses; in severe infections doses of up to 1.2 g may be given over 24 hours. Children have been given the equivalent of 9 to 27 mg of tetracycline per kg body-weight over 24 hours although the effect of tetracyclines on teeth should be considered. By intramuscular injection, the equivalent of 100 mg of tetracycline base has been given to adults up to 4 times daily.

For reports on the use of lymecycline, see Martindale 27th Edn, p. 1149.

Preparations

Lymecycline and Procaine Injection *(B.P.)*. A sterile solution of lymecycline and procaine hydrochloride, with tartaric acid and magnesium ascorbate, in Water for Injections, prepared by dissolving a dry powder, containing lymecycline, tartaric acid, and magnesium ascorbate, in a solution of procaine hydrochloride and tartaric acid immediately before use. pH 2.6 to 3. The dry powder and solvent should be stored at a temperature not exceeding 25° and protected from light; the injection decomposes and should be used immediately after preparation. For intramuscular use only.

Lymecycline Capsules *(B.P.)*. Capsules containing lymecycline. Store at a temperature not exceeding 30°.

Tetralysal *(Farmitalia Carlo Erba, UK)*. Lymecycline, available as capsules of 204 mg. (Also available as Tetralysal in *Belg., Denm., Fr., Ital., Norw., S.Afr., Swed.*).

Other Proprietary Names

Arg.—Ciclolysal, Tancilina; *Ital.*—Ciclisin, Lisinbiotic, Lisinciclina, Tralisin.

101-t

Lysostaphin. An antibiotic derived from the growth of *Staphylococcus staphylolyticus*, with a mol. wt between 20 000 and 30 000 and an isoelectric point of about pH 11.

CAS — 9011-93-2.

Lysostaphin is highly active *in vitro* against staphylococci and causes rapid lysis of the cell wall of the organism. Antigenicity may be a problem.

Methicillin-resistant *Staphylococcus aureus* appeared to be eradicated from pustules in a patient with leukaemia after an intravenous injection of lysostaphin 500 mg. However long-term follow-up was prevented by the patient's death from daunorubicin-induced heart failure.— F. R. Stark *et al.*, *New Engl. J. Med.*, 1974, *291*, 239.

Manufacturers

Mead Johnson, USA.

102-x

Mecillinam.

FL 1060; Ro 10-9070; Amdinocillin. (6*R*)-6-(Perhydroazepin-1-ylmethyleneamino)penicillanic acid.

$C_{15}H_{23}N_3O_3S = 325.4$.

CAS — 32887-01-7.

A white crystalline powder. M.p. 141° to 143°. **Soluble** 1 in 1.7 of water and 1 in 40 of alcohol (99% v/v). Slightly soluble in acetone and very slightly soluble in ether and isopropyl alcohol. A 10% solution has a pH of 4 to 6.2.

Stability in solution. A recommendation that aqueous preparations of mecillinam should be reconstituted immediately before use. For optimum stability the pH should be maintained at 4.5 to 6.— C. Larsen and H. Bundgaard, *Arch. Pharm. Chemi, scient. Edn*, 1977, *5*, 66.

Adverse Effects and Precautions. Hypersensitivity reactions may occur (see Benzylpenicillin, p.1103). Mecillinam should not be given to patients who are sensitive to penicillins or cephalosporins and should be used with caution in those with known histories of allergies.

Reduced doses may be necessary in patients with impaired renal function.

Antimicrobial Action. Mecillinam is a derivative of amidinopenicillanic acid which, unlike benzylpenicillin and related antibiotics, is very active against a wide range of Gram-negative bacteria including most of the Enterobacteriaceae. Ampicillin-resistant strains of *Escherichia coli* and *Klebsiella* spp. may be very sensitive. *Pseudomonas aeruginosa, Haemophilus influenzae*, and *Bacteroides* spp. are considered to be resistant. It is much less active against Gram-positive bacteria; *Streptococcus faecalis* is resistant.

Mecillinam interferes with the synthesis of the bacterial cell wall although not in the same manner as benzylpenicillin.

Synergism against Gram-negative organisms has been reported *in vitro* between mecillinam and the penicillins or cephalosporins, probably as a result of their differing modes of action.

A review of the antimicrobial activity of mecillinam.— D. S. Reeves, *J. antimicrob. Chemother.*, 1977, *3*, *Suppl.* B, 5.

For a study of the mechanism of action of mecillinam, see B. G. Spratt, *J. antimicrob. Chemother.*, 1977, *3*, *Suppl.* B, 13.

Mecillinam was more active than ampicillin, chloramphenicol or trimethoprim *in vitro* against 34 strains of the *Shigella* and *Salmonella* spp., and more active than ampicillin, cephaloridine, or cephalexin against 59 strains of *Escherichia coli*, 60 of *Proteus mirabilis* and 67 strains of the *Klebsiella* spp. The majority of 360 strains of enterobacteria examined were inhibited by mecillinam 2 μg or less per ml but strains of *Staphylococcus aureus, Haemophilus influenzae*, and *Pseudomonas aeruginosa* were inhibited only at high concentrations.— J. D. Williams *et al.*, *J. antimicrob. Chemother.*, 1976, *2*, 61.

Mecillinam inhibited 5, 33, 44, 53, 74, 89, and all of 92 strains of *Neisseria gonorrhoeae in vitro* at an MIC of 0.25, 0.5, 1, 2, 4, 8, and 16 μg per ml respectively.— B. A. Watts *et al.*, *J. antimicrob. Chemother.*, 1977, *3*, 331.

In a study *in vitro* beta-lactamases from Gram-negative bacteria had relatively low activity against mecillinam. Mecillinam exhibited good penetrative properties and might have substantial activity against ampicillin-resistant strains of *E. coli*.— M. H. Richmond, *J. antimicrob. Chemother.*, 1977, *3*, *Suppl.* B, 29.

Mecillinam was less active than benzylpenicillin against 115 isolates of Gram-positive bacteria *in vitro* but was generally more active against strains of *E. coli* and the *Klebsiella, Enterobacter, Citrobacter, Shigella*, and *Salmonella* spp. Strains of *Serratia*, indole-positive *Proteus*, the *Acinetobacter* spp., *H. influenzae*, and the *Bacteroides* spp., were generally resistant to mecillinam or had high MICs.— H. C. Neu, *J. antimicrob. Chemother.*, 1977, *3*, *Suppl.* B, 43.

Mecillinam hydrochloride inhibited the majority of strains of *E. coli, Kleb. aerogenes, Serratia marcescens, Pr. mirabilis*, and *Pr. vulgaris in vitro* at a concentration of 10 μg or less per ml but strains of *Pr. morgani* and *Pr. rettgeri* were more resistant. Resistance to mecillinam did not appear to be due to inactivation by beta-lactamases.— D. W. Kerry *et al.*, *J. antimicrob. Chemother.*, 1977, *3*, *Suppl.* B, 53.

Mecillinam appeared to be no more active *in vitro* than carbenicillin or cephaloridine against *E. coli, Proteus*, or *Klebsiella* spp. Mecillinam was also susceptible to beta-lactamase. However, its action on the bacterial cell wall might be complementary to that of other beta-lactam antibiotics and combinations might show enhanced activity.— M. Bakhtiar and S. Selwyn (letter), *Lancet*,

1978, *1*, 337.

Mecillinam was more active than amoxycillin *in vitro* against *E. coli* and *Klebsiella* spp. It was less effective against *Proteus* spp.— Z. Hassam (letter), *Lancet*, 1978, *1*, 445.

Further references: L. Tybring, *Antimicrob. Ag. Chemother.*, 1975, *8*, 266; L. Tybring and N. H. Melchior, *ibid.*, 271; H. C. Neu, *ibid.*, 1976, *9*, 793; G. E. Steinkraus and L. R. McCarthy, *ibid.*, 1980, *17*, 954.

Enhanced activity. Mecillinam showed enhanced activity with beta-lactam antibiotics but not with the aminoglycosides, chloramphenicol, polymyxin B, or tetracycline.— H. C. Neu, *Antimicrob. Ag. Chemother.*, 1976, *10*, 535. There was no synergy against Gram-positive cocci.— *idem*, *J. antimicrob. Chemother.*, 1977, *3*, *Suppl.* B, 43.

For a discussion on synergy and mecillinam, see J. Gray, *J. antimicrob. Chemother.*, 1977, *3*, 531. See also R. Wise, *ibid.*, 1979, *5*, 121.

Reports of enhanced activity with mecillinam and other antibiotics: E. Grunberg and R. Cleeland, *J. antimicrob. Chemother.*, 1977, *3*, *Suppl.* B, 59 (with cephazolin against *Klebsiella pneumoniae* in *mice*); D. W. Kerry *et al.*, *J. antimicrob. Chemother.*, 1977, *3*, *Suppl.* B, 53 (with cephradine against *Proteus* spp., *Providencia stuartii*, and *Serratia marcescens*); B. Chattopadhyay and I. Hall, *J. antimicrob. Chemother.*, 1979, *5*, 549 (with cephradine or amoxycillin against multi-resistant Gram-negative bacteria); W. M. Scheld *et al.*, *Antimicrob. Ag. Chemother.*, 1979, *16*, 271 (with ampicillin against *E. coli* and *Kleb. pneumoniae*); I. Trestman *et al.*, *Antimicrob. Ag. Chemother.*, 1979, *16*, 283 (with carbenicillin against *Bacteroides* spp.); R. Hone and M. Foley (letter), *J. antimicrob. Chemother.*, 1980, *6*, 410 (with ampicillin against *Proteus* spp.).

Resistance. Mecillinam resistance among urinary Enterobacteriaceae was less common than ampicillin or amoxycillin resistance. Also ampicillin-resistant or amoxycillin-resistant organisms were often sensitive to mecillinam but mecillinam-resistant organisms were not usually sensitive to these antibiotics or cephaloridine. Therapy with pivmecillinam had only a transient effect on aerobic faecal flora.— J. D. Anderson *et al.*, *Antimicrob. Ag. Chemother.*, 1976, *10*, 872.

A study *in vitro* in Enterobacteriaceae suggested that mecillinam-resistant organisms did not appear in the urinary tract during therapy with mecillinam because they had a slow growth-rate compared with mecillinam-susceptible organisms and were cleared by the flushing effect of the bladder.— J. D. Anderson *et al.*, *Antimicrob. Ag. Chemother.*, 1977, *12*, 559.

A review of the resistance of bacteria to mecillinam concluded that although cross-resistance between mecillinam and ampicillin was minimal, close monitoring of various regimens was required since resistance had developed during the prolonged treatment of salmonellal infections.— J. D. Anderson, *J. antimicrob. Chemother.*, 1977, *3*, *Suppl.* B, 89.

In a study *in vitro* in urine, resistance of strains of the *Klebsiella* and *Proteus* spp., to mecillinam was associated with increasing pH of the medium.— R. Wise *et al.*, *J. antimicrob. Chemother.*, 1977, *3*, *Suppl.* B, 113.

Absorption and Fate. Mecillinam is poorly absorbed from the gastro-intestinal tract. Peak plasma concentrations of about 6 and 12 µg per ml have been achieved half an hour after intramuscular doses of 200 and 400 mg, respectively. A plasma half-life of 1.2 hours has been reported. Between 5 and 25% of mecillinam is reported to be bound to plasma proteins. It diffuses across the placenta and has been detected in amniotic fluid. From 50 to 60% of a parenteral dose may be excreted in the urine within 6 hours and renal tubular secretion can be reduced by the concomitant use of probenecid. High concentrations are achieved in bile.

A mean peak serum concentration of 4.7 µg per ml occurred 0.43 hours after an intramuscular injection of mecillinam 273 mg given to 6 healthy subjects. The half-life was 0.97 hours.— J. D. Williams *et al.*, *J. antimicrob. Chemother.*, 1976, *2*, 61.

After the intravenous injection of mecillinam 200 or 400 mg in 9 healthy subjects, mean peak serum concentrations were about 12 and 28 µg per ml respectively, rapidly falling to less than 1 µg per ml after 2 hours. Intramuscular injection of 200 or 400 mg gave peak serum concentrations of 6 or 13 µg per ml after about 30 minutes. From 50 to 60% of a dose was excreted in the urine, mainly within 6 hours, regardless of the route of injection.— K. Roholt, *J. antimicrob. Chemother.*, 1977, *3*, *Suppl.* B, 71.

After receiving mecillinam 200 mg intravenously in 2 ml of Water for Injections, serum concentrations in 6 healthy subjects ranged from 5.7 to 9 µg per ml and had dropped to about 2 µg per ml within 1 hour of administration and to 0.8 µg per ml after 2 hours. The mean half-life of the beta-phase of elimination was about 0.8 hours.— M. Mitchard *et al.*, *J. antimicrob. Chemother.*, 1977, *3*, *Suppl.* B, 83.

Uses. Mecillinam has the same penicillanic acid nucleus as the penicillins and a substituted amidino group has been introduced at the 6-position. It is given by intravenous injection over 3 to 4 minutes, by intravenous infusion over 15 to 30 minutes, or intramuscularly in the treatment of severe Gram-negative infections, including those caused by *Salmonella typhi* and *S. paratyphi A*. For urinary-tract infections a dose of 5 mg per kg body-weight may be given every 6 to 8 hours and in severe infections 10 mg per kg may be given 6-hourly. A suggested dose in the treatment of enteric fever is 12.5 to 15 mg per kg every 6 hours; probenecid may be taken concomitantly to delay the excretion of mecillinam.

For the oral use of mecillinam as its pivaloyloxymethyl ester, see Pivmecillinam p.1204.

Mecillinam hydrochloride dihydrate ($C_{15}H_{23}N_3O_3S$, $HCl,2H_2O$=397.9) is used *in vitro* as a reference standard.

Brief reviews.— *Lancet*, 1976, *2*, 503; *ibid.*, 1978, *1*, 252 and 337; *Drug & Ther. Bull.*, 1978, *16*, 103.

The proceedings of a symposium on mecillinam.— *J. antimicrob. Chemother.*, 1977, *3*, *Suppl.* B, 1-160.

Dosage in renal failure. The use of mecillinam in patients on haemodialysis.— K. Bailey *et al.* (letter), *Br. J. clin. Pharmac.*, 1980, *10*, 177.

Further references: P. L. Svarva and T. Wessel-Aas, *Scand. J. infect. Dis.*, 1980, *12*, 303 (mecillinam for urinary-tract infections in patients with severe renal insufficiency).

Salmonellal infections. The successful use of mecillinam in 7 of 9 patients with typhoid or paratyphoid fever. Treatment was continued for 14 days with a dose of 400 mg every 6 hours apart from 2 children of 8 years given 200 mg and one adult given 600 mg.— P. D. Clarke *et al.*, *Br. med. J.*, 1976, *2*, 14. See also A. M. Geddes and P. D. Clarke, *J. antimicrob. Chemother.*, 1977, *3*, *Suppl.* B, 101.

Mention of the use of mecillinam with ampicillin in the treatment of endocarditis due to *Salmonella enteritidis*.— Shanson D.C. *et al.*, *Br. med. J.*, 1977, *1*, 612.

In 18 patients who were faecal excreters of salmonella six 14-day courses of pivmecillinam 1.2 g daily failed to eliminate the organisms from the stools and 16 courses of mecillinam 0.555 to 1.48 g daily eliminated the organisms from only 5 patients.— F. J. Nye and C. Roberts (letter), *Br. med. J.*, 1978, *2*, 1502.

Of 12 patients with enteric fever (8 typhoid fever, 4 paratyphoid fever) treated generally with mecillinam intramuscularly then pivmecillinam by mouth, only 3 became afebrile within 2 to 5 days, while a further four became afebrile in 6 to 8 days. The organisms were all sensitive. Mecillinam was not a highly effective or consistent treatment.— B. K. Mandal *et al.*, *Br. med. J.*, 1979, *1*, 586.

The use of mecillinam with amoxycillin appeared to offer no advantage over conventional therapy in the treatment of enteric fever.— M. W. McKendrick and A. M. Geddes (letter), *J. antimicrob. Chemother.*, 1979, *5*, 727.

Urinary-tract infections. Eight of 16 patients with urinary-tract infections were treated successfully with mecillinam 40 mg per Kg body-weight daily given intravenously or intramuscularly.— N. Frimodt-Møller and T. J. Ravn, *Infection*, 1979, *7*, 35.

Proprietary Preparations

Selexidin *(Leo, UK)*. Mecillinam, available as powder for preparing injections, in vials of 200 and 400 mg.

NOTE. The name Selexidin is also used as a proprietary name for Pivmecillinam Hydrochloride, p.1204.

Other Proprietary Names

Selexid (see also Pivmecillinam) *(Denm., Neth.)*.

103-r

Meclocycline Sulfosalicylate *(U.S.P.)*. GS-2989 (meclocycline); Meclocycline Sulphosalicylate. 7-Chloro-6-demethyl-6-deoxy-5β-hydroxy-6-methylenetetracycline 5-sulphosalicylate.
$C_{22}H_{21}ClN_2O_8,C_7H_6O_6S$=695.0.

CAS — 2013-58-3 (meclocycline); 73816-42-9 (sulfosalicylate).

Pharmacopoeias. In *U.S.*

Meclocycline is a tetracycline antibiotic closely related to chlortetracycline (see p.1142). It is applied topically as meclocycline sulfosalicylate.

Dermatological use.— A. Schimpf *et al.*, *Arzneimittel-Forsch.*, 1972, *22*, 1019; M. Schoog *et al.*, *ibid.*, 1022.

Preparations

Meclocycline Sulfosalicylate Cream *(U.S.P.)*. A cream containing meclocycline sulfosalicylate. Potency is expressed in terms of the equivalent amount of meclocycline. Store in airtight containers and protect from light.

Proprietary Names

Meclan *(Ortho, USA)*; Mecloderm *(Ist. Chem. Ital., Ital.)*; Meclutin Semplice *(ABC, Ital.)*; Traumatociclina *(Biomedica Foscama, Ital.)*.

185-c

Metampicillin. (6*R*)-6-(D-2-Methyleneamino-2-phenylacetamido)penicillanic acid.
$C_{17}H_{19}N_3O_4S$=361.4.

CAS — 6489-97-0.

104-f

Metampicillin Sodium. The sodium salt of metampicillin.
$C_{17}H_{18}N_3NaO_4S$=383.4.

CAS — 6489-61-8.

Metampicillin sodium 1.06 g is approximately equivalent to 1 g of metampicillin. Each g represents about 2.6 mmol (2.6 mEq) of sodium.

Metampicillin is used similarly to ampicillin in doses of 500 mg four times daily. It is hydrolysed *in vivo* to ampicillin but has some antimicrobial activity of its own. The sodium salt has been given by injection and high biliary concentrations of antibiotic have been achieved following intravenous administration.

Clinical reports.— F. Rosaschino *et al.*, *G. Mal. infett. parassit.*, 1968, *20*, 1013; G. Ginocchi and C. Radice, *Minerva med., Roma*, 1969, *60*, 5244; G. Farina and S. Zedda, *ibid.*, 1971, *62*, 1174.

Metampicillin was less active than ampicillin in serum. From studies in healthy subjects, metampicillin was found to be completely hydrolysed to ampicillin after oral administration whereas after intramuscular injection metampicillin was detected in the blood as well as ampicillin.— R. Sutherland *et al.*, *Chemotherapy, Basle*, 1972, *17*, 145.

In a study involving 35 cholecystectomised patients and 10 healthy subjects, total biliary excretion of metampicillin in the cholecystectomised patients was 8.3% of a 500-mg intravenous dose compared with 0.19% of a dose of carbenicillin 1 g intramuscularly and 0.1% of a dose of ampicillin 500 mg given by mouth or intravenously. When metampicillin was given by mouth only 0.16% of a 500-mg dose was excreted in the bile. In the healthy subjects 5.8% of the dose of metampicillin given intravenously was recovered in the duodenal juice compared with 0.04% and 0.11% after intravenous doses of ampicillin and carbenicillin respectively. Antibiotic activity in patients given metampicillin was assayed in terms of ampicillin because of its partial hydrolysis to ampicillin.— M. Pinget *et al.*, *J. antimicrob. Chemother.*, 1976, *2*, 195. See also J. M. Brogard *et al.*, *ibid.*, 363.

Proprietary Names of Metampicillin

Ampimetacil, Baldacilina, Cetinmicina, Darkepen, Demetilina, Doctamicina Oral, Italcina, Metalcor, Metampikel, Metanova, Metaval, Neo-Togram, Suvipen, Tablebiotin, Totalbiotico *(all Spain)*; Magnipen *(Midy, Fr.)*.

Proprietary Names of Metampicillin Sodium

Actuapen, Ampilprats, Ampliopenil, Co-Metampicil, Daniven, Doctamicina Inyec., Dompil, Durmetan, Fedacilina, Janopen, Lermetan, Madecilina, Maipen, Marcomycina, Mempil, Meta-Alvar, Meta-Espectral, Meta-Ferran, Meta-Framan, Metabacter, Metabiot,

Metacidan, Metaclarben, Metakes, Metam-Piror, Metamas, Metambac, Metampen, Metampicef, Metampilene, Metamplimedix, Metapenyl, Metiskia, Micinovo, Penapli, Pirobiotic, Pluriespec, Pramet, Soifamet, Tampilen, Tisquibron, Venzoquimpe, Viderpen, Vigocina (all *Spain*); Magnipen (*Midy, Fr.*; *Midy, Ital.*); Ocelina (*Roux-Ocefa, Arg.*); Suvipen (*Spedrog-Caillon, Arg.*).

105-d

Methacycline Hydrochloride (*U.S.P., B.P. 1973*).

GS 2876; Metacycline Hydrochloride; Metacyclini Chloridum; Méthylènecycline Hydrochloride; 6-Methyleneoxytetracycline Hydrochloride. 6-Demethyl-6-deoxy-5β-hydroxy-6-methylenetetracycline hydrochloride.

$C_{22}H_{22}N_2O_8$, HCl=478.9.

CAS — 914-00-1 (methacycline); 3963-95-9 (hydrochloride).

Pharmacopoeias. In *Nord.* and *U.S.*

A yellow odourless crystalline powder with a bitter taste, containing not less than 832 µg of methacycline per mg. M.p. about 240°. **Soluble** 1 in 65 to 100 of water, 1 in 80 to 300 of alcohol, and 1 in 30 of methyl alcohol; practically insoluble in chloroform and ether; soluble in dilute solutions of sodium hydroxide. A 1% solution in water has a pH of 2 to 3. **Store** in airtight containers. Protect from light.

Units. One unit of methacycline is contained in 0.001082 mg of the first International Reference Preparation (1969) of methacycline hydrochloride which contains 924 units per mg.

Adverse Effects and Precautions. As for Tetracycline Hydrochloride, p.1217.

A report of pigment deposits in the eyes and skin exposed to the light during prolonged treatment with methacycline.— K. Dyster-Aas *et al.*, *Acta derm.-vener., Stockh.*, 1974, *54*, 209.

Absorption and Fate. As for Tetracycline Hydrochloride, p.1219.

Methacycline hydrochloride is absorbed from the gastro-intestinal tract and about 80 to 90% in the circulation is bound to plasma proteins. Similarly to demeclocycline, plasma concentrations of up to 2.6 µg per ml have been reported 4 hours after a 300-mg dose. About 50% of a dose is slowly excreted unchanged in the urine.

Some 78 to 90% of methacycline was bound in the body to serum proteins. The biological half-life in serum was 14.3 hours and 60% was excreted in urine.— C. M. Kunin, *Ann. intern. Med.*, 1967, *67*, 151.

The administration of methacycline hydrochloride 300 mg every 12 hours to 9 healthy subjects resulted in mean serum concentrations of about 0.9 µg per ml after 2 hours, falling to 0.4 µg after 12 hours, rising and maintained between 1 and 2 µg after the first 24 hours' treatment. About 57 mg of the drug was recovered from the urine during the first 24 hours.— L. P. Olon and D. N. Holvey, *Clin. Med.*, 1968, *75* (Jan.), 33.

The average concentration of methacycline in lung tissue in 5 patients 8 hours after taking methacycline 300 mg was 0.83 µg per g compared with an average serum concentration of 0.64 µg per ml. In another group of 10 patients given 2 doses of 300 mg twenty and eight hours before the assay, the average lung tissue concentration was 0.98 µg per g and the average serum concentration was 1.28 µg per ml.— J. J. Timmes *et al.*, *Clin. Pharmac. Ther.*, 1971, *12*, 920.

Uses. Methacycline hydrochloride is used for the same purposes as tetracycline hydrochloride (see p.1220). It has a range of antimicrobial activity like that of demeclocycline and, similarly, is excreted more slowly than tetracycline, effective blood concentrations being maintained for longer periods.

It is administered by mouth as capsules or as the calcium chelate in a syrup. The usual adult dosage is 600 mg daily in 2 or 4 divided doses, preferably one hour before or 2 hours after meals. Up to 1.2 g daily may be given in severe infections. Children have been given 6.5 to 13 mg per kg body-weight daily but the effect of tetracyclines on teeth should be considered.

For reports on the use of methacycline hydrochloride, see Martindale 27th Edn, p. 1150.

Preparations

Methacycline Capsules (*B.P. 1973*). Capsules containing methacycline hydrochloride.

Methacycline Hydrochloride Capsules (*U.S.P.*). Capsules containing methacycline hydrochloride equivalent to 70, 140, or 280 mg of methacycline. Store in airtight containers. Protect from light.

Methacycline Hydrochloride Oral Suspension (*U.S.P.*). A suspension of methacycline hydrochloride, containing one or more suitable buffers, diluents, preservatives, colouring, dispersing, and flavouring agents. pH 6.5 to 8. It contains the equivalent of 14 mg of methacycline per ml. Store in airtight containers. Protect from light.

Proprietary Preparations

Rondomycin (*Pfizer, UK*). Methacycline hydrochloride, available as capsules of 150 mg. (Also available as Rondomycin in *Austral., Swed., Switz., USA*).

Other Proprietary Names

Belg.—Pluramycine, Rondomycine; *Fr.*—Physiomycine, Rondomycine; *Ital.*—Apriclina, Benciclina, Boscillina, Brevicillina, Ciclobiotic, Ciclum, Duecap, Duplaciclina, Duramicina, Dynamicin, Esarondil, Esquilin, Fitociclina, Franciclina, Francomicina, Gammaciclina, Globociclina, Idrossimicina, Isometa, Largomicina, Medomycin, Metabiotic, Metabioticon B.G., Metac, Metacil, Metaclin, Metaclor, Metadomus, Metagram, Metamicina, Metilenbiotic, Micociclina, Mit-Ciclina, Molciclina, Ossirondil, Paveciclina, Piziacina, Plurigram, Prontomicina, Quickmicina, Radiomicina, Rindex, Rondomicina, Sernamicina, Stafilon, Tachiciclina, Tetrabios, Tiberciclina, Ticomicina, Treis-Ciclina, Valcin, Wassermicina, Yatrociclina, Zermicina; *Spain*—Bialatan; *Switz.*—Optimycin.

NOTE. The name Adriamicina has been applied to methacycline hydrochloride (distinguish from adriamycin, see Doxorubicin, p.205).

106-n

Methicillin Sodium (*U.S.P., B.P. 1973*).

Methicillin Sod.; Meticillinum Natricum; Sodium Methicillin; Dimethoxyphenecillin Sodium; Dimethoxyphenyl Penicillin Sodium. Sodium (6*R*)-6-(2,6-dimethoxybenzamido)penicillanate monohydrate.

$C_{17}H_{19}N_2NaO_6S,H_2O$=420.4.

CAS — 61-32-5 (methicillin); 132-92-3 (sodium salt, anhydrous); 7246-14-2 (sodium salt, monohydrate).

Pharmacopoeias. In *Cz., Int., It., Jug., Nord., Roum., Rus., Turk.*, and *U.S. Jap.* has anhydrous methicillin.

A fine white crystalline powder, odourless or with a slight odour. It absorbs insignificant amounts of moisture up to about 65% relative humidity but significant amounts under damper conditions. Each g represents about 2.4 mmol (2.4 mEq) of sodium. Methicillin sodium 1.11 g is approximately equivalent to 1 g of anhydrous methicillin. The *U.S.P.* specifies not less than the equivalent of 815 µg of methicillin per mg.

Soluble 1 in 0.6 of water and 1 in 35 of alcohol; freely soluble in methyl alcohol and pyridine; slightly soluble in amyl alcohol, chloroform, ethylene chloride, and propyl alcohol; practically insoluble in ether, acetone, fixed oils, and liquid paraffin. A 1% solution in water has a pH of 5 to 7.5. A 6.0% solution is iso-osmotic with serum. Concentrated solutions should not be mixed with other antibiotics. Aqueous solutions of methicillin sodium should be used within 30 minutes of preparation or within 2 days if stored at 2° to 10°. It is unstable at a pH of less than 5 and may form a precipitate.

Store at 15° to 30° in airtight containers; if it is intended for injection, the containers should be sterile and sealed to exclude micro-organisms.

Methicillin sodium required a relative humidity of less than 55% for processing.— D. N. Gore and J. Ashwin, *J. mond. Pharm.*, 1967, (4), 365.

Incompatibility. Particulate matter was observed within 2 hours when 1 ml of commercial methicillin sodium injection was mixed with 5 ml of sterile water and 1 ml of any of the following commercial injection solutions: *levallorphan tartrate, metaraminol tartrate, prochlorperazine edisylate, promethazine hydrochloride*, and *vancomycin hydrochloride*.— R. Misgen, *Am. J. Hosp. Pharm.*, 1965, *22*, 92.

There was loss of clarity when intravenous solutions of methicillin sodium were mixed with those of *narcotic salts*.— J. A. Patel and G. L. Phillips, *Am. J. Hosp. Pharm.*, 1966, *23*, 409.

Methicillin sodium 1 g was observed to be incompatible with *tetracycline hydrochloride* 100 mg in 2 ml of water below pH 2.5, with *oxytetracycline hydrochloride* 100 mg in 2.1 ml of water at pH 2, and with *erythromycin ethylsuccinate* 100 mg in 2 ml of aqueous vehicle at pH 6. It was visually compatible when 1 g was dissolved in a solution of *chloramphenicol sodium succinate* 250 or 400 mg in 1.5 to 2 ml of water or in *lincomycin hydrochloride* 600 mg in 2 ml of an aqueous vehicle containing benzyl alcohol.— B. Lynn, *J. Hosp. Pharm.*, 1970, *28*, 71.

Reports had been received of incompatibility between methicillin sodium more than 3 g per litre and *cephalothin sodium, chloramphenicol sodium succinate*, and *lincomycin hydrochloride*.— E. A. Parker, *Am. J. Hosp. Pharm.*, 1970, *27*, 67.

A haze developed over 3 hours when methicillin sodium 4 g per litre was mixed with *methohexitone sodium* 2 g per litre in dextrose injection, with *amiphenazole hydrochloride* 600 mg per litre, or *chlorpromazine hydrochloride* 200 mg per litre in sodium chloride injection, or with *oxytetracycline hydrochloride* 1 g per litre in dextrose injection or sodium chloride injection. A crystalline precipitate occurred when methicillin sodium was mixed with *sulphadiazine sodium* 4 g per litre in dextrose injection.— B. B. Riley, *J. Hosp. Pharm.*, 1970, *28*, 228.

Methicillin underwent 15 to 20% inactivation in 5 minutes when mixed with *kanamycin* at concentrations used for intramuscular administration, though the solution remained clear.— B. Lynn (letter), *Br. med. J.*, 1971, *1*, 174.

Solutions of methicillin 2% with *hydrocortisone sodium succinate* 0.02% in sodium chloride injection, dextrose injection, or sodium chloride and dextrose injection at 25° failed to maintain a satisfactory degree of potency after 6 hours. A loss of 14 to 17% occurred which was about 3 times that which would have been expected if hydrocortisone sodium succinate had not been present.— B. Lynn, *J. Hosp. Pharm.*, 1971, *29*, 183.

Methicillin was reported to be incompatible with *ascorbic acid, atropine sulphate, canrenoate potassium, hydrocortisone sodium succinate , sulphafurazole diethanolamine, suxamethonium,* and *vitamins of the B group* in an infusion fluid.— B. Flouvat and P. Lechat, *Thérapie*, 1974, *29*, 337.

For a further list of incompatibilities including *adrenaline, aminophylline, calcium chloride, chlortetracycline, codeine, gentamicin, levorphanol, methadone, morphine, neomycin, noradrenaline, novobiocin, pentobarbitone, pethidine, polymyxin B, promazine, protein hydrolysate, sodium bicarbonate, streptomycin, thiopentone sodium,* and *vitamin-B complex*, see *Med. Lett.*, 1972, *14* (Jan.), *Suppl.*, 32.

Colistin sulphomethate sodium lost 30% of its activity 30 minutes after mixing with methicillin sodium at concentrations used for intramuscular administration.— B. Lynn, in *Clinical Use of Combinations of Antibiotics*, J. Klastersky (Ed.), London, Hodder and Stoughton, 1975, p. 24.

Stability. Ultraviolet irradiation for 2 hours had a destructive effect on methicillin sodium.— A. A. Kassem and E. H. Girgis, *Bull. Fac. Pharm., Cairo*, 1970, *9*, 157.

Stability in solution. Solutions of methicillin sodium 4 g in 5.8 ml of water retained 90% potency for about 9 days at 24° and for about 24 days at 5°.— M. H. Stolar *et al.*, *Am. J. Hosp. Pharm.*, 1968, *25*, 32.

Solutions of methicillin sodium 4 g per 500 ml, were stable for 5 hours in injections of sodium chloride, dextrose, sodium chloride and dextrose, sodium lactate, compound sodium lactate, sodium bicarbonate 1.4%, and dextran '40' 10% in sodium chloride or dextrose. Subsequently, considerable loss in potency and precipitation occurred except in sodium lactate and sodium bicarbonate. Inclusion of 10 ml of a mixture of nucleotides and nucleosides (Laevadosin) enhanced the stability of methicillin sodium, 5 g per 500 ml in sodium chloride, dextrose, sodium chloride and dextrose, and compound sodium chloride injections; loss of potency was increased in sodium lactate injection. Solutions of methicillin sodium, 10 g per 500 ml, were stable for 6 hours in Aminosol-Glucose, Aminosol-Fructose-Ethanol, and Aminosol Vitrum at 23°, and a solution containing 1 g per litre in a peritoneal dialysis solution (Dialaflex 62) was stable for up to 3 hours at 37°. A solution for intramuscular injection containing 1 g of methicillin sodium in 1.5 ml of water lost 20% potency in 7 days at 5° and 20% in 2 days at 23°.— B. Lynn, *J. Hosp. Pharm.*, 1970, *28*, 71.

The addition of 0.075% sodium bicarbonate did not exert a marked effect on pH or rate of decomposition of solutions containing methicillin sodium 1 or 10 mg per ml in 10% dextrose; satisfactory potency was retained for 5 to 6 hours. However, addition of 0.075% of sodium carbonate raised the pH to 9.4 to 9.9 and decomposition was accelerated; total inactivation was greater in the more dilute solution.— B. Lynn, *J. Hosp. Pharm.*, 1972, *30*, 81.

A buffered solution of methicillin sodium 10 mg per ml in dextrose injection lost only 5% of its potency in 24 hours at 25°. Solutions of 0.6, 2, 4, and 6 g per 100 ml in 5% Dextrose Injection *U.S.P.* and Sodium Chloride Injection *U.S.P.* retained their potency for at least 2 days at 25°.— J. F. Gallelli *et al.* (letter), *New Engl. J. Med.*, 1972, *287*, 360.

Further references: B. E. Kirschenbaum and C. J. Latiolais, *Am. J. Hosp. Pharm.*, 1976, *33*, 767.

Adverse Effects and Treatment. As for Benzylpenicillin, p.1103.

Interstitial nephritis, thought to be a hypersensitivity reaction, has occurred in patients given methicillin sodium. Blood disorders have occasionally been reported.

Blood disorders. Antiplatelet antibody was present in a woman with acute lymphoblastic leukaemia during a course of methicillin. Thrombocytopenia was subsequently sustained despite multiple platelet transfusions.— C. A. Schiffer *et al.* (letter), *Ann. intern. Med.*, 1976, *85*, 338.

A report of agranulocytosis, haemorrhagic cystitis, and acute interstitial nephritis occurring in a 24-year-old man during methicillin therapy.— M. Godin *et al.* (letter), *J. antimicrob. Chemother.*, 1980, *6*, 296.

Nephrotoxicity. Renal toxicity with fever, rash, eosinophilia, haematuria, and proteinuria occurred in 13 children given methicillin and resolved when methicillin was withdrawn. Kidney biopsy in 1 patient showed interstitial nephritis without any involvement of the glomeruli or blood vessels. Similar nephrotoxicity occurred in 2 patients given cephalothin as a substitute for methicillin indicating cross-sensitivity.— S. A. Sanjad *et al.*, *J. Pediat.*, 1974, *84*, 873.

There was evidence of haemorrhagic cystitis in 6 patients who had received methicillin 12 g per day intravenously for 8 to 21 days; two patients had also received gentamicin. Haematuria occurred in all of the patients and dysuria in 5, but both effects disappeared within 5 days of withdrawing methicillin. The haemorrhagic cystitis resolved after methicillin was replaced by cephalothin or vancomycin.— R. Bracis *et al.*, *Antimicrob. Ag. Chemother.*, 1977, *12*, 438.

For further reports of nephritis associated with the administration of methicillin, see H. A. Jensen *et al.*, *Br. med. J.*, 1971, *4*, 406; R. W. Chesney and P. J. Chesney, *Clin. Pediat.*, 1976, *15*, 1013; L. D. Sarff and G. H. McCracken (letter), *J. Pediat.*, 1977, *90*, 1031; C. M. Nolan and R. S. Abernathy, *Archs intern. Med.*, 1977, *137*, 997; J. Ditlove *et al.*, *Medicine, Baltimore*, 1977, *56*, 483; M. C. Cogan and A. I. Arieff, *Am. J. Med.*, 1978, *64*, 500; J. E. Galpin *et al.*, *Am. J. Med.*, 1978, *65*, 756.

For reference to the increased nephrotoxicity of cephalothin with an aminoglycoside antibiotic compared with methicillin and an aminoglycoside antibiotic, see Cephalothin, p.1129.

Precautions. Methicillin sodium is contra-indicated in patients known to be sensitive to penicillin and it should be given with caution to patients with known histories of allergy. It should be given cautiously to patients with impaired renal function and it has been recommended that infants should be treated cautiously.

In a study of 7 patients with cystic fibrosis and 6 healthy subjects, higher renal clearance-rates appeared to be responsible for lower serum concentrations of methicillin after a single intravenous dose in those with cystic fibrosis. Dosage might have to be increased in such patients.— S. J. Yaffe *et al.*, *J. infect. Dis.*, 1977, *135*, 828.

Sequential administration of intravenous bolus doses of streptomycin 500 mg and methicillin 1 g, over a period of 5 minutes through a subclavian vein catheter, had caused rigors in postoperative coronary bypass patients, within 30 minutes of administration. Administration of the 2 drugs separated by an interval of 4 hours appeared to avoid this.— P. C. Robinson *et al.* (letter), *Lancet*, 1978, *2*, 1056.

Antimicrobial Action. Methicillin sodium has a similar mode of action to that of benzylpenicillin but is bactericidal against both penicillinase-producing and non-penicillinase-producing staphylococci. It is also active against group A β-haemolytic streptococci, *Streptococcus viridans*, and *Str. pneumoniae*. It is virtually ineffective against *Str. faecalis*.

The minimum inhibitory concentration against staphylococci, both penicillin-resistant and non-resistant, is usually within the range of 1 to 4 μg per ml. However, its activity against penicillin-sensitive staphylococci and streptococci is about one-fiftieth of that of benzylpenicillin.

In a study of the susceptibility of the penicillinase-resistant penicillins to penicillinase of *Staphylococcus aureus*, methicillin, cloxacillin, and nafcillin were relatively resistant to penicillinase but flucloxacillin was much less resistant.— R. W. Lacey and A. Stokes, *J. clin. Path.*, 1977, *30*, 35. In a study of the relative stabilities of 5 penicillinase-stable penicillins and 5 cephalosporins to staphylococcal beta-lactamase, methicillin was the most stable, followed in descending order of stability by cloxacillin, dicloxacillin, and flucloxacillin (equal stabilities); oxacillin, cephalothin, cephradine, and cephalexin (equal); and cephazolin and cephaloridine (equal).— M. J. Basker *et al.*, *J. antimicrob. Chemother.*, 1980, *6*, 333.

There was no resistance to methicillin among 200 strains of *Staph. aureus*.— Z. A. Hassam *et al.*, *Br. med. J.*, 1978, *2*, 536.

Methicillin had similar activity against experimental endocarditis in *rabbits* whether produced by a tolerant or a nontolerant strain of *Staph. aureus*.— P. L. Goldman and R. G. Petersdorf, *Antimicrob. Ag. Chemother.*, 1979, *15*, 802.

Resistance. Resistance to methicillin has developed in both penicillinase-and non-penicillinase-producing staphylococci with cross-resistance to other penicillins, including the penicillinase-resistant penicillins, such as cloxacillin, nafcillin, and oxacillin, to the cephalosporins, and to other antibiotics including chloramphenicol, erythromycin, tetracycline, kanamycin, streptomycin, and lincomycin. This resistance is intrinsic and is unrelated to penicillinase production.

From a study of staphylococci isolated by nasal swabbing from 615 personnel in various departments of the plant engaged in the manufacture of methicillin, there was no evidence that long-term intermittent exposure to small amounts of methicillin in the atmosphere led to the development of resistance in coagulase-positive *Staph. aureus*.— K. Casson *et al.*, *Clin. Med.*, 1971, *78* (Feb.), 24.

A strain of *Staph. aureus* resistant to methicillin subcultured repeatedly at 25°, 37°, and 43° became more resistant at the first 2 temperatures but became sensitive at 43°.— S. M. Al Salihy and A. M. James (letter), *Lancet*, 1972, *2*, 331. Strains of *Staph. aureus* lost resistance to methicillin when maintained at room temperature.— W. B. Grubb and D. I. Annear (letter), *ibid.*, 1257; *ibid.*, 1973, *1*, 110.

An epidemiological study in Zurich from 1965 to 1975 of methicillin-resistant *Staph. aureus* showed that there had been a decrease in the number of resistant strains during the last 3 years.— F. H. Kayser, *Lancet*, 1975, *2*, 650.

Further references: E. J. Benner and F. H. Kayser, *Lancet*, 1968, *2*, 741; L. P. Garrod (letter), *ibid.*, 871; L. D. Sabath, *J. antimicrob. Chemother.*, 1977, *3*, *Suppl.* C, 47; W. T. Siebert *et al.*, *Sth. med. J.*, 1978, *71*, 1353; P. Vaudax and F. A. Waldvogel, *J. infect. Dis.*, 1979, *139*, 547; G. L. Archer and M. J. Tenenbaum, *Antimicrob. Ag. Chemother.*, 1980, *17*, 269; J. E. Peacock *et al.*, *Ann. intern. Med.*, 1980, *93*, 526.

Absorption and Fate. Methicillin is inactivated by acid and must be given by injection. Peak plasma concentrations are attained within ½ to 1 hour of an intramuscular injection; concentrations of 10 μg or more per ml have been reported 1 hour after a dose of 1 g. Effective concentrations are maintained for 3 to 4 hours. Up to about 40% of the methicillin in the circulation is bound to plasma proteins. It diffuses into ascitic, pleural, pericardial, and synovial fluids. There is little diffusion into the cerebrospinal fluid unless the meninges are inflamed, when concentrations of about a tenth of those in the blood can be achieved. Excretion is rapid; high concentrations are achieved in the bile, and 60% or more appears in the urine within 6 hours of a single dose of 1 g. Excretion can be delayed by probenecid.

The biological half-life of methicillin was 0.5 to 1 hour in adults, 0.9 to 3.3 hours (according to age) in infants born at term, and 1.4 to 3.3 hours (according to age) in premature infants.— W. A. Ritschel, *Drug Intell. & clin. Pharm.*, 1970, *4*, 332. See also M. Gibaldi and D. Perrier, *J. clin. Pharmac.*, 1972, *12*, 201.

Methicillin was reported to be absorbed from the peritoneal cavity.— J. S. Cheigh, *Am. J. Med.*, 1977, *62*, 555.

A study of the pharmacokinetics of methicillin in neonatal infants. Plasma clearance was directly correlated with birth weight, gestational age, and chronological age.— L. D. Sarff *et al.*, *J. Pediat.*, 1977, *90*, 1005.

Diffusion into body fluids and tissues. Following intravenous infusion, methicillin did not penetrate the aqueous humour of normal non-inflamed eyes in therapeutic amounts. Methicillin was present in effective concentrations in the intra-ocular fluids of 3 eyes with alterations in the blood-aqueous barrier.— R. E. Records, *Archs Ophthal., N.Y.*, 1966, *76*, 720.

In 11 paired samples of synovial fluid and serum obtained from children given methicillin 23 to 61 mg per kg body-weight intramuscularly or intraveneously, detectable serum and synovial-fluid concentrations were found within 30 minutes. In 4 children the serum concentration was greater than that in the synovial fluid but in the other 7 comparable or greater synovial-fluid concentrations were achieved.— J. D. Nelson, *New Engl. J. Med.*, 1971, *284*, 349.

In a study of the bone penetration of 7 antibiotics given parenterally methicillin, carbenicillin, and clindamycin were detected in bone with the greatest frequency.— J. D. Smilack *et al.*, *Antimicrob. Ag. Chemother.*, 1976, *9*, 169.

Methicillin 250 mg per kg body-weight daily given intravenously for 14 to 21 days to 10 children with osteomyelitis produced concentrations in pus ranging from 4.8 to 39.7 μg per ml (mean 18.6 μg per ml). Concentrations in bone from 9 of the children ranged from 1.2 to 45.9 μg per g (mean 12.1 μg per g). The concentrations in pus and bone equalled or exceeded the MIC and minimal bactericidal concentration (MBC) for *Staphylococcus aureus* and represented 25 and 17% of the peak serum concentration respectively. The same dose given intramuscularly to 3 similar children produced concentrations in pus of 4.5 to 11.8 μg per ml and in bone of 1.9 to 3.9 μg per g. These lower values were still equal to or greater than the MIC or MBC for *Staph. aureus*.— T. R. Tetzlaff *et al.*, *J. Pediat.*, 1978, *92*, 135.

Further references: R. H. Fitzgerald *et al.*, *Antimicrob. Ag. Chemother.*, 1978, *14*, 723 (concentrations of methicillin in cortical bone and synovial fluid).

Metabolism. Within 12 hours of the intramuscular administration of a 500-mg dose of methicillin to 6 healthy subjects, 75% was recovered unchanged in the urine with a further 7% recovered as penicilloic acid.— M. Cole *et al.*, *Antimicrob. Ag. Chemother.*, 1973, *3*, 463.

Uses. Methicillin is used only in the treatment of infections due to penicillinase-producing staphylococci. The usual dosage of methicillin sodium is 1 g intramuscularly every 4 to 6 hours; it may be given intravenously, 1 g being dissolved in 20 ml of Water for Injections and injected slowly over 3 to 4 minutes. In more severe infections up to 12 g daily can be given intravenously in divided doses by slow injection or by intermittent infusion. Higher doses have been given in staphylococcal endocarditis. A usual children's dose is 100 mg per kg body-weight daily in divided doses by intramuscular or intravenous injection. If pain is a problem, intramuscular injections may be prepared using a 0.5% lignocaine hydrochloride solution.

In staphylococcal meningitis systemic treatment has been supplemented with intrathecal injections of methicillin. The usual daily intrathecal dose is the equivalent of 5 mg of methicillin for infants from birth up to 2 years of age, 10 mg for children up to 12 years of age, and 20 mg for adults. The dose should be dissolved in sodium chloride injection 0.9% immediately before use to give a solution containing 10 mg per ml.

Doses of 0.5 to 1 g have been given daily by intra-articular injection, dissolved if necessary in a 0.5% solution of lignocaine hydrochloride, and by intrapleural injection. Doses of 500 mg have been given daily by subconjunctival injection.

In staphylococcal infections of the lung methicillin sodium has been administered by nebuliser, a dose of 500 mg being dissolved in 5 ml of sterile water and inhaled 4 times daily.

A review of the actions and uses of methicillin.— D. N. Gilbert and J. P. Sanford, *Med. Clins N. Am.*, 1970, *54*, 1113.

A guide to the use of penicillinase-resistant penicillins by the Veterans Administration Ad Hoc Interdisciplinary Advisory Committee on Antimicrobial Drug Usage.— *J. Am. med. Ass.*, 1977, *237*, 1605.

Dosage in infants and children. The suggested dose of methicillin for infants of more than 37 weeks' gestation was 25 mg per kg body-weight given intramuscularly or intravenously, by very slow bolus injection, every 12 hours for the first 48 hours of life, every 8 hours from the 3rd day to 2 weeks, then every 6 hours. For immature infants (those of less than 37 weeks' gestation) this dose should be given every 12 hours for the 1st week of life, every 8 hours from then to 4 weeks of age, and every 6 hours thereafter.— P. A. Davies, *Br. med. J.*, 1978, *2*, 676.

Further references: L. D. Sarff *et al.*, *J. Pediat.*, 1977, *90*, 1005; H. C. Spratt, *Drugs*, 1978, *16*, 226; G. H. McCracken and H. F. Eichenwald, *J. Pediat.*, 1978, *93*, 357.

Dosage in renal failure. Patients with 10 to 35% of normal kidney function could be given 1 to 2 g of methicillin every 3 to 6 hours and patients with 0 to 9% kidney function could be given 1 g intravenously every 8 hours.— D. L. Giusti, *Drug Intell. & clin. Pharm.*, 1973, *7*, 62.

The normal half-life for methicillin of 0.5 hour was increased to 4 hours in end-stage renal failure. The interval between doses should be extended from 4 hours to 8 to 12 hours in patients with a glomerular filtration-rate of less than 10 ml per minute. Concentrations of methicillin were not affected by haemodialysis or peritoneal dialysis.— W. M. Bennett *et al.*, *Ann. intern. Med.*, 1977, *86*, 754. See also *idem*, 1980, *93*, 62.

No dose change was required in patients with mild renal failure; 1 to 2 g every 8 hours was recommended in uraemia and this was also suitable during peritoneal dialysis. A dose of 1 g every 6 hours was recommended for patients undergoing haemodialysis.— G. B. Appel and H. C. Neu, *New Engl. J. Med.*, 1977, *296*, 663.

Data for predicting removal of methicillin by conventional haemodialysis.— T. P. Gibson and H. A. Nelson, *Clin. Pharmacokinet.*, 1977, *2*, 403.

Meningitis. A review of experience in 22 cases of ventricular shunt infection. *Staphylococcus epidermidis* was the infecting organism in the majority of infections and methicillin was the antibiotic most commonly used. It was given by intraventricular injection as well as systemically.— R. L. McLaurin, *Surg. Neurol.*, 1973, *1*, 191.

Preparations

Methicillin Eye Ointment. Methicillin sodium 2, liquid paraffin 25, white soft paraffin to 100. If this preparation was stored in moisture-proof containers, little loss of potency would occur in a year at room temperature.— B. Lynn, *Chemist Drugg.*, 1967, *187*, 157.

Methicillin Eye-drops. Methicillin sodium 1, phenylmercuric nitrate 0.002, sodium citrate 0.5, Water for Injections to 100. Sterilised by filtration. This preparation might be expected to lose about 4% of its initial potency in 8 days at 4° and would also be suitable for ear-drops.— B. Lynn, *Chemist Drugg.*, 1967, *187*, 157.

Methicillin Injection *(B.P. 1973).* Methicillin Sodium Injection. A sterile solution of methicillin sodium in Water for Injections, prepared by dissolving the sterile contents of a sealed container in the requisite amount of Water for Injections. The solution should be stored at 2° to 10° and used within 2 days of its preparation.

Methicillin Sodium for Injection *(U.S.P.).* A sterile mixture of methicillin sodium and either sodium edetate, or a suitable preservative and sodium citrate. Potency is expressed in terms of the equivalent amount of methicillin. The injection is prepared by the addition of diluent before use. pH 7 to 8.5 (with sodium edetate) or 6 to 8.5 (with sodium citrate).

Proprietary Preparations

Celbenin *(Beecham Research, UK).* Methicillin sodium, available as powder for preparing injections in vials of 1 g. (Also available as Celbenin in *Austral., Belg., Neth., Switz., USA*).

Other Proprietary Names

Azapen *(USA)*; Baclyn, Celpillina, Ellecillina, Esapenil BG *(all Ital.)*; Flabelline *(Fr.)*; Lucopenin *(Denm.)*; Metin *(Austral.)*; Penaureus *(Arg.)*; Pénistaph *(Fr.)*; Penysol, Sintespen, Staficyn *(all Ital.)*; Staphcillin *(Canad., Norw., USA)*.

107-h

Mezlocillin Sodium.

BAY f 1353. Sodium (6*R*)-6-[D-2-(3-mesyl-2-oxoimidazolidine-1-carboxamido)-2-phenylacetamido]penicillanate.

$C_{21}H_{24}N_5NaO_8S_2,H_2O = 579.6$.

CAS — 51481-65-3 (mezlocillin); 42057-22-7 (sodium salt, anhydrous).

A white to slightly yellow, almost odourless, crystalline substance. Each g represents about 1.7 mmol (1.7 mEq) of sodium. Readily **soluble** in water; slightly soluble in alcohol and acetone; soluble in dimethylformamide and methyl alcohol.

Adverse Effects, Treatment, and Precautions. As for Benzylpenicillin, p.1103.

Antimicrobial Action. Mezlocillin has a range of antimicrobial activity similar to, but wider than, that of carbenicillin (p.1111) and is reported to be more active than carbenicillin *in vitro*, especially against *Pseudomonas aeruginosa* and *Klebsiella* spp.

In a comparison *in vitro*, azlocillin was more active than mezlocillin against *Ps. aeruginosa* and was 8 times more active than carbenicillin against susceptible strains. Mezlocillin was more active than azlocillin against *E. coli, Klebsiella* spp., *Proteus mirabilis*, indole-positive strains of *Proteus*, and *Serratia marcescens*. Both mezlocillin and azlocillin were considerably more active than carbenicillin against *Klebsiella* spp. and were also more active against *Bacteroides fragilis* and *Haemophilus influenzae*. Carbenicillin was twice as active as mezlocillin and 4 times as active as azlocillin against *Pr. mirabilis* but mezlocillin was more active against indole-positive strains. Against *Neisseria gonorrhoeae* mezlocillin and azlocillin were generally more active than benzylpenicillin.— R. Wise *et al.*, *Antimicrob. Ag. Chemother.*, 1978, *13*, 559.

Azlocillin or mezlocillin 25 µg per ml inhibited 46 or 77% of 21 strains of *Klebsiella* spp., 68 or 96% of 47 strains of *Enterobacter*, 82 or 63% of 76 strains of *Ps. aeruginosa*, and 83 or 88% of 17 strains of *Bacteroides* respectively. By comparison, carbenicillin 25 µg per ml inhibited none of 21 strains of *Klebsiella*, 60% of the *Enterobacter*, 38% of the *Ps. aeruginosa*, and 28% of the *Bacteroides*. Against *Pr. mirabilis* up to 1.6 µg per ml of azlocillin, mezlocillin, or carbenicillin inhibited 96, 97, or 97% of 31 strains whereas against indole-positive strains of *Proteus*, 3.1 µg per ml inhibited 57, 76, or 46% of 35 strains. Mezlocillin was more active than ampicillin or carbenicillin against *Streptococcus faecalis* and inhibited all of 31 isolates at 0.8 µg or less per ml. There were differences between minimum inhibitory and minimum bactericidal concentrations with mezlocillin and azlocillin, especially against *Pseudomonas*.— K. P. Fu and H. C. Neu, *Antimicrob. Ag. Chemother.*, 1978, *13*, 930.

The activities of azlocillin, mezlocillin, and piperacillin were compared *in vitro* with those of ampicillin and ticarcillin against 290 clinical isolates of bacteria. Piperacillin and mezlocillin were the most active against *E. coli, Proteus mirabilis, Klebsiella* spp., and *Enterobacter* spp. Azlocillin was less active than piperacillin but more active than mezlocillin or ticarcillin against *Ps. aeruginosa* with a few of the gentamicin-resistant strains being relatively susceptible. All the antibiotics were similarly active against enterococci except ticarcillin which had poor activity. Azlocillin, ticarcillin, or ampicillin used with gentamicin had an additive or synergistic effect *in vitro* against strains of Enterobacteriaceae.— G. W. White *et al.*, *Antimicrob. Ag. Chemother.*, 1979, *15*, 540.

The activity of mezlocillin sodium *in vitro* against 900 clinical isolates of aerobic and anaerobic bacteria.— H. Thadepalli *et al.*, *Antimicrob. Ag. Chemother.*, 1979, *15*, 487.

See also under Piperacillin (p.1202) for the antimicrobial activity of mezlocillin.

Further references: G. P. Bodey and T. Pan, *Antimicrob. Ag. Chemother.*, 1977, *11*, 74; D. Stewart and G. P. Bodey, *ibid.*, 865; G. P. Bodey *et al.*, *ibid.*, 1978, *13*, 14; C. M. Nolan *et al.*, *Curr. ther. Res.*, 1978, *23*, 754; L. Coppens and J. Klastersky, *Antimicrob. Ag. Chemother.*, 1979, *15*, 396; C. N. Baker *et al.*, *Antimicrob. Ag. Chemother.*, 1980, *17*, 757; B. Chattopadhyay and J. C. Teli (letter), *J. antimicrob. Chemother.*, 1980, *6*, 418.

Enhanced activity. Azlocillin or mezlocillin used with gentamicin, netilmicin, or amikacin *in vitro* showed some degree of synergy against strains of *E. coli, Klebsiella, Enterobacter, Serratia, Citrobacter*, indole-positive strains of *Proteus*, and particularly against *Ps. aeruginosa*; no antagonism was observed. Azlocillin or mezlocillin and cephazolin were synergistic when used together against some strains of *Pseudomonas, Klebsiella, Citrobacter, Enterobacter*, and indole-positive strains of *Proteus* but were antagonistic against some strains of *Proteus* and *Enterobacter*.— H. C. Neu and K. P. Fu, *Antimicrob. Ag. Chemother.*, 1978, *13*, 813.

There was little if any synergy between mezlocillin and cefoxitin when tested against beta-lactamase-producing strains of Enterobacteriaceae and *Pseudomonas*, but some synergy was seen against *Bacteroides fragilis*. There was marked synergism when mezlocillin was used with clavulanic acid against beta-lactamase-producing strains of *Staphylococcus aureus, Haemophilus influenzae*, and Enterobacteriaceae, though strains of *Proteus rettgeri* and *Pr. vulgaris* showed no such effect; synergy against *B. fragilis* occurred but was not marked.— R. Wise *et al.*, *J. antimicrob. Chemother.*, 1979, *5*, 301.

Absorption and Fate. Mezlocillin is poorly absorbed from the gastro-intestinal tract.

After mezlocillin 3 g was given intravenously over 15 minutes to 9 cancer patients, a mean serum concentration of 269 µg per ml was achieved, falling to 10 µg per ml at 4 hours. The terminal half-life for mezlocillin of 66 minutes was similar to that for carbenicillin (77 minutes) and ampicillin (63 minutes). The amounts of mezlocillin, carbenicillin, and ampicillin recovered from the urine within 6 hours of a 3-g intravenous dose were 45, 80, and 61% respectively. When mezlocillin 3 g was dissolved in 100 ml of dextrose injection 5% and infused over 2 hours every 4 hours for at least 7 days in 11 febrile cancer patients, mean serum concentrations above 50 µg per ml were maintained after 3 days of treatment. Peak serum concentrations of over 100 µg per ml were achieved immediately after infusion.— B. F. Issell *et al.*, *Antimicrob. Ag. Chemother.*, 1978, *13*, 180.

Mean serum concentrations of mezlocillin of about 56, 166, and 384 µg per ml were obtained after the intravenous injection of 1, 2, and 5 g respectively given over 4 to 5 minutes to 10 healthy subjects; serum concentrations fell to 1.5, 3.9, and 13 µg per ml respectively 3 hours after administration and to 0.1, 0.1, and 2.2 µg per ml after 6 hours. The urinary recovery of mezlocillin up to 8 hours after administration increased with dose, ranging from 61% after 1 g to 69% after 5 g. The plasma half-lives of mezlocillin were 0.96, 0.79, and 1.21 hours after the 1, 2, and 5-g doses respectively.— T. Bergan, *Antimicrob. Ag. Chemother.*, 1978, *14*, 801.

Further references to pharmacokinetic studies of mezlocillin: H. Lode *et al.*, *Infection*, 1977, *5*, 163; S. J. Pancoast and H. C. Neu, *Clin. Pharmac. Ther.*, 1978, *24*, 108 (comparison with carbenicillin); T. Bergan *et al.*, *Antimicrob. Ag. Chemother.*, 1979, *16*, 651; E. Francke *et al.*, *Clin. Pharmac. Ther.*, 1979, *26*, 228; G. R. Aronoff *et al.*, *Clin. Pharmac. Ther.*, 1980, *28*, 523 (in renal impairment); J. M. Brogard *et al.*, *Antimicrob. Ag. Chemother.*, 1980, *18*, 69 (biliary elimination); N. Frimodt-Möller *et al.*, *Antimicrob. Ag. Chemother.*, 1980, *17*, 599 (varying renal function); D. Kampf *et al.*, *Antimicrob. Ag. Chemother.*, 1980, *18*, 81 (impaired renal function and dialysis).

Uses. Mezlocillin sodium is a ureido-penicillin, closely related to azlocillin sodium (p.1099), and is used in the treatment of pseudomonal infections and other infections caused by sensitive organisms. The equivalent of 2 to 5 g of mezlocillin is administered every 6 to 8 hours by intravenous injection or infusion. Doses may be given every 12 hours to patients with renal insufficiency. A 10% solution in Water for Injections is infused over 15 to 20 minutes for 5-g doses;

lower doses are injected over 2 to 4 minutes. If necessary mezlocillin may be given by intramuscular injection but single doses should not exceed 2 g.

Suggested intravenous doses of mezlocillin for children are 75 mg per kg body-weight twice daily by prolonged infusion for premature infants and neonates, and 75 mg per kg thrice daily by injection or infusion for infants and older children.

Short reviews of mezlocillin.— *Drug & Ther. Bull.*, 1980, *18*, 102; *Med Lett.*, 1981, *23*, 110.

Studies and reports on azlocillin and mezlocillin.— *Arzneimittel-Forsch.*, 1979, *29*, 1915–2031; C. J. Ellis *et al.*, *J. antimicrob. Chemother.*, 1979, *5*, 517.

Further references to the use of mezlocillin: S. J. Pancoast *et al.*, *Am. J. Med.*, 1979, *67*, 747; Z. Takase *et al.*, *Chemotherapy, Tokyo*, 1979, *27*, *Suppl.* 1, 375; H. Thadepalli and B. Rao, *Antimicrob. Ag. Chemother.*, 1979, *16*, 605; B. F. Issell and G. P. Bodey, *Antimicrob. Ag. Chemother.*, 1980, *17*, 1008.

Gonorrhoea. Cure was obtained in 45 of 46 patients with uncomplicated, previously untreated, gonorrhoea following a single intravenous injection of mezlocillin 2 g. Side-effects during injection occurred in 5 patients: dizziness (2), nausea (2), and vomiting (1). Headache developed in 1 patient, and diarrhoea in another, within 24 hours of injection.— W. Fowler and M. H. Khan, *Curr. med. Res. Opinion*, 1979, *5*, 790. See also A. Lassus and O. V. Renkonen, *Br. J. vener. Dis.*, 1979, *55*, 191 (intramuscular use).

Proprietary Preparations

Baypen *(Bayer, UK)*. Mezlocillin sodium, available as powder for preparing injections in vials each containing the equivalent of 0.5, 1 or 2 g of mezlocillin, and in infusion vials containing the equivalent of 5 g. (Also available as Baypen in *Ger.*).

108-m

Midecamycin. Mydecamycin. 5-[3,6-Dideoxy-4-*O*-(2,6-dideoxy-3-*C*-methyl-4-*O*-propionyl-α-L-*ribo*-hexopyranosyl)-3-dimethylamino-β-D-glucopyranosyloxy]-6-formylmethyl-9-hydroxy-4-methoxy-8-methyl-3-propionyloxyhexadecan-10,12-dien-15-olide.

$C_{41}H_{67}NO_{15}$=814.0.

CAS — 35457-80-8.

An odourless white crystalline powder with a bitter taste. Very slightly **soluble** in water; freely soluble in acetone, alcohol, chloroform, and ethyl acetate; very soluble in methyl alcohol.

Midecamycin is a macrolide antibiotic produced by the growth of *Streptomyces mycarofaciens* and with actions and uses similar to those of erythromycin (see p.1158). It has been given by mouth in a dose of 0.8 to 1.2 g daily in divided doses; children have been given 20 to 50 mg per kg body-weight daily.

A comparative study of midecamycin with oleandomycin and clindamycin.— H. Drugeon and A. L. Courtieu, *Acta ther.*, 1978, *4*, 39.

Proprietary Names

Medemycin *(Jap.)*; Midécacine *(Clin-Comar-Byla, Fr.)*.

109-b

Minocycline Hydrochloride *(U.S.P.)*.

6-Demethyl-6-deoxy-7-dimethylaminotetracycline hydrochloride.

$C_{23}H_{27}N_3O_7,HCl$=493.9.

CAS — 10118-90-8 (minocycline); 13614-98-7 (hydrochloride).

Pharmacopoeias. In *Braz.* and *U.S.*

A yellow odourless crystalline powder with a bitter taste, containing not less than the equivalent of 785 µg of minocycline per mg. Minocycline hydrochloride 108 mg is approximately equivalent to 100 mg of minocycline. **Soluble** in water and solutions of alkali hydroxides and carbonates; slightly soluble in alcohol; practically insoluble in chloroform and ether. A solution containing about 1% has a pH of 3.5 to 4.5. **Store** in airtight containers. Protect from light.

Units. See p.1187.

Adverse Effects and Precautions. As for Tetracycline Hydrochloride, p.1217.

Vestibular side-effects including dizziness or vertigo occur with minocycline and patients should be advised not to drive or operate machinery. Minocycline appears to have little photosensitising capacity.

A black thyroid was found post mortem in a 69-year-old man who had taken minocycline for a year up to 4 months before death. Similar effects had been seen in some *animals*.— H. D. Attwood and X. Dennett, *Br. med. J.*, 1976, *2*, 1109.

Skin pigmentation associated with minocycline therapy in 4 patients. The discoloration occurred in lesions already infected or inflamed.— N. A. Fenske *et al.*, *J. Am. med. Ass.*, 1980, *244*, 1103.

Allergy. A patient who had developed contact sensitivity to minocycline after 3 months' treatment presented the same widespread immunological response when he inadvertently received minocycline by mouth for the treatment of a urinary-tract infection 2 months later.— W. B. Shelley and C. L. Heaton, *J. Am. med. Ass.*, 1973, *224*, 125.

Intracranial hypertension. A report of benign intracranial hypertension occurring after treatment with minocycline.— F. Monaco *et al.*, *Eur. Neurol.*, 1978, *17*, 48.

Nephrotoxicity. A report of interstitial nephritis attributed to minocycline given in a dose of 250 mg four times daily for 5 days.— R. G. Walker *et al.*, *Br. med. J.*, 1979, *1*, 524. The dose was 5 times that recommended in the UK and a causal relationship was not established.— G. W. R. Hill and M. Roach, *Lederle* (letter), *ibid.*, 820.

Vestibular toxicity. Side-effects including anorexia, ataxia, dizziness or vertigo, weakness, and vomiting occurred in 17 of 19 patients given minocycline 200 to 400 mg daily either for bacteriuria or for meningococcal prophylaxis. These effects were often acute and severe but reversible and in at least 8 patients minocycline had to be withdrawn.— D. N. Williams *et al.*, *Lancet*, 1974, *2*, 744. Vestibular side-effects occurred in 4 of 120 men treated with minocycline 100 mg twice daily for 3 weeks but 15 women out of a group of 105 given the same treatment developed side-effects within the first week.— C. S. Nicol and J. D. Oriel (letter), *Lancet*, 1974, *2*, 1260. The estimated overall incidence of giddiness based on published and unpublished reports was 5%.— A. Yeadon, *Lederle* (letter), *Lancet*, 1975, *1*, 109.

A recommendation that minocycline should not be used until the frequency and severity of its vestibular side-effects have been assessed.— J. C. Allen, *Ann. intern. Med.*, 1976, *85*, 482.

Vestibular side-effects occurred during the first 72 hours of taking minocycline in 27 of 30 patients with meningococcal meningitis. Three patients with vertigo also had visual disturbances.— W. L. Fanning and D. W. Gump, *Archs intern. Med.*, 1976, *136*, 761. See also T. M. Drew *et al.*, *J. infect. Dis.*, 1976, *133*, 194; F. J. Grill *et al.*, *Drug Intell. & clin. Pharm.*, 1977, *11*, 26.

Minocycline 100 mg twice a day for 5 days produced vestibular symptoms in 24 of 45 subjects (5 of 18 men and 19 of 27 women). Six of 44 subjects given placebo experienced similar symptoms. The higher incidence in women was attributed to their higher serum-minocycline concentrations which might be a reflection of their smaller size.— W. L. Fanning *et al.*, *Antimicrob. Ag. Chemother.*, 1977, *11*, 712. In 60 healthy women who took minocycline 150 or 200 mg daily there was no significant difference in the incidence or severity of vestibular symptoms, lightheadedness, disassociation, or difficulty in concentrating. These effects were seen with either dose despite higher serum concentrations in those on the higher dose. Side-effects were not related to body-size either.— D. W. Gump *et al.*, *Antimicrob. Ag. Chemother.*, 1977, *12*, 642.

A claim that the vestibular toxicity of minocycline has not been proved.— V. A. Joy, *Lederle, USA* (letter), *New Engl. J. Med.*, 1979, *301*, 1450. Criticism of this view.— I. R. Friedlander (letter), *ibid.*

Further references: J. Lienard *et al.*, *Thérapie*, 1975, *30*, 459; J. A. Jacobson and B. Daniel, *Antimicrob. Ag. Chemother.*, 1975, *8*, 453.

Antimicrobial Action. Minocycline has a spectrum of activity and mode of action similar to that of tetracycline hydrochloride (see p.1218) but it is more active against many species. In addition it is reported to be effective *in vitro* against some tetracycline-resistant staphylococci, streptococci and certain strains of tetracycline-resistant *Escherichia coli* and *Haemophilus influenzae*.

Tetracycline-resistant strains of *E. coli*, *Salmonella typhimurium*, and unspecified *Klebsiella* bearing R-factors were more sensitive to minocycline and doxycycline *in vitro*. All of 26 strains of *Staph. aureus* with plasmids for tetracycline resistance were much more sensitive to minocycline and most showed some sensitivity to doxycycline.— G. Lebek and Z. Forter, *Schweiz. med. Wschr.*, 1974, *104*, 1124.

Of 48 strains of *Staph. aureus* which required 6.25 µg or more per ml of tetracycline for inhibition the MIC of minocycline was 0.25 µg or less per ml for 45 of the strains whereas the same concentration of doxycycline inhibited 13 of the strains.— D. A. Leigh and K. Simmons (letter), *Lancet*, 1974, *1*, 1006. Amongst 7 tetracyclines minocycline then doxycycline were the most active against strains of *Staph. aureus* and *Staph. epidermidis*; oxytetracycline was the least active.— L. D. Sabath *et al.*, *Antimicrob. Ag. Chemother.*, 1976, *9*, 962.

Of 152 tetracycline-resistant strains of *Staph. aureus* tested by disk diffusion only 33 (22%) were considered to be sensitive to minocycline.— B. Chattopadhyay and E. Harding (letter), *Lancet*, 1975, *1*, 405.

Of 169 strains of penicillin-resistant *Staph. aureus* 84.5% were sensitive to tetracycline and minocycline. However 13.5% were resistant to tetracycline but sensitive to minocycline. Also 48 of 311 isolates of Enterobacteriaceae were sensitive to minocycline but resistant to tetracycline. It was considered that the routine testing for susceptibility to the tetracycline group with tetracycline-only disks was not satisfactory.— C. Candanoza and P. D. Ellner, *Antimicrob. Ag. Chemother.*, 1975, *7*, 227. See also J. N. Minuth *et al.*, *ibid.*, 1974, *6*, 411.

Minocycline was generally more active *in vitro* than tetracycline against both tetracycline-sensitive and -resistant strains of *Haemophilus influenzae* and *Streptococcus pneumoniae* and inhibited all of the 51 strains of *H. influenzae* at a concentration of 2 µg per ml. Although minocycline was more active than tetracycline *in vitro* against strains of group A streptococci, MICs were still greater than 4 µg per ml.— M. J. Wood *et al.*, *J. antimicrob. Chemother.*, 1975, *1*, 323.

Sensitivity tests carried out on 300 isolates of *Neisseria gonorrhoeae* showed 70% sensitive to penicillin with an MIC of less than 0.1 µg per ml and 89% sensitive to minocycline with an MIC of less than 0.5 µg per ml. Nine strains were resistant to penicillin whereas 5 were resistant to minocycline and 3 had reduced sensitivity.— M. Shahidullah and P. W. Greaves, *Br. J. vener. Dis.*, 1975, *51*, 265.

All but 1 of 23 strains of *Acinetobacter calcoaceticus* were sensitive to minocycline 7 ng per ml. Although only 7 of 178 strains of *Serratia marcescens* had an MIC of 2 µg or less per ml, 44.9 and 63.5% of *Serratia marcescens* strains were inhibited by 8 and 16 µg per ml respectively of minocycline; these concentrations could be achieved in the urine with the usual doses.— E. G. Maderazo *et al.*, *Antimicrob. Ag. Chemother.*, 1975, *8*, 54. See also N. A. Kuck, *Lederle, USA*, *ibid.*, 1976, *9*, 493. Minocycline was active against *Acinetobacter anitratus* with an MIC against 43 strains of 0.4 µg or less per ml. Tetracycline was less effective.— J. Z. Montgomerie *et al.*, *Antimicrob. Ag. Chemother.*, 1976, *10*, 102.

Minocycline showed greater activity than tetracycline against 50 strains of *Bacteroides fragilis*, 48% of strains being inhibited by 0.1 µg per ml of minocycline but 14% by 0.1 µg per ml of tetracycline. With an average blood concentration of 2 to 3 µg per ml for minocycline 78% of strains would be inhibited compared with an inhibition of 60% by tetracycline in an average blood concentration of 2 to 4 µg per ml.— D. A. Leigh and K. Simmons, *Lancet*, 1975, *1*, 51. Minocycline was more active than tetracycline or doxycycline against 624 strains of anaerobic bacteria *in vitro*. At 5 µg per ml minocycline, doxycycline, and tetracycline inhibited 84, 74, and 66% respectively of 241 strains of *Bacteroides* spp.— V. Bach *et al.*, *Curr. ther. Res.*, 1978, *23*, 206. See also V. L. Sutter and S. M. Finegold, *Antimicrob. Ag. Chemother.*, 1976, *10*, 736.

Three of 6 *guinea-pigs* infected with the organism of legionnaires' disease survived following treatment with minocycline hydrochloride; this was a better response than that achieved with rifampicin, amikacin, tobramycin, or gentamicin.— P. Nash *et al.* (letter), *Lancet*,

1978, *1,* 45.

The majority of 167 strains of *Neisseria meningitidis* were inhibited by 0.256 µg per ml of minocycline, 0.064 µg per ml of cefuroxime, or 0.064 µg per ml of rifampicin.— W. Brown and R. J. Fallon, *J. antimicrob. Chemother.,* 1980, *6,* 91.

A study of the activity of minocycline *in vitro* against *Mycobacterium* spp.— M. Tsukamura, *Tubercle,* 1980, *61,* 37.

Further references: N. A. Simmons (letter), *Br. med. J.,* 1974, *1,* 158; R. E. T. McGill (letter), *Br. med. J.,* 1974, *3,* 625; T. P. Felegie *et al., Antimicrob. Ag. Chemother.,* 1979, *16,* 833.

Enhanced activity. Demonstration *in vitro* of enhanced antimicrobial activity with a combination of gentamicin and minocycline against the Enterobacteriaceae, especially *E. coli*.— R. J. Fass *et al., Antimicrob. Ag. Chemother.,* 1976, *10,* 34.

Minocycline enhanced the activity of amphotericin *in vitro* against 30 strains of *Candida albicans, Cryptococcus neoformans, Torulopsis glabrata,* and strains of *Candida* other than *albicans.* Minocycline alone had no activity against any of the strains.— M. A. Lew *et al., Antimicrob. Ag. Chemother.,* 1978, *14,* 465.

Absorption and Fate. Minocycline is readily absorbed from the gastro-intestinal tract and is not significantly affected by the presence of food. Normal doses of 200 mg followed by 100 mg every 12 hours produced plasma concentrations within the range of 1 to 3 µg per ml. It is more lipid-soluble than doxycycline and the other tetracyclines and is widely distributed in body tissues and fluids, including the cerebrospinal fluid. A higher ratio of CSF to blood concentrations has been reported with minocycline than with doxycycline. It crosses the placenta and diffuses into milk of nursing mothers. Up to 75% of minocycline in the circulation is bound to plasma proteins. It has a lower renal clearance than doxycycline with a plasma half-life ranging from 10 to 17 hours increasing following continuous administration. Only about 11% of a dose is excreted in the urine in 96 hours and about 34% is excreted in the faeces. Little minocycline is removed by dialysis. The plasma half-life tends to be prolonged in patients with severe renal impairment.

The plasma half-life of minocycline determined in 20 healthy adults was 13.7 hours, and was not dependent on the dose administered or time of administration. Plasma half-life was prolonged in patients with renal dysfunction but was not affected by hepatic dysfunction.— B. Bernard *et al., J. clin. Pharmac.,* 1971, *11,* 332. The urinary excretion of minocycline was not slowed significantly in a study of 12 patients with renal impairment.— M. C. McHenry *et al., Clin. Pharmac. Ther.,* 1972, *13,* 146. After a 200-mg intravenous dose of minocycline the serum half-life was prolonged from 14.6 to 17.3 hours in 8 patients with chronic stable renal failure (creatinine clearance less than 5 ml per minute) compared with 8 subjects with normal renal function. However, excretion appeared to be almost independent of renal function since only 0.7% of the dose was recovered over 72 hours from the urine of those with renal failure compared with 11% in the normal subjects.— D. Heaney and G. Eknoyan, *Clin. Pharmac. Ther.,* 1978, *24,* 233.

In healthy subjects absorption of minocycline was rapid and complete and the serum half-life was about 16 hours after a single oral dose of 150 mg. An average of 76% binding to serum protein was found and urinary excretion tests demonstrated that minocycline was partly metabolised. Following multiple oral doses (200 mg initially then 100 mg twice daily) steady-state serum concentrations of 2.3 to 3.5 µg per ml were reached. Administration of minocycline to patients prior to surgery revealed favourable tissue penetration, the highest concentrations being reached in the intestinal tract, liver, gall-bladder, and bile, suggesting a hepatic role in excretion. After a dosage of 100 mg twice daily in healthy subjects antibiotic concentrations were found in skin, scalp, sebum, and sweat. Minocycline was also shown to pass more effectively into the CSF than doxycycline.— H. Macdonald *et al., Clin. Pharmac. Ther.,* 1973, *14,* 852.

A study in 12 healthy subjects indicated that there were no significant differences between absorption, excretion, and concentrations of minocycline in serum and urine after administration as capsules or film-coated tablets.— A. C. Cartwright *et al., J. antimicrob. Chemother.,* 1975, *1,* 317.

Further references: R. Le Verge *et al., Thérapie,* 1976, *31,* 105; C. Simon *et al., Arzneimittel-Forsch.,* 1976, *26,* 556.

Diffusion. Minocycline concentrations in serum, saliva, sputum, pleural exudate, and lung extracts in patients with respiratory-tract infections.— D. Sommerwerck *et al., Dt. med. Wschr.,* 1978, *103,* 822.

Saliva and tears. Minocycline is more lipophilic than doxycycline, oxytetracycline, or tetracycline. Concentrations in saliva and tears known to be inhibitory to meningococci, were attained in 5 healthy subjects given minocycline 100 mg every 12 hours for 5 days. With doxycycline 100 mg every 12 hours the mean MIC for *Neisseria meningitidis* was only just reached.— P. D. Hoeprich and D. M. Warshauer, *Antimicrob. Ag. Chemother.,* 1974, *5,* 330.

Sinus secretions. D. Worgan and R. J. E. Daniel, *Scott. med. J.,* 1976, *21,* 197.

Sputum. D. MacCulloch *et al., N.Z. med. J.,* 1974, *80,* 300; T. D. Brogan *et al., J. antimicrob. Chemother.,* 1977, *3,* 247.

Uses. Minocycline hydrochloride has actions and uses similar to those of tetracycline hydrochloride (see p.1217). It has been used in the elimination of the meningococcal carrier state although the risk of vestibular disturbances may make such a use unwise.

Minocycline is normally given by mouth but may be given by slow intravenous infusion. The usual dose by either route is the equivalent of 200 mg of minocycline initially followed by 100 mg every 12 hours. Children have been given 4 mg per kg body-weight initially followed by 2 mg per kg every 12 hours but the effect of tetracyclines on teeth should be considered.

A single 300-mg dose of minocycline has been given by mouth in the treatment of male gonorrhoea.

There is controversy about the safe use of minocycline in patients with renal impairment; if used the dosage should be reduced.

Reviews of the actions and uses of minocycline: R. N. Brogden *et al., Drugs,* 1975, *9,* 251; J. C. Allen, *Ann. intern. Med.,* 1976, *85,* 482; *Drug & Ther. Bull.,* 1977, *15,* 34.

A 14-year-old boy with a granulomatous lesion caused by *Serratia marcescens* which had persisted for 5 years was successfully treated with minocycline 100 mg twice daily for 3 months. On cessation of treatment the lesion reappeared; complete clearing occurred when therapy was reinstituted.— E. Epstein and T. E. Carson, *J. Am. med. Ass.,* 1973, *223,* 670.

A report of tri-minocycline, a highly water-soluble form of minocycline, being given intravenously to 13 patients.— I. L. Kahán, *Chemotherapy, Basle,* 1978, *24,* 61.

Bronchitis. In a single-blind study involving 60 patients moderately ill with purulent exacerbations of chronic bronchitis, minocycline 200 mg twice daily for 10 days was found to be as effective as tetracycline hydrochloride 500 mg six-hourly for 10 days and its gastro-intestinal tolerance was better.— A. Pines *et al., Practitioner,* 1974, *213,* 727.

Dosage in renal failure. Minocycline was contra-indicated in patients with impaired renal function.— C. R. P. George *et al., Med. J. Aust.,* 1973, *1,* 640. See also G. B. Appel and H. C. Neu, *New Engl. J. Med.,* 1977, *296,* 663.

There appeared to be no reduction in drug clearance in a study of single and repeated doses of minocycline given to patients with various degrees of renal function.— P. G. Welling *et al., Antimicrob. Ag. Chemother.,* 1975, *8,* 532.

The normal half-life for minocycline of 12 to 15 hours was increased to 17 to 30 hours in end-stage renal failure. The interval between doses should be extended from 12 hours to 18 to 24 hours in patients with a glomerular filtration-rate (GFR) of 10 to 50 ml per minute, and to 24 to 36 hours in those with a GFR of less than 10 ml per minute. Concentrations of minocycline were not affected by haemodialysis or peritoneal dialysis.— W. M. Bennett *et al., Ann. intern. Med.,* 1980, *93,* 62.

See also under Absorption and Fate.

Gonorrhoea. Single doses of 300 or 400 mg of minocycline were given to 349 men with uncomplicated gonococcal urethritis. Of the 328 who returned 13 were treatment failures and 16 had or developed non-specific urethritis by day 29. Side-effects included dizziness in 2 patients and nausea in 3.— G. Masterton and C. B. S. Schofield, *Br. J. vener. Dis.,* 1976, *52,* 43. See also G. Masterton and C. B. S. Schofield (letter), *Lancet,* 1974, *2,* 1139.

Single oral doses of minocycline 300 mg were more effective than talampicillin 1.5 g in the treatment of uncomplicated gonococcal urethritis in 230 men. Failure-rates were 3.2% and 8.7% respectively.— A. Saeed and R. B. Roy, *Br. J. clin. Pract.,* 1979, *33,* 199.

Further references: W. C. Duncan *et al., Br. J. vener. Dis.,* 1971, *47,* 364; H. Baytch *et al., Med. J. Aust.,* 1974, *1,* 831; M. Shahidullah, *Br. J. vener. Dis.,* 1975, *51,* 97; A. Bjornberg and L. Hellgren, *Curr. ther. Res.,* 1976, *19,* 216; P. M. Waterworth *et al., Br. J. vener. Dis.,* 1979, *55,* 343; M. A. Waugh *et al., ibid.,* 411.

Prophylaxis. In a prospective study in the Far East of 1080 men exposed to the risk of gonococcal infection, postexposure prophylaxis with a single dose of minocycline 200 mg completely prevented infection by gonococci susceptible to 0.75 µg per ml of tetracycline hydrochloride, reduced the risk of infection or prolonged the incubation period in those exposed to gonococci with MICs of 1 to 2 µg per ml, did not reduce infection or prolong incubation in those exposed to gonococci resistant to 2 µg per ml, and did not increase the risk of asymptomatic infection. However, the widespread prophylactic use of minocycline for the control of gonorrhoea is probably of limited value because of the tendency of this regimen to select gonococci that are relatively resistant to tetracycline. Of 27 men with symptomatic gonorrhoea given minocycline 900 mg over 4 days, only 11 were cured.— W. O. Harrison *et al., New Engl. J. Med.,* 1979, *300,* 1074.

Malaria. Minocycline and tetracycline in the treatment of acute falciparum malaria.— E. J. Colwell *et al., Am. J. trop. Med. Hyg.,* 1972, *21,* 144.

Meningococcal carriers. After 5 men developed meningococcal disease, minocycline 100 mg was administered as suppositories every 12 hours for 5 days to 8721 recruits. No more cases developed until 4 weeks after the start of prophylaxis by which time over 50% of the recruits were new and untreated. The rate of nasopharyngeal carriage of meningococci was reduced from 68% to 35%.— R. B. Guttler and H. N. Beaty, *Antimicrob. Ag. Chemother.,* 1972, *1,* 397.

Minocycline 200, 100, and 100 mg at 12-hour intervals followed by 3 similar doses of rifampicin 600 mg to meningococcal carriers inhibited the emergence of rifampicin resistance with only 1 of 7 strains isolated after treatment being resistant. Unfortunately this strain spread.— L. F. Devine *et al., Am. J. Epidem.,* 1973, *97,* 394.

The US Public Health Service had recommended that, due to the high incidence of vestibular toxicity, minocycline should no longer be used for the prophylaxis of meningococcal disease and that rifampicin should be used instead. In view of the conflicting reports of the incidence of side-effects and because of doubts of the effectiveness of rifampicin in such infections further studies were desirable.— *Med. Lett.,* 1975, *17,* 39.

Further references: L. F. Devine *et al., Am. J. med. Sci.,* 1972, *263,* 79; T. M. Drew *et al., J. infect. Dis.,* 1976, *133,* 194.

For references to the suggestion that minocycline is more suitable than rifampicin for meningococcal prophylaxis, see Rifampicin, p.1581.

Prostatitis. Reports of the use of minocycline in the treatment of bacterial prostatitis.— D. F. Paulson and R. D. White, *J. Urol.,* 1978, *120,* 184; S. K. P. Kan and R. W. W. Kay, *Trans. R. Soc. trop. Med. Hyg.,* 1978, *72,* 522.

Minocycline appeared to be the most effective of the tetracyclines in the treatment of non-bacterial prostatitis. A 14-day course of treatment is recommended, with maintenance therapy for the following 6 weeks.— N. J. Blacklock, *Practitioner,* 1979, *223,* 318.

Skin disorders. Treatment with minocycline, 200 mg initially then 100 mg every 12 hours, was successful in 22 of 23 patients with soft tissue or skin infections caused by *Staphylococcus aureus* or β-haemolytic streptococci. One patient developed a transient macular rash which did not require treatment.— A. Hoagland and L. G. Smith, *Clin. Med.,* 1973, *80* (Apr.), 22.

Mycobacterium marinum infection in 2 patients responded to treatment with minocycline 100 mg twice daily.— N. A. Lockshin (letter), *Archs Derm.,* 1977, *113,* 987.

Acne. In a double-blind study of 16 patients with severe acne vulgaris, minocycline was as effective as doxycycline when 100 mg of either was given daily for 3 months.— F. Smit, *Dermatologica*, 1978, *157*, 186. Of 25 patients with acne vulgaris who had not responded to treatment with tetracycline 1 g daily for 6 to 8 weeks, 22 responded to minocycline 50 mg twice daily given for a similar period. No vestibular side-effects were noted.— S. I. Cullen, *Cutis*, 1978, *21*, 101.

Syphilis. Minocycline was given in an initial dose of 200 mg followed by 100 mg twice daily to 9 patients with syphilis, 5 with lymphogranuloma venereum, 6 with granuloma inguinale, and 6 with chancroid. Medication was continued for 15 days in patients with syphilis or until ulcers and buboes healed with the other diseases. Healing time averaged 15 days for lymphogranuloma venereum, 21 days for granuloma inguinale, and 16 days for chancroid. All patients with syphilis showed clearing of lesions and satisfactory response to serological tests for up to 1 year. No serious side-effects occurred.— J. E. Velasco *et al.*, *J. Am. med. Ass.*, 1972, *220*, 1323.

Urinary-tract infections. Treatment with minocycline 100 mg twice daily was compared with oxytetracycline 250 mg twice daily or tetracycline (sustained-release) 250 mg twice daily, all given for 7 days, in 505 patients with nonspecific urethritis. Of those available for assessment after 3 months, 29 of 102 given minocycline had relapsed compared with 42 of 109 given oxytetracycline and 43 of 103 who received tetracycline.— B. A. Evans, *Br. J. vener. Dis.*, 1978, *54*, 107. See also M. J. Prentice *et al.*, *Br. J. vener. Dis.*, 1976, *52*, 269.

Minocycline 50 mg four times a day for 10 days was given to 124 women with symptomatic urinary-tract infection. Of 65 women with bacteriuria who completed treatment 52 were cured. Adverse effects occurred in 24 women and necessitated discontinuation of therapy in 16. Vestibular toxicity occurred in 14 women while other side-effects reported included headache, nausea, and vomiting.— T. P. Greco *et al.*, *Curr. ther. Res.*, 1979, *25*, 193.

Further references: *Practitioner*, 1975, *214*, 110 (Report No. 190 of the General Practitioner Research Group).

Units. One unit of minocycline is contained in 0.0011587 mg of the first International Reference Preparation (1975) of minocycline hydrochloride which contains 863 units per mg.

Preparations

Minocycline Hydrochloride Capsules *(U.S.P.)*. Capsules containing minocycline hydrochloride equivalent to 50 or 100 mg of minocycline. Store in airtight containers. Protect from light.

Minocycline Hydrochloride Oral Suspension *(U.S.P.)*. A suspension of minocycline hydrochloride with one or more suitable diluents, preservatives, flavouring, and wetting agents, in an aqueous vehicle. pH 7 to 9. It contains the equivalent of 10 mg of minocycline per ml. Store in airtight containers. Protect from light.

Minocycline Hydrochloride Tablets *(U.S.P.)*. Tablets containing minocycline hydrochloride equivalent to minocycline 100 mg. Store in airtight containers. Protect from light.

Proprietary Preparations

Minocin *(Lederle, UK)*. Minocycline hydrochloride, available as tablets each containing the equivalent of 50 and 100 mg of minocycline. (Also available as Minocin in *Belg., Canad., Ital., Neth., Spain, Switz., USA*).

Other Proprietary Names

Klinomycin *(Ger.)*; Minomycin *(Austral., Jap., S.Afr.)*; Mynocine *(Fr.)*; Ultramycin *(Canad.)*; Vectrin *(USA)*.

110-x

Nafcillin Sodium *(U.S.P.)*. Nafcillinum Natricum; Nafcilina Sōdica; Sodium Nafcillin. Sodium (6*R*)-6-(2-ethoxy-1-naphthamido)penicillanate monohydrate.

$C_{21}H_{21}N_2NaO_5S,H_2O$=454.5.

CAS — 147-52-4 (nafcillin); 985-16-0 (sodium salt, anhydrous); 7177-50-6 (sodium salt, monohydrate).

Pharmacopoeias. In *Braz.*, *Int.*, and *U.S.*

A white to yellowish-white powder with not more than a slight characteristic odour. Each g represents 2.2 mmol (2.2 mEq) of sodium. Nafcillin sodium 1.1 g is approximately equivalent to 1 g of anhydrous nafcillin. The *U.S.P.* specifies not less than the equivalent of 820 μg of nafcillin per mg.

Freely **soluble** in water and chloroform; soluble in alcohol. A 3% solution in water has a pH of 5 to 7. Solutions should be refrigerated at 2° to 4° after preparation and used within 48 hours. The free acid precipitates at a pH below 5.6. Nafcillin sodium in concentrations of 2 to 30 mg per ml is stable for 24 hours at room temperature in injections of dextrose 5% and sodium chloride 0.9%. It is not stable in dextrose solution at an alkaline pH. **Store** at a temperature not exceeding 25° in airtight containers.

Incompatibility. Nafcillin was incompatible in solutions with *chlortetracycline, gentamicin, oxytetracycline, polymyxin B*, sympathomimetic agents, *tetracycline*, and *vitamin-B complex*.— *Med. Lett.*, 1972, *14*, (Jan.), *Suppl.*, 32.

A precipitate could occur within a few hours when nafcillin sodium 0.05% injection was mixed with injections of vitamin B complex or ascorbic acid; solutions in various intravenous diluents containing 0.2 to 3% nafcillin sodium were compatible for up to 24 hours. A precipitate occurred within 1 hour when a 0.05% nafcillin injection was mixed with hydrocortisone sodium succinate injection, 0.025%. There was a 14% loss in potency in 24 hours when aminophylline 500 mg per litre was added to nafcillin sodium 0.2% in dextrose injection 5%.— E. A. Parker and H. J. Levin, *Am. J. Hosp. Pharm.*, 1975, *32*, 943.

Stability in solution. Sodium bicarbonate should be added to intravenous infusions containing nafcillin sodium to prevent precipitation, though haziness would still occur.— J. M. Meisler and M. W. Skolaut, *Am. J. Hosp. Pharm.*, 1966, *23*, 557.

Nafcillin sodium 500 mg per 100 ml lost 50% activity in dextrose injection 5% after 2 days at 25° or 28 days at 5°.— J. F. Gallelli *et al.*, *Am. J. Hosp. Pharm.*, 1969, *26*, 630.

Nafcillin sodium was most stable at pH 6 and much less stable at pH 4. When buffered with citrate, it was stable in intravenous infusions for up to 24 hours at 25° provided that a pH of 5 to 8 was maintained.— E. A. Parker and H. J. Levin, *Am. J. Hosp. Pharm.*, 1975, *32*, 943.

Further references: B. E. Kirschenbaum and C. J. Latiolais, *Am. J. Hosp. Pharm.*, 1976, *33*, 767.

Adverse Effects and Treatment. As for Benzylpenicillin, p.1103.

Thrombophlebitis may occur when nafcillin sodium is given by intravenous injection, particularly in elderly patients. Increased concentrations of serum aspartate aminotransferase (SGOT) have been observed after intramuscular injection.

Blood disorders. A report of reversible agranulocytosis in a woman with endocarditis due to *Staphylococcus aureus* who received nafcillin sodium 12 g daily for 19 days. Agranulocytosis improved after nafcillin was replaced by vancomycin.— S. M. Markowitz *et al.*, *J. Am. med. Ass.*, 1975, *232*, 1150. See also D. J. Wolf and G. D. Resnick, *N.Y. St. J. Med.*, 1978, *78*, 256.

Neutropenia occurred in a man given nafcillin sodium 3 g every 4 hours for 3 days then 2 g every 4 hours, intravenously. On the 23rd day the patient developed neutropenia and fever and nafcillin therapy was discontinued; neutrophils began to reappear in the blood within 1 day. The patient had also received probenecid for the first 2 days and paracetamol and flurazepam while in hospital.— M. Sandberg *et al.*, *J. Am. med. Ass.*, 1975, *232*, 1152. See also G. R. Greene and E. Cohen, *Pediatrics*, 1978, *61*, 94; G. J. Couchonnal *et al.*, *Sth. med. J.*, 1978, *71*, 1356. A 46-year-old man who developed neutropenia together with relative eosinophilia, in association with nafcillin therapy, also did so on receiving piperacillin.— C. Wilson *et al.* (letter), *Lancet*, 1979, *1*, 1150.

Electrolyte disturbances. Hypokalaemia in one patient given nafcillin sodium 8 g daily.— J. A. Mohr *et al.*, *J. Am. med. Ass.*, 1979, *242*, 544.

Nephrotoxicity. Nephritis which had developed in a 6-year-old boy who received methicillin recurred when he was given nafcillin 150 mg per kg body-weight daily.— M. F. Parry *et al.* (letter), *J. Am. med. Ass.*, 1973, *225*, 178. The nephropathy was also exacerbated by cephalothin.— S. N. Cohen and J. E. Conte (letter), *ibid.*, 1974, *227*, 325.

Further references to interstitial nephritis associated with nafcillin: T. W. Bodendorfer (letter), *J. Am. med. Ass.*, 1980, *244*, 2609.

Precautions. Nafcillin sodium is contra-indicated in patients known to be sensitive to penicillin and it should be used with caution in patients with a known history of allergy.

False-positive results for proteinuria occurred in 2 patients; very high doses of nafcillin caused a heavy urinary sediment.— D. E. Line *et al.*, *J. Am. med. Ass.*, 1976, *235*, 1259.

Plasma clearance of nafcillin was reduced in patients with biliary obstruction or cirrhosis and lower doses might be necessary in such patients.— J. P. Marshall *et al.*, *Gastroenterology*, 1977, *73*, 1388.

Interactions. Aspirin, sulphamethoxypyridazine, and sulphaethidole inhibited the serum-binding of nafcillin *in vitro* and *in vivo*.— C. M. Kunin, *Clin. Pharmac. Ther.*, 1966, *7*, 180.

For the effect of other drugs on the antimicrobial activity of nafcillin sodium, see below under Antimicrobial Action.

Antimicrobial Action. Nafcillin sodium has an antimicrobial action similar to that of Cloxacillin Sodium, p.1149.

For a report of nafcillin being one of the most active penicillins against *Staph. aureus* and *Staph. epidermidis*, see Benzylpenicillin, p.1106.

Diminished activity. Quinine dihydrochloride decreased the antibacterial effect *in vitro* of nafcillin sodium and oxacillin sodium against *Staph. aureus*.— M. A. Toama *et al.*, *J. pharm. Sci.*, 1978, *67*, 23.

Enhanced activity. The activity of nafcillin against *Staph. aureus* was enhanced when used in conjunction with netilmicin or sissomicin.— C. Watanakunakorn and C. Glotzbecker, *Antimicrob. Ag. Chemother.*, 1977, *12*, 346.

Nafcillin sodium and gentamicin sulphate used together had enhanced activity *in vitro* against 49 of 50 strains of *Staph. aureus* isolated from patients with endocarditis.— C. U. Tuazon *et al.*, *Curr. ther. Res.*, 1978, *23*, 760. When nafcillin was used with gentamicin in *mice* infected with methicillin-resistant *Staph. epidermidis*, there was an increased death-rate compared with the use of either of the drugs alone. The antagonism was not due to drug-drug inactivation.— F. D. Lowy *et al.*, *Antimicrob. Ag. Chemother.*, 1979, *16*, 314.

Rifampicin and nafcillin sodium enhanced each others' activity *in vitro* against 12 of 20 clinical isolates of *Staph. aureus* and their activities were additive against 2.— C. U. Tuazon *et al.*, *Antimicrob. Ag. Chemother.*, 1978, *13*, 759.

Further references: R. Yogev *et al.*, *Antimicrob. Ag. Chemother.*, 1980, *17*, 461; R. Yogev and W. J. Kabat, *ibid.*, *18*, 122 (enhanced activity with nafcillin and ampicillin against ampicillin-resistant *Haemophilus influenzae*).

Resistance. As for Methicillin Sodium, p.1183.

Absorption and Fate. Nafcillin sodium is incompletely and irregularly absorbed from the gastro-intestinal tract, especially when administered after a meal. Peak plasma concentrations of 1.5 to 5 μg per ml have been reported 1 hour after a dose of 0.5 to 1 g given by mouth. After intramuscular injection it is absorbed more reliably, an injection of 500 mg producing peak plasma concentrations of 5 to 8 μg per ml within about 1 to 2 hours. By either route, plasma concentrations are lower than those achieved with the same dose of oxacillin sodium. It is widely distributed in body tissues including synovial fluid. Up to 90% of nafcillin in the circulation is bound to plasma proteins.

A high concentration of nafcillin is excreted via the bile though some reabsorption takes place in the small intestine. Only about 10% of a dose given by mouth before food and about 30% of a dose given intramuscularly is excreted in the urine.

The reversibility of the plasma-protein binding of nafcillin *in vitro*.— M. Barza *et al.*, *Antimicrob. Ag. Chemother.*, 1972, *1*, 427.

The biological half-life of nafcillin was 0.5 hour.— W. M. Bennett *et al.*, *J. Am. med. Ass.*, 1973, *223*, 991.

Nafcillin sodium with calcium carbonate was not satisfactorily absorbed following oral administration to 10 healthy subjects. Food interfered with any absorption.— C. Watanakunakorn, *Antimicrob. Ag. Chemother.*, 1977, *11*, 1007.

A report of serum concentrations achieved in infants

and children given nafcillin by intravenous infusion.— W. E. Feldman *et al.*, *J. Pediat.*, 1978, *93*, 1029. The pharmacokinetics of nafcillin administered intravenously to premature infants.— W. Banner *et al.*, *Antimicrob. Ag. Chemother.*, 1980, *17*, 691.

Nafcillin differs from most other penicillins in that it is largely eliminated by hepatic metabolism.— R. K. Roberts *et al.*, *Drugs*, 1979, *17*, 198.

Diffusion into body fluids. Nafcillin diffused poorly into the interstitial fluid and this was a reflection of its high degree of protein binding.— J. S. Tan *et al.*, *J. infect. Dis.*, 1972, *126*, 492, per J. S. Tan and S. J. Salstrom, *Antimicrob. Ag. Chemother.*, 1977, *11*, 698.

In a study of 9 patients with either staphylococcal sepsis or meningitis who received nafcillin intravenously in doses of 1 to 5 g daily, cerebrospinal fluid concentrations of nafcillin ranged from 0.13 to 88 µg per ml, while serum concentrations ranged from 5.8 to 615 µg per ml. Although there was considerable individual variation, nafcillin concentrations in the CSF usually exceeded the minimum bactericidal concentrations for *Staph. aureus* but a dose of at least 100 to 200 mg per kg body-weight daily was recommended for the treatment of meningitis caused by *Staph. aureus*.— J. G. Kane *et al.*, *Ann. intern. Med.*, 1977, *87*, 309. See also W. J. Sanders (letter), *ibid.*, 1978, *88*, 271.

Nafcillin sodium diffused into the CSF in 16 patients with non-inflamed meninges given a dose of 40 mg per kg body-weight by intravenous infusion. At 1 hour the mean CSF concentration was 0.05 µg of nafcillin per ml compared with a serum concentration of 34.4 µg per ml; at 2 hours the figures were 0.12 and 12.7 µg per ml; at 3 hours 0.09 and 4.9 µg per ml. At 4 hours detectable CSF concentrations were present in 3 of 4 patients. Large doses of nafcillin were considered to be appropriate for the prophylaxis and treatment of staphylococcal meningitis.— B. E. Fossieck *et al.*, *Antimicrob. Ag. Chemother.*, 1977, *11*, 965.

Uses. Nafcillin sodium is administered by intramuscular injection in the treatment of severe infections caused by benzylpenicillin-resistant staphylococci. It is also given by mouth in less severe infections or after preliminary parenteral injection. Mixed streptococcal or pneumococcal and staphylococcal infections may be treated with nafcillin when the staphylococci are penicillin-resistant.

The usual dose by intramuscular injection for adults is the equivalent of 500 mg of nafcillin every 4 to 6 hours and for children 25 mg per kg body-weight twice daily. Newborn infants may be given 10 mg per kg twice daily. The dose by mouth for adults is the equivalent of 0.25 to 1 g of nafcillin every 4 to 6 hours, for children 6.25 to 12.5 mg per kg four times daily, and for neonates 10 mg per kg three or four times daily, given 1 or 2 hours before meals.

Nafcillin sodium has also been given intravenously to adults in doses of 0.5 to 1 g of nafcillin every 4 hours for not more than 24 to 48 hours because of the risk of thrombophlebitis. The dose should be dissolved in 15 to 30 ml of Water for Injections or of sodium chloride injection and either injected over 5 to 10 minutes or dissolved in 150 ml of sodium chloride injection and given by slow intravenous infusion.

A guide to the use of penicillinase-resistant penicillins.— Veterans Administration Ad Hoc Interdisciplinary Advisory Committee on Antimicrobial Drug Usage, *J. Am. med. Ass.*, 1977, *237*, 1605.

Dosage in renal failure. The normal half-life for nafcillin of 0.5 hours was increased to 1.2 hours in end-stage renal failure. It could be given in usual doses to patients with renal failure. Concentrations of nafcillin were not affected by haemodialysis.— W. M. Bennett *et al.*, *Ann. intern. Med.*, 1977, *86*, 754. See also *idem*, 1980, *93*, 62. Where severe renal and hepatic impairment were associated, dosage adjustment might be necessary.— M. Rudnick *et al.*, *Clin. Pharmac. Ther.*, 1976, *20*, 413.

Data for predicting removal of nafcillin by conventional haemodialysis.— T. P. Gibson and H. A. Nelson, *Clin. Pharmacokinet.*, 1977, *2*, 403.

Further references: D. L. Giusti, *Drug Intell. & clin. Pharm.*, 1973, *7*, 62; C. R. Diaz *et al.*, *Antimicrob. Ag. Chemother.*, 1977, *12*, 98.

Endocarditis. A report of the successful use of nafcillin sodium intravenously, followed by oral antibiotic therapy, in staphylococcal endocarditis.— R. H. Parker and B. E. Fossieck, *Ann. intern. Med.*, 1980, *93*, 832.

Preparations

Nafcillin Sodium Capsules *(U.S.P.)*. Capsules containing nafcillin sodium equivalent to 250 mg of nafcillin. Store in airtight containers.

Nafcillin Sodium for Injection *(U.S.P.)*. A sterile dry mixture of nafcillin sodium and a suitable buffer, suitable for parenteral use. Potency is expressed in terms of the equivalent amount of nafcillin. The injection is prepared by the addition of diluent before use. pH 5 to 8.

Nafcillin Sodium for Oral Solution *(U.S.P.)*. Nafcillin sodium with one or more suitable buffers, colours, diluents, dispersing agents, flavours, and preservatives. Store in airtight containers. The solution is prepared by the addition of diluent before issue and contains the equivalent of 50 mg of nafcillin per ml. pH 5.5 to 7.5.

Nafcillin Sodium Tablets *(U.S.P.)*. Tablets containing nafcillin sodium equivalent to nafcillin 500 mg. Store in airtight containers. Protect from light.

Proprietary Names

Nafcil *(Bristol, USA)*; Unipen *(Wyeth, Canad.; Wyeth, USA)*.

111-r

Neomycin.

A mixture of 2 isomers, neomycins B and C, and neomycin A (neamine), an inactive component and degradation product of neomycins B and C; about 10 to 15% may be present in neomycin. Neomycin B is 2-deoxy-4-*O*-(2,6-diamino-2,6-dideoxy-α-D-glucopyranosyl)-5-*O*-[3-*O*-(2,6-diamino-2,6-dideoxy-β-L-idopyranosyl)-β-D-ribofuranosyl]-D-streptamine.

$C_{23}H_{46}N_6O_{13}$=614.6.

CAS — 1404-04-2 (neomycin); 3947-65-7 (neomycin A); 119-04-0 (neomycin B); 66-86-4 (neomycin C).

Framycetin (see p.1165) consists mainly of neomycin B with not more than 3% of neomycin C and not more than 1% of neomycin A.

112-f

Neomycin Sulphate

(B.P., B.P. Vet., Eur. P.). Neomycin Sulfate *(U.S.P.)*; Neomycini Sulfas; Neomycin; Fradiomycin Sulphate.

CAS — 1405-10-3.

Pharmacopoeias. In *Arg., Belg., Br., Braz., Cz., Eur., Fr., Ger., Hung., Ind., Int., It., Jap., Jug., Neth., Nord., Pol., Port., Roum., Rus., Swiss, Turk.*, and *U.S.*

Neomycin sulphate is a mixture of the sulphates of the antimicrobial substances produced by the growth of certain selected strains of *Streptomyces fradiae*. The *B.P.* specifies, when dried, not less than 650 units per mg; *U.S.P.* specifies not less than the equivalent of 600 µg of neomycin per mg.

Neomycin sulphate occurs as a white or yellowish-white, odourless or almost odourless, hygroscopic powder. It contains, when dried, 27 to 31% of sulphate and loses not more than 6% of its weight on drying.

Slowly **soluble** 1 in 1 of water; very slightly soluble in alcohol; practically insoluble in acetone, chloroform, and ether. A solution in water is dextrorotatory. A 10% solution in water has a pH of 5 to 7.5. Solutions are **stable** at room temperature for a year, though some darkening in colour occurs. Solutions of neomycin are **sterilised** by maintaining at 98° to 100° with a bactericide for 30 minutes or by filtration.

Incompatible in solution with some anionic substances, with which it may form a precipitate, including sodium lauryl sulphate in Aqueous Cream (*B.P.*); also incompatible with cephalothin sodium and with novobiocin sodium. **Store** at a temperature not exceeding 30° in airtight containers. Protect from light.

113-d

Neomycin Undecenoate.

Neomycin Undecylenate. The 10-undecenoate salt of neomycin.

CAS — 1406-04-8.

A yellowish-white to pale yellow, stable, waxy, unctuous powder with a candle-like odour. It contains not less than 300 mg of neomycin base per g. Practically **insoluble** in water; very soluble in alcohol; freely soluble in propylene glycol; soluble in chloroform; practically insoluble in vegetable oils.

NOTE. When Neomycin is prescribed or demanded, Neomycin Sulphate must be dispensed or supplied.

Effect of gamma-irradiation. Neomycin sulphate powder became discoloured and the resultant solutions pale yellow at 25 000 Gy and orange at 250 000 Gy. The initial potency of 666 µg per mg fell to 639 µg per mg at 25 000 Gy and to 644 µg per mg at 250 000 Gy.— *The Use of Gamma Radiation Sources for the Sterilisation of Pharmaceutical Products*, London, ABPI, 1960.

Loss of activity. Neomycin was very much less active against *Staphylococcus aureus* in the presence of magnesium trisilicate, acacia, tragacanth, sodium alginate, pectin, bentonite, and kaolin and much less active with calamine, silica (Aerosil), methylcellulose, carboxymethylcellulose, maize starch, gelatin, and polysorbate 80.— M. A. El-Nakeeb and R. T. Yousef, *Acta pharm. suec.*, 1968, *5*, 1.

The interaction between neomycin and pectin was inhibited by the presence of electrolytes. Neomycin preparations containing pectin could be expected to be as effective as the antibiotic alone.— W. A. Harris, *Australas. J. Pharm.*, 1971, *52*, S69.

Although neomycin was inactivated in plain mixtures with kaolin, products could be formulated so that neomycin was not adsorbed by the kaolin.— *Br. med. J.*, 1972, *2*, 587. An improved formulation in which the suspending agent aluminium magnesium silicate was replaced by methylcellulose, edetic acid by magnesium chloride, and the pH of the mixture raised to 5.5.— M. Aggag *et al.*, *Mfg Chem.*, 1977, *48* (June), 39.

Sodium phosphate was successfully used to prevent the formation of insoluble complexes between soluble corticosteroid phosphate salts and neomycin sulphate in aqueous ophthalmic solutions.— J. W. McGinity and R. L. Brown, *J. pharm. Sci.*, 1975, *64*, 1528.

The antimicrobial activity of neomycin sulphate was reduced in the presence of vitamins of the B complex or ascorbic acid.— M. A. El-Nakeeb *et al.*, *Can. J. pharm. Sci.*, 1976, *11*, 85.

A study of the effect of the antibiotic and preservative on each other's binding to pharmaceutical adjuvants in mixtures containing benzalkonium chloride or chlorocresol and neomycin B sulphate.— M. A. El-Nakeeb and M. H. Ali, *Mfg Chem.*, 1976, *47* (Mar.), 37.

Preparation of sterile solution. A sterile 1% solution of neomycin sulphate for bladder irrigation could be made by dissolving neomycin sulphate in sodium chloride injection and sterilising by filtration. Autoclaving discoloured the solution but there was no significant loss of potency after 12 months by either method.— L. H. Austin (letter), *Am. J. Hosp. Pharm.*, 1972, *29*, 206.

Stability. Neomycin was cationic and became firmly bound to bentonite; it cracked emulsions prepared with sodium lauryl sulphate and precipitated certain gums from jellies. It was incompatible with hydrophilic ointment and carboxymethylcellulose jelly. Washable emulsion bases, jellies, and sorbitan ester bases (Spans 40 and 85) most readily released neomycin. Neomycin was stable for 30 days in ointments containing water but there was a slight decrease in potency after 60 days.— W. T. Hill *et al.*, *Drug Stand.*, 1955, *23*, 80.

The addition of neomycin sulphate to aqueous gels made with the free acid derivative of ethylene maleic anhydride (EMA-71, *Monsanto*), carbomer (Carbopol 934), an anionic heteropolysaccharide (Biopolymer XB-23, *General Mills*), or sodium carboxymethylcellulose caused precipitation and loss of viscosity. Methylcellulose and ethylene oxide copolymer (Polyox, *Union Carbide*) gels were unaffected. The gels could be stabilised by adsorbing the neomycin on a cation-exchange resin (Amberlite IRP-69M) before incorporation in the gel.— A. Heyd, *J. pharm. Sci.*, 1971, *60*, 1343.

There was no significant loss of potency when neomycin powder was added to each of 3 commercially available 0.5% hypromellose solutions in plastic squeezy bottles (Lacril, pH 5.9; Tearisol, pH 7.3; Isoptotears, pH 7.4) and the resulting solutions of neomycin 33 mg per ml kept at 25° for 7 days. Neomycin and Lacril produced a slightly insoluble mixture.— E. Osborn *et al.*, *Am. J. Ophthal.*, 1976, *82*, 775.

The stability of neomycin preparations was shown to be enhanced by propylene glycol and sodium metabisulphite.— N. A. Hodges and J. Singh, *J. Pharm. Pharmac.*, 1978, *30*, 737.

Units. One unit of neomycin is contained in 0.0012903 mg of the second International Reference Preparation (1974) of neomycin sulphate which contains 775 units per mg.

Collaborative assay by 11 laboratories of the material now established as the Second International Reference Preparation of Neomycin. Chemical examination in 4 or 5 laboratories showed a mean of 91.05% of neomycin B, 8.62% of neomycin C, and less than 1% of neamine.— J. W. Lightbown *et al.*, *J. biol. Stand.*, 1979, *7*, 227.

Adverse Effects. Neomycin may cause irreversible partial or total deafness when given by injection, by mouth, by enema or by instillation into cavities, or when applied as solutions or aerosols to open wounds or damaged skin. The effect is dose-related and is enhanced by renal or hepatic impairment. Progressive loss of hearing may continue after neomycin is discontinued. Reversible kidney damage may occur after systemic therapy and is also dose-related. The risk of nephrotoxicity is not great when neomycin is given by mouth in recommended doses, as neomycin is poorly absorbed.

Blood and urine of patients receiving neomycin parenterally should be examined frequently for evidence of renal damage and audiometric tests should be carried out, especially if the patients have previously been treated with streptomycin.

When given by mouth neomycin in large doses causes nausea, vomiting, and diarrhoea. Prolonged oral therapy may cause a malabsorption syndrome with steatorrhoea and diarrhoea which can be very severe. Supra-infection may occur, especially with prolonged oral treatment, and staphylococcal enterocolitis has been reported.

Neomycin has a neuromuscular blocking action similar to but stronger than that of streptomycin, gentamicin, or kanamycin, and respiratory depression and arrest has followed the instillation of neomycin into the intestines of anaesthetised patients.

Hypersensitivity reactions, usually of the delayed type, occur frequently during local treatment with neomycin but may be masked by the combined use of a corticosteroid. Cross-sensitivity with other aminoglycoside antibiotics may occur.

Allergy. Of 1205 persons with dermatitis or eczema submitted to patch testing with neomycin sulphate 40% in yellow soft paraffin, 1.7% gave a positive reaction.— E. Rudzki and D. Kleniewska, *Br. J. Derm.*, 1970, *83*, 543.

Of 4000 patients subjected to patch testing in 5 European clinics 3.6% of males and 3.7% of females showed positive reactions to neomycin sulphate 20% in soft paraffin.— H. Bandmann *et al.*, *Archs Derm.*, 1972, *106*, 335.

Of 2175 subjects who were patch-tested with a preparation containing neomycin sulphate 20%, only 2 out of 22 who had reactions were judged to have clear-cut contact allergy. All the other reactions were described as being of a non-allergic irritant type.— J. J. Leyden and A. M. Kligman, *J. Am. med. Ass.*, 1979, *242*, 1276.

Further references: K. Wereide, *Acta derm.-vener., Stockh.*, 1970, *50*, 114; L. Förström and V. Pirilä, *Contact Dermatitis*, 1978, *4*, 312, per *Abstr. Hyg.*, 1979, *54*, 494.

Colitis. *Clostridium difficile*-associated colitis in a patient treated with neomycin responded to treatment with metronidazole.— R. P. Bolton, *Br. med. J.*, 1979, *2*, 1479.

Malabsorption syndrome. Lactose malabsorption and reduction in disaccharidases in the small bowel was induced after 3 days' therapy with neomycin sulphate, 8 g daily. Histological study of the bowel mucosa suggested that neomycin had a direct toxic action.— G. D. Cain *et al.*, *Archs intern. Med.*, 1968, *122*, 311.

Further references: A. I. Rogers *et al.*, *J. Am. med. Ass.*, 1966, *197*, 185; G. F. Longstreth and A. D. Newcomer, *Mayo Clin. Proc.*, 1975, *50*, 284.

Ototoxicity. A brief review of the occurrence of deafness after the use of neomycin by a variety of routes.— E. S. Harpur (letter), *Pharm. J.*, 1977, *1*, 494.

Complete loss of eighth cranial nerve function with total deafness, vertigo, and nystagmus in a 9-year-old girl was attributed to systemic absorption of neomycin following its topical application with dimethyl sulphoxide.— J. K. Herd *et al.*, *Pediatrics*, 1967, *40*, 905.

Three patients became deaf and developed acute renal failure, and 1 also developed muscular weakness and apnoea after their orthopaedic wounds had been irrigated with solutions containing neomycin. Treatment included haemodialysis.— J. E. Davia *et al.*, *Archs intern. Med.*, 1970, *125*, 135.

Of 13 patients with liver disease who had been given neomycin by mouth, 6 developed irreversible deafness. Total doses ranged from 84 to 4500 g. Neomycin could cause deafness when used to irrigate wounds and burns, by inhalation for bronchiectasis, and by application in the ear.— J. Ballantyne, *J. Lar. Otol.*, 1970, *84*, 967.

The Boston Collaborative Drug Surveillance Program monitored consecutively 32 812 medical inpatients. Drug-induced deafness occurred in 7 of 802 patients given neomycin.— J. Porter and H. Jick, *Lancet*, 1977, *1*, 587.

The Committee on Safety of Medicines had issued a warning on the use of aerosol preparations of neomycin. Deafness had occurred following the use of such preparations in the treatment of extensive skin damage from burns or other causes.— *Lancet*, 1977, *1*, 1115.

A reminder of the increased risk of drug-induced deafness in patients with perforation of the tympanic membrane when otitis externa is treated topically with preparations containing aminoglycoside antibiotics such as framycetin and neomycin. It is important to ensure that there is no perforation before such preparations are prescribed.— Committee on Safety of Medicines, *Current Problems Series No. 5*, 1981.

Overdosage. A patient who was inadvertently given 6 g of neomycin by intramuscular injection for hepatic coma developed anuria but was managed successfully by haemodialysis.— F. A. Krumlovsky *et al.*, *Ann. intern. Med.*, 1972, *76*, 443.

A fatality preceded by deafness in a patient inadvertently given 8 g of neomycin intramuscularly instead of by mouth.— L. D. Lowry *et al.*, *Ann. Otol. Rhinol. Lar.*, 1973, *82*, 876.

Treatment of Adverse Effects. Patients who develop renal failure may be treated with haemodialysis or peritoneal dialysis although the rate of removal of neomycin is slow. The neuromuscular blocking activity of neomycin may sometimes be reversed by neostigmine or a calcium salt and corticosteroids have been given to treat sensitivity reactions.

Precautions. Neomycin is contra-indicated for intestinal disinfection when an obstruction is present and in patients with a known history of allergy to neomycin. It should be used with great care in patients with kidney or liver disease and in those with impaired hearing. The topical use of neomycin in patients with extensive skin damage or perforated tympanic membranes may result in deafness (see Adverse Effects, above). The parenteral use of neomycin is no longer recommended. Intraperitoneal instillation of neomycin may precipitate respiratory paralysis in patients who have received neuromuscular blocking agents.

Prolonged local use should be avoided as it may lead to skin sensitisation. Neomycin by mouth and possibly the parenteral administration of other aminoglycosides such as gentamicin, might cause immediate skin sensitivity reactions in patients previously sensitised by the topical use of neomycin.

As with streptomycin (see p.1214), neomycin should be used with caution in patients receiving other drugs with neuromuscular blocking activity, anticoagulants, anti-emetics, and other drugs which are ototoxic.

Neomycin, taken by mouth, has been reported to impair the absorption of other drugs including phenoxymethylpenicillin and digoxin; the efficacy of oral contraceptives might be reduced.

A 7-month-old child who had received six 100-mg doses of neomycin on the day before anticipated surgery developed respiratory depression and cyanosis after a saline enema, possibly due to increased absorption of neomycin caused by the enema.— G. F. Marx *et al.*, *Can. Anaesth. Soc. J.*, 1965, *12*, 415.

A recommendation that the dose of neomycin for topical treatment should not exceed 1 g daily for 7 days. Higher or more prolonged dosage would appear to be ototoxic.— C. Diamond, *Adverse Drug React. Bull.*, 1978, Apr., 244.

Effect on blood estimations. Neomycin could interfere biologically with chemical estimations for cholesterol in the blood to produce erroneous lowered results.— *Drug & Ther. Bull.*, 1972, *10*, 69.

Interactions. For reports of other compounds affecting the antimicrobial activity of neomycin, see Antimicrobial Action, below.

Pregnancy and the neonate. Deafness in the infant of a mother given neomycin during pregnancy has been reported.— J. M. Forrest, *Med. J. Aust.*, 1976, *2*, 138.

Antimicrobial Action. Neomycin has a mode of action and spectrum of activity similar to those of streptomycin sulphate (p.1214) and kanamycin sulphate (p.1175). It is bactericidal and effective against staphylococci and a wide range of Gram-negative bacteria including *Escherichia coli*, *Klebsiella*, *Haemophilus influenzae*, *Proteus*, *Salmonella*, and *Shigella*. *Mycobacterium tuberculosis* is sensitive. Neomycin is most active in alkaline media.

The minimum inhibitory concentrations of neomycin have been reported to range from 0.5 to 8 μg per ml.

Diminished activity. In concentrations of 30 μg or more per ml heparin decreased *in vitro* the antibacterial effect of neomycin 1 μg per ml against *Staphylococcus aureus*.— W. P. Raab and J. Windisch, *Arzneimittel-Forsch.*, 1973, *23*, 1326.

Aspirin decreased the antibacterial effect *in vitro* of neomycin sulphate against *Staph. aureus* and *E. coli*.— M. A. Toama *et al.*, *J. pharm. Sci.*, 1978, *67*, 23.

For reports of various compounds decreasing the activity of neomycin, see above under Loss of Activity.

Enhanced activity. Sensitivity studies carried out on *Staph. aureus* and *Pseudomonas aeruginosa* demonstrated that caffeine and theophylline enhanced the antimicrobial activity of neomycin against these organisms *in vitro*.— B. G. Charles and B. D. Rawal, *Lancet*, 1973, *1*, 971.

Urea might enhance the antimicrobial activity of neomycin against staphylococci and *Ps. aeruginosa*.— B. W. Burt and G. Dempsey, *Pharm. J.*, 1977, *2*, 255.

Resistance. Resistance to neomycin and the other aminoglycoside antibiotics, apart from streptomycin, is acquired slowly. It is often associated with the plasmid-mediated production of bacterial enzymes. Frequent and long-term use has led to resistant staphylococci. Strains of *Escherichia coli* resistant to neomycin have been isolated from the urine of patients given kanamycin and resistant *Proteus* strains have been isolated from the faeces of patients given neomycin by mouth.

There is almost complete cross-resistance between neomycin, kanamycin, paromomycin, and framycetin. Cross-resistance with gentamicin has also been reported.

In 11 of 14 patients who had taken neomycin for at least 3 months for hypercholesterolaemia, coliform bacteria from the gut were resistant to several antimicrobial agents and the resistance was transferable to *E. coli*.— M. V. Valtonen *et al.*, *Br. med. J.*, 1977, *1*, 683.

Resistance of salmonellae. Of 400 strains of *Salmonella* isolated from patients in the USA during 1967, 5 were resistant to neomycin sulphate. Assessment of resistance was based upon a zone of inhibition of 11 mm or less using disks containing 30 μg of neomycin sulphate.— S. A. Schroeder *et al.*, *J. Am. med. Ass.*, 1968, *205*, 903.

Absorption and Fate. Neomycin is poorly absorbed from the alimentary tract, about 97% of an orally administered dose being excreted unchanged in the faeces. Doses of 3 to 4 g by mouth produce peak plasma concentrations of up to 4 μg per ml and absorption is similar after administration by enema. It is, however, rapidly absorbed after intramuscular injection, doses of 0.5 to 1 g producing a plasma concentration of about 20 μg per ml. Absorption has also been reported to occur from the peritoneum, respiratory tract, bladder, wounds, and inflamed skin.

Once neomycin is absorbed it is rapidly excreted by the kidneys in active form; 30 to 50% of a parenteral dose has been detected in the urine.

No difference in absorption of neomycin, assessed by urinary excretion, was observed in 7 healthy subjects given 2 g in a fasting or non-fasting state and no difference in absorption was observed in subjects given neomycin by mouth or as an enema. Antacids did not affect gastro-intestinal absorption nor did gastro-intestinal ulcerative disease. Prolonging the enema retention time or giving a prior cleansing enema did not affect rectal absorption.— K. J. Breen *et al., Ann. intern. Med.*, 1972, *76*, 211.

The biological half-life of neomycin was 2 hours.— W. M. Bennett *et al., J. Am. med. Ass.*, 1973, *223*, 991. In premature infants it was 3.7 to 5.4 hours (according to age).— W. A. Ritschel, *Drug Intell. & clin. Pharm.*, 1970, *4*, 332.

Systemic absorption of neomycin from a wound irrigation solution containing neomycin 1% occurred in 10 patients undergoing hip surgery. Serum neomycin reached concentrations which have been associated with toxic reactions.— A. J. Weinstein *et al., J. Am. med. Ass.*, 1977, *238*, 152.

Uses. Neomycin sulphate is administered topically in the treatment of infections of the skin and eye due to susceptible staphylococci and other organisms. Neomycin undecenoate or sulphate is used in ear-drops.

To prevent the development of resistant strains, another antibacterial agent such as bacitracin, polymyxin B, or chlorhexidine is sometimes used in conjunction with neomycin.

A cream containing neomycin sulphate and chlorhexidine hydrochloride has been used for application to the nostrils in the treatment of staphylococcal nasal carriers but resistant organisms have developed.

Because neomycin sulphate is poorly absorbed from the gastro-intestinal tract, it has been given by mouth for the suppression of bacterial growth in the intestine before abdominal surgery although the development of resistant organisms may be encouraged and supra-infection may occur; it is used similarly, with other antibacterial agents, in neutropenic patients. Neomycin is given to patients with hepatic encephalopathy to suppress ammonia-forming bacteria in the gastro-intestinal tract and may also be used in the treatment of infective diarrhoea caused by *Escherichia coli*.

For pre-operative use, 1 g of neomycin sulphate is given by mouth every 4 hours for 6 doses or more but for no longer than 3 days; if time is short, 1 g may be given hourly for 4 hours and then every 4 hours. For the treatment of intestinal infections a total daily dosage of 50 to 80 mg per kg body-weight may be given in 3 or 4 divided doses. Children have been given up to approximately 100 mg per kg daily in divided doses.

As an adjunct in the management of hepatic coma, 4 to 12 g may be given daily in divided doses; prolonged administration may cause malabsorption.

Neomycin sulphate was formerly administered by intramuscular injection for the treatment of systemic or urinary-tract infections but it has been replaced by equally effective and less toxic antibiotics.

Neomycin has also been used as the palmitate.

Dialysis. Infection during peritoneal dialysis had been eliminated by the adoption of 2 measures: the prophylactic administration of neomycin by mouth, and the percutaneous use of thin stylet catheters for only 2 or 3 days each and then re-inserted as necessary. Before these changes, when protective isolation of the patient had been employed, the incidence of peritonitis was nearly 50%. Invariably this was caused by enteric organisms. Since starting to use neomycin, 2 g daily for 3 days, both the need for protective isolation and the use of tetracycline in the dialysis fluid (12.5 mg per litre) had been abandoned as unnecessary.— F. D. Schwartz *et al., J. Am. med. Ass.*, 1967, *199*, 79.

There was no difference in the incidence of peritonitis and of significant asymptomatic infection in patients given neomycin 500 mg every 6 hours for 48 hours or placebo in a study of patients undergoing 95 peritoneal dialyses.— B. K. Sharma *et al., Am. J. med. Sci.*, 1971, *262*, 175.

Dosage in renal failure. The use of neomycin should be avoided in uraemic patients.— G. B. Appel and H. C. Neu, *New Engl. J. Med.*, 1977, *296*, 722.

Enteritis. Neomycin 100 mg per kg body-weight daily was given by mouth for various periods to 113 infants to terminate *Escherichia coli* diarrhoeal disease. Bacteriological relapse occurred in 7 of 56 infants treated for an average of 3 days and in 14 of 57 treated for 10 days.— J. D. Nelson, *Pediatrics*, 1971, *48*, 248.

In a controlled study of 77 patients with acute gastroenteritis, treatment with a mixture containing kaolin and neomycin was less effective than kaolin alone.— M. T. Everett, *J.R. Coll. gen. Pract.*, 1973, *23*, 183.

Hypercholesterolaemia. A reappraisal of neomycin in the treatment of hypercholesterolaemia. Neomycin has been shown to decrease plasma concentrations of cholesterol by 20 to 30% and has been reported to be effective even in some patients with resistant familial hypercholesterolaemia. The usual dose of 2 g daily is gradually decreased when possible to as little as 500 mg daily taken at bedtime. Administration for from 2 weeks to 8 years has been reported and has generally been well tolerated, with transient diarrhoea and abdominal cramps in one-third to one-half of patients usually subsiding after 10 to 14 days. However, neomycin is potentially toxic and the small amount absorbed from the gastro-intestinal tract is excreted through the kidneys. It should not be given to patients whose renal function is compromised but can be used safely in selected high-risk patients with hypercholesterolaemia providing that frequent monitoring for undesirable side-effects is undertaken.— P. Samuel, *New Engl. J. Med.*, 1979, *301*, 595. Neomycin should only be used in patients with familial type II hyperlipidaemia unresponsive to diet and who are unable to take alternative agents.— S. Meisel and R. Rate (letter), *ibid.*, 1980, *302*, 233. Reply.— P. Samuel (letter), *ibid.*

Further references to neomycin in hypercholesterolaemia: *Drug & Ther. Bull.*, 1980, *18*, 25; *Med. Lett.*, 1980, *22*, 65.

Skin infections. Trophic plantar ulcers in leprosy patients were treated with an antibiotic spray (Polybactrin), antibiotic cream (Cicatrin), and antibiotic powder (Cicatrin). Treatment with the spray with either the cream or powder gave the best results. Of 17 ulcers treated, only 1 showed no improvement.— I. A. Susman, *Lepr. Rev.*, 1967, *38*, 213.

It was considered that topical neomycin preparations were ineffective in the treatment and prophylaxis of skin infections.— *Med. Lett.*, 1973, *15*, 101.

An extensive review of the topical use of neomycin and other antibiotics such as bacitracin, gramicidin, polymyxin B, and the tetracyclines for the prophylactic and therapeutic control of infections in superficial wounds and skin abrasions. The proper use of topical preparations containing these antibiotics was generally considered safe and effective.— V. Anderson, *Int. J. Derm.*, 1976, *15* (No.2), *Suppl.*, 1-118. See also *Br. med. J.*, 1977, *1*, 738.

Corticosteroid-antibiotic combinations are recommended for the management of secondarily infected dermatoses although long-term topical use of antibiotics should be avoided. A neomycin-corticosteroid preparation is suggested for *Staphylococcus aureus* infections. The allergenicity of neomycin is considered to be exaggerated; the majority of contact allergies follow prolonged application to chronically inflamed skin but brief or intermittent use does not appear to carry a high risk of sensitisation. There is no evidence that wide-spread use of neomycin might lead to cross-resistance to gentamicin.— J. J. Leyden and A. M. Kligman, *Br. J. Derm.*, 1977, *96*, 179. Agreement with this view. The short-term use of neomycin, especially in children, appears to carry little risk of sensitisation and for dermatoses infected with *Staph. aureus* neomycin is usually the antibiotic of choice. Prolonged use should be avoided as should any application of neomycin to eczema or ulcers of the lower leg.— *Br. med. J.*, 1977, *1*, 1303. See also R. F. A. Becke, *Drugs*, 1977, *14*, 394.

The application of neomycin or other antibiotics to infected ulcers is generally not necessary and their use is discouraged.— M. R. Sather *et al., Drug Intell. & clin. Pharm.*, 1977, *11*, 154.

Further references: *Br. med. J.*, 1977, *1*, 1494.

Suppression of intestinal flora. Infection from endogenous bacteria was prevented in 16 patients with burns who received the following treatment for an average of 24 days; neomycin sulphate 500 mg with erythromycin 500 mg every six hours by mouth or nasogastric tube and nystatin 500 000 units every 8 hours.— F. Jarrett *et al., J. Am. med. Ass.*, 1977, *237*, 2179.

Neomycin has been substituted for framycetin and is given prophylactically with 2 other oral non-absorbable antibiotics, colistin and nystatin (the NEOCON regimen), to patients with acute non-lymphoblastic leukaemia who are also nursed in protective isolation. The Royal Marsden Hospital leukaemia unit now suggests the following regimen for these patients: one tablet twice daily of neomycin sulphate 500 mg, colistin sulphate 1.5 million units, and nystatin 500 000 units; nystatin as syrup 100 000 units twice daily; chlorhexidine obstetric cream 1% to vagina and vulva twice daily; and lozenges of amphotericin 10 mg, sucked four times daily; chlorhexidine mouth-washes (0.02% aqueous) are used only if necessary.— J. G. Watson and B. Jameson (letter), *Lancet*, 1979, *1*, 1183.

Analysis of 41 consecutive cases of peritonitis in 29 patients with terminal renal failure on peritoneal dialysis, revealed that the intestinal flora is a relatively rare source of peritonitis. The use of non-absorbable intestinal antibiotics is accordingly not advisable.— H. J. Kolmos and K. E. H. Andersen (letter), *Lancet*, 1979, *1*, 1355.

See also under Surgical Infection Prophylaxis, below.

Surgical infection prophylaxis. A technique for preparing patients for large-bowel surgery involving flushing out the entire gastro-intestinal tract with a solution of electrolytes was evaluated. The time for preparation was reduced from several days to 2 to 3 hours and the addition of neomycin 1 mg per ml to the irrigant eliminated *E. coli* and *Streptococcus faecalis*.— J. Hewitt *et al., Lancet*, 1973, *2*, 337.

The incidence of wound infection was 6 of 76 (7.9%) when wounds were sprayed during closure with neomycin, bacitracin, and polymyxin B (Polybactrin or Rikospray) compared with 8 of 39 (20.5%) when washed with sterile saline or 0.02% chlorhexidine. For contaminated wounds (endodermal cavities) the difference was significant.— S. J. Hildred and C. J. Henderson, *Br. med. J.*, 1977, *2*, 869.

The frequency of postoperative pelvic infection following vaginal hysterectomy was 16% in a group of 50 patients for whom a topical aerosol spray containing neomycin sulphate, polymyxin B sulphate, and bacitracin zinc (Sterispray) was used prophylactically, and 34% in a similar group using a placebo spray.— V. C. Wright *et al., Can. med. Ass. J.*, 1978, *118*, 1395.

A conclusion that systemic antimicrobial therapy, given at the time of operation only, and antiseptics used locally should replace oral prophylaxis before surgery.— *Lancet*, 1978, *2*, 1132.

Comment on the controversy over the choice of antimicrobial agent for pre-operative preparation of the colon. In a controlled study of 53 patients undergoing colorectal surgery, those given neomycin and metronidazole pre-operatively fared better than those who received neomycin and erythromycin. All patients received a single intravenous dose of cephaloridine at induction.— A. V. Pollock and M. Evans (letter), *New Engl. J. Med.*, 1980, *303*, 1066.

For reviews and discussions on surgical infection prophylaxis see under Prophylactic Use of Antibiotics, p.1081.

Urinary-tract infections. In a double-blind study a sterile solution of neomycin sulphate 0.2% in saline was more effective than sterile saline in preventing bacteriuria following catheterisation. The solutions (40 ml) were instilled into the bladder before removal of the catheter, or if the catheter was left indwelling it was clamped for 15 minutes and the procedure repeated daily.— L. Clark, *Med. J. Aust.*, 1973, *1*, 1034.

A randomised controlled study in 187 catheterised patients failed to demonstrate a reduction of urinary-tract infections in 89 who were irrigated with a solution of neomycin sulphate 0.004% and polymyxin B sulphate 0.002% in physiological saline using a triple-lumen closed catheter system. Infecting organisms in those who underwent irrigation were significantly more resistant to the antibiotics used than were those recovered from 98 patients who were not irrigated.— J. W. Warren *et al., New Engl. J. Med.*, 1978, *299*, 570. See also A. M. Haldorson *et al., Antimicrob. Ag. Chemother.*, 1978, *14*, 368.

Further references: K. F. Fairley *et al., Lancet*, 1967, *2*,

427; F. Hinman and F. O. Belzer, *J. Urol.*, 1969, *101*, 477.

Preparations containing a corticosteroid and neomycin sulphate which are used mainly for their anti-inflammatory effects are described in the section on Corticosteroids, p.446..

Creams

NCP Cream. Neomycin sulphate 2 mg, chlorhexidine hydrochloride 1 mg, polymyxin B 1 mg, cetomacrogol emulsifying wax q.s., water to 1 g. A prophylactic cream for the treatment of burns.—J.S. Cason and E.J.L. Lowbury, *Lancet*, 1960, *2*, 501.

Neomycin Cream *(B.P.C. 1973).* Neomycin sulphate 500 mg, chlorocresol 100 mg, disodium edetate 10 mg, cetomacrogol emulsifying ointment 30 g, and freshly boiled and cooled water 69.39 g. A phosphate buffer may be included. Store in a cool place in well-closed containers which prevent evaporation and contamination.

Dental Preparations

Dental Paste for Dry Socket. Neomycin sulphate 800 mg, paramethasone acetate 16 mg, water 2 ml, zinc oxide 10 g, macrogol '4000' 15 g, and macrogol '1500' 5 g. Each 500-mg application contained 12.5 mg of neomycin sulphate and 250 µg of paramethasone acetate. A piece of paste was moulded into the previously isolated and dried tooth socket. When stored in a well-closed container in a cool place and protected from light the paste retained its activity for at least 12 months. Encouraging results had been claimed.—C.W. Shuttleworth, *Br. dent. J.*, 1967, *122*, 234.

Dental Root-canal Paste. The following paste had antibiotic and antifungal properties, and was effective in sterilising infected root canals in an average of 2 dressings. There should be little risk of hypersensitivity. Neomycin sulphate 2 g, polymyxin B sulphate 100 mg, bacitracin 500 mg, nystatin 500 000 units, macrogol basis to 10 g.—G.B. Winter, *Br. dent. J.*, 1966, *120*, 11.

Dusting-powders

Neomycin and Bacitracin Dusting-powder *(Nord. P.).* Conspergens Topicini. Neomycin sulphate 250 mg, bacitracin 500 mg, and sterilised absorbable dusting-powder 99.25 g.

Ear-drops

Bacitracin, Neomycin and Polymyxin Ear Drops *(A.P.F.).* Neomycin sulphate 50 mg, bacitracin 10 000 units, polymyxin B sulphate 100 000 units, propylene glycol to 10 ml. These ear-drops should be freshly prepared, stored at a temperature not exceeding 8°, protected from light, and used within 1 week.

Neomycin and Polymyxin B Sulfates and Hydrocortisone Otic Solution *(U.S.P.).* Neomycin and Polymyxin B Sulfates and Cortisol Otic Solution. A sterile solution containing neomycin sulphate, polymyxin B sulphate, and hydrocortisone. It may contain one or more suitable buffers, dispersing agents, and solvents. Potency is expressed in terms of the equivalent amounts of neomycin and polymyxin B. When no strength is specified a solution containing in each ml the equivalent of 3.5 mg of neomycin, the equivalent of 10 000 units of polymyxin B, and hydrocortisone 10 mg is supplied. pH 2 to 4.5. Store in airtight containers. Protect from light.

Neomycin and Polymyxin B Sulfates and Hydrocortisone Otic Suspension *(U.S.P.).* Neomycin and Polymyxin B Sulfates and Cortisol Otic Suspension. A suspension of neomycin sulphate, polymyxin B sulphate, and hydrocortisone. It may contain one or more suitable buffers, dispersing agents, and preservatives. Potency is expressed in terms of the equivalent amounts of neomycin and polymyxin B. When no strength is specified a suspension containing in each ml the equivalent of 3.5 mg of neomycin, the equivalent of 10 000 units of polymyxin B, and hydrocortisone 10 mg is supplied. pH 3 to 5.5. Store in airtight containers. Protect from light.

Elixirs

Neomycin Elixir *(B.P.C. 1973).* Neomycin Mixture; Neomycin Sulphate Mixture. Neomycin sulphate 200 mg, benzoic acid 20 mg, saccharin sodium 9 mg, disodium edetate 5 mg, citric acid monohydrate q.s., sorbitol solution 3.85 ml, compound tartrazine solution 0.06 ml, freshly boiled and cooled water to 10 ml. The mixture may be lime-flavoured; the compound tartrazine solution may be replaced by any other suitable food grade dye or dyes approved for use in food in the country concerned. If the mixture is recently prepared, the disodium edetate may be omitted. If necessary, add sufficient citric acid monohydrate to produce a pH of 4 to 5. Store in a cool place. Protect from light. The mixture contains 400 mg (approx. 250 000 units) of neomycin sulphate in each 20 ml. *Dose.* Children: up to 1 year, 2.5 to 10 ml every 6 hours; 1 to 5 years, 10 to 20 ml every 6 hours.

Eye Ointments

Bacitracin, Neomycin and Polymyxin Eye Ointment *(A.P.F.).* Neomycin sulphate 5 mg, bacitracin zinc 400 units, polymyxin B sulphate 5000 units, Eye Ointment Base *A.P.F.* 1 g. Prepared aseptically.

Neomycin and Polymyxin B Sulfates and Bacitracin Zinc Ophthalmic Ointment *(U.S.P.).* A sterile eye ointment containing neomycin sulphate, polymyxin B sulphate, and bacitracin zinc. Potency is expressed in terms of the equivalent amounts of neomycin, polymyxin B, and bacitracin. Store in airtight containers.

Neomycin and Polymyxin B Sulfates, Bacitracin Zinc, and Hydrocortisone Ophthalmic Ointment *(U.S.P.).* A sterile eye ointment containing neomycin sulphate, polymyxin B sulphate, bacitracin zinc, and hydrocortisone. Potency is expressed in terms of the equivalent amount of neomycin, polymyxin B, and bacitracin. Store at 15° to 30° in airtight containers.

Neomycin Eye Ointment *(B.P.C. 1973).* A sterile eye ointment containing neomycin sulphate in Eye Ointment Basis. *U.S.P.* (Neomycin Sulfate Ophthalmic Ointment) specifies the equivalent of 0.35% of neomycin.

Neomycin Sulfate and Dexamethasone Sodium Phosphate Ophthalmic Ointment *(U.S.P.).* A sterile eye ointment containing neomycin sulphate and dexamethasone sodium phosphate. Potency is expressed in terms of the equivalent amounts of neomycin and dexamethasone phosphate. When no strength is specified an ointment containing in each g the equivalent of 3.5 mg of neomycin and the equivalent of 500 µg of dexamethasone phosphate is supplied. Store at 15° to 30°.

Neomycin Sulfate and Prednisolone Sodium Phosphate Ophthalmic Ointment *(U.S.P.).* A sterile eye ointment containing neomycin sulphate and prednisolone sodium phosphate. Potency is expressed in terms of the equivalent amounts of neomycin and prednisolone phosphate. When no strength is specified an ointment containing in each g the equivalent of 3.5 mg of neomycin and the equivalent of 2.5 mg of prednisolone phosphate is supplied. Store at 15° to 30°.

Eye-Drops

Bacitracin, Neomycin and Polymyxin Eye Drops *(A.P.F.).* Neomycin sulphate 50 mg, bacitracin 5000 units, polymyxin B sulphate 50 000 units, boric acid 150 mg, chlorbutol 50 mg, Water for Injections to 10 ml. Prepared aseptically. These eye-drops should be freshly prepared, stored below 25°, protected from light, and used within 1 week.

Neomycin and Polymyxin B Sulfates and Gramicidin Ophthalmic Solution *(U.S.P.).* A sterile solution in an iso-osmotic aqueous vehicle containing in each ml the equivalent of 1.75 mg of neomycin and 5000 units of polymyxin B, with gramicidin 25 µg; it contains one or more suitable buffers, dispersing agents, and preservatives. pH 4.7 to 6. Store at a temperature not exceeding 40° in airtight containers.

Neomycin and Polymyxin B Sulfates Ophthalmic Solution *(U.S.P.).* A sterile solution containing in each ml the equivalent of 3.5 mg of neomycin and the equivalent of 5000 or 16 250 units of polymyxin B; it may contain one or more suitable buffers, irrigants, preservatives, and dispersing agents. pH 5 to 7. Store at a temperature not exceeding 40° in airtight containers.

Neomycin Eye Drops *(A.P.F.).* Neomycin sulphate 500 mg, sodium acid phosphate 700 mg, sodium phosphate 700 mg, sodium chloride 400 mg, disodium edetate 10 mg, phenylmercuric nitrate 2 mg, Water for Injections to 100 ml. Sterilised by maintaining at 98° to 100° for 30 minutes. Store in a cool place. Protect from light.

Neomycin Eye-drops *(B.P.C. 1973).* NEO. A sterile solution containing up to 0.5% of neomycin sulphate, with 0.7% of sodium acid phosphate, 0.7% of sodium phosphate, and 0.002% of phenylmercuric acetate or nitrate, in water. It may also contain 0.01% of disodium edetate. Sterilised by filtration or by maintaining at 98° to 100° for 30 minutes. Protect from light.

Neomycin Sulfate and Dexamethasone Sodium Phosphate Ophthalmic Solution *(U.S.P.).* A sterile aqueous solution of neomycin sulphate and dexamethasone sodium phosphate; it may contain one or more suitable buffers, dispersing agents, and preservatives. Potency is expressed in terms of the equivalent amounts of neomycin and dexamethasone phosphate. When no strength is specified a solution containing in each ml the equivalent of 3.5 mg of neomycin and the equivalent of 1 mg of dexamethasone phosphate is supplied. pH 6 to 8. Store at a temperature not exceeding 40° in airtight containers. Protect from light.

Oculoguttae Topicini *(Nord. P.).* Neomycin sulphate 500 mg, bacitracin 1 g, sodium chloride 800 mg, and Water for Injections 97.7 g. Prepared aseptically.

Insufflations

Bacitracin, Neomycin and Polymyxin Insufflation *(A.P.F.).* Neomycin sulphate 50 mg, bacitracin zinc 5000 units, polymyxin B sulphate 50 000 units, lactose, sterilised, to 10 g. Prepared aseptically. Store below 25° in airtight containers.

Mixtures

Neomycin Mixture CF *(A.P.F.).* Neomycin Mixture for Children. Neomycin sulphate 250 mg, disodium edetate 2.5 mg, syrup 1 ml, concentrated chloroform water 0.1 ml, water to 5 ml. *Dose.* 5 to 10 ml given 4 times daily is a suitable dose for a child weighing 20 kg.

Neomycin Sulfate Oral Solution *(U.S.P.).* A solution containing neomycin sulphate equivalent to 17.5 mg of neomycin per ml; it may contain one or more suitable colouring and flavouring agents and preservatives. pH 5 to 7.5. Store in airtight containers. Protect from light.

Ointments

Neomycin and Bacitracin Ointment *(B.P.C. 1973).* Neomycin sulphate 500 mg, bacitracin zinc 50 000 units, liquid paraffin 10 g, white soft paraffin to 100 g. Store in airtight containers. The ointment may be expected to retain its potency for 2 years provided that the moisture content does not exceed 0.2%. The moisture content may be expected to be below this figure when *B.P.* materials are used.

Neomycin Sulfate Ointment *(U.S.P.).* An ointment containing neomycin sulphate equivalent to 3.5 mg of neomycin per g.

Neomycin and Polymyxin B Sulfates and Bacitracin Zinc Ointment *(U.S.P.).* It contains in each g the equivalent of 3 mg of neomycin, 8000 units of polymyxin B, and 400 units of bacitracin or the equivalent of 3.5 mg, 5000 units, and 400 units respectively; it may contain 1% of hydrocortisone acetate.

Unguentum Topicini *(Nord. P.).* Neomycin sulphate 500 mg, bacitracin 1 g, wool fat 10 g, and yellow soft paraffin 88.5 g.

Unguentum Topicini cum Hydrocortisono *(Dan. Disp.).* Neomycin sulphate 500 mg, bacitracin 1 g, hydrocortisone 1 g, wool fat 10 g, and yellow soft paraffin 87.5 g. Prepared aseptically. Store in a cool place. Protect from light. Use within 1 year of preparation.

Solutions

Neomycin and Polymyxin B Sulfates Solution for Irrigation *(U.S.P.).* A sterile aqueous solution containing the equivalent of 40 mg of neomycin and 200 000 units of polymyxin B per ml. It may contain a suitable preservative. pH 4.5 to 6. Store in airtight containers. For use, after dilution, for bladder irrigation.

Suspensions

Neomycin Sulphate, Bacitracin, and Hydrocortisone Acetate Suspension *(Hadassah Univ. Hosp.).* Neomycin sulphate 1 g, bacitracin 1 g, hydrocortisone acetate 500 mg, sterile methylcellulose solution (2%) 50 ml, sterile water to 100 ml. Prepared aseptically. Used for burns.

Tablets

Neomycin Tablets *(B.P.).* Tablets containing neomycin sulphate. Store at a temperature not exceeding 30°. Protect from light. *U.S.P.* (Neomycin Sulfate Tablets) specifies the equivalent of 150, 175, or 350 mg of neomycin. Store in airtight containers.

NOTE. Proprietary preparations containing a corticosteroid and neomycin sulphate which are used mainly for their anti-inflammatory effects are described in the section on Corticosteroids, p.446.

Audicort *(Lederle, UK).* Ear-drops containing in each ml neomycin undecenoate equivalent to neomycin 3.5 mg and undecenoic acid 7 mg, triamcinolone acetonide 1 mg, and benzocaine 50 mg. For bacterial or fungous infections of the ear.

Cicatrin (known in some countries as Cicatrex or Cicatrene) *(Calmic, UK).* **Aerosol Spray** consisting of a pressurised spray of 100 g providing 3 g of dry powder, each g of which contains neomycin sulphate 16 500 units, bacitracin zinc 1250 units, glycine 60 mg, and L-cysteine 12 mg, in a basis of absorbable dusting-powder. **Cream** containing in each g neomycin sulphate 3300 units, bacitracin zinc 250 units, glycine 10 mg, L-cysteine 2 mg, and DL-threonine 1 mg. **Powder** of the same composition as the cream.

Dispray Antibiotic Powder Spray *(Stuart, UK).* A sterile aerosol spray of 110 g containing 1.2 g of powder, providing neomycin sulphate 650 000 units, polymyxin B sulphate 165 000 units, and bacitracin zinc 10 000 units, with propellent. For the prevention of infection during surgery and the treatment of infected cuts.

Graneodin *(Squibb, UK).* **Ointment** and **Ophthalmic Ointment** each containing neomycin sulphate equivalent to neomycin 2.5 mg and gramicidin 250 μg per g in a basis of white wax, white soft paraffin, and arachis oil.

Gregoderm Ointment *(Unigreg, UK: Vestric, UK)*. Contains in each g neomycin sulphate 4 mg, polymyxin B sulphate 7250 units, hydrocortisone 10 mg, and nystatin 100 000 units.

Kaomycin *(Upjohn, UK)*. A suspension containing in each 5 ml neomycin sulphate 53 mg and kaolin 1.03 g (suggested diluent, water). For bacterial diarrhoea caused by neomycin-susceptible organisms. *Dose*. Adults: 30 to 60 ml four times daily; children over 2 years: 10 to 20 ml; infants under 2 years: 5 to 10 ml. Adults dosage is based on giving a minimum of 1.2 g neomycin sulphate per day.

Maxitrol Eye-drops *(Alcon, UK: Farillon, UK)*. Contain in each ml neomycin sulphate equivalent to neomycin 3.5 mg, polymyxin B sulphate 6000 units, with dexamethasone 0.1%, in a basis containing hypromellose 0.5%. **Maxitrol Eye Ointment**. Contains in each g neomycin sulphate equivalent to neomycin 3.5 mg, polymyxin B sulphate 6000 units, with dexamethasone 0.1%.

Minims Neomycin Sulphate *(Smith & Nephew Pharmaceuticals, UK)*. Sterile eye-drops containing neomycin sulphate 0.5%, available in single-dose disposable applicators.

Mycifradin Sterile Powder *(Upjohn, UK)*. Neomycin sulphate, available as powder for preparing injections in vials of 500 mg. (Also available as Mycifradin in *Austral., Canad., S.Afr., USA*).

Myciguent *(Upjohn, UK)*. Preparations containing neomycin sulphate 0.5%, available as **Ointment** and as **Ophthalmic Ointment**. (Also available as Myciguent in *Austral., Canad., S.Afr., USA*).

Neo-Cortef *(Upjohn, UK)*. **Eye-Ear Drops** and **Eye-Ear Ointment** each containing neomycin sulphate 0.5% and hydrocortisone acetate 1.5%; **Lotion** containing neomycin sulphate 0.5% and hydrocortisone acetate 1%; and **Ointment** containing neomycin sulphate 0.5% and hydrocortisone acetate 1 or 2.5%.

Neosporin Eye Drops *(Calmic, UK)*. Contain in each ml neomycin sulphate 1700 units, gramicidin 25 units, and polymyxin B sulphate 5000 units.

Nivemycin *(Boots, UK)*. Neomycin sulphate, available as **Eye-drops** and **Ointment** each containing 0.5%; as **Elixir** containing 100 mg in each 5 ml; and as **Tablets** of 500 mg.

Otoseptil *(Napp, UK)*. Ear-drops containing in each ml neomycin undecenoate equivalent to neomycin 670 μg, tyrothricin 1 mg, hydrocortisone 1 mg, and ethylene oxide polyoxypropylene glycol condensate 10 mg. For bacterial and fungous infections of the ear.

Otosporin *(Calmic, UK)*. Ear-drops containing in each ml neomycin sulphate 3400 units, polymyxin B sulphate 10 000 units, and hydrocortisone 10 mg.

Polybactrin *(Calmic, UK)*. Pressurised sterile powder spray containing in each 115 ml neomycin sulphate 495 000 units, bacitracin zinc 37 500 units, and polymyxin B sulphate 150 000 units, with propellents. For wound sepsis associated with surgery.

Polybactrin Soluble GU *(Calmic, UK)*. Vials each containing, as a sterile powder, neomycin sulphate 20 000 units, bacitracin 1000 units, and polymyxin B sulphate 75 000 units for solution in sodium chloride 0.9%. For irrigating the bladder.

Tampovagan N *(Norgine, UK)*. Pessaries each containing neomycin sulphate 20 mg. For vaginal infections resistant to other forms of therapy. *Administration*. 2 pessaries to be inserted at night. (Also available as Tampovagan N in *Austral., S.Afr.*).

Tribiotic (formerly known as Rikospray Antibiotic) *(Riker, UK)*. A sterile aerosol spray containing in 110 g neomycin sulphate 500 000 units, bacitracin zinc 10 000 units, and polymyxin B sulphate 150 000 units. For the prevention of bacterial infection during and after surgery and for infected skin conditions.

Unidiarea *(Unigreg, UK: Vestric, UK)*. Capsules each containing neomycin sulphate 200 mg, clioquinol 125 mg, and activated attapulgite 80 mg. For diarrhoea.

Other Proprietary Names

Arg.—Neomas Bowers; *Austral.*—Neomate, Neopt, Neosulf, Quintress-N, Siguent Neomycin; *Belg.*—Fradyl; *Canad.*—Herisan Antibiotic, Neocin; *Ger.*—Bykomycin, Myacyne; *S.Afr.*—Emelmycin, Neo-Gelicil, Neopan; *Spain*—Biofradin, Burn-Gel, Dermonalef, Larmicin, Neointestin; *Switz.*—Filmaseptic; *USA*—Neobiotic, Otobiotic.

Neomycin sulphate was also formerly marketed in Great Britain under the proprietary name Neomin (*Glaxo*). Preparations containing neomycin or neomycin sulphate were also formerly marketed under the proprietary names Biotren, Carmycin (both *Carlton Laboratories*), Dermamed Ointment (*Medo-Chemicals*), Donnagel with Neomycin (*Robins*), Framyspray (*Fisons*), Ivax (*Boots*), Neobacrin (*Glaxo*), Neotulle (*Fisons*), Neovax (*Norton*), Polynorm Ointment (*Norma*), and Duobac, Tribactric Dusting Powder, and Trisep (all *Stuart*).

114-n

Netilmicin Sulphate.

Sch-20569; *N*-Ethyl Sissomicin. 4-*O*-[(2*S*,3*S*)-3-Amino-6-aminomethyl-3,4-dihydro-2*H*-pyran-2-yl]-2-deoxy-6-*O*-[3-deoxy-4-*C*-methyl-3-methylamino-β-L-arabinopyranosyl]-1-*N*-ethyl-D-streptamine sulphate. $(C_{21}H_{41}N_5O_7)_2,5H_2SO_4$=1441.5.

CAS — 56391-56-1 (netilmicin); 56391-57-2 (sulphate).

A semi-synthetic derivative of sissomicin. Netilmicin sulphate 1.5 g is approximately equivalent to 1 g of netilmicin.

For the effect of ticarcillin on netilmicin, see Gentamicin Sulphate, p.1166.

Adverse Effects, Treatment, and Precautions. See Gentamicin Sulphate, p.1166.

Dizziness following treatment with netilmicin was reported in 1 patient and nephrotoxic effects in 5 of 38 patients treated.— F. J. Buckwold *et al.*, *Can. med. Ass. J.*, 1979, *120*, 161.

Comparative studies indicated that there was no significant difference between the toxicities of netilmicin and amikacin.— B. V. Bock *et al.*, *Antimicrob. Ag. Chemother.*, 1980, *17*, 217; M. Barza *et al.*, *ibid.*, 707.

Antimicrobial Action. Netilmicin has antimicrobial activity similar to that of gentamicin (see p.1168) and sissomicin (see p.1209). It is reported to be more active than gentamicin against some strains of Enterobacteriaceae but less active against *Pseudomonas aeruginosa*. Netilmicin appears to be resistant to some of the bacterial enzymes which inactivate gentamicin and it is active against some gentamicin-resistant isolates. It is considered to be active against fewer gentamicin-resistant Gram-negative organisms than amikacin, but because of different enzyme susceptibilities netilmicin may be effective where amikacin is not.

Like amikacin, netilmicin was active against gentamicin-resistant isolates of Enterobacteriaceae that produced aminoglycoside-adenylating enzymes. It was ineffective against strains, some of them susceptible to amikacin, gentamicin, or tobramycin, that produced aminoglycoside-acetylating enzymes. Most gentamicin-resistant strains of *Pseudomonas* were resistant to netilmicin.— S. A. Kabins *et al.*, *Antimicrob. Ag. Chemother.*, 1976, *10*, 139.

Of 342 clinical isolates all *Staphylococcus aureus*, 92% of *Escherichia coli*, 93% of *Klebsiella pneumoniae*, and 92% of *Enterobacter* were inhibited by 0.8 μg per ml of netilmicin but only 78% of *Pseudomonas aeruginosa* were inhibited by 3.1 μg per ml. Most isolates of enterococci, *Serratia marcescens*, and *Providencia* were not inhibited by 3.1 μg per ml. Activity *in vitro* was decreased by sodium, calcium, and magnesium and was increased at an alkaline pH.— K. P. Fu and H. C. Neu, *Antimicrob. Ag. Chemother.*, 1976, *10*, 526.

Netilmicin was less active than tobramycin or gentamicin against 100 isolates of *Ps. aeruginosa* but was more active than tobramycin and as active as gentamicin against 131 isolates of *E. coli*, 116 of *Kleb. pneumoniae* and 49 of the *Enterobacter* spp. All 3 antibiotics had a similar activity against 68 isolates of the *Proteus* spp. but netilmicin was active against a few isolates of *Klebsiella* and *Serratia* that were resistant to both gentamicin and tobramycin.— P. Chadwick *et al.*, *Antimicrob. Ag. Chemother.*, 1977, *12*, 301.

In a comparative study of the activity of netilmicin, gentamicin, tobramycin, amikacin, and kanamycin *in vitro*, netilmicin was generally the most active against strains of *E. coli*, *Proteus mirabilis*, and the *Klebsiella* spp. that were resistant to gentamicin or tobramycin.— R. P. Mouton and M. C. J. de Kok-Broeren, *J. antimicrob. Chemother.*, 1977, *3*, 393.

Netilmicin *in vitro* was as active as tobramycin or amikacin and more active than sissomicin or gentamicin against 163 strains of *Klebsiella*, and less active than gentamicin, tobramycin, or sissomicin against 94 strains of *Ps. aeruginosa*. Netilmicin had an MIC of 0.7 μg per ml against 21 strains of *Enterobacter* spp. and 58 strains of *Pr. mirabilis* and an MIC of 1 μg or less per ml against 90% of 178 strains of *E. coli*.— J. Klastersky *et al.*, *Antimicrob. Ag. Chemother.*, 1977, *12*, 503.

A study *in vitro* indicated the need for a separate standardised netilmicin disk from that used for gentamicin in disk susceptibility tests.— V. Habwe and S. Shadomy, *Antimicrob. Ag. Chemother.*, 1978, *13*, 1046.

Netilmicin had an MIC of 0.25, 0.5, 1.0, 2, and 4 μg per ml *in vitro* against 6, 29, 63, 79, and 81 of 83 isolates of *Serratia marcescens*. Amikacin sulphate had an MIC *in vitro* of 0.5, 1.0, 2, and 4 μg per ml against 2, 55, 77, and 82 of the strains and gentamicin inhibited 16, 27, 29, 30, and 40 of the strains at 0.25, 0.5, 1.0, 4, and 8 μg per ml.— C. M. Nolan and P. G. Fox, *Curr. ther. Res.*, 1978, *23*, 78.

The activities of netilmicin, amikacin, gentamicin, sissomicin, and tobramycin were compared *in vitro* against 104 strains of Gram-negative bacteria susceptible to gentamicin and 75 resistant to gentamicin. Netilmicin had a similar activity to gentamicin against susceptible isolates of the *Enterobacter* spp. and *E. coli* but had a similar activity to amikacin against resistant isolates of *E. coli*. Netilmicin was the most active drug against both the susceptible and resistant strains of the *Klebsiella* spp. Amikacin and netilmicin had similar activities against susceptible strains of *Ps. aeruginosa* but were less active than tobramycin or gentamicin; amikacin was the most active against the resistant strains while netilmicin was the second most active. Netilmicin was less active than gentamicin, sissomicin, or amikacin against susceptible strains of *Serratia marcescens* but was the most active against drug resistant strains.— V. Habwe and SShadomy, *J. antimicrob. Chemother.*, 1979, *5*, 73.

Further references: C. Watanakunakorn, *Antimicrob. Ag. Chemother.*, 1976, *10*, 382; M. I. Marks *et al.*, *ibid.*, 399; K. P. Fu and H. C. Neu, *ibid.*, 511; D. J. Briedis and H. G. Robson, *ibid.*, 592; R. D. Meyer *et al.*, *ibid.*, 677; K. N. Brown *et al.*, *ibid.*, 768; G. H. Miller *et al.*, *ibid.*, 827; D. J. Flournay, *ibid.*, 864; V. Dhawan *et al.*, *ibid.*, 1977, *11*, 64; B. R. Meyers and S. Z. Hirschman, *ibid.*, 118; R. J. Kantor and C. W. Norden, *ibid.*, 126; J. A. Smith *et al.*, *ibid.*, 362; I. Phillips *et al.*, *ibid.*, 402; T. C. Eickhoff and J. M. Ehret, *ibid.*, 791; D. Stewart *et al.*, *ibid.*, 1017; G. Greenstone *et al.*, *Chemotherapy, Basle*, 1978, *24*, 29; J. D. Siegel *et al.*, *Antimicrob. Ag. Chemother.*, 1979, *15*, 246.

Enhanced activity. The activities of benzylpenicillin and netilmicin were enhanced *in vitro* against 28 strains of *Streptococcus faecalis* when used together; the enhanced activity was similar to that of benzylpenicillin and gentamicin. This was confirmed in a study in *rabbits* with endocarditis caused by organisms resistant or susceptible to streptomycin.— O. M. Korzeniowski *et al.*, *Antimicrob. Ag. Chemother.*, 1978, *13*, 430.

Absorption and Fate. The absorption and fate of netilmicin is similar to that of gentamicin (see p.1170).

In a comparative study 13 healthy subjects were given netilmicin or gentamicin 1 mg per kg body-weight intramuscularly and intravenously. After intramuscular injection, mean peak serum concentrations were 3.76 μg per ml for each antibiotic; there was less individual variation with netilmicin but the peak concentration was achieved more slowly. After intravenous administration over 3 to 5 minutes netilmicin disappeared from serum more rapidly than gentamicin, had a greater volume of distribution, less variability in elimination half-life, and less was recovered in the urine.— L. J. Riff and G. Moreschi, *Antimicrob. Ag. Chemother.*, 1977, *11*, 609. See also J. A. Jahre *et al.*, *Clin. Pharmac. Ther.*, 1978, *23*, 591; M. Chung *et al.*, *Antimicrob. Ag. Chemother.*, 1980, *17*, 184.

A mean peak serum concentration of 16.56 μg per ml was achieved 3 minutes after the intravenous infusion of netilmicin 2 mg per kg body-weight over 30 minutes in 10 healthy subjects. Of the dose infused, 39% was excreted in the urine during the first 8 hours.— B. R. Meyers *et al.*, *Antimicrob. Ag. Chemother.*, 1977, *12*, 122.

In a study of 42 male patients aged 48 to 85 years some with impaired renal function, netilmicin given in doses of 1 or 2 mg per kg body-weight showed a biphasic distribution pattern. It appeared to equilibrate between the serum and extravascular tissues and fluids within 1 to 2 hours of administration. The mean serum half-life (β-phase) of netilmicin in patients with a creatinine clearance greater than 100 ml per minute, between 50 and 100 ml per minute, and less than 50 ml per minute was 2.3, 5.0, and 10.3 hours respectively after the intravenous injection of netilmicin 1 mg per kg and 2.1,

6.2, and 12.9 hours respectively after a similar 2 mg per kg dose. Dosage in patients with renal impairment could be based on creatinine status or clearance. Serum concentrations of netilmicin remained above the MIC for most organisms susceptible to netilmicin for up to 8 hours after a does in patients with normal renal function and for at least 12 hours in those with impaired renal function.— P. G. Welling *et al., Antimicrob. Ag. Chemother.*, 1977, *12,* 328.

The elimination half-life of netilmicin ranged from 2.14 to 2.40 hours in 12 healthy subjects with normal renal function after netilmicin 2 or 3 mg per kg body-weight was given intramuscularly or by intravenous infusion over a period of 30 minutes. Of the injected dose, 60 to 70% and 80 to 90% were recovered in the urine during the first 6 and 24 hours respectively after administration. The elimination half-life of netilmicin after 2 mg per kg was given intramuscularly to 18 patients with varying degrees of renal function ranged from 1.94 to 2.43 hours in 6 patients [creatinine clearance rate (CCR): greater than 100 ml per minute], from 3.35 to 7.30 hours in 3 patients (CCR: 50 to 100 ml per minute), and from 5.17 to 26.09 hours in 9 patients (CCR: 10 to 49 ml per minute); the elimination half-life ranged from 16.22 to 29.48 hours in 6 patients (CCR less than 10 ml per minute) who required haemodialysis and received a similar dose. The urinary elimination of netilmicin was inversely related to the degree of renal impairment and although peak serum concentrations of netilmicin increased with greater renal impairment the difference was not significant. There was a decrease in the mean serum concentration of netilmicin of about 63% during a dialysis session of 7 to 8 hours in the 6 patients who required haemodialysis.— G. Humbert *et al., Antimicrob. Ag. Chemother.*, 1978, *14,* 40.

Mean peak serum concentrations of netilmicin which occurred immediately after a one-hour intravenous infusion of 2 mg per kg body-weight in 50 ml of sodium chloride injection were 10.8 μg per ml in 7 healthy subjects with a creatinine clearance (CCR) of 70 ml per minute or more, 8.7 μg per ml in 7 patients with a CCR between 70 and 25 ml per minute, and 8.6 μg per ml in 6 patients with a CCR between 25 and 4 ml per minute; estimated serum half-lives were 2.7, 10.0, and 31.9 hours respectively and the percentages of the dose recovered in the urine within 24 hours of administration were about 70, 41, and 15% respectively. There was a positive correlation between the CCR and the overall elimination-rate constant and the serum clearance for netilmicin. In 5 anephric patients who received the same dose before undergoing a 5-hour haemodialysis session the mean peak serum concentration was 9.2 μg per ml immediately after infusion and during haemodialysis the clearance of netilmicin was positively correlated with the plasma flow-rate. It was estimated that about 50% of the dose of netilmicin might be lost during haemodialysis. Suggestions were given for dosage adjustments for patients with renal impairment.— F. C. Luft *et al., Antimicrob. Ag. Chemother.*, 1978, *14,* 403.

The pharmacokinetics of netilmicin were studied in 101 neonates. Mean peak serum concentrations which occurred 30 minutes after intramuscular administration were directly related to birth-weight and gestational age and ranged from 5.6 to 6.9 μg per ml after 3 mg per kg body-weight and from 7.8 to 8.4 μg per ml after 4 mg per kg. Six hours after administration mean serum concentrations had fallen to 2.3 to 3.5 μg per ml with the higher concentrations after the 4-mg per kg dose. Serum half-lives of netilmicin ranged from 3.4 to 4.7 hours. The pharmacokinetics of netilmicin were similar after intravenous and intramuscular administration. Average concentrations in urine after intramuscular administration of 3 and 4 mg per kg were 46 and 69 μg per ml respectively during the first 3 hours after administration and 29 and 103 μg per ml during the next 3 hours.— J. D. Siegel *et al., Antimicrob. Ag. Chemother.*, 1979, *15,* 246.

Further references: J. -C. Pechere *et al., Clin. Pharmacokinet.*, 1978, *3,* 395; *idem, Clin. Pharmac. Ther.*, 1978, *23,* 677; J. -C. Pechere and R. Dugal, *Clin. Pharmacokinet.*, 1979, *4,* 170; M. Wenk *et al., Eur. J. clin. Pharmac.*, 1979, *16,* 331; H. Michalsen and T. Bergan, *Antimicrob. Ag. Chemother.*, 1981, *19,* 1029.

Uses. Netilmicin is a semisynthetic aminoglycoside antibiotic which has been used similarly to gentamicin (see p.1170). It has been given intramuscularly or intravenously in doses of 4 to 6 mg per kg body-weight daily in two divided doses in the treatment of Gram-negative infections. Up to 7.5 mg per kg may be given daily in divided doses every 8 hours in severe infections. Dosage should be reduced in patients with renal impairment.

Proceedings of a conference on netilmicin.— *Clin. Trials J.*, 1980, *17,* 242–411.

A clinical cure was achieved in all of 27 patients with Gram-negative infections who received netilmicin 4.5 to 7.5 mg per kg body-weight per day in divided doses every 8 hours by intravenous or intramuscular injection. Those patients who had a creatinine clearance rate (CCR) above 50 ml per minute excreted from 80 to 100% of the dose within 8 hours of administration and patients with a CCR of 30 to 50 ml per minute excreted 30 to 80% of the dose. Of 21 patients who had audiograms one had evidence of ototoxicity and of 25 patients assessed, 4 had nephrotoxicity. Serum concentrations of alkaline phosphatase were raised in 9 of 21 patients but there was no clinical evidence of hepatobiliary toxicity.— A. P. Panwalker *et al., Antimicrob. Ag. Chemother.*, 1978, *13,* 170.

Netilmicin 2 or 2.5 mg per kg body-weight (reduced in renal failure) given intravenously every 8 hours produced a cure in 24 of 40 patients with Gram-negative bacterial infections and a favourable response in a further 8. Of 4 patients who had organisms in which resistance to netilmicin developed during treatment, 3 were treatment failures. Eight of 37 patients evaluated developed renal insufficiency.— D. R. Snydman *et al., Antimicrob. Ag. Chemother.*, 1979, *15,* 50.

Further references: P. H. Edelstein and R. D. Meyer, *J. antimicrob. Chemother.*, 1978, *4,* 495; T. Edén *et al., Curr. ther. Res.*, 1978, *24,* 96; F. J. Buckwold *et al., Can. med. Ass. J.*, 1979, *120,* 161; R. L. Herting *et al., Arzneimittel-Forsch.*, 1981, *31,* 366.

Dosage. There was no evidence of drug accumulation in 11 patients with malignant neoplasms who received netilmicin 60 mg per m^2 body-surface by continuous infusion in 250 ml of dextrose injection every 6 hours after an initial dose of 60 mg per m^2 administered intravenously in 50 ml over 0.5 hours. A mean of 55% of a dose of netilmicin administered intramuscularly was excreted in the urine within 6 hours by 10 similar patients who received 50 mg per m^2, and a mean of 45% was excreted in the urine when they received the same dose by intravenous infusion. There was no evidence of ototoxicity in 11 patients who had had an audiogram.— B. -S. Yap *et al., Antimicrob. Ag. Chemother.*, 1977, *12,* 717.

A report on high-dose netilmicin therapy.— C. O. Solberg *et al., J. antimicrob. Chemother.*, 1980, *6,* 133.

Dosage in infants and children. There was evidence of accumulation of netilmicin in 12 low-birth-weight infants (less than 2 kg) who received 4 mg per kg body-weight every 12 hours for an average of 6.4 days and on discontinuation serum concentrations declined in a biphasic manner having a short serum half-life of 6.5 hours followed by a longer half-life of 62.4 hours. It was considered that the pharmacokinetics of netilmicin were similar to those of gentamicin and that a dose of 3 mg per kg given every 12 hours should give serum concentrations in the therapeutic and safe range.— J. D. Siegel *et al., Antimicrob. Ag. Chemother.*, 1979, *15,* 246.

Further references: P. Henriksson *et al., Curr. ther. Res.*, 1978, *24,* 108.

See also under Absorption and Fate.

Dosage in renal failure. It was suggested that netilmicin 2 mg per kg body-weight given every 8 or 12 hours intramuscularly or by intravenous infusion (over 30 to 60 minutes) would be a suitable dose for patients with normal renal function and that the interval between doses should be extended for patients with renal insufficiency; a dose of 2 mg per kg given after each haemodialysis session would be sufficient to produce effective antibiotic concentrations in patients undergoing haemodialysis twice weekly.— G. Humbert *et al., Antimicrob. Ag. Chemother.*, 1978, *14,* 40.

Further references: M. Jonsson *et al., J. int. med. Res.*, 1978, *6,* 226; N. Frimodt-Möller *et al., Antimicrob. Ag. Chemother.*, 1979, *16,* 406.

See also under Absorption and Fate.

Urinary-tract infections. All of 25 patients with acute pyelonephritis had negative urine and blood cultures after 24 hours of therapy with netilmicin 1.5 to 2.5 mg per kg body-weight given by intravenous infusion over 20 minutes or intramuscularly every 8 hours (dosage was reduced to 0.7 mg per kg in renal insufficiency). Two patients, one of whom developed ototoxicity, were changed to other antibiotics and of the remaining 23 patients who had therapy for 7 to 12 days 19 were bacteriologically and clinically cured 9 to 50 days after the end of treatment. Five patients developed evidence of nephrotoxicity during therapy and three patients, one with impaired renal function, developed ototoxicity.— I. Trestman *et al., Antimicrob. Ag. Chemother.*, 1978, *13,* 832.

A cure was obtained in 20 of 29 patients with complicated urinary-tract infections 7 days after receiving netilmicin 2 mg per kg body-weight intramuscularly every 12 hours for 7 to 10 days. Of 28 similar patients who received amikacin 7.5 mg per kg intramuscularly every 12 hours, 16 were cured.— S. Maigaard *et al., Antimicrob. Ag. Chemother.*, 1978, *14,* 544.

In a study in 58 patients with symptomatic urinary-tract infections netilmicin 2 mg per kg body-weight twice daily was as effective as gentamicin 1 mg per kg thrice daily. Both drugs were given by intramuscular injection.— C. E. Cox, *Curr. ther. Res.*, 1979, *25,* 603. See also M. O. Loveless *et al., ibid.*, 595.

Further references: L. Weissbach *et al., Dt. med. Wschr.*, 1978, *103,* 1961; P. Chadwick *et al., Can. med. Ass. J.*, 1978, *119,* 1189.

Proprietary Preparations

Netillin *(Kirby-Warrick, UK).* Netilmicin sulphate, supplied as solution for injection containing the equivalent of netilmicin 10 mg per ml in ampoules or vials of 1.5 ml, 50 mg per ml in ampoules or vials of 1 ml, and 100 mg per ml in ampoules or vials of 1, 1.5, or 2 ml.

Other Proprietary Names

Certomycin *(Ger.).*

115-h

Novobiocin.

Streptonivicin. 4-Hydroxy-3-[4-hydroxy-3-(3-methylbut-2-enyl)benzamido]-8-methylcoumarin-7-yl 3-*O*-carbamoyl-5,5-di-*C*-methyl-4-*O*-methyl-α-L-*lyxo*-hexopyranoside.
$C_{31}H_{36}N_2O_{11}$=612.6.

CAS — 303-81-1.

An antimicrobial substance produced by the growth of *Streptomyces niveus* or related organisms, or by any other means. Unlike other antibiotics produced by actinomycetes, novobiocin is a weak dibasic acid and forms salts with bases.

It occurs as a white to cream-coloured amorphous powder or pale yellow crystals.

Practically **insoluble** in water at a pH below 7.5; soluble in alcohol, acetic acid, amyl acetate, dioxan, ethyl acetate, and methyl alcohol; practically insoluble in chloroform and ether. Insoluble salts are formed with heavy metals, organic bases, and basic antibiotics such as amikacin, erythromycin, kanamycin, neomycin, and streptomycin. **Incompatible** with dextrose in solution. The dry powder is stable at room temperature when **protected** from light.

116-m

Novobiocin Calcium *(B.P. 1973).*

Calcium Novobiocin; Novobiocinum Calcicum. The calcium salt of novobiocin.
$(C_{31}H_{35}N_2O_{11})_2Ca$=1263.3.

CAS — 4309-70-0.

Pharmacopoeias. In *Int.*

A white or yellowish-white, odourless, crystalline powder with a sweet taste and bitter after-taste. It contains not less than 850 units per mg of the dried substance. Novobiocin calcium 1.03 g is approximately equivalent to 1 g of novobiocin.

Soluble 1 in 300 of water, 1 in 8 of alcohol, 1 in 60 of acetone, 1 in 100 of butyl acetate, 1 in 1100 of chloroform, 1 in 450 of ether, and 1 in 8 of methyl alcohol. A 2.5% suspension in water has a pH of 7 to 8.5. **Store** in a cool place in airtight containers. Protect from light.

117-b

Novobiocin Sodium *(B.P. 1973).*

Novobiocinum Natricum; Sodium Novobiocin. The monosodium salt of novobiocin.
$C_{31}H_{35}N_2NaO_{11}$=634.6.

CAS — 1476-53-5.

Pharmacopoeias. In *Fr., Ind., Int., It., Rus.,* and *Swiss.*

A white or yellowish-white, odourless, hygroscopic, crystalline powder with a sweet taste and bitter after-taste, containing not less than 850 units per mg of the dried substance. Each g represents 1.6 mmol (1.6 mEq) of sodium. Novobiocin sodium 1.04 g is approximately equivalent to 1 g of novobiocin.

Soluble 1 in 5 of water, 1 in 7 of alcohol, and 1 in 3 of methyl alcohol; practically insoluble in acetone, chloroform, and ether; freely soluble in glycerol and propylene glycol; slightly soluble in butyl acetate. A 2.5% solution in water has a pH of 7 to 8.5.

Incompatible with dextrose solutions, which should not be used as diluents, and with basic antibiotics such as amikacin, erythromycin, kanamycin, lincomycin, neomycin, spiramycin, streptomycin, and viomycin. Solutions for injection are prepared aseptically. **Store** in a cool place in airtight containers; if it is intended for injection, the containers should be sterile and sealed to exclude micro-organisms. Protect from light.

Incompatibility. A precipitate was formed when novobiocin sodium solution was mixed with *dextrose injection, 5% dextrose in sodium chloride injection,* or *lactated Ringer's solution.* Precipitates were also formed within 4 hours when novobiocin sodium in sodium chloride injection was mixed with solutions of the following: *calcium gluconate, chloramphenicol, corticotrophin, dimenhydrinate, erythromycin gluceptate, heparin, hydrocortisone sodium succinate, oxytetracycline hydrochloride, ristocetin, tetracycline hydrochloride,* and *vancomycin hydrochloride.*— H. R. Grant, *Hosp. Pharmst,* 1962, *15,* 67.

There was loss of clarity when intravenous solutions of novobiocin sodium were mixed with those of *adrenaline hydrochloride, calcium gluconate, chloramphenicol sodium succinate, corticotrophin, dextrose, erythromycin gluceptate, heparin sodium, hydrocortisone sodium succinate, insulin, magnesium sulphate, narcotic salts, noradrenaline acid tartrate, procaine hydrochloride, protein hydrolysate, streptomycin sulphate, tetracycline hydrochloride,* or *vancomycin hydrochloride.* Novobiocin sodium was incompatible in injections of 5% *dextrose, laevulose, invert sugar, lactated Ringer's solution, sodium lactate,* or *ammonium chloride.*— J. A. Patel and G. L. Phillips, *Am. J. Hosp. Pharm.,* 1966, *23,* 409.

Novobiocin was incompatible with *ajmaline, aminophylline, atropine sulphate, soluble barbiturates, calcium chloride, canrenoate potassium, calcium gluceptate, dextran, meclofenoxate, metaraminol tartrate, potassium chloride, prochlorperazine, sulphafurazole diethanolamine, suxamethonium, thiopentone sodium, vitamins of the B group,* and *vitamins of the B group with vitamin C* in an infusion fluid.— B. Flouvat and P. Lechat, *Thérapie,* 1974, *29,* 337.

Loss of activity. Novobiocin sodium was very much less active against *Staphylococcus aureus* in the presence of magnesium carbonate, magnesium oxide, calamine, methylcellulose, sodium alginate, pectin, polysorbate 80, and less active with bismuth subcarbonate, calcium carbonate, magnesium trisilicate, zinc oxide, acacia, carmellose sodium, maize starch, gelatin, macrogol 4000, and propylene glycol.— M. A. El-Nakeeb and R. T. Yousef, *Acta pharm. suec.,* 1968, *5,* 1.

Stability. A study of the antibacterial activity and relative stability of novobiocin in various ointment bases.— E. Stempel *et al., Am. J. Pharm.,* 1958, *130,* 116.

When protected from light, the solid (novobiocin sodium) was stable for 2 years at temperatures up to 37°. Solutions of a concentration of 6.25% or less might be stable for several months in a refrigerator or for about 1 month at room temperature. Concentrated solutions became coloured, particularly above 20° and in the presence of air. Light had little effect on potency but irradiation with u.v. light accelerated loss of potency. Loss was accelerated by increase of temperature and pH and in the presence of certain heavy metals, phosphates, and possibly sulphates. Novobiocin sodium was soluble in water at alkaline pH values but was precipitated as the free acid at acid pH values. Suspensions of novobiocin (free acid) were sufficiently stable to meet the requirements for shelf-life of pharmaceutical products.— M. J. Busse *et al., J. Pharm. Pharmac.,* 1959, *11,* 250T.

In aqueous suspension, amorphous novobiocin was metastable and was slowly converted to a more stable but biologically inactive crystalline form. The rate of conversion was increased with temperature and concentration but could be retarded by the addition of methylcellulose, alginates, or povidone. The calcium salt was amorphous, biologically active, and stable in aqueous suspension. The crystalline sodium salt was also active, possibly because it was precipitated as the amorphous acid in the stomach.— J. D. Mullins and T. J. Macek, *J. Am. pharm. Ass., scient. Edn,* 1960, *49,* 245.

Units. One unit of novobiocin is contained in 0.001031 mg of the first International Standard Preparation (1965) of novobiocin acid which contains 970 units per mg.

Adverse Effects. Novobiocin produces many side-effects. Nausea, colic, vomiting, and diarrhoea frequently occur but are usually not sufficiently severe to necessitate stopping treatment. Sensitisation reactions are common with courses lasting more than 1 week and symptoms include urticarial and maculopapular skin eruptions, often with fever. Erythema multiforme has been reported. Eosinophilia, leucopenia, thrombocytopenia, and occasionally haemolytic anaemia have occurred. Total and differential blood counts should be made routinely during treatment.

A yellow pigment which may appear in the plasma of patients treated with novobiocin is a metabolite of the drug, which may interfere with the determination of serum bilirubin. In a few cases, novobiocin appears to have produced some degree of liver dysfunction with raised serum-bilirubin concentration; this is a special risk in neonates.

Precautions. Novobiocin should not be given to children under 6 months of age. Care is necessary in the administration of novobiocin during pregnancy, particularly just before childbirth. Routine blood counts should be made during treatment.

Antimicrobial Action. Novobiocin appears to act in several ways; one mechanism is interference with the synthesis of bacterial cell walls. In high concentrations it is bactericidal against highly susceptible species.

It is active against Gram-positive micro-organisms such as *Staphylococcus aureus, Corynebacterium diphtheriae,* and *Streptococcus pneumoniae.* Of the Gram-negative bacteria, *Haemophilus influenzae, Neisseria gonorrhoeae,* and *N. meningitidis* are sensitive. Streptococci and *Proteus vulgaris* are variable in their reaction to novobiocin. *Pseudomonas pseudomallei* may be sensitive at high concentrations. *Escherichia coli, Ps. aeruginosa, Klebsiella, Salmonella,* and *Shigella* spp. are resistant to novobiocin.

The usual minimum inhibitory concentration of novobiocin for sensitive strains of Gram-positive bacteria has been reported to range from 0.1 to 4 µg per ml.

Novobiocin suppressed the multiplication of herpes virus *in vitro* and was found to have greater activity at an acid pH. Novobiocin enhanced the activity of idoxuridine against herpes virus and vaccinia virus and the emergence of resistant herpes virus appeared to be delayed.— T. Chang and L. Weinstein, *Antimicrob. Ag. Chemother.,* 1970, 165.

The antimicrobial activity of novobiocin was enhanced in alkaline urine.— S. A. Kabins, *J. Am. med. Ass.,* 1972, *219,* 206.

Novobiocin and rifampicin enhanced the activity of each other *in vitro* against 17 of 18 strains of *Salmonella typhi.*— D. C. Shanson and T. Leung, *J. antimicrob. Chemother.,* 1976, *2,* 81.

For a report of various compounds decreasing the activity of novobiocin sodium, see Loss of Activity, above.

Resistance. Many species of bacteria are capable of developing resistance to novobiocin. *Staphylococcus aureus* readily develops resistance both *in vitro* and *in vivo.*

Absorption and Fate. Novobiocin given as the calcium or sodium salt is absorbed from the gastro-intestinal tract, giving maximum plasma concentrations of about 10 µg per ml within 1 to 4 hours of a dose equivalent to about 250 mg. Over 90% of novobiocin in the circulation is bound to plasma proteins.

Novobiocin is excreted mainly in the bile from which it is repeatedly reabsorbed and eventually excreted in the faeces. No more than 3% is excreted in the urine. It diffuses into the pleural and ascitic fluids but not into the cerebrospinal fluid unless the meninges are inflamed.

It is excreted in milk.

Some 95.5% of novobiocin in the body was bound to serum proteins. The half-life in serum was 2.3 hours and 1.5 to 3.3% was excreted in urine.— C. M. Kunin, *Ann. intern. Med.,* 1967, *67,* 151. See also J. G. Wagner and R. E. Damiano, *J. clin. Pharmac.,* 1968, *8,* 102.

Uses. There appears to be little reason for the continued use of novobiocin as alternative therapy for susceptible infections is usually safer. Apart from being used in staphylococcal infections, it has formed part of the treatment of melioidosis due to *Ps. pseudomallei.*

Novobiocin is given by mouth as the sodium or calcium salt in doses of 250 mg (of base) every 6 hours. Children have been given 30 mg per kg body-weight daily. Novobiocin sodium has also been given by intravenous infusion in doses equivalent to 500 mg of novobiocin.

Combinations of novobiocin with tetracycline and novobiocin with sulphamethizole have been condemned by some authorities.

Preparations

Novobiocin Mixture *(B.P.C. 1973).* Novobiocin Syrup. A suspension of novobiocin calcium, of specified particle size, in a suitable flavoured vehicle which may be coloured. pH 6.5 to 7.5. Store in a cool place. Protect from light. When a dose of less than 5 ml is prescribed, the mixture should be diluted to 5 ml with syrup. Such dilutions must be freshly prepared and not used more than 2 weeks after issue.

Novobiocin Tablets *(B.P. 1973).* Tablets containing novobiocin calcium or novobiocin sodium. They may be coated.

Proprietary Preparations

Albamycin T *(Upjohn, UK).* Capsules each containing novobiocin sodium equivalent to novobiocin 125 mg and tetracycline hydrochloride equivalent to 125 mg of tetracycline. **Albamycin T Paediatric.** A suspension (supplied as granules for preparation with water before use) containing in each 5 ml novobiocin calcium equivalent to novobiocin 62.5 mg and tetracycline 62.5 mg.

Other Proprietary Names

Albamycin *(Belg., USA)*; Cathomycine *(Fr.)*; Catomicina *(Spain)*; Novobioplast *(Spain)*; Robiocina *(Ital., Spain).*

Preparations containing novobiocin calcium or novobiocin sodium were also formerly marketed in Great Britain under the proprietary names Albamycin, Albamycin GU, and Albamycin, Sterile *(Upjohn).*

118-v

Oleandomycin Phosphate.

3-(2,6-Dideoxy-3-*O*-methyl-α-L-*arabino*-hexopyranosyloxy)-8,8-epoxymethano-11-hydroxy-2,4,6,10,12-pentamethyl-9-oxo-5-(3,4,6-trideoxy-3-dimethylamino-β-D-*xylo*-hexopyranosyloxy)tetradecan-13-olide phosphate.

$C_{35}H_{61}NO_{12},H_3PO_4$=785.9.

CAS — 3922-90-5 (oleandomycin); 7060-74-4 (phosphate).

The phosphate of an antimicrobial substance produced by the growth of *Streptomyces antibioticus.*

A white almost odourless crystalline powder with a potency of not less than 775 µg of oleandomycin base activity per mg. **Soluble** 1 in 2.5 of water and 1 in 3 of alcohol; slightly soluble in ether. A 5% solution in water has a pH of 3 to 4. Solutions in water are stable at room temperature over a pH range of 2 to 9. **Store** in airtight containers.

Loss of activity. Vitamins of the B group and ascorbic acid reduced the antimicrobial activity *in vitro* of oleandomycin phosphate.— M. A. El-Nakeeb *et al., Can. J. pharm. Sci.,* 1976, *11,* 85.

Units. One unit of oleandomycin is contained in 0.001176 mg of the first International Standard

Preparation (1964) of oleandomycin chloroform adduct which contains 850 units per mg.

Oleandomycin is an antibiotic with actions and uses similar to those of erythromycin (see p.1158). It has antimicrobial activity weaker than that of erythromycin; cross-resistance occurs between oleandomycin and the other macrolides.

Oleandomycin phosphate has been used in the treatment of susceptible infections but more effective antibiotics are generally preferred. It has been given by mouth or by slow intravenous infusion in a dose of 1 to 2 g daily in divided doses; in children 30 to 50 mg per kg bodyweight daily has been recommended. The intramuscular route is rarely used and such injections are painful unless a local anaesthetic is added to the solution; intramuscular doses in adults have ranged from 0.6 to 2 g daily in divided doses.

Oleandomycin has also been given by mouth as the triacetyl ester, triacetyloleandomycin (see p.1228).

The administration of oleandomycin could interfere with measurements of urinary 17-hydroxycorticosteroids.— J. M. Rosenberg and I. S. Kampa, *Drug Intell. & clin. Pharm.*, 1973, *7*, 33.

Oleandomycin phosphate and tetracycline had a synergistic bacteriostatic action against *Escherichia coli*. There was no synergism between oleandomycin and erythromycin, lincomycin, or chloramphenicol.— C. M. Won and E. R. Garrett, *J. pharm. Sci.*, 1973, *62*, 1087.

Further references: E. Semenitz, *J. antimicrob. Chemother.*, 1978, *4*, 455 (antibacterial activity).

Proprietary Names

Matromycin, Mittamycin (both *Jap.*); Oleandocyn (*Pfizer, Ger.*) (see also under Triacetyloleandomycin); Taocin-P (*Jap.*); Triolmicina (oleandomycin) (*Ripari-Gero, Ital.*).

119-g

Oxacillin Sodium *(U.S.P.)*.

Oxacillinum Natricum; Oxacillinum Natrium; Sodium Oxacillin; (5-Methyl-3-phenyl-4-isoxazolyl)penicillin Sodium. Sodium (6*R*)-6-(5-methyl-3-phenylisoxazole-4-carboxamido)penicillanate monohydrate.

$C_{19}H_{18}N_3NaO_5S,H_2O = 441.4$.

CAS — 66-79-5 (oxacillin); 1173-88-2 (sodium salt, anhydrous); 7240-38-2 (sodium salt, monohydrate).

Pharmacopoeias. In *Braz., Cz., Int., Roum., Rus., Turk.*, and *U.S.*

A fine white crystalline powder, odourless or with a slight odour, with a bitter taste. Each g represents about 2.3 mmol (2.3 mEq) of sodium. Oxacillin sodium 1.1 g is approximately equivalent to 1 g of anhydrous oxacillin. The *U.S.P.* specifies the equivalent of 815 to 950 µg of oxacillin per mg.

Soluble 1 in 3.5 of water and 1 in 90 of alcohol; freely soluble in dimethyl sulphoxide; slightly soluble in dehydrated alcohol, chloroform, methyl acetate, and pyridine; practically insoluble in acetone, ether, ethyl acetate, ethylene chloride, and light petroleum. A 3% solution in water has a pH of 4.5 to 7.5. A 6.64% solution is iso-osmotic with serum.

Solutions containing 16% in Water for Injections are stable for 3 days at 21° and for 7 days when stored in a refrigerator. Solutions containing up to 2 mg per ml in dextrose or sodium chloride injections may be expected to lose not more than 10% of their activity in 6 hours when stored at 21°. **Store** at 15° to 30° in airtight containers.

Incompatibility. Oxacillin sodium was incompatible with *stearic acid*. A dry mixture lost potency on storage.— H. Jacobson and G. Reier, *J. pharm. Sci.*, 1969, *58*, 631.

Oxacillin was incompatible in intravenous solutions with *gentamicin, metaraminol, nitrofurantoin, noradrenaline, novobiocin, oxytetracycline, pentobarbitone, phenobarbitone, polymyxin B, protein hydrolysate, sulphadiazine, tetracycline,* and *vitamin-B complex*.— *Med. Lett.*, 1972, *14* (Jan.), *Suppl.*, 32.

Oxacillin was reported to be incompatible with *ascorbic acid, canrenoate potassium, suxamethonium,* and *vitamins of the B group with vitamin C* in an infusion fluid.— B. Flouvat and P. Lechat, *Thérapie*, 1974, *29*, 337.

Stability. Ultraviolet irradiation for 2 hours had a destructive effect on oxacillin sodium.— A. A. Kassem and E. H. Girgis, *Bull. Fac. Pharm., Cairo*, 1970, *9*, 157.

Stability in solution. There was a reduction of 12% in the availability of oxacillin from a solution in 5% dextrose in normal saline over a period of 12 hours.— J. N. Bair and D. P. Carew, *Bull. parent. Drug Ass.*, 1965, *19*, 153.

The activity of solutions of oxacillin sodium in either sucrose 10% or dextrose 5% at 37° was negligible after 24 hours.— M. S. Simberkoff *et al.*, *New Engl. J. Med.*, 1970, *283*, 116.

Oxacillin sodium, buffered with phosphate, was stable for 24 hours at 21° to 25° when added to injections of dextrose 5% or sodium chloride 0.9%.— D. Chatterji *et al.*, *Am. J. Hosp. Pharm.*, 1975, *32*, 1130. See also B. E. Kirschenbaum and C. J. Latiolais, *ibid.*, 1976, *33*, 767; C. J. Latiolais, *ibid.*, 1120.

There was no significant loss of potency when oxacillin for injection was added to 3 commercially available 0.5% hypromellose solutions in plastic squeezy bottles (Lacril, pH 5.9; Tearisol, pH 7.3; Isoptotears, pH 7.4), and the resulting solutions, containing oxacillin 66 mg per ml, kept at 25° for 7 days.— E. Osborn *et al.*, *Am. J. Ophthal.*, 1976, *82*, 775.

Adverse Effects and Treatment. As for Benzylpenicillin, p.1103.

Increased serum concentrations of aspartate and alanine aminotransferases (SGOT and SGPT), associated with hepatitis, have been reported during intravenous treatment with oxacillin sodium. Neutropenia has also occurred. Haematuria, albuminuria, and uraemia have followed the administration of large doses to infants.

Blood disorders. Neutropenia occurred during treatment with oxacillin 200 mg per kg body-weight daily by intravenous injection in 4 children aged from 9 months to 15½ years. In one child the dose was increased to 400 mg per kg daily. Neutrophil counts increased in each patient after the withdrawal of oxacillin.— J. M. Leventhal and A. B. Silken, *J. Pediat.*, 1976, *89*, 769.

Further reports of neutropenia attributed to treatment with oxacillin.— J. Y. Chu *et al.*, *J. Pediat.*, 1977, *90*, 668; I. Brook, *Sth. med. J.*, 1977, *70*, 565; D. W. Ortbals and J. J. Marr, *ibid.*, 1245; J. A. Fallon *et al.*, *Acta haemat.*, 1978, *59*, 163.

A report of agranulocytosis which developed in an 18-year-old man while receiving oxacillin sodium 12 g daily by intravenous injection over a 3-week period.— J. B. Kahn (letter), *J. Am. med. Ass.*, 1978, *240*, 2632; R. D. Scalley and R. D. Roark, *Drug Intell. & clin. Pharm.*, 1977, *11*, 420.

Colitis. For reference to diarrhoea and toxin-producing *Clostridium difficile* associated with oxacillin, see Dicloxacillin Sodium, p.1154.

Hepatotoxicity. Three patients developed fever or nausea and vomiting and abnormal liver function with elevation of serum aspartate aminotransferase (SGOT) while receiving oxacillin sodium intravenously. Symptoms subsided when the drug was withdrawn. A hypersensitivity reaction was suggested as a possible cause of this liver dysfunction.— W. E. Dismukes, *J. Am. med. Ass.*, 1973, *226*, 861.

An increase in serum concentrations of aspartate and alanine aminotransferases (SGOT and SGPT) was reported in a 23-year-old man on the 8th day of treatment for bacterial endocarditis with oxacillin 16 g daily by intravenous injection. The concentrations increased further until the 19th day of treatment, but fell rapidly when oxacillin was discontinued, although they remained elevated during the patient's stay in hospital.— I. Klein and H. Tobias, *Am. J. Gastroent., N.Y.*, 1976, *65*, 546.

A retrospective study of records of 54 patients who had received oxacillin by intravenous injection at a daily dosage greater than 6 g indicated that 8 had developed hepatitis during treatment with oxacillin, the symptoms occurring at 2 to 21 days after the beginning of treatment. Normal liver function had returned when oxacillin was withdrawn. Symptoms started to resolve in 2 patients still receiving oxacillin. The total dose before onset of hepatitis ranged from 16 to 300 g.— I. M. Onorato and J. L. Axelrod, *Ann. intern. Med.*, 1978, *89*, 497. Criticisms.— L. J. D'Angelo (letter), *ibid.*, 1979, *90*, 442. Reply.— J. L. Axelrod and I. M. Onorata, *ibid.* A further report of hepatitis in a 24-year-old man following the administration of a total of 324 g oxacillin intravenously over 27 days to treat *Staph. aureus* endocarditis. Hepatotoxicity was reversed when nafcillin was given instead of oxacillin.— C. Taylor *et al.* (letter), *ibid.*, 857.

Further references: R. N. Olans and L. B. Weiner, *J. Pediat.*, 1976, *89*, 835; A. H. Bruckstein and A. A. Attia, *Am. J. Med.*, 1978, *64*, 519; A. Denny *et al.* (letter), *Ann. intern. Med.*, 1979, *90*, 277.

Nephrotoxicity. Renal failure with acute interstitial nephritis and eosinophilia occurred in a patient given oxacillin by mouth.— J. R. Burton *et al.*, *Johns Hopkins med. J.*, 1974, *134*, 58.

Further references: D. B. Tillman *et al.*, *Archs intern. Med.*, 1980, *140*, 1552.

Neurotoxicity. A neurotoxic reaction to oxacillin occurred in a 37-year-old diamorphine addict with impaired renal function.— A. J. Malone *et al.* (letter), *New Engl. J. Med.*, 1977, *296*, 453.

For a report of convulsions associated with oxacillin therapy in 1 patient, see Benzylpenicillin, p.1105.

Precautions. Oxacillin sodium is contra-indicated in patients known to be sensitive to penicillin and it should be given with caution to patients with known histories of allergy. It should be used with caution in newborn infants and in patients with hepatic dysfunction.

In healthy infants given a single dose of oxacillin 578 mg per m² body-surface by stomach tube during the first week after birth, maximum serum concentrations of 26.2 µg per ml were recorded 2 hours after administration. Elimination then became much more rapid at 2 to 4 weeks of age. In premature infants, elimination of oxacillin was still retarded at 2 months of age.— G. -A. von Harnack *et al.*, *Dt. med. Wschr.*, 1965, *90*, 1433.

Interactions. Aspirin, sulphamethoxypyridazine, and sulphaethidole inhibited the serum-binding of oxacillin *in vitro* and *in vivo*. The oral absorption of oxacillin also appeared to be diminished by the sulphonamides.— C. M. Kunin, *Clin. Pharmac.Ther.*, 1966, *7*, 180.

For the effects of other drugs on the antimicrobial activity of oxacillin sodium, see below under Antimicrobial Action.

Antimicrobial Action. Oxacillin sodium has a range of antimicrobial activity similar to that of cloxacillin sodium (see p.1149).

In an *in vitro* study, flucloxacillin was bactericidal against 88% of 26 penicillin-resistant isolates of *Staph. aureus* at 0.4 µg per ml and against all of them at 6.2 µg per ml; cloxacillin was bactericidal against 81% of the isolates at 0.8 µg per ml and against all at 12.5 µg per ml; and oxacillin was bactericidal against 88% of the isolates at 0.2 µg per ml and against all at 1.6 µg per ml.— M. G. Bergeron *et al.*, *Am. J. med. Sci.*, 1976, *271*, 13.

Diminished activity. Quinine dihydrochloride decreased the antibacterial effect *in vitro* of nafcillin sodium and oxacillin sodium against *Staph. aureus*.— M. A. Toama *et al.*, *J. pharm. Sci.*, 1978, *67*, 23.

Enhanced activity. The activity *in vitro* of oxacillin against *Staph. aureus* was enhanced when used in conjunction with netilmicin or sissomicin.— C. Watanakunakorn and C. Glotzbecker, *Antimicrob. Ag. Chemother.*, 1977, *12*, 346.

Ampicillin and oxacillin enhanced the activity of each other *in vitro* against 7 strains of enterococci. A bacteriological cure was obtained in one patient with enterococcal endocarditis who received ampicillin sodium together with oxacillin.— J. Garau and S. A. Kabins, *J. antimicrob. Chemother.*, 1979, *5*, 31.

Resistance. As for Methicillin Sodium, p.1183.

Of 30 isolates of *Staph. aureus* 19 were tolerant to the bactericidal effect of oxacillin or cephalothin but none was tolerant to gentamicin. Tolerance was unrelated to phage type and was said to occur when a strain had a low minimum inhibitory concentration but a very high minimum bactericidal concentration.— J. J. Bradley *et al.*, *Antimicrob. Ag. Chemother.*, 1978, *13*, 1052.

Absorption and Fate. Oxacillin sodium is more stable in acid gastric secretion than benzylpenicillin or methicillin but is less stable than phenoxymethylpenicillin. Absorption is reduced by food in the stomach or small intestine and is less than with cloxacillin or dicloxacillin. Peak plasma concentrations of 3 to 6 µg per ml are

achieved 1 hour after a dose of 500 mg given before food. Following the intramuscular injection of 500 mg peak plasma concentrations of about 10 μg per ml are achieved after 30 minutes. Doubling the dose can double the plasma concentration. About 93% of the oxacillin in the circulation is bound to plasma proteins.
Some 23% to 30% of an oral dose and 40% of an intramuscular dose is rapidly excreted in the urine. Oxacillin is also excreted in the bile. It diffuses into pleural, synovial, and amniotic fluids and has been detected in cord serum and milk; it does not penetrate well into normal cerebrospinal fluid.
Serum concentrations are enhanced if probenecid is given.

The biological half-life of oxacillin was reported to be 0.7 hours in adults, 1.1 hours in children, 1.5 hours in infants born at term, and 1.2 to 1.6 hours (according to age) in premature infants.— W. A. Ritschel, *Drug Intell. & clin. Pharm.*, 1970, *4*, 332. Half-lives of 0.5 hours.— C. M. Kunin, *Ann. intern. Med.*, 1967, *67*, 151. A range of 0.4 to 0.7 hours.— K. L. Duchin and R. W. Schrier, *Clin. Pharmacokinet.*, 1978, *3*, 58.

The reversibility of the plasma-protein binding of oxacillin *in vitro*.— M. Barza *et al.*, *Antimicrob. Ag. Chemother.*, 1972, *1*, 427.

Oxacillin was reported to be absorbed from the peritoneal cavity.— J. S. Cheigh, *Am. J. Med.*, 1977, *62*, 555.

Diffusion into body fluids and tissues. Concentrations of oxacillin in cortical bone in 22 patients who received 1 g intravenously before undergoing total hip arthroplasty ranged from 0.3 to 14.5 μg per g (mean 2.1 μg per g) 1 hour after administration. There was no consistent relationship between concentrations of oxacillin in cortical bone and those in serum. Concentrations of oxacillin in synovial tissue of 14 patients ranged from 0.3 to 5.6 μg per g(mean 1.8 μg per g).— R. H. Fitzgerald *et al.*, *Antimicrob. Ag. Chemother.*, 1978, *14*, 723.

For details of the accumulation of oxacillin sodium in burn crusts in patients receiving prophylactic treatment for burns, see Sodium Fusidate, p.1211.

Metabolism. About 49% of a 500-mg dose of oxacillin was metabolised. Within 12 hours of the dose being taken by 6 healthy subjects 33% was recovered in the urine, 16% as penicilloic acid.— M. Cole *et al.*, *Antimicrob. Ag. Chemother.*, 1973, *3*, 463.

Oxacillin was metabolised to a slightly less potent antibacterial compound that probably accumulated in patients with renal impairment.— H. H. W. Thijssen and H. Mattie, *Antimicrob. Ag. Chemother.*, 1976, *10*, 441.

Plasma concentrations. After intravenous infusion of oxacillin sodium 250 mg hourly for 3 hours in healthy subjects, the average plasma concentration of oxacillin fell from 9.7 μg per ml at the end of the infusion to 0.16 μg per ml 2 hours later. The rate of renal clearance of oxacillin was 226.8 ml per minute. In 15 hours the total amount excreted in the urine was 55.5% for oxacillin as compared with 73.3% for dicloxacillin and 62% for cloxacillin.— J. E. Rosenblatt *et al.*, *Archs intern. Med.*, 1968, *121*, 345.

In 5 children (age 1 week to 2 years) with staphylococcal infection given oxacillin sodium 25 mg per kg body-weight intramuscularly peak serum concentrations, 30 minutes after administration, ranged from 45 to 86 μg per ml with a mean elimination half-life of 78 minutes. After 7 to 10 days, treatment was changed to cloxacillin 25 mg per kg by mouth four times daily with peak concentrations, 1 to 2 hours after administration, of 28 to 80 μg per ml and a mean elimination half-life of 71 minutes.— G. J. Burckart *et al.*, *Am. J. Hosp. Pharm.*, 1978, *35*, 1380.

Further references: Z. Modr *et al.*, *Čas. Lék. česk.*, 1967, *106*, 945.

For details of plasma concentrations in infants, see under Precautions.

Uses. Oxacillin sodium is used for the treatment of infections due to staphylococci resistant to benzylpenicillin; it is also used for mixed streptococcal or pneumococcal and staphylococcal infections when the staphylococci are penicillin-resistant. It is less well absorbed from the gastro-intestinal tract and has slightly less activity against penicillinase-producing staphylococci than cloxacillin.
Oxacillin sodium is administered by mouth preferably 1 or 2 hours before meals. Adults should be given the equivalent of 0.5 to 1 g of oxacillin every 4 to 6 hours for 5 days or more depending on the severity of the infection. Children weighing less than 40 kg should be given the equivalent of 50 to 100 mg per kg body-weight daily in 4 to 6 divided doses.
Oxacillin is given by intramuscular injection in doses of 0.25 to 1 g every 4 to 6 hours. The same dose is given by slow intravenous injection in 5 to 10 ml of Water for Injections or sodium chloride injection 0.9%, or by intravenous infusion.
A dose of 25 mg per kg body-weight daily in divided doses by injection has been suggested for newborn and premature infants but it should be used with caution.

A guide to the use of penicillinase-resistant penicillins.— Veterans Administration Ad Hoc Interdisciplinary Advisory Committee on Antimicrobial Drug Usage, *J. Am. med. Ass.*, 1977, *237*, 1605.

Oxacillin 4 to 12 g daily given intravenously for up to 18 days followed by dicloxacillin 1 to 2 g daily by mouth for up to 23 days cured 4 patients with renal carbuncle. Cures were also obtained in a patient who received gentamicin with oxacillin for 14 days and another who received one course of oxacillin and ampicillin and a second course of dicloxacillin and ampicillin.— M. Schiff *et al.*, *Ann. intern. Med.*, 1977, *87*, 305.

Dialysis. For details of a study of oxacillin, ampicillin, and tetracycline given to patients undergoing dialysis, see Ampicillin, p.1096.

Dosage in renal failure. Two of 3 patients with staphylococcal septicaemia and acute renal failure were successfully treated with oxacillin in doses of 5 to 25 g daily and a total dose of up to 918 g. Secondary candidiasis in 1 patient was controlled with amphotericin in a dosage of 400 μg per kg body-weight at intervals of 48 to 72 hours. One patient developed polyneuritis. Renal failure was not a contra-indication to high doses of oxacillin.— E. Schröder *et al.*, *Dt. med. Wschr.*, 1966, *91*, 1035.

Patients with anuria and a creatinine clearance of 10 ml or less per minute should be given 1 g of oxacillin intravenously every 4 to 6 hours. Patients with both kidney and liver disorders should receive lower doses because of the rapid metabolism of oxacillin in the liver. Haemodialysis did not remove oxacillin.— D. L. Giusti, *Drug Intell. & clin. Pharm.*, 1973, *7*, 62.

Data for predicting removal of oxacillin by conventional haemodialysis.— T. P. Gibson and H. A. Nelson, *Clin. Pharmacokinet.*, 1977, *2*, 403.

The normal half-life for oxacillin of 0.4 hour was increased to 0.5 to 1 hour in end-stage renal failure. It could be given in usual doses to patients with renal failure. Concentrations of oxacillin were not affected by haemodialysis or peritoneal dialysis.— W. M. Bennett *et al.*, *Ann. intern. Med.*, 1980, *93*, 62. See also G. B. Appel and H. C. Neu, *New Engl. J. Med.*, 1977, *296*, 663.

Osteomyelitis. Chronic bacterial osteomyelitis of the spine was successfully treated in 4 patients by a modified technique of closed suction and irrigation with a 0.2% solution of oxacillin sodium in sodium chloride injection 0.9%. To each litre of irrigating fluid 60 ml of Alevaire (containing tyloxapol 0.125%) was added as a wetting agent to aid penetration into necrotic tissues and bone. After debridement of the sinus tract, irrigation was started at a rate of 1 litre every 12 hours, and was usually continued for 7 to 10 days. In addition, 2 patients were given lincomycin hydrochloride, 500 mg four times daily, starting 2 days before irrigation and continuing for a total of 3 weeks. The sensitivity of the infecting organism in 1 patient changed after 3 days' treatment, and methicillin sodium was later successfully substituted for oxacillin.— E. O. Leventen, *J. Am. med. Ass.*, 1966, *196*, 761.

Preparations

Oxacillin Sodium Capsules *(U.S.P.)*. Capsules containing oxacillin sodium equivalent to 125, 250, or 500 mg of oxacillin. Store at 15° to 30° in airtight containers.

Oxacillin Sodium for Injection *(U.S.P.)*. A sterile dry mixture of oxacillin sodium and one or more suitable buffers. Potency is expressed in terms of the equivalent amount of oxacillin. Store at 15° to 30°. The injection is prepared by the addition of diluent before use. pH of a 3% solution 6 to 8.5.

Oxacillin Sodium for Oral Solution *(U.S.P.)*. Oxacillin sodium with one or more suitable buffers, colouring and flavouring agents, preservatives, and stabilisers. Store at 15° to 30°. The solution is prepared by the addition of diluent before issue, and contains the equivalent of 25 or 50 mg of oxacillin per ml. pH 5 to 7.5.

Proprietary Names
Bactocill *(Beecham, USA)*; Bristopen *(Bristol, Fr.)*; Cryptocillin *(Hoechst, Ger.)*; Penistafil *(Antibioticos, Spain)*; Penstapho *(Bristol, Belg.*; *Bristol Italiana Sud, Ital.)*; Pro-Staphlin *(Lundbeck, Denm.)*; Prostaphlin *(Bristol, Canad.*; *Bristol, USA)*; Stapenor *(Bayer, Ger.)*.

120-f

Oxytetracycline Calcium *(U.S.P.)*.
The calcium salt of 5β-hydroxytetracycline.
$C_{44}H_{46}CaN_4O_{18}$=958.9.

CAS — 15251-48-6 (xCa).

Pharmacopoeias. In *U.S.*

A yellow to light brown crystalline powder. It contains 8 to 14% of water and not less than 865 μg of oxytetracycline per mg of anhydrous material. Oxytetracycline calcium 1.04 g is approximately equivalent to 1 g of oxytetracycline.
Practically **insoluble** in water; soluble in dilute solutions of sodium hydroxide. A 2.5% suspension in water has a pH of about 6 to 8. **Store** in a cool place in airtight containers. Protect from light.

121-d

Oxytetracycline Dihydrate *(B.P., B.P. Vet., Eur. P.)*.
Oxytetracycline *(U.S.P.)*; Oxytetracyclini Dihydras; 5-Hydroxytetracycline; Ossitetracíclina Biidrato; Terrafungine. 5β-Hydroxytetracycline dihydrate.
$C_{22}H_{24}N_2O_9,2H_2O$=496.5.

CAS — 79-57-2 (anhydrous); 6153-64-6 (dihydrate).

Pharmacopoeias. In *Arg.*, *Br.*, *Cz.*, *Eur.*, *Fr.*, *Ger.*, *Hung.*, *It.*, *Jug.*, *Neth.*, *Nord.*, *Pol.*, *Rus.*, *Swiss*, and *U.S.*

The dihydrate of oxytetracycline, an antimicrobial substance produced by the growth of certain strains of *Streptomyces rimosus*, or by any other means. It occurs as an odourless yellow to tan-coloured crystalline powder with a slightly bitter taste. The *B.P.* specifies that it contains not less than 950 units per mg, calculated with reference to the anhydrous substance. The *U.S.P.* specifies not less than 832 μg of oxytetracycline per mg. Stable in air but darkens on exposure to strong sunlight. Oxytetracycline dihydrate 1.08 g is approximately equivalent to 1 g of oxytetracycline.
Soluble 1 in 4150 of water, 1 in 66 of dehydrated alcohol, and 1 in 6250 of ether; sparingly soluble in alcohol; practically insoluble in chloroform; soluble in dilute acids and alkalis. A solution in dilute hydrochloric acid is laevorotatory. A 1% suspension in water has a pH of 5 to 7.5. It deteriorates in solutions having a pH of less than 2 and is rapidly destroyed by alkalis. **Store** in airtight containers. Protect from light.

122-n

Oxytetracycline Hydrochloride *(B.P., B.P. Vet., Eur. P., U.S.P.)*.
Oxytetracyclini Hydrochloridum; Chlorhydrate de Terrafungine. 5β-Hydroxytetracycline hydrochloride.
$C_{22}H_{24}N_2O_9,HCl$=496.9.

CAS — 2058-46-0.

Pharmacopoeias. In *Arg.*, *Aust.*, *Belg.*, *Br.*, *Cz.*, *Eur.*, *Fr.*, *Ger.*, *Hung.*, *Ind.*, *Int.*, *It.*, *Jug.*, *Neth.*, *Nord.*, *Rus.*, *Swiss*, *Turk.*, and *U.S.*
Jap. specifies dihydrate.

A yellow, odourless, hygroscopic, crystalline powder with a bitter taste. The *B.P.* specifies that it contains not less than 880 units per mg of anhydrous oxytetracycline hydrochloride. The *U.S.P.* specifies that it contains not less than 835 µg of oxytetracycline per mg of anhydrous substance. Oxytetracycline hydrochloride 1.08 g is approximately equivalent to 1 g of oxytetracycline. It decomposes above 180°. It darkens on exposure to sunlight or to moist air above 90°, but there is little loss of potency.

Soluble 1 in 2 of water, 1 in 45 of alcohol, and 1 in 45 of methyl alcohol; less soluble in dehydrated alcohol; soluble in propylene glycol; practically insoluble in chloroform and ether. A 1% solution in water has a pH of 2.3 to 2.9.

Solutions in water become turbid on standing owing to hydrolysis and precipitation of oxytetracycline base. Oxytetracycline hydrochloride deteriorates in solutions having a pH of less than 2 and is rapidly destroyed by alkalis.

Solutions for injection are prepared aseptically. **Store** in airtight containers. If it is intended for injection the containers should be sterile and sealed to exclude micro-organisms. Protect from light.

Incompatibility has been reported with alkalis, aminophylline, amphotericin, ampicillin sodium, soluble barbiturates, benzylpenicillin, carbenicillin sodium, cefapirin sodium, cephaloridine, cephalothin sodium, cephazolin sodium, cloxacillin sodium, erythromycin salts, iron dextran injection, methicillin sodium, novobiocin sodium, oxacillin sodium, phenytoin sodium, sodium bicarbonate, sulphadiazine sodium, and sulphafurazole diethanolamine. Incompatibility has also been reported, generally less consistently, with calcium chloride, calcium gluconate, chloramphenicol sodium succinate, heparin, hydrocortisone sodium succinate, lactated Ringer's injection, protein hydrolysate, and sodium lactate, and, depending on the diluent, with amikacin sulphate.

Effect of gamma-irradiation. For the effect of gamma-irradiation on oxytetracycline, see Chlortetracycline Hydrochloride, p.1142.

Epimerisation. Oxytetracycline epimerised much less readily than tetracycline in aqueous solution at pH 4.— D. A. Hussar *et al.*, *J. Pharm. Pharmac.*, 1968, *20*, 539.

Incompatibility. Oxytetracycline was incompatible with *calcium chloride, calcium gluconate, calcium gluceptate, heparin, hydroxyzine, metaraminol tartrate, methylprednisolone sodium succinate, prochlorperazine, promethazine, suxamethonium, thiopentone sodium,* and *vitamins of the B group* in an infusion fluid.— B. Flouvat and P. Lechat, *Thérapie*, 1974, *29*, 337.

Further references: H. R. Grant, *Hosp. Pharmst*, 1962, *15*, 67; J. A. Patel and G. L. Phillips, *Am. J. Hosp. Pharm.*, 1966, *23*, 409; J. M. Meisler and M. W. Skolaut, *Am. J. Hosp. Pharm.*, 1966, *23*, 557; B. Lynn, *Chemist Drugg.*, 1967, *187*, 157; B. B. Riley, *J. Hosp. Pharm.*, 1970, *28*, 228; E. A. Parker, *Am. J. Hosp. Pharm.*, 1970, *27*, 327; J. Jacobs *et al.*, *J. clin. Path.*, 1973, *26*, 742.

Stability in solution. Oxytetracycline in dextrose injection 5% at pH 3.22 lost 17% activity in 12 hours, increasing to 25% after 24 hours.— J. N. Bair and D. P. Carew, *Bull. parent. Drug Ass.*, 1965, *19*, 153.

A study of the effects of pH and temperature on the degradation of oxytetracycline in aqueous solutions. Maximum stability occurred at pH 2.— B. Vej-Hansen *et al.*, *Arch. Pharm. Chemi, scient. Edn*, 1978, *6*, 151.

Further references: A. Sina *et al.*, *Can. J. pharm. Sci.*, 1974, *9*, 44.

Units. One unit of oxytetracycline is contained in 0.0011364 mg of the second International Standard Preparation (1966) of oxytetracycline base dihydrate which contains 880 units per mg.

Adverse Effects and Precautions. As for Tetracycline Hydrochloride, p.1217.

Oxytetracycline is less likely than other older tetracyclines to stain the teeth of children.

Oxytetracycline was more likely to cause local irritation of the oropharyngeal or oesophageal mucosa than other tetracyclines.— *Br. med. J.*, 1974, *2*, 663.

In a study involving 7 geriatric patients given parenteral nutrition with an amino acid solution and dextrose, infusions of oxytetracycline 1 g daily produced a negative nitrogen balance within 1 or 2 days and very high peak blood concentrations. A dose of 500 mg had the same effect on nitrogen balance. Folic acid supplements for those with folate deficiency prevented this effect. Doxycycline 100 mg by infusion daily had only slight if any effect on nitrogen balance.— J. Korkeila, *Ann. clin. Res.*, 1974, *6*, 25.

A 68-year-old man developed thrombocytopenic purpura while taking oxytetracycline. He recovered after withdrawal of oxytetracycline.— N. G. Kounis, *J. Am. med. Ass.*, 1975, *231*, 734.

Interactions. Oxytetracycline appeared to have a hypoglycaemic effect in 2 insulin-dependent diabetic patients.— J. B. Miller (letter), *Br. med. J.*, 1966, *2*, 1007.

Nephrotoxicity. Oxytetracycline was not recommended in patients with poor renal function. Two patients developed uraemia following treatment with oxytetracycline, which improved when treatment was stopped. Oxytetracycline should not be given intravenously in doses in excess of 1 g daily and should never be given to pregnant women.— O. M. Edwards *et al.*, *Br. med. J.*, 1970, *1*, 26.

Absorption and Fate. As for Tetracycline Hydrochloride, p.1219.

Some 20 to 35% of oxytetracycline was bound in the body to serum proteins. The half-life in serum was 9.6 hours and 70% was excreted in urine.— C. M. Kunin, *Ann. intern. Med.*, 1967, *67*, 151.

Studies in 36 subjects with normal or impaired renal function demonstrated that in normal subjects the half-life in serum was 9.3 hours and that the urinary clearance was 82% of the glomerular filtration. In those subjects with impaired kidney function urinary excretion decreased in proportion to the decrease in glomerular filtration and so lengthened the half-life in serum. In 3 patients with a creatinine clearance rate between 0 and 2 ml per minute, the mean serum half-life of oxytetracycline was reduced from 54 to 12 hours by haemodialysis.— G. Mérier *et al.*, *Schwiez. med. Wschr.*, 1970, *100*, 1442.

Bioavailability. A review of the bioavailability of oxytetracycline.— W. G. Crouthamel *et al.*, *J. Am. pharm. Ass.*, 1975, *NS15*, 461.

Diffusion. A study of the tissue concentrations of oxytetracycline in man following intravenous administration.— F. Legler and K. Schwemmle, *Arzneimittel-Forsch.*, 1974, *24*, 185.

Sputum. The average sputum concentration of oxytetracycline in 9 patients with acute exacerbations of chronic chest disease was 1 µg per ml after receiving oxytetracycline 500 mg 4 times daily for 4 days; the corresponding serum concentration was 3.7 µg per ml.— T. D. Brogan *et al.*, *J. antimicrob. Chemother.*, 1977, *3*, 247. See also D. MacCulloch *et al.*, *N.Z. med. J.*, 1974, *80*, 300.

For a report of the content of antibiotic in sputum being increased when bromhexine is given in addition to oxytetracycline, see Bromhexine Hydrochloride, p.688.

Pregnancy and the neonate. The concentration of oxytetracycline in foetal blood was one-quarter that of the maternal blood.— P. Demers *et al.*, *Can. med. Ass. J.*, 1968, *99*, 849.

Uses. Oxytetracycline has the antimicrobial activity and uses described for tetracycline hydrochloride (see p.1218).

The calcium salt is used in aqueous oral suspensions, the dihydrate in tablets and intramuscular injections, and the hydrochloride in capsules and intramuscular or intravenous injections. Doses are expressed confusingly as oxytetracycline or as the calcium salt, the hydrochloride, or the dihydrate; in practice this appears to make little difference.

Oxytetracycline hydrochloride is usually given in doses of up to 3 g daily by mouth or up to 2 g daily by intravenous infusion. Children have been given 25 to 50 mg per kg body-weight daily by mouth and up to 20 mg per kg daily by injection but the effect of tetracyclines on teeth should be considered.

For the possible use of oxytetracycline in treating doxorubicin-induced cardiotoxicity, see Doxorubicin, p.206.

Dosage in renal failure. The use of oxytetracycline should be avoided in patients with even mild renal failure; doxycycline may be used if necessary.— G. B. Appel and H. C. Neu, *New Engl. J. Med.*, 1977, *296*, 663.

For a comparison of oxytetracycline and doxycycline in patients with renal failure, see Doxycycline Hydrochloride, p.1156.

Leptospirosis. Oxytetracycline, 500 mg six-hourly for 10 days, was successful in the treatment of a 47-year-old man with leptospirosis.— S. N. Sinha, *Practitioner*, 1969, *202*, 273. See also R. W. R. Russell, *Lancet*, 1958, *2*, 1143.

Skin disorders. *Acne.* In a double-blind study in 28 patients with acne, oxytetracycline and doxycycline appeared to be equally effective in reducing the number of lesions to about 55% of the original number, within 4 weeks. Patients received during the first 4 weeks either oxytetracycline 250 mg thrice daily, or doxycycline 100 mg daily; during the second period of 4 weeks the doses were reduced to once daily and every third day respectively; during the third period of 4 weeks the patients received the lower dosage of the alternative treatment. Some patients relapsed on the lower doses.— L. Juhlin and S. Lidén, *Br. J. Derm.*, 1969, *81*, 154.

No significant difference was found between systemic treatment for acne with either oxytetracycline or zinc sulphate during a 12-week double-blind study in 37 patients.— G. Michaëlsson *et al.*, *Br. J. Derm.*, 1977, *97*, 561.

Further references: L. Stankler, *Br. J. clin. Pract.*, 1979, *33*, 137.

Toxoplasmosis. Toxoplasmosis in a young man responded partially to a 3-week course of oxytetracycline; pyrimethamine and sulphadiazine were not helpful; prolonged symptomatic relief was later obtained after a month's course of oxytetracycline with prednisolone. An adequately long course of tetracycline was suggested as treatment.— A. Fertig *et al.*, *Br. med. J.*, 1977, *1*, 1064. Adequate proof of the beneficial effect of oxytetracycline was lacking.— P. L. Grossman and J. S. Remington (letter), *Br. med. J.*, 1977, *1*, 1664. See also F. J. Nye, *J. antimicrob. Chemother.*, 1979, *5*, 244.

Trachoma. Cervical swabs were positive for *Chlamydia trachomatis* in 282 of 1009 women attending a clinic for sexually transmitted diseases. Swabs from the eyes of 33 of 103 neonates with conjunctivitis were positive. Swabs became negative in 18 of 24 infants treated with oxytetracycline eye ointment daily for 1 month.— D. Hobson and E. Rees, *Postgrad. med. J.*, 1977, *53*, 595.

Further references: S. Darougar *et al.*, *Br. J. Ophthal.*, 1980, *64*, 37; *idem*, 291.

Urinary-tract infections. In a study of different dosage regimens of oxytetracycline in patients with nongonococcal urethritis the highest cure-rate measured at 3 months was 87.5% in 200 patients given 250 mg four times daily for 21 days compared with 72% in 169 patients given 500 mg four times daily for 10 days and 55% in 132 patients given 500 mg thrice daily for 5 days.— J. John, *Br. J. vener. Dis.*, 1971, *47*, 266.

In a study of 33 patients with urinary-tract infections treated with oxytetracycline 250 mg four times daily it was the bactericidal activity of the urine, not of the serum, that determined the failures and cures.— T. A. Stamey *et al.*, *New Engl. J. Med.*, 1974, *291*, 1159.

Vaginitis. During a placebo-controlled study of treatment regimens for *Gardnerella vaginalis* (*Haemophilus vaginalis*) vaginitis in 30 patients, sensitivity tests *in vitro* demonstrated that of 47 of the strains isolated 35 were sensitive to tetracycline. Four of 10 infected women treated with oxytetracycline 500 mg twice daily for 7 days were assessed as clinical failures on the first follow-up visit; the other 6 showed clinical cure although the culture was still positive in 3 (heavy growth in 1 and moderate in 2), the organisms being resistant to oxytetracycline *in vitro*. Five of these patients attended 4 weeks later; all were clinically cured and the organism was not isolated. Although tests *in vitro* had shown a relative insensitivity, better results were obtained with metronidazole.— M. J. Balsdon *et al.*, *Lancet*, 1980, *1*, 501.

Preparations

Capsules

Oxytetracycline Capsules *(B.P.)*. Caps. Oxytetracyc. Capsules containing oxytetracycline hydrochloride. The *B.P.* requires 70% dissolution in 45 minutes. Store at a temperature not exceeding 30°.

Oxytetracycline Hydrochloride Capsules *(U.S.P.)*. Capsules containing oxytetracycline hydrochloride. Potency is expressed in terms of the equivalent amount of anhydrous oxytetracycline. Store in airtight containers. Protect from light.

Injections

Oxytetracycline and Procaine Injection *(B.P. 1958)*. Oxytetracycline Hydrochloride and Procaine Hydrochloride Injection. A sterile solution of oxytetracycline hydrochloride and procaine hydrochloride in Water for

Injections; it may contain suitable buffering and stabilising agents. It is prepared by dissolving the sterile contents of a sealed container in Water for Injections. Store at not more than 4° and use within 5 days. For intramuscular injection.

Oxytetracycline Hydrochloride for Injection *(U.S.P.)*. A sterile dry mixture of oxytetracycline hydrochloride and a suitable buffer. Potency is expressed in terms of the equivalent amount of anhydrous oxytetracycline. The injection is prepared by the addition of diluent before use. pH of a 2.5% solution 1.8 to 2.8.

Oxytetracycline Injection *(B.P.)*. Inj. Oxytetracyc.; Oxytetracycline Hydrochloride Injection. A sterile solution of oxytetracycline hydrochloride in Water for Injections. It is prepared by dissolving the sterile contents of a sealed container in the requisite amount of Water for Injections. The sealed container also contains a suitable buffering agent. Store at a temperature not exceeding 4° and use within 72 hours. For intravenous injection only, as a well-diluted solution.

Oxytetracycline Injection *(U.S.P.)*. A sterile solution of oxytetracycline dihydrate with or without suitable anaesthetics, antoxidants, buffers, complexing agents, preservatives, and solvents. pH 8 to 9. It contains the equivalent of 50 or 125 mg of anhydrous oxytetracycline per ml.

Suspensions

Oxytetracycline Calcium Oral Suspension *(U.S.P.)*. A suspension of oxytetracycline calcium with one or more suitable buffers, preservatives, suspending, colouring, flavouring, and stabilising agents. It contains *N*-acetyl glucosamine. pH 5 to 8. It contains the equivalent of 25 mg of anhydrous oxytetracycline per ml. Store in airtight containers. Protect from light.

Tablets

Oxytetracycline Tablets *(B.P.)*. Tablets containing oxytetracycline dihydrate. The tablets are coated. The *B.P.* requires 70% dissolution in 45 minutes.

Oxytetracycline Tablets *(U.S.P.)*. Tablets containing oxytetracycline dihydrate equivalent to 250 mg of anhydrous oxytetracycline. Store in airtight containers. Protect from light.

Proprietary Preparations containing Oxytetracycline and its Salts

Abbocin *(Abbott, UK)*. Oxytetracycline, available as tablets each containing 250 mg of the dihydrate.

Berkmycen *(Berk Pharmaceuticals, UK)*. Oxytetracycline, available as **Capsules** each containing 250 mg of the hydrochloride and as **Tablets** each containing 250 mg of the dihydrate.

Chemocycline *(Consolidated Chemicals, UK)*. Oxytetracycline, available as **Syrup** (supplied as powder for preparation with water before use) containing in each 5 ml oxytetracycline calcium equivalent to oxytetracycline 125 mg and as **Tablets** each containing oxytetracycline dihydrate 250 mg.

Galenomycin *(Galen, UK)*. Oxytetracycline, available as tablets each containing 250 mg of the dihydrate.

Imperacin *(ICI Pharmaceuticals, UK)*. Oxytetracycline dihydrate, available as tablets of 250 mg.

Oxymed *(Unimed, UK)*. Oxytetracycline, available as tablets each containing 250 mg of the dihydrate.

Oxymycin *(DDSA Pharmaceuticals, UK)*. Oxytetracycline, available as tablets each containing 250 mg of the dihydrate.

Terra-Bron *(Pfizer, UK)*. A liquid preparation containing in each 5 ml oxytetracycline calcium equivalent to oxytetracycline 250 mg, ephedrine hydrochloride 7.5 mg, and ipecacuanha liquid extract 0.03 ml (suggested diluent, syrup). For bronchitis. *Dose.* 5 ml every 6 hours.

Terra-Cortril Ear Suspension *(Pfizer, UK)*. A suspension containing in each ml oxytetracycline hydrochloride equivalent to oxytetracycline 5 mg, hydrocortisone acetate 15 mg, and polymyxin B sulphate 10 000 units in a controlled-viscosity gel-like basis.

Terra-Cortril Nystatin Cream *(Pfizer, UK)*. Contains in each g oxytetracycline calcium equivalent to oxytetracycline 30 mg, hydrocortisone 10 mg, and nystatin 100 000 units.

Terra-Cortril Spray *(Pfizer, UK)*. A pressurised spray containing in each 30 ml oxytetracycline hydrochloride equivalent to anhydrous oxytetracycline 150 mg and hydrocortisone 50 mg.

Terra-Cortril Topical Ointment *(Pfizer, UK)*. Contains in each g oxytetracycline hydrochloride equivalent to oxytetracycline 30 mg and hydrocortisone 10 mg in a basis containing soft paraffin.

Terramycin *(Pfizer, UK)*. Preparations for oral administration, available as **Capsules** each containing oxytetracycline hydrochloride equivalent to oxytetracycline 250 mg; as **Syrup** containing in each 5 ml oxytetracycline calcium equivalent to oxytetracycline 125 mg (suggested diluent, syrup); and as **Tablets** each containing oxytetracycline dihydrate equivalent to oxytetracycline 100 and 250 mg. (Also available as Terramycin in *Austral., Canad., Ger., Neth., S.Afr., Switz., USA*).

Terramycin Intramuscular *(Pfizer, UK)*. A dry powder in vials for the preparation of 2 ml of a solution for intramuscular injection containing in each ml oxytetracycline hydrochloride equivalent to oxytetracycline 50 mg and magnesium chloride 50 mg, with 2% procaine hydrochloride.

Terramycin Ophthalmic Ointment with Polymyxin B Sulphate *(Pfizer, UK)*. Contains in each g oxytetracycline hydrochloride equivalent to oxytetracycline 5 mg and polymyxin B sulphate 10 000 units in a soft paraffin basis.

Terramycin Topical Ointment *(Pfizer, UK)*. Contains in each g oxytetracycline hydrochloride equivalent to oxytetracycline 30 mg in a soft paraffin basis.

Terramycin SF *(Pfizer, UK)*. Capsules each containing oxytetracycline hydrochloride equivalent to oxytetracycline 250 mg, ascorbic acid 75 mg, thiamine mononitrate 2.5 mg, riboflavine 2.5 mg, and nicotinamide 25 mg. *Dose.* 1 or 2 capsules 4 times daily.

Unimycin *(Unigreg, UK: Vestric, UK)*. Capsules each containing oxytetracycline hydrochloride 250 mg.

Other Proprietary Names for Oxytetracycline and Oxytetracycline Hydrochloride

Arg.—Terraven; *Austral.*—Bramcycline, Oxycycline; *Belg.*—Terraject, Terramycine, Terraven, Vendarcin; *Fr.*—Gynamousse, Terramycine; *Ger.*—Macocyn, Terravenös, Tetra-Tablinen; *Ital.*—Proteroxyna, Terramicina; *Neth.*—Vendarcin; *S.Afr.*—Betacycline, Inoxtet, Lenocyclin, Oxim, Oxypan, Oxytet, Roxy, Tetramel; *Spain*—Crisamicin, Elaciclina, Geobiotico (see also Doxycycline), Huberbiotic, Humusmycin, Terramicina, Terramyfar; *Swed.*—Oxy-Dumocyclin, Oxytetral; *Switz.*—Oxylag, Oxy-Rivo, Terravenös, Vendarcin; *USA*—Uri-Tet.

Oxytetracycline dihydrate was also formerly marketed in Great Britain under the proprietary names Oppamycin (*Oppenheimer*, now *LRC Products*), Oxydon (*RP Drugs*), and Stecsolin (*Squibb*). Oxytetracycline calcium and dihydrate were also formerly marketed in Great Britain under the proprietary name Clinimycin (*Glaxo*). In some countries it was marketed as Clinmycin.

Clinimycin is also a synonym for clindamycin (see p.1144).

123-h

Paromomycin Sulphate *(B.P.C. 1973)*.

Paromomycin Sulfate (*U.S.P.*); Amminosidina Solfato; Aminosidinum Sulfuricum; Catenulin. 4-*O*-(2-Amino-2-deoxy-α-D-glucopyranosyl)-2-deoxy-5-*O*-[3-*O*-(2,6-diamino-2,6-dideoxy-β-L-idopyranosyl)-β-D-ribofuranosyl]-D-streptamine sulphate. $C_{23}H_{45}N_5O_{14}, xH_2SO_4$=615.6 (paromomycin).

CAS — 7542-37-2 (paromomycin); 1263-89-4 (sulphate).

NOTE. Aminosidin Sulphate (Crestomycin Sulphate) produced by the growth of *Streptomyces chrestomyceticus* was shown by R.T. Schillings and C.P. Schaffner (*Antimicrob. Ag. Chemother.*, 1961, 274) to be identical with paromomycin sulphate.

Monomycin, an antibiotic, isolated from *Streptomyces circulatus* var. *monomycini* (see *Extra Pharmacopoeia 26th Edn*, p. 1386) is considered to be identical with paromomycin.

Pharmacopoeias. In *It.* and *U.S.*

A mixture of the sulphates of the antimicrobial substances produced by the growth of certain strains of *Streptomyces rimosus* forma *paromomycinus*.

A creamy-white to light yellow, odourless or almost odourless, hygroscopic, amorphous powder with a saline taste containing not less than 675 μg or units per mg, calculated on the dried material. The *B.P.C. 1973* specifies not less than 23 to 26% of sulphate. One million units of paromomycin are approximately equivalent to 1 g of paromomycin base.

Soluble 1 in 1 of water, practically insoluble in alcohol, chloroform, and ether; soluble in dilute acids and solutions of alkali hydroxides. A solution in water is dextrorotatory. A 3% solution in water is clear and has a pH of 5 to 7.5. **Store** in airtight containers.

Loss of activity. Paromomycin was much less active against *Staphylococcus aureus* in the presence of bentonite, magnesium trisilicate, pectin, and tragacanth, and less active with acacia, carmellose, kaolin, methylcellulose, polysorbate 80, silica, and sodium alginate.— M. A. El-Nakeeb and R. T. Yousef, *Acta pharm. suec.*, 1968, *5*, 1.

Units. One unit of paromomycin is contained in 0.001333 mg of the first International Reference Preparation (1965) of paromomycin sulphate which contains 750 units per mg.

Adverse Effects and Precautions. As for Neomycin Sulphate, p.1189.

Ototoxicity. The Boston Collaborative Drug Surveillance Program monitored consecutively 32 812 medical inpatients. Drug-induced deafness occurred in 1 of 75 patients given paromomycin.— J. Porter and H. Jick, *Lancet*, 1977, *1*, 587.

Antimicrobial Action. Paromomycin sulphate has an antimicrobial spectrum similar to that of neomycin sulphate (p.1189). It is active *in vitro* against *Actinomyces bovis* and is directly amoebicidal against *Entamoeba histolytica*.

Studies *in vitro* demonstrated that paromomycin sulphate 5, 10, or 20 μg per ml significantly reduced or inhibited the transfer of the tetracycline resistance R-factor between *Escherichia coli* and *Salmonella pullorum*. It was suggested that the emergence of tetracycline-resistant pathogens could be prevented by the presence of paromomycin in low concentrations.— A. Buogo and P. Cattaneo, *J. pharm. Sci.*, 1978, *67*, 35.

Resistance. There is cross-resistance between paromomycin, kanamycin, and neomycin.

Absorption and Fate. Paromomycin is poorly absorbed from the gastro-intestinal tract and most of the dose is eliminated in the faeces.

Uses. Paromomycin sulphate is administered by mouth in the treatment of intestinal amoebiasis. A recommended dose is the equivalent of 25 to 30 mg of paromomycin per kg body-weight daily in 3 doses for 5 to 10 days. Paromomycin has also been effective in the treatment of tapeworm infestation.

It has been used in the treatment of dysentery and, similarly to neomycin, in enteritis and in the suppression of intestinal flora both pre-operatively and in the management of hepatic coma.

Dosage in renal failure. The use of paromomycin in patients with varying renal function.— A. Novarini *et al.*, *Clin. Nephrol.*, 1975, *4*, 23.

Tapeworm infestation. Paromomycin, 20 to 50 mg per kg body-weight daily for 3 or 4 days, was effective in clearing infestation due to *Taenia saginata* and *T. solium* in 91 of 92 patients. Good results had also been obtained against *Hymenolepis nana* infections.— A. Ulivelli (letter), *Lancet*, 1968, *1*, 696.

For other reports of the use of paromomycin, see Martindale 27th Edn, pp. 1166-7.

Preparations

Paromomycin Sulfate Capsules *(U.S.P.)*. Capsules containing paromomycin sulphate equivalent to 250 mg of paromomycin. Store in airtight containers.

Paromomycin Sulfate Syrup *(U.S.P.)*. A syrup containing paromomycin sulphate and one or more suitable solvents, flavouring agents, colouring agents, preservatives, and buffers. pH 7.5 to 8.5. It contains the equivalent of 25 mg of paromomycin per ml. Store in airtight containers.

Proprietary Names

Aminoxidin *(Farmalabor, Ital.)*; Gabbromicina *(Montedison, Arg.)*; Gabbromycin *(Farmitalia, Ger.)*; Gabbroral *(Montedison, Arg.; Montedison, Belg.; Farmalabor, Ital.)*; Gabromicina *(Spain)*; Gabroral *(Spain)*; Humagel *(Parke, Davis, Fr.)*; Humatin *(Parke, Davis, Belg.; Parke, Davis, Fr.; Parke, Davis, Ger.; Parke, Davis, Ital.; Substantia, Neth.; Parke, Davis, Spain; Parke, Davis, Swed.; Parke, Davis, Switz.; Parke, Davis, USA)*; Paramicina *(Ragionieri, Ital.)*; Sinosid *(SIFI, Ital.)*.

Paromomycin sulphate was formerly marketed in Great Britain under the proprietary name Humatin (*Parke, Davis*).

124-m

Penamecillin. Wy 20788. Acetoxymethyl (6*R*)-6-(2-phenylacetamido)penicillanate.
$C_{19}H_{22}N_2O_6S=406.5$.

CAS — 983-85-7.

A white or creamy-white odourless powder. M.p. about 107°. Practically **insoluble** in water; soluble in chloroform.

Penamecillin has actions and uses similar to those of benzylpenicillin (see p.1102) and is given in doses of 350 mg every 8 hours. It should not be given for severe, chronic, or deep-seated infections.

For reports of comparisons of penamecillin with phenoxymethylpenicillin, see Report No. 104 of the General Practitioner Research Group, *Practitioner*, 1967, *198*, 568; J. Gomez and G. Gomez, *Br. J. clin. Pract.*, 1967, *21*, 183.

Proprietary Preparations

Havapen *(Wyeth, UK)*. Penamecillin, available as tablets of 350 mg.

125-b

Penethamate Hydriodide *(B.P.C. 1954)*. Diethylaminoethyl Penicillin G Hydroiodide. 2-Diethylaminoethyl (6*R*)-6-(2-phenylacetamido)penicillanate hydriodide.
$C_{22}H_{31}N_3O_4S,HI=561.5$.

CAS — 3689-73-4 (penethamate); 808-71-9 (hydriodide).

A fine white odourless powder with a bitter taste. **Soluble** 1 in 100 of water; soluble in alcohol, acetone, and methyl alcohol; practically insoluble in ether. A 1% solution in water has a pH of 5.5 to 7. **Store** in a cool dry place in sterile containers.

Penethamate hydriodide was formerly used by intramuscular injection similarly to benzylpenicillin (see p.1107).

Proprietary Names

Bronchocilline *(Bellon, Switz.)*; Iodocillina *(Lusofarmaco, Ital.)*.

126-v

Penicillin O Sodium. Almecillin Sodium; Sodium Penicillin O. Sodium (6*R*)-6-[2-(allylthio)acetamido]-penicillanate.
$C_{13}H_{17}N_2NaO_4S_2=352.4$.

CAS — 87-09-2 (penicillin O); 7177-54-0 (sodium salt).

A white crystalline powder with an onion-like odour and taste. Readily **soluble** in water.

Penicillin O sodium was formerly used similarly to benzylpenicillin (see p.1107).

127-g

Penimepicycline. N^2-[4-(2-Hydroxyethyl)piperazin-1-ylmethyl]tetracycline (6*R*)-6-(2-phenoxyacetamido)penicillanate.
$C_{45}H_{56}N_6O_{14}S=937.0$.

CAS — 4599-60-4.

Penimepicycline is the phenoxymethylpenicillin salt of a tetracycline compound with the expected actions of these antibiotics. It has been given by mouth in doses of 1.5 g daily in 2 divided doses; 500 mg has been given intramuscularly twice daily.

Proprietary Names

Criseosil *(Montedison, Arg.)*; Mucosiris *(Osiris, Arg.)*; Penetracyn *(Midy, Ital.)*; Peniltetra 500 *(Panther-Osfa, Ital.)*; Pénétracyne *(Midy, Fr.)*; Prestociclina *(Chemil, Ital.)*; Pulmobiotic *(Miluy, Spain)*; Tetrabiomar *(Bio-Mar, Spain)*; Ultrabiotic *(Infal, Spain)*.

128-q

Penimocycline. Bo 725. (6*R*)-6-{2-[(4*S*,4a*S*,5a*S*,6*S*,12a*S*)-4-Dimethylamino-1,4,4a,5,5a,6,11,12a-octahydro-3,6,10,12,12a-pentahydroxy-6-methyl-1,11-dioxonaphthacene-2-carboxamidomethylamino]-2-phenylacetamido}penicillanic acid.
$C_{39}H_{43}N_5O_{12}S=805.9$.

CAS — 16259-34-0.

The penimocycline molecule combines the structures of tetracycline and ampicillin. It has been used as an antibiotic in doses of 2 to 4 g daily.

Proprietary Names

Intraxium *(Bottu, Fr.)*.

129-p

Phenethicillin Potassium *(B.P., U.S.P.)*.

Phenethicillin Pot.; Pheneticillinum Kalicum; Penicillin B; Potassium Phenethicillin; Potassium α-Phenoxyethylpenicillin. A mixture of the D(+)- and L(−)-isomers of potassium (6*R*)-6-(2-phenoxypropionamido)penicillanate.
$C_{17}H_{19}KN_2O_5S=402.5$.

CAS — 147-55-7 (phenethicillin); 132-93-4 (potassium salt).

Pharmacopoeias. In *Br.*, *Int.*, *Jap.*, and *U.S.* which specifies 55 to 75% of the L(−)-isomer.

A white or almost white, fine crystalline powder with a slightly sulphurous odour and a bitter taste. Each g represents about 2.5 mmol (2.5 mEq) of potassium. Phenethicillin potassium 1.1 g is approximately equivalent to 1 g of phenethicillin. It absorbs insignificant amounts of moisture at 25° at relative humidities up to about 65%, but under damper conditions it absorbs significant amounts.

Soluble 1 in 1.5 of water, 1 in 85 of alcohol, and 1 in 800 of dehydrated alcohol; slightly soluble in chloroform; practically insoluble in ether. A 10% solution in water has a pH of 5.5 to 7.5. **Store** in airtight containers.

Stability. Optimum stability for phenethicillin potassium in aqueous solution was provided by maintaining the pH between 6 and 6.5 with a suitable buffer, such as a citrate which had no effect on the rate of hydrolysis at this pH. Phosphate ions had a catalytic action on the hydrolysis of phenethicillin.— M. A. Schwartz *et al.*, *J. pharm. Sci.*, 1962, *51*, 523.

Stability in acid. The half-life of a 0.1% solution of phenethicillin potassium in 50% aqueous alcohol at pH 1.3 and 35° was about 160 minutes.— B. Lynn, *Chemist Drugg.*, 1967, *187*, 134.

Adverse Effects and Treatment. As for Benzylpenicillin, p.1103.

A 31-year-old pharmacist developed a generalised urticarial reaction within 10 minutes of taking a single dose of phenethicillin potassium. The reaction persisted for several hours. In subsequent skin tests the patient was hypersensitive to penicilloyl-polylysine at a dilution of 10^{-10}M, but not to penicillin, phenethicillin, penicilloate, or penilloate.— M. J. Fellner *et al.*, *J. Am. med. Ass.*, 1967, *202*, 909.

Colitis. A report of colitis in association with phenethicillin.— P. de Mulder *et al.* (letter), *Lancet*, 1978, *2*, 1151.

Precautions. As for Phenoxymethylpenicillin, p.1200.

Antimicrobial Action. Phenethicillin potassium has a range of activity similar to that of benzylpenicillin (see p.1105) and phenoxymethylpenicillin (see p.1200). It is less effective than phenoxymethylpenicillin against pneumococci, haemolytic streptococci, non-penicillinase-producing staphylococci, and neisseriae. Phenethicillin is slightly less susceptible to penicillinase than phenoxymethylpenicillin.

Absorption and Fate. Phenethicillin potassium is more resistant to inactivation by the acid of gastric secretions and is more completely absorbed than benzylpenicillin from the gastro-intestinal tract following administration by mouth. Absorption is generally rapid but can be variable. Peak plasma concentrations, of about 3 µg per ml, have been observed within 1 hour of a 250-mg dose, but the concentration declines to a low level in 4 hours. About 75% is bound to plasma protein. Distribution in the body is similar to that with phenoxymethylpenicillin and there is little diffusion into the CSF unless the meninges are inflamed. Up to 60% of the dose is excreted in the urine within 6 hours.

Metabolism. About 31% of a 500-mg dose of phenethicillin was metabolised. Within 12 hours of the dose being taken by 6 healthy subjects, 72% was recovered in the urine, about 22% as penicilloic acid.— M. Cole *et al.*, *Antimicrob. Ag. Chemother.*, 1973, *3*, 463.

Uses. Phenethicillin potassium is given by mouth for the treatment of infections similar to those for which phenoxymethylpenicillin (see p.1200) is used. Though it produces higher blood concentrations than phenoxymethylpenicillin it is less active against some bacteria.

The usual dosage is the equivalent of 250 mg of phenethicillin every 6 hours but doses of up to 500 mg may be given for more severe infections. Children under 2 years of age may be given one quarter the adult dose and from 2 to 10 years, one half the adult dose. Doses should preferably be taken ½ to 1 hour before food.

Preparations

Phenethicillin Capsules *(B.P.)*. Capsules containing phenethicillin potassium. Potency is expressed in terms of the equivalent amount of phenethicillin. Store at a temperature not exceeding 30°.

Phenethicillin Elixir *(B.P.C. 1973)*. Phenethicillin Syrup. A solution of phenethicillin potassium in a suitable coloured flavoured vehicle. pH 5.2 to 6.2. It is prepared freshly by dissolving a powder consisting of the dry mixed ingredients in the specified volume of water. Store in a cool place. When a dose less than 5 ml is prescribed, the elixir should be diluted to 5 ml with syrup. The elixir and diluted elixir must be freshly prepared and used within 1 week of preparation. The elixir should not lose more than 10% potency in a week at 15°.

Phenethicillin Potassium for Oral Solution *(U.S.P.)*. A dry mixture of phenethicillin potassium, with or without one or more suitable buffers, colouring and flavouring agents, and preservatives. The solution is prepared by the addition of diluent before issue. When reconstituted it contains the equivalent of 25 mg of phenethicillin per ml.

Phenethicillin Potassium Tablets *(U.S.P.)*. Tablets containing phenethicillin potassium equivalent to 250 mg of phenethicillin. Store in airtight containers.

Phenethicillin Tablets *(B.P.)*. Tablets containing phenethicillin potassium. Potency is expressed in terms of the equivalent amount of phenethicillin. The tablets may be flavoured with peppermint oil.

Proprietary Preparations

Broxil *(Beecham Research, UK)*. Phenethicillin potassium, available as **Capsules** containing the equivalent of 250 mg of phenethicillin; as **Syrup** (supplied as powder for preparation with water before use) containing the equivalent of 125 mg of phenethicillin in each 5 ml (suggested diluent, syrup); and as scored **Tablets** containing the equivalent of 250 mg of phenethicillin. (Also available as Broxil in *Neth.*, *S.Afr.*).

Other Proprietary Names

Altocillin *(Ital.)*; Bendralan *(Spain)*; Esterloven *(phenethicillin iodide) (Spain)*; Metilpen *(Ital.)*; Optipen *(Austral.)*; Penicilloral *(phenethicillin sodium) (Ital.)*; Penorale *(Ital.)*; Pensig *(Austral.)*; Syncillin *(USA)*.

130-n

Phenoxymethylpenicillin *(B.P., B.P. Vet., Eur. P.)*.

Penicillin V *(U.S.P.)*; Phenoxymethylpenicillinum; Phenoxymethyl Penicillin; Phénomycilline. (6*R*)-6-(2-Phenoxyacetamido)penicillanic acid.
$C_{16}H_{18}N_2O_5S=350.4$.

CAS — 87-08-1.

Pharmacopoeias. In *Arg.*, *Aust.*, *Br.*, *Eur.*, *Fr.*, *Ger.*,

Int., It., Jap., Jug., Neth., Pol., Roum., Rus., Swiss, Turk., and *U.S.*

Phenoxymethylpenicillin is an antimicrobial acid produced by the growth of certain strains of *Penicillium notatum* or related organisms on a culture medium containing an appropriate precursor, or by any other means. It is a white odourless crystalline powder. The *B.P.* specifies that it contains not less than 95% of total penicillins and not less than 92% of phenoxymethylpenicillin.

Soluble 1 in 1700 of water, 1 in 7 of alcohol, and 1 in 6 of acetone; soluble in chloroform and glycerol; practically insoluble in fixed oils and liquid paraffin. A 0.5% suspension in water has a pH of 2.4 to 4. **Store** in airtight containers.

131-h

Phenoxymethylpenicillin Calcium *(B.P. Vet., B.P. 1973).*

Phenoxymethylpenicillin Calc.; Phenoxymethylpenicillinum Calcicum; Penicillin V Calcium. The dihydrate of the calcium salt of phenoxymethylpenicillin.

$(C_{16}H_{17}N_2O_5S)_2Ca,2H_2O$=774.9.

CAS — 147-48-8 (anhydrous).

Pharmacopoeias. In *Int.*

A white finely crystalline powder; odourless or with a slight characteristic odour and with a slightly bitter taste. Each g of phenoxymethylpenicillin calcium represents about 1.3 mmol (2.6 mEq) of calcium. Phenoxymethylpenicillin calcium 1.11 g is approximately equivalent to 1 g of phenoxymethylpenicillin.

Slowly **soluble** 1 in 120 of water; practically insoluble in fixed oils and liquid paraffin. A 0.5% solution in water has a pH of 5 to 7.5. **Store** in airtight containers.

132-m

Phenoxymethylpenicillin Potassium *(B.P., B.P. Vet.).*

Penicillin V Potassium (*U.S.P.*); Phenoxymethylpenicillin Pot.; Phenoxymethylpenicillinum Kalicum; Phenoximethylpenicillinkalium; Fenoximetilpenicilina Potássica V. The potassium salt of phenoxymethylpenicillin.

$C_{16}H_{17}KN_2O_5S$=388.5.

CAS — 132-98-9.

Pharmacopoeias. In *Br., Braz., Cz., Ind., Int., It., Jap., Nord., Pol.*, and *U.S.*.

A white odourless crystalline powder with slightly bitter taste. Each g of phenoxymethylpenicillin potassium represents about 2.6 mmol (2.6 mEq) of potassium. Phenoxymethylpenicillin potassium 1.11 g is approximately equivalent to 1 g of phenoxymethylpenicillin.

Soluble 1 in 1.5 of water and 1 in 150 of alcohol; practically insoluble in acetone, ether, fixed oils, and liquid paraffin. A 0.5% solution in water has a pH of 5 to 7.5. The optimum pH for stability of solutions in water is 5.3 to 5.4; at this pH, a solution loses about 20% of its activity in 7 days. **Store** in airtight containers.

Effect of gamma-irradiation. Phenoxymethylpenicillin (free acid) was unchanged in colour at 25 000 Gy and became brown at 250 000 Gy. Its solution in aqueous sodium bicarbonate became pale yellow at 25 000 Gy and brown at 250 000 Gy. The potency fell to 99% of the original potency at 25 000 Gy and to 97% at 250 000 Gy.— *The Use of Gamma Radiation Sources for the Sterilisation of Pharmaceutical Products*, London, ABPI, 1960.

Loss of activity. The activity of phenoxymethylpenicillin against *Staphylococcus aureus* was very much reduced in the presence of zinc oxide and reduced to a lesser extent in the presence of magnesium carbonate, magnesium oxide, calamine, acacia, tragacanth, methylcellulose, sodium alginate, maize starch, gelatin, macrogol 4000, and propylene glycol.— M. A. El-Nakeeb and R. T. Yousef, *Acta pharm. suec.*, 1968, *5*, 1.

Stability. Ultraviolet irradiation for 2 hours had no effect on phenoxymethylpenicillin or its potassium salt.— A. A. Kassem and E. H. Girgis, *Bull. Fac. Pharm., Cairo*, 1970, *9*, 157.

Stability in solution. Benzylpenicillin, phenoxymethylpenicillin, and dicloxacillin formed complexes in solution with *sucrose* and their degradation-rates were increased. Ampicillin was only slightly affected by sucrose.— S. L. Hem *et al., J. pharm. Sci.*, 1973, *62*, 267. Accelerated degradation of benzylpenicillin sodium, ampicillin sodium, carbenicillin sodium, and phenoxymethylpenicillin potassium in neutral and alkaline sucrose solutions was due to a nucleophilic displacement reaction with the formation of sucrose penicilloate esters. These esters might be antigenic and their presence should be avoided by maintaining the pH of solutions of penicillins and sucrose at 6 to 6.5.— H. Bundgaard and C. Larsen, *Int. J. Pharmaceut.*, 1978, *1*, 95.

Units. One unit of phenoxymethylpenicillin was contained in 0.00059 mg of the first International Standard Preparation (1957) which contained 1695 units per mg. The International Standard was discontinued in 1968.

Adverse Effects and Treatment. These are similar to those of benzylpenicillin (see p.1103). Phenoxymethylpenicillin is usually well tolerated but may occasionally cause transient nausea and diarrhoea.

The effects of penicillins on the mouth flora.— *Br. med. J.*, 1971, *2*, 63.

Allergy. A 29-year-old woman suffered anaphylaxis after taking a single tablet of phenoxymethylpenicillin; she had previously tolerated penicillin.— J. Simmonds *et al., Br. med. J.*, 1978, *2*, 1404.

Colitis. A 12-year-old girl with no history of adverse reactions to penicillin developed pseudomembranous colitis after a short course of phenoxymethylpenicillin.— H. E. Larson *et al., Br. med. J.*, 1977, *1*, 1246. A report of 5 patients who suffered acute bloody diarrhoea associated with administration of ampicillin, amoxycillin, or phenoxymethylpenicillin. Pseudomembranous colitis was excluded and it was believed that the diarrhoea was allergic in origin. Symptoms resolved within a day or so of stopping the penicillin and were associated with petechiae in the mouth and oropharynx of one patient and submucosal haemorrhage of the stomach and duodenum of a second, suggesting that the patients might also have allergic vasculitis in areas other than the colon.— R. B. Toffler *et al., Lancet*, 1978, *2*, 707. Two further patients with colitis after taking phenoxymethylpenicillin.— I. G. Barrison and S. P. Kane (letter), *ibid.*, 843.

Hepatotoxicity. A severe systemic reaction with liver impairment occurred in a patient given phenoxymethylpenicillin.— L. Beeley *et al.* (letter), *Lancet*, 1976, *2*, 1297. See also L. I. Goldstein and K. G. Ishak, *Archs Path.*, 1974, *98*, 114.

Precautions. Phenoxymethylpenicillin is contra-indicated in patients known to be hypersensitive to penicillin and it should be used with caution in patients with known histories of allergy. It is not recommended for chronic, severe, or deep-seated infections such as subacute bacterial endocarditis, meningitis, or syphilis.

In a study of 13 infants coeliac disease, but not diarrhoea, impaired the absorption of phenoxymethylpenicillin.— P. Bolme *et al., Acta paediat. scand.*, 1977, *66*, 573. See also A. E. Davis and R. C. Pirola, *Australas. Ann. Med.*, 1968, *17*, 63.

Interactions. The average serum concentration of penicillin in 5 healthy subjects given a 250-mg dose of phenoxymethylpenicillin was reduced by more than 50% after 8 days' dosage with neomycin 12 g daily. The average 24-hour recovery of penicillin in the subjects' urine was reduced by a similar amount. Phenoxymethylpenicillin administered to the same subjects 6 days after withdrawl of neomycin produced the expected serum concentrations.— S. H. Cheng and A. White, *New Engl. J. Med.*, 1962, *267*, 1296.

Aspirin, sulphamethoxypyridazine, and sulphaethidole inhibited the serum-binding of phenoxymethylpenicillin *in vitro* and *in vivo*.— C. M. Kunin, *Clin. Pharmac. Ther.*, 1966, *7*, 180.

For a report of chloroquine diminishing the antibacterial action of phenoxymethylpenicillin, see below under Antimicrobial Action.

Pregnancy and the neonate. In 6 women 38 to 40 weeks pregnant, the administration of phenoxymethylpenicillin 653 mg every 8 hours caused a reduction of 32% in the urinary excretion of oestrogen and a reduction of 48% in the plasma concentrations of oestriol.— M. Pulkkinen and K. Willman (letter), *Br. med. J.*, 1971, *4*, 48.

Antimicrobial Action. Phenoxymethylpenicillin has a range of antimicrobial activity similar to that of benzylpenicillin (see p.1105) and a similar mode of action. However, it is slightly less active against streptococci and much less active against Gram-negative micro-organisms including gonococci. It is inactivated by penicillinase.

Diminished activity. Chloroquine phosphate decreased the antibacterial effect *in vitro* of benzylpenicillin and phenoxymethylpenicillin against *Staphylococcus aureus*.— M. A. Toama *et al., J. pharm. Sci.*, 1978, *67*, 23.

Resistance. As for Benzylpenicillin, p.1106.

Resistance of streptococci. Penicillin-resistant strains of streptococci were found in 23 of 24 children receiving prophylactic phenoxymethylpenicillin for rheumatic fever, in 14 of 23 receiving benzathine penicillin injections monthly, and in 15 of 25 control children attending an orthopaedic clinic who had not received penicillin within 6 months.— D. Bentley *et al., Antimicrob. Ag. Chemother.*, 1970, 277.

Absorption and Fate. Phenoxymethylpenicillin is more resistant to inactivation by the acid of gastric secretions and is more completely absorbed than benzylpenicillin from the gastro-intestinal tract following administration by mouth. Absorption is usually rapid, but peak serum concentrations are variable; peak serum concentrations of about 0.7 μg per ml have been observed following a dose of 125 mg and 3 to 5 μg per ml following 250 to 500 mg. The biological half-life of phenoxymethylpenicillin in serum is about 30 minutes and about 55 to 80% is protein bound. Phenoxymethylpenicillin diffuses across the placenta; it also diffuses into ascitic, pericardial, pleural, and synovial fluids. There is little diffusion into the cerebrospinal fluid unless the meninges are inflamed. The calcium and potassium salts are better absorbed than the free acid. Some 20 to 35% of a dose appears in the urine within 24 hours. Only small concentrations are excreted in the bile.

Following a dose of phenoxymethylpenicillin potassium 500 mg to 4 men, concentrations of 22 to 69 μg per ml were present in the urine after 6 hours.— J. Birner, *J. pharm. Sci.*, 1970, *59*, 757.

Phenoxymethylpenicillin was not absorbed well in patients with gluten-sensitive enteropathy.— A. Breckenridge, *Acta pharmac. tox.*, 1971, *29, Suppl.* 3, 225.

In a crossover study in 6 healthy subjects the mean amount of phenoxymethylpenicillin recovered in the urine 6 hours after administration of a 250-mg dose was almost 3 times that of benzylpenicillin after a similar dose.— P. E. Gower *et al., J. antimicrob. Chemother.*, 1975, *1*, 187.

A report of the bioavailability of various preparations of phenoxymethylpenicillin.— W. G. Crouthamel, *J. Am. pharm. Ass.*, 1977, *NS 17*, 243.

The absorption of phenoxymethylpenicillin in children.— P. Bolme and M. Eriksson, *Scand. J. infect. Dis.*, 1978, *10*, 223.

Diffusion into body tissues. Concentrations of phenoxymethylpenicillin in tonsillar tissue correlated with those in the serum in a study of 39 patients given the potassium salt 2 or 3 hours before tonsillectomy.— H. Beckmann *et al., Münch. med. Wschr.*, 1975, *117*, 1405.

Metabolism. About 57% of a dose of phenoxymethylpenicillin 500 mg was metabolised when given to 6 healthy subjects. Within 12 hours about 26% of the dose was recovered unchanged in the urine and about 34% was excreted as penicilloic acid.— M. Cole *et al., Antimicrob. Ag. Chemother.*, 1973, *3*, 463.

A study in 12 healthy subjects indicated that phenoxymethylpenicillin potassium underwent decomposition to the extent of about 30% in the upper gastro-intestinal tract probably during exposure to the acid gastric contents and was thought to produce the biologically inactive penicilloic acid which was more slowly absorbed than phenoxymethylpenicillin potassium and had a considerably longer half-life.— K. Hellström *et al., Clin. Pharmac. Ther.*, 1974, *16*, 826.

Uses. Phenoxymethylpenicillin is used in the treatment of mild to moderate infections caused by susceptible Gram-positive organisms in a dose of 125 to 500 mg every 4 to 6 hours, depending on the severity of the infection. Children may be given the following doses every 6 hours: up to 1 year, 62.5 mg; 1 to 5 years, 125 mg; and 6 to 12 years, 250 mg. Parenterally administered benzylpenicillin is preferable in the treatment of severe acute infections.

To prevent the recurrence of rheumatic fever, phenoxymethylpenicillin may be administered in doses of 125 mg every 12 hours.

Phenoxymethylpenicillin is administered by mouth, either as the free acid or as its potassium or calcium salt, preferably 30 minutes before food.

Dosage in infants and children. A suggested dose of phenoxymethylpenicillin for older infants was 60 mg per kg body-weight daily.— *Br. med. J.*, 1980, *280*, 703.

Dry socket. For a comparison of phenoxymethylpenicillin and clindamycin hydrochloride in the control of infection after dental surgery, see Clindamycin Hydrochloride, p.1146.

Haemophilus infections. Phenoxymethylpenicillin was emphatically contra-indicated in genuine *Haemophilus influenzae* infections; it was 16 times less active than ampicillin, only half as well absorbed, and 80% was bound to plasma proteins.— L. P. Garrod (letter), *Br. med. J.*, 1973, *3*, 290.

Pharyngitis. Bacteriological follow-up of 331 children treated with about 480 mg of phenoxymethylpenicillin or with nafcillin daily for 10 days for pharyngitis due to group A streptococci revealed that the infection persisted in 39 children. Relapse occurred in 11 of these 39 children.— B. J. Rosenstein *et al.*, *J. Pediat.*, 1968, *73*, 513.

Treatment of acute streptococcal pharyngitis in 300 children was as effective with phenoxymethylpenicillin administered by mouth for a full course of 10 days as parenteral administration of procaine and benzathine penicillin.— I. S. Colcher and J. W. Bass, *J. Am. med. Ass.*, 1972, *222*, 657. Comments and criticism.— P. I. Nieburg (letter), *ibid.*, 1973, *223*, 800; B. Phibbs (letter), *ibid.*, 801. A reply.— J. W. Bass (letter), *ibid.*, 1973, *224*, 1038.

Phenoxymethylpenicillin potassium 30 mg per kg body-weight daily is the treatment of choice in infants and children with group A streptococcal pharyngitis.— G. H. McCracken and H. F. Eichenwald, *J. Pediat.*, 1978, *93*, 357.

For a report of failure of penicillin to eradicate group A streptococci, see Benzathine Penicillin, p.1102.

Rheumatic fever prophylaxis. References: J. P. Phair *et al.*, *Am. J. Dis. Child.*, 1973, *126*, 48.

For reports of the use of phenoxymethylpenicillin in the prophylaxis of rheumatic fever, see Prophylactic Use of Antibiotics, p.1080.

Staphylococcal infections. No difference in the efficacy of phenoxymethylpenicillin, phenethicillin, and lincomycin was found in a comparative trial in 221 patients who were treated for superficial staphylococcal infections. Penicillin-resistant staphylococci were isolated from one-half the lesions.— D. J. E. Price *et al.*, *Br. med. J.*, 1968, *3*, 407. Comments.— R. J. Fallon (letter), *ibid.*, 1968, *4*, 55.

Streptococcal infections, other. Of 220 children with scarlet fever, half received phenoxymethylpenicillin and the remainder ampicillin, in doses of 60 and 125 mg respectively for children 1 to 4 years of age, and twice this dose for those aged 5 to 13 years. Treatment was continued for 10 days. Phenoxymethylpenicillin was superior in reducing the period of fever, hastening the elimination of bacteria, and reducing streptococcal recurrence. Side-effects, particularly skin rashes, were more numerous in those who received ampicillin.— J. Strom, *Acta paediat., Stockh.*, 1968, *57*, 285.

Prophylaxis. Phenoxymethylpenicillin 250 mg daily, as a single dose, was usually necessary and effective prophylaxis for recurrent attacks of erysipelas.— *Br. med. J.*, 1979, *1*, 999.

Preparations of Phenoxymethylpenicillin and its Salts

Penicillin V for Oral Suspension *(U.S.P.)*. A dry mixture of phenoxymethylpenicillin with or without one or more suitable buffers, suspending, colouring, and flavouring agents. Store in airtight containers. The suspension is prepared by the addition of diluent before issue and contains the equivalent of 25, 50, or 208.3 mg of phenoxymethylpenicillin per ml. pH 2 to 4.

Penicillin V Potassium for Oral Solution *(U.S.P.)*. A dry mixture of phenoxymethylpenicillin potassium. It may contain one or more suitable buffers, preservatives, and colouring, flavouring, and suspending agents. Store in airtight containers. The solution is prepared by the addition of diluent before issue and contains the equivalent of 25 or 50 mg of phenoxymethylpenicillin per ml. pH 5 to 7.5.

Penicillin V Tablets *(U.S.P.)*. Tablets containing phenoxymethylpenicillin 125, 300, or 500 mg. Store in airtight containers.

Phenoxymethylpenicillin Elixir *(B.P.C. 1973)*. Penicillin V Elixir; Phenoxymethylpenicillin Solution; Phenoxymethylpenicillin Syrup. A solution of phenoxymethylpenicillin potassium in a suitable coloured flavoured vehicle. It is prepared freshly by dissolving granules of the dry mixed ingredients in the specified quantity of water. Store in a cool place and use the elixir or diluted elixir within 1 week. Loses not more than 20% potency in a week at 15°. When a dose less than 5 ml is prescribed, the elixir should be diluted to 5 ml with syrup. Such dilutions must be freshly prepared.

Phenoxymethylpenicillin Mixture *(B.P.C. 1973)*. Penicillin V Mixture. A suspension of phenoxymethylpenicillin, phenoxymethylpenicillin calcium, or phenoxymethylpenicillin potassium in a suitable flavoured oily vehicle, which may be coloured. Store in a cool place. When a dose less than 5 ml is prescribed, the mixture should be diluted to 5 ml with fractionated coconut oil. Such dilutions must be freshly prepared and not used more than 2 weeks after issue.

Phenoxymethylpenicillin Potassium Capsules *(B.P.)*. Penicillin VK Capsules. Capsules containing phenoxymethylpenicillin potassium. Potency is expressed in terms of the equivalent amount of phenoxymethylpenicillin. The *B.P.* requires 70% dissolution in 45 minutes. Store at a temperature not exceeding 30°.

Phenoxymethylpenicillin Potassium Tablets *(B.P.)*. Penicillin VK Tablets. Tablets containing phenoxymethylpenicillin potassium. Potency is expressed in terms of the equivalent amount of phenoxymethylpenicillin. The tablets may be film-coated. The *B.P.* requires 70% dissolution in 45 minutes. Penicillin V Potassium Tablets (*U.S.P.*) contain the equivalent of 125, 250, and 500 mg of phenoxymethylpenicillin. Store in airtight containers.

Proprietary Preparations

Apsin VK *(Approved Prescription Services, UK)*. Phenoxymethylpenicillin potassium, available as **Syrup** (supplied as granules for preparation with water before use) containing in each 5 ml the equivalent of 125 or 250 mg of phenoxymethylpenicillin (suggested diluent, syrup) and as **Tablets** each containing the equivalent of 250 mg phenoxymethylpenicillin.

Co-Caps Penicillin V-K *(Co-Caps, UK)*. Phenoxymethylpenicillin potassium, available as capsules of 250 mg.

Crystapen V *(Glaxo, UK)*. **Suspension** containing in each 5 ml phenoxymethylpenicillin calcium equivalent to 125 mg of phenoxymethylpenicillin (suggested diluent, fractionated coconut oil); **Syrup** (supplied as granules for preparation with water before use) containing in each 5 ml phenoxymethylpenicillin potassium equivalent to 125 and 250 mg of phenoxymethylpenicillin (suggested diluent, syrup); and **Tablets** each containing phenoxymethylpenicillin potassium equivalent to 250 mg of phenoxymethylpenicillin.

Distaquaine V-K *(Dista, UK)*. Phenoxymethylpenicillin potassium, available as **Elixir** (supplied as granules for preparation with water before use) containing the equivalent of 62.5 mg of phenoxymethylpenicillin in each 5 ml (suggested diluent, syrup); as **Syrup** (supplied as granules for preparation with water before use) containing the equivalent of 125 and 250 mg in each 5 ml (suggested diluent, syrup); and as scored **Tablets** containing the equivalent of 125 or 250 mg. (Also available as Distaquaine V-K in *Austral.*, *S.Afr.*).

Econocil VK *(DDSA Pharmaceuticals, UK)*. Phenoxymethylpenicillin potassium, available as **Capsules** each containing the equivalent of phenoxymethylpenicillin 250 mg and as **Tablets** each containing the equivalent of 125 or 250 mg.

Icipen *(ICI Pharmaceuticals, UK)*. Phenoxymethylpenicillin potassium, available as scored tablets each containing the equivalent of 300 mg of phenoxymethylpenicillin.

Penicillin V Potassium *(Lilly, UK)*. Phenoxymethylpenicillin potassium, available as paediatric syrup (supplied as granules for preparation with water before use) containing the equivalent of phenoxymethylpenicillin 62.5 mg in each 5 ml (suggested diluent, syrup).

Stabillin V-K *(Boots, UK)*. Phenoxymethylpenicillin potassium, available as **Elixir 62.5**, **Elixir 125**, and **Elixir 250** (supplied as granules for preparation with water before use) containing the equivalent of phenoxymethylpenicillin 62.5, 125, and 250 mg respectively in each 5 ml and as **Tablets** containing the equivalent of phenoxymethylpenicillin 250 mg.

Ticillin V-K *(Ticen, Eire)*. Phenoxymethylpenicillin potassium, available as oral solution containing the equivalent of 125 mg of phenoxymethylpenicillin in each 5 ml.

V-Cil-K *(Lilly, UK)*. Phenoxymethylpenicillin potassium, available as **Capsules** of 250 mg; as **Pedipacs** (single-dose sachets) each containing 125 mg; as **Syrup** (supplied as granules for preparation with water before use) containing 125 or 250 mg in each 5 ml (suggested diluent, syrup); and as **Tablets** of 125 and 250 mg; all strengths expressed as phenoxymethylpenicillin. (Also available as V-Cil-K in *NZ*, *S.Afr.*).

Other Proprietary Names of Phenoxymethylpenicillin

Belg.—Oracilline; *Canad.*—Penbec-V; *Fr.*—Oracilline; *Ital.*—Fenospen, Tripapenicillina; *Neth.*—Acipen-V; *S.Afr.*—Penoral, Veekay; *Switz.*—Pengrocill, Widocillin; *USA*—V-Cillin.

NOTE. The name Oracilline is also used as a proprietary name for Benzathine Phenoxymethylpenicillin (see p.1102).

Phenoxymethylpenicillin was formerly marketed in Great Britain under the proprietary name Penicillin-V-Lilly (*Lilly*).

Other Proprietary Names of Phenoxymethylpenicillin Calcium

Austral.—Pfipen V (see also under Phenoxymethylpenicillin Potassium and Hydrabamine Phenoxymethylpenicillin); *Denm.*—Calcipen; *Norw.*—Calcipen; *Swed.*—Penicals; *Switz.*—Brunocillin, Calcipen.

Other Proprietary Names of Phenoxymethylpenicillin Potassium

Arg.—Cliacil, Pen-Oral, Pentid; *Austral.*—Abbocillin-VK, Bramcillin, Cilicaine VK, Compocillin VK, Crystapen VK, Falcopen VK, LPV, Pfipen V (see also under Phenoxymethylpenicillin Calcium and Hydrabamine Phenoxymethylpenicillin), Propen VK, PVK, PVO, Rocilin, Viraxacillin-V; *Belg.*—Orpenic, Peni-oral, Pentabs; *Canad.*—Ledercillin VK, Nadopen-V, Novopen-VK, PVF K, V-Cillin K, VC-K 500; *Denm.*—Fenoxcillin, Primcillin, Rocilin, Vepicombin; *Fr.*—Ospen; *Ger.*—Antibiocin, Arcasin, Beromycin, DuraPenicillin, Isocillin, Ispenoral, Megacillin (see also under Benzylpenicillin, Clemizole Penicillin, and Procaine Penicillin), Ospen, Pencompren, Pencompren-Mio; *Norw.*—Apocillin, Femepen, Fenoxypen, Rocilin; *NZ*—Compocillin VK, Crystapen VK, DQVK; *S.Afr.*—Copen, Darocillin, Deltacillin, Fenoxypen, Incil-VK, Jatcillin, Novo-VK, Nutracillin; *Swed.*—Apopen, Calciopen, Fenoxypen, Kåvepenin, Roscopenin, Vepen; *Switz.*—Cliacil, Fenoxypen Novo, Monocillin (see also under Benzathine Phenoxymethylpenicillin), Ospen, Penadur VK, Stabicilline(see also under Benzathine Phenoxymethylpenicillin); *USA*—Betapen-VK, Dowpen VK, Ledercillin VK, Paclin VK, Penapar VK, Pen-Vee-K, Pfizerpen VK, Robicillin VK, Ro-Cillin VK, Uticillin VK, V-Cillin K, Veetids.

NOTE. The name Ospen is also used as a proprietary name for Benzathine Phenoxymethylpenicillin (see p.1102). The name Uticillin is used as proprietary name for Carfecillin Sodium (see p.1114).

Phenoxymethylpenicillin potassium was also formerly marketed in Great Britain under the proprietary names CVK (*Abbott*), GPV (*Galen*), and Norcillin (*RP Drugs*). Preparations containing phenoxymethylpenicillin potassium were also formerly marketed under the proprietary names Tonsillin (*Winthrop*) and V-Cil-K Sulpha (*Lilly*).

133-b

Piperacillin Sodium. CL 227193; T-1220. Sodium (6*R*)-6-[D-2-(4-ethyl-2,3-dioxopiperazine-1-carboxamido)-2-phenylacetamido]penicillanate.
$C_{23}H_{26}N_5NaO_7S$=539.5.

CAS — 61477-96-1 (piperacillin); 59703-84-3 (sodium salt).

A white crystalline powder. Piperacillin sodium 1.04 g is approximately equivalent to 1 g of piperacillin. Each g

of piperacillin sodium represents 1.85 mmol (1.85 mEq) of sodium.
Soluble 1 in 1.4 of water and methyl alcohol and 1 in 5 of alcohol. M.p. 180°.

Adverse Effects, Treatment, and Precautions. As for Benzylpenicillin, p.1103.

For a report of neutropenia and eosinophilia associated with piperacillin, see Nafcillin Sodium, p.1187.

Antimicrobial Action. Piperacillin is a substituted ampicillin with antimicrobial activity similar to that of carbenicillin (p.1111) but generally reported to be more active *in vitro*, especially against *Pseudomonas aeruginosa* and other Gram-negative organisms.

Piperacillin had a similar antimicrobial spectrum to carbenicillin but was more active *in vitro* against *Pseudomonas aeruginosa, Klebsiella pneumoniae, Proteus* spp., and *Serratia marcescens*. At 12.5 µg per ml, 85% of 300 strains of *Ps. aeruginosa* were inhibited by piperacillin compared with only 6% inhibited by carbenicillin. The minimum bactericidal concentration (MBC) of piperacillin against penicillinase-producing strains of *Kleb. pneumoniae, Pr. vulgaris,* and *Ps. aeruginosa* was at least 4 to 8 times higher than the minimum inhibitory concentration (MIC). In *mice*, piperacillin was more effective than ampicillin or carbenicillin against *Kleb. pneumoniae* or *Ps. aeruginosa* but was less active than ampicillin against *E. coli*.— K. Ueo *et al., Antimicrob. Ag. Chemother.*, 1977, *12*, 455.

Piperacillin had a broad spectrum of activity against Gram-negative bacilli and Gram-positive and -negative cocci. In general the MIC and MBC was very similar with only a slight inoculum effect apart from some strains of *Ps. aeruginosa* when a large inoculum was associated with a large increase in MBC. There was cross-resistance between piperacillin, carbenicillin, and ampicillin.— L. Verbist, *Antimicrob. Ag. Chemother.*, 1978, *13*, 349.

In a study *in vitro* involving about 3600 clinical isolates including *Kleb. pneumoniae, Ps. aeruginosa,* Enterococci, *Serratia marcescens, Bacteroides fragilis, Enterobacter* spp., and *Proteus* spp., the activity of piperacillin was compared with that of other antibiotics. Apart from *E. coli*, piperacillin inhibited 90% or more of the isolates in each group at 64 µg per ml. The antibacterial spectrum was similar to that of gentamicin. Generally the MIC and MBC were close but with 16 isolates of *Ps. aeruginosa* the MICs for piperacillin and carbenicillin were 32 µg per ml and 512 µg per ml respectively whereas MBCs were 512 µg per ml for both antibiotics.— D. J. Winston *et al., Antimicrob. Ag. Chemother.*, 1978, *13*, 944.

Piperacillin was generally more active *in vitro* than ticarcillin or carbenicillin against 612 isolates of aerobic bacteria including 100 of *Pseudomonas* spp., 104 of *E. coli*, 84 of *Proteus* spp., 77 of *Staphylococcus aureus* and 54 of the *Klebsiella* spp.— I. Roy *et al., Curr. ther. Res.*, 1978, *23*, 200.

The activity *in vitro* of piperacillin against 577 isolates was compared with that of mezlocillin, azlocillin, carbenicillin, ticarcillin, and amoxycillin. In general piperacillin was the most active antibiotic against *E. coli, Klebsiella* spp., *Serratia marcescens, Enterobacter* spp., *Pr. mirabilis,* and *Ps. aeruginosa*. Except against *Ps. aeruginosa* and *Pr. mirabilis*, when mezlocillin was less active, piperacillin and mezlocillin had similar MICs. Piperacillin was 8 times more active than carbenicillin against indole-positive strains of *Proteus* and 16 times more active against most other isolates.— G. P. Bodey and B. Le Blanc, *Antimicrob. Ag. Chemother.*, 1978, *14*, 78.

Studies *in vitro* concluded that a 100-µg piperacillin disk was satisfactory for susceptibility testing of organisms by the single-disk agar diffusion technique and that the same zone standards applied as those for tests with a 100-µg carbenicillin disk.— A. L. Barry *et al., Antimicrob. Ag. Chemother.*, 1979, *16*, 378.

Further reports of the antimicrobial activity of piperacillin and comparisons with other antibiotics: V. T. Bach *et al., Curr. ther. Res.*, 1977, *22*, 583 (anaerobic bacteria); K. P. Fu and H. C. Neu, *Antimicrob. Ag. Chemother.*, 1978, *13*, 358 (Gram-negative bacteria); W. L. George *et al., ibid.*, 484 (Gram-negative); K. Iida *et al., ibid., 14*, 257 (mechanism of action against *E. coli*); R. Wise *et al., ibid.*, 549 (Gram-positive and Gram-negative; *Bacteroides fragilis*); G. M. Dickinson *et al., ibid.*, 919 (Gram-negative); G. R. G. Monif *et al., ibid.*, 643 (Gram-negative bacteria and *Bacteroides fragilis*); S. E. Milne and P. M. Waterworth, *J. antimicrob. Chemother.*, 1978, *4*, 247 (Gram-negative); L. O. Gentry *et al., Curr. ther. Res.*, 1979, *26*, 158 (Gram-negative); J. E. McGowan and P. M. Terry, *Antimicrob. Ag. Chemother.*, 1979, *15*, 137 (Gram-negative); P. P. Shah *et al., ibid.*, 346 (Gram-negative); C. Thornsberry *et al., J. antimicrob. Chemother.*, 1979, *5*, 137 (*Neisseria gonorrhoeae* and *Haemophilus influenzae*); C. N. Baker *et al., Antimicrob. Ag. Chemother.*, 1980, *17*, 757 (*N. gonorrhoeae* and *H. influenzae*).

See also, Mezlocillin Sodium p.1184.

Enhanced activity. Enhanced activity against isolates of *Ps. aeruginosa* was demonstrated *in vitro* when piperacillin, ticarcillin, or carbenicillin were used with gentamicin, tobramycin, or amikacin.— P. Chanbusarakum and P. R. Murray, *Antimicrob. Ag. Chemother.*, 1978, *14*, 505.

Absorption and Fate.

Peak serum concentrations of piperacillin in 12 healthy subjects immediately after bolus intravenous injections of piperacillin 15, 30, and 60 mg per kg body-weight were 138, 205, and 520 µg per ml respectively. The half-life ranged from 1.3 to 1.5 hours and was similar for all doses. About 42% of the dose appeared in the urine 24 hours after administration of 15 mg per kg and 70% after 60 mg per kg. When piperacillin was given by intravenous infusion over 2 hours corresponding peak serum concentrations were about 24, 64, and 143 µg per ml and occurred 1 to 2 hours after administration.— M. A. L. Evans *et al., J. antimicrob. Chemother.*, 1978, *4*, 255.

In healthy subjects mean peak serum concentrations of piperacillin of about 71, 199, 331, and 452 µg per ml were obtained immediately after intravenous injection over a 3-minute period of 1, 2, 4, and 6 g respectively, falling to 0.9, 4.7, 17.7, and 32.8 µg per ml after 3 hours; the mean half-lives were 36, 54, 61, and 63 minutes. About 49 to 64% of the dose was recovered unchanged in the urine within 2 hours and about 74 to 89% within 24 hours. Following intramuscular injection of 0.5, 1, and 2 g mean peak serum concentrations of about 5, 13, and 30 µg per ml were obtained 30 to 50 minutes after administration and half-lives were 60, 69, and 81 minutes respectively. About 57 to 59% was recovered in the urine within 24 hours. Probenecid 1 g given by mouth about 1 hour before intramuscular administration of piperacillin increased peak serum concentrations and the terminal half-life by about 30%, but the 24-hour urinary excretion of piperacillin was similar.— T. B. Tjandramaga *et al., Antimicrob. Ag. Chemother.*, 1978, *14*, 829.

Further references to pharmacokinetic studies of piperacillin: V. K. Batra *et al., Clin. Pharmac. Ther.*, 1979, *26*, 41; E. L. Francke *et al., Antimicrob. Ag. Chemother.*, 1979, *16*, 788; B. R. Meyers *et al., Antimicrob. Ag. Chemother.*, 1980, *17*, 608 (comparison with carbenicillin and ticarcillin).

Uses. Piperacillin sodium is used similarly to carbenicillin sodium (p.1112) and has been given intramuscularly or intravenously in the treatment of pseudomonal and other Gram-negative infections in doses equivalent to 100 to 300 mg of piperacillin per kg body-weight daily.

Long-term eradication of the causative pathogen was achieved in 14 of 20 patients with uncomplicated urinary-tract infections when they were given piperacillin sodium 2 g every 12 hours by intramuscular injection in 6.6 ml of a 0.25% solution of lignocaine for 6 to 8 days.— E. Schoutens *et al., Curr. ther. Res.*, 1979, *26*, 848.

Piperacillin sodium was used to treat 20 serious Gram-negative infections in 19 patients in doses ranging from 4 g daily in a patient with chronic renal failure to 22 g daily, given in divided doses every 4 to 6 hours. Doses were administered intravenously by infusion over 20 minutes in 5% dextrose. Clinical and bacteriological response-rates were 75% and 70% respectively; 5 infections were cured and 15 improved. Of the 8 patients infected with *Pseudomonas aeruginosa* only 4 were cured or improved and 2 died as a result of their infection. Strains of*Pseudomonas* resistant to piperacillin developed in 2 patients during treatment, suggesting that it might be unwise to use piperacillin alone in serious Gram-negative infections, especially those due to *Ps. aeruginosa*.— G. L. Simon *et al., Antimicrob. Ag. Chemother.*, 1980, *18*, 167.

Further references to the use of piperacillin sodium: A. S. Prince and H. C. Neu, *J. Pediat.*, 1980, *97*, 148 (pulmonary disease in cystic fibrosis); S. Sander *et al., Chemotherapy, Basle*, 1980, *26*, 141 (urinary-tract infection); H. Thadepalli *et al., Chemotherapy, Basle*, 1980, *26*, 377; D. J. Winston *et al., Am. J. Med.*, 1980, *69*, 255.

Proprietary Preparations

Pipril *(Lederle, UK)*. Piperacillin sodium, available as powder for preparing injections, in vials containing the equivalent of piperacillin 1 and 2 g and infusion bottles containing the equivalent of 4 g. (Also available as Pipril in *Ger.*).

Other Proprietary Names

Pentcillin *(Jap.)*.

134-v

Pirbenicillin Sodium. CP-33994-2. Sodium (6*R*)-6-{D-2-[2-(isonicotinimidoylamino)acetamido]-2-phenylacetamido}penicillanate.
$C_{24}H_{25}N_6NaO_5S$=532.5.

CAS — 55975-92-3 (pirbenicillin); 55162-26-0 (sodium salt).

A substituted ampicillin with a range of antimicrobial activity similar to that of carbenicillin (see p.1111) but reported to be 8 to 16 times more active *in vitro* against strains of *Pseudomonas aeruginosa*. It is less active than carbenicillin against *Proteus* spp. Pirbenicillin sodium has been given by intravenous injection.

Antimicrobial activity.— J. A. Retsema *et al., Antimicrob. Ag. Chemother.*, 1976, *9*, 975; T. Murakawa and L. D. Sabath, *ibid.*, 1977, *11*, 1; C. E. Lopez *et al., ibid.*, 441; R. Wise *et al., J. antimicrob. Chemother.*, 1977, *3*, 175; D. Greenwood *et al., ibid.*, 185; R. Wise *et al., Antimicrob. Ag. Chemother.*, 1978, *13*, 559.

The clinical pharmacology of pirbenicillin.— W. E. Grose *et al., Curr. ther. Res.*, 1976, *20*, 604.

Seven patients with severe *Pseudomonas aeruginosa* infections unresponsive to other treatment were given pirbenicillin 250 mg per kg body-weight daily in 4 divided doses by slow intravenous injection in combination with tobramycin 3 to 5 mg per kg daily in 3 divided doses; 3 patients recovered, and 3 died.— M. Laverdiere *et al., Curr. ther. Res.*, 1977, *21*, 464.

Manufacturers

Pfizer, USA.

188-t

Pivampicillin. Pivaloyloxymethyl (6*R*)-6-(α-D-phenylglycylamino)penicillanate.
$C_{22}H_{29}N_3O_6S$=463.5.

CAS — 33817-20-8.

Pivampicillin 1.3 g is approximately equivalent to 1 g of ampicillin.

135-g

Pivampicillin Hydrochloride. MK 191. The hydrochloride of pivampicillin.

$C_{22}H_{29}N_3O_6S,HCl$=500.0.

CAS — 26309-95-5.

Pharmacopoeias. In *Nord.* which permits a variable content of isopropyl alcohol.

A white crystalline hygroscopic powder with a bitter taste. Pivampicillin hydrochloride 1.43 g is approximately equivalent to 1 g of ampicillin. **Soluble** 1 in 2 of water and 1 in 1.5 of chloroform; very slightly soluble in ether.

Adverse Effects, Treatment, and Precautions. As for Ampicillin, p.1092. Gastro-intestinal effects appear to be more common when pivampicillin is taken on an empty stomach.

Ampicillin concentrations in serum, urine, and urogenital tissue were determined in 64 patients given pivampicillin 700 mg by mouth pre-operatively. Absorption of pivampicillin was significantly reduced after 1 hour in patients who received pre-operative medication with atropine and pethidine.— O. Alfthan and O. V. Renkonen, *Arzneimittel-Forsch.*, 1975, *25*, 1831.

For reduced absorption in coeliac disease, see below under Absorption and Fate.

Antimicrobial Action. Pivampicillin has the antimicrobial activity of ampicillin *in vivo* (see p.1093).

Absorption and Fate. Pivampicillin is acid-stable and is readily absorbed from the gastro-intestinal tract. It is rapidly and almost completely hydrolysed to ampicillin in tissues and blood to produce plasma and urine concentrations of ampicillin greater than those achieved with equivalent doses of ampicillin. Unlike ampicillin the absorption of pivampicillin has been reported not to be significantly affected by food. Peak plasma-ampicillin concentrations occur at 1 to 1.5 hours and following doses equivalent to 250 and 500 mg of ampicillin, peak concentrations of about 5 and 9 μg per ml have been reported. The majority of ampicillin obtained from pivampicillin is excreted in the urine, where up to about 70% is excreted within 6 hours.

When 8 volunteers received ampicillin trihydrate 250 mg and pivampicillin equivalent to 250 mg of ampicillin by mouth in a crossover study on 4 separate days, the peak serum-ampicillin concentrations 1 hour after pivampicillin were 5.07 and 5.28 μg per ml fasting and with food respectively, and 2 hours after ampicillin were 2.1 and 1.7 μg per ml respectively. Urinary excretion 8 hours after pivampicillin was 69% in fasting subjects and 82% with food compared with 46 and 41% after ampicillin. In another crossover study, ampicillin peak serum concentrations after pivampicillin equivalent to 500 mg of ampicillin were 9.1 μg per ml in fasting subjects and 8.6 μg per ml when given with food, but were 10.3 μg per ml after 30 minutes in subjects given ampicillin sodium, 500 mg intramuscularly. The corresponding urinary excretion values after 8 hours were 77% with food, 54% fasting, and 67% after intramuscular ampicillin.— M. C. Jordan *et al.*, *Antimicrob. Ag. Chemother.*, 1970, 438.

In 50 healthy volunteers the mean peak serum concentrations after 250 mg were 1.7 μg per ml at 1.5 hours for ampicillin and 4.8 μg per ml at 1 hour for pivampicillin equivalent to ampicillin 250 mg; after 500 mg the concentrations were 2.7 μg per ml at 2 hours for ampicillin and 8.4 μg per ml at 1.5 hours for pivampicillin. After doses of 250 and 500 mg the average urinary concentrations in 24 hours ranged from 35 to 37% for ampicillin and 56 to 71% for pivampicillin. The absorption of pivampicillin was unaffected by administration with milk or after food, but food depressed the absorption of ampicillin.— E. L. Foltz *et al.*, *Antimicrob. Ag. Chemother.*, 1970, 442.

In 10 healthy males absorption of pivampicillin, ampicillin anhydrous, and ampicillin trihydrate averaged 82%, 53%, and 49%. In 6 healthy males the extent of absorption of pivampicillin by mouth was similar to that of ampicillin by intramuscular injection. Whereas the distribution, metabolism, and excretion of pivampicillin was not dose-dependent the extent of absorption appeared to diminish with increasing doses. Similarities in the values obtained for renal clearance and serum half-life of pivampicillin by mouth and ampicillin by mouth and parenterally, supported the view that pivampicillin was hydrolysed to ampicillin, possibly as it was being absorbed.— J. C. K. Loo *et al.*, *Clin. Pharmac. Ther.*, 1974, *16*, 35.

In 8 healthy female subjects ingestion of pivampicillin with food delayed the absorption by about 1 hour compared to absorption following ingestion in the fasting state.— P. J. Neuvonen *et al.*, *J. int. med. Res.*, 1977, *5*, 71.

The absorption of penicillin esters including pivampicillin was reported to be reduced in patients with coeliac disease, perhaps due to a deficiency of enzymes necessary for hydrolysis to the absorbable form.— R. L. Parsons *et al.*, *Br. J. clin. Pharmac.*, 1977, *4*, 267.

Further references: W. Daehne *et al.*, *Antimicrob. Ag. Chemother.*, 1970, 431; E. R. Hultberg and B. Backelin, *Scand. J. infect. Dis.*, 1972, *4*, 149; M. F. Michel and O. Driessen, *Ned. Tijdschr. Geneesk.*, 1974, *118*, 1508; H. Knothe *et al.*, *Arzneimittel-Forsch.*, 1974, *24*, 951; P. J. Little and B. A. Peddie, *Med. J. Aust.*, 1974, *2*, 598; C. Simon *et al.*, *Dt. med. Wschr.*, 1974, *99*, 137; M. W. Kunst and H. Mattie, *Antimicrob. Ag. Chemother.*, 1975, *8*, 11; B. Lund *et al.*, *Clin. Pharmac. Ther.*, 1976, *19*, 587.

Bioavailability. A gastroscopic and pharmacological study of the disintegration time and absorption of pivampicillin capsules and tablets.— H. Hey *et al.*, *Br. J. clin. Pharmac.*, 1979, *8*, 237. See also H. Hey *et al.*, *Arch. Pharm. Chemi, scient. Edn*, 1979, *7*, 169; E. J. Didriksen and B. Nielsen, *ibid.*, 1980, *8*, 121 (bioavailability of reformulated tablets).

Uses. Pivampicillin has the actions and uses of ampicillin (see p.1095) and may be given in doses of 0.5 to 1 g twice daily with milk or food. In gonorrhoea a single dose of 1.5 to 2 g has been given, often in association with probenecid 1 g.

A review of pivampicillin.— J. B. Wilcox *et al.*, *Drugs*, 1973, *6*, 94. See also H. C. Neu, *ibid.*, 1975, *9*, 81.

The treatment of respiratory and urinary-tract infections with pivampicillin.— P. Dano and P. F. Hansen, *Chemotherapy, Basle*, 1973, *18*, 63.

Bronchitis. A comparison of pivampicillin and tetracycline in the treatment of exacerbations of chronic bronchitis.— A. Pines *et al.*, *Chemotherapy, Basle*, 1974, *20*, 361.

Dosage in infants and children. A crossover study in 11 infants and children of the comparative absorption of pivampicillin and ampicillin confirmed that pivampicillin is better absorbed than ampicillin. Following oral administration of equimolar doses of suspensions to 4 children aged 8 to 11 months and 7 aged over 12 months, however, pivampicillin produced relatively lower serum-ampicillin concentrations in those below the age of 12 months whereas this was not the case for ampicillin. Although the implications of these findings were unclear and further study was needed in more children, it might be that children aged less than 12 months required higher doses of pivampicillin to attain serum-ampicillin concentrations as high as those in older children and adults.— L. Pedersen-Bjergaard and K. E. Petersen, *Clin. Pharmacokinet.*, 1977, *2*, 451.

Gonorrhoea. Pivampicillin 1.4 g with probenecid 1 g as a single dose taken with 100 to 150 ml of water was given to 535 patients with gonorrhoea and of those followed there were only 2 probable failures and 3 to 6% had defaulted.— A. -S. Malmborg *et al.*, *Acta derm.-vener., Stockh.*, 1973, *53*, 501. Similar satisfactory results were achieved in 243 patients with uncomplicated gonorrhoea given pivampicillin 1.4 g with probenecid 1 g or ampicillin 2 g with probenecid 1 g.— L. Forström, *Br. J. vener. Dis.*, 1974, *50*, 61.

Further references: L. Forström and A. Lassus, *Br. J. vener. Dis.*, 1972, *48*, 510; A. -S. Malmborg *et al.*, *Chemotherapy, Basle*, 1973, *18*, 262; R. B. Hunton *et al.*, *N.Z. med. J.*, 1974, *80*, 205; K. O. Alausa *et al.*, *W. Afr. J. Pharmac. Drug Res.*, 1976, *3*, 31; V. L. Ongom *et al.*, *E. Afr. med. J.*, 1977, *54*, 674; M. A. Waugh and K. C. Nayyar, *Clin. Trials J.*, 1977, *14*, 152.

Urinary-tract infections. In 25 elderly patients with urinary-tract infections given pivampicillin 700 mg (equivalent to ampicillin 500 mg) thrice daily for a week mean serum concentrations 2 hours and 6 hours after a dose were 5.7 and 1.5 μg per ml respectively; the mean concentration in urine was 546 μg per ml. In 20, bacteria were eliminated from the urine. In 11 of the 20 from whom a further culture was obtained 8 days later, 4 had relapsed and 6 had infection with a fresh organism.— M. Peromet *et al.*, *Curr. ther. Res.*, 1974, *16*, 201.

Ampicillin 25 mg per kg body-weight and pivampicillin, equivalent to ampicillin 12.5 mg per kg, every 6 hours were equally effective in the treatment of urinary-tract infections in 17 children. A mean peak serum-ampicillin concentration of about 13 μg per ml was achieved in 6 children given pivampicillin compared with about 8 μg per ml in 8 children given double the dose of ampicillin.— O. J. Moe *et al.*, *Scand. J. infect. Dis.*, 1977, *9*, 31.

Further references: K. J. Berg and T. E. Wideroe, *Chemotherapy, Basle*, 1973, *18*, 130; L. B. Nilsson, *ibid.*, *19*, 115; I. Aaraas *et al.*, *J. antimicrob. Chemother.*, 1977, *3*, 227.

Proprietary Preparations

Pondocillin *(Burgess, UK)*. Pivampicillin, available as **Suspension** (supplied as powder for preparation before use) containing 162 mg in each 5 ml and as **Tablets** each containing 500 mg. (Also available as Pondocillin in *Belg.* (hydrochloride), *Denm.*, *Neth.*, *Norw.*, *Swed.*, *Switz.*).

Other Proprietary Names of Pivampicillin and Pivampicillin Hydrochloride

Arg.—Centurina, Oxidina; *Belg.*—Pivatil; *Fr.*—Pondocil; *Ger.*—Berocillin, Maxifen; *Ital.*—Pivascel, Pondocillina; *Spain*—Acerum, Bensamin, Brotalcilina, Centurina, Co-Pivam, Crisbiotic, Devonian, Diancina, Inacilin, Isvitrol, Kesmicina, Lanzabiotic, Lervipan, Penimenal, Pibena, Piva Efesal, Pivabiot, Pivacid, Pivacilin-Base, Pivadilon, Pivam-Piror, Pivamboi, Pivaminol, Pivamkey, Pivapen, Pivastol, Piviotic, Tam-Cilin, Tryco, Vampi-Framan.

136-q

Pivmecillinam.

FL 1039; Ro 10-9071; Amdinocillin Pivoxil. Pivaloyloxymethyl (6*R*)-6-(perhydroazepin-1-ylmethyleneamino)penicillanate.

$C_{21}H_{33}N_3O_5S = 439.6$.

CAS — 32886-97-8.

137-p

Pivmecillinam Hydrochloride.

$C_{21}H_{33}N_3O_5S,HCl = 476.0$.

CAS — 32887-03-9.

A white crystalline powder with a bitter taste. Very **soluble** in water. Pivmecillinam 1.35 g and pivmecillinam hydrochloride 1.46 g are each approximately equivalent to 1 g of mecillinam.

Adverse Effects. Hypersensitivity reactions to pivmecillinam may occur (see Benzylpenicillin, p.1103). Gastro-intestinal disturbances and urticarial rashes have been reported.

Treatment of Adverse Effects. See Benzylpenicillin, p.1105.

Precautions. Pivmecillinam should not be given to patients who are sensitive to penicillins or cephalosporins and should be used with caution in those with known histories of allergies. Reduced doses may be necessary in patients with impaired renal function.

Pivmecillinam 1.2 to 2.4 g daily by mouth greatly reduced *E. coli* and other Enterobacteriaceae of gut flora.— H. Knothe, *Arzneimittel-Forsch.*, 1976, *26*, 427.

Antimicrobial Action. Pivmecillinam has the antimicrobial activity of mecillinam to which it is hydrolysed *in vivo* (see p.1180).

Studies *in vitro* suggested that uncomplicated urinary-tract infections produced by Micrococcaceae might be expected to respond to treatment with pivmecillinam 400 mg four times daily but urinary-tract infections produced by faecal streptococci would not. A disk containing mecillinam 50 μg might be more accurate in antibiotic sensitivity tests than the 10 μg disk previously used.— J. D. Anderson *et al.*, *J. antimicrob. Chemother.*, 1976, *2*, 351.

Absorption and Fate. Pivmecillinam is well absorbed from the gastro-intestinal tract and is rapidly hydrolysed in tissues and blood to the active drug mecillinam (see p.1180). The presence of food in the stomach does not appear to have a significant effect on absorption. Peak plasma concentrations of mecillinam of up to 5 μg per ml have been achieved 1 to 2 hours after a 400-mg dose of pivmecillinam. Up to a dose of 800 mg, doubling the dose approximately doubles the plasma concentration. Plasma half-lives from about 1 to 1.4 hours have been reported.

About 45% of a dose may be excreted in the urine as mecillinam, mainly within the first 6 hours of a dose.

Mean serum-mecillinam concentrations of 3.93, 3.48, 1.3, and 0.74 μg per ml were achieved 1, 2, 4, and 6 hours respectively after pivmecillinam 400 mg was given to 22 patients with urinary-tract infections. Urine concentrations of mecillinam at 6 hours ranged from 37 to 787 μg per ml (mean 187 μg per ml) in 33 patients.— R. Wise *et al.*, *Chemotherapy, Basle*, 1976, *22*, 335.

The mean peak serum-mecillinam concentration in 6 healthy subjects after pivmecillinam 200 mg was 1.43 μg per ml and after 400 mg 2.5 μg per ml. When a similar dose was taken following pivmecillinam 1.6 g daily for 6 days, or after probenecid 1g, mean peak serum-mecillinam concentrations were 2.7 μg and 3.8 μg per ml respectively. The mean serum half-life of the 200-mg dose was 1.2 hours. Mecillinam was not accumulated in young subjects but this might not be so in elderly patients. Lower peak serum concentrations were observed in resting than in ambulant subjects.— J. Andrews *et al.*, *Br. J. clin. Pharmac.*, 1976, *3*, 627.

The mean peak serum concentrations of mecillinam in 6 healthy young subjects after receiving pivmecillinam 6.5 mg per kg body-weight in an oral solution or 400 mg as capsules, were 2.2 and 2.4 μg per ml respectively and occurred 1.5 and 1.7 hours respectively after administration. The corresponding half-lives of mecillinam were

0.82 and 0.92 hours. About 25% of the doses by mouth were recovered in the urine 6 hours after administration.— J. D. Williams *et al.*, *J. antimicrob. Chemother.*, 1976, *2*, 61. In 6 patients over 65 years of age with urinary-tract infections who also received pivmecillinam 400 mg every 8 hours as capsules there was no significant difference between the peak serum concentrations of mecillinam after the first dose and rates of absorption compared with the younger subjects but the mean serum elimination half-life was 3.97 hours. Mean urinary concentrations of mecillinam in 3 patients were below 100 µg per ml 7 hours after administration and it was considered that an increase of dosage might be necessary in the treatment of urinary-tract infection in the elderly.— A. P. Ball *et al.*, *ibid.*, 1978, *4*, 241.

The pharmacokinetics of pivmecillinam were studied in 13 healthy subjects and 12 patients with coeliac disease. The coeliac disease had no effect on absorption. In fasting subjects plasma concentrations of mecillinam after a dose of pivmecillinam 600 mg followed a pattern similar to ampicillin concentrations after ampicillin 500 mg. Estimated peak plasma concentrations of 3.91 µg per ml of mecillinam at 1.44 hours correlated with 4.54 µg per ml of ampicillin at 1.73 hours. Food delayed absorption.— R. L. Parsons *et al.*, *Br. J. clin. Pharmac.*, 1977, *4*, 267.

Pharmacokinetic studies of mecillinam and pivmecillinam. A mean peak serum concentration of 5.1 µg per ml was achieved 0.86 hours after a single dose of pivmecillinam hydrochloride 400 mg was taken as tablets by 10 healthy fasting subjects. Results were similar when pivmecillinam was given in solution or as capsules. From 40 to 45% of a dose was excreted in the urine within 6 hours. A further study in 11 subjects indicated that the absorption of pivmecillinam was not significantly affected when it was taken immediately after a meal. Four metabolites, 3 of them inactive, were found in urine after a single dose of 600 mg was given to healthy subjects.— K. Roholt, *J. antimicrob. Chemother.*, 1977, *3*, *Suppl.* B, 71.

The mean peak serum concentration of mecillinam achieved after pivmecillinam hydrochloride 400 mg was taken by 6 healthy subjects was 1.9 µg per ml and occurred 1 to 2.5 hours after administration; serum concentrations remained above 1 µg per ml for about 3.5 hours and the mean half-life of the beta-phase of elimination was 1.06 hours.— M. Mitchard *et al.*, *J. antimicrob. Chemother.*, 1977, *3*, *Suppl.* B, 83.

Uses. Pivmecillinam is the pivaloyloxymethyl ester of mecillinam (see p.1180), to which it is hydrolysed on absorption, and is used in the treatment of Gram-negative infections. Doses of pivmecillinam are expressed in a confusing manner since no differentiation is made between the hydrochloride and the base. In urinary-tract infections the usual dose is 200 to 400 mg of pivmecillinam hydrochloride taken three to four times daily; children may be given about 20 to 40 mg of pivmecillinam base per kg body-weight daily. Up to 2.4 g daily for 14 days has been recommended for salmonellal infections; carriers may receive the same dose for 2 to 4 weeks.

Pivmecillinam should preferably be taken with food.

The hydrochloride is used in tablets and the base in suspensions for oral use.

For parenteral administration mecillinam (see p.1181) is used.

The proceedings of a symposium on mecillinam and pivmecillinam.— *J. antimicrob. Chemother.*, 1977, *3*, *Suppl.* B, 1-160. See also *Chemotherapy, Tokyo*, 1977, *25*, 1-356.

Brief reviews of pivmecillinam.— *Lancet*, 1978, *1*, 252 and 337; *Drug & Ther. Bull.*, 1978, *16*, 103.

Bronchitis. Amoxycillin 500 mg alone or with pivmecillinam 400 mg was compared to pivmecillinam 200 mg with amoxycillin 250 mg, all given thrice daily for 10 days to 132 patients with exacerbations of chronic bronchitis. Significantly greater improvement was reported in those patients who received the higher dose of combined treatment when assessed 7 and 11 days after starting treatment and relapses occurred more frequently in those patients who received amoxycillin alone.— A. Pines *et al.*, *J. antimicrob. Chemother.*, 1977, *3*, *Suppl.* B, 141.

Dosage in renal failure. After an oral dose of pivmecillinam the urinary excretion of mecillinam was markedly delayed in 3 patients with impaired renal function; the interval between doses should be increased in such patients. Peak serum concentrations were achieved more slowly but were higher in 5 patients on maintenance haemodialysis compared with 12 patients with normal renal function and 3 with impaired function.— M. Ekberg *et al.*, *Scand. J. infect. Dis.*, 1978, *10*, 127.

Salmonellal infections. Pivmecillinam 300 mg given 4 times daily for 28 days to 12 chronic *Salmonella* carriers followed when necessary after 5 weeks by 1.2 g four times daily for a further week. Of 8 patients who appeared to have been cured 1 year after treatment, 1 had been cured after cholecystectomy during treatment and 2 had been cured only after receiving both courses of treatment and undergoing cholecystectomy.— M. Jonsson, *J. antimicrob. Chemother.*, 1977, *3*, *Suppl.* B, 103.

A comparative study of pivmecillinam and co-trimoxazole in the treatment of enteric fever.— A. P. Ball *et al.*, *J. Infect.*, 1979, *1*, 353.

Urinary-tract infections. Of 30 girls (aged 6 to 12 years) with recurrent bacteriuria produced by *E. coli*, 19 were cured 3 months after receiving pivmecillinam 400 mg thrice daily for 7 days. Cures had previously been obtained with co-trimoxazole in 9 of 17 of the girls and with ampicillin in 6 of 15. One girl developed a mild erythematous rash while taking pivmecillinam but this subsided after completion of treatment.— E. R. V. Jones and A. W. Asscher, *J. antimicrob. Chemother.*, 1975, *1*, 193.

In a comparative study of patients with urinary-tract infections who received amoxycillin 375 mg or pivmecillinam 400 mg thrice daily for 10 days, cures were obtained in 123 of 142 and in 105 of 113 patients respectively. There was a significant increase in multiresistant strains of Enterobacteriaceae isolated after treatment with amoxycillin but not after pivmecillinam. In a further 92 similar patients dosage with pivmecillinam 200 mg was as effective as the 400 mg dose and produced a lower incidence of side-effects.— B. Bresky, *J. antimicrob. Chemother.*, 1977, *3*, *Suppl.*B, 121. See also J. Ishigami, *ibid.*, 129; D. Höffler, *Dt. med. Wschr.*, 1978, *103*, 1108.

In a multicentre study pivmecillinam 400 mg given 4 times daily was considered to be as effective as co-trimoxazole 960 mg given twice daily for 7 days in the treatment of 46 patients with symptoms of cystitis.— D. Guttmann, *J. antimicrob. Chemother.*, 1977, *3*, *Suppl.* B, 137. In a double-blind study pivmecillinam 600 mg and co-trimoxazole 480 mg were equally effective when given twice daily for 6 days in the treatment of 46 patients with bacteriuria.— T. Damsgaard *et al.*, *J. antimicrob. Chemother.*, 1979, *5*, 267.

Pivmecillinam was significantly more effective than pivampicillin in the treatment of urinary-tract infections produced by the Enterobacteriaceae.— I. Aaraas *et al.*, *J. antimicrob. Chemother.*, 1977, *3*, 227. A 3-day course of pivmecillinam was as effective as a 7-day course in a study of 125 women with acute cystitis.— B. T. Marsh and A. P. Menday, *J. int. med. Res.*, 1980, *8*, 105. See also J. F. Donald and D. M. D. Rimmer, *ibid.*, 112. It was considered that an 8-day course of pivmecillinam would be more effective bacteriologically than a 4-day course for the treatment of urinary-tract infections in hospital in-patients.— D. C. Shanson *et al.* (letter), *J. antimicrob. Chemother.*, 1980, *6*, 682.

Further references: P. D. Clarke *et al.*, *J. antimicrob. Chemother.*, 1977, *3*, 169; R. Wise *et al.*, *ibid.*, *Suppl.* B, 113; W. Brumfitt *et al.*, *Scand. J. infect. Dis.*, 1979, *11*, 275 (comparison with cephradine in pregnant and non-pregnant women).

Proprietary Preparations

Selexid *(Leo, UK)*. **Suspension** (supplied as granules for preparation with water before use) available in single-dose sachets each containing pivmecillinam 100 mg and **Tablets** each containing pivmecillinam hydrochloride 200 mg. (Also available as Selexid in *Denm., Neth.*).

NOTE. The name Selexid is also used as a proprietary name for Mecillinam (see p.1181).

Other Proprietary Names

Melicin *(Jap.)*; Selexidin *(see also Mecillinam) (Swed.)*.

139-w

Polymyxin B Sulphate *(B.P., Eur. P.)*.

Polymyxin B Sulfate *(U.S.P.)*; Polymyx. B Sulph.; Polymyxini B Sulfas. A mixture of the sulphates of certain polypeptides produced by the growth of certain strains of *Bacillus polymyxa* or obtained by other means.

CAS — 1404-26-8 (polymyxin B); 1405-20-5 (sulphate).

Pharmacopoeias. In *Arg., Belg., Br., Braz., Eur., Fr., Ger., Int., It., Jap., Jug., Neth., Nord., Swiss, Turk.,* and *U.S.*; *U.S.* also includes Sterile Polymyxin B Sulfate.

A white or buff-coloured, hygroscopic powder, odourless or with a slight odour. The *B.P.* specifies that it contains not less than 6500 units per mg when dried; it loses not more than 6% of its weight on drying. The *U.S.P.* specifies not less than 6000 units per mg and a loss on drying of not more than 7%.

Very **soluble** in water; slightly soluble in alcohol; practically insoluble in ether. A 2% solution in water has a pH of 5 to 7. Solutions are **sterilised** by filtration. It is **stable** in the dry state. Aqueous solutions should be used within 3 days. It is rapidly inactivated by strong acids and alkalis and its activity is inhibited by ferrous, cobaltous, manganous, and magnesium ions. **Incompatible** with cefapirin sodium, cephalothin sodium, and cephazolin sodium.

Store in a cool place in airtight containers; if it is intended for injection the containers should be sterile and sealed to exclude micro-organisms. Protect from light.

Effect of gamma-irradiation. One sample of polymyxin B sulphate was unchanged in appearance at 25 000 Gy and off-white at 250 000 Gy while the potency fell from 8750 units per mg to 8450 and 8350 units per mg respectively. No abnormal spots were noted when a sample exposed to 25 000 Gy was chromatographed.— *The Use of Gamma Radiation Sources for the Sterilisation of Pharmaceutical Products*, London, ABPI, 1960.

Incompatibility. A haze or precipitate was observed within an hour when an average dose of polymyxin B sulphate was mixed in dextrose injection with *cephalothin sodium, chloramphenicol sodium succinate, chlortetracycline hydrochloride, nitrofurantoin sodium,* or *prednisolone sodium phosphate. Tetracycline hydrochloride* injection was also incompatible because of its acidity.— J. M. Meisler and M. W. Skolaut, *Am. J. Hosp. Pharm.*, 1966, *23*, 557.

A precipitate was formed when a solution of polymyxin B 250 000 units in 1.5 ml of water was mixed with a solution of *cloxacillin sodium*. There was no precipitate when the solution of polymyxin B was added to *ampicillin sodium* 500 mg in 1.5 ml of water, but a precipitate formed if the concentration of ampicillin was reduced by one-half.— B. Lynn, *Chemist Drugg.*, 1967, *187*, 157.

Polymyxin B sulphate 200 mg per litre was physically compatible for 24 hours in a buffered solution of *benzylpenicillin*.— E. A. Parker, *Am. J. Hosp. Pharm.*, 1969, *26*, 543. There was visual compatibility for 1 hour when *benzylpenicillin sodium* 1 million units was dissolved in a solution of polymyxin B sulphate 250 000 units in 1.5 to 2 ml of water.— B. Lynn, *J. Hosp. Pharm.*, 1970, *28*, 71.

A haze developed over 3 hours when polmyxin B sulphate 2 million units per litre was mixed with *amphotericin* 200 mg per litre in dextrose injection, or with *heparin* 20 000 units per litre in sodium chloride injection; an immediate precipitate was formed when they were mixed in dextrose injection. A yellow colour was produced with *chlorothiazide* 2 g per litre in dextrose injection.— B. B. Riley, *J. Hosp. Pharm.*, 1970, *28*, 228.

For a list of incompatibilities including *benzylpenicillin, kanamycin, methicillin, nafcillin, phenytoin,* and *protein hydrolysate*, see *Med. Lett.*, 1972, *14* (Jan.), *Suppl.*, 32.

Units. One unit of polymyxin B is contained in 0.000119 mg of the second International Standard Preparation (1969) of polymyxin B sulphate which contains 8403 units per mg.

NOTE. The available forms of polymyxin B sulphate are generally less pure than the International Standard Preparation and doses are sometimes stated in terms of pure polymyxin base; 100 mg of pure polymyxin B is considered to be equivalent to 1 million units (1 mega unit).

Adverse Effects. Neurotoxic reactions including dizziness, ataxia, and sensory disturbances of the face and extremities are fairly common following the parenteral administration of polymyxin B sulphate and appear to be dose-related. Reversible neuromuscular blockade resulting in respiratory paralysis has occurred especially in patients with impaired renal function. Serious dose-related nephrotoxicity can develop and produce haematuria, proteinuria, and tubular necrosis. Meningeal irritation may follow the intrathecal administration of polymyxin B when given in doses of 50 000 to 100 000 units. Other side-effects include fever and skin rashes; pain following intramuscular injection can be severe and may not be controlled by the use of local anaesthetics.

Electrolyte disturbances. Severe hypochloraemia, hypokalaemia, hyponatraemia, and nitrogen retention developed in 57 adults with acute leukaemia given 107 courses of treatment with polymyxin B. Hypocalcaemia was evident in most patients whose serum calcium was determined. The toxicity was related to the duration of treatment.— V. Rodriguez *et al.*, *Clin. Pharmac. Ther.*, 1970, *11*, 106.

Ototoxicity. Intratympanic application of a 0.1% solution of polymyxin B sulphate appeared to be harmless in *guinea pigs*, but concentrations of 0.2 to 2.5% produced sensory cell degeneration in the cochlea, ranging from loss of a few hair cells to complete destruction of the organ of Corti. Other less toxic drugs might be safer where prolonged local therapy for chronic otitis media is required.— A. Kohonen and J. Tarkkanen, *Acta otolar.*, 1969, *68*, 90.

A reminder of the increased risk of drug-induced deafness in patients with perforation of the tympanic membrane when otitis externa is treated topically with preparations containing polymyxins. It is important to ensure that there is no perforation before such preparations are prescribed.— Committee on Safety of Medicines, Current Problems Series No. 5, February 1981.

Treatment of Adverse Effects. Most of the adverse effects of polymyxin B are reversible although recovery may be slow. Patients with respiratory paralysis can be treated with artificial respiration and calcium salts. Neostigmine has been used with conflicting results and probably has no place in the treatment of such patients.

High blood concentrations of polymyxin B have been reported not to be reduced substantially by dialysis.

For a report of the successful use of exchange transfusion in the treatment of colistin overdosage, see Colistin Sulphomethate Sodium, p.1150.

Precautions. Polymyxin B sulphate should not be given to patients with a history of hypersensitivity to the polymyxins. Reduced dosage should be employed in patients with impaired renal function. Because polymyxin may give rise to muscular weakness and respiratory depression, patients should be constantly supervised during parenteral therapy; special care is required for patients with myasthenia gravis and those who have received neuromuscular blocking agents, general anaesthetics, or drugs such as colistin or gentamicin and the other aminoglycosides which are neurotoxic. It should be used cautiously if other potentially nephrotoxic drugs are used.

Ear-drops containing polymyxin B or colistin should not be used in patients with perforated ear-drums.

The administration of polymyxin B by aerosol could cause bronchospasm.— E. C. Rosenow, *Ann. intern. Med.*, 1972, *77*, 977.

For the antagonism of polymyxin B sulphate by calcium and magnesium, see below.

Antimicrobial Action. Polymyxin B and the other polymyxin antibiotics (see p.1085) act primarily by binding to and changing the permeability of the bacterial cytoplasmic membrane. Polymyxin B has a bactericidal action on most Gram-negative bacilli except *Proteus* spp. It is particularly effective against *Pseudomonas aeruginosa*, *Escherichia coli*, *Enterobacter*, and *Klebsiella* spp. Of the other Gram-negative organisms, *Haemophilus influenzae*, *Bordetella pertussis*, *Salmonella*, and *Shigella* spp. are sensitive. Classical *Vibrio cholerae* is sensitive but the *eltor* biotype is resistant. *Serratia marcescens* and *Bacteroides fragilis* are usually resistant. It is not active against *Neisseria gonorrhoeae*, *N. meningitidis*, fungi, and Gram-positive bacteria.

In the presence of large amounts of serum, polymyxin B is reported to lose about 50% of its activity *in vitro*. Most sensitive organisms are inhibited by 0.1 to 0.2 units per ml.

The inactivation of endotoxin by polymyxin B.— M. S. Cooperstock, *Antimicrob. Ag. Chemother.*, 1974, *6*, 422.

Polymyxin B inhibited all of 12 strains of *Coccidioides immitis in vitro* at a concentration of 10 µg per ml. Fungistatic activity was demonstrated in *mice* infected with the organism.— M. S. Collins and D. Pappagianis, *Antimicrob. Ag. Chemother.*, 1976, *10*, 318.

Polymyxin B showed slight activity *in vitro* against *Acanthamoeba* spp.— R. J. Duma and R. Finley, *Antimicrob. Ag. Chemother.*, 1976, *10*, 370.

Polymyxin B protected *Pr. mirabilis in vitro* against usually bactericidal concentrations of benzylpenicillin.— I. J. Sud and D. S. Feingold, *Antimicrob. Ag. Chemother.*, 1978, *14*, 916.

Addition of sodium chloride or sucrose to media used for testing the activity of polymyxin B against *Ps. aeruginosa* protected whole cells against lysis but not against death. It was suggested that cell death was due to a progressive and specific increase in membrane permeability to ions and that this might be a process distinct from lysis. Care should therefore be exercised when using cell lysis as an indicator of polymyxin activity since this might vary with the media used.— R. M. Klemperer *et al.*, *Antimicrob. Ag. Chemother.*, 1979, *15*, 147.

For a report of carbenicillin with polymyxin B showing an additive or slightly antagonistic effect against *Ps. aeruginosa*, see Carbenicillin Sodium, p.1111.

Diminished activity. Physiological concentrations of calcium present in serum inhibited the antibacterial activity *in vitro* of polymyxin B against *Ps. aeruginosa*.— S. D. Davis *et al.*, *J. infect. Dis.*, 1971, *124*, 610.

The bactericidal action of polymyxin B was antagonised by calcium and magnesium and it was suggested that interaction of the divalent cations with the cell wall prevented access of the antibiotic to the cytoplasmic membrane.— C. -C. H. Chen and D. S. Feingold, *Antimicrob. Ag. Chemother.*, 1972, *2*, 331.

Enhanced activity. Urea might enhance the antimicrobial activity of polymyxin against staphylococci and *Ps. aeruginosa*.— B. W. Burt and G. Dempsey, per *Pharm. J.*, 1977, *2*, 255.

The activities of polymyxin B and rifampicin were enhanced when used together *in vitro* against 52 isolates of *Serratia marcescens*.— R. C. Ostenson *et al.*, *Antimicrob. Ag. Chemother.*, 1977, *12*, 655.

Resistance. Bacteria do not readily acquire resistance to polymyxin B, but when resistance does occur *in vitro* there is complete cross-resistance between polymyxin B and colistin. Resistant strains of *Pseudomonas aeruginosa* have occasionally been reported.

A strain of *Ps. aeruginosa* cultured *in vitro* developed resistance to polymyxin B and cross-resistance to carbenicillin and gentamicin. However, sensitivity to chloramphenicol, erythromycin, and especially tetracycline was increased.— M. R. W. Brown *et al.* (letter), *Lancet*, 1972, *2*, 86.

Absorption and Fate. Polymyxin B sulphate is not absorbed from the gastro-intestinal tract, except in the newborn, but only a small proportion of an oral dose appears unchanged in the faeces. It is not absorbed through the intact skin.

A single dose of 250 000 units of polymyxin B given intramuscularly produces plasma concentrations of 2.4 units or less per ml within 1 hour, but after repeated doses every 4 hours for 5 days concentrations of 5 to 10 units per ml have been achieved. There is no diffusion into the CSF.

Polymyxin B sulphate is excreted mainly by the kidneys, up to 60% being recovered in the urine, but there is a considerable time lag before an effective concentration is built up in the urine.

Polymyxin B was only bound to a limited extent to serum proteins in the body. The half-life in serum was 6 hours.— C. M. Kunin, *Ann. intern. Med.*, 1967, *67*, 151.

Uses. Polymyxin B as the sulphate is used by intravenous or sometimes by intramuscular injection in the treatment of systemic and urinary-tract infections due to susceptible organisms which are resistant to other less toxic antibiotics, particularly *Pseudomonas aeruginosa*. Meningitis has been treated by intrathecal injections. Polymyxin B sulphate, often in association with neomycin (see p.1190) and bacitracin (see p.1100), is applied topically in the treatment of skin and eye infections and solutions are used for bladder irrigation.

It has been given orally for the treatment of intestinal infections with conflicting results.

In systemic infections the usual dose is 15 000 to 25 000 units per kg body-weight daily by slow intravenous infusion. Infants have been given up to 40 000 units per kg daily by intramuscular or intravenous injection. Doses should be reduced in patients with renal impairment. Intramuscular administration is not recommended routinely but doses of 25 000 to 30 000 units per kg have been given daily. In meningeal infections a dose of 50 000 units in 1 ml of 0.9% sodium chloride injection is given daily by intrathecal injection to adults and 20 000 units daily to children under 2 years of age; daily doses as high as 200 000 units have been given to adults.

Doses of up to 6 million units daily have been given by mouth to adults and 40 000 units per kg thrice daily to children. In eye infections doses of up to 10 000 units daily have been injected subconjunctivally and 0.1 to 0.25% solutions have been administered as drops.

A brief review of the polymyxins.— D. Andrews, *Can. J. Hosp. Pharm.*, 1978, *31*, 215.

Eight of 12 patients with nosocomial infections due to multiple-resistant strains of *Serratia marcescens* had a favourable response to treatment with polymyxin B given intravenously and rifampicin taken by mouth 2 hours before each infusion of polymyxin B. Three patients died and one of the deaths was associated with supra-infection with *Proteus mirabilis*. Another patient developed jaundice which regressed when the antibiotics were withdrawn.— R. C. Ostenson *et al.*, *Antimicrob. Ag. Chemother.*, 1977, *12*, 655.

Dosage in renal failure. In patients with oliguria, intervals between doses of polymyxin B should be increased to every 3 to 4 days.— C. M. Kunin, *Ann. intern. Med.*, 1967, *67*, 151.

Further references: G. B. Appel and H. C. Neu, *New Engl. J. Med.*, 1977, *296*, 663.

Eye infections. A recommendation that treatment of patients with a presumed infective corneal condition in the absence of bacteriological evidence should include polymyxin because of its action against *Ps. aeruginosa*, the most virulent organism in the cornea. Treatment with chloramphenicol alone was considered to be incorrect.— D. O. Crompton (letter), *Med. J. Aust.*, 1978, *1*, 444.

Meningitis. A report of the intrathecal administration of polymyxin B in 2 patients with *Pseudomonas* meningitis following craniofacial surgery.— G. W. Geelhoed and A. S. Ketcham, *J. Surg. Oncol.*, 1973, *5*, 365.

Pneumonia. *Prophylaxis.* Polymyxin B 2.5 mg per kg body-weight daily in 6 divided doses administered as an aerosol sprayed into the pharynx and tracheal tube, if present, was compared with placebo in 744 patients admitted to a respiratory-surgical intensive care unit. Placebo and polymyxin cycles alternated every 2 months. The incidence of *Ps. aeruginosa* colonisation in the upper respiratory tract was 1.6% during polymyxin therapy and 9.7% during placebo administration. Pneumonia due to *Pseudomonas* occurred in 3 during polymyxin and 17 during placebo cycles.— J. M. Klick *et al.*, *J. clin. Invest.*, 1975, *55*, 514. Polymyxin B was administered in the same dose by aerosol to 292 patients during their stay of about 5 days in a respiratory-surgical intensive care unit and admitted over a period of 7 months; 11 acquired pneumonia although in only 1 patient was this due to *Ps. aeruginosa*. Ten of the cases of pneumonia were due to polymyxin-resistant organisms and out of the group of 11 patients, 7 died. The continuous use of polymyxin B aerosol appeared to be dangerous.— T. W. Feeley *et al.*, *New Engl. J. Med.*, 1975, *293*, 471.

Preparations

Polymyxin B Sulfate Otic Solution *(U.S.P.)*. A sterile solution of polymyxin B sulphate containing 10 000 units per ml; it may contain hydrocortisone 0.5% and one or more suitable buffers and preservatives. Store in airtight containers. Protect from light. pH 3.8 to 4.3 if it contains acetic acid.

Polymyxin Ear Drops *(A.P.F.)*. Polymyxin B sulphate 100 000 units, propylene glycol 2 ml, freshly boiled and cooled water to 10 ml. Protect from light.

Polymyxin Eye Drops *(A.P.F.)*. Polymyxin B sulphate 150 000 units, sodium chloride 90 mg, phenylmercuric nitrate 200 μg, Water for Injections to 10 ml. Prepared aseptically or sterilised by filtration. These eye-drops must be freshly prepared, stored below 25°, protected from light, and used within 1 month.

Polymyxin Injection *(B.P.C. 1973)*. Polymyxin B Sulphate Injection. A sterile solution of polymyxin B sulphate, prepared by dissolving, shortly before use, the sterile contents of a sealed container in the requisite amount of Water for Injections or of sodium chloride injection. The injection should be used within 24 hours of its preparation.

Sterile Polymyxin B Sulfate *(U.S.P.)*. A grade of polymyxin B sulphate for injection, in vials of 500 000 units.

For other preparations containing polymyxin B sulphate, see under Neomycin Sulphate, p.1191..

Proprietary Preparations

Aerosporin *(Calmic, UK)*. Polymyxin B sulphate, available as sterile powder for solution before use in vials of 500 000 units. (Also available as Aerosporin in *Austral., Canad., Switz., USA*).

Ototrips *(Consolidated Chemicals, UK)*. Ear-drops (supplied as powder for preparation with water before use) containing in each vial polymyxin B sulphate 16 000 units, bacitracin 20 000 units, and trypsin 25 000 *N.F.* units, with sodium chloride 27 mg and gelatin 15 mg. For ear infections.

Polyfax *(Calmic, UK)*. **Ointment** and **Ophthalmic Ointment** each containing polymyxin B sulphate 10 000 units and bacitracin zinc 500 units per g, in a soft paraffin basis.

For other proprietary preparations containing polymyxin B sulphate, see under Neomycin Sulphate, p.1191..

140-m

Pristinamycin. RP 7293. A mixture of 2 antimicrobial substances produced by the growth of *Streptomyces pristinaspiralis*.

CAS — 11006-76-1.

A pale yellow odourless powder with a bitter taste. Sparingly **soluble** in water; soluble in most organic solvents. It is inactivated by alkalis.

Pristinamycin is an antibiotic of the streptogramin group, having 2 components, a macrocyclic lactone and a cyclopeptide lactone. They have a synergistic action.— D. Videau, *Annls Inst. Pasteur Lille*, 1965, *108*, 602, per *J. Am. med. Ass.*, 1965, *193* (July 12), A200.

Pristinamycin is an antibiotic with properties similar to those of erythromycin (see p.1158) and with a similar antimicrobial spectrum. Partial cross-resistance has been demonstrated *in vitro* between pristinamycin and erythromycin but not between pristinamycin and spiramycin. It has been used in the treatment of staphylococcal and other susceptible infections in a dose of 2 to 4 g daily in divided doses. Children have been given 50 to 100 mg per kg body-weight daily.

Proprietary Names

Pyostacine *(Specia, Belg.; Specia, Fr.)*.

141-b

Procaine Penicillin *(B.P., B.P. Vet.)*.

Penicillin G Procaine *(U.S.P.)*; Procaine Penicil.; Procaini Benzylpenicillinum; Benzylpenicillin Novocaine; Procaine Benzylpenicillin; Procaine Penicillin G. Procaine (6*R*)-6-(2-phenylacetamido)penicillanate monohydrate; 2-(4-Aminobenzoyloxy)ethyldiethylammonium (6*R*)-6-(2-phenylacetamido)penicillanate monohydrate. $C_{13}H_{20}N_2O_2,C_{16}H_{18}N_2O_4S,H_2O=588.7$.

CAS — 54-35-3 (anhydrous); 6130-64-9 (monohydrate).

Pharmacopoeias. In all pharmacopoeias examined except *Chin., Eur.,* and *Neth.*

A white, odourless or almost odourless, crystalline powder containing not less than 96% of total penicillins and 37.5 to 40.5% of procaine. Procaine penicillin 300 mg is approximately equivalent to 200 mg of benzylpenicillin (300 000 units).

Soluble 1 in 200 of water, 1 in 30 of alcohol, and 1 in 60 of chloroform; slightly soluble in acetone and fixed oils; very slightly soluble in amyl acetate and ether. A 30% suspension in water has a pH of 5 to 7.5.

Buffered aqueous suspensions of procaine penicillin are more stable than benzylpenicillin solutions, since only the proportion of procaine penicillin in solution is subject to deterioration. Suitably buffered suspensions stored at a temperature not exceeding 20° and protected from light may be expected to retain their potency for at least 18 months. It is rapidly inactivated by acids, alkali hydroxides, and oxidising agents.

Store at a temperature not exceeding 30° in airtight containers. If intended for injection, the the containers should be sterile and sealed to exclude micro-organisms.

The stability of procaine penicillin in oleaginous preparations containing colloidal silica.— H. Zia *et al.*, *Can. J. pharm. Sci.*, 1974, *9*, 117.

Delayed absorption. Absorption of procaine penicillin could be delayed by the use of an oily vehicle gelled with 2% aluminium monostearate; in addition, procaine penicillin in small particles (less than 5 μm) was absorbed more slowly than when in larger particles.— F. H. Buckwalter and H. L. Dickison, *J. Am. pharm. Ass., scient. Edn*, 1958, *47*, 661.

Storage. A depot injection of procaine penicillin had satisfactory rheological properties when fresh and after storage for 2 years at 5°. Storage at higher temperatures increased the yield value and made the product impossible to inject from its disposable syringe pack after 3 weeks at 37°. Elevated temperature storage could not be used to predict shelf-life in this case.— J. C. Boylan and R. L. Robison, *J. pharm. Sci.*, 1968, *57*, 1796.

Adverse Effects and Treatment. As for Benzylpenicillin, p.1103.

Severe reactions with symptoms of severe anxiety and agitation, psychotic reactions, including visual and auditory disturbances, tachycardia and hypertension, cyanosis, and a sensation of impending death have occasionally been reported with procaine penicillin and may be due to accidental intravascular injection. Procaine has been implicated as a cause of these reactions, especially after high doses.

Induration may develop at the site of injection.

A pseudoanaphylactic reaction occurred in 3 patients given inadvertent infusions of procaine penicillin.— J. E. Galpin *et al.*, *Ann. intern. Med.*, 1974, *81*, 358.

A report of 14 patients who developed severe non-allergic reactions after treatment with aqueous procaine penicillin administered intramuscularly. The reactions were characterised by auditory disturbances, fear of impending death, and grand mal seizures or violent behaviour, tachycardia, and an increase in blood pressure. Treatment with phenobarbitone produced rapid recovery in all patients.— T. F. Downham and D. P. Ramos, *Mich. Med.*, 1973, *72*, 223. Seven patients experienced an acute non-allergic reaction to procaine penicillin. As well as the fear of impending death the patients showed acute depersonalisation.— H. E. Menke and L. Pepplinkhuizen (letter), *Lancet*, 1974, *2*, 723.

Of 920 patients receiving procaine penicillin 4.8 g, there were 18 toxic reactions. In 26 patients plasma-procaine concentrations measured immediately after injection ranged from 3.6 to 11 μg per ml but 30 minutes later were less than 1.0 μg per ml. As the initial procaine concentrations had been shown to produce similar reactions in studies with procaine injection, the reactions to procaine penicillin were considered to be due to the immediate release of toxic quantities of procaine after injection. The concentration of free procaine in the mixture before injection did not appear to be significant.— R. L. Green *et al.*, *New Engl. J. Med.*, 1974, *291*, 223.

Ischaemia. Irreversible ischaemic gangrene occurred in a one-year-old child, and a hand had to be amputated, after the unintentional intra-arterial injection of procaine penicillin.— S. Sengupta, *Aust. N.Z. J. Med.*, 1976, *6*, 71. See also H. Schanzer *et al.*, *J. Am. med. Ass.*, 1979, *242*, 1289.

Further references to the inadvertent intra-arterial injection of procaine penicillin: W. Gordon and J. Dove, *S.Afr. med. J.*, 1972, *46*, 1833.

Skin reactions. Toxic epidermal necrolysis occurred in a 1-year-old child after treatment with procaine penicillin intramuscularly and a penicillin suspension.— K. M. Stein *et al.*, *Br. J. Derm.*, 1972, *86*, 246.

Precautions. As for Benzylpenicillin, p.1105. It should not be given to patients known to be hypersensitive to procaine. Procaine penicillin should be given with care to infants who appear to be especially susceptible to local reactions. It is best avoided in neonates.

Procaine penicillin should not be used as the sole treatment for severe acute infections.

Absorption and Fate. Procaine penicillin is slowly absorbed after intramuscular injection, and produces antibacterial concentrations of penicillin in plasma lower than those following an equivalent dose of benzylpenicillin, but maintained for 12 to 24 hours in most patients.

Uses. Procaine penicillin is administered by deep intramuscular injection to create a depot from which benzylpenicillin is slowly liberated. It has the same antimicrobial action as benzylpenicillin (see p.1105) and is used for similar purposes in doses of 300 mg once or twice daily. It is suitable for domiciliary treatment, but because of the relatively low blood concentrations produced, its use should be restricted to infections caused by micro-organisms that are highly sensitive to penicillin.

In the treatment of gonorrhoea 4.8 g is given as a single dose with probenecid, usually 1 g, taken at the same time. Patients with early syphilis are given procaine penicillin 600 mg, or occasionally 1.2 g, daily for 8 to 10 days or for longer in late syphilis. Children with congenital syphilis have been given 10 to 50 mg per kg body-weight daily for 10 days.

For the treatment of severe acute infections, when an immediate high concentration of penicillin in the blood is necessary, benzylpenicillin may be injected simultaneously with procaine penicillin. The duration of detectable amounts of penicillin in the serum has been still further prolonged by intramuscular injection of procaine penicillin in oil with aluminium monostearate (PAM)—a suspension of procaine penicillin in an oily vehicle to which 2% of aluminium monostearate has been added.

Actinomycosis. For the use of procaine penicillin in actinomycosis, see under Benzylpenicillin, p.1108.

Arthritis, gonococcal. Procaine penicillin, 1.2 g given 12-hourly by intramuscular injection for 3 to 7 days, together with probenecid, 500 mg four times daily, and followed by phenoxymethylpenicillin by mouth for 2 patients, was used successfully in the treatment of 3 women with gonococcal arthritis. Surgical intervention was necessary for 1 patient.— A. Fam *et al.*, *Can. med. Ass. J.*, 1973, *108*, 319.

Procaine penicillin 600 mg intramuscularly twice daily for up to 10 days was as effective as the same dose of procaine penicillin intramuscularly plus benzylpenicillin intravenously for 3 days in the treatment of gonococcal arthritis.— D. E. Trentham *et al.*, *J. Am. med. Ass.*, 1976, *236*, 2410.

See also under Benzylpenicillin, p.1108.

Endocarditis, prophylaxis. Procaine penicillin 1 g twice daily was recommended from the onset of labour for prophylaxis against subacute bacterial endocarditis in women with rheumatic or congenital heart disease.— *Br. med. J.*, 1969, *3*, 518.

For other recommendations for the use of procaine penicillin in the prophylaxis of bacterial endocarditis, see Benzylpenicillin, p.1108.

Gonorrhoea. The US Public Health Service recommended procaine penicillin 4.8 g with probenecid 1 g as one regimen for the treatment of uncomplicated gonorrhoea in both men and women. Procaine penicillin could also be used in other gonococcal infections.— *Morb. Mortal.*, 1979, *28*, 13. See also *Neisseria gonorrhoeae and gonococcal infections*, Report of a WHO Scientific Group, *Tech. Rep. Ser. Wld Hlth Org. No. 616*, 1978.

Single-dose antibiotic therapy was effective in 108 episodes of gonorrhoea in 100 prepubertal children aged between 14 months and 14 years. Probenecid 25 mg per kg body-weight (maximum dose 1 g) was given with procaine penicillin 100 mg per kg (maximum dose 4.8 g) intramuscularly or amoxycillin trihydrate 50 mg per kg (maximum dose 3.5 g) by mouth.— J. D. Nelson *et al., J. Am. med. Ass.*, 1976, *236*, 1359.

Further references: K. K. Holmes *et al., J. infect. Dis.*, 1973, *127*, 455; *J. Am. med. Ass.*, 1973, *226*, 616; V. S. Rajan *et al., Br. J. vener. Dis.*, 1978, *54*, 398; D. A. Lebedeff and E. B. Hochman, *Ann. intern. Med.*, 1980, *92*, 463 (rectal gonorrhoea).

See also under Ampicillin, p.1096, and Choice of an Antibiotic, p.1078.

Leptospirosis. Most patients with serologically proven leptospirosis responded promptly to treatment with procaine penicillin 5 g initially, followed by 2.5 to 3 g daily, then 1.5 g for a total course of 5 to 7 days.— H. Nicholls (letter), *Br. med. J.*, 1973, *4*, 301.

Relapsing fever, louse-borne. A single intramuscular injection of penicillin given in an aluminium monostearate suspension to 12 patients with louse-borne relapsing fever produced a slower response than did a single intravenous dose of tetracycline given to 13 patients, but only 1 patient given penicillin developed a reaction compared with all the patients given tetracycline.— R. H. Knaack *et al., Ethiop. med. J.*, 1972, *10*, 15.

For a report of the use of procaine penicillin in the treatment of louse-borne relapsing fever, see Tetracycline Hydrochloride, p.1221.

Syphilis. Treatment with penicillin was likely to lead to healing of lesions in primary syphilis and in most cases of secondary, early latent, or early congenital syphilis. About 5 or 6% of patients with early syphilis required retreatment and all but 1 or 2% were cured. Late complications of syphilis were not markedly affected by penicillin treatment. Erythromycin and the tetracyclines were also employed in the treatment of syphilis.— Report of a WHO Scientific Group, *Tech. Rep. Ser. Wld Hlth Org. No. 455*, 1970.

The aim of treatment of congenital syphilis in infants was to achieve a penicillin concentration of 30 ng per ml in serum and CSF. A dose of 10 mg per kg body-weight of procaine penicillin daily for 10 days or a single dose of 37.5 mg per kg of benzathine penicillin was considered adequate in active syphilis without neurological involvement. If there was neurological involvement then 50 mg per kg of procaine penicillin should be used.— G. H. McCracken and J. M. Kaplan, *J. Am. med. Ass.*, 1974, *228*, 855.

A 60-year-old man with neurosyphilis given procaine penicillin 600 mg daily had serum concentrations of 1.2 μg of benzylpenicillin per ml and negligible concentrations in the cerebrospinal fluid. After therapy was changed to benzylpenicillin intravenously every 4 hours concentrations in the cerebrospinal fluid were satisfactory. — F. W. Yoder, *J. Am. med. Ass.*, 1975, *232*, 270.

In 1976 the US Public Health Service recommended procaine penicillin 600 mg daily by intramuscular injection for 8 days in the treatment of primary, secondary, or latent syphilis of less than one year's duration, extended to 15 days in late syphilis. Infants with congenital syphilis and abnormal CSF may be given 50 mg per kg body-weight daily for at least 10 days.— *Obstet. Gynec.*, 1976, *48*, 727. See also *Med. Lett.*, 1977, *19*, 105; R. D. Catterall, *Br. J. Hosp. Med.*, 1977, *17*, 585.

Further references: O. Idsøe *et al., Bull. Wld Hlth Org.*, 1972, *47, Suppl.*, 5.

See also under Yaws.

Yaws. For the eradication of yaws, mass treatment should consist of a single intramuscular injection of procaine penicillin with aluminium monostearate (PAM) to all patients with active disease, 1.2 g being given to adults and 600 mg to children under 15 years of age; one-half these doses should be given to all other members of the community to control latent infection.— C. J. Hackett, *Trans. R. Soc. trop. Med. Hyg.*, 1967, *61*, 148. See also Fifth Report of WHO Expert Committee on Venereal Infections and Treponematoses, *Tech. Rep. Ser. Wld Hlth Org. No. 190*, 1960.

Yaws has much in common with syphilis and it may be difficult to distinguish between them. Even though there may be a history of treatment for yaws, patients in whom the diagnosis is uncertain especially pregnant women, should be treated again with procaine penicillin 600 mg daily for 10 days.— *Br. med. J.*, 1979, *1*, 912.

Preparations

Aqueous Injections

Fortified Procaine Penicillin Injection *(B.P.)*. Procaine Benzylpenicillin with Benzylpenicillin Injection. A sterile suspension of procaine penicillin in a solution of benzylpenicillin potassium or benzylpenicillin sodium in Water for Injections; it contains suitable dispersing agents and may contain a suitable buffering agent. It is prepared by adding the requisite amount of Water for Injections to the sterile contents of a sealed container which contains a mixture of 5 parts of procaine penicillin and 1 part of benzylpenicillin potassium or benzylpenicillin sodium together with dispersing agents and possibly a buffering agent. Store at 2° to 8° and use within 7 days, or, if a buffering agent is present, within 14 days; if stored at temperatures approaching 20°, it should be used within 24 hours or, if a buffering agent is present, within 4 days. For intramuscular injection only.

Procaine Penicillin Injection *(B.P.)*. Procaine Benzylpenicillin Injection. A sterile suspension of procaine penicillin in Water for Injections containing suitable buffering and dispersing agents. Protect from light at a temperature not exceeding 20°; under these conditions it may be expected to retain its potency for at least 18 months. For intramuscular injection only.

Sterile Penicillin G Procaine Suspension *(U.S.P.)*. A sterile suspension of procaine penicillin in Water for Injections with one or more suitable suspending or dispersing agents and buffers and a suitable preservative. It may contain procaine hydrochloride up to 2% and may contain one or more suitable stabilisers. It contains the equivalent of not less than 300 000 units of benzylpenicillin per ml or per container. Store at 2° to 8°.

Oily Injection

Sterile Penicillin G Procaine with Aluminum Stearate Suspension *(U.S.P.)*. PAM; Procaine Penicillin in Oil with Aluminium Monostearate. A sterile suspension of procaine penicillin in a refined vegetable oil with one or more suitable dispersing and hardening agents. It contains the equivalent of 300 000 units of benzylpenicillin per ml.

Proprietary Preparations

Bicillin *(Brocades, UK)*. Vials each containing Fortified Procaine Penicillin Injection consisting of procaine penicillin 3 g (3 million units) and benzylpenicillin sodium 600 mg (1 million units) (supplied as powder for preparing intramuscular injections). *Dose.* 400 000 units (procaine penicillin 300 mg with benzylpenicillin sodium 60 mg) every 12 or 24 hours.

NOTE. Bicillin is used in some countries as a name for preparations of benzathine penicillin (see p.1102)..

Depocillin *(Brocades, UK)*. Procaine penicillin (supplied as powder for solution before use), available in vials of 3 g. **Depocillin Aqueous.** A brand of Procaine Penicillin Injection containing 300 mg per ml, in vials of 10 ml.

Other Proprietary Names

Arg.—Penicil Dermol; *Austral.*—Aquacaine G, Aquacillin, Cilicaine Syringe, Megacillin (see also under Benzylpenicillin, Clemizole Penicillin, and Phenoxymethylpenicillin); *Canad.*—Ayercillin, Wycillin; *Neth.*—Depocilline Vloeibaar; *NZ*—Cilicaine Syringe; *S.Afr.*—Hostacillin, Novocillin; *Spain*—Aqucilina, Farmaproina, Klaricina, Penifasa '900', Sanciline Procaina '300'; *USA*—Crysticillin AS, Duracillin AS, Pfizerpen AS, Wycillin.

Pessaries containing procaine penicillin, sulphanilamide, and sulphathiazole were formerly marketed in Great Britain under the proprietary name Tampovagan PSS (*Norgine*).

142-v

Propicillin Potassium *(B.P. 1973)*.

Propicillin Pot.; Propicillinum Kalicum; Potassium α-Phenoxypropylpenicillin. A mixture of the D(+)- and L(−)-isomers of potassium (6*R*)-6-(2-phenoxybutyramido)penicillanate.

$C_{18}H_{21}KN_2O_5S$=416.5.

CAS — 551-27-9 (propicillin); 1245-44-9 (potassium salt).

Pharmacopoeias. In *Int.*

A white or almost white hygroscopic finely crystalline powder with a faint unpleasant odour and a bitter taste. Each g represents about 2.4 mmol (2.4 mEq) of potassium. Propicillin potassium 1.1 g is approximately equivalent to 1 g of propicillin.

Soluble 1 in 1.2 of water, 1 in 25 of alcohol, and 1 in 65 of dehydrated alcohol; very slightly soluble in acetone and isopropyl alcohol; practically insoluble in carbon tetrachloride, chloroform, ether, and light petroleum. A 10% solution in water has a pH of 5 to 7. Solutions are stable for at least 7 days at room temperature when buffered at pH 6. **Store** below 25° in airtight containers.

The half-life of 0.1% solution of propicillin potassium in 50% aqueous alcohol at pH 1.3 and 35° was about 160 minutes.— B. Lynn, *Chemist Drugg.*, 1967, *187*, 134.

Propicillin potassium was hygroscopic and required a relative humidity of less than 45% for processing and close control of moisture content.— D. N. Gore and J. Ashwin, *J. mond. Pharm.*, 1967, (4), 365.

The actions of propicillin, a phenoxypenicillin, are similar to those of benzylpenicillin (see p.1102) and its range of antimicrobial activity is similar to that of phenoxymethylpenicillin (see p.1200) although it is less active.

Propicillin is relatively stable in acid gastric secretion and its absorption is generally rapid but can be variable. Peak plasma concentrations of about 3 μg per ml have occurred 1 hour after a dose of 250 mg. Up to 90% is bound to plasma proteins. Distribution in the body and excretion is similar to that described under Phenoxymethylpenicillin, p.1200.

Propicillin has been given by mouth, as the potassium salt, for the treatment of infections similar to those for which phenoxymethylpenicillin (see p.1200) is used. Doses equivalent to 0.5 to 1.5 g of propicillin have been used daily in divided doses.

The biological half-life of propicillin was 0.5 to 1 hour.— W. A. Ritschel, *Drug Intell. & clin. Pharm.*, 1970, *4*, 332.

Metabolism. About 32% of a 500-mg dose of propicillin was metabolised. Within 12 hours of the dose being taken by 6 healthy subjects about 66% was recovered in the urine, 21% as penicilloic acid.— M. Cole, *Antimicrob. Ag. Chemother.*, 1973, *3*, 463.

Preparations

Propicillin Elixir *(B.P.C. 1973)*. Propicillin Syrup. A solution of propicillin potassium in a suitable coloured flavoured vehicle. pH 5.5 to 6.5. It is freshly prepared by dissolving a powder consisting of the dry mixed ingredients in the specified volume of water. When a dose less than 5 ml is prescribed, the elixir should be diluted to 5 ml with syrup. The elixir and diluted elixir must be freshly prepared and used within 1 week of preparation. Store in a cool place. The elixir should not lose more than 15% of its potency in a week at 15°.

Propicillin Tablets *(B.P. 1973)*. Tablets containing propicillin potassium. Potency is expressed in terms of the equivalent amount of propicillin. They may be flavoured with peppermint oil.

Proprietary Names

Baycillin *(Bayer, Ger.)*; Bayercillin *(Bayer, Ital.)*; Bayercilline *(Bayer, Belg.)*; Delprosyn *(Gist-Brocades, Neth.)*; Oricillin *(Grünenthal, Ger.; Grünenthal, Switz.)*.

Propicillin potassium was formerly marketed in Great Britain under the proprietary name Ultrapen (*Pfizer*).

143-g

Puromycin. L 3123; CL 13 900; P 638. 3′-[2-Amino-3-(4-methoxyphenyl)propionamido]-3′-deoxy-*NN*-dimethyladenosine.

$C_{22}H_{29}N_7O_5$=471.5.

CAS — 53-79-2.

NOTE. Puromycin was at first called achromycin in the scientific literature but in 1953 this name became a trade-name for tetracycline hydrochloride.

An antibiotic produced by the growth of *Streptomyces albo-niger*. It is a colourless crystalline basic substance which forms salts with acids. **Soluble** in water. It has generally been used as the hydrochloride (CL 16 536, $C_{22}H_{29}N_7O_5$,2HCl=544.4).

Puromycin has been used experimentally because of its ability to inhibit protein synthesis.

Effect on memory. By interfering with the development of protein puromycin was considered to decrease the memory span.— B. F. Brown, *Sci. Horiz.*, 1967, (May), 13.

144-q

Ribostamycin Sulphate. SF 733 *(ribostamycin)*. 2-Deoxy-4-*O*-(2,6-diamino-2,6-dideoxy-α-D-glucopyranosyl)-5-*O*-β-D-ribofuranosyl-D-streptamine sulphate.
$C_{17}H_{34}N_4O_{10},xH_2SO_4$=454.5 (ribostamycin).

CAS — 25546-65-0 (ribostamycin); 53797-35-6 (sulphate).

An aminoglycoside antibiotic derived from *Streptomyces ribosidificus* or prepared synthetically. A white or yellowish powder, odourless or almost odourless, and with a bitter taste. **Soluble** in water; practically insoluble in organic solvents. A 25% aqueous solution has a pH of about 7.

Ribostamycin sulphate has actions and uses similar to those of kanamycin sulphate (see p.1175), and has been given in a dose of 25 mg per kg body-weight daily intramuscularly in 2 divided doses.

The antibacterial spectrum of ribostamycin against 161 strains of Gram-negative bacilli was identical with that of kanamycin. It was slightly less active than kanamycin against sensitive strains.— E. Yourassowsky and M. P. B. Linden, *Arzneimittel-Forsch.*, 1976, *26*, 184.

Proprietary Names
Ibistacin *(Ibi, Ital.)*; Ribastamin *(Morrith, Spain)*; Ribomycine *(Delalande, Fr.)*; Ribostamin *(Delalande, Ital.)*; Vistamycin *(Jap.)*.

145-p

Rifamide. Rifamycin B *NN*-diethylamide.
$C_{43}H_{58}N_2O_{13}$=810.9.

CAS — 2750-76-7.

An odourless orange-yellow crystalline powder with a bitter taste. M.p. about 170°.
It has been used as the sodium salt, which is **soluble** about 1 in 7 of water at pH 7. A solution for injection loses up to about 10% of its activity during storage at 25° for 2 years.

Antimicrobial Action. Rifamide has a bactericidal action against Gram-positive organisms, and *Mycobacterium tuberculosis* is often inhibited by 0.2 μg per ml. *Bacteroides* and *Neisseria* spp. and *Haemophilus influenzae* are reported to be susceptible to low concentrations. Concentrations of 10 to 100 μg per ml are required to inhibit the growth of other Gram-negative micro-organisms. Resistance to rifamide has been found in staphylococci, but there does not appear to be cross-resistance with other antibiotics.

References: B. C. Stratford and S. Dixson, *Med. J. Aust.*, 1966, *1*, 1; P. Cavanagh (letter), *Br. med. J.*, 1969, *1*, 317; J. D. Williams and J. Andrews, *ibid.*, 1974, *1*, 134.

Absorption and Fate. Rifamide is irregularly absorbed from the gastro-intestinal tract. The intramuscular injection of 150 mg produces peak plasma concentrations of about 1 μg per ml. The biological half-life is 1 to 2 hours and 70 to 80% of a dose is bound to plasma proteins. About 80% of a dose is excreted in the bile.

Uses. Rifamide is a rifamycin antibiotic which was formerly used in the treatment of susceptible infections of the respiratory and biliary tracts. It was given by intramuscular injection, usually with lignocaine hydrochloride, in doses of 150 mg as the sodium salt 2 to 4 times daily.

Infections of the biliary tract. References: B. C. Stratford, *Med. J. Aust.*, 1966, *1*, 7; P. G. Bevan and J. D. Williams, *Br. med. J.*, 1971, *3*, 284.

Proprietary Names
Rifocin M *(Lepetit, Austral.)*.

Rifamide was formerly marketed in Great Britain under the proprietary name Rifocin M (*Lepetit*).

146-s

Rifamycin Sodium *(B.P., Eur. P.)*. Rifamycinum Natricum; Rifamycin SV Sodium; Rifamicina.
$C_{37}H_{46}NNaO_{12}$=719.8.

CAS — 6998-60-3 (rifamycin); 15105-92-7 (sodium salt).

Pharmacopoeias. In *Br., Eur., Fr., Ger., It.,* and *Neth.*

The monosodium salt of rifamycin SV, a substance obtained by chemical transformation of rifamycin B which is produced during growth of certain strains of *Streptomyces mediterranei*. Rifamycin SV may also be obtained directly from certain mutants of *Streptomyces mediterranei*. Rifamycin sodium contains not less than 900 units per mg. A brick-red, almost odourless, fine or slightly granular powder, containing 12 to 17% of water. **Soluble** in water; freely soluble in dehydrated alcohol and methyl alcohol; soluble in chloroform; practically insoluble in ether. A 5% solution has a pH of 6.5 to 7.5. Solutions for injection are **sterilised** by filtration. **Store** in airtight containers. If it is intended for injection the containers should be sterile and sealed to exclude micro-organisms. Protect from light.

Units. One unit of rifamycin is contained in 0.001127 mg of the first International Reference Preparation (1967) of rifamycin sodium which contains 887 units per mg.

Adverse Effects. Some gastro-intestinal side effects have occurred following injections of rifamycin sodium. High doses may produce alterations in liver function. Skin reactions have rarely been reported.

Antimicrobial Action. Rifamycin sodium has a similar antimicrobial action to rifamide (see above); it is reported to be less active.

Rifamycin was effective *in vitro* against the amoeba *Naegleria fowleri*.— Y. H. Thong *et al.* (letter), *Lancet*, 1977, *2*, 876.

Absorption and Fate. Rifamycin sodium is not effectively absorbed from the gastro-intestinal tract. Plasma concentrations of about 1.5 μg per ml have been achieved 1 hour after a dose of 250 mg by intramuscular injection. It is excreted mainly in the bile and only small amounts appear in the urine.

References: G. Acocella *et al.*, *Gut*, 1968, *9*, 536.

Uses. Rifamycin sodium has been used in the treatment of infections caused by Gram-positive bacteria and in the treatment of tuberculosis. It has been given by intramuscular injection in doses of 250 mg.

Reference to the use of rifamycin in the treatment of herpes zoster.— L. Bruni *et al.*, *J. int. med. Res.*, 1980, *8*, 1.

Meningitis. Three neonates with meningitis due to *Flavobacterium meningosepticum* were given effective treatment with rifamycin 20 mg per kg body-weight every 12 hours by intramuscular or slow intravenous injection; rifamycin 2 to 5 mg daily in sodium chloride injection 2 ml was also instilled into the ventricles to treat ventriculitis. Treatment was continued although jaundice lasting for from 4 to 8 weeks occurred in 2 patients. Hydrocephalus occurred in all 3 patients and in 1 patient development was delayed by neurological defect.— E. L. Lee *et al.*, *Archs Dis. Childh.*, 1976, *51*, 209. See also I. Rios *et al.*, *Antimicrob. Ag. Chemother.*, 1978, *14*, 444.

Proprietary Names
Rifobac *(Liade, Spain)*; Rifocin *(Lepetit, Ital.; Lepetit, Switz.)*; Rifocina *(Lepetit, Spain)*; Rifocine *(Lepetit, Belg.; Lepetit, Fr.; Lepetit, Neth.)*.

148-e

Ristocetin. A mixture of 2 antimicrobial substances produced by the growth of *Nocardia lurida* (Actinomycetaceae).

CAS — 1404-55-3.

White or light tan-coloured crystals or powder. Very **soluble** in water; practically insoluble in organic solvents.

Ristocetin was formerly used in the treatment of severe staphylococcal infections unresponsive to other antibiotics but has been superseded by less toxic antibiotics.

A specific test for diagnosis of von Willebrand's disease using ristocetin.— H. Gralnick, *J. Am. med. Ass.*, 1977, *238*, 1625.

Ristocetin sulphate when added to plasma samples from 22 patients accelerated the thrombin clotting time in 20.— A. Aronstam *et al.*, *J. clin. Path.*, 1978, *31*, 1106.

149-l

Rolitetracycline *(U.S.P.)*. PMT; Pyrrolidinomethyltetracycline. N^2-(Pyrrolidin-1-ylmethyl)tetracycline.
$C_{27}H_{33}N_3O_8$=527.6.

CAS — 751-97-3.

Pharmacopoeias. In *Jap.* and *U.S.*

A light yellow crystalline powder with a characteristic musty amine-like odour, containing not less than 900 μg per mg, calculated on the anhydrous basis. M.p. about 163°. Rolitetracycline 275 mg is approximately equivalent to 250 mg of tetracycline hydrochloride.
Soluble 1 in 1.1 of water and 1 in 200 of alcohol; slightly soluble in dehydrated alcohol; soluble in acetone; very slightly soluble in ether. A 1% solution has a pH of 7 to 9. Solutions for injection are prepared aseptically immediately before use. **Store** in airtight containers. Protect from light.

150-v

Rolitetracycline Nitrate. Pyrrolidinomethyltetracycline Nitrate Sesquihydrate.
$C_{27}H_{33}N_3O_8,HNO_3,1\frac{1}{2}H_2O$=617.6.

CAS — 20685-78-3 (anhydrous); 26657-13-6 (sesquihydrate).

Pharmacopoeias. In *Jap.*

A yellow crystalline powder. **Soluble** 1 in 40 of water.

Loss of activity. Storage for 30 days at 37° and 100% relative humidity resulted in the almost complete loss of activity of rolitetracycline.— V. C. Walton *et al.*, *J. pharm. Sci.*, 1970, *59*, 1160.

Stability in solution. Solutions in water of both rolitetracycline nitrate and base were more than 50% hydrolysed to tetracycline in 3 hours at 25°.— D. W. Hughes *et al.* (letter), *J. Pharm. Pharmac.*, 1974, *26*, 79.

Reconstituted injections of rolitetracycline base lost 15% of their original antibiotic content in 21 to 25 hours when stored at 5° (the manufacturers' recommendation was 2° to 10°). Injections of the nitrate lost 15% of their content 1.5 to 3.5 hours after reconstitution and more than 60% in 8 to 20 hours when stored at 25° (the manufacturers' recommended storage at 21°). The major decomposition product was tetracycline.— W. L. Wilson *et al.*, *Can. J. pharm. Sci.*, 1976, *11*, 126.

Further references: E. Pawelczyk *et al.*, *Pol. J. Pharmac. Pharm.*, 1977, *29*, 431.

Units. One unit of rolitetracycline is contained in 0.001004 mg of the first International Standard Preparation (1968) which contains 996 units per mg.

Adverse Effects and Precautions. As for Tetracycline Hydrochloride, p.1217.
Shivering and more rarely rigor may be associated with the first few injections of rolitetracycline in infections due to organisms highly sensitive to tetracyclines. Injections may be followed by a peculiar taste sensation, often similar to ether. Rapid intravenous injection may cause transient giddiness, hot flushes, reddening of the face and, occasionally, peripheral circulatory failure.
Staphylococcal enterocolitis has followed treatment with rolitetracycline.
Symptoms of myasthenia gravis have been exacerbated by the intravenous administration of rolitetracycline.

A report of the accidental intra-arterial injection of rolitetracycline in one infant causing arteriolar obstruction followed by gangrene of the affected limb.— J. M. Wynne, *Archs Dis. Childh.*, 1978, *53*, 396.

Absorption and Fate. As for Tetracycline Hydrochloride, p.1219.
Rolitetracycline is not absorbed from the gastro-intestinal tract. When administered by injection about 50% of rolitetracycline in the circulation is bound to plasma proteins. Peak plasma concentrations of about 4 to 6 μg per ml have been reported 1 hour after a dose of 350 mg given intramuscularly and after 24 hours concentrations of up to 0.8 μg per ml are still present. Peak concentrations of about 11 μg per ml have been observed after repeated doses. About 50% of a dose is excreted in the urine.

The biological half-life of rolitetracycline was variously reported as 4.5 to 7 hours; in renal failure this might be increased to 4 to 5 days.— W. A. Ritschel, *Drug Intell.*

& clin. Pharm., 1970, *4*, 332. See also F. Reubi, *Klin. Wschr.*, 1967, *45*, 285.

Diffusion. Peak concentrations in bile of 45 and 310 μg per ml occurred 2 to 3 hours after an intravenous injection of 275 mg of rolitetracycline was given to 2 patients. Concentrations gradually declined and reached levels of 2.8 and 28 μg per ml after 12 hours.— G. Acocella *et al.*, *Gut*, 1968, *9*, 536.

Uses. Rolitetracycline has antimicrobial activity and uses similar to those of tetracycline hydrochloride (see p.1218). It has been given as the base or nitrate by deep intramuscular injection, usually with a local anaesthetic, or by slow intravenous injection or infusion. Treatment with an oral tetracycline should be substituted as soon as possible.

Adults may be given an intramuscular dose of up to 350 mg once daily, increased to 12-hourly in severe infections. Similar doses are given by slow intravenous injection over at least one minute or by infusion. Extravasation into subcutaneous tissues should be avoided.

Children have been given 10 to 15 mg per kg body-weight daily in one or 2 doses by either route but the effect of tetracyclines on teeth should be considered.

For reports on the uses of rolitetracycline, see Martindale 27th Edn, p. 1177.

Preparations

Rolitetracycline for Injection *(U.S.P.)*. A sterile dry mixture of rolitetracycline with one or more suitable buffers. If intended for intramuscular injection it contains one or more suitable anaesthetics. The injection is prepared by the addition of diluent before use. pH 3 to 4.5.

Proprietary Names

Bristacin *(Bristol, Neth.)*; Farmaciclina *(hydrochloride) (Selvi, Ital.)*; Reverin *(Hoechst, Arg.; Hoechst, Austral.; Hoechst, Belg.; Hoechst, Canad.; Hoechst, Denm.; Hoechst, Ital.; Hoechst, Neth.; Hoechst, S.Afr.; Hoechst, Switz.)*; Tetralidina*(Ital Suisse, Ital.)*; Transcycline *(Hoechst, Fr.)*.

Preparations containing rolitetracycline nitrate were formerly marketed in Great Britain under the proprietary name Tetrex-PMT (*Bristol*).

151-g

Rosaramicin. Rosamicin; Sch 14947. 12,13-Epoxy-6-formylmethyl-3-hydroxy-4,8,12,14-tetramethyl-9-oxo-5-(3,4,6-trideoxy-3-dimethylamino-β-D-*xylo*-hexopyranosyloxy)heptadec-10-en-15-olide.
$C_{31}H_{51}NO_9$=581.7.

CAS — 35834-26-5.

Rosaramicin is a macrolide antibiotic derived from *Micromonospora rosaria*. It has an antimicrobial spectrum similar to that of erythromycin (see p.1158) but is generally more active than erythromycin against Gram-negative bacteria. Several salts and esters of rosaramicin are also under study.

Absorption and fate. Higher prostate concentrations of antibiotic were achieved when rosaramicin 250 mg every 6 hours for 4 doses was given to 9 patients with benign prostatic hyperplasia than when erythromycin 250 mg as the gluceptate was given similarly to 9 further patients.— A. Baumueller *et al.*, *Antimicrob. Ag. Chemother.*, 1977, *12*, 240.

Antimicrobial action. Rosaramicin had an MIC of 1.6 μg per ml against 29 strains of *Bacteroides fragilis* and had similar activity to josamycin, clindamycin, and metronidazole. Erythromycin was less active. Rosaramicin and clindamycin had similar bactericidal activity, less than that of metronidazole and greater than that of josamycin and erythromycin.— J. Santoro *et al.*, *Antimicrob. Ag. Chemother.*, 1976, *10*, 188.

Josamycin and rosaramicin were considered comparable to erythromycin in their action *in vitro* against some aerobic Gram-positive cocci. They were inferior to clindamycin against anaerobes.— S. Shadomy *et al.*, *Antimicrob. Ag. Chemother.*, 1976, *10*, 773.

Rosaramicin was more active *in vitro* than ampicillin, chloramphenicol, or erythromycin against 15 strains of *Haemophilus influenzae* and inhibited all 15 at a concentration of 0.5 μg per ml. Rosaramicin had an MIC of 0.25 μg or less per ml against 25 strains of *Neisseria meningitidis*, being as active as benyzlpenicillin, but more active than rifampicin, minocycline, erythromycin, or chloramphenicol. At a concentration of 0.03 μg per ml 94, 46, 12, and 6% of 50 strains of *N. gonorrhoeae* were inhibited by rosaramicin, benzylpenicillin, erythromycin, and tetracycline respectively. Rosaramicin had an MIC of 0.03 μg per ml against a strain of penicillinase-producing *N. gonorrhoeae*.— C. C. Sanders and W. E. Sanders, *Antimicrob. Ag. Chemother.*, 1977, *12*, 293.

Rosaramicin was active *in vitro* against *Chlamydia trachomatis*, the MIC against 15 strains being 0.05 μg per ml and against 1 strain 0.25 μg per ml. These figures were comparable with those for tetracycline and 2 to 10 times smaller than those for erythromycin.— C. -C. Kuo *et al.*, *Antimicrob. Ag. Chemother.*, 1977, *12*, 80. Rosaramicin was more active than tetracycline, erythromycin, or benzylpenicillin *in vitro* against 30 isolates of *Chlamydia trachomatis* and inhibited 43 and 100% of the strains at concentrations of 0.01 and 0.1 μg per ml respectively.— T. F. Smith and H. E. Washton, *Antimicrob. Ag. Chemother.*, 1978, *14*, 493.

Rosaramicin inhibited all of 54 strains of beta-lactamase-positive *Neisseria gonorrhoeae* at a concentration of 0.25 μg per ml and erythromycin inhibited all the strains at 2 μg per ml; both antibiotics were more active than josamycin, clindamycin, or benzylpenicillin. Activities were similar against 77 beta-lactamase-negative strains except that benzylpenicillin was considerably more active than rosaramicin against the more sensitive strains, but required 2 μg per ml to inhibit all the strains.— J. W. Biddle and C. Thornsberry, *Antimicrob. Ag. Chemother.*, 1979, *15*, 243. See also J. R. Dillon *et al.* (letter), *J. antimicrob. Chemother.*, 1978, *4*, 477; B. B. Diena and L. Eidus (letter), *Can. med. Ass. J.*, 1978, *119*, 1009.

The activity of rosaramicin was compared with erythromycin and clindamycin *in vitro* against 208 strains of anaerobic bacteria. Rosaramicin was generally more active than erythromycin against Gram-negative bacteria and as active against Gram-positive bacteria. Clindamycin was generally more active than rosaramicin. At achievable serum concentrations 69, 65, and 94% of the strains were inhibited by rosaramicin, erythromycin, and clindamycin respectively.— Y. -Y. Kwok *et al.*, *J. antimicrob. Chemother.*, 1979, *5*, 61.

Alkalinisation of the media consistently and significantly increased the antibacterial activity of rosaramicin and erythromycin against 311 strains of bacteria representing common urinary-tract pathogens, except for erythromycin against strains of *Proteus*. At pH 8 rosaramicin was 2- to 6-fold more active than erythromycin against strains of Enterobacteriaceae, but was of similar activity against *Pseudomonas aeruginosa* and less active against group D streptococci.— T. C. Eickhoff and J. M. Ehret, *Antimicrob. Ag. Chemother.*, 1979, *16*, 69.

Further references: G. H. Wagman *et al.*, *J. Antibiot., Tokyo*, 1972, *25*, 641; J. A. Waitz *et al.*, *J. Antibiot., Tokyo*, 1972, *25*, 647; C. C. Crowe and W. E. Sanders, *Antimicrob. Ag. Chemother.*, 1974, *5*, 272; V. L. Sutter and S. M. Finegold, *Antimicrob. Ag. Chemother.*, 1976, *9*, 350; J. R. DiPersio and T. L. Krafczyk, *Antimicrob. Ag. Chemother.*, 1978, *14*, 274; S. Feltham *et al.* (letter), *J. antimicrob. Chemother.*, 1979, *5*, 731; T. F. Smith, *Antimicrob. Ag. Chemother.*, 1979, *16*, 106.

Manufacturers
Schering, USA.

152-q

Sissomicin Sulphate. Antibiotic 6640; Sch 13475 (sissomicin); Sisomicin Sulfate *(U.S.P.)*. 4-*O*-[(2*S*,3*S*)-3-Amino-6-aminomethyl-3,4-dihydro-2*H*-pyran-2-yl]-2-deoxy-6-*O*-(3-deoxy-4-*C*-methyl-3-methylamino-β-L-arabinopyranosyl)-D-streptamine sulphate.
$(C_{19}H_{37}N_5O_7)_2,5H_2SO_4$=1385.4.

CAS — 32385-11-8 (sissomicin); 53179-09-2 (sulphate).

Pharmacopoeias. In *U.S.*

Sissomicin is an antibiotic produced by *Micromonospora inyoensis* and closely related to gentamicin C_{1A}.

The sulphate is a white to yellowish-brown hygroscopic substance. It contains not less than 580 μg of sissomicin per mg. Sissomicin sulphate 1.5 g is approximately equivalent to 1 g of sissomicin. Very readily **soluble** in water, practically insoluble in alcohol. A 4% solution is dextrorotatory and has a pH of 3.5 to 5.5. **Store** in airtight containers.

Adverse Effects, Treatment, and Precautions. See Gentamicin Sulphate, p.1166.

Antimicrobial Action. Sissomicin has antimicrobial activity similar to that of gentamicin (see p.1168) and there is cross-resistance between the two antibiotics.

Studies *in vitro* suggested that tobramycin was more active than gentamicin, kanamycin, or sissomicin against *Pseudomonas* spp., whilst sissomicin and gentamicin were most active against *Serratia* spp. Against other species differences were slight. *In vivo* sissomicin was the most active of the 4 antibiotics.— J. A. Waitz *et al.*, *Antimicrob. Ag. Chemother.*, 1972, *2*, 431. See also C. C. Crowe and E. Sanders, *ibid.*, 1973, *3*, 24.

In a comparative study *in vitro* sissomicin showed little activity against gentamicin-resistant Gram-negative rods and MICs against gentamicin-sensitive rods were generally higher than those of gentamicin.— F. A. Drasar *et al.*, *Br. med. J.*, 1976, *2*, 1284. Comment.— R. Wise and D. S. Reeves (letter), *Br. med. J.*, 1977, *1*, 288.

For the relative absence of effect of sissomicin against gentamicin-resistant *Pseudomonas aeruginosa* and *Serratia marcescens*, see R. D. Meyer *et al.*, *Lancet*, 1976, *1*, 580. See also M. I. Marks *et al.*, *Antimicrob. Ag. Chemother.*, 1976, *10*, 399.

In a study *in vitro* of the susceptibility of *Staphylococcus aureus* and *Staph. epidermidis* to 65 antimicrobial agents with antistaphylococcal activity, rifampicin was the most active overall. Amongst 11 aminoglycosides, sissomicin was the most active.— L. D. Sabath *et al.*, *Antimicrob. Ag. Chemother.*, 1976, *9*, 962.

Sissomicin was more active *in vitro* than netilmicin against 35 strains of *Staph. aureus*. The activity *in vitro* of nafcillin or oxacillin against *Staph. aureus* was enhanced when used in conjunction with netilmicin or sissomicin. The activity of netilmicin and sissomicin also appeared to be enhanced by nafcillin and oxacillin.— C. Watanakunakorn and C. Glotzbecker, *Antimicrob. Ag. Chemother.*, 1977, *12*, 346.

Carbenicillin and sissomicin were synergistic when used together *in vitro* against *Pseudomonas* isolates whereas ampicillin and sissomicin were antagonistic when used against *Proteus morganii*.— M. I. Marks *et al.*, *Antimicrob. Ag. Chemother.*, 1978, *13*, 753.

The activities of benzylpenicillin or ampicillin were enhanced when used together with sissomicin or netilmicin *in vitro* against 35 strains of enterococci.— C. Watanakunakorn and C. Glotzbecker, *J. antimicrob. Chemother.*, 1978, *4*, 539.

For a comparison of the effect of sissomicin sulphate, netilmicin, and streptomycin on the activity of benzylpencillin on enterococci, see Benzylpenicillin, p.1106.

Further references: M. Scheer, *Arzneimittel-Forsch.*, 1976, *26*, 772; P. Naumann *et al.*, *Dt. med. Wschr.*, 1976, *101*, 1277; I. Phillips *et al.*, *J. antimicrob. Chemother.*, 1977, *3*, 403.

Absorption and Fate. The absorption and fate of sissomicin is similar to that of gentamicin (see p.1170).

After intramuscular doses of sissomicin 20 and 40 mg per m^2 body-surface mean peak serum concentrations achieved after 1 hour were 2.5 and 4 μg per ml respectively; within 6 hours the urinary excretion was 49 and 61%. After an intravenous injection of 30 mg per m^2, mean peak serum concentrations of 5.1 μg per ml were achieved after ½ hour.— V. Rodriguez *et al.*, *Antimicrob. Ag. Chemother.*, 1975, *7*, 38.

In a comparative study of the pharmacokinetics of gentamicin, sissomicin, and tobramycin in doses of 1 mg per kg body-weight sissomicin gave the highest serum concentration of 4.66 μg per ml and the serum-concentration curve exceeded that of the other 2 antibiotics.— H. Lode *et al.*, *Antimicrob. Ag. Chemother.*, 1975, *8*, 396.

The pharmacokinetics of sissomicin were studied in 10 healthy subjects given doses of 1 mg per kg body-weight intramuscularly or intravenously as an infusion in 250 ml of dextrose injection over 30 minutes. Peak serum-sissomicin concentrations of 3.08 μg per ml at 1 hour after intramuscular injection and 7.12 μg per ml 30 minutes after infusion were obtained. No serum concentration was detectable at 24 hours following either route. About 34% of the intramuscular dose was excreted in the urine during the first 8 hours and about 6% during the next 16; comparable figures for the intravenous dose were about 30 and 4%. The half-life for the beta phase was 2.63 hours following intramuscular administration and 2.55 hours following intravenous administration.— B. R. Meyers *et al.*, *Antimicrob. Ag. Chemother.*, 1976, *10*, 25.

A study of the concentrations of sissomicin in the lumbar and ventricular cerebrospinal fluid after intramuscular or intrathecal injection.— P. Veyssier *et al.*, *Nouv. Presse méd.*, 1978, *7*, 731.

Further references: C. Simon *et al.*, *Int. J. clin. Pharmac. Biopharm.*, 1978, *16*, 145; J. -C. Pechere and R. Dugal, *Clin. Pharmacokinet.*, 1979, *4*, 170.

Uses. Sissomicin is an aminoglycoside antibiotic which has been used, as the sulphate, similarly to gentamicin (see p.1170) in the treatment of Gram-negative infections. A suggested dose is the equivalent of 3 mg of sissomicin per kg body-weight daily given intramuscularly or intravenously in 3 divided doses. Dosage should be reduced in patients with renal impairment.

Reports of the actions and uses of sissomicin.— W. Marget and G. Gruenwaldt (Ed.), *Infection*, 1976, *4*, *Suppl.* 4, S283-S514.

After carbenicillin and a cephalosporin had failed in the treatment of 139 febrile episodes in 120 cancer patients, 61% of those given sissomicin by continuous intravenous infusion responded compared with 46% of those given sissomicin by intermittent infusion. The difference was not significant.— R. Feld *et al.*, *Am. J. med. Sci.*, 1977, *274*, 179.

Dosage in infants and children. Sissomicin 4.5 mg per kg body-weight daily, in divided doses every 8 hours was administered intravenously over 30 minutes, for 5 to 26 days to 11 children aged 2 weeks to 18 years with serious bacterial infections. There was a clinical cure in 10 and a bacteriological cure in 8. Nine of the children also received other antibiotics. One child who had received treatment for 26 days developed reversible nephrotoxicity.— M. I. Marks *et al.*, *Antimicrob. Ag. Chemother.*, 1978, *13*, 753.

References to the use of sissomicin in severe neonatal infections.— P. Henriksson *et al.*, *Acta paediat. scand.*, 1977, *66*, 317.

Dosage in renal failure. The mean serum half-life of sissomicin after an intramuscular injection of 1 mg per kg body-weight was 2.23 hours in 10 healthy subjects; 8 hours in 11 patients with a creatinine-clearance rate [CCR] of 20 to 80 ml per minute; about 22.6 hours in 6 patients with a CCR of 5 to 20 ml per minute and about 57 hours in 7 patients with a CCR of less than 5 ml per minute. The corresponding percentages of the dose recovered in the urine within 24 hours were about 87, 55, 28 and 1.7% respectively. The mean serum half-life was 8.54 hours in 7 patients during an 8-hour haemodialysis session. It was suggested that in uraemic patients the dose should be 1 mg per kg given at intervals equal to 3 times the serum half-life or a normal dose should be given followed every 12 hours by a sustaining dose related to the CCR. The serum half-life could be estimated by multiplying the serum creatinine concentration in mg per 100 ml by a factor of 3 to 5.— A. Leroy *et al.*, *J. antimicrob. Chemother.*, 1976, *2*, 373.

Further references: J. -C. Pechère *et al.*, *Antimicrob. Ag. Chemother.*, 1976, *9*, 761; S. Roth *et al.*, *Eur. J. clin. Pharmac.*, 1976, *10*, 357; T. P. Gibson and H. A. Nelson, *Clin. Pharmacokinet.*, 1977, *2*, 403; G. B. Appel and H. C. Neu, *New Engl. J. Med.*, 1977, *296*, 663.

Urinary-tract infections. Sissomicin in doses of 0.5, 0.75, and 1 mg per kg body-weight intramuscularly thrice daily for 7 days cleared lower urinary-tract infections in 36 male patients. A very high degree of relapse occurred with the lower doses.— P. G. Welling *et al.*, *J. clin. Pharmac.*, 1974, *14*, 567.

In 40 patients with bacterial infections sissomicin in doses ranging from 1.5 to 3.75 mg per kg body-weight daily intramuscularly was effective in urinary-tract infections. Granular casts and traces of protein in urine appeared transiently in 22% of the patients.— J. Klastersky *et al.*, *J. clin. Pharmac.*, 1975, *15*, 252.

Administration of sissomicin as a single daily dose of 2 mg per kg body-weight was less effective than 1 mg per kg twice daily in the treatment of urinary-tract infections.— J. Klastersky *et al.*, *J. clin. Pharmac.*, 1977, *17*, 520.

Further references: R. R. Bailey and B. Peddie, *N.Z. med. J.*, 1978, *87*, 91.

Preparations

Sisomicin Sulfate Injection *(U.S.P.)*. A sterile solution of sissomicin sulphate in Water for Injections. It may contain one or more suitable buffers, chelating agents, and preservatives. Potency is expressed in terms of the equivalent amount of sissomicin. pH 2.5 to 5.5.

Proprietary Names

Baymicin *(Bayer, Ital.; Bayer, S.Afr.)*; Baymicine *(Bayer, Belg.; Bayer, Fr.)*; Extramycin *(Bayer, Ger.; Bayer, Switz.)*; Mensiso *(Menarini, Ital.)*; Pathomycin *(Byk Essex, Ger.)*; Siseptin *(Scherag, S.Afr.)*; Sismine *(Schering, Belg.)*; Sisolline *(Cétrane, Fr.)*; Sisomin *(Essex, Ital.; Schering, Switz.)*; Sisomina *(Essex, Arg.)*.

154-s

Sodium Fusidate *(B.P.)*.

Fusidate Sodium; SQ 16360. The sodium salt of fusidic acid. $C_{31}H_{47}NaO_6=538.7$.

CAS — 751-94-0.

Pharmacopoeias. In *Br.*

A white or almost white, odourless or almost odourless, slightly hygroscopic, crystalline powder with a bitter taste.

Soluble 1 in 1 of water, 1 in 1 of alcohol, and 1 in 350 of chloroform; practically insoluble in acetone and ether. An aqueous solution is dextrorotatory. A 1.25% solution in water had a pH of 7.5 to 9. **Store** in airtight containers. Protect from light.

Adverse Effects and Precautions. Apart from mild gastro-intestinal upsets sodium fusidate appears to be well tolerated when given by mouth. Skin rashes have been reported. Treatment with sodium fusidate has been associated with jaundice and changes in liver function have occasionally been noted but normal liver function was restored when treatment was stopped. Fusidates should be given with caution to patients with impaired liver function.

Venospasm and thrombophlebitis has occurred in patients given diethanolamine fusidate intravenously. To reduce this it is recommended that solutions be buffered and that the solution should be given as a slow infusion into a large vein where there is a good blood-flow.

Treatment with sodium fusidate and erythromycin was associated with the development of tunnel vision in a patient with diphtheroid endocarditis. The visual impairment resolved when sodium fusidate was withdrawn.— G. Jackson and K. Saunders, *Br. Heart J.*, 1973, *35*, 931.

Hepatotoxicity. In a retrospective study of patients with staphylococcal bacteraemia, jaundice developed during treatment in 38 of 112 patients given fusidic acid (in 32 of 66 given the intravenous preparation with or without oral treatment) compared with 2 of 101 patients given other antimicrobial agents. It was suggested that since the jaundice was reversible the continuing use of this drug would seem to be justified but that the intravenous preparation should be diluted to a volume of 500 ml or the maximum volume compatible with the clinical condition of the patient and infused slowly over at least 6 to 8 hours, that liver function should be monitored regularly in any patient receiving the drug by this route, and that oral medication be given as soon as possible.— M. W. Humble *et al.*, *Br. med. J.*, 1980, *280*, 1495. Comments.— C. F. H. Vickers and A. P. Menday (letter), *ibid.*, *281*, 308; R. R. H. Coombs (letter), *ibid.*; J. Talbot and L. Beeley (letter), *ibid.*

Interactions. Studies *in vitro* and in *rats* indicated that cholestyramine could bind sodium fusidate and interfere with its absorption from the gastro-intestinal tract.— W. H. Johns and T. R. Bates, *J. pharm. Sci.*, 1972, *61*, 730 and 735.

Fusidic acid might interfere with fluorimetric estimations of plasma hydrocortisone.— J. Millhouse, *Adverse Drug React. Bull.*, 1974, Dec., 164.

For a report of hydrocortisone diminishing the activity of fusidic acid, see under Antimicrobial Action.

Antimicrobial Action. Sodium fusidate inhibits bacterial protein synthesis and it may be bacteriostatic or bactericidal. It is highly active against *Staphylococcus aureus*, including strains that are resistant to the penicillins and to other antibiotics. Streptococci are less sensitive but *Corynebacterium diphtheriae* and *Clostridium* spp. are sensitive. Among the Gram-negative bacteria the *Neisseria* spp. are sensitive; *Bacteroides fragilis* is less sensitive. It has some activity against *Mycobacterium tuberculosis*.

Sodium fusidate has been reported to inhibit the growth of *Staph. aureus* in concentrations of 0.03 to 0.16 µg per ml and of streptococci in concentrations of up to 16 µg per ml.

For a brief discussion of fusidic acid, see p.1084.

Fusidic acid inhibited 12 of 14 strains of *Bacteroides fragilis in vitro* at a concentration of 2 µg per ml and all 14 at 8 µg per ml; the addition of serum to the medium raised the MIC considerably for most strains.— J. Stirling and S. Goodwin (letter), *J. antimicrob. Chemother.*, 1977, *3*, 523.

Sodium fusidate had an MIC of 0.5, 0.25, 0.12, 0.06, 0.03, and 0.015 µg per ml against 100, 98, 94, 85, 55, and 19 of 100 strains of meningococci *in vitro*.— R. S. Miles and A. Moyes, *J. clin. Path.*, 1978, *31*, 355.

Sodium fusidate had an MIC of up to 1 µg per ml against 114 strains of *Clostridia* spp. and an MIC of up to 2 µg per ml against 41 isolates of other species of anaerobic Gram-positive rods. All of 156 strains of *Bacteroides* were inhibited over a range of concentrations of 0.06 to 8 µg per ml, but up to 16 µg per ml was required to inhibit strains of *B. fragilis* and up to 32 µg per ml to inhibit strains of *B. thetaiotaomicron* and *Fusobacterium necrophorum*. Sodium fusidate inhibited all of 130 anaerobic cocci at a concentration of up to 8 µg per ml.— G. E. Steinkraus and L. R. McCarthy, *Antimicrob. Ag. Chemother.*, 1979, *16*, 120.

Diminished activity. The antibacterial activity *in vitro* of fusidic acid against *Staph. aureus* was markedly decreased in the presence of hydrocortisone.— W. P. Raab, *Br. J. Derm.*, 1971, *84*, 582.

Resistance. Bacterial resistance to sodium fusidate is readily acquired in the laboratory and has been reported to occur during treatment, especially when topical preparations have been used in hospital skin wards.

Resistance to fusidic acid developed within 5 days in a boy with staphylococcal septicaemia. Fusidic acid should always be used with another antibiotic.— A. W. Goodwin *et al.* (letter), *Lancet*, 1973, *2*, 1504.

In a study in Birmingham between 1967 and 1975 strains of *Staph. aureus* resistant to fusidic acid emerged during 1967 in dermatology wards and increased despite restrictions on the topical use of the antibiotic. In contrast, resistance to fusidic acid was low in burns wards.— G. A. J. Ayliffe *et al.*, *J. clin. Path.*, 1977, *30*, 40.

Of 200 strains of *Staph. aureus* 7 were resistant to sodium fusidate.— Z. A. Hassam *et al.*, *Br. med. J.*, 1978, *2*, 536. See also H. Roser, *Münch. med. Wschr.*, 1974, *116*, 1849.

Further references: W. C. Noble and J. Naidoo, *Br. J. Derm.*, 1978, *98*, 481.

Absorption and Fate. Sodium fusidate is absorbed from the gastro-intestinal tract. A single 500-mg dose produces plasma concentrations of about 30 µg per ml after 2 to 4 hours in fasting subjects. Milk has been reported to delay absorption. Higher concentrations may occur with repeated doses; concentrations of up to 144 µg per ml have been reported after treatment with 1.5 g daily for 4 days. About 95% of sodium fusidate in the circulation is bound to plasma proteins. It is widely distributed in body tissues and fluids but it does not diffuse into the cerebrospinal fluid when the meninges are not inflamed. Concentrations have been detected in the foetal circulation and in the milk of nursing mothers.

Sodium fusidate is excreted in the bile and about 2% appears unchanged in the faeces; metabolites have been detected in the bile. Little is excreted in the urine or removed by dialysis.

The biological half-life of fusidic acid was 4 to 6 hours.— W. A. Ritschel, *Drug Intell. & clin. Pharm.*, 1970, *4*, 332.

The absorption of sodium fusidate was increased in patients with coeliac disease.— R. L. Parsons *et al.*, *J. antimicrob. Chemother.*, 1975, *1*, 39.

The absorption of fusidate preparations.— R. Wise *et al.*, *Br. J. clin. Pharmac.*, 1977, *4*, 615.

Diffusion. *Bone and connective tissue.* References: G. Hierholzer *et al.*, *Arzneimittel-Forsch.*, 1966, *16*, 1549.

Brain. Fusidic acid seemed to penetrate well into intracranial pus.— J. de Louvois *et al.*, *Br. med. J.*, 1977, *2*, 985.

Burn crusts. In patients given fusidic acid as tablets or solution by mouth in the prophylactic treatment of burns, the antibiotic was found in the burn crusts in a concentration considerably higher than that in the serum. In other patients with burns given oxacillin sodium or benzylpenicillin sodium, oxacillin accumulated in the crusts to a lesser extent but in concentrations greater than serum concentrations, while benzylpenicillin concentrations were much higher in serum than in the crusts.— B. Sørensen *et al.*, *Acta chir. scand.*, 1966, *131*, 423.

Eye. Study of 18 patients having cataract extractions showed that sodium fusidate was present in therapeutic concentrations in the aqueous humour after doses of 500 mg thrice daily for 3 days. As sodium fusidate binds with protein, a higher concentration might be expected in the inflamed eye.— A. J. Chadwick and B. Jackson, *Br. J. Ophthal.*, 1969, *53*, 26. See also J. Williamson *et al.*, *ibid.*, 1970, *54*, 126.

Skin. Tests *in vitro* showed that sodium fusidate and fusidic acid penetrated human skin when applied locally and that absorption was increased by the addition of dimethyl sulphoxide or salicyclic acid.— C. F. H. Vickers, *Br. J. Derm.*, 1969, *81*, 902.

Uses. Sodium fusidate, alone or in conjunction with other antibiotics, is used in the treatment of infections due to staphylococci, especially strains resistant to other antibiotics. It is often used in conjunction with various penicillins. Although, there is evidence of antagonism with such mixtures, they may still be bactericidal.

The usual dose of sodium fusidate is 500 mg by mouth every 8 hours. In severe infections 3 g daily may be given. Children may be given 20 to 40 mg per kg body-weight daily; an aqueous suspension of fusidic acid (p.1166) is available for oral use and 250 mg of fusidic acid is stated to be equivalent therapeutically to 175 mg of sodium fusidate. To reduce gastro-intestinal disturbances, doses may be taken with meals.

In severe infections the equivalent of 500 mg of sodium fusidate as diethanolamine fusidate (p.1155) is given thrice daily by slow intravenous infusion over not less than 6 hours. Each 500-mg dose is administered as a buffered solution (pH 7.5) diluted to 500 ml with sodium chloride injection or other suitable intravenous solution. For children and adults weighing less than 50 kg a dose of 6 to 7 mg per kg body-weight of diethanolamine fusidate thrice daily has been recommended.

Sodium fusidate is used as an ointment (2%) in the local treatment of skin infections. A sterile gel of fusidic acid (2%) is used for the treatment of abscesses. Topical use may lead to problems of resistance.

In 15 of 18 children, aged from 18 months to 15 years, with cystic fibrosis, treatment with fusidic acid, 800 mg daily for the younger patients and 1 g daily for older patients (23 to 50 mg per kg body-weight), in conjunction with lincomycin 1 g daily proved highly successful in 18 of 21 treatments in eliminating staphylococcal infection which had lasted from 1 month to 9 years; 2 treatments were unsuccessful and 1 was doubtful. Treatment was unsuccessful when fusidic acid was given in conjunction with phenoxymethylpenicillin 1 g daily, cloxacillin 1 g daily, chloramphenicol 750 mg daily, or novobiocin 500 mg or 1 g daily.— G. L. T. Wright and J. Harper, *Lancet*, 1970, *1*, 9.

Two patients with severe staphylococcal infection were treated successfully with intravenous fusidic acid for 59 and 33 days and received a total of 88.5 and 49.5 g of fusidic acid. To avoid venospasm and thrombosis, heparin 500 units and hydrocortisone 25 mg were added to each 250-ml infusion of fusidic acid.— I. J. Copperman, *Br. J. clin. Pract.*, 1972, *26*, 83.

For the use of sodium fusidate in the treatment of infected arterial or venous shunts, see Cloxacillin Sodium, p.1150.

Abscess. Sterile fusidic acid gel was introduced into the abscess cavity (after incision and curetting) on a single occasion in 87 patients and sodium fusidate ointment dressings were applied daily after similar pretreatment in a further 71 patients. Mean healing times were 4.8 and 9.9 days respectively. A similar significant reduction of healing times occurred in each subgroup of patients analysed according to the size and site of abscess. *Staphylococcus aureus* was responsible for 82% of the infections and was resistant to penicillin and ampicillin in 49%.— I. C. Ritchie, *Br. med. J.*, 1972, *2*, 381.

There was more rapid healing of 23 abscesses all packed with 5 g of a preparation of fusidic acid 2% gel (Fucidin Caviject) compared to the healing of 20 packed with fusidic acid-impregnated wick.— A. Franklin and R. F. Calver (letter), *Lancet*, 1973, *2*, 573. See also *idem*, *Practitioner*, 1974, *212*, 388.

There was no significant difference between the mean time to healing in 17 patients who had a 2% fusidic acid gel introduced into abscess cavities compared with 22 similar patients who also received flucloxacillin 250 mg four times daily by mouth.— J. Kotowski, *Practitioner*, 1979, *222*, 269.

Abscess of the CNS. Fusidic acid was the drug of choice in the treatment of spinal and post-traumatic intracranial abscesses due to *Staphylococcus aureus*.— J. de Louvois *et al.*, *Br. med. J.*, 1977, *2*, 985.

Dosage in renal failure. The dosage interval of sodium fusidate was not affected in renal failure.— P. Sharpstone, *Br. med. J.*, 1977, *2*, 36.

Effect on leucocyte migration. Sodium fusidate inhibited leucocyte migration (leucotaxis) *in vitro*.— A. Forsgren and D. Schmeling, *Antimicrob. Ag. Chemother.*, 1977, *11*, 580.

Osteomyelitis. Fusidic acid with benzylpenicillin or erythromycin was considered the most effective treatment in 38 patients with acute osteomyelitis. The failure-rate was reduced to 10.5% with this treatment compared with 18.7, 14.5, and 27% for benzylpenicillin and tetracycline, benzylpenicillin and cloxacillin, and miscellaneous antibiotics.— N. J. Blockey and T. A. McAllister, *J. Bone Jt Surg.*, 1972, *54B*, 299.

Preparations

Sodium Fusidate Capsules *(B.P.)*. Sod. Fusidate Caps. Capsules containing sodium fusidate. Store at a temperature not exceeding 30°.

Sodium Fusidate Gauze Dressing *(D.T.F.)*. Cotton gauze of leno weave impregnated with a white soft paraffin and wool fat basis containing sodium fusidate 2%, sterilised. It is supplied in 10-cm squares as single pieces.

Proprietary Preparations

Fucidin *(Leo, UK)*. Enteric-coated tablets each containing sodium fusidate 250 mg. **Fucidin Ointment**. Contains sodium fusidate 2%. **Fucidin H Ointment**. Contains, in addition, hydrocortisone acetate 1%. (Also available as Fucidin in *Austral.*, *Denm.*, *Neth.*, *Norw.*, *S.Afr.*, *Switz.*).

Fucidin Intertulle *(Leo, UK)*. A sterile gauze dressing impregnated with ointment containing sodium fusidate 2%.

Other Proprietary Names

Fucidine *(Belg., Fr., Ger., Spain)* (see also Diethanolamine Fusidate).

155-w

Spectinomycin.

Actinospectacin; M 141; U 18409. Decahydro-4a,7,9-trihydroxy-2-methyl-6,8-bis(methylamino)-4*H*-pyrano[2,3-*b*][1,4]benzodioxin-4-one.

$C_{14}H_{24}N_2O_7$=332.4.

CAS — 1695-77-8.

An antimicrobial substance produced by the growth of *Streptomyces spectabilis*. It occurs as a white amorphous powder, **soluble** in water.

156-e

Spectinomycin Hydrochloride.

Spectinomycin dihydrochloride pentahydrate.

$C_{14}H_{24}N_2O_7,2HCl,5H_2O$=495.4.

CAS — 21736-83-4 (anhydrous); 22189-32-8 (pentahydrate).

Pharmacopoeias. In *Braz. U.S.* includes Sterile Spectinomycin Hydrochloride.

A white to pale buff crystalline powder with a slight characteristic odour and taste. Spectinomycin hydrochloride 1.5 g is approximately equivalent to 1 g of spectinomycin. Freely **soluble** in water; very slightly soluble in acetone; practically insoluble in alcohol, chloroform, and ether. A 1% solution in water has a pH of 3.8 to 5.6. A 5.66% solution in water is iso-osmotic with serum.

157-l

Spectinomycin Sulphate.

$C_{14}H_{24}N_2O_7,H_2SO_4,4H_2O$=502.5.

CAS — 23312-56-3 (anhydrous).

A white to pale buff crystalline powder. Freely **soluble** in water; very slightly soluble in alcohol, acetone, and chloroform.

An aqueous solution of spectinomycin hydrochloride iso-osmotic with serum (5.66%) caused 3% haemolysis of erythrocytes cultured in it for 45 minutes.— C. Sapp *et al.*, *J. pharm. Sci.*, 1975, *64*, 1884.

Stability. The stability of spectinomycin was a function of pH and temperature. No significant degradation occurred in 0.1M hydrochloric acid and at pH 4.65 for over 43 days at 30°, but degradation was significant in alkaline solution. Spectinomycin should be stable enough for practical purposes below pH 5.— E. R. Garrett and G. R. Umbreit, *J. pharm. Sci.*, 1962, *51*, 436.

Units. One unit of spectinomycin is contained in 0.00149 mg of the first International Reference Preparation (1975) which contains 671 units per mg.

Adverse Effects and Precautions. Nausea and vomiting, headache, dizziness, fever, and slight pruritus and urticaria have occasionally occurred with single doses of spectinomycin hydrochloride. Mild to moderate pain has been reported in a few patients following intramuscular injections. Alterations in kidney and liver function and a decrease in haemoglobin and blood count have occasionally been observed with repeated doses. Spectinomycin should not be used to treat syphilis.

Healthy subjects given up to 8 g of spectinomycin hydrochloride daily for 5 days showed no evidence of ototoxicity, hepatotoxicity, or nephrotoxicity.— E. Novak *et al.*, *J. clin. Pharmac.*, 1974, *14*, 442. See also *idem*, *J. infect. Dis.*, 1974, *130*, 50.

Spectinomycin ototoxicity.— M. Akiyoshi *et al.*, *Jap. J. Antibiotics*, 1976, *29*, 771. See also T. Iwasawa, *ibid.*, 1977, *30*, 117.

Dosage in renal failure. Spectinomycin should not be used in patients with mild renal failure.— G. B. Appel and H. C. Neu, *New Engl. J. Med.*, 1977, *296*, 663.

Interactions. For the effect of spectinomycin on lithium, see Lithium Carbonate, p.1539.

Antimicrobial Action. Spectinomycin shows activity against a wide range of Gram-positive and Gram-negative organisms but its main effect is against *Neisseria gonorrhoeae*, most strains of which are inhibited by less than 7.5 to 20 µg per ml. It acts by inhibiting bacterial protein synthesis.

The majority of 100 strains of *Bacteroides fragilis* were inhibited *in vitro* by spectinomycin at a concentration of 16 µg per ml. Although the MIC was not significantly affected by the inoculum size, type of medium, or presence of serum it was markedly increased at low pH and diminished at high pH. Studies *in vitro* suggested that *Bacteroides fragilis* slowly acquired resistance to spectinomycin.— I. Phillips and C. Warren, *J. antimicrob. Chemother.*, 1975, *1*, 91. The addition of clindamycin or metronidazole had little effect.— R. Wise *et al.* (letter), *ibid.*, 439. Spectinomycin was not a potent inhibitor of *Bacteroides fragilis* or other clinically significant anaerobes and would probably not be effective in the treatment of anaerobic infection.— J. E. Rosenblatt and A. M. Gerdts, *Antimicrob. Ag. Chemother.*, 1977, *12*, 37.

The action of spectinomycin on *Neisseria gonorrhoeae*.— M. E. Ward, *J. antimicrob. Chemother.*, 1977, *3*, 323.

The activity of 9 aminoglycosides and spectinomycin was tested *in vitro* against 351 strains of Enterobacteriaceae, 34 of *Pseudomonas aeruginosa*, 38 gentamicin-sensitive and 42 gentamicin-resistant strains of the *Pseudomonas* spp., 20 of the *Acinetobacter* spp., 17 of *Haemophilus influenzae* and 41 strains of *Neisseria gonorrhoeae*; spectinomycin inhibited 63, 0, 32, 0, 55, 100, and 100% of the strains respectively at a concentration of 16 μg per ml.— I. Phillips *et al.*, *J. antimicrob. Chemother.*, 1977, *3*, 403.

Further references: R. J. Fass and R. B. Prior, *Antimicrob. Ag. Chemother.*, 1977, *12*, 551.

Resistance. Resistant gonococci have been reported. Resistance to spectinomycin has also developed amongst other bacteria.

A strain of *Neisseria gonorrhoeae* resistant to spectinomycin at concentrations greater than 2048 μg per ml was isolated from a 26-year-old man with urethritis.— C. Thornsberry *et al.*, *J. Am. med. Ass.*, 1977, *237*, 2405.

Studies *in vitro* indicated that resistance of strains of the *Bacteroides* spp. to spectinomycin emerged at a relatively low rate but resistant streptococci emerged more frequently.— M. S. Osman and R. H. George (letter), *J. antimicrob. Chemother.*, 1978, *4*, 95.

Absorption and Fate. Spectinomycin is rapidly absorbed following the intramuscular injection of the hydrochloride. A 2-g dose produces peak plasma concentrations of about 100 μg per ml at 1 hour while a 4-g dose produces peak concentrations of about 160 μg per ml at 2 hours. Therapeutic plasma concentrations are maintained for up to 8 hours. Spectinomycin is excreted in an active form in the urine and up to 100% of a dose has been recovered within 48 hours. Mean half-lives of up to 2.5 hours have been reported.

Uses. Spectinomycin is used as the hydrochloride in the treatment of gonorrhoea when penicillin or tetracycline treatment is ineffective or inadvisable. It is administered by intramuscular injection as a single dose equivalent to 2 g of spectinomycin. A dose of 4 g for females is sometimes recommended.

Spectinomycin sulphate is used for agricultural and veterinary purposes.

Gonorrhoea. The US Public Health Service recommended spectinomycin 2 g in one intramuscular injection as an alternative to penicillins or tetracycline for the treatment of men and women with uncomplicated gonococcal infections. For patients with disseminated infection caused by penicillinase-producing *Neisseria gonorrhoeae*, spectinomycin 2 g given intramuscularly twice daily for 3 days was the treatment of choice.— *Morb. Mortal.*, 1979, *28*, 13. See also *Neisseria gonorrhoeae and gonococcal infections*, Report of a WHO Scientific Group, *Tech. Rep. Ser. Wld Hlth Org. No. 616*, 1978.

Some references on the use of spectinomycin in the treatment of gonorrhoea: W. W. Karney *et al.*, *New Engl. J. Med.*, 1977, *296*, 889; I. A. Porter and H. W. Rutherford, *Br. J. vener. Dis.*, 1977, *53*, 115; N. J. Fiumara, *J. Am. med. Ass.*, 1978, *239*, 735; M. S. Siegel *et al.*, *J. infect. Dis.*, 1978, *137*, 170; M. Sands, *J. Am. med. Ass.*, 1980, *243*, 1143; H. H. Neumann (letter), *ibid.*, *244*, 1437.

Reviews Med. Lett., 1971, *13*, 105; R. N. Brogden and G. S. Avery, *Drugs*, 1972, *3*, 314; *Drug & Ther. Bull.*, 1974, *12*, 22; *Lancet*, 1974, *2*, 1239; W. M. McCormack and M. Finland, *Ann. intern. Med.*, 1976, *84*, 712.

Urinary-tract infections. Spectinomycin 2 g intramuscularly as a single dose or repeated once or twice at 12-hourly intervals was effective in the treatment of 18 of 27 men with urethritis due to *Ureaplasma urealyticum*. It was ineffective in urethritis due to *Chlamydia trachomatis*. Streptomycin had originally been used in this study but because of dizziness spectinomycin was used instead.— W. R. Bowie *et al.*, *Lancet*, 1976, *2*, 1276. See also L. K. Pickering *et al.*, *Am. J. med. Sci.*, 1977, *274*, 291.

Preparations

Sterile Spectinomycin Hydrochloride *(U.S.P.)*. A grade of spectinomycin hydrochloride for injection. It has a potency of not less than 603 μg of spectinomycin per mg.

Trobicin *(Upjohn, UK)*. Spectinomycin hydrochloride, available as powder for preparing injections, in vials each containing the equivalent of spectinomycin 2 g, supplied with ampoules of solvent containing benzyl alcohol 0.9%, for preparing 5 ml of solution for injection. (Also available as Trobicin in *Austral.*, *Belg.*, *Canad.*, *Denm.*, *Ital.*, *Jap.*, *Norw.*, *S.Afr.*, *Switz.*, *USA*).

Other Proprietary Names

Delspectin *(Neth.)*; Kempi *(Spain)*; Stanilo *(Ger.)*; Togamycin *(Arg.)*; Trobicine *(Fr.)*.

158-y

Spiramycin.

IC 5902; NSC 64393. A mixture of basic antimicrobial substances produced by the growth of *Streptomyces ambofaciens* and consisting of Spiramycin I, $C_{45}H_{78}N_2O_{15}$=887.1 (about 63%), Spiramycin II, $C_{47}H_{80}N_2O_{16}$=929.2 (about 24%), and Spiramycin III, $C_{48}H_{82}N_2O_{16}$=943.2 (about 13%).

CAS — 8025-81-8.

NOTE. The stated molecular formulas for the spiramycins may vary.

Pharmacopoeias. Jap. includes Acetylspiramycin.

A white or slightly yellowish amorphous powder with a slight odour and a bitter taste. It contains about 2700 units per mg, calculated with reference to the dried substance.

Soluble 1 in 50 of water; very soluble in alcohol and chloroform; practically insoluble in light petroleum; soluble in dilute acids. When dry it is **stable** to light and air.

Units. One unit of spiramycin is contained in 0.0003125 mg of the first International Reference Preparation (1962) which contains 3200 units per mg.

Adverse Effects. There have been only a few reports of untoward reactions following the use of spiramycin; these include nausea, vomiting, diarrhoea, epigastric pain, and skin sensitisation.

A 27-year-old man developed acute colitis on the fifth day of taking spiramycin 500 mg four times daily for 5 days for a tooth infection. A barium enema showed marked spasm, nodularity, and micro-ulcerations in the descending colon. All complaints disappeared within 24 hours of stopping the antibiotic.— G. M. Decaux and C. Devroede (letter), *Lancet*, 1978, *2*, 993.

Antimicrobial Action. Spiramycin has antimicrobial activity similar to but less potent that that of erythromycin (see p.1158); it is also less potent than oleandomycin (see p.1195). There is evidence of cross-resistance between spiramycin and the other macrolides.

Absorption and Fate. Spiramycin is irregularly absorbed from the gastro-intestinal tract and is widely distributed in the tissues. A dose of 1 g produces blood concentrations of approximately 1 μg per ml after 2 to 3 hours; peak blood concentrations are maintained for 4 to 6 hours after a single dose. High tissue concentrations are achieved and persist long after the plasma concentration has fallen to low levels. From 12 to 16% of the maternal blood concentration has been reported in the amniotic fluid; it does not diffuse into the cerebrospinal fluid to an appreciable extent.

Spiramycin is slowly eliminated; substantial amounts are excreted in the bile and about 10% in the urine. High concentrations appear in the milk of nursing mothers.

Uses. Spiramycin is a macrolide antibiotic which is given by mouth and has been used similarly to erythromycin (see p.1159) in the treatment of susceptible infections. The adult dose is 2 to 4 g daily, usually in 2 divided doses. Children have been given 50 to 100 mg per kg body-weight daily.

The spiramycin salt of difetarsone (see p.977) is used as an amoebicide and anthelmintic.

Spiramycin is used in some countries as an additive for animal feeding stuffs. The adipate is also used in veterinary practice.

A study indicating that usual therapeutic doses of spiramycin improved colour vision.— J. Laroche and C. Laroche, *Annls pharm. Fr.*, 1972, *30*, 433. See also *idem*, 1970, *28*, 333.

Toxoplasmosis. For a report of the use of spiramycin, 2 g daily, in conjunction with pyrimethamine and prednisolone in the treatment of toxoplasmosis, see T. G. Ramsell and B. A. Gamero, *Br. J. Ophthal.*, 1967, *51*, 282. See also B. Hoernli *et al.*, *Archs Ophthal.*, *N.Y.*, 1978, *96*, 62.

Spiramycin 2 to 3 g daily in divided doses for 3 weeks, repeated at 2-weekly intervals, was given to pregnant women with toxoplasmosis and reduced the overall incidence of foetal infections when compared with an untreated group of mothers but did not influence significantly the course of established foetal toxoplasmosis.— G. Desmonts and J. Couvreur, *New Engl. J. Med.*, 1974, *290*, 1110. Comment on the problem of congenital toxoplasmosis. Spiramycin therapy has been suggested for pregnant women found to convert serologically from negative to positive, but the detection and avoidance of a single case would be very costly.— *Lancet*, 1980, *1*, 578.

Discussions on the treatment of toxoplasmosis including the use of spiramycin.— T. C. Jones, *Drug Ther.*, 1977, *7*, 31, per *Int. pharm. Abstr.*, 1978, *15*, 163; R. J. Scott, *Trop. Dis. Bull.*, 1978, *75*, 809; F. J. Nye, *J. antimicrob. Chemother.*, 1979, *5*, 244; D. G. Fleck, *ibid.*, *Suppl.* A, 87.

Proprietary Names

Rovamicina *(Farmalabor, Ital.)*; Rovamycin *(Rhone-Poulenc, Denm.*; *Rhône-Poulenc, Norw.*; *Leo Rhodia, Swed.)*; Rovamycine *(Rhodia, Arg.*; *Specia, Belg.*; *Rhône-Poulenc, Canad.*; *Specia, Fr.*; *Rhône-Poulenc, Ger.*; *Specia, Neth.*; *Rhodia, Spain*; *Specia, Switz.)*; Selectomycin *(Grünenthal, Ger.)*.

Spiramycin was formerly marketed in Great Britain under the proprietary name Rovamycin (*May & Baker*).

159-j

Streptoduocin. Combined Streptomycin; Dihydrostreptomycin-Streptomycin. A mixture of equal parts of dihydrostreptomycin sulphate and streptomycin sulphate.

CAS — 8027-25-6.

A white to yellowish-white, odourless, hygroscopic powder. Freely **soluble** in water; practically insoluble in alcohol, chloroform, and ether.

Streptoduocin was formerly used in an unsuccessful attempt to reduce the toxicity of each ingredient.

160-q

Streptomycin.

Estreptomicina. 4-*O*-[2-*O*-(2-Deoxy-2-methylamino-α-L-glucopyranosyl)-5-deoxy-3-*C*-formyl-α-L-lyxofuranosyl]-*NN'*-diamidino-D-streptamine.

$C_{21}H_{39}N_7O_{12}$=581.6.

CAS — 57-92-1.

NOTE. Under the name Streptomycin, *Mex. P.* and *Span. P.* include the calcium chloride complex, the hydrochloride, the phosphate, and the sulphate.

An antimicrobial organic base produced by the growth of certain strains of *Streptomyces griseus*, or by any other means.

NOTE. The *B.P.* directs that when Streptomycin is prescribed or demanded, Streptomycin Sulphate (see below) be dispensed or supplied. The quantity of streptomycin specified is interpreted as referring to streptomycin base, and the amount corresponding to 1 g of this is 1.25 g of streptomycin sulphate.

161-p

Streptomycin Calcium Chloride *(B.P. 1953)*.

$(C_{21}H_{39}N_7O_{12},3HCl)_2,CaCl_2$=1492.9.

Pharmacopoeias. In *Mex.* and *Span.* See also above under Streptomycin.

A sterile white hygroscopic solid containing not less than 600 units (microgram equivalents of streptomycin base) per mg. Streptomycin calcium chloride 1.28 g is approximately equivalent to 1 g of streptomycin. Very **soluble** in water; practically insoluble in alcohol, chloroform, and ether. A 5% solution in water is iso-osmotic with serum. When mixed with sulphates, calcium sulphate is precipitated.

162-s

Streptomycin Hydrochloride *(B.P. 1953).*

$C_{21}H_{39}N_7O_{12},3HCl=691.0$.

CAS — 6160-32-3.

Pharmacopoeias. In *Mex.* and *Span.* See also above under Streptomycin.

A sterile white solid containing not less than 600 units (microgram equivalents of streptomycin base) per mg. Streptomycin hydrochloride 1.19 g is approximately equivalent to 1 g of streptomycin. Very **soluble** in water; practically insoluble in alcohol, chloroform, and ether.

163-w

Streptomycin Sulphate *(B.P., B.P. Vet., Eur. P.).* Streptomycini Sulfas; Sulfato de Estreptomicina.

$(C_{21}H_{39}N_7O_{12})_2,3H_2SO_4=1457.4$.

CAS — 3810-74-0.

Pharmacopoeias. In *Arg., Aust., Belg., Br., Braz., Cz., Eur., Fr., Ger., Hung., Ind., Int., It., Jap., Jug., Mex., Neth., Nord., Pol., Roum., Rus., Span., Swiss,* and *Turk.*
U.S. includes Sterile Streptomycin Sulfate.

A white or almost white hygroscopic powder, odourless or with a slight odour, and with a slightly bitter taste. It contains not less than 720 units per mg calculated on the dried substance. It loses not more than 7% of its weight on drying. Streptomycin sulphate 1.25 g is approximately equivalent to 1 g of streptomycin.
Very **soluble** in water; practically insoluble in alcohol, acetone, chloroform, and ether. A 25% solution in water has a pH of 4.5 to 7. **Incompatible** with acids and alkalis. **Store** at a temperature not exceeding 30° in airtight containers. If it is intended for injection, the containers should be sterile and sealed to exclude micro-organisms.
Stability. Streptomycin salts are stable when dry for at least 2 years at room temperature but some loss in potency occurs at higher temperatures. The rate of deterioration increases in the presence of moisture but is otherwise unaffected by light and air.
In solutions of pH between 3 and 7, the salts retain their potency for several weeks at room temperature, though some discoloration may occur, and for longer periods when stored at temperatures not exceeding 4°. At elevated temperatures, loss in potency is fairly rapid, about 50% being lost at pH 6.5 in about 4 hours at 95°. Outside the optimum pH range, deterioration is also fairly rapid; at 28° about 50% of the potency is lost in 12 days at pH 9.5 and in 4 days at pH 0.8.
The changes in colour that occur when solutions are exposed to light are not necessarily accompanied by loss of activity, but solutions should preferably be stored in the dark.
In addition to being inactivated by acids and alkalis, streptomycin is apparently inactivated by oxidising and reducing agents and urea and other carbonyl-containing compounds, as well as by cysteine and other sulphydryl-containing substances.

CAUTION. *Streptomycin may cause severe dermatitis in sensitised persons, and pharmacists, nurses, and others who handle the drug frequently should wear masks and rubber gloves.*

Effect of gamma-irradiation. Streptomycin sulphate powder became cream-coloured at 25 000 Gy and pale brown at 250 000 Gy. Solutions became pale yellow at 25 000 Gy and pale brown at 250 000 Gy. The initial potency of 742 units per mg fell to 720 at 25 000 Gy and to 706 at 250 000 Gy.— *The Use of Gamma Radiation Sources for the Sterilisation of Pharmaceutical Products,* London, ABPI, 1960.

Incompatibility. Incompatible, on the basis of immediate precipitation, with *amaranth, sodium alginate, carmellose sodium,* and *sodium lauryl sulphate.*— *J. Am. pharm. Ass., pract. Pharm. Edn,* 1952, *13,* 658.

The increase in colour of a solution of streptomycin sulphate in the presence of *procaine hydrochloride* was due to a reaction between the carbonyl group of the streptomycin and the *p*-amino group of the procaine.— A. V. Puccini and A. J. Spiegel, *J. pharm. Sci.,* 1962, *51,* 496.

There was loss of clarity when intravenous solutions of streptomycin sulphate were mixed with those of *amylobarbitone sodium, calcium gluconate, chlorothiazide sodium, erythromycin gluceptate, heparin sodium, nitrofurantoin sodium, noradrenaline acid tartrate, novobiocin sodium, pentobarbitone sodium, phenobarbitone sodium, phenytoin sodium, quinalbarbitone sodium, sodium bicarbonate, sulphadiazine sodium,* or *sulphafurazole diethanolamine.*— J. A. Patel and G. L. Phillips, *Am. J. Hosp. Pharm.,* 1966, *23,* 409.

A haze developed over 3 hours when streptomycin sulphate 4 g per litre was mixed with *amphotericin* 200 mg per litre in dextrose injection 5%, crystals were produced with *methohexitone sodium* 2 g per litre or *sulphadiazine sodium* 4 g per litre in sodium chloride injection 0.9%, and an immediate precipitate occurred with *heparin* 20 000 units per litre in dextrose injection 5% and sodium chloride injection 0.9%.— B. B. Riley, *J. Hosp. Pharm.,* 1970, *28,* 228.

Loss of activity. The following salts materially decreased the activity of streptomycin: sodium and potassium chloride, sodium sulphate, sodium tartrate, Sørensen's buffer, and ammonium acetate. The salts present in defibrinated sheep blood and human serum caused no demonstrable loss in activity. Streptomycin activity decreased with decreasing pH.— S. Berkman *et al., J. Bact.,* 1947, *53,* 567.

Inorganic ions, especially calcium and magnesium, inhibited the activity of streptomycin.— K. E. Price *et al., Antibiotics Chemother.,* 1957, *7,* 672.

Streptomycin was very much less active against *Staphylococcus aureus* in the presence of magnesium trisilicate, acacia, tragacanth, carmellose, sodium alginate, pectin, bentonite, and kaolin and less active with calamine, zinc oxide, methylcellulose, maize starch, gelatin, and polysorbate 80.— M. A. El-Nakeeb and R. T. Yousef, *Acta pharm. suec.,* 1968, *5,* 1.

When intramuscular injections of streptomycin and *benzylpenicillin* were mixed, both drugs lost about 30% of their potency within 30 minutes. Streptomycin lost 24% of its potency within 15 minutes with *carbenicillin.* Ampicillin, cloxacillin, and methicillin also lost some potency when mixed with streptomycin.— B. Lynn and A. Jones, *Beecham Research, Advances in Antimicrobial and Antineoplastic Chemotheraphy,* Vol. I, pt 1, Munich, Urban and Schwarzenberg, 1972, 701.

The antimicrobial activity of streptomycin sulphate was reduced in the presence of *vitamins* of the *B complex* or *ascorbic acid.*— M. A. El-Nakeeb *et al., Can. J. pharm. Sci.,* 1976, *11,* 85.

A study of the effect of the antibiotic and preservative on each other's binding to pharmaceutical adjuvants in mixtures containing benzalkonium chloride or chlorocresol and streptomycin sulphate.— M. A. El-Nakeeb and M. H. Ali, *Mfg Chem.,* 1976, *47,* (Mar.), 37.

Quinine dihydrochloride decreased the antibacterial effect *in vitro* of streptomycin sulphate and dihydrostreptomycin sulphate against *Staph. aureus* and *E. coli.*— M. A. Toama *et al., J. pharm. Sci.,* 1978, *67,* 23.

Units. One unit of streptomycin is contained in 0.001282 mg of the second International Standard Preparation (1958) of streptomycin sulphate which contains 780 units per mg.

Adverse Effects. Streptomycin sulphate is not appreciably absorbed from the gastro-intestinal tract and systemic toxic effects are unlikely to occur after administration of streptomycin by mouth.
Minor toxic effects such as paraesthesia in and around the mouth, vertigo, headache, and lassitude sometimes occur after intramuscular injection and are more common in ambulant patients than in patients confined to bed. Pain and irritation are sometimes felt at the site of injection.
Hypersensitivity reactions may occur, usually during the first 4 weeks of treatment. Sensitisation is common among nurses, pharmacists, and others who handle streptomycin, and may lead to dermatitis sometimes associated with periorbital swelling and conjunctivitis; hypersensitivity through inhalation of streptomycin may occur.
More serious toxic effects arise from the selective toxic action of the antibiotic on the eighth cranial nerve, especially the vestibular branch, and consist of vertigo and tinnitus and sometimes deafness which may be permanent. The occurrence of vestibular disturbances appears to be related to the total daily dosage, blood concentrations of streptomycin, the age of the patient, renal efficiency, and a hereditary predisposition. These disturbances are more common in patients over 40 years of age than in younger persons. Ototoxicity has been observed in infants whose mothers had been given streptomycin during pregnancy.
Kidney damage has been reported after large doses.
Lupus erythematosus may occur during treatment and there have been rare reports of aplastic anaemia and agranulocytosis.

Allergy. Acute haemolytic anaemia and renal failure developed in a 45-year-old man shortly after he injected himself with streptomycin and ampicillin. Antibodies to streptomycin were demonstrated. He had used streptomycin repeatedly over the previous 15 years.— J. M. -L. Letona *et al., Br. J. Haemat.,* 1977, *35,* 561.

For reference to the incidence of intolerance to streptomycin, see Isoniazid, p.1572.

Blood disorders. Episodes of haemolytic anaemia occurred on 139 occasions in 63 patients with a deficiency of glucose-6-phosphate dehydrogenase. Of 119 acute episodes 46 were believed to be precipitated by drugs, 1 of them by streptomycin.— E. R. Burka, *Ann. intern. Med.,* 1966, *64,* 817.

Spontaneous transient inhibition of blood-clotting factor V occurred in a patient. Streptomycin might have been implicated in this effect, as it might have been in 5 of 7 other patients who were known to have had the same inhibition.— D. I. Feinstein *et al., Ann. intern. Med.,* 1973, *78,* 385.

Eye changes. Streptomycin might cause optic neuritis, optic atrophy, toxic amblyopia, loss of vision, and scotoma.— H. I. Silverman, *Am. J. Optom.,* 1972, *49,* 335.

A study indicating that usual therapeutic doses of streptomycin interfere with colour vision.— J. Laroche and C. Laroche, *Annls pharm. fr.,* 1972, *30,* 433. See also *idem,* 1970, *28,* 333.

Industrial toxicity. Streptomycin, 10 to 15 mg per m^3 produced changes in the upper respiratory tract, including atrophic processes in the mucosa, and reduced sensitivity and olfactory function in workers engaged in streptomycin production. Increased sensitivity to streptomycin and actinomycin occurred in 38.1 and 17.6% of workers respectively. Occupational dermatitis was also observed. The recommended maximum atmospheric concentration of industrial premises should be 100 μg per m^3.— I. M. Trakhtenberg *et al., Gig. Truda prof. Zabol.,* 1967, *11,* 38, per *Bull. Hyg., Lond.,* 1967, *42,* 617.

Ototoxicity. A review of the ototoxicity of streptomycin and related antibiotics with investigations into the mechanisms causing this effect.— J. Ballantyne, *J. Lar. Otol.,* 1970, *84,* 967.

Ototoxic symptoms developed in 37 patients who had received streptomycin as the sulphate or pantothenate, dihydrostreptomycin sulphate, or kanamycin. Treatment lasted 5 to 14 days for two-thirds of the patients, the total dose of antibiotic being less than 20 g in most cases, and 10 g or less in 22 cases. Daily dosage was usually 1.5 to 2 g daily equivalent to 20 to 28 mg per kg body-weight. Impaired renal function was present in two-thirds of the patients. The daily dose of these antibiotics in patients with normal kidney function should not exceed 1 g per 70 kg body-weight or 15 mg per kg; the maximum serum concentration should then not exceed about 25 μg per ml, and should fall below 5 to 10 μg per ml before the next injection. The dosage in obese patients should be reduced, as well as in those with impaired renal function, since higher concentrations of streptomycin would occur in the extracellular fluid of an obese person than in a person of ordinary build.— P. Erlanson and A. Lundgren, *Acta med. scand.,* 1964, *176,* 147.

In the foetus. G. C. Robinson and K. G. Cambon, *New Engl. J. Med.,* 1964, *271,* 949; E. Varpela *et al., Scand. J. resp. Dis.,* 1969, *51,* 101, per *Abstr. Hyg.,* 1970, *45,* 693.

Skin reactions. Seven cases of toxic epidermal necrolysis had been reported associated with the use of streptomycin.— E. D. Lowney *et al.*, *Archs Derm.*, 1967, *95*, 359.

Treatment of Adverse Effects. Those who handle streptomycin should wear rubber gloves and face-masks. Some of the symptoms of hypersensitivity may be relieved by the administration of antihistamines.

Before commencing streptomycin therapy, it may be advisable to perform intradermal skin tests to determine whether the patient is hypersensitive, or has been sensitised previously. Haemodialysis or peritoneal dialysis has been recommended for oliguric patients who have been given streptomycin.

The neuromuscular blocking action of streptomycin may sometimes be reversed by neostigmine or a calcium salt.

Precautions. If streptomycin is administered to patients with impaired liver or kidney function, great care and frequent determinations of the blood concentrations are required to ensure that toxic concentrations are not reached. Patients with impaired renal function, the elderly, and newborn and premature infants should be given reduced doses of streptomycin as their excretion of the antibiotic is diminished. If it is given to women during pregnancy, the eighth cranial nerve of the foetus may be damaged. Owing to its ototoxic effects streptomycin should not be given to patients with diseases of the ear although it has been used to treat Ménière's disease. It should not be given to patients sensitised to it unless desensitisation has been carried out successfully. Anaphylactic reactions have been precipitated by skin tests in hypersensitive patients.

In order to diminish the development of resistant strains of the micro-organism, streptomycin should not be used alone in the treatment of tuberculosis.

Streptomycin has a weak neuromuscular blocking action and may enhance the neuromuscular blocking activity of such drugs as suxamethonium or tubocurarine and general anaesthetics; it should be used with caution in patients with myasthenia gravis. Anti-emetics may mask the early symptoms of ototoxicity and patients receiving these drugs should be given streptomycin with care. Care should also be taken when patients are given streptomycin and other drugs such as ethacrynic acid that have been associated with ototoxicity. Due to alterations in endogenous vitamin K, patients taking streptomycin may need to have their dose of oral anticoagulant reduced.

There was an approximate 20% increase in the free fraction of streptomycin in the serum of patients with kwashiorkor.— N. Buchanan and L. A. Van der Walt, *S.Afr. med. J.*, 1977, *52*, 522.

Sequential administration of intravenous bolus doses of streptomycin 500 mg and methicillin 1 g, over a period of 5 minutes through a subclavian vein catheter, had caused rigors in postoperative coronary bypass patients, within 30 minutes of administration. Administration of the 2 drugs separated by an interval of 4 hours appeared to avoid this.— P. C. Robinson *et al.* (letter), *Lancet*, 1978, *2*, 1056.

Effect on blood estimations. Streptomycin could interfere technically with chemical estimations for urea in the blood to produce erroneous lowered results.— *Drug & Ther. Bull.*, 1972, *10*, 69.

Antimicrobial Action. Streptomycin inhibits protein synthesis in the bacterial cell. It has bacteriostatic and bactericidal activities, depending on its concentration, particularly against *Mycobacterium tuberculosis* and Gram-negative bacteria including *Escherichia coli, Klebsiella pneumoniae, Enterobacter* spp., *Neisseria gonorrhoeae, N. meningitidis*, and some species of *Proteus, Salmonella*, and *Shigella*. It is also effective against *Yersinia pestis, Haemophilus influenzae, Francisella tularensis, Brucella* spp., and a few strains of *Pseudomonas aeruginosa*. Some strains of staphylococci are sensitive but it is ineffective against most other Gram-positive cocci and bacilli; *Streptococcus faecalis* is invariably resistant but may be inhibited by streptomycin in conjunction with penicillin. *Bacteroides* spp., rickettsias, fungi, and viruses are resistant to streptomycin.

It is most active in a slightly alkaline medium.

The minimum inhibitory concentration of streptomycin has been reported to be 2 to 4 µg per ml for *E. coli*, 1 to 2 µg per ml for *Klebsiella* spp., 16 to 64 µg per ml for *Ps. aeruginosa*, 4 to 16 µg per ml for *Salmonella* spp., and 0.5 µg per ml for *M. tuberculosis*.

Streptomycin was found to inhibit the growth of a variety of yeasts in concentrations of 20 to 100 µg per ml.— M. Richards and F. R. Elliott (letter), *Nature*, 1966, *209*, 536.

In Calcutta, sensitivity tests of 149 strains of *Vibrio cholerae* to streptomycin sulphate showed that the MIC for 144 strains ranged from 1 to 8 µg per ml.— L. M. Prescott *et al.*, *Bull. Wld Hlth Org.*, 1968, *39*, 967.

Further references: I. Phillips *et al.*, *J. antimicrob. Chemother.*, 1977, *3*, 403.

Diminished activity. Antagonism has been reported between streptomycin and chloramphenicol.— P. J. Sanderson (letter), *Lancet*, 1978, *2*, 210.

For reports of various compounds decreasing the activity of streptomycin, see above under Loss of Activity.

Enhanced activity. Penicillin and other antibiotics which inhibited cell wall synthesis such as bacitracin, cephalothin, cycloserine, vancomycin, and several semisynthetic penicillins enhanced the activity of streptomycin against *Str. faecalis*. Synergy was not detected when there was a high degree of resistance to streptomycin. It was considered that streptomycin was normally ineffective because it could not penetrate the bacteria and that this was reversed by the other antibiotics.— R. C. Moellering *et al.*, *J. Lab. clin. Med.*, 1971, *77*, 821.

The activity of streptomycin *in vitro* against *E. coli* was enhanced when used with human serum.— B. S. Dutcher *et al.*, *Antimicrob. Ag. Chemother.*, 1978, *13*, 820.

For a comparison of the effect of netilmicin, sissomicin, and streptomycin on the activity of benzylpenicillin on enterococci, see Benzylpenicillin, p.1106.

Resistance. Many strains of bacteria initially sensitive to streptomycin become resistant during therapy. Resistance in non-tuberculous infections may develop within 2 or 3 days of instituting treatment, whereas in tuberculosis the slower rate of multiplication of the infecting organisms may delay development of complete resistance for a few weeks. The emergence of resistant strains may be delayed by combining the streptomycin therapy with the administration of other antibiotics or other chemotherapeutic agents.

There is complete cross-resistance between streptomycin and dihydrostreptomycin, and partial cross-resistance between streptomycin, neomycin, kanamycin, and paromomycin.

A strain of *Mycobacterium smegmatis* was found to carry a streptomycin-resistant R-factor and was also found to possess a more stable resistance which did not inactivate the antibiotic.— W. D. Jones and H. L. David, *Tubercle*, 1972, *53*, 35.

In a study of the susceptibility of 200 strains of *Ps. aeruginosa* to streptomycin, resistance was classified into high-level or low-level forms. High-level resistance was infrequent and could have been due to R-factor inactivation or streptomycin-resistant ribosomes. The majority of resistant strains were classified as low-level and were associated with a diminished uptake of streptomycin.— J. T. Tseng *et al.*, *Antimicrob. Ag. Chemother.*, 1972, *2*, 136.

A report of 2 forms of resistance in *M. tuberculosis* to streptomycin; a stable resistance that did not inactivate streptomycin and a transducible inactivating type.— W. D. Jones *et al.*, *Tubercle*, 1974, *55*, 73.

In a continuing study of primary drug resistance of tuberculosis in the USA, 271 of 3146 cultures of *M. tuberculosis* from newly-diagnosed untreated patients were resistant to antitubercular agents. Resistance-rates ranged from 3.4 to 18.7% according to geographical area and resistance was most frequently seen to streptomycin (5.1%) compared with isoniazid (4.4%), PAS (1.3%), ethionamide (0.8%), ethambutol (0.7%), rifampicin and capreomycin (0.3%), viomycin and cycloserine (0.2%), and kanamycin (0.1%).— D. E. Kopanoff *et al.*, *Am. Rev. resp. Dis.*, 1978, *118*, 835.

For reports of resistance to streptomycin in the treatment of tuberculosis, see Tuberculostatics and Tuberculocides, p.1564.

Absorption and Fate. Streptomycin is not appreciably absorbed or inactivated in the gastro-intestinal tract and most of a dose administered by mouth is excreted unchanged in the faeces.

After intramuscular injection, maximum concentration in the blood is reached in 0.5 to 2 hours but the time taken and the concentration attained, which may be as high as 40 or 50 µg per ml after a dose of 0.5 to 1 g, vary considerably. A minimum effective plasma concentration is about 10 µg per ml. Following intramuscular injection of 1 g of streptomycin, therapeutic plasma concentrations may persist for 8 hours or longer, and significant amounts may still be present after 24 hours. The biological half-life of streptomycin is about 2½ hours in young adults, but may be considerably longer in premature and newborn infants and in adults over 40 years of age. About one-third of streptomycin in the circulation is bound to plasma proteins.

A high plasma concentration is achieved for the first hour after intravenous injection but after that concentrations are no higher than those from an equal dose given by intramuscular injection. Little is absorbed by inhalation. Topical application is not recommended since penetration does not usually occur and the risks of local reactions and sensitisation are high.

Streptomycin does not readily pass into the cerebrospinal fluid but detectable amounts have been reported in patients with inflamed meninges.

Streptomycin diffuses rapidly into most body tissues and is present in the extracellular fluid. It does not readily enter red blood cells and does not penetrate thick-walled abscesses, but significant amounts are found in tuberculous cavities. It diffuses into pleural, pericardial, and synovial effusions. After intramuscular injection, some streptomycin diffuses into the eye, mostly into the aqueous humour. Streptomycin diffuses across the placenta and is found in foetal blood and in amniotic fluid in concentrations about one-half those in maternal blood. It has been detected in breast milk.

Excretion is by glomerular filtration. The rate of excretion varies in different individuals and the concentration of streptomycin in the urine is often very high with about 30 to 90% of a dose usually being excreted within 24 hours in subjects with healthy kidneys. Concentrations may exceed 300 µg per ml after a 500-mg dose and 1 mg per ml after a 1-g dose. There is some secretion into bile following parenteral administration and concentrations of 10 to 20 µg per ml have been detected after large doses. High concentrations are excreted in the faeces following administration by mouth and small concentrations may be observed following large doses given by injection.

References: C. M. Kunin, *Ann. intern. Med.*, 1967, *67*, 151; W. A. Ritschel, *Drug Intell. & clin. Pharm.*, 1970, *4*, 332.

Uses. Streptomycin is mainly used in the treatment of tuberculosis, in conjunction with other drugs such as isoniazid (p.1574), sodium aminosalicylate (p.1583), ethambutol (p.1570), and rifampicin (p.1580) and may be classified as a first-line or primary antituberculous agent. In pulmonary tuberculosis it is effective in the early stages or when the disease is progressing rapidly; it is of less value in chronic tuberculosis with fibrotic lesions.

Streptomycin and penicillin have a synergistic action against bacteria and are used together in the treatment of subacute bacterial endocarditis caused by *Streptococcus faecalis*; it may also be useful in peritonitis, but should not be given by intraperitoneal injection to patients who have recently received neuromuscular blocking agents.

Streptomycin is effective in the treatment of plague, tularaemia, and, in conjunction with tetracycline, in brucellosis. It has been given by mouth in the treatment of infections of the intestine and more rarely prior to abdominal surgery but other agents are preferred.

Streptomycin is used as the sulphate and is given by intramuscular injection as a solution containing the equivalent of 1 g of the base dissolved in 1.25, 3.25, or 4.25 ml of Water for Injections. Intravenous administration is not advisable because it produces high and potentially toxic blood concentrations.

The initial treatment for young adults with tuberculosis is 0.75 to 1 g of streptomycin daily by intramuscular injection, with other primary agents. Doses of 20 to 30 mg per kg body-weight daily have been recommended for premature and full-term infants but for not more than 10 days. Older children have been given up to 40 mg per kg daily in divided doses although for long-term treatment 20 mg per kg is usually recommended.

In general, for patients over 40 years of age the dose of streptomycin should not exceed 750 mg daily and for those over 60 years of age it should not exceed 500 mg because of the greater risk of vestibular disturbance. In patients with renal impairment, the initial dose should produce peak plasma concentrations no greater than 40 to 50 μg per ml at 1 hour. Thereafter a dose of 500 mg every 3 to 4 days may be adequate.

For the treatment of tuberculous meningitis, normal doses are given by intramuscular injection. In addition, both isoniazid (up to 10 mg per kg body-weight daily) and aminosalicylate are given by mouth. Other agents such as ethambutol and rifampicin may be substituted for streptomycin or aminosalicylate. Many authorities consider that intrathecal injections are not necessary, but others advise a course of 10 or more doses in severe meningitis. The intrathecal dose in adults should not exceed 100 mg daily, dissolved in at least 10 ml of sodium chloride injection or cerebrospinal fluid. Children have been given 1 mg per kg body-weight to a maximum dose of 50 mg.

For the treatment of non-tuberculous infections, the usual dose is 1 g daily for not more than 5 to 10 days because of the possibility of inducing drug resistance; higher doses are recommended in the treatment of plague and tularaemia.

Intrapleural injections of streptomycin 0.5 to 1 g in 20 to 50 ml of sodium chloride injection have occasionally been used but should be given with extreme caution because of the possibility of respiratory depression, especially in patients recently given neuromuscular blocking agents or general anaesthetics.

For reviews of the actions and uses of streptomycin and other aminoglycoside antibiotics, see Gentamicin Sulphate, p.1171.

Brucellosis. For reports of the use of streptomycin and tetracycline in the treatment of brucellosis, see Tetracycline Hydrochloride, p.1220.

Cholera. For a comparison of streptomycin and other drugs in the treatment of cholera, see Tetracycline Hydrochloride, p.1220.

Dosage. For detailed dosage recommendations, see under Ototoxicity in the section on Adverse Effects.

Dosage in infants and children. The suggested dose of streptomycin for infants of more than 37 weeks' gestation was 7.5 mg per kg body-weight given intramuscularly every 12 hours for the first 48 hours of life increased thereafter to 10 mg per kg every 12 hours. For immature infants (those of less than 37 weeks' gestation), 7.5 mg per kg could be given every 12 hours for the 1st week then 10 mg per kg every 12 hours.— P. A. Davies, *Br. J. Hosp. Med.*, 1972, *8*, 13. See also L. Herngren *et al.*, *Scand. J. infect. Dis.*, 1977, *9*, 301.

Dosage in renal failure. The normal half-life for streptomycin of 2.5 hours was increased to 100 to 110 hours in end-stage renal failure. The interval between doses should be extended from 12 hours to 24 hours in patients with a glomerular filtration-rate (GFR) above 50 ml per minute, to 24 to 72 hours in those with a GFR of 10 to 50 ml per minute, and to 72 to 96 hours in those with a GFR of less than 10 ml per minute. Concentrations of streptomycin were affected by haemodialysis.— W. M. Bennett *et al.*, *Ann. intern. Med.*, 1977, *86*, 754. See also *idem*, 1980, *93*, 62. Blood concentrations could also be altered by peritoneal dialysis.— P. Sharpstone, *Br. med. J.*, 1977, *2*, 36.

After a loading dose of 1 g streptomycin could be given in a dose of 0.5 to 1 g every 2 or 3 days to patients with a creatinine clearance of 20 to 30 ml per minute, and 0.5 g every 3 or 4 days to those with a clearance of 5 ml per minute. In haemodialysis 0.5 g every 3 or 4 days could be given, and 0.25 g after dialysis.— J. S. Cheigh, *Am. J. Med.*, 1977, *62*, 555.

Data for predicting removal of streptomycin by conventional haemodialysis.— T. P. Gibson and H. A. Nelson, *Clin. Pharmacokinet.*, 1977, *2*, 403.

Hypercalcaemia. Malignant hypercalcaemia associated with primary hepatocellular carcinoma in a 45-year-old man was refractory to treatment with phosphates, glucagon, and saline infusions. There was a transient response to intra-arterial injection of mitomycin. Streptomycin 1 or 1.5 g daily by intramuscular injection produced a prompt reduction in serum-calcium concentration and a slow significant decrease in serum-alkaline phosphatase concentration. These values rose again when the streptomycin was stopped.— W. E. W. Roediger *et al.*, *Postgrad. med. J.*, 1975, *51*, 399.

Leprosy. Twenty-five patients with typical lepromatous leprosy were given daily intramuscular injections of streptomycin sulphate 1 g, together with isoniazid 300 mg daily by mouth. Maximum response occurred after 3 to 6 months' treatment.— A. B. A. Karat *et al.*, *Lepr. Rev.*, 1967, *38*, 163. See also *idem*, 25.

Further references: S. R. Pattyn and E. Saerens, *Lepr. Rev.*, 1978, *49*, 275.

Ménière's disease. The neurotoxic effect of streptomycin was used therapeutically in Ménière's disease. The usual dose was 1 g thrice daily for 3 to 4 weeks or until the caloric response disappeared in the more seriously affected labyrinth. Ataxia often occurred and could be more disabling than the original disease. The treatment should not be given to patients over 50 years of age or to those with unilateral disease.— *Br. med. J.*, 1970, *1*, 614.

Mycetoma. For reference to the successful antibacterial therapy of actinomycetoma using regimens incorporating streptomycin, see Co-trimoxazole, p.1465.

Plague. In a study of 10 patients with *Yersinia pestis* infection (plague) who were randomly assigned to treatment with streptomycin or co-trimoxazole for 10 days, all patients survived. Streptomycin was given in a dose of 1 g twice daily by intramuscular injection (patients weighing less than 25 kg received half this dose). Co-trimoxazole was given intravenously for 3 to 5 days and then by mouth. Those treated with streptomycin had a shorter duration of fever and fewer complications and it was considered that streptomycin should remain the drug of choice.— T. Butler *et al.*, *J. infect. Dis.*, 1976, *133*, 493. See also *idem*, 1977, *136*, 317.

A 28-year-old woman who had contracted plague in her 5th month of pregnancy was successfully treated with streptomycin 500 mg by intramuscular injection every 8 hours for 5 days. The pregnancy went to full term without complications.— J. M. Mann and R. Moskowitz, *J. Am. med. Ass.*, 1977, *237*, 1854.

For further references to the use of streptomycin in plague, see Tetracycline Hydrochloride, p.1221.

Tuberculosis, pulmonary. For reports on the use of streptomycin in the treatment of pulmonary tuberculosis, see p.1565.

Tuberculous meningitis. Children with tuberculous meningitis were given as standard treatment: streptomycin 40 mg per kg body-weight daily by intramuscular injection; isoniazid 20 mg per kg daily by mouth; PAS 250 mg per kg daily by mouth, and prednisolone 2 mg per kg by mouth for 30 days. In addition, some received intrathecal injections of streptomycin 2 mg per kg to a maximum dose of 25 mg daily for 5 doses then alternate days for 5 doses; some also received hydrocortisone 10 to 25 mg. After 6 weeks, deaths occurred less frequently in those given intrathecal injections but up to 4 years later there was no difference in death-rates in the 3 groups. However, poor recoveries occurred more frequently in those children who received only the standard treatment.— I. Freiman and J. Geefhuysen, *J. Pediat.*, 1970, *76*, 895. See also J. Lorber, *Br. med. J.*, 1960, *1*, 1309.

Tularaemia. Streptomycin was the treatment of choice for tularaemia, and the recommended dosage was 1 g twelve-hourly by intramuscular injection for 7 to 10 days. If this was contra-indicated, tetracycline 500 mg six-hourly by mouth could be given for 10 to 14 days or demeclocycline 300 mg eight-hourly by mouth. A live vaccine preparation could be given prophylactically in those likely to be exposed to *Francisella tularensis*.— W. E. Herrell, *Clin. Med.*, 1968, *75* (Apr.), 62.

Uveitis. Subconjunctival injection of streptomycin 250 to 500 mg (total dose) was suggested for topical treatment of uveitis in children.— E. C. Cowan, *Practitioner*, 1970, *204*, 72.

Preparations

Paediatric Streptomycin Elixir *(B.P.C. 1973)*. Paediatric Streptomycin Mixture. Streptomycin sulphate 157 mg, citric acid monohydrate 5 mg, sodium citrate 45 mg, methyl hydroxybenzoate 6.5 mg, amaranth solution 0.01 ml, sucrose 3.75 g, freshly boiled and cooled water to 5 ml. *Dose.* 5 ml (equivalent to about 125 mg of streptomycin base).

Sterile Streptomycin Sulfate *(U.S.P.)*. A grade of streptomycin sulphate for injection. It has a potency of not less than 650 μg and not more than 850 μg of streptomycin per mg.

Streptomycin Mixture CF *(A.P.F.)*. Streptomycin Elixir for Infants. Streptomycin sulphate 157 mg, sodium citrate 45 mg, citric acid monohydrate 5 mg, methyl hydroxybenzoate 5 mg, syrup 4 ml, amaranth solution 0.01 ml, water to 5 ml. *Dose.* 5 ml (equivalent to 125 mg of streptomycin base).

Streptomycin Sulphate Injection *(B.P.)*. Streptomycin Injection. A sterile solution of streptomycin sulphate in Water for Injections containing suitable stabilising agents; it may contain a suitable buffering agent. Potency is expressed in terms of the equivalent amount of streptomycin. pH 5 to 6.5. Protect from light and store at a temperature not exceeding 20°; under these conditions it may be expected to retain its potency for at least 18 months. *U.S.P.* (Streptomycin Sulfate Injection) specifies the equivalent of 400, 420, or 500 mg of streptomycin per ml.

Proprietary Preparations

Streptomycin Sulphate *(Glaxo, UK)*. Streptomycin sulphate, available as powder for preparing injections, in vials containing the equivalent of 1 g of streptomycin base.

Other Proprietary Names

Ger.—Solvo-strept S; *Ital.*—Strycin; *S.Afr.*—Darostrep, Novostrep; *Spain*—Dif-Estrepto E, Estrepto E, Estreptomade, Neodiestreptobap.

Streptomycin sulphate was also formerly marketed in Great Britain under the proprietary name Orastrep (*Dista*).

164-e

Sulbenicillin Sodium. α-Sulfobenzylpenicillin Sodium; Sulfocillin Sodium. The disodium salt of (6*R*)-6-(2-phenyl-2-sulphoacetamido)penicillanic acid.

$C_{16}H_{16}N_2Na_2O_7S_2$=458.4.

Sulbenicillin sodium produced commercially usually contains 75% of D(−) and 25% of L(+) isomers.

A white to yellow crystalline powder. Each g represents about 4.4 mmol (4.4 mEq) of sodium. Sulbenicillin sodium 1.1 g is approximately equivalent to 1 g of sulbenicillin. Very **soluble** in water; sparingly soluble in alcohol; soluble in methyl alcohol; practically insoluble in acetone and chloroform.

Stability in solution. A study on the stability of sulbenicillin sodium in large-volume parenteral fluids. Sulbenicillin sodium was most stable within the pH range of 5 to 7. Degradation occurred in association with amines and amino acids.— H. Fukuchi *et al.*, *Drug Intell. & clin. Pharm.*, 1978, *12*, 418.

Adverse Effects, Treatment, and Precautions. As for Benzylpenicillin, p.1103.

Sulbenicillin or its major metabolite α-sulphobenzylpenicilloic acid caused inhibition of platelet aggregation and release of serotonin from platelets *in vitro*, the metabolite producing a greater effect. It was suggested that the action of α-sulphobenzylpenicilloic acid might produce unexpected bleeding when uraemic patients received large doses of sulbenicillin.— Y. Ikeda *et al.*, *Antimicrob. Ag. Chemother.*, 1978, *13*, 881.

Antimicrobial Action. Sulbenicillin has an antibacterial action similar to that of Carbenicillin Sodium, p.1111.

Sulbenicillin inhibited 3, 40, 44, 46, 61, 91 and all of 92 strains of *Neisseria gonorrhoeae in vitro* at an MIC of 0.016, 0.03, 0.06, 0.25, 0.5, 1 and 2 µg per ml respectively.— B. A. Watts *et al.*, *J. antimicrob. Chemother.*, 1977, *3*, 331.

Sulbenicillin was less active than gentamicin sulphate or dibekacin against 218 strains of *Pseudomonas aeruginosa in vitro* but more active against 29 strains of *Ps. maltophilia* and 10 of *Ps. cepacia*.— K. Tsuchiya and M. Kondo, *Takeda, Jap.*, *Antimicrob. Ag. Chemother.*, 1978, *13*, 536.

Further reference: K. Tsuchiya *et al.*, *J. Antibiot., Tokyo*, 1971, *24*, 607.

Uses. Sulbenicillin sodium has actions and uses similar to those of Carbenicillin Sodium, p.1110, and has been given by intramuscular and intravenous injection in similar doses.

A review of sulbenicillin.— *Japan med. Gaz.*, 1973, *10* (Feb. 20), 4.

The pharmacokinetics of sulbenicillin and carbenicillin were found to be very similar when they were compared in a study of 13 patients, 8 of them with impaired renal function.— I. Hansen *et al.*, *Clin. Pharmac. Ther.*, 1975, *17*, 339.

References to the use of sulbencillin sodium: J. Kjellander *et al.*, *Scand. J. infect. Dis.*, 1978, *10*, 235 (pseudomonal infections); A. Montanari *et al.*, *Int. J. clin. Pharmac. Biopharm.*, 1980, *18*, 225 (in renal failure).

Proprietary Names

Lilacillin *(Jap.)*; Sulbenil *(Gist-Brocades, Neth.)*.

165-l

Sulphomyxin Sodium *(B.P. 1973)*. Sulfomyxin Sodium. A mixture of sulphomethylated polymyxin B and sodium bisulphite.

CAS — 1405-52-3 (sulphomyxin); 58253-07-9 (sodium salt).

A white almost odourless powder with a bitter taste containing not less than 5000 units per mg. **Soluble** 1 in less than 1 of water and 1 in 750 of alcohol. A 2% solution in water has a pH of 6 to 8. Solutions for injection are prepared aseptically. **Store** in a cool place in airtight containers. If intended for injection the containers should be sterile and sealed to exclude micro-organisms. Protect from light.

Units. One unit of sulphomyxin is contained in 0.000174 mg of the first British Standard Preparation (1968) of sulphomyxin sodium which contains 5759 units per mg.

Uses. Sulphomyxin sodium has actions and antimicrobial activity resembling those of polymyxin B (see p.1204). It has been given in a dose of up to 2 million units daily in divided doses in place of polymyxin B when intramuscular administration is required.

Preparations

Sulphomyxin Injection *(B.P. 1973)*. A sterile solution of sulphomyxin sodium in Water for Injections. It is prepared by dissolving the sterile contents of a sealed container in the requisite amount of Water for Injections. Store at 2° to 10° and use within 48 hours of preparation.

Sulphomyxin sodium was formerly marketed in Great Britain under the proprietary name Thiosporin (*Wellcome*)..

166-y

Talampicillin Hydrochloride.

BRL 8988. Phthalidyl (6*R*)-6-(α-D-phenylglycylamino)penicillanate hydrochloride.

$C_{24}H_{23}N_3O_6S,HCl=518.0$.

CAS — 47747-56-8 (talampicillin); 39878-70-1 (hydrochloride).

A white to off-white hygroscopic powder with a slight characteristic odour and a bitter persistent taste. Talampicillin hydrochloride 1.48 g is approximately equivalent to 1 g of ampicillin. **Soluble** 1 in 4 of water, 1 in 2 of chloroform, and 1 in 2 of methyl alcohol; practically insoluble in ether. A 1% solution in water has a pH of 3.0 to 4.5.

167-j

Talampicillin Napsylate.

Phthalidyl (6*R*)-6-(α-D-phenylglycylamino)penicillanate naphthalene-2-sulphonate.

$C_{24}H_{23}N_3O_6S,C_{10}H_8O_3S=689.8$.

CAS — 71953-01-0.

A white to pale yellow hygroscopic powder with a slight characteristic odour and a bitter taste. Talampicillin napsylate 1.33 g is approximately equivalent to 1 g of talampicillin hydrochloride. Practically **insoluble** in water and ether; soluble 1 in 3 of chloroform, 1 in 2 of methyl alcohol, and 1 in 4 of methylene chloride.

Adverse Effects and Treatment. As for Ampicillin, p.1092.

Diarrhoea has been reported to occur less frequently with talampicillin.

A report of rash occurring in an 18-year-old man with infectious mononucleosis given talampicillin.— J. Morris (letter), *Lancet*, 1976, *1*, 423.

A 47-year-old man suffered anaphylaxis after taking a single tablet of talampicillin; he had previously tolerated penicillin.— J. Simmonds *et al.*, *Br. med. J.*, 1978, *2*, 1404.

Precautions. As for Ampicillin, p.1093.

The use of talampicillin is best avoided in patients with impaired kidney or liver function.

Antimicrobial Action. Talampicillin has the antimicrobial action of ampicillin *in vivo*. It possesses no intrinsic activity and requires to be hydrolysed to ampicillin.

Absorption and Fate. Talampicillin is readily absorbed from the gastro-intestinal tract and is rapidly hydrolysed to release ampicillin and to produce earlier and higher peak plasma-ampicillin concentrations than equivalent doses of ampicillin. A dose of 250 mg of talampicillin hydrochloride produces a peak plasma-ampicillin concentration of 4.7 µg per ml in about 40 minutes. Overall absorption appears to be unaffected by the presence of food in the stomach.

Over 70% of absorbed ampicillin is excreted in the urine.

Hydrolysis also releases the phthalidyl moiety of talampicillin and this is metabolised to 2-hydroxymethylbenzoic acid which is excreted in the urine.

Studies in healthy volunteers showed that the mean peak serum-ampicillin concentration in fasting persons was reached within 1 hour of dosage with talampicillin and was about twice as high as that attained with an equivalent dose of ampicillin. Dosage after food reduced and delayed the peak concentration but overall absorption was unaffected. A mean peak concentration of 800 mg of ampicillin per litre of urine was found during the first 2 hours of collection when talampicillin 390 mg was given to 10 fasting volunteers; 47% of the dose was recovered in the urine in 6 hours. Among 40 patients with urinary-tract infections given talampicillin 390 mg thrice daily or 750 mg twice daily for 7 days the mean total antibiotic recovery was 42%, with a wide variation among individuals. The incidence of diarrhoea was less with talampicillin.— D. A. Leigh *et al.*, *Br. med. J.*, 1976, *1*, 1378.

In a study in 32 healthy subjects a mean peak serum-ampicillin concentration of 4.65 µg per ml was achieved 40 minutes after a dose of talampicillin hydrochloride 250 mg equivalent to ampicillin 169 mg was given to fasting subjects, and 3.26 µg per ml at 60 minutes when not fasting. Comparable peaks of 2.46 µg per ml at 90 minutes and 1.46 µg per ml at 120 minutes were achieved in fasting and non-fasting subjects respectively after a dose of ampicillin 250 mg. Recovery from the urine in 24 hours was 91, 92, 60, and 41% respectively.— K. H. Jones, *Br. med. J.*, 1977, *2*, 232.

Further references: J. P. Clayton *et al.*, *Antimicrob. Ag. Chemother.*, 1974, *5*, 670; L. Verbist, *Antimicrob. Ag. Chemother.*, 1976, *10*, 173; J. M. T. Hamilton-Miller and W. Brumfitt, *J. antimicrob. Chemother.*, 1979, *5*, 699 (bioavailability study comparing brands of ampicillin with talampicillin).

Uses. Talampicillin is the phthalidyl ester of ampicillin and has the actions and uses of ampicillin (see p.1091). It is given by mouth as the hydrochloride or napsylate and doses of the napsylate are expressed in terms of the hydrochloride. The usual dose is 250 to 500 mg of the hydrochloride thrice daily; children may be given half the adult dose. Under 2 years 3 to 7 mg per kg body-weight may be given thrice daily. A single dose of 1.5 to 2 g is used in the treatment of gonorrhoea.

A review of talampicillin.— *Drug & Ther. Bull.*, 1976, *14*, 27. See also *ibid.*, 1977, *15*, 65.

In a multicentre comparative study, talampicillin hydrochloride 250 mg thrice daily was shown to be as effective as ampicillin 250 mg four times daily in the treatment of bacterial infections of the respiratory tract, urinary tract, and skin and soft tissue. Side-effects occurred more frequently with talampicillin; the incidence of diarrhoea was less with talampicillin than with ampicillin, but other gastro-intestinal disturbances were more common.— E. T. Knudsen and J. W. Harding, *Br. J. clin. Pract.*, 1975, *29*, 255. A comparative study of talampicillin and ampicillin in 607 patients.— G. Jaffé *et al.*, *Practitioner*, 1976, *216*, 455.

Talampicillin was used to treat 69 episodes of acute infections of the respiratory tract, urinary tract, and soft tissue in 65 hospitalised patients. Doses of 250 mg to 1 g were given every 8 hours for 7 to 10 days depending on the severity of infection. A good clinical response was obtained in 64 of the episodes. Ampicillin-resistant organisms which were not present at the start of therapy were identified during treatment in 3 patients. One patient developed severe diarrhoea and talampicillin therapy was stopped.— B. E. Bourke *et al.*, *Br. J. clin. Pract.*, 1979, *33*, 231.

Further references: D. A. Leigh *et al.*, *Br. med. J.*, 1976, *1*, 1378; *Br. J. clin. Pract.*, 1980, *34*, 136.

Gonorrhoea. A single dose ot talampicillin 1.5 g without probenecid given to 81 patients with acute uncomplicated gonorrhoea resulted in a failure-rate in the 71 followed up of only 4.2%. This compared favourably with results previously achieved when amoxycillin, ampicillin, or pivampicillin were given with probenecid.— R. R. Wilcox, *Br. J. vener. Dis.*, 1976, *52*, 184. Similar satisfactory results. When talampicillin 1.48 g with probenecid 1 g was given to 245 men with gonorrhoea there were only 4 treatment failures.— J. D. Price *et al.*, *ibid.*, 1977, *53*, 113.

Talampicillin 1.5 g with probenecid 2 g and ampicillin 3 g with probenecid 2 g were equally effective in the treatment of gonococcal urethritis. There were 2 recurrences in 95 men given ampicillin and 3 in 98 men given talampicillin.— S. Al-Egaily *et al.*, *Br. J. vener. Dis.*, 1978, *54*, 243.

Proprietary Preparations

Talpen *(Beecham Research, UK)*. **Syrup** and **Syrup Forte** (supplied as powder for preparation with water before use) containing talampicillin napsylate equivalent to talampicillin hydrochloride 125 and 250 mg respectively in each 5 ml (suggested diluent, syrup) and **Tablets** containing talampicillin hydrochloride 250 mg.

Other Proprietary Names

Penbritin-T *(S. Afr.)*; Yamacillin *(Jap.)*.

168-z

Tetracycline

(U.S.P., B.P.C. 1973). A hydrated form of (4*S*,4a*S*,5a*S*,6*S*,12a*S*)-4-dimethylamino-1,4,4a,5,5a,6,11,12a-octahydro-3,6,10,12,12a-pentahydroxy-6-methyl-1,11-dioxo-naphthacene-2-carboxamide.

$C_{22}H_{24}N_2O_8=444.4$.

CAS — 60-54-8 (anhydrous); 6416-04-2 (trihydrate).

Pharmacopoeias. In *Jap.*, *Roum.*, *Rus.*, and *U.S.*

An antimicrobial substance produced by the growth of certain strains of *Streptomyces aureofaciens* or by the catalytic reduction of chlortetracycline. A yellow, odourless or almost odourless, crystalline, amphoteric powder with a bitter taste. It loses up to 13% of moisture when dried and contains not less than 1000 units per mg calculated on the anhydrous substance. Tetracycline (anhydrous) 1 g is approximately equivalent to 1.08 g of tetracycline hydrochloride.

Soluble 1 in 2500 of water and 1 in 50 of alcohol; freely soluble in dilute acids and, with decomposition, in solutions of alkali hydroxides; practically insoluble in chloroform and ether. A 1% suspension in water has a pH of 3.5 to 6. It darkens in strong sunlight in a moist atmosphere. It is inactivated at a pH below 2 and slowly destroyed at pH 7 and above. **Store** in airtight containers. Protect from light.

169-c

Tetracycline Hydrochloride *(B.P., Eur. P., U.S.P.).* Tetracyclini Hydrochloridum.

$C_{22}H_{24}N_2O_8,HCl=480.9$.

CAS — 64-75-5.

Pharmacopoeias. In *Aust., Belg., Br., Braz., Cz., Eur., Fr., Ger., Hung., Ind., Int., It., Jap., Jug., Neth., Nord., Pol., Port., Roum., Rus., Swiss, Turk.,* and *U.S.*

A yellow, odourless, hygroscopic, crystalline, amphoteric powder with a bitter taste. The *B.P.* specifies not less than 950 units per mg calculated on the dried substance; *U.S.P.* specifies not less than 900 µg per mg.

Soluble 1 in 10 of water and 1 in 100 of alcohol; soluble in methyl alcohol and in aqueous solutions of alkali hydroxides and carbonates; practically insoluble in acetone, chloroform, and ether. A 1% solution in water has a pH of 1.8 to 2.8. Solutions in water become turbid on standing owing to hydrolysis and precipitation of tetracycline. Solutions for injection are prepared aseptically. Tetracycline hydrochloride darkens in moist air when exposed to strong sunlight. Its potency is reduced in solutions having a pH below 2 and it is slowly destroyed in solutions at pH 7 and above.

Store in airtight containers. If intended for injection, the containers should be sterile and sealed to exclude micro-organisms. Protect from light.

Incompatibility has been reported with alkalis, amikacin sulphate, aminophylline, amphotericin, ampicillin sodium, soluble barbiturates, benzylpenicillin, carbenicillin sodium, cefapirin sodium, cephaloridine, cephalothin sodium, cephazolin sodium, chlorothiazide sodium, cloxacillin sodium, dimenhydrinate, erythromycin salts, heparin, hydrocortisone sodium succinate, methicillin sodium, nitrofurantoin sodium, novobiocin sodium, phenytoin sodium, sodium bicarbonate, sulphadiazine sodium, sulphafurazole diethanolamine, and warfarin sodium.

Incompatibility has also been reported, generally less consistently, with calcium chloride, calcium gluconate, chloramphenicol sodium succinate, and methyldopate hydrochloride.

The addition of bromelains to the core of enteric-coated tetracycline hydrochloride tablets improved absorption of tetracycline, resulting in increased plasma and urine concentrations.— G. Renzini and M. Varengo, *Arzneimittel-Forsch.*, 1972, *22,* 410.

The effect of vehicle on tetracycline applied to the eye.— J. Y. Massey *et al., Am. J. Ophthal.*, 1976, *81,* 151.

Effect of gamma-irradiation. Sterilisation of tetracycline ophthalmic ointments by gamma-irradiation.— R. A. Nash, *Bull. parent. Drug Ass.*, 1974, *28,* 181.

The sterilisation of tetracycline hydrochloride by gamma-irradiation.— G. P. Jacobs, *Pharm. Acta Helv.*, 1977, *52,* 302.

Epimerisation. Epimerisation at carbon atom 4 of tetracycline occurred at pH 2 to 6, producing a ratio of epimer to tetracycline of 0.6:1 in 24 hours. The epiisomers were less active therapeutically. Alkaline degradation occurred but tetracyclines were fairly stable to oxidation.— H. S. Carlin and A. J. Perkins, *Am. J. Hosp. Pharm.*, 1968, *25,* 270.

Incompatibility. Aqueous tetracycline solutions showed maximum degradation, by air and light, in the presence of *riboflavine* 0.01 to 0.1%. Maximum degradation at 37° and pH 4.5, in the absence of light, occurred with riboflavine 1%. Ascorbic acid suppressed the degradation of tetracycline by riboflavine.— L. J. Leeson and J. F. Weidenheimer, *J. pharm. Sci.*, 1969, *58,* 355.

For a list of incompatibilities including *adrenaline, aminophylline, calcium salts, chlorpromazine, colistin sulphomethate sodium, corticotrophin, nafcillin, noradrenaline, oxacillin, prochlorperazine, protein hydrolysate injection, streptomycin,* and *vitamin-B complex,* see *Med. Lett.*, 1972, *14* (Jan.), *Suppl.*, 32.

When reconstituted with bacteriostatic water for injection and mixed with 500 ml of Ringer's injection or lactated Ringer's injection, each with 40 mmol of potassium chloride added, tetracycline hydrochloride 500 mg, as Achromycin Intravenous (*Lederle*), maintained at least 90% of its stated potency for 24 hours at ambient conditions and for 48 hours when refrigerated. Under these conditions chelation with calcium salts was not a problem, confirming that tetracycline can be given in compound sodium lactate injection.— M. Roach, *Lederle* (letter), *Pharm. J.*, 1978, *1,* 143.

Further references: H. R. Grant, *Hosp. Pharmst*, 1962, *15,* 67; J. A. Patel and G. L. Phillips, *Am. J. Hosp. Pharm.*, 1966, *23,* 409; J. M. Meisler and M. W. Skolaut, *ibid.*, 557; B. Lynn, *Chemist Drugg.*, 1967, *187,* 157; B. B. Riley, *J. Hosp. Pharm.*, 1970, *28,* 228; E. A. Parker, *Am. J. Hosp. Pharm.*, 1970, *27,* 327; J. Jacobs *et al., J. clin. Path.*, 1973, *26,* 742.

Loss of activity. Tetracycline was very much less active against *Staphylococcus aureus* in the presence of magnesium carbonate, magnesium oxide, magnesium trisilicate, carmellose sodium, bentonite, and kaolin and less active with calcium carbonate, calamine, acacia, tragacanth, methylcellulose, and sodium alginate.— M. A. El-Nakeeb and R. T. Yousef, *Acta pharm. suec.*, 1968, *5,* 1.

The effects of various additives on the adsorption of tetracycline by magnesium trisilicate and milk *in vitro.*— N. A. Daabis *et al., Pharmazie*, 1976, *31,* 125.

A study of the effect of the antibiotic and preservative on each other's binding to pharmaceutical adjuvants in mixtures containing benzalkonium chloride or chlorocresol and tetracycline hydrochloride.— M. A. El-Nakeeb and M. H. Ali, *Mfg Chem.*, 1976, *47* (Mar.), 37.

Stability. Tetracycline hydrochloride lost 10% potency when stored for 2 months at 37° and 66% relative humidity. The presence of citric acid increased the degradation of tetracycline hydrochloride to anhydrotetracycline and epianhydrotetracycline when stored under the same conditions.— V. C. Walton *et al., J. pharm. Sci.*, 1970, *59,* 1160.

Stability in solution. Tetracycline hydrochloride in intravenous solutions of pH 3 to 5 was chemically stable for 6 hours, but had lost 8 to 12% potency in 24 hours at room temperature.— E. A. Parker, *Am. J. Hosp. Pharm.*, 1967, *24,* 434.

Tetracycline hydrochloride 1 g per 100 ml lost 50% activity in dextrose injection after 14 days at 25°.— J. F. Gallelli *et al., Am. J. Hosp. Pharm.*, 1969, *26,* 630.

Tetracycline hydrochloride 970 mg per litre was stable in sodium chloride injection for 24 hours. The pH of the mixture was 3.1.— R. L. Nedich, *Bull. parent. Drug Ass.*, 1973, *27,* 228.

A study on the effects of pH on the degradation of tetracycline in aqueous solution at 60°. Maximum stability occurred at about pH 3.— B. Vej-Hansen and H. Bundgaard, *Arch. Pharm. Chemi, scient. Edn*, 1978, *6,* 201.

See also above under Incompatibility.

Units. One unit of tetracycline is contained in 0.00101833 mg of the second International Standard Preparation (1970) of tetracycline hydrochloride which contains 982 units per mg.

Adverse Effects. The side-effects of tetracycline hydrochloride are common to all tetracyclines. Gastro-intestinal effects including nausea, vomiting, and diarrhoea are common especially with high doses and most are attributed to irritation of the mucosa. Oral candidiasis, vulvovaginitis, and pruritus ani occur due to overgrowth with *Candida albicans* and there may be overgrowth of resistant coliform organisms, such as *Pseudomonas* spp. and *Proteus* spp., causing diarrhoea. The most serious supra-infection is by resistant staphylococci, causing a fulminating enteritis with dehydration and, occasionally, death; this complication is rare, except after abdominal surgery, especially gastrectomy.

Therapeutic doses given to patients with renal disease increase the severity of uraemia with increased excretion of nitrogen and losses of sodium and the development of anorexia, nausea, vomiting, and weakness, accompanied by acidosis and hyperphosphataemia. These effects are related to the dose and the severity of renal impairment and are probably due to the anti-anabolic effects of the tetracycline.

Severe and sometimes fatal hepatotoxicity associated with fatty changes in the liver and pancreatitis has been reported in pregnant women given tetracycline intravenously for pyelonephritis, and in other patients with renal impairment or those given high doses.

Haemolytic anaemia, eosinophilia, neutropenia, and thrombocytopenia have been reported rarely.

Vitamin deficiency may occur especially with prolonged dosage.

Tetracyclines are deposited in deciduous and permanent teeth causing discoloration, enamel hypoplasia, and reduced mineralisation. They are also deposited in calcifying areas in bone and the nails and when given in therapeutic doses to young infants or women during the late stages of pregnancy tetracyclines interfere with bone growth. An increase in intracranial pressure, which may be associated with a bulging fontanelle in infants, has been reported in patients given tetracyclines.

Allergic reactions to tetracycline and its analogues have been reported and cross-sensitisation is common; photosensitivity of the skin and nails has occurred, especially after demeclocycline, and onycholysis may be associated with nail discoloration. Local irritation can occur when tetracyclines are given parenterally and thrombophlebitis may follow intravenous injections. A Herxheimer-like reaction has been reported in patients with relapsing fever treated with tetracycline.

The use of out-of-date tetracyclines has been associated with the development of a reversible Fanconi-type syndrome characterised by polyuria and polydipsia with nausea, vomiting, proteinuria, glycosuria, acidosis, and aminoaciduria. These effects have been attributed to the presence of degradation products epitetracycline, epianhydrotetracycline, and anhydrotetracycline, resulting from exposure to acid, moisture, and heat.

A malignant lymphoepithelioma occurred in a schoolgirl after 2 years of treatment with tetracycline for acne.— L. Sadoff and T. Eckberg (letter), *Lancet*, 1973, *1,* 675.

Myospherulotic lesions, which appeared to be composed of shrunken distorted erythrocytes, were associated with the packing of cavities, following ENT surgery, with soft paraffin-based ointments containing tetracycline.— *Lancet*, 1978, *2,* 358.

A report of irregular menses and amenorrhoea associated with the administration of tetracycline in the treatment of acne.— S. P. Stone (letter), *J. Am. Acad. Derm.*, 1979, *1,* 151.

Allergy. A fatal anaphylactic reaction in a 25-year-old man after a single intravenous injection of tetracycline.— C. V. Singh *et al., Anaesthesia*, 1977, *32,* 268.

Blood disorders. Prothrombin activity was modestly or markedly reduced in 14 patients given tetracycline intravenously.— R. L. Searcy *et al., Clin. Res.*, 1964, *12,* 230.

Folate deficiency with megaloblastic anaemia was associated with tetracycline 250 mg which had been given twice daily for 3 years.— C. C. Jones, *Ann. intern. Med.*, 1973, *78,* 910.

Deposition in bones and teeth. In a study in 505 children aged 3 to 5 years (born May 1966 to May 1969) tetracycline deposits were present in the teeth of 67, 72, and 71% respectively of those 3, 4, and 5 years old, compared with 76, 73, and 67% in a study 5 years earlier (D. J. Stewart, *Br. dent. J.*, 1968, *124,* 318). It was estimated that 23% of the children in the study would show discoloration of their permanent teeth. A plea was made for the manufacture of paediatric preparations to be discontinued except for those of oxytetracycline (less liable to cause discoloration) for use in special circumstances.— D. J. Stewart, *Br. med. J.*, 1973, *3,* 320.

Agreement to withdraw all paediatric preparations of tetracyclines from the Australian market.— *Aust. J. Pharm.*, 1977, *58,* 275. See also *FDA Drug Bull.*, 1978, *8,* 23.

Further references: K. L. Baker and E. Storey, *Med. J. Aust.*, 1970, *1*, 109; E. Storey, *Drugs*, 1973, *6*, 321; C. E. Renson, *British Dental Association* (letter), *Br. med. J.*, 1977, *2*, 892.

Effect on the gastro-intestinal tract. Oesophageal ulceration was associated with the ingestion of tetracycline or doxycycline capsules in 3 patients. Capsules taken at night were believed to have lodged in the oesophagus.— T. D. Crowson *et al.*, *J. Am. med. Ass.*, 1976, *235*, 2747. See also K. S. Channer and D. Hollanders, *Br. med. J.*, 1981, *282*, 1359.

Of 1517 hospital in-patients in a Boston Collaborative Drug Surveillance Program who received tetracycline none developed colitis.— R. R. Miller and H. Jick, *Clin. Pharmac. Ther.*, 1977, *22*, 1.

Excessive flatulence with alternating diarrhoea and constipation in a patient appeared to be due to a water-soluble metabolite of tetracycline fed to animals for growth promotion or veterinary treatment and present in food.— H. M. Anthony, *Br. med. J.*, 1977, *2*, 1632.

Erythema multiforme. Tetracycline had been implicated in the Stevens-Johnson syndrome.— D. B. Coursin, *J. Am. med. Ass.*, 1966, *198*, 113.

Eye changes. A report of transient myopia due to tetracycline.— *Adverse Drug React. Bull.*, 1972, Oct., 112.

Hepatotoxicity. Six non-pregnant women died after receiving tetracycline 1 to 3 g daily by intravenous injection. At post mortem a foamy type of fatty change in the liver was evident. Death was attributed to tetracycline in 4 patients, and 2 others were considered to have died from pre-existing disease which could have been adversely affected by hepatic dysfunction. Pyelonephritis might predispose the liver to fatty changes.— R. L. Peters *et al.*, *Am. J. Surg.*, 1967, *113*, 622.

Three children with obstructive renal disorders given tetracycline developed lethargy, jaundice, and liver and kidney failure. One child recovered when tetracycline was withdrawn and 2 died. Biopsy demonstrated fatty infiltration. These findings emphasised the hazards of giving tetracycline intravenously to children with impaired renal function.— J. D. Lloyd-Still *et al.*, *J. Pediat.*, 1974, *84*, 366.

Further references: M. A. Schiffer, *Am. J. Obstet. Gynec.*, 1966, *96*, 326, per *Int. pharm. Abstr.*, 1967, *4*, 27.

Intracranial hypertension. A 7-year-old boy developed benign intracranial hypertension after treatment with tetracycline. The hypertension subsided when tetracycline was stopped. Symptoms were first apparent after only four 250-mg doses of tetracycline and persisted until tetracycline was discontinued.— J. C. Maroon and J. Mealy, *J. Am. med. Ass.*, 1971, *216*, 1479.

Further reports of benign intracranial hypertension associated with the use of tetracycline in adolescent and adult patients of both sexes.— G. D. Ohlrich and J. G. Ohlrich, *Med. J. Aust.*, 1977, *1*, 334; B. N. J. Walters and S. S. Gubbay, *Br. med. J.*, 1981, *282*, 19; M. G. Pearson *et al.* (letter), *ibid.*, 568; D. J. Meacock and R. L. Hewer (letter), *ibid.*, 1240.

Lupus erythematosus. Tetracycline had been implicated in the provocation of lupus erythematosus in 3 patients.— C. A. Domz *et al.*, *Ann. intern. Med.*, 1959, *50*, 1217.

Nephrotoxicity. Tetracycline could produce 3 types of renal disease: acute renal failure without oliguria in patients with fatty liver or pancreatitis, a Fanconi-like syndrome, and uraemia in patients with impaired renal function.— H. T. Lew and S. W. French, *Archs intern. Med.*, 1966, *118*, 123.

Of 158 patients referred to a renal unit with acute deterioration of renal function, 48 had received treatment with tetracyclines in the previous 2 weeks. Of these 3 had acute renal failure on admission and recovered after treatment with peritoneal dialysis. Of the other 45, 11 were uraemic although they had not previously shown signs of renal failure.— N. Ribush and T. Morgan, *Med. J. Aust.*, 1972, *1*, 53.

Further references: *Br. med. J.*, 1972, *3*, 370; M. E. Phillips *et al.*, *Br. med. J.*, 1974, *2*, 149; *Lancet*, 1978, *2*, 558.

Neuromuscular blockade. For reports of respiratory paralysis after the administration of tetracyclines to unanaesthetised myasthenic patients, see C. B. Pittinger *et al.*, *Anesth. Analg. curr. Res.*, 1970, *49*, 487.

Photosensitivity. Tetracycline photosensitivity was observed in a 17-year-old girl. Quantitative determination showed that tetracycline was concentrated in the dermatitic areas of the skin.— S. I. Cullen *et al.*, *Archs Derm.*, 1966, *93*, 77.

Photosensitivity accounted for 35% of the 235 adverse reactions to tetracyclines recorded by the Australian Registry. It was more frequent with the longer acting forms such as demeclocycline, doxycycline, and methacycline.— *Med. J. Aust.*, 1972, *1*, 435.

Porphyria-like skin changes in 5 patients taking tetracycline and exposed to the sun.— J. H. Epstein *et al.*, *Archs Derm.*, 1976, *112*, 661.

Reports of onycholysis, usually associated with photosensitivity, in patients receiving tetracycline.— C. V. Sanders *et al*, *Sth. med. J.*, 1976, *69*, 1090; M. S. Rothstein (letter), *Archs Derm.*, 1977, *113*, 520; H. Baker (letter), *Br. med. J.*, 1977, *2*, 519.

Skin reactions. Five cases of toxic epidermal necrolysis had been reported associated with the use of tetracyclines.— E. D. Lowney *et al.*, *Archs Derm.*, 1967, *95*, 359.

A 30-year-old man developed an acneform eruption on 3 occasions after treatment with tetracycline.— S. F. Bean, *Br. J. Derm.*, 1971, *85*, 585.

In 3 patients fixed drug reactions occurred 2 to 4 days after starting tetracycline therapy.— S. T. Brown (letter), *J. Am. med. Ass.*, 1974, *227*, 801.

Further references to skin reactions associated with tetracycline: J. F. Walter and K. D. Macknet, *Archs Derm.*, 1979, *115*, 1087 (cutaneous osteomas).

See also under Erythema Multiforme and Photosensitivity (above).

Supra-infection. In a double-blind study, 111 patients with respiratory infections (36 of whom were receiving antibiotics at the start of the study) were given tablets of tetracycline 250 mg or tetracycline 250 mg with nystatin 250 000 units in a dosage of 2 tablets 4 times daily for 10 days. It was found that though the addition of nystatin suppressed the growth of *Candida* in the faeces it did not lead to any significant reduction in the incidence of gastro-intestinal symptoms, but the incidence of symptoms such as pruritus ani was reduced.— *Br. med. J.*, 1968, *4*, 411 (Report to the Research Committee of the British Tuberculosis Association by the Clinical Trials Subcommittee,). Criticisms.— G. Holti (letter), *ibid.*, 829; H. I. Winner (letter), *ibid.*, 1969, *1*, 186; D. D. Adams (letter), *ibid.*, 122; K. M. Citron *et al.* (letter), *ibid.*, 575; G. Holti (letter), *ibid.*, 781; H. I. Winner (letter), *ibid.*, 782.

Precautions. The tetracyclines with the exception of doxycycline are generally contra-indicated in patients with renal impairment. Care must be taken when liver function is impaired. Potentially hepatotoxic drugs should not be given with tetracyclines nor should compounds such as methoxyflurane that can be nephrotoxic.

The use of tetracyclines in pregnancy should be avoided. When administered to women during the latter half of pregnancy, to nursing mothers, or during childhood up to the age of 12 years, permanent discoloration of the child's teeth may occur. Symptoms of myasthenia gravis may be exacerbated by tetracyclines. Absorption of tetracyclines is diminished by milk, alkalis, aluminium hydroxide, and the salts of other trivalent and divalent cations including calcium, iron, and magnesium, when these are taken concomitantly.

Doses of anticoagulants may need to be reduced when patients are given tetracyclines.

Tetracyclines should not be given to patients with known hypersensitivity to any of this group of antibiotics.

Because of possible antagonism of the action of the penicillins by predominantly bacteriostatic tetracyclines it has been recommended that the two types of antibiotic should not be given concomitantly, especially when a rapid bactericidal action is necessary.

Although the reduction in partial oxygen pressure of the blood after intravenous injections of doxycycline and rolitetracycline could be considered to be within normal limits, the intravenous administration of tetracyclines to patients with hypoxaemia and arterial cyanosis should be carried out very slowly and with great care.— H. Krekeler *et al.*, *Arzneimittel-Forsch.*, 1971, *21*, 1637.

Whereas chlortetracycline and demeclocycline interfere with colour vision, tetracycline itself does not.— J. Laroche and C. Laroche, *Annls pharm. fr.*, 1972, *30*, 433.

A report of cross-sensitivity between tetracycline and dipyrone in a patient who experienced attacks of fixed eruption after either drug.— J. S. Pasricha and S. R. Shukla, *Br. J. Derm.*, 1979, *101*, 361.

Interactions. Reports of the diminished absorption of tetracyclines when taken with *iron salts*: P. J. Neuvonen *et al.*, *Br. med. J.*, 1970, *4*, 532; F. J. A. Bateman, *Pfizer* (letter), *Br. med. J.*, 1970, *4*, 802; N. J. Greenberger, *Ann. intern. Med.*, 1971, *74*, 792; P. J. Neuvonen *et al.* (letter), *Br. J. clin. Pharmac.*, 1975, *2*, 94. *sodium bicarbonate:* W. H. Barr *et al.*, *Clin. Pharmac. Ther.*, 1971, *12*, 779. *zinc:* K. -E. Andersson *et al.*, *Eur. J. clin. Pharmac.*, 1976, *10*, 59. *bismuth salicylate:* K. S. Albert *et al.*, *J. pharm. Sci.*, 1979, *68*, 586. See also P. J. Neuvonen, *Drugs*, 1976, *11*, 45.

Tetracyclines could interfere technically with laboratory estimations for catecholamines in the urine to produce erroneous raised results.— *Drug & Ther. Bull.*, 1972, *10*, 69. See also J. Millhouse, *Adverse Drug React. Bull.*, 1974, Dec., 164.

Tetracyclines should not be administered concurrently with other potentially hepatotoxic drugs. These included erythromycin estolate, triacetyloleandomycin, chloramphenicol, sulphonamides, aminosalicylic acid, isoniazid, chlorpromazine and other phenothiazine derivatives, phenytoin and other anticonvulsants, cinchophen, phenylbutazone, chlorpropamide, methyltestosterone, phenindione, and chlorothiazide.— H. F. Dowling and M. H. Lepper, *J. Am. med. Ass.*, 1974, *188*, 307.

Cimetidine. Evidence that cimetidine can interfere with the absorption of tetracycline.— J. J. Cole *et al.* (letter), *Lancet*, 1980, *2*, 536. In a single-dose crossover study 6 healthy subjects received tetracycline 500 mg as tablets with either placebo or cimetidine 400 mg. The mean peak plasma-tetracycline concentration and the area under the concentration-time curve were reduced by 40% and the 72-hour urinary tetracycline excretion was diminished by about 30%, these changes all being significant. When multiple doses of cimetidine (400 mg every 8 hours and at bedtime) or placebo were given for 6 days and the tetracycline administered on the fifth day of dosing, the within-subject variability of plasma and urinary tetracycline concentrations increased, and there was no significant effect on mean peak plasma concentration, area under the concentration-time curve, or 72-hour tetracycline excretion.— H. J. Rogers *et al.* (letter), *ibid.*, 694. A further study indicating that cimetidine does not affect the absorption of tetracycline.— M. Garty and A. Hurwitz, *Clin. Pharmac. Ther.*, 1980, *28*, 203.

Diuretics. When 1957 patients were screened for increases in blood-urea-nitrogen concentrations, rises were confined to those patients receiving diuretics in addition to tetracycline therapy. Patients on diuretic therapy should be given alternative antibiotics.—A report from the Boston Collaborative Drug Surveillance Program, *J. Am. med. Ass.*, 1972, *220*, 377. A study in 8 patients with chronic bronchitis showed that in 6 the blood-urea-nitrogen concentrations rose after treatment with tetracycline with or without diuretics. It was suggested that this rise might be due to the inhibition of protein formation during tetracycline therapy.— H. J. P. M. Dijkhuis and A. J. van Meurs (letter), *ibid.*, 1973, *223*, 441.

Lithium carbonate. For the effect of tetracycline on lithium carbonate, see Lithium Carbonate, p.1539.

Phenformin. Precipitation of phenformin-induced lactic acidosis by tetracycline in a 76-year-old patient with maturity-onset diabetes and bacteriuria. It was recommended that tetracycline should not be given to patients receiving biguanide drugs.— A. Aro *et al.* (letter), *Lancet*, 1978, *1*, 673.

Pregnancy and the neonate. For a report of congenital abnormalities associated with the use of a tetracycline during pregnancy, see Clomocycline, p.1148.

Antimicrobial Action. The group of tetracycline antibiotics have a broad spectrum of antimicrobial activity (see p.1085) and act by interfering with bacterial protein synthesis. They are active against a large number of Gram-positive and Gram-negative pathogenic bacteria, including some which are resistant to penicillin, and are mainly bacteriostatic.

In addition to the staphylococci, streptococci, and Enterobacteriaceae, organisms sensitive to tetracyclines in the concentrations usually achieved after oral doses include *Bacillus anthracis*, *Bordetella*, *Brucella*, *Haemophilus*, *Vibrio*, and *Yersinia* spp., *Calymmatobacterium granulomatis*, *Francisella tularensis*, *Mycoplasma pneumoniae*, *Neisseria gonorrhoeae*, *Pasteurella multocida*, and *Treponema pallidum* and some other spirochaetes. Chlamydiae, rickettsiae, *Coxiella burnettii*, *Actinomyces* spp., and *Plasmodium falciparum* are also sensitive. The Gram-negative bacteria *Serratia marcescens*, most *Proteus* spp., and *Pseudomonas aeruginosa* are usually resistant but *Ps. pseudomallei* is sensitive. Fungi, yeasts, and true viruses are also resistant. The tetracyclines are more active in an acid medium.

MICs for tetracycline against 68 strains of *H. influenzae* ranged from 0.12 to 16 μg per ml.— J. D. Williams and J. Andrews, *Br. med. J.*, 1974, *1*, 134.

Tetracycline was active *in vitro* against *Chlamydia trachomatis*, the MIC against 16 strains ranging from 0.02 to 0.5 μg per ml.— C. -C. Kuo *et al.*, *Antimicrob. Ag. Chemother.*, 1977, *12*, 80.

Tetracycline was effective *in vitro* against the amoeba *Naegleria fowleri*.— Y. H. Thong *et al.* (letter), *Lancet*, 1977, *2*, 876. See also K. K. Lee *et al.*, *Antimicrob. Ag. Chemother.*, 1979, *16*, 217.

Tetracycline inhibited about 97.1, 98.5, 98.8, and 100% of 517 non-beta-lactamase producing strains of *Neisseria gonorrhoeae* at concentrations of 0.5, 1, 2, and 4 μg per ml respectively. Of 13 beta-lactamase-producing strains about 54, 77, and 100% were inhibited at concentrations of 0.5, 1, and 2 μg per ml respectively.— P. D. Duck *et al.*, *Antimicrob. Ag. Chemother.*, 1978, *14*, 788.

Minocycline was more active than tetracycline or doxycycline against 624 strains of anaerobic bacteria *in vitro*. At 5 μg per ml minocycline, doxycycline, and tetracycline inhibited 84, 74, and 66% respectively of 241 strains of *Bacteroides* spp.— V. Bach *et al.*, *Curr. ther. Res.*, 1978, *23*, 206. See also O. A. Okubadejo *et al.*, *Br. med. J.*, 1973, *2*, 212; V. L. Sutter and S. M. Finegold, *Antimicrob. Ag. Chemother.*, 1976, *10*, 736; P. C. Appelbaum and S. A. Chatterton, *Antimicrob. Ag. Chemother.*, 1978, *14*, 371.

Using agar dilution tests tetracycline inhibited all of 17 strains of *Mycobacterium fortuitum* at a concentration of 16 μg per ml but only 29% of 7 strains of *M. chelonei*.— D. F. Welch and M. T. Kelly, *Antimicrob. Ag. Chemother.*, 1979, *15*, 754.

Tetracycline was the most active of 16 antibiotics against 14 strains of *Pasteurella multocida* and had a median MIC of 0.09 μg per ml and a median MBC of 3.12 μg per ml.— D. L. Stevens *et al.*, *Antimicrob. Ag. Chemother.*, 1979, *16*, 322.

In a study *in vitro* of the activity of 20 antimicrobial agents against *Campylobacter fetus* subsp. *jejuni* clindamycin, doxycycline, and gentamicin were the most active agents but only doxycycline, tetracycline, and gentamicin were active against all the strains at concentrations attainable in serum with standard dosage.— M. Walder, *Antimicrob. Ag. Chemother.*, 1979, *16*, 37.

Enhanced activity. Urea might enhance the antimicrobial activity of tetracycline against staphylococci and *Ps. aeruginosa*.— B. W. Burt and G. Dempsey, *Pharm. J.*, 1977, *2*, 255.

The activity of tetracycline *in vitro* against *E. coli* was enhanced when used with human serum.— B. S. Dutcher *et al.*, *Antimicrob. Ag. Chemother.*, 1978, *13*, 820.

Synergism occurred against some strains of *Staphylococcus aureus* when the activity of tetracycline was tested *in vitro* with actinomycin D or mitomycin.— J. Y. Jacobs *et al.*, *Antimicrob. Ag. Chemother.*, 1979, *15*, 580.

Resistance. Resistance to the tetracyclines is usually plasmid-mediated and may be transferable. It generally develops relatively slowly in susceptible organisms but the incidence of resistance to these antibiotics has risen with their continued use so that resistant strains of the majority of sensitive species have now been reported. An organism resistant to one of the tetracyclines is usually resistant to all other members of the group although some tetracycline-resistant staphylococcal, streptococcal, and Gram-negative organisms may be sensitive to minocycline.

Administration of tetracycline-containing feeds to farm *animals* led within 3 to 5 months to an increase in tetracycline-resistant intestinal bacteria in the farm workers. Antibiotic-supplemented feeds contributed to the selection of human resistant strains of bacteria; this form of animal treatment should be re-evaluated.— S. B. Levy *et al.*, *New Engl. J. Med.*, 1976, *295*, 583.

A survey of the use of tetracycline in the community and its possible relation to the excretion of tetracycline-resistant bacteria.— M. H. Richmond and K. B. Linton, *J. antimicrob. Chemother.*, 1980, *6*, 33.

Resistance of coliforms. Faecal *Escherichia coli* resistant to tetracycline were found in 4 of 18 patients before treatment with tetracycline 250 mg four times daily for 10 days and in all patients 4 to 7 days after treatment. Multiple resistance to ampicillin, chloramphenicol, streptomycin, and sulphonamide occurred. Treatment of other patients with ampicillin or sulphadimidine produced an insignificant increase in *E. coli* resistance. By 5 weeks the effects of treatment had worn off.— N. Datta *et al.*, *Lancet*, 1971, *1*, 312. See also M. V. Valtonen *et al.*, *Br. J. Derm.*, 1976, *95*, 311.

Resistance of Haemophilus. Plasmid mediated R-factors the same as those from the Enterobacteriaceae had been detected in strains of *Haemophilus influenzae* producing resistance to ampicillin and tetracycline.— R. Laufs *et al.*, *Dt. med. Wschr.*, 1978, *103*, 658.

Resistance of pneumococci. Of 1528 strains of pneumococci isolated in 21 laboratories in the UK 13% were resistant to tetracycline; of 1515 group A streptococci 36% were resistant. There was wide geographical variation.— Report of an Ad-hoc Study Group on Antibiotic Resistance, *Br. med. J.*, 1977, *1*, 131. See also P. A. Boswell and G. E. Hillier (letter), *Br. med. J.*, 1977, *1*, 446.

Of 866 strains of *Str. pneumoniae* 59 (6.8%) were resistant to tetracycline; this was significantly lower than the incidence of resistance (13%) in an earlier study. Of 952 strains of *H. influenzae* 26 (2.7%) were resistant to tetracycline.— A. J. Howard *et al.*, *Br. med. J.*, 1978, *1*, 1657.

Further references: A. Percival *et al.*, *Lancet*, 1969, *1*, 998; K. V. Gopalakrishna and P. I. Lerner, *Am. Rev. resp. Dis.*, 1973, *108*, 1007; M. Bullen and D. Hansman (letter), *Lancet*, 1975, *1*, 466.

Resistance of salmonellae. Of 400 strains of *Salmonella* isolated from patients in USA during 1967, 12.5% were resistant to tetracycline; 31.4% of *S. typhimurium* strains were resistant. Assessment of resistance was based upon a zone of inhibition of 11 mm or less, using disks containing 30 μg of tetracycline hydrochloride.— S. A. Schroeder *et al.*, *J. Am. med. Ass.*, 1968, *205*, 903.

Resistance of strains of *Salmonella typhi* and *S. typhimurium* to tetracycline had been reported in India, Malaysia, Thailand, and Vietnam.— *Chronicle Wld Hlth Org.*, 1975, *29*, 30.

The decrease in tetracycline resistance in *Salmonella* of human and porcine origin that has occurred in the Netherlands since 1974, appears to coincide with the legislative ban by the EEC on incorporation of tetracycline in animal feeds.— W. J. van Leeuwen *et al.*, *Antimicrob. Ag. Chemother.*, 1979, *16*, 237.

Resistance of staphylococci. Transferable resistance to tetracycline was observed amongst strains of *Staphylococcus aureus* grown on milk, cheese, and cream.— R. W. Lacey and R. Didcock (letter), *Lancet*, 1973, *1*, 825.

Periodic surveys in a general hospital indicated a decline in the proportions of patients with strains of *Staph. aureus* in their noses resistant to tetracycline, erythromycin, kanamycin, methicillin, and novobiocin. This was associated with a large reduction in the use of tetracycline, but no overall reduction in the use of antibiotics. Replies from microbiologists in 20 British hospitals also confirmed published reports of a reduced incidence of resistant hospital strains of *Staph. aureus*. No similar reduction was noted in a hospital for diseases of the skin where tetracyclines are commonly used. A dramatic fall in tetracycline-resistant and multiresistant *Staph. aureus* was noted in a burns unit (where tetracycline was rarely used) associated with unusually low numbers of patients and little antibiotic use; this was reversed when both increased, the increase in novobiocin- and tetracycline-resistant strains probably being due to selection by treatment with erythromycin.— G. A. J. Ayliffe *et al.*, *Lancet*, 1979, *1*, 538.

Further references: E. Schön *et al.*, *Rev. czech. Med.*, 1972, *18*, 1; Z. A. Hassam *et al.*, *Br. med. J.*, 1978, *2*, 536.

Resistance of streptococci. The incidence of tetracycline-resistant strains of beta-haemolytic streptococci fell, in south-west Essex, from 35% in 1965 to 9% in 1972.— M. H. Robertson, *Br. med. J.*, 1973, *4*, 84. There was no fall in the Glasgow area.— R. J. Fallon (letter), *ibid.*, 300.

Of 1176 strains of group A streptococci isolated in Japan in the period 1972 to 1974, 241 were resistant to tetracycline, 234 to tetracycline and chloramphenicol, 427 to tetracycline, chloramphenicol, erythromycin, oleandomycin, josamycin, midecamycin, and lincomycin, and 19 to chloramphenicol alone. Seven of 83 strains of group B streptococci were resistant to tetracycline and chloramphenicol and 26 to tetracycline alone. It was considered that because resistance to a single macrolide antibiotic was rare and that acquisition of resistance to tetracycline and/or chloramphenicol appeared to be a prerequisite for resistance to macrolide antibiotics, restriction of the use of tetracycline and chloramphenicol would lead to a decline in the frequency of macrolide-antibiotic resistance.— Y. Miyamoto *et al.*, *Antimicrob. Ag. Chemother.*, 1978, *13*, 399.

Further references: J. Brorson *et al.*, *Br. J. Derm.*, 1972, *86*, 449; M. Nakae *et al.*, *Antimicrob. Ag. Chemother.*, 1977, *12*, 427.

See also Resistance of Pneumococci, above.

Resistance of Vibrio cholerae. During the first 6 months of the fourth cholera epidemic in Tanzania, determination of the MICs of 110 isolates of *Vibrio cholerae* taken from 102 patients, revealed rapid emergence of resistance to tetracycline, which was used extensively for both prophylaxis and treatment. Whereas all isolates were fully sensitive to tetracycline during the first month 76% were resistant (MIC greater than 100 μg per ml) after 5 months of extensive use. Tetracycline resistance, however, was not the only factor which led to continued excretion of *V. cholerae* since the concentration of tetracycline in the faeces may reach considerably more than 100 μg per ml and although some patients with isolates with MICs above 100 μg per ml continued to excrete *V. cholerae* after tetracycline treatment, several did not. The MICs of isolates taken from 8 resistant patients measured both before and after tetracycline therapy did not change indicating that resistance did not develop *in vivo*. The results reaffirmed the view that resistance of *V. cholerae* to chemotherapeutic agents is complex and that further studies are needed before resistance to chemotherapeutic agents *per se* can be blamed for failure of chemotherapy. Resistance to chloramphenicol, which was used less than tetracycline, developed more slowly. Resistance to nitrofurantoin, neomycin, ampicillin, and sulphadimidine (which were not used in the outbreak) also developed more slowly.— F. S. Mhalu *et al.*, *Lancet*, 1979, *1*, 345. This is one of the first examples of a widespread outbreak of R plasmid-carrying strains of *V. cholerae*. The appearance of resistance to tetracycline demonstrates the way in which plasmid-mediated resistance can emerge and rapidly spread under the heavy selection pressure of mass prophylaxis.— K. J. Towner *et al.* (letter), *ibid.*, *2*, 147.

A report on antimicrobial susceptibility of *Vibrio cholerae* El Tor from Zaire and Rwanda.— J. Colaert *et al.* (letter), *Lancet*, 1979, *2*, 849.

Absorption and Fate. The tetracyclines are incompletely and irregularly absorbed from the gastro-intestinal tract. The degree of absorption is diminished by the soluble salts of divalent and trivalent metals, with which tetracyclines form stable complexes and to a variable degree by milk or food. It has been recommended that tetracyclines should be given before food. Sodium metaphosphate may enhance the absorption of tetracycline.

As a rule, doses of 250 to 500 mg by mouth every 6 hours produce therapeutically effective plasma concentrations of tetracycline ranging from 1 to 3 μg per ml and 1.5 to 5 μg per ml respectively. Intravenous injections of 250 to 500 mg produce plasma concentrations of 15 to 20 μg per ml at 0.5 hours falling to 4 to 10 μg per ml at 1 to 2 hours, though at 12 hours 1 to 3 μg per ml may still be present. Intramuscular doses of 100 mg yield plasma concentrations of up to 2 μg per ml and 250-mg doses up to 3.6 μg per ml at 3 to 4 hours.

In the circulation, tetracyclines are bound to plasma proteins in varying degrees, and figures have been reported ranging from 20 to 35% for oxytetracycline, from 24 to 65% for tetracycline, and from 41 to 90% for demeclocycline. They are widely distributed throughout the body tissues and fluids. Concentrations in cerebrospinal fluid are relatively low, but may be raised if the meninges are inflamed. Tetracyclines appear in the milk of nursing mothers where concentrations may be 60% or more of those in the plasma. They diffuse across the placenta and appear in the foetal circulation in concentrations of about 25 to 75% of those in the maternal blood. Only small amounts appear in saliva, tears, and intra-ocular fluids. Tetracyclines are retained at sites of new bone formation and recent calcification, in developing teeth, and in some injured soft tissues.

The biological half-life of tetracycline has been reported to be 8.5 hours; comparable figures reported for other tetracyclines are chlortetracycline 5.5 hours, demeclocycline 12 hours, doxycycline 15 to 17 hours, methacycline 15 hours, minocycline 17 to 19 hours, and oxytetracycline 9.5 hours.

The tetracyclines are excreted in the urine and in the faeces. Renal clearance is by glomerular filtration and concentrations in the urine of up to 300 μg per ml of tetracycline may be reached 2 hours after a dose is taken and be maintained for about 6 to 12 hours. Up to 60% of an intravenous dose and rather less of a dose by mouth is eliminated in the urine but only about 10 to 15% of a dose of chlortetracycline is eliminated in the urine.

The tetracyclines are excreted in the bile where concentrations 5 to 20 times those in plasma can occur. Since there is some reabsorption complete elimination is slow. Considerable quantities occur in the faeces after administration by mouth and lesser amounts after administration by injection.

In a study of 170 men and 142 women given various antibiotics, blood concentrations following tetracycline 370 mg were 19% higher in the females at 2 hours and 21.5% higher at 6 hours.— R. Scotti, *Chemotherapy, Basle*, 1973, *18*, 205.

The renal excretion of tetracycline and doxycycline was enhanced by rendering the urine alkaline and was probably the result of altered tubular reabsorption.— J. M. Jaffe *et al.*, *J. Pharmacokinet. Biopharm.*, 1973, *1*, 267.

In a comparative study involving 4 healthy subjects the calculated mean plasma half-lives of tetracycline, oxytetracycline, doxycycline, and minocycline were 11.7, 8.75, 16.9, and 11 hours respectively. Tetracycline and oxytetracycline had a much larger volume of distribution than the other two antibiotics.— R. Green *et al.*, *Eur. J. clin. Pharmac.*, 1976, *10*, 245.

Absorption. A discussion of factors affecting the absorption of tetracyclines.— P. J. Neuvonen, *Drugs*, 1976, *11*, 45.

No difference in either rate or extent of tetracycline absorption after administration by mouth was found between 5 elderly patients with achlorhydria and 5 controls. It was suggested that previous reports of reduced absorption in patients with elevated gastric pH may have resulted from using poorly formulated preparations.— P. A. Kramer *et al.*, *Clin. Pharmac. Ther.*, 1978, *23*, 467.

See also under Precautions (above).

Bioavailability. A review of the bioavailability of tetracycline.— T. D. Sokoloski *et al.*, *J. Am. pharm. Ass.*, 1975, *NS15*, 709.

Bioavailability tests *in vivo* of tetracycline should cover a period of 96 hours. Absorption from a capsule and 2 film-coated tablets did not show any significant differences until after 6 hours.— C. M. Davis *et al.*, *Am. J. med. Sci.*, 1973, *265*, 69.

The bioavailability of tetracycline from tablets and suspension was found to be similar.— P. Fisher *et al.*, *Br. J. clin. Pharmac.*, 1980, *9*, 153.

Diffusion. A study indicating that tetracycline rapidly enters red blood cells *in vitro*.— H. W. Jun and B. H. Lee, *J. pharm. Sci.*, 1980, *69*, 455.

Milk.— J. A. Knowles, *J. Pediat.*, 1965, *66*, 1068.

Bile.— G. Acocella *et al.*, *Gut*, 1968, *9*, 536.

Sputum.— C. G. C. MacArthur *et al.*, *J. antimicrob. Chemother.*, 1978, *4*, 509.

Protein binding. A report that the protein binding of tetracycline was significantly reduced in malnutrition and probably accounted for its more rapid elimination by the kidneys in such patients.— A. K. Shastri and K. Krishnaswamy, *Clinica chim. Acta*, 1976, *66*, 157.

Further references: I. W. Kellaway and C. Marriott, *Can. J. pharm. Sci.*, 1978, *13*, 90.

Uses. The tetracyclines have a wide spectrum of activity and have been used in the treatment of a large number of infections caused by susceptible organisms. With the emergence of bacterial resistance and the development of other antibacterial agents their use may be restricted increasingly to the treatment of rickettsial infections, including typhus, Rocky Mountain spotted fever, and Q fever; chlamydial infections, including psittacosis, lymphogranuloma venereum, trachoma, and inclusion conjunctivitis; and mycoplasmal infections, especially those caused by *Mycoplasma pneumoniae*. Tetracyclines are also used in the treatment of brucellosis, plague, tularaemia, malabsorption syndromes such as tropical sprue and Whipple's disease, urinary-tract infections, especially non-specific urethritis, and are given in low doses in the long-term treatment of severe acne.

Tetracyclines are not recommended in the treatment of streptococcal sore throat. They are used, however, in the management of chronic bronchitis to prevent acute exacerbations due to susceptible organisms.

The tetracyclines are used effectively in the treatment of cholera and reduce fluid requirements. Relapsing fever responds to treatment with tetracycline but a Herxheimer-like reaction appears to be a frequent complication; it has been given alone or in conjunction with quinine in the management of malaria especially when resistant to chloroquine. Tetracyclines have also been given in the treatment of amoebic dysentery, often with an amoebicide, and in the treatment of balantidiasis.

In penicillin-sensitive patients tetracyclines have been of value in the treatment of staphylococcal and streptococcal infections where tetracycline resistance is not a problem, and may also be used in such patients in certain stages of syphilis, and in yaws, gonorrhoea, actinomycosis, anthrax, and leptospirosis.

Tetracycline has been used topically in the treatment of chlamydial infections of the eye.

In the treatment of systemic infections the tetracyclines are usually administered by mouth; in severe acute infections they may be given by slow intravenous infusion or by intramuscular injection; parenteral therapy should be substituted by oral administration as soon as practicable.

In children, the effects on teeth should be considered and tetracyclines only used when absolutely essential.

The usual adult dosage of tetracycline hydrochloride is 250 or 500 mg every 6 hours preferably one hour before or 2 hours after meals; up to 3 g daily may be given if necessary. Children have been given 10 to 50 mg per kg body-weight daily by mouth. Tetracycline base is used in oral suspensions.

In severe infections, tetracycline hydrochloride may be administered by slow intravenous infusion every 12 hours as a solution containing not more than 0.5%. The usual dose is 1 g daily but up to 2 g daily has been given to patients with normal renal function; children may be given 10 to 20 mg per kg body-weight daily.

Administered intramuscularly as a solution containing not more than 5%, tetracycline hydrochloride is given in a dosage of 200 to 800 mg for adults and 5 to 25 mg per kg body-weight for children daily, in divided doses with a maximum of 250 mg daily. As intramuscular injections are painful, procaine is usually included in the solution.

Tetracyclines, apart from doxycycline, should generally be avoided in patients with renal impairment.

Reports and reviews of the actions and uses of the tetracyclines.— W. R. Wilson, *Mayo Clin. Proc.*, 1977, *52*, 635; M. Barza and R. T. Schiefe, *Am. J. Hosp. Pharm.*, 1977, *34*, 49; D. S. Reeves *et al.*, *Br. med. J.*, 1978, *2*, 410; *Bull. N.Y. Acad. Med.*, 1978, *54*, 141; I. Chopra *et al.*, *J. antimicrob. Chemother.*, 1981, *8*, 5.

References to slow-release preparations of tetracycline.— A. Pines *et al.*, *Br. J. clin. Pract.*, 1972, *26*, 475; *Drug & Ther. Bull.*, 1972, *10*, 63.

The use of tetracycline labelled with technetium-99m in detecting the location and extent of the necrotic tissue in acute cardiac infarctions.— B. L. Holman *et al.*, *New Engl. J. Med.*, 1974, *291*, 159.

Tetracycline 250 mg thrice daily for 2 weeks, then twice daily, resulted in improvement in a patient with panniculitis of the lower legs. The beneficial effect was thought to be due to the anti-lipase activity of tetracycline.— H. L. Chan, *Br. J. Derm.*, 1975, *92*, 351.

'Seal finger' infection due to an unidentified organism and contracted by hunters handling seals and polar bears could be controlled within 7 days by tetracycline given by mouth; erythromycin, penicillin, and sulphonamide were ineffective.— B. Beck and T. G. Smith (letter,), *Can. med. Ass. J.*, 1976, *115*, 105. See also E. Sargent (letter), *J. Am. med. Ass.*, 1980, *244*, 437.

Tetracycline was considered the treatment of choice in cat scratch fever but it should not be given prophylactically.— *Br. med. J.*, 1978, *1*, 427.

A report of the successful management of pneumothorax in 2 patients with the intrapleural instillation of 500 mg of tetracycline dissolved in 50 ml of sodium chloride injection.— R. C. Goldszer *et al.*, *J. Am. med. Ass.*, 1979, *241*, 724. See also under Malignant Effusions (below).

Amoebiasis. For reports on the use of tetracycline hydrochloride in conjunction with chloroquine phosphate and diloxanide furoate in the treatment of intestinal amoebiasis, see Diloxanide Furoate, p.978.

Aphthous ulcers. Tetracycline relieved the pain in aphthous ulceration probably by reducing secondary infection. The contents of a 250-mg capsule in water were used as a mouth-wash 3 or 4 times daily.— A. D. Macalister, *Drugs*, 1973, *5*, 453.

In a double-blind study in 20 patients with recurrent aphthous ulcers 5 ml of syrup containing tetracycline hydrochloride 125 mg and amphotericin 25 mg, used as a mouthwash thrice daily, was significantly more effective than placebo in relieving pain and reducing the incidence of new ulcers.— A. M. Denman and A. A. Schiff, *Br. med. J.*, 1979, *1*, 1248.

Brucellosis. Tetracycline was the most widely recommended antibiotic in the treatment of brucellosis. The daily dose for adults was 1 to 2 g by mouth for 3 weeks or longer. If a relapse occurred, therapy should be repeated for a further 2 to 3 weeks. If the infection was severe and there were demonstrable local lesions, such as those due to *Brucella suis* or *Br. melitensis*, tetracycline could be administered parenterally together with streptomycin 1 g daily for 2 weeks.— Fifth Report of the Joint FAO/WHO Expert Committee on Brucellosis, *Tech. Rep. Ser. Wld Hlth Org. No. 464*, 1971, 35.

Recommended treatment for both acute and chronic brucellosis was tetracycline 2 to 3 g daily by mouth for 3 to 4 weeks.— P. D. Welsby and C. C. Smith, *Br. J. Hosp. Med.*, 1978, *19*, 20.

The successful use of tetracycline with streptomycin and rifampicin in a man with *Brucella melitensis* endocarditis.— D. S. Pratt *et al.*, *Am. J. Med.*, 1978, *64*, 897.

Further references: J. D. Coghlan and H. J. A. Longmore, *Practitioner*, 1973, *211*, 645; M. G. Robertson (letter), *J. Am. med. Ass.*, 1973, *225*, 750; *Br. med. J.*, 1981, *282*, 1180.

Chlamydial infections. A review of the treatment of genital and eye infections caused by chlamydias. Tetracyclines were considered highly effective but erythromycin was recommended for the treatment of pregnant or lactating women or young children.— *Drug & Ther. Bull.*, 1978, *16*, 37. See also E. M. C. Dunlop, *J. antimicrob. Chemother.*, 1977, *3*, 377; *Lancet*, 1978, *1*, 192; S. J. Richmond and J. D. Oriel, *Br. med. J.*, 1978, *2*, 480; J. Schachter, *New Engl. J. Med.*, 1978, *298*, 490; M. R. Hammerschlag, *New Engl. J. Med.*, 1978, *298*, 1083.

In a study of 64 women with genital cultures containing *Chlamydia trachomatis*, 20 took tablets containing tetracycline, chlortetracycline, and demeclocycline (Deteclo) twice daily for 21 days and the remainder took a similar dose for 7 days. All cultures were negative after treatment.— M. A. Waugh and K. C. Nayyar, *Br. J. vener. Dis.*, 1977, *53*, 96. See also W. M. McCormack *et al.*, *New Engl. J. Med.*, 1979, *300*, 123.

For further references to the use of tetracycline in chlamydial infections, see A. J. Abrams, *J. Am. med. Ass.*, 1968, *205*, 199 (lymphogranuloma venereum); J. P. Anderson and F. A. J. Bridgwater, *Br. J. Dis. Chest*, 1968, *62*, 155 (ornithosis); G. D. W. McKendrick *et al.*, *Lancet*, 1973, *2*, 1255 (psittacosis).

See also under Trachoma and Urinary-tract Infections.

Cholera. Tetracycline or chloramphenicol, intravenously or by mouth, in doses of 250 or 500 mg every 6 hours, produced satisfactory clinical responses in patients with cholera. The higher dose, administered for 3 days, was necessary to ensure freedom from bacteriological relapses. The emergence of resistant strains was considered likely.— WHO Expert Committee on Cholera, Second Report, *Tech. Rep. Ser. Wld Hlth Org. No. 352*, 1967.

Tetracycline 250 to 750 mg six-hourly for 2 to 4 days

and chloramphenicol 250 to 750 mg six-hourly for 2 days, or 250 to 500 mg six-hourly for 3 days caused a significant reduction in the duration of diarrhoea and of positive stool cultures, in stool volume, and in intravenous fluid requirements in a study of 318 patients with cholera. Streptomycin was less effective, and paromomycin was considered of little value. Similar studies in 238 children, weighing less than 15 kg, using tetracycline 125 to 250 mg six-hourly for 2 to 4 days, chloramphenicol 125 to 500 mg six-hourly for 2 to 3 days, streptomycin 500 mg six-hourly for 2 to 3 days, and paromomycin 125 mg six-hourly for 2 to 3 days, or 250 mg six-hourly for 3 days, suggested that for children tetracycline was the drug of choice; chloramphenicol was less effective and streptomycin and paromomycin were of little value.— J. Lindenbaum *et al.*, *Bull. Wld Hlth Org.*, 1967, *36*, 871; *idem*, *37*, 529.

The results of a study of 42 patients, from whose stools *Vibrio cholerae* had been cultured, indicated that treatment with tetracycline, chloramphenicol, or sulphamethoxazole with trimethoprim hastened the elimination of the organism from the intestinal tract. For elimination of *V. cholerae* from all patients, 4 days' therapy with tetracycline, 2 g daily, or 4 tablets of sulphamethoxazole with trimethoprim daily, or 7 days' therapy with chloramphenicol 2 g daily was necessary. In 5 of 40 patients who had 3 consecutive daily negative stool cultures and who received a purge, a positive stool culture was obtained subsequently.— R. A. Gharagozloo *et al.* (preliminary communication), *Br. med. J.*, 1970, *4*, 281. See also W. M. McCormack *et al.*, *Bull. Wld Hlth Org.*, 1968, *38*, 787.

After tetracycline had been administered in doses of 0.25 to 1 g daily for 3 days to cholera carriers there was a significant decrease in the number of vibrio excretors in the next 5 days. When the drug was withdrawn the number of excretors rose again.—Report of a Joint ICMR-GWB-WHO Cholera Study Group, Calcutta, India, *Bull. Wld Hlth Org.*, 1971, *45*, 451.

Prophylaxis. A recommendation that tetracycline 250 mg four times daily should be given prophylactically when travel into an area where there is an epidemic of cholera is unavoidable, and should be continued for 2 days after leaving the area.— A. G. Higginson, *Practitioner*, 1979, *223*, 529.

For a study comparing sulfadoxine with tetracycline in the therapy of cholera contacts, see Sulfadoxine, p.1470.

Diarrhoea. Severe antibiotic-associated diarrhoea in 3 patients was not controlled by stopping the antibiotics or by symptomatic treatment. It did respond when tetracycline 250 mg four times daily was taken by mouth.— R. DeJesus and W. W. Peternel, *Gastroenterology*, 1978, *74*, 818. Vancomycin is preferable to tetracycline in the treatment of antibiotic-associated colitis.— R. Toshniwal *et al.*, *Antimicrob. Ag. Chemother.*, 1979, *16*, 167.

See also Cholera and Dysentery.

Dialysis. For details on a study of tetracycline, ampicillin, or oxacillin administered to patients undergoing dialysis, see Ampicillin, p.1096.

Dosage in renal failure. Tetracycline hydrochloride should be avoided in patients with even mild renal failure; doxycycline may be used if necessary.— G. B. Appel and H. C. Neu, *New Engl. J. Med.*, 1977, *296*, 663.

Data for predicting removal of tetracyclines by conventional haemodialysis.— T. P. Gibson and H. A. Nelson, *Clin. Pharmacokinet.*, 1977, *2*, 403. Haemodialysis has been reported to clear tetracycline from blood to a lesser extent than creatinine and urea. Peritoneal dialysis does not appear to remove significant amounts either.— A. S. Watanabe, *Drug Intell. & clin. Pharm.*, 1977, *11*, 407.

Further references: W. M. Bennett *et al.*, *Ann. intern. Med.*, 1977, *86*, 754; J. S. Cheigh, *Am. J. Med.*, 1977, *62*, 555.

Dysentery. A report of the successful use of a single 2.5-g dose of tetracycline hydrochloride in patients with diarrhoea attributed to *Shigella* spp. Some of the organisms eradicated were resistant to tetracycline *in vitro*.— L. K. Pickering *et al.*, *J. Am. med. Ass.*, 1978, *239*, 853. See also N. D. W. Lionel *et al.*, *J. trop. Med. Hyg.*, 1969, *72*, 170.

Effect on leucocyte migration. Tetracyclines inhibited leucocyte migration (leucotaxis) *in vitro*.— A. Forsgren and D. Schmeling, *Antimicrob. Ag. Chemother.*, 1977, *11*, 580.

Endocarditis. Experience gained in treating 6 patients with Q-fever endocarditis suggested that the most satisfactory therapy was probably tetracycline given in a dose of 2 g daily for a month and thereafter in a dose of 1 g daily for 6 months or a year.— A. Kristinsson and H. H. Bentall, *Lancet*, 1967, *2*, 693.

Gonorrhoea. Of 57 patients with gonorrhoea treated with 500 mg of a sustained-release preparation of tetracycline then 250 mg twice daily for 5 days 47 were cured and of these 7 developed non-gonococcal urethritis.— P. S. Silver, *Br. J. vener. Dis.*, 1975, *51*, 48.

A comparison of the treatment of gonorrhoea with tetracycline 1.5 g initially then 500 mg four times daily to a total of 9 g or single doses of spectinomycin 2 or 4 g in 4043 men and women. The minimum cure-rate for anogenital gonorrhoea was 94% with either drug although the response to spectinomycin was poor in men with oropharyngeal infection.— W. W. Karney *et al.*, *New Engl. J. Med.*, 1977, *296*, 889. See also W. M. McCormack, *ibid.*, 934.

Tetracycline has been effective in the treatment of gonorrhoea when compliance is good but it is not recommended for use in the Western Pacific or East Asia where tetracycline-resistant gonococci are a problem. A suggested dose is 500 mg four times daily by mouth for 4½ days. The effectiveness of this dose against incubating syphilis is unknown.— *Neisseria gonorrhoeae and gonococcal infections*, Report of a WHO Scientific Group, *Tech. Rep. Ser. Wld Hlth Org. No. 616*, 1978. The same dose of tetracycline hydrochloride, taken for 5 days, is one regimen recommended for uncomplicated gonococcal infections by the US Public Health Service and may be used in patients allergic to penicillin; single-dose therapy is ineffective. Penicillin-resistant infections should be treated with spectinomycin.— *Morb. Mortal.*, 1979, *28*, 13.

Tetracycline is less effective than either procaine penicillin or ampicillin (plus probenecid) for treating rectal gonorrhoea in men.— D. A. Lebedeff and E. B. Hochman, *Ann. intern. Med.*, 1980, *92*, 463.

Tetracyclines by mouth may be supplemented by the insertion of 125-mg tetracycline hydrochloride suppositories once daily for 4 days in the treatment of anorectal gonorrhoea.— H. H. Neumann (letter), *J. Am. med. Ass.*, 1980, *244*, 1437.

Herpetiform ulcers. Symptomatic relief could be obtained in acute herpes infections of the mouth by using a mouth-wash prepared by adding the contents of a 250-mg capsule to warm water. Alternatively a liquid preparation could be given four times daily in doses of 250 mg rinsed around the mouth before swallowing.— A. D. Macalister, *Drugs*, 1973, *5*, 453. See also T. Lehner, *Br. dent. J.*, 1967, *122*, 15; W. R. Tyldesley, *ibid.*, 1973, *135*, 449.

Malaria. For rapid control of symptoms and asexual parasitaemia, quinine should be used in addition to tetracycline in the treatment of non-immune or moderately ill patients with chloroquine-resistant falciparum malaria.— E. J. Colwell (letter), *J. R. Soc. trop. Med. Hyg.*, 1973, *67*, 612.

Further references: E. J. Colwell *et al.*, *J. Am. med. Ass.*, 1972, *220*, 684; A. B. G. Laing (letter), *Trans. R. Soc. trop. Med. Hyg.*, 1972, *66*, 956.

Malignant effusions. Comment on the instillation of tetracycline for the management of malignant effusions.— *Lancet*, 1981, *1*, 198.

Tetracycline was successfully used in the management of cardiac tamponade secondary to malignant pericardial effusion in 6 patients. A solution of 0.5 to 1 g of tetracycline hydrochloride dissolved in 20 ml of sterile saline was instilled intrapericardially, the cannula flushed with a further 30 ml of saline, and the whole procedure repeated every 48 to 96 hours until total sclerosis occurred or no more fluid could be drained.— S. Davis *et al.*, *New Engl. J. Med.*, 1978, *299*, 1113.

It was recommended that 15 ml of lignocaine hydrochloride solution 1% should be added when tetracycline, 1 g in 60 ml of sodium chloride solution 0.9%, is administered intrapleurally.— G. N. Fox (letter), *J. Am. med. Ass.*, 1979, *242*, 1362.

For reports on the use of tetracycline by instillation in the treatment of pleural effusions, see P. G. Jenkins and W. D. Shelp, *J. Am. med. Ass.*, 1974, *230*, 587; H. W. Wallach, *Chest*, 1975, *68*, 510.

Malignant neoplasms. The results of a retrospective study of 218 patients with tumours of the larynx or nasopharynx, who had subsequently died, suggested that the addition of tetracyclines to their treatment had prolonged the survival of some patients. Inhibition of mitochondrial protein synthesis by the tetracyclines was proposed as a possible mechanism of this effect.— J. A. Leezenberg *et al.*, *Eur. J. clin. Pharmac.*, 1979, *16*, 237.

Diagnosis. An account of the pre-operative use of tetracycline in conjunction with u.v. light to delineate brain tumours in 45 patients.— W. E. Goldhahn, *Arzneimittel-Forsch.*, 1967, *17*, 139.

The detection of gastric carcinoma using the tetracycline fluorescence test.— F. Bobien, *Münch. med. Wschr.*, 1967, *109*, 1503.

Bladder tumours were diagnosed in patients given tetracycline when epithelial cells radiated a bright yellow fluorescence.— M. Kafkas, *J. Urol.*, 1977, *117*, 581.

Melioidosis. Patients with pulmonary melioidosis caused by *Pseudomonas pseudomallei* responded rapidly to treatment with tetracycline. The dosage was 3 g daily for at least 30 days, or until lung cavities had closed and chest X-rays were either normal or revealed only stable residual scars.— M. Spotnitz *et al.*, *J. Am. med. Ass.*, 1967, *202*, 950.

A report of the successful use of massive doses of tetracycline in a patient with chronic melioidosis.— K. V. Smith *et al.*, *Med. J. Aust.*, 1975, *2*, 479.

Meningitis. The successful treatment of 2 infants with meningitis caused by strains of *Mycoplasma hominis* sensitive to chloramphenicol and tetracycline in one and gentamicin and tetracycline in the other.— M. Gewitz *et al.*, *Archs Dis. Childh.*, 1979, *54*, 231.

Pelvic inflammatory disease. In a randomised study 120 women with acute pelvic inflammatory disease were given tetracycline 1.5 g initially then 500 mg four times daily for 10 days, while a further 62 received procaine penicillin 4.8 g intramuscularly and probenecid 1 g by mouth followed by ampicillin 500 mg four times daily for 10 days. Both regimens were equally effective. Mild nausea was reported with ampicillin; 4 women in the tetracycline group had to transfer to penicillin as a result of nausea and vomiting.— F. G. Cunningham *et al.*, *New Engl. J. Med.*, 1977, *296*, 1380.

Plague. Prompt treatment was essential in human plague especially in the pneumonic type where it was necessary to start specific treatment within 15 hours of overt illness if it was to have a favourable effect on the outcome of the disease. Tetracycline was the recommended treatment for bubonic and pneumonic plague. It should be given in a dosage of 4 to 6 g daily during the first 48 hours. Intravenous therapy, in conjunction with treatment by mouth if tolerated, was essential for the treatment of severely ill patients. Streptomycin, though effective, caused severe intoxication and should be given with other antibiotics, in doses of 500 mg intramuscularly 4-hourly for 2 days, followed by 500 mg six-hourly until clinical improvement had occurred. Chloramphenicol given in a dose of 50 to 75 mg per kg body-weight had also been given by mouth up to a total dose of 20 to 25 g. Sulphadiazine 12 g daily for 4 to 7 days had reduced mortality in bubonic plague but not in the pneumonic disease. Less severe infections had been treated with a 4-g initial dose, 2 g four-hourly until the temperature was normal, and 500 mg four-hourly to complete a course of 7 to 10 days.— *Tech. Rep. Ser. Wld Hlth Org. No. 447*, 1970.

Pneumonia. Tetracyclines were ineffective in preventing or treating bacterial pneumonia complicating viral pneumonia in 35 patients.— C. Ellenbogen *et al.*, *Am. J. Med.*, 1974, *56*, 169.

Q fever. Tetracycline was effective *in vitro* against *Coxiella burnetii* but it appeared to have little effect on the recovery-rate of the average patient with Q fever.— G. L. Brown, *Br. med. J.*, 1973, *2*, 43.

See also under Endocarditis.

Reiter's disease. Tetracycline, 250 mg six-hourly for about 7 days, was recommended, together with rest, to control the genital infection but not the arthritic aspect of Reiter's disease.— *Br. med. J.*, 1969, *4*, 576.

Relapsing fever, louse-borne. In 10 patients with louse-borne relapsing fever, treatment with tetracycline, 250 mg intravenously, was rapidly effective in achieving disappearance of spirochaetes but was followed by severe haemodynamic changes. Shortly after the disappearance of the spirochaetes from peripheral blood the patients became confused and restless with pyrexia and increased heart-rate, blood pressure, and respiration-rate. The increase in the blood pressure was transient but the other symptoms were more persistent. Some 1 to 2 hours later the central venous pressure and the arterial pressure fell to be followed by a rise in the central venous pressure, in most cases to the levels from which it had fallen but in some cases to pathologically high levels. It was suggested that the changes might explain why deaths sometimes occurred during the early treatment of louse-borne relapsing fever.— E. H. O. Parry *et al.*, *Lancet*, 1967, *1*, 81. The reaction could be controlled by hydrocortisone given in a dose of at least 4.5 mg per kg body-weight intravenously and supplemented by prednisone in a dose of 1.5 mg per kg by mouth daily for at least 48 hours and then gradually reduced.— G. E. Breen (letter), *ibid.*, 158.

The successful use of a combination of tetracycline and procaine penicillin in the treatment of louse-borne relapsing fever in 160 patients.— S. Y. Salih and D.

Mustafa, *Trans. R. Soc. trop. Med. Hyg.*, 1977, *71*, 49.

In an evaluation of single-dose antibiotic regimens in patients with louse-borne relapsing fever due to *Borrelia recurrentis*, 21 patients were given either tetracycline or erythromycin by mouth and 30 received either tetracycline 250 mg intravenously or procaine penicillin 600 mg intramuscularly. Although tetracycline given intravenously was superior to procaine penicillin, the treatment of choice was considered to be a single 500-mg dose of tetracycline or erythromycin by mouth. In 15 similar patients given paracetamol 650 mg, hydrocortisone sodium succinate 500 mg intravenously, or no drug 2 hours before and 2 hours after a dose of erythromycin, rigor was not prevented although defervescence occurred earlier in those given hydrocortisone. The best management of a possible Jarisch-Herxheimer reaction was considered to be the prophylactic infusion of sodium chloride injection to prevent hypotension.— T. Butler *et al.*, *J. infect. Dis.*, 1978, *137*, 573.

Skin disorders. *Acne.* A review of the pathogenesis and treatment of acne vulgaris, including the systemic use of tetracycline and erythromycin in moderate to severe acne. Doses may vary from 250 mg twice daily in moderate acne to 1 g or more daily in severe acne. Treatment for at least 6 months is recommended, during which time dosage may be reduced.— W. J. Cunliffe, *Br. med. J.*, 1980, *280*, 1394. The systemic dose of tetracycline in acne usually varies from 250 mg to 2 g daily. Erythromycin may be useful when tetracycline is contra-indicated or ineffective. Topical tetracycline may be effective in some patients with mild acne; its main disadvantage is yellow discoloration of the skin and fluorescence under 'black light' used in discotheques.— *Med. Lett.*, 1980, *22*, 31.

In 13 patients with acne treated for 3 months with tetracycline 250 mg daily there was significant clinical improvement associated with a mean serum-tetracycline concentration of 1.98 µg per ml. The free fatty acid and cholesterol content of the skin lipids fell and the triglyceride content rose. There was no significant change in the bacterial count. It was suggested that tetracycline acted by inhibition of extracellular lipases.— W. J. Cunliffe *et al.*, *Br. med. J.*, 1973, *4*, 332.

In 13 patients with acne vulgaris, given tetracycline hydrochloride 800 mg daily for 5 days then 100 mg daily for about 2 months, strains of *Escherichia coli* resistant to tetracycline were found in 80% of faecal samples during treatment compared with only 27% of samples before treatment. Patients having multiresistant strains rose from 18% to 48%.— M. V. Valtonen *et al.*, *Br. J. Derm.*, 1976, *95*, 311.

Tetracycline in high doses of up to 2 g daily was effective in patients with the most severe forms of acne, although one patient with conglobated acne took 3.5 g daily for the first 3 months of treatment and still required 1 g daily 22 months later. It was suggested that liver, kidney, and haematological functions should be monitored during high-dose treatment.— R. L. Baer *et al.*, *Archs Derm.*, 1976, *112*, 479.

Further references: Ad Hoc Committee on the Use of Antibiotics in Dermatology, *Archs Derm.*, 1975, *111*, 1630; R. Jackson, *Can. med. Ass. J.*, 1976, *115*, 838; K. Liddell, *Practitioner*, 1978, *221*, 783; M. I. Marks, *Drugs*, 1978, *16*, 202; J. E. Rasmussen, *Pediat. Clins N.Am.*, 1978, *25*, 285; W. J. Cunliffe *et al.*, *Br. J. Derm.*, 1979, *101*, 321; A. A. Fisher, *Cutis*, 1980, *25*, 474.

Perioral dermatitis. Perioral dermatitis resulting from the use of potent topical corticosteroids may be cured in most patients by a 6-to 8-week course of systemic tetracyclines.— *Lancet*, 1980, *1*, 75. A suggested course of treatment is oxytetracycline 250 mg twice daily for 4 weeks, followed by a further month's treatment with one tablet daily, and the withdrawal of all topical corticosteroids as soon as possible.— *Br. med. J.*, 1980, *280*, 136.

Rosacea. In a study of tetracycline therapy in rosacea, patients received tetracycline 250 mg twice daily or a placebo for 1 month. All patients then received this dose of tetracycline for a further month. At the end of the first month 47 had improved, 28 having received tetracycline and 19 the placebo. There was no improvement in 31, of whom 23 had received the placebo and 8 tetracycline. In the second month, 17 of the 23 patients who showed no improvement with the placebo cleared when given tetracycline. Only 6 of the 78 patients failed to show improvement by the end of the trial. A number of patients required small maintenance doses of tetracycline to prevent relapse.— I. B. Sneddon, *Br. J. Derm.*, 1966, *78*, 649.

A dose of tetracycline of 250 mg once daily is usually adequate in the treatment of rosacea; it might have to be taken permanently.— *Br. med. J.*, 1978, *2*, 750.

Further references: A. G. Knight and C. F. H. Vickers, *Br. J. Derm.*, 1975, *93*, 577.

Sprue. *For reports of the use of tetracycline in the treatment of tropical sprue and other malabsorption syndromes, see Martindale 27th Edn,* p. 1192.

Surgical infection prophylaxis. Irrigation of appendicectomy wounds with tetracycline 250 mg in sodium chloride injection 50 ml reduced the incidence of infection from 7 of 30 control patients to 3 of 41 treated patients.— E. A. Benson *et al.* (letter), *Lancet*, 1973, *2*, 322.

For a similar report of tetracycline reducing the duration of fever in patients undergoing appendicectomy for perforated appendix, see Ampicillin, p.1097.

Syphilis. The US Public Health Service recommended tetracycline hydrochloride 500 mg taken four times daily for 15 days as one regimen for the treatment of early syphilis in patients who were allergic to penicillin.— *Obstet. Gynec.*, 1976, *48*, 727.

Toxoplasmosis. For reference to tetracyclines in the treatment of toxoplasmosis, see Oxytetracycline, p.1197.

Trachoma. In a study in which 1300 children with trachoma were treated with 1% ointments of tetracycline hydrochloride or chlortetracycline there was no conclusive evidence of the superior efficacy of either preparation. Administration was by twice-daily applications on 5 consecutive days every 4 weeks for 6 months. The initial cure-rate was high, but during a 4-year follow-up it was found that 1 year after withdrawal of treatment the relapse-rate was about 25%. The use of 2 courses did not have any significantly greater effect than 1 course of treatment.— F. A. Assaad *et al.*, *Bull. Wld Hlth Org.*, 1968, *38*, 565.

Tetracycline 1% in polyvinyl alcohol 1.4% was considered a suitable alternative to tetracycline in oil for use as eye-drops in trachoma.— M. M. O. Beiram, *Sudan med. J.*, 1970, *8*, 215, per *Trop. Dis. Bull.*, 1971, *68*, 1115.

The WHO-recommended scheme for the control of communicable ophthalmia consisted of the application of a tetracycline eye ointment to both eyes once, or preferably twice, daily for 5 days each month for 3, or preferably 6 months. It should form the basis of mass control programmes although other methods are under investigation.— B. R. Jones *et al.*, *Br. J. Ophthal.*, 1976, *60*, 492.

Intermittent once-daily application to the eyes of an oily suspension or an ointment containing tetracycline, oxytetracycline, or chlortetracycline was almost as effective as twice-daily application in the treatment of trachoma and has been responsible for improvement of cure-rates, particularly in the Sudan. The prevalence of active trachoma in rural areas fell from 39.9% to 4.7% after treatment; among children under 10 years of age the prevalence rate fell from 54% to 7.2%. Treatment was also effective among schoolchildren in Afghanistan, Ethiopia, Iraq, Kuwait, and Syria. The incidence of impairment of vision and blindness due to trachoma fell from 10.2% to 0.9% in one area of Ethiopia although the prevalence of active trachoma there dropped from 73.6% to 61.2% after treatment.— *Chronicle Wld Hlth Org.*, 1976, *30*, 97.

Immediate intensive treatment with tetracycline 1% eye-drops was recommended in the treatment of trachoma inclusion conjunctivitis (TRIC) ophthalmia neonatorum. The drops should be instilled every minute for half an hour, every 5 minutes for one hour, and then hourly until clinical cure. After a few days the drops can be changed to tetracycline eye ointment used every 2 to 4 hours.— C. A. Brown, *Practitioner*, 1978, *220*, 16.

Further references: C. R. Dawson *et al.*, *Lancet*, 1967, *2*, 961; G. W. Csonka and E. D. Coufalik, *Postgrad. med. J.*, 1977, *53*, 592.

Urinary-tract infections. A review of the management of nongonococcal urethritis (preferred to the term non-specific urethritis). The main causes of nongonococcal urethritis are *Chlamydia trachomatis* and *Ureaplasma urealyticum* (formerly called 'T-strain' mycoplasma) and tetracyclines are the antimicrobial agents of choice, the recommended regimen being tetracycline 250 mg four times daily for 2 weeks. Shorter courses of treatment, especially if less than one week, are almost certainly suboptimal. Erythromycin is the antibiotic of choice for patients intolerant of tetracyclines and for pregnant women.— J. D. Oriel, *Drugs*, 1979, *18*, 398. An earlier review.— J. C. Simopoulos, *Br. J. vener. Dis.*, 1977, *53*, 230.

A triple tetracycline preparation (Deteclo) was given in a dose of 300 mg twice daily for 21 days to 107 patients with non-specific urethritis. Of those followed up 1 patient failed to respond when seen after 1 month, 5 after 2 months, and 6 after 3 months—an estimated failure-rate of 11.9%.— M. N. Bhattacharyya and R. S. Morton, *Br. J. vener. Dis.*, 1973, *49*, 521. In a study involving 756 patients with non-specific urethritis, triple tetracycline (Deteclo) 300 mg taken twice daily for 3 weeks was more effective than treatment with oxytetracycline or doxycycline.— O. P. Arya *et al.*, *Br. J. vener. Dis.*, 1978, *54*, 414.

In a comparative study of 86 patients with acute urinary-tract infections, treatment with doxycycline or minocycline offered no advantage over the use of tetracycline phosphate complex.— W. J. Mogabgab and B. Pollock, *Curr. ther. Res.*, 1977, *22*, 172.

A report of a study in 59 women with uterine chlamydial infections given oxytetracycline 250 mg four times daily or doxycycline 100 mg daily for 5 to 7 days. The results of this small study suggested that short courses of tetracycline are as apparently effective in eradicating chlamydia from the cervix as 21-day courses.— J. Hunter *et al.* (letter), *Lancet*, 1979, *2*, 848.

See also Chlamydial Infections (above).

Vaginitis. For a report on the use of a tetracycline in *Gardnerella vaginalis (Haemophilus vaginalis)* vaginitis, see Oxytetracycline, p.1197.

Preparations

Capsules

Tetracycline Capsules *(B.P.).* Capsules containing tetracycline hydrochloride. The *B.P.* requires 70% dissolution in 45 minutes. Store at a temperature not exceeding 30°. *U.S.P.* (Tetracycline Hydrochloride Capsules) specifies 50, 100, 125, 250, or 500 mg. Store in airtight containers. Protect from light.

Eye Ointments

Tetracycline Hydrochloride Ophthalmic Ointment *(U.S.P.).* A sterile eye ointment containing tetracycline hydrochloride 1%.

Injections

Tetracycline and Procaine Injection *(B.P.C. 1973).* A sterile solution of tetracycline hydrochloride and procaine hydrochloride in Water for Injections, prepared by dissolving the sterile contents of a sealed container in the requisite amount of Water for Injections; the sealed container also contains suitable buffering and stabilising agents. The injection deteriorates on storage and should be used within 24 hours of preparation.

Tetracycline Hydrochloride for Injection *(U.S.P.).* A sterile dry mixture of tetracycline hydrochloride; one form contains magnesium chloride or magnesium ascorbate and one or more suitable buffers and may contain one or more suitable preservatives, solubilising, stabilising, and anaesthetic agents; the other form contains one or more suitable stabilising agents. If it contains an anaesthetic agent it is intended for intramuscular use only. A 1% solution has a pH of 2 to 3. Protect from light. The injection is prepared by the addition of diluent before use.

Tetracycline Injection *(B.P.).* Tetracycline Hydrochloride Injection. A sterile solution of tetracycline hydrochloride in Water for Injections, prepared by dissolving the sterile contents of a sealed container in the requisite amount of Water for Injections; the sealed container also contains a suitable buffering agent. A 10% injection has a pH of 2 to 3. The injection should be stored at a temperature not exceeding 4° and used within 72 hours of preparation. For intravenous use only in a well-diluted solution.

Mixtures

Tetracycline Mixture *(B.P.C. 1973).* Tetracycline Mouth-bath; Tetracycline Elixir; Tetracycline Syrup. A suspension of tetracycline in a suitable coloured flavoured vehicle. When a dose less than 5 ml is prescribed, the mixture should be diluted to 5 ml with syrup. Such dilutions must be freshly prepared and not used more than 2 weeks after issue. Store in a cool place. Protect from light. *Dose.* The equivalent of tetracycline hydrochloride, every 6 hours: children under 1 year, 25 to 62.5 mg; 1 to 5 years, 62.5 to 125 mg; 6 to 12 years, 250 mg. When used as a mouth-bath 10 ml containing the equivalent of 250 mg of tetracycline hydrochloride is held in the mouth for 2 or 3 minutes thrice daily.

Solutions

Tetracycline Hydrochloride for Topical Solution *(U.S.P.).* A dry mixture of tetracycline hydrochloride with 4-epitetracycline hydrochloride and sodium metabisulphite, with a suitable aqueous vehicle. Store in airtight containers. Protect from light. The solution is prepared by the addition of the diluent before issue and contains 2.2 mg of tetracycline hydrochloride per ml. pH 2.8 to 4.4.

Suspensions

Tetracycline for Oral Suspension *(U.S.P.).* A dry mixture of tetracycline with one or more suitable colouring, flavouring, and suspending agents. Store in airtight containers. Protect from light. The suspension is prepared by the addition of diluent before issue and contains the equivalent of 50 mg of tetracycline hydrochloride per ml. pH 4.0 to 6.5.

Tetracycline Hydrochloride Ophthalmic Suspension *(U.S.P.)*. A sterile suspension of tetracycline hydrochloride 1% in a suitable oil. Store in airtight containers. Protect from light.

Tetracycline Oral Suspension *(U.S.P.)*. A suspension of tetracycline with or without one or more suitable buffers, preservatives, stabilising, and suspending agents; pH 3.5 to 6.0. It contains the equivalent of 25 mg of tetracycline hydrochloride per ml. Store in airtight containers. Protect from light.

Tablets

Tetracycline Tablets *(B.P.)*. Tablets containing tetracycline hydrochloride. They are coated. The *B.P* requires 70% dissolution in 45 minutes. *U.S.P.* (Tetracycline Hydrochloride Tablets) specifies 250 or 500 mg. Store in airtight containers. Protect from light.

Proprietary Preparations

Achromycin *(Lederle, UK)*. Preparations for oral use, available as **Capsules** and **Tablets** each containing 250 mg of tetracycline hydrochloride; as **Syrup** containing tetracycline equivalent to tetracycline hydrochloride 125 mg in each 5 ml (suggested diluent, syrup); and as **Powder** (tetracycline hydrochloride). (Also available as Achromycin in *Austral., Canad., Denm., Ger., Neth., Norw., S.Afr., Swed., Switz., USA*).

Achromycin *(Lederle, UK)*. Preparations containing tetracycline hydrochloride for topical use, available as **Eye/Ear Ointment** containing 1%; as **Ointment** containing 3%, with hydroxybenzoates, in a basis of soft paraffin and wool fat; and as **Ophthalmic Oil Suspension** containing 1% in sesame oil.

Achromycin Intramuscular *(Lederle, UK)*. Tetracycline hydrochloride, available in vials of 100 mg with procaine hydrochloride 40 mg and magnesium chloride 46.84 mg, buffered with ascorbic acid 250 mg, for solution before use.

Achromycin Intravenous *(Lederle, UK)*. Tetracycline hydrochloride buffered with ascorbic acid (625 or 1250 mg), in vials of 250 and 500 mg, for solution before use.

Achromycin V Capsules *(Lederle, UK)*. Each contains tetracycline equivalent to 250 mg of the hydrochloride, buffered with sodium metaphosphate. **Achromycin V Syrup**. Contains in each 5 ml tetracycline equivalent to tetracycline hydrochloride 125 mg, buffered with citric acid and sodium citrate (dilution not recommended). (Also available as Achromycin V in *Austral., Canad., Switz., USA*).

Chymocyclar *(Armour, UK)*. Capsules each containing tetracycline hydrochloride 250 mg and, in an enteric-coated core, proteolytic activity (provided by a concentrate of trypsin and chymotrypsin) 50 000 Armour units. For bacterial infections. *Dose*. 1 or 2 capsules 4 times daily, 30 minutes before meals.

Co-Caps Tetracycline *(Co-Caps, UK)*. Tetracycline hydrochloride, available as capsules of 250 mg.

Deteclo *(Lederle, UK)*. **Tablets** each containing tetracycline hydrochloride 115.4 mg, chlortetracycline hydrochloride 115.4 mg, and demeclocycline hydrochloride 69.2 mg, and **Syrup** (supplied as powder for preparation with water before use) containing the equivalent of one-quarter of the above amounts in each 5 ml (dilution not recommended). *Dose*. 1 tablet or 20 ml of syrup every 12 hours; children, 5 to 9 years, 5 ml of syrup twice daily; 9 to 15 years (less than 40 kg) 5 ml three times daily; 9 to 15 years (more than 40 kg) 10 ml twice daily.

Economycin *(DDSA Pharmaceuticals, UK)*. Tetracycline hydrochloride, available as **Capsules** and **Tablets** of 250 mg.

Mysteclin *(Squibb, UK)*. **Capsules** each containing tetracycline hydrochloride 250 mg and nystatin 250 000 units; **Syrup** containing in each 5 ml tetracycline hydrochloride equivalent to tetracycline 125 mg and amphotericin 25 mg (suggested diluent, syrup); and **Tablets** each containing tetracycline hydrochloride 250 mg and nystatin 250 000 units. For bacterial infections in patients liable to candidiasis. *Dose*. 1 capsule, 10 ml of syrup, or 1 tablet 4 times daily; children, approximately 1 to 2 ml of syrup per kg body-weight daily.

Sustamycin Capsules *(MCP Pharmaceuticals, UK)*. Each contains tetracycline hydrochloride 250 mg in a sustained-release basis. *Dose*. 2 capsules initially, then 1 every 12 hours.

Tetrabid-Organon *(Organon, UK)*. Sustained-release capsules each containing tetracycline hydrochloride 250 mg and fumaric acid ($C_4H_4O_4$=116) 33 mg. *Dose*. 2 capsules initially, then 1 capsule every 12 hours.

Tetrachel *(Berk Pharmaceuticals, UK)*. **Capsules** and **Tablets** each containing tetracycline hydrochloride 250 mg, and **Syrup** containing in each 5 ml tetracycline equivalent to 125 mg of the hydrochloride (suggested diluent, syrup). (Also available as Tetrachel in *Neth., USA*).

Tetracyn *(Pfizer, UK)*. Tetracycline hydrochloride, available as **Capsules** and **Tablets** each containing the equivalent of tetracycline 250 mg. (Also available as Tetracyn in *Austral., Canad., USA*).

Tetracyn Intramuscular *(Pfizer, UK)*. Tetracycline hydrochloride, available in vials containing the equivalent of tetracycline 100 mg with procaine hydrochloride 40 mg, magnesium chloride 100 mg, and ascorbic acid 250 mg, for solution before use.

Tetracyn S.F *(Pfizer, UK)*. Capsules each containing tetracycline hydrochloride equivalent to tetracycline 250 mg, ascorbic acid 75 mg, thiamine mononitrate 2.5 mg, riboflavine 2.5 mg, and nicotinamide 25 mg. *Dose*. 1 capsule 4 times daily.

Other Proprietary Names for Tetracycline and Tetracycline Hydrochloride

Arg.— Acromicina, Ciclotetryl, Omnaze, Pervasol, Steclin; *Austral.*— Austramycin, Austramycin V, Hostacycline, Hydracycline, Panmycin M, Panmycin P, Polycycline, Quadcin, Quatrax, Steclin-V, Tetracap, Tetracyn-V, Tetramykoin; *Belg.*— Hostacycline; *Canad.*— Bio-Tetra, Cefracycline, Medicycline, Novotetra, T-Caps, Tetracrine, Tetralean, Triacycline; *Denm.*— Dumocyclin, Tetranovin; *Fr.*— Florocycline, Sifacycline (cyclohexylsulphamate); *Ger.*— Akne-Pyodron Kur, Hostacyclin, Remicyclin, Steclin, Supramycin N, Tefilin, Tetrabakat, Tetrablet, Tetracitro, Tetralution; *Ital.*— Acromicina, Ambramicina, Archiciclina, Binicap (see also tetracycline phosphate complex), Calociclina, Ibicyn, Tetrabioptal, Tetraplus, Ultraciclina, Unitetra; *Jap.*— NC; *Neth.*— Tetrarco; *Norw.*— Dumocyclin; *S.Afr.*— Cyclabid, Gammatet, Hostacycline, Riocyclin, Steclin-V; *Spain*— Acromicina, Ambramicina, Bristaciclina, Fermentmycin, Friciclin, Hostaciclina, Roviciclina, Sanbiotetra, Teciclina, Teclinazets, Tetra-B, Tetra-Liser, Tetraciclene, Tetralen, Tetrarco Simple, Zyler; *Switz.*— Diocyclin, Grocyclin, Hostacyclin, Mephacyclin, Tetramavan, Tetrarco LA, Tetraseptin, Tetrasuiss, Tetrivo Bicaps, Triphacyclin; *USA*— Bristacycline, Centet, Cyclopar, Panmycin, Piracaps, Retet, Retet-S, Robitet, Sumycin, Topicycline, U-Tet.

Tetracycline hydrochloride was also formerly marketed in Great Britain under the proprietary names Oppacyn (*Oppenheimer*, now *LRC Products*), Steclin (*Squibb*), and Totomycin (*Boots*).

170-s

Tetracycline Phosphate Complex *(U.S.P.)*.

CAS — 1336-20-5.

Pharmacopoeias. In *U.S. Jap. P.* includes Tetracyclini Metaphosphas ($C_{22}H_{24}N_2O_8$,HPO_3,1/5$NaPO_3$=544.8).

A yellow crystalline powder with a faint characteristic odour and a potency of not less than 750 µg per mg, as tetracycline hydrochloride, calculated on the anhydrous substance. **Soluble** 1 in 31 of water, 1 in 130 of alcohol, and 1 in 100 of methyl alcohol; very slightly soluble in acetone. **Store** in airtight containers. Protect from light.

Small amounts of anhydrotetracycline and epianhydrotetracycline were found in newly manufactured tetracycline phosphate preparations. Storage in warm humid conditions increased the percentage of these degradation products.— V. C. Walton *et al., J. pharm. Sci.*, 1970, *59*, 1160.

Tetracycline phosphate complex has the same actions and uses as tetracycline hydrochloride (see p.1217) but has been claimed to be more readily absorbed. It has been given in doses equivalent to 250 to 500 mg of tetracycline hydrochloride.

The administration of tetracycline phosphate complex, 500 mg every 12 hours to 10 healthy subjects resulted in mean serum concentrations of about 1.5 µg per ml after 2 hours, falling to 0.64 µg after 12 hours, rising and maintained between 2 and 4 µg after the first 24 hours' treatment. About 95 mg of the drug was recovered from the urine during the first 24 hours.— L. P. Olon and D. N. Holvey, *Clin. Med.*, 1968, *75* (Jan.), 33.

Tissue concentrations of tetracycline following the administration of tetracycline complex by mouth.— G. Racz, *Curr. ther. Res.*, 1971, *13*, 553.

Preparations

Tetracycline Phosphate Complex Capsules *(U.S.P.)*. Capsules containing tetracycline phosphate complex equivalent to tetracycline hydrochloride 50, 100, 125, 250, or 500 mg. Store in airtight containers. Protect from light.

Tetracycline Phosphate Complex for Injection *(U.S.P.)*. A sterile dry mixture of tetracycline phosphate complex and magnesium chloride or magnesium ascorbate and one or more suitable buffers. It may contain one or more suitable preservatives, anaesthetic, solubilising, and stabilising agents. Potency is expressed in terms of the equivalent amount of tetracycline hydrochloride. The injection is prepared by the addition of diluent before use. A 1% solution has a pH of 2 to 3.

Proprietary Preparations

Tetrex *(Bristol-Myers Pharmaceuticals, UK)*. Tetracycline phosphate complex, available as capsules each containing the equivalent of 250 mg of tetracycline hydrochloride. (Also available as Tetrex in *Austral., Belg., Canad., Ital., S.Afr., Switz., USA*).

Other Proprietary Names

Austral.—Hostacycline-P; *Fr.*—Hexacycline; *Ital.*—Binicap (see also tetracycline hydrochloride), Conciclina; *S.Afr.*—Hostacycline-P; *Spain*—Biocheclina, Bristaciclina Retard, Ciclindif Infantil, Tetramin, Tetrazetas Retard; *Swed.*—Tetradecin Novum.

171-w

Thiamphenicol *(B.P.)*.

CB 8053; Win 5063-2; Dextrosulphenidol; Tiamfenicolo; Thiophenicol. 2,2-Dichloro-*N*-[(αR,βR)-β-hydroxy-α-hydroxymethyl-4-mesylphenethyl]acetamide.

$C_{12}H_{15}Cl_2NO_5S$=356.2.

CAS — 15318-45-3.

NOTE. Racephenicol is the racemic form of thiamphenicol.

Pharmacopoeias. In *Br.* and *It.*

A fine white to yellowish-white odourless crystalline powder with a bitter taste. M.p. 163° to 167°. Slightly **soluble** in water, ether, and ethyl acetate; soluble in methyl alcohol; sparingly soluble in dehydrated alcohol and acetone; very slightly soluble in chloroform; freely soluble in dimethylformamide and acetonitrile; very soluble in dimethylacetamide. A solution in dehydrated alcohol is dextrorotatory; a solution in dimethylformamide is laevorotatory. A saturated solution in water has a pH of 5.8 to 7.5. **Store** in airtight containers. Protect from light.

172-e

Thiamphenicol Glycinate Hydrochloride.

Thiamphenicol Aminoacetate Hydrochloride; Tiamfenicolo Glicinato Cloridrato. (2*R*,3*R*)-2-(2,2-Dichloroacetamido)-3-hydroxy-3-(4-mesylphenyl)propyl glycinate hydrochloride.

$C_{14}H_{18}Cl_2N_2O_6S$,HCl=449.7.

CAS — 2393-92-2 (thiamphenicol glycinate).

Pharmacopoeias. In *It.*

A sterile, white to slightly yellow, odourless, crystalline powder with a bitter taste. Thiamphenicol glycinate hydrochloride 1.26 g is approximately equivalent to 1 g of thiamphenicol. Freely **soluble** in water; slightly soluble in alcohol; practically insoluble in chloroform and ether. A 5% solution in water has a pH of 3 to 4.5. **Store** in a cool place in airtight containers. Protect from light.

Thiamphenicol was incompatible with *canrenoate potassium, hydrocortisone sodium succinate*, and *hydroxydione succinate* in an infusion fluid.— B. Flouvat and P. Lechat, *Thérapie*, 1974, *29*, 337.

Adverse Effects, Treatment, and Precautions. As for Chloramphenicol, p.1137.

Thiamphenicol is probably more liable to cause

reversible depression of the bone marrow than chloramphenicol but there have been fewer reports of aplasia so far.

Doses of thiamphenicol should be reduced in patients with renal impairment.

Blood disorders. References to the haematological side-effects of thiamphenicol: E. Gluckman *et al.*, *Nouv. Presse méd.*, 1971, *79*, 1385; J. P. Kaltwasser *et al.*, *Arzneimittel-Forsch.*, 1974, *24*, 190; *idem*, 343 and 561; J. P. Kaltwasser *et al.*, *Klin. Wschr.*, 1973, *51*, 347; R. Franceschinis, *Arzneimittel-Forsch.*, 1974, *24*, 944; A. Cornet *et al.*, *Sem. Hôp. Paris*, 1974, *50*, 1567.

Peripheral neuritis. Reports of peripheral neuritis due to thiamphenicol.— *Japan med. Gaz.*, 1977, *14* (Dec. 20), 12; Y. Shinohara *et al.*, *Eur. Neurol.*, 1977, *16*, 161.

Antimicrobial Action. Thiamphenicol has a broad spectrum of activity resembling that of chloramphenicol (see p.1138) although in general it is less active.

Cross-resistance has been reported between thiamphenicol and chloramphenicol.

Thiamphenicol inhibited 97.5, 99.6, and 100% of 517 strains of *Neisseria gonorrhoeae* at concentrations of 2, 4, and 8 μg per ml respectively and inhibited 76.9 and 100% of 13 beta-lactamase-producing strains of *N. gonorrhoeae* at concentrations of 2 and 4 μg per ml respectively.— P. D. Duck *et al.*, *Antimicrob. Ag. Chemother.*, 1978, *14*, 788.

Absorption and Fate. Thiamphenicol is absorbed from the gastro-intestinal tract following oral administration and serum concentrations of 3 to 6 μg per ml have been achieved 2 hours after a 500-mg dose. Concentrations from about 7 to 13 μg per ml have been reported one hour after 500 mg administered intramuscularly.

Thiamphenicol has been reported to diffuse into the cerebrospinal fluid, across the placenta, into breast milk, and to penetrate well into purulent and mucous sputum. Unlike chloramphenicol (see p.1139), 50 to 70% of an oral dose of thiamphenicol is excreted unchanged in the urine in 24 hours; only 5 to 10% is conjugated with glucuronic acid in the liver. It is also excreted in the bile.

Plasma concentrations, half-life, and urinary excretion of thiamphenicol were studied in 13 healthy subjects, 19 patients with cirrhosis of the liver, and 16 with acute viral hepatitis. Disturbed liver function did not influence the metabolism or excretion of the drug. High doses of heparin seemed to decrease the activity of thiamphenicol.— H. P. Menz *et al.*, *Arzneimittel-Forsch.*, 1974, *24*, 99.

In patients with renal failure the half-life of thiamphenicol was prolonged to 13.5 hours during the interval between dialysis treatment. During haemodialysis the half-life was still 2 to 3 times longer than in patients with normal renal function.— H. P. Menz *et al.*, *Arzneimittel-Forsch.*, 1974, *24*, 102.

The absorption and excretion of thiamphenicol palmitate in *rats* and humans.— D. D. Bella *et al.*, *Arzneimittel-Forsch.*, 1974, *24*, 836.

The pharmacokinetics of thiamphenicol were unaltered by peritoneal dialysis in anephric patients.— K. I. Furman *et al.*, *Antimicrob. Ag. Chemother.*, 1976, *9*, 557.

Concentrations of thiamphenicol in diseased kidneys.— T. A. Plomp *et al.*, *Infection*, 1978, *6*, 171.

Pregnancy and the noenate. The placental transfer of thiamphenicol.— T. A. Plomp *et al.*, *Eur. J. Obstet. Gynec. reprod. Biol.*, 1977, *7*, 383.

Uses. Thiamphenicol has been used similarly to chloramphenicol (see p.1139) in the treatment of susceptible infections. The usual adult dose is 1.5 g daily by mouth in divided doses; up to 3 g daily has been given initially in severe infections. Equivalent doses may be administered by intramuscular or intravenous injection as the more water-soluble glycinate which has also been given by aerosol inhalation.

Thiamphenicol palmitate is used in liquid preparations for oral use.

The proceedings of a symposium on the metabolism, pharmacokinetics, toxicity, actions, immunosuppressant effects, and uses of chloramphenicol and thiamphenicol.— *Postgrad. med. J.*, 1974, *50* (Oct.), *Suppl.*, 5.

A report on the use of thiamphenicol as an immunosuppressant in patients with nephritis.— D. E. Richmond, *Aust. N.Z. J. Med.*, 1979, *9*, 670.

Beneficial results with thiamphenicol in patients with non-sporing anaerobic infections.— B. M. Limson *et al.*, *Curr. ther. Res.*, 1981, *29*, 438.

Gonorrhoea. Most of the 580 patients with gonococcal urethritis appeared to be free from infection 5 days after receiving a single dose of thiamphenicol 2.5 g by mouth. Of the 11 who did not respond, some carried a gonococcal strain resistant to thiamphenicol.— E. Heinke, *Postgrad. med. J.*, 1972, *48* (Jan.), *Suppl.*, 54.

Prostatitis. Of 10 patients with chronic bacterial prostatitis who received thiamphenicol 500 mg every 8 hours for 6 weeks, 8 had a good or excellent response to treatment. Mean concentrations of thiamphenicol in blood and ejaculate were 5.3 and 2.3 μg per ml respectively 2 hours after the start of therapy and 7.3 and 13.9 μg per ml respectively after 24 hours.— T. A. Plomp *et al.*, *J. antimicrob. Chemother.*, 1978, *4*, 65. See also T. A. Plomp *et al.*, *Chemotherapy, Basle*, 1979, *25*, 254.

Salmonellal infections. A report on the use of thiamphenicol 1.5 or 2 g daily for typhoid and paratyphoid fever.— B. M. Limson *et al.*, *Curr. ther. Res.*, 1975, *17*, 335.

Proprietary Names

Flumucil *(as glycine acetylcysteinate) (Inpharzam, Belg.)*; Glitisol *(also as palmitate) (Zambon, Ital.)*; Hyrazin, Neomyson, Rincrol, Thiamcol *(all Jap.)*; Thiophénicol *(Midy, Fr.)*; Urfamycin *(Montpellier, Arg.; Rio, S.Afr.; Zambon, Spain)*; Urfamycine *(Inpharzam, Belg.; Inpharzam, Ger.; Inpharzam, Neth.; Inpharzam, Switz.)*.

173-l

Ticarcillin Sodium.

BRL 2288; Ticarcillin Disodium. The disodium salt of (6*R*)-6-[(*R*)-2-carboxy-2-(3-thienyl)acetamido]penicillanic acid.

$C_{15}H_{14}N_2Na_2O_6S_2$=428.4.

CAS — 34787-01-4 (ticarcillin); 4697-14-7; 29457-07-6 (both disodium salt).

Pharmacopoeias. In *U.S.* as Sterile Ticarcillin Disodium.

A white to pale yellow hygroscopic powder. Each g represents about 4.7 mmol (4.7 mEq) of sodium. Ticarcillin sodium 1.1 g is approximately equivalent to 1 g of ticarcillin. The *U.S.P.* specifies not less than the equivalent of 800 μg of ticarcillin per mg.

Freely **soluble** in water. A solution in water containing about 1% has a pH of 6 to 8. A 50% aqueous solution retains more than 90% of its potency for 24 hours at 25° and for 7 days at 5°. **Store** in a cool place in airtight containers.

Incompatibility. Gentamicin sulphate was reported to be gradually inactivated when mixed with ticarcillin sodium in a solution of 5% dextrose.— B. Lynn, in *Clinical Use of Combinations of Antibiotics*, J. Klastersky (Ed.), London, Hodder and Stoughton, 1975, 24.

Stability in solution. The half-life of an 0.1% solution of ticarcillin sodium at pH 2 was approximately 45 minutes at 37°. Ticarcillin in a 2% solution at 25° retained 94% of its potency for 24 hours in sodium chloride injection, 97% in dextrose injection, 101% in sodium chloride and dextrose injection, and 89% in sodium lactate injection. Though aqueous solutions were considered to be stable it was recommended that solutions for injection be used within 30 minutes due to the formation of polymers.— B. Lynn, *Eur. J. Cancer*, 1973, *9*, 425.

Adverse Effects, Treatment, and Precautions. As for Carbenicillin Sodium, p.1111.

Blood disorders. A haemorrhagic diathesis had been seen following ticarcillin.— K. Andrassy *et al.* (letter), *New Engl. J. Med.*, 1975, *292*, 109. See also C. H. Brown *et al.*, *Antimicrob. Ag. Chemother.*, 1975, *7*, 652.

Interactions. Ticarcillin inactivated gentamicin to a greater degree than carbenicillin in patients with renal failure.— F. R. Ervin *et al.*, *Antimicrob. Ag. Chemother.*, 1976, *9*, 1004. Stability tests *in vitro* indicated that ticarcillin caused significantly less inactivation of aminoglycoside antibiotics, particularly amikacin and netilmicin, than did carbenicillin.— L. K. Pickering and P. Gearhart, *Antimicrob. Ag. Chemother.*, 1979, *15*, 592. A report of reduced serum concentrations of ticarcillin and gentamicin in patients receiving the 2 antibiotics together as compared with each of the drugs given together with cephalothin.— J. Murillo *et al.*, *J. Am. med. Ass.*, 1979, *241*, 2401.

See also under Antimicrobial Action (below).

Neurotoxicity. A report of neurotoxicity associated with ticarcillin administration in a patient with renal failure.— M. C. Kallay *et al.* (letter), *Lancet*, 1979, *1*, 608. Criticism; the dosage used was excessive for a patient with renal failure. Seven patients with both renal and hepatic failure have been treated with ticarcillin and neurotoxicity has never been encountered.— H. C. Neu (letter), *ibid.*, 981.

Antimicrobial Action. Ticarcillin is bactericidal and has a mode of action and range of activity similar to that of carbenicillin (see p.1111) but is reported to be 2 to 4 times more active against *Pseudomonas aeruginosa*.

Ticarcillin is inactivated by penicillinase. As with carbenicillin, some strains of *Pseudomonas* may develop resistance fairly rapidly and cross-resistance between the two antibiotics is usual.

The antimicrobial action of ticarcillin can be enhanced by gentamicin (see p.1168) or by tobramycin (see p.1226).

In a study of 23 antibiotics, ticarcillin was the most effective against 24 strains of *Haemophilus influenzae* and against 7 strains of *Neisseria meningitidis*.— L. D. Sabath *et al.*, *Antimicrob. Ag. Chemother.*, 1970, 53.

Ticarcillin inhibited 89% of *Pseudomonas* strains in a concentration of 100 μg per ml and was 2 to 4 times more active than carbenicillin. Indole-positive strains of *Proteus* were inhibited by 10 μg or less per ml and 87% of *Enterobacter*, 87% of *Pr. mirabilis*, and 80% of *Escherichia coli* were inhibited by 25 μg per ml of ticarcillin. *Klebsiella pneumoniae* and *Serratia* were resistant. Ticarcillin showed synergy with gentamicin. Ticarcillin was 10 to 20 times less active than ampicillin against Gram-positive organisms. Among the enterococci tested, 46% were resistant to 25 μg per ml of ticarcillin.— H. C. Neu and E. B. Winshell, *ibid.*, 385.

Ticarcillin was more active than carbenicillin and BL-P 1654 against strains of *Staph. aureus, E. coli, Ps. aeruginosa,* and *Enterobacter, Klebsiella,* and *Proteus* spp. It was less effective than BL-P 1654 against *Staph. epidermidis*. Except for enterococci and *Staph. epidermidis* ticarcillin was considered to be 2 to 4 times more active than carbenicillin.— T. C. Eickhoff and J. M. Ehret, *Antimicrob. Ag. Chemother.*, 1976, *10*, 241.

For further comparisons of the activities of ticarcillin and carbenicillin, see P. C. Fuchs *et al.*, *Am. J. med. Sci.*, 1977, *274*, 255; R. B. Prior and R. J. Fass, *Antimicrob. Ag. Chemother.*, 1978, *13*, 184 (*Ps. aeruginosa*); J. W. Pearman *et al.*, *Med. J. Aust.*, 1978, *1*, 452 (*Ps. aeruginosa*); J. D. King *et al.*, *J. clin. Path.*, 1980, *33*, 297 (*Ps. aeruginosa*).

Ticarcillin inhibited 5, 30, 44, 45, 59, 71, and all of 92 strains of *Neisseria gonorrhoeae in vitro* at an MIC of 8, 16, 30, 125, 250, 500 and 1000 ng per ml respectively.— B. A. Watts *et al.*, *J. antimicrob. Chemother.*, 1977, *3*, 331.

Further references: R. Sutherland *et al.*, *Antimicrob. Ag. Chemother.*, 1970, 390; G. P. Bodey and B. Deerhake, *Appl. Microbiol.*, 1971, *21*, 61; H. C. Neu and E. B. Winshell, *ibid.*, 66; E. R. Wald *et al.*, *Antimicrob. Ag. Chemother.*, 1975, *7*, 336.

For a report of piperacillin being more active than ticarcillin or carbenicillin against 612 isolates of aerobic bacteria, see Piperacillin Sodium, p.1202.

For further comparative studies of the activity *in vitro* of ticarcillin and other antibiotics, see Azlocillin Sodium, p.1099 and Mezlocillin Sodium, p.1184.

Activity against anaerobic bacteria. Ticarcillin inhibited the majority of 258 strains of anaerobic bacteria at 128 μg per ml, including 40 of 42 strains of *Bacteroides fragilis*.— V. L. Sutter and S. M. Finegold, *Antimicrob. Ag. Chemother.*, 1976, *10*, 736.

A comparative evaluation of ticarcillin, carbenicillin, and benzylpenicillin *in vitro* against anaerobic organisms. All 3 antibiotics appeared to be generally equally effective except against some *Bacteroides* spp. where ticarcillin appeared to be the most effective.— I. Roy *et al.*, *Antimicrob. Ag. Chemother.*, 1977, *11*, 258.

Reports of the comparable activity of ticarcillin and carbenicillin against *Bacteroides* spp. *in vitro*.— D. K. Henderson *et al.*, *Antimicrob. Ag. Chemother.*, 1977, *11*, 679; J. A. G. Rodriguez *et al.* (letter), *J. antimicrob. Chemother.*, 1978, *4*, 284.

Enhanced activity. A synergistic effect was observed against *Ps. aeruginosa* when ticarcillin was administered with either gentamicin or polymyxin B.— P. Acred *et* *al., Antimicrob. Ag. Chemother.*, 1970, 396. A similar effect with tobramycin.— K. R. Comber *et al., Antimicrob. Ag. Chemother.*, 1977, *11*, 956. With acetylcysteine.— M. F. Parry and H. C. Neu, *J. clin. Microbiol.*, 1977, *5*, 58.

There was no synergistic effect against 11 of 45 strains of *Ps. aeruginosa* when ticarcillin was used *in vitro* with gentamicin, tobramycin, or amikacin. The MICs of individual drugs gave no indication of the degree of synergism to be expected and it was considered that screening with a particular pair of drugs was not a reliable guide to the activities of other pairs.— H. S. Heineman and W. M. Lofton, *Antimicrob. Ag. Chemother.*, 1978, *13*, 827.

The activity *in vitro* of ticarcillin was enhanced against 11 of 20 strains of *Ps. aeruginosa* by sub-bactericidal concentrations of amikacin. All the strains were susceptible to amikacin alone and ticarcillin was active against 16. Sub-bactericidal concentrations of ticarcillin enhanced the activity of amikacin against 10 of the strains.— T. T. Yoshikawa and S. A. Shibata, *Antimicrob. Ag. Chemother.*, 1978, *13*, 997.

Clavulanic acid generally enhanced the activity of ticarcillin *in vitro* against ticarcillin-resistant strains of *E. coli, Kleb. pneumoniae,* the *Citrobacter* spp., and a strain of each of *Salmonella enteritidis* and *Pr. mirabilis* but generally had no effect on the activity of ticarcillin against ticarcillin-resistant strains of *Ps. aeruginosa* and one of *Serratia marcescens*. The activity of ticarcillin and clavulanic acid used together *in vitro* was variable against strains of the *Enterobacter* and the *Pseudomonas* spp. It was considered that beta-lactamases which were R-factor mediated with primary penicillin activity were the most susceptible to inhibition by clavulanic acid.— J. W. Paisley and J. A. Washington, *Antimicrob. Ag. Chemother.*, 1978, *14*, 224.

Absorption and Fate. Ticarcillin sodium is not absorbed from the gastro-intestinal tract. After the intramuscular injection of the equivalent of ticarcillin 1 g approximate plasma concentrations of 31 µg per ml at 30 minutes, 16 µg per ml at 2 hours, and 3 µg per ml at 6 hours have been recorded. Doubling the dose can double the concentration. About 45% of a dose is bound to plasma proteins and a plasma half-life of 70 minutes has been reported. Ticarcillin is excreted by glomerular filtration and tubular secretion. Concentrations of 2 to 4 mg per ml are achieved in the urine after the intramuscular injection of the equivalent of 1 or 2 g; about 80% of a dose is excreted within 12 hours.

After 3 g of ticarcillin by intravenous injection a plasma concentration of 190 µg per ml has been reported at 15 minutes, falling to about 52 µg per ml at 2 hours, and 14 µg per ml at 4 hours. Increasing the dose or giving probenecid by mouth concomitantly produces higher plasma concentrations. A urinary concentration of 10 mg per ml has followed the intravenous injection of 5 g.

Distribution of ticarcillin in the body is similar to that of carbenicillin and concentrations have been detected in interstitial, cerebrospinal, pleural, and peritoneal fluids and also in sputum and bile.

In healthy adults who received a single intramuscular injection of 1 g of ticarcillin, a peak serum concentration of 35 µg per ml was reached and in the following 6 hours 72% of the dose was excreted in the urine. After an intravenous injection of 1 g of ticarcillin a peak serum concentration of 100 µg per ml was measured but fell rapidly to 2 µg per ml at 6 hours. It was not active by mouth. When ticarcillin was administered with probenecid more prolonged serum concentrations were achieved.— R. Sutherland and P. J. Wise, *Antimicrob. Ag. Chemother.*, 1970, 402. A similar study. Ticarcillin was administered intravenously to 5 patients in doses of 5 and 10 g in dextrose injection over a period of 15 minutes. The average serum concentration 1 hour after the 10-g dose was 480 µg per ml, falling to 20 µg per ml after 6 hours. Following the 5-g dose, the average serum concentration was 310 µg per ml after 1 hour, 170 µg per ml after 2 hours, and negligible after 6 hours. Most of the dose was excreted in the urine within 8 hours.— J. Klastersky *et al., J. clin. Pharmac.*, 1974, *14*, 172.

Binding of ticarcillin with serum proteins could not be demonstrated using 2 techniques of ultrafiltration.— U. Ullmann (letter), *J. antimicrob. Chemother.*, 1976, *2*, 213.

Studies in healthy subjects indicated that the serum half-life of ticarcillin following rapid intravenous infusion of 1, 2, 5, or 10 g was 72.4 minutes. The average steady-state serum concentrations resulting from continuous intravenous infusions of either 1 or 2 g per hour following a loading dose of 1 g (total dose 5 g) were 105 and 125 µg per ml respectively.— A. Dalhoff and D. Hoffler, *J. int. med. Res.*, 1977, *5*, 307.

The pharmacokinetics of ticarcillin in patients with normal and impaired renal function.— D. Höffler *et al., Dt. med. Wschr.*, 1978, *103*, 931.

Further references to pharmacokinetic studies of ticarcillin: V. Rodriguez *et al., Antimicrob. Ag. Chemother.*, 1973, *4*, 31; C. Simon *et al., Dt. med. Wschr.*, 1974, *99*, 2460; R. D. Libke *et al., Clin. Pharmac. Ther.*, 1975, *17*, 441; J. D. Nelson *et al., Pediatrics*, 1978, *61*, 858; B. R. Meyers *et al., Antimicrob. Ag. Chemother.*, 1980, *17*, 608.

Diffusion into body fluids and tissues. Ticarcillin diffused into interstitial fluid. This diffusion was related to the amount of protein binding.— J. S. Tan and S. J. Salstrom, *Antimicrob. Ag. Chemother.*, 1977, *11*, 698.

Concentrations of ticarcillin in serum, muscle, and fat after a single intravenous dose.— F. D. Daschner *et al., Antimicrob. Ag. Chemother.*, 1980, *17*, 738.

Metabolism. About 15% of a 1-g dose of ticarcillin, given intramuscularly to 6 healthy subjects, was metabolised to penicilloic acid and recovered in the urine within 12 hours. The remainder of the dose was excreted unchanged.— M. Cole *et al., Antimicrob. Ag. Chemother.*, 1973, *3*, 463.

Uses. Ticarcillin sodium has actions and uses similar to those of carbenicillin sodium (see p.1110) and is indicated in the treatment of severe Gram-negative infections, especially those due to *Pseudomonas aeruginosa*. The usual adult dose is the equivalent of 15 to 20 g of ticarcillin daily in divided doses every 4 to 8 hours although 3 g has been given every 3 hours in very severe infection. It is administered by slow intravenous injection over 3 to 4 minutes or by infusion over 30 to 40 minutes. Children may be given 200 to 300 mg per kg body-weight daily in divided doses.

The concomitant administration of probenecid 1 g thrice daily by mouth may achieve higher and more prolonged serum concentrations of ticarcillin but is not recommended in patients with impaired renal function. Doses of ticarcillin may need to be reduced in renal failure.

As with carbenicillin, ticarcillin may be used with gentamicin (see p.1170) or tobramycin (see p.1227) but the injections must be administered separately because of possible inactivation by ticarcillin.

In the treatment of uncomplicated urinary-tract infections the usual dose is the equivalent of 3 to 4 g in divided doses daily intramuscularly or by slow intravenous injection. Children have been given 50 to 100 mg per kg body-weight daily. If intramuscular injections prove painful they may be prepared using a 0.5% solution of lignocaine hydrochloride.

As an adjunct to systemic use, ticarcillin may be given by intra-articular injection in doses of 500 mg to 1 g, by intrapleural injection in doses of 1 g daily, and by local irrigation as a 0.2% solution. The equivalent of ticarcillin 500 mg dissolved in 3 to 5 ml of water may be nebulised and inhaled 3 to 4 times daily.

Reviews of ticarcillin.— C. D. Peterson *et al., Drug Intell. & clin. Pharm.*, 1977, *11*, 482; *Med. Lett.*, 1977, *19*, 17; *Chemotherapy, Tokyo*, 1977, *25*, 2389-2931; *Drug & Ther. Bull.*, 1980, *18*, 11; R. N. Brogden *et al., Drugs*, 1980, *20*, 325..

Ticarcillin in conjunction with cephalothin or gentamicin provided effective antibiotic treatment in granulocytopenic cancer patients.— S. C. Schimpff *et al., Antimicrob. Ag. Chemother.*, 1976, *10*, 837. A similar study suggested that ticarcillin used with gentamicin rather than with cephalothin might be a useful initial antimicrobial regimen for empirical therapy of febrile episodes in such patients.— J. Murillo *et al., ibid.*, 1978, *13*, 992.

Further references to the use of ticarcillin in granulocytopenic cancer patients: L. J. Love *et al., Am. J. Med.*, 1979, *66*, 603 (with gentamicin, amikacin, or netilmicin).

Anaerobic infections. Reports of the use of ticarcillin in the treatment of anaerobic infections: D. Webb *et al., Archs intern. Med.*, 1978, *138*, 1618; E. L. Westerman *et al., Am. J. med. Sci.*, 1978, *276*, 159; G. K. M. Harding *et al., J. infect. Dis.*, 1980, *142*, 384.

Dosage in infants and children. Using the results of pharmacokinetic studies in 54 newborn infants the following dosage regimens for ticarcillin by intramuscular injection were suggested for babies with normal renal function: an initial injection of 100 mg per kg bodyweight followed by 75 mg per kg every 8 hours for those weighing less than 2 kg in the first week of life. For small babies over 1-week-old and those heavier than 2 kg in the first 2 weeks of life 75 mg per kg could be given every 4 or 6 hours and after 2 weeks the larger babies could be given 100 mg per kg every 4 hours.— J. D. Nelson *et al., J. Pediat.*, 1975, *87*, 474.

Further references: G. H. McCracken and H. F. Eichenwald, *J. Pediat.*, 1978, *93*, 357.

Dosage in renal failure. Ticarcillin 1 g was given intravenously to 3 patients immediately after haemodialysis, to 3 patients at the beginning of haemodialysis, and to 2 patients undergoing peritoneal dialysis. Haemodialysis removed ticarcillin rapidly; clearance was slower with peritoneal dialysis and adequate therapeutic serum concentrations should persist for up to 3 peritoneal dialysis cycles. A dose of 1 g intravenously every 8 to 12 hours would maintain a serum concentration of 50 µg per ml. Doses during haemodialysis of 1 g every four hours and during peritoneal dialysis of 1 g every six hours were recommended to maintain this concentration.— R. Wise *et al., Antimicrob. Ag. Chemother.*, 1974, *5*, 119.

The normal half-life for ticarcillin of 1 to 1.5 hours was increased to 16 hours in end-stage renal disease. The interval between doses should be extended from 4 to 6 hours to 8 to 12 hours in patients with a glomerular filtration-rate (GFR) of more than 50 ml per minute, to 12 to 24 hours in those with a GFR of 10 to 50 ml per minute, and to 24 to 48 hours in those with a GFR of less than 10 ml per minute. Alternatively, doses could be reduced to 75%, 50%, and 25% respectively. Concentrations of ticarcillin were affected by haemodialysis or peritoneal dialysis.— W. M. Bennett *et al., Ann. intern. Med.*, 1980, *93*, 62.

Further references: M. F. Parry and H. C. Neu, *J. infect. Dis.*, 1976, *133*, 46; G. B. Appel and H. C. Neu, *New Engl. J. Med.*, 1977, *296*, 663.

Pseudomonal infections. The use of ticarcillin 174 to 307 mg per kg body-weight in the treatment of 27 patients with serious Gram-negative infections. Five of 8 patients with pseudomonal pneumonia, 9 of 12 with other pneumonias, and 5 of 6 with other pseudomonal infections improved or were cured. Supra-infection occurred in 2 patients, bleeding was prolonged in 2 patients, eosinophilia occurred in 13, and hypokalaemia in 2.— F. R. Ervin and W. E. Bullock, *Antimicrob. Ag. Chemother.*, 1976, *9*, 94.

An overall response-rate of 81% was achieved when 64 patients with serious Gram-negative infections, mainly caused by *Ps. aeruginosa*, were treated with ticarcillin, sometimes in association with gentamicin. In systemic infections 3 g of ticarcillin or 50 mg per kg body-weight was given every 4 hours by intravenous infusion over 1½ to 2 hours. A similar intravenous dose or 1 g intramuscularly was given every 6 hours in urinary-tract infections. Pulmonary infections responded less frequently than septicaemia or urinary-tract infections.— M. F. Parry and H. C. Neu, *J. infect. Dis.*, 1976, *134*, 476.

Ticarcillin alone, gentamicin alone, or the 2 antibiotics given concomitantly all produced similar response-rates in patients with cystic fibrosis and acute respiratory symptoms attributed to *Ps. aeruginosa*.— M. F. Parry *et al., J. Pediat.*, 1977, *90*, 144.

For a report on the use of ticarcillin with tobramycin in the treatment of severe infections mainly due to *Ps. aeruginosa*, see Tobramycin, p.1228.

Urinary-tract infections. Ticarcillin 1 g intramuscularly every 6 hours for 5 to 7 days was used to treat 17 patients with urinary-tract infections. Of the 15 who completed treatment 12 responded satisfactorily. Pain at the injection site was a problem.— R. Wise and D. S. Reeves, *Chemotherapy, Basle*, 1974, *20*, 45.

Preparations

Sterile Ticarcillin Disodium *(U.S.P.)*. An injection grade of ticarcillin sodium.

Ticar *(Beecham Research, UK)*. Ticarcillin sodium, available as powder for preparing injections, in vials each containing the equivalent of 1, 3, and 5 g of ticarcillin, and in infusion bottles containing the equivalent of 5 g. (Also available as Ticar in *Canad., USA*).

Other Proprietary Names
Aerugipen *(Ger.)*; Tarcil *(Austral.)*; Ticarpen *(Neth., Switz.)*.

174-y

Tobramycin *(B.P., U.S.P.)*. 47663; Nebramycin Factor 6. 6-*O*-(3-Amino-3-deoxy-α-D-glucopyranosyl)-2-deoxy-4-*O*-(2,6-diamino-2,3,6-trideoxy-α-D-*ribo*-hexopyranosyl)-D-streptamine.
$C_{18}H_{37}N_5O_9$=467.5.

CAS — 32986-56-4.

Pharmacopoeias. In *Br.* and *U.S.*

An antibiotic substance produced by the growth of *Streptomyces tenebrarius* or by any other means. It contains not more than 8% of water. The *B.P.* specifies not less than 930 units of tobramycin per mg and the *U.S.P.* specifies not less than 900 μg per mg, both calculated on the anhydrous basis.

A white or almost white hygroscopic powder. **Soluble** 1 in 1.5 of water and 1 in 2000 of alcohol; practically insoluble in chloroform and ether. A solution in water is dextrorotatory. A 10% solution in water has a pH of 9 to 11. **Store** at a temperature not exceeding 25° in airtight containers.

It is used as tobramycin sulphate, a solution of tobramycin in sulphuric acid adjusted to pH 5.8.

Tobramycin was stable for several weeks at pH 1 to 11 at temperatures from 5° to 37°; it could be autoclaved without loss of potency. Tobramycin combined with carbenicillin, other penicillins, and cephalosporins and should not therefore be mixed with them. Calcium and magnesium ions inhibited the activity of tobramycin against *Pseudomonas*; the clinical significance was uncertain.— J. L. Dienstag and H. C. Neu, *Clin. Med.*, 1975, *82* (Dec.), 13.

Tobramycin sulphate was physically compatible with most intravenous fluids and the solutions were stable for at least 24 hours at 25°. Tobramycin was incompatible with heparin and probably with the penicillins and cephalosporins.— R. F. Bergstrom *et al.*, *Am. J. Hosp. Pharm.*, 1975, *32*, 887.

Solutions of tobramycin sulphate and clindamycin phosphate are reported to be unstable in dextrose injection, see p.1147.

Units. One unit of tobramycin is contained in 0.00112613 mg of the first British Standard Preparation (1974) of tobramycin which contains 888 units per mg.

Adverse Effects, Treatment, and Precautions. As for Gentamicin Sulphate, p.1166.

Anaemia, granulocytopenia, thrombocytopenia, and abnormal liver-function tests have been reported. Plasma concentrations of tobramycin should not exceed 12 μg per ml.

Cross-sensitivity between tobramycin and neomycin has been reported.

Of 3506 patients given tobramycin, 136 developed drug-related adverse reactions. These included 21 with ototoxicity (auditory in 7, vestibular in 9, and both in 5), 53 with nephrotoxicity, 18 with hypersensitivity and skin reactions, and 12 with hepatotoxicity. The effects were usually reversible. Risk factors for ototoxicity and nephrotoxicity included the total dose given, the presence of impaired renal function, and the use of other ototoxic and nephrotoxic drugs.— C. L. Bendush *et al.*, *Lilly, Med. J. Aust.*, 1977, *2*, *Suppl.* 3, 22.

Symposium reports of *animal* and clinical studies comparing the toxicity of tobramycin with that of other aminoglycoside antibiotics.— *J. antimicrob. Chemother.*, 1978, *4*, *Suppl.* A, 1-101.

A study of 20 patients with burns and 8 healthy subjects demonstrated that glomerular filtration-rate was increased in those with burns, especially the younger patients, and that the plasma half-life of tobramycin was consequently reduced. Creatinine clearance should be monitored and the interval between doses of tobramycin, and other aminoglycosides with predominantly urinary excretion, reduced, if necessary, to maintain adequate plasma concentrations.— P. Loirat *et al.*, *New Engl. J. Med.*, 1978, *299*, 915.

The mean half-life for tobramycin of 67.3 minutes, after intramuscular injection in 4 children with kwashiorkor, was shorter than that in normal subjects and was reduced to only 50.2 minutes on recovery.— N. Buchanan and C. Eyberg (letter), *S. Afr. med. J.*, 1978, *53*, 273.

Nephrotoxicity. Case reports of 2 patients who developed renal failure (fatal in 1) after concomitant treatment with tobramycin and cephalothin. Tobramycin and carbenicillin had been given on more than 30 occasions without convincing evidence of nephrotoxicity.— J. S. Tobias *et al.* (letter), *Lancet*, 1976, *1*, 425. Criticism. Tobramycin and clindamycin had been used on 40 occasions without nephrotoxicity.— P. Gillett *et al.* (letter), *ibid.*, 1976, *1*, 547.

In 38 consecutive patients given either gentamicin or tobramycin, the effect on renal function was compared by measuring serum-creatinine concentrations and endogenous creatinine clearance. In general, tobramycin appeared to be less nephrotoxic than gentamicin but monitoring of renal function and serum-tobramycin concentrations is necessary.— G. Kahlmeter *et al.*, *J. antimicrob. Chemother.*, 1978, *4*, *Suppl.* A, 47. See also under Gentamicin Sulphate, p.1167.

Further references: A. Coca *et al.*, *Postgrad. med. J.*, 1979, *55*, 791.

For reference to the increased nephrotoxicity of cephalothin with tobramycin or gentamicin compared with methicillin and either of the aminoglycoside antibiotics, see Cephalothin, p.1129.

Neuromuscular blockade. Paralysis occurred following the postoperative infusion of tobramycin in a 59-year-old man who had previously received tubocurarine during anaesthesia. The neuromuscular blockade was reversed successfully by neostigmine and atropine.— P. M. Waterman and R. B. Smith, *Anesth. Analg. curr. Res.*, 1977, *56*, 587.

Ototoxicity. A review of tobramycin ototoxicity.— H. C. Neu and C. L. Bendush, *J. infect. Dis.*, 1976, *134*, *Suppl.*, S206.

In 3 patients given tobramycin for pseudomonal infections cochlear function was rapidly and reversibly depressed at serum-tobramycin concentrations of 7.4 to 15.6 μg per ml. The relationship with long-term ototoxicity of the aminoglycosides was not clear.— P. Wilson and R. T. Ramsden, *Br. med. J.*, 1977, *1*, 259.

A report of permanent complete bilateral loss of peripheral vestibular function during therapy with tobramycin in 2 patients with normal renal function.— E. A. Baarsma and E. Rijntjes, *J. Lar. Otol.*, 1979, *93*, 725.

There were no signs of vestibular dysfunction in 53 children (average age of 11.8 years) who received a total of 170 courses of tobramycin 10 mg per kg body-weight given daily for 10 to 14 days. A 10-year-old girl who received 9.85 mg per kg daily for 10 days with a maximum serum-tobramycin concentration of 3.8 μg per ml had a transient high-tone hearing loss which did not reappear during 3 further courses of tobramycin. The risk of ototoxic effects using 10 mg per kg daily in children with normal kidney function appeared to be minimal but further studies were required before this dosage could be recommended for adults.— J. Thomsen *et al.*, *J. antimicrob. Chemother.*, 1979, *5*, 257.

Antimicrobial Action. Tobramycin is bactericidal and has an antimicrobial spectrum and minimum inhibitory concentrations similar to those of gentamicin (see p.1168) but is reported to be 2 to 4 times more active against *Pseudomonas aeruginosa* and less active against *Serratia marcescens*. An enhanced effect has been reported when tobramycin is used with carbenicillin or ticarcillin against *Ps. aeruginosa* and with benzylpenicillin against *Streptococcus faecalis*.

It is more active in an alkaline medium.

A concentration of 6.25 μg per ml of tobramycin *in vitro* inhibited 90% of strains of *Ps. aeruginosa* and 80% were inhibited by 1.56 μg per ml. Of 25 *Staphylococcus aureus* strains 85% were inhibited by 1.56 μg per ml and 100% by 6.25 μg per ml; 5 of these strains were methicillin-resistant and 3 kanamycin-resistant. Tobramycin 6.25 μg per ml was also effective against 92% of *Escherichia coli* strains, 72% of *Enterobacter* spp., 88% of *Klebsiella* spp., and 64% of *Proteus* spp. although it was not so effective against *Pr. mirabilis*, nor against *Serratia marcescens* and *Providencia* or *Salmonella* strains.— J. Dienstag and H. C. Neu, *Antimicrob. Ag. Chemother.*, 1972, *1*, 41.

Tobramycin 100 ng per ml inhibited 80% of 100 isolates of *Ps. aeruginosa* from patients with malignant neoplasms whereas gentamicin sulphate in a similar concentration inhibited only 4%. A concentration of 1.56 μg per ml of tobramycin was effective against most Gram-negative organisms.— G. P. Bodey and D. Stewart, *Antimicrob. Ag. Chemother.*, 1972, *2*, 109.

The mean MIC for 119 strains of *Pseudomonas* was 0.52±0.42 μg per ml for tobramycin and 2.26±1.9 μg per ml for gentamicin.— M. R. Britt *et al.*, *Antimicrob. Ag. Chemother.*, 1972, *2*, 236.

Tobramycin at a concentration of up to 3.12 μg per ml inhibited 23% of 26 isolates of gentamicin-resistant *Ps. aeruginosa* compared with 4% for sissomicin and none for amikacin, netilmicin, and gentamicin. However 8% of isolates, were inhibited by up to 12.5 μg per ml of amikacin. Enhanced activity was observed with combinations of carbenicillin with tobramycin, sissomicin, or amikacin.— M. I. Marks *et al.*, *Antimicrob. Ag. Chemother.*, 1976, *10*, 399.

The activity of 9 aminoglycosides and spectinomycin were tested *in vitro* against 351 strains of Enterobacteriaceae, 34 of *Ps. aeruginosa*, 38 gentamicin-sensitive and 42 gentamicin-resistant strains of the *Pseudomonas* spp., 20 of the *Acinetobacter* spp., 17 of *Haemophilus influenzae*, and 41 strains of *Neisseria gonorrhoeae*; tobramycin inhibited 95, 94, 98, 5, 80, 100, and 48% of the strains respectively at a concentration of 4 μg per ml.— I. Phillips *et al.*, *J. antimicrob. Chemother.*, 1977, *3*, 403.

Further references: P. M. Waterworth, *J. clin. Path.*, 1972, *25*, 979; P. Bégué *et al.*, *Nouv. Presse méd.*, 1973, *2*, 2655; A. V. Reynolds *et al.*, *Br. med. J.*, 1974, *3*, 778; I. B. R. Duncan and J. L. Penner, *Can. med. Ass. J.*, 1975, *113*, 29; E. T. Houang and E. McKay-Ferguson (letter), *Lancet*, 1976, *1*, 423.

For a comparison of the activities of tobramycin, amikacin, sissomicin, and gentamicin against 408 strains of Gram-negative rods, see Gentamicin, p.1168.

Diminished activity. Physiological concentrations of calcium in serum antagonised the *in vitro* activity of tobramycin against *Ps. aeruginosa* but not *E. coli*. Gentamicin appeared to be more affected by the addition of serum than tobramycin.— S. D. Davis and A. Iannetta, *Antimicrob. Ag. Chemother.*, 1972, *1*, 466.

Enhanced activity. An evaluation *in vitro* of tobramycin showed that it had a similar antibacterial range to gentamicin but was generally more active at similar concentrations. Tobramycin together with carbenicillin was more active against *Ps. aeruginosa*, *E. coli*, and *Staph. aureus*. A solution of tobramycin 10 μg per ml with carbenicillin 200 or 400 μg per ml showed no loss of tobramycin activity after 24 hours at 37°; with 600 μg per ml of carbenicillin there was no loss for 6 hours but a decrease of 90% by 24 hours; and with 800 μg there was a 50% decrease of tobramycin activity after 2 hours. However, serum concentrations of carbenicillin greater than 400 μg per ml seldom occurred.— M. E. Levison *et al.*, *Antimicrob. Ag. Chemother.*, 1972, *1*, 381.

The antimicrobial activity of tobramycin or gentamicin against Gram-negative rods was not significantly enhanced *in vitro* by carbenicillin or cephalothin with the exception of *Ps. aeruginosa* and *Providencia*.— J. Klastersky *et al.*, *Am. J. med. Sci.*, 1973, *266*, 13, per *Int. pharm. Abstr.*, 1974, *11*, 332.

The enhanced activity of a combination of tobramycin with ticarcillin was similar to that of gentamicin and carbenicillin although, because of the difference in activity of the individual antibiotics, tobramycin with ticarcillin was about 4 times more active *in vitro* against *Ps. aeruginosa*. The enhanced effect was also demonstrated in experimental infections in *mice*.— K. R. Comber *et al.*, *Antimicrob. Ag. Chemother.*, 1977, *11*, 956.

For a report of no synergism against 11 of 45 strains of *Ps. aeruginosa* when ticarcillin was used with tobramycin, see Ticarcillin, p.1225.

Resistance. There is evidence for transferable resistance similar to that which occurs with gentamicin (see p.1169) although tobramycin is inactivated by fewer bacterial enzymes. Cross-resistance occurs between gentamicin and tobramycin but it may not be complete for *Pseudomonas aeruginosa*.

Clinical isolates of gentamicin-resistant bacteria were also resistant to tobramycin. Resistance to tobramycin was also noted in 4 strains of *Ps. aeruginosa* in which gentamicin resistance had been induced.— J. L. Brusch, *Antimicrob. Ag. Chemother.*, 1972, *1*, 280.

Transferable resistance to tobramycin was associated with the enzymatic acetylation of tobramycin in *Klebsiella pneumoniae* and *Enterobacter cloacae* isolated from burn wounds.— B. H. Minshew *et al.*, *Antimicrob. Ag. Chemother.*, 1974, *6*, 492.

Mucoid strains of *Ps. aeruginosa* isolated from patients with cystic fibrosis were more resistant *in vitro* to carbenicillin, flucloxacillin, or tobramycin and more sensitive to tetracycline than non-mucoid strains isolated simultaneously from the same sputa.— J. R. W. Govan and J. A. M. Fyfe, *J. antimicrob. Chemother.*, 1978, *4*, 233.

Absorption and Fate. Tobramycin is poorly absorbed from the gastro-intestinal tract. Following intramuscular administration peak plasma concentrations are achieved within half to 1 hour and concentrations of about 4 μg per ml have been reported following doses of 100 mg. After injection tobramycin has been detected in body fluids but concentrations in the cerebrospinal fluid are low even when there is meningeal inflammation. It crosses the placenta and small amounts have been detected in breast milk. A plasma half-life of 2 hours has been reported.

Most of a dose is excreted by glomerular filtration in the urine within 24 hours. Tobramycin is readily removed by haemodialysis; removal by peritoneal dialysis is relatively slow.

A review of the clinical pharmacokinetics of tobramycin and other aminoglycoside antibiotics.— J. -C. Pechere and R. Dugal, *Clin. Pharmacokinet.*, 1979, *4*, 170.

Intramuscular injections of tobramycin produced average peak serum concentrations of 1.14, 2.09, and 2.71 μg per ml in 1 hour after doses of 25, 50, and 75 mg respectively, and the corresponding urine concentrations were 12.28, 21, and 54 μg per ml, mostly during the 12 hours after injection.— H. R. Black and R. S. Griffith, *Antimicrob. Ag. Chemother.*, 1970, 314.

When tobramycin 100 mg was administered intramuscularly to 10 fasting volunteers serum concentrations reached a peak of 3.77 and 3.75 μg per ml at 30 minutes and 1 hour respectively. Following intravenous injections peak serum concentrations of 5.5 and 6.02 μg per ml were achieved at 30 minutes following doses of 1 mg and 1.5 mg per kg body-weight respectively. The half-life after an intramuscular injection was 2 hours and after an intravenous injection 1.3 hours. Serum concentrations of gentamicin after similar doses were generally higher.— B. R. Meyers and S. Z. Hirschman, *J. clin. Pharmac.*, 1972, *12*, 321.

Similar serum concentrations were achieved following intravenous infusions and intramuscular injections of tobramycin and gentamicin.— C. Regamey *et al.*, *Clin. Pharmac. Ther.*, 1973, *14*, 396.

Tobramycin given as a slow bolus intravenous injection over 2.5 to 3 minutes to 5 healthy subjects in a standard dose of 80 mg produced a peak serum concentration of about 11 μg per ml within 5 minutes. A dose of 1 mg per kg body-weight produced a slightly lower peak of about 10 μg per ml. The regression curves for both doses were similar.— B. C. Stratford *et al.*, *Lancet*, 1974, *1*, 378.

In a study of 35 patients with stable renal function (creatinine-clearance rate (CCR): 22 to 128 ml per minute) who received tobramycin, serum concentrations of tobramycin fell in 2 phases after the final dose. The first-phase half-lives correlated well with CCR, but the half-life of the second phase (mean 146 hours) which began about 24 hours after the final dose did not. A two-compartment model was used to predict serum and tissue concentrations of tobramycin. It was considered that tissue accumulation and release might be a major source of variation in tobramycin disposition.— J. J. Schentag *et al.*, *Antimicrob. Ag. Chemother.*, 1978, *13*, 649.

Tobramycin was detected in the serum and urine of an 80-year-old man with normal renal function for 11 days after the end of treatment with tobramycin. A 2-compartment open model for describing the pharmacokinetics of tobramycin might be inadequate.— G. Kahlmeter *et al.*, *J. antimicrob. Chemother.*, 1978, *4*, *Suppl.* A, 5.

The pharmacokinetics of tobramycin in obese patients.— R. A. Blouin *et al.*, *Clin. Pharmac. Ther.*, 1979, *26*, 508.

Absorption and fate in infants and children. In 40 children given tobramycin 5 mg per kg body-weight daily in 3 divided doses by intramuscular injection, the mean serum concentration was 2.77 μg per ml one hour after injection, falling to 0.4 μg per ml after 8 hours. The serum half-life was about 4.5 hours.— F. J. Da Nobrega *et al.*, *Curr. ther. Res.*, 1977, *21*, 741.

Further references: J. L. Hoecker *et al.*, *J. infect. Dis.*, 1978, *137*, 592; D. Bratlid and J. E. Fuglesang, *Scand. J. infect. Dis.*, 1979, *11*, 73.

Diffusion. *Eye.* Following a single dose of tobramycin 10 mg by subconjunctival injection, therapeutically effective concentrations were achieved in aqueous humour whilst negligible concentrations were reached after intramuscular injection of tobramycin 80 or 100 mg.— A. Petounis *et al.*, *Br. J. Ophthal.*, 1978, *62*, 660.

Tobramycin concentrations of 3 to 4 μg per ml were achieved in the aqueous humour of patients with cataract 1 hour after the intravenous infusion of 1 mg per kg body-weight, compared with peak serum concentrations of 2.93 to 3.70 μg per ml half an hour after administration. After the intramuscular injection of a similar dose peak concentrations in the aqueous humour were only 0.22 to 0.32 μg per ml four hours after injection. Variable concentrations occurred in the aqueous humour of 4 patients after the subconjunctival injection of tobramycin 10 or 20 mg.— F. P. Furgiuele *et al.*, *Am. J. Ophthal.*, 1978, *85*, 121.

Synovial fluid. The concentration of tobramycin in synovial fluid ranged from 60 to 105% that of simultaneous serum concentrations in 6 patients with non-traumatic joint effusions 90 or 120 minutes after they received tobramycin 1 to 1.5 mg per kg body-weight intramuscularly.— T. H. Dee and F. Kozin, *Antimicrob. Ag. Chemother.*, 1977, *12*, 548.

Other tissues and fluids. For further reports of diffusion into tissues and body fluids see: W. H. Hall *et al.*, *J. infect. Dis.*, 1977, *135*, 957; J. S. Tan and S. J. Salstrom, *Antimicrob. Ag. Chemother.*, 1977, *11*, 698 (interstitial fluid); D. N. Gerding *et al.*, *Ann. intern. Med.*, 1977, *86*, 708 (ascitic fluid); U. Kroening *et al.*, *Infection*, 1978, *6*, 231 (lung); C. B. Williams *et al.*, *Urology*, 1979, *13*, 589 (prostate); M. R. Alexander *et al.*, *Chest*, 1979, *75*, 675 (bronchial secretions); G. Mombelli *et al.*, *Antimicrob. Ag. Chemother.*, 1981, *19*, 72 (bronchial secretions).

Pregnancy and the neonate. Concentrations of tobramycin in the breast milk of one patient were 0.6 and 0.58 μg per ml one and 8 hours respectively after the intramuscular injection of 80 mg, with corresponding serum concentrations of 4.2 and 0.8 μg per ml.— M. Uwaydah *et al.*, *J. antimicrob. Chemother.*, 1975, *1*, 429.

Tobramycin 2 mg per kg body-weight was given intramuscularly to 35 pregnant women before abortion. Foetal assay showed transplacental diffusion, tobramycin being detected in foetal serum, kidney, urine, and amniotic fluid. Low concentrations were detected in the cerebrospinal fluid of 9 of 15 foetuses of less than 17 weeks gestation; none was found in the CSF of older foetuses. The placental mean concentration of 1.4 μg per g for at least 24 hours was considered to be sufficiently high to suggest tobramycin for the treatment of placental infections.— B. Bernard *et al.*, *Antimicrob. Ag. Chemother.*, 1977, *11*, 688.

Protein binding. Tobramycin did not exhibit any protein binding in studies *in vitro* of human serum under controlled physiological conditions using an ultra-filtration technique.— R. C. Gordon *et al.*, *Antimicrob. Ag. Chemother.*, 1972, *2*, 214. See also U. Ullmann (letter), *J. antimicrob. Chemother.*, 1976, *2*, 213.

Uses. Tobramycin is an aminoglycoside antibiotic with actions and uses similar to those of gentamicin (see p.1166).It is used as the sulphate, mainly in the treatment of pseudomonal infections.

As with gentamicin, tobramycin may be used with carbenicillin or ticarcillin; the injections should be administered separately.

The usual dose for adults and children is the equivalent of 3 to 5 mg of tobramycin per kg body-weight daily in divided doses every 6 or 8 hours. It is given by intramuscular injection, or by intravenous infusion over 20 to 60 minutes in 50 to 100 ml of diluent or proportionately less for children. It has also been given by direct intravenous injection in concentrations of not more than 1 mg per ml. Treatment should generally continue for not longer than 7 to 10 days because of the increased risk of nephrotoxicity and ototoxicity. Plasma concentrations should not exceed 12 μg per ml. Doses are reduced for patients with impaired renal function. After a loading dose of 1 mg per kg, subsequent doses are reduced or the intervals between them prolonged according to the serum-creatinine concentration or the creatinine clearance.

A review of the actions and uses of tobramycin.— R. N. Brogden *et al.*, *Drugs*, 1976, *12*, 166-200.

See also under Gentamicin (p.1171) for general reviews of the aminoglycoside antibiotics.

The proceedings of symposiums on the actions and uses of tobramycin.— *J. infect. Dis.*, 1976, *134*, *Suppl.* (Aug.), S1-S234; *Med. J. Aust.*, 1977, *2*, *Suppl.* 3, 1-40.

Comparative reviews of tobramycin and gentamicin.— W. S. Burkle, *Drug Intell. & clin. Pharm.*, 1976, *10*, 43; *Med. Lett.*, 1980, *22*, 85.

Tobramycin used with clindamycin was considered to be effective in the treatment of febrile episodes in 22 patients with leukaemia. Three patients died after superinfection with *Candida albicans*. In 5 patients in whom there was no improvement after 72 hours addition of co-trimoxazole to the regimen produced a clinical improvement within 48 hours.— R. H. Falk *et al.*, *J. antimicrob. Chemother.*, 1977, *3*, 317. See also G. P. Bodey *et al.*, *Am. J. Med.*, 1979, *67*, 608 (with carbenicillin).

For a report of the use of tobramycin with cephalothin in patients with severe infections and blood diseases, see Cephalothin, p.1130.

Dosage. A recommendation that tobramycin be given every 6 hours in a total daily dose of 6 mg per kg body-weight when administered by intravenous bolus injection.— A. P. Gillett *et al.*, *J. infect. Dis.*, 1976, *134*, *Suppl.* (Aug.), S110.

In a study of 20 patients with acute leukaemia and neutropenia, doses of tobramycin calculated from a nomogram for gentamicin (G.E. Mawer *et al. Br. J. clin. Pharmac.*, 1974, *1*, 45) produced higher serum concentrations of tobramycin during the first hour after administration compared with tobramycin 80 mg given every 8 hours intravenously. It was suggested that the latter regimen might be insufficient and larger doses could safely be given. There was no evidence of accumulation of drug 8 hours after administration with the conventional regimen and low concentrations of gentamicin were only occasionally detected with the nomogram-assisted regimen.— J. S. Tobias *et al.*, *J. antimicrob. Chemother.*, 1977, *3*, 305.

The clinical evaluation of a pharmacokinetic model for determining individual dosage requirements of tobramycin.— R. J. Cipolle *et al.*, *J. clin. Pharmac.*, 1980, *20*, 570.

Dosage in infants and children. A dose of 2 mg per kg body-weight could be given every 12 hours for up to 10 days to neonates without accumulation. This dose produced peak serum concentrations of 4.5 to 5.5 μg per ml. Over 90% of coliform organisms and *Pseudomonas* spp. were susceptible *in vitro* to 5 μg per ml of tobramycin.— J. M. Kaplan *et al.*, *Am. J. Dis. Child.*, 1973, *125*, 656.

A suggested dose of tobramycin for infants of more than 37 weeks' gestation is 2.5 mg per kg body-weight given intramuscularly or by very slow bolus intravenous injection every 12 hours for the first 48 hours of life and then every 8 hours. For immature infants (those of less than 37 weeks' gestation) this dose should be given every 12 hours for the first week of life and then every 8 hours.— P. A. Davies, *Br. med. J.*, 1978, *2*, 676. See also H. C. Spratt, *Drugs*, 1978, *16*, 226.

The recommended tobramycin dose of 3 to 5 mg per kg body-weight daily results in unacceptably low serum concentrations in infants and children. Studies of tobramycin kinetics at 3 dosage regimens in 15 infants and children aged 3 weeks to 10 years, indicated that 7.5 mg per kg daily in 3 divided doses is the most suitable regimen for starting tobramycin therapy in infants aged more than 3 weeks and in children, if peak serum concentrations of 3 to 8 μg per ml are to be attained.— D. A. Kafetzis *et al.* (letter), *Lancet*, 1978, *2*, 1264. Following pharmacokinetic studies in 50 children aged 2 to 18 it was felt that tobramycin should be administered to children at a dose of 8 to 10 mg per kg body-weight daily intravenously, given every 4 to 6 hours. Because of inter-patient variation serum concentrations should be monitored. Tobramycin was administered over a period of 30 to 60 minutes to avoid neuromuscular blockade with subsequent cessation of respiration, particularly in infants.— L. K. Pickering and T. G. Cleary (letter), *Lancet*, 1979, *1*, 102.

Further references: G. H. McCracken and J. D. Nelson, *J. Pediat.*, 1976, *88*, 315; H. Yoshioka *et al.*, *Infection*, 1979, *7*, 180.

Dosage in renal failure. Tobramycin could be given in doses of 1 mg per kg body-weight by intramuscular injection every 12 to 24 hours to patients with renal failure, the dose being varied according to blood concentrations or serum-creatinine concentrations.— A. W. Derrington, *Med. J. Aust.*, 1974, *2*, 571.

Peritoneal dialysis decreased the serum half-life of tobramycin to the extent that, to maintain bactericidal serum concentrations, a loading dose should be given followed by either a similar dose every third half-life or by half the dose every half-life.— R. F. Malacoff *et al.*, *Antimicrob. Ag. Chemother.*, 1975, *8*, 574.

After a loading dose of 1 mg per kg body-weight tobramycin could be given in a dose of 1 to 1.5 mg per kg at a frequency (in hours) of 6 times the serum-creatinine concentration in mg per 100 ml; for those with a creatinine clearance of 5 ml per minute 0.1 mg per kg could be given every 8 hours; 1 mg per kg could be given after dialysis.— J. S. Cheigh, *Am. J. Med.*, 1977, *62*, 555.

Data for predicting removal of tobramycin by conventional haemodialysis.— T. P. Gibson and H. A. Nelson, *Clin. Pharmacokinet.*, 1977, *2*, 403.

The normal half-life for tobramycin of 2.5 hours was increased to 56 hours in end-stage renal failure. The interval between doses should be extended from 8 hours to 8 to 12 in patients with a glomerular filtration-rate (GFR) above 50 ml per minute, to 12 to 24 hours in those with a GFR of 10 to 50 ml per minute, and 24 to 48 hours in those with a GFR of less than 10 ml per minute; alternatively doses should be reduced to 75 to 100%, 50 to 75%, and 25 to 50% of normal respectively. Concentrations of tobramycin were affected by haemodialysis or peritoneal dialysis; 4 to 5 mg could be added to each litre of peritoneal dialysate to obtain satisfactory serum concentrations.— W. M. Bennett *et al.*, *Ann. intern. Med.*, 1980, *93*, 62.

Further references: L. D. Bechtol and H. R. Black, *Am. J. med. Sci.*, 1975, *269*, 317; G. B. Appel and H. C. Neu, *New Engl. J. Med.*, 1977, *296*, 663.

Eye infections. For reports of the penetration of tobramycin into the aqueous humour after intramuscular or intravenous injection and the concentrations achieved after subconjunctival injections, see Absorption and Fate (above).

Gram-negative infections, miscellaneous. Tobramycin was used by intravenous infusion or by intramuscular injection to treat 52 infections with Gram-negative organisms in 51 patients; 17 were urinary-tract infections, 13 bacteraemia, and 13 acute pyelonephritis. In 41 infections there was an immediate satisfactory response, although 2 patients with mixed infections and 1 patient with meningitis due to *Serratia* spp. required carbenicillin in addition and a further patient was also given cephazolin sodium; 7 patients who responded developed superinfection later. In 10 patients there was no response to tobramycin.— T. J. Marrie *et al.*, *Can. med. Ass. J.*, 1977, *117*, 138.

Further references: G. Jaffe *et al.*, *Antimicrob. Ag. Chemother.*, 1974, *5*, 75; E. D. Carmalt *et al.*, *Am. J. med. Sci.*, 1976, *271*, 285; R. L. Perkins *et al.*, *Am. J. med. Sci.*, 1976, *271*, 297; R. Feld *et al.*, *J. infect. Dis.*, 1977, *135*, 61; L. D. Edwards *et al.*, *Curr. ther. Res.*, 1978, *24*, 599.

For a report of the successful treatment of severe Gram-negative infections using gentamicin or tobramycin in association with cephamandole, see Cephamandole, p.1132.

Meningitis. A suggested lumbar intrathecal or intraventricular dose of tobramycin in Gram-negative bacillary meningitis was 5 mg every 18 to 24 hours in addition to systemic treatment. Concentrations in the ventricles were very low after intrathecal injection.— A. B. Kaiser and Z. A. McGee, *New Engl. J. Med.*, 1975, *293*, 1215 (but see also under Gentamicin Sulphate, p.1172).

Pseudomonal infections. Tobramycin was given to 13 children with cystic fibrosis and chronic pulmonary infections due to *Ps. aeruginosa*. The initial dose was 125 mg per m^2 body-surface daily increased in 9 to 250 mg per m^2 by intramuscular injection in 4 divided doses; 8 of the high dose group also received tobramycin by aerosol, 100 mg in 2 ml of saline being inhaled twice daily. *Ps. aeruginosa* was eradicated in 5 of the high-dose patients but 1 month after discontinuing treatment all patients were re-infected. All patients showed some clinical improvement.— G. E. Hoff *et al.*, *Scand. J. infect. Dis.*, 1974, *6*, 333.

Carbenicillin and tobramycin produced a favourable response in 9 of 10 children with cystic fibrosis suffering from *Ps. aeruginosa* infections.— P. Déry, *J. Am. med. Ass.*, 1977, *237*, 1415.

In a study of 82 patients with severe Gram-negative infections, mainly due to *Ps. aeruginosa*, 37 of 40 patients responded favourably to ticarcillin and tobramycin compared with 30 of 42 who responded to carbenicillin and gentamicin. The doses used in patients with normal renal function were: ticarcillin 300 mg per kg body-weight daily or carbenicillin 450 mg per kg daily, intravenously, and tobramycin or gentamicin 4.5 mg per kg daily by intravenous or intramuscular injection, all given for at least 5 days.— M. F. Parry and H. C. Neu, *Am. J. Med.*, 1978, *64*, 961.

Surgical infection prophylaxis. Three of 37 patients given tobramycin 160 mg and lincomycin 600 mg by intramuscular injection with premedication for abdominal surgery and again 8 hours later developed wound infection. This was significantly less than the incidence of 16 of 38 similar control patients receiving no prophylaxis and of 15 of 38 similar patients who received applications of povidone-iodine after closing the peritoneum and after inserting skin sutures. The tobramycin and lincomycin regimen was considered suitable for routine prophylaxis against coliforms, bacteroides, and *Pseudomonas* bacteria likely to be encountered in colorectal surgery R. B. Galland *et al.*, *Lancet*, 1977, *2*, 1043.

Urinary-tract infections. Tobramycin 1.2 mg per kg body-weight daily was given intramuscularly either 8- or 12-hourly to 32 patients with recurrent urinary-tract infections. The cure-rate of 78.1% after therapy had dropped to 65.6% 15 days later.— F. P. Queiroz *et al.*, *Am. J. med. Sci.*, 1976, *271*, 29.

Further references: R. R. Bailey and B. Peddie, *Med. J. Aust.*, 1977, *2*, *Suppl.* 3, 34.

Preparations

Tobramycin Injection *(B.P.)*. A sterile solution of tobramycin in Water for Injections containing sufficient sulphuric acid to adjust the pH to 3.5 to 6. It may contain a suitable stabilising agent. It is sterilised by filtration. Potency is expressed in terms of the equivalent amount of tobramycin. *U.S.P.* (Tobramycin Sulfate Injection) specifies the equivalent of 10 or 40 mg of tobramycin per ml.

Nebcin (formerly known as Obracin) *(Lilly, UK)*. Tobramycin sulphate, available as an injection containing the equivalent of 10 mg of tobramycin per ml, in vials of 2 ml, and the equivalent of 40 mg per ml, in vials of 1 and 2 ml. (Also available as Nebcin in *Austral., Canad., S.Afr., USA*).

Other Proprietary Names

Brulamycin *(Hung.)*; Gernebcin *(Ger.)*; Nebcina *(Denm., Norw., Swed.)*; Nebcine *(Fr.)*; Nebicina *(Ital.)*; Obracin *(Belg., Neth., Switz.)*; Tobra *(Arg.)*; Tobracin *(Jap.)*; Tobradistin *(Spain)*; Tobrex *(USA)*.

175-j

Triacetyloleandomycin *(B.P.C. 1968)*.

Troleandomycin. The triacetyl ester of oleandomycin.

$C_{41}H_{67}NO_{15}$=814.0.

CAS — 2751-09-9.

A white odourless crystalline powder, containing not less than 800 units per mg. Triacetyloleandomycin 1.18 g is approximately equivalent to 1 g of oleandomycin. Slightly **soluble** in water and ether; soluble 1 in 10 of alcohol and 1 in 1 of chloroform. A 1% solution in alcohol (50%) has a pH of 7 to 8.5.

Units. One unit of triacetyloleandomycin is contained in 0.0012 mg of the first International Reference Preparation (1962) which contains 833 units per mg.

Adverse Effects. Reported side-effects include hypersensitivity reactions and gastro-intestinal disturbances. After administration of triacetyloleandomycin for 2 weeks or more, hepatotoxicity with transient disturbances of liver function and jaundice, as described for erythromycin estolate (see p.1161), have occurred.

Precautions. As for Erythromycin Estolate, p.1161.

Triacetyloleandomycin should not generally be administered for longer than 10 days unless tests of liver function are made frequently. It should not be given to patients with impaired liver function or to patients who have developed jaundice or other symptoms of liver toxicity during previous treatment with triacetyloleandomycin.

Interactions. The administration of triacetyloleandomycin could interfere with measurements of urinary 17-hydroxycorticosteroids.— J. M. Rosenberg and I. S. Kampa, *Drug Intell. & clin. Pharm.*, 1973, *7*, 33.

A report of acute ergotism being associated with a combination of *dihydroergotamine* and triacetyloleandomycin.— A. Franco *et al.*, *Nouv. Presse méd.*, 1978, *7*, 205.

The concurrent administration of triacetyloleandomycin and *oral contraceptives* may increase the risk of jaundice present when either agent is given alone.— J. -P. Miguet *et al.* (letter), *Ann. intern. Med.*, 1980, *92*, 434.

For the effect of triacetyloleandomycin on serum-*theophylline* concentrations, see Aminophylline, p.343.

For the effect of triacetyloleandomycin on *carbamazepine*, see Carbamazepine, p.1246.

Antimicrobial Action. Triacetyloleandomycin has a range of activity similar to but, in general, less effective than that of erythromycin (see p.1158). There is evidence of cross-resistance between triacetyloleandomycin and the other macrolides.

Absorption and Fate. Triacetyloleandomycin is more rapidly and completely absorbed from the gastro-intestinal tract than is oleandomycin, to which it is hydrolysed *in vivo*. Peak plasma-oleandomycin concentrations of about 2 µg per ml are attained 2 hours after a single dose of 500 mg, and detectable amounts are present in plasma after 12 hours. It is excreted in the urine and bile; about 20% of the dose can be recovered in active form from the urine.

The mean ratio of antibiotic concentration in tonsillar tissue to the concentration in serum was significantly higher in 6 patients given triacetyloleandomycin for 2 days pre-operatively than in 6 further patients given similar doses of erythromycin.— S. Georgiew *et al.* (letter), *J. antimicrob. Chemother.*, 1978, *4*, 472.

Uses. Triacetyloleandomycin is a macrolide antibiotic and has been given by mouth in the treatment of susceptible infections but more effective antibiotics are generally preferred. The usual adult dose is the equivalent of 1 to 2 g daily of oleandomycin in divided doses. Children have been given the equivalent of 30 to 50 mg per kg body-weight daily.

Asthma. Five of 10 children with apparently intractable asthma showed significant improvement and reduced need for steroids after treatment with triacetyloleandomycin 15 mg per kg body-weight daily. One patient was withdrawn from study because of liver toxicity.— *J. Am. med. Ass.*, 1969, *210*, 1010. See also I. H. Itkin and M. L. Menzel, *J. Allergy*, 1970, *45*, 146; S. L. Spector *et al.*, *J. Allergy & clin. Immunol.*, 1974, *54*, 367, per *J. Am. med. Ass.*, 1975, *232*, 1084; R. S. Zeiger *et al.*, *J. Allergy & clin. Immunol.*, 1980, *66*, 438; S. J. Szefler *et al.*, *ibid.*, 447.

Proprietary Names

Aovine *(Wyeth, Belg.)*; Cetilmin *(Lafare, Ital.)*; Isotriacin *(ISOM, Ital.)*; Micotil *(Magis, Ital.)*; Oleandom *(Coli, Ital.)*; Oleandocyn *(Pfizer, Ger.)* (see also Oleandomycin Phosphate); TAO *(Pfizer, Austral.; Roerig, Belg.; Pfizer, Fr.; Pfizer, Ital.; Pfizer, S.Afr.; Hispano Quimica, Spain; Roerig, USA)*; Treis-Micina *(Ecobi, Ital.)*; Treolmicina *(Guidi, Ital.)*; Triacet *(Ausonia, Ital.)*; Triocetin *(OFF, Ital.)*; Triolan *(Ital Suisse, Ital.)*; Viamicina *(Benvegna, Ital.)*; Wytrion *(Wyeth, Switz.)*.

Triacetyloleandomycin was formerly marketed in Great Britain under the proprietary name Evramycin (*Wyeth*).

176-z

Tyrothricin. Tirotricina.

CAS — 1404-88-2.

Pharmacopoeias. In *Arg., Braz., Fr.,* and *Swiss.*

An antimicrobial substance produced by the growth of *Bacillus brevis* Dubos. It is a mixture consisting chiefly of gramicidin (about 20 to 25%) and tyrocidine (about 60% to 80%), the latter being usually present as the hydrochloride. Both components are mixtures of polypeptides. Tyrothricin occurs as a white, greyish-white, or brownish-white, almost odourless and tasteless powder.

Practically **insoluble** in water; soluble 1 in 15 of alcohol and propylene glycol; freely soluble in glacial acetic acid; sparingly soluble in acetone; practically insoluble in chloroform and ether. It forms stable aqueous solutions in the presence of certain cationic and nonionic surfactants; formaldehyde may also be used as a solubilising agent. Solutions in propylene glycol or macrogols may be **sterilised** by autoclaving. The powder is **stable** in air and withstands heating at 100° for 1 hour.

Adverse Effects and Precautions. The parenteral administration of tyrothricin causes haemolysis and liver and kidney damage and it should never be given by injection. It is also intensely irritating to the meninges and has given rise to chemical meningitis. It damages the sensory epithelium of the nose and instances of prolonged loss of smell have occurred after its use as a nasal spray or instillation. Tyrothricin should not be instilled into the nasal cavities or into closed body cavities.

Erythema multiforme. Tyrothricin had been implicated in the Stevens-Johnson syndrome.— D. B. Coursin, *J. Am. med. Ass.*, 1966, *198*, 113.

Uses. Tyrothricin is unsuitable for systemic treatment. It is readily inactivated *in vivo*, and it is dangerously toxic when administered intravenously.

Tyrothricin is active *in vitro* against many Gram-positive bacteria. It has been used either alone or in conjunction with other antibacterial agents in the local treatment of infections of the skin and mouth.

Preparations

Tyrothricin and Hydrocortisone Lotion *(Guy's Hosp.)*. Tyrothricin 75 mg, hydrocortisone (micronised) 500 mg, chlorocresol 50 mg, cetomacrogol emulsifying wax 500 mg, industrial methylated spirit '74 OP' 2 ml, Tween '80' 0.04 ml, propylene glycol 9 ml, water 88 ml.

Tyrothricin and Hydrocortisone Lotion *(St. John's Hosp.)*. Tyrothricin 0.1, hydrocortisone 0.5, cetomacrogol emulsifying wax 2, liquid paraffin 5, glycerol 5, methyl hydroxybenzoate 0.15, propyl hydroxybenzoate 0.02, water to 100.

Tyrothricin Lotion *(Guy's Hosp.)*. Tyrothricin 100 mg, industrial methylated spirit '74 OP' 2.5 ml, Tween '80' 0.05 ml, propylene glycol 12.5 ml, water to 100 ml.

Proprietary Preparations

Tyrosolven *(Warner, UK)*. Lozenges each containing tyrothricin 1 mg, benzocaine 5 mg, and cetylpyridinium chloride 1 mg. For infections of the mouth and throat. *Dose.* 1 lozenge to be sucked every hour until relief is obtained, then every 3 hours; not more than 8 in 24 hours.

Tyrozets *(Merck Sharp & Dohme, UK)*. Lozenges each containing tyrothricin 1 mg and benzocaine 5 mg. For infections of the mouth and throat. *Dose.* 1 lozenge to be sucked every 3 hours; not more than 8 in 24 hours.

For another proprietary preparation containing tyrothricin, see under Neomycin Sulphate, p.1192.

Other Proprietary Names

Ginotricina *(Ital.)*; Hydrotricine *(Belg., Ital.)*; Rinotricina, Solutricina *(both Ital.)*; Solutricine *(Fr.)*.

A preparation containing tyrothricin was also formerly marketed in Great Britain under the proprietary name Tetrazets (*Merck Sharpe & Dohme*).

177-c

Vancomycin Hydrochloride *(B.P., U.S.P.)*.

Vancomycini Hydrochloridum.

CAS — 1404-90-6 (vancomycin); 1404-93-9 (hydrochloride).

Pharmacopoeias. In *Br.*, *Int.*, and *U.S.*, which also includes Sterile Vancomycin Hydrochloride.

An amphoteric glycopeptide antimicrobial substance produced by the growth of certain strains of *Streptomyces orientalis*, or by any other means. A light brown, odourless powder with a bitter taste containing not less than 900 units per mg, calculated on the anhydrous substance. One million units of vancomycin are approximately equivalent to 1 g of vancomycin.

Soluble 1 in 10 of water and 1 in 700 of alcohol; practically insoluble in chloroform; slightly soluble in ether. Urea increases its solubility in neutral aqueous solution. A 5% solution in water has a pH of 2.5 to 4.5. It may be precipitated from solutions by heavy metals and from acid solutions by ammonium chloride and sodium chloride.

Store in sterile containers, sealed to exclude micro-organisms. Solutions are most stable at pH 3 to 5; they should be stored in a refrigerator.

Incompatibility. There was loss of clarity when intravenous solutions of vancomycin hydrochloride were mixed with those of *aminophylline, amylobarbitone sodium, benzylpenicillin, chloramphenicol sodium succinate, chlorothiazide sodium, dexamethasone sodium phosphate, heparin sodium, hydrocortisone sodium succinate, methicillin sodium, nitrofurantoin sodium, novobiocin sodium, pentobarbitone sodium, phenobarbitone sodium, phenytoin sodium, quinalbarbitone sodium, sodium bicarbonate, sulphadiazine sodium*, or *sulphafurazole diethanolamine*.— J. A. Patel and G. L. Phillips, *Am. J. Hosp. Pharm.*, 1966, *23*, 409.

Vancomycin was incompatible with *soluble barbiturates* and *vitamins of the B group with vitamin C* in an infusion fluid.— B. Flouvat and P. Lechat, *Thérapie*, 1974, *29*, 337.

Further references: *Med. Lett.*, 1972, *14* (Jan.), *Suppl.*, 32.

Stability in solution. Vancomycin hydrochloride 500 mg per 100 ml retained 100% activity in both dextrose injection and sodium chloride injection at 5° after 28 days. At 25° the activity fell to 97% and 85% respectively.— J. M. Mann *et al.*, *Am. J. Hosp. Pharm.*, 1971, *28*, 760.

There was no significant loss of potency when vancomycin for injection was dissolved in water, added to each of 3 commercially available 0.5% hypromellose solutions in plastic squeezy bottles (Lacril, pH 5.9; Tearisol, pH 7.3; Isoptotears, pH 7.4), and the resulting solutions of vancomycin 31 mg per ml kept at 25° for 7 days. The relative potency of vancomycin varied according to the hypromellose solution used.— E. Osborn *et al.*, *Am. J. Ophthal.*, 1976, *82*, 775.

Units. One unit of vancomycin is contained in 0.000993 mg of the first International Standard Preparation (1963) of vancomycin sulphate which contains 1007 units per mg.

Adverse Effects. Thrombophlebitis has been a common complication of vancomycin therapy; it may be minimised by slow intravenous injection of a dilute solution of the antibiotic, and by using different veins in rotation.

Febrile reactions with rigors and macular rashes have occurred; eosinophilia, anaphylactic reactions, and alterations in kidney function have also been reported. High blood concentrations of vancomycin or prolonged treatment may produce deafness which may be irreversible; it is sometimes preceded by tinnitus which must be regarded as a sign to discontinue treatment.

Profound neutropenia in an 11-year-old girl given vancomycin therapy.— H. H. Kesarwala *et al.* (letter), *Lancet*, 1981, *1*, 1423. See also C. D. R. Borland and W. E. Farrar (letter), *J. Am. med. Ass.*, 1979, *242*, 2392.

Precautions. Vancomycin should not usually be given to patients with renal disease and uraemia or with a history of deafness or to patients who have experienced a hypersensitivity reaction to vancomycin. If it must be given doses should be controlled by frequent determinations of the serum concentration, which should not exceed 25 µg per ml; monitoring of auditory function is advised, especially in elderly patients. Haematological status and kidney and liver function should be assessed periodically in all patients.

The concurrent use of other ototoxic or nephrotoxic drugs should be avoided.

Pregnancy and the neonate. If given during pregnancy vancomycin might cause damage to the eighth cranial nerve of the foetus.— G. M. Stirrat, *Prescribers' J.*, 1973, *13*, 135.

Antimicrobial Action. Vancomycin is an antibiotic which acts by interfering with bacterial cell wall synthesis. Most of the Gram-positive bacteria are sensitive to vancomycin but Gram-negative organisms, mycobacteria, and fungi are highly resistant.

The minimum inhibitory concentration of vancomycin has been reported to range from 0.2 to 6 µg per ml. In adequate concentrations it has bactericidal activity.

Strains of *Clostridium difficile* isolated from patients with pseudomembraneous colitis or diarrhoea were sensitive *in vitro* to vancomycin at concentrations well below those found in the faeces of patients with diarrhoea given 125 mg every 6 hours.— D. W. Burdon *et al.*, *J. antimicrob. Chemother.*, 1979, *5*, 307.

Vancomycin inhibited all of 100 strains of methicillin-resistant *Staphylococcus epidermidis* at a concentration *in vitro* of 3.12 µg or less per ml. Enhanced activity was demonstrated with vancomycin in association with cephamandole, cephalothin, or rifampicin.— M. E. Ein *et al.*, *Antimicrob. Ag. Chemother.*, 1979, *16*, 655.

For a study of the activity of gentamicin used with vancomycin against methicillin-resistant isolates of *Staph. epidermidis*, see Gentamicin Sulphate, p.1168.

Diminished activity. Antagonism occurred against some strains of *Staphylococcus aureus* when the activity of vancomycin was tested *in vitro* with daunorubicin or doxorubicin.— J. Y. Jacobs *et al.*, *Antimicrob. Ag. Chemother.*, 1979, *15*, 580.

Enhanced activity. A report of the synergism of vancomycin and streptomycin as well as of vancomycin and gentamicin against enterococci.— C. Watanakunakorn and C. Bakie, *Antimicrob. Ag. Chemother.*, 1973, *4*, 120. See also G. L. Mandell *et al.*, *Am. J. med. Sci.*, 1970, *259*, 346.

When used together *in vitro*, vancomycin and rifampicin showed enhanced activity against 5 of 20 isolates of *Staph. aureus*; their activities were additive against one strain.— C. U. Tuazon *et al.*, *Antimicrob. Ag. Chemother.*, 1978, *13*, 759.

Resistance. Sensitive bacteria do not readily acquire resistance to vancomycin. A few strains of *Staphylococcus aureus* have been reported to be naturally resistant to 5 µg or more per ml of vancomycin.

A report of group G streptococci exhibiting tolerance to vancomycin.— J. T. Noble *et al.* (letter), *Lancet*, 1980, *2*, 982.

Absorption and Fate. Vancomycin is not absorbed from the gastro-intestinal tract; therapeutically effective blood concentrations are maintained by intravenous injection of 500 mg every 6 hours or 1 g every 12 hours. Serum concentrations of vancomycin have been reported to range from 5 to 14 µg per ml following a dosage of 500 mg every 6 hours.

The antibiotic diffuses into pleural, pericardial, ascitic, and synovial fluids, but does not readily penetrate the cerebrospinal fluid unless the meninges are inflamed. It has been reported to diffuse across the placenta in *animals*. About 90% of the dose is excreted in urine. Vancomycin is not removed by haemodialysis or peritoneal dialysis.

Some 10% of vancomycin was bound in the body to serum proteins. The half-life in serum was 6 hours and 30 to 100% was excreted in urine.— C. M. Kunin, *Ann. intern. Med.*, 1967, *47*, 151.

Peak serum concentrations of vancomycin were 660 and 460 ng per ml in 2 of 5 anephric subjects undergoing haemodialysis thrice weekly, after receiving 500 mg four times daily by mouth for 4 days; concentrations were not assayable in the remaining subjects.— C. S. Bryan and W. L. White, *Antimicrob. Ag. Chemother.*, 1978, *14*, 634.

Further references to pharmacokinetic studies of vancomycin: J. R. Torres-R. *et al.* (letter), *J. antimicrob. Chemother.*, 1979, *5*, 475 (diffusion in tissues); D. J. Krogstad *et al.*, *J. clin. Pharmac.*, 1980, *20*, 197; U. B. Schaad *et al.*, *J. Pediat.*, 1980, *96*, 119.

Uses. Vancomycin hydrochloride is used in patients critically ill with staphylococcal or streptococcal infections resistant to the commonly used antibiotics and for patients who are allergic to penicillin. It has been recommended as an alternative to penicillin in the prophylaxis of bacterial endocarditis.

Vancomycin hydrochloride is administered intravenously, in dilute solution; it is irritating to the venous endothelium and may cause pain at the site of injection. It is administered by mouth in the treatment of staphylococcal enterocolitis and pseudomembranous colitis.

The usual adult dose is the equivalent of 500 mg of vancomycin every 6 to 8 hours by intravenous infusion, or 2 g daily by continuous intravenous infusion. Children may be given up to 45 mg per kg body-weight daily by intravenous infusion.

For the preferred method of intermittent infusion, a concentrated solution containing the equivalent of 500 mg of vancomycin in 10 ml of Water for Injections is added to 100 to 200 ml of dextrose injection or of sodium chloride injection and the diluted solution infused over 20 to 30 minutes.

For continuous intravenous infusion, the equivalent of 1 to 2 g is added to a sufficiently large volume of dextrose or sodium chloride solution to permit the daily dose to be given over a period of 24 hours.

In the treatment of colitis, the equivalent of up to 500 mg has been given by mouth every 6 hours. To guard against accumulation, regular determinations should be made of the concentrations of vancomycin in the blood; a concentration of 10 to 20 μg per ml should be maintained.

Reviews of the actions and uses of vancomycin.— J. E. Geraci, *Mayo Clin. Proc.*, 1977, *52*, 631; A. L. Esposito and R. A. Gleckman, *J. Am. med. Ass.*, 1977, *238*, 1756; F. V. Cook and W. E. Farrar, *Ann. intern. Med.*, 1978, *88*, 813.

Colitis. Findings of *Clostridium difficile* toxin in the stools of 6 patients with chronic inflammatory bowel disease during symptomatic relapse. Five of the 6 patients obtained a beneficial response to vancomycin therapy, and the sixth was controlled with corticosteroids, sulphasalazine, and bowel rest. Stool toxin should be assayed in patients with symptomatic inflammatory bowel disease unresponsive to standard medical therapy, irrespective of previous antibiotic therapy. This will allow selection of a sub-group of patients who may benefit from vancomycin therapy.— J. T. LaMont and Y. M. Trnka, *Lancet*, 1980, *1*, 381. See also R. P. Bolton *et al.*, *ibid.*, 383. Comment.— *ibid.*, 402.

Pseudomembranous colitis. Administration of vancomycin 500 mg by mouth every 6 hours for at least 7 days had a rapidly beneficial effect in 9 patients with antibiotic-induced colitis; the concentration of toxin in the gut was rapidly reduced, and bowel habits returned to normal within 10 days of the start of therapy. Serum assays indicated that absorption of vancomycin was insignificant despite the inflammatory bowel lesion and high intraluminal concentrations of vancomycin. Long-term follow-up of the patients indicated no recurrence on discontinuation of vancomycin. Unfortunately, parenteral administration of vancomycin to another patient who could not receive it by mouth did not reduce the titre of cytopathic toxin in the stool and no vancomycin could be detected in the patient's colostomy effluent after 5 days of treatment.— F. Tedesco *et al.*, *Lancet*, 1978, *2*, 226.

Of 44 patients with postoperative diarrhoea 16 had *Clostridium difficile* and faecal toxins in their stools while 5 had *Cl. difficile* without faecal toxins. The patients were treated with vancomycin 125 mg six-hourly for 5 days or with a placebo. The organism was eliminated from all except one of 12 treated with vancomycin but from only one of 9 given placebo. Clinical response followed removal of the organism and its toxin. Patients without the organism or its toxin did not improve.— M. R. B. Keighley *et al.*, *Br. med. J.*, 1978, *2*, 1667.

Three patients with pseudomembranous colitis were treated successfully with vancomycin 2 g daily by mouth but subsequently relapsed within 7, 27, and 28 days respectively of the cessation of therapy.— W. L. George *et al.*, *New Engl. J. Med.*, 1979, *301*, 414. See also R. G. Finch *et al.* (letter), *Lancet*, 1979, *2*, 1076.

Reports of the successful use of vancomycin in patients with pseudomembranous colitis, or similar conditions, attributed to: *Ampicillin*.— R. Modigliani and J. C. Delchier (letter), *Lancet*, 1978, *1*, 97. *Clindamycin*.— H. E. Larson *et al.* (letter), *Lancet*, 1978, *2*, 48. *Lincomycin*.— T. J. Marrie *et al.*, *Can. med. Ass. J.*, 1978, *119*, 1058. *Cephalosporins*.— J. G. Bartlett *et al.*, *J. Am. med. Ass.*, 1979, *242*, 2683.

A suggestion that an adequate dose of vancomycin for pseudomembranous colitis is 125 mg every six hours for 5 days.— A. H. V. Schapira and P. H. P. Dyson (letter), *Lancet*, 1980, *2*, 204. Metronidazole 400 mg thrice daily for 7 to 10 days is an effective and well-tolerated treatment for *Cl. difficile* colitis, and should be considered as an alternative to the vastly more expensive vancomycin.— R. P. Bolton (letter), *ibid.*, 428.

Death of a patient with pseudomembranous colitis despite eradication of *Cl. difficile* and its toxin by vancomycin.— P. C. Hawker *et al.*, *Br. med. J.*, 1981, *282*, 109.

Staphylococcal enterocolitis. References: M. Y. Khan and W. H. Hall, *Ann. intern. Med.*, 1966, *65*, 1.

Dosage in renal failure. A 1-g dose would maintain safe and therapeutic serum concentrations for 10 to 14 days in adult oliguric patients, even those receiving intermittent haemodialysis.— D. D. Lindholm and J. S. Murray, *New Engl. J. Med.*, 1966, *274*, 1047.

In 6 anuric patients given vancomycin 1 g by intravenous infusion, serum concentrations in excess of 2.5 μg per ml were maintained for about 7 days. Vancomycin was only minimally removed during haemodialysis. For anuric patients, vancomycin 1 g every 7 days was necessary to maintain adequate serum antibiotic concentrations for the treatment of staphylococcal infections. Some accumulation of vancomycin might occur over several weeks' treatment.— S. Eykyn *et al.*, *Br. med. J.*, 1970, *3*, 80.

In 25 patients with end-stage renal disease a dose of 1 g of vancomycin every 14 days produced plasma concentrations that were effective against *Staph. aureus* and were considered effective for prophylaxis of staphylococcal infection in external arteriovenous shunts. Up to 54 g had been given over 2 years without ill effect.— A. J. Morris and R. T. Bilinsky, *Am. J. med. Sci.*, 1971, *262*, 87.

Data for predicting removal of vancomycin by conventional haemodialysis.— T. P. Gibson and H. A. Nelson, *Clin. Pharmacokinet.*, 1977, *2*, 403.

The normal half-life for vancomycin of 6 to 8 hours was increased to 200 to 250 hours in end-stage renal failure. The interval between doses should be extended from 24 hours to 24 to 72 hours in patients with a glomerular filtration-rate (GFR) above 50 ml per minute, to 72 to 240 hours in those with a GFR of 10 to 50 ml per minute, and to 240 hours in those with a GFR of less than 10 ml per minute. Concentrations of vancomycin were not affected by haemodialysis or peritoneal dialysis.— W. M. Bennett *et al.*, *Ann. intern. Med.*, 1980, *93*, 62.

Mention of data indicating that vancomycin passes into the peritoneal cavity and may be removed by peritoneal dialysis. The dosage of vancomycin in patients undergoing peritoneal dialysis should be adjusted on the basis of serum concentrations.— D. A. Silverman (letter), *New Engl. J. Med.*, 1981, *304*, 361..

Further references: G. B. Appel and H. C. Neu, *New Engl. J. Med.*, 1977, *296*, 663; J. S. Cheigh, *Am. J. Med.*, 1977, *62*, 555; R. C. Moellering *et al.*, *Ann. intern. Med.*, 1981, *94*, 343 (a nomogram for dosage).

Endocarditis. A 61-year-old woman with enterococcal endocarditis developed pruritus and urticaria when treatment with benzylpenicillin and then ampicillin was begun. However she responded to therapy with vancomycin hydrochloride 500 mg intravenously every 8 hours and streptomycin sulphate 1 g daily. Studies with 18 group D streptococcal isolates demonstrated that vancomycin and streptomycin together exerted a synergistic action *in vitro*.— G. O. Westenfelder *et al.*, *J. Am. med. Ass.*, 1973, *223*, 37.

Vancomycin hydrochloride failed to eradicate *Staphylococcus aureus* in a man with endocarditis. The minimum inhibitory concentration was 0.78 μg per ml but the minimum bactericidal concentration was 25 μg per ml.— V. Gopal *et al.*, *J. Am. med. Ass.*, 1976, *236*, 1604.

High doses of vancomycin were not effective in 2 children with bacteraemia and endocarditis caused by *Staph. aureus*. The addition of rifampicin resulted in rapid and sustained clinical improvement.— R. J. Faville *et al.*, *J. Am. med. Ass.*, 1978, *240*, 1963.

Further references: C. K. Friedberg *et al.*, *Archs intern. Med.*, 1968, *122*, 134; R. E. Van Scoy *et al.*, *Mayo Clin. Proc.*, 1977, *52*, 216; E. W. Hook and W. D. Johnson, *Am. J. Med.*, 1978, *65*, 411.

Prophylaxis. A recommendation that vancomycin can be used prophylactically in patients allergic to penicillin who are at risk of developing bacterial endocarditis. A dose of 1 g may be infused intravenously over 30 to 60 minutes before dental procedures and surgery of the upper respiratory tract. In patients undergoing surgery of the gastro-intestinal and genito-urinary tracts streptomycin 1 g by intramuscular injection should also be administered.—Report of the Committee on Prevention of Rheumatic Fever and Bacterial Endocarditis of the American Heart Association, *Circulation*, 1977, *56*, 139A. Hypotension had occurred in patients given vancomycin 1 g pre-operatively in 10 ml of solution over 10 minutes but was avoided by the administration of a dilute solution (0.25 to 0.5%) over 30 minutes. Frequent monitoring of blood pressure and heart-rate was recommended.— P. Newfield and M. F. Roizen, *Ann. intern. Med.*, 1979, *91*, 581.

See also under Prophylactic Use of Antibiotics, p.1080.

Meningitis. Two children with meningitis due in one to *Staph. aureus* and in the other to *Flavobacterium meningosepticum* responded to treatment with vancomycin. The recommended dose is 40 mg per kg body-weight daily intravenously to a maximum of 2 g daily. Intrathecal therapy with 20 mg daily should only be added if the CSF is not sterile after 48 hours.— H. B. Hawley and D. W. Gump, *Am. J. Dis. Child.*, 1973, *126*, 261.

Further references: J. L. Ryan *et al.*, *Am. J. Med.*, 1980, *68*, 449 (intrathecal vancomycin and rifampicin by mouth in enterococcal meningitis).

Suppression of intestinal flora. A study in 38 patients with leukaemia who received gentamicin, vancomycin, and nystatin (GVN) or gentamicin and nystatin for prophylactic suppression of intestinal flora, indicated that vancomycin could be safely omitted from the GVN regimen provided that microbiological monitoring was performed to detect the emergence of resistant organisms. Tolerance was improved when vancomycin was omitted.— J. F. Bender *et al.*, *Antimicrob. Ag. Chemother.*, 1979, *15*, 455.

See also under Gentamicin Sulphate, p.1172.

Preparations

Sterile Vancomycin Hydrochloride *(U.S.P.)*. A grade of vancomycin hydrochloride for injection, in packs containing the equivalent of 500 mg of vancomycin.

Vancomycin Hydrochloride for Oral Solution *(U.S.P.)*. The solution is prepared by the addition of diluent before issue. pH after reconstitution 2.5 to 4.5. Potency is expressed in terms of the equivalent amount of van comycin. Store in airtight containers.

Vancomycin Injection *(B.P.)*. Vancomycin Hydrochloride Injection. A sterile solution of vancomycin hydrochloride in Water for Injections, prepared by dissolving, immediately before use, the sterile contents of a sealed container in Water for Injections.

Proprietary Preparations

Vancocin *(Lilly, UK)*. Vancomycin hydrochloride, available as powder for preparing solutions for intravenous infusion, in vials each containing the equivalent of 500 mg of vancomycin. Also available, for oral use, in bottles containing the equivalent of 10 g of vancomycin; when mixed with 115 ml of water each 6 ml provides approximately 500 mg of vancomycin. (Also available as Vancocin in *Austral., Belg., Canad., Denm., Norw., S.Afr., Switz., USA*).

Other Proprietary Names

Diatracin *(Spain)*.

178-k

Virginiamycin.

Antibiotic 899; SKF 7988; Virgimycin. A mixture consisting principally of 2 antimicrobial substances, virginiamycin M_1, and virginiamycin S_1, produced by the growth of *Streptomyces virginiae* or by any other means.

CAS — 11006-76-1; 21411-53-0 (virginiamycin M_1); 23152-29-6 (virginiamycin S_1).

Very slightly **soluble** in water.

Adverse Effects. Virginiamycin may cause gastro-intestinal irritation and vomiting. A few instances of hypersensitivity have been observed.

A study indicating that usual therapeutic doses of virginiamycin interfere with colour vision.— J. Laroche and C. Laroche, *Annls pharm. Fr.*, 1972, *30*, 433. See also *idem*, 1970, *28*, 333.

Antimicrobial Action. Virginiamycin is active against staphylococci and some streptococci; *Neisseria gonorrhoeae* and *Haemophilus influenzae* are reported to be sensitive.

An *in vitro* study indicated that strains of *Streptococcus faecalis* could transfer erythromycin-resistance to group A, B, and D streptococci. Large scale use of macrolide antibiotics and virginiamycin for growth promotion in animal husbandry could lead to a reservoir of macrolide-resistant group-D streptococci indigenous in animals which could transfer resistance to the virulent group A and group B streptococci.— J. D. A. van Embden *et al.* (letter), *Lancet*, 1978, *1*, 655.

Absorption and Fate. Virginiamycin is rapidly absorbed from the gastro-intestinal tract, and is excreted in the urine and faeces.

In 2 volunteers given radioactive virginiamycin peak plasma and urinary concentrations were achieved about 4 hours after the dose; about 15 to 20% of the dose was excreted within 24 hours.— B. Boon *et al.*, *Thérapie*, 1973, *28*, 367.

Uses. Virginiamycin is used for the treatment of infections due to sensitive organisms, particularly Gram-positive cocci. The usual dose by mouth is 2 to 4 g daily in divided doses. Children have been given 50 mg per kg body-weight. It has been applied locally in a dusting-powder (2%), ointment (0.5%), or by instillation as a suspension (0.5%).

Virginiamycin is used as an additive for animal feeding stuffs.

Proprietary Names

Stafilomicina *(Smith Kline & French, Ital.)*; Staphylomycine *(RIT, Belg.*; *Smith Kline & French, Fr.*; *Smith Kline & French, Neth.)*; Staxidin *(Smith Kline & French, Spain)*.

Peroxides

5901-f

Hydrogen Peroxide Solution (3 per cent)

(B.P., Eur. P.). Hydrogen Peroxide Topical Solution *(U.S.P.)*; Dilute Hydrogen Peroxide Solution; Hydrogenii Peroxidum Dilutum; Hydrogen Peroxide Solution (10-volume).

CAS — 7722-84-1 (H_2O_2).

Pharmacopoeias. In all pharmacopoeias examined except *Braz., Ind.*, and *Int. Turk.* specifies 3 to 3.5% w/v.

An aqueous solution containing 2.5 to 3.5% w/v of H_2O_2 (= 34.01) corresponding to about 10 times its volume of available oxygen. It may be stabilised for a limited time by adding a suitable stabilising agent. The *U.S.P.* permits up to 0.05% of a suitable preservative or preservatives.

A colourless almost odourless liquid which on dilution has a slightly acid taste. It decomposes in contact with oxidisable organic matter and with certain metals, and also if allowed to become alkaline.

Incompatible with reducing agents, including organic matter and oxidisable substances, and with alkalis, iodides, permanganates, and other stronger oxidising agents. Its decomposition is increased by metallic salts, light, agitation, and heat, as well as by metals. It is comparatively stable in the presence of a slight excess of acid.

Store in a cool place in bottles closed with glass stoppers, paraffined corks, or plastic or protected metal screw caps. Solutions not containing a stabiliser should be stored in a cool place. Protect from light.

5902-d

Hydrogen Peroxide Solution (6 per cent)

(B.P.). Hydrogen Peroxide Solution; Hydrogen Peroxide Solution (20-volume); Hydrog. Perox. Soln.; Liquor Hydrogenii Peroxidi; Liq. Hydrog. Perox.; Hydrogen Dioxide Solution; Soluté Officinal d'Eau Oxygénée; Wasserstoffsuperoxydlösung; Solución de Bióxido de Hidrogeno; Oxydol.

Pharmacopoeias. In *Br.* and *Ind.*

An aqueous solution containing 5 to 7% w/v of H_2O_2 corresponding to about 20 times its volume of available oxygen. It may be stabilised for a limited period by adding a suitable stabilising agent.

A colourless odourless liquid which on dilution has a slightly acid taste. It decomposes rapidly in contact with oxidisable organic matter and with certain metals, and also if allowed to become alkaline.

Incompatibility and **Storage.** As for Hydrogen Peroxide Solution (3 per cent) (above).

NOTE. The *B.P.* directs that when Hydrogen Peroxide is prescribed or demanded, Hydrogen Peroxide Solution (6 per cent) be dispensed or supplied.

5903-n

Hydrogen Peroxide Solution (27 per cent)

(B.P., Eur. P.). Hydrogenii Peroxidum 27 per centum; Strong Hydrogen Peroxide Solution; Strong Hydrog. Perox. Soln.; Hydrogen Peroxide Solution (100-volume); Hydrogenii Peroxidum; Perossido D'Idrogeno Soluzione; Solutio Hydrogenii Peroxydati.

Pharmacopoeias. In *Br., Eur., Ger., It., Neth.*, and *Turk.*

An aqueous solution containing 26 to 28% w/w (about 30% w/v) of H_2O_2, corresponding to about 100 times its volume of available oxygen. It may contain a suitable stabilising agent.

A colourless almost odourless liquid. It decomposes vigorously in contact with oxidisable organic matter and with certain metals, and also if allowed to become alkaline.

Incompatibility and **Storage.** As for Hydrogen Peroxide Solution (3 per cent) (above). Strong solutions of hydrogen peroxide are more stable than the weaker solutions and, when properly stored, should lose not more than about 0.5% of their original hydrogen peroxide content in a year. The stopper or cap should be provided with a vent.

5904-h

Hydrogen Peroxide Solution (30 per cent)

(B.P., Eur. P.). Hydrogenii Peroxidum 30 per centum.

Pharmacopoeias. In *Arg., Belg., Br., Eur., Fr., Ger., It., Neth., Nord., Pol., Roum., Span.*, and *Swiss. Aust.* specifies 30 to 32%, *Cz.* 28 to 32%, *Hung.* 27.5 to 32%, and *Jug.* 28 to 31%. *U.S.* specifies Hydrogen Peroxide Concentrate 29 to 32%.

An aqueous solution containing 29 to 31% w/w of H_2O_2, corresponding to about 110 times its volume of available oxygen. It may contain a suitable stabilising agent.

A colourless almost odourless liquid. It decomposes vigorously in contact with oxidisable organic matter and with certain metals and also if allowed to become alkaline.

Other industrial strengths of hydrogen peroxide solution are manufactured, including 35% w/w, 50% w/w, and 85% w/w.

Incompatibility and **Storage**. As for Hydrogen Peroxide Solution (27 per cent).

Adverse Effects and Precautions. Strong solutions of hydrogen peroxide produce irritating 'burns' on the skin and mucous membranes with a white eschar, but the pain disappears in about an hour. Continued use of hydrogen peroxide as a mouth-wash may cause reversible hypertrophy of the papillae of the tongue.

It is dangerous to inject hydrogen peroxide into closed body cavities from which the released oxygen has no free exit. Colonic lavage with solutions of hydrogen peroxide as weak as 0.75% has been followed by gas embolism and by gangrene of the intestine.

Maximum permissible atmospheric concentration of hydrogen peroxide 1 ppm.

Hydrogen peroxide could interfere with the Clinitest and Labstix qualitative urine tests for glucose to produce false positive results.— *Drug & Ther. Bull.*, 1972, *10*, 69.

Uses. Hydrogen peroxide is used as a disinfectant and deodorant. It owes its action to its ready release of oxygen when applied to tissues, but the effect lasts only as long as the oxygen is being released and is of short duration; in addition the antimicrobial effect of the liberated oxygen is reduced in the presence of organic matter.

Hydrogen peroxide usually as a 6% solution is used to cleanse wounds; the effervescence of oxygen detaches dead tissue and pockets of bacteria from inaccessible parts. However, injection into closed body cavities is dangerous (see adverse effects). Adhering and blood-soaked dressings may be released by the application of a solution of hydrogen peroxide.

A 1.5% solution of hydrogen peroxide has been used as a mouthwash in the treatment of acute stomatitis and as a deodorant gargle. In dentistry, hydrogen peroxide has been used to clean septic sockets and root canals.

Hydrogen peroxide ear-drops have been used for the removal of wax. They are prepared by diluting a 6% solution of hydrogen peroxide with 3 parts of water preferably just before use.

For bleaching hair and delicate fabrics hydrogen peroxide 6% should be neutralised or rendered faintly alkaline and diluted with an equal volume of water. In some countries cosmetic product regulations limit the concentration of hydrogen peroxide in hair care products to 12.1%.

Strong solutions (27 per cent and 30 per cent) of hydrogen peroxide are used for the preparation of weaker solutions.

Hydrogen peroxide and other peroxides have many industrial uses as bleaching and oxidising agents.

Disinfection of respirators. Nebulised hydrogen peroxide disinfected mechanical ventilators; not all nebulisers effectively nebulised hydrogen peroxide.— P. A. Judd *et al., Lancet*, 1968, *2*, 1019; G. Spencer *et al.* (letter), *ibid.*, 1144.

Disinfection of rooms. Hydrogen peroxide aerosols were dispersed in rooms over a period of 5 minutes at a temperature of 20° to 22° and a relative humidity of 21 to 29%; hydrogen peroxide concentrations were 20 to 31 mg per m^3. Influenza virus A2 was isolated from 12 of 27 air samples taken before disinfection and from none of 24 taken 40 minutes after disinfection.— B. P. Fedyaev *et al., Zh. Mikrobiol. Epidem. Immunobiol.*, 1972, *9*, 137, per *Abstr. Hyg.*, 1973, *48*, 252.

Preparations

Hydrogen Peroxide Ear Drops *(B.P., A.P.F.).* Auristillae Hydrogenii Peroxidi. Hydrogen peroxide solution (6 per cent) 25 ml, water to 100 ml. *A.P.F.* specifies freshly boiled and cooled water.

Proprietary Preparations

Genoxide *(Interox, UK).* A brand of Hydrogen Peroxide Solution (3 per cent).

Hioxyl *(Quinoderm, UK).* Hydrogen peroxide, available as cream containing 1.5%.

Other Proprietary Names

Brintoverilte, Caroxin *(*see also under Urea Hydrogen Peroxide*)* *(*both *Denm.).*

5905-m

Benzoyl Peroxide.

Hydrous Benzoyl Peroxide *(U.S.P.).* Dibenzoyl peroxide.

$C_{14}H_{10}O_4$=242.2.

CAS — 94-36-0.

Pharmacopoeias. In *Braz.* and *U.S.*

A white granular powder with a characteristic odour. Sparingly **soluble** in water and alcohol; soluble in acetone, chloroform, and ether.

Benzoyl peroxide decomposes at a rate which increases with rise of temperature and it may explode at temperatures higher than 60° or cause fires in the presence of reducing substances. For safety, benzoyl peroxide is moistened with about 26% w/w of water. **Store** in original container, treated to reduce static charges, at room temperature. Unused material should not be returned to its original container but should be destroyed with sodium hydroxide solution. Protect from light.

CAUTION. *Benzoyl peroxide may decompose violently if subjected to grinding.*

Stability. Benzoyl peroxide 35% and dicalcium phosphate 65% mixed powder was stable for at least 8 weeks at 60° and 27 weeks at 49°. A spectrophotometric method showed that stability was reduced in cream and lotion preparations and a minimum of 90% potency was retained for only 3 weeks in 2 commercial lotions and 5 weeks in a commercial cream stored at 46°.— M. P. Gruber and R. W. Klein, *J. pharm. Sci.*, 1967, *56*, 1505.

At both 30° and 40° benzoyl peroxide was destroyed within 1 month in formulations containing alcohol and acidic chelating agents. Substitution of acetone for alcohol, removal of the chelating agents, and adjustment of the pH of gel preparations with sodium hydroxide enhanced stability.— J. N. Bollinger *et al., J. pharm. Sci.*, 1977, *66*, 718.

Adverse Effects. Application of benzoyl peroxide may produce an initial stinging effect. Contact sensitisation has been reported in some patients using preparations containing benzoyl peroxide.

Maximum permissible atmospheric concentration 5 mg per m^3.

Of 50 patients studied, 38 demonstrated sensitivity to gel preparations containing benzoyl peroxide 5%; patch tests using a 1% solution of benzoyl peroxide in acetone on 10 of the sensitive subjects showed the sensitivity to be retained for at least 3 months.— J. J. Leyden and A. M. Kligman, *Contact Dermatitis*, 1977, *3*, 273.

A report of an unusual unpleasant body odour in one patient attributed to the topical use of benzoyl peroxide.— P. Molberg (letter), *New Engl. J. Med.*, 1981, *304*, 1366.

Uses. Benzoyl peroxide has keratolytic properties and may have some antimicrobial action. It is used in the treatment of acne, usually in topical preparations containing 5 to 10% which may also contain 2 to 5% of sulphur.

Benzoyl peroxide is also used as a bleaching agent in the food industry and as a catalyst in the plastics industry.

Acne. A brief discussion of the use of benzoyl peroxide for the treatment of acne.— J. W. Melski and K. A. Arndt, *New Engl. J. Med.*, 1980, *302*, 503. See also R. N. Brogden *et al.*, *Drugs*, 1974, *8*, 417; W. J. Cunliffe, *Br. med. J.*, 1980, *280*, 1394.

In a double-blind study in 196 patients with acne, 5.5% benzoyl peroxide lotion, 5.5% benzoyl peroxide lotion plus 0.25% halquinol (Loroxide), or a similar lotion containing also hydrocortisone 0.5% (Loroxide-HC) were more effective than a placebo preparation when each were used 4 times daily for 4 weeks; clinical evaluation favoured the preparation containing halquinol.— M. Ede, *Curr. ther. Res.*, 1973, *15*, 624.

In a double-blind 12-week study slightly more reduction in facial lesions was reported among 44 patients with acne applying tretinoin solution 0.025% twice daily than among those using a lotion containing benzoyl peroxide 5%; initially tretinoin appeared to exacerbate the condition causing hidden lesions to erupt.— J. H. Bucknall and P. N. T. Murdoch, *Curr. med. Res. Opinion*, 1977, *5*, 266. An 8-week study completed by 60 of 69 patients with moderately severe facial acne showed that treatments with benzoyl peroxide gel 5% or with a cream containing tretinoin 0.05% were equally effective in reducing numbers of lesions. No serious side-effects were reported for either preparation.— B. S. Belknap, *Cutis*, 1979, *23*, 856.

Earlier reports of the use of creams containing benzoyl peroxide and sulphur in various strengths in the treatment of acne.— W. E. Pace, *Can. med. Ass. J.*, 1965, *93*, 252; R. D. Wilkinson *et al.*, *Can. med. Ass. J.*, 1966, *95*, 28.

Ulcers. Uncontrolled studies showed that benzoyl peroxide either in a 20% oil/water emulsion, or in a 50% paste with water and containing 0.5% of a colloidal aluminium magnesium silicate, or both preparations, used in succession, aided the healing of cutaneous ulcers in 115 of 133 patients. Treatment was discontinued in 5 patients who developed irritant or contact dermatitis. The application of a protective ointment to tissue surrounding the ulcer during treatment was recommended.— W. E. Pace, *Can. med. Ass. J.*, 1976, *115*, 1101.

Preparations

Benzoyl Peroxide Gel *(U.S.P.)*. Contains benzoyl peroxide in a suitable gel basis. pH 3.5 to 6. Store in airtight containers.

Benzoyl Peroxide Lotion *(U.S.P.)*. A lotion containing benzoyl peroxide in a suitable basis. Store in airtight containers.

Proprietary Preparations

AcetOxyl *(Stiefel, UK)*. Benzoyl peroxide, available as a gel containing 2.5 or 5% in an acetone basis. (Also available as AcetOxyl in *Canad.*).

Acnegel *(Kirby-Warrick, UK)*. Contains benzoyl peroxide 5%. **Acnegel Forte.** Contains benzoyl peroxide 10%.

Benoxyl 5 *(Stiefel, UK)*. **Cream** and **Lotion** each containing benzoyl peroxide 5%. **Benoxyl 5 with Sulphur** contains in addition sulphur 2%. **Benoxyl 10. Lotion** containing benzoyl peroxide 10%. **Benoxyl 10 with Sulphur. Cream** and **Lotion** each containing benzoyl peroxide 10% and sulphur 5%. **Benoxyl 20. Lotion** containing benzoyl peroxide 20%. For acne. (Also available as Benoxyl in *Austral.*, *Canad.*).

Debroxide 5 *(Alcon, UK: Farillon, UK)*. Benzoyl peroxide, available as a gel containing 5%. **Debroxide 10.** Contains benzoyl peroxide 10%.

Panoxyl 5 Acne Gel *(Stiefel, UK)*. Contains benzoyl peroxide 5% in a gel basis. **Panoxyl 10 Acne Gel.** Contains benzoyl peroxide 10%. (Also available as Panoxyl in *Austral.*, *Ger.*, *Norw.*, *Switz.*, *USA*).

Vanair *(Carter-Wallace, UK)*. Cream containing benzoyl peroxide 10% and colloidal sulphur 2.5%. For acne.

Other Proprietary Names

Austral.—Acnacyl; *Canad.*—Benzagel, Dermoxyl, Oxyderm, Persa-Gel; *Denm.*—Benoxid; *Ger.*—Akne-Aid; *NZ*—Kerolyte; *USA*—Benzac, Benzagel, Clearasil, Dermodex, Desquam-X, Fostex BPO, Persadox, Teen, Xerac BP.

5906-b

Magnesium Peroxide *(B.P.C. 1949)*. Magnesium Perhydrolum.

CAS — 1335-26-8; 14452-57-4.

Pharmacopoeias. In *Arg.*, *Aust.*, *Cz.*, *Ger.*, *Hung.*, *Neth.*, *Port.*, *Roum.*, *Rus.*, *Span.*, and *Swiss*, most of which specify about 25% of MgO_2 (6.5% available oxygen).

A white odourless tasteless powder containing not less than 15% of MgO_2 (=56.30) (4.5% available oxygen). Practically **insoluble** in water, but is gradually decomposed by it with the evolution of oxygen; practically insoluble in alcohol; slowly soluble in dilute acids with the formation of H_2O_2. It decomposes on heating. **Store** in a cool place in airtight containers. Protect from light.

Magnesium peroxide is used as a deodorant and disinfectant, mainly as an ingredient of dentifrices.

Proprietary Names

Ozovit *(Pascoe, Ger.)*.

5907-v

Potassium Permanganate *(B.P., Eur. P., U.S.P.)*. Pot. Permang.; Kalii Permanganas; Kalium Hypermanganicum; Kalium Permanganicum.

$KMnO_4$=158.0.

CAS — 7722-64-7.

Pharmacopoeias. In all pharmacopoeias examined except *Int.*

Odourless dark purple or almost black crystals or granular powder, almost opaque by transmitted light and with a blue metallic lustre by reflected light and with a sweet astringent taste and a disagreeable astringent after-taste. It decomposes, with a risk of explosion, in contact with certain organic substances.

Soluble 1 in 16 of water and 1 in 3.5 of boiling water giving purple solutions. An acidified solution in water is readily reduced by hydrogen peroxide, by easily oxidisable substances, and by organic matter. **Incompatible** with iodides, reducing agents, and most organic substances. **Store** in well-closed containers avoiding contact with organic substances.

WARNING. *The Council of the Pharmaceutical Society of Great Britain advises pharmacists not to supply materials likely to be used for making fireworks, including permanganates, to children under any circumstances, and recommends that potassium permanganate should be sold only to persons who are, or appear to be, 18 years of age or over.*

Adverse Effects. The crystals and concentrated solutions of potassium permanganate are caustic and even fairly dilute solutions are irritant to tissues. Repeated use of dilute solutions may cause corrosive burns.

Symptoms of poisoning following ingestion of potassium permanganate include nausea, vomiting of a brownish coloured material, corrosion, oedema, and brown coloration of the buccal mucosa, liver and kidney damage, and cardiovascular depression. The fatal dose is probably about 10 g and death may occur up to 1 month from the time of poisoning.

The insertion into the vagina of potassium permanganate in the form of tablets, crystals, or a douche, for its supposed abortifacient action, causes corrosive burns, severe vaginal haemorrhage, and perforation of the vaginal wall, leading to peritonitis. Vascular collapse may occur.

Methaemoglobinaemia in 2 patients associated with potassium permanganate ingestion.— M. C. Mahomedy *et al.*, *Anaesthesia*, 1975, *30*, 190.

Treatment of Adverse Effects. Poisoning from the ingestion of potassium permanganate should be treated immediately with milk to delay absorption. The circulation should be maintained with infusions of plasma or suitable electrolyte solutions, but care is necessary as anuria may occur. Burns and ulcers of the mucous membranes should be treated by repeated copious washing with water.

The brown stain caused by solutions can be removed from the skin by oxalic or by sulphurous acid.

Uses. Potassium permanganate possesses oxidising properties which in turn confer disinfectant and deodorising properties. It is also astringent. Though bactericidal *in vitro* its clinical value as a bactericide is minimised by its rapid reduction in the presence of body fluids.

It is used as a 1 in 1000 solution in water as a cleansing application to ulcers or abscesses and as a 1 in 4000 solution as a gargle or mouthwash; freshly prepared solutions should be used. Solutions of similar strengths are used as wet dressings and in baths in eczematous conditions and acute dermatoses especially where there is secondary infection. A 1% solution has been used in bromhidrosis, in mycotic infections such as athlete's foot, and in poison ivy dermatitis. A 5% solution has a powerful styptic action.

A 0.02% solution in water can be employed as a stomach wash-out in the treatment of poisoning by morphine, opium, and strychnine; its use should be followed by evacuation of the stomach. It is of no value in poisoning by atropine, cocaine, or the barbiturates.

Potassium permanganate has been widely used as a first-aid treatment in snake bite but it is of no value for this purpose, though a solution will destroy any venom lying free on the surface of the skin.

Preparations

Potassium Permanganate Tablets for Topical Solution *(U.S.P.)*. Potassium Permanganate Tablets for Solution. Solution tablets containing potassium permanganate. Store in airtight containers.

5908-g

Sodium Perborate *(B.P.)*. Sod. Perbor.; Natrii Perboras.

$NaBO_2,H_2O_2,3H_2O$=153.9.

CAS — 7632-04-4 (anhydrous); 10042-94-1 (hydrate).

Pharmacopoeias. In *Br.*, *Fr.*, *Ind.*, *Port.*, and *Span.*

Odourless or almost odourless, colourless prismatic crystals or a white powder, stable in crystalline form, with a saline taste.

Soluble 1 in 40 of water, gradually decomposing into sodium metaborate and hydrogen peroxide with the evolution of oxygen; the oxygen is evolved more rapidly if the solution is warmed. Its decomposition is accelerated by even the weakest acids and by enzymes and other catalysts. Solutions in water are alkaline to litmus. **Store** in a cool place in airtight containers. Protect from light.

Adverse Effects. Frequent use of tooth-powders containing sodium perborate may cause blistering and oedema. Hypertrophy of the papillae of the

tongue has also been reported.
The effects of swallowed sodium perborate are similar to those of boric acid (see p.337).

Uses. Sodium perborate is a mild disinfectant and deodorant. It readily releases oxygen in contact with oxidisable matter and has been used in aqueous solutions for purposes similar to weak solutions of hydrogen peroxide. Vincent's infection may be treated by the application of a paste made with water or glycerol; the paste is retained in the mouth for 5 minutes and then rinsed out.
Sodium perborate has also been used, mixed with 2 to 4 parts of calcium carbonate, as a tooth-powder. A 2% solution freshly prepared is used as a mouth-wash.
Sodium perborate is also used in the formulation of household detergents. The less soluble $NaBO_2,H_2O_2$ known as sodium perborate monohydrate is also used in denture cleaners and detergent preparations.

A study of the absorption of boron after use of sodium perborate mouthwash [Bocosept] indicated that there was little risk of boron poisoning. Blood concentrations of boron did not exceed 320 ng per ml. Boron did not appear to be absorbed by the oral mucosa but was probably absorbed from the intestine after ingestion of residual amounts from the mouth.— L. Edwall *et al.*, *Eur. J. clin. Pharmac.*, 1979, *15*, 417. See also H. Dill *et al.*, *Int. J. clin. Pharmac. Biopharm.*, 1977, *15*, 16.

Proprietary Preparations

Bocasan (known in some countries as Amosan, Bocosept, and Kavosan) *(Cooper, UK)*. A powder in sealed sachets containing sodium perborate monohydrate 68.635% buffered with anhydrous sodium hydrogen tartrate 29.415%, and flavoured with peppermint oil and menthol. The contents of 1 sachet in 30 ml of water are used as a mouth-wash in the treatment of gingivitis, Vincent's infection, and other periodontal conditions.

5909-q

Sodium Percarbonate *(B.P.C. 1949).*

$Na_2CO_3,1\frac{1}{2}H_2O_2$=157.0.

A white crystalline powder. **Soluble** 1 in 9 of water, gradually decomposing into sodium carbonate and hydrogen peroxide with the evolution of oxygen. **Store** in a cool place in airtight containers. Protect from light.

Sodium percarbonate has properties similar to those of sodium perborate and has been used for the same purposes, but since its decomposition products are more alkaline the perborate is usually preferred.

5910-d

Urea Hydrogen Peroxide. Carbamide Peroxide; Hydroperite; Urea Peroxide.

$NH_2.CO.NH_2,H_2O_2$=94.07.

CAS — 124-43-6.

Pharmacopoeias. In *Hung.*

White crystals or a crystalline powder, consisting of equimolecular proportions of hydrogen peroxide and urea, which yields about 35% of H_2O_2.
Soluble 1 in 2.5 of water. It decomposes in air into urea, oxygen, and water. **Incompatible** with alcohol and ether, which cause partial decomposition. **Store** in a cool place. Protect from light.

Adverse Effects.

A preparation containing urea hydrogen peroxide 10% in anhydrous glycerol was applied to a periodontal abscess thrice daily and used as a mouth-wash. After 96 hours the patient developed a black hairy tongue which returned to normal when treatment was discontinued.— A. E. Michanowicz and J. P. Michanowicz, *Oral Surg.*, 1964, *18*, 459.

Uses. Urea hydrogen peroxide is used for the extemporaneous preparation of hydrogen peroxide. It has been employed for infections of the ear, mouth, and skin. Preparations containing urea hydrogen peroxide 6.5% in glycerol are used to soften ear wax.

Preparations

Carbamide Peroxide Topical Solution *(U.S.P.)*. Carbamide Peroxide Solution. A solution of urea hydrogen peroxide in anhydrous glycerol, containing the equivalent of 2.82 to 3.98% w/w of hydrogen peroxide. pH 4 to 7.5. Store at a temperature not exceeding 40° in airtight containers. Protect from light.

Exterol *(Dermal Laboratories, UK)*. Urea hydrogen peroxide, available as ear-drops containing 5%. For the softening of hardened wax.

Other Proprietary Names

Caroxin (see also under Hydrogen Peroxide) *(Norw.)*; Debrox *(Canad., USA)*; Gly-Oxide *(Canad., USA)*; Murine *(USA)*; Proxigel *(USA)*.

Urea hydrogen peroxide was formerly marketed in Great Britain under the proprietary name Lapural *(Laporte)*.

5911-n

Zinc Permanganate *(B.P.C. 1949).* Zinc. Permang.

$Zn(MnO_4)_2,6H_2O$=411.3.

CAS — 23414-72-4 (anhydrous).

Brownish-black iridescent deliquescent crystals. **Soluble** 1 in 3 of water (usually leaving some residue). **Incompatible** with iodides, reducing agents, and most organic substances. **Store** in airtight containers. Protect from light.

CAUTION. *Zinc permanganate is liable to explode spontaneously and if the stopper of a bottle containing it becomes stuck, the bottle should be wrapped in a cloth before removal of the stopper is attempted.*

Zinc permanganate possesses the oxidising properties of the potassium salt but is more astringent and is readily reduced.

5912-h

Zinc Peroxide *(B.P. 1953).* Medicinal Zinc Peroxide.

CAS — 1314-22-3.

Pharmacopoeias. In *Arg., Fr., Port.*, and *Span.* (all not less than 35%).

A mixture of zinc peroxide, zinc oxide, and zinc hydroxide, containing not less than 60% of ZnO_2 (=97.38). It is a fine white or faintly yellow odourless powder. Practically **insoluble** in water and organic solvents; readily soluble in dilute mineral acids. **Incompatible** with oxidising and reducing agents. **Store** in a cool place in airtight containers.

Uses. The action of zinc peroxide is similar to that of hydrogen peroxide. Applied locally as a 40% suspension it has been used for disinfecting, deodorising, and promoting the healing of burns, wounds and various ulcers and lesions. It has been used as a bleaching agent in dental practice.

Preparations

Zinc Peroxide Cream *(Roy. Marsden Hosp.)*. Zinc peroxide 1 g, zinc oxide 5 g, wool fat 2 g, calcium hydroxide solution 1 ml, arachis oil 8 ml. It should be freshly prepared. Shelf-life 21 days.

Phenytoin and some other Anticonvulsants

6600-k

Anticonvulsant drugs are used chiefly in the treatment of various types of epilepsy.

Epilepsy has been described as a chronic condition characterised by more or less frequent recurrence of seizures, associated with loss or disturbance of consciousness and usually with convulsive or other body movements and correlated with abnormal EEG discharges.

There have been numerous attempts at classification; a proposed classification of epileptic seizures divides epilepsy into generalised and partial. Generalised seizures include 'absences' (*petit mal*), tonic-clonic seizures (*grand mal*), and myoclonic seizures; and partial (focal) seizures include those with motor, sensory, or autonomic symptoms, and those of complex symptomatology including *temporal lobe* or *psychomotor* seizures.

The anticonvulsant drugs include the *hydantoins* (ethotoin, methoin, and phenytoin), carbamazepine, valproic acid, the *oxazolidines* (dimethadione, paramethadione, and troxidone), the *succinimides* (ethosuximide, methsuximide, and phensuximide), primidone, and phenobarbitone (see p.814), the *acetylureas* (phenacemide and pheneturide), some *benzodiazepine* compounds (clonazepam; diazepam—see p.1523; and nitrazepam—see p.808), acetazolamide (see p.582), and corticotrophin (see under Corticosteroids, p.453).

For comments on the actions and relative merits of anticonvulsant drugs in the different forms of epilepsy see under phenytoin (p.1243) as well as the individual drug monographs.

Publications: *Antiepileptic Drugs*, D.M. Woodbury *et al.* (Ed.), New York, Raven Press, 1980; *The Treatment of Epilepsy*, J.H. Tyrer (Ed.), Lancaster, England, MTP Press, 1980.

Pregnancy and the neonate. Comment on epilepsy and pregnancy including a discussion on the teratogenic risks of anticonvulsants. Compounds like troxidone may have serious effects and are best avoided. Congenital malformations in man have not been reported with sodium valproate, though in *animals* it has induced teratogenic effects. The risk that the foetus will develop harelip, cleft palate, or congenital heart lesions is increased by 2 or 3 if the mother is treated during pregnancy with phenytoin, either alone or in association with phenobarbitone, primidone, or carbamazepine. This risk of major and minor malformations may also be related in part to the maternal epilepsy and other variables, including maternal age, diabetes, social class, family history of malformations, incidence of twins, and obstetric complications. On balance, the teratogenic risk of anti-epileptic drugs seems small and does not justify discouraging a woman who needs treatment with them from having a child, nor does it justify changing a satisfactory drug regimen when the epilepsy is well controlled. A woman having treatment for epilepsy who wants to embark on pregnancy should ideally be on a single drug with its serum concentration in the optimum range; but if control has been achieved with an association of anticonvulsants the patient should be encouraged to continue with the same regimen because the risks to the foetus and mother may be greater from uncontrolled fits than from the drugs.— *Br. med. J.*, 1980, *281*, 1087. See also *Pediatrics*, 1979, *63*, 331; *Br. med. J.*, 1981, *283*, 515; A. H. Bardy *et al.* (letter), *ibid.*, 1405 (criticism).

Surveys and comments on the association between anticonvulsant therapy and congenital malformations: A. V. Bird (letter), *Lancet*, 1969, *1*, 311; J. Elshove and J. H. M. Van Eck, *Ned. Tijdschr. Geneesk.*, 1971, *115*, 1371; B. D. Speidel and S. R. Meadow, *Lancet*, 1972, *2*, 839; J. South (letter), *ibid.*, 1154; C. R. Lowe, *ibid.*, 1973, *1*, 9; E. V. Kuenssberg and J. D. E. Knox (letter), *ibid.*, 198; J. H. D. Millar and N. C. Nevin (letter), *ibid.*, 328; J. Fedrick, *Br. med. J.*, 1973, *2*, 442; J. D. Niswander and W. Wertelecki (letter), *Lancet*, 1973, *1*, 1062; A. A. E. Starreveld-Zimmerman *et al.* (letter), *ibid.*, 1973, *2*, 48; S. Livingston *et al.* (letter), *ibid.*, 1265; R. R. Monson *et al.*, *New Engl. J. Med.*, 1973, *289*, 1049; J. E. Barry and D. M. Danks (letter), *Lancet*, 1974, *2*, 48; R. M. Hill *et al.*, *Am. J. Dis. Child.*, 1974, *127*, 645; J. F. Annegers *et al.*, *Archs Neurol., Chicago*, 1974, *31*, 364; G. Blennow *et al.* (letter), *Lancet*, 1975, *1*, 449; R. C. Andersen, *J. Pediat.*, 1976, *89*, 318; S. Shapiro *et al.*, *Lancet*, 1976, *1*, 272; J. W. Hanson and D. W. Smith (letter), *ibid.*, 1976, *1*, 692; J. F. Annegers *et al.*, *Int. J. Epidemiol.*, 1978, *7*, 241.

For controversy concerning the role of phenytoin in congenital abnormalities, see Phenytoin, p.1238.

For reference to foetal head growth retardation in the children of mothers given carbamazepine during pregnancy, see Carbamazepine, p.1246.

For a report of a suspected link between valproic acid and human dysmorphism, see p.1257.

6601-a

Phenytoin *(B.P.C. 1973, U.S.P.).*

Diphenylhydantoin; Fenitoína; Phenytoinum; Phenantoinum. 5,5-Diphenylhydantoin; 5,5-Diphenylimidazolidine-2,4-dione.

$C_{15}H_{12}N_2O_2$=252.3.

CAS — 57-41-0.

Pharmacopoeias. In *Aust.*, *Braz.*, *Cz.*, *Ger.*, *Hung.*, *Int.*, *Jap.*, *Nord.*, *Roum.*, *Swiss*, *Turk.*, and *U.S.*

A white, or almost white, odourless or almost odourless, tasteless, crystalline powder. M.p. about 295° with decomposition. Phenytoin 0.92 g is approximately equivalent to 1 g of phenytoin sodium. Practically **insoluble** in water; slightly soluble in alcohol; soluble in hot alcohol; soluble 1 in 500 of chloroform and 1 in 600 of ether; soluble in solutions of alkali hydroxides. **Store** in airtight containers.

6602-t

Phenytoin Sodium *(B.P., B.P. Vet., Eur. P., U.S.P.).*

Phenytoin Sod.; Phenytoinum Natricum; Diphenin; Fenitoína Sódica; Soluble Phenytoin; Diphenylhydantoin Sodium; Sodium Diphenylhydantoin.

$C_{15}H_{11}N_2NaO_2$=274.3.

CAS — 630-93-3.

Pharmacopoeias. In *Arg.*, *Br.*, *Braz.*, *Chin.*, *Eur.*, *Fr.*, *Ger.*, *Ind.*, *It.*, *Jap.*, *Mex.*, *Neth.*, *Pol.*, *Span.*, and *U.S.* *U.S.* also includes Sterile Phenytoin Sodium.

A white, odourless, slightly hygroscopic crystalline powder which on exposure to air absorbs carbon dioxide with the liberation of phenytoin. **Soluble** in water and alcohol; practically insoluble in chloroform and ether. A 5% solution in water is alkaline to phenolphthalein. In aqueous solution it is partly hydrolysed to the base and turbidity develops which only dissolves if the reaction of the solution is adjusted to pH 11.7. Solutions are **sterilised** by filtration. **Store** in airtight containers.

Incompatible with amikacin sulphate, cefapirin sodium, clindamycin phosphate, and many other drugs. It is recommended that phenytoin sodium be not mixed with other drugs or with infusion solutions.

The average solubilities of phenytoin in phosphate buffer pH 7.4 at 25° and 37° were about 1 in 50 000 and 1 in 33 000 respectively. Using buffer solutions the apparent dissociation constant (pKa′) was calculated as 8.06.— P. A. Schwartz *et al.*, *J. pharm. Sci.*, 1977, *66*, 994.

Bioavailability. A review of the clinical pharmacokinetic and therapeutic implications due to variations in bioavailability of phenytoin formulations.— P. J. Neuvonen, *Clin. Pharmacokinet.*, 1979, *4*, 91. See also *Med. Lett.*, 1980, *22*, 49.

Incompatibility. Particulate matter was observed within 2 hours when 1 ml of commercial phenytoin sodium injection was mixed with 5 ml of sterile water and 1 ml of any of the following commercial injection solutions: aminophylline, benzylpenicillin potassium, chloramphenicol sodium succinate, diphenhydramine hydrochloride, dimenhydrinate, erythromycin gluceptate, hydroxyzine hydrochloride, kanamycin sulphate, levallorphan tartrate, metaraminol tartrate, methylphenidate hydrochloride, oxytetracycline hydrochloride, phenobarbitone sodium, phenylephrine hydrochloride, phytomenadione, procainamide hydrochloride, prochlorperazine edisylate, promazine hydrochloride, promethazine hydrochloride, tripelennamine hydrochloride, sulphafurazole diethanolamine, tetracycline hydrochloride, vancomycin hydrochloride.— R. Misgen, *Am. J. Hosp. Pharm.*, 1965, *22*, 92.

There was loss of clarity when intravenous solutions of phenytoin sodium were mixed with those of aminophylline, benzylpenicillin, cephalothin sodium, chloramphenicol sodium succinate, dimenhydrinate, diphenhydramine hydrochloride, erythromycin gluceptate, hydroxyzine hydrochloride, insulin, kanamycin sulphate, lincomycin hydrochloride, metaraminol tartrate, narcotic salts, noradrenaline acid tartrate, oxytetracycline hydrochloride, pentobarbitone sodium, phenobarbitone sodium, phenylephrine hydrochloride, phytomenadione, procaine hydrochloride, prochlorperazine maleate, promethazine hydrochloride, quinalbarbitone sodium, streptomycin sulphate, sulphafurazole diethanolamine, tetracycline hydrochloride, tripelennamine hydrochloride, or vancomycin hydrochloride.— J. A. Patel and G. L. Phillips, *Am. J. Hosp. Pharm.*, 1966, *23*, 409.

Discussions and condemnation of the giving of phenytoin sodium in sodium chloride injection.— *Drug Intell. & clin. Pharm.*, 1973, *7*, 418 and 419. Phenytoin sodium solutions 1 mg per ml required for slow intravenous infusion were more stable and less likely to form crystals when they had been prepared with lactated Ringer's injection or with sodium chloride injection than when mixed with solutions containing dextrose 5%; such mixtures should be prepared immediately before use.— J. L. Bauman *et al.*, *ibid.*, 1977, *11*, 646.

A recommendation that phenytoin can be given by intravenous infusion in a 5% solution of dextrose in water.— E. M. Sellers and H. Kalant, *New Engl. J. Med.*, 1976, *294*, 757. Criticisms of phenytoin dosage recommendations and instructions for diluting.— R. E. Marks (letter), *ibid.*, *295*, 109; D. J. Mehlman and M. E. Egorin (letter), *ibid.*; R. De Forest (letter), *ibid.* Reply.— E. M. Sellers and H. Kalant (letter), *ibid.* Despite the warning on the package insert precipitation of phenytoin from dilute solutions made in 5% solution of dextrose was slow and far from complete; when freshly prepared such solutions were appropriate for intravenous infusion.— D. J. Greenblatt and R. I. Shader (letter), *ibid.*, 1078. On testing, nonvisible crystals had developed within an hour.— J. L. Bauman and J. K. Siepler (letter), *ibid.*, 1977, *296*, 111. See also S. Schondelmeyer *et al.* (letter), *ibid.*

Sodium chloride injection and solutions of sodium chloride 0.45% in small volumes appeared to be suitable vehicles for the intravenous infusion of phenytoin. Dextrose injection or lactated Ringer's injection were unsuitable.— J. C. Cloyd *et al.*, *Am. J. Hosp. Pharm.*, 1978, *35*, 45.

Adverse Effects. Side-effects of phenytoin sodium are of fairly frequent occurrence, and include nausea, vomiting, constipation, ataxia, slurred speech, diplopia, nystagmus, and mental confusion, together with headache, dizziness, transient nervousness, and insomnia. Some of these effects may disappear with continued treatment at reduced dosage.

Tenderness and hyperplasia of the gums is a frequent occurrence particularly in younger patients; hirsutism is a less frequent effect, but is most noticeable in young females.

There have been a number of reports of rickets, reduced bone density, and osteomalacia in patients taking phenytoin, probably due to the induction by phenytoin of liver enzymes involved in the metabolism of vitamin D. Polyarthropathy, fever, hepatitis, and lymphadenopathy have occasionally occurred. Hyperglycaemia may occur.

Leucopenia, thrombocytopenia, pancytopenia, granulocytopenia, and agranulocytosis have been reported. Megaloblastic anaemia following prolonged use usually responds to treatment with folic acid.

Skin rashes, sometimes accompanied by fever, are common, particularly in children; these may resemble measles. More serious skin reactions include lupus erythematosus and erythema multiforme, and the occurrence of bullous, exfoliative, or purpuric rash is an indication for withdrawing phenytoin.

Overdosage may lead to hypotension, coma, and respiratory depression.

For a discussion of the possible adverse effect of anticonvulsants, including phenytoin, on the foetus, see p.1235; see also under Pregnancy and the Neonate, below.

Intravenous injections of phenytoin sodium are irritant and may cause phlebitis. Depression of cardiac conduction, and the occurrence of ventricular fibrillation and heart block have been reported. Rapid injection may also cause hypotension and central nervous system depression.

The clinical efficacy and toxicity of phenytoin showed considerable variation from person to person in relation to blood and tissue concentrations but were fairly consistent in individual patients. Most patients had blurred vision and nystagmus at blood-phenytoin concentrations of 20 µg per ml, ataxia and unsteady gait at 30 µg per ml, and lethargy at more than 40 µg per ml.— H. Kutt, *Ann. N.Y. Acad. Sci.*, 1971, *179*, 704.

In a group of mentally retarded epileptics who were mainly taking phenytoin sodium in large doses, facial changes, thickening of the skull, and raised alkaline phosphatase activity occurred, possibly as a result of the effect of phenytoin in increasing tissue proliferation.— E. B. Lefebvre *et al.*, *New Engl. J. Med.*, 1972, *286*, 1301. See also H. Kutt and S. Louis, *ibid.*, 1316. Scepticism.— D. C. Poskanzer (letter), *ibid.*, *287*, 721; G. Nellhaus (letter), *ibid.*; N. T. Griscom (letter), *ibid.* A reply.— E. B. Lefebvre (letter), *ibid.*

Coarsening of facial features compared with their identical twins was associated in 2 patients with prolonged treatment for epilepsy.— M. A. Falconer and S. Davidson, *Lancet*, 1973, *2*, 1112. Thickening of the heel pad associated with long-term phenytoin therapy.— K. R. Kattan, *Am. J. Roentg.*, 1975, *124*, 52.

A study indicating that anticonvulsant drug toxicity could not be attributed to low plasma concentrations of zinc. Plasma concentrations of copper were elevated in those patients receiving anticonvulsants.— G. D. Schott and H. T. Delves (letter), *Br. J. clin. Pharmac.*, 1978, *5*, 279.

Allergy. A review of 38 patients with phenytoin hypersensitivity. Thirty-five of the reactions occurred within the first 2 months of therapy, and were usually preceded by fever and dermatitis. In 25 patients, there was a licheniform or morbilliform eruption, which progressed to erythema multiforme or Stevens-Johnson syndrome in 7; in a further 3 erythema multiforme or Stevens-Johnson syndrome occurred without dermatitis preceding. Fever was the second most common manifestation (14 patients), followed by lymphadenopathy (9 patients), which was associated with a rash in all and with fever in all but one. Eosinophilia occurred in 8 patients and was associated with lymphadenopathy in all, with fever in 6, and with abnormal liver function tests in 6. Liver function tests were abnormal in 13 patients and blood counts were abnormal in 12 patients (leucopenia in 6, thrombocytopenia in 2, anaemia in 6, and increased atypical lymphocytes in 1). Two patients had serum sickness, 2 had albuminuria, and 1 had renal failure. It was concluded that prompt recognition of possible hypersensitivity reactions with early drug withdrawal and appropriate therapy, including corticosteroids when indicated, may reduce morbidity.— F. Haruda, *Neurology, Minneap.*, 1979, *29*, 1480. See also H. E. Booker, *Epilepsia*, 1975, *16*, 171 (idiosyncratic reactions).

Individual reports of allergic reactions possibly associated with phenytoin: S. R. Targan *et al.*, *Ann. intern. Med.*, 1975, *83*, 227 (disseminated intravascular coagulation with purpura fulminans, exfoliative dermatitis, hepatitis, cutaneous vasculitis, and microangiopathic haemolytic anaemia); A. S. Bayer *et al.* (letter), *Ann. intern. Med.*, 1976, *85*, 475 (miliary chest infiltrates and severe hypoxaemia, extensive dermatitis, hepatitis); J. R. Michael and W. E. Mitch, *J. Am. med. Ass.*, 1976, *236*, 2773; A. J. Wilensky (letter), *ibid.*, 1977, *237*, 2600 (both: reversible renal failure, myositis, fever, lymphadenopathy, exfoliative dermatitis, and hepatitis); B. N. Agarwal *et al.*, *Nephron*, 1977, *18*, 249 (acute renal failure with rash and fever); L. J. McCarthy and J. C. Aguilar (letter), *Lancet*, 1977, *2*, 932 (fatal hypersensitivity); K. J. Sheth *et al.*, *Pediatrics*, 1977, *91*, 438 (nephritis); L. R. Hyman *et al.*, *J. Pediat.*, 1978, *92*, 915 (nephritis).

Diabetogenic effect. In 6 healthy young men given phenytoin 200 mg thrice daily for 3 days the amount of insulin in the blood after infusion of dextrose decreased and blood-glucose concentrations were increased; it was probable that phenytoin had caused a decrease in pancreatic secretion of insulin. It was likely that certain subjects were particularly sensitive to this effect of phenytoin.— C. Malherbe *et al.*, *New Engl. J. Med.*, 1972, *286*, 339.

Phenytoin was not considered to cause carbohydrate intolerance as measured by the serum-immunoreactive insulin and blood-glucose response during glucose tolerance tests in 16 patients with epilepsy taking phenytoin and in 6 control subjects.— C. M. Castleden and A. Richens (letter), *Lancet*, 1973, *2*, 966.

Individual reports of hyperglycaemia in patients given phenytoin: B. H. Peters and N. A. Samaan, *New Engl. J. Med.*, 1969, *281*, 91; E. M. Goldberg, *Diabetes*, 1969, *18*, 101.

Effects on the blood. Subnormal serum-folate concentrations were found in one-half of 52 patients with chronic epilepsy who had been treated for 5 to 25 years with phenytoin 200 to 700 mg daily; most of the patients had also been given phenobarbitone and primidone. Twenty patients had neurological involvement. There was no significant difference in serum-folate concentrations between patients with or without neuropathy. Administration of folic acid 5 mg daily or a placebo for 3 months to 12 patients with nerve involvement produced no measurable improvement in their neuropathy.— S. J. Horwitz *et al.*, *Lancet*, 1968, *1*, 563.

In 75 children with epilepsy, most of whom were taking anticonvulsants, serum-folate concentrations and red-cell-folate concentrations were subnormal in 59% and 58% respectively. These low values correlated with hepatic microsomal enzyme activity (assessed by excretion of D-glucaric acid in urine) and with the daily dose of anticonvulsants. It was suggested that folate deficiency resulted from accelerated metabolism of folate consequent upon induction of liver enzymes by anticonvulsants. It might also explain the reduction in phenytoin concentrations (with consequent increase in the incidence of fits) in patients when given folic acid: prolonged administration of inducers (e.g. phenytoin) of liver enzymes would lead to increased demand for folate which might be a necessary cofactor for the metabolism of phenytoin. Folic acid supplements could then lead to increased metabolism of phenytoin.— J. D. Maxwell *et al.*, *Br. med. J.*, 1972, *1*, 297.

Although reduced folate values were detected in a study of 44 patients given phenytoin the effect was not found to be dose-dependent.— A. D. Korezyn *et al.*, *J. Neurol.*, 1974, *207*, 151.

Of 14 patients taking anticonvulsants (phenytoin in 13, usually with other anticonvulsants) 11 had evidence of megaloblastic erythropoiesis. Only 2 had evidence of vitamin B_{12} or folate deficiency, as assessed by abnormal suppression in the deoxyuridine test. Megaloblastic changes or macrocytosis were mediated by biochemical pathways other than the conversion of deoxyuridylate to thymidylate.— S. N. Wickramasinghe *et al.*, *Br. med. J.*, 1975, *4*, 136. See also I. Yaar, *Harefuah*, 1973, *85*, 256, per *J. Am. med. Ass.*, 1973, *226*, 1260.

Inspection of the blood picture of 96 mentally handicapped patients receiving anticonvulsant drug therapy revealed that although a considerable proportion had low serum and red cell folate values, only 1 patient had macrocytic anaemia; folate depletion was not incriminated in 5 patients with hypochromic anaemia. The macrocytic anaemia sometimes noted in epileptic patients undergoing anticonvulsant therapy might represent inadequate nutrition rather than an effect of the anticonvulsants.— M. Rose and I. Johnson, *Lancet*, 1978, *1*, 1349. It has long been recognised that additional nutritional deficiency may sometimes precipitate megaloblastic anaemia, as may pregnancy. However, nutritional deficiency is not present in many patients and in view of the high incidence of macrocytosis, megaloblastic haemopoiesis, and low serum and red cell folate in non-anaemic treated epileptics, there can be little doubt that the drugs also play a role in the occasional anaemia.— E. H. Reynolds and M. Laundy (letter), *ibid.*, 1978, *2*, 682. Reply; the findings do not support the belief that long-term anticonvulsant therapy leads through a progression of abnormalities to megaloblastic anaemia due to folate depletion. The vast majority of such patients have low folates but neither anaemia nor macrocytosis, suggesting that we are dealing with something different.— M. Rose and I. Johnson (letter), *ibid.*, 994. Further comments and criticisms.— J. A. Child (letter), *ibid.*, 160; C. Hawkins (letter), *ibid.*, 317.

Further studies into folate deficiency and its relevance in patients receiving anticonvulsants: D. Labadarios *et al.*, *Br. J. clin. Pharmac.*, 1978, *5*, 167.

Studies into the interaction between phenytoin and folate: C. D. Gerson *et al.*, *Gastroenterology*, 1972, *63*, 246; C. M. Houlihan *et al.*, *Gut*, 1972, *13*, 189; M. Furlanut *et al.*, *Clin. Pharmac. Ther.*, 1978, *24*, 294; R. G. Strauss *et al.*, *Obstet. Gynec.*, 1978, *51*, 682 (in pregnancy); K. A. Makki *et al.*, *Br. J. clin. Pharmac.*, 1980, *9*, 304P.

Individual reports of *megaloblastic anaemia* in patients receiving anticonvulsants including phenytoin: N. Berlyne *et al.*, *Br. med. J.*, 1955, *1*, 1247; S. Shah (letter), *Lancet*, 1966, *1*, 1422 (in one patient during pregnancy); E. H. Reynolds *et al.*, *Lancet*, 1968, *1*, 394; D. G. Wells (letter), *ibid.*, 146; A. Dvilansky and E. Lehman (letter), *New Engl. J. Med.*, 1972, *287*, 990; J. Pinkhas *et al.* (letter), *J. Am. med. Ass.*, 1973, *224*, 246 (death of thalassaemic patient).

Agranulocytosis. A report of agranulocytosis with marked phagocytosis of myeloid precursors by marrow histiocytes associated with phenytoin 300 mg daily in one patient.— M. -F. Tan (letter), *Ann. intern. Med.*, 1976, *84*, 710. See also W. A. Parker and R. J. Gumnit, *Neurology, Minneap.*, 1974, *24*, 1178.

Aplastic anaemia. A report of reversible pure red cell aplasia in a 19-year-old woman, probably associated with phenytoin therapy.— K. I. Pritchard *et al.*, *Can. med. Ass. J.*, 1979, *121*, 1491. See also Y. -G. Jeong *et al.*, *J. Am. med. Ass.*, 1974, *229*, 314; S. Livingston and L. L. Pauli (letter), *ibid.*, *230*, 211; P. C. Huijgens *et al.*, *Acta haemat.*, 1978, *59*, 31.

Haemophilia, acquired. A report of 2 patients in whom the appearance of circulating anticoagulants against antihaemophilic factor might have been associated with phenytoin therapy. One patient had also received penicillin.— M. -C. Poon *et al.*, *Blood*, 1977, *49*, 477.

Haemolytic anaemia. An episode of haemolytic anaemia occurred in a patient with a deficiency of glucose-6-phosphate dehydrogenase.— E. R. Burka, *Ann. intern. Med.*, 1966, *64*, 817. Phenytoin did not cause haemolysis in Chinese patients with glucose-6-phosphate dehydrogenase deficiency.— T. K. Chan *et al.*, *Br. med. J.*, 1976, *2*, 1227.

Leukaemia. Three cases of leukaemia developed after several years' treatment with hydantoin derivatives; hydantoins might be a factor in multifactorial aetiology of leukaemia.— R. Wildhack, *Münch. med. Wschr.*, 1973, *115*, 1275, per P. Lechat *et al.*, *Thérapie*, 1975, *30*, 381.

Thrombocytopenia. An analysis of blood dyscrasias reported to the Swedish Adverse Drug Reaction Committee for the 5-year period 1966-70 showed that thrombocytopenia attributable to phenytoin had been reported on 3 occasions. It was estimated that reported figures represented one-third of the true frequency.— L. E. Böttiger and B. Westerholm, *Br. med. J.*, 1973, *3*, 339.

After receiving phenytoin as single drug therapy for 8 years a patient developed thrombocytopenia. The phenytoin was stopped and the platelet count rose rapidly. Primidone was successfully substituted.— R. W. Fincham *et al.*, *Ann. Neurol.*, 1979, *6*, 370.

Effects on bones. Following early reports by F. Schmid (*Fortschr. Med.*, 1967, *85*, 381) and R. Kruse (*Mschr. Kinderheilk.*, 1968, *116*, 378) of bone disorders in patients receiving anticonvulsant therapy, C.E. Dent *et al.* (*Br. med. J.*, 1970, *4*, 69) recorded osteomalacia in 4 epileptic patients receiving long-term anticonvulsant therapy. A. Richens and D.J.F. Rowe (*Br. med. J.*, 1970, *4*, 73) then reported a study of 160 adults with grand mal epilepsy, all but 3 of whom were receiving 1 or more of the major anticonvulsant drugs, phenytoin, phenobarbitone, primidone, and pheneturide; serum-calcium concentrations were below 90 µg per ml in 36 patients. Serum alkaline phosphatase was raised in 47 patients. Hypocalcaemia was related to multiple drug therapy, and then occurred most commonly in those receiving pheneturide and was progressively less frequent in those receiving primidone, phenytoin, and phenobarbitone. They concluded that these abnormalities were probably the result of vitamin-D deficiency, the anticonvulsants accelerating the breakdown of vitamin D by liver enzyme induction. Similar findings were reported in children by J. Hunter *et al.* (*Br. med. J.*, 1971, *4*, 202) who considered 6 of the 105 children studied to have biochemical osteomalacia. The findings were confirmed by a number of other workers including J. Linde *et al.* (*Br. med. J.*, 1971, *3*, 433) and C. Christiansen *et al.* (*Br. med. J.*, 1973, *4*, 695). These studies were carried out in Europe, but T.J. Hahn *et al.* (*New Engl. J. Med.*, 1972, *287*, 900 and 1975, *292*, 550) found that they were also applicable to America despite the higher mean daily vitamin D intake and higher incidence of exposure to sunlight. A suggestion by S. Livingston (*J. Am. med. Ass.*, 1973, *224*, 1634) that development of osteomalacia in some of the reported cases might be due to inadequate nutrition and inactivity was refuted by K.G. Tolman *et al.* (*Pediatrics*, 1975, *56*, 45) in a survey of 289 severely retarded in-patients. Tolman *et al.* found an increased incidence of osteomalacia in those receiving anticonvulsant medication with no other differences in the variables which might influence bone mineralisation, such as age, physical activity, sunshine exposure, and vitamin D intake. Moreover, the prevalence increased from 47% after 5 years to 67% after 10 years, and the incidence did not appear to be prevented by usual supplemental doses of cholecalciferol. C. Christiansen *et al.* (*Br. med. J.*, 1973, *4*, 695) provided treatment for 3 months with ergocalciferol 2000 units daily and calcium lactate providing 390 mg of calcium daily, and increased bone mineral mass in 116 patients by about 4%. These data were confirmed by P. Peterson *et al.* (*Clin. Pharmac. Ther.*, 1976, *19*, 63) who obtained positive calcium balance with cholecalciferol 2000 units daily. Disturbingly, Peterson *et al.* found that the requirement of vitamin D in their institutionalised control patients was unexpectedly high although lower than in those receiving anticonvulsants. In a review on the subject T.J. Hahn (*Drugs*, 1976, *12*, 201) has discussed the controversy surrounding the need to give prophylactic vitamin-D therapy to seizure patients, and described a regimen of prophylactic vitamin-D supplementation with 10 000 units of ergocalciferol weekly, only in patients who have been on therapy for 6 months or longer; the dose of supplemental vitamin D is always adjusted on the basis of individual requirements and response.

Further references: T. C. B. Stamp *et al.*, *Br. med. J.*, 1972, *4*, 9 (calcifediol in osteomalacia unresponsive to ergocalciferol); C. D. Marsden *et al.*, *Br. med. J.*, 1973, *4*, 526 (severe osteomalacia with widespread myopathy); J. Silver *et al.*, *Archs Dis. Childh.*, 1974, *49*, 344 (rickets in epileptic children); L. Mosekilde and F. Melsen, *Acta med. scand.*, 1976, *199*, 349 (bone changes); D. P. Addy, *Archs Dis. Childh.*, 1976, *51*, 972 (rickets in children with tuberous sclerosis given anticonvulsants); J. Trabulus *et al.* (letter), *Ann. intern. Med.*, 1976, *84*, 709 (masking of hypocalcaemic tetany by phenytoin); K. H. Krause *et al.*, *Dt. med. Wschr.*, 1977, *102*, 1872 (diagnosis of osteomalacia); J. L. Winnacker *et al.*, *Am. J. Dis. Child.*, 1977, *131*, 286 (diagnosis of rickets); G. Pylypchuk *et al.*, *Can. med. Ass. J.*, 1978, *118*, 635 (minimal bone loss in adults); R. K. Marya *et al.*, *Nutrition and Metabolism*, 1979, *23*, 167 (benefit of sunshine); M. Davie *et al.*, *Clin. Sci.*, 1979, *57*, Sept 6P (no enhanced cholecalciferol metabolism; effect on 25-OHD remains to be considered); T. O. Wahl *et al.*, *Clin. Pharmac. Ther.*, 1981, *30*, 506 (gastro-intestinal calcium absorption).

Granulomata. Multiple noncaseating bone-marrow granulomata developed in a black alcoholic and diabetic patient after treatment with phenytoin for 4 weeks. He had no recent history of bone lesions. Symptoms and signs abated within 2 weeks of withdrawing phenytoin.— H. V. Wu and M. Kosmin (letter), *Ann. intern. Med.*, 1977, *86*, 663.

Hypomagnesaemia. Mean serum-magnesium concentrations in 226 patients with epilepsy were significantly lower than in 95 controls; the difference was greatest in those taking phenytoin with or without other anticonvulsants.— C. Christiansen *et al.* (letter), *Br. med. J.*, 1974, *1*, 198. Significant hypomagnesaemia could not be detected. There was, however, increased variance, indicating that there is some important effect on magnesium metabolism.— S. H. Katz *et al.* (letter), *ibid.*, 1976, *1*, 341. See also M. J. Stewart (letter), *ibid.*, 649.

Effects on the eyes. Partial or total external ophthalmoplegia was reported in 3 patients after excessive doses of phenytoin and primidone. In a further patient, phenytoin only had been taken.— D. N. Orth *et al.*, *J. Am. med. Ass.*, 1967, *201*, 485. See also R. H. Spector *et al.*, *Neurology, Minneap.*, 1976, *26*, 1031.

Effects on the gums. A study suggesting that phenytoin-induced deficiency of salivary IgA can result in increased susceptibility to gingival inflammation and ultimately gingival hyperplasia.— J. A. Aarli, *Epilepsia*, 1976, *17*, 283. Severe criticism of the design of the study.— P. C. Reade, *Drugs*, 1977, *14*, 395.

Phenytoin-induced overgrowth of gum tissue, which sometimes almost buries the teeth in soft tissue, occurs most often and more severely in children than in adults. Not only is the appearance unattractive, but dental hygiene becomes difficult, and tooth decay and periodontal disease often result. Dentists sometimes remove the excess tissue surgically but it often grows back.— *J. Am. med. Ass.*, 1980, *243*, 1038. Results of a small study demonstrating that folate supplementation may help to alleviate or prevent gingival hyperplasia in patients receiving long-term phenytoin therapy.— F. Inoue and J. V. Harrison (letter), *Lancet*, 1981, *2*, 86.

Effects on the kidneys. For reference to nephritis and renal failure in patients given phenytoin, see Allergy, above.

Effects on lipid metabolism. Four patients with epilepsy who were not adequately controlled with usual doses of phenytoin were found to have high serum-triglyceride and cholesterol concentrations with low serum-phenytoin concentrations. Low-fat diets and clofibrate restored control of seizures. Another patient maintained on phenytoin 100 mg twice daily showed signs of phenytoin toxicity when serum-cholesterol concentrations decreased from 2.3 to 1.82 mg per ml and serum-phenytoin concentrations increased from 15 to 32 µg per ml.— D. R. Reimer and S. Nagaswami (letter), *New Engl. J. Med.*, 1973, *289*, 808.

In 9 patients with epilepsy (previously untreated) given phenytoin 300 to 450 mg daily serum concentrations of cholesterol were significantly increased after 3 months' treatment and remained elevated during continued treatment for the 12 months of study.— R. Pelkonen *et al.*, *Br. med. J.*, 1975, *4*, 85. Experience with thousands of epileptic patients on various drug regimens, including phenytoin, had indicated an exceedingly low incidence of coronary heart disease. Clinical evidence of metabolic or endocrine disorders unequivocally due to phenytoin had been rare.— S. Livingston (letter), *ibid.*, 1976, *1*, 586.

Effects on the liver. Acute parenchymal hepatic disease developed in a 46-year-old Negro who had received phenytoin sodium, 300 mg daily, for 5 weeks. The condition was associated with high fever and generalised muscle pain and tenderness and subsided slowly when phenytoin was withdrawn.— U. Harinasuta and H. J. Zimmerman, *J. Am. med. Ass.*, 1968, *203*, 1015. See also W. A. Parker and C. A. Shearer, *Neurology, Minneap.*, 1979, *29*, 175. See also under Allergy, above.

Changes in liver function tests were noted in 11 epileptic patients who had received phenytoin for many years. Liver biopsies revealed few uni- or paucicellular necroses in 5 of the 11. None of the biopsies showed signs of permanent liver damage.— N. O. Jacobsen *et al.*, *Acta med. scand.* 1976, *199*, 345.

A report of prolonged cholestatic liver disease in an 11-year-old boy given phenytoin.— C. B. Campbell *et al.*, *Dig. Dis. Scis*, 1977, *22*, 255.

Liver size was increased in 21 epileptic patients who had taken anticonvulsants, mainly phenytoin, for at least one year when compared with 28 controls. Liver weight gave a linear correlation between *in vivo* and *in vitro* studies of drug metabolism except in those with the most severe distortion of liver structure.— H. I. Pirttiaho *et al.*, *Br. J. clin. Pharmac.*, 1978, *6*, 273.

A cohort study of patients with very severe epilepsy and an increased mortality rate, provided no evidence of an increase in liver tumours.— S. J. White *et al.*, *Lancet*, 1979, *2*, 458. Updating of a previous 40-year review of the patients who died in 4 mental hospitals did not reveal an association between prolonged usage of various anticonvulsant and tranquillising drugs and liver cancer.— J. Jancar (letter), *ibid.*, 1980, *1*, 484.

Results of a study in 63 epileptic children indicated that phenobarbitone and phenytoin therapy may be continued despite transient elevations in transaminase values, and that liver biopsies are not warranted in such children.— H. W. Aiges *et al.*, *J. Pediat.*, 1980, *97*, 22.

Effects on lymphoid tissue. A discussion on benign lymphadenopathy or pseudolymphoma, a rare side-effect of phenytoin, and its association, if any, with true lymphoma. It seems likely that an aetiological relationship exists between phenytoin treatment and true lymphoma. Nevertheless, the possibility of this side-effect should not, on present evidence, deter those concerned in the management of epilepsy from prescribing phenytoin.— *Lancet*, 1971, *2*, 1071. Evidence of depressed immunological function in patients given phenytoin.— T. C. Sorrell *et al.*, *ibid.*, 1233. See also P. J. Grob and G. E. Herold, *Br. med. J.*, 1972, *2*, 561; J. Seager *et al.*, *Lancet*, 1975, *2*, 632; A. Fontana *et al.*, *ibid.*, 1976, *2*, 228.

The lymphocyte count in peripheral blood was significantly reduced in 11 patients taking phenytoin compared with 18 healthy controls. This might be associated with the possible increased risk of malignant lymphoma in patients taking phenytoin.— L. Brandt and P. G. Nilsson (letter), *Lancet*, 1976, *1*, 308. Lymphocytosis had been observed.— A. Higashi *et al.* (letter), *ibid.*, 1976, *2*, 44. There was an insignificant rise in the lymphocyte count in 17 children given phenytoin for about 6 months.— J. Saeger (letter), *ibid.*, 1205.

Immunologic studies in a 28-year-old woman with phenytoin-induced pseudolymphoma syndrome did not support the suggestion that the syndrome resulted from a delayed hypersensitivity reaction.— E. N. Charlesworth, *Archs Derm.*, 1977, *113*, 477.

Studies into the possible association between phenytoin and malignant lymphomas: F. P. Li *et al.*, *Cancer*, 1975, *36*, 1359.

Effects on mental state. A 30-year-old woman developed a delayed idiosyncratic psychosis while taking phenytoin 100 mg four times a day. The serum-phenytoin concentration was 3.2 µg per ml. After therapy with phenytoin was discontinued the patient recovered and psychotic symptoms disappeared.— C. E. McDanal and W. M. Bolman, *J. Am. med. Ass.*, 1975, *231*, 1063.

Effects on the nervous system. Progressive neurological deterioration, thought at first to be a degenerative central nervous system disease, was observed in 9 patients receiving long-term hydantoin therapy. Symptoms included cerebellar signs of nystagmus and ataxia, and signs of more diffuse encephalopathy, including impaired intellectual performance, bizarre behaviour, increased seizure frequency, impaired speech, and EEG changes. On stopping the hydantoins, 6 patients improved neurologically and 3 did not deteriorate further.— J. M. Vallarta *et al.*, *Am. J. Dis. Child.*, 1974, *128*, 27.

A report of word reversal associated with phenytoin.— B. H. Fookes (letter), *Lancet*, 1975, *2*, 134.

In a retrospective study 70 of 131 (53%) mentally subnormal epileptics being treated with long-term phenytoin had clinical signs of toxicity which abated, at least partly, on dosage reduction, 122 (93%) had abnormal pneumoencephalographic recordings, and 18 patients became permanently unable to walk. There were significantly more EEG abnormalities in these patients than in 68 epileptics not given phenytoin. It was considered that the best method of ensuring safe and effective treatment of epileptics on multiple therapy was to monitor drug concentrations and EEGs.— M. Iivanainen and M. Viukari (letter), *Lancet*, 1977, *1*, 860. See also J. B. Selhorst *et al.*, *Archs Neurol., Chicago*, 1972, *27*, 453; P. D. Horne, *J. Ir. med. Ass.*, 1973, *66*, 147; N. R. Ghatek *et al.*, *Neurology, Minneap.*, 1976, *26*, 818.

Dyskinesias. An account of a variety of dyskinesias in 6 epileptic patients with toxic plasma concentrations of phenytoin and other anticonvulsants, and a review of previously reported patients with anticonvulsant-induced dyskinesias. Phenytoin, carbamazepine, primidone, and phenobarbitone may cause asterixis. Phenytoin, but not other anticonvulsants, may cause orofacial dyskinesias, limb chorea, and dystonia in patients given excessive doses. These dyskinesias are similar to those induced by neuroleptics and may be related to the dopamine antagonist properties of phenytoin.— D. Chadwick *et al.*, *J. Neurol. Neurosurg. Psychiat.*, 1976, *39*, 1210.

Individual reports of dyskinesias (mainly choreoathetosis) in patients receiving phenytoin alone or with other anticonvulsants: E. Shuttleworth *et al.*, *J. Am. med. Ass.*, 1974, *230*, 1170; D. L. McLellan and M. Swash, *Br. med. J.*, 1974, *2*, 204; K. W. G. Heathfield (letter), *ibid.*, 507; M. H. Bellman and L. Haas (letter), *ibid.*, *3*, 256; E. G. Chalhub *et al.*, *Neurology, Minneap.*, 1976, *26*, 494; S. Zinsmeister and R. E. Marks, *Am. J. Dis. Child.*, 1976, *130*, 75; K. Luhdorf and M. Lund, *Epilepsia*, 1977, *18*, 409; S. Rasmussen and M. Kristensen, *Acta med. scand.*, 1977, *201*, 239; C. L. Opida *et al.*, *Ann. Neurol.*, 1978, *3*, 186; F. Mauguiere *et al.*, *Eur. Neurol.*, 1979, *18*, 116; R. J. Stark, *Med. J. Aust.*, 1979, *1*, 156.

Peripheral neuropathy. Patients receiving long-term phenytoin treatment may develop a predominantly sensory polyneuropathy that is usually mild and rarely causes symptoms. The incidence is uncertain, but signs of peripheral nerve disorders, such as depression of tendon reflexes, are found increasingly often in those receiving prolonged treatment.— Z. Argov and F. L. Mastaglia, *Br. med. J.*, 1979, *1*, 663. See also R. E. Lovelace and S. J. Horwitz, *Archs Neurol., Chicago*, 1968, *18*, 69; B. H. Dobkin, *Archs Neurol., Chicago*, 1977, *34*, 189 (reversible subacute peripheral neuropathy).

Effects on neuromuscular transmission. Myasthenia gravis associated with phenytoin.— J. Brumlik and R. S. Jacobs, *Can. J. neurol. Sci.*, 1974, *1*, 127.

Effects on respiratory function. Pulmonary function loss with phenytoin.— D. R. Hazlett *et al.*, *Chest*, 1974, *66*, 660.

Effects on sexual function. Anticonvulsants diminish sexual potency and fertility in young male epileptics. Phenytoin is excreted in human semen in small quantities and this may possibly affect sperm morphology and motility.— *Br. med. J.*, 1979, *2*, 1118.

Plasma concentrations of free testosterone were reduced in male epileptics receiving anticonvulsants.— J. Dana-Haeri *et al.*, *Br. med. J.*, 1982, *284*, 85.

Effects on the skin. The incidence of skin rash in children taking phenytoin for the first time was correlated with the plasma-phenytoin concentration; those with rash had a lower concentration of the metabolite *p*-hydroxyphenytoin, but the role of metabolism was not known.— J. T. Wilson *et al.*, *Br. med. J.*, 1978, *1*, 1583.

Individual reports of adverse skin reactions associated with phenytoin therapy: N. Hurwitz, *Br. med. J.*, 1969, *1*, 539 (erythema multiforme); R. B. Jenkins and A. C. Ratner (letter), *New Engl. J. Med.*, 1972, *287*, 148 (acne); J. A. Bosso and G. M. Chudzik, *Drug Intell. & clin. Pharm.*, 1973, *7*, 336 (Stevens-Johnson syndrome); K. P. Dawson, *Archs Dis. Childh.*, 1973, *48*, 239 (fatal morbilliform rash; macular rash); L. E. Gately and M. A. Lam, *Ann. intern. Med.*, 1979, *91*, 59 (fatal toxic epidermal necrolysis); S. J. Spechler *et al.*, *ibid.*, 1981, *95*, 455 (cholestasis and toxic epidermal necrolysis).

Lupus erythematosus. Four children who had been taking anticonvulsants had lupus-like disease; 11 of 48 other asymptomatic children had significant antinuclear antibodies.— D. H. Beernink and J. J. Miller, *J. Pediat.*, 1973, *82*, 113, per *Drug Intell. & clin. Pharm.*, 1973, *7*, 186.

Overdosage. Intoxication with phenytoin sodium had been diagnosed in 13 children over a 5-year period. Signs and symptoms included nystagmus, ataxia, mental disturbances, slurred speech, and dilated pupils. Some of the children had had gross ataxia for some time before admission to hospital. In only 1 patient had the diagnosis been correct.— H. Patel and J. U. Crichton, *J. Pediat.*, 1968, *73*, 676, per *Abstr. Wld Med.*, 1969, *43*, 238.

A 5-year-old child recovered without neurological damage after inadvertently receiving phenytoin 500 mg daily for 3 weeks.— A. W. Pruitt *et al.*, *Clin. Pharmac. Ther.*, 1975, *18*, 112.

Further references to phenytoin overdosage: M. D. Rawson, *Neurology, Minneap.*, 1968, *18*, 1009 (raised CSF protein and CNS damage); M. Wand and J. A. Mather, *New Engl. J. Med.*, 1972, *286*, 88 (phenytoin-contaminated cannabis and a botulism-like syndrome); M. A. Gill *et al.*, *West. J. Med.*, 1978, *128*, 246 (kinetics in overdosage); J. T. Wilson *et al.*, *J. Pediat.*, 1979, *95*, 135 (prolonged toxicity in a child).

Porphyria. Administration of phenytoin exacerbated experimental porphyria in *rats* but the validity of the test must depend on clinical observation.— A. A. -B. Badawy (letter), *Lancet*, 1978, *1*, 1361.

Pregnancy and the neonate. An account of 5 unrelated children born to epileptic mothers treated with hydantoin anticonvulsants and who were found to have a similar broad multi-system pattern of abnormalities, including craniofacial defects, nail and digital hypoplasia, prenatal onset growth deficiency, and mental deficiency. This altered pattern of morphogenesis is distinct from other recognised disorders and has been reported only in the offspring of women using hydantoins, thus justifying the term 'foetal hydantoin syndrome'.— J. W. Hanson and D. W. Smith, *J. Pediat.*, 1975, *87*, 285. Results of a prospective study of 35 infants exposed prenatally to the hydantoins indicated that 11% had sufficient features to be classified as having the foetal hydantoin syndrome, and an additional 31% displayed some features compatible with the prenatal effects of hydantoins. These conclusions were supported by a case-control study of 104 infants whose mothers had convulsive disorders and were treated with hydantoins continuously throughout pregnancy, identified from the Collaborative Perinatal Project of the National Institute of Neurological and Communicative Disorders and Stroke (*The Collaborative Perinatal Study: The Women and their Pregnancies*, K.R. Niswander and M. Gordon, Ed., Philadelphia, W.B. Saunders, 1972). The divergent results, that it may be the epilepsy rather than the drug exposure which is responsible for the increased risk of malformations which S. Shapiro *et al.* (*Lancet*, 1976, *1*, 272) derived from the same study may be due to the variant methods of the respective analyses.— J. W. Hanson *et al.*, *ibid.*, 1976, *89*, 662. Both the prospective and the case-control studies are open to bias. The clinical observation that certain children, exposed *in utero* to phenytoin, have hypoplasia of the distal phalanges or fingernails (a well-defined and otherwise rather rare phenomenon) is noteworthy and deserves further study, but many of the other dysmorphic features are common, and on the present evidence it remains to be established that hydantoin anticonvulsants are teratogenic to human beings.— S. Shapiro *et al.*, *ibid.*, 1977, *90*, 673. Reply.— J. W. Hanson and D. W. Smith (letter), *ibid.*, 674. Further criticism.— H. C. Miller (letter), *ibid.*, 675. Reply.— J. W. Hanson and D. W. Smith (letter), *ibid.*

Individual reports of abnormalities in the infants of mothers given phenytoin, either alone or in association with other anticonvulsants, during pregnancy: T. W. Pendergrass and J. W. Hanson (letter), *Lancet*, 1976, *2*, 150; S. Sherman and N. Roizen (letter), *ibid.*, 517 (both foetal hydantoin syndrome and neuroblastoma); R. Corcoran and M. W. Rizk (letter), *Lancet* 1976, *2*, 960 (multiple malformations); M. Waziri *et al.*, *Am. J. Dis. Child.*, 1976, *130*, 1022 (multiple malformations); W. W. Tunnessen and E. H. Lowenstein (letter), *J. Pediat.*, 1976, *89*, 154 (glaucoma and foetal hydantoin syndrome); W. A. Blattner *et al.*, *J. Am. med. Ass.*, 1977, *238*, 334 (cleft lip and palate; malignant mesenchymoma at 18 years of age); W. Pinto *et al.*, *Am. J. Dis. Child.*, 1977, *131*, 452 (abnormal genitalia); S. A. Bustamante and L. C. Stumpff, *Am. J. Dis. Child.*, 1978, *132*, 978 (foetal hydantoin syndrome in triplets); C. S. Hoyte and F. A. Billson, *Br. J. Ophthal.*, 1978, *62*, 3 (optic nerve hypoplasia in 7 children); R. S. Wilson *et al.*, *J. Pediat. Ophthal. Strabis.*, 1978, *15*, 137 (multiple malformations and ocular defects); T. -S. Yang *et al.*, *Obstet. Gynec.*, 1978, *52*, 682 (multiple malformations); R. W. Allen *et al.*, *J. Am. med. Ass.*, 1980, *244*, 1464 (foetal hydantoin syndrome, neuroblastoma, and haemorrhagic disorder); A. N. W. Evans *et al.*, *Practitioner*, 1980, *224*, 315 (foetal hydantoin syndrome); W. F. Taylor *et al.* (letter), *Lancet*, 1980, *2*, 481 (foetal hydantoin syndrome and extrarenal Wilms' tumour); W. E. Truog *et al.*, *J. Pediat.*, 1980, *96*, 112 (foetal hydantoin syndrome, haemorrhagic disease, and persistent foetal circulation); L. T. Ehrenbard and R. S. K. Chaganti (letter), *Lancet*, 1981, *2*, 97 (foetal hydantoin syndrome and neuroblastoma).

For a general comment on epilepsy and pregnancy and references to surveys on the incidence of congenital malformations in the infants of epileptic women, see p.1235.

Lactation. Methaemoglobinaemia in an infant might have been caused by phenytoin in the mother's milk.— E. Finch and J. Lorber, *J. Obstet. Gynaec. Br. Commonw.*, 1954, *61*, 833.

The neonate. In a prospective study of 16 neonates born to epileptic mothers treated with anticonvulsant drugs, 7 had a severe coagulation defect similar to that in vitamin K deficiency, 1 had a mild defect, and 8 were normal. The mothers of the affected infants had received phenobarbitone or primidone in addition to phenytoin, whereas those of 3 of the unaffected infants had not received a barbiturate or primidone. Similarly, all of 11 previously reported infants with neonatal bleeding had been exposed to a barbiturate or a drug metabolised to a barbiturate and, furthermore, the prothrombin-time has been reported as prolonged in neonates born to mothers treated with barbiturates during pregnancy or labour. This suggests that the coagulation defect may be due to barbiturate treatment of the mother, but this may possibly be more severe if phenytoin or another anticonvulsant is given in addition. Two of the 16 infants in the study had clinical evidence of bleeding, which stopped soon after administration of vitamin K_1, but in some cases bleeding has continued despite treatment with vitamin K_1. It is therefore recommended that the prothrombin-time of cord-blood be measured at delivery, and if it is less than 10%, or if there is any evidence of bleeding during the neonatal period, treatment with infusions of fresh frozen plasma or concentrates of factors II, VII, IX, and X be considered in addition to intravenous administration of vitamin K_1. Treatment of the mother with vitamin K_1 may prevent the coagulation defect in the neonate and thus be the best form of prophylaxis. It could be given as vitamin K_1 tablets throughout the month before delivery, and intravenously during labour.— K. R. Mountain *et al.*, *Lancet*, 1970, *1*, 265. See also A. D. Griffiths (letter), *ibid.*, 1981, *2*, 1296.

A report of hypocalcaemia in 2 infants at term whose mothers had been receiving anticonvulsants.— B. Friis and H. Sardemann, *Archs Dis. Childh.*, 1977, *52*, 239.

In a study of 11 169 children and 11 169 controls included in a survey of childhood cancers the mothers of children who developed cancer reported about 25% more illnesses during pregnancy than the mothers of the control children. An examination of the drugs given, particularly phenytoin and isoniazid, showed little difference between the 2 groups and did not therefore support an association between the drugs given and the subsequent development of cancer.— B. M. Sanders and G. J. Draper, *Br. med. J.*, 1979, *1*, 717.

Treatment of Adverse Effects. The stomach should be emptied by aspiration and lavage. The use of activated charcoal as an adjunct to gastric lavage has been recommended. Supportive therapy alone may then suffice for patients who are not severely poisoned (for general guidelines to the symptomatic therapy of drug overdosage, see Phenobarbitone, p.812).

In patients on long-term phenytoin therapy, vitamin-D supplements are given to prevent rickets and osteomalacia (see under Adverse Effects, Effects on Bones, above) and folic acid is given to combat folate deficiency (see under Adverse Effects, Effects on the Blood, above).

Activated charcoal. For comment on the *in vitro* adsorption of phenytoin by activated charcoal, see Activated Charcoal, p.79.

Dialysis and haemoperfusion. A study of plasma-phenytoin concentrations in a patient undergoing haemodialysis suggested that additional replacement of phenytoin after haemodialysis was unnecessary. The benefit of haemodialysis as a treatment for phenytoin overdose was open to doubt.— D. S. Adler *et al.*, *Clin. Pharmac. Ther.*, 1975, *18*, 65.

The efficiency of haemodialysis in the treatment of a patient reported to have taken an overdose of 10 g of phenytoin was calculated to be 10%. Plasma concentrations reached a maximum of 34 µg per ml 6 hours after ingestion and did not change significantly for 24 hours, despite haemodialysis. About 350 mg of phenytoin was removed by haemodialysis and 1.05 g by gastric lavage.— D. Rubinger *et al.* (letter), *Br. J. clin. Pharmac.*, 1979, *7*, 405.

A review of data from 2 patients with phenytoin overdosage treated with charcoal haemoperfusion. Phenytoin has a relatively small volume of distribution, and haemoperfusion, particularly at high drug concentrations, should contribute significantly to total drug removal.— S. Pond *et al.*, *Clin. Pharmacokinet.*, 1979, *4*, 329. Lack of benefit.— R. W. Baehler *et al.*, *Archs intern. Med.*, 1980, *140*, 1466.

Peritoneal dialysis did not appreciably enhance the elimination of phenytoin in a 3-year-old boy with phenytoin intoxication. The effectiveness of peritoneal dialysis for phenytoin poisoning should be seriously questioned. The child died of septicaemia, which emphasises the potential hazards of peritoneal dialysis.— P. A. Czajka *et al.*, *J. clin. Pharmac.*, 1980, *20*, 565.

Precautions. Phenytoin should be given with caution to patients with hepatic disease. Vitamin-D supplements may be necessary for some patients on long-term therapy (for further details see Effects on the Bones, under Adverse Effects).

For the use of phenytoin in pregnancy and lactation see under Pregnancy and the Neonate, under Adverse Effects.

Intravenous phenytoin must be given slowly and extravasation must be avoided. Phenytoin should not be given intravenously to patients with bradycardia, heart block, or Stokes-Adams syndrome, and should be used with caution in patients with hypotension and severe myocardial insufficiency; electrocardiographic monitoring is recommended during intravenous therapy.

Since phenytoin is extensively bound to plasma proteins it can be displaced by drugs competing for protein-binding sites, thus liberating more free (pharmacologically active) phenytoin into the plasma. This is reported to be of little clinical significance because this free phenytoin is extensively distributed into the tissues and is excreted in the urine, so that the actual concentration in the plasma remains more or less unchanged. When plasma concentrations of phenytoin are being monitored, however, relatively lower total plasma-phenytoin concentrations will be found to be effective since there is less bound (pharmacologically inactive) phenytoin available for measurement. Drugs reported to displace phenytoin from plasma protein-binding sites include aspirin and salicylic acid, diazoxide, halofenate, phenylbutazone, sulphonamides, tolbutamide, and valproic acid; drugs which effect lipid concentrations, such as clofibrate and heparin, may also influence binding by changing lipid availability.

A much more serious type of interaction stems from the fact that phenytoin metabolism, being saturable, is susceptible to a relatively minor degree of inhibition. Toxic concentrations of phenytoin readily develop in patients given drugs which inhibit phenytoin metabolism. Drugs that have been reported to inhibit the metabolism of phenytoin include some antibiotics, some other anticonvulsants, some antihistamines, coumarin anticoagulants, disulfiram, dextropropoxyphene, isoniazid, methylphenidate, some phenothiazines, phenylbutazone and phenyramidol, tricyclic antidepressants and viloxazine, and possibly benzodiazepines. Particularly marked inhibition has been reported for chloramphenicol, dicoumarol, isoniazid, sulphaphenazole, and sulthiame. Phenylbutazone and valproic acid appear both to inhibit phenytoin metabolism and to displace it from plasma proteins.

Folic acid has been reported to induce the metabolism of phenytoin and, in turn, phenytoin influences that of folic acid but the evidence for this interaction is inconclusive (for further details of the interaction between phenytoin and folate, see Effects on the Blood, under Adverse Effects); carbamazepine and phenytoin may also mutually enhance one another's metabolism. Phenytoin is a potent enzyme inducer, and induces the metabolism of a number of drugs, including some antibiotics (notably, doxycycline), anticoagulants, corticosteroids and metyrapone, misonidazole, quinidine, and sex hormones (notably, oral contraceptives). Phenytoin also influences the metabolism of vitamin D and may induce rickets or osteomalacia, which is why patients on long-term phenytoin therapy may need vitamin-D supplements (see above). Induction or inhibition has been variously reported for alcohol and phenobarbitone.

Drugs with an epileptogenic potential, such as tricyclic antidepressants (see amitriptyline, p.112) or phenothiazines (see chlorpromazine, p.1512) may diminish the pharmacological action of phenytoin. The hypotensive properties of dopamine and the cardiac depressant properties of drugs such as lignocaine or propranolol may be dangerously enhanced by intravenous administration of phenytoin.

Phenytoin may interfere with blood-calcium and blood-sugar estimations, with protein-bound iodine estimations, and with dexamethasone and metyrapone tests.

Forty-one years of experience, including over 1000 epileptic patients who took part in competitive athletics, has indicated that tolerable dosages of anticonvulsant medications rarely interfere with performance. Of at least 20 000 patients prescribed phenytoin, many continuously for 30 to 40 years, standard dosages caused fatigue during routine daily activities in only a few.— S. Livingston, *J. Am. med. Ass.*, 1978, *240*, 59.

Phenytoin, carbamazepine, and sodium valproate in appropriate doses may not as such impair driving skills, but epilepsy itself dictates the practice of driving.— T. Seppala *et al.*, *Drugs*, 1979, *17*, 389.

Interactions. A detailed review of drug interactions with phenytoin.— E. Perucca and A. Richens, *Drugs*, 1981, *21*, 120.

Acidity. Of 40 patients stabilised on phenytoin and then given sodium bicarbonate 4 g daily for a week and ammonium chloride 7.5 to 9 g daily for a week, 4 had increased seizures while taking sodium bicarbonate and 6 had evidence of phenytoin toxicity while taking ammonium chloride. These changes could not be correlated with changes in the concentration of phenytoin in serum or the CSF.— N. Matti *et al.*, *Behav. Neuropsychiat.*, 1969, *1*, (Nov.), 13.

Alcohol. Phenytoin, given in a dose of 100 mg thrice daily for 3 days, was eliminated more rapidly (mean 16.3 hours) from the blood of 15 heavy drinkers than from 76 controls (mean 23.5 hours).— *J. Am. med. Ass.*, 1968, *206*, 1709.

Much greater intersubject variability in phenytoin plasma half-life in *alcoholics*.— P. Sandor *et al.*, *Clin. Pharmac. Ther.*, 1980, *27*, 283.

Further references: P. Sandor *et al.*, *Clin. Pharmac. Ther.*, 1981, *30*, 390.

Alcohol and disulfiram. Administration of *disulfiram* 400 mg daily to 4 patients who had received prolonged treatment with phenytoin resulted in rises of 100 to 500% in serum concentrations of phenytoin over a period of 9 days. It required about 3 weeks after withdrawal of disulfiram before the serum concentrations of phenytoin returned to normal.— O. V. Olesen, *Acta pharmac. tox.*, 1966, *24*, 317.

A 49-year-old woman with chronic alcoholism and epilepsy receiving phenytoin 300 mg daily and disulfiram 250 mg daily developed a series of grand mal seizures on withdrawal of disulfiram. The plasma-phenytoin concentration 4 hours after a dose was 3.9 µg per ml, compared with 13.1 µg per ml while taking disulfiram, and although fits were controlled during the following 4 weeks by the administration of diazepam, phenobarbitone, and phenytoin 800 mg daily, signs of phenytoin toxicity appeared. At this point the plasma-phenytoin concentration was 54.8 µg per ml but was finally stabilised at 18 µg per ml with a dose of 500 mg daily.— D. J. Birkett *et al.*, *Med. J. Aust.*, 1977, *2*, 467.

Further references: E. Kiørboe, *Epilepsia*, 1966, *7*, 246; J. Dry and A. Pradalier, *Thérapie*, 1973, *28*, 799.

Anaesthetic agents. A 10-year-old girl with epilepsy who had been treated with phenytoin 100 mg thrice daily for 5 years and who had lateral nystagmus developed symptoms of phenytoin intoxication following anaesthesia with *halothane*. The plasma concentration of phenytoin 72 hours after anaesthesia was 41 µg per ml. It was suggested that temporary liver dysfunction was responsible for impaired metabolism of phenytoin.— J. M. Karlin and H. Kutt, *J. Pediat.*, 1970, *76*, 941.

Antibiotics. In patients taking phenytoin, 250 mg daily, the administration of 2 g of *chloramphenicol* daily caused a considerable rise in the concentration of phenytoin in the serum, and its half-life was prolonged. Chloramphenicol, 3 g and 1.5 g given intravenously to 2 patients, prolonged the half-life of phenytoin from 10.5 to 22 hours and from 9 to 12.5 hours respectively.— L. K. Christensen and L. Skovsted, *Lancet*, 1969, *2*, 1397. Serum-phenytoin concentrations in a patient taking 400 mg daily increased from 7 to 24 µg per ml on being given chloramphenicol 2 g intravenously every 6 hours, and nystagmus became apparent. Phenytoin was withdrawn for a few days, then treatment was started again at a dose of 300 mg daily 3 days before treatment with chloramphenicol finished; this produced a serum concentration of 13 µg per ml. After chloramphenicol was stopped the serum-phenytoin concentration 15 days later had fallen to 3 µg per ml.— R. E. Ballek *et al.* (letter), *Lancet*, 1973, *1*, 150. Increased serum concentrations of phenytoin and phenobarbitone developed on administration of chloramphenicol to a patient previously stabilised on anticonvulsant medications. It was calculated that concomitant administration of chloramphenicol reduced phenytoin clearance by about 50% and phenobarbitone clearance by about 40%.— J. R. Koup *et al.*, *Clin. Pharmac. Ther.*, 1978, *24*, 571. See also J. Q. Rose *et al.*, *J. Am. med. Ass.*, 1977, *237*, 2630; C. W. Greenlaw, *Drug Intell. & clin. Pharm.*, 1979, *13*, 609.

Following addition of *oxacillin* by mouth to the therapeutic regimen of a burnt epileptic woman who was taking phenytoin by mouth, her plasma-phenytoin concentrations showed a very marked drop and she developed status epilepticus. It was considered that the oxacillin might have interfered with the absorption of phenytoin.— R. W. Fincham *et al.*, *Neurology, Minneap.*, 1976, *26*, 879.

For the effect of phenytoin on *doxycycline*, see Doxycycline Hydrochloride, p.1155.

Anticoagulants. Studies in 6 healthy volunteers showed that serum-phenytoin concentrations were increased by a mean of 126% when *dicoumarol* was given concurrently. Considerable increases in the half-life of phenytoin in blood were also noted. It was suggested that dicoumarol could inhibit the hydroxylation of phenytoin in the liver. Phenindione had not been found to interfere with the metabolism of phenytoin.— J. M. Hansen *et al.*, *Lancet*, 1966, *2*, 265.

A patient maintained on phenytoin, 100 mg thrice daily, was given *warfarin* and developed nystagmus and behavioural side-effects which disappeared when phenytoin was withdrawn.— N. O. Rothermich (letter), *Lancet*, 1966, *2*, 640.

For the effects of phenytoin on dicoumarol, see Dicoumarol, p.771.

Anticonvulsants. R. Buchanan *et al.* (*Pediatrics*, 1969, *43*, 114) reported a reduction in the blood concentrations of phenytoin in 5 patients who had taken *phenobarbitone* for 28 days and M. Kristensen *et al.* (*Acta med. scand.*, 1969, *185*, 347) reported the more rapid clearance of intravenously administered phenytoin after pretreatment with phenobarbitone. H. Kutt (*Ann. N.Y. Acad. Sci.*, 1971, *179*, 704) found slightly lower concentrations of phenytoin in 44 patients taking phenobarbitone concomitantly than in 37 taking phenytoin alone. Plasma concentrations of phenytoin remained unchanged in 11 patients when phenobarbitone was added to their treatment, fell in 9, and rose in 6. P.L. Morselli (*Ann. N.Y. Acad. Sci.*, 1971, *179*, 88) found that concentrations of phenytoin fell when phenobarbitone was added, and discussed the effects of genetic factors, age, pregnancy, concomitant disease, and exposure to alcohol, other drugs, and chemicals. P.A. Toseland (*Thérapie*, 1973, *28*, 993) in a 6-year-study in 908 patients found no increase in the metabolism of phenytoin. Phenytoin and phenobarbitone have been widely used concomitantly and there seems no reason to suggest any alteration though perhaps patients should be carefully observed if the relative doses of the 2 drugs are changed. For the effect of phenytoin on phenobarbitone and *primidone*, see under the respective drugs.

The blood half-life of phenytoin given to 5 patients before and after 9 days' treatment with *carbamazepine* 600 mg daily was reduced from 10.6 to 6.4 hours. In 7 patients taking phenytoin 400 mg daily, the addition of carbamazepine 600 mg daily reduced the serum-phenytoin concentration in 3.— J. M. Hansen *et al.*, *Clin. Pharmac. Ther.*, 1971, *12*, 539. For the effect of phenytoin on carbamazepine, see Carbamazepine, p.1246.

Eight of 20 patients (40%) receiving phenytoin and *sulthiame* had serum-phenytoin concentrations in excess of 25 µg per ml compared with 15 of 116 patients (13%) not receiving sulthiame. A 20-year-old woman taking phenytoin, ethosuximide, phenobarbitone, and sulthiame had a serum-phenytoin concentration of 42 µg per ml which dropped to 17 µg per ml within 15 days when sulthiame was withdrawn. Unless facilities were available for monitoring serum concentrations sulthiame should not be added to phenytoin treatment.— A. Richens and G. W. Houghton (letter), *Lancet*, 1973, *2*, 1442. See also *idem*, *Br. med. J.*, 1973, *2*, 544; *idem*, *Br. J. clin. Pharmac.*, 1974, *1*, 59.

Investigations in 9 patients demonstrated that *pheneturide* inhibited phenytoin metabolism.— G. W. Houghton and A. Richens, *Br. J. clin. Pharmac.*, 1974, *1*, 344P.

Considerably increased plasma-phenobarbitone concentrations on concomitant administration of *methsuximide* to patients receiving phenobarbitone or primidone, and even more markedly increased concentrations of phenytoin. In turn, plasma concentrations of *N*-desmethylmethsuximide, the active metabolite of methsuximide, appeared to be raised by phenobarbitone and phenytoin.— B. Rambeck, *Epilepsia*, 1979, *20*, 147.

During studies *in vitro sodium valproate* displaced significant amounts of phenytoin from serum proteins of epileptic patients, and from the serum of normal subjects which had been incubated with phenytoin.— S. Lecchini *et al.*, *Farmaco, Edn prat.*, 1978, *33*, 80. Studies in 5 patients with epilepsy confirmed previous reports from studies *in vitro* that phenytoin and valproic acid competed for serum protein-binding sites.— G. Gatti *et al.*, *ibid.*, 1979, *34*, 46.

Results of a study in 7 healthy subjects suggested that *valproic acid* may have 2 separate and opposing effects on phenytoin disposition: displacement of phenytoin from plasma protein-binding sites (and possibly from storage sites in tissues), and reduced clearance of free phenytoin by inhibiting its metabolism in the liver. The first effect would be expected to enhance phenytoin elimination, shorten half-life, and increase the systemic clearance of total drug, while the second would be expected to have the opposite effect in each case. The overall result of the interaction would depend on the combination of the 2 opposing trends. In the 7 subjects studied, despite the marked fall in total serum phenytoin concentration, free drug increased significantly, the increase being sufficiently marked to be potentially clinically important. An important implication is that in the presence of valproic acid, total serum phenytoin concentrations may grossly underestimate the concentration of free drug, and be misleading.— E. Perucca *et al.*, *Clin. Pharmac. Ther.*, 1980, *28*, 779.

Further studies into the interaction between phenytoin and valproic acid: A. Monks *et al.*, *Br. J. clin. Pharmac.*, 1978, *6*, 487; A. Monks and A. Richens, *Clin. Pharmac. Ther.*, 1980, *27*, 89; R. Dahlquist *et al.*, *Br. J. clin. Pharmac.*, 1979, *8*, 547; G. M. Frigo *et al.*, *ibid.*, 553; J. Bruni *et al.*, *Neurology*, 1980, *30*, 1233.

Individual reports of an interaction between phenytoin and valproic acid: A. Bardy *et al.* (letter), *Lancet*, 1976, *2*, 1297 (increased seizure frequency; phenytoin toxicity on sodium valproate withdrawal); S. I. Johannessen, *Arzneimittel-Forsch.*, 1977, *27*, 1083 (toxic phenytoin concentrations on sodium valproate addition); P. Silberstein, *Med. J. Aust.*, 1977, *1*, 95 (reduced phenytoin concentrations and status epilepticus; increased phenytoin concentrations and toxicity); J. C. Sackellares *et al.*, *Epilepsia*, 1979, *20*, 697 (stupor).

For a suggestion that concomitant administration of phenytoin may enhance sodium valproate-associated liver damage, see Sodium Valproate, p.1256.

Antidepressants. Plasma-phenytoin concentrations rose in 2 epileptic patients also receiving *imipramine* 75 mg daily for about 3 months for endogenous depression. In one patient the concentration gradually increased over several weeks to more than twice the pretreatment figure and he showed mild signs of phenytoin intoxication which remitted after imipramine was stopped.— E. Perucca and A. Richens (letter), *Br. J. clin. Pharmac.*, 1977, *4*, 485.

For the effect of phenytoin on *amitriptyline*, see Amitriptyline Hydrochloride, p.112. For the effect of anticonvulsant therapy on *nortriptyline*, see Nortriptyline Hydrochloride, p.127.

Antidiabetic agents. In 17 epileptics maintained on phenytoin for at least 3 months who were given *tolbutamide* 500 mg twice or thrice daily, there was a transient mean increase of 44.6% in the plasma concentration of free phenytoin whereas the total plasma concentration of phenytoin fell by about 10%. The increase in free phenytoin was possibly due to displacement from binding sites by tolbutamide; this was confirmed by *in vitro* experiments.— H. Wesseling and I. Mols-Thürkow, *Eur. J. clin. Pharmac.*, 1975, *8*, 75.

For the effect of phenytoin on tolbutamide, see Tolbutamide, p.860.

Antihistamines. A young woman developed drowsiness, ataxia, diplopia, tinnitus, and episodes of occipital headaches associated with vomiting after concomitant administration of phenytoin sodium and *chlorpheniramine*. Chlorpheniramine might have delayed the hepatic metabolism of phenytoin thereby increasing the plasma concentrations.— R. N. H. Pugh *et al.* (letter), *Br. J. clin. Pharmac.*, 1975, *2*, 173.

Agranulocytosis in a 17-year-old male given *cimetidine* and phenytoin had some characteristics of agranulocytosis reported for each drug. Cimetidine and phenytoin may be synergistic with respect to haematological toxicity.— E. Sazie and J. P. Jaffe (letter), *Ann. intern. Med.*, 1980, *93*, 151. See also F. H. Al-Kawas *et al.* (letter), *ibid.*, 1979, *90*, 992.

In 4 patients taking phenytoin and other anticonvulsant drugs (doses unchanged) the plasma-phenytoin values rose by 13 to 33% when *cimetidine* was given concomitantly.— D. J. Hetzel *et al.*, *Br. med. J.*, 1981, *282*, 1512. See also P. J. Neuvonen *et al.* (letter), *ibid.*, *283*, 501; G. J. Algozzine *et al.* (letter), *Ann. intern. Med.*, 1981, *95*, 244.

Antihypertensives and diuretics. In 2 patients plasma-phenytoin concentrations were raised by *frusemide* given concomitantly and in 1 patient by *propranolol*.— M. J. Eadie and J. H. Tyrer, *Anticonvulsant Therapy*, London, Churchill Livingstone, 1974, p. 64. For the effect of phenytoin on frusemide, see Frusemide, p.597.

A report of severe osteomalacia in 2 active young women taking *acetazolamide* in association with phenytoin or primidone and phenobarbitone.— L. E. Mallette (letter), *New Engl. J. Med.*, 1975, *293*, 668. See also I. Matsuda *et al.*, *J. Pediat.*, 1975, *87*, 202; L. E. Mallette, *Archs intern. Med.*, 1977, *137*, 1013.

In 2 children with hypoglycaemia and convulsions, phenytoin 17 and 29 mg per kg body-weight daily failed to produce therapeutic serum concentrations when *diazoxide* was given concomitantly. When diazoxide was withdrawn phenytoin 6.6 and 10 mg per kg daily was effective.— T. F. Roe *et al.*, *J. Pediat.*, 1975, *87*, 480.

Antineoplastics. Plasma concentrations of phenytoin fell during antineoplastic therapy with *cisplatin* and *bleomycin*. Primidone and phenobarbitone concentrations were unaffected. Mucosal damage may have reduced the absorption of phenytoin.— R. W. Fincham and D. D. Schottelius, *Ther. Drug Monit.*, 1979, *1*, 277.

For the effect of phenytoin on *streptozocin*, see Streptozocin, p.226.

Aspirin and other anti-inflammatory analgesics. When *phenyramidol*, 400 mg thrice daily, was given to 5 healthy volunteers who were receiving phenytoin, 100 mg thrice daily, the mean biological half-life of phenytoin was increased from 26 to 55 hours; serum concentrations were correspondingly elevated from an average of 6.6 to 12 µg of phenytoin per ml 12 hours after administration.— H. M. Solomon and J. J. Schrogie, *Clin. Pharmac. Ther.*, 1967, *8*, 554.

Vertigo, anorexia, vomiting, irreversible cerebellar damage in 2 patients receiving phenytoin, following concurrent administration of *phenylbutazone*.— M. B. Kristensen, *Clin. Pharmacokinet.*, 1976, *1*, 351. Treatment for 3 days with *aspirin, tolfenamic acid*, and *paracetamol* had no significant effect on serum concentrations of phenytoin or carbamazepine in 13 epileptic patients receiving continuous antiepileptic therapy. *Phenylbutazone* significantly lowered serum concentrations of phenytoin but not carbamazepine. When *phenylbutazone* was given for 2 weeks to 6 patients serum concentrations of phenytoin decreased in the first 2 days then increased and after 2 weeks were significantly higher than initial concentrations. It was concluded that aspirin, paracetamol, and tolfenamic acid could be used in moderate doses by epileptics taking phenytoin and carbamazepine. The use of phenylbutazone was not recommended although some patients did tolerate it well.— P. J. Neuvonen *et al.*, *Eur. J. clin. Pharmac.*, 1979, *15*, 263.

An epileptic woman stabilised on phenytoin and primidone developed phenytoin intoxication on receiving *azapropazone*. Azapropazone was considered to have competed for the hepatic metabolism of phenytoin.— C. J. C. Roberts *et al.*, *Postgrad. med. J.*, 1981, *57*, 191.

Evidence of displacement of phenytoin from plasma binding sites by *salicylate*.— D. G. Fraser *et al.*, *Clin. Pharmac. Ther.*, 1980, *27*, 165. Observations that aspirin induces a fall in total serum-phenytoin concentration, possibly due to a redistribution reaction with the displaced phenytoin diffusing out of the plasma into the extravascular water until a new equilibrium is attained. Extrapolation to the clinical situation suggested that modification of the dose of phenytoin would not be necessary.— J. W. Paxton, *ibid.*, 170. Results of a study in 10 healthy subjects who had achieved steady-state plasma-phenytoin concentrations, indicated that although high-dose salicylate administration induced displacement of phenytoin from plasma proteins, this was unlikely to be of clinical significance.— R. F. Leonard *et al.*, *Clin. Pharmac. Ther.*, 1981, *29*, 56.

Benzodiazepines. In patients treated with phenytoin the administration of a benzodiazepine drug could precipitate phenytoin intoxication.— F. J. E. Vajda *et al.* (letter), *Br. med. J.*, 1971, *1*, 346. Investigation in 8 patients demonstrated that *diazepam* and *chlordiazepoxide* appeared to be weak inducing agents of phenytoin metabolism.— G. W. Houghton and A. Richens, *Br. J. clin. Pharmac.*, 1974, *1*, 344P.

Absence of effect of *clonazepam* on serum concentrations of phenytoin, phenobarbitone, or carbamazepine.— S. I. Johannessen *et al.*, *Acta neurol. scand.*, 1977, *55*, 506. For the effect of phenytoin and phenobarbitone on clonazepam, see Clonazepam, p.1249.

Phenytoin intoxication in 2 patients on concurrent administration of diazepam.— H. J. Rogers *et al.*, *J. Neurol. Neurosurg. Psychiat.*, 1977, *40*, 890.

Cardiac glycosides. For the effects of phenytoin on digoxin and digitoxin, see Digoxin, p.534 and Digitoxin, p.541.

Corticosteroids. For the effect of phenytoin on corticosteroids, see Corticosteroids, p.450.

Levodopa. For the effect of phenytoin on levodopa, see Levodopa, p.885.

Lipid-regulating agents. Halofenate reduced the protein binding of phenytoin *in vitro*.— F. E. Karch *et al.* (letter), *Br. J. clin. Pharmac.*, 1977, *4*, 625.

See also under Adverse Effects (Effects on Lipid Metabolism), above.

Lithium. For the effect of phenytoin on lithium, see Lithium Carbonate, p.1539.

Local anaesthetics. For the effects of phenytoin on *bupivacaine* and *lignocaine*, see Bupivacaine Hydrochloride, p.911 and Lignocaine Hydrochloride, p.903.

Misonidazole. For the effect of phenytoin on misonidazole, see Misonidazole, p.1729.

Narcotic analgesics. Blood-phenytoin concentrations were elevated into the toxic range in a patient taking *dextropropoxyphene* concomitantly.— H. Kutt, *Ann. N.Y. Acad. Sci.*, 1971, *179*, 704. See also B. S. Hansen *et al.*, *Acta neurol. scand.*, 1980, *61*, 357.

For the effect of phenytoin on *methadone*, see Methadone Hydrochloride, p.1016.

Neuroleptics. Increased serum concentration of phenytoin in one patient given concomitant *chlorpromazine*, but no change in another 4.— G. W. Houghton and A. Richens, *Int. J. clin. Pharmac. Biopharm.*, 1975, *12*, 210. See also J. H. Siris *et al.*, *N.Y. St. J. Med.*, 1974, *74*, 1554.

A reduction of serum-phenytoin concentration was reported in 1 patient when he was given *loxapine succinate* 20 mg daily in addition to phenytoin 400 mg daily.— G. M. Ryan and P. A. Matthews (letter), *Drug Intell. & clin. Pharm.*, 1977, *11*, 428.

Toxic concentrations of phenytoin in 2 patients were associated with concomitant administration of *thioridazine*.— F. M. Vincent (letter), *Ann. intern. Med.*, 1980, *93*, 56.

For the effects of phenytoin on neuroleptics, see Chlorpromazine Hydrochloride, p.1512, Haloperidol, p.1533, and Thioridazine, p.1560.

Quinidine. For the effect of phenytoin on quinidine, see Quinidine, p.1371.

Sex hormones. In 15 of 23 women taking phenytoin plasma concentrations of sex-hormone binding globulin were elevated above the range found in a reference group of 68 women. The clinical significance was not clear but it might prove useful as a measure of enzyme induction in patients taking anticonvulsants.— A. Victor *et al.*, *Br. med. J.*, 1977, *2*, 934.

For the effects of phenytoin on *oral contraceptives*, see Oral Contraceptives, p.1405. For the effect of phenytoin on *conjugated oestrogens*, see Conjugated Oestrogens, p.1429.

Sodium glutamate. For a possible effect of phenytoin on sodium glutamate, see Sodium Glutamate, p.59.

Sulphonamides. In 6 patients the mean half-life of phenytoin was increased from 12.8 to 19.2 hours when *co-trimoxazole* was given concomitantly. Therapeutic doses of *sulphaphenazole, sulphadiazine*, and *sulphamethizole* inhibited the metabolism of phenytoin, but sulphadimethoxine, sulphamethoxypyridazine, and sulphamethoxydiazine did not.— J. M. Hansen *et al.* (letter), *Br. med. J.*, 1975, *2*, 684. See also J. Mølholm Hansen *et al.*, *Acta med. scand.*, 1979, *624*, 106.

Sympathomimetics. The serum concentrations of phenytoin sodium and primidone were more than doubled in a 5-year-old boy when *methylphenidate* was added to his treatment. The serum concentration of phenobarbitone was also increased but to a lesser degree. No similar effect was seen in 2 other children who were receiving smaller doses of phenobarbitone and phenytoin.— L. K. Garrettson *et al.*, *J. Am. med. Ass.*, 1969, *207*, 2053. Methylphenidate 10 mg thrice daily given in a controlled study over 6-week periods to 11 epileptic patients aged 15 to 53 years was considered to have no significant effect on their plasma-anticonvulsant concentrations.— H. J. Kupferberg *et al.*, *Clin. Pharmac. Ther.*, 1972, *13*, 201.

For the effect of phenytoin on *dopamine*, see Dopamine Hydrochloride, p.9.

Thyroid preparations. For the effect of phenytoin on *thyroxine*, see Thyroxine Sodium, p.1502.

Tuberculostatics. A report from the Boston Collaborative Drug Surveillance Program that about 25% of the recipients of phenytoin who also receive *isoniazid*, experience toxic effects on the CNS, whereas the frequency in patients receiving phenytoin without isoniazid is only about 3%. When isoniazid is added to the therapeutic regimen of a patient receiving phenytoin, a reduction in the dose of phenytoin should be anticipated. Specific guidelines for the dosage reduction have not been established, therefore plasma concentrations should be monitored.— R. R. Russell *et al.*, *Chest*, 1979, *75*, 356. Further references: H. Kutt *et al.*, *Am. Rev. resp. Dis.*, 1970, *101*, 377; R. W. Brennan *et al.*, *Neurology, Minneap.*, 1970, *20*, 687; J. Johnson (letter), *Br. med. J.*, 1975, *1*, 152.

Vitamins. Folic acid reduced the serum concentrations of phenytoin in 50 folate-deficient patients who were taking phenytoin, but with the exception of 1 patient the frequency of fits was not affected.— E. M. Baylis *et al.* (preliminary communication), *Lancet*, 1971, *1*, 62. For the effects of phenytoin on serum-folate concentrations see under Adverse Effects (Effects on the Blood), above.

Pyridoxine reduced concentrations of phenytoin in serum in 7 patients.— O. Hansson and M. Sillanpaa (letter), *Lancet*, 1976, *1*, 256.

For the effects of phenytoin on vitamin D see under Adverse Effects (Effects on Bones), above.

Interference with diagnostic tests. Phenytoin might interfere with estimation of barbiturates in the blood.— J. Millhouse, *Adverse Drug React. Bull.*, 1974, Dec., 164.

A study of 10 patients who received phenytoin and 20 healthy subjects who did not, indicated that therapeutic serum-phenytoin concentrations displaced thyroid hormones from binding proteins thus increasing free hormone concentrations and reducing serum-total-hormone concentrations. The concentration of free thyroxine was increased to a greater extent than free tri-iodothyronine, this being reflected by an increased urinary excretion of unconjugated thyroxine. However, serum-free-hormone concentrations, which were considered to determine the thyroid status of a patient, remained within the euthyroid range.— J. F. Finucane and R. S. Griffiths, *Br. J. clin. Pharmac.*, 1976, *3*, 1041.

In 42 patients taking anticonvulsants (phenytoin, sometimes with phenobarbitone or carbamazepine) serum concentrations of total thyroxine, free thyroxine, and free tri-iodothyronine were significantly depressed compared with controls; there was no clinical evidence of hypothyroidism.— P. P. B. Yeo *et al.*, *Br. med. J.*, 1978, *1*, 1581. Criticism.— J. Finucane (letter), *ibid.*, 1978, *2*, 357.

For the effect of phenytoin on some estimations of blood-theophylline concentrations, see Aminophylline, p.343.

Withdrawal. Of 148 children who had been free from seizures for 4 years on anticonvulsant drugs 36 relapsed when treatment was gradually withdrawn. The EEG was of limited value in indicating the likely success of withdrawal, which was greatest in those with early age of onset and prompt control of seizures. Relapse-rates according to type of seizure were: grand mal 8%, febrile and petit mal 12%, psychomotor 25%, multiple seizures 40%, and Jacksonian 53%.— J. Holowach *et al.*, *New Engl. J. Med.*, 1972, *286*, 169.

Absorption and Fate. Phenytoin is slowly but almost completely absorbed from the gastro-intestinal tract; the rate of absorption is variable and its bioavailability can differ markedly with different pharmaceutical formulations. Small particles are better absorbed than large particles and, in particular, the use of calcium sulphate as an excipient has been reported to reduce the bioavailability of phenytoin very considerably. Large doses are more slowly absorbed than small doses and intramuscular doses are more slowly absorbed than oral doses.

Phenytoin is extensively metabolised in the liver to its primary metabolite, 5-(4-hydroxyphenyl)-5-phenylhydantoin, which is inactive. It is excreted in the urine, mainly as its hydroxylated metabolite, either free or in conjugated form. Phenytoin hydroxylation is capacity-limited, and is therefore readily inhibited by agents which compete for its metabolic pathways.

Phenytoin is widely distributed throughout the body and is extensively bound to plasma protein. It has a very variable, dose-dependent half-life, but the mean appears to lie somewhere within the range of 17 to 22 hours following oral administration of therapeutic doses. The therapeutic and adverse effects of phenytoin have been correlated with plasma concentrations: in general, the anticonvulsant effect of phenytoin is obtained at concentrations of 10 to 20 μg per ml (40 to 80 μmol per litre), while concentrations above 20 μg per ml are associated with progressively severe signs of toxicity. Phenytoin crosses the blood-brain barrier and the placental barrier, and small amounts are excreted in milk.

General reviews and comments on the pharmacokinetics of phenytoin: M. J. Eadie, *Clin. Pharmacokinet.*, 1976, *1*, 52; G. Alvan, *ibid.*, 1978, *3*, 155; A. Richens, *ibid.*, 1979, *4*, 153; *idem*, 1980, *5*, 402; G. Tognoni *et al.*, *ibid.*, 1980, *5*, 105.

Absorption. Phenytoin absorption was increased by the presence of food. It was suggested that phenytoin should always be taken in the same relationship to meals.— A. Melander *et al.*, *Eur. J. clin. Pharmac.*, 1979, *15*, 269.

Further references: C. Balabaud *et al.* (letter), *Br. J. clin. Pharmac.*, 1979, *8*, 369 (influence of dietary protein and carbohydrate on phenytoin metabolism); M. C. Kennedy and D. N. Wade, *Br. J. clin. Pharmac.*, 1979, *7*, 515 (effect of ileojejunal bypass); D. Jung *et al.*, *Clin. Pharmac. Ther.*, 1980, *28*, 479 (effect of dose on absorption).

Metabolism and pharmacokinetics. Following oral administration of phenytoin 100 mg thrice daily for 3 days to 68 healthy male and female subjects, the mean half-life of phenytoin was estimated to be 22 hours, with a range of 7 to 42 hours. Considerably longer half-lives of 72.5 and 55 hours in a further 2 subjects were excluded because it was considered they might be 'slow metabolisers' of phenytoin, or could have an inability to parahydroxylate phenytoin. The mean half-life in Negro males in the study (26.5 hours) was significantly longer than that in Caucasian males (18.5 hours). Results of a further study in 10 subjects indicated that the half-life of phenytoin is dose-dependent, which may be explained by saturation of a rate-limiting enzyme in the metabolism of the drug.— K. Arnold and N. Gerber, *Clin. Pharmac. Ther.*, 1970, *11*, 121.

Investigations in epileptic patients indicated that increasing the daily dose of phenytoin caused a lengthening of the half-life and a reduction in the ratio of its major metabolite to unchanged phenytoin thus indicating that phenytoin hydroxylation was saturable.— G. W. Houghton and A. Richens, *Br. J. clin. Pharmac.*, 1974, *1*, 155.

The pharmacokinetics and bioavailability of phenytoin in 6 healthy male subjects following single doses of 300 mg (4 mg per kg body-weight) by mouth and intravenously, and repeated doses of 300 mg daily by mouth for 14 days. A steady-state plasma concentration of 10 μg per ml was not achieved in any of the subjects, indicating that in many individuals doses exceeding 4 mg per kg would be required to obtain therapeutic concentrations. Variations in bioavailability and elimination rates prevented accurate prediction of steady-state concentrations; monitoring of plasma-phenytoin concentrations might therefore be of special importance. The mean plasma elimination half-life was about 17 hours after oral or intravenous administration, and lengthened to a mean of about 19 hours after chronic administration.— R. Gugler *et al.*, *Clin. Pharmac. Ther.*, 1976, *19*, 135.

Study of plasma concentrations of 5-(4-hydroxyphenyl)-5-phenylhydantoin in phenytoin-treated patients.— C. Hoppel *et al.*, *Clin. Pharmac. Ther.*, 1977, *21*, 294. Two metabolites of phenytoin 5-(3,4-dihydroxyphenyl)-5-phenylhydantoin and 5-(3-methoxy-4-hydroxyphenyl)-5-phenylhydantoin were identified in the urine of 2 subjects who had received phenytoin 300 mg.— K. K. Midha *et al.*, *J. pharm. Sci.*, 1977, *66*, 1596. See also K. S. Albert *et al.*, *Res. Commun. chem. Path. Pharmac.*, 1974, *9*, 463; E. Perucca *et al.*, *Clin. Pharmac. Ther.*, 1978, *24*, 46; J. P. Allen *et al.*, *ibid.*, 1979, *26*, 445.

A kinetic study of a family of phenytoin hypometabolisers.— M. R. Vasko *et al.*, *Clin. Pharmac. Ther.*, 1980, *27*, 96. See also N. Gerber *et al.*, *Ann. intern. Med.*, 1972, *77*, 765 (hypometabolism); D. W. Hawkins *et al.*, *Neurology, Minneap.*, 1976, *26*, 343 (hypermetabolism).

Further references to the pharmacokinetics of phenytoin: A. J. Handley, *Br. med. J.*, 1970, *3*, 203 (intravenous); K. Siersbaek-Nielsen *et al.* (letter), *ibid.*, 1971, *1*, 231 (intravenous); L. Lund *et al.*, *Eur. J. clin. Pharmac.*, 1974, *7*, 81; J. D. Robinson *et al.*, *Br. J. clin. Pharmac.*, 1975, *2*, 345; L. K. Garrettson and W. J. Jusko, *Clin. Pharmac. Ther.*, 1975, *17*, 481; G. W. Houghton *et al.*, *Br. J. clin. Pharmac.*, 1975, *2*, 251 (age, height, weight, and sex); G. Gatti *et al.*, *Farmaco, Edn prat.*, 1977, *32*, 470 (intravenous); J. Q. Rose *et al.*, *Int. J. clin. Pharmac. Biopharm.*, 1978, *16*, 547 (smokers and non-smokers); E. A. De Leacy *et al.*, *Br. J. clin. Pharmac.*, 1979, *8*, 33 (sex, smoking habits, alcohol and oral contraceptive use); I. E. Leppik *et al.*, *New Engl. J. Med.*, 1979, *300*, 481 (increased clearance in infectious mononucleosis); B. Andoh *et al.*, *Br. J. clin. Pharmac.*, 1980, *9*, 282P (Negroes and Caucasians).

Plasma concentrations. Individual doses of phenytoin sodium ranging from 200 to 500 mg daily were required in 50 patients to maintain a serum-phenytoin concentration within the therapeutic range of 10 to 20 μg per ml. The dose requirement correlated most strongly with body-surface, a dose of about 200 mg per m^2 body-surface daily being calculated, but this relationship accounted for only 33% of the total variance of phenytoin dosage requirements. The use of body-surface was a better guide to individual dose than body-weight but was not much more successful than the common practice of prescribing 300 mg daily for all adult patients.— M. H. Barot *et al.*, *Br. J. clin. Pharmac.*, 1978, *6*, 267.

Studies directed at relating therapeutic response to plasma concentrations of phenytoin, with the aim of individualising dosage regimens: T. M. Ludden *et al.*, *Clin. Pharmac. Ther.*, 1977, *21*, 287; E. Martin *et al.*, *J. Pharmacokinet. Biopharm.*, 1977, *5*, 579; T. M. Ludden *et al.*, *ibid.*, 1978, *6*, 399; P. W. Mullen, *Clin. Pharmac. Ther.*, 1978, *23*, 228; P. W. Mullen and R. W. Foster, *J. Pharm. Pharmac.*, 1979, *31*, 100; T. M. Ludden (letter), *ibid.*, 1980, *32*, 152; S. Vozeh and F. Follath, *Eur. J. clin. Pharmac.*, 1980, *17*, 33.

Protein binding. In 15 healthy subjects with therapeutic blood concentrations of phenytoin (16 μg per ml) the proportion of phenytoin not bound to plasma proteins was 8% at room temperature. The proportion was similar in plasma from epileptic patients under treatment with phenytoin and was increased by about 60% at 37°. The unbound proportion (at room temperature) in plasma from 13 neonates was 10.6%; this might explain the clinical effectiveness of phenytoin in infants at doses less than those needed to produce therapeutic concentrations in adults. A patient with uraemia had 30% unbound phenytoin.— L. Lund *et al.*, *Ann. N.Y. Acad. Sci.*, 1971, *179*, 723. See also M. M. Reidenberg *et al.*, *New Engl. J. Med.*, 1971, *285*, 264 (reduced binding in uraemia).

The main metabolite, *p*-hydroxyphenytoin, was about 81 to 84% protein bound.— G. J. Conard *et al.*, *J. pharm. Sci.*, 1971, *60*, 1642.

There was little interindividual difference in the extent of plasma-protein binding or the CSF-plasma ratio of phenytoin in 8 patients with epilepsy treated solely with phenytoin.— L. Lund *et al.*, *Clin. Pharmac. Ther.*, 1972, *13*, 196. See also N. Barth *et al.*, *Clin. Pharmacokinet.*, 1976, *1*, 444.

Studies in 97 volunteers indicated that the amount of phenytoin not bound to plasma proteins was not significantly different in pregnant women (mean 11.6%), women taking oral contraceptives (9.9%), healthy men (10.6%), and healthy women (11%), but was increased in patients with renal disease (15.8%), hepatic disease (15.9%), or hepatorenal disease (15.6%).— W. D. Hooper *et al.*, *Clin. Pharmac. Ther.*, 1974, *15*, 276. An *in vitro* study of the binding of phenytoin to serum protein in 16 healthy drug-free women, 12 healthy women on combined oral contraceptive preparations, and 16 healthy pregnant women during the first and the last trimesters of pregnancy. Women on oral contraceptives and those in the first trimester of pregnancy had normal phenytoin binding, but the binding of phenytoin to serum proteins was considerably reduced in the last 3 months of pregnancy.— M. Ruprah *et al.* (letter), *Lancet*, 1980, *2*, 316. Comment.— R. Leonard (letter), *ibid.*, 1312. Reply.— M. Ruprah *et al.* (letter), *ibid.*, 1981, *1*, 97.

Saliva concentrations. Measurements of total and unbound plasma concentrations and salivary concentrations of phenytoin were carried out in 17 epileptic patients receiving 90 to 400 mg daily and in 6 patients with chronic renal failure on haemodialysis as well as 1 patient with a renal transplant in rejection given 200 to 500 mg daily. Salivary concentrations correlated with free plasma concentrations and could be used to monitor phenytoin therapy in patients with normal as well as abnormal renal function where the proportion of unbound to bound phenytoin was increased.— F. Reynolds *et al.*, *Lancet*, 1976, *2*, 384. See also J. W. Paxton *et al.* (letter), *ibid.*, 639.

The saliva concentration was about 10% of the serum concentration of unbound phenytoin.— J. W. Paxton *et al.*, *Eur. J. clin. Pharmac.*, 1977, *11*, 71.

Further studies on concentrations of phenytoin in saliva: J. C. Mucklow and C. T. Dollery, *Br. J. clin. Pharmac.*, 1978, *6*, 75 (to assess patient compliance); J. W. Paxton and S. Foote (letter), *Br. J. clin. Pharmac.*, 1979, *8*, 508 (aberrantly high concentrations); G. W. Rylance *et al.*, *Archs Dis. Childh.*, 1979, *54*, 801 (in children); J. W. Paxton and J. B. Wilcox, *J. Pharm. Pharmac.*, 1980, *32*, 586 (for bioavailability studies); G. W. Rylance and T. A. Moreland, *Archs Dis. Childh.*, 1981, *56*, 637 (no relationship between dose and saliva concentration nor between saliva concentration and convulsion control); C. Knott *et al.*, *Br. med. J.*, 1982, *284*, 13 (in the presence of valproate).

Pregnancy and the neonate. In a study of 14 patients the plasma clearance of phenytoin, phenobarbitone, and carbamazepine was generally increased during pregnancy and immediately after delivery although there were considerable individual fluctuations. The concentration of the active metabolite carbamazepine epoxide relative to that of carbamazepine was increased during pregnancy.— M. Dam *et al.*, *Clin. Pharmacokinet.*, 1979, *4*, 53. Further references: K. I. Mygind *et al.*, *Acta neurol. scand.*, 1976, *54*, 160; C. M. Lander *et al.*, *Neurology, Minneap.*, 1977, *27*, 128; M. J. Landon and M. Kirkley, *Br. J. Obstet. Gynaec.*, 1979, *86*, 125.

For studies on the protein binding of phenytoin in pregnancy, see under Protein Binding, above.

Lactation. Data suggesting a rather limited transport capacity of the mammary glands for phenytoin, which is probably exceeded at relatively low plasma concentrations. Phenytoin concentrations in the breast milk and colostrum of 2 women on chronic anticonvulsant therapy were significantly below those in the maternal plasma, and increasing the maternal plasma concentration of phenytoin from 5.5 μg per ml to 8.4 μg per ml did not lead to a corresponding increase in the phenytoin concentration of breast milk.— B. L. Mirkin, *J. Pediat.*, 1971, *78*, 329.

The concentrations of anticonvulsant drugs in serum and breast milk were measured in 9 lactating women with epilepsy. Concentrations in maternal serum were phenytoin, 2.1 to 5.7 μg per ml, phenobarbitone, 2.5 to 42 μg per ml, primidone, 0.8 to 15.7 μg per ml, carbamazepine, 3.2 to 6.2 μg per ml, and ethosuximide, 18 to 39 μg per ml. Concentrations in milk were phenytoin 0.5 to 1.4 μg per ml, phenobarbitone, 0.5 to 33 μg per ml, primidone, 0.5 to 6.7 μg per ml, carbamazepine 0.8 to 3.8 μg per ml, and ethosuximide, 18 to 24 μg per ml. The ratio of drug concentration in milk to that in serum was about 18% for phenytoin, 45% for phenobarbitone, 80% for primidone, 39% for carbamazepine, and 78% for ethosuximide.— S. Kaneko *et al.* (letter), *Br. J. clin.*

Pharmac., 1979, *7*, 624.

The neonate. The pharmacokinetics of phenytoin given intravenously as the sodium salt to 30 newborn and young infants. The plasma half-life of phenytoin was prolonged and variable in premature infants. At term the half-life was less prolonged and less variable and this pattern of reduction continued in the children aged 2 to 96 weeks. Protein binding appeared to be diminished in infants under 12 weeks of age but thereafter binding was similar to that in the adult. Maintenance treatment with 4 mg per kg body-weight every 12 hours in the first week of life in full-term and premature infants produced some toxic plasma concentrations. No fixed dose could be recommended from these results for infants aged up to 2 weeks although some full-term infants could achieve therapeutic though variable plasma concentrations with 5.9 mg per kg every 24 hours. Most children aged 2 weeks or more would require doses of at least 8 mg per kg every 24 hours with the interval between doses being decreased from 12 to 6 or 8 hours.— P. M. Loughnan *et al.*, *Archs Dis. Childh.*, 1977, *52*, 302.

Kinetics of placentally transferred phenytoin and its *p*-hydroxylated metabolites in newborn infants.— A. Rane *et al.*, *Br. J. clin. Pharmac.*, 1979, *8*, 465. See also A. Rane *et al.*, *Clin. Pharmac. Ther.*, 1974, *15*, 39.

Further references to the metabolism of phenytoin in neonates: M. J. Painter *et al.*, *J. Pediat.*, 1978, *92*, 315; *idem*, *Neurology, Minneap.*, 1979, *29*, 542.

Uses. Phenytoin sodium is an anticonvulsant used to control tonic-clonic or grand mal and psychomotor or partial (focal) seizures. It is believed to stabilise rather than elevate the seizure threshold and to limit the spread of seizure activity.

The dose of phenytoin should be adjusted to the needs of the individual patient to achieve adequate control of seizures; this usually requires plasma concentrations of 10 to 20 µg per ml (40 to 80 µmol per litre). It has been recommended that children should be weighed regularly as weight loss may presage signs of overt toxicity. The suggested initial dose is 100 mg thrice daily progressively increased at intervals of a few days to a maximum of 600 mg daily; the usual maintenance dose is 300 to 400 mg daily. A suggested initial dose for children is 5 mg per kg body-weight daily in 2 or 3 divided doses; a suggested maintenance dose is 4 to 8 mg per kg body-weight daily.

Since phenytoin has a long plasma half-life, a twice-daily dosage regimen is adequate to maintain an effective plasma concentration and is preferred because improved compliance has been associated with twice-daily dosage regimens. Once-daily regimens, usually given at night, are also suitable in some patients receiving brands of phenytoin known to have a slow rate of dissolution. Different commercially available brands of phenytoin can vary in their bioavailability and in their rates of dissolution, therefore patients should be maintained on the initial form used for stabilisation, and the need for restabilisation must be understood if a change is envisaged.

The practice of starting phenytoin therapy with initial small doses means that over a week may be required before therapeutic plasma concentrations are established. Some authorities therefore prefer to give an initial loading dose in order to reach the recommended plasma concentrations sooner. A suggested oral loading dose is 12 to 15 mg per kg body-weight divided into 2 or 3 doses given over about 6 hours, followed by 100 mg thrice daily on the following days.

In order to lessen gastric irritation, phenytoin should be taken with at least half a tumblerful of water and may be taken with or after food. The time and manner of taking phenytoin should be standardised for the patient since variations might affect absorption with consequent fluctuations in the plasma concentrations.

If the patient is already taking other anticonvulsant drugs, the transition to phenytoin sodium should be made gradually, with some overlapping in dosage, since too rapid withdrawal of these drugs may lead to an increase in frequency of seizures; similarly if patients are transferred from phenytoin to another anticonvulsant the transition should be gradual. Phenytoin may be given in association with other anticonvulsants, such as phenobarbitone, but single-drug therapy is generally preferred unless the patient is suffering from 2 different forms of epilepsy which require control by different drugs.

In the treatment of status epilepticus 150 to 250 mg of phenytoin sodium may be given by slow intravenous injection at a uniform rate of not more than 50 mg per minute; a further 100 to 150 mg may be given 30 minutes later if necessary. A suggested intravenous dose for children is 5 mg per kg body-weight as one dose or divided into 2 doses. Deaths have been caused by the over-rapid intravenous injection of phenytoin sodium (for further details, see under Administration, below). Phenytoin sodium is only very slowly absorbed from the intramuscular site therefore intramuscular injections are not appropriate for the emergency arrest of status epilepticus although they may be used to maintain or establish therapeutic plasma concentrations of phenytoin in patients who are unconscious or otherwise unable to take phenytoin by mouth. Owing to the slower absorption of phenytoin from intramuscular sites, patients stabilised on the oral route require an increase in the intramuscular dose of about 50%, at least initially; on transfer back to the oral route lower doses should be given initially, to allow for continued absorption of the residual phenytoin in the intramuscular sites (for further details, see under Administration, below).

The suggested dose of phenytoin sodium for the prophylactic control of seizures in neurosurgery is 100 to 200 mg by intramuscular injection 3 or 4 times daily.

Phenytoin is also a class I anti-arrhythmic agent (see p.1370); it is used in the treatment of cardiac arrhythmias, particularly those associated with digitalis intoxication; it is of little or no value in cardiac arrhythmias caused by acute or chronic heart disease. The usual dose is 3.5 to 5 mg per kg body-weight administered by slow intravenous injection at a uniform rate of not more than 50 mg per minute; this dose may be repeated once if necessary. Electrocardiographic monitoring is recommended.

Publications relating to anticonvulsant therapy, including phenytoin: *The Treatment of Epilepsy*, J.H. Tyrer (Ed.), Lancaster, England, MTP Press, 1980.

Action. A review of theories on the mode of action of anticonvulsants including phenytoin. In contrast to phenobarbitone and troxidone, phenytoin does not raise the threshold for minimal electroshock seizures, but it strikingly limits the development of maximal seizure activity, and reduces the spread of seizure activity from a discharging focus without necessarily influencing the focus itself. This may explain why phenytoin may be very effective in controlling grand mal attacks clinically but is less so in preventing minor seizures from a focal discharge. Phenytoin, phenobarbitone, and other anticonvulsants with a phenyl ring that are effective against grand mal seizures also modify the pattern of maximal tonic-clonic electroshock seizures by abolishing the tonic phase. The clonic phase may be exaggerated and prolonged, but the EEG shows a reduced voltage and frequency of convulsive discharges.— E. H. Reynolds, *Br. J. Hosp. Med.*, 1978, *19*, 505.

Administration and dosage. From a study in 97 adults and 125 children, the average child up to 10 years of age needs a larger dose (11 mg per kg body-weight daily) of phenytoin to achieve a plasma-phenytoin concentration of 15 µg per ml than do persons over 14 years of age (6.5 mg per kg daily); the position of children aged 11 to 13 years is intermediate. To reduce the risk of overdosage a dose of 4 to 5 mg per kg might be used initially in both children and adults.— M. J. Eadie *et al.*, *Proc. Aust. Ass. Neurol.*, 1973, *10*, 53.

With the exception of one 16-year-old female (who developed nystagmus, ataxia, and mental confusion) a loading dose of 1 g of phenytoin sodium was well tolerated by 53 adolescent and adult patients when given 2-hourly in divided doses (400, 300, and 300 mg) over a 4-hour period whereas 4 of a further 8 patients became nauseated on receiving single doses of 1 g. Of the 60 patients who tolerated phenytoin 18% experienced side-effects but these were mild and transient.— B. J. Wilder *et al.*, *Clin. Pharmac. Ther.*, 1973, *14*, 797.

A detailed investigation of partially-controlled epileptic patients indicated that when the serum concentration of phenytoin reached 5 to 10 µg per ml it was then appropriate to adjust the dosage by small steps of about 25 mg to achieve therapeutic concentrations of 10 to 20 µg per ml. Fifteen patients received a phenytoin-tolerance test to predict a daily maintenance dose for a desired steady-state but this was not considered essential; for the test the last regular dose of phenytoin was given at 10 pm on the preceding night; other drugs were given at the usual dosage during the test. At 10 am on the following day 6 tablets of phenytoin sodium 100 mg were given by mouth. No more phenytoin was given for 48 hours and venous blood samples taken after 1, 2, 4, 12, 24, 36, and 48 hours were used to calculate elimination-rates and theoretical daily doses.— G. E. Mawer *et al.*, *Br. J. clin. Pharmac.*, 1974, *1*, 163.

Nomograms for phenytoin dosage: A. Richens and A. Dunlop, *Lancet*, 1975, *2*, 247; L. Lund and G. Alván (letter), *ibid.*, 1305; A. Richens and A. Dunlop (letter), *ibid.*; D. G. Lambie *et al.*, *Lancet*, 1976, *2*, 386.

Studies and comments on the suitability of once and twice daily dosage of phenytoin: A. F. Haerer and R. A. Buchanan, *Neurology, Minneap.*, 1972, *22*, 1021; R. A. Buchanan *et al.*, *J. Pediat.*, 1973, *83*, 479; D. A. Cocks *et al.*, *Br. J. clin. Pharmac.*, 1975, *2*, 449.

For a recommendation that phenytoin should always be given at the same time in relation to food, see under Absorption and Fate, above.

Intramuscular. After an investigation in 11 patients the following regimen was recommended for the transfer of phenytoin by mouth to the intramuscular route: the dosage should be increased by 50% in order to maintain constant concentrations of phenytoin in the plasma and of its principal metabolite in the urine; on returning patients to phenytoin by mouth a dose equivalent to 50% of the original dose by mouth should be administered for the same period as that during which the intramuscular route was used. It was believed that this regimen might be valid following transfer of phenytoin to the intramuscular route for periods of up to 19 days.— B. J. Wilder *et al.*, *Clin. Pharmac. Ther.*, 1974, *16*, 507. Eight epileptic patients who received phenytoin intramuscularly once daily for 1 week in a dose 50% greater than their oral dose followed by a return to oral therapy for 1 week at half the original oral dose did not show undue fluctuations in plasma-phenytoin concentrations, indicating that such a regimen was suitable for patients requiring intramuscular therapy. In 4 patients who received the same intramuscular regimen in divided doses daily the plasma concentrations began to rise, within 1 week corresponding to the increase in dose and falling only gradually during the final oral stage, suggesting that the intramuscular regimen on the 50% larger dose should not exceed a 1-week period and supporting the use of a once-daily injection.— B. J. Wilder and R. E. Ramsay, *ibid.*, 1976, *19*, 360.

By giving an initial intravenous dose of phenytoin 10.7 mg per kg body-weight, infused at 25 mg per minute (slower rates for infants), followed immediately by an intramuscular loading dose of 12.7 mg per kg distributed over varied sites followed by daily intramuscular maintenance doses of 8.6 mg per kg therapeutic plasma concentrations of phenytoin were achieved in two-thirds of 98 patients most of whom were unconscious. About one-third needed an adjustment of the maintenance dose. When the change to administration by mouth was made, the initial oral doses were reduced to allow for the continuing release of phenytoin from the intramuscular sites.— D. Perrier *et al.*, *Ann. intern. Med.*, 1976, *85*, 318.

Anticonvulsants should not be given intramuscularly in emergency situations because of slowness of absorption and relatively low peak serum concentrations.— T. R. Browne, *Am. J. Hosp. Pharm.*, 1978, *35*, 1048.

Intravenous. Sudden marked sinus bradycardia, hypotension and syncope occurred in 4 of 15 young healthy subjects during intravenous administration of phenytoin 250 mg at a rate of 35 to 40 mg at 60-second intervals; in all 4 the arrhythmia occurred after about 105 to 120 mg had been given, and responded to atropine. Patients should be carefully monitored and anti-arrhythmic drugs should be available even when the rate of intravenous injection is slow.— S. A. Barron (letter), *New Engl. J. Med.*, 1976, *295*, 678. The rate of administration was excessive; it should be given so that 50 mg was given continuously over 60 seconds, timing the rate with the second hand of a watch, so that 300 mg would be given as an intravenous infusion over 6 minutes. Administration of aliquots of 35 to 40 mg at 60-second intervals might have led to higher cardiac concentrations resulting in the arrhythmias.— P. E.

Cooper (letter), *ibid.*, 1078. See also R. E. Cranford *et al.*, *Neurology, Minneap.*, 1978, *28*, 874.

Reports of adverse responses, including fatalities, following intravenous phenytoin: Grissom J.H. *et al.*, *Br. med. J.*, 1967, *4*, 34; G. L. Gellerman and C. Martinez, *J. Am. med. Ass.*, 1967, *200*, 337; A. H. Unger and H. J. Sklaroff, *ibid.*, 335; H. Kutt (letter), *ibid.*, *201*, 210; S. Zoneraich *et al.*, *Am. Heart J.*, 1976, *91*, 375.

The manufacturers of commercial preparations of phenytoin sodium do not recommend dilution of intravenous solutions of phenytoin sodium owing to the risk of precipitation of the crystals. Nevertheless, some sources report that they have diluted the intravenous preparation. For controversy over this practice see under Incompatibility, above.

Rectal. Lack of efficacy of phenytoin suppositories in anti-epileptic treatment.— L. Kvan and S. Johannessen, *Acta neurol. scand.*, 1976, *54*, 103.

Administration in children. Reviews and comments on the management of epilepsy in children: D. P. Addy, *Br. med. J.*, 1978, *2*, 811; B. Bower, *Br. J. Hosp. Med.*, 1978, *19*, 8; *Br. med. J.*, 1979, *2*, 1.

Dosage. Evidence of relatively little fluctuation in serum concentrations in infants and children given phenytoin every 12 hours by mouth.— W. E. Dodson, *Clin. Pharmac. Ther.*, 1980, *27*, 704.

Administration in the elderly. A marked increase of phenytoin clearance occurred in people over 65 years of age compared with those under 45 years of age. Phenytoin clearance correlated inversely with phenytoin binding and plasma albumin, both of which were found to be reduced in the elderly.— M. J. Hayes *et al.*, *Br. J. clin. Pharmac.*, 1975, *2*, 73.

Evidence of increased plasma-phenytoin concentrations with age.— G. W. Houghton *et al.*, *Br. J. clin. Pharmac.*, 1975, *2*, 251.

Administration in hepatic failure. In situations such as hepatic failure which decrease both protein binding and hepatic clearance, plasma-phenytoin concentrations must be carefully monitored to avoid toxicity during continued administration.— J. L. Anderson *et al.*, *Drugs*, 1978, *15*, 271. For comments on the relevance of free and bound phenytoin in relation to plasma-phenytoin monitoring, and the significance of impaired hepatic metabolism of phenytoin, see under Precautions (above).

Further references: T. F. Blaschke *et al.*, *Clin. Pharmac. Ther.*, 1975, *17*, 685 (acute viral hepatitis and phenytoin).

Administration in renal failure. The administration of phenytoin sodium by mouth or intravenously to 20 uraemic patients with seizures produced lower plasma concentrations of phenytoin than in 20 non-uraemic patients with seizures, but plasma concentrations of 4-hydroxyphenytoin were much higher in the uraemic patients.— J. M. Letteri *et al.*, *New Engl. J. Med.*, 1971, *285*, 648. The proportion of phenytoin not bound to plasma proteins was 2 to 4 times greater in uraemic patients than in normal patients, probably due to a qualitative change in the plasma proteins.— M. R. Blum *et al.* (letter), *ibid.*, 1972, *286*, 109. Studies in 9 healthy subjects and 11 patients with renal failure, of the impaired plasma protein binding of phenytoin in uraemia. The displacement effect of salicylic acid was considerably less marked in plasma from uraemic subjects indicating that displacing drugs should not be expected to cause a significant further decrease of plasma binding of phenytoin in uraemia.— I. Odar-Cederlöf and O. Borgå, *Clin. Pharmac. Ther.*, 1976, *20*, 36. Reduced clearance and increased plasma concentrations of hydroxylated metabolite in uraemic subjects.— O. Borgå *et al.*, *Clin. Pharmac. Ther.*, 1979, *26*, 306.

Phenytoin can be given in usual doses to patients in renal failure. Concentrations of phenytoin are not affected by haemodialysis.— W. M. Bennett *et al.*, *Ann. intern. Med.*, 1977, *86*, 754. See also *idem*, 1980, *93*, 286.

A study in 7 patients undergoing long-term haemodialysis who received phenytoin suggested that supplemental doses of phenytoin were not needed as the amount of phenytoin removed by haemodialysis was not clinically significant.— E. Martin *et al.*, *J. Am. med. Ass.*, 1977, *238*, 1750. Haemodialysis affected the protein binding of phenytoin.— W. H. Steele *et al.*, *Eur. J. clin. Pharmac.*, 1979, *15*, 69.

A study demonstrating that in end-stage renal disease the enzyme-multiplied immunoassay gives falsely high results for serum-phenytoin concentrations.— E. D. Burgess *et al.*, *Ann. intern. Med.*, 1981, *94*, 59.

For comments on the relevance of free and bound phenytoin in relation to plasma-phenytoin monitoring, see under Precautions, above.

Alcoholism. A regimen incorporating phenytoin for the management of alcohol-withdrawal seizures.— M. J. Finer (letter), *J. Am. med. Ass.*, 1971, *215*, 119. A criticism of such regimens and comments on the inappropriate nature of phenytoin for alcohol-withdrawal seizures.— P. K. Gessner (letter), *ibid.*, *216*, 887. Support for the use of phenytoin in alcohol withdrawal.— H. P. Adams (letter), *ibid.*, *218*, 598. Further criticism, and a review of the ineffectiveness of phenytoin in alcohol withdrawal.— P. K. Gessner (letter), *ibid.*, 1972, *219*, 1072. Phenytoin in association with chlordiazepoxide for alcohol detoxification in patients with a history of convulsions in adulthood.— R. Sampliner and F. L. Iber, *ibid.*, 1974, *230*, 1430. Further references to phenytoin being given for alcohol-withdrawal symptoms: E. Rothstein, *Am. J. Psychiat.*, 1973, *130*, 1381.

A comment that phenytoin is not effective in treating seizures induced by alcohol withdrawal, even though it may accelerate the normalisation of ethanol-induced electrolyte imbalances.— M. Linnoila *et al.*, *Drugs*, 1979, *18*, 299.

Anorexia and obesity. Of 10 patients with *compulsive eating* 9 showed improvement after treatment with phenytoin 100 mg two to four times daily. Nine of the 10 had EEG abnormalities.— R. S. Green and J. H. Rau, *Am. J. Psychiat.*, 1974, *131*, 428. A double-blind study in 7 obese patients showed that phenytoin was no more effective than placebo in producing weight loss.— F. L. Greenway *et al.*, *Curr. ther. Res.*, 1977, *21*, 338. See also L. Levitz and T. Weiss (letter), *Am. J. Psychiat.*, 1976, *133*, 1093.

Anxiety. Phenytoin sodium, 100 mg twice daily, given for 4 weeks to patients with *anxiety neurosis* had no significant effect when compared with similar patients given a placebo.— W. G. Case *et al.*, *Am. J. Psychiat.*, 1969, *126*, 254. In a double-blind crossover study in 30 patients with anxiety neurosis, treatment with 100 mg of phenytoin sodium thrice daily for 3 weeks was more effective than a 5-mg dose thrice daily.— J. H. Stephens and J. W. Schaffer, *Psychopharmacologia*, 1970, *17*, 169, per *Abstr. Wld Med.*, 1970, *44*, 781. See also W. J. Turner, *Int. J. Neuropsychiat.*, 1967, *3*, 94.

In a preliminary study phenytoin was shown to have a short-term effect in decreasing the anxiety and depression of *child-abusing* parents, but did not affect attitudes towards the children.— S. Rosenblatt *et al.*, *Curr. ther. Res.*, 1976, *19*, 332.

Behaviour disorders. A double-blind study in 50 delinquent boys failed to show that phenytoin sodium, 100 mg twice daily, was significantly better than a placebo in its effects on *disruptive and disturbed behaviour*.— M. M. Lefkowitz, *Archs gen. Psychiat.*, 1969, *20*, 643, per *J. Am. med. Ass.*, 1969, *208*, 2518. In a double-blind study in 47 retarded boys, aged 9 to 14, treatment with phenytoin 100 mg twice daily led to marked improvement in several parameters evaluated, with a trend to improvement in others.— J. B. Goldberg and A. A. Kurland, *J. nerv. ment. Dis.*, 1970, *150*, 133, per *Clin. Med.*, 1970, *77* (Nov.), 37. Further references: J. G. Millichap and G. W. Fowler, *Pediat. Clins N.Am.*, 1967, *14*, 767; J. G. Millichap, *Ann. N.Y. Acad. Sci.*, 1973, *205*, 321.

A comment that the hydantoins and carbamazepine may help to prevent attacks of *explosive rage* in patients who do not have seizures but in whom there is EEG evidence of a seizure focus.— F. A. Elliott, *Practitioner*, 1976, *217*, 51.

Cardiac disorders. A review of the cardiac effects of phenytoin. Phenytoin is highly effective against both atrial and ventricular arrhythmias caused by digitalis toxicity, for which it should be considered one of the drugs of choice. For the most part it is ineffective against atrial arrhythmias and not markedly effective against ventricular arrhythmias associated with acute or chronic cardiac disease. In the latter, phenytoin is usually only considered after other anti-arrhythmic therapy has failed. Studies on the mechanisms responsible for the anti-arrhythmic effects of phenytoin are, as yet, inconclusive, but there is good evidence that its actions differ from those of the commonly used drugs with local anaesthetic effects. The extent to which it exerts therapeutically relevant direct effects on the heart remains to be demonstrated, and there is good evidence that its CNS effects may be of prime importance to its therapeutic efficacy.— A. L. Wit *et al.*, *Am. Heart J.*, 1975, *90*, 397.

Myocardial infarction. In a collaborative study 283 patients received phenytoin 300 to 400 mg daily for a year after myocardial infarction; the death-rate in these patients was no different from that in 285 similar patients (untreated) receiving 3 to 4 mg daily. Palpitations were more common in the untreated group. In 1 of the 6 hospitals participating, ventricular extrasystoles occurred in 7% of the treated group and in 19% of the untreated group, and there were 10 deaths in 64 patients with plasma concentrations below 10 µg per ml compared with none in 32 patients with concentrations of 10 µg or more per ml. It was possible that wide variations in plasma concentrations masked a beneficial effect.—Collaborative Group, *Lancet*, 1971, *2*, 1055. Criticism of the design of the study.— D. J. Bleifer *et al.* (letter), *ibid.*, 1972, *1*, 495.

Results of a prospective, randomised, open study in 150 patients who had had a myocardial infarction, did not demonstrate any reduction in the incidence of instantaneous or sudden deaths in patients given long-term phenytoin therapy, compared with control patients. Deaths in the treatment group were not associated with low plasma concentrations. Phenytoin therapy showed no beneficial effects on mortality and was associated with a high incidence of side-effects.— T. Peter *et al.*, *Br. Heart J.*, 1978, *40*, 1356.

The concentration of high-density lipoproteins (HDL) and of apolipoprotein A-I was increased in patients taking phenytoin 200 to 300 mg daily; the total serum-cholesterol concentration was not increased. A negative association between HDL concentrations and coronary heart disease had been reported and raised the possibility of the use of phenytoin prophylactically.— E. A. Nikkilä *et al.*, *Br. med. J.*, 1978, *2*, 99. See also *idem*, *Acta med. scand.*, 1978, *204*, 517.

Epilepsy. A review of the drug treatment of epilepsy. Once the need for therapy has been established, it should be started with a small dose of one drug. The choice of drug is still debatable but, for grand mal and partial seizures, possibly rests between *phenytoin* and *carbamazepine*. Although phenytoin is probably more toxic in the long-term, carbamazepine is much more expensive, whereas *phenobarbitone* and *primidone* are effective, but soporific, and may affect behaviour, especially in children. *Clonazepam* causes drowsiness and tolerance may develop, but it may be useful in myoclonic epilepsy or where anxiety is prominent. *Sodium valproate* may also be useful for myoclonic epilepsy. The evidence on which to make a rational choice for petit mal is even more sparse. Until recently most physicians have started with *ethosuximide*. Claims that *sodium valproate* is superior have yet to be substantiated. It is essential for the patient to understand the implications of starting therapy, particularly the need to take it regularly and no more than twice daily. Recurrence of seizures because of poor compliance and resultant withdrawal effects is an underestimated hazard. It may be safer to avoid medication altogether than to take it irregularly. If seizures continue despite achieving optimum serum concentrations of one drug it is still uncertain whether the addition of another drug will give further protection. An alternative and probably preferable measure is to substitute a different drug. There may be no significant difference in group response to different drugs but this does not exclude the possibility of a different individual response. In patients with more than one seizure type, such as grand mal and petit mal, two drugs may be necessary, each specific for one seizure type.— E. H. Reynolds, *Lancet*, 1978, *2*, 721.

Advice on the choice of drugs in epilepsy. *Phenytoin* is the drug of first choice in tonic-clonic (grand mal) seizures, but has the disadvantage of causing gingival hyperplasia, coarse facies, acne, and hirsutism, and it may therefore be kinder to use an alternative drug such as *carbamazepine* in adolescent girls. If phenytoin alone is ineffective, a change to carbamazepine should be made, and if this fails the two should be given together. Only if success has not then been achieved should *phenobarbitone* or *primidone* be tried. Although *sodium valproate* will control grand mal seizures, it is probably not as effective as the standard drugs. *Clonazepam* is very sedative and has no place in major epilepsy. Partial (focal) seizures may occur in the absence of grand mal, but in a large proportion of patients there is secondary generalisation of the paroxysmal activity to give rise to tonic-clonic seizures. The same range of drugs is used to treat partial (focal) seizures as is recommended for primary grand mal, but in the doses required to control partial (focal) seizures, particularly temporal lobe (or psychomotor) seizures, *carbamazepine* has the advantage that it is less likely to produce the toxic confusional state to which patients with focal brain damage are so susceptible. It has been claimed that carbamazepine improves mood and behaviour, this is probably due to its substitution for more toxic drugs. Although carbamazepine is much more expensive than phenytoin or phenobarbitone, the total annual cost is justifiable for effective control. *Sodium valproate* has a poor effect on partial (focal) seizures, and therefore has no place in therapy. *Clonazepam* is much too sedative in the doses necessary for effective control. Temporal lobe absences are frequently mistaken for petit mal, but the distinction is important because true petit mal responds well to *sodium valproate* or *ethosuximide*, while temporal lobe absences do not. It is too early to say whether sodium valproate is as effective as ethosuximide in petit mal, but it does have the advantage that it is also active against the grand mal seizures which co-exist in about one-third of patients. In childhood, a variety of syndromes occur in which myoclonic jerks are prominent. These have responded poorly to the traditional drugs, but *sodium valproate* and *clonazepam* are particularly helpful. Sodium valproate should be tried first as children tolerate it much better than clonazepam. Occasional brief myoclonic jerks trouble some patients with major epilepsy, particularly first thing in the morning, but generally they respond well to either drug. The association of clonazepam and sodium valproate has occasionally produced stupor and is therefore better avoided.— A. Richens, *Prescribers' J.*, 1978, *18*, 125. See also *idem*, *Recent Adv. clin. Pharmac.*, 1978, *1*, 147.

A view that carbamazepine is superior to phenytoin in controlling psychomotor (temporal lobe) seizures, whereas phenytoin is superior to carbamazepine in controlling major motor (grand mal) convulsions.— S. Livingston *et al.* (letter), *Neurology, Minneap.*, 1978, *28*, 101.

Further reviews and comments on epilepsy and its treatment: D. F. Scott, *Br. J. Hosp. Med.*, 1978, *20*, 178 (temporal lobe epilepsy); *Drug & Ther. Bull.*, 1979, *17*, 89; M. J. Eadie, *Drugs*, 1979, *17*, 213; A. Hopkins, *Br. J. Hosp. Med.*, 1979, *22*, 265 (uncontrolled epilepsy); *Med. Lett.*, 1979, *21*, 25; J. K. Penry and M. E. Newmark, *Ann. intern. Med.*, 1979, *90*, 207; *Br. med. J.*, 1980, *280*, 812.

Single drug or combination therapy for epilepsy.— E. H. Reynolds and S. D. Shorvon, *Drugs*, 1981, *21*, 374.

Reports on the merits of single-drug therapy for epilepsy: E. H. Reynolds *et al.*, *Lancet*, 1976, *1*, 923; S. D. Shorvon and E. H. Reynolds, *Br. med. J.*, 1977, *1*, 1635; S. D. Shorvon *et al.*, *ibid.*, 1978, *1*, 474; S. D. Shorvon and E. H. Reynolds, *ibid.*, 1979, *2*, 1023; D. J. Gannaway and G. E. Mawer (letter), *Lancet*, 1981, *1*, 217; M. P. Feely and M. N. Callaghan (letter), *ibid.*, 847.

A study on the risk of relapse after stopping anticonvulsant therapy in children with epilepsy.— R. Emerson *et al.*, *New Engl. J. Med.*, 1981, *304*, 1125.

Post-traumatic epilepsy. A review of the incidence of post-traumatic epilepsy caused by blunt head injuries, with special reference to the work of B.Jennett (*Epilepsy after Non-missile Head Injuries*, London, Heinemann, 1975 and *Develop. Med. Child Neurology*, 1973, *15*, 56). The decision on prophylaxis depends on risk factors and the circumstances of the patient such as his age and career, and whether he must drive. The duration of treatment should also depend on the risk factor and the patient's circumstances, but it seems prudent to continue for at least 2 years, after which the drug should always be tailed off slowly. We still do not know whether prophylactic medication decreases the risk of developing late epilepsy.— *Br. med. J.*, 1978, *2*, 229.

Data from a retrospective study in 62 patients considered to confirm that treatment with phenytoin decreases the incidence of post-traumatic epilepsy. Only 5 of 50 patients given phenytoin developed epilepsy of late onset, whereas 6 of 12 untreated patients did.— R. N. W. Wohns and A. R. Wyler, *J. Neurosurg.*, 1979, *51*, 507.

Preliminary results of a double-blind study into the role of phenytoin in reducing postoperative epilepsy following cranial surgery.— J. B. North *et al.*, *Lancet*, 1980, *1*, 384. Criticisms.— A. E. Richardson and D. Uttley (letter), *ibid.*, 650; P. P. R. Clarke (letter), *ibid.*

Sleep seizures. Care should be exercised in using anticonvulsants to suppress sleep seizures; by adversely altering sleep patterns they could make attacks worse.— F. B. Gibberd and M. C. Bateson, *Br. med. J.*, 1974, *2*, 403.

Beneficial effect of phenytoin or carbamazepine in 6 young adults with unusual sleep walking episodes characterised by screaming or unintelligible vocalisations, complex (often violent) automatisms, and ambulation.— T. A. Pedley and C. Guilleminault, *Ann. Neurol.*, 1977, *2*, 30.

Status epilepticus. For comments on the management of status epilepticus, see Diazepam, p.1525.

Febrile convulsions. For the role of anticonvulsants in the treatment and prevention of febrile convulsions in children, see Diazepam, p.1525.

Hiccup. Phenytoin 200 mg given intravenously over 5 minutes abolished persistent refractory hiccup within 1 hour. Treatment was continued with 100 mg four times daily intramuscularly then by mouth for 10 days without recurrence.— D. Petroski and A. N. Patel (letter), *Lancet*, 1974, *1*, 739.

Hypertension. In a double-blind crossover study 20 patients with mild hypertension were given phenytoin 100 mg thrice daily or a placebo. Thirty minutes after administration of phenytoin there was a fall in systolic blood pressure, but no sustained hypotensive effect was seen after administration for 2 weeks. It was concluded that the hypotensive effect of phenytoin is transient, and of no therapeutic use in hypertension.— J. M. Sullivan and H. S. Solomon, *J. clin. Pharmac.*, 1977, *17*, 607.

Metabolic and endocrine disorders. Treatment with phenytoin in 2 patients with *Cushing's syndrome* produced improvement over several months, but neither patient completely recovered normal adrenocortical function. It was suggested that microsomal enzyme induction by phenytoin hastened hydrocortisone turnover and inhibited the hypothalamic feedback system.— E. E. Werk *et al.* (letter), *New Engl. J. Med.*, 1967, *276*, 877.

Both phenytoin 100 mg every 6 hours for 9 days and diazoxide 100 mg every 8 hours for 7 days raised the blood-sugar concentrations in a patient with a benign insulinoma and symptoms of *hypoglycaemia*, and improved the ratio of insulin to blood sugar.— M. S. Cohen *et al.* (letter), *Lancet*, 1973, *1*, 40. See also F. D. Hofeldt *et al.*, *Diabetes*, 1974, *23*, 192; J. E. Stambaugh and D. C. Tucker, *Diabetes*, 1974, *23*, 679; J. Mirouze *et al.*, *Thérapie*, 1976, *31*, 605. Further references to phenytoin in *disorders of carbohydrate metabolism:* S. R. Levin *et al.*, *Diabetes*, 1973, *22*, 194 (detection of glucose intolerance), per *J. Am. med. Ass.*, 1973, *224*, 644; W. Jubiz and M. L. Rallison, *Archs intern. Med.*, 1974, *134*, 418 (glycogen storage disease).

The symptoms of the syndrome of *inappropriate antidiuretic hormone secretion* in a 68-year-old woman were successfully treated with demeclocycline 300 mg four times daily, but gastro-intestinal side-effects resulted in discontinuation of therapy. Control of symptoms was then maintained by phenytoin 100 mg twice daily.— A. Tanay *et al.*, *Ann. intern. Med.*, 1979, *90*, 50.

Muscular disorders. Phenytoin sodium in doses of 100 mg thrice daily would relieve or abolish the symptoms of myotonia in muscular dystrophy.— J. N. Walton, *Br. med. J.*, 1969, *3*, 639. See also T. L. Munsat, *Neurology, Minneap.*, 1967, *17*, 359.

Phenytoin in doses of 1 g for the first day followed by 300 to 400 mg daily for two 6-week periods increased muscle strength in a 47-year-old man with prednisolone-induced muscle weakness.— L. Z. Stern *et al.* (letter), *J. Am. med. Ass.* 1973, *223*, 1287.

Neuralgias and neuropathies. Four of 5 patients with *trigeminal neuralgia* obtained complete relief of previously intractable pain after treatment with phenytoin sodium, 100 mg, three or four times daily by mouth or by intramuscular injection. Continued treatment kept 2 patients free of pain for 10 months and 1 year respectively.— A. Chinitz *et al.*, *Am. J. med. Sci.*, 1966, *252*, 62. In the treatment of trigeminal neuralgia the initial dose of phenytoin was usually 100 mg twice or thrice daily increased up to 800 mg daily if required. Relief might be partial or complete. After a week free of pain the dose was decreased and an attempt made to withdraw treatment which was re-instituted at the first hint of relapse. Concomitant treatment with carbamazepine was also useful.— *Br. med. J.*, 1972, *2*, 583.

Two patients with *dysaesthesia* believed to be due to thalamic infarction responded to treatment with phenytoin.— F. K. Cantor, *Br. med. J.*, 1972, *4*, 590.

Treatment with phenytoin led to no improvement in visual acuity or visual fields in 15 patients with visual impairment after acute, presumably ischaemic, *optic neuropathy*.— C. Ellenberger *et al.*, *Archs Ophthal., N.Y.*, 1974, *91*, 435, per *J. Am. med. Ass.*, 1974, *228*, 1599.

Phenytoin 1 g in divided doses for the first day then 300 mg daily relieved facial pain in a man with the *Wallenberg* or *posterior inferior cerebellar artery syndrome*.— E. K. Mladinich (letter), *J. Am. med. Ass.*, 1974, *230*, 372.

Results of a double-blind crossover study in which phenytoin and placebo were administered for 23 weeks each to 12 insulin-dependent diabetic patients, indicated that phenytoin has no role in the treatment of *diabetic symmetric polyneuropathy*. Phenytoin was noted to raise the blood sugar.— C. D. Saudek *et al.*, *Clin. Pharmac. Ther.*, 1977, *22*, 196.

Schizophrenia. In a controlled study 76 Negro patients with chronic *schizophrenia* were treated with phenytoin or placebo after the withdrawal of phenothiazines. Patients deteriorated on phenytoin or placebo though phenytoin had some effect on some parameters.— A. M. Simopoulos *et al.*, *Archs gen. Psychiat.*, 1974, *30*, 106. See also under Adverse Effects (Effects on Mental State), above.

Skin disorders. *Epidermolysis bullosa.* A favourable but variable clinical response to phenytoin was achieved in patients with recessive dystrophic epidermolysis bullosa. Treatment with phenytoin was begun with a dose of about 3 mg per kg body-weight daily, taken by mouth in 2 divided doses, and the dose adjusted every 10 to 14 days until a blood concentration of at least 8 µg per ml was attained. A reduction in blisters and erosions of more than 45% was achieved in 12 of 17 patients. Studies *in vitro* suggested that the favourable response to phenytoin might result from an inhibition of collagenase expression.— E. A. Bauer *et al.*, *New Engl. J. Med.*, 1980, *303*, 776.

Scleroderma. Encouraging results with phenytoin in 5 patients with localised linear scleroderma.— K. H. Neldner, *Cutis*, 1978, *22*, 569.

Spasticity. Following initial promising results in an open trial, a placebo-controlled double-blind crossover study was carried out to assess phenytoin in association with chlorpromazine to alleviate spasticity in conditions such as multiple sclerosis. Both phenytoin alone and chlorpromazine alone were effective, but the greatest benefit was obtained with the association of both. Phenytoin was given in doses of 200 mg daily increased to 300 to 500 mg daily after a week and chlorpromazine hydrochloride was given in doses of 25 mg daily initially increased in steps of 25 mg each week to 150 mg daily where tolerated.— S. L. Cohan *et al.*, *Archs Neurol.*, 1980, *37*, 360.

Tetany. Phenytoin 250 mg intravenously or 100 mg by mouth thrice daily and at bedtime eliminated tetany, tetanic equivalents, and a strongly positive Trousseau test in 6 patients with hypocalcaemia due to hypoparathyroidism or pseudohypoparathyroidism, and in 1 with hypocalcaemia and hypomagnesaemia due to malabsorption.— M. Schaaf and C. A. Payne, *New Engl. J. Med.*, 1966, *274*, 1228.

Tinnitus. For the use of phenytoin to alleviate tinnitus, see Carbamazepine, p.1248.

Preparations of Phenytoin and Phenytoin Sodium

Extended Phenytoin Sodium Capsules *(U.S.P.)*. Capsules containing phenytoin sodium. The *U.S.P.* requires not more than 40% dissolution at 30 minutes, 50% at 60 minutes, and not less than 70% at 120 minutes. Store in airtight containers.

Phenytoin Capsules *(B.P.)*. Phenytoin Sodium Capsules. Capsules containing phenytoin sodium. Store at a temperature not exceeding 30°.

Phenytoin Injection *(B.P.)*. Phenytoin Sodium Injection; Soluble Phenytoin Injection. A sterile solution of phenytoin sodium 4.75 to 5.25% containing propylene glycol 40% v/v and alcohol 10% v/v in Water for Injections. It is sterilised by filtration. pH 11.5 to 12.1. Store at a temperature not exceeding 25°. Protect from light. Solutions which have developed a haze or precipitate should not be used.

Phenytoin Mixture *(B.P.C. 1973)*. Phenytoin Suspension. A suspension of phenytoin in a suitable coloured flavoured vehicle. When a dose less than 5 ml is prescribed, the mixture should be diluted to 5 ml with syrup. Such dilutions must be freshly prepared and not used more than 2 weeks after issue.

Phenytoin Oral Suspension *(U.S.P.)*. A suspension of phenytoin in a suitable vehicle. Store in airtight containers. Avoid freezing.

Phenytoin Tablets *(B.P.)*. Phenytoin Sodium Tablets. Tablets containing phenytoin sodium. They are sugar-coated.

Phenytoin Tablets *(U.S.P.)*. Tablets containing phenytoin. They may be chewed.

Prompt Phenytoin Sodium Capsules *(U.S.P.)*. Capsules containing phenytoin sodium. The *U.S.P.* requires 85% dissolution in 30 minutes. Store in airtight containers. Not for once-daily dosing.

Sterile Phenytoin Sodium *(U.S.P.)*. Sterile phenytoin sodium suitable for parenteral use. A 5% solution in the solvent provided has a pH of 10 to 12.3.

Proprietary Preparations of Phenytoin and Phenytoin Sodium

Epanutin *(Parke, Davis, UK)*. **Capsules** each containing 25, 50, or 100 mg of phenytoin sodium; and **Suspension** containing 30 mg of phenytoin in each 5 ml (suggested diluent, syrup). (Also available as Epanutin in *Belg., Ger., Neth., Norw., S.Afr., Spain, Swed., Switz.*).

Epanutin with Phenobarbitone Capsules *(Parke, Davis, UK)*. Each contains phenytoin sodium 100 mg and phenobarbitone 50 mg.

Epanutin Infatabs *(Parke, Davis, UK)*. Phenytoin, available as scored chewable tablets of 50 mg.

Epanutin Ready Mixed Parenteral *(Parke, Davis, UK)*. A solution containing phenytoin sodium 50 mg per ml in a vehicle containing propylene glycol 40%, alcohol 10%, and Water for Injections, adjusted to pH 12, in ampoules of 5 ml. Protect from light. For intramuscular or intravenous injection; do not dilute with infusion solutions.

Garoin *(May & Baker, UK)*. Scored tablets each containing phenytoin sodium 100 mg and phenobarbitone sodium 50 mg.

Other Proprietary Names

Arg.—Epamin, Pyoredol; *Austral.*—Dilantin, Phentoin; *Belg.*—Diphantoine; *Canad.*—Dantoin, Dilantin; *Denm.*—Difhydan, Fenytoin; *Fr.*—Di-Hydan, Pyorédol, Solantyl; *Ger.*—Phenhydan, Zentropil; *Ital.*—Dintoina; *Jap.*—Hydantol; *Neth.*—Diphantoine; *Norw.*—Epinat, Fenytoin; *S.Afr.*—Toin Unicelles; *Spain*—Labopal, Neosidantoina; *Swed.*—Difhydan, Fenantoin, Lehydan; *Switz.*—Antisacer, Epilantin, Phenhydan, Tacosal; *USA*—Dilantin, Diphenylan, Ditan.

6603-x

Albutoin. Bax 422Z. 3-Allyl-5-isobutyl-2-thiohydantoin.

$C_{10}H_{16}N_2OS=212.3$.

CAS — 830-89-7.

Albutoin is a hydantoin anticonvulsant with general properties similar to those of phenytoin (p.1235). It has been studied in doses of 0.1 to 2.4 g daily.

Albutoin was given in daily doses of 0.1 to 2.4 g (average 725 mg) to 142 non-ambulatory patients with grand mal epilepsy inadequately controlled by other medication; 108 patients achieved a 50% or greater reduction in seizure frequency and 31 became free of seizures; a few patients achieved these results without other anticonvulsants concomitantly.— C. H. Carter, *Clin. Med.*, 1971, *78* (Jan.), 33.

Evaluation of albutoin in a population of institutionalised patients. In a dosage of 600 mg daily albutoin was no more effective than placebo in preventing excess seizures. A dose of 1.2 g daily was about as effective as phenobarbitone 150 mg daily. Anorexia, nausea, and vomiting occurred in nearly 15% of the patients receiving albutoin 1.2 g daily.— J. J. Cereghino *et al.*, *Clin. Pharmac. Ther.*, 1974, *15*, 406.

Further references: J. G. Millichap and W. R. Ortiz, *Neurology, Minneap.*, 1967, *17*, 162; J. R. Green *et al.*, *ibid.*, 1969, *19*, 1207.

6604-r

Beclamide. Benzchlorpropamide. *N*-Benzyl-3-chloropropionamide.

$C_{10}H_{12}ClNO=197.7$.

CAS — 501-68-8.

Colourless crystals with a slightly acid taste. Sparingly **soluble** in water.

Adverse Effects. Side-effects include dizziness, nervousness, gastro-intestinal distress, and occasionally a skin rash or transitory leucopenia.

Uses. Beclamide is reported to be an anticonvulsant for the management of behaviour disorders in non-epileptic subjects and in grand mal and psychomotor epilepsy.

Beclamide is given in a dosage of 1.5 to 4 g daily in divided doses. Suggested doses for children are: less than 5 years of age, 0.75 to 1 g daily; 5 to 10 years of age, 1.5 g daily.

Studies of plasma concentrations and the excretion of beclamide in healthy subjects.— H. Leach *et al.*, *Br. J. clin. Pharmac.*, 1975, *2*, 377P.

Behaviour disorders. References to the use of beclamide in behaviour disorders: S. A. Price and D. A. Spencer, *J. ment. Subnorm.*, 1967, *13*, 75; B. Melin, *ibid.*, 1970, *16*, 119; D. A. Sime and F. P. D. Easby, *Br. J. ment. Subnorm.*, 1974, *20*, 90.

Epilepsy. References to the use of beclamide in epilepsy: J. Hoenig *et al.*, *J. Am. med. Ass.*, 1956, *161*, 1195; D. S. Sharpe *et al.*, *Br. med. J.*, 1958, *1*, 1044; N. Kaye *et al.*, *ibid.*, 1959, *1*, 627; J. Wilson *et al.*, *ibid.*, 1275; J. Puech *et al.*, *Presse méd.*, 1962, *70*, 1015.

Proprietary Preparations

Nydrane *(Rona, UK)*. Beclamide, available as scored tablets of 500 mg. (Also available as Nydrane in *Austral.*).

Other Proprietary Names

Neuracen *(Ger.)*; Nidrane *(Arg.)*; Posedrine *(Belg., Fr., Ital., Spain, Switz.)*; Seclar *(Arg.)*.

6605-f

Carbamazepine *(B.P., U.S.P.)*.

Carbamazepinum; G 32883. 5*H*-Dibenz[*b,f*]azepine-5-carboxamide.

$C_{15}H_{12}N_2O=236.3$.

CAS — 298-46-4.

Pharmacopoeias. In *Br.*, *Braz.*, *Jap.*, and *U.S.*

A white or yellowish-white, almost odourless, crystalline powder; tasteless or with a slightly bitter taste. M.p. 189° to 193°.

Practically **insoluble** in water and ether; soluble 1 in 10 of alcohol and 1 in 10 of chloroform; soluble in acetone. **Store** in airtight containers.

Adverse Effects. Fairly common side-effects of carbamazepine, particularly in the initial stages of therapy, include dizziness, drowsiness, and ataxia. These effects may be minimised by starting therapy with a low dose. Drowsiness and disturbances of cerebellar and oculo-motor function (with ataxia, nystagmus, and diplopia) are also symptoms of excessive plasma concentrations of carbamazepine, and may disappear with continued treatment at reduced dosage.

Gastro-intestinal symptoms are reported to be less common, and include dry mouth, gastric distress and abdominal pain, nausea and vomiting, anorexia, and diarrhoea or constipation.

Generalised erythematous rashes, which may be severe, occur in about 3% of patients given carbamazepine, and may necessitate withdrawal of treatment. Photosensitivity reactions, urticaria, exfoliative dermatitis, erythema multiforme and the Stevens-Johnson syndrome, and lupus erythematosus have also been reported.

Occasional reports of blood disorders include agranulocytosis, aplastic anaemia, eosinophilia, leucopenia, leucocytosis, thrombocytopenia, and purpura. Abnormalities of liver and kidney function, and jaundice have occurred.

Other adverse effects reported include paraesthesia, headache, heart block, congestive heart failure, water intoxication, and dyskinesias with asterixis.

Overdosage leads to drowsiness, confusion, delirium, stupor, coma, and death. Other symptoms are dizziness, ataxia, nystagmus, nausea and vomiting, agitation, tremor, dyskinesias, abnormal reflexes, hypertension or hypotension.

For a discussion of the possible adverse effects of anticonvulsants, including carbamazepine, on the foetus, see p.1235; see also under Pregnancy and the Neonate, below.

Carbamazepine was associated with decreased taste sensitivity in 1 patient.— H. Rollin, *Ann. Otol. Rhinol. Lar.*, 1978, *87*, 37.

A report of twice-daily fevers associated with carbamazepine in a 62-year-old woman.— C. R. Stewart *et al.* (letter), *New Engl. J. Med.*, 1980, *302*, 1262.

Allergy. Eosinophilia and asthma associated with treatment with carbamazepine.— T. Lee *et al.*, *Br. med. J.*, 1981, *282*, 440. See also S. A. Cullinan and G. C. Bower, *Chest*, 1975, *68*, 580.

Effects on the blood. A study confirming the high incidence of low folate concentrations in the serum of patients receiving phenytoin, and providing evidence that patients receiving carbamazepine also develop low serum-folate concentrations.— P. Reizenstein *et al.*, *Scand. J. Haematol.*, 1973, *11*, 158.

Agranulocytosis. A report of agranulocytosis associated with carbamazepine in a 61-year-old man. He had a positive reaction with anti-lymphoid leukaemia antiserum during recovery.— C. W. I. Owens *et al.*, *Postgrad. med. J.*, 1980, *56*, 665.

Aplastic anaemia. Details of aplastic anaemia in 2 patients given carbamazepine for trigeminal neuralgia. It is felt that the close temporal relationship between the administration of carbamazepine and the development of aplastic anaemia casts strong suspicion on carbamazepine.— G. W. K. Donaldson *et al.*, *Br. J. clin. Pract.*, 1965, *19*, 699. See also J. D. Spillane, *Practitioner*, 1964, *192*, 71. Further references: W. R. Fellows, *Headache*, 1969, *9*, 92. Criticism of reports of carbamazepine-associated aplastic anaemia, and the view that a causative role of carbamazepine in the development of aplastic anaemia is not conclusively proved.— S. Livingston *et al.*, *Neurology, Minneap.*, 1978, *28*, 101.

Leucopenia. Leucopenia in an immunosuppressed renal transplant patient appeared to be associated with carbamazepine therapy.— J. G. Gerber *et al.*, *Sth. med. J.*, 1979, *72*, 81.

Thrombocytopenia. A 79-year-old woman who had taken carbamazepine 200 mg six-hourly for the pain of trigeminal neuralgia developed thrombocytopenia. When treatment was stopped the patient's platelet count returned to normal.— J. Pearce and M. A. Ron (letter), *Lancet*, 1968, *2*, 223.

Effects on the endocrine system. Five patients who had been taking carbamazepine in doses above 700 mg daily and who had blood-carbamazepine concentrations above 8.3 µg per ml had hyponatraemia (mean 132 mmol per litre). There was a potential risk of water intoxication.— D. A. Henry *et al.*, *Br. med. J.*, 1977, *1*, 83. Two patients developed water intoxication while taking carbamazepine. In one patient it recurred on challenge. Special care was necessary when carbamazepine was given to elderly patients or those with cardiovascular disease. If symptoms consistent with water intoxication occurred the plasma-sodium concentration and osmolality should be checked.— W. P. Stephens *et al.*, *ibid.*, 754. Water intoxication occurred in a 45-year-old woman taking carbamazepine; the condition regressed when the dose was reduced.— M. G. Ashton *et al.*, *ibid.*, 1977, *1*, 1134. No evidence of hyponatraemia or change of serum osmolality was found in 28 children under treatment with carbamazepine.— I. Helin, *ibid.*, 1977, *2*, 558. Hyponatraemia in a 65-year-old woman taking carbamazepine was associated with an inappropriately high plasma concentration of argipressin.— N. J. Smith *et al.*, *ibid.*, 804. The ability to excrete a water load was reduced in 10 of 12 healthy subjects given carbamazepine 600 mg daily for 7 days. Plasma-argipressin concentrations were reduced indicating that the mechanism was not increased by secretion of antidiuretic hormone.— W. P. Stephens *et al.*, *ibid.*, 1978, *1*, 1445.

Results of a study in epileptic subjects suggest that phenytoin counteracts the antidiuretic action of carbamazepine by lowering its serum concentration rather than by inhibiting the release of antidiuretic hormone, as originally suggested by P. Sordillo *et al.* (*Archs intern. Med.*, 1978, *138*, 299). The best rational approach to prevent excessive water retention may be to monitor serum-carbamazepine concentrations.— E. Perucca and A. Richens, *Br. J. clin. Pharmac.*, 1980, *9*, 302P.

Further references to inappropriate secretion of antidiuretic hormone associated with carbamazepine therapy: K. M. Flegel and C. H. Cole, *Ann. intern. Med.*, 1977, *87*, 722; E. Perucca *et al.*, *J. Neurol. Neurosurg. Psychiat.*, 1978, *41*, 713; A. N. Singh (letter), *Can. med. Ass. J.*, 1978, *118*, 24.

Effects on the eyes. On rare occasions lenticular opacities have been associated with carbamazepine.— *Med. Lett.*, 1976, *18*, 63.

Effects on the heart. Bradycardia occurred in an 85-year-old woman following administration of carbamazepine 1 g daily. She had no history of heart failure but her conduction tissue could have been affected by malignant metastasis or post-radiation fibrosis. Caution should be observed in patients with a defective conducting system.— L. Herzberg (letter), *Lancet*, 1978, *1*, 1097. A further case.— D. V. Hamilton (letter), *ibid.*, 1365.

In 4 patients with AV conduction disturbances, with pacemakers, carbamazepine delayed the resumption of idioventricular activity after a break in pacemaker stimulation. Carbamazepine should not be given to patients with grade II or III AV block.— B. Beermann and O. Edhag, *Br. med. J.*, 1978, *2*, 171.

Report and comment on 2 elderly patients who developed heart block on receiving carbamazepine.— *Med. J. Aust.*, 1979, *1*, 574.

A 33-year-old man who had been taking phenytoin, phenobarbitone, and thioridazine for 4 years, developed congestive heart failure on addition of carbamazepine. He recovered on discontinuing carbamazepine and administration of frusemide 100 mg over 48 hours. At no time were his electrolytes abnormal. The pathogenesis of congestive heart failure was considered to be most likely due to the chemical similarity of carbamazepine to the tricyclic antidepressants, which are known to cause cardiovascular complications, but the possible additive effect of thioridazine and carbamazepine may also have played a part.— C. F. Terrence and G. Fromm, *Ann. Neurol.*, 1980, *8*, 200.

Effects on the kidneys. A 59-year-old man with trigeminal neuralgia unresponsive to carbamazepine 200 mg four times daily was relieved by taking twice this dose. Three weeks later he had oliguria and when seen 5 weeks after starting the higher dose had a blood-urea concentration of 2.85 g per litre. The renal failure was considered due to acute tubular necrosis. Three other cases of oliguria, dysuria, or haematuria had been reported.— D. P. Nicholls and M. Yasin (letter), *Br. med. J.*, 1972, *4*, 490.

Effects on the liver. Hepatic encephalopathy leading to coma and death occurred in a 14-year-old girl with epilepsy after she had taken carbamazepine 400 mg daily in addition to phenobarbitone, for about 6 months.— P. Zucker *et al.*, *J. Pediat.*, 1977, *91*, 667. See also I. D. Ramsay, *Br. med. J.*, 1967, *4*, 155; W. R. Fellows, *Headache*, 1969, *9*, 92.

A study indicating that carbamazepine is relatively free of serious adverse effects, including hepatotoxicity.— R. L. Huf and R. J. Schain, *J. Pediat.*, 1978, *93*, 884.

Granulomatous hepatitis secondary to carbamazepine.— M. Levy *et al.*, *Ann. intern. Med.*, 1981, *95*, 64.

Effects on the lungs. Acute hypersensitivity pneumonitis was reported in a 16-year-old boy receiving carbamazepine and may have developed because of a concomitant infection.— W. C. Stephan *et al.*, *Chest*, 1978, *74*, 463.

See also under Allergy, above.

Effects on the muscles. Dystonia in brain-damaged children, associated with carbamazepine.— C. J. Crosley and P. T. Swander, *Pediatrics*, 1979, *63*, 612.

A report of transient dystonia associated with treatment with carbamazepine in 4 patients.— D. Jacome (letter), *J. Am. med. Ass.*, 1979, *241*, 2263.

Effects on the nervous system. A study of 3 patients with acute carbamazepine intoxication whose symptoms included equilibrium disorders, gait and speech disturbances, drowsiness, gaze nystagmus, depressed optokinetic nystagmus, and disturbances of smooth pursuit eye movement. The symptoms disappeared on stopping carbamazepine. It was felt that carbamazepine affects structures within the brain stem as well as the cerebellum.— Y. Umeda and E. Sakata, *Ann. Otol. Rhinol. Lar.*, 1977, *86*, 318.

Dyskinesias. For an account of dyskinesias associated with anticonvulsants and mention of asterixis associated with carbamazepine, see Phenytoin, p.1237.

Effects on sexual function. Anticonvulsants diminish sexual potency and fertility in young male epileptics.— *Br. med. J.*, 1979, *2*, 1118.

Effects on the skin. Carbamazepine has been implicated in the Stevens-Johnson syndrome.— D. B. Coursin, *J. Am. med. Ass.*, 1966, *198*, 113.

A report of a 72-year-old man with a pigmented purpuric rash due to carbamazepine. The eruption was seen on the trunk and limbs and was maximal on the legs; there was also oedema of the lower legs and forearms. Within a day of stopping the drug, the rash and oedema began to improve and after 3 weeks a little fine scaling and pigmentation on the lower legs were all that remained.— R. R. M. Harman (letter), *Br. J. Derm.*, 1967, *79*, 500.

A woman with a history of seborrhoeic dermatitis and a possible skin reaction to phenytoin, developed widespread dermatitis, in some places exfoliative in character, on receiving carbamazepine.— G. R. Ford and L. Bieder, *N.Z. med. J.*, 1968, *68*, 386.

Carbamazepine may cause photosensitivity.— *Med. Lett.*, 1980, *22*, 64.

Lupus erythematosus. A skin eruption in a 63-year-old woman was undoubtedly caused by the administration of carbamazepine as it disappeared spontaneously on stopping the drug and promptly recurred when treatment was resumed. The clinical picture suggested lupus erythematosus or dermatomyositis.— J. R. Simpson, *Br. med. J.*, 1966, *2*, 1434.

Overdosage. Overdosage with carbamazepine (5.8 g) in a 16-year-old boy resulted in profound stupor and encephalopathy which was similar to a postictal state.— M. Salcman and C. E. Pippenger (letter), *J. Am. med. Ass.*, 1975, *231*, 915.

Massive carbamazepine overdosage in a 15-year-old girl was typical of anticholinergic toxicity; she became wild, requiring restraints, and apparently experiencing hallucinations. She was treated with bile suction, forced catharsis, and general supportive therapy and recovered within 48 hours.— C. A. Smoot and D. I. Wood, *J. Am. osteop. Ass.*, 1977, *76*, 758.

An unusual case of carbamazepine poisoning with a near fatal relapse after 2 days.— R. A. de Zeeuw *et al.*, *Clin. Toxicol.*, 1979, *14*, 263.

Pregnancy and the neonate. Follow-up of 133 pregnant epileptic women indicated that administration of carbamazepine alone and with phenobarbitone was associated with foetal head growth retardation; no catch-up growth occurred by the age of 18 months. Phenytoin alone was not associated with small head circumference, but phenytoin with phenobarbitone was. It suggested the low-dose monotherapy with phenytoin is a good choice for the control of epilepsy in pregnancy.— V. K. Hiilesmaa *et al.*, *Lancet*, 1981, *2*, 165.

Individual reports of abnormalities in the infants of women given carbamazepine either alone, or in association with other anticonvulsants, during pregnancy: W.F. Taylor *et al.* (letter), *Lancet*, 1980, *2*, 481 (with phenytoin; foetal hydantoin syndrome and extrarenal Wilms' tumour).

For a general comment on epilepsy and pregnancy and references to surveys on the incidence of congenital malformations in the infants of epileptic women, see p.1235.

Water intoxication. For reports of water intoxication associated with carbamazepine see under Effects on the Endocrine System, above.

Treatment of Adverse Effects. The stomach should be emptied by aspiration and lavage. The use of activated charcoal as an adjunct to gastric lavage has been suggested. Supportive therapy alone may then suffice for patients who are not severely poisoned (for general guidelines to the symptomatic therapy of drug overdosage, see Phenobarbitone, p.812).

ECG monitoring is recommended to detect arrhythmias or conduction defects.

Activated charcoal. For the use of activated charcoal to reduce the absorption of carbamazepine, see Activated Charcoal, p.79.

Precautions. It has been recommended that carbamazepine should be avoided in patients with atrioventricular conduction abnormalities unless paced. Carbamazepine should be given with caution to patients with a history of cardiac, hepatic, or renal disease. It should also be given with caution to patients with a history of blood disorders, and frequent blood counts are recommended.

Owing to the similarity of its structure to that of other tricyclic compounds (see Amitriptyline Hydrochloride, p.112) carbamazepine should be given with caution to patients with latent psychosis, and the risk of agitation and confusion in the elderly should be considered. Since carbamazepine has mild anticholinergic properties caution should be observed in patients with raised intra-ocular pressure, and, owing to the similarity of its structure to that of phenothiazines (see Chlorpromazine Hydrochloride, p.1512) patients should be examined periodically for eye changes.

For the use of carbamazepine in pregnancy, see p.1235. It has been recommended that mothers taking carbamazepine should not breast feed their infants.

Carbamazepine is extensively bound to plasma proteins and is therefore susceptible to interactions with drugs liable to compete for similar binding sites; for a comment on the relevance of this type of interaction, see Phenytoin, Precautions, p.1238.

The metabolism of carbamazepine is reported to be less susceptible to inhibition by other drugs than that of phenytoin, nevertheless, dextropropoxyphene, erythromycin, and triacetyloleandomycin have been found to inhibit its metabolism, resulting in raised plasma concentrations.

Carbamazepine is a hepatic enzyme inducer and induces its own metabolism as well as that of a number of other drugs, including some antibiotics (notably, doxycycline), anticoagulants, and sex hormones (notably, oral contraceptives). It may also enhance the metabolism of folic acid; carbamazepine and phenytoin may also mutually influence one another's metabolism. The metabolism of carbamazepine is similarly enhanced by enzyme inducers such as phenobarbitone.

Because of the structural similarity to tricyclic antidepressants, it has been suggested that carbamazepine should not be given to patients taking a monoamine oxidase inhibitor or within 14 days of stopping such treatment.

Carbamazepine may interfere with some urinary steroid tests.

For a comment on carbamazepine and driving, see Phenytoin, p.1239.

Interactions. Carbamazepine is an enzyme inducer in man.— J. M. Hansen *et al.*, *Clin. Pharmac. Ther.*, 1971, *12*, 539.

Antibiotics. Eight epileptic patients controlled with carbamazepine suffered signs of carbamazepine intoxication when given *triacetyloleandomycin*.— C. Dravet *et al.* (letter), *Lancet*, 1977, *1*, 810. Further details of the interaction between triacetyloleandomycin and carbamazepine, and a report of a similar response in 2 patients given *erythromycin* in addition to carbamazepine. Triacetyloleandomycin or other macrolide antibiotics should not be given to patients receiving carbamazepine.— E. Mesdjian *et al.*, *Epilepsia*, 1980, *21*, 489.

For the effect of carbamazepine on *doxycycline*, see Doxycycline Hydrochloride, p.1155.

Anticoagulants. For the effect of carbamazepine on *warfarin*, see Warfarin Sodium, p.777.

Anticonvulsants. A study of 123 patients receiving carbamazepine alone (30), with *phenytoin* (48), with *phenobarbitone* (18), and with phenytoin and phenobarbitone (27). The plasma-carbamazepine concentrations were higher in those given carbamazepine alone compared with those given phenytoin and/or phenobarbitone.— J. Christiansen and M. Dam, *Acta neurol. scand.*, 1973, *49*, 543.

Evidence that concomitant administration of phenytoin with carbamazepine may increase the brain concentrations of the active metabolite of carbamazepine.— M. L. Friis *et al.*, *Eur. J. clin. Pharmac.*, 1978, *14*, 47. See also M. L. Friis and J. Christiansen, *Acta neurol. scand.*, 1978, *58*, 104.

For the effect of carbamazepine on *phenytoin*, see Phenytoin, p.1239, for the effect on *primidone*, see Primidone, p.1254, and for the effect on *valproic acid*, see Sodium Valproate, p.1257.

Antihistamines. Plasma concentrations of carbamazepine were increased when a patient was also given *cimetidine*.— N. Telerman-Toppet *et al.* (letter), *Ann. intern. Med.*, 1981, *94*, 544.

Aspirin and other anti-inflammatory analgesics. For the effect of *aspirin*, *phenylbutazone*, *paracetamol*, and *tolfenamic acid* on carbamazepine, see Phenytoin, p.1240.

Benzodiazepines. For the effect of carbamazepine on *clonazepam*, see Clonazepam, p.1249.

Cardiac glycosides. For the effect of carbamazepine on *digitalis*, see Digoxin, p.534.

Lithium. For the effect of carbamazepine on lithium, see Lithium Carbonate, p.1539.

Narcotic analgesics. Dextropropoxyphene hydrochloride 65 mg thrice daily given to 5 patients being treated with carbamazepine alone or with other anticonvulsants increased plasma-carbamazepine concentrations and decreased plasma clearance in all patients. The oxidation of carbamazepine was probably inhibited.— M. Dam and J. Christiansen (letter), *Lancet*, 1977, *2*, 509. See also M. Dam *et al.*, *Acta neurol. scand.*, 1977, *56*, 603; B. S. Hansen *et al.*, *ibid.*, 1980, *61*, 357.

Pituitary hormones. For the effect of carbamazepine on *desmopressin*, see Desmopressin, p.1266.

Porphyria. A study in *rats* indicated that carbamazepine should be regarded as potentially hazardous for patients with a hereditary hepatic porphyria.— G. H. Blekkenhorst *et al.* (letter), *Lancet*, 1980, *1*, 1367. Criticisms of extrapolating data obtained from *animal* experiments to the treatment of human disease.— M. J. Brodie (letter), *ibid.*, *2*, 86; A. Gorchein (letter), *ibid.*, 152.

Absorption and Fate. Carbamazepine is slowly but fairly completely absorbed from the gastro-intestinal tract; the rate of absorption is variable and its bioavailability can differ markedly with different pharmaceutical formulations.

Carbamazepine is extensively metabolised in the liver and one of its primary metabolites, carbamazepine-10,11-epoxide has been reported to have about one-third of the anticonvulsant activity of carbamazepine. Carbamazepine is excreted in the urine almost entirely in the form of its metabolites.

Carbamazepine is widely distributed throughout the body and is extensively bound to plasma proteins. It has the property of inducing its own metabolism so that the plasma half-life after administration of single doses to previously untreated subjects, which has been variously estimated to range from about 18 to over 60 hours, may be considerably reduced on repeated administration. Estimations of the plasma half-life of carbamazepine on repeated administration range from about 10 to over 35 hours; it appears to be considerably shorter in children than in adults. Moreover, the metabolism of carbamazepine is readily induced by drugs, such as phenobarbitone, which induce hepatic microsomal enzymes.

The therapeutic and adverse effects of carbamazepine have been correlated with plasma concentrations: in general, the anticonvulsant effect of carbamazepine is obtained at plasma concentrations of 4 to 12.5 μg per ml (16 to 50 μmol per litre), while concentrations above this are associated with progressively severe signs of toxicity.Carbamazepine crosses the blood-brain barrier and the placental barrier, and is excreted in milk.

General reviews and comments on the pharmacokinetics of carbamazepine: L. Bertilsson, *Clin. Pharmacokinet.*, 1978, *3*, 128.

Absorption. Carbamazepine absorption was increased in the presence of food.— R. H. Levy *et al.*, *Clin. Pharmac. Ther.*, 1975, *17*, 657.

Metabolism and pharmacokinetics. Carbamazepine-10,11-epoxide was identified as a metabolite of carbamazepine in the urine of 3 volunteers who had received 400 mg of carbamazepine.— A. Frigerio *et al.*, *J. pharm. Sci.*, 1972, *61*, 1144.

Carbamazepine-10,11-epoxide and 10,11-dihydro-10,11-dihydroxy-5*H*-dibenz[*b,f*]azepine-5-carboxamide and its glucuronide were urinary metabolites of carbamazepine in man. Iminostilbene and its glucuronide were also found in *rat* urine.— J. Csetenyi *et al.* (letter), *J. Pharm. Pharmac.*, 1973, *25*, 340.

No relationship was found in 14 epileptic patients between changes in serum concentrations of carbamazepine and its active metabolite carbamazepine-10,11-epoxide and changes in dosage. Carbamazepine and its metabolite had CSF concentrations from 19 to 34% and 34 to 71% of serum concentrations respectively and an inverse relationship was observed.— S. I. Johannessen *et al.*, *Br. J. clin. Pharmac.*, 1976, *3*, 575.

Following oral administration of carbamazepine 200 mg to 2 healthy fasting subjects peak plasma concentrations occurred in 6 to 8 hours and remained constant for about 24 hours before declining over the subsequent 6 days. The plasma half-life was about 36 hours.— L. Palmér *et al.*, *Clin. Pharmac. Ther.*, 1973, *14*, 827. See also M. D. Rawlins *et al.*, *Eur. J. clin. Pharmac.*, 1975, *8*, 91 (half-lives of 24 to 46 hours following single doses in 8 healthy subjects).

Following administration of single doses of carbamazepine to 4 patients the plasma half-lives ranged from 18.5 to 54.7 hours, whereas following administration of repeated doses the half-lives ranged from 16.4 to 26.6 hours. The data suggest that carbamazepine induces its own metabolism during repeated administration.— M. Eichelbaum *et al.*, *Eur. J. clin. Pharmac.*, 1975, *8*, 337.

Half-lives of carbamazepine ranging from 5.0 to 13.6 hours in patients also receiving other anticonvulsants. The data indicated that it is the epoxide-diol pathway that is induced during long-term therapy. Concomitant therapy with primidone, phenytoin, phenobarbitone, ethosuximide, or methsuximide further induces carbamazepine metabolism.— M. Eichelbaum *et al.*, *Clin. Pharmac. Ther.*, 1979, *26*, 366.

A study on the induction by carbamazepine of its own metabolism. Initial induction was noted as soon as 1 or 2 days after starting a multiple-dose study and additional self-induction was noted after about 2 weeks.— P. J. McNamara *et al.*, *J. Pharmacokinet. Biopharm.*, 1979, *7*, 63.

Further references to the half-life of carbamazepine and its ability to induce its own metabolism: E. Rey *et al.*, *Int. J. clin. Pharmac. Biopharm.*, 1979, *17*, 90 (in children); L. Bertilsson *et al.*, *Clin. Pharmac. Ther.*, 1980, *27*, 83 (in children).

Plasma concentrations. Comment on the monitoring of plasma concentrations of carbamazepine. The concentration of the metabolite, carbamazepine-10,11-epoxide, which has approximately one-third of the activity of carbamazepine, is usually much lower than that of carbamazepine, therefore it is not generally necessary to measure the metabolite. Present evidence suggests that plasma concentrations of 4 to 12.5 μg per ml (16 to 50 μmol per litre) are associated with optimum control of fits in a majority of patients. Carbamazepine can be absorbed erratically, and its rate of metabolism is variable and can be increased by other drugs, therefore a good case can be made for routine monitoring of carbamazepine concentrations. Timing of the sample in relation to dose is important because carbamazepine has a relatively short half-life of 8 to 19 hours on repeated administration.— A. Richens and S. Warrington, *Drugs*, 1979, *17*, 488. A similar view in relation to children where steady-state concentrations are less than 20% those expected from single-dose pharmacokinetic studies and in whom carbamazepine has a relatively short half-life of 4.1 to 18.3 hours.— G. W. Rylance and T. A. Moreland, *Archs Dis. Childh.*, 1980, *55*, 89.

Studies directed at relating therapeutic response to plasma concentrations of carbamazepine, with the aim of individualising dosage regimens: F. Monaco *et al.*, *Neurology, Minneap.*, 1976, *26*, 936 (therapeutic concentrations of 4 to 10 μg per ml); A. Rane *et al.*, *Clin. Pharmac. Ther.*, 1976, *19*, 276 (in children); B. Terhaag *et al.*, *Int. J. clin. Pharmac. Biopharm.*, 1978, *16*, 607 (traces in bile); R. Huf and R. J. Schain, *J. Pediat.*, 1980, *97*, 310 (in children); J. A. Wada *et al.*, *Epilepsia*, 1978, *19*, 251 (syrup bioavailability); R. J. Höppener *et al.*, *Epilepsia*, 1980, *21*, 341 (transient fluctuations); E. Perucca *et al.*, *Clin. Pharmacokinet.*, 1980, *5*, 576 (correlation between dose and serum concentration).

Protein binding. The mean amount of carbamazepine not bound, *in vitro*, to plasma proteins from 24 healthy subjects was 18.2%; the mean amount not bound in plasma from 54 patients taking carbamazepine was 26.9% (range 7.9 to 60%). There was no significant difference in binding capacity between plasma from patients with renal disease and that from healthy subjects but the plasma from patients with liver disease bound a slightly lower percentage of carbamazepine than did normal plasma.— W. D. Hooper *et al.*, *Clin. Pharmac. Ther.*, 1975, *17*, 433. See also M. D. Rawlins *et al.*, *Eur. J. clin. Pharmac.*, 1975, *8*, 91 (70 to 74% protein binding in 8 healthy subjects).

Saliva concentrations. In 15 children saliva concentrations and plasma concentrations of carbamazepine were well correlated, provided contamination by unabsorbed drug was avoided. Saliva concentrations of 1.3 to 3.55 μg per ml were considered comparable with therapeutic plasma concentrations of 4.25 to 11.8 μg per ml.— G. W. Rylance *et al.* (letter), *Br. med. J.*, 1977, *2*, 1481.

Excellent linear correlation between steady-state carbamazepine concentration in saliva and plasma occurred in 7 patients receiving carbamazepine. The mean saliva/plasma ratio was 0.26 (range 0.25 to 0.28).— H. G. M. Westenberg *et al.*, *Clin. Pharmac. Ther.*, 1978, *23*, 320.

Further studies on concentrations of carbamazepine in saliva: L. Hendeles *et al.*, *J. Allergy clin. Immunol.*, 1977, *60*, 335; S. Pynnönen, *Acta pharmac. tox.*, 1977, *41*, 465; J. W. Paxton and R. A. Donald, *Clin. Pharmac. Ther.*, 1980, *28*, 695; J. J. MacKichan *et al.*, *Br. J. clin. Pharmac.*, 1981, *12*, 31.

Pregnancy and the neonate. A study indicating that carbamazepine penetrates the placenta in early human pregnancy. The highest concentrations of carbamazepine were contained in foetal liver and kidney, with rather low values in foetal brain and lungs. In paediatric autopsy material carbamazepine seemed to accumulate in the cerebral cortex, heart, liver, and kidney. The concentration in milk was about 60% of the respective plasma value. According to the observations of the mothers taking carbamazepine and breast feeding, there were no discernible adverse effects on the infants.— S. Pynnönen *et al.*, *Acta pharmac. tox.*, 1977, *41*, 244. See also S. Pynnönen and M. Sillanpää (letter), *Lancet*, 1975, *2*, 563.

A study of the pharmacokinetics of carbamazepine in the neonate and the child. Absorption was very variable and the plasma half-life was considerably shorter than in adults, with a range of less than 3 to over 15 hours.— E. Rey *et al.*, *Int. J. clin. Pharmac. Biopharm.*, 1979, *17*, 90.

Further references to carbamazepine in pregnancy, lactation, and the neonate: A. Rane *et al.*, *Eur. J. clin. Pharmac.*, 1975, *8*, 283 (transplacental diffusion); J. R. Niebyl *et al.*, *Obstet. Gynec.*, 1979, *53*, 139 (pregnancy and lactation); S. Kaneko *et al.* (letter), *Br. J. clin. Pharmac.*, 1979, *7*, 624 (lactation).

See also under Phenytoin, Absorption and Fate, p.1241.

Uses. Carbamazepine is an anticonvulsant used to control grand mal and psychomotor or partial (focal) seizures. Its mode of action in epilepsy is not fully understood but some of its actions resemble those of phenytoin (p.1242) and although it does not superficially appear to have any chemical similarity in fact its 3-dimensional structure is similar.

The dose of carbamazepine should be adjusted to the needs of the individual patient to achieve adequate control of seizures; this usually requires plasma concentrations of 4 to 12.5 μg per ml (16 to 50 μmol per litre). The suggested initial dose is 100 to 200 mg once or twice daily gradually increased to a usual maintenance dose of 0.8 to 1.2 g daily in 2 to 4 divided doses; up to 1.6 g daily may occasionally be necessary. Dosage increments of 200 mg daily are recommended. Suggested daily doses for children are: up to 1 year of age, 100 to 200 mg; 1 to 5 years, 200 to 400 mg; 5 to 10 years, 400 to 600 mg; 10 to 15 years, 600 mg to 1 g.

Since carbamazepine has a long plasma half-life, a twice-daily dosage regimen is usually adequate to maintain an effective plasma concentration and is preferred because improved compliance has been associated with twice-daily dosage regimens. A low initial dose of carbamazepine is recommended to minimise side-effects.

Withdrawal of carbamazepine or transition to or from another type of anticonvulsant therapy should be made gradually to avoid precipitating an increase in the frequency of seizures.

Carbamazepine is also used in the treatment of trigeminal neuralgia. The suggested initial dose is 100 mg twice daily increased by 200 mg daily (100 mg every 12 hours) to a maximum of 1.2 g daily. The usual maintenance dose is 400 to 800 mg daily in 2 to 4 divided doses; when pain relief has been obtained attempts should be made to reduce and ultimately discontinue the therapy, until another attack occurs.

Carbamazepine should be taken with food. The time and manner of taking carbamazepine should be standardised for the patient since variations might affect absorption with consequent fluctuations in the plasma concentrations.

Administration. The mean fluctuation of carbamazepine in plasma of patients receiving the drug twice and thrice daily has been found to be similar whereas the fluctuation is reduced by dividing the daily dosage into 4. It has been concluded that a single daily dose is inadequate and 2 daily doses are appropriate in most cases, but some patients may benefit from more frequent dosing to avoid side-effects.— L. Bertilsson, *Clin. Pharmacokinet.*, 1978, *3*, 128.

A study of 43 epileptic patients who were receiving carbamazepine, usually thrice daily, together with other anticonvulsants, and who were suffering from intermittent carbamazepine-induced side-effects which corresponded to fluctuations in the plasma concentrations of carbamazepine. It was concluded that administration of carbamazepine with other anticonvulsants results in a distinct decrease in its half-life so that 4 daily doses might be required.— R. J. Höppener *et al.*, *Epilepsia*, 1980, *21*, 341.

Administration in children. A comment that when children are given carbamazepine instead of phenytoin, primidone, or phenobarbitone for epilepsy, the change for the better in alertness, gaiety, and scholastic performance is at times remarkable.— B. D. Bower, Epilepsy in Childhood and Adolescence, in *The Treatment of Epilepsy*, J.H. Tyrer (Ed.), Lancaster, England, MTP Press, 1980.

A report on the satisfactory long-term use of carbamazepine in children. No serious side-effects were encountered in 61 children given carbamazepine for up to 5 years. Carbamazepine is considered to qualify as a first-choice anticonvulsant for children with major motor seizures. It was given in a dosage of 10 mg per kg body-weight in 2 divided doses initially, gradually increased if necessary to a maximum of 35 mg per kg daily in 3 divided doses; dose changes were made at 2-week intervals and some subjects continued to receive other anticonvulsants, principally phenytoin or phenobarbitone. The therapeutic range of serum concentrations was found to be 3 to 15 μg per ml.— R. Huf and R. J. Schain, *J. Pediat.*, 1980, *97*, 310.

Administration in renal failure. The dose of carbamazepine should be reduced in patients with a glomerular filtration-rate of less than 10 ml per minute.— W. M. Bennett *et al.*, *Ann. intern. Med.*, 1980, *93*, 286.

For the use of carbamazepine in uraemic neuropathy, see under Neuralgias and Neuropathies, below.

Affective disorders. A report on 3 years of experience with carbamazepine in a double-blind placebo-controlled study of 24 manic-depressive patients. Carbamazepine was observed to have antimanic as well as antidepressant and prophylactic effects in affective illness. Carbamazepine was given in an initial dose of 200 mg twice daily, gradually increased to a total of 0.6 to 1.6 g daily. The patients appeared to respond to doses that achieved blood concentrations between 7 and 12 μg per ml, similar to the high therapeutic range for epilepsy.— J. C. Ballenger and R. M. Post, *Am. J. Psychiat.*, 1980, *137*, 782.

Alcoholism. Evidence from a multicentre placebo-controlled study, that carbamazepine may help to alleviate withdrawal symptoms in ambulant alcoholics. The patients also received hypnotics and vitamins of the B group.— S. -E. Björkqvist *et al.*, *Acta psychiat. scand.*, 1976, *53*, 333. Conflicting reports on the role of carbamazepine in alcohol withdrawal: C. Carlsson and L. Pettersson, *Int. Z. klin. Pharmak.*, 1972, *5*, 403; H. Gammer, *Läkartidningen*, 1976, *73*, 2819. For controversy over the role of anticonvulsants of the phenytoin type in alcoholism, see Phenytoin, p.1243.

Cardiac disorders. Further evaluation is necessary to document the anti-arrhythmic effects of carbamazepine, and to determine the plasma concentration range necessary for such effects.— R. L. Woosley and T. Z. Rumboldt, *Recent Adv. clin. Pharmac.*, 1978, *1*, 93 to 122.

Further references to the anti-arrhythmic action of carbamazepine: A. Sanabria *et al.*, *Nouv. Presse méd.*, 1976, *5*, 431.

Epilepsy. Reports and studies on carbamazepine in epilepsy: S. Livingston *et al.*, *J. Am. med. Ass.*, 1967, *200*, 204; J. J. Cereghino *et al.*, *Neurology, Minneap.*, 1974, *24*, 401; A. S. Troupin *et al.*, *Neurology, Minneap.*, 1974, *24*, 863; J. J. Cereghino *et al.*, *Clin. Pharmac. Ther.*, 1975, *18*, 733; E. A. Rodin *et al.*, *J. nerv. ment. Dis.*, 1976, *163*, 41; A. S. Troupin *et al.*, *Neurology, Minneap.*, 1977, *27*, 511; C. B. Dodrill and A. S. Troupin, *ibid.*, 1023.

For comments on the role of carbamazepine in epilepsy, see Phenytoin, p.1243.

See also Administration in Children, above.

Gilles de la Tourette's syndrome. A 9-year-old boy with severe Gilles de la Tourette's syndrome obtained marked improvement on receiving carbamazepine 100 mg thrice daily.— E. G. Lutz, *Am. J. Psychiat.*, 1977, *134*, 98.

Metabolic and endocrine disorders. Seven of 9 patients with diabetes insipidus responded to treatment with carbamazepine 600 mg daily in divided doses for 7 days then increased if necessary to 1.2 g daily. One patient achieved a partial response but with ataxia and limb pain; reduction of the dose to 800 mg daily and the addition of clofibrate produced a desirable response.— J. K. Wales, *Lancet*, 1975, *2*, 948.

Oral therapy with carbamazepine, which sensitises the kidney to the effects of vasopressin, has been used in diabetes insipidus but it is much less active than desmopressin and is not effective in severe forms.— J. S. Jenkins, *Practitioner*, 1979, *222*, 312.

Further references to carbamazepine in diabetes insipidus: J. P. Radó, *Br. med. J.*, 1973, *3*, 479; R. N. Bickler (letter), *Lancet*, 1976, *2*, 749; L. Czako and F. A. Laszlo, *Int. J. clin. Pharmac. Biopharm.*, 1975, *11*, 58.

See also under Adverse Effects, Effects on the Endocrine System, above.

Multiple sclerosis. Carbamazepine in a dose of 400 to 600 mg daily controlled tonic seizures in 4 patients with multiple sclerosis.— Y. Kuroiwa and H. Shibasaki (letter), *Lancet*, 1967, *1*, 116. See also M. L. E. Espir and M. E. Walker (letter), *ibid.*, 280.

Carbamazepine, initially 200 mg daily, increased by 200 mg every other day until an effective dose or a maximum of 1.2 g daily was reached, brought dramatic and persistent relief from pain in 4 of 6 patients with multiple sclerosis.— M. L. Albert, *New Engl. J. Med.*, 1969, *280*, 1395.

Carbamazepine 200 mg by mouth 4 times daily controlled intractable hiccup in a patient with acute multiple sclerosis.— D. A. McFarling and J. O. Susac (letter), *J. Am. med. Ass.*, 1974, *230*, 962.

Carbamazepine in divided doses of up to 1.2 g daily for short periods effectively controlled bouts of paroxysmal itching in 3 patients with multiple sclerosis.— P. O. Osterman, *Br. J. Derm.*, 1976, *95*, 555.

Muscular disorders. In a 62-year-old woman with generalised muscle weakness and absence of tendon reflexes, relief from pain was achieved with carbamazepine 400 mg before sleep and prednisone 60 mg daily.— I. Winspur (letter), *Lancet*, 1970, *1*, 85.

Increased tonus of flexor and extensor muscles in patients with myotonic dystrophy was relieved by carbamazepine.— A. Jusic and D. Stimak, *Fortschr. Neurol. Psychiat.*, 1972, *40*, 105, per *J. Am. med. Ass.*, 1972, *220*, 1028.

Neuralgias and neuropathies. In a double-blind trial 70 patients with *trigeminal neuralgia* were given carbamazepine, 100 to 200 mg three or four times daily, or a placebo for alternate fortnights for a total of 8 weeks. Carbamazepine was significantly more effective than the placebo in reducing the severity of pain and the number of paroxysms.— F. G. Campbell *et al.*, *J. Neurol. Neurosurg. Psychiat.*, 1966, *29*, 265. Complete or satisfactory relief of trigeminal neuralgia was obtained by 20 of 30 patients treated with carbamazepine for an average of 13 months. The drug had only minor effects in 6 patients with postherpetic neuralgia but was effective in 2 patients with *tabetic neuralgia*. It was of no benefit in 4 patients with *atypical facial pain*.— J. M. Killian and G. H. Fromm, *Archs Neurol., Chicago*, 1968, *19*, 129. Of 55 patients with typical or atypical trigeminal neuralgia 46 were relieved, usually within 1 to 2 days, by carbamazepine. Of 15 patients with non-neuralgic facial pain 8 obtained relief. Of the 54 patients who obtained relief and were given maintenance treatment 37 remained free of pain in an observation period of 2 to 5½ years.— P. Rasmussen and J. Riishede, *Acta neurol. scand.*, 1970, *46*, 385. In adequate doses carbamazepine will control at least 75% of patients with trigeminal neuralgia.— M. Anthony, *Drugs*, 1979, *18*, 122.

Four patients with *glossopharyngeal neuralgia* improved within 24 hours of the start of treatment with carbamazepine. The pain returned immediately the treatment was withdrawn but disappeared when it was recommenced.— K. A. Ekbom and C. E. Westerberg, *Archs Neurol., Chicago*, 1966, *14*, 595. Failure of carbamazepine, initially effective, in recurrence of glossopharyngeal neuralgia.— J. R. Rees and P. G. Bicknell (letter), *Br. med. J.*, 1979, *1*, 754. Carbamazepine, in doses similar to those used in trigeminal neuralgia, is the treatment of choice for glossopharyngeal neuralgia, although it is less effective.— M. Anthony, *Drugs*, 1979, *18*, 122.

In 7 patients with *tabes dorsalis*, severe lightning pain was relieved within 1 to 3 days after treatment with carbamazepine 400 to 800 mg daily; pain recurred when treatment ceased.— K. Ekbom, *Archs Neurol., Chicago*, 1972, *26*, 374. See also D. Alarcón-Segovia and M. A. Lazcano (letter), *J. Am. med. Ass.*, 1968, *203*, 57.

Carbamazepine 600 mg produced relief from pain for 48 hours in 4 wounded soldiers with *paraesthesia* who were developing tolerance to narcotics. Although the pain had returned to its former intensity within 96 hours an increased dose of 1.2 g was effective in 2 patients.— M. L. Albert (letter), *New Engl. J. Med.*, 1974, *290*, 693.

Carbamazepine 400 to 600 mg daily was recommended for patients with disabling *phantom limb phenomena*.— F. Elliott *et al.*, *New Engl. J. Med.*, 1976, *295*, 678.

Five patients with severe *uraemic neuropathy* and on haemodialysis reported relief from pain after 1 or 2 weeks of treatment with carbamazepine 100 to 300 mg twice daily.— Z. Zarday and R. J. Soberman (letter), *Ann. intern. Med.*, 1976, *84*, 296.

Severe painful paraesthesia in the lower limbs of a patient with *amyloidosis* was relieved by administration of carbamazepine 200 mg thrice daily.— J. L. Bada *et al.* (letter), *New Engl. J. Med.*, 1977, *296*, 396.

A favourable report of the use of carbamazepine for the relief of *metatarsophalangeal pain* (*Morton's neuralgia*) in 2 patients.— R. J. Guiloff, *Br. med. J.*, 1979, *2*, 904.

Raynaud's syndrome. Symptoms of Raynaud's disease disappeared during treatment with carbamazepine 300 mg daily in a 31-year-old patient with nocturnal complex partial seizures, migraine, and Raynaud's disease.— J. R. Merikangas and R. Auchenbach (letter), *Lancet*, 1977, *2*, 1186.

Sleep apnoea. Carbamazepine 1.2 g daily controlled partial seizures in a patient with sleep apnoea syndrome. His wife reported that within a week of starting carbamazepine his snoring and attacks of breath-holding stopped.— G. B. Murray (letter), *J. Am. med. Ass.*, 1977, *238*, 212.

Tinnitus. One hundred and twenty-five patients with incurable and intolerable tinnitus were given lignocaine 1 to 2 mg per kg body-weight intravenously and divided into 5 groups according to whether they obtained excellent, good, partial, unilateral, or no significant relief from their tinnitus. They were then given carbamazepine (or phenytoin if unable to tolerate carbamazepine), and a high proportion of those who had responded to the lignocaine test were found to have a correspondingly good response to the anticonvulsants. Of 91 who had a good to excellent response to lignocaine, 51 had a good to excellent response to anticonvulsant therapy. Carbamazepine was given in initial doses of 100 mg thrice daily very gradually increased to usual doses of 0.6 to 1 g daily, and phenytoin in initial doses of 100 mg daily very gradually increased to usual doses of 400 mg daily.— P. S. Melding and R. J. Goodey, *J. Lar. Otol.*, 1979, *93*, 111.

Preparations

Carbamazepine Tablets *(B.P.)*. Tablets containing carbamazepine.

Carbamazepine Tablets *(U.S.P.)*. Tablets containing carbamazepine. Store in airtight containers.

Tegretol *(Geigy, UK)*. Carbamazepine, available as a **Syrup** containing 100 mg in each 5 ml (suggested diluent, an equal volume of tragacanth mucilage) and as **Tablets** of 100 mg and scored tablets of 200 and 400 mg. (Also available as Tegretol in *Arg., Austral., Belg., Canad., Denm., Fr., Ital., Neth., Norw., S.Afr., Spain, Switz., USA*).

Other Proprietary Names

Convuline *(Austral.)*; Hermolepsin *(Swed.)*; Karbamazepin *(Denm., Norw.)*; Nordotol *(Denm.)*; Tegretal, Timonil *(bothGer.)*.

6606-d

Clonazepam *(U.S.P.)*. Ro 5-4023. 5-(2-Chlorophenyl)-1,3-dihydro-7-nitro-2*H*-1,4-benzodiazepin-2-one.

$C_{15}H_{10}ClN_3O_3$=315.7.

CAS — 1622-61-3.

Pharmacopoeias. In *U.S.*

A light yellow powder with a faint odour. M.p. about 239°. Practically **insoluble** in water; slightly soluble in alcohol and ether; sparingly soluble in acetone and chloroform. **Store** at room temperature in airtight containers. Protect from light.

Dependence. Prolonged use of clonazepam may lead to the development of dependence of the barbiturate-alcohol type (see p.792).

It has a low liability for abuse.

Withdrawal. Two patients with temporal lobe epilepsy receiving clonazepam associated with phenobarbitone in one and phenobarbitone and carbamazepine in the other, developed psychotic episodes on withdrawal of their anticonvulsant therapy, that were attributed to clonazepam. Both patients had daily seizures without mental changes during the first 3 days of withdrawal, and on the fourth and fifth days respectively they became seizure-free and presented an acute dysphoric state characterised by childish excitement, severe anxiety, outbursts of aggressiveness, and hallucinations with religious preoccupations and sexual fantasies; one patient had fine tremor of both hands. Plasma concentrations of phenobarbitone and carbamazepine were at the lower limit of the therapeutic range, but those of clonazepam were not detectable. The psychiatric changes disappeared only when clonazepam was readministered and reached a plasma concentration of about 5 to 7 ng per ml.— V. A. Sironi *et al.*, *J. Neurol. Neurosurg. Psychiat.*, 1979, *42*, 724.

Adverse Effects, Treatment, and Precautions. As for Diazepam, p.1520. Salivary or bronchial hypersecretion may cause respiratory problems in children.

Concomitant administration of hepatic enzymes inducers, such as phenobarbitone or phenytoin, may enhance the metabolism of clonazepam.

Concomitant administration of alcohol may affect the patient's response to clonazepam and is not recommended. Clonazepam may enhance the effects of central nervous system depressants, and may reduce the patient's ability to drive vehicles or operate machinery.

In a double-blind crossover study 14 of 18 patients with generalised or partial epilepsy inadequately controlled by existing medication had improved control when clonazepam was added to their treatment; in a further open study 19 of 21 patients had improved control. The initial dosage was 1 mg thrice daily increased after 2 weeks to 2 mg thrice daily further increased according to response, usually to a maximum of 12 mg daily. Most patients could tolerate 3 to 6 mg daily without unduly severe side-effects. Side-effects included drowsiness (26 patients), giddiness (18), aggression (6), irritability (6), and diplopia (1). There were no significant changes in biochemical, haematological, and urinary parameters studied. In 12 patients taking phenytoin (dosage unchanged) mean plasma-phenytoin concentrations fell from 20.5 to 14.1 µg per ml after 2 months' treatment with clonazepam. Of 5 patients from whom clonazepam was suddenly withdrawn 2 developed status epilepticus and one developed frequent major seizures.— V. E. Edwards and M. J. Eadie, *Proc. Aust. Ass. Neurol.*, 1973, *10*, 61.

Details of experience with clonazepam which has led to the view that it is less effective than diazepam in the treatment of childhood myoclonic epileptic seizures, and much more toxic.— S. Livingston and L. L. Pauli (letter), *Archs Neurol., Chicago*, 1976, *33*, 731.

Clonazepam, gradually increased to 6 mg daily was given to 27 newly-diagnosed epileptics. Side-effects appeared in 26 patients and included drowsiness, disturbances of gait, and behavioural and mental changes; 8 patients discontinued treatment because of side-effects, and 5 for other reasons. Phenytoin given in addition to patients whose seizures were inadequately controlled, lowered the plasma concentrations of clonazepam.— O. Sjö *et al.*, *Eur. J. clin. Pharmac.*, 1975, *8*, 249.

Fever of unknown origin occurred in an 18-year-old man 6 months after he began treatment with clonazepam 500 µg twice daily, increased to thrice daily after 3 months. His temperature returned to normal within 2 days of withdrawal of clonazepam.— R. Gray and L. N. Folkerts (letter), *Drug Intell. & clin. Pharm.*, 1977, *11*, 367.

Effects on the blood. A report of thrombocytopenia in a 52-year-old woman following a few weeks' treatment with clonazepam 0.5 to 1 mg twice daily; the patient had also been receiving phenytoin 150 mg daily.— R. M. Veall and H. C. Hogarth (letter), *Br. med. J.*, 1975, *4*, 462. See also S. Livingston and L. L. Pauli (letter), *Archs Neurol., Chicago*, 1976, *33*, 731.

Effects on mental state. Serious psychiatric symptoms associated with the use of clonazepam in children.— O. Hansson and B. Tonnby, *Läkartidningen*, 1976, *73*, 1209, per *Int. pharm. Abstr.*, 1977, *14*, 221.

See also above for mention of aggression and irritability in patients taking clonazepam.

Interactions. Concurrent administration of *carbamazepine* was found to reduce the half-life of clonazepam by induction of its metabolism.— A. A. Lai *et al.*, *Clin. Pharmac. Ther.*, 1978, *24*, 316. Both *phenobarbitone* and *phenytoin* reduced the half-life of clonazepam by induction of its metabolism. Neither drug affected the protein binding of clonazepam.— K. -C. Khoo *et al.*, *ibid.*, 1980, *28*, 368.

For the effect of concomitant administration of clonazepam and *sodium valproate*, see Sodium Valproate, p.1257.

Overdosage. A 2-year-old child who ingested about 60 mg of clonazepam completely recovered within 3 to 4 days. Gastric lavage was performed within an hour of ingestion and though drowsiness and ataxia rapidly set in the child needed no other treatment. Ataxia was manifested for up to 72 hours.— P. F. Bladin, *Med. J. Aust.*, 1973, *1*, 683.

During the 24 hours after admission to hospital with an overdose of clonazepam, a 4-year-old boy cycled 7 times between alert agitation and unresponsive coma with pinpoint pupils. He had received naloxone by injection, and magnesium sulphate and charcoal by mouth. The possibility of enterohepatic recycling was considered to have been prevented by the charcoal and the catharsis, but the possibility of an active metabolite was considered.— T. R. Welch *et al.*, *Clin. Toxicol.*, 1977, *10*, 433.

Urinary incontinence. Urinary incontinence developed in 2 elderly patients given clonazepam.— A. Williams and M. Gillespie, *Ann. Neurol.*, 1979, *6*, 86.

Withdrawal. See under Dependence, above.

Absorption and Fate. For an account of the absorption and fate of a benzodiazepine, see Diazepam, p.1522.

Clonazepam is extensively metabolised, its principal metabolite being 7-aminoclonazepam, which probably has little anticonvulsant activity; minor metabolites are acetamide and hydroxylated derivatives. It is excreted in the urine almost entirely as its metabolites in free or conjugated form. It is about 50% bound to plasma protein and estimations of its plasma half-life range from about 20 to 40 hours, and occasionally up to 60 hours.

Clonazepam crosses the placental barrier.

The pharmacokinetics of clonazepam.— E. Eschenhof, *Arzneimittel-Forsch.*, 1973, *23*, 390.

Peak blood concentrations of clonazepam occurring 1 to 2 hours after administration of a single 2-mg dose by mouth ranged from 6.5 to 13.5 ng per ml. The apparent half-life ranged from 18.7 to 39 hours. Less than 0.5% was excreted as unchanged clonazepam.— S. A. Kaplan *et al.*, *J. pharm. Sci.*, 1974, *63*, 527. See also J. A. F. de Silva *et al.*, *ibid.*, 520.

A study of the pharmacokinetics of clonazepam in 8 healthy subjects following single oral and intravenous doses, and repeated oral administration. Clonazepam was rapidly absorbed, with peak plasma concentrations obtained within 4 hours in all subjects. The plasma half-life ranged from 19 to 60 hours and was not significantly altered in 5 of the subjects after repeated administration for 15 days.— A. Berlin and H. Dahlström, *Eur. J. clin. Pharmac.*, 1975, *9*, 155.

Attempts to correlate plasma concentrations of clonazepam and its principal metabolite, 7-aminoclonazepam, with side-effects, in 27 newly diagnosed epileptic patients. At a usual daily dose of clonazepam 6 mg, the average plasma concentrations of both drug and metabolite were about 50 ng per ml (with an individual range of 30 to about 80 ng per ml). In general, no correlation could be found between plasma concentrations and side-effects, although serious dysphoria did appear to be associated with the higher concentrations in some patients. Withdrawal symptoms, which occurred in 4 of 13 patients who stopped clonazepam, were associated with much higher concentrations of the metabolite.— O. Sjö *et al.*, *Eur. J. clin. Pharmac.*, 1975, *8*, 249.

A study indicating that the rate of acetylation of 7-aminoclonazepam to 7-acetamidoclonazepam in the biotransformation of clonazepam is determined by acetylator phenotype.— M. E. Miller *et al.*, *Clin. Pharmac. Ther.*, 1981, *30*, 343.

Pregnancy and the neonate. Seven days after starting therapy with clonazepam for epileptic seizures in a pregnant woman, a child in excellent clinical condition was delivered by elective caesarean section. Plasma concentration measurements confirmed *animal* work indicating that clonazepam crosses the placental barrier. The development of the child during the first 7 days after birth was normal.— G. de Groot *et al.*, *IRCS med. Sci.*, 1977, *5*, 589.

Uses. Clonazepam is a benzodiazepine compound similar to diazepam (p.1523), with marked anticonvulsant properties.

It is used in the treatment of all types of epilepsy and seizures. Treatment is initiated with small doses which are progressively increased to an optimum dose according to the response of the patient. The usual daily doses, given in 3 or 4 divided doses, are: infants, 0.5 to 1 mg; children 1 to 5 years, 1 to 3 mg; children 5 to 12 years, 3 to 6 mg; adults, 4 to 8 mg.

In status epilepticus clonazepam is given by intravenous injection over about 30 seconds. The usual dose is 500 µg for infants and children and 1 mg for adults, repeated if required. It may also be given by slow intravenous infusion, in sodium chloride infusion, dextrose 5 or 10% infusion, or sodium chloride 0.45% and dextrose 2.5% infusion.

Withdrawal of clonazepam or transition to or from another type of anticonvulsant therapy should be made gradually to avoid precipitating an increase in the frequency of seizures.

Action. A review of clonazepam, including comments on its possible mode of action. Generalised EEG abnormalities are more readily suppressed than focal abnormalities, and clonazepam often limits the spread of discharge while not suppressing the primary focus. These observations may be explained by the ability of benzodiazepines to enhance polysynaptic inhibitory processes at all levels of the CNS. The ultimate mechanism presumably involves actions on neurotransmitters or cell membranes (or both). It has been suggested that clonazepam may act by mimicking the effects of the neurotransmitter glycine, or by increasing the concentration of serotonin at synaptic sites.— T. R. Browne, *New Engl. J. Med.*, 1978, *299*, 812. See also *idem*, *Archs Neurol., Chicago*, 1976, *33*, 326.

Chorea. Clonazepam was effective in suppressing choreiform movements in 3 patients with Huntington's chorea, 3 with non-familial chorea, and 1 with senile chorea. It was not effective in 1 patient with chorea (possibly senile chorea). Effective doses ranged from 3.5 to 5.5 mg daily.— J. B. Peiris *et al.*, *Med. J. Aust.*, 1976, *1*, 225.

Dyskinesias. Clonazepam had been given to 42 patients with drug-induced dyskinesia in doses of 0.5 to 1 mg twice or thrice daily with consistent improvement.— P. M. O'Flanagan (letter), *Br. med. J.*, 1975, *1*, 269. Disappointing results with clonazepam in 18 patients with tardive oral dyskinesia.— G. Sedman (letter), *ibid.*, 1976, *2*, 583.

Epilepsy. Reports and studies on clonazepam in epilepsy.— H. Gastaut *et al.*, *Epilepsia*, 1971, *12*, 197 (status epilepticus); V. E. Edwards and M. J. Eadie, *Proc. Aust. Ass. Neurol.*, 1973, *10*, 61; P. F. Bladin, *Med. J. Aust.*, 1973, *1*, 683; C. Y. Huang *et al.*, *ibid.*, 1974, *2*, 5; C. Fazio *et al.*, *Archs Neurol., Chicago*, 1975, *32*, 304; M. J. Carson and C. Gilden, *Develop. Med. Child. Neurol.*, 1975, *17*, 306; F. Bang *et al.*, *Epilepsia*, 1976, *17*, 321; B. Mikkelsen *et al.*, *Archs Neurol., Chicago*, 1976, *33*, 322; P. Bielmann *et al.*, *Int. J. clin. Pharmac. Biopharm.*, 1978, *16*, 268.

For comments on the role of clonazepam in epilepsy, see Phenytoin, p.1243.

Gilles de la Tourette's syndrome. Partial relief of Gilles de la Tourette's syndrome with clonazepam.— M. Gonce and A. Barbeau, *Can. J. neurol. Sci.*, 1977, *4*, 279.

Migraine. Disappolnting results with clonazepam in migraine prophylaxis.— P. Stensrud and O. Sjaastad, *Headache*, 1979, *19*, 333.

Myoclonus. Clonazepam 4 to 12 mg daily by mouth given to 6 patients with myoclonus and 1 mg given intravenously to 1 similar patient produced marked improvement in 3, although in 1 this only lasted 1 to 2 months, and slight improvement in 3. The response was similar to that from 5-hydroxytryptophan and was probably due to increased brain concentrations of serotonin.— D. Chadwick *et al.*, *Lancet*, 1975, *2*, 434.

Narcolepsy. For a beneficial response to clonazepam in cataplexy, see Clomipramine Hydrochloride, p.116.

Neuralgia. Clonazepam in daily doses of 1.5 to 3 mg was very effective for prevention of pain attacks in 4 of 6 patients with Sluder's syndrome and 9 of 14 with trigeminal neuralgia.— S. Smirne and G. Scarlato, *Med. J. Aust.*, 1977, *1*, 93.

Further references: J. E. Court and C. S. Kase, *J. Neurol. Neurosurg. Psychiat.*, 1976, *39*, 297 (trigeminal neuralgia).

Porphyria. Convulsions in a young woman with acute intermittent porphyria were controlled by clonazepam 6 mg daily and oral contraceptives. It is considered that if clonazepam is found to be porphyrogenic in high doses, the only safe therapy for chronic seizure management would be bromide.— J. A. Garcia-Merino and J. J. Lopez-Lozano (letter), *Lancet*, 1980, *2*, 856.

Restless legs syndrome. In 5 patients the restless legs syndrome had been abolished or greatly relieved by clonazepam; a typical dose was 1 mg as a single or divided doses in the evening.— W. B. Matthews (letter), *Br. med. J.*, 1979, *1*, 751. See also D. Boghen, *Ann. Neurol.*, 1980, *8*, 341.

Beneficial results with clonazepam in the uraemic restless legs syndrome.— D. J. Read *et al.*, *Br. med. J.*, 1981, *283*, 885.

Stiff-man syndrome. Clonazepam 6 mg daily was effective in the management of fluctuating muscular rigidity and spasm (stiff-man syndrome) in a woman who had previously required up to 40 mg of diazepam daily.— U. Westblom (letter), *J. Am. med. Ass.*, 1977, *237*, 1930.

Preparations

Clonazepam Tablets *(U.S.P.).* Tablets containing clonazepam. The *U.S.P.* requires 80% dissolution in 60 minutes. Store at room temperature in airtight containers. Protect from light.

Rivotril *(Roche, UK).* Clonazepam, available as an **Injection** containing 1 mg per ml, in ampoules of 1 ml (supplied with 1-ml ampoules of Water for Injections) and as scored **Tablets** of 0.5 and 2 mg. (Also available as Rivotril in *Arg., Austral., Belg., Canad., Denm., Fr., Ger., Ital., Neth., Norw., S.Afr., Spain, Switz.*).

Other Proprietary Names

Clonopin *(USA)*; Iktorivil *(Swed.)*.

6607-n

Dimethadione. BAX 1400Z; AC 1198. 5,5-Dimethyloxazolidine-2,4-dione.

$C_5H_7NO_3$=129.1.

CAS — 695-53-4.

Dimethadione is a metabolite of troxidone (p.1255). It has been used similarly.

6608-h

Dipropylacetamide. Valpromide. 2-Propylvaleramide.

$C_8H_{17}NO$=143.2.

CAS — 2430-27-5.

A white odourless crystalline powder with a bitter taste. M.p. about 125°. Practically **insoluble** in water.

Dipropylacetamide is the amide of valproic acid (see p.1256). It is used in the treatment of various psychotic disorders including depression and mania, and in convulsive disorders. The recommended dosage is 0.3 to 1.8 g daily in divided doses.

Proprietary Names

Depamide *(Labaz, Fr.; Sigmatau, Ital.; Labaz, Spain)*; Vistora *(Vita, Spain)*.

6609-m

Doxenitoin. SKF 2599. 5,5-Diphenylimidazolidin-4-one.

$C_{15}H_{14}N_2O$=238.3.

CAS — 3254-93-1.

Crystals. M.p. 183° to 187°. Practically **insoluble** in water; soluble in glacial acetic acid; less soluble in alcohol, chloroform, and ethyl acetate.

Doxenitoin was formerly used in the treatment of psychomotor, petit mal, and other forms of epilepsy. It was given in doses of 400 to 600 mg daily.

6610-t

Eterobarb. DMMP; Dimethoxymethylphenobarbital; EX 12-095. 5-Ethyl-1,3-bis(methoxymethyl)-5-phenylbarbituric acid.

$C_{16}H_{20}N_2O_5$=320.3.

CAS — 27511-99-5.

Eterobarb is an anticonvulsant with general properties similar to those of phenobarbitone (p.811). It has been reported to cause less sedation than phenobarbitone.

In 2 studies in patients with partial seizures with complex symptomatology with or without secondary generalisation, eterobarb in a mean dose of 5.8 or 6.7 mg per kg body-weight daily caused an average 59% reduction in seizures in 19 of 28 patients without secondary generalisation and an average 70% reduction in all of those with secondary generalisation.— B. B. Gallagher *et al.*, *Neurology, Minneap.*, 1975, *25*, 399.

Manufacturers

Merrell-National, USA.

6611-x

Ethosuximide *(B.P., U.S.P.)*. PM 671; H 940.

2-Ethyl-2-methylsuccinimide.

$C_7H_{11}NO_2$=141.2.

CAS — 77-67-8.

Pharmacopoeias. In *Br., Chin., Nord.,* and *U.S.*

A white or off-white, powder or waxy solid, odourless or with a characteristic odour and with a slightly bitter taste. M.p. 46° to 52°. **Soluble** 1 in 4.5 of water and 1 in less than 1 of alcohol, chloroform, and ether; very slightly soluble in light petroleum. **Store** in airtight containers.

Stability. The kinetics of hydrolysis of ethosuximide.— G. J. Yakatan and T. Fan, *Drug Dev. ind. Pharm.*, 1977, *3*, 315.

Adverse Effects. Gastro-intestinal side-effects including nausea, vomiting, anorexia, gastric upset, and abdominal pain occur fairly frequently. Other side-effects which may occur include headache, fatigue, lethargy, drowsiness, dizziness, ataxia, hiccup, and euphoria. Abnormal renal and liver function values, dyskinesias, personality changes, depression, psychosis, and skin rashes, and lupus erythematosus have also been reported.

Ethosuximide is less liable to induce serious blood disorders than troxidone, but eosinophilia, leucopenia, agranulocytosis, thrombocytopenia, pancytopenia, and aplastic anaemia have occasionally been reported. Erythema multiforme has also been reported.

Effects on the blood. Fatal *bone-marrow aplasia* occurred in a girl given ethosuximide.— L. B. Mann and H. A. Habenicht, *Bull. Los Ang. neurol. Soc.*, 1962, *27*, 173.

A 9-year-old girl with epilepsy who had been treated with phenobarbitone for 3 years developed *granulocytopenia* and *thrombocytopenia* about 2 months after starting concomitant treatment with ethosuximide. The ethosuximide was stopped and she rapidly improved after treatment with prednisone, phenobarbitone sodium, and tetracycline.— E. Koutsoulieris (letter), *Lancet*, 1967, *2*, 310.

Fatal *agranulocytosis* in a 7-year-old boy after treatment with ethosuximide.— J. F. Spittler, *Klin. Pediat.*, 1974, *186*, 364.

Effects on the eyes. Mention of one patient experiencing photophobia on ethosuximide.— E. S. Goldensohn *et al.*, *J. Am. med. Ass.*, 1962, *180*, 840.

Effects on the gastro-intestinal tract. Very severe gastro-intestinal symptoms occurred in 2 patients, aged 40 and 26, with idiopathic epilepsy who had been treated with ethosuximide for a week and 10 months respectively. Both had epigastric pain sufficiently severe to suggest cardiac infarction or perforation of a viscus. In 1 patient this was associated with occipital headache and in the other peripheral paraesthesias.— C. W. Burke (letter), *Lancet*, 1964, *2*, 966.

Effects on the skin. A report of the *Stevens-Johnson syndrome* developing after 3 weeks' treatment with ethosuximide.— A. Taaffe and C. O'Brien, *Br. dent. J.*, 1975, *138*, 172.

Extrapyramidal effects. A 15-year-old girl developed dyskinetic movements of the face, arms, and legs within hours of taking ethosuximide. They lasted for several hours and were stopped within minutes of intravenous administration of diphenhydramine.— G. J. Kirschberg, *Archs Neurol., Chicago*, 1975, *32*, 137.

Lupus erythematosus. Systemic lupus erythematosus developed in a 5-year-old girl who had been treated with ethosuximide, 1.25 g daily in divided doses, for 2 years. Two other similar cases were briefly described.— S. Livingston *et al.*, *J. Am. med. Ass.*, 1968, *204*, 731.

Ethosuximide was responsible for the development of systemic lupus erythematosus and scleroderma in a 16-year-old Chinese girl. The symptoms resolved on withdrawal of the drug.— P. C. Teoh and H. L. Chan, *Archs Dis. Childh.*, 1975, *50*, 658.

Treatment of Adverse Effects. The stomach should be emptied by aspiration and lavage, and supportive therapy given (for general guidelines to the symptomatic therapy of drug overdosage, see Phenobarbitone, p.812).

Precautions. Ethosuximide should be used with extreme caution in patients with impaired hepatic or renal function.

Regular blood counts, tests of liver function, and examinations of the urine should be made during treatment with ethosuximide.

For a comment on anticonvulsant therapy and driving, see Phenytoin, p.1239.

Interactions. Addition of ethosuximide to *phenobarbitone* therapy caused a dramatic increase in the incidence of absence seizures in a 9-year-old boy. The possibility of a drug interaction was considered, or the particular sub-type of epilepsy may have been worsened by ethosuximide.— A. B. Todorov *et al.*, *Archs Neurol., Chicago*, 1978, *35*, 389. For raised plasma concentrations of *phenobarbitone* and *phenytoin* in patients given concomitant *methsuximide* therapy, see Phenytoin, p.1239.

In 4 of 5 patients given *valproic acid* in addition to their ethosuximide therapy, plasma concentrations of ethosuximide increased to toxic values. It was not determined whether the effect was transient because the dose of ethosuximide was reduced to diminish side-effects, and the patients were subsequently controlled on valproic acid alone.— R. H. Mattson and J. A. Cramer, *Ann. Neurol.*, 1980, *7*, 583.

Results of a study in 6 healthy subjects indicated that concomitant administration of *carbamazepine* speeds the metabolism of ethosuximide.— J. W. Warren *et al.*, *Clin. Pharmac. Ther.*, 1980, *28*, 646.

Porphyria. Succinimides have been reported to precipitate attacks of porphyria.— *Drug & Ther. Bull.*, 1976, *14*, 55.

Pregnancy and the neonate. Ethosuximide is recommended for the treatment of petit mal epilepsy in women of childbearing age because of its proven efficacy and relatively low teratogenic potential; trimethadione and paramethadione are potentially more hazardous to the foetus and should not be used.— S. Fabro and N. A. Brown (letter), *New Engl. J. Med.*, 1979, *300*, 1280.

For a general comment on epilepsy and pregnancy, and references to surveys on the incidence of congenital malformations in the infants of epileptic women, see p.1235.

Absorption and Fate. Ethosuximide is readily absorbed from the gastro-intestinal tract and extensively hydroxylated in the liver to its principal metabolite which is reported to be inactive. It is excreted in the urine mainly in the form of its metabolites either free or in conjugated form but about 20% is also excreted as unchanged ethosuximide.

Ethosuximide is widely distributed throughout the body, but is not significantly bound to plasma proteins. A half-life of about 60 hours has been reported for adults with a shorter half-life of about 30 hours in children.

The therapeutic effects of ethosuximide have been correlated with plasma concentrations: in general, the anticonvulsant effect of ethosuximide is obtained at plasma concentrations of 40 to 100 μg per ml (about 300 to 700 μmol per litre). Ethosuximide crosses the blood-brain barrier and the placental barrier, and is excreted in milk.

Metabolism and pharmacokinetics. A study in 5 children showed that though gastro-intestinal absorption of ethosuximide was quicker from a syrup than from a capsule, equivalent peak plasma concentrations from each occurred about 3 to 7 hours after administration. The mean half-lives for syrup and capsule were 33.4 and 29.7 hours respectively. Half-life correlated with body-weight and ethosuximide appeared to be uniformly distributed throughout the body.— R. A. Buchanan *et al.*, *J. clin. Pharmac.*, 1969, *9*, 393.

About 20% of a dose of ethosuximide given to a healthy subject was excreted unchanged in the urine within 60 hours and the plasma half-life was 48 hours, suggesting a considerable metabolism of ethosuximide.— E. van der Kleijn *et al.*, *J. Pharm. Pharmac.*, 1973, *25*, 324.

3-Hydroxyethosuximide was identified as a major urinary metabolite of ethosuximide in humans.— P. G. Preste *et al.*, *J. pharm. Sci.*, 1974, *63*, 467.

Plasma concentrations. Monitoring of plasma-ethosuximide concentrations with the aim of improved epileptic control in 70 patients. Of 33 patients who were initially completely controlled, only 9% had plasma-ethosuximide concentrations below 40 μg per ml, and none were below 30 μg per ml. Attempts were therefore directed at achieving concentrations above 40 μg per ml by increasing the dose or by encouraging improved compliance. The total number of patients whose seizures were completely controlled or who achieved practical control rose from 45 (64%) to 57 (81%). Only 3 of the 70 patients had an increased seizure frequency, and 19 had a significant increase in plasma-ethosuximide concentrations.— A. L. Sherwin *et al.*, *Archs Neurol., Chicago*, 1973, *28*, 178.

In 46 epileptic patients steady-state plasma concentrations of ethosuximide were proportional to dose when expressed on a body-weight basis, regardless of age. In female patients the plasma concentration increased more rapidly with dose than in males. Apart from methylphenobarbitone, which tended to raise plasma concentrations of ethosuximide, other anticonvulsants including phenobarbitone had no effect when taken concurrently. To achieve a plasma concentration in the middle of the therapeutic range of 40 to 100 μg per ml a dose of 30 mg per kg body-weight daily was suggested. In individual patients the relationship between dose and plasma concentration was curvilinear, successive dose increments of equal size producing progressively greater increases in plasma concentrations.— G. A. Smith *et al.*, *Clin. Pharmacokinet.*, 1979, *4*, 38.

Saliva concentrations. Because ethosuximide is not bound to plasma protein, the concentration in saliva should equal the concentration in plasma. A study in 3 patients indicated that saliva can be used instead of plasma for monitoring therapy with ethosuximide.— M. G. Horning *et al.*, *Clin. Chem.*, 1977, *23*, 157.

Pregnancy and the neonate. A study of the pharmacokinetics of ethosuximide in a pregnant woman and her infant. The infant was not breast fed and the half-life of elimination of the transplacentally acquired ethosuximide in the neonate was calculated to be 41.3 hours. The ratio of breast milk to maternal serum concentration was approximately 1. It was predicted that total daily exposure to ethosuximide as a result of nursing would be 12.8 to 38.4 mg.— J. R. Koup *et al.*, *Epilepsia*, 1978, *19*, 535.

Ethosuximide concentrations in breat milk and in the plasma of a nursing mother and her infant.— A. Rane and R. Tunell, *Br. J. clin. Pharmac.*, 1981, *12*, 855.

See also under Phenytoin, p.1241.

Uses. Ethosuximide is a succinimide anticonvulsant used in the treatment of petit mal epilepsy; its mode of action is not fully understood. It may be used in conjunction with other anticonvulsants, such as phenobarbitone, phenytoin, or primidone when petit mal co-exists with grand mal or other forms of epilepsy. Occasionally this combined treatment may increase the incidence of grand mal attacks, necessitating a readjustment of the medication used for controlling the major seizures. Change-over from existing medication should be made gradually.

A concentration of 40 to 100 μg per ml (about 300 to 700 μmol per litre) of plasma appears to be generally necessary. The initial dose for patients under 6 years of age is 250 mg daily and for patients of 6 years and over 500 mg daily . The dosage is then adjusted by increments, usually of 250 mg every 4 to 7 days, according to the response of the patient. Strict supervision is necessary if the dose exceeds 1 g daily for a child of up to 6 years or 1.5 g daily for an adult.

A review of ethosuximide: *Antiepileptic Drugs*, D.M. Woodbury *et al.* (Ed.), New York, Raven Press, 1972.

Administration. In a controlled double-blind study involving 20 healthy subjects steady-state plasma concentrations and urinary excretion were the same following administration of ethosuximide on a once-daily or a thrice-daily basis.— J. R. Goulet *et al.*, *Clin. Pharmac. Ther.*, 1976, *20*, 213.

Administration in children. Transfer of 9 children with petit mal epilepsy from a multiple to a single daily dosage regimen of ethosuximide did not interfere with seizure control or lead to increased side-effects.— R. A. Buchanan *et al.*, *Clin. Pharmac. Ther.*, 1976, *19*, 143.

Administration in renal failure. The dose of ethosuximide should be reduced in patients with a glomerular filtration-rate of less than 10 ml per minute.— W. M. Bennett *et al.*, *Ann. intern. Med.*, 1980, *93*, 286.

Behaviour disorders. Ethosuximide, 250 mg daily, given to 27 children with atypical EEG records and specific learning problems, produced dramatic changes in intellectual functioning.— W. L. Smith and T. C. Weyl, *Curr. ther. Res.*, 1968, *10*, 265.

Epilepsy. Individual reports and studies on ethosuximide in petit mal: K. W. G. Heathfield and E. C. O. Jewesbury, *Br. med. J.*, 1961, *2*, 565; *idem*, 1964, *2*, 616; S. Livingston *et al.*, *J. Am. med. Ass.*, 1962, *180*, 822; E. S. Goldensohn *et al.*, *ibid.*, 840; E. Kiorboe *et al.*, *Epilepsia*, 1964, *5*, 83; A. W. Weinstein and R. J. Allen, *Am. J. Dis. Child.*, 1966, *111*, 63; T. R. Browne *et al.*, *Neurology, Minneap.*, 1975, *25*, 515.

For comments on the role of ethosuximide in epilepsy, see Phenytoin, p.1243.

Narcolepsy. A patient with severe *cataplexy*, who was having at least 1 attack every day, obtained immediate remission when given ethosuximide.— H. Garland, *Practitioner*, 1962, *189*, 461.

Preparations

Ethosuximide Capsules *(B.P.)*. Capsules containing ethosuximide. Store at a temperature not exceeding 30°.

Ethosuximide Capsules *(U.S.P.)*. Capsules containing ethosuximide as a solution in macrogol 400 or other suitable solvent. Store in airtight containers.

Ethosuximide Elixir *(B.P.)*. Ethosuximide Syrup. A solution of ethosuximide in a suitable flavoured vehicle which may be coloured. Store at a temperature not exceeding 25°. When a dose less than, or not a multiple of, 5 ml is prescribed, the elixir should be diluted to 5 ml, or a multiple, with syrup. Such dilutions must be freshly prepared unless a suitable preservative is added to the diluent, in which case it may be recently prepared.

Proprietary Preparations

Emeside *(Laboratories for Applied Biology, UK)*. Ethosuximide, available as **Capsules** of 250 mg and as **Syrup** containing 250 mg in each 5 ml (suggested diluent, syrup), with a choice of flavouring, black currant or orange.

Zarontin *(Parke, Davis, UK)*. Ethosuximide, available as **Capsules** of 250 mg and as **Syrup** containing 250 mg in each 5 ml (suggested diluent, syrup). (Also available as Zarontin in *Arg., Austral., Belg., Canad., Fr., Ital., Neth., S.Afr., Spain, USA*).

Other Proprietary Names

Ethymal *(Belg., Neth.)*;Petinimid *(Switz.)*; Petnidan, Pyknolepsinum *(Ger.)*; Simatin *(Switz.)*; Suxinutin *(Ger., Swed., Switz.)*; Thetamid *(Ital.)* Zarondan *(Denm., Norw.)*.

6612-r

Ethotoin *(B.P. 1973)*. Ethotoinum. 3-Ethyl-5-phenylhydantoin.

$C_{11}H_{12}N_2O_2$=204.2.

CAS — 86-35-1.

Pharmacopoeias. In *Roum.*

A white, almost odourless, almost tasteless, crystalline powder. M.p. about 90°. Practically **insoluble** in water; soluble 1 in 4 of dehydrated alcohol, 1 in 1.5 of chloroform, and 1 in 25 of ether.

The dissolution rate of ethotoin was increased by either forming a co-precipitate or physical mixture with povidone 25 000 or by preparing a solid dispersion in macrogol 6000.— A. S. Geneidi *et al.*, *J. pharm. Sci.*, 1978, *67*, 114.

Adverse Effects, Treatment, and Precautions. As for Phenytoin, p.1235.

Paranoid symptoms have been reported in patients receiving phenacemide concomitantly with ethotoin.

Although ethotoin is reported to be less toxic than phenytoin, and to induce less ataxia, gum hypertrophy, and hirsutism than phenytoin, it is also less effective.

Pregnancy and the neonate. A report of bilateral cleft lip and cleft palate in a 32-week premature infant whose mother had been taking ethotoin 500 mg four times daily and methylphenobarbitone 100 mg four times daily for many years.— M. Zablen and N. Brand (letter), *New Engl. J. Med.*, 1977, *297*, 1404. See also *idem*, 1978, *298*, 285.

Absorption and Fate. For an account of the absorption and fate of a hydantoin, see Phenytoin, p.1241.

The half-life of ethotoin is shorter than that of phenytoin and its metabolites are reported to be inactive; accordingly several doses are required throughout the day.

Metabolism and pharmacokinetics. A study in epileptic subjects indicating that only a small fraction of ethotoin is eliminated unchanged, and that saturation of the elimination capacity is approached above a concentration of about 8 μg per ml. On repeated administration plasma concentrations tended to decrease in the first week possibly due to auto-induction of metabolism. Since the dose-dependent kinetics of ethotoin make it probable that toxic manifestations may occur with only minor dosage increases, monitoring of the plasma concentration appears to be just as important as for phenytoin.— O. Sjö *et al.*, *Clin. exp. Pharmac. Physiol.*, 1975, *2*, 185. For a study in which dose-dependent kinetics of ethotoin were not detected, see Methoin, p.1251.

The plasma half-life of ethotoin ranged from 5 to 11 hours after oral administration of 0.5 or 2 g to epileptic subjects; it was the same for the 2 dose levels in the same individual. Studies of urinary metabolites indicated that it is metabolised by hydroxylation of the phenyl ring, followed by conjugation with glucuronic acid, and by *N*-de-ethylation followed by enzymatic ring-opening to form 2-phenylhydantoic acid.— W. Yonekawa *et al.*, *Pharmacologist*, 1975, *17*, 193.

Uses. Ethotoin is a hydantoin anticonvulsant with actions and uses similar to those of phenytoin (p.1242), but it is less effective.

Ethotoin is given in an initial dosage of 1 g daily, increased by 500 mg at intervals of several days to 2 to 3 g daily, given in 4 to 6 divided doses after meals. A suggested dose for children is 500 mg daily gradually increased to 1 to 2 g daily.

Preparations

Ethotoin Tablets *(B.P. 1973)*. Tablets containing ethotoin.

Peganone *(Abbott, UK)*. Ethotoin, available as scored tablets of 500 mg. (Also available as Peganone in *Austral., Denm., Norw., Swed., Switz., USA*).

6613-f

Methoin *(B.P. 1973)*. Methoinum; Mephenetoin; Mephenytoin *(U.S.P.)*; Methantoin; Phenantoin. 5-Ethyl-3-methyl-5-phenylhydantoin.

$C_{12}H_{14}N_2O_2$=218.3.

CAS — 50-12-4.

Pharmacopoeias. In *Aust., Cz., Ind., Nord., Pol.,* and *U.S.*

Colourless, odourless, tasteless, lustrous plates or a white crystalline powder. M.p. 136° to 140°. **Soluble** 1 in 1400 of water, 1 in 15 of alcohol, 1 in 3 of chloroform, and 1 in 90 of ether; soluble in aqueous solutions of alkali hydroxides.

Adverse Effects, Treatment, and Precautions. As for Phenytoin, p.1235.

The incidence of minor side-effects, especially gum hyperplasia and hirsutism, appears to be lower than with phenytoin, but the risk of serious skin reactions, blood dyscrasias, hepatitis, and lymphadenopathy is greater. Methoin has a sedative effect in some patients.

Frequent blood counts should be made during treatment with methoin and treatment should be stopped if the neutrophil count falls below 1600 per mm^3. Patients should be instructed to report a sore throat, fever, skin rash, nausea, bleeding, or jaundice.

Methoin should not be given with troxidone.

Generalised lymphadenopathy and the nephrotic syndrome associated with methoin administration.— C. Snead *et al.*, *Pediatrics*, 1976, *57*, 98.

Effects on the blood. *Agranulocytosis* attributed to methoin had been reported in 17 cases, 7 of which were fatal.— P. MacArthur, *Lancet*, 1952, *1*, 592.

Haemolytic anaemia in association with a positive reaction to the Coombs' test has been reported in patients taking methoin.— I. Snapper *et al.*, *Ann. intern. Med.*, 1953, *39*, 619, per M. G. Robinson and M. Foadi, *J. Am. med. Ass.*, 1969, *208*, 656.

For a comment on the risk of *aplastic anaemia* associated with methoin, see under Epilepsy, below.

Absorption and Fate. For an account of the absorption and fate of a hydantoin, see Phenytoin, p.1241.

Some of the side-effects of methoin may be due to the metabolite, 5-ethyl-5-phenylhydantoin (also termed nirvanol), the toxicity of which is recognised.

Metabolism and pharmacokinetics. Single-dose studies of the pharmacokinetics of methoin and ethotoin in epileptic subjects. Both methoin and ethotoin were readily absorbed but whereas the mean half-life of methoin in 5 subjects was estimated to be 6.8 hours and that of its active metabolite, 5-ethyl-5-phenylhydantoin to be 95.8 hours, the mean half-life of ethotoin in another 5 subjects was only 5.1 hours. Despite the report of O. Sjö *et al.* (*Clin. exp. Pharmac. Physiol.*, 1975, *2*, 185) dose dependency was not seen for ethotoin over a wide range of serum concentrations.— A. S. Troupin *et al.*, *Ann. Neurol.*, 1979, *6*, 410.

Plasma concentrations. Combined serum concentrations of methoin and its active metabolite, nirvanol, in the 25 to 40 µg per ml range are associated with good seizure control without clinical intoxication. Some patients will benefit from lower serum concentrations, or be able to tolerate higher concentrations, but with higher serum concentrations paradoxical intoxication, characterised by an increase in seizures without associated appreciable increase in anticonvulsant side-effects, is a possible complication.— A. S. Troupin *et al.*, *Epilepsia*, 1976, *17*, 403.

Uses. Methoin is a hydantoin anticonvulsant with actions and uses similar to those of phenytoin (p.1242), but it is more toxic. Because of its potential toxicity it is given only to patients unresponsive to other treatment.
Methoin is given in a daily divided dosage beginning with 50 to 100 mg and increasing by about 50 mg weekly until the optimum dose is reached, which is usually between 200 and 600 mg daily for an adult and 100 and 400 mg daily for a child.

Epilepsy. A retrospective evaluation of methoin in 93 epileptic out-patients. Side-effects frequently associated with phenytoin were absent, but drowsiness, an occasional rash, and a single, fatal case of aplastic anaemia were found. Performance on psychological tests of cognitive-attentional skills showed a modest improvement during methoin administration. It was considered that the drug merits wider employment in refractory seizure problems, but vigilant follow-up is required owing to the potential danger of aplastic anaemia.— A. S. Troupin *et al.*, *Epilepsia*, 1976, *17*, 403.

Preparations

Mephenytoin Tablets *(U.S.P.)*. Tablets containing methoin.

Methoin Tablets *(B.P. 1973)*. Tablets containing methoin.

Proprietary Names

Mesantoin *(Sandoz, Austral.; Sandoz, Canad.; Sandoz, Swed.; Sandoz, Switz.; Sandoz, USA)*; Sedantoinal *(Sandoz, Spain)*.

Methoin was formerly marketed in Great Britain under the proprietary name Mesontoin (*Sandoz*).

6614-d

Methsuximide *(U.S.P.)*. PM 396; Mesuximide. *N*,2-Dimethyl-2-phenylsuccinimide.
$C_{12}H_{13}NO_2$=203.2.

CAS — 77-41-8.

A white to greyish-white crystalline powder; odourless or with a slight odour. M.p. 50° to 56°. **Soluble** 1 in 350 of water, 1 in 3 of alcohol, 1 in less than 1 of chloroform, and 1 in 2 of ether. **Store** in airtight containers.

Stability. The kinetics of hydrolysis of methsuximide.— G. J. Yakatan and T. Fan, *Drug Dev. ind. Pharm.*, 1977, *3*, 315.

Adverse Effects, Treatment, and Precautions. Side-effects from methsuximide are similar to those described under Ethosuximide, p.1250; gastro-intestinal effects, drowsiness, ataxia, and dizziness are the most frequent. Periorbital hyperaemia, diplopia, insomnia, and sweating may occur. Erythema multiforme has been reported.

Effects on bones. In a 22-year-old woman, who had taken methsuximide 900 mg daily for 2 years then 450 mg daily for about 4 years, osteomalacia was confirmed by X-ray and metabolic studies. Dietary intake of vitamin D was normal and no other cause for the disease was evident. After discontinuation of methsuximide X-ray improvement was observed within 2 months.— C. J. Aponte and M. P. Petrelli (letter), *J. Am. med. Ass.*, 1973, *225*, 1248.

Interactions. For the effect of methsuximide on phenobarbitone, primidone, and phenytoin, see Phenytoin, p.1239.

Overdosage. An 18-year-old girl who ingested about 10 g of methsuximide was still deeply comatose 60 hours later though the plasma half-life of methsuximide was only 3 hours and the concentration at 64 hours was 2 µg per ml. However a metabolite of methsuximide, *N*-desmethylmethsuximide, was present in the serum in concentrations of 44 µg per ml at 14 hours and 38 µg per ml at 60 hours.— S. B. Karch, *J. Am. med. Ass.*, 1973, *223*, 1463. See also V. Gellman, *Manitoba med. Rev.*, 1965, *45*, 141.

Pregnancy and the neonate. Fatal haemorrhage developed shortly after birth in an infant whose mother had been treated with metharbital and methsuximide during pregnancy. The infant had been given phytomenadione after birth — W. A. Bleyer and A. L. Skinner, *J. Am. med. Ass.*, 1976, *235*, 626.

Absorption and Fate. Methsuximide is readily absorbed from the gastro-intestinal tract. Peak concentrations in plasma are reached in 1 to 4 hours. A half-life of 2.6 to 4 hours has been reported. Less than 1% of a dose has been reported to be recovered unchanged in the urine; metabolites have been detected.

In 17 patients taking methsuximide mean concentrations in plasma of the metabolite *N*-desmethylmethsuximide were 700 times those of the parent drug. The metabolite had anticonvulsant properties almost equal to those of the parent drug and was probably responsible for the therapeutic effect; concentrations below 10 µg per ml appeared to be ineffective and those above 40 µg per ml were toxic.— J. M. Strong *et al.*, *Neurology, Minneap.*, 1974, *24*, 250. See also R. J. Porter *et al.*, *ibid.*, 1977, *27*, 375; B. Rambeck, *Epilepsia*, 1979, *20*, 147.

A study in *dogs* of the pharmacokinetics of 2-methyl-2-phenylsuccinimide (*N*-desmethylmethsuximide) which is the major metabolite of methsuximide (obtained by *N*-demethylation).— M. R. Dobrinska and P. G. Welling, *J. pharm. Sci.*, 1977, *66*, 688.

Uses. Methsuximide is a succinimide anticonvulsant with general properties similar to those of ethosuximide (p.1251). It is less effective than ethosuximide in petit mal, but is also effective in psychomotor epilepsy.
The usual initial dosage is a single dose of 300 mg daily by mouth, and this is increased by 300 mg at weekly intervals to an optimum dosage, according to the patient's response. The suggested maximum daily dose is 1.2 g although daily doses of up to 3.6 g have been given. Children under the age of 6 years may be given 150 mg daily for the first week increased by 150 mg at weekly intervals to 1.2 g.

References: *Antiepileptic Drugs*, D.M. Woodbury *et al.* (Ed.), New York, Raven Press, 1972.

Preparations

Methsuximide Capsules *(U.S.P.)*. Capsules containing methsuximide. Store at a temperature not exceeding 40° in airtight containers.

Proprietary Names

Celontin *(Parke, Davis, Austral.; Parke, Davis, Belg.; Parke, Davis, Canad.; Parke, Davis, Ital.; Parke, Davis, S.Afr.; Parke, Davis, USA)*; Petinutin *(Parke, Davis, Ger.; Parke, Davis, Switz.)*.

Methsuximide was formerly marketed in Great Britain under the proprietary name Celontin (*Parke, Davis*).

6615-n

Paramethadione *(U.S.P., B.P. 1973)*. Paramethad. 5-Ethyl-3,5-dimethyloxazolidine-2,4-dione.
$C_7H_{11}NO_3$=157.2.

CAS — 115-67-3.

Pharmacopoeias. In *Ind.* and *U.S.*

A clear colourless liquid with a characteristic aromatic odour. Sparingly **soluble** in water; freely soluble in alcohol, chloroform, and ether. A 2.5% solution in water has a pH of 4 to 7.5. **Store** in airtight containers.

Adverse Effects, Treatment, and Precautions. As for Troxidone, p.1255.

Absorption and Fate. Like troxidone (see p.1256), paramethadione is readily absorbed from the gastro-intestinal tract and is metabolised to an active *N*-demethylated metabolite which is slowly excreted in the urine.

Serum concentrations of paramethadione and its major metabolite 5-ethyl-5-methyl-2,4-oxazolidinedione were measured after a single dose of 300 mg in 3 healthy fasted subjects. Paramethadione was rapidly absorbed and metabolised; a mean peak serum concentration of 6 µg per ml was achieved at 1 hour and decreased to 0.3 µg per ml at 48 hours. The metabolite was detectable within 1 hour and serum concentrations gradually increased to 8.4 µg per ml at 32 hours.— D. J. Hoffman and A. H. C. Chun, *J. pharm. Sci.*, 1975, *64*, 1702.

Uses. Paramethadione is an oxazolidinedione anticonvulsant with actions and uses similar to those of troxidone (p.1256).
The initial dose of paramethadione is 900 mg daily in divided doses, increased by steps of 300 mg at intervals of one week, according to the patient's response, to 1.8 g daily in divided doses; sources in the USA state a maximum dose of 2.4 g daily. Suggested initial doses of paramethadione for children are: less than 2 years of age, 300 mg daily; 2 to 6 years, 600 mg daily.

Preparations

Paramethadione Capsules *(B.P. 1973)*. Capsules containing paramethadione.

Paramethadione Capsules *(U.S.P.)*. Capsules containing paramethadione. Store in airtight containers.

Paramethadione Oral Solution *(U.S.P.)*. A solution in dilute alcohol (63 to 67%) containing 282 to 318 mg of paramethadione in each ml. Store in airtight containers. Protect from light.

Proprietary Preparations

Paradione *(Abbott, UK)*. Paramethadione, available as capsules of 300 mg. (Also available as Paradione in *Austral., Belg., Canad., Fr., USA*).

6616-h

Phenacemide *(U.S.P.)*. Phenacemidum; Carbamidum Phenylaceticum. (Phenylacetyl)urea.
$C_9H_{10}N_2O_2$=178.2.

CAS — 63-98-9.

Pharmacopoeias. In *Pol.* and *U.S.*

An odourless or almost odourless, tasteless, white or almost white, crystalline powder. M.p. about 213°. Very slightly **soluble** in water, alcohol, chloroform, and ether; slightly soluble in acetone and methyl alcohol. **Store** in airtight containers.

Adverse Effects. Adverse effects associated with phenacemide include nausea, vomiting, anorexia, weight loss, headaches, drowsiness, dizziness, paraesthesia, skin rashes, liver and kidney damage, bone-marrow depression, and severe personality changes.

Effects on the kidneys. Greatly increased serum-creatinine concentrations in the absence of elevated blood-urea-nitrogen values or any other evidence of renal disease occurred in 3 patients receiving phenacemide and other anticonvulsants for uncontrollable psychomotor epilepsy. Similar results were found in *rats* and *rabbits* given phenacemide.— R. K. Richards *et al.*, *Clin. Pharmac. Ther.*, 1978, *23*, 430.

Precautions. Phenacemide should be avoided in severe renal or hepatic disease. It should be used with extreme caution in patients with a history of personality disorders. Extreme caution is also necessary if phenacemide is given with any anticonvulsant known to cause similar side-effects; in particular paranoid symptoms have been reported in patients receiving phenacemide concomitantly with ethotoin.
Urine tests and tests of liver function should be made before and during treatment with phenacemide. Frequent blood counts should be carried out, particularly in the initial stages of therapy, and patients receiving phenacemide should be instructed to report immediately symptoms of infection or bleeding tendency, such as sore throat or easy bruising.

Absorption and Fate. Phenacemide is readily absorbed from the gastro-intestinal tract, and extensively metabolised in the liver to inactive metabolites which are excreted in the urine.
It has been reported to have a duration of action of about 5 hours following a single dose.

Uses. Phenacemide is an acetylurea anticonvulsant used in the treatment of epilepsy, especially in the psychomotor type of seizure; it is of less value in grand mal or petit mal or in mixed seizures. It should be employed only in patients whose seizures are impossible to control with other recognised anticonvulsants.
The dosage of phenacemide is usually 500 mg thrice daily, this dose being gradually increased until the symptoms are adequately controlled. The average dose for adults seldom exceeds 2 to 3 g daily. For children 5 to 10 years old, half the adult dose is given.
Withdrawal of phenacemide or transition to or from another type of therapy should be made gradually to avoid precipitating an increase in the frequency of seizures.

Preparations

Phenacemide Tablets *(U.S.P.)*. Tablets containing phenacemide.

Proprietary Names
Phenurone *(Abbott, USA)*; Phetylureum *(Katwijk, Neth.)*.

6617-m

Pheneturide. Ethylphenacemide; S 46. (2-Phenylbutyryl)urea.
$C_{11}H_{14}N_2O_2$=206.2.

CAS — 90-49-3.

A white crystalline powder. Practically **insoluble** in water and ether; slightly soluble in alcohol; very soluble in acetic acid.

Adverse Effects. Pheneturide was reported to be less likely to cause toxic effects than phenacemide (see above), to which it is chemically related. Side-effects associated with pheneturide include anorexia, ataxia, leucopenia, rashes, and increase in serum alkaline phosphatase. Increase in existing personality disturbances has been reported. Aplastic anaemia has also been reported.

Investigations in a total of 403 patients showed that the mean serum-calcium concentration in patients receiving pheneturide 550 mg daily was significantly lower than in patients receiving other anticonvulsants. The mean serum-folate concentration was also significantly lower in patients receiving pheneturide, while the 24-hour urinary output of D-glucaric acid, measured as an index of liver enzyme induction, was highest in this group.— A. N. Latham *et al.*, *J. clin. Pharmac.*, 1973, *13*, 337.

A syndrome resembling systemic lupus erythematosus might occur during therapy with pheneturide.— *Adverse Drug React. Bull.*, 1973, Dec., 140.

A 23-year-old epileptic who had been taking phenobarbitone and phenytoin developed generalised pruritus 3 weeks after phenytoin was replaced by pheneturide; vesiculation, exfoliation, lymphadenopathy, and splenomegaly followed. The condition regressed when pheneturide was withdrawn and prednisolone was given.— J. W. Rassam and G. Anderson (letter), *Br. med. J.*, 1975, *2*, 139.

Precautions. Pheneturide should be avoided in severe renal or hepatic disease.

Interactions. For the effect of pheneturide on *phenytoin*, see p.1239.

Pregnancy and the neonate. For a general comment on epilepsy and pregnancy and references to surveys on the incidence of congenital malformations in the infants of epileptic women, see p.1235.

Uses. Pheneturide is an acetylurea anticonvulsant which has been used in the treatment of grand mal and psychomotor epilepsy. It was reported to have a slight stimulant action.

The suggested adult dose was 0.6 to 1 g daily. Suggested doses for children were: 6 months to 2 years, 50 mg daily; 2 to 5 years, 100 to 200 mg daily; 6 to 10 years, 200 to 600 mg daily.

A study of the pharmacokinetics of pheneturide. It was concluded that the disposition of pheneturide follows one-compartment first-order kinetics. Pheneturide is completely metabolised and may induce its own metabolism. Because of its slow absorption and long half-life (a mean of 8 and 54 hours respectively; mean clearance 2.5 litres per hour), a daily dosage regimen results in a continuous steady-state concentration with almost no fluctuations.— R. L. Galeazzi *et al.*, *J. Pharmacokinet. Biopharm.*, 1979, *7*, 453.

Epilepsy. Forty-four patients with psychomotor epilepsy unresponsive to other drugs were treated for 5 to 48 months with pheneturide in a dose of 200 mg daily, increasing by 200 mg every 4 days to 200 mg thrice daily and, if necessary, 4 or 5 times daily. Complete control of seizures was obtained in 9 patients, reduced frequency in 7, but no change occurred in 14. Side-effects, most frequently drowsiness and ataxia, necessitated withdrawal of the treatment from 14 patients. Raised alkaline phosphatase activity was found in 7 patients.— C. J. Vas and M. J. Parsonage, *Acta neurol. scand.*, 1967, *43*, 580, per *Abstr. Wld Med.*, 1968, *42*, 537.

A 12-month retrospective study of 30 children with epilepsy showed that the addition of pheneturide to their therapy in an initial dosage of 100 mg twice or thrice daily increasing to 200 mg twice or thrice daily reduced the frequency of fits.— J. C. Bowe and B. J. Shersby, *Br. J. clin. Pract.*, 1973, *27*, 174.

Regret at the withdrawal of pheneturide from sale and supply in Great Britain.— P. K. P. Harvey *et al.* (letter), *Br. med. J.*, 1979, *2*, 444.

Proprietary Names
Benuride *(Sapos, Switz.)*.

Pheneturide was formerly marketed in Great Britain under the proprietary name Benuride (*Bengué*). A preparation containing pheneturide, phenytoin, and phenobarbitone was formerly marketed under the proprietary name Trinuride (*Bengué*).

6618-b

Phensuximide *(B.P.C. 1973, U.S.P.)*. Fensuximid. *N*-Methyl-2-phenylsuccinimide.
$C_{11}H_{11}NO_2$=189.2.

CAS — 86-34-0.

Pharmacopoeias. In *Cz.*, *Nord.*, and *U.S.*

A white to off-white, odourless or almost odourless, tasteless, crystalline powder. M.p. 68° to 74°. **Soluble** 1 in 250 of water, 1 in 20 of alcohol, 1 in 1.5 of chloroform, and 1 in 35 of ether. **Store** in airtight containers.

Stability. The kinetics of hydrolysis of phensuximide.— G. J. Yakatan and T. Fan, *Drug Dev. ind. Pharm.*, 1977, *3*, 315.

Adverse Effects, Treatment, and Precautions. As for Ethosuximide, p.1250.

Anorexia, nausea, dizziness, and drowsiness are the most frequent side-effects. Urinary frequency and evidence of renal damage with haematuria has occurred occasionally.

Effects on the blood. A woman taking phensuximide 500 mg six times daily together with phenobarbitone showed signs of megaloblastic anaemia after 10 weeks. It responded to folic acid. The patient had a previous history which indicated that her bone marrow was unduly sensitive to anticonvulsant drugs.— A. Doig and J. B. Stanton, *Br. med. J.*, 1961, *2*, 998.

Absorption and Fate. Phensuximide is readily absorbed from the gastro-intestinal tract. Peak concentrations in plasma are reached in 1 to 4 hours. The half-life in plasma appears to be about 4 hours. It is excreted in the urine and in the bile. About 27% of a dose has been recovered from the urine chiefly as the *p*-hydroxyphenyl derivative.

Uses. Phensuximide is a succinimide anticonvulsant with actions similar to, but less potent than, those of ethosuximide. It is used in the treatment of petit mal.

The initial daily dose for adults and children of 6 years of age and older is 0.5 to 1 g in divided doses increasing by 500 mg daily at intervals of 2 or 3 weeks to a total not exceeding 3 g daily. For children up to 6 years of age the usual initial dose is 250 mg twice daily increasing by 250 mg at intervals of 2 to 3 weeks to 1.5 g daily.

References: *Antiepileptic Drugs*, D.M. Woodbury *et al.* (Ed.), New York, Raven Press, 1972.

Preparations

Phensuximide Capsules *(B.P.C. 1973)*. Capsules containing phensuximide.

Phensuximide Capsules *(U.S.P.)*. Capsules containing phensuximide. Store in airtight containers.

Phensuximide Oral Suspension *(U.S.P.)*. A suspension containing phensuximide. Store in airtight containers.

Proprietary Names
Milontin *(Parke, Davis, Austral.; Parke, Davis, Canad.; Parke, Davis, USA)*; Succitimal *(Katwijk, Neth.)*.

6619-v

Primidone *(B.P., B.P. Vet., U.S.P.)*. Primidon.; Primidonum; Hexamidinum; Primaclone. 5-Ethylperhydro-5-phenylpyrimidine-4,6-dione.
$C_{12}H_{14}N_2O_2$=218.3.

CAS — 125-33-7.

NOTE. The name Hexamidine is also applied to a compound with antibacterial and fungistatic properties, see p.567.

Pharmacopoeias. In *Arg.*, *Br.*, *Braz.*, *Chin.*, *Ind.*, *Int.*, *Jap.*, *Jug.*, *Nord.*, *Pol.*, *Rus.*, *Turk.*, and *U.S.*

A white odourless crystalline powder with a slightly bitter taste. M.p. 279° to 284°. **Soluble** 1 in 2000 of water and 1 in 170 of alcohol; practically insoluble in most other organic solvents.

Adverse Effects. Undesirable side-effects caused by primidone are drowsiness, ataxia, nausea, vomiting, vertigo, irritability, headache, visual disturbances, and general malaise or fatigue, and occasionally skin eruptions; they are usually transitory or mild and may disappear with continued therapy, possibly with reduced dosage.

Adverse effects which occur only rarely include personality changes, oedema, thirst, polyuria, and impaired sexual function. Serious toxic reactions are rare but megaloblastic anaemia has been reported; it usually responds to treatment with folic acid, there being no necessity to discontinue primidone therapy.

Leucopenia and thrombocytopenia have been reported rarely.

See also under Phenobarbitone, p.812.

A 71-year-old man who took primidone 750 mg daily for 4 years developed lymphadenopathy, megaloblastic anaemia, and thyroid enlargement. Primidone was stopped and phenobarbitone, folic acid, and ferrous sulphate administered. The anaemia responded to the folic acid and iron. The lymph nodes were smaller within a week of stopping primidone and 2 weeks later they were not palpable. The thyroid remained slightly enlarged even after 9 months.— A. O. Langlands *et al.*, *Br. med. J.*, 1967, *1*, 215. A study on the influence of primidone on thyroid function in 30 children receiving long-term treatment indicated that according to the TRH test the children were euthyroid although primidone may stimulate hepatocellular thyroxine breakdown.— W. Schönberger *et al.*, *Dt. med. Wschr.*, 1979, *104*, 915.

Effects on the blood. *Thrombocytopenia* occurred in 1 patient in association with the ingestion of primidone.— W. A. Parker (letter), *Ann. intern. Med.*, 1974, *81*, 559.

Primidone has been reported to cause *aplastic anaemia*.— R. H. Girdwood, *Drugs*, 1976, *11*, 394.

Effects on the nervous system. Severe flapping tremor, resembling uraemic encephalopathy, with drowsiness and cerebellar signs, was associated with high serum-primidone concentrations in an epileptic woman with poor renal function. The metabolites of primidone, phenobarbitone and phenylethylmalonamide were not considered to be implicated because the condition resolved before their blood concentrations dropped. Although the woman had also been prescribed cimetidine 6 weeks previously this drug has not been associated with a flapping tremor.— M. B. Forman *et al.* (letter), *Lancet*, 1979, *2*, 1250.

Effects on the skin. A 70-year-old woman in whom primidone had precipitated toxic epidermal necrolysis developed the condition again a year later when she was inadvertently given 300 mg of phenobarbitone.— G. Stüttgen, *Br. J. Derm.*, 1973, *88*, 291.

Lupus erythematosus. Symptoms resembling those of systemic lupus erythematosus developed in a woman taking primidone, 500 mg thrice daily. She improved when the treatment was withdrawn.— G. K. Ahuja and G. A. Schumacher, *J. Am. med. Ass.*, 1966, *198*, 669.

Overdosage. In 2 cases of acute primidone toxicity due to overdosage the CNS depression and dysequilibrium were considered due to primidone rather than to the metabolite phenobarbitone. In one patient a urine specimen contained masses of shimmering white crystals; the crystalluria persisted during the first 24 hours after admission; crystalluria may be useful in identifying primidone overdosage.— J. Brillman *et al.*, *Archs Neurol., Chicago*, 1974, *30*, 255.

Further references to primidone overdosage.— M. S. Kappy and J. Buckley, *Archs Dis. Childh.*, 1969, *44*, 282; D. N. Bailey and P. I. Jatlow, *Am. J. clin. Path.*, 1972, *58*, 583 (massive crystalluria); J. C. Cate and R. Tenser, *Clin. Toxicol.*, 1975, *8*, 385.

Pregnancy and the neonate. A report of possible primidone embryopathy in 2 siblings born to an epileptic mother who took primidone during both pregnancies.— N. L. Rudd and R. M. Freedom, *J. Pediat.*, 1979, *94*, 835.

The neonate. A mother who had taken primidone 250 mg twice daily throughout pregnancy gave birth to an infant who showed abnormal tremor for several days. Primidone was present in the blood and urine of the infant.— G. Martinez and R. D. Snyder, *Neurology, Minneap.*, 1973, *23*, 381.

For a general comment on epilepsy and pregnancy, and

references to surveys on the incidence of congenital malformations in the infants of epileptic women, see p.1235, and for a study demonstrating an increased incidence of vitamin-K responsive coagulation defect in the infants of mothers given barbiturates or drugs which metabolise to barbiturates, see p.1238. See also under Phenobarbitone, p.814.

Treatment of Adverse Effects. As for Phenobarbitone, p.812.

Precautions. As for Phenobarbitone, p.813.
Conversion of primidone to phenobarbitone may be inhibited by concomitant administration of isoniazid, and acetazolamide may reduce the absorption of primidone.
Since induction of the foetal liver enzyme system may result in vitamin-K deficiency, vitamin-K supplements may be given for the last month of pregnancy to minimise the risk of haemorrhage in the newborn.

Administration in hepatic failure. For a report of coma in a patient receiving phenobarbitone and primidone who developed acute hepatitis, see Phenobarbitone, p.813.

Interactions. *Anticonvulsants.* Initially raised serum-primidone concentrations on concomitant administration of *sodium valproate*.— A. Windorfer *et al.*, *Acta paediat. scand.*, 1975, *64*, 771.

In a study of 58 patients neither age nor sex had a significant effect on the dose of primidone required to produce a given plasma-phenobarbitone concentration. Plasma-phenobarbitone concentrations were significantly increased in 52 and 13 patients also taking *phenytoin* or *carbamazepine* respectively.— M. J. Eadie *et al.*, *Br. J. clin. Pharmac.*, 1977, *4*, 541. The concentration of serum-phenobarbitone increased in a 16-year-old epileptic taking phenytoin and primidone, when the dose of phenytoin was increased. When the primidone dose was raised, serum-phenobarbitone concentration rose further and the patient became drowsy. Serum-phenytoin concentrations reached toxic values. After phenytoin was withdrawn for 3 days and the dose lowered, serum concentrations of phenytoin and phenobarbitone declined.— L. K. Garrettson and M. Gomez (letter), *Br. J. clin. Pharmac.*, 1977, *4*, 693. See also E. H. Reynolds *et al.*, *Br. med. J.*, 1975, *2*, 594. For a study in children suggesting that phenytoin has no effect on primidone metabolism, see under Absorption and Fate (below).

In 2 of 3 patients studied there was evidence of an interaction between *acetazolamide* and primidone. It was considered that acetazolamide might interfere with the absorption of primidone in susceptible patients. In one of the patients peak serum concentrations were merely delayed but in the other both primidone and its metabolites were nearly undetectable, after administration of primidone with acetazolamide.— G. B. Syversen *et al.*, *Archs Neurol., Chicago*, 1977, *34*, 80.

For the effect of *methsuximide* on primidone, see Phenytoin, p.1239.

Corticosteroids. For the effect of primidone on corticosteroids, see Corticosteroids, p.450.

Diuretics. For an interaction with acetazolamide, see under Anticonvulsants, above.

Tuberculostatics. Inhibition of primidone metabolism by *isoniazid* in one patient.— G. Sutton and A. J. Kupferberg, *Neurology, Minneap.*, 1975, *25*, 1179.

For other details of drug interactions relevant to primidone, see Phenobarbitone, p.813.

Absorption and Fate. Primidone is readily absorbed from the gastro-intestinal tract and is reported to have a relatively short plasma half-life of about 10 hours, compared with those of its principal metabolites, phenylethylmalonamide (estimated to have a plasma half-life in the region of 24 to 48 hours) and phenobarbitone (see p.814).
Although primidone and phenylethylmalonamide have been shown to have anticonvulsant properties in *animals* their role in the management of epilepsy, compared with that of phenobarbitone, is unclear. In patients receiving primidone, therefore, plasma-phenobarbitone concentrations are generally used to monitor therapy.
Whereas phenobarbitone is fairly extensively bound to plasma proteins, primidone and phenylethylmalonamide are negligibly bound.
Primidone crosses the blood-brain and the placental barriers and is excreted in breast milk.

Metabolism and pharmacokinetics. In 6 healthy volunteers given primidone 500 mg in the fasting state the half-life of primidone was 10 to 12 hours. No phenobarbitone was detected in the serum within 48 hours but all the volunteers had side-effects which included giddiness, drowsiness, nystagmus, lack of concentration, and slurred speech. In 30 patients taking primidone but no barbiturate the mean serum-primidone concentration was 9.2 µg per ml and the mean serum-phenobarbitone concentration was 31 µg per ml. Serum concentrations of primidone increased progressively from a mean of 3.2 to a mean of 14.7 µg per ml with increasing daily doses from 0.25 to 1.25 g.— H. E. Booker *et al.*, *Epilepsia*, 1970, *11*, 395.

There was significant correlation between brain and plasma concentrations of primidone in 8 patients with epilepsy undergoing temporal lobectomy, 6 of whom had received primidone and 2 of whom had received phenobarbitone, together with other anticonvulsant therapy prior to operation. The brain : plasma ratios varied from 0.35 : 1 to 0.91 : 1.— F. Vajda *et al.*, *Clin. Pharmac. Ther.*, 1974, *15*, 597.

A study of the kinetics of primidone metabolism and excretion in 12 children aged 7 to 14 years during long-term administration. Results indicated that the plasma half-life of primidone does not differ from that in adults and simultaneous administration of phenytoin has no detectable effect on the primidone half-life or the mean serum concentrations of phenobarbitone. An average of about 5% appeared to be metabolised to phenobarbitone which agreed with *animal* studies but was lower than the estimate of O.V. Olesen and M. Dam (*Acta neurol. scand.*, 1967, *43*, 348) of 24.5% in adult patients. The rate of metabolism of primidone to phenobarbitone appeared to be variable which might explain therapeutic and toxicity problems in some patients.— R. E. Kauffman *et al.*, *Clin. Pharmac. Ther.*, 1977, *22*, 200.

Plasma concentrations. Most of the anticonvulsant activity of primidone rests with phenobarbitone and therefore measuring phenobarbitone will give the best estimate of the drug's effect.— A. Richens and S. Warrington, *Drugs*, 1979, *17*, 488.

Saliva concentrations. It seems likely that saliva can be used for indirect estimation of the plasma-primidone concentration, but whether saliva is a useful fluid for monitoring primidone therapy depends very much on the reliability of salivary-phenobarbitone concentration measurements.— M. Danhof and D. D. Breimer, *Clin. Pharmacokinet.*, 1978, *3*, 39.

Pregnancy and the neonate. Decreased blood concentrations of primidone and phenobarbitone were noted during pregnancy in a woman receiving primidone and carbamazepine; they rose again after delivery. A similar effect was not noted for carbamazepine. Both drugs achieved concentrations in the breast milk of less than half that in the maternal serum and the woman observed no difference in the infant's behaviour during and after breast feeding for 5 weeks.— J. R. Niebyl *et al.*, *Obstet. Gynec.*, 1979, *53*, 139.

See also under Phenytoin, p.1241.

Uses. Primidone is an anticonvulsant which is partially metabolised to phenobarbitone and is used in the treatment of grand mal and psychomotor or partial (focal) seizures.
For adults and for children over 9 years, the initial dosage is usually 125 to 250 mg daily increased by 125 to 250 mg at intervals of 3 to 7 days to a usual dose of 0.75 to 1.5 g daily, with a maximum of 2 g daily. Children up to 2 years are usually maintained on 250 to 500 mg daily, children aged 2 to 5 years on 500 to 750 mg daily, and children aged 6 to 9 years on 0.75 to 1 g daily.
The daily dosage is usually divided into 2 amounts, given morning and evening.
Withdrawal of primidone or transition to or from another type of anticonvulsant therapy should be made gradually to avoid precipitating an increase in the frequency of seizures.

A detailed review of primidone: *Antiepileptic Drugs*, D.M. Woodbury *et al.* (Ed.), New York, Raven Press, 1972.

Administration in hepatic failure. See under Precautions, above.

Administration in renal failure. The interval between doses of primidone should be extended from 8 hours to 8 to 12 hours in patients with a glomerular filtration-rate of 10 to 50 ml per minute, and to 12 to 24 hours in those with a glomerular filtration-rate of less than 10 ml per minute. Concentrations of primidone were affected by haemodialysis.— W. M. Bennett *et al.*, *Ann. intern. Med.*, 1977, *86*, 754. See also *idem*, 1980, *93*, 286.

Cardiac disorders. A report of a woman with the long QT syndrome and a temporal lobe seizure, in whom primidone has been successful in suppressing potentially lethal arrhythmias during a 2-year follow-up. Primidone also shortened the QT interval in 2 affected relatives, and further clinical investigations are considered warranted.— D. L. DeSilvey and A. J. Moss, *Ann. intern. Med.*, 1980, *93*, 53.

Epilepsy. A crossover study aimed at detecting differences between primidone and phenobarbitone. Fourteen of 21 epileptic subjects experienced fewer tonic-clonic seizures on primidone than on phenobarbitone, 4 had more frequent attacks, and the remainder no change. Primidone was superior to phenobarbitone in controlling this type of seizure, but there was no significant difference in the frequency of the minor (partial and absence) attacks on the 2 treatments.— J. Oxley *et al.*, *Br. J. clin. Pharmac.*, 1979, *7*, 414P.

Further references to primidone in epilepsy.— E. A. Rodin *et al.*, *J. nerv. ment. Dis.*, 1976, *163*, 41 (comparison with carbamazepine).

For comments on the role of primidone in epilepsy, see Phenytoin, p.1243.

Tremor. Successful treatment of benign familial tremor (essential tremor) in 12 patients with primidone; the effect was considered largely due to phenylethylmalonamide.— M. D. O'Brien *et al.*, *Br. med. J.*, 1981, *282*, 178. Comments.— L. J. Findley *et al.* (letter), *ibid.*, *283*, 234; G. Procaccianti *et al.* (letter), *ibid.*, 558.

Preparations

Primidone Mixture *(B.P.)*. Primidone Suspension. A suspension of primidone in a suitable flavoured vehicle. When a dose less than, or not a multiple of, 5 ml is prescribed, the mixture should be diluted to 5 ml, or a multiple, with syrup. Such dilutions must be freshly prepared and not used more than 2 weeks after issue. A diluted mixture which may be used wihin 3 months of preparation may be prepared by using a diluent of the following composition: methyl hydroxybenzoate 150 mg, propyl hydroxybenzoate 15 mg, carmellose sodium '50' 1 g, sucrose 20 g, freshly boiled and cooled water to 100 ml.

Primidone Oral Suspension *(U.S.P.)*. Contains 4.5 to 5.5% of primidone in a suitable aqueous vehicle; pH 5.5 to 7. Store in airtight containers. Protect from light.

Primidone Tablets *(B.P., U.S.P.)*. Tablets containing primidone.

Proprietary Preparations

Mysoline (known in some countries as Mylepsin and Mylepsinum) *(ICI Pharmaceuticals, UK)*. Primidone, available as **Suspension** containing 250 mg in each 5 ml (suggested diluent, as for Primidone Mixture) and as scored **Tablets** of 250 mg. (Also available as Mysoline in *Austral., Belg., Canad., Denm., Fr., Ital., Neth., Norw., S.Afr., Spain, Switz., USA*).

Other Proprietary Names

Dilon *(Arg.)*; Liskantin *(Ger.)*; Majsolin *(Jug.)*; Midone *(Austral.)*; Prosoline *(Israel)*; Resimatil *(Ger.)*; Sertan *(Canad.)*.

A preparation containing primidone and phenytoin sodium was formerly marketed in Great Britain under the proprietary name Mysoline with Phenytoin Tablets *(ICI Pharmaceuticals)*.

6621-f

Sulthiame *(B.P.)*. Sultiame. 4-(Tetrahydro-2*H*-1,2-thiazin-2-yl)benzenesulphonamide *SS*-dioxide.
$C_{10}H_{14}N_2O_4S_2$=290.4.

CAS — 61-56-3.

Pharmacopoeias. In *Br.*

A white odourless crystalline powder with a slightly bitter taste. M.p. 185° to 188°. **Soluble** 1 in 2000 of water, 1 in 350 of alcohol, 1 in 700 of chloroform, and 1 in 500 of ether; readily soluble in alkaline solutions.

Adverse Effects. Toxic effects from sulthiame which have been most frequently reported are ataxia, anorexia, and paraesthesias of the face and extremities; hyperpnoea and dyspnoea provoked by metabolic acidosis occur frequently, especially in children. Headache, giddiness, nausea, loss of weight, and psychic changes also occur. Abdominal pain, depression, skin rash, drooling, increased frequency of fits, insomnia, leucopenia, and

status epilepticus have also been reported.
Overdosage is associated with crystalluria.

The administration of sulthiame to 54 patients produced the following severe and prolonged side-effects in some patients: ataxia, drowsiness, confusion, headache, psychotic reactions, vertigo, dysarthria, blurring of vision, nausea or vomiting, insomnia, dyspnoea, paraesthesias, papular rash, and ptosis. In other patients, the effects were transitory.— H. Garland and D. Sumner, *Br. med. J.*, 1964, *1*, 474. All but 6 of the patients were also taking primidone. It appeared that the concomitant use of sulthiame and primidone could lead to severe side-effects.— *idem*, 1043. Experience of sulthiame in children under the age of 12 years had shown that side-effects had been neither so severe nor so frequent as those described in adult patients by Garland and Sumner (see above). Ataxia, confusion, headache, dysarthria, or blurring of vision attributable to sulthiame had not occurred.— T. T. S. Ingram (letter), *ibid.*, 769.

Side-effects in a long-term trial of sulthiame included loss of weight in 37 patients, ataxia, drowsiness, and paraesthesias.— M. C. Liu, *Br. J. Psychiat.*, 1966, *112*, 621.

Effects on the kidneys. A 24-year-old male epileptic received, for 3 months, 400 mg daily of sulthiame in addition to his usual treatment with phenytoin sodium and phenobarbitone. He developed acute renal failure which gradually remitted. A biopsy specimen showed many proximal convoluted tubules with necrosis and sloughing of the tubular epithelium.— A. Aviram *et al.* (letter), *Lancet*, 1965, *1*, 818.

Erythema multiforme. A 14-year-old boy developed the Stevens-Johnson syndrome after 6 months' treatment with sulthiame.— A. Taaffe and C. O'Brien, *Br. dent. J.*, 1975, *138*, 172.

Overdosage. A 17-year-old boy who attempted suicide by swallowing about 4 g of sulthiame developed about 6 hours later symptoms of poisoning which included vomiting, severe headache, vertigo, ataxia, and hyperpnoea. Associated with the latter was a temporary rise in the urinary pH which probably prevented serious crystalluria and renal damage.— G. J. Rockley, *Br. med. J.*, 1965, *2*, 632.

A 43-year-old man who was given phenytoin, primidone, and sulthiame for epilepsy secondary to cortical atrophy, attempted suicide by taking approximately 100 sulthiame tablets. Though an alcoholic, the patient had not taken alcohol beforehand. He recovered completely in less than 24 hours during which time he showed marked but transient catatonia, hypotension, and some disorientation.— L. J. Mykyta, *Med. J. Aust.*, 1968, *2*, 118.

A 21-year-old woman who took 4 g of sulthiame developed symptoms of metabolic acidosis together with hyperventilation. She was successfully treated with intravenous infusions of dextrose with 300 mmol (300 mEq) of sodium bicarbonate given over 24 hours.— G. Stockdill and A. R. Lorimer, *Br. J. clin. Pract.*, 1971, *25*, 331.

Pregnancy and the neonate. Sulthiame did not appear to have been implicated as a cause of malformation in the foetus.— *Br. med. J.*, 1973, *1*, 796.

Treatment of Adverse Effects. In acute poisoning the stomach should be emptied by emesis or by aspiration and lavage. The urine should be rendered alkaline to prevent crystalluria. Forced alkaline diuresis may hasten the elimination of sulthiame (for details, see Phenobarbitone, p.812).

Precautions. Sulthiame should be used with caution in patients with renal disease.
Plasma concentrations of phenobarbitone and phenytoin are increased by concomitant administration of sulthiame.

Interactions. For the effect of sulthiame on *phenobarbitone*, see Phenobarbitone, p.814, and for the effect on *phenytoin*, see Phenytoin, p.1239.

Interference with diagnostic tests. Sulthiame might interfere with estimation of barbiturates in the blood.— J. Millhouse, *Adverse Drug React. Bull.*, 1974, Dec., 164.

Absorption and Fate. Sulthiame is readily absorbed from the gastro-intestinal tract and is excreted chiefly in the urine.

In 5 subjects given radioactive sulthiame excretion was chiefly in the urine. About 60% of excreted material was unchanged sulthiame; a metabolite without anticonvulsant properties was also present.— S. Diamond and L. Levy, *Curr. ther. Res.*, 1963, *5*, 325.

In 4 patients receiving long-term sulthiame treatment peak concentrations in serum occurred 1 to 5 hours after a dose. In 36 patients who had taken 3 to 14.5 mg per kg body-weight daily for at least 6 months concentrations in serum ranged from 0.5 to 12.5 μg per ml. In 27 patients 17 to 69% (mean 32%) of the dose was recovered unchanged in the urine in 24 hours.— O. V. Olesen, *Acta pharmac. tox.*, 1968, *26*, 22.

Uses. Sulthiame is a carbonic anhydrase inhibitor which is used as an anticonvulsant in all forms of epilepsy except petit mal. It is usually given in conjunction with other anticonvulsants.
Sulthiame is given in initial doses of 100 mg twice daily gradually increased to 200 mg thrice daily. A suggested dose for children is 3 to 5 mg per kg body-weight daily in equal divided doses, gradually increased to 10 to 15 mg per kg daily in equal divided doses.

Behaviour disorders. In a double-blind crossover study in 42 patients (aged 6 to 38 years) with severe behaviour disorders, sulthiame 300 to 600 mg daily reduced the incidence, but not the type, of disturbed behaviour. It did not affect the frequency of seizures in 25 epileptic patients who continued to take their previous anticonvulsants.— W. R. Moffat *et al.*, *Br. J. Psychiat.*, 1970, *117*, 673.

Epilepsy. Of 55 patients with temporal lobe epilepsy treated with phenytoin, 45 obtained a large measure of control when sulthiame in daily dosages of 200 to 800 mg was added to their anticonvulsant therapy. Three patients showed no significant improvement. Minor side-effects, including paraesthesia and gastric symptoms, occurred initially in about one-third of the patients, and the severity of these effects caused withdrawal of sulthiame therapy in 7 patients.— P. Mann *et al.*, *Med. J. Aust.*, 1967, *2*, 729. See also M. C. Liu, *Br. J. Psychiat.*, 1966, *112*, 621.

Acetazolamide and sulthiame are carbonic anhydrase inhibitors and are moderately effective against the tonic-extensor phase of maximal electroshock seizures in *rodents*, but ineffective against threshold pentetrazol seizures. Acetazolamide is transiently effective in children against generalised seizures (absences). Sulthiame probably owes much of its clinical effectiveness to inhibition of the hepatic metabolism of other anticonvulsant drugs given concurrently.— B. S. Meldrum, Mode of Action of Anticonvulsant Drugs: Biochemical Effects, in *The Treatment of Epilepsy*, J.H. Tyrer *et al.* (Ed.), Lancaster, England, MTP Press, 1980.

Preparations

Sulthiame Tablets *(B.P.)*. Tablets containing sulthiame. They are film-coated.

Ospolot *(Bayer, UK)*. Sulthiame, available as **Suspension** containing 50 mg in each 5 ml (suggested diluent, for short-term storage, tragacanth mucilage), as **Tablets** of 50 mg, and as scored tablets of 200 mg. (Also available as Ospolot in *Austral., Denm., Ger., Ital., Neth., S.Afr., Spain*).

6622-d

Troxidone *(B.P.)*. Troxid.; Trimethadione *(U.S.P.)*; Trimethadionum; Trimethinum. 3,5,5-Trimethyloxazolidine-2,4-dione.

$C_6H_9NO_3$=143.1.

CAS — 127-48-0.

Pharmacopoeias. In *Braz., Br., Cz., Fr., Ind., Int., It., Jap., Mex., Neth., Nord., Rus., Turk.*, and *U.S.*

Colourless or white granular crystals with a slightly camphoraceous odour. M.p. 45° to 47°. **Soluble** 1 in 13 of water and 1 in 2 of alcohol; freely soluble in chloroform and ether. A 4.22% solution in water is iso-osmotic with serum. **Store** in a cool place in airtight containers.

An aqueous solution of troxidone iso-osmotic with serum (4.22%) caused 100% haemolysis of erythrocytes cultured in it for 45 minutes.— E. R. Hammarlund and K. Pedersen-Bjergaard, *J. pharm. Sci.*, 1961, *50*, 24.

Adverse Effects. Many adverse effects of troxidone are serious and call for prompt discontinuation of therapy. Common side-effects include drowsiness, which may subside on continuation of therapy, and photophobia and hemeralopia (blurring of vision in bright light), which is more frequent in adults and may respond to reduced dosage.
Other side-effects include nausea and vomiting, gastric distress, abdominal pain, anorexia, weight loss, hiccups, malaise, insomnia, vertigo, headache, alopecia, paraesthesias, changes in blood pressure, precipitation of grand mal seizures, and personality changes. Blood disorders include neutropenia (which does not call for withdrawal of therapy providing it remains moderate), thrombocytopenia, pancytopenia, agranulocytosis, and aplastic anaemia. Lymphadenopathy, a lupus erythematosus syndrome, the nephrotic syndrome, and hepatitis may also occur. Skin rashes may lead to exfoliative dermatitis and erythema multiforme. A syndrome resembling myasthenia gravis has also been reported.
Characteristic congenital malformations have been associated with the use of troxidone in pregnancy.
Symptoms of acute overdosage include drowsiness, nausea, dizziness, ataxia, visual disturbances, and coma.

Pseudolymphoma developed in a patient taking paramethadione and phenobarbitone, and in a second patient taking troxidone and phenytoin.— N. A. Bercel and H. H. Henstell, *Bull. Los Ang. neurol. Soc.*, 1970, *35*, 21, per *Clin. Med.*, 1971, *78* (Feb.), 44.

Effects on the kidneys. Of 12 children treated with troxidone, 8 showed microscopic urinary abnormalities, microscopic haematuria, and granular casts.— J. G. Millichap and B. H. Kirman, *Lancet*, 1953, *1*, 1074.

For a review of reports of the nephrotic syndrome due to troxidone and paramethadione and discussion of the treatment and prevention of the syndrome, see AMA Council on Drugs, *J. Am. med. Ass.*, 1967, *202*, 893. See also P. Kincaid-Smith, *Practitioner*, 1978, *220*, 862.

Effects on the skin. *Erythema multiforme* in a boy given troxidone and phenobarbitone.— J. L. Leblanc and A. Feldman, *Can. med. Ass. J.*, 1961, *85*, 200.

Troxidone might have been responsible for a case of *toxic epidermal necrolysis* in a boy proved post mortem to be suffering from encephalitis.— A. Lyell, *Br. J. Derm.*, 1967, *79*, 662.

Troxidone might cause a skin reaction resembling *lupus erythematosus*.— J. L. Verbov, *Br. J. clin. Pract.*, 1968, *22*, 229. See also D. H. Beernink and J. J. Miller, *J. Pediat.*, 1973, *82*, 113.

Myasthenia gravis. An 8-year-old girl with epilepsy developed a myasthenic reaction with weakness of bulbar and respiratory muscles during treatment with troxidone in a dosage of up to 1.8 g daily. Other medication consisted of methylphenobarbitone 64 mg daily and primidone 500 mg daily. A severe crisis with respiratory failure followed a major convulsion. She responded to edrophonium and neostigmine and remission was complete 6 months after troxidone had been withdrawn.— H. E. Booker *et al.*, *J. Am. med. Ass.*, 1970, *212*, 2262. See also H. de C. Peterson, *New Engl. J. Med.*, 1966, *274*, 506.

Pregnancy and the neonate. An account of the offspring of 3 mothers who took troxidone during pregnancy. The children were considered to have a specific phenotype associated with intra-uterine exposure to troxidone which was termed 'the foetal troxidone syndrome'. Common features of the foetal troxidone syndrome included mild mental retardation, speech difficulty, V-shaped eyebrows, epicanthus, low-set backward sloped ears with anteriorly folded helix, palatal anomaly, and teeth irregularities. Less common features included intra-uterine growth retardation, short stature, microcephaly, cardiac anomaly, ocular anomaly, hypospadias, inguinal hernia, and simian crease.— E. H. Zackai *et al.*, *J. Pediat.*, 1975, *87*, 280.

Comment on the high incidence of congenital malformations associated with the use of troxidone in pregnancy. It is stressed that troxidone and paramethadione should be abandoned for petit mal epilepsy in the fecund woman. Ethosuximide is recommended as a drug of proved efficacy and low relative teratogenic potential.— S. Fabro and N. A. Brown (letter), *New Engl. J. Med.*, 1979, *300*, 1280.

Further references to troxidone and congenital malformations: D. W. Smith, *Am. J. Dis. Child.*, 1977, *131*, 1337; G. L. Feldman *et al.*, *ibid.*, 1389; A. S. Goldman and S. J. Yaffe, *Teratology*, 1978, *17*, 103; R. C. Rosen and E. S. Lightner, *J. Pediat.*, 1978, *92*, 240.

For a general comment on epilepsy and pregnancy, including mention that compounds like troxidone should be avoided during pregnancy, see p.1235.

Treatment of Adverse Effects. The stomach should be emptied by aspiration and lavage, and supportive therapy given (for general guidelines to the symptomatic therapy of drug overdosage, see Phenobarbitone, p.812).

Precautions. Troxidone is contra-indicated in patients with severe hepatic or renal disease or with severe blood dyscrasias. It should be used with caution in patients with disease of the retina or optic nerve and should be withdrawn if scotomata occur.

Frequent examinations of blood, urine, and hepatic function should be carried out in patients receiving troxidone, and therapy should be withdrawn promptly at signs of renal or hepatic dysfunction, severe neutropenia or other blood dyscrasias, or drug hypersensitivity. Patients receiving troxidone should be instructed to report immediately symptoms of infection or bleeding tendency, such as sore throat or easy bruising.

Troxidone should also be discontinued, at least temporarily, on the appearance of any skin disorder, however mild.

Administration of troxidone in pregnancy has been associated with a high incidence of congenital malformations.

Absorption and Fate. Troxidone is readily absorbed from the gastro-intestinal tract and extensively metabolised in the liver to its active metabolite, dimethadione, which is reported to be primarily responsible for the activity of troxidone on chronic administration.

Troxidone is very slowly excreted in the urine, over a period of several days, almost entirely in the form of dimethadione.

Troxidone is reported not to be significantly bound to plasma proteins.

Some correlation has been found between plasma concentrations of dimethadione exceeding 700 µg per ml and therapeutic response.

Metabolism and pharmacokinetics. A gas chromatographic procedure for the measurement of troxidone and its major metabolite, dimethadione, in serum.— H. E. Bocker and B. Darcey, *Clin. Chem.*, 1971, *17*, 607.

Metabolism in *animals*.— H. -H. Frey and R. Schulz, *Acta pharmac. tox.*, 1970, *28*, 477.

Plasma concentrations. A study of the pharmacokinetics of dimethadione following administration of troxidone to patients with petit mal. It was concluded that dimethadione is responsible for the anticonvulsant effect of troxidone. Considerable variation was noted in dimethadione concentrations but above 700 µg per ml, 8 of 10 patients were free from episodes, while at a concentration lower than 700 µg per ml, 14 of 27 were free from episodes. A study following withdrawal from 4 patients indicated that dimethadione remains in the body for very long periods of time, with concentrations of 100 µg per ml still present a month after withdrawal. Alkalinisation of the urine with sodium bicarbonate increased the rate of elimination.— B. N. Jensen, *Dan. med. Bull.*, 1962, *9*, 74. See also H. R. Chamberlin *et al.*, *Neurology, Minneap.*, 1965, *15*, 449.

Uses. Troxidone is an oxazolidinedione anticonvulsant used in the treatment of petit mal refractory to other treatment; where there are associated grand mal seizures it may be given in association with a suitable grand mal anticonvulsant, such as phenytoin.

The initial dose of troxidone is 900 mg daily in divided doses, increased by steps of 300 mg at intervals of one week, according to the patient's response, to 1.8 g daily in divided doses; sources in the USA state a maximum dose of 2.4 g daily. Suggested initial doses of troxidone for children are: less than 2 years of age, 300 mg daily; 2 to 6 years, 600 mg daily.

Withdrawal of troxidone or transition to or from another type of anticonvulsant therapy should be made gradually to avoid precipitating an increase in the frequency of seizures.

A review of the pharmacology of the oxazolidinediones.— C. D. Withrow, Oxazolidinediones, in *Antiepileptic Drugs: Mechanisms of Action*, G.H. Glaser *et al.* (Ed.), New York, Raven Press, 1980, p. 577.

Preparations

Paediatric Troxidone Tablets *(B.P.C. 1973)*. Tablets containing troxidone. They may contain suitable flavouring. Protect from light. The tablets should be crushed or chewed before swallowing.

Trimethadione Capsules *(U.S.P.)*. Capsules containing troxidone. Store at 15° to 30° in airtight containers.

Trimethadione Oral Solution *(U.S.P.)*. An aqueous solution of troxidone. pH 3 to 5. Store at 15° to 30° in airtight containers.

Trimethadione Tablets *(U.S.P.)*. Tablets containing troxidone. Store at a temperature not exceeding 25° in airtight containers.

Troxidone Capsules *(B.P.)*. Capsules containing troxidone.

Proprietary Preparations

Tridione *(Abbott, UK)*. Troxidone, available as capsules of 300 mg. (Also available as Tridione in *Austral., Belg., Denm., Ger., S.Afr., Spain, Switz., USA*).

Other Proprietary Names

Trimedone *(Canad.)*; Trioxanona *(Spain)*.

6623-n

Valproic Acid.

Abbott 44089. 2-Propylvaleric acid; 2-Propylpentanoic acid.

$C_8H_{16}O_2$=144.2.

CAS — 99-66-1.

6624-h

Sodium Valproate *(B.P.)*.

Valproate Sodium; Abbott 44090. Sodium 2-propylvalerate; Sodium 2-propylpentanoate.

$C_8H_{15}NaO_2$=166.2.

CAS — 1069-66-5.

Pharmacopoeias. In *Br.*

A white or almost white, odourless or almost odourless, crystalline, deliquescent, powder with a saline taste. **Soluble** 1 in 5 of water and of alcohol. **Store** in airtight containers.

Adverse Effects. Nausea, vomiting, gastro-intestinal irritation, increased appetite and excessive weight gain, drowsiness, ataxia, oedema, and transient alopecia with regrowth of curly hair, have been reported with valproic acid or its sodium salt. Tremor, reversible prolongation of bleeding time, and thrombocytopenia may occur, particularly with high doses.

Liver dysfunction including hepatic failure has occasionally been reported, usually in the first few months of treatment, and calls for withdrawal of valproic acid; there have been fatalities. Pancreatitis has also been reported.

For a discussion of the possible adverse effects of anticonvulsants, including valproate, on the foetus, see p.1235; see also under Pregnancy and the Neonate, below.

Rare side-effects reported in association with valproic-acid therapy include incoordination, dizziness, irritability, diplopia, spots before eyes, rash, headache, leucopenia, enuresis, insomnia, depression, psychosis, confusional state, hallucinations, paraesthesias, asterixis, hyperactivity, curly hair, and hypersalivation.— T. R. Browne, *New Engl. J. Med.*, 1980, *302*, 661.

A possible association of reduced serum concentrations of IgA with sodium valproate.— P. H. Joubert *et al.*, *S. Afr. med. J.*, 1977, *52*, 642.

Alopecia and curly hair. Five out of 250 patients developed curly hair during treatment with sodium valproate 1 g daily; in 3 patients this effect followed temporary alopecia.— P. M. Jeavons *et al.* (letter), *Lancet*, 1977, *1*, 359.

Anorexia and increased appetite. Both anorexia and increased appetite (with weight gain) have been reported in association with sodium valproate therapy.— R. M. Pinder *et al.*, *Drugs*, 1977, *13*, 81.

Increased appetite and excessive weight gain occurred in 44 of 100 epileptic children treated with sodium valproate. Other side-effects included: transient gastro-intestinal disturbances (20 patients), transient nocturnal enuresis (7), transient hair loss (6), severe lassitude (9), and aggressive behaviour (4).— J. Egger and E. M. Brett, *Br. med. J.*, 1981, *283*, 577. Comments.— T. K. Daneshmend (letter), *ibid.*, 1189; J. Egger and E. M. Brett (letter), *ibid.*

Effects on the blood. Studies on the plasma of healthy subjects, and platelet-function tests in 23 patients taking sodium valproate indicated that sodium valproate inhibited the secondary phase of aggregation. The bleeding time in all 23 patients studied was, however, normal. It was advisable to measure the bleeding time and platelet count of patients taking sodium valproate before major surgery.— S. G. N. Richardson *et al.* (letter), *Br. med. J.*, 1976, *1*, 221. There was evidence of haemorrhagic side-effects among 20 patients receiving sodium valproate as an anticonvulsant.— H. von Voss *et al.* (letter), *ibid.*, 1976, *2*, 179.

Sodium valproate depressed fibrinogen concentrations in a 16-year-old boy. Concentrations rose on withdrawal of sodium valproate.— B. M. Dale *et al.* (letter), *Lancet*, 1978, *1*, 1316. Indirect evidence corroborating the report that sodium valproate can cause depletion of fibrinogen.— J. G. Nutt *et al.* (letter), *ibid.*, 1978, *2*, 636. Criticism. Examination of fibrinogen concentrations in 20 epileptic patients on valproate and 20 on other anticonvulsant drugs showed no significant difference between the 2 groups. Fibrinogen concentrations were depressed within the low-normal range but there was no significant correlation with any one specific drug.— R. M. Hutchinson *et al.* (letter), *ibid.*, 1309.

Reduced plasma-fibrinogen concentrations in 9 patients receiving valproic acid in addition to other anticonvulsants, were considered to be evidence of a direct, dose-related hepatotoxic effect.— N. M. Sussman and L. W. McLain, *J. Am. med. Ass.*, 1979, *242*, 1173.

Neutropenia. Reversible neutropenia in a 3-month-old child given sodium valproate. No antibodies against granulocytes were detected and it was suggested that sodium valproate can induce a biochemical syndrome similar to that of the ketotic hyperglycinaemias.— J. Jaeken *et al.* (letter), *Archs Dis. Childh.*, 1979, *54*, 986.

Thrombocytopenia. A report of thrombocytopenia, with platelet-bound auto-antibody, in a 6-year-old child receiving sodium valproate 2 g daily.— R. M. Sandler *et al.*, *Br. med. J.*, 1978, *2*, 1683. Platelet-bound antibody (without thrombocytopenia) in 4 of 31 patients taking sodium valproate. Checking of platelet counts and monitoring of serum concentrations of sodium valproate were recommended when the dose of sodium valproate was increased.— *idem*, 1979, *2*, 1476.

Transient thrombocytopenia occurred during respiratory infections in a 7-year-old child receiving sodium valproate 25 to 35 mg per kg body-weight daily. The anticonvulsant was not withdrawn.— A. P. Cole, *Develop. Med. Child Neurology*, 1978, *20*, 487.

Further reports and comments on reduced platelet counts in patients taking sodium valproate: D. A. Winfield *et al.*, *Br. med. J.*, 1976, *2*, 981; R. E. Raworth and G. Birchall (letter), *Lancet*, 1978, *1*, 670; A. N. Neophytides *et al.*, *Ann. Neurol.*, 1979, *5*, 389; R. D. Eastham and J. Jancar (letter), *Br. med. J.*, 1980, *280*, 186.

Effects on the liver. A report of liver disease associated with administration of sodium valproate in 5 patients, 4 of whom were children; 3 of the patients died. Although evidence of a causal relationship can only be circumstantial, similarities in the patients included: occurrence in childhood (except in one case), 3 to 6 months' treatment before onset of symptoms, and frequent accompaniment by other side-effects of sodium valproate (hair loss, thrombocytopenia) which though well-recognised, are rare in clinical practice; swollen cheeks (the meaning of which is uncertain) were noted in 2 patients, and in one previously described. In addition, there were close resemblances between the features of the liver in 2 patients and in those previously reported. The mechanism of liver damage is considered to be idiosyncrasy or a hypersensitivity reaction, possibly due to an idiosyncratic metabolic pathway for sodium valproate, producing increased proportions of toxic metabolites. If this were the case, concomitant use of enzyme-inducing agents, such as phenobarbitone or phenytoin might increase the severity of the lesion. Sodium valproate is a very useful drug, and toxicity as described is probably very rare, but the following precautions are recommended: avoidance in patients with altered liver function, regular measurement of liver function, and consideration of hepatotoxicity when a patient, especially a child, becomes ill a few months after starting treatment with sodium valproate. It may also be advisable to avoid concomitant administration with enzyme-inducing anticonvulsants, such as phenobarbitone and phenytoin.— S. Ware and G. H. Millward-Sadler, *Lancet*, 1980, *2*, 1110. Comment.— *ibid.*, 1119. A report of a 17-year-old girl who died as a result of acute hepatic failure probably related to sodium valproate.— G. Le Bihan *et al.* (letter), *ibid.*, 1298.

Further reports and comments on hepatotoxicity associated with sodium valproate administration: F. J. Suchy *et al.*, *New Engl. J. Med.*, 1979, *300*, 962; R. K. Mathis *et al.* (letter), *ibid.*, *301*, 436; J. S. Partin *et al.* (letter), *ibid.*, 436; G. Jacobi *et al.* (letter), *Lancet*, 1980, *1*, 712; P. B. Mortensen (letter), *ibid.*, *2*, 856.

See also under Effects on the Blood, above.

Effects on mental state. A psychotic reaction with confusion, bizarre behaviour (vacant stare, unintelligible shouting), and hallucinations occurred in a 14-year-old boy after taking sodium valproate 1.6 g daily for 14 days. He later tolerated 800 mg daily.— M. H. Bellman and E. M. Ross (letter), *Br. med. J.*, 1977, *1*, 1662.

Effects on the nervous system. Doses of 1 or 1.5 g daily of valproic acid were associated with adverse effects on the central nervous system in 6 healthy subjects. These effects included sedation (3 subjects), difficulty in concentrating (3), malaise (2), stammering or slurred speech (2), and frequent bad dreams (1). They were not seen when 500 mg daily was taken.— T. A. Bowdle *et al.* (letter), *New Engl. J. Med.*, 1979, *301*, 435.

Evidence that secondary hyperammonaemia not due to liver disease, may occur in patients taking valproic acid, and this may explain why some patients become stuporous or comatose while taking this drug.— D. L. Coulter and R. J. Allen (letter), *Lancet*, 1980, *1*, 1310. A view that these concentrations of ammonia in the blood are not harmful.— J. Jaeken *et al.* (letter), *ibid.*, *2*, 260. Hyperammonaemia has now been recorded in several other children, with no evidence of liver damage, who had become lethargic and who improved when the dosage of valproate was reduced. Although the degree of hyperammonaemia so far has only been modest, it is comparable to concentrations found in some patients with Reye's syndrome.— D. L. Coulter (letter), *ibid.* A report of 2 children who had encephalopathy during valproate therapy; in one the possibility of hyperammonaemia could be inferred and the other had unequivocal evidence of hyperammonaemia.— J. A. Sills *et al.* (letter), *ibid.*

Tremor occurred in 4 patients taking sodium valproate and other anticonvulsants.— N. M. Hyman *et al.*, *Neurology, Minneap.*, 1979, *29*, 1177.

Extrapyramidal effects. An extrapyramidal syndrome, unresponsive to benztropine or benzhexol, developed in a 52-year-old man with schizophrenia given a therapeutic trial of sodium valproate 1 to 2 g daily.— A. Lautin *et al.*, *Br. med. J.*, 1979, *2*, 1035. Administration of sodium valproate to a man with dystonic movements of the neck and spine produced a severe subjective and objective deterioration in his symptoms which returned to their previous severity on withdrawal of the drug.— D. J. Dick and M. Saunders (letter), *ibid.*, 1980, *280*, 189.

Hyperglycinaemia. Hyperglycinaemia associated with sodium valproate.— J. Jaeken *et al.* (letter), *Lancet*, 1977, *2*, 617. See also K. Bartlett (letter), *ibid.*, 716; B. Wolf (letter), *Lancet*, 1978, *2*, 369.

Nonketotic hyperglycinaemia should not be considered to be a contra-indication to the use of sodium valproate. Two patients with this condition received sodium valproate without any increase in the concentrations of glycine in the CSF (considered to be the cause of encephalopathy in nonketotic hyperglycinaemia). One patient developed neutropenia.— K. MacDermot *et al.*, *Pediatrics*, 1980, *65*, 624.

Overdosage. A 23-year-old man receiving phenobarbitone and phenytoin became increasingly lethargic over the following 5 days when valproic acid 750 mg thrice daily was added to his treatment. On the sixth day all drugs were withdrawn and over the next 3 hours he became comatose and died. Post mortem revealed massive pulmonary oedema. Since the dose exceeded the recommended initial dose of valproic acid of 15 mg per kg body-weight daily, the patient's death was considered to be the direct result of an overdose.— J. P. Tift (letter), *New Engl. J. Med.*, 1980, *303*, 394. Comment.— T. R. Browne (letter), *ibid.*

Pancreatitis. Pancreatitis in 2 children might have been associated with valproic acid therapy.— P. R. Camfield *et al.* (letter), *Lancet*, 1979, *1*, 1198. A report of pancreatitis in an adult, associated with administration of sodium valproate.— M. J. Murphy *et al.* (letter), *ibid.*, 1981, *1*, 41. A report of a third case of pancreatitis in childhood due to valproic acid.— M. Sasaki *et al.* (letter), *ibid.*, 1196.

Further references to pancreatitis associated with valproate therapy: P. B. Batalden *et al.*, *Pediatrics*, 1979, *64*, 520.

Pregnancy and the neonate. Studies in *mice* suggest that valproic acid is a more potent teratogen than phenytoin, and as potent a teratogen as troxidone. It is possible, however, that the *animal* data on valproic acid represent an exaggeration of the risk to the human population.— N. A. Brown *et al.* (letter), *Lancet*, 1980, *1*, 660. As part of a prospective study on pregnant epileptic women and their children, 12 women have been recorded who took valproic acid usually in association with phenytoin or carbamazepine; only one used valproic acid alone. No malformations or other anomalies were encountered in the 12 infants either at birth or during follow-up which ranges from 2 months to 4 years. Although the series is too small to justify conclusions about the teratogenic potential of valproic acid in man, 2 groups of patients are now being allowed to continue valproic acid during pregnancy, namely women who are already pregnant and are taking the drug, and those for whom valproic acid was considered essential to control the seizures before they became pregnant.— V. K. Hiilesmaa *et al.* (letter), *ibid.*, 883.

Possibly the first report of a suspected causal link between valproic acid and human dysmorphism.— B. Dalens *et al.* (letter), *J. Pediat.*, 1980, *97*, 332. Comment.— R. G. Dickinson and N. Gerber (letter), *ibid.*, 333.

The neonate. Two reports of neonatal hyperglycinaemia following sodium valproate ingestion during pregnancy.— S. Similä *et al.* (letter), *Archs Dis. Childh.*, 1979, *54*, 985.

Treatment of Adverse Effects. The stomach should be emptied by aspiration and lavage, although it has been suggested that gastric lavage may be of limited value in view of the rapid absorption of valproic acid. Supportive therapy alone may then suffice for patients who are not severely poisoned (for general guidelines to the symptomatic therapy of drug overdosage, see Phenobarbitone, p.812).

A 19-month-old child weighing 11.08 kg ingested about 2.25 g of sodium valproate. He became lethargic and irritable; an emetic and activated charcoal were given without producing improvement. Three hours after ingestion the child was unconscious and the clinical picture resembled that of opiate overdose. Naloxone 10 µg per kg body-weight intravenously reversed the coma. A second dose of naloxone was required since the child relapsed 20 minutes after the first dose.— G. S. Steiman *et al.* (letter), *Ann. Neurol.*, 1979, *6*, 274.

Precautions. Patients should be monitored for platelet function before and during valproic acid therapy and before elective surgery; valproic acid should be withdrawn if patients develop bruising or bleeding. Liver function tests should also be carried out before starting therapy, during the first 6 months of therapy, and when dosage is being increased. Valproic acid should be discontinued if signs of liver dysfunction occur, and should not be given to patients with pre-existing liver disease. It has also been recommended that pancreatic function be monitored.

For the use of valproic acid in pregnancy, see p.1235; see also under Adverse Effects, above.

Valproic acid is extensively bound to plasma proteins and is therefore susceptible to interactions with drugs liable to compete for similar binding sites; for a comment on the relevance of this type of interaction, see Phenytoin, Precautions, p.1238.

Concomitant administration of hepatic enzyme inducers, such as phenobarbitone or phenytoin, may enhance the metabolism of valproic acid whereas, in turn, valproic acid has been reported to cause rises in phenobarbitone (and primidone) concentrations in plasma. The interaction between valproic acid and phenytoin is complex and involves inhibition of phenytoin metabolism as well as competition for protein binding sites. Caution is recommended when administering valproic acid with other drugs liable to interfere with blood coagulation, such as aspirin or warfarin. Valproic acid may enhance the effects of central nervous system depressants (including alcohol), and may reduce the patient's ability to drive vehicles or operate machinery.

Sodium valproate may cause false positives in urine tests for diabetes mellitus.

For a comment on valproate and driving, see Phenytoin, p.1239.

Interactions. Sodium valproate did not induce liver enzymes when given to 8 epileptic patients in doses of 600 to 800 mg daily.— J. Oxley *et al.* (letter), *Br. J. clin. Pharmac.*, 1979, *8*, 189.

Valproic acid was bound *in vitro* to albumin in serum and was displaced from these binding sites by *palmitic acid*.— A. Monks and A. Richens (letter), *Br. J. clin. Pharmac.*, 1979, *8*, 187.

A report of *in vitro* equilibrium dialysis experiments indicating that *salicylate* and *phenylbutazone* displace valproate from its binding sites on human serum albumin at therapeutic concentrations, whereas *warfarin* and *carbamazepine* do not. Judging from the characteristics of the binding it was considered that *ibuprofen, ethacrynic acid*, and *clofibrate* could also be expected to compete with valproate for binding sites on albumin.— J. S. Fleitman *et al.*, *J. clin. Pharmac.*, 1980, *20*, 514.

Alcohol. Variable effects of alcohol on the metabolism of sodium valproate in *animals*.— T. B. Vree and E. Van der Kleijn, *Pharm. Weekbl. Ned.*, 1977, *112*, 313.

Anticonvulsants. Comment on reports of absence status in patients taking *clonazepam* and sodium valproate simultaneously. Since some patients with refractory absence seizures have an excellent response to this combination of drugs, it would be improper to conclude that clonazepam and valproic acid should never be given together.— T. R. Browne (letter), *New Engl. J. Med.*, 1978, *299*, 812.

Evidence that *carbamazepine* enhances the hepatic metabolism of sodium valproate.— T. A. Bowdle *et al.*, *Clin. Pharmac. Ther.*, 1979, *26*, 629. See also M. I. Reunanen *et al.*, *Curr. ther. Res.*, 1980, *28*, 456.

For the effect of sodium valproate on *ethosuximide*, see Ethosuximide, p.1250, for the effect on *phenobarbitone*, see Phenobarbitone, p.814, for the effect on *phenytoin*, see Phenytoin, p.1239, and for the effect on *primidone*, see Primidone, p.1254.

Porphyria. A study in *rats* indicated that sodium valproate should be regarded as potentially hazardous for patients with a hereditary hepatic porphyria.— G. H. Blekkenhorst *et al.* (letter), *Lancet*, 1980, *1*, 1367. Criticisms of extrapolating data obtained from *animal* experiments to the treatment of human disease.— M. J. Brodie (letter), *ibid.*, *2*, 86; A. Gorchein (letter), *ibid.*, 152.

A report of a young woman in whom an acute episode of acute intermittent porphyria was induced by sodium valproate.— J. A. Garcia-Merino and J. J. Lopez-Lozano (letter), *Lancet*, 1980, *2*, 856. See also M. Doss *et al.* (letter), *ibid.*, 1981, *2*, 91.

See also under Uses.

Absorption and Fate. Valproic acid is rapidly and completely absorbed after oral administration; the rate of absorption is delayed by administration after food or as enteric-coated tablets.

Valproic acid is extensively metabolised in the liver and some of its metabolites have been reported to have anticonvulsant properties; it is excreted in the urine almost entirely in the form of its metabolites.

Valproic acid is extensively bound to plasma protein. Estimations of the plasma half-life of valproic acid range from about 9 to 21 hours, with a mean of about 12 or 13 hours. It does not appear to have the property of enhancing its own metabolism therefore the half-life on chronic administration is not shorter than that following single doses, but its metabolism is induced by drugs such as phenobarbitone which induce hepatic microsomal enzymes.

A limited correlation has been found between the therapeutic effects of valproic acid and minimum plasma concentrations of about 50 µg per ml (approximately 350 µmol per litre).

Valproic acid crosses the blood-brain barrier and the placental barrier, and small amounts are excreted in milk.

General reviews and comments on the pharmacokinetics of valproic acid.— R. Gugler and G. E. von Unruh, *Clin. Pharmacokinet.*, 1980, *5*, 67.

Absorption. A study involving one subject indicated that the lag time for the appearance of valproic acid in plasma was prolonged from 2 to 4.5 hours when enteric-coated tablets were given after a standard breakfast instead of on an empty stomach. The peak concentration was delayed from 3.0 to 7.5 hours, but the bioavailability was not affected by food.— U. Klotz and K. H. Antonin, *Clin. Pharmac. Ther.*, 1977, *21*, 736.

Further studies on the absorption and bioavailability of valproic acid, including enteric-coated formulations.— S.

I. Johannessen and O. Henriksen, *Acta neurol. scand.*, 1979, *60*, 371; A. H. C. Chun *et al.*, *J. clin. Pharmac.*, 1980, *20*, 30.

Metabolism. 2-Propylglutaric acid, 5-hydroxy-2-propylvaleric acid, 3-keto-2-propylvaleric acid, and dehydrodipropylacetic acid were found in the urine of patients receiving sodium valproate. In 4 patients the excretion of succinic acid, glutaric acid, 2-hydroxyglutaric acid, and adipic acid was greatly increased.— W. Kochen *et al.*, *Arzneimittel-Forsch.*, 1977, *27*, 1090.

In 11 patients receiving maintenance sodium valproate therapy, 3-keto-, 4-hydroxy-, and 5-hydroxy-sodium valproate had been detected as urinary metabolites in addition to the glucuronide of sodium valproate.— H. Schäfer and R. Lührs, *Arzneimittel-Forsch.*, 1978, *28*, 657.

Further metabolic studies on valproic acid: T. Kuhara *et al.*, *Eur. J. Drug Metab. Pharmacokinet.*, 1978, *3*, 171.

Pharmacokinetics. A crossover study of the bioavailability and pharmacokinetics of sodium valproate in 6 healthy subjects following administration of 400 mg intravenously, 600 mg by mouth as enteric-coated tablets, and 600 mg by mouth as a solution. Sodium valproate was almost completely absorbed after oral administration. It had an average initial half-life of about 1 hour after intravenous injection and a terminal half-life, regardless of the route of administration, of 8.7 to 21.5 hours (average about 12.2 hours).— U. Klotz and K. H. Antonin, *Clin. Pharmac. Ther.*, 1977, *21*, 736.

Results of a study of the pharmacokinetics of valproic acid after oral and intravenous administration in 6 healthy subjects, indicated that absorption following oral administration is rapid and complete, and kinetic parameters are similar for both routes of administration. Half-lives ranged from about 10 to 15 hours with a mean of 12.7 after oral administration and 12.8 after intravenous administration. The mean apparent volume of distribution was only 147 ml per kg body-weight, which was considered to be partially due to its high degree of plasma protein binding.— E. Perucca *et al.*, *Br. J. clin. Pharmac.*, 1978, *5*, 313. A study using the same protocol showed considerably higher serum clearance of valproic acid in epileptic patients also taking phenytoin and phenobarbitone.— *idem*, 495.

Further studies of the pharmacokinetics of valproic acid: R. Gugler *et al.*, *Eur. J. clin. Pharmac.*, 1977, *12*, 125; J. Bruni *et al.*, *Clin. Pharmac. Ther.*, 1978, *24*, 324; G. W. Mihaly *et al.*, *Eur. J. clin. Pharmac.*, 1979, *16*, 23; A. C. Mehta *et al.*, *J. clin. Hosp. Pharm.*, 1980, *5*, 329; T. A. Bowdle, *Clin. Pharmac. Ther.*, 1980, *28*, 486.

Plasma concentrations. A study on the relationship between serum concentrations of valproic acid and clinical response permitted the conclusion that serum concentrations of 300 to 350 µmol per litre have a superior clinical effect to that of lower concentrations. It is still an open question whether higher serum concentrations may provide even better results.— L. Gram *et al.*, *Epilepsia*, 1979, *20*, 303.

A review of the monitoring of plasma concentrations. The action of sodium valproate may not be accurately reflected by its serum concentration, and the suggested range of 350 to 700 µmol per litre (50 to 100 µg per ml) has yet to be validated by a prospective study.— A. Richens and S. Warrington, *Drugs*, 1979, *17*, 488.

Further studies directed at relating therapeutic response to plasma concentrations of valproic acid with the aim of individualising dosage regimens.— A. Baruzzi *et al.*, *Int. J. clin. Pharmac. Biopharm.*, 1977, *15*, 403; W. Fröscher *et al.*, *Fortschr. Med.*, 1979, *97*, 1464; G. J. Schapel *et al.*, *Eur. J. clin. Pharmac.*, 1980, *17*, 71.

Protein binding. The mean amount of valproic acid not bound to plasma proteins was 8.4% in 16 healthy subjects as against 17.5% in 24 patients with renal disease. In patients with renal disease there was a good correlation between valproic acid not bound to plasma proteins and serum-creatinine concentration but a poor correlation with total protein or albumin concentration in plasma.— R. Gugler and G. Mueller, *Br. J. clin. Pharmac.*, 1978, *5*, 441.

Evidence that the protein binding of sodium valproate in human plasma is greatly reduced in conditions of uraemia. The extent to which binding is impaired shows considerable interindividual variation.— D. Brewster and N. C. Muir, *Clin. Pharmac. Ther.*, 1980, *27*, 76.

Further references to valproic acid and protein binding: J. Bruni *et al.*, *Neurology, Minneap.*, 1980, *30*, 557 (uraemia).

See also under Precautions, above.

Saliva concentrations. Unlike phenytoin, sodium valproate therapy could not be monitored by measuring concentrations in saliva since it had a low pKa value of 4.6.— D. Schmidt (letter), *Lancet*, 1976, *2*, 639.

Pregnancy and the neonate. Study of one neonate demonstrated that sodium valproate readily crosses the placenta. It is excreted in breast milk at a concentration between 5 and 10% of that in maternal serum; absorption by the infant from the breast milk appears to be insignificant.— F. W. Alexander (letter), *Archs Dis. Childh.*, 1979, *54*, 240. See also R. G. Dickinson, *J. Pediat.*, 1979, *94*, 832.

Uses. Valproic acid is an anticonvulsant used in the treatment of various forms of epilepsy, including petit mal. Its mode of action in epilepsy is not fully understood but may involve a modification of the behaviour of gamma-aminobutyric acid in the brain.

Valproic acid can be given as its sodium salt (sodium valproate) or as valproic acid itself. The dose of sodium valproate or valproic acid should be adjusted to the needs of the individual patient to achieve adequate control of seizures; a limited correlation with plasma concentrations has indicated that plasma concentrations of valproic acid above 50 µg per ml (approximately 350 µmol per litre) are usually necessary.

A suggested initial dose of sodium valproate in Great Britain is 600 mg daily in divided doses, increased every 3 days by 200 mg daily to a usual range of 1 to 1.6 g daily; further increases to a maximum of 2.6 g daily may be necessary if adequate control has not been achieved after 2 weeks. A suggested initial dose for children weighing more than 20 kg is 400 mg daily (irrespective of weight) in divided doses, gradually increased until control is achieved, with a usual range of 20 to 30 mg per kg daily; children weighing less than 20 kg may be given 20 mg per kg daily, which may be increased to 50 mg per kg in severe cases. It has been recommended that a dose of 50 mg per kg body-weight should only be exceeded in patients whose plasma concentrations are being monitored, and that plasma concentrations of 200 µg per ml (approximately 1400 µmol per litre) should be exceeded only with caution and with monitoring of haematological function. Valproic acid is employed in the USA in doses similar to the British doses of sodium valproate for children.

Withdrawal of sodium valproate or valproic acid or transition to or from another type of anticonvulsant therapy should be made gradually to avoid precipitating an increase in the frequency of seizures.

Sodium valproate and valproic acid should be taken with or after food and should be swallowed whole with a little water; in particular it has been recommended that aerated water should be avoided with sodium valproate. A low initial dose is recommended to minimise gastric intolerance. The time of taking valproic acid and its salts should be standardised for the patient since variations might lead to inappropriate fluctuations in the plasma concentrations.

Action. A review of valproic acid, including comments on its possible mode of action. Valproic acid has been shown to increase total brain and cerebellar concentrations of the inhibitory neurotransmitter gamma-aminobutyric acid (GABA), but elevation of total brain concentrations of GABA may not be the only or even the principal mechanism of action of valproic acid, since this is not routinely obtained in clinical practice, and some forms of experimental seizures are blocked by doses that do not elevate total brain concentrations of GABA. Other possible mechanisms include a selective increase in GABA concentrations in some parts of the brain, enhancement of the postsynaptic inhibition of GABA, competitive inhibition of its re-uptake in synapses, decrease in the brain concentrations of aspartate or cyclic guanine monophosphate, production of oxidised fatty acids simulating the ketogenic dietary regimen, and hyperpolarisation of neurones by increased potassium conductance.— T. R. Browne, *New Engl. J. Med.*, 1980, *302*, 661 and 1421. See also C. Garvin (letter), *ibid.*, *303*, 394.

Further reviews: R. M. Pinder *et al.*, *Drugs*, 1977, *13*, 81; *Drug & Ther. Bull.*, 1981, *19*, 93.

Administration. Sodium valproate given rectally by enema or suppository in doses of 400 and 600 mg controlled 2 patients with intractable tonic-seizure status epilepticus not responding properly to oral therapy.— F. J. E. Vajda *et al.* (letter), *Lancet*, 1977, *1*, 359. See also *idem*, *Neurology, Minneap.*, 1978, *28*, 897.

Adrenal disorders. Beneficial results with sodium valproate, with reduction of very high circulating concentrations of adrenocorticotrophic hormone (ACTH), in 6 patients suffering from Nelson's syndrome, suggested that the disease might arise from a relative deficiency in the gamma-aminobutyric-acid transmission system within the hypothalamus. Excessive skin pigmentation was reduced in 5 of the patients, and 3 developed increased energy; disappearance of polyuria and polydipsia in one patient was also of interest. Some patients obtained amelioration of headaches, suggesting that sodium valproate may also inhibit pituitary enlargement. The addition of diazepam produced no significant beneficial effect. Since Nelson's syndrome is a clinical sequela of bilateral adrenalectomy for Cushing's disease, the possibility is being investigated that some patients with Cushing's disease might also respond to sodium valproate with a lowering of plasma ACTH and hence plasma cortisol (hydrocortisone).— M. T. Jones *et al.*, *Lancet*, 1981, *1*, 1179. Results suggesting that sodium valproate is unable to lower ACTH in patients with Cushing's disease.— B. Allolio *et al.* (letter), *ibid.*, 1982, *1*, 171.

Alcoholism. The prevention of alcohol-withdrawal symptoms with sodium valproate.— D. G. Lambie *et al.*, *Aust. N.Z. J. Psychiat.*, 1980, *14*, 213.

Chorea. Sodium valproate 0.6 to 1.2 g daily failed to benefit 5 patients with chorea (3 with Huntington's disease).— J. A. R. Lenman *et al.*, *Br. med. J.*, 1976, *2*, 1107. A report of 5 patients with chorea who failed to respond to sodium valproate and one (who was also taking diazepam 15 mg daily) who obtained an excellent response.— G. M. Yuill (letter), *ibid.*, 1562. Further comment.— P. J. Schechter (letter), *ibid.*

A 19-year-old woman with Sydenham's chorea responded rapidly to treatment with valproic acid 250 mg twice daily.— R. S. McLachlan (letter), *Br. med. J.*, 1981, *283*, 274.

Further references: D. S. Bachman *et al.*, *Neurology, Minneap.*, 1977, *27*, 193.

Dyskinesias. Evidence of a beneficial effect of sodium valproate in neuroleptic-induced tardive dyskinesia.— M. Linnoila *et al.*, *Br. J. Psychiat.*, 1976, *129*, 114. See also *idem*, *Int. Drug Ther. Newslett.*, 1976, *11*, 33; D. E. Casey and J. P. Hammerstad, *J. clin. Psychiat.*, 1979, *40*, 483.

No beneficial effect in 25 schizophrenic patients with tardive dyskinesia given sodium valproate 600 mg daily together with their usual neuroleptics.— A. C. Gibson, *Br. J. Psychiat.*, 1978, *133*, 82. No objective effect with sodium valproate 1.2 g daily on parkinsonism or levodopa-induced dyskinesias in a double-blind crossover study of 12 patients.— P. A. Price *et al.*, *J. Neurol. Neurosurg. Psychiat.*, 1978, *41*, 702.

For a report of sodium valproate exacerbating neuroleptic-induced tardive dyskinesia, see under Adverse Effects (Effects on the Nervous System), above.

Epilepsy. Reports and studies on valproic acid in epilepsy: P. M. Jeavons and J. E. Clark, *Br. med. J.*, 1974, *2*, 584; A. R. Manhire and M. Espir (letter), *ibid.*, 1974, *3*, 808; A. Richens and S. Ahmad, *ibid.*, 1975, *4*, 255; S. E. Barnes and B. D. Bower, *Develop. Med. Child Neurology*, 1975, *17*, 175; P. M. Jeavons *et al.*, *ibid.*, 1977, *19*, 9; J. W. Lance and M. Anthony, *Archs Neurol., Chicago*, 1977, *34*, 14; *idem*, *Med. J. Aust.*, 1977, *1*, 911; P. Silberstein, *ibid.*, 1977, *1*, 95; R. H. Briant *et al.*, *N.Z. med. J.*, 1978, *88*, 479; G. F. A. Harding *et al.*, *Epilepsia*, 1978, *19*, 555 (photosensitive epilepsy); R. H. Mattson *et al.*, *Ann. Neurol.*, 1978, *3*, 20; S. Livingston *et al.* (letter), *J. Am. med. Ass.*, 1979, *241*, 1892; E. P. G. Vining *et al.*, *Am. J. Dis. Child.*, 1979, *133*, 274; J. Bruni *et al.*, *Neurology, Minneap.*, 1980, *30*, 42; D. L. Coulter *et al.*, *J. Am. med. Ass.*, 1980, *244*, 785.

For comments on the role of valproic acid in epilepsy, see Phenytoin, p.1243.

Febrile convulsions. In a study in 108 children, aged 6 to 42 months, over 184 six-month periods, the incidence of febrile convulsions was significantly reduced by sodium valproate (in a dose of 20 to 30 mg per kg body-weight daily, designed to produce a concentration in plasma of 60 µg or more per ml) or phenobarbitone (4 to 5 mg per kg daily to produce a concentration of 16 µg or more per ml), compared with no treatment.— S. J. Wallace and J. A. Smith, *Br. med. J.*, 1980, *280*, 353 and 612. Criticisms and comments.— A. Herxheimer (letter), *ibid.*, 642; J. B. P. Stephenson (letter), *ibid.;* P. M. Jeavons (letter), *ibid.*, 863.

Further references to valproic acid and febrile convulsions: A. J. Williams *et al.*, *Clin. Pediat.*, 1979, *18*, 426; E. Ngwane and B. Bower, *Archs Dis. Childh.*, 1980, *55*, 171.

For the role of anticonvulsants in the treatment and prevention of febrile convulsions in children, see also Diazepam, p.1525.

Myoclonus. There was a marked reduction in involuntary movements when valproic acid was added to the phenytoin and clonazepam being taken by a 52-year-old woman with action myoclonus. A similar patient became free of seizures when treated with the same regimen. Measurement of 5-hydroxyindoleacetic acid concentrations in the cerebrospinal fluid before and after the introduction of valproic acid suggested that this anticonvulsant might increase the activity of serotonin-containing neurones in the central nervous system, possibly by disinhibition.— S. Fahn (letter), *New Engl. J. Med.*, 1978, *299*, 313.

Sodium valproate 1 g daily suppressed postanoxic action myoclonus (Lance-Adams syndrome) in one patient. However, this treatment produced severe uncontrollable yawning. Lowering the dose of sodium valproate stopped the yawning. Addition of pimozide to full dosage of sodium valproate also stopped the yawning.— R. D. Rollison *et al.* (letter), *Archs Neurol.*, 1979, *36*, 253.

Pain. A comment that there is clinical evidence that sodium valproate with amitriptyline can have a beneficial effect on the pain of shingles.— M. Mehta (letter), *Br. med. J.*, 1979, *1*, 346.

Porphyria. The severity and frequency of convulsive crises and symptoms of acute intermittent porphyria in a 14-year-old epileptic boy were both reduced when treatment with phenobarbitone and phenytoin was replaced by sodium valproate 70 mg per kg body-weight daily.— R. Biagini *et al.*, *Archs Dis. Childh.*, 1979, *54*, 644.

For *animal* studies suggesting that sodium valproate is potentially hazardous in porphyria, and for reports of induction of porphyria in patients, see Precautions, above.

Schizophrenia. As sodium valproate was reported to raise brain concentrations of gamma-aminobutyric acid it should be studied for an effect in schizophrenia.— L. M. Koran (letter), *Lancet*, 1976, *2*, 1025.

Of 8 schizophrenic patients given sodium valproate, one experienced an abrupt exacerbation on only 750 mg and was dropped from the study, 5 deteriorated dramatically, one showed no change, and one showed minimal improvement. Caution is recommended when using sodium valproate for convulsions in patients with a history of schizophrenia.— A. Lautin *et al.*, *IRCS Med. Sci.*, 1979, *7*, 569.

Preparations of Sodium Valproate

Sodium Valproate Elixir *(B.P.).* Sodium Valproate Syrup. A solution of sodium valproate in a suitable flavoured vehicle which may be coloured.

Sodium Valproate Tablets *(B.P.).* Tablets containing sodium valproate.

Epilim *(Labaz Sanofi, UK).* Sodium valproate, available as **Syrup** containing 200 mg in each 5 ml and as enteric-coated **Tablets** of 200 and 500 mg. (Also available as Epilim in *Austral.*, *S.Afr.*).

Epilim syrup changed colour going from red to yellow when diluted with syrup preserved with sulphur dioxide or sodium metabisulphite.— *Chemist Drugg.*, 1978, *210*, 444.

Other Proprietary Names of Valproic Acid and Sodium Valproate

Convulex *(Belg., Ger., Switz.)*; Convulexette *(Belg.)*; Depakene *(Jap., USA)*; Depakin *(Ital.)*; Depakine *(Belg., Fr., Neth., Spain, Switz.)*; Deprakine *(Denm.)*; Ergenyl *(Ger.)*; Logical (magnesium valproate) *(Arg.)*; Orfiril *(Denm., Ger.)*; Propymal *(Neth.)*.

Pholcodine and some other Cough Suppressants

5600-s

The drugs described in this section are used primarily to suppress irritant unproductive cough however, few have been shown to be effective by controlled trials. Drugs with marked analgesic effects which are also used to suppress cough, such as codeine (p.1005), diamorphine (p.1009), and methadone (p.1016), are described in the section on Narcotic Analgesics.

A cough suppressant may occasionally be given in conjunction with an expectorant but there is little evidence to support the use of such a mixture. Antihistamines may also be used but undue sedation would occur if they were used in doses that have been reported to suppress cough.

A long review of the analgesic and cough suppressant effects of codeine and its alternatives, including benzonatate, carbetapentane, chlophedianol, dextromethorphan, dimethoxanate, noscapine, pholcodine, pipazethate, isoaminile, oxeladin, and sodium dibunate.— N. B. Eddy *et al.*, *Codeine and its Alternates for Pain and Cough Relief*, Geneva, World Health Organization, 1970; *idem*, *Bull. Wld Hlth Org.*, 1969, *40*, 639 and 721.

Further references, discussions and reviews: J. S. Templeton, *Br. med. J.*, 1970, *3*, 633; *Tech. Rep. Ser. Wld Hlth Org. No. 495*, 1972; E. Wilkes, *Prescribers' J.*, 1974, *14*, 98; *Br. med. J.*, 1976, *2*, 493; *Br. med. J.*, 1977, *1*, 1374; D. T. D. Hughes, *Br. med. J.*, 1978, *1*, 1202; *Med. Lett.*, 1979, *21*, 103.

5601-w

Pholcodine (*B.P., Eur. P.*).

Pholcod.; Pholcodinum; Morpholinylethylmorphine; MEM. O^3-(2-Morpholinoethyl)morphine monohydrate. $C_{23}H_{30}N_2O_4,H_2O$=416.5.

CAS — 509-67-1 (anhydrous).

Pharmacopoeias. In *Br., Eur., Fr., Ger., Int., It.,* and *Neth.*

Colourless crystals or a white or almost white, odourless, crystalline powder with a very bitter taste. M.p. about 99°.

Soluble 1 in 50 of water and 1 in 3 of dehydrated alcohol; very soluble in acetone and chloroform; slightly soluble in ether; soluble in dilute hydrochloric acid. A solution in alcohol is laevorotatory. **Incompatible** with chlorocresol. Solutions are **sterilised** by maintaining at 98° to 100° for 30 minutes with a bactericide or by filtration. **Store** in airtight containers.

5602-e

Pholcodine Tartrate (*B.P.C. 1963*).

Pholcod. Tart. Pholcodine di(hydrogen tartrate) trihydrate. $C_{23}H_{30}N_2O_4,2C_4H_6O_6,3H_2O$=752.7.

An odourless white crystalline powder with a bitter taste. **Soluble** 1 in 8 of water; very slightly soluble in alcohol; slightly soluble in chloroform and ether. A 7.5% solution in water has a pH of 3.1 to 3.5.

Adverse Effects. Nausea and drowsiness occasionally occur. Restlessness, excitement, and ataxia may occur after large doses. A toxic dose in children is reported to be about 200 mg.

Uses. Pholcodine is a cough suppressant with mild sedative but little analgesic action; it can relieve local irritation of the respiratory tract for about 4 to 5 hours. Its depressant effects on the respiration are less than those of morphine.

Pholcodine is used for the relief of unproductive cough. It is administered by mouth, usually as a linctus or syrup, in a dose of 5 to 15 mg for adults, 5 mg for children over 2 years, and 2.5 mg for children under 2 years. The tartrate has been given in doses of 10 to 30 mg.

The citrate has also been used.

Preparations

Pholcodine Citrate Syrup (*B.P.C. 1959*). Syr. Pholcod. Cit. Pholcodine 8 mg, citric acid monohydrate 80 mg, chloroform spirit 0.6 ml, syrup to 4 ml. *Dose.* 2 to 4 ml.

Pholcodine Linctus (*A.P.F.*). Pholcodine 5 mg, citric acid monohydrate 50 mg, concentrated chloroform water 0.15 ml, compound amaranth solution 0.1 ml, glycerol 1 ml, syrup to 5 ml. *Dose.* 5 to 10 ml.

Pholcodine Linctus CF (*A.P.F.*). Pholcodine Linctus for Children. Pholcodine 2.5 mg, citric acid monohydrate 25 mg, concentrated chloroform water 0.1 ml, compound amaranth solution 0.05 ml, glycerol 0.5 ml, syrup to 5 ml. *Dose.* Children over 2 years, 10 ml; children under 2 years, 5 ml.

Pholcodine Linctus (*B.P.*). Pholcodine 5 mg, citric acid monohydrate 50 mg, chloroform spirit 0.375 ml, compound tartrazine solution 0.05 ml, amaranth solution 0.005 ml, syrup to 5 ml. Protect from light. When a dose less than or not a multiple of 5 ml is prescribed, the linctus should be diluted to 5 ml, or a multiple, with syrup. Such dilutions must be freshly prepared and not used more than 2 weeks after issue.

Strong Pholcodine Linctus (*B.P.*). Pholcodine 10 mg, citric acid monohydrate 100 mg, chloroform spirit 0.4 ml, alcohol (90%) 0.35 ml, compound tartrazine solution 0.1 ml, amaranth solution 0.01 ml, syrup to 5 ml. Protect from light. When a dose less than or not a multiple of 5 ml is prescribed, the linctus should be diluted to 5 ml, or a multiple, with syrup. Such dilutions must be freshly prepared and not used more than 2 weeks after issue.

Proprietary Preparations

Copholco (*Rorer, UK*). A cough linctus containing in each 5 ml pholcodine 5.63 mg, menthol 1.41 mg, cineole 0.0026 ml, and terpin hydrate 2.82 mg, in a colloidal basis. *Dose.* 10 ml without water 4 or 5 times daily; children, over 5 years, 2.5 to 5 ml.

Copholcoids (*Rorer, UK*). Pastilles each containing pholcodine 4 mg, menthol 2 mg, cineole 0.004 ml, and terpin hydrate 16 mg. *Dose.* 1 or 2 pastilles 3 or 4 times daily; children, over 5 years, 1 pastille every 4 hours up to a maximum of 3 in 24 hours.

Dia-Tuss (*Rona, UK*). Pholcodine, available as a sugar-free linctus containing 10 mg in each 5 ml (suggested diluent, Sorbitol Solution, non-crystallising).

Expulin (*Galen, UK*). Linctus containing in each 5 ml pholcodine 5 mg, ephedrine hydrochloride 8 mg, chlorpheniramine maleate 2 mg, and menthol 1.1 mg. For cough associated with congestion. *Dose.* 10 to 15 ml every 6 hours; children, 2 to 6 years, 2.5 to 5 ml; 6 to 12 years, 5 to 10 ml.

Falcodyl (*Norton, UK: Vestric, UK*). A syrup containing in each 5 ml pholcodine 4 mg and ephedrine hydrochloride 4 mg. For cough with bronchospasm. *Dose.* 10 ml thrice daily, children 2.5 to 5 ml.

Pavacol-D Cough Mixture (*WB Pharmaceuticals, UK: Boehringer Ingelheim, UK*). A sugar-free linctus containing in each 5 ml pholcodine 5 mg, papaverine hydrochloride 1 mg, tolu balsam, clove oil, ginger tincture, anise oil, capsicum tincture, peppermint oil, alcohol, and chloroform (suggested diluent, Sorbitol Solution). For cough. *Dose.* 5 to 10 ml as required; children, 2.5 to 5 ml three to five times daily.

PEM (*Loveridge, UK*). Linctus containing in each 5 ml pholcodine 5 mg, ephedrine hydrochloride 10 mg, guaiphenesin 12.5 mg, and menthol 1.25 mg. For cough. *Dose.* 5 to 10 ml thrice daily.

Pholcomed (*Medo Chemicals, UK*). Linctus containing in each 5 ml pholcodine 5 mg and papaverine hydrochloride 1.25 mg. For cough. *Dose.* 10 to 15 ml three or four times daily; children, 2.5 to 5 ml. *Pholcomed Diabetic.* A linctus containing the above amounts in a sugar-free basis..

Pholcomed Forte Linctus (*Medo Chemicals, UK*). Contains in each 5 ml pholcodine 19 mg and papaverine hydrochloride 5 mg. **Pholcomed Forte Diabetic Linctus.** A linctus containing the above amounts in a sugar-free basis. *Dose.* 5 ml thrice daily.

Pholtex (*Riker, UK*). A mixture containing in each 5 ml pholcodine 15 mg and phenyltoloxamine 10 mg, both in the form of ion-exchange resin complexes for sustained release (suggested diluent, syrup or tragacanth mucilage). Cough suppressant. *Dose.* 5 ml twice or thrice daily; children, 2.5 to 5 ml.

Rubelix (*Pharmax, UK*). A cough syrup containing in each 5 ml pholcodine 4 mg and ephedrine hydrochloride 6 mg (suggested diluent, syrup). For cough. *Dose.* 10 ml three or four times daily; children, 2.5 to 5 ml.

Sancos (*Sandoz, UK*). A linctus containing in each 5 ml pholcodine 5 mg, glycerol 750 mg, and syrup 5.25 g (suggested diluent, syrup). For unproductive cough. *Dose.* 10 ml every 3 or 4 hours; children, 2.5 to 5 ml.

Sancos Co (*Sandoz, UK*). Linctus containing in each 5 ml pholcodine 5 mg, pseudoephedrine hydrochloride 20 mg, chlorpheniramine maleate 2 mg, glycerol 600 mg, and syrup 5.25 g (suggested diluent, syrup). For cough with associated nasal or bronchial congestion. *Dose.* 10 to 15 ml every 6 hours; children, 2 to 6 years, 2.5 to 5 ml; 6 to 12 years, 5 to 10 ml.

Triocos (*Wander, UK*). Syrup containing in each 5 ml pholcodine 5 mg, pseudoephedrine hydrochloride 20 mg, chlorpheniramine maleate 2 mg, glycerol 600 mg, and syrup 5.25 g. For cough associated with nasal or bronchial congestion. *Dose.* 10 to 15 ml every 6 hours; children, 2 to 6 years, 2.5 to 5 ml; 6 to 12 years, 5 to 10 ml.

Triopaed (*Wander, UK*). Syrup containing in each 5 ml pholcodine 4 mg, glycerol 750 mg, and syrup 5.25 g (suggested diluent, syrup). Cough suppressant. *Dose.* Children, 2 to 6 years, 5 ml every 6 hours; over 6 years, 5 to 10 ml.

Valledrine Cough Linctus (*May & Baker, UK*). Contains in each 5 ml pholcodine citrate equivalent to pholcodine 4 mg, trimeprazine tartrate 2.5 mg, and ephedrine hydrochloride 7.5 mg (suggested diluent, syrup). *Dose.* 5 to 10 ml twice or thrice daily; children, 2 to 5 years, 2.5 ml; 5 to 10 years, 2.5 to 5 ml.

Other Proprietary Names

Adaphol (*Austral.*); Codisol (*Denm.*); Duro-Tuss (*Austral.*); Homocodeina Jarabe (*Spain*); Lantuss, Pectolin, Pholcolin, Pholcolin Red, Pholtrate, Pholtussin, Sedlingtus, Tussinol (all *Austral.*); Tussokon (*Swed.*).

5603-l

Alloclamide Hydrochloride.

264-CE. 2-Allyloxy-4-chloro-*N*-(2-diethylaminoethyl)benzamide hydrochloride. $C_{16}H_{23}ClN_2O_2,HCl$=347.3.

CAS — 5486-77-1 (alloclamide); 5107-01-7 (hydrochloride).

Crystals. M.p. 125° to 127°. **Soluble** in dehydrated alcohol.

A cough suppressant; 75 to 100 mg has been given daily in divided doses.

Proprietary Names

Tuselin Jarabe (*Liade, Spain*).

5604-y

Aminothiazoline Camphorate.

2-Amino-2-thiazoline camphorate. $(C_3H_6N_2S)_2,C_{10}H_{16}O_4$=404.5.

CAS — 1779-81-3 (aminothiazoline); 2387-58-8 (camphorate).

Crystals. M.p. 186° to 188°. **Soluble** in water; practically insoluble in alcohol and ether.

Aminothiazoline camphorate has been used as a cough suppressant in doses of 200 mg three or four times daily.

5605-j

Benzonatate (*U.S.P.*).

KM 65; Benzonatine. 3,6,9,12,15,18,21,24,27-Nonaoxaoctacosyl 4-butylaminobenzoate. $C_{13}H_{18}NO_2(OCH_2CH_2)_nOCH_3$, where *n* has an average value of 8.

CAS — 104-31-4 (where n = 8).

Pharmacopoeias. In *U.S.*

A clear, pale yellow, viscous liquid with a faint

characteristic odour and a bitter numbing taste. **Soluble** 1 in less than 1 of water, alcohol, chloroform, and ether. **Store** in airtight containers. Protect from light.

Adverse Effects. Drowsiness, headache, dizziness, gastro-intestinal disturbances, nasal congestion, hypersensitivity, and skin rash have been reported. Convulsions have also been reported. Benzonatate has local anaesthetic properties and may produce numbness of the mouth, tongue and pharynx.

Uses. A cough suppressant stated to act both centrally and peripherally. The usual dose for adults is 100 mg three to 6 times daily; children under 10 years may be given 8 mg per kg body-weight daily in divided doses. Benzonatate is reported to act within 20 minutes and its effects are reported to last for 3 to 8 hours.

The use of benzonatate in the treatment of cough.— F. Gregoire *et al., Can. med. Ass. J.*, 1958, *79*, 180.

Hiccup. Intractable hiccup in 6 patients was relieved within 20 minutes following the administration of benzonatate.— C. M. Ayres, *Dis. nerv. Syst.*, 1966, *27*, 397.

Preparations

Benzonatate Capsules *(U.S.P.).* Capsules containing benzonatate. Store in airtight containers. Protect from light.

Proprietary Names

Tessalin *(Ciba, Norw.)*; Tessalon *(Ciba, Canad.; Ciba, Neth.; Ciba, Swed.; Ciba-Geigy, Switz.; Endo, USA).*

5640-k

Bibenzonium Bromide. Diphenetholine Bromide; ES132. [2-(1,2-Diphenylethoxy)ethyl]trimethylammonium bromide.
$C_{19}H_{26}BrNO$=364.3.

CAS — 59866-76-1 (bibenzonium); 15585-70-3 (bromide).

Bibenzonium bromide is a cough suppressant which is stated to act on the cough centre and to be free from analgesic and sedative effects. It is used in the treatment of unproductive cough in doses of 20 to 30 mg.

Proprietary Names

Bractos *(Volpino, Arg.)*; Lysobex *(Bracco, Ital.)*; Rea-Tos Jarabe *(Rocador, Spain)*; Sedobex *(Continental Pharma, Belg.).*

5606-z

Butamyrate Citrate. Abbott 36581; HH 197; Butamirate Citrate. 2-(2-Diethylaminoethoxy)ethyl 2-phenylbutyrate dihydrogen citrate.
$C_{18}H_{29}NO_3,C_6H_8O_7$=499.6.

CAS — 18109-80-3 (butamyrate); 18109-81-4 (citrate).

Butamyrate citrate is an antitussive. The usual dose is 6 mg three to five times daily; children have been given 8 to 12 mg daily in divided doses.

Proprietary Names

Pertix-Hommel *(Hommel, Ger.)*; Sincodix *(Beta, Arg.)*; Sinecod *(Hommel, Belg.; Karlspharma, Ger.; Bonomelli-Hommel, Ital.; Abello, Spain; Hommel, Switz.).*

5607-c

Carbetapentane Citrate. Pentoxyverine Citrate; UCB 2543. 2-(2-Diethylaminoethoxy)ethyl 1-phenylcyclopentane-1-carboxylate dihydrogen citrate.
$C_{20}H_{31}NO_3,C_6H_8O_7$=525.6.

CAS — 77-23-6 (carbetapentane); 23142-01-0 (citrate).

Pharmacopoeias. In *Chin.*

A white or almost white odourless crystalline powder. M.p. 90° to 95°. Very **soluble** in water and chloroform; soluble in alcohol; practically insoluble in ether.

Uses. Carbetapentane citrate is a cough suppressant; it is reported to diminish bronchial secretions. It is given in divided doses of 25 to 150 mg daily.

The broncholytic effect of carbetapentane was demonstrated in patients with obstructive lung disease, but was less than that of orciprenaline.— E. Krieger, *Arzneimittel-Forsch.*, 1972, *22*, 389.

Proprietary Names

Atussil *(Squibb, Fr.)*; Germapect *(Thiemann, Ger.)*; Sedotussin *(citrate or hydrochloride) (UCB, Ger.)*; Toclase *(citrate or hydrochloride) (UCB, Arg.; UCB, Denm.; UCB, Norw.; UCB, Swed.)*; Tuclase *(citrate or hydrochloride) (UCB, Belg.; UCB, Ital.; UCB, Neth.)*; Tussa-Tablinen *(Sanorania, Ger.).*

5608-k

Chlophedianol Hydrochloride. Clofedanol Hydrochloride; SL 501; Bayer B186. 2-Chloro-α-(2-dimethylaminoethyl)-α-phenylbenzyl alcohol hydrochloride.
$C_{17}H_{20}ClNO,HCl$=326.3.

CAS — 791-35-5 (chlophedianol); 511-13-7 (hydrochloride).

Soluble in water and alcohol; sparingly soluble in ether.

Adverse Effects and Precautions. Nausea, vomiting, excitation, irritability, nightmares and hallucination may occur. Anticholinergic effects, urticaria, and other hypersensitivity reactions have also been reported. Chlophedianol should be used with care in conjunction with other centrally-acting drugs.

Uses. Chlophedianol hydrochloride is a centrally-acting cough suppressant with mild local anaesthetic properties; it is given in doses of 25 mg.

Proprietary Names

Detigon *(Bayer, Arg.; Bayer, Ital.)*; Eletuss *(Serpero, Ital.)*; Eutus 24 *(Eufarma, Ital.)*; Farmatox *(Cifa, Ital.)*; Gen-Tos *(Morgens, Spain)*; Pectolitan *(Kettelhack Riker, Ger.)*; Prontosed *(Francia Farm., Ital.)*; Tigonal *(IBP, Ital.)*; Tuxidin *(Gazzini, Ital.)*; Ulotos *(Riker, Arg.).*

5609-a

Clobutinol Hydrochloride. KAT 256. 2-(4-Chlorobenzyl)-3-(dimethylaminomethyl)butan-2-ol hydrochloride.
$C_{14}H_{22}ClNO,HCl$=292.2.

CAS — 14860-49-2 (clobutinol); 1215-83-4 (hydrochloride).

Adverse Effects. Drowsiness, dizziness, insomnia, nausea, abdominal discomfort, and sputum reduction.

Uses. Clobutinol hydrochloride is a cough suppressant given in doses of 40 to 80 mg thrice daily; doses of 20 mg have been given by subcutaneous, intramuscular, or intravenous injection.

In 10 healthy volunteers given clobutinol 40 mg by mouth peak plasma concentrations of 160 to 220 ng per ml occurred after 2 hours. Renal and faecal elimination accounted for 80 to 90% and 3% respectively of the administered dose.— A. Zimmer *et al., Arzneimittel-Forsch.*, 1977, *27*, 2011.

References: N. B. Eddy *et al., Codeine and its Alternates for Pain and Cough Relief*, Geneva, World Health Organization, 1970; *Tech. Rep. Ser. Wld Hlth Org. No. 495*, 1972.; M. Loos, *Arzneimittel-Forsch.*, 1973, *23*, 331.

Proprietary Names

Lomistat *(Boehringer Sohn, Spain)*; Silomat *(Boehringer, Arg.; Boehringer Ingelheim, Belg.; Boehringer Ingelheim, Denm.; Badrial, Fr.; Thomae, Ger.; Boehringer Ingelheim, Ital.; Jap.; Boehringer Ingelheim, Norw.; Boehringer Ingelheim, S.Afr.; Boehringer Ingelheim, Swed.; Boehringer Sohn, Switz.).*

5610-e

Cloperastine Hydrochloride. 1-[2-(4-Chlorobenzhydryloxy)ethyl]piperidine hydrochloride.
$C_{20}H_{24}ClNO,HCl$=366.3.

CAS — 3703-76-2 (cloperastine); 14984-68-0 (hydrochloride).

A white crystalline powder with a bitter taste. M.p. about 152°. Freely **soluble** in water, alcohol, and chloroform; slightly soluble in ether.

Adverse Effects. Dry mouth and drowsiness may occur.

Uses. An antitussive agent with an effect similar to that of codeine; it also has some antihistaminic effect. It is given in doses of 10 to 20 mg thrice daily.

Cloperastine fendizoate ($C_{20}H_{24}ClNO,C_{20}H_{14}O_4$ = 648.2) is used similarly; 177 mg of cloperastine fendizoate is approximately equivalent to 100 mg of cloperastine hydrochloride.

Proprietary Names

Hustazol *(Jap.).*

5611-l

Coltsfoot Flower *(B.P.C. 1934).* Tussilaginis Flos; Farfarae Flores.

Pharmacopoeias. In *Port.* and *Swiss.*

The dried flowering shoots of *Tussilago farfara* (Compositae).

5612-y

Coltsfoot Leaf *(B.P.C. 1934).* Tussilaginis Folium; Farfarae Folia; Huflattichblätter.

Pharmacopoeias. In *Aust., Ger., Pol.,* and *Port.*

The dried leaves of *T. farfara.*

Coltsfoot flower has been used, as a liquid extract (1 in 1; alone or diluted with syrup), as a demulcent to relieve chronic and irritable cough. Coltsfoot leaf has been used similarly as a decoction (1 in 20 in doses of 60 ml).

5634-t

Dextromethorphan *(U.S.P.).* (+)-3-Methoxy-9a-methylmorphinan.

$C_{18}H_{25}NO$=271.4.

CAS — 125-71-3.

Pharmacopoeias. In *U.S.*

A practically white or slightly yellow odourless crystalline powder. M.p. 109.5° to 112.5°. Dextromethorphan 7.3 mg is approximately equivalent to 10 mg of dextromethorphan hydrobromide. Practically **insoluble** in water; freely soluble in chloroform. **Store** in airtight containers.

5613-j

Dextromethorphan Hydrobromide *(B.P., U.S.P.).* Dextromethorphanium Bromide. Dextromethorphan hydrobromide monohydrate.

$C_{18}H_{25}NO,HBr,H_2O$=370.3.

CAS — 125-69-9 (anhydrous); 6700-34-1 (monohydrate).

Pharmacopoeias. In *Br., Braz., It., Jap.,* and *U.S.*

A white or almost white crystalline powder, odourless or with a faint odour, and a bitter taste. M.p. about 125° with decomposition. **Soluble** 1 in 60 to 65 of water and 1 in 10 of alcohol; freely soluble in chloroform with the separation of water; practically insoluble in ether. A solution in hydrochloric acid is dextrorotatory. A 2% solution in water has a pH of 5.2 to 6.5. **Store** in airtight containers.

Adverse Effects. Dextromethorphan hydrobromide occasionally causes drowsiness, dizziness, excitation, mental confusion, and gastro-intestinal disturbances. Very high doses may produce respiratory depression.

There have been a few instances of abuse of dextromethorphan, but there does not appear to be any evidence of dependence of the morphine type.

A toxic psychosis characterised by hyperactive behaviour, extreme pressure of thought, and marked visual and auditory hallucinations, developed in a 23-year-old drug addict who had taken dextromethorphan 300 mg. The patient likened this experience to the effects of lysergide.— ADodds and E. Revai (letter), *Med. J. Aust.*, 1967, *2*, 231.

A 22-month-old girl developed ataxia and excitability after taking about 120 ml of a cough syrup containing 360 mg of dextromethorphan hydrobromide. Her ataxia was rapidly reversed by naloxone 60 µg intravenously. The excitability resolved within 8 hours.— W. L. Shaul *et al.*, *Pediatrics*, 1977, *59*, 117.

Dependence. After investigations into the prevalence and incidence of abuse of dextromethorphan, it was concluded that there was no evidence to warrant its international control as a narcotic.— Sixteenth Report of WHO Expert Committee on Drug Dependence, *Tech. Rep. Ser. Wld Hlth Org. No. 407*, 1969.

Dextromethorphan was capable of producing very slight psychic dependence but not physical dependence of the morphine type.— Seventeenth Report of WHO Expert Committee on Drug Dependence, *Tech. Rep. Ser. Wld Hlth Org. No. 437*, 1970.

Precautions. Dextromethorphan should be administered with caution to patients with liver disease and to asthmatic patients.

Absorption and Fate. Dextromethorphan is well absorbed from the gastro-intestinal tract. It is metabolised in the liver and excreted as unchanged dextromethorphan and demethylated morphinan compounds.

After administration of dextromethorphan hydrobromide 30 mg by mouth to 6 subjects, the average plasma concentrations of its major metabolites dextrorphan and conjugates were about 21 ng per ml, about 107 ng, and about 368 ng per ml after 15 minutes, 30 minutes, and 60 minutes respectively with a peak of about 381 ng per ml after 2 hours.— G. Ramachander *et al.*, *J. pharm. Sci.*, 1977, *66*, 1047.

Uses. Dextromethorphan is a cough suppressant which is used similarly to pholcodine, often together with an antihistamine in the treatment of unproductive cough. It has no analgesic or sedative properties.

It is administered by mouth, usually in the form of syrup or lozenges. The dose of dextromethorphan hydrobromide for adults is 15 to 30 mg, for children 6 to 12 years 6.75 mg, and for infants over 1 year, about 3.5 mg; these doses may be repeated up to four times daily.

A review of the paediatric use of cough syrups containing dextromethorphan or codeine.— S. Segal *et al.*, *Pediatrics*, 1978, *62*, 118, per *Int. pharm. Abstr.*, 1979, *16*, 417.

Preparations

Dextromethorphan Hydrobromide Syrup *(U.S.P.)*. A syrup containing dextromethorphan hydrobromide. Store in airtight containers. Protect from light.

Dextromethorphan Tablets *(B.P. 1973)*. Dextromethorphan Tab. Tablets containing dextromethorphan hydrobromide. The tablets are sugar-coated.

Proprietary Preparations

Cosylan *(Parke, Davis, UK)*. Dextromethorphan hydrobromide, available as syrup containing 13.5 mg in each 5 ml.

Dexylets *(Parke, Davis, UK)*. Lozenges each containing dextromethorphan hydrobromide 2.5 mg and phenylephrine hydrochloride 500 µg. For cough. *Dose.* 1 lozenge as required; not more than 10 in 24 hours.

Muflin Syrup *(Concept Pharmaceuticals, UK)*. Contains in each 5 ml dextromethorphan hydrobromide 10 mg, pheniramine maleate 7.5 mg, sodium citrate 130 mg, and citric acid monohydrate 20 mg (suggested diluent, syrup). For cough. *Dose.* 5 to 10 ml three or four times daily; children, up to 6 years, 2.5 to 5 ml; 6 to 12 years, 5 ml.

Paranorm Paediatric Cough Syrup *(Wallace Mfg Chem., UK: Farillon, UK)*. Contains in each 10 ml dextromethorphan hydrobromide 5.5 mg, ephedrine hydrochloride 4 mg, guaiphenesin 20 mg, and glycerol 500 mg. *Dose.* Children, 10 ml every 4 hours; infants, 6 to 12 months, 5 ml.

Syrtussar *(Armour, UK)*. A syrup containing in each 5 ml dextromethorphan hydrobromide 10 mg and pheniramine maleate 7.5 mg (suggested diluent, syrup). For cough. *Dose.* Adults, 5 to 10 ml three or four times daily; children, 2.5 to 5 ml.

Tancolin *(Ashe, UK)*. A flavoured linctus containing in each 5 ml dextromethorphan hydrobromide 2.62 mg, theophylline 15 mg, sodium citrate 99.56 mg, citric acid monohydrate 45.85 mg, ascorbic acid 12.35 mg, and glycerol 655 mg.

Unitussin *(Unimed, UK)*. Mixture containing in each 5 ml dextromethorphan hydrobromide 5 mg, ammonium chloride 100 mg, ipecacuanha liquid extract 0.02 ml, chloroform 0.01 ml, and menthol 0.5 mg. Expectorant.

Other Proprietary Names

Arg.—Pectobron, Romilar; *Canad.*—Balminil D.M., Broncho-Grippol-DM, Deca-Toux, Demo-Cineol Antitussive syrup, DM Syrup, Robidex, Sedatuss, Tussorphan; *Jap.*—Dextphan; *Ital.*—Canfodion, Romilar, Sedotus, Tussistop, Val Atux; *Spain*—Romilar.

5614-z

Dextrorphan. (+)-9a-Methylmorphinan-3-ol.
$C_{17}H_{23}NO$=257.4.

CAS — 125-73-5.

Dextrorphan is a cough suppressant which is less potent than dextromethorphan of which it is a metabolite (see above). Dextrorphan does not have the marked analgesic properties of its isomer levorphanol (see p.1015).

5615-c

Dimemorfan Phosphate. AT 17. (+)-3,9a-Dimethylmorphinan phosphate.
$C_{18}H_{25}N,H_3PO_4$=353.4.

CAS — 36309-01-0 (dimemorfan); 36304-84-4 (phosphate).

A white or yellowish-white odourless crystalline powder with a bitter astringent taste. M.p. about 265° with decomposition. Sparingly **soluble** in water and methyl alcohol; practically insoluble in acetone, alcohol, chloroform, and ether; soluble in hydrochloric acid and in glacial acetic acid.

Adverse Effects. Anorexia, nausea, and dry mouth.

Uses. Dimemorfan is structurally related to dextromethorphan hydrobromide (see p.1261) and has similar antitussive properties. It is given in doses of 10 to 20 mg.

Pharmacology in animals.— Y. Kasé *et al.*, *Arzneimittel-Forsch.*, 1976, *26*, 353; *idem*, 361.

Proprietary Names
Astomin *(Jap.)*.

5616-k

Dimethoxanate Hydrochloride. 2-(2-Dimethylaminoethoxy)ethyl phenothiazine-10-carboxylate hydrochloride.
$C_{19}H_{22}N_2O_3S,HCl$=394.9.

CAS — 477-93-0 (dimethoxanate); 518-63-8 (hydrochloride).

Dimethoxanate hydrochloride is a cough suppressant with local anaesthetic and spasmolytic properties given in doses of 25 to 50 mg. Its effects are reported to last for 3 to 7 hours. Adverse effects include nausea, slight drowsiness, and skin rash.

Proprietary Names
Cothera *(Inibsa, Spain)*; Cotrane *(Clin-Midy, Belg.; Midyfarm, Fr.)*; Tussizid *(Nagel, Ital.)*.

5617-a

Drotebanol. Oxymethebanol. 3,4-Dimethoxy-9a-methylmorphinan-6β,14-diol.
$C_{19}H_{27}NO_4$=333.4.

CAS — 3176-03-2.

White or almost white crystals or crystalline powder with a slightly bitter taste. M.p. about 169°. Practically **insoluble** in water; freely soluble in alcohol and chloroform; soluble in acetone; very slightly soluble in ether.

Adverse Effects. Anorexia, dry mouth, nausea, vomiting, constipation or diarrhoea, dizziness, and headache.

Uses. Drotebanol is a narcotic antitussive agent given in doses of 2 mg thrice daily. It has also been given subcutaneously or intramuscularly in similar doses.

Proprietary Names
Metebanyl *(Jap.)*.

5618-t

Ethyl Orthoformate. Éther de Kay; Triethoxymethane. Triethyl orthoformate.
$C_7H_{16}O_3$=148.2.

CAS — 122-51-0.

A colourless liquid. B.p. about 145°. Slightly **soluble** in water with decomposition; soluble in alcohol.

Ethyl orthoformate is a cough suppressant. It is reported to be a respiratory antispasmodic and is administered by mouth or rectally.

Proprietary Names
Aethone *(Cochard, Belg.; Laboratoires Biologiques de l'Île-de-France, Fr.)*; Orthoformyl *(Cochard, Belg.)*.

5619-x

Fedrilate. UCB 3928; Fedrilatum. 1-Methyl-3-morpholinopropyl perhydro-4-phenylpyran-4-carboxylate.
$C_{20}H_{29}NO_4$=347.5.

CAS — 23271-74-1.

Fedrilate is a cough suppressant given in doses of 50 mg three or four times daily; children, 10 mg thrice daily.

Proprietary Names
Tussapax *(UCB, S.Afr.)*; Tussefan *(ICN, Neth.)*.

5620-y

Fominoben Hydrochloride. PB 89. 3′-Chloro-2′-[*N*-methyl-*N*-(morpholinocarbonylmethyl)aminomethyl]-benzanilide hydrochloride.
$C_{21}H_{24}ClN_3O_3,HCl$=438.5.

CAS — 18053-31-1 (fominoben); 24600-36-0 (hydrochloride).

A white powder. M.p. 206° to 208°. Slightly **soluble** in water.

Fominoben hydrochloride is a cough suppressant and respiratory stimulant given in doses of 160 mg twice or thrice daily by mouth or 40 to 80 mg twice or thrice daily by slow intravenous injection.

The metabolism and excretion of fominoben hydrochloride.— A. Zimmer, *Arzneimittel-Forsch.*, 1973, *23*, 317 and 1798.

The use of fominoben hydrochloride in patients with tuberculosis, chronic bronchitis, and other respiratory-tract diseases.— J. Heitmann, *Arzneimittel-Forsch.*, 1973, *23*, 329; M. Loos, *ibid.*, 331; E. R. Köhler, *ibid.*, 351; H. Schneiderhan, *ibid.*, 353; O. Jahn and J. Kolle, *ibid.*, 355; G. Huber, *ibid.*, 359; F. Arch, *ibid.*, 363.

In 11 patients given fominoben hydrochloride intravenously mean systolic and diastolic blood pressures at rest and during exercise were reduced. Mean alveolar ventilation was reduced by 9% at rest but was unchanged during exercise.— G. Koch, *Arzneimittel-Forsch.*, 1976, *26*, 438.

The biotransformation of fominoben hydrochloride.— A. Zimmer *et al.*, *Arzneimittel-Forsch.*, 1978, *28*, 688.

In 10 healthy subjects given radioactive fominoben hydrochloride 160 mg by mouth a mean peak plasma concentration of 4.3 µg per ml occurred 2 hours after administration. After 96 hours 65% and 23% to 26% of the administered radioactivity had been excreted in the urine and faeces respectively. Following administration of a tablet containing fominoben 160 mg and etofylline 300 mg to the same subjects similar values for fominoben plasma concentrations and excretion were obtained.— R. Jauch and A. Zimmer, *Arzneimittel-Forsch.*, 1978, *28*, 693.

An improvement of pulmonary haemodynamics was observed in 10 patients with chronic obstructive lung diseases given fominoben 160 mg and etofylline 300 mg thrice daily for 8 to 32 days.— G. Siemon and R. Thoma, *Arzneimittel-Forsch.*, 1978, *28*, 698.

Proprietary Names
Finaten *(Finadiet, Arg.)*; Noleptan *(Thomae, Ger.)*; Terion *(Lusofarmaco, Ital.)*.

5621-j

Hydrocotarnine Hydrochloride. 5,6,7,8-Tetrahydro-4-methoxy-6-methyl-1,3-dioxolo[4,5-*g*]isoquinoline hydrochloride monohydrate.
$C_{12}H_{15}NO_3,HCl,H_2O=275.7$.

CAS — 550-10-7 (hydrocotarnine); 5985-55-7 (hydrochloride, anhydrous).

Pharmacopoeias. In *Jap.*

White to yellowish, odourless crystals or crystalline powder with a bitter taste. **Soluble** 1 in 3 of water and 1 in 70 of alcohol; practically insoluble in ether. A 5% solution has a pH of 4 to 6.

Hydrocotarnine hydrochloride has actions and uses similar to those of noscapine (see below), to which it is chemically related.

5622-z

Isoaminile Citrate.

4-Dimethylamino-2-isopropyl-2-phenylvaleronitrile dihydrogen citrate.
$C_{16}H_{24}N_2,C_6H_8O_7=436.5$.

CAS — 77-51-0 (isoaminile); 28416-66-2 (citrate).

Adverse Effects. Dizziness, nausea, constipation, and diarrhoea have been reported.

There have been some instances of abuse of isoaminile but little evidence of physical dependence of the morphine type.

Isoaminile citrate was responsible for a fixed drug eruption in 1 patient.— J. A. Savin, *Br. J. Derm.*, 1970, *83*, 546.

Uses. Isoaminile citrate is a cough suppressant which is used in doses of 40 mg similarly to pholcodine (see p.1260) in the treatment of unproductive cough. It has no analgesic or sedative properties and does not depress the respiration.

The base, isoaminile, is administered in the form of capsules. The dose of the base is approximately one-half that of the citrate.

Isoaminile has also been used as the cyclamate.

Comparison with codeine. In a double-blind crossover study completed by 78 patients with cough due to various conditions, better relief was obtained by treatment with isoaminile 45 to 90 mg every 4 hours for 3 to 4 days than with codeine phosphate 15 to 30 mg given similarly; children received reduced doses.—Report No. 85 of the General Practitioner Research Group, *Practitioner*, 1966, *196*, 436.

Proprietary Preparations of Isoaminile and Some of its Salts

Dimyril Linctus *(Fisons, UK)*. Contains isoaminile citrate 40 mg in each 5 ml.

Other Proprietary Names

Peracan *(Belg.)*; Peracon (citrate or cyclamate) *(Arg., Denm., Ger., Ital., Neth., Norw., S.Afr., Swed., Switz.)*; Perogan (citrate or cyclamate) *(Spain)*; Sedotosse (citrate) *(Ital.)*.

5623-c

Levopropoxyphene Napsylate *(U.S.P.)*.

(−)-1-Benzyl-3-dimethylamino-2-methyl-1-phenylpropyl propionate naphthalene-2-sulphonate monohydrate.
$C_{22}H_{29}NO_2,C_{10}H_8O_3S,H_2O=565.7$.

CAS — 2338-37-6 (levopropoxyphene); 5714-90-9 (napsylate, anhydrous); 55557-30-7 (napsylate, monohydrate).

Pharmacopoeias. In *U.S.*

A white almost odourless powder with a bitter taste. M.p. 158° to 165° with a range of not more than 4°. Levopropoxyphene napsylate 1.66 g is approximately equivalent to 1 g of levopropoxyphene. Very slightly **soluble** in water; soluble 1 in 17 of alcohol and 1 in 2 of chloroform; soluble in acetone and methyl alcohol. A solution in chloroform is laevorotatory. **Store** in airtight containers.

Adverse Effects. Headache, drowsiness, dizziness, nausea, vomiting, urinary urgency, skin rash, diarrhoea and visual disturbances may occur.

Uses. Levopropoxyphene napsylate is a cough suppressant given in doses equivalent to 50 to 100 mg of levopropoxyphene; unlike its dextroisomer dextropropoxyphene, it has no analgesic activity. Its effects last for about 4 hours.

Preparations

Levopropoxyphene Napsylate Capsules *(U.S.P.)*. Capsules containing levopropoxyphene napsylate. Potency is expressed in terms of the equivalent amount of levopropoxyphene. Store in airtight containers.

Levopropoxyphene Napsylate Oral Suspension *(U.S.P.)*. A syrup containing levopropoxyphene napsylate. Potency is expressed in terms of the equivalent amount of levopropoxyphene. Store in airtight containers and avoid freezing. Protect from light.

Proprietary Names

Novrad *(Lilly, USA)*; Sotorni (levopropoxyphene dibudinate)*(Ravensberg, Ger.)*.

5624-k

Morclofone Hydrochloride. 4′-Chloro-3,5-dimethoxy-4-(2-morpholinoethoxy)benzophenone hydrochloride.
$C_{21}H_{24}ClNO_5,HCl=442.3$.

CAS — 31848-01-8 (morclofone); 31848-02-9 (hydrochloride).

Morclofone hydrochloride is a antitussive agent given in doses of 400 to 600 mg daily. It is given by mouth and rectally by suppository.

Proprietary Names

Medicil *(Medici, Ital.)*; Plausitin *(Montedison, Arg.; Carlo Erba, Ital.)*.

5625-a

Noscapine *(B.P., Eur. P., U.S.P.)*.

Noscapinum; Narcotine; L-α-Narcotine. (3*S*)-6,7-Dimethoxy-3-[(5*R*)-5,6,7,8-tetrahydro-4-methoxy-6-methyl-1,3-dioxolo[4,5-*g*]isoquinolin-5-yl]phthalide.
$C_{22}H_{23}NO_7=413.4$.

CAS — 128-62-1.

Pharmacopoeias. In *Br., Eur., Fr., Ger., Int., It., Jap., Neth., Swiss, Turk.*, and *U.S.*

Noscapine is an alkaloid obtained from opium. It occurs as colourless odourless tasteless crystals or as a fine white crystalline powder. M.p. 174° to 176° with decomposition.

Practically **insoluble** in water at 20°, very slightly soluble at 100°; slightly soluble in alcohol and ether; soluble in acetone and chloroform; soluble in strong acids to give readily hydrolysable salts. Solutions in organic solvents are laevorotatory; aqueous acidic solutions are dextrorotatory. **Store** in airtight containers.

5626-t

Noscapine Hydrochloride *(B.P., Eur. P.)*.

Noscapini Hydrochloridum; Noscapinium Chloride; Narcotine Hydrochloride.
$C_{22}H_{23}NO_7,HCl,H_2O=467.9$.

CAS — 912-60-7 (anhydrous).

Pharmacopoeias. In *Br., Eur., Ger., It., Jug., Neth.*, and *Nord.* (all with H_2O); *Hung.* and *Swiss* (both with $2H_2O$); *Fr.* and *Jap.* (both with xH_2O).

Colourless odourless crystals or a fine white crystalline powder, hygroscopic, and with a bitter taste. M.p. about 200° with decomposition.

Soluble 1 in 4 of water and 1 in 8 of alcohol; freely soluble in chloroform; soluble in methyl alcohol; sparingly soluble in acetone; practically insoluble in ether. A solution in hydrochloric acid is dextrorotatory. A 2% solution in water has a pH not below 2.4. Aqueous solutions may deposit the base on standing. **Store** in airtight containers.

Adverse Effects. Side-effects include slight drowsiness, dizziness, headache, nausea, allergic rhinitis, conjunctivitis, and skin rash.

Absorption and Fate. Noscapine is well absorbed from the gastro-intestinal tract.

The kinetics of metabolism, urinary excretion, and distribution of noscapine.— K. P. Nayak *et al.*, *J. pharm. Sci.*, 1965, *54*, 191.

The biological half-life of noscapine was 0.147 hours.— W. A. Ritschel, *Drug Intell. & clin. Pharm.*, 1970, *4*, 332.

Uses. Noscapine is a cough suppressant which is used similarly to pholcodine (see p.1260) in the treatment of unproductive cough. It has weak bronchodilator properties and stimulates the respiration. Noscapine has no analgesic or sedative properties and it does not produce euphoria. Its use is unlikely to lead to dependence.

The usual dose is 15 to 30 mg three or four times daily, but single doses of up to 60 mg may be given. The effect lasts for up to 4 hours.

Noscapine embonate is sometimes used.

Cough. Noscapine, in a dose of 15 to 60 mg daily, had a beneficial suppressant effect in 50 of 54 trials carried out in 51 patients with cough due to various pulmonary conditions. Side-effects occurred in 6 patients and included drowsiness, difficulty in clearing secretions, and headache. Gradual loss of effectiveness was noted in 3 patients.— M. S. Segal *et al.*, *Dis. Chest*, 1957, *32*, 305.

Preparations of Noscapine and Some of its Salts

Noscapine Linctus *(A.P.F.)*. Noscapine 15 mg, citric acid monohydrate 50 mg, water 0.5 ml, concentrated chloroform water 0.1 ml, tartrazine solution 0.1 ml, syrup to 5 ml. *Dose.* 5 ml.

Noscapine Linctus *(B.P.)*. Linct. Noscap. Noscapine 15 mg, citric acid monohydrate 50 mg, freshly boiled and cooled water 0.5 ml, chloroform spirit 0.375 ml, compound tartrazine solution 0.015 ml, syrup to 5 ml. Store at a temperature not exceeding 25°. When a dose less than or not a multiple of 5 ml is prescribed, the linctus may be diluted to 5 ml, or a multiple, with syrup. Such dilutions must be freshly prepared and not used more than 2 weeks after issue.

For a report of incompatibility when Noscapine Linctus was prepared with or diluted with syrup preserved with hydroxybenzoates, see under Sucrose, p.61.

Proprietary Names of Noscapine and Some of its Salts

Bequitusin (hydrochloride with embonate) *(Cecef, Spain)*; Capval (resin complex or hydrochloride) *(Dreluso, Ger.)*; Dru Tosse *(Virgiliano, Ital.)*; Finipect *(Mepros, Neth.)*; Longactin (resin complex) *(Dumex, Norw.)*; Longatin *(Dumex, Denm.; Dumex, Swed.)*; Lyobex retard (resin complex or hydrochloride) *(Lappe, Ger.)*; Narcotos *(Pierre Bardin, Arg.)*; Narcotussin (hydrochloride) *(Biologici Italia, Ital.)*; Nipaxon *(Leo, Swed.)*; Nitepax *(MPS Lab., S.Afr.)*; Noscapect (hydrochloride) *(Roter, Belg.; Roter, Neth.)*; Noscatuss *(Fisons, Canad.)*; Rode Hoestsiroop (hydrochloride) *(Daro, Neth.)*; Tucotine (hydrochloride) *(Sanders-Probel, Belg.)*; Tusscapine *(Fisons, USA)*; Tussicare (base with embonate) *(Wolfs, Belg.)*; Tussinil (hydrochloride with embonate) *(Pental, Spain)*.

Noscapine was formerly marketed in Great Britain under the proprietary name Coscopin *(Duncan, Flockhart)*.

5627-x

Oxeladin Citrate. 2-(2-Diethylaminoethoxy)ethyl 2-ethyl-2-phenylbutyrate dihydrogen citrate. $C_{20}H_{33}NO_3,C_6H_8O_7=527.6$.

CAS — 468-61-1 (oxeladin); 52432-72-1 (citrate).

A white crystalline powder with a bitter numbing taste. **Soluble** in water.

Oxeladin citrate is a cough suppressant which depresses the activity of the cough reflex. It is given in doses of 40 mg twice or thrice daily.

Proprietary Names

Antusel *(Lema, Arg.)*; Dorex-retard *(Woelm, Ger.)*; Frenotos *(Disprovent, Arg.)*; Neobex *(Lampugnani, Ital.)*; Paxeladine *(Beaufour, Belg.; Beaufour, Fr.)*; Pectamol *(Malesci, Ital.)*; Pectamon *(Hässle, Swed.)*; Tussilisin *(Ibirn, Ital.)*; Tussilong *(Restan, S.Afr.)*.

5628-r

Picoperine Hydrochloride. Picoperidamine Hydrochloride; TAT-3. *N*-(2-Piperidinoethyl)-*N*-(2-pyridylmethyl)aniline hydrochloride. $C_{19}H_{25}N_3,HCl=331.9$.

CAS — 21755-66-8 (picoperine); 24699-40-9 (hydrochloride).

White crystals or crystalline powder, odourless or with a slight characteristic odour, and with a bitter taste. M.p. about 184°.

Adverse Effects. Anorexia, nausea, constipation, drowsiness, headache, and mild palpitations.

Uses. Picoperine hydrochloride is an antitussive agent. The tasteless palmitate is similarly used.

Pharmacology in *animals*.— Y. Kasé *et al.*, *Arzneimittel-Forsch.*, 1969, *19*, 1916.

Proprietary Names

Coben, Coben-P (palmitate) (both *Jap.*).

5629-f

Pipazethate Hydrochloride.

Piperestazine Hydrochloride; LG 254. 2-(2-Piperidinoethoxy)ethyl pyrido[3,2-*b*][1,4]benzothiazine-10-carboxylate hydrochloride. $C_{21}H_{25}N_3O_3S,HCl=436.0$.

CAS — 2167-85-3 (pipazethate); 6056-11-7 (hydrochloride).

A white crystalline powder. Very **soluble** in water; soluble in alcohol and methyl alcohol; practically insoluble in acetone and benzene. A 2% solution in water has a pH of about 5.4.

Adverse Effects. Pipazethate hydrochloride may occasionally cause drowsiness, nausea, vomiting, restlessness, insomnia, and urticaria. Tachycardia has been reported.

A healthy 4-year-old child became somnolent and agitated, with convulsions, followed by coma, 1 hour after swallowing an unknown number of tablets containing pipazethate; cardiac arrhythmias also developed. She recovered completely after treatment with diazepam for the convulsions, intravenous infusion of sodium bicarbonate to control acidosis, and lignocaine to control arrhythmias. Phenytoin was also given prophylactically.— O. A. da Silva and M. Lopez, *Clin. Toxicol.*, 1977, *11*, 455.

Uses. Pipazethate is a cough suppressant which has been used similarly to pholcodine (see p.1260) in the treatment of unproductive cough. It has been suggested that it acts on the central cough centre. It does not depress the respiration. It acts in 10 to 30 minutes and the effects last for 4 to 6 hours.

Pipazethate hydrochloride has been given in doses of 20 to 40 mg thrice daily.

Favourable reports on the cough suppressant effects of pipazethate hydrochloride.— F. J. Prime, *Br. med. J.*, 1961, *1*, 1149; K. D. Phillips and E. W. Guillaume, *Practitioner*, 1961, *186*, 238; S. H. Goodman, *Practitioner*, 1961, *187*, 803; A. B. Amler and C. B. Rothman, *J. new Drugs*, 1963, *3*, 362.

Pipazethate 40 to 70 mg daily was no better than a placebo in relieving coughs induced by a spray of citric acid monohydrate in 41 persons, or chronic cough in 70 patients, most of whom had tuberculosis.— B. J. Vakil *et al.*, *Clin. Pharmac. Ther.*, 1966, *7*, 515.

Proprietary Names

Lenopect *(Draco, Swed.)*; Selvigon *(Homburg, Ger.)*; Selvjgon *(Armour, Ital.)*; Toraxan *(Unifa, Arg.)*.

Pipazethate hydrochloride was formerly marketed in Great Britain under the proprietary name Selvigon *(Smith Kline & French)*.

5630-z

Piperidione. NU 1510. 3,3-Diethylpiperidine-2,4-dione. $C_9H_{15}NO_2=169.2$.

CAS — 77-03-2.

Piperidione is a centrally-acting cough suppressant with sedative properties. It has been given in doses of 100 to 200 mg.

Proprietary Names

Sedulon *(Roche, Swed.)*.

5631-c

Prenoxdiazin Hydrochloride. HK 256. 3-(2,2-Diphenylethyl)-5-(2-piperidinoethyl)-1,2,4-oxadiazole hydrochloride. $C_{23}H_{27}N_3O,HCl=397.9$.

CAS — 982-43-4.

Prenoxdiazin hydrochloride is an antitussive agent given in doses of 100 mg. Prenoxdiazin benzhydrate is also used.

References: K. Harsányi *et al.*, *Arzneimittel-Forsch.*, 1966, *16*, 615 (synthesis); L. Tardos and I. Erdély, *ibid.*, 617 (pharmacology); M. Hankovszky and A. Károlyi, *ibid.*, 622 (clinical use).

Proprietary Names

Libexin (also as benzhydrate) *(Chinoin, Hung.; Chiesi, Ital.)*; Lomapect (also as benzhydrate) *(TAD, Ger.)*; Tibexin *(Christiaens, Belg.)*; Varoxil *(Padro, Spain)*.

5632-k

Sodium Dibunate. L 1633. Sodium 2,6-di-*tert*-butylnaphthalene-1-sulphonate. $C_{18}H_{23}NaO_3S=342.4$.

CAS — 14992-58-6 (dibunate); 14992-59-7 (sodium dibunate).

Sodium dibunate is a cough suppressant claimed to have central actions and also to depress the transmission of afferent cough impulses. It is given in doses of 30 to 60 mg.

Proprietary Names

Becantal *(Labaz, Spain)*; Becantex *(Labaz, Belg.; Labaz, Fr.; Labaz, Neth.)*; Bechisan *(Sidus, Ital.)*; Bexedan (chlorcyclizine dibunate) *(UCB, Ital.)*; Licolen (chlorcyclizine dibunate) *(Molteni, Ital.)*.

The name naftoclizine has been used for chlorcyclizine dibunate.

5633-a

Zipeprol Hydrochloride. CERM 3024. 1-Methoxy-3-[4-(β-methoxyphenethyl)piperazin-1-yl]-1-phenylpropan-2-ol dihydrochloride. $C_{23}H_{32}N_2O_3,2HCl=457.4$.

CAS — 34758-83-3 (zipeprol); 34758-84-4 (hydrochloride).

A white powder with a bitter taste. **Soluble** in water; practically insoluble in ether.

Zipeprol hydrochloride is an antitussive agent which is stated to exert its effect by relieving bronchial spasm; 150 to 300 mg may be given daily in divided doses.

Studies on the metabolism and excretion of zipeprol hydrochloride in acid urine in 4 healthy subjects.— A. H. Beckett and R. Achari, *J. Pharm. Pharmac.*, 1976, *28, Suppl.*, 57P.

Following administration of 175 and 200 mg doses by mouth to 3 healthy subjects with their urine maintained at an acid pH zipeprol was rapidly and extensively metabolised, 1 to 5% of the dose being excreted in the urine as unchanged drug. Two *N*-dealkylated metabolites accounted for about 19 to 38% of the dose; excretion rates of these metabolites fell sharply when the pH of the urine was allowed to rise.— A. H. Beckett and R. Achari, *J. Pharm. Pharmac.*, 1977, *29*, 589. Identification of a further metabolic product of zipeprol in man.— *idem*, 645. See also *idem*, 253.

Zipeprol was mainly metabolised by *N*-dealkylation, oxidation, hydroxylation, and methylation, but was partially eliminated unchanged.— M. Constantin and J. F. Pognat, *Arzneimittel-Forsch.*, 1978, *28*, 64.

Proprietary Names

Respilène *(Winthrop, Fr.)*; Respirex *(Inibsa, Spain)*; Talasa *(Andromaco, Arg.)*; Zitoxil *(Farmochimica Italiana, Ital.)*.

Pituitary and Hypothalamic Hormones

5920-h

The pituitary gland or hypophysis is composed of the adenohypophysis and neurohypophysis. The adenohypophysis consists of the anterior lobe and the neurohypophysis of the posterior lobe and the neural stalk, above which lies the hypothalamus. The anterior lobe is linked to the hypothalamus by a portal vascular system but there is no vascular link between the posterior lobe and the hypothalamus.

The following hormones are secreted by the anterior lobe of the pituitary: adrenocorticotrophic hormone, p.1265; the gonadotrophic hormones, follicle-stimulating hormone, p.1269, and luteinising hormone, p.1270; growth hormone, p.1270; lactogenic hormone or prolactin, p.1275; thyroid-stimulating hormone or thyrotrophin, p.1278; the status of melanocyte-stimulating hormone, p.1272, in man is uncertain.

The octapeptide hormones oxytocin and vasopressin are synthesised in the hypothalamus. They become associated with a carrier protein, neurophysin, and are then transported down nerve fibres to the posterior pituitary where they are stored until required. The release of oxytocin and vasopressin appears to be controlled mainly by nervous reflex responses.

The secretion of anterior pituitary hormones, in which the hypothalamus plays a major part, is regulated by a complex interaction between stimulatory and inhibitory neural and hormonal influences. Transmitter substances are secreted within neurones of the hypothalamus, stored in the median eminence, and released into the hypophyseal portal system to reach the anterior pituitary. Extracts of the hypothalamus which contain these substances have been shown to inhibit or stimulate the release of specific anterior pituitary hormones. Conventionally these transmitters are referred to as 'factors' and when their structure is known and they are well established as physiological regulators of anterior pituitary hormone secretion, they are called hormones. The following hypothalamic hormones and factors are described below: gonadotrophin-releasing hormone or gonadorelin, p.1267; growth-hormone-release-inhibiting hormone or somatostatin, p.1277; melanocyte-stimulating-hormone-release-inhibiting factor or melanostatin, p.1272; thyrotrophin-releasing hormone or protirelin, p.1276.

The synthesis and release of hypothalamic hormones may be controlled by feedback mechanisms involving target organ hormones, pituitary hormones, and possibly the hypothalamic hormones themselves, as well as by excitatory or inhibitory impulses from different parts of the brain. These impulses may be mediated by dopamine, acetylcholine, gamma-aminobutyric acid, or other neurotransmitters; the hypothalamic hormones and other peptides such as substance P, enkephalins, and endorphins may act as transmitters or modulators in the hypothalamus.

Nomenclature. Several different names are used to describe these hormones since a comprehensive system of nomenclature is not yet in general use. The greatest confusion exists with the hypothalamic hormones or factors which are often described in terms of the pituitary hormone the release of which they inhibit or stimulate, as with growth-hormone-release-inhibiting hormone. Because of the length of such composite words, abbreviations consisting of initial letters e.g. GH-RIH or GH-RIF are commonly employed. Some form of approved name has been used for each hormone or factor described below in preference to these abbreviations or detailed names which are, however, provided as synonyms.

Reviews of the actions of pituitary hormones: A. P. Somlyo and A. V. Somlyo, *Pharmac. Rev.*, 1970, *22*, 249; A. G. Davies, *Br. med. J.*, 1972, *2*, 282; C. A. Hardisty and D. S. Munro, *Practitioner*, 1978, *221*, 499.

Reviews of the actions of the hypothalamic hormones: *Br. med. J.*, 1972, *1*, 65; J. S. Jenkins, *ibid.*, 1972, *2*, 99; R. Guillemin, in *Chemistry and Biology of Peptides, Proceedings of the Third American Peptide Symposium*, J. Meienhofer (Ed.), Ann Arbor, Ann Arbor Science Publishers 1972, p. 585; R. Hall, *Br. J. Hosp. Med.*, 1973, *9*, 109; G. M. Besser, *Br. med. J.*, 1974, *3*, 560 and 613; J. B. Martin *et al.*, *Lancet*, 1975, *2*, 393; J. C. Buckingham, *J. Pharm. Pharmac.*, 1977, *29*, 649; A. V. Schally, *Science*, 1978, *202*, 18; R. Guillemin, *Science*, 1978, *202*, 390; *Pharmacology of the Hypothalamus*, B. Cox *et al.* (Ed.), London, Macmillan, 1978.

An account of pituitary diseases.— J. A. Strong, *Br. med. J.*, 1976, *1*, 640. See also L. Alexander, *Practitioner*, 1977, *218*, 532.

The assessment of hypothalamic, pituitary, and adrenal function.— J. S. Jenkins, in *Clinical Medicine and Therapeutics*, P. Richards and H. Mather (Ed.), Oxford, Blackwell, 1977, p. 178.

A review of the processes responsible for removing biologically active peptide hormones from the circulation.— H. P. J. Bennett and C. McMartin, *Pharmac. Rev.*, 1978, *30*, 247.

A review of brain peptides.— D. T. Krieger and J. B. Martin, *New Engl. J. Med.*, 1981, *304*, 876; *idem*, 944.

5921-m

Adrenocorticotrophic Hormone. ACTH; Corticotrophin.

CAS — 9002-60-2.

Adrenocorticotrophic hormone, which is secreted from the anterior lobe of the pituitary, is a polypeptide which stimulates development of the adrenal cortex and secretion of the corticosteroids but does not affect the adrenal medulla. Overproduction of the hormone induces adrenal hyperplasia with the associated disorders of adrenocortical hyperfunction such as Cushing's syndrome.

Secretion of adrenocorticotrophic hormone or corticotrophin from the pituitary is controlled by a hypothalamic releasing factor (CRF), which has not yet been identified, and by the inhibitory effect of circulating corticosteroids. Somatostatin (p.1277) may also inhibit its release.

The actions and clinical uses of adrenocorticotrophic hormone are described under Corticotrophin, p.486.

5922-b

Desmopressin. [1-(3-Mercaptopropionic acid),8-D-arginine]-vasopressin.

$C_{46}H_{64}N_{14}O_{12}S_2$=1069.2.

CAS — 16679-58-6.

5923-v

Desmopressin Acetate. The monoacetate trihydrate of desmopressin.

$C_{46}H_{64}N_{14}O_{12}S_2,C_2H_4O_2,3H_2O$=1183.3.

CAS — 62288-83-9 (anhydrous); 62357-86-2 (trihydrate).

Adverse Effects and Precautions. As for Vasopressin Injection, p.1278.

The pressor activity of desmopressin is about 2000 times less than that of argipressin and it is well tolerated.

Paranoid psychosis after desmopressin therapy for Alzheimer's dementia.— G. B. Collins *et al.* (letter), *Lancet*, 1981, *2*, 808.

Absorption and Fate. Desmopressin is absorbed from the nasal mucosa.

Confirmation that desmopressin acetate given intranasally induces antidiuresis, in patients with diabetes insipidus, over approximately 12 hours (consistently exceeding this).— P. R. Blackett *et al.*, *Clin. Pharmac. Ther.*, 1981, *29*, 793.

References: P. T. Pullan *et al.*, *Clin. Endocr.*, 1978, *9*, 273.

Uses. Desmopressin as the acetate is used similarly to Vasopressin Injection (p.1279) in the diagnosis and treatment of cranial diabetes insipidus. It has greater antidiuretic activity, a more prolonged action, and slight pressor activity compared with vasopressin or lypressin (p.1272). It is given as a solution intranasally and by injection.

In the control of diabetes insipidus, desmopressin acetate is used intranasally in usual doses of 10 to 20 µg once or twice daily; children may be given 5 to 10 µg once or twice daily. It may also be administered intramuscularly or intravenously in a dose of 1 to 4 µg once daily; a dose of 0.4 µg may be used in children. Single intranasal or intramuscular doses are given in the diagnosis of diabetes insipidus and to test renal function.

Desmopressin acetate, by intravenous infusion, is given to boost concentrations of factor VIII prior to surgical procedures in patients with mild to moderate haemophilia or von Willebrand's disease. It has also been given intravenously as a test of fibrinolytic response.

Reports and reviews of the actions and uses of desmopressin.— I. Vávra *et al.*, *Lancet*, 1968, *1*, 948; J. K. Murdoch, *Can. pharm. J.*, 1978, *111*, 301; *Med. Lett.*, 1978, *20*, 26; M. E. Kosman, *J. Am. med. Ass.*, 1978, *240*, 1896; *ibid.*, 1979, *241*, 360.

There was a significant rapid release of plasminogen activator in the plasma of 5 healthy subjects given desmopressin.— A. M. A. Gader *et al.* (preliminary communication), *Lancet*, 1973, *2*, 1417.

In 12 of 20 healthy subjects desmopressin 4 µg intravenously in the morning caused an increase in plasma-cortisol concentrations, and in the remaining 8 the cortisol concentration decreased, following the diurnal rhythm. In a further 10 patients given desmopressin 80 µg intranasally no effect was seen on plasma cortisol concentrations.— J. P. Rado and E. Juhos, *J. clin. Pharmac.*, 1976, *16*, 333.

The effect of desmopressin in a patient with Bartter's syndrome.— J. P. Rado *et al.*, *Int. J. clin. Pharmac. Biopharm.*, 1978, *16*, 22.

Administration. A report of 2 new modes (a metered-dose nasal spray and a gelatin-based sublingual lozenge) of administration of desmopressin. A study in 12 patients with confirmed cranial diabetes insipidus indicated that the methods produced a similar antidiuresis and duration of action to that produced by administration by 'rhinyle'. The patients in general preferred the nasal spray method.— A. Grossman *et al.*, *Br. med. J.*, 1980, *280*, 1215.

Coagulation disorders. Desmopressin produced a therapeutically effective rise in factor VIII activity in a study of 12 patients with mild or moderate haemophilia or with von Willebrand's disease who were undergoing dental extractions or surgical procedures and who were also given tranexamic acid. Experience with these 12 patients, only 2 of whom required treatment for postoperative bleeding complications, indicated that optimum conditions for dental extractions were basal concentrations of factor VIII activity of 8 to 10% [normal was considered to be 56 to 148%] and a dose of desmopressin of 0.4 µg per kg body-weight intravenously starting at the time of surgery and repeated twice every 12 hours. If the patients required major surgery then basal concentrations of 10 to 20% or more would be required.— P. M. Mannucci *et al.*, *Lancet*, 1977, *1*, 869. See also *ibid.*, 889. Water retention occurred in one patient when large doses of desmopressin (0.5 µg per kg body-weight) were given intravenously every 12 hours.— G. Lowe *et al.* (letter), *ibid.*, 1977, *2*, 614. Water intoxication could be avoided by careful instructions to limit water intake and simple monitoring.— G. I. C. Ingram and P. J. Hilton (letter), *ibid.*, 721. Another 5 patients were managed successfully with doses of 0.4 µg per kg of desmopressin intravenously. Resistance developed with repeated doses. Water retention would not be expected with 0.5 µg per kg but might be attributed to sensitivity.— P. M. Mannucci *et al.* (letter), *Lancet*, 1977, *2*, 1171.

The administration of desmopressin intranasally in 2 doses of 1 μg per kg body-weight produced some improvement of the haemostatic indexes in a patient with severe haemophilia. There was no change in factor-VIII activity.— A. H. Sutor *et al.* (letter), *Lancet*, 1978, *1*, 446.

Desmopressin 0.2 μg per kg body-weight infused intravenously into 5 patients with haemophilia B shortened the prothrombin time and increased the activity of factors VIII and XII without affecting the activity of factor IX. Desmopressin might be of use in haemorrhagic episodes in patients with haemophilia B.— I. Kobayashi *et al.* (letter), *Lancet*, 1978, *1*, 615.

Studies on a man with mild haemophilia, covered for elective surgery with desmopressin and tranexamic acid, confirmed that the boost in factor VIII activities was less with each successive infusion of desmopressin. Allowance should be made for this when giving factor VIII after desmopressin.— F. E. Boulton and A. Smith (letter), *Lancet*, 1979, *2*, 535.

Further references: W. Theiss and E. Sauer, *Dt. med. Wschr.*, 1977, *102*, 1769; C. Menon *et al.* (letter), *Lancet*, 1978, *2*, 743; R. W. Slee (letter), *Br. dent. J.*, 1978, *145*, 295.

Depression. In a double-blind placebo-controlled study, 4 severely depressed patients with major affective illness, were given 60 to 160 μg of desmopressin daily for 3 to 7 weeks, intranasally by the use of a calibrated catheter. During the active drug periods 3 of the 4 patients showed significant improvement in cognitive function, and 2 of these patients also had significant elevation of mood and amelioration of other affective symptoms. The mood elevation may have occurred because the patients could think more clearly and organise information better, but there was no clear correlation between cognitive enhancements and clinical change. Brief hyponatraemia, temporally unassociated with behavioural change occurred in 2 patients.— P. W. Gold *et al.* (preliminary communication), *Lancet*, 1979, *2*, 992 and 1202.

Diabetes insipidus. Reviews of desmopressin in diabetes insipidus: *Drug & Ther. Bull.*, 1976, *14*, 81; *Br. med. J.*, 1977, *1*, 1050; J. S. Jenkins, *Practitioner*, 1979, *222*, 312.

In a study over 8 to 19 months desmopressin 1.25 to 10 μg given intranasally twice daily to 10 children with diabetes insipidus due to deficiency in antidiuretic hormone returned the urine production and drinking pattern to normal in all children without any side-effects.— A. S. Aronson *et al.*, *Acta paediat. scand.*, 1973, *62*, 133. Desmopressin, given intranasally in doses of 5 to 15 μg in the morning and 2.5 to 7.5 μg at night, was considered to be the treatment of choice in children with diabetes insipidus.— D. J. Becker and T. P. Foley, *J. Pediat.*, 1978, *92*, 1011.

In 7 patients with cranial diabetes insipidus, treatment with desmopressin 2 or 3 μg intravenously or 20 μg intranasally produced a marked antidiuresis lasting for 10 hours or more. Treatment was ineffective in 2 patients with nephrogenic diabetes insipidus.— C. R. W. Edwards *et al.*, *Br. med. J.*, 1973, *3*, 375.

Desmopressin 20 μg given intranasally had a greater antidiuretic effect than the same dose of lypressin in a study of 14 patients with hypothalamic diabetes insipidus. Its effect lasted for about 18 hours compared with about 2 hours for lypressin. A prolonged effect was also observed when desmopressin 0.5 to 1 μg was given intravenously. There were no side-effects nor was there a diminution of activity in 24 patients given desmopressin intranasally for up to 26 months.— K. Irmscher *et al.*, *Dt. med. Wschr.*, 1974, *99*, 2431.

In 8 patients with severe central diabetes insipidus desmopressin 5, 10, and 20 μg as a nasal spray produced antidiuresis for 8 to 20 hours. The response to all 3 dosages was identical in 6 patients but 20 μg gave a longer response in 2. One patient developed a headache after 10 but not after 5 μg. No side-effects were noted during the subsequent 6 months of therapy when 3 patients received 5 or 10 μg every 18 hours, 3 received 5 μg every 12 hours, and 2 received 5 or 10 μg every 8 hours.— A. G. Robinson, *New Engl. J. Med.*, 1976, *294*, 507. In addition to variable interpatient responses to desmopressin, changes had occurred in the same patient. Desmopressin might be able to enhance its own metabolism thus increasing dosage requirements; in 3 patients who had previously received carbamazepine therapy enhanced metabolism had also been noted.— J. P. Radó (letter), *New Engl. J. Med.*, 1976, *295*, 393.

Patients with diabetes insipidus who required high doses of chlorpropamide or carbamazepine for antidiuresis were less likely to respond to desmopressin.— J. P. Radó *et al.*, *J. clin. Pharmac.*, 1976, *16*, 518.

Desmopressin reduced urine volume and fluid intake in 9 of 11 patients with lithium-induced polyuria and polydipsia.— E. Widerlöv *et al.* (letter), *Lancet*, 1977, *2*, 1080.

Further references: K. -E. Andersson and B. Arner (letter), *Br. med. J.*, 1971, *3*, 111; D. Oravec and B. Lichardus (letter), *ibid.*, 1972, *4*, 114; M. K. Ward and T. R. Fraser, *Br. med. J.*, 1974, *3*, 86; R. Kauli and Z. Laron, *Archs Dis. Childh.*, 1974, *49*, 482; J. M. Parkin (letter), *ibid.*, 1975, *50*, 84; W. N. P. Lee *et al.*, *Am. J. Dis. Child.*, 1976, *130*, 166; J. R. Short and A. Isles, *Med. J. Aust.*, 1976, *1*, 756; J. J. Graham *et al.*, *Med. J. Aust.*, 1977, *2*, 113; C. A. Kikugawa *et al.*, *Am. J. Hosp. Pharm.*, 1977, *34*, 1013; W. E. Cobb *et al.*, *Ann. intern. Med.*, 1978, *88*, 183; L. Czako *et al.*, *Int. J. clin. Pharmac. Biopharm.*, 1978, *16*, 10.

Enuresis. A pilot study of desmopressin 5 to 10 μg given intranasally to 20 enuretic children aged 6 to 15 years and resistant to other therapy. Eleven children became completely dry, 4 were dry on 5 or 6 nights a week, and 5 failed to respond.— S. B. Dimson (letter), *Lancet*, 1977, *1*, 1260.

Further references: M. Birkasova *et al.*, *Pediatrics*, 1978, *62*, 970.

Lumbar-puncture headache. Results of a double-blind crossover study completed by 9 healthy subjects suggested that intramuscular injection of desmopressin 6 μg might reduce the frequency and/or intensity of headaches following lumbar puncture. However, the difference between desmopressin and placebo saline injections was not statistically significant.— E. Widerlöv and L. Lindström (letter), *Lancet*, 1979, *1*, 548. A technique involving tilting the patient prevents the development of such headaches.— J. D. Easton (letter), *ibid.*, 974. See also W. F. Durward and H. Harrington (letter), *Lancet*, 1976, *2*, 1403; A. Sakula (letter), *ibid.*, 1977, *1*, 146.

In a double-blind study involving 79 patients, prophylactic intranasal administration of desmopressin had no significant effect on the incidence of headache or on the consumption of analgesics following lumbar puncture or pneumoencephalography compared with a placebo.— P. E. Hansen and J. H. Hansen, *Acta neurol. scand.*, 1979, *60*, 183.

In a double-blind study in 50 patients undergoing lumbar puncture, desmopressin 4 μg intramuscularly 4 hours before puncture then 12-hourly for a total of 3 doses did not decrease the incidence of headache but significantly reduced the severity. Desmopressin might also be of value for established headache.— J. M. A. Cowan *et al.*, *Br. med. J.*, 1980, *280*, 224.

A controlled study indicating that 24 hours of bed rest does not reduce the incidence of lumber puncture headache.— P. A. T. Carbaat and H. van Crevel, *Lancet*, 1981, *2*, 1133.

Further comments on headache following lumbar puncture and on methods to reduce the incidence: F. R. Smith *et al.* (letter), *Lancet*, 1980, *1*, 1245; J. W. Paulley (letter), *ibid.*, *2*, 33; R. H. Gerner (letter), *ibid.*

Memory. Desmopressin failed to have any beneficial effect on the impairment of memory arising from severe head injuries in 6 men, aged 24 to 36 years, injured in road traffic accidents 3 to 8 years previously, none of whom had diabetes insipidus. A subsequent course of lypressin also failed to have any beneficial effect.— J. S. Jenkins *et al.* (letter), *Lancet*, 1979, *2*, 1245. See also N. Koch-Henriksen and H. Nielsen (letter), *ibid.*, 1981, *1*, 38 (lypressin); J. S. Jenkins *et al.* (letter), *ibid.*, 39 (desmopressin or desglycinamide arginine vasopressin [DGAVP]).

Renal-function test. Desmopressin is effective for the assessment of urine-concentrating ability. There was no significant difference between the effect of 2 μg intramuscularly and 40 μg intranasally given overnight; the intranasal dose has also been given at 9 a.m., the bladder being emptied at that time and a second urine specimen being obtained 5 to 9 hours later.— J. P. Monson and P. Richards, *Br. med. J.*, 1978, *1*, 24. Urine-concentrating ability was reduced with advancing age.— J. P. Monson and P. Richards (letter), *Br. med. J.*, 1978, *1*, 1054.

Experience in 32 adults suggests that desmopressin is as effective as vasopressin tannate for assessing urinary concentration; a dose of 40 μg intranasally was suggested at 8 a.m. after 12 hours' water deprivation.— K. Delin *et al.*, *Br. med. J.*, 1978, *1*, 757. Intranasal administration of desmopressin is used routinely and the result checked using the intramuscular route if technical difficulties arise. Maximum concentration of the urine was not achieved when desmopressin 4 μg was given intravenously.— K. Delin *et al.* (letter), *Br. med. J.*, 1979, *1*, 888.

The intramuscular injection of desmopressin 4 μg is suitable for assessing renal concentrating ability in sedentary subjects or hospital inpatients.— J. R. Curtis and B. A. Donovan, *Br. med. J.*, 1979, *1*, 304.

A study indicating that a test of urinary osmolality using desmopressin before and after 14 hours of total restriction of fluid intake is a safe, convenient, and reliable means of estimating renal concentrating capacity in patients treated with lithium.— K. Asplund *et al.* (letter), *Lancet*, 1979, *1*, 491. See also P. Vestergaard and H. E. Hansen, *Acta psychiat. scand.*, 1980, *61*, 152.

Further references: A. S. Aronson and N. W. Svenningsen, *Archs Dis. Childh.*, 1974, *49*, 654; E. Scheitza, *Arzneimittel-Forsch.*, 1975, *25*, 260; E. Scheitza *et al.* (letter), *New Engl. J. Med.*, 1976, *295*, 393; S. D. Somerfield and A. G. Hocken, *N.Z. med. J.*, 1977, *86*, 472.

Sickle-cell disease. Preliminary but encouraging results with desmopressin in 3 patients with severe sickle-cell anaemia. Desmopressin administered intranasally was used to induce hyponatraemia, which resulted in a reduction in mean corpuscular haemoglobin concentration, a decreased degree of sickling, and an increase in oxygen affinity. Sustained treatment appears to reduce the frequency of crises and acute induction of hyponatraemia appears to shorten their duration.— R. M. Rosa *et al.*, *New Engl. J. Med.*, 1980, *303*, 1138. Although results in 4 patients confirmed that hyponatraemia could be induced in hospital and that the use of desmopressin acetate rather than vasopressin was essential, the number of hospital admissions for sickle-cell crisis was not altered nor was the length of hospital stay during crises. There were also neurological complications. Anorexia and listlessness occurred in 3 of the 4 patients, hallucinations in 2, and a grand mal seizure in 1.— M. Leary and N. Abramson (letter), *ibid.*, 1981, *304*, 844. Reply.— F. H. Epstein *et al.* (letter), *ibid.*

Proprietary Preparations

DDAVP *(Ferring, UK)*. Desmopressin acetate, available as **Injection** containing 4 μg per ml, in ampoules of 1 ml, and as **Solution** containing 100 μg per ml, supplied with a catheter (rhinyle) for intranasal administration. (Also available as DDAVP in *Canad., USA*).

Other Proprietary Names

Dav Ritter *(Switz.)*; Minirin *(Austral., Ger., Ital., Norw., Swed.)*; Minurin *(Denm.)*.

5924-g

Felypressin. Phelypressine; PLV2. [2-L-Phenylalanine,8-L-lysine]-vasopressin.
$C_{46}H_{65}N_{13}O_{11}S_2$=1040.2.

CAS — 56-59-7.

Felypressin is a vasopressor agent with actions similar to those of Vasopressin Injection (p.1278). Its antidiuretic effects are less than those of vasopressin. It is used as a vasoconstrictor in local anaesthetic injections for dental use when sympathomimetic agents should be avoided (see Prilocaine Hydrochloride, p.920).

The administration of felypressin raised the blood pressure in over 50% of 53 women undergoing operation for vaginal prolapse with halothane anaesthesia. One-third of the patients had bradycardia, 1 had cardiac collapse, and another sustained atrial fibrillation.— A. Dahl, *Nord. Med.*, 1968, *79*, 119, per *J. Am. med. Ass.*, 1968, *203* (Mar. 4), A238.

For a review of the use of felypressin in local anaesthetic injections, see *Drug & Ther. Bull.*, 1970, *8*, 38.

If a patient receiving tricyclic antidepressants required the injection of a local anaesthetic with a vasoconstrictor during dental treatment, the use of a solution containing prilocaine 3% and felypressin 0.03 unit per ml was acceptable and did not risk the precipitation of a dangerous hypertensive episode.— V. Goldman (letter), *Br. med. J.*, 1971, *1*, 175.

In 11 normotensive patients with reduced renal blood flow associated with cirrhosis of the liver, infusions of felypressin at the rate of 0.001 to 0.016 units per minute increased renal and intrarenal blood flow in only 1 of 6 patients in whom the blood pressure was not concomitantly increased, but increased renal and intrarenal blood flow in 3 of 5 patients in whom blood pressure was concomitantly raised by at least 5 mmHg.— M. C. Kew *et al.*, *Gut*, 1972, *13*, 293.

For earlier reports of the clinical uses of felypressin, see Extra Pharmacopoeia 26th Edn, p. 1502.

Proprietary Names

Octapressin *(Astra, UK)*.

5925-q

Gonadorelin *(B.P.).* Hoe471; Gonadoliberin; Luliberin; Gonadotrophin-releasing Hormone; GnRH; LH/FSH-RH; LH-RH; LH/FSH-RF; LH-RF. 5-Oxo-L-prolyl-L-histidyl-L-tryptophyl-L-seryl-L-tyrosylglycyl-L-leucyl-L-arginyl-L-prolylglycinamide.
$C_{55}H_{75}N_{17}O_{13}$=1182.3.

CAS — 33515-09-2; 34973-08-5 (diacetate, anhydrous); 52699-48-6 (diacetate, tetrahydrate); 51952-41-1 (xHCl).

A decapeptide obtained from the hypothalamus or by synthesis. A white or faintly yellowish-white powder. It contains not less than 85% of peptide, not more than 6% of acetic acid, and 3 to 7% of water. **Soluble** 1 in 25 of water, 1 in 50 of methyl alcohol, and 1 in 25 of 1% v/v acetic acid; soluble in alcohol.

Gonadorelin acetate and hydrochloride have been described.

Stability. Gonadorelin stored at 4° in nonsterile solutions of 0.9% sodium chloride or 1% glycine was inactive at 23 or 27 weeks respectively. Similar solutions stored at −20° retained their activity for about a year.— W. C. Dermondy and J. R. Reel (letter), *New Engl. J. Med.*, 1976, *295,* 173. This loss of activity was probably due to bacterial contamination of the solutions. Gonadorelin in lyophilised form and as a sterile solution retained its activity when stored at 4° and 40° for 18 months.— J. Sandow *et al.* (letter), *New Engl. J. Med.*, 1977, *296,* 885.

Adverse Effects. Abdominal pain, nausea, headache, and menorrhagia have been reported to occur in patients given gonadorelin.

Transient amaurosis in a patient with pituitary macroadenoma after intravenous gonadorelin and protirelin.— A. Cimino *et al.* (letter), *Lancet,* 1981, *2,* 95. See also under Protirelin, p.1276.

Absorption and Fate. Gonadorelin has a plasma half-life of only a few minutes after intravenous injection and about half of a dose has been reported to be excreted in the urine as metabolites within one hour.

Gonadotrophin-releasing hormone has been detected in milk in concentrations of 0.1 to 3.0 nanograms per ml. Thyrotrophin-releasing hormone appears in smaller concentrations.— T. Baram *et al.*, *Science,* 1977, *198,* 300.

Further references: T. W. Redding *et al.*, *J. clin. Endocr. Metab.*, 1973, *37,* 626; B. Pimstone *et al.*, *J. clin. Endocr. Metab.*, 1977, *44,* 356.

Uses. Gonadorelin is a hypothalamic releasing hormone which stimulates the synthesis of follicle-stimulating hormone (p.1269) and luteinising hormone (p.1270) in the anterior lobe of the pituitary as well as their release. Gonadorelin secretion is controlled by several factors including circulating sex hormones.

Gonadorelin is used, sometimes with clomiphene (p.1406), in the diagnosis of hypothalamic-pituitary-gonadal dysfunction. It is also given with protirelin (p.1276) in the assessment of pituitary function. The usual dose of gonadorelin is 100 µg by intravenous injection. The subcutaneous, intramuscular, and intranasal routes have also been used.

Gonadorelin has been given in the treatment of sterility due to an absence or deficiency of gonadotrophins and in cryptorchidism but because of its short half-life repeated doses may be necessary. Analogues of gonadorelin with a more prolonged action are being developed as well as inhibitory analogues with potential contraceptive activity.

Reviews of the action and uses of gonadorelin: S. M. McCann, *New Engl. J. Med.*, 1977, *296,* 797. See also L. J. Valenta and J. C. Zolman (letter), *ibid.*, *297,* 725; S. M. McCann (letter), *ibid.; Drug & Ther. Bull.*, 1978, *16,* 10; G. Fink, *Br. med. Bull.*, 1979, *35,* 155.

A significant increase in the plasma concentration of growth hormone occurred in 6 of 16 patients with active acromegaly after they were given gonadorelin 25 µg intravenously. Protirelin had a similar effect in 4 of the 6 patients.— G. Faglia *et al.*, *J. clin. Endocr. Metab.*, 1973, *37,* 338.

Gonadorelin was effective when given intranasally to 5 male subjects and increased plasma-luteinising hormone concentrations in them all. Follicle-stimulating hormone concentrations were increased in 2 of the subjects.— H. G. Solbach and W. Wiegelmann (letter), *Lancet,* 1973, *1,* 1259. Similar results from intranasal administration, but a dose of 2.5 mg was required to give the same results as 100 µg given intravenously.— D. R. London *et al.* (letter), *ibid.*, 1450. In 10 amenorrhoeic women, intranasal administration of 2 mg of gonadorelin produced an LH and FSH response broadly comparable with that produced by 100 µg given intravenously.— S. Jeppsson *et al.* (letter), *Br. med. J.*, 1973, *4,* 231.

Gonadorelin 500 µg self-administered subcutaneously every 8 hours in 12 hypogonadal male patients with hypothalamic or pituitary dysfunction produced a rise in circulating androgen concentrations in all patients.— C. H. Mortimer *et al.*, *Br. med. J.*, 1974, *4,* 617.

The response to gonadorelin was diminished in patients with anorexia nervosa in whom weight loss was severe and basal gonadotrophins low.— R. L. Palmer *et al.*, *Br. med. J.*, 1975, *1,* 179. In 3 patients with anorexia nervosa and secondary amenorrhoea, ovulation was induced by the long-term use of gonadorelin 500 µg thrice daily. In 2 patients normal corpus luteum function was achieved by the prior use of chorionic gonadotrophin.— S. J. Nillius and L. Wide, *ibid.*, 1975, *3,* 405. See also *Lancet,* 1979, *2,* 563.

When gonadorelin 200 or 400 µg was given as an infusion over 2 minutes to 7 healthy subjects there was no change in heart-rate or significant effect on cortical activity.— H. Ashton *et al.*, *Br. J. clin. Pharmac.*, 1976, *3,* 523.

A study of the biological activity of the potent gonadorelin analogue D-Trp^6-Pro^9-NEt-LHRH ($LHRH_A$) in healthy men and hypogonadotrophic subjects previously unresponsive to 100 µg of synthetic gonadorelin. All subjects responded to $LHRH_a$ and the analogue had an augmented ability to discharge gonadotrophins and to sustain their release when compared with gonadorelin.— W. F. Crowley *et al.*, *New Engl. J. Med.*, 1980, *302,* 1052.

[D-Leu^6]-des-Gly-NH_2^{10} pro-ethylamide GnRH, a synthetic analogue of gonadorelin, was shown in *mice* to produce striking protection from histologically detectable cyclophosphamide-induced testicular damage.— L. M. Glode *et al.*, *Lancet,* 1981, *1,* 1132.

Contraception. The intranasal use of a gonadorelin analogue, buserelin [(6-*O-tert*-butyl-D-serine)-des-10-glycinamide-gonadorelin ethylamide, $C_{60}H_{86}N_{16}O_{13}$ = 1239.4], as a contraceptive agent. In 27 regularly menstruating women daily doses of 400 or 600 µg, starting on the first day of menstrual bleeding, inhibited ovulation during all but 2 of 89 treatment months. The 2 women with initial evidence of ovulation had technical problems with their nasal spray bottles. Side-effects were temporary local nasal irritation in 4, and short-lived headaches during the first week of treatment in 3. Six of the 27 women became amenorrhoeic during the treatment but had no symptoms of oestrogen deficiency and menstrual bleeding returned rapidly after discontinuation. No dysfunctional uterine bleeding occurred.— C. Bergquist *et al.*, *Lancet,* 1979, *2,* 215. See also S. J. Nillius *et al.*, *Contraception,* 1978, *17,* 537; C. Bergquist *et al.*, *Contraception,* 1979, *19,* 497.

Gonadorelin 2 mg twice daily by the intranasal route appeared to inhibit ovulation, as indicated by hormone measurements, throughout the latter half of the cycle of 16 women.— R. F. Lambe *et al.* (letter), *Lancet,* 1979, *2,* 801.

Reversible inhibition of testicular steroidogenesis and spermatogenesis by a potent gonadorelin agonist, D-Trp^6-Pro^9-*N*-ethylamide-LHRH ($LHRH_A$), in normal men.— R. Linde *et al.*, *New Engl. J. Med.*, 1981, *305,* 663.

Further references: D. Gonzalez-Barcena *et al.*, *Lancet,* 1977, *2,* 997.

Cryptorchidism. Gonadorelin in an estimated dose of 1.2 mg was given intranasally in 6 divided doses daily for 4 weeks to 46 boys with 61 undescended testes and compared in a double-blind study with placebo in 38 boys with 51 undescended testes. Twenty-three testes descended in the treated boys and one in the control boys. There was improvement in the position of 17 testes in the treated group and 7 testes in the control group. When gonadorelin was continued for an additional 2 to 6 weeks only 3 of 15 boys who had not responded to 4 weeks' therapy achieved complete testicular descent. Response to gonadorelin was poor when the testes could not be palpated before therapy.— R. Illig *et al.*, *Lancet,* 1977, *2,* 518. Patients should be chosen carefully for their ability to respond to gonadorelin.— W. Hamilton (letter), *ibid.*, 874 and 940. Evidence for an intact hypothalamic pituitary gonadal system being required for testicular descent and a suggestion that therapy might need to be continued after descent.— F. Hadziselimovic *et al.* (letter), *Lancet,* 1977, *2,* 1125.

Testicular descent and cessation of retractility occurred within 3 days in 2 of 4 boys given gonadorelin 100 or 500 µg subcutaneously thrice daily for 3 days.— M. C. White and J. Ginsburg (letter), *Lancet,* 1977, *2,* 1361.

Five of 13 prepubertal boys with unilateral cryptorchidism achieved descent of the testis after intranasal administration of gonadorelin 500 µg twice daily for 1 week, compared to 2 of 9 similar boys who received 200 µg six times daily.— P. Pirazzoli *et al.*, *Archs Dis. Childh.*, 1978, *53,* 235.

Complete testicular descent was achieved in 4 of 11 prepubertal cryptorchid boys who received a synthetic analogue of gonadorelin [(6-D-leucine)-des-10-glycinamide-gonadorelin ethylamide, $C_{59}H_{84}N_{16}O_{12}$ = 1209.4] intranasally.— J. Happ *et al.*, *Fert. Steril.*, 1978, *29,* 552.

A discussion on the therapy of cryptorchidism concluded that gonadorelin appeared to have no particular advantage over chorionic gonadotrophin.— *Lancet,* 1978, *1,* 1344.

Further references: J. Happ *et al.*, *Fert. Steril.*, 1978, *29,* 546.

Depression. A single intramuscular injection of gonadorelin 500 µg produced a striking response in 8 patients with depression caused by prolonged severe stress. Depressive symptoms resolved, and feelings of normal functioning with normal coping, were restored within 12 to 48 hours of the injection. The responses were usually preceded by drowsiness. Little or no effect was noted in a further 19 patients with primary unipolar or bipolar affective disorder, except that they too experienced improved sleep on the night following the injection.— G. A. German and H. G. Stampfer (letter), *Lancet,* 1979, *2,* 789. In a single-blind placebo-controlled study involving 30 depressed patients and 23 healthy control subjects no mood changes were noted in the patients or the controls after either gonadorelin or placebo.— J. D. Amsterdam *et al.* (letter), *Lancet,* 1979, *2,* 1138.

Diagnosis of hypothalamic and pituitary dysfunction. In 155 patients with hypothalamic-pituitary-gonadal dysfunction, of whom 137 were clinically hypogonadal, an intravenous injection of 100 µg of gonadorelin produced an LH response in all except 16 and an FSH response in all except 10. It was not possible to differentiate between hypothalamic and pituitary causes of hypogonadism but repeated administration of gonadorelin might restore fertility.— C. H. Mortimer *et al.*, *Br. med. J.*, 1973, *4,* 73. See also J. C. Marshall *et al.*, *ibid.*, 1972, *4,* 643.

An evaluation of the capability of gonadorelin for restoration of the pituitary gonadotrophin reserve in patients with hypogonadotrophic hypogonadism. Repeated administration of gonadorelin was of value in the diagnosis of hypogonadism due to hypothalamic dysfunction.— Y. Yoshimoto *et al.*, *New Engl. J. Med.*, 1975, *292,* 242.

Diagnosis of constitutional delayed puberty in 7 boys was suggested by finding a luteinising hormone and follicle-stimulating hormone response after intravenous administration of gonadorelin 100 µg given over 30 seconds. However, patients with isolated gonadotrophin deficiency would also respond to gonadorelin.— J. Sagel *et al.*, *Postgrad. med. J.*, 1975, *51,* 611.

Fifty-six women with amenorrhoea and 14 with anovulatory cycles were given the gonadorelin test (100 µg intravenously) and 24 were also given the clomiphene test (2 mg per kg body-weight daily, to the nearest 50 mg, for 7 days). Most patients responded to gonadorelin with significant increases in LH and FSH. Exaggerated responses occurred in those with gonadal dysgenesis or premature ovarian failure. Patients unresponsive to gonadorelin failed to respond to clomiphene. All patients with anovulatory cycles responded to gonadorelin and to clomiphene, while 7 of 13 with amenorrhoea and a normal response to gonadorelin responded to clomiphene.— J. Ginsburg *et al.*, *Br. med. J.*, 1975, *3,* 130.

Further references: P. G. Crosignani *et al.*, *Obstet. Gynec.*, 1975, *46,* 15; Z. Dickerman *et al.*, *Fert. Steril.*, 1976, *27,* 162; J. C. Feore and M. L. Taymor, *Fert. Steril.*, 1976, *27,* 1240; R. T. Kirkland *et al.*, *J. Pediat.*, 1976, *89,* 941; B. Cantor *et al.*, *Fert. Steril.*, 1977, *28,* 526; W. N. Spellacy *et al.*, *Fert. Steril.*, 1977, *28,* 733; F. I. Reyes *et al.*, *Fert. Steril.*, 1977, *28,* 1175; J. Van Campenhout *et al.*, *Am. J. Obstet. Gynec.*, 1977, *127,* 723; G. S. Jones *et al.*, *Am. J. Obstet. Gynec.*, 1977, *129,* 760; F. Peters *et al.*, *Dt. med. Wschr.*, 1978, *103,* 898.

For reference to the functional evaluation of pituitary reserve in patients with the amenorrhoea-galactorrhoea syndrome utilising gonadorelin, levodopa, or chlorpromazine, see Chlorpromazine Hydrochloride, p.1515.

Infertility. A positive pituitary response to 12.5 μg of gonadorelin given intravenously was observed in 15 of 21 women with secondary amenorrhoea who had not responded to clomiphene given in a total dose of up to 750 mg. The 21 women were then treated with clomiphene 100 mg over 5 days followed 6 to 7 days later by gonadorelin 50 μg infused intravenously over 4 hours. Ovulation was induced in 12 of the 15 women who had responded to the test dose and 2 of these became pregnant. Ovulation did not occur in the women who had shown no initial pituitary response.— P. J. Keller, *Lancet*, 1972, *2*, 570. See also P. J. Keller, *Am. J. Obstet. Gynec.*, 1973, *116*, 698.

The use of gonadorelin to induce ovulation in contraceptive-induced anovulation.— J. Zanartu *et al.*, *Br. med. J.*, 1974, *1*, 605.

Induction of ovulation in a woman with hypothalamic anovulatory infertility, by intermittent self-administration of gonadorelin 1 μg per minute for 3.4 minutes every 62.5 minutes into the subcutaneous tissue of the abdominal wall via a scalp vein needle, using a programmed battery operated syringe driver. This method of treatment simulates the endogenous episodic secretion of gonadorelin thereby reducing the risks of ovarian hyperstimulation and multiple pregnancies.— E. J. Keogh *et al.* (letter), *Lancet*, 1981, *1*, 147.

Further references: S. J. Nillius *et al.*, *Am. J. Obstet. Gynec.*, 1975, *122*, 921; K. Huang, *Fert. Steril.*, 1976, *27*, 65.

Male infertility. Gonadorelin 500 μg twice daily intramuscularly for 6 months produced an increase in spermatozoa in 3 of 4 azoospermic patients but the highest count was still below 6 million per ml. Three of 6 oligospermic patients had more than 10 million spermatozoa per ml after 3 months but this figure decreased in the following 3 months of therapy. Motility and normal forms increased in all patients. No wives became pregnant.— A. Zárate *et al.*, *Fert. Steril.*, 1973, *24*, 485.

Further references: *Br. med. J.*, 1979, *2*, 1169.

Precocious puberty. Encouraging preliminary results in 5 girls given the gonadorelin analogue, D-Trp^6-Pro^9-NEt-LHRH (LHRH$_A$) for the treatment of idiopathic precocious puberty.— F. Comite *et al.*, *New Engl. J. Med.*, 1981, *305*, 1546. Benefit in one girl using a similar analogue, (D-Trp^6)-LH-RH.— Z. Laron *et al.*, *Lancet*, 1981, *2*, 955.

Preparations

Gonadorelin Injection *(B.P.)*. A sterile solution of gonadorelin in Water for Injections containing suitable stabilising agents; it may be prepared by dissolving the contents of a sealed container (Gonadorelin for Injection) in the specified solvent before use. Potency is expressed in terms of the content of peptide. pH 4.5 to 5.5. Store in a cool place. Protect from light.

Proprietary Preparations

HRF Ayerst *(Ayerst, UK)*. Gonadorelin, available as powder for preparing injections, in vials of 100 and 500 μg; supplied with 2-ml ampoules of diluent. (Also available as HRF Ayerst in *Belg.*, *S.Afr.*).

Relefact LH-RH *(Hoechst, UK)*. Gonadorelin, available as an injection containing 100 μg per ml, in ampoules of 1 ml. (Also available as Relefact LH-RH in *Ger.*).

Relefact LH-RH/TRH *(Hoechst, UK)*. An injection containing in each ml gonadorelin 100 μg and protirelin 200 μg, in ampoules of 1 ml. *Dose.* 1 ml by intravenous injection.

Other Proprietary Names

Lutamin *(Jap.)*; Relisorm L *(Ital.)*; Stimu-LH *(Fr.)*.

5926-p

Gonadotrophic Hormones

The anterior lobe of the pituitary gland secretes hormones which stimulate the normal functioning of the gonads and the secretion of sex hormones in both men and women. Two gonadotrophins are produced, *follicle-stimulating hormone* (FSH) and *luteinising hormone* or *interstitial-cell-stimulating hormone* (LH; ICSH). The pituitary secretion of FSH and LH is regulated by a complex interaction between the hypothalamic releasing hormone, gonadorelin (p.1267), and both positive and negative feedback effects of circulating sex hormones on the pituitary and hypothalamus. This control system is also influenced by the pituitary hormone prolactin (p.1275).

Gonadotrophins are also produced by the placenta. These are more easily obtained than the hormones from the pituitary and have therefore been extensively used in medicine. A gonadotrophin with predominantly luteinising properties is obtained from the urine of pregnant women (chorionic gonadotrophin) and one with predominantly follicle-stimulating properties is obtained from the urine of postmenopausal women (menotrophin). A gonadotrophin with predominantly follicle-stimulating properties has also been obtained from the serum of pregnant mares (serum gonadotrophin).

The functional relationship of the gonadotrophic hormones is complicated.

In a normal menstrual cycle follicle-stimulating hormone stimulates the development and maturation of the follicles and ova. As the follicle develops it produces oestrogen in increasing amounts which at mid-cycle stimulate the release of luteinising hormone. This causes rupture of the follicle with ovulation and converts the follicle into the corpus luteum which secretes progesterone.

In men, follicle-stimulating hormone has a role in spermatogenesis while luteinising hormone stimulates the interstitial cells of the testis to secrete testosterone, which in turn has a direct effect on the seminiferous tubules. Spermatogenesis has been reported to promote the secretion of a selective FSH suppressor, inhibin.

The gonadotrophins and thyrotrophin (p.1278) are glycoproteins and are each composed of alpha and beta subunits which have little or no biological activity on their own. The alpha subunits of FSH, LH, thyrotrophin, and chorionic gonadotrophin are considered to have essentially identical amino-acid sequences. The beta subunits differ in structure, although there are similarities between the beta subunits of LH and chorionic gonadotrophin. The activity of these hormones can therefore be considered to be a characteristic of the beta subunit even though alpha and beta subunits are both required for activity.

Proceedings of a symposium on the use of gonadotrophic hormones.— *J. reprod. Med.*, 1978, *21*, *Suppl.*, 189–218.

Accounts of the pituitary control of gonadal activity: K. M. Henderson, *Br. med. Bull.*, 1979, *35*, 161 (ovarian); G. A. Lincoln, *Br. med. Bull.*, 1979, *35*, 167 (testicular).

Infertility. For a review of the use of gonadotrophins for the treatment of infertility in men and in women with amenorrhoea and little or no evidence of endogenous oestrogen activity, see Agents Stimulating Gonadal Function in the Human, *Tech. Rep. Ser. Wld Hlth Org. No. 514*, 1973.

For reports of the use of gonadotrophic hormones in the treatment of infertility, see Follicle-stimulating Hormone, p.1270.

5927-s

Chorionic Gonadotrophin *(B.P., B.P. Vet.)*.

Chorion. Gonadotr.; Gonadotrophinum Chorionicum; CG; Choriogonadotrophin; Chorionic Gonadotropin *(U.S.P.)*; HCG; Human Chorionic Gonadotrophin; PU; Pregnancy-urine Hormone.

CAS — 9002-61-3.

Pharmacopoeias. In *Aust.*, *Br.*, *Braz.*, *Chin.*, *Hung.*, *Ind.*, *It.*, *Jap.*, *Jug.*, *Nord.*, *Swiss*, *Turk.*, and *U.S.*

A preparation of a glycoprotein substance secreted by the placenta and obtained from the urine of pregnant women. It is a white or almost white amorphous powder containing not less than 1500 units per mg. The *B.P.* specifies a sterile preparation.

Soluble in water; practically insoluble in alcohol, acetone, and ether. **Store** at a temperature not exceeding 20° in airtight containers sealed to exclude micro-organisms and protected from light; under these conditions it may be expected to retain its potency for not less then 3 years. The *U.S.P.* specifies storage at 2° to 8°.

Units. 5300 units of human chorionic gonadotrophin for bioassay are contained in approximately 2 mg (with lactose 5 mg) in one ampoule of the second International Standard Preparation (1963).

650 units of human chorionic gonadotrophin for immunoassay are contained in approximately 70 μg (with human albumin 5 mg) in one ampoule of the first International Reference Preparation for Immunoassay (1975).

70 units of the alpha subunit of human chorionic gonadotrophin for immunoassay are contained in approximately 70 μg (with human albumin 5 mg) in one ampoule of the first International Reference Preparation for Immunoassay (1975).

70 units of the beta subunit of human chorionic gonadotrophin for immunoassay are contained in approximately 70 μg (with human albumin 5 mg) in one ampoule of the first International Reference Preparation for Immunoassay (1975).

An account of a new reference preparation of human chorionic gonadotrophin and its alpha and beta subunits.— R. E. Canfield and G. T. Ross, *Bull. Wld Hlth Org.*, 1976, *54*, 463. See also Thirtieth Report of WHO Expert Committee on Biological Standardization, *Tech. Rep. Ser. Wld Hlth Org. No. 638*, 1979.

See above for reference to the alpha and beta subunits of gonadotrophic hormones.

Adverse Effects and Precautions. Side-effects that have been reported include headache, tiredness, changes in mood, oedema, and pain on injection. Treatment for cryptorchidism may produce precocious puberty. Gynaecomastia has been reported. Ovarian hyperstimulation may occur (see Follicle-stimulating Hormone, p.1269).

Chorionic gonadotrophin should be given with care to patients in whom fluid retention might be a hazard as in asthma, epilepsy, migraine, or cardiac or renal disorders. Allergic reactions may occur and patients suspected to be susceptible should be given skin tests before treatment. It should not be given to patients with disorders that might be exacerbated by androgen release.

A 17-year-old boy who received chorionic gonadotrophin 3000 units twice weekly for 6 weeks developed, after 3 months, a slipped capital femoral epiphysis probably related to rapid growth spurt.— P. J. Hirsch and S. A. Hirsch, *J. Am. med. Ass.*, 1976, *235*, 751.

Uses. Chorionic gonadotrophin is produced in the placenta and is found in the blood and urine of pregnant women; its action is predominantly that of the pituitary luteinising hormone. In the male, it stimulates the interstitial cells of the testes and consequently the secretion of androgens.

In women it is given to induce ovulation after follicular development has been stimulated with follicle-stimulating hormone (see p.1270) in the treatment of infertility due to absent or low concentrations of gonadotrophins. Duration of therapy varies but the total dose is in the region of 5000 or 10 000 units, by intramuscular injection. It has also been tried in the treatment of metropathia haemorrhagica, in the prevention and treatment of habitual abortion, and in secondary amenorrhoea.

In males it has been used in the treatment of cryptorchidism in doses of 500 to 4000 units thrice weekly by intramuscular injection. It has also been given for hypogonadism in doses of 4000 units thrice weekly.

Chorionic gonadotrophin has been used in the treatment of obesity but there is no evidence to support its value.

The chemical, immunological, and biological properties of human chorionic gonadotrophin.— G. T. Ross, *Am. J. Obstet. Gynec.*, 1977, *129*, 795.

After thrice-weekly injections of chorionic gonadotrophin 1000 units for 6 weeks, the prostaglandin concentration of the seminal fluid increased in 21 of 24 men with deficient semen, indicating the presence of functioning Leydig cells.— H. -C. Sturde and K. Böhm, *Arzneimittel-Forsch.*, 1971, *21*, 986.

Chorionic gonadotrophin, 1500 to 3000 units daily for 4 or more injections, was stated to be effective in the treatment of affective disorders and tension with depression.— W. Bujanow (letter), *Br. med. J.*, 1972, *4*, 298.

The effect of chorionic gonadotrophin on testicular androgen production in 16 men with chronic renal failure undergoing regular dialysis.— K. Rager *et al.*, *J. Reprod. Fert.*, 1975, *42*, 113, per *J. Am. med. Ass.*, 1975, *232*, 1415.

The use of the testosterone response to the daily intramuscular injection of chorionic gonadotrophin 1000 units for 3 days as a test for abnormal sexual development.— D. B. Grant *et al.*, *Archs Dis. Childh.*, 1976, *51*, 596. See also D. A. Adamopoulos *et al.*, *Br. med. J.*, 1978, *1*, 1177.

See also under Pituitary-function Test below.

Chorionic gonadotrophin was detected in a plasma pool from 13 normal men. Concentrations detected in individual plasma samples from 12 of 16 subjects (10 men and 6 nonpregnant women) ranged from 4.4 to 361 pg per ml (median concentration 19 pg per ml).— A. Borkowski and C. Muquardt, *New Engl. J. Med.*, 1979, *301*, 298. Comment.— J. L. Vaitukaitis, *ibid.*, 324.

Evidence that Profasi, *Serono* brand of chorionic gonadotrophin produces strikingly less pain on intramuscular injection than Pregnyl, *Organon* brand.— J. A. Heady *et al.* (letter), *Lancet*, 1980, *2*, 198. Another preparation, Gonadotraphon LH (*Paines and Byrne*) is not painful. Investigation has shown that it is the solvent supplied with Pregnyl which causes the pain.— R. Newill (letter), *ibid.*, 417.

Asthma. Encouraging results were obtained in 37 asthmatic boys following administration of chorionic gonadotrophin.— C. Grimaldi, *Practitioner*, 1967, *198*, 559.

In 7 male patients with a mean age of 14 years suffering from severe asthma and growth retardation, a 3-month course of 1500 units of chorionic gonadotrophin injection thrice weekly increased weight, height, and skeletal and sexual maturation, but relief of asthma was not seen.— S. Sanders and A. P. Norman, *Practitioner*, 1973, *210*, 690.

Cryptorchidism. A discussion on the use of chorionic gonadotrophin or gonadorelin for the treatment of cryptorchidism.— *Lancet*, 1978, *1*, 1344.

Gonadotrophin therapy was more effective for bilateral than unilateral undescended testes, the former requiring only a short course of 3 injections, in comparison with a course of 20 for the latter. Optimum results were obtained in patients 2 to 5 years old. The treatment was successfully used in causing the descent of 81 of 350 testes.— R. M. Ehrlich *et al.*, *J. Urol.*, 1969, *102*, 793.

Eunuchoidism. A 19-year-old youth with primary pituitary insufficiency which induced a eunuchoid state responded to treatment with chorionic gonadotrophin 2000 units thrice weekly by intramuscular injection. During the first 2 weeks, secondary sexual characteristics developed and the genitalia increased in size. Biopsy of the testis showed the onset of spermatogenesis after 12 days of treatment. When 12.5 units of human follicle-stimulating hormone was given thrice weekly in addition to chorionic gonadotrophin for 8 weeks, genital development was accelerated and more advanced histological changes ensued.— B. Lytton and N. Kase, *New Engl. J. Med.*, 1966, *274*, 1061.

A 38-year-old man who had had a total hypophysectomy received injections of chorionic gonadotrophin, 5000 units weekly for 5 months postoperatively, with the successful production and maintenance of spermatogenesis.— L. Weinrauch (letter), *Med. J. Aust.*, 1968, *1*, 74.

A patient with secondary hypogonadism and severe oligospermia had an increase in sperm concentration and motility after treatment with chorionic gonadotrophin.— E. Meinhard *et al.*, *Br. med. J.*, 1973, *3*, 577.

Infertility. References to the induction of ovulation using clomiphene and chorionic gonadotrophin.— G. I. Swyer *et al.*, *Br. J. Obstet. Gynaec.*, 1975, *82*, 794; A. Lopata *et al.*, *Fert. Steril.*, 1978, *30*, 27; W. H. James, *Br. med. J.*, 1980, *281*, 711 (low proportion of males in infants conceived after induction of ovulation).

Pituitary-function test. In 15 healthy men the intramuscular injection of 2000 units of chorionic gonadotrophin caused an increase in plasma concentrations of 17β-hydroxy androgens (17-OHA) with a mean increase of 109% in 24 to 72 hours; a second injection 3 days later caused a further increase in 4 of 7 men. In 8 boys with cryptorchidism given intramuscular injections of 2000 units twice weekly, 17-OHA values rose slowly. In patients with panhypopituitarism, 2 injections caused a rise in the initially low concentrations of 17-OHA to within the normal range. In patients with gonadotrophin deficiency, the response was variable. Patients with Klinefelter's syndrome showed a positive response. The HCG test alone could not be used to distinguish different forms of hypogonadism.— D. C. Anderson *et al.*, *Clin. Endocr.*, 1972, *1*, 127.

Sickle-cell disease. Peak and mean foetal haemoglobin concentrations were raised when a mother with sickle-cell thalassaemia was treated with chorionic gonadotrophin in a dose of up to 10 000 units daily. A similar peak was seen in a patient who did not receive chorionic gonadotrophin.— A. I. Sutnick *et al.*, *J. Am. med. Ass.*, 1968, *206*, 1795.

Transient increases in the concentration of haemoglobin F were observed in 2 patients with sickle-cell disease after treatment with chorionic gonadotrophin.— E. Beutler (letter), *J. Am. med. Ass.*, 1969, *207*, 2284.

Ulcerative colitis. One man and 7 women, aged 23 to 40 years, who had suffered with ulcerative colitis for 10 days to 3 years, benefited from intramuscular injections of human gonadotrophin, 500 to 6000 units weekly, for 2 to 7 months. None relapsed during 3 to 29 months.— S. M. Talaat, *Am. J. dig. Dis.*, 1968, *13*, 907, per *Abstr. Wld Med.*, 1969, *43*, 738.

Use as a tumour marker. There was a high correlation between the degree of malignancy and elevated titres of chorionic gonadotrophin, measured by radioimmunoassay for the beta subunit of the hormone, in patients with trophoblastic neoplasms.— D. A. Boyes *et al.*, *Can. med. Ass. J.*, 1977, *117*, 753.

Further references: T. H. Maugh, *Science*, 1977, *197*, 543; B. Nørgaard-Pedersen *et al.* (letter), *Lancet*, 1978, *2*, 1042; J. L. Vaitukaitis, *New Engl. J. Med.*, 1979, *301*, 324; E. E. Fraley *et al.*, *ibid.*, 1370.

Preparations

Chorionic Gonadotrophin Injection *(B.P.)*. A sterile solution of chorionic gonadotrophin in Water for Injections, prepared by dissolving, immediately before use, the sterile contents of a sealed container (Chorionic Gonadotrophin for Injection) in the requisite amount of Water for Injections. The sealed container may also contain added inert substances. pH of a 1% solution is 6 to 8. Several other pharmacopoeias have a similar injection.

Chorionic Gonadotropin for Injection *(U.S.P.)*. A sterile dry mixture of chorionic gonadotropin with suitable diluents and buffers; it may contain an antimicrobial agent. Its solution has a pH of 6 to 8.

Jap. P. has a similar preparation.

Proprietary Preparations

Gonadotraphon LH *(Paines & Byrne, UK)*. Chorionic gonadotrophin, available as powder for preparing injections in ampoules of 500, 1000, and 5000 units, with solvent.

Pregnyl *(Organon, UK)*. Chorionic gonadotrophin, available as powder for preparing injections, in ampoules of 500, 1500, and 5000 units, with solvent. (Also available as Pregnyl in *Austral., Denm., Ital., Neth., Norw., S. Afr., Switz.*).

Profasi *(Serono, UK)*. Chorionic gonadotrophin, available as powder for preparing injections in ampoules each containing 500, 1000, 2000, or 5000 units, supplied with 1-ml ampoules of sodium chloride injection. (Also available as Profasi in *Ital., Neth., S.Afr., Switz., USA*).

Other Proprietary Names

Antuitrin S *(Austral., Canad.)*; A.P.L. *(Austral., Canad., Ital., S.Afr., USA)*; Choragon *(Ger.)*; Choriomon *(Switz.)*; Coriantin *(Ital.)*; Endocorion *(Arg.)*; Follutein *(USA)*; Gonadex *(Swed., Switz., USA)*; Gonadotrafon LH *(Ital.)*; Harvatropin *(USA)*; Neogonadil *(Ital.)*; Physex *(Denm., Norw.)*; Predalon, Pregnesin (both *Ger.*); Primogonyl *(Austral., Ger., S.Afr., Switz.)*.

5930-b

Follicle-stimulating Hormone. Follitropin; Follotropin; FSH.

CAS — 9002-68-0.

Pharmacopoeias. In *Br.*, *It.*, and *U.S.* as preparations.

A purified standardised extract of the urine of postmenopausal women, containing primarily the follicle-stimulating hormone with varying concentrations of luteinising hormone. It may also be prepared from pituitary glands (human pituitary gonadotrophin; HPG).

Menotrophin (*B.P.*) is a dry sterile preparation of a glycoprotein fraction obtained from human postmenopausal urine and containing urinary derivatives of follicle-stimulating hormone and luteinising hormone. It is an off-white or slightly yellow powder containing not less than 40 units of follicle-stimulating hormone activity per mg and about 1 unit of luteinising hormone activity per unit of follicle-stimulating hormone activity. **Soluble** in water. A 1% solution in water has a pH 6 to 8. **Sterilise** by filtration. **Store** at a temperature not exceeding 25° in containers sealed to exclude micro-organisms. Protect from light. Under these conditions it may be expected to retain its potency for not less than 3 years.

Menotropins (*U.S.P.*) contains not less than 40 units of follicle-stimulating hormone and not less than 40 units of luteinising hormone per mg; store at 2° to 8° in airtight containers. Menotropina (*It. P.*) is a similar preparation.

NOTE. Urofollitrophin is the name given to a preparation of follicle-stimulating hormone extracted from human menopausal urine and possessing no luteinising hormone activity.

Human follicle-stimulating hormone exists in monomeric, dimeric, and tetrameric forms, with molecular weights of approximately 17 000, 34 000, and 68 000 respectively.— C. J. Gray (letter), *Nature*, 1967, *216*, 1112.

For evidence that follicle-stimulating hormone obtained from the urine of postmenopausal women differed chemically from the therapeutically similar substance obtained from human postmortem pituitary glands, see W. R. Butt, 1970, per J. K. Butler, *Postgrad. med. J.*, 1972, *48*, 27. For immunological differences, see M. L. Taymor and T. Tamada, *J. clin. Endocr. Metab.*, 1967, *27*, 709.

Units. 54 units of human urinary follicle-stimulating hormone and 46 units of human urinary luteinising hormone are contained in approximately 1 mg (with lactose 5 mg) in one ampoule of the first International Standard Preparation for Bioassay (1974).

10 units of human pituitary follicle-stimulating hormone and 25 units of human pituitary luteinising hormone are contained in approximately 500 µg (with lactose 1.25 mg) in one ampoule of the first International Reference Preparation for Bioassay (1974).

A highly purified preparation of human pituitary follicle-stimulating hormone has been obtained and its use in immunoassay is to be studied.— Thirtieth Report of WHO Expert Committee on Biological Standardization, *Tech. Rep. Ser. Wld Hlth Org. No. 638*, 1979.

Adverse Effects. Follicle-stimulating hormone when given with luteinising hormone may cause sensitivity reactions and dose-related ovarian hyperstimulation varying from mild ovarian enlargement and abdominal discomfort to severe hyperstimulation with ovarian rupture and intraperitoneal haemorrhage. There may be ascites, pleural effusion, oliguria, hypotension, and arterial thrombo-embolism. Fatalities have been reported.

Swelling of pre-existing pituitary tumours leading to visual field defects may occur during pregnancy in women treated for infertility.

There is a risk of multiple births, with a reported incidence of about 30%.

Pregnancy and the neonate. There was a 15% incidence of multiple delivery in 66 infants whose mothers had received human menopausal gonadotrophin at or shortly before conception for ovulation induction. There were one major and 5 minor malformations, an incidence close to expected frequencies.— S. Harlap (letter), *Lancet*, 1976, *2*, 961.

Precautions. Follicle-stimulating hormone should not be given to pregnant patients. Use should be avoided in patients with intracranial lesions, adrenal or thyroid disorders, or ovarian cysts or enlargement. It should be used with caution in patients who might demonstrate hypersensitivity. There may be a diminished effect in patients with hyperprolactinaemia.

Interactions. A controlled study in 4 anovulatory women showed that ethinyloestradiol, given in a dose of 100 µg daily for 10 days commencing 5 days before the administration of human menopausal gonadotrophin and chorionic gonadotrophin, inhibited ovulation.— A. Jacobson and J. R. Marshall (letter), *Lancet*, 1968, *2*, 286.

Uses. Follicle-stimulating hormone followed by chorionic gonadotrophin is used in the treatment of anovulatory infertility due to insufficient gonadotrophins. Follicle-stimulating hormone is administered to induce follicular maturation and endometrial proliferation, and is followed by treatment with chorionic gonadotrophin to stimulate ovulation and corpus luteum formation. It is considered that follicle-stimulating hormone alone does not produce full follicular maturation; a preparation containing follicle-stimulating hormone and luteinising hormone (human menopausal gonadotrophin; HMG) in an equal number of units is usually used. Clomiphene (p.1406) can also be used to induce ovulation; amenorrhoeic women with hyperprolactinaemia may be treated with bromocriptine (p.894).

The dosage and schedule of treatment must be determined according to the needs of each patient; it is usual to monitor response by studying the patient's urinary oestrogen excretion. Follicle-stimulating hormone may be given daily by intramuscular injection in a dose of 75 units with 75 units of luteinising hormone, until an adequate response, judged on the basis of daily oestrogen determinations, is achieved, followed after 1 or 2 days by chorionic gonadotrophin (see p.1268). Alternatively, three doses may be given on alternate days followed by chorionic gonadotrophin on the eighth day.

Infertility. A detailed analysis was made of 78 pregnancies and births resulting from the induction of ovulation in 68 patients with long-term sterility. All women received treatment with chorionic gonadotrophin and follicle-stimulating hormone with luteinising hormone except 2 who were given clomiphene citrate and follicle-stimulating and luteinising hormones. The pregnancies resulted in 122 births, including 47 single, 23 twin, 5 triplet, 2 quadruplet, and 1 sextuplet set. Ten women developed mild or severe hyperstimulation and 3 of 4 children with major malformations were born to mothers who suffered hyperstimulation. The hyperstimulation syndrome was characterised by an abnormal hormone excretion and disturbances in the normal homoeostasis of the body. Intra-uterine growth and postnatal development of the children born after treatment were normal. The abortion-rate was 29% and the foetal and neonatal death-rate was 27%.— M. Hack *et al.*, *J. Am. med. Ass.*, 1970, *211*, 791.

Anovulatory infertility in 59 patients was treated according to a treatment-orientated diagnostic classification of their amenorrhoea. Patients with oestrogen deficiency who did not respond to clomiphene and who did not have raised serum concentrations of follicle-stimulating hormone or prolactin were treated with follicle-stimulating hormone with luteinising hormone and chorionic gonadotrophin; 11 of 12 patients subsequently conceived. Six similar patients in whom weight loss was a problem were encouraged to increase their weight and 5 conceived without the use of gonadotrophins, although 2 were given clomiphene to correct luteal deficiency when menstruation had resumed.— M. G. R. Hull *et al.*, *Br. med. J.*, 1979, *1*, 1257.

Further references: E. T. Tyler, *J. Am. med. Ass.*, 1968, *205*, 16; A. D. Tsapoulis and A. C. Crooke, *Lancet*, 1968, *2*, 1321; A. C. Crooke *et al.*, *ibid.*, 180; *Br. med. J.*, 1972, *4*, 167; Human Pituitary Advisory Committee, *Med. J. Aust.*, 1975, *2*, 549; J. D. Ellis and J. G. Williamson, *Br. J. Obstet. Gynaec.*, 1975, *82*, 52; J. Evans and L. Townsend, *Am. J. Obstet. Gynec.*, 1976, *125*, 321; D. Rabinowitz *et al.*, *New Engl. J. Med.*, 1979, *300*, 126; G. Oelsner *et al.*, *Fert. Steril.*, 1978, *30*, 538; C. M. March *et al.*, *Obstet. Gynec.*, 1979, *53*, 8.

Male infertility. In 11 infertile men with severe oligospermia, treatment with follicle-stimulating and luteinising hormones increased the sperm count in 5 patients and definitely improved the motility of spermatozoa in 7. The wives of 2 patients in the latter group subsequently became pregnant.— J. M. Danezis and L. Batrinos, *Fert. Steril.*, 1967, *18*, 788, per *J. Am. med. Ass.*, 1968, *203* (Jan. 15), A212.

Ovarian-function test. As a test of ovarian function prior to induction of ovulation, patients were given by injection 3 ampoules of follicle-stimulating hormone 75 units with luteinising hormone 75 units daily for 3 days. Where ovarian function could be stimulated, a rise in urinary oestrone occurred and reached a peak 3 to 4 days after the treatment. The urinary oestrone concentration 2 days after treatment was compared with the concentration prior to treatment; increases of 6 to 40 µg per 24 hours were considered satisfactory and an increase of 41 µg or more per 24 hours indicative of ovarian over-responsiveness. Of 11 patients adjudged satisfactory by the test, 10 subsequently ovulated when treated with either clomiphene or gonadotrophin.— R. I. Cox *et al.*, *Lancet*, 1966, *2*, 888.

Preparations

Menotrophin Injection *(B.P.)*. A sterile solution of menotrophin in Water for Injections prepared by dissolving, immediately before use, the contents of a sealed container (Menotrophin for Injection) in the requisite amount of Water for Injections. pH 6 to 8. The sealed container may contain added inert substances.

Menotropins for Injection *(U.S.P.)*. A sterile freeze-dried mixture of menotropins *U.S.P.* and suitable excipients; it may contain an antimicrobial agent. pH of the reconstituted solution 6 to 7.

Pergonal *(Serono, UK)*. Ampoules each containing, as powder for preparing solutions, follicle-stimulating hormone 75 units and luteinising hormone 75 units with lactose 10 mg, supplied with 1-ml ampoules of sodium chloride injection. (Also available as Pergonal in *Austral., Ger., Neth., S.Afr., USA*).

Other Proprietary Names

Humegon *(Austral., Belg., Denm., Fr., Ger., Neth., Norw., S.Afr., Swed., Switz.)*; Néo-Pergonal *(Fr.)*.

5931-v

Luteinising Hormone.
Human Interstitial-cell-stimulating Hormone; Lutropin.

CAS — 9002-67-9; 39341-83-8 (human).

Units. 77 units of human pituitary luteinising hormone for immunoassay are contained in approximately 11.6 µg (with human albumin 1 mg and lactose 5 mg) in one ampoule of the first International Reference Preparation for Immunoassay (1974).

See also under Follicle-stimulating Hormone, above.

Preparations to replace the international reference preparation of human pituitary luteinising hormone for immunoassay are being considered. Highly purified alpha and beta subunits of human pituitary luteinising hormone are also being studied for their suitability as international reference materials.— Thirtieth Report of WHO Expert Committee on Biological Standardization, *Tech. Rep. Ser. Wld Hlth Org. No. 638*, 1979.

Luteinising hormone is extracted from the pituitary or urine of postmenopausal women. It is used together with follicle-stimulating hormone in the induction of follicular maturation in women being treated for failure of ovulation. Chorionic gonadotrophin (p.1268) has the actions of luteinising hormone and is the form in which it is generally used for other purposes.

5932-g

Serum Gonadotrophin *(B.P., B.P. Vet.)*.
Gonadotr. Seric.; PMSG; Pregnant Mares' Serum Gonadotrophin.

Pharmacopoeias. In *Aust.*, *Br.*, *Jap.*, and *Turk. Jap.* specifies not less than 1000 units per mg.

A dry sterile preparation of the glycoprotein fraction obtained from the plasma of mares in their sixtieth to seventy-fifth day of pregnancy, that stimulates the formation of follicles in the mammalian ovary.

A white or pale grey amorphous powder containing not less than 900 units per mg, calculated with reference to the dried substance, and losing not more than 10% of its weight on drying. **Soluble** in water. **Store** in a cool place in containers sealed to exclude micro-organisms and protect from light; under these conditions it may be expected to retain its potency for not less than 2 years.

Units. 1600 units of equine serum gonadotrophin for bioassay, obtained from the serum of pregnant mares, is contained in approximately 800 µg (with lactose 5 mg) in one ampoule of the second International Standard Preparation (1966).

Uses. Serum gonadotrophin has actions similar to those of follicle-stimulating hormone (p.1269). Its clinical value is doubtful. Doses have ranged from 500 units intramuscularly weekly, to 3000 units daily.

Preparations

Serum Gonadotrophin Injection *(B.P.)*. A sterile solution of serum gonadotrophin prepared by dissolving, immediately before use, the contents of a sealed container (Serum Gonadotrophin for Injection) in the requisite amount of Water for Injections. The sealed container may contain added inert substances and buffering agents. pH of a solution containing 5000 units per ml 6 to 8.

Jap. P. includes a similar preparation.

Gonadotraphon FSH *(Paines & Byrne, UK)*. Serum gonadotrophin, available as dry powder in ampoules of 1000 units, with solvent.

Other Proprietary Names

Anteron *(Ger., S.Afr.)*; Eleagol *(Arg.)*; Gestyl *(Austral., Switz.)*; Primantron *(Austral.)*; Seragon *(Ger.)*; Seriomon *(Switz.)*.

Serum gonadotrophin was also formerly marketed in Great Britain under the proprietary name Gestyl (*Organon*).

5933-q

Growth Hormone.
CB-311; HGH; STH; Somatotrophin; Somatropin. H-Phe-Pro-Thr-Ile-Pro-Leu-Ser-Arg-Leu-Phe-Asp-Asn-Ala-Met-Leu-Arg-Ala-His-Arg-Leu-His-Gln-Leu-Ala-Phe-Asp-Thr-Tyr-Gln-Glu-Phe-Glu-Glu-Ala-Tyr-Ile-Pro-Lys-Glu-Gln-Lys-Tyr-Ser-Phe-Leu-Gln-Asn-Pro-Gln-Thr-Ser-Leu-Cys-Phe-Ser-Glu-Ser-Ile-Pro-Thr-Pro-Ser-Asn-Arg-Glu-Glu-Thr-Gln-Gln-Lys-Ser-Asn-Leu-Gln-Leu-Leu-Arg-Ile-Ser-Leu-Leu-Leu-Ile-Gln-Ser-Trp-Leu-Glu-Pro-Val-Gln-Phe-Leu-Arg-Ser-Val-Phe-Ala-Asn-Ser-Leu-Val-Tyr-Gly-Ala-Ser-Asn-Ser-Asp-Val-Tyr-Asp-Leu-Leu-Lys-Asp-Leu-Glu-Glu-Gly-Ile-Gln-Thr-Leu-Met-Gly-Arg-Leu-Glu-Asp-Gly-Ser-Pro-Arg-Thr-Gly-Gln-Ile-Phe-Lys-Gln-Thr-Tyr-Ser-Lys-Phe-Asp-Thr-Asn-Ser-His-Asn-Asp-Asp-Ala-Leu-Leu-Lys-Asn-Tyr-Gly-Leu-Leu-Tyr-Cys-Phe-Arg-Lys-Asp-Met-Asp-Lys-Val-Glu-Thr-Phe-Leu-Arg-Ile-Val-Gln-Cys-Arg-Ser-Val-Glu-Gly-Ser-Cys-Gly-Phe-OH.

$C_{990}H_{1529}N_{263}O_{299}S_7$=22 124.

CAS — 9002-72-6; 12629-01-5 (human); 37267-05-3 (sheep).

A water-soluble protein from the anterior pituitary with an iso-electric point at pH 4.9. Human growth hormone consists of a single polypeptide chain of 191 amino acids. It is destroyed by boiling and by proteolytic enzymes.

The synthesis of human growth hormone fragments with growth-promoting activity.— F. Chillemi *et al.*, *Nature New Biol.*, 1972, *238*, 243.

Two immunoreactive components were identified in plasma or pituitary extracts of human growth hormone and named 'big' HGH and 'little' HGH. Little HGH was eluted as a globular protein of molecular weight 22 000 from Sephadex gel following filtration. Big HGH was less retarded by the gel and was considered to have twice the molecular weight. Big HGH made up 24 to 37% of the total circulating material in healthy subjects and 8 to 14% in acromegalic patients. Big HGH had much less activity in a radioreceptor assay than in the radioimmunoassay in both subjects and patients whereas there was no difference with little HGH.— P. Gorden *et al.*, *Science*, 1973, *182*, 829.

The synthesis of human growth hormone in bacterial cells using synthetic DNA fragments and human pituitary material.— *J. Am. med. Ass.*, 1979, *242*, 701.

The amino-acid sequence of human growth hormone.— C. H. Li, *Can. med. Ass. J.*, 1979, *120*, 575.

Units. 0.35 unit of human growth hormone for immunoassay is contained in approximately 175 µg (with sucrose 5 mg and buffer salts) in one ampoule of the first International Reference Preparation for Immunoassay (1968).

Adverse Effects and Precautions. Antibodies have been formed in some patients. Because of the diabetogenic effect of growth hormone it should not be given to patients with diabetes mellitus.

Hypothyroidism has been reported during treatment with growth hormone.

Absorption and Fate. After intravenous injection growth hormone has a half-life of about 30 minutes.

References: M. L. Parker *et al.*, *J. clin. Invest.*, 1962, *41*, 262; B. J. Boucher (letter), *Nature*, 1966, *210*, 1288.

Pregnancy and the neonate. Human growth hormone administered intravenously to 14 healthy pregnant women 270 and 10 minutes before delivery was not transferred across the placenta to the foetus.— Z. Laron *et al.*, *Acta endocr., Copenh.*, 1966, *53*, 687, per *J. Am. med. Ass.*, 1967, *199* (Feb. 13), A206.

Uses. Growth hormone is secreted by the anterior lobe of the pituitary. It promotes skeletal, visceral, and general body growth, stimulates protein anabolism, and affects fat and mineral metabolism. The hormone has a diabetogenic action on carbohydrate metabolism.

Growth hormone secretion is dependent on neural and hormonal influences including a hypothalamic release-inhibiting hormone (Somatostatin, p.1277), a hypothalamic releasing factor (GHRF), not yet identified, and monoamines.

Somatomedins, formerly called sulphation factors, are polypeptides thought to mediate the effects of growth hormone on skeletal growth; they are formed in the liver and possibly the kidney.

Growth hormone is species specific, only that of human origin being effective in man.

In man, deficient secretion of growth hormone during the years of active body growth results in pituitary dwarfism. Overproduction of growth hormone before growth is complete results in gigantism. If it occurs after cessation of growth when the epiphyses have closed, it causes acromegaly, in which the features become coarse and the hands and feet become enlarged.

Growth hormone is given by injection in the treatment of pituitary dwarfism following assessment of pituitary function. Doses of 0.5 unit per kg body-weight have been given weekly by intramuscular injection in 2 or 3 divided doses.

Reviews of the actions and uses of growth hormone: *Lancet*, 1967, *1*, 257; J. A. Strong, *Practitioner*, 1968, *200*, 502; K. J. Catt, *Lancet*, 1970, *1*, 933; *Br. med. J.*, 1971, *2*, 236; *ibid.*, 1971, *3*, 547; J. M. Tanner, *Nature*, 1972, *237*, 433; *Med. J. Aust.*, 1972, *2*, 457; *Med. Lett.*, 1977, *19*, 57; R. Shields, *Nature*, 1977, *267*, 308; P. C. Sizonenko, *Postgrad. med. J.*, 1978, *54*, *Suppl.* 1, 91; R. D. G. Milner, *Archs Dis. Childh.*, 1979, *54*, 733; D. W. Golde *et al.*, *Ann. intern. Med.*, 1980, *92*, 650; *Br. med. J.*, 1980, *280*, 270.

A review of somatomedins.— M. C. Stuart and L. Lazarus, *Med. J. Aust.*, 1975, *1*, 816. See also M. M. Rechler and S. P. Nissley, *Nature*, 1977, *270*, 665.

The measurement of serum concentrations of somatomedin-C by radioimmunoassay appeared to be a useful adjunct to existing methods for the diagnosis of acromegaly. In 57 fasting acromegalic patients the mean serum concentration of immunoreactive somatomedin-C was 6.8 units per ml, 10 times the mean value in 48 healthy subjects, and was found to correlate significantly with clinical indicators of disease activity.— D. R. Clemmons *et al.*, *New Engl. J. Med.*, 1979, *301*, 1138. Somatomedin-C is probably identical to insulin-like growth factor I (IGF-I).— W. H. Daughaday, *ibid.*, 1175.

The intravenous infusion of pentagastrin resulted in a prompt and significant increase in plasma concentrations of growth hormone in 7 healthy male subjects; prolactin concentrations were not affected. This growth hormone-releasing property suggests a potential role for gastrin tetrapeptide as a local neurotransmitter in the hypothalamic-pituitary system. The peptide may be related to the growth hormone-releasing factor that has not yet been identified.— W. Domschke *et al.* (letter), *New Engl. J. Med.*, 1980, *303*, 458.

Effect on metabolism. A review of the mechanism of the diabetogenic effects of growth hormone.— J. Bornstein *et al.*, *Postgrad. med. J.*, 1973, *49* (Mar.), *Suppl.*

The intravenous infusion of 4 mg of growth hormone over 30 minutes increased mean systemic concentrations of the hormone to 92.6 ng per ml. Plasma-glucose concentrations decreased by 9.5% and plasma concentrations of free fatty acids by 21.2% during the first hour. After 2 hours the free fatty acid concentrations rose to 145% of basal concentration. Intra-arterial perfusion did not produce early insulin-like effects nor stimulate lipolysis. Slight increases in growth-hormone concentrations had significant metabolic effects, including a 30% decrease in skeletal muscle sugar uptake and conversion of potassium output to uptake.— S. E. Fineberg and T. J. Merimee, *Diabetes*, 1974, *23*, 499, per *J. Am. med. Ass.*, 1974, *229*, 1368.

In a follow-up study of 26 dwarfs deficient in growth hormone, metabolic similarities to diabetic patients including grossly abnormal glucose tolerance and hyperlipidaemia were still apparent 10 years later. Unlike diabetics, retinopathy had not occurred and the prevalence of arteriosclerosis and hypertension was considerably lower in the dwarfs. Growth hormone may be one of the factors involved in clinical diabetic complications.— T. J. Merimee, *New Engl. J. Med.*, 1978, *298*, 1217. See also A. I. Winegrad and D. A. Greene, *ibid.*, 1250; R. W. Stout (letter), *ibid.*, *299*, 663.

Studies in 6 patients with isolated growth hormone deficiency demonstrated that insulin binding to monocytes was increased in such patients when compared with 8 controls. Insulin binding fell after treatment with growth hormone. These changes in binding were accompanied by similar changes in sensitivity to insulin.— V. Soman *et al.*, *New Engl. J. Med.*, 1978, *299*, 1025. The data on insulin binding in growth hormone deficiency are questionable and the study is being repeated.— P. Felig (letter), *ibid.*, 1980, *303*, 1120.

Further references: Z. Laron *et al.*, *Helv. paediat. Acta*, 1968, *23*, 37; M. Zachmann, *Schweiz. med. Wschr.*, 1969, *99*, 1125, per *J. Am. med. Ass.*, 1969, *209*, 1555; J. F. Aloia *et al.*, *Metabolism*, 1977, *26*, 787.

Hand-Schüller-Christian disease. Five patients with Hand-Schüller-Christian disease were given growth hormone 2 units thrice weekly by intramuscular injection for 15 months to 2 years. All responded with a significant increase in growth-rate, which was greater in the 1st year than in the 2nd.— G. D. Braunstein *et al.*, *New Engl. J. Med.*, 1975, *292*, 332.

Obesity. A brief review of the use of growth hormone as therapy for obesity.— R. S. Rivlin, *New Engl. J. Med.*, 1975, *292*, 26.

Pituitary dwarfism. Fifteen children with growth-hormone deficiency were treated for at least 2 years with highly purified human growth hormone, 2 mg intramuscularly thrice weekly, increased to 4 mg thrice weekly if the growth-rate fell below 6 cm per year. Thyroid hormone was also given when necessary. During the first 6 months, the growth-rate increased twofold or more, but fell to or below the initial level when treatment was stopped. During the 1st and 2nd years, the average increases in height were 9 and 8.4 cm respectively. Seven children were given a third year of therapy and the average increase was 7 cm; increases of 7.8 and 7.2 cm occurred during the 4th and 5th years respectively in 1 child whose treatment was continued.— L. F. Soyka *et al.*, *J. clin. Endocr. Metab.*, 1970, *30*, 1.

In 12 children with hypopituitary dwarfism, growth occurred at a faster rate in 10 when they received growth hormone 0.1 unit per kg body-weight thrice weekly together with fluoxymesterone 2.5 mg per m^2 daily than when they received growth hormone alone.— M. H. MacGillivray *et al.*, *J. Am. med. Ass.*, 1972, *221*, 551.

A report of the first 5 years of a national study of the administration of growth hormone for 6 months in each year to patients with growth-hormone deficiency. The deficiency was idiopathic in 76% of the 151 patients and secondary to organic disease in 17%. The response was greater in younger patients and was dose-related; it was less in the later courses than during the 1st year but diminution was not progressive. Growth velocity increased in 9 of 11 patients with a decreased growth response when given fluoxymesterone.— H. Guyda *et al.*, *Can. med. Ass. J.*, 1975, *112*, 1301.

In a study of 17 children with growth abnormalities growth hormone was given and withheld for alternating 3-month periods; some patients also received testosterone enanthate monthly. It was concluded that such children should receive growth hormone continuously throughout puberty and ideally until growth ceases.— J. M. Tanner *et al.*, *J. Pediat.*, 1976, *89*, 1000. See also A. Aynsley-Green *et al.*, *J. Pediat.*, 1976, *89*, 992.

A positive response in 2 children to growth hormone given for 18 months with an increase in growth-rate. Both children had congenital rubella with growth-hormone deficiency as well as deafness and retinopathy.— M. A. Preece *et al.*, *Lancet*, 1977, *2*, 842.

The efficacy of a depot gel preparation of growth hormone was evaluated in 15 children, aged between 7 and 15 years, with growth hormone deficiency. Plasma concentrations were measured in 6 patients following a single intramuscular injection of growth hormone 2 units, either in aqueous solution or in 15% gelatin solution (growth hormone gel). The peak plasma concentration of growth hormone was lower but more prolonged following administration of growth hormone gel. Studies in 6 patients indicated that intramuscular injection of growth hormone gel 2 units twice weekly is as effective as an aqueous solution of growth hormone 2 units thrice weekly, although the response to growth hormone treatment from either preparation is less in the second 12 months of therapy. A further 9 patients who were given growth hormone 0.3 units per kg body-weight weekly also showed diminished response to growth hormone in the second year of treatment. Use of a depot gel may reduce the amount of hormone and the frequency of injection required but does not solve the problem of a waning response to the long-term administration of growth hormone.— B. Lippe *et al.*, *Archs Dis. Childh.*, 1979, *54*, 609.

A study refuting the suggestion by W. Hamilton (*Archs Dis. Childh.*, 1979, *54*, 971) that human growth hormone provided in the UK by the Medical Research Council causes disproportionate osseous maturation for height gained, with ultimate stunting.— R. D. G. Milner *et al.*, *Archs Dis. Childh.*, 1980, *55*, 461.

Further references: P. H. Henneman, *J. Am. med. Ass.*, 1968, *205*, 828; A. Pertzelan *et al.*, *Clin. Endocr.*, 1976, *5*, 15; A. G. Kenien *et al.*, *J. Pediat.*, 1978, *92*, 491; D. Rudman *et al.*, *New Engl. J. Med.*, 1981, *305*, 123; M. A. Preece, *Br. med. J.*, 1981, *283*, 1145.

Turner's syndrome. A 14-year-old girl with Turner's syndrome and with normal concentrations of growth hormone grew 0.23 cm per month during about a year of observation. In the following year, during which she received growth hormone 10 mg weekly, the rate of growth was 0.5 cm per month; and in the third year, during which she received conjugated oestrogens 625 µg daily, the rate of growth was 0.3 cm a month.— M. Tzagournis, *J. Am. med. Ass.*, 1969, *210*, 2373.

A 9-year-old girl with Turner's syndrome and growth hormone deficiency grew only 2.3 cm during a year of observation. The next year she received growth hormone 5 units thrice weekly and grew 6.4 cm with bone age advancing proportionately.— C. G. D. Brook (letter), *New Engl. J. Med.*, 1978, *298*, 1203.

Proprietary Preparations

Crescormon *(KabiVitrum, UK)*. Human growth hormone, available as sterile powder in vials of 4 units (about 2 mg), with 2-ml ampoules of sodium chloride injection. Store at 5°. (Also available as Crescormon in *Denm., Norw., S.Afr., Swed., Switz., USA*).

Nanormon *(Nordisk-UK, UK)*. Human growth hormone, available as sterile powder in vials of 4 units (about 1.5 mg), with 2-ml ampoules of Water for Injection. Store at 2° to 8°. (Also available as Nanormon in *Denm., Norw.*).

Other Proprietary Names

Asellacrin *(USA)*; Grorm*(Ger., Ital.)*; Somacton *(porcine) (Ger.)*; Somatotrope Choay *(bovine) (Fr.)*.

5934-p

Lypressin.

LVP. [8-L-Lysine]-vasopressin.
$C_{46}H_{65}N_{13}O_{12}S_2$=1056.2.

CAS — 50-57-7.

A stable, water-soluble, polypeptide which is usually prepared synthetically, or may be extracted from the posterior pituitary of pigs.

Units. 7.7 units of lysine-vasopressin are contained in approximately 23.4 µg of synthetic peptide (with albumin 5 mg and citric acid) in one ampoule of the first International Standard Preparation (1978).

5935-s

Lypressin Injection *(B.P., Eur. P.)*. Lypressini Solutio Iniectabilis.

Pharmacopoeias. In *Br., Eur., Fr., Ger., It.,* and *Neth.*

A clear colourless sterile aqueous solution of lypressin. It contains a suitable buffering agent such as sodium acetate and a suitable antimicrobial preservative such as chlorbutol, and may be rendered iso-osmotic with blood by the addition of sodium chloride. **Sterilised** by filtration. pH 3.7 to 4.3. **Store** in sterile containers sealed to exclude micro-organisms at 2° to 25° and avoid freezing. Under these conditions it may be expected to retain its potency for not less than 2 years from the date of manufacture.

Adverse Effects, Treatment, and Precautions. As for Vasopressin Injection, p.1278.

Nasal congestion with ulceration of the nasal mucosa has been reported occasionally following its use. Hypersensitivity reactions are less with synthetic lypressin than with other forms of vasopressin prepared from animals.

Uses. Lypressin has the actions and uses of Vasopressin Injection (see p.1279). In the treatment of diabetes insipidus, lypressin is administered in a nasal spray in doses of 2.5 to 10 units 3 to 7 times daily. It is rapidly absorbed from the nasal mucosa; a peak antidiuretic effect has been reported within 30 minutes to 2 hours but its action is less prolonged than that of desmopressin (p.1265).

Lypressin has been given by intramuscular injection to assess hypothalamic-pituitary-adrenal function with conflicting results.

Diabetes insipidus. Lypressin, administered as a nasal spray, effectively and safely controlled diabetes insipidus in 3 patients who had earlier reacted allergically to preparations of antidiuretic hormone of *animal* origin. In 1 patient the use of oily injections of vasopressin tannate had led to an extensive maculopapular eruption and pruritus. In the other 2 patients the use of posterior pituitary insufflation had been associated with allergic rhinitis and asthma, and with rectal tenesmus, respectively.— N. Mimica *et al., J. Am. med. Ass.*, 1968, *203,* 802.

Further references: S. B. Bronstein *et al., J. Am. med. Ass.*, 1969, *208,* 1481; *Med. Lett.*, 1972, *14,* 98.

Memory. Lypressin about 16 units daily intranasally for 3 days was associated with improved responses to tests of learning and memory in 12 subjects when compared with a placebo given to 11.— J. J. Legros *et al.* (letter), *Lancet,* 1978, *1,* 41. Another placebo group should be run to evaluate the reliability of the findings.— L. W. Poon (letter), *Lancet,* 1978, *1,* 557.

For poor results with lypressin in memory impairment, see Desmopressin, p.1266.

Pituitary-adrenal function. Since some healthy subjects had failed to respond to the lypressin test of hypothalamic-pituitary-adrenal function and since almost half those given the test experienced side-effects its use was abandoned.— A. B. Myles and J. R. Daly, *Corticosteroids and ACTH Treatment,* London, Arnold, 1974, p. 35.

Further references: M. M. Webb-Peploe *et al., Lancet,* 1967, *1,* 195; J. S. Mackay *et al.* (letter), *ibid.*, 1967, *2,* 211; J. R. Tucci *et al., Ann. intern. Med.*, 1968, *69,* 191, per *J. Am. med. Ass.*, 1968, *206* (Sept. 30), A154.

For a comparison of the effects of pyrogen, lypressin, and insulin on pituitary-adrenal function, see Pyrogens, p.1671.

Preparations

Lypressin Nasal Solution *(U.S.P.).* A solution of synthetic lypressin in a suitable diluent; it contains suitable preservatives and is supplied in packages which permit administration as a nasal spray in controlled dosage. pH 3 to 4.3.

Syntopressin Spray *(Sandoz, UK).* A nasal spray containing 50 units of lypressin in each ml and providing a dose of 2.5 units with each squeeze of the plastic bottle. Store in a cool place.

Other Proprietary Names

Diapid *(Fr., USA)*; Postacton *(Ger., Swed.).*

NOTE. Lypressin is also marketed in some countries under the names Vasopresina, Vasopressin, and Vasopressine.

5936-w

Melanocyte-stimulating Hormone. B Hormone; Chromatophore Hormone; Intermedin; Melanotropin; MSH; Pigment Hormone.

CAS — 9002-79-3.

A polypeptide isolated from the pars intermedia of the pituitary of fish and amphibia.

Melanocyte-stimulating hormone has been isolated in two chemically distinct forms. Alpha-melanocyte-stimulating hormone (α-MSH) is probably an artifact resulting from the degradation of adrenocorticotrophic hormone. Beta-melanocyte-stimulating hormone (β-MSH) comprises 18 amino acids in most species but 22 in man; it is considered to be formed by the degradation of the much larger molecule, beta-lipotrophin (β-LPH), which has 91 amino acids and the same heptapeptide core as adrenocorticotrophic hormone. Beta-lipotrophin has been identified in the pituitary in man; it is probably synthesised by the same cells as adrenocorticotrophic hormone and the two hormones may be secreted together.

Melanocyte-stimulating hormone causes dispersal of melanin granules in the skin of fish and amphibia and allows adaptation to the environment.

Its release is inhibited by melanostatin; there is also evidence for a hypothalamic releasing factor (MRF).

Discussions on melanocyte-stimulating hormone and beta-lipotrophin: A. J. Kastin *et al., Mayo Clin. Proc.*, 1976, *51,* 632; *Br. med. J.*, 1977, *1,* 533; A. J. Thody, *Adv. Drug Res.*, 1977, *11,* 23; J. D. Brown and R. P. Doe, *J. Am. med. Ass.*, 1978, *240,* 1273; C. H. Li, *Can. med. Ass. J.*, 1979, *120,* 575.

The intramuscular injection of daily doses of 20 to 40 mg of beta-melanocyte-stimulating hormone induced or aggravated tremor and impaired muscular strength, posture, gait, and other movements in 6 patients with Parkinson's disease. Abdominal cramps and diarrhoea, which appeared initially, faded in 5 patients but persisted in the sixth. Pigmentation of the skin, particularly over the face and arms, was increased.— G. C. Cotzias *et al., New Engl. J. Med.*, 1967, *276,* 374.

For the physiological effects of melanocyte-stimulating hormone in women with amenorrhoea, see A. J. Kastin *et al., Lancet,* 1968, *1,* 1007.

Studies in 5 patients with hypopituitarism showed normal concentrations of immunoreactive beta-melanocyte-stimulating hormone (β-MSH) in the plasma and CSF; it was suggested that β-MSH was produced by and secreted from neural tissue.— S. Shuster *et al., Br. med. J.*, 1977, *1,* 1318. See also S. Shuster *et al., Lancet,* 1973, *1,* 463; M. Sandler *et al.* (letter), *ibid.*, 612.

5937-e

Melanostatin. MIF; Intermedin-inhibiting Factor; Melanocyte-stimulating-hormone-release-inhibiting Factor; Melanotropin Release-inhibiting Factor.

CAS — 9083-38-9.

A peptide obtained from the hypothalamus.

There is conjecture about the structure of melanostatin. It has been considered to be a tripeptide, L-prolyl-leucyl-L-glycinamide (PLG) based on extraction from the bovine hypothalamus or a polypeptide, tocinoic acid, based on the ring structure of synthetic oxytocin but tocinoic acid is an unlikely candidate since its activity has not been confirmed.

References on the structure of melanostatin: R. M. Nair *et al., Biochem. biophys. Res. Commun.*, 1971, *43,* 1376; A. Bower *et al., Biochem. biophys. Res. Commun.*, 1971, *45,* 1185; A. V. Schally *et al.*, in *Pharmacology of the Hypothalamus,* B. Cox *et al.* (Ed.), London, Macmillan, 1978, p. 161.

Uses. Melanostatin is the active principle of the hypothalamus which inhibits the release of melanocyte-stimulating hormone (see above) in animals. However, there is little evidence of its activity in man. It has been tried in the treatment of depression and parkinsonism but with little benefit.

Depression. The use of melanostatin as an anti-depressant.— R. H. Ehrensing and A. J. Kastin, *Archs gen. Psychiat.*, 1974, *30,* 63.

Parkinsonism. A report of symptomatic improvement in 3 previously untreated patients with Parkinson's disease, when they were given melanostatin (tripeptide) 50 mg daily by mouth for 2 months.— A. J. Kastin and A. Barbeau, *Can. med. Ass. J.*, 1972, *107,* 1079. Melanostatin (tripeptide) enhanced the action of levodopa.— A. Barbeau, *Lancet,* 1975, *2,* 683. In a double-blind study involving 19 patients with Parkinson's disease, there was no significant improvement when melanostatin (tripeptide) in doses increasing to 1 to 1.5 g daily by mouth was compared with placebo.— A. Barbeau *et al., Can. med. Ass. J.*, 1976, *114,* 120.

Manufacturers

Abbott, USA.

5938-l

Ornipressin. [8-L-Ornithine]-vasopressin.

$C_{45}H_{63}N_{13}O_{12}S_2$=1042.2.

CAS — 3397-23-7.

Ornipressin is a synthetic derivative of vasopressin with similar actions (see p.1278). It is reported to be a strong vasoconstrictor with only weak antidiuretic properties and has been used to reduce bleeding during surgery. A solution containing 5 units in 20 to 60 ml of sodium chloride injection or local anaesthetic solution has been infiltrated into the area involved.

Ornipressin was used in 333 cases of plastic surgery. Vasoconstriction commenced in 2 to 3 minutes and lasted at least an hour. Ornipressin could be used with halothane. A dose of 10 units in 50 ml was suggested.— G. H. Buck, *Wien. med. Wschr.*, 1971, *121,* 691, per *Int. pharm. Abstr.*, 1974, *11,* 22.

In 12 subjects undergoing anaesthesia with nitrous oxide or nitrous oxide and halothane, ornipressin 5 units intravenously increased peripheral vascular resistance and mean arterial blood pressure and reduced heart-rate and cardiac output. There was no dysrhythmia.— A. J. Coleman and L. W. Baker, *Br. J. Anaesth.*, 1973, *45,* 511.

The use of ornipressin, 5 units in 50 ml of solution containing lignocaine 2%, was recommended for surgery of the scalp.— R. C. Shiell (letter), *Med. J. Aust.*, 1973, *1,* 144.

Pancuronium slightly enhanced the pressor effect of local injections of ornipressin given to gynaecological surgical patients.— A. Guzmán and J. Boada, *Farmaco, Edn prat.*, 1979, *34,* 561.

Proprietary Names

Por 8 *(Sandoz, Austral.; Sandoz, Ger.; Sandoz, S.Afr.; Sandoz, Switz.).*

5940-g

Oxytocin. [3-L-Isoleucine,8-L-leucine]-vasopressin.

$C_{43}H_{66}N_{12}O_{12}S_2$=1007.2.

CAS — 50-56-6.

A cyclic polypeptide with all the amino acids except glycine being in the L-form. The oxytocic principle of the posterior lobe of the pituitary body. It may be prepared by a process of fractionation from the glands of oxen or other mammals or by synthesis.

5941-q

Oxytocin Citrate.

$C_{43}H_{66}N_{12}O_{12}S_2,C_6H_8O_7$=1199.3.

5942-p

Oxytocin Injection *(B.P., B.P. Vet., Eur. P., U.S.P.).* Oxytocini Injectio; Oxytocini Solutio Iniectabilis; Alpha-Hypophamine; Oxytocin.

Pharmacopoeias. In *Br., Eur., Fr., Ger., Hung., Ind., It., Jap., Jug., Neth., Pol.,* and *U.S.* (no strength specified); in *Arg., Cz., Int., Nord.,* and *Turk.* (which specify 10 units per ml); in *Swiss* (which specifies 1, 5, and 10 units per ml).

A clear, colourless, sterile, aqueous solution containing the oxytocic principle of the posterior lobe of the pituitary body, which may be prepared from the glands of oxen or other mammals or by synthesis. The *B.P.* specifies that it contains not more than 1 unit of vasopressor activity per 20 units of oxytocic activity. The solution has a pH of 3 to 4.5.

The solution is **sterilised** by filtration. When **stored** at 2° to 8° it may be expected to retain its potency for not less than 3 years from the date of manufacture and when kept at a temperature not exceeding 25° it may be expected to retain its potency for not less than 2 years.

The *B.P.* requires that the label states the animal source of the oxytocin, or that it is synthetic.

Incompatibility. Oxytocin 0.5 *U.S.P.* unit was 'physically incompatible' with plasmin 200 mg, or warfarin sodium 10 mg in 100 ml of dextrose injection.— R. D. Dunworth and F. R. Kenna, *Am. J. Hosp. Pharm.*, 1965, *22*, 190.

Oxytocin was incompatible with sodium bisulphite and solutions lost 80% of their activity over 6 hours.— C. H. Chang *et al.*, *Can. J. Hosp. Pharm.*, 1972, *25*, 152.

Stability. Based on information received from the manufacturer, oxytocin injection (synthetic) was stable for 5 years at temperatures not exceeding 25°.— R. R. Wolfert and R. M. Cox, *Am. J. Hosp. Pharm.*, 1975, *32*, 585.

Units. 12.5 units of oxytocin for bioassay are contained in approximately 21.4 µg of synthetic peptide (with human albumin 5 mg) in one ampoule of the fourth International Standard Preparation (1978).

Adverse Effects. Excess oxytocin may cause violent uterine contractions leading to uterine rupture and extensive laceration of the soft tissues, foetal bradycardia and arrhythmias, and perhaps foetal or maternal death.

Maternal deaths from severe hypertension and subarachnoid haemorrhage have occurred. Postpartum haemorrhage and fatal hypofibrinogenaemia have been reported but may be due to obstetric complications.

Water retention and intoxication with convulsions, coma, and even death may follow oxytocin especially when given intravenously in large doses or over prolonged periods.

Anaphylactic and other allergic reactions, pelvic haematomas, and nausea and vomiting may occur. The use of oxytocin of natural origin may occasionally produce reactions similar to those of vasopressin (see p.1279).

There are reports of neonatal jaundice associated with the use of oxytocin in the management of labour.

A report of 2 studies comparing oxytocin with dinoprostone in the induction and augmentation of labour. There was a greater increase in resting uterine tone, contractions, and incoordinate activity with oxytocin in the induction study. In the augmentation group the duration of labour, basal uterine tone, frequency of contractions, nausea, vomiting, ketosis, and late foetal bradycardia were significantly greater with oxytocin than dinoprostone.— J. Kelly and A. M. Flynn (letter), *Br. med. J.*, 1974, *4*, 101.

The cardiovascular effects of oxytocin were studied in 26 women undergoing elective termination of pregnancy. Forty seconds after a bolus intravenous injection of oxytocin 0.1 unit per kg body-weight, mean arterial pressure had decreased by about 30% and total peripheral resistance by about 50%. However, heart-rate was increased by about 30%, stroke volume by about 25%, and cardiac output by about 50%. There were no significant cardiovascular changes when oxytocin was infused in dilute solution.— F. R. Weis *et al.*, *Obstet. Gynec.*, 1975, *46*, 211.

Haemorrhage. In a study of 3674 normal deliveries the incidence of postpartum haemorrhage was increased (5.5%) in those in whom labour was induced by amniotomy and oxytocin, compared with the incidence (3.4%) in spontaneous labour.— P. R. S. Brinsden and A. D. Clark, *Br. med. J.*, 1978, *2*, 855. The incidence of postpartum haemorrhage in primigravidas was 5.1% in spontaneous labour, 7.5% in augmented labour, 8.2% in those given dinoprostone gel, and 10.3% in induced labour; for multigravidas the figures were 2.5, 5.8, 5.6, and 7.3%.— I. Z. MacKenzie (letter), *Br. med. J.*, 1979, *1*, 750. See also P. R. Brinsden and A. D. Clark (letter), *Br. med. J.*, 1979, *1*, 1147.

Postpartum haemorrhage was not increased in 164 primagravidas in whom labour was induced by oxytocin, but was possibly increased in 143 multigravidas.— D. D. Mathews (letter), *Br. med. J.*, 1978, *2*, 1162. Haemorrhage was reduced by continuing to give oxytocin intravenously for an hour after delivery.— M. Thiery (letter), *Br. med. J.*, 1978, *2*, 1162.

Further references: J. L. Hallum (letter), *Br. med. J.*, 1968, *4*, 705.

Jaundice. Hyperbilirubinaemia occurred in 6 of 97 babies born to mothers who had not received any oxytocic agent compared with 18 of 103 babies whose mothers had been given some oxytocic treatment.— A. Ghosh and F. P. Hudson (letter), *Lancet*, 1972, *2*, 823. Reducing the dose of oxytocin used for induction had virtually eliminated neonatal hyperbilirubinaemia of unknown origin in one hospital.— A. Ghosh and F. P. Hudson (letter), *Br. med. J.*, 1973, *3*, 636.

The increasing incidence of neonatal jaundice coincided with the introduction of active management of labour but no association was found between the use of oxytocin and the development of jaundice.— N. Campbell *et al.*, *Br. med. J.*, 1975, *2*, 548. See also A. A. Calder *et al.*, *Lancet*, 1974, *2*, 1339.

There were no significant differences in the incidence of hyperbilirubinaemia between 9418 infants delivered after unstimulated labour, 980 after oxytocin-induced labour, and 2768 after oxytocin-augmented labour.— E. A. Friedman and M. R. Sachtleben, *Br. med. J.*, 1976, *1*, 198. Similar reports of oxytocin having no effect on neonatal bilirubin: D. C. Davidson *et al.* (letter), *Br. med. J.*, 1973, *4*, 106; E. A. Friedman and M. R. Sachtleben (letter), *Lancet*, 1974, *2*, 600; H. G. Gray and R. Mitchell (letter), *Lancet*, 1974, *2*, 1144; S. R. Gould *et al.*, *Br. med. J.*, 1974, *3*, 228; M. Thiery *et al.* (letter), *Lancet*, 1975, *1*, 161; P. Boylan, *Br. med. J.*, 1976, *2*, 564; B. Alderman and J. Beazley (letter), *ibid.*, 818.

Serum-bilirubin concentrations were not significantly different in 54 infants delivered spontaneously and after the use of oxytocin to accelerate labour (28 infants), but were increased in 99 infants delivered after amniotomy and the use of oxytocin.— W. C. Chew and I. L. Swann, *Br. med. J.*, 1977, *1*, 72.

Analysis of neonatal jaundice in 12 461 single births confirmed a higher incidence in those given oxytocin, independent of gestational age at birth, sex, race, epidural analgesia, method of delivery, and birth weight, each of which was also associated with jaundice.— L. Friedman *et al.*, *Br. med. J.*, 1978, *1*, 1235. Further reports of neonatal jaundice after the induction or augmentation of labour by oxytocin.— D. P. Davies *et al.*, *Br. med. J.*, 1973, *3*, 476; B. Alderman and J. M. Beazley (letter), *Br. med. J.*, 1974, *3*, 624; I. Chalmers *et al.*, *Br. med. J.*, 1975, *2*, 116; J. M. Beazley and B. Alderman, *Br. J. Obstet. Gynaec.*, 1975, *82*, 265; J. H. Drew and W. H. Kitchen, *J. Pediat.*, 1976, *89*, 657; W. C. Chew, *Br. med. J.*, 1977, *2*, 679.

In 40 infants delivered after oxytocin-induced labour the packed cell volume of cord blood, the erythrocyte deformability index (a determinant of erythrocyte life span), the plasma-haptoglobin concentration, and the plasma osmolality were significantly reduced while the plasma-bilirubin concentration and the plasma lactate dehydrogenase activity were significantly increased, compared with 40 infants delivered after spontaneous labour and 15 delivered by caesarean section. Oxytocin *in vitro* had a time-related and dose-related effect on erythrocyte deformability.— P. C. Buchan, *Br. med. J.*, 1979, *2*, 1255.

Uterine hypertonus. Reports of uterine hypertonus or rupture in patients given oxytocin buccally in doses of 600 to 4000 units: P. M. Leney (letter), *Br. med. J.*, 1964, *2*, 689; H. O. Nicholson (letter), *ibid.*, 876; E. M. O'Dwyer (letter), *ibid.*, 1133.

The incidence of tetanic contractions, baseline hypertonus, or bigeminy was greater in women in whom labour was induced by oxytocin or dinoprostone, or augmented by oxytocin, than in controls. More variable and late foetal heart-rate decelerations occurred in stimulated labours, especially in those involving oxytocin.— E. A. Friedman and M. R. Sachtleben, *Am. J. Obstet. Gynec.*, 1978, *130*, 403.

Further references: M. R. Peyser and R. Toaff, *Obstet. Gynec.*, 1972, *40*, 371; D. A. Grimes *et al.*, *Am. J. Obstet. Gynec.*, 1978, *130*, 591.

Water intoxication. A 24-year-old woman developed acute dilutional hyponatraemia and coma during a mid-trimester abortion when oxytocin 150 units was given by constant intravenous infusion in 5 litres of dextrose injection over 41 hours. There was gradual recovery after the infusion was stopped and all fluids withheld. Restriction of fluid intake was recommended during oxytocin infusion. The antidiuretic effect of oxytocin was dose-related and because of the high dose required to induce abortion in the second trimester prostaglandin infusion could be preferable.— A. J. Ahmad *et al.*, *Postgrad. med. J.*, 1975, *51*, 249.

A 24-year-old woman who received 36 units of oxytocin in 6.5 litres of dextrose injection over 18 hours had a grand mal convulsion 15 minutes before delivery; the plasma-sodium concentration was 117 mmol per litre. The infant was also hyponatraemic and had repeated generalised convulsions which resolved only after treatment with 1.8% sodium chloride intravenously with fluid restriction.— R. H. Schwartz and R. W. A. Jones, *Br. med. J.*, 1978, *1*, 152. The infant might have suffered asphyxia during the mother's convulsion. Hyponatraemia (as low as 120 mmol per litre) was not uncommon in the newborn.— S. Ware (letter), *ibid.*, 362. Two further cases of water intoxication after the use of oxytocin and large volumes of fluid.— M. F. Vere and S. M. Sellers (letter), *ibid.*

In 50 infants born to mothers in whom labour had been induced with oxytocin, hyponatraemia, hypo-osmolality, and enhanced osmotic fragility of erythrocytes was observed at birth, and serum-bilirubin concentrations were significantly higher 72 hours after birth than in 50 control infants. Dextrose injection, used as the vehicle for oxytocin infusion, may further aggravate these changes. Infants with cord serum-sodium concentrations of less than 125 mmol per litre and/or osmolality of less than 260 mmol per kg body-weight were at risk of developing jaundice and should be considered for prophylactic administration of phenobarbitone.— S. Singhi and M. Singh, *Archs Dis. Childh.*, 1979, *54*, 400. See also S. Singhi and M. Singh (letter), *Br. med. J.*, 1977, *2*, 1028.

Further references: A. A. Lilien, *Obstet. Gynec.*, 1968, *32*, 171; W. Bilek and P. Dorr, *Can. med. Ass. J.*, 1970, *103*, 379; P. B. B. Gatenby, *J. Ir. med. Ass.*, 1975, *68*, 283; D. B. Morgan *et al.*, *Br. J. Obstet. Gynaec.*, 1977, *84*, 6.

Precautions. Oxytocin should not be given to women with severe toxaemia, hypertonic uterine dysfunction, or a predisposition to uterine rupture as in patients of high parity or with uterine scar from previous caesarean section. It should not be given for induction before the head is engaged. Placenta praevia, major cephalopelvic disproportion, malposition of the foetus, or obvious foetal distress are also contra-indications.

Care is necessary in the use of oxytocin in patients being treated with pressor agents for hypotension, as severe hypertension has been stated to occur. For the induction of labour oxytocin should be infused slowly in dilute solution since bolus injections may cause severe hypotension with an increase in heart rate, stroke volume, and cardiac output. The infusion volume should be low in patients with cardiovascular disorders.

It is inadvisable to employ 2 routes of administration simultaneously.

Oestrogens intensify and progesterone may diminish the effect of oxytocin on the uterus.

In normal conscious subjects the cardiovascular effects of oxytocin would be minimal, but in patients under halothane anaesthesia there is danger in using oxytocin because of the hypotension produced. This danger also exists with other hypotensive drugs when they are used with halothane.— A. M. Hernandez, *Br. med. J.*, 1964, *2*, 571.

A 29-year-old pregnant woman with congenital aortic stenosis who was given oxytocin parenterally during therapeutic abortion developed heart failure and died. Autopsy revealed an extensive myocardial infarction. Extreme care should be taken when more than 2 units per minute of oxytocin are given intravenously to pregnant women with heart disease.— M. Robinson *et al.*, *J. Am. med. Ass.*, 1967, *200*, 378.

Water intoxication occurred in 2 patients given intra-amniotic injections of sodium chloride and oxytocin infusion. It was considered that patients receiving this combination must have fluid intake restricted at the beginning of the oxytocin infusion.— D. R. Gupta and N. H. Cohen, *J. Am. med. Ass.*, 1972, *220*, 681.

When oxytocin is to be administered before the membranes are ruptured it is considered that the infusion should be slowed when the time for rupturing is reached to prevent the rapid conversion of the hypotonic uterus to the tetanic state, with possible fatal result for the foetus.— J. M. Gate (letter), *Br. med. J.*, 1974, *2*, 118.

Of 658 consecutive deliveries 325 were spontaneous, 148 occurred after amniotomy, 143 after low-dose oxytocin (not more than 32 milliunits per minute), and 42 after high-dose oxytocin. The incidence of foetal distress, 5-minute Apgar score of less than 8, admission to special nursery, and rapid contractions was greater in those receiving oxytocin, particularly in high doses. Careful monitoring of the foetus is essential.— W. A. Liston and A. J. Campbell, *Br. med. J.*, 1974, *3*, 606. Criticism.— G. Chamberlain (letter), *ibid.*, 684.

Interactions. Oxytocin appeared to modify the effect of suxamethonium in 5 patients. Neuromuscular block of the non-depolarising type occurred but was slower in onset than the depolarising blockade normally produced by suxamethonium. Total respiratory depression was more prolonged than expected normally; recovery might be hastened by neostigmine.— R. J. H. Hodges *et al.*, *Br. med. J.*, 1959, *1*, 413.

Laboratory studies showed that the effects of oxytocin on uterus tissue were reduced by progesterone and its metabolite pregnanolone. Pregnanolone was found to have greater inhibitory activity than progesterone.— L. Gyermek (letter), *Lancet*, 1968, *2*, 1195.

Absorption and Fate. Oxytocin is rapidly absorbed from the mucous membranes when administered buccally or intranasally. It is metabolised by the liver and kidneys.

Uses. Oxytocin causes contraction of the uterus, the effect varying with the period in the menstrual cycle in which it is given and depending on whether or not the uterus is pregnant and on the stage of pregnancy. The response is greatest in the later stages of pregnancy. Small doses increase the tone and amplitude of the uterine contractions; large or repeated doses result in tetany lasting for 5 to 10 minutes. Oxytocin also stimulates the smooth muscle associated with the secretory epithelium of the lactating breast causing the ejection of milk but having no direct effect on milk secretion. It has little pressor or antidiuretic action.

Oxytocin is used for the induction and maintenance of labour, to control postpartum bleeding and uterine hypotonicity in the third stage of labour, and to promote lactation in cases of faulty milk ejection. It is also used in missed abortions.

It is administered parenterally as Oxytocin Injection, intranasally as a spray, and in the form of a buccal tablet as oxytocin citrate.

For the induction of labour, oxytocin 2 to 5 units in one litre of Dextrose Intravenous Infusion 5% may be given by slow intravenous infusion at an initial rate of 1 to 2 milliunits per minute and then gradually increased until a contraction pattern similar to that of normal labour is achieved. Foetal heart-rate and uterine contractions should be monitored continuously. To overcome uterine inertia in labour, 1 to 5 units similarly diluted may be given by intravenous infusion at a rate of 30 drops per minute until the inertia is overcome. Doses of 2 to 5 units may be administered by subcutaneous or intramuscular injection or by slow intravenous injection to control postpartum haemorrhage; it is used for this purpose with ergometrine maleate.

In missed abortion 10 to 20 units in 500 ml of Dextrose Intravenous Infusion 5% is infused at the rate of 10 to 30 drops per minute and increased by 10 to 20 units per 500 ml every hour to a maximum of 100 units per 500 ml.

Doses equivalent to 100 to 200 units of oxytocin have been given by buccal administration every half hour for induction of labour to a maximum limit of from 3000 to 4400 units. However, as absorption from this route is irregular and results unpredictable, oxytocin should preferably be given by intravenous infusion if required for induction.

Oxytocin spray is used to facilitate lactation; the usual dose is 2 to 4 units intranasally several minutes before suckling.

An oxytocin challenge test has been used in pregnant patients at high-risk; oxytocin is infused until a contraction-rate of 3 per 10 minutes is achieved and the occurrence of late or variable decelerations of foetal heart-rate monitored. A negative response is considered to be indicative of foetal well-being although false-negative tests have been reported.

Reports and reviews on the actions of oxytocin: M. P. Embrey and J. C. Moir, *J. Obstet. Gynaec. Br. Commonw.*, 1967, *74*, 648; G. M. Mitchell, *Practitioner*, 1968, *200*, 147; *Br. med. J.*, 1969, *2*, 619.

In 7 men, rapid intravenous injection of 2 units of oxytocin significantly raised the concentrations of follicle-stimulating hormone in serum and caused a slight fall in the concentrations of luteinising hormone.— J. J. Legros and P. Franchimont (letter), *Lancet*, 1968, *2*, 735.

Unlike the prostaglandins, the use of oxytocin to induce labour was associated with a significant increase in plasma-cortisol concentrations.— A. H. Gowenlock *et al.*, *Br. J. Obstet. Gynaec.*, 1975, *82*, 215.

Studies in 11 patients undergoing mid-trimester abortion showed only limited correlation between uterine activity and plasma concentrations of oxytocin; it was considered that there was individual myometrial sensitivity to oxytocin.— A. Vasicka *et al.*, *Am. J. Obstet. Gynec.*, 1977, *127*, 171.

Abortion. A technique of inducing abortion in mid-trimester in 30 women by giving urea intra-amniotically and oxytocin intravenously.— I. Craft and B. Musa, *Lancet*, 1971, *2*, 1058.

In a study of 682 patients given intra-amniotic instillations of sodium chloride 20% for mid-trimester abortion, the administration of oxytocin 10 units per hour intravenously starting within 2 hours of the sodium chloride significantly reduced the mean abortion time and the incidence of complications when compared with those given no oxytocin or given oxytocin later.— N. H. Lauersen and J. D. Schulman, *Am. J. Obstet. Gynec.*, 1973, *115*, 420, per *Int. pharm. Abstr.*, 1974, *11*, 724.

The use of oxytocin and dinoprostone for 19 late first and second trimester pregnancies.— T. M. Coltart and M. J. Coe (letter), *Lancet*, 1975, *1*, 173. See also J. M. Beazley and J. F. B. Clarke (letter), *ibid.*, 335; *idem*, *Br. J. clin. Pract.*, 1980, *34*, 329.

Administration. Many of the disadvantages of regulating and maintaining an accurate rate of infusion of injections of oxytocin were overcome by using a variable-speed infusion pump.— J. MacVicar and P. W. Howie, *Lancet*, 1967, *2*, 1339.

Gastric atony. Use of oxytocin in gastric atony.— M. Hashmonai *et al.*, *Br. J. Surg.*, 1979, *66*, 550.

Induction of labour. Studies in 61 pregnant women showed that labour could be more rapidly induced with an oxytocin infusion in women whose plasma-progesterone concentration was low (mean 96 ng per ml) than in those with a high concentration of progesterone (140 ng per ml).— E. D. B. Johansson (letter), *Lancet*, 1968, *2*, 570.

In 290 of 2272 deliveries, labour was induced by intravenous injection of synthetic oxytocin started before or at amniotomy. Oxytocin was administered from a solution containing 0.5 unit in 500 ml of dextrose injection at the rate of 20 drops per minute, equivalent to 1.32 milliunits per minute, and increased every 15 minutes to a maximum of 60 drops per minute and the strength of the solution to 5 units per 500 ml. Delivery occurred within 12 hours in 220 patients. Of 13 caesarean sections necessary, 4 were regarded as due to failure of the method of induction. The method greatly reduced the hazards of induction of labour. There was an increased incidence of postpartum haemorrhage.— M. E. Pawson and S. C. Simmons, *Br. med. J.*, 1970, *3*, 191. The indiscriminate use of oxytocin intravenously in all patients at the time of amniotomy was deprecated.— C. J. Carr (letter), *ibid.*, 348. Further comments.— E. G. Robertson (letter), *ibid.*, 405.

Oxytocin 0.05 unit per ml and dinoprostone 5 μg per ml were equally effective in the induction of labour in 300 patients in a double-blind study; 73% of patients in each group were delivered or achieved a 6-cm dilatation of the cervix within 12 hours of the start of infusion.— J. M. Beazley and A. Gillespie, *Lancet*, 1971, *1*, 152. See also M. G. Elder, *Br. J. Obstet. Gynaec.*, 1975, *82*, 674; A. A. Calder and M. P. Embrey, *Br. J. Obstet. Gynaec.*, 1975, *82*, 728.

A monitoring system to indicate patients requiring skilled attention during labour.— R. H. Philpott and W. M. Castle, *J. Obstet. Gynaec. Br. Commonw.*, 1972, *79*, 592. Of 624 primigravidas (excluding those with antepartum haemorrhage, eclampsia, multiple pregnancy, or malpresentation) 22% passed an 'alert line' and 11% passed an 'action line' and were given active management consisting of lumbar epidural block, pelvic assessment, intravenous fluids and carbohydrates, and oxytocin stimulation consisting of infusion at the rate of 10 drops per minute of oxytocin solution 2.5 units per litre in dextrose solution, increased if necessary by 10 drops each half hour until adequate uterine contractions were established. Oxytocin stimulation was continued for 6 hours provided foetal distress did not occur. Using this technique the proportion of those delivered in less than 12 hours was increased from 57.5 to 94.7% (compared with an earlier group managed conventionally), caesarean section was reduced from 9.9 to 2.6%, and perinatal deaths from 5.8 to 0.6%.— *idem*, 599. See also *Br. med. J.*, 1972, *4*, 126.

In a programme of active management of labour, stimulation by artificial rupture of the membranes was followed an hour later by an infusion of oxytocin. A solution containing 10 units per litre was started at a rate of 10 drops per minute and increased every 15 minutes to a maximum of 60 drops per minute and to a maximum total of 1 litre. Of 1000 consecutive primigravidas 550 received oxytocin and only 7 were in labour for more than 12 hours because of treatment failure.— K. O'Driscoll *et al.*, *Br. med. J.*, 1973, *3*, 135. Criticism, particularly of inadequate relief of pain.— J. S. Crawford (letter), *ibid.*, 453. General criticism.— J. W. K. Ritchie and R. O. Robinson (letter), *ibid.*, 539; G. Roberts (letter), *ibid.*, 540.

The incidence of low infant Apgar scores (less than 6) in 533 spontaneous deliveries was 7% compared with 5.5% in 200 deliveries induced by amniotomy and low-dose oxytocin (less than 16 milliunits per minute) and 7.4% in 310 deliveries induced by amniotomy and oxytocin in higher doses.— B. Alderman (letter), *Br. med. J.*, 1974, *4*, 44. See also M. B. McNay *et al.*, *Br. med. J.*, 1977, *1*, 347; J. Leeson and A. Smith (letter), *ibid.*, 707; I. Chalmers *et al.* (letter), *ibid.*; A. Lynch (letter), *ibid.*, 708; D. Meagher and K. O'Driscoll (letter), *ibid.*

In 160 women (77 primiparous) oxytocin was given intravenously to induce labour, after amniotomy, in increasing dosage. The total dose of oxytocin varied considerably and the time to the onset of regular contractions varied according to the Bishop score. Once cervical dilatation of 5 cm was achieved a dose of 7 milliunits per minute was adequate for the maintenance of labour.— J. M. Beazley *et al.*, *Br. med. J.*, 1975, *2*, 248.

In a controlled retrospective study involving 32 women with spontaneous labour, 31 induced by amniotomy, and 38 induced by amniotomy and oxytocin no significant differences occurred between the groups in respect to maternal complications during labour or neonatal problems. The children at 5 years old underwent intelligence tests, gross and fine motor tests, and auditory and visual tests but no differences were found relative to the method of birth.— W. G. McBride *et al.*, *Med. J. Aust.*, 1977, *2*, 456.

Further references: J. M. Beazley and A. Kurjak, *Lancet*, 1972, *2*, 348; J. Studd *et al.*, *Br. med. J.*, 1975, *2*, 545; J. Seitchik *et al.*, *Am. J. Obstet. Gynec.*, 1977, *127*, 223; *Br. med. J.*, 1979, *2*, 407.

For references to the intranasal administration of oxytocin for the induction of labour, see Martindale 27th Edn, p. 1260.

Buccal administration. In a double-blind study in 44 primigravidas, there was no evidence that oxytocin, 200 units given thrice daily as buccal tablets from the 38th week of pregnancy, had any effect on uterine activity in late pregnancy or labour.— T. H. Coltart and T. G. Nash (letter), *Br. med. J.*, 1974, *3*, 467.

The use of buccal oxytocin with or without artificial rupture of membranes for induction during labour produced no problems when used by skilled general medical practitioners.— G. A. Richmond, *J.R. Coll. gen. Pract.*, 1977, *27*, 406.

Further references: T. Bakke, *Nord. Med.*, 1971, *85*, 273; J. A. Chalmers and A. Prakash, *Am. J. Obstet. Gynec.*, 1971, *111*, 227; A. Cordano and V. Kraus, *Obstet. Gynec.*, 1972, *39*, 247.

Lactation. The use of oxytocin nasal spray to enhance lactation in women who had given birth prematurely.— H. Ruis *et al.*, *Br. med. J.*, 1981, *283*, 340.

Oxytocin challenge test. Haemorrhage occurred after two oxytocin challenge tests; the patient was found to have a major placenta praevia.— K. H. Ng and W. P. Wong (letter), *Br. med. J.*, 1976, *2*, 698.

Neonatal hyperbilirubinaemia was associated with an oxytocin challenge test in the mother before labour. This test should be used with caution in women whose babies might be at risk from hyperbilirubinaemia.— D. Peleg and J. A. Goldman (letter), *Lancet*, 1976, *2*, 1026.

The oxytocin challenge test (OCT) was performed on 399 occasions in 305 women with pregnancies at risk and a gestational age of 36 weeks or more. Oxytocin 1 milliunit per minute was given by infusion pump and increased every 5 to 10 minutes until a contraction-rate of 3 per 10 minutes was achieved. Less than 10% of late or variable decelerations of foetal heart-rate (FHR) was judged negative; 10 to 29% was judged equivocal; and 30% or more was judged positive. The finding of a positive or equivocal response to the OCT was considered a prediction of decelerations of the FHR during parturition, though the type of risk might vary. The OCT merited continued usage and refinement.— H. Schulman *et al.*, *Am. J. Obstet. Gynec.*, 1977, *129*, 239.

Reports of foetal death despite negative oxytocin challenge tests.— R. G. Marcum (letter), *Am. J. Obstet. Gynec.*, 1977, *127*, 894; R. P. Lorenz and J. S. Pagano, *Am. J. Obstet. Gynec.*, 1978, *130*, 232; R. Dittman and J. Belcher (letter), *New Engl. J. Med.*, 1978, *298*, 56.

Further references: M. Ray *et al.*, *Am. J. Obstet. Gynec.*, 1972, *114*, 1; R. K. Freeman, *Am. J. Obstet. Gynec.*, 1975, *121*, 481; A. B. Weingold *et al.*, *Am. J. Obstet. Gynec.*, 1975, *123*, 466; R. K. Freeman *et al.*, *Obstet. Gynec.*, 1976, *47*, 8; G. Farahani *et al.*, *Obstet. Gynec.*, 1976, *47*, 159; J. T. Parer and J. F. Afonso, *Am. J. Obstet. Gynec.*, 1977, *127*, 204; S. G. Gabbe *et al.*, *Am. J. Obstet. Gynec.*, 1977, *129*, 723; T. F. Baskett and E. A. Sandy, *Br. J. Obstet. Gynaec.*, 1977, *84*, 39; T. F. Baskett and E. A. Sandy, *Obstet. Gynec.*, 1979, *54*, 365.

Porphyria. Mention of the successful use of oxytocin for caesarean section in a woman with porphyria and for whom ergometrine was accordingly contra-indicated.— S. C. Allen and G. A. D. Rees, *Br. J. Anaesth.*, 1980, *52*, 835.

Postpartum haemorrhage. In a study in 148 patients who had received oxytocin infusions during the first and second stages of labour and who had received epidural analgesia, blood loss at delivery was similar in those given ergometrine 500 µg intravenously or oxytocin 5 units intravenously; the incidence of nausea, retching, and vomiting was 46% in those receiving ergometrine and nil in those receiving oxytocin. Oxytocin was preferable to ergometrine particularly in patients with heart disease, pre-eclampsia, hypertension, phaeochromocytoma, thyrotoxicosis, and coronary insufficiency.— J. E. Moodie and D. D. Moir, *Br. J. Anaesth.*, 1976, *48*, 571.

In a study in 88 primigravidas who had spontaneous delivery, oxytocin 10 units intravenously was as effective as ergometrine 500 µg intravenously in preventing third stage uterine haemorrhage at delivery. Vomiting or retching occurred in 13% of the mothers who received ergometrine.— D. D. Moir and A. B. Amoa, *Br. J. Anaesth.*, 1979, *51*, 113.

Further references: B. Sorbe, *Obstet. Gynec.*, 1978, *52*, 694.

See also under Adverse Effects above.

Schizophrenia. Oxytocin was stated to be effective in the treatment of acute schizophrenia and, to a lesser degree, in chronic schizophrenia; 10 to 15 units intravenously or 20 to 25 units intramuscularly was given daily for 6 to 10 days.— W. Bujanow (letter), *Br. med. J.*, 1972, *4*, 298.

Preparations

Oxytocin Nasal Solution *(U.S.P.)*. A solution of synthetic oxytocin in a suitable diluent; it contains suitable preservatives. pH 3.7 to 4.3.

Oxytocin Tablets *(B.P.)*. Tablets of synthetic oxytocin. They contain not more than 1 unit of vasopressor activity per 20 units of oxytocic activity. Store at a temperature not exceeding 25°; under these conditions they may be expected to retain their potency for at least 3 years from the date of manufacture. The tablets should be allowed to dissolve slowly in the mouth.

Syntocinon *(Sandoz, UK)*. Oxytocin Injection containing 1 unit of synthetic oxytocin per ml, in ampoules of 2 ml; 5 units per ml in ampoules of 1 ml; and 10 units per ml in ampoules of 1 and 5 ml. **Syntocinon Nasal Spray.** A solution of synthetic oxytocin containing 40 units per ml, providing 2 units with each squeeze of the container. (Also available as Syntocinon in *Arg., Austral., Belg., Canad., Denm., Fr., Ger., Ital., Neth., Norw., S.Afr., Switz., USA*).

Other Proprietary Names

Orasthin *(Ger.)*; Partocon *(Ger., Swed.)*; Pitocin *(Austral., Belg., Canad., Denm., Ger., Norw., S.Afr., USA)*; Piton-S *(Neth.)*.

Synthetic oxytocin was also formerly marketed in Great Britain under the proprietary name Pitocin (*Parke, Davis*).

5943-s

Powdered Pituitary (Posterior Lobe) *(B.P.C. 1973)*.

Powdered Pituit. (Post. Lobe); Pituitarium Posterius Pulveratum; Pituitary; Posterior Pituitary; Hypophysis Cerebri Pars Posterior; Hypophysis Sicca; Ipofisi Posteriore.

Pharmacopoeias. In *Arg., Aust., It.,* and *Turk.* (which specify not less than 1 unit of oxytocic activity per mg), and *Jug.* (no strength specified).

A yellowish-white or grey amorphous powder with a characteristic odour, prepared from the posterior lobes of mammalian pituitary bodies and containing not less than 800 units of specific oxytocic activity per g. Partly **soluble** in water. **Store** in a cool place in airtight containers.

When issued for use as an antidiuretic it is assayed by the method given in Appendix 18 of the *B.P.C. 1973*, the strength being expressed as units (antidiuretic) per g.

Adverse Effects, Treatment, and Precautions. Similar to those for Oxytocin Injection (p.1273) and for Vasopressin Injection (p.1278). Allergic rhinitis, asthma, and alveolitis have occasionally been reported following the use of Pituitary (Posterior Lobe) Insufflation. The major protein contained in the preparation is neurophysin (p.1265) and nearly all patients treated have antineurophysin antibodies.

Uses. Powdered pituitary (posterior lobe) has oxytocic, pressor, antidiuretic, and hyperglycaemic actions and has generally been replaced by preparations with more specific actions such as Oxytocin Injection (p.1274) and Vasopressin Injection (p.1278). It has been administered by insufflation in the treatment of diabetes insipidus in doses of 60 to 90 units daily but desmopressin (p.1265) is preferred.

For references to the use of posterior pituitary preparations, see Martindale 27th Edn, p. 1261.

Preparations

Pituitary (Posterior Lobe) Injection *(B.P.C. 1968)*. Inj. Pituit. Post.; Pituitary Liquid Extract; Injectio Pituitarii Posterioris; Pituitary Injection; Extract of Pituitary (Posterior Lobe); Posterior Pituitary Injection; Pituitrinum pro Injectionibus. A sterile aqueous extract of powdered pituitary (posterior lobe) adjusted to contain 10 units of oxytocic activity per ml and to pH 3 to 4. Sterilised by autoclaving or by filtration after the addition of a suitable bactericide. Store at as low a temperature as possible above its freezing-point.

Stability. The injection could be stored with a maximum loss of 5% of its activity, as follows: refrigerator, 3 to 4 years; 6° to 15°, 1 year; 15° to 20°, 6 months.— A. T. Nielsen, *Dansk Tidsskr. Farm.*, 1959, *33*, 1, per *Am. J. Hosp. Pharm.*, 1959, *16*, 137.

Pituitary (Posterior Lobe) Insufflation *(B.P.C. 1973)*. Pituitary Snuff. Powdered pituitary (posterior lobe) adjusted with lactose to contain 300 units of antidiuretic activity per g. Store in a cool place in airtight containers.

Posterior Pituitary Injection *(U.S.P.)*. A sterile solution, in a suitable diluent, of material containing the polypeptide hormones derived from the posterior lobes of mammalian pituitary bodies. It is standardised in respect of oxytocic and pressor activity. pH 2.5 to 4.5. Avoid freezing.

Proprietary Preparations

Di-Sipidin *(Paines & Byrne, UK)*. Pituitary (Posterior Lobe) Insufflation, available as capsules each containing not less than 30 antidiuretic units. (Also available as Di-Sipidin in *Austral., Ital., Switz.*).

Other Proprietary Names

Endopituitrina, Piton, Pituidrol *(all Ital.)*; Pituitrin *(USA)*; Thymophysin *(Ger.)*.

5944-w

Prolactin.

Galactin; Lactogenic Hormone; Lactotropin; LMTH; LTH; Luteomammotropic Hormone; Luteotrophic Hormone; Mammotropin.

CAS — 9002-62-4; 12585-34-1 (sheep); 56832-36-1 (ox); 9046-05-3 (pig).

A water-soluble protein from the anterior pituitary. Sheep prolactin has a molecular weight of about 25 000 and an isoelectric point at pH 5.7. Its activity is readily destroyed by proteolytic enzymes and by cysteine.

The entire amino-acid sequence of linear human prolactin has been reported by B. Shome and A.F. Parlow (*J. clin. Endocr. Metab.*, 1977, *45*, 1112); it consists of 198 amino-acid residues, only 16% of the sequence corresponding with that of human growth hormone and only 13% with that of human placental lactogen.

Units. One unit of ovine prolactin for bioassay is contained in 0.04545 mg of the second International Standard Preparation (1962) which contains 22 units per mg.

0.65 unit of human prolactin for immunoassay is contained in approximately 20 µg (with human albumin 1 mg and lactose 5 mg) in one ampoule of the first International Reference Preparation for Immunoassay (1978).

Uses. In *animals*, prolactin has a wide variety of actions and is involved in reproduction, parental care, feeding of the young, electrolyte balance, and growth and development. In humans it has a definite role with other hormones in lactation; oxytocin (p.1274) stimulates milk ejection. Relatively high concentrations of prolactin have been found in amniotic fluid. Placental lactogen has been shown to have prolactin-like activity.

Hyperprolactinaemia, sometimes accompanied by galactorrhoea, occurs in many patients with gonadal disorders and may be associated with amenorrhoea in women and impotence in men. More than 70% of patients with pituitary adenomas have been reported to secrete excessive amounts of prolactin.

The hypothalamus can both stimulate and inhibit prolactin secretion by the anterior pituitary; the inhibitory influence is predominant and is thought to be mediated through a dopaminergic system. The hypothalamic inhibitory factor (PIF or PRIF) is probably dopamine; noradrenaline and gamma-aminobutyric acid are also inhibitory as are dopaminergic agents such as bromocriptine. Although protirelin (p.1276) has prolactin-releasing activity, there is evidence for the existence of a separate hypothalamic releasing factor (PRF). Prolactin secretion may also be stimulated by methyldopa, reserpine, metoclopramide, and tranquillisers of the phenothiazine or butyrophenone type.

Reviews of prolactin: D.F. Horrobin, *Prolactin: Physiology and Clinical Significance*, Lancaster, Medical and Technical Publishing, 1973; D.F. Horrobin, *Prolactin*, Lancaster, Medical and Technical Publishing, 1974; A. S. McNeilly, *Postgrad. med. J.*, 1975, *51*, 231; *Br. med. J.*, 1975, *4*, 188; G. Strauch and H. Bricaire, *Thérapie*, 1975, *30*, 509; G. Tolis and H. G. Friesen, *Can. med. Ass. J.*, 1976, *115*, 709; J. Senior, *Pharm. J.*, 1977, *1*, 80; *Br. med. J.*, 1977, *2*, 846; A. G. Frantz, *New Engl. J. Med.*, 1978, *298*, 201; *Lancet*, 1979, *2*, 234; D. F. Horrobin, *Drugs*, 1979, *17*, 409.

The relation of prolactin to breast cancer.— F. Smithline *et al.*, *New Engl. J. Med.*, 1975, *292*, 784.

A discussion of the multifactorial regulation of prolactin secretion. Prolactin release in response to one or more stimuli, including catecholamines and indolamines, might depend upon several mechanisms employing different regulatory factors.— H. A. Zacur *et al.*, *Lancet*, 1976, *1*, 410.

In 6 women with hyperprolactinaemia and galactorrhoea, serum-prolactin concentrations were not affected by the infusion of phentolamine or propranolol.— J. A. Board *et al.*, *Am. J. Obstet. Gynec.*, 1977, *127*, 285.

A 19-year-old woman who had twice developed stress-induced breast engorgement had a marked increase in prolactin concentration after insulin-induced hypoglycaemia and after protirelin; the response to hypoglycaemia was inhibited by cyproheptadine while the response to protirelin was not. This suggested serotonin-mediated stress release of prolactin at a functional level above the pituitary.— B. Corenblum and M. Whitaker, *Br. med. J.*, 1977, *2*, 1328.

Mention of prolactin in relation to male sexual function.— J. D. Horowitz and A. J. Goble, *Drugs*, 1979, *18*, 206.

A discussion on hyperprolactinaemia and the diagnosis of prolactin-secreting pituitary adenomas.— *Lancet*, 1980, *1*, 517.

Effect of prolactin given intramuscularly. Sheep prolactin administered by intramuscular injection to 5 healthy subjects in a dose of 8 mg and compared with a placebo reduced the water and sodium excretion significantly and raised plasma-sodium concentration. Individual urinary pH variations were observed and there was an insignificant reduction in potassium excretion. All 5 experienced muscle aches and malaise, 4 noted thirst, and 3 had a craving for salt.— D. F. Horrobin *et al.*, *Lancet*, 1971, *2*, 352.

Controlled studies in 3 subjects given sheep prolactin 8 mg intramuscularly demonstrated the presence of antidiuretic hormone in their urine which could account for the renal retention effect of prolactin.— M. S. Manku *et al.* (letter), *Lancet*, 1972, *1*, 1243.

Daily intramuscular injections of prolactin, 600 to 900 µg per kg body-weight daily for 3 to 6 weeks, provoked an erythropoietic response in 2 patients with chronic bone-marrow failure, but not in 2 patients with acute failure.— J. H. Jepson and E. E. McGarry, *J. clin. Pharmac.*, 1974, *14*, 296.

Proprietary Names

Ferolactan *(Bioindustria, Ital.)*; Prolatte *(Fabo, Ital.)*.

5945-e

Protirelin. Abbott-38579; Lopremone; Thyroliberin; Thyrotrophin-releasing Hormone; TRF; TRH. L-Pyroglutamyl-L-histidyl-L-prolinamide; 5-Oxo-L-prolyl-L-histidyl-L-prolinamide.

$C_{16}H_{22}N_6O_4$=362.4.

CAS — 24305-27-9.

A tripeptide obtained from the hypothalamus or by synthesis.

Adverse Effects. Protirelin given by intravenous injection may cause nausea, a desire to micturate, flushing, dizziness, and a strange taste. These effects have been attributed to contraction of smooth muscles by the bolus injection. Hypoglycaemia has been reported. Nausea has followed administration by mouth.

Epileptic seizures induced by protirelin in a patient with a history of convulsions.— K. Maeda and K. Tanimoto (letter), *Lancet*, 1981, *1*, 1058.

Bronchospasm in an asthmatic boy given protirelin intravenously.— R. G. McFadden *et al.* (letter), *Lancet*, 1981, *2*, 758.

Transient amaurosis and headache after protirelin injection.— P. L. Drury *et al.* (letter), *Lancet*, 1982, *1*, 218.

Effect on the cardiovascular system. A significant increase in arterial blood pressure and heart-rate occurred about 1 minute after rapid intravenous injection of protirelin 200 µg. The effect lasted less than 5 minutes. Other haemodynamic parameters were unchanged. A direct stimulant effect on the smooth muscle of arteries was suggested.— H. A. Abplanalp, *Arzneimittel-Forsch.*, 1976, *26*, 271.

Effect on the central nervous system. Mild euphoria, relaxation, and a sense of increased energy unrelated to thyrotrophin response or somatic effects occurred in a controlled study in 10 healthy women given protirelin.— I. C. Wilson *et al.*, *Archs gen. Psychiat.*, 1973, *29*, 15, per *J. Am. med. Ass.*, 1973, *225*, 325.

Intravenous infusions of protirelin 600 µg had no significant cortical activity in 8 healthy subjects.— H. Ashton *et al.*, *Br. J. clin. Pharmac.*, 1976, *3*, 523.

Effect on sexual function. On questioning, 7 of 16 women reported a sensation of mild vaginal sexual arousal occurring 1 to 3 minutes after intravenous injection of protirelin. Four women also experienced urinary sensations, and 3 described an urge to urinate with no sexual component.— M. Blum and M. Pulini (letter), *Lancet*, 1980, *2*, 43. A report of a penile-urethral sensation associated with thyroid-releasing hormone [sic].— P. J. Green (letter), *ibid.*, 199.

Hypercholesterolaemia. Five of 8 patients had elevated serum-cholesterol concentrations after treatment for 2 to 15 months with protirelin 10 to 40 mg daily.— M. J. E. van der Vis-Melsen and J. D. Wiener (letter), *Br. med. J.*, 1973, *4*, 419.

Precautions. Protirelin should be given with care to patients with cardiac insufficiency or severe hypopituitarism. Patients with obstructive airways disease should be given protirelin by mouth rather than injection. Protirelin is best avoided in early pregnancy due to its effect on smooth muscle.

In 2 patients with adrenal medullary phaeochromocytomas, following a standard protirelin test using 200 µg the thyrotrophin response was impaired, which could have led to a misdiagnosis of thyrotoxicosis.— D. C. Linch and E. J. Ross (letter), *Lancet*, 1979, *1*, 210. A report of a similar patient with a normal response. An impaired thyrotrophin response to protirelin is not an invariable finding in patients with phaeochromocytoma.— W. J. Kalk and E. Rogaly (letter), *ibid.*, 1079. See also R. Reid *et al.* (letter), *ibid.*

Interactions. A brief review of drugs influencing the response to protirelin. The secretion of thyrotrophin appears to be modulated by dopaminergic and noradrenergic pathways at both the hypothalamic and pituitary level. Dopamine and bromocriptine have depressed the response to protirelin; levodopa is a powerful depressant. Partial depression has been reported after the administration of chlorpromazine, thioridazine, and phentolamine, all of which have alpha-receptor blocking properties. Beta-receptors do not appear to be involved in the thyrotrophin response to protirelin whereas the antiserotonin agent, cyproheptadine, has an inhibitory effect. Aspirin and corticosteroids with predominantly glucocorticoid activity have also depressed the response. An enhanced response to protirelin has been seen after the administration of theophylline. Oestrogens may also increase the response in men but not usually in women; when combined with a progestogen a slightly depressed response has been reported.— B. -A. Lamberg and A. Gordin, *Ann. clin. Res.*, 1978, *10*, 171.

Lithium diminished the thyroid response to protirelin.— U. B. Lauridsen *et al.*, *J. clin. Endocr. Metab.*, 1974, *39*, 383.

Absorption and Fate. Protirelin is absorbed from the buccal and nasal mucosa and from the upper part of the gastro-intestinal tract. It is rapidly metabolised and excreted in the urine.

Protirelin disappeared rapidly from the plasma of 8 male subjects who were given 400 µg intravenously; over 90% was removed within 20 minutes, with a half-life of about 5.3 minutes. Protirelin was rapidly metabolised in plasma and possibly the tissues. About 5.5% of the dose was excreted in the urine, mostly within 30 minutes.— R. M. Bassiri and R. D. Utiger, *J. clin. Invest.*, 1973, *52*, 1616.

Uses. Protirelin is a hypothalamic releasing hormone which stimulates the release of thyrotrophin (p.1278) from the anterior lobe of the pituitary. It also has prolactin-releasing activity (see p.1275).

Protirelin is used in the assessment of the hypothalamic-pituitary-thyroid axis in the diagnosis of mild hyperthyroidism, primary hypothyroidism, and ophthalmic Graves' disease. A normal thyrotrophin response excludes thyrotoxicosis and primary hypothyroidism. The response to protirelin is generally used in preference to the thyrotrophin stimulation test (p.1278) for differentiating between primary and secondary hypothyroidism. Protirelin is given with gonadorelin (p.1267) in the assessment of anterior pituitary function.

Protirelin is given intravenously usually in doses of 200 µg. A qualitative response may be achieved by giving 40 mg by mouth to fasting patients.

A review of thyrotropin-releasing hormone.— I. M. D. Jackson, *New Engl. J. Med.*, 1982, *306*, 145.

A review of the diagnostic use of protirelin.— B. -A. Lamberg and A. Gordin, *Ann. clin. Res.*, 1978, *10*, 171.

Details of the simultaneous assessment of both the thyroid and pituitary reserve using protirelin.— L. Shenkman *et al.*, *Lancet*, 1972, *1*, 111.

Protirelin 200 µg given intravenously to 5 subjects had no effect on human growth hormone or luteinising hormone, although the plasma-hydrocortisone concentrations fell steadily. Plasma-prolactin concentration rose sharply.— M. L'Hermite *et al.*, *Lancet*, 1972, *1*, 763.

Plasma concentrations of growth hormone were increased in 10 of 16 patients with active acromegaly after they were given protirelin 200 µg intravenously.— G. Faglia *et al.*, *J. clin. Endocr. Metab.*, 1973, *37*, 338.

The plasma concentration of thyrotrophin was raised in normal pregnancy but the response to protirelin was unchanged.— V. Kannan *et al.*, *Obstet. Gynec.*, 1973, *42*, 547.

A single dose of protirelin 160 mg was considered to have a small but significant euphoriant psychotropic effect in 10 healthy female subjects in a double-blind study.— T. A. Betts *et al.*, *Br. J. clin. Pharmac.*, 1976, *3*, 469.

Lactation, suppressed in 4 women by bromocriptine, was re-established by protirelin 250 µg intravenously, followed by dosage by mouth.— E. S. Canales, *Am. J. Obstet. Gynec.*, 1977, *128*, 695.

A study of protirelin tartrate as a direct stimulant of the central nervous system.— M. Ogashiwa and K. Takeuchi, *Int. J. clin. Pharmac. Biopharm.*, 1979, *17*, 145.

Further references: R. Hall *et al.*, *Br. med. J.*, 1970, *2*, 274; *Lancet*, 1972, *1*, 782; A. J. Prange *et al.*, *Archs gen. Psychiat.*, 1973, *29*, 28; *Br. med. J.*, 1973, *3*, 465; J. M. Hershman, *New Engl. J. Med.*, 1974, *290*, 886; *Drug & Ther. Bull.*, 1974, *12*, 31; N. D. Barnes, *Archs Dis. Childh.*, 1975, *50*, 497; R. Mornex and F. Berthezene, *Thérapie*, 1975, *30*, 475.

Behaviour disorders. The administration of protirelin 200 µg intravenously to a 15-year-old boy with a behaviour disorder undergoing investigations for gigantism induced a calm and reasonable state which lasted for 9 to 10 hours.— C. M. Tiwary *et al.* (letter), *Lancet*, 1972, *2*, 1086.

Depression. In a controlled study of 5 patients with depression given protirelin 500 µg intravenously daily for 3 days, 4 patients showed a marked and 1 a mild improvement which lasted for a few hours to several weeks.— A. J. Kastin *et al.* (preliminary communication), *Lancet*, 1972, *2*, 740. See also A. J. Prange *et al.*, *Lancet*, 1972, *2*, 999; M. J. E. van der Vis-Melsen and J. D. Wiener (letter), *Lancet*, 1972, *2*, 1415.

In 5 patients with the alcohol-withdrawal syndrome protirelin had an antidepressant effect only on the day of injection.— P. T. Loosen *et al.*, *Arzneimittel-Forsch.*, 1976, *26*, 1164.

Reports of the ineffectiveness of protirelin in depression.— C. Q. Mountjoy *et al.*, *Lancet*, 1974, *1*, 958; A. Coppen *et al.*, *Lancet*, 1974, *2*, 433; A. A. Sugerman *et al.*, *Curr. ther. Res.*, 1976, *19*, 94; O. Benkert and K. H. Lücke, *Arzneimittel-Forsch.*, 1976, *26*, 1162.

Diagnosis of depression. Data from 10 patients suggesting that the magnitude of the protirelin-induced thyrotrophin response may be useful in the differentiation of bipolar and unipolar depressed patients.— M. S. Gold *et al.* (letter), *Lancet*, 1979, *2*, 411. These findings could not be confirmed.— N. Bjørum and C. Kirkegaard (letter), *Lancet*, 1979, *2*, 694; J. D. Amsterdam *et al.* (letter), *ibid.*, 904.

Findings of a controlled study in 58 female depressive patients matched with 42 healthy female controls indicated that the deficient thyrotrophin response to protirelin, when present, is useful in the differentiation of bipolar and unipolar disorder in females.— J. Mendlewicz *et al.* (letter), *Lancet*, 1979, *2*, 1079. Criticism.— C. Kirkegaard and N. Bjørum (letter), *ibid.*, 1980, *1*, 152.

Thyrotrophin responses to protirelin were significantly less in 13 patients with primary unipolar depression than those in 5 patients with secondary depression, even after clinical recovery.— G. M. Asnis *et al.* (letter), *Lancet*, 1980, *1*, 424.

Further references: W. Pühringer *et al.* (letter), *Lancet*, 1975, *1*, 1344; I. Extein *et al.* (letter), *New Engl. J. Med.*, 1980, *302*, 923; P. T. Loosen and A. J. Prange (letter), *ibid.*, *303*, 224.

Diagnosis of hypothalamic and pituitary dysfunction. In a study of 76 patients with pituitary-hypothalamic disease given protirelin 200 µg intravenously, 7 of 35 patients with acromegaly, 12 of 26 with other pituitary lesions, and 7 of 15 patients with hypothalamic lesions responded normally. However, 13 of the 15 patients with hypothalamic lesions had a delayed response and this could be used in diagnosis.— R. Hall *et al.*, *Lancet*, 1972, *1*, 759.

An evaluation of the protirelin stimulation test in assessing pituitary thyrotrophin reserve in 8 healthy subjects and 20 patients with hypopituitarism.— R. A. Hajjar *et al.*, *Archs intern. Med.*, 1973, *132*, 836, per *J. Am. med. Ass.*, 1974, *227*, 97.

The use of protirelin in 100 patients enabled the detection of, and differentiation between, hormonal abnormalities due to hypothalamic and pituitary disease, by assessment of thyrotrophic hormone and lactogenic hormone secretory reserves.— P. J. Synder *et al.*, *Ann. intern. Med.*, 1974, *81*, 751.

Diagnosis of pituitary adenomas. Testing with chlorpromazine and protirelin could be of diagnostic value in distinguishing between those patients with galactorrhoea and amenorrhoea produced by pituitary tumours, idiopathic disease or other causes. Testing with protirelin alone was of no diagnostic value.— A. E. Boyd *et al.*, *Ann. intern. Med.*, 1977, *87*, 165.

In 14 infertile women with hyperprolactinaemia the impaired prolactin responses to stimulation with protirelin 200 µg intravenously or metoclopramide 10 mg intravenously were reliable and clinically useful aids to diagnosis. Suppression tests using levodopa or bromocriptine were less reliable.— E. A. Cowden *et al.*, *Lancet*, 1979, *1*, 1155. The protirelin test is an unreliable discriminant for prolactinoma.— D. Handelsman *et al.* (letter), *Lancet*, 1979, *2*, 581. A similar view.— J. G. M. Klijn *et al.* (letter), *ibid.*

Effect in euthyroid and hypothyroid patients. In a study with 14 healthy subjects, intravenous injection of protirelin acetate (TRH) 50 µg or more caused a variable but significant rise in serum concentrations of thyrotrophin (TSH), the peak effect occurring after about 20 minutes. Side-effects included nausea, a flushing sensation, a desire to micturate, a peculiar taste, and tightness in the chest. After administration of 1 mg or more of TRH by mouth, peak TSH concentrations occurred after 2 hours, but a consistent rise in TSH occurred only after administration of 20 mg or more. Rises in serum protein-bound iodine followed increases in TSH.— B. J. Ormston *et al.*, *Br. med. J.*, 1971, *2*, 199.

Protirelin acetate 200 µg in 2 ml of saline given to 45 healthy subjects produced a rise in serum thyrotrophin. In 24 patients with hypothyroidism, the increase in thyrotrophin following the same dose of protirelin was greater than in the controls; this was not the case in 2 patients with preclinical hypothyroidism. Thyrotrophin concentrations following protirelin 200 µg given to 33 patients with hyperthyroidism did not reach those seen in the control subjects.— B. J. Ormston *et al.*, *Lancet*, 1971, *2*, 10.

Two patients had no response to protirelin 200 µg in spite of being euthyroid. The decision to treat patients who had not responded to protirelin as thyrotoxic should not be based on that test alone.— N. F. Lawton *et al.*, *Lancet*, 1971, *2*, 14. A study in 11 euthyroid patients not responding to intravenous protirelin indicated that oral administration of protirelin, to provide depot stimulation, is a useful diagnostic test for euthyroid patients with impaired thyrotrophin reserve but euthyroid function.— J. J. Stuab *et al.* (letter), *Lancet*, 1979, *1*, 209. Comment.— C. Kirkegaard *et al.* (letter), *ibid.*, 556.

The responses of 11 euthyroid patients with Graves' disease to protirelin were compared with the results of the tri-iodothyronine (T_3) suppression test. Of 5 patients whose thyroid uptake of radio-iodine could not be suppressed, 2 had large increases in serum thyrotrophin in response to protirelin 31 µg or 500 µg and 3 had poor responses. In 6 patients whose radio-iodine uptake was suppressible by tri-iodothyronine there were responses to protirelin. Patients with Hashimoto's thyroiditis or normal glands had exaggerated responses to protirelin. No correlation was found between the responses and the course of the exophthalmos.— P. S. Franco *et al.*, *Metabolism*, 1973, *22*, 1357.

Subclinical hypothyroidism or premyxoedema could be diagnosed by an exaggerated response to protirelin; 88 of 100 patients suspected of having premyxoedema had an exaggerated response compared with none of 20 controls.— J. Alaghband-Zadeh *et al.*, *Lancet*, 1977, *2*, 998.

Evidence that a protirelin dose of 1 µg per kg bodyweight intravenously is the ideal dose for the protirelin test in children. Higher doses do not give any more clinical information.— S. Zabransky (letter), *Lancet*, 1980, *2*, 864.

Neurological diseases. Protirelin given to 5 patients with parkinsonism produced improvement in well-being for several hours after an injection in 2 of the 3 who were also taking levodopa.— J. A. McCaul *et al.* (letter), *Lancet*, 1974, *1*, 735.

There were impaired prolactin responses to chlorpromazine and protirelin in patients with Huntington's chorea when compared with controls. This might be of value in early detection of the disorder and suggested that there was a dopaminergic influence.— M. R. Hayden *et al.*, *Lancet*, 1977, *2*, 423. Experience with bromocriptine (a dopaminergic agonist) in patients with Huntington's chorea did not show any evidence of dopaminergic hypersensitivity.— R. J. Chalmers *et al.* (letter), *ibid.*, 824.

Results of a study indicating that protirelin is effective against ataxia of spinocerebellar degeneration.— I. Sobue *et al.* (letter), *Lancet*, 1980, *1*, 418.

Beneficial effect of protirelin on spinal trauma in *cats*, indicating therapeutic potential in man.— A. I. Faden *et al.*, *New Engl. J. Med.*, 1981, *305*, 1063.

Schizophrenia. In a preliminary study of protirelin 200 and 400 µg a rapid beneficial effect was produced in 4 schizophrenic women.— I. C. Wilson *et al.* (letter), *Lancet*, 1973, *2*, 43.

Two of 3 patients with chronic schizophrenia deteriorated when treated with protirelin. Similar results were reported (K.E. Davis *et al.*, *Am. J. Psychiat.*, 1975, *132*, 951) with 7 of 9 treated patients deteriorating.— L. B. Bigelow *et al.* (letter), *Lancet*, 1975, *2*, 869.

Thyroid cancer. Protirelin 10 to 40 mg daily by mouth for periods of 8 to 15 days did not stimulate radio-iodine uptake in the radionuclide treatment of 4 patients with metastases from thyroid carcinoma.— R. Mornex and F. Berthezene, *Thérapie*, 1975, *30*, 475.

Proprietary Preparations

TRH-Roche *(Roche, UK)*. Protirelin, available as an **Injection** containing 100 µg per ml, in ampoules of 2 ml, and as scored **Tablets** of 40 mg.

See Gonadorelin, p.1268, for a preparation containing protirelin and gonadorelin..

Other Proprietary Names

Antepan *(Ger.)*; Inithyran *(Denm.)*; Relefact *(USA)*; Relefact TRH *(Canad., Ger.)*; Relisorm T *(Ital.)*; Stimu-TSH *(Fr.)*; Thypinone *(USA)*; Thyrefact *(Denm., Swed.)*; Tiregan *(Spain)*; Trhelea *(Arg.)*.

5946-l

Somatostatin.

GHRIF; GHRIH; Growth-hormone-release-inhibiting Hormone; Somatotrophin-release-inhibiting Factor. Ala-Gly-Cys-Lys-Asn-Phe-Phe-Trp-Lys-Thr-Phe-Thr-Ser-Cys cyclic (3→14) disulphide.

$C_{76}H_{104}N_{18}O_{19}S_2$ (sheep, cyclic) = 1637.9.

CAS — 51110-01-1; 38916-34-6 (sheep, cyclic); 40958-31-4 (sheep, linear).

A polypeptide obtained from the hypothalamus or by synthesis. The naturally occurring form has a cyclic structure; a non-native linear form is also used.

The isolation and structure of somatostatin from *sheep*.— P. Brazeau *et al.*, *Science*, 1973, *179*, 77.

Uses. Somatostatin is a hypothalamic release-inhibiting hormone which inhibits the release of growth hormone (p.1270) from the anterior pituitary. The intravenous infusion of 100 µg or more of somatostatin has reduced circulating concentrations of growth hormone in patients with acromegaly. It may also inhibit the release of thyrotrophin (p.1278) and corticotrophin (p.486) from the pituitary.

Somatostatin appears to have a role in the regulation of pancreatic, duodenal, and gastric secretions since it has been detected in the pancreas and alimentary tract and has been found to inhibit the secretion of several substances including glucagon, insulin, and gastrin.

It has a very short duration of action and several analogues of somatostatin have been produced in an attempt to prolong its activity as well as making its inhibitory effects more specific.

Reviews of the actions and possible uses of somatostatin: *Lancet*, 1974, *1*, 1148; P. C. Sizonenko, *Postgrad. med. J.*, 1978, *54*, *Suppl.* 1, 91.

Cyclic somatostatin blocked the thyrotrophin response to protirelin but not prolactin release.— D. Carr *et al.*, *Br. med. J.*, 1975, *3*, 67.

When somatostatin 250 or 375 µg was given as an infusion over 10 minutes to 7 healthy subjects there was a decrease in heart-rate of about 10 beats per minute. There was no significant effect on cortical activity.— H. Ashton *et al.*, *Br. J. clin. Pharmac.*, 1976, *3*, 523.

A study *in vitro* suggesting that somatostatin may act as a neurotransmitter or modulator in the *rat* brain.— L. L. Iversen *et al.*, *Nature*, 1978, *273*, 161.

Results of a study in 11 healthy subjects suggested that somatostatin decreases urinary calcium excretion and may aid in the regulation of the calcium balance of the body.— P. E. Lins *et al.* (letter), *Lancet*, 1978, *2*, 687.

Results in patients with impaired liver function due to alcoholic cirrhosis indicate that somatostatin is metabolised in the liver to some extent.— S. Munkgaard *et al.* (letter), *New Engl. J. Med.*, 1981, *304*, 1429.

A comparison of prosomatostatin (Pro-SS), a 28-aminoacid peptide, with somatostatin on the glucose, growth hormone, and prolactin responses to arginine.— M. D. Rodriguez-Arnao *et al.*, *Lancet*, 1981, *1*, 353.

Acromegaly. After a bolus injection of linear somatostatin 250 µg followed by a constant infusion of 500 µg over 45 minutes there was an immediate decrease in circulating growth hormone in 5 patients with acromegaly. Concentrations returned to basal level within 60 minutes of the cessation of the infusion. Insulin concentrations decreased rapidly within 15 minutes and remained low during the infusion. Plasma glucose also decreased, though more slowly, reaching a minimum concentration at the end of the infusion.— S. S. C. Yen *et al.*, *New Engl. J. Med.*, 1974, *290*, 935. See also P. Brazeau and R. Guillemin, *ibid.*, 963.

Further references: G. M. Besser *et al.*, *Br. med. J.*, 1974, *4*, 622; G. Schaison *et al.*, *Nouv. Presse méd.*, 1976, *5*, 629; N. Faure *et al.*, *Can. med. Ass. J.*, 1977, *117*, 478.

Carcinoid syndrome. The symptoms of a patient with a carcinoid tumour were controlled with methyldopa and somatostatin before surgery. During surgical manipulation of the tumour 3 hypotensive episodes were quickly corrected with bolus intravenous injections of somatostatin. Somatostatin was twice given postoperatively to control hypotensive crises.— L. Thulin *et al.* (letter), *Lancet*, 1978, *2*, 43.

Somatostatin had a beneficial effect on bronchial constriction in a patient with carcinoid syndrome. Bronchial resistance was reduced for more than 90 minutes after the intravenous injection of somatostatin 250 µg.— R. Klapdor (letter), *New Engl. J. Med.*, 1980, *303*, 464.

Further references: J. C. Frölich *et al.*, *New Engl. J. Med.*, 1978, *299*, 1055; M. J. Nissenblatt (letter), *ibid.*, 1979, *300*, 624; L. Thulin *et al.* (letter), *ibid.*; Z. T. Bloomgarden *et al.* (letter), *ibid.*; K. Dharmsathaphorn *et al.*, *Ann. intern. Med.*, 1980, *92*, 68.

Effect on blood sugar. A review of somatostatin and its possible role in carbohydrate homoeostasis and the treatment of diabetes mellitus.— J. E. Gerich, *Archs intern. Med.*, 1977, *137*, 659.

An intravenous infusion of cyclic somatostatin in 10 patients with insulin-dependent diabetes decreased plasma concentrations of glucose and glucagon by about 25% and 50% respectively. Linear somatostatin given subcutaneously had a transient effect. Somatostatin with insulin abolished post-meal hyperglycaemia in 4 diabetic patients and the combination was more effective than insulin alone.— J. E. Gerich *et al.*, *New Engl. J. Med.*, 1974, *291*, 544. See also *idem*, 1975, *292*, 985.

Results following 5-hour infusion of linear somatostatin at a rate of 500 to 720 µg per hour into 8 subjects with maturity-onset diabetes controlled by dietary regimen alone suggested that glucagon was not essential for the development and maintenance of fasting hyperglycaemia. Somatostatin accentuated hyperglycaemia, hyperketonaemia, and hyperaminoacidaemia which argued against its use in maturity-onset diabetics with residual insulin secretion.— W. V. Tamborlane *et al.*, *New Engl. J. Med.*, 1977, *297*, 181.

A study in an infant born to an insulin-dependent diabetic mother suggested that somatostatin may have a role in suppressing hyperinsulinism in such infants.— E. Mallet *et al.* (letter), *Lancet*, 1980, *1*, 776.

Further references: C. H. Mortimer *et al.*, *Lancet*, 1974, *1*, 697; K. Lundbaek *et al.*, *Lancet*, 1976, *1*, 215; U. Keller (letter), *ibid.*, 644; J. Wahren and P. Felig, *Lancet*, 1976, *2*, 1213; M. J. del Guercio *et al.*, *Diabetes*, 1976, *25*, 550; J. L. Botha *et al.*, *S. Afr. med. J.*, 1977, *51*, 872; P. Raskin and R. H. Unger, *New Engl. J. Med.*, 1978, *299*, 433; R. S. Sherwin and P. Felig (letter), *ibid.*, 1366; A. J. Barnes *et al.* (letter), *ibid.*, 1367; R. H. Unger (letter), *ibid.*

Effect on coagulation. Intravenous infusions of cyclic somatostatin in doses of 3.4 to 6 µg per minute for 5.25 to 6 hours in 4 healthy subjects impaired platelet aggregation in all 4. Subjective side-effects including abdominal pain, dizziness, and diarrhoea occurred in the 3 subjects who received doses higher than 3.4 µg per minute. It appeared that somatostatin might be involved in a specific intravascular coagulation process.— G. M. Besser *et al.*, *Lancet*, 1975, *1*, 1166. See also E. Carmina *et al.* (letter), *New Engl. J. Med.*, 1976, *294*, 226.

The infusion of linear or cyclic somatostatin in 8 patients, 7 with diabetes, had no apparent effect on coagulation or platelet function.— C. H. Mielke *et al.*, *New Engl. J. Med.*, 1975, *293*, 480.

Effect on gastro-intestinal tract. A study of the gastrin-inhibiting effects of cyclic somatostatin in man.— S. R. Bloom *et al.*, *Lancet*, 1974, *2*, 1106.

Cyclic somatostatin inhibited gastric acid release in *dogs;* this was considered to be due to a direct action on the gastric parietal cell.— A. A. J. Barros D'Sa *et al.*, *Lancet*, 1975, *1*, 886. For similar results on pepsin and gastric acid inhibition in *cats*, see A. Gomez-Pan *et al.*, *ibid.*, 888.

Cyclic somatostatin 250 µg intravenously as a bolus followed by 250 µg as an infusion over 1 hour inhibited the release of cholecystokinin due to the intraduodenal instillation of olive oil.— W. Schlegel *et al.*, *Lancet*, 1977, *2*, 166.

A 24-hour infusion of cyclic somatostatin dramatically reduced faecal losses in a patient with Verner-Morrison syndrome with the full watery diarrhoea, hypokalaemia, and achlorhydria sequence, high serum concentrations of vasoactive intestinal polypeptide, and a pancreatic tumour. On withdrawal of the somatostatin, however, a marked rebound effect occurred.— S. Bonfils *et al.* (letter), *Lancet*, 1979, *2*, 476.

Further references: J. H. Walsh *et al.*, *Ann. intern. Med.*, 1979, *90*, 817.

Haemorrhage. *Alimentary tract.* Administration of somatostatin 250 µg as a bolus injection followed by 250 µg per hour at a constant rate intravenously for 48 to 120 hours, stopped bleeding caused by peptic ulcer disease in 9 of 13 patients. Of the other 4 patients; rebleeding occurred in 2 and was controlled in one by a second course of somatostatin; a short bleeding episode, associated with endoscopic manipulation, occurred during therapy in the third; only in the fourth was bleeding not definitely controlled by somatostatin infusion. No side-effects were noted, not even after infusion for 120 hours in some of the patients.— L. Kayasseh *et al.* (letter), *Lancet*, 1978, *2*, 833. See also G. Tydén *et al.* (letter), *New Engl. J. Med.*, 1978, *299*, 1466; G. Tydén *et al.*, *ibid.*, 1979, *301*, 46.

Bolus injection of somatostatin 250 µg followed by continuous infusion of 250 µg per hour for 20 to 67 hours, controlled acute bleeding ulcers in about 4 hours, in 5 of 9 patients in whom bleeding could not be controlled by cimetidine.— B. Limberg and B. Kommerell (letter), *Lancet*, 1979, *2*, 1361.

Somatostatin had no beneficial effect in 5 patients with bleeding oesophageal varices.— S. Raptis and C. Zoupas (letter), *New Engl. J. Med.*, 1979, *300*, 736.

Results of a randomised controlled study of sequential design, comparing cimetidine and somatostatin for the treatment of severe and persistent gastro-intestinal bleeding due to peptic ulcer in patients unsuitable for emergency surgery. Bleeding was stopped by somatostatin in 8 out of 10 patients, whereas cimetidine stopped bleeding in only 1 out of 10 patients. Thus cimetidine failed to control peptic ulcer bleeding, whereas somatostatin is suitable for conservative treatment in patients who are unsuitable for surgery, and when stabilisation of the circulation and patient's general condition will decrease the risk of later surgery. Cyclic somatostatin was given as an intravenous bolus injection of 250 µg followed by infusion of 250 µg per hour for 48 to 120 hours.— L. Kayasseh *et al.*, *Lancet*, 1980, *1*, 844. Doubt as to whether it can be concluded from the data presented, that somatostatin may be suitable for the control of peptic ulcer bleeding.— R. J. S. Thomas and J. F. Forbes (letter), *ibid.*, *2*, 200. Reply.— L. Kayasseh *et al.* (letter), *ibid.*, 861. Further reports and comments.— B. Limberg and B. Kommerell (letter), *ibid.*, 916; D. P. Mikhailidis *et al.* (letter), *ibid.*, 1981, *1*, 274.

Pancreatic disorders. *Endocrine tumours.* Somatostatin inhibited insulin secretion from non-malignant insulinomas in 2 patients.— S. E. Christensen *et al.* (letter), *Lancet*, 1975, *1*, 1426.

The activity of somatostatin in suppressing the insulin response to tolbutamide in patients with hyperinsulinism due to pancreatic hyperplasia but not to insulinoma could be used as a diagnostic test. Suppression would also occur in healthy subjects.— J. L. Del Arbol *et al.* (letter), *Lancet*, 1978, *1*, 281. The test might not be able to differentiate uniformly between the normal function of pancreatic beta-cells and insulinoma or between hyperplasia and neoplasia of the islet-cells.— F. Van Kersen (letter), *Lancet*, 1978, *1*, 557. See also F. Escobar-Jimenez *et al.* (letter), *ibid.*, 1150.

A report of dramatic improvement of skin lesions in 2 patients with glucagonomas following infusion of cyclic somatostatin.— J. Sohier *et al.* (letter), *Lancet*, 1980, *1*, 40.

For preliminary results with an octapeptide analogue of somatostatin in patients with pancreatic endocrine tumours, see R. G. Long *et al.*, *Lancet*, 1979, *2*, 764.

Pancreatitis. Preliminary findings which suggest that somatostatin may be beneficial in the treatment of acute pancreatitis.— B. Limberg and B. Kommerell (letter), *New Engl. J. Med.*, 1980, *303*, 284. See also K. -H. Usadel *et al.* (letter), *ibid.*, 999.

Manufacturers

Ayerst, USA; Wyeth, USA.

5947-y

Thyrotrophin. TSH; Thyroid-stimulating Hormone; Thyrotrophic Hormone; Thyrotropin.

CAS — 9002-71-5.

A glycoprotein from the anterior pituitary with a mol. wt in man of between 24 000 and 30 000. Its activity is destroyed by proteolytic enzymes and by cysteine.

Studies on the structure of bovine thyrotrophin. The linear amino-acid sequence of the α and β chains has been determined except for the assignment of some amides.— B. Shome *et al.*, *J. biol. Chem.*, 1971, *246*, 833; T. -H. Liao and J. G. Pierce, *ibid.*, 850.

Units. One unit of bovine thyrotrophin for bioassay is contained in 13.5 mg of the first International Standard Preparation (1954).

0.15 unit of human thyroid-stimulating hormone for immunoassay is contained in approximately 46 µg (with human albumin 1 mg and lactose 5 mg) in one ampoule of the first International Reference Preparation for Immunoassay (1974).

Although the first International Reference Preparation for Immunoassay (1974) contained some luteinising hormone and lost some biological activity when kept for various periods at ambient temperatures, it had been accepted since no better material was available and there was an urgent need for a standard. Due to the varying potency estimates from different assays this preparation was not calibrated against the standard preparation for bovine thyrotrophin and the potency was based on approximate values. A more suitable reference preparation for immunoassay was to be established as soon as possible.— Twenty-sixth Report of WHO Expert Committee on Biological Standardization, *Tech. Rep. Ser. Wld Hlth Org. No. 565*, 1975. See also *Tech. Rep. Ser. Wld Hlth Org. No. 638*, 1979.

Adverse Effects. Infrequent side-effects include nausea, vomiting, headache, urticaria, transitory hypotension, and cardiac arrhythmias. Swelling of the thyroid has followed high doses. Allergic reactions have occurred. There may be menstrual irregularities.

An allergic reaction to thyrotrophin.— C. H. Kirkpatrick *et al.*, *J. Allergy & clin. Immunol.*, 1973, *51*, 296.

Precautions. Thyrotrophin is contra-indicated in patients with coronary thrombosis or adrenal insufficiency and should be given cautiously to patients with angina pectoris, heart failure, or hypopituitarism, and to those receiving corticosteroids.

Uses. Thyrotrophin is a glycoprotein secreted by the anterior lobe of the pituitary and with an alpha subunit essentially the same as that of the gonadotrophins (p.1268). Its main actions are to increase the iodine uptake by the thyroid and the formation and secretion of the thyroid hormones. It may produce hyperplasia of thyroid tissue. Thyrotrophin secretion is controlled by a hypothalamic releasing hormone (Protirelin, p.1276) and by circulating thyroid hormones; somatostatin (p.1277) may inhibit the release of thyrotrophin.

Thyrotrophin is used in the diagnosis of mild forms of hypothyroidism and to differentiate between primary and secondary hypothyroidism (but see Protirelin); the secondary form due to pituitary dysfunction responds to thyrotrophin. Because of the sensitivity of patients with hypopituitarism adrenal function should always be assessed before giving thyrotrophin. It may also be used to evaluate thyroid medication.

Thyrotrophin increases the uptake of radio-iodine by the thyroid and so is used as an adjunct in the treatment of certain types of thyroid cancer. This effect is also made use of in the detection of metastases from thyroid carcinoma and to counteract the effect of Aqueous Iodine Solution on radio-iodine uptake.

The usual dose is 10 units daily by intramuscular or subcutaneous injection.

It was generally accepted that maternal thyrotrophin did not cross the placenta.— S. Q. Cohlan, *N.Y. St. J. Med.*, 1964, *64*, 493. A review.— J. B. E. Baker, *Pharmac. Rev.*, 1960, *12*, 37.

A study of the effects of exogenous thyrotrophin on endogenous thyrotrophin and the thyroid response in 20 patients with hypothyroidism and in 53 euthyroid patients.— J. C. Nelson *et al.*, *Ann. intern. Med.*, 1972, *76*, 47.

A brief discussion of the thyrotrophin stimulation test in the differential diagnosis of primary and secondary hypothyroidism.— C. W. H. Havard and M. Boss, *Br. med. J.*, 1974, *3*, 678.

There was complete regression of a hyperfunctioning thyroid nodule after the patient was given thyrotrophin 10 units daily by intramuscular injection for 3 days.— H. Kammer and M. O. Loveless, *J. nucl. Med.*, 1978, *19*, 1149.

Thyroid–pituitary interaction.— P. R. Larsen, *New Engl. J. Med.*, 1982, *306*, 23.

Proprietary Preparations

Thytropar *(Armour, UK).* Thyrotrophin from bovine anterior pituitary glands, available as powder for preparing subcutaneous or intramuscular injections, in vials of 10 units. (Also available as Thytropar in *Austral.*, *Canad.*, *S.Afr.*, *Switz.*, *USA*).

Other Proprietary Names

Actyron *(Norw., Swed.)*; Ambinon *(Belg., Neth.)*; Thyratrop, Thyreostimulin *(both Ger.)*; Thyréostimuline *(Fr.)*.

5948-j

Vasopressin. ADH; Antidiuretic Hormone.

CAS — 11000-17-2.

The pressor principle of the posterior lobe of the pituitary gland. It may be prepared by extraction or by synthesis.

NOTE. In some countries Lypressin is marketed under the names Vasopresina, Vasopressin, and Vasopressine.

5949-z

Argipressin. AVP; 8-Arginine-vasopressin.

Cys-Tyr-Phe-Gln-Asn-Cys-Pro-Arg-Gly-NH_2 cyclic (1→6) disulphide.

$C_{46}H_{65}N_{15}O_{12}S_2$=1084.2.

CAS — 113-79-1.

Vasopressin from most mammals including man but excluding pig. Lypressin (p.1271) is vasopressin from pig.

Units. 8.2 units of arginine-vasopressin for bioassay are contained in approximately 20 µg of synthetic peptide (with human albumin 5 mg and citric acid) in one ampoule of the first International Standard Preparation (1978).

5950-p

Vasopressin Injection *(B.P., U.S.P.).* Vasopressini Injectio; Beta-Hypophamine; Vasopressin.

Pharmacopoeias. In *Arg.*, *Ind.*, and *Nord.* (which specify 10 units per ml); in *Cz.* (which specifies 5 or 10 units per ml); in *Br.*, *It.*, *Jap.*, *Jug.*, and *U.S.* (no strength specified); in *Swiss* (which specifies 5, 10, and 20 units per ml); and in *Int.* and *Turk.* (which specify 20 units per ml).

A sterile aqueous solution with a faint characteristic odour containing the pressor principle of the posterior lobe of the pituitary gland, prepared from the glands of oxen or other mammals, including pigs. *U.S.P.* allows synthetic vasopressin. It contains not more than 1.2 units of oxytocic activity per ml. The solution has a pH of 3 to 4.

Sterilised by filtration. **Store** at 2° to 8° and avoid freezing when it may be expected to retain its potency for not less than 3 years from the date of manufacture. When kept at a temperature not exceeding 25° it may be expected to retain its potency for not less than 2 years.

Vasopressin Injection contained variable proportions of argipressin and lypressin. K. Adamsons and others (*Endocrinology*, 1958, *63*, 679) stated that argipressin was less stable than lypressin.— D. Barltrop, *Lancet*, 1963, *2*, 276.

Adverse Effects. Large doses of Vasopressin Injection may give rise to marked pallor, nausea, eructation, cramp, and a desire to defaecate. In women it may cause uterine cramps of a menstrual character. Hyponatraemia with water retention and signs of water intoxication can occur.

Hypersensitivity reactions have occurred and include urticaria, fever, bronchial constriction, and neurodermatitis. Shock has been reported and may be due to foreign protein.

The most dangerous side-effect of Vasopressin Injection is that it may constrict coronary arteries. Chest pain, myocardial ischaemia, and infarction have occurred and fatalities have been reported.

A report of severe but reversible cardiac toxicity in a 35-year-old patient given vasopressin intravenously to treat oesophageal haemorrhage. There were signs of severe myocardial injury and haemodynamic toxicity.— B. M. Beller *et al.*, *Am. J. Med.*, 1971, *51*, 675, per *Int. pharm. Abstr.*, 1973, *10*, 758.

Gangrene occurred in 2 patients after the extravasation of vasopressin given by intravenous infusion. Amputation was necessary in one patient and the other developed clostridial sepsis and died.— R. A. Greenwald *et al.*, *Gastroenterology*, 1978, *74*, 744.

Ventricular tachycardia and fibrillation developed in a patient with no history of cardiac disorder after she had received vasopressin 20 units intravenously over 15 minutes.— K. J. Kelly *et al.*, *Ann. intern. Med.*, 1980, *92*, 205.

Treatment of Adverse Effects. The antidiuretic effects on water retention and sodium imbalance may be treated by water restriction and a temporary withdrawal of vasopressin.

A report of the localised intravenous and intra-arterial administration of guanethidine in the treatment of a patient with extravasation of vasopressin. The intra-arterial administration of guanethidine was considered to have helped to avoid necrotic changes.— M. C. Crocker (letter), *New Engl. J. Med.*, 1981, *304*, 1430.

Precautions. Vasopressin Injection should not be used in patients with vascular disease or chronic nephritis with nitrogen retention. It should be given with care to patients with asthma, epilepsy, migraine, heart failure, or other conditions which might be aggravated by water retention. Fluid intake should be adjusted to avoid hyponatraemia and water intoxication.

Resistance. After 20 years of treatment with vasopressin injection a patient with hypothalamic diabetes insipidus developed resistance associated with a high titre of antibodies.— N. G. Soler *et al.*, *Archs intern. Med.*, 1979, *139*, 677.

Uses. Vasopressin Injection has a direct antidiuretic action on the kidney. It also constricts peripheral vessels and causes contraction of the smooth muscle of the intestine, gall-bladder, and urinary bladder. It has practically no oxytocic activity.

Vasopressin Injection is used in the treatment and diagnosis of diabetes insipidus due to a deficiency in antidiuretic hormone. It is ineffective in nephrogenic diabetes insipidus. It should not be used to raise the blood pressure. It has also been used in the treatment of abdominal distension, but other measures are preferred. It is sometimes given to remove gas in abdominal visualisation procedures. Because it decreases hepatic blood flow and portal venous pressure it has been used in the treatment of bleeding oesophageal varices, but with variable results.

In the treatment of diabetes insipidus to control polyuria, Vasopressin Injection is usually administered subcutaneously or intramuscularly in doses of 0.25 to 1 ml (5 to 20 units) and must be given at least twice daily. It has also been given, well diluted, by the intravenous route, and has been used intranasally, but lypressin (p.1272) or desmopressin (p.1265) may be preferred. Because its actions last only a few hours its main use is in the diagnosis of diabetes insipidus.

A comparison of plasma-vasopressin measurements with a standard indirect test in the differential diagnosis of polyuria.— R. L. Zerbe and G. L. Robertson, *New Engl. J. Med.*, 1981, *305*, 1539.

Reports and reviews on the actions and uses of vasopressin: J. S. Aldrete *et al.*, *Mayo Clin. Proc.*, 1966, *41*, 399; Y. J. Silva *et al.*, *J. Am. med. Ass.*, 1969, *210*, 1065 (circulatory pressures); W. P. Dyck, *Am. J. dig. Dis.*, 1973, *18*, 33 (pancreatic exocrine secretion); R. M. Hays, *New Engl. J. Med.*, 1976, *295*, 659; J. S. Jenkins, *Practitioner*, 1979, *222*, 312 (kidney).

A hypothesis that vasopressin plays a neuroregulatory role in the pathophysiology of affective illness, particularly manic-depressive disorders.— P. W. Gold *et al.*, *Lancet*, 1978, *1*, 1233. Comment.— D. de Wied (letter), *ibid.*, 1978, *2*, 273.

Data which do not support the concept that an acute or chronic excess of vasopressin makes an important contribution to the regulation of blood pressure.— P. L. Padfield *et al.*, *New Engl. J. Med.*, 1981, *304*, 1067.

Haemorrhage. A discussion on vasopressin in the control of gastro-intestinal bleeding.— C. A. Athanasoulis, *New Engl. J. Med.*, 1980, *302*, 1117.

In 260 patients, 0.5 to 0.75 unit of vasopressin injected submucosally into the cervix provided adequate haemostasis, without cardiovascular effects or complications. Doses of more than 1 unit caused cardiovascular changes.— C. A. Harper *et al.*, *Obstet. Gynec.*, 1967, *30*, 70, per *J. Am. med. Ass.*, 1967, *201* (July 17), A155.

Control of massive bleeding from oesophageal varices was achieved in 4 of 17 patients with hepatic cirrhosis or extrahepatic portal vein block by infusion of vasopressin in 5% dextrose solution into the superior mesenteric artery at the rate of 0.2 unit per minute for 10 minutes, repeated in doses of up to 0.8 unit per minute if required. Initial control only was obtained in 7 other patients. Six patients survived to leave hospital, 3 of these following surgical intervention with ligation of varices. The treatment was not recommended because of the high rate of complications including the risk of bacterial invasion.— I. M. Murray-Lyon *et al.*, *Gut*, 1973, *14*, 59.

Continuous peripheral intravenous infusion of vasopressin was as effective as infusion into the superior mesenteric artery in the control of variceal haemorrhage and there were fewer catheter-related complications.— W. C. Johnson *et al.*, *Ann. Surg.*, 1977, *186*, 369.

A report of discouraging preliminary results with vasopressin in the management of bleeding oesophageal varices.— G. Fourtanier *et al.*, *Thérapie*, 1977, *32*, 283.

The intravenous infusion of vasopressin 0.4 unit per minute markedly reduced haematuria and transfusion requirements in a 15-year-old boy with massive bleeding due to haemorrhagic cystitis after treatment with cyclophosphamide. Bleeding recurred when attempts were made to reduce the dose of vasopressin.— R. E. Pyeritz *et al.*, *J. Urol.*, 1978, *120*, 253.

A 3-year retrospective study of the treatment of 70 episodes of gastro-intestinal bleeding in 65 patients. Vasopressin was given by constant arterial infusion in a dose of 0.2 unit per minute, increased to 0.4 unit per minute if bleeding did not stop. Haemorrhage was completely controlled in 43% of variceal bleeds, 67% of episodes of haemorrhagic gastritis, 45% of bleeding ulcers, and 62% of patients with bleeding colons. The infusion was usually tapered off over 24 to 48 hours; the overall incidence of relapse after initial control was 16%. Major complications occurred in 22 patients and especially those with cirrhosis.— L. M. Sherman *et al.*, *Ann. Surg.*, 1979, *189*, 298.

Further references to the intra-arterial infusion of vasopressin in the control of bleeding from the alimentary tract.— M. Nusbaum *et al.*, *Archs Surg., Chicago*, 1968, *97*, 1005; D. C. Morello *et al.*, *Am. J. Surg.*, 1972, *123*, 160; M. Nusbaum *et al.*, *Am. J. Surg.*, 1972, *123*, 165; A. G. Lerner *et al.*, *Pediatrics*, 1973, *51*, 126; M. E. Gordon *et al.* (letter), *Ann. intern. Med.*, 1973, *79*, 451; T. H. Covey and A. E. Baue, *Angiology*, 1974, *25*, 54; M. Nusbaum *et al.*, *Archs Surg., Chicago*, 1974, *108*, 342; H. O. Conn *et al.*, *Gastroenterology*, 1975, *68*, 211; J. Cavaluzzi *et al.*, *Am. J. Roentg.*, 1976, *127*, 672; W. C. Johnson and W. C. Widrich, *Am. J. Surg.*, 1976, *131*, 481; S. Kaufman *et al.*, *Am. J. Roentg.*, 1977, *128*, 567; G. Davis *et al.*, *Am. J. Roentg.*, 1977, *128*, 733.

Kidney biopsy. Subcutaneous injection of vasopressin, 5 to 15 units, prior to kidney biopsy increased the density of contrast, diminished urinary flow, and eliminated any gas in the colon in front of the kidney. Continuous intravenous infusion of contrast medium was not necessary.— B. Lindqvist, *Acta med. scand.*, 1967, *181*, 97, per *Drug Intell.*, 1967, *1*, 195.

Memory. Vasopressin had a beneficial effect on amnesia in 4 patients.— J. C. Oliveros *et al.* (letter), *Lancet*, 1978, *1*, 42. Two patients with severe amnesia induced by alcohol did not respond to vasopressin.— D. R. Blake *et al.* (letter), *Lancet*, 1978, *1*, 608. In a placebo-controlled study vasopressin nasal spray had a beneficial effect on memory in a chronic alcoholic patient with Korsakoff syndrome.— A. LeBoeuf *et al.* (letter), *Lancet*, 1978, *2*, 1370.

Further references: *Lancet*, 1979, *1*, 418.

Ovarian-function test. In 89 normally menstruating women, the uterine response to vasopressin was positive during menstruation, became less during the proliferative phase, and shifted to negative at midcycle. At the beginning of the secretory phase, the negative response reverted to positive. It was considered that the vasopressin response could be used for evaluating ovarian function and detecting ovulation.— E. M. Coutinho and A. C. V. Lopes, *Am. J. Obstet. Gynec.*, 1968, *102*, 470, per *J. Am. med. Ass.*, 1968, *206*, 2364.

Release of corticosteroids. In healthy adults, vasopressin and lypressin given by intramuscular injection increased plasma-corticosteroid concentrations similarly but increases in the concentrations of growth hormone followed only in some of them.— D. Czarny *et al.*, *Lancet*, 1968, *2*, 126.

A new Pitressin preparation with less marked corticotrophin-releasing effect *in vitro*.— J. Julesz *et al.* (letter), *Lancet*, 1981, *2*, 253. For details of the change in composition of Pitressin, see below.

Release of growth hormone. Vasopressin Injection given after an overnight fast by intramuscular injection, in a dose of 10 units in adults and 0.3 unit per kg bodyweight up to 5 units in children, increased the concentrations of growth hormone in serum. Maximum responses were attained between 30 to 120 minutes after the injection was given. A release of growth hormone did not occur in 4 patients with hypopituitarism.— J. J. Gagliardino *et al.*, *Lancet*, 1967, *1*, 1357.

Proprietary Preparations

Pitressin *(Parke, Davis, UK)*. Synthetic vasopressin (argipressin), available as injection containing 20 units per ml in ampoules of 1 ml. (Also available as Pitressin in *USA* and some other countries).

NOTE. Pitressin formerly consisted of Vasopressin Injection (*B.P.*).

Other Proprietary Names

Pos-Hipon *(Arg.)*.

5951-s

Vasopressin Tannate

The water-insoluble tannate of the pressor principle of the posterior lobe of the pituitary.

Adverse Effects, Treatment, and Precautions. As for Vasopressin Injection, above. Intramuscular injections of vasopressin tannate in oil can be painful.

In an evaluation of the long-term treatment of diabetes insipidus with posterior pituitary preparations, injections of vasopressin tannate produced gluteal infiltrates. One patient developed chronic hyponatraemia, hypervolaemia, and hypertension.— J. K. Van De Ree and F. Schwarz, *Ned. Tijdschr. Geneesk.*, 1971, *115*, 1186, per *Int. pharm. Abstr.*, 1972, *9*, 47.

Uses. Vasopressin tannate has the actions described under Vasopressin Injection. As its effects last for about 36 to 72 hours, it is used in the treatment of diabetes insipidus. It has been given intramuscularly in oily suspension in doses of 0.3 to 1 ml, equivalent to 1.5 to 5 units of pressor activity at intervals of about 1 to 3 days as required. It must not be administered intravenously and should be warmed and thoroughly shaken before use.

Proprietary Names

Pitressin Tannaat *(Substantia, Neth.)*; Pitressin Tannat *(Parke, Davis, Ger.; Parke, Davis, Norw.)*; Pitressin Tannate *(Parke, Davis, Austral.; Parke, Davis, Belg.; Parke, Davis, S.Afr.; Parke, Davis, Switz.; Parke, Davis, USA)*.

Preservatives and Antoxidants

6630-d

Deterioration in pharmaceutical products during storage may result from chemical changes brought about by acidity or alkalinity, heat, light, moisture, and oxygen, and by microbial contamination. Deterioration may also result from chemical reactions between the active ingredients and other constituents of a preparation and the container or closure.

Changes caused by oxygen can often be minimised by replacing the oxygen with an inert gas such as nitrogen or even removing the atmosphere entirely and keeping under vacuum, or by the inclusion of an antoxidant. Changes caused by the growth of bacteria and fungi can be prevented by sterilising the product or, less effectively, by the inclusion of an antimicrobial preservative. Changes due to chemical reactions and to microbial contamination are also retarded by storing at low temperatures.

Changes resulting from reactions with the container or closure can only be prevented by careful selection of the container and closure for a particular preparation; since such reactions cannot always be predicted, thorough testing should be carried out, particularly where plastic or rubber is used.

Antimicrobial Preservatives. Antimicrobial preservatives are included in preparations to kill or inhibit the growth of micro-organisms that may be present in the ingredients or that are introduced either in the process of preparation or during use. Preparations containing water are particularly susceptible to spoilage by micro-organisms. Preservatives should have a rapid effect at low concentrations against a wide range of pathogenic micro-organisms such as *Pseudomonas aeruginosa, Salmonella* spp., *Escherichia coli, Staphylococcus aureus, Candida albicans,* and *Aspergillus niger*. Their concentrations in preparations should be lethal rather than inhibitory.

The choice of a suitable preservative for a preparation depends on pH, compatibility with other ingredients, the route, dose and frequency of administration of the preparation, partition coefficients with ingredients and containers or closures, degree and type of contamination, concentration required, and rate of antimicrobial effect.

Pharmaceutical preparations which require an antimicrobial preservative may be classified in 2 groups.

The first group consists of those preparations, such as injections, eye-drops, eye ointments, irrigation solutions for introduction into body cavities, preparations for application to wounds, and any other preparations that are required to be dispensed as sterile products and kept in multidose containers. The function of a preservative in a preparation of this group is to maintain sterility in order to ensure that the preparation is safe for injection or instillation. Preservatives which have been used in this group of preparations include:

benzalkonium chloride, p.549, benzyl alcohol, p.39, cetrimide, p.551, chlorbutol, p.1285, chlorhexidine, p.554, chlorocresol, p.558, cresol, p.559, hydroxybenzoates, p.1282, phenethyl alcohol, p.1288, phenol, p.570, phenoxyethanol, p.1288, phenylmercuric nitrate, p.1289.

The second group consists of those preparations which are not dispensed as sterile products and includes the majority of preparations intended for oral or external use. The function of a preservative in a preparation of this group is to inhibit the growth of those micro-organisms which may be introduced during preparation and use, although special care to avoid contamination should be taken in preparing, dispensing, diluting, and packaging such products. The effective preservation of creams and other preparations which may be applied to broken or inflamed skins is especially important.

Preservatives should not be included in preparations to mask microbial contamination that may arise from unsatisfactory processes of preparation, inadequate packaging, or unsuitable conditions of storage.

Other preservatives which have been used, in addition to those in this section, include: alcohols, p.35, chloroform, p.745, formaldehyde, p.563, glycerol, p.706, sugars p.60.

A detailed review of the preservation of emulsions against microbial attack.— D. I. Wedderburn, *Adv. pharm. Sci.*, 1964, *1*, 195.

A discussion of the use and kinetics of preservatives in pharmaceutical preparations.— H. S. Bean, *J. Soc. cosmet. Chem.*, 1972, *23*, 703.

The proceedings of a colloquium on the use of antimicrobial agents as preservatives in pharmaceutical preparations.— *J. appl. Bact.*, 1978, *44*, *Suppl.*, Si-Slv.

Effect of gamma-irradiation. The effect of gamma-irradiation on several aqueous preservative solutions.— T. J. McCarthy, *Pharm. Weekbl. Ned.*, 1978, *113*, 698.

Enhanced effect. Studies of the additive and synergistic effects shown by mixtures of some commonly used antimicrobial substances *in vitro*.— P. G. Hugbo, *Can. J. pharm. Sci.*, 1976, *11*, 17 and 66.

Haemolysis. The haemolysis of erythrocytes by commonly used preservatives.— H. C. Ansel and D. E. Cadwallader, *J. pharm. Sci.*, 1964, *53*, 169.

Incompatibility. A review and discussion of the interaction of nonionic surfactants with preservatives and a survey of the physicochemical and biological methods of determining interactions.— M. S. Parker and M. Barnes, *Soap Perfum. Cosm.*, 1967, *40*, 163. See also D. Coates, *Mfg Chem.*, 1973, *44*, (Aug.), 41.

A review of the incompatibilities of preservatives.— J. B. Murray and G. Smith, *Pharm. J.*, 1968, *1*, 87.

Reviews of interactions with suspending agents: D. Coates, *Mfg Chem.*, 1973, *44* (Oct.), 34; *idem*, (Dec.), 19.

Preservatives in eye-drops. Reviews of the use of preservatives in formulating eye-drops: T. F. J. Tromp *et al.*, *Pharm. Weekbl. Ned.*, 1975, *110*, 465; *idem*, 485.

References: M. R. W. Brown and D. A. Norton, *J. Soc. cosmet. Chem.*, 1965, *16*, 369; R. M. E. Richards, *Australas. J. Pharm.*, 1967, *48*, S96.

Preservatives in topical preparations. A review and explanation of the rationale of preserving creams and lotions.— H. S. Bean, *Pharm. J.*, 1967, *2*, 289. A discussion and review of the clinical aspects of microbial contamination of topical preparations.— J. A. Savin, *ibid.*, 285.

Mathematical models for calculating the concentration of preservatives available in the water of emulsions.— H. S. Bean *et al.*, *J. Pharm. Pharmac.*, 1969, *21*, *Suppl.*, 173S; A. G. Mitchell and S. J. A. Kazmi, *Can. J. pharm. Sci.*, 1975, *10*, 67.

A review of the principles of cosmetic preservation and preservatives commonly used.— W. E. Rosen and P. A. Berke, *J. Soc. cosmet. Chem.*, 1973, *24*, 663. See also B. Croshaw, *ibid.*, 1977, *28*, 3.

The influence of factors such as pH, emulsifier, and ageing on the preservative requirements of oil-in-water emulsions.— G. Jacobs *et al.*, *J. Soc. cosmet. Chem.*, 1975, *26*, 105.

For other reviews, see Martindale, 27th Edn, p. 1272.

Skin reactions. A report of the contact sensitising potential of 23 preservatives and disinfectants used on the skin.— F. N. Marzulli and H. I. Maibach, *J. Soc. cosmet. Chem.*, 1973, *24*, 399.

Sorption. By plastics. A study of the stability of solutions of preservatives stored in polyethylene, polyvinyl chloride, and glass containers. Polyethylene was unsuitable for aromatic alcohols and chlorocresol. Benzalkonium chloride and chlorhexidine acetate were removed to the least extent by all the containers. The addition of 0.1% sodium metabisulphite reduced the instability of 0.1% sorbic acid in polyvinyl chloride and glass containers.— T. J. McCarthy, *Pharm. Weekbl. Ned.*, 1970, *105*, 557. In a further study polyethylene was shown to be unsuitable for substituted phenols, phenylmercuric nitrate, and benzoic acid.— *idem*, 1139.

Further references: K. Kakemi *et al.*, *Chem. pharm. Bull., Tokyo*, 1971, *19*, 2523.

Sorption. By rubber. The loss of preservatives in the presence of 3 types of rubber closures was investigated. The preservatives tested were benzyl alcohol, phenethyl alcohol, and methyl hydroxybenzoate. Aqueous buffered solutions of each were filled into multidose vials and stoppered with natural, neoprene, and butyl rubber closures. Sorption was least with butyl rubber and greatest with neoprene rubber closures. Some extractives from the butyl rubber were leached into the preservative solutions.— L. Lachman *et al.*, *J. pharm. Sci.*, 1963, *52*, 241 and 244.

Stability. The instability of antimicrobial preservatives.— L. Lachman, *Bull. parent. Drug Ass.*, 1968, *22*, 127.

Antoxidants. Many pharmaceutical preparations deteriorate on storage because of oxidation of the active or other ingredients on exposure to atmospheric oxygen. Examples of substances susceptible to oxidation are unsaturated oils and fats, vitamins, phenols, adrenaline, and apomorphine; some drugs such as physostigmine first degrade by hydrolysis to form colourless products which are subsequently oxidised to form coloured compounds; plastic and rubber, used in containers and closures, also tend to oxidise on storage. Many of the oxidation reactions which occur in pharmaceutical preparations are considered to be 'autoxidation' reactions. These are chain reactions which are often initiated by ultraviolet radiation in the presence of a trace of oxygen and which involve the formation of highly reactive free radicals; the reactions are often catalysed by the presence of heavy-metal ions. These chain reactions can be inhibited by the addition of very small amounts of substances known as *antoxidants*.

Antoxidants may be classified in 3 groups. The first group, sometimes known as *true antoxidants* and also known as 'anti-oxygens', consists of those substances which probably inhibit oxidation by reacting with free radicals and thus block the chain reaction. They are effective against autoxidation but not in reversible oxidation (redox) reactions. Examples are the alkyl gallates, butylated hydroxyanisole, butylated hydroxytoluene, nordihydroguaiaretic acid, and the tocopherols.

The second group consists of those substances known as *reducing agents*; these substances have a lower redox potential than the drug or adjuvants which they are intended to protect and are therefore more readily oxidised than the drug. They are effective against oxidising agents. Reducing agents may act also by reacting with free radicals. Examples of reducing agents are ascorbic acid, isoascorbic acid, the potassium and sodium salts of sulphurous acid, and sodium formaldehyde sulphoxylate.

The third group consists of substances known as *antoxidant synergists*; these substances usually have little antoxidant effect themselves but probably enhance the action of antoxidants in the first group by reacting with those heavy-metal ions which catalyse oxidation. Examples of synergists are citric acid, edetic acid and its salts, lecithin, tartaric acid, and thiodipropionic acid. Mixtures of true antoxidants or true antoxidants and reducing agents may also show synergism.

The choice of a suitable antoxidant for a preparation depends on the route, dose and frequency of administration, the chemical and physical properties of the other ingredients and the container and closure. It is rarely possible to predict the effectiveness of various antoxidants in a particular preparation; the choice of concentration required should be determined by experiment.

A review of oxidation mechanisms and antoxidants in cosmetics and pharmaceuticals.— J. P. Ostendorf, *J. Soc. cosmet. Chem.*, 1965, *16*, 203.

A review of the use and rationale of antoxidants and

chelating agents as stabilisers in liquid dosage forms.— L. Lachman, *Drug Cosmet. Ind.*, 1968, *102* (Jan.), 36.

A general review of developments in the field of antoxidants.— L. Chalmers, *Soap Perfum. Cosm.*, 1971, *44*, 29.

A review of the uses and efficacy of some antoxidants and synergists.— *Fd Add. Ser. Wld Hlth Org. No. 3*, 1972.

Background toxicological information.— *Fd Add. Ser. Wld Hlth Org. No. 5*, 1974.

Several compounds related to phenolic antoxidants including nordihydroguaiaretic acid, butylated hydroxyanisole, gallic acid, and propyl gallate enhanced the inhibitory activity of amphotericin against various species of yeasts *in vitro*.— F. A. Andrews *et al.*, *J. antimicrob. Chemother.*, 1979, *5*, 173. See also W. H. Beggs *et al.*, *Antimicrob. Ag. Chemother.*, 1978, *13*, 266; W. H. Beggs *et al.* (letter), *J. antimicrob. Chemother.*, 1980, *6*, 291 (amphotericin methyl ester).

Temporary estimated acceptable daily intake of tertiary butylhydroquinone (THBQ): up to 500 µg per kg body-weight as tertiary butylhydroquinone, butylated hydroxyanisole, butylated hydroxytoluene, or the sum of all three.— Twenty-first Report of the Joint FAO/WHO Expert Committee on Food Addivites, *Tech. Rep. Ser. Wld Hlth Org. No. 617*, 1978.

Adverse effects. A small outbreak of toxic methaemoglobinaemia in a paediatric ward was thought to be due to the antoxidants (butylated hydroxyanisole, butylated hydroxytoluene and propyl gallate) used to preserve the oil in a soybean infant feed formula.— M. Nitzan *et al.*, *Clin. Toxicol.*, 1979, *15*, 273.

Preservatives in Food. *Antimicrobials.* In Great Britain, the antimicrobial preservatives which may be added to foods are controlled by The Preservatives in Food Regulations 1979 (SI 1979: No. 752) as amended (SI 1980: No. 931; SI 1982: No. 15) and The Preservatives in Food (Scotland) Regulations 1979 [SI 1979: No. 1073 (S.96)] as amended [SI 1980: No. 1232 (S.95)]. Under these regulations the term 'preservative' is defined as 'any substance which is capable of inhibiting, retarding, or arresting the growth of micro-organisms or any deterioration of food due to micro-organisms or of masking the evidence of any such deterioration' but does not include any permitted antoxidant, artificial sweetener, bleaching agent, colouring matter, emulsifier, improving agent, solvent, stabiliser, or miscellaneous additive; or vinegar; any soluble carbohydrate sweetening matter; potable spirits or wines, herbs, spices, hop extract or flavouring agent when used for flavouring purposes; sodium chloride; or any substance added to food by the process of curing known as smoking.

The permitted preservatives, the use of each of which is limited to particular specified foods, generally in specified maximum proportions, are benzoic acid (or its calcium, sodium, or potassium salt), diphenyl, ethyl hydroxybenzoate (or sodium ethyl hydroxybenzoate), formaldehyde (derived from wrappings or as additive to dimethicone), hexamine, methyl hydroxybenzoate (or sodium methyl hydroxybenzoate), nisin, *o*-phenylphenol (or its sodium salt), propionic acid (or its sodium, potassium, or calcium salt), propyl hydroxybenzoate (or sodium propyl hydroxybenzoate), sodium nitrate (or potassium nitrate), sodium nitrite (or potassium nitrite), sorbic acid (or its sodium, potassium, or calcium salt), sulphur dioxide (or sodium sulphite, sodium acid sulphite, sodium metabisulphite, potassium metabisulphite, calcium sulphite, or calcium acid sulphite), and thiabendazole.

Preservatives for use in animal feeding stuffs are controlled by the Fertilisers and Feeding Stuffs Regulations 1973 (SI 1973: No. 1521) as amended (SI 1976: No. 840; SI 1977: No. 115).

A discussion of the problems associated with the use of food preservatives.— A. G. Lloyd and J. J. P. Drake, *Br. med. Bull.*, 1975, *31*, 214.

Antoxidants. In Great Britain, the antoxidants which may be added to foods are controlled by The Antioxidant in Food Regulations, 1978 (SI 1978: No. 105) as amended (SI 1980: No. 1831) and The Antioxidants in Food (Scotland) Regulations, 1978 [SI 1978: No. 492 (S.47)] as amended [SI 1980: No. 1886 (S.173)].

Under these regulations the term 'antioxidant' is defined as 'any substance which is capable of delaying, retarding, or preventing the development in food of rancidity or other flavour deterioration due to oxidation but does not include any permitted artificial sweetener, bleaching agent, colouring matter, emulsifier, improving agent, miscellaneous additive, preservative, stabiliser, solvent, or esters of ascorbic acid with straight-chain C_{14} and C_{18} fatty acids used to dilute or dissolve colouring matter'.

The antoxidants permitted in foods include: ascorbic acid, calcium ascorbate, sodium ascorbate, ascorbyl palmitate, extracts of natural origin rich in tocopherols, synthetic α-, γ-, or δ-tocopherol, some alkyl gallates, butylated hydroxyanisole, and butylated hydroxytoluene. There is some debate about the continued use of ethoxyquin.

Certain antoxidants may only be added to the following foods:(i) butter, butter fat, dried cream, dried cheese, dried whey, and dried whey derivatives for use as ingredients in the preparation of food intended for sale for human consumption; (ii) anhydrous edible oils and fats and vitamin oils and concentrates other than preparations of vitamin A or vitamin-A esters containing more than 30 000 microgrammes retinol equivalents per g; (iii) any permitted emulsifier or permitted stabiliser containing combined fatty acids whether polymerised or not; (iv) essential oils and isolates from the concentrates of essential oils; (v) potato powder, potato flakes, and potato granules; (vi) shelled walnuts; (vii) apples and pears; (viii) chewing-gum base; (ix) chewing gum prepared from the base containing its permitted antoxidant; and (x) preparations of vitamin A and vitamin-A esters containing more than 30 000 microgrammes retinol equivalents per g. The antoxidants and the maximum proportions permitted in the 10 classes of foods are

(a) propyl gallate, octyl gallate, or dodecyl gallate or any mixture of these, 100 ppm in (i) calculated on the milk fat content, (ii), and (iii), and 1000 ppm in (iv);

(b) butylated hydroxyanisole, butylated hydroxytoluene or any mixture of these, 25 ppm in (v), 33.3 ppm for every 1000 microgrammes retinol equivalents per g in (x), 70 ppm of each and 140 ppm of an equal mixture of both in (vi), 200 ppm in (i) calculated on the milk fat content, (ii), and (iii), and 1000 ppm in (iv);

(c) butylated hydroxytoluene, 200 ppm in (ix) and 1000 ppm in (viii); and

(d) ethoxyquin 3 ppm in (vii).

Mixtures of the 2 types of antoxidants, (a) and (b), may be used provided each is within the limits specified and that the total amount does not exceed 1000 ppm in the case of (iv). Diphenylamine may be in or on (vii) at a concentration not exceeding 10 ppm if used solely as a scald inhibitor.

These antoxidants should not be used in foods intended for babies or young children except for preparations of vitamin A and vitamin-A esters for use as ingredients in the preparation of such foods where butylated hydroxyanisole, butylated hydroxytoluene, or any mixture of these may be used in a proportion not exceeding 0.35 ppm for every 1000 microgrammes retinol equivalents per g.

The Food Additives and Contaminants Committee recommended in their 1974 Report on the Antioxidant in Food Regulations 1966 and 1974 (FAC/REP/18, London, HM Stationery Office) that ascorbyl diacetate, included in the EEC Directive on Antioxidants, be not permitted in the UK. The other recommendations of this Committee have been incorporated in The Antioxidants in Food Regulations, 1978.

Antoxidants for use in animal feeding stuffs are controlled by the Fertilisers and Feeding Stuffs Regulations 1973 (SI 1973: No. 1521) as amended (SI 1976: No. 840; SI 1977: No. 115).

6631-n

The Alkyl Gallates

The alkyl esters of gallic acid (3,4,5-trihydroxybenzoic acid).

The lower alkyl gallates are moderately soluble in water but very sparingly soluble in oils and fats. With increasing molecular weights, water solubilities decrease and solubilities in oils and fats increase. The gallates are dissolved in fixed oils by warming the mixture to 70° to 80° and in solid fats by warming until the fat is just melted.

Adverse Effects. Alkyl gallates may cause skin reactions.

Background toxicological information.— *Fd Add. Ser. Wld Hlth Org. No. 5*, 1974.

Absorption and Fate. Gallate esters are hydrolysed to gallic acid in the body and excreted in the urine as free acid or 4-*O*-methylgallic acid and its glucuronide.

Uses. The alkyl gallates are used as antoxidants in oils, fats, foods, cosmetics, and perfumes. They are also effective in inhibiting the development of peroxides in ethers, paraldehyde, and similar substances. Their effectiveness may be enhanced by the addition of a syngergist such as citric acid, phosphoric acid or lecithin.

Rancidity in most oils is prevented by the addition of up to 0.1% of propyl gallate (or other alkyl gallate), the amount required depending upon the degree of unsaturation of the oil. The addition of 0.002% to ether prevents the formation of peroxides and 0.01% retards the oxidation of paraldehyde. In Great Britain, the use of alkyl gallates in foods is controlled by The Antioxidant in Food Regulations—see above.

A review of the uses and efficacy of alkyl gallates as antoxidants. Allergic responses to skin contact with gallate dusts have been reported.— *Fd Add. Ser. Wld Hlth Org. No. 3*, 1972.

6632-h

The Hydroxybenzoates

The hydroxybenzoates are esters or salts of *p*-hydroxybenzoic acid.

The esters are tasteless, odourless, inert, stable, and of low toxicity but they are not very soluble in water, their solubility decreasing, with a corresponding increase in their solubility in oily media, with increase in molecular weight. The methyl ester is usually employed in concentrations of 0.1 to 0.2% in aqueous preparations, while the higher esters are used in near-saturated solutions. The sodium derivatives are more soluble in water than are the esters themselves but they cannot be used in acid or neutral solutions at a concentration higher than the corresponding free ester. The esters are usually incorporated in the preparation as a solution in boiling water, but in non-aqueous preparations they may be added dissolved in acetone, alcohol, melted fats and oils, glycerol, or propylene glycol.

The preservative activity of the hydroxybenzoates is reduced in the presence of nonionic surfactants.

Effect of freeze-drying. A report of the loss of hydroxybenzoate preservatives (methyl-and propyl-hydroxybenzoate) during freeze drying. The loss is dependent on the vacuum of the system, the length of drying cycle, the temperature of the product, and the amount and chemical entity of the materials present. Analysis of hydroxybenzoate-containing freeze-dried products for both active ingredient and preservative appears warranted.— K. P. Flora *et al.*, *J. Pharm. Pharmac.*, 1980, *32*, 577.

Incompatibility. Interaction between methyl or propyl hydroxybenzoate and sucrose esters could be due to hydrogen and hydrophobic bonding.— C. Valdez *et al.*, *J. pharm. Sci.*, 1968, *57*, 2093.

Adverse Effects. Dilute solutions of hydroxybenzoates may be painful and cause irritation when applied to the eye. Hypersensitivity reactions have occurred after the application of preparations containing hydroxybenzoates to the skin. Hypersensitivity reactions have also been reported after parenteral or oral administration. Cross-sensitivity occurs between the hydroxybenzoates.

Background toxicological information.— *Fd Add. Ser. Wld Hlth Org. No. 5,* 1974.

A study in neonates with hyperbilirubinaemia indicated that methyl hydroxybenzoate in a solution of gentamicin increased the concentration of free unconjugated bilirubin in serum by interfering with the binding of bilirubin to serum proteins; gentamicin had no significant effect. Further assessment was required to determine the risk in these patients.— C. J. Loria *et al.*, *J. Pediat.*, 1976, *89*, 479, per *Int. pharm. Abstr.*, 1977, *14*, 339.

Allergy. A review of the contact sensitivity of the hydroxybenzoates.— O. J. Lorenzetti and T. C. Wernet, *Dermatologica*, 1977, *154*, 244.

Four patients with chronic contact dermatitis resistant to treatment gave strong positive reactions to hydroxybenzoates by closed patch testing. All showed marked cross-sensitivity to methyl, ethyl, propyl, and butyl hydroxybenzoates. When treatment with topical steroids in hydroxybenzoate-free formulations was substituted, complete recovery occurred eventually. The incidence of this reaction was found to be 0.8% in a 2-year study with 273 consecutive patients suffering from long-standing inflammatory skin conditions. A 5% hydroxybenzoate ointment was used for patch testing under occlusion for 48 hours.— W. F. Schorr, *J. Am. med. Ass.*, 1968, *204*, 859.

Of 100 patients with allergic contact dermatitis, 3 gave positive reactions to patch testing with a mixture of 3 hydroxybenzoates 5% in soft paraffin.— A. A. Fisher *et al.*, *Archs Derm.*, 1971, *104*, 286.

Of 4000 patients subjected to patch testing in 5 European clinics 1.3% of males and 2.3% of females showed positive reactions to mixed hydroxybenzoates 15% in soft paraffin.— H. Bandmann *et al.*, *Archs Derm.*, 1972, *106*, 335.

Of 75 patients with recurrent urticaria and angio-oedema of more than 4 months' duration, 44 were found to be sensitive to sodium benzoate or *p*-hydroxybenzoic acid, alone or in conjunction with aspirin or azo dyes, or both.— A. -M. Ros *et al.*, *Br. J. Derm.*, 1976, *95*, 19. See also G. Michaëlsson *et al.*, *Archs Derm.*, 1974, *109*, 49. See also Tartrazine, p.431.

A hydrocortisone preparation containing methyl and propyl hydroxybenzoates caused bronchospasm and pruritus when given intravenously to an asthmatic patient. Intravenous challenge and intradermal tests elicited hypersensitivity reactions although patch tests did not.— J. E. Nagel *et al.*, *J. Am. med. Ass.*, 1977, *237*, 1594.

Further references: W. F. Schorr and A. H. Mohajerin, *Archs Derm.*, 1966, *93*, 721; I. L. Schamberg, *ibid.*, 1967, *95*, 626; S. Epstein, *Ann. Allergy*, 1968, *26*, 185; D. Kleinhaus and W. Knoth, *Z. Haut- u. GeschlKrankh.*, 1973, *48*, 699.

Uses. The hydroxybenzoates are used as preservatives in a wide variety of cosmetic and pharmaceutical preparations. They are not suitable bactericides for injections or ophthalmic solutions.

The hydroxybenzoates are active against moulds, fungi, and yeasts, but less active against bacteria. The higher esters are the most effective, but are limited by lower solubility. Unlike benzoic and sorbic acids, the hydroxybenzoates are active at pH 7 to 9. Mixtures of 2 or more esters are likely to be more effective than the use of a single ester, since in this way a higher total concentration of preservative can be obtained in the solution and, in addition, the mixture may be active against a wider range of organisms.

The hydroxybenzoates are used in concentrations of up to 0.2% as preservatives in food, up to 0.3% in various enzyme preparations and up to 1% in liquid foam headings but their numbing effect on the mouth may be a disadvantage. In Great Britain, the use of hydroxybenzoates in food is controlled by the Preservatives in Food Regulations—see p.1282.

Estimated acceptable daily intake of ethyl, methyl, and propyl hydroxybenzoates: up to 10 mg per kg body-weight, as the sum of ethyl, methyl, and propyl hydroxybenzoates.— Seventeenth Report of the Joint FAO/WHO Expert Committee on Food Additives, *Tech. Rep. Ser. Wld Hlth Org. No. 539,* 1974.

Use as preservatives. A review of antimicrobial agents, including hydroxybenzoates, used in cosmetics.— I. R. Gucklhorn, *Mfg Chem.*, 1970, *41*, (Dec.), 50.

The use of hydroxybenzoates to preserve dextrose/sucrose solutions and the effect of adding hydroxybenzoates to skin cleansing preparations containing hexachlorophane.— E. E. Boehm and D. N. Maddox, *Mfg Chem.*, 1972, *43*, (Aug.), 21.

The effect of pH and temperature on the hydrolysis of methyl, ethyl, propyl, and butyl hydroxybenzoates.— S. M. Blaug and D. E. Grant, *J. Soc. cosmet. Chem.*, 1974, *25*, 495.

Methyl, ethyl, propyl, and butyl hydroxybenzoates, used as preservatives in oral liquid preparations, were found to partition into flavouring oils. The partitioning effect depended on the concentration of the oils, pH of the aqueous medium, and the nature of other additives. Depletion of the hydroxybenzoates from the aqueous phase could lower their concentration below that required for preservative action.— P. B. Chemburkar and R. S. Joslin, *J. pharm. Sci.*, 1975, *64*, 414.

Phenol was formed when 2 strains of *Pseudomonas aeruginosa* were incubated with sterile butyl, ethyl, methyl, and propyl hydroxybenzoates. *Klebsiella aerogenes* metabolised *p*-hydroxybenzoic acid to phenol.— R. Nakamori *et al.* (letter), *J. pharm. Sci.*, 1975, *64*, 1071.

Use in ophthalmic solutions. *For a discussion on the inadequacy of hydroxybenzoates for preserving ophthalmic solutions, see Martindale 27th Edn,* p. 1273.

Proprietary Preparations of Mixed Hydroxybenzoates

Nipacombin SK *(Nipa, UK).* A mixture of sodium salts of the higher esters of *p*-hydroxybenzoic acid.

Nipasept *(Nipa, UK).* A mixture of the methyl, ethyl, and propyl esters of *p*-hydroxybenzoic acid.

Nipasept Sodium *(Nipa, UK).* A water-soluble form of Nipasept.

Nipastat *(Nipa, UK).* A mixture of the methyl, ethyl, propyl, and butyl esters of *p*-hydroxybenzoic acid.

Topanol *(ICI Petrochemicals, UK).* A range of antoxidants.

See also entries under individual monographs.

6633-m

Ascorbyl Palmitate *(U.S.N.F.).* Vitamin C Palmitate.

L-Ascorbic acid 6-palmitate; 3-Oxo-L-gulofuranolactone 6-palmitate.

$C_{22}H_{38}O_7$=414.5.

CAS — 137-66-6.

Pharmacopoeias. In *U.S.N.F.*

A white to yellowish-white powder or crystals with a characteristic odour. M.p. 107° to 117°. Very slightly **soluble** in water, chloroform, ether, and vegetable oils; soluble in alcohol. A solution in methanol is dextrorotatory. **Store** in a cool place in airtight containers.

Ascorbyl palmitate is used as an antoxidant in food.

A review of the uses and efficacy of ascorbyl palmitate as an antoxidant and synergist.— *Fd Add. Ser. Wld Hlth Org. No. 3,* 1972.

Estimated acceptable daily intake of ascorbyl palmitate: up to 1.25 mg per kg body-weight.— Seventeenth Report of the Joint FAO/WHO Expert Committee on Food Additives, *Tech. Rep. Ser. Wld Hlth Org. No. 539,* 1974.

Background toxicological information.— *Fd Add. Ser. Wld Hlth Org. No. 5,* 1974.

6634-b

Benzoic Acid *(B.P., U.S.P.).* Acidum Benzoicum; Benzoesäure.

$C_6H_5.CO_2H$=122.1.

CAS — 65-85-0.

Pharmacopoeias. In all pharmacopoeias examined except *Eur.*, *Fr.*, and *Neth.*

Colourless light feathery crystals or white scales or powder with a slight characteristic odour. M.p. 121.5° to 123.5°; somewhat volatile at moderate temperatures; freely volatile in steam; it sublimes on heating.

Soluble 1 in 300 to 350 of water, 1 in 20 of boiling water, 1 in 3 of alcohol, 1 in 5 of chloroform, 1 in 3 of ether, 1 in 30 of carbon disulphide; freely soluble in acetone; soluble in glycerol; very soluble in fats and oils. A solution in water is acid to methyl red. **Incompatible** with ferric salts and salts of heavy metals.

The solubility of benzoic acid in water was increased in the presence of citric acid or sodium acetate.— S. Bolton, *J. Am. pharm. Ass., scient. Edn,* 1960, *49*, 237.

Benzoic acid was adsorbed by light kaolin; adsorption was maximal at about pH 5.— C. D. Clarke and N. A. Armstrong, *Pharm. J.*, 1972, *2*, 44.

The Pharmaceutical Society's Department of Pharmaceutical Sciences found no loss of active constituent or detectable deterioration of the container when benzoic acid 0.1% aqueous solution was stored for 8 weeks in polyvinyl chloride bottles.— *Pharm. J.*, 1973, *1*, 100.

Effect of gamma-irradiation. A study of the effect of gamma-irradiation on aqueous solutions of benzoic acid.— T. J. McCarthy, *Pharm. Weekbl. Ned.*, 1978, *113*, 698.

Adverse Effects. Allergic reactions to benzoic acid have been reported. Large doses may produce gastric irritation.

Allergy. Of 100 patients with asthma undergoing provocation tests with benzoic acid, 47 showed positive reactions.— L. Rosenhall and O. Zetterström, *Tubercle*, 1975, *56*, 168.

Of 75 patients with recurrent urticaria and angio-oedema of more than 4 months' duration, 44 were found to be sensitive to sodium benzoate or *p*-hydroxybenzoic acid, alone or in conjunction with aspirin or azo dyes, or both.— A. -M. Ros *et al.*, *Br. J. Derm.*, 1976, *95*, 19. See also G. Michaëlsson *et al.*, *Archs Derm.*, 1974, *109*, 49.

There was no significant objective or subjective skin response to two 500-mg daily doses of benzoic acid or of lactose in a double-blind study of 150 dermatological inpatients.— A. Lahti and M. Hannuksela (letter), *Lancet*, 1981, *2*, 1055. See also under Hypersensitivity in Tartrazine, p.431.

Absorption and Fate. When taken by mouth, benzoic acid is rapidly absorbed from the gastro-intestinal tract. It is conjugated with glycine in the liver to form hippuric acid which is rapidly excreted in the urine within 12 hours; up to 97% may be excreted in the first 4 hours. When taken in large doses, some benzoic acid may be excreted as benzoylglucuronic acid.

Uses. Benzoic acid has antibacterial and antifungal properties and, in a concentration of 0.1%, it is a moderately effective preservative for pharmaceutical preparations providing that the pH is not above 5; above this pH it is much less effective since its antimicrobial properties are due to the undissociated acid. It is used as a preservative in certain acid food products.

It was formerly employed as a urinary antiseptic, usually in the form of one of its salts. Applied externally, it has antimycotic properties and Compound Benzoic Acid Ointment is used for the treatment of fungous infections of the skin.

Estimated acceptable daily intake: up to 5 mg per kg body-weight, as the sum of benzoic acid and sodium and potassium benzoate.— Seventeenth Report of the Joint FAO/WHO Expert Committee on Food Additives, *Tech. Rep. Ser. Wld Hlth Org. No. 539,* 1974.

Background toxicological information.— *Fd Add. Ser. Wld Hlth Org. No. 5,* 1974.

A review of oral and topical therapy, including the use of benzoic acid ointment, for common superficial and cutaneous fungal infections.— L. E. Millikan, *Postgrad. Med.*, 1976, *60*, 52, per *Int. pharm. Abstr.*, 1977, *14*, 847.

Otitis externa. A solution of benzoic acid 0.5% and salicylic acid 0.5% in alcohol 30% instilled before and after swimming was successful in preventing or reducing the frequency of attacks of otitis externa in patients who suffered recurrent attacks, particularly after swimming.— I. H. McKee (letter), *Br. med. J.*, 1969, *2*, 251.

Preparations

Benzoic and Salicylic Acids Ointment *(U.S.P.)*. Contains benzoic acid and salicylic acid, in the ratio of about 2:1, in a suitable ointment basis. Store at a temperature not exceeding 30°.

Benzoic Acid Solution *(B.P., A.P.F.)*. Liq. Acid. Benz. Benzoic acid 5 g, propylene glycol 75 ml, freshly boiled and cooled water to 100 ml.

About 2% of this solution may be added to mixtures having a slightly acid reaction to prevent the growth of micro-organisms.

Compound Benzoic Acid Ointment *(B.P.)*. Ung. Acid. Benz. Co.; Benzoic Acid Compound Ointment; Benzoic Acid Ointment Compound *(A.P.F.)*; Benzoic and Salicylic Acid Ointment; Whitfield's Ointment. Benzoic acid 6% and salicylic acid 3% in emulsifying ointment. Store at a temperature not exceeding 25°.

NOTE. Whitfield's original formula was that of Compound Benzoic Acid Ointment (*B.P.C. 1934*), i.e. benzoic acid 5%, salicylic acid 3%, white soft paraffin 27.6%, and coconut oil 64.4%.

Proprietary Preparations

Aserbine *(Bencard, UK)*. **Cream** containing benzoic acid 0.024%, malic acid 0.36%, salicylic acid 0.006%, propylene glycol 1.7%, and hexachlorophane 0.015%; and **Solution** containing benzoic acid 0.15%, malic acid 2.25%, salicylic acid 0.037%, and propylene glycol 40%. For burns, varicose ulcers, and bedsores.

Daily application of Aserbine to gravitational ulcers in 46 patients resulted in complete healing of ulcer with scab shedding in 30% and healing with scab retained in 17%. The rate of healing appeared to be much better with the smaller ulcers. The commonest side-effect was irritation of the surrounding skin in 13% of patients.—Report No. 87 of the General Practitioner Research Group, *Practitioner*, 1966, *196*, 578.

Malatex *(Norton, UK: Vestric, UK)*. **Cream** containing benzoic acid 0.024%, malic acid 0.36%, salicylic acid 0.006%, and propylene glycol 1.7%; and **Solution** containing benzoic acid 0.15%, malic acid 2.25%, salicylic acid 0.0375%, and propylene glycol 40%. For bedsores, burns, and varicose and indolent ulcers.

6635-v

Benzyl Hydroxybenzoate *(B.P.)*. Benzylparaben. Benzyl *p*-hydroxybenzoate.

$C_{14}H_{12}O_3$=228.2.

CAS — 94-18-8.

Pharmacopoeias. In *Br.*

A fine white to creamy-white, odourless or almost odourless, crystalline powder. M.p. about 112°. Practically **insoluble** in water; soluble 1 in 2.5 of alcohol, 1 in 1 of acetone, 1 in 6 of ether, 1 in 70 of glycerol, and 1 in 8 of propylene glycol; soluble in arachis oil and in solutions of alkali hydroxides.

For the general properties and uses of the hydroxybenzoates, see p.1282.

Proprietary Preparations

Nipabenzyl *(Nipa, UK)*. A brand of benzyl hydroxybenzoate.

6636-g

Bronopol. 2-Bromo-2-nitropropane-1,3-diol.

$C_3H_6BrNO_4$=200.0.

CAS — 52-51-7.

A white or almost white, slightly hygroscopic, crystalline powder, odourless or with a faint characteristic odour. M.p. about 130°. **Soluble** 1 in 4 of water, 1 in 2 of alcohol, 1 in 7 of propylene glycol, and 1 in 100 of glycerol; slightly soluble in oils. Solutions in water have a pH of 5 to 7. Solutions in water are stable at low pH but when exposed to light, especially under alkaline conditions, they may become yellow or brown. Formaldehyde and nitrites are amongst the decomposition products produced. There is no apparent correlation between change of colour and loss of antimicrobial activity. **Incompatible** with sulphydryl compounds or with aluminium or iron containers but stable in contact with tin or stainless steel. Unstable in anhydrous solutions of glycerol. Anionic or nonionic surfactants and 50% serum are stated to cause little or no inactivation.

The stability of bronopol.— D. M. Bryce and R. Smart, *J. Soc. cosmet. Chem.*, 1965, *16*, 187.

Although bronopol showed little adsorption on to several powders widely used in pharmaceutical and cosmetic preparations, the alkaline pH of the aqueous suspensions of some of these powders adversely affected its antibacterial activity. A similar effect was obtained with some thickening agents.— J. A. Myburgh and T. J. McCarthy, *Cosmet. Toilet.*, 1978, *93* (Feb.), 47.

Effect of gamma-irradiation. A study of the effect of gamma-irradiation on aqueous solutions of bronopol.— T. J. McCarthy, *Pharm. Weekbl. Ned.*, 1978, *113*, 698.

Adverse Effects. Bronopol may be irritant to skin and eyes at concentrations greater than 1%.

A review including the toxicology of bronopol.— D. M. Bryce *et al.*, *J. Soc. cosmet. Chem.*, 1978, *29*, 3.

Bronopol had come into use as a preservative for cosmetic products, but was too toxic to allow consideration for use in liquid oral medicines.— M. S. Parker, *Pharm. J.*, 1979, *1*, 92.

Uses. Bronopol is an antimicrobial agent which is active against a wide range of bacteria, including *Pseudomonas aeruginosa*, but is less active against moulds and yeasts. Its activity does not vary much over the range pH 5 to 8. Concentrations of 0.02 to 0.05% are bacteriostatic. Bronopol has been used as a preservative in shampoos, cosmetics, and suppositories.

Reviews.— I. R. Gucklhorn, *Mfg Chem.*, 1970, *41* (Jan.), 42. Correction.— M. D. Potter (letter), *ibid.*, *41*, (Mar.), 44; *Cosmet. Toilet.*, 1977, *92* (Mar.), 87; D. M. Bryce *et al.*, *J. Soc. cosmet. Chem.*, 1978, *29*, 3.

It was suggested that the mode of action of bronopol was the oxidation of the thiol groups of bacterial cell constituents to disulphides.— R. J. Stretton and T. W. Manson, *J. appl. Bact.*, 1973, *36*, 61.

Manufacturers

Boots, UK.

6637-q

Butyl Hydroxybenzoate *(B.P.)*. Butylis Paraoxybenzoas; Butylparaben *(U.S.N.F.)*. Butyl *p*-hydroxybenzoate.

$C_{11}H_{14}O_3$=194.2.

CAS — 94-26-8.

Pharmacopoeias. In *Br.* and *Jap.* Also in *U.S.N.F.*

Odourless or almost odourless colourless crystals or white crystalline powder; it is tasteless but produces numbness of the tongue. M.p. 68° to 72°. Very slightly **soluble** in water (1 in 5000) and boiling water; soluble 1 in 1 of alcohol; freely soluble in acetone and ether; soluble 1 in about 1 of propylene glycol, 1 in 250 of glycerol, and 1 in 20 of arachis oil; soluble in solutions of alkali hydroxides.

The solubility of butyl hydroxybenzoate in a variety of aliphatic alcohols over a temperature range of 25 to 40°.— K. S. Alexander *et al.*, *J. pharm. Sci.*, 1977, *66*, 42.

For the general properties and uses of the hydroxybenzoates, see p.1282.

The acceptable daily intake of butyl hydroxybenzoate could not be determined from the toxicological data available.— *Fd Add. Ser. Wld Hlth Org. No. 5*, 1974.

Proprietary Preparations

Nipabutyl *(Nipa, UK)*. A brand of butyl hydroxybenzoate.

6638-p

Butylated Hydroxyanisole *(B.P., U.S.N.F.)*.

BHA. 2-*tert*-Butyl-4-methoxyphenol.

$C_{11}H_{16}O_2$=180.2.

CAS — 25013-16-5.

Pharmacopoeias. In *Br.*, *Fr.*, *It.*, and *Swiss.* Also in *U.S.N.F.* *Br.* permits not more than 15% of 3-*tert*-butyl-4-methoxyphenol; *Fr.* permits not more than 10%; *It.* permits not more than 1%; *Swiss* describes 3-*tert*-butyl-4-methoxyphenol and permits the presence of 2-*tert*-butyl-4-methoxyphenol; *U.S.N.F.* has no specific limit for 3-*tert*-butyl-4-methoxyphenol.

A white or almost white crystalline powder or a yellowish-white waxy solid with an aromatic odour and a slightly bitter burning taste. It contains a variable proportion of 3-*tert*-butyl-4-methoxyphenol.

Practically **insoluble** in water; soluble 1 in 4 of alcohol, 1 in 2 of chloroform, 1 in 1.2 of ether, 1 in 2 of propylene glycol, 1 in 3 of arachis oil, 1 in 100 of liquid paraffin, and 1 in 4 of lard; soluble in solutions of alkali hydroxides. **Incompatible** with oxidising agents and ferric salts. **Protect** from light.

Adverse Effects. Hypersensitivity reactions have occurred following the application of preparations containing butylated hydroxyanisole to the skin.

Background toxicological information.— *Fd Add. Ser. Wld Hlth Org. No. 5*, 1974.

Allergy. Patch testing of 6 patients with contact dermatitis showed that 3 were sensitive to butylated hydroxyanisole present as an antoxidant in foods and topical preparations.— J. Roed-Petersen and N. Hjorth, *Br. J. Derm.*, 1976, *94*, 233.

Further references: C. L. Menenghini *et al.*, *Dermatologica*, 1971, *143*, 137; H. Degreef and L. Verhoeve, *Contact Dermatitis*, 1975, *1*, 269.

Absorption and Fate. Butylated hydroxyanisole is absorbed from the gastro-intestinal tract and may be stored in body fat following large doses. Up to 77% has been reported to be excreted in the urine as the glucuronide and less than 1% as unchanged drug within 24 hours of ingestion.

A study *in vitro* indicated that following ingestion of usual doses, butylated hydroxyanisole was highly bound to plasma proteins.— R. El-Rashidy and S. Niazi, *J. pharm. Sci.*, 1978, *67*, 967.

Studies in 2 healthy subjects given butylated hydroxyanisole 100 mg indicated that the bioavailability and rate of absorption may differ greatly between subjects. In both of the subjects less than 1% of the administered dose was excreted in the urine as unchanged drug within 24 hours.— R. El-Rashidy and S. Niazi, *J. pharm. Sci.*, 1979, *68*, 103.

Uses. Butylated hydroxyanisole is used as an antoxidant for oils and fats either alone or with a gallate and a synergist such as citric or phosphoric acid.

It may be dissolved in many oils at room temperature, or by warming slightly; it dissolves readily in molten fats. Care should be taken not to incorporate air in the oil or fat while dissolving the antoxidant. Up to 200 ppm of butylated hydroxyanisole or of butylated hydroxytoluene, or a mixture of these, may be used for the preservation of fixed oils, fats, or vitamin oil concentrates in pharmaceutical practice (see p.1282).

A review of the uses and efficacy of butylated hydroxyanisole as an antoxidant and synergist.— *Fd Add. Ser. Wld Hlth Org. No. 3*, 1972.

Temporary estimated acceptable daily intake: up to 500 µg per kg body-weight, as butylated hydroxyanisole, butylated hydroxytoluene, or the sum of both. A multigeneration reproduction study was required.— Twentieth Report of the Joint FAO/WHO Expert Committee on Food Additives, *Tech. Rep. Ser. Wld Hlth Org. No. 599*, 1976. The temporary estimated acceptable daily intake was as butylated hydroxyanisole, butylated hydroxytoluene, tertiary butylhydroquinone, or the sum of all three.— Twenty-first Report of the Joint FAO/WHO Expert Committee on Food Additives, *Tech. Rep. Ser. Wld Hlth Org. No. 617*, 1978.

Antimicrobial action. A report of butylated hydroxyanisole having antiviral activity.— P. Wanda *et al.*, *Antimicrob. Ag. Chemother.*, 1976, *10*, 96.

Studies *in vitro* indicated that butylated hydroxyanisole had a marked antimicrobial activity against *Clostridium perfringens* and consistently inhibited its growth at a concentration of 200 ppm. An enhanced effect was obtained when butylated hydroxyanisole was used in conjunction with nitrite, sorbic acid or esters of *p*-hydroxybenzoic acid. The presence of a lipid or surfactant greatly reduced the antimicrobial activity of butylated hydroxyanisole.— K. J. Klindworth *et al.*, *J. Fd Sci.*, 1979, *44*, 564, per *Abstr. Hyg.*, 1979, *54*, 985.

Proprietary Preparations

Embanox *(May & Baker, UK).* A range of antoxidants including **Embanox BHA**, a brand of butylated hydroxyanisole; **Embanox 2,** containing butylated hydroxanisole 18%, butylated hydroxytoluene 20% in vegetable oil; **Embanox 3,** containing butylated hydroxyanisole 20%, propyl gallate 6%, citric acid 4%, in propylene glycol; **Embanox 4,** containing butylated hydroxyanisole 20%, citric acid 20% in propylene glycol; **Embanox 5,** containing butylated hydroxyanisole 20% in vegetable oil; and **Embanox 6,** containing butylated hydroxyanisole 20%, propyl gallate 10%, citric acid 10%, propylene glycol, vegetable oil, and fatty acid monoglyceride. **Embanox 7** consists of butylated hydroxyanisole 66.7% and dodecyl gallate 33.3%. **Embanox EC30M** is an emulsifiable formulation containing butylated hydroxyanisole 22.5%, butylated hydroxytoluene 7.5%, acetylated monoglycerides, and polysorbate 80.

Nipantiox 1-F *(Nipa, UK).* A brand of butylated hydroxyanisole.

Tenox *(Eastman, UK).* A range of antoxidants including **Tenox BHA**, a brand of butylated hydroxyanisole; **Tenox 2,** containing butylated hydroxyanisole 20%, propyl gallate 6%, and citric acid 4%, in propylene glycol; **Tenox 4,** containing butylated hydroxyanisole 20%, and butylated hydroxytoluene 20%, in maize oil; **Tenox 4A,** containing butylated hydroxyanisole 30% in maize oil; **Tenox 6,** containing butylated hydroxyanisole 10%, butylated hydroxytoluene 10%, propyl gallate 6%, citric acid 6%, glyceryl mono-oleate 28%, maize oil 28%, and propylene glycol 12%; **Tenox 7,** containing butylated hydroxyanisole 28%, propyl gallate 12%, citric acid 6%, and glyceryl mono-oleate 20% in propylene glycol; **Tenox A,** containing butylated hydroxyanisole 40% and citric acid 8% in propylene glycol; and **Tenox R,** containing butylated hydroxyanisole 20% and citric acid 20% in propylene glycol.

Proprietary Preparations of Similar Compounds

Embanox TBHQ *(May & Baker, UK).* A brand of 2-*tert*-butylhydroquinone ($C_{10}H_{14}O_2$ = 166.2). **Embanox 101** contains 2-*tert*-butylhydroquinone 20% and citric acid 10% in propylene glycol. **Embanox 102** contains 2-*tert*-butylhydroquinone 10% and butylated hydroxyanisole 10% in vegetable oil. **Embanox 106** contains 2-*tert*-butylhydroquinone 10%, butylated hydroxyanisole 20%, citric acid 10%, propylene glycol, vegetable oil, and fatty acid monoglyceride.

Tenox TBHQ *(Eastman, UK).* A brand of 2-*tert*-butylhydroquinone. **Tenox 20** contains 2-*tert*-butylhydroquinone 20% and citric acid 10% in propylene glycol; **Tenox 20A** contains 2-*tert*-butylhydroquinone 20%, citric acid 3%, maize oil 30%, glyceryl mono-oleate 32% and propylene glycol 15%; **Tenox 22** contains 2-*tert*-butylhydroquinone 6%, butylated hydroxyanisole 20%, and citric acid 4%, in propylene glycol; **Tenox 26** contains 2-*tert*-butylhydroquinone 6%, butylated hydroxyanisole 10%, butylated hydroxytoluene 10%, citric acid 6%, maize oil 28%, glyceryl mono-oleate 28%, and propylene glycol 12%; **Tenox 27** contains 2-*tert*-butylhydroquinone 12%, butylated hydroxyanisole 28%, citric acid 6%, glyceryl mono-oleate 20%, and propylene glycol 34%.

6639-s

Butylated Hydroxytoluene *(B.P., U.S.N.F.).*

Butylhydroxitoluenum; BHT. 2,6-Di-*tert*-butyl-*p*-cresol.

$C_{15}H_{24}O$=220.4.

CAS — 128-37-0.

Pharmacopoeias. In *Br., Fr.,* and *Nord.* Also in *U.S.N.F.*

Tasteless, colourless crystals or white crystalline powder, odourless or with a faint odour. F.p. not lower than 69.2°.

Practically **insoluble** in water, glycerol, propylene glycol and solutions of alkali hydroxides; soluble 1 in 4 of alcohol, 1 in 1.1 of chloroform, 1 in 0.5 of ether, 1 in 5 of liquid paraffin, and 1 in 3 of fixed oils.

Adverse Effects. Hypersensitivity reactions have occurred following the application of preparations containing butylated hydroxytoluene to the skin.

Maximum permissible atmospheric concentration 10 mg per m³.

Background toxicological information.— *Fd Add. Ser. Wld Hlth Org. No. 5,* 1974.

Allergy. Three patients with contact dermatitis were found to be sensitive to the presence of butylated hydroxytoluene in foods and topical preparations.— J. Roed-Petersen and N. Hjorth, *Br. J. Derm.,* 1976, *94,* 233.

Absorption and Fate. Butylated hydroxytoluene is readily absorbed from the gastro-intestinal tract. It is metabolised and excreted in the urine mainly as the glucuronides of oxidation products. About one-half of a dose is excreted within 24 hours.

The main metabolites of butylated hydroxytoluene in man were the glucuronide of an aldehyde compound resulting from the oxidation of all 3 alkyl groups and minor amounts of di-*t*-butyl-4-hydroxybenzoic acid and its glucuronide.— J. W. Daniel *et al., Food & Cosmet. Toxicol.,* 1967, *5,* 475; *idem, Biochem. J.,* 1968, *106,* 783. The carboxylic acid of butylated hydroxytoluene and its ester glucuronide were the only major metabolites detected in human urine, though their occurrence required further verification. The aldehyde compound isolated by J.W. Daniel *et al.* could not be found.— G. M. Holder *et al.* (letter), *J. Pharm. Pharmac.,* 1970, *22,* 375.

Uses. Butylated hydroxytoluene is used similarly to butylated hydroxyanisole, p.1284 as an antoxidant for oils and fats.

A review of the uses and efficacy of butylated hydroxytoluene as an antoxidant and synergist.— *Fd Add. Ser. Wld Hlth Org. No. 3,* 1972.

Temporary estimated acceptable daily intake: up to 500 µg per kg body-weight, as butylated hydroxytoluene, butylated hydroxyanisole, or the sum of both. An adequate carcinogenicity study was required.— Twentieth Report of the Joint FAO/WHO Expert Committee on Food Additives, *Tech. Rep. Ser. Wld Hlth Org. No. 599,* 1976. The temporary estimated acceptable daily intake was as butylated hydroxyanisole, butylated hydroxytoluene, tertiary butylhydroquinone, or the sum of all three.— Twenty-first Report of the Joint FAO/WHO Expert Committee on Food Additives, *Tech. Rep. Ser. Wld Hlth Org. No. 617,* 1978.

Antiviral action. Butylated hydroxytoluene inactivated lipid-containing viruses *in vitro.*— W. Snipes *et al., Science,* 1975, *188,* 64. See also P. Wanda *et al., Antimicrob. Ag. Chemother.,* 1976, *10,* 96.

Use in food. The Food Additives and Contaminants Committee recommended that, on the grounds of safety, butylated hydroxytoluene could continue to be used as a stabiliser for solvents used in food.— *Report on the Review of Solvents in Food,* FAC/REP/25, Ministry of Agriculture, Fisheries and Food, London, HM Stationery Office, 1978.

Proprietary Preparations

Anullex BHT *(BTP Cocker Chemicals, UK).* A brand of butylated hydroxytoluene.

Embanox BHT *(May & Baker, UK).* A brand of butylated hydroxytoluene.

For antoxidant mixtures containing butylated hydroxytoluene, see under Butylated Hydroxyanisole, p.1285.

Butylated hydroxytoluene was also formerly marked in Great Britain under the proprietary name Tenox BHT *(Eastman).*

6640-h

Chlorbutol *(B.P.).*

Chlorobutanol *(Eur. P., U.S.N.F.)*; Chlorbutanolum; Chlorobutanolum; Acetone-Chloroforme; Chlorbutanol; Chlorbutanolum Hydratum; Chloretone; Trichlorbutanolum; Alcohol Trichlorisobutylicus. 1,1,1-Trichloro-2-methylpropan-2-ol hemihydrate.

$C_4H_7Cl_3O,\frac{1}{2}H_2O$=186.5.

CAS — 57-15-8 (anhydrous); 6001-64-5 (hemihydrate).

Pharmacopoeias. In *Aust., Belg., Chin., Cz., Hung., Ind., Jug., Nord., Pol., Span.,* and *Swiss* (all with ½H_2O). In *Arg., Braz., Int., Mex., Port.,* and *U.S.N.F.* (anhydrous or with ½H_2O).

Br., Eur., Fr., Ger., It., and *Neth.* have separate monographs for anhydrous and hemihydrate. *Jap.* permits up to 6% of water. *Turk.* has anhydrous.

Colourless or white crystals with a musty, somewhat camphoraceous odour and taste. It is volatile at ordinary temperatures. M.p. about 76° to 79°; anhydrous chlorbutol melts at about 95°. B.p. about 167°.

Soluble 1 in 130 of water, 1 in 0.6 of alcohol, 1 in 3 of chloroform, 1 in 8 to 10 of glycerol, 1 in 30 of liquid paraffin, 1 in 12 of olive oil; freely soluble in volatile oils; very soluble in ether and propylene glycol. A 2% suspension in water is neutral to litmus. It forms liquid mixtures with menthol, phenazone, phenol, salol, and thymol. **Store** in a cool place in airtight containers. Protect from light.

In the presence of magnesium trisilicate 1%, chlorbutol 0.5% had no antibacterial activity against *Staphylococcus aureus.* Bentonite 1% and carmellose 1% both reduced its activity by between 20 and 30%.— R. T. Yousef *et al., Can. J. pharm. Sci.,* 1973, *8,* 54.

Effect of gamma-irradiation. The potency and pH of chlorbutol solution fell after very low doses of gamma-irradiation, and an amorphous yellow precipitate and acetone were formed at doses of up to 25 000 Gy.— L. J. Rasero and D. M. Skauen, *J. pharm. Sci.,* 1967, *56,* 724.

Haemolysis. Total haemolysis occurred when erythrocytes were cultured for 45 minutes in a 0.5% solution of chlorbutol in sodium chloride injection. Only slight haemolysis occurred when the strength was reduced to 0.37%.— H. C. Ansel and D. E. Cadwallader, *J. pharm. Sci.,* 1964, *53,* 169.

Sorption. Chlorbutol diffused out of a 0.5% aqueous solution stored in polyethylene containers. Losses increased with time, storage temperature, and area of polyethylene in contact with the solution. After 10 weeks, 0.5% chlorbutol solution stored at about 20° in polyethylene containers of 15 to 60 ml was not bactericidal to *Pseudomonas aeruginosa,* but storage at 6° to 8° was satisfactory in containers of 15 to 120 ml.— W. T. Friesen and E. M. Plein, *Am. J. Hosp. Pharm.,* 1971, *28,* 507.

Storage tests of contact lens solutions in plastic containers indicated that chlorbutol could be sorbed by polyethylene and polypropylene leading to almost complete loss of preservative.— N. E. Richardson *et al., J. Pharm. Pharmac.,* 1977, *29,* 717. Comments.— H. D. Blackburn *et al.* (letter), *ibid.,* 1978, *30,* 666. See also N. E. Richardson *et al., Pharm. J.,* 1979, *2,* 462.

Chlorbutol was reversibly sorbed from aqueous solution into contact lenses manufactured from polyhydroxyethylmethacrylate.— N. E. Richardson *et al., J. Pharm. Pharmac.,* 1978, *30,* 469.

Stability. The half-life at 25° for chlorbutol in a solution buffered at pH 3 was calculated to be 90 years whereas at pH 7.5 it was 0.23 year. Similarly, the decomposition in aqueous solution when heated for 30 minutes at 115° was calculated to be 13% at pH 5 and 58% at pH 6.— A. D. Nair and J. L. Lach, *J. Am. pharm. Ass., scient. Edn,* 1959, *48,* 390.

A 0.5% solution of chlorbutol with a pH of 5 to 6 lost 10% of its potency when stored for six weeks at 25° to 30°. Neutral or alkaline solutions were less stable.— N. V. Patwa and C. L. Huyck, *J. Am. pharm. Ass.,* 1966, *NS6,* 372.

Polysorbate 20 and lauromacrogol [1000] reduced the rate of hydrolysis of chlorbutol at pH 9.2 but macrogol 4000 had no effect.— R. A. Anderson and A. H. Slade, *J. Pharm. Pharmac.,* 1966, *18,* 640.

Adverse Effects. Acute poisoning with chlorbutol may produce central nervous system depression with weakness, loss of consciousness, and depressed respiration.

Symptoms of chlorbutol intoxication developed in a 40-year-old man with a history of alcoholism who had been taking between 6 and 10 sedative capsules daily each containing chlorbutol 150 mg and salicylamide 300 mg. During treatment the elimination half-life of chlorbutol was found to be 13.2 days.— T. Borody *et al., Med. J. Aust.,* 1979, *1,* 288.

Allergy. A report of a hypersensitivity reaction to chlorbutol used to preserve heparin injection.— S. Dux *et al.* (letter), *Lancet,* 1981, *1,* 149.

Treatment of Adverse Effects. Empty the stomach by aspiration and lavage. The respiration should be assisted until spontaneous breathing is fully restored.

Uses. Chlorbutol has antibacterial and antifungal properties and it is used at a concentration of 0.5% as a preservative in injections and in eye-drops. At this concentration it is close to its

saturation point at low temperatures, and crystallisation may occur. It is unstable in alkaline solution, it is more stable in acid solution at room temperature and it decomposes appreciably on autoclaving or steaming.
Chlorbutol has been used as a mild sedative and local analgesic as well as in motion sickness but other compounds are preferred. It has also been used as a dusting powder, in nose drops and as a dental preparation for exposed or infected pulps.
The use of chlorbutol in cosmetics and toiletries is restricted in Great Britain under the Cosmetic Products Regulations 1978 (SI 1978: No. 1354).

Preparations

Unguentum Chlorbutoli *(Dan. Disp.).* Rektol. Chlorbutol 3 g, mercurous chloride 3 g, tannic acid 1.5 g, liquid paraffin 14 g, yellow soft paraffin 23 g, wool fat 52.5 g, water 3 g.

Unguentum Chlorbutoli Benzocaini *(Dan. Disp.).* Rektol med Benzokain. Chlorbutol 3 g, mercurous chloride 3 g, benzocaine 10 g, tannic acid 1.5 g, water 3 g, liquid paraffin 14 g, yellow soft paraffin 20.5 g, wool fat 45 g.

6641-m

Cinnamic Acid *(B.P.C. 1973).* Cinnam. Acid; Cinnamylic Acid. *trans*-3-Phenylpropenoic acid.
$C_6H_5.CH{:}CH.CO_2H = 148.2$.

CAS — 621-82-9.

Colourless crystals with a faint balsamic odour and a burning taste. M.p. 132° to 134°. Very slightly **soluble** in water; soluble 1 in 6 of alcohol, 1 in 15 of chloroform, and 1 in 15 of ether; freely soluble in acetone and oils. A saturated solution in water is acid to methyl red.

Cinnamic acid has antibacterial and antifungal properties similar to those of benzoic acid (see p.1283). It is used with benzoic acid as an ingredient of Opiate Squill Pastilles to simulate the flavour of tolu.

6642-b

Dehydroacetic Acid *(U.S.N.F.).* Methylacetopyronone. 3-Acetyl-3,4-dihydro-6-methyl-2*H*-pyran-2,4-dione (keto form); 3-Acetyl-4-hydroxy-6-methyl-2*H*-pyran-2-one (enol form).
$C_8H_8O_4 = 168.1$.

CAS — 520-45-6 (keto form); 771-03-9 (enol form).

Pharmacopoeias. In *U.S.N.F.*

A white odourless crystalline powder with a faint acid taste. M.p. 109° to 111°. Very slightly **soluble** in water; soluble 1 in 35 of alcohol and 1 in 5 of acetone; soluble in solutions of alkalis.

Effect of gamma-irradiation. A study of the effect of gamma-irradiation on aqueous solutions of dehydroacetic acid.— T. J. McCarthy, *Pharm. Weekbl. Ned.*, 1978, *113*, 698.

Dehydroacetic acid is an antimicrobial agent and it inhibits the growth of many bacteria, fungi, and yeasts. Dehydroacetic acid is used in the preservation of cosmetics and shampoos. It has been used in toothpastes to depress oral enzyme activity and has been included in antifungal packaging material.

6643-v

Diethyl Pyrocarbonate. DEPC.
$C_6H_{10}O_5 = 162.1$.

CAS — 1609-47-8.

A clear colourless liquid with a fruity odour. B.p. 155°. **Soluble** 1 in 160 of water; very soluble in alcohol, esters, and fixed oils; soluble in glycerol and glycols. **Incompatible** with amines, phenols, and carboxylic acids, forming esters, and with some plastics and rubber. It decomposes in aqueous solution, forming alcohol and carbon dioxide. It loses 100% of its potency in 4 hours at 22° to 25° and pH 3; a rise in pH increases the rate of hydrolysis. In alcoholic solution it decomposes with the formation of diethyl carbonate. **Store** in airtight containers.

Adverse Effects and Treatment. Diethyl pyrocarbonate is corrosive to the skin and dilute solutions and vapours are irritant to the eyes and to mucous membranes. It may be removed from the skin by applying dilute ammonia solution or sodium bicarbonate.

Since there was the risk of the carcinogen diethylurethane being produced with ammonium ions, diethyl pyrocarbonate could not be recommended for use in food.— *Review of the Preservatives in Food Regulations 1962,* Food Additives and Contaminants Committee Report, Ministry of Agriculture, Fisheries and Food, London, HM Stationery Office, 1972. See also Seventeenth Report of the Joint FAO/WHO Expert Committee on Food Additives, *Tech. Rep. Ser. Wld Hlth Org. No. 539,* 1974..

Background toxicological information.— *Fd Add. Ser. Wld Hlth Org. No. 5,* 1974.

Uses. Diethyl pyrocarbonate is a preservative which is mainly effective against yeast. It was formerly used for the preservation of soft drinks and wine.

6644-g

Diphenyl. Phenylbenzene. Biphenyl.
$C_{12}H_{10} = 154.2$.

CAS — 92-52-4.

A white crystalline powder with a characteristic odour. M.p. about 69°. Practically **insoluble** in water; soluble in alcohol, ether, and fats.

Diphenyl has fungistatic properties but it is only effective against a limited number of moulds; it does inhibit the growth of those species of *Penicillium* that cause the decay of citrus fruits and it is employed for impregnating the material used for wrapping citrus fruits. Maximum permissible atmospheric concentration 0.2 ppm.

Though primarily used for treating wrappers for fruit, diphenyl penetrated into the skin of the fruit and might consequently be included in food or drink prepared from the fruit.— Sixth Report of the Joint FAO/WHO Expert Committee on Food Additives, *Tech. Rep. Ser. Wld Hlth Org. No. 228,* 1962.

Adverse effects, including nausea, vomiting, and irritation of the eyes and nose occurred in workers exposed to diphenyl.— E. Weil *et al., Archs Mal. prof. Méd. trav.*, 1965, *26,* 405, per *Bull. Hyg., Lond.*, 1966, *41,* 146.

Maximum acceptable daily intake of diphenyl: 125 µg per kg body-weight.— Report of the 1972 Joint FAO/WHO Meeting on Pesticide Residues in Food, *Tech. Rep. Ser. Wld Hlth Org. No. 525,* 1973.

Nine workers exposed to diphenyl developed toxic symptoms which included headache, nausea, diffuse abdominal pain, aching of limbs, and general fatigue. Six had liver damage and 1 of the 6 workers who also had psychic symptoms, somnolence, icterus, ascites, and oedema of the legs died with yellow liver atrophy.— I. Häkkinen *et al., Archs envir. Hlth,* 1973, *26,* 70, per *Abstr. Hyg.*, 1973, *48,* 721.

6645-q

Dodecyl Gallate *(B.P.).* Dodecyl Gall.; Laurylum Gallicum; Lauryl Gallate. Dodecyl 3,4,5-trihydroxybenzoate.
$C_{19}H_{30}O_5 = 338.4$.

CAS — 1166-52-5.

Pharmacopoeias. In *Aust.* and *Br.*

A white or creamy-white, odourless, tasteless powder. M.p. 96° to 97.5°.
Practically **insoluble** in water; soluble 1 in 3.5 of alcohol, 1 in 2 of acetone, 1 in 60 of chlorofrom, 1 in 4 of ether, 1 in 1.5 of methyl alcohol, 1 in 60 of propylene glycol, 1 in 7 of castor oil, and 1 in 30 of arachis oil. **Incompatible** with iron salts. **Store** in airtight containers and avoid contact with metals. Protect from light.

For the general properties and uses of the alkyl gallates, see p.1282.

Background toxicological information.— *Fd Add. Ser. Wld Hlth Org. No. 5,* 1974.

Temporary estimated acceptable daily intake: up to 200 µg per kg body-weight as dodecyl, octyl, or propyl gallate or their sum.— Twentieth Report of the Joint FAO/WHO Expert Committee on Food Additives, *Tech. Rep. Ser. Wld Hlth Org. No. 599,* 1976.

Sensitivity to the presence of dodecyl gallate was reported in a patient with contact dermatitis.— J. Roed-Petersen and N. Hjorth, *Br. J. Derm.*, 1976, *94,* 233.

Proprietary Preparations

Progallin LA *(Nipa, UK).* A brand of dodecyl gallate.
Progallin BU is a brand of butyl gallate.

For other preparations containing dodecyl gallate in mixtures with other antoxidants, see under Butylated Hydroxyanisole, p.1285..

6646-p

Ethoxyquin. 6-Ethoxy-1,2-dihydro-2,2,4-trimethylquinoline.
$C_{14}H_{19}NO = 217.3$.

CAS — 91-53-2.

An oily liquid, light amber in colour when freshly prepared but tending to polymerise and darken in colour on exposure to light and air. Practically **insoluble** in water; soluble in organic solvents, oils, and fats.

Ethoxyquin has been used as an antoxidant for the prevention of common scald of apples and pears during storage at a concentration of up to 3 ppm.

Maximum acceptable daily intake of ethoxyquin: 60 µg per kg body-weight.— Report of the 1972 Joint FAO/WHO Meeting on Pesticide Residues in Food, *Tech. Rep. Ser. Wld Hlth Org. No. 525,* 1973.

A report of 2 cases of contact dermatitis attributed to ethoxyquin.— D. Burrows, *Br. J. Derm.*, 1975, *92,* 167.

Proprietary Names

Santoquin *(Monsanto, USA).*

6647-s

Ethyl Gallate *(B.P.).* Ethyl 3,4,5-trihydroxybenzoate.
$C_9H_{10}O_5 = 198.2$.

CAS — 831-61-8.

Pharmacopoeias. In *Br.*

A white to creamy-white odourless crystalline powder. M.p. 151° to 154°.
Soluble 1 in 500 of water, 1 in 3 of alcohol, 1 in 3 of ether, and 1 in 3 of propylene glycol; practically insoluble in arachis oil. Aqueous solutions more concentrated (up to about 3%) than is indicated by its solubility can be prepared by boiling with water and cooling. **Incompatible** with alkalis and iron salts. **Store** in airtight containers and avoid contact with metals. Protect from light.

The solubility of ethyl gallate in macrogols and in solutions of macrogol ether surfactants.— L. S. C. Wan, *Can. J. pharm. Sci.*, 1972, *7,* 25.

Ethyl gallate has the general properties and uses of the alkyl gallates, see p.1282.

Proprietary Preparations

Progallin A *(Nipa, UK).* A brand of ethyl gallate.

6648-w

Ethyl Hydroxybenzoate *(B.P.).* Aethylum Hydroxybenzoicum; Ethylis Paraoxybenzoas; Ethylparaben *(U.S.N.F.).* Ethyl *p*-hydroxybenzoate.
$C_9H_{10}O_3 = 166.2$.

CAS — 120-47-8.

Pharmacopoeias. In *Br., Chin., Fr.,* and *Jap.* Also in *U.S.N.F.*

Odourless or almost odourless colourless crystals or white crystalline powder; it is tasteless but produces numbness of the tongue. M.p. 115° to 118°.
Soluble 1 in 1500 of water, 1 in 2 of alcohol, 1 in 1.2 of acetone, 1 in 10 of chloroform, 1 in 3.5 of ether, 1 in 200 of glycerol, 1 in 4 of propylene glycol, and 1 in 100 of arachis oil; soluble in solutions of alkali hydroxides. A saturated solution in water is acid to litmus.

The solubility of ethylhydroxybenzoate in a variety of aliphatic alcohols over a temperature range of 25 to 40°.— K. S. Alexander *et al., J. pharm. Sci.*, 1977, *66,* 42.

For the general properties and uses of the hydroxybenzoates, see p.1282.

Estimated acceptable daily intake of ethyl hydroxybenzoate: up to 10 mg per kg body-weight, as the sum of ethyl, methyl, and propyl hydroxybenzoates. Further biochemical studies in man and *animals* were desirable.— Seventeenth Report of the Joint FAO/WHO Expert Committee on Food Additives, *Tech. Rep. Ser. Wld Hlth Org. No. 539,* 1974.

Background toxicological information.— *Fd Add. Ser. Wld Hlth Org. No. 5,* 1974.

Proprietary Preparations

Nipagin A *(Nipa, UK).* A brand of ethyl hydroxybenzoate.

6649-e

Gallic Acid. Acid. Gall.; Acide Pyrogallolcarbonique; Gallussäure. 3,4,5-Trihydroxybenzoic acid monohydrate.
$C_7H_6O_5,H_2O=188.1$.

CAS — 149-91-7 (anhydrous).

NOTE. Care should be taken to avoid confusion with inorganic gallates, e.g. sodium gallate, $NaGaO_2$.

Pharmacopoeias. In *Port., Span.,* and *Swiss.*

White or pale brown, odourless, acicular or prismatic crystals. **Soluble** 1 in 100 of water, 1 in 3 of boiling water, 1 in 6 of alcohol, 1 in 5 of acetone, 1 in 100 of ether, and 1 in 10 of glycerol; practically insoluble in chloroform. **Incompatible** with alkalis, ferric salts, heavy metals, and oxidising agents. **Protect** from light.

Gallic acid has been used as an antoxidant for oils and fats. The properties and uses of alkyl gallates are described on p.1282.

6650-b

Isoascorbic Acid. Erythorbic Acid. 3-Oxo-D-glucofuranolactone.
$C_6H_8O_6=176.1$.

CAS — 89-65-6.

A white or almost white crystalline powder. M.p. 164° to 171°. **Soluble** 1 in 3 of water and 1 in 20 of alcohol. **Store** in airtight containers. Protect from light.

Isoascorbic acid is used as an antoxidant in emulsions of fats and oils. It has little or no vitamin-C potency.

A review of the uses and efficacy of isoascorbic acid as an antoxidant and synergist. In practice ascorbic acid was more effective.— *Fd Add. Ser. Wld Hlth Org. No. 3,* 1972.

Estimated acceptable daily intake of isoascorbic acid: up to 5 mg per kg body-weight.— Seventeenth Report of the Joint FAO/WHO Expert Committee on Food Additives, *Tech. Rep. Ser. Wld Hlth Org. No. 539,* 1974.

Background toxicological information.— *Fd Add. Ser. Wld Hlth Org. No. 5,* 1974.

6651-v

Methyl Hydroxybenzoate *(B.P.).* Methyl Hydroxybenz.; Methyl Parahydroxybenzoate *(Eur. P.)*; Methylis Parahydroxybenzoas; Methylparaben *(U.S.N.F.)*; Methylis Oxybenzoas; Methylis Paraoxibenzoas; Metagin; Metilparabeno. Methyl *p*-hydroxybenzoate.
$C_8H_8O_3=152.1$.

CAS — 99-76-3.

Pharmacopoeias. In *Aust., Belg., Br., Braz., Eur., Fr., Ger., Hung., Ind., It., Jap., Jug., Mex., Neth., Nord., Pol., Port., Roum., Span., Swiss,* and *U.S.*

Colourless crystals or a fine, white, crystalline powder; odourless or with a faint odour, it is tasteless but produces a slight burning sensation of the mouth and tongue, followed by local numbness. M.p. 125° to 128°. **Soluble** 1 in 400 to 500 of water, 1 in 20 of boiling water, 1 in 3 to 3.5 of alcohol, 1 in 3 of acetone, 1 in 40 of chloroform, 1 in 10 of ether, and 1 in 3 of propylene glycol; soluble 1 in 40 of warm vegetable oils and 1 in 60 of warm glycerol, giving clear solutions on cooling; slightly soluble in carbon tetrachloride; freely soluble in methyl alcohol and solutions of alkali hydroxides. **Incompatible** with alkalis and iron salts. **Protect** from light.

Effect of gamma-irradiation. A study of the effect of gamma-irradiation on aqueous solutions of methyl hydroxybenzoate.— T. J. McCarthy, *Pharm. Weekbl. Ned.,* 1978, *113,* 698.

Hydrolysis. The half-life of methyl hydroxybenzoate at 25° in 0.1% buffered aqueous solution was calculated to be 6675 days at pH 6, 892 days at pH 8, and 412 days at pH 9. Autoclaving at 121° for 30 minutes led to 5.5% decomposition at pH 6 and 42% at pH 9. Aqueous solutions buffered at pH 3 and 6 were reported to be undecomposed by heating at 100° for 2 hours or at 120° for 30 minutes.— N. N. Raval and E. L. Parrott, *J. pharm. Sci.,* 1967, *56,* 274.

Inactivation. The antibacterial activity of methyl hydroxybenzoate 0.1% against *Staphylococcus aureus* was reduced by 75 to 100% by 1% of aluminium magnesium silicate, talc, polysorbate 80, and magnesium trisilicate.— R. T. Yousef *et al., Can. J. pharm. Sci.,* 1973, *8,* 54.

Solubility. The solubility of methyl hydroxybenzoate in a variety of aliphatic alcohols over a temperature range of 25 to 40°.— K. S. Alexander *et al., J. pharm. Sci.,* 1977, *66,* 42.

Sorption. By plastics. Sorption by nylon 6 (capran polyamide) of methyl and propyl hydroxybenzoates decreased their antimicrobial activity against *Aspergillus niger, Klebsiella aerogenes,* and *Pseudomonas aeruginosa.*— N. K. Patel and N. Nagabhushan, *J. pharm. Sci.,* 1970, *59,* 264.

For the general properties and uses of the hydroxybenzoates, see p.1282.

Heating at 100° for 30 minutes at pH 5 with methyl hydroxybenzoate 0.1% was ineffective in killing the spores of *Bacillus stearothermophilus.*— R. A. Anderson, *J. Hosp. Pharm.,* 1969, *26,* 48.

Estimated acceptable daily intake of methyl hydroxybenzoate: up to 10 mg per kg body-weight, as the sum of ethyl, methyl, and propyl hydroxybenzoates. Additional studies in man were desirable.— Seventeenth Report of the Joint FAO/WHO Expert Committee on Food Additives, *Tech. Rep. Ser. Wld Hlth Org. No. 539,* 1974.

Background toxicological information.— *Fd Add. Ser. Wld Hlth Org. No. 5,* 1974.

Butacaine sulphate 1% in 0.9% sodium chloride solution was found to have some antimicrobial action *in vitro,* particularly against *Escherichia coli.* The addition of butacaine sulphate enhanced the bactericidal activity of benzalkonium chloride, chlorocresol, and of methyl hydroxybenzoate.— M. A. El-Nakeeb and A. Farouk, *Can. J. pharm. Sci.,* 1976, *11,* 58.

For a report of methyl hydroxybenzoate increasing serum concentrations of bilirubin, see Hydroxybenzoates, p.1283.

Preparations

Aqua Conservans *(F.N. Belg.).* Methyl hydroxybenzoate 80 mg, propyl hydroxybenzoate 20 mg, propylene glycol 900 mg, water to 100 ml.

Hydroxybenzoates Spirits *(Adelaide Child. Hosp.).* Methyl hydroxybenzoate 6.5 g, propyl hydroxybenzoate 3.5 g, alcohol (90%) to 100 ml. Used in Sulphadiazine Mixture, p.1474, and in Aluminium Hydroxide Topical Paste, p.73.

Solutio Conservans *(Hung. P.).* Methyl hydroxybenzoate 7 g, propyl hydroxybenzoate 3 g, alcohol 90 g.

Solution for Eye-drops. Liq. pro Gutt. Methyl hydroxybenzoate 22.9 mg, propyl hydroxybenzoate 11.4 mg, purified water to 100 ml. Prepare aseptically.

NOTE. Solution for Eye-drops was included in succeeding editions of the *B.P.C.* from 1949 to 1959. It was not initially included in the *B.P.C.* 1963 but was added by amendment in December 1963 and then deleted by the *B.P.C.* Supplement 1966. Solution for Eye-drops has been shown to be unsatisfactory as a preservative for eye-drops.

Proprietary Preparations

Nipagin M *(Nipa, UK).* A brand of methyl hydroxybenzoate.

Other Proprietary Names

Methyl Chemosept *(USA).*

6652-g

Monothioglycerol *(U.S.N.F.).* α-Monothioglycerol; Thioglycerol. 3-Mercaptopropane-1,2-diol.
$C_3H_8O_2S=108.2$.

CAS — 96-27-5.

Pharmacopoeias. In *U.S.N.F.*

A colourless or pale yellow, viscous, hygroscopic liquid with a slight odour of sulphide. It contains not more than 5% of water. Specific gravity 1.241 to 1.250. Freely **soluble** in water; miscible with alcohol; practically insoluble in ether. Monothioglycerol is unstable in alkaline solutions. A 10% solution in water has a pH of 3.5 to 7. **Store** in airtight containers.

Monothioglycerol is used as an antoxidant.

6653-q

Nordihydroguaiaretic Acid. Acidum Nordihydroguaiareticum; NDGA. 4,4′-(2,3-Dimethyltetramethylene)bis(benzene-1,2-diol).
$C_{18}H_{22}O_4=302.4$.

CAS — 500-38-9.

Pharmacopoeias. In *Nord.*

A white to greyish-white crystalline powder. M.p. about 184°.

Practically **insoluble** in water; slightly soluble in hot water; soluble 1 in 4 of alcohol and 1 in 15 of ether; practically insoluble in light petroleum and toluene; practically insoluble in dilute acids but soluble in concentrated sulphuric acid; soluble in dilute alkalis, but the solution develops a bright red colour; soluble, at 30°, 1 in 140 of cottonseed oil and, at 45°, 1 in 200 of lard. **Incompatible** with alkalis and oxidising agents and discolours in the presence of metals. **Store** in airtight containers. Protect from light.

Adverse Effects. Nordihydroguaiaretic acid may occasionally cause contact dermatitis.

Background toxicological information.— *Fd Add. Ser. Wld Hlth Org. No. 5,* 1974.

Contact dermatitis due to nordihydroguaiaretic acid was reported in 6 patients and in 3 was connected with the use of a branded lanolin cream containing this antoxidant.— J. Roed-Petersen and N. Hjorth, *Br. J. Derm.,* 1976, *94,* 233.

Uses. Nordihydroguaiaretic acid has been used as an antoxidant for oils and fats at a concentration of up to 0.01%.

A review of the actions, uses, and toxicity of nordihydroguaiaretic acid.— E. P. Oliveto, *Chemy Ind.,* 1972, 677.

The available biological data were inadequate to evaluate its use as an antoxidant in food.— Seventeenth Report of the Joint FAO/WHO Expert Committee on Food Additives, *Tech. Rep. Ser. Wld Hlth Org. No. 539,* 1974.

6654-p

Octyl Gallate *(B.P.).* Octyl Gall. Octyl 3,4,5-trihydroxybenzoate.
$C_{15}H_{22}O_5=282.3$.

CAS — 1034-01-1.

Pharmacopoeias. In *Br.*

A white or creamy-white, odourless, tasteless powder. M.p. 100° to 102°.

Practically **insoluble** in water; soluble 1 in 2.5 of alcohol, 1 in 1 of acetone, 1 in 30 of chloroform, 1 in 3 of ether, 1 in 0.7 of methyl alcohol, 1 in 7 of propylene glycol, 1 in 4 of castor oil, and 1 in 33 of arachis oil. **Incompatible** with iron salts. **Store** in airtight containers and avoid contact with metals. Protect from light.

Effect of gamma-irradiation. The active oxygen number increased on storage in cod-liver oil containing octyl gallate 0.5% following irradiation, suggesting that the antoxidant action had been destroyed.— *The Use of Gamma Radiation Sources for the Sterilisation of Pharmaceutical Products,* London, ABPI, 1960.

For the general properties and uses of the alkyl gallates, see p.1282.

Background toxicological information.— *Fd Add. Ser. Wld Hlth Org. No. 4,* 1972; ibid., *No. 5,* 1974..

Temporary estimated acceptable daily intake: up to 200 μg per kg body-weight as dodecyl, octyl, or propyl gallate or their sum. Octyl gallate should not be used in beverages.— Twentieth Report of the Joint FAO/WHO Expert Committee on Food Additives, *Tech. Rep. Ser. Wld Hlth Org. No. 599,* 1976.

Proprietary Preparations

Progallin O *(Nipa, UK).* A brand of octyl gallate.

6655-s

Pentachlorophenol. PCP.
C_6HCl_5O=266.3.

CAS — 87-86-5.

White crystals with a characteristic odour. M.p. about 191°. Very slightly **soluble** in water; freely soluble in alcohol, ether, and sodium hydroxide solution. **Store** in airtight containers. Protect from light.

Adverse Effects and Treatment. As for Dinitrophenol Insecticides, p.831. The fatal dose in man is about 1 g. Pentachlorophenol and its aqueous solutions are irritant to the eyes, mucous membranes, and to the skin and may produce caustic burns.

Maximum permissible atmospheric concentration 0.5 mg per m^3.

Nine cases of pentachlorophenol poisoning, 2 of them fatal, occurred in a nursery for newborn babies. Symptoms included profuse diaphoresis, increased respiration, and metabolic acidosis, but these disappeared within hours of exchange transfusions. The poisoning was traced to the laundry, where an anti-mildew product containing sodium pentachlorophenate 22.9% and triclocarban 4% was being added to the last rinse of the nappy wash at 3 to 4 times the recommended concentration.— *Can. med. Ass. J.*, 1968, *98*, 424.

Further reports of poisoning by pentachlorophenol.— H. Bergner *et al.*, *Can. med. Ass. J.*, 1965, *92*, 448; J. B. Chapman and P. Robson, *Lancet*, 1965, *1*, 1266; M. A. D. Crawford (letter), *Lancet*, 1966, *1*, 875.

A pharmacokinetic study of poisoning with pentachlorophenol in an elderly patient suggested that forced diuresis was the treatment of preference in adults.— J. F. Young and T. J. Haley, *Clin. Toxicol.*, 1978, *12*, 41.

Aplastic anaemia due to pentachlorophenol.— H. J. Roberts (letter), *New Engl. J. Med.*, 1981, *305*, 1650.

Carcinogenicity. Hodgkin's disease and, possibly, nasal cancer among workers in the wood industry might be associated with exposure to chemical preservatives, notably pentachlorophenol.— M. H. Greene *et al.* (letter), *Lancet*, 1978, *2*, 626.

Malignant lymphoma of the histiocytic type in one patient exposed to pentachlorophenol and in 3 exposed to parachlorophenol.— L. Hardell (letter), *Lancet*, 1979, *1*, 55.

Absorption and Fate. Pentachlorophenol may be absorbed after ingestion or inhalation or through the skin. Following ingestion the majority of a dose is eliminated in the urine within 7 days as unchanged pentachlorophenol and its glucuronide with small amounts appearing in the faeces.

The pharmacokinetics and metabolism of pentachlorophenol were determined in 4 healthy male subjects after ingestion of 100 µg per kg body-weight. The dynamics of absorption and elimination could be described by a one-compartment open-system model with first-order absorption, enterohepatic circulation, and first-order elimination. The half-lives for absorption and elimination from plasma were 1.3 and 30.2 hours respectively. About 74 and 12% of the doses were eliminated in the urine as pentachlorophenol and its glucuronide , respectively, within 168 hours of ingestion. About 4% appeared in the faeces. The maximum plasma concentration obtained was 248 ng per ml. A simulation of repeated daily ingestion of 100 µg per kg indicated that pentachlorophenol would not cause cumulative toxicity even with repeated daily low-level exposures.— W. H. Braun *et al.*, *Toxic. appl. Pharmac.*, 1978, *45*, 278.

Uses. Pentachlorophenol has been used mainly as the sodium salt (C_6Cl_5NaO = 288.3), as a preservative for a wide range of industrial and agricultural products, including woods, textiles, glues and starch. It has also been used for the control of slime and algae.

A review of antimicrobial agents, including pentachlorophenol, used in cosmetics.— I. R. Gucklhorn, *Mfg Chem.*, 1970, *41* (Oct.), 49.

References to the use of pentachlorophenol or its sodium salt as a molluscicide.— L. S. Ritchie and L. A. Berríos-Durán, *Bull. Wld Hlth Org.*, 1969, *40*, 471; L. S. Ritchie *et al.*, *ibid.*, 474; *Tech. Rep. Ser. Wld Hlth Org. No. 515*, 1973.; J. V. Toledo *et al.*, *Bull. Wld Hlth Org.*, 1976, *54*, 421; *Tech. Rep. Ser. Wld Hlth Org. No. 643*, 1980..

Sodium pentachlorophenate was formerly marketed in Great Britain under the proprietary name Santobrite (*Monsanto*)..

6656-w

Phenethyl Alcohol. Phenylethyl Alcohol *(U.S.P., B.P.C. 1963)*; Phenethanolum; Benzyl Carbinol. 2-Phenylethanol.
$C_6H_5.CH_2.CH_2OH$=122.2.

CAS — 60-12-8.

Pharmacopoeias. In *Nord.* and *U.S.*

A colourless liquid with a rose-like odour and a sharp burning taste. Specific gravity 1.017 to 1.020.
Soluble 1 in 60 of water, 1 in less than 1 of alcohol, chloroform, ether, benzyl benzoate, and diethyl phthalate; slightly soluble in liquid paraffin; very soluble in glycerol, propylene glycol, and fixed oils. **Store** in a cool place in airtight containers. Protect from light.

Effect of gamma-irradiation. A study of the effect of gamma-irradiation on aqueous solutions of phenethyl alcohol.— T. J. McCarthy, *Pharm. Weekbl. Ned.*, 1978, *113*, 698.

Haemolysis. Total haemolysis occurred when erythrocytes were cultured for 45 minutes in a 0.8% solution of phenethyl alcohol in sodium chloride injection. Only slight haemolysis occurred when the strength was reduced to 0.65%.— H. C. Ansel and D. E. Cadwallader, *J. pharm. Sci.*, 1964, *53*, 169.

Sorption. There was no loss by adsorption when 30 ml of a 0.5% solution of phenethyl alcohol was filtered through sintered glass, unglazed porcelain candle, asbestos pad, or membrane filter.— N. T. Naido *et al.*, *Aust. J. pharm. Sci.*, 1972, *1*, 16.

Uses. Phenethyl alcohol has antimicrobial properties and is more active against Gram-negative than Gram-positive organisms. It is used as a preservative in ophthalmic solutions at a concentration of 0.25 to 0.5%, usually in conjunction with another bactericide. It is also used in flavouring essences and perfumes.

Antimicrobial action. Heating at 100° for 30 minutes at pH 5 with phenethyl alcohol 0.6% was ineffective in killing the spores of *Bacillus stearothermophilus*.— R. A. Anderson, *J. Hosp. Pharm.*, 1969, *26*, 48.

Solutions of fluorescein sodium 2% inoculated with *Pseudomonas aeruginosa* were sterile within 3 hours in the presence of phenylmercuric nitrate 0.002% and within 1 hour when phenethyl alcohol 0.4% was also present.— R. M. E. Richards *et al.*, *J. Pharm. Pharmac.*, 1969, *21*, 681.

In sterile ophthalmic solutions containing chlorhexidine acetate 0.01% as preservative, the time taken for the solution to become sterile after contamination with *Ps. aeruginosa* was reduced by the addition of phenethyl alcohol 0.4% from 60 to 15 minutes for pilocarpine hydrochloride solution and from 180 to 30 minutes for physostigmine salicylate solution. With phenylmercuric nitrate 0.002% as preservative the resterilisation time was reduced from 240 to 60 minutes for pilocarpine solution, from 24 hours to 90 minutes for atropine solution and from 90 to 45 minutes for physostigmine sulphate or salicylate solution. With benzalkonium chloride 0.01% the resterilisation time was reduced from 60 to 15 minutes for atropine solution but did not improve the times of 15 minutes for pilocarpine and physostigmine sulphate.— R. M. E. Richards and R. J. McBride, *J. Pharm. Pharmac.*, 1972, *24*, 145.

Phenethyl alcohol-resistant strains of *Ps. aeruginosa* were more sensitive to the actions of benzalkonium chloride, chlorhexidine acetate, and phenylmercuric nitrate than phenethyl alcohol-sensitive strains.— R. M. E. Richards and R. J. McBride, *J. pharm. Sci.*, 1972, *61*, 1075.

Phenethyl alcohol was found to be more effective than benzyl alcohol in inhibiting bacterial growth.— M. Lang and R. M. Rye, *J. Pharm. Pharmac.*, 1972, *24*, 219.

6657-e

Phenoxyethanol *(B.P.)*. Phenoxyaethanol; β-Phenoxyethyl Alcohol; Ethyleneglycol Monophenylether. 2-Phenoxyethanol.
$C_8H_{10}O_2$=138.2.

CAS — 122-99-6.

Pharmacopoeias. In *Br.*

A colourless slightly viscous liquid with a faint pleasant odour and a warm astringent taste. F.p. not lower than 12°. Wt per ml 1.105 to 1.11 g.
Soluble 1 in 43 of water, 1 in 50 of arachis oil and of olive oil; miscible with acetone, alcohol, and glycerol. Aqueous solutions are best prepared by shaking the phenoxyethanol in hot water until dissolved, cooling, and adjusting to volume. Solutions are **sterilised** by autoclaving or by filtration.
For precautions to be taken in preparing and storing antiseptic solutions, see under Phenol, p.570.

Uses. Phenoxyethanol has antibacterial properties and is effective against strains of *Pseudomonas aeruginosa* even in the presence of 20% serum. It is less effective against *Proteus vulgaris*, other Gram-negative organisms, and Gram-positive organisms. It has been used as a preservative at a concentration of 1%. A wider spectrum of antimicrobial activity is obtained with preservative mixtures of phenoxyethanol and hydroxybenzoates.
Phenoxyethanol may be used as a 2.2% solution or a 2% cream for the treatment of superficial wounds, burns, or abscesses infected by *Ps. aeruginosa*. In skin infections, derivatives of phenoxyethanol are used with either salicylic acid or zinc undecenoate.

Antimicrobial action. An evaluation of the mixture of phenoxyethanol and hydroxybenzoates (Phenonip) as a preservative.— J. E. Lucas and T. J. McCarthy, *Acta pharm. suec.*, 1970, *7*, 149.

A review of antimicrobial agents, including phenoxyethanol, used in cosmetics.— I. R. Gucklhorn, *Mfg Chem.*, 1970, *41* (Jan.), 42.

A study of the bactericidal and fungicidal activity of 1-phenoxypropan-2-ol (Propylene Phenoxetol) alone or together with benzalkonium chloride.— O. G. Clausen and I. K. Hegna, *Meddr norsk farm. Selsk.*, 1977, *39*, 197.

A solution of phenoxyethanol 2% was more active than Resiguard or chlorhexidine gluconate against 5 different species of Gram-negative bacteria grown in urine. It was considered that chlorhexidine gluconate would not be effective for the prevention of infection and cross-infection in the urinary tract when Gram-negative organisms (especially *Providencia stuarti*) were involved; phenoxyethanol might be a suitable alternative but its lack of activity against Gram-positive organisms might necessitate its being used with another antibacterial agent.— B. Thomas *et al.*, *J. clin. Path.*, 1978, *31*, 929.

Preservatives for vaccines. A review of different preservative systems compatible with 2 multiple component vaccines with particular reference to the combined use of phenoxyethanol, neomycin and streptomycin.— J. Cameron, *Develop. biol. Stand.*, 1974, *24*, 155.

Proprietary Preparations of Phenoxyethanol and Related Compounds

Phenonip *(Nipa, UK)*. Contains phenoxyethanol in conjunction with esters of hydroxybenzoic acid.

Phenoxetol *(Nipa, UK)*. A brand of phenoxyethanol. The following related compounds are also available: **Para-Chloro-Phenoxetol** (2-*p*-chlorophenoxyethanol, $C_8H_9ClO_2$ = 172.6) and **Propylene Phenoxetol** (1-phenoxypropan-2-ol, $C_9H_{12}O_2$ = 152.2).

Phytocil Cream *(Rorer, UK)*. Contains 1-phenoxypropan-2-ol 2%, 2-*p*-chlorophenoxyethanol 1%, salicylic acid 1.5%, menthol 1%, and glycerol 7% in a nonionic basis. **Phytocil Powder** contains 1-phenoxypropan-2-ol 2%, 2-*p*-chlorophenoxyethanol 1%, and zinc undecenoate 5.8%. For fungous infections of the skin.

Other Proprietary Names of Phenoxyethanol
Lanohex *(Canad.)*.

6658-l

Phenylmercuric Acetate *(B.P.C. 1973, U.S.N.F.)*. Phenylmerc. Acet.; Phenylhydrargyri Acetas; PMA. (Acetato)phenylmercury.
$C_8H_8HgO_2$=336.7.

CAS — 62-38-4.

Pharmacopoeias. In *Aust.* and *Chin.* Also in *U.S.N.F.*

A white or creamy-white, odourless or almost odourless, crystalline powder or small prisms or leaflets with a weakly metallic astringent taste. M.p. 149° to 153°.
Slightly **soluble** in water; soluble 1 in 19 of acetone, and 1 in 220 of ether. **Incompatibilities** as for phenylmercuric nitrate. **Store** in airtight containers. Protect from light.
For precautions to be taken in preparing and storing antiseptic solutions, see under Phenol, p.570.

Sorption. Solutions containing phenylmercuric acetate lost more than 30% preservative potency after 2 weeks and 66% after 12 weeks when stored in natural or pigmented polyethylene containers.— L. Lachman, *Bull. parent. Drug Ass.*, 1968, *22*, 127.

Adverse Effects and Treatment. As for Phenylmercuric Nitrate, p.1289.

Phenylmercuric acetate was considered to be unsafe as an ingredient in vaginal contraceptives.— *Am. Pharm.*, 1978, *NS18* (Aug.), 23.

Allergy. References: J. Hartung, *Berufsdermatosen*, 1965, *13*, 116, per *Bull. Hyg., Lond.*, 1965, *40*, 933; A. A. Fisher *et al.*, *Archs Derm.*, 1971, *104*, 286; F. N. Marzulli and H. I. Maibach, *J. Soc. cosmet. Chem.*, 1973, *24*, 399.

Percutaneous intoxication by fungicides. Severe bullous eruptions of the hands occurred in 5 employees handling a mercurial fungicide containing 1.5% of mercury in the form of phenylmercuric acetate and ethylmercuric chloride. Increased salivation occurred in 2 patients and a rise in concentration of mercury in the urine to 250 and 760 µg per litre respectively.— B. Jovicic, *Ann. occup. Hyg.*, 1968, *11*, 305, per *Abstr. Hyg.*, 1970, *45*, 39.

Uses. Phenylmercuric acetate has the actions and uses of phenylmercuric nitrate, p.1289; since the acetate is the more soluble it may sometimes be preferred.

Phenylmercuric acetate was shown *in vitro* to have inhibited completely the growth of the yeast *Malassezia ovalis*, which was associated with dandruff.— J. Brotherton, *Br. J. Derm.*, 1968, *80*, 749.

The MICs of phenylmercuric acetate against *Pseudomonas aeruginosa* and *Staphylococcus aureus* were 12 and 0.5 µg per ml respectively.— A. E. Elkhouly and R. T. Yousef, *J. pharm. Sci.*, 1974, *63*, 681.

For a report of phenylmercuric acetate enhancing the antimicrobial activity of hexachlorophane, see Hexachlorophane, p.566.

Spermicide. Necrospermia was found in all of 100 patients, 24 hours after they received an injection of 2 to 2.5 ml of an 0.04% solution of phenylmercuric acetate in each vas deferens during vasectomy.— J. V. Rico *et al.*, *Curr. ther. Res.*, 1979, *26*, 881.

Proprietary Names

Nylmerate Solution *(Irving, Austral.; Holland-Rantos, USA)*.

A preparation containing phenylmercuric acetate was formerly marketed in Great Britain under the proprietary name Volpar (*Duncan, Flockhart*).

6659-y

Phenylmercuric Borate. Phenylhydrargyri Boras; Hydrargyrum Phenyloboricum; Phenomerborum.
$C_6H_5.Hg.O.B(OH)_2,C_6H_5.Hg.OH = 633.2$.

CAS — 8017-88-7.

Pharmacopoeias. In *Aust., Belg., Cz., Hung., Jug., Swiss,* and *Turk.*

An equimolecular compound of phenylmercuric borate or metaborate and phenylmercuric hydroxide. It is a white odourless crystalline powder with a slightly metallic taste. M.p. about 177°. **Soluble** 1 in 300 of water, 1 in 100 of boiling water, 1 in 250 of alcohol and 1 in 50 of glycerol. A solution in water is neutral to litmus. **Store** in airtight containers and protect from light.

Adverse Effects and Treatment. As for Phenylmercuric Nitrate, p.1289.

An 18-month-old girl developed glycosuria, albuminuria, amino-aciduria, and impaired phosphate reabsorption following the application of a glycerinated solution of phenylmercuric borate to her gums for a period of 1 year. It was estimated that 320 mg of the organomercurial had been applied and mercury was excreted at a rate of 60 µg per day.— L. Rutzler, *Schweiz. med. Wschr.*, 1973, *103*, 678, per *Pharm. J.*, 1974, *1*, 471.

Phenylmercuric borate in soap was absorbed through the skin, metabolised, and excreted in the urine as inorganic mercury. Use of the soap an average of 60 times a day by nurses resulted in urinary mercury concentrations of 46 µg per litre.— M. N. Valloton and M. Lob, *Schweiz. med. Wschr.*, 1973, *103*, 1455, per *Abstr. Hyg.*, 1974, *49*, 365.

Uses. Phenylmercuric borate has actions and uses similar to those of phenylmercuric nitrate, p.1289.

The antimicrobial effects of phenylmercuric borate, alcohol 80 and 70%, and a quaternary ammonium compound (toloconium methylsulphate) were compared *in vitro* by agar diffusion and germ-holder tests. Against *Staphylococcus aureus*, phenylmercuric borate and the quaternary were both effective within 10 minutes; 80% alcohol had some effect and 70% alcohol was not effective. Against *Escherichia coli* only the phenylmercuric borate was effective within 10 minutes and 80% alcohol was only one-quarter as active.— M. Gaschen, *Pharm. Acta Helv.*, 1967, *42*, 365.

The MICs of phenylmercuric borate against *Pseudomonas aeruginosa* and *Staph. aureus* were 12 and 0.5 µg per ml respectively.— A. E. Elkhouly and R. T. Yousef, *J. pharm. Sci.*, 1974, *63*, 681.

Studies of the preservative properties of phenylmercuric borate in eye-drops against various bacteria indicated that the bactericidal activity of phenylmercuric borate was too weak for it to be a good preservative. Doubling the concentration of phenylmercuric borate from 0.002% to 0.004% had little effect on its activity.— T. F. J. Tromp *et al.*, *Pharm. Weekbl. Ned.*, 1977, *112*, 441; *idem*, 461.

Proprietary Names

Exomycol *(Geigy, Arg.; Zyma-Galen, Belg.; Zyma, Ger.; Zyma, S.Afr.)*; Gyne-Merfen *(Zyma, Ger.)*; Glycero-Merfen *(Zyma, Ger.)*; Hydro-Mercuryl *(Streuli, Switz.)*; Hydro-Merfen *(Zyma, Ger.; Zyma, Switz.)*; Mercuryl-Orange *(Streuli, Switz.)*; Merfen *(Zyma-Galen, Belg.; Zyma, Ger.; Zyma, Switz.)*; Merfène *(Riker, Fr.)*; Septiféne *(Syntex, Switz.)*; Spersasept *(Dispersa, Switz.)*.

6660-g

Phenylmercuric Nitrate *(B.P., U.S.N.F.)*.

Phenylmerc. Nit.; Phenylhydrargyri Nitras; PMN; Nitrato Fenilmercúrico. A basic phenylmercuric nitrate.
$C_6H_5.Hg.OH,C_6H_5.Hg.NO_3 = 634.4$.

CAS — 55-68-5 ($C_6H_5HgNO_3$).

Pharmacopoeias. In *Br., Braz., Ind., Int., Nord., Port., Swiss,* and *Turk.* Also in *U.S.N.F.*

Odourless white lustrous plates or crystalline powder with a weakly metallic and astringent taste. M.p. about 188° with decomposition.

Very slightly **soluble** in water; soluble 1 in 1000 of alcohol; more soluble in glycerol and fixed oils; more soluble in the presence of nitric acid or alkali hydroxide; slowly soluble 1 in 100 of propylene glycol. A solution in water has a pH of about 4.2.

Incompatible with halides with which it forms less soluble halogen compounds; on standing, solutions are liable to deposit metallic mercury and they should not be used when a precipitate is present. It is also incompatible with aluminium and other metals, ammonia and ammonium salts, and with some sulphur compounds (e.g. in rubber); its activity may be reduced in the presence of anionic emulsifying and suspending agents. **Store** in airtight containers. Protect from light.

For precautions to be taken in preparing and storing antiseptic solutions, see under Phenol, p.570.

For a note on the incompatibility of mercurials with aluminium and steel, see under Mercuric Chloride, p.939.

Inactivation. The antibacterial activity of phenylmercuric nitrate solutions was reduced by the addition of disodium edetate, and also by the addition of sodium thiosulphate.— R. M. E. Richards and J. M. E. Reary, *J. Pharm. Pharmac.*, 1972, *24, Suppl.*, 84P.

Aluminium magnesium silicate, bentonite, and magnesium trisilicate reduced the antibacterial activity of phenylmercuric nitrate against *Staphylococcus aureus* by more than 60%, while starch, talc, and kaolin reduced it by more than 30%.— R. T. Yousef *et al.*, *Can. J. pharm. Sci.*, 1973, *8*, 54.

Sorption. About 50 pharmaceutical specialities available in Sweden and containing organic mercurials were examined for loss of mercury. The mercury content was low in the products packed in polyethylene containers or in glass bottles with rubber closures. In bottles with non-rubber closures there was usually no loss or an overage of mercurial. The losses were due to adsorption into the plastic or rubber.— K. Eriksson, *Acta pharm. suec.*, 1967, *4*, 261.

Even without heat treatment there was considerable loss of phenylmercuric nitrate from solutions in eye-drop bottles with dropper units of either silicone rubber or nylon.— R. Kvamme and E. Steinnes, *Norg. Apotekerforen. Tidsskr.*, 1968, *76*, 261.

Silicone rubber teats removed up to 38% of phenylmercuric nitrate from a 0.004% solution during autoclaving. The same teats were assembled into eye-dropper units containing 10 ml of phenylmercuric nitrate 0.002% solution, and autoclaved. After 7 weeks, the percentage phenylmercuric nitrate lost from solution was less than from the 0.004% solution and greater from eye-drop bottles stored in the inverted position than in the upright position.— Pharm. Soc. Lab. Rep. No. P/69/26, 1969. See also K. Christensen and E. Dauv, *J. mond. Pharm.*, 1969, *12*, 5.

The losses by adsorption of phenylmercuric nitrate from 30 ml of 0.002% aqueous solution filtered through sintered glass, unglazed porcelain candle, asbestos pad, or membrane filter were 7.2, 100, 9, and 13% respectively. In 0.2M acetate buffer (pH 5.9) the respective losses were 2.3, 62, 11, and 3.3%. In aqueous solution with disodium edetate 0.1% the respective losses were 1.9, 77, 39, and 4%.— N. T. Naido *et al.*, *Aust. J. pharm. Sci.*, 1972, *1*, 16.

Adverse Effects and Treatment. As for Mercury, pp.937-8.

Phenylmercuric nitrate is irritant to the skin and may given rise to erythema and blistering 6 to 12 hours later. Hypersensitivity reactions have been reported.

Effect on the eyes. A cataractous lens showing the appearance of mercurialentis was removed from a patient who had used eye-drops containing 0.004% of phenylmercuric nitrate thrice daily for 4 years. It contained 1.08 ppm of mercury compared with 0.03 and 0.08 ppm respectively in 2 other lenses removed from patients because of cataracts.— J. D. Abrams and V. Majzout, *Br. J. Ophthal.*, 1970, *54*, 59.

A report of primary atypical band keratopathy in 48 patients who had used pilocarpine eye-drops containing phenylmercuric nitrate.— R. E. Kennedy *et al.*, *Trans. Am. ophthal. Soc.*, 1974, *72*, 107.

For a study into the penetration of organic mercurials into the eye, see Thiomersal, p.576.

Further references: J. D. Abrams, *Trans. ophthal. Soc. U.K.*, 1963, *83*, 263 (mercurialentis); L. K. Garron *et al.*, *Trans. Am. ophthal. Soc.*, 1976, *74*, 295 (mercurialentis).

Precautions. Eye-drops containing phenylmercuric nitrate as a preservative should not be used for prolonged periods.

For reports of various compounds reducing the antibacterial activity of phenylmercuric nitrate, see above.

Uses. Phenylmercuric nitrate has antibacterial and antifungal properties. Like other organic mercurial compounds it is bacteriostatic rather than bactericidal. Its activity is not appreciably affected by acidity or alkalinity but is reduced in the presence of body fluids.

Phenylmercuric nitrate is employed as a preservative for injection solutions in a concentration of 0.001% and for sterilisation by heating with a bactericide a concentration of 0.002% is used. It should not be included in solutions for intrathecal, intracisternal, or peridural injection, or for intravenous injection solutions where the dose exceeds 15 ml. As a preservative for some eye-drops, concentrations of 0.002% are used.

Phenylmercuric nitrate is also spermicidal and is used in some chemical contraceptives. The spermicidal activity is much reduced in a vaginal environment with a pH greater than 7.2.

The use of phenylmercuric compounds in cosmetics and toiletries is restricted in Great Britain under the Cosmetic Products Regulations 1978 (SI 1978: No. 1354).

Heating at 100° for 30 minutes at pH 5 with phenylmercuric nitrate 0.002% was not an effective method of sterilising a suspension of 2×10^4 spores per ml of *Bacillus stearothermophilus.* Heating at 100° in acetate buffer at pH 4 in the absence of phenylmercuric nitrate was more effective than heating at pH 5 or more in the presence of phenylmercuric nitrate.— R. A. Anderson, *J. Hosp. Pharm.*, 1969, *26*, 48.

A solution containing phenylmercuric nitrate 0.002% and sodium metabisulphite 0.1% was more active against *Pseudomonas aeruginosa* at an acid pH but less active at an alkaline pH than phenylmercuric nitrate alone.— R. M. E. Richards *et al.* (letter), *J. Pharm. Pharmac.*, 1972, *24*, 999.

The MICs of phenylmercuric nitrate against *Ps. aeruginosa* and *Staphylococcus aureus* were 12 and 0.5 µg per ml respectively.— A. E. Elkhouly and R. T. Yousef, *J. pharm. Sci.*, 1974, *63*, 681.

For a report of the enhancement of the action of phenylmercuric nitrate as a preservative, see Phenethyl Alcohol, p.1288.

Spermicide. At examination up to 2 to 3 weeks after receiving an injection of 2.5 ml of a 0.02% solution of phenylmercuric nitrate in the lumen of each vas deferens during vasectomy, 83 of 91 patients showed azoospermia or non-motile sperm. All the patients were azoospermic 3 months after the operation.— P. B. Ruch, *Aust. J. Hosp. Pharm.*, 1978, *8*, 16. See also D. W. Hamilton, *Med. J. Aust.*, 1977, *1*, 402; *idem*, *2*, 34.

Preparations

Phenylmercuric Nitrate Ear Drops *(A.P.F.)*. Aurist. PMN. Phenylmercuric nitrate 100 mg, propylene glycol 50 ml, freshly boiled and cooled water to 100 ml. Protect from light. Sensitisation has been reported after topical use of mercurials.

Phenylmercuric Nitrate Gel *(A.P.F.)*. See under Tragacanth, p.963.

6661-q

o-Phenylphenol. 2-Hydroxybiphenyl; *o*-Hydroxydiphenyl.

$C_{12}H_{10}O=170.2$.

CAS — 90-43-7.

A white crystalline free-flowing powder with a mildly phenolic odour. M.p. about 57°. **Soluble** 1 in 1000 of water; very soluble in most organic solvents; soluble in oils and fats.

o-Phenylphenol has antibacterial and antifungal properties and has many industrial uses as a preservative for a wide range of materials, particularly against moulds and rots. Its antimicrobial properties are similar to those of chloroxylenol (see p.558) and it is used in disinfectants; it is more active than chloroxylenol against *Pseudomonas aeruginosa*. It is used as a preservative on citrus fruits.

Maximum acceptable daily intake of *o*-phenylphenol: 1 mg per kg body-weight.— Report of the 1972 Joint FAO/WHO Meeting on Pesticide Residues in Food, *Tech. Rep. Ser. Wld Hlth Org. No. 525*, 1973.

Effect of gamma-irradiation. A study of the effect of gamma-irradiation on aqueous solutions of *o*-phenylphenol.— T. J. McCarthy, *Pharm. Weekbl. Ned.*, 1978, *113*, 698.

6662-p

Potassium Metabisulphite. Kalii Metabisulfis; Potassium Pyrosulphite; Potasio Metabisulfito.

$K_2S_2O_5=222.3$.

CAS — 4429-42-9; 16731-55-8.

White crystals or crystalline powder with a sulphurous odour. It is oxidised to sulphate in moist air. **Soluble** 1 in 2 of water forming an acid solution; practically insoluble in alcohol. With acids, sulphur dioxide is liberated. It may catch fire on trituration. **Incompatible** with oxidising agents.

Potassium metabisulphite has the actions and uses of sodium metabisulphite (see p.1291). It has been used in the Campden process for preserving fruit.

Estimated acceptable daily intake of potassium metabisulphite (as SO_2): up to 700 µg per kg body-weight.— Seventeenth Report of the Joint FAO/WHO Expert Committee on Food Additives, *Tech. Rep. Ser. Wld Hlth Org. No. 539*, 1974.

Background toxicological information.— *Fd Add. Ser. Wld Hlth Org. No. 5*, 1974.

6663-s

Potassium Sorbate *(B.P., U.S.N.F.)*. Potassium (*E,E*)-hexa-2,4-dienoate.

$C_6H_7KO_2=150.2$.

CAS — 590-00-1; 24634-61-5.

Pharmacopoeias. In *Br.* and *It.* Also in *U.S.N.F.*

White or creamy-white crystals or powder with a faint characteristic odour. M.p. about 270° with decomposition.

Soluble 1 in less than 1 of water and 1 in 70 of alcohol; soluble in propylene glycol; very slightly soluble in acetone, chloroform, and ether, and in fats and oils. A solution in water is neutral to litmus. **Store** in a cool place in airtight containers. Protect from light.

Potassium sorbate has the actions and uses of sorbic acid (see p.1292) but is more soluble in water.

Estimated acceptable daily intake: up to 25 mg per kg body-weight, as the sum of sorbic acid and its calcium, potassium, and sodium salts.— Seventeenth Report of the Joint FAO/WHO Expert Committee on Food Additives, *Tech. Rep. Ser. Wld Hlth Org. No. 539*, 1974.

Background toxicological information.— *Fd Add. Ser. Wld Hlth Org. No. 5*, 1974.

Proprietary Preparations

Sorbistat-K *(Pfizer, UK)*. A brand of potassium sorbate.

6664-w

Propyl Gallate *(B.P., U.S.N.F.)*. Propyl Gall.; Propylum Gallicum; Propylis Gallas. Propyl 3,4,5-trihydroxybenzoate.

$C_{10}H_{12}O_5=212.2$.

CAS — 121-79-9.

Pharmacopoeias. In *Aust.*, *Belg.*, *Br.*, *Cz.*, and *Nord.* Also in *U.S.N.F.*

A white to creamy-white crystalline powder, odourless or with a faint odour, and with a slightly bitter taste. M.p. 146° to 151°.

Soluble 1 in 1000 of water, 1 in 3 of alcohol, 1 in 3 of ether, 1 in 3 of propylene glycol, and 1 in 2000 of arachis oil. **Incompatible** with alkalis and iron salts. **Store** in airtight containers and avoid contact with metals. Protect from light.

The solubility of ethyl gallate, methyl gallate, and propyl gallate in macrogols and in solutions of macrogol ether surfactants.— L. S. C. Wan, *Can. J. pharm. Sci.*, 1972, *7*, 25.

For the general properties and uses of the alkyl gallates, see p.1282.

Background toxicological information.— *Fd Add. Ser. Wld Hlth Org. No. 5*, 1974.

Temporary estimated acceptable daily intake: up to 200 µg per kg body-weight as dodecyl, octyl, or propyl gallate or their sum.— Twentieth Report of the Joint FAO/WHO Expert Committee on Food Additives, *Tech. Rep. Ser. Wld Hlth Org. No. 599*, 1976.

Hypersensitivity. Contact dermatitis occurred in 5 of 10 people following topical application of propyl gallate for about 20 days.— G. Kahn *et al.*, *Archs Derm.*, 1974, *109*, 506, per *J. Am. med. Ass.*, 1974, *228*, 520.

Sunscreen agent. Propyl gallate was an effective sunscreen agent but caused sensitisation.— G. Kahn and M. C. Curry, *Archs Derm.*, 1974, *109*, 510, per *Int. pharm. Abstr.*, 1975, *12*, 980.

Proprietary Preparations

Progallin P *(Nipa, UK)*. A brand of propyl gallate.

Tenox PG *(Eastman, UK)*. A brand of propyl gallate.

Tenox S-1 contains propyl gallate 20% and citric acid monohydrate 10% in propylene glycol.

For other preparations containing propyl gallate in mixtures with other antoxidants, see under Butylated Hydroxyanisole, p.1285.

6665-e

Propyl Hydroxybenzoate *(B.P.)*. Propyl Hydroxybenz.; Propyl Parahydroxybenzoate *(Eur. P.)*; Propylis Parahydroxybenzoas; Propylparaben *(U.S.N.F.)*; Propylis Oxybenzoas; Propylis Paraoxibenzoas; Propagin. Propyl *p*-hydroxybenzoate.

$C_{10}H_{12}O_3=180.2$.

CAS — 94-13-3.

Pharmacopoeias. In *Aust.*, *Belg.*, *Br.*, *Braz.*, *Cz.*, *Eur.*, *Fr.*, *Ger.*, *Hung.*, *Ind.*, *It.*, *Jap.*, *Jug.*, *Mex.*, *Neth.*, *Nord.*, *Pol.*, *Roum.*, and *Swiss.* Also in *U.S.N.F.*

Colourless crystals or a white crystalline powder, odourless or with a faintly aromatic odour; it is tasteless but numbs the tongue. M.p. 95° to 98°.

Soluble 1 in 2500 of cold water, 1 in 400 of boiling water, 1 in 3.5 of alcohol, 1 in 3 of acetone, 1 in 4 of chloroform, 1 in 3 of ether, 1 in 140 of glycerol, 1 in 6 of propylene glycol, and 1 in 40 of fixed oils; freely soluble in methyl alcohol; readily soluble in solutions of alkali hydroxides. **Incompatible** with alkalis and iron salts.

The solubility of propyl hydroxybenzoate in a variety of aliphatic alcohols over a temperature range of 25 to 40°.— K. S. Alexander *et al.*, *J. pharm. Sci.*, 1977, *66*, 42.

For the general properties and uses of the hydroxybenzoates, see p.1282.

Estimated acceptable daily intake of propyl hydroxybenzoate: up to 10 mg per kg body-weight, as the sum of ethyl, methyl, and propyl hydroxybenzoates.— Seventeenth Report of the Joint FAO/WHO Expert Committee on Food Additives, *Tech. Rep. Ser. Wld Hlth Org. No. 539*, 1974.

Background toxicological information.— *Fd Add. Ser. Wld Hlth Org. No. 5*, 1974.

Proprietary Preparations

Nipasol M *(Nipa, UK)*. A brand of propyl hydroxybenzoate.

6666-l

Sodium Benzoate *(B.P., U.S.N.F.)*. Sod. Benz.; Sodii Benzoas; Natrii Benzoas; Natrium Benzoicum.

$C_6H_5.CO_2Na=144.1$.

CAS — 532-32-1.

Pharmacopoeias. In all pharmacopoeias examined except *Eur.*, *Fr.*, *Ger.*, and *Int.*

A white, amorphous, granular, flaky or crystalline powder; odourless or with a faint odour of benzoin, and an unpleasant, sweetish, saline taste. **Soluble** 1 in 2 of water, 1 in 90 of alcohol, 1 in 10 of glycerol. A 2.25% solution in water is iso-osmotic with serum. Solutions are **sterilised** by autoclaving or by filtration. **Incompatible** with acids, ferric salts, calcium salts, and salts of heavy metals.

Adverse Effects. As for Benzoic Acid, p.1283.

Kernicterus. Sodium benzoate in caffeine and sodium benzoate injection could uncouple bilirubin from its albumin binding sites, which might induce kernicterus. Such injections should be administered with caution, if at all, to neonates with raised bilirubin concentrations.— D. Schiff *et al.*, *Pediatrics*, 1971, *48*, 139.

The concentration of sodium benzoate in Valium injection was not considered high enough to cause neonatal hyperbilirubinaemia following administration of 10 to 20 mg diazepam (with 100 to 200 mg sodium benzoate contained in the solvent) by intramuscular injection to the mother during labour.— R. Stockmann *et ql.*, *J. int. med. Res.*, 1978, *6*, 468.

Absorption and Fate. As for Benzoic Acid, p.1283.

Uses. Sodium benzoate has the actions and uses of benzoic acid and is sometimes used as a preservative in place of benzoic acid because of its greater solubility in water. However, its activity is dependent on the concentration of undissociated benzoic acid achieved and it is not very effective above pH 5. It is also used as a corrosion inhibitor in storage solutions for surgical instruments.

Although sodium benzoate is less irritant to the gastric mucosa than benzoic acid it should not be taken on an empty stomach. It was formerly used in a dosage of 0.3 to 2 g as a urinary antiseptic but it has been superseded by more effective agents.
Because of its excretion as hippuric acid, sodium benzoate is employed in a test for liver function. For this test, 6 g dissolved in 200 ml of water is given by mouth; the hippuric acid content of the urine in the following 4 hours is usually 2.5 g or more. The test may also be carried out by the intravenous injection of 1.8 g of sodium benzoate dissolved in 20 ml of Water for Injections; 1 g or more of hippuric acid is normally excreted in the urine in 1 hour. In hepatic dysfunction, excretion of hippuric acid is usually reduced.

Estimated acceptable daily intake: up to 5 mg per kg body-weight, as the sum of benzoic acid and its potassium and sodium salts.— Seventeenth Report of the Joint FAO/WHO Expert Committee on Food Additives, *Tech. Rep. Ser. Wld Hlth Org. No. 539,* 1974.

For background toxicological information, see *Fd Add. Ser. Wld Hlth Org. No. 5,* 1974.

Hyperammonaemia. Administration of sodium benzoate 6.25 g daily for 11 days lowered plasma concentrations of ammonium and increased urinary nitrogen excretion in a 17-year-old patient with a deficiency of carbamyl phosphate synthetase. Glycine concentrations in plasma remained normal during treatment. Subsequently, administration of a single dose of sodium benzoate 250 to 350 mg per kg body-weight produced a fall in plasma ammonium and clinical improvement in 4 patients (aged 11 months to 18 years) in hyperammonaemic coma.— S. Brusilow *et al., Science,* 1980, *207,* 659.

Nonketotic hyperglycinaemia. For a report of administration of strychnine as an adjunct to sodium benzoate in the treatment of nonketotic hyperglycinaemia, see Strychnine Hydrochloride, p.320.

Preparations

Mouthwash Solution-Tablets *(B.P.).* Solvellae pro Collutorio; Solv. pro Collut.; Effervescing Mouthwash Tablets. Sodium benzoate, menthol and other aromatics in an effervescent basis. One tablet should be dissolved in 300 ml of warm water.
Store in airtight containers.

Sodium Benzoate and Chlorocresol Solution *(B.P.C. 1963).* Liq. Sod. Benz. et Chlorocresol.; Surgical Instrument Preservative Solution. Sodium benzoate 1.5 g, chlorocresol 200 mg, water to 100 ml. This solution is not intended for sterilising surgical instruments.

6667-y

Sodium Butyl Hydroxybenzoate *(B.P.).* Sodium Butylparaben. The sodium derivative of butyl *p*-hydroxybenzoate.
$C_{11}H_{13}NaO_3$=216.2.

CAS — 36457-20-2.

Pharmacopoeias. In *Br.*

A white odourless hygroscopic powder. **Soluble** 1 in 1 of water and 1 in 10 of alcohol. A 0.1% solution in water has a pH of 9.5 to 10.5. **Store** in airtight containers.

For the general properties and uses of the hydroxybenzoates, see p.1282.

Proprietary Preparations

Nipabutyl Sodium *(Nipa, UK).* A brand of sodium butyl hydroxybenzoate.

6668-j

Sodium Dehydroacetate *(U.S.N.F.).* The sodium salt of 3-acetyl-3,4-dihydro-6-methyl-2*H*-pyran-2,4-dione.
$C_8H_7NaO_4$=190.1.

CAS — 4418-26-2.

Pharmacopoeias. In *U.S.N.F.*

A white powder. It loses 8.5 to 10% of its weight when dried. **Soluble** in water.

Sodium dehydroacetate is used similarly to dehydroacetic acid (see p.1286).

6669-z

Sodium Diacetate. Sodium hydrogen diacetate.
$CH_3COONa,CH_3COOH(+xH_2O)$.

CAS — 126-96-5 (anhydrous).

A white hygroscopic crystalline powder, with an acetic odour. It may contain a slight excess of acetic acid or sodium acetate. **Soluble** 1 in 1 of water. A 10% solution has a pH of 4.5 to 5.

Sodium diacetate is used as an inhibitor of moulds and rope-forming micro-organisms in bread.

Estimated acceptable daily intake of sodium diacetate: up to 15 mg per kg body-weight.— Seventeenth Report of the Joint FAO/WHO Expert Committee on Food Additives, *Tech. Rep. Ser. Wld Hlth Org. No. 539,* 1974.

Background toxicological information.— *Fd Add. Ser. Wld Hlth Org. No. 5,* 1974.

6670-p

Sodium Ethyl Hydroxybenzoate. The sodium derivative of ethyl *p*-hydroxybenzoate.
$C_9H_9NaO_3$=188.2.

CAS — 35285-68-8.

A white hygroscopic crystalline powder. **Soluble** 1 in 2 of water and 1 in 3 of alcohol 50%. A 0.1% aqueous solution has a pH of 9.9 to 10.3. **Store** in airtight containers.

For the general properties and uses of the hydroxybenzoates, see p.1282.

Proprietary Preparations

Nipagin A Sodium *(Nipa, UK).* A brand of sodium ethyl hydroxybenzoate.

6671-s

Sodium Formaldehyde Sulphoxylate. Sodium Formaldehyde Sulfoxylate *(U.S.N.F.).* Sodium hydroxymethanesulphinate dihydrate.
$CH_3NaO_3S,2H_2O$=154.1.

CAS — 149-44-0 (anhydrous).

Pharmacopoeias. In *Fr.* Also in *U.S.N.F.*

White crystals or hard white masses with an alliaceous odour. M.p. 63° to 64°.
Soluble 1 in 3.4 of water, 1 in 510 of alcohol, 1 in 175 of chloroform, and 1 in 180 of ether. A 2% solution in water has a pH of 9.5 to 10.5. **Store** at 15° to 30°. Protect from light.

Sodium formaldehyde sulphoxylate is used as a preservative and antoxidant. It is used in the treatment of acute mercury poisoning (see p.938).

6672-w

Sodium Isoascorbate. Sodium Erythorbate. 3-Oxo-D-glucofuranolactone sodium enolate monohydrate.
$C_6H_7NaO_6,H_2O$=216.1.

CAS — 6381-77-7 (anhydrous).

A white, almost odourless, crystalline powder. **Soluble** 1 in 7 of water. A 10% solution in water has a pH of 5.5 to 8. **Store** in airtight containers. Protect from light.

Sodium isoascorbate is used as an antoxidant in the food industry.

A review of the uses and efficacy of sodium isoascorbate as an antioxidant and synergist. In practice ascorbic acid was more effective.— *Fd Add. Ser. Wld Hlth Org. No. 3,* 1972.

Estimated acceptable daily intake of sodium isoascorbate: up to 5 mg per kg body-weight.— Seventeenth Report of the Joint FAO/WHO Expert Committee on Food Additives, *Tech. Rep. Ser. Wld Hlth Org. No. 539,* 1974.

Background toxicological information.— *Fd Add. Ser. Wld Hlth Org. No. 5,* 1974.

6673-e

Sodium Metabisulphite *(B.P.).* Sodium Metabisulfite *(U.S.N.F.)*; Natrii Pyrosulfis; Disodium Pyrosulphite; Sodium Pyrosulphite; Natrium Pyrosulfurosum.
$Na_2S_2O_5$=190.1.

CAS — 7681-57-4; 7757-74-6.

Pharmacopoeias. In *Aust., Belg., Br., Chin., Cz., Hung., Ind., Int., Jap., Jug., Neth., Nord.,* and *Turk.* Also in *U.S.N.F.*
Jap. and *U.S.N.F.* also have Sodium Bisulfite, described as consisting of the acid sulphite ($NaHSO_3$ = 104.1) and the metabisulphite in varying proportions: *U.S.N.F.* specifies the equivalent of 58.5 to 67.4% of SO_2; *Jap.* specifies 64 to 67.4%. *Port. P.* and *Span. P.* have monographs for sodium bisulphite (Natrii Bisulfis, Bissulfito de Sódio, Natrii Sulphis Acidus) but this is probably the metabisulphite or a mixture of the bisulphite and the metabisulphite.
NOTE. The *U.S.N.F.* permits the use of sodium metabisulphite in place of sodium bisulphite.

Colourless prismatic crystals or a white or yellowish crystalline powder. It has a sulphurous odour and an acid saline taste. It contains not less than 95% of $Na_2S_2O_5$ and not less than 64% of SO_2. It usually contains small amounts of sodium sulphite and sodium sulphate. On exposure to air and moisture, it is slowly oxidised to sulphate with disintegration of the crystals.
Soluble 1 in 2 of water; freely soluble in alcohol; freely soluble in glycerol. A solution in water is acid to phenol red and has the odour of sulphur dioxide. A 1.38% solution in water is iso-osmotic with serum. **Incompatible** with oxidising agents and thiamine. **Store** at a temperature not exceeding 40° in well-filled airtight containers. Protect from light.

Studies of the stability and oxidation of sulphurous acid salts.— L. C. Schroeter, *J. pharm. Sci.,* 1963, *52,* 559; *idem,* 564; *idem,* 888.

Incompatibility. Sodium metabisulphite reacted with sympathomimetics and other drugs which were *o*- or *p*-hydroxybenzyl alcohol derivatives to form sulphonic acid derivatives possessing little or no activity. The most important drugs subject to this inactivating reaction were adrenaline and its derivatives. Sodium metabisulphite also inactivated chloramphenicol, but by a more complex reaction.— T. Higuchi and L. C. Schroeter, *J. Am. pharm. Ass., scient. Edn,* 1959, *48,* 535.

Adverse Effects. Gastric irritation due to liberation of sulphurous acid follows ingestion of sodium metabisulphite and other sulphites. Large doses of sulphites may cause collapse with respiratory or circulatory failure, and depression of the nervous system.
Concentrated solutions of salts of sulphurous acid are irritant to skin and mucous membranes and may occasionally cause dermatitis.
Treatment of foods with sulphites reduces their thiamine content.

A discussion of the possible mutagenicity of sulphurous acid salts.— G. Smith and M. F. G. Stevens, *Pharm. J.,* 1972, *2,* 570.

A report of toxicological studies.— *Fd Add. Ser. Wld Hlth Org. No. 5,* 1974.

Allergy. An urticarial reaction with difficulty in breathing and swallowing occurred in a 50-year-old man and was associated with ingestion of sodium bisulphite.— B. M. Prenner and J. J. Stevens, *Ann. Allergy,* 1976, *37,* 180.

Effect on food. Thiamine was destroyed by treatment with sulphites; foods that served as a significant source of thiamine, such as meat, cereals, dairy products, and nuts, should not therefore be treated with sulphites.— Sixth Report of FAO/WHO Expert Committee on Food Additives, *Tech. Rep. Ser. Wld Hlth Org. No. 228,* 1962.

Peritoneal absorption. The occurrence of toxic symptoms, typical of central nervous stimulation, following the intraperitoneal injection of dialysing fluids containing 7% of dextrose, was considered to be possibly due to sodium metabisulphite which was usually present in these solutions in a concentration of 0.05%. The intraperitoneal injection of this solution into 5 *rabbits* resulted in the death of 3 and examination of the tissues showed that appreciable absorption of metabisulphite had occurred, elimination having been slower than absorption. It was concluded that the use of sodium metabisulphite in peritoneal dialysis fluids, which might be given in large volumes, was dangerous and should be discontinued.— S. F. Halaby and A. M. Mattocks, *J. pharm. Sci.*, 1965, *54*, 52. *Animal* studies suggested that its incorporation in peritoneal dialysis fluids in concentrations up to 0.05% was unlikely to give rise to adverse effects in man, especially as less than 25% remained in dextrose solutions after autoclaving.— J. W. Wilkins *et al.*, *Clin. Pharmac. Ther.*, 1968, *9*, 328.

Absorption and Fate. Sulphites and metabisulphites are oxidised in the body to sulphate and excreted in the urine.

Uses. Sodium metabisulphite is a strong reducing agent widely used as an antoxidant in solutions especially those that contain drugs which are readily oxidised to form highly coloured decomposition products. It is often used in a concentration of 0.1% but concentrations of 0.01% to 1% have been employed. In the formulation of a pharmaceutical preparation, the minimum concentration should be chosen which will give the desired antoxidant effect. A chelating agent such as disodium edetate is sometimes added to sodium metabisulphite to remove heavy-metal ions which often catalyse autoxidation reactions.
Sodium metabisulphite is usually employed as an antoxidant in acid preparations; for alkaline preparations, sodium sulphite is usually preferred.
As an antoxidant, sodium metabisulphite has several disadvantages. It decomposes in air, especially on heating, and an appreciable amount may be lost during sterilisation before it has had time to exert its antoxidant effect; decomposition in solutions is accompanied by a fall in pH. Injections containing sodium metabisulphite should preferably be filled into containers in which the air has been replaced by an inert gas such as nitrogen. Since it may react with the rubber caps used to close multidose containers, the caps should be pretreated with sodium metabisulphite solution. Sodium metabisulphite may react, under certain conditions, with adrenaline and other drugs which are derivatives of *o*- or *p*-hydroxybenzyl alcohol, and with thiamine, dyes, and flavouring agents. Preparations containing sodium metabisulphite should therefore be thoroughly tested to determine its effect on the active constituents and other ingredients. At concentrations above about 500 ppm it imparts a noticeable taste to preparations.
Sodium metabisulphite is used as a preservative in acid solutions and syrups, its antimicrobial action being due to the presence of sulphur dioxide and sulphurous acid liberated by reaction between the metabisulphite and the acid. It is effective against most bacteria, fungi, and yeasts at acid pH in concentrations of 200 ppm or more.
Sodium metabisulphite is used in the food industry as an antimicrobial preservative and as an anti-browning agent. The Campden process for preserving fruit involves the bottling of the fruit in a cold solution of sodium metabisulphite and sealing the containers. Sodium metabisulphite is used as a reducing agent in photography.

Reviews of the uses of sodium metabisulphite, sodium sulphite, and other sulphurous acid salts as antoxidants.— L. C. Schroeter, *J. pharm. Sci.*, 1961, *50*, 891; L. C. Schroeter, *Sulfur Dioxide, Applications in Foods, Beverages, and Pharmaceuticals*, London, Pergamon Press, 1966; G. Smith and M. F. G. Stevens, *Pharm. J.*, 1972, *2*, 570.

Estimated acceptable daily intake of sodium metabisulphite (as SO_2): up to 700 µg per kg body-weight.— Seventeenth Report of the Joint FAO/WHO Expert Committee on Food Additives, *Tech. Rep. Ser. Wld Hlth Org. No. 539*, 1974.

Proprietary Preparations

Campden Fruit and Wine Preserving Tablets *(Cox, UK)*. Tablets of sodium metabisulphite each yielding at least 254 mg of available SO_2.

NOTE. Campden Tablets were conceived in England at the Chipping Campden Research Station and originally consisted of potassium metabisulphite. Each tablet then supplied 259 mg of available SO_2.— W. H. B. Denner, *MAFF, Personal Communication*, 1979.

6674-l

Sodium Methyl Hydroxybenzoate *(B.P.)*. Methyl. Hydroxybenz. Solub.; Soluble Methyl Hydroxybenzoate; Sodium Methylparaben. The sodium derivative of methyl *p*-hydroxybenzoate.
$C_8H_7NaO_3$=174.1.

CAS — 5026-62-0.

Pharmacopoeias. In *Br.*

A white, almost odourless, hygroscopic, crystalline powder; it is tasteless but produces a slight burning sensation of the mouth and tongue, followed by local numbness. **Soluble** 1 in 2 of water and 1 in 50 of alcohol; practically insoluble in fixed oils. A 0.1% solution has a pH of 9.5 to 10.5. **Store** in airtight containers.

For the general properties and uses of the hydroxybenzoates, see p.1282.

Proprietary Preparations

Nipagin M Sodium *(Nipa, UK)*. A brand of sodium methyl hydroxybenzoate.

6675-y

Sodium *o*-Phenylphenol. Sodium Biphenyl-2-yl Oxide. Sodium *o*-phenylphenolate tetrahydrate.
$C_{12}H_9NaO,4H_2O$=264.3.

CAS — 132-27-4 (anhydrous).

A buff-coloured flaked solid. Very **soluble** in water, alcohol, and acetone; soluble in propylene glycol; practically insoluble in hydrocarbons and oils. A 2% solution in water has a pH of about 11.

Sodium *o*-phenylphenol is used for similar purposes to *o*-phenylphenol, see p.1290.

Maximum acceptable daily intake of sodium *o*-phenylphenol expressed as *o*-phenylphenol: 1 mg per kg body-weight.— Report of the 1972 Joint FAO/WHO Meeting on Pesticide Residues in Food, *Tech. Rep. Ser. Wld Hlth Org. No. 525*, 1973.

6676-j

Sodium Propyl Hydroxybenzoate *(B.P.)*. Soluble Propyl Hydroxybenzoate; Sodium Propylparaben. The sodium derivative of propyl *p*-hydroxybenzoate.
$C_{10}H_{11}NaO_3$=202.2.

CAS — 35285-69-9.

Pharmacopoeias. In *Br.*

A white, odourless, tasteless, hygroscopic, crystalline powder. **Soluble** 1 in 1 of water, 1 in 50 of alcohol, and 1 in 2 of alcohol (50%); practically insoluble in fixed oils. A 0.1% solution in water has a pH of 9.5 to 10.5. **Store** in airtight containers.

For the general properties and uses of the hydroxybenzoates, see p.1282.

Proprietary Preparations

Nipasol M Sodium *(Nipa, UK)*. A brand of sodium propyl hydroxybenzoate.

6677-z

Sodium Sulphite *(B.P.C. 1973)*. Sod. Sulphite; Sodii Sulphis; Sulfito de Sódio.
$Na_2SO_3,7H_2O$=252.1.

CAS — 10102-15-5.

Pharmacopoeias. In *Port.*

Odourless or almost odourless, colourless, efflorescent crystals with a saline sulphurous taste, becoming opaque and slowly oxidised in air to sulphate.
Soluble 1 in 2 of water and 1 in 28 of glycerol; practically insoluble in alcohol. A solution in water is alkaline to litmus. On boiling a saturated aqueous solution, the anhydrous salt separates out as a crystalline powder which redissolves on cooling. **Incompatible** with most acids. **Store** in airtight containers.

Sodium sulphite is used as an antoxidant and antimicrobial preservative in alkaline preparations as described under Sodium Metabisulphite, p.1292.
Calcium sulphite is also used as a preservative.

Estimated acceptable daily intake of sodium sulphite (as SO_2): up to 700 µg per kg body-weight.— Seventeenth Report of the Joint FAO/WHO Expert Committee on Food Additives, *Tech. Rep. Ser. Wld Hlth Org. No. 539*, 1974.

Background toxicological information.— *Fd Add. Ser. Wld Hlth Org. No. 5*, 1974.

6678-c

Anhydrous Sodium Sulphite *(B.P.)*. Exsiccated Sodium Sulphite; Natrii Sulphis; Natrii Sulfis Siccatus; Sodium Sulfite; Sulfito Dissódico Sêco.
Na_2SO_3=126.0.

CAS — 7757-83-7.

Pharmacopoeias. In *Br.*, *Fr.*, *Jap.*, and *Span.*

A white odourless or almost odourless crystalline powder with a cooling, saline, sulphurous taste. It is slowly oxidised in air. **Soluble** 1 in 4 of water; practically insoluble in alcohol. Aqueous solutions are alkaline to litmus and to phenolphthalein. **Store** in airtight containers.

Anhydrous sodium sulphite has the same uses as sodium metabisulphite.

6679-k

Sorbic Acid *(B.P., U.S.N.F.)*. Acidum Sorbicum. (*E,E*)-Hexa-2,4-dienoic acid.
$C_6H_8O_2$=112.1.

CAS — 110-44-1; 22500-92-1.

Pharmacopoeias. In *Aust.*, *Belg.*, *Br.*, and *Cz.* Also in *U.S.N.F.*

A white or creamy-white crystalline powder with a faint characteristic odour and a slightly acid and astringent taste. M.p. 132° to 137°.
Soluble 1 in 700 of water, 1 in 30 of boiling water, 1 in 10 of alcohol, 1 in 7 of dehydrated alcohol, 1 in 16 of chloroform, 1 in 20 of ether, 1 in 300 of glycerol, 1 in 12 of isopropyl alcohol, 1 in 8 of methyl alcohol, 1 in 18 of propylene glycol, and about 1 in 150 of fats and fatty oils. **Store** in a cool place in airtight containers. Protect from light.

Solutions of sorbic acid 0.1% stored in polypropylene, polyvinyl chloride, polyethylene, or glass containers showed a marked loss of potency except when refrigerated or when an antoxidant such as sodium metabisulphite was also present.— T. J. McCarthy *et al.*, *Cosmet. Perfum.*, 1973, *88* (May), 43. See also T. J. McCarthy, *Pharm. Weekbl. Ned.*, 1972, *107*, 1.

Effect of gamma-irradiation. A study of the effect of gamma-irradiation on aqueous solutions of sorbic acid.— T. J. McCarthy, *Pharm. Weekbl. Ned.*, 1978, *113*, 698.

Adverse Effects. Sorbic acid is irritant to the eyes and possibly also to the skin.

Background toxicological information.— *Fd Add. Ser. Wld Hlth Org. No. 5*, 1974.

Uses. Sorbic acid has antibacterial and antifungal properties. It is active against moulds and yeasts and to a lesser degree against bacteria. It is not effective above about pH 6.5; the optimum pH is about 4.5. Its fungistatic activity is increased by the addition of acids and sodium chloride. It is used as a preservative in pharmaceutical and cosmetic preparations at a usual concentration of 0.1 to 0.2% and is sometimes preferred to other preservatives in preparations containing nonionic surfactants. It has been used in concentrations of up to 0.2% as a preservative in food and up to 0.3% in enzyme preparations and gelatin capsules. It has been reported to be a satisfactory preservative for mucilages of acacia and tragacanth and solutions of guar gum and sucrose.

Sorbic acid 0.1% as a preservative for syrup.— R. M. E. Richards (letter), *Pharm. J.*, 1972, *2*, 91.

Estimated acceptable daily intake: up to 25 mg per kg body-weight, as the sum of sorbic acid and its calcium, potassium, and sodium salts.— Seventeenth Report of the Joint FAO/WHO Expert Committee on Food Additives, *Tech. Rep. Ser. Wld Hlth Org. No. 539*, 1974.

Antimicrobial action. Sorbic acid inhibited *in vitro*, to the extent of 51%, the growth of the yeast *Malassezia ovalis*, which was associated with dandruff.— J. Brotherton, *Br. J. Derm.*, 1968, *80*, 749.

Sorbic acid proved to be a suitable preservative against most common microbial contaminants with the exception of *Bacillus cereus* which was resistant to both sorbic acid and methyl hydroxybenzoate.— G. Lenart, *Gyogyszereszet*, 1977, *21*, 408, per *Int. pharm. Abstr.*, 1979, *16*, 126.

Proprietary Preparations

Sorbistat *(Pfizer, UK)*. A brand of sorbic acid.

6680-w

Sulphur Dioxide. Sulfur Dioxide *(U.S.N.F.)*.

SO_2=64.06.

CAS — 7446-09-5.

Pharmacopoeias. In *U.S.N.F.*

A colourless non-inflammable gas with a strong suffocating odour characteristic of burning sulphur. It condenses readily under pressure to a colourless liquid which boils at about −10° and has a wt per ml of about 1.5 g.

Soluble 36 in 1 of water and 114 in 1 of alcohol by vol. at 20° and normal pressure; soluble in chloroform and ether. A solution in water is strongly acid to litmus. **Incompatible** with oxidising agents and thiamine.

Liquid sulphur dioxide is available in cylinders and siphons.

Adverse Effects. Inhalation of sulphur dioxide in high concentrations inhibits respiration and may cause death from asphyxia. Lower concentrations are irritant to the respiratory tract and conjunctivae and may lead to death from pulmonary or glottal oedema or laryngeal spasm. Atmospheric concentrations of sulphur dioxide of 500 ppm are dangerous even for short exposures. Maximum permissible atmospheric concentration 2 ppm.

Liver damage was found in 82.6% and serum abnormalities in 73% of 230 workers at a copper smelting plant who were exposed chronically to sulphur dioxide in atmospheric concentrations of 60 to 120 mg per m^3.— N. P. Sterekhova *et al.*, *Gig. Truda prof. Zabol.*, 1970, *14*, 12, per *Abstr. Wld Med.*, 1971, *45*, 542.

Studies involving 20 472 children and adults linked excessive acute respiratory disease with atmospheric pollution due to sulphur dioxide.— J. G. French *et al.*, *Archs environ. Hlth*, 1973, *27*, 129, per *Abstr. Hyg.*, 1974, *49*, 10.

A report of toxicological studies.— *Fd Add. Ser. Wld Hlth Org. No. 5*, 1974.

Reviews and discussions on the health risks of sulphur oxides and suspended particulate matter as air pollutants.— J. McK. Ellison and R. E. Waller, *Environ. Res.*, 1978, *16*, 302; *Bull. N.Y. Acad. Med.*, 1978, *54*, 983, per *Abstr. Hyg.*, 1979, *54*, 698; *J. Am. med. Ass.*, 1978, *239*, 2103; *Environmental Health Criteria 8: Sulfur oxides and suspended particulate matter*, Geneva, WHO, 1978.

Treatment of Adverse Effects. Remove the patient to fresh air. If necessary, assist the respiration until spontaneous breathing is resumed and keep the patient under observation for signs of pulmonary oedema.

Uses. Sulphur dioxide has antibacterial and antifungal properties and is used as a preservative for food; it is added in the form of gas or as sodium, potassium, and calcium metabisulphites, acid sulphites (bisulphites), or sulphites. In general, various items of food and drink intended for consumption without further cooking or dilution may contain up to 30 to 450 ppm and food and drink for cooking or dilution before consumption may contain up to 50 to 2500 ppm. Fresh fruit or fruit products may contain up to 15 to 2000 ppm. Some ingredients used in home brewing, such as finings, may contain up to 50 000 ppm.

Sulphur dioxide in the form of sulphurous acid or sodium metabisulphite is used to preserve Concentrated Raspberry Juice. Raspberry Syrup, for flavouring purposes, prepared by diluting the concentrated juice with syrup, may contain up to 420 ppm w/w of sulphur dioxide.

Sulphur dioxide was formerly used for the disinfection of rooms by fumigation. It is effective only when the air is saturated with moisture; in the absence of moisture it has little germicidal activity.

Sulphurous acid, which is a saturated solution of sulphur dioxide, is a powerful disinfectant. Mixed with 1 or 2 volumes of water or glycerol, it has been applied externally in the treatment of various parasitic skin diseases.

For information on the antoxidant properties of sulphurous acid salts, see under Sodium Metabisulphite, p.1292.

A review.— R. J. L. Allen and M. Brook, *Effects of Sulphur Dioxide in Animals and Man*, Third International Congress of Food Science and Technology, Washington, 1970.

Estimated acceptable daily intake of SO_2: up to 700 µg per kg body-weight. Additional mutagenic studies in a mammalian system and studies over longer periods in man were desirable.— Seventeenth Report of the Joint FAO/WHO Expert Committee on Food Additives, *Tech. Rep. Ser. Wld Hlth Org. No. 539*, 1974.

Sputum production. A pressurised spray of 0.25% sulphur dioxide was used by inhalation to induce the production of sputum as an aid to the bacteriological diagnosis of pulmonary tuberculosis.— J. R. Clarke and Z. M. Blacklock, *Med. J. Aust.*, 1967, *1*, 172.

Preparations

Sulphurous Acid *(B.P.C. 1949)*. Acid. Sulphuros. A colourless liquid with a strong sulphurous odour. It contains about 5% of sulphur dioxide, correspondong to about 6.5% w/w of H_2SO_3, all of which may be evolved on boiling. Wt per ml about 1.025 g. Traces of sulphates are always present. Store in a cool place in well-closed, glass-stoppered bottles.

6681-e

Thiodipropionic Acid. 3,3′-Thiodipropionic acid.

$C_6H_{10}O_4S$=178.2.

CAS — 111-17-1.

Thiodipropionic acid and its dilauryl and distearyl esters ($C_{30}H_{58}O_4S$ = 514.8 and $C_{42}H_{82}O_4S$ = 683.2) have been used as synergists for fats.

A review of the uses and efficacy of thiodipropionates as antoxidants and synergists.— *Fd Add. Ser. Wld Hlth Org. No. 3*, 1972.

Estimated acceptable daily intake (as thiodipropionic acid): up to 3 mg per kg body-weight of thiodipropionic acid or dilauryl thiodipropionate. Biochemical studies in man were required. Because studies were insufficient for the distearyl ester no acceptable daily intake (ADI) was provided.— Seventeenth Report of the Joint FAO/WHO Expert Committee on Food Additives, *Tech. Rep. Ser. Wld Hlth Org. No. 539*, 1974.

Background toxicological information.— *Fd Add. Ser. Wld Hlth Org. No. 5*, 1974.

Promethazine and other Antihistamines

6100-x

Antihistamines diminish or abolish the main actions of histamine in the body, probably by occupying the receptor sites in the effector cells to the exclusion of histamine; they do not prevent the production of histamine.

The effects of histamine are considered to be mediated by 2 sets of receptors, termed H_1 and H_2. Those effects which are mediated by the histamine H_1 receptors include the contraction of smooth muscle and the dilatation and increased permeability of the capillaries. The effects of histamine on vascular smooth muscle are mediated by the H_2 as well as the H_1 receptors. Other effects which are mediated by H_2 receptors include cardiac accelerating effects and, in particular, the stimulating action of histamine on the secretion of gastric acid.

The conventional antihistamines are histamine H_1-receptor antagonists; they have no effect on the stimulating action of histamine on the secretion of gastric acid. Most of the histamine H_1-receptor antagonists belong to the following 5 main chemical groups: ethanolamines (e.g. diphenhydramine); ethylenediamines (e.g. tripelennamine); alkylamines (e.g. chlorpheniramine); piperazines (e.g. hydroxyzine); and phenothiazines (e.g. promethazine).

Many histamine H_1-receptor antagonists have other pharmacological properties, largely independent of antihistamine activity, including anticholinergic, adrenaline-enhancing and/or adrenaline-antagonising, and serotonin-antagonising effects. Some of these properties are not generally of beneficial clinical significance and may be regarded as side-effects. Most histamine H_1-receptor antagonists cause depression of the central nervous system changing to stimulation with very large doses. Most have some local anaesthetic properties.

The secretion of gastric acid is inhibited by a class of antihistamines, with a close structural relationship to histamine, termed histamine H_2-receptor antagonists. Members of this group are burimamide (p.1299), cimetidine (p.1300), metiamide (p.1316), and ranitidine (p.1318).

Histamine, when released from the tissues, causes allergic reactions. The numerous manifestations of such reactions include asthma, hay fever, urticaria, vasomotor rhinitis, and angioneurotic oedema. Unless the agent precipitating the histamine release is permanently removed or the patient is carefully desensitised (see under Allergens and Specific Desensitisation, p.1321) a cure cannot be expected. Adrenaline and other sympathomimetic agents, antihistamines, and corticosteroids all provide temporary symptomatic relief to a greater or lesser extent, but must be administered as long as the cause of the allergy persists.

Adverse Effects of Antihistamines (H_1-Receptor Antagonists). Side-effects with antihistamines vary in incidence and severity with each patient as much as with each drug, though some of the drugs give rise to more side-effects than others. The most common effect, caused to some extent by all is sedation, varying from slight drowsiness to deep sleep, and including inability to concentrate, lassitude, dizziness, hypotension, muscular weakness, and inco-ordination. Sedative effects, when they occur, may diminish after a few days.

Other side-effects include gastro-intestinal disturbances such as nausea, vomiting, diarrhoea or constipation, and epigastric pain. Antihistamines may also produce headache, blurred vision, tinnitus, elation or depression, irritability, nightmares, anorexia, difficulty in micturition, dryness of the mouth, tightness of the chest, and tingling, heaviness, and weakness of the hands.

In infants and children, some antihistamines act as cerebral stimulants and symptoms of overdosage may include convulsions and hyperpyrexia. Symptoms of stimulation may also arise in some adults, especially after taking phenindamine, but occasionally with other antihistamines too. They include insomnia, nervousness, tachycardia, tremors, muscle twitching, and convulsions. Large doses of antihistamines may precipitate fits in epileptics.

Administration of antihistamines may occasionally cause allergy. Local application of antihistamines carries a risk of skin sensitisation with eczematous eruptions but dermatological reactions may also result from oral administration.

Blood disorders, including agranulocytosis and haemolytic anaemia, though rare, have been reported.

Systemic side-effects have been reported after topical application of antihistamines to large areas of the skin.

There have been reports suggesting a possibility of human foetal abnormalities resulting from the use of some antihistamines, especially the piperazine derivatives, but a causal relationship has largely been rejected.

Abuse. For reports of abuse of antihistamines see under the individual antihistamine monographs.

Effects on the skin. The antihistamines have a marked tendency to cause eczematous reactions when applied topically and many authorities consider that they should not be prescribed for the local treatment of skin disorders. The only logical use of antihistamines locally is in the earliest stages of insect bites and some forms of urticaria, but in both conditions oral treatment is preferable. In sunburn, prickly heat, eczema, and pruritus, histamine plays no significant part and an antihistamine effect is not indicated.— B. Russell, *Prescribers' J.*, 1965, *5*, 58. Experience over 20 years with hundreds of pruritic patients has taught that the injunction to avoid local anaesthetic or antihistamine creams or ointments, because of the risk of allergic contact sensitisation, is a counsel of perfection that has denied to many patients the relief these preparations can offer. Although antihistamines may cause allergic contact dermatitis when used topically, the risk of sensitisation is small, especially on 'normal' as opposed to eczematous skin. Provided the prescriber and patient are aware of the hazard and can react promptly if adverse reactions occur, little harm is likely to be done. Furthermore, the same negative advice in respect of local anaesthetics is out of date, and refers to the procaine series (benzocaine, amethocaine). The chemically unrelated lignocaine only rarely sensitises and is a useful antipruritic drug topically.— H. Baker (letter), *Lancet*, 1980, *2*, 863.

Four cases of toxic epidermal necrolysis had been reported associated with the use of antihistamines.—E. D. Lowney *et al., Archs Derm.*, 1967, *95*, 359.

Extrapyramidal symptoms. A review of the literature has indicated that oral dyskinesia after administration of antihistamines is rare but not unexpected.— R. P. Granacher (letter), *New Engl. J. Med.*, 1977, *296*, 516. Dystonic reactions caused by antihistamines are identical to neuroleptic-induced dystonic reactions, which are involuntary tonic muscle contractions. They occur at the onset of therapy and are self-limiting and benign. True orofacial dyskinesia, clinically indistinguishable from *tardive dyskinesia*, secondary to chronic antihistamine administration has also been described.— R. Sovner (letter), *ibid.*, 633.

For possible exacerbation of dystonic glutethimide-withdrawal symptoms by antihistamines, see Glutethimide, p.803.

Tardive dyskinesia. Tardive dyskinesia developed in a 51-year-old man after 30 years' intermittent use of antihistamines.— C. Hale and T. Heins, *Med. J. Aust.*, 1978, *1*, 112.

For other reports of extrapyramidal symptoms following administration of antihistamines, see under the individual antihistamine monographs.

Pregnancy and the neonate. Of 50 282 children born to mothers monitored by the Collaborative Perinatal Project 5401 were found to have been exposed to antihistamines, and possibly other drugs, at some time during the first 4 months of pregnancy. Although there was no constantly discernible pattern between malformation rate and antihistamine exposure a slight suggestion of association between respiratory malformation and pheniramine, between inguinal hernia and meclozine, and between inguinal hernia or genito-urinary malformation and diphenhydramine was made. Also a slight association was found between cardiovascular deformities and phenothiazines.— O. P. Heinonen *et al.*, *Birth Defects and Drugs in Pregnancy*, Littleton MA, Publishing Sciences Group, 1977, p. 322.

The percentage of malformed children among 1309 children born to mothers who had taken phenothiazines during the first 4 months of pregnancy was comparable to that in 48 973 children not so exposed. When analysed for specific malformations there was some evidence of an association with cardiovascular and possibly respiratory malformations but the finding was of doubtful import. IQ scores at 4 years were not affected.— D. Slone *et al., Am. J. Obstet. Gynec.*, 1977, *128*, 486.

For further reports of the effect of antihistamines during pregnancy, see under the individual antihistamine monographs.

Treatment of Adverse Effects. In severe overdosage the stomach should be emptied by aspiration and lavage. Emetics should not be used.

The patient should be kept quiet to minimise the excitation which occurs particularly in children. Convulsions may be controlled with diazepam given intravenously. For general guidelines to the symptomatic therapy of overdosage of central nervous system depressants, see Phenobarbitone, p.812.

Forced diuresis is of little value since antihistamines are rapidly metabolised and only traces are recovered in the urine.

A survey of 220 cases of antihistamine poisoning, including toxic effects and treatment.— K. Würmli, *Pharm. Acta. Helv.*, 1973, *48*, 200.

For references on the use of physostigmine in the treatment of antihistamine overdosage, see Physostigmine Salicylate, p.1043.

Precautions for Antihistamines (H_1-Receptor Antagonists). Ointments containing antihistamines should not be used for acute vesicular and exudative dermatoses.

Patients should be warned that antihistamines may enhance the sedative effect of central nervous system depressants including alcohol, barbiturates, hypnotics, narcotic analgesics, sedatives, and tranquillisers. Since antihistamines have some anticholinergic properties they should be used with care in conditions liable to be exacerbated or otherwise adversely affected by atropine (p.290), such as glaucoma and prostatic hypertrophy. Also the effects of anticholinergic drugs, such as atropine and tricyclic antidepressants, may be enhanced by the concomitant administration of those antihistamines possessing similar activity. It has been suggested that some antihistamines could mask warning symptoms of damage caused by ototoxic drugs, such as the aminoglycoside antibiotics. Some antihistamines have been reported to affect the metabolism of drugs in the liver.

CAUTION. *Antihistamines may cause drowsiness and dulling of mental alertness. Patients undergoing treatment with these drugs should not take charge of vehicles, other means of transport, or machinery where loss of attention may lead to accidents. Patients should abstain from alcohol.*

A report of a significant association between the use of antihistamines and motorcycle accidents.— D. C. G. Skegg *et al., Br. med. J.*, 1979, *1*, 917.

Further general studies and comments on the effects of antihistamines on driving performance.— T. Seppala *et al., Drugs*, 1979, *17*, 389.

See also under the individual antihistamine monographs.

Interactions. The Committee on Safety of Drugs suggested that patients be warned not to take alcohol while under treatment with drugs affecting the CNS, in particular, barbiturates and antihistamines.— *Chemist Drugg.*, 1968, *190*, 524.

Absorption and Fate. In general, antihistamines are readily absorbed from the gastro-intestinal tract, metabolised in the liver, and excreted usually mainly as metabolites in the urine.

The prominent mode of inactivation of histamine in most animal species was by methylation by histamine methyltransferase. Antihistamines acting on H_1-receptors had been shown to stimulate or inhibit histamine methyltransferase *in vitro* according to concentration. Similar findings had been made for the H_2-receptor antagonists burimamide and metiamide.— D. M. Shepherd *et al.*, *Digestion*, 1974, *11*, 307.

Uses of Antihistamines (H_1-Receptor Antagonists). The antihistamines are used therapeutically for palliative treatment in allergic reactions. Where the reaction is due to the release of histamine, antihistamines will usually be of value; where other substances are involved in the allergic reaction, antihistamines may still be of value by virtue of their other actions. Most antihistamines antagonise the actions of acetylcholine and produce local anaesthesia when applied locally. Some antihistamines have been demonstrated to possess both adrenaline-antagonising and adrenaline-enhancing properties.

The antihistamines improve or relieve the symptoms of seasonal hay fever in a high percentage of patients though a high dosage may be necessary in some individuals. The relief obtained is dependent on the severity and nature of the symptoms, relief being greater in the milder stages of hay fever. As in the treatment of other allergic conditions, an antihistamine with pronounced sedative side-effects and a prolonged action may be of benefit at night.

In vasomotor rhinitis, antihistamines are also beneficial. The nasal irritation and the watery discharge are most readily relieved but nasal obstruction is little affected. Where gross infection or large polypi are present these must be treated first.

Although adrenaline (p.4) must be used for acute attacks, urticaria, angioneurotic oedema, and sensitivity reactions usually respond well to the antihistamines. In urticaria, the pruritus is usually relieved a few hours after the first dose; the oedema is more resistant but a decrease in the number of lesions usually occurs subsequently. The antihistamines are effective in abolishing the urticaria and skin irritations in serum sickness but the joint symptoms are little affected. Other itching skin conditions, including pruritus ani and pruritus vulvae, the pruritus of drug rashes and jaundice, contact dermatitis, and insect bites, are often relieved by the oral administration of antihistamines. Local applications are not advised since the antihistamines give rise to skin sensitisation without being very effective by this route.

In patients with asthma, wheezing is not greatly improved by antihistamines, though coughing may be reduced. The antihistamines are useless in the treatment of acute asthmatic attacks.

Though the antihistamines were formerly considered to be beneficial in treatment of the common cold, extensive trials have shown these claims to be unsubstantiated. Antihistamines with nasal decongestant properties may however be used to inhibit nasal discharge in the common cold. They are also used as ingredients of cough linctuses.

Some of the antihistamines have a powerful anti-emetic action and are used for the prevention and treatment of motion sickness. Because all of those so far tried for motion sickness cause some drowsiness, they should never be taken as prophylactics or remedies by drivers, pilots, or those in charge of public transport and vehicles.

The antihistamines have also been used for the prevention and treatment of irradiation sickness, postoperative vomiting, the nausea and vomiting of pregnancy, and drug-induced nausea and vomiting; they have also been used for symptomatic treatment of nausea and vertigo due to Ménière's disease and other labyrinthine disturbances.

Antihistamines with sedative and anti-emetic properties are used for anaesthetic premedication. Although they may have some anticholinergic properties of their own they are usually given with an anticholinergic agent such as atropine to provide more effective reduction of salivation.

Some of the antihistamines were formerly used in the treatment of Parkinson's syndrome, but more effective drugs are now preferred.

Among adults there is considerable variation between effective individual doses, and some patients will not respond unless antihistamines are given in large doses. Children tolerate the antihistamines well, and those over the age of 12 may usually be given a full adult dose. If there is no improvement after three days of treatment with adequate dosage, it is unlikely that the patient will benefit from this form of therapy.

The antihistamines are usually given by mouth and should be taken after food to avoid gastric irritation. Antihistamines may also be given by deep intramuscular or slow intravenous injection when administration by mouth is not feasible or in the treatment of very severe allergy.

When given by mouth, most antihistamines have an onset of action in 15 to 30 minutes and are fully effective within 1 hour.

Reports and studies on inflammatory and allergic mechanisms.— E. G. McQueen, *Drugs*, 1973, *6*, 104 (role of histamine and serotonin); R. Patterson *et al.*, *New Engl. J. Med.*, 1976, *295*, 277 (classification of hypersensitivity reactions); M. Greaves *et al.*, *Br. J. Derm.*, 1977, *97*, 225 (H_1 and H_2 receptors in skin blood vessels); *Lancet*, 1980, *1*, 1226 (slow-reacting substances of anaphylaxis).

Allergy. Reviews and discussions on the actions and uses of antihistamines in allergic disorders.— D. S. Pearlman, *Drugs*, 1976, *12*, 258 (general); J. Brostoff, *Practitioner*, 1978, *220*, 532 (hay fever).

Anaphylaxis. An account of the course, mechanisms, and treatment of anaphylaxis.— J. F. Kelly and R. Patterson, *J. Am. med. Ass.*, 1974, *227*, 1431.

A review of fatal insect stings with guidelines for prophylaxis and treatment of subjects known to be at risk.— *Br. med. J.*, 1974, *2*, 345. Comments.— C. Thomson (letter), *ibid.*, *3*, 113; K. K. Nayak (letter), *ibid.*

For further reference to the use of antihistamines in the management of anaphylactic shock, see Adrenaline, p.4.

Snake bite. For reference to the role of antihistamines in the management of snake bites, see Snake Venom Antiserum, p.1608.

Motion sickness. A short review of anti-emetic drugs and the treatment of motion sickness. The stresses due to motion encountered in most civilian travel can be counteracted effectively by the antihistaminic group of antimotion sickness preparations. Examples are dimenhydrinate 50 mg, cyclizine 50 mg, and meclozine 50 mg, and doses can be given thrice daily during prolonged exposure. If the conditions are more stressful, promethazine 25 mg alone or combined with ephedrine can be given. Highly susceptible patients and very rough conditions may require hyoscine. Promethazine or hyoscine can be given intramuscularly as a therapeutic measure after motion sickness has developed.— C. D. Wood, *Drugs*, 1979, *17*, 471.

Vertigo. Comments on the use of antihistamines in the treatment of vertigo.— N. Roydhouse, *Drugs*, 1974, *7*, 297; J. S. Turner, *ibid.*, 1977, *13*, 382.

6101-r

Promethazine.
1,*N*,*N*-Trimethyl-2-(phenothiazin-10-yl)ethylamine.

$C_{17}H_{20}N_2S$=284.4.

CAS — 60-87-7.

A crystalline solid. M.p. about 60°.

6102-f

Promethazine Hydrochloride *(B.P., B.P. Vet., Eur. P., U.S.P.).*
Promethazini Hydrochloridum; Proazamine Chloride; Promethazinium Chloride; Diprazinum.

$C_{17}H_{20}N_2S,HCl$=320.9.

CAS — 58-33-3.

Pharmacopoeias. In *Arg., Aust., Belg., Br., Braz., Chin., Cz., Eur., Fr., Ger., Hung., Ind., Int., It., Jap., Jug., Neth., Nord., Pol., Rus., Swiss, Turk.,* and *U.S.*

A white or faintly yellow, odourless or almost odourless, crystalline powder with a very bitter taste. M.p. about 222° with decomposition. On prolonged exposure to air it is slowly oxidised, becoming blue in colour.

Soluble 1 in 0.6 of water, 1 in 9 of alcohol, and 1 in 2 of chloroform; practically insoluble in acetone, ether, and ethyl acetate. A 10% solution in water has a pH of 3.5 to 5. Solutions are **sterilised** by autoclaving in containers in which the air has been replaced by nitrogen or other suitable gas. **Incompatible** with alkalis and alkaline solutions such as those of aminophylline, soluble barbiturates, and phenytoin sodium. **Store** in airtight containers. Protect from light.

Incompatibility. A precipitate formed when promethazine hydrochloride was mixed with iodipamide and diatrizoic acid salts in solution.— C. Riffkin, *Am. J. Hosp. Pharm.*, 1963, *20*, 19.

There was a precipitate when an injection of diodone, meglumine and sodium diatrizoates, iodipamide meglumine, meglumine iosefamate, or meglumine and sodium iothalamates was added to promethazine hydrochloride injection.— T. R. Marshall *et al.*, *Radiology*, 1965, *84*, 536.

Particulate matter was observed within 2 hours when 1 ml of commercial promethazine hydrochloride injection was mixed with sterile water 5 ml and 1 ml of any of the following commercial injection solutions: aminophylline, benzylpenicillin potassium, chloramphenicol sodium succinate, dimenhydrinate, heparin, hydrocortisone sodium phosphate, methicillin sodium, phenobarbitone sodium, phenytoin sodium, prednisolone sodium phosphate, and sulphafurazole diethanolamine.— R. Misgen, *Am. J. Hosp. Pharm.*, 1965, *22*, 92.

There was loss of clarity when intravenous solutions of promethazine hydrochloride were mixed with those of aminophylline, benzylpenicillin, chloramphenicol sodium succinate, chlorothiazide sodium, dextran, heparin sodium, hydrocortisone sodium succinate, methicillin sodium, nitrofurantoin sodium, pentobarbitone sodium, phenobarbitone sodium, phenytoin sodium, sulphafurazole diethanolamine, or thiopentone sodium.— J. A. Patel and G. L. Phillips, *Am. J. Hosp. Pharm.*, 1966, *23*, 409.

An immediate precipitate occurred when promethazine hydrochloride 100 mg per litre was mixed with aminophylline 1 g per litre, chlorothiazide 2 g per litre, ethamivan 2 g per litre, methohexitone sodium 2 g per litre, or sulphadimidine sodium 4 g per litre in dextrose injection and sodium chloride injection. An immediate precipitate also occurred when promethazine hydrochloride was mixed with phenobarbitone sodium 800 mg per litre in sodium chloride injection, but when they were mixed in dextrose injection a haze developed over 3 hours.— B. B. Riley, *J. Hosp. Pharm.*, 1970, *28*, 228.

Cloudiness developed when promethazine hydrochloride 12.5 mg was drawn up into a syringe containing morphine sulphate 8 mg.— N. M. Fleischer (letter), *Am. J. Hosp. Pharm.*, 1973, *30*, 665.

A report of incompatibility between carbenicillin and promethazine in solution.— G. E. Otterman and D. W. Samuelson (letter), *Am. J. Hosp. Pharm.*, 1979, *36*, 1156.

Adverse Effects. As for the antihistamines in general, p.1294.

Although cardiovascular side-effects are rare, minor increases in blood pressure and occasional mild hypotension have been reported with promethazine. Leucopenia and rarely agranulocytosis and, as with other phenothiazine derivatives, jaundice and extrapyramidal reactions have also been reported.

Photosensitivity reactions have followed its use by mouth or topical application.

Studies into the effect of promethazine on performance.— C. H. Clarke and A. N. Nicholson, *Br. J. clin. Pharmac.*, 1978, *6*, 31.

Speculation as to the possible role of phenothiazines in sudden infant death.— A. Kahn and D. Blum (letter), *Lancet*, 1979, *2*, 364.

Allergy. In a modified 'repeated-insult' patch test, 25% promethazine was found to produce moderate sensitisation of the skin.— A. M. Kligman, *J. invest. Derm.*, 1966, *47*, 393.

See also Effects on the Blood, below.

Effects on the blood. Allergic agranulocytosis in a 34-year-old man attributed to promethazine therapy.— H. Engel, *Dt. med. Wschr.*, 1976, *101*, 1128.

Promethazine had been reported to cause aplastic anaemia.— R. H. Girdwood, *Drugs*, 1976, *11*, 394.

Effects on the eyes. A study indicating that usual doses of promethazine interfere with colour vision.— J. Laroche and C. Laroche, *Annls pharm. fr.*, 1972, *30*, 433.

Epileptogenic effect. Convulsions which occurred in 3 children after premedication with a preparation containing promethazine, pethidine, and hyoscine were tentatively attributed to idiosyncrasy to promethazine.— R. G. Waterhouse, *Br. J. Anaesth.*, 1967, *39*, 268.

Extrapyramidal symptoms. Risus sardonicus and bizarre movements of the jaw simulating tetanus occurred in a 9-year-old boy 5 minutes after the intramuscular injection of 50 mg of promethazine hydrochloride; the promethazine was considered responsible.— X. G. Okojie (letter), *Br. med. J.*, 1972, *4*, 796.

The Boston Collaborative Drug Surveillance Program monitored consecutively 32 812 medical inpatients. Drug-induced extrapyramidal symptoms occurred in 1 of 1194 patients given promethazine.— J. Porter and H. Jick, *Lancet*, 1977, *1*, 587.

Further references.— M. E. Dodson and R. J. Eastley, *Br. J. Anaesth.*, 1978, *50*, 1059.

Overdosage. A 12-year-old boy developed a toxic delirium, characterised by hallucinations and anxiety, 4 hours after ingestion of about 200 mg of promethazine. He was given chlorpromazine intramuscularly and recovered on arousal.— D. Leak and D. Carroll, *Br. med. J.*, 1967, *2*, 31.

Pregnancy and the neonate. In a study of 836 infants with congenital malformations there was no significant difference in the maternal usage of promethazine during the first trimester of pregnancy compared with the use in 836 controls.— G. Greenberg *et al.*, *Br. med. J.*, 1977, *2*, 853.

For further studies on the effects of phenothiazine-type and other antihistamines during pregnancy, see p.1294.

Labour. Promethazine rapidly diffused across the placenta and when 50 mg was given intravenously to 39 women before delivery, promethazine was found in umbilical vein blood in all cases. About 15 minutes after administration the maternal and foetal blood concentrations were the same. Some clinical depression of infants had been observed. Promethazine had been detected in foetal blood up to 4 hours after administration to the mother.— F. Moya and V. Thorndike, *Am. J. Obstet. Gynec.*, 1962, *84*, 1778.

Although administration of promethazine and pethidine to the mothers of 12 infants during labour had no effect on the maternal platelet function 9 of the infants had impaired platelet aggregation.— D. G. Corby and I. Schulman, *J. Pediat.*, 1971, *79*, 307.

See also under Uses.

Treatment of Adverse Effects. As for the antihistamines in general, p.1294.

Postoperative hallucinations attributed to promethazine and occurring 5 hours after the operation in a child given promethazine 20 mg together with hyoscine 1 mg for premedication, responded to treatment with chlorpromazine 25 mg every 3 hours.— I. H. Jones *et al.*, *Med. J. Aust.*, 1973, *1*, 382.

Precautions. As for the antihistamines in general, p.1294.

As for all phenothiazine derivatives it should be used cautiously in patients with hepatic diseases.

Intravenous injections of promethazine hydrochloride must be given slowly and extreme care must be taken to avoid perivascular extravasation or inadvertent intra-arterial injection, due to the risk of severe chemical irritation.

Administration in renal failure. Neurological symptoms of drug intoxication were attributed to promethazine in a patient suffering from renal failure.— G. Richet *et al.*, *Br. med. J.*, 1970, *2*, 394.

A report of promethazine-induced toxic psychosis in a patient with chronic renal failure.— C. J. McAllister *et al.*, *Clin. Nephrol.*, 1978, *10*, 191.

Anaesthesia. In 8 healthy subjects promethazine 25 mg intravenously appeared to increase the incidence of gastro-oesophageal reflux and might therefore increase the risk of regurgitation and aspiration of gastric contents during induction of and recovery from anaesthesia.— J. G. Brock-Utne *et al.*, *Br. J. Anaesth.*, 1978, *50*, 295.

Interactions. In *cats* the antihypertensive action of clonidine was antagonised by prior intra-arterial administration of some phenothiazine derivatives, including promethazine. Similar results were observed in *rats* after prior intravenous administration of phenothiazine derivatives.— P. A. van Zwieten, *J. Pharm. Pharmac.*, 1977, *29*, 229.

For a report of the effect of promethazine on the absorption of other drugs, see Diphenhydramine Hydrochloride, p.1311.

Absorption and Fate. As for the antihistamines in general, p.1295.

An account of the disposition of promethazine in man. Promethazine is highly bound to plasma proteins. Experimental results indicate that an extensive first-pass effect occurs with promethazine.— J. Quinn and R. Calvert, *J. Pharm. Pharmac.*, 1976, *28*, *Suppl.*, 59P.

Pregnancy and the neonate. For details of transplacental diffusion of promethazine, see under Adverse Effects.

Uses. Promethazine hydrochloride is a phenothiazine derivative with the properties and uses of the antihistamines (see p.1295). It has a prolonged antihistamine action. A single daily dose is usually adequate, preferably taken at night because it also has a pronounced sedative effect. It also has some anticholinergic, antiserotoninergic, and marked local anaesthetic properties.

For allergic conditions promethazine hydrochloride is usually given in a dose of 25 mg each night and if necessary this may be increased to 50 mg; it may, however, be given twice to thrice daily if required in doses of 10 to 20 mg increased as necessary. Doses for children are: up to 1 year of age 5 to 10 mg; 1 to 5 years 5 to 15 mg; older children 10 to 25 mg; if 2 doses are given in 24 hours the lower dose should be used. It may also be given in severe allergies by deep intramuscular injection in doses of 25 to 50 mg; a dose of 100 mg should not be exceeded. In extreme emergency the injection may be diluted to 0.25% with Water for Injections and given by slow intravenous injection.

Promethazine hydrochloride is also used for anaesthetic premedication; it is given by intramuscular injection with pethidine and atropine.

Doses of 50 mg have been given at night for sedation and hypnosis. It is employed as a hypnotic for children: up to 1 year of age 5 to 10 mg; 1 to 5 years 15 to 20 mg; and 6 to 10 years 20 to 25 mg. If administration by mouth is not possible half the oral dose may be given by deep intramuscular injection.

Promethazine hydrochloride is used by injection as an anti-emetic but promethazine theoclate is usually given for this purpose when the administration of tablets is possible. For the treatment of motion sickness in children the dosage of promethazine hydrochloride is: up to 1 year of age 5 to 10 mg; 1 to 5 years 10 to 15 mg; and 6 to 12 years 15 to 25 mg. It is given 30 minutes before the journey; for long journeys the dose is divided and given at intervals of 12 hours.

Promethazine hydrochloride is used in cough linctuses.

Larger doses have been given for control of parkinsonian symptoms, especially oculogyric crises.

Promethazine hydrochloride has been used locally for treatment of allergic skin conditions but systemic treatment is to be preferred. A 2% cream has been used for treatment of burns but is not recommended since it may delay healing and produce skin sensitisation.

Promethazine has also been given as the embonate.

Postoperative adhesions. For the use of promethazine with dexamethasone in the prevention of postoperative adhesions, see Dexamethasone, p.467.

Pregnancy and the neonate. The use of promethazine hydrochloride with pethidine for sedation and analgesia in more than 7500 obstetric patients.— J. J. Carroll and R. S. Moir, *J. Am. med. Ass.*, 1958, *168*, 2218. See also H. Zakut *et al.*, *Harefuah*, 1970, *78*, 61; R. H. Petrie *et al.*, *Obstet. Gynec.*, 1976, *48*, 431.

Promethazine hydrochloride 150 mg daily was given to 21 mothers with severe rhesus isoimmunisation for 3 to 24 weeks of the pregnancy. Seven of 22 babies required intrauterine transfusions, a slightly lower figure than expected without promethazine pretreatment, but its value was not confirmed.— M. A. Stenchever, *Am. J. Obstet. Gynec.*, 1978, *130*, 665. See also S. Biermé and R. Biermé (letter), *Lancet*, 1967, *1*, 574; B. D. Tait (letter), *J. Pharm. Pharmac.*, 1968, *20*, 479; J. P. Gusdon *et al.*, *Am. J. Obstet. Gynec.*, 1974, *119*, 543; A. Rubinstein *et al.*, *J. Pediat.*, 1976, *89*, 136.

See also under Adverse Effects.

Respiratory disorders. A study indicating that promethazine is of some benefit for breathlessness and exercise tolerance in pink and puffing patients with fixed airways obstruction.— A. A. Woodcock *et al.*, *Br. med. J.*, 1981, *283*, 343.

Preparations

Elixirs and Syrups

Promethazine Hydrochloride Elixir *(B.P.)*. Promethazine Elixir. A solution of promethazine hydrochloride in a suitable flavoured vehicle which may be coloured. Store at a temperature not exceeding 25°. Protect from light. When a dose less than or not a multiple of 5 ml is prescribed, the elixir should be diluted to 5 ml, or a multiple, with syrup. Such dilutions must be freshly prepared and not used more than 2 weeks after issue.

Promethazine Hydrochloride Syrup *(U.S.P.)*. A syrup containing promethazine hydrochloride. Store in airtight containers. Protect from light.

Promethazine Syrup *(F.N. Belg.)*. Promethazine hydrochloride 100 mg, ascorbic acid 200 mg, citric acid monohydrate 1 g, flavouring syrup 65 g, aqua conservans to 100 ml. Orange-flower or lemon syrups are suitable flavouring agents.

Injections

Promethazine Hydrochloride Injection *(B.P.)*. Promethazine Injection. A sterile solution of promethazine hydrochloride in Water for Injections free from dissolved air and containing suitable stabilising agents. The solution is distributed into containers, the air in which is replaced by nitrogen or other suitable gas, and sterilised by autoclaving. pH 5 to 6. Protect from light.

Promethazine Hydrochloride Injection *(U.S.P.)*. A sterile solution of promethazine hydrochloride in Water for Injections. pH 4 to 5.5. Protect from light.

Tablets

Promethazine Hydrochloride Tablets *(B.P.)*. Tablets containing promethazine hydrochloride. The tablets are sugar-coated.

Promethazine Hydrochloride Tablets *(U.S.P.)*. Tablets containing promethazine hydrochloride. Store in airtight containers. Protect from light.

Proprietary Preparations

Phenergan *(May & Baker, UK)*. Promethazine hydrochloride, available as **Elixir** containing 5 mg in each 5 ml (suggested diluent, syrup); as **Tablets** of 10 and 25 mg; and as **Solution** for injection containing 2.5% in ampoules of 1 and 2 ml. **Phenergan Cream** contains promethazine base 2% and dibromopropamidine isethionate 0.15% in a water-miscible basis. (Also available as Phenergan in *Austral., Belg., Canad., Denm., Fr., Neth., Norw., S.Afr., Switz., USA*).

Phenergan Compound Expectorant Linctus *(May & Baker, UK)*. Contains in each 5 ml promethazine hydrochloride 5 mg, ipecacuanha liquid extract 0.01 ml, potassium guaiacolsulfonate 45 mg, and citric acid monohydrate 65 mg (suggested diluent, syrup). For nasal and bronchial congestion. *Dose.* 5 to 10 ml twice or thrice daily; children, under 5 years, 2.5 ml; 5 to 10 years, 2.5 to 5 ml.

Phensedyl Cough Linctus *(May & Baker, UK).* Contains in each 5 ml promethazine hydrochloride 3.6 mg, codeine phosphate 9 mg, and ephedrine hydrochloride 7.2 mg (suggested diluent, syrup). *Dose.* 5 to 10 ml twice or thrice daily; children, 2 to 5 years, 2.5 ml; 5 to 10 years, 2.5 to 5 ml.

A 27-year-old man was dependent on Phensedyl, presumably because of its ephedrine content.— A. R. Foster (letter), *Br. med. J.*, 1974, *3*, 581.

Tixylix *(May & Baker, UK).* A linctus containing in each 5 ml promethazine hydrochloride 1.5 mg, pholcodine citrate equivalent to pholcodine 1.5 mg, and phenylpropanolamine hydrochloride 5 mg (suggested diluent, syrup). For cough in children. *Dose.* 1 to 2 years, 2.5 to 5 ml twice or thrice daily; 2 to 5 years, 5 ml; 6 to 10 years, 5 to 10 ml.

Other Proprietary Names

Arg.—Fenergan; *Austral.*—Progan, Prothazine; *Belg.*—Pelpica; *Canad.*—Histantil; *Ger.*—Atosil; *Ital.*—Fargan, Fenazil; *S.Afr.*—Lenazine, Prohist; *Spain*—Fenergan, Sayomol; *Swed.*—Lergigan; *USA*—Fellozine, Ganphen, Phencen, Promine, Quadnite, Remsed, V-Gan, ZiPan.

A preparation containing promethazine hydrochloride and butobarbitone was also formerly marketed in Great Britain under the proprietary name Sonergan (*May & Baker*).

6103-d

Promethazine Theoclate *(B.P.).*

Promethazine Chlorotheophyllinate; Promethazine Teoclate. The promethazine salt of 8-chlorotheophylline.
$C_{17}H_{20}N_2S,C_7H_7ClN_4O_2$=499.0.

CAS — 17693-51-5.

Pharmacopoeias. In *Br.*

A white or almost white odourless powder with a slightly bitter taste. Promethazine theoclate 1.5 mg is approximately equivalent to 1 mg of promethazine hydrochloride.

Very slightly **soluble** in water; soluble 1 in 70 of alcohol and 1 in 2.5 of chloroform; practically insoluble in ether. **Store** in airtight containers. Protect from light.

Adverse Effects, Treatment, and Precautions. As for the antihistamines in general, p.1294.

Although cardiovascular side-effects are rare, minor increases in blood pressure and occasional mild hypotension have been reported following administration of promethazine. Leucopenia and rarely agranulocytosis and, as with other phenothiazine derivatives, jaundice and extrapyramidal reactions have also been reported with promethazine.

Photosensitivity reactions have followed the use of promethazine by mouth or by topical application.

As with all phenothiazine derivatives it should be used cautiously in patients with hepatic diseases.

Uses. Promethazine theoclate has the general properties of promethazine hydrochloride (p.1296) but is used mainly as an anti-emetic in the prevention and treatment of motion sickness. It has also been used in irradiation sickness, postoperative vomiting, the nausea and vomiting of pregnancy, drug-induced nausea and vomiting, and for the symptomatic treatment of nausea and vertigo due to Ménière's disease and other labyrinthine disturbances.

The usual dose for an adult is 25 mg by mouth and for a child, aged 5 to 10 years, 12.5 mg. For the prevention of motion sickness, this dose is taken 1 or 2 hours before commencing the journey, and preferably at bedtime on the previous night; for treatment, the dose is taken as soon as possible, repeated the same evening and again the following evening.

Preparations

Promethazine Theoclate Tablets *(B.P.).* Tablets containing promethazine theoclate. Protect from light.

Avomine *(May & Baker, UK).* Promethazine theoclate, available as scored tablets of 25 mg. (Also available as Avomine in *Austral., S.Afr.*).

Other Proprietary Names

Meth-Zine *(Austral.).*

6104-n

Antazoline Hydrochloride *(B.P. 1973).*

Antazolini Hydrochloridum; Antazolinium Chloride; Imidamin Hydrochloride; Phenazolinum. *N*-Benzyl-*N*-(2-imidazolin-2-ylmethyl)aniline hydrochloride.
$C_{17}H_{19}N_3,HCl$=301.8.

CAS — 91-75-8 (antazoline); 2508-72-7 (hydrochloride).

Pharmacopoeias. In *Arg., Cz., Fr., Ind., Int., Jug., Nord., Pol., Port., Swiss,* and *Turk.*

A white or almost white, odourless or almost odourless, crystalline powder with a bitter taste. M.p. about 240° with decomposition.

Soluble 1 in 50 of water and 1 in 16 of alcohol; slightly soluble in chloroform; practically insoluble in ether. A 1% solution in water has a pH of 5 to 6.5. Solutions are **sterilised** by autoclaving or by filtration. **Store** in airtight containers. Protect from light.

6105-h

Antazoline Mesylate *(B.P.C. 1973).*

Antazoline Methanesulphonate.
$C_{17}H_{19}N_3,CH_3SO_3H$=361.5.

CAS — 3131-32-6.

Pharmacopoeias. In *Cz.*

A white or almost white, odourless or almost odourless powder with a bitter taste. M.p. 165° to 168°. It is slightly hygroscopic; significant amounts of moisture are absorbed at 20° at relative humidities above about 70%.

Soluble 1 in 6 of water, 1 in 7 of alcohol, and 1 in 12 of chloroform; practically insoluble in ether. A 1% solution in water has a pH of 4 to 6.5. Solutions are **sterilised** by autoclaving in sealed containers in which the air has been replaced by nitrogen or other suitable gas, or by filtration. **Store** in airtight containers. Protect from light.

6106-m

Antazoline Phosphate *(U.S.P.).*

Antazolinium Biphosphate.
$C_{17}H_{19}N_3,H_3PO_4$=363.4.

CAS — 154-68-7.

Pharmacopoeias. In *U.S.*

A white to off-white crystalline powder with a bitter taste. M.p. 194° to 198° with decomposition. **Soluble** in water; sparingly soluble in methyl alcohol; practically insoluble in ether. A 2% solution in water has a pH of 4 to 5. **Store** in airtight containers.

Adverse Effects, Treatment, and Precautions. As for the antihistamines in general, p.1294.

Allergic thrombocytopenic purpura and agranulocytosis have been reported. Transient dizziness and anorexia have followed the intravenous administration of antazoline, and cardiac arrest has occurred.

Allergy. A report of interstitial pneumonitis, with fever, rash, and dyspnoea, after antazoline; the condition recurred after challenge.— A. Pahissa *et al.*, *Br. med. J.*, 1979, *2*, 1328.

Effects on the blood. Antazoline was reported to be a haemolytic agent in subjects deficient in glucose-6-phosphate dehydrogenase but only in conjunction with other factors such as infection.— M. E. Pembrey, *Practitioner*, 1974, *213*, 647. See also E. Beutler, *Pharmac. Rev.*, 1969, *21*, 73; U. Bengtsson *et al.*, *Acta med. scand.*, 1975, *198*, 223.

Uses. Antazoline is an ethylenediamine derivative with the properties and uses of the antihistamines (see p.1295). It is one of the least active of the commonly used antihistamines and has a short duration of action. It has local anaesthetic and also some anticholinergic properties. It is claimed to be less irritating to the tissues than most other antihistamines.

Antazoline sulphate and phosphate are used locally with a vasoconstrictor, such as naphazoline nitrate or xylometazoline hydrochloride, in nasal drops and eye-drops containing 0.5%, for nasal and ocular allergies. The hydrochloride has been used similarly in eye-drops.

Antazoline has been given as the hydrochloride in doses of 100 to 300 mg daily in divided doses. Doses of up to 600 mg daily have been given for short periods in severe cases.

Antazoline has been used by mouth in the prevention and treatment of cardiac arrhythmias; it has also been administered by intramuscular or slow intravenous injection.

It has been used topically, as the hydrochloride or the mesylate, for its antipruritic effect as a 2% cream.

Antazoline hydrochloride by intramuscular and intravenous injection caused the pulse-rate to become distinguishable and breathing to start again in a young man who had been stung by a jelly-fish, genus *Physalia*. He made a normal recovery after further treatment with dimethothiazine and promethazine.— J. A. Gollan (letter), *Med. J. Aust.*, 1968, *1*, 973.

Preparations

Antazoline Tablets *(B.P. 1973).* Tablets containing antazoline hydrochloride. Protect from light in airtight containers.

Antistin-Privine *(Ciba, UK).* An aqueous iso-osmotic solution containing antazoline sulphate 0.5% and naphazoline nitrate 0.025%. For allergic conditions of the nose.

Other Proprietary Names

Antasten *(Swed.)*; Antistin *(Ger., Switz.)*; Antistina *(Denm., Spain)*; Antistine *(Canad., Fr.).*

6107-b

Azatadine Maleate.

Sch 10649. 6,11-Dihydro-11-(1-methyl-4-piperidylidene)-5*H*-benzo[5,6]cyclohepta[1,2-*b*]pyridine dimaleate.
$C_{20}H_{22}N_2,2C_4H_4O_4$=522.6.

CAS — 3964-81-6 (azatadine); 3978-86-7 (maleate).

Adverse Effects, Treatment, and Precautions. As for the antihistamines in general, p.1294.

The most frequently reported adverse effects of azatadine are sleepiness, dizziness, disturbed coordination, epigastric distress, and thickening of bronchial secretions. Haemolytic anaemia, thrombocytopenia, and agranulocytosis have also occurred. It is not yet known how azatadine compares with other antihistamines in frequency, severity, or range of adverse effects.— *Med. Lett.*, 1977, *19*, 77.

The effect of azatadine on performance.— B. Biehl, *Curr. med. Res. Opinion*, 1979, *6*, 62; D. K. Luscombe *et al.*, *Br. J. clin. Pract.*, 1980, *34*, 75.

Uses. Azatadine maleate has the properties and uses of the antihistamines (see p.1295). It also has anticholinergic and antiserotonin properties.

Azatadine maleate is given for allergic disorders in usual doses of 1 mg twice daily; if necessary 2 mg twice daily may be given. Children aged 6 to 12 years may be given 0.5 to 1 mg twice daily.

Proprietary Preparations

Optimine *(Kirby-Warrick, UK).* Azatadine maleate, available as **Syrup** containing 500 µg in each 5 ml and as scored **Tablets** of 1 mg. (Also available as Optimine in *Canad., Neth., S.Afr., USA).*

Other Proprietary Names

Idulamine *(Arg.)*; Idulian *(Fr.)*; Zadine *(Austral.).*

6108-v

Bamipine. *N*-Benzyl-*N*-(1-methyl-4-piperidyl)aniline. $C_{19}H_{24}N_2$=280.4.

CAS — 4945-47-5.

Bamipine has the general properties and uses of the antihistamines (see p.1294). It has pronounced sedative effects and also local anaesthetic properties.

It has been given as the hydrochloride in usual doses of 50 mg up to thrice daily. Higher doses of up to 400 mg daily in divided doses have also been given. Bamipine has also been applied topically as the lactate.

Proprietary Names

Soventol *(as hydrochloride and/or lactate) (Knoll, Austral.; Knoll, Belg.; Knoll, Ger.; Knoll, Ital.; Knoll, Neth.; Knoll, S.Afr.; Knoll, Switz.)*; Taumidrine *(hydrochloride) (Biosédra, Fr.)*.

6109-g

Bromodiphenhydramine Hydrochloride

(U.S.P.). Bromazine Hydrochloride; Histabromamine Hydrochloride. 2-(4-Bromobenzhydryloxy)-*NN*-dimethylethylamine hydrochloride. $C_{17}H_{20}BrNO,HCl$=370.7.

CAS — 118-23-0 (bromodiphenhydramine); 1808-12-4 (hydrochloride).

Pharmacopoeias. In *U.S.*

A white to pale buff-coloured, crystalline powder with a faint odour. M.p. 148° to 152°. **Soluble** 1 in less than 1 of water, 1 in 2 of alcohol and of chloroform, and 1 in 31 of isopropyl alcohol; practically insoluble in ether and light petroleum. **Store** in airtight containers.

Adverse Effects, Treatment, and Precautions. As for the antihistamines in general, p.1294.

Effects on the blood. A 0.052% solution of bromodiphenhydramine hydrochloride in 0.9% sodium chloride solution caused 100% haemolysis of erythrocytes cultured in it for 45 minutes.— C. J. Fievet *et al.*, *Am. J. Hosp. Pharm.*, 1971, *28*, 961.

Uses. Bromodiphenhydramine hydrochloride is an ethanolamine derivative with the properties and uses of the antihistamines (see p.1295). It has been claimed to be about twice as potent as diphenhydramine hydrochloride but to have only about one-quarter of the anticholinergic potency.

It has been given in usual doses of 25 mg three or four times daily.

Preparations

Bromodiphenhydramine Hydrochloride Capsules *(U.S.P.).* Capsules containing bromodiphenhydramine hydrochloride. Store in airtight containers.

Bromodiphenhydramine Hydrochloride Elixir *(U.S.P.).* An elixir containing bromodiphenhydramine hydrochloride with 12 to 15% of alcohol. Store in airtight containers. Protect from light.

Proprietary Names

Ambodryl *(Parke, Davis, Belg.; Parke, Davis, USA)*.

Bromodiphenhydramine hydrochloride was formerly marketed in Great Britain under the proprietary name Ambodryl *(Parke, Davis)*.

6110-f

Brompheniramine Maleate

(U.S.P.). Parabromdylamine Maleate. (±)-3-(4-Bromophenyl)-*NN*-dimethyl-3-(2-pyridyl)propylamine hydrogen maleate. $C_{16}H_{19}BrN_2,C_4H_4O_4$=435.3.

CAS — 86-22-6 (brompheniramine); 980-71-2 (maleate); 32865-01-3 (maleate, ±).

Pharmacopoeias. In *U.S.*

A white odourless crystalline powder. M.p. 130° to 135°. **Soluble** 1 in 5 of water and 1 in 15 of alcohol and of chloroform; slightly soluble in ether. A 1% solution in water has a pH of 4 to 5. **Store** in airtight containers. Protect from light.

Incompatibility. There was a precipitate when sodium and meglumine diatrizoates, iodipamide meglumine, or meglumine iosefamate injections were added to brompheniramine maleate injection.— T. R. Marshall *et al.*, *Radiology*, 1965, *84*, 536.

Adverse Effects, Treatment, and Precautions. As for the antihistamines in general, p.1294.

The effect of brompheniramine maleate on performance.— A. N. Nicholson, *Br. J. clin. Pharmac.*, 1979, *8*, 321.

Effects on the blood. A 0.4% solution of brompheniramine maleate in 0.9% sodium chloride solution caused 100% haemolysis of erythrocytes cultured in it for 45 minutes.— C. J. Fievet *et al.*, *Am. J. Hosp. Pharm.*, 1971, *28*, 961.

Agranulocytosis in a 34-year-old alcoholic man was possibly associated with brompheniramine therapy.— A. S. Hardin and F. Padilla, *J. Ark. med. Soc.*, 1978, *75*, 206.

Effects on mental state. For reports of psychotic episodes probably associated with the phenylpropanolamine content of preparations containing brompheniramine and phenylpropanolamine, see Phenylpropanolamine Hydrochloride, p.25.

Extrapyramidal symptoms. A report of 2 patients who developed oral and facial dyskinesias after long-term use of preparations for allergic rhinitis containing antihistamines (brompheniramine, chlorpheniramine, or phenindamine) and sympathomimetics. One patient improved when the preparations were discontinued. These cases best fit the category of late-onset, drug-induced (tardive) dyskinesia. The dyskinesias were thought to be associated with the antihistamines due to the structural and pharmacological similarity between them and the psychotropic phenothiazines, well-documented as causing dyskinesias.— B. T. Thach *et al.*, *New Engl. J. Med.*, 1975, *293*, 486.

Overdosage. A young boy swallowed at least 25 tablets, each of 12 mg of brompheniramine maleate. There was marked restlessness, twitchings of the limbs, periods of coma, pallor, flushing, tachycardia, dilated pupils, ataxia, incoherence, and nail-biting. He was very ill for 2 days and still unsteady and restless 5 days after the mishap. He was treated with gastric lavage and phenobarbitone.— E. Gilmore and B. H. Athreya, *New Engl. J. Med.*, 1960, *263*, 149.

Absorption and Fate. As for the antihistamines in general, p.1295.

In a man on a normal diet who was given brompheniramine maleate, 3 mg daily for 21 days, about 18% of the dose was excreted in the urine as free brompheniramine (5.4%), *N*-desmonomethylbrompheniramine (6.3%), and *N*-desdimethylbrompheniramine (5.8%) respectively.— P. Kabasakalian *et al.*, *Can. J. pharm. Sci.*, 1968, *3*, 18. See also *idem*, *J. pharm. Sci.*, 1968, *57*, 621.

Uses. Brompheniramine maleate is an alkylamine derivative with the properties and uses of the antihistamines (see p.1295). It is somewhat more potent than promethazine hydrochloride but has a shorter duration of action and less pronounced sedative effects.

Brompheniramine maleate is given usually in doses of 4 to 8 mg three or four times daily.

Children up to 3 years of age have been given 0.4 to 1 mg per kg body-weight over 24 hours in four divided doses. Children aged 3 to 6 years may be given 2 mg three or four times daily and those aged 6 to 12 years 2 to 4 mg three or four times daily.

It has also been given in severe allergies by subcutaneous, intramuscular, or slow intravenous injection; the dosage is usually 5 to 20 mg and the total dose by these routes in 24 hours should not normally exceed 40 mg. It is also used in cough mixtures.

Allergy. In a double-blind trial, 72 patients, 90% with hay fever and 10% with allergic rhinitis, were given chlorpheniramine for 1 week, brompheniramine maleate for 1 week, and whichever drug had proved the better for a third week. Both drugs were given in the form of 4-mg tablets in a dose ranging from 1 to 8 tablets daily. No major differences were demonstrated between the 2 drugs. Side-effects, the commonest being drowsiness, occurred in 23% on brompheniramine and in 14% on chlorpheniramine.—Report No. 74 of the General Practitioner Research Group, *Practitioner*, 1965, *194*, 688. See also N. Edwards *et al.*, *Practitioner*, 1973, *211*, 220.

Coryza. In a double-blind trial in patients with acute coryza, relief of symptoms was better after 48 hours in 31 patients treated with tablets each containing brompheniramine maleate 12 mg, phenylephrine hydrochloride 15 mg, and phenylpropanolamine hydrochloride 15 mg (Dimotapp LA), 1 twice daily, than in 35 given a placebo, but at the end of 1 week there was no difference between them.—Report No. 102 of the General Practitioner Research Group, *Practitioner*, 1967, *198*, 437.

Preparations

Brompheniramine Maleate Elixir *(U.S.P.).* An elixir containing brompheniramine maleate, with alcohol 2.7 to 3.3%. pH 2.5 to 3.5. Protect from light.

Brompheniramine Maleate Injection *(U.S.P.).* A sterile solution in Water for Injections. pH 6.8 to 7. Protect from light.

Brompheniramine Maleate Tablets *(U.S.P.).* Tablets containing brompheniramine maleate. Store in airtight containers.

Proprietary Preparations

Dimotane *(Robins, UK).* Brompheniramine maleate, available as **Elixir** containing 2 mg in each 5 ml (suggested diluent, syrup), and as scored **Tablets** of 4 mg.

Dimotane LA. Sustained-release tablets each containing brompheniramine maleate 12 mg. *Dose.* 1 or 2 tablets morning and evening.

See also Dimotane Expectorant, p.689.

Dimotapp Elixir *(Robins, UK).* Contains in each 5 ml brompheniramine maleate 4 mg, phenylephrine hydrochloride 5 mg, and phenylpropanolamine hydrochloride 5 mg (suggested diluent, syrup). For upper respiratory tract disorders, including rhinitis and sinusitis. *Dose.* 5 to 10 ml three or four times daily; children, 2 to 6 years, 2.5 to 5 ml and 6 to 12 years, 5 ml.

Dimotapp Elixir Paediatric *(Robins, UK).* Contains in each 5 ml brompheniramine maleate 1 mg, phenylephrine hydrochloride 2.5 mg, and phenylpropanolamine hydrochloride 2.5 mg. For upper respiratory tract disorders, including rhinitis and sinusitis. *Dose.* Children, 2 to 6 years, 2.5 to 10 ml three or four times daily; 6 to 12 years, 10 ml.

Dimotapp LA *(Robins, UK).* Sustained-release tablets each containing brompheniramine maleate 12 mg, phenylephrine hydrochloride 15 mg, and phenylpropanolamine hydrochloride 15 mg. For upper respiratory tract disorders, including rhinitis and sinusitis. *Dose.* 1 or 2 tablets morning and evening.

Other Proprietary Names

Antial *(Ital.)*; Bromolent *(Arg.)*; Dimegan *(Fr., Switz.)*; Dimetane *(Austral., Canad., S.Afr., Spain, Swed., USA)*; Drauxin *(Ital.)*; Ebalin *(Ger.)*; Gammistin *(Ital.)*; Ilvin *(Ger., Ital., Swed.)*; Pyrimetane *(Arg.)*; Veltane *(USA)*.

6111-d

Buclizine Hydrochloride.

UCB 4445. 1-(4-*tert*-Butylbenzyl)-4-(4-chlorobenzhydryl)piperazine dihydrochloride. $C_{28}H_{33}ClN_2,2HCl$=506.0.

CAS — 82-95-1 (buclizine); 129-74-8 (hydrochloride).

A white crystalline powder; slightly **soluble** in water.

Adverse Effects, Treatment, and Precautions. As for the antihistamines in general, p.1294.

For a discussion on early suggestions that foetal abnormalities might result from the use of buclizine and similar compounds, see under Meclozine Hydrochloride, p.1314.

Uses. Buclizine hydrochloride is a piperazine derivative with the properties of the antihistamines (see p.1295) but is used mainly for its anti-emetic action. It may also be used for the symptomatic treatment of allergic conditions and of vertigo. It is reported to have a prolonged antihistamine action and to have less pronounced

sedative effects than promethazine.
The usual dose is 25 to 50 mg thrice daily by mouth, the larger dose being suitable for motion sickness. For allergic conditions or nausea 25 to 50 mg daily may be adequate. Buclizine in association with analgesics is also used in migraine.

Appetite stimulation. Studies suggesting that buclizine promoted weight gain in *animals* and man.— S. T. Devare *et al.*, *J. Indian med. Prof.*, 1968, *15*, 6664; S. D. Kulkarni *et al.*, *Eur. J. Pharmac.*, 1972, *17*, 312.

Migraine. Studies and comments on the use of buclizine, alone or in combination with analgesics (as Migraleve), in migraine.— W. H. Myers, *Med. Dig., Lond.*, 1972, *17* (July), 45. Report No. 184 of the General Practitioner Research Group, *Practitioner*, 1973, *211*, 357; J. Scopa *et al.*, *Curr. ther. Res.*, 1974, *16*, 1270; P. B. Jorgensen *et al.*, *ibid.*, 1276; D. M. Merrington, *ibid.*, 1975, *18*, 222.

Proprietary Preparations

Equivert *(Pfizer, UK)*. Tablets each containing buclizine hydrochloride 25 mg and nicotinic acid 25 mg. For vertigo and recurrent headaches including migraine. *Dose.* 1 tablet thrice daily before meals.

Migraleve *(International Laboratories, UK)*. Pink tablets each containing buclizine hydrochloride 6.25 mg, paracetamol 500 mg, codeine phosphate 8 mg, and docusate sodium 10 mg, and yellow tablets each containing paracetamol 500 mg, codeine phosphate 8 mg, and docusate sodium 20 mg. For migraine. *Dose.* 2 pink tablets at the start of an attack, then 2 yellow tablets every 3 or 4 hours if required; maximum daily dose, 2 pink tablets and 6 yellow tablets.

Other Proprietary Names

Aphilan R *(Fr.)*; Bucladin-S *(USA)*; Longifene *(Belg., Neth., S.Afr., Switz.)*; Postafen *(Arg.)*.

6112-n

Burimamide. 1-[4-(Imidazol-4-yl)butyl]-3-methylthiourea.
$C_9H_{16}N_4S=212.3$.

CAS — 34970-69-9.

Burimamide is a histamine H_2-receptor antagonist (see p.1294) with actions similar to those of cimetidine (p.1300), but it is less potent by mouth.

References: J. W. Black *et al.*, *Nature*, 1972, *236*, 385; J. H. Wyllie *et al.*, *Lancet*, 1972, *2*, 1117; N. Capurro and R. Levi, *Br. J. Pharmac.*, 1973, *48*, 620; D. W. Harris *et al.*, *Br. J. Pharmac.*, 1975, *53*, 293; A. J. C. Hood *et al.*, *Br. J. Pharmac.*, 1975, *53*, 525; J. K. Siepler *et al.*, *Am. J. Hosp. Pharm.*, 1978, *35*, 141.

Manufacturers

Smith Kline & French, UK.

6113-h

Carbinoxamine Maleate *(U.S.P.)*.

2-[4-Chloro-α-(2-pyridyl)benzyloxy]-*NN*-dimethylethylamine hydrogen maleate.
$C_{16}H_{19}ClN_2O,C_4H_4O_4=406.9$.

CAS — 486-16-8 (carbinoxamine); 3505-38-2 (maleate).

Pharmacopoeias. In *U.S.*

A white odourless crystalline powder with a bitter taste. M.p. 116° to 121°. **Soluble** 1 in less than 1 of water, and 1 in 1.5 of alcohol and of chloroform; very slightly soluble in ether. A 1% solution in water has a pH of 4.6 to 5.1. **Store** in airtight containers. Protect from light.

Stability. In comparison with diphenhydramine hydrochloride, carbinoxamine maleate was very stable in aqueous solution at pH 1 to 8.— I. Tanaka *et al.*, *Arch. prac. Pharm.*, 1964, *24*, 303, per *Int. pharm. Abstr.*, 1966, *3*, 321.

Adverse Effects, Treatment, and Precautions. As for the antihistamines in general, p.1294.

Uses. Carbinoxamine maleate is an ethanolamine derivative with the properties and uses of the antihistamines (see p.1295). It is reported to be almost as potent as promethazine hydrochloride but to have less pronounced sedative effects, anticholinergic activity, and local anaesthetic properties. It has a short duration of action.
Carbinoxamine maleate is usually given in doses of 4 to 8 mg three or four times daily. The dose for children, given 3 or 4 times daily, is: 1 to 3 years of age 2 mg, 3 to 6 years 2 to 4 mg, and older children 4 mg. It is also given in cough linctuses.

Preparations

Carbinoxamine Maleate Elixir *(U.S.P.)*. An elixir containing carbinoxamine maleate with 6.5 to 8% of alcohol. pH 5 to 6.7. Store in airtight containers. Protect from light.

Carbinoxamine Maleate Tablets *(U.S.P.)*. Tablets containing carbinoxamine maleate. Store in airtight containers. Protect from light.

Davenol *(Wyeth, UK)*. A linctus containing in each 5 ml carbinoxamine maleate 2 mg, ephedrine hydrochloride 7 mg, and pholcodine 4 mg (suggested diluent, syrup). For cough. *Dose.* 5 to 10 ml three or four times daily; children up to 5 ml.

Other Proprietary Names

Allergefon *(Fr.)*; Clistin *(Arg., Austral., Ital., USA)*; Histex *(Austral.)*; Lergefin *(Spain)*; Polistine *(Neth.)*; Ziriton *(Ital.)*.

6114-m

Chlorcyclizine Hydrochloride *(B.P., U.S.P.)*.

Chlorcyclizini Hydrochloridum; Chlorcyclizinium Chloride. (±)-1-(4-Chlorobenzhydryl)-4-methylpiperazine hydrochloride.
$C_{18}H_{21}ClN_2,HCl=337.3$.

CAS — 82-93-9 (chlorcyclizine); 1620-21-9; 14362-31-3 (both hydrochloride).

Pharmacopoeias. In *Arg.*, *Br.*, *Ind.*, *Int.*, *It.*, *Turk.*, and *U.S.*

A white, odourless or almost odourless, crystalline powder with a bitter taste. M.p. about 225°. **Soluble** 1 in 2 of water, 1 in 11 of alcohol, and 1 in 4 of chloroform; practically insoluble in ether. A 1% solution in water has a pH of 4.8 to 5.5. **Store** in airtight containers. Protect from light.

Adverse Effects, Treatment, and Precautions. As for the antihistamines in general, p.1294.
For a discussion on early suggestions that foetal abnormalities might result from the use of chlorcyclizine and similar compounds, see under Meclozine Hydrochloride, p.1314.

Reports of *animal* studies showing increased enzymic activity in the liver following the administration of chlorcyclizine.— A. H. Conney *et al.*, *J. Pharmac. exp. Ther.*, 1961, *132*, 202; *idem*, *Ann. N.Y. Acad. Sci.*, 1965, *123*, 98; J. J. Burns *et al.*, *ibid.*, 273.

Absorption and Fate. As for the antihistamines in general, p.1295.

A study of the metabolism of chlorcyclizine in healthy subjects and in *rats*.— R. Kuntzman *et al.*, *J. Pharmac. exp. Ther.*, 1967, *155*, 337.

Uses. Chlorcyclizine hydrochloride is a piperazine derivative with the properties and uses of the antihistamines (see p.1295). It has a prolonged antihistamine action of similar duration to that of promethazine hydrochloride. It has anticholinergic, anti-emetic, and local anaesthetic properties.
Chlorcyclizine hydrochloride has been given in allergic conditions in doses of 50 to 100 mg once or twice daily. A 2% cream or lotion has been used topically.

Preparations

Chlorcyclizine Tablets *(B.P. 1973)*. Tablets containing chlorcyclizine hydrochloride. They may be sugar-coated.

Proprietary Names

Di-Paralene *(Abbott, Austral.; Abbott, Belg.; Abbott, Fr.; Abbott, Ital.; Abbott, Norw.; Abbott, Swed.)*; Tri-histan *(GEA, Denm.; Weiders, Norw.; GEA, Switz.)*.

A preparation containing chlorcyclizine hydrochloride was formerly marketed in Great Britain under the proprietary name Histofax *(Wellcome Consumer Division)*.

6115-b

Chloropyrilene Citrate. Chlorothen Citrate; Chloromethapyrilene Citrate; Chlorpyrilen Citrate. *N*-(5-Chloro-2-thenyl)-*N'N'*-dimethyl-*N*-(2-pyridyl)ethylenediamine dihydrogen citrate.
$C_{14}H_{18}ClN_3S,C_6H_8O_7=488.0$.

CAS — 148-65-2 (chloropyrilene); 148-64-1 (citrate).

Pharmacopoeias. In *Arg.*

A white crystalline powder, usually having a faint odour. M.p. 112° to 116°; on further heating it gradually solidifies and remelts at 125° to 140°.
Soluble 1 in 35 of water; soluble in alcohol; practically insoluble in chloroform and ether. A solution in water is acid to litmus. **Protect** from light.

Chloropyrilene citrate is an ethylenediamine derivative with the properties and uses of the antihistamines (see p.1294). It has been given in doses of 25 mg every 3 or 4 hours up to a maximum of 150 mg in 24 hours.

Proprietary Names

Panta *(Valeas, Ital.)*.

6116-v

Chlorpheniramine Maleate *(B.P., U.S.P.)*.

Chlorphenamine Maleate; Chlorprophenpyridamine Maleate. (±)-3-(4-Chlorophenyl)-*NN*-dimethyl-3-(2-pyridyl)propylamine hydrogen maleate.
$C_{16}H_{19}ClN_2,C_4H_4O_4=390.9$.

CAS — 132-22-9 (chlorpheniramine); 42882-96-2 (chlorpheniramine, ±); 113-92-8 (maleate).

Pharmacopoeias. In *Arg.*, *Br.*, *Braz.*, *Chin.*, *Jap.*, *Turk.*, and *U.S.*

A white odourless crystalline powder with a bitter taste. M.p. 130° to 135°.
Soluble 1 in 4 of water and 1 in 10 of alcohol and of chloroform; slightly soluble in ether. A 1% solution in water has a pH of 4 to 5. Solutions are **sterilised** by autoclaving after distributing in containers in which the air has been replaced by nitrogen or other suitable gas. **Incompatible** with calcium chloride, noradrenaline acid tartrate, and pentobarbitone sodium; incompatibility has been reported with kanamycin sulphate. **Store** in airtight containers. Protect from light.

Incompatibility. There was a precipitate when iodipamide meglumine injection was added to chlorpheniramine maleate injection.— T. R. Marshall *et al.*, *Radiology*, 1965, *84*, 536.

Further references.— J. A. Patel and G. L. Phillips, *Am. J. Hosp. Pharm.*, 1966, *23*, 409.

Adverse Effects. As for the antihistamines in general, p.1294.
Injections may be irritant.

A 36-year-old man with sinusitis was treated with phenylephrine locally for 4 days, with tetracycline for 10 days, and with a preparation containing chlorpheniramine for 10 days. He developed lethargy, headache, extrasystoles, and some loss of touch sensation. Chlorpheniramine had been implicated in 12 other patients with less pronounced symptoms.— D. M. Holloway (letter), *J. Am. med. Ass.*, 1969, *207*, 2103.

Effects on the blood. Chlorpheniramine given to an elderly woman to treat a wasp sting was probably responsible for agranulocytosis. She received a total of about 170 mg of chlorpheniramine.— G. Shenfield and C. J. F. Spry (letter), *Br. med. J.*, 1968, *2*, 52.

A report of chlorpheniramine-induced thrombocytopenic purpura in a 53-year-old man.— E. V. Eisner *et al.*, *J. Am. med. Ass.*, 1975, *231*, 735.

Pancytopenia in a 32-year-old black woman was attributed to chlorpheniramine; thrombocytopenia developed rapidly after a challenge dose.— P. M. Deringer and A. Manicatis (letter), *Lancet*, 1976, *1*, 432. Doubts as to whether chlorpheniramine was responsible.— C. J. F. Spry (letter), *ibid.*, 545.

Aplastic anaemia was associated in 1 patient with prolonged chlorpheniramine use.— T. Kanoh *et al.* (letter), *Lancet*, 1977, *1*, 546.

Extrapyramidal symptoms. Long-term use of chlorpheniramine caused progressive left-sided facial dyskinesia in a 57-year-old man. In the 6 weeks since chlorpheniramine had been discontinued, dramatic improvement in the facial dyskinesia had occurred.— W. A. Davis (letter), *New Engl. J. Med.*, 1976, *294*, 113.

Treatment of Adverse Effects. As for the antihistamines in general, p.1294.

Adsorption. For comment on the *in vitro* adsorption of chlorpheniramine by activated charcoal, see p.79.

Precautions. As for the antihistamines in general, p.1294.

The effect of chlorpheniramine on performance.— C. H. Clarke and A. N. Nicholson, *Br. J. clin. Pharmac.*, 1978, *6*, 31.

Interactions. For a report of the effect of chlorpheniramine on phenytoin, see Phenytoin Sodium, p.1240.

Absorption and Fate. As for the antihistamines in general, p.1295.

The metabolism of radio-labelled chlorpheniramine maleate was studied in healthy subjects. A single dose of 12 mg given by mouth to each of 6 subjects produced a mean peak plasma-chlorpheniramine concentration of about 17 ng per ml 2 hours after administration with an estimated plasma half-life of 12 to 15 hours. Metabolites of chlorpheniramine were present in the plasma for at least 48 hours. A mean of about 34% of the dose was excreted in the urine over 48 hours; less than 1% was excreted in the faeces. Two subjects were given a single dose of 4 mg intravenously and the plasma half-life was about 15 minutes during the initial decay phase and 28 hours during the secondary disappearance phase. As with oral administration about one-third of the dose was excreted in the urine after 48 hours with only small amounts appearing in the faeces. Comparison of data on faecal excretion following oral and intravenous administration indicated that chlorpheniramine may undergo enterohepatic circulation. Chlorpheniramine was extensively metabolised and unchanged drug, mono- and di-desmethylchlorpheniramine, and unidentified compounds were detected in the urine after both oral and intravenous administration. Studies *in vitro* indicated that chlorpheniramine was about 72% bound to plasma proteins.— E. A. Peets *et al.*, *J. Pharmac. exp. Ther.*, 1972, *180*, 464.

A mean biological half-life for chlorpheniramine of 30.3 hours (range 20.6 to 42.5 hours), after the administration of chlorpheniramine maleate 8 mg by mouth to 5 fasting healthy subjects, was much longer than half-lives previously reported. Frequent dosing or the use of sustained-released preparations were considered unnecessary. A duration of effect of about 24 hours was predicted for most subjects.— W. L. Chiou *et al.* (letter), *New Engl. J. Med.*, 1979, *300*, 501.

Excretion of chlorpheniramine was studied under steady-state conditions in 5 healthy subjects given chlorpheniramine maleate 8 mg with pseudoephedrine hydrochloride 120 mg as a sustained-release preparation twice daily for 8 days; 18% of a chlorpheniramine dose was excreted unchanged in the urine, 22.5% as monodesmethylchlorpheniramine, and 4.7% as didesmethylchlorpheniramine between successive doses. In 4 further healthy subjects given a single dose excretion of chlorpheniramine and metabolites was enhanced after treatment with ammonium chloride to alter the pH of the urine.— C. M. Lai *et al.*, *J. pharm. Sci.*, 1979, *68*, 1243.

Further references.— P. Kabasakalian *et al.*, *J. pharm. Sci.*, 1968, *57*, 621; *idem*, 856; J. A. Thompson and F. H. Leffert, *ibid.*, 1980, *69*, 707; A. Yacobi *et al.*, *ibid.*, 1077.

Uses. Chlorpheniramine maleate is an alkylamine derivative with the properties and uses of the antihistamines (see p.1295). It is one of the most potent of the antihistamines and generally causes less sedation than promethazine.

Chlorpheniramine maleate is given usually in doses of 4 mg three or four times daily. Higher doses of up to 36 mg daily have been given in sustained-release preparations. The dose for children up to 1 year is 1 mg twice daily; for those aged 1 to 5 years, 1 to 2 mg thrice daily; and for those aged 6 to 12 years, 2 to 4 mg three or four times daily.

In severe allergies it may be given by intramuscular, subcutaneous, or, diluted with 5 to 10 ml of blood, by slow intravenous injection over a period of 1 minute. The usual dose is 10 to 20 mg and the total dose given by these routes in 24 hours should not normally exceed 40 mg. It has been administered prophylactically to persons with a history of transfusion reactions but should not be added to the blood being transfused.

Administration in renal failure. Chlorpheniramine could be given in usual doses to patients in renal failure.— W. M. Bennett *et al.*, *Ann. intern. Med.*, 1980, *93*, 286.

Asthma. High doses (10 to 25 mg) of chlorpheniramine given intravenously produced bronchodilatation in 10 patients with bronchial asthma. In a double-blind study involving 6 of these patients the effectiveness of these doses was confirmed.— V. T. Popa, *J. Allergy & clin. Immunol.*, 1977, *59*, 54. Bronchodilatation was also produced by nebulised chlorpheniramine in children with asthma.— R. C. Groggins *et al.*, *Archs Dis. Childh.*, 1979, *54*, 163.

Urticaria. Delayed pressure urticaria in 15 patients did not respond to chlorpheniramine maleate 8 mg six-hourly or promethazine hydrochloride 50 mg eight-hourly.— T. J. Ryan *et al.*, *Br. J. Derm.*, 1968, *80*, 485.

An unfavourable report of the use of chlorpheniramine in primary acquired cold urticaria in 8 patients.— A. A. Wanderer *et al.*, *Archs Derm.*, 1977, *113*, 1375.

Chlorpheniramine maleate 4 mg immediately after food was as effective when given alone as when given with cimetidine 400 mg in 4 doses daily for the treatment of 19 patients with a history of daily spontaneous urticarias of unknown origin (chronic idiopathic urticaria).— C. A. Commens and M. W. Greaves, *Br. J. Derm.*, 1978, *99*, 675. See also R. Marks (letter), *ibid.*, 1980, *102*, 240.

Preparations

Elixirs and Syrups

Chlorpheniramine Elixir *(B.P.)*. Chlorpheniramine Syrup. A solution of chlorpheniramine maleate in a suitable flavoured vehicle which may be coloured. Store at a temperature not exceeding 25°. Protect from light. When a dose less than or not a multiple of 5 ml is prescribed, the elixir should be diluted to 5 ml, or a multiple, with syrup. Such dilutions must be freshly prepared and not used more than 2 weeks after issue.

Chlorpheniramine Maleate Syrup *(U.S.P.)*. A syrup containing 36 to 44 mg of chlorpheniramine maleate in each 100 ml and 6 to 8% of alcohol. Store in airtight containers. Protect from light.

Injections

Chlorpheniramine Injection *(B.P.)*. A sterile solution of chlorpheniramine maleate in Water for Injections free from dissolved air. It is distributed in containers, the air in which is replaced by nitrogen or other suitable gas, and sterilised by autoclaving. pH 4 to 5.2. Protect from light.

Chlorpheniramine Maleate Injection *(U.S.P.)*. A sterile solution of chlorpheniramine maleate in Water for Injections. pH 4 to 5.2. Protect from light.

Tablets

Chlorpheniramine Maleate Tablets *(U.S.P.)*. Tablets containing chlorpheniramine maleate. Store in airtight containers.

Chlorpheniramine Tablets *(B.P.)*. Tablets containing chlorpheniramine maleate.

Proprietary Preparations

Haymine *(Pharmax, UK)*. Sustained-release tablets each containing chlorpheniramine maleate 10 mg and ephedrine hydrochloride 15 mg. For allergic disorders. *Dose.* 1 tablet once or twice daily.

Piriton *(Allen & Hanburys, UK)*. Chlorpheniramine maleate, available as **Injection** containing 10 mg per ml, in ampoules of 1 ml; as **Syrup** (suggested diluent, syrup free from preservatives) containing 2 mg in each 5 ml; and as **Tablets** of 4 mg. **Piriton Duolets.** Tablets each containing 8 mg of chlorpheniramine maleate, 4 mg in an outer shell for immediate release and 4 mg in an inner core for sustained release. **Piriton Spandets.** Tablets each containing 12 mg of chlorpheniramine maleate, 4 mg in a yellow layer for immediate release and 8 mg in a white layer for sustained release. (Also available as Piriton in *Austral.*).

Other Proprietary Names

Arg.— Cloro Trimeton, Prof-N-4; *Austral.*— Allergex, Bramahist, Chloramin, Chlor-Trimeton, Histaids, Teledrin; *Belg.*— Kelargine; *Canad.*— Chlor-Tripolon, Histalon, Novopheniram; *Ger.*— Polaronil; *Ital.*— Allerton, Clorten, Lentostamin, Trimeton; *Jap.*— Atalis-D, C-Meton-S, Poracemin; *Neth.*— Methyrit; *S.Afr.*— Allergex, Chlortrimeton, Histamed (see also under Mepyramine Maleate); *Spain*— Colirio Llorens Antihistaminico; *Swed.*— Allergisan; *USA*— AL-R, Chlor-100, Chlor-Mal, Chlormene, Chlorspan, Chlortab, Chlor-Trimeton, Drize, Histaspan, Lorphen, Niratron, Teldrin.

NOTE. The name Chloramin has been applied to chloramine.

Chlorpheniramine maleate was also formerly marketed in Great Britain under the proprietary name Haynon *(R.P. Drugs)*.

6117-g

Cimetidine. SKF 92334. 2-Cyano-1-methyl-3-[2-(5-methylimidazol-4-ylmethylthio)ethyl]-guanidine.

$C_{10}H_{16}N_6S = 252.3$.

CAS — 51481-61-9.

A crystalline powder. M.p. about 142°. **Soluble** 1 in about 88 of water.

Adverse Effects. Diarrhoea, muscle pain, dizziness, and skin rashes may occasionally occur. Reversible confusional states may also occasionally occur, especially in the elderly or in seriously ill patients, such as those with renal failure. Raised serum creatinine concentrations have been regularly observed in patients receiving cimetidine but they appear to have been of no clinical significance. Other side-effects that have occasionally been reported include allergy, gynaecomastia, reversible changes in liver-function values, fever, interstitial nephritis, acute pancreatitis, cardiac arrhythmias, and loss of libido. There have been some reports of neutropenia in patients receiving cimetidine but no cause and effect relationship has been established.

Reviews of side-effects associated with cimetidine therapy.— P. G. Blain, *Adverse Drug React. Bull.*, 1980, Aug., 300.

Allergy. Three episodes of facial oedema and laryngospasm occurred in a 35-year-old woman who was taking cimetidine. Each episode began soon after a dose of cimetidine 300 mg by mouth and was relieved by the administration of corticosteroids.— L. Delaunois (letter), *New Engl. J. Med.*, 1979, *300*, 1216.

Further references.— C. L. Corbett and C. D. Holdsworth, *Br. med. J.*, 1978, *1*, 753.

Diabetogenic effect. Increases in blood-sugar concentrations occurred in 9 patients and 3 healthy subjects given cimetidine. This suggested care in treating potential or overt diabetic patients.— D. B. Jeffreys and J. A. Vale (letter), *Lancet*, 1978, *1*, 383. Criticism. Cimetidine did not appear to affect the handling of dextrose given by intravenous infusion but appeared to retard absorption following administration of dextrose by mouth.— R. L. McIsaac *et al.* (letter), *ibid.*, 551. The development of non-ketotic hyperosmolar diabetes in a 72-year-old woman with an oesophageal rupture might have been associated with cimetidine administration.— E. W. Pomare (letter), *ibid.*, 1202.

Effects on the blood. A discussion on whether administration of cimetidine is associated with granulocytopenia, including the observation that in some cases the data were inadequate for evaluation while other cases represented complex medical problems with concomitant medications and serious illnesses.— J. W. Freston, *Ann. intern. Med.*, 1979, *90*, 264.

A 56-year-old woman with Zollinger-Ellison syndrome developed agranulocytosis as a result of metiamide therapy. She subsequently received cimetidine for 6 months with no evidence of granulocytopenia.— D. Fleischer and I. M. Samloff (letter), *New Engl. J. Med.*, 1977, *296*, 342. See also W. L. Burland *et al.*, *Lancet*, 1975, *2*, 1085.

Individual reports of possible adverse effects of cimetidine on the blood.— E. R. Craven and J. M. Whittington (letter), *Lancet*, 1977, *2*, 294 (agranulocytosis); N. M. Johnson *et al.* (letter), *Lancet*, 1977, *2*, 1226 (leucopenia); M. H. Ufberg *et al.*, *Gastroenterology*, 1977, *73*, 635 (neutropenia); C. L. Corbett *et al.*, *Br. med. J.*, 1978, *1*, 753 (leucopenia); E. Gouffier *et al.*, *Nouv. Presse méd.*, 1978, *7*, 2660 (marrow aplasia); C. James and B. J. Prout (letter), *Lancet*, 1978, *1*, 987 (marrow suppression); S. A. Klotz and B. F. Kay (letter), *Ann.*

intern. Med., 1978, *88*, 579 (marrow suppression); A. López-Luque *et al.* (letter), *Lancet*, 1978, *1*, 444 (leucopenia); R. K. Teichmann *et al.*, *Chirurg.*, 1978, *49*, 397 (agranulocytosis); F. H. Al-Kawas *et al.* (letter), *Ann. intern. Med.*, 1979, *90*, 992 (agranulocytosis); C. de Galocsy and C. van Ypersele de Strihou (letter), *Ann. intern. Med.*, 1979, *90*, 274 (pancytopenia); H. K. Chang and S. L. Morrison, *Ann. intern. Med.*, 1979, *91*, 580 (marrow suppression); F. Druart *et al.*, *Dig. Dis. Scis*, 1979, *24*, 730 (marrow failure); J. Idvall (letter), *Lancet*, 1979, *2*, 159 (thrombocytopenia); G. O. Littlejohn and M. B. Urowitz (letter), *Ann. intern. Med.*, 1979, *91*, 317 (agranulocytosis); J. L. McDaniel and J. J. Stein (letter), *New Engl. J. Med.*, 1979, *300*, 864 (thrombocytopenia); R. Rate *et al.* (letter), *Ann. intern. Med.*, 1979, *91*, 795 (granulocytopenia, thrombocytopenia, and a haemolytic disorder); B. Rotoli *et al.* (letter), *Lancet*, 1979, *2*, 583 (haemolytic anaemia); M. J. Collen, *West. J. Med.*, 1980, *132*, 257 (thrombocytopenia and leucopenia); A. J. Isaacs, *Br. med. J.*, 1980, *280*, 294 (thrombocytopenia); V. M. Yates and R. E. I. Kerr (letter), *Br. med. J.*, 1980, *280*, 1453 (thrombocytopenia); E. Sazie and J. P. Jaffe (letter), *Ann. intern. Med.*, 1980, *93*, 151 (granulocytopenia); H. W. Carloss *et al.*, *Ann. intern. Med.*, 1980, *93*, 57 (granulocytopenia); B. Tonkonow and R. Hoffman (letter), *Archs intern. Med.*, 1980, *140*, 1123 (aplastic anaemia).

Effects on bones and joints. A report of 5 patients who developed severe arthritic complaints in association with cimetidine administration.— T. K. Khong and P. J. Rooney (letter), *Lancet*, 1980, *2*, 1380.

Effects on the endocrine system. Although high intravenous bolus doses of cimetidine of 200 mg or more caused rapid and sustained prolactin secretion, intravenous infusion of 500 mg at a rate of 100 mg per hour had no effect. Moreover, no measurable effects had been found in patients who had received 1 g daily by mouth for a month. These data suggest that the standard dosage of cimetidine for long-term therapy does not stimulate prolactin release in man.— G. Delitala *et al.* (letter), *Lancet*, 1978, *2*, 1054. No significant difference was noted in the prolactin concentrations of 14 patients with peptic ulcer given cimetidine 1 g daily for one month. The clinical relevance of hyperprolactinaemia in patients taking cimetidine is doubtful, particularly as prolactin is a stress-related hormone and may be raised non-specifically.— S. La Brooy *et al.*, *Gut*, 1978, *19*, A986.

Further comnments and studies on plasma-prolactin concentrations following cimetidine administration.— M. Petrillo *et al.* (letter), *Lancet*, 1977, *2*, 761; J. C. Daubresse *et al.* (letter), *ibid.*, 1978, *1*, 99; S. K. Majumdar *et al.*, *Br. med. J.*, 1978, *1*, 409; W. L. Burland *et al.* (letter), *ibid.*, 717; R. Valcavi *et al.* (letter), *Lancet*, 1978, *2*, 528; D. Rowley-Jones (letter), *ibid.*, 635; G. F. Nelis and J. G. C. Van de Meene, *Postgrad. med. J.*, 1980, *56*, 26.

The effect of cimetidine, as an anti-androgen, on the function of the hypothalamic-pituitary-gonadal axis was studied in 7 men of proven fertility who took cimetidine 1.2 g daily for 9 weeks. The sperm count was significantly reduced after cimetidine, the luteinising hormone response to gonadorelin given intravenously was reduced although plasma-testosterone concentrations were increased, and gonadotrophin responses to provocation by clomiphene were considered inadequate. Caution is necessary when cimetidine is prescribed for prolonged periods and regular sperm counts are recommended.— D. H. Van Thiel *et al.*, *New Engl. J. Med.*, 1979, *300*, 1012. Comment and criticism.— R. J. Temple *et al.*, *ibid.*, 1046. Criticism of the study and the generalisations made from results in only 7 men.— R. J. Fuentes and D. Dolinsky (letter), *ibid.*, *301*, 501. Further criticism and different findings in 8 men who took cimetidine 1 g daily for a minimum of 6 weeks. Endocrine disturbance was not proved.— M. C. White *et al.* (letter), *ibid.*, 502. Reply.— D. H. Van Thiel (letter), *ibid.*

Mention of diabetes insipidus developing in 2 patients taking cimetidine.— *Br. med. J.*, 1981, *282*, 56.

See also under Effects on Sexual Function and Gynaecomastia.

Effects on the gastro-intestinal tract. Long-term effects of cimetidine on gastric secretion.— R. J. Holden *et al.*, *Gut*, 1977, *18*, A949. Hypergastrinaemia associated with cimetidine administration.— K. D. Buchanan *et al.*, *ibid.*, 1978, *19*, A437.

Carcinoma. There have been occasional reports of gastric carcinoma in patients receiving cimetidine. No cause and effect relationship has been established and at least some of these reports may involve previously undiagnosed carcinoma, the symptoms of which were initially alleviated by cimetidine therapy, hence masking the underlying malignancy. Nevertheless J.B. Elder *et al.* (*Lancet*, 1979, *1*, 1005) have speculated that cimetidine could react with nitrites in the gut to form mononitrosocimetidine, a nitrosoguanidine, an analogue of which is a known experimental gastric carcinogen. This view and the evidence upon which it was based has been severely criticised (F.J.C. Roe, *Lancet*, 1979, *1*, 1039; W.S.J. Ruddell, *ibid.*, 1234; M.J. Hill, *ibid.*, 1235; P. Rubin, *ibid.*, 1236; P.W. Mullen, *ibid.*, 1406; M. Guslandi, *ibid.*), with comments which include a reminder that many commonly used drugs can be nitrosated to produced carcinogens. In a reply J.B. Elder *et al.* (*Lancet*, 1979, *2*, 245) reiterate their view, adding the information that nitrosocimetidine produced *in vitro* is mutagenic.

The problem of increased numbers of metabolically active bacteria invading the achlorhydric stomach, which is common to antisecretory drugs of all types, has been investigated by W.S.J. Ruddell *et al.* (*Lancet*, 1980, *1*, 672). These workers did find an increase in the total bacterial count (including an increase in the count of nitrate-reducing organisms normally found in the faeces) in samples of gastric juice from patients treated with cimetidine. In an earlier study (W.S.J. Ruddell *et al.*, *Lancet*, 1976, *2*, 1037) they found an inverse relationship between mean nitrite and hydrogen ion concentrations in fasting subjects undergoing routine gastro-intestinal investigations. This was confirmed by P. Schlag *et al.* (*Lancet*, 1980, *1*, 727) in a study attempting to establish whether nitrite and *N*-nitroso compounds in gastric juice are risk factors for carcinoma in the operated stomach. While considering that high nitrite concentrations in the resected stomach, with an increase in *N*-nitroso compounds, could be one of the factors sharing responsibility for the cancer risk to the gastric stump of the resected stomach, Schlag *et al.* also felt that other factors besides pH play a significant part in *N*-nitrosation in the operated stomach. A number of aspects of the work by Schlag *et al.* have, however, been criticised by W.S.J. Ruddell and C.L. Walters (*Lancet*, 1980, *1*, 1187). With specific reference to cimetidine G.P. Crean *et al.* (*Lancet*, 1979, *2*, 797 and *New Engl. J. Med.*, 1981, 304, 672) have reported no association between cimetidine and gastric neoplasia in long-term studies on *dogs*. Moreover in a clinical study negative findings were also obtained by T.J. Muscroft *et al.* (*Lancet*, 1981, *1*, 408). They found that cimetidine is unlikely to increase formation of intragastric *N*-nitroso compounds in subjects taking a normal diet suggesting that long-term treatment with cimetidine is unlikely to promote gastric cancer as a result of bacterial metabolic activity. This work was subsequently discussed and criticised (see R.F.McCloy and J.H. Baron, *Lancet*, 1981, *1*, 609; W.S.J. Ruddell, *ibid.*, 784; T.G. Allen-Mersh *et al.*, *ibid.*, 835; T.J. Muscroft and M.R.B. Keighley, *ibid.*, 1002). Nevertheless, a need for continued vigilance has been voiced by P.I. Reed *et al.* (*Lancet*, 1981, *2*, 550 and 553) in their studies on gastric juice *N*-nitrosamines in health and gastroduodenal disease and the property of cimetidine of raising gastric juice *N*-nitrosamine concentrations. This work was subsequently discussed and criticised by R. Brimblecombe, *Lancet*, 1981, *2*, 686; P.N. Magee, *ibid.*, 984; N.J.McC. Mortensen and W.K. Eltringham, *ibid.*; P.I. Reed *et al.*, *ibid.*, 1281; R.W. Brimblecombe, *ibid.*, 1982, *1*, 402.

Some individual reports of gastric carcinoma in patients given cimetidine.— P. I. Reed *et al.* (letter), *Lancet*, 1979, *1*, 1234; T. V. Taylor *et al.* (letter), *ibid.*, 1235; P. C. Hawker *et al.* (letter), *ibid.*, 1980, *1*, 709.

Diarrhoea. Severe colonic distension, sometimes with diarrhoea, occurred in 3 burned patients (classified as 30 to 45%) when given cimetidine for 3 to 7 days.— W. C. Watson *et al.* (letter), *Lancet*, 1977, *2*, 720.

Moderately severe and persistent diarrhoea in a 60-year-old man resulted in severe dehydration and was attributed to treatment with cimetidine.— R. Field and G. W. Meyer (letter), *New Engl. J. Med.*, 1978, *299*, 262.

Further references: W. S. J. Ruddell and M. S. Losowsky, *Br. med. J.*, 1980, *281*, 273.

Erosions. In a 43-year-old man a duodenal ulcer healed under cimetidine treatment but punctate erosive gastritis and florid duodenitis developed and persisted for 6 months. Four months after cimetidine was stopped the gastritis had disappeared but duodenitis persisted. The clinical significance was not clear.— J. Webster *et al.*, *Br. med. J.*, 1978, *1*, 20. The rise in gastric pH associated with cimetidine administration might have encouraged the growth of *Candida albicans* which could have caused the gastritis. When healing is delayed or has failed or there is evidence of erosive gastritis or duodenitis, biopsy material and stool cultures should be tested for *C. albicans*; when positive, concurrent administration of nystatin with cimetidine should be considered.— P. E. Nicholls and K. Henry (letter), *Lancet*, 1978, *1*, 1095. A further case of severe erosive duodenitis in a patient receiving cimetidine. The aetiology remained obscure.— B. Al-Nakib (letter), *ibid.*, 1979, *1*, 607. It was considered that the development of erosions might be part of the natural history of the syndrome rather than a drug-related effect.— K. D. Bardhan (letter), *ibid.*, 726.

Mention of gastric and duodenal candidiasis in a patient taking cimetidine for a prepyloric ulcer.— F. Cipollini and F. Altilia (letter), *Lancet*, 1981, *2*, 1047.

Further references.— J. Scott-Findlay (letter), *Med. J. Aust.*, 1977, *2*, 719; G. Fedeli *et al.* (letter), *Br. med. J.*, 1978, *1*, 853; B. D. Linaker and S. Hughes (letter), *ibid.*, 1278.

Intrinsic factor. In 16 patients with proven duodenal ulceration cimetidine reduced the output of intrinsic factor and its concentration in gastric secretion. The effect of long-term cimetidine treatment on the absorption of cyanocobalamin needed study.— L. P. Fielding *et al.*, *Br. med. J.*, 1978, *1*, 818. In 7 healthy men the reduction in total and peak intrinsic factor output produced by cimetidine during pentagastrin infusion was entirely accounted for by the concomitant reduction in the volume of gastric secretion.— P. C. Sharpe *et al.*, *Br. med. J.*, 1979, *1*, 1251. See also P. C. Sharpe *et al.*, *Gut*, 1977, *18*, A948.

Data suggesting that patients on long-term cimetidine therapy may malabsorb food-bound cobalamine.— W. M. Steinberg *et al.*, *Dig. Dis. Scis*, 1980, *25*, 188.

Further references.— H. J. Binder and R. M. Donaldson, *Gastroenterology*, 1978, *74*, 371.

Perforation. A 46-year-old man with a 7-year history of peptic ulcer symptoms developed a perforated duodenal ulcer after receiving cimetidine 200 mg thrice daily and 400 mg at night for 20 days. The patient may have been one of the few who do not respond to cimetidine therapy.— L. Lombardo *et al.*, *Ital. J. Gastroenterol.*, 1978, *10*, 249.

Further references.— D. J. Ellis *et al.* (letter), *Br. med. J.*, 1977, *2*, 1538.

See also under Precautions.

Phytobezoar. After treatment for 2 weeks with cimetidine 300 mg four times daily and gastric antacids (Mylanta II and Gaviscon), a 55-year-old woman obtained complete healing of an oesophageal ulcer secondary to reflux oesophagitis, but had a large phytobezoar in the fundus of her stomach.— T. W. Nichols (letter), *Lancet*, 1978, *2*, 1263.

Pyloric obstruction. Pyloric obstruction during cimetidine therapy.— W. Gazala and I. Hatim (letter), *Br. med. J.*, 1978, *1*, 722.

Effects on the heart. Severe arrhythmias (fatal in 1 patient) were associated in 2 patients with the intravenous injection of cimetidine.— J. Cohen *et al.*, *Br. med. J.*, 1979, *2*, 768. Cimetidine should be given intravenously by infusion; moreover, one patient had renal failure and the dose was too high.— S. Ahmad (letter), *ibid.*, 1369.

Further individual reports of the effects of cimetidine on the heart.— P. Reding *et al.* (letter), *Lancet*, 1977, *2*, 1227 (bradycardia with atrioventricular dissociation); D. B. Jefferys and J. A. Vale (letter), *Lancet*, 1978, *1*, 828 (bradycardia); F. Bournerias *et al.*, *Nouv. Presse méd.*, 1978, *7*, 2069 (fatal arrhythmia); M. Ligumsky *et al.* (letter), *Ann. intern. Med.*, 1978, *89*, 1008 (bradycardia and suppression of arrhythmia); B. Stimmesse *et al.*, *Nouv. Presse méd.*, 1978, *7*, 4233 (bradycardia).

The infusion of cimetidine 300 mg in 10 patients had no effect on heart-rate or sinus node function.— T. R. Engel and J. C. Luck, *New Engl. J. Med.*, 1979, *301*, 591. Criticism of conclusions based on single-dose therapy, when reports of adverse cardiac effects have involved chronic therapy.— R. Levi and J. P. Trzeciakowski (letter), *ibid.*, 1980, *302*, 235. Reply.— T. R. Engel and J. C. Luck (letter), *ibid.*

No demonstrable cardiovascular effects in peptic ulcer patients given cimetidine 400 mg four times daily for 4 weeks.— S. Saltissi *et al.*, *Br. J. clin. Pharmac.*, 1981, *11*, 497.

Similar studies.— I. O. Samuel and J. W. Dundee, *J.R. Soc. Med.*, 1979, *72*, 898; S. Warburton *et al.*, *S. Afr. med. J.*, 1979, *55*, 1125; M. J. Boyce, *Br. J. clin. Pharmac.*, 1981, *12*, 268P.

Effects on immune function. Comments and studies on the effects of cimetidine on the immune response.— C. G. A. McGregor *et al.* (preliminary communication), *Lancet*, 1977, *1*, 122; B. E. de Pauw *et al.* (letter), *ibid.*, 1977, *2*, 616; J. Avella *et al.*, *ibid.*, 1978, *1*, 624; F. G. C. Jones (letter), *ibid.*, 880; M. W. Greaves (letter), *ibid*; J. S. Goodwin (letter), *ibid.*, 934; M. D. Smith *et al.* (letter), *ibid.*, 1979, *1*, 1406; A. J. Robertson *et al.*

(letter), *ibid.*, 1979, *2*, 420.

Kidney transplants. Rejection of kidney transplant occurred in 2 children given cimetidine either for the treatment or prophylaxis of stress ulcer.— W. A. Primack (letter), *Lancet*, 1978, *1*, 824. In 6 patients treated with cimetidine from the time of operation there has been no evidence of increased susceptibility to rejection.— C. C. Doherty and M. G. McGeown (letter), *ibid.*, 1048. Cimetidine had no effect on graft rejection in 12 patients who received 800 mg daily compared with 46 who did not.— B. Charpentier and D. Fries (letter), *ibid.*, 1265. See also C. J. Rudge *et al.* (letter), *ibid.*, 1154.

Effects on the kidneys. Serum creatinine concentrations quite commonly rise in patients taking cimetidine, but this does not necessarily imply renal failure, and other tests of renal function are not usually affected.— J. G. Salway, *Prescribers' J.*, 1979, *19*, 23.

Individual reports and studies on altered creatinine concentrations associated with cimetidine.— M. Dutt *et al.*, *Gut*, 1978, *19*, A441; H. Malchow *et al.*, *Dt. med. Wschr.*, 1978, *103*, 149; M. McElligott (letter), *Lancet*, 1978, *1*, 99; R. Larsson *et al.*, *Acta med. scand.*, 1979, *205*, 87.

Acute interstitial nephritis associated with cimetidine.— W. R. McGowan and S. E. Vermillion, *Gastroenterology*, 1980, *79*, 746.

Reversible renal failure developed in a patient who had been taking cimetidine 1 g daily for about one month.— R. Seidelin, *Postgrad. med. J.*, 1980, *56*, 440.

Effects on the liver. Mention of a patient given cimetidine who developed signs of liver damage associated with hypersensitivity.— G. Bodemar and A. Walan, *Lancet*, 1978, *1*, 403. See also J. P. Villeneuve and H. A. Warner, *Gastroenterology*, 1979, *77*, 143.

Further references.— P. C. Sharpe and B. W. Hawkins, in *Cimetidine: Proceedings of the Second International Symposium on Histamine H_2-Receptor Antagonists*, W.L. Burland and M.A. Simkins (Ed.), Oxford, Excerpta Medica, 1977, p. 358 (centrilobular necrosis); H. Zuchner, *Dt. med. Wschr.*, 1977, *102*, 1788 (cholestatic hepatitis); C. L. Corbett and C. D. Holdsworth, *Br. med. J.*, 1978, *1*, 753 (raised serum aminotransferase values); D. M. McCarthy, *Gastroenterology*, 1978, *74*, 453 (possible hypersensitivity hepatic dysfunction).

Effects on the muscles. Mention of muscle cramps and weakness in association with cimetidine therapy.— R. J. M. Lane and F. L. Mastaglia, *Lancet*, 1978, *2*, 562.

Effects on the nervous system. A reversible brain stem syndrome in a 54-year-old man might have been associated with administration of cimetidine. Within 2 days of starting cimetidine 1 g daily he experienced lightheadedness and frontal headache. Over the next 10 days he suffered progressive unsteadiness with frequent falls, he suffered episodes of transient bilateral visual impairment and became deaf in his left ear; his speech became progressively dysarthric until it was unintelligible, and he had been doubly incontinent; he complained of paraesthesia. On admission to hospital his abnormal symptoms were found to be confined to the nervous system and within 5 days of stopping cimetidine his neurological status had returned to normal.— W. J. K. Cumming and J. B. Foster (letter), *Lancet*, 1978, *1*, 1096.

Of 36 critically ill patients receiving cimetidine, usually in a dose of 300 mg intravenously every six hours, 6 developed moderate to severe mental changes. Three of the 6 had both renal and hepatic failure and in all 6 serum-cimetidine concentrations estimated 5 minutes before the next dose (trough concentrations) were above 1.25 µg per ml whereas they were below 1.25 µg per ml in the other 29 evaluated, only 2 of whom had renal and hepatic failure (and both of whom were receiving low doses of cimetidine). CSF samples taken from 2 patients with mental changes and 3 without, demonstrated that cimetidine can cross the blood-brain barrier, although not freely, the CSF to serum ratio of cimetidine concentrations being about 0.24 : 1. It thus appears that cimetidine causes dose-related mental confusion and that patients with both renal and hepatic impairment are likely to have raised serum-cimetidine concentrations, presumably because neither excretory system can partially compensate for the other, and should be given reduced doses. One patient tolerated serum concentrations of cimetidine above 2 µg per ml despite having suffered significant mental changes on initial exposure; the possibility of tolerance should be studied.— J. J. Schentag *et al.*, *Lancet*, 1979, *1*, 177. Only 57 reports of confusional states in some kind of association with cimetidine had been received out of several million patients treated. Of 44 with enough information, 35 concerned elderly patients or those with serious concomitant illness that might independently have contributed. No indication of relationship with dose had emerged. Cimetidine had been used in full dosage in many patients with severe hepatic disease and the suggestion based on a single patient from a total of 5 is not considered sufficient to recommend a reduction of dosage in patients with isolated liver failure.— A. C. Flind and D. Rowley-Jones, *Smith Kline & French* (letter), *ibid.*, 379.

Individual reports of adverse neurological effects possibly associated with cimetidine and mainly in patients who were elderly, seriously ill, or had impaired renal function.— T. A. Grimson (letter), *Lancet*, 1977, *1*, 858 (confusion); J. C. Delaney and M. Ravey (letter), *Lancet*, 1977, *2*, 512 (confusion); W. Grave *et al.* (letter), *Lancet*, 1977, *2*, 719 (twitching and deepening of unconsciousness); N. Menzies-Gow (letter), *Lancet*, 1977, *2*, 928 (confusion); T. J. Robinson and T. O. Mulligan (letter), *Lancet*, 1977, *2*, 719 (confusion); C. A. Wood *et al.* (letter), *J. Am. med. Ass.*, 1978, *239*, 2550 (confusion); S. K. Agarwal (letter), *J. Am. med. Ass.*, 1978, *240*, 214 (hallucinations); M. L. Levine (letter), *J. Am. med. Ass.*, 1978, *240*, 1238 (coma); M. A. McMillen *et al.* (letter), *New Engl. J. Med.*, 1978, *298*, 284 (confusion); J. B. Spears (letter), *Am. J. Hosp. Pharm.*, 1978, *35*, 1035 (confusion); T. R. Vickery (letter), *Drug Intell. & clin. Pharm.*, 1978, *12*, 242 (confusion); C. C. Barnhart and C. L. Bowden, *Am. J. Psychiat.*, 1979, *136*, 725 (confusion); M. E. Edmonds *et al.*, *J. R. Soc. Med.*, 1979, *72*, 172 (confusion, muscular twitching and convulsions); M. B. Forman *et al.* (letter), *Lancet*, 1979, *2*, 1250 (flapping tremor resembling uraemic encephalopathy with cimetidine and primidone); J. W. Jefferson, *Am. J. Psychiat.*, 1979, *136*, 346 (depression); J. Johnson and S. Bailey, *Br. J. Psychiat.*, 1979, *134*, 315 (depression); H. G. Kinnell and A. Webb (letter), *Br. med. J.*, 1979, *2*, 1438 (paranoia and confusion); S. R. Mogelnicki *et al.*, *J. Am. med. Ass.*, 1979, *241*, 826 (confusion); B. J. Kimelblatt *et al.*, *Gastroenterology*, 1980, *78*, 791 (confusion); L. E. Adler *et al.*, *Am. J. Psychiat.*, 1980, *137*, 1112 (paranoia); A. B. Atkinson *et al.* (letter), *Lancet*, 1980, *2*, 36 (neuropathy; with captopril); T. G. Feest and D. J. Read (letter), *Br. med. J.*, 1980, *281*, 1284 (myopathy); T. J. Walls *et al.*, *Br. med. J.*, 1980, *281*, 974 (motor neuropathy); J. Totte *et al.* (letter), *Lancet*, 1981, *1*, 1047 (neurological dysfunction and metabolite).

Effects on sexual function. Three men experienced loss of libido progressing to impotence while taking cimetidine; the Committee on Safety of Medicines had received reports of 23 cases of impotence.— N. R. Peden *et al.*, *Br. med. J.*, 1979, *1*, 659. Comment; there is unlikely to be an endocrine basis for the impotence.— S. G. Barber (letter), *Br. med. J.*, 1979, *1*, 1147.

Further reports.— M. M. Wolfe (letter), *New Engl. J. Med.*, 1979, *300*, 94.

See also under Effects on the Endocrine System and Gynaecomastia.

Effects on the skin. *Alopecia.* Alopecia occurred in a 35-year-old woman taking cimetidine for duodenal ulcer. The hair loss ceased when cimetidine was stopped, and occurred again after a fresh course of treatment was begun.— S. Ahmad (letter), *Ann. intern. Med.*, 1979, *91*, 930.

Transitory alopecia and hypergonadotrophic hypogonadism during cimetidine treatment.— M. I. Vircburger *et al.* (letter), *Lancet*, 1981, *1*, 1160.

Erythrosis. Wide-spread erythrosis-like lesions in a 36-year-old man were probably induced by cimetidine.— G. Angelini *et al.* (letter), *Br. med. J.*, 1979, *1*, 1147.

Exfoliative dermatitis. A report of exfoliative dermatitis associated with the use of cimetidine.— P. L. Yantis, *Dig. Dis. Scis*, 1980, *25*, 73.

Psoriasis. Administration of cimetidine had had a beneficial effect in 3 patients with psoriasis.— A. Giacosa *et al.* (letter), *Lancet*, 1978, *2*, 1211. Several patients with psoriasis who were taking cimetidine for duodenal ulcers had obtained no benefit to their psoriasis.— E. J. Raffle (letter), *ibid.*, 1314. A report of 2 similar patients whose psoriasis had not improved.— D. I. McCallum and P. W. Grant (letter), *ibid.* A report of a patient whose psoriasis was precipitated by administration of cimetidine.— G. S. Rai and S. G. P. Webster (letter), *ibid.*, 1979, *1*, 50. See also V. M. Yates and R. E. I. Kerr (letter), *Br. med. J.*, 1980, *280*, 1453.

Stevens-Johnson syndrome. For the Stevens-Johnson syndrome in association with cimetidine see below.

Urticaria. A 46-year-old woman developed a generalised red rash with moderate pruritus after taking cimetidine for about 3 weeks. This disappeared within 48 hours of stopping cimetidine but recurred when she again took cimetidine and developed into widespread giant urticaria.— W. A. Hadfield (letter), *Ann. intern. Med.*, 1979, *91*, 128.

Effects on uric acid concentrations. Mention of a slight but consistent rise in serum-uric acid concentrations in patients taking cimetidine.— *Gut*, 1979, *20*, 68.

Fever. A febrile reaction to cimetidine.— C. Ramboer (letter), *Lancet*, 1978, *1*, 330. Another report of cimetidine-induced fever.— J. C. McLoughlin *et al.* (letter), *ibid.*, 499. Cimetidine-induced fever might be caused by blockade of histamine H_2 receptors in the thermoregulatory areas of the hypothalamus.— G. Nisticò *et al.* (letter), *ibid.*, 1978, *2*, 265.

Gynaecomastia. Five of 25 patients taking cimetidine 1.6 g daily for duodenal ulcer or severe duodenitis developed gynaecomastia after treatment for 4 to 9 months; it rapidly regressed and disappeared after completion of treatment at 12 months. Libido was temporarily reduced in one patient.— R. W. Spence and L. R. Celestin, *Gut*, 1979, *20*, 154.

Similar reports.— G. F. Delle Fave *et al.* (letter), *Lancet*, 1977, *1*, 1319 (gynaecomastia and galactorrhoea); M. C. Bateson *et al.* (letter), *ibid.*, 1977, *2*, 247 (galactorrhoea); H. M. Smedley (letter), *Lancet*, 1981, *2*, 638 (malignant breast change in a man given cimetidine and doxepin).

See also under Effects on the Endocrine System and Effects on Sexual Function.

Hypotension. Two patients experienced severe hypotension after bolus intravenous injections of 600 mg of cimetidine. No haemodynamic changes occurred when administration was changed to intravenous infusion.— W. A. Mahon and M. Kolton (letter), *Lancet*, 1978, *1*, 828. Intravenous cimetidine should be administered in infusion form to avoid hypotension.— S. Ahmad (letter), *Br. med. J.*, 1979, *2*, 1369.

See also under Effects on the Heart.

Overdosage. A patient who took about 12 g of cimetidine had slurred speech, high pulse-rate, and dilated pupils. Five hours after gastric lavage he was confused, agitated, disorientated and making staccato nonsensical conversation. He recovered from these mental symptoms the next day. There were no changes in ECG, blood indexes, liver or kidney.— P. G. Nelson (letter), *Lancet*, 1977, *2*, 928.

A patient took a 2-month course of cimetidine in one week without untoward effect; this produced a daily dose of about 12 g. His dyspepsia was relieved and his duodenal ulcer healed.— G. V. Gill (letter), *Lancet*, 1978, *1*, 99.

Four men took overdoses (5.2 to 19.6 g) of cimetidine; plasma concentrations of up to 57 µg per ml were recorded, compared with reported peak concentrations of 1 µg per ml after a single 200-mg dose. Apart from dry mouth no patient experienced untoward effects.— R. N. Illingworth and D. R. Jarvie, *Br. med. J.*, 1979, *1*, 453.

Respiratory depression associated with cimetidine overdosage.— J. B. Wilson (letter), *Br. med. J.*, 1979, *1*, 955.

Pancreatitis. A possible association between acute pancreatitis and cimetidine in one patient.— F. Arnold *et al.* (letter), *Lancet*, 1978, *1*, 382. Studies in *rats* also indicated that this might be a risk.— S. N. Joffe and F. D. Lee (letter), *ibid.*, 383. The association was doubted. Experiments in *rats* were not considered to be relevant to man.— R. L. McIsaac *et al.* (letter), *ibid.*, 551. There was no deterioration in the clinical course of acute pancreatitis in 11 patients whose treatment of alcoholic pancreatitis included continuous infusion with cimetidine 800 mg daily.— H. G. Dammann and H. J. Augustin (letter), *ibid.*, 666. *Animal* studies favouring clinical reports which dissociate acute pancreatitis and treatment with cimetidine.— S. Szabo and H. Goldman (letter), *ibid.*, 1978, *2*, 266.

Results of a study in 32 patients receiving cimetidine for duodenal ulcer showed no evidence that cimetidine damages the pancreas.— J. A. Murie *et al.* (letter), *Br. J. clin. Pharmac.*, 1980, *9*, 279.

Two patients with pancreatitis associated with cimetidine therapy.— M. L. Wilkinson *et al.* (letter), *Lancet*, 1981, *1*, 610.

Further references.— D. P. Maudgal *et al.*, *Gut*, 1977, *18*, A981.

See also under Uses.

Pregnancy and the neonate. No abnormalities were found in the male infant of a woman to whom it had been considered essential to administer cimetidine 1 g daily from the sixteenth to the twentieth week of pregnancy.— P. Zulli and Q. Di Nisio (letter), *Lancet*, 1978, *2*, 945.

Intravenous administration of cimetidine 200 mg to 20 patients in labour did not prolong labour or alter the pattern or strength of uterine contractions. It was confirmed that cimetidine crosses the placenta but there were no alterations in the rate or pattern of the foetal heart-rate.— W. A. W. McGowan, *J. R. Soc. Med.*, 1979, *72*, 902.

See also under Precautions.

Stevens-Johnson syndrome. After taking cimetidine for 25 days a 38-year-old Asian woman with a history of penicillin allergy developed the Stevens-Johnson syndrome. It was not considered ethically justifiable to confirm the association by readministering cimetidine.— A. H. Ahmed *et al.* (letter), *Lancet*, 1978, *2*, 433.

Treatment of Adverse Effects. There is no specific treatment. In recent severe overdosage with cimetidine the stomach should be emptied by aspiration and lavage. For general guidelines to the symptomatic therapy of drug overdosage, see Phenobarbitone, p.812.

In patients with renal failure cimetidine may be removed by dialysis but such measures would not be necessary in patients with normal renal function.

The use of forced diuresis in a patient who had taken an overdose of cimetidine and oxazepam.— A. W. A. M. van Rijthoven (letter), *Lancet*, 1979, *2*, 370. Concern that forced diuresis, a procedure not without risk, was used for cimetidine poisoning. Experience with 14 adults and 4 children, who had taken cimetidine alone or with alcohol and various other drugs, has not demonstrated any significant toxicity of cimetidine in overdosage. Three of 7 adults who remained completely free of symptoms had taken 20 g of cimetidine, and 3½ hours after ingestion one of these had a blood-cimetidine concentration of 45.8 mg per litre. In view of the apparent lack of toxicity of cimetidine in overdosage it is recommended that treatment should consist of gastric lavage or administration of syrup of ipecacuanha, provided that not more than 4 hours have elapsed since ingestion of the drug, followed by supportive measures and symptomatic treatment only. Forced diuresis is not recommended and, moreover, there appears to be no evidence that it enhances the excretion of cimetidine from the body.— T. J. Meredith and G. N. Volans (letter), *ibid.*, 1367.

Precautions. Before giving cimetidine to patients with gastric ulcers the possibility of malignancy should be excluded since cimetidine may mask symptoms and delay diagnosis. Cimetidine should be given in reduced dosage to patients with impaired renal function.

Cimetidine may enhance the effects of warfarin. Cimetidine may also interfere with the metabolism of some benzodiazepines (see under Diazepam, p.1522).

Intravenous injections of cimetidine should be given slowly; intravenous infusion is recommended in patients with cardiovascular impairment.

A placebo-controlled study in 6 healthy subjects indicated that infusion of cimetidine 400 mg has an influence on Romberg's test (a study of body sway, thought to be sensitive to changes in CNS function). Several of the subjects experienced transitory euphoria or mental relaxation.— J. Brynskov *et al.* (letter), *Lancet*, 1980, *1*, 1421.

Administration in children. For adverse effects associated with high doses of cimetidine in children, see under Uses (Administration in children).

Administration in the elderly. For a suggestion that elderly subjects may require reduced doses of cimetidine, see under Uses (Administration in the elderly).

Carcinoma of the stomach. Cimetidine appeared to mask signs of carcinoma of the stomach. Delays of 2 to 12 months from time of presentation with symptoms to diagnosis of tumour had occurred in 12 of 29 patients treated for adenocarcinoma of the stomach; 8 of the 12, who were all men over the age of 57 years, had been treated with cimetidine and antacids for 6 to 12 months before surgical referral; only 2 had a barium meal and none had a gastroscopy before starting treatment. Whereas the incidence of gastric carcinoma in young people is low, patients over the age of 50, especially those with dyspepsia, anaemia, or dysphagia of recent onset, require urgent investigation; they should not be prescribed cimetidine without prior radiological and/or endoscopic examination.— C. J. Stoddard *et al.* (letter), *Lancet*, 1980, *2*, 199. See also R. H. Taylor *et al.*, *ibid.*, 1978, *1*, 686; C. Murray *et al.* (letter), *ibid.*, 1092; G. Minoli *et al.* (letter), *ibid.*

Interactions. In general, cimetidine does not appear to produce significant interactions with other drugs by affecting absorption. The major method whereby it alters the disposition of other drugs appears to be by inhibition of microsomal metabolism.— H. J. Rogers *et al.* (letter), *Lancet*, 1980, *2*, 694.

Variability in the enzyme-inhibiting effect of cimetidine.— T. K. Daneshmend *et al.*, *Br. J. clin. Pharmac.*, 1981, *11*, 421P.

Aminophylline. The administration of cimetidine was associated with accumulation of theophylline to a potentially toxic concentration in a 15-year-old girl.— M. M. Weinberger *et al.* (letter), *New Engl. J. Med.*, 1981, *304*, 672. See also under Aminophylline, p.343.

Antacids. In healthy subjects antacids given after a meal probably do not interfere with the absorption of cimetidine. A study in 9 fasting patients with chronic active peptic ulcer, however, indicated that concomitant administration of an antacid preparation, containing aluminium hydroxide and magnesium hydroxide, with cimetidine lowered the amount of cimetidine absorbed.— G. Bodemar *et al.* (letter), *Lancet*, 1979, *1*, 444.

Further references.— W. L. Burland *et al.* (letter), *Lancet*, 1976, *2*, 965; G. Bodemar *et al.*, *Scand. J. Gastroenterol.*, 1977, *12*, 12; G. Bodemar *et al.*, *Gut*, 1978, *19*, A990.

Antibiotics. For the effect of cimetidine on tetracycline, see Tetracycline, p.1218.

Anticholinergics. Some reduction in the bioavailability of cimetidine on concomitant administration of *metoclopramide* and *propantheline*.— J. Kanto *et al.* (letter), *Br. J. clin. Pharmac.*, 1981, *11*, 629.

Anticoagulants. For the effect of cimetidine on anticoagulants, see Warfarin Sodium, p.778.

Anticonvulsants. In 4 patients taking phenytoin and other anticonvulsant drugs (doses unchanged) the plasma-phenytoin values rose by 13 to 33% when cimetidine was given concomitantly.— D. J. Hetzel *et al.*, *Br. med. J.*, 1981, *282*, 1512.

Antineoplastics. For the effect of cimetidine on immunosuppressants, see Carmustine, p.195.

Benzodiazepines. For the effect of cimetidine on diazepam and other benzodiazepines, see Diazepam, p.1522.

Beta-adrenoceptor blocking agents. For the effect of cimetidine on propranolol and other beta-adrenoceptor blocking agents, see Propranolol, p.1328.

Iron. For the effect of cimetidine on ferrous sulphate, see Ferrous Sulphate, p.878.

Pentagastrin. Evidence from a study on medical students that some of the somatic symptoms induced by pentagastrin can be modified by cimetidine pretreatment. Cimetidine seems to abolish sensations of body heat, and also sensations arising from the arms but not the legs. Dizziness, however, occurred considerably more frequently when pentagastrin and cimetidine were given together than when cimetidine was given alone.— A. Wade and D. Wingate, *Lancet*, 1980, *2*, 516.

Interference with diagnostic tests. A study indicating that, contrary to suggestions, cimetidine does not interfere with allergy skin testing.— J. A. Smith *et al.*, *Ann. Allergy*, 1979, *42*, 353.

Cimetidine could produce a false-positive reaction if ingested within 15 minutes of a test for detecting blood in gastric juice, using Hemoccult.— R. G. Norfleet *et al.* (letter), *New Engl. J. Med.*, 1980, *302*, 467. Dye in the cimetidine tablet may be responsible for the interference.— J. J. Schentag (letter), *ibid.*, *303*, 110. Evidence that cimetidine itself is responsible for false-positive Hemoccult reactions; the reaction appeared to be dependent on the cimetidine concentration.— A. Hauser *et al.* (letter), *ibid.*, 1981, *304*, 847. Findings that cimetidine administered by mouth in a dose of 1 g daily did not provoke a false positive reaction in the Hemoccult test for faecal occult blood.— P. Herzog and K. H. Holtermüller (letter), *ibid.*, *305*, 644.

Pregnancy and the neonate. Cimetidine was detected in the milk of a nursing mother in concentrations higher than in her plasma.— A. Somogyi and R. Gugler, *Br. J. clin. Pharmac.*, 1979, *7*, 627.

See also under Adverse Effects.

Withdrawal. There is no firm evidence that recurrences or complications of ulcer disease occur sooner or more severely in patients withdrawn from cimetidine than in patients withdrawn from other forms of treatment.— *Med. Lett.*, 1978, *20*, 77.

Reports, comments, and studies relating to withdrawal of cimetidine.— M. J. Gill and J. B. Saunders (letter), *Br. med. J.*, 1977, *2*, 1149 (perforation); B. D. Keighley (letter), *Br. med. J.*, 1977, *2*, 1022 (perforation); W. A. Wallace *et al.*, *Br. med. J.*, 1977, *2*, 865 (perforation); P. V. Turkie (letter), *Br. med. J.*, 1977, *2*, 1022 (relationship between cimetidine and perforation not established); H. J. Binder *et al.*, *Gastroenterology*, 1978, *74*, 380 (absence of rebound effect); P. Brown *et al.*, *Curr. ther. Res.*, 1978, *23*, 706 (possibility of rebound effect); O. Epstein *et al.*, *Gut*, 1978, *19*, 327 (absence of rebound effect); M. Guslandi *et al.* (letter), *Br. med. J.*, 1978, *1*, 718 (possibility of rebound effect); P. Hoste *et al.* (letter), *Lancet*, 1978, *1*, 666 (perforation in a patient who also took aspirin); J. P. Buck *et al.* (letter), *Lancet*, 1979, *2*, 42 (perforation of ulcerating adenocarcinoma); A. S. Bulman (letter), *Br. med. J.*, 1979, *1*, 409 (perforation); K. E. L. McColl (letter), *Br. med. J.*, 1979, *1*, 755 (multiple gastroduodenal ulceration).

See also under Ulcers, Gastric and Duodenal in the Uses section, below.

Absorption and Fate. Cimetidine is absorbed from the gastro-intestinal tract and peak plasma concentrations are obtained about an hour after administration on an empty stomach and about 2 hours after administration with food. The duration of action is reported to be prolonged by administration with food. Over two-thirds of a dose is excreted in the urine within 24 hours; following parenteral administration this is mainly as unchanged cimetidine, but following oral administration a portion is metabolised, mainly to the sulphoxide. Cimetidine crosses the placental barrier and is excreted in milk. It does not readily cross the blood-brain barrier.

Cimetidine 75 to 117 mg administered by intravenous infusion to 9 healthy subjects gave peak blood concentrations of 2 to 4.3 nmol per ml which declined with a half-life of about 2 hours. Up to 60% of the dose was excreted after 2.5 hours and 81 to 96% had been excreted in the urine of 8 subjects and 60% in the ninth after 24 hours. The volume of gastric juice in 7 subjects was reduced by an average of 68%, the acidity by an average of 72%, and pepsin concentration by an average of 27%. The average blood concentration of cimetidine which achieved 50% inhibition of acid output was 2 nmol per ml regardless of whether histamine or pentagastrin was used as a stimulant. Following intraduodenal administration of cimetidine 200 mg to 3 subjects peak blood concentrations of 4.8 to 6.2 nmol per ml were obtained after 30 to 90 minutes; the maximum inhibition of acid output was 75 to 95%, both volume and acidity of the gastric juice being reduced, and pepsin output was reduced by an average of 82%. Following administration of cimetidine 200 mg by mouth to 6 subjects the average peak blood concentration 45 to 75 minutes after administration was 2.8 nmol per ml. After administration intravenously, intraduodenally, or by mouth an average of 70% of cimetidine was excreted unchanged in the urine within about 24 hours, and preliminary studies in 5 subjects indicated that after intravenous or oral administration up to 19% was excreted as the sulphoxide with a further 7 to 17% as unidentified metabolite. Despite pretreatment with mepyramine all subjects who received histamine experienced flushing; this disappeared during cimetidine infusion.— W. L. Burland *et al.*, *Br. J. clin. Pharmac.*, 1975, *2*, 481.

A method for the analysis of cimetidine in blood and urine, and results obtained in 12 healthy subjects given 2 doses of cimetidine 200 mg by mouth in aqueous solution, with an interval of 7 days between doses. Urinary excretion and blood concentration values indicated that cimetidine is well absorbed; no significant difference was noted between values obtained after the 2 doses. Peak blood concentrations were obtained after a mean of about an hour after either dose, and the mean elimination half-life was 1.90 hours after the first dose and 1.72 hours after the second dose. After either dose a mean of about 58% was excreted in the urine over 24 hours.— W. C. Randolph *et al.*, *J. pharm. Sci.*, 1977, *66*, 1148.

Further references.— B. Norlander *et al.*, *Scand. J. Gastroenterol.*, 1976, *11*, *Suppl.* 38, 110 (blood concentrations); G. Bodemar *et al.*, *ibid.*, 1977, *12*, 10 (bioavailability); P. V. Pedersen and R. Miller, *J. pharm. Sci.*, 1980, *69*, 394 (pharmacokinetics and bioavailability).

Uses. Cimetidine is a histamine H_2-receptor antagonist (see p.1294). Accordingly, it inhibits gastric acid secretion, and it has also been shown to inhibit other actions of histamine mediated by H_2-receptors. It is used in gastric and duodenal ulcer, and in other conditions where inhibition of gastric acid secretion may be beneficial. The usual dose by mouth is 200 mg thrice daily with meals and 400 mg at night, increased if necessary to 400 mg four times daily (with meals and at night). In duodenal ulcer, 400 mg twice daily with breakfast and at bedtime has also been reported to be effective. Treatment should be continued initially for at least 4 weeks (6 weeks in the case of gastric ulcer). Where appropriate a maintenance dose of 400 mg may then be given once at night, or both in the morning and at night.

In reflux oesophagitis the recommended dose is 400 mg four times daily (with meals and at night) for 4 to 8 weeks, and in pathological hypersecretory conditions, such as the Zollinger-Ellison syndrome, the dose of 400 mg four times daily may also be required, occasionally increased to a total of 2 g daily. Doses of 200 mg thrice daily with meals and 400 mg at night, if necessary increased to 400 mg four times daily (with meals and at night), have been recommended for the management of patients at risk from stress-related ulceration of the upper gastro-intestinal tract, such as those with fulminant hepatic failure.

Cimetidine may also be given by slow intravenous injection in a usual dose of 200 mg every 4 to 6 hours to a maximum of 2 g daily. It may also be given diluted in solutions of electrolytes or dextrose by intravenous infusion at a rate of 100 mg per hour for 2-hour periods every 4 to 6 hours (maximum rate 150 mg per hour), or continuously at a rate of 75 mg per hour; the maximum dose by infusion should not normally exceed 2 g daily. Cimetidine may also be given by intramuscular injection in a usual dose of 200 mg every 4 to 6 hours to a maximum of 2 g daily. The dosage of cimetidine should be reduced in patients with impaired renal function; suggested doses according to creatinine clearance are: creatinine clearance of 0 to 15 ml per minute, 200 mg twice daily; creatinine clearance of 15 to 30 ml per minute, 200 mg thrice daily; creatinine clearance of 30 to 50 ml per minute, 200 mg four times daily; creatinine clearance of over 50 ml per minute, normal dosage. Blood concentrations of cimetidine are reduced by haemodialysis.

A suggested dose of cimetidine for children is 20 to 40 mg per kg body-weight daily by mouth or intravenously; some sources consider lower doses to be advisable (see below under Administration in Children).

The doses of cimetidine cited above relate to UK use. This is because, depending on the country in which it is marketed, cimetidine is supplied in different dose units; most doses in the UK are 200 to 400 mg while most doses in the USA are 300 mg. In both the UK and the USA cimetidine tablets contain the base. In the UK injection of cimetidine is stated to contain the base, although it is formulated with the aid of hydrochloride, whereas in the USA the content is expressed in terms of the hydrochloride. In effect, therefore, the preparations are similar; the doses of both are expressed in terms of the base.

In general the recommended dose of cimetidine in the USA is 300 mg four times daily (with meals and at night), but in pathological secretory conditions such as the Zollinger-Ellison syndrome the 300-mg dose may be given up to 8 times daily to give a maximum total daily dose of 2.4 g. Similar doses are recommended intramuscularly, and by slow intravenous injection over a period of not less than 2 minutes, and a similar daily dose is recommended by intravenous infusion.

Some references to pharmacological studies on cimetidine.— J. W. Black *et al.*, *Nature*, 1972, *236*, 385 (definition and antagonism of histamine H_2-receptors); R. W. Brimblecombe *et al.*, *Br. J. Pharmac.*, 1975, *53*, 435P (actions on histamine); R. W. Brimblecombe *et al.*, *J. int. med. Res.*, 1975, *3*, 86 (absence of local anaesthetic effect); R. Cano *et al.*, *Gastroenterology*, 1976, *70*, 1056 (gastric acid inhibition); K. P. Bhargava *et al.*, *Br. J. Pharmac.*, 1977, *59*, 349 (minimal role of histamine H_2-receptors in the skin); S. E. Knight *et al.*, *Gut*, 1977, *18*, A948 (effect on gastric mucosal blood flow); P. A. MacKercher *et al.*, *Ann. intern. Med.*, 1977, *87*, 676 (protection against aspirin-induced mucosal damage); B. Simon and H. Kather (letter), *Br. J. clin. Pharmac.*, 1977, *4*, 488 (inhibition of gastric acid secretion by inhibition of the histamine H_2-receptor-coupled adenylate cyclase system); E. Aadland and A. Berstad, *Scand. J. Gastroenterol.*, 1978, *13*, 193 (gastric acid and pepsin secretion after prolonged use); R. Corinaldesi *et al.*, *Acta ther.*, 1978, *4*, 199 (regularising of gastric emptying); J. A. H. Forrest *et al.*, *Gut*, 1978, *19*, A440 (long-term effects on gastric acid secretion, gastric emptying, and serum gastrin); R. J. Holden *et al.*, *Gut*, 1978, *19*, A441 (acid and pepsin secretion); K. J. Ivey and P. A. MacKercher, *Gut*, 1978, *19*, 414 (mode of reduction of gastric acid); J. M. Schöön and L. Olbe, *Gut*, 1978, *19*, 27 (gastric acid inhibition); R. Chakrabarti and S. G. Thompson (letter), *Lancet*, 1979, *2*, 962 (*in vitro* inhibition of fibrinolysis).

Reviews of the actions and uses of cimetidine.— R. N. Brogden *et al.*, *Drugs*, 1978, *15*, 93; W. Finkelstein and K. J. Isselbacher, *New Engl. J. Med.*, 1978, *299*, 992; *Drug & Ther. Bull.*, 1979, *17*, 29; R. B. McConnell, *Prescribers' J.*, 1979, *19*, 136; M. J. S. Langman, *Recent Adv. clin. Pharmac.*, 1980, *2*, 101; *Lancet*, 1981, *1*, 875.

Administration. A recommendation that cimetidine should always be taken with food for optimal effect.— R. Lawrence (letter), *Can. J. Hosp. Pharm.*, 1978, *31*, 78. Further discussion and letters: *ibid.* See also *ibid.*, 122.

With anticholinergics. In a study of 9 duodenal ulcer patients concurrent administration of propantheline bromide 15 mg with cimetidine 300 mg was noted to have an additive effect on gastric acid secretion.— M. Feldman *et al.*, *New Engl. J. Med.*, 1977, *297*, 1427. Studies in 4 patients with duodenal ulcer showed that the decrease in gastric acid secretion produced by cimetidine 1 g daily was not further reduced by the addition of atropine 2.4 mg daily.— R. E. Pounder *et al.*, *Gut*, 1977, *18*, 85.

Administration in children. Following administration of cimetidine 40 mg per kg body-weight daily, after massive intestinal resection for midgut volvulus, a 2-month-old infant developed cerebral toxicity, which resolved on withdrawal of cimetidine, and did not recur with a dose of 25 mg per kg daily. The cimetidine dose of 40 mg per kg daily might be too high for infants.— J. Thompson and J. Lilly (letter), *Lancet*, 1979, *1*, 725. Encephalopathy in a 4-year-old child might have been associated with administration of cimetidine 15 mg per kg body-weight daily.— J. F. Bale *et al.* (letter), *ibid.*

Further references to the use of cimetidine in infants and children.— A. Bacigalupo *et al.* (letter), *Lancet*, 1978, *2*, 45 (intractable vomiting and gastric bleeding associated with treatment for aplastic anaemia); Y. Chhattriwalla *et al.*, *Pediatrics*, 1980, *65*, 301 (oesophagitis and ulcers in neonates).

Administration in the elderly. A preliminary report of a marked reduction in the plasma clearance of cimetidine with increasing age.— R. Gugler and A. Somogyi (letter), *New Engl. J. Med.*, 1979, *301*, 435. In a study in 20 healthy subjects aged 22 to 84 years, the bioavailability of cimetidine appeared to be increased in the elderly subjects, possibly due to decreased clearance of the drug. It was suggested that the standard dose of cimetidine could be reduced by about 30% to 50% without loss of efficacy.— A. Redolfi *et al.*, *Eur. J. clin. Pharmac.*, 1979, *15*, 257.

Further references: A. Somogyi *et al.*, *Clin. Pharmacokinet.*, 1980, *5*, 84.

Administration in hepatic failure. Magnesium hydroxide given by nasogastric tube to 13 patients with fulminant hepatic failure was ineffective in preventing haemorrhage from gastric erosions when compared with 12 control patients. Cimetidine or, in previous cases, metiamide in doses of 150 mg infused at a rate of 100 mg per hour in dextrose 5% was significantly more effective than no treatment in preventing haemorrhage; 1 of 26 treated patients bled compared with 13 of 24 controls. Also cimetidine or metiamide effectively raised and maintained the intragastric pH above 5. A consistent effect on pH was not seen with the antacids.— B. R. D. MacDougall *et al.*, *Lancet*, 1977, *1*, 617.

Evidence to suggest that a reduction in the dosage of cimetidine in patients with compensated cirrhosis appears unwarranted.— J. Sonne *et al.*, *Clin. Pharmac. Ther.*, 1981, *29*, 191.

A retrospective survey indicating that systemic fungal infection is a rare complication of patients with fulminant hepatic failure and does not seem to be related to treatment with cimetidine.— R. J. Wyke *et al.* (letter), *Lancet*, 1981, *2*, 1236.

Further references.— R. J. Bailey *et al.*, *Gut*, 1975, *5*, 389; R. J. Bailey *et al.*, *Br. med. J.*, 1976, *2*, 678.

See also under Ulceration, stress-induced.

Administration in renal failure. In 13 patients undergoing haemodialysis, given 2 doses of cimetidine 200 mg, twelve hours apart, blood-cimetidine concentrations fell from a mean of 2.22 µg per ml before dialysis to a mean of 0.69 µg per ml after dialysis. Experience with 8 similar patients with peptic lesions suggested that a dose of cimetidine 200 mg twelve-hourly was suitable.— R. H. Jones *et al.*, *Br. med. J.*, 1979, *1*, 650.

Further references.— C. C. Doherty *et al.*, *Br. med. J.*, 1977, *2*, 1506; K. W. Ma *et al.*, *Gastroenterology*, 1978, *74*, 473; N. D. Vaziri *et al.*, *Archs intern. Med.*, 1978, *138*, 1685; G. D. Luk *et al.* (letter), *Ann. intern. Med.*, 1979, *90*, 991; P. A. L. Bjaeldager *et al.*, *Br. J. clin. Pharmac.*, 1980, *9*, 585; M. K. Dutt *et al.*, *Br. J. clin. Pharmac.*, 1981, *12*, 47.

Renal transplantation. None of 30 patients, given cimetidine prophylactically after renal transplantation, developed gastro-intestinal haemorrhage compared with 6 of 33 (1 fatality) not given cimetidine. The dosage was 200 mg intravenously every 12 hours initially, then by mouth, gradually increased to the standard dose as renal function improved.— R. H. Jones *et al.*, *Br. med. J.*, 1978, *1*, 398. Following the introduction of prophylactic cimetidine therapy no upper gastro-intestinal bleeding has occurred in a series of 93 renal transplant recipients. Moreover, none of the thirty patients originally reported has subsequently developed peptic ulceration. Routine use of prophylactic cimetidine after renal transplantation is advisable.— C. J. Rudge *et al.* (letter), *Lancet*, 1979, *1*, 562.

Disapproval of the routine use of prophylactic cimetidine after renal transplantation. Prevention of upper gastro-intestinal complications in renal transplant patients can be more logically achieved by pretransplant gastric assessment, administration of prophylactic cimetidine to those who have peptic ulcer, and use of a low-dosage rather than a high-dosage prednisolone regimen.— C. C. Doherty and M. G. McGeown (letter), *Lancet*, 1979, *1*, 778.

In a comparative study 24 renal transplant recipients received prophylactic cimetidine alone, and 27 received antacids alone. Three patients in the cimetidine group developed clinically significant ulcers whereas none in the antacid group did so. Of 182 renal transplant recipients treated with antacids alone, before this study, none had manifestations of upper gastro-intestinal ulcers. It appears that cimetidine cannot be used alone in renal transplant patients. It may have a beneficial role used judiciously with antacid therapy.— J. L. Hussey and F. O. Belzer (letter), *Lancet*, 1979, *1*, 1089.

Further reports and comments on the use of cimetidine in the management of peptic ulcer in renal failure and transplantation.— C. C. Doherty *et al.*, *Proc. Eur. Dialysis Transplant Ass.*, 1977, *14*, 386; J. Ahonen *et al.*, *ibid.*, 396.

Alkalosis. Cimetidine 300 mg given intravenously every 12 hours was considered to be a useful adjunct to haemodialysis in the control of metabolic alkalosis in a patient with renal failure who had undergone abdominal surgery.— N. D. Vaziri (letter), *Ann. intern. Med.*, 1978, *88*, 266. A similar report.— G. R. Aronoff and R. J. Hamburger (letter), *ibid.*

Further references.— B. J. Rowlands *et al.*, *Postgrad. med. J.*, 1978, *54*, 118.

Allergy. For the use of cimetidine in association with an H_1-receptor antagonist in the prophylaxis of polygeline allergy, see Polygeline, p.958.

Further references.— O. T. Tan *et al.* (letter), *Lancet*, 1979, *2*, 365 (alcohol-induced flushing).

Carcinoid syndrome. Elimination of flushing attacks associated with a metastatic gastric carcinoid tumour was achieved when diphenhydramine hydrochloride 50 mg and cimetidine 300 mg were both taken 6-hourly by a 54-year-old woman who had suffered attacks every day for the previous 22 years. Diphenhydramine alone reduced the frequency of attacks while cimetidine alone reduced their duration. Over a 6-week period on the combined treatment the patient experienced only about 2 very mild flushes weekly.— L. J. Roberts *et al.*, *New Engl. J. Med.*, 1979, *300*, 236. A 58-year-old woman with carcinoid syndrome associated with metastatic ileal carcinoid tumour was treated similarly without success.— T. D. Wingert *et al.* (letter), *ibid.*, 1980, *302*, 234. The frequency, duration, and intensity of flushing were substantially reduced by treatment with diphenhydramine 25 mg and cimetidine 300 mg, both four times daily, in a man with metastatic ileal carcinoid tumour.— J. D. Pyles *et al.* (letter), *ibid.* Comment.—

L. J. Roberts *et al.* (letter), *ibid.*, 235.

Carcinoma. Cimetidine provided useful relief of pain after 7 days in a patient with inoperable gastric carcinoma.— C. L. Welsh *et al.* (letter), *Br. med. J.*, 1977, *1*, 1413.

Reports and comments on the use of cimetidine to reduce tumour formation in *animals* and on its potential as an immunostimulator.— M. E. Osband *et al.*, *Lancet*, 1981, *1*, 636; R. R. M. Gifford *et al.*, *ibid.*, 638; I. Fraser and P. R. F. Bell (letter), *ibid.*, 900; C. Burtin *et al.* (letter), *ibid;* N. R. Peden *et al.* (letter), *ibid;* S. C. Knight (letter), *ibid.*, 901.

See also under Immunological Disorders (below).

Crohn's disease. Eight of 10 patients with Crohn's disease and who were anergic to 2,4-dinitrochlorobenzene were given cimetidine 1.2 g daily in divided doses for one month. On retesting 7 of the 8 were then found to have one or more positive skin tests at this time. No changes in clinical disease activity were observed during this period but further studies of cimetidine and other drugs which enhance T cell immune competence are indicated.— R. O. Bicks and E. W. Rosenberg (letter), *Lancet*, 1980, *1*, 552.

Cystic fibrosis. For reports of cimetidine therapy in cystic fibrosis, see under Pancreatic Insufficiency.

Gastritis and duodenitis. Gastritis and duodenitis associated with chronic duodenal ulceration appeared to be unaffected by treatment with cimetidine.— H. M. Gilmour *et al.*, *Gut*, 1978, *19*, A981.

Gastro-intestinal bleeding. Cimetidine appeared to prevent rebleeding from gastric but not duodenal ulcers in a double-blind study of 66 patients.— A. M. Hoare *et al.*, *Lancet*, 1979, *2*, 671. In a double-blind study involving patients over 65 years of age with severe upper gastro-intestinal bleeding the code was broken at 30 patients when an overall bleeding-rate of 20% was noted. Although the figures were too small for statistical analysis, no trend was noted in favour of cimetidine with or without chlorpheniramine, compared with a placebo, and the study was abandoned.— A. F. Macklon *et al.* (letter), *ibid.*, 1135.

Studies suggesting that cimetidine is not of value for the control of gastro-intestinal bleeding which is not stress-induced.— S. La Brooy *et al.*, *Gut*, 1978, *19*, A447; R. G. Pickard *et al.*, *Br. med. J.*, 1979, *1*, 661; S. M. Z. A. Siddiqi (letter), *ibid.*, 954; L. Kayasseh *et al.*, *Lancet*, 1980, *1*, 844.

For the effect of cimetidine on stress-induced bleeding, see Ulceration, stress-induced.

Headache. No significant benefit was observed in 12 patients with cluster headache receiving combined therapy with cimetidine and chlorpheniramine.— D. Russell, *J. Neurol. Neurosurg. Psychiat.*, 1979, *42*, 668.

Further references.— T. Veger *et al.* (letter), *Br. med. J.*, 1976, *2*, 585; M. Anthony *et al.*, *Headache*, 1978, *18*, 261.

Hirsutism. Preliminary results suggesting that cimetidine may have a beneficial effect in androgen-dependent hirsutism. Cimetidine 300 mg given 5 times daily for 3 months to 5 severely hirsute women decreased the rate of hair growth by a mean of 64% in 4; there was no response in the fifth patient, who was also taking phenytoin. Bleeding from the vagina occurred in 3 patients within 3 weeks of starting treatment with cimetidine.— R. A. Vigersky *et al.*, *New Engl. J. Med.*, 1980, *303*, 1042.

See also under Skin Disorders, Acne.

Hyperparathyroidism. Cimetidine has been reported by J.K. Sherwood *et al.* (*Lancet*, 1980, *1*, 616) to be of value as an adjunct to the operative management of hyperparathyroidism, but this view has been strongly criticised by H. Heath (*Lancet*, 1980, *1*, 980) *et al.* See also G. A. MacGregor (letter), *Lancet*, 1980, *1*, 980; S. Awoke and G. D. Lawrence (letter), *ibid.*, 1134; K. E. Pettengell and M. J. Grayson (letter), *ibid;* G. Graziani *et al.* (letter), *ibid.*

Results of a study in 10 patients indicated that cimetidine is of no clinical benefit in patients with primary hyperparathyroidism.— S. Ljunghall *et al.* (letter), *Lancet*, 1980, *2*, 480.

Further references.— J. Sherwood *et al.* (letter), *New Engl. J. Med.*, 1979, *300*, 200; A. I. Jacob *et al.*, *ibid.*, 1980, *302*, 671; F. J. Palmer *et al.* (letter), *ibid.*, 692; J.-L. Vanherweghem *et al.* (letter), *ibid.*, *303*, 395; A. I. Jacob and J. F. Bourgoignie (letter), *ibid.*, 396; S. Ljunghall *et al.* (letter), *ibid.*, 1178; J. K. Sherwood *et al.* (letter), *Lancet*, 1980, *1*, 1298; U. Knigge *et al.* (letter), *ibid.*, *2*, 212; C. E. Fiore *et al.* (letter), *ibid.*, 1981, *1*, 501.

Immunological disorders. Encouraging results with cimetidine in 4 patients with chronic mucocutaneous candidiasis. Cimetidine could be evaluated in other clinical situations characterised by impaired cell-mediated immunity.— J. L. Jorizzo *et al.*, *Ann. intern. Med.*, 1980, *92*, 192. Comment.— M. R. Simon (letter), *ibid.*, *93*, 152. Reply.— W. M. Sams (letter), *ibid.*

Irritable colon. Cimetidine might be of value in irritable colon; subjective improvement had occurred in 3 or 4 patients.— E. M. S. Frew (letter), *Lancet*, 1978, *1*, 279.

Mastocytosis. A report demonstrating the beneficial effect of combined treatment with H_1 and H_2 antihistamines in a 54-year-old man with mastocytosis unresponsive to H_1 antihistamines. Persisting therapeutic benefit was achieved when cimetidine 300 mg four times daily, gradually reduced to once or twice daily, was given, cyproheptadine was discontinued, and the dose of hydroxyzine tapered from 400 mg to 25 mg daily.— R. A. Simon (letter), *New Engl. J. Med.*, 1980, *302*, 231. A controlled double-blind study is needed to compare the effects of cimetidine with those of sodium cromoglycate in patients with systemic mastocytosis.— J. C. O'Laughlin and J. E. Bredfeldt (letter), *ibid.* Further comment on the relative merits of treatment with H_1 and H_2 antihistamines and with sodium cromoglycate.— K. F. Austen *et al.* (letter), *ibid.*

Further reports.— D. M. McCarthy, *Gastroenterology*, 1978, *74*, 453; B. I. Hirschowitz and J. F. Groarke, *Ann. intern. Med.*, 1979, *90*, 769; R. Linde *et al.* (letter), *ibid.*, 1980, *92*, 716.

Meckel's diverticulum. Cimetidine 300 mg by mouth 4 times daily was used successfully for the management of Meckel's diverticulum in a 27-year-old man.— R. A. Kirkpatrick (letter), *Ann. intern. Med.*, 1978, *88*, 846. Perforation of a Meckel's diverticulum in a 12-year-old boy during therapy with cimetidine. It was considered that surgery was the treatment of choice in this condition.— P. E. Minchom *et al.* (letter), *Archs Dis. Childh.*, 1980, *55*, 321.

Further references.— R. J. Petrokubi *et al.*, *Clin. nucl. Med.*, 1978, *3*, 385.

Menetrier's disease. Beneficial results with cimetidine in a patient with Menetrier's disease (a protein-losing gastropathy) given 200 mg thrice daily and 400 mg at night.— E. Krag *et al.*, *Scand. J. Gastroenterol.*, 1978, *13*, 635.

Oesophageal reflux. In a double-blind crossover study of 27 patients with symptomatic gastro-oesophageal reflux, administration of cimetidine 1.6 g daily for 6 weeks provided significant relief of pain compared with placebo, as assessed by pain frequency and antacid consumption, but the action appeared to be solely an antacid effect with no changes in mucosal sensitivity to acid and no clear-cut healing effect. Cimetidine should therefore be reserved for patients with gastro-oesophageal reflux who did not respond to antacid therapy and other simple measures, such as advice on dietary regimen and on posture.— P. Powell-Jackson *et al.*, *Lancet*, 1978, *2*, 1068. Decreased mucosal acid sensitivity in cimetidine-treated patients.— J. Behar *et al.*, *Gastroenterology*, 1978, *74*, 441.

Similar results after 6 weeks of therapy were obtained with cimetidine 1.6 g daily and with placebo in a double-blind study involving 36 patients with reflux oesophagitis but after another 6 weeks of treatment those receiving cimetidine had improved endoscopic findings and fewer complaints compared to the placebo group. It was suggested that if non-surgical treatment was indicated it must be continued for at least 6 to 12 weeks.— G. Lepsien *et al.*, *Dt. med. Wschr.*, 1979, *104*, 901.

In a double-blind study in 10 patients with gastro-oesophageal reflux cimetidine increased lower oesophageal sphincter pressure but had no demonstrable effect on oesophageal pH or reflux.— R. J. R. Goodall and J. G. Temple, *Br. med. J.*, 1980, *280*, 611.

Further references.— W. G. Thompson and R. Barr, *Gastroenterology*, 1977, *73*, 808 (Barrett's oesophagus); K. D. Bardhan (letter), *Br. med. J.*, 1978, *1*, 370 (chicken-pox oesophagitis); R. Ferguson *et al.*, *Br. med. J.*, 1979, *2*, 472 (reflux oesophagitis); I. C. E. Wesdorp *et al.*, *Gut*, 1981, *22*, 724 (Barrett's oesophagus).

Pancreatic insufficiency. From studies in 6 men with alcoholic chronic pancreatitis it was considered that if steatorrhoea and symptoms of malabsorption persisted after treatment with pancreatin, the administration of cimetidine with pancreatin and a meal might prevent inactivation of pancreatin by gastric acid and so help correct malabsorption. When given to 16 patients with active duodenal ulcer cimetidine 300 mg did not impair the normal secretion of pancreatic enzymes.— P. T. Regan *et al.*, *Mayo Clin. Proc.*, 1978, *53*, 79.

Preliminary results suggesting that cimetidine in association with propantheline may be of benefit in chronic pancreatitis.— G. S. Weinstein and P. J. Dupont (letter), *New Engl. J. Med.*, 1978, *298*, 1203. Criticism.— N. Hadas *et al.* (letter), *ibid.*, *299*, 487.

Cimetidine 300 mg intravenously four times daily was no more effective than a placebo in a double-blind study involving 27 patients with acute episodes of alcoholic pancreatitis of mild to moderate severity.— H. Meshkinpour *et al.*, *Gastroenterology*, 1979, *77*, 687.

Cimetidine had no beneficial effect on the therapeutic response to pancreatic extracts taken by mouth.— J. L. Staub *et al.* (letter), *New Engl. J. Med.*, 1981, *304*, 1364.

Further references.— J. P. Galmiche *et al.* (letter), *Lancet*, 1977, *1*, 647 (chronic pancreatitis); G. B. Porro *et al.* (letter), *Lancet*, 1977, *2*, 878 (chronic pancreatitis); P. T. Regan *et al.*, *New Engl. J. Med.*, 1977, *297*, 854 (chronic pancreatitis).

Cystic fibrosis. A preliminary study suggesting that cimetidine may help to reduce steatorrhoea in patients with cystic fibrosis.— A. S. Ahuja and N. N. Mann (letter), *Archs Dis. Childh.*, 1978, *53*, 766.

Addition of cimetidine, 150 or 200 mg by mouth 30 minutes before meals, to the enzyme therapy of 10 patients with severe pancreatic exocrine insufficiency due to cystic fibrosis resulted in a significant reduction of steatorrhoea and azotorrhoea. Lower doses of cimetidine resulted in less significant reductions.— K. L. Cox *et al.*, *J. Pediat.*, 1979, *94*, 488.

Scleroderma. In an 8-week crossover study in 15 patients with scleroderma and associated heartburn, cimetidine 300 mg four times daily gave a significantly greater relief of heartburn than an antacid. Cimetidine therapy also resulted in significant endoscopic improvement of the oesophageal mucosa.— R. J. Petrokubi and G. H. Jeffries, *Gastroenterology*, 1979, *77*, 691. See also G. F. Sciallis and H. Levenson, *Archs Derm.*, 1979, *115*, 1036.

Short-bowel syndrome. In a 36-year-old woman with short-bowel syndrome and gastric hypersecretion, cimetidine improved intraluminal digestion and intestinal absorption by reducing gastric acid and gastric-volume output resulting in decreased luminal acidity and flow. Diarrhoea was markedly reduced when she was given cimetidine 300 mg thrice daily before meals.— A. Cortot *et al.*, *New Engl. J. Med.*, 1979, *300*, 79. In 4 similar patients who had undergone extensive small-bowel resection, cimetidine by intravenous infusion significantly reduced gastric output of hydrogen ions and fluid, and reduced fractional emptying-rates after a water load.— J. P. Murphy *et al.*, *ibid.*, 80. See also D. M. McCarthy, *Gastroenterology*, 1978, *74*, 453.

Skin disorders. In a double-blind study on 12 healthy subjects cimetidine 400 mg produced a significant reduction in wheal and flare reactions to histamine. Simultaneous systemic administration of cimetidine 400 mg and chlorpheniramine 8 mg was more effective than either drug alone in inhibition of the erythematous reaction due to exogenous and endogenous histamine. It was suggested that treatment with both H_1- and H_2-histamine receptor antagonists would be more effective than either alone in histamine reactions in skin.— R. Marks and M. W. Greaves, *Br. J. clin. Pharmac.*, 1977, *4*, 367.

Acne. A study in 10 male and female acne patients indicated that cimetidine 1 g daily inhibited sebum secretion to a varying extent.— F. Lyons *et al.* (preliminary communication), *Lancet*, 1979, *1*, 1376. Comments on the anti-androgen properties of cimetidine and its potential role in acne and hirsutism.— J. L. Burton and C. R. Lovell (letter), *ibid.*, 1979, *2*, 305; S. Shuster (letter), *ibid.*, 1020.

Cimetidine 1.6 g daily was found to have no effect on sebum excretion or acne in a placebo-controlled double-blind study involving 39 patients with mild to severe acne.— H. Jones *et al.* (letter), *Lancet*, 1980, *2*, 1201.

Alopecia. For the use of cimetidine to reverse acquired tolerance to 2,4-dinitrochlorobenzene being used for the treatment of alopecia, see 2,4-Dinitrochlorobenzene, p.1703.

Herpes. Cimetidine in the treatment of herpes viral infections.— S. Van der Spuy *et al.*, *S. Afr. med. J.*, 1980, *58*, 112.

Pruritus. After successful results with cimetidine in 2 patients suffering from cholestatic pruritus, no beneficial effect could be demonstrated when cimetidine 300 mg four times daily was compared with placebo in a double-blind crossover study in 6 similar patients.— A. R. Harrison *et al.* (letter), *New Engl. J. Med.*, 1979, *300*, 433. Cimetidine 200 mg thrice daily for 2 to 4 weeks had no beneficial effect in 12 patients with polycythaemia rubra vera and pruritus.— G. L. Scott and R. J. Horton (letter), *ibid.*, 434 and 936. In a study involving 6 patients, cimetidine alone or in association with diphenhydramine had no effect on severe diffuse pruritus associated with chronic renal failure.— A. R. Zappacosta and D. Hauss (letter), *ibid.*, 1280.

Individual reports of the successful use of cimetidine to alleviate pruritus mainly in myeloproliferative disorders.— P. Easton and P. R. Galbraith (letter), *New Engl. J. Med.*, 1978, *299*, 1134 (one patient); C. E. Hess (letter), *New Engl. J. Med.*, 1979, *300*, 370 (4 patients); D. V. Schapira and J. M. Bennett (letter), *Lancet*, 1979, *1*, 726 (one patient); J. P. Aymard *et al.*, *Br. med. J.*, 1980, *280*, 151 (4 patients).

Psoriasis. For reports of various effects on psoriasis, see Adverse Effects.

Tinea capitis. For the use of cimetidine as an adjunct to griseofulvin, see Griseofulvin, p.715.

Urticaria. Chlorpheniramine maleate 4 mg immediately after food was as effective when given alone as when given with cimetidine 400 mg four times daily for the treatment of 19 patients with a history of daily spontaneous urticarias of unknown origin (chronic idiopathic urticaria).— C. A. Commens and M. W. Greaves, *Br. J. Derm.*, 1978, *99*, 675.

Nine of 10 patients with chronic urticaria had a beneficial response when cimetidine 300 mg thrice daily was added to their previous therapy of large doses of conventional antihistamines and/or corticosteroids. In all but one it was possible to discontinue corticosteroids and 5 of the 10 are off all medication and remain free from urticaria.— H. B. Kaiser *et al.* (letter), *Lancet*, 1980, *2*, 206. See also P. Phanuphak *et al.*, *Clin. Allergy.*, 1978, *8*, 429.

Individual reports of the successful use of cimetidine in urticaria.— J. W. Gerrard and C. Ko, *J. Pediat.*, 1979, *94*, 843.

Ulcer, gastric and duodenal. A number of clinical studies have established that cimetidine very effectively promotes the healing of duodenal ulcers in a large majority of patients, and that its use is associated with a low incidence of side-effects. It is generally given in a dose of 200 mg thrice daily with meals and 400 mg at night. Symptomatic relief may be expected within a few days and ulcer healing within about 6 weeks. In accordance, however, with the natural history of the disease, patients generally relapse on stopping cimetidine therapy. Further studies were therefore directed at the long-term effect of maintenance cimetidine therapy for the prevention of duodenal ulcer recurrence. It was established that maintenance therapy with doses of 400 mg at night or 400 mg twice daily will usually prevent relapse.

Beneficial results have also been obtained with cimetidine in patients with gastric ulcer, again allowing for the high incidence of recurrence on completion of a course of therapy.

Cimetidine has also been shown to be useful for the control of ulcers developing after gastric surgery.

Cimetidine has accordingly had a considerable impact on the management of peptic ulcers, but the question of whether life-long maintenance therapy (or possibly a regimen of limited courses of treatment during relapses) is better than the surgical management of a disease which is characterised by relapses has not yet been resolved, particularly in relation to younger members of society whose operative risk is low. References.— D. H. Winship, *Gastroenterology*, 1978, *74*, 402; C. G. Clark, *Br. J. clin. Pract.*, 1979, *33*, 216; *Br. med. J.*, 1979, *1*, 169.

See also under Gastro-intestinal Bleeding.

Reports and studies on the use of cimetidine for the management of ulcers following gastric surgery.— R. F. McCloy and I. M. Modlin (letter), *Lancet*, 1977, *2*, 1131; A. M. Hoare *et al.*, *Br. med. J.*, 1978, *1*, 1325; T. Kennedy and A. Spencer, *ibid.*, 1242; J. H. B. Saunders *et al.* (letter), *ibid.*, 1619; H. P. M. Festen *et al.*, *Gastroenterology*, 1979, *76*, 83; R. Gugler *et al.*, *New Engl. J. Med.*, 1979, *301*, 1077; J. G. Stage *et al.*, *Scand. J. Gastroenterol.*, 1979, *14*, 977.

Reports, studies, and comments on the acute treatment of duodenal ulcers with cimetidine.— S. J. Haggie *et al.*, *Lancet*, 1976, *1*, 983; W. S. Blackwood *et al.*, *ibid.*, 1976, *2*, 174; G. Bodemar and A. Walan, *ibid.*, 161; W. Domschke *et al.*, *Dt. med. Wschr.*, 1976, *101*, 1752; G. R. Gray *et al.*, *Gut*, 1976, *17*, 820; D. Hollander *et al.*, *Am. J. dig. Dis.*, 1976, *21*, 361; O. N. Manousos *et al.*, *J. int. med. Res.*, 1978, *6*, 381; P. Peter *et al.*, *Dt. med. Wschr.*, 1978, *103*, 1163; J. J. Villalobos *et al.*, *J. int. med. Res.*, 1978, *6*, 351; G. Fedeli *et al.*, *Dig. Dis. Scis*, 1979, *24*, 758; R. Ubilluz, *Curr. ther. Res.*, 1979, *25*, 243.

Reports, studies, and comments on the maintenance treatment of duodenal ulcers with cimetidine.— W. S. Blackwood *et al.*, *Lancet*, 1978, *1*, 626; M. J. S. Langman and K. G. Wormsley (letter), *ibid.*, 932; G. Bodemar and A. Walan, *Lancet*, 1978, *1*, 403; *idem* (letter), *Lancet*, 1980, *1*, 38; D. Martin and J. P. Miller (letter), *ibid.*, 307; *Br. med. J.*, 1978, *1*, 1435; P. C. Sharpe and C. Wastell (letter), *ibid.*, 1978, *2*, 58; J. M. Cargill *et al.*, *Lancet*, 1978, *2*, 1113; M. W. Dronfield *et al.*, *Gut*, 1978, *19*, A99; M. W. Dronfield *et al.*, *Gut*, 1979, *20*, 526; E. Gudmand-Høyer *et al.*, *Br. med. J.*, 1978, *1*, 1095; M. J. S. Langman, *Am. J. Med.*, 1978, *65*, 885; R. C. P. M. Mekel, *S. Afr. med. J.*, 1978, *54*, 1089; K. D. Bardhan *et al.*, *Gut*, 1979, *20*, 158; A. Berstad *et al.*, *Scand. J. Gastroenterol.*, 1979, *14*, 827; G. Bodemar *et al.*, *ibid.*, 1979, *14*, *Suppl.* 55, 96; A. Sonnenberg *et al.*, *Dt. med. Wschr.*, 1979, *104*, 725; K. D. Bardhan, *Br. med. J.*, 1980, *281*, 20; R. E. Pounder, *Lancet*, 1981, *1*, 29; J. H. Wyllie (letter), *ibid.*, 209.

Reports, studies, and comments on the acute treatment of gastric ulcers with cimetidine.— R. E. Pounder *et al.*, *Lancet*, 1976, *1*, 337; R. F. A. Logan and J. A. H. Forrest (letter), *ibid.*, 1976, *1*, 650; F. Frost *et al.*, *Br. med. J.*, 1977, *2*, 795; R. J. Machell *et al.* (letter), *ibid.*, 1023; A. G. Morgan *et al.*, *ibid.*, 1978, *2*, 1323; K. -F. Sewing *et al.*, *Dt. med. Wschr.*, 1978, *103*, 152; P. J. Ciclitira *et al.*, *Gut*, 1979, *20*, 730; S. J. La Brooy *et al.*, *Br. med. J.*, 1979, *1*, 1308.

Reports, studies, and comments on the maintenance treatment of gastric ulcers with cimetidine.— R. J. Machell *et al.*, *Postgrad. med. J.*, 1979, *55*, 393.

Ulceration, stress-induced. A discussion on the use of cimetidine for stress-induced gastro-intestinal bleeding.— *Br. med. J.*, 1980, *281*, 631. Comment.— D. Hetzel (letter), *ibid.*, 1348.

Cimetidine maintained the gastric pH above 4 in 28 of 39 critically ill patients and none of the 28 had any gastro-intestinal bleeding of consequence once therapy was initiated. In the remaining 11 patients cimetidine did not consistently raise the gastric pH above 4. There appears to be a high-risk group of patients, including comatose patients, those with 4 or more organ system injuries, those receiving total parenteral nutrition, those with renal failure, and those with sepsis, who may not respond to cimetidine and whose gastric pH must be regularly monitored.— L. F. Martin *et al.*, *Archs Surg., Chicago*, 1979, *114*, 492.

Usual doses of cimetidine seem to be able to prevent gastric lesions (ulcers or erosions) in patients with intracranial trauma. Of 10 patients with no history of peptic ulcer (one with a gastric erosion) admitted comatose after a head injury and given cimetidine 1 g daily intravenously, endoscopy was normal in all 10 on the sixth day. Of 10 similar control patients (again, one with a gastric erosion), 7 had gastric lesions (ulcers in 2 and erosions in 5) on the sixth day. Endoscopy on the third day had revealed 2 lesions in the cimetidine group compared with 5 in the control group.— N. Silvestri *et al.* (letter), *Lancet*, 1980, *1*, 885.

Further references.— D. H. Dunn *et al.*, *Surgery Gynec. Obstet.*, 1978, *147*, 737; M. P. Bubrick *et al.*, *Surgery, St Louis*, 1978, *84*, 510.

For comparison of cimetidine and antacids in the prophylaxis of acute gastro-intestinal bleeding, see Antacids and some other Gastro-intestinal Agents, p.71.

See also under Administration in Hepatic Failure.

Use in surgery. A preliminary report that cimetidine 400 mg, especially when given 4 to 6 hours before anaesthesia, increased the pH of gastric contents above 2.5 in women undergoing elective gynaecological surgery.— R. P. Husemeyer *et al.*, *Br. J. Anaesth.*, 1978, *50*, 1080P. See also *idem*, *Anaesthesia*, 1978, *33*, 775.

In a study involving 36 patients cimetidine 300 mg by mouth the night before surgery with 300 mg intramuscularly 90 minutes before surgery was significantly more effective in increasing gastric pH than either 2 doses of cimetidine by mouth night and morning, a single dose of cimetidine by mouth before surgery, or no additional medication.— L. Weber and C. A. Hirshman, *Anesth. Analg. curr. Res.*, 1979, *58*, 426.

Further references.— P. J. Keating *et al.*, *Br. J. Anaesth.*, 1978, *50*, 1247; *Lancet*, 1980, *1*, 465; G. Dobb (letter), *ibid.*, 709; R. Chakrabarti and S. G. Thompson (letter), *ibid.*

Zollinger-Ellison syndrome. A discussion on the treatment of the Zollinger-Ellison syndrome with cimetidine.— D. M. McCarthy, *New Engl. J. Med.*, 1980, *302*, 1344. Comment.— S. Bonfils *et al.* (letter), *ibid.*, *303*, 942. Reply.— D. M. McCarthy (letter), *ibid.*

Cimetidine 300 mg every 6 hours was used successfully in the management of 2 patients with Zollinger-Ellison syndrome and in a further 2 patients who had received earlier treatment with metiamide. The patients were symptom-free after 5 and 12 months' therapy.— D. M. McCarthy *et al.*, *Ann. intern. Med.*, 1978, *87*, 668. See also D. M. McCarthy, *Gastroenterology*, 1978, *74*, 453. Either gastrinoma excision or total gastrectomy was ultimately required in 13 patients with the Zollinger-Ellison syndrome who were initially treated with cimetidine.— S. Bonfils *et al.*, *Gut*, 1978, *19*, A981.

Individual reports on the successful use of cimetidine in the Zollinger-Ellison syndrome.— C. T. Richardson and J. H. Walsh, *New Engl. J. Med.*, 1976, *294*, 1011; T. U. Hausamen *et al.*, *Dt. med. Wschr.*, 1977, *102*, 1709; W. Larkworthy and H. L. Davies, *Postgrad. med. J.*, 1977, *53*, 749; J. L. Orchard and W. W. Peternel, *J. Am. med. Ass.*, 1977, *237*, 2221; A. M. Spiegel *et al.* (letter), *Lancet*, 1978, *1*, 881; E. Straus *et al.*, *ibid.*, 1978, *2*, 73.

Proprietary Preparations

Tagamet *(Smith Kline & French, UK).* Cimetidine, available as 2-ml **Ampoules** containing 100 mg per ml; as **Syrup** containing 200 mg in each 5 ml; and as **Tablets** of 200 mg. (Also available as Tagamet in *Arg., Austral., Belg., Canad., Denm., Fr., Ger., Ital., Neth., Norw., NZ, S.Afr., Spain, Swed., Switz., USA*).

Other Proprietary Names

Arg.— Acibilin, Cimetum, Ulcerfen, Ulcimet; *Ital.*— Cimetin, Eureceptor, Gastromet, Itacem, Tametin, Ulcomet.

6118-q

Cinnarizine. 516 MD; R 516; R 1575. 1-Benzhydryl-4-cinnamylpiperazine.

$C_{26}H_{28}N_2$=368.5.

CAS — 298-57-7.

Adverse Effects, Treatment, and Precautions. As for the antihistamines in general, p.1294.

Absorption and Fate. As for the antihistamines in general, p.1295.

The mean plasma elimination half-life of cinnarizine in 12 healthy subjects was 3.24 hours.— P. J. Morrison *et al.*, *Br. J. clin. Pharmac.*, 1979, *7*, 349.

Uses. Cinnarizine is a piperazine derivative with the properties and uses of the antihistamines (see p.1295) but it is mainly used for the symptomatic treatment of nausea and vertigo due to Ménière's disease and other labyrinthine disturbances and for the prevention and treatment of motion sickness. It acts within about 30 minutes and its effects last for about 4 hours. Sedative effects are not marked.

The usual dose is 15 to 30 mg thrice daily. Children aged 5 to 12 years may be given half the adult dose. For motion sickness a dose of 30 mg may be taken two hours before the start of the journey and 15 mg every 8 hours during the journey. Again children aged 5 to 12 years may be given half the adult dose.

Cinnarizine is also used in the management of peripheral arterial disease in doses of 75 mg twice or thrice daily.

Asthma. In a double-blind crossover study in 9 chronic asthmatics, cinnarizine 75 mg thrice daily reduced the 'asthma symptom score' by 20% or more in 5 patients compared with placebo. No side-effects were reported. It was postulated that cinnarizine antagonised calcium ion transport across the mast cell membrane and thus had a pharmacological effect similar to sodium cromoglycate.— M. B. Emanuel *et al.*, *Br. J. clin. Pharmac.*, 1979, *7*, 189.

Peripheral vascular insufficiency. After 3 months, cinnarizine 75 mg given thrice daily improved muscle capacity in 10 of 12 elderly patients with arteriosclerosis compared with an improvement in 5 of 11 control patients.— V. Schuermans *et al.*, *Arzneimittel-Forsch.*, 1971, *21*, 1541. See also A. Jageneau *et al.*, *ibid.*, 1974, *24*, 1839.

Further references: F. Ellis *et al.*, *J. int. med. Res.*, 1975, *3*, 93; M. B. Emanuel and J. A. Will, *Proc. R. Soc. Med.*, 1977, *70*, *Suppl.* 8, 7; F. Ellis and D. E. Hyams, *ibid.*, 13; A. J. Staessen, *ibid.*, 17; J. de Cree *et al.*, *ibid.*, 21; T. Di Perri *et al.*, *ibid.*, 25.

Vertigo. In a double-blind crossover trial, 63 patients suffering from vertigo were given either cinnarizine 15 to 30 mg or prochlorperazine 5 to 10 mg, thrice daily. The treatment started with the lower dose and was increased to the higher dose if there was no improvement at the end of the first week, and the drugs were crossed over at 4 weeks. No significant differences were demonstrated between the 2 drugs. Side-effects were few with both drugs, but drowsiness or lassitude occurred in 8% on cinnarizine and in 3% on prochlorperazine.—Report No. 183 of the General Practitioner Research Group, *Practitioner*, 1973, *211*, 224.

Proprietary Preparations

Stugeron *(Janssen, UK)*. Cinnarizine, available as scored tablets of 15 mg. **Stugeron Forte.** Cinnarizine, available as capsules of 75 mg. (Also available as Stugeron in *Arg., Belg., Ital., Neth., S.Afr., Spain, Switz.*).

Other Proprietary Names

Arg.—Dismaren, Folcodal, Natropas; *Belg.*—Dimitronal; *Denm.*—Sepan; *Fr.*—Midronal; *Ger.*—Cerepar, Cinnacet, Gigantēn, Stutgeron; *Ital.*—Cinazyn, Senoger, Toliman; *Jap.*—Aplactan, Aplexal, Apomiterl, Apotomin, Apsatan, Artate, Carecin, Cerebolan, Cinaperazine, Corathiem, Cysten, Denapol, Eglen, Hilactan, Hirdsyn, Izaberizin, Katoseran, Processine, Razlin, Roin, Sapratol, Sedatromin, Siptazin, Spaderizine, Torizin; *Neth.*—Cinnipirine; *Swed.*—Glanil; *Switz.*—Cerepar, Cero-Aterin.

6119-p

Clemastine Fumarate.

Meclastine Fumarate; Mecloprodin Fumarate. (+)-(2*R*)-2-{2-[(*R*)-4-Chloro-α-methylbenzhydryloxy]ethyl}-1-methylpyrrolidine hydrogen fumarate.
$C_{21}H_{26}ClNO,C_4H_4O_4$=460.0.

CAS — 15686-51-8 (clemastine); 14976-57-9 (fumarate).

Clemastine fumarate 1.34 mg is approximately equivalent to 1 mg of clemastine base.

Adverse Effects, Treatment, and Precautions. As for the antihistamines in general, p.1294.

The effect of clemastine, either taken alone or in association with alcohol, on performance: E. S. Day *et al.* (letter), *J. clin. Pharmac.*, 1972, *12*, 240; C. Bye *et al.*, *Br. J. clin. Pharmac.*, 1974, *1*, 342P; I. Hindmarch, *Curr. med. Res. Opinion*, 1976, *4*, 197; C. H. Clarke and A. N. Nicholson, *Br. J. clin. Pharmac.*, 1978, *6*, 31; H. M. Franks *et al.*, *Med. J. Aust.*, 1979, *1*, 185.

Effects on the eyes. A study indicating that usual therapeutic doses of clemastine interfere with colour vision.— J. Laroche and C. Laroche, *Annls pharm. fr.*, 1972, *30*, 433.

Absorption and Fate. As for the antihistamines in general, p.1295.

In 12 healthy subjects given clemastine fumarate by mouth peak plasma concentrations occurred after 3 to 5 hours. After intravenous injection in 3 subjects a rapid decline in plasma concentration during the first 30 minutes occurred followed by a slow rise to peak concentration 2 to 3 hours after administration. In 5 subjects given clemastine fumarate the ability to inhibit histamine flares correlated well with plasma concentration.— R. Tham *et al.*, *Arzneimittel-Forsch.*, 1978, *28*, 1017.

Uses. Clemastine fumarate has the properties and uses of the antihistamines (see p.1295). It generally causes less sedation than promethazine; it has been reported to have a duration of action of about 10 to 12 hours.

Clemastine fumarate is given by mouth for allergic conditions; the usual dose is the equivalent of 1 mg of clemastine night and morning. If necessary the equivalent of up to 6 mg daily may be given in divided doses. The dose for children up to 12 years is the equivalent of 0.5 to 1 mg night and morning according to age.

It may be given by intramuscular injection in a dose equivalent to 2 to 4 mg of clemastine daily; children may be given up to one-half this amount according to age.

Clemastine 1 mg twice daily was more effective than chlorpheniramine maleate 4 mg twice daily in inhibiting wheals due to the intradermal introduction of histamine in 6 volunteers.— A. Hedges *et al.*, *J. clin. Pharmac.*, 1971, *11*, 112.

Allergy. Clemastine was frequently effective in the symptomatic control of hay fever, allergic rhinitis, and vasomotor rhinitis in 89 patients. Optimal dosage was 1 mg twice daily for adults and 0.5 to 1 mg twice daily for children. It appeared to be effective in a few patients with allergic skin disorders and pruritus. Side-effects included drowsiness and dry mouth. One patient receiving 2 mg thrice daily experienced dizziness, prickly feelings, and general malaise.— A. Roncevich, *Curr. ther. Res.*, 1969, *11*, 625.

Clemastine 1 mg and chlorpheniramine 4 mg were considered to be equally effective for the symptomatic relief of seasonal hay fever in a study completed by 46 of 51 patients with a history of hay fever, symptoms of sneezing and nasal obstruction, and positive response to skin tests for allergic dermatoses, who took part in a double-blind randomised parallel group study.— J. M. Sherriff and M. G. Wallace, *Curr. med. Res. Opinion*, 1976, *4*, 245.

Further references: I. S. Collins and F. J. Morton, *Curr. ther. Res.*, 1968, *10*, 373; B. Grove, *Med. J. Aust.*, 1969, *1*, 1235; A. Axelsson, *Läkartidningen*, 1970, *67*, 3093; *Practitioner*, 1972, *208*, 839 (Report No. 171 of the General Practitioner Research Group); J. S. Thomas *et al.*, *Ann. Allergy*, 1977, *38*, 169; *idem*, 175; S. Jungert, *Curr. ther. Res.*, 1978, *24*, 269.

Proprietary Preparations

Tavegil *(Wander, UK)*. Clemastine fumarate, available as **Elixir** (suggested diluent, syrup or water) containing in each 5 ml the equivalent of 500 µg of clemastine and as scored **Tablets** each containing the equivalent of 1 mg of clemastine. (Also available as Tavegil in *Ger., Ital., Neth., Spain*).

Other Proprietary Names

Alagyl, Aloginan, Alphamin, Alusas, Anhistan, Benanzyl, Clemanil, Fuluminol, Fumaresutin, Histamedine, Inbestan, Kinotomin, Lacretin, Lecasol, Maikohis, Malermin-F, Marsthine, Masletine, Natarilon, Piloral, Reconin *(all Jap.)*; Tavegyl *(Arg., Austral., Belg., Denm., Fr., Hung., Jap., Norw., S.Afr., Switz.)*; Tavist *(Canad., USA)*; Telgin-G, Trabest, Xolamin *(all Jap.)*.

6120-n

Clemizole Hydrochloride. 1-(4-Chlorobenzyl)-2-(pyrrolidin-1-ylmethyl)benzimidazole hydrochloride.
$C_{19}H_{20}ClN_3,HCl$=362.3.

CAS — 442-52-4 (clemizole); 1163-36-6 (hydrochloride).

A white crystalline powder. M.p. about 246°. **Soluble** in water, alcohol, and chloroform; practically insoluble in ether.

Clemizole hydrochloride has the properties and uses of the antihistamines (see p.1294). It has moderate sedative effects and little anticholinergic activity. Clemizole hydrochloride has been given in doses of 20 to 40 mg two to four times daily; clemizole tannate has been used similarly. Clemizole hydrochloride has been given by subcutaneous, intramuscular, and slow intravenous injection. As the hydrogen sulphate it has been applied topically.

Cardiac arrhythmias. A report of the use of clemizole in the treatment of atrial flutter.— L. Cardenas *et al.*, *Archs Mal. Coeur*, 1969, *62*, 401.

Proprietary Names

Alercur *(Schering, Spain)*; Allercur *(Schering, Austral.; Schering, Switz.)*; Allerpant *(Panther-Osfa, Ital.)*; Pan-Allerg *(Borromeo, Ital.)*.

6121-h

Cyclizine *(U.S.P.)*.

1-Benzhydryl-4-methylpiperazine.
$C_{18}H_{22}N_2$=266.4.

CAS — 82-92-8.

Pharmacopoeias. In *U.S.*

A white or creamy-white almost odourless crystalline powder. M.p. 106° to 109°.

Practically **insoluble** in water; soluble 1 in 6 of alcohol and of ether, and 1 in 0.9 of chloroform. A saturated solution in water has a pH of 7.6 to 8.6. **Store** in airtight containers. Protect from light.

6122-m

Cyclizine Hydrochloride *(B.P., U.S.P.)*.

Cyclizini Hydrochloridum; Cyclizinium Chloride.
$C_{18}H_{22}N_2,HCl$=302.8.

CAS — 303-25-3.

Pharmacopoeias. In *Br., Ind., Int.,* and *U.S.*

A white, odourless or almost odourless, crystalline powder, or small colourless crystals, with a bitter taste. M.p. about 285° with decomposition. **Soluble** 1 in about 125 of water, 1 in about 120 of alcohol, and 1 in 75 of chloroform; practically insoluble in ether. A 2% solution in alcohol 2 vol. and water 3 vol. has a pH of 4.5 to 5.5. Solutions for injection are **sterilised** by autoclaving or by filtration. **Store** in airtight containers. Protect from light.

6123-b

Cyclizine Lactate.

$C_{18}H_{22}N_2,C_3H_6O_3$=356.5.

CAS — 5897-19-8.

Incompatibility. A precipitate was formed when cyclizine lactate 50 mg in 1 ml was mixed with morphine sulphate 10 mg in 1 ml in the same syringe.— I. W. Marshall, *Royal Infirmary, Edinburgh, Personal Communication*, September 1971.

Adverse Effects, Treatment, and Precautions. As for the antihistamines in general, p.1294.

For a discussion on early suggestions that foetal abnormalities might result from the use of cyclizine and similar compounds, see under Meclozine Hydrochloride, p.1314.

Studies on the effect of cyclizine on performance: M. Clubley *et al.*, *Br. J. clin. Pharmac.*, 1977, *4*, 652P; *idem*, 1979, *7*, 157.

Abuse. Three boys aged 17 each took 750 mg of cyclizine (15 tablets), and became euphoric within 30 minutes. Four hours later, 1 boy had a convulsion and fell asleep, while 2 were hallucinated. All had tachycardia (heart-rate 120 to 140 per minute) and hypertension (150/90 to 160/100 mmHg), and were disorientated and incoordinated, with widely dilated and slowly reactive pupils. Six hours after the dose the boys were orientated, euphoric, and tremulous, but vital signs were normal. Hallucinations persisted in 1, but next morning all 3 had recovered, except for some tremor.— P. H. Gott, *New Engl. J. Med.*, 1968, *279*, 596.

Allergy. In a 26-year-old man, a 50-mg dose of cyclizine for travel sickness produced, after about 12 hours, irritation and soreness of the penis, which became more severe after several hours and was followed by erythema, vesiculation, and swelling. A similar reaction occurred on 2 subsequent occasions and after a challenge dose.— W. A. D. Griffiths and R. D. G. Peachey, *Br. J. Derm.*, 1970, *82*, 616.

Effects on the liver. An 8-year-old girl developed jaundice on 2 occasions after taking cyclizine 25 mg daily. 'Hypersensitivity hepatitis' was considered responsible.— M. C. Kew *et al.* (letter), *Br. med. J.*, 1973, *2*, 307.

Pregnancy and the neonate. For studies involving the use of cyclizine during pregnancy, see under Meclozine Hydrochloride, p.1314.

Uses. Cyclizine is a piperazine derivative with the properties of the antihistamines (see p.1295) but it is used mainly for its potent anti-emetic action. It has anticholinergic activity. Sedative effects are not marked.

It is used for the prevention and treatment of motion sickness. It has also been used in irradiation sickness, postoperative vomiting, and drug-induced nausea and vomiting, and for the symptomatic treatment of vertigo due to Ménière's disease and other labyrinthine disturbances.

For the prevention of motion sickness cyclizine hydrochloride 50 mg is taken 20 to 30 minutes before departure; this dose may be repeated every 4 to 6 hours if necessary. The dosage for children of 1 to 5 years is 12.5 mg twice or thrice daily, and for those aged 6 to 12 years, 25 mg thrice daily.

Cyclizine is given by injection as the lactate in doses of 50 mg thrice daily; for the prevention of postoperative vomiting it may be injected intramuscularly about 20 minutes before the anticipated end of surgery. Children aged 1 to 5 years have been given one-quarter the adult dose and those aged 6 to 12 years one-half the adult dose.

Cyclizine hydrochloride has also been given by suppository in doses of 100 mg thrice daily; children have been given correspondingly smaller doses.

Anaesthesia. Cyclizine 50 mg, given with either atropine or pethidine by injection prior to operation, was found to be a poor pre-operative sedative. Cyclizine increased the incidence of excitatory phenomena after methohexitone anaesthesia, enhanced the soporific effect of pethidine, and reduced pre-operative emesis. Postoperative sickness was markedly reduced by cyclizine.— J. W. Dundee *et al.*, *Br. J. Anaesth.*, 1966, *38*, 50.

Further references: P. S. Marcus and J. C. Sheehan, *Anesthesiology*, 1955, *16*, 423; J. J. Bonica *et al.*, *ibid.*, 1958, *19*, 532; P. H. Lorhan, *Anesth. Analg. curr. Res.*, 1958, *37*, 247; J. W. Dundee and P. O. Jones, *Br. J. clin. Pract.*, 1968, *22*, 379.

Nausea and vomiting. Cyclizine was recommended as the anti-emetic of choice for patients with breast cancer because 50-mg intramuscular doses did not affect circulating prolactin concentrations.— M. O. Thorner *et al.* (letter), *Br. med. J.*, 1974, *3*, 467. It was doubtful whether there was sufficient evidence to justify predictions concerning the effect of anti-emetics on breast cancer growth.— P. K. Bondy and T. J. Powles (letter), *ibid.*, 1974, *4*, 228.

Preparations

Cyclizine Hydrochloride Tablets *(U.S.P.)*. Tablets containing cyclizine hydrochloride. Store in airtight containers. Protect from light.

Cyclizine Lactate Injection *(U.S.P.)*. A sterile solution in Water for Injections prepared from cyclizine with the aid of lactic acid. pH 3.2 to 4.7. Protect from light.

Cyclizine Tablets *(B.P.)*. Tablets containing cyclizine hydrochloride.

Proprietary Preparations

Marzine *(Wellcome Consumer Division, UK)*. Cyclizine hydrochloride, available as tablets of 50 mg. (Also available as Marzine in *Austral.*, *Canad.*, *Denm.*, *Fr.*, *Ital.*, *Neth.*, *Norw.*, *Swed.*, *Switz.*).

Valoid *(Calmic, UK)*. Cyclizine hydrochloride, available as scored tablets of 50 mg. **Valoid Injection.** Contains 50 mg of cyclizine lactate per ml, in ampoules of 1 ml. (Also available as Valoid in *S.Afr.*).

Other Proprietary Names

Echnatol *(Switz.)*; Maremal *(Spain)*; Marezine *(USA)*; Motozina *(Ital.)*.

6124-v

Cyproheptadine Hydrochloride *(B.P., U.S.P.)*.

Cyproheptadini Chloridum. 4-(5*H*-Dibenzo[*a*,*d*]cyclohepten-5-ylidene)-1-methylpiperidine hydrochloride sesquihydrate.

$C_{21}H_{21}N,HCl,1\frac{1}{2}H_2O=350.9$.

CAS — 129-03-3 (cyproheptadine); 969-33-5 (hydrochloride, anhydrous); 41354-29-4 (hydrochloride, sesquihydrate).

Pharmacopoeias. In *Br.*, *Jap.*, *Nord.*, and *U.S.*

A white to slightly yellow, odourless or almost odourless, crystalline powder with a slightly bitter taste. Anhydrous cyproheptadine hydrochloride 10 mg is approximately equivalent to 11 mg of cyproheptadine hydrochloride. **Soluble** 1 in 275 of water, 1 in 35 of alcohol, 1 in about 16 of chloroform, and 1 in 1.5 of methyl alcohol; practically insoluble in ether. **Store** in airtight containers.

Adverse Effects and Treatment. As for the antihistamines in general, p.1294.

Increased appetite and weight gain may occur with cyproheptadine; this effect has been used clinically.

Effects on the liver. A 25-year-old Iraqi woman developed reversible cholestatic jaundice a month after starting to take cyproheptadine hydrochloride 12 mg daily.— D. A. Henry *et al.*, *Br. med. J.*, 1978, *1*, 753. Jaundice has not occurred and liver function tests have remained normal in 20 patients with various endocrine disorders given cyproheptadine 16 to 32 mg daily for up to 9 months. The only side-effects noted have been drowsiness, which is usually transient and lasts for up to 4 weeks after starting treatment, and an increase in weight.— J. Wortsman *et al.* (letter), *ibid.*, 1217.

Overdosage. A 7-year-old boy on haemodialysis developed hallucinations when his normal dose of cyproheptadine was increased from 4 mg daily to 8 mg twice daily for 1 day, instead of to 4 mg twice daily; his condition improved gradually over 5 days, when drugs were withdrawn.— M. Berger *et al.*, *Clin. Nephrol.*, 1977, *7*, 43.

Precautions. As for the antihistamines in general, p.1294.

Interference with diagnostic tests. Cyproheptadine reduced hypoglycaemia-induced growth hormone secretion in 7 of 8 volunteers. It was suggested that if patients receiving cyproheptadine were given a pituitary function test which used growth hormone response to insulin-induced hypoglycaemia, then cyproheptadine therapy should be stopped before the test.— C. H. Bivens *et al.*, *New Engl. J. Med.*, 1973, *289*, 236.

Uses. Cyproheptadine hydrochloride has the properties and uses of the antihistamines (see p.1295). It is one of the more potent of the antihistamines though the effect is of shorter duration than that of promethazine. It has anticholinergic and pronounced serotonin-antagonising properties. It has also been used as an appetite stimulant.

It is given usually in doses equivalent to 4 mg of anhydrous cyproheptadine hydrochloride 3 or 4 times daily. Higher doses have been used to a maximum of 32 mg daily. Children may be given 250 µg per kg body-weight daily in 3 divided doses.

A discussion on the actions and uses of cyproheptadine. Cyproheptadine is a potent antagonist of histamine, acetylcholine, and serotonin. As an antihistamine it has proved disappointing in allergic disorders but its antiserotonin properties are now attracting much interest. There is evidence that serotonin is involved in the control of corticotrophin (ACTH) secretion, possibly by stimulating corticotrophin-releasing-factor secretion. Cushing's disease seems to be due to defective hypothalamic regulation of corticotrophin release from the pituitary.— *Lancet*, 1978, *1*, 367.

Further references: C. Ferrari *et al.*, *Clin. Endocr.*, 1976, *5*, 575; K. A. Halmi and B. S. Sherman, *Psychopharmac. Bull.*, 1977, *13*, 63; C. Ferrari *et al.*, *Eur. J. clin. Pharmac.*, 1979, *15*, 395.

Acromegaly. Cyproheptadine 4 mg every 6 hours for 2 days decreased plasma concentrations of growth hormone during oral glucose tolerance tests in 4 of 6 patients with acromegaly.— J. M. Feldman *et al.*, *Clin. Endocr.*, 1976, *5*, 71.

Aldosteronism. Suppression of aldosterone by cyproheptadine in idiopathic aldosteronism.— M. D. Gross *et al.*, *New Engl. J. Med.*, 1981, *305*, 181.

Appetite stimulation. Cyproheptadine is the first clinically proven appetite stimulant but indications for its clinical use are few. It has been used successfully to increase the appetite of underweight patients with pulmonary tuberculosis and may be of some limited value in the management of anorexia nervosa. Exclusion of organic causes of weight-loss is important before treatment begins.— *Lancet*, 1978, *1*, 367.

References to the use of cyproheptadine for stimulating appetite and promoting weight gain: S. S. Bergen, *Am. J. Dis. Child.*, 1964, *108*, 270; A. Drash *et al.*, *Clin. Pharmac. Ther.*, 1966, *7*, 340; R. E. Noble, *J. Am. med. Ass.*, 1969, *209*, 2054; J. N. Stiel *et al.*, *Metabolism*, 1970, *19*, 192; A. Andronic and A. DiMascio, *Curr. ther. Res.*, 1971, *13*, 40; M. V. Silbert, *S. Afr. med. J.*, 1971, *45*, 374; *Med. Lett.*, 1971, *13*, 17; P. Mainguet, *Practitioner*, 1972, *208*, 797; A. Antoon, *J. Am. med. Ass.*, 1973, *223*, 611; G. J. Pawlowski, *Curr. ther. Res.*, 1975, *18*, 673; S. C. Goldberg *et al.*, *Br. J. Psychiat.*, 1979, *134*, 67.

Carcinoid syndrome. In a patient with the carcinoid syndrome and associated myopathy, diarrhoea was considerably reduced by treatment with cyproheptadine 16 to 32 mg daily.— E. M. Berry *et al.*, *Gut*, 1974, *15*, 34.

Cushing's disease. Beneficial results were obtained following administration of cyproheptadine 4 mg twice daily increased to 8 mg thrice daily, to a 30-year-old woman with Cushing's disease and paranoid psychosis. Considerable improvement in her psychiatric symptoms might have been associated with concomitant administration of perphenazine 8 mg daily.— S. A. Middler (letter), *New Engl. J. Med.*, 1976, *295*, 394. Cyproheptadine was ineffective in the treatment of a patient with pituitary-dependent Cushing's disease and with a history of psychiatric illness. It might have precipitated an acute psychiatric episode which developed during treatment and which improved following cyproheptadine withdrawal and treatment with major tranquillisers.— C. J. Pearce *et al.* (letter), *Lancet*, 1977, *1*, 1368.

A report of 2 patients 1 of whom did not undergo remission suggesting the existence of subgroups of patients with Cushing's disease representing different causes. In responding patients relapse occurred on discontinuation of cyproheptadine but remission could again be obtained by reinstatement of therapy.— D. T. Krieger (letter), *New Engl. J. Med.*, 1976, *295*, 394.

Three of 5 patients with pituitary-dependent Cushing's disease improved when treated with cyproheptadine in doses of up to 8 mg thrice daily for at least 6 weeks. One patient who had not responded clinically improved when treatment was changed to bromocriptine 7.5 to 30 mg daily for 1 month. The addition of cyproheptadine to this treatment produced no further improvement.— J. Marek *et al.* (letter), *Lancet*, 1977, *2*, 653.

Experience in treating 2 children led to the suggestion that, partly because of weight gain, cyproheptadine is not to be regarded as an acceptable substitute for bilateral adrenalectomy in children suffering from Cushing's disease.— A. J. D'Ercole *et al.*, *J. Pediat.*, 1977, *90*, 834.

Further conflicting reports of the merits of cyproheptadine therapy in Cushing's disease.— D. T. Krieger *et al.*, *New Engl. J. Med.*, 1975, *293*, 893; J. M. Feldman, *ibid.*, 930; *Lancet*, 1975, *2*, 1135; J. B. Tyrrell *et al.* (letter), *New Engl. J. Med.*, 1976, *295*, 1137; D. T. Krieger (letter), *ibid.*, 1138; J. Allgrove *et al.*, *Br. med. J.*, 1977, *1*, 686; P. Barnes *et al.* (letter), *Lancet*, 1977, *1*, 1148; A. W. Burrows *et al.* (letter), *Br. med. J.*, 1977, *1*, 1084; D. Doyle and D. K. O'Donovan (letter), *New Engl. J. Med.*, 1977, *296*, 576; R. Scott *et al.* (letter), *ibid.*, 57.

See also under Growth Enhancement, below.

Nelson's syndrome. Cyproheptadine 12 mg daily controlled the symptoms of Nelson's syndrome (a corticotrophin-producing tumour of the pituitary) in a woman who had undergone bilateral adrenalectomy for Cushing's disease about 6 years previously.— W. Hartwig *et al.* (letter), *New Engl. J. Med.*, 1976, *295*, 394. Three of 4 patients with Nelson's syndrome had responded to cyproheptadine therapy.— D. T. Krieger (letter), *ibid.*

Cyproheptadine in doses of up to 40 mg daily was ineffective in the treatment of Nelson's syndrome in 3 patients.— J. Cassar *et al.* (letter), *Lancet*, 1976, *2*, 426.

In an adrenalectomised woman with Nelson's syndrome following bilateral adrenalectomy for Cushing's disease, remission has been maintained for 18 months after stopping prolonged treatment with cyproheptadine. When cyproheptadine was previously discontinued the patient relapsed within about 4 months.— N. Aronin and D. T. Krieger, *New Engl. J. Med.*, 1980, *302*, 453.

Dumping syndrome. Patients suffering from the dumping syndrome might obtain relief of circulatory symptoms by taking cyproheptadine 4 mg by mouth 1 to 2 hours before meals.— J. E. Lennard-Jones, *Prescribers' J.*, 1967, *7*, 7.

Extrapyramidal symptoms. Beneficial results with cyproheptadine in 3 patients with marked chorea-athetotic dyskinesia following prolonged phenothiazine therapy.— D. Goldman, *Psychopharmac. Bull.*, 1976, *12*, 7. Cyproheptadine 4 mg twice daily for up to 6 weeks failed to produce any striking improvement in 5 patients with obvious tardive dyskinesia.— G. Gardos and J. O. Cole, *ibid.*, 1978, *14*, 18.

Cyproheptadine in doses up to 42 mg daily was ineffective in controlling levodopa-induced dyskinesia in 6 patients with idiopathic parkinsonism.— P. S. Papavasiliou *et al.*, *Clin. Pharmac. Ther.*, 1978, *23*, 195.

Galactorrhoea-amenorrhoea syndrome. Cyproheptadine, 16 to 24 mg daily in divided doses for 16 weeks, was used in the treatment of the galactorrhoea-amenorrhoea syndrome in 15 women. Serum-prolactin concentrations decreased in 12 women and menstrual bleeding resumed in 10. However, galactorrhoea decreased in only 7 patients, and stopped in only 2, and ovulation did not occur in any of the patients.— J. Wortsman *et al.*, *Ann. intern. Med.*, 1979, *90*, 923. Comments on the effect of cyproheptadine on pituitary function, with particular relevance to its use in the galactorrhoea-amenorrhoea syndrome. It was considered that the treatments of choice in this syndrome are surgery and bromocriptine.— L. I. Dolman (letter), *Ann. intern. Med.*, 1979, *91*, 927.

Growth enhancement. Cyproheptadine 12 mg daily for 18 months was used to treat growth suppression due to mild Cushing's disease in a 15-year-old boy. Within 6 months of starting treatment, growth restarted, and plasma- and urine-cortisol concentrations returned to normal, and remained so 9 months after stopping cyproheptadine treatment.— D. B. Grant and S. M. Atherden, *Archs Dis. Childh.*, 1979, *54*, 466.

Further references: A. G. Kenien *et al.*, *J. Pediat.*, 1978, *92*, 491 (administration with growth hormone in hypopituitarism).

Melkersson-Rosenthal syndrome. Cyproheptadine, 8 mg thrice daily, was given to a man suffering from recurrent swelling of the face after facial palsy (the Melkersson-Rosenthal syndrome). Swelling subsided over a 6-week period and the patient remained free from symptoms for the next 3 months, but when cyproheptadine therapy was suspended, symptoms recurred within 3 weeks. They subsided after further treatment with cyproheptadine.— S. C. Loong and J. W. Lance, *Med. J. Aust.*, 1968, *2*, 671.

Orthostatic syndrome. A report of cyproheptadine being used to treat a patient with an orthostatic syndrome.— D. H. P. Streeten *et al.*, *Lancet*, 1972, *2*, 1048.

Pregnancy and the neonate. Cyproheptadine 6 to 8 mg daily was given during pregnancy to 3 women who had suffered habitual abortion due to serotonin. The pregnancies of 2 continued despite repeated bleeding and normal healthy babies were delivered. The third patient aborted but during her next pregnancy the dose was raised to 12 to 16 mg daily and at 6 months she was delivered of a live premature baby.— E. Sadovsky *et al.*, *Harefuah*, 1970, *78*, 332, per *J. Am. med. Ass.*, 1970, *212*, 1253.

Pruritus. Cyproheptadine, in doses of 4 mg three or four times daily, had been found effective in suppressing the pruritus of 12 of 17 patients with polycythaemia vera when other antihistamines had afforded only transient relief; improvement had occurred in 3 further patients.— *J. Am. med. Ass.*, 1968, *205* (Aug. 26), A27. See also H. S. Gilbert *et al.*, *Blood*, 1966, *28*, 795.

Urticaria. A favourable report of the use of cyproheptadine in primary-acquired cold urticaria in 8 patients.— A. A. Wanderer *et al.*, *Archs Derm.*, 1977, *113*, 1375.

Further references: A. A. Wanderer and E. F. Ellis, *J. Allergy & clin. Immunol.*, 1971, *48*, 365.

Preparations

Cyproheptadine Hydrochloride Syrup *(U.S.P.)*. A syrup containing cyproheptadine hydrochloride. Potency is expressed in terms of the equivalent amount of anhydrous cyproheptadine hydrochloride. pH 3.5 to 4.5. Store in airtight containers.

Cyproheptadine Hydrochloride Tablets *(U.S.P.)*. Tablets containing cyproheptadine hydrochloride. Potency is expressed in terms of the equivalent amount of anhydrous cyproheptadine hydrochloride.

Cyproheptadine Tablets *(B.P.)*. Tablets containing cyproheptadine hydrochloride. Potency is expressed in terms of the equivalent amount of anhydrous cyproheptadine hydrochloride.

Periactin *(Merck Sharp & Dohme, UK)*. Cyproheptadine hydrochloride, available as **Syrup** containing in each 5 ml the equivalent of 2 mg of anhydrous cyproheptadine hydrochloride (suggested diluent, syrup) and as scored **Tablets** each containing the equivalent of 4 mg of anhydrous cyproheptadine hydrochloride. (Also available as Periactin in *Arg., Austral., Belg., Canad., Denm., Ital., Neth., Norw., S.Afr., Spain, Swed., Switz., USA*).

Other Proprietary Names

Austral.—Antegan; *Canad.*—Vimicon; *Fr.*—Périactine; *Ger.*—Nuran, Periactinol; *Hung.*—Peritol; *Jap.*—Ifrasarl; *Spain*—Cipractin, Sigloton.

A preparation containing cyproheptadine hydrochloride was also formerly marketed in Great Britain under the proprietary name Perideca (*Merck Sharp & Dohme*).

6125-g

Deptropine Citrate. Dibenzheptropine Citrate. (1*R*,3*r*,5*S*)-3-(10,11-Dihydro-5*H*-dibenzo[*a,d*]cyclohepten-5-yloxy)tropane dihydrogen citrate.
$C_{23}H_{27}NO,C_6H_8O_7$=525.6.

CAS — 604-51-3 (deptropine); 2169-75-7 (citrate).

A white to off-white, almost odourless, microcrystalline powder with a slightly bitter acidic taste.
Very slightly **soluble** in water and alcohol; soluble 1 in 100 of methyl alcohol; practically insoluble in acetone, chloroform, and ether. **Protect** from light.

Adverse Effects, Treatment, and Precautions. As for the antihistamines in general, p.1294.
It is contra-indicated in patients with glaucoma and prostatic hypertrophy because of its marked anticholinergic effects.

Uses. Deptropine citrate has the properties and uses of the antihistamines (see p.1295). It has a prolonged action, is more potent than promethazine hydrochloride, and has marked anticholinergic and serotonin-antagonising properties.
Deptropine citrate has been given by mouth in doses of 1 mg twice daily mainly for the relief of chronic non-specific respiratory disorders. It was formerly used for these purposes as an aerosol spray. Deptropine citrate has been used by injection for premedication prior to operation.

Allergy. Deptropine citrate and chlorpheniramine maleate were found to be equally effective in patients with hay fever.—Report No. 57 of the General Practitioner Research Group, *Practitioner*, 1964, *192*, 682.

Anaesthesia. A comparison of deptropine citrate and atropine for premedication.— J. F. Cam and C. M. T. Gleave, *Br. J. Anaesth.*, 1968, *40*, 885.

Asthma and bronchitis. Deptropine citrate was used for the prophylaxis of chronic bronchitis in 71 patients. In a dose of 500 µg thrice daily it offered no advantages over a placebo.—Report No. 58 of the General Practitioner Research Group, *Practitioner*, 1964, *192*, 684.

Further references: M. C. S. Kennedy, *Br. med. J.*, 1965, *2*, 916; F. J. Prime, *Br. J. Dis. Chest*, 1968, *62*, 82; *Drug & Ther. Bull.*, 1976, *14*, 85.

Proprietary Preparations

Brontina *(Brocades, UK)*. Deptropine citrate, available as scored tablets of 1 mg.

Other Proprietary Names

Brontin *(Ital.)*; Brontine *(Belg., Neth.)*.

6126-q

Dexbrompheniramine Maleate *(U.S.P.)*.

Dexbrompheniramine is the dextrorotatory isomer of brompheniramine which is racemic.

CAS — 132-21-8 (dexbrompheniramine); 2391-03-9 (maleate).

Pharmacopoeias. In *Braz.* and *U.S.*

A white odourless crystalline powder. M.p 103° to 113°. **Soluble** 1 in 1.2 of water, 1 in 2.5 of alcohol, and 1 in 2 of chloroform; very slightly soluble in ether. A solution in dimethylformamide is dextrorotatory. A 1% solution has a pH of about 5. **Store** in airtight containers. Protect from light.

Adverse Effects, Treatment, and Precautions. As for the antihistamines in general, p.1294.

Effects on the skin. A report of the development of maculopapular rash following the ingestion of dexbrompheniramine 6 mg together with pseudoephedrine.— G. Smith and H. L. Fred, *Archs Derm.*, 1966, *94*, 200, per *Int. pharm. Abstr.*, 1966, *3*, 1667.

Extrapyramidal symptoms. A report of an acute oral and facial dystonic reaction associated with the overdose of dexbrompheniramine maleate 24 mg and pseudoephedrine sulphate 480 mg in an 18-month-old girl.— D. A. Barone and J. Raniolo (letter), *New Engl. J. Med.*, 1980, *303*, 107.

Pregnancy and the neonate. Irritability, excessive crying, and disturbed sleep patterns occurred in a 3-month-old breast-fed infant whose mother was receiving a decongestant containing dexbrompheniramine and pseudoephedrine. Discontinuation of medication and substitution of an artificial feed were associated with resumption of normal behaviour in the infant within 12 hours.— E. A. Mortimer (letter), *Pediatrics*, 1977, *60*, 780.

Uses. Dexbrompheniramine maleate is an alkylamine derivative with actions and uses similar to those of brompheniramine maleate (see p.1298). It has been given in usual doses of 2 mg four times daily but higher doses of up to 18 mg daily have also been given in sustained-release preparations.

6127-p

Dexchlorpheniramine Maleate *(U.S.P.)*.

Dexchlorpheniramine is the dextrorotatory isomer of chlorpheniramine which is racemic.

CAS — 25523-97-1 (dexchlorpheniramine); 2438-32-6 (maleate).

Pharmacopoeias. In *Nord.* and *U.S.*

A white odourless crystalline powder. M.p. 110° to 115°. **Soluble** 1 in 1.1 of water, 1 in 2 of alcohol, and 1 in 1.7 of chloroform; very slightly soluble in ether. A solution in dimethylformamide is dextrorotatory. A 1% solution in water has a pH of 4 to 5. **Store** in airtight containers. Protect from light.

Adverse Effects, Treatment, and Precautions. As for the antihistamines in general p.1294.

Effects on the eyes. A study indicating that usual therapeutic doses of dexchlorpheniramine interfere with colour vision.— J. Laroche and C. Laroche, *Annls pharm. fr.*, 1972, *30*, 433.

Uses. Dexchlorpheniramine maleate is an alkylamine derivative with actions and uses similar to those of chlorpheniramine maleate (see p.1300). It is given usually in a dose of 2 mg three or four times daily. Higher doses of up to 18 mg daily have been given in sustained-release preparations. For children the dose is 0.5 to 1 mg three or four times daily, according to age.

Preparations

Dexchlorpheniramine Maleate Syrup *(U.S.P.)*. A syrup containing dexchlorpheniramine maleate, with alcohol 5 to 7%. Store in airtight containers. Protect from light.

Dexchlorpheniramine Maleate Tablets *(U.S.P.)*. Tablets containing dexchlorpheniramine maleate. Store in airtight containers.

Proprietary Names

Afeme *(Cetus, Arg.)*; Alergitrat *(Fecofar, Arg.)*; Destral *(Tiber, Ital.)*; Isomerine *(Essex, Arg.)*; Phenamin *(Nyco, Norw.)*; Polaramin *(Schering, Denm.; Essex, Ital.; Schering, Norw.; Schering, Swed.)*; Polaramine *(Essex, Austral.; Schering, Belg.; Schering, Canad.; Cétrane, Fr.; Essex, Neth.; Scherag, S.Afr.; Essex, Spain; Schering, Switz.; Schering, USA)*.

6128-s

Dimenhydrinate *(B.P., U.S.P.)*.

Diphenhydramine Theoclate; Diphenhydramini Teoclas; Chloranautine; Anautin. The diphenhydramine salt of 8-chlorotheophylline.
$C_{17}H_{21}NO,C_7H_7ClN_4O_2$=470.0.

CAS — 523-87-5.

Pharmacopoeias. In *Arg., Br., Braz., Chin., Ind., Int., Jap.,* and *U.S.*

A white odourless crystalline powder with a bitter numbing taste. M.p. 102° to 107°.
Soluble 1 in 95 of water, 1 in 2 of alcohol, and 1 in 2 of chloroform; sparingly soluble in ether. A solution in equal parts of propylene glycol and water, with 5% benzyl alcohol, is **sterilised** by maintaining at 98° to 100° for 30 minutes. **Store** in airtight containers.

Incompatibility. Dimenhydrinate caused precipitation when mixed with solutions of tetracycline hydrochloride in dextrose injection and when mixed with novobiocin sodium in sodium chloride solution.— H. R. Grant, *Hosp. Pharmst*, 1962, *15*, 67.

Dimenhydrinate could be dispensed in aqueous alcoholic solutions within the pH range 5.4 to 8.6 and these solutions could be sterilised by autoclaving. Substances which were incompatible with solutions of dimenhydrinate included phenothiazine derivatives, reserpine, methoxamine hydrochloride, pentobarbitone sodium, thiamylal sodium, nicotinic acid, pyridoxine hydrochloride, and certain antibiotic solutions such as chloramphenicol succinate.— N. Brudney *et al.*, *Can. pharm. J.*, 1963, *96*, 470.

Particulate matter was observed within 2 hours when 1 ml of commercial dimenhydrinate injection was mixed with 5 ml of sterile water and 1 ml of any of the following commercial injection solutions: aminophylline, heparin sodium, hydrocortisone sodium succinate, hydroxyzine hydrochloride, phenobarbitone sodium, phenytoin sodium, prednisolone sodium phosphate, prochlorperazine edisylate, promazine hydrochloride, and promethazine hydrochloride.— R. Misgen, *Am. J. Hosp. Pharm.*, 1965, *22*, 92.

There was a precipitate when iodipamide meglumine injection was added to dimenhydrinate injection.— T. R. Marshall *et al.*, *Radiology*, 1965, *84*, 536.

There was loss of clarity when intravenous solutions of dimenhydrinate were mixed with those of aminophylline, ammonium chloride, amylobarbitone sodium, heparin sodium, hydrocortisone sodium succinate, hydroxyzine hydrochloride, pentobarbitone sodium, phenobarbitone sodium, phenytoin sodium, prochlorperazine maleate, or thiopentone sodium.— J. A. Patel and G. L. Phillips, *Am. J. Hosp. Pharm.*, 1966, *23*, 409.

Adverse Effects, Treatment, and Precautions. As for the antihistamines in general, p.1294.

Abuse. Hallucinations occurred in 2 men aged 20 and 22 years, after ingesting dimenhydrinate 800 mg by mouth. The second patient also experienced paranoia.— R. Malcolm and W. C. Miller, *Am. J. Psychiat.*, 1972, *128*, 1012. See also J. H. Brown and H. K. Sigmundson, *Can. med. Ass. J.*, 1969, *101*, 710.

Effects on the eyes. The effect of dimenhydrinate 100 mg and aspirin 1.28 g on visual processes was studied in 16 healthy subjects. Three doses of active drug or placebo were given at about 4 hour intervals. Both drugs affected colour discrimination and dimenhydrinate degraded night vision, reaction time, and stereopsis. The effects of aspirin were minor, but the effects produced by dimenhydrinate appeared to be of practical importance.— S. M. Luria *et al.*, *Br. J. clin. Pharmac.*, 1979, *7*, 585.

Extrapyramidal symptoms. Extrapyramidal symptoms in an 11-year-old child were associated with the administration of dimenhydrinate.— C. Cassimos *et al.*, *J. Pediat.*, 1975, *87*, 981.

See also under Overdosage (below).

Overdosage. A 24-year-old woman died after taking 7.5 g of dimenhydrinate in an attempt to procure abortion. Vomiting, vertigo, and convulsions led to coma, cyanosis, and death from respiratory failure 90 minutes later. Acute pulmonary stasis and renal tubular degeneration were observed at necropsy.— J. B. Dalgaard and J. Jakobsen, *Ugeskr. Laeg.*, 1962, *124*, 1844, per *Pharmacy Dig.*, 1963, *27*, 559.

Severe delirium similar to atropine poisoning and with possible extrapyramidal symptoms followed an overdose of dimenhydrinate. Treatment with chlordiazepoxide, benztropine, and fluids was effective in 24 hours.— J. H. Brown and H. K. Sigmundson, *Can. med. Ass. J.*, 1969, *101*, 710.

Pregnancy and the neonate. Of 50 282 children born to mothers monitored by the Collaborative Perinatal Project, 5773 were found to have been exposed to xanthines, and possibly other drugs, at some time during the first 4 months of the pregnancy. Although no association was seen between malformations and exposures to xanthines in general a relationship between cardiovascular defects and inguinal hernia and dimenhydrinate exposure (319 children) was noted.— O. P. Heinonen *et al.*, *Birth Defects and Drugs in Pregnancy*, Littleton MA, Publishing Sciences Group, 1977, p. 366.

Uses. Dimenhydrinate is diphenhydramine theoclate and has the general properties of diphenhydramine hydrochloride (see p.1311). It is used mainly as an anti-emetic in the prevention and treatment of motion sickness. It has also been used for irradiation sickness, postoperative vomiting, drug-induced nausea and vomiting, and the symptomatic treatment of nausea and vertigo due to Ménière's disease and other labyrinthine disturbances.

It is usually given by mouth in doses of 50 mg thrice daily, the first dose for preventing motion sickness being taken about 30 minutes before the journey. For treatment, 4-hourly administration may be required. Doses of 100 mg may be required but a daily total of 300 mg should not usually be exceeded. Children of 1 to 6 years may be given 12.5 to 25 mg twice or thrice daily and those of 7 to 12 years 25 to 50 mg twice or thrice daily. Similar doses may be administered rectally or intramuscularly. In extreme emergency the injection may be diluted to 0.5% with sodium chloride injection and given by slow intravenous injection.

For the prevention of postoperative vomiting, 50 mg has been injected intramuscularly before the operation, again at the end of the operation, and then 3 times at intervals of 4 hours.

Preparations

Dimenhydrinate Injection *(B.P.).* A sterile solution of dimenhydrinate in a mixture of equal volumes of propylene glycol and Water for Injections containing 5% v/v of benzyl alcohol. Sterilised by heating at 98° to 100° for 30 minutes. pH 6.8 to 7.2.

Dimenhydrinate Injection *(U.S.P.).* A sterile solution of dimenhydrinate in a mixture of propylene glycol and water. pH 6.4 to 7.2.

Dimenhydrinate Suppositories *(U.S.P.).* Suppositories containing dimenhydrinate. Store in a cool place.

Dimenhydrinate Syrup *(U.S.P.).* A syrup containing dimenhydrinate and 4 to 6% of alcohol. Store in airtight containers.

Dimenhydrinate Tablets *(B.P., U.S.P.).* Tablets containing dimenhydrinate.

Proprietary Preparations

Dramamine *(Searle, UK).* Dimenhydrinate, available as **Injection** containing 50 mg per ml with benzyl alcohol 5% and propylene glycol 50% in water, in ampoules of 1 ml, and as scored **Tablets** of 50 mg. (Also available as Dramamine in *Austral., Belg., Canad., Fr., Ger., Neth., S.Afr., Spain, USA*).

Gravol *(Pharmax, UK).* Dimenhydrinate, available as **Suppositories** containing 50 mg (children) and 100 mg (adults) and as scored **Tablets** of 50 mg. (Also available as Gravol in *Canad.*).

Other Proprietary Names

Austral.—Andrumin; *Canad.*—Nauseatol, Novodimenate, Travamine; *Denm.*— Neptusan; *Ger.*—Epha-retard, Novomina, Vomex A; *Ital.*—Amalmare, Lomarin, Valontan, Xamamina; *Neth.*—Amosyt; *Norw.*— Dromyl; *Pol.*—Aviomarine; *Spain*—Azules, Biodramina, Dramarr, Dramavir, Mareosan, Mareozina Retard, Marolin; *Swed.*—Amosyt; *Switz.*—Antemin; *USA*—Dimate, Dramocen.

6129-w

Dimethindene Maleate *(U.S.P.).*

Dimethpyrindene Maleate; Dimethylpyrindene Maleate; Su 6518. *NN*-Dimethyl-2-{3-[1-(2-pyridyl)ethyl]-1*H*-inden-2-yl}ethylamine hydrogen maleate.

$C_{20}H_{24}N_2,C_4H_4O_4=408.5$.

CAS — 5636-83-9 (dimethindene); 3614-69-5 (maleate).

Pharmacopoeias. In *U.S.*

A white to off-white crystalline powder with a characteristic odour. M.p. about 161° with decomposition. **Soluble** 1 in 63 of water, 1 in 185 of alcohol, 1 in 10 of chloroform; practically insoluble in ether. **Store** in airtight containers. Protect from light.

Adverse Effects, Treatment, and Precautions. As for the antihistamines in general, p.1294.

Uses. Dimethindene maleate is an alkylamine derivative with the properties and uses of the antihistamines (see p.1295). It is considerably more potent than promethazine but has an action which is probably of shorter duration. It is given by mouth for the symptomatic treatment of allergic conditions particularly to control pruritus.

Dimethindene maleate is given in usual doses of 1 to 2 mg up to thrice daily but sustained-release preparations are commonly used, given in doses of 2.5 mg once or twice daily. Children over 6 years of age may be given 1 mg up to thrice daily.

Proprietary Preparations

Fenostil-Retard Tablets *(Zyma, UK).* Sustained-release tablets each containing dimethindene maleate 2.5 mg. (Also available as Fenostil in *Austral., S.Afr.*).

Other Proprietary Names

Fenistil *(Belg., Denm., Ger., Ital., Neth., Norw., Spain, Swed., Switz.)*; Forhistal *(Canad., USA)*; Triten *(USA)*.

6130-m

Dimethothiazine Mesylate.

Fonazine Mesylate; IL 6302 *(dimethothiazine)*; RP 8599 *(dimethothiazine)*. 10-(2-Dimethylaminopropyl)-*NN*-dimethylphenothiazine-2-sulphonamide methanesulphonate.

$C_{19}H_{25}N_3O_2S_2,CH_3SO_3H=487.6$.

CAS — 7456-24-8 (dimethothiazine); 7455-39-2; 13115-40-7 (both mesylate).

A white crystalline powder. M.p. about 175°. Dimethothiazine mesylate 124 mg is approximately equivalent to 100 mg of dimethothiazine. Very **soluble** in water; practically insoluble in ether. **Protect** from light.

Adverse Effects, Treatment, and Precautions. As for the antihistamines in general, p.1294.

As for all phenothiazine derivatives it should be used cautiously in patients with hepatic diseases.

Uses. Dimethothiazine mesylate is a phenothiazine derivative with the properties and uses of the antihistamines (see p.1295). It has about the same activity as promethazine as an antihistamine and it is reported to be more active in its serotonin-antagonising and anti-emetic effects. Its sedative effects are less than those of promethazine.

The usual dose is the equivalent of 20 mg of dimethothiazine thrice daily, increased, if necessary, to a total of 120 mg daily. Children of 6 to 12 years of age may be given 10 mg twice daily and older children 20 mg twice or thrice daily.

Dimethothiazine has also been used in the treatment of migraine and of spasticity.

Allergy. Similar therapeutic effects and side-effects were observed with dimethothiazine, 12.5 to 25 mg thrice daily, and chlorpheniramine, 4 to 8 mg thrice daily, in a double-blind comparison in 81 patients with hay fever or allergic rhinitis.—Report No. 106 of the General Practitioner Research Group, *Practitioner*, 1967, *198*, 711. See also J. Gomez and G. Gomez, *Br. J. clin. Pract.*, 1967, *21*, 401.

Migraine. Prophylactic treatment with dimethothiazine benefited 31 of 38 patients with idiopathic migraine and 14 of 19 patients with cervical migraine. In a further 17 patients with headache due to injury, Horton's syndrome, or haemorrhage, a very good response was not obtained but only 1 showed no improvement. Side-effects included tiredness and depression.— F. Gerstenbrand, *Wien. med. Wschr.*, 1969, *119*, 429.

Spasticity. In a double-blind crossover trial in 19 patients with spastic conditions including multiple sclerosis, cerebrovascular accidents, or cervical spondylosis, dimethothiazine 100 mg daily increased over 7 weeks to 300 mg daily was apparently more effective than diazepam 10 mg daily increased over 7 weeks to 30 mg daily.—Report No. 188 of the General Practitioner Research Group, *Practitioner*, 1974, *213*, 101. See also Report No. 180 of the General Practitioner Research Group, *ibid.*, 1973, *210*, 429; D. J. Burke, *Drugs*, 1975, *10*, 112.

Proprietary Preparations

Banistyl *(May & Baker, UK).* Dimethothiazine mesylate, available as scored tablets each containing the equivalent of 20 mg of dimethothiazine. (Also available as Banistyl in *Austral., S.Afr.*).

Other Proprietary Names

Alius *(Ital.)*; Bisbermin, Bonpac, Calsekin, Migrethiazin *(all Jap.)*; Migristene *(Arg., Belg., Fr., Ger., Jap., Spain, Switz.)*; Neomestin, Normelin *(both Jap.)*; Promaquid *(Canad.)*; Yoristen *(Jap.)*.

6131-b

Diphenhydramine Hydrochloride *(B.P., U.S.P.).* Diphenhydramini Hydrochloridum; Diphenhydraminium Chloride; Benzhydraminum Hydrochloricum; Dimedrolum. 2-Benzhydryloxy-*NN*-dimethylethylamine hydrochloride. $C_{17}H_{21}NO,HCl=291.8$.

CAS — 58-73-1 (diphenhydramine); 147-24-0 (hydrochloride).

Pharmacopoeias. In *Aust., Br., Braz., Chin., Ind., Int., It., Jap., Jug., Mex., Neth., Nord., Pol., Port., Rus., Swiss, Turk.,* and *U.S.*
Jap. also includes Diphenhydramine and Diphenhydramine Tannate.

A white or almost white, odourless or almost odourless, crystalline powder with a bitter numbing taste. M.p. 167° to 172°. It slowly darkens on exposure to light.

Soluble 1 in 1 of water, 1 in 2 of alcohol, 1 in 50 of acetone, and 1 in 2 of chloroform; practically insoluble in ether. A 5% solution in water has a pH of 4 to 6. Solutions are **sterilised** by autoclaving or filtration. **Incompatible** with amphotericin, amylobarbitone sodium, cephalothin sodium, iodides, pentobarbitone sodium, phenobarbitone sodium, quinalbarbitone sodium, and thiopentone sodium. Incompatibility has also been reported with hydrocortisone sodium succinate. **Store** in airtight containers. Protect from light.

Incompatibility. A precipitate formed when diphenhydramine hydrochloride was mixed with iodipamide salts and on standing with some concentrations of diatrizoic acid salts.— C. Riffkin, *Am. J. Hosp. Pharm.*, 1963, *20,* 19. See also T. R. Marshall *et al.*, *Radiology*, 1965, *84,* 536.

Particulate matter was observed within 2 hours when 1 ml of commercial diphenhydramine hydrochloride injection was mixed with 5 ml of sterile water and 1 ml of commercial injections of phenytoin sodium or phenobarbitone sodium.— R. Misgen, *Am. J. Hosp. Pharm.*, 1965, *22,* 92.

Further references: J. A. Patel and G. L. Phillips, *Am. J. Hosp. Pharm.*, 1966, *23,* 409; J. M. Meisler and M. W. Skolaut, *Am. J. Hosp. Pharm.*, 1966, *23,* 557.

Adverse Effects and Treatment. As for the antihistamines in general, p.1294.

Abuse. Abuse of diphenhydramine preparations has been reported in Scandinavia.— *Br. med. J.*, 1979, *1,* 459.

Allergy. An anaphylactoid reaction characterised by dizziness, weakness, tightness in the chest, severe shortness of breath, and a cough producing frothy red sputum occurred in a patient who received diphenhydramine hydrochloride 25 mg by intravenous injection over a period of about 10 seconds.— W. H. Lauderdale *et al.*, *Archs intern. Med.*, 1964, *114,* 693.

Effects on the blood. A 0.575% solution of diphenhydramine hydrochloride in 0.9% sodium chloride solution caused 100% haemolysis of erythrocytes cultured in it for 45 minutes.— C. J. Fievet *et al.*, *Am. J. Hosp. Pharm.*, 1971, *28,* 961.

Diphenhydramine was reported to be a haemolytic agent in subjects deficient in glucose-6-phosphate dehydrogenase but only in conjunction with other factors such as infection.— M. E. Pembrey, *Practitioner,* 1974, *213,* 647.

Effects on the skin. Diphenhydramine could cause photosensitivity.— J. L. Verbov, *Br. J. clin. Pract.*, 1968, *22,* 229. See also E. A. Emmett, *Archs Derm.*, 1974, *110,* 249.

Extrapyramidal symptoms. An acute dystonic reaction occurred in a 4-year-old boy 2 hours after being given a second dose of diphenhydramine hydrochloride 25 mg. Rapid recovery occurred after discontinuation of the drug.— B. L. Lavenstein and F. K. Cantor, *J. Am. med. Ass.*, 1976, *236,* 291.

A report of trismus and subsequent laryngospasm following intramuscular injection of diphenhydramine.— K. A. Brait and A. J. Zagerman (letter), *New Engl. J. Med.*, 1977, *296,* 111. Comment.— R. Sovner (letter), *ibid.*, 633.

Overdosage. A 16-year-old girl developed a toxic psychosis resembling acute schizophrenia after she had ingested 500 mg of diphenhydramine hydrochloride. Throughout the reaction atropine-like autonomic symptoms were evident. She recovered her normal mental state within about 29 hours.— S. A. Nigro, *J. Am. med. Ass.*, 1968, *203,* 301.

Reports and comments on diphenhydramine overdosage and its treatment.— H. E. Hestand and D. W. Teske, *J. Pediat.*, 1977, *90,* 1017; M. Borkenstein and M. Haidvogl (letter), *ibid.*, 1978, *92,* 167; H. E. Hestand and D. W. Teske (letter), *ibid.*

Pregnancy and the neonate. There was a significant incidence of cleft palate and clefts with other defects in children whose mothers had taken diphenhydramine during pregnancy.— I. Saxén (letter), *Lancet,* 1974, *1,* 407.

For further studies on the effects of diphenhydramine and other antihistamines during pregnancy, see p.1294.

Neonatal dependence. A pregnant woman who was receiving diphenhydramine hydrochloride 150 mg daily for a pruritic rash gave birth to an infant who developed diarrhoea and generalised tremulousness 5 days later. The infant had a serum-diphenhydramine concentration of 7 µg per ml and the delay in appearance of withdrawal symptoms was considered to be due to absence of full activity of glucuronyl conjugating enzymes in the first few days of life. A response was obtained to phenobarbitone and the tremulousness did not recur on withdrawal of the phenobarbitone.— D. E. Parkin (letter), *J. Pediat.*, 1974, *85,* 580.

Precautions. As for the antihistamines in general, p.1294.

The effect of diphenhydramine on performance.— M. Burns and H. Moskowitz, *Eur. J. clin. Pharmac.*, 1980, *17,* 259.

Interactions. Diphenhydramine 50 mg intramuscularly, 10 minutes before ingestion of sodium aminosalicylate 2 g, significantly reduced the concentration of sodium aminosalicylate found in the blood 10 minutes after ingestion. Diphenhydramine also briefly affected the absorption of other drugs, namely barbitone and sulphacetamide. Promethazine has been shown to have similar effects to diphenhydramine.— J. -G. Lavigne and C. Marchand, *Clin. Pharmac. Ther.*, 1973, *14,* 404.

Myasthenia. Diphenhydramine interfered with neuromuscular transmission under experimental conditions and although it had not been implicated clinically it should be used with caution in patients with myasthenia.— Z. Argov and F. L. Mastaglia, *New Engl. J. Med.*, 1979, *301,* 409.

Absorption and Fate. As for the antihistamines in general, p.1295.

Maximum plasma-diphenhydramine concentrations ranging from 81 to 159 ng per ml were obtained 2 to 4 hours after administration of diphenhydramine hydrochloride 100 mg by mouth to 4 healthy subjects. The plasma half-life calculated over the period 4 to 24 hours after administration ranged from about 5 to 8 hours. The plasma half-life calculated for total amines gave values of about 8 to 10 hours in 3 subjects indicating that the metabolites were eliminated less rapidly than unchanged diphenhydramine. Urinary excretion of diphenhydramine metabolites was about 64% of the dose after 96 hours. Following administration of diphenhydramine hydrochloride 50 mg four times daily for 13 doses to 4 subjects plasma-diphenhydramine concentrations reached a plateau after 2 or 3 days, total amines being about twice the concentration of unchanged diphenhydramine. After the last dose the plasma half-life was about 6 hours for diphenhydramine and about 8 for total amines; the mean recovery of urinary metabolites was about 50% of the total dose, with traces detected 2 to 3 days after the last dose.— A. J. Glazko *et al.*, *Clin. Pharmac. Ther.*, 1974, *16,* 1066.

Studies in 2 healthy subjects indicated that diphenhydramine exhibits a large first-pass effect, with about 50% metabolism occurring before the drug reaches the general circulation following oral administration.— K. S. Albert *et al.*, *J. Pharmacokinet. Biopharm.*, 1975, *3,* 159.

Diphenhydramine was reported to be 98% bound to plasma proteins. The normal half-life was 4 to 7 hours.— W. M. Bennett *et al.*, *Ann. intern. Med.*, 1980, *93,* 286.

Further references: J. G. Wagner *et al.*, *J. Pharmacokinet. Biopharm.*, 1977, *5,* 161.

Uses. Diphenhydramine hydrochloride is an ethanolamine derivative with the properties and uses of the antihistamines (see p.1295). It is less potent than promethazine hydrochloride and has a shorter duration of action, but like promethazine it has pronounced sedative properties. It also has anti-emetic, anticholinergic, and local anaesthetic properties.

Diphenhydramine hydrochloride is given in usual doses of 25 to 50 mg three or four times daily. The dose for children aged 1 to 5 years is 12.5 to 25 mg three or four times daily, and for those aged 6 to 12 years 25 to 50 mg thrice daily. It has also been given in severe allergies by deep intramuscular or slow intravenous injection in usual doses of 10 to 50 mg.

Diphenhydramine hydrochloride is also used in cough mixtures. It has been used for the control of parkinsonian symptoms and for the prevention and treatment of nausea and vomiting.

It has been given with methaqualone as a hypnotic.

A 2% water-miscible cream has been used for allergic dermatoses but may cause skin sensitisation. Eye-drops have been used for ocular allergies.

Administration. In a placebo-controlled crossover study in 6 healthy subjects given diphenhydramine 50 mg intravenously and by mouth a positive correlation between plasma-diphenhydramine concentration and sedative and antihistamine effects occurred. There appeared to be a concentration range of 25 to 50 ng per ml within which there was significant antihistaminic effect without significant sedation.— S. G. Carruthers *et al.*, *Clin. Pharmac. Ther.*, 1978, *23,* 375.

Administration in renal failure. The interval between doses of diphenhydramine should be extended from 6 hours to 6 to 9 hours in patients with a glomerular filtration-rate (GFR) of 10 to 50 ml per minute, and to 9 to 12 hours in those with a GFR of less than 10 ml per minute.— W. M. Bennett *et al.*, *Ann. intern. Med.*, 1980, *93,* 286.

Allergy. Anaphylactic shock and anaphylactoid reaction: an analysis of 62 patients, 39 of whom were treated with diphenhydramine alone or in association with other therapy.— M. D. MacFarlane and M. M. McCarron, *Drug Intell. & clin. Pharm.*, 1973, *7,* 394.

Anaesthesia. Details of a technique for sedating patients with diphenhydramine, other sedatives, and analgesics prior to cardiac catheterisation.— S. A. Akdikmen *et al.*, *Anesth. Analg. curr. Res.*, 1966, *45,* 293.

Behaviour disorders. Diphenhydramine might be of some benefit in the treatment of hyperkinetic children.— *Br. med. J.*, 1973, *1,* 305.

Carcinoid syndrome. For reports of the use of diphenhydramine in carcinoid syndrome, see Cimetidine, p.1304.

Extrapyramidal symptoms. Diphenhydramine produced a dramatic response in 2 patients with oculogyric crises, in 1 patient following chlorpromazine and in the other possibly associated with amphetamine or ethylene chlorhydrin (C_2H_5ClO = 80.5).— D. Hilson and J. M. Abraham (letter), *Br. med. J.*, 1968, *1,* 381.

Differential diagnosis of tardive dyskinesia. A suggestion that diphenhydramine may be useful in the differential diagnosis of neuroleptic-induced oral-facial dyskinesia. Difficulty may arise in deciding whether certain oral-facial dyskinesias are early or late reactions and a simple method to differentiate them is to administer diphenhydramine. If the movement disorder disappears the dyskinesia is probably early-onset whereas if diphenhydramine does not relieve the symptoms the dyskinesia is more likely to be tardive.— B. D. Beitman, *Am. J. Psychiat.*, 1977, *134,* 695.

Hypnotic effect. In a drug surveillance programme, 512 patients received diphenhydramine hydrochloride as a hypnotic, usually in doses of 50 to 100 mg. In 355 patients evaluated, the response was considered good in 73%. Side-effects, which were reversible, occurred in 1.8% of patients and included vomiting in 1 patient and CNS depression in 8.— S. Shapiro *et al.*, *J. Am. med. Ass.*, 1969, *209,* 2016.

Further references: R. M. Russo *et al.*, *J. clin. Pharmac.*, 1976, *16,* 284.

Laryngitis. Mention of the use of a solution containing diphenhydramine hydrochloride 0.5%, applied to the pharynx and larynx, for non-infective laryngitis.— N. A. Punt, *Proc. R. Soc. Med.*, 1968, *61,* 1152.

Preparations

Capsules

Diphenhydramine Capsules *(B.P.).* Capsules containing diphenhydramine hydrochloride. Store at a temperature not exceeding 30°.

Diphenhydramine Hydrochloride Capsules *(U.S.P.).* Capsules containing diphenhydramine hydrochloride. Store in airtight containers.

Elixirs

Diphenhydramine and Ephedrine Elixir *(A.P.F.)*. Diphenhydramine hydrochloride 10 mg, ephedrine hydrochloride 10 mg, citric acid monohydrate 25 mg, red syrup (*A.P.F.*) 2 ml, concentrated chloroform water 0.1 ml, water to 5 ml. *Dose*. 5 to 10 ml.

Diphenhydramine Elixir *(A.P.F.)*. Diphenhydramine hydrochloride 10 mg, citric acid monohydrate 25 mg, red syrup (*A.P.F.*) 2 ml, concentrated chloroform water 0.1 ml, water to 5 ml. *Dose*. 5 to 10 ml.

Diphenhydramine Elixir *(B.P.)*. A solution of diphenhydramine hydrochloride in a suitable flavoured vehicle which may be coloured. Protect from light. When a dose less than or not a multiple of 5 ml is prescribed, the elixir should be diluted to 5 ml, or a multiple, with syrup. Such dilutions must be freshly prepared and not used more than 2 weeks after issue.

Diphenhydramine Hydrochloride Elixir *(U.S.P.)*. An elixir containing diphenhydramine hydrochloride and alcohol 12 to 15%. Store in airtight containers. Protect from light.

Injections

Diphenhydramine Hydrochloride Injection *(U.S.P.)*. A sterile solution of diphenhydramine hydrochloride in Water for Injections. pH 4 to 6.5. Protect from light.

Diphenhydramine Injection *(B.P. 1973)*. A sterile solution of diphenhydramine hydrochloride in Water for Injections. pH 5 to 6. Protect from light.

Tablets

Tablettae Coffinautini *(Nord. P.)*. Diphenhydramine and Caffeine Tablets. Each tablet contains diphenhydramine hydrochloride 50 mg and caffeine 50 mg.

Proprietary Preparations

Benadryl *(Parke, Davis, UK)*. Diphenhydramine hydrochloride, available as capsules of 25 mg. (Also available as Benadryl in *Arg., Austral., Belg., Canad., Denm., Ital., Neth., S.Afr., Spain, Swed., Switz., USA*).

Benafed *(Parke, Davis, UK)*. Syrup containing in each 5 ml diphenhydramine hydrochloride 12.5 mg, dextromethorphan hydrobromide 15 mg, pseudoephedrine hydrochloride 30 mg, ammonium chloride 125 mg, sodium citrate 57 mg, and menthol 1 mg (suggested diluent, syrup). For cough. *Dose*. 5 ml every 4 to 6 hours; children, 2 to 4 years, 1.25 ml every 6 hours; 4 to 12 years, 2.5 to 5 ml.

Benylin Day and Night Cold Treatment *(Parke, Davis, UK)*. Day-time tablets each containing paracetamol 500 mg and phenylpropanolamine hydrochloride 25 mg, and Night-time tablets each containing diphenhydramine hydrochloride 25 mg and paracetamol 500 mg. For relief of the symptoms of colds and influenza. *Dose*. 1 Day-time tablet thrice daily and 1 Night-time tablet at night.

Benylin Decongestant *(Parke, Davis, UK)*. Syrup containing in each 5 ml diphenhydramine hydrochloride 14 mg, pseudoephedrine hydrochloride 10 mg, sodium citrate 57 mg, and menthol 1.1 mg. For coughs and catarrh. *Dose*. 10 ml four times daily; children, 1 to 5 years, 2.5 ml; 6 to 12 years, 5 ml.

Benylin Expectorant *(Parke, Davis, UK)*. A flavoured syrup containing in each 5 ml diphenhydramine hydrochloride 14 mg, ammonium chloride 135 mg, sodium citrate 57 mg, and menthol 1.1 mg (suggested diluent, syrup). For cough and upper respiratory congestion. *Dose*. 5 to 10 ml every 2 or 3 hours; children, 1 to 5 years, 2.5 ml every 3 or 4 hours; 6 to 12 years, 5 ml.

Benylin Fortified Linctus *(Parke, Davis, UK)*. Contains in each 5 ml diphenhydramine hydrochloride 14 mg, dextromethorphan hydrobromide 6.5 mg, sodium citrate 57 mg, and menthol 1.1 mg (suggested diluent, syrup). For dry irritating cough. *Dose*. 10 ml every 4 hours; children, 1 to 5 years, 2.5 ml; 6 to 12 years, 5 ml.

Benylin Paediatric *(Parke, Davis, UK)*. Contains in each 5 ml diphenhydramine hydrochloride 7 mg, menthol 550 µg, and sodium citrate 28.5 mg. For cough and upper respiratory congestion. *Dose*. Children, 1 to 5 years, 5 ml every 3 hours; 6 years and over, 10 ml.

Benylin with Codeine *(Parke, Davis, UK)*. Contains in each 5 ml diphenhydramine hydrochloride 14 mg, codeine phosphate 5.7 mg, sodium citrate 57 mg, and menthol 1.1 mg (suggested diluent, syrup). For dry irritating cough. *Dose*. 10 ml every 3 or 4 hours; children, 1 to 5 years, 2.5 ml, 6 to 12 years, 5 ml.

Caladryl *(Parke, Davis, UK)*. **Cream** containing diphenhydramine hydrochloride 1%, calamine (*U.S.P.*) 8%, camphor 0.1%, and propylene glycol, in a water-miscible basis and **Lotion** containing diphenhydramine hydrochloride 1%, calamine (*U.S.P.*) 8%, camphor 0.1% and glycerol 2.5%. For skin irritation.

Globolotion *(R.P. Drugs, UK)*. Lotion containing diphenhydramine hydrochloride 1% and calamine 8%. For skin irritations.

Guanor Expectorant *(R.P. Drugs, UK)*. Contains in each 5 ml diphenhydramine hydrochloride 14 mg, ammonium chloride 135 mg, sodium citrate 57 mg, and menthol 1.1 mg. *Dose*. 5 to 10 ml every 2 or 3 hours.

Guanor Paediatric Expectorant *(R.P. Drugs, UK)*. Contains in each 5 ml diphenhydramine hydrochloride 7 mg, sodium citrate 28.5 mg, and menthol 550 µg. *Dose*. Children, 1 to 5 years, 5 ml every 3 or 4 hours; 6 to 12 years, 10 ml.

Histalix Expectorant *(Wallace Mfg Chem., UK: Farillon, UK)*. Syrup containing in each 5 ml diphenhydramine hydrochloride 14 mg, ammonium chloride 135 mg, sodium citrate 57 mg, and menthol 1.1 mg. *Dose*. 5 to 10 ml every 3 hours; children, 2.5 to 5 ml.

Histergan *(Norma, UK: Farillon, UK)*. Diphenhydramine hydrochloride, available as **Cream** containing 2%; as **Syrup** containing 10 mg in each 5 ml; and as **Tablets** of 25 mg.

Lotussin *(Searle, UK)*. Linctus containing in each 5 ml diphenhydramine hydrochloride 5 mg, dextromethorphan hydrobromide 6.25 mg, ephedrine hydrochloride 7.5 mg, and guaiphenesin 50 mg (suggested diluent, syrup). For cough and nasal congestion. *Dose*. 10 ml thrice daily; children, 1 to 5 years, 2.5 to 5 ml; 6 to 12 years, 5 to 10 ml.

Ticipect *(Ticen, Eire)*. A syrup containing in each 5 ml diphenhydramine hydrochloride 13.9 mg, ammonium chloride 135 mg, sodium citrate 56.4 mg, menthol 1 mg, and chloroform 22.5 mg. For cough and respiratory congestion. *Dose*. 5 to 10 ml every 2 or 3 hours.

Other Proprietary Names

Austral.— Alergicap, Bidramine; *Canad.*— Insomnal, Somnium; *Denm.*— Amidryl; *Ger.*— Dolestan, Halbmond, Pheramin; *Ital.*— Allergan (see also under Mepyramine Maleate), Allergina, Dermistina; *S.Afr.*— Dihydral (see also under Dihydrotachysterol); *Spain*— Teldrin (methyliodide); *Swed.*— Desentol; *Switz.*—Benocten, Cathejell, Dobacen, Felben, Neo-Synodorm, Somenox; *USA*— Lensen, Valdrene, Wehydryl.

A preparation containing diphenhydramine hydrochloride was also formerly marketed in Great Britain under the proprietary name Benylets (*Parke, Davis*).

6132-v

Diphenylpyraline Hydrochloride *(B.P., U.S.P.)*. 4-Benzhydryloxy-1-methylpiperidine hydrochloride.

$C_{19}H_{23}NO,HCl=317.9$.

CAS — 147-20-6 (diphenylpyraline); 132-18-3 (hydrochloride).

Pharmacopoeias. In *Br.* and *U.S.*

A white or almost white, odourless or almost odourless, crystalline powder. M.p. 204° to 209°. **Soluble** 1 in 1 of water, 1 in 3 of alcohol, and 1 in 2 of chloroform; practically insoluble in ether. **Store** in airtight containers. Protect from light.

Adverse Effects, Treatment, and Precautions. As for the antihistamines in general, p.1294.

Uses. Diphenylpyraline hydrochloride has the properties and uses of the antihistamines (see p.1295). It has a shorter duration of action than promethazine and it generally causes less sedation.

Diphenylpyraline hydrochloride has been given in usual doses of 3 to 4.5 mg four times daily but sustained-release preparations are more commonly used, given in doses of 5 to 10 mg twice daily. Children aged 3 to 6 years have been given 0.75 to 1.5 mg four times daily and those aged 7 years and over have been given 1.5 to 3 mg four times daily. A dose of 2.5 mg twice daily, as a sustained-release preparation, may be given to children aged 7 years and over.

Preparations

Diphenylpyraline Hydrochloride Tablets *(U.S.P.)*. Tablets containing diphenylpyraline hydrochloride. Store in airtight containers. Protect from light.

Proprietary Preparations

Histryl *(Smith Kline & French, UK)*. Diphenylpyraline hydrochloride, available as **Spansule** sustained-release capsules of 5 mg and as **Paediatric Spansule** capsules of 2.5 mg. *Dose*. 1 capsule twice daily. (Also available as Histryl in *Austral., Belg., S.Afr.*).

Lergoban *(Riker, UK)*. Tablets each containing diphenylpyraline hydrochloride 5 mg in a porous plastic basis. *Dose*. 1 or 2 tablets twice daily. (Also available as Lergoban in *Belg., Neth.*).

Other Proprietary Names

Arg.— Dayfen; *Austral.*— Allerzine, Anti-Hist, Histalert; *Belg.*— Anti-H; *Ger.*— Kolton (see also under Piprinhydrinate), Lyssipoll; *S.Afr.*— Histalert; *USA*— Diafen, Hispril.

6133-g

Doxylamine Succinate *(U.S.P.)*. Doxylaminium Succinate; Histadoxylamine Succinate.

NN-Dimethyl-2-[α-methyl-α-(2-pyridyl)benzyloxy]ethylamine hydrogen succinate.

$C_{17}H_{22}N_2O,C_4H_6O_4=388.5$.

CAS — 469-21-6 (doxylamine); 562-10-7 (succinate).

Pharmacopoeias. In *Arg.* and *U.S.*

A white or creamy-white powder with a characteristic odour. M.p. 103° to 108° with a range of not more than 3°. **Soluble** 1 in 1 of water, 1 in 2 of alcohol and of chloroform, and 1 in 370 of ether. A solution in water is acid to litmus. **Protect** from light.

Adverse Effects, Treatment, and Precautions. As for the antihistamines in general, p.1294.

Extrapyramidal symptoms. Facial dyskinesia in a 19-year-old woman might have been associated with ingestion of doxylamine.— G. R. Favis (letter), *New Engl. J. Med.*, 1976, *294*, 730. Comment.— R. Sovner (letter), *ibid.*, *296* 633.

Overdosage. For reports of overdosage with a preparation of doxylamine succinate with dicyclomine hydrochloride, see Dicyclomine Hydrochloride, p.298.

Pregnancy and the neonate. In a study in 836 infants with congenital malformations there was no significant difference in the maternal usage of doxylamine during the first trimester of pregnancy compared with the use in 836 controls.— G. Greenberg *et al.*, *Br. med. J.*, 1977, *2*, 853.

The percentage of malformed children among 1169 children born to mothers who had taken doxylamine succinate during the first 4 months of pregnancy was comparable to that in 49 113 children not so exposed. When analysed for specific malformations there was some evidence of a modest association with gastro-intestinal malformation, hypospadias, and clubfoot, but the results were not statistically significant. IQ scores at 4 years were not affected. Doxylamine succinate did not appear to be harmful to the foetus.— S. Shapiro *et al.*, *Am. J. Obstet. Gynec.*, 1977, *128*, 480.

For a review of the controversy surrounding the use of combination preparations containing dicyclomine, doxylamine, and pyridoxine in pregnancy, see Dicyclomine Hydrochloride, p.298.

Uses. Doxylamine succinate is an ethanolamine derivative with the properties and uses of the antihistamines (see p.1295). It is somewhat less potent than promethazine but has a similar duration of action. It also has pronounced sedative effects.

Doxylamine succinate has been given in usual doses of 25 mg up to 4 times daily. It has also been given with dicyclomine and pyridoxine for the nausea and vomiting of early pregnancy.

Preparations

Doxylamine Succinate Syrup *(U.S.P.)*. A syrup containing doxylamine succinate. Store in airtight containers. Protect from light.

Doxylamine Succinate Tablets *(U.S.P.)*. Tablets containing doxylamine succinate. Protect from light.

Proprietary Names

Decapryn *(Merrell-National, USA)*; Hoggar N *(Stada, Ger.)*; Mereprime *(Inibsa, Spain)*; Mereprine *(Merrell Toraude, Belg.; Merrell Toraude, Fr.; Merrell, Ger.; Inibsa, Spain; Merrell, Switz.)*; Unisom *(Leeming, USA)*.

NOTE. It is anticipated that Debendox (see p.299), will be reformulated so as to contain only doxylamine succinate 10 mg and pyridoxine hydrochloride 10 mg in each tablet.

6134-q

Embramine Hydrochloride. Mebrophenhydramine Hydrochloride. 2-(4-Bromo-α-methylbenzhydryloxy)-*NN*-dimethylethylamine hydrochloride.
$C_{18}H_{22}BrNO,HCl=384.7$.

CAS — 3565-72-8 (embramine); 13977-28-1 (hydrochloride).

Pharmacopoeias. In *Cz.*

Embramine hydrochloride is an ethanolamine derivative with the properties and uses of the antihistamines (see p.1294). It has been given in doses of up to 60 mg twice daily.

Embramine hydrochloride was given to 50 patients with various allergic conditions. The average daily dose was two 25-mg tablets and the results were excellent or good in 39 patients and fair or poor in 11 patients. The drug produced an effect within 1.5 to 2 hours and this lasted for about 12 hours. Drowsiness which was usually slight was complained of in 13 patients.— N. Mendick, *Practitioner*, 1963, *191*, 211.

Further references: A. E. R. Campbell, *Br. J. Dis. Chest*, 1963, *57*, 153; Z. Mechl *et al.*, *Vnitr. Lék.*, 1968, *14*, 277.

Proprietary Names
Bromadryl *(Cz.).*

Embramine hydrochloride was formerly marketed in Great Britain under the proprietary name Mebryl *(Smith Kline & French).*

6135-p

Halopyramine Hydrochloride. Chloropyramine Hydrochloride. *N*-(4-Chlorobenzyl)-*N'N'*-dimethyl-*N*-(2-pyridyl)ethylenediamine hydrochloride.
$C_{16}H_{20}ClN_3,HCl=326.3$.

CAS — 59-32-5 (halopyramine); 6170-42-9 (hydrochloride).

Pharmacopoeias. In *Hung.* and *Roum.*

An odourless white powder; freely **soluble** in water, alcohol, and chloroform; practically insoluble in ether. **Store** in airtight containers. Protect from light.

Halopyramine hydrochloride is an ethylenediamine derivative with the properties and uses of the antihistamines (see p.1294). It has been given in divided doses of up to 150 mg daily. It has also been given by injection.

Proprietary Names
Synopen *(Padro, Spain; Geigy, Switz.)*; Synpen *(Geigy, Ger.).*

6136-s

Histapyrrodine Hydrochloride. *N*-Benzyl-*N*-phenyl-2-(pyrrolidin-1-yl)ethylamine hydrochloride.
$C_{19}H_{24}N_2,HCl=316.9$.

CAS — 493-80-1 (histapyrrodine); 6113-17-3 (hydrochloride).

Histapyrrodine hydrochloride is an ethylenediamine derivative with the properties and uses of the antihistamines (see p.1294). It has been given in a dosage of 50 to 150 mg daily in divided doses.

Proprietary Names
Domistan *(Servier, Fr.).*

6137-w

Homochlorcyclizine. 1-(4-Chlorobenzhydryl)perhydro-4-methyl-1,4-diazepine.
$C_{19}H_{23}ClN_2=314.9$.

CAS — 848-53-3.

Homochlorcyclizine has the properties and uses of the antihistamines (see p.1294). It has been given in doses of 10 to 20 mg thrice daily. The hydrochloride has also been used in similar doses.

Proprietary Names
Attackmin, Clomon-S, Curosajin, Homadamon, Homochlo, Homoclicin, Homoclizine, Homoclomin, Homocolzine, Homoradin, Homorestar, Noikohis, Puradenin, Rimskin, Sacronal, Sankumin, Wicron *(all Jap.).*

6138-e

Hydroxyzine Embonate.

Hydroxyzine Pamoate *(U.S.P.)*. 2-{2-[4-(4-Chlorobenzhydryl)piperazin-1-yl]ethoxy}ethanol 4,4'-methylenebis(3-hydroxy-2-naphthoate).
$C_{21}H_{27}ClN_2O_2,C_{23}H_{16}O_6=763.3$.

CAS — 68-88-2 (hydroxyzine); 10246-75-0 (embonate).

Pharmacopoeias. In *U.S.*

A pale yellow almost odourless powder. Hydroxyzine embonate 170 mg is approximately equivalent to 100 mg of hydroxyzine hydrochloride. Practically **insoluble** in water, chloroform, ether, and methyl alcohol; soluble 1 in 700 of alcohol and 1 in 10 of dimethylformamide; freely soluble in 10M sodium hydroxide solution. **Store** in airtight containers.

6139-l

Hydroxyzine Hydrochloride *(U.S.P.)*.

$C_{21}H_{27}ClN_2O_2,2HCl=447.8$.

CAS — 2192-20-3.

Pharmacopoeias. In *Belg., Jap., Jug.*, and *U.S.*

A white odourless crystalline powder with a bitter taste. M.p. about 200° with decomposition. **Soluble** 1 in 1 of water, 1 in 4.5 of alcohol, and 1 in 13 of chloroform; slightly soluble in acetone; practically insoluble in ether. **Store** in airtight containers.

Incompatibility. There was loss of clarity when intravenous solutions of hydroxyzine hydrochloride were mixed with those of aminophylline, amylobarbitone sodium, benzylpenicillin, chloramphenicol sodium succinate, dimenhydrinate, heparin sodium, pentobarbitone sodium, phenobarbitone sodium, phenytoin sodium, or sulphafurazole diethanolamine.— J. A. Patel and G. L. Phillips, *Am. J. Hosp. Pharm.*, 1966, *23*, 409.

Stability. Hydroxyzine hydrochloride in aqueous solution was unstable when exposed to UV irradiation.— S. F. Pong and C. L. Huang, *J. pharm. Sci.*, 1979, *68*, 666.

Adverse Effects and Treatment. As for the antihistamines in general, p.1294.

Intramuscular injection of hydroxyzine has been reported to cause marked local discomfort.

For a discussion on early suggestions that foetal abnormalities might result from the use of hydroxyzine and similar compounds, see under Meclozine Hydrochloride, p.1314.

Necrosis caused by the accidental intra-arterial injection of hydroxyzine.— W. H. Hardesty (letter), *J. Am. med. Ass.*, 1970, *213*, 872.

Allergy. Hypersensitivity to hydroxyzine in a boy with a history of allergic reactions.— N. Massoud, *J. Pediat.*, 1978, *93*, 308.

Effects on the blood. Haemolysis associated with intravenous injection of hydroxyzine.— G. S. Linder and J. B. Dillon, *Anesth. Analg. curr. Res.*, 1967, *46*, 90.

Effects on the heart. ECG abnormalities, particularly alterations in T-waves, were associated with hydroxyzine hydrochloride therapy in elderly psychotic patients.— L. E. Hollister, *Psychopharmac. Comm.*, 1975, *1*, 61.

Pregnancy and the neonate. In 131 parturients who were given 1.2 to 1.6 mg of hydroxyzine hydrochloride per kg body-weight alone or in conjunction with 600 to 800 μg of pethidine hydrochloride per kg, Apgar scores, blood pressure, heart-rate, and respiration-rate were not adversely affected by the 2 drugs used concurrently and anxiety was adequately alleviated.— E. K. Zsigmond and R. L. Patterson, *Anesth. Analg. curr. Res.*, 1967, *46*, 275, per *J. Am. med. Ass.*, 1967, *201* (July 24), A149.

Symptoms of withdrawal in the infant of a woman who had taken hydroxyzine and phenobarbitone were attributed to hydroxyzine.— B. M. Prenner, *Am. J. Dis. Child.*, 1977, *131*, 529.

Precautions. As for the antihistamines in general, p.1294.

It was recommended that intravenous injections of hydroxyzine be given slowly to minimise the amount of haemolysis which had been found to occur *in vitro* when the drug was mixed with blood.— R. J. Trudnowski (letter), *Br. J. Anaesth.*, 1973, *45*, 303.

Interference with diagnostic tests. The administration of hydroxyzine could interfere with measurements of urinary 17-hydroxycorticosteroids.— J. M. Rosenberg and I. S. Kampa, *Drug Intell. & clin. Pharm.*, 1973, *7*, 33.

For the effect of hydroxyzine on some estimations of blood-theophylline concentrations, see Aminophylline, p.343.

Absorption and Fate. As for the antihistamines in general, p.1295.

In 4 healthy subjects given a single dose of hydroxyzine hydrochloride 100 mg mean peak plasma-hydroxyzine concentration was 82 ng per ml at a mean of 3 hours after administration. The mean half-lives of absorption and elimination were 1.02 and 2.97 hours respectively.— H. G. Fouda *et al.*, *J. pharm. Sci.*, 1979, *68*, 1456.

Uses. Hydroxyzine is a piperazine derivative with the properties and uses of the antihistamines (see p.1295). It has a shorter duration of action and causes less sedation than promethazine, but like promethazine it has pronounced sedative properties. It also has anti-emetic and anticholinergic properties. It is used as an anti-emetic and is reported to have a duration of action of 4 to 6 hours. It is also used for pre- and postoperative sedation and as an adjunct in the treatment of urticaria and dermatoses. It has also been used in the treatment of anxiety, tension, and agitation.

Hydroxyzine is given by mouth as the hydrochloride or embonate in usual doses equivalent to 25 mg of the hydrochloride 3 or 4 times daily but up to 400 mg has been given daily in divided doses. Children may be given 2 mg per kg body-weight daily in 4 divided doses. Hydroxyzine is also given by intramuscular injection as the hydrochloride in doses of 25 to 100 mg every 4 to 6 hours. Children have been given 1 mg per kg body-weight intramuscularly for pre- and postoperative sedation.

Alcohol and drug withdrawal. A study of hydroxyzine in alcohol withdrawal.— S. L. Dilts *et al.*, *Am. J. Psychiat.*, 1977, *134*, 92.

Allergy. In a double-blind study involving 43 patients with allergic rhinitis hydroxyzine in a dose gradually increased to 50 mg thrice daily provided significantly better relief than a placebo during the ragweed season.— L. Schaaf *et al.*, *J. Allergy & clin. Immunol.*, 1979, *63*, 129.

Anaesthesia. The incidence of postoperative nausea in 60 outpatients undergoing general anaesthesia for therapeutic abortion was 20% in a control group, 15% in a diazepam group, and 5% in a hydroxyzine group; treatment being given pre-operatively. The incidence of pre-operative nausea was 45 to 50% in all groups.— R. K. Wadhwa (letter), *J. Am. med. Ass.*, 1974, *227*, 557.

In a double-blind study in 140 patients undergoing surgery, diazepam 7.5 or 15 mg was generally more effective as premedication than hydroxyzine 75 or 150 mg in terms of relief of anxiety, sedation, lack of recall, and patient acceptance. The drugs were given intravenously and assessment was made by the patient and by a nurse observer.— R. H. Wender *et al.*, *Br. J. Anaesth.*, 1977, *49*, 907.

Further references: E. Mojdehi *et al.*, *Anesth. Analg. curr. Res.*, 1968, *47*, 685 (premedication in children); Y. S. Falick and B. G. Smiler, *Anesthesiology*, 1975, *43*, 472 (premedication); J. C. Gasser and J. W. Bellville, *Anesthesiology*, 1975, *43*, 599 (respiration); J. W. Bellville *et al.*, *J. clin. Pharmac.*, 1979, *19*, 290 (postoperative pain).

Anxiety and depression. A review of the treatment of anxiety with hydroxyzine.— S. F. Barranco and W. Bridger, *Curr. ther. Res.*, 1977, *22*, 217.

References to studies of hydroxyzine in anxiety or depression: I. H. Breslow, *Curr. ther. Res.*, 1968, *10*, 421; M. B. Clyne *et al.*, *Practitioner*, 1968, *201*, 496; D.

Silver *et al.*, *Curr. ther. Res.*, 1969, *11*, 663; M. Colon and J. Polderman, *Eur. J. clin. Pharmac.*, 1978, *13*, 409.

Hypnotic effect. Hydroxyzine in doses of 50 and 150 mg was not an effective hypnotic agent and had an unacceptable 'hangover' effect.— C. R. Brown *et al.*, *J. clin. Pharmac.*, 1974, *14*, 210.

Skin disorders. Of 14 patients with cholinergic urticaria who received a week's treatment with hydroxyzine, 25 mg thrice daily, brompheniramine, 4 mg thrice daily, or a placebo, 8 expressed a preference for the hydroxyzine.— M. Moore-Robinson and R. P. Warin, *Br. J. Derm.*, 1968, *80*, 794.

In a double-blind study in 33 patients with dermographism, pressure-induced wheals were reduced to a greater extent by hydroxyzine embonate 25 mg thrice daily than by chlorpheniramine maleate 4 mg thrice daily; 29 patients taking hydroxyzine had relief from itching and 16 of those taking chlorpheniramine had some relief. Side-effects included drowsiness (5 patients) and lack of concentration (1) in those taking hydroxyzine, and excessive tiredness in 2 of those taking chlorpheniramine.— C. N. A. Matthews *et al.*, *Br. J. Derm.*, 1973, *88*, 279.

Preparations of Hydroxyzine Salts

Hydroxyzine Hydrochloride Injection *(U.S.P.)*. A sterile solution in Water for Injections. pH 3.5 to 6. Protect from light.

Hydroxyzine Hydrochloride Syrup *(U.S.P.)*. A syrup containing hydroxyzine hydrochloride. Store in airtight containers. Protect from light.

Hydroxyzine Hydrochloride Tablets *(U.S.P.)*. Tablets containing hydroxyzine hydrochloride. Store in airtight containers.

Hydroxyzine Pamoate Capsules *(U.S.P.)*. Capsules containing hydroxyzine embonate. Potency is expressed in terms of the equivalent amount of hydroxyzine hydrochloride.

Hydroxyzine Pamoate Oral Suspension *(U.S.P.)*. A suspension of hydroxyzine embonate. pH 4.5 to 7. Potency is expressed in terms of the equivalent amount of hydroxyzine hydrochloride. Store in airtight containers. Protect from light.

Proprietary Preparations

Atarax *(Pfizer, UK)*. Hydroxyzine hydrochloride, available as **Syrup** containing 10 mg in each 5 ml (suggested diluent, syrup) and as **Tablets** of 10 and 25 mg. (Also available as Atarax in *Arg., Austral., Belg., Canad., Denm., Fr., Ger., Ital., Neth., Norw., Swed., Switz., USA*).

Other Proprietary Names of Hydroxyzine Salts

Belg.— Paxistil; *Ger.*— Masmoran; *Ital.*— Atazina, Neocalma, Neurozina; *S.Afr.*— Aterax; *Swed.*— Vistaril; *USA*— Sedaril, Vistaril.

Hydroxyzine embonate was formerly marketed in Great Britain under the proprietary name Equipose (*Pfizer*).

6140-v

Isothipendyl Hydrochloride *(B.P.C. 1973)*.

NN-Dimethyl-1-(pyrido[3,2-*b*][1,4]benzothiazin-10-ylmethyl)ethylamine hydrochloride.

$C_{16}H_{19}N_3S,HCl=321.9$.

CAS — 482-15-5 (isothipendyl); 1225-60-1 (hydrochloride).

A fine white odourless or almost odourless crystalline powder. M.p. about 212° with decomposition. **Soluble** 1 in 5 of water, 1 in 60 of alcohol, and 1 in 10 of chloroform; practically insoluble in ether. Solutions are **sterilised** by filtration. Aqueous solutions are sensitive to heat and light but are most stable at pH 4.5 to 5. **Protect** from light.

Adverse Effects, Treatment, and Precautions. As for the antihistamines in general, p.1294.

As for all phenothiazine derivatives it should be used cautiously in patients with hepatic diseases.

Uses. Isothipendyl hydrochloride is an azaphenothiazine derivative with the properties and uses of the antihistamines (see p.1295). It is more potent than promethazine but has a shorter duration of action and causes less sedation.

Isothipendyl hydrochloride has been given usually in doses of 4 to 8 mg three or four times daily. It has also been given in severe allergies by intramuscular or slow intravenous injection in doses of 10 mg daily.

Preparations

Isothipendyl Tablets *(B.P.C. 1973)*. Isothipendyl Hydrochloride Tablets. Tablets containing isothipendyl hydrochloride. They may be sugar-coated.

Proprietary Names

Andantol *(Homburg, Belg.; Gerda, Fr.; Homburg, Ger.; Armour, Ital.; Homburg, S.Afr.; Treupha, Switz.)*; Andanton *(Lacer, Spain)*; Nilergex *(ICI, Austral.)*.

Isothipendyl hydrochloride was formerly marketed in Great Britain under the proprietary name Nilergex (*ICI Pharmaceuticals*).

6141-g

Mebhydrolin Napadisylate *(B.P.C. 1968)*.

Diazolinum; Mebhydrolin Naphthalenedisulphonate. 5-Benzyl-1,2,3,4-tetrahydro-2-methyl-γ-carboline naphthalene-1,5-disulphonate.

$(C_{19}H_{20}N_2)_2,C_{10}H_8O_6S_2=841.1$.

CAS — 524-81-2 (mebhydrolin); 6153-33-9 (napadisylate).

Pharmacopoeias. In *Rus.*

A white or almost white, odourless, tasteless powder. Mebhydrolin napadisylate 152 mg is approximately equivalent to 100 mg of mebhydrolin. Very slightly **soluble** in water, alcohol, chloroform, and ether.

Adverse Effects, Treatment, and Precautions. As for the antihistamines in general, p.1294.

Agranulocytosis has been reported.

The effect of mebhydrolin on performance.— C. J. Roberts, *Clin. Trials J.*, 1972, *9*, 3.

Uses. Mebhydrolin napadisylate has the properties and uses of the antihistamines (see p.1295). It is less potent than promethazine, has a shorter duration of action, and causes less sedation.

Mebhydrolin napadisylate is given in doses equivalent to 50 to 100 mg of mebhydrolin base thrice daily. Children up to 10 years old may be given 50 to 200 mg of the base daily in divided doses.

Preparations

Mebhydrolin Tablets *(B.P.C. 1968)*. Mebhydrolin Napadisylate Tablets. Sugar-coated tablets, which may be coloured, containing mebhydrolin napadisylate.

Fabahistin *(Bayer, UK)*. **Suspension** containing mebhydrolin napadisylate equivalent to 50 mg of mebhydrolin in each 5 ml (suggested diluent, tragacanth mucilage) and **Tablets** each containing mebhydrolin 50 mg. (Also available as Fabahistin in *Austral., S.Afr.*).

Other Proprietary Names

Incidal *(Ital., Neth.)*; Incidaletten *(Neth.)*; Omeril *(Ger.)*.

6142-q

Meclozine Hydrochloride *(B.P.)*.

Meclozini Hydrochloridum; Meclizine Hydrochloride *(U.S.P.)*; Meclizinium Chloride. 1-(4-Chlorobenzhydryl)-4-(3-methylbenzyl)piperazine dihydrochloride.

$C_{25}H_{27}ClN_2,2HCl=463.9$.

CAS — 569-65-3 (meclozine); 1104-22-9 (hydrochloride, anhydrous); 31884-77-2 (hydrochloride, monohydrate).

Pharmacopoeias. In *Br.* and *Int. Braz., Ind., Jug., Nord.*, and *U.S.* specify the monohydrate. *Nord.* also includes meclozine base.

A white or slightly yellowish, almost odourless, tasteless, crystalline powder. M.p. 217° to 224° with decomposition. **Soluble** 1 in 1000 of water, 1 in 25 of alcohol, and 1 in 5 of chloroform; freely soluble in acid-alcohol-water mixtures and pyridine; slightly soluble in dilute acids; practically insoluble in ether. **Store** in airtight containers.

Adverse Effects, Treatment, and Precautions. As for the antihistamines in general, p.1294.

Meclozine has produced teratogenic effects in *rats* and such effects have also been produced with buclizine, chlorcyclizine, cyclizine, and hydroxyzine. There have been reports suggesting a possibility of human foetal abnormalities resulting from the administration of meclozine but numerous studies since 1962 have failed to establish this relationship in humans.

Extrapyramidal symptoms. Extrapyramidal signs in a 60-year-old woman with alcoholic liver disease given therapeutic doses of meclozine were attributed to abnormally high plasma-meclozine concentrations resulting from impaired hepatic metabolism of the drug.— J. Park *et al.*, *Clin. Toxicol.*, 1977, *11*, 117.

Pregnancy and the neonate. In 1962 meclozine had been implicated in reports of foetal malformations but a number of criteria sharply differentiated it from thalidomide: meclozine intake was associated with a variety of common malformations rather than any typical pattern; the incidence of its intake in mothers of malformed children was not significantly different from that of mothers with normal children; there was a rather high intake of meclozine (5 to 10%) in pregnancies with a normal outcome; there was no relationship between time of intake and malformation. In 5 out of 6 Swedish reports of limb deformities meclozine had not been taken until the end of limb development, and in 3 cases of myelomeningocele meclozine had only been taken at a time when the neural tube was closed. A very low incidence of dysmorphogenicity from meclozine had not been excluded but the risk, if any, was very remote.— W. Lenz, *Sth. med. J.*, 1971, *64, Suppl.* 1, 41.

Evaluation of a number of antinauseant drugs, including meclozine and cyclizine prescribed during the years 1959 to 66, for about 2000 pregnant women in the first 84 days of pregnancy, provided no evidence that either meclozine or cyclizine is associated with teratogenicity.— L. Milkovich and B. J. van den Berg, *Am. J. Obstet. Gynec.*, 1976, *125*, 244. See also W. G. McBride, *Aust. N.Z. J. Obstet. Gynaec.*, 1969, *9*, 103.

In a study in 836 infants with congenital malformations there was no significant difference in the maternal usage of meclozine during the first trimester of pregnancy compared with the use in 836 controls.— G. Greenberg *et al.*, *Br. med. J.*, 1977, *2*, 853.

In a study of 1014 infants born to mothers who had taken meclozine during the first 4 months of pregnancy, malformations were not generally greater than in 49 268 infants not so exposed; for defects of the eye and ear the risk factor for those exposed to meclozine was significant at 2.79, but the suggestion that meclozine exposure might be related to ocular malformations had to be treated with extreme caution.— S. Shapiro *et al.*, *Br. med. J.*, 1978, *1*, 483.

For clinical reports, some purporting to demonstrate and others to refute a causal association between teratogenic effects and the administration of meclozine to pregnant women, see G. I. Watson, *Br. med. J.*, 1962, *2*, 1446; R. W. Smithells, *ibid.*, 1539; M. P. Carter and F. W. Wilson, *ibid.*, 1609; C. G. Fagg, *ibid.*, 1681; T. E. Barwell, *ibid.*; J. Woodall, *ibid.*, 1682; P. L. C. Diggory and J. S. Tomkinson, *Lancet*, 1962, *2*, 1222; G. W. Mellin and M. Katzenstein, *ibid.*, 1963, *1*, 222; A. David and A. H. Goodspeed, *British Drug Houses* (letter), *Br. med. J.*, 1963, *1*, 121; G. I. Watson, *ibid.*, 122; A. F. Burry, *ibid.*, 1476; R. W. Smithells and E. R. Chinn, *ibid.*, 1964, *1*, 217; F. Petterson, *Lancet*, 1964, *1*, 675.

For further studies on the effects of meclozine and other antihistamines during pregnancy, see p.1294.

Uses. Meclozine hydrochloride is a piperazine derivative with the properties of the antihistamines (see p.1295) but is used mainly for its anti-emetic action which is potent and may last for up to 24 hours. Meclozine has anticholinergic activity. Sedative effects are not marked.

Meclozine hydrochloride is used for the prevention and treatment of motion sickness and for the relief of allergic states. It has also been used in irradiation sickness, postoperative vomiting, drug-induced nausea and vomiting, and the symptomatic treatment of nausea and vertigo due to Ménière's disease and other labyrinthine disturbances. It may also be used in vomiting of

pregnancy.
The usual dosage is 25 to 50 mg by mouth. For motion sickness the first dose is taken 1 hour before commencing travel. Children aged 6 to 12 years old have been given half the adult dose.
For severe nausea and vomiting a dose of 25 to 50 mg may be required 2 or 3 times daily.

Vertigo. In a double-blind crossover study meclozine hydrochloride was significantly more effective than placebo in treating patients with positional and continuous vestibular vertigo.— B. Cohen and J. M. B. V. deJong, *Archs Neurol., Chicago*, 1972, *27*, 129.

Preparations

Meclizine Hydrochloride Tablets *(U.S.P.)*. Tablets containing meclozine hydrochloride.

Meclozine Tablets *(B.P.)*. Tablets containing meclozine hydrochloride.

Ancoloxin *(Duncan, Flockhart, UK)*. Tablets each containing meclozine hydrochloride 25 mg and pyridoxine hydrochloride 50 mg. For nausea. *Dose*. 2 to 6 tablets daily.

Other Proprietary Names

Arg.— Bonamina; *Austral.*— Ancolan; *Belg.*— Postafene; *Canad.*— Bonamine; *Denm.*— Postafen; *Ger.*— Bonamine, Calmonal, Peremesin, Postafen; *Ital.*— Neo-Istafene; *Neth.*— Postafene, Suprimal; *Norw.*— Postafen; *S.Afr.*— Navicalm; *Spain*— Chiclida, Navicalm, Supermesin; *Swed.*— Postafen; *Switz.*— Duremesan, Peremesin; *USA*— Antivert, Bonine.

6143-p

Medrylamine. UCB 502. 2-(4-Methoxybenzhydryloxy)-*NN*-dimethylethylamine.
$C_{18}H_{23}NO_2$=285.4.

CAS — 524-99-2.

Medrylamine is an ethanolamine derivative with the properties of the antihistamines (see p.1294) but has been used only topically as a 2% ointment for the relief of allergic and pruritic skin disorders.

Proprietary Names

Postafen Salbe *(UCB, Ger.)*.

NOTE. The name Postafen is also applied to a preparation containing meclozine hydrochloride (see p.1315).

6144-s

Mepyramine Maleate *(B.P., B.P. Vet.)*.

Mepyramini Maleas; Pyranisamine Maleate; Pyrilamine Maleate *(U.S.P.)*. *N-p*-Anisyl-*N'N'*-dimethyl-*N*-(2-pyridyl)ethylenediamine hydrogen maleate.
$C_{17}H_{23}N_3O,C_4H_4O_4$=401.5.

CAS — 91-84-9 (mepyramine); 59-33-6 (maleate).

Pharmacopoeias. In *Arg., Br., Braz., Fr., Ind., Int., It., Nord., Swiss, Turk.*, and *U.S.*

A white or creamy-white, crystalline powder, odourless or with a slight odour and with a bitter taste. M.p. 99° to 103°. **Soluble** 1 in 0.5 of water, 1 in 2.5 of alcohol, 1 in 15 of dehydrated alcohol, and 1 in 1.5 of chloroform; slightly soluble in ether. A 1% solution in water has a pH of 4.7 to 5.2. Solutions are **sterilised** by autoclaving. **Incompatible** with alkalis and oxidising agents. **Store** in airtight containers. Protect from light.

Adverse Effects, Treatment, and Precautions. As for the antihistamines in general, p.1294.

Interactions. Mepyramine both prevented and reversed the blocking action of guanethidine on the cold pressor response. Caution should be exercised in the concomitant administration of the 2 drugs.— B. S. Verma and O. D. Gulati, *Proc. Congr. Int. Dermatol.*, 1968, *13* (2), 1053.

For a report of toxic encephalopathy in children associated with the administration of mepyramine and pentobarbitone, see Pentobarbitone Sodium, p.810.

Uses. Mepyramine maleate is an ethylenediamine derivative with the properties and uses of the antihistamines (see p.1295). It is less potent, has a shorter duration of action, and causes less sedation than promethazine. It has some local anaesthetic effect.
In the treatment of allergic conditions, mepyramine maleate is usually given in doses of 100 mg thrice daily; this may be increased gradually according to the response and tolerance of the patient, but the maximum daily dose should not exceed 1 g. The dose for children, given 3 or 4 times daily, is: under 3 years of age 12.5 to 25 mg, 3 to 7 years 25 to 50 mg, and older children 25 to 75 mg. In the treatment of severe allergies it may be given by deep intramuscular or, in extreme emergencies, by slow intravenous injection in doses of 25 to 50 mg.
Mepyramine has also been used for the prevention and treatment of nausea and vomiting.
A 2% cream has been employed locally for insect bites or stings, and for allergic and pruritic skin conditions, but may cause sensitisation. If large areas are treated, absorption through the skin may be sufficient to cause side-effects.

Preparations

Injectabile Mepyramini *(Nord. P.)*. Mepyramine maleate 2.5 g, sodium chloride 600 mg, Water for Injections to 100 ml. *Dan. Disp.* specifies 1% w/v benzyl alcohol as preservative.

Mepyramine Elixir *(B.P.)*. A solution of mepyramine maleate in a suitable flavoured vehicle which may be coloured. Protect from light.

Mepyramine Injection *(B.P.)*. A sterile solution of mepyramine maleate in Water for Injections. Sterilised by autoclaving. pH 4.5 to 5.5.

Mepyramine Tablets *(B.P.)*. Sugar-coated tablets containing mepyramine maleate.

Pyrilamine Maleate Tablets *(U.S.P.)*. Tablets containing mepyramine maleate.

Proprietary Preparations

Anthisan *(May & Baker, UK)*. Mepyramine maleate, available as **Cream** containing 2% in a water-miscible basis and as **Tablets** of 50 mg. (Also available as Anthisan in *Austral., Denm., Norw., S.Afr.*).

Flavelix *(Pharmax, UK)*. Elixir containing in each 5 ml mepyramine maleate 12.5 mg, ephedrine hydrochloride 10 mg, ammonium chloride 90 mg, and sodium citrate 40 mg (suggested diluent, syrup). For cough and bronchial congestion. *Dose*. 10 ml three or four times daily; children aged 1 to 5 years, 2.5 ml thrice daily; aged 5 to 10 years 5 ml thrice daily.

Other Proprietary Names

Allergan (see also under Diphenhydramine Hydrochloride)*(Switz.)*; Histamed (see also under Chlorpheniramine Maleate), Pymal (both *S.Afr.*).

6145-w

Mequitazine.

LM209. 10-(Quinuclidin-3-ylmethyl)phenothiazine.
$C_{20}H_{22}N_2S$=322.5.

CAS — 29216-28-2.

Practically **insoluble** in water; soluble in alcohol and chloroform. M.p. about 143°.

Adverse Effects, Treatment, and Precautions. As for the antihistamines in general, p.1294.
As for all phenothiazine derivatives it should be used cautiously in patients with hepatic diseases.

Uses. Mequitazine is a phenothiazine derivative with the properties and uses of the antihistamines (see p.1295). It is reported to cause less sedation than promethazine.
Mequitazine is given in usual doses of 5 mg twice daily.

Allergy. In a double-blind 7-day study involving 49 patients there was no statistical difference between the use of mequitazine 5 mg twice daily and dexchlorpheniramine 6 mg twice daily for the treatment of allergic respiratory disorders; some patients in each group responded and required no further treatment and intolerance to each drug was reported by a small number of patients. Continuing treatment at a reduced dose for a further 7 days was of benefit with mequitazine but dexchlorpheniramine was not effective at the lower dose.— H. Muler and F. Blum, *Curr. med. Res. Opinion*, 1978, *5*, 359.

A double-blind study in 48 patients with a variety of allergic disorders showed mequitazine 5 mg twice daily to be as effective treatment over 14 days as brompheniramine 12 mg twice daily, but mequitazine was less likely to cause drowsiness.— J. Blamoutier, *Curr. med. Res. Opinion*, 1978, *5*, 366.

In a double-blind study involving 40 patients mequitazine 5 mg twice daily for 14 days was shown to be more effective than a placebo for the treatment of allergic skin conditions; 4 patients taking mequitazine and 7 taking the placebo required additional topical treatment. Reports of drowsiness were similar in the 2 groups of patients.— P. Laugier and M. Orusco, *Curr. med. Res. Opinion*, 1978, *5*, 371.

Proprietary Preparations

Primalan *(Smith & Nephew Pharmaceuticals, UK)*. Mequitazine, available as tablets of 5 mg. (Also available as Primalan in *Fr.*).

Other Proprietary Names

Instotal *(Arg.)*; Metaplexan *(Ger.)*; Mircol *(Belg., Neth., Spain)*; Vigigan *(Switz.)*.

6146-e

Methapyrilene Fumarate *(U.S.P.)*.

NN-Dimethyl-*N'*-(2-pyridyl)-*N'*-(2-thenyl)ethylenediamine fumarate.
$(C_{14}H_{19}N_3S)_2,3C_4H_4O_4$=871.0.

CAS — 91-80-5 (methapyrilene); 33032-12-1 (fumarate).

Pharmacopoeias. In *U.S.*

A white or almost white crystalline powder with a slight odour. M.p. 133° to 137°. **Soluble** 1 in 20 of water and 1 in 30 of alcohol. A 5% solution in water has a pH of 3 to 4. **Store** at a temperature not exceeding 30° in airtight containers. Protect from light.

6147-l

Methapyrilene Hydrochloride *(U.S.P.)*.

Methapyrilenium Chloride; Thenylpyramine Hydrochloride.
$C_{14}H_{19}N_3S,HCl$=297.8.

CAS — 135-23-9.

Pharmacopoeias. In *Arg.* and *U.S.*

A white or almost white crystalline powder with a faint odour. M.p. 161° to 165°. **Soluble** 1 in 0.5 of water, 1 in 5 of alcohol, and 1 in 3 of chloroform; practically insoluble in ether. A solution in water has a pH of about 5.5. **Store** in airtight containers. Protect from light.

Methapyrilene is an ethylenediamine derivative with the properties and uses of the antihistamines (see p.1294). It is less potent than promethazine and has a much shorter duration of action. It has a moderate sedative effect.
It has been given as the fumarate and as the hydrochloride but following reports of carcinogenicity in *rats* exposed to 25 times the dose appropriate to man it is now little used.

Preparations

Methapyrilene Fumarate Syrup *(U.S.P.)*. A syrup containing methapyrilene fumarate, with alcohol 3.5 to 6.5%. Store at a temperature not exceeding 30° in airtight containers. Protect from light.

Methapyrilene Hydrochloride Capsules *(U.S.P.)*. Capsules containing methapyrilene hydrochloride. The *U.S.P.* requires 80% dissolution in 30 minutes. Store in airtight containers.

Methapyrilene Hydrochloride Injection *(U.S.P.)*. A sterile solution of methapyrilene hydrochloride in Water for Injections. pH 4 to 7. Protect from light.

A preparation containing methapyrilene fumarate, codeine phosphate, ephedrine hydrochloride, and ammonium chloride was formerly marketed in Great Britain under the proprietary name Histadyl EC *(Lilly)*.

6148-y

Methdilazine *(U.S.P.)*. 10-(1-Methylpyrrolidin-3-ylmethyl)phenothiazine.
$C_{18}H_{20}N_2S=296.4$.

CAS — 1982-37-2.

Pharmacopoeias. In *U.S.*

A light tan crystalline powder with a characteristic odour. M.p. 83° to 88° with a range of not more than 2°. Methdilazine 7.2 mg is the equivalent of approximately 8 mg of methdilazine hydrochloride. Practically **insoluble** in water; soluble 1 in 2 of alcohol, 1 in 1 of chloroform, and 1 in 8 of ether; freely soluble in 3M hydrochloric acid. **Store** in airtight containers. Protect from light.

Methdilazine has actions and uses similar to those of methdilazine hydrochloride. It is given in usual doses of 7.2 mg two to four times daily.

Preparations

Methdilazine Tablets *(U.S.P.)*. Tablets containing methdilazine. Store in airtight containers. Protect from light.

Proprietary Names

Tacaryl *(Westwood, USA)*.

6149-j

Methdilazine Hydrochloride *(U.S.P.)*. 10-(1-Methylpyrrolidin-3-ylmethyl)phenothiazine hydrochloride.
$C_{18}H_{20}N_2S,HCl=332.9$.

CAS — 1229-35-2.

Pharmacopoeias. In *U.S.*

A light tan crystalline powder with a slight characteristic odour. It darkens on exposure to light. M.p. 184° to 190°. **Soluble** 1 in 2 of water and of alcohol, and 1 in 6 of chloroform; practically insoluble in ether; soluble in 0.1 M hydrochloric acid and 0.1 M sodium hydroxide solution. A 1% solution in water has a pH of 4.8 to 6. **Store** in airtight containers. Protect from light.

Adverse Effects, Treatment, and Precautions. As for the antihistamines in general, p.1294.
As with all phenothiazine derivatives it should be used cautiously in patients with hepatic diseases.

Uses. Methdilazine hydrochloride is a phenothiazine derivative with the properties and uses of the antihistamines (see p.1295). It is more potent than promethazine and generally causes less sedation. It has a duration of action of 8 to 12 hours. It has serotonin-antagonising and anticholinergic properties.
Methdilazine hydrochloride is given for the symptomatic treatment of allergic conditions, particularly to control pruritus. It may also be given for pruritus of non-allergic origin. The usual dose is 8 mg twice daily and may be increased to 4 times daily if necessary. Children may be given 300 µg per kg body-weight daily in 2 divided doses.

Allergy. Ninety-six patients suffering from allergy, of whom 58% had pruritus and 27% hay fever, were studied over 2 weeks in a double-blind study designed to compare methdilazine hydrochloride with promethazine hydrochloride. The dose was usually 8 mg of the former and 20 mg of the latter, twice daily in syrup. Both drugs gave relief to about one-half the patients and there was little difference in efficacy for pruritus, but promethazine was superior to methdilazine in the relief of hay fever. Drowsiness occurred in 32% of the patients when they were taking promethazine, being twice the incidence seen with the other drug, but in spite of this the patients generally preferred it.—Report No. 25 of the General Practitioner Research Group, *Practitioner*, 1962, *188*, 803.

Migraine. Methdilazine 4 to 8 mg thrice daily was useful to prevent or reduce the frequency of migraine attacks.— J. M. Sutherland, *Drugs*, 1973, *5*, 212.

For a report of the use of methdilazine in the treatment of migraine, see Methysergide Maleate, p.669.

Preparations

Methdilazine Hydrochloride Syrup *(U.S.P.)*. A syrup containing methdilazine hydrochloride, with alcohol 6.5 to 7.5%. pH 3.3 to 4.1. Store in airtight containers. Protect from light.

Methdilazine Hydrochloride Tablets *(U.S.P.)*. Tablets containing methdilazine hydrochloride. Store in airtight containers. Protect from light.

Proprietary Names

Dilosyn *(Allen & Hanburys, Austral.; Allen & Hanburys, Canad.)*; Tacaryl *(Mead Johnson, Austral.; Pharmacia, Swed.; Westwood, USA)*; Tacryl *(Pharmacia, Denm.)*.

Methdilazine hydrochloride was formerly marketed in Great Britain under the proprietary name Dilosyn *(Duncan, Flockhart)*.

6150-q

Metiamide. SKF 92058. 1-Methyl-3-[2-(5-methylimidazol-4-ylmethylthio)ethyl]thiourea.
$C_9H_{16}N_4S_2=244.4$.

CAS — 34839-70-8.

Adverse Effects. Metiamide may cause agranulocytosis.

Acute reversible neutropenia occurred in 2 patients given metiamide.— J. A. H. Forrest *et al.* (letter), *Lancet*, 1975, *1*, 392. Bone-marrow depression due to metiamide was thought to be due to the thiourea present in the metiamide molecule, rather than to H_2-receptor blockade.— *ibid.*, 1975, *2*, 802.

A further 4 cases of metiamide-induced agranulocytosis had occurred and trials had stopped.— W. L. Burland *et al.*, *Smith Kline & French* (letter), *Lancet*, 1975, *2*, 1085.

Further references: E. J. Feldman and J. I. Isenberg, *New Engl. J. Med.*, 1976, *295*, 1178.

Uses. Metiamide is a histamine H_2-receptor antagonist (see p.1294) with actions similar to those of cimetidine (p.1303) but a shorter duration of action. It has been used in doses of 1 g daily in conditions associated with gastric hyperacidity but has been found to cause bone-marrow depression.

References to the action and uses of metiamide: R. W. Brimblecombe *et al.*, *S. Afr. med. J.*, 1974, *48*, 2253; D. M. Shepherd *et al.*, *Digestion*, 1974, *11*, 307; B. Thjodleifsson and K. G. Wormsley, *Br. med. J.*, 1974, *2*, 304; *idem*, *Gut*, 1975, *16*, 501; G. I. Barbezat *et al.*, *Gut*, 1975, *16*, 186; J. I. Isenberg, *Ann. intern. Med.*, 1976, *84*, 212; A. S. MacDonald *et al.* (preliminary communication), *Lancet*, 1976, *1*, 68; J. M. Hind and T. J. Sutton, *J. Pharm. Pharmac.*, 1977, *29*, 244; O. R. Griffith *et al.*, *Br. J. Pharmac.*, 1978, *64*, 416P.

Duodenal ulcers. References to the use of metiamide in duodenal ulcers: M. Mainardi *et al.*, *New Engl. J. Med.*, 1974, *291*, 373; G. J. Milton-Thompson *et al.*, *Lancet*, 1974, *1*, 693; R. E. Pounder *et al.*, *Br. med. J.*, 1975, *2*, 307; *Lancet*, 1975, *2*, 779; *ibid.*, 802; R. Earlam (letter), *ibid.*, 973; J. H. B. Saunders and K. G. Wormsley, *Lancet*, 1977, *1*, 765.

Zollinger-Ellison syndrome. References to the use of metiamide in the Zollinger-Ellison syndrome: M. H. Thompson *et al.* (letter), *Lancet*, 1975, *1*, 35; L. G. Halloran *et al.* (letter), *ibid.*, 281; E. R. Smith *et al.*, *Med. J. Aust.*, 1976, *1*, 1000; D. M. McCarthy *et al.*, *Ann. intern. Med.*, 1978, *87*, 668; J. K. Siepler *et al.*, *Am. J. Hosp. Pharm.*, 1978, *35*, 141.

Manufacturers

Smith Kline & French, UK.

6151-p

Oxomemazine. RP 6847; Trimeprazine *SS*-Dioxide. 10-(3-Dimethylamino-2-methylpropyl)phenothiazine 5,5-dioxide.
$C_{18}H_{22}N_2O_2S=330.4$.

CAS — 3689-50-7.

A white crystalline powder with a bitter taste. M.p. 155°. Practically **insoluble** in water; slightly soluble in alcohol; soluble in chloroform and ether.

6152-s

Oxomemazine Hydrochloride.
$C_{18}H_{22}N_2O_2S,HCl=366.9$.

CAS — 4784-40-1.

Crystals. M.p. 250°. Oxomemazine hydrochloride 11.1 mg is approximately equivalent to 10 mg of oxomemazine.

Oxomemazine is a phenothiazine derviative with the properties and uses of the antihistamines (see p.1294). It has been given both as the base and as the hydrochloride in doses equivalent to 10 to 40 mg of oxomemazine daily.

Proprietary Names

Doxergan *(Specia, Belg.; Specia, Fr.; Specia, Neth.; Specia, Switz.)*; Imakol *(Rhône-Poulenc, Ger.)*.

6153-w

Phenindamine Tartrate *(B.P.)*. Phenindamini Tartras; Phenindaminium Tartrate; Phenindamine Acid Tartrate. 1,2,3,4-Tetrahydro-2-methyl-9-phenyl-2-azafluorene hydrogen tartrate; 2,3,4,9-Tetrahydro-2-methyl-9-phenyl-1*H*-indeno-[2,1-*c*]pyridine hydrogen tartrate.
$C_{19}H_{19}N,C_4H_6O_6=411.5$.

CAS — 82-88-2 (phenindamine); 569-59-5 (tartrate).

Pharmacopoeias. In *Arg.*, *Br.*, *Ind.*, *Int.*, and *Turk.*

A white or almost white, almost odourless, voluminous powder with a bitter taste. M.p. 160° to 162°; on further heating it solidifies and melts again at about 168° with decomposition. **Soluble** 1 in 70 of water and 1 in 300 of alcohol; practically insoluble in chloroform and ether. A 1% solution in water has a pH of 3.4 to 3.9. **Store** in airtight containers. Protect from light.

Incompatibility. Incompatible with alkalis, sodium salicylate, phosphates, and oxidising substances. Solutions were unstable above pH 7 and were most stable at pH 3.5 to 5. Heating could cause phenindamine to isomerise to an inactive form.— *J. Am. pharm. Ass., pract. Pharm. Edn*, 1956, *17*, 273.

Adverse Effects, Treatment, and Precautions. As for the antihistamines in general, p.1294.
Unlike most other antihistamines phenindamine tartrate may have a stimulant effect; to avoid the possibility of insomnia it should not be given after 4 p.m.

Allergy. In a modified 'repeated-insult' patch test, 25% phenindamine tartrate was found to produce extreme sensitisation of the skin.— A. M. Kligman, *J. invest. Derm.*, 1966, *47*, 393.

Extrapyramidal symptoms. For a report of tardive dyskinesia associated with the use of phenindamine, see Brompheniramine Maleate, p.1298.

Uses. Phenindamine tartrate has the properties and uses of the antihistamines (see p.1295). It is less potent than promethazine but it does not generally produce drowsiness and may even be mildly stimulating. It has a moderate anticholinergic action.
Phenindamine tartrate is given in doses of 25 to 50 mg up to thrice daily.

Preparations

Phenindamine Tablets *(B.P.)*. Tablets containing phenindamine tartrate. They are sugar-coated.

Thephorin *(Sinclair, UK)*. Phenindamine tartrate, available as tablets of 25 mg. (Also available as Thephorin in *Austral.*, *S.Afr.*).

6154-e

Pheniramine Maleate *(B.P.).* Pheniraminium Maleate; Prophenpyridamine Maleate. *NN*-Dimethyl-3-phenyl-3-(2-pyridyl)propylamine hydrogen maleate.
$C_{16}H_{20}N_2,C_4H_4O_4$=356.4.

CAS — 86-21-5 (pheniramine); 132-20-7 (maleate).

Pharmacopoeias. In *Br.*

A white or almost white crystalline powder with a slight amine-like odour. M.p. 106° to 109°. **Soluble** 1 in 0.3 of water, 1 in 2.5 of alcohol, and 1 in 1.5 of chloroform; very slightly soluble in ether. A 1% solution in water has a pH of 4.5 to 5.5. **Store** in airtight containers. Protect from light.

Adverse Effects. As for the antihistamines in general, p.1294.

Abuse. Pheniramine aminosalicylate in doses exceeding 300 mg caused hallucinatory effects followed by exhaustion. Other side-effects were cramps, dilated pupils, anorexia, ataxia, and incoordination. In 1 patient the vision remained clouded for several days.— I. H. Jones *et al., Med. J. Aust.,* 1973, *1,* 382.

A report of transient toxic psychosis in 2 young men who had taken between 0.5 and 1 g of pheniramine aminosalicylate.— E. R. Csillag and A. A. Landauer, *Med. J. Aust.,* 1973, *1,* 653.

Overdosage. Hallucinatory effects lasting for 2 days and major fits were reported in a child who took 750 to 1500 mg of pheniramine maleate.— I. H. Jones *et al., Med. J. Aust.,* 1973, *1,* 382.

Pregnancy and the neonate. For studies on the adverse effects of pheniramine and other antihistamines during pregnancy, see p.1294.

Treatment of Adverse Effects. As for the antihistamines in general, p.1294.

Adsorption. Studies *in vitro* indicated the pheniramine is efficiently adsorbed by activated charcoal.— J. J. Boehm *et al., Clin. Toxicol.,* 1978, *12,* 523.

Overdosage. A comment that pheniramine is associated with cardiac arrhythmias in overdosage and that electrocardiographic monitoring may be necessary.— D. W. Gilmore *et al., Med. J. Aust.,* 1976, *2,* 212. See also J. Coakley (letter), *ibid., 1,* 895. The use of tacrine in a patient with pheniramine overdosage.— G. Mendelson (letter), *ibid., 2,* 110.

Precautions. As for the antihistamines in general, p.1294.

Absorption and Fate. As for the antihistamines in general, p.1295.

On average, 22.6% of an administered dose of pheniramine was excreted unchanged in the urine. Under repeated daily dosage with 37 mg of pheniramine maleate, 24.3% was excreted unchanged, 26.1% as *N*-desmonomethylpheniramine, 0.5% as *N*-desdimethylpheniramine, and about 49% was unaccounted for.— P. Kabasakalian *et al., J. pharm. Sci.,* 1968, *57,* 621.

Uses. Pheniramine is an alkylamine derivative with the properties and uses of the antihistamines (see p.1295). It is less potent than promethazine, has a shorter duration of action, and generally causes less sedation.

Pheniramine maleate has been given in doses of up to 40 mg thrice daily but sustained-release preparations are more commonly used in doses of 75 mg once or twice daily or 150 mg at night if required.

The dose for children given up to three times daily is: under 1 year of age 7.5 mg, 1 to 5 years 7.5 to 15 mg, 6 years and over 15 to 22.5 mg.

Pheniramine is also administered as the aminosalicylate ($C_{16}H_{20}N_2,C_7H_7NO_3$ = 393.5) in usual doses of 25 to 50 mg thrice daily. It has also been given as the tannate.

Proprietary Preparations

Daneral-SA Tablets *(Hoechst, UK).* Sustained-release tablets each containing pheniramine maleate 75 mg. *Dose.* 1 or 2 tablets daily.

Owing to the risk of intestinal obstruction, sustained-release preparations such as Daneral-SA, where the drug is released in transit, but the matrix ghost is often eliminated intact, should not be prescribed in patients with Crohn's disease or other intestinal disease in which strictures may form.— J. L. Shaffer *et al.* (letter), *Lancet,* 1980, *2,* 487.

Other Proprietary Names

Acovil, Acoviletas *(both Spain);* Avil *(aminosalicylate and/or maleate) (Austral., Belg., Ger., Neth., S.Afr.);* Aviletten *(aminosalicylate) (Ger.);* Avilettes *(aminosalicylate) (Austral.);* Fenamine *(aminosalicylate and/or maleate) (Austral.);* Inhiston *(Ital.).*

A preparation containing pheniramine tannate was formerly marketed in Great Britain under the proprietary name Rynabond *(Fisons).*

6155-l

Phenyltoloxamine Citrate. C 5581; Phenyltolyloxamine Citrate; PRN. 2-(2-Benzylphenoxy)-*NN*-dimethylethylamine dihydrogen citrate.
$C_{17}H_{21}NO,C_6H_8O_7$=447.5.

CAS — 92-12-6 (phenyltoloxamine); 1176-08-5 (citrate).

Phenyltoloxamine citrate is an ethanolamine derivative with the properties and uses of the antihistamines (see p.1294). It is a structural isomer of diphenhydramine (see p.1311). It has been given in doses of 25 to 50 mg three or four times daily.

Abuse. Mention of the abuse of a cough mixture containing hydrocodone with phenyltoloxamine.— Y. J. Berry (letter), *New Engl. J. Med.,* 1976, *295,* 286.

Proprietary Preparations

Phenyltoloxamine citrate is an ingredient of Rinurel, see under Phenylpropanolamine Hydrochloride, p.26.

Phenyltoloxamine is an ingredient of Pholtex: see under Pholcodine, p.1260.

6156-y

Piprinhydrinate. The diphenylpyraline salt of 8-chlorotheophylline; 4-Benzhydryloxy-1-methylpiperidine salt of 8-chlorotheophylline.
$C_{26}H_{30}ClN_5O_3$=496.0.

CAS — 606-90-6.

Piprinhydrinate is diphenylpyraline theoclate and has the general properties of diphenylpyraline hydrochloride (see p.1312). It has been given in doses of 3 to 9 mg up to thrice daily.

Proprietary Names

Colton *(Byk Liprandi, Arg.);* Kolton *(see also under Diphenylpyraline Hydrochloride) (Promonta, Belg.; Promonta, Ger.).*

6157-j

Pizotifen Malate. Pizotyline Malate; BC-105 (base). 9,10-Dihydro-4-(1-methyl-4-piperidylidene)-4*H*-benzo[4,5]cyclohepta[1,2-*b*]thiophene hydrogen malate.
$C_{19}H_{21}NS,C_4H_6O_5$=429.5.

CAS — 15574-96-6 (pizotifen).

Pizotifen malate 145 mg is approximately equivalent to 100 mg of pizotifen.

Adverse Effects, Treatment, and Precautions. As for the antihistamines in general, p.1294.

Increased appetite and weight gain may occur.

A review of the actions and uses of pizotifen. Tolerance to alcohol could be lowered by pizotifen. The effects of tranquillisers, sedatives, and some tricyclic antidepressants could be enhanced. It should not be given with monoamine oxidase inhibitors. Because of its structural similarity to tricyclic antidepressants it might antagonise the adrenergic neurone blockade induced by some antihypertensive agents.— T. M. Speight and G. S. Avery, *Drugs,* 1972, *3,* 159.

Of 47 patients with severe migraine given pizotifen 1 to 2 mg daily adverse effects were recorded in 22 patients. These reactions included weight increase (15), muscle pain or cramps (3), heavy legs or restless legs (3), fluid retention (3), drowsiness (2), more frequent milder headaches (2), facial flushing (1), reduced libido (1), exacerbation of epilepsy (1), and dreaming (2). Adverse effects necessitating withdrawal from the study occurred in 11 patients. Advantageous effects were mood elevation in 3 and increased alertness in 6.— K. M. S. Peet, *Curr. med. Res. Opinion,* 1977, *5,* 192.

Uses. Pizotifen malate has the properties of the antihistamines (see p.1295). It also has pronounced antiserotonin, antitryptamine, and weak anticholinergic properties.

Pizotifen malate is used for the prophylaxis of migranous headache. The usual dose is the equivalent of 500 µg of pizotifen thrice daily; some patients may be controlled on 500 µg daily; up to 6 mg daily has been given. It has been recommended that treatment should commence with 500 µg daily increased gradually over the following 5 days.

Reviews and comments on the action and uses of pizotifen.— T. M. Speight and G. S. Avery, *Drugs,* 1972, *3,* 159; M. Anthony and J. W. Lance, *ibid.,* 153; *Drug & Ther. Bull.,* 1976, *14,* 29.

The use of pizotifen in 3 patients to prevent or reduce the side-effects following calcitonin injections.— A. J. Crisp (letter), *Lancet,* 1981, *1,* 775.

Appetite stimulation. In a double-blind study in 40 patients with tuberculosis the mean weekly weight gain in those given pizotifen 500 µg thrice daily for 4 weeks was 890 g compared with 230 g for those given placebo.— A. Tsougranis, *Curr. ther. Res.,* 1972, *14,* 372.

Carcinoid syndrome. Pizotifen was found to stop diarrhoea and facial flushing in a patient with malignant carcinoid syndrome, the excision of whose primary tumour was followed by regression of metastatic lesions. Chlorpromazine, methysergide, and cyproheptadine were ineffective.— S. C. Loong *et al., Med. J. Aust.,* 1968, *2,* 845.

Carotodynia. A favourable report of the use of pizotifen in the treatment of 4 patients with carotodynia, a form of vascular neck and face pain.— T. J. Murray, *Can. med. Ass. J.,* 1979, *120,* 441.

Cluster headache. Patients with cluster headache who did not respond to ergotamine might be relieved by methysergide 3 to 6 mg daily or by pizotifen 1.5 to 3 mg daily for the duration of the bout.— *Br. med. J.,* 1975, *4,* 425.

Further references.— K. Ekbom, *Acta neurol. scand.,* 1969, *45,* 601.

Cushing's disease. Administration of pizotifen 500 µg thrice daily for 2 to 7 months had a beneficial effect in 4 of 5 women with Cushing's disease, without serious side-effects. On stopping pizotifen one women remained in remission for 10 months before relapsing, another relapsed 2 months after stopping, and 2 were still in remission 3 and 6 months respectively after withdrawal of pizotifen. One patient's weight increased by about 4 kg after 7 months of therapy. In patients being prepared for surgery or in those in whom other forms of therapy have failed, pizotifen may have a place.— A. Kasperlik-Zaluska *et al.* (letter), *Lancet,* 1980, *1,* 490.

Depression. A double-blind study involving 20 patients with minor to moderate depression indicated that pizotifen possessed certain antidepressant properties.— J. E. Standal, *Acta psychiat. scand.,* 1977, *56,* 276.

Further references.— W. V. Krumholz *et al., Curr. ther. Res.,* 1968, *10,* 342.

Migraine. Of 26 patients suffering from severe attacks of migraine (classical migraine in 25) treated for 8 weeks in a double-blind crossover trial with placebo or pizotifen in doses increased up to 1 mg thrice daily (in addition to any existing medication), 9 obtained complete relief or a reduction of at least one-half in the number of their attacks. Ten patients noted increased appetite, 6 a change of mood, and 5 experienced depression when active treatment ceased. Other side-effects were tiredness (5), facial flushing (1), and increased vomiting (1).— R. C. Hughes and J. B. Foster, *Curr. ther. Res.,* 1971, *13,* 63. See also J. B. Foster, *ibid.,* 1976, *19,* 66.

Further references.— F. Sicuteri *et al., Int. Archs Allergy appl. Immun.,* 1967, *31,* 78; J. W. Lance and M. Anthony, *Med. J. Aust.,* 1968, *1,* 54; O. Sjaastad and P. Stensrud, *Acta neurol. scand.,* 1969, *45,* 594; J. W. Lance *et al., Br. med. J.,* 1970, *2,* 327; J. Schaer, *Headache,* 1970, *10,* 67; B. Anselmi, *Schweiz. med. Wschr.,* 1972, *102,* 487; A. J. Krakowski and R. Engisch, *Psychosomatics,* 1973, *14,* 302; J. D. Carroll and W. P. Maclay, *Curr. med. Res. Opinion,* 1975, *3,* 68; E. R. Lawrence *et al., Headache,* 1977, *17,* 109; K. W. G. Heathfield *et al., Practitioner,* 1977, *218,* 428; K.

M. S. Peet, *Curr. med. Res. Opinion*, 1977, *5*, 192; O. Bademosi and B. O. Osuntokun, *Practitioner*, 1978, *220*, 325.

Pruritus. Beneficial results with pizotifen in 6 of 9 patients with pruritus associated with polycythaemia vera.— E. J. Fitzsimons *et al.*, *Br. med. J.*, 1981, *283*, 277.

Proprietary Preparations

Sanomigran *(Wander, UK)*. Pizotifen malate, available as tablets each containing the equivalent of 0.5 and 1.5 mg of pizotifen.

Other Proprietary Names

Mosegor *(Arg., Belg., Ger., Spain, Switz.)*; Sandomigran *(Arg., Austral., Belg., Canad., Ger., Ital., Neth., S.Afr., Spain, Switz.)*; Sandomigrin *(Swed.)*; Sanmigran *(Fr.)*.

6158-z

Propiomazine Hydrochloride *(U.S.P.)*. Wy 1359. 1-[10-(2-Dimethylaminopropyl)phenothiazin-2-yl]propan-1-one hydrochloride.

$C_{20}H_{24}N_2OS,HCl = 376.9$.

CAS — 362-29-8 (propiomazine); 1240-15-9 (hydrochloride).

Pharmacopoeias. In *U.S.*

A yellow almost odourless powder. **Soluble** 1 in less than 1 of water, 1 in 6 of alcohol, and 1 in 2 of chloroform; practically insoluble in ether. A 2% solution has a pH of 4.6 to 5.6. **Incompatible** with barbiturate salts and other alkalis. **Store** in airtight containers.

6159-c

Propiomazine Maleate. Propiomazine Hydrogen Maleate; CB 1678.

$C_{20}H_{24}N_2OS,C_4H_4O_4 = 456.6$.

CAS — 3568-23-8.

A yellow odourless microcrystalline powder with a bitter taste. Propiomazine maleate 1.3 mg is approximately equivalent to 1 mg of propiomazine and 1.1 mg of propiomazine hydrochloride. **Soluble** 1 in 500 of water, 1 in 60 of alcohol, and 1 in 140 of dehydrated alcohol. A 0.1% solution in water has a pH of 4.5 to 4.7. **Protect** from light.

Adverse Effects, Treatment, and Precautions. As for the antihistamines in general, p.1294.Local irritation may occur at the site of intravenous injection and as with all phenothiazine derivatives it should be used cautiously in patients with hepatic disease.

Effects on the blood. A 0.033% solution of propiomazine hydrochloride in 0.9% sodium chloride solution caused 100% haemolysis of erythrocytes cultured in it for 45 minutes.— C. J. Fievet *et al.*, *Am. J. Hosp. Pharm.*, 1971, *28*, 961.

Uses. Propiomazine is a phenothiazine derivative with the properties of the antihistamines (see p.1295).

It is reported to have weaker antihistamine actions and more potent central nervous depressant actions than promethazine.

It has been given by mouth as the maleate for sedation in doses equivalent to 25 mg of the base 2 to 4 times daily. It has also been given, usually by intramuscular injection, in doses of 20 mg of the hydrochloride for anaesthetic premedication and during surgical and obstetric procedures; doses of up to 40 mg have been employed. It has also been given by cautious intravenous injection care being taken to avoid extravasation.

Preparations

Propiomazine Hydrochloride Injection *(U.S.P.)*. A sterile solution in Water for Injections. pH 4.7 to 5.3. Do not use if cloudy or if a precipitate has formed. Store at 15° to 30°. Protect from light.

Proprietary Names

Largon (hydrochloride) *(Wyeth, USA)*; Propavan (maleate) *(Pharmacia, Swed.)*; Serentin (maleate) *(Midy, Ital.)*.

6160-s

Pyrathiazine Theoclate. Parathiazone Teoclate; Parathiazone Theoclate. 10-(Pyrrolidin-1-ylethyl)phenothiazine 8-chlorotheophyllinate.

$C_{18}H_{20}N_2S,C_7H_7ClN_4O_2 = 511.0$.

CAS — 84-08-2 (pyrathiazine); 14006-99-6 (theoclate).

Pyrathiazine theoclate is a phenothiazine derivative with the properties of the antihistamines (see p.1294) but has been used mainly as an anti-emetic in the treatment of motion sickness and postoperative vomiting. It has been given in doses of 25 to 100 mg daily in divided doses. For the prevention of motion sickness, 25 mg has been given 30 minutes before commencing the journey with further 25-mg doses at intervals during the journey.

Proprietary Names

Mediamer *(Hispano-Medial, Spain)*.

6161-w

Pyrrobutamine Phosphate *(U.S.P.)*. 1-[4-(4-Chlorophenyl)-3-phenylbut-2-enyl]pyrrolidine diphosphate.

$C_{20}H_{22}ClN,2H_3PO_4 = 507.8$.

CAS — 91-82-7 (pyrrobutamine); 135-31-9 (phosphate).

Pharmacopoeias. In *U.S.*

A white or almost white crystalline powder, usually with a faint odour. M.p. 127° to 131°. **Soluble** in water; soluble 1 in 20 of alcohol; practically insoluble in chloroform and ether. **Store** in airtight containers. Protect from light.

Adverse Effects, Treatment, and Precautions. As for the antihistamines in general, p.1294.

Uses. Pyrrobutamine phosphate has the properties and uses of the antihistamines (see p.1295). It has a slow onset of action and its effects last for about 10 hours.

It has been given in usual doses of 15 to 30 mg twice or thrice daily.

Proprietary Preparations

Co-Pyronil *(Lilly, UK)*. Capsules each containing pyrrobutamine phosphate 15 mg and cyclopentamine hydrochloride 12.5 mg. For allergic conditions. *Dose.* 1 capsule twice or thrice daily.

NOTE. Co-Pyronil capsules previously each contained, in addition, methapyrilene hydrochloride equivalent to methapyrilene 25 mg.

6162-e

Ranitidine. AH 19065 (hydrochloride). *NN*-Dimethyl-5-[2-(1-methylamino-2-nitrovinylamino)ethylthiomethyl]furfurylamine.

$C_{13}H_{22}N_4O_3S = 314.4$.

CAS — 66357-35-5.

Adverse Effects and Precautions. Like cimetidine, ranitidine is a histamine H_2-receptor antagonist and therefore the adverse effects that have been associated with the H_2-receptor blocking properties of cimetidine may also follow ranitidine therapy.

Ranitidine should be given in reduced dosage to patients with impaired renal function; it is removed by haemodialysis.

Effects on the blood. Reduced white cell count in 11 of 12 healthy subjects following administration of ranitidine.— P. A. Lebert *et al.*, *Clin. Pharmac. Ther.*, 1981, *30*, 539.

Effects on the endocrine system. Reversible amenorrhoea possibly associated with ranitidine.— L. Lombardo (letter), *Lancet*, 1982, *1*, 224.

Effects on the gastro-intestinal tract. Ranitidine and nitroso derivatives.— S. Detlora (letter), *Lancet*, 1981, *2*, 993.

For a review of the relevance of histamine H_2-receptor antagonists to nitrosation in the stomach, see Cimetidine, p.1301.

Interactions. Results from studies in 8 subjects suggesting that ranitidine, unlike cimetidine, does not inhibit hepatic microsomal drug oxidative function.— D. A. Henry *et al.*, *Br. med. J.*, 1980, *281*, 775.

In 5 healthy subjects taking daily subtherapeutic doses of warfarin the addition of ranitidine 200 mg twice daily for 14 days did not affect prothrombin time or plasma-warfarin concentrations.— M. J. Serlin *et al.*, *Br. J. clin. Pharmac.*, 1981, *12*, 791.

A study suggesting that ranitidine reduces liver blood flow; this would be expected to impair the hepatic elimination of drugs, such as propranolol and lignocaine, that are highly extracted by the liver.— J. Feeley and E. Guy (letter), *Lancet*, 1982, *1*, 169. Criticism.— S. L. Grainger *et al.*, *ibid.*, 398.

Pancreatitis. A study suggesting that ranitidine does not damage the exocrine pancreas.— R. Mohammed and K. Mitchell (letter), *Br. J. clin. Pharmac.*, 1981, *11*, 408.

Absorption and Fate. Ranitidine is readily absorbed from the gastro-intestinal tract. It is reported to have an elimination half-life of about 2 hours and to suppress gastric acid secretion for about 12 hours. It is excreted in the urine mainly as unchanged ranitidine with small amounts of the *N*-oxide, *S*-oxide, and desmethyl metabolites. Ranitidine is excreted in breast milk.

In 2 healthy subjects given ranitidine hydrochloride 100, 200, and 400 µg per kg body-weight on 3 separate occasions mean peak plasma-ranitidine concentrations occurred 2, 0.67, and 1 hour after administration respectively. With all 3 doses, plasma-ranitidine concentrations were measurable at 8 hours but after 24 hours they had fallen to below the detectable limit (5 ng per ml). Plasma-desmethylranitidine concentrations were not above the threshold sensitivity of the assay. Mean elimination half-lives for the 3 doses were 3.0, 2.9, and 3.9 hours respectively and more than half of the administered dose was excreted in the urine within the first 6 hours. After 48 hours about 77% of the dose was excreted as unchanged ranitidine with only about 4% appearing as desmethylranitidine.— G. W. Mihaly *et al.*, *J. pharm. Sci.*, 1980, *69*, 1155.

A study of ranitidine kinetics and dynamics in 12 healthy subjects. It was concluded that an appropriate therapeutic effect should be achieved with a dose of 80 mg every 8 hours.— P. A. Lebert *et al.*, *Clin. Pharmac. Ther.*, 1981, *30*, 539. Intravenous dose studies and comparison with cimetidine.— *idem*, 545.

Further references: D. C. Garg *et al.*, *Clin. Pharmac. Ther.*, 1981, *29*, 247 (evidence of significant first-pass metabolism); J. J. McNeill, *Br. J. clin. Pharmac.*, 1981, *12*, 411 (pharmacokinetics; elimination half-life unaffected by food).

Uses. Ranitidine is a histamine H_2-receptor antagonist (see p.1294) with actions similar to those of cimetidine (p.1303).

The usual dose is 150 mg of ranitidine (as the hydrochloride) twice daily. When appropriate, maintenance doses of 150 mg may be given at night. Reflux oesophagitis may be treated with 150 mg twice daily for up to 8 weeks. In the Zollinger-Ellison syndrome 150 mg is given thrice daily and the daily dose may be increased to 900 mg.

Ranitidine may also be given by slow intravenous injection in a usual dose of 50 mg every 6 to 8 hours or it may be given by intravenous infusion over 2 hours at 25 mg per hour and repeated at 6 to 8 hour intervals.

Some references to studies on ranitidine including mention of its increased efficacy, on a molar basis, relative to cimetidine.— J. Bradshaw *et al.*, *Br. J. Pharmac.*, 1979, *66*, 464P (histamine H_2-receptor antagonism *in vitro* and inhibition of histamine-induced gastric acid secretion in *animals*); W. Domschke *et al.* (letter), *Lancet*, 1979, *1*, 320 (inhibition of pentagastrin-stimulated gastric acid secretion in healthy subjects); N. R. Peden *et al.*, *Lancet*, 1979, *1*, 690 (inhibition of gastric secretion in patients with duodenal ulceration); N. R. Peden *et al.* (letter), *Lancet*, 1979, *2*, 199 (inhibition of pentagastrin-stimulated acid secretion in patients with duodenal ulcer); D. von Kleist *et al.* (letter), *Lancet*, 1979, *2*, 1071 (effect on gastric transmural potential differences); T. Bohman *et al.*, *Scand. J. Gastroenterol.*, 1980, *15*, 183 (inhibition of histamine-stimulated gastric acid secretion in healthy subjects); S. J. Konturek *et al.*, *Gut*, 1980, *21*, 181 (inhibition of histamine-induced gastric acid secretion in patients with chronic duodenal ulcer); R. P. Walt *et al.*, *Gut*, 1980, *21*, A898 (inhibition of meal-stimulated acid secretion); R. P. Walt *et al.*, *Gut*, 1981, *22*, 49 (inhibition of gastric acid secretion in patients with duodenal ulcer); M. Guslandi, *Br. med. J.*, 1981, *283*, 699 (lack of influence on gastric mucus secretion).

Administration in renal failure. A patient with renal failure who became agitated, confused, and delirious on cimetidine was able to tolerate ranitidine both intravenously and by mouth. He remained alert and free of mental disorder.— P. Bories *et al.* (letter), *Lancet*, 1980, *2*, 755. Comment that the dosage of cimetidine (1.2 g daily reduced to 0.6 g daily) was above that recommended in renal failure whereas the dosage of ranitidine (50 mg daily by intravenous injection for 8 days followed by 150 mg twice daily by mouth) was probably appropriate for such a condition.— P. C. Sharpe and W. L. Burland, *Smith Kline & French* (letter), *ibid.*, 924. See also G. D. Tovey, *Smith Kline & French* (letter), *Pharm. J.*, 1980, *2*, 460.

Ulcer. In an 8-week study involving 37 patients with endoscopically proven duodenal ulceration, ulcer healing occurred in 17 of 19 given ranitidine 100 mg twice daily and in 17 of 18 given cimetidine 200 mg thrice daily and 400 mg at night. The 2 patients who did not respond to ranitidine also failed to respond to later cimetidine therapy. Although concentrations of serum urea and creatinine rose slightly but significantly in patients given cimetidine, this did not occur in the ranitidine-treated group.— M. J. S. Langman *et al.*, *Br. med. J.*, 1980, *281*, 473.

Data suggesting that women with duodenal ulcer are less likely than men to achieve healing with one month of treatment with ranitidine.— N. R. Peden *et al.*, *Br. med. J.*, 1981, *282*, 866.

Further references to the use of ranitidine in the acute treatment of duodenal ulcer: J. H. B. Saunders *et al.*, *Gut*, 1980, *21*, A455; R. P. Walt *et al.*, *ibid.*, A897; R. P. Walt *et al.*, *Gut*, 1981, *22*, 319.

Ulceration, stress-induced. Following abdominal surgery life-threatening gastric hypersecretion developed in 3 patients and was resistant to cimetidine. It responded to ranitidine.— M. Danilewitz *et al.*, *New Engl. J. Med.*, 1982, *306*, 20.

Zollinger-Ellison syndrome. Ranitidine and cimetidine in the Zollinger-Ellison syndrome.— M. Mignon *et al.* (letter), *Br. J. clin. Pharmac.*, 1980, *10*, 173.

Proprietary Preparations of Ranitidine Hydrochloride

Zantac Injection *(Glaxo, UK)*. Ranitidine hydrochloride, available as solution containing in each ml the equivalent of ranitidine 10 mg, in ampoules of 5 ml. **Zantac Tablets**. Each contains ranitidine hydrochloride equivalent to ranitidine 150 mg.

6163-l

Rotoxamine Tartrate. Levocarbinoxamine Tartrate. (−)-2-[4-Chloro-α-(2-pyridyl)benzyloxy]-*NN*-dimethylethylamine hydrogen tartrate.
$C_{16}H_{19}ClN_2O,C_4H_6O_6$=440.9.

CAS — 5560-77-0 (rotoxamine); 49746-00-1 (tartrate).

A white to creamy-white odourless crystalline powder. M.p. 137° to 143°. **Soluble** 1 in 10 of water and 1 in 100 of alcohol; practically insoluble in chloroform and ether. **Store** in airtight containers.

Rotoxamine is the laevo-isomer of carbinoxamine which is the racemic mixture. Rotoxamine tartrate has the same general properties as carbinoxamine maleate (see p.1299) but it is reported to be twice as potent. It has been given as the tartrate in doses equivalent to 2 to 4 mg of rotoxamine base two to four times daily.

6164-y

Thenalidine Tartrate. Thenophenopiperidine Tartrate; Thenopiperidine Tartrate. *N*-(1-Methyl-4-piperidyl)-*N*-(2-thenyl)aniline hydrogen tartrate.
$C_{17}H_{22}N_2S,C_4H_6O_6$=436.5.

CAS — 86-12-4 (thenalidine); 16509-35-6 (tartrate).

Thenalidine tartrate has the properties and uses of the antihistamines (see p.1294). It has been given in doses of 100 to 150 mg daily in divided doses.

Agranulocytosis has been reported following its use.— D. A. Adams and S. Perry, *Br. med. J.*, 1958, *2*, 636; J. Stevenson and A. C. Kennedy, *Scott. med. J.*, 1961, *6*, 522.

Proprietary Names
Sandosten *(Sandoz, S.Afr.)*.

6165-j

Thenyldiamine Hydrochloride. Thenyldiaminium Chloride. *NN*-Dimethyl-*N'*-(2-pyridyl)-*N'*-(3-thenyl)ethylenediamine hydrochloride.
$C_{14}H_{19}N_3S,HCl$=297.8.

CAS — 91-79-2 (thenyldiamine); 958-93-0 (hydrochloride).

Pharmacopoeias. In *Arg.*

A white, almost odourless, crystalline powder. **Soluble** 1 in 5 of water, of alcohol, and of chloroform; practically insoluble in ether. A solution in water is neutral to litmus. **Protect** from light.

Thenyldiamine hydrochloride is an ethylenediamine derivative with the properties and uses of the antihistamines (see p.1294). It has been given in usual doses of 15 mg up to 6 times daily. Thenyldiamine is an isomer of methapyrilene.

Preparations

Thenyldiamine hydrochloride is an ingredient of Bronchilator, p.14, Franol Plus, p.12, and Hayphryn, p.25.

6166-z

Thiazinamium Methylsulphate. Methylpromethazinium Methylsulfuricum; Thiazinamium Metilsulfate. Trimethyl[1-methyl-2-(phenothiazin-10-yl)ethyl]ammonium methyl sulphate.
$C_{19}H_{26}N_2O_4S_2$=410.5.

CAS — 2338-21-8 (thiazinamium); 58-34-4 (methylsulphate).

Thiazinamium methylsulphate is a phenothiazine derivative with the properties and uses of the antihistamines (see p.1294). It has anticholinergic properties. It has been given in doses of 0.6 to 1.2 g daily by mouth.

References to the absorption and fate of thiazinamium methylsulphate.— J. H. G. Jonkman *et al.*, *J. Pharm. Pharmac.*, 1974, *26, Suppl.*, 63P (oral and intramuscular administration); J. H. G. Jonkman *et al.* (letter), *Lancet*, 1976, *1*, 693 (intramuscular and intravenous administration); J. H. G. Jonkman *et al.*, *Clin. Pharmac. Ther.*, 1977, *21*, 457 (oral and intramuscular administration); J. H. G. Jonkman *et al.*, *Int. J. Pharmaceut.*, 1979, *3*, 55 (rectal administration); J. H. G. Jonkman *et al.*, *J. pharm. Sci.*, 1979, *68*, 69 (rectal administration).

References to the use of thiazinamium methylsulphate in respiratory disorders.— L. E. van Bork *et al.*, *Tubercle*, 1975, *56*, 244 (generalised chronic obstructive lung disease); J. Zielinski and E. Chodosowska, *Respiration*, 1977, *34*, 31 (asthma).

Proprietary Names
Multergan *(Specia, Belg.; Specia, Fr.; Specia, Neth.)*.

6167-c

Thonzylamine Hydrochloride. Histylamine Hydrochloride. *N*-*p*-Anisyl-*N'N'*-dimethyl-*N*-(pyrimidin-2-yl)ethylenediamine hydrochloride.
$C_{16}H_{22}N_4O,HCl$=322.8.

CAS — 91-85-0 (thonzylamine); 63-56-9 (hydrochloride).

Pharmacopoeias. In *Arg.*

A white crystalline powder with a faint odour. **Soluble** 1 in 1 of water, 1 in 6 of alcohol, and 1 in 4 of chloroform; practically insoluble in ether. A solution in water has a pH of about 5 to 6. **Protect** from light.

Thonzylamine hydrochloride is an ethylenediamine derivative with the properties and uses of the antihistamines (see p.1294). It is less potent than promethazine and has a shorter duration of action. It has been given in usual doses of 50 mg to 100 mg daily.

Preparations

Thonzylamine hydrochloride is an ingredient of Biomydrin, see under Phenylephrine Hydrochloride, p.25..

Proprietary Names
Tonamil *(Ecobi, Ital.)*.

6168-k

Tolpropamine Hydrochloride. *NN*-Dimethyl-3-phenyl-3-*p*-tolylpropylamine hydrochloride.
$C_{18}H_{23}N,HCl$=289.8.

CAS — 5632-44-0 (tolpropamine); 3339-11-5 (hydrochloride).

A white crystalline powder. **Soluble** in water and alcohol; practically insoluble in chloroform and ether.

Tolpropamine hydrochloride is an alkylamine derivative with the properties of the antihistamines (see p.1294) but it has been used by topical application (1%) for the symptomatic relief of allergic and pruritic skin disorders.

Proprietary Names
Pragman *(Hoechst, Austral.; Albert-Farma, Ital.)*; Pratalgin *(Albert-Farma, Spain)*.

6169-a

Trimeprazine Tartrate *(B.P., B.P. Vet., U.S.P.)*.

Alimemazine Tartrate. *NN*-Dimethyl-2-methyl-3-(phenothiazin-10-yl)propylamine tartrate.
$(C_{18}H_{22}N_2S)_2,C_4H_6O_6$=747.0.

CAS — 84-96-8 (trimeprazine); 4330-99-8 (tartrate).

Pharmacopoeias. In *Br.*, *Braz.*, *Jap.*, and *U.S.*

A white or slightly cream-coloured odourless or almost odourless crystalline powder with a bitter taste. M.p. 159° to 163°. It darkens in colour on exposure to light. Trimeprazine tartrate 25 mg is approximately equivalent to 20 mg of trimeprazine.

Soluble 1 in 4 of water, 1 in 30 of alcohol, and 1 in 5 of chloroform; very slightly soluble in ether. A 2% solution has a pH of 5 to 6.5. Solutions in Water for Injections containing suitable stabilisers are distributed into ampoules the air in which is replaced by nitrogen or other suitable gas and **sterilised** by autoclaving. **Store** in airtight containers. Protect from light.

Adverse Effects. As for the antihistamines in general, p.1294. Acute poisoning may be associated with profound depression of the central nervous system and hypothermia. Other effects include extrapyramidal symptoms, elation or depression, nasal stuffiness, and, very rarely, agranulocytosis.

A 3½-year-old child became restless and progressively more confused and disorientated after tonsillectomy and adenoidectomy, for which trimeprazine 44 mg and hyoscine hydrobromide 200 µg had been given as premedication. The condition cleared up the next day. A week later another child showed mild confusion following trimeprazine therapy.— R. B. Roberts (letter), *Lancet*, 1959, *1*, 630.

Fatal malignant hyperpyrexia occurred in a 3-year-old child given 72 mg of trimeprazine tartrate.— D. G. Moyes, *Br. J. Anaesth.*, 1973, *45*, 1163.

Speculation as to the possible role of phenothiazines in sudden infant death, with special reference to 4 infants who had shown excessive sleep tendencies after receiving alimenazine [sic] 1 mg per kg body-weight daily and one (whose sibling had died with the sudden infant death syndrome) who developed repeated apnoeic crises after receiving promethazine.— A. Kahn and D. Blum (letter), *Lancet*, 1979, *2*, 364.

Severe respiratory and CNS depression in 2 siblings given trimeprazine tartrate in doses of 2.4 and 2.9 mg per kg body-weight respectively.— N. P. Mann, *Archs Dis. Childh.*, 1981, *56*, 481.

Treatment of Adverse Effects and Precautions. As for Chlorpromazine Hydrochloride, p.1511.

As with all phenothiazine derivatives it should be used cautiously in patients with hepatic diseases.

Absorption and Fate. As for the antihistamines in general, p.1295.

A study of the absorption and excretion of trimeprazine tartrate.— P. C. Johnson and Y. F. Masters, *J. Lab. clin. Med.*, 1962, *59*, 993.

Uses. Trimeprazine is a phenothiazine derivative with pharmacological activity intermediate between that of promethazine (see p.1296) and chlorpromazine (see p.1513). It has the histamine-antagonising properties of the antihistamines (see p.1295), more pronounced than with promethazine, and pronounced sedative and other central nervous system effects resembling those of chlorpromazine. Its adrenergic-blocking action is less than that of chlorpromazine and its anticholinergic actions are weak. It is used mainly for its marked effect in the relief of pruritus. Its effects like those of promethazine are slow in onset and are prolonged.

Trimeprazine tartrate is given by mouth for the relief of pruritus in doses of 10 to 40 mg daily for adults and 7.5 to 20 mg daily for children, in 3 or 4 divided doses. In severe cases adults have been given up to 100 mg daily. It is also used for pre-operative medication of children. The usual dose, administered about 90 minutes before operation, is 2 to 4 mg per kg body-weight by mouth. It has also been given in doses of 600 to 900 µg per kg by deep intramuscular injection. When given with barbiturates the dose of the latter should be reduced since their effect is enhanced. It may also be used in cough linctuses.

Anaesthesia. When given with hyoscine as premedication in children, the effects of trimeprazine were most marked when the dose was given 2 hours before induction of anaesthesia. A dose of 4.4 mg per kg body-weight was more effective than a smaller dose in producing amnesia and in reducing salivation; its use was associated with a greater tendency to noisy delirium and with a high frequency of postoperative pallor. Sedation was unreliable but anti-emetic effects with doses of 2.2 or 4.4 mg of trimeprazine per kg were comparable.— D. R. Davies and A. Doughty, *Br. J. Anaesth.*, 1966, *38*, 878.

Trimeprazine tartrate was preferred to diazepam as premedication in children prior to anaesthesia for adenotonsillectomy because it had greater antisialogogue and soporific effects and because blood loss was reduced.— I. U. Haq and J. W. Dundee, *Br. J. Anaesth.*, 1968, *40*, 972. A similar report showing a preference for diazepam.— N. H. Gordon and D. J. Turner, *ibid.*, 1969, *41*, 136. The amount of blood loss in children during adenotonsillectomy was similar in groups receiving trimeprazine, diazepam, or phenobarbitone sodium by mouth for premedication.— S. M. Wilson *et al.*, *ibid.*, 1973, *45*, 86.

In a detailed study of a variety of drugs used pre- and postoperatively for vomiting after adenotonsillectomy, trimeprazine 4 mg per kg body-weight by mouth to a maximum of 100 mg given pre-operatively together with dihydrocodeine phosphate 1 to 1.5 mg per kg intramuscularly postoperatively was the most effective.— B. L. Smith and M. L. M. Manford, *Br. J. Anaesth.*, 1974, *46*, 373.

Further references.— M. Dunn and M. H. Gough, *Practitioner*, 1978, *220*, 937.

Hypnotic effect. In a study of 59 patients with insomnia nitrazepam 5 mg was considered to be more effective than trimeprazine 20 mg taken at night during the first week; there was a further improvement in those taking trimeprazine after 3 weeks of treatment. Nitrazepam appeared to be more suitable for elderly patients.— O. Lingjaerde *et al.*, *Curr. ther. Res.*, 1978, *24*, 388.

Further references.— K. Kayed *et al.*, *Eur. J. clin. Pharmac.*, 1977, *11*, 163.

In children. A regimen involving a short course of trimeprazine tartrate in high dosage in order to alter the sleep pattern of children with difficulty going to sleep.— H. B. Valman, *Br. med. J.*, 1981, *283*, 423. For mention of excessive respiratory and CNS depression in children given trimeprazine, see p.1319.

Pruritus. Itching dermatoses in 83 adults and 53 children were treated with trimeprazine; adult dosage was 10 mg four times daily given in tablet form. A particularly good response was obtained in patients with atopic dermatitis and neurodermatitis. In cases of infantile eczema and juvenile atopic dermatitis the drug was given in the form of a syrup in a dosage of 10.8 to 28.8 mg daily according to age and severity of itching. Benefit was obtained in most cases. No toxic effects were noted.— T. E. Anderson and D. Chalmers, *Br. J. Derm.*, 1959, *71*, 214.

Preparations

Elixirs

Paediatric Trimeprazine Elixir *(B.P.C. 1973).* Trimeprazine Syrup. A solution containing trimeprazine tartrate 0.15% in a suitable coloured flavoured vehicle. It contains 7.5 mg of trimeprazine tartrate in 5 ml. When a dose less than, or not a multiple of, 5 ml is prescribed, the mixture should be diluted to 5 ml, or a multiple, with syrup. Such dilutions should be freshly prepared and not used more than 2 weeks after issue. Protect from light. *Dose.* Children, for the relief of pruritus, 2 months to 1 year, 5 to 7.5 mg of trimeprazine tartrate thrice daily; 1 to 5 years, 10 mg in the morning and up to 25 mg at night.

Strong Paediatric Trimeprazine Elixir *(B.P.C. 1973).* Strong Trimeprazine Syrup. A solution containing trimeprazine tartrate 0.6% in a suitable coloured flavoured vehicle. It contains 30 mg of trimeprazine tartrate in 5 ml. Protect from light. *Dose.* Children, for pre-operative medication, trimeprazine tartrate 2 to 5 mg per kg body-weight.

Injections

Trimeprazine Injection *(B.P.C. 1973).* A sterile solution of trimeprazine tartrate, with suitable stabilising agents, in Water for Injections free from carbon dioxide. pH 4.5 to 5.5 Protect from light. *Dose.* For pre-operative medication about 90 minutes before surgery, by deep intramuscular injection, trimeprazine tartrate 600 to 900 µg per kg body-weight.

Syrups

Trimeprazine Tartrate Syrup *(U.S.P.).* A syrup containing trimeprazine tartrate with alcohol 4.5 to 6.5%. Potency is expressed in terms of the equivalent amount of trimeprazine. Store in airtight containers. Protect from light.

Tablets

Trimeprazine Tablets *(B.P.).* Trimeprazine Tartrate Tablets. Tablets containing trimeprazine tartrate. They may be sugar-coated.

Trimeprazine Tartrate Tablets *(U.S.P.).* Tablets containing trimeprazine tartrate. Potency is expressed in terms of the equivalent amount of trimeprazine. Protect from light.

Proprietary Preparations

Vallergan *(May & Baker, UK).* Trimeprazine tartrate, available as **Syrup** containing 7.5 mg in each 5 ml (suggested diluent, syrup); as **Forte Syrup** containing 30 mg in each 5 ml; and as **Tablets** of 10 mg. (Also available as Vallergan in *Austral., Denm., Norw., S.Afr.*).

Vallex *(May & Baker, UK).* An expectorant linctus containing in each 5 ml trimeprazine tartrate 2.5 mg, phenylpropanolamine hydrochloride 10 mg, guaiphenesin 25 mg, menthol 1.2 mg, citric acid monohydrate 65 mg, sodium citrate 200 mg, and ipecacuanha liquid extract 0.015 ml (suggested diluent, syrup). *Dose.* 5 to 10 ml twice or thrice daily; children, 2 to 5 years, 2.5 ml; children, 5 to 10 years, 2.5 to 5 ml.

Other Proprietary Names

Nedeltran *(Neth.)*; Panectyl *(Canad.)*; Repeltin *(Ger.)*; Temaril *(USA)*; Theralen *(Swed.)*; Theralene *(Belg., Fr., Ger., Switz.)*; Variargil *(Spain)*.

6170-e

Trimethobenzamide Hydrochloride *(U.S.P.).*

N-[4-(2-Dimethylaminoethoxy)benzyl]-3,4,5-trimethoxybenzamide hydrochloride.

$C_{21}H_{28}N_2O_5,HCl=424.9.$

CAS — 138-56-7 (trimethobenzamide); 554-92-7 (hydrochloride).

Pharmacopoeias. In *U.S.*

A white crystalline powder with a slight phenolic odour. M.p. 186° to 190°. **Soluble** 1 in 2 of water, 1 in about 60 of alcohol, 1 in 67 of chloroform, and 1 in 720 of ether. Solutions are **sterilised** by autoclaving.

Adverse Effects, Treatment, and Precautions. As for the antihistamines in general, p.1294.

Pain at the site of injection and local irritation after rectal administration have been noted.

Allergy. A 4-year-old boy given 75 mg of trimethobenzamide hydrochloride intramuscularly for persistent vomiting complained of abdominal pain and developed painful swellings of the wrists and knees, with puffiness of the face and eyes. He was given an injection of adrenaline, and diphenhydramine hydrochloride 20 mg by mouth thrice daily. The swelling subsided during the following 3 days.— S. J. Nichamin, *Harper Hosp. Bull.*, 1964, *22*, 2.

Effects on the liver. A 50-year-old woman developed acute hepatitis after taking trimethobenzamide hydrochloride, 250 mg four times daily for 3 days.— I. Borda and H. Jick, *Archs intern. Med.*, 1967, *120*, 371.

Extrapyramidal symptoms. Extrapyramidal symptoms in a 2-week-old boy were possibly associated with the administration of about 300 mg of trimethobenzamide rectally over the previous 24 hours.— C. Holmes and R. J. Flaherty, *J. Pediat.*, 1976, *89*, 669.

Pregnancy and the neonate. Evaluation of a number of antinauseant drugs, including trimethobenzamide, prescribed during the years 1959 to 1966, for about 2000 pregnant women in the first 84 days of pregnancy, suggested a slight excess of severe congenital anomalies with trimethobenzamide.— L. Milkovich and B. J. van den Berg, *Am. J. Obstet. Gynec.*, 1976, *125*, 244.

Uses. Trimethobenzamide hydrochloride is an ethanolamine derivative with the properties of the antihistamines (see p.1295) but it appears to have only weak antihistamine activity. It has been used in irradiation sickness, postoperative vomiting, the nausea and vomiting of pregnancy, drug-induced nausea and vomiting, and the symptomatic treatment of nausea and vertigo due to Ménière's disease and other labyrinthine disturbances. It is of little or no value in the prevention and treatment of motion sickness.

The usual dose is 250 mg by mouth or 200 mg by deep intramuscular injection 3 or 4 times daily. It has also been given rectally, as a suppository.

Anaesthesia. Trimethobenzamide, in a dose of 200 mg, given with either atropine or pethidine by injection prior to operation, had a slight sedative effect. It enhanced the soporific effect of pethidine and reduced pre-operative emesis.— J. W. Dundee *et al.*, *Br. J. Anaesth.*, 1966, *38*, 50.

Further references.— B. Wolfson *et al.*, *Anesth. Analg. curr. Res.*, 1962, *41*, 172; A. L. Brandt *et al.*, *ibid.*, 1966, *45*, 402.

Preparations

Trimethobenzamide Hydrochloride Capsules *(U.S.P.).* Capsules containing trimethobenzamide hydrochloride. Only lactose, magnesium stearate, starch, and talc may be present as added substances.

Trimethobenzamide Hydrochloride Injection *(U.S.P.).* A sterile solution of trimethobenzamide hydrochloride in Water for Injections. pH 4.8 to 5.2.

Proprietary Names

Anaus *(Molteni, Ital.)*; Ibikin *(IBP, Ital.)*; Tigan *(Roche, Canad.; Beecham, USA)*.

6171-l

Tripelennamine Citrate *(U.S.P.).*

Tripelennaminium Citrate. *N*-Benzyl-*N'N'*-dimethyl-*N*-(2-pyridyl)ethylenediamine dihydrogen citrate.

$C_{16}H_{21}N_3,C_6H_8O_7=447.5.$

CAS — 91-81-6 (tripelennamine); 6138-56-3 (citrate).

Pharmacopoeias. In *U.S.*

A white crystalline powder. M.p. about 107°. Tripelennamine citrate 150 mg is approximately equivalent to 100 mg of tripelennamine hydrochloride. **Soluble** 1 in 1 of water; freely soluble in alcohol; very slightly soluble in ether; practically insoluble in chloroform. Solutions in water are acid to litmus. **Protect** from light.

6172-y

Tripelennamine Hydrochloride *(U.S.P., B.P. 1963).*

Tripelen. Hydrochlor.; Tripelennamini Hydrochloridum; Tripelennaminium Chloride.

$C_{16}H_{21}N_3,HCl=291.8.$

CAS — 154-69-8.

Pharmacopoeias. In *Braz., Fr., Ind., Int., Pol., Turk.,* and *U.S.*

A white odourless crystalline powder with a bitter taste. M.p. 188° to 192°. It slowly darkens on exposure to light. **Soluble** 1 in 1 of water, 1 in 6 of alcohol and of chloroform, and 1 in 350 of acetone; practically insoluble in ether and ethyl acetate. Solutions in water are practically neutral to litmus. **Protect** from light.

Incompatibility. There was loss of clarity when intravenous solutions of tripelennamine hydrochloride were mixed with those of chloramphenicol sodium succinate, phenobarbitone sodium, or phenytoin sodium.— J. A. Patel and G. L. Phillips, *Am. J. Hosp. Pharm.*, 1966, *23*, 409.

Adverse Effects, Treatment, and Precautions. As for the antihistamines in general, p.1294. Agranulocytosis has been reported.

Abuse. Mention of the abuse of tripelennamine in combination with pentazocine.— C. V. Showalter and L. Moore (letter), *J. Am. med. Ass.*, 1978, *239*, 1610.

Allergy. From patch tests carried out in 413 patients with contact dermatoses, 7 were found to be allergic to tripelennamine.— E. Epstein, *J. Am. med. Ass.*, 1966, *198*, 517.

Cutaneous absorption. A severe toxic reaction, including agitation and hallucinations, occurred in an 8-year-old child who was sprayed over the trunk and extremities with tripelennamine in the treatment of severe poison ivy poisoning. It was likely that inhalation of the fine mist of the aerosol spray contributed to the reaction but in this patient the initial reaction began 3 hours after exposure suggesting that percutaneous absorption through the multiple skin lesions probably contributed significantly. The original reaction was prolonged by treatment with diphenhydramine and promethazine.— P. G. Schipior, *J. Pediat.*, 1967, *71*, 589.

Uses. Tripelennamine is an ethylenediamine derivative with the properties and uses of the antihistamines (see p.1295). It is less potent than promethazine, has a shorter duration of action, and generally causes less sedation although drowsiness is prominent. It has anticholinergic and marked local anaesthetic properties.

Tripelennamine hydrochloride is given in usual doses of 25 to 50 mg every 4 to 6 hours. Higher doses of up to 600 mg daily have been given. A recommended dose of the hydrochloride for children is 5 mg per kg body-weight daily in 4 to 6 divided doses; the citrate is used in equivalent doses in an elixir.

Tripelennamine has also been given parenterally as the hydrochloride.

Local anaesthesia. Tripelennamine and diphenhydramine, each as a 1% solution, and lignocaine, as a 2% solution with adrenaline, were compared in a double-blind trial as local anaesthetics by injection for tooth extraction. Tripelennamine was effective in 10 out of 11 patients and gave anaesthesia for an average of 80.7 minutes, and diphenhydramine and lignocaine were both effective in 7 out of 9 and 7 patients respectively and the average duration of anaesthesia was 78.8 minutes and 151.4 minutes respectively. Either of the antihistamines was considered useful for patients allergic to the usual anaesthetics.— R. A. Meyer and W. Jakubowski, *J. Am. dent. Ass.*, 1964, *69*, 112.

Preparations

Tripelennamine Citrate Elixir *(U.S.P.)*. An elixir containing 705 to 795 mg of tripelennamine citrate per 100 ml and 11 to 13% of alcohol. Store in airtight containers. Protect from light.

Tripelennamine Hydrochloride Tablets *(U.S.P.)*. Tablets containing tripelennamine hydrochloride.

Tripelennamine Tablets *(B.P. 1963)*. Tripelen. Tab. Tablets containing tripelennamine hydrochloride.

Proprietary Names

Azaron *(Chefaro, Neth.)*; PBZ *(Geigy, USA)*; Pyribenzamine *(Ciba, Canad.)*; Sedilene *(Montefarmaco, Ital.)*.

6173-j

Triprolidine Hydrochloride *(B.P., U.S.P.)*.

295C51. (*E*)-2-[3-(Pyrrolidin-1-yl)-1-*p*-tolylprop-1-enyl]pyridine hydrochloride monohydrate.
$C_{19}H_{22}N_2,HCl,H_2O=332.9$.

CAS — 486-12-4 (triprolidine); 550-70-9 (hydrochloride, anhydrous); 6138-79-0 (hydrochloride, monohydrate).

Pharmacopoeias. In *Br.* and *U.S.*

A white crystalline powder, odourless or with a slight unpleasant odour and with a bitter taste. M.p. 118° to 121°. **Soluble** 1 in about 2 of water, 1 in about 1.5 of alcohol, 1 in less than 1 of chloroform, and 1 in 2000 of ether. A solution in water is alkaline to litmus. **Store** in airtight containers. Protect from light.

Adverse Effects, Treatment, and Precautions. As for the antihistamines in general, p.1294.

Skin eruptions resembling poikiloderma of Civatte occurred in 2 women following the administration by mouth of triprolidine hydrochloride. Eruptions reappeared on challenge and were more marked in exposed areas. One patient noticed that her rash became more marked after exposure to sunshine.— S. Alexander (letter), *Br. med. J.*, 1964, *2*, 512.

The effect of triprolidine hydrochloride on performance.— A. N. Nicholson, *Br. J. clin. Pharmac.*, 1979, *8*, 321.

Absorption and Fate. As for the antihistamines in general, p.1295.

In a study involving 16 healthy subjects triprolidine hydrochloride 3.75 mg administered as a syrup gave a mean peak plasma concentration of about 8 ng per ml, with a range of 3 to 17.4 ng per ml, 2 hours after administration. It was eliminated from plasma with a half-life of 5 hours (range 1.5 to 20 hours).— R. L. DeAngelis *et al.*, *J. pharm. Sci.*, 1977, *66*, 841.

Uses. Triprolidine hydrochloride has the properties and uses of the antihistamines (see p.1295). It is one of the more potent of the antihistamines, and its actions last for up to 12 hours. Triprolidine hydrochloride is given by mouth, the usual dose for adults being 2.5 to 5 mg thrice daily; these doses have also been given every 4 to 6 hours. The dose for children, which may be given thrice daily, is up to 1 year of age 1 mg, 1 to 6 years 2 mg, and 7 to 12 years 3 mg.

Allergy. Of 120 patients with various allergic conditions 109 obtained rapid relief after administration of sustained-release tablets containing triprolidine hydrochloride 10 mg, usually once daily at night.— G. C. Young, *Practitioner*, 1964, *193*, 664.

In a double-blind crossover study in 10 subjects with a history of allergic rhinitis, pseudoephedrine 60 mg and triprolidine 2.5 mg were equally effective, and significantly better than placebo, in reducing the rise in nasal airways resistance produced by histamine challenge to one nostril.— M. G. Britton *et al.*, *Br. J. clin. Pharmac.*, 1978, *6*, 51. See also *idem*, *Ann. Allergy*, 1979, *42*, 330.

Preparations

Triprolidine Hydrochloride Syrup *(U.S.P.)*. A syrup containing triprolidine hydrochloride with 3 to 5% of alcohol. pH 5.6 to 6.6. Store in airtight containers. Protect from light.

Triprolidine Hydrochloride Tablets *(U.S.P.)*. Tablets containing triprolidine hydrochloride. The *U.S.P.* requires 80% dissolution in 30 minutes. Store in airtight containers. Protect from light.

Triprolidine Tablets *(B.P.)*. Tablets containing triprolidine hydrochloride.

Proprietary Preparations

Actidil *(Wellcome, UK)*. Triprolidine hydrochloride, available as **Elixir** containing 2 mg in each 5 ml (suggested diluent, syrup) and as scored **Tablets** of 2.5 mg. (Also available as Actidil in *Austral., Canad., Denm., Ital., S.Afr., Swed., USA*).

Pro-Actidil *(Wellcome, UK)*. Sustained-action tablets containing triprolidine hydrochloride 10 mg. *Dose.* Adults and children over 10 years, 1 tablet swallowed whole in the early evening or 5 to 6 hours before retiring; very severe cases, 2 tablets every 24 hours. (Also available as Pro-Actidil in *Austral., Ger., Neth., S.Afr., Spain, Switz.*).

Triprolidine hydrochloride is an ingredient of Actifed preparations, see under Pseudoephedrine Hydrochloride, p.27.

Other Proprietary Names

Actidilon *(Arg., Fr.)*; Actiphyll *(Spain)*; Pro-Actidilon *(Fr.)*; Venen *(Jap.)*.

6174-z

Zolamine Hydrochloride. 194-B; WI 291. *N*-*p*-Anisyl-*N'N'*-dimethyl-*N*-(thiazol-2-yl)ethylenediamine hydrochloride.
$C_{15}H_{21}N_3OS,HCl=327.9$.

CAS — 553-13-9 (zolamine); 1155-03-9 (hydrochloride).

Odourless crystals with a slightly bitter taste. M.p. 167° to 168°. **Soluble** in water.

Zolamine hydrochloride is an ethylenediamine derivative with the properties of the antihistamines (see p.1294). It has local anaesthetic properties. It has been used as ear-drops containing 1% with euprocin hydrochloride for the relief of earache associated with otitis media. It has also been used in suppositories for the treatment of haemorrhoids.

6175-c

Allergens and Specific Desensitisation

Hay fever, allergic asthma, urticaria, contact dermatitis, and other allergic conditions are most frequently due to hypersensitivity to a foreign protein but the sensitising agent may also be a simple chemical substance.

Ingestion of many foods and drugs may give rise to allergies, as may also inhalation of pollens, animal fur, hair, or feathers, house dust, mites, mould spores, bacteria, and cosmetics. Contact with dyes, chemicals such as chromates, with nickel, turpentine, synthetic resins, antibiotics, cosmetics, paints, and certain complex plant substances, particularly oleoresins, may also cause sensitisation, and sensitisation may follow a bee or wasp sting.

Once the individual is sensitised to an allergen, ingestion or inhalation of this agent, or contact with it, may result in an antigen-antibody reaction during which histamine and substances such as serotonin are released from the body cells. This causes the allergic reaction. The anti-allergic effect of the antihistamines is due to their competition with this released histamine for the histamine receptors in the body.

Diagnosis in allergic conditions demands a comprehensive case history. Skin tests are undertaken only as a final step to confirm the sensitivities to allergens indicated by the case history, since a high proportion of the population who have no clinical allergy do in fact give positive skin test reactions as a result of sub-clinical sensitivities. Adrenaline must always be available for immediate use in case a reaction follows testing. For diagnostic purposes, the use of a large number of skin tests regardless of case history is grossly misleading. Due to their extreme sensitivity skin testing should be carried out with great care in patients with a history of allergy to wasp or bee stings.

In order to carry out skin testing a drop of a dilute solution of the suspected allergen is placed on the forearm, thigh, or back, and a drop of saline on the corresponding spot on the opposite side of the body; the skin underlying these drops is then pricked or scratched. If the patient is allergic to the suspected solution an urticarial wheal develops within 5 minutes with the test solution but not with the saline, and reaches its maximum size in about 15 minutes. The test may also be carried out by intradermal injection but this is not recommended for pollen allergens since it is more likely to give rise to systemic reactions.

Another test is the patch test in which the suspected material or solution or extract of this is applied to the skin for 24 to 48 hours. A positive reaction is shown by erythema, swelling, and sometimes vesiculation. The various regions of the body do not react alike to skin tests. The suprascapular region of the back reacts more strongly than the upper arm, the flexor surfaces more than the extensor, the upper arm more than the forearm. Hence in comparing results it is necessary to make sure that all tests are made on the same region of the body.

The results obtained from these tests are often unsatisfactory and difficult to assess; in urticaria they are of little value but in other allergies they may confirm a suggestive case history.

When an allergy is due to ingestion or inhalation of the allergen, the sensitising agent should be avoided by the patient as far as possible. Should avoidance be impossible, as is usually the case with the inhaled allergens, specific desensitisation may be attempted.

A review of allergic and hypersensitivity reactions including tests for allergens and contact sensitisers.— J. Hardy, *J. Soc. cosmet. Chem.*, 1973, *24*, 423. See also L. Wide *et al.*, *Lancet*, 1967, *2*, 1105.

Two patients had acute self-limiting unilateral brachial plexus neuropathy associated with desensitisation by subcutaneous injections of extracts of dust, pollens, and moulds in 1 and dust and mould in the other. Both received short courses of prednisone (about 11 days). Abnormal sensations disappeared slowly and normal function returned to the affected limb over a period of months.— E. R. Wolpow, *J. Am. med. Ass.*, 1975, *234*, 620.

Variations and anomalies in skin tests.— L. Kumar, *J. Lar. Otol.*, 1977, *91*, 795; K. G. Huggins and J. Brostoff (letter), *Lancet*, 1978, *2*, 149; J. M. James and F. E. R. Simons, *Can. med. Ass. J.*, 1979, *120*, 330; E. Henocq *et al.* (letter), *Lancet*, 1979, *1*, 674.

Further references: A. C. M. L. Miller, *Clin. Allergy*, 1976, *6*, 551; *idem*, 557.

Desensitisation comprises a series of subcutaneous injections of gradually increasing strengths and quantities of the allergen or allergens causing symptoms until a stage is reached (by the end of the recommended dosage scheme) when the patient remains symptom-free. Antihistamines may be given concurrently to prevent a generalised allergic reaction.

When the injections are discontinued, sensitivity may gradually return and fresh courses may have to be given at intervals for several years. Specific desensitisation is of little value in allergic dermatitis or for drug eruptions.

Allergic reactions may occur during specific desensitisation, especially in small children.

The patient should be kept under observation for at least 20 minutes (small children for at least 1 hour) after injection. The first symptoms of a general reaction are itching, especially of the palms, suffusion of the eyes, and an intense feeling of bulging or pressure in the ears. A subcutaneous injection of 0.5 ml of Adrenaline Injection should be given immediately and repeated as often as necessary until symptoms subside.

In view of the cost, the potential risk of anaphylaxis, and the theoretical possibility of immune disorders, desensitisation of patients with allergic rhinitis appeared to be justified only when antihistamines by mouth or corticosteroids intranasally had failed.— *Med. Lett.*, 1973, *15*, 55.

Desensitisation is not commonly indicated in patients with bronchial asthma but needs to be considered in 2 situations. Patients with seasonal spring and summer asthma, where pollens are the dominant precipitating agents, frequently benefit significantly from grass pollen immunotherapy which should be given before the pollen season and usually needs to be repeated for 2 or 3 consecutive years as preseasonal courses. Secondly, immunotherapy with the house dust mite should be considered in any asthmatic patient where the mite has been shown to be a dominant precipitating factor and where the asthma control is so poor that oral corticosteroids are required. Thus no patient should be committed to long-term oral corticosteroids without immunotherapy having been tried.— A. B. X. Breslin, *Drugs*, 1979, *18*, 103.

A 19-year-old girl with allergic asthma and rhinitis who had received 14 desensitisation injections without reaction suffered an anaphylactic reaction and died following the fifteenth injection.— D. A. Rands, *Br. med. J.*, 1980, *281*, 854. A similar report.— R. C. H. Pollard (letter), *ibid.*, 1429.

Further reviews and comments on the use of skin tests and desensitisation in asthma and rhinitis: R. M. Morris-Owen, *Practitioner*, 1978, *220*, 575; *Drug & Ther. Bull.*, 1979, *17*, 73.

In a 14-year study the value of hyposensitisation therapy was assessed in 130 children with perennial bronchial asthma. The children were treated with a 1 in 10 000, 1 in 5000, or 1 in 250 dilution of sensitising allergens. An untreated group acted as controls. They were followed up until the age of 16. At the end of the study 22% of those who were not treated and those who were treated with 1 in 10 000 dilution of antigens were free of asthma, compared with 62% who received the 1 in 5000 dilution and 78% receiving the 1 in 250 dilution.— D. E. Johnstone and A. Dutton, *Pediatrics*, 1968, *42*, 793, per *Abstr. Wld Med.*, 1969, *43*, 459.

For reference to the RadioImmunoSorbent Test and the RadioAllergoSorbent Test, see Iodine-125, p.1391.

House-dust allergy. A review and discussion of the limited value of hyposensitisation to house dust mites in adults.— *Br. med. J.*, 1980, *280*, 589.

Further reviews and comments on vaccines made from house dust mites: *Drug & Ther. Bull.*, 1971, *9*, 89; *ibid.*, 1976, *14*, 35; *Br. med. J.*, 1975, *3*, 263.

In a double-blind clinical study 11 asthmatic subjects allergic to house dust showed a substantial improvement in symptoms and in their need for other therapy after treatment with house-dust mite extract, compared with 11 control subjects. Of 10 patients followed up for a year, 5 remained well.— A. P. Smith, *Br. med. J.*, 1971, *4*, 204.

A double-blind study in 45 patients with asthma sensitive to house-dust mite failed to show any benefit from a course of vaccine (Migen).— J. Gaddie *et al.*, *Br. med. J.*, 1976, *2*, 561. Criticism of the selection of patients and conduct of the study.— J. O. Warner and J. F. Price (letter), *ibid.*, 945.

In a study of the effect of immunotherapy on the treatment of chronic perennial bronchial asthma, 12 of the 18 patients who completed a full course of injections with a tyrosine-adsorbed vaccine prepared from house dust mite, *Dermatophagoides pteronyssinus*, (Migen) were considered to be definitely improved in clinical symptoms and 13 patients required less oral anti-asthma treatment; 9 patients were reported to have an increase in blocking antibodies to mite antigen.— P. Choovoravech *et al.*, *Curr. med. Res. Opinion*, 1976, *4*, 330.

Desensitisation with a course of injections of *Dermatophagoides pteronyssinus* tyrosine adsorbate had a beneficial effect in 27 children with fairly severe perennial asthma and who were positive to *D. pteronyssinus* both by prick tests and by bronchial provocation. Comparison was with 24 similar children who received placebo.— J. O. Warner *et al.*, *Lancet*, 1978, *2*, 912.

A multicentre study of house dust mite extract in bronchial asthma. Of 70 patients recruited at the start of the study, 56 were observed for at least 6 months. Of 43 patients who started injections of active material 7 had side-effects severe enough to necessitate withdrawal. In patients not receiving corticosteroids the treated group did a little better than the controls but no benefit was apparent by extending treatment beyond 18 weeks. In contrast patients receiving corticosteroids given placebo injections did a little better than the treated group. In view of the marginal benefit which was found only in the patients not receiving corticosteroids it seems doubtful whether treatment in this form is suitable for general use.—Mite Allergy Subcommittee of the Research Committee of the British Thoracic Association, *Br. J. dis. Chest*, 1979, *73*, 260.

Further references: C. Bernecker (letter), *Lancet*, 1968, *2*, 1145; D. Munro-Ashman *et al.*, *Ann. Allergy*, 1971, *29*, 578; J. A. Lunn, *Practitioner*, 1972, *208*, 411; L. J. Lees, *Br. J. clin. Pract.*, 1974, *28*, 343; B. Cooper, *Br. J. clin. Pract.*, 1979, *33*, 323.

Insect sting allergy. Allergic reactions to insect stings can include urticaria, bronchospasm, laryngeal oedema, hypotension, and death. The insects whose stings most often cause anaphylactic reactions are the *Hymenoptera* spp., including bees (honey-bees), wasps, hornets, fire ants, and yellow-jackets (*Med. Lett.*, 1978, *20*, 54). It has been proposed by W.C. Light *et al.* (*J. Allergy clin. Immunol.*, 1977, *59*, 247) that treatment directed at increasing IgG antibody concentrations against venom proteins may be essential for protection in insect allergy. Acceptance of this view has been criticised by S.E. Barr (*New Engl. J. Med.*, 1978, *299*, 1135) but this criticism has been countered by L.M. Lichtenstein *et al.* (*New Engl. J. Med.*, 1978, *299*, 1136) citing their data on the protective role of IgG antibody in allergic disease (M.H. Lessof *et al.*, *Johns Hopkins med. J.*, 1978, *142*, 1). This role of IgG antibody is a relevant factor in comparison of the merits of prophylactic injection of crushed whole insect bodies, which do not raise IgG antibody concentrations, with those of pure insect venom, which do. Whole-body extracts have been reported by D. Ordman (*Int. Archs Allergy appl. Immun.*, 1965, *28*, 366), E.A. Friedman and A.V. Mascia (*Ann. Allergy*, 1968, *26*, 430), and H.L. Mueller (*Pediatrics*, 1977, *59*, 773) to be highly effective in protecting susceptible subjects against anaphylactic reactions, but K.J. Hunt *et al.* (*New Engl. J. Med.*, 1978, *299*, 157) have questioned their value in a study advocating pure bee venom. This study by Hunt *et al.* has led not only to spirited defences of whole-body insect extracts, but also to controversy over the ethics of challenge stinging in a life-endangering condition (see H.L. Mueller, *New Engl. J. Med.*, 1978, *299*, 1135; S.E. Barr, *ibid.*; M. Coleman, *ibid.*, 1136; L.M. Lichtenstein *et al.*, *ibid.*). A study of pure bee venom has subsequently been carried out by C. Abkiewicz *et al.* (*S. Afr. med. J.*, 1979, *55*, 285) after initial skin testing according to the technique of K.J. Hunt *et al.* (*Ann. intern. Med.*, 1976, *85*, 56). Of 40 patients with a history of severe systemic reactions after bee stings, who were desensitised with pure bee venom, 11 who were subsequently stung suffered only mild local reactions. The desensitisation injections caused local reactions in nearly all 40 patients, and systemic reactions (reversed by subcutaneous adrenaline or intravenous mepyramine maleate) occurred in 5. These authors concluded that although their study confirmed the efficacy and safety of pure venom testing and desensitisation for the prevention of life-threatening allergic reactions to bee stings, nevertheless, systemic and local reactions were decidedly more common than those experienced during the usual desensitisation programmes in which respiratory allergens are used, and greater care and vigilance would be required of the physician; furthermore, the optimal regimen had not yet been established but it appeared that monthly maintenance injections would be required for an unlimited period. These drawbacks made an accurate diagnosis essential in each case and patients should be carefully evaluated before a decision was made to desensitise. A criticism of the continued use of whole body extract, illustrated by 4 cases of anaphylaxis despite receiving it (T. H. Lee *et al.* (letter), *Lancet*, 1981, *2*, 301).

Further reviews, studies, and comments: F. Wortmann, *Schweiz. med. Wschr.*, 1969, *99*, 974; R. M. M. Owen, *Br. J. clin. Pract.*, 1978, *32*, 309 and 339; *idem*, 1979, *33*, 7; R. Urbanek *et al.*, *Dt. med. Wschr.*, 1978, *103*, 1656; J. A. Grant (letter), *New Engl. J. Med.*, 1979, *300*, 565; *Med. Lett.*, 1980, *22*, 37.

Poison ivy allergy. Hyposensitisation by mouth with extracts of poison ivy, oak, or sumac was a tedious procedure with limited benefit. Side-effects included gastro-intestinal disturbances, pruritus ani, and skin rashes. Intramuscular use could cause unacceptably severe reactions.— *Med. Lett.*, 1975, *17*, 52.

Ragweed allergy. A comparative study in 23 atopic subjects demonstrated that polymerised ragweed antigen provided more rapid immunisation than standard monomeric preparations, with fewer side-effects.— W. J. Metzger *et al.*, *New Engl. J. Med.*, 1976, *295*, 1160. Comment.— L. M. Lichtenstein, *ibid.*, 1195.

Further references: E. Bacal *et al.*, *J. Allergy & clin. Immunol.*, 1978, *62*, 288.

Proprietary Preparations of Allergens

Alavac (known in some countries as A.D.L. or S.D.V-R.) *(Bencard, UK)*. Adsorbed desensitising vaccines containing alum-precipitated extracts from aqueous pyridine solutions of allergens, available as **Alavac-P** prepared from 12 varieties of common grass pollens, for the prophylaxis and treatment of hay fever and pollen asthma, and as **Alavac-S** prepared to the patient's requirements from a wider range of allergens. They are available in sets of 3 vials of graded strengths providing graduated doses and single vials for maintenance; preserved with phenol 0.5% and containing aluminium hydroxide not more than 0.3%.

Albay Pure Venom *(Dome/Hollister-Stier, UK)*. Freeze-dried powder prepared from bee or wasp venom, with mannitol 2%, providing on reconstitution at full strength a solution containing venom 100 µg per ml; supplied with diluent containing in each ml albumin 300 µg, sodium chloride 9 mg, and phenol 4 mg in Water for Injections. For diagnosis and treatment of allergy to bee and wasp stings.

Allpyral-G *(Dome/Hollister-Stier, UK)*. A pyridine-extracted alum-precipitated extract from 5 common grasses suspended in sodium chloride solution 0.9% and preserved with phenol 0.4%, in sets of 3 vials. For hyposensitisation therapy. **Allpyral Specific Vaccines** are similar extracts of pollens and other inhalant allergens formulated according to each patient's requirements. **Allpyral Specific (stinging insects)**. A pyridine-extracted alum-precipitated antigen complex in aqueous suspension, prepared from the whole bodies of bees and/or wasps, in vials of graded strengths.

Allpyral-Mite Fortified House Dust *(Dome/Hollister-Stier, UK)*. A pyridine-extracted alum-precipitated extract prepared from house dust, with added house dust mites (*Dermatophagoides farinae*), suspended in sodium chloride solution 0.9% and preserved with phenol 0.4%, in sets of 3 vials of graded strengths. For hyposensitisation therapy. **Allpyral-D.** A similar vaccine prepared from house dust mites (*Dermatophagoides pteronyssinus*), in sets of 3 vials of graded strengths.

Bencard Skin Testing Solutions *(Bencard, UK)*. A range of aqueous allergen extracts for the identification of the causative allergens in hay fever, asthma, and other allergic conditions; available as solutions for prick or intradermal testing. Prick test solutions also contain glycerol 50%, sodium chloride 6%, and phenol 0.5%; solutions for intradermal use also contain a phosphate buffer and phenol 0.5%. Prick test solutions must not be used for intradermal testing.

Conjuvac Two Grass *(Dome/Hollister-Stier, UK)*. A freeze-dried extract of the allergens of timothy grass and cocksfoot grass pollens, conjugated with sodium alginate; available in a set of 12 single-dose vials of 3 graded strengths for graduated dosage, supplied with 2-ml ampoules of Water for Injections. For hyposensitisation. Also available in a set of 4 vials of the highest strengths for maintenance therapy.

Glycerinated Skin Testing Solutions *(Dome/Hollister-Stier, UK)*. A range of aqueous allergen extracts with glycerol 50% and phenol 0.4%. For allergy testing by the prick or scratch methods.

Merck Skin Testing Solutions *(E. Merck, UK)*. A range of aqueous allergen extracts containing glycerol 50% and phenol 0.4%; available in a range to match the extracts used in Norisen vaccines. For allergy testing by a modified prick test (skin) or by nasal-provocation testing.

Migen (known in some countries as Bencard A, Bencard HDM, or Tyrivac) *(Bencard, UK)*. A vaccine prepared from tyrosine-adsorbed glycerolated extract of house-dust mite (*Dermatophagoides pteronyssinus*) containing tyrosine 4% and preserved with phenol. Available in sets of 6 disposable syringes containing 0.5 ml of vaccine in graded strengths providing graduated doses and in a single (maximum) strength for maintenance. For hyposensitisation therapy when house-dust mite is the principal allergen.

Norisen *(E. Merck, UK)*. A vaccine, formulated according to each patient's requirements, prepared from aluminium-adsorbed extracts of a range of allergens, including whole-body extracts of bee, hornet, and wasp; supplied as suspensions in sodium chloride solution 0.9% with phenol 0.4% as preservative; available in sets of 3 vials of graded strengths. For hyposensitisation.

Norisen Grass *(E. Merck, UK)*. An aluminium-adsorbed extract of 6 common grass pollens, suspended in sodium chloride solution 0.9% and preserved with phenol 0.4%, in sets of 3 × 4.5-ml vials of graduated strengths. For hyposensitisation therapy.

Pharmalgen *(Pharmacia, UK)*. Freeze-dried powder prepared from bee or wasp venom, supplied with diluent providing on reconstitution a solution containing in each ml venom 100 µg, albumin 600 µg, mannitol 30 mg, sodium chloride 9 mg, and phenol 4 mg in Water for Injections. For diagnosis and treatment of allergy to bee and wasp stings.

Pollinex *(Bencard, UK)*. A tyrosine-adsorbed vaccine containing glutaraldehyde-modified extracts from 12 varieties of common grass pollens, available in sets of 3 × 0.5-ml syringes providing graduated doses. For pre-seasonal treatment of hay fever and pollen asthma.

SDV Specific Desensitising Vaccine (known in some countries as S.D.L.) *(Bencard, UK)*. An aqueous solution of allergen extracts with sodium chloride 0.9% and phenol 0.5% as preservative, formulated according to each patient's requirements from a wide range of allergens, in sets of 3 × 10-ml vials of graded strengths usually providing 18 graduated doses for subcutaneous use: the third (full strength) solution is also available (without pollen allergens) in vials of 10 ml for maintenance therapy. If, exceptionally, courses including pollen allergen are administered during the pollination season a special low-dose schedule must be followed.

Spectralgen *(Pharmacia, UK)*. Freeze-dried extracts of grass and tree pollens; all supplied in sets of 4 vials of graded strengths for intial treatment or single vials for maintenance treatment, with either NSA Diluent containing albumin, sodium chloride, and phenol, or Depot Diluent containing aluminium hydroxide, disodium edetate, sodium chloride, and phenol. **Spectralgen Pollens (Single Species).** Prepared from any of 4 common grass allergens or 3 common tree allergens. For diagnosis or hyposensitisation. **Spectralgen Pollens (4 Grass Mix).** Prepared from a mixture of the grass allergens available in the Single Species presentation. For hyposensitisation. **Spectralgen Pollens (3 Tree Mix).** Prepared from a mixture of the tree allergens available in the Single Species presentation. For hyposensitisation.

Propranolol and other Beta-adrenoceptor Blocking Agents

6300-v

Propranolol and other beta-adrenoceptor blocking agents or antagonists are competitive inhibitors of the effects of catecholamines at beta-adrenergic receptor sites (see Adrenaline and other Sympathomimetics, p.1). They are also known as beta-adrenoreceptor or beta-adrenergic blocking agents. The principal effect of beta-adrenoceptor blockade is to reduce cardiac activity by diminishing or preventing beta-adrenoceptor stimulation. By reducing the rate and force of contraction of the heart, and decreasing the rate of conduction of impulses through the conducting system, the response of the heart to stress and exercise is reduced. These properties are used in the treatment of angina pectoris to reduce the oxygen consumption and increase the exercise tolerance of the heart. They are used in the treatment of cardiac arrhythmias to block adrenergic stimulation of cardiac pacemaker potentials.

The beta-adrenoceptor blocking agents are also beneficial in the long-term treatment of hypertension but their mode of action has not yet been fully elucidated. They are generally used with thiazide diuretics and do not usually give rise to postural hypotension.

Since beta-adrenoceptor blocking agents reduce the responses to the beta-adrenoceptor stimulating effects of adrenaline they are used (in conjunction with an alpha-adrenoceptor blocking agent) in the management of phaeochromocytoma, and they have also been used for the symptomatic relief of catecholamine-provoked tremor in conditions such as anxiety or hyperthyroidism.

The actions and uses of beta-adrenoceptor blocking agents are mainly described under Propranolol Hydrochloride.

An account of beta-adrenergic receptors, their recognition and regulation.— R. J. Lefkowitz, *New Engl. J. Med.*, 1976, *295*, 323.

A review of adrenoceptors.— G. M. Lees, *Br. med. J.*, 1981, *283*, 173.

An account of beta-adrenoceptor blockade, past, present, and future. The reason that beta-adrenoceptor blocking drugs lower the blood pressure seems to be a property of their beta-receptor inhibitory action. Regardless of associated properties, the presence or absence of membrane-stabilising or sympathomimetic action, hypotensive effect is seen. A number of suggestions have been made to explain their hypotensive effect, including an effect on the CNS, an adrenergic neurone-blocking action, an anti-renin effect, an effect secondary to the reduced cardiac output, and, finally, a mechanism consequent on resetting the baroreceptors. It may be that a drug with such wide actions as a beta-receptor inhibitory drug may act to lower blood pressure by more than one mechanism. Providing patients are selected properly (excluding those with heart failure and asthma), adverse effects to beta-adrenoceptor blocking drugs are uncommon; severe adverse reactions may occur soon after initiation of therapy, even with small doses, but once therapy has been started, gradual dosage increase is most unlikely to be associated with precipitate adverse reactions. There is evidence that beta-adrenoceptor blocking drugs are of similar potency to adrenergic neurone inhibitory drugs and methyldopa. The beta-adrenoceptor blocking drugs have the advantage of the absence of postural and exercise hypotension, and possible long-term benefits in reducing the manifestations of ischaemic heart disease.— B. N. C. Prichard, *Br. J. clin. Pharmac.*, 1978, *5*, 379.

Choice and Classification of a Beta-adrenoceptor Blocking Agent. Although the clinical action of beta-adrenoceptor blocking agents seems to be a property of their beta-receptor inhibitory activity, associated properties, such as the presence or absence of cardioselectivity, membrane-stabilising (or local anaesthetic; or quinidine-like) activity, and intrinsic sympathomimetic action (ISA; or partial agonist activity) have been used (initially by J.D. Fitzgerald, *Clin. Pharmac. Ther.*, 1969, *10*, 292, and *Acta Cardiol.*, 1972, *Suppl.* 25, 199) as a basis for their classification. Accordingly, they are divided into non-cardioselective drugs (Division I) and cardioselective drugs (Division II). Both groups are then sub-divided depending on the presence or absence of membrane-stabilising activity and intrinsic sympathomimetic activity. Thus:

Division I, Group I drugs are non-cardioselective and possess both membrane activity and intrinsic sympathomimetic activity, e.g. alprenolol, p.1336, oxprenolol, p.1344;

Division I, Group II drugs are non-cardioselective and possess membrane activity but no intrinsic sympathomimetic activity, e.g. propranolol, p.1325;

Division I, Group III drugs are non-cardioselective, have no membrane activity but do possess intrinsic sympathomimetic activity, e.g. pindolol, p.1347;

Division I, Group IV drugs are non-cardioselective, and possess neither membrane activity nor intrinsic sympathomimetic activity, e.g. sotalol, p.1350, timolol, p.1351; and:

Division II, Group I drugs are cardioselective and possess both membrane activity and intrinsic sympathomimetic activity, e.g. acebutolol, p.1335;

Division II, Group II drugs are cardioselective and possess membrane activity but no intrinsic sympathomimetic activity;

Division II, Group III drugs are cardioselective, have no membrane activity but do possess intrinsic sympathomimetic activity, e.g. practolol, p.1348;

Division II, Group IV drugs are cardioselective, but possess neither membrane activity nor instrinsic sympathomimetic activity, e.g. atenolol, p.1337, metoprolol, p.1342.

A third group, Division III, describes beta-adrenoceptor blocking agents which also possess alpha-adrenoceptor blocking activity, e.g. labetalol, p.1339. The additional alpha-adrenoceptor blocking properties of labetalol confer upon it a much more rapid onset of action, some enhancement of antihypertensive effect, and a certain incidence of postural hypotension.

Since the therapeutic effectiveness of the beta-adrenoceptor blocking agents seems to depend on their beta-blocking action and since most side-effects stem from this action there is in general, little to choose between them when given in equi-effective doses. The membrane-stabilising and intrinsic sympathomimetic activities associated with some beta-adrenoceptor blocking agents are of pharmacological interest only; any clinical significance has yet to be demonstrated.

The cardioselective properties of some beta-adrenoceptor blocking agents may, however, confer upon them some advantage. Practolol was found to have a more selective action on the receptors in the heart (termed β_1 receptors) than on those in the lungs (termed β_2 receptors). This cardioselective property of practolol led to a reduced incidence of some side-effects, such as bronchospasm, which are common with the non-selective beta-adrenoceptor blocking agents. Unfortunately, its association with a series of severe sensitivity reactions has militated against its long-term use (see Adverse Effects of Practolol, p.1348). Modest cardioselective properties have also been demonstrated for other beta-adrenoceptor blocking agents (see above), but serious increases in airways resistance have, nevertheless, been associated with members of this group, including practolol itself.

A discussion on beta-adrenoceptor antagonists and methodological problems associated with assessing their effect on respiratory function. The situation remains that cardioselective beta-adrenoceptor blocking drugs must be preferred (at least on theoretical grounds) in patients with bronchial asthma or chronic obstructive airways disease. There is some evidence that non-selective drugs with intrinsic sympathomimetic (partial agonist) activity are preferable to non-selective drugs without this property, but the suggestion that these agents are as good as or better than cardioselective drugs must be regarded as unproven. It is still necessary to use all these drugs cautiously, recognising that an individual patient may suffer a deterioration of respiratory function with any beta-adrenoceptor antagonist.— D. G. McDevitt, *Br. J. clin. Pharmac.*, 1978, *5*, 97. Comments and criticisms.— W. H. Perks *et al.* (letter), *ibid.*, *6*, 171; C. R. Kumana (letter), *ibid.*, 172; V. M. S. Oh *et al.* (letter), *ibid.*, 173. Reply.— D. G. McDevitt (letter), *ibid.*, 174.

A warning that, despite their selectivity, β_1-adrenoceptor antagonists might block β_2-receptors in coronary vessels in the same way as they are able to cause bronchospasm in asthmatics by blockade of β_2-receptors in the lung as the dose increases.— M. E. Conolly (letter), *New Engl. J. Med.*, 1979, *300*, 864.

Discussion on the choice of the more cardioselective beta-blocking agents for patients who are also diabetic.— *Lancet*, 1977, *1*, 843.

Further comparative reviews: *Drug & Ther. Bull.*, 1974, *12*, 33; H. J. Waal-Manning, *Drugs*, 1976, *12*, 412; B. N. C. Prichard, *Practitioner*, 1977, *219*, 501; C. R. Kumana and G. E. Marlin, *Recent Adv. clin. Pharmac.*, 1978, *1*, 31 to 54.

Beta-adrenoceptor Blocking Therapy during Anaesthesia. Beta-adrenoceptor blocking agents alter the response of the body to stress and depress the myocardium. Some authorities have advocated temporary withdrawal prior to anaesthesia in order to provide better control of the circulatory system, but sudden withdrawal may expose the patient to severe uncontrolled angina or cardiac arrhythmias. There are also operative risks associated with uncontrolled hypertension. Anaesthesia may proceed safely under beta-adrenoceptor blockade provided that the patient is protected against bradycardia by the intravenous administration of atropine 1 to 2 mg, and provided that anaesthetic agents causing myocardial depression, such as ether, chloroform, cyclopropane, and trichloroethylene, are avoided.

Awareness by the anaesthetist that beta-adrenoceptor blocking agents are being taken is of the greatest importance.

In a study of 78 patients who underwent coronary bypass surgery and who had been receiving long-term propranolol therapy, the withdrawal of propranolol at 12 hours before surgery resulted in fewer complications during anaesthesia than withdrawal at 24 to 72 hours before surgery. The continuation of propranolol had no adverse effect on cardiac resuscitation after bypass or any adverse influence on recovery and it was recommended that propranolol therapy should continue to 6 to 12 hours before coronary bypass surgery.— S. Slogoff *et al.*, *J. Am. med. Ass.*, 1978, *240*, 1487.

We have found that the patient maintained on stable antihypertensive therapy up to and including the day of surgery has the best chance of a successful outcome. This is particularly so with hypertensive patients receiving clonidine and those on beta-receptor antagonists for the treatment of angina.— C. Prys-Roberts (letter), *Lancet*, 1979, *2*, 529.

Similar reports, comments, and recommendations: C. Prys-Roberts *et al.*, *Br. J. Anaesth.*, 1973, *45*, 671; D. G. Shand, *New Engl. J. Med.*, 1975, *293*, 449; *Med. Lett.*, 1976, *18*, 41; C. J. Kopriva *et al.*, *Anesthesiology*, 1978, *48*, 28; W. T. Edwards (letter), *New Engl. J. Med.*, 1979, *301*, 158.

Controlled hypotension. For a discussion of the use of beta-adrenoceptor blocking agents in controlled hypotension during surgery, see G. E. H. Enderby, *Postgrad. med. J.*, 1974, *50*, 572; A. P. Adams, *Br. J. Anaesth.*, 1975, *47*, 777.

Interactions. Severe bradycardia developed in a patient receiving propranolol therapy when he was given neostigmine and atropine concurrently for reversal of pancuronium blockade. The last dose of propranolol had been given 10 hours prior to induction of anaesthesia. It was suggested that in patients who had been taking propranolol, atropine should be given before neostigmine for reversal of neuromuscular blockade.— D. H. Sprague, *Anesthesiology*, 1975, *42*, 208.

6301-g

Propranolol Hydrochloride *(B.P., U.S.P.).* AY 64043; ICI 45520. (±)-1-Isopropylamino-3-(1-naphthyloxy)propan-2-ol hydrochloride. $C_{16}H_{21}NO_2,HCl=295.8$.

CAS — 525-66-6 (propranolol)[5051-22-9(+); 4199-09-1(−); 13013-17-7(±)]; 318-98-9 (hydrochloride)[13071-11-9(+); 4199-10-4(−); 3506-09-0(±)].

Pharmacopoeias. In *Br., Braz., Chin., Jap., Nord.,* and *U.S.*

A white or off-white odourless powder with a bitter taste. M.p. about 164°. It absorbs less than 1% of moisture at relative humidities of up to 80% at 25°.

Soluble 1 in 20 of water and alcohol; slightly soluble in chloroform; practically insoluble in ether. A 1% solution in water has a pH of 5 to 6. Solutions should be **sterilised** by autoclaving or by filtration. In aqueous solutions it decomposes with oxidation of the isopropylamine side-chain, accompanied by a reduction in pH and discoloration of the solution. Solutions are most stable at pH 3 and decompose rapidly when alkaline. **Protect** from light.

Stability tests on a suspension of propranolol hydrochloride for oral administration.— G. C. Brown and J. B. Kayes, *J. clin. Pharm.*, 1976, *1*, 29.

Adverse Effects. The most common side-effects of propranolol are nausea, vomiting, diarrhoea, fatigue, and dizziness. Cardiovascular effects include bradycardia, congestive heart failure, heart block, hypotension, cold extremities, Raynaud's phenomenon, and paraesthesia. Central nervous system effects include depression, hallucinations, and disturbances of sleep and vision. Bronchospasm may occur, particularly in susceptible individuals. Blood disorders and skin rashes may also occur. Other adverse effects reported include constipation, fluid retention and weight gain, muscle cramps, and dry mouth.

Side-effects may be minimised by starting treatment with a small dose and gradually increasing, although serious reactions have been reported after small doses.

In a Boston collaborative drug survey the following adverse reactions to propranolol occurred among a total of 319 hospital in-patients: pulmonary oedema (3), bradycardia and shock (3), complete heart block (1), bradycardia and angina (1), asymptomatic bradycardia (5), hypotension and syncope (5), asymptomatic hypotension (3), gastro-intestinal disturbance (3), dizziness (2), fatigue (1), fluid retention (1), 2:1 heart block (1), blurring of vision (1). In a survey of 23 published reports in which propranolol was administered by mouth to a total of 797 out-patients treated for periods of a few weeks to 6 years, the following adverse reactions were noted: gastro-intestinal disturbances (11.2%), cold extremities or exacerbation of Raynaud's phenomenon (5.8%), congestive heart failure (5.4%), sleep disturbances (4.3%), dizziness (4.1%), fatigue (3.1%), bronchospasm (2.6%), mental depression (1.6%), paraesthesias (1.5%), bradycardia (0.8%), hallucinations (0.8%), skin rash (0.8%), hypotension (0.5%), muscle cramps (0.5%), dry mouth (0.4%), heart block (0.3%), and blurring of vision (0.1%).— D. J. Greenblatt and J. Koch-Weser, *Drugs*, 1974, *7*, 118.

Other reviews of the incidence and management of adverse effects associated with propranolol and other beta-adrenoceptor blocking agents: *Br. med. J.*, 1977, *1*, 529; M. A. Riddiough, *Am. J. Hosp. Pharm.*, 1977, *34*, 465; G. L. Sanders, *Adverse Drug React. Bull.*, 1978, Feb., 240; *idem*, Apr., 247; *Lancet*, 1981, *2*, 539 (Medical Research Council Working Party on Mild to Moderate Hypertension).

Propranolol as a cause of watery nasal secretion.— L. Malm (letter), *Lancet*, 1981, *1*, 1006.

Allergy. Forty-five minutes after her first dose of propranolol hydrochloride 20 mg, a 29-year-old moderately hypertensive woman suffered severe laryngospasm and died 24 days later. Although she had previously received tablets containing tartrazine without symptoms of allergy it was believed that she had suffered an allergic reaction to the tartrazine in propranolol hydrochloride tablets although allergy to propranolol itself could not be ruled out.— S. J. Morris *et al.*, *Archs intern. Med.*, 1977, *137*, 1222.

Deafness. The Boston Collaborative Drug Surveillance Program monitored consecutively 32 812 medical inpatients. Drug-induced deafness occurred in 1 of 853 patients given propranolol.— J. Porter and H. Jick, *Lancet*, 1977, *1*, 587.

Tinnitus. Tinnitus followed the administration of propranolol in a dose of 10 mg twice daily for 4 days.— R. H. Lloyd-Mostyn (letter), *Br. med. J.*, 1969, *2*, 766.

Dupuytren's contracture. Fibrosing conditions developed in 2 patients during treatment with propranolol. Peyronie's disease [penile fibrosis] occurred in 1 and the other developed Dupuytren's contracture of both hands.— W. W. Coupland (letter), *Med. J. Aust.*, 1977, *2*, 137.

Dyskinesia. A 35-year-old woman with a history of dystonic reactions to neuroleptic drugs suffered a similar reaction when her dose of propranolol reached 600 mg twice daily. Symptoms included rolled-up eyes, clenched teeth, perspiration and salivation, distortion of body and limbs, and arching of the back.— J. P. Crawford (letter), *Br. med. J.*, 1977, *2*, 1156.

Effects on the blood. *Agranulocytosis.* A 64-year-old man with cardiac arrhythmia who received propranolol 40 mg daily with procainamide 4 g daily for 6 weeks then propranolol alone 40 mg every 4 hours for 6 days developed agranulocytosis. On cessation of propranolol therapy he recovered completely.— I. U. Nawabi and N. D. Ritz, *J. Am. med. Ass.*, 1973, *223*, 1376.

Platelet adhesiveness. Increased platelet adhesiveness associated with abrupt withdrawal of propranolol.— W. H. Frishman *et al.*, *Am. Heart J.*, 1978, *95*, 169.

References to inhibition of platelet adhesiveness by propranolol: J. R. Hampton *et al.*, *Cardiovasc. Res.*, 1967, *1*, 101; W. H. Frishman *et al.*, *Circulation*, 1974, *50*, 887.

Thrombocytopenic purpura. One case of thrombocytopenic purpura had been reported following administration of propranolol and 2 cases of non-thrombocytopenic purpura.— S. A. Stephen, *Am. J. Cardiol.*, 1966, *18*, 463.

Effects on bones and joints. A patient developed severe incapacitating pain in her hip during propranolol treatment, which was relieved when her treatment was changed to practolol.— N. -H. Areskog and L. Adolfsson, *Br. med. J.*, 1969, *2*, 601.

Effects on the circulation. Intermittent claudication was reported in 4 patients who had been treated with propranolol or practolol in doses of 120 to 300 mg daily for 3 weeks to 6 months.— J. C. Rodger *et al.*, *Br. med. J.*, 1976, *1*, 1125. Comment.— A. F. Lant and D. O. Gibbons (letter), *ibid.*, 1469.

Of 117 patients, usually with hypertension or angina, treated with a single drug (propranolol 42, practolol 19, oxprenolol 56) 22 had cold extremities before treatment; 5 were made worse; 18 patients developed cold extremities for the first time.— D. Trash *et al.* (letter), *Br. med. J.*, 1976, *2*, 527.

Vascular symptoms in patients with primary Raynaud's phenomenon were not exacerbated by propranolol or labetalol taken by mouth.— J. A. Steiner *et al.* (letter), *Br. J. clin. Pharmac.*, 1979, *7*, 401.

Bilateral incipient gangrene of the feet in 2 patients associated with the use of beta-adrenoceptor blocking agents.— D. A. O'Rourke *et al.* (letter), *Med. J. Aust.*, 1979, *2*, 88.

Further references: E. D. Frochlich *et al.*, *J. Am. med. Ass.*, 1969, *208*, 2471; P. D. McSorley and D. J. Warren, *Br. med. J.*, 1978, *2*, 1598; R. N. Fogoros (letter), *New Engl. J. Med.*, 1980, *302*, 1089.

Effects on the eyes. When 483 hypertensive patients being treated with propranolol or other hypotensive drugs were questioned about symptoms of gritty feelings, sore or red eyes, photophobia, and the need to use eye-drops, between 12 and 30% gave positive answers. There was no indication that patients taking beta-adrenoceptor blocking drugs were more likely to complain of eye symptoms than patients on other antihypertensive therapy.— C. T. Dollery *et al.*, *Br. J. clin. Pharmac.*, 1977, *4*, 295.

Ocular symptoms were reported by 14 of 71 patients when taking practolol but only by 4 of the 71 before practolol treatment. Skin rash was reported by 16 during but 8 before treatment; both ocular symptoms and rash occurred in 7 during and 1 before treatment. A similar investigation of 246 patients who had taken propranolol showed a smaller insignificant difference in the incidence of eye complaints consisting of 42 patients during and 31 patients before propranolol treatment. The overall incidence of rash was not significantly greater during propranolol treatment but 14 patients had both an eye complaint and rash during treatment compared to 4 patients before treatment.— D. C. G. Skegg and R. Doll, *Lancet*, 1977, *2*, 475.

Eye symptoms, including early cataract in 1 eye, occurred in a 70-year-old man during treatment with propranolol, and abated at the end of each course of treatment.— T. J. Halloran (letter), *J. Am. med. Ass.*, 1979, *241*, 2784.

For a statement that serious side-effects of the type induced by practolol were uncommon with other beta-adrenoceptor blocking agents, see Practolol, p.1348.

Effects on the gastro-intestinal tract. A report of retroperitoneal fibrosis associated with propranolol in one patient.— J. R. Pierce *et al.* (letter), *Ann. intern. Med.*, 1981, *95*, 244.

Effects on the heart. In 7 patients with mitral stenosis, propranolol was given during exercise and at rest. The decrease in heart-rate could have increased total diastolic time and allowed more blood to pass the mitral valve, but in practice there was a further overall decrease in cardiac performance.— G. R. Cumming and W. Carr, *Can. med. Ass. J.*, 1966, *95*, 527.

Heart failure occurred in 4 patients with atrial fibrillation and chronic rheumatic valvular disease who were given propranolol to control the ventricle-rate when digitalis failed.— N. Conway *et al.*, *Br. med. J.*, 1968, *2*, 213.

Propranolol 40 mg daily for 1 week caused an intermittent atrioventricular block in a 38-year-old man with angina pectoris.— M. Ilyas (letter), *New Engl. J. Med.*, 1972, *286*, 376.

A patient receiving propranolol developed syncopal episodes while eating or drinking.— J. Schluger *et al.*, *Chest*, 1973, *64*, 651.

Thirty-five elderly patients with severe chest pain but no ECG evidence of myocardial infarction were noted to be receiving propranolol or oxprenolol.— M. S. Pathy, *Am. Heart J.*, 1979, *98*, 168.

Severe bradycardia in 2 patients was associated with propranolol therapy.— M. M. Scheinman *et al.*, *Am. J. Med.*, 1978, *64*, 1013.

Chronic beta-blocker treatment may sometimes paradoxically be the cause of abnormal T-wave inversion.— T. M. Griffith *et al.*, *Br. med. J.*, 1982, *284*, 19. See also under Sotalol Hydrochloride, p.1350.

Effects on lipid metabolism. Of 379 men who had been regularly followed for at least 5 years as untreated controls in the Oslo study drug trial of mild hypertension, the effects of propranolol alone, prazosin alone, and propranolol in association with prazosin, were studied in 23 with a stable diastolic blood pressure of 100 mmHg or more; each patient was given each of the 3 treatments for 8-week periods in a randomised crossover trial design. Propranolol significantly reduced both high-density-lipoprotein cholesterol and the cholesterol ratio, and increased total triglycerides. Conversely, prazosin reduced total cholesterol by reducing the low-density-lipoprotein plus very-low-density-lipoprotein fraction, and had no significant effect on high-density-lipoprotein cholesterol, so that the cholesterol ratio was significantly increased; total triglycerides were also significantly reduced by prazosin. The effects on lipids of the association of propranolol and prazosin included features of both, but owing partly to opposite effects of the 2 drugs, the net effect was small and did not reach statistical significance; the only significant effect of the association was a reduced high-density-lipoprotein cholesterol value. Propranolol alone significantly raised the serum-uric-acid concentration; this was also raised after the association of propranolol and prazosin but remained within normal limits, although the propranolol-induced rise might achieve clinical importance if the association were to be given with a diuretic. The clinical importance of the observed effects of the antihypertensives on blood lipids is uncertain, but all pharmacological effects of antihypertensive drugs should be taken into consideration, particularly when embarking on life-long treatment for young people.— P. Leren *et al.*, *Lancet*, 1980, *2*, 4. Comment.— *ibid.*, 19.

Treatment with beta-blockers had no effect on plasma lipid and urate concentrations in a study of 51 hypertensive patients who had received propranolol (47 patients), atenolol (2), or metoprolol (2) for an average of 54 (range 8 to 79) months.— B. Ø. Kristensen, *Br. med. J.*, 1981, *283*, 191.

Further references: N. Tanaka *et al.*, *Metabolism*, 1976, *25*, 1071; A. Helgeland *et al.*, *Br. med. J* 1978, *2*, 403; D. Streja and D. Mymin (letter), *ibid.*, 1978, *2*, 1495; P. Bielmann *et al.* (letter), *New Engl. J. Med.*, 1980, *302*, 298.

Effects on the liver. In a 69-year-old woman receiving propranolol, serum concentrations of aspartate aminotransferase (SGOT), lactic dehydrogenase, and alkaline phosphatase rose, and returned to normal when propranolol was withdrawn.— R. Wilkinson *et al.* (letter), *Br. med. J.*, 1971, *2*, 276.

Further references: P. Munzenberger and SisterEmmanuel, *Am. J. Hosp. Pharm.*, 1971, *28*, 786.

Effects on mental state. Depression occurred in 28 of 89 patients given propranolol for cardiac arrhythmias. The incidence was highest in patients treated for periods over 3 months with doses higher than 120 mg daily.— H. J. Waal (letter), *Br. med. J.*, 1967, *2*, 50. There was no indication that an important incidence of depression was associated with propranolol administration.— J. D. Fitzgerald, *I.C.I.* (letter), *ibid.*, 372. A brief discussion of the role of beta-adrenoceptor blocking agents in causing depression.— F. A. Whitlock and L. E. J. Evans, *Drugs*, 1978, *15*, 53.

An acute brain syndrome similar to thyroid storm occurred in one patient being treated with propranolol. Symptoms, which included agitation, confusion, and paranoia, improved rapidly when propranolol was withdrawn.— D. Topliss and R. Bond (letter), *Lancet*, 1977, *2*, 1133. Another similar case.— L. Helson and L. Duque (letter), *ibid.*, 1978, *1*, 98.

Visual hallucinations or illusions occurred in 11 of 63 patients taking propranolol 80 to 320 mg daily, alone or with diuretics for hypertension.— R. Fleminger, *Br. med. J.*, 1978, *1*, 1182. In a 53-year-old woman, with a family history of schizophrenia but no personal history, schizophrenic symptoms, occurring when the dose of propranolol was increased, regressed when propranolol was withdrawn.— J. Steinert and C. R. Pugh, *ibid.*, 1979, *1*, 790.

Further references: R. D. Hinshelwood (letter), *Br. med. J.*, 1969, *2*, 445; H. S. Fraser and A. C. Carr (letter), *Br. J. Psychiat.*, 1976, *129*, 508; B. M. Kuhr, *J. clin. Psychiat.*, 1979, *40*, 198; M. L. Kurland (letter), *New Engl. J. Med.*, 1979, *300*, 366; E. S. Gershon *et al.*, *Ann. intern. Med.*, 1979, *90*, 938.

Effects on the muscles. Three patients who were taking conventional doses of propranolol or oxprenolol developed myasthenia gravis or a myasthenia-like syndrome. It was considered that beta-blocking agents were capable of enhancing a myasthenic condition.— Y. Herishanu and P. Rosenberg (letter), *Ann. intern. Med.*, 1975, *83*, 834.

Clinical myotonia occurred in a patient receiving propranolol and disappeared when treatment was stopped. Examination of biopsy material revealed a pre-existing mild dystrophia myotonica.— W. Blessing and J. C. Walsh (preliminary communication), *Lancet*, 1977, *1*, 73. See also S. Satya-Murti *et al.* (letter), *New Engl. J. Med.*, 1977, *297*, 223.

A study in 6 healthy subjects indicated that neither propranolol nor metoprolol reduced muscle strength, coordination, endurance, or perception of effort. So far, no direct explanation can be given for the clinical experience of muscle fatigue associated with beta-adrenoceptor blockade.— G. Grimby and U. Smith (letter), *Lancet*, 1978, *2*, 1318.

Proximal myopathy in a 68-year-old woman who had taken sotalol for several months persisted when sotalol was replaced by propranolol, regressed when propranolol was withdrawn, and recurred when it was again given.— J. C. Forfar, *Br. med. J.*, 1979, *2*, 1331.

A report of muscle wasting in 3 patients with thyrotoxicosis taking beta-blockers.— M. Uusitupa *et al.* (letter), *Br. med. J.*, 1980, *280*, 183.

Comment on muscle fatigue as a side-effect of beta-adrenoceptor blockade.— *Lancet*, 1980, *1*, 1285.

Effects on respiratory function. Propranolol given by intravenous injection in doses of 10 mg to healthy persons and in doses of 5 mg to asthmatics resulted in significant mean rises in airway resistance. In healthy persons the rise was not accompanied by any respiratory upset. In asthmatics there was a much greater rise in airway resistance and it usually resulted in dyspnoea, and occasionally in wheezing. Atropine sulphate in a dose of 1.2 mg by intravenous injection almost completely abolished the rise in airway resistance in normal persons and markedly reduced the rise in asthmatics.— A. G. Macdonald *et al.*, *Br. J. Anaesth.*, 1967, *39*, 919.

A drop of about 35% in specific airway conductance occurred in 5 asthmatic patients after an injection of 10 mg of propranolol whilst there was no significant effect in 10 normal subjects.— P. S. Richardson and G. M. Sterling, *Br. med. J.*, 1969, *3*, 143.

Effects on sexual function. Of 95 men treated with propranolol, 5 developed erectile dysfunction with doses of 120 mg or more daily.— S. C. Warren and S. G. Warren (letter), *Ann. intern. Med.*, 1977, *86*, 112. A further report of probable propranolol-induced reversible impotence in one patient.— R. A. Miller (letter), *Ann. intern. Med.*, 1976, *85*, 682.

See also under Peyronie's disease.

Effects on the skin. A brown discoloration of the tongue occurred in 2 patients taking propranolol for cardiac arrhythmias.— F. Raleigh, *Drug Intell. & clin. Pharm.*, 1975, *9*, 455.

Cutaneous thickening in 6 hyperthyroid patients treated with radioactive iodine and beta-blockade might have been associated with the beta-blocking therapy, with special reference to sotalol.— J. P. Michel *et al.* (letter), *Lancet*, 1979, *1*, 54.

Alopecia. A case of reversible alopecia occurred on administration of propranolol. The causal relationship was confirmed by drug challenge.— C. M. Martin *et al.*, *Am. Heart J.*, 1973, *86*, 236.

Further references: R. J. Hilder, *Cutis*, 1979, *24*, 63.

Cheilostomatitis. A 65-year-old woman with dryness and soreness of the mouth, and with ulcerations of the lower lip and buccal mucosa, had been taking propranolol for about 5 years. Symptoms subsided over 12 weeks when propranolol was withdrawn and alprenolol was given, recurred within a week on propranolol challenge, and again subsided when propranolol was withdrawn.— S. E. Tangsrud and S. Golf, *Br. med. J.*, 1977, *2*, 1385.

Erythema multiforme. Erythema multiforme developed in a patient after several months' treatment with propranolol as the sole therapy for hyperthyroidism.— B. Pimstone *et al.*, *S. Afr. med. J.*, 1969, *43*, 1203.

Necrosis. Three patients developed foot pain, with multiple areas of skin necrosis, but with palpable foot pulses, while taking beta-adrenoceptor blocking agents. The necrosis resolved when medication was withdrawn.— R. Gokal *et al.*, *Br. med. J.*, 1978, *1*, 721. See also B. I. Hoffbrand (letter), *ibid.*, 1979, *1*, 1082.

Psoriasiform eruptions. Details of 6 patients who developed reversible psoriasiform cutaneous eruptions during long-term propranolol therapy, similar to those reported after practolol.— H. A. Jensen *et al.*, *Acta med. scand.*, 1976, *199*, 363.

Further reports: P. L. Padfield *et al.* (letter), *Br. med. J.*, 1975, *1*, 626; N. J. Farr (letter), *ibid.*, 1976, *1*, 961; S. Halevy and E. J. Feuerman, *Cutis*, 1979, *24*, 95.

Urticaria. A woman developed giant urticaria following administration of propranolol 40 mg daily; the association was confirmed by rechallenge with propranolol 10 mg. Precipitation of the allergy by an additive in the tablets could not be excluded. She was successfully transferred to tolamolol therapy.— S. F. Seides *et al.*, *Chest*, 1975, *67*, 496.

Hyperkalaemia. Paradoxical changes in serum-potassium concentrations have been noted during cardiopulmonary bypass in association with non-cardioselective beta-adrenoceptor blockade.— D. W. Bethune and R. McKay (letter), *Lancet*, 1978, *2*, 380. Results confirming that beta-adrenoceptors are involved in the regulation of plasma-potassium concentrations.— E. Carlsson *et al.* (letter), *Lancet*, 1978, *2*, 424.

Further references: T. Nawar (letter), *Lancet*, 1978, *1*, 717.

Hypertension. Of 44 mental patients receiving propranolol in doses of 0.6 to 5 g daily for the treatment of psychoses, 8 developed a paradoxical rise in blood pressure; in 2 this was abrupt but in most the increase was progressive over 3 to 24 hours. The skin became pale, cold and clammy and the patients exhibited pronounced tension and outbursts of psychomotor unrest. In all cases the hypertension responded immediately to a single dose of phentolamine 15 to 30 mg intravenously, with phenoxybenzamine 10 to 20 mg daily for 3 to 4 days reducing the blood pressure to the previous low levels without discontinuing the propranolol; the other symptoms subsided with the blood pressure reduction. Most of the hypertensive episodes occurred when the propranolol dosage was increased after a previous reduction. In a few further cases when symptoms appeared phentolamine and phenoxybenzamine given together prevented the blood pressure rise despite continuing the propranolol.— I. Blum *et al.*, *Br. med. J.*, 1975, *4*, 623. Comment.— N. J. Yorkston *et al.* (letter), *ibid.*, 1976, *1*, 769.

Leaving aside the special cases of phaeochromocytoma and psychosis, the occasional fluid retention that occurs with beta-adrenoceptor blocking agents could explain the paradoxical rise in blood pressure sometimes occurring in patients receiving beta-adrenoceptor blocking drugs.— B. N. C. Prichard (letter), *Lancet*, 1977, *1*, 536.

Further references: I. Blum and A. Atsmon, *Am. Heart J.*, 1977, *93*, 802.

Hypoglycaemia. Severe hypoglycaemic episodes occurred in 2 children while taking propranolol. Both recovered after dextrose therapy. The children had been eating poorly prior to the episodes.— J. M. Feller (letter), *Med. J. Aust.*, 1973, *2*, 92. See also T. F. Mackintosh (letter), *Lancet*, 1967, *1*, 104 (operative use of propranolol).

Severe hypoglycaemia during haemodialysis occurred, after 24 hours of fasting, in a 20-year-old woman taking propranolol. The addition of dextrose to the dialysis fluid was recommended.— K. Samii *et al.* (letter), *Lancet*, 1976, *1*, 545. The use of propranolol did not appear to cause hypoglycaemia in a study of 10 hypertensive patients on chronic haemodialysis compared with 12 similar patients not taking beta-blocking agents.— H. A. Jensen *et al.* (letter), *ibid.*, 1976, *2*, 368.

Relatively selective beta-adrenoceptor blocking agents might be less likely to produce hypoglycaemia.— R. J. Newman, *Br. med. J.*, 1976, *2*, 447; S. P. Deacon (letter), *ibid.*, 587; S. P. Linton *et al.* (letter), *ibid.*, 877.

Further references to hypoglycaemia in association with propranolol: R. Wray and S. B. J. Sutcliffe (letter), *Br. med. J.*, 1972, *2*, 592; I. Lager *et al.*, *Lancet*, 1979, *1*, 458.

Diabetogenic effect. A patient taking propranolol 960 mg daily developed diabetes; the blood-sugar concentration returned to normal when propranolol was withdrawn and no further treatment was necessary.— R. J. Inglis (letter), *Br. med. J.*, 1979, *1*, 1795.

Further reports and comments on the diabetogenic effect of propranolol: S. Podolsky and C. G. Pattavina, *Metabolism*, 1973, *22*, 685; A. Antonis *et al.*, *Lancet*, 1967, *1*, 1135.

See also under Precautions.

Hypotension. A 49-year-old man with alcoholic cardiomyopathy developed severe hypotension after being given a single dose of 10 mg of propranolol by mouth for the treatment of atrial fibrillation.— J. H. N. Bett (letter), *Lancet*, 1968, *1*, 302.

A 33-year-old woman with an acute attack of intermittent porphyria, given 2 doses of 10 mg of propranolol with a 6-hour interval, developed bradycardia and hypotension.— H. L. Bonkowsky and D. P. Tschudy (letter), *Br. med. J.*, 1974, *4*, 47.

Migraine. In 2 patients propranolol appeared to have precipitated attacks of migraine.— C. J. Sharpe (letter), *Br. med. J.*, 1974, *3*, 522.

Further references: N. K. Blank and M. J. Rieder (letter), *Lancet*, 1973, *2*, 1336; R. H. Robson, *Br. Heart J.*, 1977, *39*, 1157.

Overdosage. A 45-year-old man who had taken about 2 g of propranolol in a suicide attempt showed no signs of cardiac disturbance during a 5-day stay in hospital.— W. Wermut and M. Wójcicki (letter), *Br. med. J.*, 1973, *3*, 591.

Severe cardiac disturbances occurred in a 24-year-old woman who ingested 1 g of propranolol, 100 ml of whisky, and some beer in a suicide attempt.— G. Frithz (letter), *Br. med. J.*, 1976, *1*, 769.

Fatalities following propranolol overdosage: R. Gault *et al.*, *Clin. Toxicol.*, 1977, *11*, 295; J. Kristinsson and T. Jóhannesson (letter), *Acta pharmac. tox.*, 1977, *41*, 190.

A report of generalised seizures and broadening of the QRS complex of the ECG in 2 patients following massive overdosage with propranolol. The possibility of drug-induced hypoglycaemia and other metabolic causes for the seizures was ruled out and although cerebral hypoperfusion may have contributed the second patient suffered convulsions despite an adequate blood pressure. It was suggested that the ECG changes may have been due to the membrane-stabilising effect of propranolol. Both patients recovered.— A. Buiumsohn *et al.*, *Ann. intern. Med.*, 1979, *91*, 860.

Peyronie's disease. Two patients taking propranolol developed pain in the penis on erection. Examination revealed fibrous plaques on the dorsum of the penis (Peyronie's disease). There might be an association between beta-adrenoceptor blocking agents and abnormal fibrous tissue production.— D. R. Osborne (letter), *Lancet*, 1977, *1*, 1111. Other cases.— A. A. Wallis *et al.* (letter), *ibid.*, 1977, *2*, 980; W. W. Coupland (letter), *Med. J. Aust.*, 1977, *2*, 137.

Of 146 patients with Peyronie's disease seen between January 1975 and May 1978, 19 had been on beta-adrenoceptor blocking therapy with propranolol (12), practolol (6), or both (1). None of a matched group of control patients had been taking these drugs. There might be an association between Peyronie's disease and beta-adrenoceptor blocking therapy or it might be that atherosclerosis and hypertension are the common aetiological factors.— J. P. Pryor and O. Khan (letter), *Lan-*

cet, 1979, *1*, 331. Investigation of the medical and drug history of 98 consecutive men with Peyronie's disease showed that only 5 had taken beta-adrenoceptor blocking agents before the onset of the disease. It is considered that chronic degenerative arterial disease rather than beta blockers is associated with Peyronie's disease.— J. P. Pryor and W. M. Castle (letter), *ibid.*, 1982, *1*, 917.

Shock. A 50-year-old man with a history of cardiomyopathy, congestive heart failure, and frequent atrial arrhythmias developed severe epigastric pain and diarrhoea and became profoundly collapsed after he was given 10 mg of propranolol by mouth. He made a good recovery when treated with isoprenaline. Challenge doses of 2.5 mg of propranolol produced only a soft bowel movement; 5 mg caused epigastric pain and a further bowel movement and a similar dose given 3 hours later caused epigastric pain and a fall in heart-rate. He became cyanosed and later circulatory collapse ensued. The patient recovered after intensive therapy. Because small doses of propranolol could cause profound shock and pancreatitis in susceptible individuals it was suggested that the first dose should be given in hospital.— J. A. Taylor (letter), *Lancet*, 1968, *1*, 532.

Treatment of Adverse Effects. Bradycardia and severe hypotension should be treated immediately by the intravenous injection of 1 to 2 mg or more of atropine followed, if necessary, by 25 µg of isoprenaline or 500 µg of orciprenaline by slow intravenous injection. Adrenaline has also been suggested for the treatment of hypotension.

Bronchospasm should be treated by the intravenous injection of aminophylline or by the inhalation or intravenous injection of isoprenaline.

Heart failure should be treated with digitalis and diuretic therapy.

High doses of glucagon have been found to be life-saving.

In overdosage the stomach should be emptied by aspiration and lavage, if ingestion is recent.

Recommendations for the treatment of overdosage with beta-adrenoceptor blocking agents. Gastric lavage is unlikely to prevent serious poisoning since all beta-adrenoceptor blocking drugs are absorbed rapidly. Estimation of blood concentrations may confirm poisoning but is of limited value. Although it has not been tried in gross overdosage, haemodialysis is unlikely to rid the body of propranolol, but it may be possible to dialyse beta-adrenoceptor blocking agents that are more water soluble and less protein bound. Optimum management involves intensive care facilities, and transvenous electrical pacing may be useful. Atropine 2 to 3 mg intravenously, in divided doses, should be given to reduce unopposed vagal activity. Isoprenaline should be given by intravenous infusion according to the response of the pulse and the blood pressure; massive doses may be required. Intensive care may be required for several days since the effects of beta-adrenoceptor blocking agents last longer than their half-life in the plasma. Theoretically, other catecholamines such as dopamine or dobutamine may have advantages over isoprenaline, especially in poisoning with cardioselective drugs such as atenolol or metoprolol. Glucagon intravenously may also be of value, and should be given early in severe overdosage.— *Br. med. J.*, 1978, *1*, 1010. Although isoprenaline has its merits, the dose which will increase heart-rate will also reduce diastolic blood pressure. Studies with atropine have shown that 40 µg per kg body-weight is required to abolish vagal influences on the heart after therapeutic doses of beta-adrenoceptor blocking agents; such a dose given as an intravenous bolus after propranolol or labetalol has been observed to increase significantly systolic and diastolic pressures in normal healthy males. Moreover, the same dose of atropine alone has a similar effect on blood pressure, and can substantially enhance the pressor effects of intravenous noradrenaline. Under these circumstances the usual effects of noradrenaline, causing marked reductions in heart-rate and cardiac output, do not occur. Thus, atropine, alone or after beta-adrenoceptor blocking agents, can raise blood pressure and heart-rate while maintaining cardiac output. Therefore, the use of atropine is endorsed, in doses of at least 3 mg as bolus injections. As an alternative to isoprenaline in patients who are still hypotensive, provided atropine has been given previously, graded infusions of noradrenaline are recommended to restore blood pressure.— D. A. Richards and B. N. C. Prichard (letter), *ibid.*, 1623.

Further references: *Lancet*, 1980, *1*, 803.

Individual reports. Atropine sulphate 1.2 mg intravenously given before propranolol almost completely abolished the expected rise in airway resistance in normal persons and markedly reduced the rise in asthmatics.— A. G. Macdonald *et al.*, *Br. J. Anaesth.*, 1967, *39*, 919.

A discussion of the treatment of incidental anaphylaxis in propranolol-treated patients. Ten ml of calcium gluconate 10% given intravenously was theoretically the agent of choice.— A. N. Corbascio (letter), *Clin. Pharmac. Ther.*, 1971, *12*, 559.

A report of hypoglycaemia in 2 healthy siblings after ingestion of overdoses of propranolol. A boy aged 20 months was given an intravenous injection of 30 ml of dextrose injection 50% followed by an intravenous infusion of dextrose injection 5%; his 3-year-old sister was given milk and sugar by mouth. The girl's heart-rate was normal but the boy suffered from bradycardia which could have confused the diagnosis by obscuring the tachycardia normally found in hypoglycaemia.— B. Hesse and J. T. Pedersen, *Acta med. scand.*, 1973, *193*, 551.

Following complete beta-adrenoceptor blockade with propranolol hydrochloride in anaesthetised *dogs* glucagon was superior to isoprenaline in enhancing myocardial contractility and heart-rate.— E. J. Kosinski and G. S. Malindzak, *Archs intern. Med.*, 1973, *132*, 840.

A comment on the role of beta-stimulants and glucagon in beta-blocking poisoning, and the suggestion that aminophylline may also be beneficial. Care should be taken to avoid exacerbation of hypotension during administration of aminophylline.— B. Jones (letter), *Lancet*, 1980, *1*, 1031. A case report illustrating the value of glucagon during beta-blocker poisoning (with alprenolol). Glucagon should be given in an intravenous dose of 8 to 10 mg repeated one hour later if necessary. Dopamine was used as a β_1-stimulant and a pacemaker was inserted; the use of isoprenaline is viewed with reserve.— D. Jacobsen *et al.* (letter), *ibid.* Mention of the successful use of glucagon to treat 2 patients with no recordable blood pressure due to beta-blocker poisoning, and agreement that it is the treatment of choice for beta-blocker poisoning. It is considered that 2 patients known to have died with propranolol poisoning while being treated with atropine and catecholamines, might have survived had they been given large amounts of glucagon.— R. N. Illingworth (letter), *ibid.*, *2*, 86.

See also under Oxprenolol,p.1345.

Precautions. Propranolol should not be given to patients with bronchial asthma or bronchospasm, hypoglycaemia, metabolic acidosis, sinus bradycardia, or partial heart block. It should be given to patients with congestive heart failure only when they are fully digitalised and only then with great caution. It should never be given to patients with phaeochromocytoma without concomitant alpha-adrenoceptor blocking therapy.

Propranolol may mask the symptoms of hyperthyroidism although it does not interfere with thyroid-function tests. It may also mask the symptoms of hypoglycaemia, as well as enhancing the effects of hypoglycaemic agents in patients with diabetes mellitus.

Great care should be exercised in giving propranolol to patients undergoing anaesthesia (see p.1324) and myocardial depressants such as chloroform or ether must be avoided. The effects of other myocardial depressant agents such as quinidine, procainamide, or lignocaine, and drugs which interfere with calcium transport, such as verapamil, may also be enhanced by propranolol.

The effects of propranolol are diminished by beta-adrenoceptor stimulating agents such as isoprenaline; the hypotensive effects of propranolol may be dangerously reversed and the peripheral vasoconstrictor effects enhanced by alpha-adrenoceptor stimulating agents such as noradrenaline or those with mixed alpha- and beta-adrenoceptor stimulating properties such as adrenaline; bradycardia may also occur (for further comment, see Adrenaline, p.2).

The effects of propranolol may be enhanced by adrenergic neurone blocking agents such as guanethidine or bethanidine, or catecholamine-depleting agents such as reserpine, and the hypotensive effects by diuretics.

Propranolol may enhance some of the cardiac effects of digitalis and diminish others. It has been suggested that clonidine withdrawal symptoms may be exacerbated in patients who are concurrently taking a beta-adrenoceptor blocking agent.

For comments on the withdrawal of propranolol, see below.

Cardiac disorders. Beta-adrenoceptor blocking agents are contra-indicated in the carotid sinus syndrome and possibly in the hyperactive carotid sinus reflex syndrome.— A. J. Reyes, *Br. med. J.*, 1973, *2*, 662.

A study confirming that beta-blocking agents should be prescribed only with extreme caution in heart failure of ischaemic origin.— S. H. Taylor and B. Silke, *Lancet*, 1981, *2*, 835.

Epilepsy. In patients with convulsive disorders who manifested a normal QT-time on the ECG, propranolol led to epileptiform activity on the EEG.— H. R. Ruser *et al.*, *Dte Gesundh Wes.*, 1972, *27*, 2092.

Hyperthyroidism. Propranolol treatment has masked symptoms of thyrotoxicosis (G.F. Cohen, *Lancet*, 1968, *2*, 1349, and L. Shenkman *et al.*, *J. Am. med. Ass.*, 1977, *238*, 237); it can cause errors in the Achilles reflex test for thyroid disease (H.J. Waal-Manning, *Clin. Pharmac. Ther.*, 1969, *10*, 199). Another adverse effect in hyperthyroid patients may be dangerous depression of serum-calcium concentrations (Y.K. Seedat *et al.*, *Br. med. J.*, 1970, *3*, 525). The fall in cardiac output and heart-rate associated with propranolol given intravenously has been reported by H. Ikram (*Br. med. J.*, 1977, *1*, 1505) to be insignificant in patients with uncomplicated thyrotoxicosis, but to be significant in those also suffering from heart failure, contra-indicating its use in such patients; the effect of oral propranolol was not studied. Subsequently J.S. Staffurth and R. Stott (*Br. med. J.*, 1977, *2*, 191) have reported fatalities in 2 patients with thyrotoxicosis and propranolol may have contributed to these deaths. Results of a study by A.D.B. Harrower *et al.* (*Postgrad. med. J.*, 1977, *53*, 687) have indicated that propranolol-induced impairment of glucose tolerance is unlikely to be a serious contra-indication to treatment unless the patient has diabetes in addition to hyperthyroidism.

See also under Uses.

Hypoglycaemia and diabetes mellitus. Studies in 6 healthy persons demonstrated that propranolol reduced the blood-sugar response to exercise and to hypoglycaemia. The danger of prescribing beta-adrenoceptor blocking agents for patients during treatment with hypoglycaemic agents is emphasised.— P. D. Bewsher (letter), *Lancet*, 1967, *1*, 104. The dangers of the concurrent use of insulin and propranolol may have been overestimated. Increased sweating in insulin-dependent diabetics taking propranolol is an indication of hypoglycaemia.— L. Strom (letter), *New Engl. J. Med.*, 1978, *299*, 487. A cardioselective β_1-adrenoceptor blocking agent should be used in diabetics rather than propranolol.— U. Smith and I. Lager (letter), *ibid.*, 1467. See also A. H. Barnett *et al.*, *Br. med. J.*, 1980, *280*, 976; U. Smith *et al.* (letter), *ibid.*, *281*, 1143.

Further reports and studies on the effects of propranolol and hypoglycaemic agents: W. S. Reveno and H. Rosenbaum (letter), *Lancet*, 1968, *1*, 920; G. W. Molnar and R. C. Read, *Clin. Pharmac. Ther.*, 1974, *15*, 490; R. J. McMurtry (letter), *Ann. intern. Med.*, 1974, *80*, 669; R. H. Lloyd-Mostyn and S. Oram, *Lancet*, 1975, *1*, 1213; J. Feely (letter), *Lancet*, 1977, *1*, 950.

In 20 hypertensive patients with diabetes blood-sugar concentrations rose significantly while the patients were treated with propranolol 80 mg twice daily or metoprolol 100 mg twice daily. The actual increase was relatively small and not detectable clinically in most patients.— A. D. Wright *et al.*, *Br. med. J.*, 1979, *1*, 159.

In 6 hypertensive diabetic patients studied under double-blind conditions propranolol 80 or 160 mg twice daily or metoprolol 100 or 200 mg twice daily had no significant effect on fasting plasma-glucose concentrations, glucose tolerance, or insulin response.— K. L. Woods *et al.*, *Br. med. J.*, 1980, *281*, 1321.

Further reports and comments on the administration of propranolol in diabetes mellitus: K. D. Ball and C. Thomson, *Pharm. J.*, 1979, *1*, 547; L. Gerlis and P. Wittels (letter [Hoechst]), *ibid.*, 1979, *2*, 55; M. J. Kendall and S. Roden, *J. clin. Pharm.*, 1979, *4*, 33; H. J. Waal-Manning, *Drugs*, 1979, *17*, 157.

Interactions. A discussion of interactions, including desirable interactions, between beta-adrenoceptor blocking agents and other drugs.— J. E. Crook and A. S. Nies, *Drugs*, 1978, *15*, 72.

Alcohol. Studies in 7 healthy subjects did not demonstrate decreased tolerance to alcoholic beverages after beta-adrenoceptor blockade. The elimination-rate of alcohol was not decreased after administration of therapeutic doses of propranolol for 14 days.— T. L. Svendsen *et al.*, *Eur. J. clin. Pharmac.*, 1978, *13*, 91.

In healthy subjects alcohol increased the plasma clearance-rate of propranolol and diminished its hypotensive effect.— E. A. Sotaniemi *et al.*, *Clin. Pharmac. Ther.*, 1981, *29*, 705.

Antacids. In 4 of 5 healthy subjects concomitant administration of propranolol and aluminium hydroxide mixture decreased the plasma concentration of propranolol.— J. H. Dobbs *et al.*, *Curr. ther. Res.*, 1977, *21*, 887.

Anti-arrhythmic agents. Beta-adrenoceptor blocking agents may enhance the negative inotropic action of anti-arrhythmic agents. In particular, prenylamine and verapamil should probably not be used in association with beta-blockers.— P. J. Lewis, *Prescribers' J.*, 1979, *19*, 94. A review of drugs for angina pectoris. At the larger doses of verapamil that are usually required, it may precipitate heart failure and hypotension, and its use with beta-blockers should be avoided.— P. J. B. Hubner, *ibid.*, 143.

Reports of serious adverse reactions, including some deaths, in patients stabilised on beta-adrenoceptor blocking agents who were given an oral loading dose of disopyramide (400 mg).— *Aust. J. Pharm.*, 1980, *61*, 446.

See also under interactions relating to lignocaine (below).

Anticoagulants. In 3 patients who were apparently well stabilised on long-term phenindione therapy bleeding episodes occurred after administration of propranolol.— G. H. Neilson and W. A. Seldon, *Med. J. Aust.*, 1969, *1*, 856.

Antihypertensive agents. A hypertensive response to propranolol (1 mg by slow intravenous injection) occurred in a 36-year-old Caucasian male after several days' treatment with methyldopa 500 mg six-hourly. The patient was also receiving hydralazine 50 mg six-hourly and had previously received diazoxide. Intravenous phentolamine promptly reduced the blood pressure but despite intensive therapy the patient died two months later without regaining consciousness. It was recommended that propranolol should be given with caution to patients receiving methyldopa especially if there might be high circulatory concentrations of catecholamines.— A. S. Nies and D. G. Shand, *Clin. Pharmac. Ther.*, 1973, *14*, 823.

For a report of the adverse effect of concomitant administration of high doses of clonidine with high doses of propranolol, see Clonidine Hydrochloride, p.139.

Anti-inflammatory agents. Investigations in *rats* demonstrated that propranolol could impair the anti-inflammatory action of amidopyrine, phenylbutazone, sodium salicylate, and hydrocortisone.— L. Riesterer and R. Jaques, *Helv. physiol. Acta*, 1968, *26*, 287.

Nine patients with various inflammatory responses but all with a raised erythrocyte sedimentation-rate had strikingly higher plasma-propranolol concentrations following a dose of 40 mg than had 13 healthy controls.— J. Babb *et al.* (letter), *Lancet*, 1976, *1*, 1413. See also under Absorption and Fate.

Inhibition of prostaglandin synthesis by indomethacin in 7 hypertensive patients receiving propranolol or pindolol increased diastolic blood pressure. It was considered that salicylate-like compounds and non-steroidal anti-inflammatory agents should be avoided in hypertensive patients taking beta-blocking agents.— V. Durão *et al.* (preliminary communication), *Lancet*, 1977, *2*, 1005 and 1242. Indomethacin can cause hypertension on its own; this might explain the results.— M. VandenBurg (letter), *ibid.*, 1184. Further comments: C. Davidson (letter), *ibid.*; A. Barrientos *et al.* (letter), *ibid.*, 1978, *1*, 277.

Although indomethacin produced no net effect in 19 untreated patients with essential hypertension, it blunted or reversed the antihypertensive effect of diuretic and beta-adrenoceptor blockade in 9 patients who received chlorthalidone or hydrochlorothiazide, sometimes with frusemide, and 11 patients treated with propranolol.— J. A. Lopez-Ovejero *et al.*, *Clin. Sci. & mol. Med.*, 1978, *55*, 203S.

In 15 patients whose mild essential hypertension was controlled by either propranolol or thiazide diuretics the addition of indomethacin 50 mg twice daily for 3 weeks caused an increase in blood pressure and body-weight.— J. Watkins *et al.*, *Br. med. J.*, 1980, *281*, 702. Comment that the antacid (aluminium hydroxide) taken if necessary to alleviate gastro-intestinal distress may have caused a decrease in the bioavailability of propranolol.— R. J. Mangini (letter), *ibid.*, 1353.

Chlormethiazole. Profound bradycardia in an 84-year-old woman receiving propranolol 40 mg twice daily following the second of 2 doses of chlormethiazole 192 mg.— *Med. J. Aust.*, 1979, *2*, 553.

Cimetidine. Cimetidine reduced the clearance of intravenous propranolol in 6 healthy subjects by decreasing liver blood flow and also inhibited the metabolism of propranolol taken by mouth.— J. Feely *et al.*, *New Engl. J. Med.*, 1981, *304*, 692. Correspondence: K. L. Melmon and D. W. Nierenberg, *ibid.*, 723; J. E. Jackson (letter), *ibid.*, *305*, 99; D. Lebrec *et al.* (letter), *ibid.*, 100; J. Feely *et al.* (letter), *ibid.*

Results of a study in a duodenal ulcer patient indicated that concomitant administration of cimetidine may very considerably increase the bioavailability of propranolol.— M. A. Donovan *et al.* (letter), *Lancet*, 1981, *1*, 164. Preliminary data indicating that cimetidine increases the bioavailability of labetalol and therefore presumably of other highly extracted drugs.— T. K. Daneshmend and C. J. C. Roberts (letter), *ibid.*, 565. Mean peak plasma concentrations of propranolol and metoprolol were increased significantly by concurrent administration of cimetidine. Atenolol kinetics were not affected.— W. Kirch *et al.* (letter), *ibid.*, *2*, 531. Cimetidine significantly increased plasma concentrations of propranolol in 6 patients, by reducing hepatic first-pass extraction of propranolol.— A. M. Heagerty *et al.*, *Br. med. J.*, 1981, *282*, 1917.

Corticosteroids. Studies on the effects of different beta-adrenoceptor blocking agents on cortisol determinations.— J. P. Radó and L. Végh, *Int. J. clin. Pharmac. Biopharm.*, 1977, *15*, 5.

Dantrolene. For reference to a possible interaction between beta-adrenoceptor blocking agents and dantrolene, see Dantrolene Sodium, p.989.

Digoxin. Two men with digoxin intoxication each developed progressive bradycardia within 2 hours of a single dose of 10 mg of propranolol by mouth, and both died. Bradycardia was possibly due to a synergistic action between propranolol and digoxin and could be prevented by the use of a test dose of propranolol or possibly by the routine administration of atropine with propranolol.— D. A. L. Watt, *Br. med. J.*, 1968, *3*, 413. Comments.— K. Hazell (letter), *ibid.*, 619; D. A. L. Watt (letter), *ibid.*, 1968, *4*, 58. Further comment.— M. O'Reilly *et al.* (letter), *Lancet*, 1974, *1*, 138. No antagonism was found in 15 patients though when digitalis was given alone the frequency of attacks increased.— M. H. Crawford *et al.* (letter), *ibid.*, 457.

Further references: W. Gebhardt and G. Blümchen, *Cardiologia*, 1968, *52*, 190; M. Crawford *et al.*, *Clin. Pharmac. Ther.*, 1974, *15*, 203.

Ergotamine tartrate. For a report of a possible interaction in a patient taking ergotamine tartrate and propranolol for migraine prophylaxis, see Ergotamine Tartrate, p.666.

Glucose. Propranolol could interfere biologically with chemical estimations for glucose in the blood to produce erroneous lowered results.— *Drug & Ther. Bull.*, 1972, *10*, 69.

Halofenate. Concurrent administration of halofenate with propranolol resulted in decreased plasma-propranolol concentrations which correlated with reduced beta-adrenoceptor blockade. The mechanism of the interaction was not determined.— D. H. Huffman *et al.*, *Clin. Pharmac. Ther.*, 1976, *19*, 807.

Isosorbide dinitrate. Treatment with isosorbide dinitrate and propranolol could be harmful as well as beneficial in patients with angina pectoris.— W. S. Aronow and M. A. Kaplan, *New Engl. J. Med.*, 1969, *280*, 847.

Further references: H. I. Russek, *Am. J. med. Sci.*, 1967, *254*, 406; D. J. Battock *et al.*, *Circulation*, 1969, *39*, 157; A. N. Goldbarg *et al.*, *ibid.*, *40*, 847; W. S. Aronow and H. M. Chesluk, *ibid.*, 1970, *41*, 869; W. S. Aronow and M. A. Kaplan, *Curr. ther. Res.*, 1969, *11*, 80.

Lignocaine. An increase in plasma half-life of lignocaine of up to 50% has been observed in the presence of propranolol.— *Aust. J. Pharm.*, 1974, *55*, 521.

A study demonstrating that, in healthy subjects, both prolonged infusion of lignocaine and co-administration of propranolol reduce the plasma clearance of lignocaine. It may be necessary to reduce the dosage of lignocaine when propranolol is given concomitantly and to reduce the rate of infusion when lignocaine is given for prolonged periods.— H. R. Ochs *et al.*, *New Engl. J. Med.*, 1980, *303*, 373. Two reports of the concomitant administration of propranolol possibly enhancing the toxicity of lignocaine.— C. F. Graham *et al.* (letter), *ibid.*, 1981, *304*, 1301.

Muscle relaxants. A study in *cats* demonstrated that the effects of tubocurarine and suxamethonium were enhanced by propranolol. Fasciculations due to suxamethonium were prevented.— J. E. Usubiaga, *Anesthesiology*, 1968, *29*, 484.

Monoamine oxidase inhibitors. Although it had been suggested that treatment with monoamine oxidase inhibitors should be withdrawn 2 weeks before commencing treatment with propranolol, investigations in *cats* failed to unmask any undesirable property of propranolol following monoamine oxidase inhibition.— A. M. Barrett and V. A. Cullum, *J. Pharm. Pharmac.*, 1968, *20*, 911.

Neostigmine. Severe bradycardia occurred after simultaneous administration of atropine and neostigmine, to reverse pancuronium-induced neuromuscular blockade, in a patient on long-term propranolol therapy.— D. H. Sprague, *Anesthesiology*, 1975, *42*, 208.

Nifedipine. A warning that administration of nifedipine might exacerbate the symptoms of beta-adrenoceptor blockade withdrawal, since it causes significant peripheral vasodilatation with subsequent reflex increase in sympathetic activity.— Ø. L. Pedersen and E. Mikkelsen (letter), *Lancet*, 1979, *1*, 554.

Two patients developed heart failure when nifedipine was given in addition to beta-blockers.— C. J. Anastassiades, *Br. med. J.*, 1980, *281*, 1251.

Phenazone. Impairment of phenazone clearance by propranolol.— D. J. Greenblatt, *Clin. Pharmac. Ther.*, 1977, *21*, 104.

Phenothiazines. Pretreatment of *rats* with chlorpromazine or desipramine inhibited the metabolism of propranolol *in vitro*.— D. G. Shand and J. A. Oates, *Biochem. Pharmac.*, 1971, *20*, 1720.

Caution is needed when using propranolol with phenothiazines and tricyclic antidepressants.— R. Galinsky (letter), *New Engl. J. Med.*, 1976, *295*, 281. The need for caution is accepted but there is little reported evidence of trouble with the association.— N. M. Kaplan (letter), *ibid.*

In healthy subjects given propranolol, plasma-propranolol concentrations increased after the introduction of chlorpromazine to the treatment.— R. E. Vestal *et al.*, *Clin. Pharmac. Ther.*, 1979, *25*, 19.

For the effect of propranolol on chlorpromazine, see Chlorpromazine, p.1512.

Sympathomimetics. Adrenaline and noradrenaline should not be given to patients being treated with propranolol; when the beta receptors which caused vasodilatation were blocked by propranolol, adrenaline and similar drugs could produce a powerful vasoconstrictor effect by acting on the alpha receptors.— J. Grayson (letter), *Lancet*, 1967, *1*, 788. Bradycardia and atrioventricular block occurred in a subject given adrenaline 1 hour after propranolol in a laboratory investigation.— J. Kram *et al.* (letter), *Ann. intern. Med.*, 1974, *80*, 282.

A report of a fatality occurring in a 49-year-old woman with asymptomatic hypertension on a regimen of hydrochlorothiazide 50 mg twice daily and propranolol hydrochloride 40 mg four times daily, following the instillation of one drop of 10% phenylephrine hydrochloride solution in each eye during an ophthalmological examination.— E. Cass *et al.*, *Can. med. Ass. J.*, 1979, *120*, 1261.

Tricyclic antidepressants. For comments on the possible interaction between propranolol and tricyclic antidepressants see under interactions relating to phenothiazines (above).

Verapamil. See under interactions relating to anti-arrhythmic agents (above).

Xanthines. For the effect of propranolol on theophylline, see Aminophylline, p.343.

Interference with diagnostic tests. A study indicating that a metabolite of propranolol, a conjugate of 4-hydroxypropranolol that is normally excreted in the urine, accumulates in the plasma of patients with chronic renal failure not receiving dialysis and interferes with the diazo reaction for detecting serum bilirubin to produce false-positive results. The Bilirubinometer method was not affected by this metabolite.— S. Al-Damluji and J. H. Meek, *Br. med. J.*, 1980, *280*, 1414.

See also under Corticosteroids and Glucose in Interactions (above).

Phaeochromocytoma. Pulmonary oedema occurred in 2 patients with phaeochromocytoma shortly after starting propranolol. This supported the suggestion that beta blockade should not be established before alpha blockade in such patients.— J. D. Wark and R. G. Larkins, *Br. med. J.*, 1978, *1*, 1395.

Pregnancy and the neonate. There is doubt about the use of beta-adrenoceptor blocking agents in pregnancy. There have been isolated reports of intra-uterine growth retardation, acute foetal distress in labour, and hypoglycaemia in the neonate. Although these may all be complications of hypertension in pregnancy, because of these reports beta-adrenoceptor blocking agents are not recommended as first-line treatment for hypertension in pregnancy.— M. de Swiet, *Prescribers' J.*, 1979, *19*, 59.

A study on the neonatal effects of maternal administration of acebutolol or methyldopa suggested that beta-adrenoceptor blocking agents should be used with caution during pregnancy. Blood pressure was significantly lower in 10 infants born to mothers who had received acebutolol and remained so for the first 3 days of life; heart-rate was also lower.— Y. Dumez *et al.*, *Br. med. J.*, 1981, *283*, 1077.

On current evidence beta-blocker treatment of hypertension in pregnancy appears to improve the likelihood that the foetus will be normal.— P. C. Rubin, *New Engl. J. Med.*, 1981, *305*, 1323.

Further references: M. E. Tunstall, *Br. J. Anaesth.*, 1969, *41*, 792; G. I. Fiddler (letter), *Lancet*, 1974, *2*, 722; G. R. Gladstone *et al.*, *J. Pediat.*, 1975, *86*, 962; A. Habib and J. S. McCarthy, *J. Pediat.*, 1977, *91*, 808; C. M. Cottrill *et al.*, *ibid.*, 812; S. Datta *et al.*, *Obstet. Gynec.*, 1978, *51*, 577; G. D. G. Oakley *et al.*, *Br. med. J.*, 1979, *1*, 1749.

Lactation. An estimation that the suckling infant of a woman taking propranolol 40 mg four times daily was only receiving 21 µg of propranolol over a 24-hour period.— J. H. Bauer *et al.*, *Am. J. Cardiol.*, 1979, *43*, 860.

Further references: B. Karlberg *et al.*, *Acta pharmac. tox.*, 1974, *34*, 222; P. O. Anderson and F. J. Salter (letter), *Am. J. Cardiol.*, 1976, *37*, 325; A. A. Levitan (letter), *ibid.*

Withdrawal. Reviews and comments on the withdrawal syndrome associated with beta-adrenoceptor blocking agents: *Lancet*, 1975, *2*, 592; D. G. Shand, *New Engl. J. Med.*, 1975, *293*, 449; *J. Am. med. Ass.*, 1975, *231*, 125; P. J. Ross *et al.* (letter), *Lancet*, 1979, *1*, 875; J. H. Botting and A. Gibson (letter), *ibid.*

In a retrospective analysis of a double-blind crossover efficacy study of propranolol 160 to 320 mg daily in angina pectoris it was noted that within 2 weeks of abrupt withdrawal of propranolol untoward ischaemic events occurred in 10 patients. Six had serious withdrawal complications: intermediate coronary syndrome (3), ventricular tachycardia (1), fatal myocardial infarction (1), and sudden death (1), and 4 suffered increased anginal symptoms.— R. R. Miller *et al.*, *New Engl. J. Med.*, 1975, *293*, 416.

A syndrome similar to florid thyrotoxicosis occurred in 3 patients within a week of the sudden withdrawal of propranolol 0.96 to 2 g daily for hypertension.— E. T. O'Brien (letter), *Lancet*, 1975, *2*, 819.

The effects of infusions of isoprenaline 2 µg per minute administered for 10 minutes before and after withdrawal of propranolol 40 mg four times daily over a 2-day period were studied in 6 healthy subjects. Hypersensitivity to isoprenaline was found 24 to 48 hours after propranolol withdrawal. Discontinuation of propranolol therapy for 24 hours or more before surgery might not be without risks.— H. Boudoulas *et al.*, *Ann. intern. Med.*, 1977, *87*, 433. To prevent rebound phenomena propranolol may have to be administered at reduced dosage or tapered for at least 10 to 14 days before withdrawal.— S. Nattel *et al.* (letter), *ibid.*, 1978, *89*, 288.

A withdrawal syndrome occurs with both cardioselective and nonselective beta-adrenoceptor blocking agents, and in both angina and hypertension.— B. Ø. Kristensen (letter), *Lancet*, 1979, *1*, 554.

In 4 hypertensive patients who had been taking propranolol 240 to 640 mg daily for 18 to 60 months, blood pressure and heart-rate rose and plasma concentrations of noradrenaline fell when propranolol was withdrawn; 3 patients experienced a forceful heart beat on the 3rd and 4th days after withdrawal.— T. J. B. Maling and C. T. Dollery, *Br. med. J.*, 1979, *2*, 366. Comment.— M. J. Lewis *et al.* (letter), *ibid.*, 606. Reply.— C. T. Dollery and T. J. B. Maling (letter), *ibid.*, 1074.

Similar reports and studies: R. Slome (letter), *Lancet*, 1973, *1*, 156; R. G. Diaz *et al.* (letter), *ibid.*, 1068; E. L. Alderman *et al.*, *Ann. intern. Med.*, 1974, *81*, 625; R. Allen and B. Genovese (letter), *Ann. intern. Med.*, 1975, *82*, 431.

Symptoms following withdrawal of propranolol from 100 consecutive patients undergoing coronary arteriography did not support the view that there is a propranolol withdrawal syndrome. Symptoms occurred exclusively in patients with class IV symptoms and were possibly due to loss of protection of beta-adrenoceptor blockade. There is virtually no evidence to support the view that propranolol dosage should be tapered off and no data have been presented comparing the relative merits of gradual versus abrupt withdrawal.— M. G. Myers *et al.*, *Am. Heart J.*, 1979, *97*, 298.

Similar reports and studies: J. A. Pantano and Y. C. Lee, *Archs intern. Med.*, 1976, *136*, 867; M. G. Myers and G. Wisenberg, *Chest*, 1977, *71*, 24; R. A. Shiroff *et al.*, *Am. J. Cardiol.*, 1978, *41*, 778.

Absorption and Fate. Propranolol is almost completely absorbed from the gastro-intestinal tract, but is subject to considerable first-pass metabolism. Peak plasma concentrations occur about 2 hours after a dose. It is metabolised in the liver, the metabolites being excreted in the urine together with only small amounts of unchanged propranolol; at least one of its metabolites is considered to be biologically active. The biological half-life of propranolol is longer than would be anticipated from its plasma half-life of about 3 to 6 hours. Propranolol crosses the placenta and traces are found in milk. It also crosses the blood-brain barrier. It is highly protein bound and not reported to be significantly dialysable.

A review of the clinical pharmacokinetics of propranolol.— P. A. Routledge and D. G. Shand, *Clin. Pharmacokinet.*, 1979, *4*, 73.

Plasma-propranolol concentrations varied sevenfold in subjects given doses by mouth and twofold when given doses by intravenous infusion and the estimated percentage of an oral dose reaching the systemic circulation was 16 to 60. Mean plasma half-lives were about 3 hours for 40 and 80 mg given by mouth to fasting subjects, 3 to 4 hours for 80 mg given by mouth with food, and about 2.5 hours for 10 mg given intravenously at the rate of 1.03 mg per minute. Less than 25 µg of propranolol was excreted in the urine of 4 subjects in the 7 hours following the intravenous administration of 10 mg which indicated extensive metabolism and the high calculated volume of distribution indicated concentration of propranolol in the tissues.— D. G. Shand *et al.*, *Clin. Pharmac. Ther.*, 1970, *11*, 112.

Propranolol 160 mg was given to 9 healthy subjects and although the plasma half-life was only 3.5 hours, effects on heart-rate and blood pressure persisted over the 24-hour study period.— J. Kanto *et al.*, *Acta pharmac. tox.*, 1976, *39*, 573. See also D. M. Leaman *et al.*, *J. thorac. cardiovasc. Surg.*, 1976, *72*, 67.

A very wide inter- and intra-individual variation in serum concentration was found in 9 patients with angina pectoris given propranolol 40 mg thrice daily for at least 1 week. No relationship was seen between serum concentration and either blood pressure or dose related to body-weight.— E. Vervloet *et al.*, *Clin. Pharmac. Ther.*, 1977, *22*, 853. See also A. Lehtonen *et al.*, *Eur. J. clin. Pharmac.*, 1977, *11*, 155.

In 15 healthy subjects given propranolol 80 mg every 8 hours the mean steady-state blood-propranolol concentration was 72 ng per ml (range 33 to 143 ng per ml) with a mean half-life of 3.9 hours (range 2.8 to 5.7 hours).— D. M. Kornhauser *et al.*, *Clin. Pharmac. Ther.*, 1978, *23*, 165. A similar study.— B. W. Hadzija and A. M. Mattocks, *J. pharm. Sci.*, 1978, *67*, 1307.

Slower metabolism of propranolol in malnutrition.— A. O. K. Obel and D. W. Vere, *E. Afr. med. J.*, 1978, *55*, 20, per *Trop. Dis. Bull.*, 1978, *75*, 1151.

Propranolol accumulated in blood to reach a steady-state within 48 hours of starting a dosage regimen of 80 mg every 8 hours in 5 healthy subjects.— A. J. J. Wood *et al.*, *Br. J. clin. Pharmac.*, 1978, *6*, 345.

Increased clearance of propranolol in thyrotoxicosis.— J. Feely *et al.*, *Ann. intern. Med.*, 1981, *94*, 472.

Further references: D. J. Coltart and D. G. Shand, *Br. med. J.*, 1970, *3*, 731; E. M. Phillips *et al.*, *Postgrad. med. J.*, 1973, *49*, 18; T. Walle, *J. pharm. Sci.*, 1974, *63*, 1885; R. J. Sawchuk *et al.* (letter), *Br. J. clin. Pharmac.*, 1974, *1*, 440; M. M. LeWinter *et al.*, *Clin. Pharmac. Ther.*, 1975, *17*, 709; D. G. McDevitt and D. G. Shand, *ibid.*, *18*, 708; R. Gomeni *et al.*, *J. Pharmacokinet. Biopharm.*, 1977, *5*, 183.

Diffusion into the CSF. Measurement of CSF/plasma concentrations in subjects given propranolol.— E. A. Taylor *et al.*, *Br. J. clin. Pharmac.*, 1978, *6*, 447P.

Further references: M. D. Day *et al.*, *J. Pharm. Pharmac.*, 1977, *29*, *Suppl.*, 52P (*animals*); G. Neil-Dwyer *et al.*, *Br. J. clin. Pharmac.*, 1981, *11*, 549.

First-pass effect. Individual variation in the bioavailability of propranolol was determined mainly by first-pass metabolism rather than differences in gastric emptying.— C. M. Castleden *et al.*, *Br. J. clin. Pharmac.*, 1978, *5*, 121. See also C. F. George and M. Castleden (letter), *Br. med. J.*, 1977, *1*, 47.

Propranolol in low doses blocked cardiac, vascular, and renal beta-adrenoceptors in 6 healthy subjects who received 5 doses of 5 mg every 8 hours. Blood concentrations of propranolol could not be detected satisfactorily by fluorometry; gas-liquid chromatography showed concentrations ranging from 2.3 to 8.5 ng per ml. These results confound suggestions of a threshold dose by mouth being required to overcome a first-pass effect.— R. Davies *et al.*, *Lancet*, 1978, *1*, 407. The first-pass effect of propranolol has been amply proved and has important clinical implications.— C. F. George (letter), *ibid.*, 715. The first-pass effect was accepted; it was the threshold for this effect that was being questioned.— R. Davies *et al.* (letter), *ibid.*, 827. The active metabolite must also be considered.— L. P. Balant and J. Fabre (letter), *ibid.*, 1978, *2*, 425.

A report of significant first-pass uptake of propranolol by the lungs.— D. M. Geddes *et al.*, *Br. J. clin. Pharmac.*, 1978, *5*, 354P.

Food reduced the first-pass hepatic clearance of propranolol.— A. J. McLean *et al.*, *Clin. Pharmac. Ther.*, 1981, *30*, 31.

Metabolites. After administration of propranolol 40 mg by mouth the metabolite 4-hydroxypropranolol was identified in the blood and was believed to be pharmacologically active; 4-hydroxypropranolol was not found after intravenous administration but an unidentified inactive metabolite was present in large amounts.— C. T. Dollery *et al.*, *Ann. N.Y. Acad. Sci.*, 1971, *179*, 108. See also J. D. Fitzgerald and S. R. O'Donnell, *Br. J. Pharmac.*, 1971, *43*, 222.

Plasma concentrations of propranolol and 4-hydroxypropranolol during long-term oral therapy.— L. Wong *et al.*, *Br. J. clin. Pharmac.*, 1979, *8*, 163.

Further references: C. R. Cleaveland and D. G. Shand, *Clin. Pharmac. Ther.*, 1972, *13*, 181; Y. Garceau *et al.*, *J. pharm. Sci.*, 1978, *67*, 826; T. Walle *et al.*, *Clin. Pharmac. Ther.*, 1979, *26*, 548; *idem*, 686; *idem*, 1980, *27*, 22.

Protein binding. The amount of plasma-protein binding of propranolol was not significantly altered in 7 hyperthyroid and 10 hypothyroid patients who became euthyroid after treatment.— J. G. Kelly and D. G. McDevitt, *Br. J. clin. Pharmac.*, 1977, *4*, 628P.

Studies *in vitro* demonstrated that there was an inverse relationship between α_1 acid glycoprotein concentration and the amount of unbound propranolol in plasma. The most extensive binding of propranolol was seen in plasma from patients with inflammatory diseases such as rheumatoid arthritis and Crohn's disease, all of whom had elevated plasma concentrations of α_1 acid glycoprotein. Similar results were seen with chlorpromazine. Plasma-protein binding of cationic drugs appeared to be increased in inflammatory disease because of increased concentrations of α_1 acid glycoprotein which was able to bind them.— K. M. Piafsky *et al.*, *New Engl. J. Med.*, 1978, *299*, 1435.

Comment on the significance of drug binding to α_1 acid glycoprotein.— *Lancet*, 1979, *1*, 368.

Further references: O. Borga *et al.*, *Br. J. clin. Pharmac.*, 1977, *4*, 627P; R. E. Schneider *et al.* (letter), *Lancet*, 1979, *1*, 554; B. J. Scott *et al.* (letter), *ibid.*, 930; R. E. Schneider *et al.*, *Br. J. clin. Pharmac.*, 1979, *8*, 43.

Sustained-release preparations. A comparison of the pharmacokinetics and pharmacodynamics of a long-acting capsule formulation of propranolol 160 mg with standard 40, 80, and 160 mg tablets.— J. McAinsh *et al.*, *Br. J. clin. Pharmac.*, 1978, *6*, 115.

Further references: A. P. Douglas-Jones, *J. int. med. Res.*, 1979, *7*, 221.

Uses. Propranolol reduces cardiac activity by diminishing or preventing beta-adrenoceptor stimulation. It reduces the rate and force of contraction of the heart and decreases the rate of conduction of impulses through the conducting system.

Its principal effect is to reduce the response of the heart to stress and exercise and it reduces blood pressure in patients with hypertension. It also reduces some of the responses of the body to the effects of adrenaline and isoprenaline. It has weak membrane-stabilising properties and does not possess intrinsic sympathomimetic activity but this is not of clinical significance (see p.1324). Propranolol is classified as non-cardioselective.

Propranolol is used in the treatment of cardiac arrhythmias. It is often effective in paroxysmal supraventricular tachycardia. It is used with digitalis to reduce the ventricle-rate in atrial fibrillation and flutter which are not effectively controlled by digitalis alone. It is usually effective in the control of arrhythmias associated with digoxin intoxication and, administered intravenously, in the control of arrhythmias occurring during anaesthesia. It has been used in ventricular fibrillation when counter-shock cannot be employed.

Propranolol is used to improve the tolerance to exercise in patients with angina pectoris. It has been given for the prevention of re-infarction in patients who have suffered an acute myocardial infarction.

Propranolol is also used in the treatment of hypertension, usually in conjunction with a thiazide diuretic. It does not produce postural hypotension but the full benefit of the treatment may not be evident for 6 to 8 weeks.

In hyperthyroidism, propranolol is given to reduce the heart-rate and control other symptoms of sympathetic nervous hyperactivity.

In the surgical treatment of phaeochromocytoma, propranolol may be given pre-operatively always in association with an alpha-adrenoceptor blocking agent such as phenoxybenzamine.

Propranolol hydrochloride is usually given by mouth. Dosage is largely determined by the response of the patient. In most conditions, treatment should begin with a small dose which should be gradually increased. Usually 10 to 40 mg is given by mouth three or four times a day, but the dose may be increased up to 400 mg or more daily in the treatment of angina pectoris or hypertension. In phaeochromocytoma, 60 mg daily should be given on 3 pre-operative days always in association with alpha-adrenoceptor blockade (see Precautions).

For the emergency treatment of cardiac arrhythmias, propranolol hydrochloride may be given by slow intravenous injection in a dose of 1 mg injected over a period of 1 minute, repeated if necessary every 2 minutes until a maximum total of 10 mg has been given in conscious patients and 5 mg in patients under anaesthesia. Similar doses have been used in thyrotoxic crisis. Atropine, 1 to 2 mg, should be given intravenously before propranolol is injected. Propranolol is *not* suitable for the emergency treatment of hypertension; it should never be given intravenously in hypertension.

Propranolol has also been used for some symptoms of anxiety, for migraine, and for essential tremor.

Action. A detailed review of the actions and uses of alpha- and beta-adrenoceptor blocking agents.— D. G. McDevitt, *Drugs*, 1979, *17*, 267.

Further reviews and comments on beta-adrenoceptor blocking agents: R. P. Ahlquist, *Prog. Drug Res.*, 1976, *20*, 27; *Postgrad. med. J.*, 1976, *52*, *Suppl.* 4, 1–192; *Med. Lett.*, 1977, *19*, 21; B. N. C. Prichard, *Br. J. clin. Pharmac.*, 1978, *5*, 379; D. Robertson and A. S. Nies, *Recent Adv. clin. Pharmac.*, 1978, *1*, 55; L. H. Opie, *Lancet*, 1980, *1*, 693; R. C. Wetzel (letter), *ibid.*, 1031; B. I. Hoffbrand (letter), *ibid*; A. H. Robins (letter), *ibid.*, 1357; J. M. Cruickshank (letter), *ibid.*, 1415; L. H. Opie (letter), *ibid.*, *2*, 428; W. H. Frishman, *New Engl. J. Med.*, 1981, *305*, 500.

Reports and studies on the pharmacology of propranolol: M. Guazzi *et al.*, *Clin. Pharmac. Ther.*, 1976, *20*, 304 (beta-adrenoceptor blockade); C. P. Mustchin *et al.*, *Br. med. J.*, 1976, *2*, 1229 (effect on response to carbon dioxide); T. Hanssen *et al.* (letter), *Lancet*, 1977, *2*, 309 (melatonin); H. Keltz *et al.*, *Am. J. med. Sci.*, 1977, *274*, 131 (response to carbon dioxide); D. N. Middlemiss *et al.*, *Nature*, 1977, *267*, 289 (serotonin); A. E. G. Raine and T. G. Pickering, *Br. med. J.*, 1977, *2*, 90 (reduced sympathetic activity); H. Boudoulas *et al.*, *Chest*, 1978, *73*, 146 (negative inotropic and chronotropic effects); J. Conway *et al.*, *Clin. Sci. & mol. Med.*, 1978, *54*, 119 (central action); J. I. Drayer *et al.*, *Am. J. Med.*, 1978, *64*, 187 (aldosterone); H. H. Harms *et al.*, *Br. J. clin. Pharmac.*, 1978, *5*, 19 (lipolysis, insulin release, and renin release); S. P. Deacon, *ibid.*, 123 (lipolysis); O. L. Pedersen and E. Mikkelsen (letter), *Lancet*, 1978, *2*, 1160 (uric acid excretion); J. L. Day *et al.*, *Br. med. J.*, 1979, *1*, 77 (elevation of triglycerides).

For references to effects on plasma renin, see under Hypertension.

Administration. Studies in healthy subjects indicated that more propranolol entered the general circulation following administration with food than when it was taken on an empty stomach; administration should always be standardised relative to meals.— A. Melander *et al.*, *Clin. Pharmac. Ther.*, 1977, *22*, 108. See also T. Walle *et al.*, *Clin. Pharmac. Ther.*, 1981, *30*, 790.

Comments and studies on responses to therapy with beta-adrenoceptor blocking agents in hypertensive persons of different races: Y. K. Seedat and J. Reddy, *S. Afr. med. J.*, 1971, *45*, 284; K. Jennings and V. Parsons, *Br. J. clin. Pharmac.*, 1976, *3*, *Suppl.* 3, 773; A. Reyes *et al.*, *Curr. ther. Res.*, 1978, *23*, 715; L. A. Salako *et al.*, *Eur. J. clin. Pharmac.*, 1979, *15*, 299.

Further references relating to administration: R. G. McAllister, *Clin. Pharmac. Ther.*, 1976, *20*, 517 (intravenous administration); A. Hussain *et al.*, *J. pharm. Sci.*, 1980, *69*, 1240 (nasal administration).

In children. A study of the disposition of propranolol in 7 children.— J. T. Wilson *et al.*, *Clin. Pharmac. Ther.*, 1976, *19*, 264.

In the elderly. Two hours after the administration of propranolol 40 mg, the mean peak plasma-propranolol concentration was 111 ng per ml in 9 elderly subjects and 27 ng per ml in 9 young subjects. Propranolol was eliminated from the plasma more rapidly in young subjects.— C. M. Castleden *et al.*, *Br. J. clin. Pharmac.*, 1975, *2*, 303. Comment.— R. E. Vestal, *Drugs*, 1978, *16*, 358.

A study of the relationship between age of the subject and the ability of propranolol to block the chronotropic effects of isoprenaline, supported the view that the sensitivity of beta-adrenoceptors declines with advancing age.— R. E. Vestal *et al.*, *Clin. Pharmac. Ther.*, 1979, *26*, 181.

Further references: R. E. Schneider *et al.* (letter), *Br. J. clin. Pharmac.*, 1980, *10*, 169.

Administration in gastro-intestinal disorders. The plasma-propranolol concentration in 8 patients with coeliac disease was significantly higher 1 hour after a 40-mg dose than in 12 controls. In 10 patients with Crohn's disease the concentration was significantly higher from half to 6 hours after the dose.— R. E. Schneider *et al.*, *Br. med. J.*, 1976, *2*, 794. See also R. L. Parsons *et al.* (letter), *ibid.*, 1977, *1*, 103.

Administration in hepatic failure. A study of the effects of cirrhosis on the disposition of propranolol during steady-state oral administration in 9 normal subjects and 7 with cirrhosis. There was a mean 3-fold increase in unbound propranolol concentrations in the blood in patients with cirrhosis when compared with the controls. Mean half-lives for the 2 groups were 11.2 and 4 hours respectively. Changes in systemic availability, clearance, and protein binding were proportional to the severity of the liver disease.— A. J. J. Wood *et al.*, *Clin. Pharmacokinet.*, 1978, *3*, 478. Further references: R. A. Branch *et al.*, *Br. J. clin. Pharmac.*, 1977, *4*, 630P; R. A. Branch and D. G. Shand, *Clin. Pharmacokinet.*, 1976, *1*, 264.

Effect on hepatic blood flow. Whereas the (+)-isomer of propranolol had no effect on hepatic blood flow when taken by 19 hypertensive patients, (±)-propranolol significantly reduced it. The decrease was considered to be produced by the beta-adrenoceptor blockade due to the (−)-isomer in the racemic mixture.— Y. A. Weiss *et al.*, *Br. J. clin. Pharmac.*, 1978, *5*, 457.

Administration in renal failure. In 3 patients with hypertension and impaired renal function, there was further deterioration of renal function after treatment with propranolol for 9 and 70 days respectively and with oxprenolol for 20 days; 2 patients needed dialysis. It was recommended that beta-adrenoceptor blocking agents should not be given to patients with moderately severe renal failure.— D. J. Warren *et al.*, *Br. med. J.*, 1974, *2*, 193. Criticism.— P. Kincaid-Smith and A. S. P. Hua (letter), *ibid.*, 1974, *3*, 520. In 69 patients treated for not less than 6 months with propranolol mean initial creatinine clearance was 72.3 ml per minute and final clearance 69.2 ml per minute. In no instance had there been a fall in renal function sufficient to affect the patient clinically.— F. D. Thompson and A. M. Joekes (letter), *ibid.*, 1974, *2*, 555. Two further reports of sudden deterioration in renal function after administration of propranolol to patients with chronic renal failure.— C. P. Swainson and R. J. Winney (letter), *ibid.*, 1976, *1*, 459.

Propranolol 40 to 80 mg daily rapidly reduced blood pressure to normal and reduced plasma-renin activity in 2 patients with chronic renal failure and hypertension which had been refractory in spite of regular haemodialysis. The need for nephrectomy was avoided.— S. B. Moore and F. J. Goodwin, *Lancet*, 1976, *2*, 67.

The pharmacokinetics and effects of propranolol in terminal uraemic patients. Preliminary data suggested that, because of the greater systemic availability of the drug and reduced hepatic clearance, lower doses of propranolol should be given to patients with renal failure not yet undergoing dialysis. Although haemodialysis itself does not appear to contribute to removal of propranolol, marked fluctuations were noted in blood concentrations owing to variations in the hepatic elimination capacity and the apparent volume of distribution; no alteration in plasma protein binding was noted. Propranolol should be used with great caution and in low doses in patients with chronic renal failure.— G. Bianchetti *et al.*, *Clin. Pharmacokinet.*, 1976, *1*, 373. A similar study.— D. T. Lowenthal *et al.*, *Clin. Pharmac. Ther.*, 1974, *16*, 761.

Massive retention of propranolol metabolites in patients undergoing maintenance haemodialysis.— W. J. Stone and T. Walle, *Clin. Pharmac. Ther.*, 1980, *28*, 449.

A study indicating that there is no pharmacokinetic reason to amend the dosage of propranolol in patients with renal failure.— A. J. J. Wood *et al.*, *Br. J. clin. Pharmac.*, 1980, *10*, 561.

Further references: A. Lindner *et al.*, *Ann. intern. Med.*, 1978, *88*, 457.

See also Renal Osteodystrophy under Hypertension.

Administration in respiratory insufficiency. A study of propranolol and other beta-adrenoceptor blocking agents in asthma, and the warning that no beta-adrenoceptor blocking agent, even if claiming to be cardioselective, is absolutely safe for the asthmatic patient.— P. B. S. Decalmer *et al.*, *Br. Heart J.*, 1978, *40*, 184.

Further reports and comments: K. N. V. Palmer (letter), *Br. med. J.*, 1977, *1*, 841; V. M. S. Oh *et al.*, *Br. J. clin. Pharmac.*, 1978, *5*, 107.

Alcoholism. Reviews of propranolol in alcohol withdrawal: C. Carlsson, *Postgrad. med. J.*, 1976, *52*, *Suppl.* 4, 166.

In a double-blind study involving 64 male alcoholics, 32 received propranolol 40 to 160 mg daily for 3 days and 32 received placebo prior to acute alcohol administration. Subsequent tests demonstrated that propranolol did not block or significantly modify the effects of acute alcohol ingestion on objective measurements of mood and cognitive function in alcoholics.— J. H. Mendelson *et al.*, *Clin. Pharmac. Ther.*, 1974, *15*, 571. Some beneficial effects of propranolol in mild to moderately severe alcohol withdrawal.— E. M. Sellers *et al.*, *ibid.*, 1976, *19*, 115.

Further reports: P. Tyrer (letter), *Lancet*, 1972, *2*, 707; D. M. Gallant *et al.*, *J. clin. Pharmac.*, 1973, *13*, 41; D. H. Zilm *et al.* (letter), *Ann. intern. Med.*, 1975, *83*, 234; C. Carlsson and B. G. Fasth, *Br. J. Addict.*, 1976, *71*, 321; H. Teräväinen and A. Larsen, *J. Neurol. Neurosurg. Psychiat.*, 1976, *39*, 607; E. M. Sellers *et al.*, *J. Stud. Alcohol*, 1977, *38*, 2096.

Anaesthesia. An evaluation of propranolol in the prevention of cardiac overactivity and cardiac arrhythmias during halothane anaesthesia.— M. Johnstone, *Br. J. Anaesth.*, 1966, *38*, 516.

Propranolol 1 to 2 mg was given intravenously to 115 patients during or after cardiovascular surgery under halothane anaesthesia. In 141 episodes of cardiac irregularities, it was usually effective in causing reversion to normal sinus rhythm within 1 to 3 minutes.— A. McClish *et al.*, *Can. med. Ass. J.*, 1968, *99*, 388.

Further references: J. Hellewell and M. W. Potts, *Br. J. Anaesth.*, 1966, *38*, 794; K. Fukushima *et al.*, *ibid.*, 1968, *40*, 53; R. G. Merin, *Anesth. Analg. curr. Res.*, 1972, *51*, 617; A. Romagnoli and P. B. Sabawala, *Clin. Pharmac. Ther.*, 1974, *15*, 217.

Anxiety. The (+)-isomer of propranolol (dexpropranolol) which caused no β-blockade had no effect on anxiety in a double-blind crossover pilot study of 10 patients indicating that the anti-anxiety effect observed previously with (±)-propranolol was due to its beta-blocking activity and not to a central action.— J. A. Bonn and P. Turner (letter), *Lancet*, 1971, *1*, 1355. See also P. J. Tyrer and M. H. Lader, *Br. J. clin. Pharmac.*, 1974, *1*, 379; *idem*, 387.

In a crossover study in 6 patients with chronic anxiety and mainly somatic symptoms and 6 further patients with mainly psychic symptoms given successively propranolol, diazepam, or placebo, patient preference and psychiatric rating favoured diazepam for the whole group, but in the patients with somatic symptoms the response to diazepam and propranolol was comparable.— P. J. Tyrer and M. H. Lader, *Br. med. J.*, 1974, *2*, 14.

Infusion of isoprenaline could be used to detect which anxiety-prone patients would respond to propranolol since such infusions precipitated anxiety attacks in susceptible patients.— D. G. Sherman and J. D. Easton (letter), *Lancet*, 1976, *2*, 911. See also J. D. Easton and

D. G. Sherman, *Archs Neurol., Chicago*, 1976, *33*, 689.

Comment on the value of beta-blockade to counteract stage-fright among musicians. Although beta-blockade could counteract the physical effect, the mental component remained a problem.— T. A. Brantigan *et al.* (letter), *Lancet*, 1978, *2*, 896. Criticism of the use of propranolol to combat stage-fright.— C. Swartz (letter), *ibid.*, 1105.

A report on beneficial effects with propranolol in some forms of acute pathological panic states.— J. F. Heiser and D. DeFrancisco, *Am. J. Psychiat.*, 1976, *133*, 1389.

Further references: C. Brewer (letter), *Lancet*, 1972, *2*, 435; A. W. Webster (letter), *ibid.*, 542; W. N. Stone *et al.*, *Archs gen. Psychiat.*, 1973, *29*, 620; P. C. Bryan *et al.* (letter), *Br. J. clin. Pharmac.*, 1974, *1*, 82; R. Kellner *et al.*, *J. clin. Pharmac.*, 1974, *14*, 301; M. G. Bamber (letter), *Lancet*, 1980, *2*, 1308.

Cardiac disorders. *Angina pectoris.* Reviews of the use of propranolol in the management of angina pectoris: H. B. Kay, *Drugs*, 1977, *13*, 276; J. A. Cairns, *Can. med. Ass. J.*, 1978, *119*, 477; G. D. Plotnick, *J. Am. med. Ass.*, 1978, *239*, 860; H. Ikram, *Drugs*, 1979, *18*, 130.

Of 35 patients with angina 19 of 29 who were sexually active experienced anginal pain during intercourse. After basic advice all were given beta-blocking agents. Patients experiencing pain became free from pain (6 also needed isosorbide dinitrate) and 4 resumed sexual activity.— G. Jackson, *Br. med. J.*, 1978, *2*, 16.

In a comparative study involving 16 patients with stable angina pectoris, single doses of propranolol, oxprenolol, practolol, tolamolol, and metoprolol were generally equally effective in the treatment of exercise-induced angina. A beneficial effect occurred within one hour and persisted for at least 8 hours.— U. Thadani *et al.*, *New Engl. J. Med.*, 1979, *300*, 750.

Preliminary report on an interim follow-up of a multicentre study to which 768 patients with stable angina pectoris were admitted for a comparative study of surgical against medical treatment. Patients randomised to treatment with bypass surgery did not have a significantly higher survival-rate at 2 years than those allotted to treatment without bypass surgery. This agrees with the finding of M.L. Murphy *et al.* (*New Engl. J. Med.*, 1977, *297*, 621) but, unlike their finding, a significantly higher survival-rate was noted in patients with three-vessel disease who underwent surgery. There was a significant decrease in the proportion of patients in the surgical group treated with beta-adrenoceptor blocking agents but no change in the medical group.—European Coronary Surgery Study Group, *Lancet*, 1979, *1*, 889. Similar studies: M. L. Murphy *et al.*, *New Engl. J. Med.*, 1977, *297*, 621; *ibid.*, 1464–70; N. de Soyza *et al.*, *Ann. intern. Med.*, 1978, *89*, 10; F. E. Kloster *et al.*, *New Engl. J. Med.*, 1979, *300*, 149. Second Interim Report by the European Coronary Surgery Study Group, *Lancet*, 1980, *2*, 491.

In a double-blind study involving 16 patients with severe exertional angina pectoris the incidence of pain and consumption of glyceryl trinitrate were significantly decreased by nifedipine 30 or 60 mg daily compared with placebo, but a significantly greater reduction was produced by propranolol 240 or 480 mg daily. Although the higher dose of propranolol had no additional benefit over the lower dose, the higher dose of nifedipine was significantly more effective than the lower. Combination of the 2 drugs in the higher doses produced further significant improvement.— P. Lynch *et al.*, *Br. med. J.*, 1980, *281*, 184.

Further references: J. D. Fitzgerald, *Postgrad. med. J.*, 1976, *52*, 770; S. G. Warren *et al.*, *Am. J. Cardiol.*, 1976, *37*, 420; B. Pugh *et al.*, *ibid.*, 1978, *41*, 1291; H. Halkin *et al.*, *Eur. J. clin. Pharmac.*, 1979, *16*, 387.

Cardiac arrhythmias. Reviews of anti-arrhythmic drugs, including propranolol: J. L. Anderson *et al.*, *Drugs*, 1978, *15*, 271; *Med. Lett.*, 1978, *20*, 113.

In a study of 12 patients with stable ventricular ectopic beats given propranolol and dexpropranolol, it was shown that suppression of ventricular ectopic beats by propranolol was closely related to beta-adrenoceptor blockade and not to its quinidine-like effect.— D. J. Coltart *et al.*, *Br. med. J.*, 1971, *1*, 490. In a study involving dexpropranolol, the dextro-isomer of alprenolol, and practolol it was concluded that both beta-blocking activity and membrane (quinidine-like) activity were drug actions capable of suppressing ectopic cardiac rhythms.— E. Smith *et al.*, *Guy's Hosp. Rep.*, 1971, *120*, 9, per *Abstr. Wld Med.*, 1971, *45*, 836.

Propranolol was the drug of choice in the treatment of regular supraventricular tachycardia with normal QRS complexes in Wolff-Parkinson-White syndrome. Maintenance doses of propranolol hydrochloride, 10 to 30 mg three or four times daily by mouth, might be useful in the prevention of arrhythmias. In some cases combined treatment with quinidine may be necessary.— E. K. Chung, *J. Am. med. Ass.*, 1977, *237*, 376. See also *idem*, *Am. J. Med.*, 1977, *62*, 252.

Syncopal attacks in a patient with Wolff-Parkinson-White syndrome following administration of propranolol.— E. M. Berry and Y. Hasin, *Chest*, 1978, *73*, 873.

Further references: P. H. Dworkin *et al.*, *Archs Dis. Childh.*, 1973, *48*, 382 (in children); C. Z. Naggar and S. Alexander (letter), *New Engl. J. Med.*, 1976, *294*, 903; K. Wang *et al.*, *Archs intern. Med.*, 1977, *137*, 161; P. C. Gillette *et al.*, *J. Pediat.*, 1978, *92*, 141 (in children); P. Denes *et al.*, *Am. J. Cardiol.*, 1978, *41*, 1061; J. V. Nixon *et al.*, *Circulation*, 1978, *57*, 115; R. A. Winkle *et al.*, *Am. Heart J.*, 1977, *93*, 422.

Cardiomyopathy. A comparative study of 24 patients with congestive cardiomyopathy taking beta-adrenoceptor blocking agents (alprenolol, practolol, or metoprolol) in addition to digitalis and diuretics, with a similar group of 13 controls selected retrospectively who had not taken beta-blockers. The survival-rate in those also receiving beta-blockers was 83%, 66%, and 52% after 1, 2, and 3 years respectively, compared with only 46%, 19%, and 10% in those who had not received beta-blockers.— K. Swedberg *et al.* (preliminary communication), *Lancet*, 1979, *1*, 1374.

Comment on the use and hazards of beta-blockade in congestive cardiomyopathy, and the view that a controlled trial is needed before it can be recommended.— *Lancet*, 1981, *1*, 598.

Results of a double-blind controlled study of acebutolol in 15 patients argued against routine administration of beta-adrenoceptor blocking agents in congestive cardiomyopathy.— H. Ikram and D. Fitzpatrick, *Lancet*, 1981, *2*, 490.

Propranolol is standard therapy for hypertrophic obstructive cardiomyopathy.— L. H. Opie, *Lancet*, 1980, *1*, 693.

Further references: E. M. V. Williams *et al.*, *Lancet*, 1977, *2*, 850.

Fallot's tetralogy. Propranolol by mouth was often of value in milder dyspnoeic spells associated with Fallot's tetralogy and where there was less severe organic narrowing of the right-ventricular outflow tract. Propranolol intravenously was often of value during acute attacks.— G. R. Cumming (letter), *Lancet*, 1966, *2*, 1317.

Further references: B. O. Eriksson *et al.*, *Br. Heart J.*, 1969, *31*, 37.

Marfan syndrome. Prophylactic propranolol is given to patients with Marfan syndrome who are unsuitable for surgery or whose operations are delayed.— R. M. Donaldson *et al.*, *Lancet*, 1980, *2*, 1178.

Myocardial infarction. Reviews and comments on the use of beta-adrenoceptor blockade in myocardial infarction: *Drug & Ther. Bull.*, 1977, *15*, 33; *Lancet*, 1978, *2*, 1082; B. N. Singh, *Drugs*, 1978, *15*, 218; *Lancet*, 1979, *1*, 193; B. E. Sobel, *New Engl. J. Med.*, 1979, *300*, 191; *Lancet*, 1981, *1*, 873.

The platelets of hypertensive patients receiving *dl*-propranolol or *d*-propranolol aggregated less readily in response to thrombin or arachidonic acid than when they received placebo.— W. B. Campbell *et al.*, *Lancet*, 1981, *2*, 1382.

Analysis of final results, after the receipt of information previously lacking, generally confirmed that long-term treatment with beta-adrenoceptor blockade after myocardial infarction reduced mortality. Beta-blockade was recommended after anterior infarction, unless specifically contra-indicated; it should begin as soon as it was clear that serious impairment of conduction was absent, and that congestive failure was unlikely; it should probably continue for up to 2 years.—Multicentre International Study: Supplementary Report, *Br. med. J.*, 1977, *2*, 419. The earlier study, which relates to work using practolol: A Multicentre International Study, *Br. med. J.*, 1975, *3*, 735.

Propranolol 100 µg per kg body-weight was administered intravenously to 20 patients within 4 hours of the onset of suspected myocardial infarction, and followed by a total of 320 mg by mouth over the next 27 hours. Compared with 23 similar control patients the number of completed infarcts as assessed by ECG, and the number of serum-creatine kinase concentrations above the normal range was significantly reduced. The mean peak value of serum-creatine kinase concentrations was more than halved although the range, especially in the controls, was such that the difference was only of borderline significance.— R. M. Norris *et al.*, *Lancet*, 1978, *2*, 907. Criticism. An unusually high incidence of infarction in the control group may have resulted in a spuriously high beneficial effect of propranolol. A retrospective study of 50 untreated patients showed a similar rate of infarction to that cited for those treated with propranolol.— K. A. A. Fox and M. F. Oliver (letter), *ibid.*, 1979, *1*, 555. Reply.— R. M. Norris *et al.* (letter), *ibid.*, 787.

Study in 261 patients with suspected myocardial infarction showed a high incidence of serious arrhythmias, but propranolol or atenolol, in doses tolerated without causing undue hypotension, did not have a significant anti-arrhythmic effect.— J. M. Roland *et al.*, *Br. med. J.*, 1979, *2*, 518. Criticism. The recordings were made too late after the occurrence of chest pain; oral administration might have led to inadequate blood concentrations.— P. Sleight and S. Yusuf (letter), *ibid.*, 864.

A preliminary report of the double-blind randomised β-Blocker Heart Attack Trial in 3837 patients who had suffered acute myocardial infarction, indicating that patients receiving propranolol experienced a 26% lower mortality from all causes than did the control group. Overall mortality in the treated group was 7% (135 deaths) compared with 9.5% (183 deaths) in the placebo group. The study has consequently been curtailed. Patients entered the trial 5 to 21 days (average 13.8) after the onset of acute myocardial infarction and received either propranolol hydrochloride 40 mg or placebo thrice daily. A maintenance dose of 60 or 80 mg thrice daily was prescribed at follow-up 1 month later. Beneficial effects occurred primarily in the first year after infarction and were not affected by the size of infarct or the age or sex of the patient.—β-Blocker Heart Attack Study Group, *J. Am. med. Ass.*, 1981, *246*, 2073.

In a double-blind randomised study of 560 high-risk patients who had survived acute myocardial infarction, treatment for one year with propranolol significantly reduced the number of sudden cardiac deaths when compared with placebo. Treatment was started 4 to 6 days after infarction and patients received either propranolol 40 mg four times daily or placebo.— V. Hansteen *et al.*, *Br. med. J.*, 1982, *284*, 155.

Further references: H. K. Gold *et al.*, *Am. J. Cardiol.*, 1976, *38*, 689; H. S. Mueller and S. M. Ayres, *Prog. cardiovasc. Dis.*, 1977, *19*, 405; R. G. Wilcox *et al.*, *Lancet*, 1980, *2*, 765; *idem*, *Br. med. J.*, 1980, *280*, 885. The Norwegian Multicenter Study Group, *New Engl. J. Med.*, 1981, *304*, 801; P. Sleight, *ibid.*, 837; S. S. Swart *et al.* (letter), *Lancet*, 1981, *1*, 159; Å. Hjalmarson *et al.*, *Lancet*, 1981, *2*, 823.

Prinzmetal's variant angina. Although theoretically propranolol could worsen Prinzmetal's variant angina, in practice it does not appear to do so. Lower doses of propranolol do not appear to improve or worsen Prinzmetal's variant angina, but marked relief of attacks has been reported with propranolol in doses totalling 160 to 800 mg daily.— R. MacAlpin (letter), *New Engl. J. Med.*, 1976, *294*, 1007.

References: M. Guazzi *et al.*, *Br. Heart J.*, 1971, *33*, 889; *idem*, 1975, *37*, 1235.

Prosthetic valves. Propranolol reduced haemolysis in patients with an aortic prosthetic valve, probably by reducing the heart-rate.— J. T. Santinga *et al.*, *Am. Heart J.*, 1977, *93*, 197.

Causalgia. A woman with intractable causalgia of the left foot improved by more than 50% within 48 hours of starting propranolol 240 mg daily. Therapy was maintained at 240 mg daily for 3 months, then progressively reduced, with no recurrence of the problem at the 6-month follow-up. A second patient with Sudeck's atrophy with causalgia was successfully treated with propranolol.— G. Simson (letter), *J. Am. med. Ass.*, 1974, *227*, 327. Causalgia of the left arm was not relieved by propranolol, up to 360 mg daily for 10 days, in a 43-year-old patient.— C. P. Magee and H. J. Grosz (letter), *ibid.*, *228*, 826.

Further references: A. B. Pleet *et al.*, *Neurology, Minneap.*, 1976, *26*, 375.

Cerebral spasm. An *in vitro* study indicated that propranolol might be of value in the reversal of cerebral arterial spasm provided high enough concentrations could be achieved.— D. J. Boullin and J. Mohan, *Br. J. clin. Pharmac.*, 1977, *4*, 27.

Cocaine overdosage. For conflicting reports on the benefit of propranolol in acute cocaine intoxication, see Cocaine Hydrochloride, p.915.

Erythromelalgia. A woman with long-standing and worsening erythromelalgia with severe and frequent burning of the lower legs, ankles, and feet and occasional desquamation failed to respond to clonidine. Since these symptoms were the opposite of those of Raynaud's phenomenon which could be induced by beta-adrenoceptor blocking agents, treatment was tried with propranolol 10 mg thrice daily. There was a rapid and complete response which had been maintained for 3 months.— J.

L. Bada (letter), *Lancet*, 1977, *2*, 412.

Explosive rage. The form of explosive rage that often occurs as a patient emerges from coma following head injury can sometimes be controlled rather dramatically by large doses of propranolol (up to 80 mg four times daily).— F. A. Elliott, *Practitioner*, 1976, *217*, 51.

Gastro-intestinal disorders. *Carcinoid syndrome.* The frequency of spontaneous flushes in a man suffering from the carcinoid syndrome was reduced following treatment with propranolol 10 mg four times daily. The effect gradually diminished and the frequency of flushing increased. In the same patient, methysergide 1 mg thrice daily was followed by a brief improvement of diarrhoea.— R. Zeegen *et al.*, *Gut*, 1969, *10*, 617.

Diarrhoea. Propranolol was ineffective in postvagotomy diarrhoea.— T. V. Taylor *et al.*, *Lancet*, 1978, *1*, 635.

Propranolol 4 mg per kg body-weight daily for 7 days had no effect on chronic watery diarrhoea in 2 patients, one with pancreatic cholera syndrome and the other with steatorrhoea.— M. Donowitz and A. N. Charney (letter), *New Engl. J. Med.*, 1979, *300*, 201.

Further references: M. J. Coyne *et al.*, *Gastroenterology*, 1977, *73*, 971.

Dumping syndrome. Patients suffering from the dumping syndrome often obtained relief from circulatory symptoms with propranolol, 20 to 40 mg thrice daily before meals.— J. E. Lennard-Jones, *Prescribers' J.*, 1967, *7*, 7.

Spastic colon. For a study on the use of propranolol with dexamphetamine in the spastic colon syndrome, see Dexamphetamine Sulphate, p.363.

Glaucoma. A review of beta-adrenoceptor blocking agents in the management of open-angle glaucoma.— W. P. Boger, *Drugs*, 1979, *18*, 25.

The effect of propranolol on ocular tension was studied in 7 patients with open-angle glaucoma, 3 of whom had been treated previously with digoxin. Propranolol was given intravenously in a dose of 10 mg, and caused a fall in pressure that was maximal about 1 to 2.5 hours later. Subsequently, 4 patients were treated by mouth thrice daily, with doses of 5 to 40 mg, but in 3 patients the reduction in ocular pressure could not be sustained by oral therapy. The fourth patient, however, was successfully maintained on 15 mg thrice daily.— C. I. Phillips *et al.*, *Br. J. Ophthal.*, 1967, *51*, 222.

Propranolol hydrochloride eye-drops 1% significantly reduced intra-ocular pressure in 7 of 10 patients with raised pressure.— J. Vale *et al.*, *Br. J. Ophthal.*, 1972, *56*, 770.

A single-blind study in 12 patients with ocular hypertension showed that propranolol 20, 40, or 80 mg significantly reduced intra-ocular pressure in a dose-related manner.— K. Wettrell and M. Pandolfi, *Br. J. Ophthal.*, 1976, *60*, 680.

Further references: A. Ohrström and M. Pandolfi, *Am. J. Ophthal.*, 1978, *86*, 340.

Growth-hormone secretion test. For references to the use of propranolol in growth-hormone secretion tests, see Glucagon, p.705, and Levodopa, p.888.

Hepatic disorders. The effect of propranolol in reducing portal venous pressure might be useful in the prevention of recurrent bleeding caused by oesophageal varices in patients with cirrhosis.— D. Lebrec *et al.*, *Lancet*, 1980, *2*, 180. Although this use of beta-blockers in portal hypertension could have important implications, caution is needed in cirrhotics with ascites, a number of whom appear to be dependent on the renin-angiotensin system for maintaining their blood pressure.— S. P. Wilkinson (letter), *ibid.*, 429.

Long-term treatment with propranolol, in a dosage which reduced the heart-rate by about 25% (dose range, 20 to 180 mg twice daily), prevented recurrent gastro-intestinal bleeding in a controlled study of 74 patients with cirrhosis. A year after inclusion in the study 96% of treated patients were free of re-bleeding compared with 50% of the placebo group.— D. Lebrec *et al.*, *New Engl. J. Med.*, 1981, *305*, 1371.

Huntington's chorea. There was a decrease in choreiform movement and improved speech in a patient with Huntington's chorea when propranolol 20 mg four times daily was added to existing treatment with haloperidol 5 mg three or 4 times daily and hydrochlorothiazide with potassium supplements.— D. J. Martin (letter), *Drug Intell. & clin. Pharm.*, 1977, *11*, 245.

Hyperhidrosis. A recommendation that propranolol and other beta-adrenoceptor blocking agents are not suitable for the prevention of excessive sweating.— *Br. med. J.*, 1977, *2*, 876.

Hyperparathyroidism. Propranolol 120 mg daily reduced plasma concentrations of parathyroid hormone and calcium to near normal in one patient with angina and hyperparathyroidism.— J. F. Caro and A. Besarab (letter), *Lancet*, 1978, *1*, 827. Propranolol 10 mg four times daily increased to 40 mg four times daily did not control symptoms in 2 patients with probable primary hyperparathyroidism.— J. P. Monson *et al.* (letter), *ibid.*, 1979, *1*, 884.

Further references: A. Fournier *et al.* (letter), *Lancet*, 1978, *2*, 50.

See also Renal Osteodystrophy under Hypertension.

Hypertension. Reviews of the use of propranolol in hypertension: O. B. Holland and N. M. Kaplan, *New Engl. J. Med.*, 1976, *294*, 930; R. P. Ahlquist, *J. clin. Pharmac.*, 1977, *17*, 93; L. Hansson and L. Werkö, *Am. Heart J.*, 1977, *93*, 394; A. R. Lorimer and W. S. Hillis, *Adv. Med. Topics Ther.*, 1977, *3*, 218; H. J. Waal-Manning, *Drugs*, 1979, *17*, 129; B. N. C. Prichard, *Br. J. clin. Pharmac.*, 1982, *13*, 51.

Propranolol was given to 109 hypertensive patients in a dosage of 5 or 10 mg four times a day and increased, usually fortnightly, by about 25% per dose, usually until the diastolic blood pressure was controlled in the range of 80 to 100 mmHg. Six to 8 weeks were often required to reach a maximum hypotensive effect, and the dosages employed ranged from 5 mg twice daily to 1 g four times a day; some patients received this treatment for 3.5 years. Propranolol was withdrawn from 9 patients. Good control of supine blood pressure at 100 mmHg or less was achieved in 92 patients without producing postural or exercise hypotension. Propranolol was at least of similar potency to bethanidine, guanethidine, and methyldopa, and its hypotensive effect appeared to be additive to that of these drugs and to diuretics. Side-effects from propranolol included tiredness in 4 patients, cold extremities in 3, and occasional dizziness in 3. In a subjective comparison of previous therapy with bethanidine, guanethidine, or methyldopa, 26 of 31 patients felt better with propranolol therapy.— B. N. C. Prichard and P. M. S. Gillam, *Br. med. J.*, 1969, *1*, 7. Criticisms.— G. S. Humphries and D. G. Delvin (letter), *ibid.*, 445; F. J. Zacharias (letter), *ibid.*, 712.

Further references: B. N. C. Prichard *et al.*, *Br. Heart J.*, 1970, *32*, 236; F. J. Zacharias and K. J. Cowen, *Br. med. J.*, 1970, *1*, 471; C. T. Dollery and J. W. Paterson (letter), *ibid.*, 1970, *2*, 236; R. C. Tarazi *et al.*, *Am. Heart J.*, 1971, *82*, 770; R. C. Tarazi and H. P. Dustan, *Am. J. Cardiol.*, 1972, 29,, per 633 L. J. Beilin and B. E. Juel-Jensen, *Lancet*, 1972, *1*, 979; D. G. Gill (letter), *ibid.*, 1125; P. Franzen and A. Pasternack (letter), *Br. med. J.*, 1972, *3*, 763; F. J. Zacharias *et al.*, *Am. Heart J.*, 1972, *83*, 755; P. Hamet *et al.*, *Can. med. Ass. J.*, 1973, *109*, 1099; D. M. D. Lambert, *Practitioner*, 1973, *210*, 277; L. Wilson *et al.*, *Med. J. Aust.*, 1974, *1*, 212; J. W. Hollifield *et al.*, *New Engl. J. Med.*, 1976, *295*, 68; L. R. Krakoff, *ibid.*, 102; D. B. Galloway *et al.*, *Br. med. J.*, 1976, *2*, 140; J. Guevara *et al.*, *Curr. ther. Res.*, 1977, *21*, 277; B. Lindborg and L. Hansson, *Practitioner*, 1977, *218*, 435; W. A. Pettinger *et al.*, *Clin. Pharmac. Ther.*, 1977, *22*, 164; W. J. Mroczek and M. E. Davidov, *Curr. ther. Res.*, 1978, *23*, 294; M. Velasco *et al.*, *Br. J. clin. Pharmac.*, 1978, *6*, 217; M. J. Serlin *et al.*, *Clin. Pharmac. Ther.*, 1980, *27*, 586; J. Staessen *et al.* (letter), *New Engl. J. Med.*, 1980, *303*, 1121.

For a report of the MRC Working Party on Mild to Moderate Hypertension, see p.135.

In children. In 9 hypertensive children propranolol in doses of 0.6 to 6.4 mg per kg body-weight daily (average 2.5 mg per kg) reduced blood pressure and heart-rate, and was well tolerated. Five children also received a diuretic and methyldopa or hydralazine.— W. R. Griswold *et al.*, *Archs Dis. Childh.*, 1978, *53*, 594.

Further references: J. G. Mongeau *et al.* (letter), *Can. med. Ass. J.*, 1977, *116*, 589 (adolescents with essential hypertension); D. E. Potter *et al.*, *J. Pediat.*, 1977, *90*, 309 (renal transplantation).

Comparative studies. In a double-blind crossover study 20 patients with moderate to severe hypertension were given propranolol 40 mg, alprenolol 100 mg, pindolol 5 mg, or timolol 5 mg; these doses were given thrice daily and doubled if needed; mean daily doses were 176, 460, 23, and 24 mg respectively, in addition to existing medication. The fall in blood pressure in the 4 groups was broadly comparable. Heart-rate was reduced to the greatest extent in those taking propranolol or timolol. Dreams, often bizarre, occurred, particularly in patients taking pindolol; bronchospasm occurred in patients taking propranolol or timolol. In a further study in which the doses were increased in order to try to get a response in those previously resistant, patients resistant to one drug were generally resistant to others.— T. O. Morgan *et al.*, *Postgrad. med. J.*, 1974, *50*, 253.

Further references to comparative studies with other beta-adrenoceptor blocking agents: C. Davidson *et al.*, *Br. med. J.*, 1976, *2*, 7.

See also under other beta-adrenoceptor blocking agents.

In a double-blind study in 450 patients with mild hypertension propranolol, alone or in combination with hydrochlorothiazide and hydralazine or in combination with either, was compared with reserpine with hydrochlorothiazide. Reduction of diastolic blood pressure to below 90 mmHg and a reduction of at least 5 mmHg from the initial blood pressure after 6 months' treatment was achieved in 92% of patients taking propranolol with hydrochlorothiazide and hydralazine, 88% taking reserpine and hydrochlorothiazide, 81% taking propranolol and hydrochlorothiazide, 72% taking propranolol and hydralazine, and 52% taking propranolol alone. No regimen had any advantage over any other with relation to side-effects.—Veterans Administration Cooperative Study Group on Antihypertensive Agents, *J. Am. med. Ass.*, 1977, *237*, 2303.

Comparative studies with other antihypertensive agents: N. D. Vlachakis and M. Mendlowitz, *J. clin. Pharmac.*, 1976, *16*, 352 (phenoxybenzamine and hydrochlorothiazide); G. Berglund *et al.*, *Curr. ther. Res.*, 1977, *21*, 830 (hydralazine and spironolactone); P. R. Wilkinson and E. B. Raftery, *Br. J. clin. Pharmac.*, 1977, *4*, 289 (clonidine); F. G. Dunn *et al.*, *Br. J. clin. Pharmac.*, 1978, *5*, 223 (methyldopa).

For a study comparing long-term thiazide diuretic therapy with propranolol in mild to moderately severe essential hypertension, see Bendrofluazide, p.585.

Effect on plasma renin. Reviews on the antihypertensive action of beta-adrenoceptor blocking agents and the renin-angiotensin system: I. Gavras *et al.*, *Br. J. clin. Pharmac.*, 1979, *7*, *Suppl.* 2, 213S.

A review of studies aimed at elucidating the role of propranolol as an antihypertensive agent relative to plasma-renin activity.— L. R. Krakoff, *New Engl. J. Med.*, 1976, *295*, 102.

Further reviews: J. Hamer, *Br. J. clin. Pharmac.*, 1976, *3*, 425; J. R. Mitchell *et al.*, *Ann. intern. Med.*, 1977, *87*, 596.

Measurement of plasma-renin activity was used to classify 47 patients with hypertension into high, normal, and low renin groups, before treatment with propranolol. Those with high renin activity showed the greatest fall in blood pressure, usually within 24 hours, and also the greatest decrease in plasma renin activity. The normal renin group had large but variable falls in blood pressure; there was little antihypertensive effect in the low renin group and a correspondingly smaller reduction in renin activity.— F. R. Bühler *et al.*, *New Engl. J. Med.*, 1972, *287*, 1209. See also *ibid.*, 1247; *Lancet*, 1973, *1*, 243.

A study of the antihypertensive effect of propranolol in 40 patients with high-, normal- or low-renin essential hypertension. Results suggested that the antihypertensive effect of propranolol was associated with both renin-dependent and renin-independent effects.— J. W. Hollifield *et al.*, *New Engl. J. Med.*, 1976, *295*, 68.

Propranolol, like the other sympatholytic agents, methyldopa, clonidine, or guanethidine sulphate, is an inefficient antihypertensive agent in most volume-expanded (renin-suppressed) subjects. If the renin level is low emphasis should be placed on the use of diuretics to raise the renin level to normal, blood pressure control being obtained in a sizeable proportion of such patients by means of diuretic therapy alone. In the majority of hypertensive subjects, whose renin levels are normal, the emphasis should be placed on the sympatholytic agents with addition of a moderate dose of diuretic, such as hydrochlorothiazide 50 mg. A small proportion of patients with advanced renal disease and volume expansion may also have high renin levels and require aggressive diuresis and/or dialysis in association with other potent antihypertensive agents, including minoxidil.— W. A. Pettinger, *Archs intern. Med.*, 1977, *137*, 679.

Further references: G. S. Stokes *et al.*, *Br. med. J.*, 1974, *1*, 60; E. L. Bravo *et al.*, *New Engl. J. Med.*, 1975, *292*, 66; T. O. Morgan *et al.*, *Br. J. clin. Pharmac.*, 1975, *2*, 159; E. L. Bravo *et al.*, *Circulation Res.*, 1975, *36 and 37*, *Suppl.* 1, 241; B. E. Karlberg *et al.*, *Br. med. J.*, 1976, *1*, 251; F. Skrabal *et al.*, *ibid.*, 1976, *2*, 144; S. A. Atlas *et al.*, *Lancet*, 1977, *2*, 785; M. A. Weber *et al.*, *Archs intern. Med.*, 1977, *137*, 284; S. Mookherjee *et al.*, *ibid.*, 290; A. Zweifler and M. Esler, *Am. J. Cardiol.*, 1977, *40*, 105; P. Jaeger *et al.*, *J. clin. Pharmac.*, 1978, *18*, 311.

Once-daily administration. Seventeen patients with mild to moderate hypertension receiving propranolol 240 mg, metoprolol 200 mg, or acebutolol 400 mg once daily between 7 am and 8 am were studied throughout 24 hours under carefully standardised conditions. Results indicated that once-daily beta-adrenoceptor blocking therapy reduces blood pressure substantially during both sleep and physical activity throughout 24 hours. Variability in arterial pressure associated with physical activity was also reduced throughout the 24-hour period. It is not known whether the average pressure is the major factor causing damage to the arterial wall or whether peaks in pressure are important, but reduction in variability as well as reduction in pressure is a potential advantage that beta-adrenoceptor blocking agents have over diuretics and anti-adrenergic drugs which would be expected to increase variability.— R. D. S. Watson *et al.*, *Lancet*, 1979, *1*, 1210. Comment.— S. Mann *et al.* (letter), *ibid.*, 1979, *2*, 150.

Further references: A. Westerlund and L. Hansson, *Br. med. J.*, 1976, *2*, 877; A. P. Douglas-Jones *et al.*, *Eur. J. clin. Pharmac.*, 1978, *14*, 163; J. O. Woods, *Practitioner*, 1979, *223*, 834; J. C. Petrie *et al.*, *Br. med. J.*, 1980, *280*, 1573; P. Rudd *et al.*, *Curr. ther. Res.*, 1980, *27*, 29.

Renal osteodystrophy. Nine patients undergoing haemodialysis for chronic renal failure who were receiving propranolol for hypertension or angina pectoris, had lower parathyroid hormone and alkaline phosphatase concentrations in serum than 25 similar patients who were not receiving propranolol. The patients taking propranolol also had less evidence of renal osteodystrophy. Propranolol appeared to suppress the release of parathyroid hormone and might be useful in reversing or preventing renal osteodystrophy.— J. F. Caro *et al.*, *Lancet*, 1978, *2*, 451. Comments and criticisms.— D. Brancaccio *et al.* (letter), *ibid.*, 940; A. Fournier *et al.* (letter), *ibid.*, 1372. Reply to criticism.— J. F. Caro *et al.* (letter), *ibid.*, 1979, *1*, 101. Criticism of the comparability of the groups. Until prospective studies had been carried out with particular attention to the comparability of the control and treatment groups the wider use of propranolol as a treatment for the hyperparathyroidism of renal failure was premature.— J. B. Eastwood (letter), *ibid.*, 1979, *1*, 386. From a study in 9 patients it was doubtful whether propranolol had a role in the treatment of established hyperparathyroid bone disease in chronic renal failure.— K. Farrington *et al.*, *Br. med. J.*, 1980, *281*, 1320.

Further references: B. Coevoet *et al.*, *Br. med. J.*, 1980, *280*, 1344.

Renal scleroderma. A report of 3 patients who survived scleroderma renal crisis (severe uncontrolled hypertension and rapidly progressive renal failure) after intensive antihypertensive therapy. Their renal function improved and cutaneous scleroderma regressed. Vigorous antihypertensive therapy with multiple drugs was indicated in such patients before resorting to nephrectomy. Propranolol was the drug of first choice because of its renin-lowering properties.— C. Wasner *et al.*, *New Engl. J. Med.*, 1978, *299*, 873. Comment.— P. J. Cannon, *ibid.*, 886.

Further references: J. H. Felts *et al.* (letter), *J. Am. med. Ass.*, 1978, *239*, 1494.

Hyperthyroidism. An account of the management of hyperthyroidism with beta-adrenoceptor blockade. Mention is made of the value of propranolol in the pre-operative preparation for thyroidectomy and the need to continue therapy for 7 to 10 days postoperatively. Details are also given of the important role of propranolol in thyroid storm, with the caution that other general measures and antithyroid drugs must not be neglected. Those symptoms of hyperthyroidism which are improved by propranolol are listed together with its effects on the clinical signs of hyperthyroidism. The increased basal metabolic rate of hyperthyroidism is unaffected by beta-adrenoceptor blockade, but propranolol may reduce or eliminate the negative nitrogen balance. At present propranolol cannot be recommended for the sole treatment of hyperthyroidism since even in the most favourable reports the rate of remission is close to the reported spontaneous rate of remission, and patients would be subjected to the long-term metabolic effects of hyperthyroidism.— D. G. McDevitt, *Prescribers' J.*, 1977, *17*, 143.

Further reviews and comments: *Br. med. J.*, 1977, *2*, 1039; D. G. McDevitt, *Adv. Med. Topics Ther.*, 1977, *3*, 100; R. D. Utiger, *New Engl. J. Med.*, 1978, *298*, 681; M. H. Rosove (letter), *ibid.*, *299*, 45; R. D. Utiger (letter), *ibid.*, 46; R. Greene, *Prescribers' J.*, 1980, *20*, 73; *Lancet*, 1980, *1*, 184; J. Feely (letter), *ibid.*, 542.

Following a study in hyperthyroid and hypothyroid subjects, J.M. Bell *et al.* (*Br. J. clin. Pharmac.*, 1977, *4*, 79) have reported that the metabolism of propranolol does not appear to be affected by thyroid status. However, a study by S. Rubenfeld *et al.* (*New Engl. J. Med.*, 1979, *300*, 353) has emphasised the variability in plasma concentrations of propranolol in both euthyroid and hyperthyroid subjects, and the need to ensure that plasma concentrations of propranolol adequate to provide adrenoceptor inhibition are achieved. No significant changes have been noted in the plasma-protein binding of propranolol in hyperthyroidism or hypothyroidism (J.G. Kelly and D.G. McDevitt, *Br. J. clin. Pharmac.*, 1978, *6*, 123).

Reports and studies on the use of propranolol in hyperthyroidism: N. Pimstone *et al.*, *Lancet*, 1968, *2*, 1219; D. G. McLarty *et al.*, *Br. med. J.*, 1973, *2*, 332; L. A. Distiller *et al.* (letter), *Ann. intern. Med.*, 1973, *79*, 899; P. C. Teoh and J. S. Cheah, *Med. J. Aust.*, 1973, *2*, 116; M. J. Conway *et al.*, *Ann. intern. Med.*, 1974, *81*, 332; M. P. Rothberg *et al.*, *J. Am. med. Ass.*, 1974, *230*, 1017; R. Weinstein *et al.* (letter), *Ann. intern. Med.*, 1975, *82*, 540.

Mode of action. Findings in 2 groups of patients suggested that propranolol reduced the peripheral conversion of thyroxine to tri-iodothyronine.— P. Theilade *et al.* (letter), *Lancet*, 1977, *2*, 363.

Further studies: B. Ø. Kristensen and J. Weeke, *Clin. Pharmac. Ther.*, 1977, *22*, 864; N. J. Marshall *et al.*, *Nature*, 1977, *268*, 58; D. G. McDevitt *et al.*, *Br. J. clin. Pharmac.*, 1978, *6*, 297; G. J. M. Tevaarwerk *et al.*, *Can. med. Ass. J.*, 1978, *119*, 350; P. Heyma *et al.*, *Br. med. J.*, 1980, *281*, 24; M. K. Jones *et al.* (letter), *ibid.*, 453; R. T. Jung *et al.* (letter), *ibid.*, 810; N. D. S. Bax *et al.* (letter), *ibid.*, 1283.

Neonatal thyrotoxicosis. Thyrotoxicosis evident 7 days after birth in a premature child born to a thyrotoxic mother was successfully treated with propranolol, 500 µg thrice daily gradually increased to 7 mg four times daily; it was discontinued 53 days after birth. Despite vomiting which developed at 38 days and continued until the day after propranolol was stopped, the infant continued to gain weight.— K. N. Pearl and T. L. Chambers, *Br. med. J.*, 1977, *2*, 738.

Further references: C. S. Smith and N. J. Howard, *J. Pediat.*, 1973, *83*, 1046; P. J. Pemberton *et al.*, *Archs Dis. Childh.*, 1974, *49*, 813.

Thyroid storm. An 11-year-old boy with signs of thyroid storm responded dramatically to intravenous administration of propranolol 3 mg, followed by a further 3 mg two hours later. After another 2 hours he was given 30 mg by mouth and subsequently 20 mg every six hours which controlled his symptoms until propylthiouracil could take effect. Two attempts to discontinue propranolol during the first 3 weeks were unsuccessful but he was eventually withdrawn from propranolol 40 mg daily during the fifth treatment week.— M. Galaburda *et al.*, *Pediatrics*, 1974, *53*, 920.

A report of 2 patients in whom administration of propranolol failed to prevent thyroid storm.— M. Eriksson *et al.*, *New Engl. J. Med.*, 1977, *296*, 263. Criticism; the dose might have been too low.— J. J. Abrams and J. Sandler (letter), *ibid.*, 1120. Further criticisms.— S. G. Dorfman *et al.* (letter), *ibid.*; T. A. Bowdle (letter), *ibid.*, 1121. Reply.— S. Rubenfeld (letter), *ibid.* The dosage of propranolol might have been inadequate. In a study of 11 thyrotoxic patients given propranolol 40 mg four times daily the plasma-propranolol concentrations were not maintained above 50 ng per ml throughout the 6-hour dosage interval in 8, and in 4 peak concentrations were below 30 ng per ml.— R. Hellman *et al.* (letter), *ibid.*, *297*, 671.

Thyroid surgery. Following its use in 100 hyperthyroid patients undergoing subtotal thyroidectomy, propranolol alone was considered to be safe and effective in the pre-operative preparation of hyperthyroid patients, with the main advantage of increased flexibility of date of operation. The following dosage regimen was used: propranolol 40 mg every 6 hours, the patient being admitted to hospital on the fourth pre-operative day and the dose increased if necessary until the resting pulse-rate was less than 90 per minute; propranolol was continued throughout the day of operation and for 7 days subsequently. Compared with a carbimazole-treated series of patients, blood loss was less presumably because the carbimazole-treated patients had increased vascularity and size of thyroid glands owing to overtreatment. Thyroid storm was avoided by high-quality perioperative supervision with no patient undergoing the operation until the resting pulse-rate was below 90, meticulous attention being paid to the important pre-operative dose of propranolol, and prompt treatment of postoperative chest infections; if a high standard was not attainable substitution of propranolol for antithyroid drugs would be unwise.— A. D. Toft *et al.*, *New Engl. J. Med.*, 1978, *298*, 643.

Comments on the advantages of pre-operative propranolol for thyroid surgery.— W. Michie (letter), *Br. med. J.*, 1978, *1*, 106.

Further references: A. D. Toft *et al.*, *Clin. Endocr.*, 1976, *5*, 195; J. Feely *et al.* (letter), *Br. med. J.*, 1977, *2*, 1352; R. L. Ward and W. G. Paley (letter), *ibid.*, 1355; A. J. Trench *et al.*, *Anaesthesia*, 1978, *33*, 535; J. Zonszein *et al.*, *Am. J. Med.*, 1979, *66*, 411.

For the use of propranolol with potassium iodide in the pre-operative management of patients with Graves' disease, see Potassium Iodide, p.866.

Thyrotoxic hypercalcaemia. Propranolol, initially by intravenous infusion in a dose of about 10 mg per hour for 12 hours, followed by 20 or 25 mg four times daily by mouth for 3 to 4 weeks decreased serum-calcium concentrations in 2 patients with hypercalcaemia associated with hyperthyroidism.— R. K. Rude *et al.*, *New Engl. J. Med.*, 1976, *294*, 431. Criticisms.— R. A. Kaplan and M. J. Hogan (letter), *ibid.*, 1123; L. P. Georges and J. Sode (letter), *ibid.* Reply.— R. K. Rude *et al.* (letter), *ibid.*, 1124.

Hypoglycaemia. Control of severe hypoglycaemia in a patient with malignant insulinoma by administration of propranolol, and comments on its probable mode of action.— I. Blum *et al.* (letter), *New Engl. J. Med.*, 1978, *299*, 487.

Leprosy. A study into the immunostimulant effect of the addition of propranolol to the standard therapy of 12 patients with lepromatous leprosy.— R. Anderson *et al.*, *Lepr. Rev.*, 1980, *51*, 137. *In vitro* studies indicating that metoprolol, propranolol, and sotalol may be useful in the *in vivo* restoration of leucotaxis in patients with lepromatous leprosy.— R. Anderson and E. M. S. Gatner (letter), *ibid.*, 195.

Local anaesthesia. In patients who did not react to an intradermal test dose of propranolol, a 0.4% solution of propranolol was found to be a satisfactory local anaesthetic. When infiltrated around wounds the maximum effect was reached in 2 to 4 minutes and the effect lasted for about 30 minutes. When given with adrenaline, 1 in 1000, the effect lasted for more than 3 hours. When applied topically, anaesthesia was obtained within 2 to 3 minutes and lasted for about 60 minutes. With adrenaline, the effect lasted for more than 3 hours. No side-effects were noted and there was no evidence of tissue irritation.— J. N. Sinha *et al.*, *Br. J. Anaesth.*, 1967, *39*, 887.

One drop of a 0.25% solution of propranolol, instilled into the eye and repeated after 3 to 4 minutes, was found to produce satisfactory corneal anaesthesia lasting on average for about 20 minutes. The anaesthesia produced was adequate for ophthalmic procedures such as tonometry and generally 2 drops instilled at intervals of 5 minutes produced adequate anaesthesia for the removal of corneoscleral silk sutures. In operations for cataract, pterygium, and entropion 3 instillations of the drops at 5-minute intervals were adequate for operations lasting 30 to 40 minutes. The only side-effect noted was haziness of the corneal epithelium in 2 patients but this cleared within 24 hours.— K. P. Singh *et al.* (letter), *Lancet*, 1967, *2*, 158.

Menopausal symptoms. In a double-blind study involving perimenopausal women propranolol 40 mg thrice daily was no more effective than placebo in controlling hot flushes.— J. Coope *et al.*, *Br. J. Obstet. Gynaec.*, 1978, *85*, 472.

Migraine. Reviews of propranolol and other beta-adrenoceptor blocking agents in migraine: *Med. Lett.*, 1976, *18*, 55; M. Anthony, *Drugs*, 1978, *15*, 249; *Aust. J. Pharm.*, 1978, *59*, 807; E. S. Johnson, *Postgrad. med. J.*, 1978, *54*, 231.

The migraine attack-rate in 28 children given propranolol 60 mg daily for those weighing under 35 kg and 120 mg for those over 35 kg was 3.1 per 12 weeks compared to 9.3 per 12 weeks when given placebo in a double-blind study: 20 of the children were completely free from headache while on propranolol.— J. Ludvigsson (letter), *Lancet*, 1973, *2*, 799.

In an initial pilot study 41 of 49 patients with migraine received excellent benefit (more than 50% reduction in attacks) after treatment for about 6 months with propranolol, 40 mg four times daily. In a subsequent double-blind crossover study in 30 of the patients who had received excellent benefit the mean attack-rates per month in patients with classic migraine were 0.9 on propranolol and 2.1 on placebo and in patients with common migraine 0.2 and 1.5 respectively.— T. -E. Widerøe and T. Vigander, *Br. med. J.*, 1974, *2*, 699.

An excellent or good response was achieved, in an open trial, in 16 of 30 patients with migraine given single doses of propranolol 40 to 120 mg.— R. Tokola and E. Hokkanen (letter), *Br. med. J.*, 1978, *2*, 1089.

Further references: E. B. Weber and O. N. Reinmuth, *Neurology, Minneap.*, 1972, *22*, 366; R. Fogelholm (letter), *Br. med. J.*, 1972, *4*, 110; J. M. Sutherland, *Drugs*, 1973, *5*, 212; S. E. Børgesen *et al.* (letter), *Lancet*, 1974, *2*, 58; *Drug & Ther. Bull.*, 1975, *13*, 93; B. Forssman *et al.*, *Headache*, 1976, *16*, 238; A. Klimek and E. Poźniak-Patewicz, *ibid.*, 1977, *17*, 75; P. O. Behan and M. Reid, *Practitioner*, 1980, *224*, 201.

See also under Adverse Effects.

Myoclonus. Propranolol was tried in doses of 30 to 120 mg daily in the management of familial essential myoclonus in one patient. Improvement was noted at a dose of 60 mg daily and at 120 mg daily there was almost complete disappearance of myoclonus and a decrease in the amplitude of tremor.— J. M. Ferro and E. S. Calhau (letter), *Lancet*, 1977, *2*, 143.

Myopathy. Response of one patient with lipid myopathy to treatment with propanolol.— C. Martyn *et al.*, *Br. med. J.*, 1981, *282*, 1997.

Myxoedema. By giving propranolol with thyroxine in gradually increasing doses, myxoedematous patients could tolerate a high enough dose of thyroxine to correct their metabolic deficit. Treatment with thyroxine alone could result in a dangerous tachycardia or angina.— R. Greene (letter), *Br. med. J.*, 1967, *3*, 614.

Narcolepsy. Four patients with long-standing narcolepsy treated with methylphenidate were changed to therapy with propranolol 240 to 480 mg daily and this was considered to be at least as effective as methylphenidate in controlling sleep attacks. The effect of propranolol on the cataplexy, however, was variable with 1 improving, 2 remaining the same, and 1 deteriorating. In the latter 3 patients addition of a tricyclic antidepressant to propranolol essentially eliminated the cataplexy.— A. Kales *et al.*, *Ann. intern. Med.*, 1979, *91*, 741. Comments.— R. W. Clark (letter), *ibid.*, 1980, *92*, 718. A reply.— A. Kales *et al.* (letter), *ibid.*, 719.

Narcotic dependence. Contrary to previous reports, narcotic-blocking effects of propranolol could not be detected in 2 double-blind studies using doses of up to 40 mg daily; on the contrary it appeared to offer some relief from opiate withdrawal.— R. G. Jacob *et al.*, *Psychopharmacologia*, 1975, *41*, 71.

In a series of studies involving 18 narcotic-dependent subjects, propranolol failed to block diamorphine-induced euphoria, and did not precipitate or alleviate opiate withdrawal.— R. B. Resnick *et al.*, *Archs gen. Psychiat.*, 1976, *33*, 993.

Nightmares. A dose of 80 to 160 mg of propranolol or oxprenolol taken in the evening was effective in preventing bad dreams and nightmares.— L. Feldman (letter), *Med. J. Aust.*, 1976, *1*, 504.

See also under Adverse Effects.

Orthostatic hypotension. Propranolol had a beneficial effect in 3 of 5 patients with an orthostatic syndrome characterised by raised plasma-bradykinin concentrations.— D. H. P. Streeten *et al.*, *Lancet*, 1972, *2*, 1048.

A patient with orthostatic hypotension due to autonomic dysfunction was treated successfully with: tightly fitting stockings, a head-up body tilt at night, volume expansion with salt tablets and fludrocortisone, dexamphetamine for alpha-adrenergic stimulation, and propranolol for blocking beta-agonist-mediated vasodilatation and dexamphetamine-induced tachycardia. Dihydroergotamine subsequently replaced the dexamphetamine. None of the measures used alone was adequate.— K. K. P. Hui and M. E. Conolly, *New Engl. J. Med.*, 1981, *304*, 1473.

For reference to the absence of a beneficial effect of propranolol with ephedrine in orthostatic hypotension, see Ephedrine,p.12.

See also under Pindolol, p.1348.

Parkinsonism. Propranolol in doses of not less than 60 mg daily was compared with a placebo in 18 patients with parkinsonism who were also receiving levodopa. The only significant effect of propranolol was an improvement in handwriting and circle-drawing and this was not considered to be of clinical value.— C. D. Marsden *et al.* (letter), *Lancet*, 1974, *2*, 410.

For a report of the beneficial effect of concurrent administration of propranolol and levodopa in patients with parkinsonism, see Levodopa, p.887.

Phaeochromocytoma. To control tachycardia and arrhythmia during the removal of phaeochromocytoma, the following procedure was recommended. Three days before operation, phenoxybenzamine 1 mg per kg body-weight was given intravenously in 5% dextrose solution over 1 hour. Two days before operation, phenoxybenzamine was given as before and 2 hours later propranolol 40 mg was given by mouth followed after 2 hours by 80 mg or more, if necessary, to reduce the heart-rate to 80. The day before operation, phenoxybenzamine treatment was repeated and propranolol continued to reduce the heart-rate to 80 beats per minute. On the day of the operation, 1 hour before induction, premedication doses of papaveretum and hyoscine were given, then phenoxybenzamine, 50 mg intravenously, was given if the blood pressure was higher than 160/100 mmHg and propranolol was given if the heart-rate was above 90 beats per minute.— E. J. Ross *et al.*, *Br. med. J.*, 1967, *1*, 191. See also T. Himathongkam *et al.*, *J. Am. med. Ass.*, 1974, *230*, 1692.

Addition of propranolol to a pre-operative regimen using alpha-adrenoceptor blocking agents did not appear to confer any benefit on 7 patients operated on for removal of a primary phaeochromocytoma when compared with 20 patients who received the alpha-adrenoceptor blocking regimen alone.— L. B. Perry and A. B. Gould, *Anesth. Analg. curr. Res.*, 1972, *51*, 36.

See also under Precautions.

Phantom pain. Relief of phantom pain in 2 patients by the use of propranolol.— S. Ahmad (letter), *Br. med. J.*, 1979, *1*, 415.

Porphyria. Four patients with acute intermittent porphyria were relieved of tachycardia and hypertension after the administration of propranolol 40 to 400 mg daily.— A. D. Beattie *et al.*, *Br. med. J.*, 1973, *3*, 257.

Further references: A. Atsmon and I. Blum (letter), *Lancet*, 1970, *1*, 196; L. M. Flacks (letter), *ibid.*, 363; A. Atsmon *et al.*, *S. Afr. med. J.*, 1972, *46*, 311; D. Douer *et al.*, *J. Am. med. Ass.*, 1978, *240*, 766; A. S. Menawat *et al.*, *Postgrad. med. J.*, 1979, *55*, 546.

Pregnancy and the neonate. A review of the use of beta-blockers in pregnancy.— P. C. Rubin, *New Engl. J. Med.*, 1981, *305*, 1323.

Dysfunctional labour. Encouraging preliminary results were obtained with intravenous propranolol in 10 women with dysfunctional labour due to weak uterine contractions.— A. Mitrani *et al.*, *Br. J. Obstet. Gynaec.*, 1975, *82*, 651.

Foetal tachycardia. Administration of propranolol to a diabetic woman during the last 20 days of pregnancy controlled tachycardia in the infant. After birth the concentration of propranolol in the child's blood was 20% of that in the mother's.— A. Teuscher *et al.*, *Am. J. Cardiol.*, 1978, *42*, 304.

Hypertension in pregnancy. In a retrospective study the foetal outcome was considerably worse in 9 hypertensive women given propranolol and other antihypertensive agents, than in 15 given antihypertensive therapy which excluded propranolol.— B. A. Lieberman *et al.*, *Br. J. Obstet. Gynaec.*, 1978, *85*, 678.

The successful control of blood pressure by propranolol, with other agents, in 8 of 9 pregnant women; there was no effect on uterine contractions and no increased frequency of abortion or premature labour.— P. Tcherdakoff *et al.*, *Br. med. J.*, 1978, *2*, 670.

A hypertensive woman was treated with propranolol 40 mg daily throughout pregnancy without complications. Estimated intake of propranolol in breast milk by the infant was about 3 µg daily.— E. A. Taylor and P. Turner, *Postgrad. med. J.*, 1981, *57*, 427.

Further references: G. Bott-Kanner *et al.*, *Israel J. med. Scis*, 1978, *14*, 466.

Hyperthyroidism in pregnancy. Opposition to the use of propranolol for hyperthyroidism in pregnancy.— G. P. Redmond (letter), *New Engl. J. Med.*, 1978, *298*, 917. Propranolol is only indicated in thyroid storm which is particularly apt to occur during labour and delivery.— G. N. Burrow (letter), *ibid.*, 918.

A review of the management of hyperthyroidism and hypothyroidism during pregnancy.— O. M. Edwards, *Postgrad. med. J.*, 1979, *55*, 340.

For warnings concerning the use of propranolol in pregnancy see also under Precautions.

Schizophrenia. Discussion on the use of propranolol for the treatment of patients with schizophrenia.— D. G. Grahame-Smith and M. W. Orr, *Recent Adv. clin. Pharmac.*, 1978, *1*, 163 to 187. See also *Lancet*, 1980, *2*, 627; P. J. Tyrer, *Drugs*, 1980, *20*, 300.

Propranolol in an initial dose of 40 mg twice daily and increased gradually if required by no more than 80 mg daily to more than 400 mg daily produced a beneficial response when added to antipsychotic therapy in a controlled 12-week study of 14 patients with chronic schizophrenia that had not remitted during a mean of 10 years' treatment with major tranquillisers. The placebo also produced a beneficial response when added to standard therapy but this was less than with propranolol.— N. J. Yorkston *et al.*, *Lancet*, 1977, *2*, 575. Comments and criticisms.— P. J. Tyrer (letter), *ibid.*, 761; A. A. Schiff, *Squibb* (letter), *ibid.*; J. H. Gruzelier (letter), *ibid.*, 1162. A reply.— N. J. Yorkston *et al.* (letter), *ibid.*, 1082.

Propranolol reduced serum-prolactin concentrations in 4 schizophrenic patients; concentrations increased 7-fold with the addition of phenothiazines.— T. Hanssen *et al.* (letter), *Lancet*, 1978, *1*, 101.

Lack of benefit with propranolol in schizophrenia.— M. Peet *et al.*, *Br. J. Psychiat.*, 1981, *139*, 105; D. H. Myers *et al.*, *ibid.*, 118.

Sexually induced headaches. Propranolol 20 mg twice daily completely abolished severe sexually induced headaches in a 32-year-old man.— N. R. Nutt (letter), *Br. med. J.*, 1977, *1*, 1664.

Shock. Eleven patients in late septic shock refractory to conventional therapy were treated with intravenous infusions of propranolol hydrochloride 5 mg over a period of 2 to 3 hours followed by an additional 5 mg during the next 6 to 12 hours, according to response. Eight survived and it appeared that beta-adrenoceptor blockade was effective in hypodynamic shock if this was primarily due to microcirculatory failure and providing the cardiac output was not significantly decreased by the beta-adrenoceptor blockade.— J. L. Berk *et al.*, *Archs Surg., Chicago*, 1972, *104*, 46.

Tetanus. Studies in 4 patients with severe tetanus suggested that symptoms of sympathetic overactivity, including cardiac dysrhythmia, hypertension, peripheral vasoconstriction, pyrexia, and tachycardia, which occurred during intensive treatment with intermittent positive-pressure respiration, were best controlled with propranolol and bethanidine. In 2 patients, propranolol was given in small intravenous doses to control tachycardia and dysrhythmia and then by intragastric tube in maintenance doses of 10 mg every 6 to 8 hours. Bethanidine was given by intragastric tube in doses of 10 mg every 8 hours or 5 mg every 2 hours to control hypertension. The treatment was continued during the period of artificial ventilation.— C. Prys-Roberts *et al.*, *Lancet*, 1969, *1*, 542. A 73-year-old patient with tetanus had been successfully treated with propranolol and bethanidine in addition to curarisation.— J. W. Dundee and R. C. Gray (letter), *ibid.*, 779.

Further references: M. Goldman *et al.* (letter), *J. Am. med. Ass.*, 1979, *242*, 2761.

Tremor. Comment on beta-adrenoceptor blocking agents in essential tremor.— *Lancet*, 1979, *2*, 1280.

In 11 patients with essential tremor, propranolol 120 mg daily reduced the tremor by more than 50% in 6 patients and by 25 to 50% in 2 patients.— H. Pakkenberg (letter), *Lancet*, 1972, *1*, 633. Propranolol 30 to 80 mg daily reduced the tremor due to lithium but did not do so in patients also receiving tricyclic antidepressants.— L. Kirk *et al.* (letter), *ibid.*, 839. See also *idem*, 1973, *2*, 1086. Results indicating that beta-adrenoceptor blockade is ineffective in lithium-induced tremor.— J. M. Kellett *et al.*, *J. Neurol. Neurosurg. Psychiat.*, 1975, *38*, 719. Propranolol 30 to 40 mg daily controlled the lithium-induced tremor in 5 patients who had been taking lithium carbonate for 1 to 5 years. Tremor recurred in 3 patients when they stopped taking propranolol.— Y. D. Lapierre, *Can. med. Ass. J.*, 1976, *114*, 619.

Propranolol in doses ranging from 60 to 240 mg daily was effective in a double-blind study in reducing essential, familial, or senile tremor in 23 patients. There appeared to be no decrease in response over a follow-up period of 3 months to 4 years.— G. F. Winkler and R. R. Young, *New Engl. J. Med.*, 1974, *290*, 984.

A study in 4 healthy subjects and 8 patients with essential tremor indicated that single doses of propranolol suppressed catecholamine-induced tremor but did not affect essential tremor, although long-term therapy did.— R. R. Young *et al.*, *New Engl. J. Med.*, 1975, *293*, 950.

Comments on the possible mode of action of beta-adrenoceptor blocking agents in tremor.— D. Jefferson and C. D. Marsden (letter), *Lancet*, 1980, *1*, 427; O. Ljung (letter), *ibid.*, 1032; P. N. Leigh *et al.* (letter), *ibid.*, 1981, *1*, 1106.

Tardive dyskinesia. A preliminary study in psychiatric patients suggested that propranolol may be of benefit in tardive dyskinesia.— N. M. Bacher and H. A. Lewis, *Am. J. Psychiat.*, 1980, *137*, 495.

Further references: P. W. Roberts (letter), *Can. med. Ass. J.*, 1980, *123*, 1106.

Water drinking, compulsive. The use of propranolol 960 mg daily to treat compulsive water drinking in a psychiatric patient.— S. Shevitz *et al.*, *J. nerv. ment. Dis.*, 1980, *168*, 246.

Preparations

Propranolol Hydrochloride Injection *(U.S.P.)*. A sterile solution of propranolol hydrochloride in Water for Injections. pH 2.8 to 4. Protect from light.

Propranolol Hydrochloride Tablets *(U.S.P.)*. Tablets containing propranolol hydrochloride. Protect from light.

Propranolol Injection *(B.P.)*. A sterile solution of propranolol hydrochloride in Water for Injections containing citric acid monohydrate. Sterilised by autoclaving. pH 3 to 3.5. Protect from light.

Propranolol Tablets *(B.P.)*. Tablets containing propranolol hydrochloride. They may be film-coated.

Proprietary Preparations

Angilol *(DDSA Pharmaceuticals, UK)*. Propranolol hydrochloride, available as tablets of 10, 40, 80, and 160 mg.

Apsolol *(Approved Prescription Services, UK)*. Propranolol hydrochloride, available as scored tablets of 10, 40, 80, and 160 mg.

Berkolol *(Berk Pharmaceuticals, UK)*. Propranolol hydrochloride, available as scored tablets of 10, 40, 80, and 160 mg.

Inderal (known in some countries as Inderalici) *(ICI Pharmaceuticals, UK)*. Propranolol hydrochloride, available as 1-ml **Ampoules** of an injection containing 1 mg per ml and as **Tablets** of 10, 40, 80, and 160 mg. (Also available as Inderal in *Austral., Belg., Canad., Denm., Ital., Jap., Neth., Norw., S.Afr., Swed., Switz., USA*).

Inderal LA *(ICI Pharmaceuticals, UK)*. Sustained-release capsules each containing propranolol hydrochloride 160 mg. *Dose.* 1 daily, increased to 2 if necessary.

Inderetic *(ICI Pharmaceuticals, UK)*. Capsules each containing propranolol hydrochloride 80 mg and bendrofluazide 2.5 mg. For hypertension. *Dose.* 1 capsule twice daily.

Other Proprietary Names

Arg.—Blocardyl (also as dibudinate), Noloten, Oposim, Propayerst; *Austral.*—Cardinol; *Denm.*—Frekven; *Fr.*—Avlocardyl, Bétaryl propranolol phenylethylbarbiturate; *Ger.*—Dociton; *Ital.*—Beta-Neg, Tonum; *Jap.*—Caridolol, Herzul, Kemi, Pylapron, Tesnol; *Norw.*—Frekven, Pranolol, Pronovan; *Spain*—Sumial; *Swed.*—Frekvén.

6302-q

Acebutolol Hydrochloride. IL-17803A; M & B 17803A. (±)-3′-Acetyl-4′-(2-hydroxy-3-isopropylaminopropoxy)butyranilide hydrochloride.

$C_{18}H_{28}N_2O_4$,HCl=372.9.

CAS — 37517-30-9 (acebutolol, ±); 34381-68-5 (hydrochloride, ±).

A white or slightly cream powder. M.p. 141° to 144°. Acebutolol hydrochloride 111 mg is approximately equivalent to 100 mg of acebutolol.

Adverse Effects, Treatment, and Precautions. As for Propranolol Hydrochloride, p.1325.

It has been reported that acebutolol has a cardioselective action and may therefore be less likely than propranolol to cause bronchospasm, see p.1324.

In a multicentre study involving 366 hypertensive patients taking acebutolol the side-effects most often reported were lassitude, dizziness, nausea, headaches, drowsiness, skin rashes, flushing, depression, painful legs, flatulence and bradycardia.— W. L. Ashton, *Curr. med. Res. Opinion*, 1976, *4*, 442.

Allergy. Cutaneous vasculitis due to acebutolol occurred in one patient. Hypersensitivity was confirmed by sensitivity testing. Rechallenge at a later date produced no reaction to acebutolol or other beta-blockers.— R. Ashford *et al.* (letter), *Lancet*, 1977, *2*, 462.

Antinuclear factor. Development of antinuclear antibodies during acebutolol therapy.— R. J. Cody *et al.*, *Clin. Pharmac. Ther.*, 1979, *25*, 800.

Further references: M. A. Martin (letter), *Br. J. clin. Pharmac.*, 1980, *10*, 313; J. D. Wilson, *Drugs*, 1980, *19*, 292.

Effects on the eyes. Over a period of 18 months, 48 patients receiving acebutolol were given ocular examinations every 6 months. Two patients had a prickling sensation, very slight microscopic lesions were noted in 9, and results of a Schirmer test were abnormal in 6. Long-term acebutolol therapy did not appear to have harmful effects on the eyes.— C. Wagner *et al.*, *Nouv. Presse méd.*, 1978, *7*, 725.

Hypoglycaemia. In 11 healthy subjects insulin-induced hypoglycaemia was significantly enhanced and return to normoglycaemia significantly delayed by propranolol 40 mg twice daily or metoprolol 50 mg twice daily. Acebutolol 100 mg twice daily significantly enhanced hypoglycaemia but did not significantly delay return to normoglycaemia.— R. J. Newman, *Br. med. J.*, 1976, *2*, 447.

Absorption and Fate. Acebutolol is absorbed from the gastro-intestinal tract and excreted in the urine and faeces. It may be subject to enterohepatic recycling. The biological half-life of acebutolol is longer than would be anticipated from its plasma half-life of about 3 hours.

A study of the pharmacokinetics of acebutolol in 6 healthy subjects. Unlike propranolol, following intravenous administration there was little intersubject variation in plasma concentrations and urinary recovery (about 60% being recovered in 24 hours). Following administration by mouth about half the dose (given as capsules) reached the systemic circulation, plasma concentrations being variable up to 4 hours after administration and subsequently quite similar. The plasma elimination half-life was only about 3 hours after oral or intravenous administration. There was evidence of substantial non-renal elimination and renal tubular secretion.— C. M. Kaye *et al.*, *Clin. Pharmac. Ther.*, 1976, *19*, 416. See also P. J. Meffin *et al.*, *ibid.*, 1977, *22*, 557.

Further references: P. Hares *et al.* (letter), *Br. J. clin. Pharmac.*, 1977, *4*, 373.

Buccal absorption and plasma and renal elimination of acebutolol was not pH-dependent.— C. M. Kaye and A. D. Long (letter), *Br. J. clin. Pharmac.*, 1976, *3*, 196.

A study in 2 patients provided evidence that active secretion of acebutolol occurs into the bile which might produce significant enterohepatic circulation. Acebutolol probably does not form glucuronide or sulphate conjugates in the liver to any marked extent.— C. M. Kaye and V. M. S. Oh, *J. Pharm. Pharmac.*, 1976, *28*, 449.

In 10 patients given a single 300-mg dose of acebutolol the mean plasma concentrations of acebutolol and its acetyl metabolite at 2 hours were 389 and 402 ng per ml respectively; at 7 hours the concentrations were 136 and 445 ng per ml. The elimination half-life of acebutolol was about 2.5 hours; elimination of the metabolite proceeded more slowly.— A. H. Gradman *et al.*, *Circulation*, 1977, *55*, 785.

Steady-state plasma concentrations of the acetyl metabolite were 2.7 times greater than those of the unchanged drug in 7 patients with cardiac arrhythmias given acebutolol 300 or 500 mg every 6 or 8 hours. Peak plasma-acebutolol concentrations occurred at 60 to 90 minutes in 3 patients with a half-life of about 2.5 hours whilst 4 patients had irregular plasma concentration curves suggestive of erratic or delayed absorption of acebutolol from the hard gelatin capsules or from enterohepatic recycling.— R. A. Winkle *et al.*, *Br. J. clin. Pharmac.*, 1977, *4*, 519. See also R. Verbesselt *et al.*, *Boll. chim.-farm.*, 1978, *117*, 102.

There was no apparent correlation between acetylator status and the production of the active 4-acetyl metabolite of acebutolol in a study of 8 healthy subjects who took a single dose of acebutolol 400 mg. Knowledge of the acetylator status of a patient is therefore not required to determine the optimal dosage regimen of acebutolol.— A. Gulaid *et al.* (letter), *Br. J. clin. Pharmac.*, 1978, *5*, 261.

In 7 subjects given a single dose of acebutolol 400 mg peak plasma concentrations occurred 1 to 4 hours after the dose; the mean elimination half-life was about 4.3 hours. The peak concentration of the *N*-acetyl metabolite occurred 2 to 5 hours after the dose; it exceeded the concentration of acebutolol from about 2 hours after the dose; the mean half-life in 5 subjects was about 8.7 hours. There was a significant correlation between plasma concentrations of acebutolol and its metabolite and beta-blockade assessed by reduction in exercise-induced tachycardia.— M. A. Martin *et al.*, *Eur. J. clin. Pharmac.*, 1978, *14*, 383. See also R. D. S. Watson and W. A. Littler, *Br. J. clin. Pharmac.*, 1979, *7*, 557.

A study in healthy subjects of diacetolol, the major metabolite of acebutolol. Diacetolol exhibited marked cardiac beta-adrenoceptor blocking activity and persisted in the circulation for longer than acebutolol.— K. Ohashi *et al.*, *Br. J. clin. Pharmac.*, 1981, *12*, 561.

Dialysis. Unlike beta-blockers such as pindolol and propranolol, acebutolol is subject to relatively important dialysis yield.— P. Aubert *et al.*, *J. Urol. Néphrol.*, 1976, *82*, 799.

See also Uses (Administration in Renal Failure).

Diffusion into the CSF. A study in *animals* on the central uptake of beta-adrenoceptor blocking agents, including acebutolol.— M. D. Day *et al.*, *J. Pharm. Pharmac.*, 1977, *29, Suppl.*, 52P.

The penetration of acebutolol, and its major metabolite diacetolol, into CSF and saliva.— R. Zaman *et al.* (letter), *Br. J. clin. Pharmac.*, 1981, *12*, 427.

Uses. Acebutolol is a beta-adrenoceptor blocking agent (see p.1324) with uses similar to those of propranolol (see p.1329). Acebutolol is classified as cardioselective. it is used as the hydrochloride in the form of capsules containing the equivalent of 100 and 200 mg of acebutolol, as tablets containing the equivalent of 400 mg of acebutolol, and as an injection containing the equivalent of 5 mg of acebutolol in each ml.

In the treatment of hypertension the usual initial dose is 400 mg daily (at breakfast) or 200 mg twice daily, increased if necessary after 2 weeks according to the patient's response, to 800 mg once daily or 400 mg twice daily; some patients may require 800 mg in the morning and 400 mg in the evening.

The usual dose for angina pectoris is 200 mg twice daily but up to 300 mg thrice daily may be required and total daily doses of 1.2 g have been given. The usual dose for cardiac arrhythmias is 100 to 200 mg twice or thrice daily but up to 1.2 g daily in divided doses has been required. Acebutolol hydrochloride by mouth may take about 3 hours to exert its full effect.

For the emergency treatment of cardiac arrhythmias acebutolol may be given by slow intravenous injection in a dose of 25 mg, preferably over a period of 3 to 5 minutes, but more rapidly if necessary. The dose may be repeated by slow intravenous injection or by infusion preferably over an hour or more; maximum total dosages of 75 to 100 mg have been given. Response to the initial injection may take 10 minutes or longer. A dose of 5 to 15 mg intravenously is usually sufficient for the less serious arrhythmias and the effect may last for 30 to 50 minutes.

Action. A study indicating that propranolol was not cardioselective and acebutolol was not as cardioselective as practolol.— C. R. Kumana *et al.*, *Lancet*, 1975, *2*, 89.

Although acebutolol itself appears to be cardioselective, a metabolite, *N*-acetyl acebutolol, which is also a beta-blocker, is non-selective. Accumulation of this metabolite during long-term therapy by mouth may explain the lack of selectivity.— D. J. Rowlands, *Prescribers' J.*, 1980, *20*, 64.

Further studies on the cardioselectivity of acebutolol: A. J. Coleman and W. P. Leary, *Curr. ther. Res.*, 1972, *14*, 673; W. P. Leary and A. J. Coleman, *S. Afr. med. J.*, 1972, *46*, 1202; R. H. Briant *et al.*, *Br. J. Pharmac.*, 1973, *49*, 106; C. Skinner *et al.*, *Br. J. clin. Pharmac.*, 1975, *2*, 417; R. J. Newman, *Br. med. J.*, 1977, *2*, 601; M. K. Benson *et al.*, *Br. J. clin. Pharmac.*, 1978, *5*, 415; H. H. Harms *et al.*, *ibid.*, 19.

Administration in renal failure. A study involving 6 healthy subjects and 6 patients with chronic renal failure indicated that patients with chronic renal failure might require smaller doses of acebutolol. Subjects with renal failure appeared to exhibit a greater degree of non-renal elimination of acebutolol.— C. M. Kaye and J. F. Dufton (letter), *Br. J. clin. Pharmac.*, 1976, *3*, 198.

Evidence of prolongation of the half-life of acebutolol in patients with renal failure. In those undergoing haemodialysis, however, the half-life was similar to that of subjects with normal renal function.— P. Aubert *et al.*, *J. Urol. Néphrol.*, 1976, *82*, 799.

Acebutolol 400 mg in the morning effectively controlled the blood pressure of 5 of 11 patients with renal hypertension. A further 3 patients were controlled with this dose at 4 weeks but not at 12 weeks, and in the remaining 3 patients control could not be obtained with 800 mg each morning, possibly owing to weight gain reflecting subclinical salt and water retention. In 2 men with the most severe renal impairment a sharp deterioration in glomerular filtration-rate followed the introduction of acebutolol.— E. Begg *et al.*, *N.Z. med. J.*, 1979, *89*, 293.

Further references: R. Gabriel, *Br. J. clin. Pract.*, 1979, *33*, 259.

Anxiety. Acebutolol 300 mg reduced tachycardia caused by mental stress in competitive rifle shooting in 6 healthy subjects without altering concentration or skill.— D. O. Gibbons and M. Phillips (letter), *Br. J. clin. Pharmac.*, 1976, *3*, 516.

Cardiac disorders. *Angina pectoris.* A study in 18 patients with coronary insufficiency indicated that acebutolol 100 mg and propranolol 40 mg were approximately equipotent in the prophylaxis of angina attacks and in the improvement of exercise tolerance.— G. Tremblay *et al.*, *Curr. ther. Res.*, 1977, *22*, 692.

Further references: B. S. Lewis *et al.*, *S. Afr. med. J.*, 1973, *47*, 1181; P. Biron and G. Tremblay, *Eur. J. clin. Pharmac.*, 1975, *8*, 15; *idem*, *Clin. Pharmac. Ther.*, 1976, *19*, 333; J. W. Mason *et al.*, *Br. Heart J.*, 1978, *40*, 29; G. Tremblay *et al.*, *Curr. ther. Res.*, 1979, *25*, 637.

Cardiac arrhythmias. Cumulative intravenous doses of 12.5 to 50 mg of acebutolol were effective in 14 of 20 patients with various cardiac arrhythmias; they included 4 of 4 with sinus tachycardia, 2 of 3 with premature atrial beats, 3 of 4 with premature ventricular beats, 3 of 5 with atrial fibrillation, and 2 of 3 with atrial flutter. Acebutolol was ineffective in 1 patient with atrial tachycardia resistant to propranolol by mouth.— P. Biron *et al.*, *Eur. J. clin. Pharmac.*, 1975, *8*, 11. See also W. S. Aronow *et al.*, *Am. J. Cardiol.*, 1979, *43*, 106.

Acebutolol 200 mg given twice daily for 3 days to 20 patients with various cardiac disorders abolished or prevented arrhythmias or improved the patient's condition in 22 of 29 episodes of ventricular arrhythmia and in 16 of 21 episodes of supraventricular arrhythmia.— D. Burckhardt *et al.*, *Curr. med. Res. Opinion*, 1977, *4*, 496.

In 10 patients the incidence of premature ventricular contractions (PVC) was reduced in 8 by more than 50% in the first 12 hours after a single 300 mg dose of acebutolol. In 11 patients given acebutolol 300 mg eight-hourly for 5 to 10 days the incidence of PVC was reduced by 38 to 98% in a 24-hour period; in 8 patients the reduction exceeded 70%.— A. H. Gradman *et al.*, *Circulation*, 1977, *55*, 785.

Further references: W. S. Aronow *et al.*, *Clin. Pharmac. Ther.*, 1979, *25*, 149; *idem*, 1980, *28*, 28.

Myocardial infarction. Reduction of early ventricular arrhythmia by acebutolol in patients with acute myocardial infarction.— G. G. Ahumada *et al.*, *Br. Heart J.*, 1979, *41*, 654.

Hypertension. In a multicentre study of 1893 hypertensive patients, acebutolol 0.2 to 1.2 g as a single daily dose, alone or with a thiazide diuretic, provided a clinically satisfactory progressive reduction in blood pressure over 3 months in the majority of patients. Concomitant administration of diuretics enhanced the antihypertensive effect only in patients with severe hypertension. Blood pressure control was inadequate in 45 patients, and side-effects occurred in 584 patients, causing 120 to withdraw from the study.— P. G. Baker and J. Goulton, *J. int. med. Res.*, 1979, *7*, 201. A similiar report in 1007 patients.— *idem*, *Curr. med. Res. Opinion*, 1979, *6*, 50.

A double-blind crossover study in 5 hypertensive patients with a history of long-term daily ectopic activity, indicated that once-daily administration of acebutolol 400 mg resulted in a 38% decrease in the number of ectopics during 24 hours, whereas twice-daily administration of acebutolol 200 mg caused a steady reduction throughout the 24 hours amounting to 73%. Although the antihypertensive effects of once-daily and twice-daily administration of beta-blockers are similar, those with short plasma half-lives should preferably be given twice-daily in the treatment of hypertension if the presumed cardioprotective effect is to be sustained for 24 hours.— M. H. Frick and R. Kala (letter), *Lancet*, 1980, *2*, 588.

Further references: W. L. Ashton, *Curr. med. Res. Opinion*, 1977, *5*, 279; L. Hansson *et al.*, *Eur. J. clin. Pharmac.*, 1977, *12*, 89; F. Alhenc-Gelas *et al.*, *Am. J. Med.*, 1978, *64*, 1005; K. Charoenlarp and N. Jaroonvesama, *J. int. med. Res.*, 1978, *6*, 67; M. A. Martin *et al.*, *Br. J. clin. Pharmac.*, 1978, *6*, 351; C. Ongcharit *et al.*, *J. int. med. Res.*, 1980, *8*, 188.

Schizophrenia. Encouraging results were obtained following administration of acebutolol 0.2 to 1.4 g daily to hebephrenic patients.— N. T. Daskalopoulos *et al.*, *Thérapie*, 1977, *32*, 287.

Proprietary Preparations

Secadrex *(May & Baker, UK)*. Tablets each containing acebutolol hydrochloride equivalent to acebutolol 200 mg and hydrochlorothiazide 12.5 mg. For hypertension. *Dose*. One tablet daily, increased to 2 tablets if necessary.

Sectral *(May & Baker, UK)*. Acebutolol hydrochloride, available as **Capsules** containing the equivalent of 100 or 200 mg of acebutolol; as **Injection** containing the equivalent of 5 mg per ml, in ampoules of 5 ml; and as **Tablets** containing the equivalent of 400 mg. (Also available as Sectral in *Fr.*, *Neth.*, *NZ*, *S.Afr.*).

Other Proprietary Names

Neptall, Prent *(both Ger.)*; Rhodiasectral *(Arg.)*.

6303-p

Alprenolol Hydrochloride *(B.P.)*. H56/28.

(±)-1-(2-Allylphenoxy)-3-isopropylaminopropan-2-ol hydrochloride.

$C_{15}H_{23}NO_2,HCl=285.8$.

CAS — 13655-52-2 (alprenolol) [23846-72-2 (+); 23846-71-1(−); 23846-70-0(±)]; 13707-88-5 (hydrochloride) [15020-61-8(+); 15132-12-4(−); 13678-97-2(±)].

Pharmacopoeias. In *Br.* and *Nord.*

Odourless or almost odourless, colourless crystals or a white crystalline powder with a bitter numbing taste. M.p. 108° to 111°.

Soluble 1 in less than 1 of water, 1 in 2 of alcohol, and 1 in 3 of chloroform; practically insoluble in ether. A 5% solution in water has a pH of 5.5 to 6.5 **Incompatible** with alkalis. Solutions are **sterilised** by autoclaving. **Store** in airtight containers. Protect from light.

Adverse Effects, Treatment, and Precautions. As for Propranolol Hydrochloride, p.1325.

Allergy. A report of contact eczema in workers exposed to alprenolol. Alprenolol must be considered a very strong contact allergen.— L. Ekenvall and M. Forsbeck, *Contact Dermatitis*, 1978, *4*, 190.

Effects on the blood. Alprenolol-induced thrombocytopenia in 1 patient.— B. Magnusson and S. Rödjer, *Acta med. scand.*, 1980, *207*, 231.

Effects on respiratory function. A study suggesting that alprenolol affects specific airway conductance less than propranolol.— C. K. Connolly and J. C. Batten, *Br. med. J.*, 1970, *2*, 515.

Hypoglycaemia. Exercise-induced hypoglycaemia in a patient taking alprenolol and hydralazine—the hypoglycaemia was suspected on one occasion and confirmed on another.— G. Holm *et al.*, *Br. med. J.*, 1981, *282*, 1360.

Interactions. *Alcohol.* Metabolic interaction of alcohol and alprenolol in isolated *rat* liver cells.— R. Grundin, *Acta pharmac. tox.*, 1975, *37*, 185.

Anti-inflammatory agents. Studies in 5 healthy subjects showed no interaction between alprenolol and sodium salicylate.— G. Johnsson *et al.*, *Eur. J. clin. Pharmac.*, 1973, *6*, 9.

Barbiturates. A study in 5 healthy subjects indicated that pentobarbitone administration induced the metabolism of alprenolol. The decrease in plasma concentration following intravenous administration of alprenolol was insignificant, but that following oral administration was marked owing to the increased first-pass elimination.— G. Alván *et al.*, *Clin. Pharmac. Ther.*, 1977, *22*, 316.

Overdosage. For a report of the successful treatment of alprenolol poisoning, see Propranolol, p.1327.

Absorption and Fate. Alprenolol is almost completely absorbed from the gastro-intestinal tract but is subject to considerable first-pass metabolism in the liver. Peak plasma concentrations are achieved about 1 or 2 hours after a dose. Its biological half-life is longer than would be anticipated from its short plasma half-life of about 2 hours. It is excreted in the urine mainly in the form of its metabolites. It is highly protein bound.

In a study involving 16 hypertensive patients who received alprenolol 200 mg thrice daily for 6 weeks the steady-state plasma concentrations showed marked individual variation (range 11 to 141 ng per ml) as also did the degree of beta-blockade but there was significant correlation between the two factors.— P. Collste *et al.*, *Eur. J. clin. Pharmac.*, 1976, *10*, 85.

Further references: M. D. Rawlins *et al.*, *Eur. J. clin. Pharmac.*, 1974, *7*, 353.

First-pass effect. Support for the hypothesis that alprenolol is subject to significant first-pass metabolism.— G. Alván *et al.*, *J. Pharmacokinet. Biopharm.*, 1977, *5*, 193.

Protein binding. The binding of alprenolol to human serum proteins.— C. Appelgren *et al.*, *Acta pharm. suec.*, 1974, *11*, 325; K. A. Johansson *et al.*, *ibid.*, 333.

Studies *in vitro* showed that the mean free fraction of alprenolol in the plasma obtained from 23 healthy subjects was 15.8% and this correlated inversely with the α_1-acid glycoprotein concentration. No relationship was found between plasma-albumin concentration and binding.— K. M. Piafsky and O. Borgå, *Clin. Pharmac. Ther.*, 1977, *22*, 545.

Sustained-release preparations. Comparison of rapidly-disintegrating tablets with sustained-release formulations of alprenolol hydrochloride in 4 healthy subjects indicated that alprenolol hydrochloride was significantly metabolised during the passage from the intestinal lumen into the general circulation. Although metabolism was more complete when alprenolol hydrochloride was administered as sustained-release tablets the increase was not enough to render the formulation unsatisfactory.— R. Johansson *et al.*, *Acta pharm. suec.*, 1971, *8*, 59.

Uses. Alprenolol hydrochloride is a beta-adrenoceptor blocking agent (see p.1324) with uses similar to those of propranolol (see p.1329). Alprenolol is classified as non-cardioselective.

In the treatment of hypertension alprenolol hydrochloride is usually given in an initial dose of 200 mg daily, in 2 or 4 divided doses, increased weekly according to the response of the patient up to a total of 800 mg daily in divided doses. The usual dose for angina pectoris and other cardiac disorders is 50 to 100 mg four times daily.

For the emergency treatment of cardiac arrhythmias alprenolol hydrochloride may be given by slow intravenous injection in a dose of 2 mg at a rate of 1 mg per minute; the dose may be repeated after an interval of not less than 5 minutes. It has been recommended that the maximum total dose given intravenously should not exceed 20 mg.

Action. Pharmacological studies on alprenolol: *Acta pharmac. tox.*, 1967, *25*, *Suppl.* 2.

Administration in hepatic failure. The response to alprenolol which was metabolised by the liver was altered in the presence of hepatic disease.— G. L. Sanders, *Adverse Drug React. Bull.*, 1978, Feb., 240.

Anxiety. Alprenolol hydrochloride in doses of 50 and 100 mg reduced stress symptoms associated with catecholamine output in musicians about to participate in concerts.— S. Lidén and C. -G. Gottfries (letter), *Lancet*, 1974, *2*, 529.

Cardiac disorders. *Angina pectoris.* Fourteen of 21 patients with angina pectoris benefited from alprenolol 100 mg four times a day compared with 8 of the same patients given pentaerythritol tetranitrate 30 mg four times a day in a blind crossover study. Three patients on alprenolol and 5 patients on pentaerythritol were considered worse after the respective treatments. The severity of angina attacks was assessed by subjective reports from the patients and by the number of glyceryl trinitrate tablets used. Side-effects were minor.— A. Aubert *et al.*, *Br. med. J.*, 1970, *1*, 203.

Further studies: J. B. Hickie, *Med. J. Aust.*, 1970, *2*, 268; B. J. Sealey *et al.*, *Br. Heart J.*, 1971, *33*, 481; L. G. Ekelund *et al.*, *Eur. J. clin. Pharmac.*, 1973, *6*, 113; H. Ikram, *Clin. Trials J.*, 1973, *10* (2), 35; I. K. Bailey *et al.*, *Am. Heart J.*, 1976, *92*, 416.

Cardiac arrhythmias. The dextro-isomer of alprenolol was ineffective in the treatment of supraventricular arrhythmias.— J. K. Vohra *et al.*, *Br. med. J.*, 1970, *1*, 791. The dextro-isomer of alprenolol, which has membrane-stabilising activity but no beta-blocking action, was able to suppress ectopic cardiac rhythms.— E. Smith *et al.*, *Guy's Hosp. Rep.*, 1971, *120*, 9, per *Abstr. Wld Med.*, 1971, *45*, 836.

In a double-blind crossover study in 30 patients with functional cardiovascular disorders, including tachycardia and a heart-rate over 140 per minute after 6 minutes' ergometric exercise, the patients received, in conjunction with a graduated programme of physical training, either alprenolol 200 mg as a single daily dose in a sustained-release preparation or diazepam 5 mg twice daily. Alprenolol was more effective than diazepam in relief of cardiac symptoms and led to a rapid increase in exercise tolerance which was not seen with diazepam. Muscular pain in the legs occurred in 5 patients taking alprenolol and in 1 each taking diazepam or placebo.— T. Hanak, *Curr. ther. Res.*, 1978, *24*, 774.

Further references: R. E. Kerber *et al.*, *J. Am. med. Ass.*, 1970, *214*, 1849; H. G. Wilson (letter), *Med. J. Aust.*, 1970, *1*, 394; P. J. Pôntinen *et al.*, *Br. med. J.*, 1971, *4*, 723.

Cardiomyopathy. See under Propranolol Hydrochloride, p.1331.

Myocardial infarction. Of 230 patients discharged from hospital after myocardial infarction, 114 were given alprenolol 400 mg daily and 116 given placebo. During a 2-year follow-up 3 patients in the alprenolol group died suddenly compared with 11 in the placebo group and this difference was significant.— C. Wilhelmsson *et al.*, *Lancet*, 1974, *2*, 1157. In a study of 162 patients followed up for 2 years after myocardial infarction there was a significantly lower incidence of sudden death and re-infarction in the 69 given alprenolol than in the 93 controls. One sudden death and 4 re-infarctions occurred in the alprenolol group compared with 9 sudden deaths and 15 re-infarctions in the control group.— G. Ahlmark *et al.* (letter), *ibid.*, 1563. See also G. Ahlmark and H. Saetre (letter), *Br. med. J.*, 1976, *1*, 837.

In a double-blind study, 140 patients aged 65 years or less, with definite or suspected myocardial infarction, were given alprenolol 5 to 10 mg intravenously, as soon as possible, and subsequently 200 mg twice daily by mouth, as a sustained-release preparation; 142 similar patients were given placebo. Results after 6 to 12 months' follow-up indicated that alprenolol treatment started on admission significantly reduced the long-term mortality; the long-term mortality of those who dropped out of the study did not differ greatly from those who remained in, and neither their inclusion nor their exclusion affected the significance of the results. The study also initially included patients over the age of 65 years, study of their tolerance of beta-blockade being a major aim. Mortality within the first 28 days and especially the first 24 hours tended to be higher in the alprenolol group; although the difference was not significant, patients over 65 years of age were then excluded from the study. It was concluded from these preliminary results that in patients aged 65 years or less with chest pain and suspected myocardial infarction, routine alprenolol treatment, started as soon as possible, can be advocated. This recommendation does not apply to elderly patients.— M. P. Andersen *et al.*, *Lancet*, 1979, *2*, 865.

Further references: G. Lund-Larsen and E. Sivertssen, *Acta med. scand.*, 1969, *186*, 187; G. Ahlmark and H. Saetre, *Eur. J. clin. Pharmac.*, 1976, *10*, 77; L. Dintenfass and B. Lake (letter), *Lancet*, 1976, *1*, 1026; G. Myberg *et al.*, *Br. Heart J.*, 1979, *41*, 452.

Enuresis. A report of a beneficial effect of alprenolol on nocturnal enuresis in a 24-year-old woman.— B. Lake (letter), *Med. J. Aust.*, 1975, *1*, 367.

Hypertension. A study in 7 hypertensive young men indicated that long-term treatment of hypertensive subjects with alprenolol influenced haemodynamic and metabolic responses at rest and during prolonged exercise. No dissociation of the peripheral beta-adrenoceptor blocking properties was found, confirming findings in *animals* that alprenolol is a non-selective beta-adrenoceptor blocking agent.— M. Frisk-Holmberg *et al.*, *Clin. Pharmac. Ther.*, 1977, *21*, 675.

Further references: C. Furberg and G. Michaelson, *Acta med. scand.*, 1969, *186*, 447; G. Tibblin and B. Åblad, *ibid.*, 451; R. H. Bergstrand *et al.*, *Läkartidningen*, 1973, *70*, 2817; L. A. Salako *et al.*, *Curr. med. Res. Opinion*, 1979, *6*, 358; J. Tuomilehto and A. Nissinen, *Eur. J. clin. Pharmac.*, 1979, *16*, 369.

For a comparative study of alprenolol, pindolol, timolol, and propranolol in hypertension, see Propranolol Hydrochloride, p.1332.

Effect on plasma renin. In 46 patients with essential hypertension, both blood pressure and plasma-renin concentration were reduced after treatment with alprenolol, though the changes could not be correlated. Hydralazine was also given to 27 patients and produced a further reduction in blood pressure without affecting the plasma-renin concentration.— E. B. Pederson and H. J. Kornerup, *Eur. J. clin. Pharmac.*, 1977, *12*, 93.

Further references: P. Collste *et al.*, *Eur. J. clin. Pharmac.*, 1976, *10*, 89.

Preparations

Alprenolol Injection *(B.P.)*. A sterile solution of alprenolol hydrochloride in Water for Injections. Sterilised by autoclaving. pH 5 to 8. Protect from light.

Alprenolol Tablets *(B.P.)*. Tablets containing alprenolol hydrochloride. Protect from light.

Proprietary Names

Aptin *(Astra, Arg.; Astra, Austral.; Hässle, Denm.; Astra, Ger.; Byk Gulden, Ital.; Hässle, Norw.; Adcock Ingram, S.Afr.; Hässle, Swed.)*; Aptine *(Astra, Belg.; Astra, Fr.; Astra, Neth.)*; Aptol *(Astra, Switz.)*; Betacard *(Beecham, Austral.)*; Gubernal *(Geigy, Belg.; Geigy, Fr.; Ciba-Geigy, Switz.)*; Vasoton *(Astra, Arg.)*; Apllobal, Regletin, Sinalol *(all Jap.)*.

6304-s

Atenolol. ICI 66082. 2-[4-(2-Hydroxy-3-isopropylaminopropoxy)phenyl]acetamide.
$C_{14}H_{22}N_2O_3$=266.3.

CAS — 29122-68-7; 60966-51-0 (±).

Adverse Effects, Treatment, and Precautions. As for Propranolol Hydrochloride, p.1325.

It has been reported that atenolol has a cardioselective action and may therefore be less likely than propranolol to cause bronchospasm, see p.1324.

A mean daily dose of atenolol 174 (range 12.5 to 600) mg was taken by 262 patients with hypertension for a mean of 23.3 (range 2 to 52) months in a multicentre open study. Significant reductions in supine and erect blood pressures and in supine heart-rate were obtained in the majority of patients. Treatment was discontinued in 14 patients, due to side-effects in 8. Overall side-effects included cold extremities, fatigue, sinus bradycardia, dry skin and eyes and heartburn. Of 11 patients with chronic bronchitis or bronchial asthma 3 reported slight respiratory symptoms.— L. Hansson *et al.*, *Curr. ther. Res.*, 1977, *22*, 839.

Further references: *Proc. R. Soc. Med.*, 1977, *70*, *Suppl.* 5.

Effects on the gastro-intestinal tract. Severe criticism of a report by C.C. Doherty *et al.* (*Br. med. J.*, 1978, *2*, 1786) that retroperitoneal fibrosis in a 68-year-old woman might have been associated with atenolol.— M. J. Asbury, *Stuart* (letter), *Br. med. J.*, 1979, *1*, 492.

Another report of retroperitoneal fibrosis associated with atenolol.— J. N. Johnson and J. McFarland (letter), *Br. med. J.*, 1980, *280*, 864. Severe criticism and comments.— M. J. Gavin *et al.* (letter), *ibid.*, 1227; D. W. Bullimore (letter), *ibid.*, *281*, 59; W. M. Castle *et al.* (letter), *ibid.*, 311; F. L. Rose and F. Bergel (letter), *ibid.*; D. W. Bullimore (letter), *ibid.*, 564; F. L. Rose and F. Bergel (letter), *ibid.*, 745.

Effects on mental state. Of 27 patients receiving atenolol, 3 developed vivid dreams and 2 became unable to cope with work.— H. J. Waal-Manning, *Clin. Pharmac. Ther.*, 1979, *25*, 8.

Effects on the muscles. Of 27 patients receiving atenolol, 1 developed muscle cramps.— H. J. Waal-Manning, *Clin. Pharmac. Ther.*, 1979, *25*, 8.

Effects on respiratory function. In 20 patients with chronic obstructive airway disease, airway resistance was increased less by atenolol 100 mg than by propranolol 80 mg.— M. Beil and W. T. Ulmer, *Arzneimittel-Forsch.*, 1977, *27*, 419.

Effects on sexual function. Erectile dysfunction experienced by a 44-year-old man who was receiving propranolol 40 mg twice daily was reversed by substitution with atenolol 50 mg daily which also satisfactorily controlled his tachycardia.— J. Bathen (letter), *Ann. intern. Med.*, 1978, *88*, 716.

Effects on the skin. Necrosis. Multiple areas of skin necrosis on the feet of a 57-year-old man taking atenolol.— P. J. Rees (letter), *Br. med. J.*, 1979, *1*, 955.

Hypoglycaemia. In a double-blind study in 6 diabetic patients taking glibenclamide, acebutolol enhanced insulin-induced hypoglycaemia; in 6 diabetic patients on diet, propranolol enhanced insulin-induced hypoglycaemia. Propranolol and acebutolol had membrane-stabilising activity and blocking activity at β_1 and β_2 receptors. Atenolol had no membrane-stabilising activity and was specific for β_1 receptors. It did not enhance insulin-induced hypoglycaemia in either group of patients under study and might be preferable in diabetics.— S. P. Deacon *et al.*, *Br. med. J.*, 1977, *2*, 1255.

Further references: S. P. Deacon and D. Barnett, *Br. med. J.*, 1976, *2*, 272; R. Wilkinson (letter), *ibid.*, 1979, *1*, 617.

Interactions. Nifedipine. A report of severe hypotension in a patient with hypertension and angina taking atenolol when nifedipine was added to his treatment. When atenolol was withdrawn he developed unstable angina. In such situations the nifedipine should be withdrawn.— L. H. Opie and D. A. White, *Br. med. J.*, 1980, *281*, 1462.

Overdosage. A 24-year-old woman whose blood pressure was well controlled by clonidine and atenolol took 1.2 g of atenolol in a suicide attempt without significant untoward effects.— F. L. J. Shanahan and T. B. Counihan (letter), *Br. med. J.*, 1978, *2*, 773.

Absorption and Fate. Atenolol seems to be completely absorbed from the gastro-intestinal tract and is not significantly metabolised. It is excreted in the urine and its biological half-life is longer than would be anticipated from its plasma half-life of about 6 hours. Atenolol diffuses across the placenta and is excreted in breast milk. Only small amounts are reported to cross the blood-brain barrier, and it is only about 5% bound to plasma proteins.

Following intravenous administration of atenolol 50 mg to healthy subjects 100% of unchanged drug appeared in the urine indicating that atenolol was not significantly metabolised. Following administration of 50 mg by mouth absorption did not appear to be complete; bioavailability was about 63%. Following administration of 200 mg by mouth a mean of about 43% of the dose was excreted in the urine within 72 hours. Repeated administration of 200 mg daily by mouth either as a single dose or in 2 divided doses did not result in accumulation, the plasma elimination half-life after the first and the eighth days being a mean of about 6.31 hours and 6.66 hours respectively.— H. C. Brown *et al.*, *Clin. Pharmac. Ther.*, 1976, *20*, 524.

Five healthy male subjects were given atenolol 25 to 200 mg or a placebo; the reduction in heart-rate was still significant after 27 hours with the 100- and 200-mg doses.— J. D. Harry and J. Young, *Br. J. clin. Pharmac.*, 1977, *4*, 387P.

Investigations in 4 healthy subjects indicated that urinary pH had no influence on the excretion of atenolol.— C. M. Kaye (letter), *Br. J. clin. Pharmac.*, 1974, *1*, 513.

Whereas the buccal absorption of propranolol increased from 3.2% at pH 5 to 55.8% at pH 8 and 89.0% at pH 10, that of atenolol was pH-independent and less than 5%. Atenolol is considerably more hydrophilic than propranolol.— W. Schürmann and P. Turner, *Br. J. clin. Pharmac.*, 1977, *4*, 655P.

Food-induced reduction in bioavailability of atenolol.— A. Melander *et al.*, *Eur. J. clin. Pharmac.*, 1979, *16*, 327.

Further references: J. O. Malbica and K. R. Monson, *J. pharm. Sci.*, 1975, *64*, 1992; R. T. Koda *et al.*, *Clin. Pharmac. Ther.*, 1977, *21*, 108; J. D. Fitzgerald *et al.*, *Eur. J. clin. Pharmac.*, 1978, *13*, 81; O. H. Weedle *et al.*, *J. pharm. Sci.*, 1978, *67*, 1033; W. D. Mason *et al.*, *Clin. Pharmac. Ther.*, 1979, *25*, 408; E. Riva *et al.*, *Eur. J. clin. Pharmac.*, 1980, *17*, 333.

Diffusion into the CSF. Little diffusion of atenolol across the blood-brain barrier in *animals*.— M. D. Day *et al.*, *J. Pharm. Pharmac.*, 1977, *29*, *Suppl.*, 52P.

Further references: P. R. Reeves *et al.*, *Xenobiotica*, 1978, *8*, 305; P. A. van Zwieten and P. B. M. W. M. Timmermans, *J. cardiovasc. Pharmac.*, 1979, *1*, 85.

Pregnancy and the neonate. In 6 women who had taken atenolol for at least 6 days up to the time of delivery concentrations of atenolol in maternal and umbilical serum were approximately equal. In a further woman who had discontinued treatment one day before delivery atenolol was not found in maternal or umbilical serum.— A. Melander *et al.*, *Eur. J. clin. Pharmac.*, 1978, *14*, 93.

Protein binding. Results of *in vitro* studies indicate that atenolol is bound in plasma or to serum albumin to a limited extent and to a lesser degree than propranolol, with binding essentially to the albumin fraction.— H. E. Barber *et al.*, *Br. J. clin. Pharmac.*, 1978, *6*, 446P.

Uses. Atenolol is a beta-adrenoceptor blocking agent (see p.1324) with uses similar to those of propranolol (see p.1329). Atenolol is classified as cardioselective.

In the treatment of hypertension atenolol is usually given by mouth in a dose of 100 mg daily, as a single dose. The usual dose for angina pectoris is also 100 mg daily, given as single or divided doses. Additional benefit is not usually obtained from higher doses of atenolol.

For the emergency treatment of cardiac arrhythmias atenolol may be given by intravenous injection in a dose of 2.5 mg injected at a rate of 1 mg per minute, repeated if necessary every 5 minutes to a maximum total dosage of 10 mg. Alternatively atenolol may be given by intravenous infusion, a dose of 150 µg per kg bodyweight being administered over 20 minutes. The injection or infusion may be repeated every 12 hours if necessary. When control is achieved maintenance doses of 50 to 100 mg daily may be given by mouth.

Action. A detailed review of the actions and uses of atenolol.— R. C. Heel *et al., Drugs,* 1979, *17,* 425.

Further reviews and reports: *Drugs Today,* 1977, *13,* 43; *Postgrad. med. J.,* 1977, *53, Suppl.* 3, 1–181; *Aust. J. Pharm.,* 1979, *60,* 89.

Reports and studies on the pharmacology of atenolol: G. E. Marlin *et al., Br. J. clin. Pharmac.,* 1975, *2,* 151 (cardioselectivity); F. J. Conway *et al., ibid.,* 1976, *3,* 267 (cardioselectivity); J. S. Vilsvik and J. Schaaning, *Br. med. J.,* 1976, *2,* 453 (cardioselectivity); P. B. S. Decalmer *et al., Acta ther.,* 1977, *3,* 99 (cardioselectivity); H. Kather and B. Simon (letter), *Br. J. clin. Pharmac.,* 1977, *4,* 499 (lipolysis); P. L. Sharma, *Int. J. clin. Pharmac. Biopharm.,* 1977, *15,* 27 (cardiac effects); M. K. Benson *et al., Br. J. clin. Pharmac.,* 1978, *5,* 415 (cardioselectivity); S. P. Deacon, *Br. J. clin. Pharmac.,* 1978, *5,* 123 (lipolysis); W. H. Perks *et al., Br. J. clin. Pharmac.,* 1978, *5,* 101 (cardioselectivity); C. Robinson *et al., Br. Heart J.,* 1978, *40,* 14 (anti-arrhythmic effects); B. E. Strauer, *Dt. med. Wschr.,* 1978, *103,* 1785 (coronary haemodynamics); J. L. Day *et al., Br. med. J.,* 1979, *1,* 77 (triglycerides).

Administration in renal failure. In hypertensive patients with normal renal function the half-life of atenolol was about 6 hours and was increased to about 22 hours in patients with severe renal impairment, indicating that either an increased dosage interval or decreased dosage would be required in these patients.— J. Sassard *et al., Eur. J. clin. Pharmac.,* 1977, *12,* 175. See also S. H. Wan *et al., Br. J. clin. Pharmac.,* 1979, *7,* 569; B. Fluovat *et al., Br. J. clin. Pharmac.,* 1980, *9,* 379; J. McAinsh *et al., Clin. Pharmac. Ther.,* 1980, *28,* 302.

Reports that atenolol causes less deterioration in renal function than non-selective beta-adrenoceptor blocking agents, such as propranolol: R. Wilkinson (letter), *Br. med. J.,* 1979, *1,* 617; H. J. Waal-Manning and P. Bolli (letter), *ibid.,* 1082.

Administration in respiratory insufficiency. In a double-blind crossover study in patients with bronchial asthma, intravenous injection of atenolol 3 mg caused a slight increase in airways resistance when compared to a placebo. Bronchial constriction caused by atenolol was readily overcome by inhalation of salbutamol.— N. P. Boye and J. R. Vale, *Eur. J. clin. Pharmac.,* 1977, *11,* 11.

Further references: C. Carlson and K. A. Järvinen, *Allergy,* 1978, *33,* 147.

Cardiac disorders. *Angina pectoris.* The work capacity of 8 patients with angina pectoris before an attack occurred was increased by a mean of 19 and 37%, 24 hours after taking a single daily dose of atenolol 50 or 100 mg respectively and by a mean of 44% four hours after the 100-mg dose. The effect of the 100-mg dose on the heart-rate after 24 hours was about 78% of the maximum effect produced after 4 hours. It was considered that a once-daily regimen of atenolol would be effective for patients with angina pectoris starting with a 50-mg dose and increased to 100 mg if this was tolerated.— G. H. Noer and T. Ekeli, *Curr. ther. Res.,* 1978, *24,* 17.

Further references: P. Roy *et al., Br. med. J.,* 1975, *3,* 195; G. Jackson *et al., Br. Heart J.,* 1978, *40,* 998; *idem, Circulation,* 1980, *61,* 555.

Cardiac arrhythmias. A study of atenolol in 28 subjects indicated that the anti-arrhythmic properties of atenolol were similar to those of other beta-adrenoceptor blocking agents.— R. Sirbulescu, *Acta ther.,* 1977, *3,* 109.

Myocardial infarction. Evidence, from a placebo-controlled study involving 22 patients, that atenolol 100 mg daily facilitates the recovery of the ECG signs of myocardial infarction.— S. Yusuf *et al., Lancet,* 1979, *2,* 868. Results of a randomised study in 214 patients with myocardial infarction, using intravenous atenolol given within 12 hours of chest pain, indicated that early intravenous beta-blockade may produce a moderate but worthwhile reduction in mortality.— *idem,* 1980, *2,* 273.

Glaucoma. In a double-blind crossover study in 16 patients with intra-ocular pressures of or above 22 mmHg the topical application of atenolol 1, 2, or 4%(with benzalkonium chloride 0.02% and pH adjusted to 6) produced a mean maximum fall in intra-ocular pressure of 4.9, 6.1, and 6.3 mmHg respectively. The effect was evident at 1 hour, reached its maximum at 2 to 3 hours, and had disappeared after 7 hours. In 10 patients treated thrice daily for 7 days there was a sustained reduction in intra-ocular pressure with a tendency for the effect to be less at the end of the period. Pupil size, corneal sensitivity, blood pressure, and heart-rate were not affected.— K. Wettrell and M. Pandolfi, *Br. J. Ophthal.,* 1977, *61,* 334.

In a double-blind study in 8 patients with glaucoma a single dose of acetazolamide 500 mg reduced intra-ocular pressure to an insignificant extent, atenolol 50 mg reduced intra-ocular pressure significantly, and the effect of giving both drugs concomitantly was significantly greater than that of atenolol alone.— M. J. Macdonald *et al., Br. J. Ophthal.,* 1977, *61,* 345. See also M. J. Elliot *et al., ibid.,* 1975, *59,* 296.

A comparison of the reduction of intra-ocular pressure produced by atenolol 4% and adrenaline 1% eye-drops in 12 patients with intra-ocular hypertension showed that atenolol was more effective than adrenaline. No additive effect was observed when the drugs were used together.— C. I. Phillips *et al., Br. J. Ophthal.,* 1978, *62,* 296. Both atenolol and adrenaline produced a reduction in intra-ocular pressure, and combined treatment produced a fall in pressure which was greater than that observed for either drug alone.— A. Rushton, *Br. J. clin. Pharmac.,* 1979, *7,* 575.

Similar decreases in intra-ocular pressure were noted following topical application thrice daily of atenolol 2% or pilocarpine 2% in a double-blind crossover study involving 8 patients with ocular hypertension.— K. Wettrell *et al., Br. J. Ophthal.,* 1978, *62,* 292.

A brief comment on the problems associated with tolerance to atenolol eye-drops in glaucoma.— *Br. med. J.,* 1978, *1,* 460.

Further references: C. I. Phillips *et al.* (letter), *Br. med. J.,* 1976, *2,* 1448; M. J. Macdonald *et al., Br. J. Ophthal.,* 1976, *60,* 789; C. I. Phillips *et al., ibid.,* 1977, *61,* 349; R. F. Brenkman, *ibid.,* 1978, *62,* 287.

Hypertension. In a placebo-controlled crossover study completed by 14 patients with essential hypertension, blood pressure reduction by atenolol was similar to that reported in placebo-controlled studies of other beta-adrenoceptor blocking agents used in hypertension.— M. G. Myers *et al., Clin. Pharmac. Ther.,* 1976, *19,* 502.

Withdrawal of long-term therapy with atenolol in hypertensive patients.— J. Webster *et al., Br. J. clin. Pharmac.,* 1981, *12,* 211.

Further references: A. P. Douglas-Jones and J. M. Cruickshank, *Br. med. J.,* 1976, *1,* 990; E. Besterman (letter), *ibid.,* 1403; I. S. Muir (letter), *ibid.,* 1213; A. P. Douglas-Jones and J. M. Cruickshank (letter), *ibid.,* 1471; P. Lund-Johansen, *Br. J. clin. Pharmac.,* 1976, *3,* 445; T. A. Jeffers *et al., ibid.,* 1977, *4,* 523; R. G. Wilcox and J. R. A. Mitchell, *Br. med. J.,* 1977, *2,* 547; B. P. Jones *et al., Practitioner,* 1978, *220,* 149; M. H. R. Sheriff *et al., Acta ther.,* 1978, *4,* 51; D. N. Bateman *et al., Br. J. clin. Pharmac.,* 1979, *7,* 357; A. J. Marshall *et al., Postgrad. med. J.,* 1979, *55,* 537; M. Danielson and H. Lindborg, *Curr. ther. Res.,* 1980, *27,* 797; Y. K. Seedat, *Br. med. J.,* 1980, *281,* 1241; S. W. P. Mhlongo (letter), *ibid.,* 1569; J. De Giovanni (letter), *ibid.,* 1981, *282,* 225; A. D. Goldberg (letter), *ibid.;* L. T. Bannan and D. G. Beevers, *ibid.,* 1757.

Comparative studies. From multicentre studies in 67 patients with mild to moderate hypertension, 17 previously treated with beta-adrenoceptor blocking agents and 50 with methyldopa, it was concluded that atenolol 50 mg thrice daily was as effective as methyldopa 250 mg thrice daily and that atenolol 100 mg once daily might be more effective for the control of blood pressure previously poorly controlled. The incidence of side-effects, high initially and during the changes of treatment, fell when all the patients were receiving a once-daily dose of atenolol.— M. A. Basker *et al., Curr. med. Res. Opinion,* 1977, *4,* 618.

Differing views on the relative effects of atenolol and metoprolol: M. B. Comerford and E. M. M. Besterman (letter), *Br. med. J.,* 1977, *2,* 260; J. D. Harry and A. G. Shields (letter), *ibid.,* 1978, *2,* 128; J. H. Barber (letter), *ibid.,* 357; J. D. Harry (letter), *ibid.,* 640; B. M. Guyer (letter), *ibid.,* 704; T. A. Jeffers *et al., ibid.,* 1269; O. Lyngstam and L. Rydén (letter), *Lancet,* 1979, *2,* 634; M. B. Comerford and E. Besterman (letter), *Lancet,* 1980, *2,* 1196; J. D. Harry *et al., Br. J. clin. Pharmac.,* 1980, *9,* 296P.

Further controversy in relation to comparative studies of atenolol with other beta-adrenoceptor blocking agents: R. G. Wilcox, *Br. med. J.,* 1978, *2,* 383; M. Martin (letter), *ibid.,* 637; M. B. Comerford and E. Besterman (letter), *ibid.;* K. Abt (letter), *ibid.,* 1159; M. Danielsson *et al.* (letter), *ibid.;* R. G. Wilcox (letter), *ibid.,* 1160.

Further comparative studies: P. F. C. Bayliss and S. M. Duncan, *Br. J. clin. Pharmac.,* 1975, *2,* 527; J. Webster *et al., Br. med. J.,* 1977, *1,* 76; W. A. I. Rushford *et al., Acta ther.,* 1977, *3,* 117; N. M. Johnson and S. W. Clarke, *ibid.,* 1978, *4,* 147; A. S. Turner *et al., Med. J. Aust.,* 1979, *1,* 625; J. C. Petrie *et al., Br. med. J.,* 1980, *280,* 1573.

Effect on plasma renin. In 16 hypertensive patients given atenolol there was a less significant effect on plasma renin than on sympathetic responsiveness as assessed by the effect on plasma-noradrenaline concentrations.— A. Distler *et al., Am. J. Med.,* 1978, *64,* 446.

Once-daily administration. In a double-blind crossover study in 12 patients with hypertension there was comparable reduction in blood pressure after atenolol 50 mg twice daily, 100 mg twice daily, or 100 mg daily.— C. M. Castleden *et al., Postgrad. med. J.,* 1977, *53,* 679.

Further references: A. Amery *et al., Clin. Pharmac. Ther.,* 1977, *21,* 691; J. Tuomilehto *et al., Acta ther.,* 1977, *3,* 131; M. W. M. Craig *et al., Br. med. J.,* 1979, *1,* 237; P. Sleight *et al.* (letter), *ibid.,* 491; W. A. Littler and R. D. S. Watson (letter), *ibid.*

Hyperthyroidism. In a double-blind crossover study in 21 patients with hyperthyroidism, propranolol 40 mg, atenolol 50 mg, or placebo were given 4 times daily for one week in randomised order. Both atenolol and propranolol were considered to have a beneficial effect on the peripheral manifestations of hyperthyroidism and both significantly reduced heart-rate, by 29.8% and 27.1% respectively, with no significant difference between the 2 drugs.— D. G. McDevitt and J. K. Nelson, *Br. J. clin. Pharmac.,* 1978, *6,* 233.

Migraine. The use of atenolol in migraine.— P. Stensrud and O. Sjaastad, *Headache,* 1980, *20,* 204.

Pregnancy and the neonate. A study of atenolol in 13 pregnant women with severe pre-eclampsia.— K. J. Thorley *et al., Br. J. clin. Pharmac.,* 1981, *12,* 725.

Proprietary Preparations

Tenoret 50 *(Stuart, UK).* Tablets each containing atenolol 50 mg and chlorthalidone 12.5 mg. For hypertension. *Dose.* 1 tablet daily.

Tenoretic *(Stuart, UK).* Scored tablets each containing atenolol 100 mg and chlorthalidone 25 mg. For hypertension. *Dose.* 1 tablet daily.

Tenormin *(Stuart, UK).* Atenolol, available as scored tablets of 100 mg. **Tenormin LS.** Atenolol, available as tablets of 50 mg. (Also available as Tenormin in *Austral., Belg., Denm., Ger., Ital., Neth., Norw., S.Afr., Swed., Switz.*).

Tenormin Injection *(Stuart, UK).* Atenolol, available as citrate-buffered solution containing 500 µg per ml, in ampoules of 10 ml.

Other Proprietary Names

Ténormine *(Fr.).*

6305-w

Bufetolol Hydrochloride. 1-*tert*-Butylamino-3-(2-tetrahydrofurfuryloxyphenoxy)propan-2-ol hydrochloride. $C_{18}H_{29}NO_4,HCl=359.9$.

CAS — 53684-49-4 (bufetolol); 35108-88-4 (hydrochloride).

An odourless white crystalline powder with a bitter taste. M.p. about 155°. **Soluble** in water, glacial acetic acid, and methyl alcohol; sparingly soluble in alcohol and chloroform; practically insoluble in ether. **Protect** from light.

Bufetolol is a beta-adrenoceptor blocking agent with actions and uses similar to those of propranolol hydrochloride (see p.1325). It has been given in doses of 5 mg thrice daily.

Proprietary Names

Adobiol *(Jap.).*

6306-e

Bufuralol Hydrochloride. Ro 03-4787. 2-*tert*-Butylamino-1-(7-ethylbenzofuran-2-yl)ethanol hydrochloride. $C_{16}H_{23}NO_2,HCl=297.8$.

CAS — 54340-62-4 (bufuralol) [57704-15-1(±)]; 60398-91-6 (hydrochloride, ±)[57704-11-7(+); 57704-10-6(−)].

Adverse Effects, Treatment, and Precautions. As for Propranolol Hydrochloride, p.1325.

Absorption and Fate. Following absorption from the gastro-intestinal tract bufuralol is extensively metabolised and is excreted in the urine almost entirely in the form of metabolites.

Following oral administration of radioactively labelled bufuralol 20 mg to 2 healthy subjects elimination was essentially complete within 3 days. About 75% was excreted in the urine, almost entirely in the form of metabolites.— R. J. Francis *et al.*, *Eur. J. Drug Metab. Pharmacokinet.*, 1976, *1*, 113.

The pharmacokinetic and pharmacodynamic behaviour of tolamolol and bufuralol cannot be explained adequately without taking into account their active metabolites.— L. P. Balant and J. Fabre (letter), *Lancet*, 1978, *2*, 425.

Uses. Bufuralol hydrochloride is a beta-adrenoceptor blocking agent (see p.1324) with general properties similar to those of propranolol hydrochloride (see p.1329).

Action. The haemodynamic effects of bufuralol hydrochloride 20 mg intravenously were compared with those of pindolol 2 mg intravenously. Further studies are needed to determine whether bufuralol is a selective or non-selective beta-adrenoceptor blocking agent. In addition to its beta-adrenoceptor blocking effects it was considered that bufuralol may also have a direct effect on peripheral resistance.— D. Magometschnigg *et al.*, *Int. J. clin. Pharmac. Biopharm.*, 1978, *16*, 54.

Further references: J. R. Kilborn and P. Turner, *Br. J. clin. Pharmac.*, 1974, *1*, 143.

Manufacturers
Roche, UK.

6307-l

Bunitrolol. Kö 1366. 2-(3-*tert*-Butylamino-2-hydroxypropoxy)benzonitrile.
$C_{14}H_{20}N_2O_2=248.3$.

CAS — 34915-68-9.

A crystalline solid. M.p. about 164°.

Adverse Effects, Treatment, and Precautions. As for Propranolol Hydrochloride, p.1325.

Effects on respiratory function. A comparative study of bunitrolol and practolol on respiratory function.— H. M. Beumer and W. Ritter, *Respiration*, 1975, *32*, 363.

Hypoglycaemia. Absence of effect of bunitrolol on blood-sugar concentration.— H. Regula and B. Papner, *Arzneimittel-Forsch.*, 1974, *24*, 1328.

Uses. Bunitrolol is a beta-adrenoceptor blocking agent (see p.1324) with uses similar to those of propranolol (see p.1329). Bunitrolol hydrochloride has been given in doses of 10 to 20 mg twice daily in the treatment of hypertension.

Action. Doses of bunitrolol 100 to 500 µg intravenously produced a maximum effect in 5 to 20 minutes. Doses of 5 mg by mouth produced a maximum effect in 1 to 2 hours.— H. J. Gilfrich *et al.*, *Arzneimittel-Forsch.*, 1973, *23*, 768. See also H. -W. Klempt and F. Bender, *ibid.*, 1064.

Further references: *Drugs Today*, 1977, *13*, 14.

Cardiac disorders. An evaluation of the haemodynamic effects of single doses of bunitrolol 50 µg per kg body-weight given intravenously to 10 male patients with chest pain.— S. O. Banim *et al.*, *Curr. med. Res. Opinion*, 1977, *4*, 630.

Further references: H. -W. Klempt and F. Bender, *Arzneimittel-Forsch.*, 1973, *23*, 1064; K. Gloger, *ibid.*, 1975, *25*, 1300.

Hypertension. After a placebo period 18 hypertensive patients were given bunitrolol 30 mg daily for 1 week; the dose was subsequently doubled weekly, until a maximum effect was obtained, to a maximum of 240 mg daily. No significant change in blood pressure or cardiac index was seen at rest. During exercise the heart-rate fell by 25%, which was compensated by a 34% increase in stroke index, so there was little overall change in the cardiac index; blood pressure fell by about 12%.— T. Reybrouck *et al.*, *Eur. J. clin. Pharmac.*, 1977, *12*, 333.

Further references: P. Lund-Johansen, *J. cardiovasc. Pharmac.*, 1979, *1*, 77; T. Okabayashi *et al.*, *Arzneimittel-Forsch.*, 1979, *29*, 1417.

Proprietary Names of Bunitrolol Hydrochloride
Stresson *(Boehringer Ingelheim, Ger.)*.

6308-y

Bunolol Hydrochloride. W 6412A. (±)-5-(3-*tert*-Butylamino-2-hydroxypropoxy)-3,4-dihydronaphthalen-1(2*H*)-one hydrochloride.
$C_{17}H_{25}NO_3,HCl=327.9$.

CAS — 27591-01-1 (bunolol, ±)[47141-42-4(−)]; 31969-05-8 (hydrochloride, ±)[27867-05-6 (+); 27912-14-7 (−)].

Bunolol hydrochloride is a beta-adrenoceptor blocking agent (see p.1324) with properties similar to those of propranolol hydrochloride (p.1325). The dextro-isomer of bunolol has been reported to have considerably less beta-adrenoceptor blocking activity than the laevo-isomer, levobunolol (p.1341), which is the form used clinically.

Manufacturers
Warner-Lambert, USA.

6309-j

Bupranolol Hydrochloride. KL 255. 1-*tert*-Butylamino-3-(6-chloro-*m*-tolyloxy)propan-2-ol hydrochloride. $C_{14}H_{22}ClNO_2,HCl=308.2$.

CAS — 14556-46-8 (bupranolol)[61877-83-6(+); 38104-34-6(−); 70578-42-6(±)]; 15148-80-8 (hydrochloride)[53032-96-5(+); 39669-04-0(−)].

Adverse Effects, Treatment, and Precautions. As for Propranolol Hydrochloride, p.1325.

Bupranolol has been reported not to be significantly bound to plasma albumin. Bupranolol has also been reported to be metabolised in the liver under the influence of monoamine oxidase; concomitant administration with monoamine oxidase inhibitors has been contra-indicated.

Uses. Bupranolol hydrochloride is a beta-adrenoceptor blocking agent (see p.1324) with general properties similar to those of propranolol (see p.1329). It has been given in doses of 60 to 320 mg daily usually in 2 or 3 divided doses.

Action. Pharmacology of bupranolol on the isolated *guinea-pig* atrium.— J. Wagner *et al.*, *Arzneimittel-Forsch.*, 1972, *22*, 1061.

Glaucoma. Satisfactory results in glaucoma with long-term administration of bupranolol hydrochloride 1% eye-drops instilled 4 times daily.— M. Takase *et al.*, *Jap. J. Ophthal.*, 1978, *22*, 142.

Tremor. The treatment of neuroleptic-induced tremor with bupranolol.— L. Floru *et al.*, *Arzneimittel-Forsch.*, 1979, *29*, 142.

Proprietary Names
Bétadran *(Logeais, Fr.)*; Betadrenol *(Schwarz, Belg.; Pharma-Schwarz, Ger.; Melusin, Ger.; Pharma-Schwarz, Switz.)*; Monobeltin *(Norwich Eaton, Arg.)*; Ophtorenin *(Winzer, Ger.)*; Looser*(Jap.)*.

6310-q

Dexpropranolol Hydrochloride. AY 20694; ICI 47319. (+)-(*R*)-1-Isopropylamino-3-(1-naphthyloxy)propan-2-ol hydrochloride.
$C_{16}H_{21}NO_2,HCl=295.8$.

CAS — 5051-22-9 (dexpropranolol); 13071-11-9 (hydrochloride).

Dexpropranolol is the dextro-isomer of propranolol (see p.1325) and has similar membrane-stabilising effects but has little beta-adrenoceptor blocking activity.

References to dexpropranolol: G. Howitt *et al.*, *Am. Heart J.*, 1968, *76*, 736; H. Amor *et al.*, *Dt. med. Wschr.*, 1969, *94*, 2669; A. G. Wilson *et al.*, *Br. med. J.*, 1969, *4*, 399; D. Bennet *et al.*, *Thorax*, 1970, *25*, 86; J. A. Bonn and P. Turner (letter), *Lancet*, 1971, *1*, 1355; D. J. Coltart *et al.*, *Br. med. J.*, 1971, *1*, 490; E. Smith *et al.*, *Guy's Hosp. Rep.*, 1971, *120*, 9.

Manufacturers
ICI Pharmaceuticals, UK.

6311-p

Labetalol Hydrochloride. AH 5158A; Sch 15719W; Ibidomide Hydrochloride. 5-[1-Hydroxy-2-(1-methyl-3-phenylpropylamino)ethyl]-salicylamide hydrochloride; 2-Hydroxy-5-[1-hydroxy-2-(1-methyl-3-phenylpropylamino)ethyl]-benzamide hydrochloride.
$C_{19}H_{24}N_2O_3,HCl=364.9$.

CAS — 36894-69-6 (labetalol); 32780-64-6 (hydrochloride).

Adverse Effects. Since labetalol has alpha-adrenoceptor blocking properties in addition to its beta-adrenoceptor effects, postural hypotension may be associated with labetalol, particularly with high doses or in the early stages of therapy. Other side-effects reported include scalp tingling and other forms of paraesthesia, gastro-intestinal discomfort, nausea, headache, lethargy, muscular weakness and cramps, dyspnoea, failure of ejaculation, nasal stuffiness, insomnia, vivid dreams, skin rashes, and depression. A positive anti-nuclear factor test has occasionally been associated with labetalol.

Analysis of the side-effects associated with the first 3 months of labetalol therapy, in doses of up to 400 mg, in 1061 hypertensive patients was: lethargy (3.9%), dizziness (4.5%), headache (1.9%), upper gastro-intestinal tract symptoms, including nausea (2.6%), postural hypotension (0.7%), depression (0.7%), dyspnoea (1.4%), tingling sensation in skin or scalp (1.0%).— D. Harris and D. A. Richards, *Glaxo-Allenburys Research* (letter), *Br. med. J.*, 1978, *2*, 894.

Side-effects were reported by 91 of 163 patients with hypertension who received up to 6 months' therapy with labetalol at a mean initial dose of 399 mg increased to 420 mg at 4 to 6 months. Symptoms which were of sufficient severity for 29 patients to withdraw from treatment included tingling of scalp, muzzy head, tiredness, limb weakness, headaches, dizziness, gastro-intestinal effects, insomnia, and bronchospasm.— W. S. Manderson, *Practitioner*, 1979, *222*, 131.

Antinuclear factor. A positive antinuclear factor test in association with labetalol therapy.— W. J. Louis *et al.* (letter), *Lancet*, 1978, *1*, 452.

A finding of anti-mitochondrial antibodies in 7 of 90 patients on labetalol. The patients had been on labetalol for many months and were usually taking a high dose, and the anti-mitochondrial antibodies have not yet posed a clinical problem. Nevertheless, screening for anti-mitochondrial antibodies and the search for possible clinical complications seems warranted.— J. D. Wilson *et al.* (letter), *Lancet*, 1980, *2*, 312.

Further references: D. J. Pugsley *et al.*, *Br. J. clin. Pharmac.*, 1976, *3*, *Suppl.* 3, 777.

Effects on the blood. *Leucopenia.* Mention of leucopenia in a patient taking labetalol.— G. L. Sanders *et al.*, *Eur. J. clin. Pharmac.*, 1978, *14*, 301.

Effects on the eyes. *Melanin binding.* Studies in *animals* indicated that labetalol binds to ocular melanin, but no evidence of oculotoxicity was found.— D. Poynter *et al.*, *Br. J. clin. Pharmac.*, 1976, *3*, *Suppl.* 3, 711.

Effects on lipid metabolism. No significant changes were noted in plasma lipid and plasma urate concentrations in 33 patients treated with labetalol for a year.— R. J. S. McGonigle *et al.* (letter), *Lancet*, 1981, *1*, 163.

Effects on the muscles. Toxic myopathy associated with the use of labetalol.— A. Teicher *et al.*, *Br. med. J.*, 1981, *282*, 1824.

Effects on respiratory function. In 10 patients with asthma both propranolol 5 mg intravenously and labetalol 20 mg intravenously significantly reduced exercise-induced tachycardia, compared with a placebo. Patients had bronchoconstriction (assessed by forced expiratory volume and forced vital capacity) after propranolol but not after labetalol. This was consistent with blockade by labetalol of alpha-adrenoceptors in the bronchi.— C. Skinner *et al.*, *Br. med. J.*, 1975, *2*, 59.

An asthmatic woman in hospital died after receiving labetalol 400 mg which had been intended for another patient.— *Pharm. J.*, 1977, *2*, 139.

Effects on sexual function. Priapism resulting in

impotence in a patient undergoing dialysis may have been associated either with the administration of labetalol or with the uraemic condition.— M. R. Law *et al.* (letter), *Br. med. J.*, 1980, *280*, 115.

Effects on the skin. Lichen planus. An eruption resembling lichen planus developed in a 67-year-old man after taking labetalol for 12 weeks; the eruption subsided when labetalol was withdrawn and recurred 15 days after labetalol was again given. Lichenoid reactions were possibly related to beta-adrenoceptor blockade.— R. W. Gange and E. W. Jones, *Br. med. J.*, 1978, *1*, 816.

A 68-year-old woman developed a lichenoid eruption similar to both pityriasis rubra pilaris and follicular lichen planus after taking labetalol 200 to 400 mg thrice daily for several months. The rash resolved on cessation of therapy.— W. A. Branford *et al.*, *Practitioner*, 1978, *221*, 765.

A report of a hypertensive woman with scleroderma in whom a severe lichenoid skin eruption developed when she took labetalol; she was positive for anti-mitochondrial antibodies.— R. Staughton *et al.* (letter), *Lancet*, 1980, *2*, 581. The anti-mitochondrial antibodies may have been related to the scleroderma, not the labetalol.— C. J. Stevenson (letter), *ibid.*, 924.

Psoriasiform eruption. A patient who had taken labetalol 400 mg twice daily for 3 months developed a widespread scaly erythematous rash similar to that previously described in connection with other beta-blockers; the rash recurred after challenge with pure labetalol thus excluding incrimination of other ingredients of the commercial product.— A. Y. Finlay and E. Waddington (letter), *Br. med. J.*, 1978, *1*, 987. A similar report of rash in a 66-year-old woman who had taken labetalol for 13 months.— R. L. Savage *et al.* (letter), *ibid.*

Hypotension. Labetalol 1 to 2 mg per kg body-weight by intravenous bolus injection produced a poor response in 5 of 6 patients with severe hypertension but an adequate reduction in diastolic blood pressure was obtained by the additional administration of other antihypertensive drugs. In the sixth patient there was an immediate and profound depressor response following labetalol which necessitated the infusion of a pressor agent.— E. P. MacCarthy *et al.*, *Med. J. Aust.*, 1978, *1*, 399.

A comment on the incidence of postural hypotension in association with labetalol therapy. Of 57 patients treated with labetalol and a thiazide diuretic for up to 16 months, 20 had very minor symptoms of postural hypotension occurring usually 1 or 2 hours after taking the tablets. In only 5 were the effects severe enough to require a reduction in labetalol dose. This low incidence of serious postural hypotension may have reflected careful adjustment of labetalol doses, and concurrent use of a thiazide diuretic. Division of the daily dosage into 3 rather than 2 doses also reduced or abolished postural symptoms. Two patients appeared to be hypersensitive, with weakness and tachycardia in one and profound weakness and faintness in the second; their hypersensitivity may have been due to enhanced bioavailability of labetalol. This first-dose effect was similar to that seen after prazosin excepting that the patients remained sensitive to labetalol and needed only very small doses for satisfactory blood pressure control.— W. J. Louis *et al.* (letter), *Lancet*, 1978, *1*, 452.

Lupus erythematosus. Lupus-like illness in a woman taking labetalol; the condition resolved when labetalol was withdrawn.— I. D. Griffiths and J. Richardson (letter), *Br. med. J.*, 1979, *2*, 497.

SLE syndrome probably induced by labetalol.— R. C. Brown *et al.*, *Postgrad. med. J.*, 1981, *57*, 189.

Paraesthesia. Scalp tingling occurred in 2 patients receiving labetalol. In 1 patient the effect was severe enough to cause withdrawal of the drug.— A. S. P. Hua *et al.* (letter), *Lancet*, 1977, *2*, 295. One similar case of scalp tingling associated with labetalol; this patient also experienced a severe visual aura suggestive of migraine. Another patient given labetalol experienced tingling over his body, dizziness, and the desire but inability to urinate. A similar effect on urination was observed in a young diabetic with end-stage chronic renal failure given one dose of labetalol 100 mg.— R. R. Bailey (letter), *ibid.*, 720. The Committee on Safety of Medicines had received similar reports. The scalp alone was usually involved but in some instances there was widespread paraesthesia.— E. Scowen (letter), *ibid.*, 1978, *1*, 98.

A 39-year-old man developed peri-oral numbness and then tingling while taking labetalol 600 mg twice daily.— R. Gabriel (letter), *Br. med. J.*, 1978, *1*, 580.

Peyronie's disease. Peyronie's disease possibly associated with labetalol.— B. O. Kristensen, *Acta med. scand.*, 1979, *206*, 511.

Treatment of Adverse Effects. In the treatment of overdosage with labetalol, account must be taken not only of its beta-adrenoceptor blocking properties (see Propranolol, Treatment of Adverse Effects, p.1327) but also of its alpha-adrenoceptor blocking properties.

Severe hypotension may respond to placing the patient in the supine position with the feet raised. Bradycardia should be treated immediately by the intravenous injection of atropine, at least 3 mg. If further measures are required it has been recommended that noradrenaline may be preferable to the established pharmacological treatment of beta-blockade, isoprenaline. The recommended starting dose of noradrenaline is 5 to 10 μg intravenously repeated as necessary according to the patient's response; alternatively it may be given by intravenous infusion at a rate of 5 μg per minute until a satisfactory response is achieved.

The stomach should be emptied by aspiration and lavage, if ingestion of an overdose is recent.

Precautions. Owing to its beta-adrenoceptor blocking properties, as for Propranolol Hydrochloride, p.1327.

Owing to the alpha-adrenoceptor blocking properties of labetalol, postural hypotension may occur, particularly after initial doses. The effect of halothane on blood pressure may be enhanced by labetalol.

Hemiparesis with persistent paresis of the left arm developed in a 48-year-old woman given labetalol 35 mg intravenously over 2 or 3 minutes for hypertensive encephalopathy; her blood pressure fell from 250/150 to 160/95 mmHg. Labetalol should be given by slow infusion in such circumstances.— R. Solomons (letter), *Br. med. J.*, 1979, *2*, 672.

Interactions. A patient who had undergone renal transplantation and was taking methyldopa, propranolol, guanethidine, amiloride with hydrochlorothiazide, prednisolone, and azathioprine experienced a rise in blood pressure after 2 of 3 intravenous doses of labetalol.— M. Crofton and R. Gabriel, *Br. med. J.*, 1977, *2*, 737. Labetalol 1 mg per kg body-weight intravenously produced a significant fall in supine blood pressure in 10 of 17 patients with severe hypertension. Of the 7 non-responders all were receiving antihypertensive agents concurrently compared to 2 of the 10 responders.— B. P. McGarth *et al.*, *Med. J. Aust.*, 1978, *2*, 410.

Interference with diagnostic tests. In 10 hypertensive patients taking labetalol 1 to 4.8 g daily there was no evidence, when sensitive and specific radio-enzymatic methods were used, that labetalol increased plasma concentrations of noradrenaline or the urinary excretion of endogenous adrenaline or noradrenaline.— C. A. Hamilton *et al.*, *Br. med. J.*, 1978, *2*, 800.

No significant elevation of plasma concentrations of noradrenaline or adrenaline occurs after acute intravenous administration of labetalol, but it interferes with fluorimetric measurements of urinary catecholamines to cause falsely elevated values, which could lead to a misdiagnosis of phaeochromocytoma. No such interference occurs when high-pressure liquid chromatographic methods are used.— D. A. Richards *et al.* (letter), *Br. med. J.*, 1979, *1*, 685. See also under Phaeochromocytoma.

Further references: D. Harris and D. A. Richards (letter), *Br. med. J.*, 1977, *2*, 1673; R. Kolloch *et al.* (letter), *ibid.*, 1979, *1*, 268; N. J. Christensen *et al.*, *Eur. J. clin. Pharmac.*, 1978, *14*, 227.

Phaeochromocytoma. A 55-year-old woman with a predominantly adrenaline-secreting phaeochromocytoma suffered a hypertensive response to labetalol. Caution is recommended in the use of labetalol in phaeochromocytoma.— R. S. J. Briggs *et al.* (letter), *Lancet*, 1978, *1*, 1045. The effect might have been caused by alpha-adrenoceptor stimulation. Labetalol-induced tingling in the scalp had been associated with an alpha-agonist effect and in some patients this might be more widespread.— J. G. Collier (letter), *ibid.*, 1202. It was more likely that the postsynaptic alpha-blocking effects of labetalol were inadequate.— G. A. FitzGerald (letter), *ibid.*, 1259.

It was recommended that urinary 4-hydroxy-3-methoxymandelic acid and not catecholamine or metanephrine excretion should be measured when screening for phaeochromocytoma in patients being treated with labetalol.— D. A. Richards *et al.* (letter), *Br. med. J.*, 1979, *1*, 685. See also under Interactions.

Absorption and Fate. Labetalol is readily absorbed from the gastro-intestinal tract, but is subject to considerable first-pass metabolism. Peak plasma concentrations occur about 1 or 2 hours after a dose. It is metabolised in the liver, the metabolites being excreted in the urine together with only small amounts of unchanged labetalol; its major metabolite has not been found to have significant alpha- or beta-adrenoceptor blocking effects. *Animal* studies have indicated that excretion also occurs in the bile. The biological half-life of labetalol is longer than would be anticipated from its plasma half-life of about 4 hours. Labetalol crosses the placenta and is excreted in breast milk. Only very small amounts appear to cross the blood-brain barrier in *animals*. It is about 50% protein bound.

A detailed study of the metabolism of labetalol by *animals* and man.— L. E. Martin *et al.*, *Br. J. clin. Pharmac.*, 1976, *3*, *Suppl.* 3, 695.

Five patients with mild to moderate hypertension were given labetalol 100, 200, or 400 mg thrice daily and the hypotensive effect was apparent within 2 hours of administration and maximal by 4 hours. In 3 of the 5 patients the hypotensive response increased with increasing doses. There were no significant changes in pulse-rate, expiratory peak flow-rate, or plasma-renin activity. Estimates following oral and intravenous administration in one patient gave a bioavailability of 40.7%.— A. M. Breckenridge *et al.*, *Br. J. clin. Pharmac.*, 1977, *4*, 388P.

In 5 healthy subjects labetalol 100, 200, or 400 mg by mouth produced mean peak plasma concentrations of 32, 83, and 165 ng per ml respectively between 1 and 2 hours after administration, which tended to correlate with the maximum inhibition of exercise-induced tachycardia.— D. A. Richards *et al.*, *Eur. J. clin. Pharmac.*, 1977, *11*, 85.

Further references: G. L. Sanders *et al.*, *Br. J. clin. Pharmac.*, 1978, *5*, 358P; P. Lund-Johansen and O. M. Bakke, *ibid.*, 1979, *7*, 169.

Uses. Labetalol hydrochloride is an antihypertensive agent with beta-adrenoceptor blocking properties similar to those of propranolol hydrochloride (see p.1329). In addition, however, it has alpha-adrenoceptor blocking properties which reduce blood pressure by decreasing peripheral vascular resistance and, in addition, confer upon labetalol a rapid onset of action.

In the treatment of hypertension labetalol hydrochloride is usually given in an initial dose of 100 or 200 mg twice daily with food, if necessary gradually increased after about two weeks, according to the response of the patient, to 400 mg twice daily; total daily doses of 2.4 g have occasionally been required. Hospital in-patients may be given dosage increases on a daily basis where reduction of blood pressure is urgent.

For the emergency treatment of hypertension labetalol hydrochloride may be given by slow intravenous injection in a dose of 50 mg, over a period of at least 1 minute; if necessary this dose may be repeated at intervals of 5 minutes until a total of 200 mg has been given. Following bolus intravenous injection a maximum effect is usually obtained within 5 minutes and usually lasts up to 6 hours, although it may extend as long as 18 hours. Labetalol hydrochloride has also been given by intravenous infusion.

A recommended initial dose in hypotensive anaesthesia is 10 to 20 mg intravenously, with increments of 5 to 10 mg if satisfactory hypotension is not achieved after 5 minutes.

Action. A detailed review of the actions and uses of labetalol.— R. N. Brogden *et al.*, *Drugs*, 1978, *15*, 251.

Further reviews and comments: *Br. J. clin. Pharmac.*, 1976, *3*, *Suppl.* 3, 681–824; *Drugs Today*, 1977, *13*, 490; *Lancet*, 1977, *1*, 890; J. J. Brown *et al.* (letter), *ibid.*, 1147; D. A. Richards *et al.*, *Allen & Hanburys* (letter), *ibid.*; E. B. Raftery (letter), *ibid.*, 1269; W. L. Louis *et al.* (letter), *ibid.*, 1978, *1*, 452; *Drug & Ther. Bull.*, 1978, *16*, 89.

It was estimated that the alpha : beta component activity of labetalol was about 1 : 3, its action being competitive at both sites.— D. A. Richards *et al.*, *Br. J. clin. Pharmac.*, 1976, *3*, 849. See also J. Mehta and J. N. Cohn, *Circulation*, 1977, *55*, 370.

Studies in 6 normotensive subjects demonstrated that intravenously administered labetalol antagonised both the isoprenaline-induced decrease in diastolic blood pressure and the positive chronotropic effect and the noradrenaline-induced increases in systolic and diastolic blood pressure. From these responses and others previously reported for the same subjects it was concluded that the antihypertensive effect of labetalol is explained by concurrent blockade of alpha- and beta-adrenoceptors.— D. A. Richards and B. N. C. Prichard, *Clin. Pharmac. Ther.*, 1978, *23*, 253.

Further references: D. A. Richards *et al.*, *Br. J. clin. Pharmac.*, 1974, *1*, 505; G. Koch, *Am. Heart J.*, 1977, *93*, 585; D. N. W. Griffith *et al.*, *Br. J. clin. Pharmac.*, 1979, *7*, 491; D. A. Richards *et al.*, *ibid.*, 371.

Animal studies. Studies indicated that labetalol is a preferential postsynaptic alpha-adrenoceptor antagonist in the isolated *cat* spleen.— A. G. H. Blakeley and R. J. Summers, *Br. J. Pharmac.*, 1977, *59*, 643.

Administration in hepatic failure. Plasma concentrations of labetalol were similar, after intravenous administration, in patients with liver disease and in controls. After oral administration concentrations were higher in patients than in controls, due to reduced first-pass metabolism. The plasma half-life was similar in each group.— M. Homeida *et al.*, *Br. med. J.*, 1978, *2*, 1048.

Administration in renal failure. There was poor response to treatment with labetalol given intravenously in 3 patients with renal transplants and uncontrolled hypertension; a tachyphylactic response was reported in 1 patient, and only minor depressor effects in the other 2.— C. C. Anderson and R. Gabriel, *Curr. med. Res. Opinion*, 1978, *5*, 424.

Labetalol 0.4 to 2.4 g daily significantly reduced standing systolic and diastolic blood pressure and supine systolic blood pressure after 1 and 6 months' treatment respectively in 14 patients with chronic renal failure and hypertension already receiving antihypertensive therapy. Pretrial drugs were completely withdrawn with satisfactory blood pressure control in 10 patients after 4 to 6 weeks of labetalol therapy but 4 required supplementary minoxidil for adequate control.— J. G. Williams *et al.*, *Med. J. Aust.*, 1978, *1*, 225.

Administration in respiratory insufficiency. A comparison with propranolol and placebo suggested that labetalol would be less likely than propranolol to cause bronchoconstriction in asthmatic patients.— J. G. Maconochie *et al.*, *Br. J. clin. Pharmac.*, 1977, *4*, 157.

See also under Adverse Effects.

Cardiac disorders. *Cardiac arrhythmias.* A study on the anti-arrhythmic effects of labetalol.— C. Mazzola *et al.*, *Curr. ther. Res.*, 1981, *29*, 613.

Hypertension. Labetalol alone or with diuretics, and in one patient propranolol, was effective in the treatment of 15 patients admitted to hospital with poorly controlled hypertension or intolerable side-effects. Postural hypotension was not a major problem with labetalol even with doses of over 1.2 g daily.— A. Breckenridge *et al.* (letter), *Lancet*, 1977, *2*, 36.

In a 6-month study involving 22 patients with drug-resistant hypertension blood pressure was adequately controlled in 13 by the addition of labetalol, in increasing doses of 0.8 to 2.4 g daily (in 2 or 3 divided doses), to their existing medication. By the end of the study beta-adrenoceptor blocking agents and hydralazine or prazosin had been successfully withdrawn from the therapy of these 13 patients. Six patients were judged to have had an inadequate response to labetalol and 3 were withdrawn because of side-effects (postural hypotension, diarrhoea, and an erythematous rash).— T. Morgan *et al.*, *Med. J. Aust.*, 1978, *1*, 393.

Further references: B. N. C. Prichard *et al.*, *Clin. Sci. mol. Med.*, 1975, *48*, *Suppl.* 2, 97S; E. A. Rosei *et al.* (letter), *Lancet*, 1975, *2*, 1093; M. H. Frick and P. Pörsti, *Br. med. J.*, 1976, *1*, 1046; L. Hansson and B. Hänel, *Int. J. clin. Pharmac. Biopharm.*, 1976, *14*, 195; C. Harris, *Curr. med. Res. Opinion*, 1978, *5*, 618; J. Tuomilehto *et al.*, *ibid.*, 1980, *6*, 407; B. J. Milne and A. G. Logan, *Can. med. Ass. J.*, 1980, *123*, 1013; *Practitioner*, 1980, *224*, 945 (Report No. 200 of the General Practitioner Research Group); A. P. Douglas-Jones, *ibid.*, 841; J. Kane *et al.*, *ibid.*, 1981, *225*, 97.

Clonidine withdrawal. The use of labetalol to prevent hypertensive rebound after clonidine withdrawal.— T. Rosenthal *et al.*, *Eur. J. clin. Pharmac.*, 1981, *20*, 237.

Comparative studies. In a double-blind controlled study of 6 healthy subjects, the effects of labetalol 100, 200, and 400 mg on heart-rate, blood pressure, and peak expiratory flow-rate were compared with those of propranolol 40, 80, and 160 mg. Both compounds reduced heart-rates at rest and exercise with propranolol being the more potent. Similar results were achieved in the depression of peak expiratory flow-rate. Both beta-blockers also reduced systolic blood pressure; at rest there was no difference but after exercise propranolol was more potent. The mean resting diastolic pressure was reduced by labetalol in a dose-dependent manner but not by propranolol; this was accounted for by labetalol's alpha-blocking activity.— D. A. Richards *et al.*, *Br. J. clin. Pharmac.*, 1977, *4*, 15.

Further comparative studies: A. J. Barnett *et al.*, *Med. J. Aust.*, 1978, *1*, 105 (pindolol and hydralazine); J. G. Williams *et al.*, *ibid.*, 225 (a beta-adrenoceptor blocking agent and hydralazine); G. L. Sanders *et al.*, *Eur. J. clin. Pharmac.*, 1978, *14*, 301 (methyldopa); A. Dawson *et al.*, *Br. J. clin. Pharmac.*, 1979, *8*, 149 (bendrofluazide); J. S. Horvath *et al.*, *Med. J. Aust.*, 1979, *1*, 626 (bendrofluazide); A. Lehtonen, *Curr. ther. Res.*, 1979, *25*, 378 (propranolol); P. Bjerle *et al.*, *ibid.*, 1980, *27*, 516 (pindolol); D. P. Nicholls *et al.*, *Br. J. clin. Pharmac.*, 1980, *9*, 233 (propranolol); M. Thibonnier *et al.*, *ibid.*, 561 (acebutolol).

Controlled hypotension. Labetalol was used to produce controlled hypotension in 50 patients undergoing major surgery.— D. H. P. Cope and M. C. Crawford, *Br. J. Anaesth.*, 1979, *51*, 359.

Gradual reduction of blood pressure using labetalol was successfully achieved in a 43-year-old man who required reduction in blood pressure and no undue variability, in order to carry out arch aortography to confirm a suspected dissecting aneurysm of the aorta. The desired effect was achieved by using incremental infusions of labetalol, titrating the dose against the blood pressure and increasing the infusion-rate before the injection of dye to prevent any consequent rise in blood pressure.— A. M. M. Cumming and D. L. Davies (letter), *Lancet*, 1979, *1*, 929.

Effect on plasma renin. In a study involving 6 hypertensive subjects plasma renin activity decreased significantly during labetalol therapy but this effect was not dose-related, whereas the blood pressure reduction was.— M. J. Serlin *et al.*, *Br. J. clin. Pharmac.*, 1979, *7*, 165.

Further references: P. Weidmann *et al.*, *Am. J. Cardiol.*, 1978, *41*, 570.

Hypertensive crisis. Eleven patients admitted to hospital with diastolic blood pressures in excess of 130 mmHg were treated with labetalol by mouth—an initial dose of 300 mg (or 400 mg if the blood pressure exceeded 140 mmHg); subsequent doses were given 8-hourly—200 mg if the blood pressure was 120 to 130 mmHg or 100 mg if 100 to 120 mmHg. Successful control of mean blood pressure was achieved in 6 hours if the patients were supine.— R. R. Ghose *et al.*, *Br. med. J.*, 1978, *2*, 96. See also C. G. H. Maidment and R. Davies (letter), *ibid.*, 566; R. R. Ghose and W. D. Morgan (letter), *ibid.*, 772.

Further references: E. P. McCarthy *et al.*, *Med. J. Aust.*, 1978, *1*, 399; L. M. H. Wing (letter), *ibid.*, 658; W. J. Louis *et al.*, *Aust. N.Z. J. Med.*, 1978, *8*, 602.

Once-daily administration. As expected from a drug which can lower blood pressure within 2 hours of administration, labetalol is not suitable for once-daily administration. The recommended starting dose in the treatment of hypertension is 100 mg thrice daily, doubled after 1 or 2 weeks, if necessary,, and subsequently increased, if necessary in patients with more severe hypertension.— D. Harris and D. A. Richards, *Glaxo-Allenburys Research* (letter), *Br. med. J.*, 1978, *2*, 894.

Phaeochromocytoma. A report of the successful use of labetalol to control symptoms in 4 of 5 patients with phaeochromocytoma.— E. A. Rosei *et al.*, *Br. J. clin. Pharmac.*, 1976, *3*, *Suppl.* 3, 809.

Further references: G. Reach *et al.*, *Br. med. J.*, 1980, *280*, 1300; C. M. Feek and P. M. Earnshaw (letter), *ibid.*, *281*, 387.

See also under Precautions.

Pregnancy and the neonate. Beneficial results with labetalol in hypertension of pregnancy.— N. -O. Lunell *et al.*, *Br. J. clin. Pharmac.*, 1981, *12*, 345.

Tetanus. The continuous infusion over 19 days of labetalol to control adrenoceptor stimulation in a patient with severe tetanus.— J. W. Dundee and W. F. K. Morrow, *Br. med. J.*, 1979, *1*, 1121. Intermittent injections of labetalol have been found to be effective in some tetanus patients developing very high blood pressure.— M. A. K. Omar *et al.* (letter), *ibid.*, 1979, *2*, 274.

Further references: W. Hanna and G. A. C. Grell (letter), *Br. med. J.*, 1978, *2*, 772; H. Connor *et al.* (letter), *ibid.*, 1979, *2*, 502.

Proprietary Preparations

Trandate *(Allen & Hanburys, UK).* Labetalol hydrochloride, available as **Injection** containing 5 mg per ml, in ampoules of 20 ml, and as **Tablets** of 100, 200, and 400 mg. (Also available as Trandate in *Austral.*, *Fr.*, *Ger.*, *Ital.*, *Neth.*, *NZ*, *S.Afr.*, *Switz.*).

6312-s

Levobunolol Hydrochloride. (−)-Bunolol Hydrochloride; *l*-Bunolol Hydrochloride. (−)-5-(3-*tert*-Butylamino-2-hydroxypropoxy)-3,4-dihydronaphthalen-1(2*H*)-one hydrochloride.

$C_{17}H_{25}NO_3,HCl = 327.9$.

CAS — 47141-42-4 (levobunolol); 27912-14-7 (hydrochloride).

Adverse Effects, Treatment, and Precautions. As for Propranolol Hydrochloride, p.1325.

Absorption and Fate. Levobunolol is almost completely absorbed from the gastro-intestinal tract. It is excreted in the urine both unchanged and in the form of metabolites.

Following administration of a single dose of radioactively labelled levobunolol 3 mg by mouth to 5 healthy subjects absorption from the gastro-intestinal tract was rapid and virtually complete. Mean plasma concentrations of bunolol and dihydrobunolol, an active metabolite, were 3.26 and 2.4 ng per ml 0.5 and 1 hour after dosage respectively with corresponding half-lives of 6.1 and 7.1 hours; these concentrations were maintained for at least 3 hours. Bunolol glucuronide, dihydrobunolol glucuronide, and bunolol sulphate were also detected in plasma with half-lives of 9.1, 7.7, and 17.4 hours respectively. After 96 hours a mean of 77.6 and 3.1% of the administered dose had been excreted in the urine and faeces respectively.— F. J. Di Carlo *et al.*, *Clin. Pharmac. Ther.*, 1977, *22*, 858. See also F. -J. Leinweber *et al.*, *Pharmacology*, 1978, *16*, 70.

Animal studies on the metabolism of bunolol and levobunolol: F. -J. Leinweber *et al.*, *J. pharm. Sci.*, 1977, *66*, 1570; *idem*, 1978, *67*, 129; H. R. Kaplan *et al.*, *ibid.*, 132.

Uses. Levobunolol hydrochloride is a beta-adrenoceptor blocking agent (see p.1324) with uses similar to those of propranolol (see p.1329). It has been given in usual doses of 10 to 20 mg daily, in 2 or 3 divided doses.

Action. Pharmacology of bunolol and levobunolol in *animals*.— R. D. Robson and H. R. Kaplan, *J. Pharmac. exp. Ther.*, 1970, *175*, 157; H. R. Kaplan and R. D. Robson, *ibid.*, 168; R. E. Giles and M. P. Finkel, *Eur. J. Pharmac.*, 1971, *16*, 156; H. R. Kaplan and M. A. Commarato, *J. Pharmac. exp. Ther.*, 1973, *185*, 395.

Cardiac disorders. *Cardiac arrhythmias.* Following administration of a single dose of levobunolol to 22 patients, ventricular premature beats of high frequency and grade were reduced by at least 50% in 17. Reduction was over 90% in 11, being total in 9. Ventricular premature beats were exacerbated in 2 patients.— P. J. Podrid *et al.*, *Circulation*, 1977, *56*, *Suppl.* 3, 8.

Further references: W. Shapiro and J. Park, *Am. Heart J.*, 1978, *96*, 417.

Hypertension. Evaluation of the antihypertensive effect of levobunolol in doses of 1 to 5 mg thrice daily in 17 hypertensive subjects. Side-effects included insomnia (6), asthenia (1), anorexia (1), dyspnoea (1), ankle oedema (1).— E. Arce-Gomez *et al.*, *Curr. ther. Res.*, 1976, *19*, 386.

Effect on plasma renin. A study in 11 patients wtih essential hypertension and high, normal, or low plasma-renin activity showed that levobunolol significantly depressed plasma-renin activity.— H. Gavras *et al.*, *J. clin. Pharmac.*, 1977, *17*, 350.

Manufacturers

Warner-Lambert, USA.

6313-w

Metipranolol. VÚFB 6453; Methypranolum; Trimepranol. 1-(4-Acetoxy-2,3,5-trimethylphenoxy)-3-isopropylaminopropan-2-ol; 4-(2-Hydroxy-3-isopropylaminopropoxy)-2,3,6-trimethylphenyl acetate.

$C_{17}H_{27}NO_4 = 309.4$.

CAS — 22664-55-7.

Pharmacopoeias. In *Cz.*

A white odourless crystalline powder. Practically **insoluble** in water; soluble in alcohol; sparingly soluble in ether. M.p. 105 to 109°.

Adverse Effects, Treatment, and Precautions. As for Propranolol Hydrochloride, p.1325.

Hypoglycaemia. Investigations in 20 healthy subjects demonstrated that administration of metipranolol, 20 mg thrice daily for 7 days, lowered blood glucose in man. This did not appear to be mediated through hyperproduction of insulin.— J. Nedvídková and V. Felt, *Clin. Pharmac. Ther.*, 1973, *14*, 881.

Interactions. With diuretics. Antagonism of the hypokalaemic effect of chlorthalidone by metipranolol.— P. J. Neuvonen *et al.*, *Br. J. clin. Pharmac.*, 1978, *6*, 363.

Absorption and Fate. Metipranolol is absorbed from the gastro-intestinal tract and metabolised to the biologically active deacetylated form, which is subsequently further metabolised before excretion in the urine. The biological half-life of metipranolol is longer than would be anticipated from its plasma half-life of about 3 or 4 hours.

Metipranolol has a duration of action of about 12 hours despite its relatively short half-life of about 3 or 4 hours.— P. J. Pentikäinen *et al.*, *Int. J. clin. Pharmac. Biopharm.*, 1978, *16*, 279.

Uses. Metipranolol is a beta-adrenoceptor blocking agent (see p.1324) with uses similar to those of propranolol (see p.1329). In cardiac disorders it has been given in doses of 5 to 10 mg twice or thrice daily, and in hypertension it has been given in doses of 20 mg twice or thrice daily to a maximum of 40 mg thrice daily.

A comparison of metipranolol with other beta-adrenoceptor blocking agents in *animals*.— W. Bartsch *et al.*, *Arzneimittel-Forsch.*, 1977, *27*, 1022.

Hypertension. In a controlled crossover study in 18 patients with mild to moderate hypertension each patient received, in randomised order, a placebo, metipranolol 10 to 40 mg twice daily, chlorthalidone 50 mg on alternate days, and metipranolol in association with chlorthalidone, each treatment being continued for 6 weeks. Metipranolol and chlorthalidone had a similar and significant hypotensive effect which was increased when the drugs were given in association with one another. Heart-rate was decreased by metipranolol when compared with the effect of placebo or chlorthalidone. Metipranolol antagonised the hypokalaemic effect of chlorthalidone.— P. J. Neuvonen *et al.*, *Br. J. clin. Pharmac.*, 1978, *6*, 363.

Twice-daily administration. Studies indicating that metipranolol is suitable for twice-daily administration: A. J. Jounela *et al.*, *Int. J. clin. Pharmac. Biopharm.*, 1978, *16*, 183; P. J. Pentikäinen *et al.*, *ibid.*, 279.

Proprietary Names

Disorat *(Boehringer Mannheim, Ger.; Galenus Mannheim, Ger.).*

6314-e

Metoprolol Tartrate. CGP 2175; H 93/26.

(±)-1-Isopropylamino-3-[4-(2-methoxyethyl)phenoxy]propan-2-ol tartrate.

$(C_{15}H_{25}NO_3)_2,C_4H_6O_6=684.8$.

CAS — 37350-58-6 (metoprolol, ±); 56392-17-7 (tartrate, ±).

A white odourless crystalline powder with a bitter taste. M.p. about 120°.

Very **soluble** in water; soluble in alcohol and chloroform; practically insoluble in acetone and ether. **Protect** from light.

Adverse Effects. As for Propranolol Hydrochloride, p.1325.

Effects on the blood. *Platelet count.* In 10 healthy subjects administration of metoprolol tartrate 50 mg by mouth increased the peripheral platelet count.— J. Kutti *et al.* (letter), *New Engl. J. Med.*, 1976, *295*, 1079.

Further references: J. Kutti *et al.*, *Acta haemat.*, 1977, *58*, 89.

Effects on the circulation. In 10 healthy subjects a single dose of propranolol 80 mg reduced skin temperature by a mean of 1.3°. Skin blood flow and muscle blood flow before and after exercise were significantly reduced. Metoprolol 100 mg reduced muscle blood flow after exercise but to a lesser degree and had no significant effect on the other parameters. The effects of the 2 drugs were similar in normal subjects and patients with hypertension except that metoprolol reduced skin blood flow in the latter. Metoprolol had advantages over propranolol in patients with impaired peripheral circulation.— P. D. McSorley and D. J. Warren, *Br. med. J.*, 1978, *2*, 1598.

Intermittent claudication and gangrene in a 58-year-old woman was associated with metoprolol therapy. She responded to discontinuation of smoking and metoprolol, and infusion of dextran, alcohol, and phenoxybenzamine.— J. A. Vale and D. B. Jefferys (letter), *Lancet*, 1978, *1*, 1216. See also J. A. Vale *et al.* (letter), *ibid.*, 1977, *2*, 412.

Effects on the eyes. A woman developed pain and soreness of the eyes while taking metoprolol 200 mg daily; symptoms abated when metoprolol was withdrawn and recurred within 2 or 3 days when metoprolol was again given.— D. Scott (letter), *Br. med. J.*, 1977, *2*, 1221.

Effects on the gastro-intestinal tract. A report of retroperitoneal fibrosis in a patient who had been taking metoprolol and nifedipine for 11 months.— J. Thompson and D. G. Julian, *Br. med. J.*, 1982, *284*, 83.

Effects on lipid metabolism. A study in 9 hypertensive subjects indicating that metoprolol does not increase blood-triglyceride concentrations.— A. Nilsson *et al.* (letter), *Br. med. J.*, 1977, *2*, 126.

Further references: R. J. Newman, *Br. med. J.*, 1977, *2*, 601; I. W. Beinart *et al.*, *Postgrad. med. J.*, 1979, *55*, 709.

Effects on the muscles. A study in 6 healthy subjects indicated that neither propranolol nor metoprolol reduced muscle strength, coordination, endurance, or perception of effort. So far, no direct explanation can be given for the clinical experience of muscle fatigue associated with beta-adrenoceptor blockade.— G. Grimby and U. Smith (letter), *Lancet*, 1978, *2*, 1318.

Effects on respiratory function. Metoprolol-associated bronchospasm developed in a 67-year-old patient with no history of asthma.— Adverse Drug Reactions Advisory Committee, *Aust. Prescriber*, 1978, *2*, 116.

Effects on sexual function. Four of 14 men receiving metoprolol experienced disturbance of potency.— E. Arnesen, *Curr. ther. Res.*, 1978, *24*, 889.

See also under Peyronie's disease.

Effects on the skin. *Psoriasiform eruptions.* A report of eczematous and/or psoriasiform eruptions in 5 patients receiving long-term metoprolol therapy. The skin eruptions disappeared slowly within weeks or months of withdrawal of the drug.— H. A. M. Neumann *et al.* (letter), *Lancet*, 1979, *2*, 745.

Peyronie's disease. Peyronie's disease [penile fibrosis] in one patient was associated with metoprolol. Symptoms improved when metoprolol was withdrawn.— J. S. Yudkin (letter), *Lancet*, 1977, *2*, 1355.

Treatment of Adverse Effects. As for Propranolol Hydrochloride, p.1327.

Following ingestion of about 200 tablets of metoprolol 50 mg, prescribed for his father, a 19-year-old man was admitted to hospital conscious, with peripheral cyanosis and weak heart sounds, the heart-rate was 60 to 70 beats per minute, and the blood pressure was unrecordable. He was treated with infusions of electrolytes, sodium bicarbonate to correct acidosis, metaraminol 7 mg and glucagon 6 mg intravenously to raise the blood pressure followed by another intravenous dose of metaraminol (3 mg) 1 hour later after which the blood pressure stabilised at the patient's usual level. Frusemide was given to counteract fluid retention which occurred during the first 6 hours. Twelve hours after admission the patient was comfortable with no signs of cardiovascular depression. Although initial treatment included gastric lavage, measurement of the plasma concentrations indicated that most of the dose had been absorbed.— B. H. J. Möller (letter), *Br. med. J.*, 1976, *1*, 222. A similar case.— S. Sire (letter), *Lancet*, 1976, *2*, 1137.

Precautions. As for Propranolol Hydrochloride, p.1327.

It has been reported that metoprolol has a cardioselective action and therefore may be less likely than propranolol to cause bronchospasm, see p.1324.

Withdrawal. About 78 hours after withdrawal of metoprolol a 52-year-old man with 4 previous myocardial infarctions suffered a dramatic worsening of his angina pectoris, and subsequently suffered ventricular fibrillation and myocardial infarction.— T. Meinertz *et al.* (letter), *Lancet*, 1979, *1*, 270. The symptoms may have been caused by administration of nifedipine rather than by withdrawal of metoprolol.— L. Beeley and J. Talbot (letter), *ibid.*, 387. A further report.— L. C. Williams *et al.* (letter), *ibid.*, 494. Further comments: B. Ø. Kristensen (letter), *ibid.*, 554; Ø. L. Pedersen and E. Mikkelsen (letter), *ibid.*

Absorption and Fate. Metoprolol is readily and completely absorbed from the gastro-intestinal tract but is probably subject to considerable first-pass metabolism. Peak plasma concentrations occur about 1.5 hours after a single dose. It is extensively metabolised, the metabolites being excreted in the urine together with only small amounts of unchanged metoprolol; the hydroxy derivative has some biological activity. The biological half-life of metoprolol is longer than would be anticipated from its plasma half-life of about 3 or 4 hours. Metoprolol crosses the blood-brain barrier. It also crosses the placenta and is excreted in breast milk. It is only slightly bound to plasma protein.

After single or repeated doses of metoprolol 50 mg or 80 mg by mouth the elimination half-life was about 4 hours in mildly hypertensive patients which was similar to results previously obtained in healthy subjects. Peak plasma concentrations were reached about 90 minutes after administration. Metoprolol did not induce or inhibit its own metabolism.— C. Bengtsson *et al.*, *Clin. Pharmac. Ther.*, 1975, *17*, 400.

The mean ratio of the saliva concentration of oxprenolol to the plasma concentration was 0.42 in 6 healthy subjects who took oxprenolol 80 mg. The concentrations of metoprolol were greater in saliva than in plasma in a further 6 healthy subjects who took metoprolol 100 mg and there was no clear relationship between them. It was suggested that while oxprenolol diffused passively, metoprolol was actively secreted, into saliva.— C. P. Dawes *et al.*, *Br. J. clin. Pharmac.*, 1978, *5*, 217.

Peak blood concentrations of metoprolol occurred 45 to 102 minutes after a single dose of 100 mg in 7 hypertensive patients and ranged from 93 to 881 ng per ml.— S. Hunyor and G. Nyberg, *Br. J. clin. Pharmac.*, 1978, *6*, 109.

The effect of age on the pharmacokinetics of metoprolol.— C. P. Quarterman *et al.*, *Br. J. clin. Pharmac.*, 1981, *11*, 287.

Further references: C. P. Quarterman *et al.*, *Eur. J. clin. Pharmac.*, 1979, *15*, 97; D. A. Piercy (letter), *ibid.*, *16*, 219; C. P. Quarterman *et al.* (letter), *ibid.;* M. J. Kendall *et al.*, *ibid.*, 1980, *17*, 87; P. Collste *et al.*, *Clin. Pharmac. Ther.*, 1980, *27*, 441; M. G. Myers and J. J. Thiessen, *ibid.*, 756; C. -G. Regårdh and G. Johnsson, *Clin. Pharmacokinet.*, 1980, *5*, 557.

Diffusion into the CSF. A 64-year-old hypertensive woman who had been taking metoprolol 50 mg thrice daily for 2 months had a CSF-metoprolol concentration of 267 ng per ml and plasma metoprolol of 341 ng per ml. It was considered that the concentration in CSF was approximately equal to the concentration of unbound drug in plasma.— A. J. Wood (letter), *Br. J. clin. Pharmac.*, 1977, *4*, 240.

Further references: M. D. Day *et al.*, *J. Pharm. Pharmac.*, 1977, *29*, *Suppl.*, 52P.

Pregnancy and the neonate. The disposition of metoprolol in newborn infants of mothers treated with metoprolol.— P. Lundborg *et al.* (letter), *Br. J. clin. Pharmac.*, 1981, *12*, 598.

Protein binding. The binding of metoprolol to human serum proteins.— C. Appelgren *et al.*, *Acta pharm. suec.*, 1974, *11*, 325; K. A. Johansson *et al.*, *ibid.*, 333.

Uses. Metoprolol tartrate is a beta-adrenoceptor blocking agent (see p.1324) with uses similar to those of propranolol (see p.1329). It is classified as cardioselective.

In the treatment of hypertension metoprolol tartrate is usually given in an initial dose of 100 mg daily, increased weekly according to the response of the patient to 400 mg daily or 200 mg twice daily. Better control may be obtained with a twice daily dosage regimen. The usual dose for angina pectoris is 50 to 100 mg twice or thrice daily. As an adjunct in the treatment of hyperthyroidism metoprolol tartrate may be given in doses of 50 mg four times daily. In the treatment of cardiac arrhythmias the usual dose is 50 mg twice or thrice daily, increased if necessary up to 300 mg daily in divided doses.

For the emergency treatment of cardiac arrhythmias metoprolol tartrate may be given intravenously in an initial dose of up to 5 mg administered at a rate of 1 to 2 mg per minute; this may be repeated, if necessary, at intervals of 5 minutes to a total dose of 10 to 15 mg. When acute arrhythmias have been controlled, maintenance therapy with doses not exceeding 50 mg thrice daily by mouth is recommended and should be started 4 to 6 hours after intravenous therapy.

Arrhythmias may be prevented on induction of anaesthesia or controlled during anaesthesia, by the slow intravenous injection of 2 to 4 mg; further injections of 2 mg may be repeated as necessary to a maximum total dose of 10 mg.

Action. A detailed review of the pharmacological properties of metoprolol, and its therapeutic efficacy in angina pectoris and hypertension.— R. N. Brogden *et al.*, *Drugs*, 1977, *14*, 321.

Further reviews: *Aust. J. Pharm.*, 1978, *59*, 674; *Med. Lett.*, 1978, *20*, 97; *ibid.*, 1979, *21*, 24; J. Koch-Weser, *New Engl. J. Med.*, 1979, *301*, 698.

Studies on the action of metoprolol including comparative studies with other beta-adrenoceptor blocking agents: S. H. Taylor *et al.*, *Int. J. clin. Pharmac.*, 1974, *10*, 136 (comparative study); M. J. Kendall and R. A. Yates (letter), *Br. med. J.*, 1976, *1*, 1404 (haemodynamic changes); C. Davidson *et al.*, *Br. med. J.*, 1976, *2*, 7 (antihypertensive effect); R. Sannerstedt and H. Wasir, *Br. J. clin. Pharmac.*, 1977, *4*, 23 (haemodynamic changes); G. Nyberg, *ibid.*, 275 (haemodynamic changes); C. L. A. van Herwaarden *et al.* (letter), *Br. med. J.*, 1977, *1*, 1029 (catecholamine response); *idem*, *Eur. J. clin. Pharmac.*, 1977, *12*, 397 (catecholamine response); P. J. Lijnen *et al.*, *Br. J. clin. Pharmac.*, 1979, *7*, 175 (effect on renin, angiotensin, aldosterone, and catecholamines); S. B. Pearson *et al.*, *ibid.*, *8*, 143 (haemodynamic changes).

For references to effects on plasma renin, see under Hypertension.

Administration. Studies in healthy subjects indicated that more metoprolol entered the general circulation following administration with food than when it was taken on an empty stomach; administration should always be standardised relative to meals.— A. Melander *et al.*, *Clin. Pharmac. Ther.*, 1977, *22*, 108.

In the elderly. A suggestion that metoprolol might need to be given in reduced dosage or once daily to elderly patients.— M. J. Kendall *et al.* (letter), *Br. J. clin. Pharmac.*, 1977, *4*, 497.

Once-daily administration. Although metoprolol once-daily might be adequate in hypertension it might not suffice for angina and cardiac arrhythmias.— A. Lehtonen and H. Sundquist, *Curr. ther. Res.*, 1978, *23*, 131. See also under Hypertension.

Administration in renal failure. The pharmacokinetic and pharmacodynamic properties of metoprolol in patients with impaired renal function.— L. Jordö *et al.*, *Clin. Pharmacokinet.*, 1980, *5*, 169. See also K. -J. Hoffmann *et al.*, *ibid.*, 181; K. -U. Seiler *et al.*, *ibid.*, 192.

Administration in respiratory insufficiency. Neither metoprolol 50 mg nor practolol 100 mg twice daily affected the FEV_1 in 17 patients with chronic bronchial asthma and hypertension but doubling the dose of either produced a significant reduction in FEV_1. Metoprolol could be used in asthmatic patients requiring beta-adrenoceptor blockade provided the daily dose did not exceed 100 mg.— H. Formgren, *Br. J. clin. Pharmac.*, 1976, *3*, 1007.

Metoprolol may be administered with caution to patients with bronchitis and a tendency to wheezing, provided that bronchodilator therapy with a β_2-adrenoceptor stimulant such as terbutaline or salbutamol is administered concurrently. Despite this, exacerbation of asthma is likely with the dosage of β_1-adrenoceptor blocking agents usually used in the treatment of hypertension.— R. N. Brogden *et al.*, *Drugs*, 1977, *14*, 321.

Further references: G. Johnsson *et al.*, *Eur. J. clin Pharmac.*, 1975, *8*, 175; B. N. Singh *et al.*, *Clin. Pharmac. Ther.*, 1976, *19*, 493; C. Skinner *et al.*, *Br. med. J.*, 1976, *1*, 504; C. R. McGavin and I. P. Williams, *Br. J. Dis. Chest*, 1978, *72*, 327; A. S. P. Hua *et al.*, *Med. J. Aust.*, 1978, *1*, 281; D. J. M. Sinclair, *Br. med. J.*, 1979, *1*, 168.

Anaesthesia. Studies on the use of metoprolol to prevent cardiac arrhythmias during anaesthesia.— M. H. Whitehead *et al.*, *Anaesthesia*, 1980, *35*, 779; W. N. Rollason and J. G. Russell, *ibid.*, 783; A. J. Coleman and C. Jordan, *ibid.*, 972.

Anxiety. Metoprolol reduced stress-induced increase in heart-rate but not concomitant hypertension.— E. Heidbreder *et al.*, *Eur. J. clin. Pharmac.*, 1978, *14*, 391.

Cardiac disorders. *Angina pectoris.* In a double-blind crossover study in 14 patients with stable angina pectoris exercise tolerance was significantly greater when taking metoprolol 50 mg four times daily than when taking propranolol 40 mg four times daily. In a long-term study completed by 13 patients extending over a further 58 weeks exercise tolerance was maintained and no significant change occurred when the dose was changed to 100 mg twice daily. Mean serum-metoprolol concentrations at the end of the crossover study were 55.6 ng per g (range 12 to 136 ng) and 120 ng per g (range 51 to 256 ng) at the end of the long-term study. Treatment was well tolerated.— M. B. Comerford and E. M. M. Besterman, *Postgrad. med. J.*, 1976, *52*, 481.

Further references: L. G. Ekelund *et al.*, *Br. Heart J.*, 1976, *38*, 155; M. B. Comerford and E. M. M. Besterman, *Scott. med. J.*, 1977, *22*, 80; P. Bielmann and G. Leduc, *Curr. ther. Res.*, 1979, *25*, 221; F. Delage *et al.*, *Clin. Pharmac. Ther.*, 1980, *27*, 763.

Cardiomyopathy. See under Propranolol Hydrochloride, p.1331.

Myocardial infarction. In a double-blind randomised study of 1395 patients with definite or suspected acute myocardial infarction mortality was reduced by metoprolol when compared with placebo. Metoprolol 15 mg was given intravenously on arrival in hospital, followed by 100 mg twice daily by mouth for 90 days. The cumulative mortality-rate for the treatment period was 8.9% (62 deaths) in the placebo group and 5.7% (40 deaths) in the metoprolol group, a reduction in mortality of 36%.— Å. Hjalmarson *et al.*, *Lancet*, 1981, *2*, 823.

Glaucoma. Metoprolol 50 mg thrice daily for one day significantly reduced intra-ocular pressure in 11 patients with previously untreated glaucoma of one eye.— A. Alm *et al.*, *Acta Ophthalmol.*, 1979, *57*, 236.

Hypertension. In a multicentre study metoprolol 75 to 450 mg daily for 6 months was given to patients with essential hypertension. Of 76 previously untreated patients, 57 had greatly reduced diastolic blood pressure or became normotensive and of 61 uncontrolled by other drug therapy and given only metoprolol, 39 showed a good response.— S. Rosengard, *J. int. med. Res.*, 1977, *5*, 199.

After metoprolol 100 mg was given to 7 hypertensive patients, intra-arterial blood pressure fell slightly at rest and during isometric exercise and heart-rate was reduced. The reduction in blood pressure was not detected when measurement was made indirectly.— S. Hunyor and G. Nyberg, *Br. J. clin. Pharmac.*, 1978, *6*, 109.

Similar studies: A. Jäättelä and K. Pyörälä, *Br. J. clin. Pharmac.*, 1976, *3*, 655; B. -G. Hansson *et al.*, *Eur. J. clin. Pharmac.*, 1977, *11*, 239; *idem*, 247; P. Lund-Johansen and O. -J. Ohm, *Br. J. clin. Pharmac.*, 1977, *4*, 147; J. Tuomilehto and P. Pakarinen, *Curr. ther. Res.*, 1977, *21*, 257; P. Duez *et al.*, *Acta ther.*, 1978, *4*, 167; U. Klinnert, *Münch. med. Wschr.*, 1978, *120*, 1091; J. J. McNeil and W. J. Louis, *Med. J. Aust.*, 1978, *2*, 123; J. Castenfors and M. Danielsson, *Curr. ther. Res.*, 1979, *25*, 228; R. Dirix *et al.*, *Practitioner*, 1979, *222*, 713; M. Kubik *et al.*, *Clin. Pharmac. Ther.*, 1979, *25*, 25; E. J. W. Stephens and T. Duncan, *N.Z. med. J.*, 1979, *89*, 296.

Comparative studies. A double-blind crossover study in 20 patients with mild hypertension showed that 4 weeks' treatment with metoprolol 200 or 400 mg daily (in 2 doses) or atenolol 200 or 400 mg daily (in 2 doses) had similar hypotensive effects.— T. A. Jeffers *et al.*, *Br. med. J.*, 1978, *2*, 1269.

Whereas propranolol produced a sharp reduction in heart-rate and blood pressure within the first 2 weeks of a 24-week study in 28 patients with hypertension, and a further slight decrease thereafter, metoprolol produced a slower but more uniform reduction during the study. Propranolol was more effective in reducing diastolic blood pressure while metoprolol was more effective in reducing heart-rate and systolic blood pressure. It was considered that metoprolol showed greater β_1 cardioselective properties than propranolol.— A. N. Singh *et al.*, *Curr. ther. Res.*, 1978, *24*, 571.

Further comparative studies: M. B. Comerford and A. Pringle, *Practitioner*, 1976, *217*, 953 (alprenolol); E. Arnesen, *Curr. ther. Res.*, 1978, *24*, 889 (methyldopa); N. M. Johnson and S. W. Clarke, *Acta ther.*, 1978, *4*, 147 (atenolol); J. J. McNeil *et al.*, *Med. J. Aust.*, 1979, *1*, 431 (pindolol); J. D. Spence and N. A. M. Paterson, *Curr. ther. Res.*, 1979, *26*, 941 (propranolol); J. Tuomilehto and A. Nissinen, *Eur. J. clin. Pharmac.*, 1979, *16*, 369 (alprenolol and oxprenolol); M. B. Comerford and E. Besterman (letter), *Lancet*, 1980, *2*, 1196 (atenolol).

Effect on plasma renin. A study of plasma concentrations and the effects of metoprolol on blood pressure, beta-adrenoceptor blockade, and plasma renin activity in essential hypertension.— C. von Bahr *et al.*, *Clin. Pharmac. Ther.*, 1976, *20*, 130.

Once-daily administration. In a controlled study in 16 patients with hypertension metoprolol 300 mg daily as a single dose or in 3 divided doses had a comparable effect in reducing blood pressure; the variations in plasma-metoprolol concentrations were more variable after once-daily dosage and the degree of blockade (assessed by heart-rate during exercise) was more consistent after thrice-daily dosage.— T. Reybrouck *et al.*, *Br. med. J.*, 1978, *1*, 1386.

Results in healthy subjects indicating that metoprolol can attenuate the systolic blood pressure response to moderate to severe exercise over a 24-hour period provided it is given twice or possibly thrice daily with a unit dose of 100 mg.— J. D. Harry *et al.* (letter), *Lancet*, 1979, *2*, 250. In a double-blind study involving 55 hypertensive patients atenolol and metoprolol were found to be equipotent after once-daily administration.— O. Lyngstam and L. Rydén (letter), *ibid.*, 634. For other references to the comparative efficacy of atenolol and metoprolol, see Atenolol under Hypertension, p.1338.

Further references: T. J. J. M. Bloem *et al.*, *Curr. ther. Res.*, 1978, *24*, 26; B. E. Karlberg *et al.*, *Clin. Pharmac. Ther.*, 1979, *25*, 399.

Hyperthyroidism. Comparison of propranolol and metoprolol in the management of hyperthyroidism.— L. E. Murchison *et al.*, *Br. J. clin. Pharmac.*, 1979, *8*, 581.

Migraine. A report of the beneficial effect of metoprolol in 3 patients with migraine.— O. Ljung (letter), *New Engl. J. Med.*, 1980, *303*, 156.

Tremor. Metoprolol was as effective as propranolol in relieving the symptoms of a 37-year-old man with essential tremor and, unlike propranolol, did not aggravate his asthma.— T. Riley and A. B. Pleet (letter), *New Engl. J. Med.*, 1979, *301*, 663. See also C. W. Britt and B. H. Peters (letter), *ibid.*, 331.

Metoprolol, gradually increased to 50 mg thrice daily, produced a favourable response in 19 of 22 patients with long-standing essential or familial tremor. The 3 non-responders did not respond to propranolol either.— O. Ljung (letter), *New Engl. J. Med.*, 1979, *301*, 1005.

Further references: D. M. Turnbull and D. A. Shaw (letter), *Lancet*, 1980, *1*, 95.

Proprietary Preparations

Betaloc *(Astra, UK)*. Metoprolol tartrate, available as scored tablets of 50 and 100 mg. (Also available as Betaloc in *Austral.*, *Canad.*, *NZ*).

Betaloc-SA *(Astra, UK)*. Sustained-release tablets (Durules) each containing metoprolol tartrate 200 mg. *Dose.* 1 daily, increased to 2 if necessary.

Owing to the risk of intestinal obstruction, sustained-release preparations such as Betaloc-SA, where the drug is released in transit but the matrix ghost is often eliminated intact, should not be prescribed in patients with Crohn's disease or other intestinal disease in which strictures may form.— J. L. Shaffer *et al.* (letter), *Lancet*, 1980, *2*, 487.

Betaloc I.V. Injection *(Astra, UK)*. Metoprolol tartrate, available as a solution containing 1 mg per ml in ampoules of 5 ml.

Co-Betaloc *(Astra, UK)*. Scored tablets each containing metoprolol tartrate 100 mg and hydrochlorothiazide 12.5 mg. For hypertension. *Dose.* 1 to 3 tablets daily.

Lopresor *(Geigy, UK)*. Metoprolol tartrate, available as **Injection** containing 1 mg per ml in ampoules of 5 ml and as scored **Tablets** of 50 and 100 mg. (Also available as Lopresor in *Austral.*, *Belg.*, *Canad.*, *Ger.*, *Ital.*, *Neth.*, *S.Afr.*, *Switz.*).

Lopresor SR *(Geigy, UK)*. Sustained-release tablets each containing metoprolol tartrate 200 mg. *Dose.* 1 daily, increased to 2 if necessary.

Lopresoretic *(Geigy, UK)*. Tablets each containing metoprolol tartrate 100 mg and chlorthalidone 12.5 mg. For hypertension. *Dose.* One tablet daily, increased to 4 tablets if necessary.

Other Proprietary Names

Beloc *(Ger.)*; Lopressor *(USA)*; Selokeen *(Neth.)*; Seloken *(Belg., Denm., Ital., Lux., Norw., Swed.)*.

6315-l

Nadolol. SQ 11725. (2*R*,3*S*)-5-(3-*tert*-Butylamino-2-hydroxypropoxy)-1,2,3,4-tetrahydronaphthalene-2,3-diol.
$C_{17}H_{27}NO_4$=309.4.

CAS — 42200-33-9.

A white crystalline powder. **Soluble** in water; practically insoluble in lipids.

Adverse Effects, Treatment, and Precautions. As for Propranolol Hydrochloride, p.1325.

Effects on respiratory function. Near-fatal bronchospasm occurred in a young patient with asthma when given nadolol.— J. M. Raine *et al.*, *Br. med. J.*, 1981, *282*, 548.

Absorption and Fate. Nadolol is incompletely absorbed from the gastro-intestinal tract to give peak plasma concentrations about 3 or 4 hours after a dose. It does not appear to be metabolised and is excreted unchanged in the urine and the bile. The biological half-life of nadolol is longer than would be anticipated from its plasma half-life which has been variously reported as ranging from about 6 to 24 hours. It is only about 30% bound to plasma proteins and is reported to be dialysable. Nadolol is excreted in breast milk.

In 4 patients with mild hypertension given nadolol 2 mg by mouth or intravenously, the elimination half-life from plasma was an average of 10 to 12 hours (a range of 5.9 to 12.2 hours following intravenous administration, and a range of 9.6 to 14.2 hours following oral administration). This was shorter than unpublished data reporting an average terminal half-life of 17 hours for 4 healthy subjects. Calculations based on urinary excretion and plasma concentration data suggested that about 33% was absorbed after oral administration. There was evidence of biliary as well as urinary excretion since after intravenous administration about 73% was excreted in urine and 23% in faeces. Nadolol did not appear to be metabolised.— J. Dreyfuss *et al.*, *J. clin. Pharmac.*, 1977, *17*, 300. A similar study of therapeutic oral doses.— J. Dreyfuss *et al.*, *J. clin. Pharmac.*, 1979, *19*, 712.

A study of the effect of various beta-adrenoceptor blocking agents on exercise-induced changes in 9 patients with mild hypertension and 16 healthy subjects. The pharmacodynamic half-life of nadolol was about 39 hours.— R. A. Vukovich *et al.*, *Br. J. clin. Pharmac.*, 1979, *7*, *Suppl.* 2, 167S.

Pregnancy and the neonate. *lactation.* Following administration of nadolol 80 mg daily for 5 days to 12 lactating women, the mean steady-state concentration of nadolol in the breast milk was five-times higher than that in serum.— R. G. Devlin and P. M. Fleiss, *Clin. Pharmac. Ther.*, 1981, *29*, 240; R. G. Devlin *et al.*, *Br. J. clin. Pharmac.*, 1981, *12*, 393.

Uses. Nadolol is a beta-adrenoceptor blocking agent (see p.1324) with uses similar to those of propranolol (see p.1329). It is classified as non-cardioselective.

In the treatment of hypertension nadolol is usually given in an initial dose of 80 mg daily, increased weekly according to the response of the patient to 240 mg daily; some patients have required doses of 640 mg daily. In the management of angina pectoris the usual initial dose is 40 mg daily, increased weekly according to the response of the patient to usual doses of up to 160 mg daily.

Reviews of the action and uses of nadolol: R. C. Heel *et al.*, *Drugs*, 1980, *20*, 1; *Med. Lett.*, 1980, *22*, 33; W. H. Frishman, *New Engl. J. Med.*, 1981, *305*, 678.

Studies on the action of nadolol: N. K. Hollenberg *et al.*, *Br. J. clin. Pharmac.*, 1979, *7*, *Suppl.* 2, 219S (renal vascular response).

Pharmacology in *animals*.— R. J. Lee *et al.*, *Eur. J. Pharmac.*, 1975, *33*, 371; J. K. Gibson *et al.*, *J. Pharmac. exp. Ther.*, 1977, *202*, 702.

Administration in renal failure. A study in 24 patients with chronic renal failure indicated that nadolol elimination is retarded in patients with renal failure. Serum concentrations of nadolol were reduced by haemodialysis.— J. Herrera *et al.*, *Br. J. clin. Pharmac.*, 1979, *7*, *Suppl.* 2, 227S.

A study in 15 men with mild essential hypertension and slight renal impairment indicated that the addition of nadolol in effective antihypertensive doses (range 40 to 120 mg daily) to their normal medication for 10 weeks caused neither a reduction nor an increase in renal function.— H. J. Waal-Manning and C. H. Hobson, *Br. med. J.*, 1980, *281*, 423.

Cardiac disorders. *Angina pectoris.* In an initial double-blind study lasting 14 weeks in 29 patients with angina, nadolol 40 to 240 mg as a single daily dose was as effective in relieving symptoms as propranolol 10 to 60 mg four times daily. Control of angina was maintained in 23 patients for about 18 months by continued treatment with nadolol.— G. Prager, *J. int. med. Res.*, 1979, *7*, 39.

Further references: B. Furberg *et al.*, *Curr. med. Res. Opinion*, 1978, *5*, 388; G. G. Turner *et al.*, *Br. Heart J.*, 1978, *40*, 1361.

Cardiac arrhythmias. Nadolol 10 mg every 6 hours successfully controlled life-threatening cardiac arrhythmia in one patient. Quinidine, procainamide, and lignocaine had produced poor control.— R. Vukovich *et al.* (letter), *Lancet*, 1978, *1*, 162.

Hypertension. Preliminary studies of the antihypertensive effect of treatment with nadolol 40 mg to 560 mg daily in 24 of 30 patients who completed the 14-week study, showed nadolol was similar to other beta-adrenoceptor blocking agents.— G. Frithz, *Curr. med. Res. Opinion*, 1978, *5*, 383.

Further references: M. M. El-Mehairy *et al.*, *Br. J. clin. Pharmac.*, 1979, *7*, *Suppl.* 2, 199S; G. Hitzenberger, *J. int. med. Res.*, 1979, *7*, 33; K. L. Duchin *et al.*, *Clin. Pharmac. Ther.*, 1980, *27*, 57.

Comparative studies. A double-blind comparison of nadolol and propranolol in the treatment of hypertension.— M. M. El Mehairy *et al.*, *J. int. med. Res.*, 1980, *8*, 193.

Once-daily administration. A study demonstrating that once-daily dosage with nadolol is effective in essential hypertension.— L. Volicer *et al.*, *J. clin. Pharmac.*, 1979, *19*, 137.

Further references: D. A. Jackson, *Br. J. clin. Pract.*, 1980, *34*, 211.

Proprietary Preparations

Corgard *(Squibb, UK)*. Nadolol, available as tablets of 40 mg and scored tablets of 80 mg. (Also available as Corgard in *Canad., S.Afr., Switz., USA*).

Corgaretic 40 *(Squibb, UK)*. Scored tablets each containing nadolol 40 mg and bendrofluazide 5 mg.

Corgaretic 80. Scored tablets each containing nadolol 80 mg and bendrofluazide 5 mg. For hypertension. *Dose.* 1 to 2 tablets daily.

Other Proprietary Names

Solgol *(Ger.)*.

6316-y

Nifenalol. INPEA. (±)-2-Isopropylamino-1-(4-nitrophenyl)ethanol; (±)-α-[(Isopropylamino)methyl]-4-nitrobenzyl alcohol.
$C_{11}H_{16}N_2O_3$=224.3.

CAS — 7413-36-7(±); 5302-36-3(+); 5302-35-2(−).

Nifenalol is a beta-adrenoceptor blocking agent (see p.1324) with general properties similar to those of propranolol (see p.1325) that has been tried in angina pectoris and some cardiac arrhythmias.

Pretreatment with nifenalol in doses of 10, 25, and 45 mg reduced isoprenaline-induced tachycardia in 5 subjects. The effect was dose-related. However, unlike propranolol, practolol, and oxprenolol, nifenalol had no effect on the resting heart-rate.— B. M. Groden and W. S. Hillis (letter), *J. Pharm. Pharmac.*, 1972, *24*, 487.

Further references: G. Parenti *et al.*, *Cuore Circul.*, 1968, *52*, 260, per *Abstr. Wld Med.*, 1969, *43*, 357; C. Hasslacher *et al.*, *Arzneimittel-Forsch.*, 1977, *27*, 426.

Proprietary Names of Nifenalol Hydrochloride

Inpea *(Selvi, Ital.; Liade, Spain)*; Impeasel *(Roux-Ocefa, Arg.)*.

6317-j

Oxprenolol Hydrochloride *(B.P.)*. Ciba 39089; Oxyprenolol Hydrochloride. (±)-1-(2-Allyloxyphenoxy)-3-isopropylaminopropan-2-ol hydrochloride.
$C_{15}H_{23}NO_3,HCl$=301.8.

CAS — 6452-71-7 (oxprenolol) [22972-96-9 (+); 31576-00-8 (−); 22972-98-1 (±)]; 6452-73-9 (hydrochloride) [29208-41-1 (−); 22972-97-0 (±)].

Pharmacopoeias. In *Br.*

A white to slightly cream-coloured almost odourless crystalline powder with a bitter taste. M.p. 106° to 109°. **Soluble** 1 in less than 1 of water and 1 in 1.5 of alcohol; very slightly soluble in ether. A 5% solution in water has a pH of 4 to 6.

Adverse Effects. As for Propranolol Hydrochloride, p.1325.

Allergy. A report of oxprenolol-induced drug fever in a patient which was confirmed by a challenge test.— K. Hasegawa *et al.*, *Br. med. J.*, 1980, *281*, 27.

Carcinogenicity. Long-term studies in *mice* and *rats* indicated that neither pronethalol nor oxprenolol was carcinogenic. Earlier findings of a carcinogenic response to pronethalol might have been fortuitous or species-dependent, and beta-adrenoceptor blocking agents as a class should not be considered carcinogenic.— J. W. Newberne *et al.*, *Toxic. appl. Pharmac.*, 1977, *41*, 535.

Effects on the blood. *Thrombocytopenia.* A 57-year-old man taking 640 mg of a slow-release preparation of oxprenolol daily developed thrombocytopenia which resolved a week after withdrawing oxprenolol. His platelet count fell on rechallenge with a single dose of slow-release oxprenolol 320 mg. His blood pressure was subsequently controlled with propranolol with no adverse effects.— W. N. Dodds and R. J. L. Davidson (letter), *Lancet*, 1978, *2*, 683.

Effects on the eyes. A patient who had taken oxprenolol for 18 months (with clonidine, bendrofluazide, frusemide, and digoxin) developed redness of the eyes with conjunctival oedema and congestion and corneal opacities; the symptoms regressed within a week when oxprenolol was withdrawn.— M. S. Knapp and N. R. Galloway (letter), *Br. med. J.*, 1975, *2*, 557.

A 72-year-old man who had taken oxprenolol for about 7 months developed dryness of the eyes.— J. R. Clayden (letter), *Br. med. J.*, 1975, *2*, 557.

Further references: B. S. Lewis *et al.*, *S. Afr. med. J.*, 1976, *50*, 482.

Effects on the gastro-intestinal tract. Filmy abdominal adhesions were found at laparotomy in a 50-year-old woman who had taken oxprenolol for about 3 months 4 years earlier; she had not taken practolol.— S. C. Kennedy and M. Ducrow (letter), *Br. med. J.*, 1977, *1*, 1598.

Severe gastro-intestinal symptoms perhaps with obstruction of the small bowel might have been associated with oxprenolol in a patient who also had renal failure. Necropsy revealed a generalised ileus without local cause and no peritonitis.— D. W. Young *et al.* (letter), *Lancet*, 1977, *2*, 1133.

Retroperitoneal fibrosis in one patient associated with the use of oxprenolol.— D. R. McCluskey *et al.*, *Br. med. J.*, 1980, *281*, 1459.

Effects on immunological responses. A 40-year-old man taking oxprenolol developed severe chicken-pox 2 weeks after his son's attack. The possible effect of oxprenolol on immunological responses had been reported to the Committee on Safety of Medicines, who had had a report of the development of lupus erythematosus in a patient receiving oxprenolol.— L. F. W. McMahon (letter), *Br. med. J.*, 1976, *2*, 1388.

Effects on mental state. In a 66-year-old woman, with no family or personal history of schizophrenia, schizophrenic symptoms, occurring when the dose of oxprenolol was increased, regressed when the dose was reduced.— J. Steinert and C. R. Pugh, *Br. med. J.*, 1979, *1*, 790.

Effects on the muscles. A report of a myasthenia-like syndrome with weakness of ocular and limb muscles, occurring in a 67-year-old woman in association with oxprenolol therapy.— Y. Herishanu and P. Rosenberg (letter), *Ann. intern. Med.*, 1975, *83*, 834.

Effects on respiratory function. A 39-year-old man with extrinsic atopic asthma became acutely breathless and cyanosed after taking 40 mg of oxprenolol.— J. Gaddie and C. Skinner (letter), *Br. med. J.*, 1972, *1*, 749. See also A. Mithal (letter), *ibid.*, 1974, *2*, 503.

Effects on the respiratory tract. An announcement that a patient reported to have pleural thickening during oxprenolol therapy (R.L. Page, *Br. J. Dis. Chest*, 1979, *73*, 195) was subsequently found to have a malignant mesothelioma and not benign fibrosis.— *Lancet*, 1979, *1*, 1154.

Effects on the skin. *Hyperpigmentation.* A 62-year-old woman developed generalised skin pigmentation after taking oxprenolol 240 mg daily for 2 months. Pigmentation faded when oxprenolol was withdrawn and reappeared after a challenge course. Melanocyte-stimulating hormone was not considered to be involved; the reaction was probably idiosyncratic.— A. D. B. Harrower and J. A. Strong, *Br. med. J.*, 1977, *2*, 296.

Psoriasiform eruptions. A 65-year-old man had exacerbation of his psoriasis when treated with oxprenolol.— J. B. Cumberbatch (letter), *Br. med. J.*, 1974, *4*, 528.

Of 48 patients with cutaneous reactions to practolol 32 had subsequently been treated with other beta-adrenoceptor blocking agents, usually oxprenolol, for up to 30 months without the development of skin lesions.— R. H. Felix *et al.* (letter), *Br. med. J.*, 1975, *1*, 626.

Two patients developed a distinctive skin rash after treatment with oxprenolol; the lesions consisted of well-defined red rings, sometimes scaly or eroded, on the trunk, face, and limbs, with psoriasiform features on the legs in 1 patient. Histological examination showed lichenoid changes, basal cell liquefaction degeneration, intra-epidermal necrotic cells, and colloid body formation. Biopsy specimens from 2 further patients showed similar changes.— G. M. Levene and R. W. Gange (letter), *Br. med. J.*, 1978, *1*, 784.

Further references: P. J. A. Holt and E. Waddington, *Br. med. J.*, 1975, *2*, 539; W. A. Hudson and W. A. Finnis (letter), *Lancet*, 1975, *1*, 932; J. C. Leonard (letter), *ibid.*, 630.

Hyperkalaemia. Severe hyperkalaemia occurred in a patient following an overdose of oxprenolol and 15 g of potassium in the form of Navidrex-K. Such an effect would not have been expected from Navidrex-K alone and oxprenolol was considered to have added to the toxicity.— L. Hume and J. C. Forfar (letter), *Lancet*, 1977, *2*, 1182. Beta-adrenoceptor blocking agents can increase serum-potassium concentrations independently of any effect on glomerular filtration.— T. Nawar (letter), *ibid.*, 1978, *1*, 717.

Lupus erythematosus. For reference to a report of lupus erythematosus in a patient taking oxprenolol see under Effects on Immunological Responses.

Treatment of Adverse Effects. As for Propranolol Hydrochloride, p.1327.

A 62-year-old man in a state of collapse showed slow response during 35 minutes of resuscitative treatment with isoprenaline, adrenaline, calcium gluconate, and sodium bicarbonate, but responded by increase in blood pressure within 1 minute of intravenous injection of glucagon 10 mg; the patient's state was then found to be due to the ingestion of an unspecified amount of oxprenolol and diazepam.— D. E. Ward and B. Jones, *Br. med. J.*, 1976, *2*, 151.

A 39-year-old woman who had taken oxprenolol 2.5 to 3 g recovered after treatment which included gastric lavage, hydrocortisone 500 mg intravenously, assisted respiration, prolonged external cardiac massage (for about 2 hours), atropine, adrenaline, calcium gluconate, isoprenaline, sodium bicarbonate, dextran 70 injection, mannitol, dexamethasone, and antibiotics.— P. C. Mattingly (letter), *Br. med. J.*, 1977, *1*, 776.

A 38-year-old woman became unconscious and was centrally cyanosed and sweating after taking 6.08 g of oxprenolol (38 Slow Trasicor tablets) with pentazocine and paracetamol (Fortagesic) and alcohol. She recovered consciousness after naloxone 800 µg was given intravenously but cyanosis and shock persisted; further doses of naloxone had no effect and she lost consciousness. She had no recordable pulse or blood pressure for about 2 hours and atropine 1.2 mg and glucagon 2 mg and 1 mg given intravenously and an infusion of isoprenaline 30 µg per minute had no effect. However, a bolus injection of glucagon 10 mg produced vomiting, recovery of consciousness and return of pulse and blood pressure. There was transient sinus tachycardia but no arrhythmia. Within 30 minutes the blood pressure was again unrecordable and the patient lost consciousness. A bolus injection of glucagon 4 mg produced vomiting but no improvement and a further 10 mg was required to restore consciousness and blood pressure. Glucagon was then infused in dextrose injection at a rate of 3 mg per hour for 4 hours, 2 mg per hour for 3 hours, and 1 mg per hour for 5 hours. The patient's ECG was virtually normal 20 hours after the overdose. Plasma-oxprenolol concentrations had been 8.22 µg per ml 2.1 hours after ingestion and 0.5 µg per ml at 24 hours.— R. N. Illingworth, *Practitioner*, 1979, *223*, 683. See also *ibid.*, 1980, *224*, 199.

Further reports of overdosage and comments: A. Khan and J. M. Muscat-Baron, *Br. med. J.*, 1977, *1*, 552; C. Roberts and H. McNulty (letter), *ibid.*, 840; J. S. Oliver and A. A. Watson, *Medicine Sci. Law*, 1977, *17*, 279.

Precautions. As for Propranolol Hydrochloride, p.1327.

Cardiac disorders. A 58-year-old man with left ventricular failure controlled by digoxin and frusemide was given oxprenolol 20 mg. He developed circulatory collapse unresponsive to glucagon or atropine but responsive to isoprenaline. Beta-adrenoceptor blockade should be used with extreme care in patients with impaired myocardial performance.— N. H. Brooks, *Br. med. J.*, 1975, *4*, 24.

Diabetes mellitus. A diabetic patient required only one-half his previous dose of chlorpropamide during treatment with oxprenolol.— D. F. Wilson *et al.*, *Br. med. J.*, 1969, *2*, 155.

Interactions. *Sympathomimetics.* A very severe hypertensive reaction occurred in a 31-year-old hypertensive patient receiving methyldopa and oxprenolol when he was prescribed tablets containing phenylpropanolamine for a cold. Methyldopa was known to increase the pressor effects of sympathomimetic amines and the association with oxprenolol might have led to a particularly severe reaction since beta-blockade might allow an unopposed alpha constrictor response to adrenergic stimulation.— E. H. McLaren, *Br. med. J.*, 1976, *2*, 283.

Propranolol enhanced the vasoconstrictor response to noradrenaline in 8 healthy subjects; the addition of oxprenolol reversed the enhancement. This might be due to an alpha-blocking effect of oxprenolol, to a beta-agonist effect, or to a membrane-stabilising effect.— J. O'Grady *et al.*, *Eur. J. clin. Pharmac.*, 1978, *14*, 83.

Absorption and Fate. Oxprenolol is almost completely absorbed from the gastro-intestinal tract but is subject to considerable first-pass metabolism. Peak plasma concentrations occur about 1 or 2 hours after a dose. It is metabolised in the liver and almost entirely excreted in the urine; at least one of its metabolites may be biologically active. The biological half-life of oxprenolol is longer than would be anticipated from its plasma half-life of about 1.5 to 2 hours; a longer terminal half-life has also been detected. Oxprenolol diffuses across the placenta. It also crosses the blood-brain barrier.

In 7 healthy subjects given 40, 80, or 160 mg of oxprenolol the plasma half-life was approximately 80 minutes, irrespective of the dose administered.— L. Brunner *et al.*, *Eur. J. clin. Pharmac.*, 1975, *8*, 3. Following intravenous administration of oxprenolol to 6 healthy subjects a triexponential decrease in plasma concentration was noted. An initial half-life of 5 minutes, corresponding to the initial rapid-distribution phase, was followed by an intermediate half-life of about an hour; a third half-life of 4.5 hours was considered to reflect slow release from storage depots in the body. Following administration by mouth less than 30% reached the systemic circulation owing to metabolism by the liver and gut during the absorption process.— M. J. Kendall *et al.*, *Eur. J. Drug Metab. Pharmacokinet.*, 1976, *1*, 155.

Further references: C. P. Dawes *et al.*, *Br. J. clin. Pharmac.*, 1978, *5*, 217 (salivary concentrations).

Diffusion into the CSF. A study in *animals* on the central uptake of beta-adrenoceptor blocking agents, including oxprenolol.— M. D. Day *et al.*, *J. Pharm. Pharmac.*, 1977, *29*, *Suppl.*, 52P.

First-pass effect. A study in 6 healthy subjects suggesting significant pharmacokinetic differences between oxprenolol, and propranolol and other beta-adrenoceptor blocking agents. Following administration of oxprenolol by mouth peak plasma concentrations were reached after 30 to 90 minutes with wide variation in bioavailability, and the plasma half-life was about 1.94 hours; unlike propranolol the plasma half-life was not significantly different following intravenous administration, being about 2.3 hours. The first-pass effect of oxprenolol appeared to differ from that of propranolol.— W. D. Mason and N. Winer, *Clin. Pharmac. Ther.*, 1976, *20*, 401.

Metabolites. In 6 healthy volunteers oxprenolol 100 to 200 µg per kg body-weight intravenously had no effect on heart-rate, but doses of 40 to 80 mg by mouth significantly reduced the heart-rate, the effect being most evident 4 hours after a dose; this could represent the formation of an active metabolite.— A. Hedges and P. Turner (letter), *Br. med. J.*, 1973, *1*, 422.

Further references: G. A. Leeson *et al.*, *Drug Metab. & Disposit.*, 1973, *1*, 565; W. Riess *et al.*, *Xenobiotica*, 1974, *4*, 365.

Sustained-release preparations. Results of a study on 6 healthy subjects showed that oxprenolol 160 mg in a slow-release formulation produced peak plasma concentrations comparable with those of conventional oxprenolol 80 mg almost as quickly. High concentrations persisted longer with the slow-release formulation which reduced exercise-induced tachycardia for at least 14 hours compared with 8 hours for conventional oxprenolol.— M. J. West *et al.*, *Br. J. clin. Pharmac.*, 1976, *3*, 439.

Further references: C. Davidson *et al.*, *Eur. J. clin. Pharmac.*, 1976, *10*, 189; F. R. Bühler *et al.*, *Aust. N.Z. J. Med.*, 1976, *6*, *Suppl.* 3, 37; K. P. O'Brien *et al.*, *N.Z. med. J.*, 1976, *84*, 142; A. Bobik *et al.*, *Br. J. clin. Pharmac.*, 1979, *7*, 545.

Uses. Oxprenolol hydrochloride is a beta-adrenoceptor blocking agent (see p.1324) with uses similar to those of propranolol (see p.1329). It is classified as non-cardioselective.

In the treatment of hypertension oxprenolol hydrochloride is usually given initially in a dosage of 160 mg daily in 2 divided doses, increased at weekly or fortnightly intervals. In conjunction with diuretic therapy a dosage of 80 to 320 mg is usually adequate; when given alone a dose of 480 mg daily should not be exceeded.

The usual dose for angina pectoris is 120 to 480 mg daily in 3 divided doses. For cardiac arrhythmias the usual dose is 60 to 120 mg daily in 3 divided doses, increased if necessary according to the patient's response.

For the emergency treatment of cardiac arrhythmias oxprenolol hydrochloride may be given by slow intravenous injection in a dose of 2 mg repeated if necessary after 5 minutes. In resistant atrial arrhythmias a maximum cumulative dose of 16 mg may be given by slow intravenous injection. It can also be given by the intramuscular route.

A dose of 40 to 120 mg daily in 2 or 3 divided doses has been suggested for hyperthyroidism.

Action. A general review of oxprenolol and comparisons with propranolol and practolol.— C. F. George, *Prescribers' J.*, 1974, *14*, 93.

Studies of the effects of oxprenolol: T. Grandjean and J. -L. Rivier, *Br. Heart J.*, 1968, *30*, 50; G. B. Porro and A. T. Maiolo (letter), *Lancet*, 1968, *1*, 690; D. Bürgin, *Schweiz. med. Wschr.*, 1968, *98*, 940; J. -L. Rivier *et al.*, *Postgrad. med. J.*, 1970, (Nov.), *Suppl.*, 44; B. N. Singh *et al.*, *Am. J. Cardiol.*, 1971, *27*, 372; O. Ponari *et al.*, *Arzneimittel-Forsch.*, 1972, *22*, 629; A. C. Asmal *et al.*, *Postgrad. med. J.*, 1975, *51*, 173; D. N. W. Griffith *et al.*, *Br. J. clin. Pharmac.*, 1979, *7*, 491.

Administration in hepatic failure. The response to oxprenolol, which was metabolised by the liver, was altered in the presence of hepatic disease.— G. L. Sanders, *Adverse Drug React. Bull.*, 1978, Feb., 240.

Anxiety. In a 3-week double-blind trial in 29 patients with anxiety states, diazepam 15 to 35 mg daily was more effective and reduced symptoms more rapidly than oxprenolol 240 to 480 mg daily. Oxprenolol took 2 to 3 weeks to become effective.— G. Johnson *et al.*, *Med. J. Aust.*, 1976, *1*, 909.

A single dose of oxprenolol 40 mg taken 90 minutes before a concert performance significantly reduced anxiety with a significant improvement in musical performance in a double-blind crossover study of 24 musicians. Oxprenolol caused a significant reduction in pulse-rate and a slight fall in systolic blood pressure.— I. M. James *et al.*, *Lancet*, 1977, *2*, 952. Administration of oxprenolol 40 mg to 8 surgeons 1 hour before operations reduced their average heart-rate from 121 beats per minute to an average of 84 beats per minute.— G. E. Foster *et al.*, *ibid.*, 1978, *1*, 1323.

Further reports: P. R. Imhof *et al.*, *J. appl. Physiol.*, 1969, *27*, 366; P. Taggart and M. Carruthers (preliminary communication), *Lancet*, 1972, *2*, 256; W. P. McMillin (letter), *ibid.*, 1973, *1*, 1193; P. Taggart *et al.*, *ibid.*, 1973, *2*, 341; S. H. Taylor and M. K. Meeran, *Br. med. J.*, 1973, *4*, 257; W. P. McMillin, *Am. J. Psychiat.*, 1975, *132*, 965; G. Krishnan, *Curr. med. Res. Opinion*, 1976, *4*, 241; L. Siitonen and J. Jänne, *Ann. clin. Res.*, 1976, *8*, 393; S. Lehrl *et al.*, *Arzneimittel-Forsch.*, 1977, *27*, 429; L. C. Antal and C. S. Good, *Practitioner*, 1980, *224*, 755.

Cardiac disorders. *Angina pectoris.* The comparable

effectiveness of single intravenous or oral doses of propranolol, oxprenolol, and practolol under controlled conditions in 16 men with angina pectoris with ECG evidence of cardiac ischaemia, but without other complications.— U. Thadani *et al.*, *Br. med. J.*, 1973, *1*, 138. Further comparisons with propranolol: A. Pitt and S. T. Anderson, *Med. J. Aust.*, 1970, *1*, 1089; B. Sharma *et al.*, *Br. med. J.*, 1971, *3*, 152.

In a double-blind study in 18 patients oxprenolol 160 mg daily as a sustained-release tablet was as effective as propranolol 40 mg thrice daily in controlling the symptoms of angina pectoris.— P. A. Majid *et al.*, *J. int. med. Res.*, 1979, *7*, 194.

Further references to the sustained-release preparation of oxprenolol in angina pectoris: W. A. Forrest, *Br. J. clin. Pract.*, 1975, *29*, 343; P. W. Goldshaw *et al.*, *Br. J. clin. Pharmac.*, 1977, *4*, 387P; W. A. Forrest, *Curr. med. Res. Opinion*, 1978, *5*, 669.

Further references to oxprenolol in angina pectoris: G. E. Bauer and G. Michell, *Med. J. Aust.*, 1970, *1*, 170; B. Sharma *et al.*, *Postgrad. med. J.*, 1970, (Nov.), *Suppl.*, 72; W. A. Forrest, *Br. J. clin. Pract.*, 1972, *26*, 217; *idem*, *Practitioner*, 1972, *208*, 412; B. S. Lewis *et al.*, *S. Afr. med. J.*, 1972, *46*, 1209; J. Pilcher, *Postgrad. med. J.*, 1978, *54*, 663.

Cardiac arrhythmias. In 41 patients with cardiac disease treated with digitalis, diuretics, quinidine, and anticoagulants, oxprenolol, 40 to 240 mg daily, had a beneficial effect in sinus tachycardia (especially associated with emotion), paroxysmal supraventricular tachycardia, and established atrial fibrillation. In conjunction with quinidine, it effectively prevented recurrences of paroxysmal atrial fibrillation or prevented its return after counter-current. There was little effect on extrasystoles whatever the origin.— L. Scebat and J. Bensaid, *Postgrad. med. J.*, 1970, (Nov.), *Suppl.*, 86.

Myocardial infarction. Oxprenolol was used to treat 63 episodes of cardiac arrhythmias in 43 patients with acute myocardial infarction or ischaemia. Single intravenous injections were given, initially in a dose of 2 mg followed after 10 minutes by a further 4 mg and then 6 mg if the previous dose was not effective. The effects of continuous infusions of oxprenolol in a dose of 250 µg per minute were also studied. Oxprenolol successfully suppressed ventricular ectopic beats in 13 of 18 episodes and satisfactorily controlled 13 of 27 episodes of supraventricular tachycardia. It was less effective in suppressing other supraventricular arrhythmias. The most effective methods of administration were continuous intravenous infusion followed by the single intravenous injection of 6 mg. Hypotension occurred in more than 50% of patients, and oxprenolol should be given with caution to patients with low blood pressure and to patients with ventricular tachycardia.— G. Sandler and A. C. Pistevos, *Br. med. J.*, 1971, *1*, 254.

For a study suggesting that early administration of oxprenolol may not influence mortality in myocardial infarction, see Disopyramide, p.1378.

Electroconvulsive therapy. After administration of oxprenolol there was significant reduction in the mean pulse-rate before electroconvulsive therapy, after administration of the anaesthetic, and after the convulsion.— S. M. Cannicott (letter), *Br. med. J.*, 1974, *3*, 579.

Hypertension. In a clinical trial, 2211 patients aged between 25 and 65 years suffering from mild to moderate hypertension received 2 tablets each containing cyclopenthiazide 250 µg and potassium chloride 600 mg (Navidrex K) each morning and oxprenolol 80 mg twice daily, increasing fortnightly to a maximum of 480 mg daily, until control of blood pressure was achieved. Control was not achieved in 186 patients, while 89 were withdrawn because of severity of side-effects. Headache, dizziness, depression, and sleep disturbances were the most common side-effects and occurred in 264 patients. Other side-effects included gastro-intestinal disturbance in 62 patients, cardiovascular effects in 8, bronchospasm in 5, and skin rash in 4.— W. A. Forrest, *Ciba*, *Br. J. clin. Pract.*, 1973, *27*, 331. In a clinical trial in 17 patients with moderate hypertension (diastolic pressure 105 to 140 mmHg), oxprenolol 0.16 to 1.28 g daily was required to control blood pressure. One patient withdrew because of palpitations and 1 taking oxprenolol 160 mg daily complained of depression and exacerbation of duodenal ulcer pain.— A. J. Marshall and D. W. Barritt, *ibid.*, 337.

In a double-blind crossover study in 24 patients with hypertension 11 were satisfactorily controlled on oxprenolol 160 or 320 mg daily and 13 were given 480 to 960 mg daily; 11 were satisfactorily controlled on methyldopa up to 1 g daily and 13 received up to 3 g daily. There was no significant difference between the 2 treatments. It was considered that failure to respond to 320 mg or 1 g daily respectively indicated a need to add an additional antihypertensive agent.— D. W. Barritt *et al.*, *Lancet*, 1976, *1*, 503.

Further references: S. Dorph and C. Binder, *Acta med. scand.*, 1969, *185*, 443; A. Eisalo *et al.*, *Acta med. scand.*, 1969, *186*, 105; A. W. D. Leishman *et al.*, *Br. med. J.*, 1970, *4*, 342; J. D. Fitzgerald, *I.C.I.* (letter), *ibid.*, 747; J. C. M. Wilkinson (letter), *ibid.*, 802; P. A. Majid *et al.*, *Postgrad. med. J.*, 1970, (Nov.), *Suppl.*, 67; M. Motolese *et al.*, *Eur. J. clin. Pharmac.*, 1975, *8*, 21; B. J. Materson *et al.*, *Clin. Pharmac. Ther.*, 1976, *20*, 142; D. W. Barritt and A. J. Marshall, *Br. Heart J.*, 1977, *39*, 825; A. F. B. Mebadeje, *Curr. ther. Res.*, 1977, *22*, 391; G. Rowlands *et al.*, *Practitioner*, 1977, *219*, 105; W. A. Forrest, *Br. J. clin. Pract.*, 1978, *32*, 326; I. B. Davies *et al.*, *Br. J. clin. Pharmac.*, 1979, *8*, 49; S. Kalowski *et al.*, *Med. J. Aust.*, 1979, *2*, 439; J. Tuomilehto and A. Nissinen, *Eur. J. clin. Pharmac.*, 1979, *16*, 369; M. Bergström *et al.*, *Curr. ther. Res.*, 1980, *27*, 805; G. Frithz and B. Wernersson, *ibid.*, 22; A. J. Marshall *et al.*, *Br. J. clin. Pharmac.*, 1980, *10*, 217.

Effect on plasma renin. Oxprenolol and plasma renin.— R. Davies *et al.*, *Am. J. Cardiol.*, 1976, *37*, 637; L. Siitonen, *J. int. med. Res.*, 1980, *8*, 181.

Once- and twice-daily administration. In a study completed by 15 hypertensive patients satisfactory control of blood pressure was obtained with a twice-daily dosage regimen of oxprenolol (together with diuretic therapy) despite its relatively short half-life.— B. J. Materson *et al.*, *Clin. Pharmac. Ther.*, 1976, *19*, 325.

Oxprenolol as a single daily dose of a sustained-release preparation was effective in controlling blood pressure in hypertensive patients.— G. N. Volans *et al.* (letter), *Br. J. clin. Pharmac.*, 1979, *8*, 86.

A double-blind crossover study involving 23 hypertensive patients compared the effects of atenolol 100 mg once daily, sustained-release oxprenolol 160 mg once daily, and long-acting propranolol 160 mg once daily. The findings confirmed the effectiveness of atenolol and the long-acting propranolol formulation and showed them to be superior to sustained-release oxprenolol in lowering blood pressure over 24 hours. It was suggested that the present formulation of sustained-release oxprenolol may need to be reconsidered.— J. C. Petrie *et al.*, *Br. med. J.*, 1980, *280*, 1573.

Further references: C. Davidson *et al.*, *Eur. J. clin. Pharmac.*, 1976, *10*, 189; W. A. Forrest, *Br. J. clin. Pract.*, 1977, *31*, 181; R. Buoninconti *et al.*, *J. int. med. Res.*, 1979, *7*, 519; W. A. Forrest, *Br. J. clin. Pract.*, 1980, *34*, 140; *idem*, *Curr. med. Res. Opinion*, 1980, *6*, 559; *idem*, *J. int. med. Res.*, 1980, *8*, 127.

Hyperthyroidism. In a controlled double-blind crossover study of 16 patients with moderately severe thyrotoxicosis, oxprenolol 40 mg every 8 hours for 1 week was no better than placebo. The probable explanation for the failure was that oxprenolol had some inherent sympathomimetic activity.— M. G. Gibberd and J. S. Staffurth (letter), *Lancet*, 1973, *1*, 205.

Migraine. In a double-blind crossover study, oxprenolol 80 mg thrice daily for 8 weeks was ineffective in the prevention of migraine in 30 patients.— K. Ekbom and M. Zetterman, *Acta neurol. scand.*, 1977, *56*, 181.

Parkinsonism. A report of 2 elderly patients whose parkinsonism improved when they were given oxprenolol 40 mg thrice daily for angina pectoris.— M. K. Thompson (letter), *Lancet*, 1972, *2*, 388.

Oxprenolol was of no value in patients with parkinsonism who were already receiving maximum tolerated doses of levodopa.— L. E. Claveria *et al.*, *J. clin. Pharmac.*, 1975, *15*, 66. A similar report.— M. Sandler *et al.* (letter), *Lancet*, 1975, *1*, 168.

Pregnancy and the neonate. *Hypertension in pregnancy.* In a randomised study in 53 women with hypertension of pregnancy 26 were treated with oxprenolol and 27 with methyldopa in doses designed to reduce sitting diastolic blood pressure to or below 80 mmHg; hydralazine was added when necessary. Those given oxprenolol had greater plasma volume expansion, with improved placental weight and birth weight. Blood-glucose concentrations in the infants in the oxprenolol group were significantly higher than in the methyldopa group. Oxprenolol appeared to have advantages over methyldopa.— E. D. M. Gallery *et al.*, *Br. med. J.*, 1979, *1*, 1591.

Preparations

Oxprenolol Tablets *(B.P.)*. Tablets containing oxprenolol hydrochloride. They are film-coated.

Proprietary Preparations

Apsolox *(Approved Prescription Services, UK)*. Oxprenolol hydrochloride, available as tablets of 20, 40, 80, and 160 mg.

Slow-Trasicor *(Ciba, UK)*. Oxprenolol hydrochloride, available as sustained-release tablets of 160 mg. *Dose.* Initially 1 tablet in the morning, increased to 2 or 3 if necessary. (Also available as Slow-Trasicor in *S.Afr.*, *Switz.*).

Trasicor *(Ciba, UK)*. Oxprenolol hydrochloride, available as **Injection** (supplied as powder for solution before use) in ampoules of 2 mg and as **Tablets** of 20, 40, 80, and 160 mg. (Also available as Trasicor in *Arg.*, *Austral.*, *Belg.*, *Denm.*, *Fr.*, *Ger.*, *Ital.*, *Neth.*, *Norw.*, *S.Afr.*, *Spain*, *Switz.*).

Trasidrex *(Ciba, UK)*. Tablets each containing, in a sustained-release core, oxprenolol hydrochloride 160 mg and, in an outer layer, cyclopenthiazide 250 µg. For hypertension. *Dose.* Usually, 1 or 2 tablets daily.

Other Proprietary Names

Oxanol *(Spain)*; Trasacor *(Jap.)*.

6318-z

Penbutolol. 39893d; Hoe 893d. (−)-(*S*)-1-*tert*-Butylamino-3-(2-cyclopentylphenoxy)propan-2-ol.
$C_{18}H_{29}NO_2$=291.4.

CAS — 38363-40-5 (−); 38363-41-6 (+); 61914-98-5 (±).

Adverse Effects, Treatment, and Precautions. As for Propranolol Hydrochloride, p.1325.

Diabetes mellitus. During treatment of 7 hypertensive patients with penbutolol 20 to 30 mg twice daily for 3 to 8 months there was no evidence that insulin production was decreased.— B. -G. Hansson and B. Hökfelt, *Eur. J. clin. Pharmac.*, 1976, *10*, 157.

Absorption and Fate. Penbutolol is readily absorbed from the gastro-intestinal tract and peak plasma concentrations occur about 1 or 2 hours after a dose. It is extensively metabolised, the metabolites being excreted in the urine together with only small amounts of unchanged penbutolol; several of its metabilites are believed to be biologically active. The biological half-life of penbutolol is longer than would be anticipated from estimations of its plasma half-life, and a biphasic plasma half-life has been reported.

The beta-adrenoceptor blocking effects of penbutolol 20 mg were compared with those of propranolol 80 mg in a double-blind trial involving 6 healthy subjects. Penbutolol differed from propranolol in that it did not lower resting heart-rates during the 2 hours following its administration, and did not reduce systolic blood pressure at rest. The peak plasma concentration of penbutolol occurred 1 hour after oral administration and its half-life was 4.5 hours. Peak biological activity occurred at 2 hours. This might be due to an active metabolite.— J. F. Giudicelli *et al.*, *Br. J. clin. Pharmac.*, 1977, *4*, 135.

In 8 healthy subjects penbutolol 50 mg by mouth was rapidly absorbed, producing a mean peak serum concentration of 770 ng per ml after about 1 hour. The mean plasma half-lives of the fast and slow phases were 2.5 and 27 hours respectively. The apparent elimination half-life was about 27 hours, suggesting that less frequent doses would be required, compared to other beta-adrenoceptor blocking agents. About 3% of the dose was recovered unchanged from the urine over 72 hours in 7 subjects, and 9.8% in the eighth, suggesting extensive metabolism.— J. J. Vallner *et al.*, *J. clin. Pharmac.*, 1977, *17*, 231.

Further references: H. W. Jun *et al.*, *J. clin. Pharmac.*, 1979, *19*, 415; S. D. Sharma *et al.*, *Curr. ther. Res.*, 1980, *27*, 576.

Uses. Penbutolol is a beta-adrenoceptor blocking agent (see p.1324) with general properties similar to those of propranolol (see p.1329). It is classified as non-cardioselective. Penbutolol has been given as the sulphate in the treatment of hypertension and angina pectoris in an initial dose of 20 mg once daily, increased to 40 mg once or twice daily if necessary.

Action. A review of the pharmacological properties of penbutolol and its therapeutic efficacy in hypertension and angina pectoris.— R. C. Heel *et al.*, *Drugs*, 1981, *22*, 1.

Reports and studies on the pharmacology of penbutolol: R. D. Kulkarni *et al.*, *Clin. Pharmac. Ther.*, 1977, *21*, 685; P. L. Sharma and R. P. Sapru, *Int. J. clin. Pharmac. Biopharm.*, 1978, *16*, 83; *idem*, 98; G. Nyberg *et al.*, *Eur. J. clin. Pharmac.*, 1979, *16*, 381.

Cardiac disorders. *Angina pectoris.* Penbutolol 300 µg given intravenously to 6 male patients, 3 of them with mild angina pectoris, had a significant negative inotropic effect similar to that seen when propranolol 10 mg was given intravenously to 6 similar patients.— R. P. Sapru and P. L. Sharma, *Br. J. clin. Pharmac.*, 1978, *6*, 515.

Further references: J. V. Shivde and S. S. Zadgaonkar, *Curr. ther. Res.*, 1977, *22*, 501; Westheim A.S. *et al.*, *Eur. J. clin. Pharmac.*, 1978, *13*, 157.

Cardiac arrhythmias. Penbutolol was given to 28 patients with cardiac arrhythmias in an initial dose of 4 mg thrice daily, increased to a maximum of 49 mg daily if required. Ventricular arrhythmias were abolished in 14 of 21 patients, and controlled in a further 3; 2 patients were withdrawn due to side-effects including giddiness, flushing, and anorexia, and bradycardia in 1 patient. The remaining 2 did not respond. All 7 patients with supraventricular arrhythmias responded, with complete abolition in 5 and satisfactory control in 2.— P. S. Gupta and L. Thaly, *Curr. ther. Res.*, 1977, *21*, 638.

Hypertension. In a single-blind placebo-controlled crossover study penbutolol 25 to 100 mg daily for 9 weeks reduced supine diastolic pressure to less than 90 mmHg in 7 of 9 patients with essential hypertension.— V. H. Yajnik *et al.*, *J. int. med. Res.*, 1977, *5*, 236.

Further references: A. J. Coleman, *Curr. ther. Res.*, 1974, *16*, 64; B. -G. Hansson and B. Hökfelt, *Eur. J. clin. Pharmac.*, 1975, *9*, 9; *idem*, 1976, *9*, 245.

Once-daily administration. In a double-blind crossover study in 10 hypertensive patients, penbutolol 80 mg once daily significantly reduced supine and standing blood pressure and was more potent than hydrochlorothiazide 100 mg once daily. Blood pressure was still reduced 24 hours after a dose.— J. F. De Plaen *et al.*, *Br. J. clin. Pharmac.*, 1981, *12*, 215.

Further references: F. O. Müller *et al.*, *Clin. Pharmac. Ther.*, 1979, *25*, 528; M. M. Kubik and G. W. Hanks, *Eur. J. clin. Pharmac.*, 1980, *17*, 409.

Proprietary Names of Penbutolol Sulphate

Betapressin *(Hoechst, Ger.)*.

6319-c

Pindolol *(B.P.)*. LB46; Prindolol; Prinodolol.

1-(Indol-4-yloxy)-3-isopropylaminopropan-2-ol.

$C_{14}H_{20}N_2O_2=248.3$.

CAS — 13523-86-9; 68374-35-6 (+); 26328-11-0 (−); 21870-06-4 (±).

Pharmacopoeias. In *Br.*

A white or almost white, odourless or almost odourless, crystalline powder. Practically **insoluble** in water; slightly soluble in dehydrated alcohol and chloroform; sparingly soluble in methyl alcohol. **Protect** from light.

Adverse Effects, Treatment, and Precautions. As for Propranolol Hydrochloride, p.1325.

Allergy. A report of an allergic skin eruption in a patient taking pindolol; the patient was also taking digoxin and theophylline.— J. Beyreder and G. Brandstetter, *Wien. med. Wschr.*, 1973, *123*, 76, per *Int. pharm. Abstr.*, 1974, *11*, 54.

Effects on mental state. A report of a double-blind placebo-controlled crossover study of pindolol completed by 13 patients. Headaches, lethargy, and depression were associated with pindolol in 2 of the patients; 3 patients complained of bizarre dreams, which became less frequent with time.— L. J. Day *et al.*, *Practitioner*, 1977, *219*, 889.

Effects on the muscles. Administration of pindolol was associated with a high incidence of leg muscle fatigue.— S. Zetterquist *et al.*, *Curr. ther. Res.*, 1975, *17*, 139.

Fine tremor in the extremities of 5 patients during pindolol therapy was considered to have been due to its partial agonist activity.— H. Hod *et al.*, *Postgrad. med. J.*, 1980, *56*, 346.

Restless leg syndrome. A report of 1 patient in whom the restless leg syndrome occurred after commencing therapy with pindolol.— L. K. Morgan (letter), *Med. J. Aust.*, 1975, *2*, 753.

Effects on respiratory function. In 4 patients recovering from exacerbation of asthma pindolol, 200 µg intravenously or 15 mg by mouth, caused chest tightness and there was objective evidence of airways obstruction unresponsive to sympathomimetic aerosols.— K. Mattson and H. Poppius, *Eur. J. clin. Pharmac.*, 1978, *14*, 87.

Effects on the respiratory tract. A report of pulmonary fibrosis in a 55-year-old man who had taken pindolol for 7 years.— A. W. Musk and J. A. Pollard, *Br. med. J.*, 1979, *2*, 581. Comment.— P. Krupp and J. M. Crawford (letter), *ibid.*, 939.

Hypertension. Paradoxically, high doses of pindolol could cause hypertension. In 9 patients taking a mean of 48 mg daily diastolic and systolic pressure, lying and standing, was significantly higher than when taking a mean of 19 mg daily.— H. J. Waal-Manning and F. O. Simpson (letter), *Br. med. J.*, 1975, *3*, 155. There was no evidence of a paradoxical rise of blood pressure in 24 patients with essential hypertension who received pindolol in increasing doses up to 45 mg per day.— O. H. Koldsland, *Curr. ther. Res.*, 1977, *22*, 853.

For comments on paradoxical hypertension associated with administration of beta-adrenoceptor blocking agents, see Propranolol, p.1326.

Hypoglycaemia. Severe hypoglycaemia during haemodialysis occurred after 18 hours of fasting, in a 34-year-old man taking pindolol. The addition of dextrose to the dialysis fluid was recommended.— K. Samii *et al.* (letter), *Lancet*, 1976, *1*, 545.

Lupus erythematosus. A report of systemic lupus erythematosus associated with the use of pindolol.— J. Bensaid *et al.*, *Br. med. J.*, 1979, *1*, 1603.

Absorption and Fate. Pindolol is almost completely absorbed from the gastro-intestinal tract and peak plasma concentrations are obtained about 2 hours after a dose. It is only partially metabolised and is excreted in the urine both unchanged and in the form of metabolites. The biological half-life of pindolol is longer than would be anticipated from its plasma half-life of 3 or 4 hours. It is reported to be about 57% bound to plasma proteins.

A comparative review of the pharmacokinetics of pindolol and those of other beta-adrenoceptor blocking agents.— J. Meier, *Acta med. scand.*, 1977, *Suppl.*, 65.

The plasma half-life of pindolol after administration to healthy subjects by mouth was about 3.5 hours and after intravenous administration about 3 hours; the difference was not significant. About 57% was bound to plasma proteins.— R. Gugler *et al.*, *Eur. J. clin. Pharmac.*, 1974, *7*, 17.

A study in 12 hypertensive African patients indicated that the pharmacokinetics of pindolol in Africans are not dissimilar from published data on other races.— L. A. Salako *et al.*, *Eur. J. clin. Pharmac.*, 1979, *15*, 299.

Further references: R. Gugler *et al.*, *Clin. Pharmac. Ther.*, 1975, *17*, 127; Y. Weiss *et al.*, *Nouv. Presse méd.*, 1977, *6*, 927; P. Dayer *et al.*, *J. clin. Pharm.*, 1979, *4*, 87; M. Guerret *et al.*, *J. pharm. Sci.*, 1980, *69*, 1191.

Diffusion into the CSF. CSF/plasma ratios of propranolol and pindolol.— E. A. Taylor *et al.*, *Br. J. clin. Pharmac.*, 1979, *8*, 381P.

First-pass effect. A review of studies on 57 subjects indicated that the systemic bioavailability of pindolol is at least 87%. It may be concluded that in man the first-pass effect of pindolol is so low as to be negligible.— J. Meier and E. Nüesch (letter), *Br. J. clin. Pharmac.*, 1977, *4*, 371.

Uses. Pindolol is a beta-adrenoceptor blocking agent (see p.1324) with uses similar to those of propranolol (see p.1329). It is classified as non-cardioselective.

In the treatment of hypertension pindolol is usually given initially in a dosage of 5 mg twice or thrice daily, increased at weekly intervals to 45 mg daily in 2 or 3 divided doses according to the patient's response; additional benefit is rarely obtained from doses higher than 45 mg daily. A once-daily dosage regimen has been reported to be adequate for many patients. The usual dose for angina pectoris is 2.5 to 5 mg up to thrice daily.

Action. Reports and studies on the pharmacology of pindolol: J. -L. Rivier *et al.*, *Thérapie*, 1970, *25*, 245; F. C. Hugues *et al.*, *ibid.*, 1976, *31*, 179; W. H. Aellig, *Eur. J. clin. Pharmac.*, 1978, *14*, 305; M. K. Benson *et al.*, *Br. J. clin. Pharmac.*, 1978, *5*, 415; H. H. Harms *et al.*, *ibid.*, 19.

Administration in renal failure. Following administration of pindolol 40 µg per kg body-weight intravenously to 18 hypertensive patients, 9 in chronic renal failure exhibited decreased total-body and renal clearance of pindolol compared with 9 patients with normal renal function. Transfer rate-constants, distribution volumes, and non-renal clearance did not differ significantly between the 2 groups. After a single dose of pindolol 10 mg by mouth it was found that the patients with renal failure, compared with the patients with normal renal activity, effectively absorbed a decreased fraction of the dose, with increased initial rate of absorption being inversely correlated with creatinine clearance.— N. P. Chau *et al.*, *Clin. Pharmac. Ther.*, 1977, *22*, 505.

A comparative study of the pharmacokinetics of pindolol in subjects with essential hypertension suggested that when patients also had impaired renal function, the absorption of pindolol was decreased. No evidence was found for increased metabolism of pindolol in patients with reduced renal function.— D. Lavene *et al.*, *J. clin. Pharmac.*, 1977, *17*, 501.

Further references: E. E. Ohnhaus *et al.*, *Eur. J. clin. Pharmac.*, 1974, *7*, 25; A. Snell and M. Wallace (letter), *Br. med. J.*, 1974, *2*, 672; C. Heierli *et al.*, *Int. J. clin. Pharmac. Biopharm.*, 1977, *15*, 65.

Administration in respiratory insufficiency. In a study in 56 patients with chronic obstructive lung disease, the bronchial effects of single oral doses of pindolol (2.5 to 15 mg) and practolol (100 to 300 mg) were not significantly different. After intravenous administration bronchoconstriction after practolol was less pronounced than that after pindolol, but the difference was regarded as being of little clinical importance.— S. Gavrilescu and M. Pantzer, *Curr. ther. Res.*, 1978, *24*, 761.

See also under Precautions.

Anxiety. The changes in the EEG after pindolol 5 mg were similar to those produced by imipramine. Pindolol might be of use in treatment of somatic anxiety and anxiety with depression.— J. Roubicek (letter), *Br. J. clin. Pharmac.*, 1976, *3*, 661.

Cardiac disorders. *Angina pectoris.* In 12 healthy men pindolol 15 mg reduced exercise-induced tachycardia by a mean maximum of 36 beats per minute; about 40% of its activity remained 24 hours after the dose. Pindolol should be suitable for once-daily dosage in angina pectoris.— W. H. Aellig, *Eur. J. clin. Pharmac.*, 1978, *14*, 167.

Further references: P. D. Nigam and A. S. Malhotra (letter), *Br. med. J.*, 1973, *1*, 742; W. H. Aellig and K. Saameli, *Sandoz, Switz.* (letter), *ibid.*, 1973, *2*, 365; S. Zetterquist *et al.*, *Curr. ther. Res.*, 1975, *17*, 139.

Cardiac arrhythmias. Pindolol 200 to 400 µg given intravenously for 1 to 3 doses to 30 patients with cardiac arrhythmias slowed the ventricular rate within 2 hours in 13 of 14 patients with atrial fibrillation or flutter and converted 4 of these patients and 4 others with tachycardia to sinus rhythm. Premature ventricular beats of 6 or more per minute were abolished or reduced in 10 of 14 patients and premature atrial beats of 6 or more per minute were abolished in all of 3 patients.— W. S. Aronow and R. R. Uyeyama, *Clin. Pharmac. Ther.*, 1972, *13*, 15.

Glaucoma. Pindolol 1% eye-drops significantly lowered intra-ocular pressure in normal and glaucomatous eyes and were well tolerated. There was an increase in outflow facility when treatment was continued for about 1 month.— L. Bonomi and P. Steindler, *Br. J. Ophthal.*, 1975, *59*, 301.

Further references: S. E. Smith *et al.*, *Br. J. Ophthal.*, 1979, *63*, 63.

Hypertension. In the short term the plasma concentration of pindolol was the most important factor determining its antihypertensive effect; but in the long term the initial elevation of blood pressure above normal was the most important factor.— Y. A. Weiss *et al.*, *Curr. ther. Res.*, 1977, *21*, 644.

In a multicentre study, 7062 hypertensive patients aged between 12 and 89 years were treated with pindolol 7.5 to 45 mg daily, 91.6% of the patients initially receiving 15 mg as a single daily dose, for 3 to 9 weeks. Treatment was considered to be effective in 75% of the 5989 patients assessed, and satisfactory in a further 12%. Treatment was discontinued in 53 patients because of lack of effect, and 1822 (25.8%) of the patients reported side-effects which were severe enough to cause discontinuation of treatment in 507 (7.2%) patients. The most common side-effects were dizziness (8.1%), gastro-intestinal complaints (7.1%), headache (4.9%), insomnia (3.5%), lassitude (3.0%), and subjective cardiac complaints (2.6%).— J. Rosenthal *et al.*, *Br. J. clin. Pract.*, 1979, *33*, 165.

Further references: P. Bjerle *et al.* (letter), *Br. med. J.*, 1975, *4*, 284; H. J. Waal-Manning and A. J. Wood, *Med. J. Aust.*, 1975, *2*, 274; A. J. Blowers and M. A. Melvin, *Curr. med. Res. Opinion*, 1976, *4*, 368; J. P. Chalmers *et al.*, *Med. J. Aust.*, 1976, *1*, 650; R. C. Dhatariya, *Practitioner*, 1977, *218*, 570; I. Persson, *Eur.*

J. clin. Pharmac., 1977, *11*, 419; A. H. J. Hintzen *et al.*, *J. int. med. Res.*, 1978, *6*, 213; G. Nyberg *et al.*, *Lancet*, 1982, *1*, 355.

Effect on plasma renin. No correlation was found between changes in plasma-renin activity and changes in blood pressure in 26 hypertensive patients given pindolol 15 mg thrice daily.— R. Lancaster *et al.*, *Br. J. clin. Pharmac.*, 1976, *3*, 453.

Further references: S. Sonkodi *et al.*, *Therapia hung.*, 1976, *24*, 60.

Once-daily administration. In a double-blind study in 20 patients with hypertension there were no differences in effect between those given pindolol 5 mg thrice daily and those given 15 mg daily as a single dose.— G. Frithz (letter), *Br. med. J.*, 1978, *1*, 302.

Further references: M. Wilson *et al.*, *Br. J. clin. Pharmac.*, 1976, *3*, 857; Y. M. Traub and J. B. Rosenfeld, *Clin. Pharmac. Ther.*, 1977, *21*, 588.

Hyperthyroidism. Pindolol 15 and 30 mg daily given in a controlled study to 20 patients with hyperthyroidism had no effect on thyroid function. Blood pressure was not reduced but the heart-rate was decreased in a dose-dependent manner.— J. L. Schelling *et al.*, *Clin. Pharmac. Ther.*, 1973, *14*, 158.

Further references: L. Runeberg and K. -E. Kreus, *Acta med. scand.*, 1971, *189*, 423.

Migraine. Of 79 patients given pindolol 2.5 mg four times daily, 12 became free from headaches and 29 found the number of headaches was cut to half or less during the treatment. This compared with 4 headache-free out of 73 patients given clonidine and 1 of 51 patients given carbamazepine. Side-effects occurred in 15 patients on pindolol, causing 8 to abandon treatment. Constant headache, dizziness, nausea, vomiting, paraesthesia, lassitude, and exhaustion were encountered; muscle pains developed during the second and subsequent months of treatment but were relieved in 1 patient by a reduction in the dose.— M. Anthony *et al.*, *Med. J. Aust.*, 1972, *1*, 1343. See also Anthony M. and J. W. Lance, *Drugs*, 1972, *3*, 153.

Orthostatic hypotension. The successful treatment of 3 patients, with severe orthostatic hypotension because of chronic autonomic failure, with pindolol, because of its intrinsic sympathomimetic activity.— A. J. Man in't Veld and M. A. D. H. Schalekamp, *Br. med. J.*, 1981, *282*, 929. No benefit with pindolol in 1 patient.— A. C. Davidson and S. E. Smith (letter), *ibid.*, 1704. See also P. Goldstraw and D. G. Waller (letter), *ibid.*, *283*, 310. Further comments.— A. J. Man in't Veld and M. A. D. H. Schalekamp (letter), *ibid.*, 561; G. Nyberg (letter), *ibid.*, 861. Pindolol was of no benefit in 5 patients with postural hypotension due to autonomic failure associated with multiple system atrophy. In 2 of the patients it produced cardiac failure.— B. Davies *et al.* (letter), *Lancet*, 1981, *2*, 982. Comment.— A. J. Man in't Veld and M. A. D. H. Schalekamp (letter), *ibid.*, 1279.

Preparations

Pindolol Tablets *(B.P.)*. Tablets containing pindolol. Protect from light.

Proprietary Preparations

Viskaldix *(Sandoz, UK)*. Scored tablets each containing pindolol 10 mg and clopamide 5 mg. For hypertension. *Dose.* 1 tablet daily, increased if required to 3 tablets daily.

Visken *(Sandoz, UK)*. Pindolol, available as scored tablets of 5 and 15 mg. (Also available as Visken in *Arg., Austral., Belg., Canad., Denm., Fr., Ger., Ital., Lux., Norw., S.Afr., Spain, Switz.*).

Other Proprietary Names

Carvisken *(Jap.)*; Viskeen *(Neth.)*.

6320-s

Practolol *(B.P.)*. AY 21011; ICI 50172; Practololum. (±)-4′-(2-Hydroxy-3-isopropylaminopropoxy)acetanilide.

$C_{14}H_{22}N_2O_3$=266.3.

CAS — 6673-35-4; 37936-66-6(+); 37936-65-5(−); 23313-50-0(±).

Pharmacopoeias. In *Br.*, *Braz.*, and *Nord.*

A fine, white or almost white, odourless powder with a bitter taste. M.p. 141° to 144°. It absorbs insignificant amounts of moisture at 25° at relative humidities up to about 80%.

Soluble 1 in 400 of water, 1 in 40 of alcohol, and 1 in 200 of chloroform; very soluble in dilute solutions of acetic acid. Solutions are **sterilised** by autoclaving or by filtration. Aqueous solutions are most stable at pH 6. **Protect** from light.

Adverse Effects and Treatment. As for Propranolol Hydrochloride, p.1325.

Serious adverse effects on the skin, eyes, oral and nasal mucous membranes, ears, and peritoneum have been associated with practolol therapy. The changes are associated with immunological disturbances and have rarely occurred with other beta-adrenoceptor blocking agents.

Discussions of the side-effects of practolol.— *Br. med. J.*, 1975, *2*, 577; H. J. Waal-Manning, *Drugs*, 1975, *10*, 336.

By the end of 1974, 187 reports had been received of adverse effects on the eyes of patients who had been treated with practolol for periods of a few weeks to several years. Two-thirds of the reports involved diminished tear secretion and conjunctivitis; the rest involved corneal damage sometimes leading to impairment or loss of vision. There had also been several hundred reports of psoriasiform or hyperkeratotic skin reactions, and 25 complaints of deafness. Fourteen patients had developed a syndrome resembling systemic lupus erythematosus and 8 had developed an unusual form of sclerosing peritonitis. In some patients the adverse reactions were multiple and half the patients with eye changes had a rash; the mild eye changes and most of the skin reactions were reversible on withdrawal of practolol but the damage could be irreversible in the case of corneal involvement. On the basis of reports to the Committee over 10 years it seemed unlikely that similar changes would occur even after prolonged therapy with propranolol but it was too early to comment on other beta-adrenoceptor blocking agents. In addition it had been reported that abrupt cessation of practolol might lead to worsening of angina pectoris and to cardiac arrhythmia.—Committee on Safety of Medicines, *Adverse Reactions Series No. 11*, Jan. 1975.

During 1974 and 1975 ninety-five patients were reported to the Swedish Adverse Drug Reaction Committee as having had an adverse reaction to practolol involving the skin and eyes. Data on 86 of these indicated that 64 had also received at least one other beta-adrenoceptor blocking agent (alprenolol, metoprolol, oxprenolol, pindolol, or propranolol). Analysis of these 64 cases confirmed the impression that serious side-effects of the type induced by practolol were uncommon with other beta-adrenoceptor blocking agents even in patients who were unable to tolerate practolol.— A. -K. Furhoff *et al.* (letter), *Br. med. J.*, 1976, *1*, 831.

Patients who develop typical practolol-induced eye and/or skin reactions were considered to be at high risk of later developing peritonitis and should be carefully monitored. Of 11 patients with induced peritonitis, 9 had such reactions before their first abdominal symptoms and in 8 the time-lag between discontinuing practolol and the onset of these symptoms ranged from 1 to 12 months.— J. E. Idänpään-Heikkilä *et al.* (letter), *Lancet*, 1977, *2*, 1354.

Antibody specific for a practolol metabolite was present in serum from all of 24 patients who had experienced adverse reactions to practolol; it was not present in 10 patients taking other beta-blockers nor in 21 controls; it was present in some of 15 patients who had taken practolol without adverse effect. In 5 patients antibody activity was increased by challenge with practolol and one patient had an adverse reaction. Reactions to practolol might represent a hitherto unknown type of hypersensitivity reaction.— H. E. Amos *et al.*, *Br. med. J.*, 1978, *1*, 402.

Further studies into the cause of the adverse effects associated with practolol therapy: S. J. Jachuck *et al.*, *Postgrad. med. J.*, 1977, *53*, 75; H. M. Dick *et al.*, *Allergy*, 1978, *33*, 71; L. G. Dring *et al.* (letter), *Br. J. clin. Pharmac.*, 1978, *5*, 262.

Effects on the ears. In a search for late-onset side-effects in 31 patients who had taken practolol for at least a month 3 patients were identified with known rashes and one with serious otitis media.— J. Barclay *et al.*, *Br. med. J.*, 1978, *2*, 538.

Further references: R. F. McNab Jones *et al.*, *J. Lar. Otol.*, 1977, *91*, 963.

Effects on the eyes. Twenty-seven patients had been seen with ocular changes relating to the ingestion of practolol. In 19 patients a skin eruption, often psoriasiform, preceded or followed the eye changes; 15 patients had tinnitus or deafness; 3 had gut involvement; and 5 had lesions of the oral or nasal mucosa. The ocular changes, which resulted from gross reduction in tear flow, included keratoconjunctivitis sicca, conjunctival scarring, fibrosis, metaplasia, and shrinkage, and 3 patients had corneal lesions with severe visual loss. Symptoms regressed in most patients when practolol was withdrawn though some degree of reduced tear flow usually persisted. Treatment included rehydration, acetylcysteine 5 or 10% drops for their mucolytic effect, and in some patients dexamethasone 0.1% drops.— P. Wright, *Br. med. J.*, 1975, *1*, 595.

The tear-lysozyme ratio (the ratio of the concentration present to the lower limit of normality) was low in 21 patients who had taken practolol and who had the oculomucocutaneous syndrome (OCMS) and low in 31 who had taken practolol and who had not OCMS. The lysozyme ratio was also low in 5 patients who had taken tolamolol for at least a year. No reduction in lysozyme was found in 23, 26, and 23 patients who had taken respectively timolol, labetalol, and propranolol for at least 6 months, usually longer. Any patient developing a dry eye while taking a beta-adrenoceptor blocking agent should have the tear-lysozyme ratio measured; a low value, indicative of impaired function of the lachrymal gland, might precede clinical signs of adverse ocular reactions, as might high titres of antinuclear antibody and antibodies to the intercellular cement substance.— I. A. Mackie *et al.*, *Br. J. Ophthal.*, 1977, *61*, 354. See also I. A. Mackie and D. V. Seal, *Br. med. J.*, 1975, *4*, 732.

Ocular symptoms were reported by 14 of 71 patients when taking practolol but only by 4 of the 71 before practolol treatment. Skin rash was reported by 16 during but 8 before treatment; both ocular symptoms and rash occurred in 7 during and 1 before treatment. A similar investigation of 246 patients who had taken propranolol showed a smaller insignificant difference in the incidence of eye complaints—42 patients during and 31 patients before propranolol treatment. The overall incidence of rash was not significantly greater during propranolol treatment but 14 patients had both an eye complaint and rash during treatment compared to 4 patients before treatment.— D. C. G. Skegg and R. Doll, *Lancet*, 1977, *2*, 475.

Further reports and studies: A. Garner and A. H. S. Rahi, *Br. J. Ophthal.*, 1976, *60*, 684; T. van Joost *et al.*, *Br. J. Derm.*, 1976, *94*, 447.

Effects on the gastro-intestinal tract. A 56-year-old woman who had taken practolol 300 mg daily for 15 or more months, with skin rash and eye involvement, developed evanescent recurring abdominal discomfort and swelling leading eventually to emergency laparotomy. The abdomen was full of fibrinous adhesions with cocoons around the bowel. The patient developed severe chest pain and died 4 days after surgery.— W. O. Windsor *et al.*, *Br. med. J.*, 1975, *2*, 68.

A report of fibrinous peritonitis in a 57-year-old man 18 months after discontinuing practolol which he had taken for about 21 months.— D. Allan and D. Cade (letter), *Br. med. J.*, 1975, *4*, 40. A further report of sclerosing peritonitis developing in 2 patients 10 and 12 months respectively after stopping practolol.— R. C. Smith *et al.*, *Med. J. Aust.*, 1977, *2*, 394.

A report of 16 cases of peritonitis associated with practolol. Surgery, when possible, was the treatment of choice. Seven patients out of 54 taking practolol, oxprenolol, or propranolol had radiological evidence of small-bowel abnormalities; 2 were taking practolol, 2 propranolol, and 3 oxprenolol. One patient continued to take propranolol with consequent progression of the changes in the small bowel. One of the patients taking practolol and the other 5 showed regression of bowel changes when the beta-blocker was withdrawn.— A. J. Marshall *et al.*, *Q. J. Med.*, 1977, *46*, 135. Comment.— *Lancet*, 1977, *1*, 843.

The case-histories of 6 patients with sclerosing peritonitis who took practolol. Stripping of all abnormal tissue from the large and small bowel should be performed.— R. P. H. Thompson and B. T. Jackson, *Br. med. J.*, 1977, *1*, 1393.

For other clinical reports of sclerosing peritonitis in association with practolol therapy, see Martindale 27th Edn, p. 1325.

Pneumatosis coli (intestinalis). A 61-year-old man who had taken practolol in increasing doses of up to 1 g daily for 2 years developed pneumatosis coli (intestinalis) which rapidly regressed when sotalol was substituted.— S. L. Thein and P. Asquith, *Br. med. J.*, 1977, *1*, 268.

Effects on the heart and lungs. An elderly man who had taken practolol 100 mg thrice daily for about 3 years developed a psoriasiform rash, corneal perforation, and progressive dyspnoea unresponsive to bronchodilators; he developed bowel obstruction and died. Necropsy showed dense adhesive peritonitis, adhesive pericarditis, and adhesive pleurisy.— N. H. Dyer and C. C. Varley (letter), *Br. med. J.*, 1975, *2*, 443. See also D. Hunt and J. L. Frew (letter), *ibid.*, 1975, *1*, 92.

Severe respiratory disease occurred in 6 patients who had developed sclerosing peritonitis due to practolol.— A. J. Marshall *et al.*, *Lancet*, 1977, *2*, 1254. A comment that corticosteroids do not benefit the respiratory disease associated with practolol therapy once it has become chronic.— A. W. Frankland (letter), *Lancet*, 1978, *1*, 329.

See also Effects on Respiratory Function, below.

Further references: P. Bartsch and M. Reginster (letter), *Lancet*, 1977, *1*, 908; T. M. Erwteman *et al.*, *Br. med. J.*, 1977, *2*, 297; D. R. Hall *et al.*, *Thorax*, 1978, *33*, 822.

Effects on the kidneys. Severe nephrotic syndrome in a 65-year-old man was probably caused by practolol which he had taken for 3 years.— M. J. Farr *et al.*, *Br. med. J.*, 1975, *2*, 68.

Effects on the liver. A report of 2 patients with typical practolol-induced oculocutaneous lesions who also had primary biliary cirrhosis; the association was not considered fortuitous.— P. J. E. Brown *et al.*, *Br. med. J.*, 1978, *1*, 1591.

Effects on the muscles. A myasthenic syndrome in a bronchitic hypertensive patient might have been related to ingestion of practolol.— R. O. Hughes and F. J. Zacharias (letter), *Br. med. J.*, 1976, *1*, 460.

Effects on respiratory function. Administration of practolol led to the first asthmatic attack a patient had experienced for 16 years.— J. A. Bonn *et al.*, *Lancet*, 1972, *1*, 814.

See also Effects on the Heart and Lungs, above.

Effects on the skin. Psoriasiform reactions to practolol were seen in 14 patients taking practolol including 1 in whom the eruption was generalised; in 7 further patients the eruption was eczematous, lichenoid, exfoliative dermatitis, or resembled lupus erythematosus. Three patients had concomitant soreness of the eyes with ocular damage and 3 had arthralgia. Of 12 patients who subsequently took challenge doses 11 developed reactions.— R. H. Felix *et al.*, *Br. med. J.*, 1974, *4*, 321.

A report of nail dystrophy.— N. Kirkham and S. Holt, *Lancet*, 1976, *2*, 1137. See also E. Tegner, *Acta derm.-vener., Stockh.*, 1976, *56*, 493.

Further references: M. G. M. Rowland and C. J. Stevenson (letter), *Lancet*, 1972, *1*, 1130; E. S. K. Assem and R. A. Banks, *Proc. R. Soc. Med.*, 1973, *66*, 179; R. Felix and F. A. Ive (letter), *Br. med. J.*, 1974, *2*, 333; C. M. Ridley (letter), *ibid.*, 1974, *4*, 229.

Lupus erythematosus. Systemic lupus erythematosus in 3 patients was attributed to practolol which had been taken in doses of 0.6 to 1.2 g daily.— E. B. Raftery and A. M. Denman, *Br. med. J.*, 1973, *2*, 452.

Further references: G. R. Milner *et al.*, *J. clin. Path.*, 1977, *30*, 770; M. W. Stewart and S. W. Clarke, *Proc. R. Soc. Med.*, 1976, *69*, 61.

Overdosage. A 39-year-old man attempted suicide by taking 9 g of practolol; the serum concentrations 4.5 and 9.5 hours after ingestion were 40 and 58.6 µg per ml respectively (usual therapeutic concentration 1.5 µg per ml). Apart from transient slight bradycardia and transient slight hypotension he suffered no ill-effects.— P. Karhunen and G. Härtel (letter), *Br. med. J.*, 1973, *2*, 178.

Shoulder-hand syndrome. On 2 occasions the shoulder-hand syndrome, with symmetrical, hot, painful swelling of both hands, developed in a patient taking practolol and regressed when practolol was withdrawn.— W. A. Stubbs and M. B. Ablett (letter), *Br. med. J.*, 1975, *2*, 36.

Precautions. As for Propranolol Hydrochloride, p.1327.

Practolol is less likely than propranolol to affect respiratory function, and it has been employed in patients with bronchial asthma or bronchospasm.

Interactions. *Ampicillin.* In a study in 4 healthy male subjects the mean elimination half-life for practolol 400 mg by mouth was 8.6 hours. This was reduced to 6.3 hours when the subjects were receiving ampicillin 500 mg four times daily concurrently. Since a similar change was not seen when practolol was given intravenously it was considered unlikely that competitive interference with biliary excretion was the explanation.— J. G. Kelly *et al.*, *Br. J. clin. Pharmac.*, 1977, *4*, 396P.

Absorption and Fate. Practolol is completely absorbed from the gastro-intestinal tract and is excreted unchanged in the urine. Peak plasma concentrations occur 1 to 3 hours after a dose. The biological half-life of practolol is longer than would be anticipated from its plasma half-life of about 10 hours.

Comparisons of the reduction in exercise-induced tachycardia and plasma concentrations of practolol suggested that practolol has a plasma half-life of 10 to 11 hours and a pharmacological half-life of 40 to 50 hours.— S. G. Carruthers *et al.* (letter), *Br. med. J.*, 1973, *2*, 177. Criticisms.— C. R. Kumana and T. R. D. Shaw (letter), *ibid.*, 1973, *2*, 715; S. E. Smith (letter), *ibid.*

Following oral administration of incremental doses of practolol to 7 patients with essential hypertension, absorption was found to be complete and the plasma half-life was 13.2 hours. There was no detectable metabolic transformation. Excretion was entirely by the kidneys and was unaffected by changes in urinary pH from 5.4 to 8.0.— G. Bodem and C. A. Chidsey, *Clin. Pharmac. Ther.*, 1973, *14*, 26. See also C. M. Kaye *et al.*, *Br. J. Pharmac.*, 1973, *49*, 155P.

Investigations in 11 healthy male subjects indicated that practolol by mouth was rapidly, consistently, and completely absorbed; the total dose was recovered in the urine.— S. G. Carruthers *et al.*, *Clin. Pharmac. Ther.*, 1974, *15*, 497. See also *idem*, *Br. J. clin. Pharmac.*, 1974, *1*, 181P; C. R. Kumana and C. M. Kaye, *Eur. J. clin. Pharmac.*, 1974, *7*, 243.

Further references: J. D. Fitzgerald and B. Scales, *Int. J. clin. Pharmac.*, 1968, *1*, 467; D. W. Schneck *et al.*, *Clin. Pharmac. Ther.*, 1972, *13*, 685; D. Hunt *et al.*, *Br. med. J.*, 1975, *1*, 151.

Diffusion into the CSF. A study in *animals* on the central uptake of beta-adrenoceptor blocking agents, including practolol.— M. D. Day *et al.*, *J. Pharm. Pharmac.*, 1977, *29*, *Suppl.*, 52P.

Uses. Practolol is a beta-adrenoceptor blocking agent (see p.1324) with uses similar to those of propranolol (see p.1329). It is classified as cardioselective.

For the emergency treatment of cardiac arrhythmias practolol may be given by slow intravenous injection in a dose of 5 mg, repeated if necessary according to the patient's response. Total dosages of more than 20 mg are not usually required. The usual dose by mouth was 100 mg twice daily but higher doses might be needed.

Practolol is no longer recommended for long-term therapy but when its use was deemed essential it was recommended that the patient should be examined for side-effects every few weeks. Doses of 100 to 200 mg twice or thrice daily have been used for angina pectoris; daily doses of 1.2 g have been given.

In view of the adverse reactions associated with long-term practolol therapy it seemed prudent to limit its use to no more than a few weeks. If propranolol proved to be an unsatisfactory substitute oxprenolol was probably the safest of the established alternative beta-adrenoceptor blocking agents. Practolol should be replaced by another beta-adrenoceptor blocking agent even in patients who had been receiving it for a long time without adverse effects. If it proved to be the only beta-adrenoceptor blocking agent tolerated the patient should be examined and asked about symptoms every 6 to 8 weeks. Practolol remained the beta-adrenoceptor blocking agent of choice when treating dysrhythmias in acute cardiac infarction.— *Drug & Ther. Bull.*, 1975, *13*, 72. See also *ibid.*, 92.

A general review of practolol and comparisons with propranolol and oxprenolol.— G. F. George, *Prescribers' J.*, 1974, *14*, 93.

Adjunct to anaesthesia. A study in 75 patients, given atropine and anaesthetised with halothane, showed that practolol 20 mg by intravenous injection blocked sympathetic overactivity of the heart due to surgical stimuli, excess carbon dioxide, or subcutaneous injection of adrenaline 1 in 200 000. The negative chronotropic and the anti-arrhythmic actions were not associated with ECG evidence of a negative dromotropic action on the conductive tissue.— M. Johnstone, *Br. J. Anaesth.*, 1969, *41*, 130.

Further references: C. Prys-Roberts *et al.*, *Br. J. Anaesth.*, 1973, *45*, 671; W. Ryder *et al.*, *ibid.*, 745.

Administration in the elderly. Following dosage with practolol 200 mg the plasma elimination half-life of practolol was about 8.5 hours in 8 elderly patients and 7 hours in 13 young patients. Providing renal function was normal for the patient's age there was no need to reduce the dose of practolol for elderly patients.— C. M. Castleden *et al.*, *Br. J. clin. Pharmac.*, 1975, *2*, 303.

Administration in renal failure. In 13 patients with chronic renal failure (7 anephric) maintained on haemodialysis, the mean half-life of practolol, after a single 100-mg or 200-mg dose given between dialyses, was 78.2 hours (range 30.5 to 166 hours), compared with the reported mean half-life in normal subjects of 10 hours. In 5 further patients not on haemodialysis the half-life after a single 200-mg dose was 15 to 55.5 hours. In 8 patients maintained by dialysis the mean half-life was 70 hours (range 30.5 to 166 hours) when measured between dialyses and 17.1 hours (range 8 to 30 hours) when measured during a 14-hour dialysis. It was tentatively suggested that adequate blood concentrations (1.5 to 2.4 µg per ml) could be maintained by a dose of 200 mg at the beginning and end of each twice-weekly dialysis.— J. B. Eastwood *et al.*, *Br. med. J.*, 1973, *4*, 320. See also G. Bodem *et al.*, *Eur. J. clin. Pharmac.*, 1974, *7*, 249.

Administration in respiratory insufficiency. In 11 patients with asthma, practolol 20 mg intravenously given in conjunction with isoprenaline 100 µg by aerosol inhalation slightly reduced the rise in spirometric measurements and heart-rate, and prevented the fall in pO_2 in arterial blood due to the isoprenaline.— K. N. V. Palmer *et al.*, *Lancet*, 1969, *2*, 1092.

Practolol 100 mg twice daily successfully controlled a sinus tachycardia in a 63-year-old patient with severe asthma.— J. F. Beary and N. J. Fortuin (letter), *Ann. intern. Med.*, 1974, *81*, 405.

Studies in 6 healthy subjects indicated that practolol did not show absolute cardiospecific beta-adrenoceptor blockade, as significant reductions in peak flow rate occurred after vigorous exercise particularly with a 400-mg dose.— C. R. Kumana *et al.*, *Eur. J. clin. Pharmac.*, 1977, *12*, 7.

Further references: C. R. Kumana *et al.*, *Br. med. J.*, 1974, *4*, 444; M. E. Thompson *et al.*, *Clin. Pharmac. Ther.*, 1974, *16*, 750; V. M. S. Oh, *Br. J. clin. Pharmac.*, 1977, *4*, 722P.

Cardiac disorders. *Angina pectoris.* The cardiovascular effects of practolol in 8 patients with angina pectoris.— E. L. Alderman *et al.*, *Clin. Pharmac. Ther.*, 1973, *14*, 175.

Because of adverse reactions, practolol was generally unsuitable for treatment of angina or hypertension.— T. Crawford, *Committee on Safety of Medicines* (letter), *Br. med. J.*, 1976, *2*, 299.

Further references: N. -H. Areskog and L. Adolfsson, *Br. med. J.*, 1969, *2*, 601; G. Sandler and G. A. Clayton, *ibid.*, 1970, *2*, 399; C. F. George *et al.*, *ibid.*, 402; J. Le Lorier and G. Elias, *Eur. J. clin. Pharmac.*, 1976, *10*, 171.

Cardiac arrhythmias. Practolol was given to 47 patients with cardiac dysrhythmias after myocardial infarction. Initially, 5 mg was given intravenously over 2 minutes, followed by 5 mg every 2 minutes up to a total of 25 mg. In 5 patients dysrhythmia recurred within 30 to 60 minutes and an infusion of 25 to 100 mg was given over 24 hours. In 14 of 15 patients with rapid supraventricular dysrhythmias, 11 of whom had been unsuccessfully treated with digitalis, the ventricle-rate slowed within 5 minutes after practolol, and in 6 returned to sinus rhythm within 15 minutes; the effect of practolol usually lasted 90 minutes. Five of 11 patients with ventricular tachycardia resistant to lignocaine reverted to sinus rhythm after practolol, which also adequately suppressed for at least 30 minutes frequent ventricular extrasystoles in 9 of 16 patients. The effects of practolol were uncertain, but were helpful in 2 of 3 patients with persistent ventricular fibrillation resistant to counter-shock and in 1 of 2 patients with low nodal tachycardia. Only 2 patients suffered side-effects. Practolol produced a complete atrioventricular block lasting 1 minute in a patient with ventricular tachycardia and a damaged atrioventricular node. A second patient became hypotensive and confused when his ventricle-rate was reduced from 150 to 75 per minute by practolol. Atropine raised the ventricle-rate and sinus rhythm returned after counter-shock.— D. E. Jewitt *et al.*, *Lancet*, 1969, *2*, 227. See also *idem*, *Cardiovasc. Res.*, 1970, *4*, 188.

Further references: G. Gent *et al.*, *Br. med. J.*, 1970, *1*, 533; A. V. Jenkins, *Br. J. Anaesth.*, 1970, *42*, 59; J. Yahalom *et al.*, *Chest*, 1977, *71*, 592.

Myocardial infarction. For reference to studies on the prevention of myocardial infarction with long-term beta-adrenoceptor blockade, including an earlier study using practolol, see Propranolol Hydrochloride, p.1331.

Hypertension. Because of adverse reactions, practolol was generally unsuitable for the treatment of angina or hypertension.— T. Crawford, *Committee on Safety of Medicines* (letter), *Br. med. J.*, 1976, *2*, 299.

Further references: K. N. V. Palmer (letter), *Lancet*, 1970, *2*, 935; Y. Traub *et al.*, *Clin. Pharmac. Ther.*, 1973, *14*, 165; R. A. Wood *et al.*, *Clin. Trials J.*, 1973, *10* (2), 53; D. M. Chaput de Saintonge *et al.*, *Br. J. clin. Pharmac.*, 1974, *1*, 375; D. B. Galloway *et al.*, *Br. Heart J.*, 1974, *36*, 867.

Preparations

Practolol Injection *(B.P.)*. A sterile solution of practolol in Water for Injections containing citric acid monohydrate. The pH is adjusted to 6 (limits: 5.5 to 6.5) by the addition of sodium hydroxide. Sterilised by autoclaving.

Practolol Tablets *(B.P. 1973)*. Tablets containing practolol.

Eraldin (known in some countries as Dalzic) *(ICI Pharmaceuticals, UK)*. Practolol, available as injection containing 2 mg per ml, in ampoules of 5 ml. (Also available as Eraldin in *Denm., Norw., S.Afr.*).

Other Proprietary Names

Eraldina *(Swed.)*.

6321-w

Pronethalol Hydrochloride *(B.P. 1963)*. Pronetalol Hydrochloride; Compound 38174; Nethalide. 2-Isopropylamino-1-(2-naphthyl)ethanol hydrochloride.
$C_{15}H_{19}NO,HCl=265.8$.

CAS — 54-80-8 (pronethalol) [325-17-7(+); 2238-85-9(±)]; 51-02-5 (hydrochloride) [325-16-6(±)].

Pronethalol is a cardiac depressant with beta-adrenoceptor blocking actions similar to those of propranolol hydrochloride. It has shown carcinogenic effects on prolonged administration to certain species of *animals* and because of the possibility of similar effects in man it is no longer used.

Carcinogenicity. For a report of *animal* studies excluding a carcinogenic effect of pronethalol, see Oxprenolol Hydrochloride, p.1344.

6322-e

Sotalol Hydrochloride.

MJ 1999. 4′-(1-Hydroxy-2-isopropylaminoethyl)methanesulphonanilide hydrochloride.
$C_{12}H_{20}N_2O_3S,HCl=308.8$.

CAS — 3930-20-9 (sotalol) [30236-32-9(+); 30236-31-8(−); 27948-47-6 (±)]; 959-24-0 (hydrochloride) [4549-94-4(+); 4201-00-7(±)].

An off-white to pale cream crystalline powder. Freely **soluble** in water; sparingly soluble in chloroform. **Protect** from light.

Adverse Effects, Treatment, and Precautions. As for Propranolol Hydrochloride, p.1325.

Effects on the heart. Atypical ventricular tachycardia 'torsade de pointes' in a patient with chronic renal failure and hypertension was associated with administration of sotalol.— A. Kontopoulos *et al.*, *Postgrad. med. J.*, 1981, *57*, 321.

Prolonged Q-T_c intervals were seen in 29 patients taking sotalol 160 to 640 mg daily and were correlated with serum-sotalol concentrations. Since a prolonged Q-T_c interval is a risk factor for cardiac arrhythmia, ECG monitoring is recommended if sotalol is given to patients with renal insufficiency or is administered in high doses.— P. J. Neuvonen *et al.* (letter), *Lancet*, 1981, *2*, 426. Comments.— T. Pellinen *et al.* (letter), *ibid.*, 878; M. Laakso *et al.* (letter), *ibid.*, 1168. See also under Overdosage, below.

Effects on the muscles. For a report of proximal myopathy associated with sotalol, see Propranolol, p.1326.

Effects on respiratory function. Sotalol 10 mg intravenously caused a significant increase in airway resistance in 7 patients with chronic obstructive pulmonary disease although it had no such effect in 9 healthy subjects. Sotalol resembled other nonselective beta-adrenoceptor blocking agents in reducing pulmonary function and should not be used in patients suffering from obstructive lung disease.— N. -H. Areskog *et al.*, *Eur. J. clin. Pharmac.*, 1975, *8*, 403.

Effects on the skin. Cutaneous thickening in 6 hyperthyroid patients treated with radioactive iodine and beta-blockade might have been associated with the beta-blocking therapy with special reference to sotalol.— J. P. Michel *et al.* (letter), *Lancet*, 1979, *1*, 54.

Interactions. *Alcohol.* In a study of healthy subjects alcohol reduced the plasma clearance-rate of sotalol. The hypotensive effect of sotalol was increased.— (Sotaniemi, E.A. *et al.*), *Clin. Pharmac. Ther.*, 1981, *29*, 705.

Clonidine. For a report of an antagonistic effect between sotalol and clonidine, see Clonidine Hydrochloride, p.140.

Overdosage. In 2 patients who had taken overdoses of sotalol (2.4 g and 8 g respectively) the most important symptoms were hypotension, bradycardia, a prolonged Q-T interval, ventricular extrasystoles, ventricular tachycardia, and, in 1 patient, ventricular fibrillation.— E. Elonen *et al.*, *Br. med. J.*, 1979, *1*, 1184.

Absorption and Fate. Sotalol is completely absorbed from the gastro-intestinal tract and peak plasma concentrations are obtained about 2 or 3 hours after a dose. It is excreted unchanged in the urine. The biological half-life of sotalol is longer than would be anticipated from its plasma half-life of 15 to 17 hours. It is not bound to plasma proteins.

Following administration of sotalol 100 mg to 2 patients, peak plasma concentrations of 1 and 0.65 µg per ml respectively were obtained after 2 to 3 hours.— E. Besterman and C. McCarthy (letter), *Br. med. J.*, 1974, *3*, 257.

A study of the pharmacokinetics of sotalol in 8 healthy subjects and 5 hypertensive subjects. Absolute bioavailability was 100% after oral administration indicating that first-pass effects were negligible. The terminal half-life was about 17 hours and sotalol was excreted in the urine almost entirely unchanged. The data obtained after administration of single doses and after chronic administration were the same.— M. Anttila *et al.*, *Acta pharmac. tox.*, 1976, *39*, 118.

Further references: D. G. McDevitt and R. G. Shanks, *Br. J. clin. Pharmac.*, 1977, *4*, 153; K. Schnelle *et al.*, *J. clin. Pharmac.*, 1979, *19*, 516; W. J. Leahey *et al.*, *Eur. J. clin. Pharmac.*, 1980, *17*, 419.

Metabolites. Most of a dose of sotalol was excreted unchanged in the urine of *dogs* and protein binding did not occur.— K. Schnelle and E. R. Garrett, *J. pharm. Sci.*, 1973, *62*, 362.

Protein binding. No binding of sotalol to human plasma proteins.— M. Anttila *et al.*, *Acta pharmac. tox.*, 1976, *39*, 118.

Uses. Sotalol hydrochloride is a beta-adrenoceptor blocking agent (see p.1324) with uses similar to those of propranolol (see p.1329). It is classified as non-cardioselective.

In the treatment of hypertension sotalol hydrochloride is usually given in an initial dose of 160 mg daily or 80 mg twice daily, increased at fortnightly intervals according to the response of the patient. An adequate response is usually achieved with a dose range of about 160 to 600 mg daily given as a single dose, preferably on rising in the morning or given as 2 divided doses. Doses of 4 g or more daily have occasionally been recorded.

The optimum dose for angina pectoris is also about 160 to 600 mg daily. For cardiac arrhythmias it is 120 to 240 mg daily. It has been recommended that a dose of 120 to 240 mg daily may be given to reduce symptoms of sympathetic overactivity in hyperthyroidism. These doses may be taken as a single daily dose preferably on rising in the morning or in divided doses.

For the emergency treatment of cardiac arrhythmias sotalol hydrochloride may be given by slow intravenous injection in a dose of 10 to 20 mg, repeated if necessary.

Action. For reports and discussions on the pharmacology and clinical uses of sotalol, see *Advances in Beta-Adrenergic Blocking Therapy—Sotalol*, A.G. Smart (Ed.), London, Excerpta Medica, 1974.

Studies of the action of sotalol: A. J. Rice *et al.*, *Clin. Pharmac. Ther.*, 1970, *11*, 567; A. Thumala *et al.*, *Am. Heart J.*, 1971, *82*, 439; M. H. Lader and P. J. Tyrer, *Br. J. Pharmac.*, 1972, *45*, 557; D. N. W. Griffith *et al.*, *Br. J. clin. Pharmac.*, 1979, *7*, 491.

Administration in renal failure. The pharmacokinetics of sotalol were studied in 4 healthy subjects and in 6 patients with end-stage renal failure. It was considered that reduced doses of sotalol should be used during maintenance treatment in patients with advanced renal failure and that haemodialysis over 6 to 7 hours would reduce plasma-sotalol concentrations by about 20%.— T. B. Tjandramaga *et al.*, *Br. J. clin. Pharmac.*, 1976, *3*, 259.

Further references: H. K. Sundquist *et al.*, *Ann. clin. Res.*, 1975, *7*, 442; G. Berglund *et al.*, *Eur. J. clin. Pharmac.*, 1980, *18*, 321; A. D. Blair *et al.*, *Clin. Pharmac. Ther.*, 1981, *29*, 457.

See also under Effects on the Heart, above.

Anxiety. A double-blind crossover sequential trial of sotalol in 16 psychiatric out-patients, 14 of whom completed the trial, indicated that sotalol had a place in the treatment of chronic anxiety, particularly in patients with tremor as a major symptom, but was unlikely to be effective as a sole therapeutic agent. The dose range was 80 to 400 mg daily in 4 divided doses for 2 weeks and side-effects included jaundice, hallucinations (in a woman who received 600 mg daily), and respiratory difficulty.— P. J. Tyrer and M. H. Lader, *Clin. Pharmac. Ther.*, 1973, *14*, 418.

Cardiac disorders. *Angina pectoris.* In a double-blind crossover multicentre study with sotalol, 137 or 146 patients showed a significant reduction in the number of angina attacks experienced in the 6-week treatment period when sotalol was given in doses of 120 to 480 mg daily. The mean number of attacks was reduced by half in 71.2% of patients.— P. G. Gooding and E. Berman, *Postgrad. med. J.*, 1974, *50*, 734.

Cardiac arrhythmias. A study of the effect of intravenous administration of sotalol 20 mg, at a rate of 1 mg per minute, in 20 patients with cardiac arrhythmias; a maximum of 3 doses could be given at intervals of 20 minutes (maximum cumulative dose 60 mg). A beneficial effect was noted in 2 of 2 patients with sinus tachycardia and 4 of 7 with other supraventricular tachycardias. Although beta-adrenoceptor blocking agents are not generally considered to be very effective in the treatment of ventricular arrhythmias, good results were obtained in 9 of 11 patients with lignocaine-resistant ventricular arrhythmias. Life-threatening bradycardia occurred in 2 patients.— Y. Latour *et al.*, *Int. J. clin. Pharmac. Biopharm.*, 1977, *15*, 275.

A view that an intravenous dose of 10 to 20 mg of sotalol hydrochloride is only the initial starting dose, and that the range is up to 100 mg intravenously.— A. Simon, *Bristol Laboratories, USA* (letter), *Lancet*, 1980, *1*, 1356. Refusal to recommend an intravenous dose of sotalol going up to 100 mg. Bearing in mind that the dose of sotalol is likely to be somewhat similar to practolol and that practolol may be less cardiodepressant, the dose should not exceed 20 mg except in an expert coronary care unit with full haemodynamic monitoring and facilities for coping with any untoward bradycardia.— L. H. Opie (letter), *ibid.*

Further references: R. Prakash *et al.*, *Am. J. Cardiol.*, 1972, *29*, 397; A. Simon and E. Berman, *J. clin. Pharmac.*, 1979, *19*, 547.

Diabetes mellitus. Two pre-adolescent girls who had required repeated admission to hospital for episodes of severe stress-induced diabetic ketoacidosis responded well to administration of sotalol. It was considered that endogenous catecholamines played a key role in the mediation of diabetic decompensation following emotional arousal and that beta-adrenoceptor blockade could modify this.— L. Baker *et al.*, *J. Pediat.*, 1969, *75*, 19.

See also Precautions for Propranolol Hydrochloride, p.1327.

Hypertension. Studies in 12 patients with hypertension showed that sotalol given in once-daily doses in the range of 80 to 800 mg, the individual dose being determined during a titration period of about 3 weeks for each patient, could maintain the diastolic blood pressure satisfactorily for 3 months. The hypotensive action of sotalol was still evident for about 26 hours after the last dose given during the trial, although the pulse-rate had begun to rise.— R. Gabriel, *Curr. med. Res. Opinion*, 1977, *4*, 739.

Further references: L. Prescott (letter), *Br. med. J.*, 1975, *1*, 572; A. J. Jouhar, *Bristol Laboratories* (letter), *ibid.*, 1975, *2*, 38; B. N. C. Prichard (letter), *ibid.*, 275; G. Rowlands *et al.*, *Br. J. clin. Pract.*, 1977, *31*, 57; H. L. Shaw, *J.R. Coll. gen. Pract.*, 1977, *27*, 742; J. Tuomilehto *et al.*, *Curr. ther. Res.*, 1977, *21*, 668; A. Reyes *et al.*, *ibid.*, 1978, *23*, 715; J. Reynaert, *Acta ther.*, 1978, *4*, 15; L. A. Salako and A. O. Falase, *Curr. ther. Res.*, 1978, *24*, 794; L. E. du Toit, *Clin. Trials J.*, 1979, *16*, 18.

Comparative studies. In a double-blind crossover study in 30 hypertensive subjects sotalol 80 mg was shown to have equivalent antihypertensive effect to propranolol 40 mg.— G. Berglund, *Curr. ther. Res.*, 1977, *21*, 21.

Further references: H. Sundquist *et al.*, *Clin. Pharmac. Ther.*, 1974, *16*, 465 (practolol); S. V. Gajendragadkar and W. E. Clarke, *J. int. med. Res.*, 1977, *5*, 233 (methyldopa); A. P. Douglas-Jones, *Practitioner*, 1978, *220*, 804 (methyldopa); A. Lehtonen and H. Sundquist, *Curr. ther. Res.*, 1978, *23*, 131 (metoprolol); J. E. Scrazzolo and A. G. Queirol, *J. clin. Pharmac.*, 1979, *19*, 540 (methyldopa).

Once-daily administration. In 8 patients with mild or moderate hypertension satisfactory reduction of blood pressure was achieved with a once-daily dose of sotalol given at 7 a.m.— H. L. Shaw (letter), *Br. med. J.*, 1976, *2*, 46. See also under Hypertension (above).

Further references: J. Reynaert, *Curr. ther. Res.*, 1979, *26*, 799; I. Parvinen and E. Paukkala, *J. clin. Pharmac.*, 1979, *19*, 533; W. Basson and D. P. Myburgh, *ibid.*, 571; I. Parvinen and E. Paukkala, *Eur. J. clin. Pharmac.*, 1979, *15*, 293.

Proprietary Preparations

Beta-Cardone *(Duncan, Flockhart, UK)*. Sotalol hydrochloride, available as an **Injection** containing 2 mg per ml, in ampoules of 5 ml, and as scored **Tablets** of 40, 80, and 200 mg.

Sotacor *(Bristol-Myers Pharmaceuticals, UK)*. Sotalol hydrochloride, available as **Injection** containing 2 mg per ml, in ampoules of 5 ml, and as scored **Tablets** of 80 and 160 mg. (Also available as Sotacor in *Denm., Neth., S.Afr., Swed.*).

Sotazide *(Bristol-Myers Pharmaceuticals, UK)*. Scored tablets each containing sotalol hydrochloride 160 mg and hydrochlorothiazide 25 mg. For hypertension. *Dose.* 1 tablet daily, gradually increased to 4 tablets if required.

Other Proprietary Names

Betacardone *(Arg.)*; Sotalex *(Fr., Ger., Ital.)*.

6323-l

Timolol Maleate *(U.S.P.)*. Timololi Maleas; MK 950. (−)-(*S*)-1-*tert*-Butylamino-3-(4-morpholino-1,2,5-thiadiazol-3-yloxy)propan-2-ol maleate.

$C_{13}H_{24}N_4O_3S,C_4H_4O_4=432.5$.

CAS — 26839-75-8 (timolol, −)[26839-76-9(+); 47148-57-2 (±)]; 26921-17-5 (maleate, −)[26839-77-0(+); 26791-17-3(±)].

Pharmacopoeias. In *Neth.* and *U.S.*

A white or almost white, odourless or almost odourless, crystalline powder. M.p. about 200°. Freely **soluble** in water; soluble in alcohol and methyl alcohol; sparingly soluble in chloroform and propylene glycol; practically insoluble in ether and cyclohexane. A 5% solution in water has a pH of 3.5 to 4.5. A solution in N hydrochloric acid is laevorotatory. Aqueous solutions are stable up to a pH of 12. **Protect** from light.

Adverse Effects, Treatment, and Precautions. As for Propranolol Hydrochloride, p.1325.

Systemic side-effects have followed topical use of the eye-drops; mild local irritation and blurred vision have also been reported.

Effects on the eyes. A report of dryness of the eyes in a man receiving timolol in doses up to 75 mg daily. His symptoms improved immediately on withdrawal of timolol.— M. A. Frais and T. J. Bayley, *Postgrad. med. J.*, 1979, *55*, 884.

Effects on the gastro-intestinal tract. It was considered that sclerosing peritonitis in a 50-year-old man might be associated with timolol therapy.— D. C. Baxter-Smith *et al.* (letter), *Lancet*, 1978, *2*, 149. Severe criticism; it is not considered that there is any objective evidence that this is a case of sclerosing peritonitis of the practolol type.— J. F. Nancarrow, *Merck Sharp & Dohme* (letter), *ibid.*, 525.

Effects on the heart. Chronic congestive heart failure became more severe and bradycardia developed in a 72-year-old woman with severe rheumatic heart disease and atrial fibrillation after eye-drops containing timolol maleate 0.25% were substituted for her pilocarpine eye-drops.— N. A. Britman (letter), *New Engl. J. Med.*, 1979, *300*, 566.

Effects on mental state. Hallucinations associated with the use of timolol for glaucoma.— D. Yates (letter), *J. Am. med. Ass.*, 1980, *244*, 768.

Effects on respiratory function. Chronic but stable asthma in a 73-year-old woman was exacerbated and became uncontrollable after she started using timolol 0.5% eye-drops. The drops were withdrawn and pilocarpine substituted and within one week she was free of respiratory symptoms.— F. L. Jones and N. L. Ekberg (letter), *New Engl. J. Med.*, 1979, *301*, 270. Further reports of adverse effects on respiratory function associated with the use of timolol eye-drops.— S. Ahmad (letter), *Lancet*, 1979, *2*, 1028; F. L. Jones and N. L. Ekberg (letter), *J. Am. med. Ass.*, 1980, *244*, 2730.

Hypoglycaemia. Increased incidence of hypoglycaemic episodes in a diabetic woman was possibly related to the use of timolol eye-drops for glaucoma.— K. Angelo-Nielsen (letter), *J. Am. med. Ass.*, 1980, *244*, 2263.

Interactions. *Diuretics.* A study in 6 healthy subjects indicated that timolol slightly ameliorated bendrofluazide-induced hypokalaemia. The interaction should be studied over prolonged periods and in disease states to establish whether it had clinical significance.— J. Hettiarachchi *et al.*, *Clin. Pharmac. Ther.*, 1977, *22*, 58.

Myasthenia gravis. Immediate deterioration in a patient with myasthenia following topical use of timolol for glaucoma.— S. A. Shaivitz (letter), *J. Am. med. Ass.*, 1979, *242*, 1611.

Withdrawal. Withdrawal symptoms have been noted in hypertensive patients after metoprolol, timolol, and propranolol, all of which are devoid of intrinsic sympathomimetic actions.— Ø. L. Pedersen and E. Mikkelsen (letter), *Lancet*, 1979, *1*, 554.

Absorption and Fate. Timolol is almost completely absorbed from the gastro-intestinal tract but is subject to moderate first-pass metabolism. Peak plasma concentrations occur about 2 hours after a dose. It is extensively metabolised in the liver, the metabolites being excreted in the urine together with some unchanged timolol. The biological half-life of timolol is longer than would be anticipated from its plasma half-life, which has been variously estimated as ranging from about 2.5 hours to about 4.5 hours.

In a controlled crossover study of 6 healthy male subjects no significant difference in the duration of cardiac effects was noted between timolol and propranolol given intravenously in an equipotent dose.— M. R. Achong *et al.*, *Clin. Pharmac. Ther.*, 1976, *19*, 148.

After oral administration of timolol 10 mg mean peak plasma concentrations of 42.6 ng per ml were achieved about 2 hours after the dose.— O. F. Else *et al.*, *Eur. J. clin. Pharmac.*, 1978, *14*, 431. A comparison of the pharmacokinetics of timolol and propranolol. After doses of timolol maleate 5, 10, or 20 mg peak plasma concentrations occurred 1 to 4 hours after the dose; about 17% of a dose was excreted unchanged in the urine within 24 hours.— T. Ishizaki and K. Tawara, *Eur. J. clin. Pharmac.*, 1978, *14*, 7.

Differing estimations of the half-life of timolol: D. J. Tocco *et al.*, *J. pharm. Sci.*, 1975, *64*, 1879 (3 hours); *idem, Drug Metab. & Disposit.*, 1975, *3*, 361 (4.5 hours); P. Vermeij *et al.*, *J. Pharm. Pharmac.*, 1978, *30*, 53 (about 2.5 hours); O. F. Else *et al.*, *Eur. J. clin. Pharmac.*, 1978, *14*, 431 (about 4.5 to 5 hours); T. Ishizaki and K. Tawara, *Eur. J. clin. Pharmac.*, 1978, *14*, 7 (about 2.8 hours).

First-pass effect. A study indicating a moderate first-pass effect of timolol.— P. Vermeij *et al.*, *J. Pharm. Pharmac.*, 1978, *30*, 53. A study suggesting that there is significant metabolism of timolol but little first-pass effect compared to propranolol.— O. F. Else *et al.*, *Eur. J. clin. Pharmac.*, 1978, *14*, 431.

Metabolites. Metabolites of timolol in human urine.— D. J. Tocco *et al.*, *Drug Metab. & Disposit.*, 1975, *3*, 361.

Uses. Timolol maleate is a beta-adrenoceptor blocking agent (see p.1324) with uses similar to those of propranolol (see p.1329). It is classified as non-cardioselective.

Timolol maleate is usually given initially in a dose of 5 mg twice or thrice daily and the dosage increased according to the patient's response at intervals of at least 3 days; the first increase should not exceed a daily total of 10 mg in divided doses and subsequent increases should not exceed a daily total of 15 mg in divided doses.

In the treatment of hypertension the usual dose is 10 to 30 mg daily in single or divided doses but some patients may require 45 mg and a daily dosage of 60 mg should not be exceeded. The usual dose for angina pectoris is between 35 and 45 mg daily in divided doses.

Eye-drops containing timolol maleate 0.25 and 0.5% are instilled twice daily in the treatment of open-angle glaucoma. Once-daily instillation may suffice when the glaucoma has been controlled.

Action. A profile on timolol maleate.— *Aust. J. Pharm.*, 1978, *59*, 463.

Further reviews: R. N. Brogden *et al.*, *Drugs*, 1975, *9*, 164.

Immediate metabolic effects following intravenous administration of timolol in therapeutic doses closely resemble those of propranolol.— A. C. Asmal *et al.*, *Curr. ther. Res.*, 1978, *24*, 866.

Further references: M. Ulrych *et al.*, *Clin. Pharmac. Ther.*, 1972, *13*, 232 (heart-rate); Ø. L. Pedersen and E. Mikkelsen (letter), *Lancet*, 1978, *2*, 1160 (uric acid excretion).

Administration in renal failure. The mean half-life of timolol in patients with chronic renal disease was not significantly different from that of control subjects. Timolol was not significantly dialysable in patients undergoing dialysis, but 2 experienced haemodynamic complications during the haemodialysis procedure.— J. M. Pitone *et al.*, *Clin. Pharmac. Ther.*, 1977, *21*, 114.

Cardiac disorders. *Myocardial infarction.* Results of a multicentre double-blind randomised study involving 1884 patients suggesting that long-term treatment with timolol 10 mg twice daily started 7 to 28 days after myocardial infarction reduces mortality and the rate of reinfarction.—The Norwegian Multicenter Study Group, *New Engl. J. Med.*, 1981, *304*, 801. Comments.— P. Sleight, *ibid.*, 837; J. R. A. Mitchell, *Br. med. J.*, 1981, *282*, 1565; T. R. Pedersen (letter), *ibid.*, *283*, 383.

Glaucoma. A detailed review of the topical use of timolol in the treatment of glaucoma.— R. C. Heel *et al.*, *Drugs*, 1979, *17*, 38.

Further reviews: *Med. Lett.*, 1978, *20*, 109; *Lancet*, 1979, *1*, 1064; M. E. Kosman, *J. Am. med. Ass.*, 1979, *241*, 2301; *Drug & Ther. Bull.*, 1980, *18*, 13.

A report on the use of timolol eye-drops 0.1 to 0.25% instilled twice daily and increased to a maximum of 0.5% if necessary, in 37 patients with open-angle glaucoma. Timolol produced sustained reductions in intra-ocular pressure in 31 patients who used it for 3 months or longer; 7 patients used timolol for over a year. Timolol did not induce miosis, accommodative spasm, or other annoying side-effects. Systemic absorption produced a mild slowing of resting pulse-rate. In some patients timolol had an additive effect to both miotics and carbonic anhydrase inhibitors in lowering intra-ocular pressure.— W. P. Boger *et al.*, *Ophthalmology*, 1978, *85*, 259.

Timolol applied topically at a concentration of 0.5% significantly reduced the intra-ocular pressure in 5 patients with chronic uveitis and secondary glaucoma when compared with adrenaline 1% applied topically and acetazolamide given systemically. Four patients were followed up for one month and timolol 0.5% instilled once or twice daily continued to control their intra-ocular pressure.— K. M. Saari *et al.* (letter), *Lancet*, 1978, *1*, 442.

Studies on the use of timolol eye-drops in closed-angle glaucoma.— P. J. Airaksinen *et al.*, *Br. J. Ophthal.*, 1979, *63*, 822; C. I. Phillips, *ibid.*, 1980, *64*, 240.

Further references: T. J. Zimmerman and H. E. Kaufman, *Archs Ophthal., N.Y.*, 1977, *95*, 601 and 605.

Comparative studies. In a 10-week double-blind study in patients with open-angle glaucoma, eye-drops containing timolol 0.25, 0.5 and 1% were compared with eye-drops containing pilocarpine 2, 3 and 4%. Timolol reduced intra-ocular pressure at least as much as pilocarpine, and did not induce miosis, accommodative spasm or other annoying side-effects. The pulse was slowed by timolol. The 1% strength of timolol was found to have no advantage over the 0.5% strength. An initial 'escape' phenomenon was noted over the first few days of timolol therapy but significant decreases in intra-ocular pressure were still present after 10 weeks of therapy.— W. P. Boger *et al.*, *Am. J. Ophthal.*, 1978, *86*, 8.

In a 6-week double-blind crossover study, bilateral twice daily therapy with eye-drops containing timolol maleate 0.1, 0.25, and 0.5%, or eye-drops containing adrenaline hydrochloride 0.5, 1, and 2%, was compared in 36 patients with primary open-angle glaucoma or raised intra-ocular pressure. Both drugs controlled 17 patients and neither drug controlled 4. Timolol but not adrenaline was effective in 10 patients, whereas adrenaline but not timolol was effective in 2. Three patients did not complete the study. Four patients experienced significant toxicity during treatment with adrenaline but none did during treatment with timolol.— A. P. Moss *et al.*, *Am. J. Ophthal.*, 1978, *86*, 489.

Further references: R. L. Radius *et al.*, *Archs Ophthal., N.Y.*, 1978, *96*, 1003 (pilocarpine); J. Willcockson and T. Willcockson, *Curr. ther. Res.*, 1980, *27*, 538 (pilocarpine).

Hypertension. Of 12 patients with mild to moderate hypertension given timolol 10 to 60 mg and bendrofluazide 2.5 to 15 mg daily, normotension was achieved in 11 patients with 9 receiving timolol 30 mg and bendrofluazide 7.5 mg or less daily. Heart-rate was decreased in all 12 patients.— R. B. Deering *et al.*, *J. int. med. Res.*, 1977, *5*, 114.

Of 20 patients with mild or moderate hypertension given timolol in doses slowly increasing to 60 mg daily 14 were classified as responders having a decrease in mean arterial blood pressure of 10 mmHg or more.— G. Simon *et al.*, *Clin. Pharmac. Ther.*, 1978, *23*, 152.

Further references: J. A. Franciosa *et al.*, *Circulation*, 1973, *48*, 118; P. A. Poole-Wilson, *J. int. med. Res.*, 1973, *1*, 580; J. Guevara *et al.*, *Curr. ther. Res.*, 1975, *18*, 534; J. A. Franciosa and E. D. Freis, *Clin. Pharmac. Ther.*, 1975, *18*, 158; G. Lohmöller and E. D. Frohlich, *Am. Heart J.*, 1975, *89*, 437; Y. K. Seedat, *Curr. ther. Res.*, 1976, *20*, 10; A. Gillies *et al.*, *Med. J. Aust.*, 1977, *2*, 593; J. G. Nievel and J. Anderson, *Clin. Trials J.*, 1977, *14*, 164; *idem*, 173; G. Pawlowski, *Curr. ther. Res.*, 1977, *22*, 846; A. Jouve *et al.*, *Sem. Hôp. Paris*, 1978, *54*, 1363; N. B. Karatzas *et al.*, *J. int. med. Res.*, 1979, *7*, 215; O. L. Pedersen and E. Mikkelsen, *Eur. J. clin. Pharmac.*, 1979, *16*, 311; J. S. Vaicaitis, *Curr. ther. Res.*, 1980, *27*, 365; M. S. Roginsky, *ibid.*, 374; S. Oparil, *ibid.*, 527.

Comparative studies. Comparative studies of timolol with other antihypertensive agents: M. Spira, *Curr. med. Res. Opinion*, 1977, *5*, 252 (methyldopa).

Effects on plasma renin. Timolol produced a reduction in plasma-renin activity but this did not appear to be associated with its hypotensive effect since the reduction was abolished by concomitant use of hydrochlorothiazide with increased hypotensive activity.— J. Chalmers *et al.*, *Lancet*, 1976, *2*, 328. Disagreement that timolol's hypotensive action was not related to a reduction in plasma-renin activity.— M. A. Weber *et al.* (letter), *ibid.*, 1977, *1*, 367. Further comment.— F. Fyhrquist *et al.* (letter), *ibid.*, 691.

In a study involving 19 patients with essential hypertension the antihypertensive effect of timolol maleate increased as the dose was raised. This correlated with proportionally greater degrees of beta-adrenoceptor inhibition, but not with fall in plasma renin activity.— G. Simon *et al.*, *Clin. Pharmac. Ther.*, 1977, *21*, 118.

Further references: M. LeBel *et al.*, *Curr. ther. Res.*, 1978, *24*, 591; *idem*, *J. clin. Pharmac.*, 1979, *19*, 424.

Once-daily administration. In a study in 44 hypertensive patients in general practice once-daily or twice-daily treatment with timolol and bendrofluazide produced comparable control of blood pressure. Total daily doses required ranged from 10 to 50 mg of timolol and 2.5 to 12.5 mg of bendrofluazide.— D. Wheatley, *Eur. J. clin. Pharmac.*, 1978, *14*, 319.

Further references: W. P. Leary *et al.*, *Curr. ther. Res.*, 1977, *22*, 385; Alcocer L. and J. Aspe, *ibid.*, 1978, *24*, 804; I. R. Edwards and O. Else, *Eur. J. clin. Pharmac.*, 1980, *17*, 239.

Preparations

Timolol Maleate Ophthalmic Solution *(U.S.P.)*. A sterile aqueous solution of timolol maleate. pH 6.5 to 7.5. Store in airtight containers. Protect from light.

Proprietary Preparations

Betim *(Burgess, UK)*. Timolol maleate, available as scored tablets of 10 mg. (Also available as Betim in *Denm., Neth., Norw., Swed.*).

Blocadren *(Merck Sharp & Dohme, UK)*. Timolol maleate, available as scored tablets of 10 mg. (Also available as Blocadren in *Austral., Belg., Canad., Neth., Norw., S.Afr., Spain, Swed., Switz.*).

Moducren *(Morson, UK)*. Scored tablets each containing timolol maleate 10 mg, hydrochlorothiazide 25 mg, and amiloride hydrochloride 2.5 mg. For hypertension. *Dose.* 1 or 2 tablets daily.

Prestim *(Leo, UK)*. Scored tablets each containing timolol maleate 10 mg and bendrofluazide 2.5 mg. For hypertension. *Dose.* 1 or 2 tablets daily, increased to 4 tablets if necessary.

Timoptol *(Merck Sharp & Dohme, UK)*. Timolol maleate, available as eye-drops containing 0.25 or 0.5%. (Also available as Timoptol in *Austral., Fr., Neth., NZ, S.Afr.*).

Other Proprietary Names

Blocanol *(Fin.)*; Proflax *(Arg.)*; Temserin *(Ger., Greece)*; Timacor *(Denm., Fr.)*; Timoptic *(Canad., Switz., USA)*.

6324-y

Tolamolol Hydrochloride.

UK 6558-01; Tolamidol Hydrochloride. 4-[2-(2-Hydroxy-3-*o*-tolyloxypropylamino)ethoxy]benzamide hydrochloride.

$C_{19}H_{24}N_2O_4,HCl = 380.9$.

CAS — 38103-61-6 (tolamolol) [50714-52-8 (+); 50714-51-7 (−)]; 51599-37-2 (hydrochloride, ±).

Tolamolol hydrochloride is a beta-adrenoceptor blocking agent with actions similar to those of propranolol; it has been reported to have a cardioselective action. It was used in the treatment of hypertension, angina pectoris, and cardiac arrhythmias until long-term toxicity studies in *animals* revealed a possible carcinogenic effect.

Long term *animal* toxicity studies on tolamolol at doses 25 to 50 times maximum have shown possible danger of malignant tumours of breast and liver according to information provided by *Pfizer*.— P. Lund-Johansen, *Br. J. clin. Pharmac.*, 1977, *4*, 141.

Cardiac disorders. Studies of tolamolol in cardiac disorders: E. A. Amsterdam *et al.*, *Am. J. Cardiol.*, 1976, *38*, 195; D. Jewitt *et al.*, *Postgrad. med. J.*, 1976, *52*, *Suppl.* 7, 67; V. F. Miscia *et al.*, *Milit. Med.*, 1978, *143*, 629.

Hypertension. Studies of tolamolol in hypertension: K. Harno, *J. int. med. Res.*, 1977, *5*, 100; P. A. Routledge *et al.*, *Eur. J. clin. Pharmac.*, 1977, *11*, 159; *idem*, *12*, 171; N. D. Vlachakis *et al.*, *Clin. Pharmac. Ther.*, 1977, *21*, 9; N. D. Vlachakis and M. Mendlowitz, *Curr. ther. Res.*, 1979, *25*, 768.

For previous references to studies on tolamolol hydrochloride, see Martindale 27th Edn, p. 1823.

Manufacturers

Pfizer, UK.

6325-j

Toliprolol Hydrochloride.

Kö 592; ICI 45763. 1-(Isopropylamino)-3-(*m*-tolyloxy)propan-2-ol hydrochloride.

$C_{13}H_{21}NO_2,HCl = 259.8$.

CAS — 2933-94-0 (toliprolol); 306-11-6 (hydrochloride).

Adverse Effects, Treatment, and Precautions. As for Propranolol Hydrochloride, p.1325.

Uses. Toliprolol hydrochloride is a beta-adrenoceptor blocking agent (see p.1324) with general properties similar to those of propranolol hydrochloride (see p.1329). It has been given in doses of 25 to 100 mg thrice daily for angina pectoris and 10 to 20 mg thrice daily for cardiac arrhythmias.

References: R. Mendez and E. Kabela, *Lancet*, 1966, *1*, 908; R. G. Shanks *et al.* (letter), *Nature*, 1966, *212*, 88; P. Somani, *Am. Heart J.*, 1969, *77*, 63.

Proprietary Names

Doberol *(Boehringer Ingelheim, Ger.)*; Sinorytmal *(Giulini, Ger.)*.

Prostaglandins

8070-d

'Prostaglandin' was the name given by U.S. von Euler (*Klin. Wschr.*, 1935, *14*, 1182; *J. Physiol., Lond.*, 1936, *88*, 213) to a substance found in extracts and secretions from the human prostate gland and seminal vesicles which greatly lowered the blood pressure after injection into animals and stimulated the isolated intestine and uterus. This biological activity is now known to be due to several closely related compounds which are widely distributed in animal tissues. They are synthesised in the body from unsaturated fatty acids. They have also been chemically synthesised.

An important source of prostaglandins is the cortex of a Gorgonia coral, *Plexaura homomalla* or sea whip, from the Caribbean, which contains considerably higher concentrations of prostaglandins or their esters than those found in mammalian tissues.

In mammals, the most common precursor of prostaglandins is arachidonic acid, whereas eicosapentaenoic acid is a predominant precursor in fish and marine animals. The prostaglandins are all derivatives of the carbon skeleton 7-(2-octylcyclopentyl)heptanoic acid (also known as prostanoic acid). All natural prostaglandins have a double bond at position 1,2 and a hydroxyl group at position 3 of the octyl side-chain. Depending on the structure of the cyclopentane ring, the main series of prostaglandins are distinguished by the letters E, F, A, B, C, and D; the members of each series are distinguished by subscript numbers which indicate degrees of unsaturation in the side-chains—hence, those derived from eicosatrienoic acid have the subscript 1, those derived from arachidonic acid have the subscript 2, and those derived from eicosapentaenoic acid have the subscript 3, according to the degree of unsaturation of these precursors.

The E and F groups are often known as primary groups and include alprostadil (prostaglandin E_1), dinoprostone (prostaglandin E_2), prostaglandin E_3, prostaglandin $F_{1\alpha}$, dinoprost (prostaglandin $F_{2\alpha}$), and prostaglandin $F_{3\alpha}$. The A,B, and C groups (which are often known as secondary groups) are derived from the E group.

Further elucidation of the metabolism of arachidonic acid led to the important discovery of thromboxane A_2 (TXA_2) which has a fundamental role in inducing platelet aggregation and constricting arterial smooth muscle, and epoprostenol (prostacyclin; PGX; PGI_2) which, in contrast, causes vasodilatation and prevents platelet aggregation, thereby protecting the blood vessel wall from deposition of platelet aggregates.

Individual prostaglandins vary greatly in their activities and potencies; their actions also depend on the animal species and the tissues in which they are acting, and entirely opposite actions may be elicited with very small structural changes in the molecule.

The range of physiological and pharmacological activities of the prostaglandins is very wide but their fundamental actions include inhibiton or stimulation of smooth muscle contraction and inhibition of the release of noradrenaline or modulation of its effects at neuroeffector sites. They affect the uterus, the cardiovascular system, the gastro-intestinal system, the nervous system, the urinary system, and metabolic processes. It has been suggested that some of the effects of some prostaglandins are mediated within cells by activation of adenyl cyclase (adenylate cyclase) and the production of cyclic adenosine monophosphate. Prostaglandins can also be released from cells or tissues as a result of endocrine, neural, or mechanical stimuli and may themselves stimulate adenyl cyclase (adenylate cyclase).

The mode of action and many of the adverse effects of anti-inflammatory analgesics such as aspirin or indomethacin have been found to depend on the inhibition of endogenous prostaglandin synthesis. For the prophylaxis of thrombosis, attempts have been made to exploit their ability to inhibit thromboxane A_2 but avoid their associated ability to inhibit prostacyclin (epoprostenol), with the aim of reducing inappropriate coagulation within vessel walls (for further details, see Aspirin, p.240).

Synthetic analogues of prostaglandins have been developed with the aim of obtaining compounds which are more stable, have a longer duration of action, and a more specific effect. These include a methylated derivative of alprostadil (gemeprost, p.1360), the 15-methyl derivative of dinoprost (carboprost, p.1354), and the 15-methyl derivative of dinoprostone (arbaprostil, p.1353).

General reviews of prostaglandins: H. A. Gross *et al.*, *Archs gen. Psychiat.*, 1977, *34*, 1189 (neurophysiological and psychiatric implications); A. A. Mathé *et al.*, *New Engl. J. Med.*, 1977, *296*, 850 and 910 (function in the lung); *Postgrad. med. J.*, 1977, *53*, 641–67 (symposium); P. Needleman and G. Kaley, *New Engl. J. Med.*, 1978, *298*, 1122 (cardiac aspects); S. M. M. Karim and K. Hillier, *Br. med. Bull.*, 1979, *35*, 173 (reproduction); T. A. Miller and E. D. Jacobson, *Gut*, 1979, *20*, 75 (gastro-intestinal cytoprotection); S. Moncada and J. R. Vane, *New Engl. J. Med.*, 1979, *300*, 1142 (arachidonic acid metabolites); K. Hillier, *Prescribers' J.*, 1980, *20*, 142 (clinical use); *Br. med. J.*, 1981, *282*, 418 (role in obstetrics); *Lancet*, 1981, *2*, 24 (immunological aspects).

The Prostaglandins, S.M.M. Karim (Ed.), Lancaster, MTP Press, 1972; *Prostaglandins and Reproduction*, S.M.M. Karim (Ed.), Lancaster, MTP Press, 1975; *Prostaglandins: Chemical and Biochemical Aspects*, S.M.M. Karim (Ed.), Lancaster, MTP Press, 1976; *Prostaglandins: Physiological, Pharmacological and Pathological Aspects*, S.M.M. Karim (Ed.), Lancaster, MTP Press, 1976; *Practical Applications of Prostaglandins and their Synthesis Inhibitors*, S.M.M. Karim (Ed.), Lancaster, MTP Press, 1979.

8071-n

Alprostadil. U-10136; PGE_1; Prostaglandin E_1. (*E*)-(8*R*,11*R*,12*R*,15*S*)-11,15-Dihydroxy-9-oxoprost-13-enoic acid; 7-{(1*R*,2*R*,3*R*)-3-Hydroxy-2-[(*E*)-(3*S*)-3-hydroxy-oct-1-enyl]-5-oxocyclopentyl}heptanoic acid.
$C_{20}H_{34}O_5$=354.5.

CAS — 745-65-3.

Adverse Effects. Adverse effects reported following the use of alprostadil include apnoea, hypotension, headache, flushing, and transient fever and diarrhoea. Other adverse effects reported include bradycardia, tachycardia, cardiac arrest, oedema, convulsions, hypokalaemia and disseminated intravascular coagulation.

Lesions of the ductus arteriosus, possibly due to a direct effect of overstretching, were found in 3 out of 4 infants who had been treated with alprostadil for ductus-dependent cardiac problems. Although the dilating effect on the ductus arteriosus would still be useful in emergency treatment, the hazards needed evaluating.— A. J. Moulaert *et al.* (letter), *Lancet*, 1977, *1*, 703.

Effects on bones. Bone lesions resembling cortical hyperostosis occurred in 2 infants following long-term therapy with alprostadil for cyanotic congenital heart disease.— K. Ueda *et al.*, *J. Pediat.*, 1980, *97*, 834.

Uses. Alprostadil is a prostaglandin of the E series (see p.1353). It is used temporarily to maintain the patency of the ductus arteriosus in the management of congenital heart disease. It is administered by intravenous drip or constant rate infusion pump beginning with doses of 100 nanograms per kg body-weight per minute; doses should be reduced as soon as possible. Alprostadil has also been used in peripheral vascular disease.

Angiography. In 10 patients with tumours of the extremities the use of alprostadil as an adjunct in angiography improved the visualisation of small normal muscular arteries in all patients but decreased visualisation of the tumour vessels in 9. Alprostadil appeared to have little value in improving the diagnostic information obtained in angiographic studies of tumours of the extremities.— K. Jonsson *et al.*, *Am. J. Roentg.*, 1978, *130*, 7.

Blood storage. The use of alprostadil in the preparation and storage of platelet concentrates.— H. Shio and P. W. Ramwell, *Science*, 1972, *175*, 536; G. A. Becker *et al.*, *ibid.*, 538.

Cardiac disorders. A review and discussion on the diagnosis and management of congenital heart disease. The most exciting new advance in the management of congenital heart disease concerns the use of alprostadil for dilatation of the ductus arteriosus in various clinical syndromes. In patients with pulmonary atresia or severe pulmonary stenosis with ductal-dependent pulmonary blood flow, dilatation of the patent ductus with alprostadil has been shown to be extremely valuable for increasing systemic oxygen saturation and for providing clinical stabilisation until surgery can be performed. Infusion of alprostadil has also been useful in the coarctation syndrome where dilatation of the ductus arteriosus results in an increase in blood flow through the area of the coarcted segment to the lower part of the body. Side-effects of alprostadil infusion have not been a severe problem. Apnoea, which may occur in up to 10% of patients receiving an intravenous infusion, can usually be abolished by decreasing the usual infusion-rate of 100 ng per kg body-weight per minute to 25 to 50 ng per kg per minute; a febrile response, which may also develop in up to 10% of patients, is not usually a severe degree of temperature elevation and abates rapidly following discontinuation of the drug.— T. P. Graham, *Pediat. Clins N. Am.*, 1978, *25*, 707.

Further references to the use of alprostadil in congenital heart disease: R. B. Elliott *et al.*, *Lancet*, 1975, *1*, 140; N. C. Christensen and J. Fabricus (letter), *ibid.*, *2*, 406; D. J. Radford *et al.* (letter), *ibid.*, 1976, *2*, 95; M. A. Heymann and A. M. Rudolph, *Pediatrics*, 1977, *59*, 325; J. M. Neutze *et al.*, *Circulation*, 1977, *55*, 238.

Peripheral vascular disease. Alprostadil given by infusion over 72 hours in sodium chloride injection via a central venous catheter at an initial rate of 6 ng per kg body-weight per minute increased after 12 hours in the absence of side-effects to 10 ng per kg per minute to 26 patients with severe Raynaud's phenomenon and ischaemic skin changes produced appreciable symptomatic improvement in 25 and 21 reported maintained improvement after 2 weeks; reduction in pain and the severity and frequency of vasospasm were particularly noted. Side-effects were minimal but included headache (5), flushing (8), pain in the shoulder on the side of the infusion (1), mild diarrhoea (1), and symptomatic postural hypotension resolving when the infusion was stopped (1).— P. C. Clifford *et al.*, *Br. med. J.*, 1980, *281*, 1031. Comment.— A. J. M. Cleophas *et al.* (letter), *ibid.*, 1981, *282*, 1476.

Further references to alprostadil in peripheral vascular disease: H. Beitner *et al.*, *Acta derm.-vener., Stockh.*, 1980, *60*, 425; B. J. Pardy *et al.* (letter), *Lancet*, 1980, *2*, 1312.

Proprietary Preparations

Prostin VR Sterile Solution *(Upjohn, UK)*. Alprostadil, available as solution for preparing intravenous infusions, containing 500 µg per ml in dehydrated alcohol, in ampoules of 1 ml. Store in a refrigerator.

8072-h

Arbaprostil. U-42842; 15-Me-PGE_2; Methyldinoprostone; 15(*R*)-15-Methylprostaglandin E_2. (5*Z*,13*E*)-(8*R*,11*R*,12*R*,15*R*)-11,15-Dihydroxy-15-methyl-9-oxoprosta-5,13-dienoic acid; (*Z*)-7-{(1*R*,2*R*,3*R*)-3-Hydroxy-2-[(*E*)-(3*R*)-3-hydroxy-3-methyloct-1-enyl]-5-oxocyclopentyl}hept-5-enoic acid.
$C_{21}H_{34}O_5$=366.5.

CAS — 55028-70-1.

8073-m

Arbaprostil Methyl. U-38833. The methyl ester of arbaprostil.
$C_{22}H_{36}O_5$=380.5.

The stability at room temperature of arbaprostil methyl was greatly increased by dissolving in triacetin and filling into soft gelatin capsules.— S. H. Yalkowsky and T. J. Roseman, *J. pharm. Sci.*, 1979, *68*, 114.

Uses. Arbaprostil, a synthetic 15-methyl analogue of dinoprostone (see p.1357), is a prostaglandin of the E series (see p.1353). Its actions are reported to be similar to but more prolonged than those of dinoprost and dinoprostone; the presence of the methyl group delays inactivation by enzymic dehydrogenation.

Arbaprostil and its methyl ester, arbaprostil methyl, have been used in doses of about 150 µg by mouth 3 to 4 times daily to reduce gastric secretion in patients with gastric ulcer. The methyl ester of the 15(*S*)-isomer has been used similarly and has also been given for the termination of pregnancy.

Gastric and duodenal ulcer. In a double-blind trial in 20 patients with proved gastric ulcer 10 received arbaprostil 150 µg by mouth every 6 hours for 2 weeks and 10 received a placebo. The mean ulcer healing-rate was 63.3% in the treated group compared with only 17.1% in the control group. The only side-effect of arbaprostil was mild intermittent diarrhoea in the first 3 days of treatment.— W. P. Fung and S. M. M. Karim, *Med. J. Aust.*, 1976, *2*, 127. See also S. M. M. Karim (letter), *Br. med. J.*, 1974, *3*, 169; W. -P. Fung *et al.*, *Lancet*, 1974, *2*, 10 (use of arbaprostil methyl).

In a 2-week double-blind study involving 77 patients with gastro-duodenal ulcer healing of ulcers occurred in 14 of 25 given arbaprostil methyl 2 µg per kg body-weight thrice daily, in 17 of 26 given 15(*S*)-15-methylprostaglandin E_2 methyl ester (U-35960) 1.5 µg per kg thrice daily, and in 12 of 26 given a placebo. The 15(*S*)-isomer appeared to be more potent than arbaprostil methyl. Diarrhoea necessitated the reduction in dosage in some patients receiving the active medications.— K. Gibiński *et al.*, *Gut*, 1977, *18*, 636. Further study indicating that gastric ulcers appear to be totally unaffected but that duodenal ulcer healing is accelerated.— J. Rybicka and K. Gibiński, *Scand. J. Gastroenterol.*, 1978, *13*, 155. See also S. M. M. Karim *et al.*, *Br. med. J.*, 1973, *1*, 143.

Further references to arbaprostil and arbaprostil methyl in gastroenterology: C. Johansson *et al.* (letter), *Lancet*, 1979, *1*, 317; B. Kollberg and C. Johansson, *Scand. J. Gastroenterol.*, 1979, *14*, 337; S. J. Konturek *et al.*, *ibid.*, 813; W. Peterson *et al.*, *Dig. Dis. Scis*, 1979, *24*, 381; G. Vantrappen *et al.*, *Gastroenterology*, 1980, *78*, 1283.

Termination of pregnancy. References to the use of 15(*S*)-15-methylprostaglandin E_2 and its methyl ester for termination of pregnancy: S. M. M. Karim and S. S. Ratnam (letter), *Br. med. J.*, 1974, *4*, 161; W. E. Brenner *et al.*, *Fert. Steril.*, 1975, *26*, 369; S. M. M. Karim *et al.*, *Singapore J. Obstet. Gynaec.*, 1980, *11*, 7.

Manufacturers
Upjohn, UK.

8074-b

Carboprost. U-32921; 15-Me-$PGF_{2\alpha}$; Methyldinoprost; 15(*S*)-15-Methylprostaglandin $F_{2\alpha}$. (5*Z*,13*E*)-(8*R*,9*S*,11*R*,12*R*,15*S*)-9,11,15-Trihydroxy-15-methylprosta-5,13-dienoic acid; (*Z*)-7-{(1*R*,2*R*,3*R*,5*S*)-3,5-Dihydroxy-2-[(*E*)-(3*S*)-3-hydroxy-3-methyloct-1-enyl]cyclopentyl}hept-5-enoic acid.
$C_{21}H_{36}O_5$=368.5.

CAS — 35700-23-3.

8075-v

Carboprost Methyl. U-36384. The methyl ester of carboprost.
$C_{22}H_{38}O_5$=382.5.

CAS — 35700-21-1.

8076-g

Carboprost Trometamol. Carboprost Tromethamine (*U.S.P.*); U-32921E. The 2-amino-2-(hydroxymethyl)propane-1,3-diol salt of carboprost.
$C_{21}H_{36}O_5,C_4H_{11}NO_3$=489.6.

CAS — 58551-69-2.

Pharmacopoeias. In *U.S.*

A solution in alcohol is dextrorotatory. **Store** at 2° to 8°.

Adverse Effects, Treatment, and Precautions. As for Dinoprost Trometamol, p.1355.

Uses. Carboprost, a synthetic 15-methyl analogue of dinoprost (see p.1355), is a prostaglandin of the F series (see p.1353). Its actions are reported to be similar to but more prolonged than those of dinoprost (see p.1356); the presence of the methyl group delays inactivation by enzymic dehydrogenation.

For the termination of pregnancy carboprost has been given in doses of about 200 to 300 µg intramuscularly at 3-hour intervals. Carboprost has also been administered extra-amniotically in doses of about 1 mg and intra-amniotically in doses of 2.5 mg.

For vaginal administration carboprost methyl has been used. Pessaries containing 1.5 mg have been administered every 3 hours or a single sustained-release preparation containing 3 mg has been employed. An intravaginal device of silicone rubber impregnated with 0.25 to 1% of carboprost methyl has also been used to terminate pregnancy.

Termination of pregnancy. In a multicentre multinational study under the direction of the WHO 515 patients undergoing abortion at 10 to 20 weeks' gestation were given carboprost intramuscularly, 200 µg initially, then 300 µg every 3 hours for up to 30 hours. Abortion occurred in 79.3% of the patients within 24 hours and in 84.9% within 30 hours, but was judged complete in only 35%. Despite the prophylactic use of diphenoxylate and atropine there was a high incidence of vomiting and diarrhoea which rendered the procedure of limited value as a primary method. Other side-effects were cervical laceration (3 patients), flushing (14.2%), and occasional dyspnoea and chest pain.— *Am. J. Obstet. Gynec.*, 1977, *129*, 593. In a multicentre multinational study under the direction of the WHO 660 patients undergoing abortion at 10 to 20 weeks' gestation were given a single extra-amniotic injection of carboprost 920 µg. Abortion occurred in 72.6% within 24 hours and in 80.3% within 36 hours but was judged complete in only 31.7%. Diarrhoea and vomiting, though common, were generally not severe; other occasional side-effects were dyspnoea, chest pain, flushing, headache, shivering, and cervical laceration.— *ibid.*, 597. In a multicentre multinational study under the direction of the WHO 311 patients undergoing abortion at 15 to 20 weeks' gestation were given a single intra-amniotic injection of carboprost 2.5 mg. Abortion occurred in 76.4% within 24 hours and in 95.2% within 48 hours. In a second study the effect of carboprost 2.5 mg intra-amniotically was compared with that of dinoprost 40 mg intra-amniotically; the 48-hour success-rates were 95.6% and 81.7% respectively. In a third study the effect of carboprost 2.5 mg was compared with that of dinoprost 50 mg; the 48-hour success-rates were 92.8% and 86.6% respectively. Abortion was judged complete in 50 to 55% of patients in the 3 studies. Nausea and vomiting were significantly more common after carboprost than after dinoprost, but were within acceptable limits; dyspnoea, chest pain, and flushing occurred occasionally.— *ibid.*, 601.

In a multicentre multinational study under the direction of the WHO 310 patients undergoing abortion at 13 to 20 weeks' gestation were given vaginal pessaries each containing carboprost methyl 1.5 mg. These were administered at 3-hourly intervals for up to 24 hours; diphenoxylate hydrochloride 5 mg was given concomitantly with the first 3 pessaries to reduce the frequency of diarrhoea. Abortion occurred in 88.4% of patients within 24 hours and in 91.9% within 30 hours. Abortion was judged complete in 49.9% of patients, but the proportion of complete abortions was significantly higher when the gestational age of the foetus was over 16 weeks. Diarrhoea and vomiting were the most common adverse effects.— M. Bygdeman *et al.*, *Contraception*, 1977, *16*, 175, per *Int. pharm. Abstr.*, 1978, *15*, 321.

A review of the termination of abnormal intra-uterine pregnancy with prostaglandins, including carboprost.— S. M. M. Karim *et al.*, *Singapore J. Obstet. Gynaec.*, 1980, *11*, 7.

Further references to the use of carboprost and carboprost methyl for the termination of pregnancy: U. Borell *et al.*, *Contraception*, 1976, *13*, 87 (pessaries); C. A. Ballard and L. Slaughter, *ibid.*, *14*, 541 (intramuscular); N. H. Lauersen and K. H. Wilson, *Am. J. Obstet. Gynec.*, 1976, *124*, 425 (intramuscular); J. R. Dingfelder *et al.*, *ibid.*, *125*, 821 (intra-amniotic); I. Z. MacKenzie and M. P. Embrey, *Prostaglandins*, 1976, *12*, 443 (extra-amniotic); M. Bygdeman *et al.*, *Contraception*, 1977, *15*, 129 (pessaries); N. H. Lauersen and K. H. Wilson, *Am. J. Obstet. Gynec.*, 1977, *127*, 784 (impregnated vaginal silicone device); P. G. Stubblefield, *Contraception*, 1977, *15*, 175 (impregnated vaginal silicone device); C. A. Ballard *et al.*, *ibid.*, 1978, *17*, 383 (pessaries); G. Kinra *et al.*, *ibid.*, 455 (pessaries); S. Tejuja *et al.*, *ibid.*, *18*, 641 (extra- and intra-amniotic).

Menstrual induction. In 201 women with an apparently normal pregnancy and amenorrhoea of 49 days or less administration of carboprost methyl as a single vaginal pessary containing 2, 2.5, or 3 mg induced bleeding in all patients and all but 1 patient subsequently aborted. Complete abortion occurred in 76.3% of 38, 85.7% of 35, and 94.5% of 128 given the 3 dosage regimens of 2, 2.5, and 3 mg respectively. Bleeding generally started 4 to 6 hours after the start of treatment and lasted for 10 to 14 days. Vomiting and diarrhoea were common but only 4 patients developed clinical signs of endometritis.— K. Green *et al.*, *Contraception*, 1978, *18*, 551.

In 80 women with a pregnancy of less than 56 days given a single vaginal pessary containing carboprost methyl 3 mg a successful outcome (judged by evidence of sustained uterine bleeding characteristic of menses induction associated with a progressive, significant and sustained decline in HCG concentrations over a 14-day post-treatment period, a negative pregnancy test after 14 days, and no need for surgical intervention during the follow-up) occurred in 56. The successful induction of menses was associated with a more rapid increase in the plasma-carboprost concentration and a significantly higher mean concentration than in those considered as failures. The experience accumulated to date indicates that a vaginal delivery system for carboprost methyl that releases the drug faster and in a more predictable fashion than the pessary is required for the successful induction of menses.— C. H. Spilman *et al.*, *Contraception*, 1980, *21*, 353.

Further references to carboprost methyl and menstrual induction: M. Bygdeman *et al.*, *Obstet. Gynec.*, 1976, *48*, 221; S. L. Corson and R. J. Bolognese, *Fert. Steril.*, 1977, *28*, 1056; J. Robins, *ibid.*, 1048; J. H. Duenhoelter *et al.*, *Contraception*, 1978, *17*, 51.

Uterine atony. The intramuscular use of carboprost to correct post-partum uterine atony.— S. L. Corson and R. J. Bolognese, *Am. J. Obstet. Gynec.*, 1977, *129*, 918.

Preparations

Carboprost Tromethamine Injection *(U.S.P.).* A sterile solution of carboprost trometamol in aqueous solution which may contain benzyl alcohol, sodium chloride, and trometamol. Potency is expressed in terms of the equivalent amount of carboprost. pH 7 to 8. Store at 2° to 8°.

Proprietary Names
Prostin/15M *(Upjohn, Canad.; Upjohn, USA).*

8077-q

Cloprostenol Sodium *(B.P. Vet.).* ICI-80996. Sodium (±)-(*Z*)-7-{(1*R*,2*R*,3*R*,5*S*)-2-[(*E*)-(3*R*)-4-(3-chlorophenoxy)-3-hydroxybut-1-enyl]-3,5-dihydroxycyclopentyl}hept-5-enoate.
$C_{22}H_{28}ClNaO_6$=446.9.

CAS — 40665-92-7 (cloprostenol); 55028-72-3 (sodium salt).

A white or almost white amorphous hygroscopic powder. Freely **soluble** in water, alcohol, and methyl alcohol; practically insoluble in acetone. **Store** in airtight containers. Protect from light.

Uses. Cloprostenol sodium is a synthetic prostaglandin derivative of the F series (see p.1353). It is used as a luteolytic agent in veterinary medicine.

Preparations

Cloprostenol Injection *(B.P. Vet.).* A sterile solution of cloprostenol sodium in Water for Injections; it may contain suitable buffering agents. Sterilise by autoclaving or by filtration. Protect from light. Potency is expressed in terms of cloprostenol.

Proprietary Names
Estrumate *(veterinary) (ICI Pharmaceuticals, UK)*; Planate *(veterinary) (ICI Pharmaceuticals, UK).*

8078-p

Delprostenate. ONO-1052. Methyl (2*E*,5*Z*)-7-{(1*R*,2*R*,3*R*,5*S*)-2-[(*E*)-(3*R*)-4-(3-chlorophenoxy)-3-hydroxybut-1-enyl]-3,5-dihydroxycyclopentyl}hepta-2,5-dienoate.
$C_{23}H_{29}ClO_6$=436.9.

CAS — 62524-99-6.

Delprostenate is a synthetic prostaglandin derivative of the F series (see p.1353) with potential use as a luteolytic agent in veterinary medicine.

Manufacturers
Ono, Jap.

8079-s

Deprostil. AY-22469. (8*R*,12*S*)-15-Hydroxy-15-methyl-9-oxoprostanoic acid; 7-[(1*R*,2*S*)-2-(3-Hydroxy-3-methyloctyl)-5-oxocyclopentyl]heptanoic acid. $C_{21}H_{38}O_4$=354.5.

CAS — 33813-84-2.

Deprostil is a synthetic prostaglandin derivative with potential use as an anti-secretory and anti-ulcer agent.

Manufacturers
Ayerst, USA.

8080-h

16,16-Dimethylprostaglandin E_2. 16,16-Dimethyldinoprostone. (5*Z*,13*E*)-(8*R*,11*R*,12*R*,15*R*)-11,15-Dihydroxy-16,16-dimethyl-9-oxoprosta-5,13-dienoic acid; (*Z*)-7-{(1*R*,2*R*,3*R*)-3-Hydroxy-2-[(*E*)-(3*R*)-3-hydroxy-4,4-dimethyloct-1-enyl]-5-oxocyclopentyl}hept-5-enoic acid.
$C_{22}H_{36}O_5$=380.5.

CAS — 39746-25-3.

The stability at room temperature of 16,16-dimethylprostaglandin E_2 was greatly increased by dissolving in triacetin and filling into soft gelatin capsules.— S. H. Yalkowsky and T. J. Roseman, *J. pharm. Sci.*, 1979, *68*, 114.

Uses. 16,16-Dimethylprostaglandin E_2 is a synthetic prostaglandin derivative of the E series (see p.1353). It has been used for the termination of pregnancy and as an inhibitor of gastric secretion.

Gastro-intestinal disorders. The effect of 16,16-dimethylprostaglandin E_2 on meal-stimulated gastric acid secretion and serum gastrin in duodenal ulcer patients.— A. F. Ippoliti *et al.*, *Gastroenterology*, 1976, *70*, 488.

The effect of 16,16-dimethylprostaglandin E_2 on stimulated gastric secretion was examined in a controlled study of 10 healthy subjects over a 4-week period. Subjects received dimethylprostaglandin E_2 127 µg by mouth either as a capsule or liquid. Gastric stimulation was achieved by administration of histamine acid phosphate 15 µg per kg body-weight per hour for 2 hours. Results were very similar for both capsule and liquid; dimethylprostaglandin E_2 given by mouth significantly inhibited stimulated gastric secretion. After administration of the capsule the volume of gastric secretion decreased by about 37%, acid concentration by 39%, and acid output by 60%.— D. E. Wilson *et al.*, *Ann. intern. Med.*, 1976, *84*, 688.

Evidence to suggest that administration of 16,16-dimethylprostaglandin E_2 to 20 patients markedly suppressed gastric acid secretion and, in comparison to a placebo, accelerated cicatristation of duodenal but not of gastric ulcers. Two patients complained of eyes smarting, and 4 showed some excitation.— J. Rybicka and K. Gibiński, *Scand. J. Gastroenterol.*, 1978, *13*, 155.

Evidence from studies with 16,16-dimethylprostaglandin E_2 in healthy subjects, that a low oral dose of prostaglandin analogue may prevent the gastro-intestinal untoward effects of non-steroidal anti-inflammatory analgesics.— P. Müller *et al.* (letter), *Lancet*, 1981, *1*, 333.

Termination of pregnancy. Studies with the *p*-benzaldehyde semicarbazone ester of 16,16-dimethylprostaglandin E_2 for the termination of pregnancy: S. M. M. Karim and S. S. Ratnam, *Br. J. Obstet. Gynaec.*, 1977, *84*, 135; S. M. M. Karim *et al.*, *ibid.*, 269.

Menstrual induction. A report of the use of 16,16-dimethylprostaglandin E_2 as pessaries for menstrual induction in 28 pregnant women.— I. Z. Mackenzie *et al.*, *Lancet*, 1978, *1*, 1223. See also V. Lundström *et al.*, *Contraception*, 1977, *16*, 167.

8081-m

Dinoprost Trometamol. $PGF_{2\alpha}$ THAM; U-14 583E; Dinoprost Tromethamine; Prostaglandin $F_{2\alpha}$ Trometamol. The trometamol salt of (5*Z*,13*E*)-(8*R*,9*S*,11*R*,12*R*,15*S*)-9,11,15-trihydroxyprosta-5,13-dienoic acid; The 2-amino-2-(hydroxymethyl)propane-1,3-diol salt of (*Z*)-7-{(1*R*,2*R*,3*R*,5*S*)-3,5-dihydroxy-2-[(*E*)-(3*S*)-3-hydroxyoct-1-enyl]cyclopentyl}hept-5-enoic acid. $C_{20}H_{34}O_5,C_4H_{11}NO_3$=475.6.

CAS — 551-11-1 (dinoprost); 38562-01-5 (dinoprost trometamol).

A white to off-white very hygroscopic crystalline powder. Dinoprost trometamol 1.3 µg is approximately equivalent to 1 µg of dinoprost. M.p. about 100°. **Soluble** about 1 in 5 of water. Relatively insensitive to light, heat, and alkalis. **Store** in airtight containers.

The solubility of dinoprost trometamol increased 35-fold between pH 5.0 and 5.2. This sharp increase was attributed to the formation of micelles, which was found to be dependent upon both pH and concentration. At concentrations below 10 mmol per litre, the pK_a was 4.9 (monomer); in the micellar state the pK_a was 5.6.— T. J. Roseman and S. H. Yalkowsky, *J. pharm. Sci.*, 1973, *62*, 1680.

Adverse Effects. The incidence of adverse reactions to dinoprost trometamol is dose related. Nausea, vomiting, and diarrhoea occur commonly at doses required to terminate pregnancy by the intravenous route, but are less common after the extra-amniotic route for termination or the intravenous route for induction of labour. Transient cardiovascular symptoms have included flushing, shivering, headache, and dizziness; convulsions and EEG changes have also occurred rarely. Local tissue irritation and erythema may follow intravenous administration; the erythema disappears 2 to 5 hours after infusion. Temporary pyrexia and raised white-cell count may occur but generally revert to normal after termination of the infusion. Local infection may follow intra- or extra-amniotic therapy. Uterine rupture has occurred rarely.

A report of cyanosis occurring at the sites of injection of dinoprost in a patient undergoing induction of abortion. It was suggested that dinoprost was contra-indicated in patients with a history of possible peripheral vascular disturbance.— G. Roberts *et al.* (letter), *Lancet*, 1972, *2*, 425.

Side-effects were evaluated in 626 patients undergoing abortion (usually in the second trimester), using extra-amniotic or intra-amniotic dinoprost or dinoprostone, often with oxytocin. Vomiting occurred in 291, diarrhoea in 28, pyrexia in 34, transient hypotension (fall in systolic blood pressure of at least 20 mmHg) in 25, bronchospasm in 2, and blood loss exceeding 250 ml in 68 (38 lost more than 500 ml). None of 8 taking anticonvulsants developed convulsions. Of 143 patients followed 6 to 8 weeks after abortion 3 had curettage for excessive bleeding; in the remainder vaginal bleeding had ceased within 6 weeks. In 115 patients menstruation had been re-established at the time of follow-up.— I. Z. MacKenzie *et al.*, *Br. med. J.*, 1974, *4*, 683.

Four patients had been seen with unexpected cervical incompetence leading to extreme premature labour and perinatal death. Each patient had previously undergone termination of pregnancy by means of intra-amniotic injection of dinoprost.— J. Murray (letter), *Med. J. Aust.*, 1974, *2*, 717. A comparison between 204 pregnancies in 168 women who had previously undergone prostaglandin-induced abortion (dinoprostone in 129) and 612 control pregnancies showed that in the 127 pregnancies that came to term morbidity was not greatly different from that in controls. Spontaneous abortions in the study group were slightly more common than in controls and the occurrence of 2 cases of placenta praevia suggested the need for watchfulness.— I. Z. MacKenzie and K. Hillier, *Br. med. J.*, 1977, *2*, 1114.

Sudden collapse and eventual death in 2 women following the use of dinoprost intra-amniotically to induce abortion at approximately 16 weeks' gestation. The first patient, a 35-year-old woman (gravida 9, para 6, abortus 2), remained comatose for 5 months until death, which was attributed to a pulmonary embolus along with 'severe anoxic brain damage' suffered during a cardiorespiratory arrest occurring after administration of dinoprost; the second patient, a 26-year-old woman (gravida 3, para 2) remained comatose for approximately 1 month until death and the autopsy report described extensive cortical necrosis in the brain and 2 myocardial infarcts. The authors were now aware of 9 deaths following the use of dinoprost to induce abortion but the etiology for the sudden collapse is still unknown.— W. Cates and H. V. F. Jordaan, *Am. J. Obstet. Gynec.*, 1979, *133*, 398. See also W. Cates *et al.*, *ibid.*, 1977, *127*, 219.

Bronchospasm. In 10 healthy subjects the inhalation of a mean of 2.2 µmol of dinoprost caused a mean reduction (rapid and transient) of 44% in specific airway conductance; in 10 patients with reversible asthma a mean reduction (slower and prolonged) of 62% in conductance was achieved by a mean of 0.275 nmol of dinoprost. The asthmatic patients were less than 10 times more sensitive to histamine than were the controls. Dinoprostone slightly increased conductance in the controls and had a variable effect in the asthmatic patients in whom it only partly and variably counteracted the bronchoconstrictor effect of dinoprost.— A. A. Mathé *et al.*, *Br. med. J.*, 1973, *1*, 193.

In 5 of 8 healthy subjects inhaling 0.5 ml of a solution of dinoprost 50 µg per ml (as the tromethamine salt) coughing and retrosternal tightness was associated with a significant decrease in airways conductance in the absence of changes in flow-rate or FEV_1, while the remaining 3 suffered dyspnoea and wheezing associated with no change in conductance and a fall in flow-rate and FEV_1. In 5 patients with asthma marked and prolonged bronchoconstriction was generally associated with a reduction in conductance, flow-rate, and FEV_1.— K. R. Patel, *Postgrad. med. J.*, 1976, *52*, 275.

Convulsions. Convulsions occurred in 5 of 320 women who were given dinoprost intra-amniotically for the termination of pregnancy during the second trimester. The initial dose was 30 mg followed by 15 mg after 24 hours if required, and, if abortion had still not occurred, by 15 mg after another 18 hours. EEG changes were noted in 4 of 8 patients after dinoprost was administered.— R. C. Lyneham *et al.*, *Lancet*, 1973, *2*, 1003. None of 615 patients given prostaglandins for the induction of abortion had convulsions during administration. The group included 7 patients with a history of epileptic seizures who were taking anticonvulsants: 6 were given dinoprostone 0.7 to 2.8 mg in divided doses extra-amniotically and 1 was given 10 mg intra-amniotically followed by another 10 mg after 22 hours. One of these patients suffered seizures before therapy and after abortion.— I. Z. MacKenzie *et al.* (letter), *ibid.*, 1323. No convulsions were observed in a series of 319 normotensive patients given dinoprost or dinoprostone for the induction of labour or in a series of 100 patients given prostaglandins for abortion.— M. Thiery *et al.* (letter), *ibid.*, 1974, *1*, 218. A similar absence of convulsions in 380 patients given dinoprost and dinoprostone.— I. S. Fraser and C. Gray (letter), *ibid.*, 360. No similar abnormalities were observed in 9 patients given 50 mg intra-amniotically.— I. S. Fraser and C. Gray (letter), *ibid.*, 1974, *2*, 49.

Further references to convulsions and EEG changes in patients given dinoprost: R. P. Shearman *et al.*, *Br. J. Obstet. Gynaec.*, 1975, *82*, 314; A. Faden *et al.*, *Obstet. Gynec.*, 1976, *47*, 607; E. Kaplan, *S. Afr. med. J.*, 1978, *53*, 27.

Effects on the blood. In 12 patients in the second trimester of pregnancy, in whom abortion was induced by the extra-amniotic infusion of dinoprost, the prothrombin time was significantly decreased and the concentrations of factors V, VIII, and X were significantly increased. No such changes occurred in 11 patients in whom abortion was performed in the first timester by vacuum aspiration. The changes were probably related to physiological changes; in susceptible patients abortion after the first trimester might give rise to defective haemostasis or thrombo-embolism.— M. H. H. Badraoui *et al.*, *Br. med. J.*, 1973, *1*, 19.

Coagulation changes in 29 women during dinoprost-induced abortion (intra- or extra-amniotic, intravenous, or vaginal) were less than those which occurred with hypertonic sodium chloride solution.— M. H. H. Badraoui *et al.*, *Br. med. J.*, 1973, *4*, 375.

Effects on the gastro-intestinal tract. Intravenous infusion of dinoprost 280 to 860 ng per kg body-weight per minute caused abdominal colic in 8 healthy subjects, 7 of whom passed copious watery stools. Secretion of water, sodium, and chloride into the jejunal lumen 30 to 40 minutes after the start of infusion occurred in 4 subjects at doses above 560 ng per kg. There were no changes in heart-rate or blood pressure.— J. H. Cummings *et al.*, *Nature*, 1973, *243*, 169.

Hypokalaemia. Electrolyte studies in 19 women showed that intra-amniotic injection of dinoprost trometamol was regularly followed by a small decrease in serum-potassium concentration; hypokalaemia was reported in 1 patient who developed cardiac arrhythmias about an hour after injection.— R. L. Burt *et al.*, *Obstet. Gynec.*, 1977, *50*, *Suppl.*, 45S.

Lactation. Lactation lasting for a mean of 6.1 days occurred in 63 of 80 women in whom abortion had been induced by the intra-amniotic injection of dinoprost. Lactation occurred in only 1 of 36 patients in whom abortion was achieved by hysterotomy or suction curette.— I. D. Smith *et al.* (letter), *Nature*, 1972, *240*,

411.

Overdosage. Flushing, severe headache, and nausea in a 30-year-old woman following the injection of a test dose of 2.5 mg of dinoprost was possibly due to the needle not being correctly positioned in the amniotic cavity.— R. Brown (letter), *Br. med. J.*, 1974, *2*, 382. It was likely that at least part of the dose had been injected into the peritoneal cavity.— S. M. M. Karim (letter), *ibid.*, 1974, *3*, 347.

For further reports of adverse effects due to inappropriate systemic absorption of prostaglandins, including the potential hazards in the abortion of hydatidiform moles, see Dinoprostone, p.1357.

Uterine rupture. It was estimated that dinoprost given by the intra-uterine route had been used in over 5000 patients for the termination of late pregnancy, and 13 cases of cervical rupture had been reported.— S. M. M. Karim and S. S. Ratnam (letter), *Br. med. J.*, 1974, *4*, 161.

Treatment of Adverse Effects. The infusion should be slowed or discontinued if side-effects occur or if there is evidence of excessive uterine activity.

Dinoprost-induced bronchoconstriction was significantly reduced by prior inhalation of atropine but not by prior inhalation of thymoxamine or sodium cromoglycate. The effect of sodium cromoglycate in allergen-induced or exercise-induced asthma suggested that the release of dinoprost in the lung was not the primary factor in the aetiology of asthma.— K. R. Patel, *Br. med. J.*, 1975, *2*, 360.

Experiments in *animals* suggested that polyphloretin phospahte could antagonise the bronchoconstriction and changes in blood pressure caused by dinoprost.— A. A. Mathé *et al.*, *J. Pharm. Pharmac.*, 1972, *24*, 378.

Precautions. Dinoprost should not be given to patients in whom oxytocic drugs (see Oxytocin Injection, p.1273) are generally contra-indicated, or where prolonged contractions of the uterus are considered inappropriate, as, for example, in patients with a history of Caesarean section or major uterine surgery, where major degrees of cephalopelvic disproportion may be present, where foetal malpresentation is present, where there is suspicion of foetal distress, where there is a history of difficult labour or traumatic delivery, in grand multiparae with 6 or more previous term pregnancies, or in those with pelvic inflammatory disease.

Since prostaglandins enhance the effects of oxytocin use of the 2 agents together or in sequence should be carefully monitored. Dinoprost should be used with caution in patients with glaucoma or raised intra-ocular pressure, and asthma or a history of asthma.

In the induction of labour cephalopelvic relationships should be carefully evaluated before use. During infusion uterine activity, foetal status, and the progress of cervical dilatation should be carefully monitored to detect adverse responses, such as hypertonus, sustained uterine contractions, or foetal distress. In patients with a history of hypertonic uterine contractility or tetanic uterine contractions, uterine activity and the state of the foetus should be continuously monitored throughout labour. Where high-tone myometrial contractions are sustained the possibility of uterine rupture should be considered.

Foetal damage has been observed in cases of incomplete termination and the appropriate treatment for complete evacuation of the uterus should therefore be instituted whenever termination is incomplete.

Foetal damage. Four of 9 patients who received dinoprost in early pregnancy did not abort and curettage specimens showed histological damage. It was concluded that prostaglandin administration might induce vaginal bleeding but that pregnancy was not reliably terminated; gestations that continued appeared to be damaged.— A. C. Wentz and G. S. Jones, *Fert. Steril.*, 1973, *24*, 569.

Hydatidiform mole. For the hazards of prostaglandin use for abortion of hydatidiform moles, see under Dinoprostone, Overdosage, p.1357.

Uses. Dinoprost is a prostaglandin of the F series (see p.1353). It induces contraction of uterine muscle and it is used clinically as an oxytocic agent for the induction of labour, termination of pregnancy, missed abortion, hydatidiform mole, and foetal death *in utero*. It may be used at any stage of pregnancy.

Dinoprost is given intravenously or intra-amniotically as the trometamol salt. For the induction of labour the dose is the equivalent of 2.5 µg per minute of dinoprost infused intravenously, as a solution containing 15 µg per ml, for at least 30 minutes, this being subsequently maintained or increased according to the patient's response; in foetal death higher doses may be required, and an initial rate of 5 µg per minute may be used with increases at intervals of not less than 1 hour.

For the termination of pregnancy, missed abortion, or hydatidiform mole a solution containing the equivalent of 50 µg of dinoprost per ml is infused intravenously at a rate of 25 µg per minute for at least 30 minutes, then maintained, or increased to 50 µg per minute according to response; this rate should be maintained for at least 4 hours before making further increases.

For the termination of pregnancy during the second trimester, 8 ml of a solution containing the equivalent of 5 mg of dinoprost per ml is injected slowly into the amniotic sac.

Angiography. An account of the application of the vasodilating properties of dinoprost for visceral angiographic studies. Dinoprost appears to be an ideal vasodilator for use in a wide range of angiographic procedures.— D. Legge, Prostaglandins and angiography, in *Practical Applications of Prostaglandins and their Synthesis Inhibitors*, S.M.M. Karim (Ed.), Lancaster, MTP Press, 1979.

Contraception. Dinoprost, given by intravenous infusion at a rate of 12.5 to 250 µg per minute to a total of 14 to 37.5 mg, produced a marked fall in the plasma concentration of progesterone in 4 volunteers in the mid-late luteal phase of the menstrual cycle, but had no such effect in 3 patients in the early luteal phase. The high doses needed to produce an effect were associated with severe side-effects.— K. Hillier *et al.*, *Br. med. J.*, 1972, *4*, 333.

Dinoprost administration intravaginally was impractical as a luteolytic method of contraception.— W. K. C. Tom *et al.*, *Contraception*, 1972, *6*, 479. See also A. C. Wentz and G. S. Jones, *Obstet. Gynec.*, 1973, *42*, 172.

Induction of labour. Of 1044 women whose labour was induced with dinoprost or dinoprostone there were 283 women with pre-eclamptic toxaemia or hypertension. All the infants born to these 283 women were followed up for at least 1 week at which time all were normal. It was considered that there was no abnormal incidence of foetal distress.— R. G. Jacomb and H. Hinchley, *Upjohn* (letter), *Lancet*, 1974, *1*, 1226. See also I. Brosens *et al.* (letter), *ibid.*, 808.

In a double-blind study, following cervical stretching and sweeping of the foetal membranes, in association with intravaginal administration of dinoprost 50 mg (as dinoprost trometamol) in a methylcellulose gel, 20 of 40 patients went into labour before proposed induction, whereas only 3 of 40 women who underwent the same procedure in association with placebo gel did so. Although the differences did not reach significance there were more spontaneous deliveries and more labours of short duration in the prostaglandin-treated group; significantly fewer women in the prostaglandin-group required intravenous oxytocin.— A. H. MacLennan and R. C. Green, *Lancet*, 1979, *1*, 117. A reminder of the extreme sensitivity to this prostaglandin found in many patients with obstructive lung disease. Because of the risk of precipitating acute status asthmaticus this preparation should not be used if there is even the slightest hint of an obstructive lung condition.— B. D. Dubin (letter), *ibid.*, 377.

Further references: M. J. O'Sullivan *et al.*, *Obstet. Gynec.*, 1978, *51*, 77 (induction in high-risk pregnancies).

References to the use of dinoprost for induction of labour following foetal death: G. Sher, *Am. J. Obstet. Gynec.*, 1979, *134*, 493 (with urea); J. P. Lebed *et al.*, *Obstet. Gynec.*, 1980, *56*, 90 (intra-amniotic, compared with vaginal dinoprostone).

See also under Dinoprostone, p.1357.

Termination of pregnancy. In a review of studies performed under the direction of the WHO concerning the use of prostaglandins for the termination of pregnancy M. Bygdeman (*Obstet. Gynec.*, 1978, *52*, 424) concluded that the administration of prostaglandins by the *intra-amniotic* route in appropriate doses was significantly more effective than hypertonic saline for the termination of second trimester pregnancy and that intra-amniotic dinoprost was at least as safe as hypertonic saline administered by the same route. However W. Cates *et al.* (*Obstet. Gynec.*, 1978, *52*, 493) held the view that the same work had shown prostaglandins to be faster but more hazardous than hypertonic saline as intra-amniotic abortifacients. Review of other studies suggested that dilatation and evacuation was more effective, safer, and more convenient than prostaglandins for abortions after 12 weeks' gestation, especially between 13 and 16 weeks.

A review of the termination of abnormal intra-uterine pregnancy with prostaglandins (dinoprost, dinoprostone, carboprost, gemeprost, sulprostone, 2*a*,2*b*-dihomo-15(*S*)-15-methylprostaglandin $F_{2\alpha}$ and 15(*S*)-15-methylprostaglandin E_2).— S. M. M. Karim *et al.*, *Singapore J. Obstet. Gynaec.*, 1980, *11*, 7.

Abortion was successfully induced in 82 of 94 women in the first and second trimesters of pregnancy by the intra-uterine (*extra-amniotic*) instillation of prostaglandin. Doses of 200 µg of dinoprostone or 750 µg of dinoprost were instilled every 1 or 2 hours. The mean time to abortion was 22.4 hours. There was no significant difference between the effect in primigravidas and multigravidas, in the first and second trimesters, between dinoprostone and dinoprost, or between hourly and 2-hourly instillations. Vomiting occurred in 25 patients, an increase in heart-rate in 40, and an increase in blood pressure in 22. The mean white-cell count and neutrophil count rose significantly and the lymphocyte count fell significantly in 30 patients. Blood loss was below 300 ml in 85 patients and 300 to 500 ml in 9. Side-effects were considered less severe than after intravenous infusions.— M. P. Embrey *et al.*, *Br. med. J.*, 1972, *3*, 146.

Intravenous administration of dinoprost 25 to 200 µg per minute to 42 patients to induce abortion had an overall success-rate of 50%. A high and unacceptable rate of side-effects was associated with all dosage levels but especially the highest. Multiparas aborted 2.5 times more frequently than primigravidas.— G. G. Anderson *et al.*, *Contraception*, 1972, *5*, 303.

In a multicentre randomised study, dinoprost as 2 *intra-amniotic* instillations of 25 mg at 6-hour intervals in 717 women was compared with a single 200-ml instillation of hypertonic saline in 796 women. Abortion occurred within 48 hours of the first injection in 85.4 and 80.5% respectively and mean abortion times were 19.7 and 30.4 hours. There was complete abortion in about 60% in both groups. The incidence of vomiting was 1.5 and 0.4 episodes per patient and of diarrhoea 0.4 and nil respectively.— Report of a WHO Scientific Group, Advances in Methods of Fertility Regulation, *Tech. Rep. Ser. Wld Hlth Org. No. 575*, 1975, p. 34. See also *Br. med. J.*, 1976, *1*, 1357 and 1373.

A randomised study in 16 patients undergoing mid-trimester abortion showed that the time to abortion was reduced from a mean of 28.8 hours in those given urea 80 g intra-amniotically to 18.3 hours in those given urea followed by dinoprost 5 mg *intra-amniotically;* both groups received oxytocin if needed. Experience in 150 patients subsequently treated confirmed the findings and showed that the addition of dinoprost 5 mg was as effective as the earlier reported use of 10 mg.— T. M. King *et al.*, *Am. J. Obstet. Gynec.*, 1977, *129*, 817. See also R. T. Burkman *et al.*, *ibid.*, 1976, *126*, 328; L. Wellman and A. Jacobson, *Fert. Steril.*, 1976, *27*, 1374; W. B. Wilson, *Obstet. Gynec.*, 1978, *51*, 699.

Criticism of a US Public Health Service study (*Morb. Mortal.*, 1976, *25*, 370; *Family Planning Perspectives*, 1976, *8*, 275) suggesting that surgical extraction is the safest method of midtrimester abortion. Until more data becomes available most *Med. Lett.* consultants prefer intra-amniotic administration of dinoprost or saline for midtrimester abortions.— *Med. Lett.*, 1977, *19*, 25.

Results of a randomised study involving 100 women estimated to be 13 to 18 menstrual weeks' pregnant suggesting that midtrimester abortion by outpatient dilatation and evacuation appeared to be more acceptable, faster, and safer than inpatient intra-amniotic instillation of dinoprost.— D. A. Grimes *et al.*, *Am. J. Obstet. Gynec.*, 1980, *137*, 785.

Menstrual induction. Uterine bleeding occurred 2 to 5 hours after the intra-uterine administration of dinoprost 4 to 8 mg or dinoprostone 0.5 to 2 mg to 16 women during the first 2 weeks of delayed menstruation and after a positive pregnancy test. Pregnancy tests were negative after 14 days. Vomiting occurred in 6 women and uterine cramps in 12.— S. M. M. Karim (letter), *Lancet*, 1973, *2*, 794. See also P. Mocsary and A. I. Csapo (letter), *Lancet*, 1973, *2*, 683.

Of 20 pregnant women who received a single transcervical instillation of dinoprost 5 mg in 5 ml of saline between 38 and 46 days after their last menstruation, 13 successfully aborted but 7 required dilatation and curettage. Fever and pain were complications in 2 who aborted; of those who did not abort, severe haemorrhage occurred in 1 and endometritis in 3.— A. S. Lichtman *et al.*, *Contraception*, 1974, *9*, 403. A similar adverse report.— J. R. Jones *et al.*, *Prostaglandins*, 1975, *9*, 881.

In 132 primigravid women menstrual induction involving transcervical intrauterine delivery of a single dose of dinoprost 5 mg without cervical dilatation, after about 13 days of menstrual delay, did not increase the prematurity-rate in their subsequent pregnancies.— P. Mocsary and A. I. Csapo (letter), *Lancet*, 1978, *1*, 1159.

Urinary retention. Successful use of dinoprost administered intravesically via an indwelling Foley catheter in 6 of 10 patients with acute postoperative or post partum urinary retention; 4 of the 6 patients responded to a single dose of dinoprost 1 mg and the remaining 2 required a total of 3 and 4 doses respectively.— S. S. Ratnam *et al.*, *Singapore J. Obstet. Gynaec.*, 1979, *10*, 23.

Proprietary Preparations

Prostin F2 alpha *(Upjohn, UK)*. Dinoprost trometamol, available as a sterile solution containing the equivalent of 5 mg of dinoprost per ml in 0.9% benzyl alcohol solution, in ampoules of 1.5 and 5 ml for intravenous administration, and in ampoules of 4 and 8 ml for intra-amniotic administration. (Also available as Prostin F2 alpha in *Ital., Neth., S.Afr., Switz.*).

Other Proprietary Names

Amoglandin *(Denm., Norw., Swed.)*; Minprostin $F_{2\alpha}$ *(Ger.)*; Prostalmon F, Prostamodin-F *(both Jap.)*.

8082-b

Dinoprostone.

PGE$_2$; U-12062; Dinoprostonum; Prostaglandin E$_2$. (5*Z*,13*E*)-(8*R*,11*R*,12*R*,15*S*)-11,15-Dihydroxy-9-oxoprosta-5,13-dienoic acid; (*Z*)-7-{(1*R*,2*R*,3*R*)-3-Hydroxy-2-[(*E*)-(3*S*)-3-hydroxyoct-1-enyl]-5-oxocyclopentyl}hept-5-enoic acid.

$C_{20}H_{32}O_5$=352.5.

CAS — 363-24-6.

A white to off-white crystalline solid. M.p. about 65°. **Soluble** about 1 in 1000 of water; soluble in alcohol. **Incompatible** with acids and alkalis. **Store** at 4°.

Dinoprostone could be kept for long periods if prepared in concentrated alcoholic solutions in ampoules and stored at −20°. They were diluted with sterile iso-osmotic saline 24 hours before use. A personal communication from D.H. Nugteren and D.A. van Dorp recommended storage in alcoholic solutions for 1 year at −15° and in aqueous solution for a maximum of 1 week at 0° or 1 month at −15°.— H. C. Brummer (letter), *J. Pharm. Pharmac.*, 1971, *23*, 804.

The kinetics of dehydration and isomerisation of alprostadil and dinoprostone. Both were most stable at pH 3 to 4.— D. C. Monkhouse *et al.*, *J. pharm. Sci.*, 1973, *62*, 576.

Correspondence on the preparation of dinoprostone in gel, pessaries, and other formulations: M. J. Tarr and R. L. Tredree (letter), *Pharm. J.*, 1978, *2*, 497; E. L. Robins and P. R. Payne (letter), *ibid.*, 522; I. M. Sharkey and B. Corbett (letter), *ibid.*, 560; C. London and E. Mills (letter), *ibid.*, 1979, *1*, 413; D. R. Lee *et al.* (letter), *ibid.*, 523; J. M. Luff and F. G. Moore (letter), *ibid.*, 1979, *2*, 29; L. Gove (letter), *ibid.*, 274; A. S. Harris *et al.*, *ibid.*, 1980, *2*, 399; U. Ulmsten *et al.* (letter), *Lancet*, 1979, *1*, 377; F. G. Moore (letter), *ibid.*, 501; M. G. Elder and A. P. Gordon-Wright (letter), *ibid.*, 779; F. Moore and J. H. Shepherd (letter), *ibid.*, 932.

Adverse Effects, Treatment, and Precautions. As for Dinoprost Trometamol, p.1355.

Cervical tear and uterine rupture. In over 200 pregnancy terminations using dinoprostone, 3 cases of rupture of the cervix had occurred. All occurred in primigravidas of 15 to 20 weeks' gestation who had received a single intra-amniotic dose of dinoprostone 10 mg without additional stimulation by oxytocin. Lack of case reports of cervical rupture due to dinoprostone might be partly due to under-reporting and partly due to the less widespread use of dinoprostone compared with dinoprost.— I. S. Fraser (letter), *Br. med. J.*, 1974, *4*, 404.

Rupture of a uterine scar occurred in 2 women given 2.5-mg pessaries of dinoprostone to induce vaginal delivery. The presence of a uterine scar may be a contra-indication to the use of vaginal dinoprostone.— D. R. Bromham and R. S. Anderson (letter), *Lancet*, 1980, *2*, 485.

Further references: A. M. Smith (letter), *Br. med. J.*, 1975, *1*, 205; A. I. Traub and J. W. K. Ritchie (letter), *Br. med. J.*, 1979, *2*, 496; E. K. El-Etriby and E. Daw, *Postgrad. med. J.*, 1981, *57*, 265.

Convulsions. A 42-year-old woman at about 20 weeks gestation suffered a generalised epileptiform convulsion 25 minutes after the intra-amniotic injection of dinoprostone 10 mg to induce abortion. Although the patient had no abnormal neurological signs before the procedure and an electroencephalogram was normal she had suffered a generalised epileptiform convulsion 2 years earlier. It was suggested that patients with a previous history of epileptiform convulsions due to have intra-amniotic prostaglandin should receive anticonvulsant therapy and advice should be sought from a neurologist for those already receiving therapy.— J. H. Brash, *Br. J. Obstet. Gynaec.*, 1976, *83*, 665.

Effects on the blood. Dinoprostone could induce sickling in patients with sickle-cell anaemia.— A. L. Willis *et al.* (letter), *New Engl. J. Med.*, 1972, *286*, 783.

In a study of 27 patients undergoing second-trimester abortion with dinoprostone given intra-amniotically, the 9 given 5 mg of dinoprostone with hypertonic urea showed signs of intravascular coagulation. This effect was less pronounced in the 9 given the same dose with hypertonic dextrose and absent in the remaining 9 given 2 doses of 10 mg of dinoprostone alone.— I. Z. MacKenzie *et al.*, *Lancet*, 1975, *2*, 1066.

Effects on the heart. Fatal cardiac arrest possibly associated with the administration of dinoprostone 20 mg vaginally approximately 25 days earlier in an obese woman with a strong family history of cardiovascular disease.— S. P. Patterson *et al.*, *Obstet. Gynec.*, 1979, *54*, 123.

Hydatidiform mole. For the hazards of prostaglandin use for abortion of hydatidiform moles, see under Overdosage, below.

Infection. Evidence to suggest an increased risk of infection in women in whom labour was induced by dinoprostone given extra-amniotically in a cellulose derivative basis.— P. J. Callen *et al.*, *Br. J. Obstet. Gynaec.*, 1980, *87*, 513.

Jaundice. A study indicating that, unlike oxytocin, dinoprostone stimulation has no effect on neonatal serum-bilirubin concentrations.— W. C. Chew, *Br. med. J.*, 1977, *2*, 679. See also J. M. Beazley and A. R. Weekes, *Br. J. Obstet. Gynaec.*, 1976, *83*, 62.

Overdosage. In 3 patients in whom mid-trimester therapeutic abortion was attempted by the intra-amniotic infusion of urea and dinoprostone, an adverse reaction occurred, consisting of rigors, vomiting, severe abdominal pain, and an intense desire to urinate and defaecate; one patient had hypotension and another peripheral cyanosis. In 2 patients the pain followed the injection of urea.— A. H. Ross and W. L. Whitehouse (letter), *Br. med. J.*, 1974, *1*, 642. The symptoms were probably due to a relatively large dose of prostaglandins reaching the systemic circulation. No such reactions had occurred in 200 patients given urea 80 g and varying doses of dinoprost and dinoprostone. The importance of correct technique was emphasised.— I. Craft and P. Bowen-Simpkins (letter), *ibid.*, 1974, *2*, 446. Prior administration of urea would increase the rate of absorption of prostaglandins from the amniotic cavity thus producing adverse reactions. In the third patient no urea had been administered but the liquor was blood stained.— S. M. M. Karim (letter), *ibid.*, 1974, *3*, 347.

A 20-year-old woman given 20 mg of dinoprostone intra-amniotically for the expulsion of a hydatidiform mole developed profound hypotension, bradycardia, rigors, vomiting, and suprapubic pain, followed by tachycardia, pyrexia, and flushing believed to be due to the dinoprostone passing into the general circulation.— A. M. Smith (letter), *Br. med. J.*, 1974, *2*, 382. The usual extra-amniotic dose of dinoprostone was 200 µg. Because of the absence of foetal membranes in a molar pregnancy intrauterine administration of prostaglandin was similar to extra-amniotic administration. The dose of 20 mg used was thus 100 times higher than the usual extra-amniotic dose.— S. M. M. Karim (letter), *Br. med. J.*, 1974, *3*, 347.

Nausea, retching, severe abdominal pain, dizziness, difficulty in breathing with frothy, blood-stained sputum, an imperceptible pulse, and hypotension occurred in an 18-year-old woman immediately after the 'extra-amniotic' instillation of dinoprostone 200 µg to abort a hydatidiform mole. It was considered that since there is no extra-amniotic space in a hydatidiform mole the dinoprostone may have been injected directly into the maternal circulation; it was suggested that mechanical infusion pumps should be used in such circumstances.— E. McNicol and H. Gray, *Br. J. Obstet. Gynaec.*, 1977, *84*, 229.

Shock. Dramatic pyrexial and cardiovascular adverse reactions in 2 women following the intravaginal administration of dinoprostone to induce labour following intra-uterine foetal death resembled endotoxic shock.— J. P. Phelan *et al.*, *Am. J. Obstet. Gynec.*, 1978, *132*, 28.

Uterine hypertonus. Severe uterine hypertonus occurred in a patient given 3 doses of dinoprostone 500 µg at hourly intervals for the induction of labour. Pethidine 50 mg intravenously did not ease the severe pain. It was suggested that a rapid infusion of alcohol might be used to control similar occurrences.— I. S. Fraser (letter), *Lancet*, 1974, *2*, 162. See also G. Roberts and A. C. Turnbull, *Br. med. J.*, 1971, *1*, 702; J. E. Felmingham *et al.* (letter), *ibid.*, 1976, *1*, 586; M. Thiery and J. J. Amy (letter), *ibid.*, 958.

See also under Cervical Tear and Uterine Rupture, above.

Uses. Dinoprostone is a prostaglandin of the E series (see p.1353) with actions and uses similar to those of dinoprost (see p.1356).

For the induction of labour dinoprostone may be given by mouth as 500-µg tablets with about 100 ml of water in an initial dose of 1 tablet, repeated hourly. If the response is inadequate 2 tablets may be given hourly but single doses of 1.5 mg should not be exceeded. One tablet may be sufficient for maintenance.

The intravenous dose for the induction of labour is 250 nanograms per minute infused as a solution containing 1.5 µg per ml in sodium chloride injection or dextrose injection for 30 minutes, the dose being subsequently maintained or increased according to the patient's response; in foetal death higher doses may be required and an initial rate of 500 nanograms per minute may be used with increases at intervals of not less than 1 hour. The vaginal administration of dinoprostone is described below.

For the termination of pregnancy, missed abortion, or hydatidiform mole a solution containing 5 µg per ml is infused intravenously at a rate of 2.5 µg per minute for 30 minutes, then maintained or increased to 5 µg per minute; this rate should be maintained for at least 4 hours before making further increases. For the termination of pregnancy 1 ml of a solution containing 100 µg per ml may be instilled extra-amniotically through a suitable Foley catheter. Subsequent doses of 1 or 2 ml are given at intervals usually of 2 hours, according to uterine response.

Bronchospasm. Aerosols of alprostadil and dinoprostone were evaluated as bronchodilators in 32 subjects (bronchial asthma 15, chronic bronchitis 11, and normal 6). Inhalation of dinoprostone (400 ng per kg body-weight over 10 minutes) caused a significant decrease in pulmonary resistance, but the same dose of alprostadil produced no significant change. Side-effects included cough, irritation of the pharynx, and headache.— Y. Kawakami *et al.*, *Eur. J. clin. Pharmac.*, 1973, *6*, 127.

Dinoprostone administered by infusion to 10 asthmatic subjects had a slight bronchodilating effect in 4, caused bronchoconstriction in 4 and had no effect in 2. Side-effects were frequent and it was concluded that dinoprostone was unsuitable for use in the management of attacks of asthma.— A. P. Smith, *Br. J. clin. Pharmac.*, 1974, *1*, 399.

Gastro-intestinal disorders. Studies on the gastro-intestinal effects of dinoprostone: M. M. Cohen (letter), *Lancet*, 1978, *2*, 1253 (reduction of aspirin-induced faecal blood loss); C. Johansson *et al.* (letter), *Lancet*, 1979, *1*, 317; *idem*, *Gastroenterology*, 1980, *78*, 479 (reduction of indomethacin-induced faecal blood loss); M. M. Cohen *et al.*, *Gut*, 1980, *21*, 602 (reduction of aspirin-induced faecal blood loss).

Induction of labour. A favourable report of the use of dinoprostone 3-mg pessaries for the induction of labour in 502 women. If the cervix was not ripe a pessary was inserted in the evening, usually with a second pessary in the morning to induce labour. Those in whom the cervix was favourable received a single pessary for induction.— J. Shepherd *et al.*, *Br. med. J.*, 1979, *2*, 108. Comment on the role of dinoprostone vaginal pessaries in the induction of labour. It would be reassuring to have confirmation that sustained hypertonic uterine activity can be avoided by careful selection of patients and much more should be known about the effects of prostaglandin vaginal pessaries in patients with a scar in the lower uterine segment. Nevertheless, the regimen has many attractive features.— *ibid.*, 407. Mention of work by A.P. Gordon-Wright and M.G. Elder (*Br. J. Obstet. Gynaec.*, 1979, *86*, 32) where about 70% of over 500 patients went into labour without any other intervention after a single intravaginal insertion of tablets containing 4 or 5 mg of dinoprostone. Like those reported by J. Shepherd *et al.* (above), these results are not ideal and can be improved by seeking the optimum dose regimen as well as the best vehicle for release. Until these points are established it is too soon to claim that we have the best alternative to intravenous oxytocin.— M. G. Elder (letter), *ibid.*, 671. Details of some limitations to the use of prostaglandin pessaries in a busy unit. They do, however, have a valuable role in ripening the cervix and rendering it more favourable for induction by amniotomy and oxytocin infusion.— M. Sutton and P. Steer (letter), *ibid.* A brief history of prostaglandin developments for the induction of labour. The cervical ripening effect of dinoprostone was first observed in early studies with intravenous infusion in amounts insufficient to induce labour. *Intravenous* therapy was soon superseded by *extra-amniotic* infusion of dinoprostone, then by single administration of dinoprostone in a viscous cellulose-based gel into the extra-amniotic space. The most recent phase has been the adoption of *vaginal* administration of dinoprostone, either in a viscous gel or in a simple lipid-based pessary, or of tablets manufactured for oral administration. Fears that the larger dose of dinoprostone required for vaginal administration might lead to hypertonic uterine activity have not been substantiated, and there is now extensive experience of the efficacy and safety of the method. The results of vaginal administration were first reported by I.Z. MacKenzie and M.P. Embrey (*Br. med. J.*, 1977, *2*, 1381); using dinoprostone gel in 168 primigravidae with low inducibility scores, labour ensued in almost 50% without further intervention, while in the remainder the Bishop score improved significantly, making subsequent amniotomy easy and progress in labour rapid. In an analysis of 803 patients I.Z. MacKenzie and M.P. Embrey (*Br. J. Obstet. Gynaec.*, 1978, *85*, 657) found that when the cervix was ripe 65.9% of primigravidae and 87.5% of multiparae did not require formal induction of labour. The benefits are greatest when labour follows dinoprostone alone, and in such patients the frequency of caesarean section, epidural analgesia, and low Apgar scores were all reduced. Continuing experience with prostaglandin vaginal gels and pessaries has substantiated their benefits in improving prognosis and over 1500 patients have now been safely treated with dinoprostone gel, including 78 women with foetal breech presentation and 54 multigravidae previously delivered by caesarean section. The method has been adopted in many units both in Great Britain and other countries. The provision of a solitary stable dinoprostone pessary for induction of labour will have great potential, since the regimen is simple, non-invasive, and highly acceptable to patients, causing minimal inconvenience while reducing analgesic requirements and improving the prospects of labour.— M. P. Embrey (letter), *ibid.*, 793.

Comment on the bad prognostic sign of an unripe cervix in late pregnancy and the role of prostaglandins, usually dinoprostone, in ripening it. Not surprisingly, oral prostaglandin tablets have given disappointing results since systemic prostaglandin therapy is beset by the problems of rapid metabolism and side-effects. Local routes have proved much better, but extra-amniotic therapy requries an extra-amniotic catheter and comparable results have been obtained with larger doses given into the posterior vaginal fornix; the simplicity of this approach is a big advantage.— *Lancet*, 1979, *1*, 364. The view that prostaglandins synthesised and acting locally are of major importance in cervical ripening and that prostaglandin E rather than prostaglandin F is the major prostaglandin involved.— D. A. Ellwood *et al.* (letter), *ibid.*, 376.

Further references to dinoprostone for the induction of labour: P. D. Wilson, *Br. J. Obstet. Gynaec.*, 1978, *85*, 941 (oral, vaginal, and extra-amniotic routes); J. M. F. Pearce *et al.*, *Lancet*, 1979, *1*, 572 (3-mg pessaries); M. P. Embrey *et al.*, *Br. med. J.*, 1980, *281*, 901 (polymer pessaries).

After intra-uterine death. Labour was successfully induced in 15 of 20 women with missed abortion or foetal death *in utero* by the use of dinoprostone vaginal suppositories, and in the remaining 5 patients by the concomitant use of oxytocin. Nausea, vomiting, diarrhoea, chills and shaking, and fever did not necessitate withdrawal of treatment. The suppositories, each containing 20 mg, were refrigerated until required. The standard dose was one every 2 hours until delivery, with a mean dose of 90 mg.— N. H. Lauersen and K. H. Wilson, *Am. J. Obstet. Gynec.*, 1977, *127*, 609.

The use in 50 women of dinoprostone as a vaginal gel for the expulsion of a dead foetus. The dose of dinoprostone was 15 mg when the gestational age was less than 29 weeks and 5 mg for 29 weeks or more. Oxytocin was used if required.— I. Z. MacKenzie *et al.*, *Br. med. J.*, 1979, *1*, 1764.

Further references to dinoprostone for the induction of labour following intra-uterine foetal death: D. R. Kent and A. I. Goldstein, *Obstet. Gynec.*, 1976, *48*, 475 (pessaries); E. M. Southern and G. D. Gutknecht, *Obstet. Gynec.*, 1976, *47*, 602 (pessaries); A. Rutland and C. Ballard, *Am. J. Obstet. Gynec.*, 1977, *128*, 503 (pessaries); H. Schulman *et al.*, *Am. J. Obstet. Gynec.*, 1979, *133*, 742 (pessaries); J. Scher *et al.*, *Am. J. Obstet. Gynec.*, 1980, *137*, 769 (extra-amniotic instillation).

Pulmonary atresia. Oral dinoprostone therapy was used for over a month to keep the ductus arteriosus patent in a premature infant whose pulmonary circulation was ductus dependent.— J. Y. Coe and E. D. Silove (letter), *Lancet*, 1979, *1*, 1297.

Termination of pregnancy. A review of the termination of abnormal intra-uterine pregnancy with prostaglandins, including dinoprostone.— S. M. M. Karim *et al.*, *Singapore J. Obstet. Gynaec.*, 1980, *11*, 7.

Dinoprostone 10 mg administered intra-amniotically to 15 women in the mid-trimester of pregnancy induced abortion in a mean time of 26 hours 49 minutes (range 7 hours 40 minutes to 81 hours 5 minutes) whereas dinoprostone 10 mg given to 15 women in the same stage of pregnancy after the intra-amniotic infusion of urea 80 g in 80 ml of sodium chloride injection induced abortion in a mean time of 10 hours 30 minutes (range 3 hours 45 minutes to 23 hours 37 minutes).— I. Craft, *Lancet*, 1973, *1*, 1344. Reducing the dose of dinoprostone to 5 mg in 8 patients produced a similar success-rate and a lower incidence of vomiting and diarrhoea.— *idem*, 1973, *2*, 207. The use of 80 g urea with a low dose of dinoprostone (2.5 mg) for inducing abortion in patients with a mean gestation of 19 weeks.— *idem*, 1975, *1*, 1115.

Using an amended technique dinoprostone 200 µg was administered into the uterine cavity of 40 patients requiring abortion in the 12th to 18th week of pregnancy, using a fine gauge catheter inserted through a Foley catheter. The infusion was continued with 100 or 165 µg per hour and all patients aborted within 24 hours (mean 15.75 hours), only 12% requiring surgical evacuation for incomplete abortion.— M. D. Read *et al.* (letter), *Lancet*, 1974, *1*, 214.

Of 24 patients 20 aborted within 24 hours after a single extra-amniotic injection of dinoprostone 1.5 mg in a viscous vehicle; the mean abortion time was 13.5 hours. Side-effects included vomiting in 7 patients, a reaction including pallor and shivering in 1, and mild hypertension in 1; most patients required analgesic injections for painful contractions. The dinoprostone injection was prepared by adding 1.5 mg in 1.5 ml of alcohol to 7.5 ml of a 6% solution of hydroxyethylmethylcellulose previously sterilised by autoclaving.— I. Z. MacKenzie *et al.*, *Br. med. J.*, 1975, *1*, 240.

The use of dinoprostone gel extra-amniotically, repeated if necessary after 6 hours, to induce mid-trimester abortion.— D. H. Smith *et al.*, *Br. med. J.*, 1981, *282*, 2012.

Further references: A. W. F. Miller *et al.*, *Lancet*, 1972, *2*, 5; B. Alderman (letter), *ibid.*, 279; A. Gillespie, *Br. med. J.*, 1972, *1*, 150; S. M. M. Karim and G. M. Filshie, *J. Obstet. Gynaec. Br. Commonw.*, 1972, *79*, 1; K. Hillier and M. P. Embrey, *ibid.*, 14; I. Z. MacKenzie *et al.*, *ibid.*, 1974, *81*, 554; N. H. Lauersen *et al.*, *Am. J. Obstet. Gynec.*, 1975, *122*, 947.

Menstrual induction. Of 275 women with delayed menstruation owing to pregnancy, successful induction of abortion was obtained by uterine or vaginal administration of a natural prostaglandin or a prostaglandin analogue in 229 (83.3%). Side-effects were vomiting, diarrhoea, and uterine cramps usually lasting for 4 to 8 hours. Bleeding lasted for a mean of about 14 days in the successfully treated patients with slight intermittent bleeding continuing until the next menses in 19; the degree and duration of bleeding appeared to be related to the degree of menstrual delay, curettage being required by 14 patients for prolonged or excessive bleeding; blood transfusions were required in 2 patients. One patient, whose intra-uterine device was not removed before treatment, suffered acute sepsis requiring bilateral salpingectomy; subsequently the devices were always removed before treatment. Of 34 patients who were treated but subsequently found not to have been pregnant no deleterious effects were noted. The study demonstrated the safety of prostaglandin-menstrual induction which had the advantage of not generally requiring hospital admission.— I. Z. MacKenzie *et al.*, *Lancet*, 1978, *1*, 1223.

Urinary retention. Of 21 women with difficulty in micturition and chronic urinary retention 14 responded to the instillation of dinoprostone 500 µg in 40 ml of sterile water into the bladder through a urethral catheter.— M. I. Bultitude *et al.*, *Br. J. Urol.*, 1976, *48*, 631.

Proprietary Preparations

Prostin E2 Sterile Solutions *(Upjohn, UK).* Dinoprostone for preparing intravenous infusions, available as an injection containing 1 mg per ml in dehydrated alcohol, in ampoules of 0.75 ml, and 10 mg per ml in dehydrated alcohol, in ampoules of 0.5 ml; and for extra-amniotic administration, available as a solution containing 10 mg per ml in dehydrated alcohol, in ampoules of 0.5 ml with 50-ml vials of sodium chloride injection containing benzyl alcohol 0.9%. (Also available as Prostin E2 in *Canad.*, *Neth.*, *S.Afr.*).

Prostin E2 Tablets *(Upjohn, UK).* Each contains dinoprostone 500 µg.

Other Proprietary Names

Minprostin *(Denm., Norw.)*; Minprostin E_2 *(Ger.)*; Prostarmon-E *(Jap.)*.

8083-v

Doxaprost. AY-24559. (*E*)-(8*R*,12*R*)-15-Hydroxy-15-methyl-9-oxoprost-13-enoic acid; 7-{(1*R*,2*R*)-2-[(*E*)-3-Hydroxy-3-methyloct-1-enyl]-5-oxocyclopentyl}heptanoic acid.

$C_{21}H_{36}O_4$=352.5.

CAS — 51953-95-8.

Doxaprost is a synthetic prostaglandin derivative with potential use as a bronchodilator.

Manufacturers

Ayerst, USA.

8084-g

Epoprostenol.

U-53217; PGI_2; PGX; Prostacyclin; Prostaglandin I_2; Prostaglandin X. (5*Z*,13*E*)-(8*R*,9*S*,11*R*,12*R*,15*S*)-6,9-Epoxy-11,15-dihydroxyprosta-5,13-dienoic acid; (*Z*)-5-{(3a*R*,4*R*,5*R*,6a*S*)-5-Hydroxy-4-[(*E*)-(3*S*)-3-hydroxyoct-1-enyl]perhydrocyclopenta[*b*]furan-2-ylidene}valerate.

$C_{20}H_{32}O_5$=352.5.

CAS — 35121-78-9.

NOTE. In *Martindale* the term epoprostenol is used for the exogenous form and prostacyclin for the endogenous form.

8085-q

Epoprostenol Sodium.

U-53217A.

$C_{20}H_{31}NaO_5$=374.5.

CAS — 61849-14-7.

A study on the stability of epoprostenol in plasma.— K. A. Jørgensen *et al.* (letter), *Lancet*, 1979, *1*, 1352. See also K. E. H. El Tahir *et al.*, *Clin. Sci.*, 1980, *59* (Sept.), 28P.

Adverse Effects and Precautions. The incidence of adverse reactions to epoprostenol is dose-related. Side-effects commonly include hypotension, increased heart-rate, flushing, headache, and nausea and vomiting. Other side-effects reported include stomach cramps, feelings of uneasiness, pain in the legs, and hyperglycaemia.

Laryngotracheal irritation and transient coughing have followed inhalation of epoprostenol.

It has been reported that the hypotensive effects of epoprostenol are exacerbated by using acetate in dialysis fluids.

Diabetogenic effect. Observations in 3 diabetic patients showed that hyperglycaemia which might constitute a risk in patients with poorly controlled diabetes, followed the intravenous infusion of epoprostenol 5 ng per kg body-weight per minute for 72 hours. Blood-glucose concentrations were unaffected in 9 nondiabetic patients with peripheral vascular disease given similar doses of epoprostenol, and slightly increased in 7 others given 10 ng per kg per minute for 48 hours.— A. Szczeklik *et al.*, *Prostaglandins*, 1980, *19*, 959.

Interactions. When epoprostenol was used as an antithrombotic agent for dialysis procedures, hypotension was more marked in 2 patients whose blood was dialysed against an acetate bath rather than a bicarbonate bath. Dialysis had to be terminated in both patients because of a precipitous fall in blood pressure, which was associated with bradycardia in one patient. In view of the well-known vasodilatory effects of acetate it would seem reasonable to avoid the possible interaction in the future.— R. M. Zusman *et al.*, *New Engl. J. Med.*, 1981, *304*, 934.

Absorption and Fate. Prostacyclin is a product of arachidonic acid metabolism with a very short half-life. Following intravenous infusion of epoprostenol the half-life is only about 3 minutes.

A study of epoprostenol metabolites in plasma following infusion in healthy subjects. The major breakdown product was 6-keto-prostaglandin $F_{1\alpha}$.— B. Rosenkranz *et al.*, *Clin. Pharmac. Ther.*, 1981, *29*, 420.

Uses. Epoprostenol is a prostaglandin (see p.1353) which causes vasodilatation and prevents platelet aggregation.

Epoprostenol has been used as an anticoagulant in dialysis procedures, and has been studied in cardiovascular disorders, including angina pectoris and peripheral vascular disease. Epoprostenol has also been used in pre-eclampsia, and in the haemolytic-uraemic syndrome and thrombotic thrombocytopenic purpura.

Epoprostenol is given by intravenous infusion.

An account of arachidonic acid metabolism with special reference to thromboxane A_2 and prostacyclin and their role in the homoeostatic regulation of normal interactions of the platelet and vessel wall. Whereas thromboxane A_2 induces platelet aggregation and constricts arterial smooth muscle, prostacyclin prevents platelet aggregation and causes vasodilatation.— S. Moncada and J. R. Vane, *New Engl. J. Med.*, 1979, *300*, 1142.

Further reviews of the endogenous role of prostacyclin and its potential clinical applications: S. Moncada and J. R. Vane, *Pharmac. Rev.*, 1978, *30*, 293; *Lancet*, 1981, *1*, 643; S. Moncada and J. R. Vane, *Drugs*, 1981, *21*, 430.

Asthma. Results of a study in 11 asthmatic subjects indicated that epoprostenol effectively prevented bronchoconstriction induced by inhalation of a mist of distilled water and by exercise, but did not have bronchodilator activity. All subjects experienced an increase in heart-rate, this effect being particularly evident in women, in whom a significant decrease in diastolic pressure and a slight hot facial flush was also noted. Slight laryngotracheal irritation with transient coughing was also common.— S. Bianco *et al.*, *IRCS Med. Sci.*, 1978, *6*, 256. In a further 10 patients epoprostenol was ineffective in preventing bronchoconstriction induced by inhalation of a pneumoallergen.— *idem*, *Eur. J. resp. Dis.*, 1980, *61*, *Suppl.* 106, 81.

Cardiovascular disorders. *Angina pectoris.* Comment on the change in the concept of unstable angina from a mechanism involving transient increases in oxygen demand to one involving transient decreases in oxygen supply, and the potentially beneficial role of epoprostenol to end the instability.— J. S. Borer, *New Engl. J. Med.*, 1980, *302*, 1200. Intravenous infusion of epoprostenol 5 ng per kg body-weight per minute for 12 to 48 hours had a very favourable effect in 9 patients with recurrent attacks of spontaneous angina, but a dose of 5 to 10 ng per kg per minute offered no protection against anginal attacks precipitated by atrial pacing in any of 7 patients studied. Pending confirmation in a double-blind study, epoprostenol may thus be of therapeutic note in attacks of angina pectoris precipitated by reduction of oxygen delivery to the myocardium rather than by increased oxygen demand.— A. Szczeklik *et al.* (letter), *ibid.*, *303*, 881.

A study of the haemodynamic and metabolic effects of epoprostenol 2, 4, 6, and 8 ng per kg body-weight per minute in 10 male patients with coronary heart disease. The coronary and systemic effects were similar to those produced by short-acting nitrates and, together with improved pacing time to angina, indicate an acute beneficial effect. The additional effect of inhibition of platelet aggregation suggests that epoprostenol should be evaluated in unstable angina since it has been shown in experimental coronary stenoses to prevent platelet accumulation and progression to total occlusion. There were no major adverse effects during the infusion although all 10 patients had facial flushing with the 6 and 8 ng infusion levels, and some patients had mild headache at the highest infusion level; no arrhythmias were observed.— G. Bergman *et al.*, *Lancet*, 1981, *1*, 569. Comment on similar findings in haemodynamic indices but absence of improved exercise tolerance.— A. Szczeklik *et al.* (letter), *ibid.*, 1006.

Further references to epoprostenol in coronary heart disease: R. J. C. Hall and H. A. Dewar (letter), *Lancet*, 1981, *1*, 949 (potential role of local coronary arterial infusion); P. D. Hirsh *et al.*, *New Engl. J. Med.*, 1981, *304*, 685; R. M. Robertson *et al.*, *ibid.*, 998 (relevance of thromboxane).

Peripheral vascular disease. Striking clinical improvement was obtained in 5 patients with advanced arteriosclerosis obliterans of the lower limbs, following intra-arterial infusion of epoprostenol in an initial dose of 2 ng per kg body-weight per minute, increased at hourly intervals to 5 to 10 ng per kg per minute, and given for 72 hours. Pain at rest disappeared in all patients within 2 days of completing the infusion; in 3 of the 5 the necrosis completely regressed within 2 months and ulcers healed; the other 2 were considerably improved and subsequent infusions after 2 months increased this improvement. Side-effects included pain in the legs in 2 patients at the infusion-rate of 10 ng per kg per minute, reduction in systolic and diastolic blood pressure by an average of 15 mmHg, and increase in heart-rate by 5 to 20 beats per minute.— A. Szczeklik *et al.*, *Lancet*, 1979, *1*, 1111.

Six of 8 consecutive patients with end-stage peripheral arteriosclerosis and ischaemic ulcers responded to epoprostenol infusion with complete or partial healing. The effect on ulcer pain was remarkable in these 6 patients, but did not occur in a patient whose ulcer did not heal. The epoprostenol infusion was prepared in a glycine buffer at pH 10.5 at a concentration of 4 µg per ml and was given intravenously through a constant infusion pump for 12 hours daily for 3 days, in mean doses ranging from 1 to 5 ng per kg body-weight per minute. A high frequency of side-effects occurred, flushing, headache, nausea and vomiting, and general feeling of uneasiness being the most important complaints. One patient experienced these symptoms at the 1 ng per kg per minute dose, whereas another tolerated five times this amount with the same severity of symptoms.— A. G. Olsson (letter), *Lancet*, 1980, *2*, 1076. Comment on the need for controlled studies.— G. A. FitzGerald (letter), *ibid.*, 1981, *1*, 40.

Further references to epoprostenol in peripheral vascular disease: A. Szczeklik *et al.*, *Prostaglandins*, 1978, *16*, 651 (administration by aerosol inhalation).

Connective tissue disorders. A study of the effect of epoprostenol in 5 women with severe Raynaud's phenomenon associated with systemic sclerosis. Intravenous infusion of epoprostenol significantly enhanced the isoprenaline-stimulated increase in lymphocyte cyclic adenosine monophosphate.— J. D. T. Kirby *et al.*, *Lancet*, 1980, *2*, 453.

Extracorporeal circulation. A study in 11 subjects requiring regular haemodialysis indicated that continuous administration of epoprostenol 5 ng per kg body-weight per minute, by means of an infusion pump, via the dialyser inlet (arterial) line, during dialysis, enhanced the biological activity of heparin and prevented the activation and consumption of platelets. The only side-effect was mild transient facial flushing. Reduction in heparin requirements by means of epoprostenol administration should make dialysis safer, particularly for patients at risk of bleeding, while preserving the biocompatibility of the dialysis circuit. It remains to be determined whether platelet protection and heparin sparing will reduce the long-term risks of atherogenesis and osteoporosis in dialysis patients.— J. H. Turney *et al.*, *Lancet*, 1980, *2*, 219.

A report of the successful use of epoprostenol as the sole antithrombotic agent for haemodialysis in one patient with acute renal failure and 10 with chronic renal failure. With its short half-life of only about 3 to 5 minutes, and its ability to leave the clotting mechanism intact while providing adequate anticoagulation by platelet inhibition, epoprostenol was less liable to induce haemorrhage than heparin. In particular, the patient with acute renal failure had developed life-threatening bleeding from a gastro-intestinal lesion with heparin, whereas epoprostenol was associated with neither anticoagulation nor haemorrhage. Despite the advantages of epoprostenol its use was not without important hazards: symptomatic hypotension in all patients (most marked in 2 whose blood was dialysed against an acetate rather than a bicarbonate bath), and various gastro-intestinal complaints, flushing, and headache occurred in most patients. Although epoprostenol is not indicated for stable patients who can safely undergo haemodialysis with heparin, it may have a role in those at risk of bleeding. Owing to hypotension, the initial dose of 4 ng per kg per minute was reduced in all patients, in some to as little as 0.25 ng per kg per minute; it was given for periods of 34 to 240 minutes, and 2 patients underwent dialysis successfully for 240 minutes despite receiving epoprostenol for periods of only 34 and 42 minutes.— R. M. Zusman *et al.*, *New Engl. J. Med.*, 1981, *304*, 934.

Further references to the use of epoprostenol as an anticoagulant during haemodialysis and other extracorporeal circulatory procedures: A. E. S. Gimson *et al.*, *Lancet*, 1980, *1*, 173 (in fulminant hepatic failure treated by haemoperfusion); D. B. Longmore *et al.*, *Lancet*, 1981, *1*, 800 (during cardiopulmonary bypass); R. S. Arze and M. K. Ward (letter), *Lancet*, 1981, *2*, 50 (haemodialysis); J. G. Abuelo and B. S. Chang (letter), *ibid.*, 470 (haemodialysis; the need for a comparison with a group of patients not given anticoagulant).

Gastro-intestinal disorders. Prostacyclin had been found in the rectal mucosa of 16 healthy subjects. It might play an important role in the pathology of diarrhoea, proctitis, or rectal neoplasm. The action of sulphasalazine could be due to inhibition of prostacyclin synthesis.— H. Sinzinger *et al.* (letter), *Lancet*, 1978, *2*, 1253.

Obstetrics and gynaecology. A report of the successful use of infusion of epoprostenol 8 ng per kg body-weight per minute to control severe hypertension of pregnancy. The hypertension was controlled for 3 days; on the fourth day evidence of foetal distress necessitated caesarean section. The epoprostenol infusion was used to control blood pressure during the operative procedure.— J. Fidler *et al.* (letter), *Lancet*, 1980, *2*, 31.

Comment on the possible role of reduced foetal vascular prostacyclin activity in pre-eclampsia.— G. Remuzzi *et al.* (letter), *Lancet*, 1980, *2*, 310. See also R. C. Goodlin (letter), *ibid.* Reduced concentrations of prostacyclin-like activity were found in the amniotic fluid of 5 consecutive patients with pre-eclamptic toxaemia, compared with 15 uncomplicated pregnancies. A clinical trial of epoprostenol in the treatment of pre-eclampsia seems warranted.— A. Bodzenta *et al.* (letter), *ibid.*, 650. A fall has also been noted in the production of prostacyclin activity by maternal vessels.— F. Bussolino *et al.* (letter), *ibid.*, 702. Evidence of reduced foetal prostacyclin production in pre-eclampsia.— I. Downing *et al.* (letter), *ibid.*, 1374. Evidence that prostacyclin production is very low in neonates born of pregnancies complicated by chronic placental insufficiency (intrauterine growth retardation, essential hypertension, and pre-eclampsia) but is normal in those with acute placental insufficiency (abruptio placentae).— M. J. Stuart *et al.*, *ibid.*, 1981, *1*, 1126. Further references: L. O. Carreras *et al.* (letter), *ibid.*, 442; P. J. Lewis *et al.* (letter), *ibid.*, 559; C. W. G. Redman *et al.* (letter), *ibid.*, 731.

Evidence that prostacyclin is involved in excessive menstrual bleeding.— S. K. Smith *et al.*, *Lancet*, 1981, *1*, 522.

For a beneficial effect of epoprostenol in persistent foetal circulation, see under Pulmonary Vascular Disorders, below.

Ocular disorders. A study in 8 diabetic males with proliferative retinopathy, compared with 8 non-diabetic males, indicating that circulating prostacyclin may be reduced in diabetes. Although it seems unlikely that deficient production of prostacyclin is the cause of diabetic microangiopathy, it cannot yet be ruled out as a factor contributing to the risk of vascular occlusion in diabetic patients.— C. T. Dollery *et al.*, *Lancet*, 1979, *2*, 1365. A report of decreased vascular prostacyclin in juvenile-onset diabetes.— K. Silberbauer (letter), *New Engl. J. Med.*, 1979, *300*, 366.

Beneficial results with epoprostenol in 2 of 3 patients with central retinal vein occlusion. The epoprostenol was successful in 2 patients treated 24 and 48 hours after occlusion, but not in one patient treated later. It was given as epoprostenol sodium in glycine buffer at pH 10.5 and infused into the right subclavian vein at a dose of 5 ng per kg body-weight per minute for 72 hours.— H. Zygulska-Mach *et al.* (letter), *Lancet*, 1980, *2*, 1075.

Pulmonary vascular disorders. A report of dose-dependent pulmonary vasodilatation in 7 adult patients with pulmonary hypertension secondary to mitral stenosis. Increasing doses of epoprostenol of 2, 5, and 10 ng per kg body-weight per minute were given intravenously each for 30 minutes.— J. Szczeklik *et al.* (letter), *Lancet*, 1980, *2*, 1076. See also W. D. Watkins *et al.* (letter), *Lancet*, 1980, *1*, 1083.

Persistent foetal circulation. A neonate with severe and refractory hypoxaemia secondary to pulmonary vasoconstriction obtained a beneficial response to injection of epoprostenol directly into the pulmonary artery.— J. E. Lock *et al.* (letter), *Lancet*, 1979, *1*, 1343. The findings are contrary to those noted in *animals* and may reflect species difference or an unusual sensitivity to epoprostenol. Further investigation is needed before extensive clinical use.— S. Cassin *et al.* (letter), *ibid.*, 1979, *2*, 638.

Renal disorders. A suggestion that the administration of epoprostenol along with aspirin, whole blood, and fresh frozen plasma may have contributed to the recovery of a 31-year-old patient with postpartum haemolytic-uraemic syndrome with evidence of prostacyclin deficiency. Epoprostenol was given by continuous infusion.— J. Webster *et al.*, *Br. med. J.*, 1980, *281*, 271.

Failure of epoprostenol in a woman with thrombotic thrombocytopenic purpura. Adverse effects had led to a need for dosage reduction and it was considered that better control of dose-limiting toxicity might permit successful treatment of thrombotic thrombocytopenic purpura and haemolytic-uraemic syndrome.— G. T. Budd *et al.* (letter), *Lancet*, 1980, *2*, 915. Beneficial effect in one patient with thrombotic thrombocytopenic purpura following prolonged infusion with epoprostenol.— G. A. Fitzgerald *et al.*, *Ann. intern. Med.*, 1981, *95*, 319.

Manufacturers
Wellcome, UK.

8086-p

Fenprostalene. RS-84043. Methyl (±)-7-{(1*R*,2*R*,3*R*,5*S*)-3,5-dihydroxy-2-[(*E*)-(3*R*)-3-hydroxy-4-phenoxybut-1-enyl]cyclopentyl}hepta-4,5-dienoate.
$C_{23}H_{30}O_6$=402.5.

CAS — 69381-94-8.

Fenprostalene is a synthetic prostaglandin derivative of the F series (see p.1353) with potential use as a luteolytic agent.

Manufacturers
Syntex, USA.

8087-s

Fluprostenol Sodium *(B.P. Vet.)*. ICI-81008. Sodium (±)-(*Z*)-7-{(1*R*,2*R*,3*R*,5*S*)-3,5-dihydroxy-2-[(*E*)-(3*R*)-3-hydroxy-4-(3-trifluoromethylphenoxy)but-1-enyl]cyclopentyl}hept-5-enoate.
$C_{23}H_{28}F_3NaO_6$=480.5.

CAS — 40666-16-8 (fluprostenol); 55028-71-2 (sodium salt).

A white or almost white hygroscopic powder. Freely **soluble** in water, alcohol, and methyl alcohol. **Store** in airtight containers. Protect from light.

Uses. Fluprostenol sodium is a synthetic prostaglandin derivative of the F series (see p.1353). It is used as a luteolytic agent in veterinary medicine.

Preparations

Fluprostenol Injection *(B.P. Vet.)*. A sterile solution of fluprostenol sodium in Water for Injections; it may contain suitable buffering agents. Sterilise by autoclaving or by filtration. Protect from light. Potency is expressed in terms of fluprostenol.

Proprietary Names
Equimate (veterinary) *(ICI Pharmaceuticals, UK)*.

8088-w

Gemeprost. ONO-802; 16,16-Dimethyl-*trans*-Δ^2-prostaglandin E_1 methyl ester. Methyl (2*E*,13*E*)-(8*R*,11*R*,12*R*,15*R*)-11,15-dihydroxy-16,16-dimethyl-9-oxoprosta-2,13-dienoate; Methyl (*E*)-7-{(1*R*,2*R*,3*R*)-3-hydroxy-2-[(*E*)-(3*R*)-3-hydroxy-4,4-dimethyloct-1-enyl]-5-oxocyclopentyl}hept-2-enoate.
$C_{23}H_{38}O_5$=394.6.

CAS — 64318-79-2.

Uses. Gemeprost is a synthetic prostaglandin derivative of the E series (see p.1353). It has been used for the termination of pregnancy.

Termination of pregnancy. A review of the termination of abnormal intra-uterine pregnancy with prostaglandins, including gemeprost.— S. M. M. Karim *et al.*, *Singapore J. Obstet. Gynaec.*, 1980, *11*, 7.

Administration of gemeprost as pessaries containing 1 mg every 3 hours to a total of 5 doses to 50 pregnant women between 5 and 20 weeks' gestation caused complete abortion in 28 and incomplete abortion in 15; treatment was ineffective in the remaining 7. In all patients vaginal bleeding started after the insertion of the second pessary. Diarrhoea, vomiting, and fever occurred in 42, 6, and 4% of the patients respectively.— T. Wagatsuma *et al.*, *Contraception*, 1979, *19*, 591.

Menstrual induction. In a study involving pregnant women with less than 49 days of amenorrhoea complete abortion occurred in 26 of 30 given gemeprost 1-mg pessaries every 3 hours up to a total of 5 doses, in 24 of 28 undergoing suction termination under local anaesthesia, and in all of 28 undergoing suction termination under general anaesthesia. Gemeprost induced uterine bleeding in all patients but the mean duration of bleeding and the total menstrual blood loss was similar in all 3 groups.— S. K. Smith and D. T. Baird, *Br. J. Obstet. Gynaec.*, 1980, *87*, 712.

Manufacturers
May & Baker, UK.

8089-e

Luprostiol. (±)-(*Z*)-7-{(1*S*,2*R*,3*R*,5*S*)-2-[(2*S*)-3-(3-Chlorophenoxy)-2-hydroxypropylthio]-3,5-dihydroxycyclopentyl}hept-5-enoic acid.
$C_{21}H_{29}ClO_6S$=445.0.

CAS — 67110-79-6.

Luprostiol is a synthetic prostaglandin derivative of the F series (see p.1353) with potential use as a luteolytic agent in veterinary medicine.

Manufacturers
E. Merck, UK.

8090-b

Meteneprost. U-46785. (5*Z*,13*E*)-(8*R*,11*R*,12*R*,15*R*)-11,15-Dihydroxy-16,16-dimethyl-9-methyleneprosta-5,13-dienoic acid; (*Z*)-7-{(1*R*,2*R*,3*R*)-3-Hydroxy-2-[(*E*)-(3*R*)-3-hydroxy-4,4-dimethyloct-1-enyl]-5-methylenecyclopentyl}hept-5-enoic acid.
$C_{23}H_{38}O_4$=378.6.

CAS — 61263-35-2.

Uses. Meteneprost is a synthetic prostaglandin derivative. It has been used for the termination of pregnancy.

Meteneprost exhibits greater biological selectivity than 16,16-dimethyldinoprostone, together with greatly enhanced chemical stability. Of 24 second-trimester patients, treated at 0 and 8 hours with one vaginal suppository containing meteneprost 75 mg, 20 aborted within 24 hours and one at 26 hours without further therapy. Eleven patients vomited during treatment and one had 2 episodes of diarrhoea. In the other 3 patients the procedure was completed with 1 to 3 intramuscular injections of 15-methyldinoprost. Similar efficacy and low frequency of side-effects had been noted following oral administration. Results with vaginal administration for termination of very early pregnancy, and for preoperative cervical dilatation in late first trimester abortion, are also promising.— M. Bygdeman *et al.* (letter), *Lancet*, 1979, *1*, 1136.

Manufacturers
Upjohn, USA.

8091-v

Oxoprostol. M&B 33153. *trans*-2-(7-Hydroxyheptyl)-3-(3-oxo-4-phenoxybutyl)cyclopentanone.
$C_{22}H_{32}O_4$=360.5.

CAS — 69648-40-4.

Oxoprostol is a synthetic prostaglandin derivative with potential use as an inhibitor of gastric acid secretion.

Manufacturers
May & Baker, UK.

8092-g

Prostaglandin A_1. U-20305; PGA_1. (13*E*)-(8*R*,12*S*,15*S*)-15-Hydroxy-9-oxoprosta-10,13-dienoic acid; 7-{(1*R*,2*S*)-2-[(*E*)-(3*S*)-3-Hydroxyoct-1-enyl]-5-oxocyclopent-3-enyl}heptanoic acid.
$C_{20}H_{32}O_4$=336.5.

CAS — 14152-28-4; 20348-61-2 (±).

Solutions of prostaglandin A_1 0.1% in alcohol were stable for at least 2 years at 4°. When these solutions were diluted to 0.005% with sodium chloride injection to prepare an infusion the resulting solutions were chemically stable for 2 days at 4° and 1 day at 25°.— T. J. Roseman *et al.*, *Am. J. Hosp. Pharm.*, 1973, *30*, 236.

Prostaglandin A_1 is a prostaglandin of the A series (see p.1353).

The effect of prostaglandin A_1 on several vascular beds in man.— H. B. Barner *et al.*, *Am. Heart J.*, 1973, *85*, 584.

A review of the cardiovascular and renal effects of prostaglandins, including prostaglandin A_1.— J. B. Lee, *Archs intern. Med.*, 1974, *133*, 56.

Prostaglandin A_1 was administered by intravenous infusion (5 mg per 40 ml of dextrose injection) to a woman with congestive heart failure and severe hypertension (blood pressure 220/110 mmHg). At a dosage of 600 ng per kg body-weight per minute a marked diuresis occurred during the first 15 minutes with little change in blood pressure; within 2 minutes of increasing the dose to 2.4 µg per kg per minute blood pressure fell to 100/60 mmHg with a marked fall in the rate of urine flow; following gradual reduction of the dose back to 600 ng per kg per minute blood pressure and urine flow increased. The infusion was stopped after 137 minutes and within 5 minutes blood pressure levelled off at 180/120 mmHg and within several hours symptoms and signs of congestive heart failure had cleared. Prostaglandin A_1 appeared to be a promising agent for the treatment of acute hypertensive crisis with congestive heart failure.— L. M. Slotkoff, *Ann. intern. Med.*, 1974, *81*, 345.

Infusion of prostaglandin A_1 improved or corrected several metabolic abnormalities in a patient with hypertension, moderate renal insufficiency, chronic unexplained hyperkalaemia, and found to be suffering from hyporeninaemic hypoaldosteronism. It appears that a defect in renal prostaglandin synthesis had a central role in the pathophysiology of this condition.— L. H. Norby *et al.*, *Lancet*, 1978, *2*, 1118.

Manufacturers
Upjohn, USA.

8093-q

Prostaglandin A_2. PGA_2. (5*Z*,13*E*)-(8*R*,12*S*,15*S*)-15-Hydroxy-9-oxoprosta-5,10,13-trienoic acid; (*Z*)-7-{(1*R*,2*S*)-2-[(*E*)-(3*S*)-3-Hydroxyoct-1-enyl]-5-oxocyclopent-3-enyl}hept-5-enoic acid.
$C_{20}H_{30}O_4$=334.4.

CAS — 13345-50-1.

Prostaglandin A_2 is a prostaglandin of the A series (see p.1353).

A review of the cardiovascular and renal effects of prostaglandins, including prostaglandin A_2.— J. B. Lee, *Archs intern. Med.*, 1974, *133*, 56.

In 9 of 10 patients with renal failure, infusion of prostaglandin A_2 increased the renal blood flow by a mean of 50%; the glomerular filtration-rate was increased in only 5 patients by a mean of 22% and the plasma-renin activity decreased in 6 patients by a mean of 21%. The diuretic and natriuretic action was very moderate except in the one patient with acute renal failure.— A. Hornych and N. Papanicolaou, *Nouv. Presse méd.*, 1974, *3*, 2628.

8094-p

Prostaglandin D_2. PGD_2. (5*Z*,13*E*)-(8*R*,9*S*,12*R*,15*S*)-9,15-Dihydroxy-11-oxoprosta-5,13-dienoic acid; (*Z*)-7-{(1*R*,2*R*,5*S*)-5-Hydroxy-2-[(*E*)-(3*S*)-3-hydroxyoct-1-enyl]-3-oxocyclopentyl}hept-5-enoic acid.
$C_{20}H_{32}O_5$=352.5.

CAS — 41598-07-6.

Prostaglandin D_2 is a prostaglandin of the D series (see p.1353) with potential use as an antithrombotic agent.

Manufacturers
Upjohn, USA.

8095-s

Prostalene. RS-9390. Methyl (±)-(13*E*)-(8*R*,9*S*,11*R*,12*R*)-9,11,15-trihydroxy-15-methylprosta-4,5,13-trienoate; Methyl (±)-7-{(1*R*,2*R*,3*R*,5*S*)-3,5-dihydroxy-2-[(*E*)-3-hydroxy-3-methyloct-1-enyl]cyclopentyl}hepta-4,5-dienoate.
$C_{22}H_{36}O_5$=380.5.

CAS — 54120-61-5.

Uses. Prostalene is a synthetic prostaglandin derivative of the F series (see p.1353). It is used as a luteolytic agent in veterinary medicine.

Proprietary Names
Synchrocept *(Syntex, UK).*

8096-w

Sulprostone. CP-34089; SHB-286; ZK-57671; 16-Phenoxy-ω-17,18,19,20-tetranordinoprostone-methylsulphonamide. (*Z*)-7-{(1*R*,2*R*,3*R*)-3-Hydroxy-2-[(*E*)-(3*R*)-3-hydroxy-4-phenoxybut-1-enyl]-5-oxocyclopentyl]-*N*-(methylsulphonyl)}hept-5-enamide.
$C_{23}H_{31}NO_7S$=465.6.

CAS — 60325-46-4.

Uses. Sulprostone is a synthetic prostaglandin derivative of the E series (see p.1353). It has been used for the termination of pregnancy.

Termination of pregnancy. A review of the termination of abnormal intra-uterine pregnancy with prostaglandins, including sulprostone.— S. M. M. Karim *et al.*, *Singapore J. Obstet. Gynaec.*, 1980, *11*, 7.

A study of the administration of 4 dosage schedules of sulprostone intravenous infusion to 166 women between 5 and 12 weeks' of gestation. Complete abortion occurred in 7.1% of 14 patients given 1.7 µg per minute for 5 hours (total dose 0.5 mg), in 76.6% of 77 given 1.7 µg per minute for 10 hours (total dose 1 mg), in 55% of 40 given 2.8 µg per minute for 6 hours (total dose 1 mg), and in 28.6% of 35 given 4.1 µg per minute for 6 hours (total dose 1.5 mg). Common side-effects included uterine pain, nausea and vomiting, the incidence being the lowest in the group given sulprostone 1 mg over about 10 hours (the group with the highest abortifacient efficacy).— B. Schuessler *et al.*, *Contraception*, 1979, *19*, 29.

Further references to sulprostone and pregnancy termination: A. S. van den Bergh and A. A. Haspels, *Contraception*, 1978, *18*, 635; U. Gethmann *et al.*, *IRCS Med. Sci.*, 1978, *6*, 423.

Menstrual induction. A report of successful menstrual induction using sulprostone by intramuscular injection of 2 doses of 500 µg four hours apart.— A. I. Csapo *et al.* (letter), *Lancet*, 1980, *1*, 90.

Further references to sulprostone and pregnancy termination by menstrual induction: S. M. M. Karim *et al.*, *Contraception*, 1977, *16*, 377.

Proprietary Names
Nalador *(Schering, Ger.).*

8097-e

Tiaprost. Tiaprostum. (±)-(*Z*)-7-{(1*R*,2*R*,3*R*,5*S*)-3,5-Dihydroxy-2-[(*E*)-3-hydroxy-4-(3-thienyloxy)but-1-enyl]cyclopentyl}hept-5-enoic acid.
$C_{20}H_{28}O_6S$=396.5.

Tiaprost is a synthetic prostaglandin derivative of the F series (see p.1353).

Purgatives

7500-r

Purgatives (laxatives or cathartics) induce defaecation. They are widely used as self medications to satisfy the patient's desire for an altered or more regular bowel habit. Constipation can often be resolved without recourse to purgatives. An adjustment in diet to increase the content of vegetable fibre may be all that is required. Preparations such as psyllium (p.960), sterculia (p.961), methylcellulose (p.947), or bran (p.75) that increase the bulk of the faeces may be effective.

Purgatives should only be used in functional constipation that has not responded to these measures and they should be withdrawn as soon as possible. They are also used for bowel clearance before radiological examination, surgery, or childbirth.

Purgatives used in the treatment of functional constipation include phenolphthalein, senna, cascara, bisacodyl, and sodium picosulphate. In treating painful anorectal disorders, such as haemorrhoids and anal fissures, or to prevent straining at stool, lubricant purgatives such as liquid paraffin (p.1063) or docusate sodium (p.1441) may be of value. Salts of inorganic acids which are not extensively absorbed from the gastro-intestinal tract, such as sodium sulphate (p.643), retain water in the lumen of the bowel by an osmotic effect and are also used as purgatives.

Reviews of the use of purgatives and the treatment of constipation: C. Tasman-Jones, *Drugs*, 1973, *5*, 220; K. Goulston, *ibid.*, *6*, 237; *Drug & Ther. Bull.*, 1973, *11*, 77; D. E. Hyams, *Br. med. J.*, 1974, *1*, 107; E. W. Godding, *Pharm. J.*, 1975, *2*, 11, 34, 60, 81, 104, and 138; K. Rutter and D. Maxwell, *Br. med. J.*, 1976, *2*, 997; W. G. Thompson, *Can. med. Ass. J.*, 1976, *114*, 927; K. Goulston, *Drugs*, 1977, *14*, 128; H. J. Binder, *A. Rev. Pharmac. & Toxic.*, 1977, *17*, 355; R. G. Pietrusko, *Am. J. Hosp. Pharm.*, 1977, *34*, 291; N. V. Freeman, *Practitioner*, 1978, *221*, 333; W. G. Thompson, *Drugs*, 1980, *19*, 49.

Adverse Effects of Purgatives. The constant use of purgatives to induce a regular daily habit, which is commonly believed necessary for good health, may decrease the sensitivity of the intestinal mucous membranes so that larger doses have to be taken and the bowel fails to respond to normal stimuli. Thus the redevelopment of a normal habit is prevented.

The prolonged use of purgatives may produce watery diarrhoea with excessive loss of water and electrolytes, particularly potassium, muscular weakness and weight loss. Changes in the intestinal musculature associated with malabsorption, and dilatation of the bowel, similar to ulcerative colitis and to megacolon, may also occur. Cardiac and renal symptoms have been reported. Melanosis coli and discoloration of urine has followed the use of the anthraquinone purgatives.

Because the use of drastic purgatives, such as colocynth, croton oil, ipomoea, jalap, and podophyllum may be attended by severe irritation to the bowel and serious toxicity, they have mainly been replaced by purgatives of the anthraquinone group, such as senna or cascara, or by purgatives such as bisacodyl or lactulose.

Abuse. An extensive review of purgative abuse.— J. H. Cummings, *Gut*, 1974, *15*, 758.

Hypokalaemia. Reports of hypokalaemia associated with purgative abuse: N. Fleischer *et al.*, *Ann. intern. Med.*, 1969, *70*, 791; B. J. Fleming *et al.*, *Ann. intern. Med.*, 1975, *83*, 60; W. Dahlmann *et al.*, *Dt. med. Wschr.*, 1977, *102*, 1555; L. S. Basser, *Med. J. Aust.*, 1979, *1*, 47.

Osteomalacia. Osteomalacia and arthropathy in a 59-year-old woman, following prolonged abuse of purgatives.— B. M. Frier and R. D. M. Scott, *Br. J. clin. Pract.*, 1977, *31*, 17.

Pancreatic hyperplasia. Pancreatic islet cell hyperplasia associated with chronic laxative abuse in a 44-year-old man.— M. Lesna *et al.*, *Gut*, 1977, *18*, 1032.

Precautions. Purgatives should not be given to patients with intestinal obstruction, abdominal pain, nausea or vomiting. A number of purgatives are excreted in breast milk.

7501-f

Aloes *(B.P., Eur. P.)*. Aloe *(U.S.P.)*; Acibar.

CAS — 8001-97-6.

Pharmacopoeias. In *Arg., Aust., Belg., Br., Braz., Chin., Eur., Fr., Ger., Hung., Ind., It., Jap., Neth., Nord., Pol., Port., Roum., Span., Swiss, Turk.*, and *U.S. Br.* also includes Powdered Aloes.
Braz. and *Ind.* allow also Socotrine aloes.

The solid residue obtained by evaporating the liquid which drains from the cut leaves of various species of *Aloe* (Liliaceae); it is known in commerce as Cape or Barbados (Curaçao) aloes.

The *B.P.* describes Barbados aloes and Cape aloes containing not less than 28 and 18% respectively of hydroxyanthracene derivatives, calculated as anhydrous barbaloin.

Barbados aloes obtained from *Aloe barbadensis* (=*A. vera*) occurs as dark brown, opaque masses, with a conchoidal fracture; it has a strong characteristic penetrating odour reminiscent of iodoform and a nauseous bitter taste. It loses not more than 12% of its weight when dried.

Cape aloes obtained mainly from *Aloe ferox* and its hybrids occurs in dark brown masses tinged with green; it breaks with a shiny conchoidal fracture and has a strong characteristic acid odour and a nauseous bitter taste. It loses not more than 10% of its weight when dried.

Aloe (*U.S.P.*) is Cape Aloe or Curaçao Aloe, yielding not less than 50% of water-soluble extractive and losing not more than 12% of its weight when dried.

Socotrine aloes occurs as hard dark-brown or nearly black opaque masses with an uneven porous fracture and an unpleasant cheesy odour.

Zanzibar aloes occurs as livery-brown masses with a nearly smooth, slightly porous fracture and a slight odour.

Barbados and Cape aloes are partly soluble in boiling water, and practically insoluble in chloroform and ether. Powdered Barbados or Cape aloes are almost entirely soluble in alcohol 60%. **Protect** from light.

Adverse Effects and Precautions. As for Purgatives, p.1362.

The irritant action of aloes on the large intestine may cause pelvic congestion and in large doses aloes may cause nephritis.

Aloes should not be given in pregnancy; in nursing mothers it may be excreted in the milk.

Uses. Aloes is an anthraquinone purgative producing a motion within 12 hours of administration. Doses have generally been in the range of 100 to 300 mg. As it is intensely bitter it has been given in pills or tablets. Because of a tendency to cause griping, it has been used in conjunction with belladonna and carminatives. Aloes has been superseded by less toxic purgatives. It colours alkaline urine red.

Application of *Aloe vera* leaf as a domestic remedy for burns could provide a soothing effect but was not considered effective treatment.— A. G. Ship (letter), *J. Am. med. Ass.*, 1977, *238*, 1770.

The use of *Aloe vera* in cosmetics.— A. Y. Leung, *Drug Cosmet. Ind.*, 1977, *120* (June), 34.

The antifungal activity of whole-leaf powder and extracts from *Aloe arborescens* Mill subsp. *natalensis*.— K. Fujita *et al.*, *Antimicrob. Ag. Chemother.*, 1978, *14*, 132.

Preparations

Decoctions, extracts, mixtures, pills, tablets, and tinctures of aloes and tablets of aloin (see below) are described in Martindale 27th Edn, p. 1334.

7502-d

Aloin *(B.P.C. 1973)*.

CAS — 8015-61-0; 1415-73-2 (barbaloin).

Pharmacopoeias. In *Arg., Braz., Ind., Span.*, and *Swiss.*

A crystalline substance extracted from aloes and consisting almost entirely of barbaloin [10-β-D-glucopyranosyl-1,8-dihydroxy-3-hydroxymethylanthrone]. It is a pale or dull yellow, odourless or almost odourless, crystalline powder with an intensely bitter taste. It darkens on exposure to light.

Almost completely **soluble** 1 in 130 of water; soluble in alcohol and acetone; very slightly soluble in chloroform and ether. Solutions in water are neutral or not more than slightly acid to litmus. **Incompatible** with alkalis and oxidising agents.

Aloin has actions and uses similar to those of aloes but is more readily absorbed and is more likely to cause renal irritation. The urine, if alkaline, is coloured red. Doses have ranged from 13 to 60 mg.

Epidermal necrolysis. Toxic epidermal necrolysis had been reported after the ingestion of aloin.— B. Potter *et al.*, *Archs Derm.*, 1960, *82*, 903.

7503-n

Bisacodyl *(B.P., U.S.P.)*. 4,4′-(2-Pyridylmethylene)di(phenyl acetate).

$C_{22}H_{19}NO_4$=361.4.

CAS — 603-50-9.

Pharmacopoeias. In *Br., Braz., Cz., Jug.*, and *U.S.*

A white or off-white, odourless, tasteless, crystalline powder. M.p. 131° to 135°.

Practically **insoluble** in water; slightly soluble in alcohol and ether; freely soluble in chloroform; sparingly soluble in methyl alcohol. **Store** in airtight containers. Protect from light.

Adverse Effects and Precautions. As for Purgatives, p.1362.

Bisacodyl may occasionally cause severe abdominal cramps. When administered by rectum it sometimes causes irritation and repeated use may cause proctitis. Excessive purgation has also been reported. To avoid gastric irritation bisacodyl tablets are enteric-coated.

Inhalation of bisacodyl or contact with the eyes, skin, and mucous membranes should be avoided.

Absorption and Fate. Following administration by mouth a small amount is absorbed and excreted in the urine as the glucuronide, but up to 38% of the dose has been stated to be excreted in the urine in some patients. About 3% of the glucuronide appears in the bile after about 10 hours. Bisacodyl is mainly excreted in the faeces.

Bisacodyl was hydrolysed to bis(*p*-hydroxyphenyl)pyrid-2-ylmethane which was responsible for the laxative action.— R. Jauch *et al.*, *Arzneimittel-Forsch.*, 1975, *25*, 1796.

Uses. Bisacodyl is a purgative used for the treatment of constipation, for evacuation of the colon before radiological examination of the abdomen, or endoscopy, and before or after surgical operations. A solution of bisacodyl in a buffered macrogol basis may be administered together with barium enema solution. Its action is mainly in the large intestine and is probably due to intraluminal accumulation of water.

It is administered by mouth in enteric-coated tablets or by rectum in suppositories in doses of 5 to 10 mg daily. It acts within 10 to 12 hours when given after food and within 1 hour when given by rectum.

Introduction of bisacodyl or oxyphenisatin into the empty colon stimulated peristalsis, usually within 2 or 3 minutes, but the effect was delayed when faeces were present. Increased motility followed the application of bisacodyl or oxyphenisatin to the rectum but persistalsis did not occur. It was considered that bisacodyl might act by stimulating the submucosal nerve plexus and so exciting the deeper intermuscular plexus.— J. D. Hardcastle and C. V. Mann, *Gut,* 1968, *9,* 512.

A study involving 500 patients indicated that a regimen of colon cleansing, before radiological examination, using magnesium citrate followed by bisacodyl rectally and by mouth was more effective than one using castor oil and low phosphate enemas.— W. J. Dodds *et al., Am. J. Roentg.,* 1977, *128,* 57.

A thrice-weekly regimen using a faecal softener followed in 24 hours by rectal administration of a solution of bisacodyl in propylene glycol to evacuate the bowel was used successfully in the management of bowel incontinence in patients with spinal cord injuries.— R. F. Jones and G. J. L. Hall, *Med. J. Aust.,* 1979, *1,* 309.

Comment on the extreme unsuitability of suppositories for constipation in childhood.— G. S. Clayden (letter), *Lancet,* 1981, *1,* 273.

Preparations

Bisacodyl Suppositories *(B.P.).* Suppositories containing bisacodyl in a suitable basis. Store at a temperature not exceeding 30°.

Bisacodyl Suppositories *(U.S.P.).* Suppositories containing bisacodyl. Store at a temperature not exceeding 30°.

Bisacodyl Tablets *(B.P.).* Tablets containing bisacodyl. They are enteric-coated and sugar-coated.

Bisacodyl Tablets *(U.S.P.).* Tablets containing bisacodyl; they are enteric-coated. Store at a temperature not exceeding 30° in airtight containers.

Proprietary Preparations

Dulcodos *(Boehringer Ingelheim, UK).* Enteric-coated tablets each containing bisacodyl 5 mg and docusate sodium 100 mg. Laxative. *Dose.* 1 or 2 tablets at night.

Dulcolax *(Boehringer Ingelheim, UK).* Bisacodyl, available as **Children's Suppositories** each containing 5 mg; as **Suppositories** each containing 10 mg; and as enteric-coated **Tablets** of 5 mg. **Dulcolax Rectal Solution** contains bisacodyl 2.74 mg per ml in a buffered macrogol basis. (Also available as Dulcolax in *Belg., Canad., Denm., Fr., Ger., Ital., Neth., Norw., S.Afr., Swed., Switz., USA*).

Forrest X-Ray Prep Kit *(Forrest, Austral.: Schering, UK).* A kit consisting of 3 enteric-coated tablets each containing bisacodyl 5 mg; one suppository containing bisacodyl 10 mg; and a sachet of powder providing on solution magnesium citrate 12 g. For bowel preparation.

Other Proprietary Names

Austral.— Durolax, Toilex; *Canad.*— Bisacolax, Laco; *Denm.*—Perilax, Toilax; *Fr.*— Contlax; *Ger.*— Bisco-Zitron, Darmoletten, Eulaxan, Godalax, Laxagetten, Laxanin N, Laxbene, Med-Laxan, Neodrast, Obstilax forte, Serax, Stadalax, Vinco-Abführperlen; *Ital.*— Alaxa, Normalene; *Jap.*— Anan, Satolax-10; *Neth.*— Carters pilletjes, Nourilax N, Toilax; *Norw.*— Perilax, Toilax; *S.Afr.*— Perilax; *Spain*— Dulco-laxo, Sanvacual; *Swed.*— Toilax; *Switz.*— Ercolax, Laxbene, Prontolax, Rytmil, Spirolax; *USA*— Biscolax, Delco-Lax, Deficol, SK-Bisacodyl, Theralax.

7504-h

Buckthorn. Rhamnus; Bacca Spinae Cervinae; Nerprun; Espino Cerval.

Pharmacopoeias. In *Rus.* and *Span. Arg.* specifies the dried ripe fruit.

The fresh ripe fruit of buckthorn, *Rhamnus cathartica* (Rhamnaceae).

Buckthorn is a cathartic which is prone to cause severe griping; it is usually administered as a syrup. Its chief use has been in veterinary practice.

7505-m

Casanthranol. A purified mixture of the anthranol glycosides derived from cascara; practically devoid of free anthraquinones. Two active fractions have been identified as casanthranol A and casanthranol B.

CAS — 8024-48-4.

Casanthranol has purgative properties. It has been given in doses of 30 to 120 mg daily, together with a faecal softener.

7506-b

Cascara *(B.P., Eur. P.).* Casc.; Cascara Sagrada *(U.S.P.)*; Cascararinde; Sacred Bark; Rhamni Purshianae Cortex; Rhamnus Purshiana.

CAS — 8047-27-6.

Pharmacopoeias. In *Arg., Br., Belg., Braz., Eur., Fr., Ger., Int., It., Mex., Neth., Nord., Port., Span., Swiss, Turk.,* and *U.S. Br.* and *Turk.* also describe Powdered Cascara.

The dried bark of *Rhamnus purshiana* (Rhamnaceae), collected at least 1 year before use. The *B.P.* specifies that it contains not less than 8% of hydroxyanthracene derivatives of which not less than 60% consists of cascarosides, both calculated as cascaroside A.

Cascara contains the anthraquinone glycosides, cascarosides A and B (glucosides of barbaloin), cascarosides C and D (glucosides of chrysaloin), and other glucosides of anthraquinones, and not less than 23% of water-soluble extractive. It has a characteristic odour and a nauseous bitter and persistent taste. **Store** in a cool place in airtight containers. Protect from light.

Storage. Maturing during storage might be effected in 5 months and longer periods were considered unnecessary. The bark was fairly stable after drying and little difference had been found between fresh samples and others which were 8 years old.— J. W. Fairbairn, *Pharm. J.,* 1963, *1,* 271.

Adverse Effects and Precautions. As for Purgatives, p.1362.

There may be some excretion in breast milk.

Artificially high concentrations of urinary oestrogens could be recorded in patients taking purgatives containing cascara.— *Adverse Drug React. Bull.,* 1972, June, 104.

Cascara could cause red discoloration in alkaline urine.— R. B. Baran and B. Rowles, *J. Am. pharm. Ass.,* 1973, *NS13,* 139.

Uses. Cascara is an anthraquinone purgative with a mild action. The glycosides are hydrolysed by colonic bacteria and the active anthraquinones liberated in the colon, which is thereby stimulated; the stomach and small intestine are not normally affected. It is preferably given at night, a soft stool being evacuated from 6 to 8 hours later. Owing to its unpleasant taste, cascara is usually administered as an elixir, or in tablets.

Preparations

Elixirs

Cascara Elixir *(B.P.).* An aqueous extract of cascara (1 in 1) and liquorice (1 in 8) with glycerol 30% v/v and flavouring agents.

It is practically free from bitterness. *Dose.* 2 to 5 ml.

Extracts

Aromatic Cascara Fluidextract *(U.S.P.).* An aqueous extract (1 in 1) with liquorice, flavouring agents, and alcohol 20% v/v. Store at a temperature not exceeding 40° in airtight containers. Protect from light.

Cascara Dry Extract *(B.P.).* Casc. Dry Ext. A percolate (using boiling water) evaporated to dryness, containing not less than 13% of total hydroxyanthracene derivatives, of which not less than 40% is cascarosides, calculated as cascaroside A.

Store in airtight containers.

Several pharmacopoeias include similar extracts.

Cascara Liquid Extract *(B.P.).* Casc. Liq. Ext. An aqueous percolate equivalent to 1 in 1 and containing 25% v/v of alcohol (90%). *Dose.* 2 to 5 ml.

Cascara Sagrada Extract *(U.S.P.).* A percolate (using boiling water) evaporated to dryness. One g represents 3 g of cascara. Store at a temperature not exceeding 30° in airtight containers. Protect from light.

Cascara Sagrada Fluidextract *(U.S.P.).* An aqueous percolate equivalent to 1 in 1 and containing 20% v/v of alcohol. Store at a temperature not exceeding 40° in airtight containers. Protect from light.

Mixtures

Cascara and Belladonna Mixture *(B.P.C. 1973).* Mist. Casc. Co.; Compound Cascara Mixture. Cascara elixir 2 ml, belladonna tincture 0.5 ml, double-strength chloroform water 5 ml, water to 10 ml. It must be freshly prepared. *Dose.* 10 to 20 ml.

Tablets

Cascara Tablets *(B.P.).* Casc. Tab.; Cascara Sagrada Extract Tablets; Cascara Sagrada Tablets. Each contains 17 to 23 mg of total hydroxyanthracene derivatives, of which not less than 40% is cascarosides, calculated as cascaroside A. Unless otherwise specified, sugar-coated tablets are supplied. *Dose.* 1 or 2 tablets.

Cascara Tablets *(U.S.P.).* Tablets containing cascara. Store (if uncoated) in airtight containers.

Proprietary Names

Cas-Evac *(Parke, Davis, Canad.)*; Péristaltine *(Ciba, Fr.)*.

Cascara was formerly marketed in Great Britain under the proprietary name Cascara Evacuant (*Parke, Davis*).

7507-v

Cassia Pulp *(B.P.C. 1959).* Cassiae Pulpa; Cass. Pulp.

Pharmacopoeias. In *Ind.*

The aqueous percolate of crushed ripe cassia fruits (cassia pods), *Cassia fistula* (Leguminosae), evaporated to the consistence of a soft extract.

Cassia pulp is purgative owing to its content of hydroxymethylanthraquinones and is used in doses of 4 to 8 g. It is an ingredient of Senna Confection (see p.1368). It is rarely used alone.

7508-g

Colocynth *(B.P.C. 1963).* Colocynthis; Colocynth Pulp; Bitter Apple; Coloquinte; Koloquinthen; Coloquintidas.

NOTE. The synonym Bitter Apple has also been applied to the fruits of *Solanum incanum.*

Pharmacopoeias. In *Port.*

The dried pulp of the fruit of *Citrullus colocynthis* (Cucurbitaceae). It occurs in commerce in light whitish balls, about 5 cm in diameter, or in broken pieces.

Adverse Effects. As for Purgatives, p.1362.

Severe abdominal pain, vomiting, diarrhoea with blood-stained watery stools, delirium, and prostration may occur. A dose of from 4 to 6 g may be fatal. The powdered drug causes severe pain if it comes into contact with the nasal mucous membrane.

Four middle-aged or elderly women with symptoms including muscular weakness, cramps, thirst, and diarrhoea eventually admitted to having taken compound colocynth and jalap tablets for considerable periods. One patient initially diagnosed as having acute nephritis developed haematuria, oliguria, and oedema of the face and legs. In 2 others the symptoms suggested neurasthenia, Addison's disease, Conn's syndrome, and Crohn's disease. The patients were found to have hypokalaemia, and sigmoidoscopy showed the mucosa to be pale and oedematous. Three of the patients had been unable to stop taking laxatives because they felt constipated, bloated, or distended.— M. D. Rawson, *Lancet,* 1966, *1,* 1121.

Treatment of Adverse Effects. In overdosage the stomach should be emptied by inducing emesis or by aspiration and lavage. Morphine should be given intramuscularly. Atropine may assist the relief of spasm. Water and electrolyte losses should be replaced.

Precautions. As for Purgatives, p.1362. Colocynth should not be given to nursing mothers since the active principles may appear in the milk during lactation.

Uses. Colocynth has a drastic purgative action and has been used with hyoscyamus to counteract the severe griping. Colocynth has been superseded by less drastic and less toxic purgatives. It was used in doses of 120 to 300 mg.

Preparations

Various colocynth preparations, including those sometimes known as Christison's Pills, Vegetable Laxative Tablets, Alexander's Liver Pills, Gregory's Pills, and Hamilton's Pills, *are described in Martindale, 27th Edn,* p. 1336.

A preparation containing colocynth was formerly marketed in Great Britain under the proprietary name Tablax (*Wellcome*).

7509-q

Croton Oil *(B.P.C. 1949).* Oleum Crotonis; Oleum Tiglii.

CAS — 8001-28-3.

Pharmacopoeias. In *Arg., Port.,* and *Span. Chin. P.* includes fruits of *Croton tiglium.*

An oil expressed from the seeds of *Croton tiglium* (Euphorbiaceae). It is an amber-yellow, orange, or brown, viscous liquid with a nauseous odour and a taste which is at first mild but afterwards sharp and acrid. Wt per ml about 0.95 g.

Practically **insoluble** in water; soluble 1 in less than 1 of dehydrated alcohol forming a clear solution but the addition of more alcohol causes separation into 2 layers; freely soluble in carbon disulphide, chloroform, ether, light petroleum, and fixed and volatile oils. Exposure to air and light causes darkening and increases the viscosity of the oil and its solubility in alcohol. **Store** in airtight containers. Protect from light.

Croton oil is so violent a purgative that it should not now be employed. Externally, it is a powerful counter-irritant and vesicant.

Phorbol myristate acetate was the most active irritant and tumour-promoting constituent of croton oil.— J. F. Mustard and M. A. Packham, *Drugs,* 1975, *9,* 19.

Significant inhibitory activity of croton oil against P-388 lymphocytic leukaemia in *mice* was associated with a major component, phorbol 12-tiglate 13-decanoate.— S. M. Kupchan *et al., Science,* 1976, *191,* 571.

The possible mechanism of action of tumour promoters such as the phorbol diesters found in croton oil is discussed.— I. B. Weinstein and M. Wigler, *Nature,* 1977, *270,* 659.

7510-d

Danthron *(B.P., B.P. Vet., U.S.P.).*

Dantron; Dianthon; Dioxyanthrachinonum; Antrapurol; Dihydroxyanthraquinone; Chrysazin. 1,8-Dihydroxyanthraquinone.

$C_{14}H_8O_4$=240.2.

CAS — 117-10-2.

Pharmacopoeias. In *Aust., Br., Ger., Neth., Pol.,* and *U.S.*

An orange, almost odourless and tasteless, crystalline powder. M.p. 190° to 197°. It is not wetted by water and its preparations contain a wetting agent.

Practically **insoluble** in water; soluble 1 in 2500 of alcohol, 1 in 30 of chloroform, and 1 in 500 of ether; soluble in solutions of alkali hydroxides and in hot glacial acetic acid.

Adverse Effects and Precautions. Danthron colours the urine and perianal skin pink or red. The mucosa of the large intestine may be discoloured with prolonged use or high dosage. Superficial sloughing of discoloured skin may occur in incontinent patients or children wearing napkins; danthron should not be used in such patients.

Leucopenia and liver damage with deposits of IgE were reported in a 24-year-old woman taking a preparation containing danthron with docusate calcium for the treatment of chronic constipation. Neither drug alone caused changes in serum-bilirubin concentrations. Serum concentrations of bilirubin, alkaline phosphatase and SGOT returned to normal when treatment was discontinued.— K. G. Tolman *et al., Ann. intern. Med.,* 1976, *84,* 290.

Skin discoloration. Greyish-blue discoloration of the skin in a 51-year-old nurse appeared to be associated with the danthron content of Dorbanex.— C. S. Darke and R. G. Cooper, *Br. med. J.,* 1978, *1,* 1188.

Absorption and Fate. Danthron is excreted in breast milk.

Danthron given within 24 hours of induction of labour was found as the glucuronide in the urine of the mothers, with slightly less in the first urine of the infants. The meconium was not stained and there was no report of foetal catharsis in a study of 160 women, 24 of whom had taken an anthraquinone purgative during pregnancy.— A. W. Blair *et al., Archs Dis. Childh.,* 1976, *51,* 239.

Uses. Danthron is an anthraquinone purgative. It is usually given in doses of 50 to 150 mg at bedtime and is effective within 6 to 8 hours. It is often given with a wetting agent such as poloxamer 188 or docusate sodium which may increase its absorption.

Constipation. A comparison with senna.— P. G. Harris, *Practitioner,* 1966, *196,* 702.

A comparison with bisacodyl.— L. J. Christopher, *Practitioner,* 1969, *202,* 821.

Preparations

Danthron Tablets *(U.S.P.).* Tablets containing danthron.

Dorbanex *(Riker, UK).* **Capsules** each containing danthron 25 mg and poloxamer '188' 200 mg and **Liquid** containing the above amounts in each 5 ml (suggested diluent, syrup or tragacanth mucilage). For constipation. *Dose.* 1 or 2 capsules, or 5 to 10 ml of liquid, at bedtime (children, 2.5 to 5 ml of liquid); before or after surgery, 2 to 4 capsules, or 10 to 20 ml of liquid at bedtime. (Also available as Dorbanex in *Swed.*).

Dorbanex Forte Syrup *(Riker, UK).* Contains in each 5 ml danthron 75 mg and poloxamer '188' 1 g. For constipation. *Dose.* 5 ml at bedtime.

Other Proprietary Names

Bancon *(Ital.)*; Dorbane *(Canad., USA)*; Duolax *(USA)*; Fructines-Vichy (see also under Phenolphthalein) *(Fr.)*; Istizin *(Neth.)*; Modane *(Canad., USA)*; Roydan *(Canad.).*

7511-n

Euonymus *(B.P.C. 1954).* Wahoo Bark; Fusain Noir Pourpré.

The dried root-bark of *Euonymus atropurpureus* (Celastraceae).

Euonymus administered as an extract or tincture has a mild purgative action.

7512-h

Fig *(B.P.).*

Ficus; Carica.

CAS — 9001-33-6 (ficin).

The sun-dried succulent fruit of *Ficus carica* (Moraceae) containing not less than 60% of water-soluble extractive. It contains about 50% of sugars, consisting chiefly of invert sugar with some sucrose; small amounts of citric, acetic, and malic acids, and a proteolytic enzyme, ficin, are also present. **Store** in a dry place.

Fig is a mild purgative and demulcent, used medicinally as a confection or syrup, usually with senna and carminatives.

Preparations

Compound Fig Elixir *(B.P.).* Compound Fig Syrup; Compound Figs Syrup; Syrupus Ficorum Compositus; Aromatic Fig Syrup; Aromatic Syrup of Figs. Prepared from fig 32 g, compound rhubarb tincture 5 ml, senna liquid extract 10 ml, cascara elixir 5 ml, sucrose 54 g, and water to 100 ml.
Dose. 2.5 to 10 ml.

7513-m

Frangula Bark *(B.P., Eur. P.).* Alder Buckthorn Bark; Frangulae Cortex; Rhamni Frangulae Cortex; Bourdaine; Faulbaumrinde; Amieiro Negro.

CAS — 8057-57-6 (frangula extract).

Pharmacopoeias. In *Aust., Belg., Br., Cz., Eur., Fr., Ger., Hung., It., Jug., Neth., Nord., Pol., Roum., Rus., Span.,* and *Swiss. Br.* also describes Powdered Frangula Bark.

The dried bark of the stems and branches of *Rhamnus frangula* (=*Frangula alnus*) (Rhamnaceae). It contains not less than 6% of hydroxyanthracene derivatives, calculated as anhydrous glucofrangulin. It has a faint odour and a slightly bitter astringent taste. **Store** in airtight containers. Protect from light.

Frangula bark is a mild purgative with properties similar to those of cascara sagrada. It is usually employed as a liquid or as a dry extract.

Proprietary Names

Irgalax (glucofrangulin) *(Ciba-Geigy, Switz.)*; Solco-Lax *(Solco, Ger.).*

7514-b

Ipomoea *(B.P.C. 1963).* Ipomoea Root; Orizaba Jalap Root; Mexican Scammony Root; Scammony Root.

Pharmacopoeias. Radix Scammoniae of *Span. P.* is Levant scammony root, *Convolvulus scammonia.*

The dried root of *Ipomoea orizabensis* (Convolvulaceae), containing not less than 12% of resin.

7515-v

Ipomoea Resin *(B.P.C. 1963).* Ipom. Res.; Mexican Scammony Resin; Scammony Resin.

CAS — 9000-34-4.

Pharmacopoeias. In *Mex.* Resina Scammoniae of *Arg., Belg., Port., Roum.,* and *Span.* is from Levant scammony.

A mixture of glycosidal resins obtained from ipomoea. It occurs as brownish, translucent, brittle fragments or as a pale brown powder with a characteristic fragrant odour and an acrid taste.

Practically **insoluble** in water; soluble in alcohol; almost entirely soluble in ether.

Ipomoea resin has a drastic purgative action. It has been superseded by less toxic purgatives. The irritant action of ipomoea resin on the large intestine may cause pelvic congestion.

7516-g

Jalap *(B.P.C. 1963).* Jalapa; Jalap Root; Jalap Tuber; Vera Cruz Jalap; Jalapenwurzel.

Pharmacopoeias. In *Arg., Aust., Belg., Mex., Port.,* and *Span.*

Port. also includes Brazilian Jalap, the dried sliced root of *Operculina macrocarpa* (=*O. tuberosa; Ipomoea tuberosa; Piptostegia pisonis*) (Convolvulaceae), containing not less than 15% of resin.

The dried tubercles of *Ipomoea purga* (=*Exogonium purga*) (Convolvulaceae), containing not less than 10% of resin.

7517-q

Jalap Resin *(B.P.C. 1963).* Jalap Res.; Jalapenharz.

CAS — 9000-35-5.

Pharmacopoeias. In *Arg., Aust., Belg., Mex., Port., Roum.,* and *Span.*

A mixture of glycosidal resins obtained by extraction of jalap with alcohol; it contains not less than 85% ether-insoluble resin. It occurs as brownish, translucent, brittle fragments or as a pale brown powder with a slight characteristic odour and a somewhat acrid taste. Practically **insoluble** in water; soluble in alcohol.

Jalap resin has a drastic purgative action and has been used in conjunction with belladonna or hyoscyamus to counteract the griping. It has been superseded by less toxic purgatives.

Jalapin the decolorised ether-insoluble portion of jalap resin has also been used as a purgative.

7518-p

Kaladana *(B.P.C. 1949).* Pharbitis Seeds.

Pharmacopoeias. In *Jap.*

The dried seeds of the ivy-leaf morning-glory, *Ipomoea hederacea* (=*Pharbitis nil*) (Convolvulaceae), containing not less than 14% of alcohol (95%)-soluble extractive.

Kaladana is a purgative similar to jalap. Kaladana resin has also been used.

7519-s

Lactulose. 4-*O*-β-D-Galactopyranosyl-D-fructose.

$C_{12}H_{22}O_{11}$=342.3.

CAS — 4618-18-2.

A synthetic disaccharide. **Soluble** in water.

Adverse Effects. See Purgatives, p.1362.

Nausea, diarrhoea, and flatulence may occur in patients taking large doses of lactulose.

Severe hypernatraemia occurred in one patient with hepatic encephalopathy after 3 days' treatment with lactulose in a dose of about 30 g four times daily.— C. Kaupke *et al.* (letter), *Ann. intern. Med.*, 1977, *86,* 745.

Precautions. See Purgatives, p.1362.

Lactulose should not be used in patients on a galactose-free diet.

Commercial preparations contained lactose and galactose as well as lactulose and care should be taken if prescribed for a diabetic patient or patients on a galactose-free diet.— M. L. Rogers and C. W. Barrett, *Adverse Drug React. Bull.*, 1974, Aug., 156.

Diarrhoea, simulating lactose intolerance, had been seen in several children when full-strength milk foods had been re-introduced after gastroenteritis; lactulose had been identified in some proprietary milk foods and might be present in laxative amounts.— R. G. Hendrickse *et al.*, *Br. med. J.*, 1977, *1,* 1194; R. G. Hendrickse (letter), *Br. med. J.*, 1977, *2,* 187.

Uses. Lactulose is a synthetic disaccharide which is used in the treatment of constipation and in hepatic encephalopathy. When taken by mouth lactulose is probably almost completely unabsorbed from the gastro-intestinal tract; it is not affected by disaccharidase in the small intestine but in the colon it is broken down by saccharolytic bacteria into acetic and lactic acids. The acids stimulate bowel movements and exert a local osmotic effect in the colon. When larger doses are given the pH in the colon is reduced sufficiently by this acid production to cause a decrease in absorption of ammonium ions and other toxic nitrogenous compounds, so that the blood-ammonia concentration falls in patients with hepatic encephalopathy. It is usually administered as a solution containing lactulose 67% w/v and other sugars.

In the treatment of constipation, the usual initial dose is 10 to 20 g, daily for 2 to 3 days. Further daily doses may consist of 7 to 10 g. Children may be given 2.5 to 7.5 g or more according to age.

In hepatic encephalopathy, 60 to 100 g is given daily in 3 divided doses; in some patients treatment with lactulose has enabled a full protein diet to be tolerated.

Reviews of the actions and uses of lactulose: S. G. Elkington, *Gut,* 1970, *11,* 1043; G. S. Avery *et al.*, *Drugs,* 1972, *4,* 7; N. Otten, *Drug Intell. & clin. Pharm.*, 1977, *11,* 604; *Med. Lett.*, 1980, *22,* 2.

The pharmacological basis for the use of lactulose.— J. Bircher, *Drugs,* 1972, *4,* 1.

Reduction of the cholesterol saturation of bile by lactulose.— J. R. Thornton and K. W. Heaton, *Br. med. J.*, 1981, *282,* 1018.

Breath hydrogen test. The use of lactulose and breath-hydrogen appearance in the assessment of transit time in the small intestine.— G. C. Cook, *Br. med. J.*, 1978, *2,* 238.

For further references see G. Metz *et al.*, *Gut,* 1976, *17,* 397; J. M. Rhodes *et al.*, *Gut,* 1977, *18,* A985.

Constipation. In 5 elderly patients with retention of barium sulphate in the colon 2 to 6 weeks after a barium meal examination, constipation was unresponsive to conventional treatment but was relieved by 50% lactulose; 3 patients received 5 ml twice daily; 1 patient received 5 ml twice daily then thrice daily; and 1 patient received 10 ml twice daily.— B. J. Prout *et al.*, *Br. med. J.*, 1972, *4,* 530.

The use of lactulose in post-haemorrhoidectomy patients.— N. Porter, *Br. J. clin. Pract.*, 1975, *29,* 235.

The use of lactulose in the successful behavioural management of a woman with intractable constipation with no evidence of anatomical abnormality.— A. H. Yonace and J. E. Faulkner (letter), *Lancet,* 1980, *2,* 1371.

Further references: J. M. Perkin, *Curr. med. Res. Opinion,* 1977, *4,* 540; A. G. O. Crowther, *J. int. med. Res.*, 1978, *6,* 348.

Encephalopathy. A report of the clinical and biochemical effects of lactulose in 7 patients with chronic portal-systemic encephalopathy compared with those of magnesium sulphate solution administered to produce an equivalent stool response. In 6 patients, lactulose reduced the arterial ammonia concentrations. It produced a fall in the faecal pH but changes in indole and ammonia concentrations were variable and could not be correlated with the clinical condition of the patients. Clinical improvement occurred in 3 patients but 4 failed to respond.— R. Zeegan *et al.*, *Q.J. Med.*, 1970, *39,* 245.

A comparison of treatment of portal-system encephalopathy in 18 patients showed that lactulose given for from 4 to 20 days caused little improvement in 4 patients given 22.5 g daily, but 45 g daily improved the condition of 7 of 10 patients. Neomycin for 6 patients and chlortetracycline for 1 patient given after lactulose produced better improvement than lactulose alone. *Lactobacillus acidophilus* was ineffective in 6 patients.— M. Imler *et al.*, *Thérapeutique,* 1971, *47,* 237.

A brief discussion of the possible synergistic effect of lactulose and neomycin.— H. O. Conn, *Drugs,* 1972, *4,* 4.

The rectal administration of 1 litre of a 15% solution of lactulose, pH 3.8, for 1 hour reduced the arterial-ammonia concentrations in 4 patients with hepatic encephalopathy by 250 to 450 ng per ml per hour over the first 4 hours. There was prompt improvement in grade of coma. As lactulose by mouth took much longer to act it was considered that the acidic irrigation of the colon had been more important than fermentative diarrhoea.— E. S. Kersh and H. Rifkin, *Ann. intern. Med.*, 1973, *78,* 81.

Lactulose given to 80 patients with cirrhosis of the liver, 38 of whom had portal encephalopathy, reduced blood-ammonia concentrations. The optimum dose was considered to be 75 g daily in 5 doses after meals, increasing slowly from an initial 5 g five times daily.— D. Müting *et al.*, *Germ. Med.*, 1973, *3,* 43.

In a double-blind study lactulose and a preparation containing neomycin with sorbitol were found equally effective in the treatment of 33 patients with chronic portal-system encephalopathy.— H. O. Conn *et al.*, *Gastroenterology,* 1977, *72,* 573. A similar report from a study of 45 patients with acute portal-system encephalopathy.— C. E. Atterbury *et al.*, *Am. J. dig. Dis.*, 1978, *23,* 398. See also J. M. Fessel and H. O. Conn, *Am. J. med. Sci.*, 1973, *266,* 103.

Further references: *Med. Lett.*, 1976, *18,* 3.

Shigellosis. Lactulose might be effective in the treatment of shigella carriers but not in acute shigellosis.— M. M. Levine and R. B. Hornick, *Antimicrob. Ag. Chemother.*, 1975, *8,* 581.

Proprietary Preparations

Duphalac (known in some countries as Portalac) *(Duphar, UK).* Syrup containing in each 5 ml lactulose 3.35 g, lactose 300 mg, and galactose 550 mg. (Also available as Duphalac in *Austral., Belg., Denm., Fr., Ital., Norw., S.Afr., Spain, Swed., Switz.*).

Gatinar *(Wander, UK).* Syrup containing in each 5 ml lactulose 3.35 g and other sugars (lactose, galactose, tagatose, and other ketonic sugars) 1.34 g (dilution not recommended). (Also available as Gatinar in *Spain, Switz.*).

Other Proprietary Names

Bifiteral *(Belg., Ger.)*; Cephulac, Chronulac *(both Canad.* and *USA)*; Dia-colon *(Ital.)*; Lactulon *(Arg.)*; Laevilac *(Ger.)*; Monilac *(Jap.)*; Normase *(Ital.)*.

7520-h

Oxyphenisatin. Dihydroxyphenylisatin. 3,3-Bis(4-hydroxyphenyl)indolin-2-one.

$C_{20}H_{15}NO_3$=317.3.

CAS — 125-13-3.

7521-m

Oxyphenisatin Acetate *(B.P.C. 1968).* Acetphenolisatin; Diacetoxydiphenylisatin; Bisatin; Diacetyldiphenolisatin; Diasatin; Diphesatin; Isaphenin; Oxyphenisatin Diacetate.

$C_{24}H_{19}NO_5$=401.4.

CAS — 115-33-3.

Pharmacopoeias. In *Aust., Cz., Hung., Jug., Nord.,* and *Swiss.*

A white, odourless, tasteless, crystalline powder. M.p. about 245°. Practically **insoluble** in water; soluble 1 in 70 of chloroform; very slightly soluble in alcohol and ether; soluble in hot glacial acetic acid and solutions of alkalis. **Store** in airtight containers. Protect from light.

Adverse Effects and Precautions. As for Purgatives, p.1362.

Jaundice has been reported following the administration of oxyphenisatin acetate. Most cases have been in middle-aged women who have taken the drug over long periods. The concomitant administration of docusate sodium may enhance the absorption and toxicity of oxyphenisatin.

Severe abdominal cramps may occasionally occur.

Rectal administration of oxyphenisatin is reported to have been followed by sweating, vomiting, nausea, and tachycardia.

Jaundice. References to jaundice or other liver impairment associated with oxyphenisatin: T. B. Reynolds *et al.*, *New Engl. J. Med.*, 1971, *285,* 813; *Br. med. J.*, 1972, *1,* 325; C. A. Dujovne and D. W. Choeman, *Clin. Pharmac. Ther.*, 1972, *13,* 602; R. Hecker (letter), *Pharm. J.*, 1972, *2,* 224; E. Gjone and R. Stave (letter), *Lancet,* 1973, *1,* 421.

Liver damage caused by oxyphenisatin which was present in Silklax purchased by the patient from a health food shop.— P. Kotha *et al.*, *Br. med. J.*, 1980, *281,* 1530.

Lupus erythematosus. Allergic reaction to oxyphenisatin might induce or activate systemic lupus erythematosus.— D. Alarcón-Segovia, *Drugs,* 1976, *12,* 69.

Uses. Oxyphenisatin acetate is a purgative with actions and uses similar to those of bisacodyl (see p.1362). It has been administered by mouth or by rectum but is no longer permitted in some countries. It has been given in doses of 5 to 20 mg.

Oxyphenisatin 50 mg is given rectally in 2 litres of water as an enema for cleansing the large intestine and as an adjunct in barium enema examinations.

Oxyphenisatin inhibited glucose absorption from the human jejunum. The significance of this in relation to the laxative effect of oxyphenisatin was not yet clear.— S. L. Hart and I. McColl, *Br. J. Pharmac. Chemother.*, 1968, *32,* 683.

Of 73 patients given oxyphenisatin rectally, 50 received a dose of 4 mg given in such a way as to make contact with the mucosa at least 45 cm from the anal margin; 41 responded with mass peristalsis and propulsive movements in the colon within 11 to 22 minutes of contact. In an addendum it was suggested that 10 to 15 mg could be administered as an enema to enable impacted faeces to be expelled without discomfort.— J. Ritchie, *Gut,* 1972, *13,* 211.

Proprietary Preparations

Veripaque *(Sterling Research, UK).* Powder containing oxyphenisatin 50 mg in a diluent; available in tubes of 3 g. For rectal administration. (Also available as Veripaque in *Switz.*).

Other Proprietary Names

Cirotyl, Laxnormal *(both Spain).*

7522-b

Phenolphthalein *(B.P., U.S.P.).* Phenolphthal.; Fenolftaleina; Dihydroxyphthalophenone. 3,3-Bis(4-hydroxyphenyl)phthalide.

$C_{20}H_{14}O_4$=318.3.

CAS — 77-09-8.

Pharmacopoeias. In *Arg., Aust., Belg., Br., Braz., Chin.,*

Cz., Hung., It., Jug., Mex., Nord., Pol., Port., Rus., Span., Swiss, Turk., and *U.S.*

A white or yellowish-white, odourless, tasteless, crystalline or amorphous powder. It absorbs insignificant amounts of moisture at 25° at relative humidities up to about 90%. M.p. 258° to 263°.

Practically **insoluble** in water; soluble 1 in 15 of alcohol and 1 in 100 of ether; soluble in dilute solutions of alkali hydroxides, and in hot solutions of alkali carbonates, forming a red solution.

Adverse Effects and Precautions. As for Purgatives, p.1362.

Abdominal cramps may occasionally occur with phenolphthalein. Allergic reactions have been reported. Cardiac and respiratory distress have also been reported. It has occasionally caused albuminuria and the presence of free haemoglobin in the urine.

Phenolphthalein could interfere with the Acetest and Ketostix qualitative urine tests for ketones to produce a pink colour.— *Drug & Ther. Bull.*, 1972, *10*, 69.

Abuse. Osteomalacia in a 51-year-old woman was attributed to depletion of body calcium as a result of diarrhoea due to long-term phenolphthalein ingestion.— B. Frame *et al.*, *Archs intern. Med.*, 1971, *128*, 794.

Overdosage. Tablets containing 1.8 g of phenolphthalein were taken by a 3-year-old child. The stomach was washed out but after an hour she developed pulmonary oedema and became comatose. Despite treatment, 5 hours after the dose she was devoid of sphincter control, with flaccid paralysis, fixed mydriasis, intense cyanosis, and no detectable blood pressure or pulse. Death occurred after 13 hours. Postmortem examination revealed cerebral and pulmonary oedema, and phenol in the gastric juice.— L. Sarcinelli *et al.*, *Proc. Eur. Soc. Stud. Drug*, 1970, *11*, 261.

Peritoneal dialysis for 24 hours and the administration of isoprenaline was successful treatment for the hypotension, severe acidosis, pulmonary oedema, and oliguria which occurred in a 35-year-old man who had taken phenolphthalein 2 g as a chocolate laxative preparation.— N. Buchanan *et al.*, *S. Afr. med. J.*, 1976, *50*, 1060.

Skin reactions. Phenolphthalein was responsible for a fixed drug eruption in 3 patients and was strongly suspected in 2 further cases.— J. A. Savin, *Br. J. Derm.*, 1970, *83*, 546.

Bullous lesions on the hands, lips, mouth, and tongue of a 22-year-old woman were due to phenolphthalein.— W. B. Shelley *et al.*, *Br. J. Derm.*, 1972, *86*, 118.

Epidermal necrolysis. Toxic epidermal necrolysis had ben reported after the ingestion of phenolphthalein.— B. Potter *et al.*, *Archs Derm.*, 1960, *82*, 903.

Three cases of toxic epidermal necrolysis had been reported associated with the use of phenolphthalein.— E. D. Lowney *et al.*, *Archs Derm.*, 1967, *95*, 359.

Erythema multiforme. Phenolphthalein had caused fixed eruptions (eruptions recurring at the same site on re-exposure) and eruptions resembling erythema multiforme.— R. L. Baer and H. Harris, *J. Am. med. Ass.*, 1967, *202*, 710.

Absorption and Fate. Up to 15% of phenolphthalein given by mouth is absorbed. Enterohepatic circulation occurs and the active glucuronide is excreted in the bile. Some excretion occurs in the urine; alkaline faeces and urine will be coloured red.

Uses. Phenolphthalein is an irritant purgative which is usually taken at night to act in the morning; because of enterohepatic circulation its purgative effects may continue for several days.

It is usually administered in pills or tablets, or it may also be given as Liquid Paraffin and Phenolphthalein Emulsion (see p.1064). Usually a dose of 50 to 200 mg is sufficient, but bedridden patients may require up to 300 mg.

Yellow phenolphthalein, an impure form, has been claimed to be more active than phenolphthalein.

A comparison of Alophen with phenolphthalein and with aloin.— D. D. Chapman and J. J. Pittelli, *Curr. ther. Res.*, 1974, *16*, 817.

An *in vivo* study of *rat* intestines and of 6 patients with established ileostomies indicated that some of the purgative effects of phenolphthalein might be due to inhibition of water absorption in the intestines.— D. R. Saunders *et al.*, *Am. J. dig. Dis.*, 1978, *23*, 909.

Preparations

Compound Phenolphthalein Pills *(B.P.C. 1973).* Pil. Phenolphthal. Co.; Pilulae Phenaloini; Phenaloin Pills. Each contains phenolphthalein 30 mg, aloin 15 mg, and belladonna dry extract 5 mg. They are coated with a chocolate-coloured coating. *Dose.* 1 or 2 pills.

Compound Phenolphthalein Tablets *(B.P.C. 1963).* Tab. Phenolphthal. Co.; Phenaloin Tablets. Each contains phenolphthalein 30 mg, aloin 15 mg, strychnine hydrochloride 800 µg, and belladonna dry extract 5 mg. *Dose.* 1 or 2 tablets.

Phenolphthalein Tablets *(B.P.).* Tab. Phenolphthal. Tablets containing phenolphthalein. They are made with a chocolate basis; they should be chewed then swallowed.

Phenolphthalein Tablets *(U.S.P.).* Tablets containing phenolphthalein. Store in airtight containers.

Proprietary Preparations

Alophen Pill *(Parke, Davis, UK).* Each contains phenolphthalein 30 mg, aloin 15 mg, ipecacuanha 4 mg, and belladonna extract 5 mg. *Dose.* 1 to 3 pills at bedtime.

Aperient Dellipsoids D9 *(Pilsworth, UK).* Tablets each containing phenolphthalein 30 mg, aloin 15 mg, strychnine 200 µg, belladonna dry extract 5 mg, and prepared ipecacuanha 4 mg. *Dose.* 1 or 2 tablets at night.

Other Proprietary Names

Darmol *(Ger., Switz.)*; Evac-U-Gen *(USA)*; Euchessina *(Ital., Switz.)*; Fructines Vichy (see also under Danthron) *(Switz.)*; Fructine-Vichy *(Ital.)*; Laxatone *(S.Afr.)*; Laxen Busto *(Spain)*; Lilo *(Ital.)*; Prulet *(USA)*; Purganol *(Fr.)*.

A preparation containing phenolphthalein was also formerly marketed in Great Britain under the proprietary name Purgoids (*Evans Medical*).

7523-v

Podophyllum *(B.P.C. 1973, U.S.P.).* Podoph.; Podophyllum Rhizome; American Mandrake; May Apple Root.

CAS — 9000-55-9 (podophyllum); 518-28-5 (podophyllotoxin); 568-53-6 (α-peltatin); 518-29-6 (β-peltatin).

Pharmacopoeias. In *Port., Span.*, and *U.S.*

The dried rhizome and roots of *Podophyllum peltatum* (Berberidaceae). The *B.P.C. 1973* specifies that podophyllum contains not less than 4% of resin; the *U.S.P.* specifies not less than 5% of resin. The resin contains podophyllotoxin, α-peltatin, and β-peltatin.

7524-g

Indian Podophyllum *(B.P.C. 1973).* Ind. Podoph.; Indian Podophyllum Rhizome.

Pharmacopoeias. In *Chin.*

The dried rhizome and roots of *Podophyllum emodi* (=*P. hexandrum*) (Berberidaceae), containing not less than 8% of resin, which is not identical with that from podophyllum. The resin contains podophyllotoxin and demethylpodophyllotoxin and their glucosides.

7525-q

Podophyllum Resin *(B.P., U.S.P.).* Podoph. Resin; Podophylli Resina; Podophyllin.

Pharmacopoeias. In *Arg., Aust., Belg., Fr., Hung., Int., Nord., Port., Span., Swiss, Turk.*, and *U.S.* (all from podophyllum only). In *Br.* from Indian podophyllum or podophyllum. In *Ind.* from Indian podophyllum only.

A mixture of resins obtained from Indian podophyllum or from podophyllum; the *B.P.* specifies either, the *U.S.P.* specifies podophyllum. Resin from Indian podophyllum contains at least 40% podophyllotoxin, that from podophyllum only about 10%.

An amorphous powder, varying in colour from light brown to greenish-yellow or brownish-grey, with a characteristic odour and a faintly bitter taste. On exposure to light or to temperatures above 25° it becomes darker in colour.

Very slightly **soluble** in cold water; partly soluble in hot water but precipitated again on cooling; soluble completely or almost completely in alcohol; partly soluble in chloroform, ether, dilute ammonia solution, and fixed oils. A solution in alcohol is acid to litmus. **Store** in a cool place in airtight containers. Protect from light.

CAUTION. *Podophyllum resin is strongly irritant to the skin and mucous membranes and requires careful handling.*

A survey of the chemistry and biological activity of podophyllum resin.— O. Rüttimann and H. Flück, *Pharm. Acta Helv.*, 1964, *39*, 417.

Adverse Effects. As for Purgatives, p.1362.

Podophyllum resin is strongly irritant to skin and mucous membranes.

Poisoning due to systemic absorption has been reported following topical application of podophyllum resin. Polyneuritis has occurred following ingestion of large doses.

Reversible thrombocytopenia and leucopenia developed in a 15-year-old girl 4 days after initial topical treatment of condyloma acuminata with podophyllum resin 20% in tincture of benzoin. During 2 days of treatment she became lethargic and dizzy and developed tachycardia, fever, and respiratory distress, but improved clinically when treatment stopped.— G. P. Stoehr *et al.*, *Ann. intern. Med.*, 1978, *89*, 362. A similar report of use of podophyllum resin and bone marrow suppresion in a 20-year-old woman.— R. G. Rate *et al.* (letter), *ibid.*, 1979, *90*, 723.

Overdosage. A 2-year-old girl recovered after ingesting an estimated 1 g of podophyllum resin as an 8% solution in Compound Benzoin Tincture. Treatment included cimetidine 50 mg intravenously every 6 hours and diazepam intravenously when necessary to terminate convulsions. She remained in a coma for 4 days, then gradually improved, and at 10 days was fully conscious, although her reflexes were absent. On discharge she was beginning to walk, but remained areflexic.— A. N. Campbell (letter), *Lancet*, 1980, *1*, 206.

See also under Pregnancy and the Neonate, below.

Pregnancy and the neonate. Hoping to remain slim, a woman took 6 tablets daily of a preparation which contained, in each tablet, 10 mg of cascara sagrada extract, 20 mg of fucus extract, 100 mg of boldo extract, and 30 mg of podophyllum resin. These tablets were taken for 3½ weeks in the middle of the first trimester of her pregnancy and she gave birth to a small baby with multiple deformities.— J. E. Cullis (letter), *Lancet*, 1962, *2*, 511.

A 19-year-old woman who was 26 weeks pregnant was given by mistake about 1 g of podophyllum resin as a 20% solution. Vomiting was controlled with intramuscular injections of 60 mg of codeine phosphate and 20 mg of prochlorperazine edisylate. A total of 7 doses of 15 mg of morphine sulphate were given to control hyperpnoea and cough. Care was taken to replace fluid and electrolyte losses by giving dextrose injection and sodium chloride injection with supplementary potassium. No diarrhoea occurred, probably because of the morphine sulphate. The patient was discharged after 8 days and later had a normal baby at term. References were given to 4 other reports of poisoning, 3 of them fatal, and attention was drawn to the fact that this was the only patient who made a complete recovery, though 1 g was the second highest dose which had been recorded.— M. Balucani and D. D. Zellers, *J. Am. med. Ass.*, 1964, *189*, 639.

An 18-year-old pregnant woman with friable vulval warts was treated by the application of 7.5 ml of a 20% solution of podophyllum resin in Compound Benzoin Tincture under general anaesthesia. Subsequent severe peripheral neuropathy was attributed to absorption of podophyllum. The death of the foetus was probably also attributable to podophyllum.— M. J. Chamberlain *et al.*, *Br. med. J.*, 1972, *3*, 391. Applications of podophyllum in Compound Benzoin Tincture should be limited to 2 ml.— A. S. Wigfield (letter), *ibid.*, 585.

Precautions. As for Purgatives, p.1362.

Podophyllum resin should not be given during pregnancy.

Uses. Podophyllum resin has an antimitotic action and is used as a paint in the topical treatment of soft venereal and other warts. Care must be taken to avoid application to healthy tissue.

When taken by mouth podophyllum resin has a

drastic purgative action but it is highly irritant to the intestinal mucosa and produces violent peristalsis; for this reason it has been superseded by less toxic purgatives. It has no choleretic activity.

A discussion of the antimitotic actions of podophyllum resin.— F. E. Samson, *A. Rev. Pharmac. & Toxic.*, 1976, *16*, 143.

Ano-genital warts. Podophyllum resin 20% in spirit had been used [for ano-genital warts] on about 90 pregnant patients over 3 years without evidence of peripheral neuropathy or intra-uterine death.— G. Jelinek (letter), *Br. med. J.*, 1972, *3*, 699.

A paint containing podophyllum resin 50% in tincture of benzoin, applied weekly for an average of 8 weeks was used to eradicate ano-rectal warts in 26 homosexual men, but there were 11 recurrences during a follow-up period of 6 months.— O. L. A. Schlappner and E. A. Shaffer, *Can. med. Ass. J.*, 1978, *118*, 172.

Further references: *Br. med. J.*, 1972, *2*, 179; R. W. B. Scutt (letter), *ibid.*, 528; L. Forman, *ibid.*, *3*, 699.

Malignant neoplasm of the skin. A solution of podophyllum resin and salicylic acid was applied after curettage to 410 basal cell carcinomas. After a period of not less than 1 year the overall recurrence was 5.1%. On the nose and adjacent portions of the cheeks the recurrence was 13%.— L. M. Nelson, *Archs Derm.*, 1966, *93*, 457.

A cure-rate of 76% was achieved in 68 patients with carcinoma of the skin by treatment, twice daily for 14 days, with an ointment consisting of podophyllum resin 20% and linseed oil 20% in lanolin, followed by antibiotic ointment. These results were considerably better than those achieved with methotrexate/demecolcine ointment. In 14 patients treated with podophyllotoxin 5% in a linseed oil/lanolin basis the cure-rate was 80%. There was no evidence of systemic toxicity.— F. R. Bettley, *Br. J. Derm.*, 1971, *84*, 74.

Plantar warts. Plantar warts could be treated by the application of podophyllum resin 25% in Compound Benzoin Tincture.— *Br. med. J.*, 1972, *2*, 586.

Preparations

Compound Podophyllin Paint *(B.P.)*. Pig. Podoph. Co.; Podophyllin Compound Paint. Podophyllum resin 15 g, compound benzoin tincture to 100 ml.
Store in a cool place in airtight containers.
CAUTION. *This paint is very irritant to the eyes and tender parts of the skin.*

Podophyllin Paint *(A.P.F.)*. Podophyllum resin 5% in compound benzoin tincture. Podophyllin Paint Strong is a 15% solution in compound benzoin tincture.

Podophyllin Paint. Podophyllum Paint; Pig. Podoph.; Linimentum Podophyllini *(Nord. P.)*. Podophyllum resin 25% w/v in liquid paraffin. This preparation was included in the *B.P.C.* 1954 but was deleted by the *B.P.C.* Supplement 1957.

Podophyllum Resin Topical Solution *(U.S.P.)*. A solution containing 25 g of the alcohol-soluble extractive of podophyllum resin *U.S.P.* and 10 g of the alcohol-soluble extractive of Siam or Sumatra benzoin in alcohol to 100 ml. Store at a temperature not exceeding 40° in airtight containers. Protect from light.
CAUTION. *This solution is very irritant to the eyes and to mucous membranes.*

Podophyllum Tincture *(B.P.C. 1949)*. Tinct. Podoph. Podophyllum resin 3.65 g, alcohol (90%) to 100 ml. *Dose.* 0.3 to 1 ml.

Proprietary Preparations

Posalfilin *(Norgine, UK)*. Ointment containing podophyllum resin 20% and salicylic acid 25% in a fatty basis. For removal of plantar warts.

Vericap PLL *(Cuxson, Gerrard, UK)*. A dressing consisting of a strip of elastic adhesive plaster bearing a disk of ointment containing podophyllum resin 20% and linseed oil 20% in a lanolin basis, surrounded by a protective ring of felt. For plantar warts.

Other Proprietary Names

Condofil *(Ital.)*.

7526-p

Prune *(B.P.C. 1959)*. Prunus; Ameixa.

The dried ripe fruits of ***Prunus domestica*** and other species of ***Prunus*** (Rosaceae). **Store** in a dry place.

Prune has purgative and demulcent properties and is an ingredient of Senna Confection (see p.1368).

7527-s

Rhubarb *(B.P.)*. Rheum; Rhei Rhizoma; Chinese Rhubarb; Rhubarb Rhizome; Rhabarber; Ruibarbo; Rabarbaro.

Pharmacopoeias. In *Arg., Aust., Belg., Br., Braz., Chin., Cz., Fr., Ger., Hung., It., Jap., Mex., Neth., Pol., Port., Roum., Rus., Span.,* and *Swiss. Jap.* also permits *R. coreanum. Br.* and *Jap.* also describe Powdered Rhubarb.

The dried underground parts of *Rheum palmatum* or *R. officinale* (Polygonaceae) or hybrids of these species, or mixtures of these, separated from the stem, rootlets, and most of the bark. The *B.P.* specifies not less than 3% of hydroxyanthracene derivatives, calculated as rhein. Rhubarb contains anthraquinone derivatives of emodin, chrysophanol, aloe-emodin, and rhein and tannins. **Store** in airtight containers. Protect from light.

A review of the chemistry of some of the constituents of rhubarb.— A. C. Bellaart, *Pharm. Weekbl. Ned.*, 1971, *106*, 252.

Adverse Effects and Precautions. As for Purgatives, p.1362.

Uses. Rhubarb is a mild anthraquinone purgative. It differs from other anthraquinone purgatives in that it exerts an astringent action after purgation; with small doses the astringent action predominates and rhubarb is therefore also used as an astringent bitter and occasionally in the treatment of diarrhoea.

Preparations

Extracts

Rhubarb Dry Extract *(B.P.C. 1954)*. Ext. Rhei Sicc. A dry alcoholic extract prepared with alcohol (60%). Store in a cool place in airtight containers. *Dose.* 120 to 500 mg.

Rhubarb Liquid Extract *(B.P.C. 1949)*. Ext. Rhei Liq. Rhubarb 1 in 1; prepared by percolation with alcohol (60%). *Dose.* 0.6 to 2 ml. *Ger. P.* includes a similar alcoholic extract.

Infusions

Concentrated Rhubarb Infusion *(B.P.C. 1959)*. Inf. Rhei Conc. Rhubarb 1 in 2.5; prepared by percolation with alcohol (25%). *Dose.* 2 to 4 ml. Rhubarb Infusion is prepared by diluting 1 vol. of this concentrated infusion to 8 vol. with water.

Mixtures

Ammoniated Rhubarb and Soda Mixture *(B.P.)*. Mistura Rhei Ammoniata et Sodae; Mistura Rhei cum Soda; Rhubarb, Ammonia and Soda Mixture. Rhubarb 250 mg, ammonium bicarbonate 200 mg, sodium bicarbonate 800 mg, concentrated peppermint emulsion 0.25 ml, double-strength chloroform water 5 ml, water to 10 ml. It should be recently prepared. *Dose.* 10 to 20 ml.

Compound Rhubarb Mixture *(B.P.C. 1973)*. Mistura Rhei Composita; Rhubarb Compound Mixture. Compound rhubarb tincture 1 ml, light magnesium carbonate 500 mg, sodium bicarbonate 500 mg, strong ginger tincture 0.3 ml, double-strength chloroform water 5 ml, water to 10 ml. It should be recently prepared. *Dose.* 10 to 20 ml.

Paediatric Compound Rhubarb Mixture *(B.P.C. 1973)*. Mistura Rhei Composita pro Infantibus; Rhubarb Mixture for Infants. Compound rhubarb tincture 0.3 ml, light magnesium carbonate 75 mg, sodium bicarbonate 75 mg, ginger syrup 0.5 ml, double-strength chloroform water 2.5 ml, water to 5 ml. It should be recently prepared. *Dose.* Children, up to 1 year, 5 ml; 1 to 5 years, 10 ml.

Rhubarb and Soda Mixture *(A.P.F.)*. Rhubarb 250 mg, light magnesium carbonate 500 mg, sodium bicarbonate 500 mg, ginger syrup 1 ml, concentrated chloroform water 0.25 ml, water to 10 ml. *Dose.* 10 to 20 ml.

Pills

Compound Rhubarb Pills *(B.P.C. 1963)*. Pil. Rhei Co.; Pil. Aperiens. Each contains rhubarb 64.8 mg, aloes 51.8 mg, myrrh 32.4 mg, hard soap 32.4 mg, and peppermint oil 0.0049 ml, massed with liquid glucose syrup. *Dose.* 1 or 2 pills.

Powders

Compound Rhubarb Oral Powder *(B.P.)*. Compound Rhubarb Powder; Pulvis Rhei Compositus; Gregory's Powder. Rhubarb 25, heavy magnesium carbonate 32.5, light magnesium carbonate 32.5, and ginger 10. *Dose.* 0.5 to 5 g.

Tablets

Compound Rhubarb Tablets *(B.P.C. 1959)*. Tab. Rhei Co.; Tab. Aperiens. Each contains rhubarb 65 mg, aloes 52 mg, myrrh 32.5 mg, hard soap 32.5 mg, and peppermint oil 0.0049 ml. They may be coated with sugar or other suitable material. *Dose.* 1 or 2 tablets.

Rhubarb and Sodium Bicarbonate Tablets *(B.P.C. 1959)*. Tab. Rhei et Sod. Bicarb.; Tablets of Rhubarb and Soda. Each contains rhubarb 195 mg, sodium bicarbonate 97 mg, and ginger 32.5 mg. *Dose.* 1 or 2 tablets.

Tinctures

Compound Rhubarb Tincture *(B.P.)*. Co. Rhubarb Tinct.; Tinct. Rhei Co. Prepared by percolation from rhubarb 10 g, cardamom oil 0.04 ml, coriander oil 0.003 ml, glycerol 10 ml, and alcohol (60%) to 100 ml. *Dose.* Up to 15 ml daily in divided doses.

Proprietary Preparations

Pyralvex (formerly known as Peralvex) *(Norgine, UK)*. Contains 5% of anthraquinone glycosides and salicyclic acid 1%, in an alcoholic basis. For inflamed and ulcerated conditions of the mouth. *Directions.* Apply by brush 3 or 4 times daily.

7528-w

Indian Rhubarb. Rhubarb; Himalayan Rhubarb.

Pharmacopoeias. In *Ind.* as Rhubarb.

The dried rhizome of *R. emodi, R. webbianum*, or of some other related species of *Rheum*.

Indian rhubarb has a similar action to Rhubarb, for which it has been used as a substitute in doses of 0.2 to 1 g.

7529-e

Alexandrian Senna Fruit *(B.P., Eur. P.)*. Sennae Fructus; Sennae Fructus Acutifoliae; Senna Pod; Follicule de Séné; Sennesbalglein; Sene.

CAS — 8013-11-4 (senna).

Pharmacopoeias. In *Arg., Aust., Belg., Br., Eur., Fr., Ger., Hung., Ind., Int., It., Neth., Nord.,* and *Swiss.* Some have one monograph covering Alexandrian and Tinnevelly Senna Fruit. *Br.* also describes Powdered Alexandrian Senna Fruit.

The dried fruits of *Cassia senna* (=*C. acutifolia*) (Leguminosae), known in commerce as Alexandrian Senna Pods.
The principal active constituents of senna fruit are sennoside A and sennoside B, each glycoside consisting of rheindianthrone combined with 2 molecules of glucose. Alexandrian pods contain about 2.5 to 4.5% of these glycosides. The *B.P.* specifies not less than 3.6% of hydroxyanthracene derivatives calculated as sennoside B; the *Eur. P.* specifies not less than 4%. **Store** in airtight containers. Protect from light.

7530-b

Tinnevelly Senna Fruit *(B.P., Eur. P.)*. Sennae Fructus; Sennae Fructus Angustifoliae; Senna Pod; Follicule de Séné; Sennesbalglein; Sene.

Pharmacopoeias. In *Arg., Aust., Belg., Br., Eur., Fr., Ger., Hung., Ind., Int., It., Neth., Nord., Port.,* and *Swiss.* Some have one monograph covering Alexandrian and Tinnevelly Senna Fruit. *Br.* also describes Powdered Tinnevelly Senna Fruit.

The dried fruits of *Cassia angustifolia* (Leguminosae), known in commerce as Tinnevelly Senna Pods.
The principal active constituents of senna fruit are sennoside A and sennoside B, each glycoside consisting of rheindianthrone combined with 2 molecules of glucose. Tinnevelly pods contain about 1.2 to 2.5% of these glycosides. The *B.P.*

specifies not less than 2.2% of hydroxyanthracene derivatives calculated as sennoside B; the *Eur. P.* specifies not less than 2.5%. **Store** in airtight containers. Protect from light.

Adverse Effects and Precautions. As for Purgatives, p.1362.

Damage to the myenteric plexus was found in a specimen taken from a middle-aged woman who had regularly taken purgatives; similar damage occurred in *mice* given senna for a few weeks. It was suggested that the pharmacological action of senna was on myenteric neurones and that they could be damaged by prolonged treatment with senna.— B. Smith, *Gut*, 1968, *9*, 139.

Artificially high concentrations of urinary oestrogens could be recorded in patients taking purgatives containing senna.— *Adverse Drug React. Bull.*, 1972, June, 104.

Faecal peritonitis after senna preparation for barium enema.— D. Galloway *et al.*, *Br. med. J.*, 1982, *284*, 472.

Abuse. A patient with anorexia nervosa had increased her intake of senna to up to 50 tablets daily in order to obtain a regular stool. Finger clubbing in the absence of diarrhoea was believed to be associated with her ingestion of senna.— J. Prior and I. White (letter), *Lancet*, 1978, *2*, 947.

Senna abuse in one patient associated with reversible cachexia, hypogammaglobulinaemia, and finger clubbing.— D. Levine *et al.*, *Lancet*, 1981, *1*, 919.

Hypertrophic osteoarthropathy associated with excessive use of senna.— R. D. Armstrong *et al.*, *Br. med. J.*, 1981, *282*, 1836.

Absorption and Fate. There is absorption of the anthraquinones from senna preparations following hydrolysis by colonic bacteria. Excretion is by the way of the urine and the faeces as well as by way of other secretions including milk. The urine may be coloured yellow or, if alkaline, red. The faeces may be similarly coloured.

Uses. Senna fruit is an anthraquinone purgative. The glycosides are hydrolysed by colonic bacteria in the intestinal tract and the active anthraquinones liberated into the colon; the stomach and small intestine are not normally affected.

Senna fruit may be administered in the form of an infusion, 4 to 12 pods being soaked in about 150 ml of warm water for about 12 hours, but standardised preparations of senna are now generally used. Since purgation occurs 8 to 10 hours after administration, senna preparations should preferably be given at bedtime.

A concentrated senna extract, introduced into the lumen of the bowel through a colostomy, had no effect on the motility of the colon. The same extract incubated with faeces or a culture of *Escherichia coli* stimulated peristalsis in the colon. The activated senna appeared to act by contact stimulation of the submucosal nerve plexus which stimulated the deeper intramuscular plexus.— J. D. Hardcastle and J. L. Wilkins, *Gut*, 1970, *11*, 1038.

Sublaxative doses of Senokot were spasmolytic and might be of use in diverticular disorders of the elderly.— D. E. Hyams, *Br. med. J.*, 1974, *1*, 150.

The action of senna on the colon was probably due to stimulation of the myenteric plexus, direct stimulant activity and water and electrolyte secretion.— R. G. Pietrusko, *Am. J. Hosp. Pharm.*, 1977, *34*, 291. See also B. Smith, *Gut*, 1968, *9*, 139.

A comparison was made between 50 nursing mothers who were given Senokot granules either in the morning or at bedtime on the first post-partum day with a control of 50 others who received liquid paraffin or a mixture of liquid paraffin with magnesium hydroxide mixture. The senna laxative was effective in 49 of 50 mothers and their infants' bowel habits were not affected by the senna. Treatment with this form of standardised senna was more effective than the control treatment in overcoming puerperal constipation. The need for enemas or suppositories was almost entirely eliminated.— W. F. Baldwin, *Can. med. Ass. J.*, 1963, *89*, 566.

For a comparison of the laxative effects in antenatal patients and nursing mothers of a standardised senna preparation (Senokot) with other laxatives, see Sterculia, p.962.

Preparations

Compound Senna Mixture *(B.P.C. 1959).* Mist. Senn. Co.; Black Draught. Concentrated senna infusion 8.33 ml, magnesium sulphate 25 g, liquorice liquid extract 5 ml, compound cardamom tincture 10 ml, aromatic ammonia solution 5 ml, water to 100 ml. *Dose.* 30 to 60 ml.

Concentrated Senna Infusion *(B.P.C. 1959).* Inf. Senn. Conc. Prepared by percolating Alexandrian or Tinnevelly senna fruit 80 g with alcohol (20%), adding strong ginger tincture 8 ml, and adjusting to 100 ml with alcohol (20%). *Dose.* 2 to 8 ml. Senna Infusion is prepared by diluting 1 vol. of concentrated infusion to 8 vol. with water.

Senna Liquid Extract *(B.P.).* Senna Liq. Ext.; Extractum Sennae Liquidum; Ext. Senn. Liq. A 1 in 1 aqueous extract of senna fruit (Alexandrian or Tinnevelly) prepared by maceration with freshly boiled and cooled water, and containing 0.6% v/v of coriander oil and 25% v/v of alcohol (90%). *Dose.* 0.5 to 2 ml.

Senna Syrup *(B.P.C. 1959).* Syr. Senn. Senna liquid extract 25% v/v in syrup. *Dose.* 2 to 8 ml.

Senna Tablets *(B.P.).* Tablets containing the powdered pericarp of senna fruit (Alexandrian or Tinnevelly). Potency is expressed in terms of total sennosides.

Proprietary Preparations

Senokot *(Westminster, Reckitt & Colman Pharmaceuticals, UK).* A standardised preparation of senna fruit, available as **Granules** containing the equivalent of 5.5 mg of sennosides per g (calculated as sennoside B); as **Syrup** containing 1.5 mg per ml (suggested diluent, syrup); and as **Tablets** each containing 7.5 mg. *Dose.* 1 to 2 heaped 5-ml spoonfuls of granules, 10 to 20 ml of syrup, or 2 to 4 tablets; children, over 6 years, half the adult doses; 2 to 6 years, 2.5 to 5 ml of syrup. (Also available as Senokot in *Austral., Belg., Canad., Fr., Spain, USA*).

X-Prep Liquid *(Napp, UK).* Contains in each 71-ml dose standardised extract of senna fruit equivalent to 142 mg of sennosides A and B. For the preparation of the intestinal tract prior to radiography. *Dose.* 71 ml between 2 and 4 pm on the day prior to examination. (Also available as X-Prep in *Ger., USA*).

Other Proprietary Names

Bekunis *(Ger., Jap.)*; Casafru *(USA)*; Colonorm, Regulato Nr. 1 *(both Ger.)*; Sennocol *(Neth.)*; Sennokott *(Swed.)*; Senpurgin *(Ger.)*.

A standardised senna preparation was also formerly marketed in Great Britain under the proprietary name Bidrolar *(Armour)*.

7531-v

Senna Leaf *(B.P., Eur. P.).* Sennae Folium; Senna *(U.S.P.)*; Feuille de Séné; Sennesblatt; Hoja de Sen; Sene.

Pharmacopoeias. In all pharmacopoeias examined except *Chin., Cz., Pol., Roum.,* and *Turk. Br.* also describes Powdered Senna Leaf.

The dried leaflets of *Cassia senna* (=*C. acutifolia*) (Leguminosae), known in commerce as Alexandrian or Khartoum senna, or of *C. angustifolia*, known in commerce as Tinnevelly senna, or a mixture of both varieties, containing not less than 2.5% of hydroxyanthracene derivatives calculated as sennoside B. **Store** in airtight containers. Protect from light.

Senna leaf has the actions and uses of senna fruit.

Preparations

Compound Senna Tincture *(B.P.C. 1949).* Tinct. Senn. Co. Prepared by percolation from senna leaf 20 g, caraway 2.5 g, coriander 2.5 g, glycerol 10 ml, and alcohol (45%) to 100 ml. *Dose.* Single, 8 to 16 ml; repeated, 2 to 4 ml.

Senna Confection *(B.P.C. 1959).* Conf. Senn. Senna leaf, in fine powder, 100 g, coriander, in fine powder, 40 g, fig 160 g, tamarind 120 g, cassia pulp 120 g, prune 80 g, liquorice extract 15 g, sucrose 400 g, and water q.s. Prepared as directed; the product should weigh not less than 1030 g and not more than 1130 g. *Dose.* 4 to 8 g.

Senna Fluidextract *(U.S.P.).* Prepared by percolation from senna leaf (1 in 1) using a mixture of alcohol 1 part and water 2 parts. Store at a temperature not exceeding 40° in airtight containers. Protect from light.

Senna Syrup *(U.S.P.).* Senna fluidextract 25 ml, coriander oil 0.5 ml, sucrose 63.5 g, water to 100 ml. Store at a temperature not exceeding 25° in airtight containers.

Proprietary Names

Celer-X *(Gobbi-Novag, Arg.)*; Floripuran *(Scheurich, Ger.)*.

7532-g

Sennosides A and B *(U.S.P.).*

CAS — 81-27-6 (sennoside A); 128-57-4 (sennoside B); 52730-36-6 (sennoside A, calcium salt); 52730-37-7 (sennoside B, calcium salt).

Pharmacopoeias. In *U.S.*

A natural complex of anthraquinone glucosides found in senna, isolated from *Cassia angustifolia*, as calcium salts. The dried mixture contains 55 to 65% of the calcium salts.

Sennosides A and B occurs as a brownish powder. **Soluble** 1 in 35 of water; very slightly soluble in alcohol, chloroform, and ether. A 10% suspension in water has a pH of 6.3 to 7.3.

The isolation and structural definition of sennoside A_1, the optical isomer of sennoside A, from senna pods.— B. Christ, *Arzneimittel-Forsch.*, 1978, *28*, 225.

Sennosides A and B has the actions and uses of senna fruit. Daily doses of up to 30 mg have been used.

Preparations

Sennosides A and B Tablets *(U.S.P.).* Tablets containing sennosides A and B.

Senade *(Andard-Mount, UK).* Calcium sennosides A and B, available as **Syrup** containing the equivalent of 13.5 mg of sennosides A and B in each 5 ml and as **Tablets** each containing the equivalent of 13.5 mg.

Other Proprietary Names

Glysennid, Nytilax *(both USA)*; Palamkotta *(Ger.)*; Pursenid *(Spain)*; Pursennid *(Ger.)*; Pursennide *(Belg., Fr., Neth.)*.

Sennosides A and B was formerly marketed in Great Britain under the proprietary name Pursennid (*Sandoz*).

7533-q

Sodium Picosulphate. DA 1773; La 391; Picosulphol. Disodium 4,4′-(2-pyridylmethylene)di(phenyl sulphate).

$C_{18}H_{13}NNa_2O_8S_2$=481.4.

CAS — 10040-45-6.

A tasteless white microcrystalline powder. M.p. 270° to 275°. **Soluble** in water, alcohol, and acids; practically insoluble in acetone, chloroform, and ether.

Adverse Effects and Precautions. As for Purgatives, p.1362.

Absorption and Fate. Sodium picosulphate is hydrolysed by bacterial hydrolases in the colon to bis(*p*-hydroxyphenyl)pyrid-2-yl-methane which is absorbed and excreted in the urine and faeces as the glucuronide.

Uses. Sodium picosulphate is a purgative related to bisacodyl used for the treatment of constipation and for evacuation of the colon before radiological examination, surgery, or childbirth.

When taken by mouth it stimulates bowel movements following hydrolysis by colonic bacteria. Since sodium picosulphate acts within 10 to 14 hours after administration, it is usually given at bedtime as a solution in doses of 5 to 15 mg. Doses of 2.5 mg have been given to children up to 5 years of age and doses of 2.5 to 5 mg to children 5 to 10 years.

A review of sodium picosulphate.— *Drug & Ther. Bull.*, 1976, *14*, 104.

Sodium picosulphate was found to be as effective as senna (Senokot) in controlling constipation in geriatric patients.— W. J. MacLennan and A. F. W. M. Pooler, *Curr. med. Res. Opinion*, 1975, *2*, 641.

Effective outpatient preparation with sodium picosulphate for colonoscopy.— J. J. Brown and D. P. Jewell (letter), *Lancet*, 1981, *2*, 695.

Proprietary Preparations

Laxoberal *(WB Pharmaceuticals, UK: Boehringer Ingelheim, UK)*. Sodium picosulphate, available as a solution containing 5 mg in each 5 ml (suggested diluent, water). (Also available as Laxoberal in *Ger.*, and *Swed.*).

Picolax *(Ferring, Swed.: Nordic, UK)*. Powder available as 16.3-g sachets each containing sodium picosulphate 10 mg with citric acid and magnesium oxide (forming magnesium citrate in solution). For bowel preparation. *Administration.* The contents of one sachet to be taken before 8 a.m. on the day prior to the examination and repeated between 2 and 4 p.m. on the same day. The powder is dissolved in about 30 ml of water; after 5 minutes (during which heat is evolved) this solution is diluted to about 150 ml.

Other Proprietary Names

Contumax, Evacuol (both *Spain*); Guttalax *(Belg., Switz.)*; Laxante Azoxico *(Spain)*; Laxoberon *(Belg., Neth., Switz.)*; Neopax, Picolax (both *Ital.*); Skilax *(Spain)*; Totalaxan, Trali (both *Arg.*).

7534-p

Tamarind *(B.P.C. 1959)*. West Indian Tamarind.

Pharmacopoeias. In *Port.*

The fruits of *Tamarindus indica* (Leguminosae) freed from the brittle outer part of the pericarp and preserved with sugar. A dark reddish-brown moist sugary mass with a fragrant fruity odour and a sweet pleasantly acid taste; it contains tartaric acid, potassium hydrogen tartrate, 25 to 40% of invert sugar, and a small amount of nicotinic acid. **Store** in a cool place and avoid contact with copper.

Tamarind is a mild purgative. It is an ingredient of Senna Confection (see above).

7535-s

Turpeth *(B.P.C. 1949)*. Indian Jalap; Tripolium; Turpeth Root; Turbit; Turbito Vegetal.

Pharmacopoeias. In *Arg.*, *Port.*, and *Span.*

The dried root and stem of *Ipomoea turpethum* (Convolvulaceae) containing not less than 5% resin.

Turpeth resembles jalap in its action but is slower and less powerful and is given in doses of 3 to 5 g.

Quinidine and some other Anti-arrhythmic Agents

7770-x

Anti-arrhythmic agents (also termed anti-dysrhythmic agents, and formerly described as cardiac depressants) may be divided broadly into those that act on ventricular and supraventricular arrhythmias, such as quinidine (p.1370), those that act mainly on ventricular arrhythmias, such as lignocaine (p.902), and those that act on supraventricular arrhythmias, such as verapamil (p.1383). According to their different properties anti-arrhythmic agents have been classified by Vaughan Williams (E.M. Vaughan Williams, *Pharmac. Ther.*, 1975, *1*, 115; B.N. Singh and E.M. Vaughan Williams, *Cardiovasc. Res.*, 1972, *6*, 109) into different classes:

class I includes drugs which directly interfere with depolarisation of the cardiac membrane (membrane-stabilising agents); they also have local anaesthetic properties, and include: quinidine (p.1370) and quinidine-like agents—acecainide (p.1373), ajmaline (p.1373), disopyramide (p.1375), encainide (p.1378), hydroquinidine (p.1378), lorcainide (p.1378), prajmalium (p.1380), and procainamide (p.1380); lignocaine (see p.904) and lignocaine-like agents—mexiletine (p.1379), phenytoin (see p.1242), and tocainide (p.1382); miscellaneous: aprindine (p.1375) and dexpropranolol (see p.1339);

class II includes drugs with antisympathetic properties, such as propranolol (see p.1329);

class III includes drugs that prolong the duration of the cardiac action potential, such as amiodarone (p.1374) and bretylium (see p.137);

class IV includes drugs that interfere with calcium conductance, such as verapamil (not all drugs that fall into the broad general category of calcium antagonists share the same specific properties).

Based on the hypothesis that alinidine (p.1374) restricts the flow of current through anion-selective channels, J.S. Millar and E.M. Vaughan Williams (*Lancet*, 1981, *1*, 1291) have proposed alinidine (p.1374) as the prototype of a fifth class of anti-arrhythmic agents.

Many of the drugs classified in the above manner may have more than one type of anti-arrhythmic action; thus, high doses of quinidine can have a class III action; propranolol and some of the other beta-adrenoceptor blocking agents also have class I actions; amiodarone and bretylium also have class II actions; and, in addition, amiodarone also has class I actions.

Further references: E. M. Vaughan Williams, *Anti-arrhythmic Agents*, London, Academic Press, 1980.

A review of anti-arrhythmic agents.— L. H. Opie, *Lancet*, 1980, *1*, 861. Comment on new approaches to anti-arrhythmic therapy.— D. P. Zipes, *New Engl. J. Med.*, 1981, *304*, 475.

A review of the clinical electrophysiology of ventricular tachycardia.— J. A. Kastor *et al.*, *New Engl. J. Med.*, 1981, *304*, 1004.

A review of the adverse effects of anti-arrhythmic drugs.— J. B. Schwartz *et al.*, *Drugs*, 1981, *21*, 23.

7771-r

Quinidine *(B.P.C. 1949)*.
Quinidina; Chinidinum. (8*R*,9*S*)-6′-Methoxycinchonan-9-ol dihydrate; (+)-(α*S*)-α-(6-Methoxy-4-quinolyl)-α-[(2*R*,4*S*,5*R*)-(5-vinylquinuclidin-2-yl)]methanol dihydrate.

$C_{20}H_{24}N_2O_2,2H_2O$=360.5.

CAS — 56-54-2 (anhydrous); 63717-04-4 (dihydrate).

Pharmacopoeias. In *Roum.*

A dextrorotatory stereo-isomer of quinine, obtained from the bark of species of *Cinchona*. The *U.S.P.* (under Quinidine Gluconate) describes quinidine as an alkaloid that may be derived from various species of *Cinchona* and their hybrids, or from *Remijia pedunculata*, or prepared from quinine. It contains 20 to 30% of hydroquinidine, a closely allied base with similar chemical, physical, and physiological properties.

An odourless white amorphous powder or acicular crystals with a very bitter taste.

Soluble 1 in 2000 of water, 1 in 750 of boiling water, 1 in 17 of alcohol, and 1 in 70 of ether. The anhydrous alkaloid is soluble 1 in 1.6 of chloroform. Its solution in sulphuric acid has a blue fluorescence, as in the case of quinine.

7772-f

Quinidine Bisulphate *(B.P.)*.
$C_{20}H_{24}N_2O_2,H_2SO_4$=422.5.

CAS — 747-45-5.

Pharmacopoeias. In *Br.*

Colourless, odourless crystals with an intensely bitter taste. It contains not more than 15% of dihydroquinidine bisulphate. Quinidine bisulphate 234 mg is approximately equivalent to 200 mg of quinidine. **Soluble** 1 in 8 of water and 1 in 3 of alcohol; practically insoluble in ether. A solution in diluted hydrochloric acid is dextrorotatory. A 1% solution in water has a pH of 2.6 to 3.6. **Protect** from light.

7773-d

Quinidine Gluconate *(U.S.P.)*.
Quinidinium Gluconate.

$C_{20}H_{24}N_2O_2, C_6H_{12}O_7$=520.6.

CAS — 7054-25-3.

Pharmacopoeias. In *Braz.* and *U.S.*

A white odourless powder with a very bitter taste. It contains not more than 20% of dihydroquinidine gluconate. Quinidine gluconate 289 mg is approximately equivalent to 200 mg of quinidine. Freely **soluble** in water; slightly soluble in alcohol. A solution in water is dextrorotatory. **Protect** from light.

7774-n

Quinidine Polygalacturonate.
Quinidine poly(D-galacturonate) hydrate.

$C_{20}H_{24}N_2O_2,(C_6H_{10}O_7)_x,xH_2O$.

CAS — 27555-34-6 (anhydrous); 65484-56-2 (hydrate).

7775-h

Quinidine Sulphate *(B.P.)*.
Quinidine Sulfate *(U.S.P.)*; Quinidini Sulfas; Chinidinsulfate; Chinidinum Sulfuricum.

$(C_{20}H_{24}N_2O_2)_2,H_2SO_4,2H_2O$=782.9.

CAS — 50-54-4 (anhydrous); 6591-63-5 (dihydrate).

Pharmacopoeias. In all pharmacopoeias examined except *Eur.*, *Neth.*, and *Rus.*

White, odourless, acicular crystals, or fine white powder, with an intensely bitter taste, darkening on exposure to light. The *B.P.* specifies not more than 15% of dihydroquinidine sulphate; the *U.S.P.* specifies not more than 20%. When heated, 1 molecule of water is lost at 100° and the other at 120°. M.p. about 207° with decomposition. Quinidine sulphate 217 mg is approximately equivalent to 200 mg of quinidine.

Soluble 1 in 80 of water, 1 in 15 of boiling water, 1 in 10 of alcohol, and 1 in 15 of chloroform; practically insoluble in ether. A solution in diluted hydrochloric acid is dextrorotatory. A 1% solution in water has a pH of 6 to 6.8. Solutions are **sterilised** by autoclaving or by filtration. **Incompatible** with alkalis, iodides, and tannic acid. **Store** in airtight containers. Protect from light.

Adverse Effects. Quinidine and its salts commonly cause gastro-intestinal irritation with nausea, vomiting, and diarrhoea.

Hypersensitivity similar to that occurring with quinine may also occur and should be tested for in each patient by the administration of a test dose (see Uses). Reactions include anaphylaxis, fever, dyspnoea, vascular collapse, urticaria, and thrombocytopenia.

Quinidine may give rise to cinchonism (see Quinine, p.404) with tinnitus, visual disturbances, headache, hot and flushed skin, confusion, vertigo, vomiting, and abdominal pain; it is usually associated with large doses, but in idiosyncratic subjects may occur with small doses.

Quinidine may induce hypotension; this is a special risk with parenteral administration.

Quinidine is cumulative in action and inappropriately high plasma concentrations may induce heart block, extrasystoles, ventricular tachycardia, ventricular fibrillation, and sometimes death.

In a Boston Collaborative Drug Surveillance Program study 652 consecutively monitored hospital in-patients were given quinidine and 91 had adverse reactions considered severe enough to discontinue the drug. Detailed analysis of the adverse reactions in the 91 patients indicated that gastro-intestinal reactions (including nausea, vomiting, and diarrhoea) occurred in 51; arrhythmias were infrequent and occurred in 16 (considered definitely due to quinidine in 8, and usually developing within the first 3 days); drug fever in 11 (with associated hepatic granulomas in 1, and absolute or relative leucopenia in 3); skin reactions in 6; cinchonism in 6 (including tinnitus, headache, vertigo, and blurred vision); and auto-immune haemolytic anaemia in one patient was considered probably attributable to quinidine. Quinidine given alone had a 30% incidence of adverse reactions; when given with other agents, usually digitalis, the incidence was lower (11 to 17%), but the reason for this was not clear.— I. S. Cohen *et al.*, *Prog. cardiovasc. Dis.*, 1977, *20*, 151.

A review of quinidine, including mention that concurrent digitalisation does not prevent paroxysmal ventricular fibrillation.— L. H. Opie, *Lancet*, 1980, *1*, 861.

Deafness. The Boston Collaborative Drug Surveillance Program monitored consecutively 32 812 medical inpatients. Drug-induced deafness occurred in 1 of 1024 patients given quinidine.— J. Porter and H. Jick, *Lancet*, 1977, *1*, 587.

Effects on the blood. *Agranulocytosis and thrombocytopenia.* Hypoplastic anaemia and agranulocytosis (without thrombocytopenia), secondary to bone-marrow depression, developed in a 36-year-old man during treatment with digoxin 500 µg daily and quinidine sulphate 600 mg four times daily for ventricular tachycardia.— U. S. Barzel, *J. Am. med. Ass.*, 1967, *201*, 325.

An analysis of blood dyscrasias reported to the Swedish Adverse Drug Reaction Committee for the 5-year period 1966-70 showed that thrombocytopenia attributable to quinine or quinidine had been reported on 26 occasions. It was estimated that reported figures represented one-third of the true frequency.— L. E. Böttiger and B. Westerholm, *Br. med. J.*, 1973, *3*, 339.

Leucopenia and thrombocytopenia were associated with quinidine therapy in a 70-year-old woman; the serum had both antiplatelet and antileucocyte activity.— O. Castro and I. Nash (letter), *New Engl. J. Med.*, 1977, *296*, 572.

Further references: E. V. Eisner *et al.*, *J. Am. med. Ass.*, 1977, *238*, 884 (agranulocytosis); S. Rosa and R. B. Neligh, *J. Iowa med. Soc.*, 1979, *69*, 315 (thrombocytopenia); J. B. Alperin *et al.*, *Archs intern. Med.*, 1980, *140*, 266 (thrombocytopenia with pulmonary haemorrhage).

Aplastic anaemia. Pancytopenia and marrow aplasia occurred in a 66-year-old man who was taking quinidine sulphate 300 mg four times daily. Studies *in vitro* suggested that both a transient serum factor and quinidine were responsible for the aplasia.— J. G. Kelton *et al.*, *New Engl. J. Med.*, 1979, *301*, 621.

Haemolytic anaemia. Quinidine has been shown to

cause haemolytic anaemia in certain individuals with a deficiency of glucose-6-phosphate dehydrogenase.— T. A. J. Prankerd, *Clin. Pharm. Ther.*, 1963, *4*, 334. See also S. K. Ballas *et al.*, *Transfusion*, 1978, *18*, 215.

Effects on the heart. Five of 42 patients treated with quinidine, up to 1.5 g daily, suffered ventricular fibrillation or ventricular tachycardia. Another patient with acute cardiac infarction and ventricular ectopic beats developed ventricular tachycardia during quinidine treatment. Common to all these patients were enlargement of the left ventricle and ventricular ectopic beats, conditions which could, on treatment with quinidine, trigger ventricular arrhythmias.— W. Bleifeld and S. Effert (letter), *New Engl. J. Med.*, 1972, *286*, 667.

Further references: E. Kaplinsky *et al.*, *Chest*, 1972, *62*, 764 (ventricular fibrillation reversed by lignocaine); H. R. Jenzer and F. Hagemeijer, *Eur. J. Cardiol.*, 1976, *4*, 447 (torsades de pointes); R. W. Koster and H. J. Wellens, *Am. J. Cardiol.*, 1976, *38*, 519 (ventricular fibrillation).

See also under Treatment of Adverse Effects.

Effects on the liver. A report of reversible granulomatous hepatitis as a manifestation of quinidine hypersensitivity, which recurred on rechallenge. The patient also had fever, urticaria, and mild thrombocytopenia.— D. A. Bramlet *et al.*, *Archs intern. Med.*, 1980, *140*, 395.

Effects on mental state. Quinidine dementia was reported in a 72-year-old woman who had taken quinidine sulphate 400 mg and hydrochlorothiazide 50 mg regularly each day for 14 years. Symptoms included severe memory loss, confusional state, and disorientation. Improvement occurred within 24 hours of discontinuing the quinidine.— G. J. Gilbert, *J. Am. med. Ass.*, 1977, *237*, 2093.

Effects on the muscles. Skeletal-muscle enzymes became elevated in a 61-year-old man given quinidine sulphate 200 mg every 6 hours and decreased after treatment with procainamide was substituted.— M. Weiss *et al.* (letter), *New Engl. J. Med.*, 1979, *300*, 1218. The skeletal-muscle damage may have been the result of an increase in the concentration of free calcium.— J. A. Yagiela and P. WBenoit (letter), *ibid.*, *301*, 437.

For marked increases in serum concentrations of creatine phosphokinase following intramuscular injection of quinidine, see under Absorption and Fate, below.

For exacerbation of myasthenia gravis by quinidine, see under Precautions, below.

Effects on the skin. *Erythrodermia.* A patient's psoriasis steadily deteriorated to a very widespread erythrodermia when given quinidine 350 mg thrice daily for cardiac arrhythmia.— H. Baker, *Br. J. Derm.*, 1966, *78*, 161.

Lichenoid eruptions. A 61-year-old woman developed a lichen planus rash after 9 months' treatment with quinidine 300 mg twice daily, for paroxysmal auricular fibrillation. The condition cleared within 6 weeks when the drug was stopped.— I. Sarkany (letter), *Br. J. Derm.*, 1967, *79*, 123. A 51-year-old man who was taking quinidine developed a transient rash which recurred about 2 years later. He then developed a lichenoid eruption of the arms and hands, with redness and scaling of the chest. The eruption faded when quinidine treatment was stopped but recurred after a further single dose.— J. S. Pegum (letter), *ibid.*, 1968, *80*, 343.

Livedo reticularis. A 39-year-old woman developed livedo reticularis in a photosensitive distribution associated with quinidine therapy; a drug-induced lupus phenomenon could not be excluded.— D. F. Marion and C. M. Terrien, *Archs Derm.*, 1973, *108*, 100.

Photosensitivity. Photosensitivity developed in 3 patients when they had been taking quinidine sulphate for 3 to 4 months; in each patient the dermatitis cleared shortly after treatment was discontinued, and in 2 patients it developed again, in areas of skin exposed to light, within days of restarting treatment.— D. M. Pariser and J. R. Taylor, *Archs Derm.*, 1975, *111*, 1440. See also E. R. Bogoch and J. B. Ross (letter), *ibid.*, 1976, *112*, 559.

Fever. Fever (temperature 40.3°) was noted in a woman after 2 doses of quinidine sulphate 200 mg. The fever cleared within 24 hours of discontinuing the quinidine but recurred on challenge.— S. V. Savran and M. D. Flamm (letter), *New Engl. J. Med.*, 1975, *292*, 427. See also E. Grenadier *et al.*, *Practitioner*, 1979, *222*, 685.

Lupus erythematosus. A report of systemic lupus erythematosus in a 70-year-old woman who was receiving quinidine 2.4 g daily.— M. J. Kendal and C. F. Hawkins, *Postgrad. med. J.*, 1970, *46*, 729.

A middle-aged woman developed symptoms of lupus neuropathy while taking quinidine sulphate 200 mg four times daily.— M. Yudis and J. J. Meehan, *J. Am. med. Ass.*, 1976, *235*, 2000.

Vasculitis. Vasculitis has been reported in association with quinidine.— E. C. Rosenow, *Ann. intern. Med.*, 1972, *77*, 977.

Treatment of Adverse Effects. As for Quinine, p.404. The most dangerous effects of quinidine are usually those on the heart.

In clinical poisoning with quinidine the most dangerous effects are usually those on the heart. The cardiotoxicity of quinidine can assume 2 distinct forms, the first involving a failure of cardiac stimulus formation or propagation, terminating in ventricular standstill, and the second being one of abnormal stimulus formation, leading to ventricular tachyarrhythmias and terminating in ventricular fibrillation. Infusion of isoprenaline or noradrenaline is indicated in the first type of poisoning and, failing this, electrical pacing of the ventricles may be indicated, but the attempt is apt to be unsuccessful because of the high threshold of the quinidine-poisoned heart; all antifibrillatory drugs should be avoided and, except in cases of severe hypokalaemia, even potassium should be withheld. The second type of poisoning usually involves a rapid heart-rate and the aim is to moderate and control the ventricular tachycardia and prevent its deterioration into ventricular fibrillation; potassium may be a useful agent but except when used to correct pre-existing hypokalaemia, should probably be discarded in favour of an antifibrillatory drug less liable to compromise atrioventricular conduction; both propranolol and lignocaine have been used successfully, but phenytoin sodium would probably be superior to propranolol and perhaps to lignocaine under these circumstances; ventricular fibrillation may necessitate defibrillation by direct current electroshock, but ventricular contractions may resume spontaneously after brief recurring periods of fibrillation. In persons with structurally sound hearts the first type of cardiotoxicity is thought to be the most common.— R. P. Smith and R. E. Gosselin, *Ann. Rev. Pharmac. & Toxic.*, 1976, *16*, 189.

A report of the management of acute quinidine intoxication in a 16-year-old girl. Profound hypotension, resistant to standard therapeutic measures, responded favourably to an intra-aortic balloon pump.— C. Shub *et al.*, *Chest*, 1978, *73*, 173. Comment on the management of severe quinidine poisoning.— R. J. Luchi, *ibid.*, 129.

Adsorption. For comment on the *in vitro* adsorption of quinidine by activated charcoal, see p.79.

Dialysis and diuresis. A study in 4 subjects showed that the excretion of quinidine varied inversely with the pH of the urine. At a urine pH of less than 6 the average of excretion was 115 mg per litre and at a pH of more than 7.5 it was 13 mg per litre.— R. E. Gerhardt *et al.*, *Ann. intern. Med.*, 1969, *71*, 927.

Haemodialysis was used as an adjunct in the successful treatment of quinidine poisoning in a 3-year-old child. The quinidine was ingested as sustained-release tablets and after induced vomiting an estimated 1.6 g of quinidine was retained by the child. During an intensive 36-hour treatment period the child excreted 768 mg of quinidine through the kidneys and during an 8-hour period, started 12 hours after ingestion, haemodialysis almost doubled the quinidine elimination by removing an additional 145 mg.— E. W. Reimold *et al.*, *Pediatrics*, 1973, *52*, 95.

Evidence that dialysis removes quinidine metabolites well and is associated with an apparent increased clearance of quinidine.— K. A. Conrad *et al.*, *Circulation*, 1977, *55*, 1.

For comments on the limited role of dialysis and diuresis in eliminating drugs that are extensively protein bound and largely metabolised in the liver, see Quinine, pp.404-5.

Precautions. Quinidine sulphate is contra-indicated in hypersensitive patients or in patients with complete heart block or intraventricular conduction defects; it should not be given to patients with acute infection or toxic conditions, or in the presence of untreated cardiac insufficiency. It should be avoided in patients with myasthenia gravis.

Quinidine is generally contra-indicated in digitalis overdosage as it may enhance the cardiac arrhythmias; concomitant administration of quinidine with digoxin results in markedly increased plasma concentrations of digoxin.

Quinidine may enhance the effects of antihypertensive agents and vasodilators, coumarin anticoagulants, propranolol, and some skeletal muscle relaxants. Drugs with enzyme-inducing effects such as phenobarbitone, phenytoin, and rifampicin may enhance the metabolism of quinidine leading to reduced plasma concentrations. Some cardiac arrhythmias due to quinidine overdosage may be enhanced by noradrenaline. Quinidine has anticholinergic properties and may therefore diminish the cholinergic effects of agents such as neostigmine.

An initial test dose of quinidine should always be given to detect hypersensitivity.

Interactions. Studies *in vitro* indicated that *salicylic acid, phenylbutazone,* and *tolbutamide* in therapeutic concentrations significantly reduced quinidine binding to serum proteins.— E. Woo and D. J. Greenblatt, *J. pharm. Sci.*, 1979, *68*, 466.

Antacids. Decreased quinidine excretion in alkaline urine. An alkaline urine and consequent quinidine retention could lead to toxic manifestations.— R. E. Gerhardt *et al.*, *Ann. intern. Med.*, 1969, *71*, 927.

Results of a study in 4 healthy subjects indicated that aluminium hydroxide mixture does not interfere with the absorption of quinidine sulphate.— J. A. Romankiewicz *et al.*, *Am. Heart J.*, 1978, *96*, 518.

Antibiotics. A review of the actions and interactions of quinidine. Quinidine reduced the effectiveness of anticholinesterases used in the treatment of myasthenia gravis and enhanced the muscle weakness caused by antibiotics such as kanamycin, neomycin, and streptomycin.— D. M. Aviado and H. Salem, *J. clin. Pharmac.*, 1975, *15*, 477.

For a major interaction with rifampicin, see below.

Anticoagulants. A study of the factors affecting the protein binding of quinidine. Of greatest potential clinical impact was the decrease in protein binding of quinidine in patients given heparin.— K. M. Kessler *et al.*, *Clin. Pharmac. Ther.*, 1979, *25*, 204.

For the effect of quinidine on warfarin, see Warfarin Sodium, p.779.

Anticonvulsants. After a possible interaction between quinidine and anticonvulsants was noticed in 2 patients a study in 4 healthy persons was carried out. Doses of phenobarbitone or phenytoin so as to give plasma concentrations of 10 to 20 µg per ml resulted in a two- to threefold decrease in steady-state plasma-quinidine concentrations and this was considered to be due to an increased metabolism of quinidine. This interaction could result in quinidine toxicity if anticonvulsants were discontinued or in serious arrhythmias if anticonvulsants were started.— J. L. Data *et al.*, *New Engl. J. Med.*, 1976, *294*, 699.

Beta-blockers. A study indicating that concurrent propranolol administration does not significantly affect the absorption or distribution of quinidine.— R. E. Kates and M. F. Blanford, *J. clin. Pharmac.*, 1979, *19*, 378. Comment on the need for more study before the two could be used clinically.— K. M. Kessler (letter), *ibid.*, 1980, *20*, 486. Agreement.— R. E. Kates and M. F. Blanford (letter), *ibid.* Further references: K. M. Kessler *et al.*, *Am. Heart J.*, 1978, *96*, 627; H. R. Ochs *et al.*, *Pharmacology*, 1978, *17*, 301; P. Fenster *et al.*, *Clin. Pharmac. Ther.*, 1980, *27*, 450.

Quinidine may enhance the effects of hypotensive or beta-blocking agents (danger in sick-sinus syndrome).— L. H. Opie, *Lancet*, 1980, *1*, 861.

Cardiac glycosides. For a detailed review of the interaction between quinidine and digoxin, see Digoxin, p.533. For the interaction between quinidine and digitoxin, see Digitoxin, p.541.

Muscle relaxants. Quinidine sulphate enhanced suxamethonium-induced neuromuscular blockade in *cats*.— M. F. Cuthbert, *Br. J. Anaesth.*, 1966, *38*, 775.

The parenteral administration of quinidine following the use of tubocurarine resulted in the recurarisation of a surgical patient.— W. L. Way *et al.*, *J. Am. med. Ass.*, 1967, *200*, 153.

Rifampicin. Reduced plasma-quinidine concentrations with recurrence of arrhythmia in a patient given rifampicin in addition to quinidine therapy.— D. Ahmad *et al.*, *Br. J. Dis. Chest*, 1979, *73*, 409. Results of a study in 4 healthy subjects confirmed a major interaction between quinidine and rifampicin, probably as a result of increased quinidine metabolism following enzyme induction by rifampicin.— Y. Twum-Barima and S. G. Carruthers, *Clin. Pharmac. Ther.*, 1980, *27*, 290.

Interference with diagnostic tests. Quinidine might interfere with fluorimetric estimations of urinary catecholamines.— J. M. Millhouse, *Adverse Drug React. Bull.*, 1974, Dec., 164.

The administration of quinidine could interfere with measurements of urinary 17-hydroxycorticosteroids.— J.

M. Rosenberg and I. S. Kampa, *Drug Intell. & clin. Pharm.*, 1973, *7*, 33.

Myasthenia gravis. An athletic 80-year-old man given quinidine and digoxin for atrial fibrillation, which was subsequently found to be due to hyperthyroidism, developed obvious and frightening symptoms of myasthenia gravis. He noted marked improvement in his muscle strength within 4 days of stopping quinidine and taking propylthiouracil. The possibility of co-existing myasthenia gravis must be carefully excluded before using drugs that can depress the skeletal muscle motor endplate in patients with thyroid disease, since they are known to have an increased incidence of myasthenia gravis.— S. S. Stoffer *et al.* (letter), *Archs intern. Med.*, 1980, *140*, 283. See also P. Kornfeld *et al.*, *Mt Sinai J. Med.*, 1976, *43*, 10.

Pregnancy and the neonate. A report on the administration of quinidine sulphate to one woman throughout pregnancy. Concentrations in the infant's serum at delivery were similar to the mother's although amniotic fluid concentrations were raised. Quinidine diffused freely into the mother's milk and, although the infant would have received a dose far below the therapeutic dose, she was advised not to breast feed because of potential quinidine accumulation in the immature newborn liver.— L. M. Hill and G. D. Malkasian, *Obstet. Gynec.*, 1979, *54*, 366.

Absorption and Fate. Quinidine is readily and almost completely absorbed from the gastro-intestinal tract, peak plasma concentrations being achieved about 2 hours after oral administration; its bioavailability is variable, owing to first-pass metabolism in the liver.

Quinidine is metabolised in the liver to a number of metabolites, at least some of which are pharmacologically active. It is excreted in the urine, mainly in the form of its metabolites with only small amounts unchanged; the proportion of unchanged quinidine is increased in acid urine. Quinidine metabolism can be increased by agents that induce liver enzymes.

Quinidine is widely distributed throughout the body and is bound to plasma proteins. It has a plasma half-life of about 6 to 8 hours. Its therapeutic effect has been correlated with plasma concentrations within about 2 to 5 or 6 µg per ml, according to the assay technique used, progressively severe toxicity being noted at higher concentrations.

Quinidine crosses the placental barrier and is excreted in milk.

General reviews and comments on the clinical pharmacokinetics of quinidine: C. T. Ueda *et al.*, *J. Am. pharm. Ass.*, 1976, *NS16*, 413; H. R. Ochs *et al.*, *Clin. Pharmacokinet.*, 1980, *5*, 150.

Absorption and bioavailability. A controlled 4-way crossover study in 13 subjects of quinidine sulphate given by mouth as solution, capsules, and tablets, and quinidine gluconate given intramuscularly. Considerable intersubject and intrasubject variability was noted in the biological half-life of quinidine (ranging from 1.16 to 15.75 hours) regardless of dosage form or route. Any differences in the bioavailability of the different dosage forms could be biased by this, and in this study, following correction for the half-life variability only the tablet was significantly less bioavailable than the injection.— W. D. Mason *et al.*, *J. pharm. Sci.*, 1976, *65*, 1325.

A study of absolute quinidine bioavailability in 11 hospital in-patients indicated that although absorption of a quinidine salt was rapid and complete following administration by mouth, bioavailability was variable and incomplete with only 44 to 89% (average 72%) of the dose reaching the systemic circulation owing to first-pass hepatic drug metabolism.— C. T. Ueda *et al.*, *Clin. Pharmac. Ther.*, 1976, *20*, 260. See also T. W. Guentert *et al.*, *J. Pharmacokinet. Biopharm.*, 1979, *7*, 315.

Studies of the bioavailability of different quinidine formulations: W. A. Mahon *et al.*, *Clin. Pharmac. Ther.*, 1976, *19*, 566; J. P. Normand *et al.*, *Br. Heart J.*, 1976, *38*, 381; G. M. Frigo *et al.*, *Br. J. clin. Pharmac.*, 1977, *4*, 449; D. J. Greenblatt *et al.*, *Clin. Pharmac. Ther.*, 1977, *21*, 104; A. M. Soeterboek and M. Van Thiel, *Pharm. Weekbl. Ned.*, 1977, *112*, 417; T. Huynh-Ngoc *et al.*, *J. pharm. Sci.*, 1978, *67*, 1456; H. R. Ochs *et al.*, *Am. J. Cardiol.*, 1978, *41*, 770; E. J. Thompson *et al.*, *Angiology*, 1978, *29*, 251; E. Woo *et al.*, *ibid.*, 243; J. P. Amlie *et al.*, *Eur. J. clin. Pharmac.*, 1979, *16*, 45; J. -E. Eriksson *et al.*, *Acta med. scand.*, 1979, *205*, 53; D. Fremstad *et al.*, *Eur. J. clin. Pharmac.*, 1979, *16*, 107; O. M. Bakke *et al.*, *Acta med. scand.*, 1980, *207*, 183; C. V. Manion *et al.*, *Clin. Pharmac. Ther.*, 1980, *27*, 269.

Metabolism and pharmacokinetics. In 9 patients without heart failure the mean half-life of quinidine after intravenous injection was 7.8 hours; total 24-hour urinary excretion was 18.4% of the dose. After oral administration the peak concentration occurred at 2 hours; the mean half-life was 11 hours; 87% of the dose was available in the circulation. In a patient with renal failure the half-life was 9.5 to 12 hours. In a patient with cirrhosis and hepatorenal syndrome the half-life was 53 hours. In 42 patients taking quinidine sulphate or gluconate chronically the mean plasma concentration after doses of 13.2 mg per kg daily was 1.7 µg per ml in those without heart failure, and 2.8 µg per ml after doses of 11.9 mg per kg daily in those with heart failure. Mean 24-hour urinary recovery was 10.7%.— K. A. Conrad *et al.*, *Circulation*, 1977, *55*, 1.

A significantly smaller distribution volume accounted for the significantly higher plasma-quinidine concentration in 9 patients with congestive heart failure compared to 8 control subjects after the intravenous administration of quinidine gluconate.— C. T. Ueda and B. S. Dzindzio, *Clin. Pharmac. Ther.*, 1978, *23*, 158. A similar study.— W. G. Crouthamel, *Am. Heart J.*, 1975, *90*, 335. See also C. T. Ueda and B. S. Dzindzio, *Br. J. clin. Pharmac.*, 1981, *11*, 571.

The pharmacokinetics of parenteral quinidine following intramuscular injection and 15-minute intravenous infusion of quinidine base 275 to 330 mg as the lactate salt in a crossover study of 11 healthy subjects. Following intravenous administration the distribution half-life was about 3 minutes and the elimination half-life about 7 hours. Intramuscular injection was painful and raised serum creatine phosphokinase sevenfold; absorption from intramuscular injection was erratic.— D. J. Greenblatt *et al.*, *Clin. Pharmac. Ther.*, 1977, *21*, 105. See also *idem*, *J. Pharmac. exp. Ther.*, 1977, *202*, 365.

Further metabolic and pharmacokinetic studies of quinidine: P. Bolme and U. Otto, *Eur. J. clin. Pharmac.*, 1977, *12*, 73 (dose dependency); A. Fieldman *et al.*, *J. clin. Pharmac.*, 1977, *17*, 134 (cardiac effects); J. W. Mason *et al.*, *Am. J. Cardiol.*, 1977, *40*, 99 (transplant recipients); D. E. Drayer *et al.*, *Clin. Pharmac. Ther.*, 1978, *24*, 31 (plasma concentrations of quinidine and metabolites in cardiac patients with varying degrees of renal function); C. T. Ueda and B. S. Dzindzio, *Eur. J. clin. Pharmac.*, 1979, *16*, 101 (the impurity, dihydroquinone).

Plasma concentrations. A study of quinidine elimination in patients with congestive heart failure or poor renal function, using an extraction method which was specific for quinidine as opposed to a precipitation method which measured quinidine, dihydroquinidine, and their water-soluble metabolites. Therapeutic effectiveness was associated with plasma concentrations of 2.3 to 5.0 µg per ml, and ineffectiveness with lower concentrations or complicating illness.— K. M. Kessler *et al.*, *New Engl. J. Med.*, 1974, *290*, 706. A comment that the therapeutic range using the newer extraction method is considerably lower than with the older methods.— R. L. Woosley and T. Z. Rumboldt, *Recent Adv. clin. Pharmac.*, 1978, *1*, 93.

Comment on problems encountered in adjusting plasma-quinidine concentrations within the narrow therapeutic range of 4 to 6 µg per ml.— A. Richens and S. Warrington, *Drugs*, 1979, *17*, 488.

Further studies of therapeutic plasma concentrations of quinidine: H. Halkin *et al.*, *Israel J. med. Scis*, 1979, *15*, 583.

Saliva concentrations. Therapeutic drug monitoring in saliva including details of studies on saliva-quinidine concentrations. Due to the lack of information concerning the salivary concentrations of quinidine under steady state conditions, the value of saliva measurements in therapeutic monitoring is still unclear.— M. Danhof and D. D. Breimer, *Clin. Pharmacokinet.*, 1978, *3*, 39.

Protein binding. Studies of the protein binding of quinidine: D. Fremstad *et al.*, *Eur. J. clin. Pharmac.*, 1976, *10*, 441; M. Pérez-Mateo and S. Erill, *ibid.*, 1977, *11*, 225; O. G. Nilsen *et al.*, *Biochem. Pharmac.*, 1978, *27*, 871; D. E. Drayer *et al.*, *Clin. Pharmac. Ther.*, 1978, *24*, 31.

Uses. Quinidine is a class I anti-arrhythmic agent (see p.1370); it prolongs the refractory period of cardiac muscle, decreases its excitability, and decreases the conduction velocity. It also has anticholinergic properties.

Quinidine was formerly used for the conversion of atrial fibrillation, but it has been superseded for this purpose by cardioversion. It is used to maintain sinus rhythm after cardioversion of atrial fibrillation, and for the prevention of atrial and ventricular arrhythmias.

Quinidine is given by mouth as the sulphate in usual doses of 200 to 400 mg three or four times daily. In some conditions, such as atrial fibrillation, higher doses of up to 800 mg five times daily have been required initially, but when the dosage exceeds 2.5 g daily frequent monitoring of the electrocardiogram and plasma concentration is recommended. An initial test dose of 200 mg should always be given to detect hypersensitivity.

Quinidine is also given by mouth as the bisulphate, the gluconate, and the polygalacturonate, sometimes as long-acting tablets.

Quinidine has been given intramuscularly or by slow intravenous injection, but absorption from the intramuscular route is erratic, and the intravenous route is considered to be very hazardous owing to the risk of severe hypotension. Suggested parenteral doses of quinidine gluconate are: intramuscularly, 600 mg initially then 400 mg repeated up to 12 times daily if necessary; by intravenous infusion 800 mg diluted to a volume of 50 ml with 5% dextrose injection and given at a rate of 1 ml per minute with electrocardiogram and blood-pressure monitoring.

Administration. A re-evaluation of intravenous quinidine, and the view that, contrary to general opinion, well-controlled and monitored intravenous infusions of quinidine at appropriate slow rates are safe and reliable. Because quinidine is rapidly and extensively distributed to tissues, potentially toxic serum concentrations are not likely to be reached during a slow, controlled infusion of a therapeutic dose at a rate of 300 to 400 µg per kg body-weight per minute. If untoward ECG or haemodynamic effects do develop in susceptible individuals during the infusion, they can be reversed readily by stopping the infusion.— E. Woo and D. J. Greenblatt, *Am. Heart J.*, 1978, *96*, 829.

Evidence that administration of quinidine sulphate after food does not influence total systemic availability but slows the appearance in serum of unbound quinidine, and is associated with a lower incidence of side-effects compared with administration in the fasting state.— E. Woo and D. J. Greenblatt, *Clin. Pharmac. Ther.*, 1980, *27*, 188.

In the elderly. Evidence that reduced doses of quinidine are needed in the elderly.— D. E. Drayer *et al.*, *Clin. Pharmac. Ther.*, 1980, *27*, 72. See also H. R. Ochs *et al.*, *Am. J. Cardiol.*, 1978, *42*, 481.

Administration in cardiac and renal failure. Plasma-quinidine half-lives were similar in 8 patients with congestive heart failure (median 8.2 hours), 8 patients with renal failure (6.6 hours), and 9 controls (7.2 hours).— K. M. Kessler *et al.*, *New Engl. J. Med.*, 1974, *290*, 706.

Following administration of quinidine by mouth or intramuscularly to patients with congestive heart failure, peak blood concentrations were reached about 2 hours later than in healthy subjects.— W. G. Crouthamel, *Am. Heart J.*, 1975, *90*, 335.

Administration in renal failure. Quinidine could be given in usual doses to patients with renal failure. Concentrations of quinidine were affected by haemodialysis or peritoneal dialysis.— W. M. Bennett *et al.*, *Ann. intern. Med.*, 1980, *93*, 286. Decreased plasma protein binding of quinidine during haemodialysis.— K. M. Kessler and G. O. Perez, *Clin. Pharmac. Ther.*, 1981, *30*, 121.

For further studies, including evidence of higher plasma concentrations in patients with heart failure, see under Absorption and Fate, above.

Administration in hepatic failure. Indications of a significantly longer quinidine half-life in patients with cirrhosis. Maintenance quinidine dosage may have to be reduced in those with moderate to severe hepatic cirrhosis. Owing to decreased plasma protein binding in cirrhosis, total quinidine concentration measurements underestimate free quinidine concentrations in most cirrhotic patients.— K. M. Kessler *et al.*, *Am. Heart J.*, 1978, *96*, 627.

Cardiac disorders. A review of anti-arrhythmic agents, including quinidine, giving details of its uses, adverse effects, and interactions. Because of serious side-effects and the advent of more effective oral anti-arrhythmic agents, quinidine is now seldom used except before cardioversion (300 mg every 6 hours for 24 hours) to maintain sinus rhythm after cardioversion, and in selected patients for long-term oral anti-arrhythmic therapy. For conversion of atrial fibrillation it has been superseded by electrical cardioversion.— L. H. Opie, *Lancet*, 1980, *1*, 861.

Hiccup. For details of a protocol for the control of hiccups which eventually leads to oral administration of quinidine, see Chlorpromazine Hydrochloride, p.1515.

Preparations of Quinidine Salts

Quinidine Gluconate Injection *(U.S.P.)*. A sterile solution in Water for Injections containing 76 to 84 mg of quinidine gluconate in each ml.

Quinidine Sulfate Capsules *(U.S.P.)*. Capsules containing quinidine sulphate. The *U.S.P.* requires 85% dissolution in 30 minutes. Store in airtight containers. Protect from light.

Quinidine Sulfate Tablets *(U.S.P.)*. Tablets containing quinidine sulphate. The *U.S.P.* requires 85% dissolution in 30 minutes. Protect from light.

Quinidine Sulphate Tablets *(B.P.)*. Quinidine Sulph. Tab. Tablets containing quinidine sulphate. Protect from light.

Proprietary Preparations of Quinidine Salts

Kiditard *(Delandale, UK)*. Quinidine bisulphate, available as sustained-release capsules of 250 mg (equivalent to quinidine sulphate 200 mg). *Dose.* After a test dose of 1 capsule, 2 capsules morning and evening. (Also available as Kiditard in *Belg., Neth.*).

Kinidin Durules *(Astra, UK)*. Sustained-release tablets each containing quinidine bisulphate 250 mg (equivalent to quinidine sulphate 200 mg). *Dose.* After a test dose of 1 Durule, 2 to 5 Durules morning and evening, increased for fibrillation if necessary. Durules should be swallowed whole. (Also available as Kinidin Durules in *Austral.* Also available as Kinidin Duretter in *Denm., Swed.* and as Kinidin-Duriles in *Switz.*).

Owing to the risk of intestinal obstruction, sustained-release preparations such as Kinidin Durules, where the drug is released in transit but the matrix ghost is often eliminated intact, should not be prescribed in patients with Crohn's disease or other intestinal disease in which strictures may form.— J. L. Shaffer *et al.* (letter), *Lancet*, 1980, *2*, 487.

Natisédine *(Wilcox, UK: Lewis, UK)*. Quinidine phenylethylbarbiturate ($C_{32}H_{36}N_4O_5$=556.7), available as scored tablets of 100 mg. *Dose.* 1 to 3 tablets daily. (Also available as Natisédine in *Fr., Ger., Neth., Switz.*).

Quinicardine *(Wilcox, UK: Lewis, UK)*. Quinidine sulphate, available as scored tablets of 200 mg. (Also available as Quinicardine in *Spain, Switz.*).

Other Proprietary Names of Quinidine Bisulphate

Biquin *(Canad.)*; Chinidin-Duriles *(Ger.)*; Kinichron *(Switz.)*; Kinidine Durettes *(Belg., Neth.)*; Kinilentin *(Denm.)*; Quini Durules *(Arg.)*; Quinidurile *(Fr.)*.

Other Proprietary Names of Quinidine Gluconate

Duraquin *(USA)*; Gluquine *(S.Afr.)*; Quinaglute *(Canad., S.Afr., USA)*; Quinate *(Canad.)*.

Other Proprietary Names of Quinidine Polygalacturonate

Cardioquin *(Canad., Neth., Swed., USA)*; Cardioquine *(Belg., Spain, Switz.)*; Galactoquin *(Ger.)*; Galatturil-Chinidina, Naticardina, Neochinidin, Ritmocor *(all Ital.)*.

Other Proprietary Names of Quinidine Sulphate

Cin-Quin *(USA)*; Kinidine *(Canad.)*; Optochinidin retard *(Ger.)*; Quincardina *(Ital.)*; Quincardine *(Austral.)*; Quinidex *(Canad., USA)*; Quinidex LA *(Austral.)*; Quinidoxin *(Austral.)*; Quinora *(USA)*; Systodin *(Ger., Norw.)*.

Other Proprietary Names of Some Other Quinidine Salts

Quinidine arabogalactane sulphate: Longachin *(Ital.)*; Longacor *(Fr., Ital., Switz.)*; *quinidine phenylethylbarbiturate:* Natisedina *(Ital.)*; Prosedyl, Quinobarb *(both Canad.)*; Sedoquin *(Belg.)*.

7776-m

Acecainide Hydrochloride.

ASL-601; *N*-Acetylprocainamide Hydrochloride. 4'-[(2-Diethylaminoethyl)carbamoyl]acetanilide hydrochloride.
$C_{15}H_{23}N_3O_2,HCl$=313.8.

CAS — 32795-44-1 (acecainide); 34118-92-8 (hydrochloride).

Adverse Effects, Treatment, and Precautions. As for Procainamide Hydrochloride, p.1380.

It has been suggested that acecainide may be less liable to induce lupus erythematosus.

Evidence of acecainide de-acetylation to procainamide, suggesting that the greater immunological safety of acecainide may be relative rather than absolute.— G. P. Stec *et al.*, *Clin. Pharmac. Ther.*, 1980, *28*, 659.

Vasculitis. Mention of a pruritic erythematous rash in a patient given acecainide. Antinuclear antibody titres and SLE cell preparations remained negative, and in the absence of findings diagnostic of SLE, the reaction was felt to be a form of cutaneous vasculitis.— J. J. L. Lertora *et al.*, *Clin. Pharmac. Ther.*, 1979, *25*, 273.

Absorption and Fate. For the absorption and fate of acecainide, see Procainamide Hydrochloride, p.1381.

The plasma half-life of acecainide is reported to be more than twice as long as that of procainamide.

Plasma concentrations. For therapeutic and toxic plasma concentrations of acecainide, see under Uses, below.

Uses. Acecainide is the acetylated form of procainamide (see p.1382) and has the same actions and uses. It has a longer duration of action.

Acecainide has been given in doses of 500 mg four times daily increased as necessary to 6 g daily.

Peak plasma concentrations (average of 12.2 μg per ml) were obtained 1.5 to 4 hours after administration of acecainide hydrochloride 1.5 g by mouth to 9 patients with premature ventricular contractions, and were associated with significant reduction in premature contraction frequency in 6, no change in 2, and increase in 1. The results suggested that the efficacy and mode of action of the *N*-acetyl form of procainamide were similar to those of procainamide.— W. -K. Lee *et al.*, *Clin. Pharmac. Ther.*, 1976, *19*, 508.

Acecainide (*N*-acetylprocainamide) had an inferior anti-arrhythmic activity to but a longer duration than procainamide in 5 patients receiving an intravenous infusion of 500 mg of either drug over 10 minutes. Mean peak concentration and mean elimination half-life for procainamide and acecainide were 8.2 and 15.9 μg per ml and 2.4 and 6.7 hours respectively. It was considered that acecainide could be useful as an anti-arrhythmic agent.— E. Karlsson and C. Sonnhag, *Br. J. clin. Pharmac.*, 1977, *4*, 632P. See also C. Sonnhag and E. Karlsson, *Eur. J. clin. Pharmac.*, 1979, *15*, 311.

A long-term study of acecainide in 6 patients. All but one patient eventually received an 8-hourly dosage regimen; the exception could be given a 12-hourly regimen because of his satisfactory response and long plasma half-life.— J. J. L. Lertora *et al.*, *Clin. Pharmac. Ther.*, 1979, *25*, 273.

A placebo-controlled dose-ranging study of acecainide 0.5 to 1.5 g every 6 hours in 16 patients with ventricular arrhythmias. In 9 patients the frequency of arrhythmias was reduced by more than 75%. Anti-arrhythmic effects were related to dose and serum drug concentrations, concentrations of 10 to 24 μg per ml being associated with a greater than 70% reduction in arrhythmia frequency. Adverse effects were noted at concentrations ranging from 11 to 22 μg per ml—thus, there was overlapping of therapeutic and toxic concentrations.— J. Kluger *et al.*, *Am. J. Cardiol.*, 1980, *45*, 1250.

Acecainide therapy in patients with previous procainamide-induced lupus syndrome.— J. Kluger *et al.*, *Ann. intern. Med.*, 1981, *95*, 18.

Administration. In the elderly. A study of the pharmacokinetics of acecainide in the elderly. It was calculated that a dose of 5.1 g given over 24 hours would be necessary to achieve therapeutic plasma concentrations. The half-life of about 9 hours meant that the daily dose could be given in 2 divided doses, which is a major advantage over procainamide.— R. L. Galeazzi *et al.*, *Clin. Pharmac. Ther.*, 1981, *29*, 440.

Administration in cardiac and renal failure. Acecainide was reported to be 10% bound to plasma proteins. The normal half-life of 6.2 to 8 hours was increased to 42 to 70 hours in end-stage renal failure. The interval between doses should be extended and/or the dosage should be reduced in patients with a reduced glomerular filtration-rate. Concentrations of acecainide were affected by haemodialysis.— W. M. Bennett *et al.*, *Ann. intern. Med.*, 1980, *93*, 286.

Further references: G. P. Stec *et al.*, *Clin. Pharmac. Ther.*, 1979, *26*, 618 (anephric patients); R. E. Kates *et al.*, *Clin. Pharmac. Ther.*, 1980, *28*, 52 (cumulation in renal insufficiency).

Manufacturers

American Critical Care, USA.

7777-b

Ajmaline

(B.P., Eur. P.). Ajmalinum; Ajmalina; Rauwolfine. An alkaloid obtained from the root of *Rauwolfia serpentina* (Apocynaceae). (17*R*,21*R*)-Ajmalan-17,21-diol.
$C_{20}H_{26}N_2O_2$=326.4.

CAS — 4360-12-7.

Pharmacopoeias. In *Br., Cz., Eur., Fr., Ger., It., Jap.,* and *Neth. Br., Eur., Fr., Ger.,* and *Neth.* also include the monohydrate (Ajmaline Monohydrate; Ajmalinum Monohydricum).

A white or slightly yellowish, odourless or almost odourless, crystalline powder with a bitter taste. M.p. about 195° with decomposition. Practically **insoluble** in water; freely soluble in alcohol, chloroform, and glacial acetic acid; sparingly soluble in ether and methyl alcohol; soluble in dilute hydrochloric acid. A solution in diluted phosphoric acid is dextrorotatory. **Protect** from light.

7778-v

Ajmaline Monoethanolate

(B.P., Eur. P.). Ajmalinum Monoaethanolum.
$C_{20}H_{26}N_2O_2,C_2H_6O$=372.5.

CAS — 60991-48-2.

Pharmacopoeias. In *Br., Eur., Fr., Ger.,* and *Neth.*

A white or slightly yellowish crystalline powder with a slight odour characteristic of alcohol. Practically **insoluble** in water; freely soluble in alcohol, chloroform, and glacial acetic acid; sparingly soluble in ether and methyl alcohol. **Protect** from light.

Adverse Effects, Treatment, and Precautions. The adverse cardiovascular effects of ajmaline are similar to those of quinidine.

A study of the haemodynamic effects of ajmaline 50 mg intravenously in 11 patients undergoing cardiac catheterisation. Special care was required when giving ajmaline to digitalised patients or to patients with impaired intracardiac conduction.— H. Saetre *et al.*, *Eur. J. clin. Pharmac.*, 1974, *7*, 253.

Effects on the blood. Agranulocytosis. A report of granulocytopenia in 2 patients, probably caused by ajmaline.— *Japan med. Gaz.*, 1976, *13* (July 20), 12.

Effects on the liver. Liver damage in 4 patients appeared to be associated with administration of ajmaline.— K. Einarsson *et al.*, *Läkartidningen*, 1973, *70*, 1288, per *Int. pharm. Abstr.*, 1975, *12*, 153.

Myasthenia gravis. Under experimental conditions ajmaline has been shown to interfere with neuromuscular transmission. It should therefore be used with caution in patients with myasthenia.— Z. Argov and F. L. Mastaglia, *New Engl. J. Med.*, 1979, *301*, 409.

Overdosage. Recovery of a man within 21 hours of an overdosage of ajmaline. Only 4% of the ingested dose was excreted following diuresis and it was doubted whether this had any role in his recovery.— C. Almog *et al.*, *Israel J. med. Scis*, 1979, *15*, 570.

A report of a 17-month-old girl who recovered after taking an estimated 250 mg of ajmaline. Within half an hour she developed ataxic gait with clonic-tonic seizures appearing 20 minutes later. She subsequently developed loss of consciousness, apnoea, supraventricular tachycardia, left bundle-branch block, and a prolonged Q-T interval. Continuous ECG monitoring is considered mandatory in such cases. The ECG was normal after 24 hours.— G. Ben-Shachar and Y. Kishon, *Chest*, 1979, *76*, 97.

Other reports of ajmaline overdosage: W. Hager *et al.*, *Dt. med. Wschr.*, 1968, *93*, 1809; J. Noble *et al.*, *Schweiz. med. Wschr.*, 1971, *101*, 672; B. Gibb *et al.*, *Dt. GesundhWes.*, 1973, *28*, 748, per *Int. pharm. Abstr.*, 1974, *11*, 52.

Absorption and Fate. Absorption of ajmaline is reported to be unpredictable. It is mainly metabolised by the liver and has a short plasma half-life.

Uses. Ajmaline is a class I anti-arrhythmic agent (p.1370) with actions similar to those of quinidine (p.1372). It is used in the treatment of cardiac arrhythmias in usual maintenance doses of 200 to 300 mg daily. It has also been used as the hydrochloride.

A brief review of ajmaline. Ajmaline was first discovered among the rauwolfia alkaloids in 1931, and has both structural and pharmacological similarities with quinidine. Although it is proposed to be less toxic than quinidine and is widely used in Europe, it still has considerable toxicity. As with quinidine, asystole, ventricular fibrillation, and circulatory collapse have followed rapid intravenous injection. Controlled trials are needed to determine if the drug is effective and can be given without excess toxicity.— R. L. Woosley and T. Z. Rumboldt, *Recent Adv. clin. Pharmac.*, 1978, *1*, 93.

Preparations

Ajmaline Injection *(Jap. P.).* Injectio Ajmalini. A sterile solution in Water for Injections. pH 4 to 6. Protect from light.

Proprietary Names

Aritmina *(Byk Gulden, Ital.)*; Cardiorythmine (as base and/or hydrochloride) *(Eutherapie, Belg.; Servier, Fr.; Servier, Switz.)*; Gilurytmal *(Natívelle, Belg.; Giulini, Denm.; Giulini, Ger.; Giulini, Neth.; Lacer, Spain; Giulini, Swed.; Kali-Chemie, Switz.)*; Normorytmina (ajmaline 2-aminoethyl phosphate) *(Chemil, Ital.)*; Ritmos *(Inverni della Beffa, Ital.)*.

7779-g

Alinidine. ST-567; ST-567-BR (hydrobromide). *N*-Allyl-2,6-dichloro-*N*-(2-imidazolin-2-yl)aniline. $C_{12}H_{13}Cl_2N_3$=270.2.

CAS — 33178-86-8.

Alinidine resembles clonidine in chemical structure, but has been reported to differ in pharmacological action. It causes bradycardia and suppresses some types of cardiac arrhythmia. It has been suggested that its properties may represent a fifth class of anti-arrhythmic action (see p.1370).

A study in healthy subjects indicating that alinidine may be of value in patients with angina or tachyarrhythmias. Although chemically related to clonidine its effect more closely resembled that of propranolol, since it reduced exercise tachycardia which clonidine did not. Unlike propranolol, however, alinidine did not induce beta-blockade. In a dose of 80 mg alinidine reduced an exercise-induced tachycardia to the same extent as propranolol 40 mg; the 80-mg dose also significantly reduced arterial blood pressure in the standing and supine positions, and produced drowsiness and dry mouth. It was considered that 40 mg may be the preferred dose of alinidine on oral administration since this dose reduced heart-rate without adverse effects.— D. W. G. Harron *et al.*, *Lancet*, 1981, *1*, 351. Comment on a possible exacerbation of angina by alinidine. Patients given 20 or 40 mg thrice daily complained of precordial pain with a lower heart-rate at the same work-load as before treatment.— W. Ebm and H. Zilcher (letter), *ibid.*, 611.

Evidence that alinidine may represent a new, fifth class of anti-arrhythmic action.— J. S. Millar and E. M. Vaughan Williams, *Lancet*, 1981, *1*, 1291. Comment.— H. Nawrath (letter), *ibid.*, *2*, 209.

Manufacturers

Boehringer Ingelheim, UK.

7780-f

Amiodarone Hydrochloride. L 3428;

51087N. 2-Butylbenzofuran-3-yl 4-(2-diethylaminoethoxy)-3,5-di-iodophenyl ketone hydrochloride. $C_{25}H_{29}I_2NO_3$,HCl=681.8.

CAS — 1951-25-3 (amiodarone); 19774-82-4 (hydrochloride).

A white crystalline powder. M.p. about 161°. Very slightly **soluble** in water, but a 5% solution may be prepared due to autosolubilisation; soluble in alcohol; freely soluble in chloroform. A 5% solution has a pH of 3 to 4.

Adverse Effects. Prolonged treatment with amiodarone causes the development of benign yellowish-brown corneal microdeposits, sometimes associated with coloured haloes of light; these are reversible on stopping therapy.

About 10% of patients taking amiodarone develop photosensitivity reactions; slate-grey discoloration of the skin may also occur.

Adverse cardiovascular effects associated with excessive doses of amiodarone include severe bradycardia and conduction disturbances, especially in the elderly or those taking digitalis. Severe hypotension may follow intravenous administration.

Amiodarone affects thyroid function and may induce hypo- or hyperthyroidism. Other adverse effects reported include peripheral neuropathy, and extrapyramidal effects. Nausea, vomiting, a metallic taste, nightmares, vertigo, headaches, sleeplessness, and fatigue have also been reported, particularly in the initial stages of therapy.

A review of the adverse effects of anti-arrhythmic drugs, including amiodarone.— J. B. Schwartz *et al.*, *Drugs*, 1981, *21*, 23.

Alveolitis in one patient associated with amiodarone.— S. A. Riley *et al.*, *Br. med. J.*, 1982, *284*, 161.

Effects on the eyes. In an ophthalmic clinic bilateral brownish-yellow deposits in the cornea, sometimes extending into the pupillary zone, were found in 29 of 37 patients taking amiodarone; there was a correlation with the total dose and the duration of treatment, but deposits had been seen after only 20 days' treatment. The deposits disappeared within 2 or 3 months of discontinuing treatment.— J. Babel *et al.*, *Thérapie*, 1970, *25*, 331. See also J. Babel and N. Stangos, *Schweiz. med. Wschr.*, 1972, *102*, 220; T. G. Klingele *et al.* (letter), *New Engl. J. Med.*, 1981, *305*, 1587.

Effects on the heart. Sinus arrest in 2 patients during treatment with amiodarone.— B. McGovern *et al.*, *Br. med. J.*, 1982, *284*, 160.

Effects on the muscles. Return of cervical or dorsal pain in 3 patients given high doses of amiodarone.— H. Solvay and J. Van Schepdael, *Archs Mal. Coeur*, 1969, *62*, 1700.

Effects on the nervous system. Paraesthesia, ataxia, and tremor occurred in a patient treated with amiodarone 400 mg daily. These symptoms resolved slowly when treatment was changed.— F. Lustman and G. Monseu (letter), *Lancet*, 1974, *1*, 568.

A uraemic patient who had previously had an extrapyramidal reaction of a dystonic type after administration of metoclopramide, responded in the same way to amiodarone given some months later. The syndrome was reproducible and its intensity was proportional to dosage. Amiodarone should be administered with caution to patients with advanced renal failure who have an idiosyncrasy to metoclopramide.— J. Lloveras *et al.* (letter), *Lancet*, 1979, *1*, 981.

Effects on the skin. A 54-year-old woman who received amiodarone 600 mg daily for 20 months developed photosensitive skin with bluish-grey pigmentation on both exposed and non-exposed areas. Pigmentation due to lipofuscin was still present 7 months after withdrawal of the drug.— A. K. Vos *et al.*, *Ned. Tijdschr. Geneesk.*, 1972, *116*, 2404. A bluish discoloration of the nose was noted by a 54-year-old woman 9 months after starting therapy with amiodarone hydrochloride 200 to 400 mg daily. On biopsy, histiocytes were found in the dermis which contained cytoplasmic yellow-brown granules closely related to lipofuscin. The discoloration was still present 17 months after discontinuing amiodarone.— C. Delage *et al.*, *Can. med. Ass. J.*, 1975, *112*, 1205.

Necrotic tumours, diagnosed as papillomatosis (ioderma) were reported in the inguinal regions of a 67-year-old woman had taken amiodarone hydrochloride 400 mg daily for 2 years. The tumours decreased in size leaving slight hyperpigmentation when amiodarone was withdrawn and ammonium chloride given to increase the excretion of iodine.— J. E. Porters and C. F. Zantkuyl (letter), *Archs Derm.*, 1975, *111*, 1656.

Effects on thyroid function. A report of *myxoedema* in 2 women receiving long-term amiodarone therapy. Although due to iodine, amiodarone-induced hypothyroidism was not usually associated with goitre; spontaneous but slow recovery followed withdrawal of the drug.— J. Hazard *et al.*, *Nouv. Presse méd.*, 1973, *2*, 691.

Amiodarone can have profound effects on thyroid function and one complication of therapy is iodine-induced thyrotoxicosis.— K. F. Chung (letter), *Lancet*, 1979, *1*, 785. Amiodarone-induced hyperthyroidism in an 8-year-old boy.— A. Piffanelli *et al.* (letter), *ibid.*, 1350.

A report of frank thyrotoxicosis in one patient, and disturbance of thyroid function in three others, while receiving amiodarone.— S. Keidar *et al.*, *Postgrad. med. J.*, 1980, *56*, 356.

Treatment of Adverse Effects. In overdosage by mouth the stomach should be emptied by aspiration and lavage.

A beta-adrenoceptor stimulant (for example, isoprenaline) or glucagon, has been recommended for bradycardia.

Precautions. Amiodarone should not be given to patients with bradycardia or with impairment of atrioventricular conduction. It may be used with caution in patients with heart failure. The use of amiodarone should be avoided in patients with iodine sensitivity, disorders of the thyroid gland, or with a history of thyroid disorders; amiodarone interferes with thyroid-function tests. Patients taking amiodarone should avoid exposure to sunlight.

Regular ophthalmological examination is recommended during long-term therapy. ECG changes may occur in patients taking amiodarone.

Amiodarone should be used with caution with other agents liable to induce bradycardia, such as beta-blockers or calcium antagonists. The effects of warfarin may be enhanced by concomitant administration of amiodarone, and plasma concentrations of digoxin may be raised.

Amiodarone commonly caused bradycardia, particularly in the elderly, and caused changes in the ECG (e.g. prolonged Q-T interval) which were not limited to patients with angina pectoris. There was no clinical sign of impaired cardiac function. Atrioventricular conduction was not significantly affected.— J. Facquet *et al.*, *Thérapie*, 1970, *25*, 335.

An account of the oculocutaneous effects of amiodarone. Ocular deposits and dermatological abnormalities do not represent an obstacle to the prescription of amiodarone, but only require the temporary suspension of treatment or a slight reduction in dose.— P. Verin and A. Vildy, International Congress and Symposium Series No. 16, London, The Royal Society of Medicine, 1979. Comments, including views that intermittent therapy is not necessary for a relatively benign ocular side-effect when a life-threatening condition is being treated.— *ibid.*, 67-72.

Interactions. *Anticoagulants.* For the effects of amiodarone on warfarin, see Warfarin Sodium, p.778.

Cardiac glycosides. In 7 patients stabilised on digoxin, plasma-digoxin concentrations rose progressively by an average of 69% when amiodarone 200 mg thrice daily was added to their treatment.— J. O. Moysey *et al.*, *Br. med. J.*, 1981, *282*, 272.

Absorption and Fate. Amiodarone is absorbed from the gastro-intestinal tract and distributed to the tissues where it is very strongly bound so that it has a very slow turnover in the body. It is reported to have a half-life of 14 to 28 days.

During the initial days of administration amiodarone accumulates in the tissues, notably muscle and fat; excretion is noted after a few days and a steady state is reached after about a month. Some amiodarone is broken down and excreted in the urine but the majority is excreted in the bile and faeces. On stopping prolonged amiodarone therapy excretion is reported to continue for about 7 months, and a pharmacological effect is evident for 10 days to a month.

Following intravenous injection amiodarone is very rapidly redistributed into the tissues—the maximum effect is achieved within the first 15 minutes and wears off over the next 4 hours unless further injections are given.

Uses. Amiodarone is a class III anti-arrhythmic agent (see p.1370). It is used in the control of ventricular and supraventricular arrhythmias, and also in the management of angina pectoris.

Amiodarone is given as the hydrochloride in initial doses of 200 mg thrice daily for a week or more (in some patients up to 4 weeks) then is gradually reduced to a usual maintenance dosage of 200 mg daily, according to the patient's response. Some patients may respond to maintenance doses of 200 mg daily on 5 days a week or 200 mg on alternate days, whereas very rarely others may require a maintenance dose of 600 mg daily.

Amiodarone is given intravenously as the hydrochloride in doses of 5 mg per kg body-weight (doses of about 300 to 450 mg) given over a period of 30 seconds to 3 minutes; since the full effect may not be apparent for 15 minutes a second injection should not be given until at least 15 minutes after the first. Amiodarone hydrochloride may also be given by intravenous infusion usually in concentrations of 300 mg in

250 ml of dextrose injection, infused over 20 minutes to 2 hours, and repeated twice or thrice in 24 hours; concentrations weaker than 300 mg in 500 ml are not stable. For prophylactic therapy 0.45 to 1.2 g in 500 ml of dextrose injection may be infused over 24 hours.

Angina pectoris. Amiodarone was introduced as an anti-anginal drug 17 years ago when coronary vasodilatation was thought to be a primary requirement in the therapy of angina pectoris. In addition to dilating coronary arteries acutely, it also has non-competitive anti-adrenergic properties and reduces sympathetic transmitter release presynaptically. One puzzling feature is that, although the acute haemodynamic effects of amiodarone are soon over, the optimal therapeutic effect is not seen for days or weeks.— *Lancet*, 1979, *1*, 592.

Reports on amiodarone in angina pectoris: M. Vastesaeger *et al.*, *Acta cardiol.*, 1967, *22*, 483; J. Barzin and A. Fréson, *Brux. méd.*, 1969, *49*, 105; H. Solvay and J. van Schepdael, *Archs Mal. Coeur*, 1969, *62*, 1700; J. Friart and G. Rasson, *Arzneimittel-Forsch.*, 1971, *21*, 1525.

Cardiac arrhythmias. A review of anti-arrhythmic agents, including amiodarone, giving details of its uses and adverse effects. Amiodarone is an anti-arrhythmic agent with class III activity and 3 remarkable properties: efficacy against many arrhythmias, including ventricular fibrillation; a wide safety margin, including safety in the presence of severe congestive heart failure; and accumulation, so that the effect continues for 10 to 45 days after the last dose. It is especially useful in arrhythmias associated with the Wolff-Parkinson-White syndrome. Its use is likely to increase, but it has 2 main drawbacks: first, when given by mouth it takes 4 to 8 days to act although an initial regimen of 1 to 1.5 g daily can reduce this to 48 hours (experience with the parenteral form is limited); second, side-effects may be troublesome, but set against side-effects on the eyes and thyroid function is a very wide therapeutic-to-toxic ratio.— L. H. Opie, *Lancet*, 1980, *1*, 861.

Further reviews.— J. L. Anderson *et al.*, *Drugs*, 1978, *15*, 271; *Drug & Ther. Bull.*, 1981, *19*, 86; F. I. Marcus *et al.*, *Am. Heart J.*, 1981, *101*, 480.
Amiodarone in cardiac arrhythmias, International Congress and Symposium Series No. 16, London, The Royal Society of Medicine, 1979.

Reports on amiodarone and cardiac arrhythmias: M. B. Rosenbaum *et al.*, *Am. J. Cardiol.*, 1976, *38*, 934 (supraventricular or ventricular tachycardia); H. J. Wellens *et al.*, *Am. J. Cardiol.*, 1976, *38*, 189 (Wolff-Parkinson-White syndrome); D. A. Chamberlain and A. N. G. Clark, *Br. med. J.*, 1977, *2*, 1519 (Wolff-Parkinson-White syndrome); D. Leak and J. N. Eydt, *Archs intern. Med.*, 1979, *139*, 425 (refractory arrhythmias); P. J. Wheeler *et al.*, *Postgrad. med. J.*, 1979, *55*, 1 (serious arrhythmias); E. Rowland and D. M. Krikler, *Br. Heart J.*, 1980, *44*, 82 (refractory supraventricular arrhythmias); D. E. Ward *et al.*, *Br. Heart J.*, 1980, *44*, 91 (resistant paroxysmal tachycardias); J. J. Heger *et al.*, *New Engl. J. Med.*, 1981, *305*, 539 (recurrent ventricular tachycardia or ventricular fibrillation); K. Nademanee *et al.*, *Am. Heart J.*, 1981, *101*, 759 (ventricular tachyarrhythmias); J. R. Chapman and M. J. Boyd, *Br. med. J.*, 1981, *282*, 951 (intravenous therapy; refractory arrhythmias); R. I. Blandford *et al.*, *Br. med. J.*, 1981, *284*, 16 (intravenous therapy; atrial fibrillation complicating myocardial infarction).

Proprietary Preparations

Cordarone X *(Labaz Sanofi, UK)*. Amiodarone hydrochloride, available as scored tablets of 200 mg.

Other Proprietary Names

Atlansil *(Arg.)*; Cordarone *(Belg., Fr., Ital., Neth., Switz.)*; Coronovo *(Arg.)*; Trangorex *(Spain)*.

7781-d

Aprindine Hydrochloride. AC 1802; Compound 83846; Compound 99170. *N*-(3-Diethylaminopropyl)-*N*-indan-2-ylaniline hydrochloride; *NN*-Diethyl-*N'*-indan-2-yl-*N'*-phenyltrimethylenediamine hydrochloride.
$C_{22}H_{30}N_2,HCl=359.0$.

CAS — 37640-71-4 (aprindine); 33237-74-0 (hydrochloride).

Adverse Effects. Compared with quinidine, aprindine has been reported to have relatively few adverse effects on the heart, but its use has occasionally been associated with fatal agranulocytosis.

Effects on the blood. *Agranulocytosis.* Comment on agranulocytosis as an adverse effect of aprindine.— L. H. Opie, *Lancet*, 1980, *1*, 861. Criticism of bias in the reporting of agranulocytosis.— G. D. Köhler, *Madaus, Ger.* (letter), *ibid.*, 1415. Reply.— L. H. Opie (letter), *ibid.*, *2*, 689.

Individual reports of agranulocytosis associated with aprindine therapy: H. C. Bodenheimer and A. M. Samarel, *Archs intern. Med.*, 1979, *139*, 1181.

Effects on the liver. Alterations in liver function tests occurred in 2 patients within 3 weeks of starting aprindine therapy. Liver biopsy in one patient showed mild diffuse hepatitis. There was rapid resolution of liver changes on withdrawing aprindine. The reintroduction of aprindine in 1 patient was associated with the reappearance of signs of liver dysfunction but these resolved over 3 weeks even though aprindine therapy was continued.— H. F. Herlong *et al.*, *Ann. intern. Med.*, 1978, *89*, 359.

Effects on mental state. Psychosis in a woman given aprindine.— G. P. Jacobs and I. H. Pores, *Am. Heart J.*, 1980, *100*, 347.

Effects on the nervous system. Neurological side-effects associated with higher dosage of aprindine.— J. P. Van Durme *et al.*, *Eur. J. clin. Pharmac.*, 1974, *7*, 343.

Absorption and Fate. Aprindine is readily absorbed from the gastro-intestinal tract. It has a long plasma half-life, usually between 20 and 27 hours, and is extensively bound to plasma proteins. It is excreted in the urine and the bile.

Metabolism and pharmacokinetics. A study of the pharmacokinetics and metabolism of aprindine in 19 subjects. The maximum blood concentration was reached 30 minutes after intravenous administration and 75 minutes after administration by mouth; the plasma half-life was 21 hours after intravenous administration and 20 hours after administration by mouth. Metabolism after either route was by dealkylation or hydroxylation. About 15% of the dose was excreted in the urine after 24 hours and about 40% was excreted after 120 hours.— L. Dodion *et al.*, *Thérapie*, 1974, *29*, 221.

A study of the absorption, half-life, and toxicity of aprindine administered by mouth to patients with acute myocardial infarction.— F. Hagemeijer, *Eur. J. clin. Pharmac.*, 1975, *9*, 21.

Plasma concentrations. In 21 of 28 patients given aprindine good or satisfactory results were achieved with steady-state plasma concentrations ranging from 0.8 to 1.8 µg per ml.— P. L. Malini *et al.*, *Int. J. clin. Pharmac. Biopharm.*, 1979, *17*, 396. See also J. P. Van Durme *et al.*, *Eur. J. clin. Pharmac.*, 1974, *7*, 343 (minimal effective plasma concentrations ranging from 0.73 to 2.55 µg per ml).

Uses. Aprindine is a class I anti-arrhythmic agent (see p.1370) with actions similar to those of quinidine (p.1372). It is given as the hydrochloride in doses of 50 to 100 mg daily. If necessary initial doses of 150 to 200 mg daily may be given under strict surveillance for the first 2 to 3 days; initial doses of 50 mg daily are recommended for the elderly.

Cardiac disorders. A review of the long-acting anti-arrhythmic agent, aprindine, in the treatment of ventricular arrhythmias of various aetiologies. Aprindine may be especially useful in the treatment of the Wolff-Parkinson-White syndrome. To a lesser extent it may be useful in the treatment of atrial arrhythmias. Side-effects can be minimised by careful titration of the dose, and if the frequency of such serious side-effects as cholestatic jaundice and agranulocytosis remains low enough, aprindine should prove to be a useful addition to currently available anti-arrhythmic drugs.— P. Danilo, *Am. Heart J.*, 1979, *97*, 119. See also L. H. Opie, *Lancet*, 1980, *1*, 861.

Reports and studies on the anti-arrhythmic effects of aprindine: J. P. Van Durme *et al.*, *Br. J. clin. Pharmac.*, 1974, *1*, 461 (chronic premature ventricular contractions); A. F. Fasola *et al.*, *Am. J. Cardiol.*, 1977, *39*, 903 (ventricular arrhythmias); D. P. Zipes *et al.*, *Am. J. Cardiol.*, 1977, *40*, 586 (Wolff-Parkinson-White syndrome); H. L. Greene *et al.*, *Am. J. Cardiol.*, 1978, *42*, 1002 (resistant arrhythmias); J. Y. Wei *et al.*, *Ann. intern. Med.*, 1978, *89*, 6 (ventricular tachycardia); P. J. Troup and D. P. Zipes, *Am. Heart J.*, 1979, *97*, 322 (ventricular arrhythmias).

Proprietary Names

Amidonal *(Madaus, Ger.)*; Fibocil *(Lilly, USA)*; Fiboran *(Christiaens, Belg.*; *Pharmacia, Denm.*; *Sedaph, Fr.*; *Christiaens, Neth.*; *Padro, Spain)*.

7782-n

Bunaftine Citrate. *N*-Butyl-*N*-(2-diethylaminoethyl)-1-naphthamide dihydrogen citrate.
$C_{21}H_{30}N_2O,C_6H_8O_7=518.6$.

CAS — 32421-46-8 (bunaftine).

Bunaftine is used for the treatment of cardiac arrhythmias; it is a class III anti-arrhythmic agent (see p.1370). Bunaftine citrate is presented as tablets containing the equivalent of 200 mg of bunaftine for oral use. Bunaftine hydrochloride is given by intramuscular injection and is presented in vials containing the equivalent of 200 mg of bunaftine.

Cardiac disorders. A study indicating that bunaftine is a class III anti-arrhythmic agent.— R. Fenici *et al.*, *Br. Heart J.*, 1977, *39*, 787.

Further references: A. Castellucci, *Arzneimittel-Forsch.*, 1976, *26*, 241 (*animal* studies); J. L. Tamargo *et al.*, *J. Pharm. Pharmac.*, 1978, *30*, 455 (*in vitro* membrane-stabilising effects).

Proprietary Names

Bunamide *(Berenguer-Beneyto, Spain)*; Meregon *(as citrate or hydrochloride) (Malesci, Ital.)*.

7783-h

Disopyramide *(B.P.)*. SC-7031. 4-Di-isopropylamino-2-phenyl-2-(2-pyridyl)butyramide.

$C_{21}H_{29}N_3O=339.5$.

CAS — 3737-09-5.

Pharmacopoeias. In *Br.*

A white odourless powder. **Soluble** 1 in 200 of water, 1 in 10 of alcohol, 1 in 5 of chloroform, and 1 in 5 of ether. **Store** in airtight containers.

7784-m

Disopyramide Phosphate *(B.P., U.S.P.)*. SC 13957.

$C_{21}H_{29}N_3O,H_3PO_4=437.5$.

CAS — 22059-60-5.

Pharmacopoeias. In *Br.* and *U.S.*

A white or almost white odourless powder. M.p. about 205° with decomposition. Disopyramide phosphate 1.3 g is approximately equivalent to 1 g of disopyramide. **Soluble** 1 in 20 of water and 1 in 50 of alcohol; practically insoluble in chloroform and ether. A 5% solution has a pH of 4 to 5. **Store** in airtight containers. Protect from light.

Adverse Effects. The adverse effects most commonly associated with disopyramide therapy relate to its anticholinergic properties and are dose-related. They include dry mouth, blurred vision, urinary retention, and constipation. Gastro-intestinal irritation and nausea may also occur. Other adverse effects reported include skin rashes, hypokalaemia, hypoglycaemia, dizziness, fatigue, muscle aches and weakness, headache, nervousness, insomnia, and depression. There have also been rare reports of psychosis, cholestatic jaundice, and agranulocytosis. Like other anti-arrhythmic agents, disopyramide has cardiac depressant properties, and, particularly in excessive dosage, may induce cardiac arrhythmias (including ventricular tachycardia), heart failure, and hypotension.

Over-rapid intravenous injection of disopyramide may cause profuse sweating and severe cardiovascular depression.

A 75-year-old woman with atrial fibrillation suffered a grand mal convulsion followed by respiratory arrest after receiving disopyramide 150 mg intravenously over a period of 10 minutes. On recovery she complained of a dry mouth and blurred vision and it was considered that the convulsion was caused by the anticholinergic action of disopyramide, although it may have been due to a direct stimulant action.— N. M. Johnson *et al.* (letter), *Lancet*, 1978, *2*, 848. *Animal* studies and clinical experience had shown that depression of ventricular function is the primary cause of death in disopyramide intoxication. The anticholinergic action of disopyramide is weak and it does not appear to carry any special risk in epileptic patients; large intravenous doses should only be used with great caution where there is already evidence of cardiac decompensation; in atrial fibrillation and heart failure, where digoxin is felt to be contra-indicated, d.c. cardioversion is recommended as the safer alternative.— B. O'Keefe *et al.* (letter), *ibid.*, 1208.

In a 68-year-old woman with atrial tachycardia and 2:1 conduction uncontrolled by digoxin and propranolol, disopyramide 1.5 mg per kg body-weight given intravenously over 5 minutes caused atrial slowing and 1:1 conduction. It was considered that the digitalis had failed to protect the patient from the atropinic effect of disopyramide.— M. Lara *et al.*, *Br. med. J.*, 1980, *281*, 198.

Allergy. Mention of a severe allergic reaction with purpura following a test dose of disopyramide.— M. J. Katz *et al.*, *Curr. ther. Res.*, 1963, *5*, 343.

Worsening of ventricular arrhythmia and an anaphylactoid reaction occurred in a 58-year-old man after a single dose of disopyramide 300 mg by mouth. Two hours after the dose he complained of a swollen tongue and difficulty in breathing. He became cyanotic and was given diphenhydramine 25 mg intravenously, which resulted in improvement of his respiratory status.— J. G. Porterfield *et al.* (letter), *New Engl. J. Med.*, 1980, *303*, 584.

Effects on the blood. Granulocytopenia was associated on 2 occasions with the use of disopyramide phosphate in a 61-year-old man.— M. E. Conrad *et al.* (letter), *J. Am. med. Ass.*, 1978, *240*, 1857.

Effects on the eyes. Acute closed-angle glaucoma developed in a patient on the 7th day of treatment with disopyramide 100 mg thrice daily for 6 days then 200 mg thrice daily for another 6 days. After treatment with pilocarpine, physostigmine, and then surgery the patient was returned to treatment with disopyramide 100 mg four times daily.— G. E. Trope and V. M. D. Hind (letter), *Lancet*, 1978, *1*, 329.

Effects on the heart. Disopyramide given to one patient produced ventricular fibrillation and ECG abnormalities resembling those of quinidine.— J. Frieden (letter), *New Engl. J. Med.*, 1978, *298*, 975. These effects did not occur in a similar patient given disopyramide although ventricular arrhythmias and prolongation of the Q-T interval had previously developed when she had been given quinidine.— J. J. Rozanski *et al.* (letter), *ibid.*, *299*, 493.

Manifestations of acute congestive heart failure occurred in 16 of 100 patients receiving disopyramide by mouth. It was concluded that disopyramide exerts a profound negative myocardial inotropic effect and that recurrence of congestive heart failure may be precipitated in as many as 50% of those receiving disopyramide. The likelihood of this complication in patients without a history of heart failure is probably less than 5%.— P. J. Podrid *et al.*, *New Engl. J. Med.*, 1980, *302*, 614. See also M. A. Martin *et al.*, *Br. J. clin. Pharmac.*, 1980, *10*, 237.

A possible association between cardiac dysrhythmias and treatment with disopyramide in 5 patients with heart disease.— E. L. Kinney *et al.* (letter), *New Engl. J. Med.*, 1980, *302*, 1146.

In a comparative study with lignocaine, intravenous disopyramide was found to have a potent coronary constrictive activity which might be hazardous under some circumstances.— V. Kötter *et al.*, *Am. J. Cardiol.*, 1980, *46*, 469.

See also under Overdosage, below.

Effects on the liver. Intrahepatic cholestasis in one patient was associated with disopyramide 500 mg given daily for 3 days in divided doses.— T. Meinertz *et al.* (letter), *Lancet*, 1977, *2*, 828. See also N. Riccioni *et al.* (letter), *ibid.*, 1362. Further references: A. Craxi *et al.* (letter), *Ann. intern. Med.*, 1980, *93*, 150.

Abnormal liver function tests in a patient given disopyramide. Liver biopsy done 6 days after cessation of therapy showed nonspecific inflammatory changes with no intrahepatic cholestasis.— A. M. Tonkin *et al.* (letter), *Chest*, 1980, *77*, 125.

Effects on mental state. Agitation and distress leading to paranoia and auditory hallucinations developed in a patient given disopyramide. Withdrawal of the disopyramide produced a rapid and complete recovery.— R. H. Falk *et al.* (letter), *Lancet*, 1977, *1*, 858. Another similar report in 1 patient. The psychotic reaction might be due to the anticholinergic properties of disopyramide.— P. L. Padfield *et al.* (letter), *ibid.*, 1152.

Effects on the nervous system. Peripheral neuropathy affecting the feet and severe enough to prevent walking was associated with disopyramide in a 72-year-old patient. There was gradual improvement on withdrawal of disopyramide with the patient being symptom-free after 4 months.— K. D. Dawkins and J. Gibson (letter), *Lancet*, 1978, *1*, 329.

Effects on sexual function. Impotence occurred in a patient taking disopyramide. When the plasma concentration of disopyramide was reduced from 14 to 3 µg per ml the impotence was abolished without clinical deterioration.— D. J. McHaffie *et al.* (letter), *Lancet*, 1977, *1*, 859.

Effects on the skin. Disopyramide may cause photosensitivity reactions.— *Med. Lett.*, 1980, *22*, 64.

Hot flushes. Mention of 3 patients who developed hot flushes in association with disopyramide therapy.— T. E. G. Jones and R. E. Nagle (letter), *Br. med. J.*, 1977, *1*, 903.

Hypertension. Although hypotension is a more frequent effect of disopyramide, 3 of 50 patients had a hypertensive response to intravenous disopyramide.— A. M. Tonkin *et al.* (letter), *Chest*, 1980, *77*, 125.

Hypoglycaemia. An 88-year-old woman developed hypoglycaemia during disopyramide therapy. The hypoglycaemia resolved on stopping disopyramide and recurred on rechallenge.— I. J. Goldberg *et al.*, *Am. J. Med.*, 1980, *69*, 463.

Hypotension. Disopyramide 400 mg by mouth caused hypotension in a patient with cardiac failure associated with atrial flutter.— J. G. Sloman *et al.*, *Med. J. Aust.*, 1977, *1*, 176.

Overdosage. A 2-year-old boy suffered hypotension, cardiac arrhythmias, and convulsions and died 28 hours after ingestion of 600 mg of disopyramide.— A. Hutchison and H. Kilham, *Med. J. Aust.*, 1978, *2*, 335.

Prolongation of the P-R interval in a 50-year-old man was associated with administration of disopyramide. Concomitant heart failure and confusion may also have been associated with disopyramide.— A. S. Nies *et al.* (letter), *Lancet*, 1979, *1*, 330. Although the dose was within the recommended range, the toxicity was hardly surprising in view of the high plasma concentrations. It is not advisable to rely too heavily on the prescribed dose as a measure of therapeutic efficacy.— D. W. Holt and A. M. Hayler (letter), *ibid.*, 491.

Further references to disopyramide overdosage: R. S. Meltzer *et al.*, *Am. J. Cardiol.*, 1978, *42*, 1049 (atypical ventricular tachycardia); F. Powell *et al.*, *J. Irish med. Ass.*, 1978, *71*, 552 (fatality).

See also under Treatment of Adverse Effects, below.

Urinary retention. Urinary retention occurred in 4 of 7 patients given disopyramide.— S. H. Large and C. H. Todd (letter), *Lancet*, 1977, *2*, 1362. A similar effect in 2 patients.— G. R. Donald (letter), *ibid.*

Treatment of Adverse Effects. In overdosage by mouth the stomach should be emptied by aspiration and lavage.

Isoprenaline infusion is reported to be beneficial in severe hypotension; since cardiovascular collapse can occur abruptly without warning, it is recommended that the patient be prepared for an isoprenaline infusion as soon as disopyramide overdosage is suspected.

Other supportive measures include correction of hypokalaemia, assisted respiration, and electrical pacing.

It has been suggested that haemodialysis may be of value in severe overdosage.

A report of 5 cases of fatal overdosage with disopyramide. The most common clinical finding appeared to be an early loss of consciousness following an episode of respiratory arrest. Four of the patients initially responded to resuscitation but subsequently deteriorated rapidly, with cardiac arrhythmias and loss of spontaneous respiration; in 4 of the cases post-mortem examination demonstrated pulmonary congestion secondary to left ventricular failure.— A. M. Hayler *et al.*, *Lancet*, 1978, *1*, 968. *In vitro* data suggested that haemodialysis might be of value in enhancing the elimination of toxic concentrations of disopyramide.— A. Karim, *Searle, USA* (letter), *ibid.*, *2*, 214. Further comment.— J. R. Horn and M. L. Hughes (letter), *ibid.*

Recommendations, based on *animal* experiments, for the management of disopyramide overdosage: monitor arterial blood pressure continuously, preferably with an indwelling cannula, to provide immediate warning of cardiovascular collapse which may be sudden and without obvious ECG abnormalities; if disopyramide overdose is suspected set up an intravenous infusion containing a pressor agent immediately the patient is admitted to hospital, so that, in the event of a cardiovascular crisis, treatment can be initiated promptly (isoprenaline appears to be superior to the other drugs used in this situation); sudden cardiac arrhythmias may occur and may well be exacerbated by cardiodepressant drugs such as procainamide or quinidine—attention to raising the blood pressure, correcting acidosis, and the cautious use of isoprenaline are more likely to prove effective; reports suggest that, due to high endocardial threshold, patients may be refractory to transvenous ventricular pacing—isoprenaline appears to be the drug most likely to be effective when symptomatic bradycardia follows disopyramide poisoning.— A. M. Hayler *et al.* (letter), *Med. J. Aust.*, 1979, *1*, 234.

A report of the successful treatment of a 21-year-old man who had taken a reported 200 capsules of disopyramide 100 mg. It was considered that the key to the management of the patient was the prompt use of a large dose of isoprenaline following the sudden loss of blood pressure. Clinical problems subsequent to this were probably due to high-dose isoprenaline infusion and hypokalaemia. Haemoperfusion was carried out, initially using Haemacol 100, which was considered unsuitable, and subsequently using the B-D Hemodetoxifier which also gave disappointing results, possibly due to a defective column. The role of haemoperfusion remains to be established. Gastric lavage, performed when the patient was admitted, was considered to have been of benefit. Other measures included use of potassium chloride to correct hypokalaemia, and mannitol to initiate diuresis after frusemide had failed.— D. W. Holt *et al.*, *Postgrad. med. J.*, 1980, *56*, 256.

Precautions. Disopyramide is contra-indicated by mouth and intravenously in the presence of complete heart block, and intravenously in the presence of severe cardiac failure; patients with significant cardiac failure should be digitalised before receiving disopyramide by mouth.

Disopyramide should be used with caution in patients with partial heart block, in patients susceptible to hypoglycaemia (such as those with liver dysfunction), and in patients susceptible to hypokalaemia (such as those receiving potent diuretics). Disopyramide should also be used with caution in association with other cardiac depressants including beta-blockers and it is recommended that facilities for cardiac monitoring and defibrillation should be available when the injection is used. Hypotension is a special risk following intravenous administration of disopyramide; it should be injected slowly.

Dosage reduction is necessary in patients with renal or hepatic impairment; longer dosage intervals may be necessary in some cardiac disorders.

Owing to its anticholinergic properties, disopyramide should be avoided in patients with glaucoma or a tendency to urinary retention; the effects of other anticholinergic agents are enhanced by concomitant disopyramide therapy.

It has been suggested that disopyramide should be used with caution in patients with myasthenia gravis.

Interactions. Enzyme inducers such as *carbamazepine, phenobarbitone, phenytoin,* and *rifampicin* can induce the metabolism of disopyramide. Moreover, disopyramide may induce its own metabolism in some patients.— M. L. Aitio (letter), *Med. J. Aust.*, 1979, *2*, 550. See also M. -L. Aitio *et al.*, *Br. J. clin. Pharmac.*, 1981, *11*, 279.

Anti-arrhythmic agents. Data indicating that cardiac toxicity from disopyramide may add to the toxicity of lignocaine, phenytoin, procainamide, or other class I anti-arrhythmic agents.— G. Ellrodt and B. N. Singh, *Heart & Lung*, 1980, *9*, 469.

See also Lignocaine Hydrochloride, p.903.

Anticoagulants. For the effect of disopyramide on warfarin, see Warfarin Sodium, p.779.

Beta-blockers. Bradycardia with unconsciousness and severe hypotension in one patient and bradycardia and asystole in a second patient after the intravenous injection of disopyramide 20 minutes after practolol intravenously.— A. D. Cumming and C. Robertson, *Br. med. J.*, 1979, *2*, 1264. See also B. O'Keefe *et al.* (letter), *ibid.*, 1583; D. Gelipter and M. Hazell (letter), *ibid.*, 1980, *280*, 52.

In 5 patients given disopyramide by mouth in initial doses of up to 400 mg there was severe myocardial depression, hypotension, raised venous pressure, and (in 4) severe abdominal pain. Some patients were taking beta-adrenoceptor blocking agents; disopyramide should be given with caution to such patients and to patients with myocardial dysfunction, and should not be given in loading doses.— E. G. Manolas *et al.*, *Br. med. J.*, 1979, *2*, 1553.

Cardiac glycosides. Confirmation of reports that serum-digoxin concentration rises during concomitant quinidine administration. No such rise occurred when disopyramide was given.— E. B. Leakey *et al.*, *Ann. intern. Med.*, 1980, *92*, 605. See also E. G. Manolas *et al.*, *Aust. N.Z. J. Med.*, 1980, *10*, 426.

Electrolytes. Possible enhancement of the toxic effects of disopyramide on the heart by hyperkalaemia.— B. D. Maddux and R. B. Whiting, *Chest*, 1980, *78*, 654.

For a warning of the risks of hypokalaemia, see under Precautions, above.

Pregnancy and the neonate. Uterine contractions occurred 1 to 2 hours after successive oral doses of disopyramide were given to a woman who was 8 months pregnant.— R. F. Leonard *et al.*, *New Engl. J. Med.*, 1978, *299*, 84.

Disopyramide 200 mg every 8 hours was used to treat bigeminy and paroxysmal ventricular tachycardia from the 26th week of pregnancy in a 27-year-old woman. Labour was spontaneous and normal and no evidence of congenital abnormality or growth retardation was found.— E. J. Shaxted and P. J. Milton, *Curr. med. Res. Opinion*, 1979, *6*, 70.

Absorption and Fate. Disopyramide is readily and almost completely absorbed from the gastro-intestinal tract, peak plasma concentrations being attained about 1 to 3 hours after oral administration.

Disopyramide is partially dealkylated in the liver, but is excreted in the urine predominantly unchanged with only about 25% as the dealkylated metabolite (which has anti-arrhythmic and marked anticholinergic properties); the clearance of disopyramide does not appear to be influenced by urinary pH.

Disopyramide is widely distributed throughout the body and is extensively bound to plasma proteins; there is some disagreement as to factors, including dosage, which may influence protein binding. Estimations of the plasma half-life of disopyramide range from about 6 to 10 hours. The therapeutic effect of disopyramide has been correlated with plasma concentrations in the range of about 3 to 7 µg per ml.

Disopyramide crosses the placental barrier and *animal* studies have indicated that it is excreted in breast milk.

Absorption. In a study in 7 healthy subjects the bioavailability of disopyramide was comparatively high both for capsules containing the phosphate (91%) and those containing the base (83%). Clinically both preparations would probably be regarded as quite satisfactory and virtually bioequivalent.— D. K. Dubetz *et al.* (letter), *Br. J. clin. Pharmac.*, 1978, *6*, 279.

Comparative bioavailability of disopyramide phosphate after multiple dosing with standard capsules and controlled-release tablets.— G. Forssell *et al.*, *Eur. J. clin. Pharmac.*, 1980, *17*, 209.

Metabolism and pharmacokinetics. In a study involving 4 healthy subjects urinary pH was found to have no effect on the renal clearance of disopyramide. Following intravenous administration of 2 mg per kg body-weight to 2 of the subjects the total plasma-drug concentration declined biexponentially with an initial half-life of 2 to 4 minutes and an apparent terminal half-life of 5.92 to 9.20 hours. In the other 2 subjects oral ingestion of disopyramide 5 mg per kg body-weight gave peak plasma concentrations of 2.5 to 3.5 µg per ml within 1 to 1.5 hours which were sustained for about 2 to 3 hours before declining. Regardless of the route of administration more than 90% of the 72-hour urinary recovery of drug and metabolite was generally excreted in the first 24 hours, total recovery being 64.5 to 95.8% of the dose with 46.9 to 67.0% as unmetabolised drug and 11.2 to 37.2% as the *N*-deisopropyl metabolite. Renal clearance from these 4 subjects and from 3 in a previous study varied, with a decline over a 24-hour period; this was only partly explained by variation in *in vitro* plasma-protein binding as a function of total plasma concentration.— J. L. Cunningham *et al.*, *Clin. Pharmacokinet.*, 1977, *2*, 373. See also *idem* (letter), *Br. J. clin. Pharmac.*, 1978, *5*, 343.

In a study involving 3 healthy subjects little difference was found between the disposition of disopyramide 100 mg after administration by mouth or by intravenous injection. Following intravenous injection the half-life in the blood was slightly longer being about 5½ to 7½ hours while following oral administration it was about 5 to 6 hours. Whereas intestinal absorption was nearly 100% in 2 subjects it was only 50% in the third, possibly owing to genetic variation. About 80% of a dose was excreted unchanged in the urine, most within the first 8 hours following intravenous administration and between the fourth and twelfth hours following oral administration. Following either route of administration the drug was virtually totally eliminated after 72 hours, with about 20% in the urine as metabolite. In 2 subjects less than 8% of the drug was found in the faeces but in the third 23% was found after intravenous administration and 45% after oral administration; this subject had absorbed only 50% following administration by mouth and biliary elimination might have been markedly more significant. The sole metabolite of disopyramide was the monodealkylated form.— J. de Graeve *et al.*, *Thérapie*, 1977, *32*, 195.

Each of 8 healthy male subjects received the following single doses of different disopyramide preparations in randomised sequence: disopyramide 300 mg (Rythmodan capsules), disopyramide 300 mg, as the phosphate (Norpace capsules), and disopyramide 2 mg per kg body-weight as a bolus intravenous injection over 2 minutes. The mean half-life after injection was 7.79 hours. Absorption from Rythmodan capsules was significantly faster than from Norpace capsules, peak serum concentrations being achieved after 1.69 and 2.80 hours respectively with half-lives of 7.96 and 8.91 hours. Although the bioavailability of Norpace was significantly higher than that of Rythmodan it was not considered that this should normally be of any clinical significance. Urinary excretion of disopyramide after intravenous injection was almost complete within 24 hours and about 58% of the dose was excreted unchanged over 72 hours; about 51 and 55% of an oral dose of Rythmodan and Norpace were excreted respectively.— S. M. Bryson *et al.*, *Br. J. clin. Pharmac.*, 1978, *6*, 409.

Plasma concentrations. While studies relating serum concentrations of disopyramide and anti-arrhythmic activity are few, it appears that about 3 to 5 or 6 µg per ml represents the likely desirable therapeutic range.— R. C. Heel *et al.*, *Drugs*, 1978, *15*, 331. The therapeutic plasma range for disopyramide is probably in the order of 2 to 7 µg per ml.— A. Richens and S. Warrington, *ibid.*, 1979, *17*, 488.

A study of plasma concentrations of disopyramide in myocardial infarction patients. The most important clinical implication was the finding that despite a loading dose of 400 mg of disopyramide by mouth, between 18 and 170 hours were needed for most of them to achieve trough plasma concentrations surpassing the lower end of the manufacturer's recommended therapeutic range of 3.3 to 7.5 µg per ml.— K. F. Ilett *et al.*, *Clin. Pharmac. Ther.*, 1979, *26*, 1.

Individual studies directed at correlating plasma concentrations with therapeutic response: M. -L. Aitio and T. Vuorenmaa, *Br. J. clin. Pharmac.*, 1980, *9*, 149 (renal dysfunction); R. M. Hillson and E. Boyd, *J. int. med. Res.*, 1980, *8*, 314 (myocardial infarction); P. V. Luoma *et al.*, *Curr. ther. Res.*, 1980, *27*, 839 (supraventricular arrhythmia); B. Whiting *et al.*, *Br. J. clin. Pharmac.*, 1980, *9*, 67 (no evidence of a role for the metabolite).

Protein binding. A study of the binding characteristics of disopyramide in normal plasma and a discussion on the large variation in binding behaviour in earlier studies.— B. M. David *et al.* (letter), *Br. J. clin. Pharmac.*, 1980, *9*, 614.

Further studies and comments on disopyramide and plasma protein binding: P. H. Hinderling *et al.*, *J. pharm. Sci.*, 1974, *63*, 1684; Y. W. Chien *et al.*, *ibid.*, 1877; J. L. Cunningham *et al.* (letter), *Br. J. clin. Pharmac.*, 1978, *5*, 343; P. J. Meffin *et al.*, *J. Pharmacokinet. Biopharm.*, 1979, *7*, 29.

Uses. Disopyramide is a class I anti-arrhythmic agent (see p.1370) with a depressant action on the heart similar to that of quinidine (p.1372); some of its actions are reported to resemble more closely those of lignocaine (p.904). It also has anticholinergic and local anaesthetic properties. For the prevention and treatment of ventricular arrhythmias disopyramide is given by mouth as the base or the phosphate in doses of, or equivalent to, 100 to 150 mg of base every six hours with a range of 300 to 800 mg daily according to the patient's response. An initial loading dose of 200 mg may be given. Disopyramide may also be used for supraventricular arrhythmias but, in general, is less effective.

Disopyramide may be given by slow intravenous injection of the phosphate in doses equivalent to 2 mg of the base per kg body-weight to a maximum of 150 mg, at a rate not exceeding 30 mg per minute; this may be followed by 200 mg by mouth immediately on completion of the injection and every 8 hours for 24 hours; subsequently the usual maintenance dosage of 400 to 600 mg daily in divided doses may be given. If the arrhythmia recurs on completion of the intravenous injection it may be repeated once, not less than 20 minutes after the first injection; a total intravenous dose of 4 mg per kg or a maximum total of 300 mg, should not be exceeded in the first hour, nor should the total by both intravenous and oral routes exceed 800 mg in 24 hours. Alternatively, the initial intravenous injection may be followed by intravenous infusion equivalent to 0.4 mg of base per kg per hour (or 20 to 30 mg per hour) to a maximum of 800 mg daily; sodium chloride injection, dextrose injection, or compound sodium lactate injection are suitable for dilution.

Administration. In children. Intractable junctional tachycardia of over 200 beats per minute in a 6-year-old girl was controlled during the day, although brief self-terminating paroxysms still occurred in the evenings, by the administration of disopyramide 100 mg twice daily eventually increased to 100 mg four times daily. After 11 months of therapy no evidence of toxicity or side-effects had occurred.— H. Ikram and W. Chan (letter), *Med. J. Aust.*, 1978, *1*, 392.

The dose of disopyramide in children should be titrated according to the concentration in plasma. In a 2-week-old girl and a 20-month-old boy doses of 30 and 20 mg per kg body-weight respectively were needed to produce therapeutic concentrations in plasma.— D. W. Holt *et al.*, *Br. med. J.*, 1979, *2*, 1476.

Administration in cardiac failure. A study demonstrating that disopyramide given to cardiac patients in the fasting state was absorbed fairly rapidly from the gastro-intestinal tract and peak plasma concentrations were obtained within 1 to 2 hours. The half-life of about 8 hours was a little longer than that reported for healthy subjects.— K. Landmark *et al.*, *Acta med. scand.*, 1979, *206*, 385.

For lowered plasma concentrations of disopyramide following myocardial infarction, see under Absorption and Fate, above.

Administration in renal failure. The pharmacokinetics of disopyramide were studied in 6 patients with chronic renal impairment 3 of whom required routine haemodialysis but were between dialysis sessions during the study. A dose of 150 to 200 mg every 6 hours would produce the desired average plasma-disopyramide concentration of 4 µg per ml in patients without renal impairment when the half-life would be 7 to 8 hours. In severe renal impairment with a creatinine clearance of less than 8 ml per minute then the recommended dose to produce the required plasma concentration would be 150 mg daily in single or divided doses. In less severe renal failure the recommended dose was 150 mg every 12 hours or 100 mg every 8 hours. Loading dose adjustment might only be important when the reduced clearance might considerably delay the attainment of steady-state concentrations.— B. Whiting and H. L. Elliott (letter), *Lancet*, 1977, *2*, 1363.

Indications that therapeutic concentrations of disopyramide are not appreciably dialysed.— M. J. Sevka *et al.*, *Clin. Pharmac. Ther.*, 1981, *29*, 322. See also A. D. Blair *et al.*, *ibid.*, 234.

Further references to a prolonged half-life of disopyramide in renal failure: J. A. Henry *et al.*, *Br. J. clin. Pharmac.*, 1979, *7*, 427P; A. Johnston *et al.*, *ibid.*, 1980, *10*, 245.

Cardiac disorders. A review of anti-arrhythmic agents, including disopyramide, giving details of its uses and adverse effects. Disopyramide has properties and some side-effects akin to those of quinidine but some of its electrophysiological properties more closely resemble those of lignocaine, and it may help in the treatment of ventricular tachycardia where quinidine has failed. It is as effective as quinidine in reducing recurrence after electrical cardioversion and has fewer side-effects, but it is less impressive against atrial arrhythmias, except for the Wolff-Parkinson-White syndrome. Disopyramide is one of several agents used intravenously for lignocaine failure, but the risk of cardiac depression (hypotension) is greater than with lignocaine, possibly due to a mild calcium antagonist action. Like quinidine, disopyramide occasionally precipitates ventricular fibrillation and *torsade de pointes,* and when there is cardiomegaly a high first dose can cause collapse. Although the anticholinergic effect of disopyramide makes it particularly useful in the management of arrhythmias associated with sinus bradycardia, the sick-sinus syndrome may be a contra-indication (unexpectedly, bundle-branch block is not). Disopyramide is not effective in digitalis toxicity, and its use in association with quinidine, digoxin or methyldopa is inadvisable in the sick sinus syndrome. Intravenous disopyramide can substantially reduce cardiac output in beta-blocked patients; there is no interaction with lignocaine.— L. H. Opie, *Lancet,* 1980, *1,* 861.

Further reviews of disopyramide: R. C. Heel *et al., Drugs,* 1978, *15,* 331; J. Koch-Weser, *New Engl. J. Med.,* 1979, *300,* 957.

Arrhythmias. Of 48 patients with atrial fibrillation who completed a double-blind study, 24 received disopyramide 300 mg by mouth on the day before electroconversion and 500 mg daily thereafter and 24 received placebo. Of 18 patients in the disopyramide group who were successfully restored to sinus rhythm by electroconversion 13 were still in sinus rhythm after 12 weeks, whereas in the placebo group only 6 of 20 were still in sinus rhythm; this difference was significant. Side-effects in the disopyramide group included dry mouth (8 patients), disturbance of accomodation (1), and dysuria (1). Two of 4 patients who did not complete the study were in the disopyramide group: one developed recurrence of pulmonary oedema on the day following electroconversion, and the other developed low output heart failure with hypotension immediately after electroconversion; in view of a possible connection with the depressant effect of disopyramide on myocardial contraction it was recommended that it should be used with caution in patients with severe myocardial disease.— G. Härtel *et al., Clin. Pharmac. Ther.,* 1974, *15,* 551.

In a double-blind crossover study completed by 17 patients with cardiac disorders, disopyramide phosphate 100 to 200 mg by mouth, according to body-weight, 4 times daily for 8 weeks, had significant anti-arrhythmic activity. Disopyramide phosphate was effective against both ventricular and supraventricular arrhythmias, and in 10 patients ventricular ectopic beats were reduced from an average of 145 per hour to 4. One patient was withdrawn from the study due to nausea, vomiting, and diarrhoea in the first week of treatment. Other side-effects included dry mouth (4), dizziness (2), dry eyes (2), and urinary hesitancy (1).— L. A. Vismara *et al., Clin. Pharmac. Ther.,* 1974, *16,* 330.

Further references: R. A. J. Spurrell *et al., Br. Heart J.,* 1975, *37,* 861 (Wolff-Parkinson-White syndrome); D. A. Deano *et al., Chest,* 1977, *71,* 597 (intravenous therapy of ventricular and supra-ventricular arrhythmias); L. A. Vismara *et al., Am. J. Cardiol.,* 1977, *39,* 1027 (refractory ventricular tachycardia); D. G. Benditt *et al., Eur. J. Cardiol.,* 1979, *9,* 255 (recurrent ventricular tachycardia); J. Camm *et al., Br. J. clin. Pharmac.,* 1979, *8,* 441 (recurrent paroxysmal tachycardia); J. M. Desai *et al., Circulation,* 1979, *59,* 215 (bundle branch block); A. LaBarre *et al., ibid.,* 226 (caution in sinus node dysfunction); J. A. Sbarbaro *et al., Am. J. Cardiol.,* 1979, *44,* 513 (comparison with lignocaine).

Myocardial infarction. The value of disopyramide in the prophylaxis of cardiac arrhythmias was studied in open wards rather than coronary-care units over 18 months in 58 patients with 60 acute myocardial infarctions. Half the number of patients received disopyramide 100 mg as soon as possible after admission to hospital followed by 100 mg four times daily for 7 days; the remaining patients received a placebo. There were significantly fewer deaths in the treated group (1) compared with control (11), extension of infarction was significantly less with disopyramide (2) than with the placebo (11), and both ventricular and supraventricular arrhythmias were significantly reduced by disopyramide but atrioventricular block was unaffected. It was recommended that disopyramide should be given by mouth for the first 7 days after myocardial infarction to all patients not managed in an intensive-care unit.— N. Zainal *et al., Lancet,* 1977, *2,* 887. See also *ibid.,* 912. See also D. J. S. Carmichael *et al.* (letter), *ibid.,* 1185. Criticism of the analysis. The study did not justify the recommendation.— A. Pottage *et al.* (letter), *ibid.,* 1362. Risks associated with disopyramide included hypotension, seen in 3 patients given single doses of 400 mg, and further changes in conduction in patients with conduction disturbances. It was recommended that disopyramide be used in myocardial infarction with the precautions taken during procainamide or quinidine therapy.— D. Ross *et al.* (letter), *ibid.,* 1978, *1,* 330. Reply.— P. H. Kidner and E. M. M. Besterman (letter), *ibid.,* 562.

In a double-blind placebo-controlled study 157 patients with suspected myocardial infarction were given oxprenolol 40 mg thrice daily within 24 hours of the onset of symptoms, 158 similar patients were given disopyramide phosphate 150 mg thrice daily, 79 were given oxprenolol placebo, and 79 were given disopyramide placebo. The results indicated that the early use of either oxprenolol or disopyramide in patients with suspected acute myocardial infarction is unlikely to improve mortality. There was a significant excess of patients with heart failure in the disopyramide-treated group. Other reasons for withdrawal of disopyramide included acute urinary retention (4 patients), severe abdominal pain (4 patients), blurred vision (2 patients), and erythematous rashes in 2 patients which developed into a generalised exfoliative dermatitis in one.— R. G. Wilcox *et al., Lancet,* 1980, *2,* 765. Similar failure to demonstrate a reduction in mortality on administration of disopyramide after myocardial infarction.— D. P. Nicholls *et al., ibid.,* 936.

Preparations

Disopyramide Capsules *(B.P.).* Capsules containing disopyramide.

Disopyramide Phosphate Capsules *(B.P.).* Capsules containing disopyramide phosphate. Potency is expressed in terms of the equivalent amount of disopyramide.

Disopyramide Phosphate Capsules *(U.S.P.).* Capsules containing disopyramide phosphate. Potency is expressed in terms of the equivalent amount of disopyramide. The *U.S.P.* requires 80% dissolution in 20 minutes.

Proprietary Preparations

Dirythmin SA *(Astra, UK).* Disopyramide phosphate, available as sustained-release tablets each containing the equivalent of disopyramide 150 mg. *Dose.* Usual dose 2 tablets every 12 hours.

Norpace *(Searle, UK: Astra, UK).* Disopyramide phosphate, available as **Capsules** each containing the equivalent of 100 or 150 mg of disopyramide and as **Injection** containing the equivalent of 20 mg per ml, in ampoules of 5 and 7.5 ml. (Also available as Norpace in *Arg., Austral., Canad., Denm., Fin., Ger., Gib., Hong Kong, Israel, Jordan, Kenya, Malay., Mex., Neth., NZ, Nigeria, Norw., Philipp., Puerto Rico, Singapore, S.Afr., Switz., Taiwan, Tanzania, Thai., USA, Zambia*).

Rythmodan *(Cassenne, UK).* Disopyramide, available as **Capsules** of 100 and 150 mg and as **Injection** containing disopyramide phosphate equivalent to disopyramide 10 mg per ml, in ampoules of 5 ml. (Also available as Rythmodan in *Austral., Belg., Canad., Fr., Jap., Neth., S.Afr., Switz.*).

Rythmodan Retard *(Roussel, UK).* Disopyramide phosphate, available as scored sustained-release tablets each containing the equivalent of disopyramide 250 mg. *Dose.* 1 or 1½ tablets twice daily.

Other Proprietary Names

Dicorynan *(Spain)*; Durbis *(Denm., Norw., Swed.)*; Norpaso *(Arg.)*; Ritmodan *(Ital.)*; Ritmoforine *(Neth.)* Rythmodul *(Ger.).*

7785-b

Encainide Hydrochloride. MJ-9067-1. (±)-2′-[2-(1-Methyl-2-piperidyl)ethyl]-*p*-anisanilide hydrochloride. $C_{22}H_{28}N_2O_2,HCl=388.9$.

CAS — 37612-13-8; 66778-36-7 (both encainide); 66794-74-9 (hydrochloride).

Encainide is a class I anti-arrhythmic agent (see p.1370). It has been given as the hydrochloride in doses of 25 to 100 mg every 8 hours.

Encainide is an anti-arrhythmic agent with some important differences from quinidine.— L. H. Opie, *Lancet,* 1980, *1,* 861. See also J. B. Schwartz *et al., Drugs,* 1981, *21,* 23.

Encainide was an effective and well tolerated anti-arrhythmic agent in 10 of 11 patients with chronic high-frequency ventricular arrhythmias. Arrhythmias were totally suppressed in 10 patients by a range of doses of tablets containing encainide hydrochloride; patients were discharged on regimens of 25 to 100 mg every 8 hours and in 2 of the patients doses were subsequently adjusted to 50 mg every 6 hours or 75 mg every 12 hours. Encainide was generally well tolerated despite its unusual effects on the ECG—anti-arrhythmic activity was associated with marked dose-related prolongation of the P-R and Q-R-S intervals. No abnormalities in laboratory screening tests were observed during follow-up over 6 to 12 months. Transient ataxia and diplopia coincided with the abolition of arrhythmia in 2 patients. The lack of response to encainide in the eleventh patient appeared to be associated with a slow-metabolising trait. In the 10 patients who responded to treatment with encainide very variable peak plasma concentrations, ranging from 2.4 to 135 ng per ml, were achieved after a single 25-mg dose; the *O*-demethylated metabolite was detected in plasma within 2 to 3 hours. The mean elimination half-life was 2.7 hours increasing to 3.4 hours under steady-state conditions. The patient whose arrhythmia did not respond to treatment had a half-life of 7.8 hours and the *O*-demethylated metabolite was not detected until doses of 500 mg daily were given.— D. M. Roden *et al., New Engl. J. Med.,* 1980, *302,* 877. Criticism of the selection of patients. The acid test will be the efficacy and toxicity of encainide among patients with severe heart disease and recurrent malignant arrhythmias who truly require anti-arrhythmic therapy.— T. B. Graboys (letter), *ibid., 303,* 395. Reply.— D. M. Roden *et al.* (letter), *ibid.*

Further studies of encainide.— H. Kesteloot and R. Stroobandt, *Eur. J. clin. Pharmac.,* 1979, *16,* 323; M. Sami *et al., Am. J. Cardiol.,* 1979, *44,* 526.

Manufacturers

Bristol-Myers, UK; Mead Johnson, USA.

7786-v

Hydroquinidine Hydrochloride. Dihydroquinidine Hydrochloride; Hydroconchinine Hydrochloride; Dihydrochinidin Hydrochloride. (8*R*,9*S*)-10,11-Dihydro-6′-methoxycinchonan-9-ol hydrochloride.
$C_{20}H_{26}N_2O_2,HCl=362.9$.

CAS — 1435-55-8 (hydroquinidine); 1476-98-8 (hydrochloride).

Pharmacopoeias. In *Fr.*

Colourless crystals. M.p. 273° to 274°. Freely **soluble** in chloroform and methyl alcohol; less readily soluble in water and alcohol.

Hydroquinidine is an anti-arrhythmic agent with actions and uses similar to those of quinidine (see p.1370). It is given as the hydrochloride in usual maintenance doses of 150 mg three or four times daily.

The pharmacokinetics of hydroquinidine in 8 patients with congestive heart failure following the intravenous infusion of a quinidine preparation that contained 5.9% hydroquinidine as an impurity.— C. T. Ueda and B. S. Dzindzio, *Eur. J. clin. Pharmac.,* 1979, *16,* 101.

Studies in 10 healthy subjects showed that similar blood concentrations of hydroquinidine were achieved by dosage with 150 mg 6-hourly, as with 250 mg in sustained release capsules every 12 hours.— M. Maccari *et al., Farmaco, Edn prat.,* 1979, *34,* 49.

Proprietary Names

Lentoquine *(Berenguer-Beneyto, Spain).*

7787-g

Lorajmine Hydrochloride. Chloroacetylajmaline Hydrochloride; Win 11831. Ajmaline 17-chloroacetate. $C_{22}H_{27}ClN_2O_3,HCl=439.4$.

CAS — 47562-08-3 (lorajmine); 40819-93-0 (hydrochloride).

Lorajmine is an anti-arrhythmic agent which is metabolised to ajmaline (p.1373). It is given as the hydrochloride in maintenance doses of 200 to 400 mg daily. It is also given by slow intravenous injection or by infusion.

Proprietary Names

Ritmos Elle *(Inverni della Beffa, Ital.)*; Viaductor *(Servier, Fr.).*

7788-q

Lorcainide Hydrochloride. R-15889; Isocainide Hydrochloride; Socainide Hydrochloride. 4′-Chloro-*N*-(1-isopropyl-4-piperidyl)-2-phenylacetanilide hydrochloride.

$C_{22}H_{27}ClN_2O,HCl$=407.4.

CAS — 59729-31-6 (lorcainide); 58934-46-6 (hydrochloride).

Crystals. M.p. 263°.

Lorcainide is a class I anti-arrhythmic agent (see p.1370). It has been given as the hydrochloride in doses of 100 mg twice or thrice daily.

Lorcainide is a class I anti-arrhythmic agent with a structure somewhat similar to that of lignocaine, and which prolongs the duration of action potential in a manner similar to that of quinidine. It appears to be more effective during chronic therapy than on acute intravenous administration, possibly due to rapid fall in blood concentrations during distribution following an intravenous bolus. It has been suggested that it undergoes high and saturable first-pass metabolism on oral administration, and that its kinetics may be non-linear. Adverse effects include dizziness, tremor, and blurred vision during rapid intravenous injection; plasma concentration-related prolongation of the Q-R-S and P-R intervals; and significant sleep disturbances with insomnia, nightmares, vivid dreams, and increased perspiration in up to 40% of patients given oral therapy—with long-term continuation there may be some decrease in the initial sleep disturbances.— J. B. Schwartz *et al.*, *Drugs*, 1981, *21*, 23.

Further references to the use of lorcainide: H. Kesteloot and R. Stroobandt, *Archs int. Pharmacodyn. Ther.*, 1977, *230*, 225; G. Cocco and C. Strozzi, *Eur. J. clin. Pharmac.*, 1978, *14*, 105; W. Kasper *et al.*, *J. cardiovasc. Pharmac.*, 1979, *1*, 343; U. Klotz *et al.*, *Eur. J. clin. Pharmac.*, 1979, *16*, 1; C. K. Ng *et al.*, *Eur. J. clin. Pharmac.*, 1979, *15*, 241; D. P. Myburgh *et al.*, *S. Afr. med. J.*, 1980, *57*, 236.

Pharmacokinetic studies of lorcainide: U. Klotz *et al.*, *Clin. Pharmacokinet.*, 1978, *3*, 407; E. Jähnchen *et al.*, *Clin. Pharmac. Ther.*, 1979, *26*, 187; T. Meinertz *et al.*, *ibid.*, 196; U. Klotz *et al.*, *ibid.*, 221; U. Klotz *et al.*, *Int. J. clin. Pharmac. Biopharm.*, 1979, *17*, 152.

7789-p

Mexiletine Hydrochloride. Kö 1173. 1-Methyl-2-(2,6-xylyloxy)ethylamine hydrochloride.

$C_{11}H_{17}NO,HCl$=215.7.

CAS — 31828-71-4 (mexiletine); 5370-01-4 (hydrochloride).

Adverse Effects. Many adverse effects of mexiletine are related to excessive plasma concentrations and will respond to dosage reduction; the margin between therapeutic and toxic blood concentrations is, however, narrow.

Adverse effects reported are nausea, vomiting, indigestion, unpleasant taste, hiccups, light-headedness, drowsiness, confusion, dizziness, diplopia, blurred vision, nystagmus, dysarthria, ataxia, tremor, paraesthesia, convulsions, hypotension, sinus bradycardia, atrial fibrillation, and palpitations.

Serious adverse effects may be a special risk in the initial stages of intravenous therapy.

No important adverse haemodynamic effects were noted in 16 patients with valvular heart disease yet no clinical evidence of heart failure when therapeutic doses of mexiletine by intravenous injection were compared with control injections of saline. Both mexiletine and saline caused a small rise in mean pulmonary artery pressure.— N. P. S. Campbell *et al.*, *Br. Heart J.*, 1979, *41*, 182.

Overdosage. A 22-year-old man who had ingested 4.4 g of mexiletine died. Symptoms included paraesthesia of the tongue, nausea, convulsions, cyanosis, rigidity, bradycardia, and an unrecordable blood pressure. The ECG showed complete heart block; ventricular asystole was unresponsive to isoprenaline, adrenaline, electrical pacing, and cardiac massage. The blood-mexiletine concentration post mortem was 34 to 37 µg per ml compared with the therapeutic range of 1 to 2 µg per ml.— P. Jequier *et al.* (letter), *Lancet*, 1976, *1*, 429.

Treatment of Adverse Effects. Adverse cardiovascular effects of mexiletine will call for symptomatic therapy. It has been reported that *animal* studies indicate that toxic neurological effects of mexiletine may respond to diazepam.

Precautions. Mexiletine should be used with special caution in patients with sinus node dysfunction, conduction defect, bradycardia, hypotension, or cardiac, renal or hepatic failure. ECG and blood pressure monitoring should be carried out. Tremor may be increased in patients with parkinsonism.

Where withdrawal of mexiletine is appropriate, it is recommended that this should be done gradually.

Absorption of mexiletine may be delayed by concurrent administration of anticholinergics or opiates, and enhanced by concurrent administration of metoclopramide.

Interactions. Eighty-two patients in a coronary care unit were given mexiletine 600 mg on arrival, 200 mg two and four hours later, then 250 mg eight-hourly. Concentration in plasma 3 hours after the first dose varied from 0.05 to 2.09 µg per ml, and were lower in patients with *myocardial infarction* or given *narcotic analgesics*. Of patients with myocardial infarction 66% failed to achieve a therapeutic concentration of 1 µg per ml at 3 hours, and 34% and 25% failed similarly on days 2 and 3.— A. Pottage *et al.*, *Eur. J. clin. Pharmac.*, 1978, *13*, 393.

Confirmation of reports that serum-*digoxin* concentration rises during concomitant quinidine administration. No such rise occurred when mexiletine was given.— E. B. Leahey *et al.*, *Ann. intern. Med.*, 1980, *92*, 605.

Evidence that *metoclopramide* enhances and *atropine* decreases the rate of mexiletine absorption without altering the relative oral bioavailability.— L. M. H. Wing *et al.*, *Br. J. clin. Pharmac.*, 1980, *9*, 505.

For a warning that concurrent administration of *antacids* may be associated with raised plasma concentrations of mexiletine, see under Absorption and Fate, below.

Pregnancy and the neonate. A normal male child was born to a woman given mexiletine with propranolol for the control of ventricular dysrhythmias during the third trimester of pregnancy. During the first 6 hours after delivery the child had a heart-rate of only 90 beats per minute, probably due to the propranolol; it was normal thereafter. At delivery the concentration of mexiletine in the infant's serum was the same as in the mother's. The infant was breast fed and determinations on the second day and the sixth week after birth indicated that mexiletine is excreted in breast milk, but in an insufficient quantity to be measureable in the serum of the breast-fed infant. Though caution should still be exercised, mexiletine appears safe in pregnancy, and breast feeding can proceed normally.— A. D. Timmis *et al.* (letter), *Lancet*, 1980, *2*, 647.

Absorption and Fate. Mexiletine is readily and almost completely absorbed from the gastro-intestinal tract, peak plasma concentrations being obtained 2 to 4 hours after oral administration.

Mexiletine is metabolised in the liver to a number of metabolites. It is excreted in the urine, mainly in the form of its metabolites with only small amounts unchanged; there are indications that the clearance of mexiletine is decreased in alkaline urine.

Mexiletine is widely distributed throughout the body and is extensively bound to plasma proteins. It has a plasma half-life of over 10 hours. Its therapeutic effect has been correlated with plasma concentrations of 0.75 to 2 µg per ml, but the margin between therapeutic and toxic concentrations is narrow, and severe toxicity may occur within this range.

Mexiletine crosses the placental barrier; amounts appearing in breast milk, following therapeutic doses to the mother, have been reported to provide undetectable concentrations in the serum of a breast-fed infant.

Metabolism and pharmacokinetics. After administration of mexiletine by mouth and intravenously to 4 healthy subjects under acidic and normal conditions of urinary pH, 1-(4′-hydroxy-2′,6′-dimethyl)phenoxypropan-2-ol and 1-(2′-hydroxymethyl-6′-methyl)phenoxypropan-2-ol were identified as major urinary metabolites.— A. H. Beckett and E. C. Chidomere, *J. Pharm. Pharmac.*, 1977, *29*, 281.

Plasma concentrations of mexiletine fell rapidly over 2 hours, and then more slowly, after the intravenous injection of 200 mg in 5 healthy male subjects. The mean plasma elimination half-life was 11.77 hours. After mexiletine 200 mg by mouth, plasma concentrations rose slowly, reached a peak after about 2 hours, and then declined with a mean half-life of 11.40 hours.— N. P. S. Campbell *et al.* (letter), *Br. J. clin. Pharmac.*, 1978, *6*, 372.

A study of the effects of spontaneous changes in urinary pH in healthy subjects given subtherapeutic doses of mexiletine confirmed that at high urinary pH excretion and clearance of mexiletine is low and the plasma concentration is raised. Urinary pH may partly account for inter-individual differences in the pharmacokinetics of mexiletine. Urinary pH measurements may be useful during mexiletine therapy and any factors likely to cause large variations in the urinary pH, such as antacids, should be avoided.— A. Johnston *et al.*, *Br. J. clin. Pharmac.*, 1979, *8*, 349. See also M. A. Kiddie *et al.*, *Br. J. clin. Pharmac.*, 1974, *1*, 229.

Plasma concentrations. A study of the pharmacokinetics of mexiletine given in various doses by mouth or intravenously to 156 patients, 153 of whom had ischaemic heart disease, revealed great inter-patient variation. The mean plasma elimination half-life after a single intravenous dose of mexiletine 200 mg in 10 patients was 13.24 hours compared with 11.31 hours after chronic oral therapy in 30 patients. From 2 to 48% (mean 14%) of the total daily dose was excreted unchanged in the urine during the 48 hours after the last dose. In 149 patients, 79% of plasma concentrations within the range of 0.75 to 2 µg per ml were effective but 5.5% were associated with severe side-effects including hypotension, with or without bradycardia, atrio-ventricular dissociation, vomiting, tremor, and toxic confusional states. A dose of 10 to 14 mg per kg body-weight daily achieved plasma concentrations in this therapeutic range in 72% of patients. Significant increases in plasma concentration did not occur after the third day when maintenance doses of mexiletine were given.— N. P. S. Campbell *et al.*, *Br. J. clin. Pharmac.*, 1978, *6*, 103.

In 4 healthy volunteer subjects simultaneous administration of mexiletine 250 mg by intravenous infusion over 15 minutes and 400 mg by mouth rapidly produced plasma concentrations within the therapeutic range of 0.75 to 2.0 µg per ml which were maintained for 4 hours. This dosage regimen is suitable in the initial control of arrhythmias following acute myocardial infarction.— D. W. Holt *et al.*, *J. int. med. Res.*, 1979, *7*, 162.

Use of a slow-release tablet of mexiletine to maintain plasma concentrations within the therapeutic range with a 12-hourly dosage regimen.— D. M. Boyle *et al.*, *Br. J. clin. Pharmac.*, 1980, *9*, 293P.

Uses. Mexiletine is a class I anti-arrhythmic agent (see p.1370) with actions similar to those of lignocaine (p.904), to which it is structurally related. Unlike lignocaine it is suitable for oral administration.

For the prevention and treatment of ventricular arrhythmias mexiletine is given by mouth as the hydrochloride in initial doses of 400 to 600 mg, followed by 200 to 250 mg three to four times daily, starting 2 hours after the loading dose. The usual maintenance dosage of mexiletine is 600 to 800 mg daily in divided doses.

Mexiletine may be given by slow intravenous injection of the hydrochloride in doses of 100 to 250 mg at a rate of 25 mg per minute, followed by an infusion in a 5% solution of dextrose or a 0.9% solution of sodium chloride at a rate of 250 mg over 1 hour, 250 mg over the next 2 hours, and then at about 0.5 mg per minute for maintenance, according to the patient's response; when appropriate the patient may be transferred to oral therapy with doses of 200 to 250 mg of the hydrochloride 3 or 4 times daily. Alternatively, an initial intravenous dose of 200 mg at a rate of 25 mg per minute, may be followed by an oral dose of 400 mg on completion of the injection, with subsequent oral therapy as before.

A report of a symposium on mexiletine.— *Postgrad. med. J.*, 1977, *Suppl.* 1, 1–171.

Administration. In children. The dose of mexiletine in children should be titrated according to the concentration in plasma. In a 2-week-old girl and a 20-month-old boy high doses of 25 and 15 mg per kg body-weight respectively were needed to produce therapeutic concentrations in plasma.— D. W. Holt *et al.*, *Br. med. J.*, 1979, *2*, 1476.

Cardiac disorders. A review of anti-arrhythmic agents, including mexiletine, giving details of its uses and adverse effects. Mexiletine has class I activity, is similar in structure to lignocaine, and has been described as an 'oral lignocaine'. Although less toxic than procainamide, mexiletine does have some serious side-effects, especially when given intravenously to acutely ill or elderly patients. The therapeutic-to-toxic margin is low. The major therapeutic use is in the chronic oral prophylaxis of ventricular arrhythmias, especially after myocardial infarction, but as with other agents, there is no certainty that chronic oral therapy prevents ventricular fibrillation and sudden death.— L. H. Opie, *Lancet*, 1980, *1*, 861.

Further reviews of mexiletine: C. Y. C. Chew *et al.*, *Drugs*, 1979, *17*, 161; E. B. Leakey and J. T. Bigger, *Ann. intern. Med.*, 1980, *92*, 427.

Arrhythmias. Treatment with mexiletine by intravenous injection or by mouth in 59 patients with various *ventricular arrhythmias* was successful in 43 and partly successful in 12. Four patients did not respond. The dose given by slow injection varied from 30 to 300 mg followed, in patients with acute arrhythmias, by infusions of 1.5 to 3 g over 36 to 48 hours. The loading dose given by mouth of 400 to 600 mg produced peak plasma-mexiletine concentrations of 1 to 2.5 µg per ml and therapeutic concentrations of up to 2 µg per ml were readily achieved with maintenance doses of 150 to 300 mg every 6 to 8 hours. Mild toxicity, ataxia, tremor, and paraesthesia was associated with plasma concentrations of 0.8 to 3 µg per ml while severe toxicity, nausea, vomiting, dizziness, dysarthria, diplopia, drowsiness, confusion, tremor, and paraesthesia occurred within the range of 1 to 4.4 µg per ml. Cardiovascular toxicity occurred in 6 patients.— R. G. Talbot *et al.*, *Lancet*, 1973, *2*, 399. Following a preliminary evaluation in 19 patients with ventricular arrhythmias, mexiletine was given in various doses by mouth or intravenously to another 67 patients, some of whom had failed to respond to lignocaine. Ten of these patients had severe arrhythmias and a good response was obtained in 6, although in 2 this was transient; of the remaining 57 patients 32 had a good response. Maintenance treatment given by mouth to 51 patients demonstrated that doses of mexiletine below 1.2 g daily were associated with fewer side-effects but were also associated with a higher incidence of arrhythmias. The mean therapeutic plasma-mexiletine concentration was estimated as 1.33 µg per ml. Side-effects were present at a mean concentration of 2.49 µg and unacceptable effects at 3.3 µg per ml. Peak plasma concentrations were achieved between 1 and 2 hours after a dose given by mouth. Side-effects occurred in 63 patients; minor effects included nausea, nystagmus, tremor, and drowsiness. Unacceptable effects occurred in 31 patients and included bradycardia, hypotension, vomiting, confusion, and ataxia.— N. P. S. Campbell *et al.*, *ibid.*, 404.

In 4 patients with *ventricular tachycardia* refractory to previous standard drug therapy, including mexiletine, the addition of propranolol 240 mg daily to the highest dose of mexiletine that failed to produce adverse effects resulted in either greater than 80% suppression of ventricular premature depolarisations or the absence of ventricular tachycardia or both. Follow-up for 12 to 23 months has indicated that maintenance treatment has produced excellent control.— E. B. Leahey *et al.*, *Br. med. J.*, 1980, *281*, 357.

Mexiletine hydrochloride 250 mg intravenously controlled *supraventricular tachycardia* in 1 patient who had not responded to other drugs. Subsequent maintenance was with mexiletine by mouth. Beneficial results were also achieved in another 5 patients. All 6 suffered short-lived dizziness, vomiting, and hypotension from the initial parenteral dose but the first two side-effects could be controlled by the intravenous injection of prochlorperazine 12.5 mg given 5 minutes before the mexiletine injection.— H. H. Salem (letter), *Lancet*, 1977, *2*, 94. See also S. D. Slater *et al.* (letter), *Br. med. J.*, 1980, *281*, 1072; *idem*, *Br. J. clin. Pract.*, 1980, *34*, 247.

Further references: D. Jewitt *et al.*, *Postgrad. med. J.*, 1976, *52*, *Suppl.* 7, 67 (unifocal premature ventricular beats); R. G. Talbot *et al.*, *Am. Heart J.*, 1976, *91*, 58 (ventricular arrhythmias); G. Koch and B. Lindström, *Eur. J. clin. Pharmac.*, 1978, *13*, 237 (ventricular ectopic beats); J. DiMarco *et al.*, *Clin. Pharmac. Ther.*, 1980, *27*, 250 (ventricular arrhythmias).

Myocardial infarction. In a double-blind placebo-controlled study involving 344 patients mexiletine therapy reduced the prevalence of ventricular arrhythmias following myocardial infarction, but no favourable trend in mortality was observed.— D. A. Chamberlain *et al.*, *Lancet*, 1980, *2*, 1324. Criticisms.— M. F. Oliver (letter), *ibid.*, 1981, *1*, 787; S. M. Gore (letter), *ibid.*, 951.

Further references: R. W. F. Campbell *et al.*, *Lancet*, 1975, *1*, 1257; N. P. S. Campbell, *Br. Heart J.*, 1978, *40*, 796; R. W. F. Campbell, *J. cardiovasc. Pharmac.*, 1979, *1*, 43.

Proprietary Preparations

Mexitil *(Boehringer Ingelheim, UK)*. Mexiletine hydrochloride, available as **Capsules** of 50 and 200 mg and as **Injection** containing 25 mg per ml, in ampoules of 10 ml. (Also available as Mexitil in *Austral., Belg., Denm., NZ, S.Afr., Swed., Switz.*).

7790-n

Prajmalium Bitartrate. GT 1012; NPAB.

N-Propylajmalinium hydrogen tartrate.
$C_{23}H_{33}N_2O_2,C_4H_5O_6$=518.6.

CAS — 35080-11-6 (prajmalium); 2589-47-1 (bitartrate).

A white to pale yellow powder. M.p. about 133° with decomposition. **Soluble** in water; readily soluble in alcohol, glacial acetic acid, and dilute mineral acids; moderately soluble in acetone and chloroform; practically insoluble in ether.

Adverse Effects, Treatment, and Precautions. The adverse cardiovascular effects of prajmalium are similar to those of quinidine.

Effects on mental state. Confusion and disorientation in time and place occurred on 2 occasions in a 67-year-old man given prajmalium bitartrate for the control of supraventricular tachycardia; the confusion rapidly disappeared when prajmalium was withdrawn.— J. B. Lessing and I. J. Copperman, *Br. med. J.*, 1977, *2*, 675.

Uses. Prajmalium is an anti-arrhythmic agent which is the *N*-propyl derivative of ajmaline (p.1373). It is given as the bitartrate in maintenance doses of 20 mg once or twice daily.

Cardiac disorders. Evidence that prajmalium bitartrate 20 mg every 4 hours for 3 doses is an alternative to intravenous lignocaine in the treatment of ventricular arrhythmias after acute myocardial infarction.— W. -D. Bussmann *et al.*, *Am. Heart J.*, 1980, *99*, 590. See also *idem*, *Dt. med. Wschr.*, 1978, *103*, 1910.

Proprietary Names

Neo Aritmina *(Byk Gulden, Ital.)*; Neo-Gilurytmal *(Giulini, Ger.; Lacer, Spain; Giulini, Switz.)*.

7791-h

Procainamide Hydrochloride *(B.P., U.S.P.)*.

Novocainamidum; Procainamidi Hydrochloridum; Procainamidi Chloridum. 4-Amino-*N*-(2-diethylaminoethyl)benzamide hydrochloride.
$C_{13}H_{21}N_3O,HCl$=271.8.

CAS — 614-39-1.

Pharmacopoeias. In *Arg., Aust., Br., Braz., Chin., Cz., Fr., Ind., Int., It., Jap., Nord., Pol., Rus., Swiss, Turk.,* and *U.S.*

A white to tan-coloured, odourless, hygroscopic, crystalline powder. M.p. 165° to 169°. **Soluble** 1 in 0.25 of water, 1 in 2 of alcohol, and 1 in 140 of chloroform; practically insoluble in ether. A 10% solution in water has a pH of 5 to 6.5. A 5.08% solution is iso-osmotic with serum. Solutions are **sterilised** by autoclaving or by filtration. **Store** in airtight containers.

Incompatibilities. Particulate matter was observed within 2 hours when 1 ml of commercial procainamide hydrochloride injection was mixed with 5 ml of sterile water and 1 ml of commercial phenytoin sodium injection.— R. Misgen, *Am. J. Hosp. Pharm.*, 1965, *22*, 92.

There were changes in the u.v. spectrum indicating chemical change and possible incompatibility when ethacrynate sodium was added to procainamide hydrochloride in sodium chloride injection.— P. N. Catania and J. C. King, *Am. J. Hosp. Pharm.*, 1972, *29*, 141.

Stability in solution. Solutions were liable to discolour in the presence of oxygen or oxidising agents, usually without significant loss of potency.— C. Riffkin, *Am. J. Hosp. Pharm.*, 1963, *20*, 19.

Heating at 120° for 20 minutes resulted in 6% hydrolysis of procainamide hydrochloride in solution. There was no significant increase in hydrolysis during storage.— W. Wiśniewski and T. Kindlik, *Acta Pol. pharm.*, 1967, *24*, 575.

Preliminary results suggesting that procainamide should be prepared in 0.9% sodium chloride solution for maximum 24-hour stability. If dextrose 5% in water is selected as the vehicle, the stability of procainamide beyond 8 hours is uncertain.— H. L. Kirschenbaum *et al.* (letter), *Am. J. Hosp. Pharm.*, 1979, *36*, 1464.

Adverse Effects. The side-effects most frequently reported, after high dosage of procainamide, include anorexia, diarrhoea, nausea, and vomiting. Intravenous administration may cause a fall in blood pressure and, if the injection is made too rapidly, ventricular fibrillation or asystole may occur.

Following prolonged administration of procainamide, a syndrome may develop resembling systemic lupus erythematosus and is characterised by arthralgia, cutaneous lesions, pleuritic chest pain, and positive LE-cell preparations. Leucopenia and agranulocytosis have followed repeated use of procainamide. Other side-effects which have been reported include mental depression, dizziness, psychosis with hallucinations, joint and muscle pain, muscular weakness, a bitter taste, flushing, skin rashes, pruritus, and hypersensitivity leading to chills, fever, and urticaria.

Out of 488 hospitalised patients in the Boston Collaborative Drug Surveillance Program who had received procainamide, 45 experienced acute adverse effects attributed to the drug. Life-threatening reactions included heart block in 3, tachyarrhythmias in 2, and bradycardia and/or hypotension in 2. Other reactions included gastro-intestinal upsets in 19, pyrexia in 8, bradycardia and hypotension in 5, tachyarrhythmias in 3, heart block in 1, eosinophilia in 1 and urticaria in 1 patient. Eleven patients suffered from systemic lupus erythematosus or had a positive antinuclear-factor antibody titre whilst receiving procainamide prior to hospitalisation. A relationship existed between procainamide toxicity, total daily dose and duration of hospitalisation.— D. H. Lawson and H. Jick, *Br. J. clin. Pharmac.*, 1977, *4*, 507.

Alopecia. Mention of scarring baldness as a side-effect of drugs that cause lupus erythematosus, such as procainamide.— *Drug & Ther. Bull.*, 1978, *16*, 77.

Effects on the blood. Procainamide was reported to be a *haemolytic* agent in subjects deficient in glucose-6-phosphate dehydrogenase but only in conjunction with other factors such as infection.— M. E. Pembrey, *Practitioner*, 1974, *213*, 647.

The blood of a 67-year-old man who had received procainamide 1 g daily for 3 years was found to have *anticoagulant substances* which caused a slightly elevated whole-blood clotting time and a significantly prolonged plasma thrombin time and partial thromboplastin time, while prothrombin time, plasma fibrinogen and serum fibrinogen-fibrin antigen concentrations were normal. When procainamide was withdrawn the circulating anticoagulant effect was gradually reduced.— D. K. Galanakis *et al.*, *J. Am. med. Ass.*, 1978, *239*, 1873.

Agranulocytosis, aplastic anaemia, and *thrombocytopenia.* Agranulocytosis developed in a 12-year-old girl within a few days of starting procainamide therapy for a congenital heart disease. The blood count was normal within 8 days of discontinuation of the drug.— U. Gunay and G. R. Honig, *Clin. Pediat.*, 1974, *13*, 728.

Pancytopenia occurred in a 73-year-old woman taking procainamide hydrochloride.— A. Z. Bluming *et al.*, *J. Am. med. Ass.*, 1976, *236*, 2520.

A report of bone marrow granulomas and neutropenia in a 77-year-old man after receiving procainamide for 50 days.— J. Riker *et al.*, *Archs intern. Med.*, 1978, *138*, 1731.

Further reports: R. A. Prince *et al.*, *Am. J. Hosp. Pharm.*, 1977, *34*, 1362 (agranulocytosis); R. J. J. van Beek *et al.*, *Scand. J. Haematol.*, 1978, *21*, 150 (granulocytopenia and positive LE cells); I. K. Rothman, *Archs intern. Med.*, 1979, *139*, 246 (agranulocytosis and thrombocytopenia).

Effects on the kidneys. The nephrotic syndrome was reported to have been noted in patients treated with procainamide.— R. Muehrke and R. Kark, *Lancet*, 1966, *1*, 1148.

The nephrotic syndrome in a woman with procainamide-induced lupus erythematosus.— P. Zech *et al.*, *Clin. Nephrol.*, 1979, *11*, 218.

Effects on the liver. A report of fever, chills and granulomatous hepatitis in a 63-year-old man with myocardial infarction who had received lignocaine followed by procainamide. Fever subsided and serum-liver-enzyme concentrations returned to normal 24 hours after withdrawal of procainamide.— H. H. Rotmensch *et al.*, *Ann. intern. Med.*, 1978, *89*, 646.

Effects on mental state. Bizarre behaviour in a 45-year-old man was attributed to procainamide therapy.— I. D. McCrum and J. R. Guidry, *J. Am. med. Ass.*, 1978, *240*, 1265. Comment.— M. Menken (letter), *ibid.*, 1979, *241*, 1107. Reply.— I. D. McCrum and J. R. Guidry (letter), *ibid.*, 1108.

Effects on the muscles. Progressive myopathy and Sjögren's syndrome, without features of lupus, appeared in a 59-year-old Chinese-American who had been treated for 6 months with procainamide 2 g daily.— J. A. Taylor (letter), *Lancet*, 1968, *1*, 978.

For a warning concerning the possible risk of myasthenia gravis, see under Precautions, below.

Fever. Drug-induced fever which occurred in a patient after 9 days of therapy with quinidine sulphate recurred on challenge. Six days after therapy had been changed to procainamide a similar reaction developed which recurred on challenge with procainamide.— E. Grenadier *et al.*, *Practitioner*, 1979, *222*, 685.

See also under Effects on the Liver, above.

Lupus erythematosus. In a study of 20 patients on long-term procainamide treatment all 11 slow acetylators had developed antinuclear antibodies after about 5 months but only 3 of 9 rapid acetylators. Of 7 patients who subsequently developed the lupus syndrome 4 were slow and 3 were rapid acetylators. The syndrome developed after about one and 4 years of treatment respectively. Acetylation appeared to offer some protection against the induction of antinuclear antibody and the lupus syndrome.— R. L. Woosley *et al.*, *New Engl. J. Med.*, 1978, *298*, 1157. Comment.— P. Goldman and J. A. Ingelfinger, *ibid.*, 1193. The prevalence of antibodies to single-stranded DNA (sDNA) and antinuclear antibodies was compared in 44 patients receiving procainamide and 8 who were given acetylprocainamide. Both types of antibody occurred less frequently and after a longer duration of treatment in patients taking acetylprocainamide than in those taking procainamide. Antibodies to native double-stranded DNA were not seen in any of the patients. Serological abnormalities and symptoms of lupus erythematosus in a further patient, who was of rapid acetylator phenotype, subsided when acetylprocainamide was substituted for procainamide.— R. Lahita *et al.*, *New Engl. J. Med.*, 1979, *301*, 1382.

Evidence is suggestive that procainamide itself, rather than its active metabolite *N*-acetylprocainamide (acecainide), leads to the development of antinuclear antibodies and ultimately lupus erythematosus. First, acetylprocainamide has been associated with little or no lupus erythematosus reaction, and second, slow acetylators are far more likely to experience lupus erythematosus. Should these findings be substantiated it would seem reasonable to prescribe acetylprocainamide.— R. E. Bernstein (letter), *Lancet*, 1979, *2*, 1076.

Further studies and comments on lupus erythematosus and procainamide, including the role of acetylation and the possibility of a lower incidence with the acetylated metabolite acetylprocainamide (acecainide): H. G. Bluestein *et al.*, *Lancet*, 1979, *2*, 816; P. F. J. Ryan *et al.* (letter), *ibid.*, 1248; C. Sonnhag *et al.*, *Acta med. scand.*, 1979, *206*, 245.

Treatment of Adverse Effects. In overdosage by mouth the stomach should be emptied by aspiration and lavage.

Severe hypotension may be treated by placing the patient in the supine position with the feet raised. If necessary an intravenous infusion of noradrenaline acid tartrate may be given; injection of phenylephrine hydrochloride has also been suggested.

Systemic lupus erythematosus will normally respond to withdrawal of procainamide but corticosteroids may be required.

Studies in 4 healthy men showed that the renal excretion of procainamide was not affected by changes in pH.— W. Meyer *et al.*, *Eur. J. clin. Pharmac.*, 1974, *7*, 287.

Glucagon antagonised the cardiac effects of procainamide in *dogs* and might be useful in the treatment of procainamide induced cardiac toxicity.— K. Prasad and P. Weckworth, *Toxic. appl. Pharmac.*, 1978, *46*, 517.

Dialysis. Following ingestion of an estimated excess of 7 g of procainamide over her maintenance dose a 67-year-old woman with heart disease developed severe hypotension, renal insufficiency, and life-threatening cardiac toxicity. She recovered after haemodialysis which doubled procainamide clearance and increased *N*-acetylprocainamide clearance fourfold.— A. J. Atkinson *et al.*, *Clin. Pharmac. Ther.*, 1976, *20*, 585.

Precautions. As for Quinidine Sulphate, p.1371. Procainamide should preferably not be used in patients with bronchial asthma, myasthenia gravis, or systemic lupus erythematosus.

Accumulation of procainamide may occur in patients with heart failure or renal insufficiency; this may lead to impairment of hepatic function and impairment or further impairment of renal function.

Regular blood tests should be carried out in patients receiving procainamide, and screening for lupus erythematosus cells and serum antinuclear factor should be carried out before and regularly during therapy.

Procainamide may enhance the effects of antihypertensive agents, propranolol, and some skeletal muscle relaxants, and diminish those of cholinergic agents, such as neostigmine. There is cross-sensitivity between procaine and procainamide.

Grave hypotension may follow intravenous administration of procainamide; it should be injected slowly under ECG control.

Cross sensitivity to procaine. Patients allergic to procaine might have anaphylactic reactions when treated with procainamide.— *Med. Lett.*, 1974, *16*, 106.

Interactions. Evidence that procainamide and hydralazine do not interfere with one another's acetylation.— D. W. Schneck *et al.*, *Clin. Pharmac. Ther.*, 1978, *24*, 714. Evidence that procainamide and isoniazid do not interfere with one another's acetylation.— *idem*, *Pharmacology*, 1979, *18*, 34.

Cardiac glycosides. Confirmation of reports that serum-*digoxin* concentration rises during concomitant quinidine administration. No such rise occurred when procainamide was given.— E. B. Leahey *et al.*, *Ann. intern. Med.*, 1980, *92*, 605.

Muscle relaxants. Procainamide hydrochloride enhanced suxamethonium-induced neuromuscular blockade in *cats*.— M. F. Cuthbert, *Br. J. Anaesth.*, 1966, *38*, 775.

Myasthenia gravis. A 78-year-old myasthenic man who suffered a cardiac infarction was given procainamide hydrochloride 250 mg on several occasions for premature ventricular beats. After no adverse effect from the first dose, there was increasing muscle weakness with subsequent doses. Administration of edrophonium did not improve the weakness but withdrawal of procainamide started to reverse symptoms after about 3 hours.— D. A. Drachman and J. H. Skom, *Archs Neurol., Chicago*, 1965, *13*, 316.

Pregnancy and the neonate. Plasma concentrations of procainamide and *N*-acetylprocainamide were higher in the infant than in the mother after a pregnant woman received procainamide for about a week before delivery.— J. J. Lima *et al.*, *Pediatrics*, 1978, *61*, 491.

Absorption and Fate. Procainamide is readily absorbed from the gastro-intestinal tract and has a very short half-life of only about 3 hours.

Procainamide is partly acetylated in the liver and its acetylated metabolite, *N*-acetylprocainamide or acecainide (see p.1373) also has anti-arrhythmic properties, together with a longer half-life. The acetylation of procainamide is subject to genetic polymorphism. Procainamide is excreted in the urine, with about 50% as unchanged procainamide, and up to about 30% as *N*-acetylprocainamide (less in slow acetylators).

Procainamide is widely distributed throughout the body and is only about 15% bound to plasma proteins. The therapeutic effect of procainamide has been correlated with plasma concentrations of about 4 to 8 or 10 μg per ml, progressively severe toxicity being noted at higher concentrations. Procainamide crosses the placental barrier and has been reported to accumulate in the foetus.

A review of the clinical pharmacokinetics of procainamide.— E. Karlsson, *Clin. Pharmacokinet.*, 1978, *3*, 97.

Metabolism and pharmacokinetics. Plasma concentrations of procainamide in patients with normal cardiac output and normal renal function differed by up to 400% after the same dose of procainamide by mouth. Generally 75 to 95% of an oral dose was absorbed but some patients absorbed less than 50% of a dose. After intramuscular injection in 5 healthy subjects procainamide appeared in the plasma within 2 minutes and peak concentrations were reached within 25 minutes. About 14 to 16% of procainamide was bound to plasma proteins. The biological half-life in 14 subjects with normal renal function was 2.5 to 4.7 hours and plasma concentrations might fall 14 to 24% per hour. In 6 subjects 40 to 54% of a dose was excreted in the urine in 24 hours. Three-hourly administration was desirable, with the initial dose twice that of the maintenance doses.— J. Koch-Weser, *Ann. N.Y. Acad. Sci.*, 1971, *179*, 370.

Comparison of the pharmacokinetics of procainamide and *N*-acetylprocainamide after simultaneous intravenous injection in healthy subjects, all of whom were rapid acetylators. The elimination half-life of procainamide averaged 2.5 hours, whereas that of *N*-acetylprocainamide was two-and-a-half times longer at an average of 6.2 hours.— J. S. Dutcher *et al.*, *Clin. Pharmac. Ther.*, 1977, *22*, 447.

Pharmacokinetic studies of sustained-release procainamide preparations: R. Ruosteenoja *et al.*, *Curr. ther. Res.*, 1973, *15*, 707; C. Graffner *et al.*, *Clin. Pharmac. Ther.*, 1975, *17*, 414; H. Ihlen *et al.*, *Curr. ther. Res.*, 1975, *17*, 257; C. V. Manion *et al.*, *J. pharm. Sci.*, 1977, *66*, 981; W. J. Tilstone *et al.*, *Eur. J. clin. Pharmac.*, 1978, *14*, 261; P. Hore *et al.*, *Br. J. clin. Pharmac.*, 1979, *8*, 267; E. -G. V. Giardina *et al.*, *Am. J. Cardiol.*, 1980, *46*, 855.

Acetylation. Of 21 healthy subjects 9 were classified as slow acetylators of sulphadimidine and 12 as fast acetylators. The percentage of *N*-acetylprocainamide recovered from the slow acetylators after procainamide 10 mg per kg body-weight was 9.8 to 43.8% (mean 24.1%) compared with 22 to 42.6% (mean 33.7%) from the fast acetylators—a significant difference. In some subjects the classification of phenotype was probably in error; classification by the half-life of metabolism was preferable. Bimodal acetylation of procainamide was not yet established.— E. -G. V. Giardina *et al.*, *Circulation*, 1977, *55*, 388.

Further references to procainamide acetylation: E. Karlsson *et al.*, *Br. J. clin. Pharmac.*, 1974, *1*, 467; *idem*, *Eur. J. clin. Pharmac.*, 1975, *8*, 79. Gibson, T.P. *et al Clin. Pharmac. Ther.*, 1975, *17*, 395; M. M. Reidenberg *et al.*, *ibid.*, 722; W. Campbell *et al.*, *Br. J. clin. Pharmac.*, 1976, *3*, 1023; J. J. Lima *et al.*, *J. Pharmacokinet. Biopharm.*, 1979, *7*, 69.

Plasma concentrations. A review of the use of serum-procainamide concentrations as therapeutic guides. The dose required to control ventricular tachyarrhythmias varied owing to individual differences in procainamide pharmacokinetics; it should be individualised (especially in patients whose response was abnormal or difficult to evaluate) since there was a useful relationship between the serum concentration and the intensity of cardiac action. Concentrations of 4 to 10 μg per ml would correct and prevent more than 90% of arrhythmias without causing serious adverse effects, but little additional benefit was obtained above 10 μg per ml while serious toxicity increased above 12 μg per ml. The role of the relative concentration of the active metabolite *N*-acetylprocainamide, which was primarily excreted by the kidneys, had yet to be fully evaluated.— J. Koch-Weser, *Clin. Pharmacokinet.*, 1977, *2*, 389. Comment, and data suggesting that patients can safely tolerate serum concentrations of procainamide above 10 to 12 μg per ml, as long as the sum of the parent compound and its active metabolite does not exceed serum concentrations of 25 to 30 μg per ml. In the patients studied, steady state serum-procainamide concentrations of 8 to 12 μg per ml were optimal.— J. J. Lima *et al.*, *Am. J. Cardiol.*, 1979, *43*, 98.

Problems with the assay technique for measuring procainamide.— A. G. Butterfield *et al.*, *J. pharm. Sci.*, 1978, *67*, 839; M. A. F. Gadalla *et al.*, *ibid.*, 869; R. L. Nation *et al.*, *ibid.*, 1979, *68*, 532.

For therapeutic and toxic plasma concentrations of *N*-acetylprocainamide (acecainide), see also under Acecainide, p.1373.

Saliva concentrations. Therapeutic drug monitoring in saliva including details of studies on saliva-procainamide concentrations. Due to variability in the saliva-plasma ratio it is impossible to predict plasma concentrations from salivary drug concentration, but since saliva concentrations seem to reflect the drug concentrations at an active cardiac site, they may be clinically more relevant.— M. Danhof and D. D. Breimer, *Clin. Pharmacokinet.*, 1978, *3*, 39. References: R. L. Galeazzi *et al.*, *Clin. Pharmac. Ther.*, 1976, *20*, 278.

Variability of *N*-acetylprocainamide (acecainide) salivary concentrations in the elderly.— R. L. Galeazzi *et al.*, *Clin. Pharmac. Ther.*, 1981, *29*, 440.

Uses. Procainamide is a class I anti-arrhythmic agent (see p.1370); it has actions similar to those of procaine (see p.921) but they are more prolonged and its central effects are relatively less pronounced. It has a depressant action on the heart similar to that of quinidine (p.1372), and also has anticholinergic properties.

Given intravenously, procainamide is less liable to induce severe hypotension than quinidine and it may therefore be given to control lignocaine-resistant ventricular arrhythmias. It may also be used to maintain sinus rhythm after cardioversion of atrial fibrillation, and for the prevention of atrial and ventricular arrhythmias, but its value in maintenance therapy is limited by its short plasma half-life and its tendency to induce lupus erythematosus. Therapeutic plasma concentrations are 4 to 8 or 10 μg per ml.

For ventricular arrhythmias, procainamide hydrochloride is given in an initial dose by mouth of 1 g followed by 250 to 500 mg every 3 hours. In the treatment of atrial arrhythmias, an initial dose by mouth of 1.25 g is followed an hour later by 750 mg if necessary; it is then given in a dose of 0.5 to 1 g every 2 hours until the arrhythmia ceases or the limit of tolerance is reached; the maintenance dose is 0.5 to 1 g every 4 to 6 hours.

If the oral route is not suitable, procainamide hydrochloride may be given intramuscularly. A suggested intramuscular dose is 0.5 to 1 g every four to eight hours; in general the intramuscular dose required is similar to that given orally.

In emergency and under continuous ECG and blood pressure monitoring, procainamide hydrochloride may be given intravenously. The injection should be diluted in a 5% solution of dextrose to permit better control of the speed of injection, and should be given in doses of 100 mg every 5 minutes at a rate not exceeding 25 to 50 mg per minute until the arrhythmia has been suppressed or a maximum dose of 1 g has been reached. A response may be obtained after 100 to 200 mg has been given and more than 500 or 600 mg is not generally required. Therapeutic plasma concentrations may then be maintained by giving an infusion in a 5% solution of dextrose, at a rate of 2 to 6 mg per minute. When transferring to oral therapy, a period of about 3 to 4 hours should elapse between the last intravenous dose and the first oral dose.

A suggested dose for children is 50 mg per kg body-weight daily in 4 to 6 divided doses.

In order to prolong its duration of action procainamide hydrochloride is also given in the form of long-acting tablets. Procainamide has also been given as the sulphate.

Administration. The major advantage of procainamide over quinidine was a relative lack of adverse cardiovascular effects, except for hypotension when it was infused too rapidly.— *Med. Lett.*, 1974, *16*, 106.

A study demonstrating the need to give procainamide 500 mg at least every 4 hours by mouth in order to obtain satisfactory plasma concentrations.— T. R. D. Shaw *et al.*, *Br. Heart J.*, 1974, *36*, 265.

A two-infusion technique of administering procainamide in which therapeutic serum concentrations are rapidly achieved and maintained, with a loading infusion given over 1 hour followed by a maintenance infusion.— J. J. Lima *et al.*, *Am. J. Cardiol.*, 1979, *43*, 98. See also *idem*, *Eur. J. clin. Pharmac.*, 1978, *13*, 303.

In the elderly. Reduced renal clearance of procainamide in the elderly.— M. M. Reidenberg *et al.*, *Clin. Pharmac. Ther.*, 1980, *28*, 732.

Administration in cardiac, respiratory, and renal failure. Procainamide was reported to be 14 to 23% bound to plasma proteins. The normal half-life of 2.5 to 4.9 hours was increased to 5.3 to 59 hours in end-stage renal failure. The interval between doses should be extended from 3 to 4 hours to 4 hours in patients with a glomerular filtration-rate above 50 ml per minute, to 6 to 12 hours in those with a glomerular filtration-rate of 10 to 50 ml per minute, and to 8 to 24 hours in those with a glomerular filtration-rate of less than 10 ml per minute. Concentrations of procainamide were affected by haemodialysis.— W. M. Bennett *et al.*, *Ann. intern. Med.*, 1980, *93*, 286.

In 20 patients with chronic heart failure (group 1), 20 with respiratory insufficiency (group 2), and 20 with renal failure (group 3), the recovery of unchanged procainamide in the urine in 6 hours, after a 500-mg dose, was reduced compared with 20 controls; the recovery of *N*-acetylprocainamide was reduced in group 3; recovery of *p*-aminobenzoic acid and its *N*-acetyl derivative were reduced in all 3 groups; acetylation of procainamide was increased in group 1; acetylation of PABA was increased in all 3 groups. The plasma half-life was increased in all 3 groups.— P. du Souich and S. Erill, *Eur. J. clin. Pharmac.*, 1978, *14*, 21.

Further references: J. Dreyfuss *et al.*, *Clin. Pharmac. Ther.*, 1972, *13*, 366 (cardiac); T. P. Gibson *et al.*, *Clin. Pharmac. Ther.*, 1975, *17*, 321 (renal); E. -G. V. Giardina *et al.*, *Clin. Pharmac. Ther.*, 1976, *19*, 339 (cardiac).

Administration in hepatic failure. In 20 healthy subjects and 20 patients with chronic liver disease given a single dose of procainamide hydrochloride 500 mg by mouth about 64 and 33% respectively of the administered dose was excreted in the urine within 6 hours. Decreased procainamide acetylation in the patients compared to the control group was not correlated with the severity of liver disease whereas decreased procainamide hydrolysis and increased procainamide-derived aminobenzoic acid acetylation appeared to be related to the degree of hepatic impairment. It was suggested that the decrease in excretion of procainamide and its metabolites in the urine of the patients with liver disease could be due to an impairment in oral absorption since renal function was within the normal range but the variations in acetylation and hydrolysis were related to hepatic function.— P. du Souich and S. Erill, *Clin. Pharmac. Ther.*, 1977, *22*, 588.

Cardiac disorders. A review of anti-arrhythmic agents, including procainamide, giving details of its uses, adverse effects, and interactions. Procainamide has electrophysiological properties similar to those of quinidine and is likewise a class I agent. It does not prolong the Q-T interval to the same extent as quinidine and intravenously is safer; hence intravenous procainamide is one of several agents that may be tried if lignocaine fails. Oral use is limited by the short half-life and the risk of lupus, but the *N*-acetyl metabolite has also been proved to be anti-arrhythmic, has a longer half-life, and carries a lower risk of lupus.— L. H. Opie, *Lancet*, 1980, *1*, 861.

Reports and studies on the anti-arrhythmic effects of procainamide: M. V. Jelinek *et al.*, *Circulation*, 1974, *49*, 659 (ventricular arrhythmias); W. J. Mandel *et al.*, *Am. Heart J.*, 1975, *90*, 744 (Wolff-Parkinson-White syndrome); G. E. Bauer *et al.*, *Med. J. Aust.*, 1977, *2*, 733 (ventricular arrhythmias); J. A. Kastor, *Circulation*, 1977, *56*, 462 (ventricular arrhythmias); H. J. J. Wellens *et al.*, *Am. J. Cardiol.*, 1977, *40*, 579 (ventricular tachycardia); T. R. Engel *et al.*, *Clin. Pharmac. Ther.*, 1978, *24*, 274 (ventricular tachycardia).

Myocardial infarction. Procainamide hydrochloride by mouth, or intramuscularly when vomiting was troublesome, was effective in preventing ventricular arrhythmias in 37 patients who had suffered a myocardial infarction, compared with 33 others who received a placebo. A loading dose of 1 g was followed by 3-hourly doses of procainamide hydrochloride 250 mg for patients weighing less than 54 kg, 375 mg for those weighing 54 to 90 kg, or 500 mg for those heavier than 90 kg.— J. Koch-Weser *et al.*, *New Engl. J. Med.*, 1969, *281*, 1253.

The long-term use of procainamide in 39 patients recovering from myocardial infarction did not significantly reduce the incidence of sudden deaths in up to 2 years compared with controls. The high incidence of toxic effects, including elevated antinuclear antibody titre in all patients treated for 1 year or more, precluded widespread prophylactic use of procainamide.— B. D. Kosowsky *et al.*, *Circulation*, 1973, *47*, 1204.

Further references: I. Mattiasson *et al.*, *Acta med. scand.*, 1978, *204*, 27.

Muscular disorders. Symptoms of myotonia in patients with muscular dystrophy could be relieved or abolished by procainamide in doses of 250 to 500 mg three or four times daily.— J. N. Walton, *Br. med. J.*, 1969, *3*, 639.

Dysphagia in a 35-year-old woman with dystrophia myotonica improved after treatment with procainamide 500 mg thrice daily.— E. B. Casey and M. J. Aminoff, *Br. med. J.*, 1971, *2*, 443.

Preparations

Procainamide Hydrochloride Capsules *(U.S.P.)*. Capsules containing procainamide hydrochloride. Store in airtight containers.

Procainamide Hydrochloride Injection *(U.S.P.)*. A sterile solution in Water for Injections. pH 4 to 6. It should not be used if it is darker than slightly yellow or otherwise discoloured.

Procainamide Injection *(B.P.)*. A sterile solution of procainamide hydrochloride in Water for Injections containing 0.9% of benzyl alcohol and the equivalent of 0.1% of sulphur dioxide. Sterilised by autoclaving. pH 4 to 5.5.

Procainamide Tablets *(B.P.)*. Procainamide Hydrochloride Tablets. Tablets containing procainamide hydrochloride.

Proprietary Preparations

Procainamide Durules *(Astra, UK)*. Procainamide hydrochloride, available as sustained-release tablets of 500 mg. *Dose.* Usually 2 or 3 Durules thrice daily. Durules should be swallowed whole.

Owing to the risk of intestinal obstruction, sustained-release preparations such as Procainamide Durules, where the drug is released in transit but the matrix ghost is often eliminated intact, should not be prescribed in patients with Crohn's disease or other intestinal disease in which strictures may form.— J. L. Shaffer *et al.* (letter), *Lancet*, 1980, *2*, 487.

Pronestyl *(Squibb, UK)*. Procainamide hydrochloride, available as **Solution** for injection containing 100 mg per ml, with benzyl alcohol 0.9%, in vials of 10 ml, and as scored **Tablets** of 250 mg. (Also available as Pronestyl in *Arg., Austral., Belg., Canad., Denm., Fr., Ital., Neth., Norw., S.Afr., Swed., Switz., USA*).

Other Proprietary Names

Biocoryl *(Spain)*; Novocamid *(Ger.)*; Procamide *(Belg., Ital.)*; Procainamid Duriles *(Ger.)*; Procainamide Durettes *(Neth.)*; Procan SR *(USA)*; Procapan *(USA)*.

7792-m

Procainamide Sulphate *(B.P.C. 1959)*. Procainamid. Sulph. 4-Amino-*N*-(2-diethylaminoethyl)benzamide sulphate.

$(C_{13}H_{21}N_3O)_2,H_2SO_4=568.7$.

A white or yellowish-white odourless crystalline powder. **Soluble** 1 in 0.7 of water and 1 in 200 of alcohol; practically insoluble in chloroform and ether.

Procainamide sulphate has the actions and uses described under Procainamide Hydrochloride, above.

7793-b

Tocainide Hydrochloride.

W-36095. 2-Aminopropiono-2′,6′-xylidide hydrochloride.

$C_{11}H_{16}N_2O,HCl=228.7$.

CAS — 41708-72-9 (tocainide); 35891-93-1 (hydrochloride).

Adverse Effects. Adverse effects associated with tocainide are mainly neurological or on the gastro-intestinal tract. Nausea and vomiting may occur, particularly in the initial stages of therapy. Effects on the central nervous system include tremor, dizziness, lightheadedness, unsteady gait, memory impairment, decreased mental alertness, difficulty in concentration, paraesthesia, and convulsions.

Other adverse effects reported include skin rash, lupus erythematosus, exacerbation of cervical muscle spasms, sweating and hot flushes, and altered vision and hearing (tinnitus).

Bradycardia and hypotension may occur after intravenous administration of tocainide. Interstitial pneumonitis has been associated with tocainide therapy.

Effects on the lungs. Interstitial pneumonitis developed in 2 patients during tocainide therapy. Both patients recovered on withdrawal of therapy, but one required corticosteroids initially to control the symptoms.— G. M. Perlow *et al.* (letter), *Ann. intern. Med.*, 1981, *94*, 489.

Precautions. Tocainide should not be used in patients with second or third degree atrioventricular block, in the absence of a pacemaker. It should be used with caution in patients with uncompensated heart failure and in patients receiving other anti-arrhythmic agents.

Interactions. Administration of sodium bicarbonate to raise the urinary pH, decreased the renal elimination of tocainide.— D. Lalka *et al.*, *Clin. Pharmac. Ther.*, 1976, *19*, 757.

Absorption and Fate. Tocainide is readily and almost completely absorbed from the gastro-intestinal tract.

Tocainide is metabolised to a number of metabolites, and is excreted in the urine partly unchanged and partly in the form of its metabolites.

Tocainide is widely distributed throughout the body and is reported to be about 50% bound to plasma proteins. It has a plasma half-life of about 10 to 14 hours; renal clearance is reduced in alkaline urine. Its therapeutic effect has been correlated with plasma concentrations of about 6 to 10 µg per ml; a principal metabolite, lactoxylidide, has been shown to have little biological activity.

Metabolism and pharmacokinetics. A study in 6 healthy subjects indicated that tocainide is very rapidly and almost completely absorbed from the gastro-intestinal tract, administration after food decreasing peak blood concentrations but not affecting the overall absorption. The half-life was found to be about 11 hours suggesting that an 8- to 12-hourly dosage regimen is feasible. Renal clearance was considerably reduced in alkaline urine.— D. Lalka *et al.*, *Clin. Pharmac. Ther.*, 1976, *19*, 757. See also D. G. McDevitt *et al.*, *ibid.*, 396 (slightly longer half-life in patients); E. M. Wolshin *et al.*, *J. pharm. Sci.*, 1978, *67*, 1692 (8-hour terminal half-life in one healthy subject).

A study of tocainide kinetics after intravenous and oral administration in 6 healthy subjects and 16 patients with acute myocardial infarction. The elimination half-life was about 14 hours.— C. Graffner *et al.*, *Clin. Pharmac. Ther.*, 1980, *27*, 64.

Studies on the metabolism of tocainide. In 5 patients receiving long-term tocainide hydrochloride therapy (1.8 to 3.2 g daily in divided doses) a mean of 44% of the administered dose was excreted in the urine within 24 hours as free tocainide. A metabolite accounted for an additional 23% of the dose.— A. T. Elvin *et al.*, *J. pharm. Sci.*, 1980, *69*, 47. See also *idem*, *Clin. Pharmac. Ther.*, 1980, *28*, 652 (tocainide carbaminic acid glucuronide).

Details of 2 metabolites of tocainide: a glucuronide of *N*-carboxytocainide, and lactoxylidide. The average elimination half-life of lactoxylidide was about twice that of tocainide. However, although potential for lactoxylidide accumulation was shown to exist, *animal* studies indicated that it has little biological activity.— R. A. Ronfeld *et al.*, *Clin. Pharmac. Ther.*, 1980, *27*, 282.

Plasma concentrations. In 11 patients responding to tocainide therapy for frequent premature ventricular contractions, a 70% suppression of premature ventricular contractions was achieved when the plasma concentration was above 6 µg per ml; 90% suppression was achieved at plasma concentrations above 10 µg per ml. Because of the nature of the concentrations-response relationship, a disproportionate increase in plasma-tocainide concentration was required to increase response in the range of 80 to 100%, compared with that required in the range of 50 to 70%.— R. A. Winkle *et al.*, *Circulation*, 1976, *54*, 884.

Protein binding. Evidence that tocainide is about 50% bound to plasma proteins in the clinical range.— D. Lalka *et al.*, *Clin. Pharmac. Ther.*, 1976, *19*, 757.

Uses. Tocainide is a class I anti-arrhythmic agent (see p.1370) with actions similar to those of lignocaine (p.904) to which it is structurally related. Unlike lignocaine, it is suitable for oral administration.

For the treatment of ventricular arrhythmias tocainide hydrochloride 500 to 750 mg is given by slow intravenous injection or by infusion (diluted to a volume of 50 to 100 ml in dextrose or sodium chloride injection and given over 15 to 30 minutes), followed immediately by 600 to 800 mg by mouth. Maintenance therapy in a dosage of 1.2 g daily by mouth, divided into 2 or 3 doses, may be started 8 hours later. If necessary the dosage may be increased to a total of 1.8 to 2.4 g daily.

Studies of the electrophysiology of tocainide.— L. N. Horowitz *et al.*, *Am. J. Cardiol.*, 1978, *42*, 276; K. Swedberg *et al.*, *Eur. J. clin. Pharmac.*, 1978, *14*, 15; M. Schwartz *et al.*, *J. clin. Pharmac.*, 1979, *19*, 100.

Cardiac disorders. A study in 41 patients with premature ventricular contractions comparing tocainide 600 mg thrice daily with quinidine sulphate 300 mg four times daily. Neither drug met the criteria of high efficacy with a low incidence of side-effects, but quinidine was more effective, benefited a larger number of patients, and produced fewer adverse effects than tocainide. Adverse effects in the tocainide group (22) were: ataxia (9 patients), tremor (8), dizziness (6), nausea and vomiting (5), anorexia (3), visual changes (4), diarrhoea (1), personality changes (3), depression (1), disorientation (2), weakness (2), night sweats (2), rash (1), syncope (1), and pruritus (1); one patient developed changes in liver-function values which returned to normal on stopping tocainide.— J. E. Wasenmiller and W. S. Aronow, *Clin. Pharmac. Ther.*, 1980, *28*, 431. See also R. Engler *et al.*, *Am. J. Cardiol.*, 1979, *43*, 612.

Further references.— W. Ryan *et al.*, *Am. J. Cardiol.*, 1979, *43*, 285; B. Waleffe *et al.*, *ibid.*, 292; M. D. Klein *et al.*, *Chest*, 1980, *77*, 726; M. M. LeWinter *et al.*, *Am. J. Cardiol.*, 1980, *45*, 1045.

Muscular disorders. Tocainide 400 mg thrice daily had a beneficial effect on the muscular stiffness and weakness brought about by cooling, in 7 patients with paramyotonia congenita. An eighth patient aged 78 years was treated for only one day since he complained of nausea; his ECG showed no disturbances. Two patients experienced transient dizziness, anxiety, and tremor on the second day of treatment; the other 5 had no side-effects.— K. Ricker *et al.*, *J. Neurol. Neurosurg. Psychiat.*, 1980, *43*, 268.

Proprietary Preparations

Tonocard *(Astra, UK).* Tocainide hydrochloride, available as **Injection** containing 50 mg per ml, in vials of 15 ml, and as **Tablets** of 400 and 600 mg.

7794-v

Verapamil Hydrochloride *(B.P.).*

Verapamili Chloridum; Iproveratril Hydrochloride; CP 16533-1 *(verapamil)*; D 365 *(verapamil)*. 5-[*N*-(3,4-Dimethoxyphenethyl)-*N*-methylamino]-2-(3,4-dimethoxyphenyl)-2-isopropylvaleronitrile hydrochloride.

$C_{27}H_{38}N_2O_4,HCl = 491.1$.

CAS — 52-53-9 (verapamil); 152-11-4 (hydrochloride).

Pharmacopoeias. In *Br.* and *Nord.*

A white or almost white, odourless or almost odourless, crystalline powder. M.p. 141° to 144°. **Soluble** 1 in 20 of water, 1 in 25 of alcohol, and 1 in 1.5 of chloroform; practically insoluble in ether. A 5% solution in water has a pH of 4.5 to 6.5. **Protect** from light.

Adverse Effects. Administration of verapamil is commonly associated with constipation. Other adverse effects reported include nausea and vomiting, flushing, headache, and allergic reactions.

Transient heart block and hypotension have followed intravenous administration; very rarely ventricular fibrillation has been precipitated.

Overdosage with verapamil has been associated with bradycardia, hypotension, and atrioventricular dissociation; hyperglycaemia has also occurred.

Allergy. A woman prescribed verapamil felt increasingly unwell from the first dose, and complained of increasing nausea, mild headache, and aching joints. On the eighth day of therapy she complained of slightly itchy and sore eyes, and a severe headache, and was then noted to have a generalised red urticarial rash which was markedly worse in areas exposed to sunlight. She recovered on discontinuation of verapamil and 4 days of corticosteroid and antihistamine therapy.— *Med. J. Aust.*, 1979, *2*, 204.

Effects on the endocrine system. Hyperprolactinaemia and galactorrhoea associated with verapamil therapy.— L. E. Gluskin *et al.*, *Ann. intern. Med.*, 1981, *95*, 66.

Effects on the heart. In a small study, slow intravenous injections of 5 mg of verapamil relieved cardiac pain in a few patients. Congestive cardiac failure developed in 2 patients shortly after receiving verapamil. Cardiac arrhythmias developed in 3 patients during injection.— E. A. Hills and E. M. Downes (letter), *Lancet*, 1967, *2*, 1149.

Premature ventricular beats were observed before reversion to sinus rhythm in 6 patients during 7 episodes of supraventricular tachycardia treated with verapamil intravenously.— J. Vohra *et al.*, *Br. Heart J.*, 1974, *36*, 1186.

A study of the effects of verapamil on myocardial performance in coronary disease. Verapamil appeared to be a very safe agent for use in patients with coronary disease; it did not depress myocardial performance, and there was no evidence that it frequently worsened left ventricular asynergy.— J. Ferlinz *et al.*, *Circulation*, 1979, *59*, 313.

Effects on the liver. Hepatotoxicity in one patient given verapamil.— S. J. Brodsky *et al.*, *Ann. intern. Med.*, 1981, *94*, 490.

Effects on the nervous system. A report of 3 patients who complained of unusual perceptual symptoms, described as painful coldness and numbness or bursting feelings, especially in the legs, in association with verapamil therapy.— C. R. Kumana and W. A. Mahon (letter), *Lancet*, 1981, *1*, 1324.

Hypotension. A 57-year-old man with a history of 6 episodes of supraventricular tachycardia was given verapamil at the rate of 1 mg per minute intravenously to control a further episode. When 7 mg had been given he developed hypotension and asystole. He recovered after DC counter-shock treatment. The reaction might have been due to hypersensitivity or to prior treatment with practolol.— M. E. Benaim (letter), *Br. med. J.*, 1972, *2*, 169. A 46-year-old man, not taking digoxin, given verapamil 10 mg over 30 seconds developed hypotension with reduction of systolic blood pressure from 80 to 50 mmHg.— E. F. Vaughan-Neil *et al.* (letter), *ibid.*, 529.

Overdosage. A 19-year-old woman who ingested 3.2 g of verapamil developed bradycardia, hypotension, and cyanosis of the hands and feet. Because of a history of cardiac arrhythmias sympathomimetic agents were considered to be contra-indicated. She was treated, after gastric lavage, with 10 ml of 10% calcium gluconate given intravenously over 5 minutes; sinus rhythm was restored; later nodal bradycardia with an intraventricular conduction defect responded to further calcium gluconate and the patient recovered.— C. M. Perkins, *Br. med. J.*, 1978, *2*, 1127. Mention of a previous report of a 28-year-old woman who took 5.6 g of verapamil. On admission she exhibited bradycardia and pronounced hypotension, and an ECG showed atrioventricular dissociation which persisted for 7½ hours after admission. She was discharged 36 hours later. In this patient the pronounced negative inotropic effects appeared early but were short-lived. The transient hypotension responded well to infusion of sodium chloride and the administration of beta-adrenergic amines was not considered necessary in this case.— U. de Faire and T. Lundman (letter), *ibid.*, 1574. See also J. Candell *et al.*, *Chest*, 1979, *75*, 200.

A 14-year-old girl who took 2.4 g of verapamil developed cyanosis, hypotension, marked bradycardia and mental confusion. An electrocardiogram showed conduction disturbance characterised by third degree atrioventricular block. Mild metabolic acidosis and hyperglycaemia also developed. The patient recovered with symptomatic and supportive therapy.— O. A. Da Silva *et al.*, *Clin. Toxicol.*, 1979, *14*, 361.

Treatment of Adverse Effects. In overdosage by mouth the stomach should be emptied by aspiration and lavage.

Atropine or a beta-adrenoceptor agonist (for example, isoprenaline) has been recommended for prolonged atrioventricular conduction; electrical pacing may also be required.

Calcium gluconate in a dose of 10 to 20 ml of a 10% solution has been recommended for heart failure. Agents such as dopamine and dobutamine have also been suggested.

Hypotension may be treated by placing the patient in the supine position with the feet raised; infusions of dopamine, dobutamine, and noradrenaline have been suggested if necessary.

Experimental work has suggested that the positive inotropic effects of cardiac glycosides are attenuated but not nullified by verapamil, indicating that digoxin may, at least partly, reverse the depressant effects of verapamil in heart failure.— B. N. Singh *et al.*, *Drugs*, 1978, *15*, 169.

See also under Precautions, below.

Should prolonged atrioventricular conduction occur with verapamil, atropine is the antagonist of choice, though theoretically calcium gluconate might help.— *Br. med. J.*, 1981, *282*, 89. See also L. H. Opie, *Lancet*, 1980, *2*, 806. A view that calcium chloride rather than calcium gluconate is the calcium salt of choice for parenteral indications.— L. I. G. Worthley and P. J. Phillips (letter), *ibid.*, 149.

For reports of overdosage and its management, see under Overdosage, above.

Dialysis. Haemodialysis was not an effective treatment for verapamil overdosage because protein binding occurred.— B. Spiegelhalder and M. Eichelbaum, *Arzneimittel-Forsch.*, 1977, *27*, 94.

Precautions. Verapamil is contra-indicated in hypotension associated with cardiogenic shock, in marked bradycardia, in partial or complete atrioventricular block, and in uncompensated heart failure. It is also contra-indicated in the sick-sinus syndrome, although it is reported to have been used against the tachycardias of the sick-sinus syndrome under careful hospital surveillance. It should be used with caution in the acute phase of myocardial infarction.

Prolonged high dosage of verapamil has been associated with a tendency to develop cataracts in *beagle dogs*; although this appears to be specific to *beagle dogs* regular ophthalmological examination is recommended during long-term therapy.

Reduced dosage of verapamil may be required in patients with impaired liver function owing to the risk of reduced metabolism.

Severe toxicity has followed the concomitant use of verapamil and beta-adrenoceptor blocking agents, particularly by the intravenous route. Intravenous verapamil is contra-indicated in digitalis toxicity, but verapamil and digitalis may be given together by mouth in the absence of digitalis toxicity or atrioventricular block. For further details see under Interactions, below.

Interactions. Emphasis that administration of verapamil with other drugs which may inhibit the atrioventricular node such as *beta-adrenoceptor blocking agents* or *digitalis* is potentially very dangerous, especially when verapamil is given rapidly intravenously and myocardial function is impaired. Since beta-blockade abolishes the compensatory reflex tachycardia found with verapamil, and the direct cardiodepressant effects of the two are additive, hypotension and severe bradycardia have occurred in patients already receiving beta-blockers. Thus, verapamil should never be given as an intravenous bolus to patients receiving beta-blockers. In digitalis toxicity intravenous verapamil is absolutely contra-indicated because it can lethally exaggerate atrioventricular block. In the absence of digitalis toxicity or atrioventricular block there is no reason why oral verapamil and digitalis compounds should not be given together because digitalis does not inhibit the slow inward calcium ion channel.— L. H. Opie, *Lancet*, 1980, *1*, 806.

Further references.— C. B. Boothby *et al.* (letter), *Br. med. J.*, 1972, *2*, 349 (asystole on administration of verapamil after digoxin and practolol); H. Sacks and B. M. Kennelly (letter), *Br. med. J.*, 1972, *2*, 716 (heart block in 2 digitalised patients after intravenous verapamil); H. O. Klein *et al.* (letter), *New Engl. J. Med.*, 1980, *303*, 160 (raised digoxin concentrations in patients also taking verapamil); N. G. Kounis, *Br. J. clin. Pract.*, 1980, *34*, 57 (asystole after intravenous verapamil in a patient taking digoxin).

Absorption and Fate. Verapamil is almost completely absorbed from the gastro-intestinal tract, but is subject to very considerable first-pass metabolism in the liver; the oral dose required to achieve comparable plasma concentrations is about 10 times higher than the intravenous dose.

Verapamil is reported to have a plasma half-life of about 7 hours following oral administration; that of its active metabolite, norverapamil is reported to be about 9 hours. The plasma half-life of verapamil is shorter after intravenous administration and norverapamil has not been detected. Correlation between the pharmacokinetic properties and the haemodynamic and electrophysiological actions of verapamil is not direct—verapamil acts within minutes of intravenous administration but its effect may only last for less than half an hour whereas it may require 2 hours to act after oral administration with a peak effect after 5 hours. Correlation has been found between plasma concentrations and response, but the clinical state of the patient may also be an important factor.

Verapamil is very extensively bound to plasma proteins. It is mainly excreted by the kidneys in the form of its metabolites but some is also excreted in the bile into the faeces.

A review of anti-arrhythmic agents including the pharmacokinetics of verapamil.— B. N. Singh *et al.*, *Prog. cardiovasc. Dis.*, 1980, *22*, 243.

Metabolism and pharmacokinetics. The disposition of verapamil in 5 healthy subjects following intravenous or oral administration showed a bi-exponential decline with an initial rapid phase with a half-life of 18 to 31 minutes followed by a slower phase with a half-life of 161 to 442 minutes. Verapamil was about 90% bound to plasma proteins. Absorption was almost complete following oral administration, but because of extensive first pass metabolism the bioavailability was only 10 to 23%. Results indicated that oral doses had to be at least 8 to 10 times an intravenous dose to produce plasma concentrations of unchanged verapamil equal to those obtained after intravenous administation. Up to 70% of a dose was excreted in the urine within 120 hours of either form of administration with about 50% in the first 24 hours. Following intravenous administration about 9 to 16% of a dose was excreted in the faeces within 5 days.— M. Schomerus *et al.*, *Cardiovasc. Res.*, 1976, *10*, 605.

A study of the disposition kinetics of verapamil and its active metabolite, norverapamil, in patients with chronic atrial fibrillation. In the atrial fibrillation patients the half-life of verapamil was 4.9 (±3.0) hours after intravenous administration; norverapamil was not present in blood after intravenous administration. Following oral administration the half-life of verapamil was 7.2 (±4.2) hours and the half-life of norverapamil was 9.3 (±4.5) hours. It was concluded that the disappearance of verapamil in the plasma is more rapid following intravenous than oral administration, and the accumulation of norverapamil is greater than that of verapamil and may be important in influencing the clinical effect.— R. E. Kates *et al.*, *Clin. Pharmac. Ther.*, 1981, *29*, 257.

Studies suggesting that there may be reduced clearance of verapamil during long-term oral use.— R. E. Kates *et al.*, *Clin. Pharmac. Ther.*, 1981, *30*, 44; S. B. Freedman *et al.*, *ibid.*, 644; D. G. Shand *et al.*, *ibid.*, 701.

Plasma concentrations. Results of a study of the relationship between plasma-verapamil concentrations and the reduction in ventricular rate on acute intravenous administration to patients in atrial fibrillation and flutter indicated that, in addition to dose and plasma concentration, the clinical state of the patient influenced the response. The average plasma concentration of 9 responders was about 50 ng per ml, whereas 6 non-responders obtained less benefit with twice this. All the non-responders had congestive heart failure which, with its associated high endogenous catecholamine activity, could have antagonised the action of verapamil on atrioventricular nodal transmission. In the responders the decrease in ventricular rate was greatest within 5 to 10 minutes of verapamil administration, and in some patients persisted for up to 3 hours.— J. Dominic *et al.*, *Clin. Pharmac. Ther.*, 1979, *26*, 710.

Protein binding. A study of verapamil protein binding in patients and in healthy subjects. Verapamil was found to be approximately 90% bound to plasma proteins in a concentration-independent manner over the clinically observed plasma concentration range. This binding was not affected by similar concentrations of the metabolite, norverapamil, nor by end-stage renal failure or the postoperative state in coronary bypass graft patients. Changes noted in patients with reduced creatinine clearance and those undergoing cardiac catheterisation were not considered likely to be of clinical importance.— D. L. Keefe *et al.*, *Clin. Pharmac. Ther.*, 1981, *29*, 21.

Uses. Verapamil is a class IV anti-arrhythmic agent (see p.1370). It is used in the control of supraventricular arrhythmias, and also in the management of angina pectoris.

In the treatment of supraventricular tachycardias, verapamil is given by mouth as the hydrochloride in doses of 40 to 120 mg thrice daily, according to the severity of the condition and the patient's response. Suggested oral doses for children are: up to 2 years of age, 20 mg twice or thrice daily; 2 years and over, 40 to 120 mg twice or thrice daily according to age and response. Verapamil may be given intravenously as the hydrochloride in doses of 5 to 10 mg injected over a period of 30 seconds; if necessary, a further 5 mg may be injected 5 to 10 minutes after the first. Suggested intravenous doses for children are: newborn, 0.75 to 1 mg; infants, 0.75 to 2 mg; children aged 1 to 5 years, 2 to 3 mg; children aged 6 to 15 years, 2.5 to 5 mg; if necessary these doses may be repeated after 5 to 10 minutes. Smaller doses may be adequate and the injection should be stopped when a response has been obtained. Intravenous injections should be given under continuous ECG monitoring, particularly in infancy.

Verapamil hydrochloride may also be given by intravenous infusion in sodium chloride or dextrose solution at a rate of 5 to 10 mg per hour to a total of 25 to 100 mg daily.

In the management of angina pectoris, verapamil hydrochloride is given by mouth in doses of 120 mg thrice daily; some patients with angina of effort may respond to 80 mg thrice daily, but this lower dose is not likely to be effective in angina at rest or Prinzmetal's variant angina.

Administration. In children. Refractory supraventricular tachycardia in a 2½-year-old child was successfully controlled with verapamil. An initial dose of 250 µg per kg body-weight was given intravenously over 10 minutes. This produced sinus rhythm and reduced the heart-rate from 180 eventually to 120 beats per minute. Tachycardia returned about 40 minutes after the infusion. Therapy by mouth was started on the following day with 40 mg every 8 hours and normal sinus rhythm was established over 24 hours. Short bursts of tachycardia seen at follow-up one week later were eventually controlled by a final adjusted dose of 80 mg every 8 hours. Propranolol was discontinued 96 hours before verapamil was given but digoxin therapy was maintained.— D. W. Sapire *et al.*, *J. Pediat.*, 1979, *94*, 312.

Further references.— J. Soler-Soler *et al.*, *Circulation*, 1979, *59*, 876 (paroxysmal supraventricular tachycardia in infants).

Administration in hepatic failure. Investigations showing that whereas verapamil clearance was reduced in 5 patients with liver disease it was increased in 2 patients in intensive care.— B. G. Woodcock *et al.*, *Clin. Pharmac. Ther.*, 1981, *29*, 27. In patients with liver cirrhosis the intraveneous dose of verapamil should be halved and the oral dose decreased by a factor of five. A steady-state plasma concentration will not be reached until about 2 days after therapy has started.— A. Somogyi *et al.*, *Br. J. clin. Pharmac.*, 1981, *12*, 51.

Angina pectoris. In a controlled double-blind study in 16 patients with angina, verapamil 120 mg thrice daily and propranolol 100 mg thrice daily produced similar favourable results. The incidence of angina and weekly consumption of glyceryl trinitrate were significantly reduced and exercise tolerance increased. A lower dose of 40 mg thrice daily of verapamil had a similar effect but produced no objective benefit in the ECG.— G. Sandler *et al.*, *Br. med. J.*, 1968, *3*, 224. A criticism of the conclusions drawn from the statistical analysis of the results.— J. D. Proctor *et al.* (letter), *ibid.*, 1968, *4*, 515. A reply.— G. Sandler *et al.* (letter), *ibid.*, 516.

In a double-blind study in 32 patients with uncomplicated angina of effort propranolol 100 mg thrice daily and verapamil 120 mg thrice daily were comparable in reducing anginal attacks, increasing exercise tolerance, and reducing the need for glyceryl trinitrate. Both propranolol and verapamil reduced diastolic blood pressure.— B. Livesley *et al.*, *Br. med. J.*, 1973, *1*, 375. Criticism of the design of the trial and of the analysis of the results.— G. Nyberg (letter), *ibid.*, 1973, *3*, 47.

In a double-blind crossover study verapamil was significantly more effective than a placebo in the management of 12 patients in whom unstable angina at rest was attributed to coronary vasospasm and was not the result of an excessive increase in myocardial metabolic demand.— O. Parodi *et al.*, *Br. Heart J.*, 1979, *41*, 167.

A study in 28 patients with classical angina pectoris indicated that verapamil 120 mg thrice daily may be useful in the management of chronic stable angina pectoris. Side-effects were constipation requiring laxatives in 7 and prolongation of the P-R interval in 2; minor side-effects not requiring treatment were headache in 2, palpitations in 1, and sleepiness in 2.— V. B. Subramanian *et al.*, *Lancet*, 1980, *1*, 841. See also *idem*, *Postgrad. med. J.*, 1976, *52*, 143.

A comparison of verapamil in doses of 240 to 480 mg daily in 3 to 6 divided doses, with placebo, in a 9-month double-blind randomised study of 16 patients with Prinzmetal's variant angina. Ambulatory ECG monitoring was used to evaluate the response to therapy. The frequency of anginal episodes was reduced substantially during verapamil therapy and the use of glyceryl trinitrate was accordingly lessened. The number of episodes of clinical instability fell substantially during verapamil therapy and the frequency of transient ST-segment deviations was also diminished during treatment. Despite its beneficial effect on both symptoms and ischaemic ECG alterations, verapamil had only a minimal effect on the complexity of ventricular ectopic activity. Side-effects were infrequent and relatively minor (constipation in 2 patients, a slight prolongation of asymptomatic sinus pauses in 1 patient, and occasional palpitations that occurred concomitantly with an accelerated A-V junctional rhythm in 1 patient). It was concluded that verapamil is safe and effective in the therapy of variant angina pectoris.— S. M. Johnson *et al.*, *New Engl. J. Med.*, 1981, *304*, 862.

Asthma. In 9 of 10 patients, both nebulised verapamil (about 3 mg) and nebulised sodium cromoglycate (about 12 mg) significantly inhibited exercise-induced asthma, compared with saline as control. It is suggested that calcium antagonists may inhibit post-exercise bronchoconstriction by their blocking effect on calcium channels.— K. R. Patel, *Br. med. J.*, 1981, *282*, 932.

Cardiac arrhythmias. A review of anti-arrhythmic agents, including mention of verapamil. The introduction of verapamil was a major advance in the acute therapy of supraventricular arrhythmias.— L. H. Opie, *Lancet*, 1980, *1*, 861. A detailed review of the actions and uses of calcium antagonists, including verapamil. Verapamil inhibits the action potential of the upper and middle nodal regions of the heart where the slow inward calcium-ion-mediated current contributes to depolarisation. Thus, by blocking slow-channel conduction in the atrioventricular node, verapamil inhibits one limb of the re-entry circuit which is believed to underlie most paroxysmal supraventricular tachycardias. This also explains the reduction of ventricular rate in atrial flutter and fibrillation, but verapamil has negligible effects on ventricular arrhythmias probably because its first action is to cause atrioventricular block, this undesirable effect developing before it can influence ventricular arrhythmias.— *idem*, 806.

Further reviews and comments on verapamil and cardiac arrhythmias.— B. N. Singh *et al.*, *Drugs*, 1978, *15*, 169; *Med. Lett.*, 1981, *23*, 29.

The effect of verapamil, 10 mg by intravenous injection over 15 to 30 seconds, was studied in 181 patients with various arrhythmias. Of 115 patients with *atrial fibrillation* ventricular slowing occurred in 111, with regularisation of the response in 71; of 15 with *atrial flutter* conversion to sinus rhythm occurred in 4 and a decreased ventricular response in 11; of 20 with *paroxysmal supraventricular tachycardia* conversion to sinus rhythm occurred in all but there was no effect in 1 with *paroxysmal ventricular tachycardia;* there was significant slowing in 3 with *sinus tachycardia*, and conversion to sinus rhythm in 3 with *idionodal tachycardia* and 1 with *idioventricular tachycardia. Ventricular extrasystoles* were reduced or abolished in 11 of 23 patients. Response was prompt and there were no side-effects and no appreciable fall in blood pressure or precipitation or aggravation of cardiac failure.— L. Schamroth *et al.*, *Br. med. J.*, 1972, *1*, 660. Extending the work of Schamroth and others, verapamil 10 mg was given intravenously to 32 patients with *paroxysmal supraventricular tachycardia* due to a circus movement affecting the atrioventricular node; all responded promptly. In 20 patients with *atrial flutter* 5 achieved sinus rhythm while 15 had a transient increase in AV block. All of 10 patients with *reciprocating tachycardias* associated with pre-excitation syndromes achieved sinus rhythm within 2 minutes. In a further study including intracardiac measurements, 15 of 18 patients with *atrioventricular junctional tachycardias* given verapamil while in *circus-movement tachycardia* achieved sinus rhythm, and tachycardia was terminated in 7 of 8 patients with the *Wolff-Parkinson-White syndrome*. Severe hypotension occurred in 4 patients who had taken beta-blocking agents; transient bradycardia and asystole also occurred.— D. M. Krikler and R. A. J. Spurrell, *Postgrad. med. J.*, 1974, *50*, 447.

Further reports and studies on the role of verapamil in cardiac arrhythmias.— M. K. Heng *et al.*, *Am. Heart J.*, 1975, *90*, 487 (various arrhythmias); W. S. Aronow *et al.*, *Clin. Pharmac. Ther.*, 1979, *26*, 578 (atrial fibrillation and flutter); H. O. Klein *et al.*, *Archs intern. Med.*, 1979, *139*, 747 (chronic atrial fibrillation); W. S. Aronow *et al.*, *Curr. ther. Res.*, 1980, *27*, 823 (disappointing response in multifocal atrial tachycardia); S. W. Rabkin *et al.*, *Can. med. Ass. J.*, 1980, *122*, 64 (supraventricular tachyarrhythmias and co-existing chronic lung disease); R. J. Sung *et al.*, *Ann. intern. Med.*, 1980, *93*, 682 (supraventricular tachycardias); H. L. Waxman *et al.*, *Ann. intern. Med.*, 1981, *94*, 1 (paroxysmal supraventricular tachycardia and atrial fibrillation).

Anaesthetic-induced arrhythmias. On 200 occasions, verapamil had been given intravenously in a dose of 20 mg to patients who developed arrhythmias while under light anaesthesia with halothane and oxygen. It had a rapid and reliable effect in supraventricular tachycardia and ventricular arrhythmia, but had no effect on sinus tachycardia. It was not a beta-adrenergic blocking agent and therefore could be used in instances where beta-blockers were contra-indicated.— G. Brichard and P. E. Zimmermann (letter), *Lancet*, 1970, *1*, 425. Comments.— B. N. Singh (letter), *ibid.*, 563. For a fuller report, see G. Brichard and P. E. Zimmermann, *Br. J. Anaesth.*, 1970, *42*, 1005.

Hypertension. Reports and studies on verapamil in hypertension.— D. W. Brittinger *et al.*, *Dt. med. Wschr.*, 1969, *94*, 945; W. P. Leary *et al.*, *Curr. ther. Res.*, 1979, *25*, 747; G. R. J. Lewis *et al.*, *Aust. N.Z. J. Med.*, 1979, *9*, 62; K. Midtbø and O. Hals, *Curr. ther. Res.*, 1980, *27*, 830.

Hypertrophic obstructive cardiomyopathy. Verapamil was given in a daily dose of 480 to 720 mg to 22 patients with hypertrophic obstructive cardiomyopathy. After an average of 15 months (4 to 24 months) of treatment significant reductions were obtained in the QRS amplitude in the electrocardiogram and in heart volume. Follow-up catheterisation in 10 patients showed a decrease in left ventricular muscle mass in 7 patients and a slight increase in 3; coronary artery diameter decreased in 7 patients, increased in 1 and was unchanged in 2. Treatment with verapamil was considered to be superior to therapy with beta-blockers.— M. Kaltenbach *et al.*, *Br. Heart J.*, 1979, *42*, 35.

Comment on verapamil as an alternative treatment to beta-adrenoceptor blocking agents in the management of hypertrophic cardiomyopathy. In short-term studies it was not shown to reduce the number of episodes of arrhythmia.— *Br. med. J.*, 1980, *281*, 1026.

Muscular disorders. A 35-year-old man with long-standing and disabling muscle pain of unknown origin had a dramatic response to verapamil 60 mg thrice daily and obtained complete relief with a dose of 120 mg thrice daily. His 39-year-old sister who had the same condition obtained a similar response to 120 mg thrice daily which was reduced to 60 mg four times daily owing to tachycardia and extrasystoles, with no return of pain.— J. Walton (letter), *Lancet*, 1981, *1*, 993.

Preparations

Verapamil Hydrochloride Injection *(B.P.)*. A sterile solution of verapamil hydrochloride in Water for Injections. Sterilised by autoclaving. pH 4.5 to 6. Protect from light.

Verapamil Hydrochloride Tablets *(B.P.)*. Tablets containing verapamil hydrochloride. They are film-coated.

Cordilox *(Abbott, UK)*. Verapamil hydrochloride, available as 2-ml **Ampoules** of an injection containing 2.5 mg per ml, for intravenous use, and as **Tablets** of 40, 80, and 120 mg.

Other Proprietary Names

Cardimil *(S.Afr.)*; Isoptin *(Austral., Canad., Denm., Ger., Ital., Neth., Norw., S.Afr., Swed., Switz.)*; Isoptine *(Belg., Fr.)*; Isoptino *(Arg.)*; Manidon *(Spain)*; Vasolan *(Jap.)*.

Radiopharmaceuticals

5850-b

Radioactive compounds are used in medicine as sources of radiation for radiotherapy and as radioactive tracers for diagnostic purposes. They have numerous uses in research and industry.

The terms *radioisotope*, *radioactive isotope*, and *isotope* have come to be used indiscriminately when referring to those isotopes of elements which emit ionising radiations. *Radionuclide* is generally more correct as a term of general reference. The term *radioisotope* should be specifically used when discussing the different radiation-emitting isotopes of a particular element. Chemical compounds containing a radionuclide are generally referred to as *radiochemicals*, *radioactive compounds*, or, in the case of such compounds or substances for medical use, radiopharmaceuticals.

Because of different requirements for storage, handling, and disposal and because of the different methods of use, radionuclides may be categorised as *sealed* and *unsealed* sources.

Sealed radioactive sources are bonded or encapsulated to prevent the escape of the radioactive material and are used as supplied. In medicine, they are generally used by radiotherapists and kept in the custody of medical physicists. Examples of sealed radioactive sources are caesium-137 needles and tubes, various applicators for ophthalmic therapy, and high-activity sources for caesium and cobalt teletherapy units.

Unsealed sources, on the other hand, are radioactive materials usually in liquid, particulate, or gaseous form which are removed from their containers for application. All radiopharmaceuticals come within this category. They present additional hazards due to the risk of contamination by skin contact, inhalation, or ingestion.

Atomic Stucture and Isotopes. An atom is composed of a central positively charged nucleus around which, and at relatively great distances away, negatively charged electrons revolve in orbits. The electrons are arranged round the atomic nucleus in a series of 'shells' (known as the K, L, M, N . . . shells) in each of which is a limited number of orbits.

The nucleus consists of 2 main kinds of particles known as protons, each of unit positive charge, and neutrons, which are uncharged; the total number of these particles in the nucleus is known as the *mass number* (A).

Each electron carries a negative charge (1.60×10^{-19} coulomb) which is of the same size as the positive charge of the proton, so that in the neutral atom the number of electrons is equal to the number of protons in the nucleus.

The number of protons in the nucleus is known as the *atomic number* (Z), which determines the number of electrons in the extranuclear structure, and this in turn determines the chemical properties of the atom. Thus all the atoms of a particular chemical element have the same atomic number. But while the number of protons (atomic number) and thus the chemical properties of all the atoms in a given element are constant, the number of neutrons in the atoms, and thus their masses (mass numbers), may vary. These different forms of the same element are known as isotopes of the element and these isotopes differ in some of their physical properties.

Some isotopes may be stable, the differences between them arising solely from their difference in mass; others may be radioactive (*radioisotopes*), their nuclei changing spontaneously and emitting particles or electromagnetic waves, or both.

Most of the naturally occurring isotopes are stable, though there are a number which are unstable and therefore radioactive, for example, uranium-235. In addition, artificial radionuclides are prepared by converting stable nuclei into unstable forms and even naturally occurring radionuclides may be prepared by artificial means.

The symbol used for a nuclide is a development of the chemical symbol for the atom, with the mass number as a superscript and the atomic number as a subscript; thus the symbols for the 3 hydrogen isotopes—common hydrogen, deuterium, and tritium—are ${}^{1}_{1}H$, ${}^{2}_{1}H$, and ${}^{3}_{1}H$, and the symbols for the 3 naturally occurring uranium isotopes are ${}^{234}_{92}U$, ${}^{235}_{92}U$, and ${}^{238}_{92}U$; as the atomic number can be inferred from the chemical symbol it is the usual practice to omit the subscript. It is also common practice to write out the full name of the element followed by the superscript, e.g. chromium-51 for ${}^{51}Cr$.

Emissions from Radioisotopes. The 3 main types of emission from radioactive substances are *alpha particles*, *beta particles*, and *gamma-rays*. Most sources emit more than one type of radiation.

Alpha particles are positively charged particles (helium nuclei), each consisting of 2 protons and 2 neutrons. They are emitted from the nuclei of some radioactive atoms.

Beta particles (β^- or β^+) are identical with electrons or positrons but arise from the nucleus. They are emitted with great velocity and their energies are spread over a spectrum, the greatest energy being E_{max}. Positrons are similar to electrons, having a similar mass but a positive charge.

Gamma-rays are electromagnetic radiations with a wavelength much shorter than those of light. It is usual to refer to the energy of the quanta rather than the wavelengths of the radiations.

In certain cases, e.g. chromium-51, electron capture (EC) occurs, an electron from an inner shell being absorbed by the nucleus with the production of an X-ray characteristic of the daughter atom or emission of an Auger electron.

The type of emission from a radionuclide largely determines its usefulness in medicine. Those emitting α-particles are very little used partly because detection and measurement are difficult. Beta-particles penetrate relatively short distances through matter, and nuclides with weak β-emissions, such as tritium or carbon-14, cannot be detected if the sample is contained in a glass test-tube, and cannot be assayed accurately even when special devices such as thin window Geiger counters or gas flow counters are used. Special techniques such as liquid scintillation counting, where the sample solution containing the radionuclide is mixed directly with a liquid scintillator to reduce self-absorption losses, are required. Detection and measurement of γ-rays is not so difficult and γ-ray emitting radionuclides are employed in studies in which radioactivity within the tissues is detected from outside the body.

Decay of Radionuclides. A radionuclide will consist of unstable atoms which will at some time undergo an energy change with the emission of ionising radiation, those which are actually undergoing this change, and those which have undergone the change. In quantitative terms this transition occurs at a rate which is characteristic of the radionuclide and it is expressed as its half-life—the time required for the activity to fall by one-half. Many radionuclides have complex decay characteristics with several possible energies of emitted particles and radiation. Some radionuclides may be in an excited or metastable state denoted by the suffix m attached to the mass number (e.g. Technetium-99m) and undergo *isomeric transition* (IT) with the release of γ-rays.

The activity of radionuclides is measured in terms of the rate of transformation or disintegration. The unit is the becquerel (Bq) = 1 transformation per second. Up until recently the curie (Ci) was used as the unit of activity; 1 Ci = 3.7×10^{10} Bq.

Consideration of the half-life of a radionuclide is important for several reasons. Those radionuclides with half-lives in minutes or seconds may be used only if the patient is close to the production source. Those with half-lives of a few hours may be used only at a distance from the production source if they are daughter nuclides of a parent with a longer half-life. In these cases the daughter nuclide is prepared from the parent nuclide contained in a *radionuclide generator*. The generator is usually a glass or plastic column containing alumina or an ion-exchange material on which is adsorbed the parent nuclide in equilibrium with its daughter. An appropriate solution is passed through the column to elute the daughter radionuclide. Sterile generators are available for the production of indium-113m and technetium-99m.

All radionuclides except those with very long half-lives, such as carbon-14, have limited shelf lives.

Authority to Obtain and Use Radioactive Materials. The purchase and use of radioactive substances is controlled in the UK and this includes the administration of these substances. Advice may be available from the Administration of Radioactive Substances Advisory Committee.

Radiopharmaceuticals and radioactive materials for their preparation are available from several commercial sources including *Abbott*, *Mallinckrodt*, *Squibb*, and *Wellcome Reagents* as well as from *Amersham International Ltd*, Amersham, Bucks, England, HP7 9LL.

The transport by road of radioactive materials outside hospitals is governed by the Radioactive Substances (Carriage by Road) (Great Britain) Regulations, 1974 (SI 1974 : No. 1735) and the Radioactive Substances (Road Transport Workers) (Great Britain) Regulations, 1970 (SI 1970 : No. 1827) and Amendment 1975 (SI 1975 : No. 1522). Advice on carrying out these regulations is contained in a *Code of Practice for the Carriage of Radioactive Materials by Road*, Department of the Environment, London, HM Stationery Office, 1975. Additional advice is also available in a *Code of Practice for the Storage of Radioactive Material in Transit*, Departments of the Environment and Employment, London, HM Stationery Office, 1975.

A useful guide for packaging for transport is shown in Appendix K of the *Code of Practice for the Protection of Persons against Ionising Radiations arising from Medical and Dental Use*, London, HM Stationery Office, 1972.

A guide to the design, testing, and use of packaging for the safe transport of radioactive materials has been issued by the British Standards Institution (BS 3895 : 1976).

Adverse Effects of Radionuclides. The internal irradiation of tissues following the administration of radionuclides carries similar dangers to exposure to ionising radiation from an external source, and local high irradiation doses may arise if these nuclides are specifically localised in a tissue. The most serious danger is genetic damage prior to and during the reproductive period. Tissues whose cells are in a continuous state of multiplication are particularly sensitive to the effects of radiation.

Untoward effects of exposure to the larger doses of irradiation include leucopenia, anaemia, inflammation of the skin, radiation sickness, and neoplasms.

In considering the effect of a given radionuclide it is usual to calculate the dose to the organ most critically affected, and also the dose to the whole body.

Preparation of Radiopharmaceuticals. In addition to good pharmaceutical manufacturing techniques appropriate safety precautions should be taken when preparing or handling radiopharmaceuticals. Advice and information on protection from radiological hazards is available within the UK from the National Radiological Protection Board (NRPB), Harwell, Didcot, Oxfordshire, OX11 0RQ. Film monitoring badges are also available from the Board. The Committee on Radiation from Radioactive Medicinal Products has also been established for the purposes of giving advice on safety, efficacy, and quality on the radiation aspects of substances or articles covered by the Medicines Act.

Basic common safety standards are being considered within the EEC for the health protection of the general public and workers against the dangers of ionising radiation.

Reports and recommendations regarding the preparation of radiopharmaceuticals: *Guidelines for the Preparation of Radiopharmaceuticals in Hospitals,* Special Report No. 11, London, British Institute of Radiology, 1975; *The Hospital Preparation of Radiopharmaceuticals, Scientific Report Series 16,* London, Hospital Physicists' Association, 1977; *Good Pharmaceutical Manufacturing Practice Applied to the Hospital Preparation of Radiopharmaceuticals,* London, Medicines Inspectorate, DHSS, 1977; *The Handling, Storage, Use, and Disposal of Unsealed Radionuclides in Hospitals and Medical Research Establishments, A Report of ICRP Committees 3 and 4, ICRP Publication 25,* Oxford, Pergamon Press, 1977; M. Frier and S. R. Hesslewood (Ed.), *Quality Assurance of Radiopharmaceuticals, A Guide to Hospital Practice, Nuclear Medicine Communications,* London, Chapman and Hall, 1980.

Calculated absorbed doses and permissible body burdens for many radionuclides are given in *Recommendations of the International Commission on Radiological Protection, ICRP Publication 2, Report of Committee II on Permissible Dose for Internal Radiation (1959),* Oxford, Pergamon Press, 1967; *ibid., ICRP Publication 6,* Oxford, Pergamon Press, 1964. See also *ibid., ICRP Publication 9,* Oxford, Pergamon Press, 1966; G. J. Hine and R. E. Johnston (letter), *J. nucl. Med.,* 1970, *11,* 468.

Further references on protection: *Report of Committee 4 on Evaluation of Radiation Doses to Body Tissues from Internal Contamination due to Occupational Exposure, ICRP Publication 10,* Oxford, Pergamon Press, 1968; *The Assessment of Internal Contamination Resulting from Recurrent or Prolonged Uptakes, A Report of ICRP Committee 4, ICRP Publications 10A,* Oxford, Pergamon Press, 1971; *Protection of the Patient in Radionuclide Investigations, A Report Prepared for ICRP and Adopted by the Commission in 1969, ICRP Publication 17,* Oxford, Pergamon Press, 1971; *Handbook of Radiological Protection,* Part 1: Data, London, HM Stationery Office. 1971; *Code of Practice for the Protection of Persons against Ionising Radiations arising from Medical and Dental Use,* London, HM Stationery Office, 1972; *Implications of Commission Recommendations that Doses be kept as Low as Readily Achievable, A Report of ICRP Committee 4, ICRP Publication 22,* Oxford, Pergamon Press, 1973; Medical Research Council, *Criteria for Controlling Radiation Doses to the Public after Accidental Escape of Radioactive Material,* London, HM Stationery Office, 1975; C. B. Braestrup and K. J. Vikterlöf, *Manual on Radiation Protection in Hospitals and General Practice, Vol. 1, Basic Protection Requirements,* Geneva, World Health Organization, 1974; D. Frost and H. Jammet, *ibid., Vol. 2, Unsealed Sources,* Geneva, World Health Organization, 1975; *Recommendations of the International Commission on Radiological Protection, ICRP Publication 26,* Oxford, Pergamon Press, 1977.

General Uses of Radioactive Materials. Radiopharmaceuticals are used widely in many branches of medicine and surgery. The majority of applications are for the investigation and diagnosis of disease but in some circumstances they are used for therapeutic purposes.

Many investigations involve the oral or parenteral administration of radionuclides or labelled compounds, and the subsequent measurement of radioactive concentrations in organs, tissues, blood, urine, or faeces. The quantities used are always the smallest which will give the desired accuracy of measurement.

A review of nuclear medicine including a discussion of *in vivo* diagnostic procedures.— Report of a Joint IAEA/WHO Expert Committee on the Use of Ionizing Radiation and Radioisotopes for Medical Purposes (Nuclear Medicine), *Tech. Rep. Ser. Wld Hlth Org. No. 591,* 1976.

Further reviews on the uses of radiopharmaceuticals: N. D. S. Bell and P. W. Horton, *J. clin. Pharm.,* 1977, *2,* 137; M. N. Maisey, *Practitioner,* 1978, *220,* 445; L. Kreel, *Br. med. Bull.,* 1980, *36,* 205.

Storage of Radioactive Substances. Radioactive materials should be stored in specially protected areas, adequately shielded and under the control of a suitably qualified person. Shielding must protect persons in adjoining rooms and on adjacent floors as well as those in the immediate vicinity.

Care should be taken to comply with national and local regulations for protection against ionising radiations.

Disposal of Radioactive Waste. The disposal of radioactive waste in the United Kingdom is subject to control under the Radioactive Substances Act, 1960, the Radioactive Substances (Hospitals' Waste) Exemption Order 1963 (SI 1963 : No. 1833), the Radioactive Substances (Hospitals' Waste) Exemption (Scotland) Order 1963 [SI 1963 : No. 1879 (S. 96)], and Amendments 1974 [SI 1974 : No. 501 and SI 1974 : No. 487 (S.35)], and the Control of Pollution (Radioactive Waste) Regulations 1976 (SI 1976 : No. 959).

For general and detailed advice and interpretation of the regulations, see *Code of Practice for the Protection of Persons against Ionising Radiations arising from Medical and Dental Use,* London, HM Stationery Office, 1972 (A similar code of practice for the protection of persons against ionising radiations arising from research and teaching was also published in 1968).

Radiological Terms Associated with Description of Radionuclides.

Alpha particles. Nuclei of helium atoms emitted by radioactive atomic nuclei.

Annihilation. The interaction and disappearance of a positive and a negative electron with the conversion of their energy into electromagnetic radiation.

Atomic number (Z). The number of protons in the atomic nucleus.

Auger effect. The emission of an electron from an atom due to the filling of a vacancy in an inner electron shell.

Becquerel (Bq). The SI unit of activity, defined as 1 transformation per second. See also Curie (below). 1 Bq=2.7×10^{-11} Ci.

Beta particles. Electrons or positrons emitted by radioactive atomic nuclei.

Biological half-life. The time required for the amount of a particular substance to be halved by biological means, when the rate of removal is approximately exponential.

Carrier-free. A preparation in which substantially all the atoms of the activated element present are radioactive. Material of high specific activity is often loosely referred to as 'carrier-free'.

Curie (Ci). A unit of activity, defined as 3.7×10^{10} transformations per second. It is sometimes used to designate a quantity of radionuclide. The becquerel (Bq) is the SI unit of activity. 1 Ci=3.7×10^{10} Bq.

Daughter. Of a given nuclide, any nuclide that originates from it by radioactive decay.

Electron capture (EC). A mode of radioactivity decay involving the capture of an orbital electron by its nucleus.

Gamma-radiation. Electromagnetic radiation emitted in the process of a change in configuration of a nucleus or particle annihilation and having wavelengths shorter than those of X-rays.

Gray (Gy). The SI unit of absorbed dose, defined as 1 J per kg. See also rad (below). 1 Gy=100 rads.

Isomeric transition (IT). The decay of one isomer to another having a lower energy state. The transition is accompanied by the emission of gamma-radiation.

Isomers. Nuclides with the same mass number and atomic number but with nuclei having different energy states.

Isotopes. Nuclides with the same atomic number but different mass numbers.

MBq. Megabecquerel=10^6 Bq.

mCi. Millicurie=10^{-3} Ci.

Nuclide. A species of atom having a specific mass number, atomic number, and nuclear energy state.

Photon. A quantum of electromagnetic radiation.

Rad (radiation absorbed dose). A unit of absorbed dose of any ionising radiation, equal to 10^{-2} J per kg. The röntgen and the rad in soft tissue are approximately equivalent in magnitude for moderate energies. The gray (Gy) is the SI unit of absorbed dose. 1 rad=10^{-2} Gy.

Radioactive decay. The spontaneous change of a nucleus resulting in the emission of a particle or a photon.

Radioactivity. The property of certain nuclides of spontaneously emitting particles or photons or of undergoing spontaneous fission.

Radioisotope. An isotope that is radioactive.

Radionuclide. A nuclide that is radioactive.

Rem (röntgen-equivalent-man). A unit of dose equivalent, numerically equal to the absorbed dose in rads multiplied by the appropriate quality factor defining the biological effect and by any other modifying factors. Used in statements on radiation protection. The SI unit of dose equivalent known as Sievert (Sv) is the joule per kg (J kg^{-1}) equal to 100 rem.

Röntgen (R). A unit of exposure of X- or gamma-radiation, equal to 2.58×10^{-4} coulombs per kg in air. The SI unit of exposure is the coulomb per kg (C kg^{-1}). 1 C kg^{-1}=3.876×10^3 R.

Sievert (Sv). The SI unit of dose equivalent. See under Rem (above).

Specific activity. The activity per unit mass of a material containing a radioactive substance.

X-rays. Electromagnetic radiation other than annihilation radiation originating in the extranuclear part of the atom and having wavelengths much shorter than those of visible light.

For a comprehensive list of radiological terms and their definitions, see *Glossary of terms used in radiology* (BS 2597 : 1955) and *Glossary of terms used in nuclear science and technology* (BS 3455 : 1973) published by the British Standards Institution.

Radiation Data on Radionuclides.

Only those radionuclides in common use are described in this section.

The radiation data given under the radionuclides described in the following pages show the half-life, the energy of the radiation of particles in million electronvolts (MeV), and the percentage of total number of transformations which gives rise to the emission of the particular radiation. Since one transformation may give rise to more than one gamma-ray the percentages do not necessarily add up to 100%. X-rays, together with minor emissions, have been omitted unless they are a significant part of the total emission.

Nuclides which emit positrons (β^+) always give gamma-radiation of 0.51 MeV as a result of the mutual annihilation of a positron and an electron.

5851-v

Caesium-137 ($^{137}_{55}Cs$)

HALF-LIFE. 30.1 years

RADIATION EMITTED. β^- 0.512 (94.6%), 1.174 (5.4%) MeV. It also decays via barium-137m [half-life: 2.6 minutes. γ 0.662 (85.1%) MeV; X-rays (barium) 0.032 to 0.038 (~8%) MeV].

SUPPLY. Caesium-137 is not supplied in pharmaceutical dosage forms. it is supplied as teletherapy sources and, encapsulated in iridio-platinum, in the form of needles and tubes.

Uses. Caesium-137 is used in radiotherapy.

Caesium-129 as caesium chloride (^{129}Cs) has been investigated as an agent for imaging lung tumours.

5852-g

Calcium-47 ($^{47}_{20}Ca$)

HALF-LIFE. 4.54 days

RADIATION EMITTED. β^- 0.69 (82%), 1.99 (17.9%) MeV; γ 0.489 (6.8%), 0.808 (6.8%), 1.297 (75.1%) MeV.

SUPPLY. Calcium-47 is supplied as calcium chloride (^{47}Ca) in the form of an injection, iso-osmotic with serum, containing more than 7.4 megabecquerels (200 microcuries) per mg of calcium.

Uses. Calcium-47, as the chloride, is used in doses of 185 to 740 kBq (5 to 20 microcuries) administered intravenously for the investigation of calcium metabolism. It is of limited use in some aspects of calcium metabolism because its half-life is short in relation to the processes to be measured. Solutions of calcium chloride (^{47}Ca) are contaminated with small quantities of calcium-45 and scandium-47. The solution must therefore be used within a short time of receipt.

Calcium-46 has also been used as a urinary and faecal marker.

5853-q

Carbon-14 ($^{14}_{6}C$)

HALF-LIFE. 5730 years

RADIATION EMITTED. β^- 0.156 (100%) MeV.

SUPPLY. Carbon-14 is supplied in a variety of labelled organic compounds.

Uses. Many organic compounds labelled with carbon-14 are available but few are used *in vivo* except in research.

Carbon-11-labelled compounds have also been used in organ scanning.

The use of the ^{14}C-glycocholate test in the evaluation of changed bile acid metabolism in diabetic diarrhoea.— J. H. B. Scarpello *et al., Br. med. J.*, 1976, *2*, 673. See also H. Fromm and A. F. Hofmann, *Lancet*, 1971, *2*, 621; O. F. W. James *et al., Br. med. J.*, 1973, *3*, 191; S. H. Roberts *et al., Lancet*, 1977, *2*, 1193.

An assessment of the amidopyrine (^{14}C) breath test indicated that a single breath collection after a tracer dose by mouth differentiated between normal subjects and those with hepatocellular disease. The breath test was considered to be useful for screening but its advantage over other liver-function tests had yet to be shown.— J. Galizzi *et al., Gut*, 1978, *19*, 40. Results of the amidopyrine (^{14}C) breath test as an indicator of hepatic function could be affected by several factors. Reduced absorption of amidopyrine would give a falsely-low result, even in a patient with normal function; 1 patient with alcoholic cirrhosis gave a very high result, possibly due to hepatic enzyme induction by alcohol.— J. Noordhoek *et al., Eur. J. clin. Pharmac.*, 1978, *13*, 223.

A study indicating that administration of carbon-14 labelled phenylacetic oil is a reliable, simple, and rapid test for fat absorption that requires only a 5-hour urine collection. Although faecal fat continues to be the most accurate test it is cumbersome and distasteful, and requires longer time at hospital. Exposure to radioactivity is slight with complete excretion of the radioactivity in about 24 hours. Whereas conventional D-xylose tests may be affected by bacterial overgrowth, the phenylacetic oil absorption test does not seem to have this drawback.— S. M. Nasrallah and U. A. S. Al-Khalidi, *Lancet*, 1980, *1*, 229. Criticism.— D. S. Rampton and M. Sarner (letter), *ibid.*, 419.

5854-p

Chromium-51 ($^{51}_{24}Cr$)

HALF-LIFE. 27.7 days

RADIATION EMITTED. EC (100%); γ 0.320 (9.9%) MeV; X-rays (vanadium) 0.005 to 0.006 (~22%) MeV.

SUPPLY. Chromium-51 is usually supplied as sodium chromate (^{51}Cr) solutions or injections containing 9250 to 18500 megabecquerels (250 to 500 millicuries) per mg of chromium. *B.P.* and *Eur. P.* specify not less than 814 megabecquerels (22 millicuries) per mg of chromium at the date and hour stated on the label and *U.S.P.* specifies not less than 370 megabecquerels (10 millicuries) per mg of sodium chromate at the end of the expiry period. Chromium-51 is also supplied as chromic chloride (^{51}Cr) injection, iso-osmotic with serum, containing 3700 to 12 950 megabecquerels (100 to 350 millicuries) per mg of chromium, and as chromium disodium edetate (^{51}Cr) injection, containing 37 to 74 megabecquerels (1 to 2 millicuries) per mg of chromium.

Uses. Chromium-51, as Sodium Chromate (^{51}Cr) Sterile Solution, is used to label red blood cells so that red-cell survival and red-cell volume can be measured. Chromium-51 activity in the faeces can be used to estimate gastro-intestinal blood losses. Red blood cells labelled with chromium-51 and damaged by heat before reinjection have been used for spleen scanning.

As chromium disodium edetate (^{51}Cr) injection, chromium-51 is used in the determination of the glomerular filtration-rate. The usual dose is 1.295 to 11.1 MBq (35 to 300 microcuries) administered intravenously.

As chromic chloride (^{51}Cr) injection, chromium-51 is also administered intravenously in usual doses of 1.11 to 3.7 MBq (30 to 100 microcuries) for the determination of loss of serum protein into the gastro-intestinal tract.

The use of chromium-51-labelled sodium chromate in a test to indicate whether splenectomy would benefit patients with haemolytic anaemia.— A. Goldberg *et al., Lancet*, 1966, *1*, 109. The use of chromium-51-labelled erythrocytes for predicting the value of splenectomy in auto-immune haemolytic anaemia was not considered to be reliable in a study of 12 patients.— A. C. Parker *et al., Br. med. J.*, 1977, *1*, 208.

The diagnosis of constitutional hepatic dysfunction using red blood cells labelled with chromium-51.— P. D. Berk and T. F. Blaschke, *Ann. intern. Med.*, 1972, *77*, 527.

Chromium-51-labelled chromium trichloride was as useful as dichromium trioxide as an inert marker for the correction of faecal recoveries in calcium balance studies.— R. Hesp *et al., Clin. Sci.*, 1979, *57*, 89.

Preparations

Sodium Chromate Cr 51 Injection *(U.S.P.)*. A sterile solution of radioactive chromium (^{51}Cr) processed in the form of sodium chromate in Water for Injections. Sodium chloride may be added where a solution iso-osmotic with serum is required. It contains 90 to 110% of the labelled amount of ^{51}Cr as sodium chromate expressed in millicuries per ml at the time indicated on the label. The specific activity is not less than 370 MBq (10 millicuries) per mg of sodium chromate at the end of the expiry period. Use within 4 months from the date of manufacture. Other chemical forms of radioactivity do not exceed 10% of the total radioactivity. pH 7.5 to 8.5. The label indicates whether the material is intended for diagnostic or therapeutic use.

Sodium Chromate (^{51}Cr) Sterile Solution *(B.P., Eur. P.)*. Sodium Chromate (^{51}Cr) Solution; Natrii Chromatis (^{51}Cr) Solutio Sterilisata. A sterile solution of sodium chromate (^{51}Cr) made iso-osmotic with blood by the addition of sodium chloride. At the date and hour stated on the label, it contains 90 to 110% of the content of chromium-51 activity stated on the label and the specific activity is not less than 814 MBq (22 millicuries) per mg of chromium. Other chemical forms of radioactivity do not exceed 10% of the total radioactivity. pH 6 to 8. *Dose.* For labelling red blood cells in the investigation of haematological disorders, up to 7.4 MBq (200 microcuries).

5855-s

Cobalt-57 ($^{57}_{27}Co$)

HALF-LIFE. 270 days

RADIATION EMITTED. EC (100%); γ 0.014 (7.8%), 0.122 (84.8%), 0.136 (11.4%), 0.570 (0.02%), 0.72 (0.2%) MeV; X-rays (iron) 0.006 to 0.007 (~55%) MeV.

SUPPLY. Cobalt-57 is usually supplied as cyanocobalamin (^{57}Co) in the form of an aqueous solution containing 18.5 kilobecquerels (0.5 microcurie) per μg or more than 37 kilobecquerels (1 microcurie) per μg of cyanocobalamin. *U.S.P.* specifies not less than 18.5 kilobecquerels (0.5 microcuries) per μg of cyanocobalamin. It is also supplied as cyanocobalamin (^{57}Co) in the form of capsules containing 18.5 kilobecquerels (0.5 microcurie) per μg of cyanocobalamin. *U.S.P.* specifies not less than 18.5 kilobecquerels (0.5 microcurie) per μg of cyanocobalamin. Cobalt-57 is also supplied for *in vitro* diagnostic procedures as cyanocobalamin (^{57}Co) in the form of aqueous solutions containing 0.37 to 11.1 megabecquerels (10 to 300 microcuries) per μg of cyanocobalamin.

Uses. Cyanocobalamin (^{57}Co) has the action and uses of cyanocobalamin (^{58}Co) as described under Cobalt-58.

Cobalt-57-labelled bleomycin has also been used in tumour imaging.

Preparations

Cyanocobalamin (^{57}Co) Solution *(B.P., Eur. P.)*. Cyanocobalamini (^{57}Co) Solutio. A solution of cyanocobalamin (^{57}Co) which may contain a stabiliser and an antimicrobial preservative; pH 4 to 6. At the date stated on the label, it contains 85 to 115% of the content of cobalt-57 activity stated on the label, not less than 90% of the cobalt-57 is in the form of cyanocobalamin, and not more than 1% of the total activity is due to cobalt-60 together with other radionuclidic impurities. Store at a temperature not exceeding 8° and protect from light. It decomposes with an accompanying decrease in the radiochemical purity. It should be used within 3 months of the date stated on the label, and when used the radiochemical purity must be not less than 84%. *Dose.* In the investigation of the absorption and metabolism of cyanocobalamin, 37 kBq (1 microcurie).

Cyanocobalamin Co 57 Capsules *(U.S.P.)*. Capsules containing cyanocobalamin in which a portion of the molecules contain radioactive cobalt (^{57}Co) in the molecular structure. At the time stated on the label they contain 90 to 110% of the content of cobalt-57 stated on the label. The specific activity is not less than 18.5 kBq (0.5 μCi) per μg of cyanocobalamin and not less than 95% of the total radioactivity is in the form of cyanocobalamin. Protect from light. Use within 6 months from the date of standardisation.

Cyanocobalamin Co 57 Oral Solution *(U.S.P.)*. Cyanocobalamin Co 57 Solution. A solution suitable for oral administration containing cyanocobalamin in which a portion of the molecules contain radioactive cobalt (^{57}Co) in the molecular structure. It contains a suitable antimicrobial agent. pH 4 to 5.5. At the time stated on the label it contains 90 to 110% of the content of cobalt-57 stated on the label. The specific activity is not less than 18.5 kBq (0.5 μCi) per μg of cyanocobalamin and not less than 95% of the total radioactivity is in the form of cyanocobalamin. Store in airtight containers. Protect from light. Use within 6 months from the date of standardisation.

For a proprietary preparation containing cobalt-57, see Dicopac, p.528.

5856-w

Cobalt-58 ($^{58}_{27}Co$)

HALF-LIFE. 71 days

RADIATION EMITTED. β^+ 0.474 (15%) MeV; EC (85%); γ 0.511 (from β^+), 0.810 (99.4%), 0.865 (0.8%), 1.675 (0.6%) MeV; X-rays (iron) 0.006 to 0.007 (~26%) MeV.

SUPPLY. Cobalt-58 is usually supplied as cyanocobalamin (^{58}Co) in the form of an aqueous solution containing more than 37 kilobecquerels (1 microcurie) per μg of cyanocobalamin.

Uses of Radioactive Cyanocobalamin. Various preparations of cyanocobalamin labelled with either cobalt-57 or cobalt-58 are available for measurement of absorption of vitamin B_{12} in the diagnosis of pernicious anaemia and other malabsorption syndromes.

The usual dose is 18.5 to 37 kBq (0.5 to 1 microcurie) of cobalt-57 or cobalt-58 in about 1 μg of cyanocobalamin. Absorption of the vitamin can be measured directly using a scintillation counter or indirectly by measuring faecal excretion of radioactivity. If a large dose of non-radioactive cyanocobalamin is given by injection to impede uptake of the oral dose by the liver, absorption of the vitamin can be assessed by measuring the radioactivity in the urine; this is the basis of the Schilling test.

The different energies of cobalt-57 and cobalt-58 facilitate separation of the isotopes in a mixture. Advantage is taken of this to differentiate between failure of absorption due to lack of intrinsic factor (pernicious anaemia) and that due to ileal malabsorption by the simultaneous administration of cyanocobalamin (^{58}Co) and cyanocobalamin (^{57}Co) bound to gastric juice. A dual isotope kit is available for this purpose.

Cyanocobalamin (^{57}Co) of high specific activity, 0.37 to 11.1 MBq (10 to 300 microcuries) per μg of cyanocobalamin, may be used *in vitro* for vitamin B_{12} saturation analysis.

Cyanocobalamin (^{60}Co) has also been used but its use is not recommended because of its long half-life.

Preparations

Cyanocobalamin (^{58}Co) Solution *(B.P., Eur. P.)*. Cyanocobalamini (^{58}Co) Solutio. A solution of cyanocobalamin (^{58}Co) which may contain a stabiliser and an antimicrobial preservative. pH 4 to 6. At the date stated on the label, it contains 90 to 110% of the content of cobalt-58 activity stated on the label, not less than 90% of the cobalt-58 is in the form of cyanocobalamin, and not more than 1% of the total activity is due to cobalt-60 and other radionuclidic impurities. Store at a temperature not exceeding 8° and protect from light. It decomposes with an accompanying decrease in the radiochemical purity. It should be used within 3 months of the date stated on the label and when used the radiochemical purity must be not less than 84%. *Dose.* In the investigation of the absorption and metabolism of cyanocobalamin, 37 kBq (1 microcurie).

For a proprietary preparation containing cobalt-58, see Dicopac, p.528.

5857-e

Cobalt-60 ($^{60}_{27}$Co)

HALF-LIFE. 5.27 years

RADIATION EMITTED. β^- 0.318 (99.9%), 1.491 (0.1%) MeV; γ 1.173 (99.86%), 1.333 (99.98%) MeV.

SUPPLY. Cobalt-60 is supplied in several forms as a source of gamma-radiation for various clinical purposes, for industrial processes, and for research.

Uses. Cobalt-60 is used for radiotherapy in the form of alloys in large sealed sources and it has largely replaced radium for various radiological purposes.

It is also used as a radiation source for the sterilisation by gamma-irradiation of disposable syringes and catheters and surgical dressings and other surgical materials.

Cyanocobalamin (^{60}Co) was formerly used as a diagnostic aid in the detection of pernicious anaemia but, because of its long half-life, it has been superseded for this purpose by cyanocobalamin (^{58}Co) and cyanocobalamin (^{57}Co).

Sterilisation. The use of cobalt-60 in the sterilisation of various colouring agents.— B. -L. Chang *et al.*, *J. pharm. Sci.*, 1974, *63*, 758.

Preparations

Cyanocobalamin Co 60 Capsules *(U.S.P.)*. Capsules containing cyanocobalamin in which a portion of the molecules contain radioactive cobalt (^{60}Co). At the date stated on the label they contain 90 to 110% of the stated amount of cobalt-60 as cyanocobalamin. The specific activity is not less than 18.5 kBq (0.5 microcuries) per μg of cyanocobalamin. Protect from light. Use within 6 months of the date of standardisation.

Cyanocobalamin Co 60 Oral Solution *(U.S.P.)*. Cyanocobalamin Co 60 Solution. A clear, colourless to pink solution, suitable for oral administration, containing cyanocobalamin in which a portion of the molecules contain radioactive cobalt (^{60}Co), and a suitable antimicrobial agent. At the date stated on the label it contains 90 to 110% of the stated amount of cobalt-60 as cyanocobalamin. The amount of cobalt-60 as cyanocobalamin is not more than 37 kBq (1 microcurie) per ml, and the specific activity is not less than 18.5 kBq (0.5 microcurie) per μg of cyanocobalamin and not less than 95% of the total radioactivity is in the form of cyanocobalamin. pH 4 to 5.5. Protect from light. Use within 6 months of the date of standardisation.

5858-l

Gallium-67 ($^{67}_{31}$Ga)

HALF-LIFE. 78.26 hours

RADIATION EMITTED. EC (100%); γ 0.091 (3.6%), 0.185 (23.5%), 0.209 (2.6%), 0.300 (16.7%), 0.394 (4.4%) MeV; X-rays (zinc) 0.008 to 0.010 (~43%) MeV. It also decays via zinc-67m [half-life: 9.2 microseconds. γ 0.093 (37.6%) MeV; X-rays (zinc) 0.008 to 0.010 (~13%) MeV].

SUPPLY. Gallium-67 is supplied as gallium citrate (^{67}Ga) in the form of a carrier-free injection, iso-osmotic with serum, containing 18.5 to 185 megabecquerels (0.5 to 5 millicuries) per ml or 37 megabecquerels (1 millicurie) per ml.

Precautions.

Gallium scanning interfered with the measurement of anti-DNA antibodies, giving either false-positive or false-negative results depending on the radioimmunoassay used. Gallium scanning was being more frequently used in patients with fever of unknown origin and fever was often a symptom of systemic lupus erythematosus, diagnosis of which could be determined by the presence of anti-DNA antibodies.— D. Toretti *et al.*, *Ann. intern. Med.*, 1977, *86*, 309.

The radionuclide gallium-67 was found to interfere with radioenzymatic assays of aminoglycoside antibiotics. A method of overcoming this problem was described. Several other radionuclides tested did not affect the assay.— I. Bhattacharya *et al.*, *Antimicrob. Ag. Chemother.*, 1978, *14*, 448. See also K. Shannon *et al.* (letter), *J. antimicrob. Chemother.*, 1980, *6*, 285.

Reduced uptake of gallium-67 by tumours of the central nervous system was observed in patients receiving corticosteroids in larger than replacement doses. Corticosteroids did not significantly alter the sensitivity of the technetium-99m gluceptate test.— A. D. Waxman *et al.*, *J. nucl. Med.*, 1978, *19*, 480.

Pregnancy and the neonate. A 25-year-old pregnant woman had a diagnosis of Hodgkin's disease 1 week before delivery. Three weeks post partum she received gallium citrate (^{67}Ga) intravenously in a dose of 111 MBq (3 millicuries) and 48 hours later a whole-body scan showed uptake of gallium-67 by both breasts. Gallium-67 occurred in breast milk in concentrations of 2.59 kBq (70 nCi) per ml 96 and 120 hours after injection. Diagnosis of malignant breast disease by scanning was considered impossible in the postpartum period, and the administration of gallium citrate (^{67}Ga) was contra-indicated in nursing mothers.— S. M. Larson and G. L. Schall (letter), *J. Am. med. Ass.*, 1971, *218*, 257. See also R. E. Tobin and P. B. Schneider, *J. nucl. Med.*, 1976, *17*, 1055.

Uses. Gallium-67, in the form of the citrate, is concentrated in some tumours of the lymphatic system and other soft tissues, and is used in doses of 55.5 to 92.5 MBq (1.5 to 2.5 millicuries) for tumour visualisation by scanning techniques. Localisation has been reported in inflammatory lesions and gallium-67 has been used for the diagnosis of infection.

Gallium-67 as the citrate might be useful in the diagnosis of pseudohypertrophic muscular dystrophy because of its abnormal uptake.— P. Bowen *et al.* (letter), *Lancet*, 1977, *2*, 1072. During evaluation of a patient with lymphoma it was noted that gallium-67 was also taken up by muscles which had undergone physiological hypertrophic changes.— J. B. O'Connell *et al.* (letter), *Lancet*, 1980, *1*, 1083.

Improved diagnosis of sarcoidosis using an assay of angiotensin-converting enzyme in association with a gallium scan; this technique gave 3 false-negative results in 27 patients.— A. Nosal *et al.*, *Ann. intern. Med.*, 1979, *90*, 328.

Detection of neoplasms. Results of a cooperative study of the use of gallium citrate (^{67}Ga) imaging in Hodgkin's disease showed that 220 of 248 untreated patients had a positive uptake in one or more lesions, however it was considered that negative uptake at a particular site did not necessarily prove the absence of a lesion there. Of the various types of Hodgkin's disease there was a higher incidence of localisation in all except the lymphocyte-predominance type, where the uptake was slightly lower. The size of lesion most easily detected was 4 cm in diameter and none below 1 cm was successfully imaged. The technique was much less successful for abdominal lesions than for those at other sites because of uptake by the bowel and liver causing interference. In treated asymptomatic patients returning for routine follow-up a significant number of unsuspected positive lesions were observed suggesting that the gallium-67 scan has a distinctly valuable use in identifying such patients thus allowing early therapy for recurrences.— G. S. Johnston *et al.*, *J. nucl. Med.*, 1977, *18*, 692. A similar study in patients with non-Hodgkin's malignant lymphoma.— G. A. Andrews *et al.*, *ibid.*, 1978, *19*, 1013.

Further reports and comments on the use of gallium-67 for the detection of tumours: J. T. Andrews *et al.*, *Med. J. Aust.*, 1976, *2*, 170 (upper abdominal lymphomas); T. R. DeMeester *et al.*, *J. thorac. cardiovasc. Surg.*, 1976, *72*, 699 (carcinoma of the lung); B. C. Lentle *et al.*, *Can. med. Ass. J.*, 1976, *114*, 1113 (inconsistent results with primary malignant tumours); F. I. Jackson *et al.*, *Radiology*, 1977, *122*, 163 (multisystem malignant melanoma); T. Higashi *et al.*, *J. nucl. Med.*, 1977, *18*, 243 (malignant tumours of head and neck); T. Higashi *et al.*, *Radiology*, 1977, *123*, 117 (differentiation of maxillary sinus carcinoma from chronic maxillary sinusitis); C. Bekerman *et al.*, *Radiology*, 1978, *127*, 719 (childhood malignancies); H. D. Brereton *et al.*, *J. Am. med. Ass.*, 1978, *240*, 666; J. D. Bitran *et al.* (letter), *J. Am. med. Ass.*, 1979, *241*, 1106 (both small cell carcinoma of the lung); G. F. Gates, *J. nucl. Med.*, 1979, *20*, 854 (evidence of bone involvement in acute leukaemia); M. Kondo *et al.*, *Radiology*, 1979, *131*, 723 (oesophageal carcinoma).

Diagnosis of infection. Gallium-67 citrate was used successfully to identify the source of sepsis in 11 of 12 patients with septic lesions.— R. L. Littenberg *et al.*, *Ann. intern. Med.*, 1973, *79*, 403.

Gallium-67 was used to screen 68 patients for infection. Of these 37 were suspected of having deep intra-abdominal infections; 24 of 25 had negative results with gallium-67 and no histopathologic evidence of infection. Histopathology showed infection in 12 and 7 of these were correctly diagnosed using gallium-67 scintigraphy. Four of the 5 false negative results involved disease in or near the liver where gallium would normally be concentrated.— D. A. Podoloff (letter), *Ann. intern. Med.*, 1975, *82*, 848.

The use of gallium-67 scanning in pyrexia of unknown origin. Of 67 scans 50 were abnormal and 33 provided new useful information. Normal scans were of value.— A. J. W. Hilson and M. N. Maisey, *Br. med. J.*, 1979, *2*, 1330.

Further reports and comments on the use of gallium-67 for the diagnosis of infection: H. H. Caffee *et al.*, *Am. J. Surg.*, 1977, *133*, 665 (intra-abdominal abscess); N. S. Gooneratne and J. J. Imarisio, *Gastroenterology*, 1977, *73*, 1147 (decreased uptake by a bacterial hepatic abscess); H. Thadepalli *et al.*, *Chest*, 1977, *72*, 442 (pulmonary infection); S. D. Sarkar *et al.*, *J. nucl. Med.*, 1979, *20*, 833 (extrapulmonary tuberculosis); G. D. Perdue *et al.* (letter), *J. Am. med. Ass.*, 1979, *242*, 1970 (paraprosthetic infection).

Diagnosis of inflammatory lesions. Reports and comments on the use of gallium-67 in the diagnosis of inflammatory lesions.— E. B. Silberstein (letter), *Ann. intern. Med.*, 1974, *80*, 774 (dangers of false results); F. J. Tedesco *et al.*, *J. Am. med. Ass.*, 1976, *235*, 59 (colonic accumulation in pseudomembranous colitis); A. H. Niden *et al.*, *J. Am. med. Ass.*, 1977, *237*, 1206 (differential diagnosis of pulmonary embolism and pneumonitis); O. J. Rheingold *et al.*, *Dig. Dis. Scis.*, 1979, *24*, 363 (inflammatory bowel disease); J. A. Robinson *et al.*, *Ann. intern. Med.*, 1979, *90*, 198 (diagnosis of acute myocardial inflammation).

Preparations

Gallium Citrate Ga 67 Injection *(U.S.P.)*. A sterile aqueous solution, suitable for intravenous administration, of radioactive, essentially carrier-free, gallium citrate (^{67}Ga); it may contain a preservative or stabiliser. pH 4.5 to 8. At the time stated on the label it contains 90 to 110% of the labelled amount of gallium-67, as citrate. Not less than 99% of the total radioactivity is present as gallium-67 and other chemical forms of radioactivity do not exceed 15% of the total radioactivity. Use within 2 weeks of the time of manufacture.

5859-y

Gold-198 ($^{198}_{79}$Au)

HALF-LIFE. 65 hours (2.7 days)

RADIATION EMITTED. β^- 0.29 (1.2%), 0.96 (98.8%), 1.37 (0.025%) MeV; γ 0.412 (95.8%), 0.68 (1.0%), 1.09 (0.2%) MeV.

SUPPLY. Gold-198 is supplied as sterile colloidal suspensions of metallic gold stabilised with gelatin and dextrose for therapeutic or diagnostic use and containing 37 to 740 megabecquerels (1 to 20 millicuries) per mg of gold, or as gold-198 grains coated with platinum to prevent beta emission.

Adverse Effects and Precautions. Gold-198 should not be used in patients with ulcerative tumours, unhealed wounds, open cavities, or evidence of loculation.

Chromosome damage has been reported in patients given intra-articular injections of gold-198.

Striking black pigmentation of the synovial membrane observed in a woman undergoing replacement arthroplasty of the knee, and demonstrated to be due to the presence of gold in the synovium, was related to earlier intra-articular therapy with a gold-198 injection.— K. P. H. Pritzker *et al., Arthritis Rheum.*, 1980, *23*, 496.

Uses. Gold-198, as Colloidal Gold (^{198}Au) Injection with most of the activity associated with particles of diameter 5 to 20 nm, has been used in the treatment of malignant ascites and malignant pleural effusion in doses of up to 9250 MBq (250 millicuries) by intrapleural or intraperitoneal injection. However, this form of therapy is less commonly used because the patient constitutes a radiation hazard and antineoplastic agents instilled similarly appear to be equally effective. It has also been used in the treatment of rheumatoid arthritis.

The above injection has also been given intravenously in doses of 0.37 to 7.4 MBq (10 to 200 microcuries) for the measurement of liver blood flow, in liver scanning (the particles being taken up by the Kupffer cells), and for general investigations of the reticuloendothelial system. Since the gamma-ray energies are not particularly good for scanning and the radiation dose to the patient is relatively high, it has generally been superseded by more suitable agents such as technetium-99m-labelled compounds.

Gold-198 grains are used for direct implantation into tissues for various therapeutic radiation therapies.

The treatment of infantile subglottic haemangioma with a radioactive gold grain.— B. Benjamin, *Ann. Otol. Rhinol. Lar.*, 1978, *87*, 18.

Malignant neoplasms of the brain. Intrathecal colloidal gold-198 was used to prevent central nervous system leukaemia in 26 children with acute leukaemia. Of 23 who remained free of CNS recurrences, 16 were alive 3–39 months after treatment while 7 died from the underlying disease. In general 74 MBq (2 millicuries) was injected via a lumbar puncture and was well tolerated.— O. Metz *et al., Dt. med. Wschr.*, 1977, *102*, 43.

Further references: *J. Am. med. Ass.*, 1968, *206*, 751.

For a report on the use of pituitary implants of gold-198 in patients with Nelson's syndrome, see Yttrium-90, p.1400.

Malignant neoplasms of the ovary. The 5-year survival-rate in 74 patients with stage II malignant epithelial tumours of the ovary treated with intraperitoneal instillation of colloidal gold (^{198}Au) was 54.1% compared with 40% for 86 receiving external radiation. There was no significant difference for patients with stage I disease.— P. Kolstad *et al., Am. J. Obstet. Gynec.*, 1977, *128*, 617.

Further references: M. S. Piver, *Obstet. Gynec.*, 1972, *40*, 42.

Rheumatoid arthritis. Persistent knee effusions in 112 knees were treated with intra-articular injections of colloidal gold-198 in doses of 148 to 370 MBq (4 to 10 millicuries). Improvement was noted after 3 months and was at a maximum at 6 months, but recurrences were frequent after 2 years. Reactive synovitis occurred in 33% of the patients and there was an average escape of 14% of radioactive material to regional lymph nodes. A dose of 111 to 222 MBq (3 to 6 millicuries) was now used.— J. R. Topp *et al., Can. med. Ass. J.*, 1975, *112*, 1085.

Further references: M. Virkkunen *et al., Acta rheum. scand.*, 1967, *13*, 81.

Wilson's disease. The use of gold-198 in liver scans to monitor the response to penicillamine of a patient with Wilson's disease.— T. Chajek, *Postgrad. med. J.*, 1974, *50*, 56.

Preparations

Colloidal Gold (^{198}Au) Injection *(B.P., Eur. P.)*. Gold (^{198}Au) Injection; Auri Colloidalis (^{198}Au) Solutio Iniectabilis. A dark red, sterile, apyrogenic, colloidal solution of gold-198 stabilised with gelatin and containing various reducing substances such as anhydrous dextrose or dextrose monohydrate for parenteral use, or ascorbic acid. pH 4 to 8. It contains 90 to 110% of the content of gold-198 activity stated on the label at the date and hour stated on the label; about 80% of the radioactivity is present in particles within the stated range of particle size, typically 5 to 50 nm, 5 to 10 nm, and 20 to 40 nm diameter. The solution is sterilised by autoclaving. The content of gold-199 [half-life: 3.15 days; β and γ emission] does not exceed 10% of the total radioactivity. Not less than 98% of the total radioactivity is present as colloidal gold. *Dose.* In the treatment of neoplastic conditions, up to 9250 MBq (250 millicuries), by intrapleural or intraperitoneal injection.

Gold Au 198 Injection *(U.S.P.)*. A sterile colloidal solution of radioactive gold-198 stabilised with gelatin and suitable reducing agents. pH 4.3 to 7.5. It contains 90 to 110% of the labelled amount of gold-198 as colloidal gold, at the time indicated in the labelling. Use within 8 days of the date of manufacture. The label indicates whether the material is intended for diagnostic or therapeutic use. It must not be used if the colour has changed from distinctly red.

5860-g

Indium-111 ($^{111}_{49}$In)

HALF-LIFE. 67 hours (2.8 days)

RADIATION EMITTED. EC (100%); γ 0.171 (90.9%), 0.245 (94.2%) MeV; X-rays (cadmium) 0.023 to 0.027 (~84%) MeV.

SUPPLY. Indium-111 is supplied as a complex of indium (^{111}In) with bleomycin sulphate in the form of a carrier-free injection, iso-osmotic with serum, containing 40.7 MBq (1.1 millicurie) per ml. Indium-111 is also supplied as a complex of indium (^{111}In) with calcium trisodium pentetate (calcium DTPA) in the form of a carrier-free injection, iso-osmotic with serum, containing 24.05 megabecquerels (0.65 millicuries) per ml or as a complex of indium (^{111}In) with pentetic acid (DTPA) in the form of a carrier-free injection, iso-osmotic with serum, containing 37 megabecquerels (1 millicurie) per ml.

Adverse Effects.

A report of aseptic meningitis following the use of indium (^{111}In) complexed with pentetic acid in the cisternography of a patient with dementia.— G. Forster *et al., Clin. Neurol. Neurosurg.*, 1975, *78*, 289.

Uses. Indium-111 as indium (^{111}In) bleomycin injection is used for the detection of tumours in doses of 74 to 185 MBq (2 to 5 millicuries) intravenously which provide no more than 4 to 10 mg of bleomycin.

Indium-111 as indium (^{111}In) complexed with calcium trisodium pentetate is used in diagnostic scintigraphy in cerebrospinal fluid studies, cisternography, and ventriculography. The usual dose is 18.5 to 37 MBq (0.5 to 1 millicuries) administered by intrathecal, intracisternal, or intraventricular injection, or by injection into neurosurgical shunts.

Platelets labelled with indium-111-hydroxyquinoline have been used for the detection of thrombi and other haematological disorders and leucocytes similarly labelled with indium-111-hydroxyquinoline have been used in the detection of abscesses and infectious diseases.

Colloids have been prepared using indium chloride (^{111}In) solution and have been used for investigation of the lymphatic system.

Detection of thrombi. A preliminary study on the use of indium-111 labelled platelets in the diagnosis of leg-vein thrombosis. In 8 patients studied the results from this method correlated precisely with the sites of venous thrombi identified by ascending venography.— A. Fenech *et al., Br. med. J.*, 1980, *280*, 1571.

Further references: H. H. Davis *et al., Lancet*, 1978, *1*, 1185; D. A. Goodwin *et al., J. nucl. Med.*, 1978, *19*, 626.

Diagnosis of abscesses and infection. The use of indium-111-labelled leucocytes for the localisation of abscesses.— A. W. Segal *et al., Lancet*, 1976, *2*, 1056.

The diagnosis of cerebral abscesses with indium-111-labelled leucocytes.— A. M. Peters *et al.* (letter), *Lancet*, 1980, *2*, 309.

Further references: M. Thakur *et al., J. nucl. Med.*, 1977, *18*, 1014.

Diagnosis of transplant rejection. A report of the successful detection of postoperative rejection episodes following renal transplantation, using autologous platelets labelled with indium-111-hydroxyquinoline. Rejection, which occurred in 3 of 17 patients studied, was associated with deposition of labelled platelets in the transplanted kidney, as visualised by the gamma camera.— N. Smith *et al.* (letter), *Lancet*, 1979, *2*, 1241.

The use of autologous indium-111-labelled platelets helped to diagnose a probable haematoma in a patient who had received a renal transplant. Acute rejection had been suspected, to be demonstrated by abnormal platelet accumulation within the kidney, but, in fact, abnormal accumulation of platelets was found above the kidney.— A. Fenech *et al.* (letter), *Lancet*, 1980, *1*, 1250.

A study indicating that autologous indium-111-hydroxyquinoline-labelled platelets are useful in the diagnosis of chronic, as well as acute, rejection of transplanted kidneys.— C. Leithner *et al.* (letter), *Lancet*, 1980, *2*, 213.

5861-q

Indium-113m ($^{113m}_{49}$In)

HALF-LIFE. 99.5 minutes

RADIATION EMITTED. IT (100%); γ 0.392 (64.9%); X-rays (indium) 0.024 to 0.028 (~24%) MeV.

SUPPLY. Indium-113m is a daughter of tin-113 ($^{113}_{50}$Sn, half-life 115 days, γ- and X-radiation) and because of its short half-life is normally prepared just before use by elution from a sterile generator consisting of tin-113 adsorbed on an ion-exchange material contained in a column. Indium-113m is obtained by elution with a standardised dilute solution of hydrochloric acid. Columns containing 185, 370, 740, 925, 1110, 1480, 1850, and 3700 megabecquerels (5, 10, 20, 25, 30, 40, 50, and 100 millicuries) of tin-113 are available and they have a useful life of at least 6 months.

Radiopharmaceuticals of indium-113m are prepared shortly after elution to reduce loss by decay.

Uses. Indium-113m is used for labelling a variety of materials with differing physical properties suited to scanning procedures for various organs and tissues. The short half-life of indium-113m and its lack of β-emission allow large doses to be given with a small radiation dose to the patient.

High count-rates for scanning are therefore achieved.

For lung scanning, indium-113m is incorporated into particulate matter of a suitable particle size, usually 30 to 60 μm, so that when a suspension is injected intravenously the particles become trapped in lung capillaries. The most widely used are indium-113m incorporated in particles of ferric hydroxide and human serum albumin stabilised with zirconium sulphate. Care must be taken in the preparation of the injections because particles of the incorrect size may easily be produced. Ferric hydroxide appears to produce unpleasant reactions in some patients and serious reactions have occasionally been attributed to it. The usual dose is 37 to 74 MBq (1 to 2 millicuries).

A colloidal form of indium-113m can be prepared by adding ferric chloride and mannitol to the eluate from a generator and adjusting the pH to neutrality. This colloid is taken up by the reticuloendothelial cells, including the Kupffer cells of the liver, and is suitable for liver and spleen scanning. The usual dose for liver scanning is 37 to 148 MBq (1 to 4 millicuries) and up to 370 MBq (10 millicuries) is used for bone-marrow studies.

An eluted ionic chloride which labels plasma transferrin is used for location of blood 'pools', such as in the placenta or heart. The usual dose in placentography is 9.25 to 37 MBq (0.25 to 1 millicuries) and in cardiac blood pool scintigraphy about 74 MBq (2 millicuries).

A chelate of indium-113m with pentetic acid is used for brain scanning and for renal-function studies. Doses of up to 370 MBq (10 millicuries) are used.

Preparations

Indium Chlorides In 113m Injection *(U.S.P.).* A sterile aqueous solution, suitable for intravenous administration, of radioactive indium (^{113m}In) in the form of indium chloride; it may contain antimicrobial and buffering agents. pH 1.5 to 2. At the time indicated on the label it contains 90 to 110% of the stated amount of indium-113m, as the chloride. Other chemical forms of radioactivity do not exceed 5% of the total radioactivity. It contains not more than 3.7 kBq (0.1 microcurie) of tin-113 for each 37 MBq (1 millicurie) of indium-113m and not more than 18.5 kBq (0.5 microcurie) per administered dose, with similar limits for other gamma-emitting radionuclidic impurities. Use within 8 hours of manufacture.

5862-p

Iodine-123 ($^{123}_{53}$I)

HALF-LIFE. 13.2 hours

RADIATION EMITTED. EC (100%); γ 0.159 (83%), 0.347 (0.10%), 0.440 (0.35%), 0.506 (0.26%), 0.529 (1.05%), 0.539 (0.27%) MeV; X-rays (tellurium) 0.027 to 0.032 (~86%) MeV.

SUPPLY. Iodine-123 is supplied as sodium iodide (^{123}I) in the form of an injection, iso-osmotic with serum, containing 185 to 1480 megabecquerels (5 to 40 millicuries) per μg of iodine. It is also supplied as sodium iodohippurate (^{123}I) in the form of an injection, iso-osmotic with serum, containing 5.55 to 22.2 megabecquerels (150 to 600 microcuries) per mg of sodium iodohippurate.

Adverse Effects and Precautions. As for Iodine-131, p.1392.

Uses. The principal uses of iodine-123 are similar to those of iodine-131 (see p.1393). Iodine-123, as sodium iodide (^{123}I) injection is used in usual doses of 9.25 to 18.5 MBq (250 to 500 microcuries) in thyroid scanning. Sodium iodohippurate (^{123}I) injection in usual doses of 18.5 to 37 MBq (0.5 to 1 millicurie) is employed in tests of renal function.

The use of iodine-123-labelled 16-iodo-9-hexadecenoic acid ($C_{16}H_{29}IO_2$=380.3) in myocardial imaging.— N. D. Poe *et al.*, *Radiology*, 1977, *124*, 419.

The detection of atherosclerotic plaques in carotid arteries using fibrinogen labelled with iodine-123.— K. L. Mettinger *et al.*, *Lancet*, 1978, *1*, 242.

Thyroid-function tests. A review and discussion on the evaluation of diseases of the thyroid gland with the *in vivo* use of radionuclides suggesting that radionuclides delivering the lowest radiation dose, such as iodine-123, should be used whenever possible.— Task Force on Short-lived Radionuclides for Medical Applications, *J. nucl. Med.*, 1978, *19*, 107.

Further references: S. Rosenthal *et al.*, *J. nucl. Med.*, 1976, *17*, 1050; E. T. Wong and A. L. Schultz, *J. Am. med. Ass.*, 1977, *238*, 1741.

Preparations

Sodium Iodide I 123 Capsules *(U.S.P.).* Contain radioactive iodine (^{123}I) processed in the form of sodium iodide in such a manner that it is carrier-free. At the time stated on the label each capsule contains 90 to 110% of the amount of iodine-123 (as iodide) stated on the label. Other chemical forms of radioactivity do not exceed 5% of the total radioactivity. Not less than 93.3% of the total radioactivity is present as iodine-123. The capsules may contain a stabiliser. Use within 48 hours of the time of manufacture.

Sodium Iodide I 123 Solution *(U.S.P.).* A solution, suitable for oral or intravenous administration, containing radioactive iodine (^{123}I) processed in the form of sodium iodide in such manner that it is carrier-free. At the time stated on the label it contains 90 to 110% of the content of iodine-123 (as iodide) stated on the label. Other chemical forms of radioactivity do not exceed 5% of the total radioactivity. Not less than 85% of the total radioactivity is present as iodine-123. It may contain a preservative or stabiliser. If intended for intravenous use the solution is sterile. pH 7.5 to 9. Use within 48 hours of the time of manufacture.

5863-s

Iodine-125 ($^{125}_{53}$I)

HALF-LIFE. 60 days

RADIATION EMITTED. EC (100%); γ 0.035 (7%) MeV; X-rays (tellurium) 0.027 to 0.032 (138%) MeV.

SUPPLY. Iodine-125 is supplied in a large variety of forms.

Adverse Effects. As for Iodine-131, p.1392.

Pregnancy and the neonate. It was considered that the total intake of iodine by infants fed by mothers who had undergone blood-volume studies using iodine-125 at the time of delivery increased by 10 times the risk that the child would subsequently develop cancer of the thyroid.— E. P. Bland *et al.*, *Lancet*, 1969, *2*, 1039. See also A. B. W. Taylor (letter), *Br. med. J.*, 1973, *1*, 614.

Precautions. As for Iodine-131, p.1393.

It was considered that the administration of potassium iodide 60 mg at least one hour before the commencement of an investigation using ^{125}I-fibrinogen followed by 60 mg thrice weekly for the following 4 weeks to block the thyroid uptake of radio-iodine kept the radiological hazard to the thyroid to an absolute minimum.— W. R. Greig and C. R. M. Prentice (letter), *Br. med. J.*, 1978, *1*, 860.

Interference with diagnostic tests. Patients who had received a macroaggregated iodinated (^{131}I) human albumin injection for the detection of pulmonary embolisms could show false negative results to iodine-125 labelled fibrinogen tests for venous thrombosis due to the percentage increase in iodine-125 activity at the thrombus being masked by the total reading of radioactivity.— C. Warlow and A. S. Douglas (letter), *Lancet*, 1972, *2*, 1196.

Use in thyroid disorders. There was complete recovery of thyroid function in one patient more than 4 years after apparent radiodestruction with iodine-125. Long-term follow-up of such patients appeared necessary.— J. G. Turner *et al.* (letter), *Lancet*, 1977, *2*, 410.

Uses. The principal uses of iodine-125 are similar to those of iodine-131 (p.1393). Iodine-125 is not very suitable for the external counting of radioactivity in the thyroid gland because its γ-energy is weak and tissue absorption is high. However, it is very suitable for assays *in vitro* and because it has a long half-life it is preferred as a label for many compounds. It is common practice to saturate the thyroid with non-radioactive iodine when uptake of radiation by the thyroid is not desired.

Iodine-125, as iodinated (^{125}I) human fibrinogen injection, is used in a dose of 3.7 MBq (100 microcuries) to demonstrate and locate deep vein thrombosis of the leg. Iodinated (^{125}I) fibrinogen has also been used in the measurement of fibrinogen metabolism in certain disturbances of blood coagulation. To reduce the risk of transmitting serum hepatitis, the fibrinogen is obtained from plasma from small pools of donors who have been tested for hepatitis B antigen and found negative.

The use of Iodinated (^{125}I) Albumin Injection is described under Iodine-131, p.1393.

Sodium iothalamate (^{125}I) injection is used in doses of 0.185 to 1.85 MBq (5 to 50 microcuries) intravenously in the determination of glomerular filtration-rate. Sodium iodohippurate (^{125}I), specially purified to contain minimal amounts of free iodide, is given in doses of 0.185 to 1.85 MBq (5 to 50 microcuries) intravenously for the measurement of effective renal plasma flow.

Iodinated povidone (^{125}I) injection in doses of 185 to 925 kBq (5 to 25 microcuries) administered intravenously is used for the diagnosis of protein-losing gastro-intestinal disorders and for permeability studies.

Iodine-125 may also be used as a solution of sodium iodide (^{125}I), suitable for oral adminstration, in the diagnosis of thyroid disorders. The usual dose is 1.85 to 3.7 MBq (50 to 100 microcuries).

Iodinated (^{125}I) rose bengal sodium injection has been used intravenously for estimations of liver function.

Liothyronine (^{125}I) is available as a solution and as a kit for tests *in vitro* of thyroid function such as the liothyronine (T_3) uptake test. Thyroxine (^{125}I) is used similarly.

Many other compounds labelled with iodine-125 are available for *in vitro* assays to detect and estimate drugs and hormones in body fluids.

A review of the RadioImmunoSorbent Test (RIST) and the RadioAllergoSorbent Test (RAST). These tests were expensive and could only confirm, not replace, history, examination and skin tests in patients with allergic disorders. They were of most value in research, being unlikely to influence the treatment of individual patients. The RAST might become important in the standardisation of vaccines intended for hyposensitisation and for skin tests.— *Drug & Ther. Bull.*, 1976, *14*, 79.

A radioimmunoassay using iodine-125 labelled IgE anti-penicillin antibodies for the detection of penicillin allergy.— V. Ureña *et al.* (letter), *Lancet*, 1977, *1*, 1210.

Iodine-125 was involved in a radioimmunoassay for detecting schistosomiasis due to *Schistosoma mansoni*.— R. P. Pelley *et al.*, *Lancet*, 1977, *2*, 781.

The successful adaptation of the Coombs antiglobulin test for the diagnosis of immune thrombocytopenia by labelling the antiglobulin reagent with iodine-125. The modified test should be of general use in assessing antibody and complement interaction with many cell surfaces.— D. B. Cines and A. D. Schreiber, *New Engl. J. Med.*, 1979, *300*, 106.

Detection of thrombi. A review of the use of iodinated (^{125}I) fibrinogen in the diagnosis of thromboembolism. False-positive results may occur with haematomas and other conditions such as ulcers, fractures, or inflammatory exudates that cause deposition of fibrin. Little fibrinogen is taken up by thrombi more than 4 to 5 days old and in patients receiving anticoagulants and this may lead to false-negative results. The test is unreliable in the areas of the thighs and pelvis due to the large tissue mass.— *Med. Lett.*, 1978, *20*, 63.

A report of early experience with a new technique, the (^{125}I) fibrinogen sum-coincidence method, for the determination of the depth and extent of deep-vein thrombosis. Of 141 patients studied by this method the conventional (^{125}I) fibrinogen-uptake test was positive in 24, and in these the (^{125}I) fibrinogen sum-coincidence test detected and localised 28 thrombi, which was virtually in complete agreement with results by phlebography. The new technique decreases the number of phlebographies needed for detecting deep-vein thrombi after surgery, permits repeated follow-ups of detected deep-vein thrombi, and permits the monitoring of the course of even small thrombi and the effect of treatment.— U. Ulmsten *et al.* (letter), *Lancet*, 1979, *2*, 962.

Further reports and comments on the use of iodinated (^{125}I) fibrinogen in the detection of thrombi: J. R. Loudon, *Br. med. J.*, 1976, *2*, 793; R. F. Carretta *et al.*, *J. nucl. Med.*, 1977, *18*, 5; G. L. DeNardo *et al.*, *Radiology*, 1977, *125*, 765; G. K. Morris and J. R. A. Mitchell, *Br. med. J.*, 1977, *1*, 264; K. M. Moser *et al.*, *J. Am. med. Ass.*, 1977, *237*, 2195.

Malignant neoplasms of the prostate. Early results indicated that implanted seeds of iodine-125 were of use in the treatment of prostatic carcinoma. It was considered that a 15-year follow-up was needed to evaluate effectiveness.— *Med. Lett.*, 1977, *19*, 92.

Thyrotoxicosis. In a study involving 355 patients with hyperthyroidism reviewed over an average of 49 months, treatment with iodine-125 in doses ranging from 0.15 to 2.1 MBq (4 to 56 microcuries) produced a euthyroid state in 225 patients, a hypothyroid state in 119, and a hyperthyroid state in 11. Iodine-131 should be used for routine treatment.— I. R. McDougall and W. R. Greig, *Ann. intern. Med.*, 1976, *85*, 720. A disagreement that iodine-131 is the isotope of choice for the routine treatment of Graves' disease. It was considered that short-term hypothyroidism was uncommon after treatment with iodine-125.— E. C. Abbott and R. Martin (letter), *ibid.*, 1977, *87*, 797.

Further references: S. C. Werner *et al.*, *Lancet*, 1970, *2*, 681; J. K. Siemsen *et al.*, *J. nucl. Med.*, 1974, *15*, 257; P. Weidinger *et al.*, *Lancet*, 1974, *2*, 74; I. Doniach (letter), *ibid.*, 1975, *1*, 870.

Preparations

Iodinated (^{125}I) Albumin Injection *(B.P.)*. Iodinated (^{125}I) Human Albumin Injection; 125-Radio-iodinated Human Serum Albumin; IHA (^{125}I) Inj. A clear, colourless or faintly yellow, sterile, iso-osmotic saline solution of albumin which has been iodinated with iodine-125 and subsequently freed from ^{125}I iodide. pH 6.5 to 8.5. It contains not less than 1% of protein, a suitable bactericide such as benzyl alcohol, 0.9% v/v, 85 to 115% of the content of iodine-125 stated on the label at the date stated on the label, and not more than 1% of iodine-126. Other chemical forms of radioactivity do not exceed 5% of the total radioactivity. The albumin, before the addition of any carrier albumin, is uniformly iodinated to an extent that does not exceed the equivalent of 1 atom of iodine for each molecule of albumin. The solution is sterilised by filtration. Store at 2° to 8°. *Dose.* For the determination of plasma volume, 185 kBq (5 microcuries).

Iodinated I 125 Albumin Injection *(U.S.P.)*. Iodinated I 125 Serum Albumin; Radio-iodinated (^{125}I) Serum Albumin (Human). A sterile, buffered, iso-osmotic solution containing albumin radio-iodinated to the extent of not more than 1 atom of iodine for each molecule of albumin, and adjusted to provide not more than 37 MBq (1 millicurie) of activity per ml. It contains 95 to 105% of the labelled amount of iodine-125 as iodinated albumin expressed in microcuries or millicuries at the time indicated on the label; other forms of radioactivity do not exceed 3% of the total radioactivity. pH 7 to 8.5. Store at 2° to 8°. Use within 120 days of the date of completion of iodination.

Sodium Iodide (^{125}I) Solution *(B.P. 1973, Eur. P.)*. Natrii Iodidi (^{125}I) Solutio. A solution suitable for oral administration containing sodium iodide (^{125}I) and sodium thiosulphate or other suitable reducing agents. pH 7 to 10. It contains 85 to 115% of the content of iodine-125 stated on the label at the date stated on the label, and not more than 1% of the total radioactivity is due to iodine-126. It is carrier-free and the specific activity is not less than 74 MBq (2 millicuries) per microgram of iodine at the date stated on the label. *Dose.* For the investigation of thyroid disease, 185 to 925 kBq (5 to 25 microcuries).

Sodium Iodide I 125 Capsules *(U.S.P.)*. Contain radioactive iodine (^{125}I) processed in the form of sodium iodide in such manner that it is carrier-free. At the time stated on the label each capsule contains 90 to 110% of the amount of iodine-125 (as iodide) stated on the label. Other chemical forms of radioactivity do not exceed 5% of the total radioactivity. The capsules may contain a preservative or stabiliser. Use within 6 months of the date of manufacture.

Sodium Iodide I 125 Solution *(U.S.P.)*. A solution for oral or intravenous administration, containing radioactive iodine (^{125}I), processed in the form of sodium iodide in such manner that it is essentially carrier-free. It contains 85 to 115% of the labelled amount of iodine-125 as iodide at the time indicated on the label; other chemical forms of radioactivity do not exceed 5% of the total radioactivity. pH 7.5 to 9. Use within 6 months of the date of manufacture.

For proprietary preparations of iodine-125, see Some Proprietary Test Substances, p.527: Ausab; Ausria II-125; Corab; Gammadisk-Digoxin Test Kit; Havab; Lanoxitest γ; SPAC Digoxin Kit.

5864-w

Iodine-131 ($^{131}_{53}I$)

HALF-LIFE. 8.06 days

RADIATION EMITTED. β^- 0.247 (1.8%), 0.304 (0.6%), 0.334 (7.2%), 0.606 (89.7%), 0.806 (0.7%) MeV; γ 0.08 (2.4%), 0.284 (5.9%), 0.364 (81.8%), 0.637 (7.2%), 0.723 (1.8%) MeV. 1.3% of iodine-131 decays via xenon-131m [half-life: 12 days. IT (100%); γ 0.164 (2%) MeV].

SUPPLY. Iodine-131 is supplied in a large variety of forms.

Adverse Effects. Between 2 and 5% of patients treated with iodine-131 for thyrotoxicosis become hypothyroid each year so that eventually most patients will require thyroid replacement therapy. Hypoparathyroidism has also been reported. Radiation thyroiditis with soreness may develop shortly after treatment. There may be severe and potentially dangerous swelling of the thyroid especially in patients with large goitres and this has on rare occasions produced asphyxiation. Leukaemia and carcinoma of the thyroid have occasionally been reported, particularly in young patients.

In the treatment of thyroid carcinoma, the larger doses of radioactive iodine sometimes cause nausea and vomiting a few days after ingestion, which may be due to gastritis as iodine-131 is also concentrated in gastric mucosa. Large doses depress the bone marrow. Chromosomal aberrations have been reported.

Initial studies indicating an increased radiation exposure of family members of patients treated with iodine-131.— A. P. Jacobson *et al.*, *Am. J. publ. Hlth*, 1978, *68*, 225.

Carcinogenicity. Leukaemia. From a follow-up study of about 32 000 patients who had been treated for hyperthyroidism with iodine-131 or surgery or with both, it appeared that the incidence of leukaemia, up to 19 years later, was not significantly different in those given iodine-131 and in those who underwent surgery, but the incidence was higher in those who had been treated with surgery and iodine-131. The overall incidence of leukaemia was higher than that of the national population and suggested a relationship between hyperthyroidism and leukaemia.— E. L. Saenger *et al.*, *J. Am. med. Ass.*, 1968, *205*, 855. See also E. E. Pochin, *Br. med. J.*, 1960, *2*, 1545.

Although no increased incidence of leukaemia has been reported in patients previously treated with iodine-131 during childhood or adolescence, at present the number of such patients studied is insufficient to determine whether the risk is increased.— C. H. Emerson and L. E. Braverman, *New Engl. J. Med.*, 1980, *303*, 217.

Further references: A. M. Safa *et al.*, *New Engl. J. Med.*, 1975, *292*, 167; J. E. Freitas *et al.*, *J. nucl. Med.*, 1979, *20*, 847.

Thyroid. A discussion on irradiation-related thyroid cancer. It was considered that the use of iodine-131 for diagnostic purposes should be restricted to low doses for uptake studies and should be employed for thyroid imaging only when there are technical limitations to the use of technetium-99m or when documented cases of cancer require total body scanning. It was suggested that the eventual withdrawal of iodine-131 from routine use for imaging be seriously considered and technetium-99m or iodine-123 used instead.— P. G. Walfsh and R. Volpé, *Ann. intern. Med.*, 1978, *88*, 261.

A review and discussion on the adverse effects associated with thyroid irradiation. Although it is now clear that low-dose external irradiation to the thyroid is carcinogenic many studies, in contrast, have failed to reveal an association between iodine-131 therapy for hyperthyroidism and the development of thyroid cancer. It is however important to examine the differences in the settings in which the 2 sources of irradiation occur before concluding that iodine-131 therapy for hyperthyroidism is safe. It has been suggested that the lower incidence in the iodine-131 treated patients is due to the fact that the radiation dose is sufficiently high to destroy the thyroid. Another major difference between the 2 groups is the age of the patient at the time of exposure. In most reports that have associated external irradiation with carcinoma the subjects were treated at an early age whereas the widest experience with iodine-131 has been in adults; observations have indicated that the immature thyroid, probably because of the higher rate of cell mitoses is more likely to have cancer induced by radiation. Thus the impression that external irradiation is more carcinogenic to the thyroid than iodine-131 may be more apparent than real. Although recent studies have reinforced the view that the treatment of choice for older patients with hyperthyroidism is iodine-131 it is considered that this form of therapy should not be recommended for hyperthyroidism in children and adolescents.— C. H. Emerson and L. E. Braverman, *New Engl. J. Med.*, 1980, *303*, 217.

Only 4 of 3000 patients treated with iodine-131 between 1951 and 1965 have subsequently developed malignant thyroid tumours and this is no more than the expected incidence obtained from the Swedish Cancer Registry. Nevertheless continued follow-up is advisable because of the long latency period of radiation-induced thyroid tumours.— L. -E. Holm *et al.*, *New Engl. J. Med.*, 1980, *303*, 188.

Further references: A. M. Safa *et al.*, *New Engl. J. Med.*, 1975, *292*, 167; J. E. Freitas *et al.*, *J. nucl. Med.*, 1979, *20*, 847.

Cytogenetic effects. Since the radiation dose to the testes or ovary following a dose of 370 MBq (10 millicuries) of iodine-131 is similar to or less than that involved in several common roentgenographic diagnostic procedures, it seems unreasonable to deny iodine-131 treatment for hyperthyroidism to young men and non-pregnant young women on the grounds of genetic hazard alone.— J. S. Robertson and C. A. Gorman, *J. nucl. Med.*, 1976, *17*, 826.

Follow-up study of the reproductive history and the health of the offspring of 33 patients who had been treated during childhood or adolescence for papillary-follicular carcinoma of the thyroid revealed that the incidence of infertility, miscarriage, prematurity, and major congenital anomaly was not significantly different from that in the general population. It was concluded that there was no overt evidence of genetic damage in children and adolescents treated with high doses of iodine-131 for thyroid carcinoma.— S. D. Sarkar *et al.*, *J. nucl. Med.*, 1976, *17*, 460. See also A. M. Safa *et al.*, *New Engl. J. Med.*, 1975, *292*, 167; J. E. Freitas *et al.*, *J. nucl. Med.*, 1979, *20*, 847.

Although no increased incidence of birth defects or infertility has been reported in patients previously treated with iodine-131 during childhood or adolescence, at present the number of such patients studied is insufficient to determine whether the risks are increased.— C. H. Emerson and L. E. Braverman, *New Engl. J. Med.*, 1980, *303*, 217.

Effects on speech. A patient given 185 MBq (5 millicuries) of iodine-131 developed vocal chord paresis over the next 5 days. He did not completely recover until 2 months after the radio-iodine therapy.— P. W. T. Craswell, *Br. J. clin. Pract.*, 1972, *26*, 571.

Effects on the thyroid. In a follow-up study of 55 patients who were treated for hyperthyroidism with iodine-131 in doses of 111 MBq (3 millicuries) or less, the incidence of hypothyroidism was 3.7% at the end of the first year. At 5 years the incidence in 45 of the patients was 7.5%, which increased, at an average annual rate of 3.4%, to 48.1% after 17 years.— J. A. Glennon *et al.*, *Ann. intern. Med.*, 1972, *76*, 721.

A study in 13 patients showed an increase in serum concentrations of tri-iodothyronine and thyroxine following treatment with iodine-131. This might explain acute thyroid crisis in some patients treated with radio-iodine.— R. B. Shafer and F. Q. Nuttall, *Lancet*, 1975, *2*, 635.

Evidence to suggest that the incidence of hypothyroidism following usual doses of iodine-131 for toxic diffuse goitre has increased recently compared with the incidence reported about 20 to 25 years ago. Although the pathophysiology of this increase was not known with certainty, it was suggested that the decreased use of thionamide preparations and increases in dietary iodine may render the gland more radiosensitive.— S. E. Von Hofe *et al.*, *J. nucl. Med.*, 1978, *19*, 180.

Transient hypothyroidism in 10 patients after treatment with iodine-131 for hyperthyroidism. Not all patients developing hypothyroidism needed, therefore, to start lifelong treatment with thyroxine.— I. A. MacFarlane *et al., Br. med. J.*, 1979, *2*, 421. See also S. M. Shalet *et al.* (letter), *Lancet*, 1977, *2*, 1356; J. D. Veldhuis (letter), *ibid.*, 1978, *1*, 993.

See also under Carcinogenicity (above) and under Precautions.

Pregnancy and the neonate. Of 182 women who had inadvertently received radio-iodine therapy during pregnancy and had not had their pregnancies terminated the complication-rate was considered to be no greater than normal with 2 spontaneous abortions, 2 stillbirths, one infant with biliary atresia, and another with respiratory distress. However 6 infants were hypothyroid with 4 being mentally handicapped. Three of the mothers of the hypothyroid infants had received radio-iodine during the second trimester. Routine pregnancy testing should be carried out where appropriate before radio-iodine.— S. S. Stoffer and J. I. Hamburger, *J. nucl. Med.*, 1976, *17*, 146.

See also under Cytogenetic Effects (above) and under Precautions.

Precautions. The use of sodium iodide (^{131}I) is contra-indicated, even in diagnostic doses, during pregnancy and lactation. Children are very sensitive to thyroid irradiation and should not be given iodine-131. Sodium iodide (^{131}I) should not be given to patients with large toxic nodular goitres or to patients with severe thyrotoxic heart disease.

Many drugs have been reported to interfere with thyroid- or other organ-function studies and checks should be made on any treatment the patient might be receiving before any estimations are carried out.

The National Radiological Protection Board recommended regular thyroid monitoring as well as routine monitoring of skin and clothing for people working with radio-iodine. If an accident occurred thyroid uptake of radio-iodine could be blocked by giving 100 mg of stable iodine by mouth as sodium or potassium iodide or iodate. Spilled radio-iodine should be stabilised by treatment with excess sodium thiosulphate before decontamination.— *Lancet*, 1976, *1*, 133.

Increasing amounts of iodine in the diet were making the 24-hour radioactive iodine uptake test less reliable for diagnosis of hyperthyroidism as seen in one geographical area of the USA.— P. L. Hooper and R. H. Caplan, *J. Am. med. Ass.*, 1977, *238*, 411.

For a report of a macroaggregated iodinated (^{131}I) human albumin injection interfering with the iodine-125 test for venous thrombosis, see Iodine-125, p.1391.

Pregnancy and the neonate. Results from 2 mothers receiving macroaggregated iodinated (^{131}I) albumin indicated that acceptable low levels of radioactivity in breast milk were achieved within 2 weeks of the administration of the radiopharmaceutical.— J. R. Wyburn, *J. nucl. Med.*, 1973, *14*, 115.

Use in thyroid disorders. Of 33 patients who died from thyrotoxicosis 10 had received radio-iodine and in 7 patients this had been given within 3 weeks of death. It was recommended that patients with severe thyrotoxicosis should be given antithyroid compounds before and after radio-iodine.— J. L. W. Parker and D. H. Lawson, *Lancet*, 1973, *2*, 894.

A discussion of the thyroid status of 105 patients who had been treated 2 to 18 years earlier with radioactive iodine for thyrotoxicosis and of the difficulties of assessing thyroid status. Of the 85 patients who became euthyroid, 39 (46%) had elevated thyrotrophic hormone concentrations but this was no indication of potential hypothyroidism. No euthyroid patient was hypothyroid at 1 year.— W. M. G. Tunbridge *et al., Br. med. J.*, 1974, *3*, 89. From a 5-year study in 130 patients who had received iodine-131 for thyrotoxicosis it was considered that euthyroid patients with a normal serum-thyrotrophin concentration should be reviewed every 3 years, while those with a raised serum-thyrotrophin concentration, associated with a higher risk of hypothyroidism, be reviewed yearly as at present.— A. D. Toft *et al., ibid.*, 1978, *2*, 1115. The data presented did not justify the conclusions.— A. J. Hedley and J. C. G. Pearson (letter), *ibid.*, 1569. Results indicating that an isolated elevated tri-iodothyronine concentration following iodine-131 therapy for thyrotoxicosis may be associated with any clinical pattern of thyroid function and has no clear prognostic value. No specific therapy was necessary in such instances.— N. G. Soler *et al., Archs intern. Med.*, 1979, *139*, 36.

Of 43 patients treated with iodine-131 after thyroidectomy, 19 became hypothyroid. Thyroidectomy appeared to sensitise patients to radio-iodine.— W. J. Kalk *et al., Lancet*, 1978, *1*, 291.

Uses. Iodine radioisotopes are mainly used in studies of thyroid function and in the treatment of thyrotoxicosis, some forms of thyroid carcinoma, and occasionally in intractable angina pectoris. They are also used for tests on the function of the heart, kidneys, and liver, and on fat absorption or protein loss from the gastro-intestinal tract. They can be incorporated into liothyronine and thyroxine, triglycerides and fatty acids, such as triolein and oleic acid, and proteins, such as iodinated human albumin, with varying degrees of stability and with little or no change in the biological activity of the labelled molecule.

It is common practice to saturate the thyroid with non-radioactive iodine when uptake of radiation by the thyroid is not desired.

USES OF IODINATED HUMAN ALBUMIN. Human albumin iodinated with iodine-125 or iodine-131 is employed, usually in doses of 37 to 185 kBq (1 to 5 microcuries), in the determination of the plasma volume and doses of 1.85 to 3.7 MBq (50 to 100 microcuries) are employed in other circulatory investigations. Human serum albumin iodinated with iodine-125 is often preferred for these measurements, as the dose to the patient is less than with iodine-131. Both forms have also been used in ventriculography, cisternography, and myeloscintigraphy, and for the investigation of hydrocephalus and other disorders, but because of the β-energy of iodine-131 and the protein content of the injections these preparations are not usually recommended for such procedures and an injection containing indium (^{111}In) complexed with pentetic acid (see indium-111, p.1390) is generally preferred.

A form of iodinated (^{131}I) human albumin, in which the albumin is aggregated by denaturing, has been used by intravenous injection for lung scanning. The particle sizes are such that the majority of particles are trapped for a period in the lung capillaries. Doses of about 11.1 MBq (300 microcuries) have usually been employed. As the radiation dose to the patient is higher than with other labelled particles (see technetium-99m, p.1396) and the γ-energy is not very suitable for measurement with gamma scintillation cameras its use for lung scanning has been largely superseded by other agents.

USES OF SODIUM IODIDE (^{131}I). Sodium Iodide (^{131}I) Solution is given by mouth in studies of thyroid function, particularly in measurements of the uptake of iodine by the thyroid, and in thyroid scanning. The usual dose is from 0.185 to 3.7 MBq (5 to 100 microcuries). It is also used in the treatment of thyrotoxicosis in doses of 37 to 555 MBq (1 to 15 millicuries), according to the dose regimen adopted. Doses of about 3700 to 5550 MBq (100 to 150 millicuries) are employed in the treatment of malignant neoplasm of the thyroid and 370 to 1480 MBq (10 to 40 millicuries) may be used to reduce thyroid activity in patients with angina pectoris or heart failure.

Sodium iodide (^{131}I) capsules containing Sodium Iodide (^{131}I) Solution absorbed on an inert carrier are given by mouth in routine investigations of thyroid function; a colour code on the capsules identifies the activity on different days in relation to a standard.

Sodium Iodide (^{131}I) Injection is given intravenously in investigations of thyroid function, usually in a dose of 0.185 to 3.7 MBq (5 to 100 microcuries).

OTHER USES OF IODINE-131. Sodium Iodohippurate (^{131}I) Injection is used intravenously in renography in usual doses of 0.37 to 3.7 MBq (10 to 100 microcuries). A special grade of sodium iodohippurate (^{131}I) injection is available for the determination of effective renal plasma flow and is given in usual doses of 0.185 to 1.85 MBq (5 to 50 microcuries).

Rose bengal sodium (^{131}I) injection is given intravenously in tests of liver function. The usual dose is 185 to 925 kBq (5 to 25 microcuries) and for liver scintigraphy a dose of 5.55 to 11.1 MBq (150 to 300 microcuries) is employed.

An injection containing 6β-iodomethyl-19-norcholest-5(10)-en-3β-ol labelled with iodine-131 is available for adrenal scintigraphy and is given in usual doses of 18.5 to 55.5 MBq (0.5 to 1.5 millicuries).

Iodinated (^{131}I) povidone injection has been given intravenously as an aid to the diagnosis of protein-losing enteropathy.

Various solutions and test kits containing iodine-131 labelled compounds are also available for *in vitro* thyroid function studies.

For the effect of lithium carbonate increasing the uptake of iodine-131 in the thyroid, see Lithium Carbonate, p.1542.

The advantages of iodine-131-labelled sodium iodohippurate over intravenous pyelography to screen for renal hypertension.— T. M. Erwteman and J. Roos (letter), *Lancet*, 1980, *2*, 800.

Malignant neoplasm of the thyroid. A recommendation on the use of thyroid hormone and ablation with iodine-131 following surgery.— *Lancet*, 1977, *2*, 694.

A prospective study of iodine-131 following thyroidectomy in 54 patients with thyroid cancer. Ablation with iodine-131 was considered safe and effective.— G. T. Krishnamurthy and W. H. Blahd, *Cancer*, 1977, *40*, 195.

Further references: J. K. Harness *et al., Archs Surg., Chicago*, 1974, *108*, 410; B. Singh *et al., J. nucl. Med.*, 1974, *15*, 674; K. D. McCowen *et al., Am. J. Med.*, 1976, *61*, 52; S. C. N. T. Fui *et al., Br. med. J.*, 1979, *2*, 298.

Organ scanning. *Adrenal.* Location of aldosterone-producing adenomas with ^{131}I-19-iodocholesterol.— M. J. Hogan *et al., New Engl. J. Med.*, 1976, *294*, 410. See also L. M. Lieberman *et al., New Engl. J. Med* 1971, *285*, 1387; H. Kehlet *et al., Br. med. J.*, 1976, *2*, 665.

Experience with ^{131}I-6β-iodomethyl-19-norcholest-5(10)-en-3β-ol (NP-59) in 29 patients with a variety of adrenal disorders and in 4 patients without known adrenal disease indicated that the agent was particularly useful in evaluating primary aldosteronism and selected cases of Cushing's syndrome. The data also suggested that this agent has a considerable advantage over ^{131}I-19-iodocholesterol in the evaluation of adrenocortical disease.— J. M. Miles *et al., Mayo Clin. Proc.*, 1979, *54*, 321. See also U. Y. Ryo *et al., Radiology*, 1978, *128*, 157; J. E. Carey *et al., J. nucl. Med.*, 1979, *20*, 60; J. E. Freitas *et al., ibid.*, 7.

Gonads. The use of ^{131}I-6β-iodomethyl-19-norcholest-5(10)-en-3β-ol (NP 59) to demonstrate bilateral testicular Leydig cell tumours in a man with Nelson's syndrome and a Leydig cell tumour of the ovary in a woman with a virilising syndrome.— P. C. Carpenter *et al., Mayo Clin. Proc.*, 1979, *54*, 332.

Parathyroid. The use of technetium-99m and iodine-131 in the diagnosis of parathyroid adenoma in a 60-year-old woman.— K. Alagumalai *et al., Ann. intern. Med.*, 1979, *90*, 204.

Thyrotoxicosis. Sodium iodide (^{131}I) treatment in low dosage was supplemented with antithyroid drugs when necessary when given to patients with Graves' disease to prevent iodide-induced hypothyroidism. Of 85 patients studied, 46 were hyperthyroid, 33 were euthyroid, and 6 were hypothyroid on withdrawal of antithyroid drugs after 1 year. Of the 46 hyperthyroid patients 17 remained hyperthyroid at the end of the second year despite the fact that 28 had received a second dose of radioactive iodine. Low-dose treatment was not considered a satisfactory treatment for Graves' disease.— B. Rapoport *et al., J. Am. med. Ass.*, 1973, *224*, 1610. In an attempt to reduce unsatisfactory rates of residual hyperthyroidism associated with administration of low doses of radioactive iodine in Graves' disease, a gland-size related dose was used in a study involving 62 patients. One year after therapy 41 patients were euthyroid, 15 were hyperthyroid, and 6 were hypothyroid. The initial free thyroxine index might be used as a guide to the response.— C. P. Roudebush *et al., Ann. intern. Med.*, 1977, *87*, 441. Criticism of the formula used for dose calculation.— N. G. Schneeberg (letter), *ibid.*, 1978, *88*, 580. Reply.— L. J. DeGroot, *ibid.*

A retrospective study involving 229 patients with hyperthyroidism due to Graves' disease indicated that a large initial dose of sodium iodide(^{131}I) was the most effective therapy. Thyroid hormone replacement therapy was given after the hyperthyroidism had been controlled to prevent the development of hypothyroidism.— A. M. Safa and P. G. Skillern, *Archs intern. Med.*, 1975, *135*, 673.

A long-term follow-up study over 5 to 24 years was carried out on 87 patients with an original diagnosis of Graves' disease with hyperthyroidism who had been treated with iodine-131 when they were 18 years old or younger. Hyperthyroidism was controlled in all but 2, but hypothyroidism developed in 35 of 76 patients evaluated for thyroid function. There was no evidence of thyroid carcinoma or leukaemia in any patient or their 86 offspring and the fertility and spontaneous abortion-rates were no different from those of the general public.— A. M. Safa *et al.*, *New Engl. J. Med.*, 1975, *292*, 167. See also J. E. Freitas *et al.*, *J. nucl. Med.*, 1979, *20*, 847.

Preparations

Iodinated (^{131}I) Albumin Injection *(B.P.).* Iodinated (^{131}I) Human Albumin Injection; 131-Radio-iodinated Human Albumin; IHA (^{131}I) Inj. A clear, colourless or faintly yellow, sterile, iso-osmotic saline solution of albumin which has been iodinated with iodine-131 and subsequently freed from ^{131}I iodide. pH 6.5 to 8.5. It contains not less than 1% of protein, a suitable bactericide such as benzyl alcohol, 0.9% v/v, 90 to 110% of the content of iodine-131 stated on the label at the date and hour stated on the label, and not more than 55.5 MBq (1.5 millicuries) of iodine-131 per ml at the date and hour stated on the label. Other chemical forms of radioactivity do not exceed 5% of the total radioactivity. The albumin, before the addition of any carrier albumin, is uniformly iodinated to an extent that does not exceed the equivalent of one atom of iodine for each molecule of albumin. The solution is sterilised by filtration. Store at 2° to 8°. *Dose.* Plasma volume determinations, 185 kBq (5 microcuries); other investigations of the circulatory system, up to 1.85 MBq (50 microcuries).

Iodinated I 131 Albumin Aggregated Injection *(U.S.P.).* Macroaggregated Iodinated I 131 Serum Albumin. A sterile aqueous suspension of albumin which has been iodinated with iodine-131 and denatured to form aggregates of controlled particle size (not less than 90% of the particles have a diameter of 10 to 90 µm and none exceeds 150 µm). pH 5 to 6. it contains 0.3 to 3 mg of aggregated albumin per ml of suspension and 95 to 105% of the content of iodine-131 stated on the label at the time of labelling. The specific activity is 7.4 to 44.4 MBq (0.2 to 1.2 millicuries) per mg of aggregated albumin at the time stated on the label. Other chemical forms of radioactivity do not exceed 6% of the total radioactivity. Store at 2° to 8°. Use within 30 days of the date of completion of iodination. Do not use if clumping of the aggregate has occurred.

Iodinated I 131 Albumin Injection *(U.S.P.).* Iodinated I 131 Serum Albumin; Radio-iodinated (^{131}I) Serum Albumin (Human). A sterile, buffered, iso-osmotic solution containing albumin radio-iodinated to the extent of not more than 1 atom of iodine for each molecule of albumin and adjusted to provide not more than 37 MBq (1 millicurie) of activity per ml. It contains 95 to 105% of the labelled amount of iodine-131 as iodinated albumin at the time indicated on the label; other forms of radioactivity do not exceed 3% of the total radioactivity. pH 7 to 8.5. Store at 2° to 8°. Use within 30 days of the date of completion of iodination.

Iodohippurate Sodium I 131 Injection *(U.S.P.).* A sterile solution containing sodium 2-iodohippurate in which a portion of the molecules contain radioactive iodine (^{131}I) in the molecular structure. It contains 90 to 110% of the labelled amount of iodine-131 as sodium iodohippurate at the time indicated on the label. Other chemical forms of radioactivity do not exceed 3% of the total radioactivity. pH 7 to 8.5. Use within 50 days from the date of manufacture.

Macrosalb (^{131}I) Injection *(B.P. 1973).* Macrisalb (^{131}I) Injection; Macroaggregated Iodinated (^{131}I) Human Albumin Injection. A sterile iso-osmotic saline suspension of white or faintly yellow particles of human albumin which has been iodinated with iodine-131 and denatured to form insoluble aggregates having mean diameters 10 to 100 µm. pH 5 to 8.5. It contains a suitable bactericide such as benzyl alcohol 0.9% v/v and 90 to 110% of the content of iodine-131 stated on the label at the date and hour stated on the label. Store at 2° to 10°. *Dose.* 11.1 MBq (300 microcuries).

Rose Bengal Sodium I 131 Injection *(U.S.P.).* Sodium Rose Bengal I 131 Injection. A clear, deep red, sterile solution containing rose bengal sodium in which a portion of the molecules contain radioactive iodine (^{131}I) in the molecular structure; it may contain a suitable buffer. It contains 90 to 110% of the labelled amount of iodine-131 as rose bengal sodium at the time indicated on the label. Other chemical forms of radioactivity do not exceed 10% of the total radioactivity. pH 7 to 8.5. Use within 2 months from the date of manufacture.

Sodium Iodide I 131 Capsules *(U.S.P.).* Capsules containing radioactive iodine (^{131}I) processed in the form of sodium iodide in such manner that it is essentially carrier-free and contains only minute amounts of naturally occurring iodine-127. Each capsule contains 90 to 110% of the labelled amount of ^{131}I as iodide at the time indicated on the label; other chemical forms of radioactivity do not exceed 5% of the total radioactivity. They may contain a stabiliser. The label indicates whether they are intended for diagnostic or therapeutic use. Use within 2 months from the date of manufacture.

Sodium Iodide (^{131}I) Injection *(B.P.).* A sterile solution containing sodium iodide (^{131}I) and sodium thiosulphate or other suitable reducing agents. The solution is sterilised by autoclaving. It contains 90 to 110% of the content of iodine-131 activity stated on the label at the date and hour stated on the label. The specific activity is not less than 185 MBq (5 millicuries) per microgram of iodine at the date and hour stated on the label. Other chemical forms of radioactivity do not exceed 5% of the total radioactivity. pH 7 to 8.5. *Dose.* By intravenous injection at the dosage rates given under Sodium Iodide (^{131}I) Solution.

Sodium Iodide (^{131}I) Solution *(B.P., Eur. P.).* Natrii Iodidi (^{131}I) Solutio. A solution suitable for oral administration, similar to Sodium Iodide (^{131}I) Injection but unsterilised. pH 7 to 10. *Dose.* In the investigation of thyroid function, 185 to 925 kBq (5 to 25 microcuries); in the treatment of thyrotoxicosis, 185 to 555 MBq (5 to 15 millicuries), according to the patient's needs; for the ablation of normal thyroid function, 925 to 1850 MBq (25 to 50 millicuries); in the treatment of carcinoma of the thyroid, 2220 to 3700 MBq (60 to 100 millicuries), repeated after an interval if necessary.

Sodium Iodide I 131 Solution *(U.S.P.).* A solution for oral or intravenous administration containing radioactive iodine (^{131}I), processed in the form of sodium iodide in such manner that it is essentially carrier-free and contains only minute amounts of naturally occurring iodine-127. It contains 90 to 110% of the labelled amount of iodine-131 as iodide at the time indicated on the label; other chemical forms of radioactivity do not exceed 5% of the total radioactivity. It may contain a preservative or stabiliser. pH 7.5 to 9. The label indicates whether it is intended for diagnostic or therapeutic use. Use within 2 months from the date of manufacture.

Sodium Iodohippurate (^{131}I) Injection *(B.P., Eur. P.).* Natrii Iodohippurate (^{131}I) Solutio Iniectabilis. A sterile solution containing sodium 2-iodohippurate (^{131}I). It contains 90 to 110% of the content of iodine-131 activity stated on the label at the date and hour stated, of which not less than 95% is in the form of sodium 2-iodohippurate. The specific activity is 740 to 7400 MBq (20 to 200 millicuries) per g of sodium 2-iodohippurate. pH 6 to 8.5. Store in a cool place. Protect from light. The label states that the injection is not necessarily suitable for renal plasma-flow studies. *Dose.* In renography, 0.37 to 3.7 MBq (10 to 100 microcuries).

5865-e

Iridium-192 ($^{192}_{77}$Ir)

HALF-LIFE. 74 days

RADIATION EMITTED. EC (4.7%); β^- 0.250 (5.4%), 0.530 (42.6%), 0.670 (47.2%) MeV; γ 0.206 (3.4%), 0.296 (29.6%), 0.308 (30.7%), 0.316 (82.7%), 0.468 (47.0%), 0.484 (2.9%), 0.589 (4.4%), 0.604 (8.2%), 0.612 (5.3%) MeV.

SUPPLY. Iridium-192 is not supplied in pharmaceutical dosage forms. It is supplied as platinum-covered pins and wires.

Uses. Iridium-192 is used in radiotherapy.

5866-l

Iron-59 ($^{59}_{26}$Fe)

HALF-LIFE. 44.6 days

RADIATION EMITTED. β^- 0.084 (0.1%), 0.132 (1.1%), 0.274 (45.8%), 0.467 (52.7%), 1.566 (0.3%) MeV; γ 0.143 (0.8%), 0.192 (2.8%), 0.335 (0.3%), 0.383 (0.02%), 1.099 (55.8%), 1.292 (43.8%), 1.482 (0.06%) MeV.

SUPPLY. Iron-59 is supplied as ferric citrate (^{59}Fe) in the form of an injection, iso-osmotic with serum, containing 111 to 740 megabecquerels (3 to 20 millicuries) per mg of iron. *B.P.* specifies not less than 37 megabecquerels (1 millicurie) per mg of iron at the date stated on the label. Iron-59 is also supplied in the USA as ferrous citrate (^{59}Fe) injection and *U.S.P.* specifies the content as not less than 185 megabecquerels (5 millicuries) per mg of ferrous citrate on the date of manufacture.

Uses. Iron-59, in the form of ferric citrate (^{59}Fe) is used in the measurement of iron absorption and utilisation. It is given by mouth or intravenous injection in doses of 111 to 370 kBq (3 to 10 microcuries).

Iron-59, in the form of ferrous citrate (^{59}Fe) is used for similar purposes in the USA.

Iron-59 has also been used in *in vitro* radioassay tests.

There was a significant correlation between estimates of the plasma volume made by labelling albumin with iodine-125 and estimates made by labelling transferrin with iron-59 during haematological studies of 25 patients. Labelling with iron-59 could also be used in studies of plasma volume in iron-deficient patients.— C. Ricketts and I. Cavill, *J. clin. Path.*, 1978, *31*, 196.

Preparations

Ferric Citrate (^{59}Fe) Injection *(B.P.).* A clear, colourless, or faintly orange-brown, sterile solution containing iron (^{59}Fe) in the ferric state, 1% of sodium citrate, and sufficient sodium chloride to make the solution iso-osmotic with blood. pH 6 to 8. It contains 90 to 110% of the content of iron-59 stated on the label at the date stated on the label. The final content of iron-55 is not more than 2% of the total activity. The specific activity is not less than 37 MBq (1 millicurie) per mg of iron at the date stated on the label. The solution is sterilised by autoclaving. *Dose.* In the investigation of haematological disorders, 185 to 370 kBq (5 to 10 microcuries).

Ferrous Citrate Fe 59 Injection *(U.S.P.).* A sterile solution of radioactive iron (^{59}Fe) in the ferrous state complexed with citrate ion in Water for Injections; it may contain sodium chloride to render the solution iso-osmotic with blood, and bacteriostatic agents. It contains 90 to 110% of the labelled amount of iron-59 at the time indicated on the label. The specific activity is not less than 185 MBq (5 millicuries) per mg of ferrous citrate at the time of manufacture. Use within 4 months from the date of manufacture. pH 5 to 7.

5867-y

Mercury-197 ($^{197}_{80}$Hg)

HALF-LIFE. 64.4 hours

RADIATION EMITTED. EC (100%); γ 0.077 (19.2%), 0.192 (~1.1%), 0.268 (~0.1%) MeV; X-rays (gold) 0.067 to 0.080 (~73%) MeV.

SUPPLY. Mercury-197 may be supplied as chlormerodrin (^{197}Hg) in the form of an injection, containing not less than 7.4 megabecquerels (200 microcuries) per mg of chlormerodrin.

Uses. Chlormerodrin (^{197}Hg) is taken up by tubule cells in the kidney and has been widely used in renal scanning in usual doses of 3.7 to 11.1 MBq (100 to 300 microcuries), administered intravenously.

Mercury is concentrated to some extent by brain tumours, and doses of 22.2 to 111 MBq (0.6 to 3 millicuries) administered intravenously as chlormerodrin (^{197}Hg) have been used for brain scanning. Mercury has been largely superseded by other agents, such as technetium-99m.

Preparations

Chlormerodrin (^{197}Hg) Injection *(B.P. 1973, Eur. P.).* Chlormerodrini (^{197}Hg) Solutio Iniectabilis. A sterile solution containing chlormerodrin (^{197}Hg), made iso-osmotic with blood by the addition of sodium chloride. It contains 85 to 115% of the activity of mercury-197 stated on the label at the date and time stated on the label and not more than 0.2% of the total activity as mercury-203. It has a specific activity of not less than 7400 MBq (200 millicuries) per g of chlormerodrin at the date and hour stated on the label. pH 5 to 8. It may contain a bactericide. Sterilised by filtration. *Dose.* For brain scanning, 37 to 111 MBq (1 to 3 millicuries); for renal scanning, 3.7 to 11.1 MBq (100 to 300 microcuries).

Chlormerodrin Hg 197 Injection *(U.S.P.)*. A sterile solution containing chlormerodrin in which a portion of the molecules contain radioactive mercury (^{197}Hg). It contains 90 to 110% of the labelled amount of ^{197}Hg as chlormerodrin at the time indicated on the label. Other chemical forms of radioactivity do not exceed 5% of the total radioactivity. A clear, colourless solution. pH 5.5 to 8.5. Use within 14 days from the date of manufacture.

5868-j

Mercury-203 ($^{203}_{80}Hg$)

HALF-LIFE. 46.6 days

RADIATION EMITTED. β^- 0.212 (100%) MeV; γ 0.279 (81.5%) MeV; X-rays (thallium) 0.071 to 0.085 (12.8%) MeV.

SUPPLY. Mercury-203 is supplied as chlormerodrin (^{203}Hg) in sodium chloride injection containing 4.44 to 18.5 megabecquerels (120 to 500 microcuries) per mg of chlormerodrin.

Uses. Mercury-203, as chlormerodrin, has been used for similar purposes to chlormerodrin (^{197}Hg) in usual doses of 25.9 MBq (700 microcuries) for brain scanning and up to 3.7 MBq (100 microcuries) for renal scanning.

Preparations

Chlormerodrin Hg 203 Injection *(U.S.P.)*. A sterile solution containing chlormerodrin in which a portion of the molecules contain radioactive mercury (^{203}Hg). It contains 90 to 110% of the labelled amount of mercury-203 as chlormerodrin at the time indicated in the labelling. Other chemical forms of radioactivity do not exceed 5% of the total radioactivity. pH 5.5 to 8.5. The label indicates whether it is intended for diagnostic or therapeutic use. Use within 45 days from the date of manufacture.

5869-z

Phosphorus-32 ($^{32}_{15}P$)

HALF-LIFE. 14.3 days

RADIATION EMITTED. β^- 1.709 (100%) MeV.

SUPPLY. Phosphorus-32 is supplied as sodium phosphate (^{32}P) in the form of an injection containing 111 to 259 megabecquerels (3 to 7 millicuries) per mg of phosphorus in phosphate buffer. *B.P.* specifies not less than 11.1 megabecquerels (300 microcuries) per mg of orthophosphate ion.

Adverse Effects and Precautions. Because of its depressant effect on bone-marrow function, phosphorus-32, even in therapeutic doses, may produce aplastic anaemia, leucopenia, and thrombocytopenic purpura. There may be an increased incidence of acute leukaemia in patients with polycythaemia vera treated with large total doses of phosphorus-32. Nevertheless, the survival of patients with this disease after treatment with phosphorus-32 is comparable with that after any other form of treatment. Frequent examination of the blood during and after phosphorus-32 therapy is essential. Symptoms of radiation sickness have followed its use.

Special caution should be exercised when giving Sodium Phosphate (^{32}P) Injection to leukaemic patients with a red-cell count of less than 2 500 000 per mm^3. It is contra-indicated if the reticulocyte count in the presence of significant aneamia is less than 0.2% and also if the white-cell count is less than 3000 per mm^3 or the platelet count is less than 150 000 per mm^3.

Two false negative results with the ^{32}P-uptake test in patients with malignant melanomas of the choroid.— D. M. Robertson, *Br. J. Ophthal.*, 1976, *60*, 835.

Uses. Phosphorus-32, given intravenously as Sodium Phosphate (^{32}P) Injection, has a half-life of just over 14 days, but because it is metabolised and excreted, its effective half-life in the body is estimated to be only about 8 days. It is used extensively in the treatment of polycythaemia vera by intravenous injection; phosphorus-32 taken up by trabecular bone in close relation to the haemopoietic red bone marrow delivers a sufficient dose to reduce the production of red cells. The dosage varies according to the regimen adopted. A dose of up to 185 MBq (5 millicuries) may be given initially followed if necessary by doses of 111 or 148 MBq (3 or 4 millicuries) given at intervals of 2 to 3 months. Sodium phosphate (^{32}P) has also been given by mouth in doses of up to about 222 MBq (6 millicuries).

Sodium phosphate (^{32}P) is also employed in the diagnosis of malignant neoplasms especially those affecting the eye, brain, and skin.

Phosphorus-32 is also used in the palliative treatment of chronic myeloid leukaemia.

Polycythaemia vera. A discussion of the use of phosphorus-32 in the treatment of polycythaemia vera. Despite its risk it remains the method of choice particularly in older patients and those whose disease is of a severe nature.— S. M. Lewis, *Br. J. Hosp. Med.*, 1976, *16*, 125.

Further references: G. Mathé (letter), *New Engl. J. Med.*, 1978, *298*, 279; N. I. Berlin (letter), *ibid.*, 913.

Thrombocythaemia. From follow-up studies for up to 10 years in 9 patients, all under 30 years of age, with primary thrombocythaemia, treatment with long-term alkylating agents or with radioactive phosphorus to reduce the platelet count was not recommended. The condition in these patients was considered to be more benign than the secondary thrombocytosis occurring in older patients.— H. C. Hoagland and M. N. Silverstein, *Mayo Clin. Proc.*, 1978, *53*, 578.

Preparations

Sodium Phosphate (^{32}P) Injection *(B.P., Eur. P.)*. Natrii Phosphatis (^{32}P) Solutio Iniectabilis. A sterile solution of sodium phosphate (^{32}P) and sodium acid phosphate (^{32}P), and sufficient sodium chloride to render the solution iso-osmotic with blood. It contains 90 to 110% of the content of phosphorus-32 activity stated on the label at the date and hour stated on the label. Other chemical forms of radioactivity do not exceed 5% of the total radioactivity. The specific activity is not less than 11.1 MBq (300 microcuries) per mg of phosphate ion. pH 6 to 8. *Dose.* In polycythaemia vera, by intravenous injection, initial dose, 185 MBq (5 millicuries), which may be followed by a dose of 111 MBq (3 millicuries) after 3 months, according to the patient's needs.

Sodium Phosphate P 32 Solution *(U.S.P.)*. A solution suitable for oral or intravenous administration containing radioactive phosphorus (^{32}P) processed in the form of sodium phosphate; nonradioactive sodium phosphate may be added during the processing. It contains 90 to 110% of the labelled amount of phosphorus-32 as phosphate at the time indicated in the labelling. Other chemical forms of radioactivity are absent. A clear, colourless solution. pH 5 to 6. The label indicates whether it is intended for diagnostic or therapeutic use. Use within 2 months from date of manufacture. The injection may darken as a result of the effects of radiation during storage.

5870-p

Potassium-40 ($^{40}_{19}K$)

HALF-LIFE. 1.28×10^9 years

RADIATION EMITTED. EC (10.7%); β^- 1.314 (89.3%) MeV; γ 1.461 (10.7%) MeV.

SUPPLY. Potassium-40 is a naturally occurring radionuclide.

Uses. Potassium-40 occurs naturally as a very small and constant proportion of the body's total potassium. With very sensitive whole-body counters it is possible to measure the whole body potassium-40 and hence the total body potassium.

5871-s

Potassium-42 ($^{42}_{19}K$)

HALF-LIFE. 12.36 hours

RADIATION EMITTED. β^- 1.683 (0.3%), 1.995 (17.6%), 3.520 (82%) MeV; γ 0.312 (0.3%), 0.900 (0.05%), 1.021 (0.02%), 1.525 (17.9%), 1.921 (0.04%), 2.424 (0.02%) MeV.

SUPPLY. Potassium-42 is supplied as potassium chloride (^{42}K) in the form of an injection, iso-osmotic with serum, containing 592 kilobecquerels (16 microcuries) per mg of potassium.

Uses. Potassium-42, as potassium chloride (^{42}K), is given by mouth or intravenously to determine the body's total exchangeable potassium and potassium space. The usual dose is 2.59 to 5.55 MBq (70 to 150 microcuries); the higher doses in this range may be necessary if radionuclides such as sodium-24 are given for the simultaneous measurement of other mineral constituents in the body.

Potassium-43 which has a longer half-life (22 hours) has also been used to measure exchangeable potassium as well as for myocardial scanning.

5872-w

Selenium -75 ($^{75}_{34}Se$)

HALF-LIFE. 120 days

RADIATION EMITTED. EC (100%); γ 0.066 (1.1%), 0.097 (2.9%), 0.121 (15.7%), 0.136 (54.0%), 0.199 (1.5%), 0.265 (56.9%), 0.280 (18.5%), 0.401 (11.7%) MeV; X-rays (arsenic) 0.010 to 0.012 (~50%) MeV. It also decays via arsenic-75m [half-life: 16.4 milliseconds. γ 0.024 (0.03%), 0.280 (5.4%), 0.304 (1.2%) MeV; X-rays (arsenic) 0.010 to 0.012 (~2.6%) MeV].

SUPPLY. Selenium-75 is supplied as L-selenomethionine (^{75}Se) in the form of an injection containing 37 to 370 megabecquerels (1 to 10 millicuries) or 111 to 740 megabecquerels (3 to 20 millicuries) per mg of selenomethionine. *B.P.* specifies not less than 37 megabecquerels (1 millicurie) per mg of L-selenomethionine and *U.S.P.* specifies not less than 37 megabecquerels (1 millicurie) per mg of selenium at the time of manufacture. Selenium-75 is also supplied as selenonorcholestenol (^{75}Se) {6β-[(methyl[^{75}Se]-seleno)methyl]-19-norcholest-5(10)-en-3β-ol} in the form of an injection containing 74 to 740 megabecquerels (2 to 20 millicuries) per mg of selenonorcholestenol.

Uses. When injected, methionine with selenium-75 introduced in place of sulphur apparently enters the same metabolic pathways as the unaltered amino acid. Selenomethionine (^{75}Se) is concentrated by the pancreas, by the parathyroid glands, and other organs. The pancreas may be visualised by scanning methods, though since the liver also concentrates selenomethionine the technique is not a simple one. Hyperactive parathyroid glands may be localised with difficulty provided thyroid metabolism is adequately suppressed. The usual dose for pancreas and parathyroid scanning is 7.4 to 11.1 MBq (200 to 300 microcuries). L-Selenomethionine (^{75}Se) has been used to locate malignant lymphomas.

Selenium-75 in the form of 6β-[(methyl[^{75}Se]-seleno)methyl]-19-norcholest-5(10)-en-3β-ol [selenonorcholestenol (^{75}Se)] is used in adrenal scintigraphy in usual doses of 7.4 MBq (200 microcuries).

Sodium selenite (^{75}Se) was formerly used for the localisation of tumours in bone, brain, and cartilage.

Cortisol (hydrocortisone) labelled with selenium-75 is available for cortisol assays and folate labelled with selenium-75 is available for folate assays.

A discussion of radionuclide imaging of the pancreas.— M. Critchley, *Br. J. Hosp. Med.*, 1978, *20*, 129.

A comparison of selenomethionine (^{75}Se) scanning and retrograde endoscopic pancreatography for the assessment of pancreatic disease. The scan was acceptable for showing normal pancreases. Further tests were necessary if the scan showed as abnormal.— C. J. Mitchell *et al.*, *Br. med. J.*, 1976, *2*, 1307.

In a study involving 70 patients with suspected pancreatic cancer radioselenium pancreatic scans yielded a false-positive rate of over 30%. These findings confirmed those of other workers.— E. P. DiMagno *et al.*, *New Engl. J. Med.*, 1977, *297*, 737.

Because normal scans were not a reliable indicator of pancreatic normality diagnostic scanning with selenomethionine was not considered worthwhile.— P. B. Cotton *et al.*, *Br. med. J.*, 1978, *1*, 282.

Gastric distension with a carbonated liquid improved delineation of the pancreas and liver when selenomethionine (^{75}Se) was used.— M. H. Nathan and K. Domanski (letter), *J. Am. med. Ass.*, 1978, *239*, 831.

Preparations

L-Selenomethionine (^{75}Se) Injection *(B.P.)*. A sterile apyrogenic solution containing L-selenomethionine (^{75}Se). It may be made iso-osmotic with blood by the addition of sodium chloride. At the date stated on the label, it contains 90 to 110% of the content of selenium-75 activity stated on the label, of which not less than 90% is in the form of L-selenomethionine (^{75}Se). The specific activity is not less than 37 MBq (1 millicurie) per mg of L-selenomethionine. pH 4.5 to 8. Store at a temperature not exceeding 8°. Protect from light. *Dose.* For scanning the pancreas, 9.25 MBq (250 microcuries).

Selenomethionine Se 75 Injection *(U.S.P.)*. A sterile aqueous solution of L-selenomethionine. At the time stated on the label it contains 90 to 110% of the labelled amount of selenium-75, of which not less than 90% is in the form of selenomethionine. The specific activity at the time of manufacture is not less than 37 MBq (1 millicurie) per mg of selenium. It may contain not more than 3 mg of L-methionine per ml as a carrier and may contain suitable antioxidants and preservatives. pH 3.5 to 8. Store at 2° to 8° unless otherwise specified. Use within 6 months of the date of manufacture.

5873-e

Sodium-22 ($^{22}_{11}$Na)

HALF-LIFE. 2.6 years

RADIATION EMITTED. EC (9.46%); β^+ 0.546 (90.49%), 1.820 (0.05%) MeV; γ 0.511 (from β^+), 1.275 (99.95%) MeV.

SUPPLY. Sodium-22 is supplied as sodium chloride (^{22}Na) in the form of an injection, iso-osmotic with serum, containing 925 kilobecquerels (25 microcuries) per mg of sodium.

Uses. Sodium chloride (^{22}Na) has been used in the determination of the body's exchangeable sodium and sodium space in doses of 111 to 740 kBq (3 to 20 microcuries). However, the very long half-life of sodium-22, though an advantage technically, gives rise to an unacceptable radiation dose.

5874-l

Sodium-24 ($^{24}_{11}$Na)

HALF-LIFE. 15.02 hours

RADIATION EMITTED. β^- 0.284 (0.08%), 1.392 (99.92%) MeV; γ 1.369 (100%), 2.754 (99.85%), 3.861 (0.08%) MeV.

SUPPLY. Sodium-24 is supplied as sodium chloride (^{24}Na) in the form of an injection, iso-osmotic with serum, containing 12.58 megabecquerels (340 microcuries) per mg of sodium.

Uses. Sodium-24, as sodium chloride (^{24}Na) injection, is given by mouth or intravenously to determine the body's total exchangeable sodium and sodium space. The usual dose is 0.185 to 3.7 MBq (5 to 100 microcuries); the higher doses in this range may be necessary if radionuclides such as potassium-42 are given for the simultaneous measurement of other mineral constituents in the body.

The value for total exchangeable sodium is considerably smaller than that for the total body sodium due to the large amount of sodium which is inaccessible in the bones.

5875-y

Strontium-85 ($^{85}_{38}$Sr)

HALF-LIFE. 64.8 days

RADIATION EMITTED. EC (100%); γ 0.36 (0.002%), 0.88 (0.01%) MeV; X-rays (rubidium) 0.013 to 0.015 (~60%) MeV. It also decays via rubidium-85m [half-life: 0.96 microseconds. γ 0.514 (99.2%) MeV].

SUPPLY. Strontium-85 is supplied as strontium chloride (^{85}Sr) in the form of an injection containing 74 to 370 megabecquerels (2 to 10 millicuries) per mg of strontium.

Uses. Strontium isotopes are taken up by the bones and their major use has been in bone scanning. Strontium-85 has a long half-life and allows maximum clearance of radioactivity from non-tumour areas, but the radiation dose to the patient is relatively high and it is difficult to carry out repeat scans after therapy. The doses used range from 0.74 to 3.7 MBq (20 to 100 microcuries) by intravenous injection.

Strontium-87m has also been used for similar purposes.

Most lesions of bone, such as fractures, infections, and Paget's disease, show increased concentration of strontium radioisotopes, so that detection of localised concentrations is not diagnostic of malignant deposits.

The use of strontium isotopes for bone scanning, however, has in general declined and technetium-99m-labelled compounds are more commonly used.

5876-j

Strontium-90 ($^{90}_{38}$Sr)

HALF-LIFE. 28.5 years

RADIATION EMITTED. β^- 0.546 (100%) MeV. It also decays via yttrium-90—see p.1400.

SUPPLY. Strontium-90 is not supplied in pharmaceutical dosage forms. It is used as a source of beta-radiation in the form of metallic ophthalmic applicators, and as plaques and plates.

Uses. Strontium-90 is used as a source of pure β-radiation in the form of surface applicators for radiotherapeutic purposes. Like all isotopes of strontium it becomes localised in bone after ingestion but because of its long half-life it is unsuitable for diagnostic purposes.

5877-z

Sulphur-35 ($^{35}_{16}$S)

HALF-LIFE. 87.4 days

RADIATION EMITTED. β^- 0.167 (100%) MeV.

SUPPLY. Sulphur-35 is supplied as sodium sulphate (^{35}S) in the form of a carrier-free injection, iso-osmotic with serum, containing 37 to 185 megabecquerels (1 to 5 millicuries) per ml.

Uses. Sulphur-35 is used as sodium sulphate (^{35}S) injection for estimation of the extracellular fluid volume. The usual dose is 3.7 MBq (100 microcuries) administered intravenously.

5878-c

Technetium-99m ($^{99m}_{43}$Tc)

HALF-LIFE. 6.02 hours

RADIATION EMITTED. IT (100%); γ 0.141 (88.5%), 0.143 (0.03%) MeV; decays to daughter technetium-99 [half-life: 2.13 × 10^5 years. β^- 0.293 (~100%) MeV].

SUPPLY. Technetium-99m is a daughter of molybdenum-99 ($^{99}_{42}$Mo, half-life 66.2 hours) and because of its short half-life is normally prepared just before use by elution from a sterile generator consisting of molybdenum-99 adsorbed on to alumina in a plastic column. Technetium-99m as pertechnetate (^{99m} TcO_4^-) is obtained by elution with a sterile solution of sodium chloride. Columns containing 925, 1850, 2775, 3700, 4625, 5550, 7400, 9250, and 11 100 megabecquerels (25, 50, 75, 100, 125, 150, 200, 250, and 300 millicuries) of molybdenum-99 are generally available and they have a useful life of 12 to 14 days.

Radiopharmaceuticals of technetium-99m are prepared shortly after elution to reduce loss by decay.

Preparations of pyrophosphate labelled with technetium-99m as pertechnetate released free pertechnetate when stored at room temperature. It was recommended that they be stored in a refrigerator.— P. M. M. Hill (letter), *Pharm. J.*, 1975, *2*, 441. The dissociation could be prevented by making up the labelled compound shortly before injection. Refrigeration would not be needed.— P. H. Cox (letter), *ibid.*, 523. See also *idem*, 1976, *1*, 229.

Radiation decomposition of technetium-99m radiopharmaceuticals.— M. W. Billinghurst *et al.*, *J. nucl. Med.*, 1979, *20*, 138.

The effects of rubber closures on the stability of stannous ion in reagent kits for radiopharmaceuticals.— N. A. Petry *et al.*, *J. parent. Drug. Ass.*, 1979, *33*, 283.

Adverse Effects.

Technetium-99m as sulphur colloid caused itching, oedema at injection site, cough, and bronchospasm within 2 minutes of injection into 1 patient; A similar allergic reaction was observed 2 years later during a repeated liver scan with the preparation and it was considered that the reaction might have been due to the stabiliser present since no reaction followed the use of technetium-99m polyphosphate given for a bone scan some days prior to the second liver scan.— D. Krasnokuki *et al.*, *Radiologia clin.*, 1977, *46*, 307.

Collapse and loss of consciousness occurred on 2 occasions in a patient given technetium-99m labelled human serum albumin microspheres. The reaction did not occur until a few minutes after the injection, so that the technique of injecting slowly was not a suitable precaution against anaphylactic reactions.— S. J. Mather (letter), *Lancet*, 1977, *1*, 907.

Precautions.

Radionuclide scanning was ineffective in a patient with multifocal eosinophilic granuloma. An earlier similar case was discussed.— C. Eil and B. T. Adornato (letter), *Ann. intern. Med.*, 1978, *89*, 289.

Intense renal parenchymal uptake of technetium-99m-labelled pyrophosphate observed in bone scans performed in children receiving chemotherapy for various malignant diseases appeared to be associated with the administration of antineoplastic agents (cyclophosphamide, doxorubicin, and vincristine) within the preceding 7 days. Increased uptake was not observed in patients who had not received any chemotherapy within this period.— C. L. Lutrin *et al.*, *Radiology*, 1978, *128*, 165.

In 2 women arthritis of the knees caused a false-positive diagnosis of venous thrombosis when ^{99m} Tc-urokinase was used for diagnosis.— G. P. McNeill *et al.*, *Br. med. J.*, 1978, *1*, 81.

Altered body distribution of pertechnetate (^{99m}Tc) was observed in a patient with hyperaluminaemia due to therapy with an antacid preparation containing aluminium hydroxide. A repeat study performed 3 months after discontinuation of the antacids, when plasma-aluminium concentration had decreased, revealed normal distribution of pertechnetate (^{99m} Tc).— T. S. T. Wang *et al.*, *J. nucl. Med.*, 1978, *19*, 381.

Residual barium in the colon of a patient following a barium enema produced interference on a splenic scan performed with technetium-99m-labelled sulphur colloid.— S. T. Zwas and P. Braunstein, *Clin. nucl. Med.*, 1978, *3*, 202.

Pregnancy and the neonate. Samples of milk were taken from a nursing mother 4, 8, 12, and 18 hours after the injection of 74 MBq (2 millicuries) of macroaggregated albumin (^{99m}Tc). Following estimations of the total body dose to the feeding infant it was considered that the mother might resume feeding 24 hours after administration.— R. A. Berke *et al.*, *J. nucl. Med.*, 1973, *14*, 51. Results from 4 mothers receiving technetium-99m preparations indicated that acceptable low levels of radioactivity in breast milk were achieved within 2 days of the administration of the radiopharmaceutical.— J. R. Wyburn, *ibid.*, 115.

Further references: W. F. Rumble *et al.*, *J. nucl. Med.*, 1978, *19*, 913.

Uses. Because it has a short half-life and can be administered in relatively large doses, and because the energy of its γ-emission is readily detected, technetium-99m is very widely used, either as the pertechnetate or in the form of various labelled compounds, particles, and colloids for scanning bone and organs such as the brain, liver, lung, spleen, and thyroid.

Provided that it is sterile, pertechnetate (^{99m}Tc) eluted from the generator may be injected intravenously in doses of up to 740 MBq (20 millicuries) for detecting and localising tumours and other pathological lesions in the brain. It may also be used to measure cerebral blood flow. Its effectiveness depends on the fact that after clearance from the blood very little technetium-99m is retained by healthy brain tissue. Potassium perchlorate is usually given about 1 hour before injection to prevent uptake in the thyroid or choroid plexus.

Pertechnetate (^{99m}Tc) is retained by thyroid cells and it is frequently used for thyroid scanning, with the advantage that the radiation dose to the patient is smaller than occurs with iodine-131. The usual dose is 37 to 74 MBq (1 to 2 millicuries).

Pertechnetate (^{99m}Tc) may also be used for scintigraphy of the salivary glands, stomach, heart, and joints.

Macroaggregates of human albumin labelled with technetium-99m [macrosalb (^{99m}Tc)] are used in lung scanning for the detection of abnormal lung perfusion patterns in usual doses of 37 to 111 MBq (1 to 3 millicuries); following the intravenous injection of a suspension of suitable particle size, usually 10 to 100 μm, the particles become trapped in the lung capillaries enabling ischaemic areas to be defined. Labelled albumin microspheres of particle size 10 to 40 μm are used similarly.

When technetium-99m bound to human serum albumin is administered intravenously it becomes evenly distributed in the circulation and highly vascular organs or pools of blood may be readily located. Such a preparation is used in localisation of the placenta and in examination of the heart.

Technetium-99m in the form of a colloid, such as sulphur, antimony sulphide, or tin, is used for the examination of the liver, spleen, and bone marrow. The usual dose ranges are about 37 to 185 MBq (1 to 5 millicuries) in the investigation of the liver and spleen and up to 740 MBq (20 millicuries) for bone marrow. A labelled preparation of calcium phytate is also used for similar purposes.

Technetium-99m complexes of iminodiacetic acid derivatives, such as *N*-[*N′*-(2,6-dimethylphenyl)carbamoylmethyl]iminodiacetic acid (lidofenin; HIDA) and *N*-[*N′*-(2,6-diethylphenyl)carbamoylmethyl]iminodiacetic acid (etifenin; EHIDA), are employed in the investigation of hepatic function and in the imaging of the hepatobiliary system. Technetium-99m-labelled pyridoxylidene glutamate has also been used for the examination of the gall-bladder.

Various labelled preparations or complexes are used for kidney scanning. These include the succimer salt of technetium-99m given in usual doses of 37 to 185 MBq (1 to 5 millicuries) and technetium-99m as the gluceptate in doses of 370 to 555 MBq (10 to 15 millicuries). The latter has also been used for brain scanning. Other technetium-99m-labelled agents used in both brain and renal imaging are calcium gluconate and calcium trisodium pentetate (calcium DTPA). Usual doses employed for brain studies are 370 to 740 MBq (10 to 20 millicuries) and for kidney studies 74 to 740 MBq (2 to 20 millicuries).

For bone scanning various labelled phosphate compounds may be used. Technetium-99m as the methylene diphosphonate (medronate; MDP) and as the pyrophosphate is given in usual doses of about 370 to 555 MBq (10 to 15 millicuries). Technetium-99m as the pyrophosphate is also used in similar doses in cardiac scintigraphy for the detection of myocardial infarction.

Many other technetium-99m-labelled compounds have been prepared and used in different clinical studies for the examination of different organs or systems. These include bleomycin for the examination of tumours, tetracycline for myocardial infarctions, penicillamine for gall-bladders and kidneys, and iron hydroxide for lungs. Like radio-iodine, technetium-99m in various forms has been used to detect deep-vein thrombosis of the legs.

The use of technetium-99m in a patient with periarteritis nodosa and its possible diagnostic value.— J. Abramovici *et al.*, *Br. med. J.*, 1975, *1*, 373.

Polymorphonuclear cells labelled with technetium-99m were used effectively in the diagnosis of profound focal suppuration.— J. Ch. Auvergnat *et al.* (letter), *Lancet*, 1976, *2*, 852.

Scanning for soft-tissue amyloid using technetium-99m diphosphonate.— R. W. Kula *et al.* (letter), *Lancet*, 1977, *1*, 92.

The use of red blood cells labelled with technetium-99m for visualisation of blood pools.— D. Pavel *et al.*, *J. nucl. Med.*, 1977, *18*, 305.

Plasma volume measurements with technetium-99m-labelled human serum albumin.— S. S. Yang *et al.*, *J. nucl. Med.*, 1978, *19*, 804.

Detection of infarction. Reviews: A. F. Parisi *et al.*, *New Engl. J. Med.*, 1977, *296*, 368; *Br. med. J.*, 1978, *2*, 717; *Lancet*, 1978, *2*, 299.

In a study in 203 patients with suspected myocardial infarction myocardial scintigraphy, using technetium-99m stannous pyrophosphate, correlated well with other evidence of acute infarction; recognition of possible sources of interpretative error would increase its usefulness.— M. J. Cowley *et al.*, *Circulation*, 1977, *56*, 192.

Addition of dynamic sodium pertechnetate (^{99m}Tc) cardioangiography to static technetium (^{99m}Tc) stannous pyrophosphate scintigraphy for the diagnosis of suspected acute myocardial infarction helped to localise the site of infarction and provide more accurate results.— M. K. Kan *et al.*, *J. Am. med. Ass.*, 1977, *238*, 1637. See also J. T. Willerson *et al.*, *ibid.*, 1665.

Technetium-99m-pyrophosphate and thallium-201 were complementary in the detection, location and assessment of acute myocardial infarction in a study of 80 patients. No patients had false negative scans with dual imaging with both radionuclides.— H. J. Berger *et al.*, *Ann. intern. Med.*, 1978, *88*, 145. Criticism. Further studies would be needed to establish the comparative specificity of dual imaging.— B. G. Pitts (letter), *ibid.*, 844.

Further reports and comments on the use of technetium-99m-labelled agents in the detection of myocardial infarction.— D. S. Berman *et al.*, *Chest*, 1977, *71*, 349; L. M. Buja *et al.*, *Circulation*, 1977, *56*, 1016; M. J. Cowley *et al.*, *Circulation*, 1977, *56*, 192; H. Henning *et al.*, *Am. J. Cardiol.*, 1977, *40*, 147; S. C. Klausner *et al.*, *Circulation*, 1977, *56*, 173; I. S. Lowenthal *et al.*, *J. nucl. Med.*, 1977, *18*, 770; J. W. Mason *et al.*, *Am. J. Cardiol.*, 1977, *40*, 1; H. G. Olson *et al.*, *Circulation*, 1977, *56*, 181; R. Prasquier *et al.*, *Circulation*, 1977, *55*, 61; A. Righetti *et al.*, *Am. J. Cardiol.*, 1977, *39*, 43; E. H. Botvinick *et al.*, *J. nucl. Med.*, 1978, *19*, 1121; B. L. Holman *et al.*, *Am. J. Cardiol.*, 1978, *41*, 39; F. R. Malin *et al.*, *J. nucl. Med.*, 1978, *19*, 1111; D. N. Sharpe *et al.*, *Circulation*, 1978, *57*, 483; G. J. Davies *et al.*, *Br. Heart J.*, 1979, *41*, 668; S. P. Joseph *et al.*, *Br. med. J.*, 1979, *1*, 372; R. J. Kelly *et al.*, *J. nucl. Med.*, 1979, *20*, 402.

Detection of neoplasms. *Bone.* A review and discussion on the role of skeletal scanning in clinical oncology. Radionuclide imaging, because of increased sensitivity, is superior to radiology in the investigation of patients with clinical evidence of possible metastases in bone. In some cancers, such as those of the breast, lung, and prostate, and osteogenic sarcoma, which have a high predilection for spreading to bone a case may be made for scanning asymptomatic patients. Scintigraphy appears to be indicated in Ewing's sarcoma. Bone scanning, however, has no real advantage over skeletal radiology in the study of the primary tumour in osteogenic sarcoma, but all children with osteosarcoma should have a bone scan to detect distant bone metastases.— J. H. McKillop and I. R. McDougall, *Br. med. J.*, 1980, *281*, 407.

Bone scans using technetium-99m as pyrophosphate were useful in the initial staging of patients being considered for adjuvant breast cancer treatment. Serial bone scans were of use in identifying patients at high risk for early recurrence.— N. Hammond *et al.*, *Cancer*, 1978, *41*, 138. See also F. H. Gerber *et al.*, *New Engl. J. Med.*, 1977, *297*, 300.

Clinical comparisons of radiopharmaceuticals in the detection of metastases in bone.— E. Silberstein *et al.*, *J. nucl. Med.*, 1978, *19*, 161 (technetium-99m-labelled diphosphonate and pyrophosphate); I. Fogelman *et al.*, *J. nucl. Med.*, 1979, *20*, 98 (technetium-99m methylene diphosphonate and etidronate).

Bone marrow. Evaluation of bone-marrow scanning with technetium-99m-labelled sulphur colloid in 56 children with known or suspected tumours indicated that it appeared to be a useful agent for monitoring marrow alteration caused by metastases, irradiation damage, or tissue fibrosis in children receiving chemotherapy.— A. R. Siddiqui *et al.*, *J. nucl. Med.*, 1979, *20*, 379.

Brain. Of 35 patients with oat-cell carcinoma of the lung and no clinical evidence of brain involvement, brain scanning with pertechnetate (^{99m}Tc) provided new information concerning possible organ involvement in only 1 patient. It was concluded that brain scans should not be considered routine screening procedures in such patients, but that scanning in patients who already exhibit clinical evidence of brain involvement may provide useful information concerning the location and extent of such involvement.— R. E. Wittes and S. D. J. Yeh, *J. Am. med. Ass.*, 1977, *238*, 506 and 2600. A similar view.— F. Vieras (letter), *ibid.*, 2599. Comment that the imaging technique may be unsatisfactory.— E. B. Silberstein (letter), *ibid.*, 2600. Reply.— R. E. Wittes and S. D. J. Yeh (letter), *ibid.*

Clinical comparisons of radiopharmaceuticals in the detection of metastases in the brain.— J. Leveille *et al.*, *J. nucl. Med.*, 1977, *18*, 957.

Heart. Of 3 patients with metastasising carcinoma of the breast and confirmed pericardial effusion a diffuse concentration of technetium-99m pyrophosphate was observed in 2 within the myocardium. Subsequent pericardiocentesis revealed malignant cells in the pericardial fluid of these 2 patients. It was suggested that the use of labelled phosphate agents may allow early recognition of myocardial involvement in patients with disseminated neoplasm.— M. A. Quaife *et al.*, *J. nucl. Med.*, 1979, *20*, 392.

Liver. Of 21 patients with oat-cell carcinoma of the lung and no clinical evidence of liver involvement, liver scanning with a technetium-99m-labelled sulphur colloid provided new information concerning possible organ involvement in only 1 patient. It was concluded that liver scans should not be considered routine screening procedures in such patients, but that scanning in patients who already exhibit clinical evidence of liver involvement may provide useful information concerning the location and extent of such involvement.— R. E. Wittes and S. D. J. Yeh, *J. Am. med. Ass.*, 1977, *238*, 506 and 2600. Comment that the imaging technique may be unsatisfactory.— E. B. Silberstein (letter), *ibid.*, 2600. Reply.— R. E. Wittes and S. D. J. Yeh (letter), *ibid.*

Detection of thrombi. The use of macroaggregated albumin labelled with technetium-99m in lung perfusion scanning for pulmonary embolism and correlation with deep-vein thrombosis of the legs as detected by the fibrinogen uptake test.— N. L. Browse *et al.*, *Br. med. J.*, 1974, *1*, 603.

Urokinase labelled with technetium-99m was administered intravenously to 22 patients with diagnosed or suspected deep-vein thrombosis. Scanning revealed positive results in 16 and negative in 6. Venography confirmed the negative results in these 6 patients and the positive results in 11 of 12 patients from the positive group. The apparent increased uptake was considered not to be due to blood-volume effects but to uptake by the thrombus. It appeared that this technique detected both established and forming thrombi.— W. T. Millar and J. F. B. Smith (preliminary communication), *Lancet*, 1974, *2*, 695. Urokinase labelled with technetium-99m was ineffective for the visualisation of thrombi in 4 patients.— G. J. Weir *et al.*, *ibid.*, 1976, *2*, 341 and 807. The poor results could have been due to physicochemical problems associated with the labelling procedure. A modified procedure produced acceptable results.— P. H. Cox *et al.* (letter), *ibid.*, 572. See also W. T. Millar and J. F. B. Smith (letter), *ibid.*, 573.

The differential diagnosis of thrombophlebitis and dissecting popliteal (Baker's) cyst, using human serum albumin labelled with technetium-99m.— A. E. Watkins *et al.*, *Br. med. J.*, 1975, *4*, 86.

The use of red blood cells labelled with technetium-99m for the detection of deep-vein thrombosis.— W. Beswick *et al.*, *Br. med. J.*, 1979, *1*, 82.

Further reports of the use of compounds labelled with technetium-99m in the detection of deep-vein thrombosis.— V. Kempi and C. Scheele, *J. nucl. Med.*, 1976, *17*, 1096 (pertechnetate); U. Ryo *et al.*, *J. nucl. Med.*, 1977, *18*, 11 (macroaggregated albumin).

Diagnosis of transplant rejection. The differentiation of acute tubular necrosis from rejection in renal transplantation using pentetic acid labelled with technetium-99m.— K. A. McKusick *et al.*, *Ann. intern. Med.*, 1973, *78*, 827.

The clinical significance of accumulation of technetium-99m-labelled sulphur colloid in renal transplant patients.— Y. Kim *et al.*, *Radiology*, 1977, *124*, 745.

Gastric-function test. Technetium-99m had been used in studies of gastric secretion. Radioactive pertechnetate was given intravenously in 19 studies and the secretion of technetium-99m into gastric juice was shown to correlate closely with the volume of gastric secretion and to a lesser extent with acid and intrinsic-factor secretion after histamine stimulation.— W. J. Irvine *et al.*, *Lancet*, 1967, *2*, 648. See also T. V. Taylor *et al.*, *Gut*, 1977, *18*, A947.

The use of technetium-99m-labelled triethylenetetramine-polystyrene resin to assess the rate and pattern of gastric emptying.— M. C. Theodorakis *et al.*, *J. pharm. Sci.*, 1980, *69*, 568. See also G. A. Digenis *et al.*, *ibid.*, 1977, *66*, 442.

Organ scanning. Bladder. Radionuclide cystography using technetium-99m as the pertechnetate in children with vesicoureteric reflux.— D. L. Rothwell *et al.*, *Lancet*, 1977, *1*, 1072.

Bone. The use of technetium-99m as the pyrophosphate in the diagnosis of reflex sympathetic dystrophy secondary to herniated lumbar discs.— D. H. Carlson *et al.*, *Neurology, Minneap.*, 1977, *27*, 791.

Technetium-99m etidronate tin complex was used in the diagnosis of osteomyelitis in 44 children.— M. J. Gelfand and E. B. Silberstein, *J. Am. med. Ass.*, 1977, *237*, 245.

Scintigraphy of knee joints with technetium-99m as the pyrophosphate provided a possible method for following the bone changes in hyperparathyroidism.— J. Lessem *et al.* (letter), *Lancet*, 1977, *1*, 91.

Evaluation of technetium-99m (as the diphosphonate) kinetics and bone scans in patients with Paget's disease of bone before and after therapy with calcitonin.— A. Waxman *et al.*, *Radiology*, 1977, *125*, 761.

Stannous pyrophosphate labelled with technetium-99m was successfully used to diagnose sacroiliac disease in women with low-back pain.— P. Davis and B. C. Lentle, *Lancet*, 1978, *2*, 496. See also J. H. Miller and G. F. Gates, *J. Am. med. Ass.*, 1977, *238*, 2701. Scintigraphy of the sacroiliac joints using technetium-99m as the pyrophosphate was not helpful in the early diagnosis of sacroiliitis. There was wide variation in results obtained in patients with ankylosing spondylitis, 'at risk' patients with back pain, and control subjects.— H. Berghs *et al.*, *Ann. rheum. Dis.*, 1978, *37*, 190.

A study on the use of technetium-99m as the pertechnetate to assess the degree of inflammation in rheumatoid arthritis of the knee joint. It was suggested that technetium-99m joint uptake would provide a useful index of changes in disease activity.— J. Paterson *et al.*, *Ann. rheum. Dis.*, 1978, *37*, 48.

Measurement of skeletal uptake of diphosphonate after the intravenous injection of etidronate labelled with technetium-99m (Osteoscan, *Procter & Gamble, USA*) as a method for predicting the occurrence of postmenopausal osteoporosis.— I. Fogelman *et al.*, *Lancet*, 1980, *2*, 667. Comment.— O. Schaadt and H. Bohr (letter), *ibid.*, 914.

Clinical comparisons of radiopharmaceuticals in bone scanning.— J. Heerfordt *et al.*, *J. nucl. Med.*, 1976, *17*, 98; T. Rudd *et al.*, *J. nucl. Med.*, 1977, *18*, 872; T. G. Rudd *et al.*, *J. nucl. Med.*, 1979, *20*, 821.

See also under Detection of Neoplasms (above).

Brain. In more than 500 patients, angiography using sodium pertechnetate (^{99m}Tc) intravenously had demonstrated the integrity of the cerebral vasculature in all patients except 3 who had clinical evidence of irreversible brain damage. The procedure might be of value to demonstrate brain death.— J. M. Goodman *et al.*, *J. Am. med. Ass.*, 1969, *209*, 1869.

The use of technetium-99m as pertechnetate for the visualisation of cerebral arteriovenous malformations.— B. de F. Olivarius *et al.* (letter), *Br. med. J.*, 1975, *1*, 91.

Pentetic acid labelled with technetium-99m was given intravenously and the cerebrovascular perfusion studied in 1 patient. Increased activity was observed over the circle of Willis and an aneurysm of the basilar artery was confirmed by angiography and later by necropsy.— E. M. Lopez *et al.* (letter), *Lancet*, 1977, *1*, 950.

The use of perchlorate rectally in unconscious patients before brain scintigraphy with pertechnetate (^{99m}Tc).— D. Turner *et al.*, *J. nucl. Med.*, 1977, *18*, 258.

From results of a comparative evaluation of gluceptate, pertechnetate, and pentetic acid labelled with technetium-99m it was concluded that gluceptate was the agent of choice in brain imaging; it does not require the administration of perchlorate to block the salivary gland or choroid plexus, it is not affected by earlier bone studies with technetium-99m as the pyrophosphate, and highly accurate images are obtained 90 minutes after administration.— F. D. Rollo *et al.*, *Radiology*, 1977, *123*, 379.

Clinical comparisons of radiopharmaceuticals in brain imaging: G. Schall *et al.*, *Radiology*, 1971, *99*, 361; T. W. Ryerson *et al.*, *Radiology*, 1978, *127*, 429.

See also under Detection of Neoplasms (above).

Gastro-intestinal tract. Abdominal scanning was carried out in 13 infants and children with symptoms of ectopic gastric mucosa, as in Meckel's diverticulum, following the intravenous administration of pertechnetate (^{99m}Tc). Three patients were diagnosed as having Meckel's diverticulum and when surgery was carried out in 2 this was confirmed.— J. C. Leonidas and D. R. Germann, *Archs Dis. Childh.*, 1974, *49*, 21.

Abdominal scintiphotography with albumin labelled with technetium-99m was evaluated in the investigation of acute gastro-intestinal bleeding in one patient. The bleeding site was correctly located and the amount of blood lost was reasonably estimated.— J. Miskowiak *et al.* (preliminary communication), *Lancet*, 1977, *2*, 852.

Further reports of the use of technetium-99m-labelled agents in the investigation of gastro-intestinal bleeding.— J. P. Wilson *et al.*, *J. Am. med. Ass.*, 1977, *237*, 265 (pertechnetate); P. F. Winter, *J. Am. med. Ass.*, 1977, *237*, 1352 (pertechnetate).

Mention of the use of sulphur colloid labelled with technetium-99m in the diagnosis of oesophageal reflux.— *Med. Lett.*, 1980, *22*, 26.

See also under Gastric-function Test (above).

Heart. Myocardial scanning using technetium-99m as the pyrophosphate may prove useful for the early detection of cardiomyopathy in patients receiving doxorubicin.— A. K. Chacko *et al.*, *J. nucl. Med.*, 1977, *18*, 680.

Further reports of the use of technetium-99m-labelled agents for investigation of the heart: J. S. Borer *et al.*, *New Engl. J. Med.*, 1977, *296*, 839 (human serum albumin); B. L. Holman, *ibid.*, 876 (comment); R. J. Wainwright *et al.*, *Lancet*, 1979, *2*, 320 (red blood cells).

See also under Detection of Infarction (above) and Detection of Neoplasms (above).

Kidney. Renal images were recorded immediately after brain scanning in 200 patients given technetium-99m as gluceptate. Renal abnormalities were found in 22 including 11 previously unsuspected abnormalities of which 5 were of a significant nature. It was recommended that renal imaging be a routine part of a brain scan whenever gluceptate or an agent with a similar excretion pattern is used.— P. C. Kahn *et al.*, *J. nucl. Med.*, 1976, *17*, 786.

The successful evaluation of obstructive nephropathy using technetium-99m-labelled pentetic acid.— K. E. Britton *et al.*, *Lancet*, 1979, *1*, 905.

Further reports of the use of technetium-99m-labelled compounds in renal imaging: A. Taylor and L. Balner, *J. nucl. Med.*, 1978, *19*, 178 (penicillamine as an index of differential renal function); G. Kainer *et al.*, *Archs Dis. Childh.*, 1979, *54*, 931 (pentetic acid for renal function in children).

See also under Diagnosis of Transplant Rejection (above).

Liver and gall-bladder. A review of radionuclide imaging of the liver.— M. Critchley, *Br. J. Hosp. Med.*, 1978, *20*, 129.

Results of a study involving 116 patients indicated that technetium-99m-labelled pyridoxylidene glutamate scanning is more accurate for confirming a diagnosis of acute cholecystitis than oral cholecystography or ultrasonography.— R. H. L. Down *et al.*, *Lancet*, 1979, *2*, 1094. A view that iminodiacetic acid derivatives of technetium-99m are superior to the pyridoxylidene glutamate derivative, for hepatobiliary imaging.— B. Pastakia (letter), *ibid.*, 1980, *1*, 153. Further comment. The choice from among the newer scanning agents is probably unimportant because most yield up to 80% biliary excretion; the manner of performing the test is more significant.— E. A. Shaffer (letter), *ibid.*, 154.

Further reports and comments on the use of technetium-99m-labelled agents in hepatobiliary imaging: R. Stadalnik *et al.*, *Radiology*, 1976, *121*, 647 (pyridoxylidene glutamate in cholescintigraphy); R. L. MacCarty, *Am. J. Roentg.*, 1977, *129*, 23 (sulphur colloids in liver scanning); J. Papadimitriou *et al.*, *J. nucl. Med.*, 1977, *18*, 1194 (pyridoxal-phenylalanine in hepatobiliary scanning); E. Lubin *et al.*, *J. nucl. Med.*, 1978, *19*, 24 (pyridoxylidene glutamate in jaundiced patients).

See also under Detection of Neoplasms (above).

Lung. Serial X-rays and lung scans using technetium-99m macroaggregated albumin were performed in 30 bronchodilator-dependent children; 20 children had persistent perfusion defects, 5 were transiently underperfused, and 5 were normal. This technique provided information about under-perfusion that was not obtained from X-rays or by usual blood-gas studies.— J. S. Hyde *et al.*, *J. Am. med. Ass.*, 1976, *235*, 1125. See also G. F. Gates *et al.*, *Am. J. Dis. Child.*, 1976, *130*, 1222.

Muscle. Of 60 patients with either suspected or obviously devitalised muscle following acute electric burns, an abnormal muscle scan with technetium-99m as the pyrophosphate was seen in 50 and subsequent exploratory surgery confirmed these as areas of devitalised muscle. The technetium muscle scan proved to be a reliable and sensitive diagnostic adjunct not only in locating underlying damaged muscle but in better defining its anatomical extent.— J. L. Hunt *et al.*, *Archs Surg., Chicago*, 1980, *115*, 434. See also J. Hunt *et al.*, *J. Trauma*, 1979, *19*, 409.

Parathyroid. The use of technetium-99m and iodine-131 in the diagnosis of parathyroid adenoma in a 60-year-old woman.— K. Alagumalai *et al.*, *Ann. intern. Med.*, 1979, *90*, 204.

Spleen. Spleen imaging with technetium-99m-labelled erythrocytes.— R. Armas *et al.*, *Radiology*, 1979, *132*, 215.

Testis. Mention of the use of pertechnetate (^{99m}Tc) scanning in the differential diagnosis of testicular torsion and epididymo-orchitis.— N. S. Datta and T. Tanaka (letter), *J. Pediat.*, 1977, *91*, 167. See also N. S. Datta and F. S. Mishkin, *J. Am. med. Ass.*, 1975, *231*, 1060.

Preparations

Sodium Pertechnetate (^{99m}Tc) Injection (Fission) *(B.P.)*. A sterile solution containing technetium-99m as pertechnetate obtained from a preparation of molybdenum-99 extracted from uranium fission products. There are limits for the content of iodine-131, ruthenium-103, strontium-89, strontium-90, and other alpha-emitting and gamma-emitting radionuclidic impurities. In other respects it is similar to Sodium Pertechnetate (^{99m}Tc) Injection (Non-Fission) (see below).

Sodium Pertechnetate (^{99m}Tc) Injection (Non-Fission) *(B.P., Eur. P.)*. Natrii Pertechnetatis (^{99m}Tc) Sine Fissione Formati Solutio Iniectabilis. A sterile solution containing technetium-99m as pertechnetate and sufficient sodium chloride to render the solution iso-osmotic with blood. At the date and hour stated on the label, it contains 90 to 110% of the content of technetium-99m activity stated on the label. Not more than 0.01% of the radioactivity is due to radionuclides other than technetium-99m, except that molybdenum-99 may be present to the extent of 0.1% of the total radioactivity, calculated with reference to the date and the hour of administration, and that technetium-99 may be present. The injection may be obtained aseptically from a sterile preparation of molybdenum-99 or it may be sterilised by autoclaving. Molybdenum-99 is produced by the neutron irradiation of molybdenum. pH 4 to 8. *Dose.* For brain scintigraphy, 185 to 555 MBq (5 to 15 millicuries); for salivary-gland scintigraphy, 74 MBq (2 millicuries); for thyroid scintigraphy, 37 MBq (1 millicurie).

Sodium Pertechnetate Tc 99m Injection *(U.S.P.).* Sodium Pertechnetate Tc 99m Solution. A sterile solution suitable for intravenous or oral administration, containing technetium-99m in the form of sodium pertechnetate and sufficient sodium chloride to make the solution iso-osmotic. It contains 90 to 110% of the labelled amount of technetium-99m at the date and hour stated on the label. Other chemical forms of technetium-99m do not exceed 5% of the total radioactivity. If derived from molybdenum-99 formed as a result of neutron bombardment of stable molybdenum, there are limits for the content of molybdenum-99 and other gamma-emitting radionuclidic impurities. If derived from molybdenum-99 formed as a result of uranium fission, there are limits for the content of molybdenum-99, iodine-131, ruthenium-103, strontium-89, strontium-90, and all other radionuclidic impurities. A clear colourless solution. pH 4.5 to 7.5.

Technetium Tc 99m Albumin Aggregated Injection *(U.S.P.).* Technetium Tc 99m Aggregated Albumin; Technetated (^{99m}Tc) Aggregated Albumin (Human). A sterile aqueous suspension of albumin denatured to produce aggregates of controlled particle size (not less than 90% of the particles have a diameter of 10 to 90 µm and none exceeds 150 µm) labelled with technetium-99m. It is suitable for intravenous administration and contains 90 to 110% of the labelled amount of technetium-99m as aggregated albumin at the time indicated on the label. It may contain antimicrobial, reducing, chelating, and stabilising agents, buffers, and nonaggregated albumin. Other chemical forms of radioactivity do not exceed 10% of the total radioactivity. Limits for the content of other radionuclides: as for Sodium Pertechnetate Tc 99m Injection (above). A milky suspension from which particles settle on standing. pH 3.8 to 8. It should not be used if clumping of albumin is present. Store at 2° to 8°.

Technetium Tc 99m Etidronate Injection *(U.S.P.).* A sterile, clear, colourless solution, suitable for intravenous administration, of radioactive technetium (^{99m}Tc) in the form of chelate of sodium etidronate. It contains 90 to 110% of the labelled amount of technetium-99m at the time indicated on the label. Other chemical forms of radioactivity do not exceed 10% of the total radioactivity. Limits for the content of other radionuclides: as for Sodium Pertechnetate Tc 99m Injection (above). It may contain preservatives, buffering, reducing, and stabilising agents. pH 2.5 to 7.

Technetium Tc 99m Ferpentetate Injection *(U.S.P.).* Technetium Tc 99m Iron Ascorbate Pentetic Acid Complex Injection. A sterile aqueous solution, suitable for intravenous administration, of iron ascorbate-pentetic acid complexed with technetium-99m; it may contain buffers. It contains 90 to 110% of the labelled amount of technetium-99m at the time indicated on the label. Other chemical forms of radioactivity do not exceed 10% of the total radioactivity. Limits for the content of other radionuclides: as for Sodium Pertechnetate Tc 99m Injection (above). pH 4 to 5.5. Store at 2° to 8°. Protect from light. Use within 6 hours of the time of manufacture.

Technetium Tc 99m Gluceptate Injection *(U.S.P.).* Technetium Tc 99m Sodium Gluceptate Injection. A sterile aqueous solution, suitable for intravenous administration, of sodium gluceptate and stannous chloride labelled with technetium-99m; it may contain antimicrobial agents and buffers. It contains 90 to 110% of the labelled amount of technetium-99m, as stannous gluceptate complex, at the time indicated on the label. Other chemical forms of radioactivity do not exceed 10% of the total radioactivity. Limits for the content of other radionuclides: as for Sodium Pertechnetate Tc 99m Injection (above). pH 4 to 8. Store at 2° to 8°.

Technetium Tc 99m Pentetate Injection *(U.S.P.).* Technetium Tc 99m Pentetate Sodium Injection. A sterile solution, suitable for intravenous administration, of pentetic acid complexed with technetium-99m, in sodium chloride injection; it may contain buffers. It contains 90 to 110% of the labelled amount of technetium-99m at the time indicated on the label. Other chemical forms of radioactivity do not exceed 10% of the total radioactivity. Limits for the content of other radionuclides: as for Sodium Pertechnetate Tc 99m Injection (above). pH 3.8 to 7.5. Store at 2° to 8°. Use within 6 hours of the time of manufacture.

Technetium Tc 99m (Pyro- and trimeta-) Phosphates Injection *(U.S.P.).* A sterile aqueous solution, suitable for intravenous administration, of sodium pyrophosphate, sodium trimetaphosphate, and stannous chloride labelled with technetium-99m. It contains 90 to 110% of the labelled amount of technetium-99m, as phosphate, at the time indicated on the label. Other chemical forms of radioactivity do not exceed 10% of the total radioactivity. Limits for the content of other radionuclides: as for Sodium Pertechnetate Tc 99m Injection (above). pH 4 to 7. Store at 2° to 8°.

Technetium Tc 99m Pyrophosphate Injection *(U.S.P.).* A sterile aqueous solution, suitable for intravenous administration, of sodium pyrophosphate labelled with technetium-99m; it may contain antimicrobial, buffering, reducing, and stabilising agents. It contains 90 to 110% of the labelled amount of technetium-99m at the time indicated on the label. Other chemical forms of radioactivity do not exceed 10% of the total radioactivity. Limits for the content of other radionuclides: as for Sodium Pertechnetate Tc 99m Injection (above). pH 4 to 7.5. Store at 2° to 8°.

Technetium Tc 99m Sulfur Colloid Injection *(U.S.P.).* A sterile colloidal dispersion of sulphur labelled with technetium-99m, suitable for intravenous administration. It contains 90 to 110% of the labelled amount of technetium-99m as sulphur colloid at the time indicated on the label. It may contain chelating and stabilising agents and buffers. Other chemical forms of radioactivity do not exceed 8% of the total radioactivity. Limits for the content of other radionuclides: as for Sodium Pertechnetate Tc 99m Injection (above). A slightly opalescent, colourless to light tan liquid. pH 4 to 7. It should not be used if flocculent material is visible.

5879-k

Thallium-201 ($^{201}_{81}$Tl)

HALF-LIFE. 73.5 hours

RADIATION EMITTED. EC (100%); γ 0.135 (2.8%), 0.166 (0.1%), 0.167 (8.8%) MeV; X-rays (mercury) 0.065 to 0.082 (100% to 120%) MeV.

SUPPLY. Thallium-201 is supplied as thallous chloride (^{201}Tl) in the form of an injection containing more than 18 500 megabecquerels (500 millicuries) per mg of thallium or in the form of an injection containing 37 megabecquerels (1 millicurie) per ml.

Uses. Thallium-201 as a solution of thallous chloride is administered by intravenous injection for scanning the myocardium. The usual dose is 55.5 MBq (1.5 millicuries).

Detection of infarction. A review on the use of thallium scans in the evaluation of coronary heart disease. Thallium-201 scans are generally more specific than ECG stress tests for the diagnosis of coronary artery disease and false-positive results are uncommon although false-negative results have been reported in 10 to 20% of patients with more than 50% narrowing of at least one coronary artery on angiography. False-negatives may be due either to inadequate exercise because of severe angina or to global ischaemia associated with triple-vessel disease which normally produces a positive electrocardiogram. Following intravenous administration thallium is actively transported into cells and normally-perfused myocardium appears homogeneous on a scan whereas areas of myocardial ischaemia or infarction appear as defects or 'cold spots'. The radiopharmaceutical is normally administered during exercise and if a defect is observed another image is obtained after about 4 to 5 hours. Ischaemia is normally indicated by a defect seen only after exercise but a defect that persists suggests infarction; the scan alone, however, cannot distinguish between a recent and an old infarction.— *Med. Lett.*, 1979, *21*, 49.

Further reviews: *Br. med. J.*, 1978, *2*, 717.

In 23 patients with acute myocardial infarction who had undergone thallium-201 scanning there was 91% correlation between the scanning and necropsy location of infarction, and 70% correlation between the ECG and necropsy location. The size of the abnormal area detected on scanning closely reflected the extent of infarction.— F. J. T. Wackers *et al.*, *Circulation*, 1977, *56*, 72.

Further reports and comments on the use of thallium-201 in the detection of myocardial infarction: P. R. McLaughlin *et al.*, *Circulation*, 1977, *55*, 497; J. L. Ritchie *et al.*, *Circualtion*, 1977, *56*, 66; J. L. Ritchie *et al.*, *Am. J. Cardiol.*, 1978, *42*, 345; T. C. Smitherman *et al.*, *ibid.*, 177; J. L. Ritchie *et al.*, *J. nucl. Med.*, 1979, *20*, 477.

Further reports and comments on the use of thallium-201 in myocardial imaging: B. H. Bulkley *et al.*, *Chest*, 1977, *72*, 27 (diagnosis of sarcoid heart disease); B. H. Bulkley *et al.*, *Circulation*, 1977, *55*, 753 (use with technetium-99m to distinguish between ischaemic and idiopathic congestive cardiomyopathy); B. H. Greenberg *et al.*, *Am. J. Cardiol.*, 1978, *42*, 167 (evaluation of coronary bypass surgery); J. P. Finley *et al.*, *Am. J. Cardiol.*, 1978, *42*, 675 (imaging of anomalous left coronary artery arising from the pulmonary artery).

For reports and comments of dual imaging with thallium-201 and technetium-99m in the detection of myocardial infarction, see Technetium-99m, p.1397.

Detection of neoplasms. Preliminary experiments with thallium-201 as an indicator for lung neoplasms.— M. Salvatore *et al.*, *Radiology*, 1976, *121*, 487.

5880-w

Thorium-X ($^{224}_{88}$Ra). Radium-224

HALF-LIFE. 3.6 days

RADIATION EMITTED. α 5.445 (4.9%), 5.681 (95%) MeV; γ 0.24 (3.7%) MeV.

Thorium-X decays to radon-220 (thoron) with the emission of α-particles; radon-220 is itself radioactive and the decay continues through a series of radionuclides with short half-lives, finally producing stable lead-208 (thorium D).

SUPPLY. Thorium-X is a naturally occurring isotope of radium.

NOTE. In Great Britain, under the Radioactive Substances (Thorium-X) Exemption Order, 1963 (SI 1963: No. 1834) and ammendment (SI 1974: No. 500) and the Radioactive Substances (Thorium-X) Exemption (Scotland) Order, 1963 (SI 1963: No. 1880), ointments and solutions of thorium-X for medical treatment, and materials incorporating them and containing not more than 37 megabecquerels (1 millicurie) of radium-224, may be kept by hospitals, pharmacists, and doctors in their premises without registration. Provided that certain amounts are not exceeded, the disposal of waste is exempt from control.

Uses. Thorium-X was formerly used in the treatment of various skin conditions.

5881-e

Tritium ($^{3}_{1}$H). Hydrogen-3

HALF-LIFE. 12.35 years

RADIATION EMITTED. β^- 0.0186 (100%) MeV.

SUPPLY. Many organic compounds labelled with tritium are available.

Uses. Tritium, in the form of tritiated water injection, has been used to determine the total body water by a dilution technique.

Various tritiated compounds are used for *in vitro* and *in vivo* estimations.

5882-l

Xenon-133 ($^{133}_{54}$Xe)

Pharmacopoeias. In *U.S.*

HALF-LIFE. 5.25 days

RADIATION EMITTED. β^- 0.266 (0.9%), 0.346 (99.1%) MeV; γ 0.080 (0.4%), 0.081 (36.6%), 0.160 (0.05%) MeV; X-rays (caesium) 0.030 to 0.036 (~46%) MeV.

SUPPLY. Xenon-133 is supplied in the form of an injection, in which the gas is dissolved in sodium chloride injection, containing 74 000 to 370 000 megabecquerels (2 to 10 curies) per cm^3 of xenon at standard temperature and pressure or in the form of an injection containing 7.4 to 11.1 megabecquerels (200 to 300 millicuries) per mg of xenon. Xenon-133 gas is available in glass ampoules for use by inhalation after mixing with air or oxygen containing 74 000 to 370 000 megabecquerels (2 to 10 curies) per cm^3 of xenon at standard temperature and pressure. Xenon-133 gas is also available in vials, mixed with air to standard pressure, containing 7.4 to 11.1 megabecquerels (200 to 300 millicuries) per mg of xenon.

About 80% of activity might be lost during a period of 5 to 18 days after delivery of xenon-133 dissolved in saline due to uptake by rubber components in the cartridge. There might be a loss of up to 20% in plastic syringes due to sorption.— J. Keaney *et al., J. nucl. Med.*, 1971, *12*, 249, per *Int. pharm. Abstr.*, 1973, *10*, 636.

Uses. Xenon-133 is an inert gas with relatively low solubility in plasma. It is administered, usually in doses of about 37 to 185 MBq (1 to 5 millicuries), in the form of an injection in sodium chloride injection, for measurements of lung perfusion and regional blood flow. After intravenous injection, the gas is excreted promptly through the lungs.

Regional blood flow and other circulatory measurements of various regions including the brain, heart, and kidneys are carried out with 11.1 to 18.5 MBq (300 to 500 microcuries) of xenon-133 administered intra-arterially or intravenously. Blood flow in skin and muscle may be determined after administration of small intracutaneous or intramuscular injections of about 3.7 MBq (100 microcuries) xenon-133 in sodium chloride injection.

In the gaseous form, xenon-133 is mixed with air or oxygen in a bag or in a closed or open circuit spirometer to give a dose of 55.5 MBq (1.5 millicuries) of xenon-133 per litre of inhaled gas. When the administration of gas is stopped, xenon-133 is excreted promptly and completely through the lungs.

Xenon-127 has also been used in ventilation studies.

An account of the use of xenon-133 to measure liver blood flow.— S. B. Sherriff *et al., Gut*, 1977, *18*, 1027.

Regional cerebral haemodynamics during migraine and cluster headaches measured by the xenon-133 inhalation method.— F. Sakai and J. S. Meyer, *Headache*, 1978, *18*, 122.

The use of xenon-133 in ventilation studies.— R. Schor *et al., J. nucl. Med.*, 1978, *19*, 348; P. O. Alderson *et al., ibid.*, 1979, *20*, 917.

Preparations

Xenon (^{133}Xe) Injection *(B.P.)*. A sterile solution of xenon-133 made iso-osmotic with blood by the addition of sodium chloride. The injection should fill its container as completely as possible; the container should be in a form from which the injection can be extracted without the introduction of air bubbles. The content of xenon-133 is 80 to 130% of the content stated on the label at the date and hour stated on the label. pH 5 to 8. *Dose.* In studies of the circulatory system, up to 11.1 MBq (300 microcuries) by intra-arterial injection; in studies of pulmonary function, 37 to 74 MBq (1 to 2 millicuries) by intravenous injection.

Xenon Xe 133 Injection *(U.S.P.)*. A sterile iso-osmotic solution of xenon-133 in sodium chloride injection, suitable for intravenous administration. It contains 90 to 110% of the labelled amount of xenon-133, at the date and time stated on the label. Other forms of radioactivity do not exceed 5% of the total radioactivity. pH 4.5 to 8. Store at 2° to 8° in completely filled containers. Use within 5 weeks of the date of manufacture.

5883-y

Yttrium-90 ($^{90}_{39}$Y)

HALF-LIFE. 64.1 hours

RADIATION EMITTED. β^- 2.274 (~99.98%) MeV.

SUPPLY. Yttrium-90 is supplied as a suspension of colloidal yttrium (^{90}Y) silicate in aqueous solution containing 2 to 4 mg of sodium silicate per ml in the form of an injection containing 259 to 1295 megabecquerels (7 to 35 millicuries) per mg of yttrium.

Adverse Effects and Precautions. Chromosome damage has been reported in patients given intra-articular injections of yttrium-90.

A study of the effects and side-effects of radiosynovectomy with yttrium silicate (^{90}Y) on rheumatic joint cartilage indicated that changes in the human joint occur uniformly throughout the entire cartilage cell layer. It was suggested that the usual dose of 185 to 222 MBq (5 to 6 millicuries) per knee joint may be reduced to 111 to 148 MBq (3 to 4 millicuries) without diminishing therapeutic efficacy.— F. Kerschbaumer *et al., Archs orthopaed. traum. Surg.*, 1979, *93*, 95.

Uses. Yttrium-90, in the form of a colloidal suspension of yttrium silicate (^{90}Y) is suitable for instillation into pleural or peritoneal cavities in the treatment of malignant pleural effusion or malignant ascites. Doses of 370 to 1480 MBq (10 to 40 millicuries) are infused after paracentesis. Other therapies are equally effective and are generally preferred. It is also used in the treatment of arthritic conditions of joints, a dose of 185 MBq (5 millicuries) being appropriate for injection into the knee.

Yttrium-90 as yttrium oxide (^{90}Y) rods or grains have been used by implantation for the irradiation of the pituitary gland.

Pituitary ablation. Eight patients with Nelson's syndrome, all with considerable pigmentation and 1 with cranial nerve abnormalities, were treated with a pituitary implant of yttrium-90 or gold-198 or a combination of the 2, four to sixteen years after adrenal surgery. They were subsequently followed up for 3 months to 13 years: skin pigmentation became normal in 6 patients and was reduced in 2; corticotrophin concentrations became normal in 4 and were reduced in the other 2 studied; no new cranial disease or further sella expansion occurred, and remodelling of the sella was noted in 2 patients. Complications included temporary third nerve paresis (1 patient), temporary CSF leakage (1 patient), diabetes insipidus (1 patient), and gonadotrophin deficiency (1 patient).— J. Cassar *et al., Br. med. J.*, 1976, *2*, 269.

Further references: B. S. Ray *et al., J. Am. med. Ass.*, 1968, *203*, 85 (diabetic retinopathy); F. I. Akinsete *et al., Lancet*, 1973, *2*, 1050 (leucoerythroblastosis arising from carcinoma of the breast); C. W. Burke *et al., Q. J. Med.*, 1973, *42*, 693 (Cushing's disease); W. Kelly and G. F. Joplin (letter), *Br. med. J.*, 1978, *1*, 1050 (prolactin-producing pituitary tumours); J. M. Fitzpatrick *et al., Br. J. Urol.*, 1980, *52*, 301 (relief of pain in advanced prostatic carcinoma).

Rheumatoid arthritis. Irradiation with intra-articular injections of 5 ml of a colloidal suspension of yttrium-90 as the citrate, silicate, or as a resin in a dose of 185 MBq (5 millicuries) was considered as effective as synovectomy in a study of 17 patients with persistent synovitis affecting 21 knees. Irradiation appeared to give better protection than surgery against exacerbations of rheumatoid arthritis and was superior to surgery in terms of side-effects and complications, hospital stay, and nursing and physiotherapy requirements.— J. M. Gumpel and N. C. Roles, *Lancet*, 1975, *1*, 488.

It was concluded from a study of 20 patients treated with injections of yttrium-90 into knee joints that confining the patients to bed and immobilising the joint to reduce the leakage of nuclide decreased chromosome aberrations in peripheral blood lymphocytes.— D. C. Lloyd and E. J. Reeder, *Lancet*, 1978, *1*, 617. After intra-articular injection of yttrium-90 into the knee for persistent synovitis, there was no difference in the amount of isotope retained in the joint in those kept in bed and those mobilised with the joint splinted. Complete bed rest was not necessary.— J. Winfield *et al., Br. med. J.*, 1979, *1*, 986.

Further references: J. F. Bridgman *et al., Ann. rheum. Dis.*, 1971, *30*, 180; S. Jalava, *Curr. ther. Res.*, 1973, *15*, 395; *Lancet*, 1974, *1*, 346; *Br. med. J.*, 1974, *2*, 682.

Sex Hormones

9020-r

The male and female sex organs, the adrenal cortex, and the placenta produce steroidal hormones which influence the development and maintenance of the structures directly and indirectly associated with reproduction. This section describes the natural sex hormones together with synthetic compounds that possess their actions.

Of the 3 principal types of hormones involved, the *androgens* have distinct roles in the reproductive physiology of the male and the *oestrogens* and *progestogens* (progestagens) comparable roles in the female.

The androgens, exemplified by testosterone (see p.1435), are mainly concerned with the development and maintenance of the secondary male sex characters, increasing virility and libido. They also increase nitrogen and water retention and stimulate skeletal growth.

In contrast, the oestrogens, exemplified by oestradiol (see p.1425), are mainly concerned with the development and maintenance of secondary female sex characters and control the cyclical changes to which the uterus and vagina are subject during the menstrual cycle. Oestrogens are further required for maintenance of pregnancy and also have an anabolic effect on protein metabolism and water retention, though less pronounced than that of the androgens.

Progestogens, exemplified by progesterone (see p.1431), are necessary for other changes that occur in the uterus and vagina during the menstrual cycle, for development of mammary tissue, and for the maintenance of pregnancy.

The secretion of the sex hormones is controlled by the gonadotrophic hormones of the anterior lobe of the pituitary gland, but the level of secretion of the gonadotrophic hormones is in turn influenced by the hypothalamus as well as the concentration of circulating sex hormones.

Classification. The sex hormones and related compounds described in this section may be classified in the following 5 main groups on the basis of their principal pharmacological actions.

Those with pronounced oestrogenic activity include:
benzoestrol, p.1406
chlorotrianisene, p.1406
dienoestrol, p.1410
estropipate, p.1411
ethinyloestradiol, p.1411
fosfestrol, p.1414
hexoestrol, p.1415
mestranol, p.1418
methallenoestril, p.1418
oestradiol, p.1425
oestriol, p.1428
conjugated oestrogens, p.1428
oestrone, p.1429
polyestradiol, p.1431
quinestradol, p.1432
quinestrol, p.1432
stilboestrol, p.1433.

Those with pronounced androgenic properties and also anabolic properties include:
calusterone, p.1406
dehydroepiandrosterone, p.1410
fluoxymesterone, p.1413
mesterolone, p.1418
methyltestosterone, p.1420
testosterone, p.1435.

Those with pronounced anabolic properties and relatively weak androgenic properties include:
clostebol, p.1408
drostanolone, p.1410
ethyloestrenol, p.1413
methandienone, p.1418
methandriol, p.1419
methenolone, p.1419
nandrolone, p.1420
norethandrolone, p.1421
oxandrolone, p.1430
oxymesterone, p.1430
oxymetholone, p.1430
stanolone, p.1433
stanozolol, p.1433.

Those with pronounced progestational properties but little other activity include:
algestone, p.1406
allyloestrenol, p.1406
chlormadinone, p.1406
dimethisterone, p.1410
dydrogesterone, p.1411
gestronol, p.1414
hydroxyprogesterone, p.1415
medrogestone, p.1416
medroxyprogesterone, p.1416
megestrol, p.1417
norethynodrel, p.1423
progesterone, p.1431
quingestanol, p.1432.

Those with progestational, oestrogenic, and androgenic properties include:
ethisterone, p.1412
ethynodiol, p.1413
levonorgestrel, p.1424
lynoestrenol, p.1415
norethisterone, p.1421
norgestrel, p.1424.

Miscellaneous compounds with actions related to those of the sex hormones include clomiphene (p.1406), cyclofenil (p.1408), cyproterone (p.1408), and danazol (p.1409).

Adverse Effects. The adverse effects of the different groups of sex hormones are described under Norethisterone, p.1421, Oestradiol, p.1425, Progesterone, p.1431, and Testosterone, p.1436. However, the adverse effects associated with oral contraceptives are described on p.1402.

Synthetic sex hormones which have an alkyl group in the α configuration at position 17 are associated with an increased risk of liver damage (see Methyltestosterone, p.1420).

Pregnancy and the neonate. *Effects on the foetus.* A retrospective study covering 1942–72 of 76 mothers of children with transposition of the great vessels showed that 7 of 10 who had been treated with hormones during pregnancy had received a sex hormone.— E. P. Levy *et al.* (letter), *Lancet*, 1973, *1*, 611.

A retrospective study over the period of 1942–73 revealed no association between maternal hormone intake and oesophageal atresia in the infants.— T. J. David and S. E. O'Callaghan (letter), *Lancet*, 1974, *1*, 1236.

Four of 5 women who took or continued to take sex hormones during pregnancy produced children with congenital defects.— J. Robertson-Rintoul (letter), *Lancet*, 1974, *2*, 515.

Of a group of 11 468 babies, 432 were born to mothers who had a history of definite or probable administration of oestrogen or progestogen and 47 infants had one or more malformations. The risk of major malformations was considered to be 26% higher in infants exposed or probably exposed to hormones than in those not exposed; with minor malformations the risk was 33% greater.— S. Harlap *et al.* (letter), *Lancet*, 1975, *1*, 682.

Of 50 282 children born to mothers monitored by the Collaborative Perinatal Project, 1480 were found to have been exposed to progestogens or oestrogens, and possibly other drugs, at some time during the first 4 months of the pregnancy. Although no relationship between malformations in general and exposure to these sex hormones was observed the incidence of cardiovascular deformities was increased.— O. P. Heinonen *et al.*, *Birth Defects and Drugs in Pregnancy*, Littleton MA, Publishing Sciences Group, 1977, p. 388.

In a retrospective study of 104 infants with congenital heart disease 70 were identified with specified heart defects; 18 had involvement of other body systems. With respect to the 70, exposure to hormones during pregnancy had occurred in 13, compared with 2 in a series of controls—a risk factor of 6.5. Of 12 with multiple cardiac defects with involvement of other systems, 6 had been exposed to hormones.— D. T. Janerich *et al.*, *Br. med. J.*, 1977, *1*, 1058.

Pregnancy tests. The Committee on Safety of Medicines considered that hormonal pregnancy tests should not be employed for the diagnosis of pregnancy.— *Pharm. J.*, 1975, *1*, 533.

After a survey of the incidence of cleft lip and palate in Western Australia, a retrospective study revealed that in 22 of 222 cases studied mothers had received oral or parenteral pregnancy tests between the fifth and eighth weeks of gestation.— W. F. Brogan (letter), *Med. J. Aust.*, 1975, *1*, 44.

Of 836 mothers of congenitally malformed infants 73 had used hormonal pregnancy tests during the first trimester of pregnancy, compared with 35 in 836 controls. The case:control incidence ratio of 2.09 was significant. When families with a history of congenital malformation were excluded the ratio (1.91) remained significant.— G. Greenberg *et al.*, *Br. med. J.*, 1977, *2*, 853.

Negative reports.— M. Laurence *et al.* (letter), *Nature*, 1971, *233*, 495 (spina bifida or anencephaly); G. P. Oakley *et al.* (letter), *Lancet*, 1973, *2*, 256; J. Goujard and C. Rumeau-Rouquette (letter), *Lancet*, 1977, *1*, 482.

Discussions: Statement by Australian Drug Evaluation Committee on Hormonal Pregnancy Tests.— *Med. J. Aust.*, 1977, *1*, 46; *J. Am. med. Ass.*, 1977, *238*, 471; *Lancet*, 1978, *2*, 1265; D. Aarskog, *New Engl. J. Med.*, 1979, *300*, 75.

See also Norethisterone, p.1421 and Norethisterone Acetate, p.1422.

Uses. The sex hormones are primarily used for replacement therapy.

Androgens are used for replacement in hypogonadism, in the treatment of gynaecomastia, and for erythropoiesis in anaemia. They have also been used for menstrual and menopausal disorders but female hormones are generally preferred. Anabolic steroids are given in the control of conditions characterised by protein and bone wasting.

The female hormones are used for hypogonadism and during the menopause. They are sometimes maintained during the postmenopausal period although the hazards may outweigh the benefits. They are given for secondary amenorrhoea, endometriosis, uterine bleeding, other menstrual disorders, and for contraception (see Oral Contraceptives, below). They have been used in habitual or threatened abortion and for the inhibition or suppression of lactation. Treatment with the female hormones may involve replacement therapy or sustained or intermittent (cyclic) suppression of the natural hormone production via an inhibitory effect on the activity of the hypothalamus and anterior lobe of the pituitary.

A review of the actions of sex hormones.— L. Chan and B. W. O'Malley, *New Engl. J. Med.*, 1976, *294*, 1322, and 1430. See also *idem*, *Ann. intern. Med.*, 1978, *89*, 694.

The treatment of adolescent gynaecological disorders.— J. A. Jordan, *Br. med. J.*, 1977, *1*, 98.

A review on abnormal vaginal bleeding and its treatment.— J. M. Goldfarb and A. B. Little, *New Engl. J. Med.*, 1980, *302*, 666.

Contraception. A review of fertility regulation in the male; a marketable male contraceptive was unlikely to be available for several years.— D. M. de Kretser, *Bull. Wld Hlth Org.*, 1978, *56*, 353. See also J. Senior, *Pharm. J.*, 1978, *1*, 341.

See also Oral Contraceptives, below.

Sex Hormones in Neoplastic Disorders. The growth of malignant neoplasms of the breast, prostate, and endometrium is often dependent on the hormonal balance of the body. When these conditions have not responded or are no longer controlled by surgery and radiotherapy, changing the hormonal balance of the body by the administration of sex hormones may produce useful remissions.

Androgens may be used in the treatment of

women with advanced and metastatic neoplasms of the breast; fluoxymesterone (p.1414) is often used because it can be given by mouth. Androgens should not be given to men with malignant neoplasms of the prostate or breast. The anti-androgen cyproterone has been tried in prostatic carcinoma.

Oestrogens are used in the treatment of advanced metastatic neoplasms of the breast only when ovarian function has ceased. Stilboestrol (p.1434) is given but the anti-oestrogen tamoxifen (p.227) is also used. Oestrogens are also used to control inoperable and metastatic neoplasms of the prostate; stilboestrol is generally preferred.

Progestogens are used in the treatment of inoperable neoplasms of the endometrium and are given to a lesser extent in neoplasms of the breast. They have also been tried in neoplasms of the kidney and prostate. Hydroxyprogesterone hexanoate, medroxyprogesterone acetate (p.1416), megestrol acetate (p.1417), and norethisterone acetate (p.1422) have been used.

See also under Choice of Antineoplastic Agent, p.175.

9021-f

Oral Contraceptives

Oral contraceptives are only available for women although preparations for men are being evaluated. The preparations used for oral contraception can be classified into 3 types commonly known as 'combined', 'progestogen-only', and 'postcoital' and these are described below. The efficacy of the 'combined' type varies dependent upon the oestrogen and progestogen content, but the 'combined' type is more effective than the 'progestogen-only'. 'Postcoital' contraceptives are not used routinely but are very effective if given shortly after coitus.

In the *'combined'* type, also known as 'classical' or 'balanced' contraceptives, an orally active progestogen such as norethisterone or norgestrel is given in conjunction with an orally active oestrogen such as ethinyloestradiol or mestranol. The oral contraceptives of this type are described in the following pages in the monographs on their respective progestogen constituents—see under Ethynodiol Diacetate (p.1413), Lynoestrenol (p.1415), Norethisterone (p.1421), Norethisterone Acetate (p.1422), Norethynodrel (p.1423), Norgestrel (p.1424), and Levonorgestrel (p.1424). These progestogen and oestrogen combinations are administered daily usually in courses of 21 tablets from the 5th to the 25th day of the first treated cycle and thereafter repeated after intervals of 7 days for succeeding cycles. Some preparations are given for 20 days from the 5th to the 24th day of each cycle and others are given in 22-day courses.

In some preparations (*triphasic* type) the content of progestogen and oestrogen is varied at different times in the cycle. Some preparations of this type are described under Norgestrel, (p.1425).These contraceptive preparations appear to act by suppressing the mid-cycle peak of luteinising hormone and follicle-stimulating hormone, thereby inhibiting ovulation and both the progestogen and oestrogen constituents have this property. The progestogen constituent also produces thickening of the cervical mucus which is considered to render it hostile to sperm penetration. In addition, these preparations alter the endometrial pattern and may thereby prevent implantation. Transport of the ovum in the fallopian tube may also be affected.

'Progestogen-only' contraceptives appear to act mainly by rendering the cervical mucus hostile to sperm penetration but other factors may be involved. Small doses of progestogen are taken daily throughout the cycle in a continuous schedule. These preparations are less effective than the other forms of oral contraception and since their action appears to be short-lived there tends to be a greater risk of pregnancy if tablets are missed. The oral contraceptives of this type are described under the following progestogens: Ethynodiol Diacetate (p.1413), Norethisterone (p.1421), Norgestrel (p.1424), and Levonorgestrel (p.1424).

Progesterone has been given *in utero* as a depot 'progestogen-only' contraceptive; norethisterone acetate has been similarly used. Medroxyprogesterone acetate 150 mg given intramuscularly provides contraceptive cover for up to 3 months (see p.1416); norethisterone enanthate is similarly used.

'Postcoital' contraception can be effectively provided by administering large doses of oestrogen shortly after unprotected intercourse. Stilboestrol (see p.1434) is usually given for 5 days starting within 72 hours of intercourse. However, because of the potential risk to the foetus termination of pregnancy should be considered if the oestrogen is ineffective.

'Sequential' preparations are now little used. An oestrogen such as mestranol or ethinyloestradiol has been administered daily from the 5th to 20th or 21st day of the menstrual cycle and then the oestrogen in conjunction with a progestogen has been administered for the next 5 to 7 days. These preparations probably inhibit ovulation through suppression of the release of gonadotrophins from the pituitary. Another regimen that has been used consists of giving an oestrogen such as ethinyloestradiol or mestranol for 7 days per cycle followed by the oestrogen in conjunction with a progestogen for the next 15 days. For proprietary names of such preparations see under Ethinyloestradiol, p.1412 and Mestranol, p.1418.

Administration. Meticulous regularity of dosage is essential with all oral contraceptives and particularly with progestogen-only oral contraceptives. If one dose is missed it should be taken as soon as possible and the next dose taken at the usual time. Protection may be reduced if more than 36 hours elapses between doses. If 2 consecutive doses are missed, the usual dosage should be resumed as soon as possible and additional contraceptive precautions taken for the remainder of the cycle.

If breakthrough bleeding occurs, the dose should be continued. If breakthrough bleeding occurs in 2 consecutive cycles a more progestogenic preparation may be required. Sometimes withdrawal bleeding does not occur at the end of the cycle. In such cases the possibility of pregnancy should be excluded.

For reviews and discussions of the actions and uses of oral contraceptives, see Advances in Methods of Fertility Regulation, Report of a WHO Scientific Group, *Tech. Rep. Ser. Wld Hlth Org. No. 575,* 1975; *Br. med. J.,* 1976, *2,* 131; *Br. med. J.,* 1976, *2,* 1216; M. Vessey *et al., J. biosoc. Sci.,* 1976, *8,* 373; B. Law, *Practitioner,* 1977, *219,* 571; M. P. Vessey, *Br. med. J.,* 1978, *2,* 721 and 914; *Drug & Ther. Bull.,* 1979, *17,* 1; N. B. Loudon, *Practitioner,* 1979, *223,* 641; M. D. Read, *Practitioner,* 1980, *224,* 179; F. M. Graham, *Drugs,* 1981, *21,* 152; *Lancet,* 1981, *1,* 1191.

The incidences of benign thyroid swelling, thyrotoxicosis, and myxoedema were each less in women taking oral contraceptives than in controls.— *Br. med. J.,* 1978, *2,* 1531 (Royal College of General Practitioners' Oral Contraceptive Study).

A discussion on burning sensations in the oral cavity with mention of the beneficial role of cyclical oestrogen and progestagen therapy.— *Lancet,* 1978, *2,* 511.

Administration. A suggestion was made by N. Loudon (*Br. med. J.,* 1977 *2,* 521) that oral contreceptives could be started on the first, instead of the fifth, day of the cycle without the need for additional contraceptive precautions, and that a new brand could be similarly taken or taken without break after the end of the preceding course, again without additional precautions; this was supported by C. Phillips and M. Vessey (*Br. med. J.,* 1978, *2,* 1021). The Family Planning Association offered similar advice (*Pharm. J.,* 1977, *2,* 470; 1978, *1,* 532; 1978, *2,* 351).

Postcoital contraceptives. A discussion on the use of steroid hormones as 'postcoital' contraceptives.— *Lancet,* 1972, *2,* 314; Advances in Methods of Fertility Regulation, *Tech. Rep. Ser. Wld Hlth Org. No. 527,* 1973; ibid., *No. 575,* 1975; *Drug & Ther. Bull.,* 1980, *18,* 5.

For a recommended regimen for postcoital contraception see under Levonorgestrel, p.1424.

Postpartum use. Oral contraceptives could be taken 4 to 6 weeks after delivery, and as soon as possible after termination of pregnancy.— N. B. Loudon, *Practitioner,* 1979, *223,* 641.

Progestogen-only contraceptives. References to the use of progestogen-only contraceptives: Hormonal Steroids in Contraception, Reports of a WHO Scientific Group, *Tech. Rep. Ser. Wld Hlth Org. No. 386,* 1968; E. Mears *et al., Br. med. J.,* 1969, *2,* 730; H. J. E. Cox (letter), *ibid.,* 1969, *3,* 471; *Lancet,* 1971, *1,* 25; M. Karim *et al., Br. med. J.,* 1971, *1,* 200; M. P. Vessey *et al., Lancet,* 1972, *1,* 915; *Br. med. J.,* 1972, *3,* 190; *Drug & Ther. Bull.,* 1974, *12,* 9; Advances in Methods of Fertility Regulation, Report of a WHO Scientific Group, *Tech. Rep. Ser. Wld Hlth Org. No. 575,* 1975.

Adverse Effects of Oral Contraceptives. Many reports have been published of adverse effects associated with the use of oral contraceptives, the composition of which has changed with time.

There is an increased risk of thrombo-embolic disease related, at least in part, to the oestrogen content; the dose of oestrogen is therefore seldom more than 50 µg daily. The increased mortality risk factor from thrombo-embolic disease is greatest with increased age and in cigarette smokers. An increased risk of fatal myocardial infarction has been reported, the risk increasing with age; the risk may possibly be considerably higher in smokers. Other risk factors include hypertension, abnormal glucose tolerance including diabetes, and disorders of lipid metabolism.

Hypertension is associated with oral contraceptives and there may be changes in carbohydrate and lipid metabolism. Liver function can be impaired, although jaundice is rare. There appears to be a marked increase (though the incidence is still very low) in the relative risk of hepatocellular adenoma (usually benign) in women who have taken oral contraceptives for 3 years or more; the risk increases with the steroid dose, duration of use, and age. Focal nodular hyperplasia, hamartoma, and hepatic carcinoma have also occurred. Some patients may experience depression and other mental changes.

There may be gastro-intestinal side-effects, chloasma and other skin or hair changes, headache, oedema, weight gain, and breast engorgement. Spotting, breakthrough bleeding, or amenorrhoea can occur during treatment and amenorrhoea may also occur when oral contraceptives are withdrawn. Intolerance to contact lenses has been reported.

Some side-effects are considered to result from the relative balance of oestrogenic and progestogenic effects of particular products and the incidence of side-effects may be reduced by a change to a different product.

Reviews and discussions on the effects of oral contraceptives: Advances in Methods of Fertility Regulation, Report of a WHO Scientific Group, *Tech. Rep. Ser. Wld Hlth Org. No. 575,* 1975; *Med. Lett.,* 1976, *18,* 21; M. Vessey *et al., J. biosoc. Sci.,* 1976, *8,* 373; E. G. McQueen, *Drugs,* 1978, *16,* 322; R. Hoover *et al., Am. J. publ. Hlth,* 1978, *68,* 335; J. McEwan, *Br. J. Hosp. Med.,* 1979, *21,* 144.

Analysis of mortality trends in 21 countries suggested that since the introduction of oral contraceptives the relative risk of death from heart disease and hypertension, cerebrovascular disease, and all cardiovascular diseases was increased, in users, by factors of 5, 2, and 3 respectively.— V. Beral, *Lancet,* 1976, *2,* 1047.

It was estimated that in England and Wales in 1975 mortality from the use of oral contraceptives exceeded that from all complications of pregnancy and abortion. A reproductive mortality-rate, to include mortality from oral contraceptives, should replace the maternal mortality-rate.— V. Beral, *Br. med. J.,* 1979, *2,* 632.

Allergy. Hypersensitivity reactions were associated in 11 patients with the use of oral contraceptives.— C. J. Falliers (letter), *Lancet,* 1974, *2,* 515. See also D. F.

Morris (letter), *Br. med. J.*, 1974, *3*, 467; Z. Pelikan, *Ann. Allergy*, 1978, *40*, 211.

Alopecia. Reports and discussions of alopecia associated with the use of oral contraceptives.— W. A. D. Griffiths, *Br. J. Derm.*, 1973, *88*, 31; *Br. med. J.*, 1973, *2*, 499.

Amenorrhoea. Reports and discussions of amenorrhoea associated with oral contraceptives use.— R. P. Shearman, *Lancet*, 1971, *2*, 64; S. J. Steele *et al.*, *Br. med. J.*, 1973, *4*, 343; Advances in Methods of Fertility Regulation, Report of a WHO Scientific Group, *Tech. Rep. Ser. Wld Hlth Org. No. 575*, 1975; G. D. Pinkerton and H. M. Carey, *Med. J. Aust.*, 1976, *1*, 220; *idem*, 223; *Br. med. J.*, 1976, *2*, 660; K. W. Hancock *et al.*, *Br. med. J.*, 1976, *2*, 399; M. Kissi and J. A. J. Faber, *Obstet. Gynec.*, 1979, *53*, 241.

A report suggesting that oral contraceptives did not cause amenorrhoea.— H. S. Jacobs *et al.*, *Br. med. J.*, 1977, *2*, 940. Comment.— R. P. Shearman (letter), *Br. med. J.*, 1977, *2*, 1414.

In 1174 nulliparous women who stopped taking oral contraceptives in order to conceive fertility (assessed by failure to produce a live or still-born infant) was impaired, gradually returning to normal about 42 months after ceasing contraception. In 1060 parous women the effect was similar, returning to normal within about 30 months. It was not known from the study whether infertility corresponded with amenorrhoea.— M. P. Vessey *et al.*, *Br. med. J.*, 1978, *1*, 265.

Candidiasis. The incidence of vaginal *Candida albicans* in 546 women taking oral contraceptives was not greater than in 952 other women.— M. J. Goldacre *et al.*, *Br. med. J.*, 1979, *1*, 1450.

Cervical erosions. In 1498 women cervical erosions were significantly more common in those using oral contraceptives than in those using the IUD, mechanical methods, or no contraception.— M. J. Goldacre *et al.*, *Br. med. J.*, 1978, *1*, 748. Earlier references: *Br. med. J.*, 1973, *1*, 43; R. R. Dooley *et al.*, *Am. J. Obstet. Gynec.*, 1974, *118*, 971; *Br. med. J.*, 1975, *1*, 328.

Chorea. Case reports of chorea associated with oral contraceptives.— D. Riddoch *et al.*, *Br. med. J.*, 1971, *4*, 217; A. D. Malcolm (letter), *ibid.*, 491; E. T. Gamboa *et al.*, *Archs Neurol.*, *Chicago*, 1971, *25*, 112, per *Drugs*, 1972, *3*, 439; W. A. Pulsinelli and R. W. Hamill, *Am. J. Med.*, 1978, *65*, 557; P. A. Nausieda *et al.*, *Neurology*, *Minneap.*, 1979, *29*, 1605; D. J. Dove, *Am. J. Obstet. Gynec.*, 1980, *137*, 740.

Dental effects. Localised osteitis (dry socket) in the mandibular third molar (wisdom tooth) region of the mouth occurred postoperatively in 7 of 36 (19.4%) sites in 18 women taking oral contraceptives compared with 10 of 174 (5.7%) sites in 87 women not taking oral contraceptives.— J. B. Sweet and D. P. Butler, *Am. J. Obstet. Gynec.*, 1977, *127*, 518.

Radiographic changes of the mandible.— N. C. Darzenta and J. L. Giunta, *Oral Surg.*, 1977, *43*, 478.

Effects on carbohydrate metabolism. A study in women taking oral contraceptives (67 990 woman-years) or who had taken oral contraceptives (42 623 woman-years) did not suggest that the risk of developing diabetes was increased compared with that in controls (111 252 woman-years).— S. J. Wingrave *et al.*, *Br. med. J.*, 1979, *1*, 23.

Further references generally relating to impaired glucose tolerance: V. Wynn and J. W. H. Doar, *Lancet*, 1969, *2*, 761; V. Wynn *et al.*, *Lancet*, 1979, *1*, 1045; *ibid.*, 1063; L. D. Ostrander *et al.*, *J. Am. med. Ass.*, 1980, *244*, 677.

Effects on chromosomes. A significant increase in triploidy.— D. H. Carr, *Can. med. Ass. J.*, 1970, *103*, 343. See also N. F. Bishun, *Proc. R. Soc. Med.*, 1976, *69*, 353, per *Int. pharm. Abstr.*, 1976, *13*, 1180. Minimal effects.— L. R. Shapiro *et al.*, *Obstet. Gynec.*, *N.Y.*, 1972, *39*, 190, per *Int. pharm. Abstr.*, 1972, *9*, 809; D. T. Janerich *et al.*, *Br. J. Obstet. Gynaec.*, 1976, *83*, 617, per *Int. pharm. Abstr.*, 1977, *14*, 522; H. P. Klinger *et al.*, *Obstet. Gynec.*, 1976, *48*, 40, per *Int. pharm. Abstr.*, 1978, *15*, 1166; S. Harlap *et al.* (letter), *Lancet*, 1979, *1*, 1342.

See also under Pregnancy and the Neonate (below).

Effects on the endocrine system. For reports of the effects of oral contraceptives on the endocrine system, see O. J. Lucis and R. Lucis, *Bull. Wld Hlth Org.*, 1972, *46*, 443; R. D. Bulbrook *et al.*, *Lancet*, 1973, *1*, 628; R. Beckerhoff *et al.*, *Lancet*, 1973, *1*, 1218; J. M. Kjeld *et al.*, *Br. med. J.*, 1976, *2*, 1354; J. R. Givens *et al.*, *Am. J. Obstet. Gynec.*, 1976, *124*, 333; M. C. K. Browning and J. Anderson (letter), *Br. med. J.*, 1977, *1*, 107; D. R. Mishell, *Am. J. Obstet. Gynec.*, 1977, *128*, 60; M. Fern *et al.*, *Obstet. Gynec.*, 1978, *51*, 541; B. R. Carr *et al.*, *J. clin. Endocr. Metab.*, 1979, *49*, 346.

Effects on the eyes. Changes in the microvasculature of the retina.— M. Irvy and M. Oliver, *Obstet. Gynec.,N.Y.*, 1972, *39*, 909, per *Int. pharm. Abstr.*, 1973, *10*, 213. A central arterial occlusion.— B. Schutze, *Dte GesundhWes.*, 1973, *28*, 1050, per *Int. pharm. Abstr.*, 1974, *11*, 135. Retinal haemorrhage.— E. D. Svarc and D. Werner, *Am. J. Ophthal.*, 1977, *84*, 50, per *J. Am. med. Ass.*, 1977, *238*, 2650.

Absence of ophthalmic morbidity in 69 patients.— H. Wild *et al.*, *Dte GesundhWes.*, 1977, *32*, 414, per *Int. pharm. Abstr.*, 1977, *14*, 1230.

Effects on the gall-bladder. A calculated 2-fold increase in the incidence of gall-stones in women taking oral contraceptives.— *Lancet*, 1973, *1*, 1399 (Boston Collaborative Drug Surveillance Program). See also L. J. Bennion *et al.*, *New Engl. J. Med.*, 1976, *294*, 189; D. M. Small, *ibid.*, 219; K. -H. Leissner *et al.*, *Scand. J. Gastroenterol.*, 1977, *12*, 893; B. Dokert *et al.*, *Dte GesundhWes.*, 1978, *33*, 1153, per *Int. pharm. Abstr.*, 1979, *16*, 734; L. J. Bennion and S. M. Grundy, *New Engl. J. Med.*, 1978, *299*, 1221.

Effects on the gastro-intestinal tract. A discussion of small-bowel ischaemia associated with oral contraceptives, with mention of 21 cases in the literature.— *Br. med. J.*, 1978, *1*, 4.

Effects on the liver. The Boston Collaborative Drug Surveillance Program reported that of 68 women with acute hepatitis, 21 (16 of them under 25 years of age) had recently been taking oral contraceptives whereas 163 of 1142 controls had such a history. The crude risk ratio was estimated to be 2.7 but when relevant factors were considered the ratio rose to 3.3.— A. S. Morrison *et al.*, *Lancet*, 1977, *1*, 1142.

A discussion of drug-induced liver disease including mention of the Budd-Chiari syndrome associated with oral contraceptives.— H. J. Zimmerman, *Drugs*, 1978, *16*, 25. See also S. -M. Wu *et al.*, *Am. J. dig. Dis.*, 1977, *22*, 623.

Increased liver size and reduced drug-metabolising activity in women taking oral contraceptives.— M. Homeida *et al.*, *Clin. Pharmac. Ther.*, 1978, *24*, 228.

Reports and discussions of elevated values in liver-function tests.— A. Eisalo *et al.*, *Br. med. J.*, 1971, *3*, 561; A. Paton (letter), *Br. med. J.*, 1972, *1*, 632; M. B. Sammour *et al.*, *Contraception*, 1973, *7*, 403; E. Pansold *et al.*, *Dte GesundhWes.*, 1974, *29*, 470; *Br. med. J.*, 1974, *4*, 430.

See also Neoplasms, below.

Effects on the ovary. A possible association between functional ovarian cysts and progestogen-only oral contraceptives.— O. Ylikorkala (letter), *Lancet*, 1977, *1*, 1101. A negative association between ovarian cysts and the use of oral contraceptives. A Cooperative Study.— *J. Am. med. Ass.*, 1974, *228*, 68.

A histological ovarian study.— M. Maqueo *et al.*, *Contraception*, 1972, *5*, 177, per *Int. pharm. Abstr.*, 1973, *10*, 160.

See also under Neoplasms, below.

Effects on serum lipids. Reports of increased concentrations of triglycerides and cholesterol.— V. Wynn *et al.*, *Lancet*, 1969, *2*, 756; T. Stokes and V. Wynn, *Lancet*, 1971, *2*, 677; J. V. Martin *et al.*, *Lancet*, 1976, *1*, 1107; D. Hewitt *et al.*, *Can. med. Ass. J.*, 1977, *117*, 1020; R. B. Wallace *et al.*, *Lancet*, 1977, *2*, 11; V. Wynn *et al.*, *Lancet*, 1979, *1*, 1045.

Reduced concentrations of high-density-lipoprotein cholesterol.— A. C. Arntzenius *et al.*, *Lancet*, 1978, *1*, 1221; *J. Am. med. Ass.*, 1978, *239*, 692; D. D. Bradley *et al.*, *New Engl. J. Med.*, 1978, *299*, 17 (effect of progestogen component); *Lakartidningen*, 1979, *76*, 15; A. L. Nash *et al.*, *Med. J. Aust.*, 1979, *2*, 277; C. H. Hennekens *et al.*, *Circulation*, 1979, *60*, 486.

For the possible *adverse* effect of reduced concentrations of high-density-lipoprotein cholesterol, see Lipid Regulating Agents, p.408.

Effects on thyroid function. Disturbance of thyroid-function tests.— G. V-de Rodriguez *et al.*, *Obstet. Gynec.*, *N.Y.*, 1972, *39*, 779, per *Int. pharm. Abstr.*, 1973, *10*, 214; V. Chan *et al.*, *Br. med. J.*, 1972, *4*, 699.

Effects on the urinary tract. A slightly increased risk of bacteriuria in women under 50 taking oral contraceptives.— D. A. Evans *et al.*, *New Engl. J. Med.*, 1978, *299*, 536. A similar report.— M. Takahaski and D. B. Loveland, *J. Am. med. Ass.*, 1974, *227*, 762.

Effects on the uterus. A discussion as to whether changes in uterine vessels in users of oral contraceptives were biological or pathological.— *Br. med. J.*, 1977, *1*, 1119.

Effects on voice. Analysis of the vocal frequency, variability, and range in 17 women taking oral contraceptives and 13 controls showed certain changes in the voices of the treated women. Oral contraceptives should be given with caution to professional singers.— M. Dordain, *Folia phoniat.*, 1972, *24*, 86, per *Clin. Med.*, 1973, *80* (July), 34.

Galactorrhoea. Reports of galactorrhoea on discontinuing oral contraceptives.— *Br. med. J.*, 1970, *1*, 287; R. P. Shearman, *Lancet*, 1971, *2*, 64 (during treatment or on discontinuation); D. L. Kleinberg *et al.*, *New Engl. J. Med.*, 1977, *296*, 589. See also M. Lavric, *Obstet. Gynec.*, 1975, *46*, 12, per *Int. pharm. Abstr.*, 1978, *15*, 888.

Haemolytic-uraemic syndrome. An investigation of 5 women with the haemolytic-uraemic syndrome associated with oral contraceptives.— C. B. Brown *et al.*, *Lancet*, 1973, *1*, 1479.

Haemolytic-uraemic syndrome which occurred in a woman after receiving an oestrogen-containing oral contraceptive was considered to be due to a genetic predisposition.— D. Hauglustaine *et al.* (letter), *Lancet*, 1981, *1*, 328.

Headache and migraine. In patients with migraine oral contraceptive use was one of the major factors in the incidence of attacks.— E. C. G. Grant (letter), *Lancet*, 1978, *2*, 581.

Further references: E. C. G. Grant, *Br. med. J.*, 1968, *3*, 402; W. H. W. Inman and M. P. Vessey (letter), *ibid.*, 556; F. Morley (letter), *ibid;* A. Wiseman (letter), *ibid.*, 619; E. C. G. Grant and E. Mears (letter), *ibid;* J. West (letter), *ibid.*, 742; D. J. Richards, *Wyeth* (letter), *ibid.*, 743; *J. Am. med. Ass.*, 1975, *233*, 182; R. E. Ryan, *Headache*, 1978, *17*, 250.

Hypertension. Studies showing hypertension with oral contraceptives: M. P. Chidell, *Practitioner*, 1970, *205*, 58; R. J. Weir *et al.*, *Br. med. J.*, 1974, *1*, 533; D. J. Greenblatt and J. Koch-Weser, *Clin. Pharmac. Ther.*, 1974, *15*, 207; R. J. Weir, *Am. Heart J.*, 1976, *92*, 119; I. R. Fisch and J. Frank, *J. Am. med. Ass.*, 1977, *237*, 2499; *Lancet*, 1977, *1*, 624 (report of the Royal College of General Practitioners' Oral Contraceptive Study); J. A. Pritchard and S. A. Pritchard, *Am. J. Obstet. Gynec.*, 1977, *129*, 733. Discussions.— G. S. Stokes, *Drugs*, 1976, *12*, 222; *Br. med. J.*, 1978, *1*, 1570; R. J. Weir, *Drugs*, 1978, *16*, 522.

Renal failure. Hypertension leading to irreversible renal failure in one patient.— B. J. Zacherle and J. A. Richardson, *Ann. intern. Med.*, 1972, *77*, 83.

Immunosuppression. Some references to a possible effect of oral contraceptives on the immune response.— U. M. Joshi *et al.*, *Contraception*, 1971, *3*, 327; C. Hagen and A. Frøland (letter), *Lancet*, 1972, *1*, 1185; P. H. Fitzgerald *et al.* (letter), *Lancet*, 1973, *1*, 615; E. W. Barnes *et al.*, *ibid.*, 1974, *1*, 898; A. Morishima and R. T. Henrich (letter), *ibid.*, 1974, *2*, 646; R. S. Bray, *Contraception*, 1976, *14*, 417, per *Int. pharm. Abstr.*, 1977, *14*, 1248; P. S. Satoh *et al.* (letter), *New Engl. J. Med.*, 1977, *296*, 54.

Lupus erythematosus. Oral contraceptives had precipitated lupus erythematosus.— P. W. M. Copeman, *Br. J. Hosp. Med.*, 1972, *7*, 339. See also G. G. Bole *et al.*, *Lancet*, 1969, *1*, 323.

Mental changes. There was little agreement as to the incidence, nature, or cause of depressive symptoms associated with oral contraceptives; incidences of nil to 40% had been reported. Some women had pyridoxine deficiency while taking oral contraceptives. In women whose depression was troublesome, and for which there was no obvious cause, pyridoxine 50 mg daily could be given; it should be stopped after 4 weeks if no definite improvement occurred.— *Drug & Ther. Bull.*, 1978, *16*, 86.

Absence of depression.— S. J. Kutner (letter), *Lancet*, 1972, *1*, 1180; O. Fleming and C. P. Seager, *Br. J. Psychiat.*, 1978, *132*, 431.

A 10 to 40% incidence of depression.— F. J. Kane, *Am. J. Obstet. Gynec.*, 1976, *126*, 968.

References to endocrinological and metabolic aspects of mental changes associated with oral contraceptive use.— P. W. Adams *et al.*, *Lancet*, 1973, *1*, 897; R. E. Davis and B. K. Smith (letter), *ibid.*, 1245; E. C. G. Grant (letter), *Br. med. J.*, 1973, *3*, 349; A. R. Green *et al.*, *Br. J. clin. Pharmac.*, 1978, *5*, 233; D. B. Adams *et al.*, *New Engl. J. Med.*, 1978, *299*, 1145; R. M. Rose, *ibid.*, 1186; A. R. W. Forrest, *Br. med. J.*, 1979, *2*, 1403; S. E. Møller (letter), *Lancet*, 1979, *2*, 472.

Neoplasms. The effect of oral contraceptive use on the development of neoplastic disease was reviewed. Combination oral contraceptives appeared to reduce the risk of benign breast neoplasia; there was a marked increase in the relative risk of hepatocellular adenoma of the liver among women who had taken oral contraceptives for periods in excess of 3 years, the magnitude of risk increasing with the dose of steroid, duration of use, and age of user. Evidence was insufficient to establish either an adverse or beneficial effect on breast cancer, uterine fibroids, endometrial carcinoma, cervical carcinoma, pituitary adenoma, and malignant melanoma. Combined oral contraceptives may decrease ovarian cancer risk but there was insufficient evidence to draw firm conclusions. There was insufficient data available to evaluate the effect of progestogen-only oral contraceptives on the risk of neoplasia.— Steroid Contraception and the Risk of Neoplasia, Report of a WHO Scientific Group, *Tech. Rep. Ser. Wld Hlth Org. No. 619*, 1978.

Breast. In a large-scale survey the rates of hospitalisation for fibrocystic disease of the breast for non-users of oral contraceptives and users of 12 months' duration or less were similar, whereas those of users of 13 to 24 months and 25 months or over were 70 and 35% respectively of the non-users.— H. Ory *et al.*, *New Engl. J. Med.*, 1976, *294*, 419. A similar conclusion in a report of the Royal College of General Practitioners' Oral Contraceptive Study, *Lancet*, 1977, *1*, 624. See also V. A. LiVolsi *et al.*, *New Engl. J. Med.*, 1978, *299*, 381.

References to the lack of an association between oral contraceptives and neoplasms of the breast.— *Lancet*, 1973, *1*, 1399 (Boston Collaborative Drug Surveillance Program); P. E. Sartwell *et al.*, *J. natn Cancer Inst.*, 1977, *59*, 1589; J. D. Spencer *et al.*, *Br. med. J.*, 1978, *1*, 1024; J. L. Kelsey *et al.*, *Am. J. Epidem.*, 1978, *107*, 236; M. P. Vessey *et al.*, *Br. med. J.*, 1979, *1*, 1757; P. N. Matthews *et al.*, *ibid.*, 1981, *282*, 774; Royal College of General Practitioners, *ibid.*, 2089; M. P. Vessey *et al.*, *ibid.*, 2093. A view that the policy of prohibiting the use of the pill by women who have developed breast cancer should be reconsidered.— P. L. C. Diggory (letter), *Lancet*, 1981, *1*, 995.

Evidence of an increased risk of breast cancer following long-term oral contraceptive use before the first full-term pregnancy.— M. C. Pike *et al.*, *Br. J. Cancer*, 1981, *43*, 72.

Cervix. Studies suggesting an association between cervical carcinoma and oral contraceptive use.— M. R. Melamed *et al.*, *Br. med. J.*, 1969, *3*, 195; J. de Brux, *Sem. Hôp. Paris*, 1974, *50*, 1491, per *J. Am. med. Ass.*, 1974, *229*, 725; E. Peritz *et al.*, *Am. J. Epidem.*, 1977, *106*, 462; E. Stern *et al.*, *Science*, 1977, *196*, 1460; S. H. Swan and W. L. Brown, *Am. J. Obstet. Gynec.*, 1981, *139*, 52 (including role of sexual activity). Studies suggesting no assocation.— D. B. Thomas, *Obstet. Gynec., N.Y.*, 1972, *40*, 508, per *J. Am. med. Ass.*, 1973, *223*, 99; H. F. Sandmire *et al.*, *Am. J. Obstet. Gynec.*, 1976, *125*, 339, per *Int. pharm. Abstr.*, 1976, *13*, 1077; J. G. Boyce *et al.*, *Am. J. Obstet. Gynec.*, 1977, *128*, 761; H. J. A. Collette *et al.* (letter), *Lancet*, 1978, *1*, 441. A discussion.— *Lancet*, 1977, *2*, 644.

Endometrium. A retrospective study of oral contraceptive use in 117 women with endometrial cancer compared with 395 control subjects from the same population. Those who had taken the sequential oral contraceptive Oracon (ethinyloestradiol 100 µg and dimethisterone 25 mg) were estimated to have a risk of endometrial cancer 7.3 times that of other women. Those who had used combined oral contraceptives had only 50% of the incidence of endometrial cancer of nonusers; this protective effect was not seen in those who subsequently took menopausal oestrogens for 3 or more years. Patients with endometrial cancer tended to use more oestrogenic and less progestogenic preparations than did the controls but the relationship was weak and could have been due to chance.— N. S. Weiss and T. A. Sayvetz, *New Engl. J. Med.*, 1980, *302*, 551; P. Cole, *ibid.*, 575. Similar findings from a case-control study which suggest a protective effect of combined products.— D. W. Kaufman *et al.*, *New Engl. J. Med.*, 1980, *303*, 1045.
See also under Menopausal Symptoms in Oestradiol, p.1427.

Liver. A discussion of the association between liver tumours and oral contraceptives; some 200 cases had been reported.— *Br. med. J.*, 1977, *2*, 345. Estimated incidence of one benign liver tumour per 80 000 users per year.— H. Jick and R. Herman (letter), *J. Am. med. Ass.*, 1978, *240*, 828. The incidence of hepatocellular adenoma was estimated to be 1 to 1.3 per million in women not using oral contraceptives compared with 34 per million in users.— J. B. Rooks *et al.*, *J. Am. med. Ass.*, 1979, *242*, 644.

Case reports and discussions.— *J. Am. med. Ass.*, 1977, *237*, 2701; M. P. Vessey *et al.*, *Br. med. J.*, 1977, *1*, 1064; E. D. Nissen *et al.*, *Am. J. Obstet. Gynec.*, 1977, *127*, 61; *Morb. Mortal.*, 1977, *26*, 293; J. Vana *et al.*, *J. Am. med. Ass.*, 1977, *238*, 2154; H. Ellis, *Postgrad. med. J.*, 1978, *54*, 367; J. J. Gonvers *et al.*, *Schweiz. med. Wschr.*, 1978, *108*, 1899; J. M. Ham *et al.*, *Am. J. dig. Dis.*, 1978, *23*, *Suppl.*, 38S (with metastatic disease); W. J. Britton *et al.*, *Med. J. Aust.*, 1978, *2*, 223; A. Marshall and R. Smallwood, *Med. J. Aust.*, 1978, *2*, 240; W. M. Christopherson *et al.* (letter), *Lancet*, 1978, *2*, 38; C. -J. Oon *et al.* (letter), *Lancet*, 1979, *2*, 194; J. Neuberger *et al.*, *Lancet*, 1980, *1*, 273; B. L. Warren and G. D. Bellward, *Drug Intell. & clin. Pharm.*, 1979, *13*, 680 and 741.

Mention of regression of liver tumours.— D. Ross *et al.* (letter), *Ann. intern. Med.*, 1976, *85*, 203; S. Kay, *Cancer*, 1977, *40*, 1759; H. A. Edmondson *et al.*, *Ann. intern. Med.*, 1977, *86*, 180; W. L. Ramseur and M. R. Cooper, *J. Am. med. Ass.*, 1978, *239*, 1647.

Pituitary. While a high incidence of oral contraceptive use had been reported in patients with pituitary adenomas, an examination of the data from the 2 major British surveys of women using (or having used) oral contraceptives, covering about 180 000 woman-years, did not support such an association.— S. J. Wingrave *et al.*, *Br. med. J.*, 1980, *280*, 685. A similar conclusion.— C. B. Coulam *et al.*, *Fert. Steril.*, 1979, *31*, 25.

Of 42 women who underwent surgery for pituitary tumours, 30 had taken oral contraceptives, and in 24 amenorrhoea had started during or immediately after their use. Oestrogen-containing oral contraceptives might provoke the clinical expression of otherwise silent tumours.— B. M. Sherman *et al.*, *Lancet*, 1978, *2*, 1019. A contrary view.— J. F. Annegers *et al.* (letter), *Lancet*, 1978, *2*, 1384.

Skin. References to a possible association between malignant melanoma and oral contraceptive use.— V. Beral *et al.*, *Br. J. Cancer*, 1977, *36*, 804; A. B. Lerner *et al.* (letter), *New Engl. J. Med.*, 1979, *301*, 47. A contrary view.— R. G. Stevens *et al.* (letter), *New Engl. J. Med.*, 1980, *302*, 966.

Occupational exposure. Adverse effects in workers exposed to oral contraceptives: G. C. Buchanan *et al.*, *Contraception*, 1977, *16*, 351, per *Int. pharm. Abstr.*, 1978, *15*, 362; L. M. El-Semary *et al.*, *A'in Shams med. J.*, 1977, *28*, 261, per *Trop. Dis. Bull.*, 1978, *75*, 152; L. Poller *et al.*, *Br. med. J.*, 1979, *1*, 1761.

Overdosage. Minimal effects of overdosage.— A. L. Picchioni, *Am. J. Hosp. Pharm.*, 1965, *22*, 486; N. A. Wynne (letter), *Pharm. J.*, 1968, *2*, 447.

Pancreatitis. The possible association between acute pancreatitis, hyperlipoproteinaemia, and oral contraceptives.— *Br. med. J.*, 1973, *4*, 688. Case reports.— M. E. Foster and D. E. B. Powell, *Postgrad. med. J.*, 1975, *51*, 667; I. P. F. Mungall and R. V. Hague, *Postgrad. med. J.*, 1975, *51*, 855.

Porphyria. Case reports of porphyria associated with oral contraceptives.— A. W. McKenzie and U. Acharya, *Br. J. Derm.*, 1972, *86*, 453; C. J. Fowler and J. M. Ward, *Br. med. J.*, 1975, *1*, 663; A. R. Behm and W. P. Unger, *Can. med. Ass. J.*, 1974, *110*, 1052; *Br. med. J.*, 1975, *1*, 37; P. Curtis, *Br. J. clin. Pract.*, 1976, *30*, 47; G. Leonhardi *et al.*, *Dt. med. Wschr.*, 1977, *102*, 160; D. T. Roberts *et al.*, *Br. J. Derm.*, 1977, *96*, 549; L. S. Gerlis, *J. int. med. Res.*, 1978, *6*, 255 (after withdrawal).

Pregnancy and the neonate. *Ectopic pregnancy.* Progestogen ingestion for contraception in 12.6% of 238 ectopic pregnancies.— P. Liukko *et al.*, *Contraception*, 1977, *16*, 575, per *Int. pharm. Abstr.*, 1978, *15*, 460.

There was a lower incidence of ectopic pregnancy among a group of 463 women with a history of oral contraceptive use than in 406 women who had not used oral contraceptives although the difference was not significant.— G. S. Berger *et al.* (letter), *Lancet*, 1976, *2*, 961.

Further reports: J. Bonnar (letter), *Br. med. J.*, 1974, *1*, 287; K. M. Huntington (letter), *Lancet*, 1974, *1*, 360; D. F. Hawkins (letter), *Br. med. J.*, 1974, *1*, 387; R. Corcoran and R. Howard (letter), *Lancet*, 1977, *1*, 98.

Effects on the foetus. Studies showing an absence of effect.— S. C. Robinson, *Am. J. Obstet. Gynec.*, 1971, *109*, 354; C. R. Kay, *Br. J. Obstet. Gynaec.*, 1976, *83*, 608, per *Int. pharm. Abstr.*, 1977, *14*, 523; G. Greenberg *et al.*, *Br. med. J.*, 1977, *2*, 853.

Studies and discussions suggesting congenital malformations.— J. J. Nora and A. H. Nora (letter), *Lancet*, 1973, *1*, 941; J. J. Nora *et al.* (letter), *ibid.*, 1976, *1*, 313; D. T. Janerich *et al.*, *New Engl. J. Med.*, 1974, *291*, 697; J. J. Nora and A. H. Nora, *ibid.*, 731; J. J. Nora *et al.*, *J. Am. med. Ass.*, 1978, *240*, 837; K. J. Rothman and C. Louik, *New Engl. J. Med.*, 1978, *299*, 522 (increased incidence of undescended testis); P. N. Kasan and J. Andrews, *Br. J. Obstet. Gynaec.*, 1980, *87*, 545 (increased incidence of neural-tube defects).

Case reports: R. L. Kaufman (letter), *Lancet*, 1973, *1*, 1396; S. Dillon (letter), *Br. med. J.*, 1976, *2*, 1446.

Increased plasma-bilirubin concentrations in infants born to mothers who had used oral contraceptives.— Y. K. Wong and B. S. B. Wood, *Br. med. J.*, 1971, *4*, 403; J. B. McConnell *et al.*, *Br. med. J.*, 1973, *3*, 605. A contrary view.— D. Barnardo *et al.* (letter), *Br. med. J.*, 1972, *2*, 348; S. R. Gould *et al.*, *Br. med. J.*, 1974, *3*, 228.

Increased incidence of twin births in infants conceived soon after discontinuation of oral contraceptives.— K. J. Rothman, *New Engl. J. Med.*, 1977, *297*, 468. A similar report.— M. B. Bracken, *Am. J. Obstet. Gynec.*, 1979, *133*, 432. See also S. Harlap, *Br. J. Obstet. Gynaec.*, 1979, *86*, 557.

An increased incidence of pigmented skin lesions in infants born to underweight former oral contraceptive users.— S. Harlap (letter), *Lancet*, 1978, *2*, 39.

Effects on lactation. A view that oestrogens should not be used during lactation, but progestogen-only preparations may be given if non-hormonal methods are unacceptable.— S. Nilsson and K. -G. Nygren, *Res. Reprod.*, 1980, *12*, 1.

Results of a world-wide survey of doctors associated with Family Planning Associations indicated extensive use of combined oral contraceptives in lactating women, particularly in Africa, Asia, and Latin America. Combined oral contraceptives were associated with a much higher incidence of complaints about decreased milk production than progestogen-only preparations or than intrauterine devices.— R. W. Rochat *et al.*, *IPPF Med. Bull.*, 1981, *1*, 4.

A study, in 36 women, of the effects of various contraceptive preparations on the quantity and quality of human milk.— V. S. Toddywalla *et al.*, *Am. J. Obstet. Gynec.*, 1977, *127*, 245.

Further references: V. M. Barsivala and K. D. Virkar, *Contraception*, 1973, *7*, 307, per *Int. pharm. Abstr.*, 1974, *11*, 112; E. Guiloff *et al.*, *Am. J. Obstet. Gynec.*, 1974, *118*, 42.

Effects on sex ratio. Absence of effect of oral contraceptives.— K. J. Rothman and J. Liess, *New Engl. J. Med.*, 1976, *295*, 859. Earlier references: J. S. Crawford and P. Davies (letter), *Lancet*, 1973, *2*, 453 (no effect); T. L. Keserü *et al.* (letter), *Lancet*, 1974, *1*, 369 (increased proportion of females after 2 years of use). See also M. Vessey *et al.*, *J. biosoc. Sci.*, 1976, *8*, 373 (high overall incidence of males).

Rheumatic disorders. Reports of rheumatic disorders in women taking oral contraceptives.— G. G. Bole *et al.*, *Lancet*, 1969, *1*, 323; H. Spiera and C. M. Plotz (letter), *Lancet*, 1969, *1*, 571 and 898. No association.— B. J. Tarzy *et al.*, *Lancet*, 1972, *2*, 501.

A slight reduction of the incidence of rheumatoid arthritis in women who used oral contraceptives.— *Lancet*, 1978, *1*, 569 (Report of the Royal College of General Practitioners' Oral Contraceptive Study).

Possible increased risk of inflammatory disease in women taking oral contraceptives.— S. H. Swan (letter), *Lancet*, 1981, *2*, 809.

Skin disorders. Three women taking oral contraceptives developed, respectively, a fixed drug eruption, lichen simplex chronicus, and nummular eczema while taking oral contraceptives. The eruptions ceased when the oral contraceptives were withdrawn or changed.— R. J. Coskey, *Archs Derm.*, 1977, *113*, 333.

Comment on the possible association between erythema nodosum and oral contraceptives, and a detailed case report.— L. G. Darlington, *Br. J. Derm.*, 1974, *90*, 209. See also S. Bombardieri *et al.*, *Br. med. J.*, 1977, *1*, 1509.

Acanthosis nigricans in a woman taking oral contraceptives.— H. O. Curth (letter), *Archs Derm.*, 1975, *111*, 1069.

Subarachnoid haemorrhage. The risk of subarachnoid haemorrhage in smokers was 5.7 times that of non-smokers, and of current oral contraceptive users 6.5 times that of non-users. The relative risk estimate for the association of smoking and current oral contraceptive use was 21.9.— D. B. Petitti and J. Wingerd, *Lancet*, 1978, *2*, 234.

A small but not significant excess of usage of oral contraceptives in those who had died from subarachnoid haemorrhage.— W. H. W. Inman, *Br. med. J.*, 1979, *2*, 1468. Similar findings, and the view that both the relative and absolute risks of subarachnoid haemorrhage associated with the use of oral contraceptives are small and are probably associated with their hypertensive effect.— M. Thorogood *et al.*, *Br. med. J.*, 1981, *283*, 762.

Thrombo-embolic disorders. Reviews and discussions.— The Maternal and Perinatal Committee of The Health Commission of New South Wales, *Med. J. Aust.*, 1976,

1, 788; *Br. med. J.,* 1977, *2,* 918; R. P. Shearman, *Med. J. Aust.,* 1978, *1,* 75; H. M. Carey, *ibid.,* 153; L. Poller, *Br. med. Bull.,* 1978, *34,* 151; M. P. Vessey and J. I. Mann, *ibid.,* 157; K. D. MacRae, *Br. J. Hosp. Med.,* 1980, *24,* 438; B. V. Stadel, *New Engl. J. Med.,* 1981, *305,* 612 and 672; M. P. Vessey, *Br. med. J.,* 1982, *284,* 615.

The Royal College of General Practitioners' Oral Contraceptive Study was extended to June 1976 to cover about 200 000 woman-years and the effects on death-rate in Great Britain were studied. There was a significant increase in mortality due to diseases of the circulatory system but not to other causes, the ratio of mortality-rate in oral contraceptive users to controls being 4.7 to 1. This represented an increase of 1 death per 5000 users per year (or 40%) for all women irrespective of age. When age was taken into account the increase was estimated to be 1 per 3000 users aged 35 to 44 years and 1 per 700 in those aged 45 to 49 years. The mortality-rate also increased with prolonged use of oral contraceptives; 1 per 8000 for use of less than 5 years compared with 1 per 2000 for use longer than 5 years, and might increase in users who were smokers. The increased risk of cardiovascular disease and consequent death appeared to persist after oral contraceptives were withdrawn.— *Lancet,* 1977, *2,* 727. Analysis of figures from the Oxford and Family Planning Association Contraceptive Study produced similar findings. Up to the end of April 1977 there were 43 deaths among all 17 032 women in the study, 24 in those using oral contraceptives and 17 in the controls using a diaphragm or intra-uterine device and 2 in women in the oral contraceptive group dropped from the study. When cause of death was analysed there was a significant increase in death due to cardiovascular disorders, there being 9 deaths (6 occurring after oral contraception was stopped) due to such disorders in the oral contraceptive group who provided 49 681 woman-years of observation compared with none among the controls who provided 39 146 woman-years.— M. P. Vessey *et al., ibid.,* 731. The Royal Colleges of General Practitioners and of Obstetricians and Gynaecologists recommended that no change in oral-contraceptive practice was justified in women aged under 30 years. Women aged 30 years to 35 years who had taken an oral contraceptive for more than 5 years and who were cigarette smokers should reconsider their use of this form of contraception. Stopping smoking might allow them to continue oral contraception for a time. All women aged over 35 should reconsider their method of contraception. It was not possible to differentiate between preparations with various oestrogen doses.— E. V. Kuenssberg and J. Dewhurst (letter), *ibid.,* 757. The Committee on Safety of Medicines considered that a reasonable assessment of these findings could not be made, not only because of the small numbers but because the oestrogen pattern of oral contraceptives had changed and megestrol had been withdrawn during the period of study. Although the Committee recommended that no changes be made to the warnings and precautions for oral contraceptives, it emphasised the increased risks associated with age and cigarette smoking.— *ibid.,* 758.

Concern about misunderstandings and misinterpretations of the findings presented in the Royal College of General Practitioners' Oral Contraception Study on mortality among oral contraceptive users.— C. Kay (letter), *Lancet,* 1979, *2,* 521.

Further evaluation based on data up to Dec. 1979 covered 98 997 woman-years for current users, 84 811 woman-years for former users, and 138 630 woman-years for controls. The 40% higher overall mortality-rate in ever-users was confirmed; the relative risk of death from diseases of the circulatory system was 4.2. An association with smoking was confirmed, especially in those aged 35 and over. The previously reported association between risk and duration of use was no longer evident. An association between risk and parity needed confirmation.— *Lancet,* 1981, *1,* 541 (Royal College of General Practitioners' Oral Contraceptive Study). See also M. P. Vessey *et al.* (letter), *ibid.,* 549; C. R. Kay (letter), *ibid.,* 1206.

Evidence suggesing involvement of the progestogen component in the risk of thrombo-embolism.— T. W. Meade *et al., Br. med. J.,* 1980, *280* 1157. See also C. R. Kay, *J.R. Coll. gen. Pract.,* 1980, *30,* 8.

Further references to the possible mechanism of effect.— B. Åstedt *et al., Br. med. J.,* 1973, *4,* 631; L. O. Pilgeram *et al., Br. med. J.,* 1974, *3,* 556; M. P. T. Gillett and E. M. M. Besterman (letter), *Lancet,* 1974, *2,* 1387; S. Sagar *et al., Lancet,* 1976, *1,* 509; S. Wessler *et al., J. Am. med. Ass.,* 1976, *236,* 2179; T. J. Ence *et al., Metabolism,* 1976, *25,* 139, per *Int. pharm. Abstr.,* 1976, *13,* 891; J. L. Ambrus *et al., Am. J. Obstet. Gynec.,* 1976, *125,* 1057, per *Int. pharm. Abstr.,* 1977, *14,* 121; T. W. Meade *et al., Br. J. Haemat.,* 1976, *34,* 353, per *J. Am. med. Ass.,* 1977, *237,* 1161; H. Rieger *et al., Dt. med. Wschr.,* 1977, *102,* 1248; A. C. A. Carvalho *et al., J. Am. med. Ass.,* 1977, *237,* 875; J. L. Ambrus *et al., Am. J. Obstet. Gynec.,* 1977, *128,* 161; J. P. Burrow and J. K. Luce, *Postgrad. Med.,* 1977, *62,* 52, per *Int. pharm. Abstr.,* 1977, *14,* 1254; H. J. Engel *et al., Br. Heart J.,* 1977, *39,* 477; A. P. Ball and P. A. McKee, *J. Lab. clin. Med.,* 1977, *89,* 751, per *J. Am. med. Ass.,* 1977, *238,* 544; T. W. Meade *et al., Br. med. J.,* 1979, *1,* 153; J. R. Peters *et al., Lancet,* 1979, *2,* 933; M. L. Bierenbaum *et al., Am. J. Obstet. Gynec.,* 1979, *134,* 638; P. C. Buchan and H. N. Macdonald, *Br. med. J.,* 1980, *280,* 978.

See also Martindale 27th Edn, p. 1383.

Further references to oral contraceptives and thrombo-embolism: *J.R. Coll. gen. Pract.,* 1978, *28,* 393 (Royal College of General Practitioners' Oral Contraception Study); L. E. Böttiger *et al., Lancet,* 1980, *1,* 1097; *Lancet,* 1980, *1,* 1118.

Myocardial infarction. References to an increased risk of myocardial infarction associated with oral contraceptive use.— D. J. Radford and M. F. Oliver, *Br. med. J.,* 1973, *3,* 428; J. I. Mann *et al., Br. med. J.,* 1975, *2,* 241; *idem,* 1975, *3,* 631; J. I. Mann and W. H. W. Inman, *Br. med. J.,* 1975, *2,* 245; S. Shapiro, *New Engl. J. Med.,* 1975, *293,* 195; J. I. Mann *et al., Br. med. J.,* 1976, *2,* 445; F. G. Arthes and A. T. Masi, *Chest,* 1976, *70,* 574, per *J. Am. med. Ass.,* 1977, *237,* 908; C. H. Hennekens and B. MacMahon, *New Engl. J. Med.,* 1977, *296,* 1166; *Br. med. J.,* 1977, *2,* 1370; H. W. Ory, *J. Am. med. Ass.,* 1977, *237,* 2619; H. Jick *et al., J. Am. med. Ass.,* 1978, *239,* 1403; H. Jick *et al., J. Am. med. Ass.,* 1978, *240,* 2548; S. Shapiro *et al., Lancet,* 1979, *1,* 743; S. A. Adam *et al., Br. J. Obstet. Gynaec.,* 1981, *88,* 838. A study suggesting that the increased risk of myocardial infarction may persist after the discontinuation of long-term oral contraceptive use.— D. Slone *et al., New Engl. J. Med.,* 1981, *305,* 420.

Vitamin deficiency. Although vitamin concentrations might be reduced in women taking oral contraceptives vitamin supplements were not necessary in women eating a well-balanced diet.— *Med. Lett.,* 1973, *15,* 81. See also Advances in Methods of Fertility Regulation, Report of a WHO Scientific Group, *Tech. Rep. Ser. Wld Hlth Org. No. 575,* 1975.

A review of drugs and vitamin deficiency L. Ovesen, *Drugs,* 1979, *18,* 278.

Ascorbic acid. References: D. G. Kalesh *et al., Contraception,* 1971, *4,* 183, per *Int. pharm. Abstr.,* 1972, *9,* 267; M. Briggs and M. Briggs (letter), *Nature,* 1972, *238,* 277; A. B. Harris *et al.* (letter), *Lancet,* 1973, *2,* 201; A. B. Harris *et al* (letter), *Lancet,* 1975, *2,* 82.

Cobalamin. Oral contraceptives reduced serum concentrations of vitamin B_{12} in healthy young women by about 40% compared with a control group. Folate therapy did not increase vitamin B_{12} concentrations in these women.— L. F. Wertalik *et al., J. Am. med. Ass.,* 1972, *221,* 1371. No need for supplementation.— A. M. Shojania and B. Wylie, *Am. J. Obstet. Gynec.,* 1979, *135,* 129.

Folic acid. References: A. Paton (letter), *Lancet,* 1969, *1,* 418; R. R. Streiff, *J. Am. med. Ass.,* 1970, *214,* 105; *ibid.,* 137; M. E. M. Stephens *et al., Clin. Sci.,* 1972, *42,* 405, per *J. Am. med. Ass.,* 1972, *221,* 107; A. M. Shojania and G. J. Hornady, *J. Lab. clin. Med.,* 1973, *82,* 869, per *J. Am. med. Ass.,* 1974, *228,* 115; A. Gaafar *et al., Contraception,* 1973, *8,* 43, per *Int. pharm. Abstr.,* 1974, *11,* 297; M. M. Meguid and W. Y. Loebl, *Postgrad. med. J.,* 1974, *50,* 470; A. M. Shojania (letter), *Lancet,* 1975, *1,* 1198; O. Martinez and D. A. Roe, *Am. J. Obstet. Gynec.,* 1977, *128,* 255.

Pyridoxine. References: A. R. Doberenz *et al., Proc. Soc. exp. Biol. Med.,* 1971, *137,* 1100, per *Abstr. Hyg.,* 1972, *47,* 861; S. A. Price *et al., Am. J. clin. Nutr.,* 1972, *25,* 494, per *J. Am. med. Ass.,* 1972, *221,* 726; H. J. T. C. Benninck and W. H. P. Schreurs, *Contraception,* 1974, *9,* 347, per *Int. pharm. Abstr.,* 1974, *11,* 789; P. W. Adams *et al., Lancet,* 1976, *1,* 759. See also *ibid.,* 788.

Riboflavine. References: N. Sanpitak and L. Cahyutimonkul, *Lancet,* 1974, *1,* 836.

Vitamin E. References: C. C. Tangney and J. A. Driskell, *Contraception,* 1978, *17,* 499 (minimal effect), per *Int. pharm. Abstr.,* 1979, *16,* 734.

Vitamin excess. References to increased concentrations of vitamin A.— M. Briggs *et al., Contraception,* 1972, *6,* 275, per *Int. pharm. Abstr.,* 1973, *10,* 660; J. Wild *et al., Br. med. J.,* 1974, *1,* 57; I. Gal (letter), *ibid.,* 1974, *2,* 560.

Precautions. Before oral contraceptives are given the woman should undergo an appropriate medical examination and her medical history should be carefully evaluated. Regular examination is recommended during use.

Oral contraceptives are contra-indicated in patients with recurrent cholestatic jaundice or markedly impaired liver function, hormone-dependent neoplasms, uterine fibroids, previous thrombo-embolic disorders, cardiovascular disease and thrombophlebitis, severe migraine, undiagnosed vaginal bleeding, possible pregnancy, sickle-cell anaemia, or a history during pregnancy of pruritus, herpes, deteriorating otosclerosis, or idiopathic jaundice.

Oral contraceptives should be administered with caution to women with a history of diabetes mellitus, hypertension, mental depression, asthma, epilepsy, migraine, cardiac or renal dysfunction, gall-bladder disease, or other conditions influenced by fluid retention.

Administration of oral contraceptives to those undergoing surgery or prolonged bed rest may increase the risk of thrombo-embolic episodes; in nursing mothers, lactation may be reduced and oestrogen may pass to the baby in small quantities in the milk. Attacks of porphyria may be precipitated by oral contraceptives.

Increased concentrations of thyroxine-binding globulin, reflected in increased levels of protein-bound iodine, occur in patients taking oral contraceptives. While the thyroid state is generally unaffected, some tests of thyroid function give abnormal results while oral contraceptives are being taken and for up to 2 months after they are stopped. Cortisol-binding globulin may also be increased and some other laboratory test values may be affected.

The efficacy of oral contraceptives can be diminished by malabsorption and patients should be aware that this may be a hazard with vomiting and diarrhoea. There have been reports of pregnancy in women taking oral contraceptives concomitantly with anticonvulsants (barbiturates, primidone, phenytoin, and carbamazepine), rifampicin, and other antibiotics such as ampicillin. There have been suggestions that other drugs may be involved; these include analgesics (aspirin, amidopyrine, phenazone, phenacetin , phenylbutazone, oxyphenbutazone), chloramphenicol, chlorpromazine, chlordiazepoxide, diazepam, dihydroergotamine, ethosuximide, isoniazid, meprobamate, neomycin, nitrofurantoin, phenoxymethylpenicillin, promethazine, sulphamethoxypyridazine. Higher doses of hypoglycaemic agents may be needed by diabetics given oral contraceptives.

Skin reactivity to dinitrochlorobenzene was assessed in 76 women taking hormonal contraceptives. Increased sensitisation occurred in women taking progestogens either in 'combined' preparations or as depot injections but not in women taking 'sequential' preparations.— G. Gerretsen *et al., Lancet,* 1975, *2,* 347. See also *idem, Contraception,* 1979, *19,* 83.

In 611 patients followed for 2 years after hydatidiform mole evacuation, 24.6% of 65 taking oral contraceptives before gonadotrophin values had returned to normal required cytotoxic therapy for trophoblastic tumours compared with 9.3% in those not taking oral contraceptives.— M. Stone *et al., Br. J. Obstet. Gynaec.,* 1976, *83,* 913, per *Int. pharm. Abstr.,* 1977, *14,* 522. A contrary view.— R. S. Berkowitz *et al.* (letter), *Lancet,* 1980, *2,* 752. Criticism.— K. D. Bagshawe and M. Stone (letter), *ibid.,* 1250.

A study in 7 women who had undergone intestinal bypass operations showed that plasma concentrations of oral contraceptives were reduced to levels which could not be considered reliable for contraception.— E. D. B. Johansson and J. G. Krai (letter), *J. Am. med. Ass.,* 1976, *236,* 2847.

Experience in 3 women with Raynaud's syndrome suggested that 'oestrogen-progesterone' oral contraceptives were contra-indicated in that condition.— P. E. M. Jarrett (letter), *Br. med. J.,* 1976, *2,* 699.

Recommendations that women with a history of benign breast disease should not be given oral contraceptives or oestrogen replacement at the menopause and that women who develop benign breast disease while taking these compounds should stop doing so and should be monitored for an indefinite period.— P. T. Cole, *Cancer*, 1977, *39*, 1906.

But see Neoplasms under Adverse Effects, p.1403.

The effect of malnutrition on the metabolism of sex hormones in man.— J. Fishman and H. L. Bradlow, *Clin. Pharmac. Ther.*, 1977, *22*, 721.

Blood transfusion and organ transplantation. A raised ceruloplasmin concentration in the plasma of women taking oestrogens, usually in the form of oral contraceptives, had been observed increasingly in blood donors. No untoward reactions had been reported after transfusion of this blue-green plasma.— P. Wolf *et al.*, *New Engl. J. Med.*, 1969, *281*, 205. Further references: L. A. D. Tovey and G. H. Lathe, *Lancet*, 1968, *2*, 596; C. A. B. Clemetson (letter), *ibid.*, 1037.

The heart and kidneys of a woman on oral contraceptives could be used for transplants unless there was infection, disseminated malignancy, or a history of disease of the organs.— *Br. med. J.*, 1980, *281*, 727.

Diabetes. An increased risk of vascular complications in insulin-dependent diabetics taking oral contraceptives.— J. M. Steel and L. J. P. Duncan, *Contraception*, 1978, *17*, 291.

Effect on laboratory tests. A list, with references, of 38 laboratory tests which might be affected by oral contraceptives.— *Med. Lett.*, 1979, *21*, 54.

There was a reduction in erythrocyte-carbonic anhydrase-I in 15 women taking oral contraceptives and this was most pronounced in those taking preparations with low doses of oestrogen (30 µg). Assay of this enzyme could be used for the diagnosis of thyrotoxicosis. There was an implication that false-positive results could be obtained in women taking oral contraceptives.— J. A. Auton *et al.*, *Lancet*, 1976, *2*, 1385.

Interactions. Bleeding disorders were more common in women taking oral contraceptives and other drugs than in those taking oral contraceptives alone. A bleeding disturbance in a previously regular contraceptive cycle indicated that the method was no longer reliable.— E. Hempel and W. Klinger, *Drugs*, 1976, *12*, 442.

Pregnancy had been reported on 17 occasions in women taking oral contraceptives and rifampicin; on 25 occasions in those taking anticonvulsants with 23 further reports, received by the Committee on Safety of Medicines (CSM); the CSM had 38 reports of pregnancy in women also taking antibiotics.— *Br. med. J.*, 1980, *281*, 93. References: I. E. Kenyon (letter), *Br. med. J.*, 1972, *1*, 686 (anticonvulsants); L. Nocke-Finck *et al.*, *Dt. med. Wschr.*, 1973, *98*, 1521 (rifampicin); D. Janz and D. Schmidt (letter), *Lancet*, 1974, *1*, 1113 (anticonvulsants); J. L. Skolnick *et al.*, *J. Am. med. Ass.*, 1976, *236*, 1382 (rifampicin); C. B. Coulam and J. F. Annegers, *Epilepsia*, 1979, *20*, 519 (anticonvulsants); J. F. Bacon and G. M. Shenfield, *Br. med. J.*, 1980, *280*, 293 (tetracycline).

For reference to the increased bioavailability of ethinyloestradiol in women taking large doses of vitamin C, see p.1412.

Discussions of drug interactions with oral contraceptives: I. Stockley, *Pharm. J.*, 1976, *1*, 140; D. J. Back and M. L'E. Orme, *Prescribers' J.*, 1977, *17*, 137; W. C. Buss, *J. antimicrob. Chemother.*, 1979, *5*, 4; M. L'E. Orme and D. J. Back, *J. antimicrob. Chemother.*, 1979, *5*, 124.

Varicose veins. Oral contraceptives employing low doses of oestrogens were not contra-indicated in patients with varicose veins provided that there was regular follow-up, that there was no history of thrombo-embolic disorders, and that any obesity or future surgery was taken into account.— *Br. med. J.*, 1975, *1*, 726.

9022-d

Algestone Acetophenide. Alphasone Acetophenide; Dihydroxyprogesterone Acetophenide; SQ 15101. 16α,17α-(1-Phenylethylidenedioxy)pregn-4-ene-3,20-dione.

$C_{29}H_{36}O_4$=448.6.

CAS — 595-77-7 (algestone); 24356-94-3 (acetophenide).

A white or off-white, almost odourless, crystalline powder.

Algestone acetophenide is a progestational agent with actions similar to those of progesterone (see p.1431). It has been given by intramuscular injection in monthly doses of 150 mg in conjunction with oestradiol enanthate as a contraceptive.

The metabolism and excretion of algestone acetophenide and oestradiol enanthate given intramuscularly. There was greater faecal excretion of the progestogen than the oestrogen.— C. Gual *et al.*, *Contraception*, 1973, *7*, 271, per *Int. pharm. Abstr.*, 1974, *11*, 34.

For reports of the use of algestone acetophenide with oestradiol enanthate for contraception, see Martindale 27th Edn, p. 1390.

Proprietary Names of Algestone Acetophenide with Oestradiol Enanthate
Perlutal *(Promeco, Arg.)*.

9023-n

Allyloestrenol. Allylestrenol. 17α-Allylestr-4-en-17β-ol.

$C_{21}H_{32}O$=300.5.

CAS — 432-60-0.

Allyloestrenol has actions and uses similar to those of progesterone (see p.1431) and is active when given by mouth. In threatened and habitual abortion it has been given in doses of 5 to 15 mg daily. To prevent failure of nidation it has been given in doses of 10 to 20 mg daily from the 16th to the 26th day of each menstrual cycle until conception is achieved, then reduced to 10 mg daily for a minimum of 16 weeks.

Proprietary Preparations

Gestanin *(Organon, UK)*. Allyloestrenol, available as tablets of 5 mg. (Also available as Gestanin in *Austral.*, *S.Afr.*).

Other Proprietary Names

Gestanon *(Belg., Ger., Ital., Jap., Neth., Spain, Switz.)*; Gestanyn *(Swed.)*.

9024-h

Androsterone. 3α-Hydroxy-5α-androstan-17-one.

$C_{19}H_{30}O_2$=290.4.

CAS — 53-41-8.

Pharmacopoeias. In *Braz.*

A white crystalline powder. M.p. about 185°. Practically **insoluble** in water; soluble in most organic solvents.

Androsterone is a naturally occurring androgen which may be isolated from male urine. It has been synthesised.

9025-m

Benzoestrol. Benzestrol *(U.S.P.)*; Octoestrolum. 4,4'-(1,2-Diethyl-3-methyltrimethylene)diphenol.

$C_{20}H_{26}O_2$=298.4.

CAS — 85-95-0.

Pharmacopoeias. In *Rus.* and *U.S.*

An odourless white crystalline powder. M.p. 161° to 163°.

Practically **insoluble** in water and dilute mineral acids; freely soluble in alcohol, acetone, ether, methyl alcohol, and solutions of alkali hydroxides; soluble in glacial acetic acid and fixed oils; slightly soluble in diluted alcohol, chloroform, and light petroleum. A 2% solution in previously neutralised alcohol (80%) is neutral to litmus. **Store** in airtight containers. Protect from light.

Adverse Effects and Precautions. As for Oestradiol, p.1425.

Uses. Benzoestrol is a synthetic oestrogen which is not a steroid; it is structurally related to stilboestrol (see p.1433) and has actions and uses similar to those described under oestradiol (see p.1426).

It has been administered by mouth in doses of 1 to 5 mg daily.

Preparations

Benzestrol Tablets *(U.S.P.)*. Benzoestrol Tablets. Tablets containing benzoestrol. Store in airtight containers.

Tabulettae Octoestroli *(Rus. P.)*. Tablets each containing benzoestrol 1 mg.

9026-b

Calusterone. NSC 88536; U-22550; 7β,17α-Dimethyltestosterone. 17β-Hydroxy-7β,17α-dimethylandrost-4-en-3-one.

$C_{21}H_{32}O_2$=316.5.

CAS — 17021-26-0.

Adverse Effects and Precautions. As for Testosterone, p.1436.

Uses. Calusterone has actions similar to those of testosterone (see p.1436).

It is used similarly to testolactone (see p.1435) in the palliative treatment of breast cancer in postmenopausal women but is reported to have virilising effects. It is given by mouth in doses of 50 mg three to six times daily.

Calusterone is reported to increase the platelet count.

Reviews of the actions and uses of calusterone.— *Med. Lett.*, 1973, *15*, 95; R. A. Brodkin and M. R. Cooper, *Ann. intern. Med.*, 1978, *89*, 945.

Malignant neoplasm of the breast. Of 109 women with advanced neoplasm of the breast 30 had objective remissions after treatment with calusterone 200 mg daily by mouth. The average duration of therapy was 11.9 weeks and 59% survived for 1 year or more.— I. S. Goldenberg *et al.*, *J. Am. med. Ass.*, 1973, *223*, 1267.

Of 40 patients with advanced metastatic breast cancer given calusterone 200 mg daily 4 had objective regression and 13 had arrest of disease progression. Toxic effects (nausea, vomiting, oedema, liver disturbances, and androgenic effects) occurred in about 75% of the patients and led to withdrawal of treatment in 11.— J. Aslam and I. Maxwell, *Cancer Treat. Rep.*, 1977, *61*, 371.

Proprietary Names
Methosarb *(Upjohn, USA)*.

9027-v

Chlormadinone Acetate *(B.P. 1968)*. 6-Chloro-3,20-dioxopregna-4,6-dien-17α-yl acetate.

$C_{23}H_{29}ClO_4$=404.9.

CAS — 1961-77-9 (chlormadinone); 302-22-7 (acetate).

A white to creamy-white fluffy, odourless, crystalline powder. M.p. 208° to 212°. Practically **insoluble** in water; soluble 1 in 160 of alcohol, 1 in 1.5 of chloroform, 1 in 210 of ether, and 1 in 130 of methyl alcohol. **Protect** from light.

Adverse Effects. As for Progesterone, p.1431.

Because the proportion of small nodules in the breast of beagle dogs was found to be increased by continuous doses of chlormadinone acetate, the manufacture of both 'sequential' and 'progestogen-only' oral contraceptive preparations containing chlormadinone acetate was suspended in 1970.

Doses of chlormadinone acetate and megestrol acetate that were 25 times greater than the expected human dose induced mammary tumours in beagles. This was not considered to be a useful indication of carcinogenicity in women.— L. W. Nelson *et al.*, *J. Am. med. Ass.*, 1972, *219*, 1601.

Morphological changes in human oviduct epithelium induced by chlormadinone acetate and mestranol.— B. Fredricsson and N. Bjorkman, *Fert. Steril.*, 1973, *24*, 19, per *Int. pharm. Abstr.*, 1973, *10*, 600.

Both chlormadinone acetate and mestranol induced allergic dermatitis in 8 patients.— H. Adam and B. Schirmer, *Dte GesundhWes.*, 1973, *28*, 1047, per *Int. pharm. Abstr.*, 1974, *11*, 220.

Effects on blood. Coagulation factors VII and X and fibrinogen were not increased by administration of chlormadinone acetate continuously for 2 years. Changing from a 'combined' oral contraceptive to continuous chlormadinone acetate resulted in a return to normal concentrations of coagulation factors within 6 months. Thrombo-elastograph patterns and platelet aggregation were significantly worsened after 2 years, but less for platelets than with the 'combined' oral contraceptives.— L. Poller *et al.*, *Br. med. J.*, 1971, *1*, 705.

Pregnancy and the neonate. *Lactation.* Chlormadinone acetate 500 µg daily for 3 months significantly reduced the protein content of human milk in a controlled study of 40 lactating women.— M. B. Sammour *et al.*, *Fert. Steril.*, 1973, *24*, 301, per *Int. pharm. Abstr.*, 1973, *10*, 903.

Absorption and Fate. Chlormadinone acetate is readily absorbed from the gastro-intestinal tract. It is distributed in body fat from which it is slowly released.

References: Y. G. Dugwekar *et al.*, *Contraception*, 1973, *7*, 313, per *Int. pharm. Abstr.*, 1974, *11*, 33.

Uses. Chlormadinone acetate is a progestational agent with actions and uses similar to those of progesterone (see p.1431). It has been reported to have very slight oestrogenic activity. It is active by mouth and was formerly used with mestranol as a 'sequential' oral contraceptive and as a 'progestogen-only' oral contraceptive.

Proprietary Names

Cero *(Dexter, Arg.)*; Gestafortin *(E. Merck, Ger.)*; Lute-'ran *(Cassenne, Fr.)*; Menstridyl *(Syntex, Belg.)*; Progestormom *(Infal, Spain)*; Traslan *(Gramon, Arg.)*.

For other proprietary names of mestranol and mestranol with chlormadinone acetate, see under Mestranol, p.1418.

9029-q

Chlorotrianisene *(B.P., U.S.P.)*. Chlorotrian.; Chlortrianisenum; Tri-*p*-anisylchloroethylene. Chlorotris(4-methoxyphenyl)ethylene.

$C_{23}H_{21}ClO_3$=380.9.

CAS — 569-57-3.

Pharmacopoeias. In *Br.*, *Rus.*, and *U.S.*

Small white odourless crystals or crystalline powder. It exhibits polymorphism, one form melting at about 116° and the other at about 118°. **Soluble** 1 in 4200 of water, 1 in 360 of alcohol and of methyl alcohol, 1 in 7 of acetone, 1 in 1.5 of chloroform, 1 in 28 of ether, and 1 in 100 of fixed oils; practically insoluble in 2,2,4-trimethylpentane. A saturated solution in water has a pH of 5 to 7. **Store** in airtight containers.

CAUTION. *Chlorotrianisene is a powerful oestrogen. Contact with the skin or inhalation should be avoided. Rubber gloves and a face mask should be worn when handling the powder.*

Adverse Effects and Precautions. As for Oestradiol, p.1425.

Hyperlipaemia was reported in a 76-year-old man with mild adult-onset diabetes mellitus who had been treated with chlorotrianisene 12 mg daily for 10 months after prostate resection.— H. E. Sartori and G. K. Cawthorne (letter), *Drug Intell. & clin. Pharm.*, 1977, *11*, 556.

Uses. Chlorotrianisene is a synthetic non-steroidal oestrogen with properties similar to those described under oestradiol (see p.1425). It has a prolonged action.

Chlorotrianisene is given by mouth for the treatment of menopausal symptoms in a dosage of 12 to 24 mg daily for 30 days, and for symptomatic relief in malignant neoplasms of the prostate in a dosage of 24 mg daily; it has been given for suppression of lactation in a dosage of 48 mg thrice daily for 4 days or 12 mg four times daily for 7 days. The prolonged action of chlorotrianisene may make it less suitable than shorter-acting oestrogens in cyclic replacement therapy.

Preparations

Chlorotrianisene Capsules *(B.P.)*. A solution of chlorotrianisene in maize oil, enclosed in capsules. Store at a temperature not exceeding 30°.

Chlorotrianisene Capsules *(U.S.P.)*. Capsules containing chlorotrianisene. Store at a temperature not exceeding 40° and protect from cold and moisture.

Chlorotrianisene Tablets *(B.P.)*. Tablets containing chlorotrianisene.

Proprietary Preparations

Tace *(Merrell, UK)*. Chlorotrianisene, available as scored tablets of 24 mg. (Also available as Tace in *Austral., Belg., Canad., Ital., S.Afr., Spain, Switz., USA*).

Other Proprietary Names

Anisene, Clorotrisin (both *Ital.)*; Hormonisene *(Arg.)*; Merbentul *(Ger.)*; Tace FN *(Fr.)*; Triagen *(Ital.)*.

NOTE. Merbentyl is dicyclomine hydrochloride.

9030-d

Clogestone Acetate. AY 11440; 3-Acetoxychlormadinone. 6-Chloro-3β,17α-dihydroxypregna-4,6-dien-20-one diacetate.

$C_{25}H_{33}ClO_5$=449.0.

CAS — 20047-75-0 (clogestone); 3044-32-4 (acetate).

A progestogen which has been tried as an oral contraceptive. It has not been found to be very effective.

Manufacturers

Ayerst, UK.

9031-n

Clomiphene Citrate *(B.P., U.S.P.)*. Clomiphene Cit.; Clomifene Citrate; Chloramiphene Citrate; MRL 41; NSC 35770. A mixture of the *E* and *Z* isomers of 2-[4-(2-chloro-1,2-diphenylvinyl)phenoxy]triethylamine dihydrogen citrate.

$C_{26}H_{28}ClNO,C_6H_8O_7$=598.1.

CAS — 911-45-5 (clomiphene); 15690-57-0 (clomiphene, E); 15690-55-8 (clomiphene, Z); 50-41-9 (citrate); 7599-79-3 (citrate, E); 7619-53-6 (citrate, Z).

Clomiphene may be separated into its *Z* and *E* isomers, zuclomiphene and enclomiphene.

Pharmacopoeias. In *Br.*, *Braz.*, *Jap.*, *Nord.*, and *U.S.*

A white to pale yellow, odourless or almost odourless powder. It contains 30 to 50% of the *Z* isomer. M.p. about 150°. **Soluble** 1 in 900 of water, 1 in 40 of alcohol, and 1 in 800 of chloroform; freely soluble in glacial acetic acid and methyl alcohol; practically insoluble in ether. **Protect** from light.

Adverse Effects. Side-effects are related to dosage and include hot flushes resembling menopausal symptoms, transient blurring of vision, abdominal discomfort, sometimes with nausea and vomiting, and reversible ovarian enlargement and cyst formation. Slight alopecia and urticaria have occasionally been reported. There may be some abnormalities in liver function.

Some patients may experience depression, fatigue, dizziness, insomnia, headache, breast tenderness, weight gain, heavier menses, or spotting.

Reports of hydatidiform mole formation associated with clomiphene: C. I. Schneiderman and B. Waxman, *Obstet. Gynec.*, 1972, *39*, 787; G. Wajntraub *et al.*, *Fert. Steril.*, 1974, *25*, 904.

Neurological impairment with problems of gait, coordination, and use of the hands as well as a decline in intellectual function developed in a woman with breast cancer after receiving clomiphene citrate 50 mg four times daily for 6 months. Deterioration occurred over the next 8 months. There was rapid improvement when clomiphene was withdrawn.— C. M. Haskell *et al.* (letter), *Lancet*, 1977, *2*, 1227.

Cystic gynaecomastia developed in a 32-year-old man treated for 5 months with clomiphene citrate 25 mg daily for 25 days in 30.— J. H. Check, *Fert. Steril.*, 1978, *30*, 713.

Effects on the ovary. Massive ovarian enlargement and ascites occurred in a 29-year-old woman who received clomiphene citrate 50 mg daily for 5 days and, about 4 weeks later, 100 mg daily for 5 days. It was considered that the second course was administered after conception. Care should be exercised to avoid inadvertent administration of clomiphene citrate during the early stages of pregnancy.— A. Scommegna and S. R. Lash, *J. Am. med. Ass.*, 1969, *207*, 753.

Ovarian endometrial cyst formation, requiring surgery, in 4 patients treated with clomiphene citrate.— P. Gabos, *Obstet. Gynec.*, 1979, *53*, 763.

Neoplasm of the breast. Bilateral breast cancer was associated with clomiphene in 2 patients.— P. M. Bolton (letter), *Lancet*, 1977, *2*, 1176.

Neoplasm of the testis. A 28-year-old man treated over a period of 21 weeks with enclomiphene citrate 1 mg daily for oligospermia developed a teratoma and seminoma in the previously atrophied testis. It was considered possible that enclomiphene had stimulated the growth of a pre-existing neoplasm.— F. I. Reyes and C. Faiman, *Can. med. Ass. J.*, 1973, *109*, 502. See also J. P. Neoptolemos *et al.* (letter), *Lancet*, 1981, *2*, 754.

Pregnancy and the neonate. *Ectopic pregnancy.* Ectopic as well as twin intra-uterine pregnancies occurred in a patient given prednisone 2.5 mg four times daily and clomiphene 50 mg daily from the 4th to the 8th day of the cycle and who conceived during the second month.— S. Payne *et al.*, *Obstet. Gynec.*, 1971, *38*, 905, per *Int. pharm. Abstr.*, 1972, *9*, 785.

Of 21 patients with tubal pregnancies, 3 had received clomiphene. Also 2 patients with hydatidiform mole were observed in a group of pregnant women who had been given clomiphene.— D. B. Weiss and Y. Aboulafia (letter), *Lancet*, 1975, *2*, 1094.

Effects on the foetus. Anencephaly in 2 infants was associated with maternal ovulation stimulation with clomiphene.— J. L. Dyson and H. G. Kohler (letter), *Lancet*, 1973, *1*, 1256. Anencephaly might be associated with infertility and not its treatment.— W. H. James (letter), *ibid.*, 1973, *2*, 916. Clomiphene was used to induce ovulation before 1 anencephalic and 1 normal pregnancy in a woman who had already had 1 normal and 1 anencephalic pregnancy without the aid of clomiphene.— C. Barrett and C. Hakim (letter), *ibid.* See also Y. Biale *et al.*, *Acta obstet. gynec. scand.*, 1978, *57*, 483.

Two children with neural-tube defects were born to mothers who had taken clomiphene.— B. Field and C. Kerr (letter), *Lancet*, 1974, *2*, 1511. See also M. Singh *et al.*, *J. Pediat.*, 1978, *93*, 152.

Multiple congenital abnormalities occurred in an infant whose mother had received clomiphene.— P. Berman (letter), *Lancet*, 1975, *2*, 878.

Fatal congenital abnormalities affecting the respiratory tract, heart, and genito-urinary system were associated in an infant with the maternal use of clomiphene.— O. Ylikorkala (letter), *Lancet*, 1975, *2*, 1262.

There was a 13% incidence of multiple delivery in 225 infants whose mothers had received clomiphene at or shortly before conception for ovulation induction. One infant had Down's syndrome and another an imperforate anus; an incidence of malformations no greater than expected.— S. Harlap (letter), *Lancet*, 1976, *2*, 961.

Megalo-ureter, hypospadias and imperforate anus in a neonate possibly associated with the maternal ingestion of clomiphene.— F. Halal *et al.*, *Can. med. Ass. J.*, 1980, *122*, 1159.

A review of published reports indicated that the sex ratio (proportion of boys) was low among infants conceived after induction of ovulation with clomiphene or gonadotrophin or both.— W. H. James, *Br. med. J.*, 1980, *281*, 711.

Precautions. Clomiphene citrate is contra-indicated in patients with liver disease, endometrial carcinoma or ovarian cysts (other than polycystic ovary) and during pregnancy. Before starting treatment patients should be thoroughly examined to exclude liver disease, pituitary or ovarian failure, and neoplasms of the endometrium. The cause of infertility and any abnormal bleeding should be investigated. The patient should be warned of the possibility of multiple births, particularly if higher doses are used. Prolonged courses of treatment are not recommended.

Precocious or premature menopause in 2 women.— E. A. Lenton *et al.*, *Br. J. Obstet. Gynaec.*, 1979, *86*, 238.

Absorption and Fate. Clomiphene citrate is absorbed from the gastro-intestinal tract and slowly excreted through the liver into the bile. The biological half-life is reported to be 5 days. Enterohepatic recirculation takes place.

Uses. Clomiphene is chemically related to chlorotrianisene. It stimulates the secretion of pituitary gonadotrophic hormones probably by blocking the effect of oestrogens at receptor sites in the hypothalamus and pituitary.

Clomiphene is used in the treatment of anovulatory infertility. The usual dose is 50 mg of the citrate daily for 5 days, starting on or about the 5th day of the menstrual cycle or at any time if there is amenorrhoea. If ovulation occurs but is not followed by pregnancy the course may be repeated up to a total of 6 cycles. If ovulation does not occur, a course of 100 mg daily for 5 days may be given and repeated twice if necessary. If pregnancy has not occurred after 6 courses further courses are unlikely to be successful. Higher doses or prolonged treatment may lead to ovarian enlargement, but doses of up to 250 mg daily have been given. Patients with polycystic ovaries should be given the smallest possible dose. Therapy with clomiphene will not be successful unless the woman, though anovulatory, is capable of ovulation and her partner is fertile. Ovulation usually takes place 6 to 10 days after the last day of treatment.

For reviews of the actions and uses of clomiphene, see R. J. Pepperell *et al.*, *Med. J. Aust.*, 1977, *2*, 774; D. G. Limb, *Practitioner*, 1978, *221*, 917; D. T. Baird, *Prescribers' J.*, 1979, *19*, 99.

Anorexia. The use of clomiphene in anorexia nervosa: J. C. Marshall and T. R. Fraser, *Br. med. J.*, 1971, *4*, 590; P. J. V. Beaumont *et al.*, *Psychol. Med.*, 1973, *3*,

495, per *J. Am. med. Ass.*, 1974, *227*, 966.

Gynaecomastia. Relief of gynaecomastia in 18 of 19 boys given clomiphene citrate 50 mg daily reduced to 50 mg on alternate days.— A. V. Stepanas *et al.*, *J. Pediat.*, 1977, *90*, 651.

Infertility. An account of the endocrinology of female infertility.— D. T. Baird, *Br. med. Bull.*, 1979, *35*, 193.

The use of clomiphene citrate to regulate ovulation prior to donor insemination in 17 couples with male infertility.— L. J. Kaly, *Fert. Steril.*, 1976, *27*, 383, per *Int. pharm. Abstr.*, 1976, *13*, 995. See also M. F. Vere and D. N. Joyce, *Br. med. J.*, 1979, *2*, 100.

For the use of clomiphene in a regimen for the investigation and treatment of secondary amenorrhoea, see M. G. R. Hull *et al.*, *Br. med. J.*, 1979, *1*, 1257. See also J. Garcia and G. S. Jones, *Fert. Steril.*, 1977, *28*, 707, per *Int. pharm. Abstr.*, 1977, *14*, 1236.

Of 45 women 43 ovulated after courses of clomiphene citrate up to 250 mg daily for 5 days, with chorionic gonadotrophin, and 33 conceived. Of the 33, nine required more than 100 mg daily and/or more than 3 ovulatory cycles. Large doses were acceptable.— T. S. Drake *et al.*, *Fert. Steril.*, 1978, *30*, 274, per *Int. pharm. Abstr.*, 1979, *16*, 160.

Ovulation was induced and pregnancy achieved in 86% and 35.5% of 307 women treated with clomiphene citrate; results for other treatments were: cyclofenil, 71% and 23.7% in 38 women, tamoxifen, 95% and 35% in 40 women; with tamoxifen the abortion-rate was 35%.— V. Ruiz-Velasco *et al.*, *Int. J. Fert.*, 1979, *24*, 61.

Further references to clomiphene in the treatment of infertility: G. I. Swyer *et al.*, *Br. J. Obstet. Gynaec.*, 1975, *82*, 794 (with chorionic gonadotrophin); R. W. Shaw *et al.*, *Br. J. Obstet. Gynaec.*, 1975, *82*, 952 (with oestradiol benzoate), per *Int. pharm. Abstr.*, 1977, *14*, 284; E. S. Canales *et al.*, *Fert. Steril.*, 1978, *29*, 496 (with oestradiol benzoate), per *Int. pharm. Abstr.*, 1978, *15*, 1126; A. Lopata *et al.*, *Fert. Steril.*, 1978, *30*, 27 (with chorionic gonadotrophin); A. E. Schindler and A. Plenefisch, *Dt. med. Wschr.*, 1979, *104*, 1135 (with chorionic gonadotrophin); A. T. Dempsey, *Br. J. Hosp. Med.*, 1980, *24*, 48 (with chorionic gonadotrophin).

References to *enclomiphene* in the treatment of infertility: Y. S. Murthy *et al.*, *Int. J. Fert.*, 1971, *16*, 66; J. V. Campenhout *et al.*, *Am. J. Obstet. Gynec.*, 1973, *115*, 321, per *Int. pharm. Abstr.*, 1974, *11*, 676; J. F. Connaughton *et al.*, *Obstet. Gynec.*, 1974, *43*, 697.

Male infertility. Studies in 3 men showed that clomiphene citrate 200 mg daily for 5 days significantly increased plasma concentrations of follicle-stimulating hormone and luteinising hormone; the maximum effect occurred 6 days after treatment was started and persisted for 5 to 9 days after treatment was stopped.— C. M. Cargille *et al.* (letter), *Lancet*, 1968, *2*, 1298.

Clomiphene citrate, given in doses of 50 to 400 mg daily for 2 to 12 months, increased urinary gonadotrophins in 13 normal men. Low doses increased the sperm count but the higher doses produced large decreases in the count.— C. G. Heller *et al.*, *J. clin. Endocr. Metab.*, 1969, *29*, 638, per *J. Am. med. Ass.*, 1969, *208*, 2538.

Of 84 hypofertile men 27 were classified as having primary hypofertility (oligospermia and elevated concentrations of FSH) and 57 as having pregerminal hypofertility (oligospermia and normal FSH). After treatment with clomiphene citrate, 25 mg daily in 24-day cycles with 5-day rest periods, for up to 6 months a pregnancy-rate of 42% was achieved in the partners (in which no major female factor could be identified) of the second group; there was no response in the first group.— D. F. Paulson, *Fert. Steril.*, 1977, *28*, 1226, per *Int. pharm. Abstr.*, 1978, *15*, 418.

Further favourable reports of the use of clomiphene citrate.— I. F. Potts, *Med. J. Aust.*, 1968, *1*, 707; *J. Am. med. Ass.*, 1975, *231*, 907; J. A. Epstein, *Fert. Steril.*, 1977, *28*, 741, per *Int. pharm. Abstr.*, 1977, *14*, 1236; J. H. Check and A. E. Rakoff, *Fert. Steril.*, 1977, *28*, 746, per *Int. pharm. Abstr.*, 1977, *14*, 1236; J. McConnon *et al.* (letter), *Lancet*, 1979, *2*, 525.

Pituitary stimulation test. In 9 healthy men clomiphene citrate, 3 mg per kg body-weight to a maximum of 200 mg daily, caused a mean increase of 107% in serum concentrations of luteinising hormone (LH) and a mean increase of 114% in 17β-hydroxy androgens (17OHA). There was no response in LH and 17OHA values in early puberty, in panhypopituitarism, or in gonadotrophin deficiency, and LH values were unchanged in Klinefelter's syndrome. The principal use of the test was to confirm a diagnosis of gonadotrophin deficiency in adults. In the dose used side-effects included a sensation of visual flickering in most subjects, lack of concentration, disturbance of limb sensation, increased aggression, and depression.— D. C. Anderson *et al.*, *Clin. Endocr.*, 1972, *1*, 127. See also J. Newton *et al.* (preliminary communication), *Lancet*, 1971, *2*, 190.

Preparations

Clomiphene Citrate Tablets *(U.S.P.)*. Tablets containing clomiphene citrate. Protect from light.

Clomiphene Tablets *(B.P.)*. Tablets containing clomiphene citrate. Store at a temperature not exceeding 25°. Protect from light.

Proprietary Preparations

Clomid *(Merrell, UK)*. Clomiphene citrate, available as scored tablets of 50 mg. (Also available as Clomid in *Austral., Belg., Canad., Fr., Ital., Neth., S.Afr., Switz., USA*).

Serophene *(Serono, UK)*. Clomiphene citrate, available as scored tablets of 50 mg.

Other Proprietary Names

Clomivid *(Denm., Norw., Swed.)*; Clostilbegyt *(Hung.)*; Dyneric *(Ger.)*; Genozym *(Arg.)*; Omifin *(Spain)*; Prolifen *(Ital.)*.

9032-h

Clostebol Acetate. 4-Chlorotestosterone Acetate; Chlortestosterone Acetate. 4-Chloro-3-oxoandrost-4-en-17β-yl acetate.

$C_{21}H_{29}ClO_3$=364.9.

CAS — 1093-58-9 (clostebol); 855-19-6 (acetate).

Pharmacopoeias. In *Roum.*

Clostebol acetate is an anabolic steroid with actions and uses similar to those of methandienone (see p.1418). Doses of 40 mg twice weekly by intramuscular injection have been given. The hexanoate and propionate have also been used.

A report of irreversible voice changes due to clostebol in women and children.— A. Tzschoppe and G. Steude, *Dte GesundhWes.*, 1974, *29*, 1282, per *Int. pharm. Abstr.*, 1975, *12*, 343.

Proprietary Names

Alfa-Trofodermin *(Farmitalia, Ital.)*; Clostene *(SIFI, Ital.)*; Steranabol *(Farmitalia, Ger.; Farmitalia, Neth.)*.

NOTE. Steranabol Depot and Steranabol Ritardo are used as proprietary names for oxabolone cypionate.

9033-m

Cyclofenil. F 6066; ICI 48213. 4,4′-(Cyclohexylidenemethylene)bis(phenyl acetate).

$C_{23}H_{24}O_4$=364.4.

CAS — 2624-43-3.

Pharmacopoeias. In *Nord.*

A white odourless crystalline powder. M.p. 137° to 140°. Practically **insoluble** in water; soluble 1 in 250 of alcohol, 1 in 2 of chloroform, and 1 in 30 of ether.

Adverse Effects. Side-effects include gastro-intestinal effects and very occasionally hot flushes and ovarian enlargement. Cholestatic jaundice has been reported.

Precautions. As for Clomiphene Citrate, p.1407.

Uses. Cyclofenil is used similarly to clomiphene citrate (p.1407) for the induction of ovulation in the treatment of infertility and in the treatment of amenorrhoea. It appears to be less effective than clomiphene.

It is given by mouth in doses of 100 mg twice daily for 3 cycles. If there is no menstruation cycles of 200 mg twice daily can be given for 10 days separated by 20 days. Doses of 800 mg daily have been given in 5-day courses.

It has also been given in menopausal disorders.

Infertility. For a short review of the use of cyclofenil in the treatment of infertility, see Agents Stimulating Gonadal Function in the Human. *Tech. Rep. Ser. Wld Hlth Org. No. 514*, 1973.

Skin disorders. The use of cyclofenil in scleroderma.— G. Herbai *et al.*, *Acta med. scand.*, 1977, *201*, 203.

Proprietary Preparations

Rehibin *(Ferrosan, Swed.: Thames, UK)*. Cyclofenil, available as scored tablets of 100 mg.

Other Proprietary Names

Ciclifen *(Arg.)*; Fertodur *(Ger., Ital., Switz.)*; Ondogyne *(Fr., Neth.)*; Ondonid *(Austral.)*; Sexovid *(Denm., Jap., Norw., Swed.)*.

Cyclofenil was also formerly marketed in Great Britain under the proprietary name Ondonid *(Roussel)*.

9034-b

Cyproterone Acetate. SH 714. 6-Chloro-1β,2β-dihydro-3,20-dioxo-3′*H*-cyclopropa[1,2]-pregna-1,4,6-trien-17α-yl acetate.

$C_{24}H_{29}ClO_4$=416.9.

CAS — 2098-66-0 (cyproterone); 427-51-0 (acetate).

Adverse Effects. Cyproterone acetate inhibits spermatogenesis, reduces the volume of ejaculate, and causes infertility; these effects are slowly reversible. Abnormal spermatozoa may be produced. Gynaecomastia is common and permanent enlargement of the mammary glands may occur; galactorrhoea and benign nodules have been reported. There may be initial sedation and depressive mood changes. Patients may experience alterations in hair pattern, skin reactions, weight changes, headache, anaemia, gastro-intestinal disturbance, and vasomotor changes with fluctuations in blood pressure.

When given with ethinyloestradiol to women as an oral contraceptive nausea, headache, loss of libido, weight changes, depression, irregular uterine bleeding, and mastodynia have been reported.

Precautions. Cyproterone acetate is contra-indicated in patients with acute liver disorders or malignant or wasting diseases. It should not be given to patients with severe chronic depression or to those with a history of thrombo-embolic disorders. It may delay bone maturation and testicular development and so should not be given to immature youths.

It should be given with care to patients with chronic liver disease, and, since it can interfere with carbohydrate metabolism, to those with diabetes mellitus. Since anaemia has been observed blood estimations are recommended regularly during treatment. Alcohol is reported to reduce the effects of cyproterone acetate and chronic alcoholics do not respond. Depression of adrenal function has been reported.

Patients should be advised that the initial sedative effects may interfere with driving and the operation of machinery.

There were no clinical signs of severe cortisol deficiency in 13 girls with idiopathic precocious puberty treated with cyproterone acetate 80 to 160 mg per m^2 body-surface daily for up to about 6 years. However, laboratory investigation in 9 of the girls showed depressed adrenocortical activity. It was considered that cyproterone may have glucocorticoid activity which may mask the clinical symptoms of adrenocortical depression; whatever reason, these patients should carry cards and have operative adrenal coverage.— K. E. von Mühlendahl *et al.* (letter), *Lancet*, 1977, *1*, 1160.

Absorption and Fate. Cyproterone acetate is poorly absorbed from the gastro-intestinal tract. It is rapidly metabolised and slowly excreted in the faeces and urine.

In 2 men given cyproterone acetate 100 mg by mouth as a single dose, peak plasma concentrations of 100 to 150 ng per ml occurred 5 to 10 hours after administration. Absorption from the gastro-intestinal tract was poor and after 8 days 90% of the dose was eliminated in the faeces.— E. Gerhards *et al.*, *Arzneimittel-Forsch.*, 1973, *23*, 1550.

Absorption and fate of cyproterone acetate in 16 healthy subjects after receiving very low doses by mouth or intramuscularly.— D. Jentsch *et al.*, *Arzneimittel-Forsch.*, 1976, *26*, 914.

In 5 healthy men given cyproterone acetate 50 mg by mouth peak plasma concentrations of 265 to 332 ng per ml (mean 285 ng per ml) occurred 3 to 4 hours after administration.— M. Hümpel *et al.*, *Arzneimittel-Forsch.*, 1978, *28*, 319.

Uses. Cyproterone acetate has anti-androgenic and some progestogenic activity. It is used in the treatment of sexual disorders in the male. It has also been tried in the treatment of acne and hirsutism.

The usual dose is 50 mg twice daily increased if necessary after 4 weeks to 200 or 300 mg daily in divided doses until a response is achieved. Thereafter doses are gradually reduced until a suitable maintenance level is achieved.

Reviews of the actions and uses of cyproterone acetate.— *Lancet*, 1976, *1*, 1003; *Drug & Ther. Bull.*, 1977, *15*, 55.

Acne. Cyproterone acetate, 10% in dimethyl sulphoxide applied topically twice daily for 6 to 8 weeks to 12 patients with acne, had no effect on the acne or on sebum secretion.— W. J. Cunliffe *et al.*, *Br. J. Derm.*, 1969, *81*, 200.

Sebum excretion-rate was less than the control rate in 20 men receiving cyproterone acetate during treatment for sexual offences.— J. L. Burton *et al.*, *Br. J. Derm.*, 1973, *89*, 487.

No significant difference in sebum excretion-rate or improvement in acne occurred in 9 female and 5 male patients aged 15 to 27 years who had applied a suspension of cyproterone acetate 1% in Cetomacrogol Cream (Formula A) twice daily for up to 12 weeks.— R. J. Pye *et al.*, *Br. J. Derm.*, 1976, *95*, 427.

A 0.2% alcoholic solution of cyproterone acetate was applied to a balding area of scalp skin of 10 healthy male subjects for 8 months, to give a daily dose of 2 mg, a maximum of 5 times weekly. A mean reduction in sebum-excretion rate of 53% was obtained after 35 weeks.— K. D. Bingham *et al.* (letter), *Lancet*, 1979, *2*, 304.

A combination of cyproterone acetate 2 mg and ethinyloestradiol 50 µg was given to 101 women from the fifth to the twenty-fifth days of the menstrual cycles for a total of 1105 cycles. Treatment was satisfactory in 96% of those with acne, 84% of those with androgenic alopecia, 79% of those with seborrhoea, and 50% of those with mild or moderate hirsutism. None of the women became pregnant. It was suggested that this combination was the method of choice of hormonal contraception in such patients and that it was also suitable in the follow-up of high-dose cyproterone acetate treatment of severe hirsutism.— L. Moltz *et al.*, *Dt. med. Wschr.*, 1979, *104*, 1376. See also R. Palatsi *et al.*, *Acta derm.-vener., Stockh.*, 1978, *58*, 449.

Anxiety states. Pilot studies indicated that cyproterone acetate in low doses was effective in anxiety in men and in high doses was effective in women in the premenstrual syndrome.— T. M. Itil *et al.*, *Curr. ther. Res.*, 1974, *16*, 1147.

Hirsutism. Cyproterone 100 mg daily for 10 days from day 5 of the menstrual cycle alone or together with ethinyloestradiol 50 µg daily for 17 days each month, for 6 months, reduced hair growth by at least 30% in 14 of 15 hirsute female patients aged 13 to 46 years, but was not associated with a reduction in plasma-testosterone concentrations. The efficacy of cyproterone might have been due to a direct blocking action of the hair follicle.— J. A. R. Anderson and M. C. K. Browning, *Br. J. Derm.*, 1977, *97*, *Suppl.* 15, 20. A similar report in 1 patient.— F. J. Ebling *et al.*, *ibid.*, 1977, *97*, 371.

A review of cyproterone acetate for severe hirsutism. Potentially serious unwanted effects mean that it should be used only in the most severe cases of hirsutism, by a specialist.— *Drug & Ther. Bull.*, 1981, *19*, 99.

Further references: J. Hammerstein and B. Cupceancu, *Dt. med. Wschr.*, 1969, *94*, 829; C. J. Dewhurst *et al.*, *Br. J. Obstet. Gynaec.*, 1977, *84*, 119; R. Underhill and J. Dewhurst, *ibid.*, 1979, *86*, 139.

Neoplasm of the prostate. Experience in treating 55 patients with carcinoma of the prostate with cyproterone acetate for up to 4 years indicated that it might be slightly more effective than oestrogen therapy in patients who had relapsed following other hormonal therapy.— A. J. Wein and J. J. Murphy, *J. Urol.*, 1973, *109*, 68, per *J. Am. med. Ass.*, 1973, *223*, 1412. See also R. B. Smith *et al.*, *J. Urol.*, 1973, *110*, 106, per *J. Am. med. Ass.*, 1973, *226*, 493.

Puberty, precocious. Cyproterone acetate in doses of 70 to 150 mg per m^2 body-surface daily, given by mouth over periods of from 6 to 40 months was effective and preferable to depot injections of 107 to 230 mg per m^2 every 2 to 4 weeks for the treatment of precocious puberty in 29 children.— R. Kauli *et al.*, *Archs Dis. Childh.*, 1976, *51*, 202.

Sexual disorders. Cyproterone acetate in doses of 50 to 150 mg daily was used to diminish sexual responsiveness in 3 patients.— A. J. Cooper *et al.*, *Br. J. Psychiat.*, 1972, *120*, 59.

Treatment with cyproterone acetate for 6 months to 3 years was successful in 11 of 24 sexual deviants. Psychotherapy should be carried out in conjunction with chemotherapy.— E. Fahndrich, *Dt. med. Wschr.*, 1974, *99*, 234, per *J. Am. med. Ass.*, 1974, *228*, 652.

The proceedings of a short symposium on the use of cyproterone acetate in sexual disorders.— *J. int. med. Res.*, 1975, *3*, *Suppl.* 4.

Proprietary Preparations

Androcur *(Schering, UK)*. Cyproterone acetate, available as scored tablets of 50 mg. (Also available as Androcur in *Denm., Ger., Ital., Neth., Norw., Spain, Swed., Switz.*).

9035-v

Danazol *(U.S.P.)*. Win 17757. 17α-Pregna-2,4-dien-20-yno[2,3-*d*]isoxazol-17β-ol.

$C_{22}H_{27}NO_2$=337.5.

CAS — 17230-88-5.

Pharmacopoeias. In *U.S.*

A white or pale yellow crystalline powder. M.p. about 225° with decomposition. Practically **insoluble** in water and light petroleum; sparingly soluble in alcohol; freely soluble in chloroform, slightly soluble in ether; soluble in acetone. A solution in chloroform is dextrorotatory. **Store** in airtight containers. Protect from light.

Adverse Effects. Side-effects reflecting inhibition of the pituitary-ovarian axis include amenorrhoea, hot flushes, sweating, changes (usually decrease) in breast size, changes in libido, and vaginitis.

Side-effects attributable to androgenic activity include acne, oily skin or hair, hirsutism, oedema, gain in weight, deepening of the voice, and occasionally clitoral hypertrophy.

Other side-effects include gastro-intestinal disturbances, headache, dizziness, tremor, depression, sleep disorders, muscle spasm or cramp, skin rash, and occasionally elevation of liver-function test values.

Myalgia and elevated creatine phosphokinase concentrations occurred in a 40-year-old woman given danazol 200 mg twice or thrice daily to treat hereditary angioedema.— W. B. Spaulding (letter), *Ann. intern. Med.*, 1979, *90*, 854.

Danazol was associated with biochemical evidence of liver injury in 4 patients and with jaundice in one patient.— K. Pearson and H. J. Zimmerman (letter), *Lancet*, 1980, *1*, 645.

Precautions. Danazol should be used with caution in conditions which may be adversely affected by fluid retention, such as cardiac and renal disorders, migraine, or epilepsy. It should also be used with care in patients with hepatic disorders. It should not be given to women who are pregnant or breast-feeding.

Interference with thyroid-function tests.— P. R. Pannall and D. A. Maas (letter), *Lancet*, 1977, *1*, 102. See also J. I. Thorell *et al.*, *Postgrad. med. J.*, 1979, *55*, *Suppl.* 5, 33.

Impaired glucose tolerance in 14 patients after treatment with danazol 600 mg daily for 3 months.— V. Wynn, *J. int. med. Res.*, 1977, *5*, *Suppl.* 3, 25.

In 10 women taking danazol there was no change in Quick's one-stage prothrombin time compared with controls but the kaolin cephalin clotting time was significantly reduced.— T. H. Chimbira *et al.*, *Postgrad. med. J.*, 1979, *55*, *Suppl.* 5, 90.

In 19 women with endometriosis given danazol 400 to 800 mg daily there was a highly significant rise in plasma-total-cholesterol concentrations over a 6-month period. In 8 patients studied subsequently, high-density lipoprotein cholesterol fell dramatically after 2 months of treatment; since this correlates negatively with risk of coronary heart disease patients taking danazol may be at risk. Danazol should not be given for very long periods of time, at least in high-risk patients, until further studies have been carried out.— I. S. Fraser and J. K. Allen (letter), *Lancet*, 1979, *1*, 931.

Absorption and Fate. Danazol is absorbed from the gastro-intestinal tract and metabolised in the liver. A half-life of about 4.5 hours has been reported. 2-Hydroxymethylethisterone and ethisterone have been identified in the urine.

Plasma concentrations of danazol.— J. G. Lloyd-Jones and T. Williams-Ross, *J. int. med. Res.*, 1977, *5*, *Suppl.* 3, 18.

Uses. Danazol suppresses the pituitary-ovarian axis by inhibiting pituitary output of gonadotrophins. It has some androgenic activity. It is used in the treatment of endometriosis. The usual initial dose is 400 mg daily, in 2 to 4 divided doses, starting on the first day of the menstrual cycle (to exclude pregnancy); daily doses of 800 mg are also employed.

Danazol is also used in the treatment of benign breast disorders including gynaecomastia, fibrocystic breast disease, and pubertal breast hypertrophy in usual divided doses of 100 to 400 mg daily. In primary constitutional precocious puberty 100 to 400 mg daily may be given according to the child's age and weight.

Danazol has also been found to be of value in the treatment of hereditary angio-oedema.

Reports of symposia on danazol.— *J. int. med. Res.*, 1977, *5*, *Suppl.* 3, 1–127; *Postgrad. med. J.*, 1979, *55*, *Suppl.* 5, 1–95.

Possible progestational activity.— A. C. Wentz *et al.*, *Am. J. Obstet. Gynec.*, 1976, *126*, 378.

The actions and uses of danazol.— I. S. Fraser, *Scott. med. J.*, 1979, *24*, 147.

Angio-oedema. In 9 patients with hereditary angio-oedema there were 44 attacks during 47 courses of treatment with placebo and 1 attack during 46 courses of treatment with danazol 200 mg thrice daily given for 28 days or until an attack occurred. Depressed C1 esterase inhibitor activity was corrected. Side-effects were minimal—weight gain and amenorrhoea.— J. A. Gelfand *et al.*, *New Engl. J. Med.*, 1976, *295*, 1444.

Danazol 300 to 600 mg daily with a gap of 5 or 7 days every 7 days was effective in the treatment of 10 patients with hereditary angioneurotic oedema.— A. Agostoni *et al.* (letter), *Lancet*, 1978, *1*, 453.

A report on experience of treating 21 patients with hereditary angioneurotic oedema over 3½ years. Continuous administration of tranexamic acid 1.5 to 2 g daily has abolished all but the most trivial symptoms. Danazol 300 mg daily is equally successful in abolishing attacks. Premenopausal women and males are given tranexamic acid and postmenopausal women are given danazol. The only side-effect has been slight and transient weight gain with danazol. There had been 2 successful uncomplicated pregnancies and 2 more are under superivision; tranexamic acid was continued after the first trimester in all. All patients with hereditary angioneurotic oedema should be offered one or other of these treatments.— P. Naish and J. Barratt (letter), *Lancet*, 1979, *1*, 611. If oral surgery is required, tranexamic acid a week before surgery and a week post-operatively seems to be satisfactory.— P. Ward-Booth (letter), *ibid.*

An 8-year-old boy with hereditary angio-oedema remained free from attacks on danazol 200 mg every other day.— G. Tappeiner *et al.*, *Br. J. Derm.*, 1979, *100*, 207.

Of 55 patients with hereditary angio-oedema 95% were free from attacks on danazol 600 mg daily, 88% on 400 mg daily, 68% on 300 mg daily, and 11% on 200 mg daily. Short-term prophylaxis before dental procedures was achieved with 600 mg daily for 10 days.— S. W. Hosea and M. M. Frank, *Drugs*, 1980, *19*, 370.

A 24-year-old woman with hereditary angioneurotic oedema and a lupus erythematosus-like syndrome and a low level of C_1 esterase inhibitor obtained a clinical remission on administration of danazol.— R. Masse *et al.* (letter), *Lancet*, 1980, *2*, 651. A similar finding.— V. H. Donaldson and E. V. Hess (letter), *ibid.*, 1145.

Control of hereditary angio-oedema in 2 patients with danazol in doses gradually reduced to 200 mg three times a week or 300 mg weekly.— J. T. Macfarlane and D. Davies, *Br. med. J.*, 1981, *282*, 1275.

Further references: *Lancet*, 1979, *1*, 417; H. Hinter *et al.*, *Dt. med. Wschr.*, 1979, *104*, 1269; S. W. Hosea *et al.*, *Ann. intern. Med.*, 1980, *93*, 809; C. Rajagopal and J. R. Harper, *Archs Dis. Childh.*, 1981, *56*, 229.

Benign breast disease. Of 58 women with benign breast disorders (mazoplasia, mastodynia, or fibrocystic disease) 44 were markedly improved after treatment with danazol 100 to 400 mg daily for 74 to 310 days. Objective evidence of improvement was seen in 16 of 19 patients subjected to mammography. Amenorrhoea occurred in half the patients treated; other side-effects were considered trivial.— R. H. Asch and R. B. Greenblatt, *Am. J. Obstet. Gynec.*, 1977, *127*, 130.

Relief of pain and tenderness and some reduction in nodularity in 18 women with fibrocystic disease of the breast given danazol 100 to 400 mg daily.— L. J. Humphrey and N. C. Estes, *Postgrad. med. J.*, 1979, *55, Suppl.* 5, 48. Relief of pain, discomfort, heaviness, and tenderness in 6 patients with cyclical breast pain, given danazol 400 mg daily.— R. E. Mansel *et al.*, *ibid.*, 61. A favourable report of the use of danazol 400 mg daily in 27 patients with chronic cystic mastopathy.— M. Dhout *et al.*, *ibid.*, 66.

Further references: N. H. Lauerson and K. H. Wilson, *Obstet. Gynec.*, 1976, *48*, 93; W. P. Blackmore, *Int. J. med. Res.*, 1977, *5, Suppl.* 3, 101; M. F. Aksu *et al.*, *J. reprod. Med.*, 1978, *21*, 181; J. D. Brookshaw, *Postgrad. med. J.*, 1979, *55, Suppl.* 5, 52; B. Greenblatt and I. Ben-Nun, *Drugs*, 1980, *19*, 349.

Contraception. Unfavourable reports on danazol as a contraceptive.— A. C. Wentz *et al.*, *Contraception*, 1976, *13*, 619, per *Int. pharm. Abstr.*, 1978, *15*, 263; N. H. Lauersen and K. H. Wilson, *Obstet. Gynec.*, 1977, *50*, 91.

Endometriosis. Reviews and discussions.— *Med. Lett.*, 1977, *19*, 62; *Br. med. J.*, 1977, *1*, 1175; I. S. Fraser, *Med. J. Aust.*, 1978, *2*, 56; *Br. med. J.*, 1980, *281*, 889.

In 370 patients with endometriosis studied in 10 centres in the USA and treated with danazol 200 to 800 mg daily (usually 800 mg) for up to 7 months, dysmenorrhoea was relieved in 85 to 95%, pelvic pain in 70 to 89%, dyspareunia in 69 to 84%, and induration of the pouch of Douglas in 73 to 82%.— M. D. Young and W. P. Blackmore, *J. int. med. Res.*, 1977, *5, Suppl.* 3, 86.

Of 99 patients with endometriosis treated with danazol 200 mg four times daily for 3 to 18 months 39 had recurrence of symptoms when re-evaluated about 3 years after ceasing treatment. A pregnancy-rate of 46% was achieved in those desiring pregnancy or 72% if corrected to exclude those in whom an absolute sterility factor was involved. Four foetal deaths occurred in women who conceived within 3 cycles of discontinuing danazol; this might be due to endometrial thinning and abnormal placentation.— W. P. Dmowski and M. R. Cohen, *Am. J. Obstet. Gynec.*, 1978, *130*, 41.

Of 44 patients with endometriosis 7 required 600 mg daily of danazol for control; 27 were maintained on 400 mg daily, and 10 on 200 mg daily.— G. D. Ward, *Postgrad. med. J.*, 1979, *55, Suppl.* 5, 7. See also J. A. Chalmers and P. C. Shervington, *ibid.*, 44.

Further references: W. P. Dmowski and M. R. Cohen, *Obstet. Gynec.*, 1975, *46*, 147, per *Int. pharm. Abstr.*, 1978, *15*, 823; J. A. Chalmers, *Drugs*, 1980, *19*, 331.

Gynaecomastia. Danazol was given to 42 men or youths with gynaecomastia—idiopathic in 17, spironolactone-induced in 13, thyrotoxic in 1, and pubertal in 11. The dose for adults was 300 mg daily for 4 to 6 weeks, increased to 600 mg daily for 4 to 6 months, then 200 to 300 mg daily for 4 to 6 months. In adolescents the initial dose was 200 to 300 mg daily with a maintenance dose of 200 mg daily. Of the 42 patients 25 showed marked regression and 10 moderate regression.— R. Buckle, *Postgrad. med. J.*, 1979, *55, Suppl.* 5, 71. See also *idem*, *Drugs*, 1980, *19*, 356.

Infertility. Pregnancy in women with unexplained infertility after treatment with danazol.— J. G. van Dijk *et al.*, *Postgrad. med. J.*, 1979, *55, Suppl.* 5, 79. Danazol in infertility and habitual abortion.— R. B. Greenblatt, *Drugs*, 1980, *19*, 362.

See also Endometriosis, above.

Menorrhagia. Reduction of blood loss in patients with menorrhagia treated with danazol 400 mg daily.— T. H. Chimbira *et al.*, *Br. J. Obstet. Gynaec.*, 1979, *86*, 46.

Premenstrual syndrome. The possible value of danazol in the premenstrual syndrome.— J. Day, *Postgrad. med. J.*, 1979, *55, Suppl.* 5, 87.

Puberty, precocious. A favourable report on the use of danazol in 12 children (11 girls, 1 boy) with precocious puberty.— C. S. Smith and F. Harris, *Postgrad. med. J.*, 1979, *55, Suppl.* 5, 81. See also P. A. Lee *et al.*, *Johns Hopkins med. J.*, 1975, *137*, 265 (3 girls, 2 boys), per *Int. pharm. Abstr.*, 1978, *15*, 315.

Preparations

Danazol Capsules *(U.S.P.)*. Capsules containing danazol. The *U.S.P.* requires 65% dissolution in 30 minutes.

Danol Capsules *(Winthrop, UK)*. Each contains danazol 200 mg. **Danol-½ Capsules.** Each contains danazol 100 mg.

Other Proprietary Names

Cyclomen *(Canad.)*; Danatrol *(Belg., Fr., Switz.)*; Danocrine *(Austral., Denm., Fin., Norw., Swed., USA)*; Danokrin *(Aust.)*; Ladogar *(S.Afr.)*; Winobanin *(Ger.)*.

9036-g

Dehydroepiandrosterone. Dehydroisoandrosterone; Prasterone. 3β-Hydroxyandrost-5-en-17-one.
$C_{19}H_{28}O_2$=288.4.

CAS — 53-43-0.

Studies on the stability of dehydroepiandrosterone sulphate in aqueous solution.— T. Ishihara and I. Sugimoto, *Drug Dev. ind. Pharm.*, 1979, *5*, 263.

Dehydroepiandrosterone is a naturally occurring but relatively weak androgen (see under Testosterone, p.1435).

The use of a dehydroepiandrosterone sulphate loading test in the diagnosis of foetal distress in complicated pregnancies. The patients were given 50 mg in 50 ml of dextrose injection intravenously in the 35th to 42nd week of pregnancy. Plasma concentrations of oestradiol and of estetrol (produced from oestradiol by the foetus) rose in all of 17 healthy patients and 30 patients with various complications of pregnancy. In complicated pregnancies a subnormal rise in oestradiol and estetrol concentrations was suggestive of foetal distress.— D. Tulchinsky *et al.*, *New Engl. J. Med.*, 1976, *294*, 517.

The dehydroepiandrosterone test did not appear to have an advantage over existing methods of assessing placental function.— I. S. Fraser *et al.*, *Obstet. Gynec.*, 1976, *47*, 152, per *Int. pharm. Abstr.*, 1976, *13*, 932.

Proprietary Names

Astenile *(Recordati, Ital.)*; 17-Chetovis (acetate) *(Vister, Ital.)*; Deandros *(Farmochimica Italiana, Ital.)*; Mentalormon *(SIT, Ital.)*.

Dehydroepiandrosterone was formerly marketed in Great Britain under the proprietary name Diandrone *(Organon)*.

9037-q

Dienoestrol *(B.P., B.P. Vet., Eur. P.)*.

Dienoestr.; Dienestrolum; Dienoestrolum; Dienestrol *(U.S.P.)*; Dehydrostilbestrol; Oestrodienolum. *(E,E)*-4,4′-[Di(ethylidene)ethylene]diphenol.
$C_{18}H_{18}O_2$=266.3.

CAS — 84-17-3; 13029-44-2 (E,E).

Pharmacopoeias. In *Arg., Aust., Br., Braz., Eur., Fr., Ger., Hung., Ind., Int., It., Neth., Turk.*, and *U.S.* *Aust.* also includes dienoestrol diacetate, 3,4-bis(*p*-acetoxyphenyl)hexa-2,4-diene.

White or almost white, odourless, tasteless crystals or crystalline powder. M.p. 227° to 234° with a range of not more than 3°. Practically **insoluble** in water; soluble 1 in 8 of alcohol, 1 in 5 of acetone, and 1 in 15 of ether; soluble in methyl alcohol, propylene glycol, fixed oils, and solutions of alkali hydroxides; slightly soluble in chloroform. **Protect** from light.

CAUTION. *Dienoestrol is a powerful oestrogen. Contact with the skin or inhalation should be avoided. Rubber gloves and a face mask should be worn when handling the powder.*

Adverse Effects and Precautions. As for Oestradiol, p.1425.

A 70-year-old man developed gynaecomastia while exposed to the vaginal dienoestrol cream used by his wife.— C. V. DiRaimondo *et al.* (letter), *New Engl. J. Med.*, 1980, *302*, 1089.

Uses. Dienoestrol is a synthetic non-steroidal oestrogen structurally related to stilboestrol (see p.1433). It has actions and uses similar to those described under oestradiol (see p.1426). Doses of 0.5 to 5 mg daily have been given for menopausal symptoms and 15 to 30 mg daily in mammary or prostatic carcinoma. Dienoestrol is also used by local application in creams.

The use of dienoestrol cream in adhesions of the labia minora in young girls.— A. Aribarg, *Br. J. Obstet. Gynaec.*, 1975, *82*, 424, per *Int. pharm. Abstr.*, 1976, *13*, 1034.

The use of dienoestrol cream in patients undergoing irradiation of the cervix.— R. M. Pitkin *et al.*, *Obstet. Gynec.*, 1975, *46*, 243.

Menopausal symptoms. For the use of dienoestrol in the treatment of menopausal symptoms, see A. F. Connon, *Drugs*, 1973, *6*, 137.

Preparations

Dienestrol Cream *(U.S.P.)*. Dienoestrol Cream. Dienoestrol in a suitable water-miscible basis. Store in airtight containers.

Dienoestrol Tablets *(B.P.)*. Tablets containing dienoestrol. Protect from light.

Proprietary Preparations

Dienoestrol Cream *(Ortho-Cilag, UK)*. A vaginal cream containing dienoestrol 100 µg per g.

Hormofemin Cream *(Medo Chemicals, UK)*. Contains dienoestrol 0.025% in a water-miscible basis.

Other Proprietary Names

Cycladiene *(Belg., Fr.)*; DV, Estraguard (both *USA)*; Eufemine *(Belg.)*; Klianyl (acetate) *(Denm.)*; Sexadien *(Denm.)*; Sexadieno *(Spain)*.

9038-p

Dimethisterone *(B.P. 1973)*. Dimethister.; 6α,21-Dimethylethisterone. 17β-Hydroxy-6α,21-dimethyl-17α-pregn-4-en-20-yn-3-one monohydrate.
$C_{23}H_{32}O_2,H_2O$=358.5.

CAS — 79-64-1 (anhydrous); 41354-30-7 (monohydrate).

A white or almost white, odourless, tasteless, crystalline powder. M.p. about 100°, with decomposition.

Practically **insoluble** in water; soluble 1 in 3 of alcohol, 1 in 80 of arachis oil, 1 in 0.7 of chloroform, and 1 in 1 of pyridine; slightly soluble in acetone. **Store** in airtight containers. Protect from light.

Adverse Effects and Precautions. As for Progesterone, p.1431.

Pelvic pain resembling dysmenorrhoea, breast turgidity, nausea, and vertigo may occur with large doses.

Uses. Dimethisterone has actions and uses similar to those of progesterone (see p.1431). It is reported to have no significant oestrogenic or androgenic properties. It is active when given by mouth and is as effective as a similar dose of parenterally administered progesterone.

It has been used in the treatment of menstrual disorders usually in doses of 5 mg thrice daily for 10 days, starting on the 15th day of the cycle. Dimethisterone has also been given in conjunction with ethinyloestradiol as a 'sequential' oral contraceptive (see also Oral Contraceptives, p.1402).

Preparations

Dimethisterone Tablets *(B.P. 1973)*. Tablets containing dimethisterone. Protect from light.

Dimethisterone was formerly marketed in Great Britain under the proprietary name Secrosteron (*Duncan, Flockhart*).

9039-s

Drostanolone Propionate *(B.P.)*.

Dromostanolone Propionate *(U.S.P.)*. 2α-Methyl-3-oxo-5α-androstan-17β-yl propionate.
$C_{23}H_{36}O_3$=360.5.

CAS — 58-19-5 (drostanolone); 521-12-0 (propionate).

Pharmacopoeias. In *Br.* and *U.S.*

A white to creamy-white, crystalline powder, odourless or with a faint odour. M.p. 127° to 133° with a range of not more than 4°. Practically **insoluble** in water; soluble 1 in 30 of alcohol, 1 in 2 of chloroform, and 1 in 20 of ether; soluble in methyl alcohol. A solution in chloroform is dextrorotatory. **Store** in airtight containers. Protect from light.

Adverse Effects and Precautions. As for Testosterone, p.1436.

Uses. Drostanolone has anabolic and androgenic actions similar to those of methandienone (see p.1419).

Drostanolone propionate is given by intramuscular injection in an oily solution and has a prolonged duration of effect. It is used in the treatment of advanced malignant neoplasms of the breast in postmenopausal women. The usual dose is 100 mg thrice weekly.

Preparations

Dromostanolone Propionate Injection *(U.S.P.)*. A sterile solution of drostanolone propionate in a suitable oil. It contains phenol as a preservative. Protect from light.

Drostanolone Propionate Injection *(B.P.)*. Drostanolone Prop. Inj. A sterile solution of drostanolone propionate in a suitable fixed oil. Sterilised by heating at 150° for one hour. Protect from light.

Masteril *(Syntex, UK)*. Drostanolone propionate, available as an injection containing 100 mg per ml, in ampoules of 1 ml. (Also available as Masteril in *Austral., S.Afr.*).

Other Proprietary Names

Drolban *(USA)*; Masterid *(Ger., Switz.)*; Masteron *(Belg., Ital., Neth.)*; Metormon *(Spain)*; Permastril *(Fr.)*.

9040-h

Dydrogesterone *(B.P., U.S.P.)*. Dehydroprogesterone; Didrogesteron; Isopregnenone; 6-Dehydro-9β,10α-progesterone. 9β,10α-Pregna-4,6-diene-3,20-dione.
$C_{21}H_{28}O_2$=312.5.

CAS — 152-62-5.

Pharmacopoeias. In *Br.* and *U.S.*

A white to pale yellow odourless crystalline powder. M.p. 167° to 171°. Practically **insoluble** in water; soluble 1 in 40 to 52 of alcohol, 1 in 17 of acetone, 1 in 2 of chloroform, 1 in 140 of ether, 1 in 40 of methyl alcohol, and 1 in 180 of fixed oils. A solution in dioxan is laevorotatory. **Store** in airtight containers. Protect from light.

Adverse Effects. As for Progesterone, p.1431. Dydrogesterone is reported not to produce virilisation of the foetus.

Pregnancy and the neonate. *Effects on the foetus.* Anomalies of the genito-urinary tract were found in a 4-month-old baby whose mother had taken dydrogesterone 20 mg daily from the 8th to 20th week of pregnancy and 10 mg daily from then until term. She had also been given hydroxyprogesterone hexanoate 250 mg by intramuscular injection weekly from the 8th to the 20th week.— I. F. Roberts and R. J. West (letter), *Lancet*, 1977, *2*, 982.

Absorption and Fate. Dydrogesterone is absorbed from the gastro-intestinal tract. Plasma concentrations fall rapidly and about half a dose is excreted in the urine, within 24 hours.

Uses. Dydrogesterone has properties similar to those of progesterone (see p.1431) and has been used for similar purposes. However, unlike progesterone, dydrogesterone does not induce an increase in temperature or inhibit ovulation and may be preferred to other progestational agents when a contraceptive effect is not required. It does not have oestrogenic or androgenic properties.

For the treatment of amenorrhoea 10 mg is given twice daily from the 11th to 25th day of the cycle, after oestrogen priming. A similar dose is given from the 12th to 26th day for the premenstrual syndrome. In endometriosis 10 mg is given twice or thrice daily from the 5th to 25th day. The same dose has been given twice daily over the same period for dysmenorrhoea.

For the prevention or arrest of functional bleeding 10 mg is given twice daily, with appropriate oestrogen therapy. In threatened abortion 40 mg has been given immediately, then 10 mg or more 8-hourly, continued for a week after symptoms cease. Habitual abortion has been treated with 10 mg twice daily from the 11th to 25th day.

Dysmenorrhoea. In a multicentre double-blind crossover study 106 teenage girls with a history of dysmenorrhoea received dydrogesterone 10 mg or a placebo twice daily from day 5 to day 25 of each menstrual cycle for 4 cycles. Dydrogesterone produced significant reductions in backache, griping abdominal pain, moderate to severe bleeding, and the number of days aspirin was taken for analgesia; some reduction was also obtained in depression, headache, and nausea.— C. H. G. Gould, *Practitioner*, 1979, *222*, 718.

Endometriosis. Symptoms of endometriosis were relieved in 40 of 45 patients treated with dydrogesterone 5 mg twice daily for 9 months; symptoms usually subsided in 6 to 8 weeks though dyspareunia was not significantly improved until after 12 to 16 weeks. Of 19 patients with infertility 10 became pregnant after treatment.— W. I. H. Johnston, *Br. J. Obstet. Gynaec.*, 1976, *83*, 77.

Menstrual disorders. Of 50 women with premenstrual tension and low luteal-phase progesterone concentrations 16 were cured and 20 greatly improved by treatment with dydrogesterone, usually 10 mg twice daily, from the 12th to the 26th day of the cycle. Fluid retention was generally relieved and mental symptoms often relieved, but breast discomfort was rarely affected.— R. W. Taylor, *Curr. med. Res. Opinion*, 1977, *4*, *Suppl.* 4, 35. A placebo-controlled study involving 67 patients substantiated these findings.— G. D. Kerr *et al.*, *Practitioner*, 1980, *224*, 852.

Preparations

Dydrogesterone Tablets *(B.P.)*. Tablets containing dydrogesterone. Protect from light.

Dydrogesterone Tablets *(U.S.P.)*. Tablets containing dydrogesterone.

Duphaston *(Duphar, UK)*. Dydrogesterone, available as scored tablets of 10 mg. (Also available as Duphaston in *Austral., Belg., Fr., Ger., Neth., S.Afr., Spain, Swed., Switz., USA*).

Other Proprietary Names

Dabrostan *(Jug.)*; Dufaston *(Ital.)*; Gynorest *(USA)*; Terolut *(Denm., Fin., Norw.)*.

9041-m

Epioestriol. 16-Epioestriol. Estra-1,3,5(10)-triene-3,16β,17β-triol.
$C_{18}H_{24}O_3$=288.4.

CAS — 547-81-9.

Adverse Effects and Precautions. As for Oestradiol, p.1425.

Uses. Epioestriol is a naturally occurring oestrogen, closely related chemically to oestriol. It is reported to have very little oestrogenic activity.

Epioestriol was used in the treatment of acne.

Proprietary Names

Klimadoral *(Leo, Switz.)*; Ovestinon *(Organon, Spain)*.

Proprietary Names of Epioestriol Esters

Sinapause *(succinate) (Organon, Arg.)*; Synapause *(succinate) (see also under Oestriol) (Organon, Spain)*.

Epioestriol was formerly marketed in Great Britain under the proprietary name Actriol (*Organon*).

9042-b

Estropipate *(U.S.P.)*. Piperazine Oestrone Sulphate; Piperazine Estrone Sulfate. Piperazine 17-oxo-estra-1,3,5(10)-trien-3-yl sulphate.
$C_4H_{10}N_2,C_{18}H_{22}O_5S$=436.6.

CAS — 7280-37-7.

Pharmacopoeias. In *U.S.*

A fine, white to yellowish-white, crystalline powder, odourless or with a slight odour. M.p. about 190° to a light brown viscous liquid which solidifies on further heating then melts with decomposition at about 245°.

Very slightly **soluble** in water, alcohol, chloroform, and ether; soluble 1 in 500 of warm alcohol. A saturated solution in water is neutral or slightly alkaline to litmus. **Store** in airtight containers.

Adverse Effects and Precautions. As for Oestradiol, p.1425.

In a double-blind study completed by 60 women 23 took estropipate, 20 took ethinyloestradiol, and 17 placebo. Whereas significant increase in the concentration of fibrinogen and factors VII and X, and acceleration in prothrombin, cephalin, and platelet aggregation times occurred between the second and sixth months in the group taking ethinyloestradiol no such change occurred in any of these indices in the group taking estropipate either during the trial or during an 18-month follow-up period.— M. Aylward *et al.* (letter), *Br. med. J.*, 1976, *1*, 220.

Uses. Estropipate is a synthetic oestrogen conjugate with uses similar to those of oestradiol (p.1426). Its action is due to oestrone (see p.1429) to which it is hydrolysed in the body. It is active by mouth.

In menopausal disturbances and associated vaginal disorders, a dose of 1.5 to 4.5 mg is given daily. It is also used as a vaginal cream containing 0.15%.

Menopausal symptoms. A double-blind crossover study comparing estropipate with ethinyloestradiol in 79 women with menopausal symptoms. Both drugs gave similar relief of symptoms; estropipate was preferred on the grounds of safety.—Report No. 197 of the General Practitioner Research Group *Practitioner*, 1977, *218*, 573.

Estropipate was considered the drug of choice for menopausal patients for whom treatment with an oestrogen was necessary. There were conflicting views on the duration of treatment.— *J.R. Coll. gen. Pract.*, 1977, *27*, 579.

In a double-blind study in 34 menopausal patients estropipate 1.5 mg twice daily for 8 weeks had a beneficial effect on most sleep parameters but placebo had a comparable effect on mood, anxiety, and the incidence of hot flushes.— J. Thomson and I. Oswald, *Br. med. J.*, 1977, *2*, 1317.

See also under Oestradiol, p.1427.

A study indicating that estropipate 0.75 mg daily rather than 1.5 to 3 mg daily might provide adequate oestrogen replacement therapy.— J. D. Hutton *et al.*, *Lancet*, 1978, *1*, 678.

Preparations

Estropipate Tablets *(U.S.P.)*. Piperazine Estrone Sulfate Tablets. Tablets containing estropipate.

Estropipate Vaginal Cream *(U.S.P.)*. Piperazine Estrone Sulfate Vaginal Cream. Contains estropipate in a suitable cream basis.

Harmogen *(Abbott, UK)*. Estropipate, available as tablets of 1.5 mg. (Also available as Harmogen in *Switz.*).

Other Proprietary Names

Harmonet *(Denm., Swed.)*; Ogen *(Austral., Canad., USA)*; Sultrex *(Arg.)*.

9043-v

Ethinyloestradiol *(B.P., B.P. Vet., Eur. P.)*. Ethinyloestr.; Aethinyloestradiolum; Ethinyl Estradiol *(U.S.P.)*; Ethinylestradiolum; Etinilestradiol. 17α-Ethynylestra-1,3,5(10)-triene-3,17β-diol; 19-Nor-17α-pregna-1,3,5(10)-trien-20-yne-3,17β-diol.
$C_{20}H_{24}O_2$=296.4.

CAS — 57-63-6.

Pharmacopoeias. In *Arg., Aust., Br., Braz., Chin., Cz., Eur., Fr., Ger., Ind., Int., It., Jap., Jug., Neth., Nord., Port., Roum., Rus., Swiss, Turk.*, and *U.S.*

A fine, white to slightly yellowish-white, odourless, crystalline powder. There are two forms, one melts at 141° to 146° and the other at 180° to 186°.

Practically **insoluble** in water; soluble 1 in 6 of alcohol, 1 in 5 of acetone, 1 in 20 of chloroform, 1 in 4 of dioxan, and 1 in 4 of ether; soluble in fixed oils and aqueous solutions of alkali hydroxides. **Store** in a cool place in airtight containers. Protect from light.

CAUTION. *Ethinyloestradiol is a powerful oestrogen. Contact with the skin or inhalation should be avoided. Rubber gloves and a face mask should be worn when handling the powder.*

Combination tablets of norethisterone 500 µg with ethinyloestradiol 35 µg containing 4.5 µg of erythrosine (FD&C Red No. 3) as a colouring agent exhibited discoloration throughout the tablets after light studies. It was suggested that this was due to an interaction between ethinyloestradiol and erythrosine. No such effect of discoloration occurred in similar tablets containing 30 μg of Sunset Yellow FCF or in uncoloured tablets.— E. E. Kaminski *et al.*, *J. pharm. Sci.*, 1979, *68*, 368.

Adverse Effects and Precautions. As for Oestradiol, p.1425.

See also under Oral Contraceptives, p.1402.

Two patients with metastatic breast cancer given ethinyloestradiol rapidly developed irreversible and fatal hypercalcaemia considered to be due to stimulation of osteolysis by the oestrogen.— M. Cornbleet *et al.*, *Br. med. J.*, 1977, *1*, 145.

Elevation of sex hormone binding globulin by an oral contraceptive containing 50 μg of ethinyloestradiol, but not by 35 μg.— A. M. Jequier and J. R. Pogmore, *Br. J. clin. Pharmac.*, 1978, *6*, 464P (Proceedings of the British Pharmacological Society).

Erythema multiforme. A 15-year-old girl developed erythema multiforme, the Stevens-Johnson syndrome, after taking Serial-C tablets (ethinyloestradiol and megestrol acetate) for 14 weeks. She had also taken ferrous succinate and aspirin.— J. O. O'Callaghan and G. Jones, *Med. J. Aust.*, 1972, *1*, 695.

Interactions. Rifampicin increased the rate of hydroxylation of ethinyloestradiol *in vitro* and this might account for the decreased effectiveness of oral contraceptives in patients also taking rifampicin.— H. M. Bolt *et al.* (letter), *Lancet*, 1974, *1*, 1280.

In 5 volunteers mean plasma-ethinyloestradiol concentrations were increased by 16.3 and 47.6% six and 24 hours respectively after the ingestion of ascorbic acid 1 g.— D. J. Back *et al.*, *Br. med. J.*, 1981, *282*, 1516. Breakthrough bleeding possibly associated with withdrawal of high doses of vitamin C.— J. C. Morris *et al.* (letter), *ibid.*, *283*, 503. Evidence that the overall effect of a large vitamin C supplement is to convert a low-oestrogen oral contraceptive into a high-dose oral contraceptive.— M. H. Briggs (letter), *ibid.*, 1547.

See also under Oral Contraceptives, p.1406.

For the effect of ethinyloestradiol on imipramine, see Imipramine Hydrochloride, p.120.

Thrombo-embolic disorders. In a retrospective study of 111 cases of puerperal thrombo-embolism and of 641 control cases, the incidence of puerperal thrombo-embolism was 3 times higher in those women whose lactation was inhibited by ethinyloestradiol than in those who breast-fed their babies. Ethinyloestradiol was given in a total dose of 1.4 mg over 7 days.— T. N. A. Jeffcoate *et al.*, *Br. med. J.*, 1968, *4*, 19. Criticisms.— S. McPherson (letter), *ibid.*, 1969, *1*, 51. See also M. F. Oliver (letter), *Lancet*, 1967, *2*, 510.

Absorption and Fate. Ethinyloestradiol is absorbed from the gastro-intestinal tract. It is only slowly metabolised and excreted in the urine.

The pharmacokinetics of ethinyloestradiol.— E. D. Helton and J. W. Goldzieher, *Contraception*, 1977, *15*, 255, per *Int. pharm. Abstr.*, 1977, *14*, 1102.

Further references: S. Kamyab and K. Fotherby (letter), *Nature*, 1969, *221*, 360.

Pregnancy and the neonate. *Lactation.* In 4 lactating women taking an oral contraceptive containing ethinyloestradiol and megestrol acetate the concentration of ethinyloestradiol in breast milk was undetectable. In 5 women given a single 500-μg dose of ethinyloestradiol the plasma: milk ratio was 4:1.— S. Nilsson *et al.*, *Contraception*, 1978, *17*, 131, per *Int. pharm. Abstr.*, 1978, *15*, 481.

Uses. Ethinyloestradiol is a synthetic oestrogen which has actions and uses similar to those described under oestradiol (see p.1426). It is much more potent.

In menopausal symptoms, doses of 20 to 50 μg daily are given. Menopausal symptoms have been treated by the concomitant administration of ethinyloestradiol and an androgen such as methyltestosterone, in an attempt to reduce the oestrogen dose and the incidence of uterine bleeding; such treatment is not universally accepted. For the palliative treatment of malignant neoplasms of the prostate and breast doses of about 0.1 to 2 mg have been given daily.

For the treatment of primary amenorrhoea, up to 50 μg may be given thrice daily for 14 consecutive days in every 4 weeks, followed by a progestogen for the next 14 days. A wide range of doses has been used for the suppression of lactation. Recommendations have varied from 50 to 300 μg daily for the first 2 or 3 days and from 10 to 100 μg daily for the next 5 to 7 days, but oestrogens are no longer recommended for this purpose.

Functional uterine bleeding has been controlled by ethinyloestradiol but treatment with a progestogen is often preferred.

Ethinyloestradiol is also given in conjunction with ethisterone (see below) or norethisterone acetate (see p.1422) for disorders of menstruation.

Ethinyloestradiol, in conjunction with a progestational agent such as ethynodiol diacetate (see p.1413), lynoestrenol (see p.1415), norethisterone (see p.1422), norethisterone acetate (see p.1422), or levonorgestrel or norgestrel (see p.1424), is given by mouth as a contraceptive (see Oral Contraceptives, p.1402).

A comparison of the oestrogenic effect of ethinyloestradiol and mestranol.— I. A. Brosens and R. Pijnenborg, *Contraception*, 1976, *14*, 679, per *Int. pharm. Abstr.*, 1978, *15*, 228.

Acne. Ethinyloestradiol and stilboestrol reduced sebum production in 54 women, 15 of them with acne.— P. E. Pochi and J. S. Strauss, *Archs Derm.*, 1973, *108*, 210, per *J. Am. med. Ass.*, 1973, *225*, 1140.

For the use of cyproterone acetate with ethinyloestradiol in patients with acne, see Cyproterone Acetate, p.1409.

Contraception. *Postcoital contraception.* A favourable report of the use of ethinyloestradiol 5 mg daily for 5 days for postcoital contraception.— G. W. Dixon *et al.*, *J. Am. med. Ass.*, 1980, *244*, 1336. Further references: R. P. Blye, *Am. J. Obstet. Gynec.*, 1973, *116*, 1044.

Familial haemorrhagic telangiectasia. Control of epistaxis in most of 60 patients treated with ethinyloestradiol 0.5 to 1 mg daily.— D. F. N. Harrison (letter), *Lancet*, 1970, *1*, 721. See also *idem*, *Q.J. Med.*, 1964, *33*, 25.

Growth inhibition. A review of the use of oestrogen therapy to control excessive stature in tall girls.— J. D. Crawford, *Pediatrics*, 1978, *62*, 1189.

Hyperlipaemia. Ethinyloestradiol 1 μg per kg body-weight daily reduced plasma-lipid and plasma-lipoprotein concentrations in a woman with type III hyperlipoproteinaemia. This effect might have been due to the partial correction of an abnormality in the removal of very-low-density lipoprotein and its remnants.— A. Chait *et al.*, *Lancet*, 1977, *1*, 1176.

Neoplasm of the breast. In patients with advanced metastatic breast cancer, response to hormone treatment appeared to be related to the presence in the tumour of oestrogen receptors. Of 5 patients with receptors and treated with ethinyloestradiol 3 mg daily, 4 obtained objective remissions compared with 1 of 5 without receptors. All of 3 patients with receptors and treated with nandrolone phenylpropionate 25 mg three times a week obtained objective remissions.— E. Engelsman *et al.*, *Br. med. J.*, 1973, *2*, 750.

Further references: D. Quednau *et al.*, *Dt. med. Wschr.*, 1978, *103*, 2029.

See also under Stilboestrol, p.1435.

Osteoporosis. In a prospective trial in postmenopausal women, bone loss was prevented in 19 women treated for not less than 2 years with ethinyloestradiol 25 or 50 μg daily for 3 weeks in 4, while 18 untreated controls continued to lose bone. Bone loss was retarded but not prevented in 24 women treated with calcium gluconate providing 800 mg of calcium daily.— A. Horsman *et al.*, *Br. med. J.*, 1977, *2*, 789.

See also under Menopausal Symptoms in Oestradiol, p.1427 and Calcium Salts, p.621.

Preparations

Ethinyl Estradiol Tablets *(U.S.P.).* Tablets containing ethinyloestradiol.

Ethinyloestradiol Tablets *(B.P.).* Ethinyloestr. Tab. Tablets containing ethinyloestradiol. Protect from light.

Proprietary Preparations

Lynoral *(Organon, UK).* Ethinyloestradiol, available as tablets of 10 μg and 1 mg. (Also available as Lynoral in *Austral., Belg., Ger., Neth., Switz.*).

Menolet Sublets *(Marshall's Pharmaceuticals, UK).* Sublingual tablets each containing ethinyloestradiol 5 μg and methyltestosterone 5 mg.

Mixogen Tablets *(Organon, UK).* Each contains ethinyloestradiol 4.4 μg and methyltestosterone 3.6 mg. For menopausal symptoms. *Dose.* 1 or 2 tablets daily for 3 weeks out of every 4.

For Mixogen Injection see under Oestradiol Benzoate, p.1427.

Trimone Sublets *(Marshall's Pharmaceuticals, UK).* Tablets each containing ethinyloestradiol 5 μg, methyltestosterone 2.5 mg, and ethisterone 5 mg.

Other Proprietary Names

Austral.—Edrol, Estigyn, Primogyn C; *Canad.*—Estinyl; *Ger.*—Farmacyrol forte, Gynolett, Progynon C, Progynon M; *Norw.*—Etifollin; *S.Afr.*—Estinyl; *Spain*—Progynon C, Progynon M; *Swed.*—Etivex, Linoral; *Switz.*—Duramen, Eticyclin forte, Progynon C; *USA*—Estinyl, Feminone.

Other Proprietary Names of Ethinyloestradiol and Ethinyloestradiol with Lynoestrenol

Fysioquens *(Denm., Neth.)*; Normophasic *(Switz.)*; Ovanon *(Belg., Fr., Ger., Neth., Switz.)*; Ovanon 28 *(Ger.)*; Ovanone *(Denm., Swed.)*; Ovanon-E *(S.Afr.)*; Phasicon *(S.Afr.)*; Physiostat *(Fr.)*.

Other proprietary preparations containing ethinyloestradiol with progestogens are described under Ethynodiol Diacetate (see p.1413), Lynoestrenol (see p.1416), Norethisterone (see p.1422), Norethisterone Acetate (see p.1423), and Norgestrel and Levonorgestrel (see p.1425). Another proprietary preparation containing ethinyloestradiol with an androgen is described under Methyltestosterone (see p.1420).

Ethinyloestradiol was also formerly marketed in Great Britain under the proprietary name Pabendrol (*Paines & Byrne*).

Preparations containing ethinyloestradiol were also formerly marketed in Great Britain under the proprietary names Climatone (*Paines & Byrne*), Menopax (*Nicholas*), Mepilin (*Duncan, Flockhart*), and Oestradin (*Norton*).

A preparation containing ethinyloestradiol and ethinyloestradiol with megestrol acetate was formerly marketed in Great Britain under the proprietary name Serial 28 (*BDH Pharmaceuticals*).

9044-g

Ethisterone *(B.P.).* Ethisteronum; Aethisteron.; Anhydrohydroxyprogesterone; Ethinyltestosterone; Praegnin; Pregnin; Pregneninolone. 17β-Hydroxy-17α-pregn-4-en-20-yn-3-one.

$C_{21}H_{28}O_2$=312.5.

CAS — 434-03-7.

Pharmacopoeias. In *Aust., Br., Cz., Fr., Ind., Int., It., Jug., Mex., Nord., Rus., Swiss,* and *Turk.*

A white or almost white, odourless, tasteless, slightly hygroscopic, crystalline powder. M.p. 272° to 276°. Practically **insoluble** in water; soluble 1 in 1000 of alcohol, 1 in 750 of acetone, 1 in 110 of chloroform, 1 in 3000 of ether, 1 in 35 of pyridine, and 1 in 4000 of arachis oil; very slightly soluble in vegetable oils. A solution in pyridine is dextrorotatory. **Store** in airtight containers. Protect from light.

Adverse Effects and Precautions. As for Progesterone, p.1431.

Androgenic side-effects may predominate.

Pregnancy and the neonate. *Effects on the foetus.* For a report indicating that hormonal pregnancy tests, some containing ethisterone, had been found to be more frequently used in mothers who gave birth to infants with congenital malformation than in those who gave birth to normal infants, see Norethisterone Acetate, p.1422.

See also under Adverse Effects of Sex Hormones, p.1401.

Uses. Ethisterone has actions and uses similar to those of progesterone (see p.1431) but also has oestrogenic and androgenic properties and the latter may limit its usefulness. It is effective by mouth, preferably sublingually; doses of 25 to 100 mg have been given daily.

Preparations

Ethisterone Tablets *(B.P.).* Ethinyltestosterone Tablets. Tablets containing ethisterone. Protect from light.

Gestone-Oral *(Paines & Byrne, UK).* Ethisterone, available as tablets of 5, 10, and 25 mg.

Other Proprietary Names

Etherone *(Austral.)*.

Preparations containing ethisterone and ethinyloestradiol were formerly marketed in Great Britain under the proprietary names Amenorone (*Roussel*) and Paralut (*Wallace Mfg Chem.*).

9045-q

Ethyloestrenol (*B.P., B.P. Vet.*). Ethylestrenol. 17α-Ethylestr-4-en-17β-ol; 19-Nor-17α-pregn-4-en-17β-ol.
$C_{20}H_{32}O$=288.5.
CAS — 965-90-2.
Pharmacopoeias. In *Br.*

A white or almost white odourless crystalline powder. It contains not more than 4% w/w of methyl alcohol of crystallisation. M.p. about 89°. Practically **insoluble** in water; soluble 1 in 9 of alcohol, 1 in 2 of chloroform, and 1 in 6 of ether. A solution in dioxan is dextrorotatory. **Store** in a cool place. Protect from light.

Adverse Effects and Precautions. As for Testosterone (see p.1436) but it is reported to have little androgenic effect at doses normally used. High doses produce progestational effects and nausea, vomiting, fluid retention, and amenorrhoea may occur. Ethyloestrenol should be used with care in patients with liver disorders.

A report of ethinyloestradiol being mistaken for ethyloestrenol. Ethinyloestradiol was given instead of the androgen to a patient in a dose of 4 mg causing swelling of the breasts, fluid retention, and perhaps precipitating an infarction.— E. Montuschi (letter), *Lancet*, 1972, *2*, 757.

For the possible enhancement by ethyloestrenol of the effect of phenindione, see p.773.

Uses. Ethyloestrenol has anabolic actions similar to those of methandienone (see p.1419) and is used for similar purposes. It also has slight progestational activity but has little androgenic activity at doses normally used.
The usual dose is 2 to 4 mg daily.
Ethyloestrenol has been given with phenformin hydrochloride (see p.858) for fibrinolysis.

Ethyloestrenol 8 mg daily was no more effective than placebo in influencing the incidence of postoperative venous thrombosis in a group of women over the age of 40.— F. Allenby *et al.* (letter), *Lancet*, 1973, *2*, 38.
Resistance to the fibrinolytic effect of ethyloestrenol could build up within 3 to 4 weeks, and negative results would therefore be expected. Ethyloestrenol in conjunction with phenformin had produced fibrinolytic activity lasting up to 3 years.— G. R. Fearnley (letter), *ibid.*, 95.

In 31 patients given ethyloestrenol 8 mg daily for 3 months decreased fibrinolytic activity in vessel walls was significantly increased and the release capacity of fibrinolytic activators was increased. A dose of 4 mg daily was not adequate. The fibrinolytic effect was maintained by medication at the original dose.— U. Hedner *et al.*, *Br. med. J.*, 1976, *2*, 729.

Preparations

Ethyloestrenol Tablets (*B.P.*). Tablets containing ethyloestrenol. Store in a cool place. Protect from light.

Orabolin (*Organon, UK*). Ethyloestrenol, available as tablets of 2 mg. (Also available as Orabolin in *Austral., Belg., S.Afr.*).

Other Proprietary Names

Maxibolin (*Canad., USA*); Orgabolin (*Fr., Ital., Neth., Swed.*).

9046-p

Ethynodiol Diacetate (*B.P., U.S.P.*). Ethynodiol Diacet.; Etynodiol Diacetate; SC 11800. 19-Nor-17α-pregn-4-en-20-yne-3β,17β-diol diacetate.
$C_{24}H_{32}O_4$=384.5.
CAS — 1231-93-2 (ethynodiol); 297-76-7 (diacetate).
Pharmacopoeias. In *Br., Braz.*, and *U.S.*

A white or almost white, odourless, crystalline powder. M.p. 126° to 131°.
Very slightly **soluble** in water; soluble 1 in 15 of alcohol, 1 in 1 of chloroform, and 1 in 3.5 of ether; soluble in acetone; sparingly soluble in fixed oils. A solution in chloroform is laevorotatory. **Store** in airtight containers. Protect from light.

Adverse Effects and Precautions. As for Progesterone, p.1431.
See also Oral Contraceptives, p.1402.

Pregnancy and the neonate. *Effects on the foetus.* Foetal adrenal cytomegaly in a 17-week-old foetus associated with the maternal ingestion of an oral contraceptive containing ethynodiol diacetate 2 mg and mestranol 100 µg from the sixth to the fourteenth week of pregnancy.— G. S. Gau and M. J. Bennett (letter), *J. clin. Path.*, 1979, *32*, 305.

Absorption and Fate. Ethynodiol diacetate is readily absorbed from the gastro-intestinal tract and rapidly metabolised, largely to norethisterone.

The metabolites of ethynodiol diacetate in human plasma.— C. E. Cook *et al.*, *J. Pharmac. exp. Ther.*, 1973, *185*, 696.

Uses. Ethynodiol diacetate has actions and uses similar to those of progesterone (see p.1431) but is more potent. It is active by mouth and is usually given in conjunction with an oestrogen such as ethinyloestradiol or mestranol.
In the treatment of functional uterine bleeding, it has been given daily in doses of 1 or 2 mg with an oestrogen from the 5th to the 25th day of the cycle. Emergency treatment of excessive functional uterine bleeding has been treated with daily doses of 4 to 6 mg of ethynodiol diacetate. In the treatment of endometriosis, the usual dose was 2 to 4 mg daily with an oestrogen for a minimum of 9 months.
For contraception, ethynodiol diacetate is usually given in doses of 0.5 to 2 mg daily in combination with 30 or 50 µg of ethinyloestradiol for courses of 21 days starting on the 5th day of the first treated cycle, and thereafter repeated after intervals of 7 days for succeeding cycles. It is also given as a 'progestogen-only' oral contraceptive in a dose of 500 µg daily on a continuous schedule similarly to norethisterone (see p.1422).
See also Oral Contraceptives, p.1402.

Contraception. The efficacy of an oral contraceptive containing ethynodiol diacetate 500 µg was studied in 309 women for a total of 9566 cycles. Involuntary pregnancies occurred in 6 patients but this was due to patient failure in 2 cases and 1 patient had been receiving carbimazole for thyrotoxicosis. Discontinuation of treatment was mainly due to irregular breakthrough bleeding in 45 patients.— D. L. Postlethwaite, *Practitioner*, 1979, *222*, 272.

Preparations

Ethynodiol Diacetate and Ethinyl Estradiol Tablets (*U.S.P.*). Tablets containing ethynodiol diacetate and ethinyloestradiol.

Proprietary Preparations

Conova 30 (*Searle, UK*). Tablets each containing ethynodiol diacetate 2 mg and ethinyloestradiol 30 µg. For use as an oral contraceptive. *Dose.* 1 tablet daily for 21 days, commencing on the 5th day of the first treated cycle and after 7 tablet-free days for succeeding cycles.

Demulen 50 (*Searle, UK*). Tablets each containing ethynodiol diacetate 500 µg and ethinyloestradiol 50 µg. For use as an oral contraceptive. *Dose.* 1 tablet daily for 21 days, commencing on the 5th day of the first treated cycle and after 7 tablet-free days for succeeding cycles. (Also available as Demulen 50 in *Canad.*).

Femulen (*Searle, UK*). Ethynodiol diacetate, available as tablets of 500 µg. (Also available as Femulen in *S.Afr.*).

Metrulen (*Searle, UK*). Tablets each containing ethynodiol diacetate 2 mg and mestranol 100 µg. For endometriosis and uterine haemorrhage. *Dose.* 1 to 3 tablets daily. (Also available as Metrulen in *Canad.*).

Ovulen 50 (*Searle, UK*). Tablets each containing ethynodiol diacetate 1 mg and ethinyloestradiol 50 µg. For use as an oral contraceptive. *Dose.* 1 tablet daily for 21 days commencing on the 5th day of the first treated cycle and after 7 tablet-free days for succeeding cycles. (Also available as Ovulen 50 in *Neth., Switz.*).

Other Proprietary Names

Luteonorm (*Ital.*); Lutométrodiol (*Fr.*).

Other Proprietary Names of Ethynodiol Diacetate with Ethinyloestradiol

AlfamesE (*Ger.*); Anoryol (*Canad.*); Demulen (*S.Afr., Swed., USA*); Demulen-28 (*USA*); Demulen 30 (*Canad.*); Neovulen (*Denm.*); Ovulen 50-21, Ovulen 50-28 (both *Belg.*); Ovulène 50 (*Fr.*); Ovulen 0.5/50, Ovulen 1/50 (both *Austral.*); Ovulen Novum (*Norw.*).

Other Proprietary Names of Ethynodiol Diacetate with Mestranol

Etinodiene (*Ital.*); Ovulen (*Arg., Ger., Spain, USA*); Ovulen 0.5 (*Austral., Canad., Switz.*); Ovulen 1 (*Austral., Canad., Neth., Switz.*); Ovulen 2 (*Austral.*); Ovulen-21 (*S.Afr., USA*); Ovulen-28 (*USA*).

A preparation containing ethynodiol diacetate and mestranol was also formerly marketed in Great Britain under the proprietary name Metrulen M (*Searle*).

Other Proprietary Names of Ethynodiol Diacetate with Quinestrol

Soluna (*Arg.*).

9047-s

Flugestone Acetate (*B. Vet. C. 1965*). Flurogestone Acetate; SC 9880. 9α-Fluoro-11β,17α-dihydroxypregn-4-ene-3,20-dione 17-acetate.
$C_{23}H_{31}FO_5$=406.5.
CAS — 337-03-1 (flugestone); 2529-45-5 (acetate).

A white or creamy-white odourless powder. Very slightly **soluble** in water, soluble 1 in 23 of alcohol, 1 in 2.5 of chloroform, and 1 in 100 of methyl alcohol.

Flugestone acetate is a progestational agent with actions similar to those of progesterone (see p.1431). It was formerly used in sheep as a vaginal tampon for the synchronisation of oestrus.

9048-w

Flumedroxone Acetate. WG 537; 6α-Trifluoromethyl-17α-acetoxyprogesterone. 3,20-Dioxo-6α-trifluoromethylpregn-4-en-17α-yl acetate.
$C_{24}H_{31}F_3O_4$=440.5.
CAS — 15687-21-5 (flumedroxone); 987-18-8 (acetate).

A white crystalline powder. M.p. 206°. Very slightly **soluble** in water.

Flumedroxone acetate is a steroid with effects similar to those of progesterone (see p.1431). It has been used in the treatment of migraine, particularly in women.

Migraine. References: P. Hudgson *et al.*, *Br. med. J.*, 1967, *2*, 91; W. G. Bradley *et al.*, *Br. med. J.*, 1968, *3*, 531; P. O. Lundberg, *Acta neurol. scand.*, 1969, *45*, 309, per *Abstr. Wld Med.*, 1969, *43*, 868.

Proprietary Names
Demigrana (*Lövens, Swed.*).

9049-e

Fluoxymesterone (*B.P., U.S.P.*). NSC 12165; Fluoxymest. 9α-Fluoro-11β,17β-dihydroxy-17α-methylandrost-4-en-3-one.
$C_{20}H_{29}FO_3$=336.4.
CAS — 76-43-7.
Pharmacopoeias. In *Br.* and *U.S.*

A white or creamy-white, odourless, crystalline powder. M.p. about 278°. Practically **insoluble** in water; soluble 1 in 70 of alcohol and 1 in 200 of chloroform. A solution in alcohol is dextrorotatory. **Store** in airtight containers. Protect from light.

Adverse Effects and Precautions. As for Testosterone, p.1436.
Fluoxymesterone, given for prolonged periods, may cause jaundice and is contra-indicated in patients with liver disturbances.

Prostatic cancer in 2 men treated with fluoxymesterone for impotence.— P. D. Guinan *et al.*, *Am. J. Surg.*, 1976, *131*, 599, per *Int. pharm. Abstr.*, 1976, *13*, 1230.

Uses. Fluoxymesterone has actions and uses similar to those of testosterone (see p.1436). It is effective when given by mouth and is more potent than methyltestosterone.
In the treatment of male hypogonadism, fluoxymesterone is usually given in a dosage of 2 to 10 mg daily. In the palliation of inoperable neoplasms of the breast in postmenopausal women, it is given in daily doses of up to 30 mg, in divided doses. It has been given for postpartum breast engorgement in doses of 5 to 10 mg daily.
Fluoxymesterone has been administered for its anabolic effect but less virilising anabolic agents such as methandienone are usually preferred.

Anaemia. In a group of 14 patients with anaemia on maintenance haemodialysis fluoxymesterone 10 mg daily for female patients and 30 mg daily for male patients increased the mean haematocrit in 10 by at least 4 points and after 8 months 10 of the 11 who had received blood no longer required blood transfusions.— J. W. Eschbach and J. W. Adamson, *Ann. intern. Med.*, 1973, *78*, 527. See also W. R. Vogler *et al.*, *Am. J. med. Sci.*, 1971, *262*, 25, per *Int. pharm. Abstr.*, 1972, *9*, 240.

Further references: B. J. Kennedy, *J. Am. med. Ass.*, 1964, *190*, 1130.

Preparations

Fluoxymesterone Tablets *(B.P., U.S.P.)*. Tablets containing fluoxymesterone. Protect from light.

Proprietary Names

Halotestin *(Upjohn, Austral.; Upjohn, Canad.; Upjohn, Denm.; Upjohn, Fr.; Upjohn, Ital.; Upjohn, Neth.; Upjohn, Norw.; Upjohn, S.Afr.; Upjohn, Swed.; Upjohn, USA)*; Ora-Testryl *(Squibb, USA)*; Oratestin *(Hoechst, Canad.)*; Testoral (see also under Testosterone) *(Midy, Ital.)*; Ultandren *(Ciba, Ger.; Ciba, Norw.; Ciba, Switz.)*.

Fluoxymesterone was formerly marketed in Great Britain under the proprietary name Ultandren (*Ciba*).

9050-b

Flutamide. Sch 13521. α′,α′,α′-Trifluoro-4′-nitro-isobutyro-*m*-toluidide.
$C_{11}H_{11}F_3N_2O_3$=276.2.

CAS — 13311-84-7.

A yellowish crystallic powder. Practically **insoluble** in water.

Flutamide is a non-steroidal anti-androgen which has been used to improve urine flow in benign prostatic enlargement; gynaecomastia has been reported. Doses of 300 mg daily have been used.

Metabolism.— B. Katchen and S. Buxbaum, *J. clin. Endocr. Metab.*, 1975, *41*, 373.

In a double-blind trial in 30 patients with benign prostatic enlargement 15 were treated for 12 weeks with flutamide 100 mg thrice daily and 15 with placebo. There was significant improvement in the urine flow-rate and no evidence of change in residual urine volume, prostatic size, or histological appearance. Gynaecomastia occurred in 7 patients treated with flutamide.— M. Caine *et al.*, *J. Urol.*, 1975, *114*, 564.

Percutaneous absorption.— B. Katchen *et al.*, *J. invest. Derm.*, 1976, *66*, 379.

Manufacturers

Schering, USA.

9051-v

Formebolone. Formyldienolone. 11α,17β-Dihydroxy-17α-methyl-3-oxoandrosta-1,4-diene-2-carbaldehyde.
$C_{21}H_{28}O_4$=344.4.

CAS — 2454-11-7.

Formebolone is an anabolic steroid. It has been given in doses of 5 to 10 mg daily.

References: D. Gelli and E. Vignati, *J. int. med. Res.*, 1976, *4*, 96.

Proprietary Names

Esiclene *(LPB, Ital.)*; Hubernol *(Hubber, Spain)*.

9052-g

Fosfestrol.

Diethylstilbestrol Diphosphate *(U.S.P.)*; Stilboestrol Diphosphate; Phosphoestrolum. (*E*)-αβ-Diethylstilbene-4,4′-diol bis(dihydrogen phosphate); (*E*)-4,4′-(1,2-Diethylvinylene)bis(phenyl dihydrogen phosphate).
$C_{18}H_{22}O_8P_2$=428.3.

CAS — 522-40-7.

Pharmacopoeias. In *U.S.*

An off-white odourless crystalline powder. Sparingly **soluble** in water; soluble in alcohol and dilute alkalis. **Store** at a temperature not exceeding 21° in airtight containers.

9053-q

Fosfestrol Sodium.

$C_{18}H_{18}Na_4O_8P_2$=516.2.

CAS — 23519-26-8 (xNa).

Pharmacopoeias. In *Cz.* under the title Diaethylstilboestrolum Solubile.

Fosfestrol 100 mg is approximately equivalent to 121 mg of fosfestrol sodium.

Adverse Effects and Precautions. As for Oestradiol, p.1425.
Nausea and vomiting are common side-effects but may be less troublesome than with equivalent doses of stilboestrol. Following intravenous injection there may be temporary local pain in the perineal and sacral regions and at the site of bony metastases. Injections should be given slowly, with the patient lying down.

Fosfestrol and liver function.— M. Kontturi and E. Sotaniemi, *Br. med. J.*, 1969, *4*, 204.

In 126 patients treated with fosfestrol the incidence of cardiac side-effects was highest in those on continuous treatment. The duration of treatment should be reduced to a minimum. Patients older than perhaps 70 years and those with pre-existing cardiac symptoms should be excluded.— J. Otzen and E. Thybo, *Ugeskr. Laeg.*, 1977, *139*, 196, per *J. Am. med. Ass.*, 1977, *237*, 2433.

Uses. Fosfestrol or stilboestrol diphosphate is stated to require dephosphorylation before it is active. Fosfestrol and its sodium salt are used in the treatment of malignant neoplasms of the prostate.
Tablets and injections of fosfestrol sodium are available in varying strengths in different countries and in addition doses are expressed in varying ways, either as fosfestrol or as fosfestrol sodium (the tetrasodium salt). Tablets of fosfestrol are also used.
In terms of fosfestrol sodium, initial therapy for the first 5 days generally may range from 550 or 600 mg to 1.1 or 1.2 g daily by intravenous infusion in 300 ml of sodium chloride injection over one hour. In terms of fosfestrol, these doses range from 460 or 500 mg to 920 mg or 1 g. Maintenance may be with half these doses given one to four times a week. Maintenance may also be with oral therapy, daily doses ranging from 100 to 600 mg of fosfestrol sodium (approximately 80 to 500 mg of fosfestrol)

A 56-year-old man with hypercalcaemia due to parathyroid carcinoma, unresponsive to phosphate, calcitonin, mithramycin, glucagon, or antineoplastic agents, was successfully treated with fosfestrol, 1 g daily for 4 days by intravenous injection followed by 200 mg thrice daily by mouth. The injections were repeated 3 months later. It was considered that fosfestrol had a direct inhibitory effect on bone resorption.— G. Sigurdsson *et al.*, *Br. med. J.*, 1973, *1*, 27.

Neoplasm of the prostate. Comment on the disappointing progress made in the treatment of prostatic cancer and on the role of stilboestrol in its management. Stilboestrol was initially used in very high doses of, for instance, 200 mg of fosfestrol daily but since the reports of the Veterans Administration Co-operative Urologic Research Group (D.P. Byer, *Cancer*, 1973, *32*, 1126), which directed attention to problems of thrombo-embolic disease, gynaecomastia, impotence, and other adverse effects associated with oestrogen therapy, a more usual regimen has been stilboestrol 1 mg thrice daily. Some urologists are so dubious about stilboestrol, however, that they advocate bilateral orchidectomy as primary treatment.— *Lancet*, 1980, *2*, 1009.
See also under Stilboestrol, p.1435.

Preparations

Diethylstilbestrol Diphosphate Injection *(U.S.P.)*. A sterile buffered solution of fosfestrol 45 to 55 mg per ml. pH 9 to 10.5.

Honvan *(WB Pharmaceuticals, UK: Boehringer Ingelheim, UK)*. Fosfestrol sodium, available as 5-ml **Ampoules** of an injection containing 55.2 mg per ml and as **Tablets** of 100 mg. (Also available as Honvan in *Austral., Belg., Denm., Ger., Ital., Neth., Norw., S.Afr., Spain, Swed., Switz.*).

Other Proprietary Names

Fosfostilben *(Arg.)*; Honvol *(Canad.)*; ST-52 *(Fr.)*; Stilphostrol *(USA)*.

9054-p

Furazabol. Androfurazanol. 17α-Methyl-5α-androstano[2,3-*c*][1,2,5]oxadiazol-17β-ol.
$C_{20}H_{30}N_2O_2$=330.5.

CAS — 1239-29-8.

A white odourless tasteless crystalline powder. M.p. 155°. Practically **insoluble** in water; freely soluble in alcohol, acetone, chloroform, methyl alcohol, and other organic solvents.

Furazabol is an anabolic steroid. It has been given in doses of up to 6 mg daily as an anabolic agent, and up to 3 mg daily in hyperlipidaemias.

Proprietary Names

Miotolon *(Daiichi, Jap.)*.

9055-s

Gestronol Hexanoate.

Gestonorone Caproate; SH 582. 3,20-Dioxo-19-norpregn-4-en-17α-yl hexanoate.
$C_{26}H_{38}O_4$=414.6.

CAS — 1253-28-7.

Adverse Effects and Precautions. As for Progesterone, p.1431.
Local reactions have occurred at the site of injection.

Uses. Gestronol hexanoate is a long-acting progestogen. It is given in an oily solution by intramuscular injection in doses of 200 to 400 mg every 5 to 7 days for the treatment of endometrial carcinoma.
It has also been tried in the management of benign prostatic hypertrophy in doses of 200 mg weekly.

Osteoporosis. There was no evidence of bone loss over a 1-year period in 2 groups of menopausal women who received mestranol at a mean daily dose of 25 µg or gestronol hexanoate 200 mg by intramuscular injection at monthly intervals reducing to 3-monthly intervals.— R. Lindsay *et al.*, *Postgrad. med. J.*, 1978, *54*, *Suppl. 2* 50.

Neoplasms. The effects of gestronol hexanoate on the histopathology of endometrial cancer.— A. H. John *et al.*, *J. Obstet. Gynaec. Br. Commonw.*, 1974, *81*, 786, per *Int. pharm. Abstr.*, 1975, *12*, 445.

Prostatic hypertrophy. In a crossover study of 30 patients with benign prostatic hypertrophy gestronol hexanoate given for 3 months produced a significant reduction in diurnal frequency but there was no change in residual urine or the peak urine flow-rate.— J. C. Gingell *et al.* (preliminary report), *Proc. R. Soc. Med.*, 1972, *65*, 130.

Gestronol hexanoate was considered to be of no value in the management of benign prostatic hypertrophy.— *Drug & Ther. Bull.*, 1973, *11*, 75.

Further references: E. Palanca and W. Juco, *Curr. med. Res. Opinion*, 1977, *4*, 513.

Proprietary Preparations

Depostat *(Schering, UK)*. Gestronol hexanoate, available as an injection containing 100 mg per ml, in ampoules of 2 ml. (Also available as Depostat in *Belg., Fr., Ger., Ital., Neth., Norw., Spain, Swed.*).

Other Proprietary Names
Primostat *(Arg., S.Afr.)*.

9056-w

Hexoestrol *(B.P. Vet., B.P.C. 1968)*. Hexoestr.; Hexestrol; Dihydrostilboestrol; Hexanoestrol; Synestrol; Synoestrol. *meso*-4,4′-(1,2-Diethylethylene)diphenol.
$C_{18}H_{22}O_2$=270.4.

CAS — 5635-50-7; 84-16-2 (meso).

Pharmacopoeias. In *Aust., Ind., Rus.,* and *Swiss. Roum.* includes Hexoestrol Diacetate ($C_{22}H_{26}O_4$=354.4).

Odourless colourless crystals or white crystalline powder. M.p. 185° to 188°.
Very slightly **soluble** in water; soluble in alcohol, acetone, ether, propylene glycol, vegetable oils, and solutions of alkali hydroxides; slightly soluble in chloroform. Oily solutions are **sterilised** by maintaining at 150° for 1 hour. **Protect** from light.

Adverse Effects and Precautions. As for Oestradiol, p.1425.

Uses. Hexoestrol is a synthetic oestrogen which is not a steroid; it is structurally related to stilboestrol (see p.1433); it has actions and uses similar to those described under oestradiol (see p.1426). It is usually given by mouth but has also been given by intramuscular injection.
For menopausal symptoms, hexoestrol has been given by mouth, usually in doses of 1 to 5 mg daily. It has also been used in the treatment of neoplasms of the breast and prostate.
Hexoestrol dipropionate has also been used.

Proprietary Names
Cycloestrol *(Bruneau, Belg.)*; Hormoestrol *(Siegfried, Switz.)*.

Proprietary Names of Hexoestrol Dipropionate
Hormoestrol *(Siegfried, Switz.)*; Neoestrolo *(De Angeli, Ital.)*.

Proprietary Names of other Hexoestrol Esters
Sintestrol (diacetate) *(Abello, Spain)*.

9057-e

Hydroxyprogesterone Hexanoate *(B.P.)*. Hydroxyprogesterone Caproate *(U.S.P.)*; Hydroxyprogesteronum Capronicum; 17 AHPC. 3,20-Dioxopregn-4-en-17α-yl hexanoate.
$C_{27}H_{40}O_4$=428.6.

CAS — 68-96-2 (hydroxyprogesterone); 630-56-8 (hexanoate).

Pharmacopoeias. In *Br., Chin., Cz.,* and *U.S.*

A white or creamy-white crystalline powder, odourless or with a slight odour. M.p. 120° to 124°.
Practically **insoluble** in water; soluble 1 in 10 of alcohol, 1 in 0.4 of chloroform, and 1 in 10 of ether; soluble in fixed oils and esters. A solution in dioxan is dextrorotatory. Oily solutions are **sterilised** by maintaining at 150° for 1 hour. **Protect** from light.

Adverse Effects and Precautions. As for Progesterone, p.1431.
Cholestatic jaundice may occur in previously sensitised patients. There may be local reactions at the site of injection.

Pregnancy and the neonate. *Effects on the foetus.* Tetralogy of Fallot in an infant born to a mother who had received hydroxyprogesterone during pregnancy.— O. P. Heinonen *et al., New Engl. J. Med.*, 1977, *296*, 67.

Genito-urinary abnormalities in 2 infants born to women given hydroxyprogesterone hexanoate in pregnancy.— A. N. W. Evans *et al., Practitioner*, 1980, *224*, 315.

For a report of congenital hypospadias in an infant born to a mother who had received hydroxyprogesterone hexanoate during the first trimester of pregnancy, see Norethisterone, p.1421.

For a report of abnormalities of the genito-urinary tract in an infant whose mother had taken dydrogesterone and hydroxyprogesterone hexanoate during early pregnancy, see Dydrogesterone, p.1411.

Uses. Hydroxyprogesterone hexanoate has actions and uses similar to those of progesterone (see p.1431). Androgenic and oestrogenic properties are slight. It is given by intramuscular injection in oily solutions containing 125 to 250 mg per ml. It has a slow onset of action and the effects last for about 7 to 17 days.
Doses of 250 to 500 mg weekly have been given in habitual abortion.

Abortion, threatened. There was a higher incidence of abortion and it occurred earlier in a group of 255 women given hydroxyprogesterone hexanoate 500 mg intramuscularly every 7 days compared with 164 similar control patients. There was a significant correlation between the progestogen and the presence of hypogastric pain in terms of abortion-rates. Progestogen therapy for threatened abortion should be contra-indicated in women with hypogastric pain.— A. P. Camilleri and N. M. Gauci, *Obstet. Gynec.*, 1971, *38*, 893, per *Int. pharm. Abstr.*, 1972, *9*, 785.

Premature labour. In a double-blind study there were no premature deliveries in 18 women at increased risk of a premature delivery who had received hydroxyprogesterone hexanoate 250 mg intramuscularly once weekly from early in their pregnancy; in 22 control patients similarly at risk 9 had delivery at 36 weeks or less.— J. W. C. Johnson *et al., New Engl. J. Med.*, 1975, *293*, 675.

Preparations

Hydroxyprogesterone Caproate Injection *(U.S.P.)*. A sterile solution of hydroxyprogesterone hexanoate in a suitable fixed oil.

Hydroxyprogesterone Injection *(B.P.)*. A sterile solution of hydroxyprogesterone hexanoate in a suitable ester, a suitable fixed oil, or any mixture of these. Sterilised by maintaining at 150° for 1 hour. Protect from light. For intramuscular injection only.

Proluton Depot (formerly known as Primolut-Depot) *(Schering, UK)*. Hydroxyprogesterone hexanoate, available as an oily solution containing 250 mg per ml in ampoules of 1 or 2 ml and disposable syringes of 1 or 2 ml. (Also available as Proluton Depot in *Arg., Austral., Belg., Denm., Ger., Ital., Neth., Spain, Swed., Switz.*).

Other Proprietary names
Delalutin *(Canad., USA)*; Hyproval PA, Relutin (both *USA*); Idrogestene, Luteocrin depot (both *Ital.*); Pergestron *(Spain)*; Primolut-Depot *(Norw., S.Afr.)*; Proge Depot *(Jap.)*; Progestérone-Retard Pharlon *(Fr.)*; Retar-Gen P *(Arg.)*.

9058-l

Lututrin. A protein-like substance obtained from the corpus luteum of *sow* ovaries.

CAS — 1407-04-1.

Lututrin has uterine relaxing properties and has been administered in the treatment of dysmenorrhoea and threatened or habitual abortion.

9059-y

Lynoestrenol *(B.P.)*. Linestrenol; Lynenol; Lynestrenol. 19-Nor-17α-pregn-4-en-20-yn-17β-ol.
$C_{20}H_{28}O$=284.4.

CAS — 52-76-6.

Pharmacopoeias. In *Br.*

A white or almost white, odourless, tasteless, crystalline powder. M.p. 160° to 164°.
Practically **insoluble** in water; soluble 1 in 15 of alcohol and of dehydrated alcohol, 1 in 12 of acetone, 1 in 8 of chloroform, and 1 in 12 of ether. A solution in dioxan is laevorotatory. **Store** in airtight containers. Protect from light.

Chlorbutol 1%, menthol 1%, or camphor 1%, were suitable sterilising agents for 100-mg implants of lynoestrenol when heated at 80° for 20 hours. A residual content of 5 ppm of chlorbutol was found after the sterilisation procedure.— P. H. Cox and F. Spanjers, *Pharm. Weekbl. Ned.*, 1970, *105*, 681.

Adverse Effects and Precautions. As for Progesterone, p.1431.
Androgenic side-effects include hirsutism, deepening of the voice, and acne.
See also Oral Contraceptives, p.1402.

A 26-year-old woman who had been taking lynoestrenol 2.5 mg with ethinyloestradiol 50 µg (Minilyn) as an oral contraceptive for 3 years developed erythema nodosum which subsided when the Minilyn was withdrawn, reappeared when Minilyn was again given, and subsided when it was again withdrawn. However Minilyn was not considered to be responsible; there was no reaction to coded capsules containing placebo, Minilyn, lynoestrenol, or ethinyloestradiol.— A. Taaffe *et al.* (letter), *Br. med. J.*, 1977, *2*, 1353.

Effects on the liver. Reports of jaundice or liver damage associated with lynoestrenol: G. Cullberg *et al., Br. med. J.*, 1965, *1*, 695; B. A. Stoll *et al., ibid.*, 1966, *1*, 960; E. T. Heath and D. R. McTaggart, *Med. J. Aust.*, 1967, *2*, 352.

Pregnancy and the neonate. *Ectopic pregnancy.* There was one ectopic pregnancy in 3 years in women using low-dose progestogen oral contraceptives (lynoestrenol 500 µg) for an estimated 4200 woman-years.— P. Liukko and R. Erkkola (letter), *Br. med. J.*, 1976, *2*, 1257.

Absorption and Fate. Lynoestrenol is absorbed from the gastro-intestinal tract.

The pharmacokinetics of lynoestrenol.— M. Humpel *et al., Contraception*, 1977, *16*, 199.

Uses. Lynoestrenol has actions and uses similar to those of norethisterone (see p.1422). It is used mainly for contraception and is given by mouth in doses of 2.5 mg in conjunction with an oestrogen such as ethinyloestradiol for courses of 22 days starting on the 5th day of the first treated cycle, and thereafter repeated after intervals of 6 days for succeeding cycles (see also Oral Contraceptives, p.1402).
Lynoestrenol has been used with mestranol in the treatment of dysfunctional uterine bleeding and endometriosis.

Contraception. No pregnancies occurred during 3553 cycles in 361 women given lynoestrenol 500 µg daily continuously. The incidence of irregular bleeding was high in the first 2 months but then decreased. Some patients noticed a decrease in the occurrence of headaches and in others libido was increased. Five patients withdrew from the study because of increased cycle length; otherwise there were few untoward effects.— J. Ravn, *Arzneimittel-Forsch.*, 1972, *22*, 104.

The frequency of menstruation was reduced to once in 3 months in 196 women by the continuous administration of lynoestrenol 2.5 mg and ethinyloestradiol 50 µg for 84 days followed by a 6-day tablet-free period. The reduction in menstruation was welcomed by 82% of the women. Cycle control was considered to be fairly good; menstrual loss was increased in only 7 patients; weight gain was common; other side-effects were headache, dysmenorrhoea, breast discomfort, and depression. Trial had begun of a contraceptive with a reduced (30 µg) oestrogen content.— N. B. Loudon *et al., Br. med. J.*, 1977, *2*, 487.

Further references: R. Altkempes *et al., Curr. med. Res. Opinion*, 1976, *4*, 353; T. Tarkkila *et al., ibid.*, 1977, *5*, 247; S. Nummi, *ibid.*, 1978, *5*, 406.

Proprietary Preparations

Minilyn *(Organon, UK)*. Tablets each containing lynoestrenol 2.5 mg and ethinyloestradiol 50 µg. For use as an oral contraceptive. *Dose.* 1 tablet daily for 22 days, starting on the 5th day of the first treated cycle and after 6 tablet-free days for succeeding cycles.

Other Proprietary Names
Exlutena *(Swed.)*; Exluton *(Arg., Belg., Fr., Neth., S.Afr.)*; Exlutona *(Denm., Ger., Norw., Switz.)*; Orgametril *(Belg., Denm., Fr., Ger., Neth., Spain, Swed., Switz.)*.

Other Proprietary Names of Lynoestrenol with Ethinyloestradiol
Anacyclin, Anacyclin 28 (both *Ger.*); Lyndiol (*Belg., Denm., Ger., Neth., Norw., S.Afr., Swed.*); Lyndiol E (*Ital.*); Lyndiolett (*Swed.*); Mini Pregnon (*Neth.*); Ministat (*Belg., Ital., Neth.*); Neo-Lyndiol (*Spain*); Nonovulet (*Denm.*); Noracyclin (*Ger.*); Ovariostat (*Fr.*); Ovoresta (*Ger.*); Ovostat (*Belg., Neth., Switz.*); Ovostat-28 (*S.Afr.*); Ovostat-Micro (*Switz.*); Pregnon 28 (*Belg., Ger., Neth.*); Restovar (*Denm., Norw.*); Yermonil (*Ger., Switz.*).

For other proprietary names of ethinyloestradiol and ethinyloestradiol with lynoestrenol, see under Ethinyloestradiol, p.1412.

Other Proprietary Names of Lynoestrenol with Mestranol
Anacyclin 101 (*Switz.*); Lindiol 2.5 (*Arg.*); Lyndiol (*Spain, Switz.*); Lyndiol 2.5 (*Ital.*); Noracyclin 22 (*Switz.*); Orgaluton (*Neth.*).

A preparation containing lynoestrenol and mestranol was formerly marketed in Great Britain under the proprietary name Lyndiol 2.5 (*Organon*).

9061-q

Medrogestone. AY 62022; Metrogestone.
6,17α-Dimethylpregna-4,6-diene-3,20-dione.
$C_{23}H_{32}O_2$=340.5.
CAS — 977-79-7.

A white crystalline powder. Practically **insoluble** in water; soluble in most organic solvents.

Adverse Effects. As for Progesterone, p.1431.

Uses. Medrogestone is a progestational agent with actions similar to those of progesterone (see p.1431).
It is used in the treatment of functional uterine bleeding and other menstrual irregularities in doses of 5 to 10 mg daily from day 15 to day 25 of the cycle. Oestrogen therapy may also be required.

Prostatic hypertrophy. Significantly greater improvement was noted in 20 patients with benign prostatic hypertrophy when they were treated with medrogestone 50 mg twice daily for 24 weeks than when given placebo in a double-blind study. A decrease in sexual function was reported in 6 of 7 patients when taking medrogestone and 6 patients with diabetes mellitus had increased hyperglycaemia.— R. E. Rangno *et al., Clin. Pharmac. Ther.*, 1971, *12*, 658. Analysis of the study shows that there was no objective evidence of shrinkage of the gland. The reported trials of treatment with hormones do not show clinical improvement that is more than marginal.— *Br. med. J.*, 1971, *4*, 638.

Proprietary Names
Colpro (*Ayerst, Belg.*; *Ayerst, Neth.*; *Ayerst, S.Afr.*; *Ayerst, Switz.*); Colprone (*Ayerst, Canad.*; *Auclair, Fr.*; *Ayerst, Ital.*); Prothil (*Kali-Chemie, Ger.*).

9062-p

Medroxyprogesterone Acetate (*B.P., B.P. Vet., U.S.P.*). Methylacetoxyprogesterone; Metipregnone. 6α-Methyl-3,20-dioxopregn-4-en-17α-yl acetate.
$C_{24}H_{34}O_4$=386.5.
CAS — 520-85-4 (medroxyprogesterone); 71-58-9 (acetate).

Pharmacopoeias. In *Br., Braz., Chin., It., Roum.*, and *U.S.*

A white, or off-white odourless, crystalline powder. M.p. about 204°.
Practically **insoluble** in water; soluble 1 in 800 of alcohol, 1 in 50 of acetone, 1 in 10 of chloroform, and 1 in 60 of dioxan; slightly soluble in methyl alcohol and ether. A solution in dioxan is dextrorotatory. **Store** in airtight containers. Protect from light.

Adverse Effects and Precautions. As for Progesterone, p.1431.
Virilisation of the female foetus has been reported following the use of medroxyprogesterone acetate in pregnant women. Thrombo-embolisms have also been reported. Sensitivity reactions, acne, and hirsutism have occurred. Jaundice has occasionally been reported. Breast nodules, some of which were malignant and metastatic, have developed in beagle *dogs* given medroxyprogesterone acetate.
The use of injections of medroxyprogesterone acetate for long-term contraception is associated with unpredictable variation in the cycle length and menstrual bleeding. Amenorrhoea with possibly prolonged infertility may follow its withdrawal.

A WHO group concluded that there was no direct link between cervical cancer and the use of medroxyprogesterone acetate. Although there was a delay in the return of fertility after discontinuing medroxyprogesterone acetate there was no evidence of permanent infertility and no reports of breast abnormalities which could be attributed to medroxyprogesterone.— *Pharm. J.*, 1977, *2*, 106.

Of 72 women given medroxyprogesterone acetate 150 mg intramuscularly as a postpartum contraceptive while awaiting sterilisation, 19 had episodes of intermittent heavy bleeding but 69 patients were happy to have had protection.— J. Mowat, *Br. med. J.*, 1974, *2*, 306.

The use for one year of medroxyprogesterone acetate as a contraceptive had no effect on vitamin or mineral status.— K. Amatayakul *et al., Contraception*, 1978, *18*, 253, per *Int. pharm. Abstr.*, 1979, *16*, 473.

In 52 women given a single injection of medroxyprogesterone acetate 150 mg post partum after rubella vaccination, the mean number of days of post-partum bleeding was 58.5 compared with 20.8 in 52 controls. Three non-lactating women in each group had amenorrhoea. Cyclical bleeding in 15 treated women was not considered heavy.— H. M. Murphy, *Br. med. J.*, 1979, *2*, 1400. Some women given medroxyprogesterone acetate postpartum pending sterilisation suffered prolonged bleeding; if the medroxyprogesterone was delayed until a menstrual period had occurred the excess bleeding was eliminated.— M. Thiery *et al.* (letter), *Br. med. J.*, 1980, *280*, 481.

Absence of long-term effects on fertility in Thai women.— T. Pardthaisong *et al., Lancet*, 1980, *1*, 509.

Effects on carbohydrate metabolism. In a study of 37 women given medroxyprogesterone acetate intramuscularly for 1 year both glucose and insulin concentrations were increased significantly but there was no change in fasting ambulatory growth hormone. Glucose tolerance curves became abnormal in 15% of the women. There was a mean weight gain of about 3 kg.— W. N. Spellacy *et al., Fert. Steril.*, 1972, *23*, 239, per *J. Am. med. Ass.*, 1972, *221*, 211.

Absence of effect on glucose, insulin, growth hormone, and lipids.— K. Dhali *et al., Fert. Steril.*, 1977, *28*, 156.

Effects on liver function. Decrease in prothrombin activity and impaired clearance of sulphobromophthalein sodium in woman given medroxyprogesterone acetate.— F. M. Saleh and M. M. Abd-El-Hay, *Contraception*, 1977, *16*, 409, per *Int. pharm. Abstr.*, 1978, *15*, 427.

The use of medroxyprogesterone acetate postpartum in about 200 women did not adversely affect the health or the biochemical indicators of liver or lipid function in rural Thai women, with or without liver-fluke infection, over a period of 18 months.— R. A. Grossman *et al., Bull. Wld Org.*, 1979, *57*, 829.

Galactorrhoea. An investigation of 57 women who had been treated with medroxyprogesterone acetate, mostly in a total dose in excess of 500 mg, revealed that 5 had experience protracted puerperal galactorrhoea, often, though not invariably, with associated menstrual abnormalities.— R. J. Bolognese *et al., J. Am. med. Ass.*, 1967, *199*, 42.

Ischaemic colitis. Ischaemic colitis in a patient associated with 2 depot injections of medroxyprogesterone acetate.— M. D. Gelfand, *Am. J. dig. Dis.*, 1972, *17*, 275, per *Thérapie*, 1974, *29*, 15.

Neoplasms. Induction of mammary nodules in beagle *dogs* by medroxyprogesterone acetate appeared to be a species-specific effect.— M. E. Coleman *et al., Toxic. appl. Pharmac.*, 1976, *37*, 181. Acromegalic changes in beagle *dogs* following medroxyprogesterone acetate administration appeared to be species-specific.— *idem.*.

Pregnancy and the neonate. *Effects on the foetus.* Medroxyprogesterone acetate when administered to pregnant *rabbits* produced a significant number of foetuses with cleft palates and retarded development. It was considered that medroxyprogesterone might be teratogenic.— F. D. Andrew and R. E. Staples, *Toxic. appl. Pharmac.*, 1975, *33*, 196.

For a report of congenital hypospadias in an infant born to a mother who had received medroxyprogesterone during the first trimester of pregnancy, see Norethisterone, p.1421.

Absorption and Fate. Medroxyprogesterone is absorbed from the gastro-intestinal tract. It is hydroxylated in the liver.

In 7 lactating women given medroxyprogesterone acetate 150 mg the concentration of medroxyprogesterone acetate in breast milk was broadly comparable to that in plasma.— B. N. Saxena *et al., Contraception*, 1977, *16*, 605.

Uses. Medroxyprogesterone acetate has actions and uses similar to those of progesterone (see p.1431). It is active when given by mouth and may also be given by intramuscular injection in aqueous suspensions for prolonged action.
It is used for the treatment of functional uterine bleeding and secondary amenorrhoea in doses of 2.5 to 10 mg daily by mouth for 5 to 10 days starting on the assumed or calculated 16th to 21st day of the cycle.
It is given by intramuscular injection in the treatment of endometriosis when 50 mg may be given weekly or 100 mg every 2 weeks for 6 months or more. It is given in the treatment of endometrial or prostatic carcinoma usually in initial doses of up to 1 g weekly and in renal carcinoma with similar or higher initial doses given during each week; a regimen for breast carcinoma is 500 mg to 1 g daily for 28 days subsequently reduced to 500 mg twice weekly for maintenance. It has also been given for the treatment of threatened or habitual abortion in doses of 10 to 40 mg daily by mouth.
Medroxyprogesterone acetate is also given by intramuscular injection in some countries as a 'progestogen-only' contraceptive often only for short periods; 150 mg is given at the beginning of the cycle or early in the puerperium and is considered to be effective for at least 3 months. Regimens of 300 to 450 mg every 6 months have also been used.

Contraception. A dose of 300 mg of medroxyprogesterone acetate every 6 months by intramuscular injection was as effective as oral contraceptives and intra-uterine devices in a study of 991 women over 21 470 woman-months. Irregular bleeding or amenorrhoea was common but the continuation-rate was only slightly less than that with other forms of contraception. Weight gain was a side-effect.— P. C. Schwallie and J. R. Assenzo, *Contraception*, 1972, *6*, 315, per *Int. pharm. Abstr.*, 1973, *10*, 698.

Medroxyprogesterone acetate 150 mg was given intramuscularly every 3 months over 7 years for contraception in 19 204 women. Stilboestrol 500 µg or ethinyloestradiol 20 or 40 µg daily was also given on 7 to 10 days of each lunar month. Fertility returned after 14 months in 82% of 135 patients who withdrew from treatment to become pregnant.— E. B. McDaniel and T. Pardthaisong, *Contraception*, 1973, *8*, 407, per *Int. pharm. Abstr.*, 1974, *11*, 796.

A favourable report of the use of medroxyprogesterone acetate, 200 mg every 15 to 16 weeks, by injection, for contraception in 162 women, with deprived backgrounds, in Glasgow.— E. Wilson, *Br. med. J.*, 1976, *2*, 1435.

Suppression of ovulation in 14 subjects by the use of Silastic rings containing medroxyprogesterone acetate 100 or 200 mg.— M. Thiery *et al., Contraception*, 1976, *13*, 605, per *Int. pharm. Abstr.*, 1978, *15*, 269.

Of 1601 women in rural Bangladesh who had received from 1 to 12 doses of medroxyprogesterone acetate 150 mg given by intramuscular injection every 80 to 90 days for contraception 704 withdrew from the study; 253 reported that this was because of menstrual irregularities. A decrease in lactation was reported by 147 of 1020 who had received medroxyprogesterone during lactation.— L. Parveen *et al., Lancet*, 1977, *2*, 946.

In 19 875 women given medroxyprogesterone acetate 150 mg every 3 months or 450 mg every 6 months for contraception for a total of 220 530 woman-months the Pearl index [pregnancies per 100 woman-years] was 0.1069 and 0.4943 respectively.— H. J. S. Rall *et al., J. reprod. Med.*, 1977, *18*, 55, per *J. Am. med. Ass.*, 1977,

237, 2657.

Satisfactory cycle control and absence of pregnancy after 575 cycles in women given medroxyprogesterone acetate 50 mg and oestradiol cypionate 10 mg (Cyclo-Provera) by injection each month.— B. Bloch and A. H. Davies, *S.Afr. med. J.*, 1978, *53*, 846.

Further references: Advances in Methods of Fertility Regulation, *Tech. Rep. Ser. Wld Hlth Org. No. 527*, 1973; *IPPF med. Bull.*, 1977, *11*, 2; M. Smith, *Scott. med. J.*, 1978, *23*, 223; W. M. Castle *et al.*, *S. Afr. med. J.*, 1978, *53*, 842.

Contraception, male. Reduction of spermatogenesis in small groups of men given medroxyprogesterone acetate and testosterone esters.— J. F. Melo and E. M. Coutinho, *Contraception*, 1977, *15*, 627; F. Alvarez-Sanchez *et al.*, *Contraception*, 1977, *15*, 635; J. Frick *et al.*, *Contraception*, 1977, *15*, 649; J. Frick *et al.*, *Contraception*, 1977, *15*, 669; P. F. Brenner *et al.*, *Contraception*, 1977, *15*, 679.

Endometriosis. Medroxyprogesterone acetate 30 mg daily for 90 days produced improvement or remission in 35 patients with endometriosis.— K. S. Moghissi and C. R. Boyce, *Obstet. Gynec.*, 1976, *47*, 265, per *Int. pharm. Abstr.*, 1976, *13*, 935.

Hirsutism. Medroxyprogesterone acetate 100 mg was given intramuscularly every 15 days for 110 to 405 days to 24 hirsute women. Obvious diminution of hirsutism occurred in 23 patients whose improvement was maintained by continuing treatment with medroxyprogesterone by mouth.— R. F. Corrêa de Oliveira *et al.*, *Ann. intern. Med.*, 1975, *83*, 817.

The use of medroxyprogesterone acetate 10 mg thrice daily for the evaluation of hypertestosteronism in hirsute women.— B. Ettinger and I. M. Golditch, *Fert. Steril.*, 1977, *28*, 1285, per *Int. pharm. Abstr.*, 1978, *15*, 876.

Menopausal symptoms. Medroxyprogesterone acetate 150 mg monthly by intramuscular injection reduced or eliminated menopausal flushes in 51 of 57 women compared with placebo which relieved symptoms in 3 of 12 control patients. Among the side-effects were thrombophlebitis, abnormal bleeding, headache, and depression.— J. L. Bullock *et al.*, *Obstet. Gynec.*, 1975, *46*, 165.

Neoplasms. Medroxyprogesterone acetate 600 mg weekly to 300 mg daily was given by intramuscular injection in the treatment of various malignant neoplasms. Objective responses were achieved in 4 of 20 women and 2 of 2 men with breast carcinoma, 1 of 3 patients with ovarian carcinoma, 1 of 5 with malignant melanoma, none of 2 with kidney carcinoma, and 1 of 1 with testicular choriocarcinoma.— L. Sadoff, *Ann. intern. Med.*, 1973, *78*, 830.

Breast. Complete or partial remissions in 19 of 44 patients with metastatic breast disease given high doses of medroxyprogesterone acetate (1.5 g daily by intramuscular injection in 2 divided doses for up to 30 days).— F. Pannuti *et al.*, *Cancer Treat. Rep.*, 1978, *62*, 499.

Further references: F. M. Muggia *et al.*, *Ann. intern. Med.*, 1968, *68*, 328, per *J. Am. med. Ass.*, 1968, *203* (Mar. 11), A215.

Ovary. Medroxyprogesterone acetate 100 to 400 mg daily by mouth was of no significant benefit in 19 patients with recurrent and metastatic ovarian cancer.— G. D. Malkasian *et al.*, *Cancer Treat. Rep.*, 1977, *61*, 913, per *Int. pharm. Abstr.*, 1977, *14*, 1235.

Prostate. Partial remission persisting for 6 months in 2 of 10 patients with malignant disease of the prostate after treatment for about a month with high doses of medroxyprogesterone acetate (1.5 g daily in 2 divided doses).— F. Pannuti *et al.*, *IRCS Med. Sci.*, 1977, *5*, 375.

Uterus. Of 68 patients with neoplasms of the endometrium, 25 obtained remissions (12 complete, 13 partial) after treatment with medroxyprogesterone acetate. Complete remission lasted an average of 53 months. Patients without remissions were subjectively improved. The initial dose was 2 g by intramuscular injection, then 1 g weekly, maintained during the remission.— *J. Am. med. Ass.*, 1969, *209*, 1020.

Tumour regression in 16 of 44 patients with recurrent or disseminated adenocarcinoma of the endometrium treated with progestational agents, including 34 given medroxyprogesterone acetate usually 250 mg twice weekly for 8 weeks, then weekly.— J. C. Rozier and P. B. Underwood, *Obstet. Gynec.*, 1974, *44*, 60, per *Int. pharm. Abstr.*, 1978, *15*, 873.

Pickwickian syndrome. Ten male patients with Pickwickian syndrome, characterised by obesity, alveolar hypoventilation, polycythaemia, and cor pulmonale, were given medroxyprogesterone acetate 20 mg sublingually every 8 hours. There was no significant loss of weight after treatment for a mean of 7 months but after only 1 month there was significant improvement of hypoxaemia and hypercapnia which was sustained as long as treatment was continued. There was also improvement in polycythaemia and resolution of cor pulmonale. Two patients complained of impotence and another developed diabetes mellitus after treatment for 1 year.— F. D. Sutton *et al.*, *Ann. intern. Med.*, 1975, *83*, 476. See also R. McKenzie and R. K. Wadhwa, *Anesth. Analg. curr. Res.*, 1977, *56*, 133, per *J. Am. med. Ass.*, 1977, *237*, 2761.

Puberty, precocious. References to medroxyprogesterone in precocious puberty: E. J. Schoen, *J. clin. Endocr. Metab.*, 1966, *26*, 363; S. A. Kaplan *et al.*, *Am. J. Dis. Child.*, 1968, *116*, 591.

Pregnancy and the neonate. *Lactation.* Medroxyprogesterone acetate 150 mg intramuscularly every 3 months significantly raised serum-prolactin concentrations in 4 lactating women compared with 4 lactating women using non-hormonal means of contraception.— R. R. Chaudhury *et al.*, *Br. J. Pharmac.*, 1977, *59*, 433.

Sexual disorders. A report of the use of medroxyprogesterone acetate in men with a history of sex offences and antisocial behaviour.— *J. Am. med. Ass.*, 1975, *233*, 502.

Preparations

Medroxyprogesterone Acetate Tablets *(U.S.P.)*. Tablets containing medroxyprogesterone acetate.

Sterile Medroxyprogesterone Acetate Suspension *(U.S.P.)*. A sterile suspension of medroxyprogesterone acetate in a suitable aqueous vehicle; pH 3 to 7.

Proprietary Preparations

Depo-Provera *(Upjohn, UK)*. A sterile aqueous suspension of medroxyprogesterone acetate containing 50 mg per ml in vials of 1, 3, and 5 ml, and 150 mg per ml in vials of 3.3 ml. For intramuscular administration for prolonged action. (Also available as Depo-Provera in *Arg., Austral., Belg., Canad., Denm., Ital., Neth., Norw., S.Afr., Swed., Switz., USA*).

Farlutal *(Farmitalia Carlo Erba, UK)*. A sterile suspension of medroxyprogesterone acetate containing 200 mg per ml, available in vials of 2.5 and 5 ml. For intramuscular administration for prolonged action. (Also available as Farlutal or Farlutal Depot in *Belg., Fr., Ger., Ital., Neth.*).

Provera *(Upjohn, UK)*. Medroxyprogesterone acetate, available as scored tablets of 5 mg. **Provera 100 mg.** Tablets each containing medroxyprogesterone acetate 100 mg. (Also available as Provera in *Austral., Belg., Canad., Neth., Norw., S.Afr., Switz., USA*).

Other Proprietary Names

Amen, Curretab *(both USA)*; Clinovir *(Denm., Ger.)*; Depo-Clinovir *(Ger.)*; Depo-Progevera *(Spain)*; Dépo-Prodasone *(Fr.)*; Farlutal *(Belg., Fr., Ger., Ital., Neth.)*; Farlutale *(Arg.)*; Gestapuran *(Swed.)*; Luteocrin orale, Luteodione, Luteos, Lutoral, Metilgestene *(all Ital.)*; Perlutex *(Denm., Norw.)*; Prodasone *(Fr.)*; Progevera *(Spain)*.

9063-s

Megestrol Acetate *(B.P., B.P. Vet.)*.

Megestrol Acet.; BDH 1298; SC 10363. 6-Methyl-3,20-dioxopregna-4,6-dien-17α-yl acetate.

$C_{24}H_{32}O_4$=384.5.

CAS — 3562-63-8 (megestrol); 595-33-5 (acetate).

Pharmacopoeias. In *Br.* and *Chin.*

An odourless, white to creamy-white, crystalline powder. M.p. about 217°.

Practically **insoluble** in water; soluble 1 in 55 of alcohol, 1 in 0.8 of chloroform, and 1 in 130 of ether; soluble in acetone, and benzyl alcohol; slightly soluble in fixed oils. A solution in chloroform is dextrorotatory. **Protect** from light.

Adverse Effects and Precautions. As for Progesterone, p.1431.

See also Adverse Effects and Precautions for Oral Contraceptives, p.1402.

Because the proportion of tumours in the breasts of beagle *dogs* was found to be increased by megestrol acetate, the manufacture of 'combined' and 'sequential' oral contraceptives containing it was discontinued in Great Britain in 1975.

For a report of breast neoplasms in beagle *dogs* after a 2-year course of megestrol acetate given in doses up to 25 times the expected human dose, see L. W. Nelson *et al.*, *J. Am. med. Ass.*, 1972, *219*, 1601. See also *Pharm. J.*, 1975, *2*, 597; J. H. Weikel *et al.*, *Toxic. appl. Pharmac.*, 1975, *33*, 414.

Irreversible insulin-dependent diabetes mellitus developed in a middle-aged woman 6 weeks after starting treatment with megestrol acetate 40 mg four times daily.— J. C. Bottino and C. K. Tashima (letter), *Ann. intern. Med.*, 1976, *84*, 341.

Severe pain of the hands occurred in 4 women while taking megestrol acetate and melphalan; megestrol appeared to be responsible.— P. J. DiSaia and C. P. Morrow, *Am. J. Obstet. Gynec.*, 1977, *129*, 460.

Absorption and Fate. Megestrol acetate is absorbed from the gastro-intestinal tract. It is excreted mainly in the urine, but also in the faeces, in the form of the glucuronides of its metabolites.

In 5 lactating women given megestrol acetate 4 mg with ethinyloestradiol 50 µg the plasma:milk ratio of megestrol acetate was 5:4.— S. Nilsson *et al.*, *Contraception*, 1977, *16*, 615, per *Int. pharm. Abstr.*, 1978, *15*, 481.

Uses. Megestrol acetate has actions and uses similar to those of progesterone (see p.1431) but is more potent both as a progestational agent and as an inhibitor of ovulation.

It is active when given by mouth and is used in the palliative treatment or as an adjunct to other therapy in endometrial carcinoma in doses of 40 to 320 mg daily in divided doses continued for at least 2 months, and in doses of 40 mg four times a day in breast cancer.

It was formerly used with ethinyloestradiol in oral contraceptives.

For reports of the use of megestrol acetate for contraception, see Martindale 27th Edn, p. 1404.

Neoplasms. *Breast.* Megestrol acetate 40 mg four times daily given to 30 patients with progressing metastatic breast cancer produced an objective remission lasting a mean of 5.5 months in 7.— F. J. Ansfield *et al.*, *Cancer*, 1974, *33*, 907, per *J. Am. med. Ass.*, 1974, *229*, 94. A more recent report in 101 patients with breast cancer.— F. J. Ansfield *et al.*, *Cancer*, 1976, *38*, 53.

A complete or partial response was obtained in 13 of 48 patients who had malignant neoplasms of the breast, refractory to hormonal and/or combination chemotherapy, after treatment with megestrol acetate 40 mg four times daily and mitomycin 20 mg per m^2 body-surface intravenously every 4 to 6 weeks. The mean survival-time for patients who responded to treatment was 7 months compared with 2 months in non-responders. The myelosuppressive toxicity of mitomycin was cumulative and therefore smaller doses were given in subsequent courses at increasing intervals.— A. U. Buzdar *et al.*, *Cancer*, 1978, *41*, 392.

Uterus. Megestrol acetate given for at least 2 months in doses of 40 mg daily increased as the study progressed to 320 mg daily produced an objective response in 32 of 81 patients with recurrent or metastatic endometrial carcinoma. There was a partial response in 21% of patients. The best response was in patients with slow growing well-differentiated tumours.— R. B. Wait, *Obstet. Gynec.*, 1973, *41*, 129, per *Int. pharm. Abstr.*, 1974, *11*, 293. See also E. Eichner and M. Abellera, *Obstet. Gynec.*, 1971, *38*, 739, per *Int. pharm. Abstr.*, 1972, *9*, 714.

Proprietary Names

Megace *(Bristol, Canad.; Mead Johnson, USA)*; Niagestin *(Novo, Denm.; Novo, Ger.; Novo, Neth.; Novo, Norw.; Novo, Swed.; Novo, Switz.)*; Niagestine *(Novo, Belg.)*.

Preparations containing megestrol acetate with ethinyloestradiol were formerly marketed in Great Britain under the proprietary names Volidan and Volidan 21 *(Duncan, Flockhart)*.

9064-w

Mesterolone. SH 723. 17β-Hydroxy-1α-methyl-5α-androstan-3-one.
$C_{20}H_{32}O_2$=304.5.

CAS — 1424-00-6.

Pharmacopoeias. In *Nord.*

A white odourless crystalline powder. M.p. about 210°. Practically **insoluble** in water; soluble 1 in 50 of alcohol, 1 in 6 of chloroform, and 1 in 150 of ether.

Adverse Effects and Precautions. As for Testosterone, p.1436.
It is reported not to inhibit gonadotrophin secretion or spermatogenesis.

Carcinoma of the prostate gland developed in a 59-year-old man over a period of several years during which time he had taken mesterolone intermittently.— T. F. Sandeman (letter), *Med. J. Aust.*, 1975, *1*, 634.

Uses. Mesterolone is an androgen with actions and uses similar to those of testosterone (see p.1436). It is reported to have less inhibitory effect on intrinsic testicular function.
Mesterolone is used in the treatment of hypogonadism and of male infertility due to oligospermia. It is given by mouth in divided doses of 50 to 100 mg daily.

Reviews of the actions and uses of mesterolone: P. Bye, *Postgrad. med. J.*, 1975, *51*, 215.

Hypogonadism. Mesterolone 200 mg daily appeared to be an active androgen in 4 hypogonadal patients who had not previously received androgens, and in 5 of 8 previously given testosterone propionate.— E. W. Barnes *et al.* (letter), *Br. med. J.*, 1973, *1*, 234.

Infertility. Of 17 men with defective spermatogenesis given mesterolone 50 to 200 mg daily, 5 showed increased sperm counts, 1 showed increased sperm activity, and 11 showed no improvement. Of 5 eunuchoids given 200 mg daily, 3 showed no androgenic response.— G. I. M. Swyer (letter), *Br. med. J.*, 1972, *4*, 425.

Further references: B. N. Barwin *et al.*, *Practitioner*, 1973, *211*, 669; J. Mauss, *Arzneimittel-Forsch.*, 1974, *24*, 1338.

Proprietary Preparations

Pro-viron *(Schering, UK).* Mesterolone, available as scored tablets of 25 mg. (Also available as Proviron in *Arg., Austral., Belg., Fr., Ger., Ital., Neth., S.Afr., Spain, Switz.*).

Other Proprietary Names

Mestoranum *(Denm., Norw., Swed.).*

9065-e

Mestranol *(B.P., U.S.P.).* EE3ME; Compound 33355; Ethinyloestradiol-3-methyl Ether. 3-Methoxy-19-nor-17α-pregna-1,3,5(10)-trien-20-yn-17β-ol.
$C_{21}H_{26}O_2$=310.4.

CAS — 72-33-3.

NOTE. Up to 1% of mestranol occurs in Norethynodrel (*B.P.*) as normally manufactured.

Pharmacopoeias. In *Br., Braz., Cz.,* and *U.S.*

A white to creamy-white, odourless, crystalline powder. M.p. 146° to 154° with a range of not more than 4°. Practically **insoluble** in water; soluble 1 in 44 of alcohol, 1 in 23 of acetone and of ether, 1 in 4.5 of chloroform, and 1 in 12 of dioxan; slightly soluble in methyl alcohol. A solution in dioxan is dextrorotatory. **Protect** from light.

CAUTION. *Mestranol is a powerful oestrogen. Contact with the skin or inhalation should be avoided. Rubber gloves and a face mask should be worn when handling the powder.*

Adverse Effects and Precautions. As for Oestradiol, p.1425. Mestranol should be used with caution in patients with impaired liver function.
See also under Oral Contraceptives, p.1402.

Cutaneous eruptions and *in vitro* lymphocyte hypersensitivity associated with oral contraceptives and mestranol.— H. Savel *et al.*, *Archs Derm.*, 1970, *101*, 187.

A 23-year-old woman who had taken an oral contraceptive containing mestranol and norethynodrel for six months developed, 2 years later, transient acute polyneuritis affecting the feet and ankles 3 days after starting another oral contraceptive containing mestranol; this possibly represented allergic sensitisation to mestranol.— I. Eibschitz and B. Sharf (letter), *Br. med. J.*, 1974, *1*, 198.

Effect on liver function. After reviewing evidence from *animal* experiments, the Committee on Safety of Drugs concluded that mestranol caused liver damage which was sometimes severe, including on occasion the development of hepatoma, when administered to *rats* in high doses for prolonged periods. There was no evidence that the incidence of hepatic disorders was increased in women taking oral contraceptives containing mestranol.— D. A. Cahal (letter), *Lancet*, 1966, *1*, 1371.

A report of regression of focal nodular hyperplasia of the liver in a 25-year-old woman when she ceased taking mestranol with norethisterone which she had taken as an oral contraceptive preparation continuously for 5 years.— D. Ross *et al.* (letter), *Ann. intern. Med.*, 1976, *85*, 203.

Absorption and Fate. Mestranol is readily absorbed from the gastro-intestinal tract. It is slowly metabolised and excreted in the urine. The biological half-life is about 50 hours. A small proportion is also excreted in the milk of nursing mothers.

A review of the pharmacokinetics of mestranol.— E. D. Helton and J. W. Goldzieher, *Contraception*, 1977, *15*, 255, per *Int. pharm. Abstr.*, 1977, *14*, 1102.

The activity of mestranol was dependent on its demethylation to ethinyloestradiol. Studies in female patients showed that, for a given effect, the dose of mestranol required was twice that of ethinyloestradiol.— H. M. Bolt and W. H. Bolt, *Eur. J. clin. Pharmac.*, 1974, *7*, 295.

The metabolism of mestranol.— T. M. Mills *et al.*, *Am. J. Obstet. Gynec.*, 1976, *126*, 987, per *Int. pharm. Abstr.*, 1977, *14*, 853.

Pregnancy and the neonate. During 4 days following single doses of mestranol given to 4 lactating women, from 0.0002 to 0.013% of the dose was excreted in the milk. It was estimated that the regular administration of 150 µg of mestranol daily to a lactating woman could result in the excretion of 30 to 60 ng in each 100 ml of milk.— H. G. Wijmenga and H. J. van der Molen, *Acta endocr, Copenh.*, 1969, *61*, 665, per *J. Am. med. Ass.*, 1969, *209*, 2106.

Uses. Mestranol has actions similar to those of oestradiol (see p.1426) but is much more potent and is active by mouth.
The usual dose of mestranol in the treatment of disorders of menstruation is 100 µg, normally in conjunction with ethynodiol diacetate (see p.1413).
Mestranol is given by mouth as a contraceptive in conjunction with a progestational agent such as ethynodiol diacetate (see p.1413), norethisterone (see p.1422), or norethynodrel (see p.1423) (see Oral Contraceptives, p.1402).

Osteoporosis. Studies in 120 ovariectomised women showed that the rate of bone loss was reduced in all the 63 patients treated with mestranol in a mean dose of 24.8 µg daily, in a double-blind trial. Patients commencing treatment 3 to 6 years after operation showed an increase in bone density during the first 3 years which was maintained during the next 2 years. Patients receiving a placebo showed continued bone loss during the 5 years of the study.— R. Lindsay *et al.*, *Lancet*, 1976, *1*, 1038.

Review of 15 oophorectomised women after 8 years of oestrogen therapy with mestranol showed no evidence of bone loss whereas review of 14 similar women who discontinued the mestranol after 4 years showed a loss of 2.5% per year (a rate similar to that of women in the first year or two after oophorectomy); after 4 years of discontinuation they had lost all the benefits of oestrogen therapy. In a placebo-treated group of 14 similar women, the loss during the second 4-year period was significantly less than in the group whose oestrogen had been withdrawn; after the 8-year period there was no significant difference between them and the women who had received the initial 4 years of oestrogen therapy.— R. Lindsay *et al.*, *Lancet*, 1978, *1*, 1325. Review of 100 oophorectomised women, after a median follow-up period of 9 years, 58 of whom had taken mestranol and 42 placebo. Oestrogen treatment was found to protect against central, as well as peripheral, bone loss and to reduce the incidence of vertebral decompression.— R. Lindsay *et al.*, *Lancet*, 1980, *2*, 1151.

See also under Oestradiol, p.1427.

Proprietary Preparations

Syntex Menophase *(Syntex, UK).* Packs of 28 tablets, for sequential daily administration, containing 5 pink tablets each containing mestranol 12.5 µg, 8 orange tablets each containing mestranol 25 µg, 2 yellow tablets each containing mestranol 50 µg, 3 green tablets each containing mestranol 25 µg and norethisterone 1 mg, 6 blue tablets each containing mestranol 30 µg and norethisterone 1.5 mg, and 4 lavender-coloured tablets each containing mestranol 20 µg and norethisterone 750 µg. For menopausal symptoms.

A symposium on Syntex Menophase.— *Postgrad. med. J.*, 1976, *52, Suppl.* 6,.

Other Proprietary Names of Mestranol and Mestranol with Chlormadinone Acetate

Eunomin 21 *(Ger.).*

Other Proprietary Names of Mestranol and Mestranol with Norethisterone

Ortho-Novum SQ *(Belg.).*

Other proprietary preparations containing mestranol with progestogens are described under Ethynodiol Diacetate (see p.1413) and Norethisterone (see p.1422).

A preparation containing mestranol and mestranol with lynoestrenol was formerly marketed in Great Britain under the proprietary name Ovanon (*Organon*).

9066-l

Methallenoestril *(B.P.).* Methallenoestrol. 3-(6-Methoxy-2-naphthyl)-2,2-dimethylvaleric acid.
$C_{18}H_{22}O_3$=286.4.

CAS — 517-18-0.

Pharmacopoeias. In *Br.*

A white or almost white, odourless or almost odourless, crystalline powder with a slightly bitter taste. M.p. about 138°.
Very slightly **soluble** in water; soluble 1 in 10 of alcohol, 1 in 2 of chloroform, and 1 in 8 of ether; soluble in solutions of alkali hydroxides.

Adverse Effects and Precautions. As for Oestradiol, p.1425.

Uses. Methallenoestril is a synthetic oestrogen which is not a steroid. It has actions and uses similar to those of oestradiol (see p.1426) and is given by mouth.
It has been used for the treatment of menopausal symptoms in doses of 3 mg once to thrice daily. It was also used in the suppression of lactation and in prostatic neoplasms.

Preparations

Methallenoestril Tablets *(B.P.).* Tablets containing methallenoestril.

Proprietary Names

Geklimon *(GEA, Denm.)*; Vallestril *(Searle, Austral.; Searle, Canad.; Searle, Denm.; Searle, Norw.; Searle, Switz.).*

Methallenoestril was formerly marketed in Great Britain under the proprietary name Vallestril (*Searle*).

9067-y

Methandienone *(B.P., B.P. Vet.).* Metandienone; Methandrostenolone *(U.S.P.).* 17β-Hydroxy-17α-methylandrosta-1,4-dien-3-one.
$C_{20}H_{28}O_2$=300.4.

CAS — 72-63-9.

Pharmacopoeias. In *Br., Hung., Jug., Rus.,* and *U.S.*

A white or faintly yellowish-white odourless crystalline powder. M.p. 163° to 167°. Practically **insoluble** in water; soluble 1 in 2 of alcohol, 1 in less than 1 of chloroform, and 1 in 70 of ether; soluble in glacial acetic acid. A solution in alcohol is dextrorotatory. **Store** in airtight containers. Protect from light.

Adverse Effects and Precautions. As for Testosterone, p.1436.

Methandienone, given for prolonged periods, may cause jaundice and is contra-indicated in patients with liver disturbances.

Methandienone may enhance the effects of coumarin and indanedione anticoagulants and may increase plasma concentrations of oxyphenbutazone. Thyroid uptake of radio-iodine may be suppressed.

Anabolic steroids are abused by athletes.

The main possible dangers in the use of anabolic steroids by athletes for body building were impairment of liver function and carbohydrate metabolism, a decrease in the metabolism of hydrocortisone, increased blood-cholesterol concentrations, and testicular atrophy.— *Br. med. J.*, 1971, *1*, 104.

In 10 athletes taking methandienone 10 or 25 mg daily under double-blind conditions the following side-effects occurred: rise in blood pressure of 5 to 10 mmHg in 8 (2, both taking 10 mg, had rises from 130/85 to 150/110 and 120/70 to 160/90 respectively); prostatism in 1 taking 25 mg; acne in 2 (1 each taking 10 mg and 25 mg); raised serum alanine aminotransferase (SGPT) concentration in 1 taking 25 mg; reduction in libido in 1 taking 25 mg; and dizziness, headache, faintness, or lethargy in 4.— D. Freed *et al.* (letter), *Br. med. J.*, 1972, *3*, 761.

Anabolic steroids increased the hypoglycaemic effects of drugs.— *Med. Lett.*, 1973, *15*, 79.

Androgens and anabolic steroids could cause male-pattern baldness in genetically-disposed women; drugs involved included methandienone, drostanolone, and nandrolone phenylpropionate.— *Drug & Ther. Bull.*, 1978, *16*, 77.

Neoplasms. Carcinoma of the liver occurring in a patient given methandienone, see F. L. Johnson *et al.*, *Lancet*, 1972, *2*, 1273.

A benign liver adenoma developed in one patient after taking methandienone for 3 years.— L. Hernandez-Nieto *et al.*, *Cancer*, 1977, *40*, 1761.

Uses. Methandienone has actions similar to those of testosterone (see p.1436) but its anabolic properties are more pronounced than its androgenic effects. It produces increased retention of nitrogen, calcium, sodium, potassium, chloride, and phosphate, leading to an increase in skeletal weight, water retention, and increased growth of bone. It has little progestational activity.

Methandienone and other anabolic agents are given, in conjunction with an adequate diet, for conditions characterised by protein and bone wasting. However, their value has still to be proved. They are used as adjunctive therapy in the treatment of osteoporosis. Anabolic agents have produced improvement in some aplastic anaemias. They have been tried in the palliative treatment of inoperable neoplasms of the breast, especially where bone metastases have developed. Use for growth promotion in children is not generally recommended.

Methandienone is given by mouth, usually in initial doses of 5 mg daily for males and 2.5 mg daily for females, subsequently reduced to 2.5 mg every second or third day. For long-term treatment, intermittent therapy is usually adequate, courses of 6 weeks' duration being given at intervals of 2 to 4 weeks.

Anabolic steroids have a number of dangerous or undesirable side-effects. These risks far outweigh any possible slight benefit the drugs may confer in stimulating growth. They are of value in the treament of anaemia during haemodialysis, but their use in aplastic anaemia requires further study. Clinical benefit has not been shown in patients with osteoporosis, renal failure or general debility.— *Drug & Ther. Bull.*, 1979, *17*, 54.
See also under Nandrolone Phenylpropionate, p.1421.

Adjunct to athletic training. In a double-blind crossover trial in 13 male weightlifters, in training for at least a year and taking a high-protein diet, performance and body-weight were significantly increased by methandienone 10 or 25 mg daily for 6 weeks. Blood pressure increased slightly. Side-effects included acne, hypertension, headache and muzziness, urethritis, reduced sexual activity, and nausea.— D. L. J. Freed *et al.*, *Br. med. J.*, 1975, *2*, 471.

In a double-blind study in 11 athletic men in training treatment with methandienone 100 mg daily significantly increased body-weight and affected other parameters but performance was not improved.— G. R. Hervey *et al.*, *Lancet*, 1976, *2*, 699.

Anabolic steroids, usually methandienone or ethyloestrenol 15 to 25 mg daily, were taken by 20 male athletes for 18 months. No side-effects were observed. Weight increase ranged from 1.5 to 13.2% of initial body-weight. In 11 subjects tested for weight-lifting improvement there was a greater improvement when taking anabolic steroids than when not taking steroids.— A. J. Tahmindjis, *Med. J. Aust.*, 1976, *1*, 991. Comment *ibid.*, 984.

The use of anabolic steroids to enhance athletic performance was dangerous and should be discouraged.— *Med. Lett.*, 1976, *18*, 120. Criticism of the use of anabolic steroids by athletes; there was little objective evidence of the reported beneficial effect on athletic performance.— *Drug & Ther. Bull.*, 1977, *15*, 43.

See also under Adverse Effects and Precautions.

Anaemia. Review of 129 patients with aplastic anaemia; 75 were treated with androgens usually in addition to corticosteroids. Androgen therapy was considered useful and should be started as early as possible after diagnosis.— S. C. Tso *et al.*, *Q. J. Med.*, 1977, *46*, 513, per *Int. pharm. Abstr.*, 1979, *16*, 114.

A discussion of the limited use of androgens for anaemia associated with chronic renal failure.— *Br. med. J.*, 1977, *2*, 417.

Angio-oedema. Hereditary angioneurotic oedema in 2 patients had been relieved for 8 and 10 months respectively by methandienone 5 mg twice daily.— E. M. Saihan and R. P. Warin (letter), *Br. med. J.*, 1978, *1*, 367.

Contraception. In 15 healthy men given methandienone 15 mg daily for 2 months, sperm density and motility were decreased and the proportion of sperm anomalies increased; 3 men became azoospermic. Methandienone could be used as a contraceptive.— P. K. Holma, *Contraception*, 1977, *15*, 151.

Growth defects. Anabolic steroids could not replace growth hormone and they only produced growth in virilising doses which disproportionately advanced skeletal maturation, so that no final benefit was obtained.— D. Hubble, *Can. med. Ass. J.*, 1967, *97*, 1144.

Leprosy. In 14 patients with lepromatous leprosy suffering chronic lepra reaction and frequent episodes of erythema nodosum leprosum so that they were unable to tolerate sulphones or other antileprotic therapy, methandienone 25 mg intramuscularly was administered twice weekly for 2 weeks followed by 25 mg weekly for 12 weeks, their prior corticosteroid dosage being reduced concomitantly. All patients showed marked clinical improvement. In 6 the corticosteroids were discontinued and sulphone introduced without causing reactional episodes; in 4 the episodes were milder and less frequent, sulphone being tolerated in association with reduced corticosteroid therapy; the remaining 4 were also improved, tolerating sulphones in association with reduced corticosteroid therapy, but were lost to follow-up.— S. Choudhury *et al.*, *Lepr. Rev.*, 1977, *48*, 181.

Osteoporosis. A 26-month double-blind study in 26 patients with postmenopausal osteoporosis suggested that the use of methandienone prevented bone loss.— C. H. Chestnut *et al.*, *Metabolism*, 1977, *26*, 267. Comment and the view that the use of anabolic steroids in osteoporosis seems unjustified.— *Drug & Ther. Bull.*, 1979, *17*, 54.

Skin disorders. Response of psoriasis in 1 patient.— M. Sanderson (letter), *Lancet*, 1968, *1*, 1251. Absence of response in 14 of 15 patients.— A. Nyfors (letter), *Lancet*, 1969, *1*, 374.

Preparations

Methandienone Tablets *(B.P.)*. Tablets containing methandienone. Protect from light.

Methandrostenolone Tablets *(U.S.P.)*. Tablets containing methandienone. The *U.S.P.* requires 50% dissolution in 45 minutes. Store in airtight containers. Protect from light.

Proprietary Names

Andoredan *(Jap.)*; Danabol *(Canad.)*; Dianabol *(Austral., Belg., Denm., Fr., Ger., Spain, Swed., Switz., USA)*; Encephan *(Jap.)*; Lanabolin *(Switz.)*; Metabolina *(Ital.)*; Metanabol *(Pol.)*; Metastenol *(Ital.)*; Nerobol *(Hung.)*; Perbolin *(Ital.)*.

Methandienone was formerly marketed in Great Britain under the proprietary name Dianabol (*Ciba*).

9068-j

Methandriol. Methandriolum; Methylandrostendiolum; Methylandrostenediol. 17α-Methylandrost-5-ene-3β,17β-diol.

$C_{20}H_{32}O_2$=304.5.

CAS — 521-10-8.

Pharmacopoeias. In *Cz.*, *Rus.*, and *Turk.*

A white odourless crystalline powder. M.p. 199° to 206°. Practically **insoluble** in water; soluble in alcohol, ether, ethyl acetate, and methyl alcohol.

Adverse Effects and Precautions. As for Testosterone, p.1436.

Methandriol, given for prolonged periods, may cause jaundice and is contra-indicated in patients with liver disturbances.

Uses. Methandriol has anabolic and androgenic actions similar to those of methandienone (see above) and has been used for similar purposes. It is effective by mouth and has been given in doses of 50 to 150 mg daily.

Proprietary Names

Sinesex *(Wells, Ital.)*; Troformone *(Biomedica Foscama, Ital.)*.

Methandriol was formerly marketed in Great Britain under the proprietary name Stenediol (*Organon*).

9069-z

Methenolone Acetate. Metenolone Acetate; SH 567; SQ 16496. 1-Methyl-3-oxo-5α-androst-1-en-17β-yl acetate.

$C_{22}H_{32}O_3$=344.5.

CAS — 153-00-4 (methenolone); 434-05-9 (acetate).

Adverse Effects and Precautions. As for Testosterone, p.1436.

Uses. Methenolone acetate has anabolic and androgenic actions similar to those of methandienone (see above) and is used for similar purposes.

The usual adult dosage is 10 to 20 mg daily in divided doses by mouth.

Anaemia. Remission in 3 of 6 patients with pancytopenia, 2 of 4 with hypoplastic bone marrow, 1 of 5 with refractory anaemia, and 1 of 4 with myelofibrosis, after treatment with methenolone, usually 100 to 300 mg daily. Survival was not prolonged.— D. Lockner, *Acta med. scand.*, 1979, *205*, 97.

Eleven of 22 patients with aplastic anaemia responded to treatment with anabolic steroids, usually methenolone, and were alive after a mean follow-up of more than 4 years; 6 further patients showed a partial response. Five of the eleven had a relapse when the anabolic agent was withdrawn but 4 responded to further treatment. The usual initial dose of methenolone was 75 mg four times daily increased if needed to 150 mg four times daily. Treatment with anabolic agents was recommended for 2 to 3 months before bone-marrow transplantation was considered.— M. Van Hengstum *et al.*, *Br. J. Haemat.*, 1979, *41*, 323.

Proprietary Names

Primobolan *(Schering, Austral.; Schering, Belg.; Schering, Denm.; Schering, Fr.; Schering, Ger.; Schering, Norw.; Schering, S.Afr.; Schering, Spain; Schering, Swed.; Schering, Switz.)*; Primobolan S *(Schering, Ger.; Schering, Neth.; Schering, Switz.)*; Primobolan Depot *(see also under Methenolone Enanthate) (Schering, Switz.)*; Primobolan-S *(Schering, S.Afr.)*; Primonabol *(Schering, Arg.)*.

Methenolone acetate was formerly marketed in Great Britain under the proprietary name Primobolan (*Schering*).

9070-p

Methenolone Enanthate. Metenolone Enantate; Methenolone Oenanthate; NSC 64967; SH601; SQ 16374. 1-Methyl-3-oxo-5α-androst-1-en-17β-yl heptanoate.
$C_{27}H_{42}O_3$=414.6.

CAS — 303-42-4.

Methenolone enanthate has properties similar to those of methenolone acetate. Given intramuscularly in oil, it has a prolonged duration of effect. The usual adult dose is 100 mg every 2 to 4 weeks.

Proprietary Names
Primobolan Depot (see also under Methenolone Acetate) *(Schering, Austral.; Schering, Ger.; Schering, Ital.; Schering, Spain)*; Primobolan-Depot *(Schering, Belg.; Schering, Denm.; Schering, Fr.; Schering, Norw.)*.

Methenolone enanthate was formerly marketed in Great Britain under the proprietary name Primobolan Depot (*Schering*)..

9071-s

Methyltestosterone *(B.P., B.P. Vet., Eur. P., U.S.P.)*.

Methyltestost.; Methyltestosteronum. 17β-Hydroxy-17α-methylandrost-4-en-3-one.
$C_{20}H_{30}O_2$=302.5.

CAS — 58-18-4.

Pharmacopoeias. In *Aust., Br., Braz., Chin., Cz., Eur., Fr., Ger., Ind., Int., It., Jap., Jug., Mex., Neth., Nord., Pol., Roum., Rus., Span., Swiss, Turk.,* and *U.S.*

A white or slightly yellowish-white, odourless, tasteless, slightly hygroscopic, crystalline powder. M.p. 162° to 168°.

Practically **insoluble** in water; soluble 1 in 5 of alcohol, 1 in 10 of acetone, and 1 in 160 of arachis oil; freely soluble in chloroform and dioxan; soluble in methyl alcohol; sparingly soluble in fixed oils; slightly soluble in ether. A solution in alcohol is dextrorotatory. **Store** in airtight containers. Protect from light.

Solubility. The dissolution-rate of methyltestosterone was markedly increased when dispersed in macrogol 6000.— W. L. Chiou and S. Riegelman, *J. pharm. Sci.*, 1971, *60*, 1569.

Adverse Effects and Precautions. As for Testosterone, p.1436.

Methyltestosterone and other androgens or anabolic steroids with a 17α-alkyl substituent can produce a cholestatic hepatitis with jaundice especially when given in large doses or for prolonged periods. Creatinuria has also been reported. It is contra-indicated in patients with liver disturbances.

A report of very low plasma concentrations of high-density lipoprotein in a patient taking clofibrate and methyltestosterone. The effect was attributed to the androgen.— J. R. L. Masarei and W. J. Lynch (letter), *Lancet*, 1977, *2*, 827.

Effects on the liver. Peliosis hepatis developed in 7 patients on androgenic-anabolic steroid therapy, usually for bone-marrow stimulation, for periods of 2 to 27 months. Hepatic injury was a contributory cause of death in each case.— S. A. Bagheri *et al., Ann. intern. Med.*, 1974, *81*, 610.

Elevated serum-aspartate-aminotransferase (SGOT) concentrations were found in 19 of 60 patients (42 female transexuals and 18 impotent males) who had been taking methyltestosterone 50 mg thrice daily by mouth for between 2 weeks and 5 years. Liver scans in 52 patients showed abnormalities in 33. Liver biopsies from 11 patients showed histological changes in each specimen; there was evidence of early peliosis hepatis. One patient had a liver adenoma and one additional patient, not in the survey, had rupture of the liver and peliosis hepatis. The hepatotoxicity appeared to be related to the duration of methyltestosterone use.— D. Westaby *et al., Lancet*, 1977, *2*, 261.

Neoplasms of the liver. Case reports of hepatocellular carcinoma associated with methyltestosterone.— J. T. Henderson *et al.* (letter), *Lancet*, 1973, *1*, 934; G. C. Farrell *et al., lancet*, 1975, *1*, 430; M. A. Goodman and A. M. J. Laden, *Med. J. Aust.*, 1977, *1*, 220.

Reports of other liver tumours.— P. R. Boyd and G. J. Mark, *Cancer*, 1977, *40*, 1765; G. B. Coombes *et al., Br. J. Surg.*, 1978, *65*, 869.

Interactions. For the effect of methyltestosterone on imipramine, see Imipramine Hydrochloride, p.120.

Absorption and Fate. Methyltestosterone is absorbed from the gastro-intestinal tract and from the oral mucosa. It is more resistant to metabolism than testosterone (see p.1436).

Maximum serum concentrations of methyltestosterone of 24 to 39 ng per ml were reached within 1 to 2 hours of administration of a 10-mg tablet to 2 volunteers. The biological half-life was about 2.7 hours.— D. Alkalay *et al., J. pharm. Sci.*, 1972, *61*, 1746. See also D. Alkalay *et al., J. clin. Pharmac.*, 1973, *13*, 142.

Uses. Methyltestosterone has actions and uses similar to those of testosterone (see p.1436). It is effective when given by mouth; its effect is increased about 2-fold when given sublingually. When given by mouth it has one-third to one-quarter of the androgenic activity of the same weight of testosterone propionate administered intramuscularly.

In the male, methyltestosterone is generally used for maintenance therapy after the full androgenic effect has been produced by intramuscular administration of testosterone propionate or of some other ester of testosterone.

The dosage required varies considerably; suggested doses (for oral administration) are: for males, 25 to 50 mg daily; for females, 5 to 20 mg daily; for postpartum breast engorgement, 80 mg daily; for inoperable neoplasms of the breast in postmenopausal women, up to 200 mg daily.

Anaemia. For a comment on the role of androgen therapy in aplastic anaemia and anaemia during dialysis, see under methandienone (p.1419).

Angio-oedema. Methyltestosterone 10 mg sublingually significantly reduced the frequency and appeared to reduce the severity of attacks of angioneurotic oedema in 4 male patients. Concentrations of plasma C4 protein, depressed as a result of inherited biochemical abnormality, rose in all patients during treatment, in 3 to normal values. One patient developed prostatitis.— A. L. Sheffer *et al., Ann. intern. Med.*, 1977, *86*, 306.

Further references: R. M. Morris Owen (letter), *Lancet*, 1969, *1*, 574.

Impotence. Methyltestosterone 2.5 mg with thyroid 10 mg produced a favourable response in 78% of 100 patients with partial or complete impotence in a double-blind comparison with placebo which produced a similar response in 40%.— T. Jakobovits, *Fert. Steril.*, 1970, *21*, 32, per *Clin. Med.*, 1970, *77* (Oct.), 33.

Preparations

Methyltestosterone Capsules *(U.S.P.)*. Capsules containing methyltestosterone. The *U.S.P.* requires 60% dissolution in 30 minutes.

Methyltestosterone Tablets *(B.P.)*. Tablets containing methyltestosterone. Protect from light.

Methyltestosterone Tablets *(U.S.P.)*. Tablets containing methyltestosterone.

Proprietary Preparations

Plex-Hormone Tablets *(Consolidated Chemicals, UK)*. Tablets each containing methyltestosterone 5 mg, deoxycortone acetate 500 µg, ethinyloestradiol 2 µg, and tocopheryl acetate 5 mg. See also Plex-Hormone Injection, p.1438.

Virormone-Oral *(Paines & Byrne, UK)*. Methyltestosterone, available as tablets of 5, 10, 25, and 50 mg.

Other Proprietary Names

Android, Oreton Methyl, Testred, Virilon *(all USA)*; Glosso-Stérandryl *(Fr.)*; Mesteron *(Pol.)*; Metandren *(Canad., USA)*; Neo-Hombreol (see also under Testosterone Propionate) *(Belg., Neth.)*; Neohombreol M *(Swed., USA)*; Orchisterone (see also under Testosterone Propionate) *(Ital.)*; Perandren (see also under Testosterone Propionate) *(Austral.)*; Testin *(Norw.)*; Testomet *(Austral.)*; Testoviron (see also under Testosterone Propionate) *(Arg., Austral., Ital., Spain, Switz.)*; Testovis (see also under Testosterone Propionate) *(Ital.)*.

Other proprietary preparations containing methyltestosterone with an oestrogen are described under Ethinyloestradiol (see p.1412)..

Methyltestosterone was also formerly marketed in Great Britain under the proprietary name Perandren (*Ciba*).

9072-w

Nandrolone Cyclohexylpropionate. 3-Oxoestr-4-en-17β-yl 3-cyclohexylpropionate.
$C_{27}H_{40}O_3$=412.6.

CAS — 434-22-0 (nandrolone); 912-57-2 (cyclohexylpropionate).

Nandrolone cyclohexylpropionate is a long-acting anabolic agent which has been used similarly to nandrolone phenylpropionate and which is now used in veterinary medicine.

Proprietary Names
Fherbolico *(Fher, Spain)*.

9073-e

Nandrolone Decanoate *(B.P., U.S.P.)*.

Nortestosterone Decylate. 3-Oxoestr-4-en-17β-yl decanoate.
$C_{28}H_{44}O_3$=428.7.

CAS — 360-70-3.

Pharmacopoeias. In *Br.* and *U.S.*

A white to creamy-white crystalline powder, odourless or with a faint characteristic odour. M.p. 33° to 37°.

Practically **insoluble** in water; soluble 1 in 1 of alcohol; freely soluble in chloroform, ether, fixed oils, and esters; soluble in acetone, dioxan, and methyl alcohol. A solution in dioxan is dextrorotatory. Solutions in oils or ethyl oleate are **sterilised** by maintaining at 150° for 1 hour. The *B.P.* specifies **storage** at 2° to 10° in an atmosphere of nitrogen. The *U.S.P.* specifies storage at 2° to 8° in airtight containers. Protect from light.

Adverse Effects and Precautions. As for Testosterone, p.1436.

Uses. Nandrolone decanoate has anabolic and androgenic actions similar to those of methandienone (see p.1419) and is used for similar purposes. It has a longer duration of action than nandrolone phenylpropionate. The usual intramuscular dose for adults is 25 to 100 mg every 3 weeks. Higher doses may be necessary in severe conditions such as malignant neoplasm of the breast, and refractory anaemias; up to 100 to 200 mg may be required weekly.

Anaemia. In a double-blind study of 21 patients with chronic renal failure and associated anaemia, maintained on haemodialysis, nandrolone decanoate 100 mg weekly for 5 months improved the haematological condition of 17 patients. Blood transfusion requirements decreased during administration of the androgen.— E. D. Hendler *et al., New Engl. J. Med.*, 1974, *291*, 1046.

In a comparative study of 27 chronic haemodialysis patients, 9 (8 men, 1 woman) received nandrolone decanoate 200 mg intramuscularly weekly and 18 (10 men, 8 women) acted as controls. All patients received folic acid daily, and iron dextran and blood transfusions were given as required. Results indicated that nandrolone decanoate 200 mg weekly in conjunction with other haematinics had no effect on the red cell 2,3-diphosphoglycerate concentration, and no sustained effect over a period of 5 months on the packed cell volume of male chronic haemodialysis patients.— J. Goodman and A. N. Bessman, *Clin. Pharmac. Ther.*, 1975, *17*, 167.

Further references: J. S. Williams *et al., Archs intern. Med.*, 1974, *134*, 289, per *J. Am. med. Ass.*, 1974, *229*, 1120; B. D. Doane *et al., Archs intern. Med.*, 1975, *135*, 872, per *J. Am. med. Ass.*, 1975, *233*, 290.

Preparations

Nandrolone Decanoate Injection *(B.P.)*. A sterile solution of nandrolone decanoate in ethyl oleate or other suitable ester, in a suitable fixed oil, or in a mixture of these. Sterilised by maintaining at 150° for 1 hour. Protect from light. For intramuscular use only.

Nandrolone Decanoate Injection *(U.S.P.)*. A sterile solution of nandrolone decanoate in sesame oil; it contains a suitable preservative. Protect from light.

Deca-Durabolin *(Organon, UK)*. Nandrolone decanoate in oily solution for intramuscular injection containing 25 or 50 mg per ml in ampoules of 1 ml or in Orgaject disposable syringes of 1 ml, and 100 mg per ml in ampoules of 1 ml. (Also available as Deca-Durabolin in *Arg., Austral., Belg., Canad., Denm., Fr., Ger., Ital., Neth., S.Afr., Spain, Switz., USA*).

Other Proprietary Names

Anabolin LA-100 *(USA)*; Androlone-D *(USA)*; Deca-Durabol *(Norw., Swed.)*; Hybolin Decanoate *(USA)*; Methybol-Depot *(Switz.)*.

9074-l

Nandrolone Phenylpropionate *(B.P., B.P. Vet.)*.

Nandrolone Phenylprop.; Nandrolone Phenpropionate *(U.S.P.)*; 19-Norandrostenolone Phenylpropionate; Nortestosteronum Phenylpropionicum. 3-Oxoestr-4-en-17β-yl 3-phenylpropionate.

$C_{27}H_{34}O_3$=406.6.

CAS — 62-90-8.

Pharmacopoeias. In *Br., Chin., Cz.,* and *U.S.*

A white to creamy-white crystalline powder with a slight characteristic odour. M.p. 95° to 99°. Practically **insoluble** in water; soluble 1 in 20 of alcohol; soluble in chloroform, dioxan, ethyl oleate, and fixed oils. A solution in dioxan is dextrorotatory. Solutions in oils or ethyl oleate are **sterilised** by maintaining at 150° for 1 hour. **Store** in airtight containers. Protect from light.

Adverse Effects and Precautions. As for Testosterone, p.1436.

Uses. Nandrolone phenylpropionate has anabolic and androgenic actions similar to those of methandienone (see p.1419) and is used for similar purposes. It is not active when given by mouth and is administered by intramuscular injection as an oily solution; the effect lasts 7 to 10 days. The usual dose is 25 to 50 mg weekly. Higher dosage may be necessary in refractory anaemias and in malignant neoplasm of the breast.

Anaemia. Results of a prospective, randomised, double-blind study involving 21 evaluable patients, 7 with aplastic anaemia, 6 with myelofibrosis, and 8 with refractory anaemia indicated that administration of nandrolone phenylpropionate had no advantage over placebo. Of 13 patients receiving nandrolone phenylpropionate 3 responded and of 8 receiving placebo 3 responded; these responses did not correlate with the type of anaemia. Nandrolone phenylpropionate therapy appeared to be relatively free from serious toxicity with no evidence of hepatotoxicity in the total of 18 patients who eventually received the active drug; the development of Di Guglielmo's syndrome in 1 patient, evidence of acute myelogenous lymphoma involving the bone marrow within 2 years of completion of the study in another, and death from lymphoma involving the bone marrow in a third, suggested that reports linking androgen therapy with subsequent development of leukaemia should be further investigated.— R. F. Branda *et al.*, *Archs intern. Med.*, 1977, *137*, 65.

Preparations

Nandrolone Phenylpropionate Injection *(B.P.)*. Nandrolone Phenylprop. Inj. A sterile solution of nandrolone phenylpropionate in ethyl oleate or other suitable ester, in a suitable fixed oil, or in a mixture of these. Sterilised by maintaining at 150° for 1 hour. Protect from light. For intramuscular injection only.

Nandrolone Phenpropionate Injection *(U.S.P.)*. A sterile solution of nandrolone phenylpropionate in a suitable oil. Protect from light.

Durabolin *(Organon, UK)*. Nandrolone phenylpropionate, available as an injection containing 25 mg per ml, in ampoules of 1 ml and Orgaject disposable syringes of 1 ml; and 50 mg per ml in Orgaject disposable syringes of 1 ml. (Also available as Durabolin in *Austral., Belg., Canad., Denm., Fr., Ital., Neth., S.Afr., Spain, Switz., USA*).

Other Proprietary Names

Ital.—Anticatabolin, Norandrol, Sintabolin, Strabolene, Superbolin; *Norw.*—Durabol; *Spain*—Activin, Norandros; *USA*—Androlone, Hybolin Improved, Nandrolin.

Proprietary Names of some other Nandrolone Esters

Anador *(Fr.)*; Anadur *(Belg., Denm., Ger., Neth., Norw., Swed., Switz.)* (both nandrolone hexyloxyphenylpropionate, $C_{33}H_{46}O_4$ = 506.7); Dynabolon *(Fr., Ital.)* (nandrolone undecanoate, $C_{29}H_{46}O_3$ = 442.7); Anabolicus *(Spain)*; Nortesto *(Ital.)* (both nandrolone propionate, $C_{21}H_{30}O_3$ = 330.5).

9075-y

Norethandrolone *(B.P.)*.

17β-Hydroxy-19-nor-17α-pregn-4-en-3-one.

$C_{20}H_{30}O_2$=302.5.

CAS — 52-78-8.

Pharmacopoeias. In *Br.* and *It.*

A white odourless crystalline powder. M.p. about 135°.

Practically **insoluble** in water; soluble 1 in 8 of alcohol, 1 in 5 of chloroform, and 1 in 3 of methyl alcohol; very soluble in acetone; soluble in ether. A solution in methyl alcohol is dextrorotatory. **Protect** from light.

Adverse Effects. As for Testosterone, p.1436.

Because of the progestational activity of norethandrolone, amenorrhoea and uterine bleeding may result when treatment is stopped. Jaundice may develop occasionally.

A 74-year-old man was given norethandrolone 30 mg daily for 6 months. He died in hepatic coma after severe alterations of liver function which autopsy showed to be due to intrahepatic cholestasis. Anabolic steroids should be restricted in the elderly.— E. F. Gilbert *et al.*, *J. Am. med. Ass.*, 1963, *185*, 538.

Precautions. As for Testosterone, p.1436.

Norethandrolone should be used with caution in patients with impaired liver function.

It may enhance the effects of anticoagulants of the coumarin type.

Uses. Norethandrolone has anabolic and androgenic actions similar to those of methandienone (see p.1419) and is used for similar purposes. Norethandrolone has moderate progestational activity.

Norethandrolone is given by mouth in a dose of 10 to 30 mg daily.

Infertility. Norethandrolone 10 mg every 12 hours was given for 10 weeks or longer to infertile men and testosterone enanthate 200 mg was added on the first day, third week, and sixth week. A rise in the number of spermatozoa and a decrease in abnormal forms occurred following 110 of 163 of the courses.— M. J. Rowley and C. G. Heller, *Fert. Steril.*, 1972, *23*, 498, per *Int. pharm. Abstr.*, 1973, *10*, 59.

Preparations

Norethandrolone Tablets *(B.P.)*. Tablets containing norethandrolone. Protect from light.

Nilevar *(Searle, UK)*. Norethandrolone, available as tablets of 10 mg. (Also available as Nilevar in *Canad., Fr.*).

9076-j

Norethisterone *(B.P.)*.

Norethister.; Norethindrone *(U.S.P.)*; Ethinylnortestosterone; Norpregneninolone; Noretisterone. 17β-Hydroxy-19-nor-17α-pregn-4-en-20-yn-3-one.

$C_{20}H_{26}O_2$=298.4.

CAS — 68-22-4.

Pharmacopoeias. In *Br., Braz., Chin., Cz., It., Jap., Turk.,* and *U.S.*

A white or creamy-white odourless crystalline powder with a slightly bitter taste. M.p. 201° to 208°.

Practically **insoluble** in water; soluble 1 in 150 of alcohol, 1 in 80 of acetone, 1 in 30 of chloroform, and 1 in 5 of pyridine; soluble in dioxan; slightly soluble in ether; practically insoluble in fixed oils. A solution in chloroform is laevorotatory. **Protect** from light.

Adverse Effects. As for Progesterone, p.1431.

See also Adverse Effects of Oral Contraceptives, p.1402.

Doses of more than 15 mg given daily during pregnancy may produce virilisation of the foetus (for the possibility of other adverse effects on the foetus, see below under Pregnancy and the Neonate). Androgenic side-effects include hirsutism, deepening of the voice, and acne. The prolonged use of norethisterone may cause reversible disturbances of liver function.

The use of progestational agents such as norethisterone with oestrogens such as ethinyloestradiol or mestranol for contraception and other purposes is associated with effects (see p.1402) which can be related to their oestrogenic, progestational, or androgenic properties.

Effects on blood. The effects of norethisterone and mestranol (Norinyl-1 and Ortho-Novin) on blood-clotting factors were studied in 91 women. Significant rises in factor VII and factor X levels were found with both low-dose preparations from the 3rd month onwards and these changes did not appear to be dose-dependent since Norinyl-1 was one-half the strength of Ortho-Novin.— L. Poller *et al.*, *Br. med. J.*, 1968, *3*, 218. In 16 women who had not previously taken oral contraceptives, there was no evidence of adverse factors affecting clotting when given norethisterone 350 µg daily for 6 cycles; there was a tendency to reduced coagulability. There was no adverse effect on clotting in 13 women who were given norethisterone after previously taking chlormadinone acetate for at least 2 years, or in 6 women given norethisterone post partum. In 28 women given norethisterone after previously taking oestrogen/progestogen contraceptives there were significant and persistent prolongations of clotting times and improvements in platelet function.— *idem*, 1972, *4*, 391.

Effects on carbohydrate metabolism. Blood-glucose and plasma-insulin concentrations increased significantly after 6 months' treatment with norethisterone 350 µg daily in a study of 53 women. Plasma-triglyceride concentrations decreased to the same extent as in the post-partum period and did not correlate with plasma insulin.— W. N. Spellacy *et al.*, *Fert. Steril.*, 1973, *24*, 419, per *Int. pharm. Abstr.*, 1974, *11*, 105. See also *idem*, *Obstet. Gynec.*, 1975, *46*, 560, per *J. Am. med. Ass.*, 1976, *235*, 1073.

Pregnancy and the neonate. *Ectopic pregnancy.* There were 4 ectopic pregnancies in 3 years in women using low-dose progestogen oral contraceptives (norethisterone 300 µg) for an estimated 1000 woman-years.— P. Liukko and R. Erkkola (letter), *Br. med. J.*, 1976, *2*, 1257. Further reports: J. Bonnar (letter), *Lancet*, 1974, *1*, 170; *idem* (letter), *Br. med. J.*, 1974, *1*, 287; K. M. Huntington (letter), *Lancet*, 1974, *1*, 360; R. Corcoran and R. Howard (letter), *Lancet*, 1977, *1*, 98.

Effects on the foetus. Thirty-five pregnant women, given norethisterone usually in doses of 10 to 40 mg daily to prevent threatened abortion, gave birth to female infants showing masculinisation as also did 1 woman who received norethynodrel. Similarly, an examination of paediatric records and other sources showed that ethisterone had, though less frequently and severely, also been associated with masculinisation of female infants born to mothers given it to avert abortion.— L. Wilkins, *J. Am. med. Ass.*, 1960, *172*, 1028.

Of 80 infants with congenital hypospadias 5 were born to mothers who had taken progestogens during the first trimester of pregnancy. A causal relationship was suspected. Two had received medroxyprogesterone and hydroxyprogesterone hexanoate respectively for threatened abortion, and 3 had received progestogens as pregnancy tests—norethisterone, norethisterone and ethinyloestradiol, and probably either norethisterone or medroxyprogesterone respectively.— D. Aarskog, *Acta paediat. scand.*, 1970, *Suppl.*, 203.

See also under Adverse Effects of Sex Hormones, p.1401.

Precautions. As for Progesterone, p.1431.

It should be given with care to patients with liver disturbances. For precautions for oral contraceptives containing norethisterone, see p.1405.

Studies in 7 healthy women given norethisterone 350 µg daily for 3 weeks suggested that norethisterone inhibited hepatic microsomal function.— B. Field *et al.*, *Clin. Pharmac. Ther.*, 1979, *25*, 196.

Absorption and Fate. Norethisterone is absorbed from the gastro-intestinal tract and its effects last for at least 24 hours. When injected, it is detectable in the plasma after 2 days and is not completely excreted in the urine after 5 days.

The pharmacokinetics of norethisterone and norethisterone acetate.— D. J. Back *et al.*, *Br. J. clin. Pharmac.*, 1977, *4*, 729P. See also D. J. Back *et al.*, *CLin. Pharmac. Ther.*, 1978, *24*, 439 and 448.

Pregnancy and the neonate. In 5 lactating women taking norethisterone 350 µg daily the concentration of norethisterone in breast milk was about one-tenth of that in plasma.— B. N. Saxena *et al.*, *Contraception*, 1977, *16*, 605.

Uses. Norethisterone has progestational actions similar to those of progesterone (see p.1431) but is a more potent inhibitor of ovulation and in addition has weak oestrogenic and androgenic properties.

The main uses of norethisterone are in the treatment of amenorrhoea, functional uterine bleeding, endometriosis, and for contraception. It is active by mouth and is often administered in conjunction with an oestrogen such as ethinyloestradiol or mestranol.

In the treatment of primary and secondary amenorrhoea, 5 to 20 mg of norethisterone is given daily from the 5th to 25th day of the cycle. Alternatively, norethisterone may be administered in a similar dose following initial treatment with oestrogen. Withdrawal bleeding usually occurs 1 to 3 days after discontinuing treatment.

In the treatment of functional uterine bleeding, norethisterone is given in doses of 15 mg daily for 10 days.

In endometriosis the dosage is 10 or 15 mg daily for about 6 months; this may be temporarily increased to 20 to 25 mg daily, to control breakthrough bleeding.

To delay or prevent menstruation, it is usually given in doses of 15 mg daily. It has also been given to reduce premenstrual tension and to relieve dysmenorrhoea.

Norethisterone in a dose of 350 µg is given daily in a continuous regimen as an oral contraceptive. This form of contraception may reduce some of the hazards associated with the 'combination' type but the failure-rate is higher and menstrual irregularities are more frequent. Norethisterone 0.5 to 2 mg is also given as a 'combination' oral contraceptive with ethinyloestradiol 35 µg or mestranol 50 to 100 µg daily from the 5th to the 25th day of the first treated cycle, and thereafter repeated after intervals of 7 days for succeeding cycles. (See also Oral Contraceptives, p.1402).

Norethisterone is also used as the acetate and the enanthate (see below).

Contraception. Reviews of the use of norethisterone given alone as an oral contraceptive: *Med. Lett.*, 1973, *15*, 45; R. N. Brogden *et al.*, *Drugs*, 1973, *6*, 169.

The effect, in 5 women over 4 cycles, of an oral contraceptive containing norethisterone 1 mg and mestranol 50 µg (Ortho-Novin 1/50) on urinary concentrations of luteinising hormone, oestrogens, pregnanediol, and pregnanetriol.— M. Elstein *et al.*, *Br. med. J.*, 1974, *1*, 11.

A study of the use of norethisterone 350 µg daily as a contraceptive agent in a group of 70 women.— J. C. Whyte and C. S. Pooransingh, *Can. med. Ass. J.*, 1973, *109*, 295.

Menstrual suppression. Norethisterone 5 mg daily by mouth was given to 118 intellectually retarded women for periods of 2 to 30 months to suppress menstruation. Bleeding occurred in 14% of the women and was more common in the younger age groups. In 3 patients bleeding was severe.— D. R. Roxburgh and M. J. West, *Med. J. Aust.*, 1973, *2*, 310.

Osteoporosis. For the use of norethisterone in osteoporosis, see Calcium Salts, p.621.

See also under Oestradiol, p.1427 and Mestranol, p.1418.

Preparations

Norethindrone Tablets *(U.S.P.)*. Tablets containing norethisterone.

Norethindrone and Ethinyl Estradiol Tablets *(U.S.P.)*. Tablets containing norethisterone and ethinyloestradiol.

Norethindrone and Mestranol Tablets *(U.S.P.)*. Tablets containing norethisterone and mestranol.

Norethisterone Tablets *(B.P.)*. Tablets containing norethisterone. Protect from light.

Proprietary Preparations

Binovum *(Ortho-Cilag, UK)*. Packs containing 7 white tablets each containing norethisterone 0.5 mg and ethinyloestradiol 35 µg and 14 peach tablets each containing norethisterone 1 mg and ethinyloestradiol 35 µg. For use as an oral contraceptive. *Dose.* One white tablet daily starting on the first day of the first treated cycle followed by one peach tablet daily; the course is repeated after 7 tablet-free days.

Brevinor *(Syntex, UK)*. Tablets each containing norethisterone 500 µg and ethinyloestradiol 35 µg. For use as an oral contraceptive. *Dose.* 1 tablet daily for 21 days starting on the 5th day of the first treated cycle and after 7 tablet-free days for succeeding cycles. (Also available as Brevinor in *Austral.*, *S.Afr.*).

Micronor *(Ortho-Cilag, UK)*. Norethisterone, available as tablets of 350 µg. (Also available as Micronor in *Austral.*, *Canad.*, *USA*).

Noriday *(Syntex, UK)*. Norethisterone, available as tablets of 350 µg. (Also available as Noriday in *Austral.*, *S.Afr.*).

Norimin *(Syntex, UK)*. Tablets each containing norethisterone 1 mg and ethinyloestradiol 35 µg. For use as an oral contraceptive. *Dose.* 1 tablet daily for 21 days starting on the 5th day of the first treated cycle and after 7 tablet-free days for succeeding cycles.

Norinyl-1 *(Syntex, UK)*. Tablets each containing norethisterone 1 mg and mestranol 50 µg. For use as an oral contraceptive. *Dose.* 1 tablet daily for 21 days starting on the 5th day of the first treated cycle and after 7 tablet-free days for succeeding cycles. (Also available as Norinyl-1 in *Austral.*, *S.Afr.*).

Ortho-Novin 1/50 *(Ortho-Cilag, UK)*. Tablets each containing norethisterone 1 mg and mestranol 50 µg. For use as an oral contraceptive. *Dose.* 1 tablet daily for 21 days starting on the 5th day of the first treated cycle and after 7 tablet-free days for succeeding cycles.

Ovysmen *(Ortho-Cilag, UK)*. Tablets each containing norethisterone 500 µg and ethinyloestradiol 35 µg. For use as an oral contraceptive. *Dose.* 1 tablet daily for 21 days starting on the 5th day of the first treated cycle, and after 7 tablet-free days for succeeding cycles.

Primolut N *(Schering, UK)*. Norethisterone, available as tablets of 5 mg. (Also available as Primolut N in *Austral.*, *Neth.*, *Norw.*, *S.Afr.*, *Switz.*).

Utovlan *(Syntex, UK)*. Norethisterone, available as scored tablets of 5 mg.

Another proprietary preparation containing norethisterone and mestranol is described under Mestranol, (see p.1418).

Other Proprietary Names

Conceplan micro *(Ger.)*; Conludag *(Norw.)*; Gesta Plan *(Denm.)*; Micronovum *(Ger., S.Afr., Switz.)*; Mini-Pe *(Denm., Swed.)*; Norfor *(Fr.)*; Norgestin *(Ital.)*; Norluten *(Fr.)*; Norlutin *(Canad., USA)*; Nor-QD *(USA)*; Primolut *(Denm.)*; Proluteasi *(Ital.)*.

Other Proprietary Names of Norethisterone with Ethinyloestradiol

Brevicon *(Canad., Denm., Norw., USA)*; Brevinor 1 *(Austral.)*; Conceplan 21 mite *(Ger.)*; Modicon *(Austral., Neth., USA)*; Neocon *(Neth.)*; Norinyl 1+35 *(USA)*; Orthonett Novum *(Denm., Swed.)*; Ortho-Novum 1/35 *(USA)*; Ovcon-35, Ovcon-50 *(both USA)*; Ovysmen 0.5/35 *(Ger., Switz.)*; Ovysmen 1/35 *(Ger., Switz.)*.

Other Proprietary Names of Norethisterone with Mestranol

Conceplan 21, Conceplan 28 *(both Ger.)*; Conlumin *(Denm., Swed.)*; Norinyl *(Spain)*; Norinyl-2 *(Austral., Canad., USA)*; Norinyl 1+50 *(Canad., USA)*; Norinyl 1+80 *(Canad., USA)*; Orthonett *(Norw.)*; Ortho-Novin 2 mg *(S.Afr.)*; Ortho-Novum *(Switz.)*; Ortho-Novum 0.5 mg *(Canad.)*; Ortho-Novum 1/50 *(Austral., Belg., Canad., Ger., Ital., Neth., Switz., USA)*; Ortho-Novum 1/80 *(Austral., Belg., Canad., Ger., Neth., S.Afr., Switz., USA)*; Ortho-Novum 2 mg *(Austral., Canad., Ger., Ital., USA)*; Ortho-Novum 5 mg *(Canad.)*; Plan mite *(Denm.)*; Regovar *(Ital.)*.

For other proprietary names of mestranol and mestranol with norethisterone, see under Mestranol, p.1418.

A preparation containing norethisterone 1 mg and mestranol 50 µg was formerly marketed in Great Britain under the proprietary name Norinyl 1/28 (*Syntex*). A preparation containing norethisterone 2 mg and mestranol 100 µg was formerly marketed in Great Britain under the proprietary name Norinyl-2 (*Syntex*).

9077-z

Norethisterone Acetate *(B.P.)*. Norethindrone Acetate *(U.S.P.)*. 3-Oxo-19-nor-17α-pregn-4-en-20-yn-17β-yl acetate.

$C_{22}H_{28}O_3$ = 340.5.

CAS — 51-98-9.

Pharmacopoeias. In *Br.* and *U.S.*

A white or creamy-white, odourless, crystalline powder with a slightly bitter taste. M.p. about 163°.

Practically **insoluble** in water; soluble 1 in 10 to 12.5 of alcohol, 1 in 4 of acetone, 1 in less than 1 of chloroform, 1 in 2 of dioxan, and 1 in 18 of ether. A solution in dioxan is laevorotatory. **Protect** from light.

Adverse Effects and Precautions. As for Norethisterone, p.1421, which is about half as potent.

See also Adverse Effects and Precautions of Oral Contraceptives, p.1402.

Local tissue response to a silicone implant containing norethisterone acetate.— S. Jeyaseelan *et al.*, *Contraception*, 1977, *15*, 39, per *Int. pharm. Abstr.*, 1977, *14*, 1031. Endometrial histology.— D. Takkar *et al.*, *Contraception*, 1978, *17*, 103, per *Int. pharm. Abstr.*, 1978, *15*, 732.

Effects on serum lipids. Serum lipids and serum-lipoprotein fractions were measured in 8 women, aged 18 to 37 years, before and during 1 year's use of oral contraceptive tablets containing 4 mg of norethisterone acetate and 50 µg of ethinyloestradiol. After using the tablets for a year a significant rise in serum lipids, especially in low-density lipoproteins, was apparent. The effect was considered to be either indicative of androgen-like activity or of inhibition of endogenous oestrogen production.— M. Aurell *et al.*, *Lancet*, 1966, *1*, 291. Criticisms.— S. N. Herschberg (letter), *ibid.*, 816. A reply.— M. Aurell *et al.* (letter), *ibid.*

For a report of norethisterone acetate reducing plasma-triglyceride concentrations, see Uses.

Jaundice. There were 6 cases of jaundice among 107 patients with breast cancer treated with norethisterone acetate. The jaundice which was of an obstructive type was reversible when norethisterone was withdrawn.— A. O. Langlands and W. M. C. Martin (letter), *Lancet*, 1975, *1*, 584.

For further reports of jaundice associated with norethisterone acetate, see Extra Pharmacopoeia, 26th Edn, p. 1670.

Pregnancy and the neonate. The use of hormonal pregnancy tests appeared to be the only significant difference in drug treatment during pregnancy in women who gave birth to infants with meningomyelocele or hydrocephalus and those who gave birth to normal infants. Hormonal pregnancy tests, which usually contained either norethisterone acetate 10 mg and ethinyloestradiol 20 µg (Primodos) or ethisterone 50 mg and ethinyloestradiol 50 µg (Amenorone Forte), were taken by 19% of the mothers who gave birth to infants with congenital malformation and by 4% of those who gave birth to healthy infants.— I. Gal *et al.* (letter), *Nature*, 1967, *216*, 83. See also I. Gal (letter), *ibid.*, 1972, *240*, 241.

See also under Adverse Effects of Sex Hormones, p.1401.

Uses. Norethisterone acetate has the actions and uses of norethisterone (see p.1422) but is effective in about half the dosage.

In the treatment of primary and secondary amenorrhoea and in the treatment of functional uterine bleeding, daily doses of 2.5 to 10 mg have been given. In the treatment of endometriosis, an initial daily dose of 5 mg is increased every 2 weeks by 2.5 mg daily to a maintenance dose of 15 mg daily. It has been given in doses of 30 to 60 mg daily by mouth in the treatment of inoperable malignant neoplasms of the breast or as an adjunct to surgery or radiotherapy.

For contraception, it is given in doses of 0.5 to 4 mg, in each case in conjunction with ethinyloestradiol, from the 5th to the 25th day of the first treated cycle and thereafter repeated after intervals of 7 days for succeeding cycles (see also Oral Contraceptives, p.1402).

Contraception. A silicone implant containing norethisterone acetate 40 mg, implanted subdermally, provided serum concentrations of at least 800 pg per ml for up to

2 months; such concentrations had contraceptive effectiveness but did not suppress ovulation.— S. G. Hillier *et al.*, *Contraception*, 1977, *15*, 473, per *Int. pharm. Abstr.*, 1977, *14*, 1089. Minimal effects on lactation.— U. Seth *et al.*, *Contraception*, 1977, *16*, 383, per *Int. pharm. Abstr.*, 1978, *15*, 419. Efficacy in 876 women.— D. Takkar *et al.*, *Contraception*, 1978, *17*, 341, per *Int. pharm. Abstr.*, 1978, *15*, 927. Effect on pituitary-gonadal function.— S. A. Rahman *et al.*, *Contraception*, 1977, *16*, 487, per *Int. pharm. Abstr.*, 1978, *15*, 886.

Effect on serum lipids. In a study of 26 patients with various types of hyperlipoproteinaemia and 5 control subjects, norethisterone acetate 5 mg daily for 8 to 12 days or given to 2 outpatients on the 2nd day of their menstrual cycle for 28-day periods reduced the plasma-triglyceride concentrations in the 5 women and, to a lesser extent, in the 4 men with type V hyperlipoproteinaemia; it also caused a concurrent increase in post-heparin lipolytic activity. Triglyceride concentrations were reduced in 9 of 13 patients with types III and IV hyperlipoproteinaemia, most of whom had an increase in post-heparin lipolytic activity and 8 had increased triglyceride lipase activity. Female control subjects had a slight decrease in triglycerides and moderate increases in post-heparin lipolytic and triglyceride lipase activity. Male controls had no consistent response.— C. J. Glueck *et al.*, *Ann. intern. Med.*, 1971, *75*, 345. See also *idem*, *Lancet*, 1969, *1*, 1290.

Neoplasm of the breast. Norethisterone acetate produced a 41% objective remission in 154 patients with advanced breast cancer. The response in those with mainly local disease was 83% but it was poor in those with bone or visceral metastases. There was a response in 60% of those with slowly progressing disease compared with 21% in those with rapidly evolving neoplasms and disease-free periods of less than 2 years. Also 48% of those over 55 years responded compared with 27% of younger patients.— G. A. Edelstyn, *Cancer*, 1973, *32*, 1317, per *Int. pharm. Abstr.*, 1974, *11*, 630.

Skin disorders. Use in scleroderma.— A. J. Barnett *et al.*, *Australas. J. Derm.*, 1975, *16*, 45.

Preparations

Norethindrone Acetate and Ethinyl Estradiol Tablets *(U.S.P.)*. Tablets containing norethisterone acetate and ethinyloestradiol.

Norethindrone Acetate Tablets *(U.S.P.)*. Tablets containing norethisterone acetate.

Proprietary Preparations

Anovlar 21 *(Schering, UK)*. Tablets each containing norethisterone acetate 4 mg and ethinyloestradiol 50 µg. For gynaecological disorders and for use as an oral contraceptive. *Dose*. 1 tablet daily for 21 days starting on the 5th day of the first treated cycle, and after 7 tablet-free days for succeeding cycles. (Also available as Anovlar 21 in *Arg., Ger., S.Afr., Switz.*).

Controvlar *(Schering, UK)*. Tablets each containing norethisterone acetate 3 mg and ethinyloestradiol 50 µg. For menstrual disorders. *Dose*. 1 tablet daily for 21 days commencing on the 5th day of the first treated cycle, and after 7 tablet-free days for succeeding cycles.

Gynovlar 21 *(Schering, UK)*. Tablets each containing norethisterone acetate 3 mg and ethinyloestradiol 50 µg. For gynaecological disorders and for use as an oral contraceptive. *Dose*. 1 tablet daily for 21 days starting on the 5th day of the first treated cycle, and after 7 tablet-free days for succeeding cycles. (Also available as Gynovlar 21 in *Neth., S.Afr., Switz.*).

Loestrin 20 *(Parke, Davis, UK)*. Tablets each containing norethisterone acetate 1 mg and ethinyloestradiol 20 µg. For use as an oral contraceptive. *Dose*. 1 tablet daily for 21 days starting on the 5th day of the first treated cycle, and after 7 tablet-free days for succeeding cycles.

Minovlar *(Schering, UK)*. Tablets each containing norethisterone acetate 1 mg and ethinyloestradiol 50 µg. For use as an oral contraceptive. *Dose*. 1 tablet daily for 21 days starting on the 5th day of the first treated cycle, and after 7 tablet-free days for succeeding cycles. (Also available as Minovlar in *Austral.*).

Minovlar ED *(Schering, UK)*. Packs of 21 yellow tablets each containing norethisterone acetate 1 mg and ethinyloestradiol 50 µg, and 7 white inert tablets. For use as a continuous dosage oral contraceptive. *Dose*. 1 yellow tablet daily for 21 days commencing on the 1st day of the first treated cycle, then 1 white tablet daily for 7 days; the course is then repeated without a break. (Also available as Minovlar ED in *Austral., S.Afr.*).

Norlestrin *(Parke, Davis, UK)*. Tablets each containing norethisterone acetate 2.5 mg and ethinyloestradiol 50 µg. For gynaecological disorders and for use as an oral contraceptive. *Dose*. 1 tablet daily for 21 days starting on the 5th day of the first treated cycle, and after 7 tablet-free days for succeeding cycles. (Also available as Norlestrin in *Austral., Spain*).

Orlest 21 *(Parke, Davis, UK)*. Tablets each containing norethisterone acetate 1 mg and ethinyloestradiol 50 µg. For use as an oral contraceptive. *Dose*. 1 tablet daily for 21 days starting on the 5th day of the first treated cycle, and after 7 tablet-free days for succeeding cycles.

SH 420 *(Schering, UK)*. Norethisterone acetate, available as scored tablets of 10 mg. (Also available as SH 420 in *Austral., S.Afr.*).

Other Proprietary Names

Milligynon *(Fr.)*; Norlutate *(Canad., USA)*; Primolut Nor *(Arg., Austral., Belg., Fr., Ger., Ital., Spain, Swed., Switz.)*.

Other Proprietary Names of Norethisterone Acetate with Ethinyloestradiol

Anovlar *(Austral., Denm., Fr., Ital., Swed.)*; Anovlar mite *(Swed.)*; Econ *(Denm.)*; Etalontin *(Switz.)*; Etalontin 21 *(Ger.)*; Gynophase, Gynovlane *(both Fr.)*; Gynovlar *(Austral., Denm.)*; Loestrin 1/20 *(USA)*; Loestrin 1.5/30 *(Canad., USA)*; Logest 1.5/30, Logest 1/50 *(both Canad.)*; Milli Anovlar *(Fr.)*; Minestrin 1/20 *(Canad.)*; Miniphase *(Fr.)*; Neorlest 21 *(Ger.)*; Norlestrin *(Arg.)*; Norlestrin 1/50 *(Canad., USA)*; Norlestrin 2.5/50 *(Canad., USA)*; Orlest *(Austral., Switz.)*; Orlest 1 mg *(Belg., Neth.)*; Orlest 2.5 mg *(Belg., Neth.)*; Orlest 21 *(Ger.)*; Trentovlane *(Fr.)*.

Norethisterone acetate was also formerly marketed in Great Britain under the proprietary name Norlutin-A (Parke, Davis). A preparation containing norethisterone acetate and ethinyloestradiol was also formerly marketed under the proprietary name Primodos *(Schering)*.

9078-c

Norethisterone Enanthate. Norethisterone Heptanoate. 3-Oxo-19-nor-17α-pregn-4-en-20-yn-17β-yl heptanoate.

$C_{27}H_{38}O_3$=410.6.

CAS — 3836-23-5.

Norethisterone enanthate is a long-acting derivative of norethisterone which has been used similarly to medroxyprogesterone acetate (see p.1416) as a 'progestogen-only' contraceptive. The usual dose is 200 mg intramuscularly. An unacceptable pregnancy-rate has been reported after injections given every 3 months; study continues with injections given every 2 months.

Absence of effect of norethisterone enanthate on blood clotting and glucose tolerance in long-term users; a significant reduction in the high-density-lipoprotein fraction was demonstrated.— G. Howard *et al.*, *Lancet*, 1982, *1*, 423.

Contraception. A multicentre trial showed an unacceptable pregnancy-rate in patients given norethisterone enanthate 200 mg 3-monthly by injection.— G. Benagiano *et al.*, *Contraception*, 1977, *15*, 513, per *Int. pharm. Abstr.*, 1977, *14*, 1239. There was a higher incidence of menstrual abnormality with medroxyprogesterone acetate.— *idem*, 1978, *17*, 395, per *Int. pharm. Abstr.*, 1978, *15*, 1066.

No pregnancies occurred in 295 women treated with norethisterone enanthate for up to 18 months. The initial dose was 200 mg as an oily solution given intramuscularly during a menstrual period or before discharge from hospital after delivery or termination of pregnancy; 3 further injections were given 8-weekly; thereafter injections were given every 12 weeks. Drug-related discontinuations at 12 months were because of hypertension (2 patients); minor side-effects including weight gain, bloating, and various aches and pains (23); and menstrual disturbances (20).— O. F. Giwa-Osagie *et al.*, *Br. med. J.*, 1978, *1*, 1660. Criticism of the finding of no pregnancies and of very low termination-rates for amenorrhoea, and mention of contrary findings in the WHO ongoing study.— R. H. Gray (letter), *ibid.*, 1979, *1*, 343.

Ovulation within 60 days in 2 of 10 women given a single injection of norethisterone enanthate 200 mg.— K. Fotherby *et al.*, *Contraception*, 1978, *18*, 535, per *Int. pharm. Abstr.*, 1979, *16*, 465.

Proprietary Names

Noristerat *(Schering, Denm.; Schering, Ger.)*; Nur-Isterate *(Schering, S.Afr.)*.

9079-k

Norethynodrel *(B.P., U.S.P.)*. 17β-Hydroxy-19-nor-17α-pregn-5(10)-en-20-yn-3-one.

$C_{20}H_{26}O_2$=298.4.

CAS — 68-23-5.

Pharmacopoeias. In *Br., Turk.*, and *U.S.*

A white or almost white, odourless, crystalline powder. M.p. about 174° to 184° with a range of not more than 3°. The *B.P.* specifies that it contains not more than 1% of mestranol, the percentage present being stated on the label. The *U.S.P.* specifies not more than 2% of norethisterone. Practically **insoluble** in water; soluble 1 in 30 of alcohol, 1 in 7 of chloroform, and 1 in 60 of ether; soluble in acetone; very slightly soluble in light petroleum. A solution in dioxan is dextrorotatory. **Protect** from light.

Adverse Effects. As for Progesterone, p.1431, and Norethisterone, p.1421.

Thrombo-embolic disorders have occurred following the use of norethynodrel.

See also Adverse Effects of Oral Contraceptives, p.1402.

Exercise-induced abnormalities of the ST segment were increased in 12 of 13 patients treated for 2 weeks with norethynodrel and mestranol.— M. D. Jaffe, *Br. Heart J.*, 1976, *38*, 1299, per *J. Am. med. Ass.*, 1977, *237*, 1023.

Candidiasis. Vulvovaginal candidiasis occurred in 13 patients who had received norethynodrel with mestranol. Local treatment was not often effective and in 3 patients discontinuance of oral contraceptives was necessary for cure.— P. S. Porter and J. S. Lyle, *Archs Derm.*, 1966, *93*, 402.

For a study demonstrating no association between oral contraceptive use and candidiasis, see p.1403.

Precautions. As for Progesterone, p.1431.

Norethynodrel should be used with care in patients with liver disturbances.

For precautions for oral contraceptives containing norethynodrel, see p.1405.

Absorption and Fate. Norethynodrel is absorbed from the gastro-intestinal tract.

Metabolism. Norethynodrel is rapidly metabolised, in part to norethisterone.— C. E. Cook *et al.*, *J. Pharmac. exp. Ther.*, 1972, *183*, 197.

Further references: D. S. Layne *et al.*, *Biochem. Pharmac.*, 1963, *12*, 905.

Uses. Norethynodrel is a progestational agent which has actions and uses similar to those of progesterone (see p.1431). The mestranol present in some commercial samples confers slight oestrogenic activity. It is active by mouth and is given in conjunction with an oestrogen such as mestranol.

In the treatment of functional uterine bleeding and other menstrual disorders, it is given in a dosage of 5 to 10 mg daily usually from the 5th to the 24th day of the cycle; 20 to 30 mg may be required for the initial control of bleeding. In the treatment of endometriosis the usual initial dose is 5 to 10 mg daily increased to 20 mg daily and maintained for at least 6 to 9 months. Doses of up to 40 mg may be given to control breakthrough bleeding.

For contraception, it is usually given in doses of 2.5 or 5 mg with 100 or 75 µg respectively of mestranol from the 5th to the 24th day of each cycle (see Oral Contraceptives, p.1402).

There was an excellent objective response in 54 of 110 patients with fibrocystic disease of the breast who were treated with norethynodrel 5 or 10 mg with mestranol thrice daily. A further 22 patients achieved some objective remission. Weight gain was the most frequent side-effect.— I. M. Ariel, *Am. J. Obstet. Gynec.*, 1973, *117*, 453, per *J. Am. med. Ass.*, 1974, *227*, 684.

Familial haemorrhagic telangiectasia. Control in 9 patients by norethynodrel with mestranol.— H. C. Flessa and H. I. Glueck, *Archs Otolar.*, 1977, *103*, 148.

Proprietary Names of Norethynodrel with Mestranol

Conovid-E *(Searle, Austral.; Searle, S.Afr.)*; Elan

(Valeas, Ital.); Enavid *(Searle, Neth.)*; Enavid-E *(Searle, Arg.; Searle, Neth.)*; Enovid *(Searle, Canad.)*; Enovid-E *(Searle, Canad.; Searle, USA)*; Enovid 5 mg *(Searle, USA)*; Enovid-E 21 *(Searle, USA)*; Kontrazeptivum 63-ratiopharm *(Ratiopharm, Ger.)*; Novinol-21 *(Desbergers, Canad.)*; Novinol-28 *(Desbergers, Canad.)*; Ovarion *(Fher, Spain)*; Ovulen Novum *(Vita, Spain)*.

Preparations containing norethynodrel with mestranol were formerly marketed in Great Britain under the proprietary names Conovid, Conovid E, Enavid, and Enavid E *(Searle)*.

9080-w

Norgestrel *(U.S.P.)*. DL-Norgestrel; *dl*-Norgestrel; Wy 3707. (±)-13-Ethyl-17β-hydroxy-18,19-dinor-17α-pregn-4-en-20-yn-3-one. $C_{21}H_{28}O_2$=312.5.

CAS — 6533-00-2.

Pharmacopoeias. In *Chin.*, *Nord.*, and *U.S.*

A white or almost white, almost odourless crystalline powder. M.p. 205° to 212° with a range of not more than 4°. Practically **insoluble** in water; soluble 1 in 120 of alcohol, 1 in 15 of chloroform, and 1 in 400 of ether; soluble in dioxan.

9081-e

Levonorgestrel. D-Norgestrel; Wy-5104. The (−)-isomer of norgestrel.

CAS — 797-63-7.

NOTE. The name Dexnorgestrel has been used.

Pharmacopoeias. In *Nord.*

Adverse Effects and Precautions. As for Progesterone, p.1431.

See also under Oral Contraceptives, p.1402.

Norgestrel and levonorgestrel are contra-indicated in patients with markedly impaired liver function.

A sudden onset of moderate to severe papulopustular acne was noted in about 20 patients taking norgestrel in an oral contraceptive preparation, and was considered to be due to norgestrel being an androgen-dominant progestogen.— R. K. Woodward, *Archs Derm.*, 1974, *110*, 812.

A comparative study of 110 healthy women who had taken norgestrel 250 µg and ethinyloestradiol 50 µg (Neogynona) for 1 to 8 years, and 35 healthy women of similar age not taking an oral contraceptive. Results supported observations that oral contraception with this preparation increases platelet aggregation.— M. Aranda *et al.* (letter), *Lancet*, 1979, *2*, 308. Similar results in 30 women taking oral contraceptives containing oestrogens, though the measured values varied from those reported.— A. Duncan (letter), *ibid.*, 631.

Haemoglobin concentrations increased after 1 year of use of subdermal implants of levonorgestrel or norgestrienone despite increased bleeding; there was no change in blood pressure and a small increase in weight. Acne and other skin conditions increased to the same degree as in women using a copper intra-uterine device.— E. Coutinho *et al.*, *Contraception*, 1978, *18*, 335, per *Int. pharm. Abstr.*, 1979, *16*, 311.

Effect on metabolism. In 71 women given norgestrel 75 µg daily for one year there was no significant increase in weight or triglyceride or cholesterol concentrations. Blood-glucose and plasma-insulin concentrations were significantly elevated.— W. N. Spellacy *et al.*, *Am. J. Obstet. Gynec.*, 1976, *125*, 984, per *Int. pharm. Abstr.*, 1977, *14*, 138.

Increased body-weight and concentrations of total lipids and β-lipoproteins in 26 women given levonorgestrel 250 µg and ethinyloestradiol 50 µg for 6 months; there was no significant change in α-lipoproteins or pre-β-lipoproteins.— H. J. van der Steeg and J. C. Pronk, *Contraception*, 1977, *16*, 29, per *Int. pharm. Abstr.*, 1978, *15*, 477.

Pregnancy and the neonate. *Ectopic pregnancy.* There were 7 ectopic pregnancies in 3 years in women using low-dose progestogen oral contraceptives (norgestrel 30 µg) for an estimated 1600 woman-years.— P. Liukko and R. Erkkola (letter), *Br. med. J.*, 1976, *2*, 1257.

Effects on the foetus. A 23-year-old woman who had taken norgestrel and ethinyloestradiol for the first 3 months of pregnancy gave birth to an infant with a tracheo-oesophageal fistula.— O. Frost, *Br. med. J.*, 1976, *2*, 978.

Inoperable hepatoblastoma in a 7-month-old male infant might have been associated with ingestion of norgestrel 30 µg daily by the mother during the first 3 months of pregnancy.— J. Otten *et al.* (letter), *New Engl. J. Med.*, 1977, *297*, 222.

Absorption and Fate. Norgestrel and levonorgestrel are absorbed from the gastro-intestinal tract. Metabolites are excreted in the urine and faeces as glucuronide and sulphate conjugates.

After administration of norgestrel the major metabolite isolated from urine was 3α,5β-tetrahydronorgestrel which was present entirely as the D-isomer.— D. C. DeJongh *et al.*, *Steroids*, 1968, *11*, 649, per R. J. Warren and K. Fotherby, *Arzneimittel-Forsch.*, 1975, *25*, 964.

A single dose of D- or L-norgestrel 1 mg by mouth was given to 3 healthy males. Plasma concentrations were measured at 2, 8, and 24 hours and compared with those obtained after administration of norethisterone and DL-norgestrel in doses of 1 mg in a previous study. Mean plasma concentrations at 2, 8, and 24 hours were: D-norgestrel, 8.6, 1.2, 0.25 ng per ml; L-norgestrel, 8.1, 3.8, 1.3 ng per ml; DL-norgestrel, 11.1, 3.3, 1.1 ng per ml; norethisterone, 5.3, 1.1, 0.13 ng per ml. Half-lives for the periods 2 to 8 hours and 8 to 24 hours were: D-norgestrel (2 and 7 hours); norethisterone (2.7 and 5.4 hours); L-norgestrel (5.5 and 10.4 hours); DL-norgestrel (3.4 and 10.3 hours).— R. J. Warren and K. Fotherby, *Arzneimittel-Forsch.*, 1975, *25*, 964.

Gradual increases in the plasma concentrations of norgestrel when given with ethinyloestradiol might be due to increased concentrations of sex-hormone-binding globulin.— E. Weiner *et al.*, *Contraception*, 1976, *14*, 563, per *Int. pharm. Abstr.*, 1977, *14*, 1253. See also S. Nilsson *et al.*, *Contraception*, 1977, *15*, 87, per *Int. pharm. Abstr.*, 1977, *14*, 1002; A. Victor and E. D. B. Johansson, *Contraception*, 1977, *16*, 115, per *Int. pharm. Abstr.*, 1978, *15*, 314.

Serum concentrations of D-norgestrel, LH, FSH, oestradiol, and progesterone after the ingestion of norgestrel with and without oestrogen.— P. F. Brenner *et al.*, *Am. J. Obstet. Gynec.*, 1977, *129*, 133.

The concentration of D-norgestrel in milk was about 15% of that in plasma; it could not be detected in the milk of women taking only 30 µg daily.— S. Nilsson *et al.*, *Am. J. Obstet. Gynec.*, 1977, *129*, 178.

Plasma concentrations of levonorgestrel in women using an intra-uterine contraceptive device releasing levonorgestrel.— C. G. Nilsson *et al.*, *Contraception*, 1978, *17*, 569, per *Int. pharm. Abstr.*, 1979, *16*, 124.

Further references: M. Humpel *et al.*, *Contraception*, 1977, *16*, 199, per *Int. pharm. Abstr.*, 1978, *15*, 283; S. Nilsson *et al.*, *Am. J. Obstet. Gynec.*, 1977, *129*, 178, per *Int. pharm. Abstr.*, 1979, *16*, 232; M. Humpel *et al.*, *Contraception*, 1978, *17*, 207, per *Int. pharm. Abstr.*, 1978, *15*, 1186.

Uses. Norgestrel is a progestational agent with actions similar to those of progesterone (see p.1431). It is more potent as an inhibitor of ovulation than norethisterone (see p.1422) and has androgenic activity.

Levonorgestrel is the active isomer; norgestrel, the racemate, has therefore half the potency of levonorgestrel.

It is used with ethinyloestradiol 30 to 50 µg for contraception or for the control of menstrual disorders and endometriosis. Doses usually range from 150 to 250 µg of levonorgestrel or 300 to 500 µg of norgestrel, with ethinyloestradiol for 21 days commencing on the 5th day of the first cycle and thereafter repeated after an interval of 7 days for succeeding cycles. A dose of 30 µg of levonorgestrel or 75 µg of norgestrel is given daily on a continuous basis as a 'progestogen-only' contraceptive (see also Oral Contraceptives, p.1402).

Contraception. Norgestrel was given in a dosage of 75 µg daily to 144 women for up to 30 months. The incidence of pregnancy was 2 per 100 woman-years, or 1.3 if patient failure was excluded. Withdrawals from the trial totalled 94, 57 being connected with the method and 33 being related to cycle length which was very variable (6 to 88 days); more than 20% of cycles were of 17 days or less. Suspected deep leg thrombosis in 1 patient was not confirmed; 4 other patients withdrew because of pain over superficial veins in the calf or leg. In 37 patients studied, blood concentrations of globulin and cholesterol were significantly reduced. Sperm penetrability of cervical mucus was significantly reduced and was probably related to its increased content of sialic acid. Urinary excretion of pregnanediol was significantly decreased and was consistent with an absence of anovulatory effect.— P. Eckstein *et al.*, *Br. med. J.*, 1972, *3*, 195.

In 1085 women who took norgestrel 500 µg and ethinyloestradiol 30 µg for 21 days a month for 7323 cycles, the pregnancy-rate was 0.16 per 100 woman-years. In 623 women (5062 cycles) assessed, cycle length was 28 ±3 days in 98.2%; side-effects were amenorrhoea in 2.24% of cycles, 'spotting' in 8.8% (falling from 14.5% in the first cycle to less than 6%), and breakthrough bleeding in 5.2% (falling from 9.3% to 1.7%). Menstrual loss appeared to be reduced. Systolic blood pressure rose by more than 30 mmHg in 11 patients and fell by more than 30 mmHg in 9 patients. Withdrawal for medical reasons in 14% was considered a satisfactory level of acceptability.— P. G. T. Bye and M. Elstein, *Br. med. J.*, 1973, *2*, 389.

From clinical and biochemical investigations in 68 healthy young women given Biphasil, a preparation of varied composition so that they received levonorgestrel 50 µg with ethinyloestradiol 50 µg daily for 11 days, followed by levonorgestrel 125 µg with ethinyloestradiol 50 µg daily for the next 10 days, for 6 cycles, good cycle control was reported; breakthrough bleeding occurred in 1.2% of cycles, spotting in 2.8%, and amenorrhoea in 0.5%. No serious side-effects were reported.— M. H. Briggs and M. Briggs, *Curr. med. Res. Opinion*, 1977, *5*, 213.

Further references: R. N. Brogden *et al.*, *Drugs*, 1973, *6*, 169; P. Dionne and F. Vickerson, *Curr. ther. Res.*, 1974, *16*, 281; N. A. M. Bergstein, *Clin. Ther.*, 1977, *1*, 26, per *Int. pharm. Abstr.*, 1978, *15*, 466; J. N. Sartoretto *et al.*, *Contraception*, 1977, *15*, 563, per *Int. pharm. Abstr.*, 1977, *14*, 1238.

Implants. In a double-blind multicentre study 492 women received subdermal implants of levonorgestrel (about 180 mg) and 498 received norgestrienone. Pregnancy-rates at 12 months were 0.6 and 3.5% respectively. The expected effectiveness (3 to 5 years) warranted further study.— E. Coutinho *et al.*, *Contraception*, 1978, *18*, 315.

Intra-uterine device. References to the development of intra-uterine devices containing norgestrel or levonorgestrel.— C. G. Nilsson *et al.*, *Contraception*, 1976, *13*, 503, per *Int. pharm. Abstr.*, 1977, *14*, 1183; C. G. Nilsson and T. Luukkainen, *Contraception*, 1977, *15*, 295, per *Int. pharm. Abstr.*, 1977, *14*, 1190; C. G. Nilsson, *Contraception*, 1977, *15*, 379, per *Int. pharm. Abstr.*, 1977, *14*, 1079; C. G. Nilsson and P. Lahteenmaki, *Contraception*, 1977, *15*, 389, per *Int. pharm. Abstr.*, 1977, *14*, 1047; T. Luukkainen and C. G. Nilsson, *Contraception*, 1978, *18*, 451, per *Int. pharm. Abstr.*, 1979, *16*, 206.

The use of vaginal rings containing norgestrel: A. Victor and E. D. B. Johansson, *Contraception*, 1977, *16*, 137, per *Int. pharm. Abstr.*, 1978, *15*, 321.

A favourable report of the use of contraceptive vaginal rings containing norgestrel and oestriol; a longer study was planned.— D. R. Mishell *et al.*, *Am. J. Obstet. Gynec.*, 1978, *130*, 55.

Postcoital contraception. A single dose of levonorgestrel varying from 150 to 400 µg was evaluated for postcoital contraception in 4631 women treated within 3 hours of intercourse. Effectiveness was poor with the small dose but 400 µg produced a general failure-rate of 3.5 and a corrected rate of 1.7 per 100 woman-years. The main side-effects were shortening of the cycle and breakthrough bleeding.— E. Kesseru *et al.*, *Contraception*, 1973, *7*, 367, per *Int. pharm. Abstr.*, 1974, *11*, 25.

One of 608 women became pregnant after unprotected intercourse, after receiving norgestrel 2 mg and ethinyloestradiol 200 µg, in 2 divided doses, within 72 hours of exposure.— A. A. Yuzpe and W. J. Lancee, *Fert. Steril.*, 1977, *28*, 932.

Endorsement by the International Planned Parenthood Federation of the use of postcoital oral contraception after a single, unexpected, and unprotected act of sexual intercourse. The recommended regimen is ethinyloestradiol 100 µg and levonorgestrel 50 µg, followed by the same dose 12 hours later, the first dose to be taken within 72 hours of exposure to pregnancy; if the pregnancy continued there was no evidence that the regimen would cause teratogenesis. Alternatively, a copper-containing IUD could be fitted within 5 days of unprotected mid-cycle intercourse.— *Chem. Drugg.*, 1981, 955.

Neoplasm of the prostate. In 5 healthy men given

norgestrel 500 µg and ethinyloestradiol 50 µg daily for 9 days serum-testosterone concentrations fell rapidly, reaching 8% of the initial value by the 9th day. Norgestrel merited trial in the treatment of neoplasm of the prostate.— J. M. Kjeld *et al.*, *Br. med. J.*, 1977, *2*, 1261.

Preparations

Norgestrel and Ethinyl Estradiol Tablets *(U.S.P.)*. Tablets containing norgestrel and ethinyloestradiol.

Norgestrel Tablets *(U.S.P.)*. Tablets containing norgestrel.

Proprietary Preparations of Norgestrel or Levonorgestrel

Eugynon 30 *(Schering, UK)*. Tablets each containing levonorgestrel 250 µg and ethinyloestradiol 30 µg. **Eugynon 50.** Tablets each containing norgestrel 500 µg and ethinyloestradiol 50 µg. For use as oral contraceptives. *Dose.* 1 tablet daily for 21 days starting on the 5th day of the first treated cycle, and after 7 tablet-free days for succeeding cycles.

Logynon (known in some countries as Triquilar) *(Schering, UK)*. Packs of 6 brown tablets each containing levonorgestrel 50 µg and ethinyloestradiol 30 µg, 5 white tablets (distinctively marked) each containing levonorgestrel 75 µg and ethinyloestradiol 40 µg, and 10 yellow tablets containing levonorgestrel 125 µg and ethinyloestradiol 30 µg. For use as an oral contraceptive. **Logynon ED**. Packs contain in addition 7 white inert tablets (distinctively marked); for continuous dosage. *Dose.* Logynon: 1 brown tablet daily for 6 days starting on the 1st day of the first treated cycle, then 1 white (distinctively marked) tablet for 5 days, and 1 yellow tablet for 10 days; the course is repeated after 7 tablet-free days. Logynon ED: the same dosage sequence is followed, except that 1 white (distinctively marked) tablet is taken daily for 7 days in place of the tablet-free days.

Details of a possible failure of Logynon and mention of 7 further unintended pregnancies with triphasic oral contraceptives reported to the Committee on Safety of Medicines: 5 with Logynon and 2 with Trinordiol.— R. A. Fay, *Br. med. J.*, 1982, *284*, 17.

Microgynon 30 *(Schering, UK)*. Tablets each containing levonorgestrel 150 µg and ethinyloestradiol 30 µg. For use as an oral contraceptive. *Dose.* 1 tablet daily for 21 days, commencing on the 5th day of the first treated cycle, and after 7 tablet-free days for succeeding cycles. (Also available as Microgynon 30 in *Austral., Belg., Neth., Switz.*).

Microval *(Wyeth, UK)*. Levonorgestrel, available as tablets of 30 µg. (Also available as Microval in *Belg., Denm., Fr.*).

Neogest *(Schering, UK)*. Norgestrel, available as tablets of 75 µg (equivalent to levonorgestrel 37.5 µg).

Norgeston *(Schering, UK)*. Levonorgestrel, available as tablets of 30 µg.

Ovran *(Wyeth, UK)*. Tablets each containing levonorgestrel 250 µg and ethinyloestradiol 50 µg. **Ovran 30.** Tablets each containing levonorgestrel 250 µg and ethinyloestradiol 30 µg. **Ovranette**. Tablets each containing levonorgestrel 150 µg and ethinyloestradiol 30 µg. For use as oral contraceptives. *Dose.* 1 tablet daily for 21 days commencing on the 5th day of the first treated cycle, and after 7 tablet-free days for succeeding cycles.

Trinordiol *(Wyeth, UK)*. Packs of 6 brown tablets each containing levonorgestrel 50 µg and ethinyloestradiol 30 µg, 5 white tablets each containing levonorgestrel 75 µg and ethinyloestradiol 40 µg, and 10 yellow tablets each containing levonorgestrel 125 µg and ethinyloestradiol 30 µg. For use as an oral contraceptive. *Dose.* 1 brown tablet daily for 6 days starting on the 1st day of the first treated cycle, then 1 white tablet for 5 days, and 1 yellow tablet for 10 days; the course is repeated after 7 tablet-free days.

For mention of unintended pregnancies in women taking triphasic oral contraceptives, including Trinordiol, see under Logynon, above.

Other Proprietary Names of Norgestrel or Levonorgestrel

Austral.—Microlut 28, Microval-28; *Belg.*—Microlut; *Denm.*—Microluton; *Ger.*—Microlut, Mikro-30; *Norw.*—Microluton; *Swed.*—Follistrel, Microluton; *Switz.*—Microlut; *USA*—Ovrette.

Other Proprietary Names of Norgestrel or Levonorgestrel with Ethinyloestradiol

Arg.—Duoluton, Eugynon, Eugynon-CD, Microgynon, Neogynon, Neogynon CD, Nordette, Nordiol, Ovral; *Austral.*— Biphasil, Biphasil 28, Duoluton, Eugynon, Eugynon ED, Microgynon 30ED, Microgynon 50, Microgynon 50 ED, Neogynon, Neogynon ED, Nordette, Nordiol, Ovral, Sequilar ED; *Belg.*—Binordiol, Eugynon, Microgynon 50, Neogynon 21, Neo-Stediril, Sequilar, Stediril, Stediril-d; *Canad.*— Min-Ovral, Min-Ovral 28, Ovral, Ovral-28; *Denm.*—Binordiol, Eugynon, Gentrol, Gynatrol, Microgyn, Neogentrol, Neogynon, Sequilarum; *Fr.*—Adepal, Minidril, Stédiril; *Ger.*—Ediwal 21, Eugynon 21, Eugynon 28, Microgynon 21, Microgynon 28, Neogynon 21, Neogynon 28, Neo-Stediril, Perikursal 21, Sequilar 21, Sequilar 28, Stediril, Stediril-d, Stediril-d 30/150, Trinordiol 21; *Ital.*—Bivlar, Egogyn 30, Eugynon, Eugynon 28, Evanor, Evanor-d, Microgynon, Novogyn 21, Ovranet; *Neth.*—Binordiol, Eugynon, Microgynon 50, Neogynon 21, Neogynon 28, Neo-Stediril, Sequilar, Stediril, Stediril-d, Stediril-d 150/30; *Norw.*—Eugynon, Follimin, Microgynon; *S.Afr.*—Biphasil, Nordette-28, Nordiol, Normovlar ED, Ovral; *Spain*—Microgynon, Neogynona, Ovoplex; *Swed.*—Follimin, Follinett, Neovlar 21, Neovlar 28, Neovletta, Primovlar 21, Regunon, Sequilarum; *Switz.*— Binordiol, Eugynon, Microgynon 50, Neogynon 21, Neogynon 28, Neo-Stediril, Sequilar 21, Sequilar 28, Stediril, Stediril-D; *USA*—Lo/Ovral, Ovral.

9082-l

Normethandrone. Methylestrenolone; Methylnortestosterone; Normethandrolone. 17β-Hydroxy-17α-methylestr-4-en-3-one.

$C_{19}H_{28}O_2$=288.4.

CAS — 514-61-4.

Normethandrone has been given in the treatment of functional uterine bleeding and amenorrhoea. It is sometimes given with an oestrogen.

Proprietary Names

Orga-Steron *(Organon, Belg.; Organon, Neth.)*.

9083-y

Oestradiol *(B.P.C. 1968)*. Beta-oestradiol; Dihydrofolliculine; Dihydrotheelin; Dihydroxyoestrin; Estradiol *(U.S.P.)*. Estra-1,3,5(10)-triene-3,17β-diol.

$C_{18}H_{24}O_2$=272.4.

CAS — 50-28-2.

Pharmacopoeias. In *Aust., Jap., Mex., Span., Swiss, Turk.*, and *U.S.*

White or creamy-white, odourless, tasteless, hygroscopic crystals or crystalline powder. M.p. 173° to 179°.

Practically **insoluble** in water; soluble 1 in 28 of alcohol, 1 in 17 of acetone, 1 in 435 of chloroform, and 1 in 150 of ether; soluble in dioxan and solutions of alkali hydroxides; sparingly soluble in fixed oils. A solution in dioxan is dextrorotatory. Solutions in oil are **sterilised** by maintaining at 150° for 1 hour. **Store** in airtight containers. Protect from light.

A study suggesting that the use of a coprecipitate of oestradiol with povidone may increase the systemic availability of oestradiol.— D. E. Resetarits *et al.*, *Int. J. Pharmaceut.*, 1979, *2*, 113.

Adverse Effects. Oestradiol and other oestrogens give rise to side-effects which are related to their oestrogenic and their general metabolic effects. There may be undesirable uterine growth, proliferation, and withdrawal bleeding or there may be amenorrhoea. Gynaecomastia is the main side-effect in the male. There may also be sodium retention and oedema, nitrogen retention and weight gain, tenderness of the breasts, alterations in liver function, jaundice, depression, headache, and dizziness. Large doses may cause premature closure of the epiphyses. Hypercalcaemia has been reported especially when oestrogens are employed in metastatic malignant conditions. Most oestrogens produce dose-related nausea and vomiting.

Skin reactions include chloasma, rashes, and urticaria. Erythema multiforme has been reported.

Low doses of oestrogens may stimulate malignant neoplasms; high doses, however, can indirectly suppress neoplastic growth. A number of studies have shown an association between the use of oestrogens and the development of endometrial hyperplasia and cancer. This association may be prevented if progestogens are given cyclically with oestrogens. A role in precipitating breast cancer is not established. For reports of vaginal adenocarcinoma in the offspring of women given oestrogenic substances during pregnancy, see Stilboestrol, p.1434.

For the adverse effects of oestrogens used in oral contraceptives, including their effects on the incidence of thrombo-embolic conditions, see Adverse Effects of Oral Contraceptives, p.1402.

Effects on the gall-bladder. A brief discussion on the gallstone-producing capacity of oestrogen.— *Lancet*, 1977, *2*, 177. See also L. J. Bennion and S. M. Grundy, *New Engl. J. Med.*, 1978, *299*, 1221.

Neoplasms. *Breast.* Absence of association.— Casagrande J. *et al.*, *J. natn. Cancer Inst.*, 1976, *56*, 839, per *Int. pharm. Abstr.*, 1977, *14*, 17; P. E. Sartwell *et al.*, *J. natn. Cancer Inst.*, 1977, *59*, 1589.

From a study of 147 patients with breast cancer and twice that number of controls, the risk factor of developing breast cancer after high total oestrogen dosage was considered to be 2.5 compared with non-users of oestrogens.— R. K. Ross *et al.*, *J. Am. med. Ass.*, 1980, *243*, 1635. See also P. Meier and R. L. Landau, *ibid.*, 1658.

Endometrium. In a retrospective study of 317 menopausal and postmenopausal women with adenocarcinoma of the endometrium and 317 women with other gynaecological neoplasms, it was calculated that the risk of developing endometrial carcinoma was 4.5 times greater in women who had taken oestrogen.— D. C. Smith *et al.*, *New Engl. J. Med.*, 1975, *293*, 1164. See also K. J. Ryan, *ibid.*, 1199; N. S. Weiss, *ibid.*, 1200.

There were 5 cases of endometrial cancer among an estimated 1060 postmenopausal women (with intact uterus) given oestrogens (an incidence of 4.7 per 1000), compared with 1 among 1240 given oestrogen with progestogen (incidence: 0.8 per 1000) and 1 among 510 controls (incidence: 2 per 1000).— R. D. Gambrell, *J. reprod. Med.*, 1977, *18*, 301.

Of 205 women with endometrial cancer 32 had used conjugated oestrogens compared with 12 of 205 women undergoing hysterectomy for benign disease. The risk was related to dose and duration of treatment and reached 11.5-fold after 10 years.— L. A. Gray *et al.*, *Obstet. Gynec.*, 1977, *49*, 385, per *J. Am. med. Ass.*, 1977, *238*, 1096.

In 348 menopausal women who had received oestrogen treatment for 4 to 42 months the incidence of hyperplasia (among the 286 from whom satisfactory vacuum curettage specimens were obtained) was: 28% in those given oestrogen implants with progestogen by mouth for 5 days per month; 12% in those given unopposed oestrogen therapy by mouth; and 2% in those given oestrogen by mouth with progestogen. A regular bleeding pattern was no guarantee of a healthy endometrium.— D. W. Sturdee *et al.*, *Br. med. J.*, 1978, *1*, 1575. See also J. Studd *et al.* (letter), *ibid.*, 1978, *2*, 1369.

A conclusion that the association between oestrogens and endometrial cancer had been exaggerated because of a detection bias in the conventional sampling methods used in retrospective case-control studies.— R. I. Horwitz and A. R. Feinstein, *New Engl. J. Med.*, 1978, *299*, 1089. Critical comment.— G. B. Hutchison and K. J. Rothman, *ibid.*, 1129.

A case-controlled study in 901 patients confirmed the relationship between endometrial cancer and the use of oestrogens. Increasing duration of treatment and increasing dosage were associated with higher risks of cancer and cyclic use of oestrogens was found to have about the same risk as continuous use.— C. M. F. Antunes *et al.*, *New Engl. J. Med.*, 1979, *300*, 9.

Confirmation from a Group Health Cooperative with 250 000 members that long-term replacement therapy with oestrogens was strongly associated with endometrial cancer. The risk for current oestrogen users was 1 to 3% per year compared with about 0.1% in non-users. From 1975 to 1977 there was a decline in the incidence of endometrial cancer and in the use of oestrogens; the changes reflected a similar decline in the USA as a whole.— H. Jick *et al.*, *New Engl. J. Med.*, 1979, *300*, 218.

In a prospective study in 745 menopausal women over 21 736 woman-months the incidence of endometrial hyperplasia was 7% in those given low-dose oestrogens for 3 weeks in 4, 14.8% in those given high-dose oestrogens, 1.2% in those given oestrogens with added progestogens, and 14.8% after oestradiol implants

(55.8% without added progestogen, and 3% with added progestogen). There were no cases of hyperplasia in women receiving progestogen for more than 10 days each month.— M. E. L. Paterson *et al.*, *Br. med. J.*, 1980, *280*, 822.

Discussions of the association between oestrogen therapy and endometrial cancer.— *Br. med. J.*, 1977, *2*, 209; M. B. Lipsett, *J. Am. med. Ass.*, 1977, *237*, 1112; E. S. Shoemaker *et al.*, *J. Am. med. Ass.*, 1977, *238*, 1524; *Lancet*, 1977, *1*, 577; N. S. Weiss, *Ann. intern. Med.*, 1978, *88*, 410; A. Breckenridge, *Adverse Drug React. Bull.*, 1979, June, 272; *FDA Drug Bull.*, 1979, *9*, 2; *Lancet*, 1979, *1*, 1121; H. S. Jacobs, *J. R. Soc. Med.*, 1979, *72*, 797; S. B. Gusberg, *New Engl. J. Med.*, 1980, *302*, 729; M. H. Thom and J. W. W. Studd, *Br. J. Hosp. Med.*, 1980, *23*, 506.

Further references: T. M. Mack, *Pediatrics*, 1978, *62*, 1104; L. S. Levine, *ibid.*, 1178; Z. Rosenwaks *et al.*, *ibid.*, 1184; P. B. Underwood, *Gynecol. Oncol.*, 1979, *8*, 60; R. D. Gambrell *et al.*, *J. Am. Geriat. Soc.*, 1979, *27*, 389; Z. Rosenwaks *et al.*, *Obstet. Gynec.*, 1979, *53*, 403; M. H. Thom *et al.*, *Lancet*, 1979, *2*, 455; S. Shapiro *et al.*, *New Engl. J. Med.*, 1980, *303*, 485.

Pancreatitis. Pancreatitis developed in 3 women and 1 man following the administration of oestrogens. All patients had previously covert familial type V hyperlipoproteinaemia.— C. J. Glueck *et al.*, *Metabolism*, 1972, *21*, 657, per *J. Am. med. Ass.*, 1972, *222*, 230.

Porphyria. A report of porphyria cutanea tarda induced by oestrogen.— K. M. Stein *et al.*, *Obstet. Gynec.*, 1971, *38*, 755, per *Int. pharm. Abstr.*, 1972, *9*, 843.

Thrombo-embolic disorders. There was no increased risk of atherosclerotic heart disease among 1900 patients taking oestrogens. This was different with oral contraceptives.— B. MacMahon, *Lancet*, 1977, *2*, 282.

Oestrogen replacement therapy in a group of 298 post-menopausal women from the Framingham study was associated with a doubling in the incidence of coronary heart disease, mainly angina pectoris. There was no change in the mortality-rate.— T. Gordon *et al.*, *Ann. intern. Med.*, 1978, *89*, 157.

Absence of association between oestrogen usage and myocardial infarction in 220 elderly women.— R. I. Pfeffer *et al.*, *Am. J. Epidem.*, 1978, *107*, 479, per *Int. pharm. Abstr.*, 1979, *241*, 77.

Of 17 women, aged below 46 years, with myocardial infarction 9 (53%) were users of oestrogens other than oral contraceptives compared with 4 of 34 (12%) of controls. Smoking was a contributory factor.— H. Jick *et al.*, *J. Am. med. Ass.*, 1978, *239*, 1407.

No significant association between myocardial infarction and oestrogens for indications other than contraception.— L. Rosenberg *et al.*, *J. Am. med. Ass.*, 1980, *244*, 339.

See also under Oral Contraceptives, p.1404, and under Stilboestrol, p.1433.

Precautions. The use of oestrogens is contra-indicated in patients with a family or personal history of malignant neoplastic disease of the breast or genital tract (unless indicated for the treatment of the neoplasm) and in those with previous thrombo-embolic disorders, cardiovascular disease, thrombophlebitis, undiagnosed vaginal bleeding, endometriosis, disorders of lipid metabolism, or a history during pregnancy of pruritus, herpes, deteriorating otosclerosis, or idiopathic jaundice. Their use is also contra-indicated in patients with liver impairment.

Because of the risk of thrombo-embolic disorders, oestrogens should preferably be avoided for the inhibition of lactation in the puerperium, particularly in women aged over 35, or following an operative delivery.

Since oestrogens may cause hypercalcaemia and oedema they should be used with care in patients with epilepsy or heart or kidney disease. Oestrogens may precipitate porphyria in susceptible patients and may exacerbate diabetes mellitus. Oestrogens have been reported to increase the plasma concentrations of cortisol- and thyroxine-binding globulin.

Oestrogens should be avoided in pregnant women since stilboestrol (see p.1433) has been implicated in the induction of tumours in female offspring and changes in male offspring, and hormone pregnancy tests (see pp.1421-2) have been associated with congenital abnormalities.

See also Oral Contraceptives, p.1405.

Variably raised serum concentrations of cholesterol and triglycerides and usually raised concentrations of copper, iron, and the total iron binding capacity, hydrocortisone and thyroxine and PBI, all associated with an increased concentration of carrier protein, could be detected in patients taking oestrogens. Variably raised glucose and lowered serum-albumin concentrations and usually lowered serum concentrations of cholinesterase could also be detected.— *Drug & Ther. Bull.*, 1972, *10*, 69.

The continuous administration of small doses of oestrogen was not contra-indicated in women following bilateral oophorectomy and hysterectomy for endometriosis. Large doses produced vaginal endometriosis. 'Combined' or 'sequential' oral contraceptives reactivated endometriosis.— R. W. Kistner, *J. Am. med. Ass.*, 1975, *233*, 183.

Absorption and Fate. Oestradiol is absorbed from the gastro-intestinal tract and through the skin. It is partly bound to plasma proteins and is rapidly metabolised mainly in the liver to the less active oestriol and oestrone. It is excreted in the urine as sulphate and glucuronide esters together with a small proportion of unchanged oestradiol. Numerous other metabolites have been identified. Oestrogens are also secreted in bile and undergo reabsorption following hydrolysis. Oestrogens are also excreted in the milk of nursing mothers. The urinary excretion of endogenous oestradiol and its metabolites varies during the menstrual cycle.

Uses. Oestradiol is the most active of the naturally occurring oestrogenic hormones formed in the ovarian follicles under the influence of the pituitary. It controls the development and maintenance of the female sex organs, the secondary sex characteristics, and the mammary glands. It controls certain functions of the human uterus and accessory organs, particularly the proliferation of the endometrium, the development of the decidua, and the cyclic changes in the cervix and vagina. Low physiological amounts stimulate the gonadotrophic and lactogenic activities of the anterior pituitary, but large amounts depress these activities. In late pregnancy, oestradiol increases the spontaneous activity of the uterine muscle and its response to oxytocic drugs.

The additional activity of progesterone is essential for the complete biological function of the female sex organs.

Oestradiol produces systemic effects which are widespread and generalised and include sodium and water retention, and effects on the metabolism of protein, fat, glucose, calcium, and phosphorus. Hair growth, erythropoiesis, and lympholysis are also affected.

The main therapeutic use of oestradiol and other oestrogens is for replacement therapy in deficiency states, for the treatment of conditions such as primary amenorrhoea and delayed onset of puberty, and for the management of the menopausal syndrome, particularly the vasomotor disturbances (see below). They are also used for the treatment of malignant neoplasms of the prostate and of the breast of postmenopausal women. They have been used for the suppression of lactation but alternative methods, including the use of bromocriptine (see p.894), are now preferred.

Primary amenorrhoea due to ovarian dysfunction or gonadotrophin insufficiency may respond to oestrogen therapy. Secondary amenorrhoea is usually treated with cyclical oestrogen with the addition of a progestogen at the end of each cycle.

Oestrogens may be administered to control functional uterine bleeding, particularly metropathia haemorrhagica. They have also been tried in reducing male libido.

Oestrogens such as ethinyloestradiol (see p.1412) and mestranol (see p.1418) are also given with a progestogen for the control of conception (see Oral Contraceptives, p.1402). Oestrogens have also been administered alone in high doses for postcoital contraception (see Stilboestrol, p.1435). Oestradiol has been administered as tablets, implants, or by intramuscular injection. It has also been applied topically.

Oestradiol is now little used and for oral administration, compounds such as ethinyloestradiol are generally preferred; for intramuscular administration esters of oestradiol provide prolonged action.

Doses of up to 2 mg of oestradiol daily are given by mouth; up to 1.5 mg is given intramuscularly twice or thrice weekly. Doses of 20 to 100 mg are given by implantation.

A short discussion on oestrogen-replacement treatment in old age.— *Br. med. J.*, 1980, *281*, 572. See also *J. Am. med. Ass.*, 1979, *242*, 1951.

Administration. A study in 6 oestrogen-deficient women indicated that both conjugated oestrogens and oestradiol in a cream basis could be readily absorbed by the vaginal mucosa. Intravaginal application of micronised oestradiol 200 µg was considered physiologically appropriate for oestrogen replacement in deficiency states.— L. A. Rigg *et al.*, *New Engl. J. Med.*, 1978, *298*, 195. See also I. Schiff *et al.*, *Fert. Steril.*, 1977, *28*, 1063, per *Int. pharm. Abstr.*, 1978, *15* 433.

Aphthous ulcers. In a subjective assessment, oestrogens were found to be effective in healing recurrent premenstrual aphthous ulcers.— P. M. F. Bishop *et al.*, *Lancet*, 1967, *1*, 1345; R. Carruthers (letter), *ibid.*, 1967, *2*, 259.

Contraception. For a report of a study in 25 women of an oral contraceptive containing micronised oestradiol 4 mg and norethisterone 3 mg, see B. Åstedt *et al.*, *Br. med. J.*, 1977, *1*, 269.

Implanted oestradiol pellets had been used in 123 patients for contraception. Four 25-mg pellets were implanted in the abdominal wall initially, then 3, 2, and 1 at six-monthly intervals the final dosage being continued as long as the patient desired. Additional protection was recommended for the first month. There had been 2 pregnancies (other than in the first month) in 1668 cycles. Withdrawal bleeding was induced monthly by an oral progestogen for 5 to 7 days. Untoward effects were headache (1), hypermenorrhea (9), breast tenderness (7), and mild oedema (15).— R. B. Greenblatt *et al.*, *Am. J. Obstet. Gynec.*, 1977, *127*, 520.

See also under Oral Contraceptives, p.1402.

Depression. The evaluation of oestrogen therapy in severe depression.— E. L. Klaiber *et al.*, *Archs gen. Psychiat.*, 1979, *36*, 550.

Hirsutism. The regression of hirsutism due to polycystic ovaries in 5 patients after treatment with oestradiol.— R. D. Gambrell, *Obstet. Gynec.*, 1976, *47*, 569, per *Int. pharm. Abstr.*, 1977, *14*, 79.

Hyperlipidaemia. Oestrogens were considered to be of little benefit in the management of hyperlipidaemia. They had moderate hypocholesterolaemic effects, but greatly increased plasma triglycerides.— R. I. Levy and B. M. Rifkind, *Drugs*, 1973, *6*, 12.

Oestrogens might have a limited therapeutic role in women with type III hyperlipoproteinaemia that could not be controlled with diet and clofibrate therapy.— R. S. Kushwaha *et al.*, *Ann. intern. Med.*, 1977, *87*, 517.

Evidence from 25 women given synthetic or natural oestrogens did not support earlier suggestions that natural oestrogens were less likely to affect lipid metabolism.— L. Wallentin and U. Larsson-Cohn (letter), *Lancet*, 1977, *1*, 1358.

Discussion of the association between oestrogens and atheroma.— *Lancet*, 1978, *2*, 508.

See also under Oestradiol Valerate, p.1428.

Inhibition of growth. The use of oestrogens to retard growth in pubertal girls was experimental and of uncertain benefit; the best system of administration was still unknown.— *Br. med. J.*, 1975, *2*, 648.

Oestrogen therapy with 5 to 7 oestradiol pellets of 25 mg implanted every 6 months until epiphyses were almost or completely closed was effective in inhibiting growth in a study of 40 tall girls. Progestogens were used to induce cyclic withdrawal bleeding.— M. L. Colle *et al.*, *Archs Dis. Childh.*, 1977, *52*, 118. A similar report.— J. R. Bierich, *Pediatrics*, 1978, *62*, 1196, per *Int. pharm. Abstr.*, 1979, *16*, 361.

Further references: R. B. Greenblatt *et al.*, *J. clin. Endocr. Metab.*, 1966, *26*, 1185; J. D. Crawford, *Pediatrics*, 1978, *62*, 1189.

Inhibition of lactation. A recommendation for discontinuing the use of oestrogens for the inhibition or suppression of lactation.— S. J. Steele (letter), *Br. med. J.*, 1968, *4*, 578.

Oestrogens suppressed lactation but had many drawbacks—increase of lochial loss, precipitation of withdrawal bleeding, rebound lactation on withdrawal, and the risk of thrombosis. Oestrogens no longer had a place in the suppression of lactation.— *Br. med. J.*, 1977, *1*, 189.

Labour. In a comparative study of 96 pregnant women with an unfavourable cervix at term, oestradiol or oestriol in a hydroxyethylmethylcellulose gel, or the gel alone, were instilled extra-amniotically through an indwelling catheter. The only statistically significant difference was in improvement of oestriol-treated over placebo-treated women. The effect of the indwelling catheter was much greater than expected.— M. Thiery *et al.* (letter), *Lancet*, 1978, *2*, 835. See also K. Hillier and R. Wallis (letter), *ibid.*, 1377.

In 60 women, a suspension of oestradiol 150 mg in a gel basis was as effective as a dinoprostone gel in ripening the cervix before the induction of labour, and promoted less uterine activity.— P. M. Tromans *et al.*, *Br. med. J.*, 1981, *282*, 679. Comment that neonatal hyperbilirubinaemia had been observed following the administration of oestradiol extra-amniotically for the induction of labour.— S. Pedersen *et al.*, *ibid.*, 1395.

Menopausal symptoms. Low doses of oestrogen alleviate the vasomotor and vaginal atrophic symptoms of the menopause. *Osteoporosis* is retarded. Studies have shown that there may be rebound bone loss when oestrogen therapy is withdrawn, but some other work has shown that the benefits to bone may continue.

There appears to be little evidence to indicate the optimum duration of oestrogen replacement; some patients receive therapy for several months while others may be treated indefinitely. Prolonged therapy will be required for premenopausal women suffering from oestrogen deficiency due to oophorectomy or ovarian failure.

It has been reported that oestrogen given for menopausal replacement does not appear to increase the risk of thrombo-embolisms, stroke or heart disease, indeed some work indicates that there might be a protective effect.

Endometrial cancer is a hazard of replacement therapy with unopposed oestrogen, but it has been demonstrated that associated use of a progestogen can reduce oestrogen-associated endometrial proliferation and may reduce the cancer risk. Fears, have, however, been expressed that combined use of a progestogen with oestrogen may introduce a risk of thrombo-embolism, myocardial infarction, and stroke. Emphesis has, therefore, been laid on the need to use progestogens in their lowest effective dose and to select those that are least likely to induce changes in lipid metabolism.

Synthetic as well as natural oestrogens are used including ethinyloestradiol, oestradiol, and conjugated oestrogens. Local treatment has been used as an alternative to systemic treatment for vaginal atrophy but systemic effects may occur.

References: *Drug & Ther. Bull.*, 1978, *16*, 13; T. Detre *et al.*, *Ann. intern. Med.*, 1978, *88*, 373; *Ann. intern. Med.*, 1979, *91*, 921; S. Chakravarti *et al.*, *Br. med. J.*, 1979, *1*, 983; M. M. Quigley and C. B. Hammond, *New Engl. J. Med.*, 1979, *301*, 646; E. M. Grimes, *J. Am. med. Ass.*, 1980, *243*, 161; R. K. Ross *et al.*, *Lancet*, 1981, *1*, 858; *ibid.*, 1359; R. I. Horwitz *et al.*, *Lancet*, 1981, *2*, 66; M. I. Whitehead *et al.*, *New Engl. J. Med.*, 1981, *305*, 1599.

References on the effects of oestrogen replacement on bone: R. R. Recker *et al.*, *Ann. intern. Med.*, 1977, *87*, 649; L. E. Nachtigall *et al.*, *Obstet. Gynec.*, 1979, *53*, 277; B. E. C. Nordin, *Drugs*, 1979, *18*, 484; N. S. Weiss *et al.*, *New Engl. J. Med.*, 1980, *303*, 1195; S. C. Manolagas *et al.*, *Lancet*, 1979, *2*, 597; T. A. Hutchinson *et al.*, *ibid.*, 705; C. Christiansen *et al.*, *Lancet*, 1981, *1*, 459 and 1053; J. C. Stevenson *et al.*, *ibid.*, 693; R. Lindsay *et al.* (letter), *ibid.*, 729; B. L. Riggs *et al.*, *New Engl. J. Med.*, 1982, *306*, 446 (with fluoride and calcium).

See also under Mestranol, p.1418 (Osteoporosis).

Neoplasms. For details of the use of oestrogens in neoplasms of the breast, including the role of oestrogen receptors, see p.180.

Osteoporosis. See Menopausal Symptoms, above.

Premenstrual tension. Premenstrual tension was relieved by the insertion of a 75-mg or 100-mg oestradiol implant. Endometrial hyperplasia was avoided by giving norethisterone 5 mg daily for 5 days each month.— J. Studd (letter), *Br. med. J.*, 1979, *1*, 410.

Preparations

Estradiol Pellets *(U.S.P.)*. Oestradiol compressed in the form of sterile pellets with no binder, diluent, or excipient. Store in single airtight sterile containers.

Estradiol Tablets *(U.S.P.)*. Tablets containing oestradiol. Store in airtight containers. Protect from light.

Sterile Estradiol Suspension *(U.S.P.)*. Estradiol Aquosuspensoid Injection *(Jap. P.)*. A sterile suspension of oestradiol in Water for Injections.

Proprietary Preparations

Oestradiol Implants *(Organon, UK)*. Available containing 25, 50, or 100 mg of oestradiol.

Trisequens *(Organon, UK)*. Packs of 28 tablets for sequential daily administration, containing 12 blue tablets each containing oestradiol 2 mg and oestriol 1 mg, 10 white tablets each containing oestradiol 2 mg, oestriol 1 mg, and norethisterone acetate 1 mg, and 6 red tablets each containing oestradiol 1 mg and oestriol 500 µg. For oestrogen deficiency. *Administration.* Commence with one blue tablet on the 5th day of the first treated cycle.

A proprietary preparation containing oestradiol in conjunction with other oestrogens is described under Oestriol (see p.1428).

Other Proprietary Names

Dimenformon (see also under Oestradiol Benzoate) *(Belg., Neth.)*; Estrace *(Canad., USA)*; Farmacyrol *(Ger.)*; Gynoestryl, Oestrogel (both *Fr.*); Ormogamma *(Ital.)*; Ovocyclin (see also under Oestradiol Dipropionate) *(Switz.)*; Progynon *(Arg., Ital., Spain, USA)*.

9084-j

Oestradiol Benzoate *(B.P., B.P. Vet., Eur. P.)*.

Oestradioli Benzoas; Oestradiol Monobenzoate; Estradiol Benzoate *(U.S.P.)*; Estradioli Benzoas; Beta-estradiol Benzoate; Dihydroxyoestrin Monobenzoate. Estra-1,3,5(10)-triene-3,17β-diol 3-benzoate.

$C_{25}H_{28}O_3$=376.5.

CAS — 50-50-0.

Pharmacopoeias. In all pharmacopoeias examined except *Rus.*

Colourless odourless crystals or white or creamy-white crystalline powder. M.p. 190° to 198°.

Practically **insoluble** in water; slightly soluble in alcohol; soluble 1 in 50 of acetone, 1 in 500 of arachis oil, 1 in 5 of chloroform, 1 in 150 of ether, and 1 in 200 of ethyl oleate; soluble in dioxan; slightly soluble in fixed oils; practically insoluble in solutions of alkali hydroxides. A solution in dioxan is dextrorotatory. Solutions in oil are **sterilised** by maintaining at 150° for 1 hour. **Protect** from light.

Oestradiol benzoate has the actions and uses of oestradiol (p.1425). It is administered by intramuscular injection in oily solutions to provide a depot from which the drug is slowly liberated. The usual dose is 1 to 5 mg daily or at intervals of up to 14 days by intramuscular injection.

Of 14 patients with amenorrhoea and hyperprolactinaemia, usually associated with galactorrhoea, 13 failed to release luteinising hormone after receiving oestradiol benzoate 1 mg intramuscularly. The abnormality might explain the anovulation.— M. R. Glass *et al.*, *Br. med. J.*, 1975, *3*, 274. The induction of luteinising-hormone release by oestradiol benzoate for the assessment of pituitary-hypothalamic competence.— G. Weiss *et al.*, *Obstet. Gynec.*, 1976, *47*, 415.

The induction of ovulation by clomiphene and oestradiol benzoate in women unresponsive to clomiphene alone.— E. S. Canales *et al.*, *Fert. Steril.*, 1978, *29*, 496, per *Int. pharm. Abstr.*, 1978, *15*, 1126.

Preparations

Estradiol Benzoate Injection *(U.S.P.)*. A sterile solution of oestradiol benzoate in a suitable oil.

Oestradiol Benzoate Injection *(B.P.)*. Oestradiol Benz. Inj.; Oestradiol Monobenzoate Injection. A sterile solution in ethyl oleate or other suitable ester, in a suitable fixed oil, or in any mixture of these; it may contain suitable alcohols. Sterilised by maintaining at 150° for 1 hour. Protect from light; on standing solid matter may separate and it should be redissolved by warming before use. For intramuscular injection only.

Similar injections are included in several other pharmacopoeias.

Oestradiol Instillation *(A.P.F.)*. Oestradiol Nasal Drops; Oestradiol Nasal Spray. Oestradiol benzoate 8 mg, light liquid paraffin to 100 ml. Protect from light.

Proprietary Preparations

Benztrone *(Paines & Byrne, UK)*. Oestradiol benzoate, available as an injection containing 1 mg per ml, in ampoules of 1 ml, and 5 mg per ml, in ampoules of 1 and 2 ml. (Also available as Benztrone in *Ital.*).

Mixogen Injection *(Organon, UK)*. Contains in each ml oestradiol benzoate 1 mg, oestradiol phenylpropionate ($C_{27}H_{32}O_3$ = 404.5) 4 mg, testosterone propionate 20 mg, testosterone phenylpropionate 40 mg, and testosterone isocaproate 40 mg in vials of 2 ml, for intramuscular injection. *Dose.* For menopausal symptoms, 1 ml every 3 to 4 weeks.

For Mixogen Tablets see under Ethinyloestradiol, p.1412.

Other Proprietary Names

Arg.— Benzo-Gynestryl-5, Progynon B Oleoso; *Austral.*— Oestramine; *Denm.*— Follicyclin, Ovex; *Fr.*— Benzo-Gynoestryl 5, Gynécormone; *Ger.*— Ovocyclin M, Progynon B oleosum; *Ital.*— Progynon B Oleoso; *Neth.*— Dimenformon (see also under Oestradiol); *Spain*— Ovolacer, Progynon B; *Switz.*— Ovocyclin M.

9085-z

Oestradiol Cypionate.

Oestradiol Cyclopentylpropionate; Estradiol Cypionate *(U.S.P.)*. Estra-1,3,5(10)-triene-3,17β-diol 17-(3-cyclopentylpropionate).

$C_{26}H_{36}O_3$=396.6.

CAS — 313-06-4.

Pharmacopoeias. In *Braz.* and *U.S.*

A white or almost white crystalline powder, odourless or with a slight odour. M.p. 149° to 153°. Practically **insoluble** in water; soluble 1 in 40 of alcohol and 1 in 7 of chloroform; soluble in acetone and dioxan; very slightly soluble in ether; sparingly soluble in fixed oils. A solution in dioxan is dextrorotatory. **Store** in airtight containers. Protect from light.

Oestradiol cypionate has the actions and uses of oestradiol (p.1425). It is administered by intramuscular injection in oily solutions to provide a depot from which the drug is slowly liberated. It has been given in doses of 1 to 5 mg intramuscularly every 3 or 4 weeks.

Preparations

Estradiol Cypionate Injection *(U.S.P.)*. Oestradiol Cypionate Injection. A sterile solution of oestradiol cypionate in a suitable oil. Protect from light.

Proprietary Names

Depo-Estradiol Cypionate *(Upjohn, USA)*; Depofemin *(Hoechst, Denm.)*; Estradep *(Millet, Arg.)*; Neoginon Depositum *(Lusofarmaco, Ital.)*; Pertradiol *(Dexter, Spain)*.

9086-c

Oestradiol Dipropionate *(B.P.C. 1954)*.

Oestradiol Diprop.; Dihydroxyoestrin Dipropionate; Estradiol Dipropionate. Estra-1,3,5(10)-triene-3,17β-diol dipropionate.

$C_{24}H_{32}O_4$=384.5.

CAS — 113-38-2.

Pharmacopoeias. In *Arg.*, *Aust.*, *Braz.*, *Cz.*, *Ind.*, *Jug.*, and *Swiss. Hung.* includes oestradiol 17-monopropionate ($C_{21}H_{28}O_3$ = 328.5).

Small white or slightly off-white crystals, or crystalline powder. M.p. 104° to 109°. Practically **insoluble** in water; soluble 1 in 55 of alcohol; practically insoluble in solutions of alkali hydroxides; soluble in acetone, dioxan, and ether; sparingly soluble in fixed oils. Solutions in oil are **sterilised** by maintaining at 150° for 1 hour. **Protect** from light.

Oestradiol dipropionate has the actions and uses of oestradiol (p.1425). It has been administered by intramuscular injection in oily solutions to provide a depot from which the drug is slowly liberated in doses of 1 to 5 mg intramuscularly every 1 to 2 weeks, with 1 to 2.5 mg every 10 to 14 days for maintenance.

Proprietary Names

Ovocyclin (see also under Oestradiol) *(Ciba-Geigy, Switz.)*.

9087-k

Oestradiol Enanthate. Estradiol Enanthate; Oestradiol 17-Heptanoate; SQ 16150. Estra-1,3,5(10)-triene-3,17β-diol 17-heptanoate.
$C_{25}H_{36}O_3$=384.6.

CAS — 4956-37-0.

A white or off-white, crystalline powder.

Oestradiol enanthate is an oestrogen with similar properties to those of oestradiol (see p.1425). It has been administered by intramuscular injection as a solution in oil to provide a depot from which it is slowly released.

It has been tried in doses of 10 mg with algestone acetophenide as a monthly injection (see p.1406) for the control of conception.

9088-a

Oestradiol Undecanoate. Estradiol Undecylate; SQ 9993. Estra-1,3,5(10)-triene-3,17β-diol 17-undecanoate.
$C_{29}H_{44}O_3$=440.7.

CAS — 33613-02-4.

Oestradiol undecanoate has the actions and uses of oestradiol (see p.1425). It has been administered by intramuscular injection in oily solution to provide a depot from which the drug is slowly released. Doses of 100 mg every 3 weeks have been given in postmenopausal breast carcinoma and 100 to 200 mg every 2 or 3 weeks in prostatic carcinoma.

Proprietary Preparations

Trimone Retard *(Marshall's Pharmaceuticals, UK).* An injection containing in each ml oestradiol diundecanoate ($C_{40}H_{64}O_4$ = 608.9) 2.6 mg, testosterone cyclohexylpropionate ($C_{28}H_{42}O_3$ = 426.6) 67.2 mg, and hydroxyprogesterone enanthate ($C_{28}H_{42}O_4$ = 442.6) 74.9 mg in sesame oil, in ampoules of 1 ml. For prolonged-action therapy in climacteric conditions. *Dose.* 1 ml, by deep intramuscular injection, every 2 to 4 weeks.

Proprietary Names

Progynon-Retard *(Schering, Fr.)*; Progynon-Depot *(Schering, Denm.; Schering, Norw.)*; Progynon Depot 100 mg *(Schering, Ger.; Schering, Neth.; Schering, Spain).*

See also under Oestradiol Valerate.

Proprietary Names of another Oestradiol Ester

Etrosteron *(diundecanoate) (Gador, Arg.).*

Oestradiol undecanoate was also formerly marketed in Great Britain under the proprietary name Primogyn Depot 100 mg *(Schering).*

9089-t

Oestradiol Valerate.

Estradiol Valerate *(U.S.P.).* Estra-1,3,5(10)-triene-3,17β-diol 17-valerate.
$C_{23}H_{32}O_3$=356.5.

CAS — 979-32-8.

Pharmacopoeias. In *Chin.* and *U.S.*

A white crystalline powder which is odourless or has a faint fatty odour. M.p. 143° to 150°. Practically **insoluble** in water; soluble in benzyl benzoate, dioxan, methyl alcohol, and castor oil; sparingly soluble in arachis oil and sesame oil. A solution in dioxan is dextrorotatory. **Store** in airtight containers. Protect from light.

Oestradiol valerate has the actions and uses of oestradiol (see p.1425). It is administered by intramuscular injection in oily solutions containing 10 to 40 mg per ml to provide a depot from which the drug is slowly liberated. For replacement therapy doses of 5 to 40 mg are usually given every 1 to 3 weeks; smaller doses may be used for maintenance therapy. It is also given by mouth in doses of 1 or 2 mg daily usually in a cyclic regimen for menopausal symptoms.

In 16 postmenopausal women taking oestradiol valerate 2 mg [daily] for 14 weeks there was a rise in mean concentrations of factor II, X, and VII plus X complex. There was no evidence of depression of antithrombin III. There appeared to be some thrombogenic hazard.— J. Bonnar *et al., Postgrad. med. J.,* 1976, *52, Suppl.* 6, 30.

Hyperlipoproteinaemia. Administration of oestradiol valerate (Progynova), 2 mg daily for 3 months and subsequently cyclically to 17 postmenopausal women with type II hyperlipoproteinaemia, decreased mean serum-total-cholesterol by 12% and mean serum-low-density-lipoprotein cholesterol by 24%, and increased mean high-density-lipoprotein cholesterol by 12% after 3 months, this continuing to rise so that the average change at 6 months was +30%. The mean high-density-lipoprotein to low-density-lipoprotein ratio changed from 0.21 before treatment to 0.34 at 6 months. These results indicated that postmenopausal type II hypercholesterolaemia could be regarded as an additional indication for oestrogen replacement therapy.— M. J. Tikkanen *et al., Lancet,* 1978, *2,* 490. Comment.— *ibid.,* 508.

Labour. The application of oestradiol valerate 150 mg in a viscous gel to the cervix of 24 primagravid women the day before induction of labour produced a significant increase in cervical ripening compared with 24 controls given the gel alone.— A. J. Gordon and A. A. Calder, *Lancet,* 1977, *2,* 1319. Findings at variance.— I. Craft and J. Yovich (letter), *ibid.,* 1978, *2,* 208.

See also under Oestradiol, above.

Preparations

Estradiol Valerate Injection *(U.S.P.).* Oestradiol Valerate Injection. A sterile solution of oestradiol valerate in a suitable vegetable oil.

Cyclo-Progynova 1 mg (known in some countries as Cyclacur) *(Schering, UK).* Packs of 11 beige tablets each containing oestradiol valerate 1 mg and 10 light-brown tablets each containing oestradiol valerate 1 mg and levonorgestrel 250 μg. **Cyclo-Progynova 2 mg.** Packs of 11 white tablets each containing oestradiol valerate 2 mg and 10 pale brown tablets each containing oestradiol valerate 2 mg and norgestrel 500 μg. For menopausal symptoms. *Dose.* Initially, 1 beige tablet daily for 11 days (starting on the 5th day of the first treated cycle, or at any time if cycles are irregular or have ceased), followed by 1 light-brown tablet daily for 10 days; the course is repeated after 7 tablet-free days. If symptoms are not controlled, 1 white tablet daily for 11 days, followed by 1 pale brown tablet daily for 10 days.

Progynova *(Schering, UK).* Oestradiol valerate, available as tablets of 1 and 2 mg. (Also available as Progynova in *Arg., Austral., Belg., Ger., Ital., Neth., Norw., S.Afr., Spain, Switz.*).

Other Proprietary Names

Delestrogen *(USA)*; Femogex *(Canad.)*; Östrogynol sine *(Ger.)*; Primogyn Depot *(Austral., Norw., S.Afr.)*; Progynon *(Denm., Swed.)*; Progynon Depot *(Arg., Ital., Switz.)*; Progynon Depot 10 mg *(Ger., Neth., Spain)*; Progynon Depot 40 mg *(Ger.)*; Progynon-Depot *(Denm., Swed.)*; Progynova 21 Mitis *(Belg.).*

See also under Oestradiol Undecanoate.

Oestradiol valerate was also formerly marketed in Great Britain under the proprietary name Primogyn Depot 10 mg *(Schering).*

9090-l

Oestriol.

Estriol *(U.S.P.)*; Theelol. Estra-1,3,5(10)-triene-3,16α,17β-triol.
$C_{18}H_{24}O_3$=288.4.

CAS — 50-27-1.

Pharmacopoeias. In *U.S.*

A white or almost white, odourless, tasteless, crystalline powder, obtained from human placental tissue and pregnancy urine. M.p. about 280°. Practically **insoluble** in water; soluble 1 in about 500 of alcohol; soluble in acetone, chloroform, dioxan, ether, and fixed oils. A solution in dioxan is dextrorotatory. **Store** in airtight containers.

Adverse Effects and Precautions. As for Oestradiol, p.1425.

A discussion of the possible non-carcinogenicity of oestriol and its role as an oestrogen supplement for women at risk from breast or endometrial carcinoma.— A. H. Follingstad, *J. Am. med. Ass.,* 1978, *239,* 29.

Uses. Oestriol is a naturally occurring oestrogen with actions and uses similar to those of oestradiol (see p.1426); it is claimed to have a selective action on the cervix and vagina and to have relatively little effect on the endometrium. It is active when given by mouth.

It is given in doses of 250 to 500 μg daily in the treatment of menopausal symptoms. Up to 1 mg daily has been used in the treatment of dysmenorrhoea starting 14 days before the anticipated onset of symptoms.

The oestrogenic effects of oestriol.— I. Schiff *et al., Fert. Steril.,* 1978, *30,* 278, per *Int. pharm. Abstr.,* 1979, *16,* 161.

Contraception. The development of an oestriol-releasing intra-uterine device.— R. W. Baker *et al., J. pharm. Sci.,* 1978, *68,* 20.

An oral contraceptive preparation containing oestradiol and oestriol in association with norethisterone acetate is not acceptable because of bleeding problems but the metabolic advantages of micronised natural oestrogens warrant further investigation.— J. Serup *et al.* (letter), *Lancet,* 1979, *2,* 471.

Proprietary Preparations

Hormonin Tablets *(Carnrick, UK).* Each contains oestriol 270 μg, oestrone 1.4 mg, and oestradiol 600 μg. For menopausal disorders. *Dose.* ½ to 2 tablets daily.

Ovestin *(Organon, UK).* Oestriol, available as tablets of 250 μg. (Also available as Ovestin in *Austral., Belg., Denm., Fr., Ger., Ital., Neth., Switz.*).

Other Proprietary Names

Aacifemine *(Belg.)*; Holin *(Jap.)*; Hormomed *(Ger.)*; Orgestriol *(Arg.)*; Ovesterin *(Norw., Swed.)*; Triovex *(Swed.).*

Proprietary Names of other Oestriol Esters

Klimadurin *(polyoestriol phosphate) (Spain)*; Orgastyptin *(succinate) (Ger.)*; Styptanon *(succinate) (Belg., Neth., Switz.)*; Synapasa *(succinate) (Denm.)*; Synapause *(succinate) (see also under Epioestriol) (Fr., Ger., Neth., Switz.)*; Triodurin *(polyoestriol phosphate) (Swed.).*

9091-y

Conjugated Oestrogens.

Conjugated Estrogens *(U.S.P.).*

Pharmacopoeias. In *Braz.* and *U.S. U.S.* also includes Esterified Estrogens.

A mixture containing the sodium salts of the sulphate esters of the oestrogenic substances, principally oestrone and equilin, that are of the type excreted by pregnant mares, containing 50 to 65% of sodium oestrone sulphate and 20 to 35% of sodium equilin sulphate.

If it is obtained from natural sources it is a buff-coloured amorphous powder which is odourless or has a slight characteristic odour; the synthetic form is a white to light buff-coloured crystalline or amorphous powder, odourless or with a slight odour. **Soluble** in water. Conjugated oestrogens in solution are **incompatible** with ascorbic acid, protein hydrolysate, and acidic solutions. Solutions should be stored at 2° to 8° when they may be expected to remain stable for 60 days. **Store** in airtight containers.

Esterified Estrogens (*U.S.P.*) is a mixture of the sodium salts of the sulphate esters of the oestrogenic substances, principally oestrone, that are of the type excreted by pregnant mares, containing 75 to 85% of sodium oestrone sulphate and 6 to 15% of sodium equilin sulphate, the total of these being not less than 90%. A white or buff-coloured amorphous powder which is odourless or has a slight characteristic odour. **Soluble** in water. **Store** in airtight containers.

Adverse Effects and Precautions. As for Oestradiol, p.1425.

Intravenously administered conjugated oestrogens were compared with placebo in a double-blind study of the effect on capillary stability in 13 women and 14 men. No significant effect on capillary resistance to negative pressure stress or bleeding times was noted. Deep calf-vein thrombosis occurred in a 46-year-old man within 24 hours of oestrogen administration suggesting a possible relationship.— L. R. Zacharski *et al., J. Am. med. Ass.,* 1973, *224,* 1519.

In a collaborative study by the Coronary Drug Project

Group, treatment of men with a previous myocardial infarction with conjugated oestrogens 2.5 mg daily was discontinued because of suggestions of adverse trends including a greater incidence of venous thrombo-embolism and excess mortality from all cancers especially lung cancer, and a lack of evidence of a positive therapeutic effect.— Coronary Drug Project Research Group, *J. Am. med. Ass.*, 1973, *226*, 652. Data collected in follow-up for a mean of 74 months yielded no consistent evidence of carcinogenicity.— *idem*, 1978, *239*, 2758.

Exercise-induced abnormalities of the ST segment were increased in 18 of 20 patients after treatment for 2 weeks with conjugated oestrogens 10 mg daily.— M. D. Jaffe, *Br. Heart J.*, 1976, *38*, 1299, per *J. Am. med. Ass.*, 1977, *237*, 1023.

Effects on blood. In 17 postmenopausal women who had taken conjugated oestrogens 1.25 mg [daily] for 14 weeks there was a rise in mean concentrations of factor VII and X complex, but no rise in factor II and X, and no depression of antithrombin III. There appeared to be a thrombogenic hazard.— J. Bonnar *et al.*, *Postgrad. med. J.*, 1976, *52*, *Suppl.* 6, 30.

Hypercoagulability in 57.2% of 35 menopausal women taking conjugated oestrogens, compared with 14.7% in 34 controls.— J. J. Stangel *et al.*, *Obstet. Gynec.*, 1977, *49*, 314, per *J. Am. med. Ass.*, 1977, *238*, 84.

Twenty women took conjugated oestrogens 0.625 or 1.25 mg daily for 3 weeks in every 4 for 21 to 24 months. Acceleration of the prothrombin time and of clotting times in factor VII and X assays, evident at 3 months, was maintained, but there was no evidence of progression. After 12 months platelet aggregation (Chandler's tube technique—not specific) was accelerated. There were no changes in the partial thromboplastin time and in thromboelastography values—possibly due to the small number of patients.— L. Poller *et al.*, *Br. med. J.*, 1977, *1*, 935.

Transient episodes of imbalance and episodes of amaurosis fugax in a 52-year-old woman were considered due to emboli from her prosthetic heart valve, caused by conjugated oestrogens.— D. Pitcher and P. Curry, *Br. med. J.*, 1979, *2*, 244.

Effects on the gall bladder. Analysis of data obtained during the Coronary Drug Project indicated a significant increase in the development of gall-bladder disease among patients treated with conjugated oestrogens 2.5 and 5 mg daily, compared with those treated with placebo.— Coronary Drug Project Research Group, *New Engl. J. Med.*, 1977, *296*, 1185.

Effects on glucose tolerance. Comparison of the effects of conjugated oestrogens and other oestrogen/progestogen regimens on glucose tolerance.— M. Thom *et al.*, *Br. J. Obstet. Gynaec.*, 1977, *84*, 776.

Effects on the liver. Benign nodular hyperplasia of the liver in a 32-year-old woman was associated with long-term administration of moderate to high doses of conjugated oestrogens.— K. Aldinger *et al.*, *Archs intern. Med.*, 1977, *137*, 357.

Effects on serum lipids. Massive increases in serum concentrations of cholesterol and triglycerides occurred in 2 patients taking conjugated oestrogens and 1 taking an oral contraceptive.— M. E. Molitch *et al.*, *J. Am. med. Ass.*, 1974, *227*, 522.

In 12 patients with proven prostatic carcinoma, conjugated oestrogens 15 mg daily had no significant effect on serum-cholesterol concentrations but caused significant elevation of serum-triglyceride concentrations, usually with a rise in pre-β-lipoproteins.— M. Shahmanesh *et al.*, *Br. med. J.*, 1973, *2*, 512.

Further references: J. Maddock, *Postgrad. med. J.*, 1978, *54*, *Suppl.* 2, 38.

Interactions. A report of phenytoin diminishing the effect of conjugated oestrogens in a menopausal woman.— M. Notelovitz *et al.* (letter), *New Engl. J. Med.*, 1981, *304*, 788.

Neoplasm. The incidence of endometrial carcinoma among 94 women who had taken conjugated oestrogens was 57% compared with 15% in 188 controls. An estimate of the risk ratio was 7.6.— H. K. Ziel and W. D. Finkle, *New Engl. J. Med.*, 1975, *293*, 1167. An independent pathology review supported the original risk estimate of Ziel and Finkle. The revised risk estimate of 8.1 validated the original esimate of 7.6.— J. Gordon *et al.*, *New Engl. J. Med.*, 1977, *297*, 570.

In 145 women with endometrial cancer exposure to any exogenous oestrogen was found in 27% compared with 28% in 580 matched controls. The relative risk, however, was 2 for those exposed to conjugated oestrogens for any period, 4.9 for those exposed 6 months or more, 5.3 for those exposed for a year, 8.3 for those exposed for 2 years, and 7.9 for those exposed for 3 years or more. The relative risk was increased with dosage of conjugated oestrogens, and with method of administration (intermittent, cyclic, continuous).— T. W. McDonald *et al.*, *Am. J. Obstet. Gynec.*, 1977, *127*, 572.

A retrospective survey of 908 women who had received conjugated oestrogens for at least 6 months revealed 8 cases of ovarian cancer and 1 of the fallopian tube compared with an expected incidence of 3.4. The relative risk of cancer rose with increasing dose but not with duration of treatment or total accumulated dose. Four of the patients with ovarian cancer had also taken other oestrogens; in 3 stilboestrol was involved and this had been taken for one year or more.— R. Hoover *et al.* (preliminary communication), *Lancet*, 1977, *2*, 533. No association had been found between exogenous oestrogen given for 6 months or more and ovarian cancer.— J. F. Annegers *et al.* (letter), *ibid.*, 869 and 1188.

Absorption and Fate. Conjugated oestrogens are absorbed from the gastro-intestinal tract. Metabolism occurs primarily in the liver; there is some enterohepatic recycling.

In 11 postmenopausal women given conjugated oestrogens 2.5 mg daily a mean steady-state total urine-oestrogen excretion of 553.4 µg in 24 hours was achieved after 17 to 19 days of therapy.— R. N. Johnson *et al.*, *J. pharm. Sci.*, 1978, *67*, 1218.

A study of serum equilin, oestrone, and oestradiol concentrations in postmenopausal women receiving conjugated oestrogens either alone or in conjunction with norethisterone acetate. The data suggested a very long life for equilin, and hence the possibility of a prolonged oestrogen effect in both groups of women. Although exposure to conjugated oestrogens for 6 months or less has been reported to carry no increased risk of endometrial cancer, several reports had suggested a relation between conjugated oestrogen therapy and endometrial carcinoma, particularly after a year, and the apparently prolonged presence of equilin should be borne in mind. It would seem prudent to discontinue the use of equilin-containing compounds before 12 months.— P. G. Whittaker *et al.*, *Lancet*, 1980, *1*, 14. Stringent criticism, and presentation of much lower values for equilin.— C. A. Woolever and B. R. Bhavani (letter), *ibid.*, 547.

Uses. Conjugated and esterified oestrogens have actions and uses similar to those of oestradiol (see p.1426) and are used for the same purposes. For the control of various menopausal symptoms the usual dose is 0.3 to 1.25 mg daily by mouth from the 5th day of the cycle for 3 weeks then repeated similarly after a week in subsequent cycles. Amenorrhoea has been treated with doses of 1.25 to 3.75 mg daily for 21 days with a progestogen for the last 7 days.

For the palliative treatment of prostatic carcinoma, a daily dose of 3.75 to 7.5 mg has been employed. A dose of 10 mg thrice daily for at least 3 months has been used for breast carcinoma in men and postmenopausal women.

Functional uterine bleeding may be treated by giving conjugated oestrogens 25 mg by intramuscular or intravenous injection repeated if required after 6 to 12 hours.

Alopecia. The use of conjugated oestrogens in female-pattern baldness due to oestrogen deficiency.— I. I. Lubowe, *Clin. Med.*, 1972, *79* (Mar.), 25.

Aphthous ulcers. Some women with aphthous ulceration occurring before menstruation responded well to conjugated oestrogens 0.625 to 1.25 mg daily for 21 days.— H. A. Brody, *Clin. Med.*, 1972, *79* (Mar.), 18.

Contraception. Conjugated oestrogens 30 mg daily for 5 days for postcoital contraception appeared to be less effective than ethinyloestradiol 5 mg daily.— G. W. Dixon *et al.*, *J. Am. med. Ass.*, 1980, *244*, 1336.

Depression. In a double-blind study the mean depressive rating in 23 women with severe depression unresponsive to conventional treatment was significantly improved after treatment with conjugated oestrogens 5 mg daily initially, increased to 15 to 25 mg daily, compared with 17 women given a placebo. Elevated monoamine oxidase activity was significantly reduced. Side-effects were minimal.— E. L. Klaiber *et al.*, *Archs gen. Psychiat.*, 1979, *36*, 550.

Haemostasis. Despite case reports of dramatic cessation of spontaneous or traumatic bleeding after the intravenous injection of conjugated oestrogens most controlled studies had failed to confirm its usefulness. Its use in epistaxis and haemoptysis had not been rigorously studied.— M. Verstraete, *Haemostatic Drugs*, The Hague, Martinus Nijhoff, 1977, p. 74.

Intravenous doses of conjugated oestrogens significantly reduced blood loss in the urine following transurethral prostatectomy in 15 patients.— N. Gray and E. S. Palakow, *J. int. med. Res.*, 1979, *7*, 96.

Inhibition of growth. Conjugated oestrogens daily together with a progestogen daily for 5 days during the second half of the menstrual cycle were given to 41 pubescent girls for an average of 22 months. The mean estimated height restriction was 6 cm.— K. v. Puttkamer *et al.*, *Dt. med. Wschr.*, 1977, *102*, 983.

Further references: E. J. Schoen *et al.*, *Am. J. Dis. Child.*, 1973, *125*, 71, per *Int. pharm. Abstr.*, 1973, *10*, 943.

Menopausal symptoms and osteoporosis. See under Oestradiol, p.1427 and Mestranol, p.1418.

Neoplasm of the breast. Of 31 postmenopausal women with metastatic breast cancer 14 achieved a response when treated with conjugated oestrogens 2.5 mg thrice daily. The response-rate was comparable with that achieved with synthetic oestrogens, and side-effects were considered minimal.— I. E. Smith *et al.*, *Clin. Oncol.*, 1979, *5*, 159.

Preparations

Conjugated Estrogens Tablets *(U.S.P.)*. Tablets containing conjugated oestrogens.

Esterified Estrogens Tablets *(U.S.P.)*. Tablets containing esterified estrogens.

Proprietary Preparations

Premarin *(Ayerst, UK)*. Conjugated oestrogens, available as **Tablets** of 0.625, 1.25, and 2.5 mg and as **Vaginal Cream** containing 625 µg per g. (Also available as Premarin in *Austral.*, *Canad.*, *Denm.*, *Fr.*, *Ital.*, *S.Afr.*, *Switz.*, *USA*).

Prempak 0.625 *(Ayerst, UK)*. Packs of 21 maroon tablets each containing conjugated oestrogens 625 µg and 7 white tablets each containing norgestrel 500 µg. **Prempak 1.25.** Packs of 21 yellow tablets each containing conjugated oestrogens 1.25 mg and 7 white tablets each containing norgestrel 500 µg. For menopausal symptoms. *Dose.* 1 maroon or yellow tablet daily for 21 days, with 1 white tablet in addition from day 15 to day 21, and after 7 tablet-free days for succeeding cycles.

Other Proprietary Names

Arg.— Neo-Menovar; *Belg.*— Equigyne; *Canad.*— C.E.S., Oestrilin *(see also under Oestrone)*; *Fr.*— Équigyne, Prémauclair; *Ger.*— Oestro-Feminal, Presomen, Transannon; *Ital.*— Emopremarin, Equormon; *Neth.*— Equigyne; *S.Afr.*— Evoquin, Oestro-Feminal, Oestropak; *Spain*— Conestron, Equin; *Swed.*— Promarit; *Switz.*— Oestro-Feminal, Transannon; *Venez.*— Ayerogen.

Proprietary Names of Esterified Estrogens

Canad.— Climestrone, Estromed, Neo-Estrone; *USA*— Amnestrogen, Estratab, Evex, Menest.

9092-j

Oestrone *(Eur. P.)*. Estrone *(U.S.P.)*; Folliculin; Ketohydroxyoestrin; Oestronum. 3-Hydroxyestra-1,3,5(10)-trien-17-one.

$C_{18}H_{22}O_2$=270.4.

CAS — 53-16-7.

Pharmacopoeias. In *Arg.*, *Aust.*, *Braz.*, *Eur.*, *Fr.*, *Ger.*, *Hung.*, *It.*, *Mex.*, *Neth.*, *Pol.*, *Span.*, *Swiss*, *Turk.*, and *U.S.*

Odourless, tasteless, colourless crystals or white to creamy-white crystalline powder. M.p. about 260° with decomposition.

Practically **insoluble** in water; soluble 1 in 250 of alcohol, 1 in 50 of boiling alcohol and acetone at 50°, 1 in 110 of chloroform; soluble in dioxan; slightly soluble in dehydrated alcohol, ether, and solutions of alkali hydroxides. Solutions in oil are **sterilised** by maintaining at 150° for 1 hour. **Store** in airtight containers. Protect from light.

Units. The international unit for oestrone was discontinued in 1949, but continues to be used. One unit was contained in 0.0001 mg of the standard preparation.

Oestrone is a naturally occurring oestrogenic hormone with actions and uses similar to those of oestradiol (see p.1425). It has been administered by intramuscular injection in oily solutions and aqueous suspensions and in pessaries. Doses have ranged from 0.1 to 5 mg daily. Up to 0.004% of oestrone has been used in cosmetics.

In 60 men (climacteric) with endocrine impotence, better results were achieved by giving oestrone with testosterone (1:10, 1:20, or 1:50 parenterally) and oestriol (2 to 4 mg daily by mouth) than by giving testosterone alone. In a further group of elderly men satisfactory results were obtained by giving injections of oestrone, nicotinic acid, and testosterone, or oestradiol and an anabolic steroid.— J. Teter (letter), *Br. med. J.*, 1972, *4*, 114.

Studies with ^{14}C-labelled oestrone indicated that oestrone undergoes enterohepatic recirculation, that it is metabolised in the liver and intestine and that excretion is mainly as metabolites via the urine. Metabolic clearance was estimated to be about 90 litres per m^2 body-surface daily.— L. A. Pagliaro *et al.*, *J. Am. pharm. Ass.*, 1977, *NS17*, 755.

Preparations

Estrone Injection *(U.S.P.)*. Oestrone Injection. A sterile solution of oestrone in a suitable oil.

Sterile Estrone Suspension *(U.S.P.)*. A sterile suspension of oestrone in Water for Injections.

Proprietary Names

Cristallovar *(Ibi, Ital.*; *Panpharma, Switz.)*; Femogen *(Stickley, Canad.)*; Kolpon *(Organon, Austral.)*; Oestrilin (see also under Conjugated Oestrogens) *(Desbergers, Canad.)*.

A proprietary preparation containing oestrone with other oestrogens is described under Oestriol (see p.1428).

9093-z

Oxandrolone *(U.S.P.)*. 17β-Hydroxy-17α-methyl-2-oxa-5α-androstan-3-one.

$C_{19}H_{30}O_3$=306.4.

CAS — 53-39-4.

Pharmacopoeias. In *U.S.*

A white odourless crystalline powder. M.p. about 225°. Very slightly **soluble** in water; soluble 1 in about 60 of alcohol, 1 in about 70 of acetone, 1 in less than 5 of chloroform, and 1 in about 860 of ether. A solution in chloroform is laevorotatory. **Protect** from light.

Adverse Effects and Precautions. As for Testosterone, p.1436.

Oxandrolone, given for long periods, may cause jaundice and is contra-indicated in patients with liver disturbances.

Absorption and Fate. Oxandrolone is rapidly absorbed from the gastro-intestinal tract. It is excreted mainly in the urine as metabolites and unchanged oxandrolone. A small amount is excreted in the faeces.

Investigations in 6 healthy male subjects demonstrated that following oral ingestion of oxandrolone 10 mg there was rapid absorption resulting in a maximum plasma concentration of 417 ng per ml between 30 and 90 minutes. Plasma concentrations then declined in 2 phases: from 90 minutes to 4 hours with a half-life of about 33 minutes; from 4 to 48 hours the half-life was about 9 hours. Only 2.8% of the dose was excreted in the faeces whereas 60.4% was excreted in the urine within 96 hours (43.6% in the first 24 hours). Unchanged oxandrolone in the urine accounted for 28.7% of the administered dose.— A. Karim *et al.*, *Clin. Pharmac. Ther.*, 1973, *14*, 862.

Uses. Oxandrolone has anabolic and androgenic actions similar to those of methandienone (see p.1419) and is used for similar purposes.

The usual initial dose is 5 to 10 mg daily in divided doses. A dose of 2.5 to 5 mg daily is usually adequate for maintenance.

Effect on serum lipids. In 47 patients with hyperlipidaemia given oxandrolone 2.5 mg thrice daily for 2 periods of 12 and 28 weeks, plasma-cholesterol concentrations fell in 16 and triglyceride concentrations fell in 23. In 16 patients neither triglyceride nor cholesterol concentrations were significantly altered. There was a high rate of response in patients with marked elevation of pre-beta-lipoproteins. In 6 patients small elevations in serum transaminase concentration occurred in the first 4 weeks of treatment but subsided although treatment was continued.— A. E. Doyle *et al.*, *Med. J. Aust.*, 1974, *1*, 127.

During oxandrolone therapy the mean total postheparin lipolytic activity increased in 7 men with hyperlipoproteinaemia. This was considered to be due to the increase in activity of postheparin hepatic lipase and phospholipase A but not to postheparin plasma-lipoprotein lipase of which there was little increase in activity.— C. Ehnholm *et al.*, *New Engl. J. Med.*, 1975, *292*, 1314.

Serum triglycerides were significantly reduced in patients with types III, IV and V hyperlipoproteinaemia (Fredrickson classification) after oxandrolone 2.5 mg thrice daily for 7 months. In type IIb patients beta-lipoproteins were increased, suggesting that oxandrolone should not be used in this group. Type IV and V patients showed about 5% increase in body-weight.— C. L. Malmendier *et al.*, *J. clin. Pharmac.*, 1978, *18*, 42.

Growth defects. Probable accelerated vertical growth without acceleration of skeletal maturation in stunted children given oxandrolone.— T. S. Danowski *et al.*, *Clin. Pharmac. Ther.*, 1967, *8*, 548. Greater increase in linear growth than in skeletal maturation.— G. A. Limbeck *et al.*, *ibid.*, 1971, *12*, 798. A significant increase in predicted mature height in children with a bone age greater than 9 years.— H. K. Bettman *et al.*, *J. Pediat.*, 1971, *79*, 1018, per *Int. pharm. Abstr.*, 1972, *9*, 785. Acceleration of skeletal maturation greater than that of linear growth.— S. T. Jackson *et al.*, *Am. J. Dis. Child.*, 1973, *126*, 481, per *J. Am. med. Ass.*, 1973, *226*, 579. Absence of effect on growth, 12 years later, in children with Down's syndrome.— R. H. Ruvalcaba *et al.*, *J. Pediat.*, 1976, *88*, 504, per *Int. pharm. Abstr.*, 1976, *13*, 936. Acceleration of growth velocity in children with Turner's syndrome.— D. C. Moore *et al.*, *J. Pediat.*, 1977, *90*, 462, per *Int. pharm. Abstr.*, 1977, *14*, 1141. See also M. D. Urban, *J. Pediat.*, 1979, *94*, 823.

For an adverse comment on the use of anabolic steroids for growth, see Methandienone, p.1419. See also under Testosterone, p.1436.

Preparations

Oxandrolone Tablets *(U.S.P.)*. Tablets containing oxandrolone. Store in airtight containers. Protect from light.

Proprietary Names

Anavar *(Searle, USA)*; Antitriol *(Spain)*; Lonavar *(Searle, Arg.*; *Searle, Austral.*; *Dainippon, Jap.)*.

9094-c

Oxymesterone. Methandrostenediolone. 4,17β-Dihydroxy-17α-methylandrost-4-en-3-one.

$C_{20}H_{30}O_3$=318.5.

CAS — 145-12-0.

Adverse Effects and Precautions. As for Testosterone, p.1436.

Oxymesterone, given for prolonged periods, may cause jaundice and is contra-indicated in patients with liver disturbances.

Uses. Oxymesterone has anabolic and androgenic actions similar to those of methandienone (see p.1419) and has been used for similar purposes. The usual adult dose was 10 to 40 mg daily.

Proprietary Names

Anamidol *(Jap.)*; Balnimax *(Geve, Spain)*; Oranabol *(Spain)*.

Oxymesterone was formerly marketed in Great Britain under the proprietary name Oranabol 10 (*Farmitalia Carlo Erba*).

9095-k

Oxymetholone *(B.P., U.S.P.)*. 17β-Hydroxy-2-hydroxymethylene-17α-methyl-5α-androstan-3-one.

$C_{21}H_{32}O_3$=332.5.

CAS — 434-07-1.

Pharmacopoeias. In *Br.* and *U.S.*

A white to creamy-white, odourless, crystalline powder. M.p. 172° to 180°.

Practically **insoluble** in water; soluble 1 in 50 of alcohol; freely soluble in chloroform; soluble in dioxan; slightly soluble in ether. A solution in dioxan is dextrorotatory. **Protect** from light. Avoid contact with ferrous metals.

Adverse Effects. As for Testosterone, p.1436.

Liver disturbances and jaundice are common with normal doses. Leukaemia has developed in patients with aplastic anaemia treated with oxymetholone but the role of oxymetholone is not clear. Iron-deficiency anaemia may develop. Hepatic neoplasms have been reported in patients treated with oxymetholone.

Toxic confusional state and choreiform movements in a 66-year-old man given oxymetholone.— A. Tilzey *et al.*, *Br. med. J.*, 1981, *283*, 349.

Hypertriglyceridaemia and hypercholesterolaemia with angina and a left cerebral thrombosis occurred in a patient after receiving oxymetholone 100 mg daily for 5½ weeks. Serum triglyceride and cholesterol concentrations returned to normal after oxymetholone was discontinued, and angina and cerebral ischaemia did not recur.— R. D. Reeves *et al.*, *J. Am. med. Ass.*, 1976, *236*, 469.

Effects on the liver. Fatal hepatic coma associated with oxymetholone in a patient with muliple myeloma.— G. P. Young *et al.*, *Aust. N.Z. J. Med.*, 1977, *7*, 47, per *Int. pharm. Abstr.*, 1977, *14*, 1178.

Peliosis hepatis associated with oxymetholone.— G. Groos *et al.* (letter), *Lancet*, 1974, *1*, 874; E. C. McDonald and C. E. Speicher, *J. Am. med. Ass.*, 1978, *240*, 243.

Reports of various liver tumours associated with oxymetholone: M. S. Bernstein *et al.*, *New Engl. J. Med.*, 1971, *284*, 1135; F. L. Johnson *et al.*, *Lancet*, 1972, *2*, 1273; G. C. Farrell *et al.*, *ibid.*, 1975, *1*, 430; P. P. Anthony (letter), *ibid.*, 685; M. Bruguera, *ibid.*, 1295; M. Lesna *et al.*, *ibid.*, 1976, *1*, 1124; S. T. Mokrohisky *et al.* (letter), *New Engl. J. Med.*, 1977, *296*, 1411.

Leukaemia. Leukaemia in 4 patients given oxymetholone for aplastic anaemia. A causal relationship had not been proved.— I. W. Delamore and C. G. Geary, *Br. med. J.*, 1971, *2*, 743. See also A. D. Ginsburg (letter), *Ann. intern. Med.*, 1973, *79*, 914.

Of patients who present with aplastic anaemia 1 to 5% actually have leukaemia.— B. M. Camitta *et al.*, *New Engl. J. Med.*, 1982, *306*, 645.

Precautions. As for Testosterone, p.1436.

Oxymetholone is contra-indicated in patients with liver disturbances. It may enhance the actions of anticoagulants.

Uses. Oxymetholone has anabolic and androgenic actions similar to those of methandienone (see p.1419). It is used mainly in the treatment of anaemias.

The usual dosage for erythropoiesis is 1 to 5 mg per kg body-weight daily. Response may not be immediate and treatment for 3 to 6 months is suggested; maintenance dosage is often necessary. In other conditions the usual adult dose is 5 to 10 mg daily. Up to 150 mg daily has been given as an adjunct to cytotoxic therapy and radiotherapy.

Reports of oxymetholone decreasing the length of the menstrual cycle and reducing plasma concentrations of luteinising hormone and progesterone.— E. L. Klaiber *et al.*, *J. clin. Endocr. Metab.*, 1973, *36*, 142, per *Int. pharm. Abstr.*, 1974, *11*, 727; P. Cox *et al.*, *Am. J. Obstet. Gynec.*, 1975, *121*, 121, per *Drug Intell. & clin. Pharm.*, 1975, *9*, 217.

Anaemia. Only 5 of 21 patients with aplastic anaemia treated with oxymetholone 150 to 300 mg daily survived. One patient treated with fluoxymesterone died six months after the start of treatment. Few of the patients survived long enough to respond to oxymetholone.— S. Davis and A. D. Rubin, *Lancet*, 1972, *1*, 871.

Of 28 patients with aplastic anaemia treated with oxymetholone, 1 achieved a temporary complete remission and 10 achieved a partial response with appreciable improvement in the haemoglobin concentration and some increase in the white-cell count. Two patients who responded initially failed to respond when given oxymetholone again after brief withdrawal. Three patients developed leukaemia.— M. A. Mir and I. W. Delamore, *Postgrad. med. J.*, 1974, *50*, 166.

The survival rate in patients with aplastic anaemia treated with oxymetholone, with or without corticosteroids, was slightly but not significantly better than that earlier achieved with supportive therapy only.— M. A. Mir and C. G. Geary, *Postgrad. med. J.*, 1980, *56*, 322.

Further references: B. M. Camitta *et al.*, *Blood*, 1979, *53*, 504.

Sickle-cell anaemia. Six of 7 patients with sickle-cell anaemia gained a five-fold increase in urinary erythropoietin concentration with increases in erythrocyte mass of 17% to 75% after at least 2 months' treatment with oxymetholone. Serum-iron concentrations fell in all patients. Reversible liver damage occurred in 1 patient.— R. Alexanian and J. Nadell, *Blood*, 1975, *45*, 769, per *J. Am. med. Ass.*, 1975, *233*, 1325.

Preparations

Oxymetholone Tablets *(B.P.)*. Tablets containing oxymetholone. Avoid contact with ferrous metals. Protect from light.

Oxymetholone Tablets *(U.S.P.)*. Tablets containing oxymetholone.

Anapolon *(Syntex, UK)*. Oxymetholone, available as tablets of 5 mg. **Anapolon 50.** Oxymetholone, available as scored tablets of 50 mg. (Also known as Anapolon or Anapolon 50 in *Austral., Canad., S.Afr.*).

Other Proprietary Names

Adroyd *(Austral., Canad., Neth.)*; Anadrol-50 *(USA)*; Anadroyd *(Belg.)*; Anasteron *(Denm., Norw., Swed.)*; Anasteronal *(Spain)*; Nastenon *(Fr.)*; Oxitosona-50 *(Spain)*; Pardroyd *(Ger.)*; Plenastril *(Ger., Switz.)*; Synasteron *(Belg.)*; Zenalosyn *(Neth.)*.

9096-a

Pentagestrone Acetate. 3-Cyclopentyloxy-20-oxopregna-3,5-dien-17α-yl acetate.

$C_{28}H_{40}O_4$=440.6.

CAS — 7001-56-1 (pentagestrone); 1178-60-5 (acetate).

Pentagestrone acetate is a progestational agent used in the treatment of threatened and habitual abortion, and endometriosis.

Proprietary Names

Gestovis *(Vister, Ital.)*.

9097-t

Polyestradiol Phosphate. Polyoestradiol Phosphate; Leo 114.

CAS — 28014-46-2.

A water-soluble polymeric ester of oestradiol and phosphoric acid with a molecular weight of about 26 000.

Polyestradiol phosphate has actions similar to those of oestradiol (see p.1425). It has a prolonged action and is administered by deep intramuscular injection in doses of 80 to 160 mg every 4 weeks in the treatment of carcinoma of the prostate. Doses of 40 to 80 mg may be used for maintenance.

Proprietary Preparations

Estradurin Injection *(Lundbeck, UK)*. Polyestradiol phosphate, available as a powder for preparation before use, in vials of 40 mg with mepivacaine hydrochloride 5 mg, nicotinamide 25 mg, and phenylmercuric nitrate 20 µg, and in vials of 80 mg with mepivacaine hydrochloride 5 mg, nicotinamide 40 mg, and phenylmercuric nitrate 20 µg. (Also available as Estradurin in *Austral., Neth., S.Afr., Spain, USA*).

9098-x

Progesterone *(B.P., B.P. Vet., Eur. P., U.S.P.)*.

Progest.; Progesteronum; Luteal Hormone; Luteine; Pregnenedione; Progestin; NSC 9704.

Pregn-4-ene-3,20-dione.

$C_{21}H_{30}O_2$=314.5.

CAS — 57-83-0.

Pharmacopoeias. In all pharmacopoeias examined.

Colourless crystals or a white or slightly yellowish-white, odourless, tasteless, crystalline powder. There are two forms, one melts at 126° to 131° and the other, known as β-progesterone, at about 121°.

Practically **insoluble** in water; soluble 1 in 8 of alcohol, 1 in 60 of arachis oil, 1 in less than 1 of chloroform, 1 in 16 of ether, 1 in 60 of ethyl oleate, and 1 in 100 of light petroleum; sparingly soluble in acetone, dioxan, and fixed oils. A solution in dehydrated alcohol is dextrorotatory. Solutions in oil are **sterilised** by maintaining at 150° for 1 hour. **Store** in airtight containers. Protect from light.

The solubility and stability of progesterone in sesame oil or dimethicone.— B. H. Tusa and K. E. Avis, *Bull. parent. Drug Ass.*, 1972, *26*, 1.

The solubility of progesterone in water was 11 µg per ml at 30°.— D. K. Madan and D. E. Cadwallader, *J. pharm. Sci.*, 1973, *62*, 1567.

Effect of gamma-irradiation. Progesterone, at 250 000 Gy, changed from a pale cream colour to bright yellow and a resinous odour developed.— *The Use of Gamma Radiation Sources for the Sterilisation of Pharmaceutical Products*, London, ABPI, 1960.

Progesterone was discoloured, but no decomposition was apparent, after irradiation with 25 000 Gy.— G. Hortobagyi *et al.*, *Radiosterilization of Medical Products*, Vienna, International Atomic Energy Agency, 1967, p. 25.

Adverse Effects. Progesterone and progestational agents may produce virilisation of the foetus. Acne, oedema, weight gain, gastro-intestinal side-effects, gynaecomastia, headache, and depression have occurred. There may be urticaria, pruritus vulvae, candidiasis, cramps, and changes in libido, vaginal secretion, and altered menstrual patterns with unpredictable bleeding. Alterations in liver function have been reported. Jaundice appears to be rare and is similar to that occurring in pregnancy. Injections of progesterone may be painful.

An increased incidence of ectopic pregnancies has been reported in association with the use of intra-uterine devices containing progesterone.

See also Adverse Effects of Oral Contraceptives, p.1402.

Progesterone was administered subcutaneously to beagle *dogs* in varying daily doses for a period of 74 weeks. Postmortem examination of the mammary glands revealed lobular hyperplasia in most of the treated animals. Fibroadenomatous nodules were apparent in 2 of 5 animals receiving the highest doses. These nodules were well circumscribed and did not appear to be invasive.— D. K. Vallance and K. Capel-Edwards (letter), *Br. med. J.*, 1971, *2*, 221.

In *mice* exposed to a known carcinogen the incidence of carcinoma of the cervix was increased when progesterone was given concomitantly.— S. Reboud and G. Pageaut (letter), *Nature*, 1973, *241*, 398.

Progesterone dermatitis in 7 women possibly due to the earlier ingestion of progestogens.— R. Hart, *Archs Derm.*, 1977, *113*, 426.

Pregnancy and the neonate. *Ectopic pregnancy.* The reported incidence of ectopic pregnancy in women using the Progestasert intra-uterine device was 21% of the pregnancies, an incidence of 0.37 per 100 woman-years; this compared with an incidence of 0.05 or 0.06 per 100 woman-years in about 16 500 women using other intra-uterine devices in the UK.— R. Snowden (letter), *Br. med. J.*, 1977, *2*, 1600.

Of 184 pregnancies associated with the use of the Progestasert intra-uterine device 16.3% were ectopic, compared with 4.1% among 2822 pregnancies associated with the use of unmedicated intra-uterine devices and 3% among 1349 pregnancies associated with the use of copper-containing devices.— *FDA Drug Bull.*, 1978, *8*, 37.

Effects on the foetus. A report of a symposium on progesterone, progestins, and foetal development.— *Fert. Steril.*, 1978, *30*, 16.

Precautions. Progesterone should not be used during pregnancy because of the risk of virilisation of the female foetus. It should not be given to patients with missed or incomplete abortions, undiagnosed vaginal bleeding, or, unless treatment is being attempted, to patients with neoplasms of the breast. Progesterone should be used with care in patients with heart or kidney disease, asthma or epilepsy or other conditions affected by fluid retention.

Progestogens had been reported to precipitate attacks of porphyria.— *Drug & Ther. Bull.*, 1976, *14*, 55.

Absorption and Fate. Progesterone is absorbed from the gastro-intestinal tract but is rapidly inactivated in the liver and has little effect; it is absorbed when administered buccally, rectally, or vaginally, and rapidly absorbed from the site of an oily intramuscular injection. The half-life in blood is only a few minutes. It is metabolised in the liver, about 12% to pregnanediol which is excreted in the urine conjugated with glucuronic acid. Urinary excretion of pregnanediol is measured as a guide to natural progesterone secretion. Progestogens are excreted in the milk of nursing mothers.

Plasma concentrations of progesterone in healthy women.— M. H. Kim *et al.*, *J. clin. Endocr. Metab.*, 1974, *39*, 706.

Studies in 3 women showed that 10% or less of progesterone in the foetal circulation was derived from the maternal circulation.— L. Escarcena *et al.*, *Am. J. Obstet. Gynec.*, 1978, *130*, 462.

In 5 postmenopausal women given progesterone 100 mg by mouth daily for 5 days peak concentrations were present 1 to 3 hours after the last dose. Among the metabolites the concentration of pregnanediol-3α-glucuronide was most elevated, that of 17-hydroxyprogesterone least elevated, and that of 20α-dihydroprogesterone was intermediate. The concentrations of oestradiol were not significantly affected. Progesterone by mouth might be of value when synthetic progestogens had caused adverse effects.— M. I. Whitehead *et al.*, *Br. med. J.*, 1980, *280*, 825.

Uses. Progesterone is the main hormone of the corpus luteum and the placenta. It acts on the endometrium by converting the proliferative phase induced by oestrogen to a secretory phase and preparing the uterus to receive the fertilised ovum. It also suppresses uterine motility and is responsible for the further development of the breasts.

Progesterone has a catabolic action and a slight rise in basal body temperature occurs during the secretory phase of menstruation.

Progesterone and other progestogens are used in the treatment of functional uterine bleeding. They are also used, often with an oestrogen, in menstrual disorders and have been given in the treatment of neoplasms of the breast and endometrium. Some progestogens have been used in habitual and threatened abortion.

Progesterone, impregnated in an intra-uterine device, has been used (but see Adverse Effects) for contraception and progestational agents are given systemically, either alone or with an oestrogen for contraception—see Oral Contraceptives, p.1402.

Progestational agents which are active when taken by mouth are now generally preferred to progesterone.

Progesterone is usually administered by intramuscular injection as a solution in oil or as aqueous suspensions, by implantation of pellets, and as tablets for buccal administration. It may also be given as suppositories or pessaries.

In the treatment of functional uterine bleeding, doses of 5 to 10 mg are injected daily for 5 to 10 days before the expected onset of menstruation. In amenorrhoea 25 mg has been given thrice weekly for the last 2 weeks of a cycle primed with oestrogen.

In habitual abortion, progesterone has been administered from the start of pregnancy, usually in doses of 5 to 20 mg twice or thrice weekly by intramuscular injection; for threatened abortion doses of 25 to 50 mg daily have been given until pains and haemorrhage cease then reduced to 10 to 25 mg daily.

The biosynthesis, metabolism, mechanism of action, effects, uses, and toxicity of progesterone.— M. B. Aufrére and H. Benson, *J. pharm. Sci.*, 1976, *65*, 783.

A short review of the physiological action of progesterone and the pharmacological effects of some progestogens.— F. Neumann, *Schering, Ger., Postgrad. med. J.*, 1978, *54*, *Suppl.* 2, 11.

Contraception. Discussions on the use of intra-uterine devices containing progesterone for contraception.— *Br. med. J.*, 1974, *4*, 181; *Med. Lett.*, 1976, *18*, 65; *Lancet*, 1977, *1*, 1239.

Clinical experience over 1 year with an intra-uterine device containing progesterone in 150 women. Three pregnancies occurred, 2 of which were ectopic.— G. Zador *et al.*, *Contraception*, 1976, *13*, 559, per *Int. pharm. Abstr.*, 1978, *15*, 323. Absence of effect on carbohydrate and lipid metabolism.— W. N. Spellacy *et al.*, *Contraception*, 1977, *15*, 65, per *Int. pharm. Abstr.*, 1977, *14*, 996. Experience in 192 women.— L. S. Wan *et al.*, *Contraception*, 1977, *16*, 417, per *Int. pharm. Abstr.*, 1978, *15*, 427. Elevation of plasma-prolactin concentrations indicating a systemic effect.— W. N. Spellacy *et al.*, *Contraception*, 1978, *17*, 71, per *Int. pharm. Abstr.*, 1978, *15*, 733.

See also under Adverse Effects.

References relating to vaginal devices releasing progestogens.— F. G. Burton *et al.*, *Contraception*, 1978, *17*, 221, per *Int. pharm. Abstr.*, 1978, *15*, 1176; F. G. Burton *et al.*, *Contraception*, 1979, *19*, 507, per *Int. pharm. Abstr.*, 1979, *16*, 1162.

Premenstrual syndrome. Three women with long histories of repeated misdemeanours successfully pleaded diminished responsibility or mitigation due to premenstrual syndrome in crimes of manslaughter, arson, and assault, and were successfully treated with progesterone.— K. Dalton, *Lancet*, 1980, *2*, 1070. See also K. Dalton, *The Premenstrual Syndrome and Progesterone Therapy*, London, Heineman, 1977.

A study suggesting that progesterone deficiency is probably not the cause of the premenstrual syndrome and thus treatment with progesterone is illogical.— P. M. S. O'Brien *et al.*, *Br. med. J.*, 1980, *280*, 1161. Comment and criticism.— K. Dalton (letter), *ibid.*, 1980, *281*, 61; G. Sampson (letter), *ibid.*, 227; A. J. Martin and L. J. Downey (letter), *ibid.*, 562; A. W. Clare (letter), *ibid.*, 810.

Progesterone was ineffective in the premenstrual syndrome when compared with placebo.— G. A. Sampson, *Br. J. Psychiat.*, 1979, *135*, 209.

Vulvar dystrophy. Good results were achieved in 3 of 5 patients with vulvar dystrophy following the application, once or twice daily, of progesterone ointment—200 mg in about 57 g of hydrophilic ointment *U.S.P.*— E. A. Jasionowski and P. Jasionowski, *Am. J. Obstet. Gynec.*, 1977, *127*, 667.

Preparations

Progesterone Injection *(B.P.)*. A sterile solution of progesterone in ethyl oleate or other suitable ester, in a suitable fixed oil, or in any mixture of these; it may contain suitable alcohols. Sterilised by maintaining at 150° for 1 hour. Protect from light. Solid matter may separate on standing; it should be redissolved by heating before use. For intramuscular injection only.

A similar injection is included in several other pharmacopoeias.

Progesterone Injection *(U.S.P.)*. A sterile solution of progesterone in a suitable solvent.

Progesterone Intrauterine Contraceptive System *(U.S.P.)*. A sterile system containing progesterone, designed to permit gradual release of the drug.

Sterile Progesterone Suspension *(U.S.P.)*. A sterile suspension in Water for Injections. pH 4 to 7.5.

A similar injection is included in *Jap. P.* (Progesterone Aquosuspensoid Injection).

Proprietary Preparations

Cyclogest *(Collins, UK: Cox Continental, UK)*. Progesterone, available as suppositories of 200 or 400 mg; for rectal or vaginal use.

Gestone *(Paines & Byrne, UK)*. Progesterone, available as an injection containing 10 and 25 mg per ml, in ampoules of 1 ml, and 50 mg per ml in ampoules of 1 and 2 ml.

Progestasert *(Alza, USA: Polcrome, UK)*. An intrauterine device containing progesterone 38 mg and delivering progesterone to the endometrium at an average rate of 65 µg daily. For contraception. Protection is stated to be afforded for at least a year. (Also available as Progestasert in *Ital.*, *NZ*).

Other Proprietary Names

Arg.—Corlutina, Proluton; *Austral.*—Progestin, Proluton; *Canad.*—Gesterol, Progestilin; *Fr.*—Lutogyl, Progestogel, Progestosol; *Ger.*—Biograviplan Progestasert, Proluton; *Ital.*—Gestone Pabryn, Progelun, Progestolo, Proluton *Jap.*—Oophormin Luteum; *Neth.*—Progestine; *Spain*—Proluton; *Switz.*—Lutocyclin, Progestosol; *USA*—Gesterol.

Progesterone was also formerly marketed in Great Britain under the proprietary name Progesterone Implants (*Organon*). A preparation containing progesterone was also formerly marketed under the proprietary name Paralut (*Wallace Mfg Chem.*).

9099-r

Promethoestrol Dipropionate. Dimethylhexestrol Dipropionate; Methoestrol Dipropionate. 4,4′-(1,2-Diethylethylene)di(*o*-tolyl propionate).
$C_{26}H_{34}O_4$=410.6.

CAS — 130-73-4 (promethoesterol); 84-13-9 (dipropionate).

Promethoestrol dipropionate is a synthetic oestrogen with actions similar to those of oestradiol (see p.1425). A dose of 1 to 3 mg by mouth daily has been used to control menopausal symptoms.

Proprietary Names
Meprane Dipropionate *(Reed & Carnrick, USA)*.

9100-r

Quinestradol. Oestriol 3-Cyclopentyl Ether. 3-Cyclopentyloxyestra-1,3,5(10)-triene-16α,17β-diol.
$C_{23}H_{32}O_3$=356.5.

CAS — 1169-79-5.

A white crystalline powder. Practically **insoluble** in water; soluble in organic solvents and fixed oils.

Quinestradol is an oestrogen with actions similar to those of oestradiol (see p.1425) but it is claimed to have relatively less activity on breast and endometrial tissue than on the vagina.

Quinestradol may be given by mouth in capsules. The usual dosage is 500 µg once or twice daily for the relief of postmenopausal symptoms.

Acne. In a double-blind pilot study quinestradol 1 mg daily appeared to be more effective than a placebo in the treatment of acne vulgaris of young women.— P. Moroni and G. Bruni, *Arzneimittel-Forsch.*, 1976, *26*, 583.

Incontinence. In a double-blind trial, quinestradol 250 µg four times daily benefited 16 out of 18 incontinent elderly women after treatment for 4 weeks. Vaginal bleeding occurred in a further patient treated with the drug.— T. G. Judge, *Geront. clin.*, 1969, *11*, 159. A similar report.— R. M. Jameson, *Br. J. clin. Pract.*, 1969, *23*, 457.

Vaginitis. Thirty postmenopausal patients with uterine or vaginal prolapse or senile vaginitis were treated with quinestradol 250 µg twice daily for 14 days, or 500 µg twice daily for 21 days. In the latter dose vaginal symptoms were relieved with improvement in the degree of vaginal cellularity and in the glycogen content of the cells. A parallel histological response was not observed and quinestradol was not considered to be of sufficient value to recommend its clinical use.— A. M. Fisher and M. B. Wingate, *Br. J. clin. Pract.*, 1966, *20*, 193. Comments.— C. Mangioni (letter), *ibid.*, 548; F. Vischi (letter), *ibid.*, 597. Quinestradol, 250 µg twice daily for 14 days, was considered a suitable treatment for senile vaginitis.— L. Cohen, *ibid.*, 1968, *22*, 207.

Proprietary Preparations
Pentovis *(Warner, UK)*. Quinestradol, available as capsules each containing 250 µg in sesame oil.

Other Proprietary Names
Colpovis *(Ital., S.Afr.)*; Colpovister *(Spain)*.

9101-f

Quinestrol.

W 3566; Ethinyloestradiol-3-cyclopentyl Ether. 3-Cyclopentyloxy-19-nor-17α-pregna-1,3,5(10)-trien-20-yn-17β-ol.
$C_{25}H_{32}O_2$=364.5.

CAS — 152-43-2.

A white odourless powder. Practically **insoluble** in water; soluble in alcohol, chloroform, and ether.

Adverse Effects and Precautions. As for Oestradiol, p.1425.

Changes in coagulation and fibrinolysis persisting 6 weeks after the use of quinestrol for the inhibition of lactation were similar to those reported after the use of oral contraceptives and might indicate thrombogenic risk.— P. W. Howie *et al.*, *Br. J. Obstet. Gynaec.*, 1975, *82*, 968, per *Int. pharm. Abstr.*, 1977, *14*, 238.

Allergic reaction. A 30-year-old woman developed an allergic reaction, with urticaria, slight dyspnoea, and oedema, following a single dose of quinestrol by mouth for suppression of lactation.— D. A. Aitken and E. G. Daw (letter), *Br. med. J.*, 1970, *2*, 177.

Absorption and Fate. Quinestrol is absorbed from the gastro-intestinal tract and is stored in body fat. It is slowly released over several days and metabolised to ethinyloestradiol which is excreted in the urine.

Metabolism of quinestrol.— F. R. Zuleski *et al.*, *J. pharm. Sci.*, 1978, *67*, 1138.

Further references: K. I. H. Williams *et al.*, *Steroids*, 1967, *9*, 275.

Uses. Quinestrol is an oestrogen with actions and uses similar to those of oestradiol (see p.1426). It has a prolonged action.

It has been used to inhibit and suppress lactation but alternative methods, including the use of bromocriptine (see p.894), are now preferred. For inhibition a single dose of 4 mg has been given by mouth within 6 hours of delivery. A second dose was given after 4 to 6 days if lactation occurred and became persistent and troublesome. For the suppression of established lactation a dose of 4 mg was given and followed with a second dose after 48 hours.

A detailed laboratory study of the effects of quinestrol on blood chemistry, liver function, and endocrine indices.— T. S. Danowski *et al.*, *Clin. Pharmac. Ther.*, 1970, *11*, 260.

Contraception. For references to the limited usefulness of quinestrol with quingestanol acetate as a contraceptive, see F. Nudemberg *et al.*, *Fert. Steril.*, 1973, *24*, 185, per *Int. pharm. Abstr.*, 1973, *10*, 794; T. S. Danowski *et al.*, *Clin. Pharmac. Ther.*, 1973, *14*, 455; D. R. Mishell and M. Freid, *Contraception*, 1973, *8*, 37.

Inhibition of lactation. Oestrogens are no longer recommended for the inhibition of lactation. For further details, see Oestradiol, p.1426 and Stilboestrol, p.1434.

Menopausal symptoms. In a double-blind study quinestrol 100 or 200 µg once weekly was as effective as conjugated oestrogens 1.25 mg daily in 21-day cycles, for the relief of vasomotor flushes in menopausal women.— S. B. Baumgardner *et al.*, *Obstet. Gynec.*, 1978, *51*, 445.

Complete or partial response of menopausal symptoms in 35 of 40 women given quinestrol 1 mg once a month compared with 15 of 30 given a placebo.— O. E. Jaschevatzky *et al.*, *Acta obstet. gynec. scand.*, 1979, *58*, 175.

Proprietary Preparations

Estrovis *(Warner, UK)*. Quinestrol, available as tablets of 4 mg. (Also available as Estrovis in *Belg.*, *Ger.*, *Ital.*, *Neth.*, *S.Afr.*, *USA*).

Other Proprietary Names

Agalacto-Quilea, Basaquines, Eston, Qui-Lea *(all Arg.)*.

9102-d

Quingestanol Acetate. W 4540. 3-Cyclopentyloxy-19-nor-17α-pregna-3,5-dien-20-yn-17β-yl acetate.
$C_{27}H_{36}O_3$=408.6.

CAS — 10592-65-1 (quingestanol); 3000-39-3 (acetate).

A white crystalline powder. M.p. 182° to 184°

Adverse Effects. As for Progesterone, p.1431.
See also Oral Contraceptives, p.1402.

Uses. Quingestanol acetate is a progestational agent with actions similar to those of progesterone (see p.1431).

It is used as a contraceptive and for the treatment of menstrual disorders. It is given in a dose of 500 µg daily with ethinyloestradiol 50 µg for 21 days commencing on the 5th day of the first cycle and thereafter repeated after an interval of 7 days for succeeding cycles or alone as a 'progestogen-only' contraceptive in daily doses of 300 µg (see also Oral Contraceptives, p.1402.)

It has also been given, with limited usefulness, once a month as an oral contraceptive in a dose of 2.5 mg in conjunction with quinestrol 2 mg.

For clinical reports of the use of quingestanol acetate, see Martindale 27th Edn, p. 1425.

Proprietary Names
Demovis *(Vister, Ital.)*; Pilomin *(A.L., Norw.; A.L., Swed.)*.

Proprietary Names of Quingestanol Acetate with Ethinyloestradiol

Piloval *(A.L., Norw.; A.L., Swed.)*; Rélovis *(Substantia, Fr.)*.

9103-n

Stanolone *(B.P.)*. Androstanolone; Dihydrotestosterone. 17β-Hydroxy-5α-androstan-3-one.
$C_{19}H_{30}O_2$=290.4.

CAS — 521-18-6.

Pharmacopoeias. In *Br.*

An odourless white crystalline powder. M.p. 178° to 183°. Practically **insoluble** in water; soluble 1 in 20 of alcohol and 1 in 70 of ether. A solution in dioxan is dextrorotatory. **Protect** from light.

Adverse Effects and Precautions. As for Testosterone, p.1436.

Uses. Stanolone has anabolic and androgenic actions similar to those of methandienone (see p.1419). It has been given by mouth, preferably sublingually or sublabially in doses of 50 to 75 mg daily for not more than 21 days of each month.

Preparations

Stanolone Tablets *(B.P. 1973)*. Tablets containing stanolone. They may contain peppermint oil.

Proprietary Names

Anabolex *(Samil, Ital.)*; Pesomax *(Boniscontro & Gazzone, Ital.)*.

Stanolone was formerly marketed in Great Britain under the proprietary name Anabolex (*Lloyd-Hamol*).

9104-h

Stanozolol *(U.S.P.)*. Androstanazole; Methylstanazole; Win 14833. 17α-Methyl-2′*H*-5α-androst-2-eno[3,2-c]pyrazol-17β-ol.
$C_{21}H_{32}N_2O$=328.5.

CAS — 10418-03-8.

Pharmacopoeias. In *U.S.*

An odourless crystalline powder. There are 2 forms; needles melt at about 155° and prisms at about 235°. Practically **insoluble** in water; soluble 1 in about 40 of alcohol, 1 in about 75 of chloroform, 1 in 370 of ether; soluble in dimethylformamide; slightly soluble in acetone and ethyl acetate. A solution in chloroform is dextrorotatory. **Store** in airtight containers. Protect from light.

Adverse Effects and Precautions. As for Testosterone, p.1436.

Stanozolol, given for prolonged periods, may cause jaundice and should be used with caution in patients with liver disturbances.

A 66-year-old man developed jaundice after treatment for 7 months with stanozolol 10 mg daily. The histological appearance of the liver suggested cholestatic jaundice of the hypersensitivity type. The condition regressed when stanozolol was withdrawn.— S. D. Slater *et al.*, *Postgrad. med. J.*, 1976, *52*, 229.

For the enhancement of the effect of dicoumarol by stanozolol, see Dicoumarol, p.771.

Uses. Stanozolol has anabolic and androgenic actions similar to those of methandienone (see p.1419) and is used for similar purposes. The usual adult dosage is 5 mg daily by mouth; double this dose is recommended to stimulate fibrinolysis. It may be given as an aqueous suspension by intramuscular injection, in a dose of 50 mg every 2 or 3 weeks, in severe disorders and in the treatment of anaemias and neoplastic disease.

Angio-oedema. A 31-year-old man with a 13-year history of severe abdominal manifestations of angioneurotic oedema and a 3-year history of cutaneous manifestations obtained complete relief of all abdominal and cutaneous symptoms following administration of stanozolol 5 mg twice daily.— D. J. Gould *et al.* (letter), *Lancet*, 1978, *1*, 770.

Skin and fat disorders. Preliminary observations showed that treatment for up to 2½ years with inositol nicotinate 1 g thrice daily used alone or following treatment with stanozolol caused improvement in 16 patients with necrobiosis lipoidica and cleared 2 other patients; of 3 further patients given stanozolol alone, 1 found no effect and 2 some improvement.— E. L. Rhodes, *Br. J. Derm.*, 1976, *95*, 673.

In 14 patients with long-standing liposclerosis of the leg, fibrinolytic activity was increased by treatment with stanozolol 5 mg twice daily; the mean area of liposclerosis was reduced by 73%, pain was reduced, the skin became softer, and pigmentation less obvious. Five patients had been cured and 9 continued to improve. Six patients suffered intermittent cramp and 3 recurrence of migraine.— N. L. Browse *et al.*, *Br. med. J.*, 1977, *2*, 434.

In a double-blind crossover study in 34 legs of 23 patients with longstanding liposclerosis the mean area of healing under treatment with stanozolol 5 mg twice daily and elastic stockings was 155 mm^2 compared with 78 mm^2 under treatment with placebo and elastic stockings. While the difference was not statistically significant it was considered biologically important. Most patients considered they had improvement in respect of pain, heat, colour, and induration. Continued treatment had led to loss of induration and regression of pigmentation. Such treatment was considered useful in intractable cases.— K. Burnand *et al.*, *Br. med. J.*, 1980, *280*, 7. Criticism.— H. L. Muston (letter), *Br. med. J.*, 1980, *280*, 254.

Vascular disease. Continuous treatment with stanozolol 5 mg twice daily and phenformin 50 mg twice daily for 6 months in 9 patients with occlusive vascular disease failed to maintain the reduction of platelet stickiness which had been maintained for 2 to 3 years by treatment with ethyloestrenol 4 mg twice daily and phenformin 50 mg twice daily. Blood-clot lysis and plasma-fibrinogen and serum-cholesterol concentrations were however maintained at their previous values.— R. Chakrabarti *et al.*, *Lancet*, 1970, *1*, 591.

Stanozolol was not an acceptable alternative to ethyloestrenol in situations where decreased fibrinolytic activity and/or increased platelet stickiness might be encountered.— G. R. Fearnley (letter), *Br. med. J.*, 1970, *1*, 693.

In a study of 20 patients, it was found that metformin with stanozolol was as effective as phenformin with stanozolol in increasing the blood fibrinolytic activity.— I. S. Menon (letter), *Br. med. J.*, 1971, *1*, 289.

Of 16 men with idiopathic recurrent superficial thrombophlebitis and who had on average one severe attack every 8 weeks for 7.7 years, 15 had evidence of decreased fibrinolytic activity. After treatment for 6 months with stanozolol 5 mg twice daily, thrombophlebitis had ceased in 13 patients and ceased in the remaining 3 after longer treatment. Thrombophlebitis had not recurred in 11 for a mean of 12.5 months (range 3 to 24 months); in 5 in whom it recurred no further recurrence occurred after phenformin was added to their treatment.— P. E. M. Jarrett *et al.*, *Br. med. J.*, 1977, *1*, 933.

In 16 patients with severe Raynaud's syndrome and who had already undergone sympathectomy, hand blood flow, palm and index-finger temperature, and grip strength were significantly increased, and plasma-fibrinogen concentrations significantly decreased after treatment for 3 months with stanozolol 5 mg twice daily. Most patients experienced subjective improvement. Three-month courses of stanozolol, repeated after periods of 1 or 2 months, were recommended for patients in whom all other treatments had failed.— P. E. M. Jarrett *et al.*, *Br. med. J.*, 1978, *2*, 523.

For the effect of phenformin and stanozolol on fibrinolytic activity, see Phenformin, p.858.

Preparations

Stanozolol Tablets *(U.S.P.)*. Tablets containing stanozolol. Store in airtight containers. Protect from light.

Stromba *(Sterling Research, UK)*. Stanozolol, available as **Injection** containing 50 mg per ml, in 2-ml ampoules containing 1 ml, and as scored **Tablets** of 5 mg. (Also available as Stromba in *Aust., Belg., Denm., Fin., Fr., Ger., Neth., Norw., Swed., Switz.*).

Other Proprietary Names

Anasyth *(Ital.)*; Strombaject *(Belg., Fr., Ger.)*; Winstrol *(Canad., Ital., S.Afr., Spain, USA)*.

9105-m

Stilboestrol *(B.P., B.P. Vet., Eur. P.)*. Stilboestr.; Diethylstilbestrol *(U.S.P.)*; Diethylstilboestrol; Diaethylstilboestrolum; Diethylstilbestrolum; NSC 3070. (*E*)-αβ-Diethylstilbene-4-4′-diol.
$C_{18}H_{20}O_2$=268.4.

CAS — 56-53-1.

Pharmacopoeias. In *Aust., Belg., Br., Chin., Cz., Eur., Fr., Ger., Ind., Int., It., Jug., Mex., Neth., Nord., Port., Roum., Rus., Swiss, Turk.*, and *U.S.*

A white or almost white, odourless, tasteless, crystalline powder. M.p. 169° to 175° with a range of not more than 4°. It absorbs insignificant amounts of moisture at 25° at relative humidities up to about 90%.

Practically **insoluble** in water; soluble 1 in 5 of alcohol, 1 in 200 of chloroform, 1 in 3 of ether, 1 in 40 of arachis oil, and 1 in 90 of olive oil; soluble in acetone, dioxan, ethyl acetate, fixed oils, methyl alcohol, and aqueous solutions of alkali hydroxides. Solutions in oil are **sterilised** by maintaining at 150° for 1 hour. **Store** in airtight containers. Protect from light.

CAUTION. *Stilboestrol is a powerful oestrogen. Contact with the skin or inhalation should be avoided. Rubber gloves and a face mask should be worn when handling the powder.*

The dissolution of stilboestrol crystals was inhibited by most permitted food colours. Cationic dyes had a greater effect than anionic dyes.— J. Piccolo and R. Tawashi, *J. pharm. Sci.*, 1971, *60*, 1818.

The solubility of stilboestrol in water was 25 µg per ml at 30°.— D. K. Madan and D. E. Cadwallader, *J. pharm. Sci.*, 1973, *62*, 1567.

Adverse Effects. As for Oestradiol, p.1425.

Nausea is common with the high doses employed for postcoital contraception.

An increased incidence of changes in the cervix and vagina including adenitis and adenocarcinoma has been noted, particularly in the USA, in the postpubertal daughters of women who received stilboestrol or related substances during pregnancy. An increased incidence of abnormalities of the genital tract and of abnormal spermatozoa has been reported in males similarly exposed.

Severe bone-marrow changes occurred in a 71-year-old man given stilboestrol in a dose of 150 mg daily for 7 years.— A. L. Anderson and E. C. Lynch, *Archs intern. Med.*, 1980, *140*, 976.

Cardiovascular effects. There was a greater incidence of fatal and nonfatal cardiac infarctions, congestive heart failure, and cerebrovascular accidents with stilboestrol 5 mg daily when compared with placebo in 491 patients with carcinoma of the prostate. A dose of 1 mg of stilboestrol daily was considered to be effective and early results did not indicate a higher incidence of complication.— C. E. Blackard *et al.*, *Cancer*, 1970, *26*, 249, per *Drugs*, 1971, *2*, 474. See also J. C. Bailar (letter), *Lancet*, 1967, *2*, 560.

In a group of 154 patients with prostatic cancer treated with stilboestrol, chlorotrianisene, or ethinyloestradiol the incidence of cardiovascular side-effects was greatest in the stilboestrol group. There was no difference in incidence of peripheral oedema or gynaecomastia nor in mortality from cardiovascular effects.— A. Morales and B. Pujari, *Can. med. Ass. J.*, 1975, *113*, 865.

Exercise-induced abnormalities of the ST segment were increased in 16 of 18 patients after treatment for 2 weeks with stilboestrol 5 mg daily.— M. D. Jaffe, *Br. Heart J.*, 1976, *38*, 1299, per *J. Am. med. Ass.*, 1977, *237*, 1023.

Severe pain developed in a woman who took one dose of stilboestrol 5 mg for progressive osteolytic metastases. It was considered that the oestrogen had aggravated the osseous metastases.— A. Buzdar *et al.* (letter), *J. Am. med. Ass.*, 1977, *237*, 2812.

Effects on blood. Factor IX concentrations in plasma were found to be significantly higher in women receiving stilboestrol for suppression of lactation than were found in late pregnancy or in women who were lactating or in whom lactation was suppressed without the use of drugs. Stilboestrol was given in a dosage of 10 mg thrice daily for 3 days, then twice daily for 3 days, then daily for 3 days.— D. G. Daniel *et al.*, *Br. med. J.*, 1968, *1*, 801.

See also C. A. Hakim *et al.*, *ibid.*, 1969, *4*, 82.

Effects on the liver. As assessed by a modified sulphobromophthalein test in 24 healthy puerperal women 7 days after delivery, stilboestrol 30 mg daily for the first 3 days after delivery, then 20 mg daily up to the sixth day, appreciably reduced the ability of the liver to excrete dye into the bile, and reduced significantly the equivalent liver volume and plasma clearance of the dye. These effects were not seen in 21 puerperal women who received megestrol acetate in the same dosage, or in 20 women who were breast feeding. Conventional liver-function tests showed normal results in all patients.— J. Clinch and V. R. Tindall, *Br. med. J.*, 1969, *1*, 602. See also B. Gheorghescu (letter), *ibid.*, 1969, *3*, 593.

Peliosis hepatis in 2 men associated with the use of stilboestrol.— A. R. Puppala and J. A. Ro, *Postgrad. Med.*, 1979, *65*, 277.

See also under Neoplasms.

Effects on serum lipids. In 10 patients with proven prostatic carcinoma, stilboestrol 1, 7.5, or 15 mg daily had no significant effect on serum-cholesterol concentrations. In 6 of 10 patients taking 1 mg daily, serum-triglyceride concentrations remained normal but in 8 and 10 patients taking 7.5 and 15 mg respectively serum-triglyceride concentrations were significantly elevated, with a rise in pre-beta-lipoproteins.— M. Shahmanesh *et al.*, *Br. med. J.*, 1973, *2*, 512.

Neoplasms. A malignant neoplasm of the breast occurred in a man who took oestrogens for the long-term treatment of malignant neoplasm of the prostate.— W. O'Grady and R. W. McDivitt, *Archs Path.*, 1969, *88*, 162, per *J. Am. med. Ass.*, 1969, *209*, 788. See also G. Srinivasan *et al.*, *J. Ky St. med. Ass.*, 1979, *77*, 9.

Neoplasms of the endometrium after treatment with stilboestrol.— B. S. Cutler *et al.*, *New Engl. J. Med.*, 1972, *287*, 628; A. M. McCarroll *et al.*, *Br. J. Obstet. Gynaec.*, 1975, *82*, 421, per *Int. pharm. Abstr.*, 1976, *13*, 1025; G. Roberts and A. L. Wells, *Br. J. Obstet. Gynaec.*, 1975, *82*, 417, per *Int. pharm. Abstr.*, 1976, *13*, 1025; S. Krishnamurthy *et al.*, *Gynecol. Oncol.*, 1977, *5*, 291.

In a 25-year follow-up of women who participated in a study involving administration of stilboestrol during pregnancy (W.J. Dieckmann *et al.*, *Am. J. Obstet. Gynec.*, 1953, *66*, 1062) 32 of 693 who had completed a full course of stilboestrol during pregnancy and were available for follow-up developed breast cancer (4.6%) and 21 of 668 who did not receive stilboestrol also developed breast cancer (3.1%), but the difference was not statistically significant. No statistical differences were found for any other categories of disease either. The higher incidence of breast cancer in both groups was not understood but might have been related to the original selection procedure.— M. Bibbo *et al.*, *New Engl. J. Med.*, 1978, *298*, 763. The role of oestrogens in breast cancer, though highly suspect, was unproved.— K. J. Ryan, *ibid.*, 794. There remained serious cause for concern.— *FDA Drug Bulletin*, 1978, *8*, 31. Criticism of Bibbo's report.— L. C. Clark and K. M. Portier (letter), *New Engl. J. Med.*, 1979, *300*, 263. The conclusions in Dieckmann *et al.'s* report on a lack of effect on pregnancy have also been questioned recently, see below under Pregnancy and the Neonate.

Hepatic angiosarcoma developed in a 76-year-old man who had received stilboestrol 3 mg daily for 12 years.— C. Hoch-Ligeti, *J. Am. med. Ass.*, 1978, *240*, 1510.

Renal carcinoma associated with the use of stilboestrol in 2 men.— I. Nissenkorn *et al.*, *Br. J. Urol.*, 1979, *51*, 6.

See also below under Pregnancy and the Neonate.

Porphyria. Porphyria cutanea tarda developed in 2 patients, each receiving stilboestrol 5 mg daily for prostatic carcinoma. Symptoms regressed on withdrawal of the stilboestrol.— J. T. Vail, *J. Am. med. Ass.*, 1967, *201*, 671.

Pregnancy and the neonate. W.J. Dieckmann *et al.* (*Am. J. Obstet. Gynec.*, 1953, *66*, 1062) carried out a controlled study on 1646 pregnant women and concluded that stilboestrol did not significantly affect pregnancy. However, submission of the results to statistical analysis shows that stilboestrol significantly increased the incidence of abortions, neonatal deaths, and premature births.— Y. Brackbill and H. W. Berendes (letter), *Lancet*, 1978, *2*, 520.

A controlled study was carried out on the female offspring, aged 18 years or older, of mothers who had received stilboestrol at some time during their pregnancy. Of the 110 exposed women, 22% had transverse fibrous ridges of the vagina and cervix, compared with none in the 82 controls; in 56% of the exposed, portions of the vaginal mucosa failed to stain with iodine compared with 1%; and in 35% of the exposed, vaginal adenosis was present compared with 1% in the controls. In an uncontrolled study of exposed females vaginal adenosis was more frequent in those whose mothers had taken stilboestrol early in pregnancy and was not detected at all in those where stilboestrol was started in the 18th week or later. There was also a lower incidence of vaginal adenosis in those offspring who had used oral contraceptives.— A. L. Herbst *et al.*, *New Engl. J. Med.*, 1975, *292*, 334.

The Professional and Public Relations Committee of the DESAD (Diethylstilboestrol and Adenosis) Project of the Division of Cancer Control and Rehabilitation reported that of nearly 300 young females with clear-cell adenocarcinoma of the genital tract, more than 80% had been exposed *in utero* to stilboestrol-type hormones. Patients had been aged 7 to 28 years at the time of diagnosis. Doses and duration of treatment varied widely; 1.5 mg of stilboestrol daily throughout pregnancy or varying amounts for a week or more during the first trimester had shown an association. Vaginal adenosis, rare in unexposed young women, was present in about a third of those exposed in the first 4 months of pregnancy, and cervical ectropion in more than two-thirds.— *J. Am. med. Ass.*, 1976, *236*, 1107. Of 3339 women entered into the DESAD project 1340 were identified by review of their records and were considered the best population on which inferences of the effects of stilboestrol should be based; the incidence of vaginal epithelial changes was 34% in this group compared with 59 or 65% in referred (or similar) groups. From analysis of the data on 298 women for whom complete records were available, vaginal epithelial changes were most closely associated with early exposure to stilboestrol, with the total dose, and with the duration of exposure; their incidence decreased with age. No severe dysplasia or carcinoma was found in the record-review group; the risk of cancer in the first 25 years after exposure was small.— P. C. O'Brien *et al.*, *Obstet. Gynec.*, 1979, *53*, 300. Pathological findings.— S. J. Robboy *et al.*, *ibid.*, 309. See also S. J. Robboy *et al.*, *Am. J. Obstet. Gynec.*, 1981, *140*, 579.

Preliminary findings on fertility and outcome of pregnancy in a subgroup of women enrolled in the DESAD Project; 618 women who had been exposed *in utero* to stilboestrol were compared with 618 control subjects. There was no difference in fertility between the 2 groups when measured in terms of pregnancies achieved. An increased risk of unfavourable outcome of pregnancy was seen in 220 women exposed prenatally to stilboestrol compared with 224 control subjects; the relative risk was 1.69. However, of the women who became pregnant, 81% of those exposed to stilboestrol and 95% of control subjects had at least one full-term live birth.— A. B. Barnes *et al.*, *New Engl. J. Med.*, 1980, *302*, 609.

On the assumption that 1 to 10% of pregnant women in the USA were exposed to stilboestrol in 1951 to 1953 it was estimated that the risk of clear-cell adenocarcinoma of the vagina and cervix in offspring was 0.14 to 1.4 per thousand.— A. L. Herbst *et al.*, *Am. J. Obstet. Gynec.*, 1977, *128*, 43.

Of 46 women with documented exposure *in utero* to stilboestrol and 14 with probable exposure 40 had radiological evidence of changes in the uterus; in 36 the cervix showed gross anatomic changes. Of 20 with a normal uterus 4 had gross abnormal changes in the cervix. It was too early to evaluate the clinical significance of the findings.— R. H. Kaufman *et al.*, *Am. J. Obstet. Gynec.*, 1977, *128*, 51.

In 199 women with probable exposure *in utero* to stilboestrol (confirmed in 180) abnormalities of the vagina and/or cervix (assessed colposcopically) were present in 86.4%. Vaginal adenosis was present in 14.1% (or 45.2% if a more liberal definition of the vagina was used). Grade 1 cervical intra-epithelial neoplasia was present in 36 women and grade 3 neoplasia in 8; the risk of neoplasia in stilboestrol-exposed women was 4.4 to 13.3 times that in non-exposed women. There was no case of clear-cell adenocarcinoma.— W. C. Fowler and D. A. Edelman, *Obstet. Gynec.*, 1978, *51*, 459.

Development of clear-cell adenocarcinoma in a young woman after earlier negative examination emphasised the need for regular screening in women exposed *in utero* to stilboestrol.— B. Anderson *et al.*, *Obstet. Gynec.*, 1979, *53*, 293.

Some further references: E. C. Sandberg, *Am. J. Obstet. Gynec.*, 1976, *125*, 777, per *Int. pharm. Abstr.*, 1977, *14*, 471; C. M. Fenoglio *et al.*, *Am. J. Obstet. Gynec.*, 1976, *126*, 170, per *Int. pharm. Abstr.*, 1977, *14*, 371; R. F. Mattingly and A. Stafl, *Am. J. Obstet. Gynec.*, 1976, *126*, 543, per *Int. pharm. Abstr.*, 1977, *14*, 831; S. Puri *et al.*, *Am. J. Obstet. Gynec.*, 1977, *128*, 550; R. H. Kaufman and E. Adam, *Israel J. Med. Sci.*, 1978, *14*, 353; S. J. Robboy *et al.*, *Obstet. Gynec.*, 1978, *51*, 528; A. L. Herbst *et al.*, *Pediatrics*, 1978, *62*, 1151, per *Int. pharm. Abstr.*, 1979, *16*, 354.

Effect on the male foetus. A report of hypogonadism and anosmia in a 17-year-old boy whose mother had taken stilboestrol during pregnancy.— D. Hoefnagel (letter), *Lancet*, 1976, *1*, 152.

Problems in passing urine and abnormalities of the penile urethra were significantly more common in young males exposed *in utero* to stilboestrol than in controls.— B. E. Henderson *et al.*, *Pediatrics*, 1976, *58*, 505.

No cancer had been reported in the male offspring of women given synthetic hormones during pregnancy, but genital tract abnormalities (cysts of the epididymis, capsular induration, defective testicles) occurred in 41 of 163 exposed men compared with 11 of 168 controls. Sperm counts and motility were reduced.— *J. Am. med. Ass.*, 1977, *238*, 932.

In 308 males exposed *in utero* to stilboestrol the incidence of epididymal cysts was 20.8% compared with 4.9% in controls, and that of testicular hypoplasia was 8.4% compared with 1.9%. The incidence of severely pathological semen was increased.— W. B. Gill *et al.*, *J. Urol.*, 1979, *122*, 36.

Further references: M. D. Cosgrove *et al.*, *J. Urol.*, 1977, *117*, 220; W. B. Gill *et al.*, *ibid.*, 477.

Precautions. As for Oestradiol, p.1426.

Stilboestrol should not be used in pregnant patients. If it fails as a postcoital contraceptive, abortion may need to be considered.

A report of pseudocholinesterase deficiency and prolonged respiratory insufficiency after suxamethonium in a 78-year-old man. The deficiency appeared to be related to stilboestrol therapy; liver disease might have been a contributory factor.— T. L. Archer and E. C. Janowsky, *Anesth. Analg. curr. Res.*, 1978, *57*, 726.

Absorption and Fate. Stilboestrol is readily absorbed from the gastro-intestinal tract. It is slowly inactivated in the liver and excreted in the urine and faeces.

Uses. Stilboestrol is a synthetic oestrogen which is not a steroid but has actions and uses similar to those of oestradiol (see p.1426).

Stilboestrol is administered by mouth or by intramuscular injection as a solution in oil. It has also been administered in pessaries.

For the treatment of menopausal symptoms, doses of 0.1 to 2 mg by mouth daily have been given cyclically, but it is advisable to start with a low dosage and subsequently to adjust the dosage to the minimum necessary to control the symptoms.

In the treatment of secondary amenorrhoea due to ovarian insufficiency, 0.2 to 0.5 mg has been given daily during the proliferative phase of the menstrual cycle.

For the inhibition of lactation, 5 mg was formerly given twice or thrice daily initially, followed by 5 mg daily for 6 days; alternative methods, including the use of bromocriptine (see p.894), are now preferred.

Daily doses of 15 mg are used in the palliative treatment of malignant neoplasms of the breast. The usual dose in carcinoma of the prostate is 1 to 3 mg daily; higher doses have been given.

Stilboestrol has been used for postcoital contraception.

Stilboestrol has been given to *domestic animals* for growth-promoting purposes; this practice is controversial and in some countries has been banned.

Growth-hormone secretion test. Stilboestrol was given by mouth in a dosage of 5 mg twice daily for 3 days as a provocative test to assess growth-hormone reserves. Of 26 short children, 8 had low concentrations of growth hormone. The results of the test were not significantly different from those obtained using the arginine-infusion test. Side-effects included nausea, vomiting, and breast soreness.— G. E. Bacon *et al.*, *J. Pediat.*, 1969, *75*, 385, per *Abstr. Wld Med.*, 1970, *44*, 202.

Inhibition of growth. Inhibition of growth of tall girls by stilboestrol.— H. N. B. Wettenhall *et al.*, *J. Pediat.*, 1975, *86*, 602.

Inhibition of lactation. Reports and references: D. MacDonald and K. O'Driscoll, *Lancet*, 1965, *2*, 623; C. Hodge, *Lancet*, 1967, *2*, 286; G. Dalley (letter), *ibid.*, 613.

Oestrogens are no longer recommended for inhibition of lactation. For further details, see Oestradiol, p.1426.

Malignant neoplasm of the breast. In a randomised double-blind study involving 523 postmenopausal patients with either progressive inoperable or metastatic breast cancer, responsiveness to stilboestrol in doses of 1.5, 15, 150, or 1500 mg daily was studied. Regression occurred in 21% with the 1500 mg dose, 17% with 150 mg, 15% with 15 mg and 10% with 1.5 mg. No regressions occurred at any dosage in patients within the first year of menopause. In selecting the most suitable dosage, postmenopausal age and dominant site of metastases should be taken into account. It was considered that the 1500-mg dose level was applicable to patients 1 to 5 years postmenopausal with local or visceral disease or to those 10 or more years postmenopausal with local disease only. Four deaths were ascribed to drug toxicity, from pulmonary emboli and 2 with hypercalcaemia.—Report of the Cooperative Breast Cancer Group, A. C. Carter *et al.*, *J. Am. med. Ass.*, 1977, *237*, 2079. Criticism of the statistics; use of a different mathematical model yielded different conclusions.— J. T. Wittes *et al.* (letter), *J. Am. med. Ass.*, 1977, *238*, 1362.

An overall response of 38% had been achieved in 55 men with metastatic breast carcinoma treated with stilboestrol; patients with bone metastases did not respond.— G. G. Ribeiro (letter), *Br. med. J.*, 1978, *2*, 570.

Oestrogen receptors and survival in early breast cancer.— R. Croton *et al.*, *Br. med. J.*, 1981, *283*, 1289.

Malignant neoplasm of the prostate. After a consideration of 2204 patients with carcinoma of the prostate, regardless of the stage of the disease, it was found that 459 of 1103 treated with stilboestrol had died, compared with 428 of 1101 not so treated. Cardiovascular disease accounted for the death of 188 oestrogen-treated and 129 other patients. Whether doses of oestrogen lower than the 5 mg of stilboestrol given daily would produce a different result was under study. It was concluded that surgical castration and oestrogen therapy were equally effective in relieving symptoms and the psychological effects of castration would have to be balanced against the cardiovascular hazards of oestrogen therapy.— Veterans Administration Cooperative Urological Research Group, *J. Urol.*, 1967, *98*, 516, per *New Engl. J. Med.*, 1968, *278*, 848. In a report from the Veterans Administration Cooperative Urological Research Group, a daily dose of 1 mg of stilboestrol was as effective as a 5-mg dose in controlling carcinoma of the prostate but did not appear to increase the risk of death from cardiovascular disease.— J. C. Bailar *et al.*, *Cancer*, 1970, *26*, 257, per *J. Am. med. Ass.*, 1970, *213*, 1943. The current recommendation of the Group was to use stilboestrol 1 mg daily but not to institute treatment until symptoms required it.— D. P. Byar, *Bull. N.Y. Acad. Med.*, 1972, *48*, 751.

Stilboestrol 3 mg daily will reduce plasma testosterone to castration concentrations and higher doses are not justified in the management of prostatic carcinoma.— J. G. Smart, *Practitioner*, 1979, *223*, 312.

A suggestion that stilboestrol in a dose of more than 0.2 mg and less than 5 mg daily should be given when metastases of prostatic carcinoma are diagnosed, even when patients are asymptomatic. The Veterans Administration Urological Research Group have found a dose of 1 mg daily to be effective. Many workers feel that large intravenous doses of stilboestrol may be helpful when the smaller oral dose has become ineffective but this has not been confirmed. There seems little point in giving other forms of oestrogen.— *Br. med. J.*, 1979, *2*, 752.

Androgen receptors and response to hormone therapy.— R. Ghanadian *et al.* (letter), *Lancet*, 1981, *2*, 1418.

Muscular dystrophy. Stilboestrol reduced elevated serum concentrations of creatine phosphokinase and lactate dehydrogenase in 11 boys with Duchenne muscular dystrophy.— L. Cohen and J. Morgan, *Archs Neurol., Chicago*, 1976, *33*, 480, per *J. Am. med. Ass.*, 1976, *236*, 94. See also R. Dempsey *et al.*, *Clin. Pharmac. Ther.*, 1975, *18*, 104.

Postcoital contraception. Stilboestrol 25 mg twice daily was administered within 72 hours postcoitally to 1000 women for 5 days. No pregnancies occurred and there were no serious side-effects.— L. K. Kuchera, *J. Am. med. Ass.*, 1971, *218*, 562.

The use of stilboestrol to prevent conception in victims of rape.— D. Glover *et al.*, *West. J. Med.*, 1976, *125*, 331, per *Int. pharm. Abstr.*, 1977, *14*, 427.

Contraceptive failure in 3 of 200 women due to additional sexual exposure while taking stilboestrol 25 mg twice daily for 5 days for postcoital contraception.— C. R. Garcia *et al.*, *Contraception*, 1977, *15*, 445, per *Int. pharm. Abstr.*, 1977, *14*, 1039.

Further references: J. A. Board *et al.*, *Fert. Steril.*, 1973, *24*, 95, per *Int. pharm. Abstr.*, 1973, *10*, 769; *Med. Lett.*, 1973, *15*, 58; *Br. med. J.*, 1976, *2*, 961.

For a recommended regimen see under Levonorgestrel, p.1424.

Sexual disorders in males. Hormonal therapy would be appropriate in certain compulsion forms of deviant behaviour such as paedophilia. Subcutaneous implants of oestradiol have been advocated, and stilboestrol may be given by mouth in a dose of 5 mg daily until the strength of sexual drive is adequately reduced; the dose is then reduced to 1 mg daily.— D. J. Power, *Practitioner*, 1977, *218*, 805. See also *Br. med. J.*, 1980, *280*, 28.

Use in animal feeds. A discussion on the advantages and possible toxicity resulting from the use of stilboestrol in cattle production.— T. H. Jukes, *J. Am. med. Ass.*, 1974, *229*, 1920.

Concern at the continued use in the *USA*, despite a ban, of stilboestrol for the stimulation of growth of cattle.— *Drug Cosmet. Ind.*, 1980, *127* (Sept.), 18.

Preparations

Diethylstilbestrol Injection *(U.S.P.)*. Stilboestrol Injection. A sterile solution of stilboestrol in a suitable vegetable oil. Protect from light.

Diethylstilbestrol Suppositories *(U.S.P.)*. Stilboestrol Suppositories. Suppositories containing stilboestrol. Store in a cool place or at 15° to 30° in airtight containers.

Diethylstilbestrol Tablets *(U.S.P.)*. Tablets containing stilboestrol.

Stilboestrol Pessaries *(B.P.C. 1973)*. Pess. Stilboestr. Stilboestrol 500 µg with propylene glycol 0.07 ml in Glycerol Suppositories mass sufficient to fill a 4-g mould. Store in a cool place.

A.P.F. has the same strength in Glyco-Gelatin Gel.

Stilboestrol Tablets *(B.P.)*. Diethylstilbestrol Tablets. Tablets containing stilboestrol. They may be sugar-coated. Protect from light.

Proprietary Preparations

Tampovagan Stilboestrol and Lactic Acid *(Norgine, UK)*. Pessaries each containing stilboestrol 500 µg with lactic acid 5% in a macrogol basis. For senile vaginitis.

Other Proprietary Names

Cyren-A *(Ger.)*; Desma, Dicorvin *(both USA)*; Distilbene *(Belg., Fr.)*; Estilbin *(Denm.)*; Stibilium *(Canad.)*; Stilbol *(Swed.)*.

Stilboestrol was formerly marketed in Great Britain under the proprietary name Pabestrol (*Paines & Byrne*). A preparation containing stilboestrol was also formerly marketed under the proprietary name Sedestran (*Geigy*).

9106-b

Stilboestrol Dipropionate *(B.P. Vet., B.P.C. 1949)*.

Diethylstilbestrol Dipropionate. (*E*)-αβ-Diethylstilbene-4,4′-diol dipropionate.

$C_{24}H_{28}O_4$=380.5.

CAS — 130-80-3.

Pharmacopoeias. In *Aust.*, *Cz.*, *Ger.*, *Jug.*, *Pol.*, *Rus.*, and *Swiss.*

Odourless, tasteless, colourless crystals or white crystalline powder. M.p. 104° to 108°.

Slightly **soluble** in water and dilute mineral acids; soluble 1 in 100 of alcohol (90%), 1 in 6 of ether, and 1 in 45 of olive oil; freely soluble in hot alcohol, acetone, chloroform, and hot methyl alcohol; soluble in fixed oils; practically insoluble in solutions of alkali hydroxides. A suspension (1 in 100) in diluted alcohol is neutral to litmus. Solutions in oil are **sterilised** by maintaining at 150° for 1 hour. **Store** in airtight containers. Protect from light.

Effect of gamma-irradiation. Irradiation with 25 000 Gy did not alter the chemical and physical properties of stilboestrol dipropionate, and could be used as a method of sterilisation.— G. Hortobagyi *et al.*, *Radiosterilization of Medical Products*, Vienna, International Atomic Energy Agency, 1967, p. 25.

Stilboestrol dipropionate has actions and uses similar to those of oestradiol (see p.1425) and has been given by mouth usually in doses of 0.1 to 1 mg daily. It has also been given by intramuscular injection in oily solution, or applied locally in ointments.

Proprietary Names

Oestros *(Fuchs, Switz.)*; Oestrostilben *(Streuli, Switz.)*; Stilbocream *(Ford, Austral.)*.

A preparation containing stilboestrol dipropionate was formerly marketed in Great Britain under the proprietary name Stilbofax (*Wellcome*).

9107-v

Testolactone *(U.S.P.)*.

1-Dehydrotestololactone; NSC 23759; SQ 9538. *D*-Homo-17a-oxa-androsta-1,4-diene-3,17-dione.

$C_{19}H_{24}O_3$=300.4.

CAS — 968-93-4.

Pharmacopoeias. In *U.S.*

A white to off-white, practically odourless, crystalline powder. M.p. about 218°.

Soluble 1 in about 4000 of water; soluble in alcohol and chloroform; slightly soluble in benzyl alcohol; practically insoluble in ether and light petroleum. A solution in chloroform is laevorotatory. **Store** in airtight containers.

Adverse Effects and Precautions. As for Testosterone, p.1436.

Intramuscular injections may be painful.

Uses. Testolactone is a derivative of testosterone (see below) and is used in the palliative treatment of malignant neoplasms of the breast in postmenopausal women. It has no significant androgenic activity and has no erythropoietic effect.

The usual dose is 250 mg four times daily by mouth or 100 mg intramuscularly thrice weekly.

Malignant neoplasm of the breast. When given in doses of 250 mg four times daily by mouth to 32 patients with disseminated neoplasms of the breast, testolactone did not improve the regression-rate. Virilisation, hepatic and renal toxicity, or other undesirable effects were not produced.— T. J. Cantino and G. S. Gordan, *Cancer*, 1967, *20*, 458, per *Int. pharm. Abstr.*, 1967, *4*, 934.

Of 115 women with advanced neoplasm of the breast 21 had objective remissions after treatment with testolactone 1 g daily by mouth. The median duration of therapy was 12 weeks and 59% survived for 1 year or more.— I. S. Goldenberg *et al.*, *J. Am. med. Ass.*, 1973, *223*, 1267. See also *Med. Lett.*, 1970, *12*, 45.

Further references: A. N. Papaioannou and H. Volk, *Cancer Chemother. Rep.*, 1966, *50*, 323, per *Int. pharm. Abstr.*, 1967, *4*, 349.

Preparations

Sterile Testolactone Suspension *(U.S.P.)*. A sterile suspension in a suitable aqueous vehicle. pH 5 to 7.5.

Testolactone Tablets *(U.S.P.)*. Tablets containing testolactone. Store in airtight containers.

Proprietary Names

Fludestrin *(Heyden, Ger.)*; Teslac *(Squibb, Arg.; Squibb, Belg.; Squibb, Canad.; Squibb, Ital.; Squibb, USA)*.

9108-g

Testosterone *(B.P., B.P. Vet., U.S.P.)*.

Testost. 17β-Hydroxyandrost-4-en-3-one.

$C_{19}H_{28}O_2$=288.4.

CAS — 58-22-0.

Pharmacopoeias. In *Arg.*, *Aust.*, *Br.*, *Braz.*, *Mex.*, *Roum.*, *Span.*, *Swiss*, and *U.S.*

White or creamy-white, odourless, tasteless crystals or crystalline powder. M.p. 152° to 157°.

Practically **insoluble** in water; soluble 1 in 6 of dehydrated alcohol, 1 in 2 of chloroform, 1 in 100 of ether, and 1 in 150 of ethyl oleate; soluble in acetone, dioxan, and fixed oils. **Incompatible** with oxidising agents. A solution in alcohol is dextrorotatory. **Protect** from light.

Solubility. The solubility of testosterone in water was increased from about 30 µg per ml to 1.25 mg per ml in the presence of potassium laurate. Lauryltrimethylammonium and cetyltrimethylammonium bromides also solubilised testosterone in micelles.— A. L. Thakkar and N. A. Hall, *J. pharm. Sci.*, 1968, *57*, 1394.

Fast dissolution-rates were obtained with solid dispersions of testosterone in macrogol 1000, macrogol 20 000, povidone, cetomacrogol 1000, and a macrogol ester, mainly due to reduction in particle size. The povidone dispersion was unaffected by storage for 9 months but dissolution-rates for the macrogol dispersions decreased, which was attributed to coarsening of the particles.— A. Hoelgaard and N. Møller, *Arch. Pharm. Chemi, scient. Edn*, 1975, *3*, 34.

Sterilisation. Chlorbutol 1% w/w or camphor 1% w/w were suitable sterilising agents for 100-mg implants of testosterone when heated at 80° for 20 hours.— P. H. Cox and F. Spanjers, *Pharm. Weekbl. Ned.*, 1970, *105*, 681.

Adverse Effects. Testosterone and other androgens give rise to side-effects which can be related to their androgenic or anabolic activities. They include increase in nitrogen retention and skeletal weight, sodium and water retention, oedema, increased vascularity of the skin, hypercalcaemia, and increased growth of the bone. Large and repeated doses in early puberty may cause closure of the epiphyses and stop linear growth. Elderly males may become overstimulated.

In women, the inhibitory action of testosterone on the activity of the anterior pituitary results in the suppression of ovarian activity and menstruation. Continued administration of large doses, in excess of about 300 mg monthly, produces symptoms of virilism, such as male-pattern hirsutism, deepening of the voice, atrophy of the breasts and endometrial tissue, acne, and hypertrophy of the clitoris; libido is increased and lactation suppressed.

Stomatitis has been reported following the buccal or sublingual administration of testosterone.

In men, large doses suppress spermatogenesis and cause degenerative changes in the seminiferous tubules.

Androgens may accelerate the growth of malignant neoplasms of the prostate. Hepatic carcinomas have developed in some patients given androgens and anabolic steroids for prolonged periods.

Mention of gynaecomastia being associated with the use of androgens.— H. E. Carlson, *New Engl. J. Med.*, 1980, *303*, 795.

Effect on liver. Administration of testosterone 400 mg daily for 21 days to 6 healthy male subjects caused no changes in common liver parameters. Induction of the hepatic drug-metabolising system was noted.— S. G. Johnsen *et al.*, *Clin. Pharmac. Ther.*, 1976, *20*, 233.

No impairment of liver function occurred in 10 male castrates or eunuchs who had received continuous oral therapy with testosterone for up to 7.5 years.— S. G. Johnsen (letter), *Lancet*, 1978, *1*, 50.

Hepatic angiosarcoma. Results of a retrospective epidemiological study of deaths from hepatic angiosarcoma in the USA indicated that 4 of 168 were associated with long-term use of androgenic anabolic steroids (testosterone enanthate, fluoxymesterone, testosterone and methyltestosterone, and stanozolol having been administered to the 4 patients). Previously known causes (vinyl chloride, thorium dioxide, and inorganic arsenic) were associated with another 37.— H. Falk *et al.*, *Lancet*, 1979, *2*, 1120.

Precautions. Testosterone and other androgens are contra-indicated in men with carcinoma of the prostate or breast and in patients with hypercalcaemia. Their use is best avoided in patients with nephrosis. Their use is best avoided in pregnancy since virilisation of the female foetus has been reported. Use should also be avoided in lactating patients. They should also be used cautiously in patients with cardiac disorders, renal or hepatic dysfunction, epilepsy, or migraine and other conditions which would be aggravated by fluid retention.

Androgens and anabolic steroids may reduce thyroxine-binding globulin. Barbiturates may reduce the effects of testosterone by enhancing its metabolism in the liver.

The administration of oestrogens and testosterone could interfere with measurements of urinary 17-hydroxycorticosteroids.— J. M. Rosenberg and I. S. Kampa, *Drug Intell. & clin. Pharm.*, 1973, *7*, 33.

For the effect of testosterone on nortriptyline elimination, see Amitriptyline Hydrochloride, p.112.

Absorption and Fate. Testosterone is absorbed from the gastro-intestinal tract, the skin, and the oral mucosa. It is largely metabolised in the liver to the weakly androgenic androsterone and inactive etiocholanolone which are excreted in the urine mainly as glucuronides and sulphates. Testosterone absorbed from the gastro-intestinal tract is almost completely metabolised in the liver before it reaches the systemic circulation. Testosterone is extensively bound to a plasma globulin that also binds oestradiol, and a small proportion is converted to oestrogenic derivatives in the body. Only about 2% of testosterone is unbound and the plasma half-life is about 10 to 20 minutes. Testosterone is believed to be converted to the more active dihydrotestosterone in some target organs.

The metabolism of tritiated testosterone given intravenously to 3 euthyroid, 2 hyperthyroid, and 2 hypothyroid subjects. The half-life varied from 60 to 80 minutes in 1 euthyroid and the 2 hyperthyroid subjects. The elimination of metabolites was consistent with the clearance rates of 0.5 to 4.9 ml per minute for androsterone sulphate, 8.8 to 19.8 ml per minute for etiocholanolone sulphate and 73 to 350 ml per minute for the corresponding glucosiduronates.— L. Hellman and R. S. Rosenfeld, *J. clin. Endocr. Metab.*, 1974, *38*, 424, per *Int. pharm. Abstr.*, 1975, *12*, 416.

The active metabolite of testosterone in human skin during *in vitro* studies was considered to be 5α-dihydrotestosterone, produced together with androstenedione, androsterone, and other 17-oxosteroids.— J. B. Hay, *Br. J. Derm.*, 1977, *97*, 237.

Uses. Testosterone is the androgenic hormone formed in the interstitial (Leydig) cells of the testes under the control of the anterior lobe of the pituitary gland. It controls the development and maintenance of the male sex organs and the male secondary sex characteristics. A small proportion of the circulating testosterone is derived from the metabolism of less potent androgens secreted by the adrenal cortex and ovaries.

In underdeveloped or adolescent males, testosterone increases the size of the scrotum, phallus, seminal vesicles, and prostate; libido and sexual activity may also be increased.

Testosterone also produces systemic effects, such as increased retention of nitrogen, calcium, sodium, potassium, chloride, and phosphate. This leads to an increase in skeletal weight, water retention, and increased growth of bone. The skin becomes more vascular and erythropoiesis is increased.

In small doses it increases the number of spermatozoa produced but large doses inhibit the activity of the anterior lobe of the pituitary gland and suppress the formation of spermatozoa. (In women this inhibitory action results in the suppression of ovarian activity and menstruation). Testosterone is less potent than the oestrogens in inhibiting the anterior pituitary.

Testosterone and other androgens are used in the male for replacement therapy in hypogonadism, eunuchoidism, and the male climacteric. They are also used in the treatment of gynaecomastia, although they may themselves cause gynaecomastia. They are of no value in the treatment of infertility, unless this is due to sexual underdevelopment.

Androgens are used in the palliative treatment of disseminated breast cancer in postmenopausal women.

Androgens have been used to increase weight in patients suffering from emaciation or wasting diseases but less virilising anabolic agents (see under Methandienone, p.1419) are now given for this purpose. They have been given to promote growth in children of short stature but bone maturation can occur before growth has finished and so halt further growth. They have also been used in the treatment of some refractory anaemias caused by decreased erythropoiesis.

Testosterone is usually administered by implantation but may also be given by injection in aqueous suspensions, as tablets to be retained in the buccal cavity, and as suppositories. For parenteral administration testosterone propionate or other esters are generally preferred, and for oral use methyltestosterone is usually employed.

For prolonged action in the treatment of male hypogonadism, testosterone in doses of 200 to 600 mg may be implanted subcutaneously; the higher doses may result in adequate levels of testosterone for up to 8 months.

Doses of up to 1.5 g have been used in breast cancer. Alternatively doses of 10 to 30 mg daily may be given by buccal administration.

Priapism is a sign of overdosage.

Anaemia. *Aplastic.* B. M. Camitta *et al.*, *New Engl. J. Med.*, 1982, *306*, 645 and 712 (pathogenesis, diagnosis, treatment, and prognosis of aplastic anaemia).

Of 92 children with idiopathic or acquired aplastic anaemia, 61 were treated with androgens and 31 with corticosteroids or supportive therapy. Despite an initial high remission-rate (41%) in the androgen-treated group, the crude survival-rate after 5 years (26%) did not differ significantly from that of the non-androgen group (23%). The crude survival-rate appeared to be best for those with drug-induced aplasia.— D. W. O. Hughes, *Med. J. Aust.*, 1973, *2*, 361.

Long-term testosterone therapy with enanthate or cypionate, 600 to 800 mg weekly reducing to 0.2 to 1.2 g monthly, led to the complete correction of neutropenia in 20 and 24 months respectively in 2 men with rheumatoid arthritis, splenomegaly, and neutropenia (Felty's syndrome) and partial correction in a further patient with Felty's syndrome.— B. M. Wimer and M. M. Sloan, *J. Am. med. Ass.*, 1973, *223*, 671.

In renal failure. In a study of 25 patients undergoing long-term haemodialysis, 3 of whom had undergone bilateral nephrectomy, the intramuscular injection of 250 to 500 mg of testosterone caused a rise in the haemoglobin concentration. The effect was reversible and maintenance therapy was necessary. Despite iron supplements intravenously, serum-iron concentrations remained low. Side-effects included priapism in 2 men and baldness and hirsuties in a woman.— S. Shaldon *et al.*, *Br. med. J.*, 1971, *3*, 212.

Testosterone propionate 150 mg was given intramuscularly twice weekly for 5 months to 11 patients undergoing haemodialysis. There was an increase in packed cell volume and in erythropoietin in the 6 patients with some kidney tissue but not in the 5 anephric patients.— W. Fried *et al.*, *Ann. intern. Med.*, 1973, *79*, 823.

A review of the use of androgens to treat anaemia in patients with chronic renal failure undergoing haemodialysis.— M. R. Alexander, *Am. J. Hosp. Pharm.*, 1976, *33*, 242.

Sickle-cell anaemia. Either testosterone in men or progesterone in women injected once a week reduced the painful episodes of sickle-cell disease by varying degrees in 31 of 35 patients and was more effective than placebo.— W. A. Isaacs *et al.* (preliminary communication), *Lancet*, 1972, *1*, 570.

Contraception. A review of the prospects for new, reversible male contraceptives.— W. J. Bremner and D. M. de Kretser, *New Engl. J. Med.*, 1976, *295*, 1111.

See also under Testosterone Enanthate and Testosterone Propionate, below.

Eunuchism. The administration of 200 mg of micronised testosterone by mouth to 4 patients without testicular function produced normal male serum-testosterone concentrations for about 5 to 7 hours. In a double-blind study on 5 eunuchs a dose of 400 mg daily produced a positive effect on sexual ability whereas 100 mg was ineffective.— S. G. Johnsen *et al.*, *Lancet*, 1974, *2*, 1473.

Growth defects. A discussion of androgens in boys with retarded growth. It was considered that present evidence does not indicate that adult height can be increased to a significant extent, but that the hazard of disproportionally rapid bone maturation is probably not particularly great if low doses are given for limited periods.— *Br. med. J.*, 1973, *3*, 245.

The concomitant use of testosterone and growth hormone for stimulating growth in hypopituitarism.— A. Aynsley-Green *et al.*, *J. Pediat.*, 1976, *89*, 992.

For an adverse comment on the use of androgens for stimulating growth, see Methandienone, p.1419.

Inhibition of growth. The use of high doses of testosterone esters for the control of height in boys liable to be excessively tall.— M. Zachman *et al.*, *J. Pediat.*, 1976, *88*, 116, per *Int. pharm. Abstr.*, 1976, *13*, 938.

Impotence. Plasma-testosterone concentrations were not significantly different in 27 normal men, 27 with impotence, 20 with oligospermia, and 16 with azoospermia, but were significantly reduced in 21 with hypogonadism. This helped to explain why androgen therapy was not usually helpful in the treatment of impotence.— D. M. Lawrence and G. I. M. Swyer, *Br. med. J.*, 1974, *1*, 349.

Endocrine treatment of impotence was appropriate only in objective evidence of androgen deficiency.— D. R. London, *Prescribers' J.*, 1976, *16*, 139.

The endocrine basis for sexual dysfunction in men.— *Br. med. J.*, 1978, *2*, 1516. See also D. W. Lording, *Drugs*, 1978, *15*, 144; *Br. med. J.*, 1979, *2*, 1169.

See also under Testosterone Undecanoate, below.

Infertility. Androgen insensitivity was considered to be responsible for infertility in 3 unrelated phenotypically normal men.— J. Aiman *et al.*, *New Engl. J. Med.*, 1979, *300*, 223. Comment.— P. C. Walsh, *ibid.*, 253.

Liver disorders. Reduction in ascites and pedal oedema, and subjective improvement, in patients with hepatic cirrhosis treated with testosterone.— M. M. Puliyel *et al.*, *Aust. N.Z. J. Med.*, 1977, *7*, 596, per *Int. pharm. Abstr.*, 1978, *15*, 929.

See also under Testosterone Propionate, below.

Micropenis. Three prepubertal boys with micropenis and/or hypospadias massaged a 2.5% testosterone cream into the penis in an attempt to produce enlargement prior to surgery. Plasma-testosterone concentrations rose from 14, 21, and 11 ng per 100 ml to 92, 234, and 280 ng per 100 ml respectively. The 3 boys developed pubic hair but penile length did not increase significantly.— C. W. Darby *et al.* (letter), *Lancet*, 1974, *2*, 598.

For favourable reports on the use of testosterone for micropenis, see under Testosterone Cypionate and Testosterone Enanthate, below.

Preparations

Sterile Testosterone Suspension *(U.S.P.)*. A sterile suspension in an aqueous vehicle. pH 4 to 7.5.

Testosterone Implants *(B.P.)*. Testost. Implants. Sterile cylinders prepared by fusion or heavy compression of testosterone without the addition of any other substance, distributed singly in sterile containers which are sealed to exclude micro-organisms. Protect from light.

Testosterone Pellets *(U.S.P.)*. Sterile pellets consisting of compressed testosterone without the presence of any binder, diluent, or excipient. Store singly in sterile airtight containers.

Proprietary Preparations

Testoral Sublings *(Organon, UK)*. Sublingual tablets each containing testosterone 10 mg in an inert water-soluble wax basis. (Also available as Testoral in *Austral., S.Afr.*).

NOTE. Testoral is also used as a proprietary name for Fluoxymesterone, p.1414.

Testosterone Implants *(Organon, UK)*. Available containing 100 or 200 mg of testosterone.

Other Proprietary Names

Andronaq, Oreton *(both USA)*; Hydrotest *(Ital.)*; Malogen *(Canad.)*; Percutacrine Androgénique Forte *(Fr.)*; Rektandron *(Swed.)*.

9109-q

Testosterone Acetate. 3-Oxoandrost-4-en-17β-yl acetate.
$C_{21}H_{30}O_3$=330.5.

CAS — 1045-69-8.

Pharmacopoeias. In *Braz.* and *Fr.*

A white odourless crystalline powder. It occurs in 2 crystalline forms, with melting points of about 130° and 141°. Practically **insoluble** in water; soluble in dehydrated alcohol; very soluble in chloroform. **Protect** from light.

Testosterone acetate has the actions and uses of testosterone (see p.1435).

It has been given in doses of up to 40 mg daily by intramuscular injection for gynaecological disorders.

Proprietary Names

Cetovister *(Substancia, Spain)*.

9110-d

Testosterone Cypionate *(U.S.P.)*. Testosterone Cyclopentylpropionate. 3-Oxoandrost-4-en-17β-yl 3-cyclopentylpropionate.
$C_{27}H_{40}O_3$=412.6.

CAS — 58-20-8.

Pharmacopoeias. In *U.S.*

A white or creamy-white, tasteless, crystalline powder, odourless or with a slight odour. M.p. 98° to 104°. Practically **insoluble** in water; freely soluble in alcohol, chloroform, dioxan, and ether; soluble in fixed oils. A solution in chloroform is dextrorotatory. **Protect** from light.

Testosterone cypionate has the actions and uses described under testosterone (see p.1435). It is administered intramuscularly in oily solutions containing 50 to 200 mg per ml and has a prolonged duration of effect.

In the treatment of male hypogonadism, metastatic breast cancer in postmenopausal women, and for use as an anabolic agent, it is given in doses of 100 to 400 mg every 3 or 4 weeks.

Reduced postexercise ST-segment depression after treatment with testosterone cypionate.— M. D. Jaffe, *Br. Heart J.*, 1977, *39*, 1217, per *J. Am. med. Ass.*, 1978, *239*, 1568.

Anaemia. For reference to testosterone cypionate in anaemia, see under Testosterone, above.

Micropenis. Testosterone cypionate 25 mg given by intramuscular injection every 3 weeks for 3 months to 4 boys under 3 years of age with micropenis produced enlargement of the penis to normal size. There was transient acceleration of bone growth and maturation.— R. D. Guthrie *et al.*, *J. Pediat.*, 1973, *83*, 247, per *J. Am. med. Ass.*, 1973, *226*, 814.

Preparations

Testosterone Cypionate Injection *(U.S.P.)*. A sterile solution of testosterone cypionate in a suitable fixed oil. It may contain a suitable solubilising agent. Protect from light.

Proprietary Names

Andronate *(Pasadena Research Labs, USA)*; Biosterone *(Biopharm, S.Afr.)*; Ciclosterone *(Farmigea, Ital.)*; Depotrone *(Propan, S.Afr.)*; Jectatest-LA *(Reid-Provident, USA)*; Retar-Gen A *(Dispert, Arg.)*.

9111-n

Testosterone Decanoate *(B.P.)*. 3-Oxoandrost-4-en-17β-yl decanoate.
$C_{29}H_{46}O_3$=442.7.

CAS — 5721-91-5.

Pharmacopoeias. In *Br.*

White or creamy-white crystals or crystalline powder. It occurs in 2 forms melting at about 50° and about 55° respectively. Practically **insoluble** in water; very soluble in alcohol and chloroform. A solution in dioxan is dextrorotatory. **Store** in a cool place. Protect from light.

Testosterone decanoate has the actions and uses of testosterone (see p.1435). It has a prolonged duration of action. It is administered by intramuscular injection usually in association with other testosterone esters.

9112-h

Testosterone Enanthate *(B.P., U.S.P.)*.

Testosterone Heptanoate; Testosterone Oenanthate. 3-Oxoandrost-4-en-17β-yl heptanoate.
$C_{26}H_{40}O_3$=400.6.

CAS — 315-37-7.

Pharmacopoeias. In *Br., Braz., Jap.*, and *U.S.*

A white or creamy-white crystalline powder. It is odourless or has a faint odour characteristic of heptanoic acid. M.p. 34° to 39°. Practically **insoluble** in water; soluble 1 in 0.3 of alcohol, chloroform, and ether, and 1 in 0.2 of acetone; soluble in fixed oils. A solution in dioxan is dextrorotatory. **Store** in a cool place. Protect from light.

Adverse Effects and Precautions. As for Testosterone, p.1436.

A report of carcinoma of the liver occurring in association with methyltestosterone given in conjunction with testosterone enanthate.— F. L. Johnson *et al.*, *Lancet*, 1972, *2*, 1273.

Uses. Testosterone enanthate has the actions and uses of testosterone (see p.1436). It is administered intramuscularly in oily solutions containing up to 250 mg per ml and has a prolonged duration of effect.

In the treatment of male hypogonadism, metastatic breast cancer in women, and for use as an anabolic agent, it is given in doses of 100 to 400 mg every 2 to 4 weeks.

Anaemia. For reference to testosterone enanthate in anaemia, see under Testosterone, above.

Contraception. References to the study of testosterone enanthate, alone or in conjunction with other hormonal agents, as a male contraceptive.— E. Steinberger and K. D. Smith, *Fert. Steril.*, 1977, *28*, 1320; J. F. Melo and E. M. Coutinho, *Contraception*, 1977, *15*, 627, per *Int. pharm. Abstr.*, 1977, *14*, 1187; F. Alvarez-Sanchez *et al.*, *Contraception*, 1977, *15*, 635, per *Int. pharm. Abstr.*, 1977, *14*, 1186; J. Frick *et al.*, *Contraception*, 1977, *15*, 649, per *Int. pharm. Abstr.*, 1977, *14*, 1186; J. Frick *et al.*, *Contraception*, 1977, *15*, 669, per *Int. pharm. Abstr.*, 1977, *14*, 1187; P. F. Brenner *et al.*, *Contraception*, 1977, *15*, 679, per *Int. pharm. Abstr.*, 1977, *14*, 1137; E. Steinberger and K. D. Smith, *Contraception*, 1977, *16*, 261, per *Int. pharm. Abstr.*, 1978, *15*, 518.

Hypogonadism. A favourable report of the effect of testosterone enanthate on sexual function in hypogonadal men.— J. M. Davidson *et al.*, *J. clin. Endocr. Metab.*, 1979, *48*, 955, per *J. Am. med. Ass.*, 1979, *242*, 1803.

Infertility. For a reference to the use of testosterone enanthate together with norethandrolone in the treatment of male infertility, see Norethandrolone, p.1421.

Inhibition of lactation. Testosterone enanthate 360 mg had been given at delivery, especially in the USA, for the suppression of lactation.— *Br. med. J.*, 1977, *1*, 1402.

Micropenis. A report of the successful treatment of 14 boys with androgen-responsive microphallus, using testosterone enanthate. Treatment with low doses of testosterone should be considered in such patients before surgical sex reversal was contemplated.— S. Burstein *et al.*, *Lancet*, 1979, *2*, 983.

Preparations

Testosterone Enanthate Injection *(U.S.P.)*. A sterile solution of testosterone enanthate in a suitable fixed oil. *Jap. P.* has a similar preparation.

Primoteston-Depot 250 mg *(Schering, UK)*. An oily solution for intramuscular injection containing in each ml testosterone enanthate 250 mg, equivalent to 180 mg of testosterone, in ampoules of 1 ml. (Also available as Primoteston Depot in *Austral., Norw.*).

Other Proprietary Names

Androtardyl *(Fr.)*; Delatestryl *(Canad., USA)*; Enarmon Depot *(Jap.)*; Malogen LA, Testate, Testone LA, Testostroval-PA *(all USA)*; Malogex *(Canad.)*; Testinon Depot *(Jap.)*; Testo-Enant *(Ital.)*; Testoviron-Depot *(Belg., Denm., Ger., Ital., Swed., Switz.)*.

9113-m

Testosterone Isocaproate *(B.P.)*. Testosterone Isohexanoate. 3-Oxoandrost-4-en-17β-yl isohexanoate.
$C_{25}H_{38}O_3$=386.6.

CAS — 15262-86-9.

Pharmacopoeias. In *Br.*

White to creamy-white crystals or crystalline powder. M.p. about 80°. Practically **insoluble** in water; very soluble in alcohol and chloroform. A solution in dioxan is dextrorotatory. **Store** in a cool place. Protect from light.

Testosterone isocaproate has the actions and uses of testosterone, p.1435. It is usually administered by intramuscular injection in conjunction with other androgens or oestrogens.

Proprietary Preparations

Proprietary preparations containing testosterone isocaproate with an oestrogen and other androgens or with other androgens are described under Oestradiol Benzoate, p.1427, and Testosterone Undecanoate, below.

9114-b

Testosterone Phenylpropionate *(B.P., B.P. Vet.).* Testosterone Phenylprop. 3-Oxoandrost-4-en-17β-yl 3-phenylpropionate.
$C_{28}H_{36}O_3$=420.6.

CAS — 1255-49-8.

Pharmacopoeias. In *Br.*

A white to almost white crystalline powder with a characteristic odour. M.p. 114° to 117°. Practically **insoluble** in water; soluble 1 in 40 of alcohol; soluble in ethyl oleate and in fixed oils. A solution in dioxan is dextrorotatory. Solutions in oil are **sterilised** by maintaining at 150° for 1 hour. **Protect** from light.

Testosterone phenylpropionate has the actions and uses of testosterone (see p.1435) but has a prolonged duration of effect. It is administered by subcutaneous or intramuscular injection in oily solutions in doses of 5 to 25 mg once or twice weekly.

Preparations

Testosterone Phenylpropionate Injection *(B.P.).* Testosterone Phenylprop. Inj. A sterile solution of testosterone phenylpropionate in ethyl oleate or other suitable ester, in a suitable fixed oil, or in any mixture of these. Sterilised by maintaining at 150° for 1 hour. Protect from light. For intramuscular injection only.

Proprietary preparations containing testosterone phenylpropionate with an oestrogen and other androgens or with other androgens are described under Oestradiol Benzoate, p.1427, and Testosterone Undecanoate, below.

Testosterone phenylpropionate was formerly marketed in Great Britain under the proprietary name Tes. PP (*Organon*).

9115-v

Testosterone Propionate *(B.P., B.P. Vet., Eur. P., U.S.P.).*

Testosterone Prop.; Testosteroni Propionas; Testosteronum Propionicum; NSC 9166. 3-Oxoandrost-4-en-17β-yl propionate.
$C_{22}H_{32}O_3$=344.5.

CAS — 57-85-2.

Pharmacopoeias. In *Arg., Aust., Belg., Br., Braz., Chin., Cz., Eur., Fr., Ger., Hung., Ind., Int., It., Jap., Jug., Mex., Neth., Nord., Pol., Port., Roum., Rus., Span., Swiss, Turk.,* and *U.S.*

Colourless or yellowish-white crystals or a white or creamy-white odourless crystalline powder. M.p. 118° to 123°.
Practically **insoluble** in water; soluble 1 in 6 of alcohol, 1 in 4 of acetone, 1 in 35 of arachis oil, 1 in 20 of ethyl oleate, and 1 in 30 of propylene glycol; very soluble in chloroform; freely soluble in dioxan, ether, and methyl alcohol; soluble in other fixed oils. A solution in dioxan is dextrorotatory. Solutions in oil are **sterilised** by maintaining at 150° for 1 hour. **Incompatible** with alkalis and oxidising agents. **Protect** from light.

Adverse Effects and Precautions. As for Testosterone, p.1436.

Uses. Testosterone propionate has the actions and uses of testosterone (see p.1436). It has a relatively short duration of action. It is given by intramuscular injection in oily solutions or aqueous suspensions.
Treatment of hypogonadism requires up to 50 mg twice or thrice weekly. For the palliative treatment of inoperable neoplasms of the breast, 100 to 300 mg a week is given in divided doses.
Testosterone propionate is also given as buccal tablets in doses of 5 to 20 mg daily. Doses of 200 mg daily are given for inoperable neoplasms of the breast in postmenopausal women. Buccal tablets have sometimes been used for postpartum breast engorgement in doses of 40 mg daily.

Anaemia. For reference to testosterone propionate in anaemia, see under Testosterone, above.

Contraception. Seven healthy men became azoospermic after 60 days' treatment with testosterone propionate 25 mg daily by intramuscular injection. Sperm-counts returned to normal 150 days after withdrawal of treatment. The androgen had no effect on semen volume or libido.— P. R. K. Reddy and J. M. Rao, *Contraception,* 1972, *5,* 295, per *Int. pharm. Abstr.,* 1973, *10,* 153.

Liver disorders. Of 32 patients with cirrhosis of the liver who received testosterone propionate, 24 were cleared of ascites and oedema between the third and sixth week of treatment compared with 14 of 38 in a control group. The dose regimen of testosterone was 100 mg intramuscularly on alternate days for 4 weeks and then 300 mg every 3 weeks for 6 to 9 months. During the course of the study 24 patients in the control group and 11 in the treatment group died of various causes.— N. Islam and A. Islam, *Br. J. clin. Pract.,* 1973, *27,* 125.

Preparations

Testosterone Propionate Injection *(B.P.).* Testosterone Prop. Inj. A sterile solution of testosterone propionate in ethyl oleate or other suitable ester, in a suitable fixed oil, or in any mixture of these. Sterilised by maintaining at 150° for 1 hour. Protect from light. For intramuscular injection only.
A similar preparation is included in several other pharmacopoeias.

Testosterone Propionate Injection *(U.S.P.).* A sterile solution of testosterone propionate in a suitable fixed oil.

Testosterone Propionate Tablets *(U.S.P.).* Tablets containing testosterone propionate.

Proprietary Preparations

Plex-Hormone Injection *(Consolidated Chemicals, UK).* Contains in each ml testosterone propionate 20 mg, deoxycortone acetate 500 µg, oestradiol benzoate 100 µg, and tocopheryl acetate 20 mg. *Dose.* 1 ml two or three times a week for 2 weeks, then 1 ml weekly.
See also Plex-Hormone Tablets, p.1420.

Virormone *(Paines & Byrne, UK).* Testosterone propionate, available as an injection containing 10 and 25 mg per ml in ampoules of 1 ml, and 50 mg per ml in ampoules of 1 and 2 ml. (Also available as Virormone in *Ital.*).

Other Proprietary Names

Andradurin *(Swed.)*; Androxil, Testex *(both Spain)*; Neo-Hombreol *(see also under Methyltestosterone) (Neth.)*; Orchisterone *(see also under Methyltestosterone) (Ital.)*; Perandren *(see also under Methyltestosterone) (Switz.)*; Stérandryl *(Fr.)*; Testoviron *(see also under Methyltestosterone) (Arg., Austral., Ger., Ital., Spain, Swed.)*; Testovis *(see also under Methyltestosterone) (Ital.)*.

A proprietary preparation containing testosterone propionate with an oestrogen is described under Oestradiol Benzoate (see p.1427).

9116-g

Testosterone Undecanoate. 3-Oxoandrost-4-en-17β-yl undecanoate.
$C_{30}H_{48}O_3$=456.7.

Adverse Effects and Precautions. As for Testosterone, p.1436.

Uses. Testosterone undecanoate has the actions and uses of testosterone (p.1436). It is administered by mouth.
In the treatment of male hypogonadism it has been given in doses of 40 to 160 mg daily according to response.
Reports of the use of testosterone undecanoate in male hypogonadism: F. Franchi *et al., Int. J. Androl.,* 1978, *1,* 270; P. Franchimont *et al., Clin. Endocr.,* 1978, *9,* 313; M. Luisi and F. Franchi, *J. endocr. Invest.,* 1980, *3,* 305.

Proprietary Preparations

Restandol *(Organon, UK).* Testosterone undecanoate, available as capsules of 40 mg. (Also available as Restandol in *Denm.*).

Other Proprietary Names

Andriol *(Ger., Neth.)*.

Proprietary Preparations containing other Testosterone Esters

Andromar Retard 100 *(Marshall's Pharmaceuticals, UK).* A prolonged-action intramuscular injection containing testosterone cyclohexylpropionate ($C_{28}H_{42}O_3$ = 426.6) 100 mg per ml in sesame oil in ampoules of 1 ml. **Andromar Retard 200** contains 200 mg per ml in ampoules of 1 ml.

Femalone 25 *(Marshall's Pharmaceuticals, UK).* Testosterone cyclohexylpropionate, available as a solution for intramuscular injection containing 25 mg per ml, in ampoules of 1 ml.

Sustanon *(Organon, UK).* A mixture of testosterone esters in solution in oil for intramuscular injection, available as **Sustanon '100'** containing in each ml testosterone propionate 20 mg, testosterone phenylpropionate 40 mg, and testosterone isocaproate 40 mg, available in ampoules of 1 ml; and as **Sustanon '250'** containing in each ml testosterone propionate 30 mg, testosterone phenylpropionate 60 mg, testosterone isocaproate 60 mg, and testosterone decanoate 100 mg, available in ampoules of 1 ml.

Proprietary Names of other Testosterone Esters

Benzotest *(hexahydrobenzoate) (Ital.)*; Lontanyl *(hexahydrobenzylcarbonate) (Fr.)*.

9117-q

Trenbolone. Trienbolone. 17β-Hydroxyestra-4,9,11-trien-3-one.
$C_{18}H_{22}O_2$=270.4.

CAS — 10161-33-8.

Trenbolone is an anabolic agent (see Testosterone, p.1435). It has been used as the hexahydrobenzylcarbonate ($C_{26}H_{35}O_4$ = 411.6) by intramuscular injection in man and as the acetate in veterinary practice.

Proprietary Names

Finajet, Finaplix *(both acetate) (veterinary)*.

Soaps and other Anionic Surfactants

6010-a

Soaps were once defined as the sodium or potassium salts of the fatty acids but are now considered to include similar products formed by the saponification or neutralisation of fats or oils with organic or inorganic bases.

A *detergent* is any surface-active agent which concentrates at oil-water interfaces, and possesses emulsifying properties; thus it also possesses cleansing properties.

Anionic surfactants dissociate in aqueous solution to form a relatively large and complex anion, which is responsible for the surface activity, and a smaller cation which is devoid of surface-active properties. They are incompatible with cationic surfactants since the oppositely charged ions tend to neutralise each other. Anionic surfactants can be conveniently classified into several groups.

The sodium, potassium, and ammonium salts of the higher fatty acids are known as *alkali-metal and ammonium soaps*. They produce oil-in-water emulsions which are most stable at pH 10 and above; the emulsions crack in acid media because of the liberation of free fatty acids, and in the presence of calcium ions because of the formation of a calcium soap. These soaps are used mainly for their detergent properties and are also used as solubilising agents in disinfectants.

The calcium, zinc, magnesium, and aluminium salts of the higher fatty acids are known as *metallic soaps*. These soaps produce water-in-oil emulsions; the soaps are often made by chemical reaction during the preparation of the emulsion. Metallic soaps are incompatible with acids.

Amine soaps are salts of amines, such as triethanolamine, with fatty acids. They produce oil-in-water emulsions which are more stable than those made with alkali-metal soaps though they tend to crack in the presence of acids or high concentrations of ionisable salts. Like the other soaps, they are suitable only for preparations intended for external use.

Alkyl sulphates or *sulphated fatty alcohols* consist of the sodium, triethanolamine, or other salts of the sulphuric acid esters of the higher fatty alcohols; derivatives of both primary and secondary alcohols are used. They are sometimes known incorrectly as 'sulphonated fatty alcohols'. Sulphated fatty alcohols show a gradation in properties with increase in molecular weight. The lower members derived from alcohols with about 12 carbon atoms have the best wetting and penetrating properties whereas the higher member have better detergent properties; the lower members are less likely to precipitate with calcium salts. They maintain their detergent properties over a wide range of pH.

Sulphated fatty alcohols are widely used in industry and are employed in the preparation of many 'soapless' washing powders and liquids for domestic use. They are very useful for cleansing glassware. Pharmaceutical applications include the preparation of 'soapless' shampoos, toilet and cosmetic preparations, toothpastes, and toothpowders. They are also employed as ingredients of insecticides and in fruit-washing solutions.

Alkyl ether sulphates are formed by the addition of up to 6 ethylene oxide units, i.e. a short macrogol chain, to a fatty alcohol, followed by sulphation and neutralisation. They are similar in general properties to alkyl sulphates. They are said to be unaffected by hard water.

Proprietary preparations of alkyl ether sulphates are described under Sodium Lauryl Sulphate, p.1442.

Sulphated oils are prepared by treating fixed oils, e.g. castor oil, with sulphuric acid and neutralising with sodium hydroxide solution. They have similar properties to the sulphated fatty alcohols but their composition is somewhat variable.

Many *sulphonated compounds* have been produced which possess surface-active properties and are used as detergents; they include alkyl sulphonates, alkyl aryl sulphonates, and amide sulphonates. Docusate sodium (p.1440), a sulphonated dibasic acid ester, is used in medicine and pharmacy.

Ampholytic surfactants are described at the end of this section (see p.1443).

For the general properties of *cationic surfactants* see under Cetrimide, p.551.

Nonionic surfactants are described in the section on Cetomacrogol and Nonionic Surfactants (see p.370).

For the classification, uses and manufacture of synthetic detergents, see *Synthetic Detergents*, 6th Edn, A. Davidsohn and B.M. Milwidsky (Ed.), London, George Godwin, 1978.

Adverse Effects and Treatment. Anionic detergents may be irritant to the skin by removing natural oils and may produce redness, soreness, cracking and scaling and papular dermatitis. There may be some irritation of the eyes and mucous membranes. Ingestion of anionic detergents may cause gastro-intestinal irritation with nausea, diarrhoea, intestinal distension, and occasionally vomiting. Treatment is symptomatic.

Meningitis in 3 women who had received spinal anaesthesia was attributed to the use of detergent solution (Alconox) in the cleansing of syringes. Small amounts of residue were found in syringes subjected to the procedure. Alconox consisted of a blend of alkyl aryl sulphonates and fatty alcohol sulphates, with carbonates and complex phosphates.— R. B. Gibbons, *J. Am. med. Ass.*, 1969, *210*, 900.

A review of the action of soaps and detergents on the skin.— I. H. Blank, *Practitioner*, 1969, *202*, 147.

A study of the effects of ingestion of various commercial detergent products by *beagle dogs* and *pigs*.— B. A. Muggenburg *et al.*, *Toxic. appl. Pharmac.*, 1974, *30*, 134.

A detergent powder containing anhydrous soap, sodium polyphosphate 60%, and a detergent which was mainly lauryl sulphate 24% was taken in place of sugar by a family as the result of a practical joke. Adverse effects included difficulty in swallowing, heartburn, nausea, vomiting, and diarrhoea. One member of the family had superficial erosions of the distal oesophagus and gastritis; 2 others had small burns or ulcerations of the pharynx.— M. M. Berenson and A. B. Temple, *Clin. Toxicol.*, 1974, *7*, 25, per *Pharm. J.*, 1974, *2*, 533.

The anionic surfactants used in household detergents had moderate toxicity. The acute LD50 in *animals* ranged from 1 to 5 g per kg body-weight and the maximum safe amount that children could ingest had been estimated at 0.1 to 1 g per kg.— *Bulletin of the National Clearinghouse for Poison Control Centers*, 1975, Jan.–Feb.,.

6011-t

Curd Soap *(B.P.C. 1963)*. Sapo Animalis; Savon Animal; Jabon Animal; Sabão Animal.

Pharmacopoeias. In *Arg.*, *Cz.*, *Hung.*, *Port.*, and *Span.*

Prepared by heating purified solid animal fat with sodium hydroxide and water; on adding salt to the liquid, the soap separates out as a curd. It is a yellowish-white, or greyish-white, almost odourless solid or powder consisting chiefly of sodium stearate. It becomes plastic when heated but is horny and pulverisable after drying.

Slowly **soluble** in cold water; soluble in hot water; almost completely soluble in alcohol (90%).

Adverse Effects and Treatment. As for Soaps and other Anionic Surfactants, p.1439.

Uses. Curd soap was formerly used as a pill excipient for resinous substances and volatile oils.

6012-x

Hard Soap *(B.P.C. 1963)*. Sapo Durus; Castile Soap; Sapo Medicatus; Sapo Medicinalis; Savon Medicinal; Medizinische Seife; Jabon Duro; Sabão Vegetal.

Pharmacopoeias. In *Arg.*, *Aust.*, *Belg.*, *Ind.*, *Jap.*, *Mex.*, *Pol.*, *Port.*, and *Span.* All are sodium soaps. *Aust.* is made from olive oil and lard; *Belg.* from olive oil; *Pol.* from rape oil and lard; and *Arg.*, *Port.*, and *Span.* from almond oil (Sapo Amygdalinus) or olive oil (Sapo Olei Olivae).

Prepared by heating any suitable vegetable oil or oils or their fatty acids with sodium hydroxide.

It is a greyish-white, or yellowish-white, almost odourless solid or powder. **Soluble** 1 in 20 of water and 1 in 1.5 of boiling water; almost completely soluble in alcohol (90%); soluble 1 in 2 of boiling alcohol. **Incompatible** with strong acids and with soluble alkaline-earth and heavy metal salts.

Adverse Effects and Treatment. As for Soaps and other Anionic Surfactants, p.1439.

A severe allergic reaction occurred in a 33-year-old pregnant woman soon after being given an enema consisting of a proprietary brand of soap flakes in about 2 pints of water. She developed swelling of the mouth, numbness in the limbs, tightness in the chest, bronchospasm, and generalised urticaria and subsequently collapsed and became unconscious. She soon recovered consciousness with oxygen therapy, adrenaline, and chlorpheniramine and delivered a baby without any further untoward effects.— D. Smith, *Br. med. J.*, 1967, *4*, 215.

Uses. Hard soap was formerly used as a pill excipient for resinous substances and volatile oils and in the preparation of plasters.

6013-r

Potash Soap *(B.P.C. 1949)*. Sapo Kalinus; Linseed Oil Soap; Savon Potassique; Jabon de Potasio; Kaliseife.

Pharmacopoeias. In *Arg.*, *Aust.*, *Belg.*, *Cz.*, *Hung.*, *Jap.*, *Jug.*, *Nord.*, *Pol.*, *Roum.*, and *Swiss.*

Prepared by heating linseed oil with potassium hydroxide.

It is a yellowish-brown transparent soft unctous mass with a characteristic odour and alkaline taste, containing not less than 44% of fatty acids. **Soluble** 1 in 4 of water and 1 in 1 of alcohol. **Store** in airtight containers.

Adverse Effects and Treatment. As for Soaps and other Anionic Surfactants, p.1439.

Uses. Potash soap has been used in the preparation of liquid soaps.

Preparations

Potash Soap Spirit *(B.P.C. 1949)*. Spiritus Saponis Kalini (Hebra). Potash soap 65 g, lavender oil 0.31 ml, alcohol (90%) to 100 ml.

Amended Formula. Potash soap 60 g, lavender oil 0.3 ml, water 1.75 ml, industrial methylated spirit to 100 ml.—*Compendium of Past Formulae 1933 to 1966*, London, The National Pharmaceutical Union, 1969.

Spiritus Saponis Kalini *(Nord. P.)*. Prepared from linseed oil 33 g, 10M solution of commercial potassium hydroxide 17 g, alcohol q.s., acidum cocos (*Nord. P.*) q.s., and purified water q.s. Shake the linseed oil with the potassium hydroxide solution and 33 g of alcohol until clear. After standing for 24 hours, add, with shaking, acidum cocos q.s. until the mixture is just red to phenolphthalein. Add a quantity of alcohol equal to the weight of acidum cocos and sufficient water to produce 3 times the total weight of the linseed oil and acidum cocos used. Stand for 1 to 2 days in a cold place and filter. Product about 100 g, containing about 36% anhydrous soap.

Similar preparations are included in several other pharmacopoeias.

6014-f

Soft Soap *(B.P.)*. Sapo Mollis; Sap. Moll.; Green Soap; Medicinal Soft Soap; Jabon Blando; Sabão Mole.

Pharmacopoeias. In *Br., Chin., Ind., Port., Span.,* and *U.S.*
Span. specifies linseed oil and potassium hydroxide; *Port.* specifies olive oil and potassium hydroxide; *U.S.P.* includes Green Soap from vegetable oils (excluding coconut oil and palm-kernel oil) and potassium hydroxide.

Prepared by heating any suitable vegetable oil or oils, or their fatty acids, with potassium hydroxide or sodium hydroxide; the product, if prepared from oil, contains the glycerol formed during the saponification.
It is a yellowish-white to green or brown unctuous substance with a slight characteristic odour, yielding not less than 44% of fatty acids. The colour of the soap depends upon the fat used in its manufacture; chlorophyll or not more than 0.015% of a suitable green soap dye may be added to give a green colour.
Soluble 1 in 4 of water, 1 in 1 of boiling water, and 1 in 1 of alcohol. Some varieties of soft soap tend to separate as a gel from concentrated alcoholic solutions. A 5% solution is alkaline to bromothymol blue.

Adverse Effects and Treatment. As for Soaps and other Anionic Surfactants, p.1439.

A soap enema prepared inaccurately and containing perhaps 10 to 50 ml of concentrated soap solution in a litre produced inflammation of the colonic mucosa with hypotension, nausea and vomiting, and fever in a woman in active labour. The baby was stillborn. Such enemas were hazardous and of questionable value.— B. F. Pike *et al., New Engl. J. Med.,* 1971, *285,* 217.

Uses. Soft soap is used to remove incrustations in chronic scaly skin diseases such as psoriasis and to cleanse the scalp before the application of lotions. A solution in industrial methylated spirit, with the addition of solvent ether, is used to cleanse the skin. A solution of 1 part of soft soap in 20 of warm water is used as an enema to soften impacted faeces. Soap Liniment is a mild counter-irritant which is used in the treatment of sprains and bruises and to dilute more active liniments.

Preparations

Enemas

Soap Enema *(B.P.C. 1963).* Enema Saponis; Enem. Sap. Soft soap 5% w/v in water. *Dose.* 600 ml rectally.

Liniments

Soap Liniment *(B.P.C. 1973, A.P.F.).* Linimentum Saponis; Lin. Sap.; Opodeldoc. Oleic acid 4 g, potassium hydroxide solution 14 ml, alcohol (90%) (or industrial methylated spirit, suitably diluted) 70 ml, camphor 4 g, rosemary oil 1.5 ml, freshly boiled and cooled water to 100 ml. After preparation it should be allowed to stand for not less than 7 days and then filtered. pH 7.4 to 8.
A similar preparation is included in many pharmacopoeias.

Solutions

Ethereal Soap Solution *(B.P.C. 1973).* Liquor Saponis Aethereus; Liq. Sap. Aether.; Ether Soap; Solutio Saponis Aetherea. Prepared by mixing oleic acid 35 ml and alcohol (90%) (or industrial methylated spirit, suitably diluted) 15 ml and neutralising with a saturated solution of potassium hydroxide in water (1 in 1); the product is allowed to cool, lavender oil 0.21 ml is added, and the solution is diluted to 100 ml with solvent ether. Store in a cool place in airtight containers. This preparation is inflammable. Keep away from an open flame.

Sapo Liquidus *(Nord. P.).* An aqueous solution of coconut oil soap prepared by neutralising acidum cocos *(Nord. P.)* with potassium hydroxide. It contains about 28% of anhydrous potassium soap, equivalent to about 25% of fatty acid.

Soap Solution Alcoholic *(A.P.F.).* Spirit Shampoo. Soft soap 50 g, alcohol (90%) to 100 ml. Medicaments such as thymol 0.5% or coal tar solution 5% may be added.

Spirits

Soap Spirit *(B.P.).* Spiritus Saponatus; Spiritus Saponis; Sp. Sap. Soft soap 65% w/v in alcohol (90%) (or industrial methylated spirit, suitably diluted). Store at a temperature not exceeding 25°.

Tinctures

Green Soap Tincture *(U.S.P.).* Green soap *U.S.P.* 65 g, lavender oil 2 ml, alcohol to 100 ml. pH 9.5 to 11.5. Store in airtight containers.

A soap paste containing potassium iodide and myrrh resinoid, and used for therapeutic abortion, was formerly marketed in Great Britain under the proprietary name Utus.

6015-d

Aluminium Monostearate. Aluminum Monostearate *(U.S.N.F.)*; Aluminii Monostearas.

CAS — 7047-84-9 (monostearate).

Pharmacopoeias. In *Hung., Int.,* and *Jap.* Also in *U.S.N.F.*

A compound of aluminium with a mixture of solid organic acids obtained from fats and consisting mainly of variable proportions of aluminium monostearate and aluminium monopalmitate. Its aluminium content is equivalent to 14.5 to 16.5% of Al_2O_3.
It is a fine white to yellowish-white bulky powder with a faint characteristic odour. Practically **insoluble** in water, alcohol, acetone, and ether.

Uses. Aluminium monostearate forms gels with fixed or mineral oils when heated to about 60°; such gels are used to suspend medicaments in oily injections.

6016-n

Calcium Stearate *(U.S.N.F.).*

CAS — 1592-23-0 (stearate); 542-42-7 (palmitate).

Pharmacopoeias. In *Jap.* Also in *U.S.N.F.*

A compound of calcium with a mixture of solid organic acids obtained from fats, consisting mainly of variable proportions of calcium stearate and calcium palmitate. It contains the equivalent of 9 to 10.5% of CaO.
A fine, white to yellowish-white, light, bulky, unctuous powder free from grittiness with a slight characteristic odour. Practically **insoluble** in water, alcohol, acetone, and ether.

Calcium stearate is added to granules as a lubricant in tablet-making.

6017-h

Sulphated Castor Oil *(B.P.C. 1954).* Oleum Ricini Sulphatum; Ol. Ricin. Sulphat.; Sulphonated Castor Oil.

A yellow or orange-coloured viscous liquid with a faint odour, containing about 48.5% w/w of total fatty matter. Prepared by treating castor oil with sulphuric acid, washing, and neutralising with sodium hydroxide. Wt per ml 1.025 to 1.065 g. **Miscible** with water.

Sulphated castor oil is a non-irritating detergent and wetting agent and may be used to cleanse the skin when soap is contra-indicated.
It was formerly used as an emulsifying agent for oil-in-water creams and ointments, in the preparation of 'soluble' oils, and as a carrier for essential oils and water-insoluble bactericides.
It has also been used in the manufacture of soapless shampoos, liquid soaps, and deodorant sprays.

Preparations

Turkey Red Oil. Alizarine Oil. A commercial variety of sulphated castor oil; it is also prepared from other fixed oils. It is sold on the content of total fatty matter, the usual strength being 50%; it is generally strongly acid.
Turkey red oil is used in the dyeing industry as a fixing agent and as an emulsifying agent.

6018-m

Docusate Calcium *(U.S.P.).* Dioctyl Calcium Sulphosuccinate; Dioctyl Calcium Sulfosuccinate. Calcium 1,4-bis(2-ethylhexyl) sulphosuccinate.

$C_{40}H_{74}CaO_{14}S_2$=883.2.

CAS — 10041-19-7 [1,4-bis(2-ethylhexyl) sulphosuccinate]; 128-49-4 (calcium salt).

Pharmacopoeias. In *U.S.*

A white amorphous solid with the characteristic odour of octyl alcohol. **Soluble** 1 in 3300 of water, freely soluble in alcohol, chloroform, and ether; very soluble in macrogol 400 and maize oil.

Adverse Effects and Precautions. As for Docusate Sodium, p.1441.

For a report of leucopenia and liver damage occurring in a patient taking docusate calcium with danthron for chronic constipation, see Danthron, p.1364.

Absorption and Fate. As for Docusate Sodium, p.1441.

Uses. Docusate calcium is used similarly to docusate sodium as a faecal softening agent in doses of up to 240 mg daily. Children may be given 50 to 150 mg daily.

Preparations

Docusate Calcium Capsules *(U.S.P.).* Dioctyl Calcium Sulfosuccinate Capsules. Capsules containing docusate calcium. Store at 15° to 30° in airtight containers.

Proprietary Names

Surfak *(Hoechst, Canad.; Hoechst, USA).*

6019-b

Docusate Potassium *(U.S.P.).* Dioctyl Potassium Sulphosuccinate; Dioctyl Potassium Sulfosuccinate. Potassium 1,4-bis(2-ethylhexyl) sulphosuccinate.

$C_{20}H_{37}KO_7S$=460.7.

CAS — 7491-09-0.

Pharmacopoeias. In *U.S.*

A white amorphous solid with a characteristic odour suggestive of octyl alcohol. Sparingly **soluble** in water; soluble in alcohol and glycerol; very soluble in light petroleum.

Adverse Effects and Precautions. As for Docusate Sodium, p.1441.

Absorption and Fate. As for Docusate Sodium, p.1441.

Uses. Docusate potassium is used similarly to docusate sodium as a faecal softening agent in doses of up to 300 mg daily. Children aged 6 and over may be given 100 mg daily.

Preparations

Docusate Potassium Capsules *(U.S.P.).* Capsules containing docusate potassium. Store at 15° to 30° in airtight containers.

Proprietary Names

Dialose*(Stuart Pharmaceuticals, USA)*; Kasof *(Stuart Pharmaceuticals, USA)*; Rectalad Enema *(Wallace, USA).*

6020-x

Docusate Sodium *(U.S.P.).* Dioctyl Sodium Sulphosuccinate *(B.P.C. 1973)*; Dioctyl Sodium Sulfosuccinate; DSS; Sodium Dioctyl Sulphosuccinate. Sodium 1,4-bis(2-ethylhexyl) sulphosuccinate.

$C_{20}H_{37}NaO_7S$=444.6.

CAS — 577-11-7.

Pharmacopoeias. In *Arg., Ind.,* and *U.S.*

White or almost white hygroscopic waxy masses or flakes with a bitter taste and a characteristic

odour suggestive of octyl alcohol.
Slowly **soluble** 1 in 70 of water, higher concentrations forming a thick gel; soluble 1 in 3 of alcohol, 1 in 1 of chloroform, and 1 in 1 of ether; very soluble in light petroleum; freely soluble in glycerol; soluble in most organic solvents. It is stable in acid solution but hydrolyses slowly in weak alkaline solutions and rapidly above pH 9. The addition of electrolytes to aqueous solutions causes turbidity. **Store** in airtight containers.

Masking the taste. Cocoa syrup appeared to be the best vehicle for masking the taste of docusate sodium. Other flavouring agents of value were root beer, mint, wild cherry, and orange.— J. W. Ladd and F. V. Lofgren, *J. Am. pharm. Ass., pract. Pharm. Edn*, 1959, *20*, 456.

Adverse Effects. Prolonged use of docusate sodium may produce diarrhoea. Concentrations of more than 0.1% in ophthalmic preparations may cause conjunctival irritation.

Background toxicological information.— *Fd. Add. Ser. Wld Hlth Org. No. 6*, 1975.

Jaundice. A report of docusate sodium being absorbed from the gastro-intestinal tract and being cytotoxic to liver cells *in vitro*.— C. A. Dujovne and D. W. Shoeman, *Clin. Pharmac. Ther.*, 1972, *13*, 602.

Precautions. Like all laxatives, docusate sodium should not be administered when intestinal obstruction, abdominal pain, nausea or vomiting is present.
Docusate sodium may also facilitate gastro-intestinal absorption or hepatic cell uptake of other drugs, thereby enhancing their activity and possibly increasing their toxicity; it should not be used with liquid paraffin. Docusate sodium is excreted in breast milk and may cause increased bowel activity in suckling infants.

There were no well controlled studies proving the effectiveness of sulphosuccinate stool softeners. These compounds may increase the risk of hepatotoxicity from other drugs including other laxatives.— *Med. Lett.*, 1977, *19*, 45.

Effect on absorption. Studies of the increased gastro-intestinal absorption produced by docusate sodium: N. Khalafallah *et al.*, *J. pharm. Sci.*, 1975, *64*, 991 (phenolsulphonphthalein); M. Admans *et al.*, *Aust. J. pharm. Sci.*, 1976, *NS5*, 51 (phenolsulphonphthalein); M. W. Gouda *et al.*, *Can. J. pharm. Sci.*, 1978, *13*, 16 (phenolsulphonphthalein); M. Admans *et al.*, *Aust. J. pharm. Sci.*, 1976, *NS5*, 111 (tartrazine).

Effect on gastro-intestinal tract. Docusate sodium was found to break the gastric mucosal barrier after administration by mouth. This might be of clinical importance in relation to ingestion of docusate sodium alone or in combination with other agents known to damage the gastric mucosa.— K. M. Cochran *et al.*, *Gut*, 1977, *18*, A422.

Despite having treated many children with docusate sodium by mouth no gastric haemorrhage nor any other upper gastro-intestinal disturbance had been seen.— G. S. Clayden (letter), *Lancet*, 1978, *2*, 787.

Absorption and Fate. Docusate sodium is absorbed from the gastro-intestinal tract; there is significant biliary excretion. It is also excreted in breast milk.

A study of the excretion of docusate sodium in the bile after administration by mouth.— C. A. Dujovne and D. W. Shoeman, *Clin. Pharmac. Ther.*, 1972, *13*, 602.

Uses. Docusate sodium is an anionic surfactant with wetting, dispersing, detergent and emulsifying properties. It is used for its dispersing and emulsifying properties in various preparations for external use and has been used to prepare soapless shampoos. It is also spermicidal and has slight bactericidal activity; it has been reported to enhance the activity of certain phenolic and mercurial disinfectants.
Docusate sodium is also used as a faecal softening agent, sometimes in conjunction with a laxative, but there is little rationale for their use together. It is considered to ease constipation by increasing the penetration of fluid into the faeces, thereby softening them and is usually effective in 1 to 2 days. The usual daily dosage is from 50 to 300 mg given in divided doses but up to 500 mg daily has been used. Children may be given 5 mg per kg body-weight in divided doses. It has also been administered rectally in smaller doses as a 0.1% solution.
Docusate sodium has also been used, in water-miscible or oily solutions, for softening wax in the ear, and as a tablet disintegrant.

As no studies on the safety of docusate sodium were known to the Committee, the temporary estimated acceptable daily intake of 2.5 mg per kg body-weight was withdrawn.— Twenty-second Report of Joint FAO/WHO Expert Committee on Food Additives, *Tech. Rep. Ser. Wld Hlth Org. No. 631*, 1978.

Docusate sodium enhanced the activity of clotrimazole against *Candida albicans in vitro*. A similar effect might be observed with other surfactants (both anionic and nonionic) that did not contain an ethylene oxide group.— K. Iwata and H. Yamaguchi, *Antimicrob. Ag. Chemother.*, 1977, *12*, 206.

Constipation. In a controlled double-blind trial in 15 constipated elderly patients, 12 were less constipated on docusate sodium, in a dose of 100 mg thrice daily for 4 weeks, than they had been on a placebo.— C. M. Hyland and J. D. Foran, *Practitioner*, 1968, *200*, 698.

A study in 34 patients indicated that routine administration of docusate sodium by mouth did not provide significant prophylaxis against constipation.— J. Goodman *et al.*, *J. chron. Dis.*, 1976, *29*, 59, per *Int. pharm. Abstr.*, 1977, *14*, 1043.

Effect on gastric peptic activity. Studies *in vitro* indicated that docusate sodium inhibited gastric peptic activity at concentrations well below those used as a laxative.— G. S. Jodhka *et al.*, *J. pharm. Sci.*, 1976, *65*, 1319.

Softening ear wax. In a double-blind trial in 50 patients, docusate sodium 5% in maize oil (Dioctyl Ear Capsules) did not appear to have any outstanding advantages over maize oil alone in facilitating removal of ear wax.— E. H. Burgess, *Practitioner*, 1966, *197*, 811.

In a double-blind comparison of ear-drops containing docusate sodium 5% in water-miscible basis (Waxsol) and ear-drops containing turpentine oil, paradichlorobenzene, benzocaine, and chlorbutol in arachis oil (Cerumol) in 107 patients, the former was considered better for softening ear wax because of the smaller amount of water required for syringing.— *Practitioner*, 1967, *199*, 359 (Report No. 113 of the General Practitioner Research Group).

A study *in vitro* of the effects of 4 proprietary products and olive oil on the disintegration of ear wax indicated that a water-miscible solution of docusate sodium (Waxsol) was the only preparation tested that was effective.— J. I. Horowitz (letter), *Br. med. J.*, 1968, *4*, 583. See also T. Silver (letter), *ibid.*, 704; R. P. Grimshaw (letter), *ibid.*; F. de S. Donnan (letter), *ibid.*, 835.

For another comparison, see under Cerumol, p.695.

Tablet disintegrant. Docusate sodium (Aerosol OT) and di(1-methylamyl) sodium sulphosuccinate (Aerosol MA) were found to be the most effective of 21 surfactants tested as tablet disintegrants for a range of 11 tablets.— B. F. Cooper and E. A. Brecht, *J. Am. pharm. Ass., scient. Edn*, 1957, *46*, 520.

Preparations

Docusate Sodium Capsules *(U.S.P.)*. Dioctyl Sodium Sulfosuccinate Capsules. Capsules containing docusate sodium. Store at 15° to 30° in airtight containers.

Docusate Sodium Solution *(U.S.P.)*. Dioctyl Sodium Sulfosuccinate Solution. A solution containing docusate sodium. pH 5.8 to 6.9. Store in airtight containers.

Docusate Sodium Syrup *(U.S.P.)*. Dioctyl Sodium Sulfosuccinate Syrup. A syrup containing docusate sodium. pH 5.5 to 6.5. Store in airtight containers. Protect from light.

Docusate Sodium Tablets *(U.S.P.)*. Dioctyl Sodium Sulfosuccinate Tablets. Tablets containing docusate sodium.

Proprietary Preparations of Docusate Sodium and its Derivatives

Aerosol OT *(Cyanamid, UK)*. A brand of industrial docusate sodium. **Aerosol OT-B** is a powder grade of docusate sodium containing 15% of sodium benzoate. Pharmaceutical grades of docusate sodium are also available.

Anonaid TH *(ABM Chemicals, UK)*. An anionic surfactant containing a sulphosuccinate derivative in alcoholic solution.

Audinorm *(Carlton Laboratories, UK)*. Ear-drops containing docusate sodium 5% and glycerol 10%.

Dioctyl Forte *(Medo Chemicals, UK)*. Tablets each containing docusate sodium 100 mg.

Dioctyl-Medo *(Medo Chemicals, UK)*. Docusate sodium available as a **Syrup** containing 12.5 mg in each 5 ml and as scored **Tablets** of 20 mg. Also available to hospitals as **1% Concentrate** for dilution. The liquid forms are for oral administration; they have also been given rectally.

Emcol *(Witco, UK)*. A range of anionic surfactants, including a wide range of sulphosuccinate compounds.
The name Emcol is also applied to a range of cationic surfactants, see p.553.

Molcer *(Wallace Mfg Chem., UK: Farillon, UK)*. Ear-drops containing docusate sodium 5%, in a water-miscible basis.

Normax *(Bencard, UK)*. Capsules each containing docusate sodium 60 mg and danthron 50 mg. For constipation. *Dose.* 1 to 3 capsules at night. Children, 6 to 12 years, 1 capsule.

Soliwax *(Concept Pharmaceuticals, UK)*. Capsules containing docusate sodium 5% in oil. For softening wax in the ear. *Administration:* the contents of 1 capsule to be expressed into the ear several hours before syringing.

Waxsol *(Norgine, UK)*. Ear-drops containing docusate sodium 5% in a water-miscible basis. (Also available as Waxsol in *Austral.*, *S.Afr.*).

Waxsol should be used by patients on 2 successive nights prior to syringing of ears. In mild cases requiring syringing, an interval of 6 hours between instillation of Waxsol and syringing seemed to be the optimum interval.— H. Godfrey, *Norgine* (letter), *Br. med. J.*, 1969, *1*, 56.

Other Proprietary Names

Austral.—Coloxyl (see also under Poloxamers); *Belg.*—Dioctylal Forte, Rapilax; *Canad.*—Colace, Constiban, Regulex; *Denm.*—Mollax; *Jap.*—Adjust; *Spain*—Wasserlax; *USA*—Afko-Lube, Bu-Lax, Colace, Comfolax, Dilax, DioMedicone, Disonate, Doxinate.

A range of sulphosuccinates, including docusate sodium, was also formerly marketed in Great Britain under the proprietary name Manoxol (*Manchem*).

6021-r

Emulsifying Wax *(B.P.)*. Anionic Emulsifying Wax; Emulsif. Wax; Cera Emulsificans; Cetylanum.

CAS — 8014-38-8.

Pharmacopoeias. In *Br.*, *Ind.*, *Jug.*, *Nord.*, and *Swiss. Belg. P.* has cetostearyl alcohol 9 parts and sodium cetostearyl sulphate 1 part. *Ger. P.* has cetostearyl alcohol about 12.5 parts and sodium cetostearyl sulphate 1 part.
For Emulsifying Wax (*U.S.N.F.*), see under Preparations of Sorbitan Derivatives, p.378.

It is prepared from 9 parts of cetostearyl alcohol and 1 part of sodium lauryl sulphate or sodium salts of similar sulphated higher primary aliphatic alcohols.
It is an almost white or pale yellow waxy solid or flakes, becoming plastic when warm, with a faint characteristic odour. Practically **insoluble** in water, forming an emulsion; partly soluble in alcohol.

Uses. Emulsifying wax added to fatty or paraffin bases facilitates the preparation of oil-in-water emulsions which are absorbed, are non-greasy when rubbed into the skin, and protect against dirt and grease. It is a constituent of many hydrophilic ointment bases for so-called 'washable' ointments.

Preparations

Aqueous Cream *(B.P.)*. Hydrous Emulsifying Ointment; Simple Cream; Ung. Emulsif. Aquos.; Crem. Cerae Aquos. It may be prepared from emulsifying ointment 30 g, phenoxyethanol 1 g, and freshly boiled and cooled water 69 g. Store at a temperature not exceeding 25° in well-closed containers which minimise evaporation and contamination. *A.P.F.* specifies chlorocresol 100 mg and permits the addition of glycerol 5%.

Buffered Cream *(B.P.)*. Cremor Normalis; Crem. Norm. Sodium phosphate 2.5 g, citric acid monohydrate 500 mg, chlorocresol 100 mg, emulsifying ointment 30 g, and freshly boiled and cooled water 66.9 g. pH 5.7 to 6.3. Store at a temperature not exceeding 25° in well-closed containers which minimise evaporation and contamination. Aluminium containers should be internally

lacquered.
Buffered Cream Aqueous (*A.P.F.*) has a similar formula with glycerol 5%.

Emulsifying Ointment *(B.P., A.P.F., Ind. P.)*. Emulsif. Oint.; Ung. Emulsif. Emulsifying wax 3, white soft paraffin 5, and liquid paraffin 2, all by wt. Store at a temperature not exceeding 25°.

Emulsifying Ointment Soap *(Roy. Hallamshire Hosp.)*. Emulsifying wax 80 and white soft paraffin 20. For use as a soap substitute in eczema.

Proprietary Preparations

Collone HV *(ABM Chemicals, UK)*. An emulsifying wax consisting of a fatty alcohol with added saponifiable fats. **Collone SE.** An emulsifying wax similar to emulsifying wax *B.P.* **Collone SEC.** A brand of emulsifying wax *B.P.*

Crodex A *(Croda, UK)*. A brand of emulsifying wax.

Cyclochem *(Witco, UK)*. A range of anionic self-emulsifying waxes.

Cyclonette Wax *(Witco, UK)*. A brand of emulsifying wax.

Empiwax SK *(Albright & Wilson, Marchon Division, UK)*. A brand of emulsifying wax. **Empiwax SK/BP.** A brand of emulsifying wax *B.P.*

HEB Simplex (formerly known as Halden's Emulsifying Base) *(Waterhouse, UK)*. Contains 3 parts of liquid paraffin, 2 parts of white soft paraffin, and 2 parts of a mixture of higher fatty alcohols (hexadecyl and octadecyl alcohols) containing 10% of their acid esters (phosphated). **HEB Lac** is a stabilised emulsion of HEB Simplex in water.

A cream containing 5% of HEB Simplex in water had an average oil-globule size of 5 μm when homogenised, compared with 50 μm when prepared by agitation and cooling. The addition of 1% of cetostearyl alcohol or cetomacrogol might facilitate the production of a fine-texture cream.— *Chemist Drugg.*, 1968, *190*, 238.

Lanette Wax SX *(Ronsheim & Moore, UK)*. An anionic self-emulsifying wax consisting of a mixture of sodium alkyl sulphate and cetyl and stearyl alcohols, giving more viscous emulsions than those produced by emulsifying wax. **Lanette Wax SX B.P.** A brand of emulsifying wax.

Silcock's Base *(Bonfield, Eire)*. Emulsifying wax 15%, white soft paraffin 20%, methyl hydroxybenzoate 0.25%, propyl hydroxybenzoate 0.25%, and water to 100%.

6022-f

Magnesium Stearate *(B.P., Eur. P., U.S.N.F.)*. Mag. Stear.; Magnesii Stearas; Estearato de Magnésio.

CAS — 557-04-0 (stearate); 2601-98-1 (palmitate).

Pharmacopoeias. In *Arg., Aust., Br., Braz., Chin., Cz., Eur., Fr., Ger., Hung., It., Jap., Jug., Neth., Nord., Pol., Port., Roum.*, and *Swiss.* Also in *U.S.N.F*

The magnesium salt of a commercial stearic acid. It consists chiefly of a mixture of magnesium stearate and magnesium palmitate and contains 3.8 to 5% of Mg. *U.S.N.F.* describes a compound of magnesium with a mixture of solid organic acids obtained from fats consisting chiefly of magnesium stearate and magnesium palmitate, containing the equivalent of 6.8 to 8% of MgO, and losing not more than 4% of its weight when dried.

It is a fine, white, bulky, impalpable, unctuous powder, tasteless and odourless or with a faint odour of stearic acid. It adheres readily to the skin. It loses not more than 6% of its weight when dried. It is available in grades with different apparent volumes. Practically **insoluble** in water, alcohol, acetone, and ether. The filtrate from 1 g boiled for 1 minute with 20 ml of water has a pH of 6.2 to 7.4. **Incompatible** with acids and iron salts. **Store** in airtight containers.

Adverse Effects. Deaths have occurred from accidental inhalation of baby dusting powders containing magnesium stearate.

Uses. Magnesium stearate is used as a dusting-powder in skin diseases, and in cosmetics. In barrier creams the powder gives body to the cream and acts as a mechanical barrier to chemical irritants. It is dusted around fistulas to prevent excoriation. It is also added as a lubricant to the granules in tablet-making.

6023-d

Sodium Cetostearyl Sulphate. Natrium Cetylosulphuricum; Natrium Cetylstearylosulphuricum; Cetylstearylschwefelsaures Natrium.

CAS — 1120-01-0 (sodium cetyl sulphate); 1120-04-3 (sodium stearyl sulphate).

Pharmacopoeias. In *Aust., Belg., Cz., Ger.*, and *Roum.*

A mixture of approximately equal parts of sodium cetyl sulphate, $C_{16}H_{33}NaO_4S$, and sodium stearyl sulphate, $C_{18}H_{37}NaO_4S$.

It is a white or pale yellow amorphous or crystalline powder with a slight odour and a characteristic taste. **Soluble** in water, forming a foaming turbid solution; partly soluble in alcohol. **Protect** from light.

Sodium cetostearyl sulphate is used for the same purposes as sodium lauryl sulphate, see below.

Proprietary Names

Lanette E *(Deutsche Hydrierwerke, Ger.)*.

6024-n

Sodium Lauryl Sulphate *(B.P.)*. Sodium Lauryl Sulfate *(U.S.N.F.)*; Sod. Lauryl Sulph.; Natrium Lauryl Sulphuricum; Sodium Laurilsulfate.

CAS — 151-21-3.

Pharmacopoeias. In *Aust., Br., Braz., Cz., Hung., Ind., It., Jap., Jug., Pol., Roum.*, and *Swiss.* Also in *U.S.N.F.*

A mixture of sodium normal primary alkyl sulphates, consisting mainly of sodium dodecyl sulphate, $C_{12}H_{25}O.SO_2.ONa$. *B.P.* specifies that the mixture contains not less than 85% of sodium alkyl sulphates and both *B.P.* and *U.S.N.F.* specify not more than a total of 8% of sodium chloride and sodium sulphate.

It is a white or pale yellow sternutatory powder or crystals with a slight characteristic odour. **Soluble** 1 in 10 of water giving a turbid solution; partly soluble in alcohol; practically insoluble in chloroform, ether, and light petroleum. **Incompatible** with cationic materials and with acids below pH 2.5.

Hydrolysis. Practically no hydrolysis occurred in solutions of sodium lauryl sulphate at pH 4 and above. Below pH 2.5, hydrolysis to lauryl alcohol and sodium acid sulphate was accelerated; the rate of hydrolysis also varied with the temperature and the concentration.— R. R. Read and W. G. Fredell, *Drug Cosmet. Ind.*, 1959, *84*, 178.

Adverse Effects. Sodium lauryl sulphate may be irritant to the skin.

Hydrophilic ointment and sodium lauryl sulphate 1% in a similar basis produced contact irritant dermatitis when applied topically under occlusive dressings for 16 hours a day for more than 3 days.— P. R. Bergstresser and W. H. Eaglestein, *Archs Derm.*, 1973, *108*, 218, per *J. Am. med. Ass.*, 1973, *225*, 1140.

Intravenous toxicity. As a result of experiments on *animals*, it was concluded that sodium lauryl sulphate, whose adverse effects included marked toxic action on lungs, kidneys, and liver, should not be used intravenously in man.— H. F. Cascorbi *et al.*, *J. pharm. Sci.*, 1963, *52*, 803.

Uses. Sodium lauryl sulphate is an anionic emulsifying agent. It reduces surface tension and is a detergent and wetting agent, effective in both acid and alkaline solution and in hard water. It is used in medicated shampoos and as a skin cleanser. It is used in the preparation of Emulsifying Wax (see p.1441).

Magnesium lauryl sulphate is used as a lubricant in tablets.

The use of a detergent alkaline douche containing sodium lauryl sulphate, sodium perborate, and sodium borate (pH 9.3) was of benefit in patients with infectious vaginitis by relieving pruritus.— R. S. Cohen *et al.*, *Curr. ther. Res.*, 1973, *15*, 839.

Magnesium lauryl sulphate. Magnesium lauryl sulphate was equivalent to magnesium stearate as a lubricant. Tablet and capsule disintegration was faster with magnesium lauryl sulphate than with the stearate.— H. C. Caldwell and W. J. Westlake, *Can. J. pharm. Sci.*, 1973, *8*, 50.

Further references: A. M. Salpekar and L. L. Augsburger, *J. pharm. Sci.*, 1974, *63*, 289.

Proprietary Preparations of Alkyl Sulphates and Some Other Anionic Surfactants

Cycloryl 580 and 585N *(Witco, UK)*. Brands of sodium lauryl sulphate.

Empicols *(Albright & Wilson, Marchon Division, UK)*. A range of alkyl and alkyl ether sulphates including **Empicol AL30** (ammonium lauryl sulphate), **Empicol DLS** (diethanolamine lauryl sulphate), **Empicol ES** (a series of sodium lauryl ether sulphates), **Empicol LQ** (a series of monoethanolamine lauryl sulphates), **Empicol LM, LX, LZ** (series of sodium lauryl sulphates), **Empicol ML26** (magnesium lauryl sulphate), and **Empicol** TL40 (triethanolamine lauryl sulphate).

Neopon *(Witco, UK)*. A range of alkyl sulphates and alkyl ether sulphates.

Pentrones *(ABM Chemicals, UK)*. A range of anionic surfactants including **Pentrone A** (a series of fatty amine salts of alkyl aryl sulphonic acids), and **Pentrone S** (a series of sodium salts of sulphosuccinate derivatives).

Rewopols *(Rewo, UK)*. A range of anionic and nonionic surfactants. The anionic surfactants include products based on alkyl sulphates, alkyl and alkylphenol ether sulphates, derivatives of sulphosuccinates, and sulfosuccinamates, and alkyl aryl sulphonates.

Solumins *(ABM Chemicals, UK)*. A range of anionic surfactants including **Solumins FPnS** and **FXnS** (series of the sodium salts of sulphated alkyl phenoxypolyethoxyethanols), **Solumins TnS** (a series of sodium salts of sulphated ethoxylated fatty alcohols, some of which are used as detergents in surgical scrubs), and **Solumins PFN** (a series of phosphate esters of ethoxylated alkyl phenols).

Sulphonated Lorol Powder DC *(Ronsheim & Moore, UK)*. A brand of sodium lauryl sulphate, available as a spray-dried powder containing 90% of sodium alkyl sulphates. **Sulphonated Lorol Liquid TA.** Contains technical triethanolamine lauryl sulphate 40% in aqueous solution. **Sulphonated Lorol Paste.** Contains technical sodium lauryl sulphate 40 to 45% and water about 50%.

Teepol *(Shell Chemicals)*. A range of aqueous surfactant solutions based on sodium alkyl benzene sulphonate, alcohol ether sulphate, and alcohol ethoxylate.

NOTE. A grade of Teepol was described in the *B.P.C. 1949* under the name Sulphestol Solution.

Antimist solutions for spectacles. (1) Sodium chloride 1 g, glycerol 10 ml, Teepol 5 ml, water to 100 ml. (2) Teepol 25 ml, industrial methylated spirit 10 ml, water to 100 ml. A few drops of the solution were applied to the glass which was then rubbed bright; the effects lasted several hours.— *Br. med. J.*, 1961, *2*, 841.

Other Proprietary Names of Sodium Lauryl Sulphate

Anticerumen *(Spain)*.

Sodium lauryl sulphate was also formerly marketed in Great Britain under the proprietary name Maprofix Powder LK (*Onyx Chemical Co., USA*). A preparation containing triethanolamine ammonium lauryl sulphate was formerly marketed under the proprietary name ProDermide (*Kerfoot*).

6025-h

Sodium Oleate.

$C_{18}H_{33}NaO_2$=304.4.

CAS — 143-19-1.

A yellowish-white fatty solid with a faint odour of oleic acid. **Soluble** 1 in 10 of water and 1 in 20 of alcohol.

Sodium oleate has been used as an ingredient in preparations for the symptomatic relief of haemorrhoids and pruritus ani. It was also formerly used as a cholagogue.

Proprietary Preparations

Alcos-anal *(Norgine, UK)*. **Ointment** containing sodium oleate 10%, Laureth '9' 2%, and chlorothymol 0.1% and **Suppositories** each containing sodium oleate 200 mg, laureth '9' 20 mg, and chlorothymol 700 µg. For haemorrhoids and pruritus ani.

6026-m

Sodium Ricinoleate. Sodium Ricinate.

CAS — 5323-95-5.

A white or yellowish almost odourless powder consisting of a mixture of the sodium salts of the fatty acids from castor oil. **Soluble** in water and alcohol.

Sodium ricinoleate possesses surface-active properties. It has been used in toothpastes. A 2% solution has been used as a sclerosing agent.

6027-b

Sodium Stearate *(U.S.N.F.)*. Estearato de Sodio. A mixture of sodium stearate, $C_{18}H_{35}NaO_2$, and sodium palmitate, $C_{16}H_{31}NaO_2$.

CAS — 822-16-2 (stearate); 408-35-5 (palmitate).

Pharmacopoeias. In *Belg., It., Port., Span.,* and *Swiss.* Also in *U.S.N.F.*

A mixture containing not less than 90% of sodium stearate and sodium palmitate; the content of sodium stearate is not less than 40% of the total. It contains small amounts of the sodium salts of other fatty acids.

A fine white powder, soapy to the touch, with a faint tallow-like odour. Slowly **soluble** in water and alcohol; readily soluble in hot water and hot alcohol. A solution in water is alkaline to phenolphthalein. **Protect** from light.

Uses. Sodium stearate is used in the preparation of vanishing creams. It is an ingredient of Glycerin Suppositories *U.S.P.*

6028-v

Sodium Tetradecyl Sulphate. Sodium 4-ethyl-1-isobutyloctyl sulphate.

$C_{14}H_{29}NaO_4S$=316.4.

CAS — 139-88-8.

A white waxy odourless solid. **Soluble** in water, alcohol, and ether. A 5% solution in water is clear and colourless and has a pH of 6.5 to 9.

Adverse Effects. Injections outside the vein may produce sloughing, and injections into the vein, particularly in higher dosage, may be associated with pain and haemolysis. Thrombosis of injected veins may occur; occasionally this has led to pulmonary embolism. Allergic and anaphylactic reactions to sodium tetradecyl sulphate have occurred. If too much sclerosant is injected on one occasion the patient may experience thirst, shivering, headaches, and sometimes chest pain or epigastric discomfort.

A study of the local effects of intra-arterial injection of sodium tetradecyl sulphate 3% in *dogs* and *rabbits*.— W. A. L. MacGowan *et al., Br. J. Surg.*, 1972, *59*, 101.

Inadvertent intra-arterial injection of sodium tetradecyl sulphate in 5 patients resulted in severe ischaemic damage. Gangrene developed in the 3 patients who were not immediately treated with an infusion of heparin and a low-molecular-weight dextran.— E. G. Fegan and J. M. Pegum, *Br. J. Surg.*, 1974, *61*, 124.

Hair growth at the site of injection of sodium tetradecyl sulphate was noted in 3 female patients within 4 to 7 months. It was thought possibly due to improved blood supply.— C. G. Marks, *Br. J. Surg.*, 1974, *61*, 127.

Precautions. Sodium tetradecyl sulphate is contra-indicated in acute superficial thrombophlebitis or other affections in the region of the varices. As the follow-up treatment involves daily periods of walking, sodium tetradecyl sulphate should not be given to patients unable to walk. It should not be given to patients taking oral contraceptives. Sodium tetradecyl sulphate should be used with care in patients with a history of allergy.

Uses. Sodium tetradecyl sulphate is an anionic surfactant. It has sclerosing properties and is used in the treatment of varicose veins.

A 1 or 3% buffered solution containing benzyl alcohol 2% is used. A test dose of 0.5 ml of a 1% solution should be injected and the patient observed for several hours for any reaction before a larger injection is administered. Not more than 0.5 to 2 ml of a 3% solution should be injected at any one site and the total volume given at one session should not exceed 10 ml. Care is necessary to avoid injecting the solution outside the vein or sloughing may occur. For small superficial varices a 1% solution should be used. Injections may be repeated weekly.

Sodium tetradecyl sulphate is also used in disinfectant solutions as a surfactant to increase the penetration of the disinfectant.

Cystic lesions. The sclerosing action of sodium tetradecyl sulphate had been used in the management of cystic lesions in the thyroid gland.— P. G. Walfish *et al., Can. med. Ass. J.*, 1976, *115*, 35.

Hydrocele. For the use of sodium tetradecyl sulphate in the treatment of hydrocele, see under Phenol, p.571.

Oral haemangiomas. The injection of a 1% solution of sodium tetradecyl sulphate was successfully used in the non-surgical management of oral haemangiomas in 5 patients. It was considered to be superior to soaps for this purpose.— H. Baurmash and L. Mandel, *Oral Surg.*, 1963, *16*, 777, per *Am. J. Hosp. Pharm.*, 1963, *20*, 631.

Varicose veins. The use of sodium tetradecyl sulphate in Fegan's continous compression technique of injection of varicose veins was described. An injection of 0.5 ml of a 3% solution was used. Over a period of 6 years a preliminary survey of 760 treated patients showed a recurrence-rate of 15%. Provided that the correct diagnosis was made and the correct compression procedure was used, pregnancy and previous deep-vein thrombosis were not regarded as contra-indications.— W. G. Fegan, *Lancet*, 1963, *2*, 109.

Results were considered satisfactory in 81.1% of 1171 patients with varicose veins treated by compression sclerotherapy using sodium tetradecyl sulphate as the sclerosant.— D. E. Fitzgerald, *Practitioner*, 1968, *200*, 267.

For a report of the techniques employed for varicose vein treatment in an out-patient clinic using compression and injections of sodium tetradecyl sulphate, see D. J. Rhodes and G. J. Hadfield, *Practitioner*, 1972, *208*, 809.

A discussion of the respective merits of surgery and sclerosants in the treatment of varicose veins.— *Br. med. J.*, 1975, *1*, 593.

Further references.— J. Hobbs, *Archs intern. Med.*, 1977, *137*, 140; *J. Am. med. Ass.*, 1977, *237*, 848.

Variceal haemorrhage. References to the use of sodium tetradecyl sulphate as a sclerosing agent in the treatment of variceal haemorrhage: W. C. Widrich *et al., Archs Surg., Chicago*, 1978, *113*, 1331; J. Terblanche *et al., Surgery, St Louis*, 1979, *85*, 239.

Preparations

STD *(STD Pharmaceutical Products, UK)*. Sodium tetradecyl sulphate, available as a solution containing 3%, preserved with benzyl alcohol 2% and buffered to pH 7.6, for intravenous injection as a sclerosing agent, in ampoules of 1 ml and vials of 30 ml. (Also available as STD in *Austral.*).

Other Proprietary Names

Sotradecol *(USA)*; Trombovar *(Canad., Fr., Ital., Neth.)*.

Sodium tetradecyl sulphate was also formerly marketed in Great Britain under the proprietary name Trombovar (*Promedica, Fr.*).

6029-g

Zinc Oleate. Zinci Oleas.

$C_{36}H_{66}O_4Zn$=628.3.

CAS — 557-07-3.

Ointments of freshly prepared zinc oleate have been used in the treatment of chronic eczema.

6030-f

Zinc Stearate *(B.P.C. 1973, U.S.P.)*. Zinci Stearas; Zinc Stear.

CAS — 557-05-1 (stearate); 4991-47-3 (palmitate).

Pharmacopoeias. In *Arg., Aust., Fr., Ind., Pol., Swiss, Turk.*, and *U.S.*

It consists mainly of zinc stearate ($C_{36}H_{70}O_4Zn$ = 632.3) with a variable proportion of zinc palmitate ($C_{32}H_{62}O_4Zn$ = 576.2) and usually a small amount of zinc oleate. *B.P.C. 1973* specifies 10.45 to 12.45% of zinc. *U.S.P.* specifies the equivalent of 12.5 to 14% of ZnO.

It is a light, white, impalpable, amorphous powder with a faint characteristic odour. Practically **insoluble** in water, alcohol, and ether. It is neutral to moistened litmus paper.

Adverse Effects. Zinc stearate is irritant to the lungs and when inhaled it can produce a progressive pneumonitis which is often fatal, especially in infants.

Maximum permissible atmospheric concentration 10 mg per m^3.

Precautions. Zinc stearate should not be inhaled or applied to infants.

Uses. Zinc stearate is used as a soothing and protective application in the treatment of skin inflammation. It is used either alone or with other powders or in the form of a cream.

6031-d

Ampholytic Surfactants

An ampholytic (or amphoteric) surfactant possesses at least one anionic group and at least one cationic group in its molecule and can therefore have anionic, nonionic, or cationic properties depending on the pH. Ampholytic surfactants are anionic at a pH above their isoelectric point, cationic at a pH below it, and behave as zwitterions at intermediate pHs. When the strength of the cationic portion of the molecule is equivalent to that of the anionic portion the isoelectric point occurs at pH 7 and the molecule is said to be balanced. Ampholytic surfactants used include derivatives of long-chain *N*-substituted amino acids, and derivatives of imidazoline. Long-chain betaines are sometimes classed as ampholytic surfactants.

Ampholytic surfactants have the detergent properties of anionic surfactants and the disinfectant properties of cationic surfactants. Their activity depends on the pH of the media in which they are used. Ampholytic surfactants may be inactivated as disinfectants by other anionic and cationic surfactants depending on the nature of the ionic radicals of each surfactant and the pH. Ampholytic surfactants have been used generally for their disinfectant properties. Balanced ampholytic surfactants are reputed to be non-irritant to the eyes and skin and have therefore been used in baby shampoos.

The characteristics of ampholytic surfactants reviewed and compared with those of other types of surfactants.— C. D. Moore, *J. Soc. cosmet. Chem.*, 1960, *11*, 13. See also A. Schmitz and S. W. Harris, *Mfg Chem.*, 1958, *29*, 51.

A review of the use of ampholytic surfactants and

betaines as antimicrobials in cosmetics.— I. R. Gucklhorn, *Mfg Chem.*, 1969, *40* (Nov.), 35; *idem*, (Dec.), 43.

In *rabbits* a single short-term exposure of the peritoneal membrane to *N*-myristyl-β-aminopropionic acid (Deriphat 170-C) solution 0.25% accelerated peritoneal clearance of salicylate, barbiturate, and phenytoin during dialysis.— E. A. El-Bassiouni and A. M. Mattocks, *J. pharm. Sci.*, 1973, *62*, 1314.

A discussion of balanced imidazoline amphoteric surfactants, their properties and uses.— *Mfg Chem.*, 1978, *49* (Sept.), 57. See also D. Bass, *ibid.*, 1970, *41* (Aug.), 30.

Proprietary Preparations

Amphionic 25B *(ABM Chemicals, UK)*. A surfactant based on aminocarboxylic acids, for use in alkaline formulations.

Crodateric *(Croda, UK)*. A range of ampholytic surfactants based on imidazoline derivatives.

Cycloteric *(Witco, UK)*. A range of ampholytic surfactants produced by the carboxylation of alkyl imidazolines.

Rewoteric *(Rewo, UK)*. A range of ampholytic surfactants including imidazoline and alkyl-amido-betaine derivatives.

Rexoteric *(Grace, UK)*. Ampholytic surfactants based on imidazoline derivatives.

Tego *(Goldschmidt, UK)*. A range of bactericidal and fungicidal ampholytic surfactants. **Tego MHG** is dodicin hydrochloride [dodecyldi(aminoethyl)glycine hydrochloride, $C_{18}H_{40}ClN_3O_2$ = 366.0]; it is available in concentrated solution for use in hospitals as a surface disinfectant, intended mainly for use in the Tego Disinfection Technique, involving a mixing apparatus which automatically delivers the correct concentration of 1% from a spray nozzle.

A review of the properties and uses of dodicin.— F. Kornfeld, *Fette u. Seifen*, 1966, *68*, 563, per A. H. Walters, *Mfg Chem.*, 1967, *38* (Mar.), 45.

A comparison of the efficacy of solutions of dodicin (Tego 103S) 1%, alcohol 70%, and cetrimide 0.1% with chlorhexidine 0.1% in alcohol 70%, by means of bacterial counts from disinfected skin during operations, showed the alcoholic cetrimide-chlorhexidine to be the most efficient skin disinfectant.— D. B. Butler and S. C. Hopcroft, *Med. J. Aust.*, 1966, *1*, 180. Criticisms of the method of assessment used.— B. R. Frisby (letter), *ibid.*, 373. See also S. C. Hopcroft and D. B. Butler (letter), *ibid.*, 730.

Reports of contact sensitisation in workers using dodicin hydrochloride (Tego).— R. E. Bowers, *Contact Dermatitis Newslett.*, 1968, No. 4, 76; S. Fregert and I. Dahlquist, *ibid.*, 1969, No. 5, 103; C. D. Calnan, *ibid.*, 1974, No. 15, 439.

Other Proprietary Names

Deriphats *(USA)*.

A range of ampholytic surfactants was also formerly marketed in Great Britain under the proprietary name Miranol (*Venture Chemicals*).

6032-n

Some Proprietary Detergent Preparations

A list of proprietary detergent preparations approved for the cleansing and disinfection of milk containers and appliances is contained in Circular FSH 8/78, Minist. Agric. Fish. Fd, London, HM Stationery Office, 1978.

Alconox *(K & K-Greeff, UK)*. A powder consisting of alkyl aryl sulphonates, lauryl alcohol sulphates, a mixture of complex phosphates, and sodium carbonates. For cleaning laboratory and hospital equipment and instruments.

Decon 90 *(Decon Laboratories, UK)*. A liquid detergent containing anionic and nonionic surfactants with various mineral salts having complete free-rinsing properties. For cleaning and radioactive decontamination of laboratory glassware and equipment and surgical instruments.

Dri-Decon. A non-foaming powder detergent containing antibacterials and surfactants and having complete free-rinsing properties. For use in glassware and bottle washing equipment.

Pyroneg *(Diversey, UK)*. An alkaline powder detergent containing sodium carbonate, complex phosphates, and a sodium alkyl aryl sulphonate; for cleaning laboratory glassware, surgical instruments, syringes, and needles.

Detergent preparations for cleaning hospital and laboratory glassware and equipment were also formerly marketed in Great Britain under the proprietary names Liqui-Nox (*Cambrian*) and Neutrobrite (*Albright & Wilson, Eire*).

Sodium Cromoglycate and Related Anti-allergic Agents

7720-w

Sodium cromoglycate is an anti-allergic agent which is used prophylactically in allergic disorders including asthma and rhinitis. It is not absorbed from the gastro-intestinal tract and efforts have been made to find a similar substance which is absorbed when taken by mouth. Cromoglycate-like compounds, often termed chromones or cromones, which have been investigated include bufrolin, doxantrazole, and xanoxic acid. Ketotifen is an antihistamine which also has anti-allergic properties and is absorbed when taken by mouth. The use of other antihistamines in allergic conditions is described under Promethazine and other Antihistamines, p.1295.

7721-e

Sodium Cromoglycate *(B.P.).* FPL 670; Cromolyn Sodium *(U.S.P.)*; Disodium Cromoglycate; Natrii Cromoglicas. Disodium 4,4′-dioxo-5,5′-(2-hydroxytrimethylenedioxy)di(4*H*-chromene-2-carboxylate).

$C_{23}H_{14}Na_2O_{11}$=512.3.

CAS — 16110-51-3 (cromoglycic acid); 15826-37-6 (disodium salt).

Pharmacopoeias. In *Br.*, *Chin.*, *Nord.*, and *U.S.*

A white, odourless, hygroscopic, crystalline powder, tasteless at first with a slightly bitter after-taste. It loses not more than 10% of its weight on drying. **Soluble** 1 in 20 of water; practically insoluble in alcohol and chloroform. **Store** in airtight containers.

Adverse Effects. Sodium cromoglycate is generally well tolerated and reports of adverse reactions other than local irritant effects have been rare.

Inhalation of the dry powder may have a direct, often transient, irritant effect with bronchospasm, wheezing, cough, nasal congestion, and irritation of the throat, especially during or following local infection. Nausea, vomiting, headache, dizziness, hoarseness, and a bitter taste have also been reported. Some of the irritant effects may be attributed to the powder rather than the sodium cromoglycate itself. Other reactions, which have sometimes occurred after treatment for several weeks or months, include aggravation of existing asthma, urticaria, rashes, and pulmonary infiltrates with eosinophilia. Allergic reactions such as bronchospasm, laryngeal oedema, angio-oedema, and anaphylaxis have been reported rarely. Sodium cromoglycate may be inhaled with isoprenaline and for reference to the adverse effects associated with isoprenaline, see Isoprenaline Sulphate, p.15.

There may be transient irritation of the nasal mucosa following the intranasal use of sodium cromoglycate. Nausea, skin rashes, and joint pains have occurred when it is taken by mouth.

In a cooperative study, adverse reactions (excluding local irritation) occurred in only 8 of 375 asthmatic patients who had received sodium cromoglycate by inhalation for periods ranging from 2 days to 1 year. The reactions were: generalised dermatitis in 3 patients, facial dermatitis in 2, myositis in 2, and gastro-enteritis in 1. The dermatitis was usually pruritic. Reactions were reversible and all returned within a few hours or 2 days on rechallenge. Immunological tests for determining the basis of these adverse effects were not helpful.— G. A. Settipane *et al.*, *J. Am. med. Ass.*, 1979, *241*, 811.

In a comparative study of sodium cromoglycate and placebo in 12 patients with ulcerative colitis elevation of serum-aminotransferase values in 2 patients was probably not drug-related.— V. Mani *et al.*, *Lancet*, 1976, *1*, 439.

A report of severe bronchoconstriction, in a 42-year-old man with chronic asthma, provoked by sodium cromoglycate.— I. C. Paterson *et al.*, *Br. med. J.*, 1976, *2*, 916. A further report of the exacerbation of asthma by sodium cromoglycate inhalation.— J. Serup, *Acta med. scand.*, 1979, *205*, 447.

A report of pulmonary infiltrates with eosinophilia, associated with the inhalation of sodium cromoglycate. Asthmatic symptoms in a 36-year-old woman had been controlled satisfactorily until a high fever suddenly developed. Stomatitis, arthralgia of both knees, left chest pain, urticaria-like redness, and enlargement of cervical and axillary lymph nodes were noted, and pulmonary infiltration and eosinophilia were found. She responded to treatment with prednisolone but the syndrome recurred when treatment with sodium cromoglycate was continued.— *Japan med. Gaz.*, 1977, *14* (July 20), 10. See also H. Löbel *et al.* (letter), *Lancet*, 1972, *2*, 1032; L. W. Burgher *et al.*, *Chest*, 1974, *66*, 84; U. K. Repo and P. Nieminen, *Scand. J. resp. Dis.*, 1976, *57*, 1 (pulmonary infiltrations, eosinophilia, and urinary symptoms).

Marked eosinophilia, liver disease similar to primary biliary cirrhosis, and vasculitis in a 45-year-old woman were attributed to a hypersensitivity reaction to sodium cromoglycate administered by inhalation.— J. L. Rosenberg *et al.*, *Archs intern. Med.*, 1978, *138*, 989.

Oesophagitis developed in a 53-year-old woman 15 minutes after her first inhalation of sodium cromoglycate and persisted for about one hour. Symptoms were subsequently relieved by the administration of antacids before each inhalation.— R. H. Israel and J. Wood (letter), *J. Am. med. Ass.*, 1979, *242*, 2758.

Further reports of adverse effects associated with the inhalation or insufflation of sodium cromoglycate: R. Pariente, *Nouv. Presse méd.*, 1972, *1*, 883 (urticarial rash); S. H. Block, *J. Allergy & clin. Immunol.*, 1974, *53*, 243 (severe nasal congestion and wheezing); M. Rao *et al.* (letter), *J. Pediat.*, 1975, *86*, 804 (severe nasal congestion); A. L. Sheffer *et al.*, *New Engl. J. Med.*, 1975, *293*, 1220 (immunological components of hypersensitivity reactions); M. P. S. Menon and A. K. Das, *Scand. J. resp. Dis.*, 1977, *58*, 145 (generalised urticaria and provocation of an asthmatic attack after treatment for 2 months); E. E. Slater, *Chest*, 1978, *73*, 878 (peripheral eosinophilia and pericarditis with cardiac tamponade); *Med. J. Aust.*, 1979, *2*, 608 (ulceration of the lips, tongue, buccal mucosa, and pharynx, and possible oesophagitis, following nasal insufflation).

Precautions. Sodium cromoglycate should not be given to patients with known hypersensitivity to it. The precautions for isoprenaline (see p.16) should be observed for patients using sodium cromoglycate with isoprenaline.

In patients who have had systemic corticosteroid therapy reduced or discontinued this may need to be reinstated without delay if symptoms increase, during periods of stress, or where airways obstruction prevents absorption of sodium cromoglycate.

Since the action of sodium cromoglycate is prophylactic the symptoms of asthma will probably recur if it is withdrawn; it has been suggested that withdrawal should be carried out gradually over a period of a week. Where the use of sodium cromoglycate has permitted a reduction in corticosteroid dosage the dosage should be restored to at least the original amount given before administration of sodium cromoglycate.

A 14-year-old boy who died in a severe attack of nocturnal asthma had been taking sodium cromoglycate by inhalation for the preceding 4 weeks. He had suffered from persistent airway obstruction and it was considered that subjective relief derived from sodium cromoglycate therapy could have obscured the warning symptoms. He had also been treated with prednisone, the dosage of which had been reduced, perhaps to a level which was inadequate.— I. Gregg and J. Batten, *Br. med. J.*, 1969, *2*, 29.

Absorption and Fate. Sodium cromoglycate is poorly absorbed from the gastro-intestinal tract. Following inhalation as a fine powder about 8% of a dose is reported to be deposited in the lungs from where it is rapidly absorbed and excreted unchanged in the urine and bile. The majority of an inhaled dose is swallowed and excreted unchanged in the faeces.

When doses of 20 mg of sodium cromoglycate were inhaled by 12 asthmatic patients, 5 to 10% remained in the inhaler, 0.7 to 3.1% was excreted unchanged in the urine within 24 hours, and 80 to 87% was excreted unchanged in the faeces within 3 days. No metabolites were detected. Sodium cromoglycate was rapidly absorbed from the lungs to produce peak plasma concentrations of 6.5 to 12.1 ng per ml within 15 minutes and the mean plasma half-life was 81 minutes. Since approximately equal amounts of drug were excreted in the urine and faeces after an intravenous dose of about 3.8 mg, and only about 0.4% of a 20-mg dose by mouth was excreted in the urine, it was considered that about 3.2% of an inhaled dose was absorbed in the lungs. The remainder was swallowed. When given intravenously, sweating, a sensation of heat, and increased heart-rate and blood pressure were noted.— S. R. Walker *et al.*, *J. Pharm. Pharmac.*, 1972, *24*, 525. See also J. S. G. Cox *et al.*, *Br. med. J.*, 1969, *2*, 634.

A study of renal tubular function in 10 asthmatic children inhaling sodium cromoglycate. Serum-chloride concentrations were slightly raised; there was no explanation for this finding.— H. Hutchinson *et al.*, *Clin. Allergy*, 1972, *2*, 91.

Five healthy subjects inhaled sodium cromoglycate with mean particle diameters of 2, 6, and 11.7 µm. The 2-µm particles were better absorbed into the lungs than the larger particles indicating that in patients where a poor response to sodium cromoglycate was due to poor absorption a better response might be obtained using 2-µm particles.— S. H. Curry *et al.*, *Br. J. clin. Pharmac.*, 1975, *2*, 267. See also S. Godfrey *et al.*, *Clin. Sci. & mol. Med.*, 1974, *46*, 265.

Sodium cromoglycate was moderately bound (range 57 to 69%) to plasma proteins.— B. Clark *et al.*, *Fisons*, *J. Pharm. Pharmac.*, 1978, *30*, 386.

Further references to the absorption and fate of sodium cromoglycate: G. M. Shenfield *et al.*, *Br. J. clin. Pharmac.*, 1976, *3*, 583 (administration directly into the bronchi).

Uses. Sodium cromoglycate is used for the prevention of allergic reactions and is believed to act by inhibiting the release of chemical mediators from sensitised mast cells, although other mechanisms may also be involved.

It is used in the prophylactic treatment of asthma associated with allergy and in exercise-induced asthma and may also be of some benefit in intrinsic asthma. Sodium cromoglycate does not affect an established asthmatic attack thus it is not used for acute attacks including status asthmaticus. In patients taking corticosteroids for asthma it is often possible to reduce the dosage when treatment with sodium cromoglycate is started (but see Precautions, above). Sodium cromoglycate does not affect inflammatory or non-allergic symptoms of asthma and concomitant treatment with antibiotics, bronchodilators, or corticosteroids may be required.

Sodium cromoglycate is also used prophylactically in the treatment of seasonal and perennial allergic rhinitis. Eye-drops are used in the treatment of vernal keratoconjunctivitis and other allergic conditions of the eye.

It has been given by mouth, with variable results, as an adjunct in the treatment of ulcerative colitis and related diseases. Sodium cromoglycate has also been used in the prevention of food allergies.

In asthma, sodium cromoglycate is administered as a dry powder or as a nebulised solution in a usual dose of 20 mg by inhalation 4 times daily at intervals of 3 to 6 hours; in some patients 20 mg may need to be given 6 to 8 times daily. Alternatively a dose of 2 mg may be inhaled, similarly, from a metered aerosol. The maintenance of regular dosage is important. Since inhalation of the dry powder may cause bronchospasm, isoprenaline has been inhaled concomitantly; however the use of a bronchodilator, such as salbutamol, inhaled a few minutes beforehand is preferable.

For allergic rhinitis, 10 mg of sodium cromoglycate as powder is given by nasal insufflation into each nostril up to 4 times daily or a 2% solution is administered as drops or spray into each nostril 6 times daily. In ophthalmic conditions 2% eye-drops are used.

In inflammatory bowel disease or food allergy, sodium cromoglycate may be given by mouth in usual doses of 200 mg four times daily before meals; children over 2 years may be given 100 mg four times daily.

Reviews of the actions and uses of sodium cromoglycate: R. N. Brogden *et al.*, *Drugs*, 1974, *7*, 164 and 283; R. C. Godfrey and J. B. L. Howell, *ibid.*, 161; *Acta allerg.*, 1977, *32*, *Suppl.* 13, 1–115; J. W. Kerr, *Scott. med. J.*, 1977, *22*, 234; I. L. Bernstein *et al.*, *Ann. intern. Med.*, 1978, *89*, 228; L. A. Turnberg, *Topics Ther.*, 1978, *4*, 10; P. König, *Ann. Allergy*, 1979, *43*, 293.

Action. A discussion on mast cells and the mode of action of sodium cromoglycate. Mast cells are present in connective tissue throughout the body and their cytoplasmic granules contain vasoactive agents (which are also bronchoconstrictors) such as histamine, serotonin, slow-reacting substance of anaphylaxis, and prostaglandins. They also contain enzymes and other substances, such as heparin, which may be implicated in tissue damage and repair, and chemotactic mediators in some types of inflammatory reaction. These biologically active substances are released into the extracellular space when degranulation occurs in response to immunological and histochemical stimuli. Clinically, the most common trigger of degranulation appears to be a type I antigen-antibody reaction on the surface of mast cells which have been sensitised by cell-bound IgE antibody after previous exposure to antigen. In anaphylaxis large numbers of mast cells throughout the body are sensitised but more often mast-cell degranulation is confined to one or more target organs, such as the bronchi, nasal mucosa, gastro-intestinal tract, or skin, and is now widely assumed to be responsible for most of the common allergic disorders in atopic subjects. *Animal* studies showing that an IgE-mediated reaction promotes degranulation through the influx of calcium ions into mast cells and by the activation of membrane-associated enzymes provide the basis for the hypothesis that the prophylactic value of sodium cromoglycate in extrinsic asthma is related to its stabilising effect on the mast-cell membrane, thus preventing degranulation and the subsequent release of bronchoconstrictor substances. However, although there is indirect evidence for this hypothesis, it does not necessarily prove that sodium cromoglycate acts specifically or solely on mast cells. Sodium cromoglycate seems to exert more potent therapeutic effects, especially in children with extrinsic asthma, than are explained on the basis of its inhibitory effect on mast cells alone.— *Br. med. J.*, 1981, *282*, 587.

Sodium cromoglycate had been shown to inhibit the development of both immediate and late antigen-induced asthmatic reactions, whereas corticosteroids inhibited only the late response. The mode of action was believed to involve the temporary stabilisation of mast cell membranes. Sodium cromoglycate might also interact with adrenergic mechanisms or might stabilise mast cells to the effect of alpha-adrenergic receptor stimulation. A reduction in the degree of hypersensitivity to histamine had been noted in some patients, usually after prolonged use, suggesting that sodium cromoglycate might also have a direct action on bronchial smooth muscle but this could be a consequence of the anti-allergic action rather than a direct effect.— R. N. Brogden *et al.*, *Drugs*, 1974, *7*, 164.

Cromoglycate and the similar anti-allergic compounds, doxantrazole and bufrolin, might inhibit antigen-induced mediator release by interfering with calcium transport across the mast cell membrane. It was conceivable that they prevented calcium transport across the mast-cell membrane by raising intracellular concentrations of cyclic adenosine phosphate (cyclic AMP).— J. C. Foreman and L. G. Garland, *Br. med. J.*, 1976, *1*, 820. Comment.— C. J. Vardey and I. F. Skidmore, *Allen & Hanburys* (letter), *ibid.*, 1976, *2*, 369. Results indicating that cromoglycate and doxantrazole inhibit antigen-induced calcium-45 uptake in *rat* peritoneal mast cells and may exert their antisecretory effects by this mechanism. Since they also inhibit phosphodiesterase, calcium-45 uptake might be prevented indirectly by raising intracellular concentrations of cyclic AMP.— J. C. Foreman *et al.*, *Br. J. Pharmac.*, 1977, *59*, 473P.

Sodium cromoglycate is not a bronchodilator and has no anti-inflammatory or antihistaminic action.— D. C. Webb-Johnson and J. L. Andrews, *New Engl. J. Med.*, 1977, *297*, 758. A study in 20 children showed that sodium cromoglycate, inhaled in solution from an efficient nebuliser, had bronchodilator activity comparable with that of salbutamol.— J. T. N. Chung and R. S. Jones, *Br. med. J.*, 1979, *2*, 1033. A bronchodilator response to sodium cromoglycate in 2 adults.— P. Helliwell (letter), *ibid.*, 1588. Results suggesting that sodium cromoglycate does not have specific bronchodilator activity.— N. C. Thomson *et al.* (letter), *ibid.*, 1981, *282*, 1973. Evidence suggesting that, in addition to its ability to stabilise mast cells, sodium cromoglycate may also act on bronchial irritant receptors or directly on smooth muscle in asthmatic patients.— M. G. Harries *et al.*, *Lancet*, 1981, *1*, 5.

Sodium cromoglycate *in vitro* prevented or delayed the appearance of typical cytopathic effects of viruses.— K. Penttinen *et al.*, *Br. med. J.*, 1977, *1*, 82. Limited studies did not demonstrate that sodium cromoglycate had antiviral activity.— D. E. E. Loveday and R. B. M. Wenham, *ibid.*, *2*, 557.

Administration. The absence (or the presence of only minute amounts) of sodium cromoglycate in the urine in patients using 4 capsules (each 20 mg) daily suggested that in some patients insufficient was inhaled to produce benefit. Of 11 children with long-standing perennial asthma unresponsive to 3 or 4 capsules daily, 6 were improved when they used 8 capsules daily, without untoward effect.— J. M. Smith (letter), *Br. med. J.*, 1973, *2*, 303. A similar report.— N. Ure (letter), *Med. J. Aust.*, 1973, *2*, 869.

Some children can use the Intal Spinhaler satisfactorily by the age of 3 but the majority obtain little benefit until they are 5 years old. For those unable to use the Spinhaler, sodium cromoglycate can be given as a nebulised solution delivered by a compressor/nebuliser system. Administration takes up to 10 minutes and must be repeated 3 to 4 times daily. When the child has troublesome coughing and wheezing further improvement can be achieved by adding 0.5 ml of 0.5% salbutamol respirator solution to the sodium cromoglycate.— A. D. Milner, *Prescribers' J.*, 1980, *20*, 33. See also S. Bedford and J. A. Kuzemko (letter), *Br. med. J.*, 1972, *1*, 748 (successful use of Spinhaler below the age of 5); H. E. Williams and P. D. Phelan (letter), *Br. med. J.*, 1973, *2*, 488 (use of solution by inhalation, with orciprenaline); R. Vines (letter), *Med. J. Aust.*, 1974, *1*, 682 (encouraging results with oral insufflation of powder under the age of 3); E. J. Hiller *et al.*, *Archs Dis. Childh.*, 1977, *52*, 875 (successful administration of a nebulised solution under the age of 5).

For a warning that compressors used for nebuliser therapy at home should be given regular maintenance, see R. D. Steventon and R. S. E. Wilson (letter), *Lancet*, 1979, *1*, 787.

Further reports on the administration of sodium cromoglycate: A. A. Demin (letter), *Br. med. J.*, 1976, *1*, 1278 (beneficial effect of deoxyribonuclease by inhalation on the treatment of asthma with sodium cromoglycate).

Asthma. A review of the established extrinsic causes of allergic lung reactions. Hypersensitivity diseases may be classified as extrinsic or cryptogenic (usually, and less satisfactorily, termed intrinsic).— J. Pepys, *Practitioner*, 1978, *220*, 541.

A review of the treatment of asthma. A therapeutic trial of sodium cromoglycate is worthwhile if the use of a bronchodilator alone fails to control symptoms. Children and young allergic adults are most likely to benefit although a response is hard to predict and a proper trial should be performed with frequent peak expiratory flow-rate readings for several weeks before and after starting treatment with sodium cromoglycate by inhalation. Treatment should be stopped if there is no clear improvement. The combined preparation of sodium cromoglycate and isoprenaline should not be used since assessment of benefit is confused by the isoprenaline. If persistent airway narrowing or wheezing is provoked by the inhalation a sympathomimetic agent should be inhaled 15 minutes beforehand. Sodium cromoglycate is intended for regular prophylaxis and it is not desirable to reduce the daily dose to a minimum when symptoms are few.— D. W. Empey, *Br. med. J.*, 1978, *2*, 1208. A view that sodium cromoglycate should be tried in all patients with chronic perennial asthma before corticosteroid therapy is instituted; it may also have a steroid-sparing effect in steroid-dependent patients. Sodium cromoglycate is the drug of choice in the prophylactic treatment of asthmatic patients sensitive to animal danders and various occupational allergens and is one of the preferred prophylactic measures against exercise-induced asthma. Although sodium cromoglycate appears to be primarily effective in extrinsic asthma it may be of benefit in asthma without demonstrable allergens.— I. L. Bernstein *et al.*, *Ann. intern. Med.*, 1978, *89*, 228. The fact that sodium cromoglycate is still underused in asthmatic patients who are not adequately controlled with sympathomimetics and theophylline may be due to a number of factors: the setting of an unrealistic goal (e.g. total suppression of asthma), the lack of a reasonable trial (2 months at full dosage), incorrect use of the Spinhaler, or the use of inhaled corticosteroids during withdrawal from crisis corticosteroid therapy—the addition of sodium cromoglycate in such patients may allow corticosteroid dosage to be reduced subsequently or even withdrawn.— H. Guy, *Drugs*, 1980, *19*, 141.

A review of the treatment of infants and children with asthma. If symptoms are not adequately controlled with bronchodilators children over the age of 5 years should be given sodium cromoglycate by inhalation from a Spinhaler 3 or 4 times daily. Sodium cromoglycate is useful in about 70% of children with asthma. It usually blocks exercise-induced bronchoconstriction and an additional dose immediately before physical activity may be helpful. Children with the severest symptoms may require treatment with corticosteroids.— A. D. Milner, *Prescribers' J.*, 1980, *20*, 33. See also H. I. Lecks, *Clin. Pediat.*, 1977, *16*, 861; C. Green, *Practitioner*, 1979, *223*, 690; M. B. Marks, *Ann. Allergy*, 1979, *43*, 19. See also under Administration (above).

Further reviews on the treatment of asthma, including the prophylactic use of sodium cromoglycate: A. S. Rebuck, *Drugs*, 1974, *7*, 344 and 370; J. W. Paterson and J. V. Collins, *Adv. Med. Topics Ther.*, 1975, *1*, 172; I. Gregg, *Drugs*, 1977, *13*, 35; A. J. Woolcock, *Am. Rev. resp. Dis.*, 1977, *115*, 191; *Med. Lett.*, 1978, *20*, 69; G. M. Cochrane, *Practitioner*, 1979, *223*, 489.

In a long-term double-blind study of the effect of sodium cromoglycate in patients with severe asthma unresponsive to conventional therapy, patients inhaled from capsules of sodium cromoglycate 20 mg with isoprenaline 100 µg, sodium cromoglycate 20 mg, isoprenaline 100 µg, or a placebo (anhydrous sodium sulphate); the dose of 4 capsules daily initially was reduced in some patients according to response. Of those available for evaluation, the number of patients still adequately controlled at the end of 1 year was respectively 16 of 20, 10 of 15, 5 of 20, and 3 of 19. Patients with a history of allergy responded better than those with no such history. One patient taking sodium cromoglycate with isoprenaline was withdrawn early in the trial because of intolerance; otherwise the treatment was tolerated without adverse effect on serum aspartate aminotransferase (SGOT) or serum alanine aminotransferase (SGPT) values or on the haematological and urological parameters studied.—Brompton Hospital/MRC Collaborative Trial, *Br. med. J.*, 1972, *4*, 383. Results of a similar trial in Edinburgh were compared and combined. Both sodium cromoglycate regimens were superior overall to the placebo. In the second year half of the patients from both centres who continued in the trial were randomly allocated to a placebo. Whereas 50% of the patients in the placebo group relapsed only 13% in the sodium cromoglycate group did so. The number of patients who did not relapse on the placebo indicated, however, that the continued use of sodium cromoglycate was not always necessary. Results from the second-year study also endorsed the policy of allowing patients to adjust their dose of sodium cromoglycate to the lowest number of capsules that would control their symptoms.—Northern General Hospital, Brompton Hospital, and MRC Collaborative Trial, *Br. med. J.*, 1976, *1*, 361.

A study demonstrating the benefit of sodium cromoglycate in *intrinsic* asthma.— M. N. Blumenthal *et al.*, *J. Allergy & clin. Immunol.*, 1973, *52*, 104. See also F. A. Irani *et al.*, *Am. Rev. resp. Dis.*, 1972, *106*, 179. Only 3 of 20 patients with intrinsic asthma responded to treatment with sodium cromoglycate.— K. B. Saunders *et al.*, *Br. med. J.*, 1978, *1*, 1184.

Twenty-two patients with chronic asthma took sodium cromoglycate for 2.5 to 4 years without diminution of its effectiveness; in 4 patients it ceased to be effective. Of 18 patients who were receiving regular corticosteroid therapy 12 were able to discontinue it entirely and 6 required smaller less frequent doses.— J. Crisp *et al.*, *J. Am. med. Ass.*, 1974, *229*, 787. Comments.— K. G. Johnson (letter), *ibid.*, *230*, 539; W. C. Deamer, *ibid.*, 1975, *232*, 1007.

In a double-blind study of 14 asthmatic children no difference in efficacy was noted between beclomethasone dipropionate aerosol and sodium cromoglycate or between the 2 drugs used in association. A large-scale study might, however, be indicated before concluding that concurrent administration does not provide an enhanced effect.— I. Mitchell *et al.*, *Br. med. J.*, 1976, *2*, 457. In 20 children with asthma inadequately controlled by bronchodilators alone, the inhalation of betamethasone valerate 200 µg four times daily was significantly more effective, as assessed by bronchodilator dosage, symptom scores, and peak expiratory flow-rate, than sodium cromoglycate 20 mg four times daily.— S. H. Ng *et al.*, *Postgrad. med. J.*, 1977, *53*, 315.

For further comparative studies of sodium cromoglycate with other agents in the management of asthma, see G.

Hambleton *et al.*, *Lancet*, 1977, *1*, 381 (superiority of theophylline in children with chronic asthma); H. R. Gribbin and A. E. Tattersfield (letter), *ibid.*, 960 (criticism); M. Weinberger (letter), *ibid.*, 1365 (reply); D. P. Tashkin *et al.*, *Ann. Allergy*, 1977, *39*, 311 (isoprenaline, atropine, or sodium cromoglycate); A. T. Edmunds *et al.*, *Br. med. J.*, 1980, *281*, 842 (sodium cromoglycate or slow-release aminophylline; both effective in the prophylaxis of perennial asthma in children).

A suggestion that sodium cromoglycate may be of benefit in patients with asthma in whom reactions to food additives may be acting as provoking factors.— *Br. med. J.*, 1978, *1*, 669. See also A. B. X. Breslin *et al.*, *Clin. Allergy*, 1973, *3*, 71 (pretreatment with sodium cromoglycate by inhalation in allergy to the congeners in alcoholic beverages). See also under Food Allergy in Gastro-intestinal Disorders (below).

A study indicating that sodium cromoglycate helped to restore pituitary-adrenal axis function in young steroid-dependent asthmatic patients.— G. G. Shapiro *et al.*, *Chest*, 1978, *73*, 340. See also H. Kaufman *et al.*, *J. Allergy & clin. Immunol.*, 1976, *57*, 267.

Exercise-induced asthma is mainly seen in children and generally responds rapidly to inhaled bronchodilators. Attacks can often be prevented by the prior use of bronchodilators or sodium cromoglycate. If the patient is actively engaged in sport, inhalations of sodium cromoglycate can be used prophylactically.— *Br. med. J.*, 1980, *280*, 271. See also A. R. Morton and K. D. Fitch, *Med. J. Aust.*, 1974, *2*, 158; D. Wallace and M. H. Grieco, *Ann. Allergy*, 1976, *37*, 153; M. Chan-Yeung, *Chest*, 1977, *71*, 320; W. Lenney and A. D. Milner, *Archs Dis. Childh.*, 1978, *53*, 474; A. F. Racaniello (letter), *New Engl. J. Med.*, 1978, *299*, 1193.

Further references to the use of sodium cromoglycate in asthma: T. Gebbie *et al.*, *Br. med. J.*, 1972, *4*, 576; M. Silverman *et al.*, *Br. med. J.*, 1972, *3*, 378; J. S. Hyde, *Ann. intern. Med.*, 1973, *78*, 966; M. Silverman *et al.*, *Thorax*, 1973, *28*, 574; M. B. Marks, *Am. J. Dis. Child.*, 1974, *128*, 301; B. Kang *et al.*, *Br. med. J.*, 1976, *1*, 867; A. D. Clift and A. Holzel, *Ann. Allergy*, 1978, *41*, 313.

Bronchitis. Of 70 patients with chronic bronchitis who had skin sensitivity tests carried out with at least 30 allergens, 30 had 1 or more positive reactions. When these 70 patients were given sodium cromoglycate in a double-blind crossover study, there was no response in either the allergic or non-allergic patients nor was there any difference in response between either group in 24 patients given prednisone.— F. Moran, *B.T.T.A. Rev.*, 1972, *2*, 75. A similar result.—Report No. 166 of the General Practitioner Research Group, *Practitioner*, 1972, *208*, 291.

Gastro-intestinal disorders. Crohn's disease. Sodium cromoglycate 800 mg daily by mouth produced dramatic improvement in one patient with Crohn's disease refractory to sulphasalazine, corticosteroids, and metronidazole.— A. Henderson and S. Hishon (letter), *Lancet*, 1978, *1*, 109. From a double-blind crossover study in 23 patients it was concluded that sodium cromoglycate 1.2 g daily given for 6 months in addition to their usual treatment, was of no benefit when compared with placebo in the treatment of Crohn's disease.— M. J. Grundman *et al.*, *Gut*, 1978, *19*, A963. Sodium cromoglycate 800 mg daily was of no benefit in a controlled study of 25 patients with Crohn's disease whose sulphasalazine treatment had been stopped.— V. Binder *et al.*, *Gut*, 1981, *22*, 55.

Food allergy. A review of studies on the use of sodium cromoglycate for the treatment of milk and other allergies, with a detailed study of the allergens involved for 14 children aged 2 to 15 years who were given by mouth sodium cromoglycate dissolved in 30 ml of warm water, 30 minutes before meals and at bedtime. A significant protective effect on the symptoms of gastro-intestinal food allergy was shown when sodium cromoglycate was administered for 2 days prior to antigen ingestion in children whose diarrhoea had been controlled by a restricted diet. It has not proved effective when given to symptomatic children taking antigen at the time therapy was initiated.— S. Kocoshis and J. D. Gryboski, *J. Am. med. Ass.*, 1979, *242*, 1169. Criticism.— D. J. Salberg (letter), *ibid.*, 1980, *244*, 546. Reply.— S. A. Kocoshis (letter), *ibid.*

Sodium cromoglycate by mouth in a dose of 800 mg daily for a week or as a single 1-g dose before challenge, failed to protect 9 patients from their allergy to a range of substances including port wine, Bacardi, tartrazine, coconut, chocolate, aspirin, bran, and apricots. However in 4 patients with rapid asthmatic reactions, sodium cromoglycate 40 mg by inhalation gave almost immediate protection against coconut, port, tartrazine, and Bacardi, respectively.— M. G. Harries *et al.*, *Clin. Allergy*, 1978, *8*, 423. See also under Asthma (above).

In a placebo-controlled double-blind crossover study 14 of 20 subjects with food allergies obtained relief while taking sodium cromoglycate (in doses of 50 or100 mg in about 50 ml of warm water swilled around the mouth and swallowed half-an-hour before the 3 main meals and before bedtime). Four of the 14 patients, however, developed an adverse reaction to sodium cromoglycate (headaches in 2, insomnia in 1, and urticaria in 1). A further 3 of an initial 24 selected for the study also developed adverse reactions (headaches in 2 and rhinorrhoea in 1). This high figure of 7 adverse reactions in 24 subjects suggested that individuals with food allergies might be prone to adverse reactions to sodium cromoglycate.— G. A. Vaz *et al.*, *Lancet*, 1978, *1*, 1066. Comment.— R. J. T. Jarvis (letter), *ibid.*, 1978, *2*, 271. Reply.— J. W. Gerrard (letter), *ibid.*

In a double-blind controlled study 8 of 20 patients who had suffered from persistent diarrhoea for periods ranging from 3 to 30 years noted significant improvement while taking sodium cromoglycate 800 mg daily. The results suggested that food allergy may be a contributory factor in diarrhoea of unknown aetiology.— T. D. Bolin, *Gut*, 1980, *21*, 848.

Dietary elimination and subsequent challenge demonstrated evidence of food allergy in 23 of 33 migrainous subjects. Ten of the allergic patients were pretreated with oral sodium cromoglycate before a challenge. One of these had complete protection when taking sodium cromoglycate 400 mg daily for 7 days before challenge, 8 had partial or complete protection when taking 0.8 or 1.6 g, and one seemed to have no protection.— J. Monro *et al.*, *Lancet*, 1980, *2*, 1.

Further references to the use of sodium cromoglycate in food allergy: S. Freier and H. Berger, *Lancet*, 1973, *1*, 913 (intolerance to milk protein in infants; 50 mg given 4 times daily); J. Dolovich *et al.*, *Can. med. Ass. J.*, 1974, *111*, 684; P. J. Kingsley (letter), *Lancet*, 1974, *2*, 1011; J. A. Kuzemko and K. R. Simpson (letter), *Lancet*, 1975, *1*, 337; C. André *et al.* (letter), *Lancet*, 1976, *1*, 964 (20 mg before food in protein intolerance); R. M. Nizami *et al.*, *Ann. Allergy*, 1977, *39*, 102; R. Dahl, *Allergy*, 1978, *33*, 120; R. Dahl and O. Zetterström, *Clin. Allergy*, 1978, *8*, 419; J. Brostoff *et al.*, *Lancet*, 1979, *1*, 1268 (a dose of 500 mg before challenge); R. Paganelli *et al.*, *ibid.*, 1270; J. Simeon *et al.*, *Ann. Allergy*, 1979, *42*, 343 (use in hyperactive children); J. B. G. Watson and J. Timmins, *Archs Dis. Childh.*, 1979, *54*, 77.

Proctitis. A report of beneficial results in 8 patients with long-standing isolated ulcerative proctitis ('allergic proctitis': a condition which could be separated on clinical criteria—intermittent, benign course, limitation of inflammatory extent—and on immunopathological findings) when they were given sodium cromoglycate 200 mg four times daily. Doses were administered by dissolving the contents of a capsule in warm water and were taken before meals and at bedtime. All patients were receiving sulphasalazine and 3 had topical corticosteroid treatment.— P. C. M. Rosekrans *et al.*, *Gut*, 1980, *21*, 1017.

Further references: R. V. Heatley *et al.*, *Gut*, 1975, *16*, 559 (beneficial effect of sodium cromoglycate given by mouth and retention enema in chronically active proctitis).

See also under Ulcerative Colitis (below).

Ulcerative colitis. Discussions on ulcerative colitis in which sulphasalazine and corticosteroids are the mainstay of treatment. Earlier promising results with sodium cromoglycate given by mouth and by retention enema have not yet been substantiated.— *lancet*, 1978, *1*, 1190; *Drug & Ther. Bull.*, 1979, *17*, 10.

In a double-blind crossover study 12 patients with ulcerative colitis in remission or with very slight symptoms were treated for 6-month periods with sodium cromoglycate 200 mg twice daily for 2 weeks, 400 mg twice daily for 2 weeks, then 500 mg four times daily, or with placebo. The patients' sense of well-being and the sigmoidoscopic and biopsy appearances were significantly improved on sodium cromoglycate. Nausea, bitter taste, and a generalised erythematous rash, each in 1 patient, were transient. Elevation of serum-aminotransferase values in 2 patients was probably not drug-related.— V. Mani *et al.*, *Lancet*, 1976, *1*, 439.

Another report of sodium cromoglycate given by mouth having a beneficial effect in ulcerative colitis.— G. D. Cella *et al.* (letter), *Lancet*, 1976, *1*, 1129.

In a 6-month study of maintenance therapy for ulcerative colitis started by 120 patients and completed by 107, sodium cromoglycate 200 mg four times daily before meals, was greatly inferior to sulphasalazine 500 mg four times daily after meals; the 2 drugs given concomitantly in the same doses had no advantage over sulphasalazine alone. Of 37 patients in the sodium cromoglycate group 20 suffered relapses whereas only 9 of 37 in the sulphasalazine group did so; 10 of 33 in the combined-therapy group suffered relapses. Of 6 patients withdrawn because of side-effects associated with administration of sodium cromoglycate, one had severe diarrhoea, one had a rash, and 4 in the combined-therapy group suffered nausea and a bloated feeling that they had not experienced with sulphasalazine alone.— C. P. Willoughby *et al.*, *Lancet*, 1979, *1*, 119.

Further reports indicating that sodium cromoglycate taken by mouth is of no benefit in the management of ulcerative colitis: N. A. Buckell *et al.*, *Gut*, 1978, *19*, 1140; M. W. Dronfield and M. J. S. Langman, *Gut*, 1978, *19*, 1136; S. R. Gould *et al.*, *Gut*, 1978, *19*, A444; C. P. Willoughby *et al.*, *Gut*, 1978, *19*, A963; V. Binder *et al.*, *Gut*, 1981, *22*, 55.

See also under Proctitis (above).

Hay fever. See under Rhinitis, below.

Mastocytosis. In a double-blind crossover study involving 5 patients, sodium cromoglycate by mouth relieved the symptoms of systemic mastocytosis in the skin, gastro-intestinal tract, and central nervous system. Four patients took several courses of sodium cromoglycate 100 mg four times daily or placebo; courses lasted from one to 10 months. One other patient only received placebo. Of the 4 who received a total of 18 courses of sodium cromoglycate, marked improvement was seen in 3 but patients relapsed within 2 to 3 weeks of stopping treatment. Histaminuria and eosinophilia persisted despite a beneficial clinical response.— N. A. Soter *et al.*, *New Engl. J. Med.*, 1979, *301*, 465. A controlled double-blind study is needed to compare the effects of cimetidine with those of sodium cromoglycate in patients with systemic mastocytosis.— J. C. O'Laughlin and J. E. Bredfeldt (letter), *ibid.*, 1980, *302*, 231. Further comment on the relative merits of treatment with H_1 and H_2 antihistamines and with sodium cromoglycate.— K. F. Austen *et al.* (letter), *ibid.*

Ocular disorders. A brief discussion indicating that sodium cromoglycate 2% eye-drops are of value in the treatment of vernal keratoconjunctivitis and often reduce the need for corticosteroid eye-drops. They may also be of value in the treatment of marginal corneal ulcers.— *Drug & Ther. Bull.*, 1977, *15*, 25.

In a double-blind study of 22 patients with vernal catarrh, sodium cromoglycate eye-drops improved the condition of the treated eyes. A long term study of up to 2 years in 61 patients showed that keratoconjunctivitis could be controlled without topical steroids in 11 patients, and with only short periods of steroid therapy in 44 patients. Irritation, especially during exacerbation of the vernal disease, was noted in 35% of patients and was possibly due to thiomersal used as a preservative.— D. Easty *et al.*, *Trans. ophthal. Soc. U.K.*, 1971, *91*, 491.

Sodium cromoglycate eye-drops 1% were more effective than oxyphenbutazone eye ointment 10% in the treatment of marginal corneal ulcers but slightly less effective than prednisolone eye-drops.— J. I. McGill *et al.*, *Trans. ophthal. Soc. U.K.*, 1971, *91*, 501.

Eye drops containing sodium cromoglycate 2% were effective in the majority of 35 patients with recurrent allergic conjunctivitis when assessed after 1 week of treatment. Adverse effects included transient stinging on application; one patient discontinued treatment after the eyes became red and inflamed and another discontinued when the eyelids became swollen.—A Multicentre General Practitioner Study, *Practitioner*, 1979, *222*, 854.

Further reports of beneficial results with sodium cromoglycate in vernal keratoconjunctivitis.— J. Greenbaum *et al.*, *J. Allergy & clin. Immunol.*, 1977, *59*, 437 (4% solution); K. F. Tabbara and N. T. Arafat, *Archs Ophthal., N.Y.*, 1977, *95*, 2184 (children); M. El Hennawi, *Br. J. Ophthal.*, 1980, *64*, 483.

Pregnancy and the neonate. The view that sodium cromoglycate may be used during pregnancy.— M. de Swiet, *Prescribers' J.*, 1979, *19*, 59.

Renal disorders. In a 12½-year-old boy with the nephrotic syndrome remission was induced with prednisolone, but relapses occurred with the onset of the hay-fever season. Three years later a further relapse was treated with prednisolone, and sodium cromoglycate 10 mg by insufflation to each nostril 4 times daily and 40 mg by mouth with meals was given for 6 months for hay fever; hay fever recurred 3 months later and was controlled with a single intramuscular injection of methylprednisolone 20 mg. He has remained symptom-free of both the nephrotic syndrome and hay fever for 2 years without further treatment. A further 21 children with the nephrotic syndrome who responded to prednisolone were given either sodium cromoglycate 10 mg by insufflation to each nostril and 20 mg by mouth with food, or a lactose placebo for 16 weeks; prednisolone was gradually reduced, and discontinued after 8 weeks. After 16 weeks, 9 of 11 children given sodium cromoglycate had relapsed compared with 5 of 10 given placebo; the median week of relapse was 7 for sodium cromoglycate, and 15 for placebo.— R. S. Trompeter *et al.*, *Archs Dis. Childh.*, 1978, *53*, 430.

For reference to sodium cromoglycate preventing the development of glomerulonephritis in some *rabbits*, see J. Egido *et al.*, *Proc. Eur. Dialysis Transplant Ass.*, 1977, *14*, 581.

Rhinitis. A discussion on the management of patients with hay fever. For those needing treatment the choice lies between sodium cromoglycate and a topical corticosteroid, with systemic corticosteroid therapy as a last resort. Sodium cromoglycate prevents the development of symptoms in the eyes and nose when used regularly (except when exposure to pollen is not anticipated) and is available as a powder or solution for intranasal use and as eye-drops.— *Drug & Ther. Bull.*, 1979, *17*, 45.

Reports of the intranasal use of sodium cromoglycate in seasonal rhinitis (hay fever) and perennial rhinitis: J. Sunderman and W. A. Crawford, *Med. J. Aust.*, 1973, *1*, 1189 (perennial allergic rhinitis); D. J. Brain *et al.*, *J. Lar. Otol.*, 1974, *88*, 1001 (perennial rhinitis); B. T. B. Manners, *Br. J. clin. Pract.*, 1975, *29*, 153 (nasal powder or solution equally effective in hay fever); R. H. Cohan *et al.*, *J. Allergy & clin. Immunol.*, 1976, *58*, 121 (perennial allergic rhinitis); S. Craig *et al.*, *Clin. Allergy*, 1977, *7*, 569 (lack of effect in ragweed hay fever); P. W. Welsh *et al.*, *J. Allergy & clin. Immunol.*, 1977, *60*, 104 (benefit in ragweed hay fever).

Skin disorders. Allergic *urticarial* wheals, occurring in a woman during the high pollen season, responded to the topical application of the contents of insufflation capsules of sodium cromoglycate.— G. Silverman (letter), *Br. med. J.*, 1973, *3*, 502.

Pruritus in 2 patients with Hodgkin's disease was relieved by the application of sodium cromoglycate 5% in soft paraffin or propylene glycol.— A. Leven *et al.* (letter), *Br. med. J.*, 1977, *2*, 896.

In a double-blind study in 42 children with atopic *eczema* twice-daily application for 12 weeks of an ointment containing sodium cromoglycate 10% in white soft paraffin was considered more effective than a placebo (the ointment basis) in respect of inflammation, lichenification, cracking, sleep, and itching.— S. A. Haider, *Br. med. J.*, 1977, *1*, 1570. In a double-blind study in 11 patients with moderate or severe eczema the patients were to apply sodium cromoglycate 10% ointment or placebo to opposite sides of the body. Five patients failed to complete the study because of pruritus or acute flare of eczema on both sides; in the 6 who completed the study there was no significant benefit from the active treatment.— T. Thirumoorthy and M. W. Greaves (letter), *ibid.*, 1978, *2*, 500.

Treatment with sodium cromoglycate 1 g daily dissolved in water and taken in divided doses before food enabled 4 of 15 patients with *dermatitis herpetiformis* to discontinue treatment with dapsone for 9 months without relapse.— E. L. Rhodes, *Br. J. Derm.*, 1978, *99*, 581.

Further references to the use of sodium cromoglycate: P. Lip (letter), *Med. J. Aust.*, 1978, *2*, 32 (chronic leg ulcers; powder from capsules emptied into the ulcers); K. M. De Cock and M. G. Thorne, *Br. J. Derm.*, 1980, *102*, 231 (pyoderma gangrenosum).

Ulcer, aphthous. Aphthous ulcers cleared in 2 patients when given sodium cromoglycate 2.5% in a toothpaste which they used thrice daily.— M. Frost (letter), *Lancet*, 1973, *2*, 389. A toothpaste containing sodium cromoglycate 5% abolished "bad taste" without obvious origin in 3 patients although 1 relapsed when treatment was stopped.— *idem* (letter), *Br. dent. J.*, 1976, *140*, 332. The presence of a soap was needed to allow adequate oral absorption of sodium cromoglycate. The majority of patients with aphthous stomatitis who had failed to respond to the use of a toothpaste containing sodium cromoglycate responded when they used a soap mouth-wash before treatment.— *idem*, 1978, *144*, 269.

Patients had more ulcer-free days while taking sodium cromoglycate 20 mg as lozenges 4 times daily than with placebo in a double-blind crossover study over a 12-week period involving 21 patients with aphthous ulcers, but this only reached significance in the group who received placebo first. There was no significant difference between placebo and sodium cromoglycate for relief of pain. Two patients experienced a tight feeling in the chest and developed a rash on the chest while taking sodium cromoglycate.— M. J. Kowolik *et al.*, *Br. dent. J.*, 1978, *144*, 384.

Further references: D. M. Walker and A. E. Dolby (letter), *Lancet*, 1975, *1*, 1390.

Preparations

Cromoglycate Eye Drops *(A.P.F.)*. Sodium cromoglycate 2 g, sodium chloride 700 mg, benzalkonium chloride solution 0.02 ml, disodium edetate 50 mg, Water for Injections to 100 ml. Sterilised by filtration. These eye-drops should be freshly prepared.

Cromolyn Sodium for Inhalation *(U.S.P.)*. Hard gelatin capsules containing a mixture of equal parts of sodium cromoglycate and lactose. Store at a temperature not exceeding 40° in airtight containers. Protect from light.

Sodium Cromoglycate Insufflation *(B.P.)*. Sodium Cromoglycate Cartridges; Sodium Cromoglycate Inhalation. Hard gelatin capsules containing 20 to 24.4 mg of sodium cromoglycate, of specified particle size, mixed with an approximately equal amount of lactose. Store at a temperature not exceeding 30° in airtight containers. The capsules are intended to be used in an inhaler.

Proprietary Preparations

Intal *(Fisons, UK)*. Spincaps (cartridges) each containing sodium cromoglycate 20 mg for administration by inhalation by means of a specially designed inhaler (Spinhaler). **Intal Compound.** Spincaps each containing, in addition, isoprenaline sulphate 100 µg in an inert basis. **Intal Inhaler.** A pressurised spray for inhalation, providing sodium cromoglycate 1 mg in each metered dose. **Intal Nebuliser Solution.** Contains sodium cromoglycate 10 mg per ml, in ampoules of 2 ml. (Also available as Intal in *Arg., Austral., Canad., Ger., Jap., Spain, Switz., USA*).

Lomusol Nasal Spray *(Fisons, UK)*. An aqueous solution for inhalation containing sodium cromoglycate 2%, delivering approximately 2.6 mg in each metered dose. (Also available as Lomusol in *Belg., Fr., Neth.*).

Nalcrom *(Fisons, UK)*. Sodium cromoglycate, available as capsules of 100 mg for oral administration. (Also available as Nalcrom in *NZ*).

Opticrom Eye Drops *(Fisons, UK)*. Contain sodium cromoglycate 2%, with benzalkonium chloride 0.01%. (Also available as Opticrom in *Austral., Canad., Ger., NZ, Switz.*).

Rynacrom *(Fisons, UK)*. Cartridges each containing sodium cromoglycate 10 mg and lactose 10 mg for intranasal administration by means of a specially designed nasal insufflator. **Rynacrom Nasal Drops**. Contain sodium cromoglycate 2% in aqueous solution. **Rynacrom Nasal Spray**. An aqueous solution containing sodium cromoglycate 2%. (Also available as Rynacrom in *Austral., Belg., Neth., S.Afr.*).

Other Proprietary Names

Alercrom *(Arg.)*; Colimune *(Ger.)*; Cromo-Asma *(Spain)*; Frenal *(Ital.)*; Lomudal *(Belg., Denm., Fr., Ital., Neth., Norw., S.Afr., Swed., Switz.)*; Lomupren *(Ger.)*; Nasmil, Nebulasma *(both Spain)*; Opticron *(Fr.)*.

7722-l

Bufrolin Sodium. ICI 74917. Disodium 6-butyl-1,4,7,10-tetrahydro-4,10-dioxo-1,7-phenanthroline-2,8-dicarboxylate.

$C_{18}H_{14}N_2Na_2O_6$=400.3.

CAS — 54867-56-0 (bufrolin); 54545-84-5 (disodium salt).

Bufrolin sodium has anti-allergic properties resembling those of sodium cromoglycate (p.1445). It is poorly absorbed from the gastro-intestinal tract and has been administered in asthma in a dose of 1 mg by aerosol inhalation 4 times daily.

A pharmacokinetic study in asthmatic patients of bufrolin sodium administered by aerosol inhalation.— M. E. Pickup *et al.*, *Br. J. clin. Pharmac.*, 1977, *4*, 357.

Bufrolin sodium was no more effective than sodium cromoglycate in a controlled study of 32 asthmatic patients.— J. Moxham and M. McAllen, *Clin. Allergy*, 1979, *9*, 61.

Further references to bufrolin sodium: D. P. Evans *et al.* (letter), *Nature*, 1974, *250*, 592; D. P. Evans and D. S. Thomson, *Br. J. Pharmac.*, 1974, *53*, 409 (pharmacology in *animals*); N. Mygind and J. Thomsen, *Acta allerg.*, 1975, *30*, 298 (in allergic rhinitis; 500 µg into each nostril); J. S. Vilsvik and A. O. Jenssen, *Clin. Allergy*, 1976, *6*, 487 (in allergic rhinitis).

Manufacturers
ICI Pharmaceuticals, UK.

7723-y

Doxantrazole. 3-(1*H*-Tetrazol-5-yl)thioxanthen-9-one 10,10-dioxide.

$C_{14}H_8N_4O_3S$=312.3.

CAS — 51762-95-9.

Crystals. M.p. 260° to 262° with decomposition.

Uses. Doxantrazole has an anti-allergic action similar to that of sodium cromoglycate (p.1445) and, unlike sodium cromoglycate, is absorbed from the gastro-intestinal tract. It has been given by mouth in a usual dose of 200 mg thrice daily to patients with asthma but earlier encouraging results were not substantiated by more recent clinical studies. The hydrated sodium salt has also been investigated.

The anti-allergic effect of doxantrazole and doxantrazole sodium.— J. F. Batchelor *et al.*, *Wellcome Research*, *Lancet*, 1975, *1*, 1169; S. P. Haydu *et al.*, *Br. med. J.*, 1975, *3*, 283; Y. W. Cho *et al.*, *Clin. Pharmac. Ther.*, 1976, *19*, 104; C. B. B. Phillips and M. W. Greaves, *Br. J. Derm.*, 1977, *97*, *Suppl.* 15, 17; C. B. Bentley-Phillips *et al.*, *J. invest. Derm.*, 1978, *71*, 266 (cold urticaria).

A pharmacokinetic study of doxantrazole.— H. Jones and A. Bye, *J. Pharm. Pharmac.*, 1979, *31*, 730.

In a double-blind study in 14 patients with asthma, doxantrazole 200 mg thrice daily was of no significant value.— H. R. Gribbin *et al.*, *Br. med. J.*, 1979, *1*, 92. Further reports of the ineffectiveness of doxantrazole: R. Pauwels *et al.*, *Acta allerg.*, 1976, *31*, 239; *idem*, 471 (allergen-induced bronchospasm); N. H. Bluett *et al.* (letter), *Lancet*, 1977, *1*, 809 (nephrotic syndrome); H. Poppius and B. Stenius, *Eur. J. clin. Pharmac.*, 1977, *11*, 107 (exercise-induced asthma).

Manufacturers
Wellcome, UK.

7724-j

Ketotifen Fumarate. HC 20-511 *(ketotifen)*.

4-(1-Methyl-4-piperidylidene)-4*H*-benzo[4,5]-cyclohepta[1,2-*b*]thiophen-10(9*H*)-one hydrogen fumarate.

$C_{19}H_{19}NOS,C_4H_4O_4$=425.5.

CAS — 34580-13-7 (ketotifen); 34580-14-8 (fumarate).

Ketotifen fumarate 1.38 mg is approximately equivalent to 1 mg of ketotifen. Readily **soluble** in water.

Adverse Effects, Treatment, and Precautions. As for the antihistamines in general, p.1294.

Increased appetite and weight gain have been reported. A reversible fall in the platelet count has been observed in a few patients receiving ketotifen concomitantly with oral antidiabetic agents and it has been suggested that this combination should therefore be avoided.

For precautions to be observed in asthmatic patients, see sodium cromoglycate (p.1445).

Of 17 patients with asthma given ketotifen 1 mg twice daily, 11 suffered severe drowsiness necessitating withdrawal after one week; it was later withdrawn from 3 further patients for minor drowsiness. Two patients had episodes of sudden loss of balance.— K. Prowse (letter), *Br. med. J.*, 1980, *280*, 646. Drowsiness has been reported in 13.44% and dizziness in 1.77% of 7178 patients at 3-month follow-up; 245 patients (3.41%) had stopped treatment with ketotifen because of drowsiness.— W. P. Maclay, *Sandoz* (letter), *ibid.*, 1452.

Eight patients aged 6 to 34 years took overdoses of ketotifen in doses stated to range from 10 to 120 mg. Plasma concentrations of ketotifen base in 4 patients were 5 to 122 µg per ml (therapeutic range 1 to 4 µg per ml). Symptoms included drowsiness, confusion, dyspnoea, bradycardia or tachycardia, disorientation, and convulsions. Gastric lavage was performed in 6, and all recovered within 12 hours after supportive treatment.— D. B. Jefferys and G. N. Volans, *Br. med. J.*, 1981, *282*, 1755.

Absorption and Fate. Ketotifen fumarate is absorbed from the gastro-intestinal tract and, together with metabolites, is excreted in the urine and faeces.

Uses. Ketotifen has anti-allergic properties and has been used similarly to sodium cromoglycate (p.1445) in the prophylactic treatment of asthma. It also has the properties of an antihistamine (p.1295).

Ketotifen fumarate is taken by mouth in doses equivalent to 1 mg of ketotifen twice daily. If necessary the equivalent of 2 mg twice daily may be given.

Pharmacological studies of ketotifen in *animals*.— U. Martin and D. Römer, *Arzneimittel-Forsch.*, 1978, *28*, 770.

Asthma. A discussion of the actions and uses of ketotifen in asthma.— *Drug & Ther. Bull.*, 1980, *18*, 14.

Conference proceedings on ketotifen in the prophylaxis of bronchial asthma.— *Respiration*, 1980, *39*, *Suppl.* 1 1–46.

References to studies of ketotifen in asthma, some with conflicting results: J. P. Girard and M. Cuevas, *Acta allerg.*, 1977, *32*, 27; L. Craps *et al.*, *Clin. Allergy*, 1978, *8*, 373; P. Göbel, *J. int. med. Res.*, 1978, *6*, 79; R. Pauwels *et al.*, *Clin. Allergy*, 1978, *8*, 289; A. S. Weheba, *Pharmatherapeutica*, 1978, *2*, 85; B. Wüthrich and P. Radielovic, *Dt. med. Wschr.*, 1978, *103*, 1865; B. Wuethrich *et al.*, *Int. J. clin. Pharmac. Biopharm.*, 1978, *16*, 424; H. M. Beumer, *Respiration*, 1979, *37*, 271; D. Crowder and C. De H. Greenwood, *Practitioner*, 1979, *223*, 398; P. Göbel, *Pharmatherapeutica*, 1979, *2*, 153; J. Labus and V. Hlinka, *J. int. med. Res.*, 1979, *7*, 305; A. S. Weheba, *Pharmatherapeutica*, 1979, *2*, 147; B. Wüthrich, *Respiration*, 1979, *37*, 224; A. J. Dyson and A. D. Mackay, *Br. med. J.*, 1980, *280*, 360; J. M. Sherriff (letter), *ibid.*, 862; S. G. Spiro (letter), *ibid.*; A. M. Edwards (letter), *ibid.*, 1188; S. G. Spiro (letter), *ibid.*; R. Schubotz (letter), *ibid.*, 1378; J. D. Kennedy *et al.*, *ibid.*, *281*, 1458; E. Cameron (letter), *ibid.*, 1981, *282*, 147; V. Graff-Lonnevig and E. Kusoffsky, *Allergy*, 1980, *35*, 341; A. Szczeklik *et al.*, *Allergy*, 1980, *35*, 421; A. R. Tanser and J. Elmes, *Br. J. Dis. Chest*, 1980, *74*, 398; R. C. Groggins *et al.*, *Archs Dis. Childh.*, 1981, *56*, 304.

Skin disorders. References to the use of ketotifen in urticaria: K. Kuokkanen, *Acta allerg.*, 1975, *30*, 73; *idem*, 1977, *32*, 316.

Proprietary Preparations

Zaditen *(Wander, UK)*. Ketotifen fumarate, available as **Capsules** and as scored **Tablets** each containing the equivalent of ketotifen 1 mg and as **Elixir** containing in each 5 ml the equivalent of ketotifen 1 mg (recommended diluent, syrup containing hydroxybenzoate preservative). (Also available as Zaditen in *Belg.*, *Ger.*, *Lux.*, *Neth.*, *Switz.*).

7725-z

Xanoxate Sodium. Sodium Xanoxate; RS 6818; RS 7540 *(acid)*. Sodium 7-(1-methylethoxy)-9-oxo-9*H*-xanthene-2-carboxylate.

$C_{17}H_{13}NaO_5$=320.3.

CAS — 33459-27-7 (xanoxic acid); 41147-04-0 (sodium salt).

Xanoxate sodium has anti-allergic properties similar to those of sodium cromoglycate (p.1445) and in preliminary studies has been given by inhalation or by mouth in the prophylactic treatment of asthma.

References to the use of xanoxate sodium: B. Stenius *et al.*, *Scand. J. resp. Dis.*, 1978, *59*, 75 (xanoxic acid by inhalation in exercise-induced asthma).

Manufacturers

Syntex, USA.

Solvents

6500-y

The solvents described in this section are those generally without specific therapeutic uses. Also used as solvents in pharmacy and described in other sections are alcohols (p.35), benzyl benzoate (p.833), carbon tetrachloride (p.89), chloroform (p.745), fixed oils (p.694), glycerol, glycols, and macrogols (pp.706-7), paraffins (p.709), trichloroethylene (p.1063), and water (p.760).
In the UK some of the solvents described in this section are listed as prescribed dangerous substances under the Packaging and Labelling of Dangerous Substances Regulations 1978 (SI 1978: No. 209) as amended (SI 1981: No. 792).
The Solvents in Food Regulations 1967 (SI 1967: No. 1582) as amended and The Solvents in Food (Scotland) Regulations 1968 [SI 1968: No. 263 (S.23)] as amended specify the solvents that may be used in food in England and Wales and in Scotland. See also *Report on the Review of Solvents in Food*, FAC/REP/25, Ministry of Agriculture, Fisheries and Food, London, HM Stationery Office, 1978.

CAUTION. In Great Britain it is recommended that scalp lotions or shampoos containing 50% or more of alcohol or containing a more inflammable solvent should carry the following warning: 'CAUTION. *This preparation is highly flammable. Do not use it, or dry the hair, near a fire or open flame.*' Other inflammable preparations which are sold or dispensed should also carry the label: *'Highly flammable'*.

A review of problems caused by solvent impurities; and the choice of solvents for pharmaceutical analysis.— J. E. Fairbrother, *Pharm. J.*, 1979, *1*, 536.

Abuse. The inhalation of volatile solvents may lead to dependence of the volatile solvent type (Nineteenth Report of WHO Expert Committee on Drug Dependence, *Tech. Rep. Ser. Wld Hlth Org. No. 526*, 1973) and reports of the abuse of solvents may be found under Benzene (p.1451), Cyclohexane (p.1452), Kerosene (p.1454), Light Petroleum (p.1454), Toluene (p.1455), and Trichloroethane (p.1456). See also under Aerosol Propellents (p.1057).

Sudden death after sniffing solvents: a review of 110 cases.— M. Bass, *J. Am. med. Ass.*, 1970, *212*, 2075.

A report of 25 cases of clinically severe toxic polyneuropathy in young people addicted to sniffing methyl ethyl ketone-containing solvents. The peripheral motor defects took 2½ to 3 years to regress and in severe cases there were additional spastic signs. The effects were considered due to a disorder of axonal transmission which destroyed peripheral and central axons.— H. Altenkirch, *Dt. med. Wschr.*, 1979, *104*, 935.

Nephrotoxicity. References to Goodpasture's syndrome and glomerulonephritis associated with solvent abuse or exposure will be found under Trichloroethane, p.1456.

Neurotoxicity. A report of peripheral neuropathy, the primary neurological finding being segmental demyelination, in a 16-year-old boy after spray-painting his motorcycle several times in a small unventilated room. The spray paint contained acetone, dichloromethane(methylene chloride), 4-methyl-2-pentanone (methyl isobutyl ketone), 2-butanone (methyl ethyl ketone), toluene, several aliphatic acetates, and butanol.— J. AuBuchon *et al.* (letter), *Lancet*, 1979, *2*, 363. Doubt as to whether the exposure was sufficient to produce the neuropathy.— F. H. Tyrer (letter), *ibid.*, 424. The neurotoxicity may have arisen from the synergistic effects of the ketone solvents and toluene.— R. H. Goldman (letter), *ibid.*, 744. See also J. AuBuchon *et al.* (letter), *ibid.*, 1012.

See also under Abuse.

Pregnancy and the neonate. A report of an increased incidence of CNS defects in children born to mothers exposed to organic solvents during pregnancy.— P. C. Holmberg (preliminary communication), *Lancet*, 1979, *2*, 177. Criticism of the matching of exposed women and their controls. Further epidemiological evidence is needed to confirm the findings.— K. Sheikh (letter), *Lancet*, 1979, *2*, 963.

For a report of congenital abnormalities in a baby whose mother had abused solvents, see under Toluene, p.1455.

6501-j

Acetone *(B.P., U.S.P.)*. Dimethyl Ketone; 2-Propanone; Cetona.
$CH_3.CO.CH_3$=58.08.

CAS — 67-64-1.

Pharmacopoeias. In *Arg., Aust., Br., Fr., Hung., Mex., Nord., Span., Swiss,* and *U.S.*

A clear, colourless, volatile, mobile, inflammable liquid with a characteristic odour and a pungent sweetish taste. Wt per ml 0.789 to 0.791 g. B.p. about 56°. Flash-point −17° (closed-cup test). **Miscible** with water, alcohol, chloroform, ether, and most essential oils. A 50% solution in water is neutral to litmus. **Store** in a cool place in airtight containers. Protect from light.

Adverse Effects. Acetone is absorbed through the lungs and to a minor extent through the skin. Inhalation of acetone vapour causes headache, restlessness, and fatigue, leading to narcosis and unconsciousness at high concentrations. Vomiting and haematemesis may occur, and there is often a latent period of several hours. The vapour is irritant to the eyes and nose in high concentrations. Severe acute poisoning has occurred following percutaneous absorption.
Acetone is one of the solvents abused in 'glue-sniffing'.
Maximum permissible atmospheric concentration 1000 ppm.

A 42-year-old depressed man drank 200 ml of acetone and was in a coma for 12 hours. He recovered, but mild hyperglycaemia occurred during the following 4 months, and renal glycosuria was noted after 5 months.— S. Gitelson *et al.*, *Diabetes*, 1966, *15*, 810, per *J. Am. med. Ass.*, 1967, *199* (Jan. 2), 129.

Acute acetone intoxication involving 8 workers.— D. S. Ross, *Ann. occup. Hyg.*, 1973, *16*, 73.

Abuse. For reports and discussions of solvent abuse, see Solvents, p.1450.

Treatment of Adverse Effects. Remove patient to fresh air and if necessary assist respiration. Wash contaminated sites. Gastric lavage or emesis may be required. Other treatment should be symptomatic and supportive.

Absorption and Fate. Acetone is absorbed through the lungs and skin. It is mostly excreted unchanged through the lungs and in the urine. Small amounts may be oxidised to carbon dioxide or utilised in body metabolism as acetate and formate.

Uses. A ready solvent of fats, resins, and many other organic substances. It may be used in solutions for film coating tablets. It should not be used as a solvent for iodine, as the fumes formed are irritant to the eyes. On account of its low boiling point it is a suitable menstruum for extracting thermolabile substances from crude drugs. It is an ingredient of some skin preparations.

Use in food. The Food Additives and Contaminants Committee recommended that acetone be permitted for use as a solvent in food and recommended a maximum concentration of mesityl oxide in the acetone of 10 ppm.— *Report on the Review of Solvents in Food*, FAC/REP/25, Ministry of Agriculture, Fisheries and Food, London, HM Stationery Office, 1978.

6502-z

Acetonitrile. Ethanenitrile; Methyl Cyanide.
$CH_3.CN$=41.05.

CAS — 75-05-8.

A colourless liquid with an aromatic odour. Wt. per ml about 0.78 g. B.p. about 81°. Flash-point 5.6° (open-cup test), 12.8° (closed-cup test).
Freely **miscible** with water, alcohol, acetone, chloroform, carbon tetrachloride, and ethyl acetate.
Acetonitrile emits highly toxic fumes of hydrogen cyanide when heated to decomposition or when reacted with acids or oxidising agents.

Adverse Effects and Treatment. As for Stronger Hydrocyanic Acid, p.790.
Maximum permissible atmospheric concentration 40 ppm.

Absorption and Fate. See under Stronger Hydrocyanic Acid, p.790.

Uses. Acetonitrile is used as a pharmaceutical solvent.

6503-c

Amyl Acetate. A mixture of isomers, principally *iso-*, *sec-*, and *n*-amyl acetate. Amyl acetate used in pharmacy consists mainly of isoamyl acetate (3-methylbutyl acetate), perhaps with a small amount of the *sec*-isomer (2-methylbutyl acetate).
$C_7H_{14}O_2$=130.2.

CAS — 123-92-2 (iso-amyl acetate); 53496-15-4 (sec-amyl acetate); 628-63-7 (n-amyl acetate).

A colourless liquid with a sharp, fruity odour. Wt per ml about 0.87 g. B.p. about 140°. Slightly **soluble** in water; miscible with alcohol and ether.

Adverse Effects. Prolonged exposure may produce headache, fatigue, dyspnoea, depression of the central nervous system and evidence of liver or kidney damage.
Maximum permissible atmospheric concentration 100 ppm (*iso-* or *n*-amyl acetate) and 125 ppm (*sec*-amyl acetate).

Effect on cardiovascular system. Heart failure in a 27-year-old man was considered due to the use of 'methyl-cellulose' paint in an unventilated room; the solvent consisted of isomers of amyl acetate.— P. L. Weissberg and I. D. Green, *Br. med. J.*, 1979, *2*, 1113.

Uses. Amyl acetate is used as an industrial solvent.

6504-k

Aniline *(B.P.C. 1934)*. Phenylamine.
$C_6H_5.NH_2$=93.13.

CAS — 62-53-3.

A colourless or pale yellow oily liquid with a characteristic odour and an aromatic burning taste, readily darkening to brown on exposure to air and light. Wt per ml about 1.02 g. B.p. about 183°. **Soluble** 1 in 30 of water; miscible with alcohol, benzene, chloroform, ether, and oils. **Store** in airtight containers. Protect from light.

Adverse Effects. Inhalation, ingestion, or cutaneous absorption results in methaemoglobinaemia, with headache, weakness, cyanosis, stupor, and coma. Skin sensitisation, liver and kidney damage and cardiac arrhythmias may occur. Haemolysis has been reported on prolonged exposure to aniline.
Bladder papillomas have been reported in workers previously exposed to aniline. Commercial aniline may be contaminated with β-naphthylamine, a potential carcinogen.
Maximum permissible atmospheric concentration 2 ppm.

Treatment of Adverse Effects. Empty the stomach by aspiration and lavage. Wash contaminated sites. Give oxygen, with assisted respiration if necessary. Treat methaemoglobinaemia with 1 to 4 mg of methylene blue per kg body-weight intravenously as a 1% solution. Blood transfusions or exchange transfusions may be necessary in severe cases. Haemodialysis has been used to remove aniline from the circulation.

Uses. Aniline has wide industrial applications.

6505-a

Benzene *(B.P.C. 1954)*. Phenyl hydride.
C_6H_6=78.11.

CAS — 71-43-2.

NOTE. Benzene may be known as 'benzina', 'benzol', 'benzole', or 'benzolum'. However, 'benzol' is also used to describe a mixture of hydrocarbons and 'benzine' is used as a name for a commercial form of petroleum spirit.

Pharmacopoeias. In *Aust., Hung., Jug., Port.,* and *Span.*

A hydrocarbon obtained by fractional distillation of light oil of tar. It is a clear colourless inflammable liquid with a characteristic aromatic odour, which burns with a luminous smoky flame. Wt per ml 0.874 to 0.879 g. Solidifies when cooled to 0°. B.p. 79.5° to 80.5°. Flash-point about −11° (closed-cup test).

Practically **insoluble** in water; miscible with dehydrated alcohol, acetone, ether, glacial acetic acid, light petroleum, and oils. **Store** in airtight containers.

Adverse Effects. The poisonous effects of benzene are produced chiefly by inhalation of the vapour, though the risk of absorption through the skin should not be ignored. Benzene poisoning is an important industrial hazard.

Symptoms of acute poisoning following ingestion or inhalation include headache, nausea, dizziness, and irritation of mucous membranes. Large amounts cause tremors, vertigo, and CNS depression which progresses to coma and respiratory failure. Unconsciousness is frequently preceded by restlessness, excitement, or delirium. Ventricular arrhythmias may occur. Liver and kidney damage have been reported.

Chronic exposure to low concentrations of benzene vapour can have adverse effects on the gastro-intestinal tract, the central nervous system, and the bone marrow. Marrow hyperplasia with leucocytosis may precede hypoplastic changes which result in leucopenia, thrombocytopenia, and aplastic anaemia. Leukemia has also developed in exposed subjects. The early symptoms of intoxication include headache, dizziness, irritability, nausea, anorexia, pallor, and petechiae. There may be a long latent period before serious toxicity becomes evident.

Maximum permissible atmospheric concentration 10 ppm.

It was considered that the toxic effects such as aplastic anaemia attributed to benzene were due to benzene epoxide formed temporarily during the metabolism of benzene to phenol and its metabolites; administration of phenol did not induce blood disorders.— R. C. Garner, *Prog. Drug Metab.*, 1976, *1*, 77.

Reports and reviews of the effects of occupational exposure to benzene.— T. J. Haley, *Clin. Toxicol.*, 1977, *11*, 531; H. S. Cohen *et al.*, *Am. J. med. Sci.*, 1978, *275*, 124; M. G. Ott *et al.*, *Archs environ. Hlth*, 1978, *33*, 3.

Abuse. Of 110 sudden deaths associated with the sniffing of solvents in USA between 1962 and 1969, 7 were related to the use of benzene.— M. Bass, *J. Am. med. Ass.*, 1970, *212*, 2075.

For further reports and discussions of solvent abuse, see Solvents, p.1450.

Carcinogenicity. *Leukaemia.* Leukaemia in benzene workers: a study of workers exposed during 1940 to 1949.— P. F. Infante *et al.*, *Lancet*, 1977, *2*, 76. See also I. R. Tabershaw and S. H. Lamm (letter), *ibid.*, 867; P. F. Infante *et al.* (letter), *ibid.*, 868.

Further references to leukaemia associated with benzene.— M. Aksoy *et al.*, *Am. J. Med.*, 1972, *52*, 160; M. Aksoy *et al.*, *Blood*, 1974, *44*, 837; M. Aksoy and S. Erdem, *Blood*, 1978, *52*, 285; M. Aksoy (letter), *Lancet*, 1978, *1*, 441; P. F. Infante, *Tex. Rep. Biol. Med.*, 1978, *37*, 153.

Lymphoma. A report on a significant excess of deaths caused by the lymphomas in men employed in occupations involving exposure to benzene. While the possible importance of other aromatic hydrocarbons could not be excluded, this solvent was the only known chemical used by all of the occupational groups studied.— N. J. Vianna and A. Polan, *Lancet*, 1979, *1*, 1394. Calculation of proportionate mortality ratios may show that the excess in mortality from lymphomas disappears. The excess may simply be an artefact.— P. E. Enterline (letter), *ibid.*, *2*, 1021. Preliminary results from another study failed to confirm an association between lymphoma and exposure to benzene.— P. R. Smith and J. N. Lickiss (letter), *ibid.*, 1980, *1*, 719.

Treatment of Adverse Effects. If benzene is swallowed, empty the stomach by aspiration and lavage, taking care to avoid inhalation of the washings. If benzene is inhaled, remove the patient to the fresh air, and assist respiration if necessary. If eyes and skin are affected, wash thoroughly with water.

Intensive supportive therapy including repeated blood transfusions may be necessary.

Absorption and Fate. Benzene is absorbed by inhalation, ingestion, and to some extent through the skin. Some is excreted unchanged from the lungs; the remainder is either oxidised to phenol and related quinol compounds and excreted in the urine as conjugates of sulphuric or glucuronic acid, or retained in the body.

Uses. Benzene was formerly applied as a pediculicide. Its use as an industrial solvent is decreasing.

Benzene is not suitable for use as a food additive.— Twenty-third Report of Joint FAO/WHO Expert Committee on Food Additives, *Tech. Rep. Ser. Wld Hlth Org. No. 648*, 1980.

6506-t

Carbon Disulphide *(B.P.C. 1934, B. Vet. C. 1965).*

Carbonei Disulphidum; Carbon Bisulphide; Carboneum Bisulfuratum; Carbonei Sulfidum; Carboneum Sulfuratum; Schwefelkohlenstoff.

CS_2=76.13.

CAS — 75-15-0.

Pharmacopoeias. In *Aust., Nord., Pol.,* and *Span.*

A clear colourless to pale straw-coloured, volatile, highly inflammable liquid with a characteristic odour. Wt per ml about 1.264 g. B.p. 46° to 47°. Flash-point about −30° (closed-cup test).

Soluble, at 20°, in 500 parts of water; miscible with alcohol, chloroform, ether, and fixed and volatile oils. It dissolves phosphorus, sulphur, and rubber.

Store in well-filled airtight containers in a cool place. Protect from light.

The vapour mixed with air in the proportions of 1 to 50% is explosive, and can be ignited even by hot steam pipes.

Adverse Effects. Absorption takes place through the lungs and the intact skin, and the poison is cumulative. Chronic poisoning produces disturbances of peripheral nerve function and of vision. These effects are followed by a wide range of neuropsychiatric effects including emotional disorders, psychoses, and parkinsonism. There may also be effects on the kidneys and the gastro-intestinal tract. An association between exposure to carbon disulphide and coronary heart disease has been reported.

Acute poisoning may occur from ingestion or inhalation, with symptoms progressing from irritation of mucous membranes, nausea, gastro-intestinal disturbances, and headache to unconsciousness and respiratory paralysis.

Maximum permissible atmospheric concentration 10 ppm.

A report of the third international symposium on the toxicity of carbon disulphide.— J. Lieben, *Archs environ. Hlth*, 1974, *29*, 173, per *Pharm. J.*, 1975, *1*, 485.

For toxicological data, see 1971 Evaluations of some Pesticide Residues in Food, *Pestic. Residue Ser. Wld Hlth Org. No. 1*, 1972.

Health risks of carbon disulphide and measures for avoiding them.— Carbon Disulphide, *Environmental Health Criteria No. 10*, Geneva, UN/WHO, 1978.

A brief discussion of the hazards of carbon disulphide.— *Lancet*, 1980, *2*, 1347.

Effects on the adrenals. Some workers exposed to carbon disulphide had impaired adrenal, testicular, and thyroid function.— S. Maugeri *et al.*, *Medna Lav.*, 1971, *62*, 398, per *Abstr. Hyg.*, 1972, *47*, 880.

There was adrenal insufficiency in 50 of 79 patients with chronic carbon disulphide poisoning.— I. Lancranjan, *Medna Lav.*, 1973, *64*, 375, per *Abstr. Hyg.*, 1974, *49*, 1074.

Effects on blood sugar. A study showing decreased glucose tolerance in workers exposed to carbon disulphide compared with control subjects.— G. Franco *et al.* (letter), *Lancet*, 1978, *2*, 1208. See also V. Kujalová *et al.* (letter), *Lancet*, 1979, *1*, 664.

Effects on cardiovascular system. Between 1933 and 1962, an increased incidence of mortality from coronary heart disease was apparent in male workers employed in the viscose rayon industry who had suffered long-term exposure to low concentrations of carbon disulphide.— J. R. Tiller *et al.*, *Br. med. J.*, 1968, *4*, 407. Comment.— *ibid.*, 405.

Two groups, each of 343 men, were studied; one group consisted of men who had been occupationally exposed to carbon disulphide for at least 5 of the last 25 years; the others had had no such exposure. The respective incidence of various events during a 5-year follow-up was: deaths from coronary heart disease, 14 and 3; non-fatal first myocardial infarctions, 11 and 4; a history of angina, 25 and 13%; prevalence of typical angina, 12 and 5%. Causes of death other than coronary heart disease were evenly distributed between the groups.— M. Tolonen *et al.*, *Br. J. ind. Med.*, 1975, *32*, 1. After a further 3-year follow-up, at the start of which the exposure of workers to carbon disulphide was reduced and the atmospheric concentration lowered to 10 ppm, there was evidence of reduced mortality from heart disease amongst workers at risk.— M. Nurminen, *Int. J. Epidemiol.*, 1976, *5*, 179.

Further references: M. Tolonen *et al.*, *Int. Archs occup. environ. Hlth*, 1976, *37*, 249; P. G. Vertin, *J. occup. Med.*, 1978, *20*, 346.

Effects on the central nervous system. An epidemiological study of suicide-rates among nearly 5000 workers in a single viscose rayon plant exposed in varying degrees to carbon disulphide; an increased suicide-rate was observed. The onset of effects of carbon disulphide may be delayed.— T. F. Mancuso and B. Z. Locke, *J. occup. Med.*, 1972, *14*, 595.

Effects on the eye. A 5-year follow-up study of retinopathy in workers exposed to carbon disulphide indicated that the condition does not progress in those with a previous exposure of 10 years or less and in whom exposure has ceased, but may continue to progress in those who were exposed for a longer period.— K. Sugimoto *et al.*, *Int. Archs occup. environ. Hlth*, 1976, *37*, 233.

Effects on the thyroid and pituitary. Thyroid function was reduced in workers after chronic and short exposure to carbon disulphide. This effect seemed to be due to a direct toxic effect on the pituitary or hypothalamus.— A. Cavalleri *et al.*, *Medna Lav.*, 1971, *62*, 412. Serum-thyroxine concentrations were reduced in 45 workers exposed to carbon disulphide; measurement of these concentrations might be a reliable test for the early diagnosis of poisoning.— A. Cavalleri, *Archs environ. Hlth*, 1975, *30*, 85, per *J. Am. med. Ass.*, 1975, *231*, 528.

Treatment of Adverse Effects. Remove the patient from exposure and, if necessary assist respiration. Recovery may take many months.

Absorption and Fate. Carbon disulphide is rapidly absorbed when inhaled and is also absorbed through intact skin. It is partially metabolised in the body.

Uses. Carbon disulphide is used as an industrial solvent and is sometimes used, in the vapour form, as a disinfectant, insecticide, or veterinary parasiticide.

6507-x

Cyclohexane. Hexahydrobenzene; Hexamethylene.

C_6H_{12}=84.2.

CAS — 110-82-7.

A colourless liquid. Wt per ml about 0.78 g. B.p. about 81°.

Adverse Effects. Cyclohexane may irritate mucous membranes, and may also have central nervous system effects.

Maximum permissible atmospheric concentration 300 ppm.

Neurotoxicity has been associated with the straight-chain hydrocarbon *n-hexane*, and the mechanism of this effect may be identical to that of *methyl n-butyl ketone* (see Methyl Isobutyl Ketone, p.1455).

Neurotoxicity. An experimental study on the neurotoxicity of *n-hexane* metabolites.— L. Perbellini *et al.*, *Toxic. appl. Pharmac.*, 1978, *46*, 421.

Reports of peripheral neuropathy associated with *n-hexane*.— G. Abbritti *et al.*, *Br. J. ind. Med.*, 1976, *33*, 92; G. W. Paulson and G. W. Waylonis, *Archs intern. Med.*, 1976, *136*, 880; N. Rizzuto *et al.*, *J. Neurol. Scis*, 1977, *31*, 343 (industrial exposure); R. Korobin *et al.*, *Archs Neurol., Chicago*, 1975, *32*, 158; J. Towfighi *et al.*, *Neurology, Minneap.*, 1976, *26*, 238 (abuse). See also *Lancet*, 1979, *2*, 942.

Uses. Cyclohexane is used as an industrial solvent.

6508-r

Diethyl Phthalate *(B.P.C. 1973)*. Ethyl Phthalate. The diethyl ester of benzene-1,2-dicarboxylic acid.

$C_{12}H_{14}O_4$=222.2.

CAS — 84-66-2.

A clear, colourless or nearly colourless, somewhat viscous liquid with a slight odour and an acrid taste. Wt per ml about 1.117 g. B.p. about 295°. Flash-point about 117° (closed-cup test). Practically **insoluble** in water; miscible with alcohol, ether, and aromatic hydrocarbons.

Adverse Effects. Diethyl phthalate vapour is irritant to mucous membranes and, in high concentration, causes CNS depression.

Maximum permissible atmospheric concentration 5 mg per m^3.

Phthalate esters: the question of safety.— W. H. Lawrence, *Clin. Toxicol.*, 1978, *13*, 89.

The use of esters of phthalic acid as plasticisers for polythene containers might present a hazard to patients receiving blood transfusions over prolonged periods.— A. Macdonald, *J. Hosp. Pharm.*, 1974, *32*, 70.

Uses. Diethyl phthalate is used as a denaturant of alcohol, e.g. in surgical spirit, and as a solvent and plasticiser.

6509-f

Dimethyl Sulphoxide *(B.P.)*. Dimexide; Dimethyl Sulfoxide; DMSO; Methyl Sulphoxide; SQ 9453.

C_2H_6OS=78.13.

CAS — 67-68-5.

Pharmacopoeias. In *Br.*

A colourless hygroscopic viscous liquid with a slightly bitter taste; odourless or with a slight odour of dimethyl sulphide. F.p. not lower than 18.3°; b.p. 189° to 192°. Wt per ml 1.099 to 1.101 g.

Miscible with water with the evolution of heat, and with alcohol, acetone, chloroform, ether, and most organic solvents; immiscible with paraffin hydrocarbons. A 2.16% solution in water is iso-osmotic with serum. **Store** in airtight containers out of contact with plastics. Protect from light.

Carbomer 0.4% neutralised with sodium hydroxide solution was a suitable gelling agent for dimethyl sulphoxide.— Pharm. Soc. Lab. Rep. P/70/4, 1970.

Haemolysis. Dimethyl sulphoxide reduced the haemolysis of erythrocytes by phenol *in vitro*, though in high concentrations it was itself haemolytic.— H. C. Ansel and W. F. Leake, *J. pharm. Sci.*, 1966, *55*, 685.

Complete haemolysis of erythrocytes took place in aqueous dimethyl sulphoxide solutions, though the addition of 0.9% sodium chloride or iso-osmotic concentrations of other compounds prevented haemolysis in solutions containing up to 40% of dimethyl sulphoxide.— D. E. Cadwallader and J. P. Drinkard, *J. pharm. Sci.*, 1967, *56*, 583.

Dimethyl sulphoxide decreased the haemolysis of *rabbit* erythrocytes *in vitro* by preservatives, irrespective of type. The decrease was greatest at a concentration of 10 to 20% of dimethyl sulphoxide but with increasing concentration of preservative and increasing time of exposure the protective effect was reduced.— H. C. Ansel and G. E. Cabre, *J. pharm. Sci.*, 1970, *59*, 478.

Percutaneous absorption. Dimethyl sulphoxide increased the absorption of hydrocortisone and testosterone through the skin compared with an acetone basis.— H. I. Maibach and R. J. Feldmann, *Ann. N.Y. Acad. Sci.*, 1967, *141*, 423.

Percutaneous absorption of salicylic acid from hydrophilic ointment *U.S.P.* and hydrophilic petrolatum *U.S.P.* was enhanced by the addition of 15% dimethyl sulphoxide, but the absorption of sodium salicylate from hydrophilic ointment was diminished. Dimethyl sulphoxide had little effect on the release of salicylic acid or its sodium salt from macrogol ointment.— J. M. Stelzer *et al.*, *J. pharm. Sci.*, 1968, *57*, 1732.

Dimethyl sulphoxide facilitated the absorption of a polar steroid, hydrocortisone sodium succinate, through the skin in *rats*. Absorption of a lipid-soluble steroid, cortisone acetate, was not increased.— M. B. Cramer and L. A. Cates, *J. pharm. Sci.*, 1974, *63*, 793.

Adverse Effects. High concentrations applied to the skin may cause burning discomfort, itching, erythema, and occasionally vesiculation—effects resulting from marked vasodilatation. Continued use may result in maceration, scaling, and dermatitis. Nausea, vomiting, abdominal cramps, chest pain, chills, drowsiness, and hypersensitivity reactions have been reported following topical use. Administration of dimethyl sulphoxide by any route is followed by a garlic-like odour in the breath.

When given by mouth, by injection, or topically, dimethyl sulphoxide has caused lens changes in some *animals*. It has teratogenic effects in some *animals*.

When used as a penetrating basis for other drugs, dimethyl sulphoxide may enhance their toxic effects—see Precautions.

Human toxicology of dimethyl sulphoxide.— R. D. Brobyn, *Ann. N.Y. Acad. Sci.*, 1975, *243*, 497.

Dimethyl sulphoxide was capable of activating a latent virus infection within cells and could lead to the expression of differentiated functions that had been repressed by a virus or were the result of the incorporation of the viral genome. These findings were particularly apparent when dimethyl sulphoxide was present with idoxuridine or cytarabine.— R. E. Handschumacher, *Clin. Pharmac. Ther.*, 1974, *16*, 865.

In 5 healthy subjects patch tests were negative with 5% idoxuridine in white soft paraffin or 10% dimethyl sulphoxide in 0.9% sodium chloride, but were positive with undiluted dimethyl sulphoxide or with 5% idoxuridine in dimethyl sulphoxide. There was no excessive pruritus and positive reactions resolved within 24 hours of removing the patch. The tests were considered to show that dimethyl sulphoxide is a primary irritant.— R. Dawber, *Br. med. J.*, 1974, *2*, 526.

Skin irritation (as measured by changes in electrical impedance) in healthy subjects exposed to dimethyl sulphoxide increased with increasing concentrations. However, there was some evidence that repeated exposure results in adaptation and a lessening irritant effect.— K. E. Malten and J. den Arend, *Contact Dermatitis*, 1978, *4*, 80.

Effects on the eyes. Lenticular changes in *animals*.— L. F. Rubin and R. A. Mattis, *Science*, 1966, *153*, 83, per *J. Am. med. Ass.*, 1966, *197* (Aug. 15), A215; K. C. Barnett and P. R. B. Noel (letter), *Nature*, 1967, *214*, 1115. Reported adverse effects of dimethyl sulphoxide on the eye had occurred only when using doses far in excess of those likely to be used clinically.— A. D. S. Caldwell *et al.*, *Schering Chemicals* (letter), *Nature*, 1967, *215*, 1168.

A review of the literature relating to about 9800 patients who had been treated with dimethyl sulphoxide, cutaneously, or by application to the eye in concentrations of 7.5 to 66%, failed to show any evidence of lens toxicity or refractive changes due to medication with dimethyl sulphoxide.— D. M. Gordon and K. E. Kleberger, *Archs Ophthal., N.Y.*, 1968, *79*, 423. See also D. M. Gordon, *Ann. N.Y. Acad. Sci.*, 1967, *141*, 392.

Nephrotoxicity. Dimethyl sulphoxide administered by intravenous infusion to 14 patients caused haemolysis and haemoglobinuria. Infusion strengths above 10% were associated with grossly discoloured urine, but there was no evidence of significant kidney damage.— J. M. Barry and W. M. Bennett, *Clin. Pharmac. Ther.*, 1980, *27*, 273; R. S. Muther and W. M. Bennett, *J. Am. med. Ass.*, 1980, *244*, 2081.

An elderly married couple both developed changes in aspartate transaminase, hydroxybutyrate dehydrogenase, and creatine kinase, and evidence of haemolysis after receiving dimethyl sulphoxide intravenously for painful arthritic knees. The husband never became seriously ill, but the wife developed acute renal tubular necrosis, deterioration in her level of consciousness and evidence of cerebral infarction. Efforts to remove dimethyl sulphoxide failed, which was not considered surprising since it has been shown that dimethyl sulphoxide is strongly bound to plasma proteins and that clearance by haemodialysis or peritoneal dialysis is poor. It is considered that intravenous dimethyl sulphoxide is potentially dangerous and should not be used for the treatment of arthritis.— P. Yellowlees *et al.*, *Lancet*, 1980, *2*, 1004. Such side-effects have not been observed in 14 patients with amyloidosis treated with dimethyl sulphoxide both by mouth and intravenously, some for over a year. It is suggested that the effects seen may have been due to enhancement of the effects of the prochlorperazine given to both patients, and possibly the quinine given to the wife.— M. H. van Rijswijk (letter), *ibid.*, 1981, *1*, 41. Further criticisms: L. J. Knott, *Kendall Arthritis Clinic* (letter), *ibid.*, 1299; J. P. Griffin, *DHSS* (letter), *ibid.*, 1981, *1*, 41; J. C. de la Torre (letter), *ibid.*, 157. Reply, including the view that the adverse reaction was not due to enhancement of any drug action.— C. Greenfield (letter), *ibid.*, 276. A severe reaction after the infusion of dimethyl sulphoxide with cryopreserved bone marrow, but without signs of renal impairment. Reservations about the intravenous infusion of dimethyl sulphoxide merit further attention.— J. R. O'Donnell *et al.* (letter), *ibid.*, 498.

Precautions. When used as a penetrating basis for other drugs applied topically, dimethyl sulphoxide may enhance their toxic effects. High concentrations should not be applied to the eyes and should be applied with care around the eyes.

It is suggested that it should not be used during pregnancy.

Experience with dimethyl sulphoxide given by mouth and intravenously for amyloidosis, has indicated that simultaneous treatment with anticoagulants, digoxin, non-steroidal anti-inflammatory drugs, corticosteroids, and cytostatics does not appear to provide special problems. A 39-year-old woman with renal failure did, however, react with severe hypotension to the administration of carbachol and a 28-year-old man acquired a transient paralytic ileus after the administration of hyoscine butylbromide.— M. H. van Rijswijk (letter), *Lancet*, 1981, *1*, 41.

Absorption and Fate. Dimethyl sulphoxide is readily absorbed by injection, by mouth, and through the skin.

Some of the dimethyl sulphoxide is excreted unchanged in the urine and some is oxidised to dimethyl sulphone, which is more slowly excreted in the urine. The malodorous compound excreted through the lungs and producing a garlic halitosis may be methyl disulphide, methyl sulphinic acid, or allicin.

Absorption, metabolism, and fate of dimethyl sulphoxide in man. Peak serum concentrations are reached 4 hours after administration by mouth and 4 to 8 hours after topical application.— H. B. Hucker *et al.*, *J. Pharmac. exp. Ther.*, 1967, *155*, 309. After intravenous injection the elimination half-life is 4 days. After 18 days nearly all urinary excretion is complete.— K. H. Kolb *et al.*, *Ann. N.Y. Acad. Sci.*, 1967, *141*, 85.

Uses. Dimethyl sulphoxide is a highly polar substance which has exceptional solvent properties for both organic and inorganic chemicals, and is widely used as an industrial solvent.

Its reported actions include membrane penetration, anti-inflammatory effects, local analgesia, weak bacteriostasis, diuresis, vasodilatation, and dissolution of collagen.

The principal therapeutic use of dimethyl sulphoxide is as a vehicle for drugs such as idoxuridine (see p.820); it aids penetration of the drug into the skin, and so may enhance the drug's effect. It is also used to protect living cells during cold storage.

Dimethyl sulphoxide has been investigated for the treatment of renal amyloidosis, and, usually as a 50% aqueous solution for instillation, for interstitial cystitis. It has also been tried clinically for a wide range of indications including cutaneous and musculoskeletal disorders, but with little evidence of beneficial effects.

The use of dimethyl sulphoxide in cosmetic products is prohibited in the UK by the Cosmetic

Products Regulations 1978 (SI 1978: No. 1354). It is also used in veterinary medicine.

Reviews and discussions on the uses and adverse effects of dimethyl sulphoxide: *Med. Lett.*, 1980, *22*, 94; M. J. Finkel, *J. Am. med. Ass.*, 1980, *244*, 2767.

The effect of dimethyl sulphoxide on the water-binding properties of stratum corneum.— A. K. Dhall and A. B. Selkirk, *Pharm. Acta Helv.*, 1978, *53*, 172.

Failure of dimethyl sulphoxide (apart from some analgesic effect) in 24 patients with scleroderma.— S. A. Binnick *et al.*, *Archs Derm.*, 1977, *113*, 1398.

A method for estimating the whealing response of skin using dimethyl sulphoxide.— P. J. Frosch *et al.*, *Br. J. Derm.*, 1980, *103*, 263.

Amyloidosis. Following administration of dimethyl sulphoxide for more than a year, improvement in renal function and general condition was obtained in 2 patients with renal amyloidosis secondary to rheumatoid arthritis.— M. H. van Rijswijk *et al.* (letter), *Lancet*, 1979, *1*, 207.

A view that the beneficial effect of dimethyl sulphoxide on amyloidosis may be related, at least in part, to its ability to scavenge hydroxyl radicals.— D. Harman (letter), *Lancet*, 1980, *2*, 593.

Further references: *Lancet*, 1980, *1*, 1062; G. G. Glenner, *New Engl. J. Med.*, 1980, *302*, 1333.

Cerebral oedema. Elevated intracranial pressure, unresponsive to treatment with barbiturates and diuretics, was reduced to normal in 7 patients after intravenous infusion of dimethyl sulphoxide 1 g per kg body-weight. The previously refractory pressure was easily controlled by further infusions of dimethyl sulphoxide.— F. T. Waller *et al.*, *Neurosurgery*, 1979, *5*, 383.

Cryoprotection. A review of recent advances in cryobiology including the use of dimethyl sulphoxide as a cryoprotectant.— D. E. Pegg, *Practitioner*, 1978, *221*, 543.

Dimethyl sulphoxide 5% was used as a cyroprotective agent in the preparation of frozen blood platelets for subsequent transfusion in patients with leukaemia. There were no side-effects from the transfusion of small residual amounts of dimethyl sulphoxide.— C. A. Schiffer *et al.*, *New Engl. J. Med.*, 1978, *299*, 7.

Further references: P. O'Neill *et al.*, *Br. J. Ophthal.*, 1967, *51*, 13 (corneal tissue); M. O. Symes *et al.*, *Lancet*, 1968, *1*, 1052 (spleen cells).

Cystitis. A review of the use of dimethyl sulphoxide in a 50% aqueous solution for bladder instillation in the treatment of chronic interstitial cystitis concluded that it should be reserved for patients with severe symptoms who had not responded to other treatment.— *Med. Lett.*, 1978, *20*, 76.

Proprietary Names

Deltan *(Pol.; Schweiz. Serum & Impfinstitut, Switz.)*; Demsodrox *(Nezel, Spain)*; Dermialgida *(Andromaco, Spain)*; Dipirartril Topico *(Pons, Spain)*; Dromisol *(Pol.)*; Kemsol *(Horner, Canad.)*; Rimso-50 *(Research Industries Corp., USA)*.

6510-z

Dimethylacetamide. Acetyldimethylamine; DMAC. *NN*-Dimethylacetamide.
C_4H_9NO=87.12.

CAS — 127-19-5.

A colourless liquid. B.p. about 165°. Wt per ml about 0.94 g. **Miscible** with water and most organic solvents.

Adverse Effects. As for Dimethylformamide (p.1453); it may be less toxic than dimethylformamide.
Maximum permissible atmospheric concentration 10 ppm.

Uses. Dimethylacetamide is used as a solubilising agent and as a solvent in pharmaceutical products.

Cryoprotection. The use of dimethylacetamide as an alternative to dimethyl sulphoxide in protecting frozen cells.— *J. Am. med. Ass.*, 1966, *197* (Sept. 12), A36.

6511-c

Dimethylformamide. DMF. *NN*-Dimethylformamide. C_3H_7NO=73.09.

CAS — 68-12-2.

A clear colourless liquid. B.p. about 153°. Wt per ml about 0.95 g. **Soluble** in water and alcohol; miscible with most common organic solvents.

Adverse Effects. Dimethylformamide may cause ocular irritation or damage. A variety of central effects have been reported including weakness, incoordination, and hallucinations. Kidney and liver damage may occur. Loss of appetite and digestive disturbances have been reported in exposed industrial workers.
Maximum permissible atmospheric concentration 10 ppm.

Reports of disulfiram-like effects after alcohol consumption in workers exposed to dimethylformamide.— C. P. Chivers (letter), *Lancet*, 1978, *1*, 331; W. H. Lyle *et al.*, *Br. J. ind. Med.*, 1979, *36*, 63. Investigations in *rats* indicated that metabolic-acetaldehyde accumulation might be a factor in reports of intolerance to alcoholic beverages experienced by subjects following exposure to dimethylformamide; its metabolite methylformamide had similar effects.— G. K. Hanasono *et al.*, *Toxic. appl. Pharmac.*, 1977, *39*, 461.

Absorption and Fate.

The metabolism and excretion of inhaled dimethylformamide.— G. Kimmerle and A. Eben, *Int. Arch. Arbeitsmed.*, 1975, *34*, 127, per *Abstr. Hyg.*, 1975, *50*, 349.

Uses. Dimethylformamide has been used as a solvent for various drugs.

6512-k

Dioxan. Dioxane; Diethylene dioxide. 1,4-Dioxane. $C_4H_8O_2$=88.11.

CAS — 123-91-1.

NOTE. Do not confuse dioxan and dioxin (see p.1759).

A colourless hygroscopic inflammable liquid with an ethereal odour. B.p. about 101° to 103°. Wt per ml about 1.03 g. Flash-point 12° (closed-cup test). **Miscible** with water, alcohol, and ether.

CAUTION. *It is dangerous to distil or evaporate dioxan unless precautions have been taken to remove explosive peroxides.*

Adverse Effects. The vapour is irritant to the nose and eyes and high concentrations may cause nausea and vomiting. Central nervous system effects include headache, dizziness, and drowsiness. On repeated exposure, severe liver and kidney damage, including necrotic changes, can occur and may be fatal.
Maximum permissible atmospheric concentration 50 ppm.

Uses. Dioxan is a chemical reagent and industrial solvent.

6513-a

Solvent Ether *(B.P.)*. Solv. Ether; Aether Solvens; Ethyl Oxide; Ether; Diethyl Ether; Aether Aethylicus; Aether Sulphuricus; Eter.
$(C_2H_5)_2O$=74.12.

CAS — 60-29-7.

NOTE. Solvent ether is not intended for anaesthesia; only ether of a suitable quality (see p.748) should be so used.

Pharmacopoeias. An ether of similar quality is included in *Arg., Aust., Belg., Br., Cz., Hung., Ind., Jap., Jug., Mex., Nord., Pol., Port., Roum., Rus., Span., Swiss,* and *Turk. U.S.* has a monograph on Ether, with special storage requirements if for anaesthetic use.

Solvent ether is a colourless, transparent, very volatile, inflammable, very mobile liquid with a characteristic odour and a sweet burning taste. It volatilises very quickly and by so doing reduces temperature. Though ether is one of the lightest of liquids, its vapour is very heavy, being 2½ times heavier than air. Wt per ml 0.714 to 0.718 g. B.p. 34° to 36°. Flash-point about −29° (closed-cup test).
Soluble 1 in 10 of water; miscible with alcohol, chloroform, light petroleum, and fixed and volatile oils. **Store** in a cool place in airtight containers. If the containers are closed with corks these should be protected with metal foil. Protect from light.

Methylated ether for various technical purposes is prepared from industrial methylated spirit, or from duty-free alcohol with subsequent denaturation by the addition of wood naphtha. It has a wt per ml varying from 0.714 to 0.744 g. Methylated ether is unsuitable for both anaesthetic purposes and oral administration.

A British Standard Specification for a technical grade of ether (BS 579: 1957) is published by the British Standards Institution.

CAUTION. *Ether is very volatile and inflammable and mixtures of its vapour with oxygen, nitrous oxide, or air at certain concentrations are explosive. It should not be used in the presence of an open flame or any electrical apparatus liable to produce a spark; precautions should be taken against the production of static electrical discharge. Explosive peroxides are generated by the atmospheric oxidation of solvent ether and it is dangerous to distil a sample which contains peroxides.*

Adverse Effects. As for Anaesthetic Ether, p.748. Ingestion of 30 to 60 ml may be fatal.
Maximum permissible atmospheric concentration 400 ppm.

Uses. Solvent ether is used as a menstruum for exhausting drugs and as a solvent for oils, resins, and other substances. It has been used for cleaning the skin before surgical operations and for removing adhesive plaster from the skin.

Solvent ether has been tried as a topical treatment for herpes simplex virus infections with inconsistent results.

References to the use of topical ether in herpes simplex.— A. B. Sabin, *J. Am. med. Ass.*, 1977, *238*, 63; H. D. Mintun (letter), *ibid.*, 1978, *239*, 831; M. Guinan, *ibid.*, 1978, *240*, 2232; L. Corey *et al.*, *New Engl. J. Med.*, 1978, *299*, 237; M. E. Guinan *et al.*, *J. Am. med. Ass.*, 1980, *243*, 1059.

Use in food. For the recommendation of the Food Additives and Contaminants Committee on the use of ether as a solvent in foods, see Anaesthetic Ether, p.748.

6514-t

Ethyl Acetate *(U.S.N.F., B.P.C. 1934)*. Aethylis Acetas; Aethylium Aceticum; Acetic Ether; Essigäther. $CH_3.CO.O.C_2H_5$=88.11.

CAS — 141-78-6.

Pharmacopoeias. In *Cz.* and *Jug.* Also in *U.S.N.F.*

A colourless inflammable liquid with a fragrant refreshing slightly acetous odour and an acetous, burning taste. Specific gravity 0.894 to 0.898. B.p. 76° to 77.5°. Flash-point −4° (closed-cup test). **Soluble** 1 in 15 of water; miscible with alcohol, chloroform, ether, and fixed and volatile oils. **Store** at a temperature not exceeding 40° in airtight containers.

Adverse Effects. Ethyl acetate is irritant to mucous membranes. High concentrations may cause depression of the central nervous system.
Maximum permissible atmospheric concentration 400 ppm.

Uses. Ethyl acetate has been used to flavour pharmaceutical preparations. It is largely employed in industry as a solvent.

Use in food. The Food Additives and Contaminants Committee recommended that ethyl acetate be temporarily permitted for use as a solvent in food and recommended a maximum concentration of use in food as consumed of 1000 ppm. Further toxicity studies were required.— *Report on the Review of Solvents in Food*, FAC/REP/25, Ministry of Agriculture, Fisheries and Food, London, HM Stationery Office, 1978.

6515-x

Ethylmethoxyethanol. 1-Ethyl-2-methoxy-1-ethanol. 1-Methoxybutan-2-ol.
$C_5H_{12}O_2$=104.1.

A clear colourless liquid with a characteristic odour. Wt per ml 0.885 g. B.p. 137° to 138°. **Miscible** with water, alcohol, castor oil, macrogol 400, and liquid paraffin.

Uses. Ethylmethoxyethanol is a solvent for drugs for parenteral or oral use.

Proprietary Names
Soluphor CE 5151 *(BASF, Ger.)*.

6516-r

Formamide.
CH_3NO=45.04.
CAS — 75-12-7.

A colourless, oily liquid. B.p. 210°. Wt per ml, about 1.13 g.

Adverse Effects. Formamide is reported to be irritant to skin and mucous membranes.
Maximum permissible atmospheric concentration 20 ppm.

Uses. Formamide is used as a pharmaceutical solvent.

6517-f

Kerosene. Kerosine; 'Paraffin'. A mixture of hydrocarbons, chiefly members of the methane series distilled from petroleum.
CAS — 8008-20-6.

It is a colourless or pale yellow mobile oily liquid with a characteristic odour. B.p. 175° to 325°. Wt per ml about 0.8 g. An odourless grade of kerosene is described in the *B. Vet. C.* 1965 (b.p. 220° to 270°; wt per ml about 0.78 g).
Practically **insoluble** in water; soluble 1 in 2.5 of alcohol; miscible with chloroform and ether.

Adverse Effects. Ingestion leads to gastro-intestinal disturbances, cough, and sometimes drowsiness. There may be depression of the central nervous system, with weakness, dizziness, slow and shallow respiration, incoordination, restlessness, convulsions and coma. Cardiac arrhythmias have been reported. The chief danger is pneumonitis and attendant pulmonary complications resulting from the aspiration of kerosene, even very small quantities, during or shortly after swallowing. Spontaneous or induced vomiting increases the risk of aspiration.
Euphoria may follow inhalation. The course of poisoning from inhalation is similar to that following ingestion.

The toxicity of kerosene depended on the proportion of naphthenic and aromatic hydrocarbons present and these varied according to the place of origin of the parent crude oil. Kerosene was marketed in Great Britain as: (1) tractor kerosene, or vaporising oil, which contained mixed aromatic naphthenes to approximately 23% w/w in the range C_{12} to C_{15}; (2) premium or household kerosene, which contained about 7% w/w of aromatics; and (3) regular grade, which was used as aviation turbine fuel and also domestically and had an aromatic content of 15 to 20% w/w.— *Br. med. J.*, 1963, *1*, 208.

Epidermal necrolysis developed in a 12-year-old boy after wearing kerosene-soaked clothing.— R. L. Barnes and D. S. Wilkinson, *Br. med. J.*, 1973, *4*, 466. See also A. Lyell, *Br. J. Derm.*, 1967, *79*, 662.

Abuse. Reports of patients who injected themselves intravenously with kerosene- or petroleum distillate-containing products.— D. O. Green, *Clin. Toxicol.*, 1977, *10*, 283; E. M. Neeld and M. C. Limacher, *Radiology*, 1978, *129*, 36.

For further reports and discussions of solvent abuse, see Solvents, p.1450.

Nephrotoxicity. Investigation of 28 patients with glomerulonephritis pointed to an association between this condition and prolonged exposure to hydrocarbons.— S. W. Zimmerman *et al.*, *Lancet*, 1975, *2*, 199.

See also under Trichloroethane, p.1456.

Treatment of Adverse Effects. Every precaution should be taken to avoid aspiration of kerosene into the lungs. Emetics must not be used in patients who are unconscious or convulsing, or who have lost the gag reflex.
A saline cathartic should be given, whether the stomach has been emptied or not, but the use of liquid paraffin before the cathartic is controversial. *Animal* work indicates that activated charcoal may be useful.

Co-operative Kerosene Poisoning Study, Report of the Subcommittee on Accidental Poisoning of the American Academy of Pediatrics, *Pediatrics*, 1962, *29*, 648.

The use of emetics or lavage for the removal of ingested petroleum distillates was controversial. They were used successfully by some experts, when not contra-indicated, but the numbers treated were still too small to prove their efficacy or safety. The type of hydrocarbon ingested and the presence of other ingredients such as camphor, polishes, insecticides, and chlorinated hydrocarbons confused the results.— V. A. Green and B. H. Rumack, Bull. Nat. Clearinghouse Poison Control Centers, May-June, 1976.

In a retrospective study of the treatment of children who had ingested a petroleum distillate it appeared that pneumonitis was less severe in patients who had been given an emetic compared with those given gastric lavage. It was considered that the stomach should be emptied when more than 30 ml of a petroleum distillate had been taken.— R. C. Ng *et al.*, *Can. med. Ass. J.*, 1974, *111*, 537. In a further prospective study of 77 children who had ingested various hydrocarbon-containing liquids it was concluded that vomiting induced in the alert patient in the upright position does not increase the risk of aspiration pneumonitis.— R. C. Ng, *Pediat. Ann.*, 1977, *6*, 708.

Further references: L. Goldfrank *et al.*, *Hosp. Physn*, 1979, *15*, 32.

Uses. Kerosene is used as a degreaser and cleaner and as an illuminating and fuel oil in kerosene ('paraffin') lamps and stoves. The odourless grade is used as a solvent in the preparation of some insecticide sprays.

6518-d

Light Petroleum. Benzin; Petroleum Benzin; Petroleum Ether; Petroleum Spirit; Solvent Hexane; Benzinum Medicinale; Wundbenzin.

Pharmacopoeias. In *Arg.*, *Aust.*, *Ger.*, *Jap.*, *Mex.*, *Nord.*, and *Pol.* Various boiling ranges are specified.
Swiss describes Aether Petrolei, consisting mainly of pentane and hexane, and Benzinum Medicinale, consisting mainly of hexane and heptane.

NOTE. The motor fuel termed 'petrol' in the UK and 'gasoline' in the USA is a mixture of volatile hydrocarbons of variable composition containing paraffins, olefins (alkenes), cycloparaffins, and aromatic compounds.

A purified distillate of petroleum, consisting of a mixture of the lower members of the paraffin series of hydrocarbons. It is a colourless, transparent, very volatile, highly inflammable liquid with a characteristic odour. Flash-point below −17°.
Practically **insoluble** in water; soluble in dehydrated alcohol; miscible with chloroform, ether, and most fixed and volatile oils. The vapour is explosive when mixed with air. **Store** in a cool place in airtight containers. Protect from light.
Light petroleum is available in a variety of boiling ranges, including the following, which are defined in Appendix IA of the *B.P.*: 30° to 40° (wt per ml about 0.63 g), 40° to 60° (wt per ml about 0.64 g), 60° to 80° (wt per ml about 0.67 g), 80° to 100° (wt per ml about 0.70 g), 100° to 120° (wt per ml about 0.72 g), 120° to 160° (wt per ml about 0.75 g).

Adverse Effects and Treatment. As for Kerosene, p.1454. Light petroleum and petrol, being more volatile than kerosene, are more likely to be inhaled and to cause aspiration pneumonitis. The toxicity of petrol varies with its composition.

Death within 1.5 hours followed ingestion of 100 ml and 20 ml of petrol by 2 children aged 1.5 and 2 years respectively. Postmortem examination showed lung haemorrhages, cerebral oedema, and hyperaemia of most internal organs.— I. Szabó, *Arch. Tox.*, 1967, *22*, 207, per *Pharm. J.*, 1968, *1*, 212.

After inhalation of petrol, symptoms varied from headache and dizziness to convulsions, coma, and death. Octane produced rapid narcosis; olefins and cycloparaffins had a greater effect and also produced vasodilatation, hypotension, and shock; olefins produced vagal stimulation leading to miosis, salivation, bradycardia, and urinary and gastro-intestinal spasm. Cycloparaffins, and to some extent olefins, caused cardiac arrhythmias. There was further risk from the lead content.— *Br. med. J.*, 1974, *2*, 115.

Pneumonitis in a 22-year-old man who sucked about half a cup of petrol into his mouth during a siphoning procedure.— T. H. Lee and W. M. Seymour (letter), *Lancet*, 1979, *2*, 149.

Abuse. A review of gasoline sniffing.— A. Poklis and C. Burkett, *Clin. Toxicol.*, 1977, *11*, 35.

A 14-year-old boy intermittently inhaled petrol vapour for 4 months and on 1 occasion was found breathless, flushed, frightened, and hallucinated. Dependence in 15 other cases was observed; such dependence could cause sudden unconsciousness and end in death due to liver and renal necrosis.— M. F. Bethell, *Br. med. J.*, 1965, *2*, 276.

A 15-year-old boy who had been inhaling petrol vapour intermittently for over 2½ years had schizophrenia-like symptoms with hallucinations, truculent behaviour, and abnormal emotional responses.— P. D. Black, *Med. J. Aust.*, 1967, *2*, 70.

The relationship between gasoline sniffing, cardiac arrhythmias, and sudden death.— M. Bass (letter), *New Engl. J. Med.*, 1978, *299*, 203.

Lead absorption from gasoline sniffing.— A. Kaufman and W. Wiese, *Clinica pediat.*, 1978, *17*, 475. See also F. J. Coodin and R. Boeckx (letter), *New Engl. J. Med.*, 1978, *298*, 347.

For further reports and discussions of solvent abuse, see Solvents, p.1450.

Carcinogenicity. Occupational exposure to petroleum products or to their combustion products was significantly higher (36%) in 50 men with acute non-lymphocytic leukaemia than in controls (10%).— L. Brandt *et al.*, *Br. med. J.*, 1978, *1*, 553. Exposure to petroleum products seems to be associated with normal chromosomes, in contrast to chemical solvents and insecticides.— F. Mitelman *et al.* (letter), *Lancet*, 1979, *2*, 1195.

Uses. Light petroleum is used as a solvent for fats.

Use in food. The Food Additives and Contaminants Committee recommended that light petroleum solvent be temporarily permitted for use as a solvent in food provided that the unsaturated aliphatic hydrocarbon content was not more than about 0.1% w/w. Further toxicity studies were required.— *Report on the Review of Solvents in Food*, FAC/REP/25, Ministry of Agriculture, Fisheries and Food, London, HM Stationery Office, 1978.

6519-n

Methyl Chloride. Chloromethane.
CH_3Cl=50.49.
CAS — 74-87-3.

A colourless gas compressed to a colourless liquid with an ethereal odour and a sweet taste. It burns with a greenish smoky flame. B.p. about −21° to −24°. Slightly **soluble** in water; soluble in alcohol; miscible with chloroform, ether, and glacial acetic acid.

Adverse Effects. Symptoms of methyl chloride intoxication often appear after a latent period of several hours and may include weakness, confusion, dizziness, drowsiness, visual disturbances, nausea, vomiting, abdominal pain, paraesthesia, mental changes, muscle dysfunction, pulmonary oedema, convulsions and coma. The liver and kidneys may be involved.
Maximum permissible atmospheric concentration 100 ppm.

Of a crew of 15 men of a fishing trawler who were exposed to methyl chloride vapour from a leaking refrigerator, 1 died and 2 of 3 men who became mentally depressed committed suicide. Personality changes occurred in 4 cases and there was a lowered tolerance to alcohol in 5 men. Disturbances of the alimentary tract, bone marrow, heart, kidneys, and liver were noted in 5 but these were slight with no after effects. Lasting complications found in the remainder affecting the central nervous system, included fatigue, profuse sweating, tremor on exertion, pain and loss of muscle and joint function, and psychoneurosis.— *Nord. Med.*, 1965, *73*, 150, per *Pharmacy Dig.*, 1965, *28*, 315.

Further reports of poisoning from methyl chloride.— T. L. Hartman, *New Engl. J. Med.*, 1955, *253*, 552; H. C. Scharnweber *et al.*, *J. occup. Med.*, 1974, *16*, 112; L. Spevak *et al.*, *Br. J. ind. Med.*, 1976, *33*, 272.

Uses. Methyl chloride is used as a refrigerant and solvent. It was formerly used as a local anaesthetic.

6520-k

Methyl Isobutyl Ketone *(U.S.N.F.).* Hexone. 4-Methylpentan-2-one.
$C_6H_{12}O$=100.2.

CAS — 108-10-1.

A transparent, colourless, mobile, volatile liquid with a faint ketonic and camphoraceous odour. Sp. gr. not more than 0.799. B.p. 114° to 117°. Slightly **soluble** in water; miscible with alcohol and ether. **Store** in airtight containers.

Adverse Effects. The adverse effects of methyl isobutyl ketone are relatively mild although it can depress the central nervous system in high concentrations. The vapour is irritating to mucous membranes. Percutaneous absorption may occur.
Maximum permissible atmospheric concentration 100 ppm.

Neurotoxicity. When methyl isobutyl ketone and methyl ethyl ketone were replaced by *methyl n-butyl ketone* in a fabrics plant, 86 of 1157 workers developed peripheral neuropathy.— D. Billmaier *et al.*, *J. occup. Med.*, 1974, *16*, 665; N. Allen *et al.*, *Archs Neurol., Chicago*, 1975, *32*, 209. See also *Lancet*, 1979, *2*, 942.

For reports and studies of the neurotoxicity of n-hexane, see under Cyclohexane, p.1452.

Uses. Methyl isobutyl ketone has been used as an alcohol denaturant.

6521-a

Methylene Chloride *(U.S.N.F.).* Dichloromethane.

CH_2Cl_2=84.93.

CAS — 75-09-2.

Pharmacopoeias. In *U.S.N.F.*

A clear, colourless, volatile liquid with a chloroform-like odour. Specific gravity 1.320 to 1.326. B.p. 39° to 41°. Its vapour is not explosive when mixed with air. **Soluble** 1 in 50 of water; miscible with alcohol and ether. **Store** in airtight containers.

Adverse Effects. Inhalation of methylene chloride vapour may cause headache and nausea; high concentrations depress the central nervous system. Pulmonary oedema may occur. Haemolysis has been reported. Reports of chronic intoxication appear to be few, but paraesthesia has been recorded. Blood concentrations of carboxyhaemoglobin may be raised as methylene chloride is metabolised to carbon monoxide.
The liquid is irritant to the skin and the vapour irritant to the eyes.
Maximum permissible atmospheric concentration 200 ppm.

Temporary estimated acceptable daily intake of methylene chloride: up to 500 µg per kg body-weight. Long-term oral studies were required in 2 rodent species.— Twenty-third Report of Joint FAO/WHO Expert Committee on Food Additives, *Tech. Rep. Ser. Wld Hlth Org. No. 648*, 1980.

Fatal exposure to methylene chloride vapour.— S. Moskowitz and H. Shapiro, *Archs ind. Hyg. occup. Med.*, 1952, *6*, 116.

A 38-year-old man recovered after ingesting between 1 and 2 pints of a paint remover containing methylene chloride, methyl alcohol, cellulose acetate, triethanolamine, hard paraffin, and detergent (Nitromors). Such an amount had been considered lethal and initially his condition was grave. The onset of recovery was, however, rapid and induction of diuresis was considered to have played a particularly important role in preventing acute renal damage. A late effect was the development of jejunal ulceration and diverticula.— C. J. C. Roberts and F. P. F. Marshall, *Br. med. J.*, 1976, *1*, 20.

Reports of experimental and accidental exposure to methylene chloride resulting in raised blood-carboxyhaemoglobin concentrations.— R. D. Stewart *et al.*, *Science*, 1972, *176*, 295; *idem*, *Archs environ. Hlth*, 1972, *25*, 342; C. L. Hake *et al.*, *Toxic. appl. Pharmac.*, 1975, *33*, 145; P. L. Langehennig *et al.* (letter), *New Engl. J. Med.*, 1976, *295*, 1137; R. D. Stewart and C. L. Hake, *J. Am. med. Ass.*, 1976, *235*, 398; M. F. Stevenson *et al.*, *Clin. Toxicol.*, 1978, *12*, 551.

Rash, mental impairment, oedema, and temporary diabetes mellitus after exposure to a paint stripper containing methylene chloride.— N. A. Memon and A. R. Davidson, *Br. med. J.*, 1981, *282*, 1033. Personal experience of vomiting, anorexia, nausea, lassitude, urinary frequency and mental impairment lasting for up to 24 hours after exposure to a paint stripper containing methylene chloride.— B. Lee (letter), *ibid.*, 1321. Epidemiological studies showed that fears for a multisystem disorder arising from exposure to methylene chloride were unfounded.— B. A. Walker and P. L. Wyke, *I.C.I.* (letter), *ibid.*, 2057.

Uses. Methylene chloride is commonly used with other solvents in the pharmaceutical industry. Its use in cosmetics in the UK is controlled by the Cosmetic Products Regulations 1978 (SI 1978: No. 1354). It was formerly used as an anaesthetic.
Methylene chloride is widely used in paint strippers.

A mention of the experimental use of methylene chloride as an antisickling agent.— J. Dean and A. N. Schechter, *New Engl. J. Med.*, 1978, *299*, 863.

Use in food. The Food Additives and Contaminants Committee recommended that methylene chloride be temporarily permitted for use as a solvent in food provided there was a maximum concentration of use in food as consumed of 5 ppm. Amylene (2-methylbut-2-ene) was recommended as an additive at a maximum concentration in the solvent of 50 ppm. Further toxicity studies were required.— *Report on the Review of Solvents in Food*, FAC/REP/25, Ministry of Agriculture, Fisheries and Food, London, HM Stationery Office, 1978.

6522-t

Tetrachloroethane. Acetylene Tetrachloride. 1,1,2,2-Tetrachloroethane.
$C_2H_2Cl_4$=167.8.

CAS — 79-34-5.

A clear colourless liquid. B.p. 142° to 147°. Wt per ml 1.59 to 1.595 g. **Soluble** 1 in 400 of water; miscible with alcohol and ether.

Adverse Effects. Tetrachloroethane is probably the most toxic of the chlorinated hydrocarbons. Poisoning can occur through percutaneous absorption as well as ingestion or inhalation. Adverse effects include mucosal irritation, gastro-intestinal disturbances, narcosis, which may follow a latent period, haemolysis, and severe injury to liver and kidneys with jaundice, cirrhosis, liver necrosis and oliguria.
Maximum permissible atmospheric concentration 5 ppm.

For a report of 3 cases of poisoning after tetrachloroethane was given in error for tetrachloroethylene, see J. M. Ward, *Br. med. J.*, 1955, *1*, 1136.

Uses. Tetrachloroethane is used as an industrial solvent.

6523-x

Toluene *(B.P.C. 1949).* Toluol; Toluole; Methylbenzene.

C_7H_8=92.14.

CAS — 108-88-3.

A product of the distillation of coal tar. A colourless, mobile, highly inflammable liquid which burns with a smoky flame. Wt per ml about 0.87 g. B.p. 109° to 111°. Flash-point 4° (closed-cup test).
Practically **insoluble** in water; miscible with organic solvents and glacial acetic acid. **Store** in airtight containers.

Adverse Effects and Treatment. Toluene has about the same acute toxicity as benzene but is a less serious industrial hazard. Toluene may be absorbed percutaneously. It has been reported to be a common constituent of adhesives used in glue sniffing. Commercial toluene may contain benzene, and this may perhaps influence the pattern of adverse effects.
Treatment of adverse effects should be as described under Benzene, p.1451.
Maximum permissible atmospheric concentration 100 ppm.

A review of the toxicology of toluene.— J. W. Hayden *et al.*, *Clin. Toxicol.*, 1977, *11*, 549.

A report of toluene poisoning involving 29 men.— E. O. Longley *et al.*, *Archs environ. Hlth*, 1967, *14*, 481.

Abuse. Renal and hepatic damage in a man who had been sniffing cleaner containing about 80% toluene.— E. T. O'Brien *et al.*, *Br. med. J.*, 1971, *2*, 29.

A severe renal tubular defect with metabolic acidosis, a normal 'anion gap', hyperchloraemia, and a high urinary pH was associated with toluene sniffing in 2 patients.— S. M. Taher *et al.*, *New Engl. J. Med.*, 1974, *290*, 765. Metabolic acidosis with a high 'anion gap' in 2 patients who had been sniffing toluene.— C. M. Fischman and J. R. Oster, *J. Am. med. Ass.*, 1979, *241*, 1713. See also *idem*, *242*, 1491.

A report of 2 children who sniffed glue containing toluene. One of the children became comatose after an episode of 'sniffing' which lasted for several hours. Adverse effects included reduced appetite, nightmares, vertical nystagmus, and incoordination.— J. M. Watson, *Practitioner*, 1979, *222*, 845.

Convulsions in 3 patients after sniffing glue containing toluene.— M. Helliwell and M. Murphy (letter), *Br. med. J.*, 1979, *1*, 1283.

A report of psychosis associated with toluene sniffing.— M. J. Tarsh, *J. Soc. occup. Med.*, 1979, *29*, 131, per *Abstr. Hyg.*, 1980, *55*, 311.

Reversible renal damage in one patient associated with toluene sniffing.— A. M. Will and E. H. McLaren, *Br. med. J.*, 1981, *283*, 525. Progressive renal failure in another patient.— G. Venkataraman (letter), *ibid.*, 1467.

Acute encephalopathy due to toluene intoxication in 19 children.— M. D. King *et al.*, *Br. med. J.*, 1981, *283*, 663. Status epilepticus in one boy associated with toluene abuse.— C. Allister *et al.*, *ibid.*, 1156.

Further references: J. W. Knox and J. R. Nelson, *New Engl. J. Med.*, 1966, *275*, 1494; H. Z. Streicher *et al.*, *Ann. intern. Med.*, 1981, *94*, 758.

For further reports and discussions of solvent abuse, see Solvents, p.1450.

Pregnancy and the neonate. A child with nearly classic foetal alcohol syndrome was born to a woman whose major addiction was to solvents (primarily toluene). She had a 14-year history of daily solvent abuse and a 3-year history of alcohol intake of about a 6-pack of beer weekly.— C. Toutant and S. Lippmann (letter), *Lancet*, 1979, *1*, 1356.

Uses. Toluene has been used as a preservative of urine (1 ml per 100 ml of urine) for chemical examination.
It has wide industrial uses, especially in the manufacture of paint and rubber and plastic cements.

6524-r

Trichloroethane. Methylchloroform; α-Trichloroethane. 1,1,1-Trichloroethane.

$C_2H_3Cl_3$=133.4.

CAS — 71-55-6.

A colourless liquid. Practically **insoluble** in water; soluble in organic solvents. Non-inflammable.

Adverse Effects. Depression of the central nervous system is the main effect of intoxication. Dizziness, nausea, vomiting and fainting have been reported. Kidney and liver damage may occur.

Maximum permissible atmospheric concentration 350 ppm.

A man who ingested about 30 ml of trichloroethane became nauseated after 30 minutes and after an hour developed severe vomiting and diarrhoea which persisted for 6 hours. There was no liver damage. The patient was free of symptoms by the next day.— R. D. Stewart and J. T. Andrews, *J. Am. med. Ass.*, 1966, *195*, 904.

In a study of 11 subjects experimentally exposed to trichloroethane 500 ppm for 6½ to 7 hours daily for 5 days the only objective adverse response was an abnormal modified Romberg test noted in 2 of the subjects during their exposure periods.— R. D. Stewart *et al.*, *Archs environ. Hlth*, 1969, *19*, 467, per *J. Am. med. Ass.*, 1969, *210*, 573.

Fatal poisoning of a 27-year-old man who was cleaning a tank with trichloroethane. Concentrations in the tank were probably between 36 000 and 62 000 ppm.— T. R. Hatfield and R. T. Maykoski, *Archs environ. Hlth*, 1970, *20*, 279.

An account of the diagnosis and treatment of trichloroethane poisoning, illustrated by 4 cases.— R. D. Stewart, *J. Am. med. Ass.*, 1971, *215*, 1789.

For some reports of adverse effects from volatile halogenated solvents, see Refrigerants and Aerosol Propellents, p.1057.

Of 110 sudden deaths associated with the sniffing of solvents in USA between 1962 and 1969, 29 were associated with the use of trichloroethane.— M. Bass, *J. Am. med. Ass.*, 1970, *212*, 2075.

A report of the symptoms and management of trichloroethane intoxication in a 22-year-old girl who was already in end-stage renal failure due to Goodpasture's syndrome associated with a prolonged history of drug abuse which included the regular sniffing of various glues and organic solvents. Failure of renal transplantation led to a return of her solvent abuse and she inhaled 400 ml of Zoff in 36 hours. Her symptoms included persistent vomiting, extreme drowsiness and flaccidity as well as fresh bruising on her arms; she had depressed respiration and liver damage. Treatment was supportive and included lactulose, cimetidine and a high carbohydrate-low protein dietary regimen. Four hours after her last exposure to trichloroethane her regular haemodialysis was performed followed (because of initially suspected paracetamol ingestion, and also the ease of vascular access) by charcoal haemodialysis. Clinical recovery was complete within 48 hours; by 96 hours, liver function had returned to base-line, and the trichloroethane had been completely eliminated.— A. W. Nathan and P. A. Toseland (letter), *Br. J. clin. Pharmac.*, 1979, *8*, 284. For reports and discussions of Goodpasture's syndrome and glomerulonephritis in relation to exposure to solvents, see G. J. Beirne and J. T. Brennan, *Archs environ. Hlth*, 1972, *25*, 365; S. W. Zimmerman *et al.*, *Lancet*, 1975, *2*, 199; U. Ravnskov and B. Forsberg (letter), *Lancet*, 1979, *1*, 1194.

For further reports and discussions of solvent abuse, see Solvents, p.1450.

Uses. Trichloroethane has wide applications as a solvent. It is commonly used in dry cleaning. Its use in cosmetics in the UK is restricted by the Cosmetic Products Regulations 1978 (SI 1978: No. 1354).

Use in food. The Toxicity Sub-Committee of the Food Additives and Contaminants Committee recommended that trichloroethane be temporarily permitted for use as a solvent in food and recommended a maximum concentration of use in food as consumed of 5 ppm. Further toxicity studies were required. However, the Food Additives and Contaminants Committee concluded that a real case of need was lacking and recommended that trichloroethane should not be permitted for use as a solvent in food.— *Report on the Review of Solvents in Food,* FAC/REP/25, Ministry of Agriculture, Fisheries and Food, London, HM Stationery Office, 1978.

Proprietary Names

Genklene *(ICI Mond, UK).*

6525-f

White Spirit. A mixture of hydrocarbons to which a denaturant may be added.

A colourless liquid with a boiling range of 130° to 220°. Flash-point not at 32°.

A specification for mineral solvents, including white spirit, is published by the British Standards Institution (BS 245: 1976).

Adverse Effects and Treatment. As for Kerosene, p.1454.

Uses. White spirit is used as an industrial solvent.

6526-d

Xylene *(B.P.C. 1949).* Xylol; Xylole. A mixture of *o*-, *m*-, and *p*-dimethylbenzene in which the *m*-isomer predominates.

C_8H_{10}=106.2.

CAS — 1330-20-7; 108-38-3 (m-xylene); 95-47-6 (o-xylene); 106-42-3 (p-xylene).

Pharmacopoeias. In *Span.* and *Swiss.*

A colourless inflammable liquid. Wt per ml 0.85 to 0.86 g. B.p. 136° to 142°. Flash-point about 24° (closed-cup test). Practically **insoluble** in water; miscible with organic solvents and fixed oils.

Solvent naphtha (Coal Tar Solvent Naphtha) consists chiefly of xylenes and trimethylbenzenes; various fractions are available, boiling between about 120° and 200°. It should be distinguished from solvent mineral naphtha which is a petroleum product.

Adverse Effects and Treatment. The toxicity of xylene is similar to that of benzene (p.1451) but is less marked. Xylene is absorbed to some extent through the skin. Commercial xylene may contain benzene, and this may perhaps influence the pattern of adverse effects.

Treatment of adverse effects should be as described under Benzene, p.1451.

Maximum permissible atmospheric concentration 100 ppm.

Death of 1 man and prolonged unconsciousness in 2 others followed prolonged inhalation of fumes from paint in which xylene comprised more than 90% of the solvent; the total solvent comprised 34% of the paint by weight. The 2 patients who subsequently recovered were unconscious for 15 and 18 hours respectively, and both patients had transient liver cell damage, and 1 had temporary impairment of renal function.— R. Morley *et al.*, *Br. med. J.*, 1970, *3*, 442.

Uses. Xylene is used as a solvent and as a clearing agent in microscopy. It is also used in preparations to dissolve ear wax.

Proprietary Names

Cerulyse *(Chauvin-Blache, Fr.; J. Martin, Spain)*; Novo-Cerusol *(Chauvin-Blache, Switz.).*

Sulphonamides and Trimethoprim

4900-y

The sulphonamides are analogues of *p*-aminobenzoic acid. They are best known for their antibacterial activity and the sulphonamides included in this section are those generally used in the treatment of infection. Sulphonamides or derivatives of sulphonamides may have other effects sufficiently marked for them to be used clinically; the thiazides and the carbonic anhydrase inhibitors (p.581) are used for their diuretic activity and the sulphonylureas (p.844) are used for their hypoglycaemic activity.

Co-trimoxazole (p.1460), a combination of trimethoprim with sulphamethoxazole, has largely replaced the use of sulphonamides alone in the treatment of systemic infections. Other sulphonamides used in combination with trimethoprim include sulphadiazine (see Co-trimazine, p.1460), sulfametopyrazine, p.1470, sulfametrole, p.1470, sulphadimidine, p.1475, sulphamethoxypyridazine, p.1480, and sulphamoxole (see Co-trifamole, p.1459).

Reference is made in this section to long-acting sulphonamides; these include sulfadoxine, p.1470, sulfametopyrazine, p.1470, sulphadimethoxine, p.1475, sulphamethoxydiazine, p.1479, and sulphamethoxypyridazine, p.1480.

Adverse Effects of Sulphonamides. Side-effects during treatment with sulphonamides are relatively common and vary according to the particular sulphonamide used and the susceptibility of the patient; slow acetylators may be more at risk. Adverse effects are not always related to dose but they are more likely to occur with prolonged treatment. Generally, symptoms are mild but patients should be closely supervised since the onset of serious intoxication is unpredictable.

Relatively common side-effects, especially with the earlier sulphonamides such as sulphapyridine and sulphathiazole, include nausea, vomiting, diarrhoea, headache, dizziness, drug fever, and skin rashes. Cyanosis may occur, due to methaemoglobinaemia or sulphaemoglobinaemia or to the action of an oxidation product, but is rare with the more recent compounds. Other adverse effects which have been reported include acidosis, anorexia, stomatitis, goitre, hypothyroidism, arthralgia, drowsiness, fatigue, insomnia, nightmares, confusion, depression, psychosis, vertigo, ataxia, tinnitus, peripheral neuritis, and polyarteritis nodosa.

Renal complications, such as lumbar pain, dysuria, haematuria, oliguria, and anuria, may result from crystallisation of the less soluble sulphonamides, including sulfamerazine, sulphadiazine, and sulphapyridine, or the less soluble acetyl derivatives of sulphonamides in the renal tubules or urinary tract. Toxic nephrosis, which may be attributed to a hypersensitivity reaction, has also been reported.

Allergic reactions are most likely to occur 7 to 10 days after the start of treatment or on resumption of treatment in patients previously sensitised by the systemic or topical use of sulphonamides; topical use is generally contra-indicated because of the danger of sensitisation. Before treating patients with sulphonamides it is advisable that enquiries be made about previous sulphonamide treatment. Cross-sensitivity to other sulphonamides is common.

During sulphonamide treatment direct exposure to sunlight should be avoided as it facilitates development of sensitisation dermatitis. A severe form of erythema multiforme, associated with widespread lesions of the skin and mucous membranes, termed the Stevens-Johnson syndrome, which may be fatal in about 25% of cases, has occurred in patients treated with sulphonamides; the majority of reports have been associated with the use of long-acting sulphonamides. Epidermal necrolysis (Lyell's syndrome) and lupus erythematosus have also been reported.

Hepatitis has been reported and may be fatal. It may occur within 3 days of commencing sulphonamide therapy.

Blood disorders have occasionally occurred during treatment with the sulphonamides and co-trimoxazole and include agranulocytosis, aplastic anaemia, and thrombocytopenia. Leucopenia and eosinophilia have also been reported. Acute haemolytic anaemia is a rare complication occurring early in treatment; it may be associated with glucose-6-phosphate dehydrogenase deficiency or previous sensitisation to sulphonamides. Blood tests should be made frequently particularly in patients undergoing prolonged treatment; the appearance of sore throat, fever, pallor, purpura, or jaundice may be early indications of serious blood disorders.

Sulphonamides should not be given to patients who have previously shown serious toxic reactions.

For reviews of the adverse effects of sulphonamides, see L. Weinstein *et al.*, *New Engl. J. Med.*, 1960, *263*, 952; J. M. Murdoch, *Practitioner*, 1965, *194*, 26; *Br. med. J.*, 1968, *1*, 658; *Med. J. Aust.*, 1972, *1*, 435.

Toxic amblyopia in children might be caused by sulphonamides.— *Adverse Drug React. Bull.*, 1972, *Oct.*, 112.

A review of vasculitis caused by sulphonamide therapy.— D. Lehr, *J. clin. Pharmac.*, 1972, *12*, 181.

Effects on the blood. In an analysis of drug-induced disorders reported to the Swedish Adverse Drug Reaction Committee for the 10-year period 1966–75, the sulphonamides were among the 3 drugs or groups of drugs most commonly implicated. Of the 592 reports received, those attributed to sulphonamides (these included only 3 preparations: sulphamethizole with sulphamethoxypyridazine, sulphasalazine, and co-trimoxazole) were: 46 (8 fatal) of 199 reports of agranulocytosis, 11 (2 fatal) of 51 reports of aplastic anaemia, 14 of 109 reports of haemolytic anaemia, and 27 (1 fatal) of 233 reports of thrombocytopenia. Over the 10-year period there had been a shift towards the sulphonamides as causative agents and between 1971–75 sulphonamides were the most commonly reported cause of agranulocytosis, aplastic anaemia, and thrombocytopenia, and the third most common cause of haemolytic anaemia.— L. E. Böttiger *et al.*, *Acta med. scand.*, 1979, *205*, 457. An earlier study by P. Arneborn and J. Palmblad (*Acta med. scand.*), 1978, *204*, 283) of drug-induced neutropenia in the Stockholm region between 1973 and 1975 found that only 40% of cases had been reported to the Committee. During 1976 and 1977 there were 27 new episodes of drug-induced neutropenia in the Stockholm region, 13 of which were associated with sulphonamides; of the 7 patients who died, 5 had taken sulphonamides.— P. Arneborn and J. Palmblad, *Acta med. scand.*, 1979, *206*, 241.

Haemolysis. Sulphanilamide, sulphapyridine, sulphacetamide, sulphamethoxypyridazine, and sulphasalazine were reported to be haemolytic agents in subjects deficient in glucose-6-phosphate dehydrogenase but sulphafurazole only caused haemolysis in conjunction with other factors such as infection. The role of co-trimoxazole was uncertain since the only reported episodes were during infections.— M. E. Pembrey, *Practitioner*, 1974, *213*, 647.

Effects on the kidney. A review on the nephrotoxicity of the sulphonamides.— G. B. Appel and H. C. Neu, *New Engl. J. Med.*, 1977, *296*, 784.

Further references: J. R. Curtis, *Br. med. J.*, 1977, *2*, 242.

Effects on the liver. References: M. Tonder *et al.*, *Scand. J. Gastroenterol.*, 1974, *9*, 93; S. Iwarson and P. Lundin, *Acta med. scand.*, 1979, *206*, 219.

Epidermal necrolysis. Sulphonamides, taken for 2 to 14 days before the eruption, might have been responsible for 15 cases of toxic epidermal necrolysis in Britain, including 3 fatalities in patients who had received sulphamethoxypyridazine.— A. Lyell, *Br. J. Derm.*, 1967, *79*, 662.

Hiccup. Persistent hiccup in a 64-year-old man was associated with periods during which he took sulphonamides.— H. B. Eisenstadt (letter), *J. Am. med. Ass.*, 1967, *202*, 915.

Lupus erythematosus. The sulphonamides which have been implicated in causing lupus erythematosus are primarily sulphadiazine, sulphadimethoxine, sulphafurazole, sulphamethoxypyridazine, and sulphasalazine.— D. Alarcón-Segovia, *Mayo Clin. Proc.*, 1969, *44*, 664. See also P. Cohen and F. H. Gardner, *J. Am. med. Ass.*, 1966, *197*, 817.

Stevens-Johnson syndrome. A review of the association between erythema multiforme and long-acting sulphonamides.— *Br. J. Derm.*, 1968, *80*, 844. See also *Br. med. J.*, 1964, *2*, 1410.

Severe erythema multiforme was noted to occur at any time between the second and twenty-fourth days of treatment with long-acting sulphonamides and as late as 6 days after cessation of drug administration. In addition to systemic manifestations such as fever, malaise, dehydration, and general toxaemia, there were arthritis and arthralgia, and lesions affecting the respiratory, gastro-intestinal, genito-urinary, and central nervous systems. These included cough, bronchitis, pneumonia, and pleural effusion; dysphagia, haematemesis, abdominal pain, diarrhoea, and melaena; urethritis, vaginitis, albuminuria, haematuria, urinary retention, and anuria; drowsiness, confusion, coma, delirium, and abnormal deep tendon reflexes. Reports were collected of 116 cases (81 from the United States) of Stevens-Johnson syndrome associated with long-acting sulphonamides between 1957 and 1965. There were 79 cases in children under 15 years of age, with 20 deaths, and 37 in adults with 9 deaths. The US Food and Drug Administration directed that a warning statement along the following lines should be included in the package insert with long-acting sulphonamides. 'WARNING: Fatalities have occurred due to the development of Stevens-Johnson syndrome (erythema multiforme exudativum) following the use of sulfamethoxypyridazine and sulfadimethoxine. Therefore, the patient must be closely observed, and should a rash develop during therapy with these compounds, the drug should be discontinued immediately. These sulphonamides maintain a long-lasting blood concentration due to slow excretion and thus a smaller dosage than is normally employed with shorter-acting sulphonamides should be administered. Since the shorter-acting sulphonamides are effective for most of the same conditions, their use should be considered before the long-acting sulphonamides are employed'.— O. M. Carroll *et al.*, *J. Am. med. Ass.*, 1966, *195*, 691.

Severe erythema multiforme, Stevens-Johnson syndrome, occurred in the course of ulcerative colitis in 4 patients all of whom had been treated with sulphonamides. The sulphonamides involved were phthalylsulphathiazole, sulphadimidine, and sulphasalazine, and in 1 case the sulphonamide was not specified. Following treatment with corticotrophin or corticosteroids, 3 recovered from the syndrome but 1 died on the 13th day. A review of the literature showed that the Stevens-Johnson syndrome had followed treatment with sulphadiazine (3 patients), sulphadimidine (1), sulphafurazole (1), sulphamethoxydiazine (3), sulphamethoxypyridazine (19), sulphanilamide (1), and sulphathiazole (1); some patients had also received other drugs.— A. J. Cameron *et al.*, *Br. med. J.*, 1966, *2*, 1174.

Further references: J. Beveridge *et al.* (letter), *Lancet*, 1964, *2*, 593; W. D. Refshauge, *Med. J. Aust.*, 1965, *2*, 549; J. Guillén Toledo *et al.*, *Alergía, Méx.*, 1967, *15*, 8; K. Kauppinen, *Acta derm.-vener., Stockh.*, 1972, *68*, *Suppl.*, 1; H. R. Gottschalk and O. J. Stone, *Archs Derm.*, 1976, *112*, 513; Z. Rubin, *Archs Derm.*, 1977, *113*, 235.

Treatment of Adverse Effects of Sulphonamides. In cases of recent overdosage the stomach should be emptied by aspiration and lavage. If kidney function is adequate, a saline purgative, such as sodium sulphate, 30 g in 250 ml of water, may be given to promote peristalsis, and elimination of sulphonamide in the urine may be assisted by giving alkalis, such as sodium bicarbonate, and increasing the fluid intake. Severe crystalluria may require ureteric catheterisation and irrigation with warm 2.5% sodium bicarbonate solution. Treatment should be continued until it can be assumed that most of the sulphonamide has been eliminated. The majority of sulphonamides are metabolised to acetylated derivatives which retain the toxicity of the parent compound and thus more active removal may be indicated when adverse effects are very severe. Active measures suggested have included forced diuresis, haemodialysis, peritoneal dialysis, and charcoal haemoperfusion and these are discussed under the Treatment of Adverse Effects of Phenobarbitone, p.812.

Severe hypersensitivity reactions may require treatment with corticosteroids.

Precautions for Sulphonamides. In patients receiving the less soluble sulphonamides, adequate fluid intake is necessary to reduce the risk of crystalluria; the daily urine output should be 1500 ml or more. The administration of compounds which render the urine acid may increase the risk of crystalluria; the risk may be reduced with alkaline urine.

Treatment with sulphonamides should be discontinued immediately a rash appears because of the danger of severe allergic reactions such as the Stevens-Johnson syndrome. In general the sulphonamides are contra-indicated in patients with impaired hepatic function. They should be used with extreme caution in renal impairment, especially the less soluble sulphonamides and when an adequate urinary volume cannot be maintained. They should not be given to patients with a history of hypersensitivity to sulphonamides and should be used with caution in patients with allergic conditions or bronchial asthma.

Sulphonamides should not be given to infants within 1 to 2 months of birth because of the danger of producing kernicterus; for the same reason, sulphonamides, particularly of the long-acting type, should not be given to women prior to delivery and they may also be contra-indicated in nursing mothers.

In general, sulphonamides should not be applied to wounds or lesions; they may cause sensitisation.

The solution of salts of most sulphonamides are alkaline and should not be given intrathecally.

The effect of sulphonamides may be enhanced by displacement from plasma binding sites by more highly bound acidic substances; displacement may also occur in conditions such as alcoholic hepatitis, acute renal failure, and malnutrition. Conversely, sulphonamides may enhance the effects of methotrexate (p.216) and warfarin (p.776) by displacing them from binding sites.

High doses of sulphonamides have been reported to have a hypoglycaemic effect; the antidiabetic effect of the sulphonylurea compounds may be enhanced by the concomitant administration of sulphonamides.

The action of sulphonamides may be antagonised by *p*-aminobenzoic acid and compounds derived from it, particularly the procaine group of local anaesthetics. Such compounds should not be given concomitantly.

Sulphonamides could cause rust yellow to brown discoloration of the urine.— J. Karlstrand, *J. Am. pharm. Ass.*, 1977, *NS17*, 735.

Effects on laboratory tests. Sulphonamides could interfere technically with chemical estimations for urea in the blood to produce erroneous raised results.— *Drug & Ther. Bull.*, 1972, *10*, 69.

Interactions. Reports on the effects of drugs and other factors on the binding of sulphonamides to plasma.— A. H. Anton, *J. Pharmac. exp. Ther.*, 1960, *129*, 282; A. H. Anton, *Clin. Pharmac. Ther.*, 1968, *9*, 561; A. H. Anton and W. T. Corey, *Acta pharmac. tox.*, 1971, *29*, *Suppl.* 3, 134; A. W. Pruitt and P. G. Dayton, *Eur. J. clin. Pharmac.*, 1971, *4*, 59.

For a report of the effects of co-trimoxazole and sulphonamides on the half-life and metabolism of phenytoin, see Phenytoin Sodium, p.1240.

Increased risk of crystalluria. The acetylation of sulphonamides was increased by paraldehyde, with subsequent increased risk of crystalluria.— J. Thomas, *Australas. J. Pharm.*, 1967, *48*, S112.

The concomitant use of ascorbic acid in patients taking sulphonamides should be avoided since crystalluria is more likely to occur when the urine is acid.— J. Karlstrand, *J. Am. pharm. Ass.*, 1977, *NS17*, 735.

Porphyria. Sulphonamides could precipitate or aggravate porphyria.— G. A. G. Peterkin and S. A. Khan, *Practitioner*, 1969, *202*, 117.

Pregnancy and the neonate. Of 50 282 children born to mothers monitored by the Collaborative Perinatal Project 1455 were found to have been exposed to sulphonamides, and possibly other drugs, at some time during the first 4 months of the pregnancy. No association between malformations and exposure to sulphonamides was observed.— O. P. Heinonen *et al.*, *Birth Defects and Drugs in Pregnancy*, Littleton MA, Publishing Sciences Group, 1977, p. 296.

Antimicrobial Action of Sulphonamides. Sulphonamides have a similar structure to *p*-aminobenzoic acid and interfere with the synthesis of nucleic acids in sensitive micro-organisms by blocking the conversion of *p*-aminobenzoic acid to the co-enzyme dihydrofolic acid, a reduced form of folic acid; in man, dihydrofolic acid is obtained from dietary folic acid so sulphonamides do not affect human cells.

All of the sulphonamides have a similar antimicrobial spectrum. They are bacteriostatic against a wide range of Gram-negative and Gram-positive bacteria such as the Enterobacteriaceae, including *Escherichia coli* and the *Shigella* and *Salmonella* spp.; *Neisseria gonorrhoeae* and *N. meningitidis; Haemophilus influenzae* and *H. ducreyi*; some staphylococci and streptococci; *Clostridium welchii* and *Cl. tetani*;and *Bacillus anthracis*. Most strains of *Pseudomonas pseudomallei* and some strains of *Ps. aeruginosa* are sensitive to sulphonamides. Other sensitive organisms include *Actinomyces* and *Nocardia* spp., *Chlamydia trachomatis*, the protozoa *Plasmodium falciparum* and *Toxoplasma gondii*, and *Vibrio cholerae*.

See also Resistance, below.

Studies of the mode of action of sulphonamides.— J. Brandmüller and M. Wahl, *Arzneimittel-Forsch.*, 1967, *17*, 392.

A number of strains of *Aspergillus* were sensitive to sulphonamides.— B. E. Copeland and R. V. Rosvoll (letter), *J. Am. med. Ass.*, 1969, *210*, 2398.

The relationship between the antibacterial action of sulphonamides and their chemical structure.— T. H. Maren, *A. Rev. Pharmac. & Toxic.*, 1976, *16*, 309.

Sulphonamides, especially sulphamethizole, sulphafurazole, and sulphamethoxazole, were active against atypical mycobacteria *in vitro* and in infected *animals*.— J. Hejny, *Bull. int. Un. Tuberc.*, 1979, *54*, 342.

In vitro susceptibility testing of *Paracoccidiodes brasiliensis* to sulphadiazine and sulphadimethoxine.— A. Restrepo and M. D. Arango, *Antimicrob. Ag. Chemother.*, 1980, *18*, 190.

Resistance to Sulphonamides. Acquired resistance to the sulphonamides is common and has been reported in the majority of pathogenic micro-organisms sensitive to sulphonamides, including *Escherichia coli*, *Neisseria gonorrhoeae*, and *N. meningitidis*. Most strains of *Shigella sonnei* and *Streptoccus faecalis* have been reported to be resistant. Resistance in many Gram-negative bacteria may be mediated by R-plasmids. For a discussion of the factors involved in the development of resistance see Resistance to Antibiotics (p.1076).

Resistance to one sulphonamide generally involves resistance to the other sulphonamides.

For reports of resistance to sulphonamides, see Martindale 27th Edn, p. 1467.

Sensitivity Testing to Sulphonamides. The principles and methods of testing strains of micro-organisms for sensitivity to sulphonamides are similar to those described for antibiotics (p.1076). When employing the disk method care must be taken to ensure that factors inhibitory to sulphonamides, such as *p*-aminobenzoic acid or thymidine, are not present.

A warning that although the Mueller-Hinton agar used in the standard disk test is relatively free from sulphonamide inhibitors such as *p*-aminobenzoic acid, media can vary from batch to batch to produce false results of resistance *in vitro*. Specialised techniques are necessary for testing the sensitivity to sulphonamides of fastidious organisms such as meningococci.— *Med. Lett.*, 1980, *22*, 22.

Further references: A. Stokes and R. W. Lacey, *J. clin. Path.*, 1978, *31*, 165.

Absorption and Fate of Sulphonamides. Most of the sulphonamides are readily absorbed from the gastro-intestinal tract, many of them appearing in the urine within 30 minutes. Peak concentrations in the blood are usually reached within 3 or 4 hours of a dose by mouth. After injection or absorption, part of the sulphonamide, varying from less than 10 to more than 95%, is loosely bound to plasma albumin; there is also a wide range of half-lives and excretion-rates.

Most sulphonamides diffuse freely throughout the body tissues and may be detected in the urine, saliva, sweat, and bile, in the cerebrospinal, peritoneal, ocular, and synovial fluids, and in pleural and other effusions. Diffusion into cerebrospinal fluid varies considerably with different sulphonamides and for some the concentration may exceed a half of that in blood. Sulphonamides readily diffuse across the placenta. In the milk, the concentration is unlikely to affect the suckling infant unless previous sensitisation has occurred.

Sulphonamides are conjugated to varying extents, usually to the inactive N^4-acetyl derivatives, and are excreted mainly in the urine; some sulphonamides, such as sulphadimethoxine and sulphamethoxydiazine are excreted in part as soluble but inactive glucuronide.

The rate of acetylation is genetically determined in several sulphonamides, including sulphadimidine, sulphasalazine, and sulphapyridine, and there is a bimodal distribution in the population of persons who acetylate sulphonamides either slowly or rapidly. As the acetyl derivatives are inactive the duration of activity of sulphonamides, particularly of those significantly acetylated, will differ between the 2 groups.

Phthalylsulphathiazole and succinylsulphathiazole are poorly absorbed and are excreted mainly in the faeces.

Reviews of pharmacokinetic data on sulphonamides.— M. S. S. Chow and R. A. Ronfeld, *J. clin. Pharmac.*, 1975, *15*, 405; T. B. Vree *et al.*, *Clin. Pharmacokinet.*, 1980, *5*, 274.

For approximate correlations between the MIC of sulphonamides against *Escherichia coli* and their half-life, between the MIC and the degree of dissociation, between lipid solubility and half-life, between lipid solubility and MIC, and between molecular weight and degree of protein binding, see T. Struller, *Antibiotica Chemother.*, 1968, *14*, 179.

Absorption. The effect of food on the absorption of sulphonamides.— H. Macdonald *et al.*, *Chemotherapia*, 1967, *12*, 282.

Diffusion. A brief view of the penetration of sulphonamides into cerebrospinal fluid and brain tissue.— R. W. A. Barling and J. B. Selkon, *J. antimicrob. Chemother.*, 1978, *4*, 203.

Excretion. Studies of urinary excretion kinetics indicated that the excretion of sulphaethidole was inhibited by weak acids such as salicylic acid, barbitone, mandelic acid, and probenecid and also by some bases such as quinine.— S. M. Bahal, *Diss. Abstr.*, 1965, *26*, 1602, per *Int. pharm. Abstr.*, 1966, *3*, 319.

Uses of Sulphonamides. Sulphonamides are now most frequently used with trimethoprim, see Co-trimoxazole, p.1463 for an example of this combination. Their main use alone is the treatment of acute uncomplicated urinary-tract infections. The use of a sulphonamide should ideally be based on identification and sensitivity testing of the infecting organism but, with sulphonamides, results of tests *in vitro* are very dependent on the method and medium used and minimum inhibitory concentrations may be much less precise than those achieved for many antibiotics. The effect of sulphonamides is inhibited by pus and they are of little value in treating suppurative lesions.

Three sulphonamides have been given together to reduce the risk of crystalluria as the constituent sulphonamides can co-exist in solution in urine without affecting the solubility of each other.

Properties of mixed sulphonamides are similar to those of the individual sulphonamides; in general they have been replaced by the more soluble sulphonamides.

The main differences between sulphonamides relate to pharmacokinetic rather than antimicrobial properties. While long-acting sulphonamides have the advantage of reduced frequency of dosage serious side-effects have been associated with their use and their persistence in the body delays the resolution of adverse effects; in the US many long-acting sulphonamides have been withdrawn. The use of a more rapidly excreted sulphonamide should first be considered.

Sulphonamides are often of value in the treatment of infections due to *Nocardia asteroides* and have been used in the treatment of chancroid and lymphogranuloma venereum. They are used to supplement pyrimethamine in the treatment of toxoplasmosis. They are given systemically in the treatment of trachoma and inclusion conjunctivitis, supplemented by local application of tetracycline or other broad-spectrum antibiotic. The sulphonamides are used with pyrimethamine in the management of chloroquine-resistant falciparum malaria; long-acting sulphonamides have been used in leprosy.

Sulphonamides, in particular sulphadiazine, have been used in the treatment of meningococcal meningitis but resistance may be a problem and antibiotics are generally preferred.

Sulphonamides are effective against pneumococci but have been superseded by antibiotics; they should not be used to treat group A beta-haemolytic streptococcal infections since the streptococci may not be eradicated and the symptoms of infection may mask early signs of adverse effects on the blood. Sulphonamides have been used in the prevention and treatment of bacillary dysentery, but many resistant strains of *Shigella* have emerged, particularly of *Sh. sonnei*.

Sulphonamides with more specific uses include sulphasalazine, used in the management of inflammatory bowel diseases; sulphapyridine, used in dermatitis herpetiformis; silver sulphadiazine, applied topically to burns; and sulphacetamide sodium, applied in eye infections. The poorly absorbed sulphonamides such as phthalylsulphathiazole have been used pre-operatively to suppress the normal intestinal flora.

Because of the danger of the emergence of resistant strains, the prophylactic use of sulphonamides should probably be limited to the protection of contacts of patients suffering from meningococcal meningitis and to prophylaxis against recurrences of rheumatic fever in patients allergic to penicillins. Prolonged maintenance therapy is used in recurrent urinary-tract infections.

For preparations of mixed sulphonamides, see p.1486.

In sulphonamide therapy large initial doses are given to produce adequate concentrations in body tissues followed by smaller maintenance doses at regular intervals.

The initial dose is usually twice the maintenance dose and the interval between doses varies from 4 hours to 24 hours or more according to the sulphonamide being given.

Sulphonamides are usually given by mouth though parenteral administration, usually intravenously, may be necessary in patients seriously ill or unable to take or retain the sulphonamide by mouth. Administration by mouth should replace parenteral administration as soon as possible.

High concentrations of sulphonamide are achieved in urine and lower doses can be used in uncomplicated urinary-tract infections. In acute infection treatment should generally not be continued for more than 10 to 14 days.

Reviews of long-acting sulphonamides.— H. Seneca, *J. Am. med. Ass.*, 1966, *198*, 975; *Lancet*, 1967, *1*, 150.

For other reviews of the action and uses of sulphonamides, see *Br. med. J.*, 1968, *2*, 674; J. K. Seydel, *J. pharm. Sci.*, 1968, *57*, 1455; *Med. Lett.*, 1969, *11*, 21; O. L. S. Scott and M. L. Johnson, *Practitioner*, 1969, *202*, 37; R. G. Mitchell, *ibid.*, 1970, *204*, 20; *Br. med. J.*, 1970, *2*, 36; *ibid.*, 1970, *4*, 631; J. D. Williams, *Br. J. Hosp. Med.*, 1974, *12*, 722; A. P. Ball *et al.*, *Drugs*, 1975, *10*, 1; D. S. Reeves *et al.*, *Br. med. J.*, 1978, *2*, 410.

The choice of antimicrobial agents.— *Med. Lett.*, 1980, *22*, 5.

Applying theoretical kinetic principles to triple sulphonamide mixtures, minimal crystalluria and similar average serum concentrations of all 3 drugs would be achieved with a mixture of sulphadiazine, sulfamerazine, and sulphadimidine in the proportions 1:3:4 rather than the usual 1:1:1.— M. J. Taraszka and A. A. Forist, *J. pharm. Sci.*, 1968, *57*, 1379.

Crohn's disease. Sulphonamides appeared to benefit some patients with Crohn's disease.— G. T. Schmidt *et al.*, *Gut*, 1968, *9*, 7.

Enteric infections. A recommendation that a preparation of 3 sulphonamides, sulphadiazine, sulphadimidine, and sulphathiazole, with streptomycin (Streptotriad) is the best prophylactic now available for travellers' diarrhoea although it should only be used for short important trips.— A. G. Higginson, *Practitioner*, 1979, *223*, 529. See also R. S. Thubron (letter), *Br. med. J.*, 1979, *2*, 1225.

Leprosy. Long-acting sulphonamides are only weakly active against *Myobacterium leprae* and are inactive against dapsone-resistant strains; their continued use in the treatment of leprosy appears to be unjustified.— G. A. Ellard, *Lepr. Rev.*, 1974, *45*, 31. At the 10th International Leprosy Congress, Bergen, 1973 it was reported that long-acting sulphonamides had the advantage of weekly administration by mouth and some leprologists had claimed good results particularly in tuberculoid forms of the disease and its complicating neuritis, but in view of their serious side-effects they should be used with caution in mass leprosy campaigns.— *Lepr. Rev.*, 1974, *45*, 41.

Meningitis. The use of long-acting sulphonamides in certain countries for the treatment of meningococcal meningitis and the increasing incidence of resistance. With the availability of specific immunisation the need for chemoprophylaxis has declined but if a sulphonamide or antibiotic is used then a therapeutic dose should be used and treatment given only once.— Cerebrospinal Meningitis Control, Report of a WHO Study Group, *Tech. Rep. Ser. Wld Hlth Org. No. 588*, 1976.

Further references: S. Sreebhahun (letter), *Lancet*, 1967, *1*, 329; J. Stevenson, *Br. med. J.*, 1973, *2*, 411; *Lancet*, 1974, *2*, 1431; *Br. med. J.*, 1974, *3*, 295; *J. Am. med. Ass.*, 1975, *231*, 1035.

Nocardiosis. Sulphonamides are considered the treatment of choice in nocardiosis.— *Med. Lett.*, 1980, *22*, 5.

Further references: F. Cox and W. T. Hughes, *Pediatrics*, 1975, *55*, 135; G. F. Carroll *et al.*, *Am. J. clin. Path.*, 1977, *68*, 279.

Otitis media. References to the use of sulphonamides in otitis media.— S. H. Sell *et al.*, *Sth. med. J.*, 1978, *71*, 1493; C. W. Biedel, *Am. J. Dis. Child.*, 1978, *132*, 681.

Pregnancy and the neonate. The treatment of urinary-tract infection in pregnancy.— P. J. Little, *Drugs*, 1977, *14*, 390.

Sulphonamides with pyrimethamine were generally considered to be too dangerous for the treatment of toxoplasmosis in pregnant women.— H. Williams, *Postgrad. med. J.*, 1977, *53*, 614.

Urinary-tract infections. Reviews and discussions of antimicrobial agents in the treatment of urinary-tract infections.— P. J. Little, *Drugs*, 1972, *3*, 414; K. F. Fairley, *Drugs*, 1973, *6*, 417 (pyelonephritis); R. R. Bailey, *Drugs*, 1977, *13*, 137 (cystitis); A. W. Asscher, *Br. med. J.*, 1978, *1*, 1531 (cystitis); *Drug & Ther. Bull.*, 1979, *17*, 81; R. R. Bailey, *Drugs*, 1979, *17*, 219 (single-dose treatment); J. D. Anderson, *J. antimicrob. Chemother.*, 1980, *6*, 170 (single-dose treatment); *Lancet*, 1981, *1*, 26 (single-dose treatment).

Reviews of the treatment of urinary-tract infections in children.— W. F. Heale, *Drugs*, 1973, *6*, 230; J. M. Stansfeld, *Practitioner*, 1977, *218*, 59; M. H. Winterborn, *Br. J. Hosp. Med.*, 1977, *17*, 453; M. I. Marks, *Drugs*, 1978, *16*, 147.

Comment on the significance of bacteriuria and the role of long-term antibacterial therapy. No patient with urinary symptoms should receive frequent courses of full-dose antibacterial therapy or a regimen of 'rotating' antibiotics but should be referred for intravenous urography. After appropriate antibacterial treatment they should probably then begin a regimen of low-dose prophylaxis with high-fluid intake and regular and complete bladder emptying. The prognosis for adults with bacteriuria and renal scarring is not yet clear. Renal scarring is associated with bacteriuria in the presence of vesico-ureteric reflux and usually begins when the kidneys are growing, often before the age of 5. There is still no certain way of detecting patients in whom bacteriuria is benign compared with those at risk of renal damage. Population screening for bacteriuria has been extensively investigated and appears to be beneficial in early pregnancy (J.D. Williams *et al.*, in *Urinary tract infection*, W. Brumfitt and A.W. Asscher (Ed.), London, Oxford University Press, 1973, p. 103) but there is much less justification for childhood screening. In the UK, the Cardiff-Oxford Bacteriuria Study Group (*Lancet*, 1978, *1*, 889) found that although treatment of asymptomatic bacteriuria reduced infection in schoolgirls followed-up for a mean of 4 years, there was no significant difference in clinical outcome; they suggested it might be more beneficial to study girls under 5 years old. The value of screening for asymptomatic bacteriuria in children aged 3 to 7 years has been questioned by L. Righard (*Lancet*, 1980, *1*, 1369). However in the US, J.Y. Gillenwater *et al.* (*New Engl. J. Med.*, 1979, *301*, 396) in a follow-up study over 9 to 18 years of 60 schoolgirls with bacteriuria, found that screening detects those at risk of considerable morbidity from recurrent infection and a small number with major urological abnormalities. These observations emphasise the importance of detecting bacteriuria in children but do not prove that screening is the best method of doing so. An alternative approach to childhood screening is to emphasise the importance of identifying those children in whom bacteriuria gives rise to clinical illness. J.M. Smellie *et al.*, (*Br. med. J.*, 1976, *2*, 203 and *Lancet*, 1978, *2*, 175) have reported the successful long-term low-dose prophylaxis of urinary-tract infection with co-trimoxazole in children previously treated for symptomatic urinary-tract infections.— *Lancet*, 1979, *2*, 1166.

Further references: W. A. Gillespie *et al.*, *Lancet*, 1971, *2*, 675; J. Timm, *Nord. Med.*, 1971, *85*, 719; T. F. Keys, *Mayo Clin. Proc.*, 1977, *52*, 680.

Vaginitis. A sulphonamide vaginal cream (Sultrin) was ineffective in the treatment of nonspecific vaginitis and inactive *in vitro* against a probably causative organism, *Gardnerella vaginalis* (*Haemophilus vaginalis*).— T. A. Pheifer *et al.*, *New Engl. J. Med.*, 1978, *298*, 1429.

4901-j

Calcium Sulphaloxate. Calcium 4′-[(hydroxymethylcarbamoyl)sulphamoyl]phthalanilate. $(C_{16}H_{14}N_3O_7S)_2Ca = 824.8$.

CAS — 14376-16-0 (sulphaloxic acid); 59672-20-7 (calcium salt).

Calcium sulphaloxate is a sulphonamide which has been used similarly to phthalylsulphathiazole (p.1468) for its antibacterial action in the gastro-intestinal tract. Approximately 95% is claimed to remain unabsorbed in the intestine.

The usual adult dose is 1 g by mouth thrice daily.

Proprietary Preparations

Enteromide *(Consolidated Chemicals, UK)*. Calcium sulphaloxate, available as tablets of 500 mg.

Other Proprietary Names

Intestin-Euvernil *(Ger.)*.

4902-z

Co-trifamole. CN 3123. A mixture of 5 parts of sulphamoxole and 1 part of trimethoprim.

Adverse Effects, Treatment, and Precautions. As for Sulphonamides, p.1457 and Trimethoprim, p.1484.

A study of the adverse effects of co-trifamole.— M. Etzel and W. Wesenberg, *Arzneimittel-Forsch.*, 1976, *26*, 678.

In healthy subjects co-trifamole 960 mg initially then 480 mg once daily for 10 days caused a significant reduction in serum-tri-iodothyronine concentrations but did not significantly affect free thyroxine index or serum concentrations of thyroxine or thyroid-stimulating hormone. Although it could not be concluded that co-trifamole causes hypothyroidism it was suggested that tests of thyroid function should be interpreted with caution in patients on such treatment and that those on long-term therapy should have their thyroid function regularly assessed.— H. N. Cohen *et al.*, *Br. med. J.*, 1980, *281*, 646. Findings suggesting that trimethoprim does not have significant antithyroid activity, supporting the view that the sulphonamide component is responsible for the lowering of the thyroid hormone concentrations observed previously.— *idem* (letter), *Lancet*, 1981, *1*, 676.

Absorption and Fate. See Sulphamoxole, p.1480 and Trimethoprim, p.1485.

Studies of the pharmacokinetics of sulphamoxole and trimethoprim after their administration together: J. Kuhne *et al.*, *Arzneimittel-Forsch.*, 1976, *26*, 651; J. K. Seydel and E. Wempe, *ibid.*, 1977, *27*, 1521.

Uses. Co-trifamole has similar antimicrobial activity and similar uses to co-trimoxazole (p.1462). It is given in an initial dose of 960 mg (trimethoprim 160 mg and sulphamoxole 800 mg) followed by 480 mg every 12 hours and continued until 2 days after all symptoms have disappeared. A suggested dose for children, 6 to 12 years of age, is 480 to 720 mg initially followed by 240 to 480 mg every 12 hours. Lower doses may be necessary in patients with impaired renal function.

Proceedings of a symposium on co-trifamole.— Current Concepts in Antibacterial Chemotherapy Sulfamoxole/Trimethoprim (Co-trifamole), H. Knothe (Ed.), *International Congress and Symposium Series, No. 15*, London, The Royal Society of Medicine, 1980. See also: *Arzneimittel-Forsch.*, 1976, *26*, 596–683.

Studies of the antimicrobial activity of sulphamoxole/trimethoprim combinations: F. W. Kohlmann and H. Sous, *Arzneimittel-Forsch.*, 1976, *26*, 613; *idem*, 618; F. Legler, *ibid.*, 658; V. Hingst and H. -G. Sonntag, *Medsche Welt, Stuttg.*, 1979, *30*, 1199.

Clinical studies of the use of co-trifamole in the treatment of infections: M. Etzel and W. Wesenberg, *Arzneimittel-Forsch.*, 1976, *26*, 661; E. Eckstein *et al.*, *ibid.*, 665 (renal, urinary-tract); M. Etzel *et al.*, *ibid.*, 671 (bronchopulmonary, ENT); *idem*, 674 (gastro-intestinal, skin, gynaecological); H. Helwig *et al.*, *Klin. Pediat.*, 1976, *188* 518 (children; urinary-tract, bronchial, intestinal, ENT); D. Niskios *et al.*, *Therapie Gegenw.*, 1976, *115*, 646 (urinary-tract); K. Feltmann, *ibid.*, 896 (urinary-tract); W. Feldmeier, *Medsche Klin.*, 1976, *71*, 1192 (bronchopulmonary, urogenital); H. -J. Peters *et al.*, *Münch med. Wschr.*, 1977, *119*, 409 (pyelonephritis, urinary-tract); H. Frank *et al.*, *ibid.*, 1441; W. Kaldewey, *ibid.*, 1978, *120*, 1335 (urinary-tract); H. Knothe *et al.*, *Medsche Klin.*, 1978, *73*, 1780 (chronic bronchitis); R. Sanzgiri *et al.*, *Indian Pediat.*, 1978, *15*, 57 (children; respiratory-tract, gastro-intestinal tract, skin, lymphadenitis); P. C. Das, *Indian med. J.*, 1978, *71*, 75.

Proprietary Preparations

Co-Fram *(Abbott, UK)*. Co-trifamole, available as scored tablets of 480 mg.

Other Proprietary names

Nevin *(Ger.)*; Supristol *(Fr., Ger., Switz.)*.

4903-c

Co-trimazine.
A mixture of about 5 parts of sulphadiazine and 1 part of trimethoprim.

CAS — 39474-58-3.

NOTE. The product commercially available in Great Britain contains in each 500 mg sulphadiazine 410 mg and trimethoprim 90 mg.

Adverse Effects, Treatment, and Precautions. As for Sulphadiazine, p.1474 and Trimethoprim, p.1484.

Absorption and Fate. See Sulphadiazine, p.1474 and Trimethoprim, p.1485.

Mean plasma half-lives of active sulphadiazine, total sulphadiazine, and trimethoprim were 7.71, 9.18, and 12.04 hours respectively in patients with normal renal function given co-trimazine. All half-lives gradually increased with a reduction in renal function.— T. Bergan *et al.*, *Clin. Pharmac. Ther.*, 1977, *22*, 211.

In 10 healthy subjects given a single dose of sulphadiazine 800 mg with trimethoprim 160 mg, peak concentrations in serum were achieved at about 4 hours and 1 hour respectively; mean half-lives were 15.2 and 7.4 hours. The ratio of trimethoprim to sulphadiazine in serum varied from about 1:10 at 1 hour to about 1:63 at 24 hours; the ratio in urine remained fairly constant at about 1:6. About 10% of the sulphadiazine was acetylated in the serum; in the urine the mean amount of acetylated sulphadiazine rose from 21% in the first 8 hours to 41% in the period 15 to 24 hours.— F. Andreasen *et al.*, *Eur. J. clin. Pharmac.*, 1978, *14*, 57.

Serum half-lives after the oral administration of co-trimazine were, sulphadiazine 9.4 hours and trimethoprim 9.1 hours compared with half-lives after co-trimoxazole of sulphamethoxazole 10.9 hours and trimethoprim 11.6 hours. The ratios of trimethoprim: sulphonamide serum concentrations after co-trimazine or co-trimoxazole were similar but much more sulphadiazine than sulphamethoxazole was excreted in the urine in the active form.— B. Ekström *et al.*, *Infection*, 1979, *7*, 74.

A pharmacokinetic comparison in 8 healthy subjects between co-trimazine and co-trimoxazole given every 12 hours for 13 doses indicating that sulphadiazine is more suitable than sulphamethoxazole for use with trimethoprim in the treatment of urinary-tract infections. During the 12 hours after the last dose of co-trimazine 500 mg (sulphadiazine 410 mg and trimethoprim 90 mg) or co-trimoxazole 960 mg, 66% of active sulphadiazine and 13% of active sulphamethoxazole were excreted in the urine compared with 32% and 40% of the acetylated metabolites respectively. Urinary recovery of trimethoprim in the same period was 70% after co-trimazine and 58% after co-trimoxazole. The ratios of active drugs in the urine were 1:44 for trimethoprim:sulphadiazine and 1:1.1 for trimethoprim:sulphamethoxazole. About 58% of sulphadiazine was bound to plasma protein compared with 73% of sulphamethoxazole.— B. Örtengren *et al.*, *Infection*, 1979, *7*, *Suppl.* 4, S371. See also B. Örtengren *et al.*, *ibid.*, S367.

In patients given a single dose of co-trimazine or co-trimoxazole, more active sulphadiazine was excreted in the urine than active sulphamethoxazole in those with normal or reduced renal function. Unlike sulphadiazine, metabolites of sulphamethoxazole accumulated to a greater extent than either trimethoprim or active sulphamethoxazole in patients with impaired renal function and thus co-trimazine may be more suitable than co-trimoxazole for patients with renal impairment.— T. Bergan *et al.*, *Infection* 1979, *7*, *Suppl.* 4, S382.

Uses. Co-trimazine has antimicrobial activity similar to that of co-trimoxazole (p.1462) and is used in the treatment of urinary-tract infections. It is given in a dose of 500 mg (trimethoprim 90 mg and sulphadiazine 410 mg) every 12 hours for up to 14 days. Suggested doses of co-trimazine to be given to children twice daily are: 3 months to 5 years of age, 125 mg; 5 to 12 years, 250 mg. Lower doses may be necessary in patients with impaired renal function; co-trimazine is generally not recommended when creatinine clearance is below 15 ml per minute.

Proceedings of a symposium on trimethoprim/sulphonamide preparations including co-trimazine.— *Infection*, 1979, *7*, *Suppl.* 4, S309–S420.

A demonstration of enhanced activity *in vitro* with sulphadiazine and trimethoprim against *Escherichia coli* in the presence of pus.— P. N. Edmunds, *J. clin. Path.*, 1978, *31*, 162. Criticism of the study. The effect could simply be additive and the diluted pus may have lost some of its thymidine content during preparation of the plates.— R. W. Lacey and A. Stokes (letter), *ibid.*, 700. Reply.— P. N. Edmunds (letter), *ibid.*, 701.

Administration in renal failure. See under Absorption and Fate above.

Urinary-tract infections. In patients with acute pyelonephritis bacteriological cures were achieved in all of 43 who took sulphadiazine 500 mg with trimethoprim 160 mg twice daily and 32 of 38 similar patients given amoxycillin 375 mg thrice daily, both for 10 days.— P. T. Männistö and P. Lähteenmäki, *Curr. ther. Res.*, 1978, *23*, 562.

A discussion on co-trimoxazole and co-trimazine and their use in urinary infections. Co-trimazine might be preferable in patients with renal failure but it is probably more important to compare trimethoprim alone with trimethoprim/sulphonamide combinations.— *Drug & Ther. Bull.*, 1979, *17*, 97.

In a double-blind study co-trimazine 500 mg or co-trimoxazole 960 mg given every 12 hours for 14 days were equally effective in curing patients with acute uncomplicated urinary-tract infections. There was a trend towards fewer side-effects with co-trimazine but the difference was not statistically significant.— O. Skjerven and T. Bergan, *Infection*, 1979, *7*, *Suppl.* 4, S398.

Further comparative studies in patients with urinary-tract infections demonstrating similar beneficial effects with co-trimazine and co-trimoxazole.— A. Lövestead *et al.*, *Infection*, 1979, *7*, *Suppl.* 4, S401; S. Allgulander *et al.*, *ibid.*, S404; R. R. Bailey and S. Pearson, *N.Z. med. J.*, 1980, *91*, 43.

For findings that sulphadiazine 250 mg with trimethoprim 160 mg given twice daily is effective in the treatment of acute urinary-tract infections, see J. Seppänen, *Ann. clin. Res.*, 1980, *12*, *Suppl.* 25, 1–51.

Proprietary Preparations

Coptin *(Pfizer, UK)*. Co-trimazine, available as **Suspension** containing 250 mg in each 5 ml (suggested diluent, syrup) and as scored **Tablets** of 500 mg.

Other Proprietary Names of Sulphadiazine/Trimethoprim Preparations

Adiprim *(Fin.)*; Syntrizin *(Denm.)*; Triglobe *(Fr., Switz.)*; Trimin *(Swed.)*; Trobacter *(Spain)*.

4904-k

Co-trimoxazole.
A mixture of 5 parts of sulphamethoxazole and 1 part of trimethoprim.

CAS — 8064-90-2.

The injection contains sulphamethoxazole sodium 5 parts; this is formed *in situ* by interaction of sulphamethoxazole and sodium hydroxide.

Adverse Effects. As for Sulphonamides, p.1457, Sulphamethoxazole, p.1479, and Trimethoprim, p.1484.

The Stevens-Johnson and Lyell's syndromes have been reported in patients receiving co-trimoxazole. There have been conflicting reports of the incidence of deteriorating renal function during treatment with co-trimoxazole.

Precipitation of gout in 2 patients taking co-trimoxazole might have been due to the sulphonamide content.— *Br. med. J.*, 1972, *4*, 662.

From a survey of the published literature and reports to one of the manufacturers it was clear that all types of reactions to sulphonamides had been reported within 30 months of the introduction of co-trimoxazole. Three-quarters of all side-effects were related to skin or to the gastro-intestinal tract and included glossitis and stomatitis. Rashes appeared more often in older patients, possibly because of wider use in these patients and included 6 cases of erythema multiforme and 5 (3 fatal) of epidermal necrolysis. The reported incidence of rashes ranged from 1.6 to 8%; some appeared to be due to trimethoprim. Mild transient jaundice had been reported, often in patients with a history of infectious hepatitis. Blood disorders attributed to co-trimoxazole included aplastic anaemia (1 patient), megaloblastic anaemia (7), eosinophilia (5), granulocytopenia (99), agranulocytosis (9), and thrombocytopenia (42). Clinical symptoms due to folate deficiency were rare, but co-trimoxazole should not be given to patients with folate deficiency.— A. J. Salter, *Med. J. Aust.*, 1973, *1*, *Suppl.* (June 30), 70.

Analysis of reports of the early use of co-trimoxazole in 9909 patients showed gastro-intestinal side-effects in 3.3%, skin reactions in 1.5%, blood disorders in 0.8%, and other side-effects in 0.6%. Analysis of reports to the end of 1972 covered 37 914 patients estimated to cover 0.1% of the total use of co-trimoxazole. Excluding side-effects where it was not possible to assess the incidence, analysis showed gastro-intestinal side-effects in 2.9%, skin reactions in 1.32% (including exanthema, rash, erythema, urticaria, pruritus, allergic dermatitis, epidermal necrolysis—Lyell's syndrome, and erythema multiforme), blood disorders in 0.35% (including anaemia, leucopenia, neutropenia, granulocytopenia, thrombocytopenia, agranulocytosis, pancytopenia, and eosinophilia), and other side-effects in 0.48% (including headache, vertigo, renal complications, hepatic complications, sweating, weakness, insomnia, and allergic reactions). Severe side-effects were: megaloblastic anaemia (3 patients), haemolytic anaemia (1), agranulocytosis (5), pancytopenia (2), and Lyell's syndrome (2, one fatal).— L. Havas *et al.* , *Roche, Clin. Trials J.*, 1973, *10* (3), 81.

Co-trimoxazole was associated with 31 reports to the New Zealand Committee on Adverse Drug Reactions in the year 1976–7. Of the 8 due to bone-marrow depression there was one fatality. A further death resulted from epidermal necrolysis.— E. G. McQueen, *N.Z. med. J.*, 1977, *86*, 248.

Of the 29 524 medical in-patients monitored by the

Boston Collaborative Drug Surveillance Program since 1966, 649 have received co-trimoxazole. Of these, 52 patients (8%) experienced adverse effects none of which was severe and all of which were reversible. The commonest side-effects were skin rashes in 23 patients (3.5%) and upper gastro-intestinal effects in 22 (3.4%); half occurred within 3 days of starting treatment. Adverse effects were more common in female patients (10.6%) than in males (4.8%). In no patient was a deterioration in renal function attributed to co-trimoxazole.— D. H. Lawson and H. Jick, *Am. J. med. Sci.*, 1978, *275*, 53.

Allergy. Anaphylactic shock occurred in a 53-year-old woman 2 hours after taking co-trimoxazole 960 mg; she had taken co-trimoxazole 2 months previously which had been discontinued owing to development of a rash.— J. Dry *et al.*, *Thérapie*, 1975, *30*, 705.

A patient developed fatal wide-spread reactions associated with co-trimoxazole and affecting skin, lungs, kidneys, liver, pancreas, and central nervous system with probable loss of central neural control of the heart.— J. Brøckner and E. Boisen (letter), *Lancet*, 1978, *1*, 831. A similar patient recovered after intensive treatment.— W. B. Finlayson and G. Johnson (letter), *ibid.*, 1978, *2*, 682.

Further references: A. Wåhlin and N. Rosman (letter), *Lancet*, 1976, *2*, 1415; R. S. Ramaiah *et al.* (letter), *ibid.*, 1977, *1*, 604.

Effects on the blood. A study indicating that sulphamethoxazole with trimethoprim might have folate antagonistic effects in man as well as in bacteria.— J. M. England and M. Coles, *Lancet*, 1972, *2*, 1341.

The haematological hazards of co-trimoxazole.— *Lancet*, 1973, *2*, 950.

Studies in 13 patients suggested that co-trimoxazole did not depress true serum-folate concentrations; there was no definite evidence that co-trimoxazole was more liable to cause blood disorders than sulphonamides alone.— M. C. Bateson *et al.*, *Lancet*, 1976, *2*, 339.

Thrombocytopenia occurred in an 86-year-old woman who had been treated with allopurinol, dipyridamole 600 mg daily, and a 6-day course of co-trimoxazole. The thrombocytopenia was attributed to the combination of allopurinol and co-trimoxazole.— E. Raik and P. C. Vincent (letter), *Med. J. Aust.*, 1973, *2*, 468.

Acute pancytopenia due to megaloblastic arrest developed in 3 elderly patients during treatment with co-trimoxazole. Two of these patients died, one was also taking allopurinol, the other was taking digoxin, frusemide, and indomethacin in addition to co-trimoxazole and had previously received allopurinol, spironolactone, and lanatoside C.— E. A. Blackwell *et al.*, *Med. J. Aust.*, 1978, *2*, 38. Comment.— I. S. Collins (letter), *ibid.*, 26.

A 53-year-old woman developed red-cell hypoplasia after taking co-trimoxazole 960 mg twice daily for about 16 months.— M. E. M. Stephens, *Postgrad. med. J.*, 1974, *50*, 235.

A 4-year-old boy developed transient mild leucocytopenia 5 days after finishing a 14-day course of co-trimoxazole. Over the following 3 years he received another 4 courses of co-trimoxazole without adverse reactions but during the sixth course agranulocytosis developed after 8 days of therapy.— U. Lasson, *Dt. med. Wschr.*, 1977, *102*, 1287.

Mention of 13 cases of fatal aplastic anaemia or agranulocytosis in one year probably due to co-trimoxazole.— W. H. W. Inman, *Br. med. J.*, 1977, *1*, 1500.

A causal relationship between co-trimoxazole and agranulocytosis was unproved.— D. H. Lawson and D. A. Henry (letter), *Br. med. J.*, 1977, *2*, 316.

Over 7 years the Australian Adverse Drug Reactions Registry received 31 reports of thrombocytopenia related to co-trimoxazole therapy. Of these 2 patients died, 26 recovered, and the outcome was unknown in 3.— H. G. Dickson, *Med. J. Aust.*, 1978, *2*, 5.

Further references: B. Hulme and D. S. Reeves, *Br. med. J.*, 1971, *3*, 610; T. J. Stamps and A. C. B. Wicks (letter), *Br. med. J.*, 1972, *1*, 176; C. Maier and H. R. Heer, *Schweiz. med. Wschr.*, 1972, *102*, 923; T. J. Hamblin (letter), *Lancet*, 1973, *2*, 1153; A. V. L. Hill and D. N. S. Kerr, *Postgrad. med. J.*, 1973, *49*, 596; A. L. Tulloch, *J. Pediat.*, 1976, *88*, 499; A. L. Barr and M. Whineray, *Aust. N.Z. J. Med.*, 1980, *10*, 54.

Haemolysis. A patient with glucose-6-phosphate dehydrogenase deficiency developed haemolysis during treatment with co-trimoxazole.— S. K. Owusu (letter), *Lancet*, 1972, *2*, 819.

Sulphamethoxazole 90 mg per kg body-weight daily reduced the half-life of ^{51}Cr-labelled glucose-6-phosphate dehydrogenase deficient red blood cells transfused into normal recipients on 4 of 6 occasions. Trimethoprim 18 mg per kg daily did not affect survival of deficient cells.— T. K. Chan and A. J. S. McFadzean, *Trans. R. Soc. trop. Med. Hyg.*, 1974, *68*, 61.

No haemolysis was observed in 10 infants with glucose-6-phosphate dehydrogenase deficiency given co-trimoxazole. However, since haemolysis had been reported in similar patients, co-trimoxazole should be administered to such infants and children with care.— M. C. K. Chan and H. B. Wong (letter), *Lancet*, 1975, *1*, 410. See also U. Lexomboon and N. Unkurapiana, *S.E. Asian J. trop. med. publ. Hlth*, 1978, *9*, 576.

Megaloblastic anaemia. Co-trimoxazole was considered to be the main cause of megaloblastic anaemia in 4 of 112 patients studied over 2 years.— S. El Tamtamy (letter), *Lancet*, 1974, *1*, 929.

A report of megaloblastic anaemia in a patient taking co-trimoxazole daily and pyrimethamine 50 mg weekly.— A. F. Fleming *et al.* (letter), *Lancet*, 1974, *2*, 284. See also V. E. Ansdell *et al.* (letter), *ibid.*, 1976, *2*, 1257.

Further references.— P. J. Rooney and E. Housley (letter), *Br. med. J.*, 1972, *2*, 656; M. K. Chan *et al.*, *Br. J. clin. Pract.*, 1980, *34*, 187.

Effects on fertility. After receiving co-trimoxazole for suspected seminal infections, reductions in sperm count of up to 88% were noted in 14 of 40 men attending a fertility clinic.— A. Murdia *et al.* (letter), *Lancet*, 1978, *2*, 375. The effect did not appear to be due to co-trimoxazole.— J. Guillebaud (letter), *ibid.*, 523.

Effects on the gastro-intestinal tract. Pseudomembranous colitis occurred in an 80-year-old woman treated with co-trimoxazole for a urinary-tract infection after surgery for a fractured femur. The diarrhoea did not respond to neomycin with kaolin, diphenoxylate with atropine, or cholestyramine, and the patient died.— A. Cameron and M. Thomas, *Br. med. J.*, 1977, *1*, 1321.

Pseudomembranous colitis developed in 4 patients after they had received co-trimoxazole.— C. R. Pennington (letter), *New Engl. J. Med.*, 1980, *303*, 1533. Comment.— R. H. Rubin and M. N. Swartz (letter), *ibid.*, 1534.

Effects on the kidney. Deterioration in kidney function seen in 16 patients, most of whom had some pre-existing renal abnormality, was associated with the use of co-trimoxazole. Microscopic examination of tissue samples indicated acute tubular necrosis. Kidney damage in 3 of the patients was permanent and in 1 of these given a second course of treatment further irreversible damage occurred. It was recommended that co-trimoxazole should not be given to patients with a serum-creatinine concentration of more than 20 µg per ml.— S. Kalowski *et al.*, *Lancet*, 1973, *1*, 394.

Acute renal failure occurred in 2 patients given co-trimoxazole parenterally; one died. Both patients had hypoalbuminaemia reducing binding of sulphamethoxazole to plasma protein; competitive binding by penicillin and metronidazole, previously given, might also have contributed.— N. Buchanan, *Br. med. J.*, 1978, *2*, 172.

A hypersensitivity rash and acute renal failure occurred together in 4 patients who received co-trimoxazole, 2 of whom were elderly and died. The dosage was inappropriately high in relation to the patients' renal function hence accumlation of sulphonamide could have been a contributing factor. Possibly co-trimoxazole should be avoid in the elderly. Trimethoprim alone might be adequate and preferable therapy for urinary-tract infections.— J. M. Richmond *et al.* (letter), *Lancet*, 1979, *1*, 493.

A report of interstitial nephritis attributed to co-trimoxazole.— D. Saltissi *et al.*, *Br. med. J.*, 1979, *1*, 1182.

Interstitial nephritis associated with co-trimoxazole in renal transplant recipients.— E. J. Smith *et al.*, *J. Am. med. Ass.*, 1980, *244*, 360.

Further reports of deterioration in renal function after treatment with co-trimoxazole in patients with normal or impaired renal function.— *Med. J. Aust.*, 1972, *1*, 435; R. R. Bailey and P. J. Little, *ibid.*, 1976, *1*, 914; D. Shouval *et al.*, *Lancet*, 1978, *1*, 244; M. Bräutogam *et al.*, *Klin. Wschr.*, 1979, *57*, 95.

Criticism of reports of impaired renal function with co-trimoxazole.— I. S. Collins, *Wellcome, Austral.* (letter), *Med. J. Aust.*, 1976, *2*, 111; P. R. W. Tasker and H. E. de Wardener (letter), *Lancet*, 1978, *1*, 711; A. Bye and A. S. E. Fowle (letter), *ibid.*; J. P. Guignard *et al.* (letter), *ibid.*, 712.

Effects on the liver. A patient accidentally given co-trimoxazole 7.68 g daily for 2.5 days (4 times the usual twice-daily dose) developed jaundice which persisted for 2.5 weeks; liver-function tests were normal 3 months later.— A. C. B. Wicks and T. J. Stamps (letter), *Br. med. J.*, 1970, *4*, 52.

A report of hepatic necrosis which resulted in the death of a patient who had been given co-trimoxazole.— C. F. Colucci and M. L. Cicero (letter), *J. Am. med. Ass.*, 1975, *233*, 952.

Further references: D. K. Stevenson *et al.*, *Pediatrics*, 1978, *61*, 864; S. S. Nair *et al.*, *Ann. intern. Med.*, 1980, *92*, 511; A. L. Ogilvie and P. J. Toghill, *Postgrad. med. J.*, 1980, *56*, 202.

Effects on the nervous system. Acute polyneuropathy possibly associated with co-trimoxazole in one patient. Many other drugs were being taken at the time.— A. B. Grossman *et al.* (letter), *Lancet*, 1977, *2*, 616. Surgery itself might have caused the polyneuropathy.— F. M. Vincent (letter), *ibid.*, 980.

Erythema nodosum. Erythema modosum developed in a 49-year-old woman and was considered to be associated with a course of treatment with co-trimoxazole.— T. J. Delaney and B. Leppard, *Br. J. Derm.*, 1974, *90*, 205.

Immunosuppression. In 13 healthy men with tetanus antitoxin titres not greater than 1.25 and who were given co-trimoxazole 480 mg twice daily for 4 days, the antibody titres after 2 doses of tetanus vaccine were significantly less than in 10 similar vaccinated men not given the antibacterial agents.— H. Arvilommi *et al.* (letter), *Br. med. J.*, 1972, *3*, 761. See also H. Arvilommi *et al.*, *Chemotherapy, Basle*, 1976, *22*, 37.

Skin reactions. A report of 2 patients with fixed drug eruptions of the genitals associated with the use of co-trimoxazole.— M. D. Talbot, *Practitioner*, 1980, *224*, 823.

Stevens-Johnson syndrome. Twenty-eight cases of Stevens-Johnson syndrome have been reported in patients who had taken co-trimoxazole and 11 cases of erythema multiforme have been reported. The aetiological role of viral, bacterial and mycoplasmal infections and of sulphonamides and other antibacterial drugs made it difficult to establish the precise causative factor in any individual case.— L. S. Berstein and J. Cooper, *Wellcome* (letter), *Lancet*, 1978, *1*, 988.

A clear case of Stevens-Johnson syndrome in a 44-year-old woman after receiving co-trimoxazole for a urinary infection.— S. Kikuchi and T. Okazaki (letter), *Lancet*, 1978, *2*, 580.

Further reports of the Stevens-Johnson syndrome following treatment with co-trimoxazole.— J. A. C. Thorpe and A. Nysenbaum (letter), *Lancet*, 1978, *1*, 276; N. O. Azinge and G. A. Garrick, *J. Allergy & clin. Immunol.*, 1978, *62*, 125.

Treatment of Adverse Effects. As for Sulphonamides, p.1457. Bone-marrow depression due to trimethoprim may be treated with calcium folinate 3 to 6 mg intramuscularly daily for 5 to 7 days.

Precautions. As for Sulphonamides, p.1458 and Trimethoprim, p.1485.

Co-trimoxazole should not be given to patients with a history of sensitivity to it or to the sulphonamides. Because of possible interference with human folate metabolism by trimethoprim, co-trimoxazole should not be given to patients with megaloblastic anaemia. It should be avoided in those who may have megaloblastic bone-marrow changes or folic-acid deficiency such as pregnant women and patients receiving anticonvulsant drugs. Co-trimoxazole should be used with caution in patients receiving pyrimethamine or immunosuppressive therapy. Adverse effects on the blood may be more severe in malnourished or elderly patients. All patients receiving prolonged treatment with co-trimoxazole should be be given regular blood examinations.

Co-trimoxazole should be used cautiously and in reduced dosage in patients with impaired renal function. Because of the risk of crystalluria, an adequate fluid intake should be maintained and the administration of alkalis may be necessary if very large doses are used.

The absorptions of trimethoprim and sulphamethoxazole (taken as co-trimoxazole) were increased in patients with coeliac disease, small bowel diverticulosis, or Crohn's disease. There was a disproportionate increase in the plasma concentrations of trimethoprim in patients with coeliac disease or diverticulosis and peak plasma concentrations of sulphamethoxazole in patients with Crohn's disease were increased about threefold. Mean peak plasma concentrations of co-trimoxazole were reduced in healthy subjects when they also took cholestyramine.— R. L. Parsons and G. M. Paddock, *J. antimicrob. Chemother.*, 1975, *1*, *Suppl.* (Sept.), 59.

Two patients had reduced survival of transfused platelets while taking co-trimoxazole; a third patient developed thrombocytopenia. Serum from the 3 patients contained antibodies against donor platelets incubated with co-trimoxazole; the effect was against the trimethoprim component. Since co-trimoxazole is used for treatment and prophylaxis of infections in leukaemia its effect on platelets is of great importance.— F. H. J. Claas *et al.*, *Br. med. J.*, 1979, *2*, 898.

The incidences and duration of neutropenia and thrombocytopenia in 6 renal allograft recipients who received azathioprine and long-term prophylaxis (22 days or more) with co-trimoxazole were greater than in 25 similar patients who received azathioprine alone. In a further 9 patients who received azathioprine and treatment with co-trimoxazole (6 to 16 days) the incidences were not different to those in patients receiving azathioprine alone.— P. P. Bradley *et al.*, *Ann. intern. Med.*, 1980, *93*, 560.

In healthy subjects co-trimoxazole 960 mg twice daily for 10 days caused a significant reduction in free thyroxine index and in serum concentrations of thyroxine and tri-iodothyronine but did not significantly affect concentrations of thyroid-stimulating hormone. Although it could not be concluded that co-trimoxazole causes hypothyroidism it was suggested that tests of thyroid function should be interpreted with caution in patients on such treatment and that those on long-term therapy should have their thyroid function regularly assessed.— H. N. Cohen *et al.*, *Br. med. J.*, 1980, *281*, 646. Findings suggesting that trimethoprim does not have significant antithyroid activity, supporting the view that the sulphonamide component is responsible for the lowering of the thyroid hormone concentrations observed previously.— *idem* (letter), *Lancet*, 1981, *1*, 676.

Interactions. For reports of co-trimoxazole enhancing the anticoagulant effect of warfarin, see Warfarin Sodium, p.779.

Antimicrobial Action. The two components of co-trimoxazole interfere with the bacterial synthesis of tetrahydrofolic acid, an essential stage in the production of thymidine, purines, and subsequently nucleic acids. Sulphamethoxazole, like the other sulphonamides, inhibits the synthesis of dihydrofolic acid from *p*-aminobenzoic acid. Trimethoprim inhibits the action of dihydrofolate reductase and prevents the synthesis of tetrahydrofolic acid from dihydrofolic acid; although this stage also occurs in man, trimethoprim is much less active against the mammalian enzyme. Enhanced antibacterial activity has been reported when sulphamethoxazole and trimethoprim are used together *in vitro* although there is doubt as to whether sequential blockade of the bacterial synthetic pathway is responsible. The clinical relevance of this enhanced activity is uncertain especially in urinary-tract infections where inhibitory concentrations of trimethoprim appear to be dominant.

Co-trimoxazole has a wide spectrum of activity similar to that of the sulphonamides (p.1458) and trimethoprim (p.1485). It is also active against *Pneumocystis carinii*.

Action. Of 8 strains of coliform bacteria isolated from samples of infected urines all were sensitive to trimethoprim, while 4 were sensitive to sulphamethoxazole. Increased sensitivity to a mixture of these drugs was demonstrated by sulphonamide-sensitive strains only, but no bactericidal effect was observed. *In vitro* 3 of the 4 sulphonamide-resistant strains yielded trimethoprim-resistant variants in the presence of a mixture of sulphamethoxazole and trimethoprim.— D. D. Smith *et al.*, *Med. J. Aust.*, 1972, *1*, 263.

Co-trimoxazole was bacteriostatic against urinary pathogens and its use was unlikely to prevent the appearance of trimethoprim-resistant strains.— R. W. Lacey *et al.* (letter), *Lancet*, 1973, *2*, 509. See also R. W. Lacey and E. Lewis (letter), *Br. med. J.*, 1973, *4*, 165. Criticism of the experimental procedures and of the conclusions.— R. Then and P. Angehrn, *Hoffman-La Roche* (letter), *ibid.*, 1974, *1*, 78.

Reports of enhanced activity *in vitro* with sulphamethoxazole and trimethoprim.— F. W. O'Grady, *Med. J. Aust.*, 1973, *1*, *Suppl.* (June 30), 19; R. Küchler and U. J. Koch, *Chemotherapy, Basle*, 1973, *18*, 242.

Findings from an assessment *in vitro* using an experimental model of urinary infection indicated that trimethoprim alone may be as effective as co-trimoxazole in the treatment of urinary infections. Co-trimoxazole had a bacteriostatic effect against the majority of 28 urinary isolates of Enterobacteriaceae.— J. D. Anderson *et al.*, *J. clin. Path.*, 1974, *27*, 619.

Observations that sulphonamides can be moderately potent inhibitors of bacterial dihydrofolate reductase led to the hypothesis that multiple simultaneous inhibition of the enzyme might be responsible for the enhanced activity seen *in vitro* with sulphonamides and trimethoprim rather than sequential inhibition.— M. Poe, *Science*, 1976, *194*, 533.

The suggestion that sulphonamides and trimethoprim bind simultaneously to dihydrofolate reductase is not an adequate explanation of the synergistic inhibition of growth of *Escherichia coli* organisms observed.— J. J. Burchall, *Wellcome, Science*, 1977, *197*, 1300. Further criticism.— R. Then, *Roche, Switz.*, *ibid.*, 1301. Reply.— M. Poe, *ibid.* Agreement with the hypothesis of Poe. Although there may be enhanced activity with sulphamethoxazole and trimethoprim under defined conditions *in vitro*, synergy *in vivo* is only likely to occur where the local concentration of trimethoprim is sub-inhibitory.— R. W. Lacey, *J. antimicrob. Chemother.*, 1979, *5*, *Suppl.* B, 75.

Using an *in vitro* model of an infected urinary bladder and concentrations of sulphamethoxazole and trimethoprim well within those achievable therapeutically in urine, the presence of sulphonamide had no influence on the inhibitory activity of trimethoprim against *Escherichia coli*.— D. Greenwood, *J. antimicrob. Chemother.*, 1979, *5*, *Suppl.* B, 85.

Further references.— R. N. Grüneberg, *J. antimicrob. Chemother.*, 1979, *5*, *Suppl.* B, 27.

Activity against anaerobic bacteria. A study of 98 anaerobic isolates, including 38 strains of *Bacteroides fragilis*, indicated that sulphamethoxazole and trimethoprim, individually or in combination, were not active against the majority of anaerobic bacteria.— J. E. Rosenblatt and P. R. Stewart, *Antimicrob. Ag. Chemother.*, 1974, *6*, 93.

All of 28 strains of *Bacteroides fragilis* were inhibited by sulphamethoxazole at a concentration of 16 µg or less per ml (mainly 2 to 8 µg per ml) and were relatively resistant to trimethoprim (MICs of 4 to 16 µg per ml). Enhanced activity with the 2 drugs was most pronounced when they were used in equal amounts.— R. L. Then and P. Angehrn, *Antimicrob. Ag. Chemother.*, 1979, *15*, 1.

Further references.— O. A. Okubadejo *et al.*, *Br. med. J.*, 1973, *2*, 212; J. Wüst and T. D. Wilkins, *Antimicrob. Ag. Chemother.*, 1978, *14*, 384.

Activity against Enterobacteriaceae. The aminoglycosides and co-trimoxazole were the most active antimicrobial compounds against *Yersinia enterocolitica* an organism isolated with increasing frequency from children with gastro-enteritis.— S. Hammerberg *et al.*, *Antimicrob. Ag. Chemother.*, 1977, *11*, 566.

Studies *in vitro* indicated that co-trimoxazole had greater inhibitory activity than ampicillin against *Salmonella typhi* from chronic typhoid carriers.— C. M. Nolan and J. Rosenfeld, *Curr. ther. Res.*, 1977, *21*, 736.

The activities of trimethoprim and co-trimoxazole were synergistic or additive when used with gentamicin against 11 strains of *E. coli* and 10 of 12 strains of *Klebsiella pneumoniae*. Antagonism was observed once with trimethoprim and gentamicin and twice with co-trimoxazole and gentamicin against strains of *Kleb. pneumoniae*.— J. W. Paisley and J. A. Washington, *Antimicrob. Ag. Chemother.*, 1978, *14*, 656.

Activity against gonococci. Trimethoprim or sulphamethoxazole lacked antibacterial activity against 10 isolates of penicillin-resistant *Neisseria gonorrhoeae* when either was used alone but inhibitory concentrations as low as 0.31 µg per ml for trimethoprim and 5.9 µg per ml for sulphamethoxazole were achieved when they were used in combination.— T. T. Yoshikawa and S. A. Shibata (letter), *J. antimicrob. Chemother.*, 1979, *5*, 618.

In a study using 168 strains of *Neisseria gonorrhoeae*, enhanced activity for sulphamethoxazole and trimethoprim was greatest when the 2 agents were used in the ratio 1:1. Enhanced activity was minimal and antagonism sometimes occurred when they were used together in the ratio usually achievable in serum after administration by mouth (19:1).— M. F. Rein *et al.*, *Antimicrob. Ag. Chemother.*, 1980, *17*, 247.

Activity against Haemophilus. A report of enhanced activity *in vitro* with trimethoprim and sulphamethoxazole (ratio 1:20) against *Haemophilus influenzae*, including ampicillin-resistant strains.— S. Pelton *et al.*, *Antimicrob. Ag. Chemother.*, 1977, *12*, 649.

Further references.— J. D. Williams and J. Andrews, *Br. med. J.*, 1974, *1*, 134; R. Sinai *et al.*, *Antimicrob. Ag. Chemother.*, 1978, *13*, 861.

Activity against Legionella pneumophila. Sulphamethoxazole-trimethoprim had an MIC of 4.8-0.25 µg per ml against 6 isolates of the legionnaires' disease bacterium.— C. Thornsberry *et al.*, *Antimicrob. Ag. Chemother.*, 1978, *13*, 78.

Activity against Nocardia. A study *in vitro* suggested that fixed-dose commercial combinations of trimethoprim and sulphamethoxazole contained too little trimethoprim for optimum activity against isolates of *Nocardia*.— J. E. Bennett and A. E. Jennings, *Antimicrob. Ag. Chemother.*, 1978, *13*, 624.

Activity against Pseudomonas. All of 82 strains of *Pseudomonas aeruginosa* were resistant to trimethoprim and sulphamethoxazole when tested alone and together using a disk containing trimethoprim and sulphamethoxazole in the conventional ratio of 1:19. However, marked enhanced activity was demonstrated with trimethoprim and sulphamethoxazole against 22 strains of moderately-resistant *Ps. aeruginosa* in agar-plate dilution tests. Mean MICs were: trimethoprim 108 µg per ml, sulphamethoxazole 227 µg per ml, and trimethoprim with sulphamethoxazole 11.4/16.4 µg per ml. The MICs for the combination are well within concentrations achieved in urine and are also in a similar ratio. A disk containing trimethoprim and sulphamethoxazole in the ratio of 1:2 should be used for sensitivity testing of urinary isolates.— D. Grey and J. M. T. Hamilton-Miller, *J. med. Microbiol.*, 1977, *10*, 273.

All of 14 isolates of *Pseudomonas maltophilia* were susceptible *in vitro* to trimethoprim 0.09 µg per ml/sulphamethoxazole 1.78 µg per ml with a median MIC of 0.5/0.89 µg per ml. Enhanced activity was obtained against 12 of the strains when trimethoprim/sulphamethoxazole were used with carbenicillin.— T. P. Felegie *et al.*, *Antimicrob. Ag. Chemother.*, 1979, *16*, 833.

Resistance. Resistance of bacteria to sulphonamides (p.1458), including sulphamethoxazole, is common and has also been reported with trimethoprim. It is not yet clear whether the emergence of strains resistant to the components has been reduced by the use of co-trimoxazole.

A discussion on bacterial resistance to trimethoprim and sulphonamides. Within the last 10 to 15 years the incidence of resistance to sulphonamides has risen to about 25% in general practice and 50% in hospital. Organisms resistant to trimethoprim have been reported increasingly since 1970.— J. M. T. Hamilton-Miller, *J. antimicrob. Chemother.*, 1979, *5*, *Suppl.* B, 61. See also *Br. med. J.*, 1980, *281*, 571.

A report of thymine-requiring bacteria occurring in the urine or sputum of patients who had received co-trimoxazole for several months. Thymine-like compounds were present in the urine from which the mutant strains were isolated.— R. Maskell *et al.*, *Lancet*, 1976, *1*, 834. A further report of the isolation of thymine-requiring mutant bacteria resistant to trimethoprim.— O. A. Okubadejo and R. Maskell (letter), *ibid.*, 1977, *2*, 926. See also J. J. Plorde and T. Bailey (letter), *Ann. intern. Med.*, 1979, *91*, 134. See also under Sensitivity Testing.

In an 18-month study of acquired resistance to trimethoprim 133 of 4196 urinary isolates were resistant. They included 84 of 459 strains (18.3%) of *Klebsiella aerogenes*, 32 of 2210 strains (1.4%) of *Escherichia coli*, 10 of 83 strains (12%) of *Enterobacter* spp., and 7 of 334 strains (2%) of *Proteus mirabilis*. Resistance mediated by R-plasmids was rare; transferable resistance only occurred in 11 strains. Non-transferable resistance (presumably chromosomal) may be due to the production by bacteria of dihydrofolate reductase with diminished susceptibility to trimethoprim; it is potentially more serious since resistance is unlikely to disappear when the antibacterial agent is withdrawn.— W. Brumfitt *et al.* (letter), *Lancet*, 1977, *2*, 926.

Of 874 strains of *Haemophilus influenzae* 69 had an MIC for sulphamethoxazole of 32 µg or more per ml; the apparent incidence of resistance was reduced when the inoculum was reduced. Only 2 strains had an MIC for trimethoprim of 32 µg or more per ml.— A. J. Howard *et al.*, *Br. med. J.*, 1978, *1*, 1657.

Emergence of resistance to trimethoprim was monitored in 30 patients with chronic urinary-tract infections who received long-term low dosage treatment with co-trimoxazole over a period of up to 5 years. About 5% of the isolates examined were found to carry plasmids conferring transferable resistance to trimethoprim and about 17% had a resistance to trimethoprim of a non-transferable type.— K. J. Towner *et al.*, *J. antimicrob. Chemother.*, 1979, *5*, 45.

An outbreak of plasmid-mediated trimethoprim resistance in coliform bacilli was related to prior exposure to co-trimoxazole, sulphonamides, and ampicillin.— R. N. Grüneberg and M. J. Bendall, *Br. med. J.*, 1979, *2*, 7.

A report of co-trimoxazole-resistant *Shigella* in

Ontario.— R. M. Bannatyne *et al.* (letter), *Lancet*, 1980, *1*, 425. A report of a woman who acquired co-trimoxazole-resistant shigellosis in Brazil.— D. E. Taylor *et al.* (letter), *ibid.* A further report of co-trimoxazole-resistant *Shigella* in Canada.— M. Finlayson (letter), *Can. med. Ass. J.*, 1980, *123*, 718.

Further references: M. P. Fleming *et al.*, *Br. med. J.*, 1972, *1*, 726; J. R. May and J. Davies, *ibid.*, *3*, 376; S. R. M. Bushby, *Burroughs Wellcome* (letter), *ibid.*, 1973, *3*, 50; J. R. May and J. Davies (letter), *ibid.*, 407; J. G. Howe and T. S. Wilson (letter), *Lancet*, 1972, *2*, 184; A. Toivanen *et al.*, *Chemotherapy, Basle*, 1976, *22*, 97; C. A. Hart *et al.* (letter), *Lancet*, 1977, *2*, 1081; M. J. Cunningham *et al.* (letter), *Br. J. Derm.*, 1978, *99*, 597; M. C. Finlayson and F. L. Jackson (letter), *Lancet*, 1978, *2*, 375; N. Datta *et al.*, *J. antimicrob. Chemother.*, 1979, *5*, 399; M. Williams (letter), *Lancet*, 1980, *2*, 316; I. Braveny and K. Machka (letter), *ibid.*, 752; S. J. Pancoast *et al.*, *Antimicrob. Ag. Chemother.*, 1980, *17*, 263; N. Datta *et al.*, *Lancet*, 1981, *1*, 1181.

Sensitivity Testing. As for Sulphonamides, p.1458. The culture media should be free of thymidine, a specific antagonist for trimethoprim. It is also important to use a light inoculum. In the disk diffusion method of sensitivity testing the routine use of disks containing trimethoprim and sulphamethoxazole in the ratio of 1:19 has been recommended (but see below).

A recommendation that disks for sensitivity testing of urinary isolates should contain trimethoprim and sulphamethoxazole in the ratio of 1:2.— D. Grey and J. M. T. Hamilton-Miller, *J. med. Microbiol.*, 1977, *10*, 273.

A study *in vitro* indicated that the use of thymine-free and thymidine-free agar might not give a realistic assessment of the activity *in vivo* of sulphamethoxazole and trimethoprim since thymidine may possibly be present in the urine of patients.— A. Stokes and R. W. Lacey, *J. clin. Path.*, 1978, *31*, 165. A comment that sensitivity testing using thymidine-free media is an adequate guide to treatment.— R. Maskell and O. A. Okubadejo (letter), *ibid.*, 808.

A discussion on sources of error in the determination of sensitivity to co-trimoxazole and its components.— J. M. T. Hamilton-Miller, *J. antimicrob. Chemother.*, 1979, *5*, *Suppl.* B, 61.

Absorption and Fate. See sulphamethoxazole (p.1479) and trimethoprim (p.1485). When co-trimoxazole is administered, plasma concentrations of trimethoprim and sulphamethoxazole are generally in the ratio of 1:20; in urine this ratio may vary from 1:1 to 1:5. About 50% of administered trimethoprim and 50% of sulphamethoxazole is excreted in the urine in 24 hours; a larger proportion of sulphamethoxazole appears as inactive metabolite.

A review of the pharmacokinetics of trimethoprim and trimethoprim/sulphonamide preparations.— D. Reeves and P. J. Wilkinson, *Infection*, 1979, *7*, *Suppl.* 4, S330.

A review of the clinical pharmacokinetics of co-trimoxazole.— R. B. Patel and P. G. Welling, *Clin. Pharmacokinet.*, 1980, *5*, 405.

The apparent volume of distribution of trimethoprim was 5 to 6 times greater than that of sulphamethoxazole; this explained why the ratio of trimethoprim to sulphamethoxazole used clinically was higher than the optimum ratio of 1:20 *in vitro*. The half-lives of trimethoprim and sulphamethoxazole were 10.1 and 11.4 hours respectively. Peak plasma concentrations of trimethoprim in 6 healthy men after a single dose of 960 mg of co-trimoxazole were 2.7 µg per ml and 3.5 µg per ml after 15 twelve-hourly doses. Peak concentrations of unconjugated sulphamethoxazole were 40 and 90 µg per ml respectively. Suggested dose regimens in renal impairment included: the standard regimen of 960 mg of co-trimoxazole every 12 hours if the creatinine clearance exceeded 25 ml per minute; for clearances of 15 to 25 ml per minute the standard dose was used for 3 days then 960 mg daily, provided the total sulphamethoxazole concentration did not exceed 200 µg per ml.— A. S. E. Fowle, *Med. J. Aust.*, 1973, *1*, *Suppl.* (June 30), 26.

Peak-serum-nonacetylated sulphamethoxazole concentrations of between 27.9 and 45.2 µg per ml were obtained in healthy subjects 2 and 4 hours after sulphamethoxazole 800 mg in conjunction with trimethoprim 160 mg. In uraemic patients peak sulphamethoxazole concentrations were achieved at 4 or 6 hours and ranged from 18.8 to 35 µg per ml. Peak serum-trimethoprim concentrations ranging from 0.9 to 1.5 µg per ml were achieved in healthy subjects at 1 and 2 hours and similar values were obtained in uraemic patients. The serum half-lives for nonacetylated sulphamethoxazole and trimethoprim were 9.3 and 10.6 hours respectively in the healthy subjects and there was little difference when each compound was administered singly. As renal function deteriorated, the half-lives became more prolonged but both compounds were removed by haemodialysis at rates similar to the excretion in subjects with healthy kidneys. The serum-binding of unchanged sulphamethoxazole was reduced in uraemic patients and was further reduced in uraemic patients with low serum-protein concentrations; no changes were detected in the binding of trimethoprim to serum proteins. In the first 48 hours about 30% of nonacetylated sulphamethoxazole and 53% of trimethoprim were excreted in the urine. It was found that acidification of the urine increased the excretion of trimethoprim, alkalinisation decreased its excretion and increased that of free sulphamethoxazole, and renal impairment reduced the excretion of both compounds.— W. A. Craig and C. M. Kunin, *Ann. intern. Med.*, 1973, *78*, 491. See also H. Nolte and H. Buttner, *Chemotherapy, Basle*, 1973, *18*, 274.

Following single doses of co-trimoxazole 60 mg per kg body-weight administered to children aged 2 to 6 years maximum plasma concentrations were much lower than those observed in adults who had received comparable doses. The average plasma half-life for both drugs in children was generally about half of that for adults.— P. Kremers *et al.*, *Thérapie*, 1973, *28*, 117.

Administration of 960 mg of co-trimoxazole twice daily to 5 healthy subjects for 9 days gave steady-state plasma concentrations of the constituents after 3 days; for active sulphamethoxazole this was between 52.5 and 63.1 µg per ml, and for trimethoprim 1.61 and 1.91 µg per ml.— P. Kremers *et al.*, *J. clin. Pharmac.*, 1974, *14*, 112.

Seven healthy subjects who took 9 tablets of co-trimoxazole, a dose of 4.32 g, achieved in the first 8 hours mean serum concentrations of 6.12 to 8.32 µg per ml for trimethoprim and 98 to 128 µg per ml for sulphamethoxazole; at 24 hours the respective average concentrations were 2.16 and 31.70 µg per ml. This high dose could be useful in the treatment of uncomplicated gonorrhoea.— T. T. Yoshikawa and L. B. Guze, *Antimicrob. Ag. Chemother.*, 1976, *10*, 462.

In healthy subjects given 12 tablets of co-trimoxazole, elimination half-lives for trimethoprim and sulphamethoxazole were longer than those for smaller doses. Ratios of serum concentrations of trimethoprim to free sulphamethoxazole ranged from about 1:16 to 1:30 during the first 24 hours; urinary concentrations were much higher and the ratios ranged from about 1:2 to 1:4. Side-effects were severe.— R. J. Fass *et al.*, *Antimicrob. Ag. Chemother.*, 1977, *12*, 102.

Peak serum concentrations of trimethoprim and sulphamethoxazole in 6 healthy subjects occurred about 40 minutes and 2 hours respectively after an intramuscular injection of trimethoprim 4 mg per kg body-weight as the pantothenate and sulphamethoxazole 20 mg per kg.— A. Lázaro *et al.* (letter), *J. antimicrob. Chemother.*, 1978, *4*, 287.

Co-trimoxazole 960 mg was given every 8 hours by intravenous infusion over one hour to 11 cancer patients. At the end of the first infusion mean plasma concentrations for trimethoprim and free sulphamethoxazole were 3.4 and 46.3 µg per ml respectively and had fallen to 1.8 and 23.8 µg per ml at 8 hours. On the fourth day mean plasma concentrations immediately after an infusion were 8.8 µg per ml for trimethoprim and 105.6 µg per ml for sulphamethoxazole and had fallen to 5.8 and 69 µg per ml at 8 hours. The estimated half-life of 7.7 hours for trimethoprim on day 1 increased to 11.3 hours on day 4 and likewise increased for sulphamethoxazole from 8.5 to 12.8 hours. About 22% of the dose of trimethoprim appeared in the urine within 8 hours and during the same time 22% of the dose of sulphamethoxazole appeared as free sulphamethoxazole and about 10% as metabolites.— W. E. Grose *et al.*, *Antimicrob. Ag. Chemother.*, 1979, *15*, 447.

Steady-state pharmacokinetics of co-trimoxazole in healthy subjects after rectal administration.— R. Liedtke and W. Haase, *Arzneimittel-Forsch.*, 1979, *29*, 345.

For comparative studies of the pharmacokinetics of co-trimazine and co-trimoxazole, see Co-trimazine, p.1460.

Further references: M. Donike *et al.*, *Arzneimittel-Forsch.*, 1977, *27*, 2373; D. J. Morgan and K. Raymond, *Antimicrob. Ag. Chemother.*, 1980, *17*, 132.

Diffusion. A review of tissue penetration of trimethoprim and sulphonamides. Trimethoprim is widely distributed in the body with some sequestration inside cells whereas sulphonamides are more confined to the blood and extracellular fluid. After the administration of co-trimoxazole the concentration ratios of trimethoprim to sulphonamide in body fluids other than blood are usually in the range 1:2 to 1:5, with wide individual variations.— P. J. Wilkinson and D. S. Reeves, *J. antimicrob. Chemother.*, 1979, *5*, *Suppl.* B, 159.

Co-trimoxazole 960 mg given to 6 patients with cataracts gave therapeutically effective concentrations in the aqueous humour.— P. E. J. Pohjanpelto *et al.*, *Br. J. Ophthal.*, 1974, *58*, 606. See also J. D. Salmon *et al.*, *J. antimicrob. Chemother.*, 1975, *1*, 205.

Active concentrations of trimethoprim were found in all samples of vaginal fluid from 7 women who were receiving co-trimoxazole either for treatment or prophylaxis of urinary-tract infections; concentrations were often greater than in serum. Sulphamethoxazole was either undetectable or present only in very low concentrations.— T. A. Stamey and M. Condy, *J. infect. Dis.*, 1975, *131*, 261, per *Abstr. Hyg.*, 1975, *50*, 715.

Concentrations of sulphamethoxazole and trimethoprim in saliva and blood.— F. B. Eatman *et al.*, *J. Pharmacokinet. Biopharm.*, 1977, *5*, 615.

Concentrations of sulphamethoxazole and trimethoprim in middle ear fluid.— J. J. Klimek *et al.*, *J. Pediat.*, 1980, *96*, 1087.

Effect of diseases states. The absorption of sulphamethoxazole from co-trimoxazole was increased in patients with coeliac disease.— R. L. Parsons *et al.*, *J. antimicrob. Chemother.*, 1975, *1*, 39.

Pregnancy and the neonate. A brief discussion on the pharmacokinetics of co-trimoxazole in pregnancy and labour.— A. Philipson, *Clin. Pharmacokinet.*, 1979, *4*, 297.

Uses. Co-trimoxazole is used similarly to the sulphonamides (p.1458) but in a wider variety of infections, in addition to urinary-tract and lower respiratory-tract infections. Trimethoprim (p.1485) alone may be preferred to co-trimoxazole in urinary-tract infections (see also under Antimicrobial Action above).

Co-trimoxazole is usually given by mouth in a dose of 960 mg (trimethoprim 160 mg and sulphamethoxazole 800 mg) twice daily for up to 14 days; 2.88 g daily in 2 or 3 divided doses may be given in severe infections. Lower doses are given for long-term treatment and in patients with renal impairment; co-trimoxazole is generally not recommended when the creatinine clearance is less than 15 ml per minute unless facilities for haemodialysis are available.

Suggested doses of co-trimoxazole to be given twice daily to children are: from 6 weeks to 5 months of age, 120 mg; 6 months to 5 years, 240 mg; 6 to 12 years, 480 mg. Higher doses of co-trimoxazole of 120 mg per kg body-weight daily given in 2 or 4 divided doses for 14 days are used in the treatment of *Pneumocystis carinii* pneumonia; blood concentrations of sulphamethoxazole should be monitored.

Co-trimoxazole is available for parenteral use when treatment by mouth is not possible. A solution of co-trimoxazole 960 mg in 3 ml is given by deep intramuscular injection in similar doses to the oral regimen. The intramuscular route should not be used for longer than 5 successive days, or 3 days if the maximum dose is given, and should not be used in children under 6 years of age. For serious infections co-trimoxazole may be given initially by intravenous infusion as a solution diluted immediately before use in the usual dextrose or electrolyte solutions; a suggested dose is 960 mg in 250 ml twice daily, up to a maximum of 1.44 g in 500 ml twice daily, each dose infused over about 90 minutes. The maximum dose should not be given for more than 3 days. A dose of 18 mg per kg body-weight twice daily has been suggested in children.

Some reviews of and general references on the actions and uses of co-trimoxazole.— *Drugs*, 1971, *1*, 7; *J. infect. Dis.*, 1973, *128*, *Suppl.*, 425-816, per *Abstr. Hyg.*, 1974, *49*, 428; *Trimethoprim-Sulphamethoxazole in Bacterial Infections*. A Wellcome Foundation Symposium, L.S. Bernstein and A.J. Salter (Ed), Edinburgh, Churchill Livingstone, 1973, per *Abstr. Hyg.*, 1974, *49*, 429; *New Engl. J. Med.*, 1974, *291*, 624; D. S. Reeves *et al.*, *Br. med. J.*, 1978, *2*, 410; T. A. McAlister, *Scott. med. J.*, 1978, *23*, 47; G. P. Wormser and G. T. Keusch, *Ann. intern. Med.*, 1979, *91*, 420; A. M. Geddes *et al.*, *J. antimicrob. Chemother.*, 1979, *5*, *Suppl.* B,

221; *Drug & Ther. Bull.*, 1979, *17*, 66; *J. antimicrob. Chemother.*, 1979, *5*, *Suppl.* B, 1–239; *Infection*, 1979, *7*, *Suppl.* 4, S309–S420; *Med. Lett.*, 1980, *22*, 5; R. H. Rubin and M. N. Swartz, *New Engl. J. Med.*, 1980, *303*, 426.

Criticism of the unnecessarily large amount of sulphamethoxazole in co-trimoxazole.— J. K. Seydel and E. Wempe, *Arzneimittel-Forsch.*, 1977, *27*, 1521.

For reports and comments on trimethoprim as an antibacterial agent in its own right, see Trimethoprim, p.1485.

Administration in infants and children. A suggested intravenous dose of co-trimoxazole for serious infections in neonates is 18 to 24 mg per kg body-weight, diluted immediately before use with 7 to 10 volumes of physiological saline and given not more than once every 12 hours. The smaller dose is suggested for preterm infants.— P. A. Davies, *Br. med. J.*, 1978, *2*, 676.

Administration in renal failure. Co-trimoxazole was given to 20 patients with varying degrees of renal impairment to treat respiratory or urinary-tract infections.

There was no deterioration in renal function in 17 and in the other 3 factors other than co-trimoxazole might have been responsible. The dose of co-trimoxazole was based on plasma-creatinine concentrations; for a creatinine clearance above 25 ml per minute and a plasma-creatinine concentration of less than 20 µg per ml for women or 30 µg per ml for men the dose was 960 mg twice daily. With a creatinine clearance of 25 to 15 ml per minute and a plasma concentration of 20 to 45 µg per ml for women and 30 to 70 µg per ml for men the dose was 960 mg twice daily for 3 days then once daily. Where the creatinine clearance was below 15 ml per minute and the plasma concentrations were greater than 45 or 70 µg per ml respectively for women and men, the dose was 960 mg daily.— P. R. W. Tasker *et al.*, *Lancet*, 1975, *1*, 1216.

Accumulation of conjugated sulphamethoxazole was reported in 9 uraemic patients with creatinine clearances of less than 20 ml per minute.— L. Gotloib (letter), *Lancet*, 1975, *2*, 365.

Further references: W. R. Adam *et al.*, *Aust. N.Z. J. Med.*, 1973, *3*, 383; J. B. Rosenfeld *et al.*, *Med. J. Aust.*, 1975, *2*, 547; P. Sharpstone, *Br. med. J.*, 1977, *2*, 36; W. M. Bennett *et al.*, *Ann. intern. Med.*, 1980, *93*, 62.

See also under Precautions and Absorption and Fate above.

Brucellosis. Twenty patients with chronic brucellosis were treated with co-trimoxazole 1.44 g twice daily till afebrile then 960 mg twice daily for 2 months. Fever subsided in 2 to 7 days. Two patients relapsed; in the other serum agglutination titres fell or became negative in a 2-year follow-up.— P. A. Kontoyannis *et al.*, *Br. med. J.*, 1975, *2*, 480.

Further references: S. Lal *et al.*, *Br. med. J.*, 1970, *3*, 256; A. Hassan, *ibid.*, 1971, *3*, 159; L. Sueri, *G. Mal. infett. parassit.*, 1972, *24*, 3; G. Giunchi *et al.*, *ibid.*, 77; G. Barba and N. Merlo, *ibid.*, 79; *Br. med. J.*, 1972, *2*, 344; E. Williams, *ibid.*, 1973, *1*, 791; L. A. Sueri, *G. Mal. infett. parassit.*, 1973, *25*, 65, per *Abstr. Hyg.*, 1973, *48*, 904; G. K. Daikos *et al.*, *J. infect. Dis.*, 1973, *128*, *Suppl.*, 731; G. Ciaccheri and F. Ramieri, *Archo ital. Sci. med. trop. Parassit.*, 1973, *54*, 17, per *Abstr. Hyg.*, 1974, *49*, 874; G. A. Rigatos *et al.*, *Münch. med. Wschr.*, 1975, *117*, 961.

Coccidiosis. A patient with chronic coccidiosis caused by *Isospora belli* was successfully treated with co-trimoxazole 960 mg every 6 hours for 10 days followed by 960 mg twice daily for 3 weeks.— E. L. Westerman and R. P. Christensen, *Ann. intern. Med.*, 1979, *91*, 413.

Crohn's disease. Co-trimoxazole was used to treat 20 patients with Crohn's disease; some improved and this treatment was considered superior to sulphasalazine.— R. D. Montgomery (letter), *Lancet*, 1975, *2*, 1149.

Endocarditis. Co-trimoxazole appears to be a promising agent in the treatment of endocarditis due to *Pseudomonas maltophilia*.— V. L. Yu *et al.*, *Archs intern. Med.*, 1978, *138*, 1667.

Enteric infections. *Cholera.* Co-trimoxazole is as effective as tetracycline in the treatment of cholera but had no advantage over it.— C. V. Uylangco and V. B. Soriano, *J. Philipp. med. Ass.*, 1974, *50*, 111, per *Trop. Dis. Bull.*, 1975, *72*, 309.

Co-trimoxazole 960 mg twice daily for 3 days was more effective than 3 days' treatment with either chloramphenicol or tetracycline in a controlled study of 175 patients with cholera (biotype *eltor*). Co-trimoxazole also showed greater activity *in vitro*.— J. K. Dutta *et al.*, *Trans. R. Soc. trop. Med. Hyg.*, 1978, *72*, 40. Criticism of the study; tetracycline is still the agent of choice in the treatment of cholera.— W. E. Woodward (letter), *Trans. R. Soc. trop. Med. Hyg.*, 1979, *73*, 247.

For a further report of the use of co-trimoxazole in the treatment of cholera, see Tetracycline Hydrochloride, p.1221.

Shigellosis. Co-trimoxazole was superior to furazolidone in children with gastro-enteritis due to *Shigella* infection. All of 33 children given co-trimoxazole were cured and the infection eradicated within 4 days. Of 104 strains of *Shigella* all were resistant to sulphamethoxazole and 63.3% were sensitive to trimethoprim. All were sensitive to the 2 drugs together.— U. Lexomboom *et al.*, *Br. med. J.*, 1972, *3*, 23.

Co-trimoxazole was as effective as ampicillin in a study of 28 children with acute shigellosis and was also active against ampicillin-resistant strains of *Shigella*.— J. D. Nelson *et al.*, *J. Am. med. Ass.*, 1976, *235*, 1239. See also *idem*, *J. Pediat.*, 1976, *89*, 491.

Co-trimoxazole was considered to be more effective than ampicillin in a study of 19 children with shigellosis. There was a marked decrease in the sensitivity of *Shigella* spp. to ampicillin.— M. J. Chang *et al.*, *Pediatrics*, 1977, *59*, 726.

Co-trimoxazole is considered the antibacterial agent of first choice in the treatment of shigellosis. Resistance may be a problem and sensitivity tests should be performed.— *Med. Lett.*, 1980, *22*, 5.

Further references: F. A. Barada and R. L. Guerrant, *Antimicrob. Ag. Chemother.*, 1980, *17*, 961.

Typhoid fever. Despite a more prompt clinical response in typhoid fever to treatment with co-trimoxazole when compared with chloramphenicol, the incidence of persistent positive blood cultures, lack of response, relapse-rate, and carrier-rate were higher than with chloramphenicol, which remained the treatment of choice.— J. N. Scragg and C. J. Rubidge, *Br. med. J.*, 1971, *3*, 738.

Further reports suggesting that chloramphenicol is the treatment of choice in susceptible typhoid fever.— E. S. Anderson (letter), *Lancet*, 1973, *2*, 1494; M. J. Snyder *et al.*, *ibid.*, 1976, *2*, 1155; T. Butler *et al.*, *Antimicrob. Ag. Chemother.*, 1977, *11*, 645.

Only 1 of 15 chronic carriers (6 *Salmonella typhi* and 9 *S. paratyphi B*) failed to respond to 3 months' treatment with co-trimoxazole 960 mg twice daily in 10 patients and thrice daily in 5 patients. The resistant patient excreted *S. paratyphi B* 1 week after the end of treatment but none of the other 14 had positive stools during a follow-up period of 1 year.— H. Pichler and K. H. Spitzy, *Dt. med. Wschr.*, 1972, *97*, 1401, per *Germ. Med.*, 1972, *2*, 114. See also H. Schmidt *et al.*, *Dte GesundhWes.*, 1977, *32*, 563, per *Int. pharm. Abstr.*, 1977, *14*, 1240; S. Iwarson, *Scand. J. infect. Dis.*, 1977, *9*, 297.

The effect of co-trimoxazole was compared with that of chloramphenicol in 2 groups each of 50 patients with bacteriologically confirmed typhoid fever. All patients in each group responded; the mean time to defervescence was similar, but toxic symptoms (headache, confusion, disorientation, delirium, and involuntary movements) were resolved more rapidly in those treated with co-trimoxazole; 2 patients treated with chloramphenicol relapsed. The doses were: co-trimoxazole 1.92 g twice daily until defervescence, then 960 mg twice daily for 7 days; chloramphenicol 500 mg six-hourly until defervescence, then 250 mg six-hourly for 14 days.— H. V. Sardesai *et al.*, *Br. med. J.*, 1973, *1*, 82. See also A. Hassan *et al.* (letter), *ibid.*, *3*, 108 and 418.

Comparable results with co-trimoxazole or amoxycillin in the treatment of chloramphenicol-sensitive and chloramphenicol-resistant typhoid fever. Both regimens were effective but co-trimoxazole resulted in more rapid lysis of fever in infections due to chloramphenicol-sensitive strains.— R. H. Gilman *et al.*, *J. infect. Dis.*, 1975, *132*, 630.

A report recommending ampicillin or co-trimoxazole in the treatment of typhoid fever due to *S. typhi* resistant to chloramphenicol, streptomycin, sulphonamide, and tetracycline.— T. Butler *et al.*, *Antimicrob. Ag. Chemother.*, 1977, *11*, 645.

Co-trimoxazole was used successfully to treat typhoid fever in 37 children with glucose-6-phosphate dehydrogenase deficiency; only one patient showed definite signs of haemolysis.— U. Lexomboon and N. Unkurapiana, *S.E. Asian J. trop. med. publ. Hlth*, 1978, *9*, 576, per *Trop. Dis. Bull.*, 1979, *76*, 897.

Further references.— M. Kazemi *et al.*, *J. Pediat.*, 1973, *83*, 646; D. Portnoy and S. Seah, *Can. med. Ass. J.*, 1979, *120*, 1264.

Other enteric infections. A patient suffering from severe diarrhoea caused by *Salmonella typhimurium* resistant to ampicillin and chloramphenicol, had a good response to co-trimoxazole. Co-trimoxazole should be considered the antibacterial agent of choice for *S. typhimurium* in Israel, and because of growing resistance of *S. typhimurium* to ampicillin and chloramphenicol in the world, deserves worldwide consideration.— R. Enat *et al.* (letter), *Lancet*, 1978, *2*, 638.

A young man with acute gastro-enteritis due to *Plesiomonas shigelloides*, transmitted from an infected snake, was successfully treated with co-trimoxazole.— W. A. Davis *et al.*, *Sth. med. J.*, 1978, *71*, 474, per *Abstr. Hyg.*, 1978, *53*, 965.

Acute gastro-enteritis in children aged 2 months to 2 years was generally cured within 5 days of treatment with co-trimoxazole.— A. G. Billoo and A. Malik, *Curr. med. Res. Opinion*, 1978, *5*, 439.

Before culture results are available severe travellers' diarrhoea may be treated with co-trimoxazole 480 mg every 12 hours for 5 days.— *Med. Lett.*, 1979, *21*, 41.

A prolonged dysentery-like syndrome associated with repeated recovery of *Aeromonas hydrophilia* from stool cultures in a patient was relieved by the administration of co-trimoxazole 960 mg twice daily.— A. F. M. S. Rahman and J. M. T. Willoughby, *Br. med. J.*, 1980, *281*, 976.

Gonorrhoea. In a study in more than 600 patients with gonorrhoea, cure-rates for women and men respectively were 96.4 and 90.5% for those given co-trimoxazole 960 mg twice daily for 5 days; 95.3 and 95.5% for those given 1.44 g twice daily for 3 days plus a further dose of 960 mg; and 98.8 and 99% for those given 1.92 g twice daily for 2 days. There were numerous resistant or semi-resistant strains but failures were not due to resistance.— H. B. Svindland, *Br. J. vener. Dis.*, 1973, *49*, 50.

In 419 patients with gonorrhoea treated with co-trimoxazole 4.8 g in 2 equal doses 8 hours apart, the failure-rate was 1.9%. Of 319 patients treated with pivampicillin 1.4 g and probenecid 1 g the failure-rate was 0.9%. Of 9 with pharyngeal infection treated with co-trimoxazole all were cured, but 2 of 13 treated with pivampicillin did not respond. Post-gonococcal urethritis occurred in 3.4% of the first group and 7.7% of the second.— J. K. Kristensen and E. From, *Br. J. vener. Dis.*, 1975, *51*, 31.

In 271 men with uncomplicated gonorrhoea failure-rates were significantly higher in those given co-trimoxazole, either as a single dose of 4.32 g or in a dose of 2.88 g repeated after 6 hours, than in those given procaine penicillin and probenecid.— W. C. Elliott *et al.*, *J. infect. Dis.*, 1977, *135*, 939.

A suggested regimen for the treatment of uncomplicated gonorrhoea is co-trimoxazole 2.88 g, as a single dose, daily for 3 days. There are regional differences in gonococcal resistance to co-trimoxazole and further studies are needed to assess its effectiveness against beta-lactamase-producing gonococci.— *Neisseria gonorrhoeae and gonococcal infections*, Report of a WHO Scientific Group, *Tech. Rep. Ser. Wld Hlth Org. No. 616*, 1978.

There was a failure-rate of 9.1% in men with urethritis due to beta-lactamase-producing strains of gonococci who were given a single daily dose of co-trimoxazole 4.32 g for 3 consecutive days.— *Morb. Mortal.*, 1978, *27*, 10.

Co-trimoxazole 1.92 g by intramuscular injection followed 12 hours later by an oral dose of 2.88 g was used successfully in the treatment of simple gonorrhoea.— A. Lassus and O. -V. Renkonen, *Br. J. vener. Dis.*, 1979, *55*, 24.

Further references.— S. Ullman *et al.*, *Acta derm.-vener., Stockh.*, 1971, *51*, 394, per *Abstr. Hyg.*, 1972, *47*, 33; M. A. Waugh, *Br. J. vener. Dis.*, 1971, *47*, 34; A. J. Evans *et al.*, *ibid.*, 1972, *48*, 179; A. Z. Meheus *et al.*, *ibid.*, 1974, *50*, 447.

For the use of co-trimoxazole and benethamine penicillin in the treatment of gonorrhoea, see Benethamine Penicillin, p.1101.

Granuloma inguinale. Ulcers were healed and Donovan bodies eradicated within 14 days in 10 patients with granuloma inguinale who were treated with co-trimoxazole 960 mg twice daily.— B. R. Garg *et al.*, *Br. J. vener. Dis.*, 1978, *54*, 348.

Herpes. Co-trimoxazole has been used successfully for treating type 1 genital herpes simplex infections and for herpes zoster.— P. H. Gosling (letter), *Br. med. J.*, 1974, *3*, 473. Penicillin given concomitantly nullified the effect of co-trimoxazole. About 15 to 20% of patients did not respond to this treatment.— *idem*, 1975, *1*, 41.

Co-trimoxazole did not inhibit the growth of herpes simplex virus in tissue cultures. The reported clinical benefit was unexplained.— D. H. Watson and D. Haigh (letter), *Br. med. J.*, 1975, *1*, 271.

Further references.— S. M. Laird and R. B. Roy, *Br. J.*

clin. Pract., 1975, 29, 37.

Histoplasmosis. Co-trimoxazole appeared to have a beneficial effect in 2 patients with histoplasmosis due to *Histoplasma duboisii*.— J. U. Egere *et al.*, *J. trop. Med. Hyg.*, 1978, *81*, 225, per *Trop. Dis. Bull.*, 1979, *76*, 749.

Leishmaniasis. A favourable response was obtained in a patient with systemic leishmaniasis (kala-azar) after treatment with co-trimoxazole and metronidazole. Enhanced activity might have been obtained when these 2 agents were used together.— K. J. Murphy and A. C. W. Bong (letter), *Lancet*, 1981, *1*, 323. Doubt as to the diagnosis of kala-azar, and a report of a patient who did not respond to co-trimoxazole.— J. Guardia (letter), *ibid.*, 501. Doubt as to the role of co-trimoxazole. A rapid response had been obtained in a patient treated with metronidazole alone.— J. Masramon *et al.* (letter), *ibid.*, 669.

Leprosy. Following a pilot study in which the effect of co-trimoxazole 960 mg daily appeared better than conventional treatment of plantar ulcers in patients with leprosy, 68 such patients were treated with co-trimoxazole (10 were given a loading dose of 2.88 g daily for 10 days); in 17 the condition was arrested and in 30 patients it improved.— G. Tarabini-Castellani, *Medna trop.*, 1971, *47*, 236, per *Trop. Dis. Bull.*, 1972, *69*, 754.

Melioidosis. The successful use of co-trimoxazole in the treatment of pulmonary melioidosis.— J. F. John, *Am. Rev. resp. Dis.*, 1976, *114*, 1021, per *Trop. Dis. Bull.*, 1977, *74*, 300.

Meningitis. The overall mortality-rate in 108 patients with bacterial meningitis usually due to *Neisseria meningitidis*, *Streptococcus pneumoniae*, or *Haemophilus influenzae* treated with co-trimoxazole was 28%, compared with 27% in 130 treated with ampicillin, and 38.5% in 606 treated with benzylpenicillin, chloramphenicol, and sulphonamides. In a few patients studied, sulphamethoxazole and trimethoprim appeared to diffuse readily into the CSF. Co-trimoxazole was given by mouth or by intramuscular or intravenous injection in a mean dose of 56.4 mg per kg body-weight daily.— C. Lafaix *et al.*, *Advances in Antimicrobial and Antineoplastic Chemotherapy*, Vol. I/2, M. Hejzlar *et al.* (Eds), London, University Park Press, 1972, p. 1227.

Meningitis due to *Pseudomonas cepacia* in a 2-month-old infant responded promptly to co-trimoxazole after other treatment had failed.— C. P. Darby, *Am. J. Dis. Child.*, 1976, *130*, 1365.

Further references: K. G. Sabel and Å. Brandberg, *Acta paediat. scand.*, 1975, *64*, 25; K. G. Sabel, *Scand. J. infect. Dis.*, 1976, *Suppl.* 8, 86; Z. Farid *et al.* (letter), *Ann. intern. Med.*, 1976, *84*, 50; F. S. Faella *et al.*, *G. Mal. infett. parassit.*, 1979, *31*, 877, per *Abstr. Hyg.*, 1980, *55*, 696.

Mycetoma. In a study of the medical treatment of 144 patients with actinomycetoma, initially 12 received sulfadoxine, 12 received dapsone, and 12 received co-trimoxazole, for an average of 3 months. On statistical analysis the latter 2 were superior to sulfadoxine which was therefore dropped from the study. The 36 patients were then incorporated into second- and third-stage studies together with an additional 108 patients; each patient served as his own control. The following drug regimens were given: co-trimoxazole, dapsone, co-trimoxazole with streptomycin, dapsone with streptomycin, sulfadoxine with pyrimethamine and streptomycin, and rifampicin with streptomycin. Of the 144 patients, 91 (63.2%) were cured and 31 (21.5%) obtained great improvement; all infections caused by *Actinomadura pelletieri* (14), *A. madurae* (13) and *Nocardia brasiliensis* (4) were easily cured; the few cases that did not respond to treatment were among the 133 caused by *Streptomyces somaliensis*. Cures were obtained within 4 to 24 months (average about 9 months), treatment being successful even when bone involvement was advanced. Dapsone with streptomycin and co-trimoxazole with streptomycin were the most effective treatments, neither drug association being clearly superior, although certain strains appeared to respond better to one or other regimen. Good results were also obtained in the few patients treated with the other 2 regimens, making them a useful second line of therapy. Side-effects to all the drugs included moderate to severe leucopenia and/or anaemia, and reversible streptomycin-associated tinnitus developed in 3 patients. Although only 2 of 20 patients with maduromycetoma caused by *Madurella mycetomatis* were cured by griseofulvin (7 mg per kg body-weight daily in a single dose after a fatty lunch) together with penicillin, this association was considered to have an indication as an adjunct to surgery. Despite being effective *in vivo* clotrimazole was ineffective by mouth or by infiltration of the lesions with a 1% solution, and was toxic. Usual doses of the drugs given were as follows: clotrimazole 20 mg per kg body-weight thrice daily; sulfadoxine 14 mg per kg on 3 days a week; dapsone 1.5 mg per kg morning and evening; co-trimoxazole 13.8 mg per kg twice daily; streptomycin sulphate 14 mg per kg daily for a month then reduced to alternate days; rifampicin 4.3 mg per kg morning and evening; and tablets containing sulfadoxine 500 mg and pyrimethamine 25 mg at a dose of 7.5 mg per kg once or twice a week.— E. S. Mahgoub, *Bull. Wld Hlth Org.*, 1976, *54*, 303.

Further references.— E. S. Mahgoub, *Am. J. trop. med. Hyg.*, 1972, *21*, 332; *Lancet*, 1977, *2*, 23; J. M. Saksun *et al.*, *Can. med. Ass. J.*, 1978, *119*, 911.

Nocardiosis. Within 4 days, co-trimoxazole 1.44 g every 12 hours improved the condition of a 37-year-old man with systemic nocardiosis. Previous treatment with sulphadiazine and streptomycin had been unsuccessful. No undesirable side-effects were detected after 12 weeks of therapy.— A. G. Baikie *et al.* (letter), *Lancet*, 1970, *2*, 261.

A brain abscess due to *Nocardia asteroides* developed in a patient during therapy with ampicillin and sulphadiazine or sulphafurazole for pulmonary nocardiosis. The cerebral nocardiosis was treated with surgical excision and a 3-month course of co-trimoxazole. Six hours after trimethoprim 160 mg by mouth, concentrations in infected brain tissue were 5.1 µg per g.— E. G. Maderazo and R. Quintiliani, *Am. J. Med.*, 1974, *57*, 671.

A report of the failure of co-trimoxazole in invasive *Nocardia asteroides* infection.— P. J. Geiseler *et al.*, *Archs intern. Med.*, 1979, *139*, 355.

Further references.— F. V. Cook and W. E. Farrar, *Sth. med. J.*, 1978, *71*, 512.

Osteomyelitis. In 6 patients with acute osteomyelitis due to penicillin-resistant staphylococci, treatment with co-trimoxazole brought a prompt and rapid response. One or 2 doses of 480 mg were given twice daily for 28 to 147 days. The temperature returned to normal after 3 to 9 days of treatment.— J. L. Craven *et al.*, *Br. med. J.*, 1970, *3*, 201.

Otitis media. A review of the use of co-trimoxazole in the treatment of otitis media. It was of use as an alternative treatment in patients who did not respond to ampicillin or amoxycillin.— *Med. Lett.*, 1978, *20*, 59.

Further references: J. Cooper *et al.*, *Practitioner*, 1976, *217*, 804; P. A. Shurin *et al.*, *J. Pediat.*, 1980, *96*, 1081.

Pediculosis capitis. A study in 20 patients with lice infestation showed that co-trimoxazole in doses of 480 mg twice daily for 3 days caused the lice to leave infested areas during the first day, and die after leaving the body. Neither sulphamethoxazole nor trimethoprim alone had any effect and co-trimoxazole had no effect on eggs present. A second course of treatment 10 days after the first was given to free the patients from lice.— C. H. Shashindran *et al.*, *Br. J. Derm.*, 1978, *98*, 699.

Pertussis. A suggestion that co-trimoxazole 240 mg twice daily for at least 7 days should be considered for the prophylaxis of vulnerable infants exposed to whooping cough.— G. C. Arneil and T. A. McAllister (letter), *Lancet*, 1977, *2*, 33. Erythromycin was considered to offer the best prophylaxis.— E. Rabo (letter), *ibid.*, 707. Erythromycin was of value but was second choice after co-trimoxazole.— G. C. Arneil and T. A. McAllister (letter), *ibid.*, 708. See also H. Lambert, *J. antimicrob. Chemother.*, 1979, *5*, 329.

There were no cases of pertussis in 24 children at risk who had received co-trimoxazole prophylactically.— A. S. Cullen and H. B. Cullen (letter), *Lancet*, 1978, *1*, 556.

Plague. All of 50 strains of *Yersinia pestis* were sensitive to co-trimoxazole, which had been successfully used in the treatment of 12 patients.— Nguyen-Van-Ai *et al.* (letter), *Br. med. J.*, 1973, *4*, 108.

For a report of streptomycin being more successful than co-trimoxazole in the treatment of plague, see Streptomycin, p.1215.

Pneumocystis carinii pneumonia. Co-trimoxazole is the treatment of choice for infections caused by *Pneumocystis carinii*.— *Med. Lett.*, 1980, *22*, 5. See also W. T. Hughes, *New Engl. J. Med.*, 1976, *295*, 726; *idem*, 1977, *297*, 1381; D. J. Winston *et al.*, *Ann. intern. Med.*, 1980, *92*, 762.

A study in *rats* suggested that co-trimoxazole was not effective in the total eradication of *Pneumocystis carinii* and concluded that immunosuppressed patients receiving co-trimoxazole could only be protected during the time of its administration.— W. T. Hughes, *Antimicrob. Ag. Chemother.*, 1979, *16*, 333.

In adults. In a preliminary study 5 of 7 immunosuppressed adult patients recovered from *Pneumocystis carinii* pneumonia following treatment with high doses of co-trimoxazole ranging from 5.76 to 7.2 g daily; an eighth patient could not be evaluated. These results were comparable to those reported for pentamidine isethionate with the advantages of less nephrotoxicity, oral as well as parenteral administration, and greater ease of monitoring therapy.— W. K. Lau and L. S. Young, *New Engl. J. Med.*, 1976, *295*, 716. Blood concentrations following oral administration could be inadequate.— J. S. Miser *et al.* (letter), *ibid.*, 1977, *296*, 47.

Pneumonia due to *Pneumocystis carinii* in a renal transplant patient with substantial renal failure was successfully treated with co-trimoxazole in an initial dose of 3.36 g daily followed by a daily dose of 1.44 g in 3 divided doses for 14 days.— A. -M. Bourgault *et al.*, *Chest*, 1978, *74*, 91.

In children. In a study of 50 children co-trimoxazole was as effective as pentamidine in the treatment of *Pneumocystis carinii* pneumonia, was associated with far fewer adverse effects, and, unlike pentamidine, could be given by mouth. Up to 3.84 g of co-trimoxazole daily was given.— W. T. Hughes *et al.*, *J. Pediat.*, 1978, *92*, 285.

Further references.— W. T. Hughes *et al.*, *Can. med. Ass. J.*, 1975, *112*, 47S; M. Rao *et al.*, *J. Am. med. Ass.*, 1977, *238*, 2301; A. Lipson *et al.*, *Archs Dis. Childh.*, 1977, *52*, 314; M. Silverman and P. Kearney (letter), *ibid.*, 1978, *53*, 87; F. Endo *et al.* (letter), *ibid.*, 87; W. E. Larter *et al.*, *J. Pediat.*, 1978, *92*, 826.

Prophylaxis. In a 2-year double-blind study of 160 young cancer patients receiving chemotherapy which placed them at a 15% or greater risk of developing *Pneumocystis carinii* pneumonitis, none of 80 receiving trimethoprim 150 mg with sulphamethoxazole 750 mg per m^2 body-surface daily, in 2 equally divided doses at intervals of 12 hours, did so, whereas 17 of 80 who received placebo did so; 35 of the placebo patients and 36 of those receiving trimethoprim with sulphamethoxazole were studied for more than 1 year. Other infections were also less common in the active group; oral candidiasis was, however, more prevalent and 3 patients in the active group suffered disseminated candidiasis as against 1 in the placebo group.— W. T. Hughes *et al.*, *New Engl. J. Med.*, 1977, *297*, 1419.

A 2-week prophylactic course of co-trimoxazole in children with acute lymphoblastic leukaemia was unsatisfactory because it only delayed the onset of *Pneumocystis carinii* pneumonia.— L. J. Wolff and R. L. Baehner, *Am. J. Dis. Child.*, 1978, *132*, 525.

No significant prophylactic effect of co-trimoxazole in granulocytopenic patients during consolidation cancer chemotherapy.— B. Weiser *et al.*, *Ann. intern. Med.*, 1981, *95*, 436.

There was no difference in prophylaxis provided by co-trimoxazole alone or with framycetin and colistin in patients with acute leukaemia.— I. D. Starke *et al.*, *Lancet*, 1982, *1*, 5. Co-trimoxazole provided better prophylaxis than neomycin with colistin.— J. G. Watson *et al.*, *ibid.*, 6.

Failure of co-trimoxazole prophylaxis in acute leukaemia.— J. M. Wilson and D. G. Guiney, *New Engl. J. Med.*, 1982, *306*, 16.

Prostatitis. A recommendation that co-trimoxazole 960 mg twice daily be given for at least 30 days to patients with acute prostatitis due to sensitive bacteria. A similar dose is suggested for chronic prostatitis; trimethoprim is considered the agent of choice, especially because of the high concentrations achieved in prostatic fluid.— E. M. Meares, *Drugs*, 1978, *15*, 472. See also N. J. Blacklock, *Practitioner*, 1979, *223*, 318.

Further references.— E. M. Meares, *Urology*, 1978, *11*, 142; D. F. Paulson and R. D. White, *J. Urol.*, 1978, *120*, 184.

Respiratory infections. A review of the treatment of bacterial respiratory infections in infants and children.— H. C. Spratt *et al.*, *Drugs*, 1978, *16*, 115.

A double-blind study in 197 children with respiratory-tract infection showed that the routine use of antimicrobial agents (amoxycillin or co-trimoxazole) was only of marginal benefit except in the presence of streptococcal infection.— B. Taylor *et al.*, *Br. med. J.*, 1977, *2*, 552.

Bronchitis. A recommendation to use ampicillin or co-trimoxazole to treat acute exacerbations of bronchitis. Prophylaxis in chronic bronchitis is controversial but if considered necessary, tetracycline or co-trimoxazole may be used.— D. T. D. Hughes and D. W. Empey, *Practitioner*, 1979, *223*, 771. See also A. E. Tattersfield, *Br. med. J.*, 1978, *1*, 1123; *Med. Lett.*, 1980, *22*, 68.

In a double-blind study in 200 patients with acute purulent exacerbations of chronic bronchitis, co-trimoxazole 2.88 g daily was as effective as tetracycline 2 g daily in reducing purulence of sputum; clinical and bacteriological deterioration 1 month after treatment was more marked with tetracycline.— A. Pines *et al.*, *Practitioner*, 1972, *208*, 265. See also *idem*, *210*, 556.

Ampicillin 4 g taken daily for 10 days by 20 patients was as effective as co-trimoxazole 1.92 g taken daily by 21 patients in the treatment of acute exacerbations of chronic bronchitis.— J. Joly *et al.*, *J. antimicrob. Chemother.*, 1977, *3*, 429.

Further reports of co-trimoxazole and amoxycillin being equally effective in the treatment of acute bronchitis.— M. K. Tandon, *Med. J. Aust.*, 1977, *2*, 281; P. G. Carroll *et al.*, *ibid.*, 286.

Further reports comparing co-trimoxazole and amoxycillin in bronchitis.— A. Pines *et al.*, *Chemotherapy, Basle*, 1977, *23*, 58; J. Cooper *et al.* , *Wellcome, Practitioner*, 1978, *220*, 798.

Comparable results with co-trimoxazole 960 mg or cephalexin 1 g, given twice daily for 7 days, in a multicentre study of 57 patients with acute exacerbations of chronic bronchitis.— J. Cooper and F. B. McGillion, *Practitioner*, 1978, *221*, 428.

Similar beneficial results with co-trimoxazole or doxycycline in patients with acute exacerbations of chronic bronchitis.— G. J. Pandy, *Med. J. Aust.*, 1979, *1*, 264. An earlier study in which co-trimoxazole was reported to be more effective than doxycycline.—Report No. 177 of the General Practitioner Research Group, *Practitioner*, 1972, *209*, 838.

Pneumonia. In the initial treatment of pneumonia, co-trimoxazole is considered the best alternative in patients allergic to penicillin.— R. B. Cole, *Practitioner*, 1979, *223*, 765.

Rheumatoid arthritis. Co-trimoxazole 1.44 g daily was given to 9 patients with rheumatoid arthritis which had remained stable but active for more than 6 months. During treatment which lasted 6 months, hand grip improved and erythrocyte sedimentation-rate decreased.— J. L. Kalliomaki, *Curr. ther. Res.*, 1972, *14*, 22.

Skin disorders. Treatment with co-trimoxazole, in doses reduced at weekly intervals from 1.92 g daily to 480 mg daily and continued for a total of 7 weeks, was effective in reducing pustular lesions and in preventing scaling and atrophy for at least the following 6 months in 23 of 24 Nigerian patients with dermatitis cruris pustulosa et atrophicans.— W. K. Jacyk, *Br. J. Derm.*, 1976, *95*, 71.

Skin lesions due to *Mycobacterium marinum* from infected tropical fish tanks occurred in 3 patients and were successfully controlled with co-trimoxazole. Complete resolution took up to 3 months.— M. M. Black and S. J. Eykyn, *Br. J. Derm.*, 1977, *97*, 689. See also R. Kelly, *Med. J. Aust.*, 1976, *2*, 681.

Acne. In 25 patients with acne treated under double-blind conditions with co-trimoxazole 480 mg daily, the response was comparable to that in 17 patients treated with oxytetracycline.— J. A. Cotterill *et al.*, *Br. J. Derm.*, 1971, *84*, 366. See also J. W. Harcup and J. Cooper, *Practitioner* 1980, *224*, 747.

There was improvement within 12 weeks in 12 patients with pustular acne vulgaris following twice daily doses of oxytetracycline 250 mg, co-trimoxazole 480 mg, or clindamycin 75 mg, each drug being given for 2 weeks in rotation.— L. Stankler, *Br. J. clin. Pract.*, 1979, *33*, 137.

Further references: J. A. Cotterill *et al.*, *Br. J. Derm.*, 1971, *85*, 130; Y. Privat, *Advances in Antimicrobial and Antineoplastic Chemotherapy*, Vol. I/2, M. Hejzlar *et al.* (Eds), London, University Park Press, 1972, p. 1387; K. Nordin *et al.*, *Dermatologica*, 1978, *157*, 245; I. Jen, *Cutis*, 1980, *26*, 106.

Surgical infection prophylaxis. In a double-blind study co-trimoxazole 960 mg given intravenously one hour before surgery reduced wound sepsis and postoperative pulmonary complications compared with a placebo; in groups of 48 and 47 patients respectively the incidence of wound sepsis was 21 and 4% and that of pulmonary complications 49 and 19%. Trimethoprim, but not sulphamethoxazole, was concentrated in the bile.— C. Morran *et al.*, *Br. med. J.*, 1978, *2*, 462.

Further references.— D. D. Mathews *et al.*, *Br. J. Obstet. Gynaec.*, 1979, *86*, 737.

Toxoplasmosis. In 7 patients with toxoplasmosis good therapeutic results were observed with co-trimoxazole in 5 with lymphoglandular toxoplasmosis and a significant reduction in dye test titres in 6. Treatment was discontinued in 1 patient because of an allergic reaction, and 1 patient relapsed 6.5 months after the end of treatment.— R. Norrby *et al.*, *Scand. J. infect. Dis.*, 1975, *7*, 72.

Dramatic recovery in an 11½-year-old girl with generalised toxoplasmosis after she was given co-trimoxazole 480 mg twice daily for one month.— M. Williams and D. C. L. Savage (letter), *Archs Dis. Childh.*, 1978, *53*, 829.

Although clinical experience with co-trimoxazole in toxoplasmosis is very limited it could be useful, especially in toxoplasmic meningitis.— F. J. Nye, *J. antimicrob. Chemother.*, 1979, *5*, 244.

Further references.— M. LaFrenz *et al.*, *Münch. med. Wschr.*, 1973, *115*, 2057; T. Thomaidis *et al.*, *Archs Dis. Childh.*, 1977, *52*, 403.

Urethritis. In 90 patients with nongonococcal urethritis followed up for 3 months, co-trimoxazole 960 mg twice daily for 6 days had a failure-rate of 22.4%.— R. R. Willcox and R. W. Sparrow, *Acta derm.-vener., Stockh.*, 1974, *54*, 317, per *Abstr. Hyg.*, 1974, *49*, 1095.

Urinary-tract infections. A report on the use of bladder instillations of co-trimoxazole in the treatment of urinary infections.— H. J. Hachen, *Chemotherapy, Basle*, 1978, *24*, 55.

No advantage of co-trimoxazole over sulphamethoxazole alone was demonstrated in a study of 118 children with acute urinary-tract infections given either treatment in a random double-blind manner.— J. B. Howard and J. E. Howard, *Am. J. Dis. Child.*, 1978, *132*, 1085.

A discussion on the possible use of trimethoprim alone rather than in combination with a sulphonamide in the treatment of urinary-tract infections.— W. Brumfitt and J. M. T. Hamilton-Miller, *Infection*, 1979, *7*, *Suppl.* 4, S388. See also under Trimethoprim, p.1486.

A study *in vitro* of the bactericidal effect of urine from healthy subjects given co-trimoxazole indicates that the usual dose of co-trimoxazole of 960 mg every 12 hours may be higher than is necessary to treat urinary infections.— J. M. Broughall *et al.*, *Infection*, 1979, *7*, 113.

In a double-blind controlled study of 42 men with recurrent invasive urinary-tract infections a 6-week course of co-trimoxazole resulted in fewer relapses than a conventional 2-week course.— R. Gleckman *et al.*, *New Engl. J. med.*, 1979, *301*, 878.

Further references.— W. Stögmann *et al.*, *Wien. med. Wschr.*, 1971, *121*, 10; R. R. Bailey, *Chemotherapy, Basle*, 1977, *23*, 7.

Comparative studies. Patients with urinary-tract infections (321 female, 18 male) were treated under double-blind conditions with ampicillin 1 g, cephalexin 1 g, co-trimoxazole 960 mg, or trimethoprim 200 mg, every 12 hours for 7 days. Overall success-rates for the 4 regimens were 73, 69, 83, and 83% respectively. For 149 courses of treatment given to pregnant patients the success-rates were 65, 78, 85, and 82% respectively. For general practice patients the respective figures were 89, 62, 81, and 96%, and for hospital patients 67, 62, 84, and 73%. Side-effects occurred about twice as often with the first 3 regimens as with trimethoprim alone. There was no evidence of the development of resistance in those treated with trimethoprim alone.— W. Brumfitt and R. Pursell, *Br. med., J.*, 1972, *2*, 673. For another comparison with cephalexin, see P. E. Gower and P. R. W. Tasker, *ibid.*, 1976, *1*, 684. Comment.— D. Greenwood and F. O'Grady (letter), *ibid.*, 1073.

Further comparisons with ampicillin.— B. G. Wren, *Med. J. Aust.*, 1972, *1*, 261; W. Böse *et al.*, *Lancet*, 1974, *2*, 614; N. S. Ellerstein *et al.*, *Pediatrics*, 1977, *60*, 245.

In a study of 122 patients with acute urinary-tract infections, 62 of the causative organisms were resistant to sulphonamide but sensitive to co-trimoxazole. Of 82 patients treated with sulphadimidine 2 g then 1 g every 6 hours for 1 week, 52 had positive cultures after 48 to 72 hours. Treatment with co-trimoxazole 480 mg twice daily to 20 of the sulphadimidine failures and to the remaining 40 patients was successful in 58. Rash in 1 and paraesthesia in another patient were associated with co-trimoxazole.— B. Senewiratne *et al.*, *Lancet*, 1973, *2*, 225.

Comparisons with nitrofurantoin.— J. Scherwin and P. Holm, *Chemotherapy, Basle*, 1977, *23*, 282; M. Gringras and J. Cooper, *Practitioner*, 1979, *223*, 357..

Further references.— K. M. D. Coltman, *Practitioner*, 1979, *223*, 351.

For comparative studies of co-trimoxazole and co-trimazine in urinary-tract infections, see Co-trimazine, p.1460.

For a report of rifampicin with trimethoprim being more effective than co-trimoxazole in the treatment of urinary-tract infections, see Rifampicin, p.1582.

Prophylaxis. Co-trimoxazole 240 mg daily was more effective in preventing re-infections of the female urinary tract than sulphamethoxazole 500 mg daily or hexamine mandelate 500 mg four times daily plus ascorbic acid.— G. K. M. Harding and A. R. Ronald, *New Engl. J. Med.*, 1974, *291*, 597.

There were only 6 episodes of urinary-tract infection in 130 children (mostly girls) treated prophylactically for 6 to 24 months with co-trimoxazole 12 mg per kg bodyweight daily (adjusted to the nearest 60 mg). There were no serious side-effects.— J. M. Smellie *et al.*, *Br. med. J.*, 1976, *2*, 203.

Bacteriological aspects of the study.— R. N. Grüneberg *et al.*, *ibid.*, 206.

In a prospective double-blind study completed by 74 patients co-trimoxazole prophylaxis produced a highly significant reduction in the incidence of bacteriuria after prostatectomy.— N. H. Hills *et al.*, *Br. med. J.*, 1976, *2*, 498.

A study of 28 women with persistent urinary-tract infections who received 6-month courses of low-dose co-trimoxazole (240 mg daily), or nitrofurantoin 100 mg daily. Although nitrofurantoin prophylaxis is adequate for the simpler problems of re-infection, where bacteriuria persisted co-trimoxazole is indicated.— T. A. Stamey *et al.*, *New Engl. J. Med.*, 1977, *296*, 780. Comment.— S. B. Levy, *ibid.*, 813.

Of 25 children with unobstructed urinary tracts who received prophylactic therapy with low-dose nitrofurantoin or co-trimoxazole following their initial treatment for a bacteriologically proven symptomatic urinary-tract infection, none developed a further infection during the average 10-month period of prophylaxis whereas of 22 similar children who received no prophylaxis 11 developed further infections. On completion of the prophylaxis 8 of the 25 children had a further infection within 1 year whereas in the year following the initial treatment 13 of the 22 who had not received prophylaxis did so, the difference not being significant. Of children who had had a previous urinary infection, however, only 8 of 18 who received prophylaxis had a further infection within a year of completing prophylaxis whereas all of 6 in the no-prophylaxis group did so in the year following initial treatment, this difference being significant.— J. M. Smellie *et al.*, *Lancet*, 1978, *2*, 175.

A study in 32 women who suffered from recurrent urinary-tract infections indicated that thrice weekly treatment with co-trimoxazole 240 mg was effective for prophylaxis and did not predispose to colonisation or infection with trimethoprim-resistant Enterobacteriaceae.— G. K. M. Harding *et al.*, *J. Am. med. Ass.*, 1979, *242*, 1975.

Further references.— J. M. Stansfeld, *Br. med. J.*, 1975, *3*, 65; R. H. Chinn *et al.*, *ibid.*, 1976, *2*, 1411.

Single-dose regimen. A single dose of co-trimoxazole 2.88 g given to adults and 0.72, 0.96, or 1.44 g to children aged 1 to 2 years, 2 to 5 years, and 5 to 12 years respectively, was as effective in the treatment of uncomplicated urinary-tract infections as conventional 5-to 7-day courses of co-trimoxazole given every 12 hours.— R. R. Bailey and G. D. Abbott, *Can. med. Ass. J.*, 1978, *118*, 551.

Single-dose treatment with co-trimoxazole is satisfactory only for lower urinary-tract infection; recurrent infections always require further investigations.— J. Z. Shainhouse (letter), *Can. med. Ass. J.*, 1978, *119*, 308. See also R. R. Bailey and G. D. Abbott (letter), *ibid.*

Further references.— *J. Am. med. Ass.*, 1979, *241*, 1226.

Use in the compromised patient. Fourteen children aged 15 years and over undergoing chemotherapy for acute leukaemia who received co-trimoxazole 960 mg twice daily prophylactically in addition to intestinal decontamination and other routine measures, were compared with 16 similar children who acted as controls. Only 8 children in the co-trimoxazole group developed infections requiring intravenous antibiotics, compared with 15 in the control group. Moreover, the patients in the co-trimoxazole group tolerated neutropenia for considerably longer before requiring antibiotics than those in the control group, and 2 patients in the control group died of infections. The results indicated that prophylactic administration of co-trimoxazole has an important role in preventing or delaying infection in patients undergoing chemotherapy for acute leukaemia.— A. Enno *et al.*, *Lancet*, 1978, *2*, 395.

A report of the successful use of co-trimoxazole given prophylactically to patients with granulocytopenia.— M. J. Gurwith *et al.*, *Am. J. Med.*, 1979, *66*, 248.

In a study of 53 profoundly granulocytopenic patients with relapsed leukaemia who were undergoing reinduction chemotherapy, co-trimoxazole plus nystatin was as effective as gentamicin plus nystatin for prophylaxis against infection. However, co-trimoxazole plus nystatin was less effective in preventing infections of the mouth, pharynx, and oesophagus. Side-effects were fewer and compliance better with co-trimoxazole and nystatin.— J. C. Wade *et al.*, *New Engl. J. Med.*, 1981, *304*, 1057.

Further references: C. L. Hall, *Br. med. J.*, 1974, *4*, 15; M. Gurwith, *J. antimicrob. Chemother.*, 1978, *4*, 302; *Lancet*, 1978, *2*, 769; *ibid.*, 1980, *1*, 25; S. C. Schimpff, *Ann. intern. Med.*, 1980, *93*, 358.

See also under *Pneumocystis carinii* pneumonia above.

Preparations

Injections

Co-trimoxazole Intravenous Infusion *(B.P.)*. Co-trimoxazole Injection. A sterile solution prepared immediately before use by diluting Strong Sterile Co-trimoxazole Solution with 25 to 35 volumes of Dextrose Intravenous Infusion or Sodium Chloride Intravenous Infusion.

Strong Sterile Co-trimoxazole Solution *(B.P.)*. Strong Sterile Co-trimoxazole Solution for the preparation of Co-trimoxazole Intravenous Infusion. A sterile solution of sulphamethoxazole sodium (prepared by the interaction of sulphamethoxazole and sodium hydroxide) and trimethoprim in the proportion 5:1, in Water for Injections containing propylene glycol 40% v/v and suitable stabilisers. Sterilise by autoclaving. pH 9.5 to 11. Protect from light. Dilute before use.

Mixtures

Co-trimoxazole Mixture *(B.P.)*. Sulphamethoxazole and Trimethoprim Mixture; Trimethoprim and Sulphamethoxazole Mixture. A suspension containing sulphamethoxazole 8% and trimethoprim 1.6% in a suitable flavoured vehicle which may be coloured. pH 5 to 6.5. Store at a temperature not exceeding 30°. Protect from light.

Paediatric Co-trimoxazole Mixture *(B.P.)*. Paediatric Sulphamethoxazole and Trimethoprim Mixture; Paediatric Trimethoprim and Sulphamethoxazole Mixture; Co-trimoxazole Mixture Paediatric. A suspension containing sulphamethoxazole 4% and trimethoprim 0.8% in a suitable flavoured vehicle which may be coloured. pH 5 to 6.5. Store at a temperature not exceeding 30°. Protect from light. When a dose less than 5 ml is prescribed, the mixture should be diluted to 5 ml with syrup. Such dilutions must be freshly prepared and not used more than 2 weeks after issue.

Sulfamethoxazole and Trimethoprim Oral Suspension *(U.S.P.)*. A suspension containing sulphamethoxazole and trimethoprim, with not more than 0.5% of alcohol. pH 5 to 6. Store in airtight containers. Protect from light.

Tablets

Co-trimoxazole Tablets *(B.P.)*. Trimethoprim and Sulphamethoxazole Tablets. Tablets containing co-trimoxazole. They may be film-coated or sugar-coated.

Dispersible Co-trimoxazole Tablets *(B.P.)*. Dispersible Trimethoprim and Sulphamethoxazole Tablets. Tablets containing co-trimoxazole.

Paediatric Co-trimoxazole Tablets *(B.P.C. 1973)*. Paediatric Trimethoprim and Sulphamethoxazole Tablets. Tablets each containing co-trimoxazole 120 mg.

Sulfamethoxazole and Trimethoprim Tablets *(U.S.P.)*. Tablets containing sulphamethoxazole and trimethoprim. Protect from light.

Proprietary Preparations

Bactrim *(Roche, UK)*. Co-trimoxazole, available as **Adult Suspension** containing 480 mg in each 5 ml (suggested diluent, syrup); as **Drapsules** and as scored **Tablets** (dispersible) each containing 480 mg; as scored **Double Strength Tablets** each containing 960 mg; as **Paediatric Syrup** containing 240 mg in each 5 ml (suggested diluent, syrup); and as **Paediatric Tablets** each containing 120 mg. **Bactrim for Infusion.** Ampoules of 5 ml for the preparation of intravenous infusion solutions, each containing co-trimoxazole 480 mg in a vehicle containing propylene glycol 40%. **Bactrim IM Injection.** Contains co-trimoxazole 320 mg per ml, in a vehicle containing glycofurol 52%, in ampoules of 3 ml. (Also available as Bactrim in *Arg., Austral., Belg., Canad., Denm., Fr., Ger., Ital., Norw., S.Afr., Swed., Switz., USA*).

Cotrimox *(Unimed, UK)*. Co-trimoxazole, available as tablets of 480 mg.

Fectrim *(DDSA Pharmaceuticals, UK)*. Co-trimoxazole, available as dispersible **Tablets** each containing 480 mg; as dispersible **Forte Tablets** each containing 960 mg; and as **Paediatric Tablets** each containing 120 mg.

Nodilon *(Berk Pharmaceuticals, UK)*. Co-trimoxazole, available as tablets of 480 mg.

Septrin *(Wellcome, UK)*. Co-trimoxazole, available as scored **Tablets** and **Dispersible Tablets** each containing 480 mg; as scored **Forte Tablets** each containing 960 mg; as **Adult Suspension** containing 480 mg in each 5 ml; as scored **Paediatric Tablets** each containing 120 mg; and as **Paediatric Suspension** containing 240 mg in each 5 ml (suggested diluent, syrup). **Septrin for Infusion.** Ampoules of 5 ml for the preparation of intravenous infusion solutions, each containing co-trimoxazole 480 mg in a vehicle containing propylene glycol 40%. **Septrin IM Injection.** Contains co-trimoxazole 320 mg per ml, in a vehicle containing glycofurol 52%, in ampoules of 3 ml. (Also available as Septrin in *Arg., Austral., Spain*).

Other Proprietary Names

Arg.—Bacticel, Dosulfin (with antacid), Enterobacticel (with adsorbent), Lescot, Missile; *Aust.*—Eusaprim; *Austral.*—Trib; *Belg.*—Eusaprim; *Braz.*—Espectrin, Septra, Uro-Septra; *Canad.*—Septra; *Denm.*—Sulfotrim, Trisural; *Fin.*—Eusaprim; *Fr.*—Eusaprim; *Ger.*—Co-trim, Drylin, Duratrimet, Eusaprim, Kepinol, Microtrim, Omsat, Sigaprim, Sulfacet, Sulfotrimin, TMS, Trigonyl, Trimethoprim comp.-ratiopharm; *Hong Kong*—Espectrin; *Ind.*—Septran; *Jap.*—Bactramin, Baktar; *Ital.*—Abacin, Bacterial, Chemitrin, Eusaprim, Gantaprim, Gantrim, Isotrim, Magisprim, Medixin, Oxaprim, Paitrin, Septocid, Suprim, System, Teleprim, Trim, Trimesulf; *Malaysia*—Espectrin; *Neth.*—Bactrimel, Eusaprim, Sulfotrim; *Norw.*— Eusaprim, Trimetoprim-Sulfa; *Pakistan*—Septran; *Phillipp.*—Espectrin; *Singapore*—Espectrin; *S.Afr.*—Co-Trim, Mezenol, Purbac, Septran, Thoxaprim, Ultrasept; *Spain*—Abactrim, Ampliespectrum, Bactifor, Biosulten, Brogenit, Dhas, Hulin, Ixazolina, Kitaprim, Metoprin, Sinerbactin, Soifasul, Tacumil, Trisazol; *Swed.*—Eusaprim, Trimetoprim-Sulfa; *Switz.*—Eusaprim, Helveprim, Nopil, Sulfotrim; *Urug.*—Septran; *USA*—Septra.

NOTE. Abasin is used as a proprietary name for acetylcarbromal. The name Dosulfin is also used in some countries as a proprietary name for a preparation containing sulphaproxyline ($C_{16}H_{18}N_2O_4S$ = 334.4) and sulfamerazine.

4905-a

Formosulphathiazole. Formosulfathiazole; Methylenesulfathiazole; C 6257. A condensation product of sulphathiazole with formaldehyde.

CAS — 12041-72-4.

Formosulphathiazole is a sulphonamide which is used for the treatment of local intestinal infections. It is also used topically, with other antibacterial agents, in veterinary practice.

Proprietary Names

Formilae *(Quimia, Spain)*; Formo-Cibazol *(Ciba, Ger.)*; Ormidal *(Estedi, Spain)*; Sunfintestin *(Hosbon, Spain)*.

4906-t

Mafenide Acetate *(U.S.P.)*. α-Aminotoluene-*p*-sulphonamide acetate.

$C_7H_{10}N_2O_2S,C_2H_4O_2$=246.3.

CAS — 138-39-6 (mafenide); 13009-99-9 (acetate).

Pharmacopoeias. In *Braz.* and *U.S.*

A white crystalline powder with a bitter taste. M.p. 162° to 171° with a range of not more than 4°. Mafenide acetate 11.2 g is approximately equivalent to 8.5 g of mafenide. Freely **soluble** in water; sparingly soluble in alcohol. A 10% solution in water has a pH of 6.4 to 6.8. **Store** in airtight containers. Protect from light.

4907-x

Mafenide Hydrochloride. Maphenide; Benzamsulfonamide Hydrochloride; Homosulfaminum; Sulfabenzaminum. α-Aminotoluene-*p*-sulphonamide hydrochloride.

$C_7H_{10}N_2O_2S,HCl$=222.7.

CAS — 138-37-4.

Pharmacopoeias. In *Aust., Jap.*, and *Pol.*

A colourless or white odourless crystalline powder with a bitter taste. M.p. about 260°. **Soluble** 1 in 1.7 of water, 1 in 0.7 of boiling water, and 1 in 100 of alcohol; practically insoluble in chloroform and ether. A 5% solution has a pH of about 5. A 3.55% solution in water is iso-osmotic with serum. **Sterilisation** of the powder as for Sulphadimidine, p.1475. **Store** in airtight containers. Protect from light.

4908-r

Mafenide Propionate. α-Aminotoluene-*p*-sulphonamide propionate.

$C_7H_{10}N_2O_2S,C_3H_6O_2$=260.3.

Colourless crystals. M.p. 158°. **Soluble** in water.

Adverse Effects. Since mafenide is absorbed by the skin, the adverse effects seen with sulphonamides (p.1457) used systemically may occur.

Mafenide acetate cream may cause pain or a burning sensation on application to the burnt area, particularly on burns of partial skin thickness. Allergic reactions associated with a maculopapular rash, urticaria, an eczematoid reaction, contact dermatitis, and erythema multiforme have occurred. The separation of the eschar may be delayed and fungal invasion of the wound has been reported. By its action in inhibiting carbonic anhydrase mafenide may cause metabolic acidosis and hyperventilation.

Allergy. In 400 burnt patients treated with mafenide acetate the incidence of cutaneous reactions (usually localised and minor) was 9.5%. Two patients developed erythema multiforme.— H. S. Yaffee and D. P. Dressler, *Archs Derm.*, 1969, *100*, 277, per *J. Am. med. Ass.*, 1969, *209*, 1922.

Three patients developed papulovesicular eruptions after 3 to 4 weeks' treatment with mafenide acetate cream. Patch tests were positive for mafenide but not for other sulphonamides.— J. E. Velasco and J. A. Africk, *Archs Derm.*, 1971, *103*, 61, per *Drugs*, 1971, *2*, 475.

Using the Draize procedure, mafenide 5% in soft paraffin produced sensitisation of the skin in 2 of 92 subjects, while a 20% concentration sensitised between 8 and 16% of subjects tested.— F. N. Marzulli and H. I. Maibach, *J. Soc. cosmet. Chem.*, 1973, *24*, 399.

Effects on the blood. Two children rapidly developed methaemoglobinaemia after the application of mafenide acetate cream to large areas of burns; there was possibly a hereditary predisposition.— M. Ohlgisser *et al.*, *Br. J. Anaesth.*, 1978, *50*, 299.

Treatment of Adverse Effects. Allergic reactions to mafenide usually respond to the administration of a suitable antihistamine, after which treatment has sometimes been recommenced. Treatment should be discontinued at least temporarily and continuous fluid therapy given if persistent acidosis occurs; the infusion of sodium bicarbonate and assisted ventilation may be necessary.

Precautions. Mafenide should not be used on patients with a known sensitivity to sulphonamides and should be used with care in patients with impaired respiratory function or renal impairment.

Absorption and Fate. Mafenide is absorbed from wounds into the circulation and is metabolised to *p*-carboxybenzenesulphonamide which is excreted in the urine. The metabolite has no antibacterial action but retains the ability to inhibit carbonic anhydrase.

Uses. Mafenide is a sulphonamide which is not inactivated by *p*-aminobenzoic acid or by pus and serum. The acetate is used as a cream, in conjunction with debridement, for the prevention and treatment of infection, particularly by *Pseudomonas aeruginosa*, in second- and third-degree burns. It is applied to a thickness of 1 to 2 mm once or twice daily by a sterile gloved hand and, although not usually necessary, may be covered by a thin gauze dressing. Treatment is continued until healing is progressing satisfactorily or the burn site is ready for skin grafting.

Mafenide hydrochloride has also been used topically.

A 5% solution of mafenide propionate is used for the treatment of superficial eye infections and for the prevention of infection after minor eye injuries.

Bacterial resistance. From a study *in vitro* it was considered unlikely that resistance to mafenide was emerging in isolates of bacteria from burn patients since these isolates were no more resistant to mafenide than those from other patients. There was no evidence of cross-resistance between mafenide and sulphadiazine or other antimicrobial agents.— S. L. Rosenthal *et al.*, *Curr. ther. Res.*, 1978, *24*, 682.

Burns. Reviews of the use of mafenide acetate in the treatment of burns.— *Drug & Ther. Bull.*, 1971, *9*, 39; I. F. K. Muir, *Drugs*, 1971, *1*, 429; *ibid.*, 434; R. J. Moleski, *Drug Intell. & clin. Pharm.*, 1978, *12*, 28.

The following topical preparations were considered to be effective *in vitro* against many of the organisms obtained over an 18-month period from the wounds of burn patients: 0.1% gentamicin cream, 1% silver sulphadiazine, 8.5% mafenide acetate cream, and 0.2% nitrofurazone ointment. It was recommended that at least four effective topical agents should be available for clinical use.— I. A. Holder *et al.*, *J. antimicrob. Chemother.*, 1979, *5*, 455.

For a comparison of silver sulphadiazine and mafenide in the treatment of burns, see Silver Sulphadiazine, p.1469.

For earlier reports of the use of mafenide in patients with burns, see Martindale 27th Edn, p. 1469.

Preparations

Mafenide Acetate Cream *(U.S.P.)*. Mafenide acetate in a water-miscible oil-in-water cream basis, containing suitable preservatives. Potency is expressed in terms of the equivalent amount of mafenide. Store at a temperature not exceeding 40° in airtight containers. Protect from light.

Sulfamylon Cream *(Winthrop, UK)*. Contains mafenide acetate equivalent to mafenide 8.5% in a water-miscible basis. (Also available as Sulfamylon in *Arg., Austral., Canad., Denm., Fr., Swed., USA*).

Sulfomyl *(Winthrop, UK)*. Mafenide propionate, available as eye-drops containing 5%.

Other Proprietary Names of Mafenide Acetate

Mafylon *(S.Afr.)*; Napaltan *(Ger., Switz.)*.

4909-f

Noprylsulfamide. Thiasolucin; Sulphasolucin; RP 40. Disodium 1-phenyl-3-(4-sulphamoylanilino)propane-1,3-disulphonate.
$C_{15}H_{16}N_2Na_2O_8S_3$=494.5.

CAS — 576-97-6.

Noprylsulfamide is a sulphonamide used in veterinary practice.

4910-z

Paranitrosulphathiazole. 4-Nitro-*N*-(thiazol-2-yl)benzenesulphonamide.
$C_9H_7N_3O_4S_2$=285.3.

CAS — 473-42-7.

A yellow odourless powder with a slightly bitter taste. Very slightly **soluble** in water, chloroform, and ether; slightly soluble in alcohol; freely soluble in solutions of alkali hydroxides. **Protect** from light.

Paranitrosulphathiazole is a sulphonamide (p.1457) which was formerly instilled rectally in the treatment of ulcerative colitis and proctitis.

4911-c

Phthalylsulphacetamide. Sulfanilacetamidum Phthalylatum. 4′-(Acetylsulphamoyl)phthalanilic acid.
$C_{16}H_{14}N_2O_6S$=362.4.

CAS — 131-69-1.

Pharmacopoeias. In *Aust.* and *Ind.*

White or creamy-white crystals or crystalline powder with a slight odour and a slightly acid taste. M.p. 186° to 202° with decomposition. Very slightly **soluble** in water; slightly soluble in alcohol; soluble in acetone; freely soluble in solutions of alkali hydroxides. **Store** in airtight containers. Protect from light.

Phthalylsulphacetamide has actions and uses similar to those of phthalylsulphathiazole (below). It is poorly absorbed from the gastro-intestinal tract but to a greater extent than phthalylsulphathiazole or succinylsulphathiazole. The usual adult dose of phthalylsulphacetamide is 2 g thrice daily but up to 12 g daily in divided doses has been given.

Proprietary Names

Talecid *(Schering, Austral.)*; Thalacet *(Virax, Austral.)*.

4912-k

Phthalylsulphathiazole *(B.P., B.P. Vet.)*.

Phthalylsulphathiaz.; Phthalylsulfathiazolum; Phthalylsulfathiazole *(U.S.P.)*; Sulfaphtalylthiazol; Ftalilsulfatiazol; Phthalazolum. 4′-(Thiazol-2-ylsulphamoyl)phthalanilic acid.
$C_{17}H_{13}N_3O_5S_2$=403.4.

CAS — 85-73-4.

Pharmacopoeias. In *Arg., Br., Braz., Chin., Cz., Fr., Ind., Int., It., Neth., Nord., Port., Roum., Rus., Span., Swiss, Turk.*, and *U.S.*

White or yellowish-white, odourless crystals or powder with a slightly bitter taste; it darkens on prolonged exposure to light. M.p. about 275° with decomposition.

Practically **insoluble** in water, chloroform, and ether; soluble 1 in 600 of alcohol and 1 in 250 of acetone; freely soluble in dimethyl formamide and solutions of alkali hydroxides and carbonates, and in hydrochloric acid. **Protect** from light.

Adverse Effects, Treatment, and Precautions. As for Sulphonamides, p.1457.

The adverse effects that may occur with phthalylsulphathiazole are generally due to sulphathiazole (p.1484), to which phthalylsulphathiazole is hydrolysed in the large intestine. Allergic reactions may occur in patients sensitised by previous treatment with sulphonamides. The Stevens-Johnson syndrome has been reported after treatment with phthalylsulphathiazole.

Prolonged use of phthalylsulphathiazole may lead to overgrowth of *Candida* spp. Phthalylsulphathiazole may cause suppression of the synthesis of vitamins of the B group and vitamin K in the small intestine; when it is given over long periods these vitamins should be given concomitantly. The administration of liquid paraffin interferes with the action of phthalylsulphathiazole.

Absorption and Fate. Phthalylsulphathiazole is slowly hydrolysed to sulphathiazole in the large intestine and only about 5% is absorbed; concentrations of sulphonamide in the blood do not usually exceed 15 μg per ml but concentrations of up to 60 μg per ml have been reported.

Uses. Phthalylsulphathiazole has the antibacterial activity of Sulphonamides, p.1458, and is used for its bacteriostatic effect in the gastro-intestinal tract; it is preferred to succinylsulphathiazole (p.1469).

Phthalylsulphathiazole has been used in the treatment of bacillary dysentery but many strains of *Shigella* are now resistant to sulphonamides. A suggested adult dose in acute bacillary dysentery is 5 g or more daily in divided doses continuing for 24 hours after the diarrhoea ceases; infants may be given one-quarter and children one-half the adult dose. For short-term prophylaxis 1 g twice daily has been given to adults and children.

Phthalylsulphathiazole is sometimes used to reduce the bacterial count in the large bowel in patients undergoing surgery but many doubt its value. A suggested dose is 250 mg per kg body-weight 4 days before surgery, followed by 12 g daily in divided doses every 3 hours, and continued for 4 days after surgery.

Phthalylsulphathiazole has been used as an adjunct in the treatment of ulcerative colitis.

Preparations

Phthalylsulfathiazole Tablets *(U.S.P.)*. Tablets containing phthalylsulphathiazole. Protect from light.

Phthalylsulphathiazole Mixture CF *(A.P.F.)*. Phthalylsulphathiazole Mixture for Children. Phthalylsulphathiazole 500 mg, light kaolin or light kaolin (natural) 300 mg, compound tragacanth powder 100 mg, raspberry syrup 1 ml, benzoic acid solution 0.1 ml, concentrated chloroform water 0.1 ml, water to 5 ml. *Dose.* Phthalylsulphathiazole, 125 mg per kg body-weight daily in 4 to 6 divided doses.

Phthalylsulphathiazole Tablets *(B.P. 1973)*. Tablets containing phthalylsulphathiazole. Protect from light.

Proprietary Preparations

Neo-Sulfazon *(Wallace Mfg Chem., UK: Farillon, UK)*. Suspension containing in each 5 ml phthalylsulphathiazole 500 mg, kaolin 750 mg, and pectin 62.5 mg. For diarrhoea.

Thalazole *(May & Baker, UK)*. Phthalylsulphathiazole, available as tablets of 500 mg. (Also available as Thalazole in *Austral., S.Afr.*).

Other Proprietary Names

Austral.—Phthazol; *Belg.*—Ilentazol *(hydroxyquinoline derivative)*; *Canad.*—Sulfathalidine; *Fr.*—Talidine; *Ital.*—Colicitina, Enterosteril *(chlorquinaldol derivative)*, Novosulfina *(hydroxyquinoline derivative)*; *Spain*—Crematalil, Entero-Toxan *(hydroxyquinoline derivative)*, Sulfathalidin; *Swed.*—Sulftalyl; *Switz.*—Ilentazol *(hydroxyquinoline derivative)*.

4913-a

Silver Sulphadiazine.

The silver salt of N^1-(pyrimidin-2-yl)sulphanilamide.
$C_{10}H_9AgN_4O_2S$=357.1.

CAS — 22199-08-2.

Pharmacopoeias. In *Chin.*

A white powder. Practically **insoluble** in water.

The solubility of silver sulphadiazine as a function of pH.— R. U. Nesbitt and B. J. Sandmann, *J. pharm. Sci.*, 1977, *66*, 519.

Adverse Effects. Local reactions have been reported in about 2.5% of patients treated with silver sulphadiazine; the separation of the eschar may be delayed and fungal invasion of the wound may occur. Unlike mafenide acetate, the application of silver sulphadiazine is generally painless and metabolic acidosis has not been reported. Unlike silver nitrate, silver sulphadiazine does not cause staining and hypochloraemia with subsequent hyponatraemia does not occur since insufficient silver ions are released to precipitate significant amounts of chloride in the body.

Transient leucopenia has occurred although some workers consider it to be associated with the trauma of burns rather than the treatment with silver sulphadiazine.

Since significant amounts of sulphadiazine may be absorbed the adverse effects reported with sulphonamides (p.1457) given systemically may occur.

Effect on the blood. A report of leucopenia occurring in a patient with burns on the third day of treatment with silver sulphadiazine. A review of the available evidence suggests a definite association with silver sulphadiazine but unless sepsis is present there appears to be no need to stop treatment since the leucopenia is generally self-limiting.— G. L. Fraser and J. T. Beaulieu, *J. Am. med. Ass.*, 1979, *241*, 1928.

Effects on the kidney. The nephrotic syndrome occurred in a severely burnt patient after therapy with silver sulphadiazine.— C. J. Owens *et al.*, *Archs intern. Med.*, 1974, *134*, 332.

Precautions. As for Sulphonamides, p.1458.

Silver sulphadiazine cream should not generally be used on patients with a known sensitivity to sulphonamides and should be used with care in the presence of hepatic or renal impairment. Because of the possibility of kernicterus it should not be used in pregnant women near term or in newborn infants.

Absorption and Fate. Silver sulphadiazine is slowly metabolised in contact with wound exudates. Up to about 10% of the sulphadiazine may be absorbed; concentrations in blood of 10 to 20 μg per ml have been reported although higher concentrations may be achieved when extensive areas of the body are treated. Probably not more than 1% of the silver content is absorbed.

Following daily cleansing and application of 1% silver sulphadiazine cream to 12 patients with burns covering 7 to 63% of the body-surface, plasma and urinary concentrations of total sulphonamide were less than 6 μg per ml and 200 μg over a period of 24 hours, respectively. Risks of kidney damage were slight.— P. Delaveau and P. Friedrich-Noue, *Thérapie*, 1977, *32*, 563.

Uses. Silver sulphadiazine has broad antimicrobial activity against Gram-positive and Gram-negative bacteria, yeasts, and fungi. It has also been reported to be active *in vitro* against herpes virus and *Treponema pallidum*. This antimicrobial action is attributable to both silver and sulphadiazine and is not antagonised by *p*-aminobenzoic acid.

Silver sulphadiazine is used similarly to mafenide acetate (p.1467) for the prevention and treatment of infection, particularly by *Pseudomonas aeruginosa*, in severe burns. A 1% cream is usually applied daily to a thickness of 3 to 5 mm.

Silver sulphadiazine is antifungal *in vitro*, strains of *Candida, Aspergillus, Mucor*, and *Rhizopus* being inhibited by concentrations readily achieved by topical application.— T. J. Wlodkowski and H. S. Rosenkranz (letter), *Lancet*, 1973, *2*, 739.

All the species of dermatophytes tested were sensitive to 100 μg or less per ml of silver sulphadiazine.— W. T. Speck and H. S. Rosenkranz (letter), *Lancet*, 1974, *2*, 895.

Bacterial resistance. The increase in sulphadiazine resistance among Gram-negative bacilli was associated with the use of silver sulphadiazine in a burns unit; this was reversed, except in the case of *Proteus mirabilis*, when sulphonamides were withdrawn. There was evidence of transferable resistance to several antibiotics.— K. Bridges and E. J. L. Lowbury, *J. clin. Path.*, 1977, *30*, 160.

Burns. Reviews of the use of silver sulphadiazine in the treatment of burns.— J. A. Moncrief, *New Engl. J. Med.*, 1973, *288*, 444; *Med. Lett.*, 1974, *16*, 43; J. C. Ballin, *J. Am. med. Ass.*, 1974, *230*, 1184; J. Burke, *Aust. J. Hosp. Pharm.*, 1973, *3*, 147; R. J. Moleski, *Drug Intell. & clin. Pharm.*, 1978, *12*, 28.

Silver sulphadiazine 1% in a cream basis has the same silver content as a 0.475% solution of silver nitrate. Concentrations of silver ions and sulphadiazine in solution are about 12.5 μmol per litre. Both components in the complex are active against bacteria and there is some synergy with trimethoprim *in vitro*. The relative insolubility of silver sulphadiazine minimises absorption and systemic effects. In studies in burnt patients, a cream containing silver sulphadiazine 1% had no greater prophylactic value when trimethoprim 0.1% was added. Strains of Gram-positive and Gram-negative bacteria resistant to trimethoprim developed but there was no increase in resistance to sulphadiazine.— E. J. L. Lowbury *et al.*, *Injury*, 1971, *3*, 18.

Infection with *Pseudomonas aeruginosa* was much reduced when 49 patients with burns covering 10 to 80% of the body area were treated with a cream containing silver sulphadiazine. No retardation of wound healing was noted, but low serum-sodium concentrations were found up to 14 days after the burn occurred in a number of patients with extensive burns.— I. A. McDougall, *Med. J. Aust.*, 1972, *1*, 979.

Results in 22 extensively burnt patients treated with silver sulphadiazine cream 1% were compared with those in 25 treated with compresses of silver nitrate 0.5%. In a second study, results in 52 less extensively burnt patients treated with a cream containing silver nitrate 0.5% and chlorhexidine gluconate 0.2% were compared with 62 treated with silver sulphadiazine cream 1%; subsequently, results in 8 extensively burnt patients treated with the cream containing silver nitrate and chlorhexidine gluconate were compared with 17 treated with the silver sulphadiazine cream. The 3 preparations were found to be comparably effective in protecting burns from infection. Silver nitrate compresses were much less active against miscellaneous Gram-negative bacilli than the other preparations, and the morning and evening temperatures and respiration-rates of the patients treated with silver nitrate were higher than in those treated with silver sulphadiazine. *Ps. aeruginosa* and *Proteus* spp., although rare in all groups, were less common in those treated with silver nitrate compresses. Silver nitrate compresses could still give the best protection in burns of the genitalia and perineum where *Ps. aeruginosa* colonisation frequently began. The effectiveness of silver sulphadiazine was reduced in the later stages of the extensive-burns study by the emergence of resistant strains of various Gram-negative bacilli. After withdrawal of sulphonamides and silver sulphadiazine for 6 months, sensitivity in most of the Gram-negative bacilli reverted to earlier levels.— E. J. L. Lowbury *et al.*, *Br. med. J.*, 1976, *1*, 493. See also *idem*, *Lancet*, 1971, *2*, 1105.

Experimental work with zinc sulphadiazine in the treatment of pseudomonal infections in burnt *mice* and *rats*.— C. L. Fox *et al.*, *Surgery Gynec. Obstet.*, 1976, *142*, 553.

In a series of 645 patients with burns, silver sulphadiazine was statistically more effective than mafenide in terms of infection-rate and mortality-rate although neither treatment significantly decreased the rate of septicaemia when compared with a control group, some of whom were treated with other topical agents.— S. P. Pegg *et al.*, *Scand. J. plast. reconstr. Surg.*, 1979, *13*, 95.

Further references: *J. Am. med. Ass.*, 1968, *204* (May 6), A31; S. J. Dickinson, *N.Y. St. J. Med.*, 1973, *73*, 2045; J. R. Lloyd, *Archs Surg., Chicago*, 1974, *108*, 561; W. W. Monafo *et al.*, *Archs Surg., Chicago*, 1978, *113*, 397.

For the use of silver sulphadiazine in 40 patients with burns, see Gentamicin Sulphate, p.1171.

For a report of the addition of chlorhexidine to silver sulphadiazine cream reducing the staphylococcal infection-rate of burns, see p.555.

Skin disorders. Reports of the successful use of silver sulphadiazine in skin disorders.— D. Assaad *et al.*, *Can. med. Ass. J.*, 1978, *118*, 154 (epidermal necrolysis); J. M. Chadwick and T. F. Downham (letter), *Archs Derm.*, 1978, *114*, 803 (pemphigus).

Proprietary Preparations

Flamazine *(Smith & Nephew Pharmaceuticals, UK)*. Cream containing silver sulphadiazine 1% in an oil-in-water basis. (Also available as Flamazine in *Canad., Denm., Norw., S.Afr.*).

Other Proprietary Names

Flammazine *(Belg., Ger., Neth., Switz.)*; Silvadene *(USA)*; Silvazine *(Austral.)*; Silvederma *(Spain)*.

4914-t

Succinylsulphathiazole *(B.P., Eur. P.)*.

Succinylsulphathiaz.; Succinylsulfathiazolum; Succinylsulfathiazole; Succinilsolfatiazolo. 4′-(Thiazol-2-ylsulphamoyl)succinanilic acid monohydrate.

$C_{13}H_{13}N_3O_5S_2,H_2O = 373.4$.

CAS — 116-43-8 (anhydrous).

Pharmacopoeias. In *Arg., Br., Braz., Eur., Fr., Ger., Ind., Int., It., Mex., Neth., Span., Swiss* and *Turk.*

White or yellowish-white, odourless crystals or powder with a slightly bitter taste. M.p. about 190° with decomposition. It darkens on exposure to light.

Soluble 1 in 5000 of water, 1 in 150 of boiling water, 1 in 200 of alcohol, and 1 in 150 of acetone; practically insoluble in chloroform and ether; soluble in aqueous solutions of alkali hydroxides and carbonates. **Sterilisation** of the powder as for Sulphadimidine, p.1475. **Store** in airtight containers. Protect from light.

Adverse Effects, Treatment, and Precautions. As for Phthalylsulphathiazole, p.1468.

Absorption and Fate. Succinylsulphathiazole is slowly hydrolysed to sulphathiazole in the large intestine and only about 5% is absorbed; concentrations of sulphonamide in the blood do not usually exceed 40 μg per ml.

Uses. Succinylsulphathiazole has actions and uses similar to those of phthalylsulphathiazole (p.1468), though it is less active and tends to produce watery stools.

Usual adult doses of succinylsulphathiazole are in the range of 10 to 20 g daily in divided doses. As an adjunct in the treatment of ulcerative colitis 250 mg per kg body-weight daily in 6 divided doses has been suggested.

Preparations

Paediatric Succinylsulphathiazole Mixture *(B.P.C. 1973)*. Mist. Succinylsulphathiaz. pro Inf. Succinylsulphathiazole 1 g, light kaolin or light kaolin (natural) 600 mg, carmellose sodium '50' 100 mg, maize starch (as a mucilage) 200 mg, amaranth solution 0.1 ml, benzoic acid solution 0.2 ml, chloroform spirit 0.5 ml, raspberry syrup 2 ml, water to 10 ml. When prepared extemporaneously, the mixture should be recently prepared. The carmellose sodium '50', maize starch, and chloroform spirit may be replaced by compound tragacanth powder 100 mg and double-strength chloroform water 5 ml respectively. When prepared other than extemporaneously maize starch may be omitted, chloroform spirit may be replaced by double-strength chloroform water, and additional preservatives may be used. *Dose.* Children 1 to 2 years, 10 ml four times daily; 3 to 5 years, 20 ml four times daily.

Succinylsulphathiazole and Kaolin Mixture *(A.P.F.)*. Mist. Succinylsulphathiazol. et Kaolin. Succinylsulphathiazole 4 g, light kaolin or light kaolin (natural) 3 g, compound tragacanth powder 400 mg, syrup 3 ml, benzoic acid solution 0.5 ml, water to 20 ml. It should be freshly prepared. *Dose.* 20 ml.

Succinylsulphathiazole Tablets *(B.P. 1973)*. Tab. Succinylsulphathiaz. Tablets containing succinylsulphathiazole. Store in airtight containers. Protect from light.

Proprietary Preparations

Cremostrep *(Merck Sharp & Dohme, UK)*. A suspension containing in each 5 ml succinylsulphathiazole 500 mg, streptomycin sulphate equivalent to streptomycin 50 mg, and kaolin 500 mg (suggested diluent, syrup). For diarrhoea. *Dose.* 20 to 30 ml up to 6 times daily.

Other Proprietary Names

SS Thiazole *(Austral.)*; Sulfasuxidine *(Canad.)*; Thiacyl *(Fr.)*.

Succinylsulphathiazole was formerly marketed in Great Britain under the proprietary name Sulfasuxidine (*Merck Sharp & Dohme*). Preparations containing succinylsulphathiazole were also formerly marketed in Great Britain under the proprietary names Cremomycin, Cremosuxidine (both *Merck Sharp & Dohme*), and Kaovax (*Norton*).

4915-x

Sulfabenzamide. *N*-Sulphanilylbenzamide.

$C_{13}H_{12}N_2O_3S = 276.3$.

CAS — 127-71-9.

Practically **insoluble** in water; soluble 1 in 33 of alcohol and 1 in 9 of acetone.

A sulphonamide (p.1457) that has been applied topically.

4916-r

Sulfacytine.

Sulfacitine; CI-636. 1-Ethyl-N^4-sulphanilylcytosine; N^1-(1-Ethyl-1,2-dihydro-2-oxopyrimidin-4-yl)sulphanilamide.

$C_{12}H_{14}N_4O_3S = 294.3$.

CAS — 17784-12-2.

A white crystalline powder.

Adverse Effects, Treatment, and Precautions. As for Sulphonamides, p.1457.

Sulfacytine 2 g daily for 14 days had no haemolytic effects in 5 Negro subjects known to be deficient in glucose-6-phosphate dehydrogenase.— R. A. Heinrich *et al.*, *J. clin. Pharmac.*, 1971, *11*, 428.

Absorption and Fate. As for Sulphonamides, p.1458.

Sulfacytine is readily absorbed from the gastro-intestinal tract with peak blood concentrations occurring within 2 to 3 hours. A plasma half-life of 4 hours has been reported; about 85% is bound to plasma albumin. Sulfacytine is very soluble in urine within the usual acidic pH range and is rapidly excreted by the kidneys, about 90% of a dose being eliminated in 24 hours, mainly unchanged. About 10% is excreted as the acetyl derivative and a similar amount as glucuronides.

Uses. Sulfacytine is a short-acting sulphonamide which is used similarly to sulphafurazole (p.1477) in the treatment of acute urinary-tract infections. After a loading dose of 500 mg, sulfacytine 250 mg is taken four times daily for 10 days.

Urinary-tract infections. Sulfacytine did not appear to be better than sulphafurazole or other soluble sulphonamides for the treatment of urinary-tract infections; headache, nausea, pruritus, rash, dizziness, and fatigue were the most common side-effects.— *Med. Lett.*, 1976, *18*, 43.

In a double-blind study in 92 women, sulfacytine 1 g daily was as effective as sulphafurazole 4 g daily in the treatment of acute cystitis; the cure-rate was about 90% with both drugs.— P. A. Jensen and J. M. Mueller, *Curr. ther. Res.*, 1976, *19*, 573.

Further references: N. A. Moffat and F. J. Wenzel, *Curr. ther. Res.*, 1971, *13*, 286; K. E. Way, *ibid.*, 1976, *19*, 220; I. L. Goldberg *et al.*, *ibid.*, 1977, *21*, 468.

Proprietary Names

Renoquid *(Parke, Davis, USA)*.

4917-f

Sulfadoxine *(B.P., B.P. Vet.)*. Sulphormethoxine; Sulformethoxine; Sulforthomidine; Sulphorthodimethoxine; Sulfadimoxinum; Ro 4-4393.

N^1-(5,6-Dimethoxypyrimidin-4-yl)sulphanilamide.

$C_{12}H_{14}N_4O_4S=310.3$.

CAS — 2447-57-6.

Pharmacopoeias. In *Br.*, *Chin.*, and *Fr.*

A white or creamy-white odourless crystalline powder. M.p. 197° to 200°. Very slightly **soluble** in water; slightly soluble in alcohol and in methyl alcohol; practically insoluble in ether.

A solution of sulfadoxine (with trimethoprim), adjusted to pH 10 with sodium hydroxide, may be **sterilised** by autoclaving in sealed containers in which the air has been replaced by nitrogen or other suitable gas. **Protect** from light.

Adverse Effects, Treatment, and Precautions. As for Sulphonamides, p.1457.

If side-effects occur, sulfadoxine has the disadvantage that several days are required for elimination from the body. The Stevens-Johnson and Lyell's syndromes have been reported following treatment with sulfadoxine.

Absorption and Fate. Sulfadoxine is readily absorbed from the gastro-intestinal tract. High concentrations in the blood are reached in about 4 hours; the half-life in the blood is about 4 to 8 days. About 90 to 95% is reported to be bound to plasma albumin.

About 5% of sulfadoxine in the blood is present as the acetyl derivative, and 2% as the glucuronide. Sulfadoxine is very slowly excreted, only about 8% being recovered from the urine in 24 hours and about 30% in 7 days, up to 60% being excreted as the acetyl derivative and about 10% as the glucuronide.

Blood concentrations of 80 to 120 µg per ml were produced when sulfadoxine was given to children as a single dose of 25 mg per kg body-weight; the blood concentration fell to 20 to 60 µg per ml after 7 days. If a daily maintenace dose of 5 mg per kg was also given blood concentrations were maintained at 80 to 90 µg per ml. A single dose of 50 mg per kg produced a blood concentration of about 200 µg per ml which did not fall below 60 µg per ml after 7 days. Less than 10% of sulfadoxine was conjugated in the blood. About 30% of a single dose was excreted in the urine in 7 days, about 50% as the acetyl derivative and a small amount as glucuronide. Excretion in infants was delayed.— M. Vest, *Schweiz. med. Wschr.*, 1966, *96*, 920, per *Bull. Hyg., Lond.*, 1967, *42*, 89.

Blood concentrations of 130 to 200 µg per ml were achieved in 31 patients who received sulfadoxine 1.5 to 2 g weekly; the average half-life was about 7 days.— V. Haegi, *Schweiz. med. Wschr.*, 1966, *96*, 1308, per *Int. pharm. Abstr.*, 1967, *4*, 93.

Uses. Sulfadoxine is a long-acting sulphonamide with the general properties of Sulphonamides, p.1458. It has a very prolonged effect and has been used in the treatment of various infections including leprosy. It is given with pyrimethamine (p.403) in the treatment and prophylaxis of falciparum malaria resistant to other therapies.

The usual initial dose is 2 g by mouth, followed by 1 to 1.5 g weekly. Children aged 2 to 4 years may be given one-quarter of the adult doses, and children aged 5 to 8 years, one-half. In the treatment of malaria, the usual dose is 1 to 1.5 g of sulfadoxine with 50 to 75 mg of pyrimethamine; this should not be repeated for at least 7 days. For short-term prophylaxis a dose of 500 mg of sulfadoxine with 25 mg of pyrimethamine should be repeated every 7 days.

Sulfadoxine has been given, as a preparation containing 25% by deep intramuscular or slow intravenous injection. The initial dose for adults is 2.5 g followed, if necessary, by 1.5 g after 4 days. Children may be given an initial dose of 60 mg per kg body-weight followed, if necessary, by 40 mg per kg after 4 days.

A mixture of 5 parts of sulfadoxine with 1 part trimethoprim is used in veterinary medicine.

A review of the properties and uses of sulfadoxine.— H. Seneca, *J. Am. med. Ass.*, 1966, *198*, 975.

A discussion of the role of sulfadoxine in sulphonamide therapy.— *Lancet*, 1967, *1*, 150.

Enteric infections. Cholera. In a comparative placebo-controlled study 109 cholera contacts received a single dose of sulfadoxine (2 g for those aged over 14 years, 1 g for those aged 5 to 14 years, 0.5 g for those aged 1½ to 4 years), 101 received a 3-day course of tetracycline (500 mg every 12 hours for those aged over 12 years, 250 mg every 12 hours for those aged 1½ to 12 years) and 112 received placebo. Tetracycline was found to be significantly effective in reducing the load of cholera infection from the 2nd to the 6th day whereas sulfadoxine was effective from the 3rd to the 6th day. Sulfadoxine had the advantage of single dosage but the drawback of a longer lag period before it became effective. Although the treatment caused no significant adverse reactions there was less fever and diarrhoea in the tetracycline than in the sulfadoxine or placebo groups; sulfadoxine has been reported to produce skin sensitivity in some African countries. As in the earlier study (*Bull. Wld Hlth Org.*, 1971, *45*, 451) chemotherapy was again shown to have limited value in high cholera endemic areas.— B. C. Deb *et al.*, *Bull. Wld Hlth Org.*, 1976, *54*, 171.

Further references: E. J. Gangarosa *et al.*, *Bull. Wld Hlth Org.*, 1966, *35*, 669; L. Lapeyssonie *et al.*, *Bull. Acad. natn. Méd.*, 1970, *154*, 657; T. I. Francis *et al.*, *J. trop. Med. Hyg.*, 1971, *74*, 172; A. Bourgeade *et al.*, *Méd. Afr. noire*, 1972, *19*, 93, per *Trop. Dis. Bull.*, 1973, *70*, 342.

Leprosy. Sulfadoxine was used in the treatment of 17 patients with lepromatous leprosy, in a dosage increased from 0.25 to 1.5 g weekly. Clinical results were considered excellent in 10 of 13 previously untreated patients. Of 4 patients previously treated with dapsone, 2 improved and 2 developed lepra reactions. Of 17 patients with tuberculoid leprosy treated with a similar dosage, 6 of 14 previously untreated showed a good response and 3 a moderate response; 3 patients previously treated with dapsone showed considerable improvement. Side-effects included a generalised rash (1 patient), itching and burning (1), lepra reactions (2), and erythema nodosum (2). A dose of 1 g per week appeared adequate for most patients.— M. L. Gaind *et al.*, *Lepr. Rev.*, 1966, *37*, 167, per *Abstr. Wld Med.*, 1967, *41*, 186.

From experience in 17 patients given a weekly dose of sulfadoxine, it was considered that sulfadoxine was less effective than dapsone in the treatment of leprosy. Lepra reactions occurred in about two-thirds of the patients.— K. Ramanujam, *Lepr. India*, 1967, *39*, 95, per *Trop. Dis. Bull.*, 1968, *65*, 267.

Further references: V. Ekambaram and S. Venkatachari, *Lepr. India*, 1976, *48*, 24.

For an opinion that sulfadoxine is not suitable for the treatment of leprosy, see Sulphamethoxypyridazine, p.1480.

Malaria. Regimens of sulfadoxine and sulfadoxine with either chloroquine or pyrimethamine for the treatment of falciparum malaria were assessed in 65 patients whose parasitaemia had resisted treatment with chloroquine. The schizonticidal effects of a single dose of 1 g of sulfadoxine and 1.5 g of chloroquine base given in 4 divided doses during 48 hours was more rapid than that of sulphadoxine alone but the most effective regimen proved to be a single dose of 1 g of sulfadoxine and 50 mg of pyrimethamine; it was effective in 17 of 19 patients. The gametocyte count of 15 of 18 patients treated with sulfadoxine alone increased after treatment and gametocytes took between 8 and 60 days to disappear. No evidence of drug toxicity was observed with any of the regimens.— T. Harinasuta *et al.*, *Lancet*, 1967, *1*, 1117.

Treatment with sulfadoxine in conjunction with pyrimethamine failed in 4 out of 5 subjects infected with Malayan III or Thai II strains of *Plasmodium falciparum*. It was suggested that the development of cross-resistance was due to prior exposure of the parasite to a sulphone or chlorguanide.— W. Chin *et al.* (letter), *Trans. R. Soc. trop. Med. Hyg.*, 1970, *64*, 461.

Sulfadoxine 500 mg with pyrimethamine 25 mg once a week is recommended for the prophylaxis of chloroquine-resistant falciparum malaria.— *Med. Lett.*, 1979, *21*, 105.

Further references: A. B. G. Laing, *Bull. Wld Hlth Org.*, 1966, *34*, 308; A. B. G. Laing, *J. trop. Med. Hyg.*, 1968, *71*, 27; N. Al Tawil, *S.E. Asian J. trop. med. publ. Hlth*, 1978, *9*, 409.

For other reports of sulfadoxine and pyrimethamine being used in the treatment of malaria, see Pyrimethamine, p.403.

Mycetoma. For reference to the beneficial effect of sulfadoxine with pyrimethamine as second-line therapy in the medical treatment of mycetoma, see Co-trimoxazole, p.1465.

Paracoccidioidomycosis. Of 68 patients with paracoccidioidomycosis treated with sulfadoxine and studied for up to 6 years 49 were cured and 8 were clinically improved. The usual dose of sulfadoxine was 1 g daily for 10 days, then 2 g a week.— C. F. Lopes, *Medna Cutánea*, 1971, *5*, 357, per *Trop. Dis. Bull.*, 1972, *69*, 442.

Further references: M. C. Passos Filho, *Hospital, Rio de J.*, 1969, *76*, 847.

Proprietary Preparations

Fanasil (available only in certain countries; known in some countries as Fanaril, Fanasulf, Fanzil, and Fontasul) *(Roche, UK)*. Sulfadoxine, available as **Ampoules** containing 2.5 g in 10 ml and as scored **Tablets** of 500 mg.

Fansidar, which contains sulfadoxine with pyrimethamine is described on p.404.

4918-d

Sulfamerazine *(B.P. Vet., U.S.P.)*. Sulphamerazine; Sulphameraz.; Sulfamerazinum; Sulfamethyldiazine; Sulfamethylpyrimidine; Solfamerazina. N^1-(4-Methylpyrimidin-2-yl)sulphanilamide.

$C_{11}H_{12}N_4O_2S=264.3$.

CAS — 127-79-7.

Pharmacopoeias. In *Arg.*, *Aust.*, *Braz.*, *Fr.*, *Int.*, *It.*, *Jug.*, *Neth.*, *Nord.*, *Span.*, *Swiss*, and *U.S.*

A white or faintly yellowish-white, odourless or almost odourless, crystalline powder with a slightly bitter taste; it slowly darkens on exposure to light. M.p. 234° to 239° with decomposition. **Soluble** 1 in 6250 of water at 20°, 1 in 3300 of water at 37°, 1 in 300 of boiling water, 1 in 550 of alcohol, and 1 in 60 of acetone; slightly soluble in chloroform; very slightly soluble in ether; soluble in dilute mineral acids and in solutions of alkali hydroxides and carbonates. **Sterilisation** of the powder as for Sulphadimidine, p.1475. **Store** in airtight containers. Protect from light.

4919-n

Sulfamerazine Sodium. Sulphameraz. Sod.; Sulphamerazine Sodium *(B.P.C. 1959)*; Soluble Sulphamerazine; Sulfamerazinum Natricum.

$C_{11}H_{11}N_4NaO_2S=286.3$.

CAS — 127-58-2.

Pharmacopoeias. In *Aust., Braz.* and *Int.*

A white or yellowish-white odourless or almost odourless powder with a bitter taste. It slowly darkens on exposure to light; on exposure to moist air it absorbs carbon dioxide and becomes less soluble in water. Sulfamerazine sodium 1.08 g is approximately equivalent to 1 g of sulfamerazine.

Soluble 1 in 3.5 of water; slightly soluble in alcohol; practically insoluble in acetone, chloroform, and ether. A solution in water has a pH of about 9.5. A 4.53% solution is iso-osmotic with serum. Solutions are **sterilised** by distributing into ampoules, replacing the air with nitrogen or other suitable gas, sealing, and autoclaving. **Store** in airtight containers. Protect from light.

Adverse Effects, Treatment, and Precautions. As for Sulphonamides, p.1457.

Sulfamerazine has caused haematuria and persistent albuminuria in children, especially in those aged less than 6 years, even when fluid intake has been normal. The risk of crystalluria is considerable and sulfamerazine is rarely used alone.

Absorption and Fate. As for Sulphonamides, p.1458.

Sulfamerazine is readily absorbed from the gastro-intestinal tract and 60 to 80% is bound to plasma albumin. It penetrates into the cerebrospinal fluid to produce concentrations about one-half of those in the blood.

Sulfamerazine is acetylated in the body; about 15% of the sulfamerazine in the blood is in the form of the acetyl derivative. It is excreted somewhat slowly, about 40% being eliminated in the urine in 24 hours, about half being in the form of the acetyl derivative.

The biological half-life of sulfamerazine is variously reported as 16 to 40.8 hours.— W. A. Ritschel, *Drug Intell. & clin. Pharm.*, 1970, *4*, 332.

Elimination half-lifes of sulphadiazine, sulfamerazine, and sulphadimidine were 13, 12.7, and 2.3 hours respectively in a healthy subject given 330 mg of each sulphonamide as a combined suspension by mouth.— T. J. Goehl *et al., J. pharm. Sci.*, 1978, *67*, 404.

Further references: A. Traeger and G. Stein, *Int. J. clin. Pharmac. Biopharm.*, 1977, *15*, 315; B. Terhaag *et al., Int. J. clin. Pharmac. Biopharm.*, 1978, *16*, 274.

Uses. Sulfamerazine has the general properties of sulphonamides, p.1458, and has been given in a dose of 1 g every 6 hours. It is rarely used alone but is sometimes employed in conjunction with other sulphonamides—see p.1486.

Sulfamerazine is used in veterinary medicine.

Preparations

Sulfamerazine Tablets *(U.S.P.)*. Tablets containing sulfamerazine.

4920-k

Sulfametopyrazine. Solfametopirazina; Sulphalene; Sulfalene; AS 18908; Sulfamethoxypyrazine; Sulfapyrazin Methoxyne; Sulfapirazinmetossina; Solfametossipirazina. N^1-(3-Methoxypyrazin-2-yl)sulphanilamide.

$C_{11}H_{12}N_4O_3S$=280.3.

CAS — 152-47-6.

Pharmacopoeias. In *Chin.* and *It.*

A white or yellowish-white almost odourless crystalline powder with a slightly bitter taste. M.p. 175° to 178°. Practically **insoluble** in water; slightly soluble in alcohol, chloroform, and ethyl acetate; freely soluble in acetone and in dilute mineral acids and solutions of alkali hydroxides.

Adverse Effects, Treatment, and Precautions. As for Sulphonamides, p.1457.

If side-effects occur, sulfametopyrazine has the disadvantage that several days are required for its elimination from the body. It may cause the Stevens-Johnson syndrome.

Absorption and Fate. Sulfametopyrazine is readily absorbed from the gastro-intestinal tract; 60 to 80% is bound to plasma albumin. About 5 to 10% of sulfametopyrazine in the blood is in the form of the acetyl derivative. It is slowly excreted, about 70% as the acetyl derivative. The biological half-life has been reported to be about 65 hours.

In 4 persons given sulfametopyrazine in a dosage of 7 to 15.2 mg per kg body-weight, the mean half-life was 67 hours. It was bound to plasma protein to the extent of about 68%. Sulfametopyrazine and its acetyl derivative were relatively soluble at the usual urinary range of pH.— R. G. Wiegand *et al., Antimicrob. Ag. Chemother.*, 1964, 549.

Sulfametopyrazine was bound to plasma protein to the extent of 72 to 81%. Concentrations of sulfametopyrazine in cerebrospinal fluid in 2 patients were about one-third of concentrations in the blood. An initial dose of 1.25 g, followed by daily doses of 250 mg, could be expected to produce a blood concentration of 70 µg per ml.— R. L. Herting *et al., Antimicrob. Ag. Chemother.*, 1964, 554.

The mean half-life of sulfametopyrazine in the serum of children aged 3 months to 4 years was 45 hours, and in older children 73 hours. After administration by mouth, absorption of the sulphonamide was complete. The suggested dose for infants was 30 mg per kg body-weight, and for older children 20 mg per kg, once weekly. Alternatively, 20 or 12 mg per kg respectively could be given initially, followed by 6 or 3 mg per kg respectively every 24 hours for maintenance.— F. H. Dost and E. Gladtke, *Arzneimittel-Forsch.*, 1969, *19*, 1304.

The biological half-life of sulfametopyrazine is variously reported as 36 to 71.5 hours in adults, 44.2 hours in children, and 67.8 to 280 hours (according to age) in infants born at term.— W. A. Ritschel, *Drug Intell. & clin. Pharm.*, 1970, *4*, 332.

Sulfametopyrazine and trimethoprim given together in doses of 600 and 750 mg respectively for the first day then 200 and 250 mg daily for 9 days produced blood concentrations in the ratio of 10 or 20 to 1 after 10 days. Antibacterial concentrations were maintained throughout treatment.— V. de Pascale *et al., Farmaco, Edn prat.*, 1977, *32*, 228.

The pharmacokinetics of sulfametopyrazine and trimethoprim in healthy subjects following administration of a preparation containing sulfametopyrazine and trimethoprim in the ratio 4:5 (Kelfiprim).— D. S. Reeves *et al., J. antimicrob. Chemother.*, 1980, *6*, 647.

Uses. Sulfametopyrazine is a long-acting sulphonamide with the general properties and uses of Sulphonamides, p.1458. It is usually given by mouth in a single dose of 2 g once a week. For children the dose is 30 mg per kg body-weight once a week.

Sulfametopyrazine is also used with trimethoprim similarly to co-trimoxazole (p.1463).

Malaria. Reports of the use of sulfametopyrazine in the treatment of falciparum malaria.— G. Baruffa, *Trans. R. Soc. trop. Med. Hyg.*, 1966, *60*, 222; D. F. Clyde *et al., Am. J. trop. Med. Hyg.*, 1971, *20*, 804; R. L. Williams *et al., Am. J. trop. Med. Hyg.*, 1975, *24*, 734.

For reports of sulfametopyrazine being used with trimethoprim in the treatment of malaria, see Martindale 27th Edn, p. 362.

Respiratory infections. Bronchitis. In a multicentre study in 1363 patients with chronic bronchitis, 82.5% responded favourably to 2 g once weekly prophylactically. Adverse reactions occurred in 68 patients and included gastro-intestinal disturbances in 18 and skin reactions in 18.— C. S. Darke, *Med. Dig., Lond.*, 1973, Nov., 68.

Further references: C. S. Darke *et al., Br. J. Dis. Chest*, 1972, *66*, 276; A. P. Launchbury, *Pharm. J.* , 1975, *1*, 14; R. F. Willey *et al., Br. J. Dis. Chest*, 1978, *72*, 13; D. Davies and C. S. Darke, *ibid.*, 231.

Urinary-tract infections. In a multicentre clinical study in 131 patients with urinary-tract infection, sulfametopyrazine 2 g as a single dose was as effective as ampicillin 500 mg every 8 hours for 7 days.— N. Slade and S. T. Crowther, *Br. J. Urol.*, 1972, *44*, 105.

In a preliminary study, 67 of 83 (81%) patients with bacteriuria in pregnancy were cured at follow-up, 2 weeks after receiving a single 2-g dose of sulfametopyrazine; at follow-up after 6 weeks, 52 of 76 (68%) were cured. In a randomised comparative study, similar patients were given either a single 2-g dose of sulfametopyrazine, a 2-g dose followed by a further 2-g dose 4 or 5 days later, or sulphadimidine 1 g four times daily for 7 days. At follow-up after 6 weeks cures had been obtained in 30 of 45 (67%) patients, 27 of 37 (73%) patients, and 17 of 34 (50%) patients respectively.— D. S. Reeves, *J. antimicrob. Chemother.*, 1975, *1*, 171.

Proprietary Preparations

Kelfizine W *(Farmitalia Carlo Erba, UK)*. Sulfametopyrazine for weekly dosage, available as **Suspension** containing 100 mg per ml in bottles of 10 ml (paediatric) and 20 ml (adult) (suggested diluent, syrup) and as **Tablets** of 2 g to be stirred in water before use.

Other Proprietary Names

Kelfizina *(Arg., Belg., Ital., Neth.)*; Longum *(Arg., Belg., Ger., Neth.)*; Policydal *(Jap.)*.

Sulfametopyrazine was also formerly marketed in Great Britain under the proprietary name Dalysep *(Syntex)*.

4921-a

Sulfametrole. N^1-(4-Methoxy-1,2,5-thiadiazol-3-yl)sulphanilamide.

$C_9H_{10}N_4O_3S_2$=286.3.

CAS — 32909-92-5.

Sulfametrole is a sulphonamide which is used with trimethoprim in the ratio of 5 parts sulfametrole to 1 part trimethoprim, similarly to co-trimoxazole (p.1463).

Reports of the pharmacokinetics of sulfametrole with trimethoprim.— G. Brandesky and F. Takacs, *Wien. klin. Wschr.*, 1975, *87*, 611; G. Hitzenberger *et al., Int. J. clin. Pharmac. Biopharm.*, 1977, *15*, 310.

A combination of sulfametrole 20 parts with trimethoprim 1 part *in vitro* had a similar antibacterial activity to co-trimoxazole.— G. Nabert-Bock and H. Grims, *Arzneimittel-Forsch.*, 1977, *27*, 1109.

4922-t

Sulfamonomethoxine. DJ 1550; DS 36; ICI 32525; Ro 4-3476. N^1-(6-Methoxypyrimidin-4-yl)sulphanilamide monohydrate.

$C_{11}H_{12}N_4O_3S,H_2O$=298.3.

CAS — 1220-83-3 (anhydrous).

Pharmacopoeias. In *Jap.*

Odourless white or pale yellow crystals or crystalline powder. M.p. about 205°. Practically **insoluble** in water; soluble in acetone; slightly soluble in alcohol; very slightly soluble in chloroform and ether. **Protect** from light.

Sulfamonomethoxine is a sulphonamide (p.1457) which has been given in a dose of 1 g initially, then 500 mg daily.

The biological half-life of sulfamonomethoxine was 30 hours.— W. A. Ritschel, *Drug Intell. & clin. Pharm.*, 1970, *4*, 332.

There was an incidence of malarial infection of 10.2% in 127 prisoners in a malarial area given sulfamonomethoxine 1 g weekly compared with 26.5% in 158 not so treated.— B. D. Cabrera and O. L. Ramos, *S.E. Asian J. trop. med. publ. Hlth*, 1972, *3*, 501, per *Trop. Dis. Bull.*, 1973, *70*, 718.

All of 36 patients with *Plasmodium falciparum* infection were cured, without relapse, after treatment with sulfamonomethoxine 80 to 100 mg per kg body-weight over 3 days, half the total dose being given on the first day. Of 30 with resistance to chloroquine 28 were cured. The response in *P. vivax* infection was poor.— O. L. Ramos and B. D. Cabrera, *S.E. Asian J. trop. med. publ. Hlth*, 1972, *3*, 562, per *Trop. Dis. Bull.*, 1973, *70*, 718.

Proprietary Names

Daimeton *(Daiichi, Jap.)*.

4923-x

Sulfapyrazole *(B.P. Vet.)*. Ba 18605; Sulfamethylphenazole; Sulfazamet. N^1-(3-Methyl-1-phenylpyrazol-5-yl)sulphanilamide.

$C_{16}H_{16}N_4O_2S$=328.4.

CAS — 852-19-7.

A white or creamy-white, odourless or almost odourless, crystalline powder. M.p. 184° to 186°. Practically **insoluble** in water; soluble in alcohol; slightly soluble in chloroform. **Protect** from light.

Sulfapyrazole is a sulphonamide (p.1457) used in veterinary medicine.

4924-r

Sulfaquinoxaline *(B.P. Vet.)*. Sulphaquinoxaline; Sulfabenzpyrazine; Sulphaquinoxalina. N^1-(Quinoxalin-2-yl)sulphanilamide.
$C_{14}H_{12}N_4O_2S$=300.3.

CAS — 59-40-5.

Pharmacopoeias. In *Nord.*

A yellow, odourless, almost tasteless powder. Practically **insoluble** in water; very slightly soluble in alcohol and chloroform; soluble 1 in 200 of acetone; practically insoluble in ether; soluble in dilute solutions of mineral acids and in solutions of alkalis. **Store** in airtight containers. Protect from light.

Sulfaquinoxaline is a sulphonamide (p.1457) used in the treatment of coccidiosis in poultry. It has been used as an additive to veterinary feedstuffs. It has been used with warfarin in a rodenticide.

4925-f

Sulfasymazine. N^1-(4,6-Diethyl-1,3,5-triazin-2-yl)sulphanilamide.
$C_{13}H_{17}N_5O_2S$=307.4.

CAS — 1984-94-7.

Sulfasymazine is extensively bound to plasma proteins and has the general properties and uses of Sulphonamides, p.1457. It has been given in an adult dose of 1 g initially, then 500 mg twice daily.

The biological half-life of sulfasymazine was reported as 14 hours.— W. A. Ritschel, *Drug Intell. & clin. Pharm.*, 1970, *4*, 332.

Further references: A. R. Frisk and E. Hultman, *Antimicrob. Ag. Chemother.*, 1965, 672.

Proprietary Names
Prosul *(Lederle, Austral.)*.

4926-d

Sulphabromomethazine Sodium. Sodium Sulfabromomethazine. The monohydrate of the sodium salt of N^1-(5-bromo-4,6-dimethylpyrimidin-2-yl)sulphanilamide.
$C_{12}H_{12}BrN_4NaO_2S,H_2O$=397.2.

CAS — 116-45-0 (sulphabromomethazine); 3691-68-7 (sodium salt, anhydrous).

A white to light yellow, odourless or almost odourless powder. Freely **soluble** in water; slightly soluble in alcohol; very slightly soluble in acetone, chloroform, and ether. A 10% solution in water has a pH of 9.5 to 11. It may darken on exposure to light. On prolonged exposure to air it absorbs carbon dioxide with the liberation of sulphabromomethazine and becomes incompletely soluble in water. **Store** in airtight containers. Protect from light.

Sulphabromomethazine is a sulphonamide (p.1457) which is used in veterinary medicine in the treatment of bacterial infections in cattle. It is administered by mouth and by intraperitoneal injection.

4927-n

Sulphacetamide *(B.P.C. 1959)*. Sulphacetam.; Sulfacetamide; Acetosulfaminum. *N*-Sulphanilylacetamide.
$C_8H_{10}N_2O_3S$=214.2.

CAS — 144-80-9.

Pharmacopoeias. In *Arg., Aust., Cz., Fr., Ind., Neth.*, and *Pol.*

A white or yellowish-white, odourless, crystalline powder with an acid, slightly saline taste. M.p. 181° to 184°.

Soluble 1 in 150 of water, 1 in 15 of alcohol, and 1 in 7 of acetone; very slightly soluble in chloroform; slightly soluble in ether; soluble in mineral acids and solutions of alkali hydroxides and carbonates. Solutions in water are acid to litmus and sensitive to light. **Sterilisation** of the powder as for Sulphadimidine, p.1475. **Store** in airtight containers. Protect from light.

4928-h

Sulphacetamide Sodium *(B.P.)*. Sulphacetam. Sod.; Sulphacetamidum Sodium; Sulfacetamidum Natricum; Soluble Sulphacetamide; Sulfacetamide Sodium *(U.S.P.)*; Sulfacylum Natrium.
$C_8H_9N_2NaO_3S,H_2O$=254.2.

CAS — 127-56-0 (anhydrous); 6209-17-2 (monohydrate).

Pharmacopoeias. In *Arg., Br., Braz., Chin., Cz., Fr., Hung., Ind., Int., Jug., Neth., Pol., Rus., Turk.*, and *U.S.*

White or yellowish-white, odourless crystals or crystalline powder with a slightly bitter taste. It slowly darkens on exposure to light; on exposure to moist air it absorbs carbon dioxide and becomes less soluble.

Soluble 1 in 1.5 of water; slightly soluble in alcohol; sparingly soluble in acetone; practically insoluble in chloroform and ether. A 5% solution in water has a pH of 8 to 9.5; a mixture of sulphacetamide sodium and 1% sulphacetamide gives a solution in water which has a pH of about 7.4. A 3.85% solution is iso-osmotic with serum. The discoloration of solutions may be retarded by the addition of sodium metabisulphite and protection from light.

Sterilisation of the powder as for Sulphadimidine, p.1475; solutions are sterilised by autoclaving, by maintaining for 30 minutes at 98° to 100° with a bactericide, or by filtration. When solutions are sterilised by heat, hydrolysis occurs forming sulphanilamide which may be deposited as crystals, especially from concentrated solutions and under cold storage conditions. **Store** in airtight containers. Protect from light.

Bacteriostatic activity. There was no evidence that the yellow discoloration of sulphacetamide sodium solution after exposure to light impaired its activity against *Escherichia coli* and *Pseudomonas aeruginosa*.— Pharm. Soc. Lab. Rep. No. 887, 1962.

Compatibility with zinc sulphate. Precipitation occurred with a 5% solution of sulphacetamide sodium (pH 9.5) on the addition of zinc sulphate. A 5% solution prepared with sulphacetamide sodium containing 1% of sulphacetamide (pH 7.4) was compatible with 0.3% of zinc sulphate.—Pharm. Soc. Lab. Rep., *Pharm. J.*, 1955, *2*, 90.

Up to 0.5% of zinc sulphate could be incorporated without precipitation in a solution of sulphacetamide 0.5% and sulphacetamide sodium 9.5% in water, pH about 6.8.— H. E. R. Barker, *Australas. J. Pharm.*, 1955, *36*, 991. See also *ibid.*, 1954, *35*, 802.

Effect of gamma-irradiation. Sulphacetamide 10% eye-drops and 6% eye ointment were irradiated at 5000, 10 000, and 25 000 Gy. When prepared under clean conditions the irradiated preparations were sterile. There was no significant loss of potency, change in the ointment basis, or evidence of interaction between the preparations and the polyethylene tubing or gelatin capsules used for packing. The eye-drops became discoloured.— D. J. Trigger and A. D. S. Caldwell, *Pharmax*, *J. Hosp. Pharm.*, 1968, *25*, 259.

For correspondence on the possibility of sterilising sulphacetamide eye-drops by irradiation, see R. T. S. Hoile, *Pharm. J.*, 1968, *2*, 447; J. W. Hadgraft, *ibid.*, 448; K. A. Lees, *ibid.*, 476 and 546; D. Simpkins, *ibid.*, 476; D. J. Trigger, *ibid.*, 518.

Ophthalmic solutions. Tablets and powder forms of sulphacetamide sodium were stable, but ophthalmic solutions and suspensions were degraded on storage, with formation of sulphanilamide.— M. P. Gruber and R. W. Klein, *J. pharm. Sci.*, 1968, *57*, 1212.

Solutions of sulphacetamide sodium were incompatible with benzalkonium chloride. Solutions of sulphacetamide sodium 10 or 30% containing sodium metabisulphite 0.1% and infected with *Ps. aeruginosa* were not resterilised within 1 hour in the presence of phenylmercuric nitrate 0.002%, thiomersal 0.01%, chlorhexidine acetate 0.01%, or chlorocresol 0.05%. Solutions were resterilised within 1 hour in the presence of phenylmercuric nitrate 0.002% plus disodium edetate 0.05% and phenethyl alcohol 0.4%. The effect of thiomersal was less improved. Solutions were sterilised within 1 hour in the presence of chlorhexidine acetate 0.01% or chlorocresol 0.05% plus in each case either disodium edetate 0.05% or phenethyl alcohol 0.4% or both disodium edetate and phenethyl alcohol. Chlorocresol was considered the preservative of choice because it was least affected by the presence or absence of sodium metabisulphite. Resterilisation times were prolonged after storage for 7 days in the presence of phenylmercuric nitrate, thiomersal, or chlorhexidine, probably due to the formation of a complex between the preservative and sodium metabisulphite. Chlorocresol did not appear to be so affected. There was no evidence of degradation of sulphacetamide to sulphanilamide in solutions stored in the dark for 7 days.— R. M. E. Richards and R. J. McBride, *Pharm. J.*, 1973, *1*, 118.

Stability of solutions. The development of a yellowish-brown to deep reddish-brown coloration which occurred in sulphacetamide sodium solutions on keeping was thought to be due to oxidation, and was preceded by the formation of sulphanilamide by hydrolysis. Oxidation products included azobenzene-4,4′-disulphonamide and/or azoxybenzene-4,4′-disulphonamide.— P. A. Clarke, *Pharm. J.*, 1965, *1*, 375.

The rate of hydrolysis of sulphacetamide was independent of pH in the range 7.15 to 8.9, and a more acid pH caused increased discoloration. The hydrolysis reaction-rate was first order and a 0.2M to 1.0M solution had a half-life of 22 hours. Heating in an autoclave at 120° for 20 minutes or at 115° for 30 minutes resulted in a 1% loss of potency. Heating with a bactericide at 98° to 100° for 30 minutes gave a loss of less than 0.5%. Autoclaving was the method of choice.— R. A. Anderson, *Australas. J. Pharm.*, 1966, *47*, S26.

The problem of formulating a 30% solution of sulphacetamide sodium which would neither darken nor crystallise during at least 1 year's storage at room temperature in am amber glass dropper bottle containing an appreciable proportion of air was reviewed. Crystallisation was not normally a risk if the solution was not heated, exposed to light, or refrigerated, and the inclusion of sodium metabisulphite did not affect crystallisation. Unless the equivalent of 0.5% of sodium metabisulphite was added, the solutions could however discolour. Sodium thiosulphate 0.1% was a promising stabiliser, but sodium sulphite was less effective.— S. F. Forse, *Pharm. J.*, 1967, *2*, 355.

Crystals of sulphanilamide were depositied in 30% solutions of sulphacetamide sodium after steaming at 98° to 100° for 1 or 2 hours followed by 7 weeks' storage. Crystallisation could be minimised by buffering the solution to pH 9 to 9.5, though discoloration was worse at pH 8.6 than at pH 7.2. The concentration of sodium metabisulphite did not appear to affect the extent of crystallisation.— P. A. Clarke, *Pharm. J.*, 1967, *1*, 374. In further experiments, the rate of discoloration of solutions increased with increasing concentrations of sulphanilamide. Though sulphacetamide hydrolysis was independent of pH at 7.15 to 8.9, sulphanilamide was less soluble at pH 7.15 and was therefore more liable to crystallise.— *idem*, 1967, *2*, 414.

Adding 0.1% of disodium edetate to a 10% solution of sulphacetamide sodium at pH 8.8 appeared to minimise the development of colour changes on heating or storage.— H. C. Mital and J. L. Gupta, *Indian J. Pharm.*, 1968, *30*, 94.

A study of the factors affecting stability, sulphanilamide formation, colour development, and actions of antioxidants in solutions of sulphacetamide sodium. Sodium metabisulphite accelerated the hydrolytic degradation of sulphacetamide to sulphanilamide.— D. J. G. Davies *et al.*, *J. Pharm. Pharmac.*, 1970, *22*, *Suppl.*, 43S.

Storage of solutions. Avoid contact with metals, particularly copper, which causes darkening of the solutions.— A. J. Cobcroft, *Australas. J. Pharm.*, 1954, *35*, 361.

Low-density polyethylene containers were unsuitable for sulphacetamide eye-drops, which were discoloured within 1 week at 32°.— B. T. O'Boyle, *Kerfoot* (letter), *Pharm. J.*, 1973, *1*, 201.

Adverse Effects, Treatment, and Precautions. As for Sulphonamides, p.1457.

The Stevens-Johnson syndrome has been reported.

Local application of sulphacetamide sodium to the eye may cause burning or stinging but this is rarely severe enough to necessitate discontinuance of treatment. Sulphacetamide sodium ointment should not be applied to penetrating wounds of the cornea. Local anaesthetics that are esters of *p*-aminobenzoic acid may interfere with the antibacterial action of sulphacetamide sodium if used in the eye concomitantly.

Allergy. Skin sensitivity arising after the use of eye-drops or ointments containing sulphacetamide.— G. W. Beveridge, *Prescribers' J.*, 1975, *15*, 138.

Lupus erythematosus. A report of fatal systemic lupus erythematosus associated with the use of an ophthalmic preparation containing sulphacetamide sodium.— J. D. Adams, *Aust. J. Derm.*, 1978, *19*, 31.

Stevens-Johnson syndrome. A 73-year-old man who had been taking sulphamethoxazole developed the Stevens-Johnson syndrome shortly after starting treatment with sulphacetamide sodium 30% eye-drops.— Z. Rubin (letter), *Archs Derm.*, 1977, *113*, 235. See also H. R. Gottschalk and O. J. Stone, *Archs Derm.*, 1976, *112*, 513.

Absorption and Fate. As for Sulphonamides, p.1458.

Sulphacetamide is readily absorbed from the gastro-intestinal tract. It is rapidly excreted in the urine, largely unchanged.

When sulphacetamide sodium is applied to the eye high concentrations are achieved in ocular tissues and fluids; sulphonamide may be absorbed into the blood when the conjunctiva is inflamed.

The biological half-life of sulphacetamide is variously reported as 7 to 12.8 hours.— W. A. Ritschel, *Drug Intell. & clin. Pharm.*, 1970, *4*, 332.

Uses. Sulphacetamide has the general properties of sulphonamides. It was formerly used in the treatment of bacterial infections of the urinary tract.

Sulphacetamide is a constituent of mixed sulphonamide preparations for vaginal use (p.1486).

Sulphacetamide sodium is used mainly by local application in infections or injuries of the eyes. In the treatment of acute conjunctivitis and in the prophylaxis of ocular infections after injuries or burns, a 10% solution is applied every 2 hours, or a 30% solution twice daily; ointments containing 2.5, 6, or 10% are also used.

A review of the uses of sulphacetamide sodium.— L. Weinstein *et al.*, *New Engl. J. Med.*, 1960, *263*, 793.

Eye infections. Neonatal chlamydial conjunctivitis responded to treatment with sulphonamide eye-drops.— G. W. Csonka and E. D. Coufalik, *Postgrad. med. J.*, 1977, *53*, 592. See also J. E. Johnson *et al.*, *Mayo Clin. Proc.*, 1976, *51*, 574.

Ophthalmia neonatorum caused by beta-lactamase-producing gonococci in premature identical twins was successfully treated with sulphacetamide 30% eye-drops every 6 hours and erythromycin by drip feed replaced after 24 hours by cefuroxime 100 mg per kg body-weight daily intramuscularly in 3 divided doses for 7 days. The recovery of gonococci from sites other than the eye in these patients pointed to the need for systemic antigonococcal treatment in such babies.— E. M. C. Dunlop *et al.*, *Br. med. J.*, 1980, *281*, 483.

Further references: *Med. Lett.*, 1976, *18*, 70.

Skin disorders. In very chronic cases of paronychia, sulphacetamide [sodium] 15% in 50% alcohol was very useful since it was easy to apply, well tolerated, and dealt with both the bacterial and the candidal elements of the infection.— P. D. Samman, *Practitioner*, 1973, *211*, 600.

Further references: S. Olansky, *Cutis*, 1977, *19*, 852.

Preparations

Eye Ointments

Sulfacetamide Sodium Ophthalmic Ointment *(U.S.P.)*. A sterile eye ointment containing sulphacetamide sodium.

Sulphacetamide Sodium Eye Ointment *(B.P.)*. Sulphacetamide Eye Ointment; Sulphacetam. Eye Oint.; Oculent. Sulphacetam.; Sulfacetamide Eye Ointment. It contains sterile sulphacetamide sodium in a sterile basis which may consist of a mixture of liquid paraffin 1 and yellow soft paraffin 9 (by wt). *A.P.F.* specifies 10%.

Sulphacetamide Sodium Eye Ointment 6 or 10% is 'an approved eye ointment' for use in factory first-aid boxes.

Eye-drops

Sulfacetamide Sodium Ophthalmic Solution *(U.S.P.)*. A sterile solution of sulphacetamide sodium; it may contain suitable buffers, stabilisers, and antimicrobial agents. Store in a cool place in airtight containers. Protect from light.

Sulphacetamide Eye Drops *(A.P.F.)*. Gutt. Sulphacetam. Sulphacetamide sodium 10 g, sodium metabisulphite 100 mg, disodium edetate 50 mg, phenethyl alcohol 0.4 ml, phenylmercuric nitrate 2 mg, Water for Injections to 100 ml. Sterilised by autoclaving. Protect from light.

Sulphacetamide Eye Drops Strong *(A.P.F.)*. Gutt. Sulphacetam. Fort. Sulphacetamide sodium 30 g, sodium metabisulphite 100 mg, disodium edetate 50 mg, phenethyl alcohol 0.4 ml, phenylmercuric nitrate 2 mg, Water for Injections to 100 ml. Sterilised by autoclaving. Protect from light.

Sulphacetamide Sodium Eye-drops *(B.P.)*. Sulphacetamide Eye-Drops; Guttae Sulphacetamidi; SULF. A sterile solution of sulphacetamide sodium in water. When intended for use on more than one occasion they contain the equivalent of not more than 0.1% of sulphur dioxide and phenylmercuric acetate or nitrate 0.002% or thiomersal 0.01%, and should not be used later than 4 weeks after first opening the container. pH 6.6 to 8.6. Sterilised by autoclaving, maintaining at 98° to 100° for 30 minutes, or by filtration. The amount of air in the final containers should be kept to a minimum.

The *B.P.C. 1973* specified that when the strength is not specified or when Weak Sulphacetamide Eye-drops are ordered or prescribed, a solution containing 10% of sulphacetamide sodium is supplied. When Strong Sulphacetamide Eye-drops are ordered or prescribed, a solution containing 30% of sulphacetamide sodium is supplied. Store at room temperature. Protect from light.

Proprietary Preparations

Albucid *(Nicholas, UK)*. Sulphacetamide sodium, available as **Eye Drops** containing 10, 20, and 30% and as **Eye Ointment** containing 2.5 and 6% in a greasy basis and 10% in a water-miscible basis. (Also available as Albucid in *Arg., Austral., S.Afr.*).

Bleph-10 Liquifilm *(Allergan, UK)*. Eye-drops containing sulphacetamide sodium 10%. (Also available as Bleph-10 in *Canad., S.Afr., USA*).

Cortucid *(Nicholas, UK)*. A fluid water-miscible cream containing sulphacetamide sodium 10% and hydrocortisone acetate 0.5%. For inflammatory eye conditions.

Isopto Cetamide *(Alcon, UK: Farillon, UK)*. Eye-drops containing sulphacetamide sodium 15%, with hypromellose 0.5%. (Also available as Isopto Cetamide in *Austral., Canad., Neth., USA*).

Minims Sulphacetamide Sodium *(Smith & Nephew Pharmaceuticals, UK)*. Sterile eye-drops containing sulphacetamide sodium 10%, in single-use disposable applicators. (Also available as Minims Sulphacetamide Sodium in *Austral.*).

Ocusol *(Boots, UK)*. Eye-drops containing sulphacetamide sodium 5% and zinc sulphate 0.1%. For infected eye conditions.

Sulfapred *(Wallace Mfg Chem., UK: Farillon, UK)*. Eye-drops containing sulphacetamide sodium 10% and prednisolone sodium phosphate 0.5%.

Sulphacalyre *(Wallace Mfg Chem., UK: Farillon, UK)*. Eye-drops containing sulphacetamide sodium 10, 20, and 30%.

Other Proprietary Names of Sulphacetamide Sodium

Acetopt *(Austral.)*; Antebor *(Belg., Fr., Switz.)*; Blef *(Arg.)*; Buco-Albucid *(Spain)*; Cetamide *(Canad., USA)*; Isopto Cetamida *(Arg.)*; Optamide *(Austral.)*; Optosulfex *(Canad.)*; Prontamid *(Ital.)*; Sebizon *(USA)*; Sodium Sulamyd *(Canad., USA)*; Spersacet *(Switz.)*; Sulf-10 *(Canad., USA)*; Sulf-30 *(Canad.)*; Vasosulf *(S.Afr.)*.

Sulphacetamide sodium was also formerly marketed in Great Britain under the proprietary names Opulets Sulphacetamide Ointment (*Pharmax*) and Vasosulf (*Knox Laboratories* now *Cooper Vision*).

4929-m

Sulphachlorpyridazine. N^1-(6-Chloropyridazin-3-yl)sulphanilamide.

$C_{10}H_9ClN_4O_2S = 284.7$.

CAS — 80-32-0.

Sulphachlorpyridazine is a sulphonamide (p.1457) which is rapidly excreted in the urine and was formerly used in urinary-tract infections.

Proprietary Names

Durasulf *(Dessy, Ital.)*; Nefrosul *(Riker, USA)*; Sonilyn *(Mallinckrodt, USA)*; Sulfaclorazine *(Ellem, Ital.)*.

4930-t

Sulphadiazine *(B.P., B.P. Vet., Eur. P.)*.

Sulphadiaz.; Sulfadiazine *(U.S.P.)* Sulfadiazinum; Solfadiazina; Solfapirimidina. N^1-(Pyrimidin-2-yl)sulphanilamide.

$C_{10}H_{10}N_4O_2S = 250.3$.

CAS — 68-35-9.

Pharmacopoeias. In *Arg., Aust., Belg., Br., Chin., Eur., Fr., Ger., Ind., Int., It., Jug., Mex., Neth., Nord., Port., Roum., Span., Swiss, Turk.,* and *U.S.*

White, yellowish-white, or pinkish-white, odourless or almost odourless, tasteless crystals or powder, slowly darkening on exposure to light. M.p. about 255° with decomposition.

Soluble 1 in 13 000 of water at 25°, 1 in 60 of boiling water, and 1 in 300 of acetone; very slightly soluble in alcohol; practically insoluble in chloroform and ether; soluble in dilute mineral acids and in solutions of alkali hydroxides and carbonates. **Sterilisation** of the powder as for Sulphadimidine, p.1475. **Store** in airtight containers. Protect from light.

No linear correlation was found between the biological availability of sulphadiazine from tablets and their rate of dissolution *in vitro*, when 8 different brands and one control suspension were given to 10 subjects. Each received a 4-g dose of 1 preparation together with sodium bicarbonate after an overnight fast, and considerable variation of blood-total and free sulphadiazine concentrations were noted during the first 4 hours after administration.— G. R. Van Petten *et al.*, *J. clin. Pharmac.*, 1971, *11*, 27.

4931-x

Sulphadiazine Sodium *(B.P. 1968)*.

Sulphadiaz. Sod.; Soluble Sulphadiazine; Sulfadiazine Sodium *(U.S.P.)*; Sodium Sulfadiazine; Sulfadiazinum Natricum.

$C_{10}H_9N_4NaO_2S = 272.3$.

CAS — 547-32-0.

Pharmacopoeias. In *Aust., Belg., Int., Jug., Mex., Turk.,* and *U.S.*

A white or yellowish-white, odourless, almost tasteless powder. It slowly darkens on exposure to light; on exposure to moist air it absorbs carbon dioxide with the liberation of sulphadiazine and becomes incompletely soluble in water. Sulphadiazine sodium 1.09 g is approximately equivalent to 1 g of sulphadiazine.

Soluble 1 in 2 of water; slightly soluble in alcohol; practically insoluble in chloroform and ether. A 10% solution has a pH of 10 to 11. A 4.24% solution is iso-osmotic with serum. Solutions are **sterilised** by distributing into ampoules, replacing the air with nitrogen or other suitable gas, sealing, and autoclaving. **Incompatible** with acids, amikacin sulphate, cefapirin sodium, laevulose, iron salts, and salts of heavy metals. **Store** in airtight containers. Protect from light.

Incompatibility. Clarity was lost when solutions of sulphadiazine sodium were mixed with those of insulin, narcotic salts, noradrenaline acid tartrate, procaine hydrochloride, streptomycin sulphate, tetracycline hydrochloride, or vancomycin hydrochloride, or with laevulose, invert sugar, lactated Ringer's, sodium lactate, or ammonium chloride injections.— J. A. Patel and G. L. Phillips, *Am. J. Hosp. Pharm.*, 1966, *23*, 409.

A precipitate occurred within 1 hour when sulphadiazine sodium 2.5 g was added to chloramphenicol sodium succinate 1 g per litre.— E. A. Parker (letter), *Am. J. Hosp. Pharm.*, 1970, *27*, 69.

A haze developed over 3 hours when sulphadiazine sodium was mixed with amiphenazole hydrochloride in sodium chloride injection. An immediate precipitate occurred when sulphadiazine sodium was mixed with chlorpromazine hydrochloride, kanamycin sulphate, oxytetracycline hydrochloride, or tetracycline hydrochloride in dextrose injection or sodium chloride injection. A crystalline precipitate occurred when sulphadiazine sodium was mixed with lignocaine hydrochloride or methicillin sodium in dextrose injection, crystals were produced with streptomycin sulphate in sodium chloride injection, and a crystalline precipitate with gentamicin sulphate, iron dextran, lincomycin hydrochloride, metaraminol tartrate, methyldopate hydrochloride, or vitamin compound injection in dextrose injection and sodium chloride injection. A yellow colour with a precipitate developing over 3 hours occurred when sulphadiazine sodium was mixed with hydralazine hydrochloride in dextrose injection, and an immediate precipitate occurred with prochlorperazine mesylate in sodium chloride injection, but when they were mixed in dextrose injection a haze developed over 3 hours.— B. B. Riley, *J. Hosp. Pharm.*, 1970, *28*, 228.

A fine crystalline precipitate occurred when sulphadiazine sodium 40 mmol per litre was added to dextrose injection 10%.— D. Preskey and J. B. Kayes, *J. clin. Pharm.*, 1976, *1*, 39.

Adverse Effects, Treatment, and Precautions. As for Sulphonamides, p.1457.

A severe form of erythema multiforme, the Stevens-Johnson syndrome, has been reported in patients after treatment with sulphadiazine.

Because of the low solubilities of sulphadiazine and its acetyl derivative in urine, crystalluria should be guarded against; sufficient fluid should be given to maintain an adequate urine output and the urine should be rendered alkaline.

Renal complications occur more frequently with intravenous than with oral administration. Sulphadiazine sodium solution is strongly alkaline and tends to cause thrombosis of the vein; extravasation may cause sloughing and necrosis.

Sulphadiazine sodium should not be given by intrathecal or subcutaneous injection; intramuscular injections are painful.

Numerous white stone-like concretions of sulphadiazine occurred in the conjunctiva of a woman who had used sulphadiazine eye-drops for about one year.— E. A. Boettner *et al.*, *Archs Ophthal., N.Y.*, 1974, *92*, 446.

A 3-year-old girl weighing 13 kg developed crystalluria and hypoglycaemia after excessive doses of sulphadiazine—300 to 450 mg per kg body-weight per 24 hours.— A. W. Craft *et al.*, *Postgrad. med. J.*, 1977, *53*, 103.

Enhanced effect. Reports of reduced protein binding of sulphadiazine in the plasma of patients with *acute renal failure*.— F. Andreasen, *Acta pharmac. tox.*, 1973, *32*, 417. With *alcoholic hepatitis*.— M. J. Brodie and S. Boobis, *Eur. J. clin. Pharmac.*, 1978, *13*, 435. With *malnutrition*.— K. Krishnaswamy, *Clin. Pharmacokinet.*, 1978, *3*, 216.

Interactions. For the effect of sulphadiazine in slightly increasing the half-life of tolbutamide, see Tolbutamide, p.860.

Solubility in urine. The solubility of sulphadiazine in urine at pH 5.5, 6.5, and 7.5 was 130, 280, and 2000 µg per ml respectively; the solubility of the acetyl derivative at the same pH values was 200, 750, and 5120 µg per ml respectively.— D. R. Gilligan *et al.*, *J. Am. med. Ass.*, 1943, *122*, 1160.

In 7 healthy female subjects given sulphadiazine 600 mg daily by mouth for 6 days the urinary-sulphonamide concentration exceeded the experimental solubility 6 and 24 hours after the last dose in 5 and 3 patients respectively. Sulphadiazine crystals were found in the urine of 3 of the 5 patients tested at 6 hours.— P. Ylitalo and H. Vapaatalo, *Arzneimittel-Forsch.*, 1977, *27*, 1726.

Absorption and Fate. As for Sulphonamides, p.1458.

Sulphadiazine is readily absorbed from the gastro-intestinal tract, peak blood concentrations being reached 3 to 4 hours after a single dose; 20 to 55% has been reported to be bound to plasma albumin. It penetrates into the cerebrospinal fluid to produce therapeutic concentrations, usually more than half of those in the blood, within 4 hours of administration by mouth of a dose of 60 mg per kg body-weight. Up to 15% of sulphadiazine in the blood is present as the acetyl derivative.

Sulphadiazine is excreted somewhat slowly, about 50% of a single dose by mouth being eliminated in 24 hours; 15 to 40% is excreted as the acetyl derivative.

The biological half-life of sulphadiazine is variously reported as 8 to 16.8 hours.— W. A. Ritschel, *Drug Intell. & clin. Pharm.*, 1970, *4*, 332. The half-life of sulphadiazine ranges from 7 to 12 hours and that of its metabolite from 8 to 18 hours.— T. B. Vree *et al.*, *Clin. Pharmacokinet.*, 1980, *5*, 274.

Elimination half-lives of sulphadiazine, sulfamerazine, and sulphadimidine were 13, 12.7, and 2.3 hours respectively in a healthy subject given 330 mg of each sulphonamide as a combined suspension by mouth.— T. J. Goehl *et al.*, *J. pharm. Sci.*, 1978, *67*, 404.

The urinary excretion of sulphadiazine and the acetyl derivative is dependent on pH. About 30% is excreted unchanged in both fast and slow acetylators when the urine is acidic whereas about 75% is excreted unchanged by slow acetylators when the urine is alkaline.— T. B. Vree *et al.*, *Clin. Pharmacokinet.*, 1980, *5*, 274.

Bioavailability. A bioavailability study of commercially available preparations of sulphadiazine in 16 healthy subjects.— M. C. Meyer *et al.*, *J. pharm. Sci.*, 1978, *67*, 1659.

Uses. Sulphadiazine has the general properties of Sulphonamides, p.1458.

In the treatment of susceptible infections sulphadiazine may be given by mouth in an initial dose of 2 to 4 g followed by 1 g every 4 to 6 hours; a suggested dose in children is 75 mg per kg body-weight initially then 150 mg per kg daily in divided doses. In severe infections a concentration in the blood of 100 to 150 µg per ml is desirable. Sulphadiazine in doses of 2 g initially and then 0.5 to 1 g every 6 to 8 hours has been used in urinary-tract infections but is not the treatment of choice. Nocardiosis has been treated successfully with sulphadiazine. In toxoplasmosis, sulphadiazine is given with pyrimethamine (p.403).

In severe meningococcal meningitis sulphadiazine is given intravenously although meningococci resistant to sulphonamides are common and treatment with antibiotics may be preferred. Sulphadiazine sodium equivalent to sulphadiazine 1 to 1.5 g is given intravenously every 4 hours for 2 days followed by sulphadiazine by mouth; children may be given the equivalent of 50 mg per kg body-weight initially and then 100 mg per kg daily in 4 divided doses; higher doses have been given in severe infections. An oral dose of sulphadiazine 2 g daily has been given prophylactically for 3 days to contacts.

Intravenous doses of sulphadiazine sodium are given by infusion or by slow intravenous injection of a solution containing up to 5%. It may be diluted with sodium chloride injection. Sulphadiazine sodium has been given by deep intramuscular injection but great care must be exercised to prevent damage to subcutaneous tissues and the intravenous route is preferred. It must not be given intrathecally or subcutaneously. Oral administration should begin as soon as possible.

For the use of sulphadiazine with trimethoprim, see Co-trimazine, p.1460.

Sulphadiazine 1 µg per ml, a concentration capable of being achieved in saliva following oral administration, inhibited *in vitro* both plaque formation and growth of *Streptococcus mutans* considered to be implicated in dental caries.— H. G. Weld and H. J. Sandham, *Antimicrob. Ag. Chemother.*, 1976, *10*, 196. However, experience in 31 children being treated with sulphadiazine showed no beneficial effect against caries.— *idem*, 200.

Administration in renal failure. Sulphadiazine should be avoided in patients with even mild renal failure.— G. B. Appel and H. C. Neu, *New Engl. J. Med.*, 1977, *296*, 663.

Chancroid. A 27-year-old male was successfully treated for chancroid with streptomycin injection daily for 10 days and sulphadiazine 1 g four times daily for 10 weeks.— K. Harvey *et al.*, *Med. J. Aust.*, 1977, *1*, 956.

An account of an epidemic of chancroid in Greenland with 975 cases in 1977. In most cases the clinical course was uncomplicated and lesions healed within a week of starting 14 days of sulphadiazine therapy. Bubonic cases were treated with streptomycin and lymph-node aspiration as well.— L. Lykke-Olesen *et al.*, *Lancet*, 1979, *1*, 654.

Endocarditis. Endocarditis caused by *Brucella melitensis* in a patient with heart valve prostheses was successfully treated with sulphadiazine 6 g daily for 3 courses of 21 days each, together with tetracycline 2 g daily.— R. Lezaun *et al.*, *Postgrad. med. J.*, 1980, *56*, 119.

Malaria. Quinine sulphate with pyrimethamine, both for 3 days, and sulphadiazine 500 mg four times daily for 5 days is the treatment of choice in uncomplicated attacks of malaria due to chloroquine-resistant strains of *Plasmodium falciparum*. Pyrimethamine and sulphadiazine are considered to lower the rate of recurrence.— *Med. Lett.*, 1979, *21*, 105.

Meningitis. Intimate contacts of patients with meningococcal meningitis should receive sulphadiazine prophylactically for 2 to 4 days. In influenzal meningitis, treatment is only necessary if infection develops. In infants, ampicillin or chloramphenicol is preferable.— L. L. Coriell, *J. Am. med. Ass.*, 1967, *201*, 281.

In a study of 4800 men admitted to a closed community in Egypt, sulphadiazine 2 g daily for 3 days had no effect on the incidence of meningococcal carriers or of cases of meningitis. In 529 of 725 throat cultures, meningococci were isolated; 456 strains belonged to group A, and 94% of group A strains tested were resistant to sulphadiazine 10 µg per ml. During the period of 3 months 24 cases of group A meningitis occurred.— A. Hassan *et al.*, *Trop. geogr. Med.*, 1974, *26*, 87, per *Abstr. Hyg.*, 1974, *49*, 870.

Sulphadiazine sodium had an MIC of 50, 10, 5, and 1 µg per ml against 97, 86, 66, and 38 of 100 strains of meningococci *in vitro*.— R. S. Miles and A. Moyes, *J. clin. Path.*, 1978, *31*, 355.

All of 60 strains of meningococci isolated from 52 patients with meningococcal disease and 8 carriers were resistant to sulphadiazine sodium 10 µg per ml. They were all sensitive to penicillin 0.04 µg per ml, rifampicin 0.125 µg per ml, or minocycline 2 µg per ml.— M. Hassan-King *et al.*, *Trans. R. Soc. trop. Med. Hyg.*, 1979, *73*, 567.

Nocardiosis. Sulphadiazine sodium 6 g daily by mouth for 5 months was successful in the treatment of an intracranial infection with *Nocardia asteroides* which occurred in one patient secondary to head trauma. Sulphadiazine was discontinued after 5 months because of severe crystalluria.— D. M. Poretz *et al.*, *J. Am. med. Ass.*, 1975, *232*, 730.

Sulphafurazole or sulphadiazine are still considered the treatment of choice for nocardiosis.— G. P. Wormser and G. T. Keusch, *Ann. intern. Med.*, 1979, *91*, 420.

Further references: W. E. Herrell, *Clin. Med.*, 1967, *74* (May), 85; D. W. Burdon, *Br. med. J.*, 1971, *1*, 538.

Plague. The routine treatment of patients with plague with streptomycin intramuscularly 1 g daily and sulphafurazole 2 g by mouth daily was associated with a gradual increase in adenopathy, sometimes needing surgical intervention, and a period of 10 days in hospital. Adenopathy was cleared and the stay in hospital reduced to 5 days when therapy was changed to streptomycin 1 g intramuscularly and sulphadiazine 6 g by intravenous infusion on admission, with a further 1 g of streptomycin and 4 g of sulphadiazine on the following day.— N. M. Hoang and H. M. Rozendaal (letter), *J. Am. med. Ass.*, 1968, *205*, 596.

Rheumatic fever prophylaxis. Sulphadiazine 1 g once daily may be given for the continuous prophylaxis of rheumatic fever in patients at low risk of recurrences; those weighing less than 30 kg are given 500 mg daily. Sulphonamides should not be used to treat streptococcal infections since they will not eradicate the streptococcus.—Report of the Committee on Rheumatic Fever and Bacterial Endocarditis of the American Heart Association, *Circulation*, 1977, *55*, Jan. See also WHO Memorandum, *Bull. Wld Hlth Org.*, 1978, *56*, 887.

Urinary-tract infections. Findings from pharmacokinetic and clinical studies of sulphadiazine that a dose of 250 mg or 500 mg twice daily for adults or 4 mg per kg body-weight twice daily for children is adequate in the treatment of acute urinary-tract infections.— J. Seppänen, *Ann. clin. Res.*, 1980, *12*, *Suppl.* 25, 1–51.

Preparations

Sulfadiazine Sodium Injection *(U.S.P.)*. A sterile solution of sulphadiazine sodium, 237.5 to 262.5 mg per ml, in Water for Injections. pH 8.5 to 10.5. Protect from light.

Sulfadiazine Tablets *(U.S.P.)*. Tablets containing sulphadiazine. Protect from light.

Sulphadiazine Injection *(B.P.)*. Inj. Sulphadiaz. Sod. A sterile solution of sulphadiazine sodium in Water for Injections free from dissolved air; it contains the equivalent of not more than 0.1% of sulphur dioxide. It is distributed in ampoules in which the air has been replaced by nitrogen or other suitable gas, and sterilised by autoclaving. Potency is expressed in terms of the equivalent amount of sulphadiazine. pH 10 to 11. Protect from light.

Sulphadiazine Mixture *(Adelaide Child. Hosp.)*. Sulphadiazine 500 mg, tragacanth mucilage 1 ml, orange syrup 1 ml, docusate sodium 2.5 mg, hydroxybenzoates spirits 0.0005 ml, chloroform 0.0075 ml, alcohol (90%)

0.0675 ml, water to 5 ml. *Dose.* Sulphadiazine, 150 to 200 mg per kg body-weight daily in four 6-hourly doses.

Sulphadiazine Tablets *(B.P.).* Tablets containing sulphadiazine. Protect from light.

Proprietary Preparations

Sulphadiazine Sodium *(May & Baker, UK).* Available as injection containing the equivalent of 250 mg of sulphadiazine per ml, in ampoules of 4 ml. (Also available as Sulphadiazine Sodium in *Austral.*).

Other Proprietary Names of Sulphadiazine

Adiazine *(Belg., Fr.)*; Diazyl Dulcet, S-Diazine *(both Austral.)*.

4932-r

Sulphadimethoxine.

Sulfadimethoxine; Solfadimetossina; Solfadimetossipirimidina. N^1-(2,6-Dimethoxypyrimidin-4-yl)sulphanilamide.

$C_{12}H_{14}N_4O_4S=310.3$.

CAS — 122-11-2.

Pharmacopoeias. In *Br., Fr., It., Jug.,* and *Nord.*

A white, or creamy white, almost odourless, tasteless, crystalline powder. M.p. 198° to 204°. Very slightly **soluble** in water; soluble 1 in 200 of alcohol, 1 in 800 of chloroform, and 1 in 2000 of ether; soluble in dilute mineral acids and in solutions of alkali hydroxides and carbonates. **Protect** from light.

Adverse Effects, Treatment, and Precautions. As for Sulphonamides, p.1457.

If side-effects occur, sulphadimethoxine has the disadvantage that several days are required for its elimination from the body. The Stevens-Johnson syndrome has been reported following the use of sulphadimethoxine.

Effects on the blood. Sulphadimethoxine has been reported to cause haemolysis in patients with haemoglobin Zürich (an unstable haemoglobin).— E. Beutler, *Pharmac. Rev.,* 1969, *21,* 73.

Hepatitis. A patient developed granulomatous reactions in the liver and lymph nodes, with fever, skin rash, jaundice, and interstitial pneumonitis, 2 days after the administration of 2 g of sulphadimethoxine by mouth. He made a full spontaneous recovery within 3 weeks.— C. R. Espiritu *et al., J. Am. med. Ass.,* 1967, *202,* 985.

Interactions. For the effect of sulphadimethoxine in reducing protein binding of sulphonylurea compounds, see Chlorpropamide, p.853.

For the possible effect of sulphadimethoxine on the half-life of tolbutamide, see Tolbutamide, p.860.

Absorption and Fate. As for Sulphonamides, p.1458.

Sulphadimethoxine is readily absorbed from the gastro-intestinal tract. After a single dose of 2 g peak blood concentrations are reached in 4 to 6 hours; concentrations after 24 hours are still at least half the original value. About 90% of sulphadimethoxine is bound to plasma albumin. About 10% of sulphadimethoxine in the blood is present as the acetyl derivative and rather less as the glucuronide. Penetration into the cerebrospinal fluid is poor.

Sulphadimethoxine is excreted slowly in the urine, about half of a single dose being recovered in 48 hours; about 80% is excreted in the form of a relatively highly soluble glucuronide, and about 15% as the acetyl derivative. Sulphadimethoxine and its acetyl derivative are poorly soluble in urine.

The biological half-life of sulphadimethoxine is variously reported as 20.2 to 41 hours.— W. A. Ritschel, *Drug Intell. & clin. Pharm.,* 1970, *4,* 332.

Sulphadimethoxine was about 73.2% bound to human muscle tissue *in vitro.*— B. Fichtl and H. Kurz, *Eur. J. clin. Pharmac.,* 1978, *14,* 335.

Uses. Sulphadimethoxine is a long-acting sulphonamide, with the general properties of sulphonamides, p.1458. With usual doses the blood concentration of unconjugated sulphadimethoxine can be maintained at 50 to 100 μg per ml.

The initial dose is 1 or 2 g, according to the severity of the infection, followed by a dose of 0.5 to 1 g daily. A suggested dose for children is 30 mg per kg body-weight initially, followed by one-half this amount daily.

A review of sulphadimethoxine.— L. Weinstein *et al., New Engl. J. Med.,* 1960, *263,* 842.

Leprosy. For an opinion that sulphadimethoxine is not suitable for the treatment of leprosy, see Sulphamethoxypyridazine, p.1480.

For earlier clinical reports on sulphadimethoxine, see Martindale 27th Edn, p. 1478.

Preparations

Sulphadimethoxine Tablets *(B.P.).* Tablets containing sulphadimethoxine. Protect from light.

Madribon *(Roche, UK).* Sulphadimethoxine, available as scored tablets of 500 mg. (Also available as Madribon in *Austral., Belg., Canad., Denm., Fr., Ger., Ital., S.Afr., Spain, Swed., Switz.*).

Other Proprietary Names

Arg.—Lenterap; *Denm.*—Sulfoplan; *Ital.*—Bensulfa, Chemiosalfa, Crozinal, Deltin, Diasulfa, Diazinol, Dimetossilina, Fultamid, Ipersulfa, Levisul, Micromega, Neosulfamyd, Redifal, Risulpir, Ritarsulfa, Sulfabon, Sulfadomus, Sulfaduran, Sulfastop, Sulfomikron, Tempodiazina; *Pol.*—Madroxine; *S.Afr.*—Jatsulph, Lensulpha, Pansulph, Sulfathox; *Spain*— Dimetoxan, Oxazina, Sulf-reten.

4933-f

Sulphadimidine

(B.P., B.P. Vet., Eur. P.). Sulphadimid.; Sulfadimidine; Sulfadimidinum; Sulphadimethylpyrimidine; Sulphamethazine; Sulfamethazine *(U.S.P.)*; Sulfadimérazine; Sulfadimezinum; Solfametazina. N^1-(4,6-Dimethylpyrimidin-2-yl)sulphanilamide.

$C_{12}H_{14}N_4O_2S=278.3$.

CAS — 57-68-1.

NOTE. Sulfadimethylpyrimidine has been used as a synonym for sulphasomidine (see p.1483). Care should be taken to avoid confusion between the two compounds, which are isomeric.

Pharmacopoeias. In *Arg., Aust., Br., Chin., Cz., Eur., Fr., Ger., Hung., Ind., Int., It., Jug., Neth., Nord., Pol., Roum., Rus., Swiss, Turk.,* and *U.S.*

White or yellowish-white, odourless or almost odourless, crystals or powder with a slighlty bitter taste. M.p. 197° to 200°. It darkens and decomposes on exposure to light.

Very slightly **soluble** in water; soluble 1 in 200 of boiling water; soluble 1 in 120 of alcohol, 1 in 30 of acetone, 1 in 600 of chloroform, and 1 in 2500 of ether; soluble in dilute mineral acids and in aqueous solutions of alkali hydroxides and carbonates.

Sulphadimidine may be **sterilised** by reducing to a fine powder, drying at 100°, and heating in the final sealed containers so that the whole of the powder is maintained at 150° for 1 hour; the sterilised powder is not more than slightly discoloured. **Store** in airtight containers. Protect from light.

The effect of formulation and compression on the absorption of sulphadimidine tablets.— M. C. B. van Oudtshoorn *et al., J. Pharm. Pharmac.,* 1971, *23,* 583.

Mention of changes in dissolution-rate and equilibrium solubility of the hydrophobic drug sulphadimidine, brought about by the presence of hydrophilic polymers, povidone and carmellose sodium, in the dissolution medium.— *Pharm. J.,* 1978, *2,* 249.

A study on the formulation and evaluation of a sulphadimidine suspension for infants.— R. N. Nasipuri and E. O. Ogunlana, *Pharm. J.,* 1978, *2,* 258.

4934-d

Sulphadimidine Sodium

(B.P., B.P. Vet.). Sulphadimid. Sod.; Sulfadimidine Sodium; Soluble Sulphadimidine; Soluble Sulphamethazine; Soluble Sulphadimethylpyrimidine.

$C_{12}H_{13}N_4NaO_2S=300.3$.

CAS — 1981-58-4.

Pharmacopoeias. In *Aust., Br., Ind., Pol.,* and *Turk.*

White or creamy-white, odourless or almost odourless, hygroscopic crystals or powder with a bitter alkaline taste. It slowly discolours and decomposes on exposure to light; on exposure to air it absorbs carbon dioxide and becomes less soluble in water. Sulphadimidine sodium 1.08 g is approximately equivalent to 1 g of sulphadimidine.

Soluble 1 in 2.5 of water and 1 in 60 of alcohol. A 10% solution has a pH of 10 to 11. Solutions are most stable at pH 10 to 11; precipitation of sulphadimidine occurs below pH 10. Solutions are **sterilised** by distributing into ampoules, replacing the air with nitrogen or other suitable gas, sealing, and autoclaving, or by filtration into sterile ampoules in which the air is replaced by nitrogen or other suitable gas. **Incompatible** with acids, iron salts, and salts of heavy metals. **Store** in airtight containers. Protect from light.

Incompatibility. A haze developed over 3 hours when sulphadimidine sodium was mixed with amiphenazole hydrochloride in sodium chloride injection. An immediate precipitate occurred with chlorpromazine hydrochloride, promazine hydrochloride, promethazine hydrochloride, and a yellow colour with a precipitate developing over 3 hours occurred with hydralazine hydrochloride in dextrose injection or sodium chloride injection. An immediate precipitate occurred when sulphadimidine sodium was mixed with prochlorperazine mesylate in sodium chloride injection, but when they were mixed in dextrose injection a haze developed over 3 hours.— B. B. Riley, *J. Hosp. Pharm.,* 1970, *28,* 228.

Adverse Effects, Treatment, and Precautions. As for Sulphonamides, p.1457.

The Stevens-Johnson syndrome has been reported after treatment with sulphadimidine. Sulphadimidine and its acetyl derivative are relatively soluble in urine; the risk of crystalluria is therefore slight, but adequate fluid intake is recommended.

Sulphadimidine sodium should not be given intrathecally or subcutaneously; intramuscular injections are painful.

Effects on the blood. A 7-year-old boy developed acute haemolytic anaemia following a total dose of 28 g of sulphadimidine given over a period of 5 days. Recovery occurred after treatment with blood transfusion, prednisone, and penicillin intramuscularly. Hypersensitivity rather than a direct haemolytic action was thought to be the cause.— J. L. Grech and E. A. Cachia, *Br. med. J.,* 1959, *2,* 1309.

Effects on the heart. A 12-year-old African boy developed a fulminating skin lesion 2 days after sulphadimidine therapy (6 g in 2 days) and acute cardiomyopathy 28 days later. The cardiomyopathy was considered most likely to be a hypersensitivity reaction to sulphadimidine.— E. T. M. MacSearraigh and K. M. Patel, *Br. med. J.,* 1968, *3,* 33.

Solubility in urine. The solubilities of sulphadimidine and its acetyl derivative in urine at 37° were 692 and 670 μg per ml respectively at pH 6, 752 and 864 μg per ml at pH 6.4, 833 and 907 μg per ml at 6.8, 997 and 1140 μg per ml at pH 7.2, 1.445 and 1.762 mg per ml at pH 7.6, and 1.793 and 2.16 mg per ml at pH 8.— L. H. Schmidt *et al., J. Pharmac. exp. Ther.,* 1944, *81,* 17.

Absorption and Fate. As for Sulphonamides, p.1458.

Sulphadimidine is readily absorbed from the gastro-intestinal tract and about 60 to 80% is bound to plasma albumin. It penetrates into the cerebrospinal fluid, but less readily than sulphadiazine; concentrations of sulphadimidine in body fluids may be more than half those in the blood. About 40% of sulphadimidine in the blood is present as the acetyl derivative. About 50% of a dose may be excreted in the urine in 2 days, 70% being in the form of the acetyl derivative.

A study of the kinetics of the intestinal absorption of sulphadimidine.— G. L. Turco *et al., Clin. Pharmac. Ther.,* 1966, *7,* 603.

Sulphadimidine tablets, 50% of which dissolved in 1 to 5 minutes *in vitro,* were given to 9 subjects in a 3-g dose, and gave average serum concentrations of free plus acetylated sulphadimidine at 0.5, 1, 4, 10, and 24 hours of 19, 43.7, 82, 59.5, and 17.5 µg per ml respectively. Average serum concentrations of free sulphadimidine at the same times were 17.2, 37, and about 57, 32, and 8 µg per ml respectively.— M. J. Taraszka and R. A. Delor, *J. pharm. Sci.*, 1969, *58*, 207.

In 20 healthy men the biological half-life of sulphadimidine was 4 and 8.8 hours for rapid and slow acetylators respectively.— M. C. B. van Oudtshoorn and F. J. Potgieter, *J. Pharm. Pharmac.*, 1972, *24*, 357.

In 9 healthy subjects given sulphadimidine 1 g four times daily for 3 days mean plasma concentrations of unconjugated sulphadimidine on the third day were 139 µg per ml, with total sulphadimidine 205 µg per ml, and unconjugated sulphadimidine in urine 574 µg per ml. In 3 patients with renal failure and plasma-creatinine concentrations of 25 to 109 µg per ml mean plasma concentrations of unconjugated sulphadimidine on the third day were 149 µg per ml, while in 7 patients with plasma-creatinine concentrations in excess of 50 µg per ml mean urine concentrations of unconjugated sulphadimidine were 45 µg per ml, probably less than the MIC for *Escherichia coli*. In 3 patients undergoing peritoneal dialysis, for whom sulphadimidine 100 or 200 µg per ml was added to the dialysate, concentrations of unconjugated sulphonamide in plasma reached these levels in 4 or 5 days.— W. R. Adam *et al.*, *Med. J. Aust.*, 1973, *1*, 936.

Elimination half-lives of sulphadiazine, sulfamerazine, and sulphadimidine were 13, 12.7, and 2.3 hours respectively in a healthy subject given 330 mg of each sulphonamide as a combined suspension by mouth.— T. J. Goehl *et al.*, *J. pharm. Sci.*, 1978, *67*, 404.

The half-life of sulphadimidine is about 1.5 hours in fast acetylators compared with 5.5 hours in slow acetylators; half-lives for the N^4-acetyl metabolite are 5 and 7 hours respectively. The average renal clearance of the metabolite is about 7 to 20 times greater than that of the parent compound. In a fast acetylator there was no significant difference between plasma half-lives or urinary excretion when the urine was acidic compared with when it was alkaline.— T. B. Vree *et al.*, *Clin. Pharmacokinet.*, 1980, *5*, 274.

Kinetic discrimination of 3 sulphadimidine acetylation phenotypes.— D. J. Chapron *et al.*, *Clin. Pharmac. Ther.*, 1980, *27*, 104.

Bioavailability. A study on the urinary excretion of sulphadimidine following the use of coated formulations.— C. R. Kowarski *et al.*, *Pharm. Acta Helv.*, 1975, *50*, 91.

Elimination in renal impairment. In healthy adults, urinary clearance of sulphadimidine sodium was directly related to urinary pH; in 1 person, clearances were 4.2 and 12.7 ml per minute at pH 5.4 and 7.2 respectively. Urinary clearance was significantly greater in 10 patients with uraemia. Urine concentrations in 8 of the uraemic patients exceeded 60 mg per litre after a 1-g dose intravenously and were considered satisfactory for the treatment of infections due to sensitive pathogens.— D. M. Williams *et al.*, *Lancet*, 1968, *2*, 1058.

The mean renal clearance of sulphadimidine was 2.4 ml per minute in 10 uraemic patients given 1 g intravenously compared with 8.5 ml per minute in 10 healthy subjects given the same dose, and the excretion-rates were 86.9 µg per minute and 356.7 µg per minute respectively. There was less protein-bound sulphadimidine in the plasma of the uraemic patients whereas these patients had a higher concentration of acetylated sulphadimidine than did the control subjects. After 24 hours no sulphadimidine could be detected in the control subjects' plasma but 7 to 23 µg per ml was found in that of the uraemic patients.— E. Fischer, *Lancet*, 1972, *2*, 210.

Isoniazid acetylation test. Sulphadimidine, 44 mg per kg body-weight, was given by mouth as a fine suspension in water to 103 patients, of whom 52 were known slow inactivators and 51 known rapid inactivators of isoniazid. From an estimation of the free and total sulphadimidine in blood and urine collected at 6 hours, it was found that a patient might be classified as a slow inactivator of isoniazid if the proportion of acetylated sulphadimidine was less than 25% in blood, or less than 70% in urine. In rapid inactivators, the proportion of acetylated sulphadimidine was usually 25% or more in blood and 70% or more in urine.— K. V. N. Rao *et al.*, *Br. med. J.*, 1970, *3*, 495.

In 6 rapid acetylators of isoniazid given sulphadimidine 10 mg per kg body-weight by mouth the mean quotient of urinary concentration of the acetyl derivative over the urinary concentration of free sulphadimidine 4 to 6 hours later was 9.2 compared with 1.7 in 7 slow acetylators of isoniazid. Mean values over 24 hours were comparable—8.7 and 2 respectively.— J. H. Peters and L. Levy, *Ann. N.Y. Acad. Sci.*, 1971, *179*, 660.

For a simplified test for slow or rapid inactivators, using sulphadimidine, sulphapyridine, or sulphasalazine, see H. Schröder, *Br. med. J.*, 1972, *3*, 506.

Sulphadimidine remains the most useful compound for determining acetylator phenotype.— T. B. Vree *et al.*, *Clin. Pharmacokinet.*, 1980, *5*, 274.

Further references: T. Talseth and K. H. Landmark, *Eur. J. clin. Pharmac.*, 1977, *11*, 33; W. Olson *et al.*, *Clin. Pharmac. Ther.*, 1978, *23*, 204; P. du Souich *et al.*, *ibid.*, 1979, *25*, 172.

Uses. Sulphadimidine has the general properties and uses of sulphonamides, p.1458. There is some evidence that it is less active than some other sulphonamides. With regular dosage by mouth the blood concentration of unconjugated sulphadimidine can be maintained at 50 to 100 µg per ml.

In the treatment of susceptible infections sulphadimidine is given by mouth in an initial dose of up to 3 g, with a subsequent dosage of 1 g every 4 hours or 1.5 g every 6 hours. The usual dose for infections of the urinary tract is 2 g initially, followed by 0.5 to 1 g every 6 or 8 hours.

For infants from 6 months to 1 year of age the dose is one-sixth the adult dose; for children from 1 to 5 years, one-third the adult dose; from 6 to 12 years, one-half the adult dose; and 13 to 15 years, two-thirds the adult dose.

Sulphadimidine sodium may be given by deep intramuscular or slow intravenous injection, as a solution containing 1 g in 3 ml. It is not given by other parenteral routes. The parenteral dose is the same as the oral dose, but oral administration should commence as soon as possible.

Sulphadimidine has been used in the treatment of meningococcal meningitis but if a sulphonamide is to be used sulphadiazine is preferred.

Sulphadimidine has also been used with trimethoprim similarly to co-trimoxazole (p.1463).

A combination of trimethoprim 100 mg and sulphadimidine 500 mg, with either cloxacillin or lincomycin, was successfully used intravenously in 2 patients with severe *Bacteroides* septicaemia.— G. C. Hanson and R. L. Woods, *Postgrad. med. J.*, 1975, *51*, 105. See also G. C. Hanson, *ibid.*, 1974, *50*, 288.

The use of sulphadimidine with trimethoprim in patients with colitis, otitis media, and urinary-tract infections.— A. Vâta *et al.*, *Therapia hung.*, 1977, *25*, 79.

Administration in renal failure. Intraperitoneal administration of sulphadimidine at a concentration of 100 µg per ml could be used for 4 or 5 days for peritoneal infections in patients with renal failure.— W. R. Adam *et al.*, *Med. J. Aust.*, 1973, *1*, 936.

The dosage interval of sulphadimidine should be increased from 6 hours in normal patients to 12 hours in those with severe renal failure.— P. Sharpstone, *Br. med. J.*, 1977, *2*, 36.

See also under Absorption and Fate above.

Histoplasmosis. Disseminated histoplasmosis in a 10-year-old boy responded slowly to treatment with sulphadimidine.— M. K. R. Mackenjee and H. M. Coovadia, *S. Afr. med. J.*, 1976, *50*, 2015, per *Trop. Dis. Bull.*, 1977, *74*, 392.

Urinary-tract infections. Recommended doses for sulphadimidine may be too large; 500 mg every 6 hours should be adequate for simple urinary-tract infections.— D. S. Reeves *et al.*, *Br. med. J.*, 1978, *2*, 410.

Preparations

Paediatric Sulphadimidine Mixture *(B.P.C. 1973).* Sulphadimidine Mixture Paediatric; Mist. Sulphadimid. pro Inf. Sulphadimidine 500 mg, carmellose sodium '50' 50 mg, maize starch (as a mucilage) 100 mg, amaranth solution 0.05 ml, benzoic acid solution 0.1 ml, chloroform spirit 0.25 ml, raspberry syrup 1 ml, freshly boiled and cooled water to 5 ml. When prepared extemporaneously, the mixture should be recently prepared. The carmellose sodium 50, maize starch, and chloroform spirit may be replaced by compound tragacanth powder 200 mg and double-strength chloroform water 2.5 ml respectively. When prepared other than extemporaneously, maize starch may be omitted, chloroform spirit may be replaced by double-strength chloroform water 2.5 ml, and additional preservatives may be used. When a dose less than, or not a multiple of, 5 ml is prescribed, the mixture should be diluted to 5 ml, or a multiple, with chloroform water. Such dilutions must be freshly prepared and not used more than 2 weeks after issue. *Dose.* Children, 4 times daily, 6 months to 1 year, 2.5 ml; 1 to 5 years, 5 ml; 6 to 12 years, 7.5 ml. A double dose should be given initially.

Sulphadimidine Injection *(B.P.).* Sulphadimidine Sodium Injection; Sulfadimidine Injection. A sterile solution of sulphadimidine sodium in Water for Injections free from dissolved air, prepared by the interaction of sulphadimidine and sodium hydroxide; it contains the equivalent of not more than 0.1% of sulphur dioxide. It is distributed in ampoules in which the air has been replaced by nitrogen or other suitable gas and sterilised by autoclaving. pH 10 to 11. Protect from light.

Sulphadimidine Mixture CF *(A.P.F.).* Sulphadimidine Mixture for Children. Sulphadimidine 500 mg, compound tragacanth powder 150 mg, raspberry syrup 1 ml, benzoic acid solution 0.1 ml, concentrated chloroform water 0.1 ml, water to 5 ml. *Dose.* Initial, children 1 to 3 years, 10 ml and 4 to 10 years, 20 ml; subsequent doses, one-half the initial dose 4 times daily.

Sulphadimidine Tablets *(B.P.).* Tablets containing sulphadimidine. Protect from light.

Proprietary Preparations

Sulphamezathine Injection *(ICI Pharmaceuticals, UK).* Contains sulphadimidine sodium 1 g in 3 ml, in ampoules of 3 ml. (Also available as Sulphamezathine in *Austral.*).

Other Proprietary Names of Sulphadimidine

Deladine *(S.Afr.)*; Diazil *(Ital.)*; Nutradimidine *(S.Afr.)*; S-Dimidine *(Austral.)*.

4935-n

Sulphaethidole. Aethazolum; Ethazol; Sulfaethidole; Sulphaethylthiadiazole. N^1-(5-Ethyl-1,3,4-thiadiazol-2-yl)sulphanilamide.

$C_{10}H_{12}N_4O_2S_2$=284.4.

CAS — 94-19-9.

Pharmacopoeias. In *Rus.*, which also includes Sulphaethidole Sodium.

A white or yellowish-white, almost odourless, crystalline powder with a bitter taste. M.p. 186° to 190°.

Very slightly **soluble** in water; soluble 1 in 75 of alcohol, 1 in 13 of acetone, 1 in 1300 of chloroform, and 1 in 1700 of ether; slightly soluble in dilute mineral acids; freely soluble in solutions of alkali hydroxides. A 1% suspension in water has a pH of 4.4 to 4.9. **Store** in airtight containers. Protect from light.

Effect of wax on prolonged-release forms of sulphaethidole.— A. G. Cusimano and C. H. Becker, *J. pharm. Sci.*, 1968, *57*, 1104. See also P. M. John and C. H. Becker, *ibid.*, 584; Y. Raghunathan and C. H. Becker, *ibid.*, 1748.

Adverse Effects, Treatment, and Precautions. As for Sulphonamides, p.1457.

Absorption and Fate. As for Sulphonamides, p.1458.

Sulphaethidole is readily absorbed from the gastro-intestinal tract. About 2.5% of sulphaethidole in the blood and up to 10% in the urine is in the form of the acetyl derivative. Both sulphaethidole and its acetyl derivative are relatively highly soluble in urine over a wide pH range.

The biological half-life of sulphaethidole is 4.2 hours with a urinary pH of 8 and 11.4 hours at pH 5.— W. A. Ritschel, *Drug Intell. & clin. Pharm.*, 1970, *4*, 332.

Uses. Sulphaethidole has the general properties of Sulphonamides, p.1458. It has uses similar to those of sulphamethizole (p.1478) but has a longer duration of action.

Sulphaethidole has been given in sustained-release form in an initial dose for adults of 2.6 to 3.9 g followed by a maintenance dose of 1.3 to 1.95 g every 12 hours.

A review of sulphaethidole.— L. Weinstein *et al.*, *New Engl. J. Med.*, 1960, *263*, 793.

Proprietary Names

Sulfa-Perlongit *(Boehringer Ingelheim, Ger.)*.

4936-h

Sulphafurazole *(B.P.).* Sulphafuraz; Sulfafurazolum; Sulfisoxazole *(U.S.P.)*. N^1-(3,4-Dimethylisoxazol-5-yl)sulphanilamide.

$C_{11}H_{13}N_3O_3S$=267.3.

CAS — 127-69-5.

Pharmacopoeias. In *Arg.*, *Br.*, *Braz.*, *Chin.*, *Fr.*, *Ind.*,

Int., Jap., Jug., Nord., Roum., Turk., and *U.S.*

A white or yellowish-white, odourless, crystalline powder with a slight taste, becoming bitter. M.p. 194° to 199°.

Soluble 1 in 7700 of water, 1 in 50 of alcohol, 1 in 10 of boiling alcohol, 1 in 1000 of chloroform, 1 in 800 of ether, and 1 in 30 of a 5% solution of sodium bicarbonate; freely soluble in acetone; soluble in methyl alcohol and in 3M hydrochloric acid. **Store** in airtight containers. Protect from light.

The effects of various surface-active agents on the rectal absorption of sulphafurazole in *rabbits.*— K. Kakemi *et al., Chem. pharm. Bull., Tokyo,* 1967, *15,* 172.

4937-m

Acetyl Sulphafurazole.

Sulfisoxazole Acetyl *(U.S.P.). N*-(3,4-Dimethylisoxazol-5-yl)-*N*-sulphanilylacetamide.

$C_{13}H_{15}N_3O_4S$=309.3.

CAS — 80-74-0.

NOTE. Acetyl sulphafurazole is to be distinguished from the N^4-acetyl derivative formed from sulphafurazole by conjugation in the body.

Pharmacopoeias. In *U.S.*

A white to slightly yellow, tasteless, crystalline powder with a slight characteristic odour. M.p. 192° to 195°. Acetyl sulphafurazole 1.16 g is approximately equivalent to 1 g of sulphafurazole.

Practically **insoluble** in water; soluble 1 in about 180 of alcohol, 1 in 35 of chloroform, 1 in about 200 of methyl alcohol, and 1 in about 1100 of ether. **Store** in airtight containers. Protect from light.

4938-b

Sulphafurazole Diethanolamine.

Sulphafurazole Diolamine; Sulfisoxazole Diolamine *(U.S.P.).* The 2,2′-iminobisethanol salt of sulphafurazole.

$C_{11}H_{13}N_3O_3S,C_4H_{11}NO_2$=372.4.

CAS — 4299-60-9.

Pharmacopoeias. In *U.S.*

An odourless, white to off-white, fine, crystalline powder. M.p. 119° to 124°. Sulphafurazole diethanolamine 1.39 g is approximately equivalent to 1 g of sulphafurazole.

Soluble 1 in 2 of water, 1 in 16 of alcohol, 1 in 1000 of chloroform, 1 in 4 of methyl alcohol, and 1 in 250 of isopropyl alcohol; practically insoluble in ether. **Store** in airtight containers. Protect from light.

Sulphafurazole diethanolamine is **incompatible** with *aminophylline, ascorbic acid injection, cephalothin sodium, promazine hydrochloride, protein hydrolysates,* and *thiopentone sodium.* It is also reported to be incompatible with *ammonium chloride, hydroxyzine hydrochloride, insulin, narcotic analgesics, noradrenaline acid tartrate, oxytetracycline hydrochloride, phenytoin sodium, procaine hydrochloride, prochlorperazine edisylate, promethazine hydrochloride, streptomycin sulphate, tetracycline hydrochloride, vancomycin hydrochloride,* and *vitamin B complex with vitamin C;* and less consistently reported to be incompatible with *chloramphenicol sodium succinate, heparin, kanamycin sulphate,* and *methicillin sodium.*

When 1 g of sulphafurazole diethanolamine was added to 250 ml or 500 ml of dextrose 5% solution or dextrose 5% and sodium chloride solution no flocculation resulted. When added to electrolyte solutions of initial pH 4.4 to 4.6 (Baxter Travert No. 4; Sherman Electrolyte No. 48) crystallisation occurred at room temperature within 2½ hours, with a rise in pH to 5.65 and 5.75 respectively. Preliminary cooling to 20° was necessary to cause crystallisation of sulphafurazole diethanolamine added to electrolyte solutions of initial pH 6.1 to 6.6; in these instances the final pH was 4.25 to 4.9. The intensity of precipitation at any given storage temperature varied with the composition and initial pH of the basis. It was considered that fine crystal deposits might go unnoticed in a poor light, in solutions held in a high stand, or during a prolonged infusion.— A. C. Barbara *et al., New Engl. J. Med.,* 1966, *274,* 1316.

Further references: R. Misgen, *Am. J. Hosp. Pharm.,* 1965, *22,* 92; J. A. Patel and G. L. Phillips, *Am. J. Hosp. Pharm.,* 1966, *23,* 409.

Adverse Effects, Treatment, and Precautions. As for Sulphonamides, p.1457.

The Stevens-Johnson syndrome has been reported after treatment with sulphafurazole. Sulphafurazole and its acetyl derivative are relatively soluble in urine and the risk of crystalluria is generally slight, nevertheless adequate fluid intake is recommended.

Eye preparations of sulphafurazole diethanolamine should not be applied concomitantly with preparations of silver salts.

In a study of 1002 courses of treatment with sulphafurazole side-effects sufficiently severe to require treatment, reduction or discontinuation of dosage, or avoidance of further exposure occurred on 30 occasions (28 allergic) and included gastro-intestinal, dermatological, haematological, and other effects. The side-effects were not significantly dose-dependent but the risk of allergic reactions increased with increased exposure to the drug.— J. Koch-Weser *et al., Archs intern. Med.,* 1971, *128,* 399.

Effects on the blood. A 27-year-old woman was given 7 days' sulphafurazole therapy for urinary-tract infection. Initially fever subsided but recurred on the sixth day, together with a generalised fine maculopapular rash. The patient's granulocytes showed the pince-nez appearance characteristic of the Pelger-Huët anomaly. Fever subsided when sulphafurazole was withdrawn, and granulocytes were apparently normal within 6 weeks.— J. M. Kaplan and O'N. Barrett, *New Engl. J. Med.,* 1967, *277,* 421.

Sulphafurazole 8 g daily had been reported to cause haemolytic anaemia in certain individuals with a deficiency of glucose-6-phosphate dehydrogenase. The reaction was not considered clinically significant under normal circumstances (e.g. in the absence of infection). Sulphafurazole had been implicated as a causative agent in immune haemolytic anaemia.— E. Beutler, *Pharmac. Rev.,* 1969, *21,* 73. Sulphafurazole 4 g daily for 14 days had no haemolytic effects in 5 Negro volunteers known to be deficient in glucose-6-phosphate dehydrogenase.— R. A. Heinrich *et al., J. clin. Pharmac.,* 1971, *11,* 428.

Severe haemolytic anaemia occurred in an elderly Jewish woman with genetically abnormal haemoglobin, haemoglobin Hasharon, after about 20 days of treatment with sulphafurazole.— J. G. Adams *et al., Archs intern. Med.,* 1977, *137,* 1449.

Further references: E. A. Haunz *et al., J. Am. med. Ass.,* 1950, *144,* 1179; W. R. Best, *ibid.,* 1963, *185,* 286; H. E. Hamilton and R. F. Sheets, *ibid.,* 1978, *239,* 2586.

Interactions. For the effect of sulphafurazole in enhancing the action of thiopentone, see Thiopentone Sodium, p.759.

For the effect of sulphafurazole in enhancing the hypoglycaemic action of chlorpropamide and phenformin, see Chlorpropamide, p.853.

For the effect of sulphafurazole in reducing the protein binding of sulphonylurea compounds, see Chlorpropamide, p.853.

For the possible effect of sulphafurazole on the hypoglycaemic effect of tolbutamide, see Tolbutamide, p.860.

For a report of sulphafurazole enhancing the anticoagulant effect of warfarin, see Warfarin Sodium, p.779.

Salivary gland enlargement. A report of salivary gland enlargement being associated with sulphafurazole.— B. D. Nidus *et al., Ann. intern. Med.,* 1965, *63,* 663.

Absorption and Fate. As for Sulphonamides, p.1458.

Sulphafurazole is readily absorbed from the gastro-intestinal tract; about 85% is bound to plasma albumin. Sulphafurazole readily diffuses into extracellular fluid, but very little diffuses into cells. Concentrations in the cerebrospinal fluid are about one-third of those in the blood. About 30% of sulphafurazole in the blood and in the urine is in the form of the N^4-acetyl derivative.

It is excreted rapidly, up to 95% of a single dose being eliminated in 24 hours. Both sulphafurazole and its acetyl derivative are more soluble than sulphadiazine and many other sulphonamides in urine.

It is believed that acetyl sulphafurazole (the N^1-acetyl derivative) is broken down in the gastro-intestinal tract releasing sulphafurazole, with a consequent delay in absorption.

The elimination half-life of sulphafurazole was reduced from 6.3 hours under normal urine conditions to 4.4 hours under alkaline urine conditions.— A. P. Goossens and M. C. B. van Oudtshoorn (letter), *J. Pharm. Pharmac.,* 1970, *22,* 224.

The half-life of sulphafurazole after oral administration was 4.6 to 7.8 hours; after intramuscular administration, 5.0 to 7.6 hours; and after intravenous administration, 4.6 to 6.9 hours.— S. A. Kaplan *et al., J. pharm. Sci.,* 1972, *61,* 773.

Study *in vitro* of the binding of sulphafurazole to human albumin.— R. Zini *et al., Eur. J. clin. Pharmac.,* 1976, *10,* 139.

Excretion in breast milk.— R. E. Kauffman *et al., J. Pediat.,* 1980, *97,* 839.

Bioavailability. Reports in the literature indicated wide differences in the rate (but not the extent) of urinary excretion of drug after the ingestion of one proprietary brand and 2 generic brands of sulphafurazole tablets.— J. G. Wagner, *Drug Intell. & clin. Pharm.,* 1971, *5,* 115.

A review of the bioavailability of sulphafurazole.— W. L. Hayton *et al., J. Am. pharm. Ass.,* 1976, *NS16,* 617.

Uses. Sulphafurazole has the general properties and uses of sulphonamides, p.1458.

It is usually administered by mouth. A daily dose of 6 g has been reported to maintain a blood concentration of about 60 µg of free sulphafurazole per ml. In the treatment of susceptible infections sulphafurazole is given in an initial dose of 2 to 4 g followed by 1 to 2 g every 4 to 6 hours. For children, the dose is 75 mg per kg body-weight initially, followed by 150 mg per kg daily in divided doses to a maximum of 6 g daily. Acetyl sulphafurazole is tasteless and is used in liquid oral preparations of the drug; doses are expressed in terms of sulphafurazole.

Sulphafurazole may be given by subcutaneous injection or slow intravenous injection as a 5% solution prepared by diluting a 40% solution of sulphafurazole in the form of the diethanolamine salt with Water for Injections. It has also been given intramuscularly. A suggested parenteral dose for children and adults is 50 mg per kg body-weight initially, followed by 100 mg per kg daily in divided doses. Oral administration should commence as soon as possible.

Sulphafurazole diethanolamine has been used, as an ophthalmic ointment or solution containing the equivalent of 4% of sulphafurazole, in the topical treatment of susceptible eye infections.

A review of sulphafurazole.— L. Weinstein *et al., New Engl. J. Med.,* 1960, *263,* 793.

Sulphonamide therapy appeared to provide a considerable protective effect in 4 of 5 patients with chronic granulomatous disease. Studies *in vitro* showed that white blood-cells from the 5 patients gained increased bactericidal activity in the presence of sulphafurazole.— R. B. Johnston *et al., Lancet,* 1975, *1,* 824.

Administration in renal failure. The normal half-life for sulphafurazole of 3 to 7 hours was increased to 6 to 12 hours in end-stage renal failure. The interval between doses should be extended from 6 hours to 8 to 12 hours in patients with a glomerular filtration-rate (GFR) of 10 to 50 ml per minute, and to 18 to 24 hours in those with a GFR of less than 10 ml per minute. Concentrations of sulphafurazole were affected by haemodialysis and peritoneal dialysis.— W. M. Bennett *et al., Ann. intern. Med.,* 1980, *93,* 62.

Further references: J. S. Cheigh, *Am. J. Med.,* 1977, *62,* 555; G. B. Appel and H. C. Neu, *New Engl. J. Med.,* 1977, *296,* 663.

Chlamydial infections. Reports of the use of sulphafurazole in the treatment of infants with chlamydial pneumonia.— J. A. Embil *et al., Can. med. Ass. J.,* 1978, *119,* 1199; M. O. Beem *et al., Pediatrics,* 1979, *63,* 198.

Meningitis. In a retrospective review of the treatment of *Haemophilus influenzae* meningitis, streptomycin and sulphafurazole in 50 children was as effective as treatment with ampicillin in a further 61 children and might be a suitable alternative to chloramphenicol in ampicillin-resistant infections.— R. H. Meade, *J. Am. med. Ass.,* 1978, *239,* 324. Of 98 strains of *H. influenzae* type b all were inhibited *in vitro* by rifampicin 0.5 µg per ml and 95 by sulphafurazole diethanolamine 10 µg per ml.— R. M. Bannatyne and R. Cheung, *Antimicrob. Ag. Chemother.*, 1978, *13*, 969.

Nocardiosis. The treatment of choice in infections due to *Nocardia asteroides*: sulphafurazole or sulphadiazine, 8 to 10 g daily for 1 to 2 months, then sulphafurazole, 4 g daily for 1 year.— H. C. Neu *et al.*, *Ann. intern. Med.*, 1967, *66*, 274. See also G. P. Wormser and G. T. Keusch, *Ann. intern. Med.*, 1979, *91*, 420.

Otitis media. Sulphafurazole 500 mg twice daily for 3 months in a double-blind study was an effective prophylactic against otitis media in 54 children with a history of previous attacks. Greater success was noted in children less than 5 years old.— J. M. Perrin *et al.*, *New Engl. J. Med.*, 1974, *291*, 664.

Urinary-tract infections. Sulphafurazole 500 mg four times daily for 10 days was effective in the treatment of all 13 men with urethritis due to *Chlamydia trachomatis*. It was considered ineffective in urethritis due to *Ureaplasma urealyticum*.— W. R. Bowie *et al.*, *Lancet*, 1976, *2*, 1276.

Urinary-tract infection in 29 girls was considered cured in 27 (possibly in 29) after single doses of sulphafurazole 200 mg per kg body-weight.— G. Källenius and J. Winberg, *Br. med. J.*, 1979, *1*, 1175.

Further references: J. Elo *et al.*, *J. antimicrob. Chemother.*, 1978, *4*, 355.

Preparations

Sulfisoxazole Acetyl Oral Suspension *(U.S.P.)*. A suspension containing acetyl sulphafurazole. Potency is expressed in terms of the equivalent amount of sulphafurazole. pH 5 to 5.5. Store in airtight containers. Protect from light.

Sulfisoxazole Diolamine Injection *(U.S.P.)*. A sterile solution of sulphafurazole diethanolamine in Water for Injections. Potency is expressed in terms of the equivalent amount of sulphafurazole. pH 7 to 8.5. Protect from light.

Sulfisoxazole Diolamine Ophthalmic Ointment *(U.S.P.)*. A sterile eye ointment containing sulphafurazole diethanolamine. Potency is expressed in terms of the equivalent amount of sulphafurazole.

Sulfisoxazole Diolamine Ophthalmic Solution *(U.S.P.)*. A sterile solution of sulphafurazole diethanolamine. Potency is expressed in terms of the equivalent amount of sulphafurazole. pH 7.2 to 7.9. Store in airtight containers. Protect from light.

Sulfisoxazole Tablets *(U.S.P.)*. Tablets containing sulphafurazole. Protect from light.

Sulphafurazole Tablets *(B.P.)*. Tablets containing sulphafurazole. Protect from light.

Proprietary Preparations

Gantrisin Syrup *(Roche, UK)*. Contains acetyl sulphafurazole equivalent to 500 mg of sulphafurazole in each 5 ml (suggested diluent, syrup). **Gantrisin Tablets.** Each contains sulphafurazole 500 mg. (Also available as Gantrisin, containing sulphafurazole, acetyl sulphafurazole, or sulphafurazole diethanolamine, in *Austral.*, *Belg.*, *Canad.*, *Denm.*, *Ger.*, *Neth.*, *S.Afr.*, *Swed.*, *Switz.*, *USA*).

Other Proprietary Names of Sulphafurazole and its Derivatives

Austral.—Sulfazole, Urogan; *Canad.*—Novosoxazole, Sulfizole; *Fr.*—Gantrisine; *Ital.*—Pancid; *S.Afr.*—Urazole; *Spain*—Gantrisona; *USA*—Chemovag, Koro-Sulf, Lipo-Gantrisin, SK-Soxazole, Sosol, Soxa, Soxomide, Sulfagan, Sulfalar, Sulfizin, Urizole, Velmatrol.

4939-v

Sulphaguanidine *(B.P.C. 1973)*.

Sulphaguanid.; Sulfaguanidine; Sulfaguanidinum; Solfaguanidina; Sulfamidinum; Sulginum. *N'*-Amidinosulphanilamide monohydrate.

$C_7H_{10}N_4O_2S,H_2O$=232.3.

CAS — 57-67-0 (anhydrous); 6190-55-2 (monohydrate).

Pharmacopoeias. In *Arg.*, *Aust.*, *Chin.*, *Cz.*, *Fr.*, *Ger.*, *Hung.*, *Ind.*, *Int.*, *It.*, *Mex.*, *Pol.*, *Rus.*, *Span.*, *Swiss*, and *Turk.*

White or almost white, odourless or almost odourless, tasteless or slightly bitter, crystals or powder; it slowly darkens on exposure to light. M.p. 188° to 192.5°. **Soluble** 1 in 1000 of water, 1 in 10 of boiling water, and 1 in 250 of alcohol; slightly soluble in acetone; practically insoluble in ether; readily soluble in dilute mineral acids; practically insoluble in solutions of alkali hydroxides. **Store** in airtight containers. Protect from light.

For a study of the stability of sulphaguanidine suspensions, see R. D. C. Jones *et al.*, *J. pharm. Sci.*, 1970, *59*, 518.

Adverse Effects, Treatment, and Precautions. As for Sulphonamides, p.1457.

In patients with ulcerative colitis, sulphaguanidine may be absorbed into the blood stream in dangerous amounts.

Absorption and Fate. As for Sulphonamides, p.1458.

Sulphaguanidine is absorbed to a varying degree from the gastro-intestinal tract; blood concentrations of 15 to 40 µg per ml after single doses of 1 to 7 g have been reported. It is rapidly excreted in the urine, about one-third being in the form of the acetyl derivative.

Sulphaguanidine was about 55.4% bound to human muscle tissue *in vitro*.— B. Fichtl and H. Kurz, *Eur. J. clin. Pharmac.*, 1978, *14*, 335.

Uses. Sulphaguanidine is a sulphonamide (p.1457) which has been employed for the treatment of local intestinal infections, particularly bacillary dysentery, but phthalylsulphathiazole and succinylsulphathiazole are less toxic. In dysentery, sulphaguanidine has been given in a dose of 3 g three times daily for 3 days.

Preparations

Sulphaguanidine Tablets *(B.P.C. 1973)*. Tab. Sulphaguanid. Tablets containing sulphaguanidine. Store in airtight containers. Protect from light.

Guanimycin Suspension Forte *(Allen & Hanburys, UK)*. Contains in each 15 ml sulphaguanidine 1.985 g, dihydrostreptomycin sulphate 250 mg, and light kaolin 4.25 g (dilution not recommended). For bacterial infections of the gastro-intestinal tract. *Dose.* 15 ml every 4 hours; children, 1 to 4 years, 5 ml; 5 to 9 years, 5 to 10 ml; 10 to 15 years, 10 ml.

Other Proprietary Names

Ganidan *(Fr.)*; Resulfon *(Ger.)*; S-Guanidine *(Austral.)*.

4940-r

Sulphaguanole. Sulfaguanole. N^1-[(4,5-Dimethyloxazol-2-yl)amidino]sulphanilamide.

$C_{12}H_{15}N_5O_3S$=309.3.

CAS — 27031-08-9.

A pale cream crystalline powder. M.p. about 228°. Slightly **soluble** in water; soluble in hydrochloric acid and sodium hydroxide solutions.

Sulphaguanole is a sulphonamide (p.1457) which has been used similarly to sulphaguanidine in the treatment of gastro-intestinal infections. It has been given in a dose of 800 mg thrice daily on the first day, then 400 mg thrice daily.

Pharmacology of sulphaguanole in *animals*.— F. W. Kohlmann *et al.*, *Arzneimittel-Forsch.*, 1973, *23*, 172.

Maximum plasma concentrations were reached 3.5 hours after a dose of sulphaguanole. The plasma half-life was 7 hours.— R. Denk *et al.*, *Arzneimittel-Forsch.*, 1973, *23*, 187.

After administration by mouth to 14 children, 8% of a dose of sulphaguanole was absorbed and excreted within 30 hours.— E. Gladtke, *Arzneimittel-Forsch.*, 1973, *23*, 191.

Proprietary Names

Enterocura *(Nordmark-Werke, Ger.)*.

4941-f

Sulphamethizole *(B.P.)*.

Sulphamethiz.; Sulfamethizole *(U.S.P.)*. N^1-(5-Methyl-1,3,4-thiadiazol-2-yl)sulphanilamide.

$C_9H_{10}N_4O_2S_2$=270.3.

CAS — 144-82-1.

Pharmacopoeias. In *Br.*, *Fr.*, *Jap.*, *Neth.*, *Nord.*, *Swiss*, and *U.S.*

Odourless or almost odourless, colourless crystals or white or creamy-white crystalline powder with a slightly bitter taste. M.p. 208° to 212°.

Soluble 1 in 2000 of water, 1 in 60 of boiling water, 1 in 25 of alcohol, 1 in 13 to 15 of acetone, and 1 in 1900 of chloroform and ether; soluble in solutions of alkali hydroxides and in dilute mineral acids. **Sterilisation** of the powder as for Sulphadimidine p.1475. **Incompatible** with salts of heavy metals. **Store** in airtight containers. Protect from light.

Adverse Effects, Treatment, and Precautions. As for Sulphonamides, p.1457.

Crystalluria occurs very rarely but an adequate fluid intake should generally be maintained.

Effects on the blood. A review of haemolytic anaemia associated with sulphamethizole toxicity.— C. G. Berbatis *et al.*, *Aust. J. Pharm.*, 1977, *58*, 397.

Interactions. Sulphamethizole appeared to inhibit the hepatic metabolism of phenytoin, tolbutamide, and warfarin.— B. Lumholtz *et al.*, *Clin. Pharmac. Ther.*, 1975, *17*, 731.

Absorption and Fate. As for Sulphonamides, p.1458.

Sulphamethizole is readily absorbed from the gastro-intestinal tract; about 90% has been reported to be bound to plasma proteins. It is only slightly acetylated in the body and is rapidly excreted, about 60% of a dose being eliminated in the urine in 5 hours. Sulphamethizole and its acetyl derivative are readily soluble in urine over a wide pH range.

In 3 men given a 5-g dose of sulphamethizole the amount of conjugated drug in the urine was 6.2 to 11.8%.— M. Meads and M. Finland, *J. Lab. clin. Med.*, 1946, *31*, 900.

The biological half-life of sulphamethizole is 1.5 to 1.6 hours.— W. A. Ritschel, *Drug Intell. & clin. Pharm.*, 1970, *4*, 332.

In bioavailability tests, 12 to 18% of sulphamethizole excreted in the urine was acetylated.— G. L. Mattock and I. J. McGilveray, *J. pharm. Sci.*, 1972, *61*, 746.

Following administration of sulphamethizole 14.3 mg per kg body-weight to 7 healthy geriatric subjects, the mean half-life was 181 minutes and the mean blood concentration after 6 hours was 14.2 µg per ml; in 6 young subjects given the same dose, the mean values were 105 minutes and 5 µg per ml respectively.— E. J. Triggs *et al.*, *Eur. J. clin. Pharmac.*, 1975, *8*, 55.

Further references: B. A. Peddie and P. J. Little, *J. antimicrob. Chemother.*, 1979, *5*, 195.

Bioavailability. A comparative bioavailability study in 12 healthy subjects of 2 commercially available sulphamethizole suspensions.— J. D. Strum *et al.*, *J. pharm. Sci.*, 1978, *67*, 1399.

Uses. Sulphamethizole has the general properties of Sulphonamides, p.1458. It is used in the treatment of coliform infections of the urinary tract.

In Great Britain it is given in adult doses of 200 mg five times daily. In some other countries doses of 1.5 to 4 g daily are given. A suggested dose for children is 50 to 100 mg five times daily.

Sulphamethizole has been given in conjunction with the urinary analgesic phenazopyridine hydrochloride.

Of 1544 antenatal patients screened for asymptomatic bacteriuria 29 were confirmed bacteriologically positive on repeat examination and 21 had sulphonamide-sensitive organisms. Treatment of these patients with sulphamethizole 200 mg four times daily for 2 weeks produced initial clearing of the urine in all patients and 15 remained abacteriuric throughout a 6-month follow-up period after delivery.— J. Hargreaves, *Practitioner*, 1977, *218*, 718.

Preparations

Oculoguttae Sulfamethizoli *(Nord. P.)*. Sulphamethizole Eye-drops. Sulphamethizole 4.2 g, 1.0M sodium hydroxide solution 15.4 g, disodium edetate 10 mg, and Water for Injections 80.6 g. The filtered solution contains 4% w/w of sulphamethizole and is neutral or slightly alkaline; it is sterilised by autoclaving and may be preserved with phenethyl alcohol 0.5%. Protect from light.

Sulfamethizole Oral Suspension *(U.S.P.).* A buffered aqueous suspension of sulphamethizole. Protect from light. Store in airtight containers.

Sulfamethizole Tablets *(U.S.P.).* Tablets containing sulphamethizole.

Sulphamethizole Tablets *(B.P.).* Tablets containing sulphamethizole. Protect from light.

Proprietary Preparations

Urolucosil *(Warner, UK).* Sulphamethizole, available as **Suspension** containing 100 mg in each 5 ml (suggested diluent, syrup) and as scored **Tablets** of 100 mg. (Also available as Urolucosil in *Austral., Belg., Neth., Switz.*).

Other Proprietary Names of Sulphamethizole and Some of its Derivatives

Lucosil (as sulphamethizole or ammonium or monoethanolamine derivative)*(Belg., Denm., Neth., Norw., Switz.)*; Microsul, Proklar-M (both*USA*); Rufol *(Fr., Ital.)*; Salimol *(Jap.)*; S-Methizole *(Austral.)*; Sulfametin (as ammonium or calcium derivative)*(Swed.)*; Sulfapyelon *(Belg.)*; Thiosulfil *(Austral., Canad., Ital., USA)*; Urocydal *(Jap.)*; Urolex, Uroz (both *Austral.)*.

NOTE. Sulfametin was formerly the US adopted name for Sulphamethoxydiazine.

Sulphamethizole was also formerly marketed in Great Britain under the proprietary name Methisul (*R.P. Drugs*).

4942-d

Sulphamethoxazole *(B.P.).*

Sulfamethoxazole *(U.S.P.)*; Sulfisomezole. N^1-(5-Methylisoxazol-3-yl)sulphanilamide.

$C_{10}H_{11}N_3O_3S = 253.3$.

CAS — 723-46-6.

Pharmacopoeias. In *Br., Braz., Chin., Fr.,* and *U.S.*

A white or yellowish-white, odourless or almost odourless, crystalline powder with a slight taste and a bitter after-taste. M.p. 168° to 172°.

Very slightly **soluble** in water; soluble 1 in 50 of alcohol and 1 in 3 of acetone; slowly and usually incompletely soluble 1 in 2 of carbon disulphide; practically insoluble in chloroform and ether; soluble in solutions of alkali hydroxides. A 10% suspension in water has a pH of 4 to 6. **Protect** from light.

Adverse Effects, Treatment, and Precautions. As for Sulphonamides, p.1457.

The acetyl derivative of sulphamethoxazole is relatively insoluble in urine and crystalluria may be more likely to occur than with sulphadimidine or sulphafurazole; an adequate fluid intake should be maintained and the administration of alkalis may be necessary with very large doses of sulphamethoxazole.

Reports dealing with the adverse effects and precautions of sulphamethoxazole given with trimethoprim are provided under Co-trimoxazole, p.1460.

In a study of 359 courses of treatment with sulphamethoxazole side-effects sufficiently severe to require treatment, reduction or discontinuation of dosage, or avoidance of further exposure occurred on 12 occasions (11 allergic) and included gastro-intestinal, dermatological, haematological, and other effects. The side-effects were not significantly dose-dependent.— J. Koch-Weser *et al., Archs intern. Med.*, 1971, *128*, 399.

Allergy. Sulphamethoxazole provoked itching and rashes of the skin in 6 patients in 2 small series. The number of patients showing this reaction was very much higher than would ordinarily be seen in the course of therapy with sulphonamides.— J. P. Burton, *New Engl. J. Med.*, 1962, *266*, 951.

A 23-year-old man had a systemic reaction to co-trimoxazole characterised by a high fever, muscular and abdominal pains, headaches, and a stiff neck which was confirmed by rechallenge. He was subsequently challenged with trimethoprim alone without any adverse effect. It was concluded that he had had a severe serum-sickness-like reaction to sulphamethoxazole, and he was advised to avoid sulphonamides and their derivatives.— A. J. L. Clark *et al.* (letter), *Lancet*, 1980, *1*, 1030.

Effects on the blood. Agranulocytosis in 2 patients who had received sulphamethoxazole alone and in conjunction with trimethoprim was attributed to sulphamethoxazole.— I. P. Palva and O. Koivisto (letter), *Br. med. J.*, 1971, *4*, 301.

Sulphamethoxazole caused significant haemolysis in Chinese patients with glucose-6-phosphate dehydrogenase deficiency.— T. K. Chan *et al., Br. med. J.*, 1976, *2*, 1227.

Interactions. Sulphamethoxazole in large quantities could interfere with the determination of theophylline concentrations by high-pressure liquid chromatography.— S. A. McKenzie *et al., Archs Dis. Childh.*, 1978, *53*, 167.

Intracranial hypertension. Two patients aged 4½ years and 14 months respectively developed benign intracranial hypertension after completing courses of treatment with sulphamethoxazole.— L. T. Ch'ien (letter), *New Engl. J. Med.*, 1970, *283*, 47.

Absorption and Fate. As for Sulphonamides, p.1458.

Sulphamethoxazole is readily absorbed from the gastro-intestinal tract and peak plasma concentrations are reached within 4 hours. Doses of 1 g twice daily should produce blood concentrations of unconjugated sulphamethoxazole in excess of 50 µg per ml. About 65% is bound to plasma albumin and the plasma half-life is about 10 hours. About 15% of sulphamethoxazole in the blood is present as the acetyl derivative. Elimination in the urine is dependent on pH. About 25% of a single 2-g dose of sulphamethoxazole has been reported to be excreted in the urine within 8 hours, about 60% being in the form of the acetyl derivative.

A study in 10 healthy subjects indicated that urine flow and urine pH are the 2 main variables influencing the excretion and metabolism of sulphamethoxazole. When urine was maintained between pH 7 and 8, 22 to 43% of a dose was excreted unchanged in the urine over 60 hours and 31 to 72% was excreted as N^4-acetylsulphamethoxazole. With urine maintained between pH 5 and 6.5, 3.4 to 26% was excreted unchanged and 24 to 52% appeared as acetylated derivative. Although fast and slow acetylators of procainamide took part in the study, a similar classification could not be made in terms of sulphamethoxazole acetylation.— T. B. Vree *et al., Clin. Pharmacokinet.*, 1978, *3*, 319.

The pharmacokinetics of N^1-acetyl- and N^4-acetylsulphamethoxazole in healthy subjects.— T. B. Vree *et al., Clin. Pharmacokinet.*, 1979, *4*, 310.

Uses. Sulphamethoxazole has the general properties and uses of Sulphonamides, p.1458. It is principally employed in the treatment of urinary-tract infections.

The usual dose of sulphamethoxazole is 2 g initially, followed by 1 g twice daily. A total daily dose of 3 g should not be exceeded.

A suggested dose for children is 50 to 60 mg per kg body-weight initially, followed by 25 to 30 mg per kg twice daily.

Sulphamethoxazole is used with trimethoprim in Co-trimoxazole, p.1463.

Administration in renal failure. Sulphamethoxazole should be given in reduced doses to uraemic patients and should be avoided in patients undergoing peritoneal dialysis or haemodialysis.— G. B. Appel and H. C. Neu, *New Engl. J. Med.*, 1977, *296*, 663.

The normal half-life for sulphamethoxazole of 9 to 11 hours was increased to 20 to 50 hours in end-stage renal failure. Protein binding might be decreased in end-stage renal failure.— W. M. Bennett *et al., Ann. intern. Med.*, 1977, *86*, 754. See also *idem*, 1980, *93*, 62.

Urinary-tract infections. Reports suggesting a similar effect with sulphamethoxazole or co-trimoxazole in the treatment of urinary-tract infections.— J. B. Howard and J. E. Howard, *Am. J. Dis. Child.*, 1978, *132*, 1085; T. Bergan and O. Skjerven, *Infection*, 1979, *7*, 14.

Preparations

Sulfamethoxazole Oral Suspension *(U.S.P.).* A suspension containing sulphamethoxazole. Store in airtight containers. Protect from light.

Sulfamethoxazole Tablets *(U.S.P.).* Tablets containing sulphamethoxazole. The *U.S.P.* requires 50% dissolution in 20 minutes. Protect from light.

Proprietary Names

Gantanol *(Roche, Austral.; Roche, Canad.; Roche, Norw.; Roche, Spain; Roche, Switz.; Roche, USA).*

Sulphamethoxazole was also formerly marketed in Great Britain under the proprietary name Gantanol *(Roche).*

4943-n

Sulphamethoxydiazine *(B.P.).*

Sulfamethoxydiazine; Sulfameter; Sulfametin; Sulfametorinum; Sulphamethoxydin. N^1-(5-Methoxypyrimidin-2-yl)sulphanilamide.

$C_{11}H_{12}N_4O_3S = 280.3$.

CAS — 651-06-9.

Pharmacopoeias. In *Br., Chin., Cz.,* and *Roum.*

A white or yellowish-white, odourless or almost odourless, crystalline powder with a slightly bitter taste. M.p. 209° to 213°.

Practically **insoluble** in water; slightly soluble in alcohol and 2M hydrochloric acid; sparingly soluble in acetone; freely soluble in aqueous solutions of alkali hydroxides and carbonates. **Store** in airtight containers. Protect from light.

Dissolution studies on formulations of sulphamethoxydiazine.— G. P. Bettinetti *et al., Farmaco, Edn prat.*, 1973, *28*, 330.

Adverse Effects, Treatment, and Precautions. As for Sulphonamides, p.1457.

If side-effects occur, sulphamethoxydiazine has the disadvantage that several days are required for its elimination from the body. The Stevens-Johnson syndrome has been reported following treatment with sulphamethoxydiazine.

A 7-month-old child was inadvertently given 2 g of sulphamethoxydiazine daily for 3 days. She became comatose and developed severe hypoglycaemia and transient thrombocytopenia. She was treated with dextrose, mannitol, and hydrocortisone injections and was given antibiotics; she recovered.— J. Alain *et al., Presse méd.*, 1966, *74*, 2363.

A report of 3 patients who developed toxic epidermal necrolysis (Lyell's syndrome) after administration of sulphamethoxydiazine.— J. Kvasnička *et al., Br. J. Derm.*, 1979, *100*, 551.

Absorption and Fate. As for Sulphonamides, p.1458.

Sulphamethoxydiazine is readily absorbed from the gastro-intestinal tract. After a single dose peak blood concentrations are reached in 4 to 6 hours; concentrations 48 hours later are still about half of the original value; about 80% is bound to plasma albumin. It penetrates into the cerebrospinal fluid to provide concentrations about one-third of those in the blood.

About 10% of sulphamethoxydiazine is present in the blood as the acetyl derivative. Sulphamethoxydiazine is excreted in urine relatively slowly, about 70% being eliminated in 3 days. About 50% is excreted as sulphamethoxydiazine, 25% as the acetyl derivative, and the remainder as other derivatives, including the glucuronide.

There was a significant difference in the rate of absorption of 2 polymorphic forms of sulphamethoxydiazine but not in the extent of absorption.— N. Khalafallah *et al., J. pharm. Sci.*, 1974, *63*, 861.

Sulphamethoxydiazine was about 64.3% bound to human muscle tissue *in vitro*.— B. Fichtl and H. Kurz, *Eur. J. clin. Pharmac.*, 1978, *14*, 335.

A study on the effects of different types of food on the absorption of sulphamethoxydiazine.— S. Kaumeier, *Int. J. clin. Pharmac. Biopharm.*, 1979, *17*, 260.

Uses. Sulphamethoxydiazine is a long-acting sulphonamide with the general properties of Sulphonamides, p.1458. It has been given to adults in an initial dose of 1 or 1.5 g followed by 500 mg daily, preferably after breakfast. Children have been given 30 mg per kg body-weight initially followed by 10 mg per kg daily.

For reports on the use of sulphamethoxydiazine, see Martindale 27th Edn, p. 1490.

Preparations

Sulphamethoxydiazine Tablets *(B.P.).* Sulfamethoxydiazine Tablets. Tablets containing sulphamethoxydiazine. Protect from light.

Proprietary Names
Bayrena *(Bayer, Arg.; Bayer, Austral.; Bayer, Belg.; Bayer, Denm.; Bayer, Fr.; Bayer, Neth.; Bayer, S.Afr.; Bayer, Spain; Bayer, Swed.; Bayer, Switz.)*; Durenat *(Bayer, Ger.; Schering, Ger.)*; Kinecid *(Schering, Spain)*; Kirocid *(Schering, Austral.)*; Kiron *(Schering, Belg.)*; Panafil *(Riedel, Arg.)*; Sulla *(Robins, Canad.; Robins, USA)*.

NOTE. Sulphamethoxydiazine was formerly marketed in Great Britain under the proprietary name Durenate *(Bayer)*.

4944-h

Sulphamethoxypyridazine *(B.P., B.P. Vet.)*.
Sulphamethoxypyrid.; Sulfamethoxypyridazine; Sulfamethoxypyridazinum; Solfametossipiridazina. N^1-(6-Methoxypyridazin-3-yl)sulphanilamide.
$C_{11}H_{12}N_4O_3S$=280.3.

CAS — 80-35-3.

Pharmacopoeias. In *Br., Braz., Chin., Fr., Hung., Int., It., Jug., Nord.,* and *Turk.*

A white or yellowish-white, odourless or almost odourless, crystalline powder; tasteless at first but with a bitter after-taste. It slowly darkens on exposure to light. M.p. 180° to 183°.

Very slightly **soluble** in water; sparingly soluble in alcohol; soluble 1 in 25 of acetone and 1 in 400 of chloroform; soluble in methyl alcohol; practically insoluble in ether; freely soluble in dilute mineral acids and solutions of alkali hydroxides.

Solutions, prepared by the addition of sodium hydroxide to give a pH of 10, may be **sterilised** by filtration and distributed in sealed containers, the air in which is replaced by nitrogen. **Store** in airtight containers. Protect from light.

4945-m

Acetyl Sulphamethoxypyridazine.
N-(6-Methoxypyridazin-3-yl)-*N*-sulphanilylacetamide.
$C_{13}H_{14}N_4O_4S$=322.3.

CAS — 3568-43-2.

NOTE. Acetyl sulphamethoxypyridazine is to be distinguished from the N^4-acetyl derivative formed from sulphamethoxypyridazine by conjugation in the body.

Adverse Effects, Treatment, and Precautions. As for Sulphonamides, p.1457.

If side-effects occur, sulphamethoxypyridazine has the disadvantage that several days are required for its elimination from the body.

Adverse effects with sulphamethoxypyridazine are fairly common and they may be serious. There have been several reports of the Stevens-Johnson and Lyell's syndromes occurring following treatment with sulphamethoxypyridazine. It has caused death from hypersensitivity myocarditis.

Sulphamethoxypyridazine is readily soluble in urine, but the acetyl derivative is much less soluble. Adequate fluid intake should be maintained during therapy and for 2 or 3 days thereafter.

For some reports of adverse effects following treatment with sulphamethoxypyridazine, see Martindale 27th Edn, p. 1491.

Effects on the blood. Experimental evidence suggested that the administration of 2 g of sulphamethoxypyridazine might produce significant haemolysis in Negroes with a deficiency of glucose-6-phosphate dehydrogenase.— Standardization of Procedures for the Study of Glucose-6-Phosphate Dehydrogenase, *Tech. Rep. Ser. Wld Hlth Org. No. 366,* 1967.

Sulphamethoxypyridazine has been reported to cause haemolysis in patients with haemoglobin Zürich.— E. Beutler, *Pharmac. Rev.,* 1969, *21,* 73.

Haemolytic anaemia has been reported in a breast-fed infant with glucose-6-phosphate dehydrogenase deficiency; the mother was receiving sulphamethoxypyridazine.— R. L. Savage, *Adverse Drug React. Bull.,* 1976, Dec., 212.

Effects on the heart. Sulphamethoxypyridazine was considered responsible for 3 fatal cases, in elderly patients, of acute interstitial myocarditis of a type seen in drug-induced hypersensitivity reactions.— A. J. Blanchard and G. A. Mertens, *Can. med. Ass. J.,* 1958, *79,* 627.

Stevens-Johnson syndrome. Between 1958 and 1965, a total of 71 cases of erythema multiforme, the Stevens-Johnson syndrome, and epidermal necrolysis, Lyell's syndrome, associated with the use of sulphamethoxypyridazine were reported in the world medical literature.— H. Seneca, *J. Am. med. Ass.,* 1966, *198,* 975.

Absorption and Fate. As for Sulphonamides, p.1458.

Sulphamethoxypyridazine is readily absorbed from the gastro-intestinal tract. After a single dose peak blood concentrations are reached within 5 hours; about 85% is bound to plasma albumin. Concentrations of sulphamethoxypyridazine in the cerebrospinal fluid of 5 to 10% of those in the blood have been reported. About 10 to 15% of sulphamethoxypyridazine in the blood is present as the N^4-acetyl derivative.

Sulphamethoxypyridazine is excreted slowly and may be detected in the blood for up to 7 days after stopping treatment; about 25% is excreted in the urine in 24 hours, and a further 20% in the next 24 hours; 40 to 70% is excreted as the acetyl derivative and a smaller amount as glucuronide conjugate.

The biological half-life of sulphamethoxypyridazine is variously reported as 34.6 to 63 hours.— W. A. Ritschel, *Drug Intell. & clin. Pharm.,* 1970, *4,* 332.

Acetylation. Sulphamethoxypyridazine was acetylated to a much smaller extent than sulphadimidine in metabolic studies in 33 subjects who could be phenotyped as either slow or rapid 'acetylators'.— T. A. White and D. A. P. Evans, *Clin. Pharmac. Ther.,* 1968, *9,* 80.

Uses. Sulphamethoxypyridazine is a long-acting sulphonamide with the general properties of Sulphonamides, p.1458, and has been used for infections of the urinary tract in doses of 500 mg daily.

Acetyl sulphamethoxypyridazine is hydrolysed in the gastro-intestinal tract forming sulphamethoxypyridazine; it is tasteless and has been used in liquid oral preparations.

The sodium derivative of sulphamethoxypyridazine is also used.

Sulphamethoxypyridazine is also used with trimethoprim similarly to co-trimoxazole.

A review of sulphamethoxypyridazine.— L. Weinstein *et al., New Engl. J. Med.,* 1960, *262,* 842.

Dermatitis herpetiformis. Dermatitis herpetiformis in a 5-year-old boy promptly responded to a dose of 500 mg of sulphamethoxypyridazine daily, reduced to 125 mg, but the patient developed hepatitis 2 weeks after treatment started, the blood concentration of the drug being then 86 μg per ml. On withdrawal of the drug the patient slowly recovered but the dermatitis relapsed. Control of the eruption was later attained without adverse effects with sulphapyridine 500 mg thrice daily.— J. C. P. Logan and M. Childs (letter), *Br. med. J.,* 1959, *1,* 858.

Leprosy. Since *Mycobacterium leprae* shows cross-resistance between dapsone and the long-acting sulphonamides and serum concentrations of sulphamethoxypyridazine only exceed the MIC against *M. leprae* by a factor of about 4 compared with a factor of 500 in the case of dapsone, sulphamethoxypyridazine and the other long-acting sulphonamides, sulphadimethoxine and sulfadoxine, are not considered suitable for the treatment of leprosy.— M. J. Colston *et al., Lepr. Rev.,* 1978, *49,* 101.

Mycetoma. A report on African mycetomas and the successful use of dapsone and sulphamethoxypyridazine.— H. Bezes *et al., Méd. trop. Marseille,* 1979, *39,* 41, per *Trop. Dis. Bull.,* 1980, *77,* 111.

Preparations of Sulphamethoxypyridazine and Acetyl Sulphamethoxypyridazine

Sulphamethoxypyridazine Tablets *(B.P.)*. Sulfamethoxypyridazine Tablets. Tablets containing sulphamethoxypyridazine. Protect from light.

Lederkyn *(Lederle, UK)*. Sulphamethoxypyridazine, available as scored tablets of 500 mg. (Also available as Lederkyn in *Austral., Belg., Denm., Ger., Ital., Neth., Switz.* Also available as Lederkyn in *Ger., Ital., Switz.* containing acetyl sulphamethoxypyridazine.).

Other Proprietary Names of Sulphamethoxypyridazine and Acetyl Sulphamethoxypyridazine
Austral.—Midicel; *Belg.*—Minikel; *Fr.*—Sultirène; *Ital.*—Eusulfa, Ketiak, Kiron, Metazina, Microcid, Sulfadin, Sulfalex, Sulfamizina (sulphamethoxypyridazine sodium), Sulfamyd, Sulfatar, Sulforetent, Sulfo-Rit, Unisulfa; *Spain*—Aseptilex, Asey-Sulfa, Durasul, Exazol, Longisul, Midikel, Sulfa-Ulta, Sulfadepot, Sulfaintensa, Sulfo-Cidan.

Sulphamethoxypyridazine was also formerly marketed in Great Britain under the proprietary name Midicel *(Parke, Davis)*.

4946-b

Sulphamoxole.
Sulfamoxole; Sulphadimethyloxazole. N^1-(4,5-Dimethyloxazol-2-yl)sulphanilamide.
$C_{11}H_{13}N_3O_3S$=267.3.

CAS — 729-99-7.

A white crystalline powder. M.p. about 193°. Slightly **soluble** in water.

Some physical characteristics of sulphamoxole.— H. J. Dechow *et al., Arzneimittel-Forsch.,* 1976, *26,* 596.

Sulphamoxole has the general properties of Sulphonamides, p.1457, and has been given in the treatment of various infections in an adult dose of 1 g twice daily for one or two days and then 500 mg twice daily.

For the use of sulphamoxole with trimethoprim, see Co-trifamole, p.1460.

The biological half-life of sulphamoxole is variously reported as 4.4 to 10.6 hours.— W. A. Ritschel, *Drug Intell. & clin. Pharm.,* 1970, *4,* 332.

Proprietary Names
Justamil *(Anphar-Rolland, Fr.)*; Sulfmidil *(Astra, Swed.)*; Sulfuno *(Nordmark, Belg.; Ferrosan, Denm.; Nordmark-Werke, Ger.; Noristan, S.Afr.; Ferrosan, Swed.)*.

4947-v

Sulphanilamide *(B.P.C. 1968, B.P. Vet.)*.
Sulphanilam.; Sulfanilamide; Sulfanilamidum; Sulfaminum; Streptocidum; Solfammide. 4-Aminobenzenesulphonamide.
$C_6H_8N_2O_2S$=172.2.

CAS — 63-74-1.

Pharmacopoeias. In *Arg., Aust., Belg., Chin., Fr., Int., It., Mex., Nord., Pol., Port., Rus., Span.,* and *Turk.*
Rus. P. also includes Streptocidum Solubile, sodium *p*-sulphamoylanilinomethanesulphonate,
$C_7H_9N_2NaO_5S_2$=288.3.

A white, or almost white, odourless crystalline powder with a slightly bitter taste and a sweet after-taste. M.p. about 165°.

Soluble 1 in 170 of water, 1 in 2 of boiling water, 1 in 30 of alcohol, and 1 in 4 of acetone; soluble in glycerol, hydrochloric acid, and solutions of alkali hydroxides; practically insoluble in chloroform and ether. A saturated solution in water is neutral to litmus. **Sterilisation** of the powder as for Sulphadimidine, p.1475. **Store** in airtight containers. Protect from light.

Solubilisation. The solubility of sulphanilamide was increased by polysorbates 20, 60, and 80, in concentrations of 0.1 to 0.4%, the increase being greatest in the 0.4% solution. Macrogols 400, 4000, and 6000 were more effective than polysorbates, but concentrated sorbitan monolaurate had no solubilising effect.— M. N. Khawan *et al., Scientia pharm.,* 1964, *32,* 271, per *Int. pharm. Abstr.,* 1965, *2,* 939.

Adverse Effects, Treatment, and Precautions. As for Sulphonamides, p.1457.

The Stevens-Johnson syndrome has been reported after treatment with sulphanilamide.

A woman experienced acute transient myopia after applying a vaginal cream containing sulphanilamide.— M. A. Maddalena, *Archs Ophthal., N.Y.,* 1968, *80,* 186.

Uses. Sulphanilamide has the general properties of Sulphonamides, p.1458. It is now rarely used in human medicine, having been replaced by less toxic sulphonamides and antibiotics.

Sulphanilamide is used in veterinary medicine.

Proprietary Preparations

Rhinamid *(Bailly, Fr.: Bengué, UK).* Drops containing sulphanilamide 0.4%, ephedrine hydrochloride 1%, and butacaine sulphate 0.026%. An antiseptic and decongestant for conditions of the nasopharynx.

Sulphanilamide and Sulphathiazole Cream *(Ayrton, Saunders, UK).* Contains sulphanilamide 3%, sulphathiazole 3%, and glycerol 10%, in a water-miscible basis.

There was no evidence that sulphanilamide or sulphafurazole in vaginal creams were effective in most common forms of vaginitis.— *FDA Drug Bull.*, 1980, *10*, 6.

Other Proprietary Names

Belg.—Astreptine, Exoseptoplix; *Fr.*—Exoseptoplix, Tablamide; *Ger.*—Sulfonamid-Spuman; *Ital.*—Streptosil; *Spain*—Azol, Buco-Pental, Oxidermiol Sulfamida, Pental Micronizado, Sulfamida; *Switz.* Streptamin.

4948-g

Sulphaphenazole *(B.P.C. 1968).* Sulfaphenazole; Sulphaphenylpyrazol. N^1-(1-Phenylpyrazol-5-yl)sulphanilamide.

$C_{15}H_{14}N_4O_2S$=314.4.

CAS — 526-08-9.

Pharmacopoeias. In *Jug.* and *Roum.*

A white or almost white, odourless, crystalline powder. M.p. 179° to 183°.

Very slightly **soluble** in water, alcohol, chloroform, and ether; soluble in acetone, mineral acids, and solutions of alkali hydroxides. **Store** in airtight containers. Protect from light.

Adverse Effects, Treatment, and Precautions. As for Sulphonamides, p.1457.

If side-effects occur, sulphaphenazole has the disadvantage that it is slowly eliminated from the body. It may cause the Stevens-Johnson syndrome.

Interactions. For the effect of sulphaphenazole in prolonging the serum half-life of benzylpenicillin, see Benzylpenicillin, p.1107.

For the effect of sulphaphenazole in reducing protein binding of sulphonylurea compounds, see Chlorpropamide, p.853.

For the effect of sulphaphenazole in increasing the half-life of chlorpropamide, see Chlorpropamide, p.853.

For the effect of sulphaphenazole and its methyl and ethyl derivatives in increasing the half-life of tolbutamide, see Tolbutamide, p.860.

Absorption and Fate. As for Sulphonamides, p.1458.

Sulphaphenazole is readily absorbed from the gastro-intestinal tract, and up to 99% has been reported to be bound to plasma albumin. It is acetylated in the body and is slowly excreted.

The biological half-life of sulphaphenazole is variously reported as 8 to 12 hours.— W. A. Ritschel, *Drug Intell. & clin. Pharm.*, 1970, *4*, 332.

Less sulphaphenazole was bound to the plasma albumin of the foetus or neonate than to that of the adult.— C. F. Chignell *et al.*, *Clin. Pharmac. Ther.*, 1971, *12*, 897.

Uses. Sulphaphenazole has the general properties of Sulphonamides, p.1458.

The initial adult dose is 1 to 1.5 g, according to the severity of the infection, every 12 hours for 2 days; this is followed by a dose of 500 mg every 12 hours.

Preparations

Sulphaphenazole Tablets *(B.P.C. 1968).* Tablets containing sulphaphenazole.

Proprietary Names

Fenazolo *(SAM, Ital.)*; Orisul *(Ciba, Austral.; Ciba, Belg.; Ciba, Ger.; Ciba, Neth.; Ciba-Geigy, Switz.)*; Orisulf *(Ciba, NZ)*; Sulfapadil *(Padil, Ital.)*; Sulforal *(Farber-Ref, Ital.)*.

Sulphaphenazole was formerly marketed in Great Britain under the proprietary name Orisulf (*Ciba*).

4949-q

Sulphapyridine *(B.P.).* Sulphapyrid.; Sulfapyridine *(U.S.P.).* N^1-(2-Pyridyl)sulphanilamide.

$C_{11}H_{11}N_3O_2S$=249.3.

CAS — 144-83-2.

Pharmacopoeias. In *Arg.*, *Br.*, *Port.*, *Span.*, and *U.S.*

A white or yellowish-white, odourless or almost odourless, crystalline powder or granules with a very slightly bitter taste. It slowly darkens on exposure to light. M.p. 190° to 193°.

Soluble 1 in 3500 of water, 1 in 100 of boiling water, 1 in 400 to 440 of alcohol, 1 in 65 of acetone; soluble in dilute mineral acids and aqueous solutions of alkali hydroxides. **Sterilisation** of the powder as for Sulphadimidine, p.1475. **Store** in airtight containers. Protect from light.

A study of polymorphism in sulphapyridine.— M. W. Gouda *et al.*, *Drug Devel. ind. Pharm.*, 1977, *3*, 273.

EFfect of gamma-irradiation. Gamma-irradiation, even at 250 000 Gy caused little change in colour of sulphapyridine, but sufficient to bring it outside the normal specification. Tests and assay gave no indication of any change.— *The Use of Gamma Radiation Sources for the Sterilisation of Pharmaceutical Products,* London, ABPI, 1960.

4950-d

Sulphapyridine Sodium *(B. Vet. C. 1965).* Soluble Sulphapyridine.

$C_{11}H_{10}N_3NaO_2S$=271.3 (or with $1H_2O$ = 289.3).

CAS — 127-57-1 (anhydrous); 6101-41-3 (monohydrate).

Pharmacopoeias. In *Arg.*

A white or yellowish-white, odourless, crystalline powder with a very slightly bitter taste. On exposure to air, it slowly absorbs carbon dioxide with the liberation of sulphapyridine and becomes incompletely soluble in water.

Soluble 1 in 3 of water and 1 in 10 of alcohol. **Store** in airtight containers. Protect from light.

Adverse Effects, Treatment, and Precautions. As for Sulphonamides, p.1457.

Adverse effects are common, and nausea and vomiting may render continued therapy difficult. Sulphapyridine and its acetyl derivative have low solubilities in urine and crystalluria may occur; solubilities are not greatly increased with increased pH. Adequate fluid intake and the administration of alkalis are necessary.

Effects on the blood. Experimental evidence suggested that the administration of 4 g of sulphapyridine could produce significant haemolysis in Negroes and Caucasians with a deficiency of glucose-6-phosphate dehydrogenase.— Standardization of Procedures for the Study of Glucose-6-Phosphate Dehydrogenase, *Tech. Rep. Ser. Wld Hlth Org. No. 366,* 1967.

Absorption and Fate. As for Sulphonamides, p.1458.

Sulphapyridine is irregularly absorbed from the gastro-intestinal tract, and is bound to plasma albumin to the extent of 10 to 45%. It penetrates into the cerebrospinal fluid. Up to about 75% of sulphapyridine in the blood is present as the acetyl derivative. The rate of excretion appears to be irregular.

The biological half-life of sulphapyridine is 6.5 to 9.4 hours.— W. A. Ritschel, *Drug Intell. & clin. Pharm.*, 1970, *4*, 332.

Sulphapyridine is a variably acetylated drug.— *Drug & Ther. Bull.*, 1974, *12*, 21.

A brief discussion on acetylator phenotype and the pharmacokinetics of sulphapyridine.— T. B. Vree *et al.*, *Clin. Pharmacokinet.*, 1980, *5*, 274.

Uses. Sulphapyridine has the general properties of Sulphonamides, p.1458, but, because of its toxicity, the main use of sulphapyridine is in the treatment of dermatitis herpetiformis when patients do not respond to dapsone and in certain other dermatoses. It is given by mouth in a dosage of 3 or 4 g daily until no further blisters develop, and then in a dosage of 0.5 to 1 g daily.

A review on the use of sulphapyridine and dapsone in dermatology.— P. G. Lang, *J. Am. Acad. Derm.*, 1979, *1*, 479.

The favourable response of 2 young children with chronic bullous dermatosis to treatment with sulphapyridine.— N. B. Esterly *et al.*, *Archs Derm.*, 1977, *113*, 42.

Further references: S. A. M. Johnson and D. J. Cripps, *Archs Derm.*, 1974, *109*, 73.

Dermatitis herpetiformis. A review of dermatitis herpetiformis and its treatment, including the use of sulphapyridine.— S. I. Katz *et al.*, *Ann. intern. Med.*, 1980, *93*, 857.

Pemphigus. A retrospective review of patients with pemphigus seen between 1960 and 1975 showed that in 6 of 41 patients with bullous pemphigoid there was significant response to treatment with sulphapyridine or dapsone; in 5 of these patients the condition was completely controlled. Three other patients responded to treatment given together with corticosteroids and in 3 further patients response to treatment with sulphapyridine or dapsone was transient.— J. R. Person and R. S. Rogers, *Mayo Clin. Proc.*, 1977, *52*, 54.

Further references: J. R. Person and R. S. Rogers, *Archs Derm.*, 1977, *113*, 610.

Pyoderma gangrenosum. Sulphapyridine, 1 or 2 g three or four times daily, was effective, if given early in the course of the disease, in controlling the chronic indolent ulcers of pyoderma gangrenosum.— *J. Am. med. Ass.*, 1968, *206*, 2229.

Preparations

Sulfapyridine Tablets *(U.S.P.).* Tablets containing sulphapyridine. Protect from light.

Sulphapyridine Tablets *(B.P.).* Tablets containing sulphapyridine. Protect from light.

M & B 693 *(May & Baker, UK).* Sulphapyridine, available as scored tablets of 500 mg. (Also available as M & B 693 in *Austral.*, *S.Afr.*).

Other Proprietary Names of Sulphapyridine

Dagenan *(Canad.)*.

4951-n

Sulphasalazine. Sulfasalazine *(U.S.P.)*; Salicylazosulphapyridine; Salazosulfapyridine. 4-Hydroxy-4′-(2-pyridylsulphamoyl)azobenzene-3-carboxylic acid.

$C_{18}H_{14}N_4O_5S$=398.4.

CAS — 599-79-1.

Pharmacopoeias. In *U.S.*

A fine odourless bright yellow to brownish-yellowish powder. M.p. about 255° with decomposition.

Practically **insoluble** in water, chloroform, and ether; soluble 1 in 2900 of alcohol and 1 in 1500 of methyl alcohol; soluble in aqueous solutions of alkali hydroxides. **Store** in airtight containers. Protect from light.

Adverse Effects, Treatment, and Precautions. As for Sulphonamides, p.1457.

Adverse effects with sulphasalazine may be more frequent and more severe in patients who are slow acetylators.

The Stevens-Johnson and Lyell's syndromes and salicylism have been reported in patients after treatment with sulphasalazine. A pulmonary reaction with associated eosinophilia and pulmonary infiltration has occurred in some patients following the administration of sulphasalazine. Oligospermia, reversible on withdrawal of sulphasalazine, has also been reported. It should not be given to patients known to be hypersensitive to sulphonamides or salicylates.

In a group of 133 patients receiving sulphasalazine for ulcerative colitis or Crohn's disease 28 suffered side-effects. The daily dose for most of the 28 was 4 g or more and there was a correlation between side-effects and serum-sulphapyridine concentrations of more than 50 µg per ml; 24 of the 28 patients were slow acetylators and it was suggested that these were at greatest risk.— K. M. Das *et al.*, *New Engl. J. Med.*, 1973, *289*,

491. See also H. Schröder and D. A. P. Evans, *Gut*, 1972, *13*, 278; M. J. M. Van De Reijken, *Pharm. Weekbl. Ned.*, 1976, *111*, 657.

Possible cytogenetic effects with sulphasalazine.— F. Mitelman *et al.* (letter), *Lancet*, 1980, *1*, 1249.

Effects on the blood. Of 50 patients with ulcerative colitis who were receiving a mean maintenance dose of sulphasalazine 2.5 g daily, 35 were found to have one or more drug-induced red cell abnormalities. Twenty-three had red cell contraction, which correlated with dose and acetylator status, 11 had macrocytosis, 21 had elevated concentrations of methaemoglobin, and 1 had Heinz bodies.— R. E. Pounder *et al.*, *Gut*, 1975, *16*, 181.

Erythroid and megakaryocytic aplasia associated with the use of sulphasalazine in one patient.— G. E. Davies and J. Palek (letter), *Archs intern. Med.*, 1980, *140*, 1122.

Agranulocytosis. Two elderly men died with agranulocytosis after treatment which included sulphasalazine which was considered responsible; details of 4 other cases were quoted. The drug should be discontinued on the appearance of a rash and a check on the number of white cells should then be made.— J. L. Thirkettle *et al.*, *Lancet*, 1963, *1*, 1395.

Further references: N. F. Ritz and M. J. Fisher, *J. Am. med. Ass.*, 1960, *172*, 237; P. Cochrane *et al.*, *Postgrad. med. J.*, 1973, *49*, 669; W. H. W. Inman, *Br. med. J.*, 1977, *1*, 1500.

Haemolysis. A report of haemolytic anaemia during sulphasalazine therapy in 2 Negro subjects with glucose-6-phosphate dehydrogenase deficiency.— S. M. Cohen *et al.*, *J. Am. med. Ass.*, 1968, *205*, 528. See also Standardization of Procedures for the Study of Glucose-6-Phosphate Dehydrogenase, *Tech. Rep. Ser. Wld Hlth Org. No. 366*, 1967.

Haemolytic anaemia was detected in 17 of 40 patients receiving sulphasalazine for inflammatory bowel disease. Mean serum concentrations of sulphapyridine were significantly higher in patients with haemolysis. Heinz bodies were found in 8 of the 17 compared with one of the 23 patients without haemolysis; the assessment of reticulocytosis also underestimated the incidence of haemolysis.— R. L. Goodacre *et al.*, *Digestion*, 1978, *17*, 503.

Further references: A. I. Spriggs *et al.*, *Lancet*, 1958, *1*, 1039; E. Beutler, *Pharmac. Rev.*, 1969, *21*, 73; F. Kater, *Medsche Klin.*, 1974, *69*, 466.

Megaloblastic anaemia. Megaloblastic anaemia in a 68-year-old man was attributed to sulphasalazine which he had taken for 5 months; the condition regressed when sulphasalazine was withdrawn and folic acid was given.— R. E. Schneider and L. Beeley, *Br. med. J.*, 1977, *1*, 1638. Deficiency of cyanocobalamin had not been excluded.— M. Bateson (letter), *ibid.*, 1977, *2*, 190.

Further references: S. P. Kane and M. A. Boots (letter), *Br. med. J.*, 1977, *2*, 1287.

Effects on fertility. Oligospermia and infertility in 4 young male immigrants to Britain (Indian, Armenian, Ugandan Asian, and Iranian) was associated with sulphasalazine therapy for ulcerative colitis. Semen analyses rapidly improved in all 4 patients on withdrawal of sulphasalazine and 4 pregnancies occurred in 3 of the wives.— A. J. Levi *et al.*, *Lancet*, 1979, *2*, 276. Mention of a further 10 men whose infertility was caused by sulphasalazine. The effect appears to be completely reversible; it takes about 3 months for complete regeneration of spermiogenesis within the testes.— A. Toth (letter), *ibid.*, 904. See also A. Toth, *Fert. Steril.*, 1979, *31*, 538.

Further references: J. Grieve (letter), *Lancet*, 1979, *2*, 464; A. I. Traub *et al.* (letter), *ibid.*, 639; J. G. Freeman *et al.*, *Gut*, 1980, *21*, A911; S. Toovey *et al.*, *ibid.*; G. G. Birnie *et al.*, *ibid.*, A912.

Effects on the gastro-intestinal tract. Repeated episodes of fever, vomiting, and bloody diarrhoea occurred in 2 children given sulphasalazine for ulcerative colitis. Symptoms appeared to be due to the treatment rather than a flare-up of the disease.— S. L. Werlin and R. J. Grand, *J. Pediat.*, 1978, *92*, 450.

Two patients taking sulphasalazine 2 g daily experienced a metallic taste which abated when the dose was reduced to 1 g or less daily.— R. M. Ogburn, *J. Am. med. Ass.*, 1979, *241*, 837.

Effects on the liver. Reports of hepatotoxicity associated with the administration of sulphasalazine.— R. P. Sotolongo *et al.*, *Gastroenterology*, 1978, *75*, 95; R. S. Kanner *et al.*, *Am. J. dig. Dis.*, 1978, *23*, 956; J. P. Callen and R. M. Soderstrom, *Sth. med. J.*, 1978, *71*, 1159.

Effects on the nervous system. A general toxicity reaction with neurotoxicity developed in a 52-year-old patient with ulcerative colitis who was treated with sulphasalazine 1.5 g daily gradually increased to 3 g daily. Three weeks after discontinuing the drug, the patient began to recover normal gait and reflexes.— I. W. Wallace, *Practitioner*, 1970, *204*, 850.

Effects on the respiratory system. Respiratory conditions resembling pulmonary eosinophilia in 4 patients and tracheo-laryngitis with bronchospasm in 1 occurred after treatment with sulphasalazine for 2 to 5 months. One patient developed a fatal progressive fibrosing alveolitis. Dyspnoea was the dominant symptom in every case.— *Lancet*, 1974, *2*, 504. The lung damage was likely to be caused by the sulphapyridine derived from sulphasalazine.— M. Eastwood (letter), *ibid.*, 659.

Further references: D. Davies and A. MacFarlane, *Gut*, 1974, *15*, 185; T. F. Tydd and N. H. Dyer, *Med. J. Aust.*, 1976, *1*, 570; K. A. Constantinidis, *Chest*, 1976, *70*, 315; S. Berliner *et al.*, *Respiration*, 1980, *39*, 119.

Epidermal necrolysis. Fatal epidermal necrolysis [Lyell's syndrome], agranulocytosis, and erythroid hypoplasia in a 39-year-old man was associated with the use of sulphasalazine.— J. L. Maddocks and D. N. Slater, *J. R. Soc. Med.*, 1980, *73*, 587.

Folic acid deficiency. Patients with inflammatory bowel disease had impaired folic acid absorption and a high incidence of folate deficiency. Folic acid absorption was further reduced when patients were given sulphasalazine.— J. L. Franklin and I. H. Rosenberg, *Gastroenterology*, 1973, *64*, 517.

Further references: C. H. Halsted *et al.*, *New Engl. J. Med.*, 1981, *305*, 1513.

Interactions. In 5 subjects given a single dose of sulphasalazine peak serum concentrations were reduced by ferrous sulphate and delayed by calcium gluconate.— K. M. Das and M. A. Eastwood, *Scott. med. J.*, 1973, *18*, 45.

Concomitant antibiotic therapy might possibly alter the patient's response to sulphasalazine by decreasing the intestinal flora necessary for the initial breakdown of sulphasalazine.— K. M. Das and R. Dubin, *Clin. Pharmacokinet.*, 1976, *1*, 406.

For a report that concurrent administration of sulphasalazine reduced the absorption of digoxin, see Digoxin, p.534.

Lupus erythematosus. An elderly woman, a slow acetylator of sulphadimidine, taking sulphasalazine for ulcerative colitis developed symptoms suggestive of the lupus syndrome; symptoms regressed when sulphasalazine was withdrawn and recurred when it was again given.— I. D. Griffiths and S. P. Kane, *Br. med. J.*, 1977, *2*, 1188.

Further references: B. H. Jaup, *Dt. med. Wschr.*, 1978, *103*, 1211; A. J. Crisp and B. I. Hoffbrand, *J. R. Soc. Med.*, 1980, *73*, 60.

Pancreatitis. A 29-year-old woman given sulphasalazine 1 g four times daily for enteritis developed epigastric pain, sometimes radiating into the back, after 2 weeks' treatment. The symptom subsided when the drug was discontinued, but its resumption on 3 occasions produced a rise in serum amylase, followed by a rise in urinary amylase, indicating pancreatitis.— M. B. Block *et al.*, *New Engl. J. Med.*, 1970, *282*, 380.

Raynaud's syndrome. Raynaud's syndrome was associated with treatment with sulphasalazine 2 to 4 g daily, in a man with ulcerative colitis. Withdrawal of the drug and then re-introduction, on 2 occasions, resulted in successive disappearance and then reappearance of the symptoms.— J. Reid *et al.*, *Postgrad. med. J.*, 1980, *56*, 106.

Skin reactions. Following treatment of ulcerative colitis with sulphasalazine 4 g daily, a 73-year-old woman with impaired renal function developed a yellow pigmentation of the skin. Examination of the bright yellow serum showed sulphasalazine present in a concentration of 300 µg per ml (normal therapeutic concentration on a dosage of 6 g daily was 30 to 40 µg per ml). Peritoneal dialysis quickly removed the discoloration. There was no evidence of other toxic effects.— J. Yell *et al.* (letter), *Br. med. J.*, 1968, *4*, 452.

An erythematous and scaling skin eruption with fever and generalised lymphadenopathy, associated with the use of sulphasalazine, reappeared and progressed to erythrodermic psoriasis when co-trimoxazole was later inadvertently given.— C. Kennedy *et al.* (letter), *Br. med. J.*, 1979, *1*, 1356.

Absorption and Fate. Sulphasalazine is partly absorbed from the small intestine and may later enter the enterohepatic circulation but the majority of a dose passes on to the colon where it is broken down to sulphapyridine and 5-aminosalicylic acid by bacteria. Most of the sulphapyridine is absorbed and, together with its metabolites, appears in the blood 3 to 6 hours after a single dose of sulphasalazine is given to healthy subjects; a mean peak serum concentration for sulphapyridine of 21 µg per ml has been reported at 12 hours. Sulphapyridine is metabolised by acetylation, the rate being genetically determined, by hydroxylation, and by conjugation with glucuronic acid. Up to 10% of a dose of sulphasalazine is excreted unchanged in the urine and about 60% as sulphapyridine and its metabolites. About 25% of the sulphapyridine appears in the faeces and unchanged sulphasalazine may be excreted in the faeces of patients with ulcerative colitis.

The majority of 5-aminosalicylic acid is eliminated unchanged in the faeces but some appears in the blood, mainly in the free form; about 20% is excreted in the urine unchanged and in the acetylated form.

Sulphasalazine has been claimed to be concentrated in connective tissue.

A detailed review of the clinical pharmacokinetics of sulphasalazine.— K. M. Das and R. Dubin, *Clin. Pharmacokinet.*, 1976, *1*, 406.

In 10 healthy men given a single dose of 4 g of sulphasalazine mean peak serum concentrations of about 26 µg per ml were reached in 3 to 7 hours. In 9 of the men given daily doses of 4 g serum concentrations at day 5 were 4.7 to 45 µg per ml with 37 to 92 µg per ml of sulphapyridine and its metabolites—glucuronide and acetylated sulphapyridine and glucuronide. The mean half-life of sulphasalazine after single and repeated doses was 5.7 and 7.6 hours respectively. From 1.7 to 10% of sulphasalazine appeared in the urine with about 10% of sulphapyridine and about 10% of the glucuronide and about 30% of each of the acetyl derivatives. Excretion was not greatly affected by urinary pH. There was no unchanged sulphasalazine in the faeces.— H. Schröder and D. E. S. Campbell, *Clin. Pharmac. Ther.*, 1972, *13*, 539.

In 7 healthy subjects the azo-reduction of sulphasalazine and recovery of 5-aminosalicylic acid in the faeces was substantially decreased during accelerated intestinal transit. In 18 patients with severe colitis, serum-sulphapyridine concentrations were related to the diarrhoeal state and did not correlate with disease activity, suggesting that the reduced therapeutic efficacy of sulphasalazine in severe colitis may be related to accelerated intestinal transit time.— P. A. M. van Hees *et al.*, *Gut*, 1979, *20*, 300.

Further references: H. Schröder and D. A. P. Evans, *Gut*, 1972, *13*, 278; M. A. Peppercorn and P. Goldman, *Gastroenterology*, 1973, *64*, 240; H. Schröder *et al.*, *Clin. Pharmac. Ther.*, 1973, *14*, 802; H. Schröder and B. M. Schröder, *Acta pharm. suec.*, 1973, *10*, 263; K. M. Das *et al.*, *Gastroenterology* 1979, *77*, 280.

Diffusion. In 5 healthy subjects given sulphasalazine by mouth the saliva to plasma concentration ratio for sulphapyridine was 0.559 and was independent of plasma concentration and saliva pH.— T. R. Bates *et al.*, *Clin. Pharmac. Ther.*, 1977, *22*, 917. See also M. Danhof and D. D. Breimer, *Clin. Pharmacokinet.*, 1978, *3*, 39; J. M. Day and J. B. Houston (letter), *Br. J. clin. Pharmac.*, 1980, *9*, 91.

Pregnancy and the neonate. An infant was born to a mother who had taken sulphasalazine 2 g daily throughout pregnancy. Maternal serum concentrations of sulphasalazine, sulphapyridine, and the acetyl and glucuronide conjugates, were generally similar to those in umbilical cord blood and amniotic fluid.— P. A. Hensleigh and R. E. Kauffman, *Am. J. Obstet. Gynec.*, 1977, *127*, 443.

In 5 patients taking sulphasalazine 500 mg four times daily during pregnancy and the puerperium, concentrations of sulphasalazine and its metabolites in cord blood were not greatly different from those in maternal serum. No adverse effect had been seen in 10 years. In 3 patients concentrations in breast milk were lower and were not considered likely to cause harmful effects.— A. K. A. Khan and S. C. Truelove, *Br. med. J.*, 1979, *2*, 1553.

Pharmacokinetic studies indicating that concentrations of sulphasalazine and its metabolite sulphapyridine achieved in the breast milk of nursing mothers taking sulphasalazine were unlikely to present a hazard to their infants.— G. Järnerot and M. -B. Into-Malmberg, *Scand. J. Gastroenterol.*, 1979, *14*, 869; C. M. Berlin and S. J. Yaffe, *Develop. Pharmac. Ther.*, 1980, *1*, 31.

Uses. Sulphasalazine is used in the management of inflammatory bowel diseases. In ulcerative colitis it is effective in the maintenance of remissions and may be used as an adjunct to corticosteroids in the treatment of the acute phase of the disease. Sulphasalazine is also effective in the active treatment of Crohn's disease but it does not appear to be of value in maintaining remissions. The usual initial adult dose of sulphasalazine is 1 to 2 g by mouth 4 times daily; up to 12 g daily in divided doses has been given but is associated with an increased risk of toxicity. The night-time interval between doses should not exceed 8 hours. This treatment may continue for 2 to 3 weeks; on remission the dose is gradually reduced to 1.5 to 2 g daily and then generally continued indefinitely. For children doses should be proportional to body-weight; initially 40 to 60 mg per kg body-weight may be given daily in divided doses reduced to 20 to 30 mg per kg daily for the maintenance of remission.

Enteric-coated tablets have been used in patients unable to tolerate sulphasalazine but absorption may be less reliable.

Sulphasalazine is also given rectally, as suppositories, in a dose of 1 g night and morning, either alone or as an adjunct to treatment by mouth; it may also be given by enema in a dose of 3 g at bedtime.

The urine of patients taking sulphasalazine may be coloured orange-yellow.

Reviews of the actions and uses of sulphasalazine.— P. Goldman and M. A. Peppercorn, *New Engl. J. Med.*, 1975, *293,* 20; A. K. A. Khan and S. C. Truelove, The actions of sulphasalazine, in *Topics in Gastroenterology, 4,* S.C. Truelove and J.A. Ritchie (Ed.), Oxford, Blackwell, 1976.

A study of the possible use of sulphasalazine to measure mouth/caecal transit time.— M. Kennedy *et al.* (letter), *Br. J. clin. Pharmac.*, 1979, *8,* 372.

Action. Sulphasalazine was found to reduce the bacterial count of clostridia, enterobacteria, and total non-sporing anaerobes in patients with proctocolitis and it was suggested that this antibacterial effect might be related to the beneficial effect of sulphasalazine in this condition.— B. West *et al.*, *Gut,* 1974, *15,* 960. See also R. Lendrum *et al.*, *ibid.*, 344. Of 50 strains of *Escherichia coli* isolated from 40 patients treated with sulphasalazine, 49 were resistant to sulphapyridine. Of 50 strains from patients not treated with sulphasalazine, 27 were resistant.— E. M. Cooke *et al.*, *Gut,* 1974, *15,* 143.

A report associating the efficacy of sulphasalazine in ulcerative colitis with serum-sulphapyridine concentrations of 20 μg or more per ml . Such concentrations were achieved by daily doses of 3 to 4 g of sulphasalazine in rapid acetylators and by 2.5 to 3 g daily in slow acetylators.— G. O. Cowan *et al.*, *Br. med. J.*, 1977, *2,* 1057.

See also K. M. Das *et al.*, *Gut,* 1973, *14,* 631; P. Riis *et al.*, *Scand. J. Gastroenterol.*, 1979, *14,* 257.

A study in 185 patients with ulcerative colitis indicated that when patients are maintained on the same dose of sulphasalazine, the serum concentration of total sulphapyridine during remission does not influence the liability to relapse. When relapse does occur, serum concentrations of sulphapyridine fall and remain depressed until remission occurs; the fall is most pronounced in patients with colitis affecting the entire colon and least marked in patients with distal colitis.— A. K. A. Khan and S. C. Truelove, *Gut,* 1980, *21,* 706.

Studies indicating that 5-aminosalicylic acid is the active moiety of sulphasalazine in ulcerative colitis and that the other component, sulphapyridine, acts as a carrier.— A. K. A. Khan *et al.*, *Lancet,* 1977, *2,* 892; P. A. M. van Hees *et al.* (letter), *ibid.*, 1978, *1,* 277; U. Klotz *et al.*, *New Engl. J. Med.*, 1980, *303,* 1499. The results of a study in which 45 patients with proctitis were treated with suppositories containing sulphapyridine, 5-aminosalicylic acid, or placebo indicated that 5-aminosalicylic acid was the active therapeutic moiety of sulphasalazine. After 4 weeks of treatment complete clinical remission with normal rectal mucosa on sigmoidoscopy was obtained in 60% of patients given 5-aminosalicylic acid and in about 13 and 27% of those given sulphapyridine and placebo respectively.— P. A. M. van Hees *et al.*, *Gut,* 1980, *21,* 632.

The administration of salicylate as sodium salicylate enemas to patients with mild to moderate ulcerative colitis had no beneficial effect, suggesting that the 5-aminosalicylic acid moiety of sulphasalazine has some property not common to all salicylates.— M. Campieri *et al.* (letter), *Lancet,* 1978, *2,* 993. The patients might not be expected to respond since they had active disease. Aspirin by mouth or rectally should be evaluated in patients unable to tolerate sulphasalazine.— S. R. Gould (letter), *ibid.*, 1161.

Experimental findings that sulphasalazine inhibits prostaglandin metabolism but not synthesis.— J. R. S. Hoult and P. K. Moore, *Br. J. Pharmac.*, 1978, *64,* 6; P. K. Moore *et al.* (letter), *Lancet,* 1978, *2,* 98.

Studies *in vitro* showing that sulphasalazine inhibits prostaglandin synthesis in the mucosa of patients with ulcerative colitis.— P. R. Smith *et al.*, *Gut,* 1979, *20,* 802. See also A. A. Butt *et al.*, *Gut,* 1973, *15,* 344; P. R. Smith *et al.* (letter), *Lancet,* 1978, *2,* 260; D. Rachmilewitz *et al.* (letter), *ibid.*, 946; H. Sinzinger *et al.* (letter), *ibid.*, 1253.

Crohn's disease. Reviews of the treatment of Crohn's disease.— P. Brown, *Med. J. Aust.*, 1974, *1,* 269; *Br. med. J.*, 1975, *2,* 297; T. C. Northfield, *Drugs,* 1977, *14,* 198; T. C. Northfield, *Prescribers' J.*, 1979, *19,* 80; J. B. Kirsner, *J. Am. med. Ass.*, 1980, *243,* 557; *Br. med. J.*, 1980, *281,* 893.

In a multicentre comparative study of treatment for Crohn's disease, a chronic destructive inflammatory disease of the bowel, prednisone or sulphasalazine were more effective than placebo in patients with active disease; azathioprine was ineffective. Sulphasalazine may be the drug of choice for previously untreated patients; overall, it was the least toxic of the three drugs. Sulphasalazine, prednisone, or azathioprine were not of value in quiescent disease or following surgery. When sulphasalazine and prednisone were used together in actively symptomatic patients there was probably less improvement than when prednisone was used alone. Patients in remission relapsed more quickly on the combined treatment and suffered more adverse effects than those taking prednisone, suggesting that the use of sulphasalazine and prednisone in association for active Crohn's disease should be discouraged.—The National Cooperative Crohn's Disease Study, J. W. Singleton (Ed.), *Gastroenterology,* 1979, *77,* 825–944.

Further reports of the use of sulphasalazine in Crohn's disease.— F. Goldstein and M. G. Murdock, *Am. J. dig. Dis.*, 1971, *16,* 421; *Gut,* 1977, *18,* 69; A. Wenckert *et al.*, *Scand. J. Gastroenterol.*, 1978, *13,* 161.

For further references to the management of Crohn's disease, see Azathioprine, p.191, and Corticosteroids, p.453.

Pregnancy and the neonate. In 38 women with ulcerative colitis during 50 pregnancies there were no complications due to treatment with sulphasalazine and oral and/or topical corticosteroids.— H. P. McEwan, *Proc. R. Soc. Med.*, 1972, *65,* 279.

Recommendations that sulphasalazine should be continued during pregnancy if necessary for the maintenance treatment of ulcerative colitis.— J. H. Jones, *Practitioner,* 1978, *220,* 116; M. de Swiet, *Prescribers' J.*, 1979, *19,* 59.

See also Absorption and Fate.

Proctitis. A report of the use of high-fibre diet, sulphasalazine, and prednisolone sodium phosphate enemas or suppositories in haemorrhagic proctitis in 74 patients.— A. Myers *et al.*, *Postgrad. med. J.*, 1976, *52,* 224.

Further references: C. Möller *et al.*, *Clin. Trials J.*, 1978, *15,* 199.

Rheumatoid arthritis. A study of the use of sulphasalazine in the treatment of rheumatoid arthritis; sulphasalazine was given, as an enteric-coated preparation, in a dose of 0.5 g daily, increased by 0.5-g increments at weekly intervals to a maintenance dose usually of 2 g daily. Clinical scores improved, and C-reactive protein and ESR fell. Five patients developed megaloblastic anaemia and 1 neutropenia.— B. McConkey *et al.*, *Br. med. J.*, 1980, *280,* 442. Severe criticisms of this uncontrolled study.— H. L. F. Currey and D. M. Chaput de Saintonge (letter), *ibid.*, 861; D. James and J. Reeback (letter), *ibid.*. Reply.— B. McConkey (letter), *ibid.*, 862.

Scleroderma. All of 19 patients with scleroderma of 1.5 to 20 years' duration obtained subjective improvement after treatment with sulphasalazine; objective improvement occurred in several parameters and in 9 patients was marked. The dose was 1 to 7 g daily for 2 or 3 weeks, then 0.25 to 7 g daily. Side-effects were common but not severe.— N. Dover, *Israel J. med. Scis,* 1971, *7,* 1301, per *Practitioner,* 1972, *208,* 440.

In 13 patients with scleroderma of about 1 to 28 years' duration, treatment with sulphasalazine for up to 13 months produced marked improvement in 2, mild improvement in 1, some subjective improvement in 3, and no improvement in the remaining 7. Treatment was discontinued because of side-effects in 9 patients.— Z. Šťáva and M. Kobíková, *Br. J. Derm.*, 1976, *96,* 541.

Further references: A. J. Barnett *et al.*, *Aust. J. Derm.*, 1975, *16,* 55.

Ulcerative colitis. Reviews of the treatment of ulcerative colitis.— G. Watkinson, *Br. med. J.*, 1961, *1,* 147; M. A. Eastwood and K. M. Das, *Br. J. Hosp. Med.*, 1975, *13,* 142; G. Watkinson, *Practitioner,* 1976, *216,* 642; T. C. Northfield, *Drugs,* 1977, *14,* 198; *Lancet,* 1978, *1,* 1190; T. C. Northfield, *Prescribers' J.*, 1979, *19,* 80; *Br. med. J.* 1981, *282,* 1255.

Corticosteroid treatment is superior to sulphasalazine in patients with acute ulcerative colitis.— S. C. Truelove *et al.*, *Br. med. J.*, 1962, *2,* 1708. Sulphasalazine can be used for prolonged treatment after an acute attack has been controlled. A suitable dose is 500 mg four times daily, which is usually well tolerated; a few patients can not tolerate even 500 mg twice daily.— S. C. Truelove, *ibid.*, 1968, *2,* 539. If tolerated, maintenance treatment with sulphasalazine should be continued indefinitely.— A. S. Dissanayake and S. C. Truelove, *Gut,* 1973, *14,* 923.

Improvement, beginning as early as 8 days after treatment commenced, occurred in 9 of 10 patients with acute ulcerative colitis treated with sulphasalazine by enema twice daily; remissions lasted for up to 11 months. Two tablets were suspended in water to form the enema.— H. Serebro *et al.*, *Br. med. J.*, 1977, *2,* 1264. A favourable report of the use of sulphasalazine enemas (3 g in 100 ml) in the treatment of ulcerative colitis.— K. R. Palmer *et al.*, *Br. med. J.*, 1981, *282,* 1571.

In a randomised study of patients with ulcerative colitis, sulphasalazine was significantly better than sodium cromoglycate at maintaining remissions.— M. W. Dronfield and M. J. S. Langman, *Gut* 1978, *19,* 1136.

Further references: K. Rauch and H. Weiland, *Strahlentherapie,* 1972, *143,* 660; P. D. Goldstein *et al.*, *J. Pediat.*, 1979, *95,* 638; A. K. A. Khan *et al.*, *Gut,* 1980, *21,* 232.

For further references to the management of ulcerative colitis, see Azathioprine, p.191, and Corticosteroids, p.453.

Preparations

Sulfasalazine Tablets *(U.S.P.).* Tablets containing sulphasalazine.

Salazopyrin *(Pharmacia, UK: Farillon, UK).* Sulphasalazine, available as **Enema** containing 3 g in each 100 ml; as **Suppositories** of 500 mg; and as scored **Tablets** and enteric-coated (EN) tablets of 500 mg. (Also available as Salazopyrin in *Austral., Canad., Denm., Ital., Norw., S.Afr., Switz.*).

Other Proprietary Names

Azulfidine *(Arg., Ger., USA)*; Colo-Pleon *(Ger.)*; Salazopyrina *(Spain)*; Salazopyrine *(Belg., Fr., Neth.)*; Salisulf *(Ital.)*; SAS-500 *(Canad., USA)*.

4952-h

Sulphasomidine *(B.P. 1963).* Sulphasomid.; Sulfasomidine; Sulfisomidine; Sulfa-isodimérazine; Sulfaisodimidine. N^1-(2,6-Dimethylpyrimidin-4-yl)sulphanilamide. $C_{12}H_{14}N_4O_2S$=278.3.

CAS — 515-64-0.

NOTE. Sulfadimethylpyrimidine has been used as a synonym for sulphasomidine, and sulphadimethylpyrimidine is sometimes used as a synonym for sulphadimidine (p.1475). Care should be taken to avoid confusion between the two compounds, which are isomeric.

Pharmacopoeias. In *Fr., Ger.,* and *Jap.*

A white or creamy-white, odourless, finely crystalline powder which slowly darkens on exposure to light. M.p. 244° to 246°.

Slightly **soluble** in water, soluble 1 in about 60 of boiling water; slightly soluble in alcohol and acetone; very slightly soluble in chloroform and ether; readily soluble in dilute mineral acids and solutions of alkali hydroxides. **Store** in airtight containers. Protect from light.

Sulphasomidine has the general properties and uses of Sulphonamides, p.1457.

It is rapidly excreted and is soluble in acid urine; from 10 to 25% may be present as the less soluble acetyl derivative. Sulphasomidine has been given in an initial adult dose of 2 to 4 g followed by 6 g daily in divided doses every 4 or 6 hours. The sodium salt has been given by injection.

A review of the uses of sulphasomidine.— L. Weinstein *et al.*, *New Engl. J. Med.*, 1960, *263,* 793.

The biological half-life of sulphasomidine was 6 to 8

hours.— W. A. Ritschel, *Drug Intell. & clin. Pharm.*, 1970, *4*, 332.

The absorption of sulphasomidine is not affected by food.— A. Melander *et al.*, *Acta med. scand.*, 1976, *200*, 497.

Absorption studies on sulphasomidine in neonates, infants, and children.— G. Heimann *et al.*, *Arzneimittel-Forsch.*, 1978, *28*, 861.

Preparations

Sulphasomidine Tablets *(B.P. 1963).* Sulfasomidine Tablets. Tablets containing sulphasomidine. Store in airtight containers. Protect from light.

Proprietary Names

Aristamid *(also as sodium derivative) (Nordmark-Werke, Ger.)*; Elcosine *(Ciba, Fr.)*; Elkosin *(also as sodium derivative) (Ciba, Denm.; Ciba, Ger.; Ciba, Norw.; Ciba, Swed.; Ciba-Geigy, Switz.)*; Elkosina *(Ciba, Spain)*; Elkosine *(Ciba, Belg.; Ciba, Neth.)*; Isosulf *(also as sodium derivative) (A.L., Norw.)*; Pepsilphen *(Cambridge Laboratories, Austral.)*.

4953-m

Sulphathiazole *(B.P.)*. Sulphathiaz.; Sulfathiazole; Sulfathiazolum; Sulfanilamidothiazolum; Norsulfazolum; Solfatiazolo; Sulfonazolum; M & B 760. N^1-(Thiazol-2-yl)sulphanilamide.

$C_9H_9N_3O_2S_2$=255.3.

CAS — 72-14-0.

Pharmacopoeias. In *Arg., Aust., Belg., Br., Cz., Fr., Hung., Int., It., Mex., Pol., Port., Roum., Rus., Span.,* and *Swiss.*

A white or almost white, odourless or almost odourless, almost tasteless crystalline powder which slowly darkens on exposure to light. M.p. 200° to 203°.

Soluble 1 in 2500 of water, 1 in 40 of boiling water, 1 in 120 of alcohol, and 1 in 50 of acetone; practically insoluble in chloroform and ether; soluble in dilute mineral acids and solutions of alkali hydroxides and carbonates. **Sterilisation** as for Sulphadimidine, p.1475. **Store** in airtight containers. Protect from light.

Effect of gamma-irradiation. Gamma-irradiation of sulphathiazole caused a slight change of colour amounting to 5 times the normal limit at 250 000 Gy. The u.v. and i.r. absorption and the assay revealed no change but the m.p. was lowered by 2.5° and the irradiated substance was more acid in reaction.— *The Use of Gamma Radiation Sources for the Sterilisation of Pharmaceutical Products*, London, ABPI, 1960.

4954-b

Sulphathiazole Sodium *(B.P. 1953, B. Vet. C. 1965)*. Sulphathiazol. Sod.; Soluble Sulphathiazole; Sulfathiazolum Natricum.

$C_9H_8N_3NaO_2S_2,5H_2O$=367.4.

CAS — 144-74-1 (anhydrous); 6791-71-5 (pentahydrate).

Pharmacopoeias. In *Arg., Aust.,* and *Mex.* (all $1\frac{1}{2}H_2O$); in *Int.* and *Pol.* ($1\frac{1}{2}H_2O$ or $5H_2O$); and in *Rus.* ($6H_2O$).

A white or yellowish-white, odourless, almost tasteless, microcrystalline powder. It slowly darkens on exposure to light; on exposure to moist air it absorbs carbon dioxide and becomes incompletely soluble in water. Sulphathiazole sodium ($5H_2O$) 1.44 g is approximately equivalent to 1 g of sulphathiazole.

Soluble 1 in 3 of water and 1 in 20 of alcohol. A solution in water has a pH of about 9.5. A 4.82% solution is iso-osmotic with serum. Solutions are **sterilised** by distributing into ampoules, replacing the air with nitrogen, sealing, and autoclaving. **Incompatible** with acids. **Store** in airtight containers. Protect from light.

Effect of gamma-irradiation. Gamma-irradiation at 250 000 Gy changed the colour of sulphathiazole sodium to a deep chocolate-brown and a slight odour developed. The i.r. absorption and assay revealed no change but the u.v. absorption was slightly lower and the m.p. was lowered by 4°.— *The Use of Gamma Radiation Sources for the Sterilisation of Pharmaceutical Products*, London, ABPI, 1960.

Incompatibility. Magnesium chloride and calcium chloride were incompatible with sulphathiazole sodium, complexes of magnesium sulphathiazole and calcium sulphathiazole being formed.— V. H. Bruin and W. H. Oliver, *Australas. J. Pharm.*, 1957, *38*, 226.

For earlier references to the stability of sulphathiazole sodium solutions, see Extra Pharmacopoeia 26th Edn, p. 1769.

Adverse Effects, Treatment, and Precautions. As for Sulphonamides, p.1457.

Adverse effects with sulphathiazole are common. Drug fever and skin rashes are relatively frequent. The Stevens-Johnson syndrome has been reported after treatment with sulphathiazole. The acetyl derivative of sulphathiazole has a low solubility in urine and the incidence of crystalluria is high. Adequate fluid intake and administration of alkalis are essential.

Effects on laboratory tests. Sulphathiazole could interfere with the Schack and Waxler spectrophotometric assay for plasma-theophylline concentrations to give significantly false-positive elevations.— L. E. Matheson *et al.*, *Am. J. Hosp. Pharm.*, 1977, *34*, 496.

Absorption and Fate. As for Sulphonamides, p.1458.

Sulphathiazole is readily absorbed from the gastro-intestinal tract and is bound to plasma albumin to the extent of 55 to 75%. It does not readily penetrate into the cerebrospinal fluid. About 20% is acetylated in the body. Sulphathiazole is rapidly excreted, 60 to 90% being eliminated in the urine within 24 hours.

The biological half-life of sulphathiazole is variously reported as 3.4 to 3.8 hours.— W. A. Ritschel, *Drug Intell. & clin. Pharm.*, 1970, *4*, 332.

Effect of suspending agents on the bioavailability of suspensions of sulphathiazole.— H. O. Alpar and J. A. Hersey, *Farmaco, Edn prat.*, 1979, *34*, 532.

Uses. Sulphathiazole has the general properties and uses of Sulphonamides, p.1458.

It has been largely superseded by other less toxic sulphonamides and antibiotics.

A suggested dose by mouth is 2 to 3 g initially followed by 1 g every 4 or 6 hours. Sulphathiazole is used with other sulphonamides in preparations for the topical treatment of vaginal infections (see p.1486).

Sulphathiazole sodium was formerly given by intravenous injection.

Preparations

Sulphathiazole Tablets *(B.P.).* Tablets containing sulphathiazole. Protect from light.

Thiazamide *(May & Baker, UK).* Sulphathiazole, available as scored tablets of 500 mg. (Also available as Thiazamide in *S.Afr.*).

Other Proprietary Names of Sulphathiazole

Cibazol *(Ger., Switz.)*; Septozol *(Switz.)*; Sulfamul *(Canad.)*.

A preparation containing sulphathiazole was also formerly marketed in Great Britain under the proprietary name Sulfex *(Smith Kline & French)*.

4955-v

Sulphathiourea. Sulfanilthiocarbamid; Sulfanilylthiourea; Sulfathiocarbamide; Sulfanilylthioharnstoff. 1-Sulphanilyl-2-thiourea.

$C_7H_9N_3O_2S_2$=231.3.

CAS — 515-49-1.

A white, almost tasteless, crystalline powder. Very slightly **soluble** in water; slightly soluble in alcohol (90%); soluble in acetone, dilute mineral acids, and solutions of alkali hydroxides. A solution in water is acid to litmus. **Protect** from light.

Sulphathiourea is a sulphonamide (p.1457) which has been used topically.

4956-g

Sulphaurea. Sulphanilylurea; Sulfanilcarbamide; Sulphacarbamide; Urosulphanum. Sulphanilylurea monohydrate.

$C_7H_9N_3O_3S,H_2O$=233.2.

CAS — 547-44-4 (anhydrous); 6101-35-5 (monohydrate).

Pharmacopoeias. In *Rus.*

A white, odourless, almost tasteless, crystalline powder. **Soluble** 1 in 430 of water; readily soluble in boiling water; slightly soluble in alcohol; soluble in acetone, dilute mineral acids, and solutions of alkali hydroxides; practically insoluble in chloroform and ether. A solution in water is acid to litmus. **Protect** from light.

Adverse Effects, Treatment, and Precautions. As for Sulphonamides, p.1457.

Absorption and Fate. As for Sulphonamides, p.1458.

Sulphaurea is readily absorbed from the gastro-intestinal tract and most of a single dose is removed from the blood in 12 hours. It is rapidly excreted; 10 to 15% of sulphaurea in the urine is in the form of the acetyl derivative. Sulphaurea and its acetyl derivative are relatively highly soluble in urine.

Uses. Sulphaurea has the general properties and uses of Sulphonamides, p.1458. It is used in the treatment of urinary-tract infections, usually in conjunction with a urinary analgesic such as phenazopyridine. The adult dose of sulphaurea is 1 g thrice daily; children may be given one-half the adult dose.

Proprietary Preparations

Uromide *(Consolidated Chemicals, UK).* Tablets each containing sulphaurea 500 mg and phenazopyridine hydrochloride 50 mg. For urinary-tract infections. *Dose.* 2 tablets thrice daily.

Other Proprietary Names

Euvernil *(Ger., Switz.)*.

1401-c

Trimethoprim *(B.P., B.P. Vet., U.S.P.)*. Trimethoxyprim; BW 56-72. 5-(3,4,5-Trimethoxybenzyl)pyrimidine-2,4-diyldiamine.

$C_{14}H_{18}N_4O_3$=290.3.

CAS — 738-70-5.

Pharmacopoeias. In *Br., Chin.,* and *U.S.*

White or yellowish-white, odourless or almost odourless crystals or crystalline powder with a very bitter taste. M.p. 199° to 203°. **Soluble** 1 in 2500 of water, 1 in 300 of alcohol, 1 in 55 of chloroform, and 1 in 80 of methyl alcohol; soluble in benzyl alcohol; slightly soluble in acetone; practically insoluble in ether and carbon tetrachloride. **Store** in airtight containers. Protect from light.

Adverse Effects and Treatment. Side-effects reported include nausea, vomiting, headache, pruritus, and skin rash. Trimethoprim given over a prolonged period may cause a depression of haemopoiesis due to interference of the drug in the metabolism of folic acid. Injections of calcium folinate may be given to counter this effect. For reports of adverse effects of trimethoprim when used with sulphamethoxazole, see Co-trimoxazole, p.1460.

Trimethoprim-associated marrow toxicity in one patient.— J. Sheehan (letter), *Lancet*, 1981, *2*, 692.

Hypersensitivity. A 49-year-old woman developed a morbilliform rash at the end of a 10-day course of co-trimoxazole. The rash, which responded to betamethasone and dexchlorpheniramine, was considered due to trimethoprim.— G. M. Halpern (letter), *Br. med. J.*, 1972, *1*, 691.

Overdosage. Six hours after ingesting 80 tablets of trimethoprim 100 mg in a suicide attempt, a 28-year-old man vomited. Fourteen hours after ingestion he was admitted to hospital complaining of headache, swollen face, and weakness. Activated charcoal was given after gastric lavage. He was given intravenous fluids to ensure good diuresis, and during the 48 hours of observation his only complaint was mild epigastric pain after the lavage. Physically he remained normal throughout. He was estimated to have absorbed 3.2 g of trimethoprim, and the elimination of the drug followed first-order kinetics with a half-life of 11.9 hours.— K. Hoppu *et al.* (letter), *Lancet*, 1980, *1*, 778.

Precautions. Care is necessary in administering trimethoprim to patients with impaired renal function. It is suggested that regular haematological examination should be made during prolonged courses of treatment. Its use should be avoided during pregnancy.

For reports dealing with precautions for trimethoprim given with sulphamethoxazole, see Co-trimoxazole, p.1461.

Four patients with megaloblastic anaemia who were given co-trimoxazole for concurrent infections failed to respond to haematinic therapy. Reticulocytosis was suppressed in 3 patients and the fourth failed to respond clinically until the antibacterial therapy was discontinued. Thrombocytopenia and neutropenia were prominent in 2 of the patients. Trimethoprim was suspected as the agent responsible.— I. Chanarin and J. M. England, *Br. med. J.*, 1972, *1*, 651.

Further references: E. M. E. Poskitt and J. M. Parkin, *Archs Dis. Childh.*, 1972, *47*, 626.

Absorption of trimethoprim was increased in coeliac disease.— *Drug & Ther. Bull.*, 1976, *14*, 57.

For a recommendation that trimethoprim should not be given to patients between courses of antineoplastic agents because of potential bone-marrow aplasia, see Antineoplastic Agents and Immunosuppressants, p.175.

Antimicrobial Action and Resistance. Trimethoprim is active against a wide range of micro-organisms, including *Escherichia coli* and some *Klebsiella, Proteus,* and *Staphylococcus* spp.; it is also active against *Plasmodium* spp. It has no significant activity against anaerobes, *Neisseria* spp., or *Pseudomonas aeruginosa.*

It was previously considered that resistance developed rapidly when trimethoprim was used alone; these fears are now considered to have been largely unjustified, although, as with all antimicrobial agents, there are reports of resistance.

Resistance among *Plasmodium* spp. does not yet appear to be a problem. Resistance to trimethoprim with a sulphonamide is discussed under Co-trimoxazole, p.1462.

Sensitivity of *Haemophilus influenzae.*— J. D. Williams and J. Andrews, *Br. med. J.*, 1974, *1*, 134.

Two resistant strains of *Haemophilus influenzae.*— A. J. Howard *et al.*, *Br. med. J.*, 1978, *1*, 1657.

Resistance to trimethoprim occurred in 63 of 788 urinary-tract isolates of bacteria obtained from hospital patients over a 3-month period in 1975. Over a similar period in 1977, 93 of 863 isolates were resistant. The greatest increase in resistance occurred in strains of *Escherichia coli.* The proportion of isolates carrying R-factors conferring resistance to trimethoprim had increased.— S. G. B. Amyes *et al.*, *J. clin. Path.*, 1978, *31*, 850.

In a study in Finland, where trimethoprim had been used alone to treat urinary-tract infections for 5 years, the incidence of resistance to trimethoprim at 8 μg per ml ('the MIC generally used in Scandinavia to determine clinical resistance to trimethoprim') was broadly comparable with that of sulphamethoxazole:trimethoprim (20:1) at 64 μg per ml, sulphamethoxazole at 512 μg per ml, ampicillin at 32 μg per ml, and nitrofurantoin at 64 μg per ml ('the MICs used in Scandinavia to test resistance to these drugs'). *E. coli* and *Micrococcus* had a low incidence of resistance; *Proteus mirabilis* and *Klebsiella* had a high incidence; *Enterobacter, Streptococcus faecalis,* and *Staphylococcus epidermidis* showed intermediate incidence.— P. Huovinen and P. Toivanen, *Br. med. J.*, 1980, *280*, 72.

A survey of 3998 isolates of *E. coli, Klebsiella/Enterobacter* spp., and *Proteus* spp. in a 6-month period in 1978 and of 4069 of isolates in 1979 showed no overall increase in the incidence of trimethoprim resistance, but the proportion of resistance attributable to transferable R plasmids almost trebled. There was also a large increase in the proportion of resistant strains exhibiting high-level non-transferable trimethoprim resistance.— K. J. Towner *et al.*, *Br. med. J.*, 1980, *280*, 517.

A discussion of the development of trimethoprim-resistant strains of *Salmonella typhimurium.*— E. J. Threlfall *et al.*, *Br. med. J.*, 1980, *280*, 1210.

A discussion on bacterial resistance to trimethoprim.— *Br. med. J.*, 1980, *281*, 571.

Further references.— K. Fruensgaard and B. Korner, *Chemotherapy, Basle,* 1974, *20*, 97; A. Toivanen *et al.*, *Chemotherapy, Basle,* 1976, *22*, 97; D. Greenwood and F. O'Grady, *J. clin. Path.*, 1976, *29*, 162; R. N. Grüneberg and A. M. Emmerson, *J. antimicrob. Chemother.*, 1977, *3*, 453, per *Abstr. Hyg.*, 1978, *53*, 230; A. Stokes and R. W. Lacey, *J. clin. Path.*, 1978, *31*, 165; B. P. Goldstein *et al.*, *Antimicrob. Ag. Chemother.*, 1979, *16*, 736; S. J. Pancoast, *Antimicrob. Ag. Chemother.*, 1980, *17*, 263; H. E. Busk and B. Korner (letter), *Br. med. J.*, 1980, *280*, 1054; L. G. Burman (letter), *Lancet*, 1980, *1*, 1409; W. Brumfitt *et al.* (letter), *Lancet*, 1980, *1*, 1409; H. Richards and N. Datta, *Br. med. J.*, 1981, *282*, 1118.

Absorption and Fate. Trimethoprim is readily absorbed from the gastro-intestinal tract and peak concentrations in the circulation occur about 3 hours after a dose is taken. About 45% is bound to plasma proteins. Tissue concentrations are reported to be higher than serum concentrations, with particularly high concentrations occurring in the kidneys and lungs but concentrations in the cerebrospinal fluid are about one-half of those in the blood. The half-life is about 10 to 16 hours. About 40 to 50% of a dose is excreted unchanged in the urine within 24 hours, together with metabolites. Trimethoprim appears in breast milk.

The elimination half-life of trimethoprim in 2 subjects was 15 to 17 hours. Peak blood concentrations of about 2 μg per ml occurred 4 hours after trimethoprim 200 mg. The administration of 50 mg four times daily to 13 subjects for 13 weeks produced steady blood concentrations of about 0.32 to 1.84 μg per ml, depending on body-weight. Only 25 to 36% of the dose was excreted unchanged in the urine.— S. A. Kaplan *et al.*, *J. pharm. Sci.*, 1970, *59*, 358.

The half-life of trimethoprim in children aged 2 to 6 years was about 2.5 to 5 hours compared with about 10 hours in adults.— P. Kremers *et al.*, *Thérapie*, 1973, *28*, 1177.

In studies in 51 patients using varying doses of trimethoprim, the concentrations in lung tissue, bronchial secretions, and saliva were generally much higher than the serum concentration. Therapeutic concentrations were maintained for 6 to 13 hours against usual respiratory pathogens.— I. Hansen *et al.*, *Acta pharmac. tox.*, 1973, *32*, 337.

Concentrations of trimethoprim active against *Staphylococcus aureus* and Gram-negative organisms other than pseudomonas, associated with osteomyelitis were present in the porous bone and bone marrow of 11 patients 10 to 12 hours after dosage with trimethoprim 6.9 to 9.6 mg per kg body-weight daily given for 1 to 3 days.— L. M. Neilsen *et al.*, *Israel pharm. J.*, 1973, *16*, 222, per *Int. pharm. Abstr.*, 1974, *11*, 331.

The pharmacokinetics of trimethoprim with rifampicin.— J. M. T. Hamilton-Miller and W. Brumfitt, *J. antimicrob. Chemother.*, 1976, *2*, 181; G. Acocella and R. Scotti, *ibid.*, 271; A. M. Emmerson *et al.*, *ibid.*, 1978, *4*, 523.

The pharmacokinetics of trimethoprim with sulphadiazine.— T. Bergan *et al.*, *Clin. Pharmac. Ther.*, 1977, *22*, 211.

The pharmacokinetics of trimethoprim with sulfametopyrazine.— D. S. Reeves *et al.*, *J. antimicrob. Chemother.*, 1980, *6*, 647.

Trimethoprim was reported to be 40 to 70% bound to plasma proteins. The normal half-life of 8 to 15 hours was increased to 24 hours in end-stage renal failure.— W. M. Bennett *et al.*, *Ann. intern. Med.*, 1980, *93*, 62.

In 4 patients given trimethoprim 160 mg (as co-trimoxazole) concentrations in the CSF 0.5 to 1.5 hours after infusion were 20 to 44% of those in serum; in 5 patients treated by mouth concentrations in the CSF 2 to 4 hours after the dose were 13 to 34% of those in serum.— Å. Svedhem and S. Inwarson, *J. antimicrob. Chemother.*, 1979, *5*, 717.

For further reports of the absorption and fate of trimethoprim with sulphamethoxazole, see under Co-trimoxazole, p.1463.

Uses. Trimethoprim is a dihydrofolate reductase inhibitor which affects the nucleoprotein metabolism of micro-organisms by interference in the folic-folinic acid systems.

Trimethoprim has been used in conjunction with sulfametopyrazine in the treatment of chloroquine-resistant malaria but has not achieved wide acceptance. Doses of 1.5 g with sulfametopyrazine 1 g, daily for 3 days, have been used; smaller doses are generally less effective. Widespread use in areas where *P. falciparum* is sensitive to chloroquine is considered undesirable.

The antimicrobial spectrum of trimethoprim is similar to that of the sulphonamides. While sulphonamides inhibit bacterial synthesis of dihydrofolic acid from *p*-aminobenzoic acid, trimethoprim inhibits dihydrofolate reductase and thus presents the synthesis of tetrahydrofolic acid from dihydrofolic acid. The antimicrobial activity of sulphonamides may be enhanced in the presence of trimethoprim.

Trimethoprim is used in the treatment of acute urinary-tract infections; the usual dose is 200 mg twice daily; a dose of 300 mg daily is also used. Children may be given 6 to 8 mg per kg body-weight daily in 2 divided doses. For long-term prophylaxis the usual dose is 100 mg at night, with 2 to 2.5 mg per kg for children. Trimethoprim is also used in the treatment of respiratory-tract infections, in doses similar to those used in acute urinary-tract infections. Trimethoprim is also administered intravenously as the lactate in similar doses.

Trimethoprim is used in conjunction with sulphonamides in the treatment of bacterial infections. The most well known combination is co-trimoxazole (trimethoprim with sulphamethoxazole); other combinations are co-trimazine (with sulphadiazine) and co-trifamole (with sulphamoxole); trimethoprim is also used with sulfametrole or sulphadimidine, and, in veterinary practice, with sulfadoxine.

For a report of the antibacterial activity, pharmacology, and toxicity of trimethoprim and of its use in enhancing the effects of sulphonamides, see S. R. M. Bushby and G. H. Hitchings, *Br. J. Pharmac. Chemother.*, 1968, *33*, 72.

For an account of the antibacterial activity of trimethoprim, alone or in conjunction with a sulphonamide, see J. H. Darrell *et al.*, *J. clin. Path.*, 1968, *21*, 202.

For a review of the antibacterial activity, pharmacology, and clinical application of trimethoprim, alone and in conjunction with a sulphonamide, see *Br. med. J.*, 1969, *3*, 578.

The pharmacology and antimicrobial activity of trimethoprim, and its use in urinary-tract infections.— *Ann. clin. Res.*, 1978, *10*, *Suppl.* 22.

Enhanced antimicrobial effect with amikacin.— T. L. Parsley *et al.*, *Antimicrob. Ag. Chemother.*, 1977, *12*, 349.

For reports of the use of trimethoprim with sulphamethoxazole (co-trimoxazole) in the treatment of bacterial infections, see Co-trimoxazole.

Administration in renal failure. Patients in mild renal failure could receive 40 mg of trimethoprim every 12 hours while patients in uraemia or undergoing peritoneal dialysis could receive 40 mg every 24 hours.— G. B. Appel and H. C. Neu, *New Engl. J. Med.*, 1977, *296*, 663.

Enteric fever. Successful treatment of enteric fever due to *Salmonella paratyphi A* in 8 patients after treatment with trimethoprim 100 to 300 mg intravenously and by mouth every 12 hours for 14 days; one patient needed a second course.— M. W. McKendrick *et al.*, *Br. med. J.*, 1981, *282*, 364.

Malaria. *For the use of trimethoprim alone or with sulphamethoxazole or sulfametopyrazine in the treatment of malaria, see Martindale 27th Edn.*, p. 362.

Respiratory-tract infections. In a prospective randomised double-blind trial 107 patients with chest infections were given trimethoprim 100 mg twice daily for 5 days and 109 similar patients were given co-trimoxazole 600 mg twice daily. The mean response of those who received trimethoprim alone was virtually identical to that of those who received co-trimoxazole. Twenty side-effects were noted in 16 patients who received trimethoprim compared with 46 in 25 patients treated with co-trimoxazole; bad taste, sore throat, and nausea were more common with co-trimoxazole than with trimethoprim. It was considered that in the treatment of acute respiratory-tract infections trimethoprim was as effective as co-trimoxazole and produced fewer side-effects, but since there were several types of respiratory infections, these results could mask differences for certain diagnoses. Trimethoprim was as effective as co-trimoxazole in treating acute urinary-tract infections when compared in 42 patients.— R. W. Lacey *et al.*, *Lancet*, 1980, *1*,

1270; See also, *ibid.*, 1980, *2*, 326.

Urinary-tract infections. Discussions of trimethoprim and its use in urinary-tract infections.— G. P. Wormser and G. T. Keusch, *Ann. intern. Med.*, 1979, *91*, 420;; *Drug & Ther. Bull.*, 1980, *18*, 51; *Lancet*, 1980, *1*, 519; W. Brumfitt and J. M. J. Hamilton-Miller, *Br. J. Hosp. Med.*, 1980, *23*, 281; *Med. Lett.*, 1980, *22*, 69.

Trimethoprim 160 mg twice daily was as effective as co-trimoxazole 960 mg twice daily in the treatment of patients with acute urinary-tract infection. Two of 139 patients in the trimethoprim group and 4 of 129 in the co-trimoxazole group withdrew because of side-effects. Because of the risk of development of resistant strains, it was suggested that use of trimethoprim in the treatment of urinary-tract infections should be limited to out-patients.— A. Kasanen *et al.*, *Curr. ther. Res.*, 1979, *25*, 202.

Trimethoprim 100 mg was taken once daily for up to 17 months for prophylaxis by 13 patients with recurrent urinary-tract infections. All patients had negative urine cultures after 6 months of treatment. Two further patients had ceased treatment within 10 days because of side-effects or recurrence of infection. No adverse effects on haematological parameters were seen during treatment.— S. Iwarson and G. Lidin-Janson (letter), *J. antimicrob. Chemother.*, 1979, *5*, 316.

The incidence (20%) of infection with *Staphylococcus albus* (invariably resistant to sulphonamide and trimethoprim) in patients undergoing prostatectomy and treated with co-trimoxazole during catheterisation, rose to 90% when treatment was changed to trimethoprim alone.— R. Maskell and L. Pead (letter), *Lancet*, 1980, *2*, 144.

Successful treatment of 43 patients with acute pyelonephritis with sulphadiazine 500 mg with trimethoprim 160 mg twice daily for 10 days.— P. T. Männistö and P. Lähteenmäki, *Curr. ther. Res.*, 1978, *23*, 562.

In a controlled study in 40 patients with urinary-tract infections, rifampicin 600 mg with trimethoprim 160 mg (Rifaprim) as a single daily dose for 10 days was more effective than co-trimoxazole 960 mg twice daily.— T. Adachi and T. R. de Almeida, *J. int. med. Res.*, 1979, *7*, 132.

Further references.— U. J. Koch *et al.*, *Chemotherapy, Basle*, 1973, *19*, 314; A. Kasanen *et al.*, *Ann. clin. Res.*, 1974, *6*, 285; A. Kasanen *et al.*, *Scand. J. infect. Dis.*, 1974, *6*, 91; N. J. Pearson *et al.*, *Lancet*, 1979, *2*, 1205.

Proprietary Preparations

Ipral *(Squibb, UK).* Trimethoprim, available as **Paediatric Suspension** (sugar-free) containing 50 mg in 5 ml (suggested diluents, sorbitol solution, syrup, or water) and as **Tablets** of 100 and 200 mg.

Monotrim *(Duphar, UK).* Trimethoprim available as **Suspension** (sugar-free) containing 50 mg in 5 ml (suggested diluents, sorbitol solution, syrup, or water) and as scored **Tablets** of 100 mg and 200 mg. (Also available as Monotrim in *Denm.*).

Polytrim Eye Drops *(Wellcome, UK).* Contain in each ml trimethoprim 1 mg and polymyxin B sulphate 10 000 units, with thiomersal 50 µg.

Syraprim *(Wellcome, UK).* Trimethoprim, available as scored **Tablets** of 100 and 300 mg. **Syraprim Injection.** Contains trimethoprim lactate equivalent to trimethoprim 20 mg per ml, in ampoules of 5 ml for intravenous use.

Tiempe *(DDSA Pharmaceuticals, UK).* Trimethoprim, available as tablets of 100 mg.

Trimopan *(Berk Pharmaceuticals, UK).* Trimethoprim, available as **Suspension** containing 50 mg in 5 ml and scored **Tablets** of 100 and 200 mg. (Also available as Trimopan in *Denm., Fin.*).

Unitrim *(Unimed, UK).* Trimethoprim, available as tablets of 100 mg.

Other Proprietary Names

Proloprim, Trimpex *(both USA).*

Proprietary Names of Some Trimethoprim/Sulphonamide Preparations

Kelfiprim *(sulfametopyrazine)*; Kelfiprin *(sulfametopyrazine)*; Lidaprim *(sulfametrole) (Chemie-Linz, Aust.; Pharbil, Belg.; Hormonchemie, Ger.)*; Lidatrim *(sulfametrole) (Warrick, Neth.)*; Poteseptyl *(sulphadimidine) (Alkaloida Chemical Factory, Hung.)*; Trimed *(sulfametopyrazine) (Armour, Ital.)*; Trimetrol *(sulfametrole) (Essex, Belg.)*; Velaten *(sulphamethoxypyridazine) (Corvi, Ital.)*.

See also under Co-trifamole (p.1460), Co-trimazine (p.1460), and Co-trimoxazole (p.1467)..

4957-q

Preparations of Mixed Sulphonamides

For information on the actions and uses of mixed sulphonamides, see p.1458.

Sulfacombinum *(Dan. Disp.).* A powder containing sulphadiazine 33.3%, sulphadimidine 33.3%, and sulfamerazine 33.4%.

Suspensio Trisulfamidorum *(F.N. Belg.).* Trisulphonamide Mixture. Sulphadiazine 3.33 g, sulphadimidine 3.33 g, sulfamerazine 3.33 g, cinnamon syrup 40 g, glycerol 10 g, tragacanth 800 mg, methyl hydroxybenzoate 80 mg, propyl hydroxybenzoate 20 mg, alcohol 1 g, saccharin sodium 100 mg, water to 100 ml. Each 5 ml contains 500 mg of total sulphonamides.

Tablettae Sulfacombini *(Nord. P.).* Each contains sulphadiazine 166 mg, sulphadimidine 167 mg, and sulfamerazine 167 mg.

Trisulfapyrimidines Oral Suspension *(U.S.P.).* A suspension containing equal parts of sulphadiazine, sulphadimidine, and sulfamerazine; it may contain either sodium citrate or sodium lactate, and a suitable antimicrobial agent. It contains 93 to 107 mg of total sulphapyrimidines in 1 ml.

A study in 14 healthy subjects indicated several significant differences in bioavailability among 7 commercial preparations of Trisulfapyrimidines Oral Suspension.— L. K. Mathur *et al.*, *J. pharm. Sci.*, 1979, *68*, 699.

Trisulfapyrimidines Tablets *(U.S.P.).* Tablets containing equal parts of sulphadiazine, sulphadimidine, and sulfamerazine.

Trisulphonamide Tablets *(B.P.C. 1959).* Tab. Trisulphon. Each contains sulphadiazine 185 mg, sulfamerazine 130 mg, and sulphathiazole 185 mg.

Proprietary Preparations of Mixed Sulphonamides

Streptotriad *(May & Baker, UK).* Scored tablets each containing sulphadiazine 100 mg sulphadimidine 100 mg, sulphathiazole 100 mg, and streptomycin sulphate equivalent to streptomycin 65 mg. For diarrhoea and bacillary dysentery. *Dose.* Prevention, one or two tablets twice daily; treatment, 2 tablets thrice daily.

Sulphamagna *(Wyeth, UK).* A suspension containing in each 30 ml phthalylsulphathiazole 2 g, sulphadiazine 500 mg, activated attapulgite 2 g, and streptomycin sulphate equivalent to streptomycin 200 mg (suggested diluent, syrup). For diarrhoea. *Dose.* 30 ml three or four times daily.

Sulphatriad *(May & Baker, UK).* Scored **Tablets** each containing sulphadiazine 185 mg, sulfamerazine 130 mg, and sulphathiazole 185 mg, and **Suspension** (suggested diluent, syrup) containing the equivalent of 1 tablet in each 5 ml. *Dose.* For acute infections, 20 ml of suspension or 4 tablets initially, then 10 ml or 2 tablets every 4 to 6 hours; children, half the adult dose; for prevention, 5 ml or 1 tablet thrice daily; children, 7.5 to 10 ml daily.

Erythema multiforme (Stevens-Johnson syndrome) developed twice in the same patient following the administration of Sulphatriad.— J. D. G. Williams, *Practitioner*, 1963, *190*, 249.

Sultrin (Triple Sulfa) Cream *(Ortho-Cilag, UK).* A vaginal cream containing sulphacetamide 2.86%, sulfabenzamide 3.7%, and sulphathiazole 3.42% in a non-staining emollient basis. For vaginitis and cervicitis.

Sultrin Vaginal Tablets *(Ortho-Cilag, UK).* Each contains sulphacetamide 143.75 mg, sulfabenzamide 184 mg, and sulphathiazole 172.5 mg. For the treatment of vaginitis and cervicitis.

Sulphones and other Antileprotic Agents

6550-d

According to their immunological response persons suffering from leprosy can be placed into 6 different categories ranging from those with no natural defence mechanisms who develop a multibacillary form of leprosy (lepromatous leprosy) and carry massive body-loads of *Mycobacterium leprae* to those with high defence and a sparse body-load (tuberculoid leprosy). The categories are: polar lepromatous (LLp); sub-polar lepromatous (LLs); borderline lepromatous (BL); borderline (BB); borderline tuberculoid (BT); tuberculoid (TT). In patients with lepromatous leprosy the lepromin test (see under Lepromin, p.1723) is negative whereas at the tuberculoid end of the spectrum it is strongly positive. An early transitory stage, called indeterminate leprosy is also described.

Shifts between these leprosy categories cause leprosy reactions, which are responsible for much of the disability suffered by leprosy patients. Patients with other than polar lepromatous (LLp) or tuberculoid (TT) forms of leprosy may develop a Type 1 (or Lepra) reaction which in untreated patients involves a 'downgrading' towards the lepromatous end of the spectrum and in treated patients a 'reversal' or 'upgrading' towards the tuberculoid end. Patients with lepromatous forms of leprosy may develop a Type 2 (sometimes termed erythema nodosum leprosum or ENL) reaction, which generally occurs as a result of drug therapy and is associated with the massive body-load of dead bacteria. The treatment of leprosy is thus directed not only at eradicating the *Mycobacterium leprae* but also at avoiding or alleviating the reactional states.

The main agents used to and destroy the bacillus and described in this section are Clofazimine, p.1488, Dapsone, p.1489, and Thiambutosine, p.1493.

Other drugs used to destroy the bacillus include certain sulphonamides such as sulfadoxine (see p.1470), antibiotics such as rifampicin (see p.1580), and other agents used in the treatment of tuberculosis such as ethionamide (see p.1571).

Drugs used to alleviate leprosy reactions include: clofazimine (see p.1488), corticosteroids (see p.451), stibophen (see p.106), and thalidomide (see p.1760). Of these, thalidomide is of no benefit in the Type 1 (Lepra) reaction and must, of course, be avoided in fertile women with a potential for pregnancy. There is also evidence that clofazimine is not effective in Type 1 (Lepra) reactions. It is no longer considered beneficial to withhold antileprotic therapy or to reduce dosage in the Type 2 (ENL) reaction as the reaction can be effectively treated; this may also be true for the Type 1 (Lepra) reaction.

It is not yet certain how leprosy is transmitted but infectivity is only associated with untreated or lapsed multibacillary forms of leprosy. Treatment of leprosy damages or kills solid-staining viable bacilli, rendering them non-viable with a fragmented or granular appearance. The 'bacterial index' is a measure of the number of organisms per unit volume of tissue whereas the 'morphological index' is a measure of their viability. Leprosy patients with a morphological index of zero are accordingly noninfectious or 'closed', regardless of their bacterial index. Usually a patient achieves a morphological index of zero within about 6 months of effective therapy and this can be accelerated to 2 or 3 weeks by supplementation with rifampicin.

In areas where leprosy is endemic, prophylactic treatment with dapsone or related drugs (described as sulphones) has reduced the incidence of new cases but such prophylaxis has not been considered practical for large-scale routine programmes. Bacillus Calmette-Guérin Vaccine, p.1588 is also given for prophylaxis against leprosy.

Classification of leprosy according to immunity.— D. S. Ridley and W. H. Jopling, *Int. J. Lepr.*, 1966, *34*, 255. Significance of variations within the lepromatous group.— D. S. Ridley and M. F. R. Waters, *Lepr. Rev.*, 1969, *40*, 143. Histological classification and immunological spectrum of leprosy.— D. S. Ridley, *Bull. Wld Hlth Org.*, 1974, *51*, 451. The pathogenesis and classification of polar tuberculoid leprosy.— D. S. Ridley, *Lepr. Rev.*, 1982, *53*, 19.

A hypothesis on the course of *M. leprae* infection.— G. L. Stoner, *Lancet*, 1979, *2*, 994. Comment.— W. H. Jopling (letter), *Lepr. Rev.*, 1980, *51*, 269.

Reports: Report of the WHO Expert Committee on Leprosy, *Tech. Rep. Ser. Wld Hlth Org. No. 319*, 1966; *ibid., No. 459*, 1970; *ibid., No. 607*, 1977; *Leprosy in Children*, Geneva, World Health Organization, 1976; *Memorandum on Leprosy*, London, HM Stationery Office, 1977. Comment on the Final Report on the First Regional Working Group on Leprosy, Manila, Philippines, 7–12 December, 1978 (dated February, 1979). WHO Regional Office for the Western Pacific.— *Lepr. Rev.*, 1979, *50*, 326.

An account of research into the chemotherapy of leprosy.— *Bull. Wld Hlth Org.*, 1976, *53*, 425.

Proceedings of an international symposium on the epidemiology of leprosy.— O. Closs and M. Harboe (Ed.), *Lepr. Rev.*, 1981, *52*, *Suppl.* 1.

A review of recently published data (N.M. Goloschapov, *Diuciphon: Experimental and Clinical Data*, Moscow) on Diuciphon, an antileprotic drug synthesised and investigated in the USSR.— W. H. Jopling, *Lepr. Rev.*, 1981, *52*, 104.

Infectivity and prophylaxis. Six months' treatment with dapsone or 3 weeks' treatment with rifampicin rapidly reduces the number of viable bacilli in the nasal discharge of leprosy patients and such patients could virtually be considered as no longer contagious. Patients with lepromatous or borderline leprosy should receive treatment for life even after lesions are no longer active and annual checkups are desirable to check on the development of resistance. Those with tuberculoid or near-tuberculoid leprosy may in most cases stop drug therapy after regular treatment for 2 or 3 years. BCG vaccination should be offered to children or young adults (not strongly tuberculin-positive) who have been in close contact with a patient suffering from leprosy. Also dapsone which probably has some protective activity should be recommended for prophylaxis in those considered to have been at real risk because of prolonged and intimate contact with a person who had been shedding leprosy bacilli before diagnosis. The usual dose of dapsone for prophylaxis is: children up to 4 years of age 25 mg per week; 4 to 7 years 50 mg per week; 7 to 12 years 75 mg per week; 12 to 15 years 100 mg per week; patients over 15 years 200 mg per week.— *Memorandum on Leprosy*, London, HM Stationery Office, 1977.

A discussion on when leprosy patients should be considered as 'cured'. With present chemotherapy and knowledge, discharge from treatment or surveillance should not be advised in LL and BL leprosy in the interests of the patient and of the community. However, despite the continuous treatment, the patient's morale should be improved if he is told when he is considered to be no longer infective to others; a zero morphological index might be a better indication than the WHO definition which includes negative bacteriological findings. Patients who are no longer infective should be regarded as in no way different from any other sick person, and should be subject to no hospital, employment, or social restrictions.— T. F. Davey, *Lepr. Rev.*, 1978, *49*, 1.

Further references: E. M. J. Touw-Langendijk and B. Naafs, *Lepr. Rev.*, 1979, *50*, 123; V. Ekambaram, *ibid.*, 297.

Reactions. An account of the treatment of reactions in leprosy, including reasons for complete disagreement with the traditional practice of reducing effective antileprotic therapy during such reactions. Antileprotic therapy is initiated in 'downgrading' Type 1 (Lepra) reactions and continued in 'reversal' Type 1 (Lepra) reactions, and also continued in Type 2 (ENL) reactions. If anti-inflammatory drugs and stibophen are not adequate to control the reactions, corticosteroids (prednisolone 20 to 30 mg daily, usually reduced to 10 to 15 mg daily after a few days in Type 1 or Lepra reactions; prednisolone 20 to 60 mg daily for months or years in Type 2 or ENL reactions) and clofazimine (good response reported with 300 mg daily; dose not to exceed 400 to 500 mg daily) are given; since rapid control is obtained with corticosteroids whereas clofazimine takes longer, therapy can also be initiated with corticosteroids and gradually changed to clofazimine. In addition, thalidomide provides rapid, safe, and effective control of Type 2 (ENL) reactions, but its use is severely curtailed by its teratogenic properties; it is of no value in Type 1 (Lepra) reactions.— M. F. R. Waters, *Lepr. Rev.*, 1974, *45*, 337. A similar review.— D. S. Jolliffe, *Br. J. Derm.*, 1977, *97*, 345.

It was reported at the 10th International Leprosy Congress, Bergen, 1973, that the beneficial effect of clofazimine in leprosy reactions could take 8 to 12 weeks to appear and sometimes high dosages were required; in severe cases with necrotising lesions it would be necessary to administer clofazimine with corticosteroids or thalidomide until the acute phase was controlled. Clofazimine permitted withdrawal of corticosteroid in steroid-dependent cases in addition to suppressing the recurrent episodes; it also increased tolerance to dapsone in sulphone-sensitive cases while simultaneously exerting a beneficial effect on the disease process. It was a matter for serious consideration whether clofazimine could be safely used in cases of recurrent severe leprosy reaction with overt renal involvement.— *Lepr. Rev.*, 1974, *45*, 41.

A preliminary report of a study of 61 adult dapsone-sensitive men with lepromatous leprosy and recurrent leprosy reactions showed that while both clofazimine and thalidomide could generally control the reactions and increase tolerance of dapsone, thalidomide acted more rapidly. Clofazimine however exerted a longer-lasting beneficial effect which continued long after its administration was discontinued.— K. Ramanujam *et al.*, *Lepr. Rev.*, 1975, *46*, *Suppl.*, 117. Evidence that clofazimine is not effective in Type 1 Lepra reactions.— F. M. J. H. Imkamp, *ibid.*, 1981, *52*, 135.

Concurrent administration of methandienone enabled 14 patients with lepromatous leprosy and chronic ENL reactions to tolerate sulphones either without corticosteroids or with reduced doses of corticosteroids.— S. Choudhury *et al.*, *Lepr. Rev.*, 1977, *48*, 181.

Comparison of short- and long-term corticosteroid therapy in the management of reversal reaction.— B. Naafs *et al.*, *Int. J. Lepr.*, 1979, *47*, 7.

Other studies and reviews of leprosy reactions: J. M. H. Pearson and H. S. Helmy, *Lepr. Rev.*, 1973, *44*, 75; A. Carayon, *Méd. Afr. noire*, 1976, *23*, 567.

For reference to the concurrent administration of rifampicin and corticosteroids exacerbating rather than alleviating neuritis in tuberculoid leprosy, see Rifampicin, p.1578.

6551-n

Acedapsone. CI 556; DADDS. Bis(4-acetamidophenyl) sulphone.
$C_{16}H_{16}N_2O_4S$=332.4.

CAS — 77-46-3.

Pharmacopoeias. In *Braz.*

A white crystalline solid. M.p. 289° to 292°. Practically **insoluble** in water and in a mixture of benzyl benzoate and castor oil; freely soluble in dimethylformamide; slightly soluble in methyl alcohol.

Acedapsone has the actions and uses of dapsone (see p.1489) to which it is degraded probably in the viscera after slow release into the circulation. For the treatment of leprosy it is given intramuscularly as a suspension in benzyl benzoate and castor oil in a dose of 225 mg about every 70 to 77 days (or 5 times yearly) at which frequency the plasma-dapsone concentrations can be maintained above a minimum of 10 ng per ml.

Leprosy. Acedapsone should be used only when the injections can be given very regularly, and should be used in multibacillary leprosy only when an additional and effective drug with a different mechanism of action can be given.— D. A. Russell *et al.*, *Am. J. trop. Med. Hyg.*, 1975, *24*, 485.

For a regimen incorporating rifampicin with dapsone and acedapsone in the treatment of lepromatous leprosy, see Dapsone, p.1491.

Some clinical and metabolic studies of acedapsone in leprosy: C. C. Shepard *et al.*, *Am. J. trop. Med. Hyg.*, 1968, *17*, 192; J. Convit *et al.*, *Bull. Wld Hlth Org.*, 1970, *42*, 667; C. R. Boughton *et al.*, *Med. J. Aust.*, 1971, *1*, 1258; C. C. Shepard *et al.*, *Am. J. trop. Med. Hyg.*, 1972, *21*, 440; K. Ramanujam *et al.*, *Lepr. Rev.*, 1975, *46*, *Suppl.*, 85; A. R. Goss *et al.*, *Clin. exp. Pharmac. Physiol.*, 1975, *2*, 86; D. A. Russell *et al.*, *Am. J. trop. Med. Hyg.*, 1975, *24*, 485; R. Ganapati *et al.*, *Lepr. India*, 1976, *48*, 238; J. H. Peters *et al.*, *Am. J. trop. Med. Hyg.*, 1977, *26*, 127; L. C. Anand and B. S. Rathore, *Lepr. India*, 1979, *51*, 358.

Prophylaxis. Screening a population of 1500 people with a known high prevalance of leprosy identified 62 patients with active and 37 with inactive leprosy, all of whom, with 6 new cases, were then treated solely with acedapsone 225 mg by intramuscular injection every 75 days, when 66 responded. Mass prophylaxis was instituted using the above dose for adults and children over 5, and 150 mg every 75 days for children aged 6 months to 5 years. No infants born a year after the study started were given acedapsone since they had not been exposed to untreated patients. After 1 year there were 6 new patients with leprosy compared to the normal estimate of 11. In the second and third year of prophylaxis no more new patients were found.— N. R. Sloan *et al.* (preliminary communication), *Lancet*, 1971, *2*, 525. Results of continued treatment showed that the risk can be reduced to zero by 15 acedapsone injections given over 3 years, except during the first 6 months of acedapsone therapy and in those patients infected with a sulphone-resistant strain. Acedapsone cannot eradicate leprosy without the simultaneous and continuing control by adequate treatment of all multibacillary cases in the population.— D. A. Russell *et al.* (letter), *ibid.*, 1975, *2*, 771.

At the 10th International Leprosy Congress, Bergen, 1973, it was reported that chemoprophylaxis of leprosy using acedapsone had yielded satisfactory results. The value of chemoprophylaxis in the prevention of the development of lepromatous leprosy, its duration, the optimum doses, and the frequency of administration had yet to be determined.— *Lepr. Rev.*, 1974, *45*, 41.

Further references: D. A. Russell *et al.*, *Am. J. trop. Med. Hyg.*, 1979, *28*, 559; S. K. Noordeen *et al.*, *Lepr. India*, 1980, *52*, 97.

Malaria. Cycloguanil embonate given together with acedapsone in a 1:1 ratio (Dapolar) for the treatment of malaria as 3 injections at 4-monthly intervals gave complete suppression of malaria at the end of 1 year.— A. B. G. Laing, *Trans. R. Soc. trop. Med. Hyg.*, 1971, *65*, 560.

Proprietary Names

Hansolar *(Parke, Davis, USA)*.

6552-h

Achyranthes Aspera. Apamarga; Atkumah; Chirchira; Latjira. The whole plant of *Achyranthes aspera* (Amaranthaceae).

NOTE. Achyranthes (*Jap. P.*) is the root of *Achyranthes fauriei* and *A. bidentata*.

A decoction of *Achyranthes aspera* has been used in India as a diuretic. It has been tried in the treatment of leprosy and of reactional states in leprosy.

A decoction of *Achyranthes aspera*, in doses of 30 ml twice daily, was effective in the treatment of reactions in leprosy, particularly the subacute and mild type.— D. Ojha *et al.*, *Lepr. Rev.*, 1966, *37*, 115. See also D. Ojha and G. Singh, *ibid.*, 1968, *39*, 23.

6553-m

Clofazimine. B 663; G 30320. 3-(4-Chloroanilino)-10-(4-chlorophenyl)-2,10-dihydro-2-phenazin-2-ylideneisopropylamine.

$C_{27}H_{22}Cl_2N_4$=473.4.

CAS — 2030-63-9.

Dark red crystals or orange-red microcrystalline powder. M.p. about 215°. Practically **insoluble** in water; slightly soluble in alcohol and glycols; soluble in dimethylformamide and macrogol 400.

Adverse Effects. Dose-related red to brown discoloration of the skin occurs especially on areas exposed to sunlight. Discoloration tends to be more pronounced at leprotic lesions which may become mauve to black. Light-skinned subjects are especially susceptible. The generalised discoloration may disappear within a year of stopping clofazimine but it may take 5 years before the patient is free of the discoloration at the lesions. The urine may also be discoloured. Abdominal pain and diarrhoea may occasionally occur. A drying effect on the skin with scaling has also been reported.

A wide range of laboratory tests was carried out regularly on 51 patients with leprosy receiving clofazimine for periods of 2 to 8 years. The only significant undesirable laboratory changes were increases in concentrations of fasting blood sugar and of total serum bilirubin; there was also a reduction in total serum protein and some changes in leucocyte differential counts. None of these laboratory changes was associated with clinical signs of toxicity. Most of the laboratory tests revealed improvements.— R. C. Hastings *et al.*, *Int. J. Lepr.*, 1976, *44*, 287.

Allergy. A 29-year-old woman developed eosinophilic enteritis associated with peripheral eosinophilia after 3 years of treatment with clofazimine 600 mg daily; this appeared to represent a reaction to clofazimine. Despite initial reduction of dosage for 14 months followed by cessation for a further 6 months the patient had continued to suffer symptoms suggesting continuing reaction to clofazimine depots in the body.— G. H. Mason *et al.*, *Lepr. Rev.*, 1977, *48*, 175. See also K. Jagadeesan *et al.*, *Int. Surg.*, 1975, *60*, 208.

Effects on the eyes. Ten of 26 patients taking clofazimine 100 to 300 mg daily for 1 to 15 months showed corneal changes which diminished or disappeared within 2 months of withdrawing treatment. Pigmentation of the macula was observed in 1 of the 10 and in 1 other patient.— L. Öhman and I. Wahlberg (letter), *Lancet*, 1975, *2*, 933.

Two patients who had taken clofazimine 100 to 400 mg daily for 2 months (to a total dose of 20 g) for psoriasis had fine brownish lines, similar to chloroquine keratopathy, on the cornea at the end of treatment. There was no functional disturbance and the lines slowly regressed. A similar but lesser effect, possibly not drug-related, was seen in 4 further patients who had taken clofazimine.— P. -E. Wålinder *et al.*, *Br. J. Ophthal.*, 1976, *60*, 526.

Effects on the gastro-intestinal tract. A review of adverse effects of clofazimine on the gastro-intestinal tract.— W. H. Jopling, *Lepr. Rev.*, 1976, *47*, 1. Comment; significant gastro-intestinal side-effects are rare.— G. Warren (letter), *ibid.*, 343. Reply; the aim had not been to condemn clofazimine.— W. H. Jopling (letter), *ibid.*, 344.

A report of a fatal syndrome of abdominal pain, malabsorption, and intra-abdominal deposition of clofazimine crystals in one patient.— R. F. Harvey *et al.*, *Br. J. Derm.*, 1977, *97*, *Suppl.* 15, 19.

Further references: A. Bryceson (letter), *Lepr. Rev.*, 1979, *50*, 258; A. C. McDougall *et al.*, *Br. J. Derm.*, 1980, *102*, 227; E. de Bergeyck *et al.*, *Lepr. Rev.*, 1980, *51*, 221.

Precautions. In patients with impaired kidney or liver function regular tests of function are advisable during treatment.

Pregnancy and the neonate. The treatment of patients throughout pregnancy with clofazimine had produced no ill-effects in the infants. Treatment during lactation had resulted in discoloration of the milk and ruddiness of the child.—Working Party on Clofazimine, London, Sept. 1968, *Lepr. Rev.*, 1969, *40*, 21.

Antimicrobial Action. Clofazimine is bacteriostatic against *Mycobacterium* spp. Using the mouse foot-pad technique the minimum inhibitory concentration for *Mycobacterium leprae* has been estimated to lie between 0.1 and 1 µg per gram; more accurate estimation is hindered by the marked accumulation of clofazimine in the tissues.

Studies in *mice* suggest that the MIC of clofazimine for *Mycobacterium tuberculosis* is about 5 to 10 µg per gram and for *M. leprae* between 0.1 and 1 µg per gram.— L. Levy, *Am. J. trop. Med. Hyg.*, 1974, *23*, 1097.

Clofazimine had an MIC of less than 0.5µg per ml *in vitro* against 21 of 43 strains of *Mycobacterium intracellulare* and MICs of 1 and 2 µg per ml against 41 and 43 strains respectively. Clofazimine also inhibited all 5 strains of each of the following: *Mycobacterium tuberculosis*, *M. scrofulaceum*, *M. fortuitum*, and *M. chelonei* at an MIC of 0.5, 0.5, 8, and 4 µg per ml respectively.— P. Damle *et al.*, *Tubercle*, 1978, *59*, 135.

Absorption and Fate. Clofazimine is incompletely absorbed from the gastro-intestinal tract, the extent depending upon particle size and formulation. It disappears rapidly from the blood stream to become deposited in most body tissues, from which it is then slowly released. It has been estimated to have a half-life in the body of about 70 days with probably less than 1% of a dose being excreted in the urine daily. It is also excreted through sebaceous and sweat glands and in milk.

Preliminary studies in healthy subjects and in leprosy patients suggested that clofazimine is incompletely absorbed from the gastro-intestinal tract, that the clofazimine absorbed is rapidly removed from the circulation but not rapidly excreted (unless in the form of an unidentified metabolite), and that the half-life is greater than 69 days, probably considerably greater.— L. Levy, *Am. J. trop. Med. Hyg.*, 1974, *23*, 1097. Similar studies: D. K. Banerjee *et al.*, *ibid.*, 1110; R. E. Mansfield, *ibid.*, 1116.

Quantitative assessment of clofazimine in the organs of a 16-year-old boy who had discontinued prolonged clofazimine therapy 40 days before death, demonstrated heavy accumulation of the drug particularly in the reticulo-endothelial system and in the intestines (which could have been responsible for the patient's severe diarrhoea). Very low concentrations in the kidneys indicated that accumulation was proportional to the number of macrophages in the organ or tissue. Clofazimine was found in all organs studied except the brain, indicating that it did not cross the blood-brain barrier.— K. V. Desikan and S. Balakrishnan, *Lepr. Rev.*, 1976, *47*, 107.

Effect of particle size. Only about 20% of coarsely crystalline clofazimine was absorbed from the gastro-intestinal tract; about 50% in a micronised suspension was absorbed. From a suspension in oil about 85% was absorbed and from and oil-wax basis in capsules about 70%. Clofazimine was stored in the body and slowly excreted in urine, almost all as unchanged drug.— W. A. Vischer, *Lepr. Rev.*, 1969, *40*, 107.

Uses. Clofazimine, an iminophenazine dye, is an antileprotic agent with the advantage that it also has anti-inflammatory properties so that not only is it less liable than dapsone to provoke leprosy reactions but it can also be used to alleviate them (see p.1487).

Clofazimine should be used in association with other antileprotic agents and is usually given with food in doses adjusted according to body-weight and the activity of the disease.

It is given in doses of 50 to 100 mg daily or 100 mg thrice weekly during the first 4 to 6 months of long-term treatment with dapsone to prevent the development of resistance to sulphones and to prevent lepra reactions in patients with lepromatous and borderline leprosy.

In leprosy resistant to sulphones clofazimine is given in a dose of 100 mg daily, together with rifampicin 600 mg daily during the first 2 to 3 months.

For the treatment of lepra reactions clofazimine 300 mg daily for 3 months is suggested, gradually reduced, as soon as the reaction has been brought under control, to a minimum suppressant dose.

It has also been tried in the treatment of lesions caused by *Mycobacterium ulcerans* (Buruli ulcer).

Battey disease. Clofazimine was found to be of little value in the treatment of 7 patients with pulmonary tuberculosis caused by Battey Group III atypical organisms.— F. Heyworth, *Med. J. Aust.*, 1967, *1*, 106. See also B. M. Watson and J. T. Smyth, *Med. J. Aust.*, 1968, *1*, 261.

Leishmaniasis. A report of beneficial effects in 6 of 10 patients with American leishmaniasis, following clofazimine therapy.— O. Rotta *et al.*, *Anais bras. Derm. Sif.*,

1975, *50,* 197.

Leprosy. A detailed review of clofazimine in leprosy.— S. J. Yawalkar and W. Vischer, *Lepr. Rev.*, 1979, *50,* 135. Criticism.— W. F. Ross (letter), *ibid.*, 1980, *51,* 92; *idem*, 197 (correction).

A long-term study of clofazimine therapy in 17 lepromatous leprosy patients prone to repeated severe leprosy reactions. Response to treatment was slower than was usual with dapsone.— H. Plock and D. L. Leiker, *Lepr. Rev.*, 1976, *47,* 25.

Some other studies of clofazimine as an antileprotic: J. Languillon, *Méd. trop. Marseille,* 1976, *36,* 127; *Am. J. trop. Med. Hyg.*, 1976, *25,* 437 (U.S. Leprosy Panel and Leonard Wood Memorial).

For reference to the use of clofazimine in some proposed antileprotic combination regimens, see Dapsone, p.1491.

Reactions. For comments on clofazimine in the control of leprosy reactions, see p.1487.

Skin disorders. *Discoid lupus erythematosus.* Clofazimine in doses of up to 200 mg daily for 6 months produced improvement in 17 of 26 patients with discoid lupus erythematosus.— J. P. Mackey and J. Barnes, *Br. J. Derm.*, 1974, *91,* 93.

Mycosis. Clinical improvement in 3 patients with Lobo's disease (a chronic tropical mycosis) after treatment with clofazimine for 2 to 8 months.— D. Silva, *Bull. Soc. Path. exot.*, 1978, *71,* 409, per *Trop. Dis. Bull.*, 1980, *77,* 186.

Psoriasis. Pustular lesions not responsive to treatment with potassium permanganate solution or to systemic treatment with dapsone or co-trimoxazole in one patient, and controlled but not cured by maintenance doses of methotrexate in a second patient, showed rapid response to treatment with clofazimine 200 mg daily.— T. Chuaprapaisilp and T. Piamphongsant, *Br. J. Derm.*, 1978, *99,* 303.

Pyoderma gangrenosum. Clofazimine was used to treat 8 patients with pyoderma gangrenosum. Healing started within 3 to 4 days of beginning treatment.— G. Michaëlsson *et al.*, *Archs Derm.*, 1976, *112,* 344. See also E. C. Kark *et al.*, *J. Am. Acad. Derm.*, 1981, *4,* 152.

Vitiligo. Clofazimine 100 mg given daily or thrice weekly for several months and combined with exposure to sunlight was reported to have caused considerable pigmentation of vitiliginous skin in 8 white women.— S. Bor, *S. Afr. med. J.*, 1973, *47,* 1451.

Ulcers. In a controlled double-blind study of 105 patients with lesions due to *Mycobacterium ulcerans*, treatment with clofazimine 10 to 20 mg per kg body-weight daily to a maximum of 800 mg for 3 to 6 months was considered to be ineffective.— W. D. L. Revill *et al.*, *Lancet,* 1973, *2,* 873. Early encouraging reports: H. F. Lunn and R. J. W. Rees (letter), *Lancet,* 1964, *1,* 247; J. H. S. Pettit *et al.*, *Br. J. Derm.*, 1966, *78,* 187.

Clofazimine ointment 1% was used for the treatment of trophic ulcers. The dressings were left undisturbed for 4 days. Healing proceeded rapidly and with good cicatrisation despite the continued presence of viable pathogens in the exudate from the ulcers. Further investigation was recommended.— B. P. B. Ellis and E. Taube, *S. Afr. med. J.*, 1973, *47,* 378.

Proprietary Preparations

Lamprene *(Geigy, UK).* Clofazimine, available as capsules of 100 mg in an oil-wax basis. (Also available as Lamprene in *Austral., S.Afr.*).

Other Proprietary Names

Lampren *(Neth., Switz.).*

6554-b

Dapsone *(B.P., B.P. Vet., U.S.P.).* Dapsonum; DADPS; DDS; Diaphenylsulfone; Disulone; Sulphonyldianiline. Bis(4-aminophenyl) sulphone.

$C_{12}H_{12}N_2O_2S$=248.3.

CAS — 80-08-0.

Pharmacopoeias. In *Br., Braz., Chin., Fr., Ind., Int., It., Turk.*, and *U.S.*

A white or slightly yellowish-white odourless crystalline powder with a slightly bitter taste. M.p. 175° to 181°. It discolours on exposure to light but this is not accompanied by significant decomposition. **Soluble** 1 in 7000 of water and 1 in about 36 of alcohol; freely soluble in acetone; soluble in dilute mineral acids. Dapsone powder may be **sterilised** in the same way as sulphadimidine powder (see p.1475). Oily suspensions are sterilised by maintaining at 150° for 1 hour. **Protect** from light.

Adverse Effects. Most side-effects caused by dapsone are dose-related and uncommon at the low doses of up to 100 mg daily that have usually been given to treat leprosy. They include anorexia, nausea, vomiting, headache, dizziness, tachycardia, nervousness, and insomnia. Various types of skin disorders may occur including allergic dermatitis which may respond to desensitisation (see under Treatment of Adverse Effects, below), which may subside despite continued therapy, or which may occasionally become exfoliative with concurrent hepatitis, fever, and lymphadenitis; fixed drug eruptions occur in dark-skinned people. Agranulocytosis and peripheral neuritis have been reported; there are also occasional reports of psychosis. Varying degrees of dose-related haemolysis and methaemoglobinaemia occur in most subjects given more than 200 mg daily; doses of up to 100 mg daily do not cause haemolysis but subjects deficient in glucose-6-phosphate dehydrogenase are affected above about 50 mg daily. These adverse effects on the blood are probably caused by hydroxylamine derivatives produced during metabolism.

Leprosy reactions, which may complicate therapy, are not toxic effects of dapsone but changes in the category of leprosy; for further details, see p.1487.

Findings of anti-dapsone antibodies in patients receiving dapsone. Such an antibody response in a leprosy patient taking dapsone might lead to the formation of dapsone/anti-dapsone complexes, complement activation, and consequently erythema nodosum leprosum. Such complexes might also neutralise dapsone and therefore play a role in drug resistance.— P. K. Das *et al.* (letter), *Lancet,* 1980, *1,* 1309.

Allergy. A report of a fatal hypersensitivity reaction in a 17-year-old boy, three weeks after the start of therapy with dapsone 100 mg daily for erythema nodosum leprosum. The clinical symptoms and progression of illness conformed well to a 'dapsone syndrome' first described in the early 1950s. The patient had fever, dermatitis, and a striking eosinophilia during the height of his illness, and skin biopsy showed erythema multiforme. The soundness of current recommendations for beginning dapsone therapy in full dosage in patients with lepromatous leprosy is questioned.— H. M. Frey *et al.*, *Ann. intern. Med.*, 1981, *94,* 777. Comment on adverse reactions to dapsone.— *Lancet,* 1981, *2,* 184.

Effects on the blood. Comments that dapsone might interfere with the metabolism of folic acid.— L. Fry *et al.*, *Lancet,* 1967, *2,* 729; J. L. Verbov and P. Barkhan (letter), *ibid.*, 1085.

Agranulocytosis. Agranulocytosis developed in a 30-year-old woman after receiving dapsone 100 mg thrice weekly for 6 weeks for acne vulgaris.— F. C. Firkin and A. F. Mariani, *Med. J. Aust.*, 1977, *2,* 247.

Other reports: P. H. Levine and L. R. Weintraub, *Ann. intern. Med.*, 1968, *68,* 1060; A. J. Ognibene, *Ann. intern. Med.*, 1970, *72,* 521; B. McConkey (letter), *Lancet,* 1981, *2,* 525.

Effects on the eyes. See Overdosage, below.

Effects on fertility. The fertility of 2 male patients was abolished during dapsone therapy and restored some time after the drug was stopped.— J. Grieve (letter), *Lancet,* 1979, *2,* 464.

Effects on the kidneys. A 30-year-old Korean developed the nephrotic syndrome after treatment with 100 mg of dapsone daily for 3 weeks.— A. Belmont (letter), *J. Am. med. Ass.*, 1967, *200,* 262.

Renal papillary necrosis in a 51-year-old man was probably due to dapsone; he had taken 100 to 300 mg daily for about 10 years for dermatitis herpetiformis.— B. I. Hoffbrand, *Br. med. J.*, 1978, *1,* 78.

Effects on the liver. Abnormalities of liver-function tests in 3 patients taking dapsone.— D. K. Goette (letter), *Archs Derm.*, 1977, *113,* 1616.

Jaundice due to cholestasis in 2 patients and to haemolysis in a third occurred after 2 to 36 weeks of therapy with dapsone 75 to 200 mg daily.— S. P. Stone and R. M. Goodwin, *Archs Derm.*, 1978, *114,* 947.

Effects on mental state. Although psychosis is usually listed as a side-effect of dapsone it is doubtful if this can be accepted.— *Br. med. J.*, 1971, *3,* 174. Psychosis might not occur using slow-induction methods and low-dosage regimens, but in 1950 during transfer of nearly 10 000 patients from hydnocarpus oil to dapsone, many cases of psychosis occurred following induction periods of 12 weeks to attain doses of 200 mg daily.— A. S. Garrett (letter), *ibid.*, 1971, *4,* 300.

Other reports of psychosis: D. M. Sahu, *Indian J. Derm.*, 1972, *17,* 47; K. C. Verma *et al.*, *J. Indian med. Ass.*, 1973, *60,* 255.

Effects on the nervous system. A discussion on whether the use of dapsone is associated with nerve damage.— G. Warren (letter), *Lepr. Rev.*, 1980, *51,* 94.

After receiving 7.7 g of dapsone over a period of about 45 days to treat cystic acne, an 18-year-old man developed severe peripheral neuropathy. He recovered rapidly on discontinuation of dapsone, and after 2 months only mild motor and sensory deficits were demonstrable.— W. C. Koller *et al.*, *Archs Neurol., Chicago,* 1977, *34,* 644.

Further reports of peripheral neuropathy with dapsone: A. C. Saqueton *et al.*, *Archs Derm.*, 1969, *100,* 214; W. R. Hubler and H. Solomon, *ibid.*, 1972, *106,* 598; F. W. Epstein and M. Bohm, *ibid.*, 1976, *112,* 1761; E. H. Wyatt and J. C. Stevens, *Br. J. Derm.*, 1972, *86,* 521; L. Gutmann *et al.*, *Neurology, Minneap.*, 1976, *26,* 514.

Hypoalbuminaemia. Severe hypoalbuminaemia developed in 2 men with dermatitis herpetiformis after treatment for 3 and 11 years with dapsone in doses of 100 mg daily and 150 mg daily respectively. Both patients deteriorated to a point when they seemed unlikely to survive, with symptoms including massive ascites, oedema, and circulatory failure. On withdrawal of dapsone they made a rapid and complete recovery.— J. G. C. Kingham *et al.*, *Lancet,* 1979, *2,* 662. Criticism.— D. P. Jacobus (letter), *ibid.*, 1018. Reply.— J. G. C. Kingham (letter), *ibid.* See also S. Young and J. M. Marks (letter), *ibid.*, 908.

Significant hypoalbuminaemia developed in a woman with dermatitis herpetiformis after 32 months of therapy with dapsone 100 mg daily. She died 10 days after dapsone was withdrawn.— P. N. Foster and C. H. J. Swan (letter), *Lancet,* 1981, *2,* 806.

Overdosage. Three boys took large single doses of dapsone in an attempt to simplify their treatment regimens. One aged about 10 years took 500 mg without ill effect, a second aged about 16 years took 1.45 g and died about 4 days later after suffering vomiting, severe abdominal pains, haematuria, jaundice, and coma. The third, who was also about 16 years old, took 1.2 g and suffered similar symptoms but recovered within a week.— J. Sturt, *Papua New Guin. med. J.*, 1967, *10,* 97.

Permanent retinal damage occurred in a man who took 7.5 g of dapsone in a suicide attempt.— D. J. Kenner *et al.*, *Br. J. Ophthal.*, 1980, *64,* 741. Blindness (optic atrophy) and motor neuropathy after overdosage with dapsone; the conditions were not resolved 6 months later.— M. Homeida *et al.*, *Br. med. J.*, 1980, *281,* 1180. The motor neuropathy had resolved completely over the last 14 months but optic atrophy and visual impairment persisted.— T. K. Daneshmend and M. Homeida (letter), *ibid.*, 1981, *283,* 311. No evidence of impaired retinal blood flow in 7 patients taking therapeutic doses of dapsone for dermatitis herpetiformis. One patient was taking 600 mg daily.— J. N. Leonard *et al.* (letter), *Lancet,* 1982, *1,* 453.

See also under Treatment of Adverse Effects (below).

Treatment of Adverse Effects. In severe overdosage the stomach should be emptied by aspiration and lavage. Methaemoglobinaemia has been treated with intravenous injections of methylene blue 2 mg per kg body-weight, sometimes followed by intravenous injections of ascorbic acid 0.5 to 2 g. Haemolysis has been treated by infusion of concentrated human red blood corpuscles to replace the damaged cells. Supportive therapy includes administration of oxygen to alleviate hypoxia, and administration of fluids to maintain renal flow and promote the elimination of dapsone.

A report of the symptoms and treatment of accidental sulphone poisoning in 12 children, all of whom recovered. Symptoms included cyanosis (12), nausea and vomiting (9), neurological disorders (8), dyspnoea (4), jaundice (3), and renal insufficiency (2). Treatment included slow intravenous injections of methylene blue solution, 1 to 2 mg per kg body-weight, usually followed by infusions of 1 to 2 g of ascorbic acid. Two of the children received peritoneal dialysis for acute renal insufficiency and 2 others received exchange transfusions.— S. Schvartsman and E. Marcondes, *Revta Hosp. Clín. Fac. Med. Univ. S Paulo*, 1963, *18*, 345.

A detailed report of the recovery of a 2-year-old child from dapsone poisoning. Symptoms included vomiting, restlessness, and methaemoglobinaemia. Treatment included intravenous administration of 2 ml of a 1% solution of methylene blue every 8 hours, together with ascorbic acid 1 g by mouth every 4 hours. She also received sedatives, partial exchange transfusion, and fluids to promote diuresis.— J. P. Stanfield, *J. trop. Med. Hyg.*, 1963, *66*, 292.

Following high-dose administration of dapsone a 68-year-old woman developed haemolysis and methaemoglobinaemia. She was treated with intravenous fluids and diuretics to promote the elimination of the dapsone and with packed red cell infusions to replace the damaged red cells. Treatment by dialysis is not generally considered efficient and methylene blue might exacerbate the haemolytic process.— W. B. Shelley and M. I. Goldwein, *Br. J. Derm.*, 1976, *95*, 79. See also B. D. Goldstein, *Am. J. med. Sci.*, 1974, *267*, 291 (exacerbation of dapsone-induced Heinz body haemolytic anaemia following treatment with methylene blue).

A report of the recovery of 2 children from dapsone poisoning. Treatment involved administration of methylene blue which dramatically reduced the methaemoglobin concentrations and alleviated the cardiac symptoms of one child (who also received ascorbic acid intravenously).— T. J. L. Cooke, *Med. J. Aust.*, 1970, *1*, 1158.

A 45-year-old man who took about 10 g of dapsone developed methaemoglobinaemia with cyanosis, headache, confusion, and haemolysis. Methaemoglobinaemia subsided after 7 days. The initial disappearance of dapsone and monoacetyldapsone was slow, the apparent half-lives being 88 and 67 hours respectively. Activated charcoal given by mouth appeared to reduce these half-lives markedly.— E. Elonen *et al.*, *Clin. Toxicol.*, 1979, *14*, 79, per *Int. pharm. Abstr.*, 1980, *17*, 306. See also P. J. Neuvonen *et al.*, *Clin. Pharmac. Ther.*, 1980, *27*, 823.

For studies on the effect of activated charcoal on the elimination rate of dapsone, see under Adsorptive Capacity in Activated Charcoal, p.79.

Desensitisation for dapsone dermatitis. Sensitivity to dapsone could arise within a few minutes of the ingestion of the first dose of 100 mg of dapsone; more often it appeared after a few weeks of therapy on standard regimens of gradually increasing doses—100 mg twice weekly for 3 to 4 weeks, rising to 200 mg and then to 300 mg for similar periods, up to a maximum of 400 mg twice weekly for a patient weighing over 63.5 kg. To effect slow desensitisation, an aqueous solution of solapsone was prepared by dissolving 500 mg of the drug in 200 ml of water (12.5 mg in 5 ml). An initial oral dose of 5 ml was given and subsequent doses were given twice weekly; each dose was 5 ml greater than the preceding one. After the twentieth dose (100 ml containing 250 mg of solapsone) the solid drug was given in tablet form by mouth twice weekly in gradually increasing amounts. Dapsone was then substituted twice weekly for solapsone, starting with 25 mg cautiously increased until the standard dose was given. Of 52 patients, 48 were successfully desensitised (26 had recurrences of dermatitis during the desensitising course); the desensitised state was apparently permanent in 43 patients.— S. G. Browne, *Br. med. J.*, 1963, *2*, 664.

Precautions. In order to avoid permanent disability, rapid and adequate treatment is essential for patients who develop leprosy reactions (for further details, see p.1487).

Dapsone should be used with caution in patients with cardiac or pulmonary disease. Persons deficient in glucose-6-phosphate dehydrogenase are more susceptible to the haemolytic effects of dapsone. Excretion of dapsone is reduced by concurrent administration of probenecid. Rifampicin has been reported to increase the plasma clearance of dapsone.

In view of the wide-spread impression that dapsone in doses of 100 mg daily may precipitate serious reversal reaction in some patients with borderline leprosy, facilities for immediate diagnosis and adequate treatment should be readily available to patients, at risk, receiving this regimen.— S. G. Browne, *Lepr. Rev.*, 1977, *48*, 283.

See also p.1487.

Reports of Maloprim (dapsone 100 mg and pyrimethamine 12.5 mg) being dispensed mistakenly for dapsone in patients with rheumatoid arthritis or dermatitis herpetiformis and comments on the danger of high doses of pyrimethamine producing serious side-effects such as megaloblastic anaemia.— J. Marks (letter), *Lancet*, 1981, *2*, 585; P. R. Crook *et al.* (letter), *ibid.*, 760; *Pharm. J.*, 1981, *2*, 401.

Cardiac or pulmonary disease. Anaemia was more common in 43 patients given dapsone for dermatitis herpetiformis than in a control group. Haemolysis was present in most of the patients and was related to the dose given. Most of the patients who received more than 100 mg of dapsone daily had methaemoglobinaemia and sulphaemoglobinaemia. As the combination of anaemia and tissue hypoxia could be dangerous, dapsone should be used with caution in patients with cardiac or pulmonary disease.— J. J. Cream and G. L. Scott, *Br. J. Derm.*, 1970, *82*, 333.

Interactions. The efficacy of dapsone in preventing patency of mosquito-induced infection was reduced when potassium aminobenzoate was given concurrently in a dose of 4 g daily.— R. L. DeGowin *et al.*, *Bull. Wld Hlth Org.*, 1966, *34*, 671.

In 12 Ethiopian men, probenecid 500 mg with dapsone 300 mg, followed after 5 hours by a further 500-mg dose without dapsone, significantly reduced the urinary excretion of acid-labile dapsone metabolites, and to a smaller extent, of free dapsone. The blood concentrations of dapsone were raised.— C. S. Goodwin and G. Sparell, *Lancet*, 1969, *2*, 884.

Studies in *mice* have not revealed any evidence of antagonism between dapsone and rifampicin.— D. A. Russell *et al.*, *Am. J. trop. Med. Hyg.*, 1975, *24*, 485. Reports that concurrent administration of rifampicin shortens the plasma half-life of dapsone.— R. H. Gelber and R. J. W. Rees, *ibid.*, 963; S. Balakrishnan and P. S. Sheshadri, *Lepr. India*, 1979, *51*, 54, per *Trop. Dis. Bull.*, 1979, *76*, 812. Doubt as to the clinical significance of the interaction between dapsone and rifampicin.— G. Acocella and R. Conti, *Tubercle*, 1980, *61*, 171.

Antimicrobial Action. Dapsone is bacteriostatic against a wide range of bacteria but it is mainly employed for its action against *Mycobacterium leprae*. Its mechanism of action is probably similar to that of the sulphonamides since they both have a similar range of antimicrobial activity and both are antagonised by *p*-aminobenzoic acid. Using the mouse foot-pad technique the minimum inhibitory concentration for *M. leprae* has been reported to be less than 10 ng per ml; the minimum inhibitory concentration in man has been estimated to be up to 30 ng per ml.

The MIC of dapsone against *M. leprae* appeared to be less than 10 ng per ml in *mice*.— G. A. Ellard *et al.*, *Lepr. Rev.*, 1971, *42*, 101.

The relationship between the antibacterial action of sulphones and their chemical structure.— T. H. Maren, *Ann. Rev. Pharmac. Toxic.*, 1976, *16*, 309.

Data suggesting that the antimicrobial effect of dapsone on *M. leprae* is qualitatively different from its effect on other mycobacteria. Results of studies of structure-action relationships of dapsone and its analogues and derivatives in cultivable mycobacteria may not be directly applicable to *M. leprae*.— L. Levy, *Antimicrob. Ag. Chemother.*, 1978, *14*, 791.

Work on whether anti-leprosy drugs reach *Mycobacterium leprae* in peripheral nerves.— J. Boddingius and E. Stolz (letter), *Lancet*, 1981, *1*, 774.

Further references: M. F. R. Waters *et al.*, *Int. J. Lepr.*, 1968, *36*, 651; S. G. Browne, *ibid.*, 1969, *37*, 296.

Bacterial Resistance. The emergence of secondary (acquired) dapsone resistance is wide-spread, and primary dapsone resistance has been reported in areas with secondary resistance, thus establishing the infectivity of dapsone-resistant strains of *Mycobacterium leprae*. In lepromatous leprosy a specific defect in cell-mediated immunity results in the body's inability to eradicate the leprosy bacillus, and present chemotherapeutic agents also appear to be incapable of eradicating persisting viable bacilli (sometimes called 'persisters'). Patients with lepromatous forms of leprosy may therefore relapse during treatment (due to the emergence of resistant bacilli) or on the termination of years of therapy (due to the multiplication of persisting viable bacilli).

Measures to arrest the emergence of strains of *M. leprae* with secondary (acquired) resistance to dapsone, and thereby prevent the spread of primary resistance, include improved means of identifying resistant strains, the use of combined drug regimens, and measures to avoid irregular medication.

A detailed account of the problems of primary and secondary dapsone-resistant strains of *Mycobacterium leprae* and details of suitable drugs which can be given concomitantly for combination therapy.— R. J. W. Rees, *Lepr. Rev.*, 1978, *49*, 97.

Other reports and reviews on the problem of sulphone resistance in leprosy: C. L. Crawford, *Nature*, 1975, *254*, 168; B. D. Molesworth, *Lepr. Rev.*, 1975, *46*, *Suppl.*, 149; J. M. H. Pearson *et al.*, *Lancet*, 1975, *2*, 69; *Br. med. J.*, 1977, *2*, 914; T. W. Meade, *Lepr. Rev.*, 1977, *48*, 3; S. G. Browne, *ibid.*, 79; J. M. H. Pearson *et al.*, *ibid.*, 83; M. F. R. Waters, *ibid.*, 95; L. Levy *et al.*, *ibid.*, 107; L. M. Hogerzeil, *ibid.*, 123; W. H. Jopling, *ibid.*, 127; S. G. Browne, *ibid.*, 283; J. M. H. Pearson *et al.*, *ibid.*, 1979, *50*, 183; T. Warndorff (letter), *ibid.*, 1980, *51*, 261; J. M. H. Pearson *et al.* (letter), *ibid.*, 262.

Some reports of primary sulphone resistance: F. Londoño (letter), *Lepr. Rev.*, 1977, *48*, 51; J. M. H. Pearson *et al.*, *ibid.*, 129; M. F. R. Waters *et al.*, *ibid.*, 1978, *49*, 127; B. K. Girdhar *et al.*, *Lepr. India*, 1978, *50*, 352, per *Lepr. Rev.*, 1979, *50*, 176.

A rapid test for bacillary resistance to dapsone.— E. J. Ambrose *et al.*, *Lepr. India*, 1978, *50*, 131, per *Trop. Dis. Bull.*, 1979, *76*, 421.

Absorption and Fate. Dapsone is almost completely absorbed from the gastro-intestinal tract with peak plasma concentrations about 3 to 6 hours after a dose. Plasma concentrations in the region of 2 µg per ml have been reported after administration of 100 mg daily but these are subject to wide variations. The plasma half-life is subject to similar variations with reports ranging from less than 20 to over 40 hours. More than 50% of dapsone in the circulation is bound to plasma proteins and nearly 100% of its monoacetylated metabolite is bound.

Dapsone is metabolised by acetylation and *N*-oxidation, together with glucuronic acid and sulphate conjugation; acetylation exhibits genetic polymorphism and slow, intermediate, and rapid acetylators have been identified. It is widely distributed throughout the body and is subject to enterohepatic recycling so that although it is fairly rapidly excreted in the urine some traces may persist in the body for several weeks after stopping therapy.

About 70 to 90% is excreted in the urine unchanged (about 20%) and as its metabolites, in free or conjugated form. Small amounts are found in the faeces. It is excreted in milk; it may be found in the urine of breast-fed infants.

Some studies of the absorption, metabolism, and excretion of dapsone.— G. A. Ellard, *Br. J. Pharmac. Chemother.*, 1966, *26*, 212; J. O'D. Alexander *et al.*, *Br. J. Derm.*, 1970, *83*, 620; J. T. Biggs and L. Levy, *Proc. Soc. exp. Biol. Med.*, 1971, *137*, 692; Z. H. Israili *et al.*, *J. Pharmac. exp. Ther.*, 1973, *187*, 138; R. W. Riley and L. Levy, *Proc. Soc. exp. Biol. Med.*, 1973, *142*, 1168; H. Uehleke and S. Tabarelli, *Archs Pharmac.*, 1973, *278*, 55; B. Beiguelman *et al.*, *Bull. Wld Hlth Org.*, 1974, *51*, 467; K. Lammintausta *et al.*, *Int. J. clin. Pharmac. Biopharm.*, 1979, *17*, 159, per *Int. pharm. Abstr.*, 1979, *16*, 1182; R. A. Ahmad and H. J. Rogers, *Eur. J. clin. Pharmac.*, 1980, *17*, 129.

Studies following low-dose therapy: G. A. Ellard *et al.*, *Lepr. Rev.*, 1971, *42*, 101; T. Ozawa *et al.*, *Am. J. trop. Med. Hyg.*, 1971, *20*, 274.

Acetylator status. Many studies have been carried out on the acetylation of dapsone (which is bimodal since dapsone can be acetylated in both amine groups, and is subject to deacetylation). J.H. Peters *et al.*(*Am. J. trop. Med. Hyg.*, 1975, *24*, 641) have identified slow, intermediate, and rapid acetylators but, like G.A. Ellard *et al.* (*Lepr. Rev.*, 1974, *45*, 224), they have found no correlation between acetylator phenotype and variations in half-life. G.A. Ellard *et al.* (*Nature*, 1972, *239*, 159) did not consider acetylator phenotype to be of prognostic value in patients with leprosy but J.H. Peters *et al.* (*Am. J. trop. Med. Hyg.*, 1974, *23*, 222) found a higher proportion of intermediate and rapid acetylators, and also a high rate of dapsone clearance from the plasma, among a group of patients who relapsed with dapsone-resistance. However, neither R.H. Gelber and R.J.W. Rees (*Am. J. trop. Med. Hyg.*, 1975, *24*, 963) nor S. Balakrishnan and Ramu (*Lepr. India*, 1977, *49*, 59) have detected any difference in acetylator phenotype or in plasma-dapsone clearance between resistant and non-resistant subjects. Further elucidation is necessary concerning the properties of dapsone and its metabolites relative to their acetylator status.

Other studies on the variable acetylation of dapsone: R. Gelber *et al.*, *Clin. Pharmac. Ther.*, 1971, *12*, 225; J. H. Peters and L. Levy, *Ann. N.Y. Acad. Sci.*, 1971, *179*, 660; J. H. Peters *et al.*, *Am. J. trop. Med. Hyg.*, 1972, *21*, 450; J. H. Peters *et al.*, *Lepr. Rev.*, 1979, *50*, 7.

Pregnancy and the neonate. During treatment with dapsone for herpes gestationis a woman developed Heinz-body haemolytic anaemia which affected her infant. Ten days after birth, the infant's serum-bilirubin concentration and reticulocyte count fell to normal values.— D. R. Hocking, *Med. J. Aust.*, 1968, *1*, 1130.

Sulphones used for the treatment of a mother with leprosy are excreted in the milk in sufficient amounts to be of therapeutic value to the infant.— J. M. Forrest, *Med. J. Aust.*, 1976, *2*, 138.

Uses. By virtue of its cheapness and relative non-toxicity, dapsone is the principal drug used in the treatment of all forms of leprosy. The recommended dosage is 6 to 10 mg per kg body-weight weekly (about 50 to 100 mg daily, with children receiving correspondingly less). Regimens involving initial low doses have been considered to reduce the incidence of leprosy reactions but doubts have been cast on the need for this, providing prompt measures are available to control the reactions; also any merits of low-dose administration must be balanced against the increased risk of encouraging dapsone resistance, especially in the multibacillary (lepromatous) forms. In both bacteriologically negative tuberculoid and indeterminate patients dapsone in a dose of 50 mg daily is sufficient; in the initial stages of the multibacillary; (lepromatous and borderline) forms of leprosy dapsone should, however, be administered in association with another antileprotic agent such as rifampicin or clofazimine. Treatment should probably be given for about 4 or 5 years in indeterminate and tuberculoid leprosy and probably preferably for life in borderline and lepromatous leprosy.

Dapsone may also be given by intramuscular injection in a dosage of 300 to 400 mg twice weekly or 600 mg weekly; such injections are painful and can cause abscess formation.

In addition to its use in leprosy, dapsone has been found of value in dermatitis herpetiformis and other dermatoses in usual maintenance doses of 50 to 100 mg daily; as little as 50 mg weekly may be adequate but sometimes as much as 400 mg daily has been required. It is also of value in mycetoma and was formerly reported to have a beneficial effect in toxoplasmosis.

Dapsone is also used in combination regimens in the treatment of malaria (see under Chloroquine and other Antimalarials, p.394).

Gastro-intestinal disorders. Dapsone in doses of 50 mg daily or 50 and 100 mg on alternate days produced remissions in 4 of 6 patients with Crohn's disease with a fistula or rectal involvement and which had not responded to conventional treatment.— M. Ward and J. P. A. McManus (letter), *Lancet*, 1975, *1*, 1236.

Leprosy. To prevent the emergence of secondary sulphone resistance, the treatment of newly diagnosed cases of leprosy should be based on the following principles: generally dapsone should be started and maintained in full dosage, treatment should be continued regularly without interruption, and initial combined therapy should be given to lepromatous (LL) and borderline (BL, BB) cases. Dapsone remains the basis of treatment in the recommended dosage of 6 to 10 mg per kg body-weight weekly; this amounts to 50 to 100 mg daily in full-size adults, with correspondingly smaller doses for children. Dapsone injections may be given in a dose of 300 to 400 mg twice weekly or 600 mg weekly. In adult patients with bacteriologically negative tuberculoid (TT and BT) and indeterminate leprosy a dose of 50 mg daily is sufficient. The preferred combination regimen is to give dapsone in full dosage with clofazimine 100 mg daily or thrice weekly to LL and BL patients for the first 4 to 6 months of treatment followed by dapsone in unchanged dosage. Alternatively rifampicin (in a tentatively suggested dose of 300 to 600 mg daily for a minimum of 2 weeks) can be given with dapsone. Other available combinations require further clinical investigation before they can be recommended. No changes are proposed in the criteria for the release from control of inactive cases (1½ years for tuberculoid, 3 years for indeterminate, and *at least* 10 years for lepromatous and borderline cases it being advisable and important to continue the follow-up of lepromatous cases, possibly for life).— Fifth Report of the WHO Expert Committee on Leprosy, *Tech. Rep. Ser. Wld Hlth Org. No. 607*, 1977. Comment. With present chemotherapy and knowledge discharge from treatment or surveillance should not be advised in LL and BL leprosy in the interests of the patient and of the community. However, despite the continuous treatment, the patient's morale should be improved if he is told when he is considered to be no longer infective to others; a zero morphological index might be a better indication than the WHO definition which includes negative bacteriological findings. Patients who are no longer infective should be regarded as in no way different from any other sick person, and should be subject to no hospital, employment, or social restrictions.— T. F. Davey, *Lepr. Rev.*, 1978, *49*, 1. See also M. F. R. Waters *et al.*, *ibid.*, 1974, *45*, 288.

A report on recommendations of the Programme of Research on Chemotherapy of Leprosy (THELEP). Present chemotherapeutic methods for the treatment of lepromatous leprosy fail to prevent the emergence of resistant *Mycobacterium leprae* or to eradicate persisting viable bacilli, so that patients relapse either during treatment or on termination of a prolonged course of treatment. A standard protocol for chemotherapeutic trials in lepromatous leprosy has therefore been prepared in order to develop more effective therapeutic measures which would minimise the proportion of persisting *M. leprae* and prevent the multiplication of drug-resistant organisms. The protocol envisages the trial as having 2 phases: an initial short-term intensive phase lasting 3 months, followed in the same patients by a less intensive long-term phase lasting 21 months. Depending on the results of the first 2 phases a possible third phase is envisaged as follows: if no persisting *M. leprae* are detected after 24 months of treatment with one or more regimens, therapy could safely be withdrawn from half the patients, all of them thereafter being followed for a minimum of 5 years; in patients with persister bacilli detected after 24 months the effect on the persisters of a change of regimen could be measured. The following 8 potential regimens were selected for evaluation in previously untreated patients: dapsone 100 mg daily, rifampicin 600 mg daily, and clofazimine 50 or 100 mg daily for the duration of the trial (regimen A_1); identical to regimen A_1 except that prothionamide 500 mg daily is substituted for clofazimine (regimen A_2); dapsone 100 mg daily and rifampicin 600 mg daily for the duration of the trial (regimen B); dapsone 100 mg daily for the duration of the trial and a single initial dose of rifampicin 1.5 g (regimen C); dapsone 100 mg daily for the duration of the trial, a single initial dose of rifampicin 1.5 g, and clofazimine 50 or 100 mg daily for the first 3 months (regimen D_1); identical to regimen D_1 except that prothionamide 500 mg daily is substituted for clofazimine (regimen D_2); dapsone 100 mg daily for the duration of the trial, rifampicin 900 mg weekly for the first 3 months, and clofazimine 50 or 100 mg daily for the first 3 months (regimen E_1); identical to regimen E_1 except that prothionamide 500 mg daily is substituted for clofazimine (regimen E_2). In addition, 4 regimens for potential trials in patients with dapsone-resistant leprosy comprise treatment with clofazimine 50 or 100 mg daily or thiacetazone 150 mg daily, in association with rifampicin or rifampicin with prothionamide; dapsone 100 mg daily may be added to any of these regimens. The same 4 regimens supplemented with dapsone 100 mg daily were chosen for trials in patients who had already responded to an initial period of therapy with dapsone alone .— *Lepr. Rev.*, 1978, *49*, 69. A further report on the Scientific Working Group on Chemotherapy of Leprosy (THELEP). In addition to the recommendation that every patient with multibacillary leprosy should be treated with combined chemotherapy they urged that a protocol for chemotherapy trials in non-lepromatous leprosy should be developed.— *Lepr. Rev.*, 1981, *52*, 349.

Administration with clofazimine. Combined therapy of dapsone 25 to 100 mg daily in conjunction with rifampicin 300 mg daily or with clofazimine in doses varying between 300 mg daily and 200 mg weekly was considered of value in the treatment of lepromatous leprosy, and also to reduce the number and intensity of reactions.— J. C. Gatti, *Lepr. Rev.*, 1975, *46*, *Suppl.*, 155.

Administration with rifampicin. In a randomised study administration of dapsone 100 mg daily with rifampicin 600 mg daily for 6 months to 5 patients produced more rapid initial clinical improvement than in 6 similar patients who received dapsone 100 mg with placebo, although there was no discernible difference after 6 months. The incidence of ENL was similar in both groups. In those treated with dapsone alone viable *Mycobacterium leprae* were generally still found after 3 months and frequently after 6 months whereas in those who also received rifampicin they were commonly detected at 3 months but only occasionally at 6 months. Clinical, histological, and bacterial evidence indicated that dapsone with rifampicin was more effective than dapsone alone.— R. H. Gelber *et al.*, *Lepr. Rev.*, 1977, *48*, 223.

An account of a possible combined regimen for the treatment of bacteriologically positive lepromatous leprosy patients which employs the 3 most potent and well-tolerated antileprosy drugs, rifampicin, dapsone, and acedapsone, in a manner permitting the maximum amount of supervision under field conditions. Patients would be treated as in-patients for 1 to 2 weeks to receive a fully supervised course of rifampicin 600 mg daily and dapsone 100 mg daily, together with their first intramuscular injection of acedapsone 225 mg. Treatment would then be continued on an out-patient basis with a single dose of rifampicin 600 mg being swallowed once a month under supervision when the patients came to collect their supply of dapsone, which they would continue to take in a dose of 100 mg daily; once every 3 months the patients would also be given acedapsone 225 mg intramuscularly. If finances permitted, the regimen might be strengthened by giving each patient a second 600-mg dose of rifampicin each month to be swallowed on the day after the visit to the clinic.— G. A. Ellard, *Lepr. Rev.*, 1980, *51*, 199.

Further references: J. Languillon *et al.*, *Int. J. Lepr.*, 1979, *47*, 37, per *Lepr. Rev.*, 1980, *51*, 282.

High-dose therapy. A hundred patients with tuberculoid leprosy on a high-dose regimen of dapsone, 100 mg twice daily for one year, showed marked improvement within 6 weeks and the lesions disappeared within 6 to 9 months. Only 9 patients complained of side-effects including headache, anorexia, loss of taste, abdominal pains, and anaemia, and there were no relapses within the following 2 years. In a control group of 100 patients on the more conventional dose of 100 mg twice weekly, improvement was not noted before 3 months and the lesions did not disappear until after a year of treatment. There were 8 relapses and 4 patients developed wasting of the hand. It was suggested that a high-dose regimen could control the disease more rapidly, with less development of complications.— B. N. Prasad, *Lepr. Rev.*, 1971, *42*, 118.

Delayed hypersensitivity reactions ('reversal reactions') occurring in borderline leprosy could cause sudden and severe nerve damage. Reactions in 68 patients were significantly more common in those given dapsone 5 mg daily than in those given 50 mg daily. All patients with leprosy should receive 1 to 2 mg per kg body-weight daily from the start of treatment.— R. S. Barnetson *et al.*, *Lancet*, 1976, *2*, 1171. Criticism. Experience in Great Britain indicated that such reactions were less likely to happen with low than high doses. It was considered unwise to start treatment with this recommended high dose.— W. H. Jopling (letter), *ibid.*, 1977, *1*, 44.

Low-dose therapy. From a multicentre study involving 94 patients with active lepromatous leprosy at 17 institutions, twice weekly dosage for 48 weeks with dapsone 50 mg was as effective as similar treatment with clofazimine 100 mg. Lepra reactions occurred in 47 patients; 30 were taking dapsone and 17 clofazimine.— T. F. Ahrens *et al.*, *Lepr. Rev.*, 1975, *46*, 287.

Low doses of dapsone did not prevent the emergence of lepra reactions which occurred in 2 of the 5 patients on each of 5, 10, and 100 mg daily.— A. B. A. Karat, *Lepr. Rev.*, 1975, *46*, *Suppl.*, 89.

From a double-blind study carried out over 5 years dapsone doses of 3.3 mg and of 10 mg per kg body-weight weekly by mouth were considered equally effective in the treatment of lepromatous leprosy. Moderate to severe lepra reactions occurred in 8 of 11 patients on the smaller dose while reactions occurred in 5 of 10 patients on the higher dose and these tended to be more severe. Insomnia was frequently a side-effect.— K. Ramanujam *et al.*, *Lepr. Rev.*, 1975, *46*, *Suppl.*, 93.

Further references: C. G. S. Iyer *et al.*, *Lepr. India*, 1977, *49*, 372.

Monitoring of therapy. The extraordinary sensitivity of *Mycobacterium leprae* in the nose to even small doses of dapsone meant that nasal discharge was quite a sensitive guide as to whether dapsone was being taken or not.— T. F. Davey and R. J. W. Rees, *Lepr. Rev.*, 1974, *45*,

121.

Estimation of the urinary dapsone/creatinine ratio was a means whereby regularity of dapsone ingestion could be monitored although individidual patients could only be assessed reliably if their urinary dapsone/creatinine ratios under supervised treatment were known.— S. J. M. Low and J. M. H. Pearson, *Lepr. Rev.*, 1974, *45*, 218. See also G. A. Ellard, *Lepr. Rev.*, 1980, *51*, 229.
Evidence that the use of single urine samples to determine dapsone/creatinine concentrations, and hence compliance with dapsone therapy, is unreliable.— K. J. Hagan and S. E. Smith, *Lepr. Rev.*, 1979, *50*, 129.

Further tests to determine compliance with dapsone therapy: H. Huikeshoven *et al.*, *Lepr. Rev.*, 1979, *50*, 275 (enzyme-linked immunosorbent assay [ELISA] of body fluids); S. Balakrishnan, *Lepr. India*, 1980, *52*, 245 (fluorimetric screening of urine), per *Trop. Dis. Bull.*, 1980, *77*, 1040.

Prophylaxis. A double-blind trial of chemoprophylaxis in leprosy using dapsone was carried out in Chingleput, India. Over a period of 5½ years, 358 children who were in contact with active lepromatous patients were given dapsone in almost therapeutic doses and 23 developed leprosy. In a group of 360 children given a placebo who were also in contact with leprosy patients, 48 developed leprosy, representing a 52.5% reduction in incidence resulting from dapsone prophylaxis.In a trial in Culion Sanitarium, Philippines, lower doses of dapsone were given to child contacts under 10 years of age. After 3 years, 15 of 259 treated children and 26 of 251 untreated controls developed leprosy representing a 44.1% reduction of leprosy. None of the cases was lepromatous. The prophylactic value of dapsone could not be determined from these trials.— Fourth Report of the WHO Expert Committee on Leprosy, *Tech. Rep. Ser. Wld Hlth Org. No. 459*, 1970. In certain circumstances there may be a limited place for the administration of prophylactic dapsone. However, in view of the administrative, financial, and medical problems (including the slight but definite incidence of drug toxicity), and uncertainty as to the duration of the proposed prophylactic regimen and adherence to dosage regimens, the use of dapsone as a prophylactic in large-scale control programmes is not recommended.— Fifth Report of the WHO Expert Committee on Leprosy, *Tech. Rep. Ser. Wld Hlth Org. No. 607*, 1977.

Prophylactic dapsone should be recommended for those at real risk because of prolonged and intimate contact with a person who had been shedding viable leprosy bacilli before diagnosis. Usual weekly divided doses were: up to 4 years, 25 mg; 4 to 7 years, 50 mg; 7 to 12 years, 75 mg; 12 to 15 years, 100 mg; over 15 years, 200 mg.— *Memorandum on Leprosy*, London, HM Stationery Office, 1977.

Further references: S. K. Noordeen, *Lepr. India*, 1977, *49*, 504; S. K. Noordeen and P. N. Neelan, *Indian J. med. Res.*, 1978, *67*, 515.

Reactions. For reference to the management of patients suffering leprosy reactions while undergoing sulphone therapy, see p.1487.

Lupus erythematosus. Urticaria-like lesions in a patient with discoid lupus erythematosus were controlled by maintenance treatment with dapsone 150 mg daily. Earlier effective treatment with prednisone 30 mg daily caused oedema and hypertension and reduction of the dose to 20 mg daily was not effective.— C. N. A. Matthews *et al.*, *Br. J. Derm.*, 1978, *99*, 455.

A patient with urticarial vasculitis resembling systemic lupus erythematosus made slight improvement when treated with prednisone; addition of dapsone 100 mg daily led to marked clinical improvement and allowed a reduction in the dosage of prednisone.— A. S. Highet, *Br. J. Derm.*, 1980, *102*, 358.

Dapsone 25 to 100 mg daily produced a significant improvement in 4 patients with certain forms of lupus erythematosus but up to 150 mg daily was ineffective in 3 other patients. The following indications were suggested for the use of dapsone in the treatment of lupus erythematosus: vasculitic urticaria, oral ulceration, non-scarring form of discoid lupus erythematosus, and chloroquine resistance.— T. Ruzicka and G. Goerz, *Br. J. Derm.*, 1981, *104*, 53.

Malaria. For reference to the use of dapsone in conjunction with other agents for the control of malaria, see Chloroquine, p.397, Primaquine, p.401, Proguanil, p.402, Pyrimethamine, p.403, and Quinine, p.405.

Malignant disorders. Dapsone, to shorten the erythrocyte life-span, and pyrimethamine, to inhibit erythropoiesis, were used in the treatment of 5 patients with polycythaemia secondary to hypoxia.— C. D. R. Pengelly, *Lancet*, 1966, *2*, 1381.

Dapsone and sulfoxone sodium were occasionally beneficial when used alone in patients with advanced cervical and ovarian neoplasms. Dapsone appeared to enhance the effects of radiotherapy and increased the survival-rate.— J. Graham and R. Graham, *Surgery Gynec. Obstet.*, 1969, *129*, 103.

Dapsone 25 mg daily was successful in the treatment of granuloma faciale in 1 patient. Fluorouracil applied topically for 3 weeks had been effective in the patient's keratoses but not in the granuloma.— C. R. Anderson (letter), *Lancet*, 1975, *1*, 642.

Mycetoma. References to the successful use of dapsone, either alone or in association with other antibacterial therapy, in mycetoma: H. F. Vismer and J. G. L. Morrison, *S. Afr. med. J.*, 1974, *48*, 433; R. S. Rogers and S. A. Muller, *Archs Derm.*, 1974, *109*, 529.

For details of the successful antibacterial therapy of mycetoma using dapsone alone and in association with streptomycin, see Co-trimoxazole, p.1465.

Rheumatic and collagen disorders. *Animal* studies on the anti-inflammatory actions of dapsone and its related biochemistry.— K. Williams *et al.*, *J. Pharm. Pharmac.*, 1976, *28*, 555.

Chondritis. Three patients with relapsing polychondritis responded to treatment with dapsone.— V. P. Barranco *et al.*, *Archs Derm.*, 1976, *112*, 1286. A further case.— J. Martin *et al.*, *ibid.*, 1272.

Rheumatoid arthritis. Dapsone was observed to have a useful effect in rheumatoid arthritis as well as dermatitis herpetiformis. Further studies might be profitable.— T. J. Constable and B. McConkey (letter), *Lancet*, 1977, *1*, 44. See also *Pharm. J.*, 1978, *1*, 156.

Further references: B. McConkey *et al.*, *Rheumatol. Rehabil.*, 1976, *15*, 230; D. R. Swinson *et al.*, *Ann. rheum. Dis.*, 1981, *40*, 235.

Skin disorders. *Alopecia.* Regrowth of hair had been reported in 9 of 11 patients with alopecia areata after treatment with methylprednisolone 8 to 12 mg every second day and dapsone 200 mg daily for 14 days and 100 mg thereafter. Dapsone had been given in an attempt to improve the efficacy of corticosteroids at lower doses. Further evaluation of the regimen was needed.— *Br. med. J.*, 1979, *1*, 505. Lack of benefit with dapsone in patients with alopecia areata unresponsive to triamcinolone.— P. S. Friedmann *et al.*, *Br. J. Derm.*, 1981, *104*, 597.

Dermatitis herpetiformis. Reports and studies on the use of dapsone in dermatitis herpetiformis: R. Marks and M. W. Whittle, *Br. med. J.*, 1969, *4*, 772; E. Wyatt *et al.*, *Br. J. Derm.*, 1971, *85*, 511; L. Fry *et al.*, *Lancet*, 1973, *1*, 288; G. A. Ellard *et al.*, *Br. J. Derm.*, 1974, *90*, 441; D. J. Riches *et al.*, *Br. J. Derm.*, 1976, *94*, 31; S. I. Katz *et al.*, *Ann. intern. Med.*, 1980, *93*, 857; L. Fry *et al.*, *Br. J. Derm.*, 1980, *102*, 371.

Erythema elevatum diutinum. Reports and studies on the use of dapsone in erythema elevatum diutinum: D. I. Vollum, *Br. J. Derm.*, 1968, *80*, 178; S. L. Fort and O. G. Rodman, *Archs Derm.*, 1977, *113*, 819; S. I. Katz *et al.*, *Medicine, Baltimore*, 1977, *56*, 443.

Lupus erythematosus. See above.

Pemphigus. For a brief discussion on the possible mode of action of dapsone in pemphigoid, see J. R. Person and R. S. Rogers, *Mayo Clin. Proc.*, 1977, *52*, 54.

Reports and studies on the use of dapsone in pemphigus: T. Piamphongsant, *Br. J. Derm.*, 1976, *94*, 681; S. Haim and R. Friedman-Birnbaum, *Dermatologica*, 1978, *156*, 120; C. I. Harrington and I. B. Sneddon, *Br. J. Derm.*, 1979, *100*, 441.

For a reference to the use of dapsone in the treatment of bullous pemphigoid, see Sulphapyridine, p.1481.

Psoriasis. Reports and studies on the use of dapsone in psoriasis: A. L. Macmillan and R. H. Champion, *Br. J. Derm.*, 1973, *88*, 183; R. D. G. Peachey, *Br. J. Derm.*, 1977, *97*, *Suppl.* 15 64; R. Staughton, *Proc. R. Soc. Med.*, 1977, *70*, 286.

Pyoderma gangrenosum. Report on the use of dapsone in pyoderma gangrenosum: L. D. Soto, *Int. J. Derm.*, 1970, *9*, 293.

Preparations

Dapsone Injection *(Univ. Coll. Hosp.)*. Dapsone 5 g, dehydrated alcohol 40 ml, benzyl alcohol 5 ml, propylene glycol to 100 ml.
Sterilised by autoclaving; it should be tested for sterility before use. No significant loss of potency or therapeutic effect was found after storage in the dark for 9 months, though slight darkening occurred.—T.M. French, *Lepr. Rev.*, 1968, *39*, 171.

Dapsone Tablets *(B.P.)*. Tablets containing dapsone.

Dapsone Tablets *(U.S.P.)*. Tablets containing dapsone. The *U.S.P.* requires 75% dissolution in 60 minutes. Protect from light.

Proprietary Names

Avlosulfon *(ICI, Austral.; Ayerst, Canad.; ICI, Denm.; ICI, Swed.)*; D.A.P.S. *(Sintyal, Arg.)*; Dubronax *(Kela, Belg.)*.

6555-v

Ditophal *(B.P. 1963)*. 15688; ETIP: Ethyl Dithiolisophthalate. *SS'*-Diethyl dithioisophthalate.
$C_{12}H_{14}O_2S_2$=254.4.

CAS — 584-69-0.

A yellow or pale brown viscous liquid with a characteristic alliaceous odour. Wt per ml 1.17 to 1.185 g. F.p. not below −1°.
Immiscible with water; miscible with alcohol, chloroform, and ether. **Protect** from light.

Adverse Effects. The adverse effects of ditophal include local and generalised cutaneous hypersensitivity.

Uses. Ditophal is well absorbed through the skin and was formerly administered by inunction in the treatment of leprosy, its action being due to its hydrolytic product, ethyl mercaptan, a volatile foul-smelling liquid. Because resistance to ditophal develops rapidly when it is used alone, ditophal therapy was given in conjunction with oral treatment with thiambutosine or dapsone or solapsone. The dose by inunction was 5 g thrice weekly or 1.5 g daily. Ditophal has also been used in the treatment of tuberculosis of the skin, especially lupus vulgaris.

6556-g

Hydnocarpus Oil. Oleum Hydnocarpi; Chaulmoogra Oil.

CAS — 8001-74-9.

Pharmacopoeias. In *Int.* Similar oils are included in *Port.*, *Span.*, and *Turk. Ind.* allows, under the title Chaulmoogra Oil, only oil from *T. kurzii.*

NOTE. The *B.P.C. 1959* included a monograph under the title of Hydnocarpus Oil which was described as the fatty oil obtained by cold compression from the fresh ripe seeds of *H. wightiana.* Chaulmoogra Oil of the *B.P.C. 1954* was the oil from *T. kurzii.*

The fixed oil expressed from the fresh ripe seeds of *Hydnocarpus wightiana*, *H. anthelmintica*, *H. heterophylla*, and other species of *Hydnocarpus* and also *Taraktogenos kurzii* (Flacourtiuceae).
A yellow or brownish-yellow oil or soft cream-coloured fat with a slight odour and a somewhat acrid taste, containing glycerides of hydnocarpic and chaulmoogric acids. M.p. 20° to 30°. Wt per ml about 0.95 g.
Practically **insoluble** in water; almost completely soluble in hot alcohol and partly soluble in cold alcohol; soluble in carbon disulphide, chloroform, and ether. It may be **sterilised** by maintaining at 150° for 1 hour. **Store** in a cool place in well-filled containers. Protect from light.

6557-q

Ethyl Esters of Hydnocarpus Oil *(B.P.C. 1963)*. Ethyl Hydnocarpate; Ethyl Chaulmoograte; Ethylis Hydnocarpas; Oleum Hydnocarpi Aethylicum; Chaulmugrato e Hydnocarpato de Etilo. A purified mixture of the esters of the fatty acids of hydnocarpus oil. The *B.P.C. 1963* specified oil from *Hydnocarpus wightiana.*

CAS — 8028-03-3.

Pharmacopoeias. In *Span.* and *Turk.*

A colourless or faintly yellow limpid oil with a characteristic odour and a slightly acrid taste, consisting mainly of ethyl hydnocarpate, ethyl chaulmoograte, and ethyl gorlate, together with the ethyl esters of the other fatty acids of hydnocarpus oil. Wt per ml 0.9 to 0.905 g.
Practically **insoluble** in water; soluble 1 in 10 of

alcohol (90%); miscible with carbon disulphide, chloroform, ether, and light petroleum. It may be **sterilised** by maintaining at 150° for 1 hour. **Store** in a cool place in well-filled containers. Protect from light. It is liable to develop peroxides if stored in incompletely filled containers.

Hydnocarpus oil was formerly employed in the treatment of leprosy. It has generally been found to be too irritant for oral administration although it has been given by subcutaneous or intramuscular injection. It was more commonly administered by direct infiltration of the lesions for which purpose the ethyl esters of hydnocarpus oil were generally preferred; doses of 0.5 ml were initially given and then gradually increased to 7 ml weekly.

Hydnocarpus oil probably had little effect on established lepromatous leprosy, but by encouraging resolution it may have prevented some indeterminate and early borderline forms of leprosy from progressing into the lepromatous type.— T. F. Davey, *Lepr. Rev.*, 1975, *46*, 5.

Chaulmoogric acid had an MIC of 32 and 64 μg per ml *in vitro* against 24 and 34 of 43 strains of *Mycobacterium intracellulare* respectively. Chaulmoogric acid also inhibited 4 of 5 strains of each of the following: *Mycobacterium tuberculosis, M. scrofulaceum, M. fortuitum,* and *M. chelonei* at an MIC of 32, 64, 64, and 32 μg per ml respectively.— P. Damle *et al.*, *Tubercle*, 1978, *59*, 135.

6558-p

Sodium Acetosulphone. Acetosulfone Sodium; Sulfadiasulfone Sodium. Sodium 2-*N*-acetylsulphamoyl-4,4′-diaminodiphenyl sulphone.
$C_{14}H_{14}N_3NaO_5S_2$=391.4.

CAS — 80-80-8 (acetosulphone); 128-12-1 (sodium salt).

A white to pinkish-white crystalline powder. **Soluble** 1 in about 33 of water; practically insoluble in alcohol.

Sodium acetosulphone has actions and uses similar to those of dapsone (see p.1489), but only about 25% of a dose is absorbed from the gastro-intestinal tract. It has been recommended for leprosy in doses of 0.5 to 1.5 g daily increased every 2 weeks by 0.5 to 1.5 g to a maximum of 3 to 4 g daily, with rest periods of 10 to 15 days every 4 months. It has also been used in dermatitis herpetiformis.

Proprietary Names
Promacetin *(Parke, Davis, USA).*

6559-s

Sodium Glucosulphone. Glucosulfone Sodium. Disodium bis[4-(*N*-1-sulphoglucosylamino)phenyl] sulphone.
$C_{24}H_{34}N_2Na_2O_{18}S_3$=780.7.

CAS — 551-89-3 (glucosulphone); 554-18-7 (disodium salt).

Sodium glucosulphone was distributed as a mixture with about 11.5% of dextrose.
An odourless white to faintly yellow, amorphous solid with a sweet taste. Very **soluble** in water; slightly soluble in alcohol.

Sodium glucosulphone has the actions and uses of dapsone (see p.1489) to which it is converted in the body. It is not well tolerated by mouth and was given by intravenous injection in doses of 2 to 5 g daily on 6 days a week, with rest periods of 1 to 2 weeks after 1 to 3 months, to permit the haemopoietic system to recover from its haemolytic effects.

6560-h

Sodium Hydnocarpate *(B.P.C. 1949).* Sodium Chaulmoograte; Sodium Gynocardate. The sodium salt of a fraction of the acids of hydnocarpus oil.

CAS — 5587-76-8.

A fawn-coloured powder with a slight odour. **Soluble** 1 in 10 of water at 30°, yielding an alkaline solution (pH about 9); soluble in alcohol. Solutions are **sterilised** by autoclaving or by filtration.

Sodium hydnocarpate has actions similar to those of hydnocarpus oil (see above) and was formerly used for the same purpose. It has been given in pills or capsules or by injection.

6561-m

Solapsone *(B.P. 1968).* Solasulfonum; Solasulfone; Solusulfone. Tetrasodium salt of bis[4-(3-phenyl-1,3-disulphopropylamino)phenyl] sulphone.
$C_{30}H_{28}N_2Na_4O_{14}S_5(+xH_2O)$=892.8.

CAS — 133-65-3 (anhydrous).

Pharmacopoeias. In *Int.* and *It.*

An almost white, almost odourless, amorphous powder with an alkaline taste. It contains not less than 90% of $C_{30}H_{28}N_2Na_4O_{14}S_5$, calculated on the dried material; it loses 5 to 10% of moisture on drying.
Very **soluble** in water; practically insoluble in most organic solvents. A 10% solution in water has a pH of 5.5 to 7.5 and is iso-osmotic with serum. Solutions are **sterilised** by autoclaving or by filtration. It is stable in neutral or alkaline solution but decomposes in acid solution. **Store** in airtight containers.

Solapsone has the actions and uses of dapsone (see p.1489) to which it is partially metabolised. It can be given by mouth but is more commonly given by subcutaneous or intramuscular injection. For the treatment of leprosy it has been injected in doses of 1.25 to 2.5 g (2.5 to 5 ml of a 50% solution) twice weekly, but as little as 500 mg twice weekly may prove adequate providing administration is not erratic. It has been given by mouth as tablets in doses of 1.5 g daily for 1 week increased by 500 mg every third day to 3 g daily.

A study of the pharmacology of solapsone in 8 lepromatous subjects indicated that significant metabolism to dapsone occurred. Following intramuscular administration of 5 ml of solapsone 30% solution, mean plasma-dapsone concentrations were 93, 78, 48, and 40 ng per ml after 24, 48, 72, and 96 hours respectively.— R. H. Gelber *et al.*, *Lepr. Rev.*, 1974, *45*, 308; *idem*, 1975, *46*, 124. A further study of the absorption and excretion of solapsone in 6 patients. Plasma-dapsone concentrations after administration of solapsone 500 mg intramuscularly twice weekly indicated that it has a partial repository effect, and plasma concentrations were adequate for chemotherapeutic activity. Studies after a single 500-mg dose intramuscularly, however, indicated that interrupted treatment could yield dangerously low blood concentrations in some patients.— J. H. Peters *et al.*, *Lepr. Rev.*, 1975, *46*, 171.

Preparations

Solapsone Tablets *(B.P. 1968).* Tablets containing solapsone.

Strong Solapsone Injection *(B.P.C. 1968).* Inj. Solapson. Fort. A sterile solution of solapsone 50 g and anhydrous sodium carbonate 140 mg in Water for Injections to 100 ml.
When weaker solutions of solapsone for injection are specified, the strong injection is diluted to the required strength with Water for Injections by an aseptic technique.

The proprietary name Sulphetrone has been used in some countries for solapsone.

6562-b

Sulfoxone Sodium *(U.S.P.).* Sodium Sulfoxone; Aldesulfone Sodium; Sulfoxydiasulfone Sodium. Disodium salt of bis(4-sulphinomethylaminophenyl) sulphone.
$C_{14}H_{14}N_2Na_2O_6S_3$=448.4.

CAS — 144-76-3 (sulfoxone); 144-75-2 (disodium salt).

Pharmacopoeias. In *Arg.* and *U.S.*

A white to pale yellow powder with a characteristic odour, containing 73 to 81% of $C_{14}H_{14}N_2Na_2O_6S_3$ with suitable buffers and inert ingredients.
Soluble 1 in about 14 of water; very slightly soluble in alcohol, chloroform, and ether. Sodium carbonate and sodium phosphate are suitable stabilising agents for preventing deterioration through absorption of carbon dioxide. A 10% solution in water has a pH of 10.5 to 11.5. **Store** at −10° to −20° in an atmosphere of nitrogen in airtight containers. Protect from light.

Sulfoxone sodium has the actions and uses of dapsone (see p.1489). About half a dose is hydrolysed and absorbed chiefly as dapsone; the remainder is probably not absorbed. For the treatment of leprosy it is given by mouth as enteric-coated tablets, 330 mg daily being roughly equivalent to dapsone 50 mg daily. Higher doses have been given for dermatitis herpetiformis.

Following administration of sulfoxone [sodium] 330 mg to 14 patients plasma concentrations and urinary excretion of dapsone indicated that this dose is roughly equivalent to 50 mg of dapsone. Assuming complete hydrolysis to dapsone, on a molar basis, however, only a threefold increase in sulfoxone requirement would be anticipated. A difference in total dapsone excretion following sulfoxone administration as against that following dapsone administration was noted; a similar difference was also noted by M. Smith (*Lepr. Rev.*, 1949, *20*, 78) who concluded that it was due primarily to relatively poor absorption of sulfoxone from the gastro-intestinal tract.— J. H. Peters *et al.*, *Lepr. Rev.*, 1975, *46*, 171.

A 46-year-old man with dermatitis herpetiformis taking sulfoxone sodium 660 to 990 mg daily for 2 or 3 days a week ['when needed'] developed peripheral neuropathy of the thumbs and hand, without motor involvement. Similar symptoms had been seen in a further patient.— G. Volden, *Br. med. J.*, 1977, *1*, 1193.

Preparations

Sulfoxone Sodium Tablets *(U.S.P.).* Enteric-coated tablets of sulfoxone sodium. Store in airtight containers. Protect from light.

Proprietary Names
Diasone *(Abbott, Norw.; Abbott, Swed.)*; Diasone Sodium *(Abbott, USA).*

6563-v

Thiambutosine *(B.P.).* DPT; Su 1906. 1-(4-Butoxyphenyl)-3-(4-dimethylaminophenyl)thiourea.
$C_{19}H_{25}N_3OS$=343.5.

CAS — 500-89-0.

Pharmacopoeias. In *Br.*

A white or creamy-white, odourless, crystalline powder with a bitter taste. M.p. 123° to 127°.
Practically **insoluble** in water; soluble 1 in 1.5 of chloroform and 1 in 300 of ether; soluble in acetone. **Store** in airtight containers. Protect from light.

Adverse Effects. Few adverse reactions have been reported following administration of thiambutosine but an antithyroid action may occur with high doses. Skin eruptions may occur but do not generally necessitate withdrawal of the drug.

Antimicrobial Action. Thiambutosine has been reported to be bacteriostatic against *Mycobacterium leprae* with a minimum inhibitory concentration of 500 ng per ml. Acquired resistance emerges after 1 or 2 years of antileprotic monotherapy.

Demonstration of cross-resistance of *Mycobacterium leprae* to thiambutosine, thiacetazone, ethionamide, and prothionamide. These drugs should be considered as alternatives to each other when devising antileprotic drug regimens.— S. R. Pattyn and M. J. Colston (letter), *Lepr. Rev.*, 1978, *49*, 324.

Further references: J. M. B. Garrod and G. A. Ellard, *Lepr. Rev.*, 1968, *39*, 113; S. R. Pattyn, *ibid.*, 1972, *43*, 126; M. J. Colston *et al.*, *ibid.*, 1978, *49*, 101.

Absorption and Fate. Thiambutosine is poorly absorbed from the gastro-intestinal tract. Aqueous suspensions are slowly and possibly incompletely absorbed from parenteral sites. Suspensions in arachis oil appear to be more quickly absorbed after injection. It is rapidly excreted in the urine as unchanged drug and metabolites.

A study of the absorption, metabolism, and excretion of thiambutosine showed that only 10% of the dose administered by mouth was absorbed and that this small amount was metabolised to benzene-insoluble compounds and rapidly excreted in the urine. About 75% of the orally administered drug was excreted unchanged in the faeces.— G. A. Ellard and R. F. Naylor, *Lepr. Rev.*, 1961, *32*, 249.

Studies were made of the excretion of thiambutosine and its metabolites in the urine and faeces of patients given injections of a 20% aqueous suspension, of others given the drug in arachis oil, and of a third group given repeated oral doses. Absorption was slow in the first group and thiambutosine was found in the urine 4 months after injections ended. Absorption of thiambutosine from injection sites was accelerated by the use of arachis oil; the half-life of the drug in the body was 6 to 7 days. As the total excretion of thiambutosine and its metabolites never exceeded 41%, the drug was probably incompletely absorbed from the injection site. The faeces provided insignificant amounts after intramuscular injections and it was concluded that biliary excretion was not important.— G. A. Ellard, *Lepr. Rev.*, 1966, *37*, 17.

Uses. Thiambutosine has been used in the treatment of leprosy but its value is limited by the development of resistance within 1 or 2 years. It was usually given in initial doses of 1 g daily (in 2 divided doses) gradually increased to 1.5 to 2 g daily (in 2 divided doses); doses of 3 g daily have been given. Children were given 0.5 to 1.5 g daily according to age. Thiambutosine has also been given by deep intramuscular injection as a 20% suspension in oil in an initial dose of 200 mg weekly gradually increased to 1 g weekly. It has also been advocated for the treatment of dermatitis herpetiformis.

Leprosy. A study using the mouse foot-pad model indicated that the antileprotic activity of thiambutosine, thiacetazone, and thiocarlide is essentially bacteriostatic. Of the 3 drugs thiacetazone holds the most promise for adjunct use in the combination chemotherapy of leprosy. The MIC of thiambutosine against *Mycobacterium leprae* is approximately 500 ng per ml, which is similar to the peak serum concentrations reported in man after doses of 1.5 g (falling to about one-third of this value after 24 hours). This explains the weak clinical activity of thiambutosine monotherapy reported in exceptionally poor absorbers of the drug.— M. J. Colston *et al.*, *Lepr. Rev.*, 1978, *49*, 101.

Preparations

Thiambutosine Tablets *(B.P.).* Tablets containing thiambutosine. Protect from light.
Store in airtight containers.

Proprietary Names

Ciba-1906 *(Ciba, Austral.).*

Thiambutosine was formerly marketed in Great Britain under the proprietary name Ciba 1906 (*Ciba*).

6564-g

Thiazosulphone. Thiazolsulfone. 4-Aminophenyl 2-aminothiazol-5-yl sulphone.
$C_9H_9N_3O_2S_2$=255.3.

CAS — 473-30-3.

Adverse Effects. As for Dapsone, p.1489. Prolonged treatment with thiazosulphone has caused thyroid enlargement and, in young persons, the development of secondary sex characteristics before puberty.

Uses. Thiazosulphone was formerly used in the treatment of leprosy, but was found to be less effective than dapsone and other sulphones.

Sunscreen Agents

9300-g

Exposure to strong sunlight causes erythema and sunburn. There may be a rapid tanning in some people resulting from the oxidation of melanin precursors in the uppermost layers of the skin. There may also be a delayed and indirect pigmentation due to the formation of new melanin. Melanin provides some protection against further exposure, but the main protection is provided by thickening of the corneous layer. Excessive and prolonged exposure to sunlight may lead to chronic degenerative changes in the skin (premature ageing of the skin) and skin carcinogenesis.

Sunburn and sun tan are caused by ultraviolet light in the sun's rays and as ultraviolet light is not visible to the human eye the burning and tanning effects of sunlight are not necessarily related to its brightness. Ultraviolet light of wavelengths 320 to 400 nm (UVA) produces immediate direct tanning of the skin with little erythema. Ultraviolet light of wavelengths 290 to 320 nm (UVB) is about 1000 times stronger than UVA in producing erythema and is that part of the sun's spectrum that is responsible for producing sunburn. UVB also produces tanning by indirect pigmentation. The earth's surface is usually screened, by the ozone layer, from ultraviolet light of wavelengths 100 to 290 nm (UVC) from the sun. However artificial sources such as bactericidal lamps used in operating theatres can emit UVC light and it can produce erythema without tanning. Reflected ultraviolet light from snow or water adds to direct irradiation.

Sunscreen agents are of 2 types, those that are opaque and reflect most of the radiation and those that absorb a particular range of wavelengths in the ultraviolet range.

Sunscreen agents which scatter light effectively include titanium dioxide (see p.507) and zinc oxide (see p.509). Other powders used include calcium carbonate, kaolin, magnesium oxide, and talc. Powders may be dusted on to the skin or applied in an aqueous or oily basis. This type of sunscreen is usually cosmetically unappealing.

Sunscreen agents which absorb UVB light include: para-aminobenzoates, such as aminobenzoic acid (see p.1651), glyceryl aminobenzoate, and the padimates; benzophenones, such as dioxybenzone, mexenone, oxybenzone, and sulisobenzone; cinnamates, such as cinoxate; salicylates, such as benzyl salicylate, homosalate, and salol. Other compounds used as sunscreen agents include anthranilates and camphor derivatives. The benzophenones and anthranilates also absorb UVA light.

Creams and lotions containing dihydroxyacetone (see p.493) and lawsone have been employed to protect the skin by staining as well as by light absorption, and commercial grades of yellow soft paraffin (see p.1064) have been found to provide good protection but may not be cosmetically acceptable. Bergamot oil (see p.671) has also been used in suntan preparations.

The efficacy of a particular sunscreen preparation is often expressed as its sun protection factor (SPF). This is a ratio of the time required for irradiation to produce minimal perceptible erythema (minimum erythemal dose; MED) with the skin protected with the suncreen compared to the MED without protection. The scale ranges from SPF1, representing minimal protection from sunburn, but permitting suntanning to SPF 15, representing maximum protection against sunburn with permitted limited tanning.

Sunscreen agents which protect against the full spectrum of ultraviolet light are required by persons with photosensitivity or hypersensitivity to sunlight such as in vitiligo, xeroderma pigmentosum, erythropoietic protoporphyria, or porphyria cutanea tarda, for persons being treated with photosensitising drugs, or medical personnel exposed to ultraviolet bactericidal lamps.

Sunscreen agents are also used in products to promote tanning; they reduce the amount of erythemal UVB light and allow transmission of the tanning UVA light.

Reviews and discussions on sunscreen agents: G. Steinicke, *Australas. J. Pharm.*, 1971, *52*, 393 (effect of weather and altitude on intensity of ultraviolet radiation from the sun); T. B. Fitzpatrick *et al.*, *Proc. R. Soc. Med.*, 1971, *64*, 861 (use of sunscreen agents in operating rooms and in PUVA therapy); *Med. Lett.*, 1972, *14*, 27; G. A. Groves, *Aust. J. Pharm.*, 1975, *56*, 547; *idem*, 601; *idem*, 653; M. Lane-Brown, *Drugs*, 1977, *13*, 366; *Med. Lett.*, 1979, *21*, 46; D. P. Anonis, *Drug Cosmet. Ind.*, 1979, *124*, (Feb.), 44.

An evaluation of 24 sunscreen agents in desert, temperate, and alpine conditions indicated that though *aminobenzoic acid* 5% in 70 to 95% alcohol was the most effective agent in all conditions, *padimate* and *esculoside* screened off erythemal radiation better than the other agents used. Most preparations failed to guard against sunburn when the skin was washed after they were applied or when profuse sweating occurred.— M. A. Pathak *et al.*, *New Engl. J. Med.*, 1969, *280*, 1459.

Sunscreen preparations were tested in clear bright midday sunshine in Florida. *Aminobenzoic acid* 5% in alcohol and a *benzophenone* cream were found to be effective. A solution of padimate was less effective and 3 of 9 subjects complained of a burning sensation and developed erythema 30 minutes after application of the solution and exposure to sunlight.— S. I. Katz *et al.*, *Archs Derm.*, 1970, *101*, 466, per *J. Am. med. Ass.*, 1970, *212*, 493.

Red Veterinary Petrolatum had a protective factor (PF) of 2 to 19.2 against irradiation at 305 ± 15 nm. Additional applications 24 and 12 hours before exposure did not appreciably increase the PF. *Mexenone* cream 10% had a PF of 2 to 4.1 and a cream containing *benzyl salicylate* 2.75% and *benzyl cinnamate* 1.75% had a PF of 1.5 to 5.8. *Red Veterinary Petrolatum* and *mexenone* afforded no protection in some patients with photodermatoses. *Aminobenzoic acid* 5% in alcohol had a PF of 8 to 17 persisting with little reduction for 7 hours. Protection was lowered by sweating and swimming. A cream containing *dihydroxyacetone* 3% and *lawsone* 0.13% had a low PF against irradiation at 400 nm. In patients with solar keratoses a PF of 5 to 41 was afforded by *Cream ERI* (p.1497).— T. M. Macleod and W. Frain-Bell, *Br. J. Derm.*, 1971, *84*, 266.

A brief discussion of the sunscreening properties of pyridoxinate compounds.— *Mfg Chem.*, 1978, *49* (Apr.), 77.

A discussion of the proposed monograph for sunscreen products from the OTC Sunburn Treatment and Prevention Drug Review Panel of the FDA. Of 27 active sunscreen ingredients the following were considered to be both safe and effective in the specified concentrations: *aminobenzoic acid* (5–15%), *cinoxate* (1–3%), *diethanolamine p-methoxycinnamate* (8–10%), *digalloyl trioleate* (2–5%), *dioxybenzone* (3%), *ethyl 4-bis(hydroxypropyl)aminobenzoate* (1–5%), *2-ethylhexyl 2-cyano-3,3-diphenylacrylate* (7–10%), ethylhexyl p-methoxycinnamate (2–7.5%), *2-ethylhexyl salicylate* (3–5%), *glyceryl aminobenzoate* (2–3%), *homosalate* (4–15%), *lawsone* (0.25%) with *dihydroxyacetone* (2%), *menthyl anthranilate* (3.5–5%), *oxybenzone* (2–6%), *padimate* (1–5%), *padimate O* (1.4–8.0%), *2-phenyl-1H-benzimidazole-5-sulphonic acid* (1–4%), *Red Veterinary Petrolatum* (30–100%), *sulisobenzone* (5–10%), *titanium dioxide* (2–25%), *triethanolamine salicylate* (5–12%). *Allantoin* used with *aminobenzoic acid* and *5-(3,3-dimethyl-8,9,10-trinorborn-2-ylidene)-3-penten-2-one* were considered to be safe but there was insufficient data to determine their effectiveness; there was also insufficient data to determine both the safety and effectivness of *dipropylene glycol salicylate*. The following ingredients were considered to be neither safe nor effective: *2-ethylhexyl 2-(biphenyl-4-ylcarbonyl)benzoate*, *3-(4-methylbenzylidene)bornan-2-one*, and *sodium 3,4-dimethylphenylglyoxylate*. Sunscreen protection factors (SPF) required for various skin types were recommended. Tests for SPF, sweat resistance, and water resistance of sunscreen preparations were also given.— H. E. Jass, *Cosmet. Toilet.*, 1979, *94*, (Apr.), 96. See also J. Dickinson, *Aust. J. Pharm.*, 1978, *59*, 636; *Pharm. J.*, 1978, *2*, 486.

A survey of the sunscreen agents used in 197 suntan products available in Holland during the summer of 1978. Compared with the European Cosmetic Manufacturers' list of u.v. absorbers 1978, only 24 of the 60 compounds listed were identified. The 6 agents most frequently found were: *ethylhexyl p-methoxycinnamate*, *cinoxate*, *oxybenzone*, *3-(4-methylbenzylidene)bornan-2-one*, *3-benzylidene bornan-2-one*, and *2-phenyl-1H-benzimidazole-5-sulphonic acid*.— D. H. Liem and L. T. H. Hilderink, *Int. J. cosmet. Sci.*, 1979, *1*, 341.

9317-z

Benzophenone-2. 2,2′,4,4′-Tetrahydroxybenzophenone.
$C_{13}H_{10}O_5 = 246.2$.

CAS — 131-55-5.

Powder. M.p. about 195°. **Soluble** 1 in 1000 of water, 1 in 2.5 of alcohol, and 1 in 2 of methyl alcohol.

Benzophenone-2 has been used as a sunscreen agent.

Proprietary Preparations

Uvinul D-50 *(BASF, UK)*. A brand of benzophenone-2.

9318-c

Benzophenone-6. 2,2′-Dihydroxy-4,4′-dimethoxybenzophenone.
$C_{15}H_{14}O_5 = 274.3$.

CAS — 131-54-4.

Crystals or powder. M.p. 139° to 140°. Practically **insoluble** in water; slightly soluble in alcohol.

Benzophenone-6 has been used as a sunscreen agent.

Proprietary Preparations

Uvinul D-49 *(BASF, UK)*. A brand of benzophenone-6.

9319-k

Benzophenone-9. Sodium 2,2′-dihydroxy-4,4′-dimethoxy-5-sulphobenzophenone. Sodium 4-hydroxy-5-(2-hydroxy-4-methoxybenzoyl)-2-methoxybenzenesulphonate.
$C_{15}H_{13}O_8NaS = 376.3$.

CAS — 3121-60-6.

Powder. **Soluble** 1 in 20 of water, 1 in 100 of alcohol, and 1 in 50 of methyl alcohol.

Benzophenone-9 has been used as a sunscreen agent.

Proprietary Preparations

Uvinul DS-49 *(BASF, UK)*. A brand of benzophenone-9.

9320-w

Benzoresorcinol. Benzophenone-1. 4-Benzoylresorcinol; 2,4-Dihydroxybenzophenone.
$C_{13}H_{10}O_3 = 214.2$.

CAS — 131-56-6.

Powder. M.p. 144° to 145°. Practically **insoluble** in water; soluble 1 in 2.5 of alcohol and methyl alcohol; soluble in ether and glacial acetic acid.

Benzoresorcinol has been used as a sunscreen agent.

Proprietary Preparations

Uvinul 400 *(BASF, UK)*. A brand of benzoresorcinol.

9301-q

Benzyl Salicylate.
$C_{14}H_{12}O_3 = 228.2$.

CAS — 118-58-1.

A clear almost colourless oily liquid or white crystalline solid with a slight sweet, floral odour. Slightly **soluble** in water; soluble 1 in 9 of alcohol (90%) and in mineral and vegetable oils, isopropyl myristate, and acetoglycerides; miscible with ether. **Store** in a cool, dry place.

Adverse Effects. Hypersensitivity reactions to benzyl salicylate have been reported. It may cause slight smarting when applied, particularly to sensitive skins or after some sunburn has already occurred.

Skin reactions. References to skin reactions with benzyl salicylate: H. W. Rotherborg and N. Hjorth, *Archs Derm.*, 1968, *97*, 417; E. Epstein, *J. Am. med. Ass.*, 1969, *209*, 911; P. E. Osmundsen, *Dermatologica*, 1970, *140*, 65; G. Kahn, *Archs Derm.*, 1971, *103*, 497; P. E. Osmundsen and M. D. Alani, *Br. J. Derm.*, 1971, *85*, 61.

Uses. Benzyl salicylate is used as a sunscreen agent in concentrations of 2 to 7% in oils, creams, and aerosol sprays.

Manufacturers

Bush Boake Allen, UK.

9302-p

Cinoxate. 2-Ethoxyethyl *p*-methoxycinnamate.
$C_{14}H_{18}O_4$=250.3.

CAS — 104-28-9.

A viscous liquid that may have a slightly yellow tinge. B.p. about 185°. Practically **insoluble** in water; miscible with alcohols.

Adverse Effects.

Skin reactions. A report of contact dermatitis after the application of a sunscreen lotion containing cinoxate followed by exposure to sunlight.— T. F. Goodman (letter), *Archs Derm.*, 1970, *102*, 563.

Uses. Cinoxate is a sunscreen agent that is used in concentrations of 1 to 4%.

Proprietary Names

Giv-Tan F *(Givaudan, USA)*; Sundare *(Cooper, USA)*.

9321-e

Digalloyl Trioleate. The trioleic ester of 5-carboxy-2,3-dihydroxyphenyl gallate.
$C_{68}H_{106}O_{12}$=1115.6.

CAS — 17048-39-4; 27436-80-2.

Digalloyl trioleate has been used as a sunscreen agent in concentrations of 2.5% in a solid basis or 3.5% in creams.

9303-s

Dioxybenzone *(U.S.P.)*. Benzophenone-8. 2,2′-Dihydroxy-4-methoxybenzophenone.
$C_{14}H_{12}O_4$=244.2.

CAS — 131-53-3.

Pharmacopoeias. In *U.S.*

An off-white to yellow powder. It congeals at not less than 68°. Practically **insoluble** in water; freely soluble in alcohol and toluene. **Store** in airtight containers. Protect from light.

Adverse Effects.

Skin reactions. A report of contact dermatitis in a 46-year-old man after the use of a sunscreen preparation containing dioxybenzone and oxybenzone. Patch testing indicated sensitivity to dioxybenzone with a weak positive reaction to oxybenzone.— R. J. Pariser, *Contact Dermatitis*, 1977, *3*, 172.

Uses. Dioxybenzone is a sunscreen agent that is most effective in absorbing ultraviolet light with wavelengths from 300 to 380 nm but it does absorb partially from 380 to 400 nm. It is used in a concentration of 3%.

Preparations

Dioxybenzone and Oxybenzone Cream *(U.S.P.)*. Dioxybenzone and oxybenzone, 2.7 to 3.3% of each, in a suitable cream basis. Store in airtight containers.

Cyasorb UV 24 *(Cyanamid, UK)*. A brand of dioxybenzone.

9304-w

Esculoside. Esculin; Esculosidum. 6-β-D-Glucopyranosyloxy-7-hydroxycoumarin sesquihydrate.
$C_{15}H_{16}O_9,1\frac{1}{2}H_2O$=367.3.

CAS — 531-75-9 (anhydrous).

Pharmacopoeias. In *Fr.*

Esculoside is present in the bark, leaves, and seeds of the horsechestnut, *Aesculus hippocastanum* (Hippocastanaceae). It occurs as a white to slightly cream-coloured, odourless, crystalline powder with a bitter taste. Very slightly **soluble** in water; soluble 1 in 6 of boiling water and 1 in 60 of alcohol; practically insoluble in ether. Neutral and alkaline solutions have a light blue fluorescence. **Protect** from light.

Adverse Effects.

Esculoside could be toxic to human beings. Symptoms of poisoning were muscle twitching, weakness, lack of coordination, dilated pupils, vomiting, diarrhoea, paralysis, and stupor.— M. Nagy, *J. Am. med. Ass.*, 1973, *226*, 213.

Uses. Esculoside is used as a sunscreen agent, usually in lotions or creams containing 2 to 5%. It has also been used in suppositories for the treatment of haemorrhoids and has been given by mouth in a usual dose of 10 mg in the treatment of conditions associated with increased capillary fragility.

Preparations

Esculoside is an ingredient of Proctosedyl, p.474..

9322-l

Ethyl 4-Bis(hydroxypropyl)aminobenzoate.
$C_{15}H_{23}NO_4$=281.4.

CAS — 58882-17-0.

Ethyl 4-bis(hydroxypropyl)aminobenzoate has been used as a sunscreen agent in concentrations of up to 5%.

An evaluation of Amerscreen P.— L. I. Conrad, *Amerchol, USA*, *J. Soc. cosmet. Chem.*, 1976, *27*, 87.

Proprietary Preparations

Amerscreen P *(Amerchol, USA: Anstead, UK)*. A sunscreen agent comprising a mixture of isomers of ethyl 4-bis(hydroxypropyl)aminobenzoate.

9323-y

2-Ethylhexyl 2-(biphenyl-4-ylcarbonyl)benzoate.
$C_{28}H_{30}O_3$=414.5.

CAS — 75005-95-7.

A clear, greenish-yellow, highly viscous oil with a faint characteristic odour. Practically **insoluble** in water; miscible with alcohol, animal facts, or vegetable oils.

2-Ethylhexyl 2-(biphenyl-4-ylcarbonyl)benzoate has been used as a sunscreen agent in usual concentrations of 2 to 4%.

In a review of sunscreen products the OTC Sunburn Treatment and Prevention Drug Review Panel of the FDA considered 2-ethylhexyl 2-(biphenyl-4-ylcarbonyl)benzoate to be neither safe nor effective.— H. E. Jass, *Cosmet. Toilet.*, 1979, *94* (Apr.), 96.

Proprietary Preparations

Eusolex 3573 *(E. Merck, UK: BDH Chemicals, UK)*. A brand of 2-ethylhexyl 2-(biphenyl-4-ylcarbonyl)benzoate.

9324-j

Ethylhexyl *p*-Methoxycinnamate. Octyl methoxycinnamate.
$C_{18}H_{26}O_3$=290.4.

Ethylhexyl *p*-methoxycinnamate is a sunscreen agent which has been used in concentrations of up to 6.5%.

Proprietary Preparations

Piz Buin *(Greiter, Switz.: Colson & Kay, UK)*. A range of sunscreen preparations containing ethylhexyl *p*-methoxycinnamate and oxybenzone.

Other Proprietary Names

UV Sun Block, UV Sun Filter, Uvistik *(all Austral.)*.

9325-z

Etocrylene. Etocrilene; Ethyl α-cyano-β-phenylcinnamate. Ethyl 2-cyano-3,3-diphenylacrylate.
$C_{18}H_{15}NO_2$=277.3.

CAS — 5232-99-5.

Powder. M.p. about 96°. Practically **insoluble** in water; soluble 1 in 25 of alcohol and 1 in about 14 of methyl alcohol.

Etocrylene has been used as a sunscreen agent.

Proprietary Preparations

Uvinul N-35 *(BASF, UK)*. A brand of etocrylene.

9305-e

Glyceryl Aminobenzoate. Glyceryl PABA. Glyceryl 1-(4-aminobenzoate).
$C_{10}H_{13}NO_4$=211.2.

CAS — 136-44-7.

A pale yellow to amber semi-solid waxy mass or syrup with a faint aromatic odour; it liquefies and congeals very slowly. Very slightly **soluble** in water; soluble in alcohol, glycerol, ispropyl alcohol, methyl alcohol, and propylene glycol; practically insoluble in oils and fats.

Adverse Effects. As for Aminobenzoic Acid, p.1651.

Skin reactions. A patient who applied a sunscreen preparation containing glyceryl aminobenzoate developed severe dermatitis on exposure to sunlight. Glyceryl aminobenzoate was shown to be a contact allergen and a photosensitiser.— G. C. Goldman and E. Epstein, *Archs Derm.*, 1969, *11*, 447, per *J. Am. med. Ass.*, 1969, *210*, 571.

Glyceryl aminobenzoate had proved to be the most common cause of allergic dermatitis in sunscreen preparations containing aminobenzoic acid esters. Of 4 patients who developed allergic contact dermatitis after using preparations containing glyceryl aminobenzoate all had cross-sensitivity to benzocaine; cross-sensitivity was also occasionally obtained to aminobenzoic acid, paraphenylenediamine, procaine, or aniline. None of the patients had sensitivity to padimate or padimate O. Previous studies had also demonstrated that cross-sensitivity between glyceryl aminobenzoate and sulphonamides or saccharin could occur.— A. A. Fisher, *Cutis*, 1976, *18*, 495.

Uses. Glyceryl aminobenzoate is a sunscreen agent which is most effective in absorbing ultraviolet with wavelengths between 290 and 320 nm.
It is used in concentrations of 1 to 4%; being very slightly soluble in water it forms a film on the skin which is not readily removed.

Proprietary Preparations

Nipa GMPA *(Nipa, UK)*. A brand of glyceryl aminobenzoate.

Glyceryl aminobenzoate was also formerly marketed in Great Britain under the proprietary name Escalol 106 (*Van Dyk, USA*).

9306-l

Homosalate. Homomenthyl Salicylate. 3,3,5-Trimethylcyclohexyl salicylate.
$C_{16}H_{22}O_3$=262.3.

CAS — 118-56-9.

A clear almost colourless liquid. **Soluble** in alcohol, mineral and vegetable oils, isopropyl myristate, and similar fatty acid esters. **Store** in a cool, dry place.

Adverse Effects.

Skin reactions. A report of 2 patients who developed contact dermatitis to homosalate; one had used a sunscreen product (Coppertone) containing homosalate and the other patient had a boyfriend who also used the same product. The dermatitis resolved on discontinuing use of the lotion.— R. L. Rietschel and C. W. Lewis, *Archs Derm.*, 1978, *114*, 442.

Uses. Homosalate is a sunscreen agent used in concentrations of about 5 to 10%.

Proprietary Names

Heliophan *(Greeff, USA)*.

A preparation containing homosalate was formerly marketed in Great Britain under the proprietary name Antiviray (*Bush Boake Allen*).

9307-y

Lawsone. 2-Hydroxy-1,4-naphthoquinone.
$C_{10}H_6O_3$=174.2.

CAS — 83-72-7.

A dye present in henna, the dried powdered leaves of *Lawsonia* spp., or prepared synthetically.

Lawsone has been used in conjunction with dihydroxyacetone as a sunscreen agent.

For studies of the efficacy of lawsone used with dihydroxyacetone as a sunscreen agent, see Dihydroxyacetone, p.493. See also p.1495.

9308-j

Menthyl Salicylate.
$C_{17}H_{24}O_3$=276.4.

CAS — 89-46-3.

A clear yellowish syrupy liquid; odourless or with a slight fruity odour. Practically **insoluble** in water; miscible with oils and most organic solvents. **Store** in airtight containers. Protect from light.

Menthyl salicylate is used as a sunscreen agent, generally at a concentration of about 10%. However it is reported that menthyl salicylate undergoes chemical change on exposure to light, thereby considerably reducing its screening properties.

9326-c

Methyl Anthranilate. Methyl 2-aminobenzoate.
$C_8H_9NO_2$=151.2.

CAS — 134-20-3.

Crystals. M.p. about 25°. Slightly **soluble** in water; freely soluble in alcohol and ether.

Methyl anthranilate has been used in sunscreen preparations in a concentration of 5%, usually with other sunscreen agents. It is an ingredient of several essential oils.

Estimated acceptable daily intake of methyl anthranilate: up to 1.5 mg per kg body-weight and of methyl *N*-methylanthranilate: up to 200 μg per kg.— Twenty-third Report of Joint FAO/WHO Expert Committee on Food Additives, *Tech. Rep. Ser. Wld Hlth Org. No. 648*, 1980.

9309-z

Methyl Eugenol. 4-Allylveratrole. 1-Allyl-3,4-dimethoxybenzene.
$C_{11}H_{14}O_2$=178.2.

CAS — 93-15-2.

A colourless liquid. Practically **insoluble** in water; soluble in alcohol

Methyl eugenol has been used as a sunscreen agent.

9327-k

3-(4-Methylbenzylidene)bornan-2-one. 3-(4-Methylbenzylidene)camphor.
$C_{18}H_{22}O$=254.4.

CAS — 36861-47-9.

A white powder with a faint characteristic odour. M.p. 66° to 68°. **Soluble** 1 in about 4 of alcohol, arachis oil, isopropyl alcohol, or isopropyl myristate; 1 in about 8 of glycerol, 1 in about 7 of liquid paraffin, and 1 in about 25 of propylene glycol. Soluble in most fats and oils.

3-(4-Methylbenzylidene)bornan-2-one is used as a sunscreen agent in concentrations of up to 7.5%.

In a review of sunscreen products the OTC Sunburn Treatment and Prevention Drug Review Panel of the FDA considered 3-(4-methylbenzylidene)bornan-2-one to be neither safe nor effective.— H. E. Jass, *Cosmet. Toilet.*, 1979, *94* (Apr.), 96.

Proprietary Preparations

Eusolex 6300 *(E. Merck, UK: BDH Chemicals, UK)*. A brand of 3-(4-methylbenzylidene)bornan-2-one.

9310-p

Mexenone *(B.P.)*. Benzophenone-10. 2-Hydroxy-4-methoxy-4′-methylbenzophenone.
$C_{15}H_{14}O_3$=242.3.

CAS — 1641-17-4.

Pharmacopoeias. In *Br.*

A pale yellow odourless or almost odourless crystalline powder. M.p. 99° to 102°. Practically **insoluble** in water; soluble 1 in 70 of alcohol and 1 in 7 of acetone.

Uses. Mexenone has the property of absorbing ultraviolet light over a wide range of wavelengths (250 to 350 nm) and is used as a sunscreen agent in preparations to reduce the risk of sunburn and other light-induced dermatoses. It is stated to be non-irritant.

Mexenone is used in a usual concentration of 4% in a cream or a solid basis. Owing to its low solubility in water, it is not readily removed from the skin by washing or perspiration and it therefore provides prolonged protection.

Chloasma. As the chloasma induced by pregnancy or oral contraceptives was aggravated by exposure to sunlight, the use of a sunscreen cream containing mexenone was recommended.— I. B. Sneddon, *Practitioner*, 1974, *213*, 9.

Sunscreen effect. In 16 healthy persons and 10 patients with lesions of the skin apt to be worsened by sunshine, a vanishing cream containing 10% of mexenone was superior to 3 other sunscreen preparations. The 3 other preparations contained respectively 10% salol, 10% pyribenzamine, and 15% aminobenzoic acid.— J. C. Belisario, *Med. J. Aust.*, 1961, *2*, 178.

Systemic lupus erythematosus. Sunscreen creams which contained mexenone were recommended in patients with systemic lupus erythematosus whose condition was exacerbated by sunlight.— N. R. Rowell, *Br. med. J.*, 1969, *2*, 427.

Preparations

Cream ER1. Titanium dioxide 20 g, zinc oxide 6 g, kaolin 2 g, red precipitated ferric oxide 1 g, mexenone 4% cream to 100 g. A sunscreen agent.—T.M. Macleod and W. Frain-Bell, *Br. J. Derm.*, 1971, *84*, 266.

Mexenone Cream *(B.P.)*. A dispersion of mexenone in a suitable basis. pH of a dispersion (about 16%) in water 4 to 5. Store at a temperature not exceeding 25° in well-closed containers which minimise evaporation and contamination.

Uvistat *(WB Pharmaceuticals, UK: Boehringer Ingelheim, UK)*. Cream containing mexenone 4% in an oil-in-water basis. **Uvistat-L.** Contains mexenone 4% in a solid basis, for application to the lips. (Also available as Uvistat in *Austral., S.Afr.*).

Other Proprietary Names

Uvicone *(Austral.)*.

9311-s

Octabenzone. 2-Hydroxy-4-octyloxybenzophenone.
$C_{21}H_{26}O_3$=326.4.

CAS — 1843-05-6.

Pale cream to light yellow crystals or friable lumps. M.p. about 48° to 49°. Practically **insoluble** in water; soluble 1 in 33 of alcohol; freely soluble in acetone.

Octabenzone is used as a sunscreen agent.

Proprietary Preparations

Cyasorb UV 531 *(Cyanamid, UK)*. A brand of octabenzone.

9328-a

Octocrylene. 2-Ethylhexyl α-cyano-β-phenylcinnamate. 2-Ethylhexyl 2-cyano-3,3-diphenylacrylate.
$C_{24}H_{27}NO_2$=361.5.

CAS — 6197-30-4.

A viscous oil. **Immiscible** with water, miscible with alcohol and methyl alcohol.

Octocrylene has been used as a sunscreen agent.

Proprietary Preparations

Uvinul N-539 *(GAF, UK)*. A brand of octocrylene.

9312-w

Oxybenzone *(U.S.P.)*. Benzophenone-3. 2-Hydroxy-4-methoxybenzophenone.
$C_{14}H_{12}O_3$=228.2.

CAS — 131-57-7.

Pharmacopoeias. In *U.S.*

A white to off-white powder. It congeals at not less than 62°. Practically **insoluble** in water; freely soluble in alcohol and toluene. **Store** in airtight containers. Protect from light.

Oxybenzone is used as a sunscreen agent in concentrations of 1 to 4%.

Preparations

Cyasorb UV 9 *(Cyanamid, UK)*. A brand of oxybenzone.

Eusolex 4360 *(E. Merck, UK: BDH Chemicals, UK)*. A brand of oxybenzone.

Uvinul M-40 *(BASF, UK)*. A brand of oxybenzone.

See also under Dioxybenzone, p.1496, Ethylhexyl Methoxycinnamate, p.1496, and Padimate O, p.1498.

9313-e

Padimate. Padimate A; Amyl Dimethylaminobenzoate; Isoamyl Dimethylaminobenzoate. A mixture of pentyl, isopentyl, and 2-methylbutyl 4-dimethylaminobenzoates.
$C_{14}H_{21}NO_2$=235.3.

CAS — 14779-78-3.

A yellow liquid with a faint aromatic odour. Practically **insoluble** in water, glycerol, and propylene glycol. Soluble in alcohol, chloroform, isopropyl alcohol, and liquid paraffin.

Adverse Effects. As for Aminobenzoic Acid, p.1651.

Skin reactions. Whereas 19 of 32 healthy subjects developed phototoxic reactions when they applied a sunscreen containing padimate before exposure to long-ultraviolet radiation none of 18 did so when they used a sunscreen containing padimate O. In a further test the ortho-isomer of padimate was found to be a more potent photosensitiser than the para-isomer. It was considered that phototoxic reactions to padimate were more common than reported but since the reactions might be indistinguishable from sunburn, users might conclude that the sunscreen was ineffective.— K. H. Kaidbey, *Archs Derm.*, 1978, *114*, 547.

See also p.1495.

Uses. Padimate is used as a sunscreen agent. It is most effective in absorbing ultraviolet light with wavelengths between 290 and 320 nm. It is used in a usual concentration of 2.5%.

Padimate 2.5% in a basis containing yellow soft paraffin and propylene glycol was much more effective than when it was in a commercial hydrophilic basis, while mexenone 10% in a commercial cream was ineffective when these preparations were compared as sunscreen agents for 9 normal subjects.— R. P. Armati and A. Johnson, *Med. J. Aust.*, 1972, *1*, 1196.

Proprietary Preparations

Escalol 506 *(Van Dyk, USA: Black, UK)*. A brand of padimate.

SpectraBAN 4 *(Stiefel, UK)*. A lotion containing padimate 2.5% in an alcoholic basis. **SpectraBAN 15.** A lotion containing padimate 2.5% and aminobenzoic acid 5% in an alcoholic basis. (Inflammable: keep away from an open flame.)

Other Proprietary Names

Pabafilm *(Austral., USA)*; Uvosan *(Austral.)*.

Pabafilm also appears to be used as a proprietary name in some countries for Padimate O.

9314-l

Padimate O. Octyl dimethyl PABA. 2-Ethylhexyl 4-(dimethylamino)benzoate.
$C_{17}H_{27}NO_2$=277.4.

CAS — 21245-02-3.

A light yellow mobile liquid with a faint aromatic odour. Practically **insoluble** in water; soluble in alcohol, liquid paraffin, isopropyl alcohol; practically insoluble in glycerol and in propylene glycol.

Uses. Padimate O is a sunscreen agent which absorbs ultraviolet light of wavelengths 290 to 315 nm. It has been used in concentrations of 1 to 5%.

Preparations containing padimate O 3.3% or aminobenzoic acid 5% in an alcoholic basis were equally effective in preventing photoirritation in 61 patients being treated for acne vulgaris with tretinoin; some patients also received tetracycline hydrochloride.— S. I. Cullen, *Curr. ther. Res.*, 1979, *26*, 625.

Further references: R. S. Berger *et al.*, *J. Soc. cosmet. Chem.*, 1978, *29*, 641.

Proprietary Preparations

Escalol 507 *(Van Dyk, USA: Black, UK)*. A brand of padimate O.

Super Shade 15 *(Plough, UK)*. Lotion containing padimate O 7% and oxybenzone 3%.

Other Proprietary Names

Eclipse *(USA)*; Phiasol *(Austral.)*; Presun 4 *(USA)*.

Pabafilm which is a proprietary name for Padimate also appears to be used in some countries for Padimate O.

9329-t

2-Phenyl-1*H*-benzimidazole-5-sulphonic Acid.

$C_{13}H_{10}N_2O_3S$=274.3.

CAS — 27503-81-7.

A white odourless powder. Very slightly **soluble** in water.

2-Phenyl-1*H*-benzimidazole-5-sulphonic acid is used as a sunscreen agent in concentrations of 1 to 6%. Because of its low water-solubility it is also used in the form of its sodium, and mono- and triethanolamine salts.

Proprietary Preparations

Delial 10 *(Bayer, UK)*. **Cream** and **Lotion** containing 2-phenyl-1*H*-benzimidazole-5-sulphonic acid 2.8%, 3-(4-methylbenzylidene)bornan-2-one 2%, and 2-phenyl-5-methylbenzoxazole ($C_{14}H_{11}NO$ = 209.2) 1%.

Eusolex 232 *(E. Merck, UK: BDH Chemicals, UK)*. A brand of 2-phenyl-1*H*-benzimidazole-5-sulphonic acid.

9315-y

Salol *(B.P.C. 1954)*. Salicilato de Fenilo. Phenyl salicylate.

$C_{13}H_{10}O_3$=214.2.

CAS — 118-55-8.

Pharmacopoeias. In *Aust., Fr., Ind., Mex., Nord., Pol., Port., Rus., Span.,* and *Swiss.*

Colourless acicular crystals, or white crystalline powder with a faint aromatic odour recalling that of wintergreen. M.p. 42° to 43.5°.

Soluble 1 in 7000 of water, 1 in 9 of alcohol, 3 in 1 of chloroform, 3 in 1 of ether, 1 in 10 of liquid paraffin, soluble in fixed and volatile oils; very slightly soluble in glycerol. **Incompatible** with alkalis and ferric salts; liquid or soft masses are formed when it is triturated with camphor, chloral hydrate, menthol, phenacetin, and many other substances.

Adverse Effects.

Skin reactions. It had been stated that sensitisation reactions to salicylates were rare. Salol, however, in the author's personal experience has been reported by a great number of individuals to produce irritation. It was unknown if this is due to salol itself or to its hydrolysis products phenol and salicylic acid. Many of the reports could have been due to the nature of the vehicle used for salol.— G. A. Groves, *Aust. J. Pharm.*, 1975, *56*, 601.

Uses. Salol has the property of absorbing ultraviolet light over the wavelengths 290 to 330 nm and is used as a sunscreen agent in creams and lotions in concentrations of 5 to 10%. It has also been used as an enteric coating for some oral dose forms.

Salol was formerly used as an intestinal antiseptic, but effective doses were toxic owing to the liberation of phenol.

Preparations

Salol Cream Aqueous *(A.P.F.)*. Salol Cream; Sun-screen Cream. Salol 10 g, stearic acid 16 g, wool fat 2 g, triethanolamine 2 g, propylene glycol 5 ml, freshly boiled and cooled water to 100 g.

Salol Ointment (Greaseless Basis). Salol 10, macrogol ointment to 100.—*Australas. J. Pharm.*, 1956, *37*, 128.

Proprietary Names

Sola-Stick *(Hamilton, Austral.)*.

9330-l

Sodium 3,4-Dimethoxyphenylglyoxylate.

$C_{10}H_9NaO_5$=232.2.

CAS — 37891-88-6.

A white, odourless, crystalline powder. Very **soluble** in water; practically insoluble in alcohol, chloroform, or ether.

Sodium 3,4-dimethoxyphenylglyoxylate has been used as a sunscreen agent in concentrations of 2 to 4%.

Proprietary Preparations

Eusolex 161 *(E. Merck, UK: BDH Chemicals, UK)*. A brand of sodium 3,4-dimethoxyphenylglyoxylate.

9316-j

Sulisobenzone. Benzophenone-4. 5-Benzoyl-4-hydroxy-2-methoxybenzenesulphonic acid.

$C_{14}H_{12}O_6S$=308.3.

CAS — 4065-45-6.

A light yellow or light tan powder. **Soluble** 1 in 4 of water, 1 in about 3 of alcohol, and 1 in 100 of ethyl acetate.

Sulisobenzone is used as a sunscreen agent in concentrations of up to 10%.

Sunscreen effect. Sulisobenzone 10% or dioxybenzone 3% with oxybenzone 3% protected 12 fair-skinned persons exposed to germicidal u.v. radiation in an operating theatre.— J. A. Parrish *et al.*, *New Engl. J. Med.*, 1971, *284*, 1257.

Reports of sulisobenzone 10%, in a lotion, providing protection against u.v. light in patients receiving photosensitising agents: A. Satanove and J. S. McIntosh, *J. Am. med. Ass.*, 1967, *200*, 209 (thioridazine hydrochloride); C. Korenyi, *Am. J. Psychiat.*, 1969, *7*, 971 (chlorpromazine), per *Int. pharm. Abstr.*, 1969, *6*, 596.

For the use of sulisobenzone with betacarotene in the treatment of polymorphous light eruption, see under Photosensitivity in Betacarotene, p.1638.

Proprietary Preparations

Cyasorb UV 284 *(Cyanamid, UK)*. A brand of sulisobenzone.

Uvinul MS-40 *(BASF, UK)*. A brand of sulisobenzone.

Other Proprietary Names

Uval *(Canad.)*.

The name Uval is also used for a sunscreen preparation containing oxybenzone with 2-ethylhexyl *p*-methoxycinnamate.

Thyroid and other Thyroid Agents

9000-k

The main hormonal activity of the thyroid gland is dependent upon 2 active principles, thyroxine and tri-iodothyronine. These are both amino acids containing iodine and are incorporated in the glycoprotein thyroglobulin. The laevo isomer of tri-iodothyronine is liothyronine (see p.1500).

Dietary iodine, as iodide, is concentrated by the thyroid gland, and then used in the iodination of tyrosine to mono- and di-iodotyrosine, from which thyroxine and tri-iodothyronine are produced. These 2 hormones are stored in large quantities in the gland as parts of the thyroglobulin protein molecule and are released into the blood-stream after proteolysis.

The thyroid also produces calcitonin in the parafollicular cells (see p.1073).

The iodine-containing thyroid hormones are concerned with growth, development, and metabolic processes. They raise the basal metabolic rate and in some tissues stimulate oxygen consumption.

There is a close interrelation between the thyroid and other endocrine glands. The thyrotrophic hormone of the anterior lobe of the pituitary (see p.1278) is necessary for normal thyroid function.

Deficiency of thyroid secretion results in **hypothyroidism** or myxoedema; congenital thyroid deficiency leads to cretinism.

Excess of thyroid secretion results in **hyperthyroidism** (thyrotoxicosis or Graves' disease). Clinical management may include surgery, the use of iodine-131 (p.1393), or chemotherapy.

Measurement of thyroid function may be affected by drugs and disease states.

Thyroid physiology in health and disease.— J. Brown *et al., Ann. intern. Med.*, 1974, *81,* 68.

A discussion of thyroid diseases in the elderly.— M. F. Green, *Br. med. J.*, 1974, *1,* 232.

The recognition and management of thyroid disease.— B. E. W. Brownlie, *Drugs,* 1977, *14,* 376.

Feedback regulation of thyroid-stimulating hormone secretion by thyroid hormones.— P. R. Larsen, *New Engl. J. Med.*, 1982, *306,* 23.

Uses. Thyroxine (p.1502) and liothyronine (p.1500) are preferred to dried thyroid gland in the treatment of hypothyroidism. Thyroxine has a delayed effect and cumulative action, whereas the effects of liothyronine are rapid in onset and of brief duration.

Thyroid hormones are sometimes used in certain forms of thyroiditis including Hashimoto's thyroiditis.

Thyroxine is the drug of choice for routine thyroid replacement therapy.— *Med. Lett.*, 1977, *19,* 50.

A review of the use of thyroid hormones in the treatment of hypothyroidism.— W. E. Cobb and I. M. D. Jackson, *Am. J. Hosp. Pharm.*, 1978, *35,* 51.

The mechanism of action of thyroid hormone at cellular level.— K. Sterling, *New Engl. J. Med.*, 1979, *300,* 117; *idem,* 173.

Pregnancy and the neonate. A discussion of the management of hyperthyroidism and hypothyroidism during pregnancy.— O. M. Edwards, *Postgrad. med. J.*, 1979, *55,* 340. See also *Br. med. J.*, 1978, *2,* 977 (thyroid disease in pregnancy); J. Feely, *Postgrad. med. J.*, 1979, *55,* 336 (thyroid function in pregnancy); D. A. Fisher and A. H. Klein, *New Engl. J. Med.*, 1981, *304,* 702 (thyroid development and disorders in the newborn.).

9001-a

Thyroid *(U.S.P., B.P. 1973).* Thyroideum Siccum; Thyroidea; Dry Thyroid; Thyroid Extract; Thyroid Gland; Thyreoidin; Tiroide Secca; Getrocknete Schilddrüse.

Pharmacopoeias. In *Arg., Aust., Braz., Chin., Hung., Ind., Int., It., Jap., Mex., Pol., Port., Rus., Span., Turk.*, and *U.S.* Most specify about 0.2% of organically combined iodine.

Thyroid (*U.S.P.*) is the cleaned, dried, and powdered thyroid, previously deprived of connective tissue and fat, obtained from domesticated animals used for food by man. It contains 0.17 to 0.23% of iodine in thyroid combination and no iodine in inorganic or any other form. It loses not more than 6% of its weight on drying. Thyroid having a higher iodine content may be diluted as necessary by admixture with thyroid of a lower iodine content or with a suitable diluent such as dextrose, lactose, sodium chloride, starch, or sucrose.

A yellowish to buff-coloured amorphous powder with a slight characteristic meat-like odour and a saline taste.

Thyroid 60 mg is approximately equivalent to 90 µg of thyroxine sodium.

Store in a cool place in airtight containers. Protect from light.

Calcium phosphate was recommended as a diluent in preparing thyroid tablets since lactose could inhibit activity by as much as 40%. Beef thyroid was stated to be only one-half as potent as pork thyroid and this might be a major source of variation.— S. Taylor, *Lancet,* 1961, *1,* 332.

Effect of gamma-irradiation. Thyroid changed slightly in colour with irradiation of more than 10 000 Gy but free iodine was liberated increasingly above 20 000 Gy. The bacterial count could be reduced to 100 per g with doses of 13 000 to 18 000 Gy, and the thyroid was sterilised, but with some iodine loss, by 50 000 Gy.— G. Hangay *et al., Radiosterilization of Medical Products,* Vienna, International Atomic Energy Agency, 1967, p. 91.

Adverse Effects, Treatment, and Precautions. As for Thyroxine Sodium, p.1501.

A report of periodic paralysis developing in 3 patients who took thyroid tablets in an attempt to lose weight. Two patients were taking 0.6 to 1.8 g daily and the third, of Japanese origin, was taking only 120 to 240 mg daily.— R. B. Layzer and E. Goldfield, *Neurology, Minneap.*, 1974, *24,* 949.

A report of slipped capital femoral epiphysis during treatment for hypothyroidism.— A. B. Zubrow *et al., J. Bone Jt Surg.*, 1978, *60,* 256.

Neoplasm of the breast. The incidence of breast cancer was increased almost 2-fold in women who had taken thyroid for at least a year; the incidence was related to duration of treatment and was highest in nulliparous women.— C. C. Kapdi and J. N. Wolfe, *J. Am. med. Ass.*, 1976, *236,* 1124. A higher incidence of malignant disease was observed among hypothyroid women.— R. E. Hodges (letter), *ibid.*, 2743; M. Lender *et al.* (letter), *ibid.* Untreated hypothyroid women should have been used as controls.— B. O. Barnes (letter), *ibid.* A further analysis of the data from the same group of patients indicated that breast cancer and length of treatment with thyroid were both related to advancing age, and that duration of thyroid therapy did not appear to increase the risk of development of breast cancer.— P. Mustacchi and F. Greenspan, *J. Am. med. Ass.*, 1977, *237,* 1446.

A statement by the American Thyroid Association recommended that patients who were taking thyroid hormones for well-established indications should continue to take their medication. It also stressed the need for controlled studies of a possible relationship between the thyroid and cancer of the breast.— C. A. Gorman *et al., J. Am. med. Ass.*, 1977, *237,* 1459.

In a study involving 79 patients with breast cancer, no association was found between the incidence of breast cancer and thyroid hormone use.— R. B. Wallace *et al., J. Am. med. Ass.*, 1978, *239,* 958.

In a retrospective study comparing 659 women with breast cancer and 1719 control subjects, of whom 60 and 149 respectively had taken thyroid hormone, there was no evidence of an association even when thyroid supplements had been taken for more than 15 years.— S. Shapiro *et al., J. Am. med. Ass.*, 1980, *244,* 1685.

Pregnancy and the neonate. For a report suggesting an association between exposure to thyroid *in utero* and cardiac malformations, see Thyroxine Sodium, p.1501.

Uses. Thyroid produces an increase in the basal metabolic rate. It has been administered to provide the effects of thyroxine (see p.1502) and of liothyronine (see p.1500) which are the active principles.

It has been used in the treatment of adult hypothyroidism in an initial daily dose of 15 mg gradually increased up to a maintenance dose usually between 60 and 180 mg daily. Up to 600 mg has been used in some patients.

Thyroid has sometimes been given as enteric-coated tablets.

Hypothyroidism. Myxoedematous patients are seen who are being treated with apparently adequate doses of thyroid extract but who are clinically and biochemically hypothyroid. They subsequently respond to thyroxine.— W. van't Hoff *et al.* (letter), *Br. med. J.*, 1978, *2,* 200.

Studies in 40 patients whose medication was changed from thyroid to thyroxine indicated that thyroid may produce undesirably high serum concentrations of tri-iodothyronine. Thyrotoxic symptoms in 6 patients diminished or disappeared after the change to thyroxine.— I. M. Jackson and W. E. Cobb, *Am. J. Med.*, 1978, *64,* 284. Similar results in 13 of 14 children.— R. Penny and S. D. Frasier, *Am. J. Dis. Child.*, 1980, *134,* 16. See also C. T. Sawin *et al., Metabolism,* 1978, *27,* 1518.

Candidiasis. A 7-year-old boy with chronic mucocutaneous candidiasis which was resistant to prolonged treatment was found to have hypothyroidism. When doses of thyroid, up to 2 g daily, were given the skin lesions cleared though all antifungal therapy had stopped.— L. F. Martes *et al., J. Am. med. Ass.*, 1972, *221,* 156.

Thyroiditis. Twenty-seven patients with chronic thyroiditis were treated with thyroid 50 to 100 mg daily. Of these, 13 received prednisolone 20 to 30 mg daily for 4 to 6 months, and others received either chloroquine phosphate or hydroxychloroquine sulphate 100 mg daily increased to 400 mg and then decreased after 3 to 6 months. Hardness of the goitre was reduced in only 1 patient receiving thyroid alone. Prednisolone treatment generally resulted in a decrease in thyroid size, and a reduction of goitre hardness and complement fixation antibody titres. These changes were more marked after treatment with both prednisolone and chloroquine, but when prednisolone was withdrawn the complement fixation antibody titres tended to rise.— S. Ito *et al., Metabolism,* 1968, *17,* 317.

Preparations

Thyroid Tablets *(B.P. 1973).* Tablets containing thyroid. Store in a cool place in airtight containers.

Thyroid Tablets *(U.S.P.).* Tablets containing thyroid; the iodine content, in thyroid combination, is 0.17 to 0.23% of the labelled amount of thyroid. Store in airtight containers.

Proprietary Names

S-P-T *(Fleming, USA)*; Thyranon *(Organon Belge, Belg.; Organon, Neth.; Organon, Spain; Organon, Swed.)*; Thyrar *(Armour, USA)*; Thyroboline *(Choay, Fr.)*; Thyrocrine *(Lemmon, USA)*; Thyroïdine *(Labaz, Fr.)*; Tiroides *(Leo, Spain)*.

A preparation containing thyroid was formerly marketed in Great Britain under the proprietary name Thyropit (*Medo-Chemicals*).

9002-t

Acetiromate. TBF-43. 4-(4-Acetoxy-3-iodophenoxy)-3,5-di-iodobenzoic acid.

$C_{15}H_9I_3O_5$=649.9.

CAS — 2260-08-4.

White or slightly yellowish, odourless, tasteless crystals or crystalline powder. M.p. about 245° with decomposition. Practically **insoluble** in water; slightly soluble in alcohol, chloroform, and ethyl acetate; sparingly soluble in acetone; freely soluble in dimethylformamide.

Adverse Effects. Reported adverse effects include palpitations, diarrhoea, and abdominal pain.

Uses. Acetiromate, which is chemically similar to the thyroid hormones, has been used in the treatment of hypercholesterolaemia.

Proprietary Names

Adecol *(Jap.)*.

9003-x

Detrothyronine. DT 3; SKF D2623; D-Tri-iodothyronine. 4-*O*-(4-Hydroxy-3-iodophenyl)-3,5-di-iodo-D-tyrosine.
$C_{15}H_{12}I_3NO_4$=651.0.

CAS — 5714-08-9.

Detrothyronine has been used in the treatment of hypercholesterolaemia.

The hypolipidaemic and thyroid actions of sodium detrothyronine (FF-234) which was well tolerated by 10 subjects.— T. S. Danowski *et al., Clin. Pharmac. Ther.*, 1971, *12,* 126. Sodium detrothyronine ($NaDT_3$) 500 µg twice daily administered to 26 hyperlipidaemic subjects for 1 to 2 years decreased serum cholesterol concentrations by a mean of about 30%. Only slight effects attributable to thyroid hormone-like activity were seen.— *idem*, 1976, *19,* 196.

For other reports of the use of detrothyronine in hypercholesterolaemia, see D. F. Brown *et al., J. Am. med. Ass.*, 1962, *180,* 643; D. O. Mintz *et al., New Engl. J. Med.*, 1962, *266,* 808; N. B. Baroody and W. G. Baroody, *Am. J. med. Sci.*, 1962, *243,* 338.

9004-r

Dextrothyroxine Sodium *(U.S.P.).* Sodium Dextrothyroxine; D-Thyroxine Sodium; 3,5,3',5'-Tetraiodo-D-thyronine Sodium. Sodium 4-*O*-(4-hydroxy-3,5-di-iodophenyl)-3,5-di-iodo-D-tyrosinate hydrate.
$C_{15}H_{10}I_4NNaO_4(+ x\ H_2O)$=798.9.

CAS — 51-49-0 (dextrothyroxine); 137-53-1 (sodium salt, anhydrous); 7054-08-2 (sodium salt, hydrate).

Pharmacopoeias. In *U.S.*

A light yellow to buff-coloured, odourless, tasteless powder which may assume a slight pink colour on exposure to light. Loses not more than 11% of its weight on drying.

Soluble 1 in 700 of water and 1 in 300 of alcohol; soluble in solutions of alkali hydroxides and in hot solutions of alkali carbonates; practically insoluble in acetone, chloroform, and ether. A saturated solution in water has a pH of about 8.9. A solution in a mixture of sodium hydroxide solution 4% and alcohol is dextrorotatory. **Store** in airtight containers.

Adverse Effects and Treatment. As for Thyroxine Sodium, p.1501.

Other adverse effects which have been reported include neutropenia, altered liver-function test results, paraesthesia, diuresis, and skin rashes. Gall-stones have occurred in patients given dextrothyroxine

In 3798 patients with a history of myocardial infarction followed up for an average of 36 months, the number of deaths was 18.4% higher in the group of 1083 patients taking dextrothyroxine 6 mg daily to reduce hyperlipidaemia than in those taking a placebo. The mortality-rate increased progressively with duration of medication. The use of dextrothyroxine in the study was stopped.—The Coronary Drug Project Research Group, *J. Am. med. Ass.*, 1972, *220,* 996.

Precautions. As for Thyroxine Sodium, p.1501.

Dextrothyroxine is contra-indicated in patients with advanced liver or kidney disease.

Diabetes mellitus. Dextrothyroxine sodium, in doses of 2 to 8 mg daily, was given to 18 euthyroid diabetic patients. Though serum-cholesterol concentrations were reduced in all patients, there was a loss of diabetic control in 8.— W. J. Zinn and L. A. Schleissner, *Calif. Med.*, 1964, *101,* 240, per *Abstr. Wld Med.*, 1965, *37,* 262.

Interactions. For reports of enhanced anticoagulant effect in patients receiving dextrothyroxine in conjunction with dicoumarol or warfarin sodium, See Dicoumarol, p.771, and Warfarin Sodium, p.779.

Absorption and Fate. Dextrothyroxine sodium is absorbed from the gastro-intestinal tract and is bound to plasma proteins. It has been reported to be excreted in urine and faeces.

Uses. Dextrothyroxine sodium lowers the blood cholesterol concentration in patients with hypercholesterolaemia and may also reduce elevated low-density lipoprotein concentrations. It is sometimes used in type II hyperlipidaemia but this use is severely limited by cardiotoxicity. The initial dose is 1 to 2 mg daily, increased by 1 to 2 mg at monthly intervals until a satisfactory response is achieved, up to a maximum of 8 mg daily. For children, an initial daily dose of 50 µg per kg body-weight increased by up to 50 µg per kg at monthly intervals to a maximum of 4 mg daily has been suggested.

Dextrothyroxine was formerly used to treat hypothyroidism.

The limited role of dextrothyroxine in hyperlipidaemia. If it is used at all as a lipid-lowering drug, it should be reserved for the rare patient with marked hyperlipidaemia who does not respond to any other form of treatment.— *Med. Lett.*, 1976, *18,* 53. The use of dextrothyroxine is primarily for young patients, without signs or symptoms of heart disease, who cannot tolerate other treatments, or who require an additional cholesterol-lowering agent.— S. Margolis, *J. Am. med. Ass.*, 1978, *239,* 2696.

Dextrothyroxine 6 mg daily was given to 8 patients, 5 of whom had moderate hyperlipidaemia types IIa or b. After 6 weeks serum-cholesterol concentrations had fallen by an average of 15% but at the same time there was a 19% increase in cholesterol saturation of fasting-state gall-bladder bile. Dextrothyroxine might lower blood-cholesterol concentrations partly by increasing cholesterol excretion.— F. Begemann *et al.* (letter), *Lancet*, 1977, *2,* 402.

A comparison of the effect of dextrothyroxine and thyroxine on serum lipid concentrations, serum thyrotrophin concentrations, and basal metabolic rate in 27 patients with primary hypothyroidism. Daily doses of dextrothyroxine 4 mg and thyroxine 150 µg produced similar lowering of cholesterol and thyroid-stimulating hormone concentrations, and similar alterations in metabolic rate. Raising the dose of either drug produced little additional cholesterol-lowering effect.— C. A. Gorman *et al., J. clin. Endocr. Metab.*, 1979, *49,* 1.

Sprue. Of 12 patients suffering from sprue, 3 showed improvement of intestinal absorption after treatment with dextrothyroxine, 2 mg daily for 8 days followed by 4 mg daily for 8 days.— R. Rodríguez-Molina and M. Cancio, *Boln Assoc. méd. P. Rico*, 1966, *58,* 54, per *Trop. Dis. Bull.*, 1966, *63,* 1371.

Preparations

Dextrothyroxine Sodium Tablets *(U.S.P.).* Tablets containing dextrothyroxine sodium.

Choloxin *(Travenol, UK).* Dextrothyroxine sodium, available as tablets of 2 mg. (Also available as Choloxin in *Canad., S.Afr., USA*).

Other Proprietary Names

Biotirmone *(acid)*, Débétrol *(* both *Fr.)*; Dethyrona *(Spain, Switz.)*; Dethyrone *(Belg., Neth.)*; Dynothel, Eulipos *(*both *Ger.)*; Lisolipin *(Ital.)*; Nadrothyron-D *(Ger.)*.

9006-d

Liothyronine Sodium *(B.P., B.P. Vet., U.S.P.).*

Liothyronine Sod.; Liothyroninum Natricum; Sodium Liothyronine; L-Tri-iodothyronine Sodium. Sodium 4-*O*-(4-hydroxy-3-iodophenyl)-3,5-di-iodo-L-tyrosinate.
$C_{15}H_{11}I_3NNaO_4$=673.0.

CAS — 6893-02-3 (liothyronine); 55-06-1 (sodium salt).

NOTE. The abbreviation T_3 is often used for tri-iodothyronine in medical and biochemical reports..

Pharmacopoeias. In *Br., Braz., Int., It., Nord., Turk.,* and *U.S. Hung.* has liothyronine hydrochloride.

A white to buff-coloured odourless solid or crystalline powder. Liothyronine sodium 10.3 µg is approximately equivalent to 10 µg of liothyronine. Liothyronine sodium 25 µg is approximately equivalent to 60 mg of thyroid or 90 µg of thyroxine sodium. Practically **insoluble** in water, chloroform, ether, and most other organic solvents; soluble 1 in 500 of alcohol; soluble in solutions of alkali hydroxides. A solution in a mixture of hydrochloric acid and alcohol is dextrorotatory. **Store** in airtight containers. Protect from light.

Adverse Effects, Treatment, and Precautions. As for Thyroxine Sodium, p.1501. However, greater caution is required with liothyronine sodium because of its higher potency and more rapid onset of action.

Neoplasm of the breast. For reports and recommendations about breast cancer associated with thyroid hormone therapy, see Thyroid, p.1499.

Overdosage. An hour after taking 80 tablets of liothyronine 20 µg (total dose 1.6 mg), 40 tablets of brompheniramine (total dose 480 mg), and 20 tablets of clomipramine (total dose 200 mg), a 30-year-old woman arrived at hospital mentally confused but with no other signs of intoxication. Gastric lavage was performed and she was transferred to an intensive care unit, where 4 to 5 hours later she developed tachycardia (sinus rhythm 110 beats per minute) and started sweating but retained normal body temperature. Over the next 12 hours these symptoms disappeared, she became mentally orientated, and could be referred to her psychiatrist for further care. Although the laboratory findings indicated that the liothyronine overdosage had pronounced metabolic effects on thyroid hormone homoeostasis the patient had only moderate clinical signs of thyrotoxicosis, owing to the rapid clearance of liothyronine from the vascular compartment.— P. A. Dahlberg *et al.* (letter), *Lancet*, 1979, *2,* 700.

Absorption and Fate. Liothyronine sodium is almost completely absorbed from the gastro-intestinal tract. It is less readily bound to plasma proteins than thyroxine. The half-life of liothyronine in the circulation has been stated to be about 2 days.

There is limited placental transfer of tri-iodothyronine.

Absorption of liothyronine in man.— M. T. Hays, *J. clin. Endocr. Metab.*, 1970, *30,* 675.

Evidence from a study of 103 patients that liothyronine contaminating thyroxine sodium tablets did not contribute to the serum-liothyronine concentrations of patients receiving such tablets, and that their serum-liothyronine concentrations were due to extrathyroidal conversion of the administered thyroxine.— A. Kahn, *Clin. Pharmac. Ther.*, 1976, *19,* 523.

Excretion in breast milk. Significant amounts of tri-iodothyronine were excreted in the breast milk of 5 women both during late pregnancy and after delivery. The postpartum concentrations in breast milk were higher than those obtained before delivery, and were approximately twice the corresponding values for serum.— H. H. Bode *et al., Pediatrics*, 1978, *62,* 13.

Uses. Tri-iodothyronine is an active principle of the thyroid gland. It is suggested that thyroxine becomes active only through conversion to tri-iodothyronine and that this substance is probably the finally effective form of the thyroid hormone acting directly on the cellular metabolic processes. When used as a drug tri-iodothyronine is known as liothyronine. It is qualitatively similar to thyroxine in its actions but is much more potent and more rapid in onset, the effect developing within a few hours. On cessation of treatment there is a rapid return to the original metabolic state. Liothyronine is sometimes used in the treatment of thyroid-deficiency states when a rapid effect is necessary but thyroxine sodium (see p.1502) is the drug of choice for routine replacement therapy. It is usually administered as the sodium derivative preferably in 2 or 3 divided doses daily.

In adult hypothyroidism the initial daily dose is 10 to 25 µg of liothyronine sodium, increasing gradually by increments of 10 to 25 µg every 7 to 14 days to a daily dosage of up to 100 µg.

In myxoedemic coma an initial intravenous dose of 5 to 25 µg of liothyronine sodium may be used. The dose is repeated if necessary, usually at 12-hourly intervals. The minimum interval between doses is 4 hours.

A suggested initial dose for children is 5 µg daily. In children up to 1 year of age this may be increased to 20 µg. For those aged 1 to 3 years up to 50 µg may be given and for those over 3 years of age up to 100 µg may be given.

Liothyronine may be given in doses of 80 µg daily for 7 to 8 days as a test for thyrotoxicosis; the uptake of radioactive iodine is not suppressed.

Liothyronine 80 µg daily is also given with carbimazole in the treatment of thyrotoxicosis. After about a year it may be possible to discontinue the carbimazole.

Some aspects of tri-iodothyronine physiology; the significance of tri-iodothyronine in certain thyroid diseases.— H. Gharib, *J. Am. med. Ass.*, 1974, *227,* 302.

For the administration of liothyronine sodium together

with thyroxine sodium, see Thyroxine Sodium, p.1502.

Depression. Liothyronine 25 µg given daily for 2 weeks in a controlled study of euthyroid depressed patients enhanced the antidepressant activity of imipramine 150 mg daily.— A. Coppen *et al.*, *Archs gen. Psychiat.*, 1972, *26*, 234. Liothyronine in doses of 20 and 40 µg significantly enhanced the antidepressant effect of amitriptyline in a controlled study of 52 patients. This effect was more pronounced with the higher dose and in women.— D. Wheatley, *Archs gen. Psychiat.*, 1972, *26*, 229. In 33 depressed women resistant to treatment with amitriptyline in doses of up to 200 mg daily, liothyronine was given in addition in doses of 20 to 40 µg daily, resulting in improvement in 23 after 7 days; the remaining 10 did not respond. In a further 16 amitriptyline-resistant women the dose of amitriptyline was increased to 300 to 350 mg daily, and produced an improvement in 4 cases. Dysphoria and anxiety in 1 patient given liothyronine led to discontinuation. It was suggested that liothyronine is effective in patients with subclinical hypothyroidism, which contributes to depression; patients in this group had T_3 and T_4 values in the low normal range.— C. M. Banki, *Eur. J. clin. Pharmac.*, 1977, *11*, 311.

Further references.— A. J. Prange *et al.*, *Am. J. Psychiat.*, 1969, *126*, 457; B. Earle, *ibid.*, 1970, *126*, 1667; J. P. Feighner *et al.*, *Am. J. Psychiat.*, 1972, *128*, 1230; M. Steiner *et al.*, *Curr. ther. Res.*, 1978, *23*, 655; S. Tsutsui *et al.*, *J. int. med. Res.*, 1979, *7*, 138.

Hyperthyroidism. Reports of liothyronine used together with carbimazole in the treatment of thyrotoxicosis.— W. D. Alexander *et al.*, *Lancet*, 1966, *2*, 1041; *idem*, 1967, *2*, 681; P. H. Wise *et al.*, *Br. med. J.*, 1973, *4*, 143.

Hypothyroidism. In a comparative study 18 patients with Graves' disease received liothyronine 20 µg four times daily for 12 months after thyroidectomy, while 18 similar patients received no treatment after surgery. Results suggested that temporary thyroid deficiency after surgery for thyrotoxicosis may be prevented by short-term liothyronine replacement therapy, without detriment to the functional recovery of the thyroid remnant. Further studies are needed to confirm these findings, and it is emphasised that the data and conclusions do not extend to patients undergoing surgery for thyroid nodules.— T. J. Wilkin *et al.*, *Lancet*, 1979, *2*, 63.

Myxoedemic coma. Initial treatment for patients in myxoedemic coma should be with liothyronine sodium 10 to 20 µg given by intravenous injection, followed by up to 50 µg daily given by intravenous injection in small doses at 6-hourly intervals or by slow intravenous infusion.— G. A. Smart, *Prescribers' J.*, 1972, *12*, 112.

In the treatment of myxoedemic coma liothyronine sodium could be given intravenously or by mouth in an initial dose of 50 µg followed by 25 µg every 8 hours to a maximum of 100 or 125 µg in the first 24 hours. Alternatively thyroxine sodium could be given in an initial dose of 200 µg intravenously followed by 50 µg every 8 hours, or 250 µg by mouth followed by 75 µg every 8 hours. Before subsequent doses the patient should be examined for signs of hypermetabolism or cardiac decompensation. In the presence of known cardiac disease the dose should be reduced by 25% at least.— S. R. Newmark *et al.*, *J. Am. med. Ass.*, 1974, *230*, 884. Comments.— W. L. Green (letter), *ibid.*, 1975, *233*, 508; H. V. Graham and B. R. Sevier (letter), *ibid.*

A 77-year-old man in myxoedemic coma was successfully managed using liothyronine via a nasogastric tube.— J. J. Graham and P. E. Harding, *Aust. N.Z. J. Med.*, 1977, *7*, 163.

The successful use of liothyronine given intravenously to 5 patients with myxoedemic coma. The dose of liothyronine given during the first 24 hours varied from 10 to 50 µg; the total amount given intravenously ranged from 30 to 240 µg.— A. A. Khaleeli, *Postgrad. med. J.*, 1978, *54*, 825.

Obesity. A brief review of the use of thyroid hormones for obesity. Liothyronine or thyroxine should be used in physiological replacement doses only for obese patients in whom hypothyroidism can be documented clearly by clinical and laboratory criteria.— R. S. Rivlin, *New Engl. J. Med.*, 1975, *292*, 26.

A double-blind study comparing the weight loss of obese patients given a very-low-calorie liquid dietary regimen together with liothyronine sodium 20 µg thrice daily, and that of similar patients given the dietary regimen and placebo tablets. Results indicated that some obese patients who do not readily lose weight on a low-calorie dietary regimen, may have an impaired metabolic clearance rate of liothyronine and a degree of liothyronine resistance.— R. Moore *et al.*, *Lancet*, 1980, *1*, 223. Comments and criticisms.— W. H. Taylor (letter), *ibid.*, 652; G. C. Schussler (letter), *ibid.* Reply.— R. Moore *et al.* (letter), *ibid.*

For a report of hypothyroidism following the use of liothyronine for simple obesity, and a recommendation to avoid thyroid hormones for this purpose, see Thyroxine Sodium, p.1502.

Psychosis. In a controlled study 14 psychotic and 6 severely disturbed non-psychotic euthyroid children aged 3 to 6 years were given liothyronine sodium 12.5 to 75 µg daily. Exacerbation of psychotic symptoms occurred in one child and precipitation of a florid psychosis in another; one patient's condition was unchanged, otherwise liothyronine had antipsychotic and stimulating properties and was therapeutically effective in both groups of children.— M. Campbell *et al.*, *Archs gen. Psychiat.*, 1973, *29*, 602.

Preparations

Liothyronine Sodium Tablets *(U.S.P.)*. Tablets containing liothyronine sodium. Potency is expressed in terms of the equivalent amount of liothyronine. Store in airtight containers.

Liothyronine Tablets *(B.P.)*. L-Tri-iodothyronine Sodium Tablets. Tablets containing liothyronine sodium. Protect from light.

Liotrix Tablets *(U.S.P.)*. Tablets containing thyroxine sodium and liothyronine sodium in a ratio of 4 to 1. Thyroxine potency is expressed in terms of anhydrous thyroxine sodium. The label states the thyroid equivalent. Store in airtight containers.

Proprietary Preparations

Tertroxin *(Glaxo, UK)*. Liothyronine sodium, available as scored tablets of 20 µg. (Also available as Tertroxin in *Austral., Denm., S.Afr.*).

Triiodothyronine Injection *(Glaxo, UK)*. Liothyronine sodium, available as powder for preparing injections for intravenous use, in ampoules of 20 µg, with dextran.

Other Proprietary Names

Cynomel *(Fr., Switz.)*; Cytomel *(Belg., Canad., Neth., USA)*; Halotri *(Spain)*; 3-I-T-Bowers *(Arg.)*; J-Tiron *(Ital.)*; Linomel *(Arg.)*; Ro-Thyronine *(USA)*; Thybon *(liothyronine hydrochloride) (Ger.)*; Tironina *(Spain)*; Ti-Tre *(Ital.)*; Trithyrone *(DL-liothyronine) (Fr.)*.

Proprietary Names of Liotrix

Euthroid *(Parke, Davis, USA)*; Thyrolar *(Harris, Canad.*; *Armour, USA)*.

9007-n

Thyroglobulin *(U.S.P.)*. Thyroglobulin is obtained by the fractionation of thyroid glands from the hog and contains not less than 0.7% of organically bound iodine.

CAS — 9010-34-8.

Pharmacopoeias. In *U.S.*

A cream- to tan-coloured powder with a slight characteristic odour. Practically **insoluble** in water, alcohol, chloroform, carbon tetrachloride, dimethylformamide, and dilute hydrochloric acid. **Store** in airtight containers.

A discussion on the control of thyroglobulin synthesis and secretion into the circulation, including serum-thyroglobulin concentrations in thyroid diseases.— A. J. Van Herle *et al.*, *New Engl. J. Med.*, 1979, *301*, 239 and 307.

Uses. Thyroglobulin has the actions and uses of thyroid (see p.1499) and is used as tablets of 16 to 325 mg. It is equivalent in clinical effect to thyroid, on a weight basis.

Preparations

Thyroglobulin Tablets *(U.S.P.)*. Tablets containing thyroglobulin. The label states their equivalence in terms of thyroid. Store in airtight containers.

Proprietary Names

Proloid *(Substantia, Belg.*; *Parke, Davis, Canad.*; *Warner, S.Afr.*; *Parke, Davis, USA)*; Proloide *(Warner, Arg.*; *Substancia, Spain)*.

9008-h

Thyroxine Sodium *(B.P., B.P. Vet., Eur. P.)*.

Thyroxine Sod.; Thyroxinum Natricum; Levothyroxine Sodium *(U.S.P.)*; L-Thyroxine Sodium; Levothyroxinnatrium; Levothyroxinum Natricum; Tirossina; Tiroxina Sodica. Sodium 4-*O*-(4-hydroxy-3,5-di-iodophenyl)-3,5-di-iodo-L-tyrosinate hydrate.

$C_{15}H_{10}I_4NNaO_4,xH_2O = 798.9$.

CAS — 51-48-9 (L-thyroxine); 55-03-8 (sodium salt, anhydrous); 25416-65-3 (sodium salt, hydrate).

The abbreviation T_4 is often used for thyroxine in medical and biochemical reports.

Pharmacopoeias. In *Br., Braz., Eur., Fr., Ger., It., Neth., Nord., Turk.*, and *U.S.*

Ind., Int., and Jug. specify the pentahydrate. *Arg.* includes a monograph on DL-thyroxine sodium . *Aust., Mex.*, and *Swiss* include monographs on DL-thyroxine.

An odourless almost white to pale brownish-yellow, tasteless, hygroscopic, amorphous or crystalline powder. It may assume a slight pink colour on exposure to light. Thyroxine sodium 100 µg is approximately equivalent to 67 mg of thyroid or 28 µg of liothyronine sodium.

The *B.P.* specifies 6 to 12% loss of weight on drying; the *U.S.P.* specifies not more than 11%.

Soluble 1 in 700 of water (the solubility decreasing as the pH falls) and 1 in 250 to 300 of alcohol; practically insoluble in acetone, chloroform, and ether; soluble in solutions of alkali hydroxides and in hot solutions of alkali carbonates. A saturated solution in water has a pH of about 8.9. Alkaline solutions are unstable. **Store** in airtight containers. Protect from light.

Thyroxine: its isolation, structure, stereochemistry, and biosynthesis.—Symposium on Thyroxine, *Mayo Clin. Proc.*, 1964, *39*, 545-653.

Adverse Effects. If restoration of a normal metabolic-rate is attempted too rapidly, there may be tachycardia, diarrhoea, restlessness, insomnia, tremors, excitability, anginal pain, cardiac arrhythmias, headache, sweating, fever, vomiting, and excessive loss of weight. All these reactions usually disappear on reduction of dosage or temporary withdrawal of treatment. Large doses may be fatal in patients with myxoedema complicated by heart disease.

Gross overdosage has been reported to result in a clinical state resembling thyroid storm, and in collapse and coma.

An increase in heart-rate to 104 beats per minute for a few hours was the only side-effect noted after a patient accidentally took 2 mg of thyroxine sodium instead of 200 µg on 2 successive days.— *J. Am. med. Ass.*, 1966, *197*, 379.

A woman with hypothyroidism took 10 mg of thyroxine, and vomited 2 hours later. When examined 12 hours later she was still clinically euthyroid. By the fifth day she was thyrotoxic. Propranolol hydrochloride was given from day 6 to day 16. Clinical symptoms of hypothyroidism developed on day 29 and the patient resumed thyroxine therapy.— S. E. Von Hofe and R. L. Young, *J. Am. med. Ass.*, 1977, *237*, 1361.

Abuse. Features suggestive of hyperthyroidism in 4 patients were due to the surreptitious ingestion of thyroxine-containing preparations.— R. F. Harvey, *Br. med. J.*, 1973, *2*, 35.

Neoplasm of the breast. For reports and recommendations about breast cancer associated with thyroid hormone therapy, see Thyroid, p.1499.

Pregnancy and the neonate. Of 50 282 children born to mothers monitored by the Collaborative Perinatal Project 537 were found to have been exposed to thyroid or thyroxine, and possibly other drugs, at some time during the first 4 months of pregnancy. An association between exposure to these agents and cardiac malformations was detected.— O. P. Heinonen *et al.*, *Birth Defects and Drugs in Pregnancy*, Littleton MA, Publishing Sciences Group, 1977, p. 388.

Treatment of Adverse Effects. In acute overdosage empty the stomach by aspiration and lavage or by emesis, further treatment is symptomatic. The appearance of symptoms may be delayed.

Precautions. Thyroid hormones should be used with caution in patients with cardiac disease or hypertension, and in the elderly. A patient with prolonged myxoedema should be restored to normality only gradually, as some weeks are needed for mental and physical adaptation to the normal state. In pituitary myxoedema, the adrenocortical deficiency should be treated first to prevent Addisonian crisis.

Thyroxine may enhance the action of anticoagulants and liothyronine has been reported to have similar effects on tricyclic antidepressants. Diabetics receiving thyroid hormones should be monitored for increased insulin requirements. If thyroxine therapy is initiated in digitalised patients, the dose of digitalis may require adjustment.

Malabsorption of thyroxine had been described in coeliac disease.— *Drug & Ther. Bull.*, 1976, *14*, 57.

A report of hypothyroidism in a woman taking thyroxine who had had an intestinal bypass operation and whose absorption of the hormone was impaired.— F. Azizi *et al.*, *Ann. intern. Med.*, 1979, *90*, 941.

Effects on the heart. Aldosterone excretion rates and plasma-aldosterone concentrations were monitored in 10 patients being treated with incremental doses of thyroxine for myxoedema. At a dose of 200 µg, thyroxine precipitated heart failure in 2 patients, both of whose plasma-aldosterone concentrations had risen abnormally. The heart failure resolved on reduction of the dose. One of the mechanisms of heart failure in myxoedematous patients treated rapidly with thyroxine might be induction of aldosterone with consequent salt and water retention.— P. Marks *et al.*, *Lancet*, 1978, *2*, 1277. See also K. Ølgaard and K. Borup (letter), *ibid.*, 1979, *1*, 218. Sodium retention in hypothyroid patients receiving thyroxine may have a second mechanism as well as aldosterone induction. On theoretical grounds spironolactone might be useful to reduce the risk of cardiac failure.— G. Huston (letter), *ibid.*, 387.

Interactions. A 53-year-old woman being treated with quinidine sulphate and digoxin for heart disease and with thyroxine sodium 150 µg daily for hypothyroidism developed atrial flutter with 2:1 to 4:1 atrioventricular block. Treatment with digoxin was stopped, but the other drugs were continued. On the fourth day, she was given phenytoin intravenously. During the injection she developed supraventricular tachycardia (180 to 190 beats per minute) without atrioventricular block. Atrial flutter with 2:1 atrioventricular block recurred 30 minutes after the injection. Sinus rhythm was eventually restored with quinidine. Phenytoin should be given with caution to patients receiving thyroid replacement therapy because it displaced bound thyroxine from plasma protein.— M. Fulop *et al.*, *J. Am. med. Ass.*, 1966, *196*, 454. Two cogent criticisms.— S. Farzan and H. L. Gasper (letters), *ibid.*, *197*, 63.

Studies in 5 healthy subjects indicated that cholestyramine interferes with the absorption of thyroxine, that this is greatest when the two drugs are given simultaneously, and that it can be reduced by allowing about 5 hours to elapse before giving the second of the two drugs.— R. C. Northcutt *et al.*, *J. Am. med. Ass.*, 1969, *208*, 1857. See also *ibid.*, 1898.

A 61-year-old woman taking thyroxine developed supraventricular fibrillation or tachycardia on 3 occasions when imipramine was added to her treatment.— K. B. Ramanathan and C. Davidson, *Br. med. J.*, 1975, *1*, 661. For reports of liothyronine enhancing the antidepressant effect of tricyclic antidepressants, see p.1501.

An 80-year-old woman who had been taking thyroxine 300 µg daily and 2 capsules of Tuinal (each containing quinalbarbitone sodium 100 mg and amylobarbitone sodium 100 mg), for many years, became thyrotoxic on halving her nightly dose of Tuinal. She recovered after discontinuation of her thyroxine for a week and restarting at a dose of 150 µg daily. She appears to have been euthyroid on a supranormal dose of thyroxine owing to lowering of her circulating thyroid-hormone concentrations by barbiturates.— B. I. Hoffbrand (letter), *Lancet*, 1979, *2*, 903.

Absorption and Fate. Thyroxine sodium is incompletely and variably absorbed from the gastro-intestinal tract. It is almost completely bound to plasma-proteins and has a half-life in the circulation of about a week in healthy persons and slightly longer during pregnancy and in patients with myxoedema.

A large part of the thyroxine leaving the circulation is taken up by the liver. Part of a dose of thyroxine is metabolised to tri-iodothyronine. Thyroxine is excreted in the urine as free drug, deiodinated metabolites, and conjugates. Some thyroxine is excreted in the faeces.

There is limited placental transfer of thyroxine.

Reports of the peripheral conversion of both endogenous and exogenous thyroxine to tri-iodothyronine.— L. E. Braverman *et al.*, *J. clin. Invest.*, 1970, *49*, 855; K. Sterling *et al.*, *Science*, 1970, *169*, 1099; R. D. Utiger, *A. Rev. Med.*, 1974, *25*, 289; A. Kahn, *Clin. Pharmac. Ther.*, 1976, *19*, 523.

The urinary excretion of radio-labelled thyroxine.— C. S. Pittman *et al.*, *J. clin. Invest.*, 1972, *51*, 1759.

Absorption of thyroxine may be improved in the fasting subject.— K. W. Wenzel and H. E. Kirschsieper, *Metabolism*, 1977, *26*, 1.

Excretion in breast milk. Thyroxine was not considered to enter milk in significant concentrations.— R. L. Savage, *Adverse Drug React. Bull.*, 1976, (Dec.), 212. Endogenous thyroxine may be secreted into milk in amounts sufficient to mask signs of hypothyroidism in the suckling baby.— *Br. med. J.*, 1977, *2*, 1589. See also H. H. Bode *et al.*, *Pediatrics*, 1978, *62*, 13.

Uses. Thyroxine sodium is employed in the treatment of thyroid-deficiency states. Because of its delayed effect and very long half-life, the initial dose should usually be small and the amount increased at intervals of at least 2 weeks until the minimum dose required for correct metabolic balance is achieved. A single daily dose is satisfactory. Because of its irregular absorption thyroxine sodium is best taken on an empty stomach.

In hypothyroidism the initial adult dose is usually 50 µg daily and the amount increased every 2 to 4 weeks by 50 µg until the thyroid deficiency is corrected. The adult maintenance dose is commonly between 100 and 300 µg daily. When there is evidence of cardiac insufficiency, or when the patient is elderly, the initial dose may be only 12.5 to 25 µg daily. The increments may be smaller and at longer intervals in these patients.

In myxoedemic coma, in the absence of cardiac disease, 2 to 5 ml of a solution containing 100 µg per ml has been given intravenously; an additional 100 to 300 µg may be given on the next day if there is no evidence of improvement.

A suggested dose for infants is 25 to 50 µg daily. Children older than one year may be given 2.5 to 5 µg per kg body-weight daily.

Thyroxine sodium has been given with liothyronine, but this combination may make monitoring of therapy difficult.

Combination with liothyronine. In a comparison of thyroxine sodium with a combined preparation of thyroxine sodium and liothyronine sodium in 87 hypothyroid patients, thyroxine alone was preferred because side-effects occurred less frequently.— R. N. Smith *et al.*, *Br. med. J.*, 1970, *4*, 145.

In 18 children with goitre and laboratory evidence of hypothyroidism given thyroxine 40 µg with liothyronine 10 µg, the liothyronine concentrations had reached hyperthyroid values 7 to 8 hours after administration.— V. Hesse *et al.*, *Dt. med. Wschr.*, 1977, *102*, 1412.

Myxoedemic ascites in a 62-year-old man with angina pectoris responded, after a delay of about 4 weeks, to the careful introduction of liothyronine and thyroxine.— J. A. M. Turner and J. Rapoport, *Postgrad. med. J.*, 1977, *53*, 343.

Exophthalmos of thyrotoxicosis. The effect of thyroxine sodium on the exophthalmos of thyrotoxicosis was studied in patients treated with antithyroid drugs (potassium perchlorate or carbimazole) or iodine-131. Of 68 thyrotoxic patients, 13 were treated with antithyroid drugs alone, 23 with antithyroid drugs plus thyroxine sodium, 16 with iodine-131 alone, and 16 with iodine-131 plus thyroxine sodium. The dose of thyroxine sodium was 200 µg daily. Exophthalmos was measured before treatment, when the patient became euthyroid, and 3 months later. An increase in exophthalmos was recorded in each group except the group treated by iodine-131 plus thyroxine sodium in which no significant change occurred.— D. A. Koutras *et al.*, *Br. med. J.*, 1965, *1*, 493.

Hypothyroidism. Spontaneous annular choroidoretinal detachment caused by myxoedema in a 49-year-old woman was cured by treatment with thyroxine sodium, initially 50 µg daily increased slowly over 2 to 3 weeks.— J. Richardson and M. Walsh, *Br. J. Ophthal.*, 1969, *53*, 557.

Hypothalamic hypothyroidism was diagnosed in a 53-year-old man after response to protirelin. Treatment with thyroxine sodium 100 µg daily and then a maintenance daily dose of 200 µg successfully resolved features of myxoedema and prevented somnolence.— L. Shenkman *et al.*, *J. Am. med. Ass.*, 1972, *222*, 480.

The effect of intravenous thyroxine on the blood concentrations of thyroid hormones, cholesterol (reduction), cortisol, and growth hormone in 14 hypothyroid patients.— E. C. Ridgway *et al.*, *Ann. intern. Med.*, 1972, *77*, 549. A reduction in raised plasma-triglyceride concentrations.— B. R. Tulloch *et al.*, *Lancet*, 1973, *1*, 391.

In 22 previously untreated patients with hypothyroidism, adequate control (as assessed by clinical response and reduction of serum concentrations of thyrotrophic hormone to normal) was achieved by doses of 100 µg of thyroxine (13 patients), 150 µg (6), or 200 µg (3). It was probable that many patients receiving the usually recommended doses had mild hyperthyroidism. There was no indication for the concomitant use of liothyronine and thyroxine.— D. Evered *et al.*, *Br. med. J.*, 1973, *3*, 131. The persisting abnormal lipid pattern was evidence of inadequate therapy P. B. S. Fowler (letter), *ibid.*, 352.

The maintenance dose of thyroxine sodium for patients with hypothyroidism was that which just reduced the circulating thyrotrophin to within the normal range. This was usually achieved with a thyroxine concentration of 65 to 95 ng per ml and a tri-iodothyronine concentration of 1 to 1.8 ng per ml. In 89% of patients the necessary thyroxine sodium dose was between 100 and 200 µg daily.— J. M. Stock *et al.*, *New Engl. J. Med.*, 1974, *290*, 529.

Investigations of optimum daily doses of thyroxine in hypothyroid children, based on biochemical as well as clinical assessment. Doses previously recommended were too large; overtreatment may have detrimental effects on endocrine function and bone maturation.— I. Rezvani and A. M. DiGeorge, *J. Pediat.*, 1977, *90*, 291. See also V. Abbassi and C. Aldige, *J. Pediat.*, 1977, *90*, 298.

Recommendations of the Committee on Drugs of the American Academy of Pediatrics for the dosage and use of thyroxine in cretinism.— *Pediatrics*, 1978, *62*, 413.

Prescribing patterns and problems of thyroxine-replacement therapy in 2710 patients from the Scottish Automated Follow-up Register Group.— *Br. med. J.*, 1980, *281*, 969.

Patients with raised TSH concentrations and thyroid antibodies (but not either factor alone) were at some risk of hypothyroidism and could be treated with thyroxine unless contra-indicated, e.g. because of a risk of exacerbating heart disease.— W. M. G. Tunbridge *et al.*, *Br. med. J.*, 1981, *282*, 258.

The management of hypothyroidism in patients with angina should be with thyroxine usually in an initial daily dose of 25 µg. Clinical assessment should be carried out every 2 or 3 weeks when ECG recordings and measurements of serum concentrations of thyroid-stimulating hormone should be assessed. Increments of 25 µg may be given cautiously to a maximum of 150 µg daily. Dose reduction may be necessary if the severity of angina increases; indeed in some patients adequate thyroxine replacement may be prevented by the severity of the angina.— *Br. med. J.*, 1981, *282*, 1818.

For a report of the use of thyroxine and propranolol in the treatment of myxoedema, see Propranolol Hydrochloride, p.1334.

Neoplasm of the thyroid. It was recommended that thyroxine sodium 80 to 100 µg per m^2 body-surface should be given to patients with well-differentiated thyroid carcinomas after adequate surgical and radio-iodine therapy in order to suppress endogenous stimulation by thyrotrophin.— H. Creutzig *et al.*, *Dt. med. Wschr.*, 1977, *102*, 1763.

A daily dose of 220 to 250 µg of thyroxine is considered suitable for preventing the secretion of thyroid-stimulating hormone from the pituitary after treatment of thyroid cancer. Whatever dose is judged appropriate, it must be enough totally to suppress the secretion of thyroid-stimulating hormone.— B. -A. Lamberg *et al.* (letter), *Lancet*, 1977, *2*, 1290.

Obesity. A brief review of the use of thyroid hormones as therapy for obesity. Liothyronine or thyroxine should be used in physiological replacement doses only for obese patients in whom hypothyroidism can be documented clearly by clinical and laboratory criteria.— R. S. Rivlin, *New Engl. J. Med.*, 1975, *292*, 26.

A report of hypothyroidism in 5 patients who had received thyroid hormone for 1 to 9 years for the management of simple obesity. One patient was given thyroxine 150 µg daily and the other 4 an equivalent dose of liothyronine. Since the administration of exogenous thyroxine and liothyronine is of debatable value in the treatment of simple obesity and the incidence of subclinical auto-immune thyroiditis relatively common, the use of this treatment should be reconsidered.— A. Dornhorst *et al.* (letter), *Lancet*, 1981, *1*, 52.

Pregnancy and the neonate. A favourable report of the intra-amniotic injection of thyroxine 500 µg weekly for about 6 weeks to counter possible hypothyroidism in the foetus; the mother had inadvertently been given iodine-131 during pregnancy.— E. S. Lightner *et al.*, *Am. J. Obstet. Gynec.*, 1977, *127*, 487.

Respiratory distress syndrome. Thyroid hormone substitution immediately after birth may accelerate the production of lung surfactant and hence lower mortality in premature infants.— W. Schönberger *et al.* (letter), *Lancet*, 1979, *2*, 1181.

Thyroiditis. In a study of 12 patients with Hashimoto's disease given thyroxine 100 to 300 µg daily for an average period of 9.9 years, all patients became euthyroid whilst receiving thyroxine, there was a significant decrease in goitre size in 11, and in 4 the thyroid was not palpable. The protein-bound iodine fell from 31 ng per ml before treatment to 16 ng per ml six weeks after stopping thyroxine when 11 of the patients became hypothyroid despite a 5- to 16-fold increase in thyroid-stimulating hormone.— P. D. Papapetrou *et al.*, *Lancet*, 1972, *2*, 1045.

Preparations

Levothyroxine Sodium Tablets *(U.S.P.)*. Tablets containing thyroxine sodium. Potency is expressed in terms of the equivalent amount of anhydrous thyroxine sodium. Store in airtight containers. Protect from light.

Thyroxine Tablets *(B.P.)*. Thyroxine Sodium Tablets; L-Thyroxine Sodium Tablets. Tablets containing thyroxine sodium. Potency is expressed in terms of anhydrous thyroxine sodium. Protect from light.

NOTE. The *B.P. 1973* expressed potency in terms of thyroxine sodium pentahydrate 111 µg of which is equivalent to 100 µg of anhydrous thyroxine sodium.

Eltroxin *(Glaxo, UK)*. Thyroxine sodium, available as scored tablets of 50 µg and as tablets of 100 µg. Potency is expressed in terms of anhydrous thyroxine sodium. (Also available as Eltroxin in *Austral.*, *Canad.*, *Denm.*, *S.Afr.*, and *Switz.*).

Other Proprietary Names

Austral.—Oroxine, Thyroxinal; *Belg.*—Elthyrone, Euthyrox; *Canad.*—Synthroid; *Fr.*— Percutacrine Thyroxinique; *Ger.*—Euthyrox, Thevier; *Swed.*—Levaxin; *Switz.*—Eltroxine; *USA*—Cytolen, Levoid, Levothyroid, Ro-Thyroxine, Synthroid.

9009-m

Tiratricol. Triiodothyroacetic acid; Triac. [4-(4-Hydroxy-3-iodophenoxy)-3,5-di-iodophenyl]acetic acid. $C_{14}H_9I_3O_4$=622.0.

CAS — 51-24-1.

NOTE. The name Triac has also been applied to the diethanolamine salt of tiratricol.

Adverse Effects.

Hypertrophy and changes resembling human hypertrophic cardiomyopathy in the offspring of pregnant *rats* fed tiratricol diethanolamine salt.— E. G. J. Olsen *et al.*, *Lancet*, 1977, *2*, 221. See also C. Symons *et al.*, *ibid.*, 1971, *2*, 1163.

Uses. Tiratricol is a thyroid hormone with general properties similar to those of Thyroxine Sodium, p.1501. It has been stated to act more rapidly than thyroxine.

A brief review of early studies on tiratricol. Dosage and use in myxoedema. The cardiac effects of small doses.— K. Ibbertson *et al.*, *Br. med. J.*, 1959, *2*, 52.

Proprietary Names

Téatrois *(Théranol, Fr.)*; Triacana *(Ana, Fr.)*.

Tranquillisers

7000-n

The term tranquilliser is commonly used for anxiolytic sedatives, which act against anxiety, and neuroleptics, which act against psychoses.

Anxiolytic sedatives or *anti-anxiety sedatives*, formerly called *minor tranquillisers* include the benzodiazepines, the carbamates, and a number of chemically unrelated compounds such as benzoctamine, chlormezanone, and phenaglycodol. These are used in the symptomatic treatment of psychoneuroses to reduce pathological anxiety, agitation, and tension.

Neuroleptics, formerly called *major tranquillisers, ataractics*, or *antipsychotics* include the butyrophenones and related compounds, oxypertine, the phenothiazines, and the thioxanthenes. They are used mainly for the symptomatic treatment of psychoses, such as schizophrenia, mania, and senile dementia. The rauwolfia alkaloids (see p.135) were also formerly used in the treatment of psychotic states.

Lithium salts, which have no specific sedative or stimulant properties, but have an action on mania and the recurrence of manic-depressive psychosis, have been termed *antimanic agents*.

The main tranquillisers described in this section include the following groups:

Benzodiazepines:
bromazepam, p.1505; chlordiazepoxide, p.1506; clorazepate, p.1518; diazepam, p.1519; lorazepam, p.1543; medazepam, p.1545; oxazepam, p.1549; prazepam, p.1554.

Butyrophenones and related compounds:
benperidol, p.1505; droperidol, p.1526; fluspirilene, p.1531; haloperidol, p.1532; penfluridol, p.1550; pimozide, p.1552; trifluperidol, p.1563.

Carbamates:
meprobamate, p.1545; tybamate, p.1563.

Phenothiazines:
with a *dimethylaminopropyl* side-chain,
chlorpromazine, p.1509; fluopromazine, p.1527; methotrimeprazine, p.1547; promazine, p.1556.
with a *piperidine* side-chain,
pericyazine, p.1551; piperacetazine, p.1553; pipothiazine, p.1553; thioridazine, p.1559.
with a *piperazine* side-chain,
acetophenazine, p.1504; butaperazine, p.1505; carphenazine, p.1506; fluphenazine, p.1529; perphenazine, p.1551; prochlorperazine, p.1554; thiethylperazine, p.1558; thiopropazate, p.1558; thioproperazine, p.1559; trifluoperazine, p.1562.

The tranquillising and antipsychotic properties of phenothiazines in the 3 groups are qualitatively similar but those with the dimethylaminopropyl side-chain generally have more marked sedative effects. Those with a piperazine side-chain cause less hypotension, tachycardia, and drowsiness, but are most likely to cause extrapyramidal dysfunction. Those with a piperidine side-chain are least likely to cause extrapyramidal dysfunction.

Thioxanthenes:
chlorprothixene, p.1516; flupenthixol, p.1528; thiothixene, p.1561.

Other tranquillisers described which are not so readily classified include:
benzoctamine, p.1505; chlormezanone, p.1508; lithium, p.1534; loxapine, p.1544; molindone, p.1548; oxypertine, p.1550; phenaglycodol, p.1552; tetrabenazine, p.1557.

Psychotropic drugs act on psychic function, behaviour, or experience; they alter the mental state by affecting the neurophysiological and biochemical activity of the functional units of the CNS. They include: *neuroleptics*, formerly known as *major tranquillisers, ataractics* or *antipsychotics*, with effects on the psychoses and other psychiatric disorders; *anxiolytic sedatives*, formerly known as *minor tranquillisers*, reduce pathological anxiety, tension, and agitation without therapeutic effects on neurological symptoms; *antidepressants* also called *psychic energisers* or *thymoleptics*, are drugs used in the treatment of pathological depressive states; *psychostimulants* are drugs used to increase the level of alertness or of motivation; and *psychodysleptics*, also called *hallucinogens, psychotomimetics*, or *psychodelics*, are compounds that produce abnormal mental phenomena, particularly in the cognitive and perceptual spheres. The anxiolytic sedatives, the psychodysleptics, and psychostimulants have marked dependence-producing properties.— *Chronicle Wld Hlth Org.*, 1967, *21*, 463. The classification of tranquillisers, their clinical effectiveness, and their adverse clinical effects. — Research in Psychopharmacology, *Tech. Rep. Ser. Wld Hlth Org. No. 371*, 1967.

General reviews of mental disorders and drugs acting on the mental state.— M. H. Lader, *Br. J. Hosp. Med.*, 1976, *16*, 622; P. A. Berger, *Science*, 1978, *200*, 974; T. M. Itil *et al.*, *Int. Pharmacopsychiat.*, 1978, *13*, 39; M. O. Olatawura, *Bull Wld Hlth Org.*, 1978, *56*, 519.

Declaration adopted by the General Assembly of the World Psychiatric Association at the Sixth World Congress of Psychiatry, 1977.— *Br. med. J.*, 1977, *2*, 1204.

Dependence. For reviews of the dependence liability of some tranquillisers, see H. Isbell and T. L. Chruściel, *Dependence Liability of 'Non-narcotic' Drugs*, Geneva, World Health Organization, 1970; *idem*, *Bull. Wld Hlth Org.*, 1970, *43*, *Suppl.*;; H. Kalant *et al.*, *Pharmac. Rev.*, 1971, *23*, 135.

7001-h

Acepromazine Maleate *(B.P. Vet.)*. Acetylpromazine Maleate. 10-(3-Dimethylaminopropyl)phenothiazin-2-yl methyl ketone hydrogen maleate.
$C_{19}H_{22}N_2OS,C_4H_4O_4$=442.5.

CAS — 61-00-7 (acepromazine); 3598-37-6 (maleate).

Pharmacopoeias. In *Fr.*

A yellow odourless crystalline powder. M.p. 136° to 139°. Acepromazine maleate 13.5 mg is approximately equivalent to 10 mg of acepromazine.
Soluble 1 in 27 of water, 1 in 13 of alcohol, and 1 in 3 of chloroform; slightly soluble in ether and light petroleum. A 1% solution in water has a pH of 4 to 4.5. Solutions for injection are **sterilised** by autoclaving or by filtration. **Protect** from light.

Acepromazine is a phenothiazine with general properties resembling those of chlorpromazine (p.1509). It is used in conjunction with etorphine hydrochloride (see p.1012), for the immobilisation of large *animals*.

The Japanese Ministry of Health and Welfare in assessing drug efficacy considered that acepromazine maleate had no substantial evidence of bioavailability and was ineffective. The drug was ordered to be withdrawn from the Japanese market.— *Japan med. Gaz.*, 1973, *10* (Dec. 20), 1.

For a report of the accidental injection of a veterinary preparation of acepromazine with etorphine in a 41-year-old man, see Etorphine Hydrochloride, p.1012.

Proprietary Names
Plégicil *(base) (Clin-Comar-Byla, Fr.)*; Plegicil *(maleate) (Pharmacia, Denm.; Seid, Spain)*.

NOTE. Acepromazine maleate is an ingredient of Immobilon (for large animals), see Etorphine Hydrochloride, p.1012..

7002-m

Acetophenazine Maleate *(U.S.P.)*.

Acetophenazine Maleate; Acetophenazine Dimaleate; Sch 6673. 10-{3-[4-(2-Hydroxyethyl)piperazin-1-yl]-propyl}phenothiazin-2-yl methyl ketone dimaleate.
$C_{23}H_{29}N_3O_2S,2C_4H_4O_4$=643.7.

CAS — 2751-68-0 (acetophenazine); 5714-00-1 (maleate).

Pharmacopoeias. In *U.S.*

A fine yellow powder. M.p. about 165° with decomposition. **Soluble** 1 in 10 of water, 1 in 260 of alcohol, 1 in 370 of acetone, 1 in 2850 of chloroform, 1 in 6000 of ether, and 1 in 11 of propylene glycol. **Store** in airtight containers.

Adverse Effects, Treatment, and Precautions. As for Chlorpromazine, p.1509.
Extrapyramidal symptoms may be more common than the other side-effects.

Absorption and Fate. For an account of the absorption and fate of a phenothiazine, see Chlorpromazine, p.1513.

Uses. Acetophenazine maleate is a phenothiazine with actions and uses similar to those of chlorpromazine (p.1513). It has a piperazine side-chain.
The usual dose for the treatment of psychoses is 20 mg thrice daily, with a range of 40 to 120 mg daily. In severe schizophrenia doses of up to 400 to 600 mg daily have been given.

Schizophrenia. In a double-blind controlled study lasting 6 weeks, 100 men with schizophrenia were treated with 1 of 3 drugs in the following average daily doses: acetophenazine 142 mg; perphenazine 52 mg; and benzquinamide 1.26 g. Each drug produced considerable improvement, which was slightly more marked in patients with paranoid symptoms.— L. E. Hollister *et al.*, *Clin. Pharmac. Ther.*, 1967, *8*, 249.

Further references: J. E. Overall *et al.*, *Clin. Pharmac. Ther.*, 1963, *4*, 200.

Preparations

Acetophenazine Maleate Tablets *(U.S.P.)*. Tablets containing acetophenazine maleate. Store in airtight containers.

Proprietary Names
Tindal *(Schering, Denm.; Schering, USA)*; Tindala *(Schering, Swed.)*.

7003-b

Alprazolam. U 31889. 8-Chloro-1-methyl-6-phenyl-4*H*-1,2,4-triazolo[4,3-*a*][1,4]benzodiazepine.
$C_{17}H_{13}ClN_4$=308.8.

CAS — 28981-97-7.

Alprazolam is a benzodiazepine with the general properties of diazepam (p.1519). For the treatment of anxiety it has been given in doses of 0.5 to 1 mg twice or thrice daily.

References to alprazolam.— T. M. Itil *et al.*, *Curr. ther. Res.*, 1973, *15*, 603; L. F. Fabre and R. T. Harris, *ibid.*, 1974, *16*, 1010; L. F. Fabre, *ibid.*, 1976, *19*, 661; L. F. Fabre *et al.*, *J. int. med. Res.*, 1977, *5*, 26; L. F. Fabre and D. M. McLendon, *Curr. ther. Res.*, 1979, *25*, 519; D. M. McLendon and L. F. Fabre, *ibid.*, *26*, 430; G. C. Aden and S. G. Thein, *J. clin. Psychiat.*, 1980, *41*, 245; L. F. Fabre and D. M. McLendon, *Curr. ther. Res.*, 1980, *27*, 474; B. M. Maletzky, *J. int. med. Res.*, 1980, *8*, 139.

Proprietary Names
Xanax *(Upjohn, USA)*.

7004-v

Azacyclonol Hydrochloride. Azacyclonolium Chloride; MER-17. α-Phenyl-α-4-piperidylbenzyl alcohol hydrochloride.
$C_{18}H_{21}NO,HCl$=303.8.

CAS — 115-46-8 (azacyclonol); 1798-50-1 (hydrochloride).

Odourless small white crystals or crystalline powder. Stable in dry air. **Soluble** 1 in 200 of water and 1 in 1000 of alcohol; practically insoluble in acetone, chloroform, ether, and light petroleum. A saturated solution in water has a pH of 5 to 7.

Azacyclonol has been given as the hydrochloride in the treatment of psychoses in doses of 100 to 800 mg daily.

Proprietary Names
Frenquel *(Merrell Toraude, Fr.)*.

7005-g

Benactyzine Hydrochloride *(B.P.C. 1959).* 2-Diethylaminoethyl benzilate hydrochloride.
$C_{20}H_{25}NO_3,HCl=363.9$.

CAS — 302-40-9 (benactyzine); 57-37-4 (hydrochloride).

Pharmacopoeias. In *Cz.* and *Pol.*

An odourless white crystalline powder with a bitter taste. **Soluble** 1 in 14 of water and 1 in 22 of alcohol; very slightly soluble in ether. A 2% solution in water has a pH of 3.5 to 5.7.

Benactyzine possesses anticholinergic and muscle relaxant properties, exhibits a quinidine-like action on the heart, and is a local anaesthetic. It has a brief duration of action. It has been used as the hydrochloride in the management of psychoneurotic disorders in doses of 1 to 3 mg thrice daily.
Benactyzine Methobromide ($C_{21}H_{28}BrNO_3$ = 422.4) has been advocated as an antispasmodic.

Proprietary Names
Alin *(Lazar, Arg.)*; Lucidex *(Rioplatense, Arg.).*

7006-q

Benperidol.
CB 8089; R 4584; Benzperidol. 1-{1-[3-(4-Fluorobenzoyl)propyl]-4-piperidyl}benzimidazolin-2-one.
$C_{22}H_{24}FN_3O_2=381.4$.

CAS — 2062-84-2.

An off-white amorphous powder or crystals. M.p. 170° to 175°. Practically **insoluble** in water; soluble 1 in 1000 of alcohol, 1 in 4 of chloroform, 1 in 625 of ether, and 1 in 7 of acetic acid; sparingly soluble in dilute mineral acids.

Benperidol is a butyrophenone with general properties similar to those of haloperidol (p.1532). Doses of 0.25 to 1.5 mg daily have been given in the management of aberrant sexual behaviour.

Effects on sexual function. Results of a double-blind placebo-controlled crossover study demonstrated no significant difference between the effect of benperidol 1.25 mg daily, chlorpromazine 125 mg daily, or placebo, on sexual drive and arousal in 12 paedophilic sexual offenders. The only significant difference was that self-rating of frequency of sexual thoughts was lower with benperidol. The effects of benperidol are unlikely to be sufficient to control severe forms of antisocial sexually deviant behaviour.— G. Tennent *et al., Archs sex. Behav.*, 1974, *3,* 261. Current evidence is insufficient to substantiate the claim that benperidol has a specific action on sexual disorders.— *Drug & Ther. Bull.*, 1974, *12,* 12.

Psychoses. The use of benperidol in doses of up to 9 mg daily in 65 patients with psychoses, mostly of schizophrenic origin.— K. A. Flügel and W. M. Pfeiffer, *Arzneimittel-Forsch.*, 1967, *17,* 483.

Proprietary Preparations
Anquil *(Janssen, UK).* Benperidol, available as tablets of 250 µg. (Also available as Anquil in *S.Afr.*).

Other Proprietary Names
Frenactil *(Belg., Fr., Neth.)*; Glianimon *(Ger.).*

7007-p

Benzoctamine Hydrochloride. Ba 30803. *N*-(9,10-Dihydro-9,10-ethanoanthracen-9-ylmethyl)methylamine hydrochloride.
$C_{18}H_{19}N,HCl=285.8$.

CAS — 17243-39-9 (benzoctamine); 10085-81-1 (hydrochloride).

A white odourless crystalline powder with a bitter taste.

Adverse Effects. Sedation and dryness of the mouth appear to be the most common effects.

Precautions. Benzoctamine should be used with caution in patients with renal or hepatic impairment. It may impair the patient's ability to drive vehicles or take charge of other machinery.

Absorption and Fate. Benzoctamine is readily absorbed from the gastro-intestinal tract and has been reported to produce peak blood concentrations within 2 hours. It is metabolised in the liver and rapidly excreted mainly as glucuronide conjugates in the urine.

Uses. Benzoctamine hydrochloride is reported to have central and peripheral actions. It is used in the treatment of anxiety and tension states in doses of 10 to 20 mg thrice daily. Benzoctamine has also been used as the mesylate for intramuscular or slow intravenous injection.

Anaesthesia. When 30 patients were given benzoctamine as a premedicant in doses of 10, 20, and 40 mg intravenously and compared with 25 patients given diazepam 10 mg and 25 given sodium chloride injection, it was found that benzoctamine possessed a hypnotic effect similar to that of diazepam but no anxiolytic effects. It was considered to have no place in anaesthesia and was withdrawn from further study.— W. McCaughy *et al.* (letter), *Br. J. Anaesth.*, 1974, *46,* 189.

Anxiety. In a survey of 10 703 patients with moderate to severe anxiety, benzoctamine 10 mg thrice daily for 3 weeks gave symptomatic relief in 85% during the treatment period and 55% remained symptom-free for longer periods. Drowsiness was the most common side-effect.— W. A. Forrest, *Curr. ther. Res.*, 1972, *14,* 227.

In a 3-week double-blind crossover trial in 6 patients diazepam 5 to 10 mg thrice daily reduced anxiety more effectively than benzoctamine 10 to 20 mg thrice daily; the latter was no more effective that placebo.— W. R. McLeod, *Curr. ther. Res.*, 1972, *14,* 239.

In a double-blind comparison of benzoctamine and chlordiazepoxide in patients with anxiety neurosis, both drugs produced a similar therapeutic response. With both drugs, doses of 10 to 30 mg were given and 26 patients received benzoctamine compared with 29 who received chlordiazepoxide. Side-effects were more frequent in the benzoctamine group.— W. H. Lo and T. Lo, *J. clin. Pharmac.*, 1973, *13,* 48.

Benzoctamine 10 mg thrice daily was not significantly more effective than placebo in a double-blind study of 25 anxious patients.— J. S. Teja *et al., Curr. ther. Res.*, 1975, *18,* 354.

Further references.— B. J. Goldstein and D. M. Weiner, *J. clin. Pharmac.*, 1970, *10,* 19 and 194; R. L. Biddy *et al., ibid.*, 29.

Hypnotic effect. For the effect of benzoctamine on anxiety, the ability to concentrate, various stages of sleep, and plasma concentrations of growth hormone and corticosteroids, see O. O. Ogunremi *et al., Br. med. J.*, 1973, *2,* 202.

Spasticity. In 12 psychiatric patients with neurological defects causing spasticity in 1 or more limbs, benzoctamine 10 mg (but not 20 or 30 mg) reduced the latency period of the patellar reflex 2 hours after the dose.— Y. D. Lapierre *et al., Curr. ther. Res.*, 1973, *15,* 521.

Proprietary Preparations
Tacitin *(Ciba, UK).* Benzoctamine hydrochloride, available as tablets of 10 mg. (Also available as Tacitin in *Denm., Ger., Neth., Norw., S.Afr., Switz.* Tacitin is also available in *Ger., Norw., Switz.* as an injection containing benzoctamine mesylate).

Other Proprietary Names
Tacitine *(Fr.).*

7008-s

Bromazepam.
Ro 5-3350. 7-Bromo-1,3-dihydro-5-(2-pyridyl)-2*H*-1,4-benzodiazepin-2-one.
$C_{14}H_{10}BrN_3O=316.2$.

CAS — 1812-30-2.

A pale yellow crystalline solid. M.p. about 247°.

Dependence. Prolonged use of bromazepam may lead to the development of dependence of the barbiturate-alcohol type (see p.792). It has a low liability for abuse.

Adverse Effects, Treatment, and Precautions. As for Diazepam, p.1520.

Absorption and Fate. For an account of the absorption and fate of a benzodiazepine, see Diazepam, p.1522.

A study of the clinical pharmacokinetics of bromazepam in healthy subjects. Following administration of 12 mg by mouth to 10 subjects bromazepam appeared to be completely absorbed from the gastro-intestinal tract and peak plasma concentrations were obtained within 1 to 4 hours of administration. The plasma elimination half-life ranged from 7.9 to 19.3 hours (mean 11.9 hours). It was excreted in the urine almost entirely as the glucuronide conjugates of 3-hydroxybromezepam and the 3-hydroxybenzoylpyridine derivative (a mean of 27% and 40% of the dose, respectively), with a mean of only 2.3% as intact bromazepam and only 0.66% as the intact benzoylpyridine derivative. Studies of multiple daily dosing in 6 of the 10 subjects revealed similar pharmacokinetic findings.— S. A. Kaplan *et al., J. Pharmacokinet. Biopharm.*, 1976, *4,* 1.

Metabolism. The major metabolites excreted in the urine of 3 women after a single 12-mg oral dose of bromazepam were conjugated 3-hydroxylated derivatives [3-hydroxybromazepam and 2-(2-amino-5-bromo-3-hydroxybenzoyl)pyridine].— M. A. Schwartz *et al., J. pharm. Sci.*, 1973, *62,* 1776.

Further references.— J. A. F. de Silva *et al., J. pharm. Sci.*, 1974, *63,* 1440; J. Raaflaub and J. Speiser-Courvoisier, *Arzneimittel-Forsch.*, 1974, *24,* 1841.

Uses. Bromazepam is a benzodiazepine with actions and uses similar to those of diazepam (p.1523). The usual dose for the treatment of anxiety is 3 mg twice or thrice daily; in severe conditions up to 6 to 12 mg twice or thrice daily have been given.

Action. Reviews of the actions and uses of bromazepam.— *Drugs Today*, 1975, *11,* 31; *Aust. J. Pharm.*, 1976, *60,* 101.

Anxiety. Comparison of bromazepam with diazepam. Both drugs caused a similar incidence of drowsiness. Other side-effects for bromazepam included a rash and a confused mental state in 1 patient which subsided on withdrawal.— Y. D. Lapierre *et al., Curr. ther. Res.*, 1978, *23,* 475.

Further references.— K. Rickels *et al., Curr. ther. Res.*, 1973, *15,* 679.

Depression. A beneficial response to bromazepam in anxiety-depressive neurosis.— E. Shammas, *Dis. nerv. Syst.*, 1977, *38,* 201.

For comments on the use of benzodiazepines in depression, see Diazepam, p.1525.

Hypertension. Antihypertensive effects of bromazepam.— H. Pozenel *et al., Int. J. clin. Pharmac. Biopharm.*, 1977, *15,* 31; M. Masso and H. Perez, *Pharmatherapeutica*, 1979, *2,* 195.

For criticism of the use of diazepam or any other sedative drug in hypertension, see Diazepam, p.1525.

Proprietary Names
Lexatin *(Roche, Spain)*; Lexotan *(Roche, Austral.; Roche, Belg.; Roche, Denm.; Roche, Ital.; Jap.; Roche, S.Afr.)*; Lexotanil *(Roche, Arg.; Roche, Ger.; Roche, Neth.; Roche, Switz.).*

7009-w

Bromperidol. R 11333 *(*bromperidol*)*; R 46541 *(*decanoate*)*. 4-[4-(4-Bromophenyl)-4-hydroxypiperidino]-4′-fluorobutyrophenone.
$C_{21}H_{23}BrFNO_2=420.3$.

CAS — 10457-90-6.

White or yellowish amorphous or microcrystalline powder. M.p. about 156°. Very slightly **soluble** in water; soluble in dilute solutions of organic acids.

Bromperidol is a butyrophenone with general propertics similar to those of haloperidol (p.1532). It has been given in doses of about 6 to 8 mg daily in the treatment of psychosis; higher doses have also been used. It has been given intramuscularly in doses of 5 to 15 mg daily.

A symposium on bromperidol.— Acta psychiat. belg., 1978, *78,* 1–211.

Proprietary Names
Azuren *(Janssen, Belg.).*

7010-m

Butaperazine Maleate. Bayer 1362; Riker 595 *(*both butaperazine*)*; Butaperazine Dimaleate. 1-{10-[3-(4-Methylpiperazin-1-yl)propyl]phenothiazin-2-yl}butan-1-one dimaleate.
$C_{24}H_{31}N_3OS,2C_4H_4O_4=641.7$.

CAS — 653-03-2 (butaperazine); 1063-55-4 (maleate).

A yellow crystalline powder. M.p. about 195°. Butaperazine maleate 1.6 g is approximately equivalent to 1 g of butaperazine. **Soluble** in water; practically insoluble in chloroform and ether.

7011-b

Butaperazine Phosphate. Butaperazine Diphosphate. $C_{24}H_{31}N_3OS,2H_3PO_4$=605.6.

CAS — 7389-45-9.

A yellow crystalline powder. M.p. 161° to 162°. Butaperazine phosphate 1.5 g is approximately equivalent to 1 g of butaperazine. **Soluble** in water; practically insoluble in chloroform and ether.

Adverse Effects, Treatment, and Precautions. As for Chlorpromazine, p.1509.
Extrapyramidal symptoms may be more common that the other side-effects.

Interactions. *Steroids.* Plasma-butaperazine concentrations in 4 subjects were higher while they were receiving conjugated oestrogens than during control periods.— M. K. El-Yousef and D. H. Manier (letter), *J. Am. med. Ass.*, 1974, *228,* 827.

Tricyclic antidepressants. Concomitant administration of desipramine hydrochloride 150 mg or more daily and butaperazine maleate 20 mg twice daily resulted in a significant increase in plasma-butaperazine concentrations compared with concentrations achieved when butaperazine alone was given in 6 schizophrenic subjects. In 2 patients given 75 and 100 mg of desipramine daily no significant difference occurred.— M. K. El-Yousef and D. H. Manier (letter), *J. Am. med. Ass.*, 1974, *229,* 1419.

Absorption and Fate. For an account of the absorption and fate of a phenothiazine, see Chlorpromazine, p.1513.

References: D. L. Garver *et al.*, *Am. J. Psychiat.*, 1977, *134,* 304 (blood concentrations); T. B. Cooper, *Clin. Pharmacokinet.*, 1978, *3,* 14 (blood concentrations); R. C. Smith *et al.*, *Archs gen. Psychiat.*, 1979, *36,* 579 (blood concentrations).

Uses. Butaperazine is a phenothiazine with general properties similar to those of chlorpromazine (p.1513). It has a piperazine side-chain.
Butaperazine is administered by mouth as the maleate and has been given by injection as the phosphate.
The usual dose for the treatment of psychoses is 5 to 10 mg of butaperazine thrice daily, given by mouth as the maleate, to a maximum of 100 mg daily, in divided doses. It has also been given by deep intramuscular injection as the phosphate.

Schizophrenia. References to butaperazine in schizophrenia: M. L. Clark *et al.*, *Clin. Pharmac. Ther.*, 1968, *9,* 757; R. K. Brotman *et al.*, *Curr. ther. Res.*, 1969, *11,* 5; G. M. Simpson *et al.*, *J. clin. Pharmac.*, 1973, *13,* 288.

Proprietary Names
Repoise (maleate) *(Robins, USA)*; Randolectil (maleate) *(Bayer, Arg.)*.

7012-v

Camazepam. SB 5833. 7-Chloro-2,3-dihydro-1-methyl-2-oxo-5-phenyl-1*H*-1,4-benzodiazepin-3-yl dimethylcarbamate.
$C_{19}H_{18}ClN_3O_3$=371.8.

CAS — 36104-80-0.

A white crystalline powder. **Soluble** in water and alcohol.

Camazepam is a benzodiazepine with the general properties of diazepam (p.1519). The usual dose for the treatment of anxiety is 10 mg twice or thrice daily; in severe conditions up to 20 mg thrice daily has been given.

Action. Reviews of the action and uses of camazepam.— *Drugs Today*, 1977, *13,* 521.

Animal studies on the action of camazepam.— L. Merlo *et al.*, *Arzneimittel-Forsch.*, 1974, *24,* 1759; R. Ferrini *et al.*, *ibid.*, 2029.

Administration. In the elderly. A study of camazepam in elderly patients.— A. Tammaro *et al.*, *Arzneimittel-Forsch.*, 1977, *27,* 2177.

Anaesthesia. Camazepam in endoscopy.— G. Galli, *Curr. ther. Res.*, 1976, *19,* 316.

Anxiety. Studies of camazepam in the treatment of anxiety.— R. Deberdt, *Curr. ther. Res.*, 1975, *17,* 32; S. Carrara *et al.*, *Eur. J. clin. Pharmac.*, 1978, *13,* 335.

Depression. Camazepam in anxiety and depression.— M. Cesa-Bianchi *et al.*, *Arzneimittel-Forsch.*, 1974, *24,* 2032.

For comments on the use of benzodiazepines in depression, see Diazepam, p.1525.

Proprietary Names
Albego *(Sintesa, Belg.*; *Boehringer Ingelheim, Ger.*; *Simes, Ital.*; *ICN, Neth.*; *Inpharzam, Switz.)*; Limpidon *(Crinos, Ital.)*; Paxor *(Bristol, Belg.)*.

7013-g

Captodiame Hydrochloride. Captodiamine Hydrochloride. 2-(4-Butylthiobenzhydrylthio)-*NN*-dimethylethylamine hydrochloride.
$C_{21}H_{29}NS_2,HCl$=396.0.

CAS — 486-17-9 (captodiame); 904-04-1 (hydrochloride).

Captodiame hydrochloride has been given in doses of 50 mg thrice daily for the treatment of anxiety and tension.

Proprietary Names
Covatine *(Bailly, Fr.)*.

7014-q

Carphenazine Maleate *(U.S.P.)*.

Carfenazine Maleate; Wy 2445. 1-(10-{3-[4-(2-Hydroxyethyl)piperazin-1-yl]propyl}phenothiazin-2-yl)propan-1-one.
$C_{24}H_{31}N_3O_2S,2C_4H_4O_4$=657.7.

CAS — 2622-30-2 (carphenazine); 2975-34-0 (maleate).

Pharmacopoeias. In *U.S.*

A fine yellow powder, odourless or with a slight odour. M.p. 176° to 185°, with a range of not more than 3°, with decomposition. **Soluble** 1 in 600 of water and 1 in 400 of alcohol; practically insoluble in chloroform and ether. A 1% suspension in water has a pH of 2.5 to 3.5. **Store** in airtight containers. Protect from light.

Adverse Effects, Treatment, and Precautions. As for Chlorpromazine, p.1509.
Extrapyramidal symptoms may be more common than the other side-effects.

Purpura. Allergic purpura in a 67-year-old schizophrenic woman was associated with carphenazine therapy.— H. J. Corneille, *Am. J. Psychiat.*, 1965, *121,* 814.

Absorption and Fate. For an account of the absorption and fate of a phenothiazine, see Chlorpromazine, p.1513.

Uses. Carphenazine is a phenothiazine with general properties similar to those of chlorpromazine (p.1513). It has a piperazine side-chain.
Carphenazine has been given in psychoses as the maleate in usual doses of 25 to 50 mg thrice daily, to a maximum of 400 mg daily in divided doses.

Schizophrenia. Reports of the uses of carphenazine maleate in the treatment of schizophrenia: L. M. Cowley, *Dis. nerv. Syst.*, 1967, *28,* 126; M. H. Orzack *et al.*, *Psychopharmacologia*, 1967, *11,* 31; O. Vinar *et al.*, *Activitas nerv. sup.*, 1967, *9,* 353; G. Bora, *Dis. nerv. Syst.*, 1968, *29,* 695.

Preparations

Carphenazine Maleate Oral Solution *(U.S.P.)*. Carphenazine Maleate Solution. A solution containing carphenazine maleate. pH 5.8 to 6.8. Store in airtight containers. Protect from light.

Carphenazine Maleate Tablets *(U.S.P.)*. Tablets containing carphenazine maleate. Store in airtight containers. Protect from light.

Proprietary Names
Proketazine *(Wyeth, USA)*.

7015-p

Carpipramine Hydrochloride. PZ 1511. 1-[3-(10,11-Dihydro-5*H*-dibenz[*b,f*]azepin-5-yl)propyl]-4-piperidinopiperidine-4-carboxamide dihydrochloride monohydrate.
$C_{28}H_{38}N_4O,2HCl,H_2O$=537.6.

CAS — 5942-95-0 (carpipramine); 7075-03-8 (hydrochloride, anhydrous).

Carpipramine is structurally related to imipramine (p.119). It has been advocated as an adjunct in the treatment of psychoses. It is given as the hydrochloride in a usual dose equivalent to 50 mg of the base thrice daily, with a range of 50 to 400 mg daily.

References.— *Japan med. Gaz.*, 1975, *12* (Feb. 20), 6; *ibid.*, 1977, *14* (Aug. 20), 7; F. Eckmann *et al.*, *Arzneimittel-Forsch.*, 1977, *27,* 148.

Proprietary Names
Defekton *(Jap.)*; Prazinil *(Specia, Fr.)*.

7016-s

Chloracyzine Hydrochloride. Chloracizinum. 2-Chloro-10-(3-diethylaminopropionyl)phenothiazine hydrochloride.
$C_{19}H_{21}ClN_2OS,HCl$=397.4.

CAS — 800-22-6 (chloracyzine); 1045-82-5 (hydrochloride).

Pharmacopoeias. In *Rus.*

A white to slightly yellowish-white crystalline powder. M.p. 171° to 175°. Freely **soluble** in water and methyl alcohol; soluble in alcohol; practically insoluble in ether. **Store** in airtight containers. Protect from light.

Chloracyzine hydrochloride is a phenothiazine derivative which is reported to have antispasmodic actions. It has been used as a coronary vasodilator and has been given in maximum single doses of 50 mg and maximum total doses in 24 hours of 150 mg.

Cardiac disorders. Studies in *cats* indicated that the anti-anginal activity of chloracyzine might be associated with more efficient oxygen use.— I. E. Kisin, *Br. J. Pharmac.*, 1976, *58,* 189.

Preparations

Tabulettae Chloracizini Obductae *(Rus. P.)*. Chloracyzine Hydrochloride Tablets. Coated tablets each containing chloracyzine hydrochloride 15 mg.

7017-w

Chlordiazepoxide *(B.P., U.S.P.)*.

Methaminodiazepoxide. 7-Chloro-2-methylamino-5-phenyl-3*H*-1,4-benzodiazepine 4-oxide.
$C_{16}H_{14}ClN_3O$=299.8.

CAS — 58-25-3.

Pharmacopoeias. In *Br.*, *Braz.*, *Chin.*, *Cz.*, *Jap.*, *Jug.*, *Nord.*, *Roum.*, and *U.S.*

A yellow, odourless or almost odourless, crystalline powder, sensitive to sunlight. M.p. about 240°. Chlordiazepoxide 1 mg is approximately equivalent to 1.1 mg of chlordiazepoxide hydrochloride. Practically **insoluble** in water; soluble 1 in 50 of alcohol and 1 in 130 of ether; slightly soluble in chloroform. **Store** in airtight containers. Protect from light.

7018-e

Chlordiazepoxide Hydrochloride *(B.P., Eur. P., U.S.P.)*.

Chlordiazepoxidi Hydrochloridum; Methaminodiazepoxide Hydrochloride; Ro 5-0690.
$C_{16}H_{14}ClN_3O,HCl$=336.2.

CAS — 438-41-5.

Pharmacopoeias. In *Belg.*, *Br.*, *Eur.*, *Fr.*, *Ger.*, *It.*, *Neth.*, *Turk.*, and *U.S.* *U.S.* also includes Sterile Chlordiazepoxide Hydrochloride.

An odourless white or slightly yellowish crystalline powder with a very bitter taste. M.p. 212° to 218°.
Soluble 1 in 10 of water and 1 in 40 of alcohol;

practically insoluble in chloroform, ether, and light petroleum. A 5.5% solution in water is iso-osmotic with serum. A 10% solution has a pH of 2 to 3. **Store** in airtight containers. Protect from light.

Chlordiazepoxide powder was effectively sterilised by irradiation at 45 000 Gy; an unidentified degradation product was detected by thin-layer chromatography.— B. P. Jacob and K. Leupin, *Pharm. Acta Helv.*, 1974, *49*, 1 and 12, per *Pharm. J.*, 1974, *2*, 354.

Haemolysis. a 0.06% solution of chlordiazepoxide hydrochloride in 0.9% sodium chloride solution caused 100% haemolysis of erythrocytes cultured in it for 45 minutes.— C. J. Fievet *et al.*, *Am. J. Hosp. Pharm.*, 1971, *28*, 961.

Dependence. Prolonged use of chlordiazepoxide may lead to dependence of the barbiturate-alcohol type (see p.792). It has a low liability for abuse.

Abuse. Chlordiazepoxide had a moderate potential for abuse. Mild psychic and physical dependence had been reported.— H. Isbell and T. L. Chruściel, *Dependence Liability of 'Non-narcotic' Drugs*, Geneva, World Health Organization, 1970; *idem*, *Bull. Wld Hlth Org.*, 1970, *43*, *Suppl.*

Pregnancy and the neonate. Irritability and tremulousness commencing 21 days after birth, and presumed to be withdrawal symptoms, occurred in twin girls born after 36 weeks' gestation to a woman who had taken chlordiazepoxide 30 mg daily for 5 years, decreased to 20 mg daily from the 12th week of pregnancy. They improved after treatment with diazepam.— P. Athinarayanan *et al.*, *Am. J. Obstet. Gynec.*, 1976, *124*, 212.

Adverse Effects and Treatment. As for Diazepam, p.1520.

Allergy. An erythematous rash developed in a woman taking chlordiazepoxide 10 mg four times daily. The rash cleared when medication was stopped and reappeared within 24 hours of a new course of chlordiazepoxide.— H. M. Blair, *Archs Derm.*, 1974, *109*, 914.

Further references.— J. S. Ghosh (letter), *Br. med. J.*, 1977, *1*, 902.

See also under Effects on the Skin (below).

Diabetogenic effect. Chlordiazepoxide hydrochloride aggravated hyperglycaemia in an insulin-dependent woman with maturity-onset diabetes.— B. Zumoff and L. Hellman, *J. Am. med. Ass.*, 1977, *237*, 1960.

Effects on the blood. *Aplastic anaemia*. Chlordiazepoxide had been reported to cause aplastic anaemia.— R. H. Girdwood, *Drugs*, 1976, *11*, 394.

Haemolytic anaemia. A report of 2 cases of haemolytic anaemia due to chlordiazepoxide.— J. V. Dacie and S. M. Worlledge, *Prog. Hemat.*, 1969, *6*, 82.

Effects on the eyes. A double-blind crossover trial in 8 subjects showed that a single dose of 10 mg of chlordiazepoxide had no significant depressant effect on visual sensory function and coordination for up to 3 hours.— D. P. Austen *et al.*, *Br. J. physiol. Optics*, 1971, *26*, 161.

A study indicating that usual therapeutic doses of chlordiazepoxide interfere with colour vision.— J. Laroche and C. Laroche, *Annls pharm. fr.*, 1972, *30*, 433.

Effects on the liver. A woman, aged 64, suffered from a progressive, painless jaundice of 3 weeks' duration after treatment with chlordiazepoxide 10 mg thrice daily for 12 days.— D. Pickering (letter), *New Engl. J. Med.*, 1966, *274*, 1449.

Further references.— F. Clark, *Adverse Drug React. Bull.*, 1977, Oct., 232.

Effects on mental state. Seven patients with no previous history of hallucinations developed hallucinatory states after treatment with chlordiazepoxide.— D. S. Viscott, *Archs gen. Psychiat.*, 1968, *19*, 370.

Paradoxical response. In a small group study chlordiazepoxide was associated with increased interpersonal behavioural hostility when a frustration stimulus was presented to the group.— C. Salzman *et al.*, *Archs gen. Psychiat.*, 1974, *31*, 401. A conflicting report.— K. Rickels and R. W. Downing, *Am. J. Psychiat.*, 1974, *131*, 442.

Effects on the muscles. Pain at the site of injection and elevation of serum concentration of creatine phosphokinase was almost as great following intramuscular injection of the propylene glycol vehicle as after chlordiazepoxide injection. Slow absorption of chlordiazepoxide after intramuscular injection might be due to precipitation at the injection site.— D. J. Greenblatt *et al.*, *J. clin. Pharmac.*, 1976, *16*, 118. Chlordiazepoxide was about 88.8% bound to human muscle tissue *in vitro*.— B. Fichtl and H. Kurz, *Eur. J. clin. Pharmac.*, 1978, *14*, 335.

Effects on respiratory function. Chlordiazepoxide 10 mg thrice daily was administered to 6 patients who had been hospitalised for respiratory failure due to an acute exacerbation of chronic bronchitis. There was a significant increase in pCO_2 and a significant fall in forced expiratory volume. One further patient who had taken diazepam regularly before admittance had no deterioration in respiratory function.— D. G. Model and D. J. Berry, *Lancet*, 1974, *2*, 869.

Effects on the skin. A brief review of cutaneous reactions to chlordiazepoxide.— J. Almeyda, *Br. J. Derm.*, 1971, *84*, 298.

Fixed drug eruption. Chlordiazepoxide was responsible for a fixed drug eruption in 2 patients.— J. A. Savin, *Br. J. Derm.*, 1970, *83*, 546.

Photosensitivity. A report of photosensitivity probably due to chlordiazepoxide.— *Japan med. Gaz.*, 1976, *13* (Sept. 20), 9.

Purpura. Non-thrombocytopenic purpura occurred in a 65-year-old woman following administration of chlordiazepoxide for at least 12 months in irregular courses of 10 mg twice daily for about 1 week at approximately monthly intervals. The purpura reappeared within 48 hours of restarting chlordiazepoxide in a dosage of 30 mg daily.— I. J. Copperman (letter), *Br. med. J.*, 1967, *4*, 485.

Hiccups. Administration of chlordiazepoxide was associated with the development of hiccups in a 19-year-old male patient.— D. K. Winstead (letter), *Am. J. Psychiat.*, 1976, *133*, 719.

Lupus erythematosus. There was an association between a syndrome resembling lupus erythematosus and chlordiazepoxide in 8 patients.— J. H. Hicks, *Cutis*, 1973, *11*, 33.

Overdosage. There were no fatalities in 22 instances of chlordiazepoxide overdosage, even with amounts of up to 2.25 g.— L. E. Hollister, *Clin. Pharmac. Ther.*, 1966, *7*, 142.

Porphyria. Administration of chlordiazepoxide exacerbated experimental porphyria in *rats* but the validity of the test must depend on clinical observation.— A. A. -B. Badawy (letter), *Lancet*, 1978, *1*, 1361.

Further references.— R. K. Parikh and M. R. Moore, *Br. J. Anaesth.*, 1978, *50*, 1099.

Pregnancy and the neonate. *Early pregnancy*. Results of a prospective study of 19 044 live births indicated an increased incidence of defects in children of mothers exposed to chlordiazepoxide during the first 42 days of pregnancy.— L. Milkovich and B. J. van den Berg, *New Engl. J. Med.*, 1974, *291*, 1268.

Of 50 282 children born to mothers monitored by the Collaborative Perinatal Project 257 were found to have been exposed to chlordiazepoxide, and possibly other drugs, at some time during the first 4 months of the pregnancy. No association between chlordiazepoxide exposure and any type of malformation could be detected.— O. P. Heinonen *et al.*, *Birth Defects and Drugs in Pregnancy*, Littleton MA, Publishing Sciences Group, 1977, p. 335.

See also Diazepam, p.1521.

Late pregnancy and labour. A pregnant woman treated with chlordiazepoxide, 25 mg four times daily, gave birth to an infant who was 1 month premature and had sluggish reflexes and leucopenia.— S. Bitnun (letter), *Can. med. Ass. J.*, 1969, *100*, 351.

Precautions. As for Diazepam, p.1521.

As with diazepam intramuscular injections are painful and their absorption is erratic.

Interactions. *Alcohol*. A study in healthy subjects indicated that chlordiazepoxide 10 mg thrice daily for one or two weeks did not impair psychomotor performance to an extent which could cause any major risks in traffic or occupational life. Addition of alcohol, however, did so. Moreover, anxiety of the subjects was slightly increased after the association of chlordiazepoxide and alcohol.— M. Linnoila *et al.*, *Arzneimittel-Forsch.*, 1975, *25*, 1088.

Antacids. A study in 10 healthy subjects indicated that although concurrent administration of antacid (magnesium and aluminium hydroxide) delayed absorption of chlordiazepoxide it did not affect the completeness of absorption or the apparent rate of elimination.— D. J. Greenblatt *et al.*, *Clin. Pharmac. Ther.*, 1976, *19*, 234. See also *idem*, *Clin. Pharmac. Ther.*, 1977, *21*, 105; *Am. J. Psychiat.*, 1977, *134*, 559.

Cimetidine. Impaired elimination of chlordiazepoxide in subjects also receiving cimetidine.— P. V. Desmond *et al.*, *Ann. intern. Med.*, 1980, *93*, 266.

See also under Diazepam (p.1522).

Interference with diagnostic tests. In 14 euthyroid patients and 6 mildly thyrotoxic patients, administration of chlordiazepoxide in a dosage of 10 mg thrice daily for 4 weeks did not significantly affect the results of tests of thyroid iodide trapping or of thyroid hormone release. Chlordiazepoxide did not alter the commonly used tests of thyroid function.— F. Clark and R. Hall, *Br. med. J.*, 1970, *2*, 266. Similar findings.— S. D. Slater, *Br. J. clin. Pract.*, 1972, *26*, 463.

Investigations indicating that chlordiazepoxide has no significant effect on serum values for aspartate aminotransferase or alkaline phosphatase activities, values for bilirubin, albumin, or total protein, or the electrophoretic pattern for serum proteins. Although values for 17-hydroxycorticosteroids were slightly increased in addition experiments, administration of the drug was not found to have any effect on values for either 17-hydroxycorticosteroids or 17-ketosteroids in urine.— H. E. Spiegel *et al.*, *Clin. Chem.*, 1974, *20*, 1222.

Pregnancy and the neonate. *Diffusion across the placenta*. In a double-blind study in 166 women in early labour, the effect of chlordiazepoxide was compared with a placebo. Chlordiazepoxide was found to cross the placenta but no foetal or neonatal depression occurred. No significant difference between the 2 treatments was detected.— P. M. Mark and J. Hamel, *Obstet. Gynec.*, 1968, *32*, 188.

Concentrations of chlordiazepoxide in cord blood were as high as those of maternal blood in 3 of 4 infants born to mothers given chlordiazepoxide for pre-eclampsia or eclampsia; in the fourth infant the concentration was about 40% of that in maternal blood.— G. M. Stirrat *et al.* (letter), *Br. med. J.*, 1974, *2*, 729.

Absorption and Fate. For an account of the absorption and fate of a benzodiazepine, see Diazepam, p.1522.

Chlordiazepoxide has been reported to have an elimination half-life ranging from about 5 to 30 hours. Pharmacologically active metabolites include desmethylchlordiazepoxide, demoxepam, desmethyldiazepam, and oxazepam.

A detailed review of the clinical pharmacokinetics of chlordiazepoxide.— D. J. Greenblatt *et al.*, *Clin. Pharmacokinet.*, 1978, *3*, 381.

Absorption and plasma concentrations. In 8 volunteers the average peak blood concentration of chlordiazepoxide after administration of 50 mg by mouth was 1.75 µg per ml and occurred in 1 to 1.5 hours. However after intramuscular injection the average peak concentration of 1 µg per ml was delayed.— D. J. Greenblatt *et al.*, *New Engl. J. Med.*, 1974, *291*, 1116.

The biological half-life of chlordiazepoxide was found to be shorter than previously reported, and also more variable, ranging from 6.6 to 28 hours. Most of a dose was eliminated as the intermediate desmethylchlordiazepoxide. The metabolite demoxepam was not found in the plasma of any of 6 volunteers after the administration of single doses of chlordiazepoxide.— M. A. Schwartz *et al.*, *J. pharm. Sci.*, 1971, *60*, 1500.

Studies in 14 healthy subjects (7 male and 7 female) given chlordiazepoxide by intravenous infusion indicated that the apparent half-lives of distribution and elimination and the total blood clearance did not differ significantly between the sexes but that the apparent volumes of the central compartment and of the total distribution space were significantly larger in the female group. A further study in 3 subjects indicated a limited uptake of chlordiazepoxide by red blood cells.— D. J. Greenblatt *et al.*, *Clin. Pharmac. Ther.*, 1977, *22*, 893.

Further references.— H. G. Boxenbaum *et al.*, *J. Pharmacokinet. Biopharm.*, 1977, *5*, 25 (plasma concentrations); A. J. Bond *et al.*, *Br. J. clin. Pharmac.*, 1977, *4*, 51 (plasma concentrations); S. -R. Sun, *J. pharm. Sci.*, 1978, *67*, 639 (plasma concentrations and half-lives).

Metabolism. Studies of the metabolism of chlordiazepoxide.— M. A. Schwartz and E. Postma, *J. pharm. Sci.*, 1972, *61*, 123; W. R. Dixon *et al.*, *J. pharm. Sci.*, 1975, *64*, 937; R. Dixon *et al.*, *Clin. Pharmac. Ther.*, 1976, *20*, 450; G. G. Skellern *et al.*, *Br. J. clin. Pharmac.*, 1978, *5*, 483.

Plasma protein binding. A study of the CSF of 30 patients who received chlordiazepoxide hydrochloride 100 mg by mouth prior to surgical procedures indicated that simultaneous CSF concentrations of chlordiazepoxide were considerably lower than those in the plasma. Since only the unbound chlordiazepoxide in plasma has been reported to be available for diffusion into CSF (J.

Koch-Weser and E.M. Sellers, *New Engl. J. Med.*, 1976, *294*, 311 and 526; W.H. Oldendorf, *A. Rev. Pharmac.*, 1974, *14*, 239), the ratio of the concentration in CSF and plasma was used to calculate that chlordiazepoxide is about 90 to 97% protein bound. The data suggested that variations in protein binding might be responsible for differences in clinical response.— D. R. Stanski *et al.*, *Clin. Pharmac. Ther.*, 1976, *20*, 571. See also D. R. Stanski *et al.*, *Psychopharmac. Bull.*, 1977, *13*, 53.

Uses. Chlordiazepoxide is a benzodiazepine with actions and uses similar to those of diazepam (p.1523).

Chlordiazepoxide is administered by mouth as the hydrochloride and sometimes as the base. It may also be administered by intramuscular injection where the dose may be expressed in terms of the base or the hydrochloride.

The usual dose of either the base or the hydrochloride for the treatment of anxiety is 30 mg daily in divided doses; in severe conditions the dose is 40 to 100 mg daily; for elderly and debilitated patients the usual initial dose is 10 mg daily. A suggested dose for children is 5 to 20 mg daily in divided doses; another suggested dose for children is 500 μg per kg body-weight daily, in 3 or 4 divided doses.

For the control of the acute symptoms of alcohol withdrawal chlordiazepoxide hydrochloride may be given by deep intramuscular injection; the usual dose is 50 to 100 mg calculated as the base or as the hydrochloride, repeated if required within 2 to 4 hours. Intravenous administration is not usually recommended.

Action. In a study of 15 subjects with moderate to severe anxiety given chlordiazepoxide, anxiety reduction correlated with plasma concentrations of desmethylchlordiazepoxide and demoxepam but not with plasma concentrations of chlordiazepoxide.— K. -M. Lin and R. O. Friedel, *Am. J. Psychiat.*, 1979, *136*, 18.

Administration. Studies showing that the absorption of chlordiazepoxide after intramuscular injection is much slower that the same dose given by mouth.— D. J. Greenblatt *et al.*, *Eur. J. clin. Pharmac.*, 1978, *13*, 267.

In the elderly. A study on the absorption and disposition of chlordiazepoxide in young and elderly men.— R. I. Shader *et al.*, *J. clin. Pharmac.*, 1977, *17*, 709.

Administration in hepatic failure. Chlordiazepoxide therapy in hepatic insufficiency.— C. L. Mendenhall *et al.*, *Gastroenterology*, 1975, *69*, 845.

Further references.— R. K. Roberts *et al.*, *Gastroenterology*, 1978, *75*, 479; R. K. Roberts *et al.*, *Drugs*, 1979, *17*, 198.

Administration in renal failure. Chlordiazepoxide could be given in usual doses to patients with renal failure. Concentrations of chlordiazepoxide were not affected by haemodialysis.— W. M. Bennett *et al.*, *Ann. intern. Med.*, 1977, *86*, 754. See also *idem*, 1980, *93*, 286.

Alcohol and drug withdrawal. In a double-blind study 537 patients with acute alcohol withdrawal symptoms were given chlordiazepoxide, chlorpromazine, hydroxyzine, thiamine, or a placebo. Only 55 patients developed withdrawal symptoms; 2% of them were treated with chlordiazepoxide compared with 11 to 16% of the patients in the other treatment groups.— S. C. Kaim *et al.*, *Am. J. Psychiat.*, 1969, *125*, 1640, per *J. Am. med. Ass.*, 1969, *209*, 805.

Further references.— E. Rothstein, *Am. J. Psychiat.*, 1973, *130*, 1381; F. R. Funderburk *et al.*, *J. nerv. ment. Dis.*, 1978, *166*, 195; P. J. Perry *et al.*, *Clin. Pharmac. Ther.*, 1978, *23*, 535; E. M. Sellers *et al.* (letter), *Br. J. clin. Pharmac.*, 1978, *6*, 370; P. V. Desmond and S. Schenker (letter), *ibid.*, 1979, *8*, 85; B. Whiting *et al.* (letter), *ibid.*; A. Pena-Ramos and R. Hornberger, *J. clin. Psychiat.*, 1979, *40*, 361.

Anaesthesia. References to the use of chlordiazepoxide for anaesthetic premedication and basal anaesthesia.— B. J. Urban *et al.*, *Anesth. Analg. curr. Res.*, 1966, *45*, 733; W. H. K. Haslett and J. W. Dundee, *Br. J. Anaesth.*, 1968, *40*, 250; L. Gibbs *et al.*, *Anesth. Analg. curr. Res.*, 1971, *50*, 17.

Anxiety. Studies of chlordiazepoxide in anxiety.— D. Kelly *et al.*, *Br. J. Psychiat.*, 1969, *115*, 1387. Report No. 136 of the General Practitioner Research Group, *Practitioner*, 1969, *202*, 706; I. G. Podobnikar, *Psychosomatics*, 1971, *12*, 205; K. Rickels *et al.*, *Psychopharmacologia*, 1971, *20*, 128; R. S. Lipman *et al.*, *Dis. nerv. Syst.*, 1971, *32*, 240; T. P. Hackett and N. H. Cassem, *Curr. ther. Res.*, 1972, *14*, 649.

Behaviour disorders. The use of chlordiazepoxide in children with behavioural disorders.— I. A. Kraft *et al.*, *Int. J. Neuropsychiat.*, 1965, *1*, 433.

Convulsions. Administration of chlordiazepoxide hydrochloride to 28 patients with various forms of epileptic seizures resulted in a sustained reduction in frequency or cessation of seizures in 21. Of these 28 patients, 24 had previously received other anticonvulsant therapy without adequate control.— C. W. Watson *et al.*, *J. Am. med. Ass.*, 1964, *188*, 212. See also D. Goldman and G. Schynoll, *Dis. nerv. Syst.*, 1964, *25*, 52.

Depression. In a crossover study completed by 56 depressed patients chlordiazepoxide appeared to be more effective than amitriptyline. Patients with exogenous depression appeared to react more favourably to chlordiazepoxide while those with endogenous depression appeared to respond more favourably to amitriptyline.— R. Kellner, *Can. psychiat. Ass. J.*, 1973, *18*, 393.

For comments on the use of benzodiazepines for depression, see Diazepam, p.1525.

Tetanus. Beneficial results with chlordiazepoxide in tetanus.— L. A. Phillips, *Lancet*, 1965, *1*, 1097.

Tremor. Administration of chlordiazepoxide had a beneficial effect in 6 of 12 patients with essential tremor.— E. Critchley, *J. Neurol. Neurosurg. Psychiat.*, 1972, *35*, 365.

Preparations

Capsules

Chlordiazepoxide Capsules *(B.P.)*. Capsules containing chlordiazepoxide hydrochloride. Store at a temperature not exceeding 30°. Protect from light.

Chlordiazepoxide Hydrochloride Capsules *(U.S.P.)*. Capsules containing chlordiazepoxide hydrochloride. The *U.S.P.* requires 85% dissolution in 30 minutes. Store in airtight containers. Protect from light.

Injections

Sterile Chlordiazepoxide Hydrochloride *(U.S.P.)*. Chlordiazepoxide hydrochloride suitable for parenteral use. pH of a 1% solution 2.5 to 3.5. Protect from light.

Tablets

Chlordiazepoxide Hydrochloride Tablets *(B.P.)*. Tablets containing chlordiazepoxide hydrochloride; they may be film-coated. Store at a temperature not exceeding 25°.

Chlordiazepoxide Tablets *(B.P.)*. Tablets containing chlordiazepoxide. They may be film-coated or sugar-coated. Store at a temperature not exceeding 25°.

Chlordiazepoxide Tablets *(U.S.P.)*. Tablets containing chlordiazepoxide. Store in airtight containers. Protect from light.

Proprietary Preparations of Chlordiazepoxide and its Salts

Librium Ampoules *(Roche, UK)*. Each contains chlordiazepoxide hydrochloride equivalent to 100 mg of chlordiazepoxide, with 2-ml ampoules of solvent for preparing intramuscular injections. Store in a refrigerator. **Librium Capsules** each contain 5 or 10 mg of chlordiazepoxide hydrochloride. **Librium Tablets** each contain 5, 10, or 25 mg of chlordiazepoxide. (Also available as Librium in *Austral., Belg., Canad., Denm., Fr., Ger., Ital., Neth., Norw., S.Afr., Spain, Switz., USA*).

Tropium *(DDSA Pharmaceuticals, UK)*. Chlordiazepoxide hydrochloride, available as **Capsules** of 5 and 10 mg and as **Tablets** of 5, 10, and 25 mg.

Other Proprietary Names

Arg.— Diazebrum (dibudinate), Diazepina, O.C.M., Raysedan, Reposal, Sintesedan; *Canad.*— Corax, C-Tran, Medilium, Nack, Novopoxide, Relaxil, Solium, Trilium; *Denm.*— Klopoxid, Risolid; *Ger.*— Helogaphen, Multum, Zeisin; *Ital.*— Ansiacal, Benzodiapin, Cebrum, Endequil, Equibral, Labican, Liberans, Lixin, Philcorium, Psicofar, Psicoterina, Reliberan, Seren, Smail, Viansin; *Jap.*— Risachief; *Norw.*— Risolid; *Pol.*— Elenium; *S.Afr.*— Chlortran; *Spain*— Binomil, Huberplex, Normide, Omnalio; *Swed.*— Risolid; *USA*— A-Poxide, Libritabs, SK-Lygen.

Chlordiazepoxide and chlordiazepoxide hydrochloride were also formerly marketed in Great Britain under the proprietary name Calmoden (*Berk Pharmaceuticals*).

7019-l

Chlormezanone.

Chlormezanonum; Chlormethazanone. 2-(4-Chlorophenyl)-3-methylperhydro-1,3-thiazin-4-one 1,1-dioxide.
$C_{11}H_{12}ClNO_3S=273.7$.

CAS — 80-77-3.

Pharmacopoeias. In *Jap.*

A white crystalline powder with a faint characteristic odour and a slightly bitter taste. M.p. about 115°. Very slightly **soluble** in water; sparingly soluble in alcohol; freely soluble in acetone and chloroform. **Store** in airtight containers.

Adverse Effects. Drowsiness, weakness, nausea, dizziness, skin rash, flushing of the skin, depression, and dryness of the mouth have been reported. There may be difficulty in micturition. Cholestatic jaundice has occasionally occurred.

Effects on the skin. Chlormezanone in conjunction with paracetamol was strongly suspected of being responsible for a fixed drug eruption in 1 patient.— J. A. Savin, *Br. J. Derm.*, 1970, *85*, 546.

Taste perception. Loss of sense of taste in 1 patient was associated with chlormezanone and paracetamol (Muskel-Trancopal comp.).— H. Rollin, *Ann. Otol. Rhinol. Lar.*, 1978, *87*, 37.

Treatment of Adverse Effects. In recent severe overdosage the stomach should be emptied by aspiration and lavage. For general guidelines to the symptomatic therapy of overdosage with central nervous system depressants, see Phenobarbitone, p.812.

Precautions. The sedative effects of central nervous system depressants may be enhanced. If dizziness or drowsiness occurs, the patient should not drive a car or operate machinery.

Absence of significant interaction between chlormezanone 200 and 400 mg and alcohol 500 mg per kg body-weight.— T. Seppala *et al.*, *Drugs*, 1979, *17*, 389. See also M. Linnoila, *Eur. J. clin. Pharmac.*, 1973, *5*, 247.

Uses. Chlormezanone is a tranquilliser used in the treatment of anxiety and tension states. It has been claimed to be of benefit in conditions associated with muscle spasm but has not been shown to have a direct action on muscle. The usual dose for the treatment of anxiety is 200 mg thrice daily, with a range of 300 to 800 mg daily in divided doses.

As a hypnotic a dose of 400 mg at night is recommended.

Anxiety. Studies of chlormezanone in the treatment of anxiety.— F. B. Champlin *et al.*, *Clin. Pharmac. Ther.*, 1968, *9*, 11; W. G. Case *et al.*, *Am. J. Psychiat.*, 1974, *131*, 592; J. F. Donald and A. L. Molla, *J. int. med. Res.*, 1978, *6*, 105; J. M. T. Warnock, *ibid.*, 115; G. Ali-Khan, *Curr. med. Res. Opinion*, 1979, *6*, 259.

Rheumatic disease. Chlormezanone 400 mg at night improved the quality of sleep in the majority of 43 patients with sleep disturbances associated with rheumatic disease. No improvement in day-time stiffness was observed.— L. Cohen, *J. int. med. Res.*, 1978, *6*, 111. See also R. Condie, *Curr. med. Res. Opinion*, 1979, *6*, 217.

Proprietary Preparations

Trancopal *(Sterling Research, UK)*. Chlormezanone, available as tablets of 200 mg. (Also available as Trancopal in *Aust., Belg., Canad., Denm., Fin., Fr., Iceland, Ital., Neth., Norw., S.Afr., Swed., Switz., USA*).

Chlormezanone is an ingredient of Lobak (see p.270) and of Trancoprin (see p.244)..

Other Proprietary Names

Fr.—Supotran; *Ger.*— Muskel Trancopal; *Ital.*— Rexan, Rilaquil, Tanafol; *Jap.*— Chlomedinon, Myolespen, Relizon, Toyomezanon, Trancote, Transanate.

7020-v

Chlorproethazine. RP 4909. 3-(2-Chlorophenothiazin-10-yl)-*NN*-diethylpropylamine.
$C_{19}H_{23}ClN_2S$=346.9.

CAS — 84-01-5.

Chlorproethazine is a phenothiazine derivative differing chemically from chlorpromazine by the substitution of a diethyl for a dimethyl group. It has general properties similar to those of chlorpromazine (p.1509) but has been used mainly as a muscle relaxant. A recommended dosage of chlorproethazine hydrochloride by mouth is 25 to 200 mg daily (in divided portions); it has also been given by injection. Although exposure of the skin to phenothiazines has been associated with sensitivity reactions, chlorproethazine hydrochloride has also been applied topically in an ointment, with the warning to avoid direct exposure to sunlight.

References: J. Sigwald *et al.*, *Presse méd.*, 1961, *69*, 2187; S. Follin *et al.*, *ibid.*, 1962, *70*, 1982; W. B. Matthews, *Brain*, 1965, *88*, 1057.

Proprietary Names

Neuriplège (hydrochloride) (*Génévrier, Fr.*).

7021-g

Chlorpromazine *(B.P., U.S.P.).* 3(2-Chlorophenothiazin-10-yl)-*NN*-dimethylpropylamine.

$C_{17}H_{19}ClN_2S$=318.9.

CAS — 50-53-3.

Pharmacopoeias. In *Br.* and *U.S.*

A white to creamy-white powder or waxy solid, odourless or with an amine-like odour. It darkens on prolonged exposure to light. M.p. 56° to 60°. Chlorpromazine 100 mg is approximately equivalent to 111 mg of chlorpromazine hydrochloride.

Practically **insoluble** in water and dilute alkali hydroxides; soluble 1 in 2 of alcohol, 1 in less than 1 of chloroform, 1 in 1 of ether, and in dilute mineral acids. **Store** in airtight containers. Protect from light.

7022-q

Chlorpromazine Embonate. Chlorpromazine 4,4′-methylenebis(3-hydroxy-2-naphthoate).

$(C_{17}H_{19}ClN_2S)_2,C_{23}H_{16}O_6$=1026.1.

A pale yellow powder. Chlorpromazine embonate 1.44 g is approximately equivalent to 1 g of chlorpromazine hydrochloride. Very slightly **soluble** in water; soluble in acetone. Colour changes on exposure to light are less marked and less rapid than those of the hydrochloride.

7023-p

Chlorpromazine Hydrochloride *(B.P., B.P. Vet., Eur. P., U.S.P.).* Chlorpromazini Hydrochloridum; Aminazine; Cloridrato de Clorpromazina.

$C_{17}H_{19}ClN_2S,HCl$=355.3.

CAS — 69-09-0.

Pharmacopoeias. In *Arg., Belg., Br., Braz., Chin., Cz., Eur., Fr., Ger., Hung., Ind., Int., It., Jap., Jug., Neth., Nord., Pol., Port., Rus., Turk.*, and *U.S.*

An odourless white or creamy-white crystalline powder with a very bitter taste. M.p. 195° to 198°. It decomposes on exposure to air and light becoming yellow, pink, and finally violet.

Soluble 1 in 0.4 of water, 1 in 1.3 to 1.5 of alcohol, and 1 in 1 of chloroform; practically insoluble in ether. A freshly prepared 10% solution in water has a pH of 4 to 5. Solutions are **sterilised** by autoclaving after distribution into containers in which the air has been replaced by nitrogen or other suitable gas. **Incompatible** in aqueous solution with the sodium salts of barbiturates, and other alkaline solutions. Solutions may be stabilised by addition of antoxidants and stored under nitrogen. **Store** in airtight containers. Protect from light.

CAUTION. *Chlorpromazine may cause severe dermatitis in sensitised persons. Pharmacists, nurses, and others who handle the drug frequently should wear masks and rubber gloves.*

A review of the analysis of phenothiazine drugs.— J. E. Fairbrother, *Pharm. J.*, 1979, *1*, 271.

When a solution of chlorpromazine was shaken for 1 hour with a number of synthetic materials, soft plastic materials such as silicone, latex, and thin polyvinyl chloride tubing adsorbed 99, 84, and 86% of chlorpromazine respectively. Adsorption occurred with hard plastic materials, cotton wool, filter paper, and glass wool but to a lesser extent. Other lipophilic phenothiazines and thiopentone were shaken with latex and polyvinyl chloride tubing and found to be adsorbed whereas hydrophilic compounds were not. A positive relationship between temperature and adsorption was demonstrated.— G. Kriegistein *et al.*, *Arzneimittel-Forsch.*, 1972, *22*, 1538.

Incompatibility and compatibility. Chlorpromazine base was precipitated in alkaline media. The following solutions should not be mixed with chlorpromazine hydrochloride solution prior to injection; dextrose 30%, gallamine triethiodide 4%, Ringer's solution, sodium bicarbonate 1.4%, phenobarbitone sodium 10%, sodium chloride 10%, and solutions of other soluble barbiturate salts. A cloudy solution could result from mixing with a 50% solution of magnesium sulphate or with 0.9% sodium chloride solution. Chlorpromazine hydrochloride was also incompatible with solutions of ampicillin, atropine sulphate, benzylpenicillin, chloramphenicol, heparin, hydrocortisone hydrogen succinate, metaraminol, methicillin, oxytetracycline, tetracycline, thiopentone sodium, and Vitamins B and C Injection. Compatible mixtures included those with simple solutions of adrenaline 0.1%, atropine sulphate 0.05%, morphine hydrochloride 1%, pethidine hydrochloride 5%, procainamide hydrochloride 10%, procaine hydrochloride 1 and 2%, and promethazine hydrochloride 2.5%.— *Largactil in General Medicine and Anaesthesia*, 9th Edn, Dagenham, *May & Baker*, 1973, pp. 6 and 7.

An immediate precipitate occurred when chlorpromazine hydrochloride 200 mg per litre was mixed with aminophylline 1 g per litre, ampicillin sodium 2 g per litre, chlorothiazide 2 g per litre, ethamivan 2 g per litre, methohexitone sodium 2 g per litre, phenobarbitone sodium 800 mg per litre, sulphadiazine sodium 4 g per litre, and sulphadimidine sodium 4 g per litre in 5% dextrose solution and 0.9% sodium chloride solution. An immediate precipitate occurred with amphotericin 200 mg per litre in 5% dextrose solution, and a haze developed over 3 hours with chloramphenicol 4 g per litre in 0.9% sodium chloride solution, but an immediate precipitate was formed in 5% dextrose solution. A haze developed over 3 hours when chlorpromazine hydrochloride was mixed with benzylpenicillin 6 g per litre, cloxacillin sodium 1 g per litre, or methicillin sodium 4 g per litre in 0.9% sodium chloride solution.— B. B. Riley, *J. Hosp. Pharm.*, 1970, *28*, 228.

Solutions containing 2.5% of chlorpromazine hydrochloride could be diluted to 100 ml with 0.9% sodium chloride solution provided the pH of the saline solution was such that the pH of the dilution did not exceed the critical range of pH 6.7 to 6.8. With saline of pH 7 or 7.2, the final solution had a pH of 6.4.— P. F. D'Arcy and K. M. Thompson (letter), *Pharm. J.*, 1973, *1*, 28.

Morphine sulphate injection containing chlorocresol 0.2% was incompatible with chlorpromazine hydrochloride injection. Morphine injection without chlorocresol should be compatible.— J. B. Crapper, *Br. med. J.*, 1975, *1*, 33.

Adverse Effects. The side-effects of chlorpromazine include drowsiness, dryness of the mouth, nasal congestion, postural hypotension, lowering of body temperature (occasionally pyrexia), tachycardia, arrhythmias, agitation, insomnia, depression, miosis and mydriasis, convulsions, photosensitivity, skin rashes, and inhibition of ejaculation.

Jaundice of the obstructive type, and considered to be allergic in origin, has occurred in patients receiving chlorpromazine; it does not appear to be dose-related and is usually readily reversible. Chronic constipation and faecal impaction have also occurred. Urinary retention may also occasionally occur.

Various haematological disorders including agranulocytosis, leucopenia, leucocytosis, and haemolytic anaemia have occurred in patients taking chlorpromazine. Most cases of agranulocytosis have occurred within 4 to 10 weeks of starting treatment. It is advisable to beware of symptoms such as sore throat or fever and to institute white cell counts should they appear. Eosinophilia may also occur. Extrapyramidal dysfunction occurs in patients receiving phenothiazines and is largely reversible by lowering the dose, or discontinuing therapy. Extrapyramidal symptoms may also be reversed in emergency by antiparkinsonian agents, but these do not alleviate or prevent the emergence of tardive dyskinesia on long-term administration, and may mask early symptoms, with eventual exacerbation of the syndrome.

Allergic reactions include urticaria, photosensitisation and on occasions exfoliative dermatitis. Contact dermatitis can occur in people handling the drug. A lupus erythematosus-like syndrome has been reported.

The administration of large doses of chlorpromazine for prolonged periods can lead to the development of a purplish pigmentation of exposed areas of the skin and, more frequently, to the deposition of pigment in the eyes. Corneal and lens opacities have been observed in some patients.

Chlorpromazine and the other phenothiazines alter endocrine function. Patients have experienced amenorrhoea, galactorrhoea, gynaecomastia, and weight gain and there have been reports of hyperglycaemia and diabetes mellitus. There have also been reports of raised serum cholesterol concentrations.

Solutions of chlorpromazine may cause irritation at the site of injection and nodule formation may occur; inflammatory responses and gangrene have been reported. The site of injection should be altered if repeated injections are necessary. It has been suggested that pain may be reduced by the addition of a local anaesthetic such as procaine or by diluting the solution with sodium chloride injection.

Reviews and comments on the adverse effects of chlorpromazine and other psychotropic agents.— *Med. Lett.*, 1976, *18*, 89; C. F. George, *Prescribers' J.*, 1978, *18*, 75; G. M. Simpson *et al.*, *Drugs*, 1981, *21*, 138.

In 556 patients who received chlorpromazine, adverse reactions attributed to the drug occurred in 68 (12.2%). Reactions were life-threatening in 1.3%. Drowsiness or disorientation (30) and hypotension (12) were the most common adverse effects.— C. Swett, *Curr. ther. Res.*, 1975, *18*, 199.

Further references.— C. Swett, *Boston Collaborative Drug Surveillance Program, Dis. nerv. Syst.*, 1974, *35*, 509.

Allergy. Two patients, with a history of jaundice after previous dosage with the drug, developed severe abdominal pain and vomiting after doses of 25 mg of chlorpromazine by mouth. Very rare cases might occur in which jaundice following chlorpromazine therapy was allergic in origin with alarming symptoms. In these patients the drug should never be given again.— A. Rumore, *Med. J. Aust.*, 1962, *2*, 752.

In a modified 'repeated-insult' patch test, 25% chlorpromazine was found to produce strong sensitisation of the skin.— A. M. Kligman, *J. invest. Derm.*, 1966, *47*, 393.

Vasculitis has been reported in association with chlorpromazine.— E. C. Rosenow, *Ann. intern. Med.*, 1972, *77*, 977.

Severe hypotensive reactions occurred in 3 patients following the intramuscular administration of chlorpromazine. A hypersensitivity reaction was suspected since each patient had previously received chlorpromazine without any ill effect.— P. L. Man and C. H. Chen, *Br. J. Psychiat.*, 1973, *122*, 185.

Cytogenetic effects. The frequency of chromosomal aberrations in 28 patients treated with chlorpromazine or perphenazine was greater than in 41 patients and healthy persons who acted as controls.— J. Nielsen *et al.*, *Br. med. J.*, 1969, *3*, 634. There was no significant difference in the incidence of chromosomal aberrations in 6 controls and 10 patients given chlorpromazine in increasing doses up to 600 mg daily. This confirmed an earlier negative report.— M. M. Cohen *et al.*, *ibid.*, 1972, *3*, 21.

Diabetogenic effect. Studies in healthy subjects and patients with latent diabetes mellitus suggested that administration of low doses (50 or 75 mg daily by mouth) of chlorpromazine would not signficantly modify glucose tolerance or plasma insulin concentrations. However a chlorpromazine infusion (50 mg over 1 hour) could induce hyperglycaemia and inhibit insulin secretion in both groups.— G. Erle *et al.*, *Eur. J. clin. Pharmac.*, 1977, *11*, 15.

Further references.— E. Thonnard-Neumann, *Am. J. Psychiat.*, 1968, *124*, 978; C. Korenyi and B. Lowenstein, *Dis. nerv. Syst.*, 1968, *29*, 827; A. Marinow, *ibid.*, 1971, *32*, 777.

Effects on the blood. A discussion of the development of immunological and coagulation abnormalities following long-term treatment with chlorpromazine.— M. H. Zarrabi *et al.*, *Ann. intern. Med.*, 1979, *91*, 194.

Agranulocytosis. A review of 16 deaths from agranulocytosis due to phenothiazines in physically healthy chronic schizophrenics. The occurrence of agranulocytosis due to phenothiazines had been estimated to be from 1 in 3000 to 1 in 250 000. If infection developed the mortality-rate from agranulocytosis was from 20 to 50%. Agranulocytosis was unlikely in young healthy individuals.— A. Mandel and M. Gross, *Dis. nerv. Syst.*, 1968, *29*, 32, per *Int. pharm. Abstr.*, 1968, *5*, 393. See also A. V. Pisciotta, *J. Am. med. Ass.*, 1969, *208*, 1862.

Further references.— E. M. Cheongvee *et al.*, *Br. J. clin. Pract.*, 1967, *21*, 95; R. Litvak and R. Kaelbling, *Archs gen. Psychiat.*, 1971, *24*, 265; J. V. Ananth *et al.*, *Am. J. Psychiat.*, 1973, *130*, 100; J. Marcus and F. J. Mulvihill, *J. clin. Psychiat.*, 1978, *39*, 784.

Aplastic anaemia. Chlorpromazine had been reported to cause aplastic anaemia.— R. H. Girdwood, *Drugs*, 1976, *11*, 394. See also W. H. W. Inman, *Br. med. J.*, 1977, *1*, 1500.

Further references.— N. Mansour and G. O. Broun, *Archs intern. Med.*, 1967, *119*, 113.

Effects on lymphocytes. In patients treated with phenothiazines, an average of 30.8% of atypical lymphocytes was found in 28 schizophrenics and of 28.7% in 12 other patients, compared with 17.2 and 18.7% respectively in 21 schizophrenics and 23 healthy subjects who did not receive phenothiazines.— R. R. Fieve *et al.*, *Archs gen. Psychiat.*, 1966, *15*, 529, per *Abstr. Wld Med.*, 1967, *41*, 553.

Effects on platelets. The effects of chlorpromazine on blood platelets.— D. J. Boullin *et al.*, *Br. J. clin. Pharmac.*, 1975, *2*, 29.

See also under Cardiovascular Disorders in Uses (below).

Haemolytic anaemia. A report of auto-immune haemolytic anaemia provoked by chlorpromazine in a 57-year-old woman.— C. Hadnagy (letter), *Lancet*, 1976, *1*, 423.

Two girls, aged 15 and 20 years, with anorexia nervosa developed haemolytic anaemia after 2 to 3 weeks' treatment with chlorpromazine 100 mg three or four times daily; a prompt haematological response occurred when chlorpromazine was withdrawn.— J. How and R. J. L. Davidson, *Postgrad. med. J.*, 1977, *53*, 278.

Further references.— C. Swett, *Archs gen. Psychiat.*, 1975, *32*, 1416.

Effects on the endocrine system. *Pituitary and hypothalamus.* Three men who were being treated for mental illness with drug regimens that included phenothiazine derivatives (prochlorperazine, trifluoperazine, and thioridazine) developed gynaecomastia. When thioridazine was withdrawn in 1 patient the symptoms abated.— I. B. Margolis and C. G. Gross, *J. Am. med. Ass.*, 1967, *199*, 942.

A discussion of the potential danger of using phenothiazines in patients with breast cancer when the increase in serum-prolactin concentrations might have some effect on the tumour.— P. Ettigi *et al.* (letter), *Lancet*, 1973, *2*, 266. An epidemiological study demonstrating no association between neuroleptic use and breast cancer.— S. Wagner and N. Mantel, *Cancer Res.*, 1978, *38*, 2703.

Over a threefold increase in plasma-prolactin concentrations in men and women schizophrenics treated with chlorpromazine or thioridazine.— H. Y. Meltzer and V. S. Fang, *Archs gen. Psychiat.*, 1976, *33*, 279.

The majority of patients receiving chronic phenothiazine therapy have only moderately raised serum-prolactin concentrations. Of 9 patients with galactorrhoea associated with phenothiazine therapy, 6 had prolactin concentrations towards the upper end of normal and 3 had elevated concentrations ranging from 75 to 100 ng per ml.— D. L. Kleinberg *et al.*, *New Engl. J. Med.*, 1977, *296*, 589.

Hyperprolactinaemia in alcoholic patients might be exacerbated if they are treated with phenothiazines. In 5 alcoholic patients serum-prolactin concentrations were raised after treatment with promazine (to above the normal range in 3).— S. K. Majumdar (letter), *Lancet*, 1978, *2*, 101.

A study in 21 males receiving long-term phenothiazine therapy indicated no increase in pituitary size despite the theoretical risk associated with phenothiazine therapy.— S. Rosenblatt *et al.* (letter), *Lancet*, 1978, *2*, 319.

Further references.— H. Y. Meltzer *et al.*, *Psychopharmac. Bull.*, 1977, *13*, 59.

Thyroid. Serum-thyroxine concentrations were markedly depressed in 5 patients treated with phenothiazines for serious psychiatric disease. Serum-tri-iodothyronine concentrations were normal.— G. Gwinup and N. Rapp, *Am. J. clin. Path.*, 1975, *63*, 94.

Effects on the eyes. No ocular lesions like those reported to occur in psychiatric patients given long-term treatment with high doses of chlorpromazine were encountered in 44 out-patients who had taken the drug for 9 to 12 years in daily doses of about 160 mg.— L. V. Sarin *et al.*, *J. Am. med. Ass.*, 1966, *198*, 789.

Of 271 patients who had received chlorpromazine in a daily dosage of 300 mg or more for at least 2 years, 36% showed lens changes and 17% corneal changes, consisting of white and yellowish-white granules. No impairment of retinal function or abnormality of intra-ocular pressure was detected.— M. B. R. Mathalone, *Br. J. Ophthal.*, 1967, *51*, 86.

In a controlled study of schizophrenic patients, opacities of the lens, posterior cornea, or anterior cornea of the eye were more likely to appear in those treated with high doses over a 6-month period than in those who had received a low dose or placebo. The anterior corneal lesions are reversible, but follow-up revealed relatively little improvement in lenticular and posterior corneal change.— R. F. Prien *et al.*, *Archs gen. Psychiat.*, 1970, *23*, 464.

Further references.— C. G. Mason, *J. Toxic. environ. Hlth*, 1977, *2*, 977.

Effects on the gastro-intestinal tract. Postmortem reports indicated that intestinal dilatation occurred in 12% of patients from a mental hospital who had been treated with a phenothiazine derivative compared with 2% of patients from a general hospital. The mechanism of the dilatation was not known but could be related to the anticholinergic effects of phenothiazine derivatives.— V. Ritama *et al.* (letter), *Lancet*, 1969, *1*, 470.

Fatal paralytic ileus with peritonitis occurred in a 19-year-old woman who had received chlorpromazine hydrochloride 250 mg four times daily, trifluoperazine hydrochloride 10 mg four times daily, and benztropine mesylate 1 mg thrice daily. The anticholinergic effects of the 3 drugs were considered responsible.— J. Giordano *et al.*, *Sth. med. J.*, 1975, *68*, 351.

A report of necrotising colitis developing in a woman on long-term treatment with chlorpromazine.— A. M. Hay, *Dis. Colon Rectum*, 1978, *21*, 380.

Adult-onset Hirschsprung's disease (aganglionic megacolon) occurring in one patient might have been associated with phenothiazine therapy.— P. B. Lesser *et al.*, *J. Am. med. Ass.*, 1979, *242*, 747.

Effects on the heart. ECG abnormalities, including sinus tachycardia, T-wave abnormality, S-T depression, Q-T prolongation, and right bundle branch block, were found in 59 of 140 schizophrenic patients (135 men, 5 women) taking phenothiazines including chlorpromazine, thioridazine, trifluoperazine, and fluphenazine. None of the patients had shown evidence of heart disease. Exercise increased S-T depression but the abnormalities were all reversible in 48 patients. There was no significant difference between drugs.— M. V. J. Raj and R. Benson, *Postgrad. med. J.*, 1975, *51*, 65.

Cardiac arrest in a hypothyroid woman may have been due to phenothiazine sensitivity.— J. Gomez and G. Scott, *Br. J. Psychiat.*, 1980, *136*, 89.

Further references.— C. Carlsson *et al.* (letter), *Lancet*, 1966, *1*, 1208; C. S. Alexander and A. Nino, *Am. Heart J.*, 1969, *78*, 757; G. Chouinard *et al.*, *Int. J. clin. Pharmac. Biopharm.*, 1975, *11*, 327; N. O. Fowler *et al.*, *Am. J. Cardiol.*, 1976, *37*, 223; U. Elkayam and W. Frishman, *Am. Heart J.*, 1980, *100*, 397.

Effects on the kidneys. For reference to the possible impairment of concentrating capacity of the urine by the kidneys in patients receiving neuroleptic drugs, see Lithium Carbonate, p.1536.

Effects on lipid metabolism. In a series of controlled studies there was a significant incidence of raised serum-cholesterol concentrations in subjects given chlorpromazine.— M. Clark *et al.*, *Clin. Pharmac. Ther.*, 1970, *11*, 883.

Effects on the liver. Antimitochondrial antibodies were detected in the sera of 7 patients who developed jaundice after treatment with chlorpromazine; antibodies were not found in patients who did not develop jaundice, or in patients with viral hepatitis. The presence of antibodies might be of value in differential diagnosis.— M. Rodriguez *et al.*, *J. Am. med. Ass.*, 1969, *208*, 148.

Jaundice and the presence of a factor VIII inhibitor in the blood were reported in a 90-year-old man who had been given chlorpromazine 50 mg by intramuscular injection on alternate days for 2 weeks. He died in spite of treatment with blood transfusions, vitamin K, factor VIII, and cyclophosphamide.— R. L. Glazier and E. B. Crowell, *Thromb. Haemostasis*, 1977, *37*, 523.

Further references.— A. Clarke *et al.*, *Aust. N.Z. J. Med.*, 1972, *2*, 376; R. I. Russell *et al.*, *Br. med. J.*, 1973, *1*, 655.

Effects on mental state. *Catatonia.* Neuroleptic-associated catatonia in 2 patients. One patient, who had received chlorpromazine, died of pneumonia and the other, who had received haloperidol, and was subsequently given chlorpromazine after the development of catatonia, was still comatose after 7 months.— Q. R. Regestein *et al.*, *J. Am. med. Ass.*, 1977, *238*, 618. Comments. When catatonic stupor arises or substantially worsens after the beginning of treatment with neuroleptic agents a reaction to treatment should be suspected and a period of drug withdrawal should follow.— D. R. Weinberger and R. J. Wyatt (letter), *ibid.*, 1978, *239*, 1846. Reply.— Q. R. Regestein (letter), *ibid.*

Depression. A brief discussion of the role of phenothiazines and butyrophenones in causing depression.— F. A. Whitlock and L. E. J. Evans, *Drugs*, 1978, *15*, 53.

Paradoxical response. Chlorpromazine hydrochloride was more likely to have a paradoxical effect in adolescents than in adults.— M. J. L. Ellis, *Practitioner*, 1977, *218*, 818.

Sleep-walking. For reference to sleep-walking in patients receiving lithium in association with neuroleptic therapy, see Lithium Carbonate, p.1537.

Effects on sexual function. A discussion on the impairment of male sexual function by psychotropic drugs, including mention that thioridazine appears to be the worst offender.— *Br. med. J.*, 1979, *2*, 883.

Further references.— J. N. Nestoros and H. E. Lehmann, *Int. Drug Ther. Newslett.*, 1979, *14*, 21.

Priapism. Priapism due to chlorpromazine therapy could be an idiosyncratic response of the autonomic nervous system.— K. Dawson-Butterworth (letter), *Br. med. J.*, 1970, *4*, 118.

Effects on the skin. A brief review of cutaneous side-effects, especially phototoxicity, of phenothiazines.— O. Hägermark *et al.*, *Br. J. Derm.*, 1971, *84*, 605.

Lichenoid dermatitis. Lichenoid dermatitis in a 75-year-old woman was considered to be due to chlorpromazine phototoxicity.— I. Matsuo *et al.*, *Dermatologica*, 1979, *159*, 46.

Phototoxicity. Several experiments were made on about 100 patients with schizophrenia to test their sensitivity to light after varying dosage treatments with chlorpromazine. The critical dosage of chlorpromazine hydrochloride required to produce a phototoxic reaction appeared to be about 600 mg daily.— A. Satanove and J. S. McIntosh, *J. Am. med. Ass.*, 1967, *200*, 209.

Chlorpromazine caused both phototoxic and photoallergic skin reactions. In a sensitised patient a photoallergic response will be achieved with a concentration of drug that will not produce a phototoxic reaction. The two reactions can be distinguished histologically if skin tests are biopsied within 24 hours after the reaction becomes apparent. There is evidence of the reaction in the first 24 hours in phototoxicity and in 24 to 96 hours in photoallergy.— S. Epstein, *Archs Derm.*, 1968, *98*, 354.

Further references.— R. S. Day and M. Dimattina, *Chemico-biol. Interactions*, 1977, *17*, 89.

Pigmentation. The pigment found in the skin of patients treated with chlorpromazine was considered to be formed in a light-catalysed anaerobic reaction in which chlorpromazine was polymerised and deposited with melanin and hydrogen chloride liberated. The acid could account for the skin irritation. The polymer was prepared and produced a bluish-purple discoloration which faded in 3 days when injected intracutaneously into 2 volunteers.— C. L. Huang and F. L. Sands, *J. pharm. Sci.*, 1967, *56*, 259. See also M. Nejmeh and N. Pilpel, *J. Pharm. Pharmac.*, 1978, *30*, 748.

Further references.— A. H. Robins, *S. Afr. med. J.*, 1975, *49*, 1521; A. G. Smith *et al.*, *Br. J. Derm.*, 1977, *96*, 537.

Toxic epidermal necrolysis. A report of toxic epidermal

necrolysis in a 21-year-old man after treatment with chlorpromazine.— K. M. Stein *et al.*, *Br. J. Derm.*, 1972, *86*, 246.

Effects on speech. Mutism occurred in 11 patients, 9 of whom received phenothiazines. Normal speech gradually returned in 6 patients when treatment was withdrawn and some improvement occurred in 1 patient.— S. Behrman, *Br. J. Psychiat.*, 1972, *121*, 599.

Epileptogenic effect. Of 859 patients with no history of epilepsy who were treated with phenothiazines, 10 had spontaneous epileptic seizures. The seizures occurred soon after starting treatment or within a few days of a sudden increase in dosage. No seizures occurred in 669 similar patients who were not given phenothiazines. It was suggested that phenothiazines were potential epileptogenic agents.— J. Logothetis, *Neurology, Minneap.*, 1967, *17*, 869. The Boston Collaborative Drug Surveillance Program monitored consecutively 32 812 medical inpatients. Drug-induced convulsions occurred in 1 of 949 patients given chlorpromazine.— J. Porter and H. Jick, *Lancet*, 1977, *1*, 587.

Grand mal seizures followed myelography with metrizamide in a 25-year-old patient who had taken chlorpromazine 75 mg daily.— T. Hindmarsh *et al.*, *Acta radiol., Diagnosis*, 1975, *16*, 129.

Further references.— T. M. Itil and C. Soldatos, *J. Am. med. Ass.*, 1980, *244*, 1460.

Extrapyramidal effects. The Boston Collaborative Drug Surveillance Program monitored consecutively 32 812 medical inpatients. Drug-induced extrapyramidal symptoms occurred in 1 of 1067 patients given chlorpromazine, in 1 of 198 given prochlorperazine and chlorpromazine, and in 3 of 44 given trifluoperazine hydrochloride and prochlorperazine or chlorpromazine.— J. Porter and H. Jick, *Lancet*, 1977, *1*, 587.

A prolonged dystonic reaction in a woman with myxoedema given chlorpromazine 50 mg intramuscularly.— G. M. Wood and A. K. Waters, *Postgrad. med. J.*, 1980, *56*, 192.

Further references.— C. Cassimos *et al.*, *J. Pediat.*, 1975, *87*, 981.

It has been commented by S.H. Snyder (*New Engl. J. Med.*, 1979, *300*, 465) that in contrast to the hyperactivity of tardive dyskinesia, the acute extrapyramidal effects of neuroleptics usually invoke hypokinesia, as in Parkinson's disease. For details of tardive dyskinesia, see under Tardive Dyskinesia (below).

For mention of the effects of phenothiazines on speech, see Effects on Speech (above).

Tardive dyskinesia. A discussion of the problem of tardive dyskinesia, which is a syndrome, or several syndromes, of involuntary movement in psychiatric patients taking neuroleptic drugs. To meet the definition the dyskinesia must be persistent and must not have preceded the onset of neuroleptic medication. Most of the patients are chronic schizophrenics and the condition has an insidious onset with exaggerated and persistent chewing movements or variations such as sucking and smacking movements, tongue protrusion, grimacing, and grunting; it may be accompanied by more widespread choreiform movements of the neck, shoulders, and arms, and occasionally the legs and trunk. The dyskinesia is related to dose, duration of treatment, and age. At a conservative estimate, one-third of patients receiving neuroleptic medication continuously for 5 years or more will develop the syndrome. The most popular theory of its cause, is that tardive dyskinesia is due to a hypersensitivity of the post-synaptic neurone to dopamine. There is evidence for D_1 and D_2 dopamine receptors, and D_2 receptors may be those that become hypersensitive. Another theory is that tardive dyskinesia may be caused by an imbalance between the acetylcholine transmitter system and the dopamine system.— *Lancet*, 1979, *2*, 447. It is much too premature to relate tardive dyskinesia to the effect of either D_1 or D_2 dopamine receptor antagonists. Specific D_1 receptor antagonists have not been found; among the proposed selective D_2 antagonists some are known to induce tardive dyskinesias, and although others may be less likely to do so, clinical experience does not yet seem sufficient to substantiate such a claim.— J. Hyttel and I. M. Nielsen (letter), *ibid.*, 1300. Similar comments.— D. N. Bateman and P. G. Blain (letter), *ibid.*, 641; P. Jenner and C. D. Marsden (letter), *ibid.*, 900. Tardive dyskinesias appear to be associated with a form of tolerance to phenothiazine therapy. They are frequently associated with reduction in the phenothiazine dosage, and characteristically resolve when the dosage is adjusted upward; they may also develop in patients chronically maintained on a fixed dosage, and similarly respond to an increased dosage. For example, they always respond to addition of an adequate amount of haloperidol, a very potent dopaminergic blocking agent. Neuroleptic agents should only be used where their clinical efficacy is demonstrated and milder sedative agents are less beneficial, but in patients in whom they are of proven benefit they need not be discontinued because of dyskinesias.— G. J. Gilbert (letter), *ibid.*, 798. A plea for caution in the use of regular 'drug holidays', for patients requiring maintenance neuroleptic therapy, in the hope of avoiding tardive dyskinesia. Such untested treatment is inappropriate and may increase the likelihood that any emergent dyskinesia would be irreversible.— A. V. P. Mackay (letter), *ibid.*, 1018.

Further reviews and comments on tardive dyskinesia.— *Br. med. J.*, 1981, *282*, 1257.

References to studies and comments on the cause and incidence of tardive dyskinesia.— L. Gochfeld *et al.*, *Am. J. Psychiat.*, 1977, *134*, 84; G. M. Simpson *et al.*, *Psychopharmacology*, 1978, *58*, 117; W. Y. Lui, *Archs Dis. Childh.*, 1979, *54*, 150; D. V. Jeste *et al.*, *Archs gen. Psychiat.*, 1979, *36*, 585; *idem* (letter), *New Engl. J. Med.*, 1979, *301*, 1184; R. J. Bradley *et al.* (letter), *Lancet*, 1980, *1*, 320; W. A. Brown and T. P. Laughren (letter), *ibid.*, 259; W. T. Carpenter *et al.* (letter), *ibid.*, *2*, 212.

Lupus erythematosus. A report of 8 patients with systemic lupus erythematosus associated with phenothiazines out of a group of approximately 4300 patients in 2 mental hospitals.— A. J. M. Fabius and W. K. Caulhoffer, *Acta rheum. scand.*, 1971, *17*, 137.

A 38-year-old man who had taken chlorpromazine 400 mg daily for 17 months developed systemic lupus erythematosus. His condition improved 2 weeks after cessation of the drug.— E. L. Dubois *et al.*, *J. Am. med. Ass.*, 1972, *221*, 595. See also L. S. Goldman *et al.*, *Am. J. Psychiat.*, 1980, *137*, 1613.

Patients with systemic lupus erythematosus or those taking prednisone were more susceptible to extrapyramidal symptoms produced by phenothiazines or tricyclic antidepressants.— Boston Collaborative Drug Surveillance Program, *J. Am. med. Ass.*, 1973, *224*, 889.

Further references.— J. V. Ananth and K. Minn (letter), *Can. med. Ass. J.*, 1973, *108*, 680.

Overdosage. A 4-year-old child died after taking 350 mg of chlorpromazine, but adults had survived doses of up to 9.75 g.— L. E. Hollister, *Clin. Pharmac. Ther.*, 1966, *7*, 142.

Porphyria. Chlorpromazine probably did not precipitate acute porphyria.— *Drug & Ther. Bull.*, 1976, *14*, 55. See also S. C. Allen and G. A. D. Rees, *Br. J. Anaesth.*, 1980, *52*, 835.

Pregnancy and the neonate. *Early pregnancy.* In a study in 836 infants with congenital malformations there was no significant difference in the maternal usage of phenothiazine tranquillisers during the first trimester of pregnancy compared with the use in 836 controls.— G. Greenberg *et al.*, *Br. med. J.*, 1977, *2*, 853.

A prospective study involving over 10 000 pregnant women indicated an association between congenital malformation and ingestion of phenothiazines during the first 3 months after the last menstrual period.— C. Rumeau-Rouquette *et al.*, *Teratology*, 1977, *15*, 57.

The percentage of malformed children among 1309 children born to mothers who had taken phenothiazines during the first 4 months of pregnancy was comparable to that in 48 973 children not so exposed. When analysed for specific malformations there was some evidence of an association with cardiovascular and possibly respiratory malformations but the finding was of doubtful import. IQ scores at 4 years were not affected.— D. Slone *et al.*, *Am. J. Obstet. Gynec.*, 1977, *128*, 486. Of 50 282 children born to mothers monitored by the Collaborative Perinatal Project 1309 were found to have been exposed to phenothiazines, and possibly other drugs, at some time during the first 4 months of the pregnancy. A slight association between cardiovascular deformities and the phenothiazine group as a whole was noted with ventricular septal defects in particular being associated with prochlorperazine (877 exposures).— O. P. Heinonen *et al.*, *Birth Defects and Drugs in Pregnancy*, Littleton MA, Publishing Sciences Group, 1977, 322.

Late pregnancy and labour. Extrapyramidal symptoms in the child of a woman who had been given chlorpromazine 400 to 600 mg daily during pregnancy. Treatment was with diphenhydramine and some symptoms persisted for 6 months.— W. Levy and K. Wisniewski, *N.Y. St. J. Med.*, 1974, *74*, 684.

Decreased intestinal motility in 2 infants whose mothers had received chlorpromazine in late pregnancy.— C. G. Falterman and C. J. Richardson, *J. Pediat.*, 1980, *97*, 308.

See also under Precautions and Uses.

Sudden death. A report of the sudden death of a 37-year-old manic-depressive woman who had received high doses of chlorpromazine over the previous 2 days. Her death was believed to have been due to phenothiazine-induced depression of the medullary respiratory centres of the brain stem.— A. Whyman, *J. nerv. ment. Dis.*, 1976, *163*, 214. A suggestion that occasional reports of sudden death due to aspiration or asphyxiation in patients receiving phenothiazines may be due to a syndrome similar to bulbar palsy. It is not reversed by antiparkinsonian medication.— K. Solomon, *Am. J. Psychiat.*, 1977, *134*, 308.

Tardive dyskinesia. See under Extrapyramidal Effects (above).

Urinary incontinence. Urinary incontinence associated with phenothiazine and butyrophenone therapy.— H. G. Nurnberg and P. J. Ambrosini, *J. clin. Psychiat.*, 1979, *40*, 271.

Weight gain. Weight gain associated with the long-term use of psychotropic agents such as phenothiazines appears to be secondary to altered mental status and resultant appetite improvement.— P. G. Pierpaoli, *Drug Intell. & clin. Pharm.*, 1972, *6*, 89.

Treatment of Adverse Effects. In severe overdosage the stomach should be emptied by aspiration and lavage. Emetics should not be used. To counter acute hypotension the patient should be placed in the head-down position, but it has been advised that strenuous efforts need not be made to raise the blood pressure providing the patient is producing urine; where appropriate, plasma expanders may be given for severe hypotension. Some sources have advocated the cautious intravenous administration of the alpha-adrenergic sympathomimetics, noradrenaline and phenylephrine (*not* adrenaline or other pressor amines), but other sources specifically contra-indicate the use of all sympathomimetics. In general, they are probably neither desirable nor necessary. Anti-arrhythmic agents may be required for cardiac arrhythmias. Convulsions may be controlled with diazepam given intravenously.

The central nervous depression should generally be allowed to recover naturally. The low body temperature should also be allowed to recover naturally unless there is any danger of cardiac arrhythmias being induced. For general guidelines to the symptomatic therapy of overdosage with central nervous system depressants, see Phenobarbitone, p.812.

Severe extrapyramidal reactions should be treated with a slow intravenous injection of antiparkinsonian agents, such as benztropine mesylate, procyclidine hydrochloride, or some antihistamines, such as diphenhydramine hydrochloride. Diazepam may also be effective.

Anticholinergic antiparkinsonian agents do not control tardive dyskinesia associated with long-term phenothiazine (or other antipsychotic) therapy, and may exacerbate symptoms.

Chlorpromazine is not effectively removed by haemodialysis.

Adsorption. For comment on the *in vitro* adsorption of chlorpromazine by activated charcoal, see p.79.

Cardiac effects. ECG T-wave abnormalities induced in psychiatric patients by the administration of phenothiazines could be corrected by overnight fasting or the administration of 10 g of a mixture of potassium acetate, bicarbonate, and citrate each in a 10% concentration.— S. C. Alvarez-Mena and M. J. Frank, *J. Am. med. Ass.*, 1973, *224*, 1730.

Dialysis. Studies in 2 patients who were given chlorpromazine 100 mg every 6 hours by mouth for 48 hours prior to haemodialysis and 100 mg of chlorpromazine labelled with sulphur-35, 50 μCi by mouth, 2 hours prior to haemodialysis, showed little transference of chlorpromazine across the dialysing cellophane membranes. Only 1.5 to 2% of the drug was recovered; this might have been partly due to erythrocyte and protein binding. It was concluded that haemodialysis was not an effective treatment for overdosage with phenothiazines.— M. M. Avram and J. T. McGinn, *J. Am. med. Ass.*, 1966, *197*, 142.

Further references.— G. Kriegelstein *et al.*, *Arzneimittel-Forsch.*, 1972, *22*, 1538.

Extrapyramidal effects. An intravenous injection of promethazine hydrochloride 25 to 50 mg very rapidly produced complete reversion of dystonia and dyskinesia caused by phenothiazines.— A. B. Black (letter), *Med. J. Aust.*, 1966, *2*, 782.

The extrapyramidal effects of phenothiazines are considered to be due to blockade of dopaminergic receptors. Levodopa is thus ineffective in treating these effects.— K. R. Hunter, *Prescribers' J.*, 1976, *16*, 101.

Benztropine did not appear to prevent chlorpromazine-induced extrapyramidal effects; there was an incidence of 9.3% in 86 patients taking chlorpromazine and benztropine compared with 10.6% in 568 patients taking chlorpromazine alone.— C. Swett *et al.*, *Archs gen. Psychiat.*, 1977, *34*, 942.

Tardive dyskinesia. A review of the treatment and prevention of tardive dyskinesia. Several drugs including reserpine, deanol, baclofen, pyridoxine, large quantities of choline, and most recently, lecithin, have been used experimentally to treat tardive dyskinesia, with mixed results. No treatment is uniformly successful and the best prevention is to minimise use of the drugs that cause the disorder. Antipsychotic drugs can decrease the choreiform movements but since these are the drugs that cause tardive dyskinesia, most experts use them only to suppress limb and trunk movements that seriously interfere with function.— *Med. Lett.*, 1979, *21*, 34. A similar review, including mention of the use of tetrabenazine, pimozide, and clonazepam in an attempt to diminish the dyskinesias.— *Drug & Ther. Bull.*, 1978, *16*, 55.

Further references.— J. Hajioff (letter), *Br. med. J.*, 1978, *2*, 834 (use of co-dergocrine mesylate).

Gastro-intestinal disorders. Beneficial effects with domperidone in alleviating dyspepsia in schizophrenic patients receiving maintenance doses of neuroleptic drugs.— R. Deberdt, *Postgrad. med. J.*, 1979, *55*, *Suppl.* 1, 48.

Precautions. Chlorpromazine is contra-indicated in comatose patients, particularly those under the influence of alcohol, barbiturates, narcotics, or other central nervous system depressants, and in patients with bone-marrow depression. Where possible it should not be given in conjunction with drugs that might cause leucopenia such as phenylbutazone and the thiouracil derivatives.

Chlorpromazine should be used with caution in patients with cardiovascular or respiratory disease, phaeochromocytoma, or other conditions in which a sudden drop in blood pressure would be undesirable; if it is used in conjunction with other drugs likely to cause postural hypotension an adjustment of dosage may be necessary. It should be used with caution in patients with existing tachycardia or cardiac insufficiency and in patients with liver dysfunction or a history of jaundice. Phenothiazines should be used with care in patients with parkinsonism; the antiparkinsonian actions of agents such as levodopa may be diminished by concurrent administration of phenothiazines.

The anti-emetic actions of chlorpromazine may mask the symptoms of disorders such as gastro-intestinal obstruction. Chlorpromazine should be given with caution in extremes of temperature owing to its impairment of the body's temperature-regulating mechanism.

If chlorpromazine is used in obstetrics it has been recommended that it should not be given until labour is established and the cervix dilated 3 to 4 cm.

Withdrawal symptoms including nausea, vomiting, gastritis, and tremors may occur following the abrupt discontinuation of large doses.

Chlorpromazine enhances the activity of CNS depressants including alcohol, anaesthetics, hypnotics, and narcotic analgesics and doses of these agents may need to be reduced. However, the anticonvulsant properties of diazepam, phenobarbitone, phenytoin or other anticonvulsants, are not enhanced by chlorpromazine which may, conversely, lower the convulsive threshold. The phenothiazines possess an anticholinergic activity and so enhance the anticholinergic properties of drugs such as atropine and tricyclic antidepressants. The antihypertensive action of adrenergic neurone blocking agents, such as guanethidine is reduced by chlorpromazine. Chlorpromazine may raise blood-sugar concentrations which could affect diabetic control.

Patients should be examined periodically for abnormal skin pigmentation or eye-changes, and chlorpromazine withheld if necessary. Chlorpromazine should be used with care in the elderly and debilitated. Drowsiness is often experienced at the start of treatment with chlorpromazine and patients should be advised not to take charge of vehicles or other machinery during this period.

A warning that antipsychotic drugs may slightly increase the accident risk during the first 7 to 14 days of treatment, even when small doses are used for minor indications. Psychotic patients should take antipsychotic drugs regularly, because once tolerance has developed, repeated psychotic episodes may be more detrimental to driving skills than the effect of the drug itself.— T. Seppala *et al.*, *Drugs*, 1979, *17*, 389.

Interactions. The incidence of hypotension was 10.2% in 187 nonsmokers taking chlorpromazine, 7.6% in 223 smoking up to 20 cigarettes daily, 4.6% in 87 smoking 20 to 40 cigarettes daily, and nil in 18 patients smoking more than 40 cigarettes daily.— C. Swett *et al.*, *Archs gen. Psychiat.*, 1977, *34*, 661. See also C. Swett, *Psychopharmac. Bull.*, 1977, *13*, 57.

Concentrations of folate in serum and erythrocytes were lower than normal in 16 patients who took anticonvulsants, in 15 who took phenothiazines and in 7 who took tricyclic antidepressants with a benzodiazepine. All the patients showed significant induction of hepatic microsomal enzymes. Folate deficiency occurred in patients after 2 to 5 years' treatment and was greater in those treated for longer periods. It was suggested that folate deficiency due to the induction of microsomal enzymes might subsequently limit enzyme induction and hence reduce drug metabolism and could thereby lead to symptoms of toxicity in patients apparently stabilised for a number of years. The dietary intake of patients on long-term treatment with enzyme-inducing drugs might be inadequate.— D. Labadarios *et al.*, *Br. J. clin. Pharmac.*, 1978, *5*, 167. An investigation in 28 schizophrenic patients receiving long-term neuroleptic treatment with fluphenazine or flupenthixol, in some cases with chlorpromazine, showed no biochemical evidence of hepatic microsomal enzyme induction.— S. K. Majumdar and P. P. Kakad, *Postgrad. med. J.*, 1978, *54*, 789.

Further conflicting views on whether phenothiazines stimulate hepatic enzyme induction.— I. H. Stevenson *et al.* (letter), *J. Pharm. Pharmac.*, 1972, *24*, 577; T. Kolakowska *et al.*, *Br. J. clin. Pharmac.*, 1975, *2*, 25.

Adrenaline and other sympathomimetics. For comments on the interaction between adrenaline and alpha-adrenoceptor blocking agents, see Adrenaline, p.2, and Phenoxybenzamine, p.158.

For a report of the nerve uptake of noradrenaline being inhibited by chlorpromazine, see Noradrenaline Acid Tartrate, p.21.

Alcohol. Akathisia and dystonia occurred after consumption of alcohol in patients taking phenothiazines. Alcohol might lower the threshold of resistance to neurotoxic side-effects.— E. G. Lutz, *J. Am. med. Ass.*, 1976, *236*, 2422.

Antacids. Studies in 6 patients showed that chlorpromazine plasma concentrations were significantly lower after administration of chlorpromazine with an aluminium hydroxide and magnesium trisilicate antacid gel (Gelusil) than after chlorpromazine alone. *In vitro* studies indicated that chlorpromazine was highly bound to the gel.— W. E. Fann *et al.*, *J. clin. Pharmac.*, 1973, *13*, 388.

Further references.— F. M. Forrest *et al.*, *Biol. Psychiat.*, 1970, *2*, 53.

Anticoagulants. For a possible effect of chlorpromazine therapy on anticoagulant control, see Warfarin Sodium, p.776.

Aspirin and other anti-inflammatory analgesics. In 4 of 5 psychiatric patients taking chlorpromazine, serum concentrations of 'free' chlorpromazine increased when acetanilide 3 g daily was given concomitantly. The amounts of unchanged chlorpromazine excreted in the urine increased in all the patients. Salicylamide 3 g daily produced a qualitatively similar but lesser effect, but aspirin in the same dose had a negligible effect. Acetanilide, and to a lesser extent salicylamide, competed with chlorpromazine in forming hydroxy derivatives and glucuronides.— C. L. Huang and K. Hirano, *Biochem. Pharmac.*, 1967, *16*, 2023.

Benzhexol and other antiparkinsonian agents. A study of plasma-chlorpromazine concentrations in relation to clinical response. Concurrent administration of benzhexol appeared to lower chlorpromazine concentrations.— L. Rivera-Calimlim *et al.*, *Clin. Pharmac. Ther.*, 1973, *14*, 978. A placebo-controlled study indicating that benzhexol had no effect on plasma-chlorpromazine concentration.— G. M. Simpson *et al.*, *Archs gen. Psychiat.*, 1980, *37*, 205.

Beverages. In vitro findings of an interaction between the antipsychotic drugs, fluphenazine and haloperidol, and coffee or tea.— F. Kulhanek *et al.* (letter), *Lancet*, 1979, *2*, 1130. Agreement. The interaction might account for variations in blood concentrations.— S. R. Hirsch (letter), *ibid.* A study in patients receiving chlorpromazine, haloperidol, fluphenazine, or trifluoperazine indicated that limitations on coffee and tea intake in psychiatric hospitals cannot be justified on the grounds that such beverages might lower the efficacy of antipsychotic drugs.— S. Bowen *et al.* (letter), *Lancet*, 1981, *1*, 1217. Results supporting the view that coffee or tea alter the pharmacokinetics of neuroleptics by reducing the overall effect and by producing a retard drug out of the short-acting one.— F. Kulhanek and O. K. Linde (letter), *ibid.*, *2*, 359. Despite the interaction *in vitro* a study in 12 healthy subjects indicated no significant reduction in plasma concentrations of fluphenazine on concomitant ingestion of the hydrochloride with tea or coffee.— S. M. Wallace *et al.* (letter), *Lancet*, 1981, *2*, 691.

Diazoxide. For the effect of chlorpromazine on diazoxide, see Diazoxide, p.143.

Guanethidine and other adrenergic neurone blocking agents. For the effect of chlorpromazine on guanethidine, see Guanethidine Monosulphate, p.146.

Lithium. For the effect of chlorpromazine on lithium, see Lithium Carbonate, p.1539.

Phenobarbitone and other barbiturates. Phenobarbitone increased the rate of urinary chlorpromazine excretion by 10 to 81%. When epileptic patients normally receiving barbiturates and chlorpromazine had their barbiturate withdrawn for 7 days there was a 17 to 55% decrease in urinary chlorpromazine excretion. A preparation of aluminium hydroxide with magnesium hydroxide adsorbed chlorpromazine when administered simultaneously and reduced the chlorpromazine urinary excretion-rate by 10 to 45%. This effect could be reduced by giving the medications 2 hours apart.— F. M. Forrest *et al.*, *Biol. Psychiat.*, 1970, *2*, 53, per *Int. pharm. Abstr.*, 1970, *7*, 282.

Phenytoin and other anticonvulsants. A 55-year-old man who had been receiving phenytoin 300 mg daily for over 3 years and who was suffering from stable tardive dyskinesia which had been induced by haloperidol (discontinued 2 years previously) obtained amelioration of his symptoms on discontinuation of phenytoin for a week. On reintroduction of phenytoin the dyskinesia relapsed to its original severity. Phenytoin might exacerbate neuroleptic-induced dyskinesia.– J. DeVeaugh-Geiss (letter), *New Engl. J. Med.*, 1978, *298*, 457. Criticism.— P. A. Nausieda (letter), *ibid.*, 1093.

Piperazine. A child who had received piperazine for worms convulsed when given chlorpromazine several days later. Experiments in *dogs* and *goats* demonstrated that though piperazine or chlorpromazine given separately produced no ataxia, severe clonic convulsions, sometimes fatal, occurred when they were given together.— B. M. Boulos and L. E. Davis (letter), *New Engl. J. Med.*, 1969, *280*, 1245.

Propranolol and other beta-blockers. Caution is essential when giving propranolol for hypertension to patients already stabilised on phenothiazines or tricyclic antidepressants.— R. Galinsky (letter), *New Engl. J. Med.*, 1976, *295*, 281. There was little reported evidence of trouble with this association.— N. M. Kaplan (letter), *ibid.*

A study completed by 6 chronic schizophrenic patients in good general health indicated that addition of propranolol to chlorpromazine therapy raises plasma concentrations of chlorpromazine.— M. Peet *et al.* , *I.C.I. Pharmaceuticals* (letter), *Lancet*, 1980, *2*, 978.

Tricyclic antidepressants. Since phenothiazines, tricyclic antidepressants, and antiparkinsonian agents had anticholinergic properties the use of combinations of any of these drugs could produce confusion, impaired memory, hallucinations, and disorientation.— D. S. Janowsky *et al.*, *Am. J. Psychiat.*, 1972, *129*, 360.

Raised concentrations of phenothiazines caused by concomitant amitriptyline therapy.— A. Jus *et al.*, *Neuropsychobiology*, 1978, *4*, 305.

Interference with diagnostic tests. Chlorpromazine is reported to interfere with pregnancy tests, thyroid-function tests, the Coombs' test where a false-positive result can be achieved, and with adrenal medullary tests. It is also reported to interfere with estimations for serum

5-hydroxyindole-acetic acid, blood urea, urinary ketones and steroids, urinary porphobilinogen, and vitamin B_{12}.

Phenothiazines could cause a pink to red or red-brown discoloration of the urine.— L. H. Block and P. P. Lamy, *Am. prof. Pharm.*, 1968, *34* (Feb.), 27.

Myasthenia gravis. Exacerbation of myasthenia gravis by chlorpromazine.— M. P. McQuillen *et al.*, *Archs Neurol.*, 1963, *8*, 286.

Further references.— Z. Argov and Y. Yaari, *Brain Res.*, 1979, *164*, 227.

Pregnancy and the neonate. *Diffusion across the placenta.* Chlorpromazine and its metabolites were found in the maternal plasma and urine, in the foetal plasma and amniotic fluid, and in neonatal urine after doses of 50 to 100 mg of chlorpromazine were given intramuscularly to pregnant women shortly before delivery.— S. E. F. O'Donoghue (letter), *Nature*, 1971, *229*, 124.

If given in high doses over a long period during pregnancy, chlorpromazine might cause damage to the retina of the foetus.— G. M. Stirrat, *Prescribers' J.*, 1973, *13*, 135. *Animal* studies on accumulation of chorio-retino-toxic drugs in the foetal eye.— N. G. Lindquist *et al.*, *Acta pharmac. tox.*, 1970, *28*, *Suppl.* 1, 64.

Excretion in breast milk. Preliminary data suggesting that in mothers taking chlorpromazine, concentrations can be higher in milk than in maternal plasma and might be associated with drowsiness and lethargy in the infant.— D. H. Wiles *et al.* (letter), *Br. J. clin. Pharmac.*, 1978, *5*, 272.

See also under Adverse Effects and Uses.

Temperature variations. Chlorpromazine might accidentally produce hypothermia in the elderly and it should therefore be used with care, especially in winter, for patients who were not under regular medical supervision, and the dose should always be kept to the minimum.— Amulree, *Abstr. Wld Med.*, 1968, *42*, 333.

There is a risk of hypothermia occurring during swimming in patients taking phenothiazine drugs.— J. Johnson (letter), *Br. med. J.*, 1969, *1*, 711.

Death from heat stroke, during a heat wave, of a 32-year-old man taking chlorpromazine 225 mg daily.— F. Ellis (letter), *Br. med. J.*, 1976, *2*, 474.

Withdrawal. Each of 4 groups of 10 patients was given 1 of the following drugs: chlorpromazine, thioridazine, chlorprothixene, or perphenazine. When the drug was suddenly withdrawn, gastro-intestinal symptoms developed within 1 to 2 days and lasted for up to 8 days. The symptoms, which included nausea, vomiting, malaise, and abdominal pain, occurred in 3 patients given 0.9 to 1 g of chlorpromazine daily, in 3 given 100 to 300 mg of thioridazine daily, and in 1 given 450 mg of chlorprothixene daily.— P. Haden, *Can. med. Ass. J.*, 1964, *91*, 974. Withdrawal symptoms on stopping antipsychotic drugs appear to occur in between 17% and 75% of patients. Typically they start in the first few days, reach a maximum during the first week, and disappear by the end of the second week. They do not appear to be dose-related. Drugs with marked anticholinergic properties such as chlorpromazine and thioridazine have the highest rates of withdrawal symptoms, whereas the weaker anticholinergic agents, in particular the piperazine phenothiazines, rarely produce withdrawal symptoms unless antiparkinsonian drugs are withdrawn simultaneously. The withdrawal symptoms usually consist of one or more of the following: nausea, vomiting, diarrhoea, perspiration, restlessness, insomnia, rhinorrhoea, headaches, increased appetite, and giddiness.— G. Gardos *et al.*, *Am. J. Psychiat.*, 1978, *135*, 1321.

Within a month of stopping chlorpromazine, which she had taken for 6 years for schizophrenia, a 28-year-old woman developed symptoms usually associated with Gilles de la Tourette syndrome. Within the first month she had sudden brief twitches of facial muscles, these spread to her shoulders and arms and within a few months she had spontaneous vocalisations in the form of barking and clicking sounds. During the next year manifestations of both Gilles de la Tourette syndrome and schizophrenia were well controlled by haloperidol.— H. L. Klawans *et al.*, *Neurology, Minneap.*, 1978, *28*, 1064.

A 21-year-old woman who had taken phenothiazines for most of her life since the age of 5, initially probably for school refusal, subsequently for obsessional symptoms and later, in association with large doses of oxazepam, for anxiety, was admitted to hospital following a small overdose of chlorpromazine. Her state of consciousness was apparently unimpaired following the overdose but she became progressively more agitated and after initial treatment with thioridazine was eventually diagnosed as suffering from probable drug-induced organic psychosis. On recovery from the toxic psychosis she was considered to be free of psychotic symptoms. A few weeks later, however, she developed symptoms of schizophrenia and over subsequent months her illness gradually evolved into a typical schizophrenic picture. Although schizophrenia may have been insidiously developing and she had a number of aetiological factors for schizophrenia, it was also considered that her chronic phenothiazine therapy could have played a role.— I. Sale and H. Kristall, *Aust. N.Z. J. Psychiat.*, 1978, *12*, 73.

Absorption and Fate. Chlorpromazine is readily absorbed from the gastro-intestinal tract but is subject to considerable first-pass metabolism in the gut wall. It is also extensively metabolised in the liver and is excreted in the urine and faeces in the form of numerous active and inactive metabolites; there is evidence of enterohepatic recycling. Owing to the first-pass effect, plasma concentrations following oral administration are much lower than those following intramuscular administration. Moreover, there is very wide intersubject variation in plasma concentrations of chlorpromazine; no simple correlation has been found between plasma concentrations of chlorpromazine and its metabolites, and their therapeutic effect. Paths of metabolism of chlorpromazine include hydroxylation and conjugation with glucuronic acid, *N*-oxidation, oxidation of a sulphur atom, and dealkylation. Although the plasma half-life of chlorpromazine has been reported to be only a few hours, it has a very prolonged terminal elimination phase of up to about 3 weeks. Its duration of therapeutic effect can range from a few days to several weeks or possibly longer.

Chlorpromazine is very extensively bound to plasma proteins. It is widely distributed in the body and crosses the blood-brain barrier to achieve higher concentrations in the brain than in the plasma. Chlorpromazine and its metabolites also cross the placental barrier and are excreted in milk (see under Precautions).

A review of the literature on the absorption and fate of chlorpromazine. Blood and urinary studies by and large favour a fairly short sojourn of the bulk of chlorpromazine in the body. For the blood studies this is in the range of 2 to 3 days and for the urinary studies up to about 18 days. There is no doubt, however, that chlorpromazine brings about changes that can persist much longer than this after drug discontinuation. The exact relationship of persisting therapeutic effects to administered chlorpromazine is uncertain. There is the possibility that minute amounts of chlorpromazine and/or metabolites persist at active sites in slowly reversible or relatively irreversible ways. It also seems that some chlorpromazine is stored in adipose tissue and slowly mobilised after stopping chlorpromazine administration.— R. B. Lacoursiere and H. E. Spohn, *J. nerv. ment. Dis.*, 1976, *163*, 267.

A review of the problems encountered in the monitoring of plasma-antipsychotic drug concentrations with specific reference to chlorpromazine, thioridazine, butaperazine, haloperidol, thiothixene, perphenazine, and penfluridol. Owing to wide variations between concentrations and response, routine monitoring remained of research interest only.— T. B. Cooper, *Clin. Pharmacokinet.*, 1978, *3*, 14.

In 6 of 8 patients maximum plasma concentrations of chlorpromazine were noted 15 or 30 minutes after intramuscular injection of chlorpromazine 50 mg; in the other 2 maximum concentrations were not reached until 4 hours after injection. Following administration of 100 mg by mouth peak plasma concentrations usually occurred after 2 to 3 hours with a relatively rapid reduction over the next 3 to 6 hours, compared with relatively stable concentrations for 12 to 36 hours after intramuscular injection in 4 subjects, indicating relatively slow absorption. The absorption of chlorpromazine following administration by mouth appeared to be about 25% of that given intramuscularly; following repeated administration the bioavailability decreased, possibly owing to increased metabolism in the gastro-intestinal lumen or in the intestinal wall. Fainting occurred in 5 of 6 patients whose plasma concentrations of unchanged chlorpromazine exceeded 100 ng per ml following single oral or intramuscular doses but tolerance of these same concentrations was noted in 2 of these 5 patients on the thirty-third day of repeated administration.— S. G. Dahl and R. E. Strandjord, *Clin. Pharmac. Ther.*, 1977, *21*, 437.

A study of the pharmacokinetics of chlorpromazine following oral administration of a single dose to 4 healthy subjects. Chlorpromazine began to appear in the systemic circulation after a mean of less than half an hour, and continued to be absorbed for about 3 hours. The harmonic mean terminal elimination half-life was 17.7 hours (range 6.64 to 118.9 hours). In 3 of the 4 subjects about 65% of the total excreted chlorpromazine appeared in the urine during the first 6 hours; excretion rapidly declined after the first 18 hours, with little or no chlorpromazine being detected in the 48- to 72-hour urine sample.— L. R. Whitfield *et al.*, *J. Pharmacokinet. Biopharm.*, 1978, *6*, 187.

Further references.— S. H. Curry *et al.*, *Br. J. Pharmac.*, 1972, *44*, 370P (plasma concentrations); A. Raskin, *J. nerv. ment. Dis.*, 1974, *159*, 120 (sex-linked differences); L. Rivera-Calimlim, *Psychopharmac. Bull.*, 1975, *11*, 76 (plasma concentrations); T. Kolakowska *et al.*, *Psychopharmacology*, 1976, *49*, 101 (plasma concentrations); D. H. Wiles *et al.*, *Psychol. Med.*, 1976, *6*, 407 (plasma concentrations); O. T. McKeown *et al.*, *Br. J. Psychiat.*, 1977, *131*, 172 (plasma concentrations); P. L. Man and C. H. Chen, *Psychosomatics*, 1978, *19*, 151 (plasma concentrations); P. R. A. May and T. Van Putten, *Archs gen. Psychiat.*, 1978, *35*, 1081 (plasma concentrations); L. Rivera-Calimlim, *Commun. Psychopharmac.*, 1978, *2*, 215 (plasma concentrations); B. Wode-Helgodt *et al.*, *Acta psychiat. scand.*, 1978, *58*, 149 (plasma and CSF concentrations); L. Rivera-Calimlim *et al.*, *Clin. Pharmac. Ther.*, 1979, *26*, 114 (plasma concentrations); L. A. Hershey *et al.*, *Clin. Pharmac. Ther.*, 1980, *27*, 257 (plasma concentrations).

Metabolism. An analytical report giving concentrations of 11 metabolites of chlorpromazine in chronic schizophrenic patients.— P. N. Daul *et al.*, *J. pharm. Sci.*, 1972, *61*, 581.

Investigations in 86 chronic schizophrenic patients indicated that patients judged to be under good control had relatively higher concentrations of the active metabolite 7-hydroxychlorpromazine in their plasma whereas in patients who were poorly controlled the inactive chlorpromazine sulphoxide predominated.— A. V. P. Mackay *et al.*, *Br. J. clin. Pharmac.*, 1974, *1*, 425.

Further references.— A. G. Bolt *et al.*, *J. pharm. Sci.*, 1966, *55*, 1205; N. West *et al.* (letter), *J. pharm. Sci.*, 1971, *60*, 953; N. R. Schooler *et al.*, *Psychopharmac. Bull.*, 1975, *11*, 30.

First-pass metabolism. Animal studies indicating first-pass metabolism of chlorpromazine in the gut.— S. H. Curry *et al.*, *Br. J. Pharmac.*, 1971, *42*, 403.

Further references.— M. Gibaldi and D. Perrier, *Drug Metab. Rev.*, 1974, *3*, 185.

Plasma protein binding. Chlorpromazine is highly bound to plasma protein, varying from 91.8 to 97% over the range of clinical blood concentrations (0.01 to 1 μg per ml). Binding is easily reversed.— S. H. Curry, *J. Pharm. Pharmac.*, 1970, *22*, 193.

Studies on the protein binding of phenothiazines, using bovine serum albumin, indicated that chlorpromazine has the highest affinity, followed in order by trifluoperazine, perphenazine, fluphenazine, and promazine. These results indicated that the order of binding affinity was based on the hydrophobicity of the phenothiazine, with the more hydrophobic molecules being more strongly bound.— H. Zia and J. C. Price, *J. pharm. Sci.*, 1975, *64*, 1177.

Further references.— M. H. Bickel, *J. Pharm. Pharmac.*, 1975, *27*, 733 (red cell, albumin, and lipoprotein binding); D. L. Garver *et al.*, *Archs gen. Psychiat.*, 1976, *33*, 862 (red cell binding); K. M. Piafsky *et al.*, *New Engl. J. Med.*, 1978, *299*, 1435 (α_1 acid glycoprotein binding).

Uses. Chlorpromazine has a wide range of activity arising from its depressant actions on the central nervous system and its alpha-adrenergic blocking and weaker anticholinergic activities. It is a dopamine inhibitor; it inhibits prolactin-release-inhibitory factor, considered to be dopamine, thus stimulating the release of prolactin. The turnover of dopamine in the brain is also increased.

Chlorpromazine possesses sedative and tranquillising properties but patients usually develop tolerance rapidly to the sedation. It has anti-emetic, antipruritic, serotonin-blocking, and weak antihistaminic properties and slight ganglion-blocking activity. It inhibits the heat regulating centre so that the patient tends to acquire the temperature of his surroundings. Chlorpromazine is analgesic and can relax skeletal muscle. Its actions on the autonomic system produce vasodilatation, hypotension, and tachycardia. Salivary and gastric secretions are reduced.

Chlorpromazine is widely used in the management of psychotic conditions. It controls excitement, agitation, and other psychomotor disturbances in schizophrenic patients and reduces the manic phase of manic-depressive conditions. It is used to control hyperkinetic states and aggression and is sometimes given in other psychiatric conditions for the control of anxiety and tension. Within an hour of a dose by mouth or 30 minutes of an intramuscular injection patients become apathetic, drowsy, and occasionally euphoric.

Chlorpromazine is anti-emetic and is used to control the nausea and vomiting of a variety of diseases and that caused by various drugs. It does not appear to be of benefit in motion sickness.

Chlorpromazine is effective in the alleviation of intractable hiccup. The sedative and anti-emetic properties of chlorpromazine are useful in the treatment of drug dependence. It has also been used for the management of alcohol withdrawal symptoms but compounds such as diazepam are now preferred.

Chlorpromazine has been given alone or in conjunction with pethidine and sometimes promethazine as premedication for surgical or diagnostic procedures. It was usually given by mouth or by intramuscular injection. When the schedule was administered intravenously the effects became more pronounced and produced what was termed enhanced or facilitated anaesthesia where the dose of anaesthetic could be considerably reduced or where no anaesthetic was required. Such procedures have, however, been associated with dangerous degrees of hypotension. Postoperative nausea and vomiting is reduced by chlorpromazine.

Since analgesic requirements are reduced by chlorpromazine it is used as an adjunct in the management of severe pain especially in malignant disease. It has also been used as an adjunct in the treatment of tetanus and is given to control acute intermittent porphyria.

Chlorpromazine is administered as the hydrochloride by mouth or injection, and as the embonate by mouth as a concentrated suspension in doses equivalent to those of the hydrochloride, and as the base rectally by suppository.

Dosage varies both with the individual and with the purpose for which the drug is being used. In most patients oral treatment may be used from the start, commencing with a dosage of 25 to 50 mg thrice daily and increasing as necessary; the usual daily maintenance dose ranges from 25 to 100 mg thrice daily. Psychotic patients may require daily doses of up to 1 g or more.

For parenteral use, deep intramuscular injection is preferable. Subcutaneous injection is contra-indicated and intravenous injection is usually limited to anaesthesia and severe hiccups; the injection must be diluted before intravenous administration. After injection of chlorpromazine, patients should remain in the supine position for at least 30 minutes. It is fairly well tolerated for short periods and is especially useful during the initial stages of treatment in psychiatric cases. The usual dose by injection is 25 to 50 mg repeated as required 3 or 4 times in 24 hours.

In the treatment of mild alcohol withdrawal, agitated patients may be given 25 to 50 mg intramuscularly, repeated if necessary, with subsequent doses of 25 to 50 mg thrice daily by mouth. Patients with less severe withdrawal symptoms may be given 30 to 75 mg daily in divided doses by mouth. Chlorpromazine should not be given to stuporous patients.

As an adjunct to the treatment of tetanus, 25 to 50 mg has been given intramuscularly 3 or 4 times daily.

If intractable hiccup does not respond to 25 to 50 mg three or four times daily by mouth for 2 to 3 days then 25 to 50 mg should be administered intramuscularly and if this fails 25 to 50 mg in 500 to 1000 ml of sodium chloride injection should be infused slowly, with the patient supine, and careful monitoring of the blood pressure; cloudy solutions should not be infused.

In the pre-operative medication before the administration of a general anaesthetic, 25 to 50 mg of chlorpromazine hydrochloride with 50 to 100 mg of pethidine hydrochloride has been given by intramuscular injection.

If the oral and parenteral routes are not suitable chlorpromazine is administered rectally and suppositories containing 100 mg of chlorpromazine base are employed; this has an effect comparable with 40 to 50 mg of the hydrochloride by mouth or 25 mg intramuscularly. Up to 4 suppositories may be given in 24 hours.

During the first few days of treatment, patients taking chlorpromazine should be advised not to drive vehicles or to use machinery.

For children over 5 years of age, one-third to one-half the adult dose may be given, and below this age a dose of 500 µg per kg body-weight may be given 4 times daily.

Action. Reviews, reports, and studies on the processes involved in psychosis and the mode of action of chlorpromazine and other antipsychotic agents in its control.— D. A. Bender (letter), *Lancet*, 1976, *2*, 427 (serotonin); D. J. Boullin and M. W. Orr, *Br. J. clin. Pharmac.*, 1976, *3*, 929 (serotonin); J. Korf and H. M. van Praag, *Am. J. Psychiat.*, 1976, *133*, 1171 (dopamine); *J. Am. med. Ass.*, 1977, *238*, 2113 (adenylate cyclase blockade); E. J. Sachar *et al.*, *Psychopharmac. Bull.*, 1977, *13*, 60 (prolactin); P. Seeman, *Biochem. Pharmac.*, 1977, *26*, 1741 (membrane receptors); P. H. Gruen *et al.*, *Archs gen. Psychiat.*, 1978, *35*, 108 (prolactin); F. A. Henn, *Lancet*, 1978, *2*, 293 (dopamine); H. Y. Meltzer (letter), *Lancet*, 1978, *1*, 1151 (dopamine blockade); F. Owen *et al.*, *Lancet*, 1978, *2*, 223 (dopamine receptors); D. V. Jeste *et al.* (letter), *Lancet*, 1979, *2*, 850 (dopamine β-hydroxylase); J. A. Smith *et al.*, *J. Pharm. Pharmac.*, 1979, *31*, 246 (melatonin); A. A. Mathé *et al.*, *Lancet*, 1980, *1*, 16 (prostaglandins).

Administration. A study demonstrating the feasibility of a twice-daily dosage regimen of chlorpromazine or trifluoperazine on weekdays only, with omission of the tranquilliser at weekends. Patients on alternate-day regimens relapsed. Whereas most patients could be maintained without medication for up to 6 weeks, relapses occurred within 6 months in 6 of 9.— C. -P. Chien and A. DiMascio, *Behav. Neuropsychiat.*, 1971, *3*, 5. See also Precautions (Withdrawal).

Criticism of the administration of high doses of antipsychotic therapy early in treatment. A double-blind study comparing loading against standard doses of haloperidol has demonstrated that for the average decompensated schizophrenic patient a moderate dose is sufficient to start the reintegrative process, which cannot be accelerated by loading doses. A patient can be started on a sufficient but moderate dose with therapeutic response and side-effects being carefully monitored. If there was no progress after 3 or 4 days a gradual increase in dosage would be indicated. The completely refractory patient, however, deserves a trial on high doses of potent phenothiazines or haloperidol.— S. E. Ericksen *et al.* (letter), *New Engl. J. Med.*, 1976, *294*, 1296.

Guidelines for the rapid amelioration of acute psychosis.— A. S. Mason and R. P. Granacher, *Dis. nerv. Syst.*, 1976, *37*, 547; *Int. Drug Ther. Newslett.*, 1977, *12*, 5. Comments.— R. H. Culpan and F. A. Whitlock, *Drugs*, 1978, *15*, 239.

Some reviews and comments on the advantages of using long-acting depot preparations of neuroleptics.— D. A. W. Johnson, *Br. J. Hosp. Med.*, 1977, *17*, 546; *Drug & Ther. Bull.*, 1979, *17*, 41. See also under clopenthixol decanoate (p.1517), flupenthixol decanoate (p.1528), fluphenazine decanoate and fluphenazine enanthate (p.1530), and fluspirilene (p.1531).

In children. A report of phenothiazine intoxication in 30 children as a complication of phenothiazine treatment. It was considered that a large number had received excessive doses.— B. Duffy, *Med. J. Aust.*, 1971, *1*, 676.

Data suggesting that impaired gut absorption or accelerated metabolism, of chlorpromazine, may occur in children.— L. Rivera-Calimlim *et al.*, *Clin. Pharmac. Ther.*, 1977, *21*, 115.

In the elderly. An intramuscular injection of 100 mg of chlorpromazine is potentially dangerous in elderly or debilitated patients. Postural hypotension with brain softening, myocardial infarction, syncope with trauma, and irreversible shock and death could occur. The sedative and hypotensive effects of chlorpromazine 100 mg by injection are equivalent to 400 to 500 mg by mouth.— P. S. Nemetz (letter), *Br. med. J.*, 1969, *1*, 186.

Phenothiazines, particularly those with aliphatic side-chains, such as chlorpromazine, and piperidine side-chains, such as thioridazine may produce a sudden drop in blood pressure, often when a person assumes an upright position. Elderly subjects, who may already have elevated blood pressure with loss of elasticity of the arterial wall, are more sensitive to the hypotensive effect, which predisposes them to episodes of cerebrovascular insufficiency or syncopal episodes which may lead to falls and resultant fractures. These drugs may also cause tachycardia and arrhythmias, to which elderly subjects may be predisposed. The elderly are also increasingly sensitive to the neurological side-effects of psychotropic drugs; extrapyramidal side-effects associated with neuroleptic use are common in the elderly, and tardive dyskinesia is seen more often in elderly females than males.— C. Salzman *et al.*, *N.Y. St. J. Med.*, 1976, *76*, 71.

Isolated symptoms of tardive dyskinesia consisting of rhythmic involuntary rocking movements of the abdominal muscles and trunk occurred in 2 elderly women, one of whom had been receiving high doses of thioridazine and the other of haloperidol over a period of time.— F. Lemere (letter), *J. Am. med. Ass.*, 1977, *238*, 306.

Further references.— F. J. Ayd, *J. Am. med. Ass.*, 1961, *175*, 1054; G. W. Paulson, *Geriatrics*, 1968, *23*, 105; M. A. Raskind *et al.*, *3ibid.*, 1976, *31*, 51; G. Chouinard *et al.*, *Am. J. Psychiat.*, 1979, *136*, 79.

Administration in hepatic failure. There was no difference in the plasma clearance and cerebral effects of chlorpromazine in 24 patients with cirrhosis compared with matched controls. The susceptibility to chlorpromazine of some patients with cirrhosis was probably due to increased sensitivity of cerebral neurones and not to impaired liver metabolism.— J. D. Maxwell *et al.*, *Clin. Sci.*, 1972, *43*, 143, per *J. Am. med. Ass.*, 1972, *222*, 726.

Further references.— A. E. Read *et al.*, *Br. med. J.*, 1969, *3*, 497.

Administration in renal failure. Chlorpromazine could be given in usual doses to patients in renal failure, but a reduction in dose or an increase in the interval between doses might be necessary if excessive sedation occurred in patients with a glomerular filtration-rate of less than 10 ml per minute. Concentrations of chlorpromazine are not affected by haemodialysis or peritoneal dialysis.— W. M. Bennett *et al.*, *Ann. intern. Med.*, 1977, *86*, 754. See also *idem*, 1980, *93*, 286.

Chlorpromazine in total doses of 0.1 to 1 g given over periods of 2 to 7 days induced toxic psychoses in 4 patients with chronic renal failure requiring haemodialysis. In a fifth patient toxic psychosis was associated with administration of promethazine.— C. J. McAllister *et al.*, *Clin. Nephrol.*, 1978, *10*, 191.

Alcohol and drug withdrawal. *Alcohol.* Chlorpromazine and mesoridazine each produced improvement which was most marked in the first week, in a controlled study of 40 patients in alcohol withdrawal states. Agitation, tremor, anxiety, and hallucinations were relieved or reduced.— J. B. Frost, *Can. psychiat. Ass. J.*, 1973, *18*, 385, per *J. Am. med. Ass.*, 1974, *227*, 576.

Narcotic analgesics. Chlorpromazine in a daily dose of 2.2 mg per kg body-weight in divided doses at 6-hourly intervals by mouth or injection was effective in relieving all the symptoms of diamorphine withdrawal in 178 infants born to diamorphine-addicted mothers. The dose of chlorpromazine was gradually reduced over 10 to 40 days.— C. Zelson *et al.*, *Pediatrics*, 1971, *48*, 178, per *Int. pharm. Abstr.*, 1972, *9*, 746. See also J. Kahn *et al.*, *J. Pediat.*, 1969, *75*, 495; *Med. Lett.*, 1973, *15*, 47.

Anaesthesia. References to the use of chlorpromazine for premedication and other anaesthetic procedures.— C. R. Hitchcock *et al.*, *J. Am. med. Ass.*, 1966, *195*, 71 (gastric freezing); A. G. Warren and P. M. Taylor, *Lepr. Rev.*, 1973, *44*, 83 (corrective surgery in leprosy); *Med. Lett.*, 1977, *19*, 26 (minor painful procedures); G. T. Watts (letter), *Lancet*, 1979, *1*, 615 (prevention of postoperative ileus).

Anorexia nervosa. The use of chlorpromazine in anorexia nervosa.— P. Dally and W. Sargant, *Br. med. J.*, 1966, *2*, 793.

Behaviour disorders. References to the use of chlorpromazine in hyperactive children.— H. Brummit, *Psychosomatics*, 1968, *9*, 157; J. G. Millichap, *J. Am. med. Ass.*, 1968, *206*, 1527; L. M. Greenberg *et al.*, *Am. J. Psychiat.*, 1972, *129*, 532; J. G. Millichap, *Ann. N.Y. Acad. Sci.*, 1973, *205*, 321.

Cardiovascular disorders. Beneficial effect of chlorpromazine in heart failure in patients with myocardial infarction.— U. Elkayam *et al.*, *Chest*, 1977, *72*, 623. Intravenous injection of chlorpromazine, diluted to 2.5 mg per ml with saline, at a rate of 2.5 mg every 5 minutes until recovery was complete or a total dose of 25 mg had been reached, was used to treat 5 patients with pulmonary oedema who did not respond to conventional treatment. As soon as vasodilatation was apparent a bolus dose of frusemide 40 mg was given intravenously. Four of the 5 patients recovered fully.— E. Romano and A. Gullo, *Lancet*, 1980, *1*, 1000. In 9 patients with severe hypertension a single dose of chlorpromazine 50 mg intramuscularly and frusemide 50 mg intravenously with bedrest resulted in a gradual and adequate reduction in blood pressure and pulse-rate. Maintenance therapy, by mouth, with a diuretic and beta-blocker was started 4 to 8 hours after parenteral treatment.— R. J. Young *et al.*, *Br. med. J.*, 1980, *280*, 1579. Comment.— P. E. Nielsen *et al.* (letter), *ibid.*, *281*, 873.

Prophylaxis. Chlorpromazine may diminish the activating effect of red cells on platelets and hence inhibit their aggregation as thrombi. This may protect against coronary thrombosis. Epidemiological studies might support or invalidate this view.— G. V. R. Born (letter), *Lancet*, 1979, *1*, 822. Comment.— C. S. Foster (letter), *ibid.*, 1249. Reply.— G. V. R. Born (letter), *ibid.*, 1413.

Further references.— J. Zahavi and G. Schwartz (letter), *Lancet*, 1978, *2*, 164.

Cholera. Administration of chlorpromazine to 11 cholera patients with severe purging significantly reduced loss of fluid over 4 successive 8-hour periods compared with 20 similar control patients. Four of the patients received chlorpromazine 1 mg per kg body-weight intramuscularly, 4 received 4 mg per kg intramuscularly, and 3 received 1 mg per kg by mouth. After 32 hours, purging virtually stopped in those given the higher dose of chlorpromazine. In a few of the lower-dose patients a rebound purging occurred after the initial effect but was controlled by a second dose. Patients receiving chlorpromazine were mildly sedated, more comfortable, and had no nausea or vomiting. No hypotension occurred in these well-hydrated patients but this risk needs evaluation before the widespread use of chlorpromazine in cholera can be recommended.— G. H. Rabbani *et al.* (preliminary communication), *Lancet*, 1979, *1*, 410. Comment.— D. R. Nalin (letter), *ibid.*, 988.

Animal studies.— I. Lönnroth *et al.*, *Med. Biol.*, 1977, *55*, 126.

Dementia. In a double-blind crossover study, 50 elderly patients with dementia were given chlorpromazine, average dose 137.5 mg daily, or a placebo for periods of 3 weeks. In 8 patients, agitation, overactivity, restiveness, or noisiness were slightly worse when the placebo was taken, and in 11 incontinence deteriorated. There were no significant differences in effects of the treatments on idleness and insomnia. The results suggested that only about 20% of elderly patients with dementia would benefit from chlorpromazine.— R. Barton and L. Hurst, *Br. J. Psychiat.*, 1966, *112*, 989, per *Abstr. Wld Med.*, 1967, *41*, 311.

Depression. Results of a double-blind study completed by 99 patients with primary depressive disorders showed that chlorpromazine and imipramine were equally effective when given in a dosage of 100 mg daily for 2 days then 200 mg daily for 19 days. Phenothiazines may be more effective in depression than has been assumed.— E. S. Paykel *et al.*, *Br. J. Psychiat.*, 1968, *114*, 1281. Comment on the role of chlorpromazine in depression.— J. A. G. Watt (letter), *Br. med. J.*, 1980, *281*, 308.

Diagnostic use. *Huntington's chorea.* There were impaired prolactin responses to chlorpromazine and protirelin in patients with Huntington's chorea when compared with controls. This might be of value in early detection of the disorder and suggested that there was a dopaminergic influence.— M. R. Hayden *et al.*, *Lancet*, 1977, *2*, 423. Experience with bromocriptine (a dopaminergic agonist) in patients with Huntington's chorea did not show any evidence of dopaminergic hypersensitivity.— R. J. Chalmers *et al.* (letter), *ibid.*, 824.

Pituitary reserve. A comparison of the functional evaluation of pituitary reserve in patients with the amenorrhoea-galactorrhoea syndrome utilising gonadorelin, levodopa, or chlorpromazine.— A. Zárate *et al.*, *J. clin. Endocr. Metab.*, 1973, *37*, 855. Testing with chlorpromazine and protirelin could be of diagnostic value in distinguishing between those patients with galactorrhoea and amenorrhoea produced by pituitary tumours, idiopathic disease or other causes.— A. E. Boyd *et al.*, *Ann. intern. Med.*, 1977, *87*, 165.

Endocrine disorders. *Acromegaly.* Chlorpromazine 100 to 200 mg given daily for 3 to 6 months produced no improvement in 8 patients with acromegaly.— R. C. Dimond *et al.*, *J. clin. Endocr. Metab.*, 1973, *36*, 1189, per *Int. pharm. Abstr.*, 1974, *11*, 390. A similar report.— T. W. AvRuskin *et al.*, *J. clin. Endocr. Metab.*, 1973, *37*, 380, per *Int. pharm. Abstr.*, 1974, *11*, 759.

Extrapyramidal effects. *Hemiballismus.* Beneficial responses were obtained in 11 patients with acute hemiballismus following administration of chlorpromazine to 3 and haloperidol to 8. None of the patients died.— H. L. Klawans *et al.*, *New Engl. J. Med.*, 1976, *295*, 1348.

Gilles de la Tourette's syndrome. Chlorpromazine 500 to 700 mg daily controlled Gilles de la Tourette's syndrome in a 14-year-old boy, unable to tolerate haloperidol owing to the development of paranoid ideation and depersonalisation.— J. Feldman (letter), *Am. J. Psychiat.*, 1977, *134*, 99.

Headache. Comment on the beneficial response of cluster headache to chlorpromazine therapy. In view of the toxicity of prednisone and lithium carbonate, and the apparently greater effectiveness of chlorpromazine, it may be the preferred drug for prophylaxis of cluster headaches.— V. S. Caviness and P. O'Brien, *New Engl. J. Med.*, 1980, *302*, 446. See also *idem*, *Headache*, 1980, *20*, 128.

Hiccup. Details of a protocol for treating hiccups. Any metabolic abnormality should be corrected, then granulated sugar should be swallowed dry; if this is successful the sugar should be repeated if hiccups recur. If the sugar is not successful, pass nasogastric tube, decompress stomach, then irritate pharynx; if successful, repeat if hiccups recur. If not successful, give chlorpromazine 25 to 50 mg intravenously, and if succcessful maintain on chlorpromazine by mouth for 10 days. If the intravenous chlorpromazine is not successful initially, repeat up to 3 times, and if eventually successful, maintain on chlorpromazine by mouth for 10 days. If chlorpromazine is not successful, give metoclopramide 10 mg intravenously every 4 hours, and if this is successful maintain on metoclopramide by mouth for 10 days. If metoclopramide is not successful, give quinidine 200 mg by mouth 4 times daily, and if this is not successful, carry out left phrenic nerve-block then crush.— B. W. A. Williamson and I. M. C. Macintyre, *Br. med. J.*, 1977, *2*, 501.

Hypoglycaemia. Chlorpromazine was given to control hypoglycaemia in a woman with malignant insulinoma.— A. E. Lambert *et al.* (letter), *Br. med. J.*, 1972, *3*, 701.

Nausea and vomiting. Phenothiazine derivatives with anti-emetic activity act primarily in blocking the chemoreceptor trigger zone, but there is little impact on the vomiting centre, which accounts for the fact that they have not proved particularly useful in treating motion sickness. The potent and selective action on the chemoreceptor trigger zone has many useful clinical applications in conditions such as uraemia, carcinomatosis, radiation sickness, and in helping to counteract the nauseating effects of many drugs. There has been no convincing demonstration of a greater anti-emetic efficacy of one phenothiazine congener over another, but chlorpromazine is regarded as less suitable than some newer compounds because of the greater risk of jaundice. Advantages of the newer compounds are partly offset by a greater likelihood of inducing extrapyramidal side-effects.— D. Gibbs, *Br. med. J.*, 1976, *2*, 1489. As a generalisation it seems that phenothiazines with a piperazine side-chain (prochlorperazine, perphenazine, thiethylperazine, and trifluoperazine) are more effective as anti-emetics than those with dimethylaminopropyl side-chains (such as chlorpromazine).— J. W. Dundee, *Adv. Med. Topics Ther.*, 1977, *3*, 166.

Further reviews and comments.— C. D. Wood, *Drugs*, 1979, *17*, 471.

Pain. Comment on the analgesic use of psychotropic agents.— *J. Am. med. Ass.*, 1978, *240*, 1225.

Porphyria. Chlorpromazine is a good tranquilliser for patients with porphyria.— G. Dean, *Practitoner*, 1978, *221*, 219.

Pregnancy and the neonate. A discussion on anti-nauseant drugs including their use during pregnancy.— G. J. Milton-Thompson, *Practitioner*, 1979, *223*, 516.

Lactation. Chlorpromazine might be used for induction of lactation or relactation. Doses of 25 to 100 mg thrice daily produced good results in India and Vietnam.— R. E. Brown, *Pediatrics*, 1977, *60*, 117.

Neonatal drug withdrawal. For the administration of chlorpromazine to infants born to diamorphine-dependent mothers, see Alcohol and Drug Withdrawal (above).

Respiratory distress syndrome. A report of beneficial results with chlorpromazine in the respiratory distress syndrome.— E. F. Diamond and V. R. DeYoung, *J. Am. med. Ass.*, 1966, *196*, 584.

See also under Adverse Effects and Precautions.

Psychosis. *Aggression.* Chlorpromazine is the most commonly used drug in the control of psychotic hostility. It can be given by deep intramuscular injection in a dose of 50 to 100 mg according to the size and excitability of the patient; a further injection can be given after 1 or 2 hours if necessary. A single dose can sometimes cause marked hypotension but toxic side-effects are otherwise uncommon with use over a short period of time. An appropriate dose for the elderly, who tolerate the drug less well, would be 25 mg. Manic patients may require much larger doses or the use of an alternative drug, such as haloperidol.— D. J. Williams, *Prescribers' J.*, 1978, *18*, 34. A comment that the advice is applicable to patients unaccustomed to tranquillising drugs; chronic psychiatric patients who become acutely aggressive and unmanageable may require considerably higher doses. For an acutely disturbed patient already used to tranquillisers an initial intramuscular dose of haloperidol equivalent to his usual total daily intake of neuroleptics is recommended. Approximate equivalents of these drugs are: haloperidol 10 mg; chlorpromazine 400 mg; trifluoperazine 15 mg; thioridazine 300 mg; pimozide 3 mg. If no quietening in behaviour supervenes, a second intramuscular dose two to three times larger is given after 2 hours. As soon as the aggressive behaviour begins to subside, drugs are given every 4 to 6 hours, preferably by mouth for humane reasons, and as elixir since patients may conceal tablets or capsules and spit them out up to an hour later. Rapid reduction in dosage may be necessary therefore slow-release (depot) injections should be avoided in the acute stage.— A. C. Carr and M. Lader, *ibid.*, 147.

Further references.— *Br. med. J.*, 1978, *1*, 1229; P. Storey, *Practitioner*, 1978, *220*, 217.

Drug-induced psychosis. Sedation with chlorpromazine was effective when required in a study of 60 hospital admissions due to reactions to lysergide.— J. A. H. Forrest and R. A. Tarala, *Lancet*, 1973, *2*, 1310.

Mania. For a response to haloperidol in a manic patient resistant to chlorpromazine up to 4 g daily, see Haloperidol, p.1534.

Schizophrenia. A detailed account of schizophrenia including theories as to its underlying cause.— R. J. Baldessarini, *New Engl. J. Med.*, 1977, *297*, 988. See also T. J. Crow, *Br. J. Hosp. Med.*, 1978, *20*, 532.

Detailed reviews of antipyschotic drugs, including mention of the introduction of chlorpromazine.— J. Delay *et al.*, *Annls méd.-psychol.*, 1952, *110*, 112; J. M. Davis and R. Casper, *Drugs*, 1977, *14*, 260; D. A. W. Johnson, *Drugs*, 1977, *14*, 291.

Further reviews.— *Drug & Ther. Bull.*, 1977, *15*, 57; P. Hall, *Practitioner*, 1977, *219*, 493; T. R. E. Barnes and P. K. Bridges, *Practitioner*, 1978, *221*, 513; D. G. Grahame-Smith and M. W. Orr, *Recent Adv. clin. Pharmac.*, 1978, *1*, 163 to 187.

In a collaborative study, 838 patients with chronic schizophrenia were treated with chlorpromazine in a dose of 0.3 or 2 g daily or with a placebo. The higher dose of chlorpromazine was significantly more effective than the low dose or placebo in patients under 40 years of age. In older patients and patients who had been in hospital longer, the high dose was no more effective than the low dose and produced a greater number of serious side-effects.— R. F. Prien and J. O. Cole, *Archs gen. Psychiat.*, 1968, *18*, 482.

In controlled trials, the phenothiazines promazine and mepazine are clearly inferior to chlorpromazine. No difference could be detected between all other anti-psychotic agents and chlorpromazine in overall therapeutic efficacy. Further inspection of original studies reveals that all antipsychotics produce consistent changes on the same symptom dimensions. The similarity of these results is quite noteworthy. The comparability and efficacy and the nature of their action suggests that they share a specific common mechanism of action.— J. M. Davis and R. Casper, *Drugs*, 1977, *14*, 260. See also L. E. Hollister *et al.*, *Archs gen. Psychiat.*, 1974, *30*, 94.

From a study of 374 schizophrenic patients allocated, under double-blind conditions, to receive chlorpromazine or placebo after discharge from hospital the monthly risks of relapse were 3.7 and 11.7% respectively after 1 year, and 2.1 and 5% after 2 or 3 years.— G. E. Hogarty and R. F. Ulrich, *Archs gen. Psychiat.*, 1977, *34*, 297.

A few patients with acute schizophrenia appeared to be resistant to phenothiazines and thioxanthines. Sensitivity appeared to be restored by ECT.— D. L. McNeill (letter), *Br. med. J.*, 1977, *2*, 127. See also K. Smith *et al.*, *J. nerv. ment. Dis.*, 1967, *144*, 284.

A study in young male schizophrenic patients indicated that although antipsychotics appeared to be the treatment of choice for most patients in the early stages, some seemed to benefit from being off drugs in relation to long-term clinical improvement.— M. Rappaport *et al.*, *Int. Pharmacopsychiat.*, 1978, *13*, 100.

Further references.— H. E. Spohn *et al.*, *Archs gen. Psychiat.*, 1977, *34*, 633.

For earlier reports of the use of chlorpromazine in schizophrenia, see Martindale 27th Edn, p. 1527.

Scorpion sting. Three children with scorpion stings were successfully sedated with chlorpromazine, in 1 patient administered intravenously and in the other 2 patients intramuscularly [no doses stated]. All 3 children responded dramatically within minutes, though the first patient had failed to respond to a total of 160 mg of phenobarbitone.— H. L. Masco (letter), *J. Am. med. Ass.*, 1970, *212*, 2122.

Shock. Chlorpromazine was given intravenously as an alpha-blocking agent to overcome vasoconstriction and enable correction of hypovolaemia in 5 patients with cardiogenic shock.— K. M. Pagliero *et al.*, *Br. J. Surg.*, 1973, *60*, 201.

Speculation that chlorpromazine 50 mg intramuscularly every 8 hours might reduce the incidence and intensity of septic shock.— D. A. B. Hopkin, *Lancet*, 1978, *2*, 1193.

Further references.— H. S. Loeb *et al.*, *Archs intern. Med.*, 1969, *124*, 354.

Spasticity. For the use of chlorpromazine hydrochloride with phenytoin sodium in the treatment of spasticity in neurological disorders, such as multiple sclerosis, see Phenytoin, p.1244.

Temperature disorders. Heat stroke. The main aim of treatment in heat stroke is to reduce body temperature rapidly. The patient should be placed in a cool air-conditioned room, clothing removed, and ice-packs applied. Convulsions and shivering were prevented by the intravenous infusion of 200 ml of dextrose injection containing 100 mg each of chlorpromazine, pethidine, and promethazine. A double dose was sometimes used and occasionally hypnotic drugs were necessary.— S. Shibolet *et al.*, *Q.J. Med.*, 1967, *36*, 525.

See also Water, p.1670.

Hypothermia. A treatment regimen, including chlorpromazine, for the prevention of brain damage in submersion hypothermia.— A. W. Conn, *Can. med. Ass. J.*, 1979, *120*, 397.

Preparations

Elixirs and Syrups

Chlorpromazine Elixir *(B.P.).* Chlorpromazine Syrup. A solution of chlorpromazine hydrochloride in a suitable flavoured vehicle which may be coloured. When a dose less than or not a multiple of 5 ml is prescribed, the elixir should be diluted to 5 ml, or a multiple, with syrup. Such dilutions must be freshly prepared and not used more than 2 weeks after issue. Protect from light.

Chlorpromazine Hydrochloride Syrup *(U.S.P.).* A syrup containing chlorpromazine hydrochloride 190 to 210 mg in each 100 ml. Store in airtight containers. Protect from light.

Injections

Chlorpromazine Hydrochloride Injection *(U.S.P.).* A sterile solution of chlorpromazine hydrochloride, 23.75 to 26.25 mg per ml, in Water for Injections. pH 3 to 5. Protect from light.

Chlorpromazine Injection *(B.P.).* A sterile solution of chlorpromazine hydrochloride in Water for Injections free from dissolved air; it contains suitable buffering and stabilising agents. pH 5 to 6.5. Protect from light.

An injection of chlorpromazine with pethidine and promethazine, Compound Injection of Pethidine (*Gt Ormond St Child. Hosp.*), for the pre-operative medication of young children is described under Pethidine Hydrochloride (see p.1028)..

Suppositories

Chlorpromazine Suppositories *(B.P.).* Contain chlorpromazine in a suitable basis. Store at a temperature not exceeding 30°. Protect from light.

Chlorpromazine Suppositories *(U.S.P.).* Suppositories containing chlorpromazine. Store at 15° to 30°. Protect from light.

Tablets

Chlorpromazine Hydrochloride Tablets *(U.S.P.).* Tablets containing chlorpromazine hydrochloride. The *U.S.P.* requires 80% dissolution in 30 minutes. Protect from light.

Chlorpromazine Tablets *(B.P.).* Tablets containing chlorpromazine hydrochloride. The tablets are film-coated or sugar-coated.

Proprietary Preparations

Chloractil *(DDSA Pharmaceuticals, UK).* Chlorpromazine hydrochloride, available as tablets of 25 and 50 mg.

Dozine Syrup *(R.P. Drugs, UK).* Chlorpromazine hydrochloride, available as syrup containing 25 mg in each 5 ml.

Largactil *(May & Baker, UK).* Chlorpromazine hydrochloride, available as **1% Solution** for injection in ampoules of 5 ml; as **2.5% Solution** for injection in ampoules of 1 and 2 ml; as **Syrup** containing 25 mg in each 5 ml (suggested diluent, syrup); as **Tablets** of 10, 25, 50, and 100 mg; and as **Suppositories** each containing 100 mg of the base. **Largactil Forte Suspension.** Contains in each 5 ml chlorpromazine embonate equivalent to chlorpromazine hydrochloride 100 mg. (Also available as Largactil in *Austral., Belg., Canad., Denm., Fr., Ital., Neth., Norw., S.Afr., Spain, Switz.*).

Other Proprietary Names

Arg.— Ampliactil, Aspersinal; *Austral.*— Procalm, Promacid, Protran; *Canad.*— Chlorprom, Chlor-Promanyl; *Denm.*— Prozil; *Ger.*— Megaphen; *Ital.*— Prozin; *Norw.*— Hibanil; *S.Afr.*— Klorazin; *Swed.*— Hibernal, Klorpromex; *Switz.*— Chlorazin; *USA*— Promachlor, Thorazine.

NOTE. The name Protran has also been applied to meprobamate and the name Pro-Tran has been applied to promazine hydrochloride.

A preparation containing chlorpromazine hydrochloride was also formerly marketed in Great Britain under the proprietary name Amargyl (*May & Baker*).

7024-s

Chlorprothixene *(U.S.P.).* N 714; Ro 4-0403.

(*Z*)-3-(2-Chlorothioxanthen-9-ylidene)-*NN*-dimethylpropylamine.

$C_{18}H_{18}ClNS = 315.9$.

CAS — 113-59-7.

Pharmacopoeias. In *Cz.* (as the hydrochloride), in *Nord.* which also includes the hydrochloride, and in *U.S.*

A yellow, tasteless, crystalline powder with a slight amine-like odour. M.p. 96.5° to 101.5°. **Soluble** 1 in 1700 of water, 1 in 29 of alcohol, 1 in 2 of chloroform, 1 in 14 of ether, and 1 in 18 of acetone. **Incompatible** with alkalis, acids, phenobarbitone, and thiopentone sodium. **Store** in airtight containers. Protect from light.

Stability. The photochemical stability of *cis* and *trans* isomers of tyicyclic neuroleptic drugs including chlorprothixene.— A. Li Wan Po and W. J. Irwin, *J. Pharm. Pharmac.*, 1980, *32*, 25.

Adverse Effects, Treatment, and Precautions. As for Chlorpromazine, p.1509.

Effects on the liver. A 59-year-old man receiving chlorprothixene (for the second time) for acute mania developed severe obstructive jaundice within a few days; he was also taking chlorpropamide, digoxin, and diuretics; chlorprothixene was considered the most likely cause of the jaundice, though chlorpropamide could not be excluded.— D. G. S. Ruddock and J. Hoenig (letter), *Br. med. J.*, 1973, *1*, 231.

Effects on mental state. Hallucinatory dreams after an initial dose of chlorprothixene taken for postherpetic neuralgia.— G. A. Farber and J. W. Burks, *Sth. med. J.*, 1974, *67*, 808.

Effects on sexual function. Chlorprothixene was a possible cause of impotence.— A. J. Cooper, *Postgrad. med. J.*, 1972, *48*, 548.

Interactions. *Clonidine.* For the effect of chlorprothixene on clonidine, see Clonidine Hydrochloride, p.140.

Overdosage. A 1-year-old child survived a dose of 1.075 g of chlorprothixene, and adults had survived after taking 8 g.— L. E. Hollister, *Clin. Pharmac. Ther.*, 1966, *7*, 142.

Withdrawal. A 9-year-old boy with mild choreoathetotic cerebral palsy, mild mental retardation, and a severe behaviour problem, who had been taking chlorprothixene 150 mg daily for about a year developed restlessness and insomnia the day after its abrupt withdrawal. Nausea and vomiting occurred on the fourth day, followed on the sixth day by severe extrapyramidal disorders. The vomiting, which occurred after meals, persisted until the twentieth day after withdrawal, and the extrapyramidal movements were still present on the twenty-eighth day, when neuroleptic therapy was resumed owing to the severity of his behaviour problem. Control of the abnormal involuntary movements was attained within 24 hours of resuming neuroleptic therapy.— L. E. Yepes and B. G. Winsberg, *Am. J. Psychiat.*, 1977, *134*, 574.

Absorption and Fate. For an account of the absorption and fate of a thioxanthene, see Flupenthixol, p.1528.

Metabolism. Studies on the metabolism of chlorprothixene in *animals* and man. In addition to the major metabolite chlorprothixene-sulphoxide, 2 further urinary metabolites were identified, namely *N*-desmethylchlorprothixene-sulphoxide and chlorprothixene-sulphoxide-*N*-oxide.— J. Raaflaub, *Arzneimittel-Forsch.*, 1967, *17*, 1393.

Further references: L. -G. Allgén *et al.*, *Experientia*, 1960, *16*, 325.

Uses. Chlorprothixene is a thioxanthene with general properties similar to those of the phenothiazine, chlorpromazine (p.1513). The usual dose for the treatment of psychoses is 25 to 50 mg three or four times daily; in acute psychoses doses of up to 600 mg daily have been given. It may also be given intramuscularly in doses of 25 to 50 mg three or four times daily.

A suggested oral dose for children is 1 to 2 mg per kg body-weight daily in divided doses. Sources in the U.K. recommend 15 mg three or four times daily for children over 6 years of age while sources in the U.S.A. recommend 10 to 25 mg three or four times daily for children over 6 years of age.

Chlorprothixene 30 to 45 mg daily in divided doses, has also been advocated for non-psychotic emotional disturbances in adults, such as anxiety and tension. In general, however, neuroleptics are only suitable for such purposes in resistant conditions, where more appropriate agents, such as the benzodiazepines (see Diazepam, p.1523) have proved ineffective. If their use is judged to be necessary, treatment should be directed at low dosages given on a short-term basis.

Chlorprothixene should be given in reduced dosage to elderly patients.

Pain. Of 30 patients with postherpetic neuralgia 25 were given chlorprothixene 50 mg by mouth every 6 hours and 5 with severe neuralgia were given an additional 100 mg initially by intramuscular injection. Complete pain relief was experienced within 72 hours by 27 patients (within 24 hours by 11).— G. A. Farber and J. W. Burks, *Sth. med. J.*, 1974, *67*, 808.

Preparations

Chlorprothixene Injection *(U.S.P.).* A sterile solution in Water for Injections, prepared with the aid of hydrochloric acid. pH 3 to 4. Protect from light.

Chlorprothixene Oral Suspension *(U.S.P.).* A suspension containing chlorprothixene. pH 3.5 to 4.5. Store in airtight containers. Protect from light.

Chlorprothixene Tablets *(U.S.P.).* Tablets containing chlorprothixene. Protect from light.

Proprietary Preparations

Taractan *(Roche, UK).* Chlorprothixene, available as tablets of 15 and 50 mg. (Also available as Taractan in *Austral., Belg., Denm., Fr., Ger., Ital., Neth., Switz., USA*).

Other Proprietary Names

Tarasan *(Canad.)*; Truxal (as base, acetate, citrate, or hydrochloride) *(Belg., Denm., Ger., Neth., Norw., S.Afr., Swed., Switz.)*; Truxaletten (base and hydrochloride) *(Ger., Switz.)*; Truxaletter (hydrochloride) *(Norw.)*; Truxalettes (hydrochloride) *(Belg.)*.

7025-w

Clobazam. HR 376; HR 4723; LM 2717.
7-Chloro-1-methyl-5-phenyl-1*H*-1,5-benzodiazepine-2,4(3*H*,5*H*)-dione.
$C_{16}H_{13}ClN_2O_2$=300.7.

CAS — 22316-47-8.

Practically **insoluble** in water; sparingly soluble in alcohol; freely soluble in acetone and chloroform.

Dependence. Prolonged use of clobazam may lead to the development of dependence of the barbiturate-alcohol type (see p.792). It has a low liability for abuse.

Withdrawal symptoms in 2 patients on withdrawal of clobazam.— H. Petursson and M. H. Lader, *Br. med. J.*, 1981, *282*, 1931.

Adverse Effects, Treatment, and Precautions. As for Diazepam, p.1520.

The effect of clobazam on psychomotor performance.— I. Hindmarch and A. C. Parrott, *Arzneimittel-Forsch.*, 1978, *28*, 2169. See also *idem*, *Br. J. clin. Pharmac.*, 1979, *8*, 325; I. Hindmarch and A. C. Gudgeon, *ibid.*, 1980, *10*, 145.

Interactions. *Alcohol.* A study demonstrating interaction between clobazam and alcohol.— K. Taeuber *et al.*, *Br. J. clin. Pharmac.*, 1979, *7*, *Suppl.* 1, 91S.

Absorption and Fate. For an account of the absorption and fate of a benzodiazepine, see Diazepam, p.1522.

It has been reported that unlike the 1,4-benzodiazepines such as diazepam, clobazam, a 1,5-benzodiazepine, is not hydroxylated at the 3-position.

Absorption and plasma concentrations. A study of the pharmacokinetics of single and multiple doses of clobazam. At least 87% of an oral dose was absorbed with peak plasma concentrations occurring after 1 to 4 hours. The terminal half-life was estimated to be about 18 hours with a considerably longer half-life for the metabolite.— W. Rupp *et al.*, *Br. J. clin. Pharmac.*, 1979, *7*, *Suppl.* 1, 51S.

Further references: B. J. Hunt *et al.*, *Br. J. clin. Pharmac.*, 1974, *1*, 174P (plasma concentrations); J. J. Vallner *et al.*, *J. clin. Pharmac.*, 1978, *18*, 319 (plasma concentrations and half-life); J. J. Vallner *et al.*, *J. clin. Pharmac.*, 1980, *20*, 444 (plasma concentrations); G. Tedeschi *et al.* (letter), *Br. J. clin. Pharmac.*, 1981, *11*, 619 (adults and children); D. J. Greenblatt *et al.*, *Br. J. clin. Pharmac.*, 1981, *12*, 631 (age and sex differences).

Metabolism. The kinetics and metabolism of clobazam in *animals* and man. Unlike the 1,4-benzodiazepines clobazam is not hydroxylated at the 3-position.— M. Volz *et al.*, *Br. J. clin. Pharmac.*, 1979, *7*, *Suppl.* 1, 41S.

Following administration of clobazam 20 mg to a healthy subject a peak plasma-clobazam concentration of 510 ng per ml occurred after 1.5 hours and the elimination half-life during the terminal (β) phase was 22 hours. Peak concentration of desmethylclobazam, an active metabolite, occurred after 48 hours.— D. J. Greenblatt, *J. pharm. Sci.*, 1980, *69*, 1351.

Further references: P. Hunt *et al.*, *J. Pharm. Pharmac.*, 1979, *31*, 448.

Plasma protein binding. Mention that at least 10% of clobazam is not protein bound.— W. Rupp *et al.*, *Br. J. clin. Pharmac.*, 1979, *7*, *Suppl.* 1, 51S.

Uses. Clobazam is a benzodiazepine with actions and uses similar to those of diazepam (p.1523). The usual dose for the treatment of anxiety is 20 to 30 mg daily given in divided doses or as a single dose at night; in severe conditions up to 60 mg daily has been given.

Reviews, comments, and symposia on clobazam: *Br. J. clin. Pharmac.*, 1979, *7*, *Suppl.* 1, 1S–155S; *Drug & Ther. Bull.*, 1979, *17*, 65; R. N. Brogden *et al.*, *Drugs*, 1980, *20*, 161.

Action. A view that the pharmacological profile of clobazam, which is a 1,5-benzodiazepine, differs from that of the 1,4-benzodiazepines, such as chlordiazepoxide and diazepam, in that it displays a wide separation of psychosedative or 'tranquillising' properties, from impairment of motor coordination, and that this is associated with a relative lack of muscle relaxant activity.— G. W. Hanks, *Hoechst*, *Br. J. clin. Pharmac.*, 1979, *7*, *Suppl.* 1, 151S.

Further references: R. G. Borland and A. N. Nicholson, *Br. J. clin. Pharmac.*, 1975, *2*, 215; J. R. Wittenborn, *ibid.*, 1979, *7*, *Suppl.* 1, 61S; J. R. Wittenborn *et al.*, *ibid.*, 69S; I. Hindmarch, *ibid.*, 77S; A. N. Nicholson, *ibid.*, 83S; B. Biehl, *ibid.*, 85S.

Pharmacological and toxicity studies in *animals*.— F. Barzaghi *et al.*, *Arzneimittel-Forsch.*, 1973, *23*, 683; S. Fielding and I. Hoffmann, *Br. J. clin. Pharmac.*, 1979, *7*, *Suppl.* 1, 7S; H. J. Gerhards, *ibid.*, 23S; E. Schütz, *ibid.*, 33S.

Anxiety. In a double-blind study clobazam 20 to 80 mg daily was shown to be as effective as diazepam 10 to 40 mg daily in the treatment of anxiety. The incidence of side-effects was similar, with sleepiness and sedation being more frequently reported.— J. Mendels *et al.*, *J. clin. Pharmac.*, 1978, *18*, 353. Similar results were obtained in neurotic patients, using daily doses of clobazam 30 to 40 mg and diazepam 15 to 20 mg.— D. R. Doongaji *et al.*, *ibid.*, 358.

A review of some clinical studies on clobazam. In 15 studies comparing it with diazepam there was an equal incidence of drowsiness in 2, more drowsiness with clobazam in 5, and more drowsiness with diazepam in 8.— D. Koeppen, *Br. J. clin. Pharmac.*, 1979, *7*, *Suppl.* 1, 139S.

Further references: K. D. Charalampous *et al.*, *Curr. ther. Res.*, 1977, *21*, 779; P. T. Donlon *et al.*, *ibid.*, *22*, 894; O. Laudano *et al.*, *J. clin. Pharmac.*, 1977, *17*, 441; K. Sandler *et al.*, *Curr. ther. Res.*, 1977, *21*, 114; J. Ananth and N. Van Den Steen, *ibid.*, 1979, *26*, 119; I. Hindmarch, *Eur. J. clin. Pharmac.*, 1979, *16*, 17; H. P. Schjønsby *et al.*, *J. int. med. Res.*, 1979, *7*, 404; P. A. Botter, *Curr. med. Res. Opinion*, 1980, *6*, 593.

Hypnotic effect. Clobazam shortened sleep-onset latency in a double-blind study in 6 healthy subjects who took 10 or 20 mg before retiring. Although subjects reported a sense of less wakefulness the morning after ingestion of clobazam, there was no effect on observed total-sleep time and clobazam was considered to be of use in the management of disturbed sleep when impaired performance the next day would be unacceptable.— A. N. Nicholson *et al.*, *Br. J. clin. Pharmac.*, 1977, *4*, 567. Clobazam 20 mg taken at night for 6 nights by 10 healthy subjects in a double-blind crossover study produced no significant effect on psychomotor performance and car-driving ability on the morning following ingestion in 8 subjects. Subjects reported improved sleep induction and quality of sleep.— I. Hindmarch *et al.*, *ibid.*, 573. From the results of a study involving 161 patients it was concluded that clobazam had very little hypnotic activity.— C. M. Kesson *et al.*, *Br. J. clin. Pharmac.*, 1978, *6*, 243.

Proprietary Preparations

Frisium *(Hoechst, UK)*. Clobazam, available as capsules of 10 mg. (Also available as Frisium in *Belg.*, *Ger.*, *Ital.*).

Other Proprietary Names

Castilium *(Port.)*; Frisin *(Chile)*; Karidium *(Arg.)*; Noiafren *(Spain)*; Sentil *(Kor.)*; Urbadan *(Arg., Braz., Col., Ecuad., Guat., Mex., Peru, Port., Urug.)*; Urbanol *(S.Afr.)*; Urbanyl *(Fr., Switz.)*.

7026-e

Clomacran Phosphate. SKF 14336. 3-(2-Chloro-9,10-dihydroacridin-9-yl)-*NN*-dimethylpropylamine dihydrogen phosphate.
$C_{18}H_{21}ClN_2,H_3PO_4$=398.8.

CAS — 5310-55-4 (clomacran); 22199-46-8 (phosphate).

Clomacran is a member of the acridane chemical group which has a close structural similarity to the phenothiazine group. It has actions similar to those of chlorpromazine (p.1509) and has been given as the phosphate in doses of up to 600 mg daily for the treatment of schizophrenia.

Anxiety. In a double-blind trial involving 115 anxious neurotic out-patients, clomacran in doses of 100 to 150 mg daily was less effective as an anti-anxiety agent than chlordiazepoxide 40 to 60 mg daily. Side-effects were more severe with clomacran though fewer patients were affected.— K. Rickels *et al.*, *J. clin. Pharmac.*, 1972, *12*, 46.

Mania. Disappointing results with clomacran phosphate, given in doses of up to 1.2 g daily, in 8 patients with mania or hypomania. Only one patient showed improvement and she had a major epileptic attack at the dose of 1.2 g daily.— J. G. Edwards and G. M. Simpson, *Curr. ther. Res.*, 1969, *11*, 115.

Schizophrenia. In a comparison with chlorpromazine for the treatment of chronic schizophrenia, clomacran was equally effective at a dose level of 150 mg daily.— W. G. Case *et al.*, *Curr. ther. Res.*, 1971, *13*, 337.

A polymorphic light eruption developed in 10 of 27 schizophrenic patients given clomacran phosphate in doses of up to 500 mg daily.— R. F. H. Needham and W. J. Blignault, *Med. J. Aust.*, 1969, *2*, 550.

Further references: H. Freeman and M. R. Oktem, *Curr. ther. Res.*, 1966, *8*, 395; G. M. Simpson *et al.*, *ibid.*, 447; L. J. Hekimian *et al.*, *ibid.*, 1967, *9*, 17; W. G. Case and K. Rickels, *ibid.*, 477; M. P. Bishop and D. M. Gallant, *J. clin. Pharmac.*, 1967, *7*, 342; J. L. Claghorn *et al.*, *Psychosomatics*, 1967, *8*, 212; H. Freeman *et al.*, *Curr. ther. Res.*, 1968, *10*, 537; O. T. Nikolovski *et al.*, *ibid.*, 178; W. T. Lampe, *ibid.*, 300; M. P. Bishop *et al.*, *ibid.*, 447; J. E. Overall *et al.*, *J. clin. Pharmac.*, 1969, *9*, 328; B. J. Goldstein and S. Jacobsen, *Dis. nerv. Syst.*, 1969, *30*, 37; T. A. Ban *et al.*, *Curr. ther. Res.*, 1974, *16*, 971; J. C. Pecknold *et al.*, *Int. J. clin. Pharmac. Biopharm.*, 1975, *11*, 299; A. Torres-Ruiz *et al.*, *Curr. ther. Res.*, 1979, *26*, 127.

Manufacturers

Smith Kline & French, USA.

7027-l

Clopenthixol Decanoate. 2-{4-[3-(2-Chlorothioxanthen-9-ylidene)propyl]piperazin-1-yl}ethyl decanoate.
$C_{32}H_{43}ClN_2O_2S$=555.2.

A yellowish oily liquid. Practically **insoluble** in water; soluble in alcohol, chloroform, and ether.

7028-y

Clopenthixol Hydrochloride. Cloperphenthixan Hydrochloride. 2-{4-[3-(2-Chlorothioxanthen-9-ylidene)propyl]piperazin-1-yl}ethanol dihydrochloride.
$C_{22}H_{25}ClN_2OS,2HCl$=473.9.

CAS — 982-24-1 (clopenthixol); 633-59-0 (hydrochloride).

Clopenthixol hydrochloride 11.8 mg is approximately equivalent to 10 mg of clopenthixol. Freely **soluble** in water; sparingly soluble in alcohol; practically insoluble in organic solvents.

Stability. The photochemical stability of *cis* and *trans* isomers of tricyclic neuroleptic drugs, including clopenthixol.— A. Li Wan Po and W. J. Irwin, *J. Pharm. Pharmac.*, 1980, *32*, 25.

Adverse Effects, Treatment, and Precautions. As for Chlorpromazine, p.1509.

Absorption and Fate. For an account of the absorption and fate of a thioxanthene, see Flupenthixol, p.1528.

Uses. Clopenthixol is a thioxanthene with general properties similar to the phenothiazine, chlorpromazine (p.1513). Clopenthixol is administered as the hydrochloride usually by mouth or as the longer-acting decanoate by deep intramuscular injection. Doses of the hydrochloride are expressed in terms of the base, and of the decanoate in terms of the ester.

The usual dose of the hydrochloride for the treatment of psychoses is the equivalent of 25 to 50 mg of the base thrice daily; in severe schizophrenia up to 250 mg daily has been given. It has also been given intramuscularly. The long-acting decanoate should be given by deep intramuscular injection in an initial test dose of 100 mg. According to the patient's response over the following week, this may be followed by doses of 200 to 400 mg every 2 to 4 weeks. Shorter dosage intervals or greater amounts may be required according to the patient's response. If doses greater than 400 mg are considered necessary they should be divided between 2 separate injection sites. In patients already taking antipsychotic agents by mouth, the dosage should be gradually reduced on starting clopenthixol decanoate injections. In those being transferred from depot injections of phenothiazines, clopenthixol decanoate 200 mg is considered to be equivalent to fluphenazine decanoate 25 mg. Patients displaying agitation or aggression during therapy with flupenthixol may be better controlled by clopenthixol; clopenthixol decanoate 200 mg is considered to be equivalent to flupenthixol decanoate 40 mg.

Anxiety. A favourable report of clopenthixol decanoate in a patient with intractable obsessional neurotic illness.— B. Grant (letter), *Br. med. J.*, 1979, *2*, 501.

Psychoses. Favourable comment on the use of clopenthixol decanoate in 90 patients with psychosis.— B. Blake (letter), *Br. med. J.*, 1979, *2*, 48.

Schizophrenia. The administration of clopenthixol in doses up to 250 mg daily to 12 chronic schizophrenics demonstrated moderate antipsychotic activity with marked sedation and a consistent hypotensive effect, but very slight extrapyramidal effects. At higher doses side-effects appeared, sedation was less, and the antipsychotic effects were reduced.— A. A. Sugerman *et al.*, *Curr. ther. Res.*, 1966, *8*, 220.

Clopenthixol 50 mg thrice daily was compared with chlorpromazine, 100 mg thrice daily, and a placebo in 54 patients with schizophrenia. Both clopenthixol and chlorpromazine treatments were associated with changes in the objective behaviour of the patients. Of the patients who received clopenthixol, parkinsonism occurred in 2 and normal menstruation returned in 3 women after 4 years of chlorpromazine-induced amenorrhoea.— S. K. Kordas *et al.*, *Br. J. Psychiat.*, 1968, *114*, 833.

Proprietary Preparations

Clopixol Injection *(Lundbeck, UK: Farillon, UK).* Contains *cis*-(*Z*)-clopenthixol decanoate 200 mg per ml in thin vegetable oil, in ampoules of 1 ml.

Other Proprietary Names

Ciatyl *(Ger.)*; Sordinol *(Belg., Denm., Ital., Neth., Norw., S.Afr., Swed., Switz.)*.

7029-j

Clorazepate Dipotassium.

AH 3232; Abbott 35616; CB 4306. Compound of potassium 7-chloro-2,3-dihydro-2-oxo-5-phenyl-1*H*-1,4-benzodiazepine-3-carboxylate with potassium hydroxide.

$C_{16}H_{11}ClK_2N_2O_4$=408.9.

CAS — 57109-90-7.

A fine, practically odourless, light yellow powder. Clorazepate dipotassium 15 mg is approximately equivalent to 13 mg of clorazepate monopotassium. Very **soluble** in water; practically insoluble in organic solvents.

7030-q

Clorazepate Monopotassium.

Abbott 39083; CB 4311. Potassium 7-chloro-2,3-dihydro-2-oxo-5-phenyl-1*H*-1,4-benzodiazepine-3-carboxylate.

$C_{16}H_{10}ClKN_2O_3$=352.8.

CAS — 5991-71-9.

A fine, practically odourless, off-white powder. Very **soluble** in water; practically insoluble in organic solvents.

Dependence. Prolonged use of clorazepate may lead to the development of dependence of the barbiturate-alcohol type (see p.792). It has a low liability for abuse.

Dependence and withdrawal. A report of withdrawal convulsions from benzodiazepines in 4 patients, involving clorazepate (1), oxazepam (1), and lorazepam (2).— T. R. Einarson (letter), *Lancet*, 1980, *1*, 151. A comment that 2 of these patients were also taking trifluoperazine, which has known epileptogenic potential. A patient has been seen, however, who suffered a grand-mal seizure 4 days after stopping lorazepam 5 mg daily alone; lorazepam had been taken for 2 years in a daily dose of 5 to 15 mg.— P. Tyrer (letter), *ibid.*

Adverse Effects, Treatment, and Precautions. As for Diazepam, p.1520.

Studies on the effect of clorazepate on performance.— I. Hindmarch and A. C. Parrott, *Br. J. clin. Pharmac.*, 1979, *8*, 325; M. H. Lader *et al.*, *ibid.*, 1980, *9*, 83.

Effects on the liver. A report of jaundice and hepatic necrosis associated with clorazepate administration.— J. L. W. Parker, *Postgrad. med. J.*, 1979, *55*, 908.

Effects on mental state. *Paradoxical response.* A paradoxical rage reaction occurred in a 24-year-old man with mild anxiety symptoms who had taken 75 mg of clorazepate dipotassium in 8 hours. This reaction did not occur when intermittent low doses of diazepam were given.— F. E. Karch, *Ann. intern. Med.*, 1979, *91*, 61.

Interactions. *Alcohol.* Interactions between clorazepate and alcohol.— M. Staak *et al.*, *Int. J. clin. Pharmac. Biopharm.*, 1979, *17*, 205. See also M. Staak *et al.*, *Int. J. clin. Pharmac.*, 1980, *18*, 283.

Antacids. A study in 15 healthy subjects indicated that concurrent administration of clorazepate dipotassium with a magnesium and aluminium antacid tended to retard clorazepate absorption producing lower peak plasma concentrations of desmethyldiazepam; overall absorption and the elimination half-lives of clorazepate and desmethyldiazepam were unaffected.— A. H. C. Chun *et al.*, *Clin. Pharmac. Ther.*, 1977, *22*, 329.

Further references: R. I. Shader *et al.*, *Clin. Pharmac. Ther.*, 1978, *24*, 308.

Overdosage. A 26-year-old female patient recovered from an overdose of clorazepate dipotassium 600 mg by mouth. She received gastric lavage 150 minutes after ingestion of the dose and suffered from drowsiness, nystagmus, and ataxia. She was discharged 48 hours after admission with no residual neurological signs. Gastric lavage, maintenance of adequate fluid intake, and observation appeared to be adequate treatment while awaiting spontaneous recovery.— B. W. Hancock and J. F. Martin (letter), *Br. J. clin. Pharmac.*, 1974, *1*, 512.

Pregnancy and the neonate. Malformations in the infant of a mother who had taken clorazepate during the first trimester of pregnancy.— D. A. Patel and A. R. Patel (letter), *J. Am. med. Ass.*, 1980, *244*, 135.

See also under Absorption and Fate.

Absorption and Fate. For an account of the absorption and fate of a benzodiazepine, see Diazepam, p.1522.

Clorazepate is converted by the acid of the stomach to desmethyldiazepam.

Absorption and plasma concentrations. Clorazepate was rapidly converted, in the stomach, to desmethyldiazepam; in achlorhydria conversion in the blood was rapid with a half-life of clorazepate of less than 10 minutes.— P. F. Cooper (letter), *Pharm. J.*, 1974, *1*, 277.

A peak plasma-desmethyldiazepam concentration of 379 ng per ml occurred 45 minutes after administration of clorazepate dipotassium 15 mg to a healthy subject.— D. J. Greenblatt, *J. pharm. Sci.*, 1978, *67*, 427.

Further references: C. W. Abruzzo *et al.*, *J. Pharmacokinet. Biopharm.*, 1977, *5*, 377 (at varying gastric pH); M. Staak and A. Moosmayer, *Arzneimittel-Forsch.*, 1978, *28*, 1187 (plasma concentrations and metabolites); A. J. Wilensky *et al.*, *Clin. Pharmac. Ther.*, 1978, *24*, 22 (plasma concentrations and half-life); H. R. Ochs *et al.*, *ibid.*, 1979, *26*, 449 (absorption).

Pregnancy and the neonate. *Diffusion across the placenta.* The mean transport fraction across the placenta of diazepam was 40% and of desmethyldiazepam 38%, but only 11% for clorazepate.— M. Guerre-Millo *et al.*, *Eur. J. clin. Pharmac.*, 1979, *15*, 171.

Further references: R. Gaja *et al.*, *Revue fr. Gynec. Obstet.*, 1975, *70*, 751; E. Rey *et al.*, *Eur. J. clin. Pharmac.*, 1979, *15*, 181.

Excretion in breast milk. Desmethyldiazepam was found in small amounts in milk and in the blood of breast-fed infants when clorazepate was given to women who were breast-feeding.— E. Rey *et al.*, *Eur. J. clin. Pharmac.*, 1979, *15*, 181.

Uses. Clorazepate is a benzodiazepine with actions and uses similar to those of diazepam (p.1523). The usual dose for the treatment of anxiety is 15 mg daily, at night, of the dipotassium salt, which is equivalent to 13 mg daily of the monopotassium salt. Higher doses are recommended in the USA where the usual dose is 26 mg daily of the monopotassium salt, with a range of 13 to 52 mg daily and reduced doses for elderly or debilitated patients.

Action. Clorazepate is converted by acid in the stomach into desmethyldiazepam; in achlorhydria the conversion takes place during the process of absorption. Its pharmacology is therefore primarily that of desmethyldiazepam, the major metabolite of diazepam.— *Drug & Ther. Bull.*, 1974, *12*, 35. See also *Med. Lett.*, 1972, *14*, 85.

Further references: M. Patay *et al.*, *Thérapie*, 1975, *30*, 679.

Alcohol and drug withdrawal. Studies involving clorazepate in alcohol withdrawal.— S. L. Dilts *et al.*, *Am. J. Psychiat.*, 1977, *134*, 92.

Anaesthesia. *Anaesthetic premedication.* Studies of clorazepate for anaesthetic premedication.— A. Malavaud and M. Rebouillat, *Anesth. Analg. Réanim.*, 1971, *28*, 247; A. R. Cohen *et al.*, *Br. J. Anaesth.*, 1978, *50*, 821.

Anxiety. Clorazepate dipotassium 15 mg at night and diazepam 5 mg thrice daily were equally effective for psychic and somatic anxieties in a double-blind study of 54 patients with chronic anxiety.— G. D. Burrows *et al.*, *Med. J. Aust.*, 1977, *2*, 525.

Further references: G. Holmberg and B. Livstedt, *Arzneimittel-Forsch.*, 1972, *22*, 916; J. J. Ricca, *J. clin. Pharmac.*, 1972, *12*, 286; A. J. Cooper *et al.*, *Br. J. Psychiat.*, 1973, *123*, 475; S. I. Feurst, *Curr. ther. Res.*, 1973, *15*, 449; K. D. Charalampous *et al.*, *J. clin. Pharmac.*, 1973, *13*, 114; R. V. Magnus, *Br. J. clin. Pract.*, 1973, *27*, 449; S. H. Curry, *Clin. Pharmac. Ther.*, 1974, *16*, 192; R. V. Magnus *et al.*, *Dis. nerv. Syst.*, 1977, *38*, 819; L. F. Fabre *et al.*, *J. int. med. Res.*, 1979, *7*, 147.

Convulsions. Clorazepate dipotassium was given in doses of 0.4 to 2 mg per kg body-weight daily to 59 epileptic patients whose seizures were not controlled by standard treatments. Response was excellent in 20 patients, principally those with generalised minor attacks. Four patients showed a partial response. In 35 patients response was negative. None of 14 patients with psychomotor seizures responded to clorazepate treatment.— H. E. Booker, *J. Am. med. Ass.*, 1974, *229*, 552.

Clorazepate dipotassium was used in doses of 22.5 mg or more daily in 17 patients with temporal lobe epilepsy. In 8 patients depression, irritability, and aggressive behaviour occurred during clorazepate therapy.— R. G. Feldman (letter), *J. Am. med. Ass.*, 1976, *236*, 2603. Behavioural disturbances have been observed in epileptic patients after seizures had been controlled with anticonvulsant medication regardless of type.— S. Livingston *et al.* (letter), *J. Am. med. Ass.*, 1977, *237*, 1561.

Further references: A. S. Troupin *et al.*, *Neurology, Minneap.*, 1979, *29*, 458.

Hypnotic effect. The hypnotic effects of desmethyldiazepam and clorazepate dipotassium were studied in 6 healthy subjects; 10 mg of desmethyldiazepam was considered equivalent to 15 mg of clorazepate dipotassium.— A. N. Nicholson *et al.*, *Br. J. clin. Pharmac.*, 1976, *3*, 429.

Proprietary Preparations

Tranxene *(Boehringer Ingelheim, UK).* Clorazepate dipotassium, available as capsules of 15 mg. (Also available as Tranxene in *Austral., Belg., Canad., Fr., Neth., NZ, S.Afr., USA*).

Other Proprietary Names

Arg.—Covengar, Enadine, Justum, Moderane, Tencilan, Tranxilium *(all dipotassium)*; *Belg.*—Belseren, Uni-tranxene *(both dipotassium)*; *Denm.*—Tranxen *(dipotassium)*; *Ger.*—Tranxilium *(dipotassium)*; *Ital.*—Transene *(dipotassium)*; *Norw.*—Tranxilen *(dipotassium)*; *Spain*—Nansius, Tranxilium *(both dipotassium)*; *Swed.*—Tranxilen *(dipotassium)*; *Switz.*—Tranxilium *(dipotassium)*; *USA*—Azene *(monopotassium)*.

7031-p

Clothiapine.

Clotiapine; HF 2159. 2-Chloro-11-(4-methylpiperazin-1-yl)dibenzo[*b*,*f*][1,4]thiazepine.

$C_{18}H_{18}ClN_3S$=343.9.

CAS — 2058-52-8.

Clothiapine has actions similar to those of chlorpromazine (p.1509) and has been given in doses of 40 to 120 mg daily for the treatment of psychoses. It may also be given by deep intramuscular injection.

Beneficial results in acute schizophrenia with clothiapine 40 mg four times daily initially intramuscularly and subsequently by mouth. Side-effects included some decreases in haemoglobin values and white cell counts.— T. Buchan *et al.*, *S. Afr. med. J.*, 1977, *51*, 237.

Proprietary Names

Entumin *(Sandoz, Ital.)*; Entumine *(Wander, Switz.)*;

Etomine *(Sandoz, S.Afr.)*; Etumina *(Sandoz, Arg.; Sandoz, Spain)*; Etumine *(Wander, Belg.; Sandoz, Fr.)*.

7032-s

Cloxazolam. CS-370. 10-Chloro-11b-(2-chlorophenyl)-2,3,7,11b-tetrahydro-oxazolo[3,2-*d*][1,4]benzodiazepin-6(5*H*)-one.
$C_{17}H_{14}Cl_2N_2O_2$=349.2.

CAS — 24166-13-0.

A white, odourless, tasteless, crystalline powder. Practically **insoluble** in water; slightly soluble in acetone, dehydrated alcohol, and ethyl acetate; sparingly soluble in chloroform; freely soluble in glacial acetic acid. M.p. about 200° with decomposition.

Cloxazolam is a benzodiazepine with actions and uses similar to those of diazepam (p.1519). It has been given in doses of 3 to 12 mg daily for the treatment of anxiety.

Results of a double-blind placebo-controlled study in 8 healthy subjects comparing diazepam and cloxazolam. Cloxazolam 2 mg was approximately equivalent to diazepam 5 mg. The effect of cloxazolam could still be observed after 8 hours and it was considered that a dosage regimen of cloxazolam 2 mg twice daily should suffice.— B. Saletu *et al.*, *Curr. ther. Res.*, 1976, *20*, 510.

Proprietary Names

Enadel, Sepazon (both *Jap.*); Tolestan *(Roemmers, Arg.)*.

7033-w

Cyamemazine. RP 7204; Cyamepromazine. 10-(3-Dimethylamino-2-methylpropyl)phenothiazine-2-carbonitrile.
$C_{19}H_{21}N_3S$=323.5.

CAS — 3546-03-0.

Cyamemazine is a phenothiazine with general properties similar to chlorpromazine (p.1509). It has been used in the management of neuropsychiatric disorders and as an adjunct in the treatment of psychoses. The usual dose is 200 to 300 mg daily, with a range of 50 to 600 mg daily; the recommended daily dosage is given in 2 portions with the larger amount at night. It may also be given by intramuscular injection in doses of 25 to 200 mg daily.

Cyamemazine should be given in reduced dosage to elderly patients; the parenteral route is not recommended for the elderly.

Proprietary Names

Tercian *(Théraplix, Fr.)*.

7034-e

Cyclarbamate. C 1428; Cyclopentaphen. Cyclopentylidenedimethyl bis(phenylcarbamate).
$C_{21}H_{24}N_2O_4$=368.4.

CAS — 5779-54-4.

Cyclarbamate is a carbamate with general properties similar to those of meprobamate (p.1545). It was formerly given in doses of 0.5 to 1.5 g daily in divided doses for muscular spasms.

7036-y

Diazepam *(B.P., U.S.P.)*. LA 111; Ro 5-2807; Wy 3467. 7-Chloro-1,3-dihydro-1-methyl-5-phenyl-2*H*-1,4-benzodiazepin-2-one.

$C_{16}H_{13}ClN_2O$=284.7.

CAS — 439-14-5.

Pharmacopoeias. In *Br., Braz., Chin., Cz., Jap., Jug., Nord.*, and *U.S.*

A white or yellow, odourless or almost odourless, crystalline powder, tasteless at first with a bitter after-taste. M.p. 131° to 135°.

Soluble 1 in 333 of water, 1 in 25 of alcohol, 1 in 2 of chloroform, and 1 in 39 of ether. **Store** in airtight containers. Protect from light.

Formulation of injection. Adverse cardiac effects in animals given diazepam intravenously in propylene glycol solvent.— D. S. Pearl and R. A. Gillis, *Toxic. appl. Pharmac.*, 1976, *37*, 100. Indications that macrogol 400 is less detrimental.— J. A. Quest *et al.*, *ibid.*

There was a high incidence of pain on injection in 56 patients who received a single intravenous injection of diazepam in the original solvent of propylene glycol/alcohol/benzoic acid and in 58 who received a similar injection in a new formulation with Cremophor EL as the solvent. Venous thickening on the 4th or 5th day, suggestive of thrombophlebitis, was not significantly different at 9 and 4% respectively. Arm tenderness at 4 weeks was significantly different at 29 and 10%.— H. Siebke *et al.*, *Br. J. Anaesth.*, 1976, *48*, 1187.

Dilution of diazepam injection with dextrose injection, sodium chloride injection, Ringer's Injection (*U.S.P.*), or Lactated Ringer's Injection (*U.S.P.*) to concentrations of 5 mg in 40 ml or 5 mg in 50 ml produced solutions which were compatible and stable in all 4 diluents for 6 to 8 and 24 hours respectively.— M. E. Morris, *Am. J. Hosp. Pharm.*, 1978, *35*, 669.

Further references: D. P. Crankshaw and C. Raper, *J. Pharm. Pharmac.*, 1971, *23*, 313; G. W. Burton *et al.* (letter), *Br. med. J.*, 1974, *3*, 258; J. Gerritsen *et al.*, *Pharm. Weekbl. Ned.*, 1975, *110*, 277; K. Korttila *et al.*, *Acta pharmac. tox.*, 1976, *39*, 104; M. A. K. Mattila *et al.*, *Br. J. Anaesth.*, 1979, *51*, 891; A. S. Olesen and M. S. Hüttel, *ibid.*, 1980, *52*, 609.

Stability. Studies on the photochemical decomposition of diazepam.— P. J. G. Cornelissen *et al.*, *Int. J. Pharmaceut.*, 1978, *1*, 173.

A report of the extensive adsorption of diazepam to plastic tubing during continuous infusion.— J. MacKichan *et al.* (letter), *New Engl. J. Med.*, 1979, *301*, 332.

Dependence. Prolonged use of diazepam may lead to the development of dependence of the barbiturate-alcohol type (see p.792). It has a low liability for abuse.

Abuse. Diazepam has a moderate potential for abuse.— H. Isbell and T. L. Chruściel, *Dependence Liability of 'Non-narcotic' Drugs*, Geneva, World Health Organization, 1970; *idem*, *Bull. Wld Hlth Org.*, 1970, *43*, *Suppl.*

A retrospective analysis covering a 4- to 5-year period of postmortem medicolegal records from 27 centres in the United States and Canada revealed that of 914 deaths due to drug overdose in which diazepam was involved a defined history of diazepam abuse was found in only 17. There was a history of diamorphine abuse in 190 and evidence of alcohol abuse or misuse in 179. In only 2 cases was diazepam implicated as the sole drug responsible for the death.— B. S. Finkle *et al.*, *J. Am. med. Ass.*, 1979, *242*, 429.

A retrospective study of the development of psychiatric illness in 51 male drug abusers. At the end of 6 years, 6 of 11 patients who used stimulants (mainly amphetamine or methylphenidate by the end of the study) had been diagnosed as schizophrenic; 8 of 14 patients who used depressants (mainly barbiturates, benzodiazepines, and sedative hypnotics) had anxiety and depression and 5 had attempted suicide. Very little psychological change was apparent in 26 patients who abused opiates.— A. T. McLellan *et al.*, *New Engl. J. Med.*, 1979, *301*, 1310. Comment.— H. G. Pope, *ibid.*, 1341.

Dependence and withdrawal. A discussion on the dependence potential of the benzodiazepines. Although drug-dependence units usually have several patients who abuse benzodiazepines, in view of the extensive worldwide usage of the benzodiazepines serious physical dependence must be uncommon. The dependence status of patients on normal therapeutic doses is not known and many of the mild withdrawal symptoms are indistinguishable from the symptoms of anxiety states. Return of the original symptoms on withdrawal reflects the symptomatic nature of the drug therapy. Nevertheless, in some patients withdrawal is associated with features untypical of anxiety states, severe headaches and abrupt weight-loss being the most upsetting. Withdrawal syndromes from therapeutic doses of benzodiazepines are generally mild but include poor appetite, trembling, nausea, insomnia, numbness, faintness, weakness, vomiting, and lack of energy; in addition, many patients become dysphoric. Normal-dosage dependence should be suspected when a patient repeatedly tries to wean himself from a benzodiazepine and restarts the drug because of headache, dysphoria, or symptoms unrelated to the initial anxiety syndrome.— *Lancet*, 1979, *1*, 196. Analysis of data from 15 evaluations of 5 benzodiazepines indicated that rebound insomnia (a worsening of sleep compared with base-line values) occurred after withdrawal of short-term nightly administration of triazolam, nitrazepam, and flunitrazepam. It was attributed to the short and intermediate half-lives of these drugs. Withdrawal of short-term nightly administration of diazepam and flurazepam, which have longer half-lives, was not associated with similar rebound insomnia. Conclusive evidence as to whether rebound insomnia occurs with long-acting benzodiazepines would require studies evaluating withdrawal over longer periods. As has been previously suggested, rebound insomnia might occur with long-acting benzodiazepines when they have been taken for lengthy periods in high doses. It is also suggested that rebound anxiety, an analogue of rebound insomnia, may occur when certain short-or intermediate-acting benzodiazepines are given during the day and their duration of action is exceeded by the interval between doses.— A. Kales *et al.*, *J. Am. med. Ass.*, 1979, *241*, 1692.

Further reviews and comments on the dependence potential of benzodiazepines: B. M. Maletzky and J. Klotter, *Int. J. Addict.*, 1976, *11*, 95; *Drug & Ther. Bull.*, 1977, *15*, 85; M. Peet and L. Moonie (letter), *Br. med. J.*, 1977, *1*, 714; M. M. Glatt (letter), *Lancet*, 1978, *2*, 1205; D. J. Greenblatt and R. I. Shader, *Drug Metab. Rev.*, 1978, *8*, 13; J. Marks, *The Benzodiazepines: Use, Overuse, Misuse, Abuse*, Lancaster, MTP, 1978; Committee on the Review of Medicines, *Br. med. J.*, 1980, *280*, 910; *Drug & Ther. Bull.*, 1980, *18*, 97; *FDA Drug Bull.*, 1980, *10*, 2; *Pharm. J.*, 1980, *1*, 384.

Diazepam withdrawal symptoms have generally been associated with abrupt discontinuation of doses greater than 30 mg daily, but mild withdrawal symptoms of the barbiturate-alcohol type, without convulsions, have been reported by D. Haskell (*J. Am. med. Ass.*, 1975, *233*, 135) in patients who have taken diazepam in doses as low as 15 mg daily for 4 to 6 months. Convulsions have been reported by I. Vyas and M.W.P. Carney (*Br. med. J.*, 1975, *4*, 44) following the abrupt withdrawal of 30 mg daily given over 3 years, and A. Rifkin *et al.* (*J. Am. med. Ass.*, 1976, *236*, 2172) have reported convulsions following withdrawal of this dose given over only 3 months, although A. Ecker (*J. Am. med. Ass.*, 1977, *237*, 765) suggested the alternative diagnosis of stress convulsions. Major convulsions on 2 occasions in one patient have followed withdrawal of diazepam 100 and 150 mg daily according to C.F. Essig (*J. Am. med. Ass.*, 1966, *196*, 714) and dependence on a dose of up to 500 mg daily has been reported by A.W. Clare (*Br. med. J.*, 1971, *4*, 340) in a phobic woman who substituted alcohol when diazepam was not available. A withdrawal syndrome involving precipitous weight loss and orthostatic pulse-rate increase has been described by J.S. Pevnick *et al.* (*Archs gen. Psychiat.*, 1978, *35*, 995) in a man with a history of opiate addiction who had taken 30 to 45 mg of diazepam daily for 20 months; the withdrawal syndrome characteristically occurred 5 to 9 days after stopping diazepam. M.L. De Bard (*Am. J. Psychiat.*, 1979, *136*, 104) has reported psychosis, coma, and seizure, with the diagnosis of organic brain syndrome, in a man who had taken diazepam 80 mg daily for several years, and advises against long-term prescribing and abrupt discontinuation of diazepam. Psychosis was also noted by M.W. Dysken and C.H. Chan (*Am. J. Psychiat.*, 1977, *134*, 573) on withdrawal from a man who had taken diazepam 15 to 30 mg daily for about 7 years; they emphasise that dependence is a function, not only of daily dosage, but also of time, and comment that patients at risk include alcoholics given diazepam to relieve anxiety associated with the withdrawal of alcohol. Control of psychotic withdrawal symptoms may be obtained by reinstitution of diazepam and S.H. Preskorn and L.J. Denner (*J. Am. med. Ass.*, 1977, *237*, 36) recommend that these drugs should be withdrawn slowly. Psychological changes have also followed withdrawal of high-dose diazepam therapy for the treatment of tetanus and, again, J. Malatinsky *et al.* (*Postgrad. med. J.*, 1975, *51*, 860) have recommended gradual withdrawal.

On gradual withdrawal of chronic normal-dose benzodiazepine therapy from 16 patients (including 10 taking diazepam 10 to 30 mg daily) H. Petursson and M.H. Lader (*Br. med. J.*, 1981, *283*, 643) still noted what they considered to be a true withdrawal syndrome and not merely a revival of the original anxiety symptoms. In most cases the withdrawal symptoms were indistinguishable from those observed on withdrawal of higher doses.

Further individual reports of diazepam dependence: P. Agrawal, *Can. psychiat. Ass. J.*, 1978, *23*, 35; S. W. Acuda and J. Muhangi, *E. Afr. med. J.*, 1979, *56*, 76; F. Miller and J. Nulsen, *J. Nerv. ment. Dis.*, 1979, *167*, 637; A. Khan *et al.*, *N.Z. med. J.*, 1980, *92*, 94; A.

Winokur *et al.*, *Archs gen. Psychiat.*, 1980, *37*, 101; P. Tyrer *et al.*, *Lancet*, 1981, *1*, 520.

For a critical analysis of published reports of psychological and physical dependence on benzodiazepines, see J. Marks, *The Benzodiazepines: Use, Overuse, Misuse, Abuse*, Lancaster, MTP, 1978, p. 81.

For reports of neonatal dependence on diazepam see Pregnancy and the Neonate (below).

Pregnancy and the neonate. Hypertonia and hyperreflexia, in an infant born to a mother who had taken diazepam 10 mg every other day for the last 4 months of pregnancy, possibly represented withdrawal symptoms.— E. Mazzi, *Am. J. Obstet. Gynec.*, 1977, *129*, 586. Three infants born to mothers who had taken diazepam in doses of from 10 to 20 mg daily during the last few months of pregnancy, showed tremors during the first 6 hours of life, and required treatment with phenobarbitone to reduce the incidence of tremors. One child subsequently died at home; the death was attributed to the infant sudden death syndrome.— J. L. Rementería and K. Bhatt, *J. Pediat.*, 1977, *90*, 123.

See also under Adverse Effects and Treatment, Precautions, Absorption and Fate, and Uses.

Adverse Effects. The side-effects of diazepam and the other benzodiazepines are usually mild and infrequent. Drowsiness, light-headedness, and ataxia are the most common and are often dose-dependent. Elderly and debilitated patients are especially susceptible to these reactions. Diazepam can induce amnesia which may sometimes be considered as a side-effect.

Other effects occasionally observed include hypotension, some respiratory depression, nausea and constipation, changes in salivation, blurred vision and diplopia, dysarthria, skin rashes, urinary retention, incontinence, mental depression, tremor, headache, confusion, slurred speech, vertigo, and changes in libido. There have been isolated reports of blood disorders and jaundice. Overdosage produces central nervous system depression and coma.

The benzodiazepines sometimes produce paradoxical reactions, especially in high dosage or in severely disturbed patients and may provoke excitement and dysphoria instead of sedation.

Withdrawal reactions may occur with benzodiazepines, see Dependence (above).

There have been reports of an association between infant cleft lip and palate, and maternal use of diazepam, but other studies have found no significant association between congenital malformations and maternal ingestion of benzodiazepines. Administration of diazepam in late pregnancy has been associated with intoxication of the neonate.

Intravenous injections of diazepam may be painful and can cause thrombophlebitis.

Allergy. A 9-year-old boy developed slight wheezing 18 hours after an intravenous injection of diazepam 5 mg. After an intramuscular injection of diazepam 5 mg 3 days later he became cyanotic within an hour, with wheezing, increased respiratory-rate, and abnormal blood gases. This was considered to be an immediate allergic reaction.— M. Z. Blumberg and S. Young, *Pediatrics*, 1974, *54*, 811.

A 28-year-old woman with a history of allergy to various substances, including chlordiazepoxide, developed an allergic reaction after a 10-mg intramuscular dose of diazepam.— L. Milner, *Br. med. J.*, 1977, *1*, 144. A similar report.— R. H. Falk (letter), *ibid.*, 287. The solvent, Cremophor EL, might have caused the allergy.— D. Blatchley (letter), *ibid.* A suggestion that solubilisation with Cremophor EL might promote hypersensitivity reactions to previously safe drugs.— A. Padfield and J. Watkins (letter), *ibid.*, 575. Of 1500 patients given intravenous injections of diazepam in soya oil only one allergic reaction had been noted, and the cause had been doubtful.— O. von Dardel *et al.* (letter), *ibid.*, 773.

Further references: J. S. Ghosh (letter), *Br. med. J.*, 1977, *1*, 902; M. S. Hüttel *et al.*, *Br. J. Anaesth.*, 1980, *52*, 77.

See also Cremophor EL, p.373.

See also under Effects on the Eyes (below).

Convulsions. A 10-year-old girl with a history of various epileptic seizures was given diazepam 8 mg by slow intravenous injection. Abnormal spike-and-wave tracings on the EEG were abolished and replaced by spike waves characteristic of a major epileptic attack. Similar attacks occurred for 20 minutes and were accompanied by cries, apnoea, unconsciousness, tonic spasms, and incontinence.— P. F. Prior *et al.* (letter), *Lancet*, 1971, *2*, 434.

See also under Uses.

Cytogenetic effects. Chromosome analysis performed on peripheral blood of 20 healthy young adults before and after a single 12- to 20-mg intravenous dose of diazepam revealed no significant increase in chromosomal aberrations due to diazepam.— B. J. White *et al.*, *J. Am. med. Ass.*, 1974, *230*, 414.

A report of preliminary animal studies suggesting that diazepam may have a tumour-growth-promoting effect.— D. F. Horrobin *et al.* (letter), *Lancet*, 1979, *1*, 978. Severe criticism; the reported effects have not been confirmed in another laboratory.— J. Genest, *Clinical Research Institute of Montreal*, *ibid.*, 1306. Oxazepam was found to have no significant influence on the tumour growth, or the survival-time, of tumour-bearing *rats*.— A. Guaitani *et al.* (letter), *ibid.*, 1147. Results of a 2-year study on substantial numbers of *animals* do not support the suggestion that diazepam may either cause or promote tumour growth.— M. R. Jackson and P. A. Harris, *Roche* (letter), *ibid.*, 1981, *1*, 104. Further correspondence: D. F. Horrobin (letter), *ibid.*, 277; M. R. Jackson and P. A. Harris, *Roche* (letter), *ibid.*, 445; E. Boyland (letter), *ibid.*

Evaluation of diazepam from data previously collected during a multicentre breast cancer screening programme, the Breast Cancer Detection Demonstration Project, failed to demonstrate a relation between diazepam use and breast cancer.— R. A. Kleinerman *et al.* (letter), *Lancet*, 1981, *1*, 1153. See also D. W. Kaufman *et al.*, *Lancet*, 1982, *1*, 537.

Effects on the blood. Diazepam has been reported to cause aplastic anaemia.— R. H. Girdwood, *Drugs*, 1976, *11*, 394.

Benzodiazepines had been alleged to cause both leucopenia and leucocytosis in addition to eosinophilia.— J. G. Edwards, *Practitioner*, 1977, *219*, 117.

Effects on the brain. Five patients on maintenance haemodialysis developed encephalopathy attributed to flurazepam and diazepam.— L. Taclob and M. Needle, *Lancet*, 1976, *2*, 704. Dramatic reversal of the clinical symptoms of dialysis encephalopathy in 4 patients by administration of diazepam 5 mg thrice daily.— A. M. Nadel and W. P. Wilson, *Neurology, Minneap.*, 1976, *26*, 1130.

See also under Convulsions and Effects on Mental State.

Effects on the endocrine system. Plasma-testosterone concentrations were significantly increased in men taking diazepam 10 to 20 mg daily for 2 weeks.— A. E. Argüelles and J. Rosner (letter), *Lancet*, 1975, *2*, 607.

Four patients with galactorrhoea taking benzodiazepines all had normal serum-prolactin concentrations. A causal relationship between benzodiazepines and either galactorrhoea or abnormalities of prolactin secretion has yet to be established.— D. L. Kleinberg *et al.*, *New Engl. J. Med.*, 1977, *296*, 589. A 55-year-old man who had increased his diazepam intake to 80 to 140 mg daily developed bilateral gynaecomastia. The gynaecomastia resolved on withdrawal of the diazepam.— H. J. Moerck and G. Magelund (letter), *Lancet*, 1979, *1*, 1344. Diazepam does not affect plasma-prolactin concentrations.— J. D. Wilson *et al.* (letter), *Br. med. J.*, 1979, *1*, 123.

Raised serum-oestradiol concentrations in 5 men with diazepam-associated gynaecomastia.— D. Bergman *et al.* (letter), *Lancet*, 1981, *2*, 1225.

Further references: W. P. Tormey *et al.* (letter), *Br. J. clin. Pharmac.*, 1979, *8*, 90.

Effects on the eyes. A brown ring occurred on the lens of a woman who had taken moderate doses of diazepam for 3 years.— H. Pau, *Klin. Mbl. Augenheilk.*, 1974, *164*, 446, per P. Lechat *et al.*, *Thérapie*, 1975, *30*, 381.

A study indicating that usual therapeutic doses of diazepam interfere wtih colour vision.— J. Laroche and C. Laroche, *Annls pharm. fr.*, 1972, *30*, 433.

Allergic conjunctivitis occurred in 4 women after taking diazepam 5 to 10 mg. Three of them also experienced sensitivity to light.— E. G. Lutz, *Am. J. Psychiat.*, 1975, *132*, 548.

A report of angle closure glaucoma possibly associated with diazepam administration.— S. W. Hyams and C. Keroub, *Am. J. Psychiat.*, 1977, *134*, 447.

Effects on the heart. In a study of 6 patients given diazepam 2.5 mg intravenously every 30 seconds to a total dose of 12.5 to 17.5 mg there was a significant reduction in cardiac output and stroke volume and an increase in heart-rate and peripheral resistance.— J. L. Jenkinson *et al.*, *Br. J. Anaesth.*, 1974, *46*, 294.

Further references: J. S. Barrett and E. B. Hey, *J. Am. med. Ass.*, 1970, *214*, 1323; A. B. S. Mitchell *et al.*, *Postgrad. med. J.*, 1972, *48*, 436.

Effects on the liver. Diazepam could cause cholestasis.— K. G. Tolman, *Med. J. Aust.*, 1977, *2*, 655.

Effects on mental state. Five-minute speech recordings after administration of diazepam, chlordiazepoxide, lorazepam, triazolam, and flurazepam indicated disorganisation of thought, shown by incomprehensible remarks and incomplete sentences.— L. A. Gottschalk, *Curr. ther. Res.*, 1977, *21*, 192.

In healthy subjects diazepam depressed pupillary response and inhibited performance recall.— J. A. Kotzan, *J. pharm. Sci.*, 1978, *67*, 956. In 20 healthy subjects diazepam 10 mg daily tended to impair acquisition, but improve recall of information, and to reduce reaction time.— R. Liljequist *et al.*, *Eur. J. clin. Pharmac.*, 1978, *13*, 339.

Further references: E. O. Clark *et al.*, *Archs Neurol., Chicago*, 1979, *36*, 296.

Depression. Deepening depression was associated with diazepam therapy in 8 patients. In 7 subjects suicidal thoughts and impulses occurred, and 2 made serious attempts to kill themselves; 2 others succeeded. Most patients were receiving 5 mg three or four times a day.— H. F. Ryan *et al.*, *J. Am. med. Ass.*, 1968, *203*, 1137. Comment.— F. A. Whitlock and L. E. J. Evans, *Drugs*, 1978, *15*, 53.

Paradoxical response. An aberrant response to diazepam occurred in 6 patients within days of starting treatment with 40 to 60 mg daily. Symptoms included tremulousness, confusion, apprehension, insomnia, depression, and a compulsion to commit suicide against the patient's will. The symptoms cleared when diazepam was withdrawn. Two of the patients were over 65 years old and all but one (who had a postmeningitic convulsive disorder) had significant vascular disease. It is strongly recommended that physicians adhere to the maximum recommended dosages of diazepam, and be aware of the possibility that peripheral vascular disease and age may be a factor in the appearance of cumulative toxic effects.— R. C. W. Hall and J. R. Joffe, *Am. J. Psychiat.*, 1972, *129*, 738.

A review of reports in the literature associating benzodiazepines with aggression. There is little conclusive evidence to show that the benzodiazepines are associated with an increase in aggression. Indeed, what data there are tend to point in the opposite direction. The major obstacle to progress is the lack of both subjective and objective measures of hostility and aggression.— A. Bond and M. Lader, Benzodiazepines and Aggression, in *Psychopharmacology of Aggression*, M. Sandler (Ed.), New York, Raven Press, 1979, p. 173.

Effects on respiratory function. Moderate hypoventilation with increased pCO_2, decreased arterial pH, reduced tidal air and minute volume respiration, and increased respiration-rate occurred in 9 superficially anaesthetised patients given diazepam 10 mg per 20 kg body-weight intravenously.— M. Maspoli, *Schweiz. med. Wschr.*, 1967, *97*, 320, per *J. Am. med. Ass.*, 1967, *200* (Apr. 10), A 239.

Excessive secretion of saliva and bronchopneumonia occurred in 3 children given high doses of diazepam for epilepsy.— J. M. Killian and G. H. Fromm, *Develop. Med. Child Neurology*, 1971, *13*, 32, per *Abstr. Wld Med.*, 1971, *45*, 536.

Further references: R. Huch and A. Huch (letter), *Lancet*, 1974, *2*, 1267.

Extrapyramidal effects. Benzodiazepines can precipitate tardive dyskinesia.— A. H. Rosenbaum and J. R. de la Fuente (letter), *Lancet*, 1979, *2*, 900.

Hypotension. Diazepam was given to 25 patients in status epilepticus by intravenous injection and arrested continuous seizure activity in 16 patients. Hypotension developed in 6 patients, of whom 5 had also been given phenobarbitone by intramuscular injection because diazepam gave an inadequate response. Moderate falls in blood pressure occurred in 4 patients within an hour of the injection of 2.5 to 60 mg of diazepam. Two patients who were given large doses of diazepam with phenobarbitone and paraldehyde developed severe hypotension which was fatal in 1 case. Respiratory depression in 1 patient was easily controlled.— D. S. Bell, *Br. med. J.*, 1969, *1*, 159. Occasional hypotensive reactions in seriously ill people should not be allowed to detract from the value of diazepam as the drug of choice in the control of severe fits and the prevention of status epilepticus.— J. Bowe (letter), *ibid.*, 439. Diazepam was considered safe and the drug of choice in the treatment of status epilepticus if the patient had not been given any anticonvulsant therapy in the previous 6 hours and if the dose of diazepam did not exceed 40 mg per hour.— S. N. Sinha (letter), *ibid.*, 440. See also D. C. Taylor and C. Ounsted (letter), *ibid.*; D. S. Bell (letter), *ibid.*, 714.

In patients given diazepam intravenously prior to cardiac surgery, blood pressure fell from 95 to 80 mmHg, pO_2 fell from 85 to 66 mmHg, and in 2 of 50 patients amnesia occurred lasting 36 hours.— S. M. Lyons and R. S. J. Clarke (letter), *Br. med. J.*, 1971, *4*, 229.

Further references: R. B. Falk *et al.*, *Anesthesiology*, 1978, *49*, 149.

Overdosage. Serious poisoning following even large overdoses of benzodiazepines is extremely rare.— *Med. Lett.*, 1976, *18*, 60.

Following ingestion of 40 tablets of diazepam 10 mg and 2 tablets of doxepin hydrochloride [sic] a 27-year-old man developed coma, bullous and vesicular skin eruption, and eccrine sweat gland and sweat duct necrosis. Coma with bullae and eccrine sweat gland necrosis had subsequently been seen in a second case of diazepam overdose.— A. J. Varma *et al.*, *Archs intern. Med.*, 1977, *137*, 1207.

A report of 2 patients who recovered fully within about 48 hours of taking an estimated 450 to 500 mg and 2 g of diazepam, respectively. Initial blood concentrations of diazepam and its metabolites were 10 to 100 times higher than those associated with therapeutic doses. The rapid recovery was considered to be due to adaptation or tolerance to diazepam and its metabolites.— D. J. Greenblatt *et al.*, *J. Am. med. Ass.*, 1978, *240*, 1872.

A retrospective analysis covering a 4- to 5-year period of postmortem medicolegal records from 27 centres in the United States and Canada revealed 914 deaths due to drug overdose in which diazepam was involved but in only 2 of these cases was diazepam implicated as the sole drug responsible for the death.— B. S. Finkle *et al.*, *J. Am. med. Ass.*, 1979, *242*, 429.

Further references: R. Berger *et al.*, *Clin. Pediat.*, 1975, *14*, 842 (cardiac arrest).

Porphyria. Studies in *animals* indicating that diazepam had no porphyrinogenic effect.— R. K. Parikh and M. R. Moore, *Br. J. Anaesth.*, 1978, *50*, 1099. Acute intermittent porphyria in a 62-year-old man with alcoholic cirrhosis associated with the administration of diazepam.— D. R. Stone and E. S. Munson (letter), *ibid.*, 1979, *51*, 809.

Pregnancy and the neonate. *Early pregnancy.* Analysis of 278 mothers of children with various malformations carried out at the Center for Disease Control, Atlanta, demonstrated a significant fourfold risk of cleft lip with or without cleft palate in infants whose mothers had taken diazepam during the first trimester of pregnancy.— M. J. Safra and G. P. Oakley, *Lancet*, 1975, *2*, 478. A similar analysis in Finland of 599 children with oral clefts compared with 590 controls produced a significant association between oral clefts and intake of benzodiazepines during the first trimester.— I. Saxén and L. Saxén (letter), *ibid.*, 498. Of 836 mothers of congenitally malformed infants 33 had used benzodiazepines during the first trimester of pregnancy, compared with 21 in 836 controls. The case: control incidence ratio of 1.57 was not significant.— G. Greenberg *et al.*, *Br. med. J.*, 1977, *2*, 853. See also Chlordiazepoxide, p.1507.

Further references: J. J. Wallner, *Arch. Gynaek.*, 1973, *214*, 83; I. Saxén, *Int. J. Epidemiol.*, 1975, *4*, 37.

Individual reports of malformations in infants of mothers who had taken diazepam during pregnancy: E. J. Istvan, *Can. med. Ass. J.*, 1970, *103*, 1394; C. A. D. Ringrose (letter), *ibid.*, 1972, *106*, 1058.

Late pregnancy and labour. In a study in 18 infants born to mothers who had received 30 mg or less of diazepam (low-dose) in the 15 hours before delivery, none had low Apgar scores attributable to diazepam, 1 had a rectal temperature below 35°, 2 were reluctant to feed, and 1 had hypotonia. By contrast, in 14 infants whose mothers had received more than 30 mg of diazepam (high-dose) in the 15 hours before delivery, 10 had low Apgar scores, 8 had a low rectal temperature, 10 needed tube-feeding, and 12 had hypotonia. In 1 low-dose infant and 7 high-dose infants subjected to cold stress, the metabolic response was less than in 6 control infants whose mothers had not received diazepam. Cord-blood concentrations of diazepam and desmethyldiazepam were generally higher than maternal values. In 2 high-dose infants concentrations of diazepam rose after delivery possibly due to release from body stores. In 5 high-dose infants, concentrations of desmethyldiazepam rose after delivery and in many cases scarcely fell after 7 days. Care was necessary when diazepam was given in pre-eclampsia.— J. E. Cree *et al.*, *Br. med. J.*, 1973, *4*, 251.

The administration of diazepam to neonates had no effect on serum bilirubin compared with controls but concentrations rose in the treated babies when diazepam was stopped.— F. Heubel and G. Mühlberger, *Dt. med. Wschr.*, 1971, *96*, 1142. In view of the wide variation in metabolism and excretion of diazepam in the neonate doses higher than 10 to 20 mg were not recommended for the mother during labour. Competitive inhibition of the conjugation of bilirubin might lead to hyperbilirubinaemia.— J. Kanto *et al.* (letter), *Br. med. J.*, 1974, *1*, 641. In 93 infants born to mothers who received diazepam during labour, the mean serum bilirubin concentration was increased by 6.3 µg per ml at 48 hours of age and 7.2 µg per ml at 72 hours. This effect would probably only be of importance in small premature infants.— J. H. Drew and W. H. Kitchen, *J. Pediat.*, 1976, *89*, 657. The concentration of sodium benzoate in Valium injection was not considered high enough to cause neonatal hyperbilirubinaemia following administration of 10 to 20 mg diazepam (with 100 to 200 mg sodium benzoate contained in the solvent) by intramuscular injection to the mother during labour.— R. Stockmann *et al.*, *J. int. med. Res.*, 1978, *6*, 468.

Hypotonia, difficulty in sucking, and hypothermia characteristic of the floppy-infant syndrome occurred in a newborn infant whose mother had taken diazepam 2 mg thrice daily on and off for the last 3 months of pregnancy to a total dose of 110 mg. An additional dose of 10 mg had been given rectally at delivery. The infant improved as the high serum concentrations of diazepam (about 550 nmol per litre on day 12) and desmethyldiazepam (about 700 nmol per litre on day 12) fell. Neonatal disturbances had been observed in other children whose mothers had taken diazepam late in pregnancy.— C. Gillberg (letter), *Lancet*, 1977, *2*, 244. No such effect on 2 infants whose mother had taken large doses of diazepam throughout pregnancy and during labour.— K. Haram (letter), *ibid.*, 612. Criticism. Two similar cases (of the floppy-infant syndrome), one involving diazepam and nitrazepam and the other nitrazepam alone.— A. N. P. Speight (letter), *ibid.*, 878. The floppy infant syndrome had not occurred in 30 pregnancies where the mothers had received oxazepam in doses of up to 75 mg daily.— K. A. D. Drury *et al.* (letter), *ibid.*, 1126.

Comment on the hazards of diazepam in labour which include loss of the beat-to-beat variation of the foetal heart. This may reflect a loss of adaptive ability of the foetal heart and circulatory system, or possibly a depression of the cardiac reflex centres in the brain.— J. M. B. Burn (letter), *Br. med. J.*, 1978, *1*, 1216.

Further references: S. Y. Yeh *et al.*, *Obstet. Gynec.*, 1974, *43*, 363; R. J. Rowlatt (letter), *Br. med. J.*, 1978, *1*, 985; A. N. W. Evans *et al.*, *Practitioner*, 1980, *224*, 315.

The neonate. Acute retention of urine in 3 neonates was possibly associated with diazepam and phenobarbitone or phenytoin given to control convulsions.— M. J. Levene, *Archs Dis. Childh.*, 1977, *52*, 975.

See also under Dependence, Treatment of Adverse Effects, Precautions, Absorption and Fate, and Uses. For an adverse effect associated with administration of diazepam by umbilical artery catheter see Thrombo-embolic Effects (below).

Tardive dyskinesia. See under Extrapyramidal Effects (above).

Thrombo-embolic effects. Of 44 patients given a single intravenous dose of diazepam 10 mg three had phlebitis, 5 thrombosis, and 2 thrombophlebitis 2 to 3 days later; thrombosis was present in 17 after 7 to 10 days.— J. E. Hegarty and J. W. Dundee, *Br. med. J.*, 1977, *2*, 1384. See also under Formulation of Injection (above).

Skin pallor occurred within half an hour and discoloration and oedema of the forearm and hand rapidly followed in an 11-month-old child after the accidental intra-arterial injection of diazepam into the brachial artery. Pallor of the legs followed by oedema and cyanosis of the legs occurred in a 2-day-old infant given diazepam by umbilical artery catheter.— J. D. M. Gould and S. Lingan, *Br. med. J.*, 1977, *2*, 298.

A report of the accidental intra-arterial injection of diazepam in 2 patients with suggestions for the management of such accidents. Experience suggested that the clinical signs of ischaemia and gangrene may not occur until days after the event.— M. Rees and J. Dormandy, *Br. med. J.*, 1980, *281*, 289.

Treatment of Adverse Effects. There is no specific treatment. In recent severe overdosage with the benzodiazepines the stomach should be emptied by aspiration and lavage. Recovery usually follows symptomatic treatment. Dialysis is of no value. For general guidelines to the symptomatic therapy of overdosage with central nervous system depressants, see Phenobarbitone, p.812.

Physostigmine is effective in reversing diazepam-induced hypnosis, but should be used with care due to the possibility of side-effects.— G. R. Avant *et al.*, *Ann. intern. Med.*, 1979, *91*, 53. See also J. Di Liverti *et al.*, *J. Pediat.*, 1975, *86*, 106. Failure of physostigmine with atropine in reversing diazepam sedation.— J. G. Garber *et al.*, *Anesth. Analg. curr. Res.*, 1980, *59*, 58. For comments on the hazards of physostigmine in the treatment of drug overdosage, see Physostigmine Salicylate, p.1043.

The apparent reversal of diazepam toxicity by naloxone. The mechanism was not understood.— E. F. Bell, *J. Pediat.*, 1975, *87*, 803. A study suggesting that a large dose of naloxone may relieve respiratory depression following diazepam by reducing depression of carbon dioxide sensitivity.— C. Jordan *et al.*, *Br. J. Anaesth.*, 1979, *51*, 570P.

Pregnancy and the neonate. Since there appeared to be prolonged release of diazepam from tissue stores in infants whose mothers had been given diazepam during labour it was considered that exchange transfusion would be only partly successful in removing diazepam from infants.— B. O'Connell *et al.* (letter), *Br. med. J.*, 1973, *4*, 610.

Precautions. Caution should be observed when giving diazepam to elderly or debilitated patients who are specially sensitive to its side-effects, and to patients with arteriosclerosis, renal, hepatic, or respiratory dysfunction. Diazepam should not be given to patients with acute closed-angle glaucoma.

Diazepam is not suitable for the treatment of psychotic patients, nor is it an antidepressant. It may induce paradoxical reactions in severely disturbed patients or when given in excessive dosage.

Withdrawal of diazepam from patients who have been receiving it in high dosage or for prolonged periods of time should be gradual (see Dependence). Patients may experience an increase in the frequency and severity of attacks of grand mal epilepsy either during treatment with diazepam or following its abrupt withdrawal.

Some reports have indicated that the use of diazepam in early pregnancy is associated with an increased incidence of infant cleft lip and palate, other reports, however, have found no significant association between maternal diazepam use and foetal malformations. Maternal use of diazepam in late pregnancy may be associated with foetal intoxication since diazepam readily crosses the placenta. Diazepam is also excreted in breast milk.

Diazepam may enhance the effects of central nervous system depressants, and may reduce the patient's ability to drive vehicles or operate machinery. Alcohol may alter the patient's response to diazepam.

Intravenous injections of diazepam must be given slowly to avoid the risk of hypotension and apnoea; intramuscular injections should be given deeply, they are painful, and their absorption is erratic; raised serum creatine phosphokinase activity following intramuscular injection may interfere with the diagnosis of myocardial infarction.

A study of 57 persons killed or injured while driving cars, motorcycles, or cycles suggested that the risk of serious accident was increased about 5-fold in those receiving prescriptions for tranquillisers (benzodiazepines or phenothiazines) in the 3 months prior to the accident. There was a significant association between the use of antihistamines and motorcycle accidents.— D. C. G. Skegg *et al.*, *Br. med. J.*, 1979, *1*, 917. Details of the 5 patients listed did not substantiate an association between the use of minor tranquillisers and an increased risk of road accidents.— F. A. Whitlock (letter), *ibid.*, 1979, *2*, 670.

Further comments and studies on whether benzodiazepines and/or the condition for which they are prescribed are associated with increased road accidents: A. Landaver (letter), *Br. med. J.*, 1979, *2*, 207; I. Hindmarch (letter), *Br. med. J.*, 1979, *2*, 671; T. Seppala *et al.*, *Drugs*, 1979, *17*, 389; R. Honkanen *et al.*, *Br. med.*

J., 1980, *281*, 1309.

Anaesthesia. Amnesia frequently followed intravenous administration of diazepam in sedative doses. Loss of memory was dense for 10 minutes and mild impairment occurred for up to 30 minutes after injection. Care was therefore necessary with ambulatory patients.— J. A. Thornton and P. F. R. Clarke (letter), *Br. med. J.*, 1970, *2*, 732. Correlation of plasma-diazepam concentrations with clinical effects and a warning that a secondary peak after several hours could be associated with delayed recovery.— E. S. Baird and D. M. Hailey, *Br. J. Anaesth.*, 1972, *44*, 803.

Further references: P. R. F. Clarke, *Br. J. Anaesth.*, 1970, *42*, 690; J. Dundee (letter), *Br. med. J.*, 1970, *2*, 732; J. M. Gregg *et al.*, *J. oral Surg.*, 1974, *32*, 651; K. Korttila and M. Linnoila, *Anesthesiology*, 1975, *42*, 685; *idem*, *Br. J. Anaesth.*, 1975, *47*, 457; T. Seppälä *et al.*, *Br. J. clin. Pharmac.*, 1976, *3*, 831; D. M. Jones *et al.*, *Br. J. clin. Pharmac.*, 1978, *6*, 333.

Interactions. Drowsiness as a side-effect of diazepam or chlordiazepoxide, was less frequent in smokers than in non-smokers. Nicotine, a hepatic enzyme inducer, might increase the metabolism of diazepam and chlordiazepoxide.—Report from the Boston Collaborative Drug Surveillance Program, *New Engl. J. Med.*, 1973, *288*, 277. No difference between smokers and non-smokers in plasma elimination half-lives or steady-state concentrations of diazepam.— U. Klotz *et al.*, *J. clin. Invest.*, 1975, *55*, 347. Tobacco smoking has no significant effect on the metabolism of chlordiazepoxide and therefore the smaller incidence of excessive sedation in smokers cannot be explained in terms of increased metabolism.— P. V. Desmond *et al.* (letter), *New Engl. J. Med.*, 1979, *300*, 199.

Alcohol. Reviews and comments on interactions between alcohol and diazepam: E. M. Sellers and M. R. Holloway, *Clin. Pharmacokinet.*, 1978, *3*, 440; M. Linnoila *et al.*, *Drugs*, 1979, *18*, 299.

In a double-blind crossover study in 40 healthy students diazepam 5 mg thrice daily increased choice reaction and attention and slightly increased coordination, but subjects drove faster and made more mistakes. When alcohol 500 mg per kg body-weight was added reaction was reduced, but subjects drove more slowly and made fewer mistakes.— M. Linnoila *et al.*, *Br. J. clin. Pharmac.*, 1974, *1*, 176P. A further study suggested that the impairment of skills associated with driving was due to an interaction between alcohol and diazepam itself, rather than its metabolites.— E. S. Palva and M. Linnoila, *Eur. J. clin. Pharmac.*, 1978, *13*, 345.

Conflicting views on the effect of alcohol on diazepam: S. L. Hayes *et al.*, *New Engl. J. Med.*, 1977, *296*, 186; R. Bernstein and J. S. Holcenberg (letter), *ibid.*, 1006; W. E. Boden (letter), *ibid.*; S. L. Hayes *et al.* (letter), *ibid.*; S. M. MacLeod *et al.*, *Eur. J. clin. Pharmac.*, 1977, *11*, 345; D. J. Greenblatt *et al.*, *Psychopharmacology*, 1978, *57*, 199; U. Laisi *et al.*, *Eur. J. clin. Pharmac.*, 1979, *16*, 263; E. M. Sellers *et al.*, *Clin. Pharmac. Ther.*, 1980, *27*, 286; *idem*, *28*, 638; E. H. Ellinwood *et al.*, *Clin. Pharmac. Ther.*, 1981, *30*, 534.

Antacids. In a study in 4 groups of 50 women undergoing minor gynaecological surgery the sedative effect of a single 10-mg oral dose of diazepam appeared to be enhanced by Aluminium Hydroxide Mixture 40 ml or 0.3M sodium citrate 30 ml, and reduced by Magnesium Trisilicate Mixture 30 ml. In 67 patients in whom plasma-diazepam concentrations were measured Aluminium Hydroxide Mixture appeared to promote early absorption.— S. G. Nair *et al.*, *Br. J. Anaesth.*, 1976, *48*, 1175.

Evidence to suggest that co-administration of diazepam with antacids reduces the rate of absorption of diazepam but does not reduce the extent of absorption.— D. J. Greenblatt *et al.*, *Clin. Pharmac. Ther.*, 1978, *24*, 600.

Anticoagulants. Reduced plasma binding of diazepam and desmethyldiazepam and increases in the free concentrations without changes in the total blood or plasma concentrations occurred immediately following heparin intravenously. Further studies were needed to assess the clinical relevance.— P. A. Routledge *et al.*, *Clin. Pharmac. Ther.*, 1980, *27*, 528.

For the effect of diazepam on phenprocoumon, see Phenprocoumon, p.774.

Atropine and other anticholinergic agents. Injections of atropine 600 µg reduced the absorption of diazepam. The effect of intravenous injection was more pronounced than the effect of intramuscular injection.— J. A. S. Gamble *et al.*, *Br. J. Anaesth.*, 1976, *48*, 1181.

A study in healthy subjects suggesting that the action of diazepam and atropine might be antagonistic rather than mutually enhancing.— P. Holland *et al.*, *Br. J. clin. Pharmac.*, 1978, *5*, 367P.

Cimetidine. A study in 4 healthy subjects indicated that plasma concentrations of diazepam are raised by concomitant administration of cimetidine.— U. Klotz *et al.* (letter), *Lancet*, 1979, *2*, 699. A pharmacokinetic study in 6 healthy subjects confirmed that the disposition of diazepam is altered by cimetidine. Plasma clearance of diazepam was reduced and elimination half-life increased when a single intravenous injection of diazepam was given after treatment with cimetidine for one day; 5 of the 6 subjects experienced pronounced sedation. The elimination half-life of desmethyldiazepam was also prolonged by cimetidine in 2 patients. Patients receiving benzodiazepines in association with cimetidine should be monitored closely.— U. Klotz and I. Reimann, *New Engl. J. Med.*, 1980, *302*, 1012. Comment on the differing metabolism of the benzodiazepines and on the effect of cimetidine on the clearance of benzodiazepines.— R. L. Ruffalo and J. F. Thompson (letter), *ibid.*, *303*, 753. See also U. Klotz and I. Reimann (letter), *ibid.*, 754.

Disulfiram. A study suggesting that concurrent administration of disulfiram inhibits chlordiazepoxide biotransformation. It is thought that diazepam disposition will be similarly affected, but that benzodiazepines metabolised by conjugation, such as oxazepam, may be less susceptible to inhibition of biotransformation.— E. M. Sellers *et al.*, *Clin. Pharmac. Ther.*, 1977, *21*, 117. See also S. M. MacLeod *et al.*, *ibid.*, 1978, *24*, 583.

ECT. Benzodiazepine tranquillisers should not be given to alleviate anxiety in patients about to undergo electroconvulsive therapy as these tranquillisers possess anticonvulsant properties and may seriously modify or abort the induced fit.— *Lancet*, 1977, *2*, 594. No effect on ECT.— R. C. Bowen, *J. clin. Pharmac.*, 1978, *18*, 280.

Lithium. Hypothermia occurred on 4 occasions in a patient treated with lithium carbonate and diazepam, but not when either drug was given alone.— G. J. Naylor and A. McHarg, *Br. med. J.*, 1977, *2*, 22.

Metoclopramide. In groups of 10 or 12 patients, the absorption of a 10-mg oral dose of diazepam was significantly hastened when metoclopramide 10 mg was given intravenously at the same time; absorption was significantly reduced when morphine 10 mg was given intramuscularly 1 hour earlier; pethidine 100 mg intramuscularly 1 hour earlier had a similar, but lesser, effect; absorption was significantly reduced by atropine 600 µg intravenously given at the same time and, to a lesser degree, by atropine 600 µg intramuscularly.— J. A. S. Gamble *et al.*, *Br. J. Anaesth.*, 1976, *48*, 1181.

Further references: J. W. Dundee and J. A. S. Gamble (letter), *Lancet*, 1975, *1*, 1032.

Muscle relaxants. For the effects of diazepam on muscle relaxants, see Gallamine Triethiodide, p.991, and Suxamethonium Chloride, p.997.

Penicillamine. Exacerbation of intravenous diazepam-induced phlebitis by oral penicillamine.— R. D. Brandstetter *et al.*, *Br. med. J.*, 1981, *283*, 525.

Phenytoin and other anticonvulsants. For the effect of diazepam on phenytoin, see Phenytoin Sodium, p.1240. For the effect of concomitant administration of a benzodiazepine and sodium valproate, see Sodium Valproate, p.1257.

Tricyclic antidepressants. In 40 depressed patients treated with tricyclic antidepressants and/or electroconvulsive therapy, the addition of diazepam 20 mg daily was shown to retard the improvement of patients receiving tricyclics, but had no effect on those given electroconvulsive therapy.— R. C. Bowen, *J. clin. Pharmac.*, 1978, *18*, 280. See also under ECT (above).

Tuberculostatics. Prolongation of diazepam half-life by *isoniazid* and marked reduction of diazepam half-life by *rifampicin*.— H. R. Ochs *et al.*, *Clin. Pharmac. Ther.*, 1981, *29*, 671.

Interference with diagnostic tests. Diazepam was found to depress thyroid uptake of iodine-131 in some patients.— R. F. Harvey (letter), *Br. med. J.*, 1967, *2*, 52. In 12 euthyroid patients and 6 patients with thyrotoxicosis the administration of diazepam, 5 mg thrice daily for 4 weeks, did not significantly alter the results of tests of thyroid iodine trapping and binding, but there was an increase in the 1-hour thyroid uptake of ^{131}I in the euthyroid group. No change in concentrations of thyroid stimulating hormone occurred. It was not necessary to withdraw diazepam prior to the investigation of a patient with suspected thyroid disease.— F. Clark *et al.*, *Br. med. J.*, 1971, *1*, 585.

Diazepam was given to 14 patients to control excessive motor activity without masking diagnostic features of the EEG.— J. F. Laguna and J. Korein, *Archs Neurol.*, *Chicago*, 1972, *26*, 265.

A study in 98 female patients suggesting that erroneous results using maximum treadmill exercise electrocardiography tests for the diagnosis of coronary artery disease may occur in patients receiving diazepam.— J. W. Linhart *et al.*, *Circulation*, 1974, *50*, 1173.

See also Chlordiazepoxide, p.1507.

Mountain sickness. A plea that sedatives should not be given at altitude. Since diazepam, and possibly other sedatives blunt the hypoxic ventilatory response, sleep hypoxaemia might be exacerbated.— J. R. Sutton *et al.* (letter), *Lancet*, 1979, *1*, 165.

Myasthenia gravis. The benzodiazepines could make myasthenia worse.— *Drug & Ther. Bull.*, 1977, *15*, 29.

Pregnancy and the neonate. *Diffusion across the placenta.* Diazepam 5 mg labelled with carbon-14 was given intramuscularly to 8 healthy pregnant women about to undergo abortions. The 12- to 16-week-old foetuses were removed at 1, 2, or 6 hours after injection. Concentrations in the cord blood were twice those of the maternal blood. The highest concentrations at 1 hour were: cord blood, 47.5 ng per ml; placenta, 39 ng per g; foetal liver, 31 ng per g; foetal brain, 29 ng per g. Low enzyme activity was detected in the liver which was capable of metabolising about 3% of added diazepam.— J. Idänpään-Heikkilä *et al.*, *Clin. Pharmac. Ther.*, 1971, *12*, 293.

Studies of the concentrations of diazepam and its metabolites (desmethyldiazepam, oxazepam, and its glucuronide) in the plasma of 5 infants whose mothers had received 10 to 15 mg of diazepam daily for 6 to 21 days before delivery indicated that the metabolism and excretion of diazepam in the newborn was subject to wide variation; concentrations might be high enough to be active for 10 days.— J. Kanto *et al.* (letter), *Br. med. J.*, 1974, *1*, 641.

In vitro studies indicated that foetal liver microsomes could metabolise diazepam from the 13th week of gestation, forming desmethyldiazepam and *N*-methyloxazepam. It was suggested that metabolites might accumulate in the foetal liver, as the placenta would be less permeable to them than to diazepam.— E. Ackermann and K. Richter, *Eur. J. clin. Pharmac.*, 1977, *11*, 43.

Further references: J. E. Idänpään-Heikkilä *et al.*, *Am. J. Obstet. Gynec.*, 1971, *109*, 1011; R. W. Shannon *et al.*, *Br. J. clin. Pract.*, 1972, *26*, 271; R. Erkkola *et al.* (letter), *Br. med. J.*, 1974, *3*, 472; M. Mandelli *et al.*, *Clin. Pharmac. Ther.*, 1975, *17*, 564; J. A. S. Gamble *et al.*, *Br. J. Obstet. Gynaec.*, 1977, *84*, 588; K. Haram *et al.*, *Clin. Pharmac. Ther.*, 1978, *24*, 590; K. Haram and O. M. Bakke, *Br. J. Obstet. Gynaec.*, 1980, *87*, 506; C. B. McAllister, *Br. J. Anaesth.*, 1980, *52*, 423; R. L. Nation, *Clin. Pharmacokinet.*, 1980, *5*, 340.

Excretion in breast milk. After 4 days' treatment with diazepam, 10 mg thrice daily given for 6 days to 3 nursing mothers immediately after childbirth, concentrations of 491 ng per ml were found in the mothers' plasma, 51 ng per ml in the milk, and 172 ng per ml in the children's plasma; concentrations of the metabolite, *N*-desmethyldiazepam were 340 ng, 28 ng, and 243 ng per ml respectively. On the 6th day concentrations of diazepam and *N*-desmethyldiazepam had increased in the mothers' plasma to 601 ng and 483 ng per ml and in the milk to 78 ng and 52 ng per ml, but had decreased in the children to 74 ng and 31 ng per ml. Because of possible competition for conjugation causing hyperbilirubinaemia, babies should not be breast fed if the mother was receiving diazepam.— R. Erkkola and J. Kanto (letter), *Lancet*, 1972, *1*, 1235. A similar study. Diazepam 10 mg daily may safely be given to a mother who is breast-feeding, but if large doses are needed breast-feeding should be discontinued.— R. Brandt, *Arzneimittel-Forsch.*, 1976, *26*, 454.

Further references: M. J. Patrick *et al.* (letter), *Lancet*, 1972, *1*, 542; A. P. Cole and D. M. Hailey, *Archs Dis. Childh.*, 1975, *50*, 741; J. T. Wilson *et al.*, *Clin. Pharmacokinet.*, 1980, *5*, 1.

See also under Dependence, Adverse Effects and Treatment, Absorption and Fate, and Uses.

Absorption and Fate. Diazepam is readily and completely absorbed from the gastro-intestinal tract, peak plasma concentrations occurring within about 30 to 90 minutes of oral administration; the rate of absorption is age-related and tends to be delayed in the elderly. Absorption is erratic following intramuscular administration and lower peak plasma concentrations are obtained compared with those following oral administration. Diazepam crosses the blood-brain barrier and is highly lipid soluble; these properties qualify it for intravenous use in short-term anaesthetic procedures, since it acts promptly on the brain, and its initial effects decrease rapidly as it is redistributed into fat depots and tissues.

Diazepam has a biphasic half-life with an initial rapid distribution phase followed by a prolonged terminal elimination phase of 1 or 2 days; its action is further prolonged by the even longer half-life of 2 to 5 days of its principal active metabolite, desmethyldiazepam (nordazepam), the relative proportion of which increases in the body on long-term administration. No simple correlation has been found between plasma concentrations of diazepam and its metabolites, and their therapeutic effect.

Diazepam is extensively metabolised in the liver and, in addition to desmethyldiazepam, its active metabolites include methyloxazepam, oxazepam, and temazepam. It is excreted in the urine, mainly in the form of its metabolites, either free or in conjugated form. There is no biliary excretion. Diazepam is very extensively bound to plasma proteins.

The plasma half-life of diazepam is prolonged in neonates, in the elderly, and in patients with kidney or liver disease; sex differences have also been suggested in the response to diazepam. In addition to crossing the blood-brain barrier, diazepam and its metabolites also cross the placental barrier and are excreted in breast milk.

A detailed account of the clinical pharmacokinetics of diazepam.— M. Mandelli *et al.*, *Clin. Pharmacokinet.*, 1978, *3*, 72.

Further reviews: D. J. Greenblatt *et al.*, *Int. J. clin. Pharmac. Biopharm.*, 1978, *16*, 177.

Absorption and plasma concentrations. In a double-blind study 14 of 29 patients admitted to hospital for acute anxiety were treated with diazepam 20 mg daily for at least 5 days. The minimal effective steady-state plasma concentration was found to be about 400 ng per ml and the degree of diazepam effect was directly proportional to plasma concentrations and reciprocal clearance values of diazepam and its metabolite desmethyldiazepam.— H. H. Dasberg *et al.*, *Clin. Pharmac. Ther.*, 1974, *15*, 473.

Mean peak serum-diazepam concentrations in 6 healthy subjects given diazepam 20 mg intravenously, intramuscularly, and by mouth were 1600, 290, and 490 ng per ml respectively, 15, 60, and 30 minutes after administration. Clinical effects were related to serum concentrations. Significant amounts of the metabolite, desmethyldiazepam, were not produced.— L. Hillestad *et al.*, *Clin. Pharmac. Ther.*, 1974, *16*, 479. Studies in 7 healthy subjects showed cumulation in the serum of diazepam and desmethyldiazepam when diazepam was given daily by mouth for up to 2 weeks. The mean biological half-life of diazepam in 3 subjects was 54 hours.— L. Hillestad *et al.*, *ibid.*, 485.

In 4 subjects given a single 5 mg dose of diazepam, peak plasma concentrations occurred between 0.5 and 1.5 hours after administration and ranged from 64 to 160 ng per ml.— R. C. Bourne *et al.*, *Br. J. Pharmac.*, 1978, *63*, 371P.

In a study of 36 patients who had received diazepam 2 to 30 mg daily for periods from one month to 10 years, plasma-diazepam concentrations were directly related to dose and inversely related to age. Most of the patients were also receiving other drugs. There was a close association between the plasma concentrations of diazepam and its metabolite desmethyldiazepam and both concentrations were independent of the duration of therapy. Plasma-diazepam concentration ranges were 0.02 to 1.01 µg per ml, and plasma-desmethyldiazepam concentration ranges were 0.055 to 1.765 µg per ml.— D. M. Rutherford *et al.*, *Br. J. clin. Pharmac.*, 1978, *6*, 69.

Nine patients requiring artificial ventilation were given diazepam 10 mg intravenously every 4 hours for up to 22 days; their plasma-diazepam concentrations rose over the first 6 days and reached a mean plateau value of 700 ng per ml in 8 to 10 days. The concentration of the metabolite desmethyldiazepam rose progressively throughout administration. Similar results occurred in 3 patients given 5-mg doses, with a mean plateau value of 400 ng per ml. When diazepam was discontinued plasma concentrations fell with a half-life of 2 to 4 days for diazepam and 4 to 8 days for the metabolite.— J. A. S. Gamble *et al.*, *Br. J. Anaesth.*, 1976, *48*, 1087.

Mean plasma concentrations of 170 ng per ml of diazepam and 317 ng per ml of desmethyldiazepam were measured in 19 patients given diazepam in a mean dose of 11 mg daily for 2 to 4 weeks.— A. J. Bond *et al.*, *Br. J. clin. Pharmac.*, 1977, *4*, 51.

Concentrations of diazepam and desmethyldiazepam in the plasma during long-term diazepam therapy.— D. J. Greenblatt *et al.*, *Br. J. clin. Pharmac.*, 1981, *11*, 35.

Further references: J. A. F. de Silva *et al.*, *J. pharm. Sci.*, 1966, *55*, 692; D. E. Schwartz *et al.*, *Arzneimittel-Forsch.*, 1966, *16*, 1109; J. A. S. Gamble *et al.*, *Br. J. Anaesth.*, 1973, *45*, 926 and 1085; G. J. DiGregorio *et al.*, *Clin. Pharmac. Ther.*, 1978, *24*, 720; P. Hunt *et al.*, *J. Pharm. Pharmac.*, 1979, *31*, 448; J. J. de Gier *et al.*, *Br. J. clin. Pharmac.*, 1980, *10*, 151; D. J. Greenblatt *et al.*, *Clin. Pharmac. Ther.*, 1980, *27*, 301; C. Hallstrom *et al.*, *Br. J. clin. Pharmac.*, 1980, *9*, 333; C. A. Naranjo *et al.*, *ibid.*, 265; S. Nakano *et al.*, *Clin. Pharmac. Ther.*, 1980, *27*, 274 and 370.

Biliary excretion. In a study in 4 patients, who had undergone biliary surgery, biliary excretion of diazepam was insufficient to account for an enterohepatic circulation of the drug.— P. W. Eustace *et al.*, *Br. J. Anaesth.*, 1975, *47*, 983.

Further references: U. Klotz *et al.*, *Eur. J. clin. Pharmac.*, 1976, *10*, 121; W. A. Mahon *et al.*, *Clin. Pharmac. Ther.*, 1976, *19*, 443; R. Sellman *et al.*, *Eur. J. clin. Pharmac.*, 1977, *12*, 209.

Metabolism. A study in children and adults of the effect of diazepam dosage on its metabolism and excretion.— J. Kanto *et al.*, *Int. J. clin. Pharmac. Biopharm.*, 1978, *16*, 258.

Further references: J. Besic *et al.*, *Acta pharm. jugosl.*, 1977, *27*, 13.

For a study indicating benzodiazepine metabolism in the small intestine, see Flurazepam, p.802.

Plasma protein binding. A study in which the amount of diazepam estimated as being bound to plasma proteins was 98%.— H. G. Giles (letter), *Br. J. clin. Pharmac.*, 1977, *4*, 711.

Further studies and comments on the plasma protein binding of diazepam and other benzodiazepines.— T. Sjodin *et al.*, *Biochem. Pharmac.*, 1976, *25*, 2131; J. J. Vallner, *J. pharm. Sci.*, 1977, *66*, 447; J. G. Abel *et al.*, *Clin. Pharmac. Ther.*, 1979, *26*, 247; P. A. Routledge *et al.*, *ibid.*, 1980, *27*, 282; P. A. Routledge *et al.*, *Br. J. clin. Pharmac.*, 1981, *11*, 245.

Pregnancy and the neonate. A brief discussion of the metabolism of diazepam in the newborn.— D. R. Cook, *Drugs*, 1976, *12*, 212.

Clinical pharmacokinetics of benzodiazepines in neonates and infants: age-related differences and therapeutic implications.— P. L. Morselli *et al.*, *Clin. Pharmacokinet.*, 1980, *5*, 485.

See also under Dependence, Adverse Effects and Treatment, Precautions, and Uses.

Uses. Diazepam is a benzodiazepine tranquilliser with anticonvulsant, sedative, muscle relaxant, and amnesic properties. It is used in the treatment of anxiety and tension states, as a sedative and premedicant, in the control of muscle spasm, as in tetanus, and in the management of alcohol withdrawal symptoms.

It is of value in patients undergoing orthopaedic procedures, endoscopy, and cardioversion. When given by mouth diazepam may be beneficial in the treatment of some patients with epilepsy and it is the recommended treatment, when given by slow intravenous injection, for the control of status epilepticus. Diazepam is used in dentistry either to calm the patient or it is given parenterally to sedate the patient during the dental procedure.

The usual dose by mouth for mild anxiety states is 2 mg thrice daily increasing in severe states to 15 to 30 mg daily in divided doses. Doses of 5 to 10 mg may be given at night as a hypnotic; higher doses have been used for the induction of sleep, however it has been suggested that the prolonged duration of action of diazepam and its major metabolite, desmethyldiazepam, may qualify it for a 24-hour tranquillising regimen given as a single dose at night. In muscle spasm 2 to 15 mg may be given daily in divided doses increased in severe spastic disorders, such as cerebral palsy, to up to 60 mg daily.

Diazepam may also be given rectally as suppositories in doses similar to those by mouth.

Diazepam is also given by deep intramusuclar or slow intravenous injection; it is advisable to keep the patient in the supine position for at least an hour after administration. Intravenous injection should be carried out slowly at a recommended rate of 1 ml of a 0.5% solution (5 mg) per minute. Solutions for intravenous infusion may be prepared by adding 40 mg of diazepam as a 0.5% solution to not less than 500 ml of sodium chloride injection or dextrose injection; such solutions should be freshly prepared and used within 6 hours. Absorption following intramuscular injection is erratic and provides lower blood concentrations than those following oral administration.

In severe anxiety or acute muscle spasm diazepam 10 mg may be given intramuscularly or intravenously and repeated after 4 hours. Patients with tetanus may be given 100 to 300 µg per kg body-weight intravenously and repeated every 1 to 4 hours; alternatively, a continuous infusion of 3 to 10 mg per kg every 24 hours may be used or similar doses may be given by nasoduodenal tube. Considerably higher doses have also been used for tetanus. In status epilepticus 150 to 250 µg per kg is given by intramuscular or intravenous injection and repeated if required after 30 to 60 minutes. Once the patient is controlled recurrence of seizures may be prevented by a slow infusion (maximum total of 3 mg per kg over 24 hours). Facilities for respiratory assistance must be available. The usual dose in minor surgical procedures and dentistry is 200 µg per kg by injection adjusted to the patient's requirements.

A suggested sedative dose for children is 40 to 200 µg per kg body-weight up to 3 or 4 times daily. Dosage recommendations are not generally given for infants since they may be unable to metabolise diazepam, but a parenteral dose of 40 to 200 µg per kg given once only has been used. A suggested parenteral regimen for children with status epilepticus or severe recurrent seizures is 200 to 300 µg per kg body-weight or 1 mg per year of age; if necessary these doses may be repeated 30 minutes or 1 hour later; they may be followed by intravenous infusion or suppositories if necessary. Facilities for respiratory assistance must be available.

Elderly and debilitated patients should be given one-half the usual adult dose.

The metabolite desmethyldiazepam is also used (see p.1548).

Action. A brief account of *animal* studies on the mode of action of benzodiazepines with special reference to their possible interaction with specific receptor sites in the brain.— L. L. Iversen, *Nature*, 1978, *275*, 477.

Theories of anxiety and benzodiazepine receptors.— *Lancet*, 1981, *2*, 237.

Comment on therapeutic differences between benzodiazepines and their complex interrelationships. Since diazepam, chlordiazepoxide, clorazepate, and medazepam are all metabolised at least in part to desmethyldiazepam, it is hardly surprising that they overlap considerably in pharmacological properties on repeated administration. Very small amounts of temazepam are formed from diazepam; like lorazepam and oxazepam, it has little or no active metabolites.— *Drug & Ther. Bull.*, 1978, *16*, 46.

A review of the choice of treatment for anxiety. Preparations containing an antidepressant and a sedative could not be recommended on pharmacological grounds since the dosage schedule for depression consisted of regular dosage until relief of depression followed by regular maintenance dosage whereas that for anxiety consisted of intermittent dosage, according to symptoms, for as brief a period as possible.— P. Tyrer, *Practitioner*, 1977, *219*, 479. See also J. Prutting (letter), *New Engl. J. Med.*, 1979, *300*, 372. A defence of the combined use of amitriptyline and chlordiazepoxide.— J. Cohen (letter), *ibid.*, 1164.

Further reviews and comments: P. Tyrer, *Adv. Med. Topics Ther.*, 1975, *1*, 242; G. Bignami, *A. Rev. Pharmac. & Toxic.*, 1976, *16*, 329; G. D. Burrows, *Drugs*, 1976, *11*, 209; *Med. Lett.*, 1977, *19*, 49; J. L. Howard and G. T. Pollard, *Drugs Today*, 1978, *14*, 473; E. M. Sellers, *Can. med. Ass. J.*, 1978, *118*, 1533; P. Tyrer, *Br. med. J.*, 1978, *2*, 1008; I. H. McKee (letter), *ibid.*, 1296; C. Gill (letter), *ibid.*; C. Bellantuono *et al.*, *Drugs*, 1980, *19*, 195.

For comment on the use of benzodiazepines in the

management of anxiety, see under Anxiety (below).

Administration. The influence of the route of administration on the clinical action of diazepam.— R. A. E. Assaf *et al.*, *Anaesthesia*, 1975, *30*, 152.

Significantly greater plasma-diazepam concentrations were found when the same dose of diazepam was administered intramuscularly into the buttock by doctors than by nurses. This might have been due to shallow injection into fat by the nurses, with little absorption from the organic solvent.— J. W. Dundee *et al.* (letter), *Lancet*, 1974, *2*, 1461. Comment on the poor, erratic, and incomplete absorption of diazepam and chlordiazepoxide following intramuscular injection.— C. B. Tuttle, *Am. J. Hosp. Pharm.*, 1977, *34*, 965.

Increased serum concentrations of diazepam had been reported when the dose was taken 1 to 3 hours after food. This effect was not associated with an increase in plasma binding or changes in free fatty acid status.— U. Klotz *et al.* (letter), *Br. J. clin. Pharmac.*, 1977, *4*, 85.

The pharmacokinetics of diazepam following multiple-dose oral administration in healthy subjects. Single daily administration of the total daily dose at bedtime may represent a satisfactory dosage regimen.— F. B. Eatman *et al.*, *J. Pharmacokinet. Biopharm.*, 1977, *5*, 481.

In children. Solution of diazepam 1 mg per kg body-weight given rectally to 3 children produced plasma concentrations broadly comparable with those produced by the same dose of the same solution given intramuscularly to a further 3 children.— A. Meberg *et al.*, *Eur. J. clin. Pharmac.*, 1978, *14*, 273. A study indicating that very high blood concentrations of diazepam, comparable to those following intravenous administration, could be obtained in children following rectal instillation of diazepam solution. The blood concentrations tended, however, to be variable.— O. Dulac *et al.*, *J. Pediat.*, 1978, *93*, 1039.

Further references: A. Langslet *et al.*, *Acta paediat. scand.*, 1978, *67*, 699 (neonates).

In the elderly. Comments that benzodiazepines should be used with caution in elderly patients. Increased sensitivity to benzodiazepine derivatives in elderly patients is well documented. This phenomenon is not explained simply by age-related changes in benzodiazepine distribution and clearance, it varies among the different benzodiazepine derivatives, and can be influenced by such factors as the sex of the patient.— D. J. Greenblatt and R. I. Shader (letter), *New Engl. J. Med.*, 1979, *300*, 1054. See also D. J. Greenblatt *et al.*, *Int. J. clin. Pharmac. Biopharm.*, 1978, *16*, 177.

Further references: U. Klotz *et al.*, *J. clin. Invest.*, 1975, *55*, 347; C. Salzman *et al.*, *J. Am. Geriat. Soc.*, 1975, *23*, 451 (use in elderly males); U. Klotz *et al.*, *Arzneimittel-Forsch.*, 1976, *26*, 1265 (increased elimination half-life in the elderly); M. M. Reidenberg *et al.*, *Clin. Pharmac. Ther.*, 1978, *23*, 371 (increased sensitivity in the elderly); R. F. Johnson *et al.*, *J. pharm. Sci.*, 1979, *68*, 1320 (similar plasma-protein binding in the elderly); S. M. MacLeod *et al.*, *J. clin. Pharmac.*, 1979, *19*, 15 (study of age and gender-related differences).

Administration in hepatic failure. A study in 17 patients with chronic liver disease indicated that they required doses of diazepam about one-third lower than healthy subjects for premedication.— R. A. Branch *et al.*, *Gut*, 1976, *17*, 975. Comment.— *Br. med. J.*, 1977, *1*, 1241.

A study of the disposition of diazepam and its major metabolite desmethyldiazepam in 9 patients with cirrhosis, 5 with hepatic fibrosis and 1 with chronic hepatitis indicated that at least 2 steps in the metabolism of diazepam are impaired in patients with liver disease. The last step in the metabolism (glucuronidation of oxazepam) appeared to be unchanged since H.J. Shull *et al.*(*Ann. intern. Med.*, 1976, *84*, 420) had reported a normal disposition of oxazepam in patients with viral hepatitis and cirrhosis.— U. Klotz *et al.*, *Clin. Pharmac. Ther.*, 1977, *21*, 430.

Further references: I. M. Murray-Lyon *et al.*, *Br. med. J.*, 1971, *4*, 265; U. Klotz *et al.*, *J. clin. Invest.*, 1975, *55*, 347; P. B. Andreasen *et al.*, *Eur. J. clin. Pharmac.*, 1976, *10*, 115; J. B. McConnell *et al.*, *Gut*, 1977, *18*, A988.

Administration in renal failure. Diazepam could be given in usual doses to patients with renal failure. Concentrations of diazepam were not affected by haemodialysis.— W. M. Bennett *et al.*, *Ann. intern. Med.*, 1977, *86*, 754. See also *idem*, 1980, *93*, 286.

Further references: L. Kangas *et al.*, *Clin. Nephrol.*, 1976, *5*, 114 (protein binding in renal failure); H. R. Ochs *et al.*, *Br. J. clin. Pharmac.*, 1981, *12*, 829 (kinetics in renal insufficiency or hyperthyroidism).

Administration in respiratory insufficiency. A study in 8 healthy subjects indicated significantly depressed ventilatory response 15 and 30 minutes after intramuscular injection of diazepam 10 mg; a tendency to return towards control values at 60 minutes might be attributable to acute tolerance. In situations where diazepam is administered and hypoxia might be anticipated supplementary oxygen might be advisable. No significant effect was noted on hypercapnic ventilatory response after 70 to 130 minutes possibly owing to the time that had elapsed.— S. Lakshminarayan *et al.*, *Clin. Pharmac. Ther.*, 1976, *20*, 178.

A discussion on the effects of diazepam on ventilatory function, and its use for the symptomatic relief of breathlessness in the 'pink and puffing' type of patient with chronic bronchitis and emphysema, who unlike the 'blue and bloated' type, often keep their arterial blood gases near normal for many years. In view of the hazards to patients with carbon dioxide retention, diazepam should not be prescribed for the breathless patient with chronic bronchitis and emphysema, without a preliminary check on the arterial blood gases.— *Lancet*, 1980, *2*, 242.

Further references: M. K. Tandon, *Aust. N.Z. J. Med.*, 1976, *6*, 561; A. A. Woodcock *et al.*, *Br. med. J.*, 1981, *283*, 343.

Alcohol and drug withdrawal. *Alcohol.* A report of the management of the alcohol withdrawal syndrome including the use of diazepam in 3463 patients.— T. R. Marvin, *Minn. Med.*, 1970, *53*, 999. See also W. F. Spenader and B. V. Schwamberger, *Illinois med. J.*, 1971, *140*, 508.

Severe delirium tremens in 34 patients was treated with diazepam or paraldehyde. Half received diazepam 10 mg intravenously initially, then 5 mg every 5 minutes to induce a calm state which was maintained by intramuscular injections of 5 to 10 mg every 1 to 4 hours. The other 17 patients received paraldehyde 10 ml rectally in 20 ml cottonseed oil every 30 minutes followed by rectal maintenance doses of 5 or 10 ml every 2 to 4 hours. Requirements were very variable with induction dosage ranging from 15 to 215 mg diazepam or 10 to 175 ml paraldehyde. Patients with complications (pneumonia, pancreatitis, hepatitis) required twice the dose needed to induce calm in patients with delirium tremens alone. Those given diazepam were calmed in less than half the time needed with paraldehyde. Mean duration of delirium tremens was 56 hours. Serious adverse reactions, including 2 deaths, occurred in 9 of 17 patients treated with paraldehyde; there was none with diazepam.— W. L. Thompson *et al.*, *Ann. intern. Med.*, 1975, *82*, 175. Comments and criticisms.— L. W. Gray (letter), *ibid.*, 852; W. L. Thompson and W. C. Maddrey (letter), *ibid.*; M. C. Ruddy (letter), *ibid.*, *83*, 279; W. L. Thompson and W. C. Maddrey (letter), *ibid.*

Narcotic analgesics. Diazepam given to 85 adolescents dependent on diamorphine reduced the duration and severity of physiological withdrawal symptoms.— I. F. Litt *et al.*, *J. Pediat.*, 1971, *78*, 692. Diazepam was only moderately effective in reducing the withdrawal symptoms in patients dependent on methadone.— P. E. Rubin *et al.*, *Drug Intell. & clin. Pharm.*, 1973, *7*, 129.

Diazepam 1 to 2 mg was given intramuscularly every 8 hours to infants born to diamorphine-dependent mothers. Neonatal withdrawal symptoms were controlled within 24 to 72 hours when diazepam was gradually withdrawn.— G. Nathenson *et al.*, *Pediatrics*, 1971, *48*, 523.

Anaesthesia. A favourable review of the use of diazepam for minor procedures such as bronchoscopy, gastro-intestinal endoscopy, angiography, cardioversion, and some forms of dental treatment. Dose requirements usually lie between 10 to 40 mg and the margin between sedation and general anaesthesia is very narrow. Although it has a good safety record, respiratory depression may follow intravenous use, especially in debilitated patients and those with hypoxaemia, therefore resuscitation facilities should be at hand. Diazepam has a long duration of action and out-patients should be escorted home after the procedure, and warned not to drive or drink alcohol during the ensuing day; doses greater than 25 mg should not be given to out-patients. Because of its anti-analgesic properties it should not be given alone for painful procedures and when a procedure is likely to be painful adequate doses of an analgesic must be given before giving diazepam.— *Drug & Ther. Bull.*, 1976, *14*, 19. The limitations of sedatives for sedation and analgesia for minor painful procedures.— *Med. Lett.*, 1977, *19*, 26. In a comparative study involving 316 consecutive patients requiring endoscopy, 98 were randomly allocated to no preparation, 93 to throat analgesia with 10% lignocaine, and 125 were given diazepam 10 mg. Acceptability scores were highest in those given no preparation; those given local anaesthesia had a longer introduction time. It is concluded that proper instruction and a personal approach in the endoscopy room remain the best preparation for upper gastrointestinal endoscopy and that sedation is not usually beneficial.— G. F. Nelis (letter), *Lancet*, 1980, *2*, 861. The fact that some patients describe the discomfort of endoscopy as intolerable means that the procedure should not be attempted 'in cold blood'.— *Lancet*, 1980, *2*, 1064.

A detailed account of the pharmacokinetics of diazepam used for intravenous anaesthesia.— M. M. Ghoneim and K. Korttila, *Clin. Pharmacokinet.*, 1977, *2*, 344.

Further reviews: *Drug & Ther. Bull.*, 1979, *17*, 19.

Reports and studies on the use of diazepam in general anaesthesia: H. N. Konchigeri, *Clin. Pharmac. Ther.*, 1977, *21*, 108 (cardiac surgery); S. P. Kothary and E. K. Zsigmond, *ibid* (with ketamine); A. P. F. Jackson *et al.*, *Br. J. Anaesth.*, 1978, *50*, 375 (with ketamine).

Reports and studies on the use of diazepam in diazanalgesia (a benzodiazepine associated with a powerful narcotic): J. Vernhiet *et al.*, *Br. J. Anaesth.*, 1978, *50*, 165 (with fentanyl).

Anaesthetic premedication. In a study in 240 patients, premedication with a combination of droperidol 2.5 mg with diazepam 5 mg produced better relief of anxiety, sedation, amnesia, and acceptance by patient and physician than either droperidol 10 mg or diazepam 10 mg alone. Larger doses of droperidol with diazepam increased the frequency of anxiety and larger doses of diazepam with droperidol might increase sedation.— G. P. Herr *et al.*, *Br. J. Anaesth.*, 1979, *51*, 537.

Pethidine 1 mg per kg body-weight, diazepam 250 µg per kg, and flunitrazepam 20 µg per kg intramuscularly were compared as premedicants in a double-blind study in 145 children, aged up to 15 years, undergoing otolaryngological surgery. All drugs were anxiolytic in the children 5 years and older, but diazepam was less effective in children under 5 years.— L. Lindgren *et al.*, *Br. J. Anaesth.*, 1979, *51*, 321.

In a double-blind crossover study in 18 healthy subjects, diazepam 70 or 140 µg per kg body-weight (a total dose of about 5 or 10 mg) given intravenously had no effect on lower oesophageal sphincter pressure; after 280 µg per kg pressure was increased. Diazepam does not therefore appear to increase the risk of regurgitation and pulmonary aspiration when used pre- or postoperatively.— T. R. Weihrauch *et al.*, *Gut*, 1979, *20*, 64.

Further references: W. H. Forrest *et al.*, *Anesthesiology*, 1977, *47*, 241; R. H. Wender *et al.*, *Br. J. Anaesth.*, 1977, *49*, 907; T. Goroszeniuk *et al.*, *Br. med. J.*, 1980, *281*, 486; L. Lindgren *et al.*, *Br. J. Anaesth.*, 1980, *52*, 283.

For earlier reports on diazepam for premedication, see Martindale 27th Edn, p. 1534.

Cardiac catheterisation. An intravenous infusion of diazepam (27 µg per kg body-weight per minute for 15 minutes) to 7 patients undergoing cardiac catheterisation produced a decrease in systemic and pulmonary arterial pressures; effects on cardiac output, vascular resistance, and oxygen consumption were variable.— G. D'Amelio *et al.*, *Eur. J. clin. Pharmac.*, 1973, *6*, 61. See also W. Markiewicz *et al.*, *J. clin. Pharmac.*, 1976, *16*, 637.

Further references: J. E. Dalen *et al.*, *Anesthesiology*, 1969, *30*, 259; T. E. J. Healy, *Anaesthesia*, 1969, *24*, 537.

Cardioversion. Three groups, each of 50 patients, were given anaesthetics prior to DC cardioversion; the agents used were: diazapam in a mean dose of 320 µg per kg body-weight, thiopentone 3.7 mg per kg, and propanidid 4.6 mg per kg. Diazepam had minimal effects on blood pressure and might be of value in patients with cardiac disease; apnoea was infrequent but amnesia was poor. Thiopentone caused a transient fall in blood pressure; periods of apnoea exceeding 30 seconds occurred in 25 patients; thiopentone was preferable to diazepam in patients in good physical condition. Propanidid caused greater hypotension which was unlikely to be dangerous but this and a high incidence of excitation rendered it less suitable.— R. Orko, *Br. J. Anaesth.*, 1976, *48*, 257.

Dentistry. Diazepam 120 to 320 µg per kg body-weight, in doses up to 20 mg, was given intravenously in solutions containing 5 mg per ml at the rate of 1 ml per minute and induced suitable sedation prior to local analgesia in 105 patients undergoing dental treatment. Cavity preparation time was decreased in these patients but post-operative recovery was slow.— R. A. Dixon *et al.*, *Br. J. Anaesth.*, 1973, *45*, 202.

Further references: G. D. Allen *et al.*, *J. Am. dent. Ass.*, 1976, *92*, 744; R. A. Dixon *et al.*, *Br. J. Anaesth.*, 1980, *52*, 517.

For earlier reports on the use of diazepam in dentistry, see Martindale 27th Edn, p. 1535.

Endoscopy. When given with atropine for premedication, diazepam was as effective as morphine for endoscopy.

The only significant difference in response was that the conscious level was lower in those given diazepam.— R. Ludlam and J. R. Bennett, *Lancet*, 1971, *2*, 1397.

In 100 patients undergoing cystoscopy and related procedures good operating conditions were achieved in 45 by premedication with diazepam 10 mg by mouth 2 hours before surgery and induction of anaesthesia with pentazocine 1 mg per kg body-weight and diazepam 20 to 40 mg intravenously; 34 patients required supplements of nitrous oxide, and 21 required nitrous oxide and alphadolone with alphaxalone.— T. G. C. Smith *et al.*, *Br. J. Anaesth.*, 1977, *49*, 509.

Further references: C. E. Blackard *et al.*, *Minn. Med.*, 1970, *53*, 11; B. S. Millman and L. D. Bridenbaugh, *Bull. Mason Clin.*, 1971, *25*, 89; P. Brown *et al.* (letter), *Lancet*, 1972, *1*, 270; S. Rao *et al.*, *Clin. Pharmac. Ther.*, 1972, *13*, 150; A. W. Duncan and A. M. Barr, *Br. J. Anaesth.*, 1973, *45*, 1150; P. Metz and J. O. Halveg, *Anaesthesia*, 1974, *29*, 92; P. J. Cook *et al.*, *Gut*, 1974, *15*, 842; H. P. Sherr and A. E. Cocco, *Am. J. med. Sci.*, 1974, *267*, 151; H. I. Le Brun, *Gut*, 1976, *17*, 655; C. Birt *et al.*, *Gut*, 1977, *18*, A940; H. G. Giles *et al.*, *Can. med. Ass. J.*, 1978, *118*, 513.

Gynaecology. Diazepam, 10 mg given by intravenous injection 5 minutes before the intravenous injection of pethidine and promethazine, allowed minor gynaecological operations to be performed under excellent conditions in 1132 out of 1200 patients aged 16 to 78 years. No adverse reactions or complications were reported and patients slept for 4 to 5 hours.— J. A. Goldman *et al.*, *Br. J. Anaesth.*, 1972, *44*, 381.

Labour. In a small study in multiparous women diazepam 300 µg per kg body-weight intramuscularly did not reduce the requirement for pethidine during labour but was considered to have improved the quality of pain relief without affecting the neonate. A dose of 200 µg per kg had no effect on pain relief.— J. M. Davies and M. Rosen, *Br. J. Anaesth.*, 1977, *49*, 601.

Further references: C. H. de Boer and S. S. Chau (letter), *Lancet*, 1967, *2*, 1256; E. A. Friedman *et al.*, *Obstet. Gynec.*, 1969, *34*, 82.

Analgesia. Diazepam 10 mg per 60 kg body-weight, had no significant effect on the sensitivity to tibial pressure pain of 5 patients as measured by algesimetry.— J. D. Morrison, *Br. J. Anaesth.*, 1970, *42*, 838.

Diazepam had a variable effect on pain threshold.— G. M. Hall *et al.*, *Br. J. Anaesth.*, 1974, *46*, 50.

Anxiety. Comment on the use of psychotropic drugs to alleviate stress, with particular reference to the nationwide survey in the USA by G.D. Mellinger *et al.* (*Archs gen. Psychiat.*, 1978, *35*, 1045). Among other findings it appears that men with high levels of distress tend to increase their alcohol consumption rather than take drugs, whereas the opposite trend was evident in women. It is not known whether patients with psychic distress turn to alcohol if denied drugs, therefore caution should be exercised in exhorting doctors to cut down their prescribing of psychotropic drugs, since the problems of alcohol abuse are far greater.— *Lancet*, 1978, *2*, 1347.

With a reasoned approach to treatment, acute and chronic anxiety can be diminished by medications, particularly the benzodiazepines. Patients should expect that treatment will be of limited duration and will diminish but not eradicate the disorder. For situational or phobic anxiety, occasional use is indicated. For persistent symptoms, the use of anxiolytics for periods of exacerbation may be effective, although patients often report sustained improvement with maintenance treatment.— J. F. Rosenbaum, *New Engl. J. Med.*, 1982, *306*, 401.

Studies and reports on the use of diazepam in anxiety: G. R. Sprogis, *Curr. ther. Res.*, 1966, *8*, 490; A. McDowall *et al.*, *Br. J. Psychiat.*, 1966, *112*, 629; N. S. Capstick *et al.*, *Br. J. Psychiat.*, 1965, *111*, 517; G. Dhanani (letter), *Br. med. J.*, 1972, *2*, 587; D. Kelly *et al.*, *Br. J. Psychiat.*, 1973, *122*, 419; M. B. Weber, *Curr. ther. Res.*, 1973, *15*, 210 (anxiety and tension headache); H. H. Dasberg *et al.*, *Clin. Pharmac. Ther.*, 1974, *15*, 473; G. Krishnan, *Curr. med. Res. Opinion*, 1976, *4*, 241; L. Lasagna, *Am. J. Psychiat.*, 1977, *134*, 656; K. Rickels, *Clin. Ther.*, 1977, *1*, 106; H. Ashton *et al.*, *Br. J. clin. Pharmac.*, 1978, *5*, 141; A. Villalobos, *Curr. ther. Res.*, 1978, *23*, 243; L. F. Fabre *et al.*, *J. int. med. Res.*, 1979, *7*, 147; C. Z. Tansella *et al.*, *Br. J. clin. Pharmac.*, 1979, *7*, 605.

Phobias. The effect of diazepam on the psychotherapy of phobias was studied in 17 patients who were treated in a controlled manner, either 1 hour after taking diazepam 100 µg per kg body-weight or placebo or 4 hours after diazepam or placebo. All the patients improved when exposed to their phobias, improvement being significantly greater in those given diazepam.— I. M. Marks *et al.*, *Br. J. Psychiat.*, 1972, *121*, 493. The addition of diazepam to the flooding technique for the treatment of agoraphobia was considered beneficial in 4 patients.— D. Johnston and D. Gath, *ibid.*, 1973, *123*, 463.

A study in agoraphobic patients indicated that diazepam is a mild palliative during group exposure in that it reduces tension but does not affect the overall response to treatment.— J. Hafner and I. Marks, *Psychol. Med.*, 1976, *6*, 71.

In children with acute and situational anxiety, as in school phobia, anxiolytics may well impair function in between the acute, but short-lived stress periods, and are probably therefore to be avoided.— J. S. Werry, *Drugs*, 1979, *18*, 392.

Further references: W. O. McCormick, *Can. psychiat. Ass. J.*, 1973, *18*, 33; *Br. med. J.*, 1974, *4*, 63 and 177.

Cardiac disorders. *Myocardial infarction.* Administration of diazepam 10 mg intravenously followed an hour later by 15 mg by mouth this dose being repeated every 8 hours for 3 days, produced safe, pleasant sedation in patients with myocardial infarction, and reduced the need for analgesics. Catecholamine excretion was reduced, suggesting that diazepam causes a lower stress reaction.— M. Melsom *et al.*, *Br. Heart J.*, 1976, *38*, 804.

Further references: A. Formanek *et al.*, *Radiology*, 1976, *121*, 541; R. A. Dixon *et al.*, *Br. Heart J.*, 1980, *43*, 535; B. W. Johansson, *Acta med. scand.*, 1980, *207*, 47.

Convulsions. Diazepam is the recommended treatment for controlling status epilepticus. An immediate dose of 10 mg is usually given intravenously followed if required by a further 20 mg. Once the fits are controlled an infusion of 5 mg of diazepam is usually given hourly until all signs of cerebral abnormality have subsided.— *Br. med. J.*, 1974, *3*, 737. See also *Med. Lett.*, 1979, *21*, 25.

Further reviews of the use of diazepam and other benzodiazepines in status epilepticus and epilepsy: *Drug & Ther. Bull.*, 1971, *9*, 87; M. J. Eadie and J. H. Tyrer, *Anticonvulsant Therapy*, Edinburgh, Churchill Livingstone, 1974; *Drug & Ther. Bull.*, 1976, *14*, 89.

Febrile convulsions. A review of febrile convulsions. Intravenous diazepam is the drug of choice to control febrile convulsions, but phenytoin or paraldehyde can be given if the attacks continue despite intravenous diazepam.— *Drug & Ther. Bull.*, 1978, *16*, 97.

The long-term management of children with fever-associated seizures.—Summary of an NIH Consensus Statement, *Br. med. J.*, 1980, *281*, 277.

Further reviews and comments: *Lancet*, 1979, *1*, 139.

Following their first febrile convulsive episode 83 children were given diazepam as a 5-mg suppository every 8 hours when the rectal temperature was above 38.5° and 73 children were given phenobarbitone about 3.5 mg per kg body-weight daily. During the year of treatment the incidence of new febrile convulsions in both groups were about 15%, indicating that intermittent administration of diazepam during febrile episodes only was as effective as continuous long-term phenobarbitone treatment.— F. U. Knudsen and S. Vestermark, *Archs Dis. Childh.*, 1978, *53*, 660. After finding that most mothers can diagnose their children as unwell at least 6 hours before the actual fever occurs, a policy of intermittent diazepam therapy has now been implemented. Diazepam is immediately administered in doses of 600 to 800 µg per kg body-weight daily (in 3 divided doses) at the first sign of impending illness, and continued for 2 to 3 days after complete recovery. This regimen is maintained until 5 years of age. All those concerned with the child are instructed in the correct procedure and constant availability of the drug is ensured.— G. Dianese (letter), *ibid.*, 1979, *54*, 244.

Further references: R. Calderon-Gonzalez and A. Mireles-Gonzalez, *J. Am. med. Ass.*, 1968, *204*, 544; F. U. Knudsen, *Acta paediat. scand.*, 1977, *66*, 563; F. U. Knudsen, *Archs Dis. Childh.*, 1979, *54*, 855; J. Lorber and R. Sunderland (letter), *Lancet*, 1980, *2*, 1080.

Depression. A review of the literature on benzodiazepines in depressive disorders. Twenty double-blind controlled studies were inspected in which a benzodiazepine was compared with a tricyclic or a monoamine-oxidase inhibitor, sometimes with a placebo in addition. Benzodiazepines did not appear to be effective in combating symptoms of endogenous depression, although they appeared to combat some of the symptoms of non-endogenous depressive disorders, including depressed mood. Thus, they are not 'classic' antidepressants, but can elevate the depressed mood that occurs secondary to anxiety.— A. F. Schatzberg and J. O. Cole, *Archs gen. Psychiat.*, 1978, *35*, 1359. See also *Med. Lett.*, 1978, *20*, 49; C. Ballantuono *et al.*, *Drugs*, 1980, *19*, 195.

A study of patients seeking marital and sexual counselling revealed that those with depression had more often been inappropriately prescribed diazepam and similar drugs than antidepressants. This is a matter for concern since depression can result in suicide.— E. L. Gullick and L. J. King, *J. Affect. Dis.*, 1979, *1*, 55.

Epilepsy. See Convulsions (above).

Extrapyramidal effects. Diazepam 10 mg given by intravenous injection alleviated the dystonic reactions to fluphenazine enanthate and haloperidol.— A. D. Korczyn and G. J. Goldberg, *Br. J. Psychiat.*, 1972, *121*, 75.

Short-term improvement in a chronic movement disorder was noted in a patient given diazepam 5 mg by intravenous injection. Further treatment with diazepam given by mouth had no beneficial effect.— W. Heffron and M. P. McQuillen (letter), *Br. J. Psychiat.*, 1973, *122*, 122.

Diazepam 5 mg thrice daily was administered to 13 patients with phenothiazine-induced akathisia which had not responded to diphenhydramine hydrochloride 25 mg thrice daily. The akathisia was reduced or abolished in 10 of the 13 patients within 3 days. Diazepam was withdrawn from the other 3 patients because of drowsiness.— P. T. Donlon, *Psychosomatics*, 1973, *14*, 222.

Intravenous administration of diazepam 5 to 7.5 mg immediately controlled drug-induced extrapyramidal symptoms in 7 children; satisfactory but slower results were obtained in 2 children given diazepam by mouth.— C. R. Rainier-Pope, *S.Afr. med. J.*, 1979, *55*, 328. See also J. M. Darmady, *Archs Dis. Childh.*, 1974, *49*, 328.

Hiccup. Hiccups worsened in 3 patients when given diazepam 10 or 20 mg intravenously. When it was found that the patients had a history of convulsions standard anticonvulsant therapy was instituted in 2 of the patients and the hiccups were controlled.— R. G. Fariello and R. Mutani (letter), *Lancet*, 1974, *2*, 1201.

Hypertension. There are no well-controlled trials demonstrating that diazepam or any other sedative drug is of benefit in the treatment of hypertension or as an adjunct to the treatment of hypertension.— *Med. Lett.*, 1974, *16*, 96.

Hypnotic effect. Studies in 6 healthy male subjects on the immediate and residual effects of diazepam and its metabolites on performance concluded that diazepam 5 to 10 mg, temazepam 10 to 20 mg, or oxazepam 15 to 30 mg could be appropriate for occasional use as hypnotics when impaired performance the next day must be avoided. Because of its long-acting metabolite, desmethyldiazepam, doses of diazepam should not be repeated more frequently than every 48 hours when performance is important.— C. H. Clarke and A. N. Nicholson, *Br. J. clin. Pharmac.*, 1978, *6*, 325.

Further references: A. N. Nicholson *et al.*, *Br. J. clin. Pharmac.*, 1976, *3*, 533; A. N. Nicholson and B. M. Stone, *Br. J. clin. Pharmac.*, 1979, *7*, 463.

Muscular and rheumatic disorders. In a double-blind crossover study in 24 patients with rheumatoid arthritis, 1 week's treatment with diazepam 5 mg thrice daily in addition to standard anti-inflammatory therapy was no more effective in relief of pain or other symptoms than placebo. Seven patients failed to complete the study.— J. D. Vince and D. Kremer, *Practitioner*, 1973, *210*, 264. Reduced morning stiffness on addition of diazepam to indomethacin at night.— D. Hobkirk *et al.*, *Rheumatol. Rehabil.*, 1977, *16*, 125.

For the use of diazepam to prevent suxamethonium-induced muscle pain, see Suxamethonium Chloride, p.997.

See also Spasticity (below).

Pregnancy and the neonate. See also under Dependence, Adverse Effects and Treatment, Precautions, and Absorption and Fate.

Eclampsia. A brief discussion of the use of diazepam in pre-eclampsia and eclampsia.— B. M. Hibbard and M. Rosen, *Br. J. Anaesth.*, 1977, *49*, 3.

Sixteen women with eclampsia were treated with diazepam; all had convulsions and were unconscious. Convulsions ceased within 30 minutes in 13 patients and in all within 4 hours. There was one maternal death but no other maternal complications. Two mothers had been delivered before admission; there were 2 stillbirths (1 macerated) and 12 live births (by caesarean section if not delivered within 12 hours). Of the 12 live births 11 had Apgar scores of 7 to 8. Diazepam 40 mg was given intravenously followed by an infusion of 40 mg in 540 ml of 5% dextrose at a rate of 30 to 40 drops per minute, increased if necessary; 20 to 40 mg was given intravenously every 4 to 6 hours for 24 hours after delivery, followed by 10 mg by mouth every 6 hours for a week.— P. Kawathekar *et al.*, *Curr. ther. Res.*, 1973,

15, 845.

Criticism of low-dose long-term use of diazepam in mild pre-eclampsia. Not only is enough known about the harmful effects of benzodiazepines on the foetus to contra-indicate their use in this context, but there is no rationale for their use in the first place. It is irrational to assume that because diazepam is a useful anticonvulsant, in fulminating pre-eclampsia and eclampsia, that smaller, tranquillising, doses might be useful in pre-eclampsia. Moreover, doses of diazepam far in excess of a reasonable anticonvulsant dose are often prescribed in fulminating pre-eclampsia, presumably in the false belief that diazepam is an antihypertensive agent.— A. N. P. Speight (letter), *Br. med. J.*, 1978, *1*, 1420.

Labour. For the use of diazepam during labour, see Anaesthesia (above).

Neonatal drug withdrawal. For the administration of diazepam to infants born to diamorphine-dependent mothers see Alcohol and Drug Withdrawal (above).

Tetanus neonatorum. For the use of diazepam in neonatal tetanus, see Tetanus (below).

Raised intracranial pressure. A study indicating that diazepam is suitable both as an induction anaesthetic and as a post-operative sedative in patients with head injuries, without danger of increasing cerebral blood flow and consequently raising intracranial pressure.— S. Cotev and M. Shalit, *Anesthesiology*, 1975, *43*, 117.

Schizophrenia. In at least 25 schizophrenic patients, diazepam 5 mg thrice daily greatly relieved auditory hallucinations which were uncontrolled by phenothiazines alone or in conjunction with antidepressants.— B. M. Irvine and F. Schaechter (letter), *Med. J. Aust.*, 1969, *1*, 1387.

Diazepam had a beneficial effect in schizophrenic patients, possibly due to a γ-aminobutyric-acid-mimetic action.— M. Trabucchi and G. Ba (letter), *Lancet*, 1975, *2*, 868.

Spasticity. A review on diazepam in the treatment of spasticity. Diazepam is useful alone or as adjunct therapy for spasticity, especially in patients with lesions affecting the spinal cord and occasionally in patients with cerebral palsy.— R. R. Young and P. J. Delwaide, *New Engl. J. Med.*, 1981, *304*, 96.

Spasmodic torticollis. Spasmodic torticollis in 2 patients responded promptly to the intravenous injection of diazepam 5 to 10 mg.— S. Ahmad and M. K. Meeran (letter), *Br. med. J.*, 1979, *1*, 127.

Tetanus. Eight children with tetanus recovered when given diazepam 9 mg per kg body-weight daily in addition to standard treatment.— G. Gedioğlu *et al.* (letter), *Lancet*, 1973, *2*, 454.

Five patients with severe tetanus were treated with diazepam and phenobarbitone. Large doses of diazepam were used, at times 480 mg daily, and all 5 patients became comatose for periods of 13 to 21 days. Treatment continued during the coma. All 5 patients recovered. Prolonged coma was considered to be a side effect of diazepam rather than a toxic effect and should not contra-indicate its use in the management of tetanus.— K. A. Odusote *et al.*, *Trop. geogr. Med.*, 1976, *28*, 194.

High-dose diazepam as a continuous intravenous infusion of 20 to 40 mg per kg body-weight daily and intragastric phenobarbitone 10 to 15 mg per kg daily in 4 divided doses were given to 19 neonates with tetanus; 7 infants also required intermittent positive-pressure ventilation, of whom 2 died. The main side-effects were severe drowsiness, coma, and apnoeic episodes which were reversed by reduction of diazepam dosage. At follow-up 2 of the 17 survivors were mentally retarded, probably due to cerebral hypoxia during severe tetanic spasms.— B. H. Khoo *et al.*, *Archs Dis. Childh.*, 1978, *53*, 737. A further study of the use of diazepam in the treatment of 10 infants with tetanus neonatorum.— S. Singhi and P. Singhi (letter), *Archs Dis. Childh.*, 1979, *54*, 650. Comment.— B. H. Khoo *et al.* (letter), *ibid.*, 651.

Further references: R. G. Hendrickse and P. M. Sherman, *Br. med. J.*, 1966, *2*, 860; D. Femi-Pearse, *ibid.*, 862; A. T. Phatak and S. H. Shah, *Clin. Pediat.*, 1970, *9*, 573; M. J. Kendall and S. W. Clarke, *Br. med. J.*, 1972, *1*, 354; J. Thomas *et al.*, *Bull. Soc. Path. exot.*, 1972, *65*, 373; K. F. Tempero, *Am. J. med. Sci.*, 1973, *266*, 4; N. T. Vassa *et al.*, *Postgrad. med. J.*, 1974, *50*, 755; P. M. Smythe *et al.*, *Br. med. J.*, 1974, *1*, 223; A. Joseph and B. M. Pulimood, *Indian J. med. Res.*, 1978, *68*, 489.

Tremor. A brief review of the use of drugs, including diazepam, in essential tremor.— *Drug & Ther. Bull.*, 1974, *12*, 85.

A study involving 12 patients with essential tremor in which diazepam was found not to be significantly better than placebo.— T. J. Murray, *Can. med. Ass. J.*, 1976, *115*, 892.

Vertigo. A brief note on the use of chlordiazepoxide, diazepam, and some phenothiazines in the treatment of dizziness.— J. S. Turner, *Drugs*, 1977, *13*, 382. See also W. P. R. Gibson, *Practitioner*, 1978, *221*, 718.

Preparations

Diazepam Capsules *(B.P.)*. Capsules containing diazepam. Store at a temperature not exceeding 30°. Protect from light.

Diazepam Injection *(B.P.)*. A sterile solution of diazepam in Water for Injections or other suitable solvent. Sterilised by filtration. pH 6.2 to 7. Protect from light.

Diazepam Injection *(U.S.P.)*. A sterile solution in a suitable vehicle. pH 6.2 to 6.9. Protect from light.

Diazepam Tablets *(B.P.)*. Tablets containing diazepam. Protect from light.

Diazepam Tablets *(U.S.P.)*. Tablets containing diazepam. The *U.S.P.* requires 85% dissolution in 30 minutes. Store in airtight containers. Protect from light.

Proprietary Preparations

Atensine *(Berk Pharmaceuticals, UK)*. Diazepam, available as scored tablets of 2, 5, and 10 mg.

Diazemuls *(KabiVitrum, UK)*. Diazepam, available as 2-ml ampoules of an injection containing 5 mg per ml, dissolved in the lipid phase of an oil-in-water emulsion based on fractionated soya oil. For intravenous injection; may be diluted with dextrose infusions or Intralipid. (Also available as Diazemuls in *Norw.*).

Evacalm *(Unimed, UK)*. Diazepam, available as tablets of 2 and 5 mg.

Solis *(Galen, UK)*. Diazepam, available as capsules of 2 and 5 mg.

Tensium *(DDSA Pharmaceuticals, UK)*. Diazepam, available as tablets of 2, 5, and 10 mg.

Valium *(Roche, UK)*. Diazepam, available in 2-ml and 4-ml **Ampoules** of an injection containing 5 mg per ml; as **Capsules** of 2 and 5 mg; as **Suppositories** each containing 5 or 10 mg; as sugar-free **Syrup** containing 2 mg in each 5 ml (suggested diluent, syrup or sorbitol solution); and as scored **Tablets** of 2, 5, and 10 mg. (Also available as Valium in *Arg.*, *Austral.*, *Belg.*, *Canad.*, *Denm.*, *Fr.*, *Ger.*, *Ital.*, *Neth.*, *Norw.*, *S.Afr.*, *Spain*, *Switz.*, *USA*).

Valrelease *(Roche, UK)*. Diazepam, available as sustained-release capsules of 10 mg. Anxiolytic. *Dose.* 1 capsule daily in the early evening.

Other Proprietary Names

Arg.— Amiprol, Armonil, Best, Cuadel, Dipezona, Gradual, Gubex, Lembrol, Plidan, Saromet, Somasedan; *Austral.*— Ducene, Lorinon, Pro-Pam; *Canad.*— D-Tran, E-Pam, Meval, Neo-Calme, Novodipam, Paxel, Serenack, Stress-Pam, Vivol; *Denm.*— Apozepam, Stesolid; *Fin.*— Diapam; *Ind.*— Calmpose; *Ital.*— Aliseum, Ansiolin, Avex, Eridan, Noan, Quetinil, Quievita, Tranquirit, Valitran, Vatran; *Jap.*— Euphorin, Sedaril, Sonacon; *Neth.*— Stesolid; *Norw.*— Stesolid, Vival; *Pol.*— Relanium; *S.Afr.*— Cyclopam, Diatran, Dipam, Dizam, Doval, Notense, Pax, Relivan X, Scriptopam; *Spain*— Diaceplex, Drenian; *Swed.*— Apozepam, Stesolid.

Diazepam was also formerly marketed in Great Britain under the proprietary name Sedapam (*Duncan, Flockhart*).

7037-j

Dixyrazine. UCB 3412. 2-(2-{4-[2-Methyl-3-(phenothiazin-10-yl)propyl]piperazin-1-yl}ethoxy)ethanol.
$C_{24}H_{33}N_3O_2S$=427.6.

CAS — 2470-73-7.

A white to slightly greyish or yellowish powder with a bitter taste.

Very slightly **soluble** in water; soluble in alcohol, acetic acid, acetone, chloroform, ether, and methyl alcohol. **Protect** from light.

Dixyrazine is a phenothiazine with general properties similar to those of chlorpromazine (p.1509). It has a piperazine side-chain. Various doses have been advocated for psychiatric disorders usually ranging from 12.5 to 75 mg daily.

Proprietary Names

Esucos *(UCB, Arg.; UCB, Belg.; UCB, Denm.; UCB, Fr.; UCB, Ger.; UCB, Ital.; UCB, Neth.; UCB, Norw.; UCB, S.Afr.; UCB, Swed.; UCB, Switz.)*; Roscal *(Rosco, Denm.)*.

7038-z

Droperidol *(U.S.P.)*. R 4749. 1-{1-[3-(4-Fluorobenzoyl)propyl]-1,2,3,6-tetrahydro-4-pyridyl} benzimidazolin-2-one.
$C_{22}H_{22}FN_3O_2$=379.4.

CAS — 548-73-2.

Pharmacopoeias. In *U.S.*

A white to light tan-coloured amorphous or microcrystalline powder which gradually darkens on exposure to light. M.p. 144° to 148°. Practically **insoluble** in water; soluble 1 in 140 of alcohol, 1 in 4 of chloroform, and 1 in 500 of ether. Solutions may be **sterilised** by autoclaving. **Incompatible** with solutions of methohexitone, propanidid, and thiopentone. **Store** at 8° to 15° in an atmosphere of nitrogen in airtight containers. Protect from light.

Adverse Effects. As for Haloperidol, p.1532.

Pain has been reported at the site of injection.

A brief review of toxic effects of droperidol and fentanyl citrate in a fixed dose combination.— *Med. Lett.*, 1974, *16*, 42.

Extrapyramidal effects. In a double-blind trial involving 100 healthy women undergoing gynaecological procedures, droperidol 5 mg used as premedicant caused an increase in tremor and no significant decrease in nausea. Postoperative anxiety appeared to increase.— F. R. Ellis and J. Wilson, *Br. J. Anaesth.*, 1972, *44*, 1288.

Extrapyramidal symptoms were reported in a 10-year-old boy 3 hours after an intravenous injection of droperidol 10 mg.— K. L. De Silva *et al.*, *Practitioner*, 1973, *211*, 316.

A 41-year-old man developed an acute dystonic reaction following intravenous administration of droperidol 10 mg in divided doses over 10 minutes. He developed severe perioral spasms, protruded his tongue and grimaced markedly; his eyes rotated upwards and to the right and seemed fixed in that position; his neck became rigid, his mandible protruded forward, and he bit his tongue; his entire face seemed to be in spasm and he became plethoric; he remained fully conscious, could breath deeply and move his unanaesthetised extremities on command, but was unable to speak. Within a minute of intravenous administration of diphenhydramine 75 mg all signs of the extrapyramidal reaction resolved.— C. M. Patton, *Anesthesiology*, 1975, *43*, 126.

Further references: V. M. Rivera *et al.*, *Anesthesiology*, 1975, *42*, 635; L. J. Dupre and P. Stieglitz, *Br. J. Anaesth.*, 1980, *52*, 831.

Treatment of Adverse Effects. As for Chlorpromazine, p.1511.

Precautions. As for Chlorpromazine, p.1512. See also Haloperidol, p.1532.

Severe dystonic reactions have followed the use of droperidol; it should therefore be used with extreme care in susceptible patients, such as children, adolescents, and the elderly. Droperidol should not be given to patients with severe depression as it may aggravate their symptoms. If narcotic analgesics or other central depressants are required post-operatively following the use of droperidol then they should be given in reduced dosages. Droperidol has a longer duration of action than narcotic analgesics such as fentanyl and phenoperidine, therefore, during concurrent use, repeat doses of droperidol must not be given when only the narcotic analgesic is required, since this would lead to accumulation of droperidol and overdosage.

Severely impaired psychomotor performance for at least 10 hours after droperidol administration. Droperidol is probably not suitable as an anaesthetic for outpatients.— K. Korttila and M. Linnoila, *Br. J. Anaesth.*, 1974, *46*, 961.

In 8 healthy subjects droperidol 5 mg intravenously appeared to increase the incidence of gastro-oesophageal reflux and might therefore increase the risk of regurgitation and aspiration of gastric contents during induction and recovery from anaesthesia.— J. G. Brock-Utne *et al., Br. J. Anaesth.*, 1978, *50*, 295. See also *idem*, 1976, *48*, 699.

Interactions. A preparation of droperidol and fentanyl citrate enhanced the depressant effects of barbiturates and narcotic analgesics and anaesthetic misuse of such drugs might produce potentially fatal respiratory depression which might not always be immediately obvious after surgery.— E. Bloomquist (letter), *J. Am. med. Ass.*, 1971, *218*, 1301.

Anticholinergic agents. Droperidol appeared to have a mild atropinic action and enhanced the effect of atropine on heart-rate.— P. Parmentier and P. Dagnelie, *Br. J. Anaesth.*, 1979, *51*, 775.

Monoamine oxidase inhibitors. For a report of enhancement of the effects of droperidol by phenelzine, see Phenelzine Sulphate, p.130.

Myasthenia gravis. Although droperidol has not been implicated clinically, it has been shown experimentally to interfere with neuromuscular transmission, and should be used with caution in patients with myasthenia.— Z. Argov and F. L. Mastaglia, *New Engl. J. Med.*, 1979, *301*, 409.

Phaeochromocytoma. Intravenous administration of droperidol 1.25 mg to a 13-year-old boy with phaeochromocytoma caused severe hypertension which was easily controlled by phenoxybenzamine.— K. Sumikawa and Y. Amakata, *Anesthesiology*, 1977, *46*, 359.

Absorption and Fate. For a detailed account of the absorption and fate of a butyrophenone, see Haloperidol, p.1533.

Droperidol has been reported to have an initial plasma half-life of 10 minutes and a terminal plasma half-life of about 2 hours. It is extensively bound to plasma proteins.

A study of the absorption, metabolism, and excretion of droperidol in healthy subjects following intramuscular and intravenous administration. Droperidol was so rapidly absorbed from the intramuscular site that a response almost equivalent to that following intravenous administration could be expected. Droperidol was extensively metabolised and of 75% excreted in the urine less than 1% was unchanged. About 22% was recovered in the faeces, about 50% of this as unchanged droperidol; this high faecal recovery suggests biliary excretion of a portion of the dose. Droperidol had an initial half-life of about 10 minutes and terminal half-life of an average of 2.2 hours (range 120 to 163 minutes).— W. A. Cressman *et al., Anesthesiology*, 1973, *38*, 363. See also M. M. Ghoneim and K. Korttila, *Clin. Pharmacokinet.*, 1977, *2*, 344.

Uses. Droperidol is a butyrophenone with actions similar to those of haloperidol (p.1533). The duration of action of droperidol has been variously reported to last from about 2 to 4 hours to up to as long as 6 or 7 hours; alteration of consciousness may last 12 hours or longer. It is used in conjunction with an analgesic such as fentanyl citrate (p.1013) or phenoperidine hydrochloride (p.1029) to maintain the patient in a state of neuroleptanalgesia in which he is calm and indifferent to his surroundings and able to cooperate with the surgeon. The longer duration of action of droperidol must be kept in mind when using it in association with these narcotic analgesics. Droperidol is also used as a premedicant. It has also been used as an anti-emetic, and for the control of agitated patients in acute psychoses.

Droperidol is administered by mouth or by injection; generally only a single dose is required. The recommended dose is 5 to 20 mg by mouth. For premedication 2.5 to 10 mg may be administered intramuscularly 30 to 60 minutes pre-operatively. As an adjunct to general anaesthesia up to 15 mg may be administered intravenously, followed by 1.25 to 2.5 mg, usually intravenously, if required for maintenance. A suggested dose for anaesthetic use in children is 62.5 to 300 µg per kg body-weight.

Droperidol should be used in reduced dosage in the elderly.

Anaesthesia. A brief review of the use of droperidol in association with high-dose fentanyl for anaesthesia.— *Lancet*, 1979, *1*, 81. Comments and corrections.— G. M. Hall and A. Holdcroft (letter), *ibid.*, 268; A. M. Florence (letter), *ibid.*; M. Johnstone (letter), *ibid.*, 378.

For further comments on the use of droperidol in association with fentanyl and a warning that droperidol has a considerably longer duration of action than fentanyl, see Fentanyl Citrate, Administration, p.1013.

Studies on the use of droperidol in anaesthesia.— P. J. F. Baskett *et al., Br. J. Anaesth.*, 1969, *41*, 684 (with phenoperidine and nitrous oxide in children); J. W. Mostert *et al., Br. J. Anaesth.*, 1970, *42*, 501 (in chronic renal failure); J. G. Whitwam and W. J. Russell, *Br. J. Anaesth.*, 1971, *43*, 581 (cardiovascular effects); L. Becsey *et al., Anesthesiology*, 1972, *37*, 536 (for ketamine anaesthesia); B. Kay, *Anesth. Analg. curr. Res.*, 1973, *52*, 970 (with fentanyl in neonates and infants); T. P. Graham *et al., Am. Heart J.*, 1974, *87*, 287 (with fentanyl, cardiac catheterisation in children); R. D. Wilson *et al., Sth. med. J.*, 1974, *67*, 765 (in children, for ketamine anaesthesia); L. D. Becker *et al., Anesthesiology*, 1976, *44*, 291 (with fentanyl and nitrous oxide); H. I. Le Brun, *Gut*, 1976, *17*, 655 (with fentanyl in endoscopy); R. J. Prescott *et al., Lancet*, 1976, *1*, 1148 (with atropine for premedication); D. G. Whalley *et al., Br. J. Anaesth.*, 1976, *48*, 1207 (with phenoperidine in dentistry); A. A. Birch and W. H. Boyce, *Anesthesiology*, 1977, *47*, 70 (use with dopamine); J. R. Fozard and M. L. M. Manford, *Br. J. Anaesth.*, 1977, *49*, 1147 (oral premedication, with atropine, in children); F. J. Tornetta, *Anesth. Analg.*, 1977, *56*, 496 (premedication); J. T. Conner *et al., Br. J. Anaesth.*, 1978, *50*, 463 (premedication with fentanyl or morphine); G. P. Herr *et al., Br. J. Anaesth.*, 1979, *51*, 537 (premedication with diazepam).

Pregnancy and the neonate. The administration of droperidol 10 mg thirty minutes before elective caesarean section eliminated awareness during anaesthesia. Neonatal respiration was not delayed and there was some reduction in the amount of postoperative pain.— A. M. Smith and W. T. McNeil (letter), *Br. med. J.*, 1969, *1*, 572.

In a double-blind study involving normal obstetric patients in labour, no significant difference was noted in sedation obtained with droperidol 5 mg intramuscularly, given to 48 patients, and promethazine 25 to 50 mg intramuscularly, given to 17 and 35 patients respectively. Pethidine was given on request to control pain and no serious maternal or foetal side-effects were noted.— G. P. Pettit *et al., Milit. Med.*, 1976, *141*, 316.

See also under Anaesthesia.

Psychoses. Droperidol in 10- or 20-mg doses had been used on more than 100 occasions for the treatment of acute schizophrenic episodes, attacks of manic behaviour, the control of violent aggression in epileptics, and the sedation of severe emotional disturbances in autistic or brain-damaged patients.— T. S. Davies and M. White (letter), *Br. med. J.*, 1975, *2*, 559.

Of 24 patients with severe agitation or aggression treated with droperidol in individually determined doses of from 2.5 to 12.5 mg by intramuscular injection in an open clinical trial, 22 showed a marked clinical improvement. An acute dystonic reaction occurred in 1 patient and orthostatic hypotension occurred in 2 patients.— R. P. Granacher and D. D. Ruth, *Curr. ther. Res.*, 1979, *25*, 361.

Further references: E. Cocito *et al., Arzneimittel-Forsch.*, 1970, *20*, 1119; K. E. Neff *et al., Dis. nerv. Syst.*, 1972, *33*, 594; A. M. H. van Leeuwen *et al., J. nerv. ment. Dis.*, 1977, *164*, 280; M. E. Burns, *J. int. med. Res.*, 1980, *8*, 31.

Preparations

Droperidol Injection *(U.S.P.).* A sterile solution in Water for Injections prepared with the aid of lactic acid. pH 3 to 3.8. Protect from light.

Droleptan *(Janssen, UK).* Droperidol, available as an **Injection** containing 5 mg per ml, in ampoules of 2 ml (dilution not recommended); as **Liquid** containing 1 mg per ml; and as scored **Tablets** of 10 mg. (Also available as Droleptan in *Austral., Fr.*).

Droperidol is an ingredient of Thalamonal (see p.1013).

Other Proprietary Names

Dehydrobenzperidol *(Arg., Belg., Denm., Ger., Neth., Switz.)*; Dridol *(Norw., Swed.)*; Inapsin *(S.Afr.)*; Inapsine *(Canad., USA)*; Sintodian *(Ital.)*.

7039-c

Emylcamate. KABI 925; MK 250. 1-Ethyl-1-methylpropyl carbamate.
$C_7H_{15}NO_2$=145.2.

CAS — 78-28-4.

A white crystalline powder with a slight camphoraceous odour. M.p. 56° to 58°. **Soluble** 1 in 250 of water; freely soluble in alcohol and ether.

Emylcamate is a carbamate with general properties similar to those of meprobamate (p.1545). It was formerly used as an anxiolytic and muscle relaxant in doses of 200 mg three or four times daily.

7040-s

Fluanisone *(B.P. Vet.).* Haloanisone; MD 2028. 4′-Fluoro-4-[4-(2-methoxyphenyl)piperazin-1-yl]butyrophenone.
$C_{21}H_{25}FN_2O_2$=356.4.

CAS — 1480-19-9.

An almost white to buff-coloured, odourless or almost odourless, crystalline powder. M.p. 72° to 76°. Practically **insoluble** in water; soluble 1 in 12 of alcohol, 1 in 1 of chloroform, and 1 in 22 of ether; soluble in dilute solutions of organic acids. Solutions for injection are **sterilised** by autoclaving or by filtration. **Store** in airtight containers. Protect from light.

Fluanisone is a butyrophenone with general properties similar to those of haloperidol (p.1532). It has been given in psychiatric disorders in doses of 2.5 mg twice or thrice daily; higher doses have been given intramuscularly. Fluanisone is also used in veterinary medicine as a tranquilliser and for anaesthetic premedication.

Proprietary Names

Sedalande *(Delalande, Belg.;Delalande, Fr.; Delalande, Ger.; Delalande, Switz.)*.

7041-w

Fluopromazine.

Triflupromazine *(U.S.P.).* *NN*-Dimethyl-3-(2-trifluoromethylphenothiazin-10-yl)propylamine.
$C_{18}H_{19}F_3N_2S$=352.4.

CAS — 146-54-3.

Pharmacopoeias. In *U.S.*

A pale amber viscous oily liquid which forms into large irregular crystals during prolonged storage. Practically **insoluble** in water. **Store** in airtight containers. Protect from light.

7042-e

Fluopromazine Hydrochloride.

Triflupromazine Hydrochloride *(U.S.P.).*
$C_{18}H_{19}F_3N_2S,HCl$=388.9.

CAS — 1098-60-8.

Pharmacopoeias. In *U.S.*

A white to pale tan crystalline powder with a slight characteristic odour. M.p. 170° to 178°. **Soluble** 1 in less than 1 of water and of alcohol and 1 in 1.7 of chloroform; soluble in acetone; practically insoluble in ether. A 2% solution in water has a pH of 4.1. If the pH is raised to 6.4 the free base is precipitated. **Protect** from light.

Adverse Effects, Treatment, and Precautions. As for Chlorpromazine, p.1509.

Absorption and Fate. For an account of the absorption and fate of a phenothiazine, see Chlorpromazine, p.1513.

Uses. Fluopromazine hydrochloride is a phenothiazine with actions and uses similar to those of chlorpromazine (p.1513).

The usual initial dose by mouth in psychotic patients is 100 to 150 mg daily of fluopromazine hydrochloride with maintenance doses of 30 to 150 mg daily. For a more rapid effect 60 to 150 mg may be given daily by intramuscular injection.

For the control of nausea and vomiting the usual dose by mouth is 20 to 30 mg daily; by injection, 5 to 15 mg may be given intramuscularly and repeated after 4 hours if necessary; a dose of 1 mg to a maximum total daily dose of 3 mg may be given intravenously. Elderly or debilitated patients should be given 2.5 mg intramuscularly. A suggested dose for children is 200 µg per kg body-weight daily up to a maximum of 10 mg daily by mouth or intramuscularly.

Preparations of Fluopromazine and Fluopromazine Hydrochloride

Triflupromazine Hydrochloride Injection *(U.S.P.)*. A sterile solution of fluopromazine hydrochloride in Water for Injections. pH 4.5 to 5.2. Protect from light.

Triflupromazine Hydrochloride Tablets *(U.S.P.)*. Tablets containing fluopromazine hydrochloride. Protect from light.

Triflupromazine Oral Suspension *(U.S.P.)*. A suspension containing fluopromazine. Potency is expressed in terms of the equivalent amount of fluopromazine hydrochloride. Store in airtight containers. Protect from light.

Proprietary Names

Psyquil *(Squibb, Fr.; Heyden, Ger.)*; Siquil *(Squibb, Belg.; Squibb, Neth.; Squibb, NZ; Squibb, Switz.)*; Vesprin *(Squibb, Canad.; Squibb, USA)*.

7043-l

Fluoresone. ANP 215; Floretione. Ethyl 4-fluorophenyl sulphone.
$C_8H_9FO_2S = 188.2$.

CAS — 2924-67-6.

Fluoresone has been used in neuropsychiatric disorders in doses of 400 to 600 mg daily.

Proprietary Names

Bripadon *(Anphar-Rolland, Fr.)*; Caducid *(IFI, Ital.)*.

7044-y

Flupenthixol Decanoate.
2-{4-[3-(2-Trifluoromethylthioxanthen-9-ylidene)propyl]piperazin-1-yl}ethyl decanoate.
$C_{33}H_{43}F_3N_2O_2S = 588.8$.

CAS — 2709-56-0 (flupenthixol); 30909-51-4 (decanoate).

A yellow oil with a slight odour. Sp. gr. 0.95. Very slightly **soluble** in water; soluble in alcohol; freely soluble in chloroform and ether. **Store** in a cool place. Protect from light.

7045-j

Flupenthixol Hydrochloride.
Flupenthixol Dihydrochloride; Flupentixol Dihydrochloride; N 7009. 2-{4-[3-(2-Trifluoromethylthioxanthen-9-ylidene)propyl]piperazin-1-yl}ethanol.
$C_{23}H_{25}F_3N_2OS,2HCl = 507.4$.

CAS — 2413-38-9.

A white or yellowish-white powder. Flupenthixol hydrochloride 1.17 mg is approximately equivalent to 1 mg of flupenthixol. **Soluble** in water and alcohol.

Stability. Studies on the decomposition of flupenthixol hydrochloride in aqueous solution.— R. P. Enever *et al.*, *J. pharm. Sci.*, 1979, *68*, 169. See also A. Li Wan Po and W. J. Irwin (letter), *Pharm. J.*, 1978, *2*, 430; *J. Pharm. Pharmac.*, 1980, *32*, 25.

Adverse Effects and Treatment. As for Chlorpromazine, p.1509.
Extrapyramidal symptoms are the most common side-effect. Restlessness and insomnia may occur, and depressive reactions have been reported.

Effects on mental state. *Paradoxical response.* A report of 3 patients with resistant schizophrenia who exhibited apparently paradoxical reactions to high doses of long-acting depot preparations of the antipsychotics flupenthixol decanoate or fluphenazine decanoate.— T. R. E. Barnes and P. K. Bridges, *Br. med. J.*, 1980, *281*, 274. Comments.— S. Brown (letter), *ibid.*, 453; W. R. Guirguis and S. E. Bawden (letter), *ibid.*, 617. Reply.— T. Barnes and P. K. Bridges (letter), *ibid.*, 1068.

Extrapyramidal effects. *Tardive dyskinesia.* A rise in the incidence of tardive dyskinesia in 374 schizophrenic patients was associated with the introduction of depot fluphenazine and depot flupenthixol therapy.— A. C. Gibson, *Br. J. Psychiat.*, 1978, *132*, 361.

Overdosage. Experience with 28 cases of flupenthixol poisoning failed to show serious toxicity.— P. Crome *et al.* (letter), *Br. med. J.*, 1978, *1*, 859.

Urinary incontinence. Nocturnal enuresis in 4 young women was associated with depot injections of antipsychotic agents. One was receiving flupenthixol.— A. Shaikh (letter), *Br. med. J.*, 1978, *1*, 1698.

Weight gain. Two patients experienced pronounced weight gain during treatment with flupenthixol decanoate.— D. Rice (letter), *Br. J. Psychiat.*, 1973, *123*, 613.

Precautions. As for Chlorpromazine, p.1512.
Flupenthixol is not recommended for excitable or overactive patients.

A study of the effects of flupenthixol, alone or with alcohol, on driving performance.— M. Linnoila *et al.*, *Arzneimittel-Forsch.*, 1975, *25*, 1088.

Interactions. An investigation in 28 schizophrenic patients receiving long-term neuroleptic treatment with fluphenazine or flupenthixol, in some cases with chlorpromazine, showed no biochemical evidence of hepatic microsomal enzyme induction.— S. K. Majumdar and P. P. Kakad, *Postgrad. med. J.*, 1978, *54*, 789. Evidence to suggest induction of microsomal enzyme activity by flupenthixol.— S. A. Salem *et al.*, *Br. J. clin. Pharmac.*, 1980, *9*, 313P.

Lithium. For a possible interaction between flupenthixol and lithium, see Lithium Carbonate, p.1539.

Temperature variations. Because of reports of fatal hyperthermia in mentally handicapped patients receiving fluphenazine enanthate during a heat-wave in Australia, the UK manufacturers of fluphenazine decanoate and of flupenthixol decanoate recommended that these compounds should not be used in the mentally handicapped. A check of the original reports has shown that most fatalities occurred in patients also taking antiparkinsonian agents which decrease sweating.— M. J. Craft (letter), *Br. med. J.*, 1977, *1*, 835.

Absorption and Fate. Flupenthixol is readily absorbed from the gastro-intestinal tract and is probably subject to first-pass metabolism in the gut wall. It is also extensively metabolised in the liver and is excreted in the urine and faeces in the form of numerous metabolites; there is evidence of enterohepatic recycling. Owing to the first-pass effect, plasma concentrations following oral administration are much lower than those following estimated equivalent doses of the intramuscular depot preparation. Moreover, there is very wide intersubject variation in plasma concentrations of flupenthixol, but in practice, no simple correlation has been found between plasma concentrations of flupenthixol and its metabolites, and the therapeutic effect. Paths of metabolism of flupenthixol include sulphoxidation, side-chain *N*-dealkylation, and glucuronic acid conjugation. It is widely distributed in the body, and crosses the blood-brain barrier.
The decanoate ester of flupenthixol is very slowly absorbed from the site of intramuscular injection and is therefore suitable for depot injection. It is gradually released into the blood stream where it is rapidly hydrolysed to flupenthixol.

A detailed account of pharmacokinetic studies on flupenthixol and flupenthixol decanoate.— A. Jørgensen, *Drug Metab. Rev.*, 1978, *8*, 235.

Absorption and distribution. A study of the pharmacokinetics of flupenthixol and flupenthixol decanoate in 10 schizophrenic women who had been receiving either the oral or the depot preparation for at least 6 months. Peak values of radioactivity were obtained 3 to 8 hours after oral administration of radioactively labelled flupenthixol 1 mg to 5 of the women but secondary peaks were seen in all cases. In 3 of the subjects the serum concentration subsequently fell very slowly, while in 2 the fall was rather steep; the half-life of total radioactivity was several days. Following intramuscular administration of flupenthixol decanoate 28 or 40 mg in the other 5 women, the serum concentrations were noted to build up rather slowly with maximum values seen 11 to 17 days after injection, indicating a very slow release of the radioactive substance from the site of injection. A plateau was reached around and just after the time of maximum concentration, and was estimated to last within 20% of the maximum, for about 2 weeks. Concentrations in the CSF 11 days after injection were 29 to 55% of the corresponding serum concentrations.— A. Jørgensen and C. G. Gottfries, *Psychopharmacologia*, 1972, *27*, 1.

Small, but not unimportant, amounts of flupenthixol reached the foetuses of 5 women treated with oral or intramuscular forms of flupenthixol during pregnancy. Amounts in the mothers' milk were about 30% higher than those in their serum and were considered to be of no importance unless the neonate differs considerably from the adult in metabolism of, or sensitivity to, flupenthixol.— L. Kirk and A. Jørgensen, *Psychopharmacology*, 1980, *72*, 107.

Slow decline, over a period of several months, of plasma drug and prolactin concentrations after discontinuation of depot neuroleptic therapy with flupenthixol decanoate.— B. Wistedt *et al.* (letter), *Lancet*, 1981, *1*, 1163.

Metabolism. *Animal* studies on the metabolism of flupenthixol and flupenthixol decanoate.— A. Jørgensen *et al.*, *Acta pharmac. tox.*, 1969, *27*, 301; *idem*, 1971, *29*, 339.

Uses. Flupenthixol is a thioxanthene with general properties similar to those of the phenothiazine, chlorpromazine (p.1513). Unlike chlorpromazine, a certain activating effect has been ascribed to flupenthixol and, accordingly, it is not indicated in overactive patients. Flupenthixol is administered as the hydrochloride by mouth or as the longer-acting decanoate ester by deep intramuscular injection.
The usual dose of the hydrochloride for the treatment of psychoses is 3 to 9 mg twice daily; the maximum recommended dose is a total of 18 mg daily. The long-acting decanoate should be given by deep intramuscular injection in an initial test dose of 20 mg. According to the patient's response over the following 5 to 10 days, this may be followed by doses of 20 to 40 mg at intervals of 2 to 4 weeks. Shorter dosage intervals or greater amounts may be required according to the patient's response. If doses greater than 40 mg are considered necessary they should be divided between 2 separate injection sites. In patients already taking antipsychotic agents by mouth, the dosage should be gradually reduced on starting flupenthixol decanoate injections. In those being transferred from depot injections of phenothiazines, flupenthixol decanoate 40 mg is considered to be equivalent to fluphenazine decanoate 25 mg.
The standard injections of flupenthixol decanoate are available in doses of 20 mg and 40 mg contained in volumes of 1 ml and 2 ml respectively. There is, however, also a concentrated injection available, which contains flupenthixol decanoate 100 mg in 1 ml, i.e. it is five times more concentrated. This injection is indicated for patients who require high-dose therapy with flupenthixol decanoate in single doses of 100 mg or more. Doses of the concentrated injection greater than 200 mg should be divided between 2 injection sites.
Flupenthixol has also been given as the hydrochloride by mouth, for the treatment of depression, with or without anxiety. The usual dose is 1 mg twice daily, increased by increments of 500 µg to a maximum of 3 mg daily. The last dose should be given no later than 4 p.m. and if no effect has been noted within 1 week of administration of the maximum dose, the treatment should be withdrawn.
Flupenthixol should be given in reduced dosage to elderly patients.

Action. Patients taking α-flupenthixol [(*Z*)-flupenthixol] showed a significantly greater improvement after three weeks than patients who were taking equal doses of β-flupenthixol [(*E*)-flupenthixol] or a placebo, in a study of 45 patients suffering from acute schizophrenic illnesses. The α-isomer had more effect on the positive symptoms of the disease (hallucinations, delusions and thought disorder) but this difference was less apparent for the negative symptoms (psychomotor retardation, poverty of speech and disturbances of affect).— T. J. Crow *et al.*, *Br. J. clin. Pharmac.*, 1977, *4*, 648P. See also P. M. Cotes *et al.*, *ibid.*, 651P. There is evidence that distribution of the 2 isomers across the blood-brain barrier is similar.— T. J. Crow and E. C. Johnstone (letter), *Lancet*, 1978, *1*, 1050.

A comment that flupenthixol is a D_1 receptor antagonist.— P. Jenner and C. D. Marsden (letter), *Lancet*, 1979, *2*, 900.

Animal studies on the pharmacology of flupenthixol and some reference neuroleptics, including chlorpromazine and fluphenazine.— I. M. Nielsen *et al.*, *Acta pharmac. tox.*, 1973, *33*, 353.

Administration. In the elderly. Despite statements to the contrary fluphenazine decanoate and flupenthixol decanoate have a definite place in the treatment of paranoid psychosis in the elderly provided there is no serious degree of dementia and adequate community facilities are available.— T. Whitehead (letter), *Br. med. J.*, 1975, *2*, 502.

Anxiety. A study of flupenthixol in doses of up to 1 mg twice daily, for the treatment of anxiety.— I. Ovhed, *Curr. med. Res. Opinion*, 1976, *4*, 144.

Behaviour disorders. Extremely low tolerance to frustration in 6 patients was relieved by flupenthixol decanoate 10 to 12 mg every 2 weeks by deep intramuscular injection.— P. M. O'Flanagan (letter), *Br. med. J.*, 1974, *3*, 258.

For the use of flupenthixol decanoate in the treatment of disturbed adolescent girls, see Fluphenazine Decanoate, p.1530.

Depression. Flupenthixol in low doses (1 to 4.5 mg daily) is an effective antidepressant and appears to have relatively few side-effects. It is not yet established whether it differs qualitatively from other antidepressants.— *Drug & Ther. Bull.*, 1978, *16*, 43.

Further reviews and comments: C. Brewer (letter), *Br. med. J.*, 1977, *2*, 523.

Studies of flupenthixol in the treatment of depression: P. Hall and J. Coleman (letter), *Br. J. Psychiat.*, 1973, *122*, 120; J. P. R. Young *et al.*, *Br. med. J.*, 1976, *1*, 1116; D. A. W. Johnson, *Acta psychiat. scand.*, 1979, *59*, 1.

Schizophrenia. Ten of 11 chronic schizophrenic patients improved when flupenthixol decanoate 20 to 40 mg every 1 to 3 weeks was substituted for previous treatment. Two other patients became manic and had to be withdrawn from the study.— P. Hall and J. Coleman (letter), *Br. J. Psychiat.*, 1972, *120*, 241.

A report of 111 schizophrenic patients given flupenthixol 20 to 80 mg by intramuscular injection weekly for 3 weeks, 100 of whom continued as outpatients when their symptoms were controlled. Extrapyramidal side-effects were mild and occurred in 32% of patients, akathisia occurred once, and 8 patients became depressed.— M. W. P. Carney (letter), *Br. J. Psychiat.*, 1972, *121*, 458.

There was a definite improvement in symptoms (hallucinations, delusions, withdrawal, apathy, depression) in 14 patients receiving flupenthixol decanoate on average 40 mg every 3 weeks by intramuscular injection. The patients had had a poor response to previous medication. Antiparkinsonian treatment, started at the same time as flupenthixol, could be withdrawn in most cases after the first few injections.— H. R. Trueman and M. G. Valentine, *Br. J. Psychiat.*, 1974, *124*, 58.

Further references: P. J. Reiter, *Br. J. Psychiat.*, 1969, *115*, 1399; J. Bruck and H. Guss, *Wien. med. Wschr.*, 1971, *121*, 110; G. Nistico *et al.*, *J. clin. Pharmac.*, 1974, *14*, 476; R. De Smedt *et al.*, *Acta ther.*, 1977, *3*, 155; H. B. Kelly *et al.*, *Int. Pharmacopsychiat.*, 1977, *12*, 54; A. Knights *et al.*, *Br. J. Psychiat.*, 1979, *135*, 515; R. Pinto *et al.*, *Acta psychiat. scand.*, 1979, *60*, 313.

High-dose therapy. Results of a 12-week double-blind study involving 23 female schizophrenic patients who had been resistant to previous therapy, demonstrated no significant difference between those given flupenthixol decanoate 40 mg every 2 weeks, and those given 200 mg every 2 weeks. Those in the high-dose group experienced significantly more extrapyramidal side-effects compared with scores before the trial, and 3 of 4 who experienced excessive salivation were in the high-dose group. Although plasma concentrations varied considerably, they were consistently higher in the high-dose group, and there was improvement in the mental state of a sub-group of patients in the high-dose group, who may have been resistant for pharmacokinetic reasons.— R. G. McCreadie *et al.*, *Br. J. Psychiat.*, 1979, *135*, 175.

Proprietary Preparations

Depixol Injection *(Lundbeck, UK: Farillon, UK)*. Contains *cis*-(*Z*)-flupenthixol decanoate 20 mg per ml in thin vegetable oil, in ampoules of 1 and 2 ml and disposable syringes of 1 and 2 ml. **Depixol-Conc. Injection.** Contains *cis*-(*Z*)-flupenthixol decanoate 100 mg per ml in thin vegetable oil, in ampoules of 1 ml.

Depixol Tablets *(Lundbeck, UK: Farillon, UK)*. Each contains flupenthixol hydrochloride equivalent to 3 mg of flupenthixol.

Fluanxol *(Lundbeck, UK: Farillon, UK)*. Flupenthixol hydrochloride, available as tablets each containing the equivalent of 500 µg of flupenthixol. (Also available as Fluanxol in *Belg., Denm., Fr., Ger., Neth., Norw., S.Afr., Swed., Switz.*).

Other Proprietary Names of Flupenthixol Salts and Esters

Émergil *(hydrochloride) (Fr.)*; Fluanxol Depot *(decanoate) (Belg., Denm., Ger., Neth., Norw., S.Afr., Swed., Switz.)*; Fluanxol Retard *(decanoate) (Fr.)*.

7046-z

Fluphenazine Decanoate *(B.P.)*.

2-{4-[3-(2-Trifluoromethylphenothiazin-10-yl)propyl]-piperazin-1-yl}ethyl decanoate.
$C_{32}H_{44}F_3N_3O_2S = 591.8$.

CAS — 69-23-8 (fluphenazine); 5002-47-1 (decanoate).

Pharmacopoeias. In *Br.*

A pale yellow viscous liquid or a yellow crystalline oily solid with a faint ester-like odour. Fluphenazine decanoate 12.5 mg is approximately equivalent to 10.75 mg of fluphenazine hydrochloride. Practically **insoluble** in water; miscible with dehydrated alcohol, chloroform, and ether; soluble in fixed oils. Oily solutions are **sterilised** by filtration. **Protect** from light.

7047-c

Fluphenazine Enanthate *(B.P., U.S.P.)*.

Fluphenazine Heptanoate. 2-{4-[3-(2-Trifluoromethylphenothiazin-10-yl)propyl]piperazin-1-yl}ethyl heptanoate.
$C_{29}H_{38}F_3N_3O_2S = 549.7$.

CAS — 2746-81-8.

Pharmacopoeias. In *Br.* and *U.S.*

A pale yellow to yellow-orange, clear to slightly turbid, viscous liquid or a yellow crystalline oily solid with a faint ester-like odour. Fluphenazine enanthate 12.5 mg is approximately equivalent to 11.6 mg of fluphenazine hydrochloride.

Practically **insoluble** in water; soluble 1 in less than 1 of alcohol and of chloroform and 1 in 2 of ether; soluble in fixed oils. Oily solutions are **sterilised** by filtration. **Stable** in air at room temperature but unstable in strong light. **Store** in airtight containers. Protect from light.

7048-k

Fluphenazine Hydrochloride *(B.P., U.S.P.)*.

Triflumethazine Hydrochloride. 2-{4-[3-(2-Trifluoromethylphenothiazin-10-yl)propyl]piperazin-1-yl}ethanol dihydrochloride.
$C_{22}H_{26}F_3N_3OS,2HCl = 510.4$.

CAS — 146-56-5.

Pharmacopoeias. In *Br., Braz., Chin.*, and *U.S.*

A white or almost white, odourless, crystalline powder with a bitter taste. M.p. above 225°, with a range of not more than 5°.

Soluble 1 in 10 or less of water; slightly soluble in alcohol, acetone, and chloroform; practically insoluble in ether. A 5% solution in water has a pH of 1.9 to 2.3. **Store** in airtight containers. Protect from light.

Adverse Effects. As for Chlorpromazine, p.1509.

Extrapyramidal symptoms may be more common than the other side-effects.

Severe depressive reactions have been reported in patients given the long-acting fluphenazine esters. Pain can occur at the site of injection.

In a study of the side-effects of fluphenazine decanoate in 140 patients, 34% experienced side-effects which were mild in 15%, moderate in 11%, and severe in 8%. The main side-effects were akathisia in 34 patients, parkinsonian symptoms in 27, and blurred vision in 10.— D. A. W. Johnson, *Br. J. Psychiat.*, 1973, *123*, 519.

Local or allergic reactions were not observed following deltoid injection of depot fluphenazine, 0.25 to 1 ml, on over 500 occasions.— M. A. Amdur (letter), *J. Am. med. Ass.*, 1974, *230*, 1634.

Results of a double-blind crossover study in 7 evaluable patients indicated an important incidence of akinesia, involuntary movement, autonomic disturbances, and drowsiness in the first few hours following injection of fluphenazine decanoate and in the first 2 days following injection of fluphenazine enanthate.— S. H. Curry *et al.* (letter), *Lancet*, 1979, *1*, 331.

For comments on the different forms of fluphenazine, see Administration, under Uses.

Effects on the endocrine system. A 33-year-old schizophrenic man developed inappropriate secretion of antidiuretic hormone 2 days after the intramuscular injection of fluphenazine enanthate 50 mg.— J. L. G. de Rivera (letter), *Ann. intern. Med.*, 1975, *82*, 811. Criticism and comments.— J. S. Zuniga and T. Hazan (letter), *Ann. intern. Med.*, 1975, *83*, 735; J. L. G. de Rivera (letter), *ibid.*, 736; P. J. Phillips and R. W. Pain (letter), *ibid.*

Effects on mental state. In a study in 32 schizophrenic patients fluphenazine decanoate was shown to cause less impairment of the subjects' ability to perform complex learning tasks than chlorpromazine, trifluoperazine, or thioridazine.— J. S. Gillis and S. C. Parkison, *Curr. ther. Res.*, 1977, *22*, 349.

Depression. Sixteen patients, initially diagnosed as schizophrenics, developed severe depression after an injection of fluphenazine enanthate or decanoate. Five suicides were attributed to the depression. Careful supervision in the follow-up period was essential after treatment with these drugs.— R. de Alarcon and M. W. P. Carney, *Br. med. J.*, 1969, *3*, 564. Comments.— J. Johnson (letter), *ibid.*, 718; N. W. Imlah (letter), *ibid.*, 1969, *4*, 49.

Paradoxical response. Of 80 schizophrenic patients treated with normal doses of phenothiazines, 9 developed dramatic exacerbations of their psychosis associated with akathisia while taking piperazine phenothiazines, mainly fluphenazine enanthate. The exacerbation was reversed by biperiden. It was considered that the extrapyramidal actions of the tranquillisers could produce mental symptoms which resembled an exacerbation of schizophrenia.— T. Van Putten *et al.*, *Archs gen. Psychiat.*, 1974, *30*, 102, per *J. Am. med. Ass.*, 1974, *227*, 459.

A report of 3 patients with resistant schizophrenia who exhibited apparently paradoxical reactions to high doses of long-acting depot preparations of the antipsychotics flupenthixol decanoate or fluphenazine decanoate.— T. R. E. Barnes and P. K. Bridges, *Br. med. J.*, 1980, *281*, 274. Comments.— S. Brown (letter), *ibid.*, 453; W. R. Guirguis and S. E. Bawden (letter), *ibid.*, 617. Reply.— T. Barnes and P. K. Bridges (letter), *ibid.*, 1068.

Effects on the nervous system. A 49-year-old man developed a syndrome similar to bulbar palsy, with absent gag reflexes, following treatment with fluphenazine enanthate. Such a syndrome could be responsible for occasional reports of sudden death due to aspiration or asphyxiation in patients receiving phenothiazines. It is not reversed by antiparkinsonian medication.— K. Solomon, *Am. J. Psychiat.*, 1977, *134*, 308.

Extrapyramidal effects. Severe unpredictable extrapyramidal symptoms, which were not fully responsive to antiparkinsonian drugs, were an additional reaction in schizophrenics who were treated with fluphenazine enanthate or fluphenazine decanoate.— M. Segal and D. H. Ropschitz, *Br. med. J.*, 1969, *4*, 169.

Acute dystonia affecting the face occurred in 2 patients taking fluphenazine hydrochloride 5 mg at night.— X. G. Okojie (letter), *Br. med. J.*, 1972, *4*, 796.

Studies in 6 patients receiving fluphenazine decanoate every 4 weeks for control of schizophrenia indicated that signs of parkinsonism were most severe in the third week after the injection; this was at variance with suggestions of 3 to 5 days after injection as the peak period.— P. Lamb *et al.* (letter), *Lancet*, 1976, *1*, 484.

A suggestion that more extrapyramidal side-effects are associated with fluphenazine enanthate than with the decanoate.— J. Kane *et al.*, *Am. J. Psychiat.*, 1978, *135*, 1539.

Further references: A. A. Bartholomew, *Med. J. Aust.*,

1967, *2*, 66; D. J. Safer and R. P. Allen, *Biol. Psychiat.*, 1971, *3*, 237; R. N. Allan and H. C. White, *Br. med. J.*, 1972, *1*, 221; L. Rose (letter), *ibid.*, 441; R. J. M. Crawford and T. J. Robinson (letter), *ibid.*; J. B. Dillon (letter), *ibid.*, 807; R. Schilkrut *et al.*, *Arzneimittel-Forsch.*, 1978, *28*, 1494.

See also Overdosage (below).

Tardive dyskinesia. A rise in the incidence of tardive dyskinesia in 374 schizophrenic patients was associated with the introduction of depot fluphenazine and depot flupenthixol therapy.— A. C. Gibson, *Br. J. Psychiat.*, 1978, *132*, 361.

Further references: A. C. Gibson (letter), *Br. med. J.*, 1978, *2*, 434.

Nausea and vomiting. Severe nausea and vomiting associated with fluphenazine therapy was successfully treated with benztropine.— C. E. McDanal and R. A. Markoff, *Hawaii med. J.*, 1978, *37*, 268.

Overdosage. A patient who took about 30 fluphenazine 2.5 mg tablets was treated by gastric lavage. Twenty hours after hospital admission he experienced difficulty in breathing due to spasm of the respiratory muscles; other very severe extrapyramidal side-effects were also present. Muscle spasm was controlled by diazepam.— F. M. Ladhani (letter), *Med. J. Aust.*, 1974, *2*, 26.

A syndrome marked by features of catatonia and parkinsonism developed in 3 patients taking high doses of fluphenazine; differentiation from worsening schizophrenia was important. The syndrome responded to treatment with amantadine.— A. J. Gelenberg and M. R. Mandel, *Archs gen. Psychiat.*, 1977, *34*, 947. See also L. Grunhaus *et al.*, *J. clin. Psychiat.*, 1979, *40*, 99.

Pregnancy and the neonate. Four weeks after delivery, an infant born to a schizophrenic woman who had received fluphenazine decanoate intramuscularly every 3 weeks throughout pregnancy, developed mild extrapyramidal symptoms. He had been breast fed for 5 days. The extrapyramidal symptoms responded readily to administration of diphenhydramine by mouth.— M. F. Cleary, *Am. J. Psychiat.*, 1977, *134*, 815.

Tardive dyskinesia. See under Extrapyramidal Effects (above).

Urinary incontinence. Nocturnal enuresis in 3 young women was associated with fluphenazine decanoate therapy.— A. Shaikh (letter), *Br. med. J.*, 1978, *1*, 1698.

Treatment of Adverse Effects. As for Chlorpromazine, p.1511.

In 8 patients who were receiving fluphenazine enanthate injections every 2 or 3 weeks, an attempt was made, under double-blind conditions, to replace benzhexol (given to reduce extrapyramidal side-effects of fluphenazine) with a placebo. Four patients developed severe reactions which indicated their continued need of benzhexol. Periodic review of the need for and dose of benzhexol was however justified.— L. Grove and J. L. Crammer, *Br. med. J.*, 1972, *1*, 276.

A 49-year-old man suffered a very severe parkinsonian syndrome associated with depression after receiving (in addition to amitriptyline and diazepam) fluphenazine decanoate 150 mg over 5 weeks with no antiparkinsonian medication. Both his parkinsonian symptoms and his depression responded remarkably to treatment with antiparkinsonian drugs.— A. H. Fry and A. W. Beard, *Practitioner*, 1977, *218*, 874.

Precautions. As for Chlorpromazine, p.1512.

A report of dystonic reaction to fluphenazine causing risk to a patient while swimming.— M. W. Dysken and J. M. Davis (letter), *Br. med. J.*, 1978, *2*, 1164.

Interactions. In 6 male schizophrenics fluphenazine decanoate, 25 mg intramuscularly monthly for at least 12 months, did not affect hepatic microsomal enzyme activity as assessed by urinary D-glucaric acid excretion.— A. N. Latham *et al.* (letter), *Br. J. clin. Pharmac.*, 1974, *1*, 277.

Alcohol. Tests in 10 volunteers showed that the administration of alcohol (as 500 ml of beer) 8 hours after taking fluphenazine hydrochloride 1 mg led to impairment of concentration, performance, reaction-speed, and other parameters.— A. Doenicke and W. Sigmund, *Arzneimittel-Forsch.*, 1964, *14*, 907.

Beverages. For controversy on a possible interaction between neuroleptic therapy and tea or coffee, see Chlorpromazine, p.1512.

Clonidine. Delirium in a 33-year-old man, was considered to have been caused by concomitant administration of clonidine and fluphenazine decanoate.— R. M. Allen and A. Flemenbaum, *J. clin. Psychiat.*, 1979, *40*, 236.

Vitamins. Increase in manic behaviour necessitating increase in dosage with fluphenazine followed treatment with ascorbic acid to reduce Vitamin-C deficiency in a patient with steady-state fluphenazine plasma-concentrations.— M. W. Dysken *et al.* (letter), *J. Am. med. Ass.*, 1979, *241*, 2008.

Temperature variations. A 21-year-old man receiving depot injections of fluphenazine decanoate every 2 weeks died of heat stroke during a moderate heat-wave.— N. T. Forbes and E. L. Gordon, *J. Forens. Sci.*, 1976, *21*, 667. See also M. J. Craft (letter), *Br. med. J.*, 1977, *1*, 835.

Withdrawal. Reduction of very high doses of fluphenazine was associated with development of severe extrapyramidal symptoms which resolved on administration of antiparkinsonian therapy and on raising the fluphenazine dosage.— N. Polvan, *Dis. nerv. Syst.*, 1970, *Suppl.* 9, 48.

Further references: N. Capstick, *Acta psychiat. scand.*, 1980, *61*, 256.

Absorption and Fate. For an account of the absorption and fate of a phenothiazine, see Chlorpromazine, p.1513.

Fluphenazine decanoate and fluphenazine enanthate are very slowly absorbed from the site of subcutaneous or intramuscular injection. They both gradually release fluphenazine into the body and are therefore suitable for use as depot injections.

The plasma half-life of fluphenazine after a single dose was 14.7 hours in 1 patient given the hydrochloride by mouth and 14.9 and 15.3 hours in 2 patients given the hydrochloride by intramuscular injection. The half-life was 3.6 and 3.7 days in 2 patients given the enanthate intramuscularly and 9.6 and 6.8 days in 2 patients given the decanoate intramuscularly. Fluphenazine sulphoxide and 7-hydroxyfluphenazine were identified in the urine and faeces.— S. H. Curry *et al.*, *Br. J. clin. Pharmac.*, 1979, *7*, 325. See also *idem* (letter), *Lancet*, 1978, *1*, 1217.

Slow decline, over a period of several months, of plasma drug and prolactin concentrations after discontinuation of chronic treatment with fluphenazine decanoate.— B. Wistedt *et al.* (letter), *Lancet*, 1981, *1*, 1163.

Further references: D. H. Wiles and M. G. Gelder, *Br. J. clin. Pharmac.*, 1979, *8*, 565; L. E. Tune *et al.*, *Am. J. Psychiat.*, 1980, *137*, 80.

Animal studies on the relative rates of absorption of fluphenazine decanoate and enanthate, from intramuscular sites: J. Dreyfuss *et al.*, *J. pharm. Sci.*, 1976, *65*, 502.

Plasma protein binding. For the comparative protein binding of fluphenazine and other phenothiazines, see Chlorpromazine, p.1513.

Uses. Fluphenazine is a phenothiazine with actions and uses similar to those of chlorpromazine (p.1513). It has a piperazine side-chain. Fluphenazine is administered as the hydrochloride usually by mouth or as the longer-acting decanoate or enanthate esters by intramuscular or sometimes subcutaneous injection.

The usual dose of the hydrochloride for the treatment of psychoses is 1 to 5 mg daily in single or divided doses; in severe schizophrenia up to 20 mg daily has been given. Treatment is sometimes started with intramuscular injections of 1.25 mg of the hydrochloride.

The long-acting decanoate or enanthate esters of fluphenazine are usually given by deep intramuscular injection. The onset of action is usually within 1 to 3 days of injection and significant effects on psychosis are usually evident within 2 to 4 days. The initial dose of fluphenazine decanoate or enanthate is 12.5 mg intramuscularly given to patients in hospital to assess the extrapyramidal effects. A dose of 25 mg is then given every 2 weeks with subsequent adjustments in the amounts and the dosage interval according to the patient's response. Although the usual dose is 25 mg every 2 weeks, the amounts required may range from 12.5 to 100 mg and the intervals required may range from 1 or 2 weeks to 5 or 6 weeks. If doses greater than 50 mg are considered necessary cautious increments should be made in steps of 12.5 mg.

Fluphenazine hydrochloride has also been given in doses of 1 to 2 mg daily, increased if necessary to 2 to 4 mg daily, for non-psychotic emotional disturbances, such as anxiety and tension. In general, however, neuroleptics are only suitable for such purposes in resistant conditions where more appropriate agents, such as the benzodiazepines (see Diazepam, p.1523) have proved ineffective. If their use is judged to be necessary, treatment should be directed at low dosages given on a short-term basis.

Fluphenazine should be given in reduced dosage to elderly patients.

Administration. A study substantiating earlier findings of a higher incidence of side-effects in patients receiving long-term intramuscular fluphenazine decanoate therapy than in those receiving fluphenazine by mouth.— A. Rifkin *et al.*, *Archs gen. Psychiat.*, 1977, *34*, 1215. See also D. C. Watt (letter), *Lancet*, 1978, *2*, 1045.

A study of the plasma concentrations of fluphenazine following intramuscular injection of 25 mg of the decanoate in 2 subjects and intramuscular injection of 25 mg of the enanthate in a further 2 subjects. The decanoate gave an early peak in keeping with its use in acute psychotic states whereas the enanthate gave its highest concentrations after 2 to 5 days.— S. H. Curry *et al.* (letter), *Lancet*, 1978, *1*, 1217.

In the elderly. Despite statements to the contrary fluphenazine decanoate and flupenthixol decanoate have a definite place in the treatment of paranoid psychosis in the elderly provided there is no serious degree of dementia and adequate community facilities are available.— T. Whitehead (letter), *Br. med. J.*, 1975, *2*, 502.

Fluphenazine decanoate 12.5 mg every 2 weeks is usually adequate to control disturbed behaviour in elderly patients and meets the social need for treatment.— M. F. Green (letter), *Br. med. J.*, 1977, *2*, 1027.

Alcohol and drug withdrawal. A report of fluphenazine decanoate being of benefit in alcoholism.— E. H. Bennie and H. G. Kinnell (letter), *Lancet*, 1975, *2*, 1303.

Anxiety. Fluphenazine as a depot preparation, in fortnightly doses of 12.5 mg, had been successfully used for the treatment of refractory anxiety.— A. R. Cook (letter), *Br. med. J.*, 1976, *2*, 700.

Further references: H. Hakkarainen, *Headache*, 1977, *17*, 216 (tension headache).

Behaviour disorders. Ten adolescent girls, disturbed, violent, and aggressive, had been treated for up to a year with fluphenazine decanoate 12.5 to 25 mg or flupenthixol decanoate 20 to 40 mg with benefit both at weekly to monthly intervals; 3 had been able to cease treatment.— M. S. Perinpanayagam and R. A. Haig (letter), *Br. med. J.*, 1977, *1*, 835. See also H. G. Kinnell (letter), *ibid.*, 1977, *2*, 578.

Further references: E. Arnold and D. W. Maginn, *Med. J. Aust.*, 1967, *1*, 758.

Chorea. In a double-blind study in 9 patients, fluphenazine decanoate injection was more effective than a placebo in reducing chorea.— C. F. Terrence, *Curr. ther. Res.*, 1976, *20*, 177.

Further references: J. R. Whittier and C. Korenyi, *Int. J. Neuropsychiat.*, 1968, *4*, 1.

Pain. For references to the use of fluphenazine in neurological pain, see Amitriptyline Hydrochloride, p.114.

Schizophrenia. In the treatment of 91 patients with schizophrenia, a dosage of 25 mg of fluphenazine enanthate by injection every 3 or 4 weeks produced fewer side-effects than 12.5 mg weekly. The best results were achieved in patients with paranoid schizophrenia. Eighteen patients discontinued treatment, in 9 of them because of extrapyramidal side-effects. Acute side-effects were controlled by procyclidine, benzhexol, or promethazine, as appropriate. Fluphenazine enanthate was a useful long-term prophylactic measure against relapse in the chronic paranoid schizophrenic and to a lesser extent in the hebephrenic schizophrenic.— M. W. P. Carney (letter), *Br. med. J.*, 1969, *1*, 121.

Of 70 patients with schizophrenia treated with fluphenazine enanthate or decanoate 46 were being adequately controlled. Reasons for discontinuing treatment included depression, severe extrapyramidal side-effects, excessive drowsiness, lack of cooperation, and inadequate response or psychotic relapse.— G. O. Dubourg (letter), *Br. med. J.*, 1972, *3*, 703.

Patients with chronic schizophrenia controlled for at least 8 weeks by fluphenazine decanoate 25 mg or more per month were studied under double-blind conditions. Of 38 whose continued treatment for 9 months was a placebo 66% relapsed, compared with 8% whose continued treatment consisted of fluphenazine decanoate, usually 25 mg once a month. When the period of observation was continued for a further 6 months, 2 or 3 more of those treated with active medication relapsed, giving an overall relapse-rate of 14 to 17%. Fewer patients receiving active treatment needed antidepressants. Patients receiving fluphenazine tended to need more treatment for parkinsonism but the difference was not significant. Because the trial included only those who had already been controlled for at least 8 weeks it was considered that the proportion of patients in whom fluphenazine decanoate would fail to provide adequate long-term control would be more than 30%.— S. R. Hirsch *et al.*, *Br. med. J.*, 1973, *1*, 633 (Report to the MRC Committee on Clinical Trials in Psychiatry). Criticisms.— G. R. Daniel and A. A. Schiff, *Squibb* (letter), *ibid.*, 1973, *2*, 244.

The relapse-rate in 1 year in patients in remission from schizophrenia was 68% (15 of 22) when taking placebo compared with 10% (5 of 51) in those taking fluphenazine hydrochloride or decanoate. Maintenance treatment should therefore be given for at least a year. Eight of 23 patients given fluphenazine decanoate had their medication withdrawn because of akinesia. Study was necessary to see whether a dose less than 12.5 mg every 2 weeks would be adequate.— A. Rifkin *et al.*, *Archs gen. Psychiat.*, 1977, *34*, 43.

Further references: T. Jovanović and A. Marković, *Br. J. Psychiat.*, 1972, *120*, 223; D. A. W. Johnson and H. Freeman, *Practitioner*, 1972, *208*, 395; S. H. Curry and L. Adamson (letter), *Lancet*, 1972, *2*, 543; A. Keskiner, *Curr. ther. Res.*, 1973, *15*, 305; S. L. Carder and J. Snibbe, *ibid.*, 589; P. F. Marriott *et al.*, *Med. J. Aust.*, 1973, *2*, 957; G. Weiser *et al.*, *Wien. med. Wschr.*, 1973, *123*, 227; H. Christodoulidis, *Curr. ther. Res.*, 1974, *16*, 311; F. S. Abuzzahab, *Psychopharmac. Bull.*, 1977, *13*, 71; R. A. Devito *et al.*, *J. clin. Psychiat.*, 1978, *39*, 26; P. Marriott and A. Hiep, *ibid.*, 206; F. Quitkin *et al.*, *Archs gen. Psychiat.*, 1978, *35*, 889; G. E. Hogarty *et al.*, *ibid.*, 1979, *36*, 1283; A. Knights *et al.*, *Br. J. Psychiat.*, 1979, *135*, 515; R. Pinto *et al.*, *Acta psychiat. scand.*, 1979, *60*, 313; M. Raskind *et al.*, *Am. J. geriat. Soc.*, 1979, *27*, 459.

High-dose therapy. A review of megadose therapy with fluphenazine using dosage regimens ranging from 0.8 to 1.2 g daily (equivalent to chlorpromazine 40 to 60 g daily). Three studies in chronic schizophrenics who were long-term hospital in-patients showed some improvement with megadose therapy. In acute patients, however, who had not responded to at least 6 weeks of standard treatment but who had been in hospital for less than 2 months, a better response was obtained in those given 30 mg daily than in those given 1.2 g daily, indicating that schizophrenics should not be considered refractory after only 6 weeks of treatment. The value of megadose therapy in long-term patients remains problematic since a limited degree of improvement may not be worth the increased risk of tardive dyskinesia. One remarkable finding in all studies is that such enormous doses are relatively well tolerated; the increase in extrapyramidal side-effects, typically seen as the dose approaches 30 mg daily, reaches a plateau or diminishes.— A. Rifkin and F. Quitkin, *Bull. N.Y. Acad. Med.*, 1978, *54*, 869.

Further references: F. J. Ayd, *Int. Drug Ther. Newslett.*, 1972, *7*, 25; F. N. I. Fawzy *et al.* (letter), *Br. med. J.*, 1972, *2*, 114; G. M. Simpson (letter), *ibid.*, 1972, *3*, 293; F. Quitkin *et al.*, *Archs gen. Psychiat.*, 1975, *32*, 1276; A. Rifkin *et al.*, *Archs gen. Psychiat.*, 1971, *25*, 398; H. A. McClelland *et al.*, *Archs gen. Psychiat.*, 1976, *33*, 1435; P. T. Donlon *et al.*, *J. clin. Psychiat.*, 1978, *39*, 800; E. W. Fünfgeld and F. Kulhanek, *Arzneimittel-Forsch.*, 1978, *28*, 1489.

Preparations of Fluphenazine Salts and Esters

Elixirs and Oral Solutions

Fluphenazine Hydrochloride Elixir *(U.S.P.)*. An elixir containing fluphenazine hydrochloride and alcohol 13.5 to 15%. pH 5.3 to 5.8. Store in airtight containers. Protect from light.

Fluphenazine Hydrochloride Oral Solution *(U.S.P.)*. An aqueous solution of fluphenazine hydrochloride. pH 4 to 5. To be diluted before use. Store in airtight containers. Protect from light.

Injections

Fluphenazine Decanoate Injection *(B.P.)*. A sterile solution of fluphenazine decanoate in sesame oil. Sterilised by filtration. For intramuscular use only. Protect from light.

Fluphenazine Enanthate Injection *(B.P.)*. A sterile solution of fluphenazine enanthate in sesame oil. Sterilised by filtration. For intramuscular use only. Protect from light.

Fluphenazine Enanthate Injection *(U.S.P.)*. A sterile solution in a suitable vegetable oil.

Fluphenazine Hydrochloride Injection *(U.S.P.)*. A sterile solution in Water for Injections. pH 4.8 to 5.2. Protect from light.

Tablets

Fluphenazine Hydrochloride Tablets *(U.S.P.)*. Tablets containing fluphenazine hydrochloride. Store in airtight containers.

Fluphenazine Tablets *(B.P.)*. Tablets containing fluphenazine hydrochloride. They are sugar-coated.

Proprietary Preparations of Fluphenazine Salts and Esters

Modecate *(Squibb, UK)*. Fluphenazine decanoate, available as **Injection** containing 25 mg per ml in sesame oil, in ampoules of 0.5, 1, and 2 ml, disposable syringes of 1 and 2 ml, and vials of 10 ml; also available as **Concentrate Injection** containing 100 mg per ml, in ampoules of 0.5 and 1 ml. (Also available as Modecate in *Austral.*, *Fr.*, *S.Afr.*, *Spain*).

Moditen *(Squibb, UK)*. Fluphenazine hydrochloride, available as tablets of 1, 2.5, and 5 mg. (Also available as Moditen in *Belg.*, *Canad.*, *Fr.*, *Neth.*, *Switz.*).

Moditen Enanthate Injection *(Squibb, UK)*. A long-acting injection containing fluphenazine enanthate 25 mg per ml in sesame oil, in ampoules of 1 ml and vials of 10 ml. (Also available as Moditen Enanthate in *Canad.*).

Other Proprietary Names of Fluphenazine Salts and Esters

Austral.—Anatensol; *Belg.*—Anatensol, Permitil, Sevinol; *Denm.*—Pacinol; *Fr.*—Moditen Retard; *Ger.*—Dapotum, Lyogen, Omca; *Ital.*—Anatensol; Moditen Depot; *Jap.*—Anatenazine; *Neth.*—Anatensol; *Norw.*—Pacinol, Siqualone; *S.Afr.*—Anatensol; *Spain*—Eutimox; *Swed.*—Pacinol, Siqualone; *Switz.*—Dapotum, Lyogen; *USA*—Permitil, Prolixin.

7049-a

Fluspirilene.

McN-JR-6218; R 6218. 8-[4,4-Bis(4-fluorophenyl)butyl]-1-phenyl-1,3,8-triazaspiro[4.5]decan-4-one.

$C_{29}H_{31}F_2N_3O$=475.6.

CAS — 1841-19-6.

A white to yellowish amorphous or crystalline powder. M.p. about 190°. Practically **insoluble** in water; freely soluble in chloroform; sparingly soluble in acetone; slightly soluble in alcohol and ether.

Adverse Effects. The side-effects of fluspirilene, such as sedation, extrapyramidal symptoms, and tardive dyskinesia, which are the result of its pharmacological action, are similar to those of chlorpromazine (p.1509).

Sedation may be less likely than with chlorpromazine, whereas extrapyramidal reactions may be more common, occurring within about 6 to 12 hours of injection and disappearing within about 48 hours. Restlessness, excitement, and electrocardiogram changes have also been noted.

Other side-effects include skin rashes and nodules at the site of injection.

Of 24 patients who had been given fluspirilene injections weekly, 8 had deep subcutaneous lumps at the injection site; in a further 4 patients increased pressure was necessary to give the injection. Biopsy in one patient showed necrosis probably caused by precipitation of crystalline fluspirilene.— R. G. McCreadie *et al.*, *Br. med. J.*, 1979, *1*, 523.

Treatment of Adverse Effects. As for Chlorpromazine, p.1511.

Precautions. As for Chlorpromazine, p.1512.

Absorption and Fate. Fluspirilene is slowly absorbed after intramuscular injection of a microcrystalline aqueous suspension, detectable blood concentrations being reached within 4 hours of injection. It is rapidly metabolised on release from the injection site and the main metabolite, which is 4,4-bis(4-fluorophenyl)butyric acid obtained by *N*-dealkylation, is excreted in the urine.

Uses. Fluspirilene is a member of the diphenylbutylpiperidine group of antipsychotic agents which are structurally similar to the butyrophenones (see haloperidol, p.1532). When given by deep intramuscular injection it has a prolonged duration of action which lasts for about a week, with a range of 5 to 15 days.

The usual dose of fluspirilene for the treatment of schizophrenia is 2 mg weekly by deep intramuscular injection, increased by 2 mg weekly according to the patient's response. The usual maintenance dose is 2 to 8 mg weekly but in resistant conditions up to 12 mg weekly may be required. The maximum recommended dose is 20 mg weekly. Accumulation of fluspirilene, with signs of overdosage, may be managed by omission of one in 4 or 5 weekly injections.

Action. Studies on the mode of action of fluspirilene.— N. -E. Andén *et al.*, *Eur. J. Pharmac.*, 1970, *11*, 303; P. A. J. Janssen *et al.*, *Arzneimittel-Forsch.*, 1970, *20*, 1689.

Anxiety and depression. Fluspirilene 2 to 4 mg weekly given intramuscularly to 8 resistant neurotic patients was reported to be of value in patients with paranoid, depressive, or phobic symptoms associated with behavioural irritability, but not for patients whose symptoms were entirely subjective.— E. H. Bennie (letter), *Br. med. J.*, 1976, *1*, 1404.

Four patients with anxiety neurosis, anxiety state, or anorexia nervosa responded favourably to fluspirilene.— M. Trimble (letter), *Br. med. J.*, 1977, *2*, 1541.

Further references: J. Pach and W. Waniek, *Arzneimittel-Forsch.*, 1976, *26*, 1189; F. Goffioul *et al.*, *Acta Ther.*, 1977, *3*, 319.

Schizophrenia. A review of fluspirilene in the treatment of schizophrenia.— *Drug & Ther. Bull.*, 1977, *15*, 59.

Studies of fluspirilene in the treatment of schizophrenia.— J. St-Laurent *et al.*, *Curr. ther. Res.*, 1972, *14*, 599; R. G. Bankier, *J. clin. Pharmac.*, 1973, *13*, 44; K. Winter *et al.*, *Br. J. clin. Pract.*, 1973, *27*, 377; S. D. Soni, *Curr. med. Res. Opinion*, 1977, *4*, 645; G. Pinard and D. Rosales, *Curr. ther. Res.*, 1980, *27*, 419.

Proprietary Preparations

Redeptin *(Smith Kline & French, UK)*. Fluspirilene, available as an injection containing 2 mg per ml, in ampoules of 1 and 3 ml, and vials of 6 ml.

Other Proprietary Names

Imap *(Arg., Belg., Canad., Denm., Ger., Neth., Norw., Switz.)*.

7050-e

Halazepam.

Sch 12041. 7-Chloro-1,3-dihydro-5-phenyl-1-(2,2,2-trifluoroethyl)-2*H*-1,4-benzodiazepin-2-one.

$C_{17}H_{12}ClF_3N_2O$=352.7.

CAS — 23092-17-3.

Halazepam is a benzodiazepine with general properties similar to those of diazepam (p.1519). It has been given in doses of 40 mg two to four times daily for the treatment of anxiety.

The uses and toxicity of halazepam.— *Drugs of the Future*, 1978, *3*, 109.

Further references: *Drugs Today*, 1975, *11*, 191.

Administration. In the elderly. A study on the effects of halazepam and diazepam on the motor coordination of geriatric subjects.— M. A. Gagnon *et al.*, *Eur. J. clin. Pharmac.*, 1977, *11*, 443.

Alcohol and drug withdrawal. Study of the efficacy of halazepam in alleviating anxiety in 10 patients with chronic alcoholism.— K. Y. Ota *et al.*, *Curr. ther. Res.*, 1971, *13*, 463.

Anxiety. Results of a double-blind placebo-controlled study completed by 125 anxious patients comparing diazepam 20 mg daily with halazepam 160 mg daily. Highly anxious patients improved significantly more on both active drugs than on placebo but less anxious patients did particularly poorly on halazepam. In future studies halazepam should be used in a daily dosage not in excess of 120 mg for most anxious patients and a daily dose of 160 mg should be reserved only for those with rather severe and incapacitating symptoms.— K. Rickels *et al.*, *Psychopharmacology*, 1977, *52*, 129.

Further references: W. E. Fann *et al.*, *Curr. ther. Res.*, 1974, *16*, 1281; R. Kellner *et al.*, *J. clin. Pharmac.*, 1978, *18*, 203; S. Zisook *et al.*, *J. clin. Psychiat.*, 1978, *39*, 683; S. Zisook and P. J. Rogers, *Curr. ther. Res.*,

1978, *23,* 502; S. Zisook *et al., Curr. ther. Res.,* 1978, *23,* 403.

Manufacturers
Schering, USA.

7051-l

Haloperidol *(B.P., U.S.P.).* Haloperidolum; R 1625. 4-[4-(4-Chlorophenyl)-4-hydroxypiperidino]-4′-fluorobutyrophenone.
$C_{21}H_{23}ClFNO_2$=375.9.

CAS — 52-86-8.

Pharmacopoeias. In *Br., Braz., Chin., Fr., Jap., Nord.,* and *U.S.*

A white to faintly yellowish, odourless, tasteless, amorphous or microcrystalline powder. M.p. 147° to 152°.

Practically **insoluble** in water; soluble 1 in 50 to 60 of alcohol, 1 in 15 to 20 of chloroform, 1 in 200 of ether, 1 in 55 of ethyl acetate, 1 in 200 of isopropyl alcohol, and 1 in 55 of methyl alcohol. A saturated solution is neutral to litmus. Solutions are **sterilised** by filtration. **Store** in airtight containers. Protect from light.

Haloperidol was a weak monovalent base which formed a stable hydrochloride. In the presence of 1% lactic acid or tartaric acid, stable solutions in water could be prepared containing up to 20 mg per ml. Solutions for oral administration containing 2 mg of haloperidol per ml could be prepared by dissolving in purified water with a slight excess of lactic acid. The solution should be protected from sunlight or bright daylight and could be preserved with methyl hydroxybenzoate 0.19%. Solutions for intramuscular or intravenous injections containing 5 mg per ml could be prepared by dissolving in Water for Injections containing 0.5% of lactic acid. Methyl hydroxybenzoate 500 µg and propyl hydroxybenzoate 50 µg per ml could be added as preservative. The solution should be sterilised by filtration and stored in 1-ml amber glass ampoules. The solution had a pH of about 3.2 and was slightly hypo-osmotic. Haloperidol preparations were stable except that when exposed to light, solutions became discoloured after a few hours of exposure and deposited a greyish-red precipitate after several weeks.— P. J. A. W. Demoen, *J. pharm Sci.,* 1961, *50,* 350.

Adverse Effects. The side-effects of haloperidol, such as sedation, extrapyramidal symptoms, and tardive dyskinesia, which are a result of its pharmacological action, are similar to those of chlorpromazine (p.1509).

Extrapyramidal symptoms may be more common than those associated with chlorpromazine, whereas it may be less likely to cause hypotension, has fewer adverse effects on the heart, and causes less sedation.

Occasional photosensitive skin reactions have been reported. Adverse effects on the liver are not common, but an increased incidence has been reported with very high doses.

Effects on the blood. *Agranulocytosis.* Although severe haematological effects are rare, agranulocytosis has been reported in association with haloperidol.— *Med. Lett.,* 1975, *17,* 11.

Further references: N. R. Cutler and J. F. Heiser, *J. Am. med. Ass.,* 1979, *242,* 2872.

Effects on the endocrine system. Galactorrhoea has been reported in patients taking haloperidol.— G. M. Besser and C. R. W. Edwards, *Br. med. J.,* 1972, *2,* 280.

Inappropriate secretion of antidiuretic hormone in a woman taking haloperidol.— F. Matuk and K. Kalyanaraman, *Archs Neurol.,* 1977, *34,* 374. See also V. Peck and L. Shenkman, *Clin. Pharmac. Ther.,* 1979, *26,* 442.

Further references: A. Forsman and R. Öhman, *Curr. ther. Res.,* 1978, *24,* 179; E. D. Caine *et al., J. nerv. ment. Dis.,* 1979, *167,* 504; R. Öhman *et al., Curr. ther. Res.,* 1980, *27,* 137.

Effects on the eyes. There was a risk that the butyrophenones might cause opacities of the cornea and lens or pigmentation.— *Japan med. Gaz.,* 1974, *11* (Feb. 20), 10.

Effects on the heart. Aside from occasionally causing some mild hypotension, haloperidol does not cause adverse cardiovascular effects. Unlike many phenothiazine neuroleptics, it rarely produces ECG changes.— F. Ayd, *J. clin. Psychiat.,* 1978, *39,* 807.

A study in 25 schizophrenic patients in good physical health, demonstrated a high degree of cardiovascular safety for healthy subjects who require treatment with moderate doses of haloperidol intramuscularly at intervals of 30 minutes. Nevertheless, it is prudent to assume that the risk of cardiovascular effects may be greater in elderly psychotic patients, and all patients who are medically ill, particularly with cardiovascular disease.— P. T. Donlan *et al., Am. J. Psychiat.,* 1979, *136,* 233.

Cardiac arrhythmias in a 21-year-old man following rapid tranquillisation with haloperidol.— D. Mehta *et al., Am. J. Psychiat.,* 1979, *136,* 1468.

Effects on the liver. Cholestatic hepatitis has occurred in patients taking haloperidol.— *Med. Lett.,* 1975, *17,* 11.

Raised serum alkaline phosphatase concentrations in 7 of 10 patients receiving very high doses of haloperidol.— R. G. McCreadie and I. M. MacDonald, *Br. J. Psychiat.,* 1977, *131,* 310.

Further references: J. Gerlach *et al., Acta psychiat. scand.,* 1974, *50,* 410.

Effects on mental state. Akathisia (a desire to keep moving), dysphoria, and anxiety in healthy subjects given single doses of haloperidol 5 mg.— B. G. Anderson *et al.* (letter), *New Engl. J. Med.,* 1981, *305,* 643.

Catatonia. A syndrome marked by features of catatonia and parkinsonism developed in 5 patients taking high doses of haloperidol; differentiation from worsening schizophrenia was important. The syndrome responded to treatment with amantadine.— A. J. Gelenberg and M. R. Mandel, *Archs gen. Psychiat.,* 1977, *34,* 947.

Further references: D. R. Weinberger and M. J. Kelly, *J. nerv. ment. Dis.,* 1977, *165,* 263; Q. R. Regestein *et al., J. Am. med. Ass.,* 1977, *238,* 618.

Depression. Three patients given haloperidol for Gilles de la Tourette's syndrome suffered severe dysphoria, with symptoms which included sadness, crying, loss of energy, depression, despondency, drowsiness, lack of motivation, and substantial weight gain. Among a group of 72 patients treated, 3 others experienced similar, though less well documented responses to haloperidol.— E. D. Caine and R. J. Polinsky, *Am. J. Psychiat.,* 1979, *136,* 1216.

Encephalopathy. A report of encephalopathy in a 19-year-old man in association with high-dose haloperidol therapy; he had also received lithium, but similar forms of encephalopathy have also been noted in patients receiving high-dose haloperidol alone.— H. R. Veits, *Milit. Med.,* 1978, *143,* 201.

Paranoia. Administration of haloperidol 10 mg daily to a 14-year-old boy with Gilles de la Tourette's syndrome was associated with episodes of paranoid ideation and depersonalisation.— J. Feldman (letter), *Am. J. Psychiat.,* 1977, *134,* 99.

Effects on the nervous system. Neurological symptoms of drug intoxication was attributed to haloperidol in 3 patients suffering from renal failure.— G. Richet *et al., Br. med. J.,* 1970, *2,* 394.

A severe neurotoxic reaction occurred in a 74-year-old thyrotoxic patient given haloperidol.— K. Hamadah and A. F. Teggin (letter), *Lancet,* 1974, *2,* 1019. A similar report.— S. Yosselson and A. Kaplan (letter), *New Engl. J. Med.,* 1975, *293,* 201.

Effects on sexual function. Comment on the possible impairment of male sexual function by butyrophenones.— J. D. Horowitz and A. J. Goble, *Drugs,* 1979, *18,* 206.

Extrapyramidal effects. The Boston Collaborative Drug Surveillance Program monitored consecutively 32 812 medical in-patients. Drug-induced extrapyramidal symptoms occurred in 2 of 154 patients given a butyrophenone.— J. Porter and H. Jick, *Lancet,* 1977, *1,* 587.

A report of 2 patients receiving haloperidol who developed respiratory distress, possibly due to laryngeal dystonia; one had become cyanotic. The symptoms were alleviated by administration of diphenhydramine and did not recur on maintenance benztropine therapy.— J. A. Flaherty and H. W. Lahmeyer, *Am. J. Psychiat.,* 1978, *135,* 1414.

An acute dystonic syndrome in a 12-year-old girl given sodium cromoglycate with haloperidol 1.5 mg twice daily. Control was with diazepam 7.5 mg given intravenously.— M. L. P. Gross (letter), *Lancet,* 1980, *2,* 479. See also under Uses (Administration in Children).

Further references: J. Wålinder and A. Carlsson (letter), *Br. med. J.,* 1973, *1,* 551; D. E. Huttenbach (letter), *Am. J. Psychiat.,* 1977, *134,* 820.

Tardive dyskinesia. Tardive dyskinesia developed in a 57-year-old woman after receiving haloperidol at a dose never exceeding 10 mg daily for 30 weeks. The symptoms disappeared within 12 weeks of withdrawal of haloperidol.— G. L. Stimmel, *Am. J. Hosp. Pharm.,* 1976, *33,* 961.

A double-blind crossover study of the incidence of tardive dyskinesia in 16 elderly psychiatric patients during and following treatment with haloperidol and other antipsychotic agents.— J. Gerlach and H. Simmelsgaard, *Psychopharmacology,* 1978, *59,* 105.

Further references: L. K. Petty and C. J. Spar, *Am. J. Psychiat.,* 1980, *137,* 745.

Hyperpyrexia. A 30-year-old man receiving high-dose parenteral haloperidol therapy for withdrawal symptoms following barbiturate and methaqualone abuse, developed fatal hyperthermia.— D. J. Greenblatt *et al., J. clin. Psychiat.,* 1978, *39,* 673.

Hypotension. For a comment on the mild degree of hypotension associated with haloperidol therapy, see under Effects on the Heart (above).

Overdosage. Symptoms in 2 young siblings who took an overdose of haloperidol included hypothermia; unexpected bradycardia was considered to be associated with the hypothermia.— J. V. K. Scialli and W. E. Thornton, *J. Am. med. Ass.,* 1978, *239,* 48.

Three children admitted to hospital with haloperidol overdosage had become drowsy, restless, and confused. They had marked extrapyramidal symptoms which included slurred speech, difficulty in swallowing, parkinsonian face, contracted masseter muscles, opisthotonus, hand tremors, and akathisia. The symptoms subsided within a few hours of biperiden administration.— C. A. Sinaniotis *et al., J. Pediat.,* 1978, *93,* 1038.

About 36 hours after taking an estimated 15 to 20 mg of haloperidol a 22-month-old child suffered a severe hypertensive episode that required 5 days' therapy with hydralazine. Because of the delayed onset and the severity of the hypertension children should be observed in the hospital for at least 2 days after taking an overdose of haloperidol.— D. G. Cummingham, *J. Pediat.,* 1979, *95,* 489. For another report mentioning hypertension in a child following haloperidol administration, see under Uses (Administration in Children).

Pregnancy and the neonate. *Early pregnancy.* There was no evidence of teratogenicity in a study of 98 pregnant women who had been treated for up to several weeks with haloperidol 600 µg twice daily for hyperemesis gravidarum. Ninety patients had received haloperidol during the first trimester.— A. V. Waes and E. Van de Velde, *J. clin. Pharmac.,* 1969, *9,* 224.

In a retrospective survey 31 women who had borne children with severe reduction deformities did not recall taking haloperidol during pregnancy.— J. W. Hanson and G. P. Oakley (letter), *J. Am. med. Ass.,* 1975, *231,* 26. Comment.— *ibid.,* 69.

Individual reports of malformations in infants exposed to haloperidol.— P. Dieulangard *et al., Bull. Féd. Socs Gynéc. Obstét. Lang. fr.,* 1966, *18,* 85; A. E. Kopelman *et al., J. Am. med. Ass.,* 1975, *231,* 62.

See also under Precautions.

Sudden death. A woman admitted to hospital with acute psychosis died suddenly following attempts at rapid tranquillisation with high doses of haloperidol. She received 50 mg on the first day, 70 mg on the second, and 140 mg on the third. On the fourth day she was given 80 mg over 4 hours; 2 hours later she died.— R. Ketai *et al., Am. J. Psychiat.,* 1979, *136,* 112.

Tardive dyskinesia. See under Extrapyramidal Effects (above).

Treatment of Adverse Effects. As for Chlorpromazine, p.1511.

Precautions. As for Chlorpromazine, p.1512.

Severe dystonic reactions have followed the use of haloperidol, particularly in children and adolescents. It should therefore be used with extreme care in children. Haloperidol may also cause severe neurotoxic reactions in patients with hyperthyroidism. Haloperidol must be used with extreme caution in patients receiving lithium.

Haloperidol, given in five 500-µg doses over 36 hours, had little effect on low-speed tests of driving ability.— T. A. Betts *et al., Br. med. J.,* 1972, *4,* 580.

Hyperthyroidism. A 43-year-old woman with hyperthyroidism and an acute psychosis developed a severe dystonic reaction to haloperidol therapy. She was salivating and tremulous and complained of difficulty in swallowing fluids and solid foods and subsequently died of aspiration asphyxia. Several reports in the literature suggest that hyperthyroidism enhances the neurotoxic effects of haloperidol. Moreover, the development of a severe extrapyramidal reaction to haloperidol may suggest undiagnosed hyperthyroidism.— M. F. Weiner, *Am. J. Psychiat.*, 1979, *136*, 717.

Interactions. *Anticoagulants.* For a possible effect of haloperidol on anticoagulant control, see Phenindione, p.773.

Beverages. For controversy on a possible interaction between neuroleptic therapy and tea or coffee, see Chlorpromazine, p.1512.

Lithium. For possible interactions between haloperidol and lithium, see Lithium Carbonate, p.1539.

Methyldopa. For a report of dementia in 2 patients receiving methyldopa following concurrent administration of haloperidol, see Methyldopa, p.153.

Phenytoin and other anticonvulsants. A 55-year-old man who had been receiving phenytoin 300 mg daily for over 3 years and who was suffering from stable tardive dyskinesia which had been induced by haloperidol (discontinued 2 years previously) obtained amelioration of his symptoms on discontinuation of phenytoin for a week. On reintroduction of phenytoin the dyskinesia relapsed to its original severity. Phenytoin might exacerbate neuroleptic-induced dyskinesia.— J. DeVaugh-Geiss (letter), *New Engl. J. Med.*, 1978, *298*, 457. Criticism.— P. A. Nausieda *et al.* (letter), *ibid.*, 1093.

Evidence to suggest that concomitant anticonvulsant medication (phenobarbitone and phenytoin) significantly reduces plasma-haloperidol concentrations. Plasma concentrations of the anticonvulsants were not affected.— M. Linnoila *et al.*, *Am. J. Psychiat.*, 1980, *137*, 819.

Myasthenia gravis. Although haloperidol has not been implicated clinically, it has been shown experimentally to interfere with neuromuscular transmission, and should be used with caution in patients with myasthenia.— Z. Argov and F. L. Mastaglia, *New Engl. J. Med.*, 1979, *301*, 409.

Pregnancy and the neonate. *Excretion in breast milk.* Concentrations of haloperidol in the expressed breast milk of a woman receiving haloperidol were similar to observed therapeutic plasma concentrations in pharmacokinetic studies.— R. B. Stewart *et al.*, *Am. J. Psychiat.*, 1980, *137*, 849. See also L. J. Whalley *et al.* (letter), *Br. med. J.*, 1981, *282*, 1746.

See also under Adverse Effects.

Absorption and Fate. Haloperidol is readily absorbed from the gastro-intestinal tract. It is metabolised in the liver and is excreted in the urine and faeces; there is evidence of enterohepatic recycling. Owing to the first-pass effect of metabolism in the liver, plasma concentrations following oral administration are lower than those following intramuscular administration. Moreover, there is wide intersubject variation in plasma concentrations of haloperidol, but in practice, no simple correlation has been found between plasma concentrations of haloperidol and its therapeutic effect. Paths of metabolism of haloperidol include oxidative *N*-dealkylation. Haloperidol has been reported to have a plasma half-life ranging from about 13 to nearly 40 hours; its plasma half-life is prolonged during the night. Haloperidol is very extensively bound to plasma proteins. It is widely distributed in the body and crosses the blood-brain barrier.

Peak plasma-haloperidol concentrations of up to 1.5% of a 2-mg tritiated dose were detected at 3 to 6 hours in 4 healthy subjects and 4 schizophrenic patients. About 26% was excreted in the urine by the healthy subjects and 20% by the patients in the first 5 days; by the third day about 15% had been excreted in the faeces. The amount excreted in the urine increased to 29% in the schizophrenic patients after 29 days treatment with haloperidol.— P. C. Johnson *et al.* (preliminary report), *Int. J. Neuropsychiat.*, 1967, *3*, *Suppl.* 1, S24.

Studies in 36 healthy men using radioactive haloperidol showed that after a 2-mg intramuscular injection, peak plasma concentrations were reached within 20 minutes. The half-life was 20.7 hours (range 12.8 to 35.5 hours).— W. A. Cressman *et al.*, *Eur. J. clin. Pharmac.*, 1974, *7*, 99.

A study in 10 healthy subjects demonstrated that haloperidol has a serum half-life ranging from about 10 to 19 hours following intravenous administration, and 12 to 36 hours following oral administration. It had an oral bioavailability of about 60%. In addition to evidence of enterohepatic recycling of the drug, there was some evidence of extrahepatic metabolism.— A. Forsman and R. Öhman, *Curr. ther. Res.*, 1976, *20*, 319. A study in psychiatric in-patients demonstrated that the biological half-life of haloperidol was of the same order as in healthy subjects; elimination was slower during the night. Bioavailability may have been as high as 70%. Measurement of plasma concentrations suggested that a therapeutic concentration in serum could be 3 to 10 ng per ml for many patients, but for some, considerably higher concentrations could be required, possibly due to pharmacodynamic variations.— *idem*, 1977, *21*, 396.

Further references: A. Coutselinis *et al.*, *Clin. Chem.*, 1977, *23*, 900 (plasma concentrations in acute intoxication); T. B. Cooper, *Clin. Pharmacokinet.*, 1978, *3*, 14 (plasma concentrations); S. E. Ericksen *et al.*, *Psychopharmac. Bull.*, 1978, *14*, 15 (plasma concentrations); G. Bianchetti *et al.*, *Int. J. clin. Pharmac.*, 1980, *18*, 324 (plasma concentrations).

Metabolism. 4-Fluorobenzoylpropionic acid and 4-fluorophenylaceturic acid were identified as urinary metabolites of haloperidol; neither appeared to have antipsychotic activity.— A. Forsman *et al.*, *Curr. ther. Res.*, 1977, *21*, 606.

Plasma protein binding. Haloperidol was about 92% bound to plasma proteins.— A. Forsman and R. Öhman, *Curr. ther. Res.*, 1977, *21*, 245.

Further references: F. J. Rowell *et al.*, *Br. J. clin. Pharmac.*, 1981, *11*, 377.

Uses. Haloperidol is a butyrophenone with actions and uses similar to those of the phenothiazine, chlorpromazine (p.1513). Haloperidol 2 mg is reported to be approximately equivalent in action to chlorpromazine 100 mg.

The usual dose for the treatment of psychoses is 0.5 to 5 mg twice or thrice daily. In severe psychoses or resistant patients doses of up to 100 mg daily may be required; in very high dose therapy doses of 200 mg daily have been used. For the control of acute conditions haloperidol may be given intramuscularly in doses of 2 to 10 mg, subsequent doses of 5 mg may be given up to every hour until symptoms are controlled; dosage intervals of 4 to 8 hours may be adequate. Up to 30 mg intramuscularly may be required for the emergency control of very severely disturbed patients, and considerably higher doses have been employed for mania.

For the control of nausea and vomiting the usual dose of haloperidol by mouth is 1 mg twice daily. The usual intramuscular dose is 1 to 2 mg every 12 hours. Haloperidol has also been given intravenously.

Haloperidol is used in the management of Gilles de la Tourette's syndrome; a suitable dosage is reported to be up to about 10 mg daily, but requirements vary considerably and the dose must be very carefully adjusted to obtain the optimum response.

Doses of 500 µg twice daily have also been used for non-psychotic emotional disturbances, such as anxiety and tension. In general, however, like phenothiazines, the butyrophenones are only suitable for such purposes in resistant conditions, where more appropriate agents, such as the benzodiazepines (see Diazepam, p.1523) have proved ineffective. If their use is judged to be necessary, treatment should be directed at low dosages given on a short-term basis.

A suggested dose of haloperidol for the management of behaviour disorders in disturbed and schizophrenic children is 50 µg per kg bodyweight daily (in 2 divided doses). There are no recommended doses in the USA for children under 12 years of age.

Haloperidol should be used in reduced dosage in the elderly; doses on the lower end of the scale are also advised for adolescents.

Haloperidol decanoate is under study.

Action. A detailed review of the actions and uses of haloperidol. On a weight for weight basis, haloperidol is more potent than chlorpromazine; chlorpromazine has a greater propensity than haloperidol to cause sedation, anticholinergic, and cardiovascular effects, and to alter the convulsive threshold, but haloperidol has a greater propensity than chlorpromazine to cause extrapyramidal reactions. Single daily doses of haloperidol seldom cause more side-effects than the same amount of drug taken in divided doses daily.— F. J. Ayd, *J. clin. Psychiat.*, 1978, *39*, 807.

Haloperidol 10 mg is approximately equivalent to chlorpromazine 400 mg.— A. C. Carr and M. Lader, *Prescribers' J.*, 1978, *18*, 147.

Administration. *In children.* Irreversible dystonia occurred in a 5-year-old hyperactive girl given treatment for 7 weeks with haloperidol 2 mg to 2.8 mg daily in divided doses; the dangers of giving haloperidol to children with self-limiting disease were discussed.— W. Shields and P. F. Bray, *J. Pediat.*, 1976, *88*, 301. Severe extrapyramidal and hypothalamic reactions developed in 2 adolescents given high doses of haloperidol. Symptoms included hyperthermia, semicoma, raised blood pressure and tachycardia, and generalised rigidity with cogwheeling and drooling.— B. Geller and D. E. Greydanus, *J. clin. Psychiat.*, 1979, *40*, 102. See also under Adverse Effects.

See also under Gilles de la Tourette's syndrome (below).

In the elderly. Haloperidol is especially useful in the treatment of the older aggressive patient.— D. J. Williams, *Prescribers' J.*, 1978, *18*, 34.

Further comments: G. Silverman (letter), *Br. med. J.*, 1977, *2*, 318; B. Pitt, *Practitioner*, 1978, *220*, 199.

In a 6-week double-blind study involving 56 psychogeriatric patients, thioridazine 40 to 89 mg daily was compared with haloperidol 1 to 2 mg daily. Both drugs produced significant improvement in the patients' symptoms but the improvement in memory scores tended to be greater with haloperidol.— H. J. Rosen, *J. clin. Psychiat.*, 1979, *40*, 17. In a 12-week double-blind study involving 40 psychogeriatric patients, thioridazine 75 to 450 mg daily was compared with haloperidol 1.5 to 6 mg daily. Both drugs produced significant improvement in the patients' symptoms but the improvement with thioridazine tended to be greater than with haloperidol in most ratings.— L. M. Cowley and R. S. Glen, *ibid.*, 411.

Further studies: J. Gerlach and H. Simmelsgaard, *Psychopharmacology*, 1978, *59*, 105.

Administration in renal failure. Haloperidol could be given in usual doses to patients with renal failure.— W. M. Bennett *et al.*, *Ann. intern. Med.*, 1977, *86*, 754. See also *idem*, 1980, *93*, 286.

Administration in respiratory insufficiency. Comment on the advantage of haloperidol as an antipsychotic agent in patients with compromised pulmonary function but a warning that the dosage is often much lower than for patients with normal respiratory function.— J. A. Davis (letter), *J. Am. med. Ass.*, 1979, *241*, 1575.

Further references: M. K. Tandon, *Aust. N.Z. J. Med.*, 1976, *6*, 561.

Alcohol and drug withdrawal. *Alcoholism.* A study of haloperidol for the control of alcohol withdrawal symptoms.— M. L. Palestine and E. Alatorre, *Curr. ther. Res.*, 1976, *20*, 289.

Barbiturates. Beneficial results were obtained with haloperidol in the management of barbiturate withdrawal.— R. Snyder, *Milit. Med.*, 1977, *142*, 885.

Anxiety. Studies of haloperidol in the treatment of anxiety: D. J. Lord and C. B. Kidd, *Med. J. Aust.*, 1973, *1*, 586; S. M. Channabasavanna *et al.*, *Curr. ther. Res.*, 1978, *24*, 381; M. G. Budden, *Curr. med. Res. Opinion*, 1979, *5*, 759.

Behaviour disorders. Studies of haloperidol for behaviour disorders: P. Barker and I. A. Fraser, *Br. J. Psychiat.*, 1968, *114*, 855; G. F. J. Goddard (letter), *Br. med. J.*, 1973, *1*, 481; S. W. Grabowski, *Curr. ther. Res.*, 1973, *15*, 856.

See also under Administration in Children (above).

Chorea. Chorea associated with systemic lupus erythematosus in an 11-year-old boy responded rapidly to haloperidol 500 µg twice daily.— L. F. Kukla *et al.*, *Archs Dis. Childh.*, 1978, *53*, 345.

See also under Administration in Children (above).

Further references: J. Axley, *J. Pediat.*, 1972, *81*, 1216 (rheumatic chorea).

For a report of haloperidol with lithium being effective in Huntington's chorea, see Lithium Carbonate, p.1542. For a beneficial effect on the addition of propranolol to a haloperidol regimen, see Propranolol, p.1332.

Extrapyramidal effects. Haloperidol in a dose of up to 1.5 mg daily with benztropine produced a slight response which was sustained on placebo in 2 of 11 patients with torticollis, torsion dystonia, or choreoathetosis. Haloperidol was not considered effective in clinical dyskinesias.— J. A. McCaul and G. M. Stern (letter), *Lancet*, 1974, *1*, 1058.

Hemiballismus. Beneficial responses were obtained in 11 patients with acute hemiballismus following administration of chlorpromazine to 3 and haloperidol to 8. None of the patients died.— H. L. Klawans *et al.*, *New Engl. J. Med.*, 1976, *295*, 1348.

Further references: G. J. Gilbert, *J. Am. med. Ass.*, 1975, *233*, 535; G. F. Tegtmeyer (letter), *ibid.*, *234*, 1223; M. J. Davis (letter), *ibid.*, 1976, *235*, 2812; G. J. Gilbert (letter), *ibid.*, 1976, *236*, 1576.

Tardive dyskinesia. Haloperidol and tetrabenazine had a significant effect in reducing the frequency of oral dyskinesia in a study of 13 psychotic patients with tardive dyskinesia who were treated for 18 weeks.— H. Kazamatsuri *et al.*, *Am. J. Psychiat.*, 1973, *130*, 479.

Further references: H. Kazamatsuri *et al.*, *Archs gen. Psychiat.*, 1972, *27*, 100; D. Tarsy *et al.*, *Am. J. Psychiat.*, 1977, *134*, 1032; D. N. Bateman *et al.*, *Br. J. Psychiat.*, 1979, *135*, 505.

See also under Adverse Effects.

Torticollis. A preliminary report of improvement in 7 of 9 patients with torticollis treated with amantadine 100 mg thrice daily and haloperidol 500 µg four times daily increased to a maximum of 14 mg daily where required.— G. J. Gilbert (letter), *Lancet*, 1972, *2*, 234.

Gilles de la Tourette's syndrome. Experience in treating over 250 patients with Gilles de la Tourette's syndrome has indicated that some can only tolerate very gradual dosage increments of haloperidol. Whereas increments of 250 µg per day every 4 days is generally successful in most patients, this sub-group of patients should receive very gradual dosage increments such as 250 µg per day every 3 to 4 weeks.— A. K. Shapiro and E. Shapiro (letter), *J. Am. med. Ass.*, 1977, *238*, 29.

In a study of children and adolescents with Gilles de la Tourette's syndrome, a positive response to haloperidol was generally associated with plasma concentrations of 1 to 4 ng per ml. No relationship could be demonstrated for those with psychoses. Plasma concentrations of haloperidol bore no apparent relationship to the dose given.— P. L. Morselli *et al.*, *Ther. Drug Monit.*, 1979, *1*, 35.

For a comment on the transfer of patients with Gilles de la Tourette's syndrome from haloperidol to lecithin therapy, see Lecithins, p.55.

Further references: M. Boris (letter), *J. Am. med. Ass.*, 1968, *205*, 648; E. M. Craven (letter), *ibid.*, 1969, *210*, 134; J. N. DiGiacomo *et al.*, *J. nerv. ment. Dis.*, 1971, *152* 115; A. K. Shapiro *et al.*, *Archs gen. Psychiat.*, 1973, *28*, 92; M. Feinberg and B. J. Carroll, *Archs gen. Psychiat.*, 1979, *36*, 979.

Hiccup. In several patients haloperidol 5 mg given thrice daily by mouth or parenterally was successful in promptly halting persistent hiccup.— A. D. Korczyn (letter), *Br. med. J.*, 1971, *2*, 590.

Nausea and vomiting. In 17 patients with nausea and/or vomiting due to their antineoplastic treatment, marked relief was obtained in 5 and moderate relief in 7 after treatment with haloperidol, usually 1 mg thrice daily. The effect of haloperidol lasted about 5 hours.— D. A. Plotkin *et al.*, *Curr. ther. Res.*, 1973, *15*, 599.

A study in 65 postoperative patients demonstrated that haloperidol 2 mg intramuscularly has a rapid onset of action in postoperative vomiting (within 30 minutes of injection) but its activity decays over the following 4 hours at this dosage. Droperidol 5 mg intramuscularly had a slow onset of action, only reaching peak effectiveness 3 or 4 hours after administration, but had a prolonged anti-emetic action during the interval of 4 to 24 hours after administration. Prochlorperazine 10 mg intramuscularly had an onset and duration of action intermediate between the other two drugs. Use of haloperidol in association with droperidol might be more effective than any one compound alone.— E. A. Loeser *et al.*, *Can. Anaesth. Soc. J.*, 1979, *26*, 125.

Further references: F. J. Tornetta, *Anesth. Analg. curr. Res.*, 1972, *51*, 964 (postoperative vomiting); R. S. Christman *et al.*, *Curr. ther. Res.*, 1974, *16*, 1171 (gastro-intestinal disorders); M. D. Barton *et al.*, *Anesthesiology*, 1977, *42*, 508 (postoperative vomiting).

Psychoses. In an evaluation of a rapid treatment regimen, 24 patients with acute psychoses were given haloperidol intramuscularly in a dosage of: 5 mg initially followed by 10 mg every 30 minutes until satisfactory remission of symptoms occurred or a maximum of 55 mg had been given; or 5 mg initially followed by 5 mg every hour for up to 2 hours, or until remission occurred. No significant difference in response was noted between the 2 groups and results were therefore combined. Eleven of the 24 patients obtained marked improvement within 3 hours but there was wide variation in the dosage required, improvement occurring in 5 after 15 mg, 3 after 35 mg, and one each after 10, 25, and 45 mg; another 5 patients obtained marked improvement within 72 hours. Side-effects were moderate or mild and in no case required termination of the protocol. Side-effects evaluated were: extrapyramidal reactions (4 patients in each group), which were treated with benztropine 2 mg intramuscularly followed by oral benztropine as necessary; blurred vision (2 patients in each group, 2 of whom had received benztropine); dizziness (1 patient in the high-dose group); possible hypotension (1 patient in the high-dose group); and drowsiness (6 patients in the high-dose group and 2 patients in the moderate-dose group). A limitation of this preliminary study is the absence of a drug-free control group, and the proper dosage and duration of medication required following remission are still uncertain. The very rapid treatment must not allow the patient or family to deny the potential gravity of the illness, and where prolonged stays in hospital can be avoided and continuing care transferred to a more convenient location, continuity must be ensured.— W. H. Anderson *et al.*, *Am. J. Psychiat.*, 1976, *133*, 1076. See also W. H. Anderson and J. C. Kuehnle (letter), *New Engl. J. Med.*, 1976, *295*, 173.

Severe criticism of the hazardous practice of concomitantly administering benztropine parenterally with haloperidol in rapid treatment procedures. Antiparkinsonian drugs should only be used in the event of a dystonic or a parkinsonian reaction.— L. Evans (letter), *Med. J. Aust.*, 1978, *1*, 567.

Further references to the use of parenteral haloperidol in psychiatric emergencies: F. Sangiovanni *et al.*, *Am. J. Psychiat.*, 1973, *130*, 1155; M. L. Gerstenzang and T. V. Krulisky, *Dis. nerv. Syst.*, 1977, *38*, 581; B. A. Stotsky, *ibid.*, 967; P. T. Donlon *et al.*, *Am. J. Psychiat.*, 1979, *136*, 273; J. T. Hopkin *et al.*, *Curr. ther. Res.*, 1980, *27*, 620.

Aggression. For a detailed account of a dosage regimen for haloperidol in the acutely disturbed chronic psychiatric patient, see Chlorpromazine, p.1515.

Drug-induced psychosis. Haloperidol in a dose of 1 mg thrice daily increased as required and given for 1 month to 8 patients significantly decreased the incidence of sustained flashbacks due to lysergide and reduced their intensity and duration.— D. Moskowitz, *Milit. Med.*, 1971, *136*, 754, per *Int. pharm. Abstr.*, 1972, *9*, 273.

Mania. There was no evidence of hepatic or renal dysfunction in a 39-year-old man given haloperidol, 29 mg hourly for 5 weeks for control of the manic phase of his psychosis. The blurred vision noted became normal when the drug was discontinued. This patient did not respond to chlorpromazine in doses up to 4 g daily.— R. McMurdo (letter), *Med. J. Aust.*, 1972, *2*, 1506.

A patient in the manic stage of manic-depressive psychosis was given haloperidol 100 mg and benzhexol 15 mg daily. Haloperidol dosage was increased to 500 mg daily and held for 8 weeks. Although the patient did not respond adequately to treatment he suffered no apparent side-effects, having received 27 g of haloperidol.— N. James (letter), *Med. J. Aust.*, 1973, *2*, 518.

Schizophrenia. In 25 patients with chronic schizophrenia, haloperidol in doses up to 10 mg thrice daily by mouth was more effective in controlling symptoms than chlorpromazine in doses up to 100 mg thrice daily by mouth. Procyclidine hydrochloride was successfully used to control symptoms of extrapyramidal dysfunction.— H. Rompel and H. Segal, *J. int. med. Res.*, 1978, *6*, 126.

A comparative study of *high-dose* haloperidol therapy with standard doses of chlorpromazine, in chronic drug-resistant male schizophrenic patients. For 3 months haloperidol 100 mg daily was administered to 10 patients, and chlorpromazine 600 mg daily was administered to 8 patients. The patients were followed-up for a further 3 months. There were no serious extrapyramidal effects at the high doses, but most of those on the *high-dose* haloperidol showed a deterioration in ward behaviour, possibly related to drowsiness, and developed raised serum alkaline phosphatase concentrations; in the follow-up period these side-effects disappeared on discontinuation of haloperidol or reduction in dosage. One patient on haloperidol who had been a continuous in-patient for 27 years with a main problem of apathy, spontaneously asked to become a day-patient although he subsequently sought readmission. Haloperidol in high dosage appeared to produce beneficial changes in the mental state of some chronic schizophrenics.— R. G. McCreadie and I. M. MacDonald, *Br. J. Psychiat.*, 1977, *131*, 310.

Further references: G. Chouinard *et al.*, *Curr. ther. Res.*, 1973, *15*, 473 (with methyldopa); D. M. Engelhardt *et al.*, *J. clin. Psychiat.*, 1978, *39*, 834 (comparison with thiothixene).

Rheumatoid arthritis. Evidence for an antirheumatic action of haloperidol 1.5 mg daily.— M. G. Grimaldi (letter), *Br. J. clin. Pharmac.*, 1981, *12*, 579.

Stuttering. In a controlled study of 36 patients with a stuttering impediment, haloperidol in an average dose of 0.75 to 1.5 mg thrice daily and orphenadrine 50 mg thrice daily, to reduce the side-effects of haloperidol, led to a significant improvement after 4 weeks in 10 of 12 patients. No further improvement was noted in the patients treated for a further 4 weeks although the initial improvement was maintained. Side-effects which included dry mouth, blurred vision, drowsiness, and depression occurred in patients given either the active medication or a placebo.— P. G. Wells and M. T. Malcolm, *Br. J. Psychiat.*, 1971, *119*, 603.

Haloperidol was given to 18 stutterers for 3 weeks. Of these, 4 patients showed a substantial improvement, 6 showed a lesser improvement, and 8 deteriorated. The mean dose of haloperidol was 2.5 mg daily. Side-effects occurring were drowsiness, poor concentration, restlessness, visual and eye disturbances, other extrapyramidal symptoms, and depression.— P. T. Quinn and C. Peachey, *Med. J. Aust.*, 1973, *2*, 809.

Further references: P. G. Wells (letter), *Med. J. Aust.*, 1974, *2*, 613; M. Kalotkin *et al.*, *Am. J. Psychiat.*, 1976, *133*, 331; T. J. Murray *et al.*, *Br. J. Psychiat.*, 1977, *130*, 370.

Tardive dyskinesia. For the use of haloperidol in tardive dyskinesia, see under Extrapyramidal Effects (above).

Preparations

Haloperidol Injection *(B.P.)*. A sterile solution of haloperidol in Water for Injections; the pH may be adjusted to 2.8 to 3.6 by the addition of sodium hydroxide. Sterilised by autoclaving. Protect from light.

Haloperidol Injection *(U.S.P.)*. A sterile solution of haloperidol in Water for Injections, prepared with the aid of lactic acid; it may contain a suitable preservative. pH 3 to 3.8. Protect from light.

Haloperidol Oral Solution *(U.S.P.)*. Haloperidol Solution. A solution of haloperidol in water prepared with the aid of lactic acid. pH 2.75 to 3.75. Store in airtight containers. Protect from light.

Haloperidol Tablets *(B.P.)*. Tablets containing haloperidol.

Haloperidol Tablets *(U.S.P.)*. Tablets containing haloperidol. Store in airtight containers. Protect from light.

Proprietary Preparations

Haldol *(Janssen, UK)*. Haloperidol, available as **Injection** containing 5 mg per ml, in ampoules of 1 and 2 ml; as **Liquid** for oral use containing 2 mg per ml; as **Liquid Concentrate** containing 10 mg per ml (suggested diluent, water); and as scored **Tablets** of 1.5, 5, 10, and 20 mg. (Also available as Haldol in *Belg., Canad., Fr., Ger., Neth., Norw., Swed., Switz., USA*).

Serenace *(Searle, UK)*. Haloperidol, available as **Capsules** of 500 µg; as **Injection** containing 5 mg per ml in ampoules of 1 ml, and 10 mg per ml in ampoules of 2 ml; as **Liquid** for oral use containing 2 mg per ml (may be diluted 50% with either water or syrup); and as scored **Tablets** of 1.5, 5, 10, and 20 mg. (Also available as Serenace in *Austral., Jap., S.Afr.*).

Other Proprietary Names

Arg.— Halopidol; *Denm.*— Serenase; *Ger.*— Sigaperidol; *Ital.*— Serenase; *Jap.*— Brotopon, Einalon S, Halosten, Linton, Peluces.

7052-y

Homofenazine Hydrochloride. D 775. 2-{Hexahydro-4-[3-(2-trifluoromethylphenothiazin-10-yl)propyl]-1,4-diazepin-1-yl}ethanol dihydrochloride. $C_{23}H_{28}F_3N_3OS,2HCl=524.5$.

CAS — 3833-99-6 (homofenazine); 1256-01-5 (hydrochloride).

Homofenazine hydrochloride is a phenothiazine with general properties similar to those of chlorpromazine (p.1509). It has been used in the management of neuropsychiatric disorders in doses of 3 mg twice or thrice daily.

References: G. Pernhaupt and R. Quatember, *Wien. med. Wschr.* 1970, *120*, 737.

Proprietary Names

Pasaden *(Homburg, Belg.; Homburg, Ger.; Farmades, Ital.)*.

7053-j

Hydroxyphenamate. Oxyfenamate; Al 0361; P 301. 2-Hydroxy-2-phenylbutyl carbamate.
$C_{11}H_{15}NO_3$=209.2.

CAS — 50-19-1.

A white crystalline powder. **Soluble** 1 in 40 of water; soluble in alcohol and chloroform.

Hydroxyphenamate is a carbamate with general properties similar to those of meprobamate (p.1545). It has been used in the treatment of anxiety and tension states in doses of 200 mg thrice daily.

Proprietary Names
Listica *(Armour-Montagu, Fr.).*

7054-z

Imiclopazine Hydrochloride. Chlorimpiphenine Hydrochloride; P 4241. 1-(2-{4-[3-(2-Chlorophenothiazin-10-yl)propyl]piperazin-1-yl}ethyl)-3-methylimidazolidin-2-one dihydrochloride.
$C_{25}H_{32}ClN_5OS,2HCl$=559.0.

CAS — 7224-08-0 (imiclopazine); 7414-95-1 (hydrochloride).

Imiclopazine hydrochloride is a phenothiazine with general properties similar to those of chlorpromazine (p.1509). It has a piperazine side-chain. It was formerly used in the management of psychoneuroses and psychoses and was given in doses of 5 to 20 mg daily.

7055-c

Ketazolam.

U-28774. 11-Chloro-8,12b-dihydro-2,8-dimethyl-12b-phenyl-4*H*-[1,3]oxazino[3,2-*d*][1,4]benzodiazepine-4,7(6*H*)-dione.
$C_{20}H_{17}ClN_2O_3$=368.8.

CAS — 27223-35-4.

Dependence, Adverse Effects, Treatment, and Precautions. As for Diazepam, p.1519.

Side-effects associated with ketazolam included dry mouth, nasal congestion, blurred vision, dizziness, and drowsiness.— L. F. Fabre and R. T. Harris, *Curr. ther. Res.*, 1974, *16*, 848.

Effects on the skin. Skin rash in a patient taking ketazolam.— L. F. Fabre *et al.*, *J. int. med. Res.*, 1976, *4*, 50.

Absorption and Fate. For an account of the absorption and fate of a benzodiazepine, see Diazepam, p.1522.

Animal studies have indicated that ketazolam is extensively metabolised and that its metabolites include diazepam and desmethyldiazepam.

Following administration of ketazolam to *rats* metabolites included: oxazepam, 3-hydroxydiazepam, desmethyldiazepam, diazepam, and 4′-hydroxydiazepam.— F. S. Eberts *et al.*, *Pharmacologist*, 1976, *18*, 153.

Uses. Ketazolam is a benzodiazepine with general properties similar to those of diazepam (p.1523). In the treatment of anxiety it is given in a usual dose of 30 mg daily, at night, with a range of 15 to 60 mg daily, either in divided doses or a single dose at night.

A brief discussion on the actions and uses of ketazolam.— *Drug & Ther. Bull.*, 1980, *18*, 94.

Alcohol and drug withdrawal. Studies of ketazolam in the treatment of anxiety in patients with alcoholism.— D. M. Gallant *et al.*, *Curr. ther. Res.*, 1973, *15*, 123; L. A. Gottschalk *et al.*, *Psychopharmac. Bull.*, 1978, *14*, 39.

Anxiety. In a 4-week double-blind trial in 113 anxious patients ketazolam, up to 75 mg at bedtime, was compared with placebo and with diazepam, up to 15 mg thrice daily. A total of 15 patients did not complete the trial, 2 on ketazolam, 3 on diazepam, and 10 on placebo. Ketazolam was as effective as diazepam in relieving anxiety and both were superior to placebo.— L. F. Fabre *et al.*, *Curr. ther. Res.*, 1978, *24*, 875.

Further references: C. L. Bowden, *Curr. ther. Res.*, 1978, *24*, 170; K. Rickels *et al.*, *Clin. Pharmac. Ther.*, 1978, *23*, 127; L. F. Fabre and D. M. McLendon, *Curr. ther. Res.*, 1979, *25*, 710; K. Rickels *et al.*, *J. clin. Pharmac.*, 1980, *20*, 581; *Br. J. clin. Pract.*, 1980, *34*, 107.

Proprietary Preparations

Anxon *(Beecham Research, UK).* Ketazolam, available as capsules of 15 or 30 mg.

Other Proprietary Names

Contamex *(Ger.)*; Loftran *(Canad.)*; Solatran *(Belg., Switz.)*; Unakalm *(Belg.).*

7056-k

Lenperone Hydrochloride. AHR-2277. 4′-Fluoro-4-[4-(4-fluorobenzoyl)piperidino]butyrophenone hydrochloride.
$C_{22}H_{23}F_2NO_2,HCl$=407.9.

CAS — 24678-13-5 (lenperone); 24677-86-9 (hydrochloride).

Lenperone is a butyrophenone with general properties similar to those of haloperidol (p.1532). It has been given as the hydrochloride in doses of 15 to 60 mg daily for the treatment of psychoses; doses of up to 90 mg and more have also been used.

Anxiety. Lenperone 6 to 24 mg taken daily was considered to be superior to a placebo and of similar efficacy to diazepam 10 to 40 mg daily in a 28-day study of 140 patients with anxiety. Sixty-one patients did not complete the study.— L. F. Fabre and D. M. McLendon, *Curr. ther. Res.*, 1977, *22*, 900. See also L. F. Fabre and R. T. Harris, *Curr. ther. Res.*, 1976, *19*, 328.

Schizophrenia. In a double-blind study in 29 patients with chronic schizophrenia there was no significant difference between the effects of lenperone in increasing doses up to 175 mg daily and those of chlorpromazine up to 1.05 g daily. Side-effects of lenperone included sedation, oculogyric crisis, orthostatic hypotension, an urticarial skin eruption, and reversible ECG changes.— D. H. Mielke *et al.*, *Curr. ther. Res.*, 1975, *18*, 636.

A comparative study of lenperone and chlorpromazine in schizophrenia. Side-effects in the lenperone group included excitement and agitation (1 patient); depressive affect (1 patient); increased motor activity (1 patient); insomnia (2 patients); abnormal liver function (2 patients); syncope and dizziness (1 patient); hypotension (1 patient); rigidity (1 patient); and dystonic symptoms (1 patient).— J. Digiacomo *et al.*, *Curr. ther. Res.*, 1977, *22*, 605.

Lenperone given for 4 weeks in doses increased at 3-day intervals from 15 mg daily to a maximum of 60 mg daily was evaluated in 10 patients with acute schizophrenia. Total remission was reported in 2 patients and substantial improvement in 3. All patients became drowsy during treatment; other main side-effects were dry mouth in 7 patients, tremor (4), and restlessness (3). Increase in libido, dizziness, insomnia, rigidity, blurred vision, agitation, and increased sweating and salivation were also reported by 1 or 2 patients. The mean standing diastolic blood pressure fell from 67 to 61 mmHg during the study.— B. R. S. Nakra *et al.*, *Curr. med. Res. Opinion*, 1977, *4*, 529.

Further references: G. L. Sathananthan *et al.*, *Curr. ther. Res.*, 1974, *16*, 844; M. Harris, *J. clin. Pharmac.*, 1975, *15*, 187; B. Woggon *et al.*, *Int. Pharmacopsychiat.*, 1977, *12*, 113.

Manufacturers
Robins, USA.

5057-h

Lithium Carbonate *(B.P., U.S.P.).*

Lithium Carb.; CP 15467-61.
Li_2CO_3=73.89.

CAS — 554-13-2.

Pharmacopoeias. In *Br., Braz., Cz., Eur., Fr., Ger., Neth., Nord., Port., Roum., Span., Swiss,* and *U.S.*

A white odourless granular powder with a slightly alkaline taste. M.p. about 618°. Each g represents 27 mmol (27 mEq) of lithium.

Soluble 1 in 100 of water and 1 in 140 of boiling water; very slightly soluble in alcohol; soluble with effervescence in dilute mineral acids. A saturated solution is alkaline to litmus.

Adverse Effects. Side-effects of lithium are dose-related and the margin between the therapeutic and toxic dose is narrow. Those occurring during the early stages of therapy may be lessened by initiating therapy at the lower end of the therapeutic scale so that patients may adapt to lithium therapy, only raising the dose if it is necessary to achieve or maintain a response. These initial side-effects include nausea and loose stools, fine hand tremor, polyuria, and mild thirst, and they may settle as treatment progresses, although fine hand tremor in particular, which resembles essential tremor, may remain a problem.

Toxic effects may be expected at serum-lithium concentrations of about 1.5 mmol per litre, although they can appear at lower concentrations. They call for immediate withdrawal of treatment and should always be considered very seriously. All patients suffering from lithium intoxication have mental and neuromuscular symptoms and about half have gastro-intestinal symptoms.

Mild symptoms of lithium intoxication include slight apathy, sluggishness, drowsiness and lethargy, reduced concentration, muscular weakness, ataxia, troublesome but regular hand tremor, and slight muscle twitchings. Moderate symptoms include apathy, sluggishness, drowsiness, lethargy and sleepiness, difficulty with speech, irregular tremor, obvious myoclonic twitchings and muscular weakness, and ataxia; the patient looks ill, pinched, drawn, grey, and cold. Severe intoxication is associated with seriously impaired consciousness, including ‘coma vigil’ (where the patient can react when spoken to but only by moving the head or the eyes), hyperreflexia, convulsions and epileptic seizures, kidney, brain, and heart damage; a death-rate of 10 to 15% has been reported in association with lithium poisoning, with permanent neurological or renal sequelae in another 10 to 15%. Recovery does not usually occur until some time after serum-lithium concentrations have been reduced.

Other side-effects associated with lithium therapy include indigestion, weight gain and oedema (which should not be treated with diuretics), acne and exacerbation or precipitation of psoriasis, leucocytosis, headache, cogwheel rigidity (in the absence of other extrapyramidal symptoms and unresponsive to antiparkinsonian therapy), cardiac arrhythmias and T-wave changes, occasional hypothyroidism and hyperthyroidism (requiring appropriate therapy), nephrogenic diabetes insipidus (which is usually reversible on discontinuation of therapy), and occasional renal lesions in patients who have received long-term lithium therapy. Other side-effects reported include dry mouth, constipation, metallic taste, blurred vision, stuffy nose, tinnitus, flushing, feelings of unreality, stiffness of limbs, and aching of the body.

Reviews, reports, and discussion of adverse effects caused by lithium.— *Br. med. J.*, 1977, *2*, 346; H. E. Hansen and A. Amdisen, *Q.J. Med.*, 1978, *47*, 123; P. Vestergaard *et al.*, *Acta psychiat. scand.*, 1980, *62*, 193.

Abuse. Mention of lithium carbonate as a drug of abuse.— B. Lipkin (letter), *Br. med. J.*, 1977, *1*, 1411.

Cogwheel rigidity. Findings of definite cogwheel rigidity, that was not alleviated by antiparkinsonian medication, in 2 of 38 patients receiving lithium therapy. Fine and rapid tremor usually of mild to moderate severity was noted in 17 of the patients.— J. Kane *et al.*, *Am. J. Psychiat.*, 1978, *135*, 851. Slight to moderate cogwheel rigidity was noted in 28 of 79 patients treated with lithium, either alone or with tricyclic antidepressants. Cogwheeling did not appear to be related to concomitant tricyclic therapy. Apart from a lithium tremor (which is not thought to be extrapyramidal) other extrapyramidal symptoms associated with cogwheeling were rare in this study. This raises the possibility that cogwheel rigidity associated with lithium may not result from an effect of the basal ganglia.— G. M. Asnis *et al.*, *ibid.*, 1979, *136*, 1225.

Further references.— S. Shopsin and S. Gershon, *Am. J. Psychiat.*, 1975, *132*, 536; R. D. Bien (letter), *Am. J. Psychiat.*, 1976, *133*, 1093.

Cytogenetic effects. In 3 psychiatric patients treated with lithium there was a significantly higher frequency of breaks and hypodiploid cells than in samples from healthy patients of the same age.— U. Friedrich and J. Nielsen (letter), *Lancet*, 1969, *2*, 435. There was no statistical difference in the frequency of chromosome aberrations between a group of patients treated with lithium and a control group.— P. Genest and A. Villeneuve, *ibid.*, 1971, *1*, 1132.

Further references.— R. De La Torre and E. Krompotic, *Teratology*, 1976, *13*, 131.

Diabetogenic effect. A possible association between lithium and acute-onset diabetes mellitus in 2 patients.— B. B. Johnston (letter), *Lancet*, 1977, *2*, 935. A similar finding.— J. Craig *et al.* (letter), *ibid.*, 1028.

Increased serum concentrations of lithium were associated with hyperglycaemia in an insulin-dependent diabetic man suffering from mania.— R. Waziri and J. Nelson, *J. clin. Psychiat.*, 1978, *39*, 623.

Further references.— B. Shopsin *et al.*, *Archs gen. Psychiat.*, 1972, *26*, 566; M. Martinez-Maldonado and J. Terrell, *Archs intern. Med.*, 1973, *132*, 881.

Effects on the blood. Irreversible inhibition of choline transport in red blood cells by lithium.— C. Lingsch and K. Martin, *Br. J. Pharmac.*, 1976, *57*, 323. Further references.— G. Lee *et al.*, *Br. J. clin. Pharmac.*, 1974, *1*, 365; R. S. Jope *et al.* (letter), *New Engl. J. Med.*, 1978, *299*, 833.

Leucocytosis. A reversible and apparently harmless leucocytosis was observed in patients treated with lithium.— B. Shopsin *et al.*, *Clin. Pharmac. Ther.*, 1971, *12*, 923.

A view that chronic myeloid leukaemia, which developed in a woman who had been taking lithium for 11 months, might have been associated with her lithium therapy.— R. T. S. Jim (letter), *Blood*, 1979, *53*, 1031; *idem* (letter), *Ann. intern. Med.*, 1980, *92*, 262.

Acute monocytic leukaemia developed in a 26-year-old woman 5 months after the start of treatment with lithium carbonate. Her serum-lithium concentration had been maintained between 0.7 and 1 mmol per litre.— W. P. Hammond and F. Appelbaum (letter), *New Engl. J. Med.*, 1980, *302*, 808. Criticism of the conclusion that lithium may have induced leukaemia.— D. L. Longo (letter), *ibid.*, *303*, 283. A report of 2 patients in whom acute myeloid leukaemia developed during treatment with lithium.— J. L. Nielsen (letter), *ibid.*

Effects on bones and joints. Although a study in 37 postmenopausal female patients suggested that lithium did not cause acceleration of bone-loss in mature subjects it was recommended on the basis of positive *animal* results that lithium should be used with caution in patients of immature bone structure.— N. J. Birch *et al.*, *Br. J. clin. Pharmac.*, 1977, *4*, 649P.

Contrary to reports on *animal* studies, findings in 12 psychiatric patients receiving long-term lithium carbonate therapy did not reveal any gross abnormalities in serum calcium or phosphorus concentrations or in renal phosphorus handling.— G. O. Perez *et al.*, *Clin. Pharmac. Ther.*, 1977, *21*, 449.

Further references.— S. J. Choi and M. A. Taylor (letter), *Lancet*, 1976, *2*, 1080; P. C. Baastrup *et al.*, *Acta psychiat. scand.*, 1978, *57*, 124.

Effects on the electrolyte balance. A report of the effect of lithium carbonate on sodium balance and distribution.— L. Baer *et al.*, *Archs gen. Psychiat.*, 1970, *22*, 40.

Following the administration of lithium carbonate in a dose of 1.2 to 1.8 g daily for 2 weeks there was a significant decrease in total body-potassium concentration in 12 of 13 depressed patients and a significant increase in 6 of 7 manic patients.— D. L. Murphy and W. E. Bunney, *J. nerv. ment. Dis.*, 1971, *152*, 381. Hyperkalaemia in a woman given lithium.— F. C. Goggans, *Am. J. Psychiat.*, 1980, *137*, 860.

Details of the effects of lithium on plasma concentrations of calcium and magnesium with special emphasis on their variations as a predictive factor for therapeutic outcome.— J. S. Carman *et al.* (letter), *Lancet*, 1974, *2*, 1454; J. Crammer (letter), *Lancet*, 1975, *1*, 215; N. Bjørum *et al.* (letter), *ibid.*, 1243. See also under Effects on Bones and Joints (above).

Effects on the endocrine system. *Adrenals.* There was a strong negative correlation between lithium concentrations and cortisol concentrations in serum.— L. Eroğlu *et al.* (letter), *Br. J. clin. Pharmac.*, 1979, *8*, 89.

Further references.— E. J. Sachar *et al.*, *Archs gen. Psychiat.*, 1970, *22*, 304; R. Noyes *et al.*, *Compreh. Psychiat.*, 1971, *12*, 337; K. A. Halmi *et al.*, *Clin. Pharmac. Ther.*, 1972, *13*, 699.

Parathyroid. A possible association between lithium, hypercalcaemia, and hyperparathyroidism in 6 patients.— T. A. T. Christensson (letter), *Lancet*, 1976, *2*, 144.

Another report of lithium producing a mild hyperparathyroidism in manic-depressive patients. This was considered to be a biochemical syndrome without clinical features, requiring neither withdrawal nor surgery.— C. Christiansen *et al.* (letter), *Lancet*, 1976, *2*, 969. See also G. A. MacGregor (letter), *Lancet*, 1977, *2*, 1129.

Thyroid. Hypothyroidism occurred in 20 of 93 females and 2 of 56 males treated with lithium. It was recommended that thyroid function should be monitored during the first 12 to 16 weeks of treatment with lithium.— A. Villeneuve *et al.* (letter), *Lancet*, 1973, *2*, 502. Another 19 patients were known to have become hypothyroid while taking lithium.— G. G. Lloyd *et al.* (letter), *ibid.*, 619.

Of 200 patients receiving long-term lithium therapy 10 developed hypothyroidism and 3 developed hyperthyroidism. The patients with hypothyroidism were treated with thyroxine while they continued lithium therapy. Two patients with hyperthyroidism were treated with carbimazole and lithium was withdrawn while the third continued lithium therapy and was successfully treated with propylthiouracil.— M. Serry and D. Serry (letter), *Med. J. Aust.*, 1976, *1*, 505. See also G. Linstedt *et al.*, *Br. J. Psychiat.*, 1977, *130*, 452.

Further references.— J. Merry (letter), *Br. med. J.*, 1977, *2*, 765 and 894 (hyperthyroidism); G. Pallisgaard and P. K. Frederiksen, *Acta med. scand.*, 1978, *204*, 141 (thyroiditis); H. Perrild *et al.*, *Br. med. J.*, 1978, *1*, 1108 (hypothyroidism); J. Todd and T. C. Jerram, *Br. J. clin. Pract.*, 1978, *32*, 201 (hyperthyroidism); J. T. Cho *et al.*, *Am. J. Psychiat.*, 1979, *136*, 115 (hypothyroidism); D. Preodor *et al.*, *J. nerv. ment. Dis.*, 1979, *167*, 186 (hypothyroidism); V. I. Reus *et al.*, *Am. J. Psychiat.*, 1979, *136*, 724 (hyperthyroidism); B. E. W. Brownlie *et al.*, *Aust. N.Z. J. Med.*, 1980, *10*, 62.

For previous references to the effects of lithium on thyroid function, see Martindale, 27th Edn, p. 1545.

Effects on the eyes. Five of 44 patients developed exophthalmos after receiving lithium for at least 6 months. Four of 56 patients who were already receiving lithium showed an increase in ocular measurement after further treatment. Of the 91 patients who did not develop exophthalmos 67 were euthyroid before lithium therapy but hypothyroidism developed in 12 during treatment.— R. L. Segal *et al.*, *New Engl. J. Med.*, 1973, *289*, 137. See also under Effects on the Endocrine System (above).

Bilateral papilloedema in a 29-year-old woman appeared to be associated with lithium therapy.— A. Lobo *et al.*, *J. nerv. ment. Dis.*, 1978, *166*, 526.

Effects on the gastro-intestinal tract. A patient with mania was found to have regional ileitis during treatment with lithium carbonate. Abdominal symptoms abated after intestinal resection, apart from severe diarrhoea which persisted despite the dose of lithium being lowered. The diarrhoea ceased when lithium was withdrawn.— J. Varsamis and R. R. Wand (letter), *Lancet*, 1972, *2*, 1322.

In a double-blind crossover trial in 30 healthy male volunteers, various lithium salts were given twice daily by mouth as ordinary and slow-release tablets each containing 24 mmol of lithium. There was no significant difference between salts and side-effects were dependent upon the lithium ion. Slow-release tablets resulted in less nausea but considerably more diarrhoea.— K. O. Borg *et al.*, *Acta pharm. suec.*, 1974, *11*, 133.

Effects on the heart. A review of the literature on the cardiovascular effects of lithium. Therapeutic doses produce reversible T-wave depression, rarely inversion, not unlike that seen in hypokalaemia. Sinus node dysfunction or ventricular arrhythmias have been reported rarely; their occurrence should prompt a search for lithium intoxication or associated electrolyte abnormalities. Alleged cardiotoxic manifestations involving hypotension and cardiovascular collapse invariably follow days of coma caused by the neurological effects of lithium overdosage. Lithium does not appear to be contra-indicated in patients with heart disease when there are clear psychiatric indications for its use, since the cardiotoxicity of other psychotropic agents which would be required probably exceeds that of lithium. If it is used in patients with cardiac arrhythmias, electrocardiographic monitoring is essential in order to detect any possible, although unlikely, aggravation of the arrhythmia.— A. G. Tilkian *et al.*, *Am. J. Med.*, 1976, *61*, 665.

Individual reports of adverse effects of lithium on the heart.— R. G. Demers and G. R. Heninger, *J. Am. med. Ass.*, 1971, *218*, 381 (T-wave depression); T. M. Tangedahl and G. T. Gau, *New Engl. J. Med.*, 1972, *287*, 867 (premature ventricular contractions); J. R. Wilson *et al.*, *New Engl. J. Med.*, 1976, *294*, 1223 (sinus-node abnormalities); C. M. Jaffe, *Am. J. Psychiat.*, 1977, *134*, 88 (atrioventricular block); A. Hagman *et al.*, *Acta med. scand.*, 1979, *205*, 467 (sinus-node dysfunction).

Effects on the kidneys. Comment on polyuria associated with lithium therapy and the risk of chronic nephropathy.— *Lancet*, 1979, *2*, 619. Further comment, with special reference to the meeting on Lithium Treatment and Kidney Damage, arranged by the biological section of the World Psychiatric Association, Copenhagen, 1979. The risk of lithium nephropathy in the absence of lithium toxicity appears to be small. It is mandatory for those who may have pre-existing renal damage, and perhaps a history of nephritic illness, to be assessed before treatment, and if there is impaired function the assessment should be repeated at intervals during treatment. With these precautions the risk of serious progressive renal damage is likely to be slight.— *ibid.*, 1056. See also S. P. Tyrer *et al.* (letter), *ibid.*, 1980, *1*, 94.

Further reviews and comments.— *Drug & Ther. Bull.*, 1979, *17*, 27; H. E. Hansen, *Drugs*, 1981, *22*, 461.

Findings of chronic renal lesions in 13 of 14 patients receiving lithium carbonate and suffering from acute intoxication or diabetes insipidus.— J. Hestbech *et al.*, *Kidney Int.*, 1977, *12*, 205, per *Drugs*, 1979, *17*, 67.

A study of 19 patients treated with lithium, 41 treated with lithium and neuroleptic drugs, 25 treated with neuroleptic drugs alone, and 30 healthy subjects indicated that long-term lithium therapy impairs renal concentrating capacity, indicating irreversible kidney damage. Even short-term lithium therapy reduced the concentrating capacity in most patients. Lithium therapy should thus be regarded as a risk factor for surgical operations since patients might pass several litres of hypo-osmotic urine daily for which it is difficult to compensate parenterally. Neuroleptic drugs also appeared to reduce the concentrating capacity but it was not known whether the effect was reversible.— G. Bucht and A. Wahlin (letter), *Lancet*, 1978, *1*, 778. While maximum concentrating ability may be impaired by lithium there might not necessarily be gross polyuria; with proper surveillance lithium therapy is unlikely to cause serious problems during surgery.— W. R. Cattell *et al.* (letter), *ibid.*, 1978, *2*, 44. Reply.— G. Bucht and A. Wahlin (letter), *ibid.*, 580.

A unique lesion was found in renal biopsy specimens from 5 patients who had been receiving lithium for periods of 4 months to 9 years.— G. D. Burrows *et al.* (letter), *Lancet*, 1978, *1*, 1310. Additional data on the lithium-induced kidney lesion, which develops very soon after lithium is started, and is absent in kidney sampled a year after lithium has been stopped. The site of the lesion is where the vasopressin receptors are thought to be and hence it may be the pathological basis of the vasopressin-resistant diabetes-insipidus-like syndrome seen in some patients taking lithium regularly.— P. Kincaid-Smith *et al.* (letter), *ibid.*, 1979, *2*, 700.

Urine volumes, plasma-creatinine concentrations, and creatinine clearance in 106 patients taking lithium carbonate 0.25 to 2 g daily, and renal-function study in 30, did not support the suggestion that long-term lithium treatment impaired renal function.— R. P. Hullin *et al.*, *Br. med. J.*, 1979, *1*, 1457. See also D. Kimbrell *et al.* (letter), *ibid.*, 1979, *2*, 1145; H. James *et al.* (letter), *ibid.*, 1980, *280*, 46; N. J. Birch and R. P. Hullin (letter), *ibid.*, 1148; A. Coppen and W. R. Cattell (letter), *ibid.*, *281*, 61.

Nephrotic syndrome with minimal changes associated with lithium therapy in one patient.— A. V. Richman *et al.*, *Ann. intern. Med.*, 1980, *92*, 70.

Further studies and reports on the effects of lithium on the kidneys.— H. E. Hansen *et al.*, *Proc. Eur. Dialysis Transplant Ass.*, 1977, *14*, 518; N. M. Simon *et al.* (letter), *Ann. intern. Med.*, 1977, *86*, 446; P. H. Baylis and D. A. Heath, *ibid.*, 1978, *88*, 607; T. R. P. Price and P. J. Beisswenger (letter), *ibid.*, 576; A. J. M. Donker *et al.*, *Clin. Nephrol.*, 1979, *12*, 254; R. Hällgren *et al.*, *Br. J. Psychiat.*, 1979, *135*, 22; H. E. Hansen *et al.*, *Acta med. scand.*, 1979, *205*, 593; *idem*, *Q. J. Med.*, 1979, *48*, 577; J. Hestbech and M. Aurell (letter), *Lancet*, 1979, *1*, 212; P. Vestergaard (letter), *ibid.*, 491; M. Aurell and J. Hestbech (letter), *ibid.*, 882; K. J. MacDonald *et al.*, *N.Z. med. J.*, 1979, *90*, 323; P. D. Miller *et al.*, *Am. J. Med.*, 1979, *66*, 797; C. Neu *et al.*, *J. clin. Psychiat.*, 1979, *40*, 460; E. Z. Rabin *et al.*, *Can. med. Ass. J.*, 1979, *121*, 194; P. Vestergaard *et al.*, *Acta psychiat. scand.*, 1979, *60*, 504; L. Wallin and C. Alling, *Br. med. J.*, 1979, *2*, 1332; P. Vestergaard (letter), *ibid.*, 1980, *280*, 113; R. H. Gerner *et al.*, *Am. J. Psychiat.*, 1980, *137*, 834; H. E. Hansen *et al.*, *Q. J. Med.*, 1980, *192* 577.

For reference to the use of desmopressin to test renal function in patients receiving lithium therapy, see Desmopressin, p.1266.

Effects on mental state. There was no difference in memory impairment between 72 depressed patients receiving prolonged lithium therapy and 100 receiving tricyclic antidepressants. Both groups complained of significantly greater memory impairment than did healthy controls.— A. Coppen *et al.* (letter), *Lancet*, 1978, *1*, 448.

A study into the effect of lithium therapy on the creative ability of 24 manic-depressive artists. Twelve artists reported increased artistic productivity, 6 reported unaltered productivity, and 6 reported lowered productivity. There is reason to assume that manic-depressive persons with other kinds of creative work also respond individually as regards the effect of successful lithium prophylaxis on productivity.— M. Schou, *Br. J. Psychiat.*, 1979, *135*, 97.

Further references.— B. Boettcher (letter), *Med. J. Aust.*, 1974, *2*, 796; D. B. Jarrett *et al.* (letter), *ibid.*, 1975, *1*, 21; G. Johnson (letter), *ibid.*, 183; L. L. Judd *et al.*, *Archs gen. Psychiat.*, 1977, *34*, 355; M. J. Friedman *et al.*, *Am. J. Psychiat.*, 1977, *134*, 1123; D. Preodor *et al.*, *ibid.*, 1047; R. Telford and E. P. Worral, *Br. J. Psychiat.*, 1978, *133*, 424; D. Kropf and B. Müller-Oerlinghausen, *Acta psychiat. scand.*, 1979, *59*, 79.

Sleep-walking. Ten of 114 patients receiving treatment with lithium in association with a neuroleptic exhibited somnambulistic-like episodes. The neuroleptics involved were chlorpromazine, fluphenazine, haloperidol, perphenazine, thioridazine, and thiothixene. Since sleep-walking occurs out of slow-wave sleep, which is increased by lithium and some neuroleptics, it was considered that the therapy was responsible. The occurrence of grand mal seizures in 2 patients was probably unrelated. Eliminating the evening doses of neuroleptics and lithium may be helpful; if sleep-walking persists the daily dosage of neuroleptic should be reduced where possible; the addition of a stage IV suppressant drug, such as diazepam, may be helpful.— Charney. D.S. *et al.*, *Br. J. Psychiat.*, 1979, *135*, 418.

Effects on the nervous system. A report of definite lithium-induced neurotoxicity in 3 patients and possible lithium-induced neurotoxicity in 2. Comparison of the behavioural ratings of these 5 patients with 30 non-toxic lithium-treated patients suggested that marked psychotic symptoms and intense anxiety might be associated with increased vulnerability to the development of lithium neurotoxicity.— A. P. West and H. Y. Meltzer, *Am. J. Psychiat.*, 1979, *136*, 963.

Further references.— H. T. Pi and F. G. Surawicz, *Clin. Toxicol.*, 1978, *13*, 479.

Effects on sexual function. Erectile impotence has been described after the use of lithium in manic-depressive psychosis. The mechanism is unknown.— P. Turner, *Prescribers' J.*, 1978, *18*, 94.

Effects on the skin. *Acne.* A 28-year-old woman with manic depression developed severe acneform eruptions on the face and shoulders after she had been receiving lithium carbonate in a daily dose of 900 mg for 1 month. The eruptions subsided 3 weeks after the cessation of drug therapy.— R. Ruiz-Maldonado *et al.* (letter), *J. Am. med. Ass.*, 1973, *224*, 1534.

Further references.— Y. Kusumi, *Dis. nerv. Syst.*, 1971, *32*, 853; F. W. Yorder, *Archs Derm.*, 1975, *111*, 396; H. Okrasinski, *Dermatologica*, 1977, *154*, 251.

Folliculitis. A report on folliculitis in patients being treated with lithium carbonate. The eruption remitted when therapy was discontinued; it remitted partially in some patients who continued to take lithium.— S. B. Kurtin (letter), *J. Am. med. Ass.*, 1973, *223*, 802.

Further references.— D. F. Klein *et al.*, *Am. J. Psychiat.*, 1973, *130*, 1018.

Pruritus. A woman with a manic-depressive illness who had been taking lithium carbonate 900 mg daily followed by 1.2 g on alternate days developed pruritic dermatitis which was relieved by sodium sulfoxone 165 mg twice daily for 3 days. However, the serum-lithium concentrations fell and manic symptoms returned until extra doses of lithium carbonate were given.— R. E. Posey (letter), *J. Am. med. Ass.*, 1972, *221*, 1517.

Psoriasis. Exacerbation of psoriasis was reported in 3 patients who were receiving treatment with lithium for affective disorders.— A. Skott *et al.*, *Br. J. Derm.*, 1977, *96*, 445.

Further references.— N. J. Lowe and H. B. Ridgway, *Archs Derm.*, 1978, *114*, 1788; I. Skoven and J. Thormann, *ibid.*, 1979, *115*, 1185.

Stomatitis. A 36-year-old patient who was receiving lithium carbonate and chlorpromazine developed inflammation of the oral mucosa which rapidly improved when lithium carbonate was discontinued. However resumption of lithium carbonate treatment in capsule form caused no recurrence of symptoms and it was suggested that lithium carbonate could cause contact stomatitis.— C. E. Muniz and D. H. Berghman (letter), *J. Am. med. Ass.*, 1978, *239*, 2759.

Effects on speech. Dysarthria occurring in a 70-year-old patient taking 0.8 to 1.2 g of lithium carbonate daily was severe when the serum-lithium concentration was 1.4 mmol per litre and barely detectable when the concentration was 0.7 mmol per litre.— K. Solomon and R. Vickers, *J. Am. med. Ass.*, 1975, *231*, 280. See also B. Johnels *et al.* (letter), *Br. med. J.*, 1976, *2*, 642.

Effects on taste perception. Of 450 patients treated with lithium about 5% complained of impaired taste of butter; celery and other foods were also involved.— J. M. Himmelhoch and I. Hanin (letter), *Br. med. J.*, 1974, *4*, 233.

Effects on the teeth. Epidemiological and *animal* studies have demonstrated a dental caries-inhibitory effect of lithium. The high caries increment in patients receiving lithium carbonate may be a result of impaired salivary secretion which overcomes any local caries-inhibitory effect of lithium.— A. J. Rugg-Gunn (letter), *Br. dent. J.*, 1979, *146*, 136.

Further references.— A. Gillis (letter), *Br. med. J.*, 1978, *2*, 1717.

Epileptogenic effect. A grand mal seizure occurred in a 22-year-old woman with a history of febrile convulsions who had been treated with lithium carbonate 300 mg thrice daily for 4 days for control of mania. The concentration of lithium in the serum after 2 days' treatment was 0.75 mmol per litre and on the morning of the seizure was 0.78 mmol. It seemed necessary to achieve therapeutic blood concentrations of lithium more slowly in patients with a history of convulsions.— R. Demers *et al.* (letter), *Lancet*, 1970, *2*, 315.

Further references.— D. Mayfield and R. G. Brown, *J. psychiat. Res.*, 1966, *4*, 207; S. R. Platman and R. R. Fieve, *Br. J. Psychiat.*, 1969, *115*, 1185; C. C. Pfeiffer *et al.*, *J. clin. Pharmac.*, 1969, *9*, 298; R. A. Brumback *et al.*, *Pediatrics*, 1975, *56*, 831.

Extrapyramidal effects. Extrapyramidal symptoms in 2 patients receiving lithium carbonate which worsened following administration of orphenadrine.— P. Tyrer *et al.*, *Br. J. Psychiat.*, 1980, *136*, 191.

See also under Cogwheel Rigidity and Effects on Speech (both above).

Lupus erythematosus. A controlled study of 50 patients who had been taking lithium carbonate for 2 months to 10 years indicated that antinuclear antibodies were more common in patients taking lithium carbonate than in controls. The absence of anti-DNA antibodies indicated that they did not have true systemic lupus erythematosus but patients ingesting lithium might be at risk.— A. P. Presley *et al.*, *Br. med. J.*, 1976, *2*, 280.

Of 100 psychiatric patients 25 had antinuclear antibodies in their serum; of 7 taking lithium carbonate 4 had antinuclear antibodies. Drug treatment, particularly with lithium, could be a causal factor.— E. C. Johnstone and K. Whaley, *Br. med. J.*, 1975, *2*, 724. See also *idem*, *Br. J. clin. Pharmac.*, 1975, *2*, 377P.

Oedema. Oedema was associated with lithium treatment in 5 patients.— H. C. Stancer and R. Kivi (letter), *Lancet*, 1971, *2*, 985. See also A. Coppen and D. M. Shaw, *Lancet*, 1967, *2*, 805.

Overdosage. Lithium poisoning occurred in 8 patients given 600 mg of lithium carbonate daily. Early signs of poisoning included drowsiness, coarse tremor or muscle twitching, vomiting, and diarrhoea. Later developments were dominated by CNS involvement; impairment of consciousness, coarse tremor, and fasciculations were prominent. Epileptic seizures, hyper-extension of limbs, lateral rotation of the head, one-sided extensor plantar reflex, and conjugate lateral deviation of the eyes were seen in some patients. Kidney dysfunction, indicated by oliguria and moderate increases in the blood concentrations of urea or creatinine, occurred in 7 patients. ECG changes were seen in 3 patients, and atrial flutter and arrhythmia developed in 1 patient during the day before death. Serum concentrations were usually above 2 to 3 mmol per litre during severe lithium intoxication. Administration of sodium chloride 10 to 12 g daily or potassium chloride 2 to 4 g daily failed to affect the rate at which serum-lithium concentrations diminished.— M. Schou *et al.*, *Am. J. Psychiat.*, 1968, *125*, 520.

A report of 23 patients with lithium intoxication and a review of 100 cases of lithium intoxication in the literature. Lithium intoxication developed gradually in most patients and was characterised by mental and neurological symptoms, while gastro-intestinal symptoms were seen in only 2 patients. The initial symptoms were decreased alertness or slight apathy followed by muscular rigidity and/or muscular fasciculation with varying localisation, and slight ataxia. The symptoms worsened gradually and impaired consciousness, more severe fasciculation and coarse irregular tremor of the limbs and worsening ataxia developed. The severest state of lithium intoxication was characterised by a stupor-like impairment of consciousness or 'coma vigil' and spontaneous or latent twitching movements of the limbs, body, and head, often simulating a state of agitation in some patients and epilepsy in others. In most patients symptoms progressed despite stopping lithium with reduction in serum-lithium concentrations. There was no clear-cut relationship between the serum-lithium concentration and the severity of symptoms, and the length of exposure to the raised serum-lithium concentration and individual tolerance appear to play a role. Serum-lithium concentrations of 1.5 to 2.5 mmol per litre 12 hours after the last dose of lithium are usually accompanied by slight or moderate symptoms of intoxication; concentrations of 2.5 to 3.5 mmol per litre are to be regarded as serious, and concentrations above 3.5 mmol per litre are to be regarded as life-threatening. Knowledge about the mechanism of lithium intoxication is still sparse but a decrease in renal function appears to play a role and water loss may be one of the main precipitating factors.— H. E. Hansen and A. Amdisen, *Q.J. Med.*, 1978, *47*, 123.

Further references.— B. von Hartitzsch *et al.*, *Br. med. J.*, 1972, *4*, 757; F. A. Herrero, *J. Am. med. Ass.*, 1973, *226*, 1109; P. Juul-Jensen and M. Schou (letter), *Br. med. J.*, 1973, *4*, 673; S. Lavender *et al.*, *Postgrad. med. J.*, 1973, *49*, 277; E. A. Wolpert, *Am. J. Psychiat.*, 1977, *134*, 580; L. H. Warick, *West. J. Med.*, 1979, *130*, 259.

Pregnancy and the neonate. *Effects on the foetus.* Congenital abnormalities were observed in 6% of 88 infants born to mothers taking lithium carbonate during at least the first trimester of pregnancy. This incidence was considered to be no greater than that observed in the general population of infants.— M. D. Goldfield and M. R. Weinstein, *Am. J. Obstet. Gynec.*, 1973, *116*, 15. Infants born to 143 mothers who took lithium during pregnancy had a higher than expected ratio of cardiovascular anomalies to all anomalies.— M. R. Weinstein and M. D. Goldfield, *Am. J. Psychiat.*, 1975, *132*, 529. See also J. J. Nora *et al.* (letter), *Lancet*, 1974, *2*, 594.

In a retrospective study of 118 infants born to mothers who had taken lithium during the first trimester of pregnancy, 5 were stillborn and 7 died within the first week of life; of these 12, malformations were present in 6 and also in 3 others. Six of the 9 malformations involved the cardiovascular system; 1 was unilateral microtia; 1 was single umbilical artery with bilateral hypoplasia of maxilla; and 1 was stenosis of aqueduct with hydrocephalus, spina bifida with sacral meningomyelocele, and bilateral talipes equinovarus with paralysis. The incidence of malformations was much lower than indicated by *animal* studies.— M. Schou *et al.*, *Br. med. J.*, 1973, *2*, 135. Follow-up of 60 children, aged 5 years or more, who had been exposed to lithium throughout or during the first trimester of pregnancy and who were apparently normal at birth. Compared with their siblings who had not been exposed, no increased frequency of physical or mental anomalies was noted among the lithium children.— M. Schou, *Acta psychiat. scand.*, 1976, *54*, 193.

Individual reports of adverse effects in infants exposed to lithium before birth.— K. Karlsson *et al.* (letter), *Lancet*, 1975, *1*, 1295 (goitre); P. W. Nars and J. Girard, *Am. J. Dis. Child.*, 1977, *131*, 924 (goitre); A. Rane *et al.*, *J. Pediat.*, 1978, *93*, 296 (cardiovascular malformations); E. M. Mizrahi *et al.*, *J. Pediat.*, 1979, *94*, 493 (nephrogenic diabetes insipidus).

Effects on the mother. A 30-year-old woman who was given lithium carbonate in late pregnancy developed a toxic condition during delivery, apparently due to haemodynamic and metabolic alterations. She was lethargic after delivery and became incoherent and incontinent, with lithium concentrations in serum of up to 4.4 mmol per litre. She was successfully treated with carefully monitored massive diuresis with frusemide and mannitol. The infant had a high serum-lithium concentration (2.4 mmol per litre) with clinical signs of cyanosis and flaccid muscle tone which gradually improved.— G. D. Wilbanks *et al.*, *J. Am. med. Ass.*, 1970, *213*, 865.

In 4 healthy pregnant women given test doses of lithium carbonate, lithium clearances fell significantly after delivery. In 1 manic-depressive woman lithium clearance rose during pregnancy. Frequent assessments of serum-lithium concentrations were necessary during pregnancy and immediately after delivery so that the dose might be adjusted to avoid inadequate control during pregnancy or toxicity after delivery.— M. Schou *et al.*, *Br. med. J.*, 1973, *2*, 137.

Throughout pregnancy a manic-depressive woman required lithium carbonate, 1.5 g daily to maintain the serum lithium at 0.4 mmol per litre yet in the 24 hours following delivery signs of acute lithium poisoning developed with a serum-lithium concentration of 3.57 mmol per litre which fell to zero 9 days after the withdrawal of lithium. The body-fluid changes of pregnancy and a concomitant salt-free dietary regimen were thought to be contributory factors. The child was also suffering from lithium intoxication and required exchange transfusion; serum-lithium had fallen to zero by the twelfth day although accompanying hypotonia took longer to disappear. Neither mother nor child displayed electrolyte abnormalities.— M. Piton *et al.*, *Thérapie*, 1973, *28*, 1123.

A 36-year-old woman who had been taking lithium carbonate 800 mg daily became pregnant and the dose had progressively to be reduced to 400 mg to maintain therapeutic serum concentrations; the dose required returned to 800 mg daily after delivery. The infant's serum concentration of lithium (about 0.3 μmol per ml) at delivery fell rapidly and then rose again and was maintained at about 0.1 μmol per ml during breast feeding. The concentration of lithium in breast milk was about half that in maternal serum. Breast feeding was discouraged and stopped at 10 weeks.— P. A. Sykes *et al.*, *Br. med. J.*, 1976, *2*, 1299.

Effects on the neonate. Hypotonia, poor sucking, and poor respiration in a newborn infant was attributed to lithium toxicity; the concentration of lithium in cord blood was 0.32 mmol per litre. The mother had been taking 800 mg of lithium carbonate daily, yielding serum-lithium concentrations of 0.06 to 0.2 mmol per litre.— J. K. Stothers *et al.* (letter), *Br. med. J.*, 1973, *3*, 233. See also W. W. Tunnessen, *J. Pediat.*, 1972, *81*, 804.

See also under Precautions and Absorption and Fate.

Weight gain. A discussion of weight gain associated with lithium.— R. J. Kerry (letter), *Br. med. J.*, 1974, *2*, 441.

Evidence that patients gaining excessive amounts of weight during lithium therapy can lose weight by means of a calorie-controlled dietary regimen. Because electrolyte balance is important in the avoidance of lithium side-effects, it should be emphasised that weight loss can and should occur with a normal intake of sodium chloride.— G. M. Dempsey *et al.*, *Am. J. Psychiat.*, 1976, *133*, 1082.

Treatment of Adverse Effects. In the case of recent severe overdosage the stomach should be emptied by aspiration and lavage. As a result of the narrow margin between therapeutic and toxic serum concentrations, however, lithium poisoning may also develop during the course of therapeutic lithium administration.

Early lithium poisoning in patients with normal renal function may be treated by discontinuation of lithium and forced diuresis as described under phenobarbitone (p.812). Otherwise prolonged haemodialysis should be initiated without delay; peritoneal dialysis is less effective and only appropriate if haemodialysis facilities are not available.

Administration of sodium chloride is not recommended since it does not adequately enhance lithium excretion and may cause hypernatraemia.

The excretion of lithium was increased by osmotic diuresis with urea, and the administration of sodium bicarbonate, acetazolamide, and aminophylline. Frusemide, bendrofluazide, ethacrynic acid, ammonium chloride, spironolactone, potassium chloride, or water diuresis did not affect lithium excretion. A sodium-poor diet led to decrease and extra dietary sodium chloride led to increase of lithium excretion; the changes took place relatively slowly.— K. Thomsen and M. Schou, *Am. J. Physiol.*, 1968, *215*, 823.

A report of 23 patients with lithium intoxication and review of 100 cases of lithium intoxication in the literature. Administration of sodium chloride failed to enhance lithium excretion, and treatment with large volumes of sodium solutions should be avoided because of the risk of developing hypernatraemia due to water-losing nephritis in lithium-intoxicated patients. Fluid therapy or forced diuresis treatment should only be recommended in those with early symptoms of lithium intoxication, normal renal function, and when it is certain that the serum-lithium concentration has been raised for only a few days and is not above 2.5 mmol per litre. Serum-lithium concentrations should be determined at short intervals to assure that the concentration falls to 1 mmol per litre within 30 hours. If these criteria cannot be fulfilled dialysis should be initiated. Haemodialysis is considered the most effective way to remove lithium ions from an intoxicated patient. It must be carried out for a long period (10 to 12 hours) and repeated if necessary to ensure the removal of sufficient amounts of lithium from the body. Serum-lithium concentrations must be determined at short intervals after dialysis to ensure that the concentration remains low, a serum-lithium concentration of less than 1 mmol per litre six to eight hours after stopping dialysis being considered evidence of adequate treatment. Peritoneal dialysis gives a slower removal of lithium ions and should be used only if haemodialysis facilities are not available. The most effective way to prevent lithium intoxication is by regular control of 12-hour serum-lithium concentrations, and assessment of renal function and concentrating ability during therapy; daily control of 12-hour serum-lithium concentrations should be carried out where water and electrolyte balance may be disturbed.— H. E. Hansen and A. Amdisen, *Q. J. Med.*, 1978, *47*, 123.

Two patients developed hypernatraemia and hyperosmolality when treated with compound sodium lactate injection for lithium toxicity. The patients improved when the infusion was withdrawn and chlorothiazide, previously given to control polyuria and polydipsia, was re-introduced.— J. Mann *et al.*, *Br. med. J.*, 1978, *1*, 1522. Acute lithium intoxication in a 40-year-old man was successfully treated by intravenous infusion of sodium chloride injection, sodium bicarbonate injection 8.4%, and mannitol 10%.— J. M. Shneerson, *Br. J. clin. Pract.*, 1978, *32*, 232. See also Diuresis (below).

Further references.— R. Gaind and B. M. Sarand (letter), *Lancet*, 1970, *1*, 197 (lactate infusion); G. K. Spring, *Dis. nerv. Syst.*, 1974, *35*, 351 (phenytoin for seizures).

Control of lithium-induced side-effects at therapeutic concentrations.— J. M. Kellett *et al.*, *J. Neurol. Neurosurg. Psychiat.*, 1975, *38*, 719 (poor results with practolol and propranolol on tremor); R. P. Juhl *et al.*, *Am. J. Hosp. Pharm.*, 1976, *33*, 843 (hydrochlorothiazide for nephrogenic diabetes insipidus); Y. D. Lapierre, *Can. med. Ass. J.*, 1976, *114*, 619 (beneficial results with propranolol on tremor); G. Chambers *et al.*, *Br. med. J.*, 1977, *2*, 805 (bendrofluazide for thirst and polyuria); E. Widerlöv *et al.* (letter), *Lancet*, 1977, *2*, 1080 (desmopressin for thirst and polyuria).

For reference to the use of linoleic acid in the form of safflower oil in the treatment of lithium-induced neurotoxicity, see Safflower Oil, p.697.

Aspiration and lavage. A report of delayed absorption of lithium in intoxication. It was suggested that gastric lavage should be performed in addition to forced diuresis and dialysis.— H. Jensen and J. Ladefoged, *Eur. J. clin. Pharmac.*, 1975, *8*, 285.

Dialysis. A 57-year-old man who was treated with 1.6 g of lithium carbonate daily as a sustained-release preparation became drowsy and had a serum-lithium concentration of 3.17 mmol per litre. He became comatose and developed muscle tremor and hypotension with oliguria; the ECG showed changes. Haemodialysis for 17½ hours reduced the lithium concentration to 1.6 mmol per litre but his condition did not improve and he died. As lithium was distributed in the water phase of the body, frequent or continuous dialysis over a long period was necessary to reduce toxic concentrations in intracellular fluid and to remove lithium from the bones.— J. B. Hawkins and P. R. Dorken (letter), *Lancet*, 1969, *1*, 839.

A patient who had received lithium carbonate, 1.5 to 2.4 g daily for 10 years, developed renal failure and lithium intoxication with drowsiness and coma. The serum concentration of lithium was about 3 mmol per litre. Haemodialysis for 6½ hours reduced the lithium concentration to 0.7 mmol per litre. Four days after dialysis the lithium concentration in the serum was 0.4 mmol and 0.1 mmol per litre in the cerebrospinal fluid. The patient regained full consciousness after 5 days with no permanent after-effects.— A. Amdisen and H. Skjoldborg (letter), *Lancet*, 1969, *2*, 213.

Haemodialysis was much more effective than peritoneal dialysis for the treatment of acute lithium intoxication in a 62-year-old man with a serum-lithium concentration of 4.2 mmol per litre. Frusemide 1.5 g daily had no diuretic effect and renal biopsy demonstrated kidney damage, the patient remaining oliguric for 10 days.— P. Allain *et al.*, *Thérapie*, 1973, *28*, 1135.

Diuresis. Forced alkaline diuresis for 48 hours was successfully used to treat a 49-year-old man suffering from lithium intoxication, with a serum-lithium concentration of 4 mmol per litre. Keeping urinary pH above 7, volumes of 500 ml of either M/6 lactate, 1.26% sodium bicarbonate, or 5% laevulose, were given intravenously every hour with potassium supplements. There was some rebound during the first 24 hours. Although less efficient than haemodialysis, the method used was as effective as peritoneal dialysis when renal function was not impaired, and carried less risk of complications.— J. A. H. Forrest, *Postgrad. med. J.*, 1975, *51*, 189.

Precautions. The margin between the therapeutic and the toxic concentration of lithium is narrow, therefore it should be given under close medical supervision, and serum concentrations should be monitored regularly under controlled conditions, see Absorption and Fate (below). Unless deemed essential, lithium should be avoided in patients with any significant cardiovascular or renal impairment. It is contra-indicated in severe renal disease, in debilitated or dehydrated patients, and in those with sodium depletion; it is reported to be contra-indicated in Addison's disease.

Patients receiving lithium therapy should be taught to recognise the symptoms of early toxicity and, should these occur, to discontinue therapy and request medical aid at once. Among other factors, lithium requirements may change during fever, infection, and when mood swings occur. Patients should also be instructed to take their tablets at exactly the stipulated time, and not to compensate for an omitted dose by subsequently taking a double dose. Reduction in sodium intake increases the amount of lithium retained by the kidneys leading to a rise in serum-lithium concentrations; therefore, patients should avoid low-salt dietary regimens or other dietary changes which may reduce sodium intake, or circumstances which may cause excessive sodium loss such as those leading to excessive sweating, or diarrhoea, with resultant dehydration. Conversely, increased sodium intake increases the amount of lithium excreted by the kidneys, leading to reduced serum-lithium concentrations; therefore, sodium-containing medicaments, such as sodium bicarbonate in indigestion mixtures or 'fruit salts', should not be given concomitantly with lithium salts. Concurrent administration of diuretics with lithium exerts a paradoxical antidiuretic effect in patients receiving lithium, and diuretics are normally contra-indicated in patients receiving lithium therapy; nevertheless, cautious use has been made of this interaction to raise serum-lithium concentrations in refractory hospital in-patients with low serum-lithium concentrations and lithium-induced diabetes insipidus.

Patients receiving lithium should be examined periodically for abnormal thyroid function, since goitre and hypothyroidism may develop. Lithium should be used with particular care in the elderly. Impaired driving performance may occur in patients receiving lithium.

An increased incidence of cardiovascular abnormalities has been noted in the infants of women given lithium during the first 3 months of pregnancy. In pregnant women the dosage requirements of lithium can vary very abruptly, particularly immediately after delivery. The infants of women given lithium during late pregnancy may develop lithium intoxication. Lithium is excreted in breast milk.

Impaired driving performance in patients receiving lithium. The subjects usually felt that their performance had improved which might increase the driving risk.— T. Seppala *et al.*, *Drugs*, 1979, *17*, 389.

A warning that if patients with lithium-induced polyuria must not take fluids by mouth before an operation they should be given intravenous fluids the night before the operation.— M. Schou, *Br. med. J.*, 1981, *283*, 1253 and 1528.

Acidosis. Lithium treatment might make patients more susceptible to metabolic acidosis.— J. W. Jefferson, *Ann. intern. Med.*, 1978, *88*, 434.

Blood donation. It was considered that patients being treated with lithium would be acceptable as blood donors. The amount present in donor's blood at steady-state concentrations would have no biological significance when diluted in the recipient.— R. K. Gupta and S. Montgomery (letter), *Lancet*, 1975, *1*, 860.

Interactions. *Adrenaline and other sympathomimetics.* Lithium carbonate 1.2 g given daily for 7 to 10 days to 8 patients with manic depression depressed the pressor effects of *noradrenaline* in 7. Sensitivity to tyramine was unaffected.— W. E. Fann *et al.*, *Clin. Pharmac. Ther.*, 1972, *13*, 71.

A woman who had been stabilised on lithium treatment for 15 months developed lithium toxicity within a few days of being given *mazindol* 2 mg daily.— M. S. Hendy *et al.*, *Br. med. J.*, 1980, *280*, 684.

Alcohol. In tests on psychomotor skills lithium tended to antagonise the effects of alcohol, except on coordination where the effects were additive. The combination would therefore be dangerous in drivers.— M. Linnoila *et al.*, *Eur. J. clin. Pharmac.*, 1974, *7*, 337. In 23 healthy subjects therapeutic lithium concentrations did not affect positive subjective experiences from alcohol.— L. L. Judd *et al.*, *Archs gen. Psychiat.*, 1977, *34*, 463 and 615. Alcohol usually exacerbates lithium-induced tremor.— J. B. Loudon (letter), *Br. J. Hosp. Med.*, 1978, *19*, 294.

Antacids. Administration of *sodium bicarbonate* with lithium led to considerably reduced blood-lithium concentrations. On stopping the practice at least 2 patients developed toxic concentrations of lithium.— C. McSwiggan (letter), *Aust. J. Pharm.*, 1978, *59*, 6.

Antibiotics. Raised blood-lithium concentrations and signs of lithium toxicity developed in a woman receiving maintenance lithium therapy when she was treated with *spectinomycin* for gonorrhoea.— *Int. Drug Ther. Newslett.*, 1978, *13*, 15.

In a 30-year-old woman who had taken lithium carbonate for about 3 years with a stable serum-lithium concentration of 0.5 to 0.84 mmol per litre, that value rose to 1.7 mmol per litre and to 2.74 mmol per litre 2 and 4 days respectively after beginning a course of *tetracycline*.— A. J. McGennis, *Br. med. J.*, 1978, *1*, 1183. The toxicity might have been due to a low sodium intake possibly aggravated by tetracycline-induced diarrhoeal sodium loss.— U. Malt (letter), *ibid.*, 1978, *2*, 502.

Aspirin and other anti-inflammatory agents. In 3 psychiatric patients and 4 healthy subjects steady-state plasma-lithium concentrations were elevated by a mean of 59% and 30% respectively during treatment with *indomethacin* 50 mg thrice daily. Renal lithium clearance was suppressed (in the 7) by a mean of 31%, possibly by a prostaglandin-sensitive mechanism.— J. C. Frölich *et al.*, *Br. med. J.*, 1979, *1*, 1115.

Increased plasma-lithium concentrations in healthy subjects given concomitant *diclofenac*.— I. W. Reimann and J. C. Frölich, *Clin. Pharmac. Ther.*, 1981, *30*, 348.

Benzodiazepines. Hypothermia occurred on 4 occasions in a patient treated with lithium carbonate and *diazepam*, but not when either drug was given alone.— G. J. Naylor and A. McHarg, *Br. med. J.*, 1977, *2*, 22.

Diuretics. A brief discussion on the antidiuretic effect of diuretics when used with lithium.— S. MacNeil *et al.* (letter), *Lancet*, 1975, *1*, 1295.

The renal clearance of lithium in 18 patients after a single 600-mg dose was 20.2 ml per minute compared with 15.4 ml per minute in 16 patients under treatment with *hydroflumethiazide* 25 mg daily or *bendrofluazide* 2.5 mg daily; the reduction in clearance was significant. In 12 patients for whom paired observations were available the respective clearances of 19.8 and 15.7 ml per minute were not significantly different. Thiazides, and probably other diuretics, should be given with care to patients taking lithium, as the reduction in clearance might raise lithium concentrations to toxic values.— V. Petersen *et al.*, *Br. med. J.*, 1974, *3*, 143.

A 66-year-old man well controlled on lithium carbonate had symptoms of lithium toxicity and a serum-lithium concentration of 2.4 mmol per litre a week after starting to take *amiloride* and *hydrochlorothiazide*. The symptoms regressed only slowly when the diuretics were withdrawn.— A. C. Macfie (letter), *Br. med. J.*, 1975, *1*, 516.

Analysis of published data from up to 13 patients receiving concurrent lithium carbonate and *chlorothiazide* therapy indicated that to obtain the same concentration of lithium in serum as had been achieved without chlorothiazide the daily lithium dose should be reduced by about 40% in patients given chlorothiazide 500 mg daily, and by about 60% or 70% in those receiving 0.75 to 1 g daily. Care should be taken to define adequate renal function in patients intended for this association.— J. M. Himmelhoch *et al.*, *Clin. Pharmac. Ther.*, 1977, *22*, 225.

In a study of 5 healthy subjects receiving lithium 300 mg thrice daily, there were no significant changes in serum-lithium concentrations when *frusemide* 40 mg daily was given concurrently for 2 weeks. However, concurrent administration of *hydrochlorothiazide* 50 mg daily resulted in a significant increase in serum-lithium concentrations.— J. W. Jefferson and N. H. Kalin, *J. Am. med. Ass.*, 1979, *241*, 1134.

Two patients with a manic depressive disorder well stabilised on lithium carbonate had toxic serum-lithium concentrations following the administration of diuretics.— R. J. Kerry *et al.*, *Br. med. J.*, 1980, *281*, 371. See also J. W. Jefferson (letter), *ibid.*, 1217.

Further references.— T. P. Detre *et al.*, *Am. J. Psychiat.*, 1977, *134*, 149 (synergistic use); B. M. Maletzky, *J. clin. Psychiat.*, 1979, *40*, 317 (synergistic use).

ECT. A 32-year-old man receiving treatment with lithium carbonate 2.4 g daily together with chlorprothixene 800 mg daily, and having a serum-lithium concentration of 1.09 mmol per litre, suffered severe encephalopathy following ECT. It was suggested that while serum concentrations were below toxic concentrations tissue concentrations of lithium might be high and these should be reduced before ECT was given.— J. Hoenig and R. Chaulk (letter), *Can. med. Ass. J.*, 1977, *116*, 837. See also G. Jephcott and R. J. Kerry, *Br. J. Anaesth.*, 1974, *46*, 389.

Methyldopa. Concomitant administration of methyldopa appeared to induce signs of lithium toxicity in a patient stabilised on lithium carbonate.— G. J. Byrd (letter), *J. Am. med. Ass.*, 1975, *233*, 320. See also J. B. O'Regan (letter), *Can. med. Ass. J.*, 1976, *115*, 385.

Further references.— G. J. Byrd, *Clin. Toxicol.*, 1977, *11*, 1; E. Osanloo and J. H. Deglin (letter), *Ann. intern. Med.*, 1980, *92*, 433.

Muscle relaxants. For the effect of lithium on neuromuscular blockade, see Pancuronium Bromide, p.994, and Suxamethonium Chloride, p.997.

Neuroleptics. From studies in 9 physically healthy, chronic mental patients, it was found that lithium was excreted more rapidly during *chlorpromazine* treatment than when it was administered alone.— I. Sletten *et al.*, *Curr. ther. Res.*, 1966, *8*, 441.

In 4 manic patients given lithium carbonate and high doses of *haloperidol*, acute toxic reactions consisting of weakness, lethargy, fever, tremulousness, increasing confusion, and extrapyramidal symptoms occurred. After withdrawal of the drugs 2 patients experienced permanent sequelae including a cerebellar-parkinsonian reaction with dementia, and the other 2 showed persistent dyskinesias and parkinsonism.— W. J. Cohen and N. H. Cohen, *J. Am. med. Ass.*, 1974, *230*, 1283. See also J. B. Loudon and H. Waring (letter), *Lancet*, 1976, *2*, 1088. In a retrospective study of 425 patients who had taken *haloperidol* and lithium carbonate simultaneously adverse reactions in these patients were similar to those in patients given either drug alone, and no patients developed the syndrome described by W.J. Cohen and N.H. Cohen (above).— P. C. Baastrup *et al.*, *J. Am. med. Ass.*, 1976, *236*, 2645.

Marked parkinsonism in a woman receiving *flupenthixol decanoate* in addition to lithium. A second woman, given *haloperidol* in addition to lithium, noticed tingling in her fingers and episodes of marked pallor or cyanosis of the fingers; she then developed marked retrosternal pain and the haloperidol was stopped.— A. West (letter), *Br. med. J.*, 1977, *2*, 642.

In 7 healthy subjects given lithium carbonate 300 mg thrice daily for 7 days significantly decreased plasma-chloropromazine concentrations occurred after a single dose of *chlorpromazine* 100 mg by mouth compared to values obtained in the same subjects before lithium treatment.— L. Rivera-Calimlim *et al.*, *Clin. Pharmac. Ther.*, 1978, *23*, 451.

In 2 patients with mania being treated with *chlorpromazine*, together with *haloperidol* in one, in addition to lithium therapy, withdrawal of these drugs was associated with the onset of profuse lithium-induced vomiting. Concomitant administration of chlorpromazine or haloperidol with lithium may be useful not only for their antimanic action but also for their anti-emetic action; their withdrawal may therefore be followed by a phase of nausea and vomiting occurring later than expected in the course of lithium therapy. In one patient administration of metoclopramide to control the vomiting was associated with extrapyramidal disturbances.— R. Rosser and A. Herxheimer (letter), *Lancet*, 1979, *2*, 97. Chlorpromazine facilitates lithium loss in the urine so that when it is withdrawn not only is the anti-emetic effect lost but also plasma-lithium concentrations abruptly rise, leading to nausea and vomiting. Much lithium is lost in the vomitus so that plasma-lithium concentrations may not reflect the high concentrations present when the patient originally became ill.— G. E. Pakes (letter), *ibid.*, 701.

Severe neurotoxic symptoms in 4 women given *thioridazine* in association with lithium.— G. K. Spring, *J. clin. Psychiat.*, 1979, *40*, 135.

Further references.— S. H. Preskorn *et al.*, *J. clin. Psychiat.*, 1978, *39*, 756; G. Bucht and A. Wahlin, *Acta med. scand.*, 1980, *207*, 309.

Phenytoin and other anticonvulsants. A report of severe CNS toxicity in a patient, possibly with minimal brain damage, taking phenytoin, phenobarbitone, and lithium carbonate 2 to 2.4 g daily; his serum-lithium concentration was 0.8 mmol per litre.— J. Speirs and S. R. Hirsch, *Br. med. J.*, 1978, *1*, 815. Polydipsia, polyuria, and tremor in a patient taking lithium carbonate and phenytoin (each in doses to provide therapeutic concentrations) ceased when the phenytoin was replaced by carbamazepine.— W. A. G. MacCallum, *ibid.*, 1980, *280*, 610. Comments.— E. Perucca and A. Richens (letter), *ibid.*, 863; K. Ghose (letter), *ibid.*, 1122.

Sodium. Increasing the sodium in the diet in a controlled study of 3 patients with manic-depression increased the excretion of lithium, reducing blood concentrations, and increased the urine volume.— R. G. Demers and R. L. Harris, *Dis. nerv. Syst.*, 1972, *33*, 372.

Further references.— R. G. Demers and G. R. Heninger, *Am. J. Psychiat.*, 1971, *128*, 132; L. Baer *et al.*, *Archs gen. Psychiat.*, 1973, *29*, 823; R. K. Arthur (letter), *Med. J. Aust.*, 1975, *2*, 918.

See also under Antacids, above.

Tricyclic antidepressants. Tricyclic drugs usually exacerbate lithium-induced tremor.— J. B. Louden (letter), *Br. J. Hosp. Med.*, 1977, *18*, 578.

For the effect of lithium on amitriptyline, see Amitriptyline Hydrochloride, p.113.

Multiple sclerosis. A report of a patient with a clinical diagnosis of multiple sclerosis, the onset of which was closely associated with initiation of lithium therapy. Although K. Kemp *et al.* (*Dis. nerv. Syst.*, 1977, *38*, 210) have successfully used a short course of lithium to treat a patient with multiple sclerosis complicated by a manic illness, lithium should be used with the utmost caution where psychotic illness is complicated by organic neurological disturbance.— P. K. Newman and M. Saunders, *Postgrad. med. J.*, 1979, *55*, 701.

Myasthenia gravis. Following addition of lithium carbonate to her haloperidol an 18-year-old woman with severe mania developed classical manifestations of severe myasthenia gravis.— R. P. Granacher (letter), *Am. J. Psychiat.*, 1977, *134*, 702.

Further references.— J. F. Neil *et al.*, *Archs gen. Psychiat.*, 1976, *33*, 1090.

Pregnancy and the neonate. Although lithium has been shown to be teratogenic to *mice* and *rats* the evidence in man is less clear-cut. The malformation-rate is slightly increased and, while not of the order to justify therapeutic abortion, it seems wise to avoid lithium during the first 3 months of a planned pregnancy. Lithium does not appear to have toxic effects on the foetus *in utero*, and a long-term follow-up of children to the age of 5 years has not shown any cognitive or behavioural abnormalities ascribable to lithium. During pregnancy, plasma clearance of lithium rises steadily up to the time of delivery and then abruptly falling to normal; hence without any change of dosage, plasma concentrations will rise after delivery, and there has been a report of post-partum coma associated with a high serum-lithium concentration, although no lithium was given after delivery. Infants born to mothers receiving lithium during the last month of pregnancy have been reported to be flaccid, cyanosed, and occasionally hypothermic. Lithium is present in breast milk and the infant's serum concentration is a third to a half the mother's; if the infant develops an infection or diarrhoea the concentration may rise sharply, and it may be wiser to avoid breast feeding. If lithium has to be administered during pregnancy, and the indications should be pressing, the blood concentration should be checked frequently and the drug given in divided doses to avoid transient peaks; it is important to avoid sodium depletion (produced by the use of diuretics, for example), as lithium is thereby retained.— I. F. Brockington, *Prescribers' J.*, 1979, *19*, 66.

See also under Adverse Effects and Absorption and Fate.

Temperature variations. A report of lithium toxicity in a 60-year-old man after dieting and sauna baths, despite warning, at a health farm.— C. M. Tonks, *Br. med. J.*, 1977, *2*, 1396. Further references.— A. L. Granoff and J. M. Davis, *J. clin. Psychiat.*, 1978, *39*, 103; H. T. Pi and F. G. Surawicz, *Clin. Toxicol.*, 1978, *13*, 479.

Withdrawal. A 58-year-old woman who had been taking lithium carbonate 0.8 to 1.6 g daily for 6 years developed an acute confusional state when lithium was withdrawn in 400-mg stages every 3 weeks. Slow withdrawal over a period of months might be necessary.— D. G. Wilkinson, *Br. med. J.*, 1979, *1*, 235. See also M. Yuce (letter), *ibid.*, 1020.

Absorption and Fate. Lithium is readily and completely absorbed from the gastro-intestinal tract when taken in solution as one of its salts; when taken in the form of tablets small amounts are lost in the faeces (up to about 15%). Peak plasma concentrations are obtained about 2 hours after ingestion, and lithium is fairly evenly distributed throughout the body over a period of several hours, with higher concentrations occurring in the bones, the thyroid gland, and portions of the brain, than in the serum. Lithium is excreted in the kidneys and can be detected in sweat and saliva. It is not bound to plasma proteins. It crosses the placenta and is excreted in breast milk. It is reported to have a biological half-life ranging from about 7 to 20 hours during the daytime; this value is considerably extended during the night and in those with impaired renal function.

Following administration of lithium salts there is wide intersubject variation between both the plasma concentrations obtained following a given dose, and between those required for therapeutic effect. Plasma concentrations also vary considerably according to factors such as the bioavailability of the lithium preparation taken, renal function, the dietary regimen of the patient, the patient's state of health, the time at which the blood sample is taken, and concomitant medication, such as sodium salts or diuretics. Moreover, there is only a narrow margin between the therapeutic and the toxic plasma concentration of lithium. Therefore, not only is individual titration of lithium dosage essential to ensure constant appropriate plasma concentrations for the patient involved, but the conditions under which the actual blood samples are taken for monitoring must be carefully controlled. In practice, serum-lithium concentrations may be monitored by means of the 12-hour standard serum-lithium estimation (12h-stSLi), which is defined as the lithium ion concentration in the serum from a blood sample drawn in the morning exactly 12 hours (±30 minutes) after the last dose of lithium in a patient who has been taking his daily lithium requirement in 2 or more divided doses and who has been taking all his tablets at the scheduled hours during the past 48 hours (A. Amdisen, *Dan. med. Bull.*, 1975, *22*, 277). Under such conditions the usual therapeutic plasma concentrations of lithium are 0.6 to 1.2 mmol per litre, with a reported range of 0.3 to 1.3 mmol per litre. At 1.5 mmol or more per litre, toxic effects may be expected.

A detailed account of the clinical pharmacokinetics of lithium and the special requirements for carefully monitoring serum-lithium concentrations during therapy.— A. Amdisen, *Clin. Pharmacokinet.*, 1977, *2*, 73. See also J. Gaillot *et al.*, *J. Pharmacokinet. Biopharm.*, 1979, *7*, 579; F. Nielsen-Kudsk and A. Amdisen, *Eur. J. clin. Pharmac.*, 1979, *16*, 271; A. Amdisen, *Ther. Drug Monit.*, 1980, *2*, 73.

Further references.— M. Serry (letter), *Lancet*, 1969, *1*, 1267 (variable excretion by manic patients); G. L. Almy and M. A. Taylor, *Archs gen. Psychiat.*, 1973, *29*, 232 (urinary retention by manic patients); E. M. Caffey and R. F. Prein, *Am. J. Psychiat.*, 1976, *133*, 567 (concentrations for prophylaxis of depression); T. B. Cooper and G. M. Simpson, *Am. J. Psychiat.*, 1976, *133*, 440 (24-hour lithium concentrations); R. W. Mason *et al.*, *Clin. Pharmacokinet.*, 1978, *3*, 241 (half-life in schizophrenic patients); B. Terhaag *et al.*, *Int. J. clin. Pharmac. Biopharm.*, 1978, *16*, 333 (plasma and CSF concentrations); J. Cox *et al.* (letter), *Med. J. Aust.*, 1979, *1*, 622 (control with low plasma concentrations); K. White *et al.*, *Int. Pharmacopsychiat.*, 1979, *14*, 185 (plasma, red cell, and CSF concentrations); P. J. Goodnick *et al.*, *Clin. Pharmac. Ther.*, 1981, *29*, 47 (increased half-life with longer duration of therapy).

Bioavailability and bioequivalence. Reviews, comments, and studies on the relative bioavailability and bioequivalence of different salts of lithium and different brands of the same lithium salt.— A. C. Altamura *et al.*, *Eur. J. clin. Pharmac.*, 1977, *12*, 59; R. I. Poust and A. G. Mallinger (letter), *ibid.*, 1978, *13*, 463; A. C. Altamura *et al.* (letter), *ibid.*, 464; E. H. Bennie *et al.*, *Br. J. clin. Pharmac.*, 1977, *4*, 479; R. P. Hullin (letter), *Br. med. J.*, 1977, *1*, 1349; H. Godfrey (letter), *Pharm. J.*, 1977, *1*, 460; T. B. Cooper *et al.*, *Am. J. Psychiat.*, 1978, *135*, 917; D. P. Thornhill, *Eur. J. clin. Pharmac.*, 1978, *14*, 267; B. P. Wall *et al.*, *Aust. J. pharm. Sci.*, 1978, *7*, 57; G. Johnson *et al.*, *Med. J. Aust.*, 1979, *2*, 382; T. E. Needham *et al.*, *J. pharm. Sci.*, 1979, *68*, 952.

Plasma and red blood cell concentrations. Some studies, comments, and reviews on the significance of the ratio between lithium concentrations in the plasma and in the red blood cells for the management of lithium therapy.— J. L. Marini, *Br. J. Psychiat.*, 1977, *130*, 139; J. J. Ratey and A. G. Mallinger, *ibid.*, *131*, 59; J. Rybakowski *et al.*, *Clin. Pharmac. Ther.*, 1977, *22*, 465; E. Sacchetti *et al.* (letter), *Lancet*, 1977, *1*, 908; G. N. Pandey *et al.*, *Clin. Pharmac. Ther.*, 1978, *24*, 343; B. B. Johnston *et al.*, *Br. J. Psychiat.*, 1979, *134*, 482; T. A. Ramsey *et al.*, *Archs gen. Psychiat.*, 1979, *36*, 457.

Plasma and saliva concentrations. Some studies on the correlation between plasma and saliva concentrations of lithium.— U. Groth *et al.*, *Clin. Pharmac. Ther.*, 1974, *16*, 490; C. Neu and A. Di Mascio, *Psychopharmac. Bull.*, 1977, *13*, 55; M. Shimizu and D. F. Smith, *Clin. Pharmac. Ther.*, 1977, *21*, 212; J. -L. Evrard *et al.*, *Acta psychiat. scand.*, 1978, *58*, 67; P. Ravenscroft *et al.*, *Archs gen. Psychiat.*, 1978, *35*, 1123; A. Sims *et al.*, *Br. J. Psychiat.*, 1978, *132*, 152; Man. P.L., *Psychosomatics*, 1979, *20*, 758; E. Othmer *et al.*, *J. clin. Psychiat.*, 1979, *40*, 525; H. Vlaar *et al.*, *Acta psychiat. scand.*, 1979, *60*, 423; A. W. Rosman *et al.*, *Am. J. Hosp. Pharm.*, 1980, *37*, 514.

Pregnancy and the neonate. An analysis of figures from various sources showed that the breast milk of 8 mothers taking lithium had lithium concentrations of about one-half those of maternal serum. The lithium concentration of the infants' serum was one-half to one-third that of the maternal serum.— M. Schou and A. Amdisen, *Br. med. J.*, 1973, *2*, 138.

A healthy infant with normal neonatal blood concentrations of thyroxine and of thyrotrophin was born to a mother given lithium carbonate from the 11th week of pregnancy. There was no placental barrier to the diffusion of lithium ions, but the concentration of lithium in the amniotic fluid was higher than in the umbilical cord venous blood.— A. V. P. Mackay *et al.*, *Br. med. J.*, 1976, *1*, 878. See also H. Fries (letter), *Lancet*, 1970, *1*, 1233.

See also under Adverse Effects and Precautions.

Uses. Lithium carbonate is used as a source of lithium ions which may act by competing with sodium ions at various sites in the body. The mechanism by which it exerts its effect in affective disorders is not known. It is used in the prophylaxis and treatment of mania and in the prophylaxis of manic depression and depression.

The usual dose of lithium carbonate for prophylactic therapy is 0.6 to 1.2 g daily. The initial dose given is adjusted after 5 to 7 days by amounts of 200 to 400 mg daily according to the results of serum-lithium estimations obtained under strictly controlled conditions (the 12h-stSLi, see Absorption and Fate for details). During the initial stages of lithium therapy, serum-lithium concentrations must then be checked at least once a week to ensure that they remain within the usual therapeutic range of 0.6 to 1.2 mmol per litre; when consistent concentrations have been achieved, estimations may be made monthly and, eventually, every 2 months.

In the acute treatment of mania and hypomania up to 1.5 to 2 g daily may be given for the first 5 to 7 days, together with close checks on the 12h-stSLi to maintain the serum-lithium concentration within the optimum range of 0.6 to 1.2 mmol per litre. The dose must be reduced rapidly once the acute phase has passed.

The range between the toxic and the therapeutic concentration of lithium is narrow and efforts must be made to avoid toxic peaks in an otherwise therapeutic serum concentration. To this end the daily dosage should preferably be divided into at least 2 portions, which must always be taken at exactly the stipulated time of day, and the patient must be warned never to compensate for an omitted dose by subsequently taking a double dose. Similarly, lithium should preferably be taken after food to avoid an initial high absorption peak. Various formulations of lithium carbonate tablets are available which are not necessarily bioequivalent, and it is essential that patients should not be switched between these without special control of their serum-lithium concentrations.

Patients must also be taught to recognise the symptoms of early lithium intoxication (which may be expected at concentrations of 1.5 mmol per litre or more) in order to omit further doses of lithium and seek medical care. Patients must similarly be warned that the following may affect lithium dosage requirements: intercurrent illnesses, including urinary-tract infections, manic or depressive phases, changes in dietary regimen, changes in temperature, pregnancy, and concomitant medication (in particular, sodium-containing preparations and diuretics). For further details see under Precautions (above).

The dosage of lithium should be reduced in elderly or light-weight patients. Other lithium salts have been used as a source of lithium ions and these include the acetate, aspartate, gluconate, orotate, and sulphate.

General publications, reviews and discussions on the pharmacology and toxicology of lithium.— A. I. M. Glen, *Adv. Med. Topics Ther.*, 1976, *2*, 190; M. Schou, *A. Rev. Pharmac. & Toxic.*, 1976, *16*, 231; K. Ghose, *Br. J. Hosp. Med.*, 1977, *18*, 578; A. Coppen (letter), *ibid.*, 1978, *19*, 294; *Archs gen. Psychiat.*, 1979, *36*, 833; A. H. Rosenbaum *et al.*, *Mayo Clin. Proc.*, 1979, *54*, 401; *Handbook of Lithium Therapy*, F.N. Johnson (Ed.), Lancaster, MTP, 1980; *Med. Lett.*, 1980, *22*, 17; D. P. Srinivasan and R. P. Hullin, *Br. J. Hosp. Med.*, 1980, *24*, 466; *Drug & Ther. Bull.*, 1981, *19*, 21.

Some studies into the mode of action of lithium.— R. Ebstein *et al.*, *Nature*, 1976, *259*, 411; L. L. Judd *et al.*, *Archs gen. Psychiat.*, 1977, *34*, 346 and 615; A. E. Halaris and E. M. DeMet (letter), *Lancet*, 1978, *1*, 670; G. R. Heninger, *Archs gen. Psychiat.*, 1978, *35*, 228; J. E. Hesketh *et al.*, *Br. J. clin. Pharmac.*, 1978, *5*, 323; R. S. Jope *et al.*, *New Engl. J. Med.*, 1978, *299*, 833; W. R. Millington *et al.* (letter), *ibid.*, 1979, *300*, 196; G. J. Naylor *et al.* (letter), *Lancet*, 1981, *2*, 1175 (a possible mode of action and a suggestion that methylene blue may exert a similar beneficial effect).

Administration. Detailed recommendations for the management of lithium administration, with special reference to the monitoring of serum-lithium concentrations using the 12h-stSLi, which is the concentration of lithium ions in serum or plasma of a blood sample drawn in the morning, before the first lithium dose of the day, 12(±0.5) hours after the evening dose, from a patient complying completely with treatment in regard to dosage, dose regimen, and dose timing, taking the dosage in more than one dose per day (even for the controlled sustained-release tablets), and who is in steady-state equilibrium of dosage and excretion. Based on a study of the 12h-stSLi of 79 patients on successful long-term treatment, the therapeutic range of serum-lithium concentrations is 0.3 to 1.3 mmol per litre. The highest and lowest responders differ by a factor of about 3 in respect to the 12h-stSLi, while the corresponding factor for daily dose is about 7 (ranging from 8 to 54 mmol of lithium ions daily). Based on clinical experience, the therapeutic concentration at which intoxication may occur is 1.5 mmol per litre. With a patient commencing long-term treatment, whose concentration requirements are unknown, the adjustment should aim at 0.8 to 1.0 mmol per litre, because a majority of patients are seriously disturbed by adverse reactions at the upper end of the therapeutic range, before the adaptation period has elapsed; only patients suffering from relapse should subsequently be pushed to the upper concentrations. The 12h-stSLi should then be checked once a week over the following months, monthly over the next 6 months, and every second month thereafter. In addition the patient should be trained to recognise the symptom association of poisoning of moderate intensity: speech difficulty, irregular tremor, myoclonic twitchings, muscular weakness, and ataxia which calls for immediate discontinuation of the treatment and referral to the physician for control of the 12h-stSLi.— A. Amdisen, Lithium, in *Therapeutic Relevance of Drug Assays*, F.A. de Wolff *et al.* (Ed.), Leiden University Press, 1979, p. 63. A view that satisfactory plasma-lithium concentrations can be obtained with a once-daily dosage of a slow-release preparation of lithium carbonate.— K. Ghose, *Br. J. Hosp. Med.*, 1977, *18*, 578; A. Coppen (letter), *ibid.*, 1978, *19*, 294.

In children. A warning that lithium should only be given to the young with extreme caution; it should not be given to children under 12 years of age unless there are special indications. Although aggressive behaviour in young people is an indication for lithium this should be when it is hyperaggressive, occurring in an adolescent over 12 years of age, and not amenable to other means of treatment. In these circumstances short-term therapy for up to 6 months could be beneficial and the child may respond to lower doses than those recommended; long-term therapy in the young should be avoided.— B. Lena (letter), *Br. med. J.*, 1979, *1*, 685.

References to the use of lithium in children.— L. L. Greenhill *et al.*, *Archs gen. Psychiat.*, 1973, *28*, 636; R. A. Brumback and W. A. Weinberg, *Am. J. Dis. Child.*, 1977, *131*, 1122; J. Youngerman and I. Canino, *Archs gen. Psychiat.*, 1978, *35*, 216.

In the elderly. In a study, 82 psychiatric out-patients were given lithium daily to give a plasma concentration of 1 mmol per litre. It was considered necessary to reduce the daily weight-related lithium dose by 50% over the age range of 20 to 79 years to compensate for an age-related decrease in lithium excretion and to reduce lithium side-effects to a level comparable to that acceptable in younger patients.— D. S. Hewick *et al.*, *Br. J. clin. Pharmac.*, 1977, *4*, 201.

Further references.— J. R. Foster *et al.*, *J. Geront.*, 1977, *32*, 299.

Administration in renal failure. Lithium carbonate could be given in usual doses to patients with a glomerular filtration-rate of more than 50 ml per minute but should be avoided in patients with a glomerular filtration-rate of less than 50 ml per minute. Concentrations of lithium carbonate were affected by haemodialysis and peritoneal dialysis; plasma concentrations rose after dialysis as re-equilibration with tissue stores occurred.— W. M. Bennett *et al.*, *Ann. intern. Med.*, 1980, *93*, 286.

Individual reports. A 47-year-old woman with hypomania and on regular haemodialysis, intolerant of lithium carbonate by mouth, was successfully controlled by the addition of lithium chloride 1 mmol per litre to the dialysate solution; plasma concentrations were maintained at 0.8 to 0.9 mmol (0.8 to 0.9 mEq) per litre.— W. F. Oakley *et al.*, *Postgrad. med. J.*, 1974, *50*, 511.

A 25-year-old woman who suffered an episode of hypomania during maintenance haemodialysis was successfully treated with lithium carbonate 600 mg by mouth following each dialysis.— W. R. Procci, *J. nerv. ment. Dis.*, 1977, *164*, 355.

Alcohol and drug abuse. *Alcoholism.* A study involving 15 alcoholic patients with bipolar affective disorders and given lithium showed that 8 were free of their affective disorder for 6 or more months and that 5 were free of alcoholism. It was considered that lithium might be effective against symptoms of alcoholism in only a subgroup of alcoholics with affective symptoms or that it might have anti-alcoholic activity different to its antimanic or antidepressant activity.— L. D. Young and M. H. Keeler (letter), *Lancet*, 1977, *1*, 144.

Further references.— N. S. Kline *et al.*, *Am. J. med. Sci.*, 1974, *268*, 15; J. C. Wren *et al.*, *Clin. Med.*, 1974, *81* (Jan.), 33; J. Merry *et al.*, *Lancet*, 1976, *2*, 481; E. M. Sellers *et al.*, *Clin. Pharmac. Ther.*, 1976, *20*, 199; L. L. Judd *et al.*, *Archs gen. Psychiat.*, 1977, *34*, 463.

Drug abuse. In 3 patients lithium carbonate blocked the effects of amphetamine or phenmetrazine. Its use was suggested as a prophylactic in amphetamine abusers.— A. Flemenbaum, *Am. J. Psychiat.*, 1974, *131*, 820.

In a double-blind study in 8 non-psychotic subjects with histories of narcotic abuse, lithium carbonate did not block either the euphoric or the miotic effects of morphine.— D. R. Jasinski *et al.*, *Science*, 1977, *195*, 582.

Further references.— A. Flemenbaum *et al.*, *Compreh. Psychiat.*, 1979, *20*, 91.

Anaesthesia. Studies in *animals* suggested that lithium might be useful as a premedicant.— B. I. Diamond *et al.* (letter), *Lancet*, 1977, *2*, 1229.

A review of the potential hazards and therapeutic applications of lithium in anaesthetics.— H. S. Havdala *et al.*, *Anesthesiology*, 1979, *50*, 534.

Asthma. Two patients with asthma and manic-depressive psychosis obtained relief of their asthmatic symptoms as well as their psychoses on receiving lithium therapy.— S. J. Nasr and R. W. Atkins, *Am. J. Psychiat.*, 1977, *134*, 1042.

Behaviour disorders. Self-mutilation was controlled in a severely subnormal patient when given lithium carbonate 500 mg thrice daily for 6 days a week to produce a steady plasma concentration of 0.9 mmol per litre. This improvement was maintained for 5 years up to the time of the report.— A. F. Cooper and H. C. Fowlie (letter), *Br. J. Psychiat.*, 1973, *122*, 370.

Results of a double-blind placebo-controlled study in 66 non-psychotic inmates of a medium security institution with histories of chronic aggressive behaviour, indicated that lithium reduced aggressive behaviour.— M. H. Sheard *et al.*, *Am. J. Psychiat.*, 1976, *133*, 1409.

Further references.— M. H. Sheard (letter), *Nature*, 1971, *230*, 113 (aggression); S. D. Morrison *et al.*, *J. Am. med. Ass.*, 1972, *220*, 1668 (aggression); T. Van Putten and J. Alban, *J. nerv. ment. Dis.*, 1977, *164*, 218 (hysteria).

Drug-induced psychoses. The hyperkinesia due to levodopa treatment for parkinsonism was abolished in one patient given lithium 12 to 16 mmol daily without any deterioration in parkinsonian symptoms and was reduced in another given lithium 2 mmol daily but with some deterioration in symptoms.— P. Dalén and G. Steg (letter), *Lancet*, 1973, *1*, 936. See also W. Braden, *Am. J. Psychiat.*, 1977, *134*, 808.

Lithium carbonate was successfully used to control the mental changes which occurred when prednisone in excess of 15 to 20 mg daily was taken by a woman being treated for lymphoma.— F. P. Siegal (letter), *New Engl. J. Med.*, 1978, *299*, 155.

Further references.— W. E. Falk *et al.*, *J. Am. med. Ass.*, 1979, *241*, 1011 (corticotrophin-induced psychoses).

Blood disorders. Determination of the blood-leucocyte concentrations of 12 nonpsychotic patients who had been receiving long-term lithium carbonate therapy, compared with 71 normal controls studied previously, indicated that lithium induces increase in neutrophil pool sizes and their effective production by the bone marrow without impairing migration into skin lesions. Lithium might prove useful in the treatment of neutropenic patients but in view of its toxicity should not be accepted as a neutropoietic agent until its effects were known to be of sufficient magnitude to be beneficial.— G. Rothstein *et al.*, *New Engl. J. Med.*, 1978, *298*, 178.

In a study involving 6 healthy subjects who took lithium carbonate 300 mg thrice daily for up to 4 weeks, circulating granulocytes and granulocyte-marrow reserves increased significantly. It was considered that the lithium-induced granulocytosis was not merely a redistribution but was probably due to increased granulocyte production.— R. S. Stein *et al.*, *Ann. intern. Med.*, 1978, *88*, 809.

A study *in vitro* on murine haematopoiesis indicated that lithium augments granulopoiesis as a result of its effect on the pluripotent stem cell (CFU-S or colony-forming units in spleen).— L. J. Levitt and P. J. Quesenberry, *New Engl. J. Med.*, 1980, *302*, 713. Comments.— *Lancet*, 1980, *2*, 626.

Further references.— W. R. Friedenberg and J. J. Marx, *Cancer*, 1980, *45*, 91.

Adjunct to cancer chemotherapy. Lithium carbonate 1 g daily initially then adjusted to give a serum-lithium concentration of 0.7 to 0.9 mmol per litre had a beneficial effect on the blood picture in 6 leukaemic patients who had just had aplasia induced. The risk of infection might be reduced by lithium.— D. Charron *et al.* (letter), *Lancet*, 1977, *1*, 1307. Discussion on the granulocytic effects of lithium and its potential benefits in cancer.— G. Tisman and S. -J. GWu (letter), *ibid.*, 1977, *2*, 251. Administration of lithium carbonate to induce granulocytosis in a 64-year-old woman in remission from acute leukaemia might have been associated with relapse of her leukaemia.— L. E. Orr and J. F. McKernan (letter), *ibid.*, 1979, *1*, 449.

In 13 patients receiving combined cancer chemotherapy mainly for breast and lung cancer the effect on granulocyte count of courses of lithium carbonate 300 mg thrice daily was compared with that of courses of placebo (patients acting as their own controls). During lithium administration the decrease in granulocyte count was less in 14 of 18 paired comparisons suggesting that concomitant lithium administration might permit chemotherapy doses to be increased.— R. S. Stein *et al.*, *New Engl. J. Med.*, 1977, *297*, 430. Comment on the potential risk of stimulating marrow activity during cytotoxic drug administration.— A. I. Meisler (letter), *ibid.*, 1179. Reply.— R. S. Stein (letter), *ibid.*, 1180.

Lithium reduced the risk of infection and infection-related death in patients with advanced small-cell lung cancer who were receiving chemotherapy and radiotherapy. Of 45 such patients, 20 were given lithium carbonate 300 mg thrice daily between cycles of intensive chemotherapy; lithium was not given during radiotherapy. Patients who received lithium had significantly fewer episodes of neutropenia and fever and fewer infection-related deaths than the controls; they also required fewer reductions of their chemotherapy doses and fewer delays in treatment. Side-effects reported by patients receiving lithium carbonate were weakness in 16, nausea or vomiting in 14, dysphagia in 9, lethargy in 7, and mucositis in 2; one patient developed a coarse tremor and, another, reversible diabetes insipidus. Toxicity was not related to the serum concentration of lithium.— G. H. Lyman *et al.*, *New Engl. J. Med.*, 1980, *302*, 257. Comment on methodological problems in the study.— D. L. Coleman and R. I. Horwitz (letter), *ibid.*, 1365. Reply.— G. H. Lyman *et al.* (letter), *ibid.*

A woman with severe marrow hypoplasia, induced by chemotherapy and irradiation, had a short-term beneficial response to treatment with lithium carbonate 300 mg thrice daily. A rapid recurrence of symptoms, after a 4-month interval when transfusions were not needed, suggested that stimulation of the stem cells by lithium had ceased.— N. J. Vogelzang and D. H. Frenning (letter), *New Engl. J. Med.*, 1980, *303*, 525. Comment that conclusions regarding the effect of lithium on haematopoiesis need to be made with caution.— G. J. Carlson (letter), *ibid.* Reply.— L. J. Levitt and P. J. Quesenberry (letter), *ibid.*, 526.

Further references.— R. Catane *et al.* (letter), *New Engl. J. Med.*, 1977, *297*, 452; D. J. Charron *et al.* (letter), *ibid.*, 1979, *301*, 557; R. S. Stein *et al.*, *Blood*, 1979, *54*, 636; U. Visca *et al.* (letter), *Lancet*, 1979, *1*, 779; G. Bandini *et al.* (letter), *ibid.*, 1980, *2*, 926; G. A. R. Young (letter), *ibid.*, 1249; G. Bandini (letter), *ibid.*, 1981, *1*, 152; P. G. Steinherz *et al.*, *J. Pediat.*, 1980, *96*, 923.

Aplastic anaemia. Lithium given to 2 patients with aplastic anaemia increased their neutrophil count. Although in one patient this effect was only transient, the other achieved a normal neutrophil count and was being maintained on dose of 250 mg of lithium carbonate thrice daily.— A. J. Barrett *et al.* (letter), *Lancet*, 1977, *1*, 202. See also *idem* (letter), *Lancet*, 1977, *2*, 1357.

Striking haematological improvement occurred in a 58-year-old woman with aplastic anaemia that had been resistant to treatment, 2 weeks after she started to take lithium carbonate 300 mg thrice daily.— S. F. Blum (letter), *New Engl. J. Med.*, 1979, *300*, 677.

Drug-induced leucopenia. Lithium increased the white blood cell counts of 3 schizophrenic patients with persistent leucopenia.— R. Yassa *et al.*, *Am. J. Psychiat.*, 1978, *135*, 1423.

See also under Adjunct for Cancer Chemotherapy (above).

Felty's syndrome. Administration of lithium increased absolute granulocyte counts in 8 patients with Felty's syndrome (rheumatoid arthritis and granulocytopenia).— R. C. Gupta *et al.*, *Am. J. Med.*, 1976, *61*, 29. See also *idem*, *Arthritis Rheum.*, 1975, *18*, 179.

Two patients with Felty's syndrome were treated with lithium carbonate 900 mg per day. Neither patient showed a significant or sustained increase in granulocyte count.— R. A. Kaplan (letter), *Ann. intern. Med.*, 1976, *84*, 342.

Leukaemia. A 60-year-old woman with hairy-cell leukaemia that failed to respond to splenectomy, had an unequivocal and sustained improvement in haemoglobin concentration and platelet count in response to treatment with lithium carbonate.— S. F. Blum (letter), *New Engl. J. Med.*, 1980, *303*, 464. See also W. J. Paladine *et al.* (letter), *ibid.*, 1981, *304*, 1237. See also under Adjunct to Cancer Chemotherapy (above).

Cholera syndrome. Lithium carbonate, given in a dose of 300 mg every 12 hours, substantially reduced diarrhoea in a patient with pancreatic cholera syndrome secondary to metastatic non-beta islet-cell carcinoma which had become unresponsive to streptozocin. Lithium may have inhibited the action of vasoactive intestinal peptide on the mucosa of the small intestine.— S. J. Pandol *et al.*, *New Engl. J. Med.*, 1980, *302*, 1403. Lithium carbonate, given to a similar patient, was associated with an immediate explosive exacerbation of the syndrome.— D. Y. Graham (letter), *ibid.*, *303*, 1063. Reply.— S. J. Pandol *et al.* (letter), *ibid.*, 1064.

Chorea. Striking improvement occurred in 3 of 6 patients with Huntington's chorea when given lithium 24.3 mmol (24.3 mEq) daily in addition to the neuroleptics they were already receiving. A patient with tardive dyskinesia also improved.— P. Dalén (letter), *Lancet*, 1973, *1*, 107. See also B. Mattsson (letter), *Lancet*, 1973, *1*, 718.

There was no improvement in 9 patients with Huntington's chorea when given lithium in a double-blind controlled study.— M. J. Aminoff and J. Marshall, *Lancet*, 1974, *1*, 107. See also J. S. Carman *et al.* (letter), *Lancet*, 1974, *1*, 811.

In a double-blind crossover study involving 6 patients with Huntington's chorea, lithium and haloperidol were effective, only when given together, in controlling this condition when irritability and angry outbursts were prominent.— D. P. Leonard *et al.* (letter), *Lancet*, 1974, *2*, 1208.

Results of a double-blind crossover study in 6 patients with Huntington's chorea indicated that lithium has no beneficial effect in this condition.— P. Vestergaard *et al.*, *Acta psychiat. scand.*, 1977, *56*, 183.

Depression. Evidence of a reduced need for ECT in depressive patients given prophylactic lithium therapy.— E. H. Bennie (letter), *Br. med. J.*, 1978, *1*, 578. See also J. Mendels, *Am. J. Psychiat.*, 1976, *133*, 373 (responsive subgroups).

Eight patients with a major depressive disorder, who had not responded to tricyclic antidepressants alone, obtained remarkable relief of depression within 48 hours of the addition of lithium carbonate.— C. dé Montigny, *Br. J. Psychiat.*, 1981, *138*, 252.

A Medical Research Council study on continuation therapy with lithium and amitriptyline in unipolar depressive illness.— *Psychol. Med.*, 1981, *11*, 409. Comment.— *Lancet*, 1981, *2*, 563.

References to lithium in depression.— R. R. Fieve *et al.*, *Am. J. Psychiat.*, 1968, *125*, 487 (comparison with imipramine); R. F. Prien *et al.*, *Archs gen. Psychiat.*, 1973, *29*, 420 (comparison with imipramine); A. Coppen *et al.*, *Br. J. Psychiat.*, 1978, *133*, 206 (comparison with mianserin); A. J. Gelenberg and G. L. Klerman, *J. nerv. ment. Dis.*, 1978, *166*, 365 (comparison with amitriptyline); E. P. Worall *et al.*, *Br. J. Psychiat.*, 1979, *135*, 255 (administration with tryptophan).

See also under Mania and Manic-depressive Psychoses (below).

Diabetes insipidus, nephrogenic. Findings that lithium carbonate was ineffective and had serious side-effects in the treatment of inappropriate secretion of antidiuretic hormone.— J. N. Forrest *et al.*, *New Engl. J. Med.*, 1978, *298*, 173.

Further references.— M. G. White and C. D. Fetner, *New Engl. J. Med.*, 1975, *292*, 390; J. N. Forrest, *ibid.*, 423; N. Hendler *et al.* (letter), *ibid.*, 1976, *294*, 446; R. S. Baker *et al.*, *J. Pediat.*, 1977, *90*, 480; E. Casado de Frias *et al.*, *J. Pediat.*, 1980, *96*, 153.

Epilepsy. Lithium carbonate was given for 6 weeks in doses sufficient to maintain serum-lithium concentrations at 0.6 to 1.25 mmol per litre to 16 patients with severe epilepsy, 15 of whom were poorly controlled. Seizure frequency was reduced in 10 and increased only in 1 patient.— C. W. Erwin *et al.*, *Archs gen. Psychiat.*, 1973, *28*, 646.

Extrapyramidal effects. Lithium carbonate was given in increasing doses to 11 patients with torticollis, torsion dystonia, or choreoathetosis. Some improvement was observed in 3 patients with torticollis but 2 of these did not deteriorate when given placebo. Lithium was not considered effective in clinical dyskinesias.— J. A. McCaul and G. M. Stern (letter), *Lancet*, 1974, *1*, 1058.

Lithium was not considered to be beneficial in parkinsonism in a pilot study of 21 patients.— J. A. McCaul and G. M. Stern (letter), *Lancet*, 1974, *1*, 1117.

Tardive dyskinesia. Lithium carbonate 0.9 to 1.2 g daily with doxepin 50 mg thrice daily produced a complete remission in a patient with tardive dyskinesia.— R. H. Ehrensing (letter), *Lancet*, 1974, *2*, 1459.

Slight improvement following lithium administration in 6 patients with tardive dyskinesia. Most of them retained significant symptoms of tardive dyskinesia.— F. A. Reda *et al.*, *Am. J. Psychiat.*, 1975, *132*, 560.

Lithium-induced aggravation of tardive dyskinesia.— E. L. Crews and A. E. Carpenter, *Am. J. Psychiat.*, 1977, *134*, 933.

Gilles de la Tourette's syndrome. Administration of lithium carbonate to 2 male patients with Gilles de la Tourette's syndrome. Complete remission of symptoms was obtained in one and the second was markedly improved.— F. S. Messiha *et al.*, *Clin. Pharmac. Ther.*, 1977, *21*, 111.

Headache. Lithium has been reported to be prophylactic in both episodic and chronic cluster headache. It is considered to be the only reliably effective treatment for cluster headache and, although relatively few patients have been treated, it has succeeded where conventional therapy has failed. Amitriptyline appears to have some synergism with lithium; it has been possible, by adding amitriptyline 75 mg each 24 hours, to reduce the dose of lithium below the level that causes adverse effects and still retain the same control of cluster headache.— G. M. Wyant and E. M. Ashenhurst, *Can. Anaesth. Soc. J.*, 1979, *26*, 38.

An account of beneficial preliminary results with lithium in cluster headache but evidence that lithium exacerbates common and classical migraine.— R. C. Peatfield, *J. R. Soc. Med.*, 1981, *74*, 432.

Further reviews and comments.— M. Anthony, *Drugs*, 1979, *18*, 122; *Med. Lett.*, 1979, *21*, 78.

Studies and reports on lithium in cluster headache.— K. Ekbom, *Opusc. Med.*, 1974, *19*, 148; L. Kudrow, in *Current Concepts in Migraine Research*, R. Green (Ed.), New York, Raven Press, 1978, p. 159; J. Lieb and A. Zeff, *Br. J. Psychiat.*, 1978, *133*, 556.

Hyperthyroidism. Lithium carbonate 0.8 or 1.2 g daily to produce serum-lithium concentrations of 0.5 to 1.5 mmol per litre was given for 6 months as the sole treatment to 11 patients with Graves' disease. Within 2 weeks 8 patients became euthyroid and by 6 weeks all patients were euthyroid and remained so during treatment. When lithium was stopped 7 patients became hyperthyroid within 1 to 14 weeks. Although lithium reduced the hyperthyroidism it had no significant effect on the course of the disease.— J. H. Lazarus *et al.*, *Lancet*, 1974, *2*, 1160.

In 24 patients with newly diagnosed thyrotoxicosis there was no significant difference in response between 13 treated with methimazole 40 mg daily and 11 treated with lithium carbonate to maintain a serum-lithium concentration of 0.5 to 1.3 mmol per litre. Side-effects associated with lithium made treatment impracticable.— O. Kristensen *et al.*, *Lancet*, 1976, *1*, 603.

Studies in 16 patients with thyrotoxicosis showed that lithium carbonate 400 mg daily for a week before and a week after a standard dose of iodine-131 caused significant retention of the iodine-131 by the thyroid, compared with 16 controls. The technique could be useful in young patients where the total body radiation dose must be kept to a minimum.— J. G. Turner *et al.*, *Lancet*, 1976, *1*, 614. The 24- to 48-hour thyroidal uptake drop was much reduced and the mean iodine-131 uptake at 48 hours, of tracer amounts given by mouth, was significantly higher in 11 thyrotoxic patients after they had received treatment for 10 to 14 days with lithium carbonate 0.9 to 1.5 g daily, compared with the uptake in these patients when they were not given lithium.— K. Bakker *et al.* (letter), *ibid.*, 1135. Lithium carbonate in doses of 400 mg daily was effective as an adjunct to carbimazole in the initial management of severe thyrotoxicosis. Lithium unlike iodine did not delay subsequent radio-iodine therapy.— J. G. Turner and B. E. W. Brownlie (letter), *ibid.*, 1976, *2*, 904.

Further references.— R. Temple *et al.*, *J. clin. Invest.*, 1972, *51*, 2746; R. Temple *et al.*, *Mayo Clin. Proc.*, 1972, *47*, 872; H. Gerdes *et al.*, *Dt. med. Wschr.*, 1973, *98*, 1551.

Infection. Two patients with recurrent herpes simplex infections experienced remissions whilst being treated with lithium carbonate.— J. Lieb (letter), *New Engl. J. Med.*, 1979, *301*, 942.

Mania and manic depressive psychoses. A series of papers on the status of lithium in the prophylaxis and therapy of affective disorders.— *Archs gen. psychiat.*, 1979, *36*, 833. Comment.— *Lancet*, 1979, *2*, 1168.

Further reviews and comments.— R. R. Fieve, *Drugs*, 1977, *13*, 458; A. J. Poole *et al.*, *J.R. Soc. Med.*, 1978, *71*, 890.

For previous references to the effects of lithium in mania and manic-depressive psychoses, see Martindale, 27th Edn, pp. 1548–9.

Myasthenia gravis. A theory that myasthenia gravis may respond to lithium therapy.— D. F. Horrobin (letter), *Ann. intern. Med.*, 1979, *90*, 719.

See also under Precautions.

Organic brain impairment. A woman with multiple sclerosis and recurrent affective illness, either associated with or uncovered by the multiple sclerosis, had a beneficial response to lithium.— D. B. Mehta (letter), *Am. J. Psychiat.*, 1976, *133*, 236.

See also under Precautions.

Premenstrual syndrome. A study demonstrating that neither lithium nor chlorthalidone was more effective than placebo for the relief of premenstrual tension.— B. Mattsson and B. v. Schoultz, *Acta psychiat. scand.*, 1974, *Suppl.* 255, 75. See also M. Steiner *et al.*, *ibid.*, 1980, *61*, 96.

Schizophrenia. In a multicentre study of 83 patients classified as excited schizo-affectives, lithium was inferior to chlorpromazine in the treatment of highly active patients but as effective as chlorpromazine in mildly active patients. There was no significant difference in side-effects.— R. F. Prien *et al.*, *Archs gen. Psychiat.*, 1972, *27*, 182. Encouraging preliminary results with lithium in schizophrenia. Further study is merited.— P. E. Alexander *et al.*, *Am. J. Psychiat.*, 1979, *136*, 283.

Further references.— F. T. Miller and H. Libman, *Biol. Psychiat.*, 1979, *14*, 706.

Tardive dyskinesia. See under Extrapyramidal Effects (above).

Vertigo. Results of a year long double-blind placebo-controlled crossover study completed by 26 patients with vertigo indicated that lithium had no advantage over placebo therapy.— J. Thomsen *et al.*, *Clin. Otolaryngol.*, 1979, *4*, 119.

Preparations

Lithium Carbonate Capsules *(U.S.P.)*. Capsules containing lithium carbonate. The *U.S.P.* requires 60% dissolution in 30 minutes.

Lithium Carbonate Tablets *(B.P.)*. Lithium Carb. Tab. Tablets containing lithium carbonate.

Lithium Carbonate Tablets *(U.S.P.)*. Tablets containing lithium carbonate. The *U.S.P.* requires 60% dissolution in 30 minutes.

Slow Lithium Carbonate Tablets *(B.P.)*. Slow Lithium Carb. Tab. The tablets are formulated to release lithium carbonate over a period of several hours.

Proprietary Preparations

Camcolit *(Norgine, UK)*. Lithium carbonate, available as tablets of 250 mg and scored tablets of 400 mg. (Also available as Camcolit in *Austral.*, *S.Afr.*).

Liskonum *(Smith Kline & French, UK)*. Lithium carbonate, available as scored sustained-release tablets of 450 mg.

Phasal *(Pharmax, UK)*. Lithium carbonate, available as sustained-release tablets of 300 mg.

Priadel *(Delandale, UK)*. Lithium carbonate, available as scored controlled-release tablets of 400 mg. (Also available as Priadel in *Austral.*, *Neth.*, *S.Afr.*).

Other Proprietary Names

Arg.—Ceglution, Litilent; *Austral.*—Lithicarb, Manialith; *Belg.*—Hypnorex, Lithuril, Maniprex; *Canad.*—Carbolith, Lithane, Lithizine; *Denm.*—Lithionit *(sulphate)*; *Fr.*—Lithium Oligosol, Neurolithium *(both gluconate)*, Téralithe; *Ger.*—Hypnorex, Lithium-Duriles *(sulphate)*, Lithiumorotat *(orotate)*, Mikroplex Lithium *(gluconate)*, Quilonum *(acetate)*, Quilonum retard; *Norw.*—Lithionit *(sulphate)*; *S.Afr.*—Lentolith, Quilonum Retard; *Spain*—Plenur; *Swed.*—Lithionit *(sulphate)*; *Switz.*—Hypnorex, Lithiofor *(sulphate)*, Quilonorm *(acetate)*, Quilonorm-retard; *USA*—Eskalith, Lithane, Lithobid, Lithonate, Lithotabs.

7058-t

Lithium Citrate *(U.S.P.)*. Lithii Citras.

$C_6H_5Li_3O_7,4H_2O = 282.0$.

CAS — 919-16-4 (anhydrous); 6080-58-6 (tetrahydrate).

Pharmacopoeias. In *Nord.* and *U.S.*

A white, odourless, somewhat deliquescent, crystalline powder with a slightly saline taste. Each g represents about 10.6 mmol (10.6 mEq) of lithium.

Soluble 1 in 2 of water; practically insoluble in alcohol and ether. A 5% solution in water has a pH of 7 to 10. **Store** in airtight containers.

Lithium citrate has actions and uses similar to those of lithium carbonate (p.1535). It is given in doses calculated to provide the same serum-lithium concentrations as those specified under lithium carbonate.

Preparations

Lithium Citrate Syrup *(U.S.P.)*. Prepared from lithium citrate or from lithium hydroxide to which an excess of citric acid has been added. Potency is expressed in terms of the lithium content. pH 4 to 5. Store in airtight containers.

Tablettae Lithii Citratis *(Nord. P.)*. Lithium Citrate Tablets. Each contains 500 mg of lithium citrate.

Litarex *(Weddel, UK)*. Lithium citrate, available as sustained-release tablets of 564 mg. (Also available as Litarex in *Denm.*, *Neth.*, *Norw.*, *Swed.*, *Switz.*).

Other Proprietary Names

Arthri-Sel *(Fr.)*; Lithonate-S *(USA)*.

7059-x

Lithium Hydroxide *(U.S.P.)*.
$LiOH,H_2O$=41.96.

CAS — 1310-65-2 (anhydrous); 1310-66-3 (monohydrate).

Pharmacopoeias. In *U.S.*

A white solid which loses 41.0 to 43.5% of its weight on drying. **Soluble** in water yielding strongly alkaline solutions; slightly soluble in alcohol. **Store** in airtight containers.

Lithium hydroxide is used in the preparation of lithium citrate syrup.

7060-y

Lorazepam.

Wy-4036. 7-Chloro-5-(2-chlorophenyl)-1,3-dihydro-3-hydroxy-2*H*-1,4-benzodiazepin-2-one.
$C_{15}H_{10}Cl_2N_2O_2$=321.2.

CAS — 846-49-1.

A white odourless powder. M.p. 166° to 168°. Practically **insoluble** in water; soluble in alcohol, acetone, and glacial acetic acid.

Dependence. Prolonged use of lorazepam may lead to the development of dependence of the barbiturate-alcohol type (see p.792). It has a low liability for abuse.

Abuse. A 42-year-old-alcoholic man who had consumed 2 to 3 bottles of whisky daily, subsequently took very large quantities of lorazepam. Withdrawal symptoms and his erratic behaviour were the same as when he had misused alcohol.— R. Fox (letter), *Lancet*, 1978, *2*, 681. Criticism.— T. V. A. Harry, *Wyeth* (letter), *ibid.*, 1045. Reply.— R. Fox (letter), *ibid.*

Dependence and withdrawal. A report of withdrawal convulsions from benzodiazepines in 4 patients, involving clorazepate (1), oxazepam (1), and lorazepam (2).— T. R. Einarson (letter), *Lancet*, 1980, *1*, 151. A comment that 2 of these patients were also taking trifluoperazine, which has known epileptogenic potential. A patient has been seen, however, who suffered a grand-mal seizure 4 days after stopping lorazepam 5 mg daily alone; lorazepam had been taken for 2 years in a daily dose of 5 to 15 mg.— P. Tyrer (letter), *ibid.*

Further references J. R. de la Fuente *et al.*, *Mayo Clin. Proc.*, 1980, *55*, 190; J. G. Howe, *Br. med. J.*, 1980, *280*, 1163; R. B. Stewart *et al.*, *Am. J. Psychiat.*, 1980, *137*, 1113.

Adverse Effects, Treatment, and Precautions. As for Diazepam, p.1520.

Lorazepam 2.5 mg produced a greater and longer impairment of psychomotor performance than diazepam 10 mg or medazepam 15 mg in a double-blind crossover study in 10 healthy subjects. It was recommended that patients should not drive or operate machinery for 24 hours after administration of lorazepam 2.5 mg.— T. Seppala *et al.*, *Br. J. clin. Pharmac.*, 1976, *3*, 831. See also K. P. Stoller *et al.*, *Anesthesiology*, 1976, *45*, 565.

Further references: I. Hindmarch and A. C. Gudgeon, *Br. J. clin. Pharmac.*, 1980, *10*, 145.

Effects on the eyes. A study of 17 patients with glaucoma given lorazepam 1 or 2 mg daily for 100 days. No significant changes in ocular pressure were noted except for an initial transient hypotensive effect in some patients. It appears that lorazepam can be used without risking raised intra-ocular pressure or any anticholinergic effects.— N. Calixto and J. André de Costa Maia, *Curr. ther. Res.*, 1975, *17*, 156.

A study indicating that usual therapeutic doses of lorazepam strongly interfere with colour vision.— J. Laroche and C. Laroche, *Annls pharm. Fr.*, 1977, *35*, 173.

Effects on mental state. *Paradoxical response.* A report of a paradoxical reaction in a 22-year-old female who became extremely agitated and distressed after receiving lorazepam 3 mg.— R. D. Goldney, *Med. J. Aust.*, 1977, *1*, 139.

See also Overdosage (below).

Effects on respiratory function. No respiratory depression was reported when lorazepam was given in doses of 1.33 mg or 4 mg by intramuscular injection to 6 healthy subjects.— J. C. Gasser *et al.*, *Clin. Pharmac. Ther.*, 1975, *18*, 170.

In a double-blind study in 11 subjects lorazepam 1 or 2.5 mg had no depressant effect on the ventilatory response to carbon dioxide; there was a slight respiratory stimulant effect.— M. E. Dodson *et al.* (letter), *Br. J. Anaesth.*, 1976, *48*, 611.

Interactions. *Pyrimethamine.* For a report of mild liver toxicity in patients taking pyrimethamine and lorazepam concomitantly, see Pyrimethamine, p.402.

Overdosage. A 6-year-old boy who had ingested not more than 30 mg (probably considerably less) of lorazepam was drowsy and ataxic and developed marked hallucinations persisting intermittently for 9 hours.— D. I. Jeffrey and M. F. Whitfield (letter), *Br. med. J.*, 1974, *4*, 719. See also P. Vlachos *et al.*, *Toxicol. Lett.*, 1978, *2*, 109.

Porphyria. A study in *rats* indicated that lorazepam would probably not elicit an acute attack in susceptible porphyric individuals.— G. H. Blekkenhorst *et al.* (letter), *Lancet*, 1980, *1*, 1367. Criticisms of extrapolating data obtained from *animal* experiments to the treatment of human disease.— M. J. Brodie (letter), *ibid.*, *2*, 86; A. Gorchein (letter), *ibid.*, 152. Reply.— G. H. Blekkenhorst and L. Eales (letter), *ibid.*, 1250.

Pregnancy and the neonate. Concentrations of lorazepam in cord plasma in 26 neonates were slightly lower than in maternal plasma. Lorazepam was slowly excreted by infants. In a study of 53 infants born to 51 mothers with hypertension treated with lorazepam and antihypertensives, oral treatment with lorazepam had little effect on the neonate other than delay in establishment of breast feeding. Lorazepam intravenously reduced the Apgar score at birth, increased the necessity for assisted respiration, and increased neonatal hypothermia and poor suckling. Premature infants had a very high incidence of depressed respiration, hypothermia, and feeding problems, regardless of route of administration. The use of lorazepam intravenously, and before 37 weeks of gestation, should be limited to hospitals with facilities for intensive neonatal care.— A. G. L. Whitelaw *et al.*, *Br. med. J.*, 1981, *282*, 1106. Comment.— M. Johnstone (letter), *ibid.*, 1973. Reply.— A. Whitelaw (letter), *ibid.*

See also under Absorption and Fate.

Thrombo-embolic effects. Of 40 patients given a single intravenous dose of lorazepam 4 mg three had thrombosis 2 to 3 days later and 6 had thrombosis 7 to 10 days later. The incidence was lower than in those given diazepam.— J. E. Hegarty and J. W. Dundee, *Br. med. J.*, 1977, *2*, 1384.

Absorption and Fate. For an account of the absorption and fate of a benzodiazepine, see Diazepam, p.1522.

Lorazepam has been reported to have an elimination half-life ranging from about 11 to 16 hours, and to have no pharmacologically active metabolites.

Absorption from the intramuscular site is more rapid and complete than is the case for diazepam.

Absorption and plasma concentrations. Studies in 4 healthy subjects given a single intravenous injection of lorazepam 5 mg suggested that the elimination half-life was about 13 hours; 69% of the dose was recovered from urine as the glucuronide.— D. J. Greenblatt *et al.*, *J. clin. Pharmac.*, 1977, *17*, 490. Further studies in 15 healthy subjects given lorazepam up to 10 mg daily by mouth for 26 weeks. With a dose of 6 mg daily, the mean steady-state plasma concentration was 88 ng per ml of lorazepam, and 170 ng per ml of the glucuronide; and with a daily dose of 10 mg the respective plasma concentrations were 164 and 266 ng per ml.— *idem*, 495. Following administration of lorazepam 4 mg into the deltoid muscles of 6 healthy subjects rapid absorption occurred (mean apparent absorption half-life of about 20 minutes) with peak plasma concentrations ranging from 49.6 to 82.7 ng per ml after 1 to 3 hours. An average of nearly 50% of the dose was recovered from the urine as the glucuronide during the first 24 hours and only about 0.3% as free lorazepam. The mean elimination half-life of 13.6 hours was similar to reported values following oral administration.— *idem*, *Clin. Pharmac. Ther.*, 1977, *21*, 222. In 6 and 7 healthy subjects given lorazepam 2 and 4 mg respectively by intravenous, intramuscular, or oral administration apparent elimination half-life was about 14 to 16 hours and about 65 to 79% of the administered dose was excreted in the urine within 72 hours as the glucuronide.— *idem*, *J. pharm. Sci.*, 1979, *68*, 57.

Further references: H. W. Elliott *et al.*, *Clin. Pharmac. Ther.*, 1971, *12*, 468 (plasma concentrations); R. Verbeeck *et al.*, *Br. J. clin. Pharmac.*, 1976, *3*, 1033 (plasma half-life); D. J. Greenblatt *et al.*, *J. Pharmacokinet. Biopharm.*, 1979, *7*, 159 (half-lives).

Metabolism. Following administration of lorazepam 2 mg to 8 healthy subjects peak pooled plasma-lorazepam concentrations of 16.9 ng per ml were obtained after 2 hours at which time the clinical effects appeared to be maximum. Urinary excretion accounted for an average of about 88% of the dose, 86% (75% of the total dose) being as the major metabolite, lorazepam glucuronide; minor metabolites included a hydroxylated derivative, a quinazolinone derivative, and a quinazoline carboxylic acid. About 7% of the dose was recovered from the faeces but it was not established whether this was unabsorbed lorazepam or metabolites.— D. J. Greenblatt *et al.*, *Clin. Pharmac. Ther.*, 1976, *20*, 329.

Further references: H. W. Elliott, *Br. J. Anaesth.*, 1976, *48*, 1017.

Plasma protein binding. *In vitro* studies have indicated that lorazepam is approximately 85% bound to plasma proteins.— R. Verbeeck *et al.*, *Br. J. clin. Pharmac.*, 1976, *3*, 1033.

Pregnancy and the neonate. *Diffusion across the placenta.* Evidence to suggest that lorazepam does not appear to cross the placental barrier as readily as diazepam. Foetal concentration of lorazepam rarely exceeded that of the mother and following delivery the neonates were able to metabolise lorazepam at the same rate as the mother.— R. J. McBride *et al.*, *Br. J. Anaesth.*, 1979, *51*, 971. See also J. Kanto *et al.*, *Acta pharmac. tox.*, 1980, *47*, 130.

Slow conjugation and elimination of lorazepam by the neonate.— A. J. Cummings and A. G. L. Whitelaw, *Br. J. clin. Pharmac.*, 1981, *12*, 511.

See also under Precautions.

Uses. Lorazepam is a benzodiazepine with actions and uses similar to those of diazepam (p.1523). The usual dose by mouth for the treatment of anxiety is 2 to 6 mg daily in 2 to 4 divided doses with the largest dose taken at night; in severe conditions up to 8 to 10 mg daily has been given.

Lorazepam may also be given intramuscularly or preferably intravenously as a sedative or for premedication. Recommended parenteral doses of lorazepam are: for anxiety, 25 to 30 µg per kg body-weight; for premedication, 50 µg per kg.

Reviews and comments on lorazepam: *Drug & Ther. Bull.*, 1973, *11*, 27; D. J. Greenblatt and R. I. Shader, *New Engl. J. Med.*, 1978, *299*, 1342; D. E. Galinsky (letter), *ibid.*, 1979, *300*, 1054; D. J. Greenblatt and R. I. Shader (letter), *ibid.*; *Med. Lett.*, 1978, *20*, 31; B. Ameer and D. J. Greenblatt, *Drugs*, 1981, *21*, 161.

Action. The molecular structure and kinetic profile of lorazepam resemble those of oxazepam. No metabolites of quantitative importance have been discovered other than the pharmacologically inactive glucuronide conjugate.— D. J. Greenblatt and R. I. Shader, *New Engl. J. Med.*, 1978, *299*, 1342.

Administration. Despite poor water solubility intramuscular injection of lorazepam in 6 healthy subjects was found to be painless.— D. J. Greenblatt *et al.*, *Clin. Pharmac. Ther.*, 1977, *21*, 222.

Serum concentrations of lorazepam were similar whether the drug was given intramuscularly or by mouth preoperatively.— M. J. Diamond (letter), *Br. J. Anaesth.*, 1978, *50*, 730.

In the elderly. A study indicating that in healthy subjects lorazepam elimination is not affected by increasing age, but plasma drug binding decreases significantly with ageing.— J. W. Kraus *et al.*, *Gastroenterology*, 1977, *73*, 1228. See also J. W. Kraus *et al.*, *Clin. Pharmac. Ther.*, 1978, *24*, 411.

Reduced total clearance of lorazepam in the elderly.— D. J. Greenblatt, *Clin. Pharmac. Ther.*, 1979, *25*, 227.

Administration in hepatic failure. A study indicating that both cirrhosis and hepatitis decrease the plasma binding of lorazepam and tend to depress its clearance but the latter effect was not statistically significant.— J. W. Kraus *et al.*, *Gastroenterology*, 1977, *73*, 1228. See also J. W. Kraus *et al.*, *Clin. Pharmac. Ther.*, 1978, *24*, 411.

Administration in renal failure. Following repeated dosage of lorazepam in 2 patients with renal failure the half-life was greatly prolonged.— R. K. Verbeeck *et al.* (letter), *Br. J. clin. Pharmac.*, 1981, *12*, 749.

Alcohol and drug withdrawal. Withdrawal symptoms of 21 chronic alcoholic patients were successfully controlled by an initial intramuscular injection of lorazepam, usually 5 mg, followed by an average daily dose of 7 mg by mouth.— I. N. Hosein *et al.*, *Curr. med. Res. Opinion*, 1978, *5*, 632.

Anaesthesia. A summary of the important differences between diazepam and lorazepam in anaesthesia. As a premedicant diazepam 10 mg produces a degree of sedation comparable to lorazepam 2 to 2.5 mg; lorazepam has a duration of action 3 to 4 times greater than that of equivalent doses of diazepam; although diazepam by mouth has an earlier onset of action than following intramuscular injection this does not apply to lorazepam. These effects occur in parallel with plasma concentrations of the drugs. Both drugs are slowly excreted from the body, plasma concentrations remaining increased for 24 to 48 hours. Whereas desmethyldiazepam, the main metabolite of diazepam has an appreciable hypnotic action and accumulates following repeated administrations, this does not apply to lorazepam. A second peak concentration of both drugs may occur 5 to 8 hours after administration. In equivalent intravenous doses both drugs commonly produce anterograde amnesia which is not wholly dependent on sedation. Premedication with lorazepam will consistently reduce the undesirable emergence effect of ketamine, while diazepam is unreliable in this respect; in contrast, intravenous injection of diazepam near the end of a ketamine anaesthesia will reduce emergence sequelae, whereas lorazepam is not suitable for this purpose.— J. W. Dundee *et al.*, *Br. J. Anaesth.*, 1979, *51*, 439. A similar review including the comment that diazepam has a much more rapid onset of action following intravenous injection. Diazepam reaches peak sedation 2 to 3 minutes after intravenous injection, whereas lorazepam requires 15 to 30 minutes. The reason for the difference is not known, but may be associated with the greater lipid-solubility of diazepam. Whereas intravenous diazepam is suitable for procedures such as endoscopy and dental work to be performed without anaesthesia, lorazepam is not used in this way because its action comes on too slowly.— *Drug & Ther. Bull.*, 1979, *17*, 19.

A warning that although lorazepam is excellent for certain anaesthetic procedures it is too long-acting for day-case procedures.— P. Simpson (letter), *Br. med. J.*, 1978, *2*, 703. See also T. W. Ogg, *ibid.*, 1980, *281*, 212.

References to the use of lorazepam in anaesthetic procedures: J. Wilson and F. R. Ellis, *Br. J. Anaesth.*, 1973, *45*, 738 (premedication); J. A. O. Magbagbeola, *ibid.*, 1974, *46*, 449 (premedication); D. V. Heisterkamp and P. J. Cohen, *ibid.*, 1975, *47*, 79 (premedication); R. S. Cormack *et al.*, *ibid.*, 1976, *48*, 813 (premedication); J. W. Dundee *et al.*, *Curr. med. Res. Opinion*, 1976, *4*, 290 (postoperative sedation); M. Johnstone, *Anaesthesia*, 1976, *31*, 868 (ketamine anaesthesia), per *J. Am. med. Ass.*, 1977, *237*, 164; J. K. Lilburn *et al.*, *Br. J. Anaesth.*, 1976, *48*, 1125 (ketamine anaesthesia); S. K. Pandit *et al.*, *Anesthesiology*, 1976, *45*, 495 (anterograde amnesia); N. J. Paymaster, *Curr. med. Res. Opinion*, 1976, *4*, 388 (premedication); R. S. Cormack *et al.*, *Br. J. Anaesth.*, 1977, *49*, 351 (premedication); J. W. Dundee *et al.*, *ibid.*, 1047 (premedication); K. A. George and J. W. Dundee, *Br. J. clin. Pharmac.*, 1977, *4*, 45 (amnesic effect); S. Galloon *et al.*, *Br. J. Anaesth.*, 1977, *49*, 1265 (premedication); J. K. Lilburn *et al.*, *Br. J. clin. Pharmac.*, 1977, *4*, 641P (ketamine anaesthesia); W. Wassenaar *et al.*, *Br. J. Anaesth.*, 1977, *49*, 605 (premedication); M. E. Dodson and R. J. Eastley, *ibid.*, 1978, *50*, 1059 (premedication); J. M. Hewitt and A. M. Barr, *ibid.*, 1149 (premedication); R. R. Pagano *et al.*, *ibid.*, 471 (premedication).

Anxiety. Studies of lorazepam in the treatment of anxiety: L. A. Gottschalk *et al.*, *Clin. Pharmac. Ther.*, 1972, *13*, 323; A. N. Singh and B. Saxena, *Curr. ther. Res.*, 1974, *16*, 149; S. G. Olgiati, *ibid.*, 1975, *17*, 13; M. Sim *et al.*, *Br. J. clin. Pract.*, 1975, *29*, 304; T. Battelli *et al.*, *Curr. med. Res. Opinion*, 1976, *4*, 185; P. Gómez-Lozano, *Curr. ther. Res.*, 1976, *19*, 469; A. M. Kasick *et al.*, *ibid.*, 292; J. C. D. Lameiras, *Curr. med. Res. Opinion*, 1976, *4*, 411; A. J. Gross, *Curr. ther. Res.*, 1977, *22*, 597; H. A. McClelland *et al.*, *Am. J. Psychiat.*, 1977, *134*, 25; P. Gómez-Lozano, *J. int. med. Res.*, 1978, *6*, 186; B. M. Saxena *et al.*, *Curr. ther. Res.*, 1979, *25*, 150; A. N. Singh and B. M. Saxena, *ibid.*, *26*, 260.

Convulsions. Control of status epilepticus in 22 of 25 patients given lorazepam 4 mg by slow intravenous injection followed by a second dose after 15 minutes if necessary.— J. E. Walker *et al.*, *Ann. Neurol.*, 1979, *6*, 207.

Hypnotic effect. In a double-blind crossover study of 15 chronic insomniacs lorazepam 2 to 4 mg was approximately equivalent in hypnotic activity to flurazepam 30 mg. Side-effects were relatively frequent after the 4-mg dose and consisted of headache, drowsiness, lack of drive, dizziness, and tinnitus.— R. I. H. Wang *et al.*, *Clin. Pharmac. Ther.*, 1976, *19*, 191.

Further references: P. J. Brown *et al.*, *J. clin. Pharmac.*, 1975, *15*, 752; D. H. Long and R. J. Eltringham, *Anaesthesia*, 1977, *32*, 649.

Nausea and vomiting. Lorazepam 4 to 5 mg given intravenously immediately before cancer chemotherapy had a beneficial effect as an adjunct to standard anti-emetic therapy with perphenazine 5 mg given an hour beforehand, in 7 patients who had established a pattern of distressing vomiting at the time of their 3- or 4-weekly treatments; 4 of the patients had developed anticipatory vomiting. Although sleepy, they were awake enough to use a bowl if they did vomit. Lorazepam 2 mg by mouth up to every 4 hours was prescribed to keep patients asleep, but was rarely needed; standard parenteral anti-emetics were prescribed as required. Vomiting was reduced to a maximum of twice, in all but one patient, and anticipatory vomiting was abolished in 3 of 4.— J. Maher (letter), *Lancet*, 1981, *1*, 91.

Proprietary Preparations

Ativan (known in some countries as Tavor or Temesta) *(Wyeth, UK)*. Lorazepam, available as scored tablets of 1 and 2.5 mg. (Also available as Ativan in *Austral.*, *Canad.*, *S.Afr.*, *USA*).

Ativan Injection *(Wyeth, UK)*. Lorazepam, available as solution containing 4 mg per ml, in ampoules containing 1 ml. Store below 8°; protect from light.

Preparation of injection. The contents (1 ml) of the 2-ml ampoule may be diluted with 1 ml of either Water for Injections or sodium chloride injection immediately before administration; if the intramuscular route is used, the dilution should always be made.

Other Proprietary Names

Arg.— Aplacasse, Emotival, Kalmalin, NIC, Sedatival, Sidenar, Trapax; *Braz.*— Lorax; *Ital.*— Control, Lorans, Quait, Securit; *Jap.*— Wypax; *Port.*— Lorenin; *Spain*— Orfidal, Placidia, Sedarkey.

7061-j

Loxapine. CL 62362; SUM 3170. 2-Chloro-11-(4-methylpiperazin-1-yl)dibenz[*b,f*][1,4]oxazepine.

$C_{18}H_{18}ClN_3O = 327.8$.

CAS — 1977-10-2.

7062-z

Loxapine Succinate. CL 71563; Oxilapine.

$C_{18}H_{18}ClN_3O,C_4H_6O_4 = 445.9$.

CAS — 27833-64-3.

A white crystalline solid. Loxapine succinate 34 mg is equivalent to 25 mg of loxapine.

Adverse Effects. The side-effects of loxapine, such as sedation and extrapyramidal symptoms, which are the result of its pharmacological action, are similar to those of chlorpromazine (p.1509). Tardive dyskinesia may also be expected.

Extrapyramidal symptoms may be more common than those associated with chlorpromazine.

Other side-effects reported include nausea and vomiting, weight gain and loss, dyspnoea, ptosis, hyperpyrexia, headache, paraesthesia, flush, polydipsia, and agitation.

Loxapine succinate was given for 4 weeks to 13 patients with acute schizophrenia or acute exacerbations of chronic schizophrenia. The average daily dose of loxapine was 23.2 mg in week 1 and 26.8 mg daily in week 4. Side-effects occurred in all patients and included drowsiness in 10 and extrapyramidal symptoms in 2. Other side-effects included headache, dry mouth, dizziness, fatigue, tingling, nausea, agitation, lactation, palpitations, and inhibition of ejaculation.— E. Ucer and P. Casey, *Curr. ther. Res.*, 1979, *25*, 144.

Extrapyramidal effects. A report on the successful use of loxapine by intramuscular injection in 12 acutely psychotic patients. Episodes of acute dystonia occurred in 3 patients.— K. Fruensgaard and K. Jensen, *Curr. ther. Res.*, 1976, *19*, 164.

Loxapine succinate in capsules, or hydrochloride as liquid concentrate, was effective in the treatment of 17 young adult patients with acute schizophrenia in an open 4-week study. Doses varied from 10 to 250 mg daily. Dystonia and constipation were the most frequent side-effects occurring in 13 and 7 patients respectively.— J. L. Thomas, *Curr. ther. Res.*, 1979, *25*, 371.

Overdosage. Rhabdomyolysis and acute renal failure in a young man following overdosage with loxapine succinate.— C. W. Tam *et al.*, *Archs intern. Med.*, 1980, *140*, 975.

Treatment of Adverse Effects. As for Chlorpromazine, p.1511.

Precautions. As for Chlorpromazine, p.1512.

Interactions. Phenytoin. For the effect of loxapine on serum-phenytoin concentrations, see Phenytoin, p.1240.

Absorption and Fate. Loxapine is readily absorbed from the gastro-intestinal tract. It is very rapidly and extensively metabolised, with the possibility that one or more of its metabolites may be pharmacologically active; excretion occurs mainly in the first 24 hours. It is mainly excreted in the urine, in the form of its conjugated metabolites, with smaller amounts appearing in the faeces as unconjugated metabolites. The major metabolite of loxapine is hydroxyloxapine, which is conjugated to the glucuronide or sulphate; other metabolites include hydroxyloxapine-*N*-oxide, loxapine-*N*-oxide, and hydroxydesmethylloxapine. Loxapine is widely distributed and *animal* studies have indicated that it crosses the blood-brain barrier.

A comparative study of oral and intramuscular forms of loxapine in 10 schizophrenic patients. There was no difference in clinical action or side-effects between the 2 routes. Higher plasma concentrations were achieved following intramuscular administration indicating that bioavailability following oral administration is reduced by a first-pass effect.— G. M. Simpson *et al.*, *Psychopharmacology*, 1978, *56*, 225.

Further references: T. B. Cooper and R. G. Kelly, *J. pharm. Sci.*, 1979, *68*, 216.

Uses. Loxapine is a dibenzoxazepine with antipsychotic actions similar to those of chlorpromazine (p.1513). It is given by mouth as the hydrochloride or the succinate and by intramuscular injection as the hydrochloride, but the doses are expressed in terms of the base.

The usual dose by mouth for the treatment of psychoses is 20 to 50 mg daily initially, in 2 to 4 divided doses, increased over the next 7 to 10 days to 50 to 100 mg daily or more; the maximum recommended dose is 250 mg daily. For the control of acute conditions it is given by intramuscular injection in doses of 12.5 to 50 mg at intervals of 4 to 6 hours or longer.

Loxapine should be given in reduced dosage to elderly patients.

Action. A review of the properties and efficacy of loxapine.— R. C. Heel *et al.*, *Drugs*, 1978, *15*, 198.

Further reviews: *Drugs Today*, 1978, *14*, 245.

Administration. In children. In a double-blind comparative study, loxapine was shown to be as effective as haloperidol in the treatment of adolescent schizophrenia (patients aged 13 to 18 years); both treatments were better than a placebo. Extrapyramidal side-effects and sedation occurred with all treatments.— D. Pool *et al.*, *Curr. ther. Res.*, 1976, *19*, 99.

Anxiety and depression. In a double-blind comparative study in 56 patients over 4 weeks loxapine or diazepam were more effective than a placebo in the treatment of anxiety. The average daily doses used were loxapine 9.6 mg and diazepam 17.5 mg.— A. Villalobos, *Curr. ther. Res.*, 1978, *23*, 243. A comparative study of chlordiazepoxide, loxapine and placebo in 135 patients with anxiety some of whom also had neurotic depression, failed to demonstrate that loxapine 8 to 16 mg taken daily for up to 6 weeks was of use in anxious neurotic patients. Loxapine frequently produced less improvement than placebo.— K. Rickels *et al.*, *Curr. ther. Res.*, 1978, *23*, 111.

Behaviour disorders. Loxapine was as effective as thioridazine in the treatment of chronic psychoses associated with either organic brain syndrome or mental retardation.— E. Lourido and A. Santa Cruz, *Curr. ther. Res.*, 1979, *25*, 681. See also M. Versiani *et al.*, *J. int. med. Res.*, 1980, *8*, 22.

Schizophrenia. Loxapine given in maximum doses of 150 mg daily was as effective as chlorpromazine 1.5 g daily in a double-blind trial in 54 patients with acute schizophrenia.— R. M. Steinbook *et al.*, *Curr. ther.*

Res., 1973, *15*, 1.

Loxapine succinate or thioridazine hydrochloride taken for 1 to 4 weeks produced significant and comparable degrees of improvement in 29 and 27 patients respectively with acute schizophrenia. The only important difference between the 2 treatments was in ratings for thought disturbance and anxiety-depression, patients who received loxapine showing the greater improvement. Orthostatic hypotension, syncope and dizziness, constipation and dry mouth occurred more frequently in those patients who took thioridazine while hypertension, drowsiness, dermatological effects, and extrapyramidal effects were more common in those who took loxapine.— M. Kramer *et al.*, *Curr. ther. Res.*, 1978, *23*, 619.

A marked or moderate improvement was obtained in 12 of 15 patients who received loxapine succinate 10 to 197 mg per day for 4 weeks and some improvement was apparent within 48 hours of the start of therapy. Two of 17 patients withdrew from treatment due to side-effects, 1 after developing a severe dystonic reaction and the other after prolonged sedation after a single 10 mg dose. Other side-effects included extrapyramidal effects, sedation and anticholinergic effects.— S. Zisook *et al.*, *Curr. ther. Res.*, 1978, *24*, 415.

Loxapine was as effective as trifluoperazine in a 12-week controlled double-blind study in 64 hospitalised chronic schizophrenic patients. The dose of loxapine was usually between 20 and 90 mg daily. Extrapyramidal disorders and a sedative effect were the most common side-effects with loxapine.— S. Seth *et al.*, *Curr. ther. Res.*, 1979, *25*, 320.

Further references: D. M. Gallant *et al.*, *Curr. ther. Res.*, 1973, *15*, 205; B. Brauzer *et al.*, *J. clin. Pharmac.*, 1974, *14*, 455; K. D. Charalampous *et al.*, *Curr. ther. Res.*, 1974, *16*, 829; M. L. Clark *et al.*, *J. clin. Pharmac.*, 1975, *15*, 286; B. C. Schiele, *Dis. nerv. Syst.*, 1975, *36*, 361; C. D. Van der Velde and H. Kiltie, *Curr. ther. Res.*, 1975, *17*, 1; D. F. Moore, *ibid.*, *18*, 172; A. S. Mahal *et al.*, *ibid.*, 1976, *20*, 84; G. M. Simpson and Z. Cuculic, *J. clin. Pharmac.*, 1976, *16*, 60; G. Chouinard *et al.*, *Curr. ther. Res.*, 1977, *21*, 73; N. P. V. Nair *et al.*, *ibid.*, *22*, 628; M. L. Clark *et al.*, *Dis. nerv. Syst.*, 1977, *38*, 7; K. Fruensgaard *et al.*, *Curr. med. Res. Opinion*, 1978, *5*, 601; T. A. Wittkopp, *J. clin. Psychiat.*, 1978, *39*, 154; T. Sharma, *Curr. ther. Res.*, 1979, *25*, 366; R. B. Cornfield and G. L. Hogben, *ibid.*, *26*, 900; N. F. Leone, *ibid.*, 515; D. M. Moriarty *et al.*, *ibid.*, 408; J. Selkin, *ibid.*, 908.

See also under Administration in Children.

Parenteral route. Loxapine 12.5 to 50 mg administered intramuscularly twice or thrice daily as the hydrochloride for 5 days was considered to be an effective method of initiating treatment in 20 patients with acute schizophrenia. Patients were also given loxapine by mouth after 3 days and by the sixth day of treatment, loxapine was given by mouth only. Side-effects experienced only during parenteral administration of loxapine were hypotension, nausea, vomiting, dizziness, light headedness, muscle twitches, vertigo, fatigue, anorexia and headache. Other side-effects were similar to those produced after administration by mouth.— C. D. Van Der Velde, *Curr. ther. Res.*, 1978, *23*, 367.

Further references: K. Fruensgaard *et al.*, *Acta psychiat. scand.*, 1977, *56*, 256; J. Paprocki and M. Versiani, *Curr. ther. Res.*, 1977, *21*, 80; R. A. O'Connell and J. A. Lieberman, *ibid.*, 1978, *23*, 236; G. A. Dean and D. M. Gallant, *ibid.*, 1979, *25*, 721; G. Sakalis and S. Gershon, *ibid.*, 330; P. Deniker *et al.*, *J. clin. Psychiat.*, 1980, *41*, 23.

Proprietary Names

Daxolin (hydrochloride or succinate) *(Dome, USA)*; Loxapac (also as succinate) *(Lederle, Arg.; Lederle, Austral.; Lederle, Belg.; Lederle, Denm.; Lederle, Neth.; Lederle, S.Afr.)*; Loxitane (hydrochloride or succinate) *(Lederle, USA)*.

7063-c

Mebutamate. W 583. 2-*sec*-Butyl-2-methyltrimethylene dicarbamate.
$C_{10}H_{20}N_2O_4$=232.3.

CAS — 64-55-1.

A white crystalline powder with a bitter taste. Slightly **soluble** in water.

Mebutamate is a carbamate with general properties similar to those of meprobamate (p.1545). It has been suggested for use as an adjunct in the treatment of hypertension in doses of 300 mg three or four times daily.

Proprietary Names

Axiten *(Zambon, Ital.)*; Butatensin *(Benvegna, Ital.)*; Capla *(Inibsa, Spain)*; Ipotensivo Vita *(Vita, Ital.)*; Mebutina *(Formenti, Ital.)*; No-Press *(Janus, Ital.)*; Prean *(Chemil, Ital.)*; Sigmafon *(Lafare, Ital.)*; Vallene *(Farmasimes, Spain)*.

7064-k

Medazepam.

Ro 5-4556. 7-Chloro-2,3-dihydro-1-methyl-5-phenyl-1*H*-1,4-benzodiazepine.
$C_{16}H_{15}ClN_2$=270.8.

CAS — 2898-12-6.

Pharmacopoeias. In *Nord.*

A white to greenish-yellow, almost odourless, crystalline powder. M.p. 100° to 103°. Practically **insoluble** in water; soluble 1 in 8 of alcohol, 1 in 1 of chloroform, and 1 in 5 of ether.

Dependence. Prolonged use of medazepam may lead to the development of dependence of the barbiturate-alcohol type (see p.792). It has a low liability for abuse.

Adverse Effects, Treatment, and Precautions. As for Diazepam, p.1520.

Absorption and Fate. For an account of the absorption and fate of a benzodiazepine, see Diazepam, p.1522.

Medazepam is extensively metabolised to desmethyldiazepam.

A review of the pharmacokinetics of medazepam.— D. M. Hailey and E. S. Baird, *Br. J. Anaesth.*, 1979, *51*, 493.

Absorption and plasma concentrations. Mean plasma concentrations of 63 ng per ml of medazepam were measured in 20 patients given medazepam in a mean dose of 27 mg a day for 2 to 4 weeks. Mean diazepam concentrations were 28 ng per ml and desmethyldiazepam concentrations were 706 ng per ml.— A. J. Bond *et al.*, *Br. J. clin. Pharmac.*, 1977, *4*, 51.

Uses. Medazepam is a benzodiazepine with actions and uses similar to those of diazepam (p.1523).

The usual dose for the treatment of anxiety is 5 to 10 mg twice or thrice daily; in severe conditions up to 40 mg daily has been given.

Reviews of medazepam.— *Drug & Ther. Bull.*, 1971, *9*, 93; *Aust. J. Pharm.*, 1978, *59*, 512.

Action. Pharmacological studies of medazepam: F. Augustin and M. Bergener, *Arzneimittel-Forsch.*, 1969, *19*, 736; W. Berg and H. Flegel, *ibid.*, 740; W. D. Matthews and J. D. Connor, *J. Pharmac. exp. Ther.*, 1977, *201*, 613.

Anaesthesia. *Anaesthetic premedication.* In a double-blind study of premedication in 150 women, medazepam 10 mg produced less drowsiness than diazepam 10 mg but the latter was preferred by patients. Nausea and vomiting were more frequent during the first hour postoperatively in patients given medazepam.— R. A. E. Assaf *et al.*, *Br. J. Anaesth.*, 1975, *47*, 464.

Anxiety. Studies of medazepam in the treatment of anxiety: L. Bolzani and G. Slivar, *Int. Pharmacopsychiat.*, 1969, *2*, 197; R. J. Kerry and C. M. McDermott, *Br. med. J.*, 1971, *1*, 151; J. T. Silverstone *et al.*, *Br. J. clin. Pract.*, 1971, *25*, 172; P. Baume and J. Cuthbert, *Aust. N.Z. J. Med.*, 1973, *3*, 457; N. C. Moore, *Psychopharmacology*, 1977, *52*, 103.

Behaviour disorders. Medazepam 5 to 60 mg daily was given for 8 weeks to 24 emotionally disturbed mentally retarded children to correct their behavioural disturbances: some improvement was noted in all the patients. Improvement also occurred in 13 children given medazepam for an additional 4 to 5 weeks for recurrence of symptoms.— E. Ucer, *Curr. ther. Res.*, 1968, *10*, 187.

Proprietary Preparations

Nobrium *(Roche, UK)*. Medazepam, available as capsules of 5 and 10 mg. (Also available as Nobrium in *Arg., Belg., Denm., Fr., Ger., Ital., Neth., Norw., S.Afr., Spain, Switz.*).

Other Proprietary Names

Arg.— Elbrus, Navizil (dibudinate), Nivelton, Siman, Templane; *Austral.*— Raporan; *Denm.*— Anxitol; *Ital.*— Benson, Lerisum; *Jap.*— Azepamid, Metonas, Narsis, Tranquilax, Resmit; *Spain*— Megasedan.

7150-z

Melperone Hydrochloride. FG 5111; Methylperone Hydrochloride; Metylperone Chloride. 4′-Fluoro-4-(4-methylpiperidino)butyrophenone hydrochloride.
$C_{16}H_{22}FNO,HCl$=299.8.

CAS — 3575-80-2 (melperone); 1622-79-3 (hydrochloride).

Melperone is a butyrophenone with general properties similar to those of haloperidol (p.1532). For the treatment of psychoses it is given as the hydrochloride in doses of up to 100 mg three or four times daily. In acute conditions it may be given intramuscularly in doses of 25 to 50 mg up to 3 or 4 times daily.

Alcohol and drug withdrawal. A study of melperone in alcoholism.— C. Carlsson and B. Gullberg, *Int. J. clin. Pharmac. Biopharm.*, 1978, *16*, 331.

Chorea. Melperone produced only slight changes in 7 patients with Huntington's chorea when it was substituted for conventional treatment.— B. Mattsson and K. Boman (letter), *Lancet*, 1974, *2*, 1323.

Proprietary Names

Buronil (as base, hydrochloride, or palmitate) *(Lepetit, Belg.; Ferrosan, Denm.; Lepetit, Neth.; Ferrosan, Norw.; Ferrosan, Swed.)*; Eunerpan (base) *(Nordmark-Werke, Ger.)*.

7065-a

Mephenoxalone. OM 518. 5-(2-Methoxyphenoxymethyl)oxazolidin-2-one.
$C_{11}H_{13}NO_4$=223.2.

CAS — 70-07-5.

A white crystalline powder. Practically **insoluble** in water; soluble in alcohol.

Mephenoxalone has actions similar to those of meprobamate (see below). It has been used in doses of 400 mg three or four times daily in the treatment of anxiety or to relieve muscle spasm.

Proprietary Names

Control-OM *(Om, Switz.)*; Dorsiflex *(Medial, Neth.; Syntex, Switz.)*; Riself *(Gibipharma, Ital.)*; Xérène *(Martinet, Fr.)*.

7066-t

Meprobamate *(B.P., Eur. P., U.S.P.)*.

Meprobam.; Meprobamatum; Meprotanum. 2-Methyl-2-propyltrimethylene dicarbamate.
$C_9H_{18}N_2O_4$=218.3.

CAS — 57-53-4.

Pharmacopoeias. In *Arg., Belg., Br., Braz., Chin., Cz., Eur., Fr., Ger., Ind., Int., It., Jug., Neth., Pol., Port., Roum., Rus., Swiss, Turk.*, and *U.S.*

Odourless or almost odourless, colourless crystals or white crystalline powder with a bitter characteristic taste. M.p. 103° to 107°.

Soluble 1 in 240 of water, 1 in 7 of alcohol, 1 in 80 of chloroform, and 1 in 70 of ether; freely soluble in acetone. A saturated solution in water is neutral or slightly acid. **Store** in airtight containers.

Dependence. Prolonged use of meprobamate may lead to the development of dependence of the barbiturate-alcohol type (see p.792).

Abuse. Meprobamate has a high potential for abuse.— H. Isbell and T. L. Chruściel, *Dependence Liability of 'Non-narcotic' Drugs*, Geneva, World Health Organization, 1970. See also *idem*, *Bull. Wld Hlth Org.*, 1970, *43*, *Suppl.*

Withdrawal. Abstinence symptoms reported after the abrupt withdrawal of high doses of meprobamate included insomnia, vomiting, tremors, muscle twitches, anxiety, headache, ataxia, convulsions, and psychotic behaviour at times resembling delirium tremens.— C. F. Essig, *J. Am. med. Ass.*, 1966, *196*, 714.

Adverse Effects. Drowsiness is the most frequent side-effect of meprobamate. Other effects include nausea, vomiting, diarrhoea, paraesthesia, weakness, and central effects such as headache, excitement, dizziness, ataxia, and disturbances of vision. There may be hypotension, tachycardia, and cardiac arrhythmias. Hypersensitivity reactions occur occasionally. These may be limited to skin rashes, urticaria, and purpura or may be more severe with angioneurotic oedema, bronchospasm, or anuria. Erythema multiforme has been reported.

Blood disorders including agranulocytosis, eosinophilia, leucopenia, thrombocytopenia, and aplastic anaemia have occasionally been reported. Symptoms of porphyria may be exacerbated.

Withdrawal of meprobamate from patients who have been receiving it in high dosage or for prolonged periods of time should be gradual (see Dependence).

Allergy. Purpuric eruptions developed on the ankles, legs, thighs, and buttocks of a 67-year-old man treated with carbromal and pentobarbitone. The eruption improved after cessation of treatment, but reappeared after administration of meprobamate. There appeared to be cross-sensitivity between meprobamate and carbromal.— W. C. Peterson and K. P. Manick, *Archs Derm.*, 1967, *95*, 40.

Cross-sensitivity could occur between meprobamate and mephenesin and carisoprodol.— J. Verbov, *Br. J. clin. Pract.*, 1973, *27*, 310.

Effects on the blood. A 65-year-old woman who had taken meprobamate 0.8 to 1.2 g daily for 1 year developed pancytopenia and died despite treatment with prednisone, antibiotics, and transfusions of fresh blood.— C. Anastassiades (letter), *Br. med. J.*, 1971, *1*, 349.

Effects on the eyes. A study indicating that usual therapeutic doses of meprobamate interfere with colour vision.— J. Laroche and C. Laroche, *Annls pharm. fr.*, 1972, *30*, 433.

Overdosage. Of 773 admissions to Massachusetts General Hospital between 1962 and 1975 for psychotropic drug overdosage, meprobamate was implicated in 50. Serious intoxication was common and 2 patients died, one of whom had ingested an estimated 12 to 20 g, apparently with no other drugs. Hypotension was common and not always correlated with the depth of coma, indicating that it is not necessarily a consequence of CNS depression. Patients with meprobamate overdosage appear to be susceptible to cardiac failure and pulmonary oedema therefore care must be taken to avoid over-hydration. The questionable efficacy and the potential for life-threatening intoxication are important drawbacks to the clinical use of this drug.— M. D. Allen *et al.*, *Clin. Toxicol.*, 1977, *11*, 501.

Further references: R. K. Maddock and H. A. Bloomer, *J. Am. med. Ass.*, 1967, *201*, 999 (plasma concentrations in overdosage); S. Felby, *Acta pharmac. tox.*, 1970, *28*, 334 (plasma concentrations in overdosage).

Pregnancy and the neonate. In a prospective study of 19 044 live births the incidence of severe congenital defects was compared in mothers who had presented with anxiety, tension, or mild depression, and who had received meprobamate, chlordiazepoxide, other drugs, or no drugs during or just before the pregnancy. Considering the first 42 days of pregnancy the rates of defects were: when meprobamate was prescribed 12.1 per 100 live births, chlordiazepoxide 11.4, other drugs 4.6, and no drug 2.6. Considering the later stages of pregnancy there was no significant difference in the rate of defects between the 4 groups. In the meprobamate group 5 of the children with abnormalities had congenital heart disease.— L. Milkovich and B. J. van den Berg, *New Engl. J. Med.*, 1974, *291*, 1268. In prospective English and French studies of 63 and 239 women respectively who had received meprobamate, chlordiazepoxide, and other tranquillisers during the first 13 weeks of pregnancy, there were significantly more malformed children (4 of 71) born to French mothers who had received meprobamate than to those who had not. None of these were cardiac abnormalities. However 3 of the mothers had had previous unsuccessful pregnancies. The incidence of malformations in the English group was not significant. In these studies malformations were defined as those present at birth or seen within the first 6 weeks of life compared with the L. Milkovich and B.J. van den Berg study which covered the first 5 years. Congenital heart disease would therefore not be so easily detected.— D. L. Crombie *et al.* (letter), *ibid.*, 1975, *293*, 198.

Of 50 282 children born to mothers monitored by the Collaborative Perinatal Project, 356 were found to have been exposed to meprobamate, and possibly other drugs, at some time during the first 4 months of the pregnancy. Although a slight association between hypospadias and meprobamate exposure was noted no relationship to other types of malformation could be detected.— O. P. Heinonen *et al.*, *Birth Defects and Drugs in Pregnancy*, Littleton MA, Publishing Sciences Group, 1977, p. 335. See also S. C. Hartz *et al.*, *New Engl. J. Med.*, 1975, *292*, 726.

Individual reports of malformations in infants of mothers who had taken meprobamate during pregnancy: M. J. Adrian, *Bull. Féd. Socs Gynéc. Obstét. Lang. fr.*, 1963, *15*, 121; J. Gauthier, *Pédiatrie*, 1965, *20*, 489; J. R. Daube and S. M. Chow, *Neurology, Minneap.*, 1966, *16*, 179; C. A. D. Ringrose (letter), *Can. med. Ass. J.*, 1972, *106*, 1058.

Treatment of Adverse Effects. There is no specific treatment. In severe overdosage with meprobamate the stomach should be emptied by aspiration and lavage; this should be thorough as relapse after initial recovery has been attributed to incomplete gastric emptying and delayed absorption. Recovery generally follows symptomatic treatment (for general guidelines to symptomatic therapy, see Phenobarbitone, p.812), but in very severe overdosage, blood concentrations may be reduced by a regimen of forced diuresis (see again Phenobarbitone) or by haemodialysis. Peritoneal dialysis is inadequate.

The stomach of a woman who died of meprobamate overdosage was found to contain about 25 g of meprobamate despite gastric lavage. Treatment should include gastric lavage through a wide calibre tube.— E. H. Jenis *et al.*, *J. Am. med. Ass.*, 1969, *207*, 361. A 56-year-old woman was still deeply comatose 40 hours after ingestion of 36 g of meprobamate, despite gastric lavage, haemodialysis, and supportive therapy. Upon surgical operation a tarry mass weighing 140 g was removed from the stomach; it contained 24.9 g of meprobamate. She recovered following further haemodialysis.— H. S. Schwartz, *New Engl. J. Med.*, 1976, *295*, 1177.

A warning that expansion of plasma volume in hypotension due to meprobamate poisoining may cause pulmonary oedema.— F. Lhoste *et al.* (letter), *New Engl. J. Med.*, 1977, *296*, 1004.

Adsorption. For comment on the *in vitro* adsorption of meprobamate by activated charcoal, see p.79.

Dialysis and haemoperfusion. A beneficial result with charcoal haemoperfusion.— P. Crome *et al.*, *Postgrad. med. J.*, 1977, *53*, 698. The use of resin haemoperfusion in a patient following meprobamate overdosage.— W. E. Hoy *et al.*, *Ann. intern. Med.*, 1980, *93*, 455.

A detailed report of the successful use of haemodialysis in a woman with severe meprobamate overdosage. Drug removal was in excess of forced diuresis and metabolic degradation, but because of the rapidity of metabolic degradation it is felt that haemodialysis should be reserved for special cases. It is suggested that candidates for haemodialysis should have severe clinical intoxication with hypotension or respiratory failure, and either compromised normal excretory routes (for example, renal failure or liver disease), or progressive clinical deterioration.— P. I. Lobo *et al.*, *Clin. Nephrol.*, 1977, *7*, 73.

Further references: D. O. Castell and J. Sode, *Illinois med. J.*, 1967, *131*, 298 (peritoneal dialysis); D. E. Mouton *et al.*, *Am. J. med. Sci.*, 1967, *253*, 706 (peritoneal dialysis).

Diuresis. Forced diuresis with physiological saline precipitated pulmonary oedema in a 23-year-old woman who had taken an overdose of meprobamate.— J. A. Axelson and J. F. Hagaman (letter), *New Engl. J. Med.*, 1977, *296*, 1481.

Further references: A. J. Rice *et al.*, *J. Lab. clin. Med.*, 1972, *80*, 56 (*animal* study).

Precautions. Meprobamate should not be given to patients with acute intermittent porphyria. Although meprobamate has anticonvulsant properties, it may induce convulsions in patients with a history of epilepsy.

It may lower the tolerance to alcohol and other depressants of the central nervous system. Meprobamate may induce the hepatic microsomal enzymes involved in drug metabolism.

Meprobamate may cause drowsiness and patients should not drive vehicles or operate machinery where loss of attention could lead to accidents.

A study of the metabolism of meprobamate in human subjects suggested that chronic administration stimulates its metabolism.— J. F. Douglas *et al.*, *Proc. Soc. exp. Biol. Med.*, 1963, *112*, 436. Two patients receiving large doses of meprobamate for prolonged periods of time excreted meprobamate more slowly than subjects given single doses. This did not exclude the possibility of meprobamate enhancing its own metabolism.— L. E. Hollister and G. Levy, *Chemotherapia*, 1964, *9*, 20.

Interactions. Alcohol. Acute alcohol ingestion reduced the elimination-rate of meprobamate from the blood in a study of 4 subjects. It was suggested that this was due to the inhibition of hepatic microsomal metabolism.— E. Rubin *et al.*, *Am. J. Med.*, 1970, *49*, 801. A further study in 8 subjects indicated that chronic alcohol ingestion increased the elimination-rate of meprobamate from blood. There was no alteration in urinary excretion. It was considered that this effect was at least partly due to enhanced microsomal metabolism.— P. S. Misra *et al.*, *ibid.*, 1971, *51*, 346.

Further references: J. R. Ashford *et al.*, *J. Stud. Alcohol.*, 1975, *Suppl.* 7, 140; J. M. Cobby *et al.*, *ibid.*, 162.

Tricyclic antidepressants. For the effect of meprobamate in increasing the concentration of unbound desipramine in plasma, see Desipramine Hydrochloride, p.117.

Interference with diagnostic tests. The administration of meprobamate could interfere with measurements of urinary steroids.— *Adverse Drug React. Bull.*, 1972, June, 104.

Porphyria. Administration of meprobamate exacerbated experimental porphyria in *rats* but the validity of the test must depend on clinical observation.— A. A. -B. Badawy (letter), *Lancet*, 1978, *1*, 1361.

Absorption and Fate. Meprobamate is readily absorbed from the gastro-intestinal tract and peak concentrations in the plasma occur after 1 to 2 hours. Meprobamate is widely distributed. About 90% or more of a dose is excreted in the urine mainly as a hydroxylated metabolite and its glucuronide conjugate. Less than 10% appears in the faeces. Meprobamate has a half-life reported to range from about 6 to 16 hours.

It diffuses across the placenta and appears in the milk of nursing mothers at concentrations of up to 4 times those in the maternal plasma.

The elimination of meprobamate was found to be variable following administration of 800 mg to 12 healthy subjects, the half-life ranging from 6.4 to 16.6 hours (mean 11.3 hours). Considerably longer half-lives of 24 and 48 hours respectively were found following abrupt discontinuation in 2 subjects who had been receiving high doses for prolonged periods of time.— L. E. Hollister and G. Levy, *Chemotherapia*, 1964, *9*, 20.

Meprobamate was found to have a half-life of 7 hours in a study of one subject.— L. Martis and R. H. Levy, *J. pharm. Sci.*, 1974, *63*, 834.

Bioavailability. No statistically significant differences could be found in the relative bioavailability of meprobamate 400 mg tablets made by 11 different manufacturers.— M. C. Meyer *et al.*, *J. pharm. Sci.*, 1978, *67*, 1290.

Uses. Meprobamate belongs to the carbamate group of tranquillisers. It has some anticonvulsant and muscle relaxant properties. It is used in the treatment of anxiety and tension but has largely been superseded by the benzodiazepines (see Diazepam, p.1523).

Meprobamate has sometimes been used as a muscle relaxant and was tried in petit mal epilepsy (but see Precautions).

The usual dose is 400 mg thrice daily to a maximum of 2.4 g daily. Children have been given 25 mg per kg body-weight daily in divided doses.

Administration in hepatic failure. Meprobamate elimination is reported to be prolonged in patients with chronic liver disease.— R. K. Roberts *et al.*, *Drugs*, 1979, *17*, 198.

Administration in renal failure. The interval between doses of meprobamate should be extended from 6 hours to 9 to 12 hours in patients with a glomerular filtration-rate of 10 to 50 ml per minute, and to 12 to 18 hours in those with a glomerular filtration-rate of less than 10 ml per minute. Concentrations of meprobamate are affected by haemodialysis and peritoneal dialysis.— W. M. Bennett *et al.*, *Ann. intern. Med.*, 1977, *86*, 754. See also *idem*, 1980, *93*, 286.

Muscular disorders. Groups of about 30 patients with

musculoskeletal symptoms (pain, spasm, cramp) and anxiety were treated, under double-blind conditions, with tablets of aspirin 325 mg, meprobamate 200 mg, aspirin plus meprobamate, or placebo, each in a dose of 2 tablets thrice daily for 3 days. Aspirin relieved pain but not anxiety; meprobamate relieved anxiety and, to a lesser extent, pain.— M. M. Gilbert and H. H. Koepke, *Curr. ther. Res.*, 1973, *15*, 820.

Preparations

Meprobamate Injection *(U.S.P.)*. A sterile solution in a suitable solvent. pH 5.5 to 7.5.

Meprobamate Oral Suspension *(U.S.P.)*. A suspension containing meprobamate. Store in airtight containers.

Meprobamate Tablets *(B.P.)*. Tablets containing meprobamate.

Meprobamate Tablets *(U.S.P.)*. Tablets containing meprobamate. The *U.S.P.* requires 60% dissolution in 30 minutes.

Proprietary Preparations

Equanil *(Wyeth, UK)*. Meprobamate, available as tablets of 200 mg and as scored tablets of 400 mg. (Also available as Equanil in *Austral., Canad., Denm., Fr., S.Afr., USA*).

Meprate *(DDSA Pharmaceuticals, UK)*. Meprobamate, available as tablets of 200 and 400 mg.

Milonorm *(Wallace Mfg Chem., UK: Farillon, UK)*. Meprobamate, available as tablets of 400 mg.

Miltown *(Pharmax, UK)*. Meprobamate, available as scored tablets of 400 mg. (Also available as Miltown in *Canad., Spain, Switz., USA*).

Tenavoid *(Burgess, UK)*. Tablets each containing meprobamate 200 mg and bendrofluazide 3 mg. For the premenstrual syndrome. *Dose.* 1 tablet thrice daily for 5 to 7 days before each period.

Other Proprietary Names

Arg.— Distoncur, Meprin, Placidon, Sycropaz; *Austral.*—Mepron; *Belg.*— Oasil, Pertranquil, Probamyl, Procalmadiol, Quaname; *Canad.*— Lan-Dol, Meditran, Mep-E, Meprospan, Neo-Tran, Novomepro, Quietal; *Denm.*— Restenil; *Fr.*— Procalmadiol; *Ger.*— Aneural, Cyrpon, Dystoid forte, Meprocompren, Meprosa, Miltaun, Miltaunetten, Urbilat; *Ital.*— Meprodiol, Miltaun, Oasil, Perequil, Quanil, Sedoquil, Selene, Stensolo; *Norw.*— Meproban, Restenil; *S.Afr.*— Meposed, Pantranquil; *Spain*— Ansiowas, Dapaz, Ecuanil, Mepavlon, Oasil; *Swed.*— Restenil; *Switz.*— Meprodil, Oasil, Pertranquil, Probamyl, Quaname; *USA*— Mepriam, Meprospan, SK-Bamate.

Meprobamate was also formerly marketed in Great Britain under the proprietary names Mepavlon (*ICI Pharmaceuticals*) and Tised (*Ticen, Eire*).

7067-x

Mesoridazine Benzenesulphonate. Mesoridazine Besylate *(U.S.P.)*; Mesuridazine Benzenesulphonate; NC 123; TPS 23. 10-[2-(1-Methyl-2-piperidyl)ethyl]-2-(methylsulphinyl)phenothiazine benzenesulphonate.
$C_{21}H_{26}N_2OS_2,C_6H_6O_3S=544.7$.

CAS — 5588-33-0 (mesoridazine); 32672-69-8(benzenesulphonate).

Pharmacopoeias. In *U.S.*

A white to pale yellow, almost odourless, crystalline powder. M.p. about 178° with decomposition. **Soluble** 1 in 1 of water, 1 in 11 of alcohol, 1 in 3 of chloroform, and 1 in 6300 of ether; freely soluble in methyl alcohol. A freshly prepared 1% solution in water has a pH of 4.2 to 5.7. **Store** in airtight containers. Protect from light.

Adverse Effects, Treatment, and Precautions. As for Chlorpromazine, p.1509.

Interactions. *Phenytoin and other anticonvulsants.* For the effect of phenytoin and phenobarbitone on plasma-mesoridazine concentrations in patients receiving thioridazine, see under Thioridazine, p.1560.

Overdosage. Death of 2 patients from overdosage with mesoridazine; they had taken about 2.5 and 8 g respectively; death was apparently due to cardiac arrhythmias.— P. T. Donlon and J. P. Tupin, *Archs gen. Psychiat.*, 1977, *34*, 955.

Absorption and Fate. For an account of the absorption and fate of a phenothiazine, see Chlorpromazine, p.1513.
Mesoridazine is a metabolite of thioridazine (p.1559).

Plasma concentrations of mesoridazine and its metabolites following intramuscular administration: L. A. Gottschalk *et al.*, *Psychopharmac. Bull.*, 1975, *11*, 33.

Uses. Mesoridazine is a phenothiazine with actions and uses similar to those of chlorpromazine (p.1513). It has a piperidine side-chain and is a metabolite of thioridazine (p.1559). Mesoridazine is usually given as the benzenesulphonate but the doses are expressed in terms of the base. The usual dose for the treatment of psychoses is 50 mg thrice daily; doses of up to 400 mg daily have been given. It may also be given intramuscularly in an initial dose of 25 mg repeated after 30 to 60 minutes if necessary; up to 200 mg daily has been given.

Alcohol and drug withdrawal. Studies of mesoridazine in the treatment of alcoholism: J. B. Frost, *Can. psychiat. Ass. J.*, 1973, *18*, 385; I. Lowenstam, *J. chron. Dis.*, 1975, *28*, 431.

Psychoses. There is no evidence that mesoridazine offers any advantage over other phenothiazines.— *Med. Lett.*, 1975, *17*, 68.

Studies of mesoridazine in the treatment of schizophrenia and other psychoses: F. Gerstenbrand and J. Grunberger, *Wien. med. Wschr.*, 1970, *120*, 732; *Med. Lett.*, 1971, *13*, 4 and 18; M. V. McIndoo, *Sth. med. J.*, 1971, *64*, 592; R. M. Ritter and P. A. Tatum, *J. clin. Pharmac.*, 1972, *12*, 349; T. A. Hamid and W. J. Wertz, *Am. J. Psychiat.*, 1973, *130*, 689; S. E. Goldstein, *Curr. ther. Res.*, 1974, *16*, 316; G. Gardos *et al.*, *Comprehensive Psychiat.*, 1978, *19*, 517; *idem*, 527; G. Kinon *et al.*, *Curr. ther. Res.*, 1979, *25*, 534.

Preparations

Mesoridazine Besylate Injection *(U.S.P.)*. A sterile solution of mesoridazine benzenesulphonate in Water for Injections. Potency is expressed in terms of the equivalent amount of mesoridazine. pH 4 to 5. Protect from light.

Mesoridazine Besylate Oral Solution *(U.S.P.)*. A solution containing mesoridazine benzenesulphonate. Potency is expressed in terms of the equivalent amount of mesoridazine. To be diluted before use. Store at a temperature not exceeding 25° in airtight containers. Protect from light.

Mesoridazine Besylate Tablets *(U.S.P.)*. Tablets containing mesoridazine benzenesulphonate. Potency is expressed in terms of the equivalent amount of mesoridazine.

Proprietary Names

Imagotan *(Sandoz, Spain)*; Serentil *(Sandoz, Canad.; Boehringer Ingelheim, USA)*.

7068-r

Methotrimeprazine *(B.P. Vet., U.S.P.)*. Levomepromazine; RP 7044; SKF 5116. (−)-*NN*-Dimethyl-3-(2-methoxyphenothiazin-10-yl)-2-methylpropylamine.
$C_{19}H_{24}N_2OS=328.5$.

CAS — 60-99-1.

Pharmacopoeias. In *Braz.* and *U.S.*

A fine white almost odourless crystalline powder. M.p. about 126°. Practically **insoluble** in water; soluble 1 in 2 of chloroform and 1 in 10 of methyl alcohol; sparingly soluble in alcohol, but freely soluble in boiling alcohol; freely soluble in ether. A solution in chloroform is laevorotatory. **Protect** from light.

7069-f

Methotrimeprazine Hydrochloride.
$C_{19}H_{24}N_2OS,HCl=364.9$.

CAS — 4185-80-2.

Methotrimeprazine hydrochloride 1.11 g is approximately equivalent to 1 g of methotrimeprazine. Very **soluble** in water and alcohol. A 2% solution in water has a pH of about 4.8. **Incompatible** with alkaline solutions.

7070-z

Methotrimeprazine Maleate. Levomepromazine Maleate; Methotrimeprazine Hydrogen Maleate.
$C_{19}H_{24}N_2OS,C_4H_4O_4=444.5$.

CAS — 7104-38-3; 17086-29-2.

Pharmacopoeias. In *Cz., Jap.,* and *Roum.*

A white odourless crystalline powder. M.p. about 187° with decomposition. Methotrimeprazine maleate 1.35 g is approximately equivalent to 1 g of methotrimeprazine. Very slightly **soluble** in water; slightly soluble in alcohol; soluble in chloroform; practically insoluble in ether. An 0.3% solution in water has a pH of 4.3. **Protect** from light.

Adverse Effects, Treatment, and Precautions. As for Chlorpromazine, p.1509, and Promethazine and other Antihistamines, p.1294.
Methotrimeprazine may cause severe postural hypotension therefore patients receiving large initial doses or those receiving injections should be kept lying down. It should not be given to patients being treated with antihypertensive agents.
Pain at the site of injection is common.

Effects on the blood. *Agranulocytosis.* Three patients developed agranulocytosis during treatment with methotrimeprazine.— J. V. Ananth *et al.*, *Can. med. Ass. J.*, 1970, *102*, 1286.

Aplastic anaemia. Fatal pancytopenia was reported in a psychiatric woman patient given methotrimeprazine.— N. Garzotto *et al.*, *Br. J. Psychiat.*, 1976, *129*, 443.

Haemolysis. It was recommended that intravenous injections of methotrimeprazine be given slowly to minimise the amount of haemolysis which had been found to occur *in vitro* when the drug was mixed with blood.— R. J. Trudnowski (letter), *Br. J. Anaesth.*, 1973, *45*, 303.

Absorption and Fate. For an account of the absorption and fate of a phenothiazine, see Chlorpromazine, p.1513.

In a study involving a total of 5 psychiatric patients peak plasma concentrations of methotrimeprazine were noted 1 to 4 hours after administration by mouth and 30 to 90 minutes after injection into the gluteal muscle. About 50% of orally administered drug reached the systemic circulation. Although the metabolite methotrimeprazine sulphoxide could not be detected after a single intramuscular injection it was found in concentrations higher than unmetabolised methotrimeprazine after single and multiple oral dosage, both substances reaching a steady state in the plasma within 7 days of starting multiple dose oral therapy. Fluctuations in plasma concentration during multiple dose oral therapy indicated that until the correlation between acute side-effects and peak plasma concentration of methotrimeprazine had been further studied the total daily dose should be divided into 2 or 3 portions when larger doses of methotrimeprazine were given by mouth.— S. G. Dahl, *Clin. Pharmac. Ther.*, 1976, *19*, 435.

In 8 psychiatric patients given methotrimeprazine 50 to 350 mg daily the plasma half-life showed wide variation, from 16.5 to 77.8 hours, and did not correlate with the dose given.— S. G. Dahl *et al.*, *Eur. J. clin. Pharmac.*, 1977, *11*, 305.

Metabolism. Identification of metabolites of methotrimeprazine in plasma and urine of psychiatric patients.— S. G. Dahl and M. Garle, *J. pharm. Sci.*, 1977, *66*, 190.

Further references: A. De Leenheer and A. Heyndrickx, *J. pharm. Sci.*, 1972, *61*, 914; S. G. Dahl and H. Refsum, *Eur. J. Pharmac.*, 1976, *37*, 241.

Uses. Methotrimeprazine is a phenothiazine with pharmacological activity similar to that of both chlorpromazine (p.1513) and promethazine (p.1296). It has the histamine-antagonist properties of the antihistamines together with central nervous system effects resembling those of chlorpromazine. It has marked analgesic properties.
Methotrimeprazine has been given by mouth as the maleate in usual doses of 25 to 50 mg daily for the treatment of psychoses or as an adjunct to analgesics in the management of severe chronic pain; the daily dosage was usually divided into 3 portions with a larger portion taken at night. Doses of 100 to 200 mg have been given to patients in bed; gradual increase to doses of up to 1 g daily has been reported for severe psychoses.
Although the parenteral route is poorly tolerated, methotrimeprazine has also been given by intramuscular injection as the hydrochloride, usually for analgesia. The usual dose is 10 to 20 mg intramuscularly every 4 to 6 hours and patients should remain in bed for at least the first few doses; doses of up to 40 to 50 mg have been given. It is not suitable for subcutaneous administration and although some sources have reported its use by intravenous infusion this route is not generally recommended. Methotrimeprazine has also been given intramuscularly for anaesthetic premedication.
Elderly subjects were given reduced doses of methotrimeprazine.
Methotrimeprazine has also been used as the embonate.

Cardiac disorders. A double-blind study of analgesic treatment with methotrimeprazine in acute myocardial infarction. It was considered that the analgesic peak effect of methotrimeprazine 12.5 mg was equivalent to that of pethidine 50 mg.— O. Davidsen *et al., Acta med. scand.*, 1979, *205*, 191.

Preparations

Methotrimeprazine Injection *(U.S.P.)*. A sterile solution in Water for Injections prepared with the aid of hydrochloric acid. pH 3 to 5. Protect from light.

Proprietary Names

Levonormal *(Jap.)*; Levoprome *(Lederle, USA)*; Minozinan *(Specia, Belg.; Specia, Neth.; Specia, Switz.)*; Neurocil *(Bayer, Ger.)*; Nozinan *(Rhodia, Arg.; Specia, Belg.; Rhône-Poulenc, Canad.; Rhone-Poulenc, Denm.; Specia, Fr.; Farmalabor, Ital.; Specia, Neth.; Mekos, Norw.; Leo Rhodia, Swed.; Specia, Switz.)*; Procrazine *(Jap.)*; Sinogan *(Rhodia, Spain)*; Sofmin *(Jap.)*; Tisercin *(EGYT, Hung.)*; Veractil *(Rhône-Poulenc, Norw.)*.

Methotrimeprazine hydrochloride and methotrimeprazine maleate were formerly marketed in Great Britain under the proprietary name Veractil (*May & Baker*).

7071-c

Metiapine. 2-Methyl-11-(4-methylpiperazin-1-yl)dibenzo[*b,f*][1,4] thiazepine.
$C_{19}H_{21}N_3S=323.5$.

CAS — 5800-19-1.

Metiapine has been given in doses of about 50 to 300 mg daily for the treatment of schizophrenia; larger doses have also been tried.

Toxicology of metiapine in *animals*.— J. P. Gibson and J. W. Newberne, *Toxic. appl. Pharmac.*, 1973, *25*, 212; J. P. Gibson *et al., ibid.*, 220.

In 20 patients with acute schizophrenia given metiapine in doses of up to 600 mg daily objective assessment showed significant improvement chiefly in the area of cognitive disorganisation. However only 2 of the 20 achieved marked therapeutic benefit. Marked drowsiness occurred in 75% of the patients and hypotension and tachycardia in about half the patients; marked extrapyramidal symptoms also occurred.— A. Flemenbaum, *Curr. ther. Res.*, 1973, *15*, 470.

A double-blind crossover study on 10 chronic schizophrenics to compare metiapine and chlorpromazine showed little difference in efficacy. One patient responded to metiapine and not to chlorpromazine. Extrapyramidal side-effects were more marked with metiapine.— G. M. Simpson *et al., J. clin. Pharmac.*, 1973, *13*, 408.

A double-blind study was carried out in 90 patients with acute schizophrenia who were given either metiapine 25 to 600 mg daily, chlorpromazine 0.05 to 1.2 g, or a combination of secbutobarbitone 15 to 180 mg and atropine sulphate 0.17 to 2.04 mg daily for 28 days. Both metiapine and chlorpromazine were about equally effective in achieving clinical improvement and were more effective than the combination. Subjective and extrapyramidal side-effects and ECG changes were more frequent with metiapine.— M. Kramer *et al., Curr. ther. Res.*, 1975, *18*, 839.

A study indicating that metiapine and chlorpromazine were equally effective in the treatment of acute schizophrenic patients. Side-effects included tachycardia in 6 patients treated with metiapine.— R. M. Steinbook *et al., J. clin. Pharmac.*, 1975, *15*, 700.

Further references: G. M. Simpson *et al., Curr. ther. Res.*, 1971, *13*, 257; D. M. Gallant *et al., ibid.*, 734; M. Kramer *et al., ibid.*, 1973, *15*, 465.

Manufacturers

Merrell-National, USA.

7072-k

Molindone Hydrochloride.

EN 1733A. 3-Ethyl-6,7-dihydro-2-methyl-5-(morpholinomethyl)indol-4(5*H*)-one hydrochloride.
$C_{16}H_{24}N_2O_2,HCl=312.8$.

CAS — 7416-34-4 (molindone); 15622-65-8 (hydrochloride).

A white crystalline powder. Freely **soluble** in water and alcohol.

Adverse Effects. The side-effects of molindone, such as sedation and extrapyramidal symptoms, which are the result of its pharmacological action, are similar to those of chlorpromazine (p.1509). Tardive dyskinesia may also be expected.

Extrapyramidal symptoms may be more common than those associated with chlorpromazine.

Other side-effects reported include nausea, weight gain and, in particular weight loss, agitation, hyperactivity, euphoria, depression, skin rashes, and abnormal liver-function tests. Leucopenia and leucocytosis have occasionally been reported. Transient ECG changes have occasionally been noted.

Reports of galactorrhoea associated with molindone.— J. L. Kahn, *Am. J. Psychiat.*, 1979, *136*, 1617; C. E. Wesp *et al., ibid.*, 975.

Treatment of Adverse Effects and Precautions. As for Chlorpromazine, p.1511.

Absorption and Fate. Molindone is readily absorbed from the gastro-intestinal tract, peak concentrations of unchanged molindone being obtained within about 1 to 2 hours of administration. It is rapidly and extensively metabolised and a very large number of metabolites have been identified. It is excreted in the urine and faeces almost entirely in the form of its metabolites. The pharmacological effect from a single dose by mouth is reported to last for 24 to 36 hours.

Uses. Molindone is an indole derivative with antipsychotic actions similar to those of chlorpromazine (p.1513). It is given as the hydrochloride by mouth or intramuscularly.

The usual dose of molindone hydrochloride by mouth for the treatment of psychoses is 50 to 75 mg daily initially, increased within 3 or 4 days to 100 mg daily; in severe conditions doses of up to 225 mg daily may be required. The maintenance dosage can range from 15 to 225 mg daily. The recommended daily dosage may be divided into 2 to 4 portions or given as a once-daily dosage regimen. For the control of acute conditions it has been given by intramuscular injection.

Molindone should be given in reduced dosage to elderly patients.

Schizophrenia. A long-term study of molindone hydrochloride given in doses of up to 200 mg daily to 23 chronic schizophrenic in-patients. The duration of the study ranged from 6 to 19 months. The general response was similar to that with the patients' previous and subsequent antipsychotic medication but some patients responded worse and others better. Although 5 patients gained weight another 5 lost substantial amounts indicating that molindone could be of benefit in overweight patients.— R. Kellner *et al., Curr. ther. Res.*, 1976, *20*, 686.

Beneficial results with intramuscular injection of molindone in doses of up to 50 mg twice daily. It seemed reasonable to assume that higher daily doses would be tolerated if a suitable preparation were available.— D. H. Mielke and D. M. Gallant, *Curr. ther. Res.*, 1977, *22*, 356.

Further references: M. Campbell *et al., Curr. ther. Res.*, 1971, *13*, 28 (in children); G. M. Simpson *et al., J. clin. Pharmac.*, 1971, *11*, 227; F. S. Abuzzahab, *J. clin. Pharmac.*, 1973, *13*, 226; *idem*, 422.

Weight loss. Nine severely ill hospitalised chronic schizophrenics (7 obese and 2 underweight) were given molindone 20 to 60 mg daily instead of their usual treatment; 8 received molindone for 3 months and one patient for only one month because of poor control of her schizophrenia. All patients lost weight ranging from 0.9 to 16.8 kg with a mean loss of 7.6 kg representing 8.5% of initial body weight. Molindone should be investigated as a treatment for obese schizophrenic patients.— G. Gardos and J. O. Cole, *Am. J. Psychiat.*, 1977, *134*, 302. See also D. M. Gallant *et al., Curr. ther. Res.*, 1973, *15*, 915.

Proprietary Names

Lidone *(Abbott, USA)*; Moban *(Endo, S.Afr.; Endo, USA)*.

7073-a

Moperone Hydrochloride. R 1658; Moperone Chloride; Methylperidol Hydrochloride. 4′-Fluoro-4-(4-hydroxy-4-*p*-tolylpiperidino)butyrophenone hydrochloride.
$C_{22}H_{26}FNO_2,HCl=391.9$.

CAS — 1050-79-9 (moperone); 3871-82-7 (hydrochloride).

Moperone is a butyrophenone with general properties similar to those of haloperidol (p.1532). For the treatment of psychoses it has been given as the hydrochloride in doses of 10 to 60 mg daily.

References: W. A. Cook, *Med. J. Aust.*, 1966, *2*, 117.

Proprietary Names

Luvatren *(Cilag-Chemie, Denm.; Cilag-Chemie, Ital.; Yamanouchi, Jap.; Cilag-Chemie, Neth.; Cilag-Chemie, Norw.; Cilag-Chemie, Swed.; Cilag-Chemie, Switz.)*; Luvatrena *(Cilag, Ger.)*; Luvatrene *(Cilag-Chemie, Belg.)*.

7035-l

Nordazepam. Demethyldiazepam; *N*-Desmethyldiazepam; Desmethyldiazepam; Nordiazepam; A 101. 7-Chloro-1,3-dihydro-5-phenyl-2*H*-1,4-benzodiazepin-2-one.
$C_{15}H_{11}ClN_2O=270.7$.

CAS — 1088-11-5.

A white or pale yellow crystalline powder. M.p. about 216°. Practically **insoluble** in water; slightly soluble in alcohol and chloroform.

Nordazepam is a benzodiazepine with actions and uses similar to those of diazepam (p.1519). It is the principal metabolite of diazepam. It has been given in doses of 5 mg twice daily for the treatment of anxiety.

Hypnotic effect. The hypnotic effects of nordazepam and clorazepate dipotassium were studied in 6 healthy subjects; 10 mg of nordazepam was considered equivalent to 15 mg of clorazepate dipotassium.— A. N. Nicholson *et al., Br. J. clin. Pharmac.*, 1976, *3*, 429.

Further references: D. Perbellini *et al., Thérapie*, 1975, *30*, 667.

Proprietary Names

Demadar *(Volpino, Arg.)*; Madar *(Ravizza, Ital.)*.

7074-t

Oxaflumazine Disuccinate. 10-(3-{4-[2-(1,3-Dioxan-2-yl)ethyl]piperazin-1-yl}propyl)-2-trifluoromethylphenothiazine disuccinate.
$C_{26}H_{32}F_3N_3O_2S,2C_4H_6O_4=743.8$.

CAS — 16498-21-8 (oxaflumazine); 7450-97-7 (disuccinate).

Oxaflumazine is a phenothiazine with general properties similar to those of chlorpromazine (p.1509). It has a piperazine side-chain. The recommended initial dose of the disuccinate for the treatment of psychoses is 150 to 600 mg daily, with doses of up to 200 mg daily for maintenance therapy.

Proprietary Names

Oxaflumine *(Diamant, Fr.)*.

7075-x

Oxanamide. 2,3-Epoxy-2-ethylhexanamide.
$C_8H_{15}NO_2=157.2$.

CAS — 126-93-2.

A white, odourless or almost odourless, tasteless, crystalline powder. **Soluble** 1 in 100 of water.

Oxanamide is a tranquilliser with actions similar to those of meprobamate (p.1545). It was also reported to have muscle relaxant properties. It was formerly used in the treatment of anxiety and tension in doses of 400 mg four times daily.

7076-r

Oxazepam *(U.S.P.)*. Wy 3498. 7-Chloro-1,3-dihydro-3-hydroxy-5-phenyl-2*H*-1,4-benzodiazepin-2-one.
$C_{15}H_{11}ClN_2O_2$=286.7.
CAS — 604-75-1.

Pharmacopoeias. In *Braz., Cz., Nord.,* and *U.S.*

A creamy white to pale yellow, almost odourless powder. M.p. 200° to 205°. Practically **insoluble** in water; soluble 1 in 220 of alcohol, 1 in 270 of chloroform, and 1 in 2200 of ether; soluble in dioxan. A 2% suspension in water has a pH of 4.8 to 7.

Dependence. Prolonged use of oxazepam may lead to the development of dependence of the barbiturate-alcohol type (see p.792). It has a low liability for abuse.

Dependence and withdrawal. A report of oxazepam dependence eventually controlled by phenelzine.— S. M. Hanna, *Br. J. Psychiat.*, 1972, *120*, 443. Comment.— T. V. A. Harry, *Wyeth* (letter), *ibid.*, *121*, 235.

A report of withdrawal convulsions from benzodiazepines in 4 patients, involving clorazepate (1), oxazepam (1), and lorazepam (2).— T. R. Einarson (letter), *Lancet*, 1980, *1*, 151. A comment that 2 of these patients were also taking trifluoperazine, which has known epileptogenic potential. A patient has been seen, however, who suffered a grand-mal seizure 4 days after stopping lorazepam 5 mg daily alone; lorazepam had been taken for 2 years in a daily dose of 5 to 15 mg.— P. Tyrer (letter), *ibid.*

A 24-year-old man who had taken oxazepam 15 mg every 4 hours and 30 mg at night, for 2 years had withdrawal reactions when he suddenly stopped taking the drug. The symptoms which included increasing restlessness, rigidity of the limbs, stiffness of the joints, and a feeling of having great energy with impaired concentration resolved when he resumed taking oxazepam. He later stopped taking oxazepam by gradually reducing the dose without withdrawal symptoms.— G. Mendelson (letter), *Lancet*, 1978, *1*, 565 and 888.

Further references: J. W. Selig, *J. Am. med. Ass.*, 1966, *198*, 951.

Adverse Effects, Treatment, and Precautions. As for Diazepam, p.1520.

Cytogenetic effects. Oxazepam was found to have no significant influence on the tumour growth, or the survival-time, of tumour-bearing *rats*.— A. Guaitani *et al.* (letter), *Lancet*, 1979, *1*, 1147.

Effects on the eyes. A study indicating that usual therapeutic doses of oxazepam strongly interfere with colour vision.— J. Laroche and C. Laroche, *Annls pharm. Fr.*, 1977, *35*, 173.

Interactions. *Alcohol.* Alcohol-induced delay in oxazepam absorption.— H. J. Mallach *et al.*, *Arzneimittel-Forsch.*, 1975, *25*, 1840.

Overdosage. A 2-year-old girl was admitted to hospital 18 hours after taking 90 mg of oxazepam. She was apathetic and lethargic, though she showed paradoxical excitation. Reflexes were depressed and her face was oedematous. Her gait was ataxic. By the third hospital day the deep-tendon reflexes had returned to normal, and the ataxia disappeared slowly over 8 days, but at discharge, 2 weeks later, there was still slight facial puffiness.— P. M. Shimkin, *J. Am. med. Ass.*, 1966, *196*, 662.

A 45-year-old man, who ingested large doses [not stated] of oxazepam in an attempted suicide, went into a deep coma and had an apparent blood-glucose concentration of 1.68 g per 100 ml and an electrolyte imbalance. It was later discovered that oxazepam gave a positive reaction for glucose. The patient's condition did not improve until the fourth day when exchange transfusion was carried out. The importance of diagnosis of this pseudohyperglycaemic non-ketoacidotic coma and the dangers of insulin administration were emphasised.— M. S. Zileli *et al.* (letter), *J. Am. med. Ass.*, 1971, *215*, 1986. Tests indicated that lactose present as a filler in oxazepam preparations could have accounted for the false high blood-glucose concentration.— H. E. Spiegel and D. Enthoven (letter), *ibid.*, 1972, *220*, 1499. The effect of lactose could not be corroborated.— J. D. Teller (letter), *ibid.*, *222*, 209.

Fatal rhabdomyolysis (paroxysmal idiopathic myoglobulinuria) with hyperkalaemia and anuria occurred in a man after ingestion of oxazepam 6 g.— B. Goertz *et al.*, *Dt. med. Wschr.*, 1978, *103*, 121.

A 24-year-old man remained in a light sleep for 24 hours after drinking heavily over 40 hours then swallowing an estimated 2.4 g of oxazepam. A review of the literature confirms the belief that benzodiazepines are extremely safe drugs when taken in high doses.— K. Solomon, *N.Y. St. J. Med.*, 1978, *78*, 91.

Pregnancy and the neonate. See under Absorption and Fate.

Absorption and Fate. For an account of the absorption and fate of a benzodiazepine, see Diazepam, p.1522.

Oxazepam has been reported to have a half-life ranging from about 6 to 25 hours. It is the ultimate pharmacologically active metabolite of diazepam and is itself largely metabolised to the inactive glucuronide; small amounts are excreted unchanged.

Absorption and plasma concentrations. An account of the pharmacokinetics of oxazepam. Absorption of oxazepam is probably complete and in healthy subjects half-lives ranging from about 6 to 25 hours have been obtained.— G. Alván and I. Odar-Cederlöf, *Acta psychiat. scand.*, 1978, *Suppl.* 274, 47.

Further references: H. Pelzer and D. Maas, *Arzneimittel-Forsch.*, 1969, *19*, 1652 (blood concentrations); J. A. Knowles and H. W. Ruelius, *Arzneimittel-Forsch.*, 1972, *22*, 687 (plasma concentrations and half-life).

Biliary excretion. Following administration of oxazepam 45 mg to 2 subjects who had undergone cholecystectomy less than 0.1% of a dose was found in the bile.— H. J. Shull *et al.*, *Ann. intern. Med.*, 1976, *84*, 420. Increased biliary excretion and possible enterohepatic recycling in uraemic subjects.— G. Alván and I. Odar-Cederlöf, *Acta psychiat. scand.*, 1978, *Suppl.* 274, 47.

Pregnancy and the neonate. *Diffusion across the placenta.* A study on the placental passage of oxazepam and its metabolism in 12 women given a single dose of oxazepam 25 mg during labour. Oxazepam was readily absorbed and peak plasma concentrations were in the same range as those reported in healthy males and non-pregnant females given the same dose although the plasma half-life (range 5.3 to 7.8 hours in 8 subjects studied) was shorter than that reported for non-pregnant subjects. Oxazepam was detected in the umbilical vein of all 12 patients with the ratio between umbilical to maternal vein concentration of oxazepam reaching a value of about 1.35 and remaining constant beyond a dose-delivery time of 3 hours. All of the babies had a normal Apgar score value. The oxazepam plasma half-life in the newborns was about 3 to 4 times that in the mothers although in 3 the plasma concentration of oxazepam conjugate rose during the first 6 to 10 hours after delivery indicating the ability of the neonate to conjugate oxazepam.— G. Tomson *et al.*, *Clin. Pharmac. Ther.*, 1979, *25*, 74.

Further references: G. Tomson *et al.*, *Acta psychiat. scand.*, 1978, *Suppl.* 274, 75; R. L. Nation, *Clin. Pharmacokinet.*, 1980, *5*, 340; L. Kangas *et al.*, *Eur. J. clin. Pharmac.*, 1980, *17*, 301.

Uses. Oxazepam is a benzodiazepine with actions and uses similar to those of diazepam (p.1523). The usual dose for the treatment of anxiety is 15 to 30 mg three or four times daily; in severe conditions up to 180 mg daily has been given. A suggested initial dose for elderly or debilitated patients is 10 mg three or four times daily.

Oxazepam has also been used as the hemisuccinate.

Administration. Neither the rate nor the extent of oxazepam absorption was reduced by food intake.— A. Melander, *Clin. Pharmacokinet.*, 1978, *3*, 337.

Further references: A. Melander *et al.*, *Acta pharmac. tox.*, 1977, *40*, 584.

In children. Numerous authors have employed oxazepam in paediatric psychiatry. Dosage varied according to age, indication, and individual response but normally a dose of about 1 mg per kg body-weight daily in divided doses proved adequate.— R. Deberdt, *Acta psychiat. scand.*, 1978, *Suppl.* 274, 104.

In the elderly. Oxazepam elimination appears to be unaffected by age.— R. E. Vestal, *Drugs*, 1978, *16*, 358.

Administration in hepatic failure. Seven patients with acute viral hepatitis, 6 with cirrhosis of the liver, and 16 age-matched healthy control subjects received oxazepam 15 or 45 mg by mouth. Urinary excretion rates and plasma elimination patterns were unaltered in patients with acute and chronic parenchymal liver disease. In a chronic study, oxazepam 15 mg was administered thrice daily by mouth for 2 weeks to 2 healthy subjects and to 2 patients with cirrhosis and did not appear to accumulate in any of the four.— H. J. Shull *et al.*, *Ann. intern. Med.*, 1976, *84*, 420.

Further references: H. J. Shull *et al.*, *Gastroenterology*, 1975, *69*, 866; G. R. Wilkinson, *Acta psychiat. scand.*, 1978, *Suppl.* 274, 56; E. M. Sellers *et al.*, *Clin. Pharmac. Ther.*, 1979, *26*, 240.

Administration in renal failure. Increased half-life of oxazepam in patients with renal failure.— I. Odar-Cederlöf *et al.*, *Acta pharmac. tox.*, 1977, *40 Suppl.* 1, 52.

Alcohol and drug withdrawal. Studies involving oxazepam in alcohol withdrawal.— G. Pernhaupt, *Wien. med. Wschr.*, 1972, *122*, 233; Å. Bliding, *Br. J. Psychiat.*, 1973, *122*, 465; H. Guthy, *Therapie Gegenw.*, 1976, *115*, 1365.

Anaesthesia. References to the use of oxazepam for basal anaesthesia and anaesthetic premedication: B. J. Urban *et al.*, *Anesth. Analg. curr. Res.*, 1966, *45*, 733; J. Kanto *et al.*, *Int. J. clin. Pharmac. Biopharm.*, 1979, *17*, 26.

Anxiety. Oxazepam in a dosage of 15 mg thrice daily was given to 48 patients suffering from anxiety states. Patients received plain uncoated tablets which were coloured green, red, and yellow, each for a period of 1 week. Though the differences in responses to treatment with the 3 colours of tablets were not significant, green tablets appeared to be the most effective for symptoms of anxiety, and yellow the most effective for depressive symptoms.— K. Schapira *et al.*, *Br. med. J.*, 1970, *2*, 446.

Further references: *Practitioner*, 1967, *199*, 356 (Report No. 112 of the General Practitioner Research Group); R. V. de Silverio *et al.*, *J. clin. Pharmac.*, 1969, *9*, 259; *Br. J. clin. Pract.*, 1970, *24*, 323; S. Maneksha and T. Harry, *ibid.*, 1974, *28*, 65; J. R. Lion, *J. clin. Psychiat.*, 1979, *40*, 70.

Convulsions. Studies of oxazepam in epilepsy.— H. O. C. Lou, *Neurology, Minneap.*, 1968, *18*, 986.

Hypnotic effect. Oxazepam 30 or 45 mg significantly increased total sleep time and reduced the time awake in 6 healthy subjects when compared to placebo and had a more pronounced effect than diazepam 10 mg. Subjects reported impaired wakefulness on awakening after overnight ingestion of the 45-mg dose.— A. N. Nicholson and B. M. Stone (letter), *Br. J. clin. Pharmac.*, 1978, *5*, 469.

Further references: W. Ehrenstein *et al.*, *Arzneimittel-Forsch.*, 1972, *22*, 421.

Preparations

Oxazepam Capsules *(U.S.P.)*. Capsules containing oxazepam.

Oxazepam Tablets *(U.S.P.)*. Tablets containing oxazepam.

Proprietary Preparations

Serenid-D (known in some countries as Serax, Serenal, Serepax, Seresta, Serpax) *(Wyeth, UK)*. Oxazepam, available as tablets of 10 mg and as tablets of 15 mg.
Serenid Forte. Oxazepam, available as capsules of 30 mg.

NOTE. Serenal is also used as a proprietary name for Oxazolam.

Other Proprietary Names

Adumbran *(Arg., Austral., Ger., Ital., S.Afr., Spain)*; Aplakil *(Spain)*; Benzotran *(Austral.)*; Enidrel *(Arg.)*; Isodin *(Ital.)*; Limbial *(Ital.)*; Murelax *(Austral.)*; Nesontil *(Arg.)*; Nulans (hemisuccinate) *(Ital.)*; Oxepam *(Fin.)*; Praxiten *(Arg., Aust., Ger.)*; Psiquiwas *(Spain)*; Purata *(S.Afr.)*; Quen *(Ital.)*; Quilibrex *(Ital.)*; Sedokin *(Ital.)*; Sobile *(Spain)*; Sobril *(Norw., Swed.)*; Wakazepam *(Jap.)*.

7077-f

Oxazolam. Oxazolazepam. 10-Chloro-2,3,7,11b-tetrahydro-2-methyl-11b-phenyloxazolo[3,2-*d*][1,4]benzodiazepin-6(5*H*)-one.
$C_{18}H_{17}ClN_2O_2$=328.8.
CAS — 24143-17-7.

A white or almost white, almost odourless and tasteless, crystalline powder. M.p. about 187°. Practically **insoluble** in water; slightly soluble in alcohol; soluble in chloroform; sparingly soluble in acetone and ethyl acetate.

Oxazolam is a benzodiazepine with actions and uses similar to those of diazepam (p.1519). It has been given in doses of 10 to 20 mg thrice daily for the treatment of anxiety.

Proprietary Names
Convertal *(Roemmers, Arg.)*; Hializan *(Pharmainvesti, Spain)*; Serenal (see also under Oxazepam) *(Sankyo, Jap.)*.

7078-d

Oxypertine.

Win 18501. 5,6-Dimethoxy-2-methyl-3-[2-(4-phenylpiperazin-1-yl)ethyl]indole. $C_{23}H_{29}N_3O_2$=379.5.

CAS — 153-87-7.

A white crystalline powder. Slightly **soluble** in water and alcohol.

Adverse Effects. The side-effects of oxypertine, such as sedation and extrapyramidal symptoms, which are the result of its pharmacological action, are similar to those of chlorpromazine (p.1509). Tardive dyskinesia may also be expected.
Other side-effects include nausea and vomiting, eosinophilia, and insomnia. Abnormal liver-function tests and severe hypotension have also been reported.

Marked reduction in blood pressure in one patient and paralytic ileus in another, following administration of oxypertine.— *Japan med. Gaz.*, 1978, *15* (May 20), 12.

Treatment of Adverse Effects. As for Chlorpromazine, p.1511.

Precautions. As for Chlorpromazine, p.1512.
Some sources have recommended that since oxypertine has been observed in *animal* studies to release small amounts of catecholamines, it should be avoided in patients taking monoamine oxidase inhibitors. For comments on the possibility of interactions between monoamine oxidase inhibitors and direct-acting catecholamines, such as adrenaline and noradrenaline, which are metabolised by catechol *O*-methyltransferase, see Adrenaline, p.2.

Uses. Oxypertine has antipsychotic actions similar to those of chlorpromazine (p.1513). The usual dose of oxypertine for the treatment of psychoses is 80 to 120 mg daily in divided doses. The maximum recommended dose is 300 mg daily although higher doses have been used. Doses of 10 mg three or four times daily have also been used for non-psychotic emotional disturbances such as anxiety and tension. In general, however, neuroleptics are only suitable for such purposes in resistant conditions, where more appropriate agents, such as the benzodiazepines (see Diazepam, p.1523) has proved ineffective. If their use is judged to be necessary treatment should be directed at low dosages given on a short-term basis.

Anaesthesia. In a randomised study in 185 patients oxypertine 20 mg given on the evening before surgery and on the morning of surgery produced relief of anxiety comparable with that produced by the drug usually used for sedation on the evening before surgery and papaveretum 10 mg and atropine 600 µg about 1 hour before surgery.— I. T. Davie and K. B. Slawson, *Br. J. Anaesth.*, 1976, *48*, 915.

Further references: I. T. Davis and K. B. Slawson, *Br. J. Anaesth.*, 1973, *45*, 927; W. Norris and P. G. M. Wallace, *Br. J. Anaesth.*, 1973, *45*, 1222.

Anxiety and depression. Studies of oxypertine given in doses of about 10 to 20 mg thrice daily for anxiety and/or depression.— *Practitioner*, 1971, *206*, 822 (Report No. 161 of the General Practitioner Research Group); F. J. Wadzisz, *Br. J. Psychiat.*, 1972, *121*, 507; J. A. Bonn, *Postgrad. med. J.*, 1972, *48* (Sept.), *Suppl.*, 24; M. Sim *et al.*, *J. int. med. Res.*, 1978, *6*, 4.

Schizophrenia. Of 9 patients with chronic schizophrenia treated with oxypertine in daily doses of up to 120 mg, in only 1 was treatment successful and this patient developed Cushing's syndrome.— G. Pascalis and B. Chauvot, *Thérapie*, 1968, *23*, 975.

A double-blind controlled trial in 38 men with chronic schizophrenia of long standing indicated that oxypertine had equivalent psychotropic activity to chlorpromazine. A placebo was given for 4 weeks and was followed by either chlorpromazine, usually 100 mg, or oxypertine, usually 40 mg, thrice daily for 12 weeks. Side-effects with oxypertine treatment included vomiting (3 patients), tachycardia (6), akathisia and hand tremor (1), and dystonic reactions (1).— C. D. Neal *et al.*, *Curr. ther. Res.*, 1969, *11*, 367.

In a study of oxypertine 68 to 480 mg daily given to 33 schizophrenic patients and thiothixene 5 to 48 mg daily given to 38 schizophrenic patients, thiothixene was found to be superior in treating those with paranoid schizophrenia while oxypertine was more effective in depressed schizophrenic patients.— L. E. Hollister *et al.*, *Clin. Pharmac. Ther.*, 1971, *12*, 531.

Proprietary Preparations
Integrin *(Sterling Research, UK)*. Oxypertine, available as **Capsules** of 10 mg and scored **Tablets** of 40 mg.

Other Proprietary Names
Equipertine *(Belg., Fr., Neth.)*; Forit *(Ger., Switz.)*; Opertil *(Denm., Fin., Neth., Norw.)*.

7079-n

Pecazine Hydrochloride.

Mepazine Hydrochloride; P 391. 10-(1-Methyl-3-piperidylmethyl)phenothiazine hydrochloride monohydrate. $C_{19}H_{22}N_2S,HCl,H_2O$=364.9.

CAS — 60-89-9 (pecazine); 2975-36-2 (hydrochloride, anhydrous).

Pecazine is a phenothiazine with general properties similar to those of chlorpromazine (p.1509). It has a piperidine side-chain. It has been given as the hydrochloride, in doses equivalent to 12.5 to 25 mg of base, about 3 times daily by mouth; it has also been given intramuscularly as the acetate.

7080-k

Penfluridol.

R 16341. 1-[4,4-Bis(4-fluorophenyl)butyl]-4-(4-chloro-3-trifluoromethylphenyl)piperidin-4-ol. $C_{28}H_{27}ClF_5NO$=524.0.

CAS — 26864-56-2.

A white or almost white crystalline or microcrystalline powder. M.p. 104° to 109°. Practically **insoluble** in water; very soluble in alcohol, acetone, and chloroform; freely soluble in ether. **Store** in airtight containers. Protect from light.

Adverse Effects. The side-effects of penfluridol, such as sedation, extrapyramidal symptoms, and tardive dyskinesia, which are the result of its pharmacological action, are similar to those of chlorpromazine (p.1509).
Extrapyramidal symptoms may be more common than those associated with chlorpromazine, whereas it may be less likely to cause sedation.

Effects on the endocrine system. Penfluridol 100 mg weekly for 6 weeks raised plasma-prolactin concentrations in 7 chronic schizophrenic males, but had no significant effect on plasma-testosterone concentrations. There were no correlations between individual changes in prolactin and testosterone concentrations. None of the patients complained of sexual difficulties.— R. S. Nathan *et al.* (letter), *Lancet*, 1980, *2*, 94. Comment.— R. T. Rubin (letter), *ibid.*, 370.

Treatment of Adverse Effects. As for Chlorpromazine, p.1511. The prolonged duration of action of penfluridol should be borne in mind.

Precautions. As for Chlorpromazine, p.1512.

Absorption and Fate. Although penfluridol is absorbed from the gastro-intestinal tract, peak plasma concentrations are not achieved until about 12 to 24 hours after a dose by mouth. The initial peak plasma concentration is followed by a rapid decrease over the next 36 hours, probably due to tissue redistribution, followed by a slower decline over the next 120 hours. Penfluridol, accordingly, has a very long duration of action, and *animal* studies have indicated that this is partly related to its storage in, and slow release from, adipose tissue.
There is evidence of enterohepatic recycling, and penfluridol is mainly excreted unchanged in the faeces, with small amounts appearing in the urine as the metabolite 4,4-bis(4-fluorophenyl)butyric acid, which is obtained by *N*-dealkylation.

In a double-blind study of 22 schizophrenic patients who had been given regular weekly doses of 30, 60, or 120 mg of penfluridol for 12 weeks to determine steady-state plasma concentrations, the maximum mean plasma concentration of penfluridol was reached within 12 hours of the last dose; the plasma concentration then fell rapidly during the following 36 hours, and more slowly to a still detectable steady-state concentration 7 days after dosage.— S. F. Cooper *et al.*, *Clin. Pharmac. Ther.*, 1975, *18*, 325. See also D. M. Gallant *et al.*, *Am. J. Psychiat.*, 1974, *131*, 699.

Further references: S. F. Cooper *et al.*, *Int. Pharmacopsychiat.*, 1975, *10*, 78 (plasma concentrations).

Uses. Penfluridol is a member of the diphenylbutylpiperidine group of antipsychotic agents, which are structurally similar to the butyrophenones (see haloperidol, p.1532). Following administration by mouth it has a prolonged duration of action which lasts for about a week.
The usual dose of penfluridol for the treatment of psychoses is 20 to 60 mg weekly. Doses of up to 120 mg weekly may be required in resistant conditions.

Schizophrenia. A brief review of the merits of a once-weekly oral preparation for schizophrenia.— *Lancet*, 1978, *2*, 879. Comment.— A. A. Schiff, *Squibb* (letter), *ibid.*, 1101.

Results of a 3-week double-blind study completed by 29 of 33 schizophrenic patients requiring in-patient therapy, indicated that penfluridol is as effective as chlorpromazine in the treatment of schizophrenia, except for patients with very acute symptoms. Twenty-one of the 29 patients completed a 10-week follow-up study as out-patients. The mean dose of penfluridol was 102 mg weekly (range 80 to 120 mg weekly), and chlorpromazine 650 mg daily (range 100 to 900 mg daily). Five penfluridol patients required reduction of dose because of drowsiness (2), extrapyramidal effects (2), and weakness (1); 5 chlorpromazine patients also required dose reduction because of drowsiness. Two penfluridol patients were readmitted to hospital because of depression. Four chlorpromazine patients and 1 penfluridol patient left the study because of drowsiness. Supplementary chlorpromazine was required by 3 patients receiving penfluridol. Penfluridol was considered to be of similar efficacy as chlorpromazine, and to cause less drowsiness but more extrapyramidal effects.— G. Chouinard *et al.*, *J. clin. Pharmac.*, 1977, *17*, 162. See also G. Chouinard and L. Annable, *Am. J. Psychiat.*, 1976, *133*, 820.

No significant difference was found between penfluridol given weekly by mouth and fluphenazine decanoate given intramuscularly every 2 weeks in preventing relapse, during a 52-week trial in 56 schizophrenic patients who had reached a clinical plateau.— F. Quitkin *et al.*, *Archs gen. Psychiat.*, 1978, *35*, 889. See also J. L. Claghorn *et al.*, *J. clin. Psychiat.*, 1979, *40*, 107.

Further references: D. M. Gallant *et al.*, *Am. J. Psychiat.*, 1974, *131*, 699; K. Y. Ota *et al.*, *J. clin. Pharmac.*, 1974, *14*, 202; G. Nistico *et al.*, *ibid.*, 476; A. A. Kurland *et al.*, *ibid.*, 1975, *15*, 611; L. Jacobsson *et al.*, *Acta psychiat. scand.*, 1976, *54*, 113; A. Jus *et al.*, *J. clin. Pharmac.*, 1976, *16*, 298; N. M. James and A. F. Montague, *N.Z. med. J.*, 1977, *85*, 53; E. Kingstone *et al.*, *J. clin. Pharmac.*, 1977, *17*, 252; G. De Backer-Dierick and M. Van Elsacker-Van Essche, *Curr. ther. Res.*, 1978, *24*, 193; P. T. Donlon and J. E. Meyer, *J. clin. Psychiat.*, 1978, *39*, 582; M. J. Iqbal *et al.*, *ibid.*, 375.

Proprietary Names
Semap *(Johnson, Arg.; Janssen, Belg.; Janssen, Denm.; Janssen-Le Brun, Fr.; Janssen, Ger.; Janssen, Neth.; Janssen, Switz.)*.

7081-a

Perazine Dimalonate. Pemazine Dimalonate; P 725 *(Perazine)*. 10-[3-(4-Methylpiperazin-1-yl)propyl]phenothiazine dimalonate.
$C_{20}H_{25}N_3S,2C_3H_4O_4$=547.6.

CAS — 84-97-9 (perazine); 14777-25-4 (dimalonate).

Perazine dimalonate is a phenothiazine with general properties similar to those of chlorpromazine (p.1509). It has a piperazine side-chain. It has been given in usual doses equivalent to 50 to 300 mg of the base daily. It has also been given intramuscularly.

References: O. Nieschulz, *Arzneimittel-Forsch.*, 1967, *17,* 190 and 334.

Proprietary Names
Taxilan *(Promonta, Belg.; Promonta, Ger.; Byk, Neth.).*

7082-t

Pericyazine. Propericiazine; RP 8909; SKF 20716. 10-[3-(4-Hydroxypiperidino)propyl]phenothiazine-2-carbonitrile.
$C_{21}H_{23}N_3OS$=365.5.

CAS — 2622-26-6.

A yellow almost odourless crystalline powder. M.p. 115°.

Practically **insoluble** in water; soluble in alcohol and acetone; freely soluble in chloroform; slightly soluble in ether. **Protect** from light.

Adverse Effects, Treatment, and Precautions. As for Chlorpromazine, p.1509.

Sedation is marked. Postural hypotension may also be marked, particularly after intramuscular injection.

Effects on sexual function. Persistent priapism occurred in a 37-year-old man after starting to take pericyazine 25 mg thrice daily. The condition responded to treatment with benztropine but residual thrombosis caused impotence.— M. P. Osborne, *Postgrad. med. J.*, 1974, *50,* 523.

Absorption and Fate. For an account of the absorption and fate of a phenothiazine, see Chlorpromazine, p.1513.

Uses. Pericyazine is a phenothiazine with actions and uses similar to those of chlorpromazine (p.1513). It has a piperidine side-chain.

The usual dose for the treatment of psychoses is 15 to 30 mg daily; the daily dosage may be given in 2 portions, the larger amount in the evening. In severe psychoses doses of up to 75 mg daily have been given. It has also been given by intramuscular injection in doses of 10 mg repeated twice or thrice in 24 hours if necessary; up to 20 mg has been given for acute agitation.

A suggested initial daily dose by mouth for children is 500 µg per year of age.

Elderly subjects should be given reduced doses.

Anxiety. The use of pericyazine in anxiety or in conditions associated with anxiety: *Practitioner*, 1967, *198,* 139 (Report No. 99 of the General Practitioner Research Group).

Schizophrenia. A study of pericyazine in the treatment of schizophrenia: J. C. Barker and M. Miller, *Br. J. Psychiat.*, 1969, *115,* 169.

Proprietary Preparations

Neulactil *(May & Baker, UK).* Pericyazine, available as **Syrup** containing 2.5 mg in each 5 ml (suggested diluent, syrup); as **Forte Syrup** containing 10 mg in each 5 ml; and as scored **Tablets** of 2.5, 10, and 25 mg. (Also available as Neulactil in *Austral., Denm., Norw., S.Afr.*).

Other Proprietary Names
Aolept *(Ger.)*; Apamin *(Jap.)*; Nemactil *(Spain)*; Neuleptil *(Arg., Belg., Canad., Fr., Ital., Neth., Switz.).*

7083-x

Perimetazine. 1-[3-(2-Methoxyphenothiazin-10-yl)-2-methylpropyl]piperidin-4-ol.
$C_{22}H_{28}N_2O_2S$=384.5.

CAS — 13093-88-4.

Adverse Effects, Treatment, and Precautions. As for Chlorpromazine, p.1509.

Uses. Perimetazine is a phenothiazine with general properties similar to those of chlorpromazine (p.1513). It has a piperidine side-chain. The usual dose for the treatment of psychoses is 100 to 250 mg daily. Doses of 10 to 100 mg daily have been used for non-psychotic emotional disturbances such as neurotic states. In general, however, phenothiazines are only suitable for such purposes in resistant conditions, where more appropriate agents, such as the benzodiazepines (see Diazepam, p.1523) have proved ineffective. If their use is judged to be necessary treatment should be directed at low dosages on a short-term basis.

Proprietary Names
Leptryl (also for the hydrochloride) *(Bellon, Fr.).*

7084-r

Perphenazine *(B.P., B.P. Vet., U.S.P.).* Perphenazinum. 2-{4-[3-(2-Chlorophenothiazin-10-yl)propyl]piperazin-1-yl} ethanol.
$C_{21}H_{26}ClN_3OS$=404.0.

CAS — 58-39-9.

Pharmacopoeias. In *Br., Cz., Jap.,* and *U.S. Jap. P.* also includes the maleate.

A white or creamy-white odourless or almost odourless powder with a bitter taste. M.p. 94° to 100°.

Practically **insoluble** in water; soluble 1 in 20 of alcohol, 1 in 1 of chloroform, 1 in 80 of ether, and 1 in 13 of acetone; soluble in dilute hydrochloric acid. Solutions are **sterilised** by autoclaving. **Store** in airtight containers. Protect from light.

Adverse Effects, Treatment, and Precautions. As for Chlorpromazine, p.1509.

Extrapyramidal symptoms may be more common than the other side-effects. Severe dystonic reactions have followed the use of perphenazine particularly in children and adolescents.

Cytogenetic effects. There was no significant difference in the incidence of chromosomal aberrations in 6 controls and 9 patients given perphenazine in increasing doses up to 48 mg daily. An earlier report of damage was suspect.— M. M. Cohen *et al.*, *Br. med. J.*, 1972, *3,* 21.

Effects on the blood. Haemolytic anaemia. A paranoid schizophrenic patient developed haemolytic anaemia while receiving 16 and later 8 mg of perphenazine daily.— P. J. Dally, *Practitioner*, 1970, *205,* 390.

Effects on the heart. The incidence (about 24% in the fasting state) of depolarisation abnormalities on the ECG in patients taking perphenazine or perphenazine with amitriptyline was increased after a glucose load.— G. Chouinard and L. Annable, *Archs gen. Psychiat.*, 1977, *34,* 951.

Epileptogenic effect. The Boston Collaborative Drug Surveillance Program monitored consecutively 32 812 medical inpatients. Drug-induced convulsions occurred in 1 of 60 patients given amitriptyline and perphenazine.— J. Porter and H. Jick, *Lancet*, 1977, *1,* 587.

Extrapyramidal effects. In a young woman with oculogyric crisis due to perphenazine 10 mg, the administration of atropine 600 µg and pethidine 50 mg produced complete remission of symptoms within 10 minutes.— J. J. Kimerling and S. R. Patel (letter), *Br. med. J.*, 1967, *4,* 554.

Severe spontaneous bucco-oro-lingual dyskinesia due to 2.5 mg of perphenazine given by intramuscular injection before and after an eye operation in a 17-year-old girl, was relieved within seconds by an intravenous injection of 5 mg of diazepam. No further attacks were seen after a further 5 mg of diazepam given intramuscularly.— D. M. Davies (letter), *Lancet*, 1970, *1,* 567.

Three patients developed acute extrapyramidal symptoms after treatment for nausea by a single dose of perphenazine. Benztropine mesylate intravenously gave complete relief of symptoms.— P. D. Ramsden and D. L. Froggatt (letter), *Br. med. J.*, 1972, *1,* 246.

Severe torticollis developed in a 19-year-old girl given perphenazine syrup in the early stages of jaundice. Severe extrapyramidal side-effects were also seen in a jaundiced boy given normal doses of prochlorperazine. Patients with liver disease were considered to be at special risk.— A. Paton (letter), *Br. med. J.*, 1974, *3,* 344.

An acute dystonic reaction, with symptoms of tetany and tetanus, but without extrapyramidal symptoms, occurred in an 8-year-old boy who had received four 5-mg doses of perphenazine in about 36 hours. The condition responded to diazepam.— W. D. Smith and M. A. Tobias, *Br. J. Anaesth.*, 1976, *48,* 703.

Further references: D. A. Heath and J. M. McGarry (letter), *Br. med. J.*, 1967, *1,* 363; E. C. B. Keat and P. J. Toghill (letter), *ibid.*, 1967, *3,* 867; B. K. Mandal and P. Sengupta (letter), *ibid.*, 1972, *1,* 441; M. H. Bellman, *Archs Dis. Childh.*, 1974, *49,* 664.

Absorption and Fate. For an account of the absorption and fate of a phenothiazine, see Chlorpromazine, p.1513.

Perphenazine 5 or 6 mg administered intravenously had a plasma half-life from 8.4 to 12.3 hours in a study of 4 schizophrenic patients and 4 healthy subjects. Considerable fluctuations in plasma-perphenazine concentrations were observed 3 to 5 hours after administration before the exponential elimination phase. A dose of 6 mg by mouth in 4 healthy subjects failed to produce a detectable plasma concentration and only low plasma concentrations of its sulphoxide metabolite could be detected; this was attributed to a marked first-pass effect. Systemic availability was variable and poor in 4 schizophrenic patients given perphenazine 12 mg thrice daily. However, it was considered that oral therapy should be on an 8-hour dosage regimen. Intramuscular injection of perphenazine enanthate 50 or 100 mg every 2 weeks gave plasma-perphenazine concentrations similar to those after continuous oral administration but with a high initial absorption within 2 to 3 days associated with the most serious neurological and sedative side-effects.— C. E. Hansen *et al.*, *Br. J. clin. Pharmac.*, 1976, *3,* 915. See also T. B. Cooper, *Clin. Pharmacokinet.*, 1978, *3,* 14.

Details of perphenazine enanthate, a long-acting ester of perphenazine, suitable for depot injection.— *Drugs Today,* 1978, *14,* 120.

Uses. Perphenazine is a phenothiazine with actions and uses similar to those of chlorpromazine (p.1513). It has a piperazine side-chain. The usual dose for the treatment of psychoses is 4 to 8 mg thrice daily; in severe psychoses doses of up to 64 mg daily have been permitted. It may be given by intramuscular injection for the immediate relief of acute psychotic symptoms in an initial dose of 5 to 10 mg and 5-mg doses may be given if necessary at 6-hourly intervals to a maximum of 15 to 30 mg daily.

For the control of nausea and vomiting the usual dose by mouth is 4 mg thrice daily but up to 8 mg thrice daily may be required. The usual intramuscular dose is 5 mg; occasionally 10 mg may be required.

Elderly subjects should be given reduced doses.

Perphenazine is not recommended for use in children.

Perphenazine has also been used as the enanthate.

Psychoses. A study in 44 acutely psychotic patients indicated that, on the basis of global improvement and reduction in target symptom severity, perphenazine and haloperidol were equally effective. Treatment was administered by intramuscular injection, usually every 8 hours for 2 days; the mean total doses of perphenazine and haloperidol were 27.6 and 25.7 mg respectively. Extrapyramidal reactions occurred in 8 patients and necessitated withdrawal of treatment in 3.— C. H. Fitzgerald, *Curr. ther. Res.*, 1969, *11,* 515.

Further references: A. M. P. Kellam and K. S. Jones, *Acta psychiat. scand.*, 1971, *47,* 174; J. Korf and H. M. van Praag, *Am. J. Psychiat.*, 1976, *133,* 1171.

Preparations

Injections

Perphenazine Injection *(B.P.).* A sterile solution of perphenazine in Water for Injections free from dissolved air; it contains suitable buffering and stabilising agents. Sterilised by autoclaving in an atmosphere of nitrogen. pH 4.5 to 5.5. Protect from light.

Perphenazine Injection *(U.S.P.)*. A sterile solution in Water for Injections prepared with the aid of citric acid. pH 4.2 to 5.6. Protect from light.

Oral Solutions and Syrups

Perphenazine Oral Solution *(U.S.P.)*. Perphenazine Solution. Contains perphenazine. Protect from light.

Perphenazine Syrup *(U.S.P.)*. A syrup containing perphenazine. Protect from light.

Tablets

Perphenazine Tablets *(B.P.)*. Sugar-coated tablets containing perphenazine.

Perphenazine Tablets *(U.S.P.)*. Tablets containing perphenazine. Store in airtight containers.

Proprietary Preparations

Fentazin *(Allen & Hanburys, UK)*. Perphenazine, available as **Injection** containing 5 mg per ml in ampoules of 1 ml; as **Concentrate** for hospital use containing 10 mg in each 5 ml for preparing dilutions with syrup free from preservatives and as **Tablets** of 2, 4, and 8 mg.

Other Proprietary Names

Decentan *(also as enanthate) (Ger., Ital., Spain)*; F-Mon *(Jap.)*; Perfenil *(Ital.)*; Phenazine *(Canad.)*; Trilafon *(also as enanthate) (Austral., Belg., Canad., Denm., Ital., Neth., Norw., S.Afr., Spain, Swed., Switz., USA)*; Trilifan *(Fr.)*.

7085-f

Phenaglycodol. 2-(4-Chlorophenyl)-3-methylbutane-2,3-diol.
$C_{11}H_{15}ClO_2$=214.7.

CAS — 79-93-6.

A crystalline solid. Practically **insoluble** in water; soluble in alcohol and oils.

Phenaglycodol was formerly used in doses of 300 mg three or four times daily for the relief of anxiety. Side-effects included drowsiness, dizziness, nausea, ataxia, and skin rashes. Gynaecomastia was also reported.

Studies of phenaglycodol in anxiety and depression demonstrating no advantage over placebo.— B. Brauzer and B. J. Goldstein, *J. clin. Pharmac.*, 1972, *12*, 280; K. Rickels *et al.*, *Curr. ther. Res.*, 1975, *17*, 23.

Proprietary Names

Felixyn *(Radiumfarma, Ital.)*.

7086-d

Phenprobamate. MH 532; Proformiphen. 3-Phenylpropyl carbamate.
$C_{10}H_{13}NO_2$=179.2.

CAS — 673-31-4.

Phenprobamate is a carbamate with general properties similar to those of meprobamate (p.1545). It has been given as an anxiolytic and muscle relaxant in doses of 400 to 800 mg thrice daily.

A report of the metabolism of phenprobamate.— F. Schatz and U. Jahn, *Arzneimittel-Forsch.*, 1966, *16*, 866.

Proprietary Names

Actiphan, Nelaxan, Palmita, Paraquick *(all Jap.)*; Gamaquil *(Pharmacia, Denm.; Siegfried, Ger.; Mekos, Norw.; Mekos, Swed.; Siegfried, Switz.)*.

7087-n

Pimozide.

R 6238. 1-{1-[4,4-Bis(4-fluorophenyl)butyl]-4-piperidyl}benzimidazolin-2-one.
$C_{28}H_{29}F_2N_3O$=461.6.

CAS — 2062-78-4.

A colourless microcrystalline powder. M.p. 214° to 218°. Practically **insoluble** in water; soluble 1 in 140 of alcohol, 1 in 5 of chloroform, and 1 in 500 of ether; slightly soluble in solutions of mineral and organic acids.

Adverse Effects. The side-effects of pimozide, such as sedation, extrapyramidal symptoms, and tardive dyskinesia, which are a result of its pharmacological action, are similar to those of chlorpromazine (p.1509).

Extrapyramidal symptoms may be more common than those associated with chlorpromazine, whereas it may be less likely to cause sedation.

Other side-effects include skin rashes; glycosuria and altered liver-function tests have also been reported.

Allergy. Facial swelling and oedema of the eyelids in a schizophrenic patient taking pimozide.— P. A. Morris *et al.*, *Br. J. Psychiat.*, 1970, *117*, 683.

Effects on mental state. *Aggression.* An abrupt onset of aggression and violence occurred in 4 of 14 patients being treated with high doses of pimozide for chronic schizophrenia.— T. R. E. Barnes *et al.*, *Proc. R. Soc. Med.*, 1977, *70, Suppl.* 10, 44.

Extrapyramidal effects. *Tardive dyskinesia.* Mention of a patient in whom pimozide induced mild facial-lingual dyskinesias within a period of weeks or months.— S. Hirsch (discussion), *Proc. R. Soc. Med.*, 1977, *70, Suppl.* 10, 37.

Sudden death. A report of 3 fatalities possibly associated with the use of pimozide in patients initially thought to have died as a result of cardiac disorders.— *Med. J. Aust.*, 1974, *2*, 875.

Treatment of Adverse Effects. As for Chlorpromazine, p.1511.

Precautions. As for Chlorpromazine, p.1512.

Withdrawal. Three patients who had been taking pimozide had epileptiform fits 13 to 31 days after the dose of pimozide had been reduced or treatment stopped. In the absence of any other obvious reason a possible connection with pimozide has to be considered.— E. A. Burkitt and M. Faulkner (letter), *Br. med. J.*, 1972, *3*, 643.

Absorption and Fate. Pimozide is readily absorbed from the gastro-intestinal tract. Peak plasma concentrations have been reported 3 to 6 hours after oral administration, followed by an initial rapid decline, then a subsequent very slow terminal phase. Pimozide accordingly has a very long plasma half-life of about 2 days or more.

Animal studies have indicated that pimozide is metabolised in the liver and excreted in the urine and faeces, both unchanged and in the form of metabolites. The major path of metabolism of pimozide is *N*-dealkylation. *Animal* studies have also indicated that it is widely distributed in the body, but with a large proportion of the dose stored in the liver and considerably lower concentrations elsewhere, including the brain.

Uses. Pimozide is a member of the diphenylbutylpiperidine group of antipsychotic agents, which are structurally similar to the butyrophenones (see Haloperidol, p.1532). It is used in the treatment of psychoses. Treatment is usually started with 4 to 10 mg daily which may be given as a single dose, and the dose increased, if necessary, up to 20 mg daily. The usual dose range is 2 to 20 mg daily.

Administration. Pimozide had a mean plasma half-life of 55 hours after a multiple-dose regimen of 6 mg daily for 4 days and 53 hours after a single dose of 24 mg. The incidence of extrapyramidal effects was similar with both dose schedules. It was suggested that a single weekly dose might be useful.— R. G. McCreadie *et al.* (letter), *Br. J. clin. Pharmac.*, 1979, *7*, 533.

Anorexia nervosa. Since it had been suggested that anorexia could be related to a dopaminergic-receptor hyperactivity, pimozide 4 mg thrice daily for a month was used to treat an anorexic youth. Dramatic improvement occurred within 3 weeks. He gained 9 kg in weight and lost his obsession with his weight. Signs such as bradycardia and overactivity also disappeared.— F. Plantey (letter), *Lancet*, 1977, *1*, 1105.

Anxiety. Studies of pimozide in the treatment of anxiety using doses of 2 to 4 mg daily.— *Practitioner*, 1972, *208*, 836 (Report No. 170 of the General Practitioner Research Group); A. K. Kenway, *Br. J. clin. Pract.*, 1973, *27*, 67; *Practitioner*, 1975, *215*, 230 (Report No. 193 of the General Practitioner Research Group).

Behaviour disorders. A double-blind study on 30 disturbed male adolescents indicated that pimozide was more effective than placebo in alleviating anxiety and improving social behaviour. The initial dose of 2 mg pimozide daily was gradually increased by 1 mg until a satisfactory response was obtained or limiting side-effects occurred, the maximum used being 8 mg. Two subjects on pimozide became lethargic and were withdrawn from the study.— J. B. Goldberg and A. A. Kurland, *J. clin. Pharmac.*, 1974, *14*, 134.

Extrapyramidal effects. *Tardive dyskinesia.* Beneficial effects with pimozide in patients with tardive dyskinesia.— A. C. Gibson, *Proc. R. Soc. Med.*, 1977, *70, Suppl.* 10, 34.

Further references: P. F. Claveria *et al.*, *J. neurol. Scis*, 1975, *24*, 393.

See also under Adverse Effects (above).

Gilles de la Tourette's syndrome. Pimozide in doses of up to 12 mg daily was as effective as haloperidol in a small controlled study of 5 patients with Gilles de la Tourette's syndrome and had fewer side-effects.— M. S. Ross and H. Moldofsky (letter), *Lancet*, 1977, *1*, 103.

Malignant melanoma. Administration of pimozide appeared to induce a partial remission in a postmenopausal woman with metastatic malignant melanoma. It was given in a dose of 4 mg daily for the first week, 8 mg daily for the second, and 12 mg daily subsequently. Side-effects included lethargy, and dry mouth and eyes.— R. N. Taub and M. A. Baker (letter), *Lancet*, 1979, *1*, 605.

Psychoses. Five patients with monosymptomatic psychosis, each having a single hypochondriacal complaint of delusional intensity, rapidly gained a remission when treated with pimozide 2 to 6 mg each morning. There was no improvement in a sixth patient who was considered to have a personality disorder.— B. E. J. Riding and A. Munro (letter), *Lancet*, 1975, *1*, 400. See also T. M. Reilly (letter), *ibid.*, 1385.

Further references: A. Munro, *Archs Derm.*, 1978, *114*, 940; J. Sneddon, *Practitioner*, 1980, *224*, 97.

Mania. Improvement without sedation was obtained during a classical manic episode in 5 patients with recurrent manic-depressive psychoses given pimozide 8, 6 and 4 mg daily on successive days. There was a tendency to relapse on a fixed daily dose of 4 mg but 2 patients were controlled by increasing the dose to 8 mg twice daily. The response was considered to be better than that achieved with fenfluramine.— J. Cookson and T. Silverstone (letter), *Br. J. clin. Pharmac.*, 1976, *3*, 942.

Schizophrenia. Of 20 patients with chronic schizophrenia stabilised on neuroleptic medication and transferred under double-blind conditions to once-daily dosage with pimozide 17 maintained their status or improved, compared with 10 of 20 transferred to trifluoperazine and 7 of 20 transferred to a placebo. The dose of pimozide was 2 to 12 mg (mean 6.3 mg) and that of trifluoperazine 5 to 30 mg (mean 17.5 mg).— H. S. Gross, *Curr. ther. Res.*, 1974, *16*, 696. In a similar double-blind study, 12 of 22 patients remained the same or improved when transferred to pimozide compared to 16 of 22 given trifluoperazine. Side-effects occurred more frequently with pimozide, leading to withdrawal of 4 patients.— F. Kline *et al.*, *ibid.*, 1977, *21*, 768.

In a long-term study comparing pimozide and fluphenazine those on fluphenazine showed the largest improvement up to 6 months but for those remaining in the study for longer than a year there was a trend in favour of pimozide.— F. S. Abuzzahab, *Psychopharmac. Bull.*, 1977, *13*, 72.

Pimozide up to 60 mg daily was given to 16 acutely schizophrenic patients. Only 5 patients were suitable for discharge after 28 days' treatment, and the treatment was ineffective in a further 5. Extrapyramidal symptoms in 8 patients responded to antiparkinsonian therapy.— B. Shopsin and G. Selzer, *Curr. ther. Res.*, 1977, *21*, 755. In a study on the use of high-dose pimozide in 16 acutely agitated chronic schizophrenic patients, an initial single dose of 20 mg daily was rapidly increased to the maximum tolerated, but no more than 60 mg daily. In 3 patients, additional doses of pimozide 5 or 10 mg were given every hour until a calming effect developed or a maximum of 60 mg had been given. The treatment was effective in 14 patients, and 13 completed the 4-week study. The mean daily dose was 35 mg; side-effects were mainly extrapyramidal.— S. Piyakulmala *et al.*, *ibid.*, 1977, *22*, 453.

In a double-blind study of 18 chronic institutionalised patients no significant difference was found in the degree of increased socialisation between placebo and pimozide-treated groups.— E. J. McInnes *et al.*, *N.Z. med. J.*, 1978, *87*, 170.

In an uncontrolled study, 12 patients with schizophrenia of long duration took a placebo for 1 week, then up to 16 mg of pimozide daily followed by a mean maintenance dose of 6 mg for up to 9 weeks. Improvement occurred in 6 patients during the second week of the study with progressive improvement thereafter. The 4 patients who failed to improve during the first 2 weeks remained unchanged at the end of the study or in the case of 2 patients deteriorated with treatment. The main symptoms that improved were apathy, social withdrawal, thought disorders, depression and motor retardation. Side-effects experienced were dryness of the mouth, nausea, somnolence, weakness and parkinsonism.— C. S. Stier *et al.*, *Curr. ther. Res.*, 1978, *23*, 632.

A double-blind study comparing oral pimozide with injected fluphenazine in schizophrenic patients indicated that initially side-effects were similar but after 1 year they were considerably less in the group receiving oral therapy. There was evidence that reduction in side-effects on the oral preparation was due to the patients' adjustment of their own tablet dosage.— D. C. Watt (letter), *Lancet*, 1978, *2*, 1045.

Further references: A. K. Kenway and H. C. Masheter, *Br. J. clin. Pract.*, 1971, *25*, 69; P. Janssen *et al.*, *J. clin. Pharmac.*, 1972, *12*, 26; Y. D. Lapierre and J. Lavallee, *Curr. ther. Res.*, 1975, *18*, 181; I. Falloon *et al.*, *Psychol. Med.*, 1978, *8*, 59; J. Fleischhauer, *Arzneimittel-Forsch.*, 1978, *28*, 1491; D. Garton and T. Silverstone, *Curr. med. Res. Opinion*, 1979, *5*, 799; A. J. Cheadle and H. L. Freeman, *ibid.*, *6*, 35; G. S. Stirling, *ibid.*, 331; R. G. McCreadie *et al.*, *Br. J. Psychiat.*, 1980, *137*, 510.

Tardive dyskinesia. See under Extrapyramidal Effects (above).

Proprietary Preparations

Orap *(Janssen, UK)*. Pimozide, available as scored tablets of 2, 4, or 10 mg. (Also available as Orap in *Arg., Austral., Belg., Canad., Denm., Fr., Ger., Ital., Neth., Norw., S.Afr., Spain, Switz.*).

Other Proprietary Names

Opiran *(Fr.)*.

7088-h

Pinazepam. 7-Chloro-1,3-dihydro-5-phenyl-1-(prop-2-ynyl)-2*H*-1,4-benzodiazepin-2-one.
$C_{18}H_{13}ClN_2O=308.8$.

CAS — 52463-83-9.

Pinazepam is a benzodiazepine with actions and uses similar to those of diazepam (p.1519). It is reported to be metabolised to desmethyldiazepam. It has been given in doses of 5 to 10 mg twice daily for the treatment of anxiety.

Pharmacology in *animals*.— F. Scrollini *et al.*, *Arzneimittel-Forsch.*, 1975, *25*, 934; P. M. Boselli and F. Scrollini, *Boll. chim.-farm.*, 1977, *116*, 363; F. Scrollini *et al.*, *Arzneimittel-Forsch.*, 1978, *28*, 423.

Proprietary Names

Domar *(Zambeletti, Ital.)*; Duna *(Zambeletti, Spain)*.

7089-m

Pipamazine *(B.P.C. 1963)*. SC 9387. 1-[3-(2-Chlorophenothiazin-10-yl)propyl]piperidine-4-carboxamide.
$C_{21}H_{24}ClN_3OS=402.0$.

CAS — 84-04-8.

A white or creamy-white almost odourless crystalline powder. **Soluble** 1 in 500 of water, 1 in 60 of alcohol, 1 in 5 of chloroform, and 1 in 200 of ether.

Adverse Effects, Treatment, and Precautions. As for Chlorpromazine, p.1509.

Uses. Pipamazine has general properties similar to those of chlorpromazine, p.1513. It has a piperidine side-chain. It has been used as an anti-emetic in doses of 5 mg in the morning and 10 mg at night.

7090-t

Pipamperone Hydrochloride. Floropipamide Hydrochloride. 1-[3-(4-Fluorobenzoyl)propyl]-4-piperidinopiperidine-4-carboxamide dihydrochloride.
$C_{21}H_{30}FN_3O_2,2HCl=448.4$.

CAS — 1893-33-0 (pipamperone); 2448-68-2 (hydrochloride).

Pipamperone hydrochloride 1.2 mg is approximately equivalent to 1 mg of pipamperone.

Pipamperone is a butyrophenone with general properties similar to those of haloperidol (p.1532). It is given as the hydrochloride for the treatment of psychoses in doses equivalent to 40 to 120 mg of the base thrice daily.

Effects on the heart. A report of 3 cases of cardiac disturbances in schizophrenic patients taking pipamperone.— *Japan med. Gaz.*, 1975, *12* (Nov. 20), 12.

Proprietary Names

Dipiperon *(Janssen, Belg.; Janssen, Denm.; Janssen-Le Brun, Fr.; Janssen, Ger.; Janssen, Neth.; Janssen, Switz.)*; Piperonil *(Lusofarmaco, Ital.)*; Propitan *(Jap.)*.

7091-x

Piperacetazine *(U.S.P.)*. PC 1421. 10-{3-[4-(2-Hydroxyethyl)piperidino]propyl-}phenothiazin-2-yl methyl ketone.
$C_{24}H_{30}N_2O_2S=410.6$.

CAS — 3819-00-9.

Pharmacopoeias. In *U.S.*

A yellow granular powder. M.p. 102° to 106°. Practically **insoluble** in water; soluble 1 in 11 of alcohol, 1 in 1.3 of chloroform, 1 in 1200 of ether, and 1 in 25 of dilute hydrochloride acid. **Store** in airtight containers. Protect from light.

A rapid urine colour test for the detection of piperacetazine.— F. M. Forrest and I. S. Forrest, *Curr. ther. Res.*, 1972, *14*, 689.

Adverse Effects, Treatment, and Precautions. As for Chlorpromazine, p.1509.
Extrapyramidal side-effects are reported to occur more frequently with piperacetazine than with other piperidine phenothiazines.

Effects on the blood. *Aplastic anaemia.* Fatal aplastic anaemia developed in a patient being treated with piperacetazine.— K. -Y. Yeung and M. Corn (letter), *Ann. intern. Med.*, 1974, *81*, 411.

Effects on the liver. Abnormalities in liver function in 7 of 18 patients with chronic schizophrenia treated with piperacetazine.— R. T. Rada and P. T. Donlon, *Curr. ther. Res.*, 1974, *16*, 124.

Absorption and Fate. For an account of the absorption and fate of a phenothiazine, see Chlorpromazine, p.1513.

Uses. Piperacetazine is a phenothiazine with actions and uses similar to those of chlorpromazine (p.1513). It has a piperidine side-chain.
The usual initial dose for the treatment of psychoses is 10 mg two to four times daily by mouth increased if necessary over 3 to 5 days to a maximum of 160 mg daily. For the control of acute symptoms it was formerly given intramuscularly in doses of 2 to 8 mg.

Administration. *In the elderly.* Beneficial results with piperacetazine in doses of up to 45 mg daily in 50 elderly patients with organic brain syndrome. Side-effects included excitement and agitation (4 patients), toxic confusional states (3 patients), drowsiness (5 patients), and faintness and dystonic symptoms which responded to reduced dosage (1 patient).— S. E. Goldstein and F. Birnbom, *J. Am. Geriat. Soc.*, 1976, *24*, 355.

Anxiety. Piperacetazine was no more effective than a placebo in the treatment of 40 anxious neurotic patients.— Y. D. Lapierre and M. Lee, *Curr. ther. Res.*, 1976, *19*, 105.

Schizophrenia. In a comparative study of 26 patients piperacetazine was as effective as chlorpromazine in the management of aggressive uncontrollable schizophrenic patients. Piperacetazine 2 mg per ml and chlorpromazine 25 mg per ml were given intramuscularly, 1 ml initially followed by 1 to 2 ml in 1 hour then 1 to 4 ml every 4 hours to a maximum of 72 hours. The average total doses of piperacetazine and chlorpromazine were about 8 mg and 130 mg respectively.— R. B. Leonard and A. S. Kulkarni, *Clin. Med.*, 1973, *80* (May), 32.

Further references: D. M. Gallant and M. P. Bishop, *Curr. ther. Res.*, 1972, *14*, 10; A. Kiev *et al.*, *ibid.*, 376; A. C. Johnson and A. S. Kulkarni, *Am. J. Psychiat.*, 1973, *130*, 603; R. T. Rada and P. T. Donlon, *Curr. ther. Res.*, 1974, *16*, 124.

Preparations

Piperacetazine Tablets *(U.S.P.)*. Tablets containing piperacetazine. Protect from light.

Proprietary Names

Quide *(Dow, Canad.; Dow, USA)*.

7092-r

Pipothiazine. Pipotiazine; RP 19366. 10-{3-[4-(2-Hydroxyethyl)piperidino]propyl}-*NN*-dimethylphenothiazine-2-sulphonamide.
$C_{24}H_{33}N_3O_3S_2=475.7$.

CAS — 39860-99-6.

7093-f

Pipothiazine Palmitate. Pipotiazine Palmitate; IL-19552; RP 19552.
$C_{40}H_{63}N_3O_4S_2=714.1$.

CAS — 37517-26-3.

7094-d

Pipothiazine Undecenoate. Pipothiazine Undecylenate; Pipotiazine Undecenoate; RP 19551.
$C_{35}H_{51}N_3O_4S_2=641.9$.

CAS — 22178-11-6; 42573-55-7.

Adverse Effects, Treatment, and Precautions. As for Chlorpromazine, p.1509.

Absorption and Fate. For an account of the absorption and fate of a phenothiazine, see Chlorpromazine, p.1513.
Pipothiazine palmitate and undecenoate are very slowly absorbed from the site of intramuscular injection. They both gradually release pipothiazine into the body and are therefore suitable for use as depot injections.

Pharmacokinetic and pharmacological studies of some pipothiazine esters in *animals*.— L. Julou *et al.*, *Thérapie*, 1973, *28*, 491. See also P. A. Lambert and J. Midenet, *ibid.*, 561.

Pharmacokinetics of pipothiazine in patients with schizophrenia.— P. J. De Schepper *et al.*, *Arzneimittel-Forsch.*, 1979, *29*, 1056.

Uses. Pipothiazine is a phenothiazine with general properties similar to those of chlorpromazine (p.1513). It has a piperidine side-chain. Pipothiazine itself is usually administered by mouth; the longer-acting palmitate and undecenoate esters are given by intramuscular injection.
The usual dose of pipothiazine for the treatment of psychoses is 10 to 20 mg daily in a single dose; in severe psychoses higher doses have been given for brief periods. In acute conditions treatment is sometimes started with intramuscular injections of 10 to 20 mg daily in one or two injections.
The long-acting palmitate and undecenoate esters of pipothiazine are given by deep intramuscular injection. The usual dose of both the palmitate and the undecenoate is 75 mg intramuscularly, given at average intervals of 4 weeks for the palmitate and 2 weeks for the undecenoate; in the case of both esters the amounts required may range from 25 to 200 mg.
Pipothiazine should be given in reduced dosage to elderly patients.

Psychoses. A review of pipothiazine and pipothiazine palmitate and undecenoate in the treatment of schizophrenia, manic depression, and other psychoses.— F. J. Ayd, *Int. Drug Ther. Newslett.*, 1972, *7*, 1. See also *Acta psychiat. scand.*, 1973, *Suppl.* 241, 1–138.

Schizophrenia. Pipothiazine palmitate was useful in the control of symptoms of chronic schizophrenia and other psychiatric disorders in 206 patients who were not responding well to their previous maintenance therapy. Doses of 12.5 to 200 mg were given as a depot intramuscular injection at monthly intervals, the mean initial dose being 50 mg and the mean dose after 12 to 18 months of treatment being 65 mg. Side-effects (mainly extrapyramidal symptoms) occurred in 141 patients. Therapy was discontinued because of extrapyramidal side-effects (5 patients), general malaise (1 patient) and galactorrhoea (1 patient).— R. E. Johnston and F. Niesink, *J. int. med. Res.*, 1979, *7*, 187.

Further references: A. Villeneuve *et al.*, *Curr. ther. Res.*, 1972, *14*, 696; G. M. Simpson and V. Varga, *ibid.*, 1975, *17*, 276; G. Chouinard *et al.*, *J. clin. Pharmac.*, 1978, *18*, 148; T. M. Itil *et al.*, *Curr. ther. Res.*, 1978, *24*, 689; A. Schlosberg and M. Shadmi, *ibid.*, *23*, 642; A. N. Singh and B. Saxena, *ibid.*, 1979, *25*, 121; A. Villeneuve and P. Fontaine, *ibid.*, 1980, *27*, 411.

Proprietary Names

Lonseren *(Rhodia, Spain)*; Mi-Lonseren *(Rhodia, Spain)*; Piportil *(Specia, Belg.*; *Specia, Fr.*; *Specia, Neth.*; *Rhodia, Spain)*; Piportyl *(Rhodia, Arg.*; *Rhone-Poulenc, Denm.*; *Rhône-Poulenc, Norw.)*.

7095-n

Prazepam *(U.S.P.)*. W 4020. 7-Chloro-1-(cyclopropylmethyl)-1,3-dihydro-5-phenyl-2*H*-1,4-benzodiazepin-2-one.

$C_{19}H_{17}ClN_2O = 324.8$.

CAS — 2955-38-6.

Pharmacopoeias. In *U.S.*

A white to off-white crystalline powder. M.p. 143° to 148° with a range of not more than 3°. **Soluble** in alcohol, chloroform, and dilute mineral acids. **Store** in airtight containers. Protect from light.

Dependence. Prolonged use of prazepam may lead to the development of dependence of the barbiturate-alcohol type (see p.792). It has a low liability for abuse.

Adverse Effects, Treatment, and Precautions. As for Diazepam, p.1520.

Absorption and Fate. For an account of the absorption and fate of a benzodiazepine, see Diazepam, p.1522.

Prazepam is a precursor of desmethyldiazepam.

In 5 healthy men given a single dose of 25 mg of ^{14}C-labelled prazepam, peak radioactivity in the blood was reached in about 6 hours and fell gradually over the next 18 hours. The concentration of unconjugated material in the blood was about twice that of glucuronides. About 22% of the dose was excreted in the urine in 48 hours and about 7% in the faeces. Of the material excreted in the urine 4% was unconjugated (1.2% was desalkylprazepam), 83.7% was present as glucuronides (3-hydroxyprazepam glucuronide 40.7%, oxazepam glucuronide 29.7%), and 5.2% as sulphates. Unchanged prazepam was not detected.— F. J. DiCarlo *et al.*, *Ann. N.Y. Acad. Sci.*, 1971, *179*, 487. See also *idem*, *Clin. Pharmac. Ther.*, 1970, *11*, 890.

Following administration of prazepam 20 mg to 12 healthy subjects, considerable variation was noted in the plasma concentrations of desmethyldiazepam, which appears to be responsible for the pharmacological activity of prazepam. The appearance of desmethyldiazepam was not always first order and peak plasma-desmethyldiazepam concentrations were noted as little as 2.5 hours and as long as 72 hours after administration. If the clinical response to prazepam is dependent on the plasma concentration of desmethyldiazepam, the rate of onset of clinical effects could vary considerably after a single dose of prazepam. The elimination half-life in the 12 subjects was similarly very variable, ranging from 29 to 193 hours, with a mean of 69 hours.— M. D. Allen *et al.*, *J. clin. Pharmac.*, 1979, *19*, 445.

Further references: M. T. Smith *et al.*, *Eur. J. clin. Pharmac.*, 1979, *16*, 141.

Uses. Prazepam is a benzodiazepine with actions and uses similar to those of diazepam (p.1523). The usual dose for the treatment of anxiety is 10 mg thrice daily; in severe conditions up to 60 mg daily has been given.

Reviews and comments on the actions and uses of prazepam: D. J. Greenblatt and R. I. Shader, *New Engl. J. Med.*, 1978, *299*, 1342; D. E. Galinsky (letter), *ibid.*, 1979, *300*, 1054; D. J. Greenblatt and R. I. Shader (letter), *ibid.*

Action. Studies in fasting subjects given single doses of prazepam 20 mg indicated that, like clorazepate, prazepam is a precursor for desmethyldiazepam, and is not therefore pharmacokinetically unique.— D. J. Greenblatt and R. I. Shader (letter), *Lancet*, 1978, *1*, 720.

Administration. In the elderly. A study on the pharmacokinetics of prazepam in young and elderly subjects.— M. D. Allen *et al.*, *Clin. Pharmac. Ther.*, 1980, *28*, 196.

Alcohol and drug withdrawal. Prazepam 10 to 20 mg thrice daily caused greater symptomatic improvement than a placebo in the first 2 weeks of a double-blind trial involving 50 patients suffering from anxiety following withdrawal of narcotic drugs. No significant difference between drug and placebo was apparent during the third week of treatment.— A. A. Sugerman *et al.*, *J. clin. Pharmac.*, 1971, *11*, 383.

Further references: J. W. Shaffer *et al.*, *J. clin. Pharmac.*, 1968, *8*, 392 (alcohol).

Anxiety. Studies of prazepam in the treatment of anxiety.— J. H. Weir, *J. clin. Psychiat.*, 1978, *39*, 841; L. F. Fabre *et al.*, *Curr. ther. Res.*, 1979, *25*, 527; *idem*, *J. int. med. Res.*, 1979, *7*, 147.

Spasticity. In a controlled study of 16 patients with multiple sclerosis and spastic paraplegia prazepam in an optimum dose of 5 to 25 mg daily significantly reduced muscle spasm in 9. Drowsiness and muscle weakness were common in the first week.— I. M. Levine *et al.*, *Neurology, Minneap.*, 1969, *19*, 510, per *Abstr. Wld Med.*, 1969, *43*, 831.

Preparations

Prazepam Tablets *(U.S.P.)*. Tablets containing prazepam. Store in airtight containers. Protect from light.

Centrax *(Warner, UK)*. Prazepam, available as scored tablets of 10 mg. (Also available as Centrax, formerly known as Verstran, in *USA*).

Other Proprietary Names

Demetrin *(Ger., S.Afr., Spain, Switz.)*; Equipaz *(Arg.)*; Lysanxia *(Fr.)*; Prazene *(Ital.)*; Reapam *(Neth.)*.

7096-h

Prochlorperazine *(U.S.P.)*. Prochlorpemazine. 2-Chloro-10-[3-(4-methylpiperazin-1-yl)propyl]-phenothiazine.

$C_{20}H_{24}ClN_3S = 373.9$.

CAS — 58-38-8.

Pharmacopoeias. In *Braz.* and *U.S.*

A clear, pale yellow, viscous liquid, sensitive to light. Very slightly **soluble** in water; freely soluble in alcohol, chloroform, and ether. **Store** in airtight containers. Protect from light.

7097-m

Prochlorperazine Edisylate *(U.S.P.)*.

Prochlorperazine Edisilate; Prochlorperazine Ethanedisulphonate. Prochlorperazine ethane-1,2-disulphonate.

$C_{20}H_{24}ClN_3S,C_2H_6O_6S_2 = 564.1$.

CAS — 1257-78-9.

Pharmacopoeias. In *U.S.*

A white to very light yellow odourless crystalline powder. Prochlorperazine edisylate 7.5 mg is approximately equivalent to 5 mg of prochlorperazine.

Soluble 1 in 2 of water and 1 in 1500 of alcohol; practically insoluble in chloroform and ether. Solutions in water are acid to litmus. **Store** in airtight containers. Protect from light.

7098-b

Prochlorperazine Maleate *(B.P., U.S.P.)*.

Prochlorperaz. Mal.; Prochlorpemazine Maleate; Prochlorperazine Dihydrogen Maleate; Prochlorperazine Dimaleate; Prochlorperazini Maleas.

$C_{20}H_{24}ClN_3S,2C_4H_4O_4 = 606.1$.

CAS — 84-02-6.

Pharmacopoeias. In *Br.*, *Braz.*, *Cz.*, *Fr.*, *Int.*, *Jap.*, *Roum.*, and *U.S.*

A white or pale yellow, almost odourless, crystalline powder with a slightly bitter taste. M.p. 198° to 203°. Prochlorperazine maleate 8 mg is approximately equivalent to 5 mg of prochlorperazine.

Practically **insoluble** in water, alcohol, and ether; slightly soluble in warm chloroform. A saturated solution in water is acid to litmus. **Store** in airtight containers. Protect from light.

7099-v

Prochlorperazine Mesylate *(B.P.)*.

Prochlorperazine Methanesulphonate; Prochlorperazini Mesylas; Prochlorperazine Dimethanesulphonate.

$C_{20}H_{24}ClN_3S,2CH_3SO_3H = 566.1$.

CAS — 51888-09-6.

Pharmacopoeias. In *Br.* and *Int.*

A white or almost white odourless powder with a slightly bitter taste. M.p. about 242°. Prochlorperazine mesylate 7.6 mg is approximately equivalent to 5 mg of prochlorperazine.

Soluble 1 in less than 0.5 of water and 1 in 40 of alcohol; slightly soluble in chloroform; practically insoluble in ether. A 2% solution in water has a pH of 2 to 3. Solutions are **sterilised** by autoclaving in containers in which the air has been replaced by nitrogen or other suitable gas. **Protect** from light.

Incompatibility. Particulate matter was observed within 2 hours when 1 ml of commercial prochlorperazine edisylate injection was mixed with sterile water 5 ml and 1 ml of any of the following commercial injection solutions: aminophylline, benzylpenicillin potassium, chloramphenicol sodium succinate, dexamethasone phosphate, dimenhydrinate, heparin, methicillin sodium, phenobarbitone sodium, phenytoin sodium, prednisolone sodium phosphate, and sulphafurazole diethanolamine.— R. Misgen, *Am. J. Hosp. Pharm.*, 1965, *22*, 92.

Prochlorperazine edisylate 10 mg per litre was compatible with buffered benzylpenicillin for 24 hours.— E. A. Parker, *Am. J. Hosp. Pharm.*, 1969, *26*, 543.

Loss of clarity when solutions of prochlorperazine were mixed with those of calcium gluconate, chlorothiazide sodium, heparin, hydrocortisone sodium succinate, nitrofurantoin sodium, pentobarbitone sodium, and thiopentone sodium.— J. A. Patel and G. L. Phillips, *Am. J. Hosp. Pharm.*, 1966, *23*, 409.

Prochlorperazine hydrochloride was reported to be incompatible with benzylpenicillin, pentobarbitone sodium, and phenobarbitone sodium.— J. M. Meisler and M. W. Skolaut, *Am. J. Hosp. Pharm.*, 1966, *23*, 557.

An immediate precipitate occurred when prochlorperazine mesylate 100 mg per litre was mixed with aminophylline 1 g per litre or with ampicillin sodium 2 g per litre in dextrose injection and sodium chloride injection, or with ethamivan 2 g per litre in sodium chloride injection. An immediate precipitate also occurred with phenobarbitone sodium 800 mg per litre, sulphadiazine sodium 4 g per litre, or sulphadimidine sodium 4 g per litre in sodium chloride injection, but when they were mixed in dextrose injection a haze developed over 3 hours. A haze developed over 3 hours when prochlorperazine mesylate was mixed with amphotericin 200 mg per litre or methohexitone sodium 2 g per litre in dextrose injection, or with benzylpenicillin 6 g per litre, chloramphenicol 4 g per litre, or chlorothiazide 2 g per litre in sodium chloride injection.— B. B. Riley, *J. Hosp. Pharm.*, 1970, *28*, 228.

Adverse Effects, Treatment, and Precautions. As for Chlorpromazine, p.1509.

Extrapyramidal symptoms may be more common than the other side-effects. Severe dystonic reactions have followed the use of prochlorperazine, particularly in children and adolescents. It should therefore be used with extreme care in children. Pain may occur at the site of injection.

Effects on the blood. *Aplastic anaemia.* Prochlorperazine has been reported to cause aplastic anaemia.— R. H. Girdwood, *Drugs*, 1976, *11*, 394.

Effects on mental state. *Catatonia.* Twenty-four hours after she had received the last of 3 injections of prochlorperazine given over a period of 6 days, a 34-

year-old woman lapsed into a catatonic-like stupor. This was reversed within minutes of intravenous injection of diphenhydramine hydrochloride 50 mg. A relapse 4 hours later was again reversed within minutes of intravenous diphenhydramine hydrochloride in a dose of 25 mg. Five such recurrences over the next 36 hours were relieved in each instance by diphenhydramine hydrochloride 10 mg intravenously. Permanent relief was obtained after administration of benztropine mesylate 2 mg twice daily for several days.— T. Riley *et al.*, *Postgrad. Med.*, 1976, *60*, 171.

Epileptogenic effect. The Boston Collaborative Drug Surveillance Program monitored consecutively 32 812 medical inpatients. Drug-induced convulsions occurred in 1 of 2869 patients given prochlorperazine.— J. Porter and H. Jick, *Lancet*, 1977, *1*, 587.

Extrapyramidal effects. Spasm of the muscles of the neck, extensor rigidity of the back, and carpopedal spasms occurred in a 14-year-old girl after taking 30 mg of prochlorperazine and in a 12-year-old boy after 100 mg administered over 12 hours as suppositories. Symptoms were abolished in 1 patient within a few minutes of an injection of 10 mg of diphenhydramine hydrochloride.— B. Z. Berk (letter), *Lancet*, 1969, *1*, 776.

A 20-year-old woman who had received oral prochlorperazine for 2 days for the treatment of postoperative nausea, developed stiffness and spasms of jaw, neck, arm, and pectoral muscles, which were relieved by an intravenous injection of benztropine mesylate 2 mg.— A. H. Qizilbash, *Can. med. Ass. J.*, 1973, *108*, 171.

Dyskinesia with involuntary jaw movements, similar to lockjaw, occurred in a 26-year-old pilot the day after he had used prochlorperazine suppositories for the treatment of gastroenteritis.— J. B. Lorenzo and E. A. Nisonger, *U.S. Navy Med.*, 1975, *66*, 6.

The Boston Collaborative Drug Surveillance Program monitored consecutively 32 812 medical inpatients. Drug-induced extrapyramidal symptoms occurred in 9 of 3013 patients given prochlorperazine. Also 1 patient out of 198 given prochlorperazine and chlorpromazine experienced extrapyramidal symptoms.— J. Porter and H. Jick, *Lancet*, 1977, *1*, 587.

Further references: R. T. Bush, *N.Z. med. J.*, 1966, *65*, 229; S. Lamont (letter), *Br. J. Anaesth.*, 1972, *44*, 539; K. L. De Silva *et al.*, *Practitioner*, 1973, *211*, 316.

Hypoparathyroidism. Five patients with untreated hypoparathyroidism suffered a severe dystonic reaction within 5 to 31 hours of an intramuscular injection of prochlorperazine in a dose of 10 mg for adults and 130 to 160 μg per kg body-weight for children. After being given vitamin D_2 to establish normocalcaemia, 2 of 3 patients challenged with prochlorperazine suffered milder reactions than before. One patient with idiopathic latent tetany suffered a severe reaction when given perphenazine. Caution was recommended in giving phenothiazine derivatives to patients with hypoparathyroidism and it was suggested that any acute reaction to such a drug should prompt investigation for some form of latent tetany.— M. Schaaf and C. A. Payne, *New Engl. J. Med.*, 1966, *275*, 991.

Interactions. *Narcotic analgesics.* For the effect of prochlorperazine on morphine, see Morphine, p.1019.

Interference with diagnostic tests. Prochlorperazine affected the estimation of urinary 17-oxo-steroids and 17-oxogenic-steroids.— *Adverse Drug React. Bull.*, 1972, June, 104.

Pregnancy and the neonate. *Early pregnancy.* Evaluation of a number of antinauseant drugs, including prochlorperazine prescribed during the years 1959 to 66 for about 2000 pregnant women in the first 84 days of pregnancy, provided no evidence that prochlorperazine is associated with teratogenicity.— L. Milkovich and B. J. van den Berg, *Am. J. Obstet. Gynec.*, 1976, *125*, 244. See also M. M. Nelson and J. O. Forfar, *Br. med. J.*, 1971, *1*, 523.

The percentage of malformed children among 1309 children born to mothers who had taken phenothiazines during the first 4 months of pregnancy was comparable to that in 48 973 children not so exposed. When analysed for specific malformations there was some evidence of an association with cardiovascular and possibly respiratory malformations but the finding was of doubtful import. IQ scores at 4 years were not affected.— D. Slone *et al.*, *Am. J. Obstet. Gynec.*, 1977, *128*, 486. Of 50 282 children born to mothers monitored by the Collaborative Perinatal Project 1309 were found to have been exposed to phenothiazines, and possibly other drugs, at some time during the first 4 months of the pregnancy. A slight association between cardiovascular deformities and the phenothiazine group as a whole was noted with ventricular septal defects in particular being associated with prochlorperazine (877 exposures).— O. P. Heinonen *et al.*, *Birth Defects and Drugs in Pregnancy*, Littleton MA, Publishing Sciences Group, 1977, p. 322.

Further studies: J. Winberg, *Svenska Läkartidn.*, 1964, *61*, 890 (no association).

Individual reports of malformations in exposed infants: G. Hall, *Med. J. Aust.*, 1963, *1*, 449 (limb deformities); R. Freeman (letter), *ibid.*, 1972, *1*, 606 (limb deformities).

Absorption and Fate. For an account of the absorption and fate of a phenothiazine, see Chlorpromazine, p.1513.

Uses. Prochlorperazine is a phenothiazine with actions and uses similar to those of chlorpromazine (p.1513). It has a piperazine side-chain.

Depending on the country or the manufacturer, doses of prochlorperazine are expressed either as the base or the salt. Most doses in Great Britain, including the rectal doses, are expressed in terms of the salt, while most doses in the USA are apparently expressed in terms of the base. As a result there is a disparity in the dosage recommendations for these countries, with the USA doses apparently tending to be higher.

In Great Britain the usual dose for the treatment of psychoses is 50 to 100 mg of the maleate daily in divided doses; US sources recommend higher doses in severe conditions. In Great Britain, when intramuscular injection is necessary, prochlorperazine may be given by deep intramuscular injection in a dose of 12.5 to 25 mg of the mesylate twice or thrice daily. In the USA prochlorperazine is given by deep intramuscular injection as the edisylate in doses equivalent to 10 to 20 mg of base and repeated every 4 to 6 hours.

For the control of nausea and vomiting, in Great Britain the usual dose by mouth is 5 to 10 mg of the maleate thrice daily, whereas in the USA it is also given as the maleate, but in doses equivalent to 5 to 10 mg of the base, thrice daily. In Great Britain the usual intramuscular dose for nausea and vomiting is 12.5 mg of the mesylate; in the USA the edisylate may be given in doses equivalent to 5 to 10 mg of the base. In Great Britain the rectal dose is given in suppositories as the base, but in a dose equivalent to 25 mg of the maleate; in the USA it is 25 mg of the base, twice daily. There are similar problems with children's doses and owing to the risk of severe extrapyramidal reactions, prochlorperazine should be administered with extreme caution in children, in particular it is not recommended for those weighing less than 10 kg. In Great Britain a suggested oral dosage regimen for the mesylate, which is contained in the syrup, in children is: 1 to 5 years, 2.5 mg twice daily; 6 to 12 years, 5 mg twice or thrice daily; at 13 to 16 years the lower adult range may be given up to a maximum of 20 mg daily. In Great Britain suggested rectal doses of the base, calculated as the equivalent of the maleate, are: 1 to 2 years, half a 5-mg suppository once or twice daily; 2 to 5 years, half a 5-mg suppository twice or thrice daily; 6 to 12 years, half a 5-mg suppository thrice daily or one 5-mg suppository twice daily. Similar rectal doses in the USA are expressed as the base and are accordingly higher. Special care should be taken not to supply or administer one 25-mg suppository in mistake for half a 5-mg suppository (i.e. 2.5 mg). In the USA a suggested dose for children is 100 μg of the base per kg body-weight by mouth 4 times daily; half this amount may be given intramuscularly; an intramuscular dose of 135 μg of the base per kg given once only has also been proposed.

For adults only, sources in the USA have also proposed the intramuscular or intravenous use of prochlorperazine edisylate to control severe nausea and vomiting in anaesthetic procedures, with the warning that hypotension may follow the intravenous use of prochlorperazine.

Prochlorperazine is also used in Great Britain in the treatment of vertigo including that due to Ménière's disease in doses of 15 to 30 mg of the maleate daily. For acute migraine a single dose of 20 mg of prochlorperazine maleate may be given followed, if required, by a further 10 mg. Doses of 5 to 10 mg of the maleate up to 3 or 4 times daily have also been used for non-psychotic emotional disturbances, such as anxiety and tension. In general, however, neuroleptics are only suitable for such purposes in resistant conditions, where more appropriate agents, such as the benzodiazepines (see Diazepam, p.1523) have proved ineffective. If their use is judged to be necessary, treatment should be directed at low dosages given on a short-term basis.

Prochlorperazine should be given in reduced dosage to elderly patients.

Nausea and vomiting. Individual studies of prochlorperazine in nausea and vomiting: P. A. Bardfeld, *J. Am. med. Ass.*, 1966, *196*, 796; H. W. C. Ward (letter), *Br. med. J.*, 1973, *2*, 52.

Preparations

Injections

Prochlorperazine Edisylate Injection *(U.S.P.).* A sterile solution of prochlorperazine edisylate in Water for Injections, containing the equivalent of 4.75 to 5.25 mg of prochlorperazine in each ml. pH 4.2 to 6.2. Protect from light.

Prochlorperazine Injection *(B.P.).* Prochlorperazine Mesylate Injection. A sterile solution of prochlorperazine mesylate in Water for Injections free from dissolved air, containing suitable buffering and stabilising agents. Sterilised by autoclaving in an atmosphere of nitrogen or other suitable gas. pH 5.5 to 6.5. Protect from light.

Oral Solutions and Syrups

Prochlorperazine Edisylate Oral Solution *(U.S.P.).* Prochlorperazine Edisylate Solution. A solution containing prochlorperazine edisylate. Potency is expressed in terms of the equivalent amount of prochlorperazine. To be diluted before use. Store in airtight containers. Protect from light.

Prochlorperazine Edisylate Syrup *(U.S.P.).* A syrup containing, in each 100 ml, prochlorperazine edisylate equivalent to 92 to 108 mg of prochlorperazine. Store in airtight containers. Protect from light.

Suppositories

Prochlorperazine Suppositories *(U.S.P.).* Suppositories containing prochlorperazine. Store at a temperature not exceeding 37° in airtight containers; protect unwrapped suppositories from exposure to sunlight.

Tablets

Prochlorperazine Maleate Tablets *(U.S.P.).* Tablets containing prochlorperazine maleate. Potency is expressed in terms of the equivalent amount of prochlorperazine. Protect from light.

Prochlorperazine Tablets *(B.P.).* Tablets containing prochlorperazine maleate. Protect from light.

Proprietary Preparations

Stemetil *(May & Baker, UK).* Prochlorperazine mesylate, available as **Solution for Injection** containing 1.25%, in ampoules of 1 and 2 ml, and as **Syrup** containing 5 mg in each 5 ml (suggested diluent, syrup). **Stemetil Suppositories.** Each contains prochlorperazine equivalent to 5 or 25 mg of prochlorperazine maleate. **Stemetil Tablets.** Prochlorperazine maleate, available as tablets of 5 mg and scored tablets of 25 mg. (Also available as Stemetil in *Austral., Belg., Canad., Denm., Ital., Neth., Norw., S.Afr., Switz.*).

Vertigon Spansule *(Smith Kline & French, UK).* Prochlorperazine maleate, available as sustained-release capsules, each containing the equivalent of 10 or 15 mg of prochlorperazine.

Other Proprietary Names

Anti-Naus *(Austral.)*; Compazine *(Austral., USA)*; Mitil *(S.Afr.)*; Nibromin-A *(Jap.)*; Témentil *(Fr.)*.

7100-v

Promazine Embonate. Promazine Pamoate. *NN*-Dimethyl-3-(phenothiazin-10-yl)propylamine 4,4′-methylenebis(3-hydroxy-2-naphthoate).
$(C_{17}H_{20}N_2S)_2,C_{23}H_{16}O_6$=957.2.

CAS — 58-40-2 (promazine).

Promazine embonate 1.5 g is approximately equivalent to 1 g of promazine hydrochloride.

7101-g

Promazine Hydrochloride *(B.P., U.S.P.).* Propazinum.
$C_{17}H_{20}N_2S,HCl$=320.9.

CAS — 53-60-1.

Pharmacopoeias. In *Br., Rus.*, and *U.S.*

A white or slightly yellow, odourless or almost odourless, slightly hygroscopic, crystalline powder with a bitter taste. M.p. 172° to 182° with a range of not more than 3°. It is affected by air and light and traces of heavy metals. Decomposed solutions may be coloured pink, red, or blue.

Soluble 1 in 1 of water, 1 in 2 of alcohol, and 1 in 2 of chloroform; practically insoluble in ether. A 5% solution in water has a pH of 4.2 to 5.4. Solutions are **sterilised** by autoclaving or filtration and distributed in ampoules in which the air is replaced by nitrogen or other suitable gas. **Store** in airtight containers. Protect from light.

Incompatibility. Particulate matter was observed within 2 hours when 1 ml of commercial promazine hydrochloride injection was mixed with sterile water 5 ml and 1 ml of any of the following commercial injection solutions: *aminophylline, benzylpenicillin potassium, chloramphenicol sodium succinate, dimenhydrinate, heparin, hydrocortisone sodium succinate, menaphthone sodium bisulphite, phenobarbitone sodium, phenytoin sodium, prednisolone sodium phosphate,* and *sulphafurazole diethanolamine.*— R. Misgen, *Am. J. Hosp. Pharm.*, 1965, *22,* 92.

Promazine 100 mg was 'physically incompatible' with *chlortetracycline* 50 mg, *fibrinogen* 200 mg, *plasmin* 200 mg, *penicillin* 1.2 g, *pentobarbitone sodium* 20 mg, *sodium bicarbonate* 375 mg, *sulphafurazole* 400 mg, *thiopentone sodium* 250 mg, or *warfarin sodium* 10 mg, in 100 ml of dextrose 5% injection.— R. D. Dunworth and F. R. Kenna, *Am. J. Hosp. Pharm.*, 1965, *22,* 190.

An immediate precipitate occurred when promazine hydrochloride 200 mg per litre was mixed with *aminophylline* 1 g per litre, *chlorothiazide* 2 g per litre, *ethamivan* 2 g per litre, *methohexitone sodium* 2 g per litre, or *sulphadimidine sodium* 4 g per litre in dextrose 5% injection or sodium chloride 0.9% injection, or with *phenobarbitone sodium* 800 mg per litre in sodium chloride 0.9% injection.— B. B. Riley, *J. Hosp. Pharm.*, 1970, *28,* 228.

Stability. The degradation-rate of promazine hydrochloride in solution was at a minimum at pH 6.5.— H. O. Ammar *et al.*, *Pharmazie*, 1975, *30,* 368.

Adverse Effects, Treatment, and Precautions. As for Chlorpromazine, p.1509.

Postural hypotension is more marked, particularly after parenteral administration. There have been reports of cardiovascular reactions when pethidine and promazine were used in obstetrics. Thrombophlebitis has followed intravenous injections.

Effects on the blood. *Aplastic anaemia.* Promazine has been reported to cause aplastic anaemia.— R. H. Girdwood, *Drugs*, 1976, *11,* 394.

Interactions. *Adsorbents.* Absorption of promazine hydrochloride was delayed and reduced when its administration was preceded by a dose of an antidiarrhoeal mixture containing activated attapulgite 3 g, colloidal activated attapulgite 900 mg, and citrus pectin 300 mg in 30 ml.— D. L. Sorby and G. Liu, *J. pharm. Sci.*, 1966, *55,* 504. When promazine hydrochloride solution and activated attapulgite or charcoal suspensions were given simultaneously without prior equilibration, the effect of the adsorbents on absorption of promazine was negligible.— D. L. Sorby, *ibid.*, 1968, *57,* 1604.

Pregnancy and the neonate. An increased incidence of neonatal jaundice coincided with the increased use of promazine. A decrease in the incidence of jaundice was noted 3 months after the total withdrawal of the drug from the hospital.— E. John, *Med. J. Aust.*, 1975, *2,* 342.

Absorption and Fate. For an account of the absorption and fate of a phenothiazine, see Chlorpromazine, p.1513.

Plasma protein binding. For the comparative protein binding of promazine and other phenothiazines, see Chlorpromazine, p.1513.

Uses. Promazine is a phenothiazine with actions and uses similar to those of chlorpromazine (p.1513). It has been given as the hydrochloride in doses of 50 to 100 mg up to four times daily for the treatment of psychoses; higher doses have been given, and a maximum daily dose of 1 g has been specified. For the control of nausea and vomiting it has been given in doses of 25 to 50 mg up to four times daily. Similar doses of the hydrochloride have also been given intramuscularly. Promazine hydrochloride has been used parenterally in anaesthesia, usually intramuscularly but also by cautious intravenous injection in concentrations not exceeding 25 mg per ml.

Promazine is also available as an oral suspension of the embonate.

Promazine should be given in reduced dosage to elderly subjects.

Sickle-cell anaemia. The third episode of haematuria, with associated avascular necrosis of the head of the femur, in a woman with sickle-cell haemoglobin C disease was successfully treated with promazine 100 mg daily with subsequent addition of dapsone 25 to 50 mg daily. Five weeks after discontinuing therapy, bleeding recurred and was again treated by promazine and dapsone. On maintenance therapy she remained free from symptoms for 8 months.— R. A. Lewis, *Br. J. clin. Pract.*, 1967, *21,* 139.

Preparations

Promazine Hydrochloride Injection *(U.S.P.).* A sterile solution of promazine hydrochloride in Water for Injections. pH 4 to 5.5. Protect from light.

Promazine Hydrochloride Oral Solution *(U.S.P.).* Promazine Hydrochloride Solution. A solution containing promazine hydrochloride. pH 5 to 5.5. Store in airtight containers. Protect from light.

Promazine Hydrochloride Syrup *(U.S.P.).* A syrup containing promazine hydrochloride. Store in airtight containers. Protect from light.

Promazine Hydrochloride Tablets *(U.S.P.).* Tablets containing promazine hydrochloride. Store in airtight containers. Protect from light.

Promazine Injection *(B.P.).* A sterile solution of promazine hydrochloride in Water for Injections free from dissolved air and containing suitable buffering and stabilising agents. Sterilised by autoclaving under nitrogen or other suitable gas. pH 4.4 to 5.2. Protect from light.

Promazine Tablets *(B.P.).* Tablets containing promazine hydrochloride. The tablets are sugar-coated.

Proprietary Preparations

Sparine (known in some countries as Liranol) *(Wyeth, UK).* Promazine hydrochloride, available as **Solution** for injection containing 50 mg per ml, in ampoules of 1 and 2 ml, and as **Tablets** of 25, 50, and 100 mg. **Sparine Suspension.** Contains in each 5 ml promazine embonate equivalent to promazine hydrochloride 50 mg (suggested diluent, syrup). (Also available as Sparine in *Austral., Canad., Denm., S.Afr.*).

Other Proprietary Names

Calmotal *(Ital.)*; Neuroplegil *(Ital.)*; Prazine *(Belg., Neth., Switz.)*; Promabec *(Canad.)*; Promanyl *(Canad.)*; Protactyl *(Ger., Norw.)*; Talofen *(Ital.)*.

7102-q

Prothipendyl Hydrochloride. D 206; Phrenotropin. *NN*-Dimethyl-3-(pyrido[3,2-*b*][1,4]benzothiazin-10-yl)propylamine hydrochloride monohydrate.
$C_{16}H_{19}N_3S,HCl,H_2O$=339.9.

CAS — 303-69-5 (prothipendyl); 1225-65-6 (hydrochloride, anhydrous).

A crystalline powder. M.p. 108° to 112°. Prothipendyl hydrochloride 47.6 mg is approximately equivalent to 40 mg of prothipendyl. Freely **soluble** in water and methyl alcohol; practically insoluble in ether and light petroleum. **Incompatible** with phenobarbitone. **Protect** from light.

Adverse Effects, Treatment, and Precautions. As for Chlorpromazine, p.1509.

Uses. Prothipendyl is an azaphenothiazine with general properties similar to those of chlorpromazine (p.1513). It has been given as the hydrochloride in doses equivalent to 40 mg of the base up to thrice daily in psychoneuroses, and up to 240 to 960 mg daily in psychoses.

Schizophrenia. Absence of useful antipsychotic action of prothipendyl in schizophrenia.— A. A. Sugerman and J. Herrmann, *Curr. ther. Res.*, 1966, *8,* 487; G. M. Simpson and J. W. S. Angus, *ibid.*, 1967, *9,* 265.

Proprietary Names

Dominal *(Homburg, Ger.; Homburg, Neth.).*

Prothipendyl hydrochloride was formerly marketed in Great Britain under the proprietary name Tolnate *(Smith Kline & French).*

7103-p

Ripazepam. CI683; Pyrazapon. 1-Ethyl-4,6-dihydro-3-methyl-8-phenylpyrazolo[4,3-*e*][1,4]diazepin-5(1*H*)-one.
$C_{15}H_{16}N_4O$=268.3.

CAS — 26308-28-1.

Ripazepam is structurally related to the benzodiazepines and has been given in doses of 40 to 80 mg daily for the treatment of anxiety.

Action. The pharmacology of ripazepam, a pyrazolodiazepine.— *Drugs Today*, 1975, *11,* 208.

Anxiety. In a double-blind trial 30 anxious patients were given ripazepam 40 or 80 mg daily or a placebo. After 2 weeks patients receiving ripazepam showed improvement in anxiety symptoms, compared to placebo. After 1 week no difference was seen between the two doses of ripazepam, but after 2 weeks patients receiving 80 mg daily were better than those receiving 40 mg. Side-effects were nausea and vertigo, leading to discontinuation of 1 patient in each ripazepam group; 2 patients receiving placebo discontinued because of lack of improvement.— J. J. Schneyer *et al.*, *J. clin. Pharmac.*, 1976, *16,* 377.

Manufacturers

Parke, Davis, USA.

7104-s

Spiclomazine Hydrochloride. Clospirazine Hydrochloride; APY-606. 8-[3-(2-Chlorophenothiazin-10-yl)propyl]-4-thia-1,8-diazaspiro[4.5]decan-2-one hydrochloride.
$C_{22}H_{24}ClN_3OS_2,HCl$=482.5.

CAS — 24527-27-3 (spiclomazine); 27007-85-8 (hydrochloride).

Spiclomazine hydrochloride is a phenothiazine with general properties similar to those of chlorpromazine (p.1509). It has a piperidine side-chain. It has been given in doses of 50 to 150 mg thrice daily in the treatment of psychoses.

Proprietary Names

Diceplon *(Jap.).*

7105-w

Spiperone. Spiroperidol; R 5147. 8-[3-(4-Fluorobenzoyl)propyl]-1-phenyl-1,3,8-triazaspiro[4.5]decan-4-one.
$C_{23}H_{26}FN_3O_2$=395.5.

CAS — 749-02-0.

Spiperone is a butyrophenone with general properties similar to those of haloperidol (p.1532). Doses of 0.5 to 4.5 mg daily have been recommended in the treatment of schizophrenia.

The pharmacology of neuroleptic drugs.— P. A. J. Janssen *et al.*, *Arzneimittel-Forsch.*, 1965, *15,* 104 and 1196; *idem*, 1966, *16,* 339. See also *idem*, 1967, *17,* 841.

Proprietary Names

Spiropitan *(Jap.).*

7106-e

Sulforidazine. Sulphoridazine. 10-[2-(1-Methyl-2-piperidyl)ethyl]-2-methylsulphonylphenothiazine.
$C_{21}H_{26}N_2O_2S_2$=402.6.

CAS — 14759-06-9.

Adverse Effects, Treatment, and Precautions. As for Chlorpromazine, p.1509.

Absorption and Fate. For an account of the absorption and fate of a phenothiazine, see Chlorpromazine, p.1513.
Sulforidazine is a metabolite of thioridazine

Uses. Sulforidazine is a phenothiazine with actions and uses similar to those of chlorpromazine (p.1513). It has a piperidine side-chain and is a metabolite of thioridazine (p.1559). It has been given in doses of 50 to 100 mg thrice daily for the treatment of psychoses.

Proprietary Names
Inofal *(Sandoz, Ger.).*

7107-l

Sulpiride. *N*-(1-Ethylpyrrolidin-2-ylmethyl)-2-methoxy-5-sulphamoylbenzamide.
$C_{15}H_{23}N_3O_4S$=341.4.

CAS — 15676-16-1.

Adverse Effects. The side-effects of sulpiride, such as sedation and extrapyramidal symptoms, which are the result of its pharmacological action, are similar to those of chlorpromazine (p.1509). Tardive dyskinesia may also be expected.
Sleep disturbances, overstimulation, and agitation may occur. There is also a risk of hypertension.

Effects on the endocrine system. A report of reversible galactorrhoea occurring in 12 patients following the administration of sulpiride.— G. Cahen *et al., Nouv. Presse méd.*, 1970, *79*, 1545, per *Int. pharm. Abstr.*, 1973, *10*, 579.

Effects on mental state. Sulpiride usually in doses of 300 to 600 mg daily was given to 44 psychiatric in-patients for 30 days. Clinical imrovement was seen only after a longer period of administration. The main side-effects were sleep disturbance, overstimulation, and agitation.— D. Bente *et al., Arzneimittel-Forsch.*, 1974, *24*, 107.

Hypertension. Sulpiride 100 mg by mouth caused an attack of hypertension in 6 of 26 hypertensive patients; in 4 it induced a rise in urinary excretion of vanillylmandelic acid and catecholamines. A transient rise in blood pressure and catecholamines after administration of sulpiride occurred in 3 patients who were found to have a phaeochromocytoma; another patient probably had a phaeochromocytoma. The means by which sulpiride provoked hypertension were not known but appeared to be due to a noradrenergic effect. Sulpiride should be avoided during the treatment of phaeochromocytoma, and prescribed with great care in hypertensive patients.— P. Corvol *et al., Sem. Hôp. Paris*, 1974, *50*, 1265, per *J. Am. med. Ass.*, 1974, *228*, 1605.

Treatment of Adverse Effects. As for Chlorpromazine, p.1511.

Precautions. As for Chlorpromazine, p.1512.
Sulpiride should not be administered to patients with phaeochromocytoma and only with caution to patients with hypertension.

Sulpiride may affect driving skills less than chlorpromazine.— T. Seppala *et al., Drugs*, 1979, *17*, 389. See also T. Seppala, *Archs int. Pharmacodyn. Thér.*, 1976, *223*, 311.

Absorption and Fate. Sulpiride is absorbed from the gastro-intestinal tract and excreted in the urine and faeces. It is reported to have a plasma half-life of about 8 or 9 hours. *Animal* studies have indicated that it does not readily cross the placental barrier.

The pharmacokinetics of intravenous and oral sulpiride in healthy subjects.— F. -A. Wiesel *et al., Eur. J. clin. Pharmac.*, 1980, *17*, 385.

Uses. Sulpiride has antipsychotic properties similar to those of chlorpromazine (p.1513). It also has an anti-emetic action and inhibits gastrin secretion. It may be given by mouth or intramuscularly.
Recommended doses for the treatment of psychoses are 600 to 800 mg daily in divided doses intramuscularly, followed by 1.2 to 1.6 g daily by mouth and subsequently reduced to 400 to 800 mg daily for maintenance.
Sulpiride has also been given in doses of 100 to 200 mg daily for neurosis, migraine (particularly of digestive origin), and functional intestinal spasms; 150 to 300 mg daily has been given for gastric and duodenal ulcers.

Action. Behavioural studies in *animals* indicated that the psychopharmacological profile of sulpiride was different from those of known psychotropic agents.— O. Fontaine *et al., Thérapie*, 1975, *30*, 573. Neuro-endocrinological studies in *animals*.— A. Soulairac *et al., ibid.*, 597.

A study in *animals* suggesting that the central pharmacological activity of sulpiride and sultopride resides in the (−)-enantiomers and that this activity occurs at central dopamine receptors not dependent on adenylate cyclase for functional activity.— P. Jenner *et al., J. Pharm. Pharmac.*, 1980, *32*, 39.

Further references: P. T. Männistö *et al., Arzneimittel-Forsch.*, 1978, *28*, 76 (effect on serum prolactin); P. Jenner and C. D. Marsden (letter), *Lancet*, 1979, *2*, 900 (D_2 receptor antagonism).

Alcohol and drug withdrawal. Nalorphine-induced withdrawal symptoms in *monkeys* treated with morphine for 15 days were controlled by intramuscular administration of sulpiride 30 mg per kg body-weight. Sulpiride was not a pharmacological replacement for morphine.— J. Mercier and P. Etzensperger, *Thérapie*, 1975, *30*, 221. Studies in *dogs* have indicated that sulpiride can suppress the morphine-withdrawal syndrome.— A. De Permentier (letter), *Med. J. Aust.*, 1976, *1*, 98.

Relatively low doses of sulpiride induced extrapyramidal syndromes in heroin addicts.— D. De Maio *et al., Neuropsychobiology*, 1978, *4*, 36.

A diamorphine addict given cyamemazine 1.8 g and sulpiride 4.8 g intravenously, over 48 hours for detoxification, developed hypertonia and malignant hyperthermia and died.— G. Bleichner *et al.* (letter), *Lancet*, 1981, *1*, 386.

Behaviour disorders. Sulpiride had no effect on the restlessness associated with mental retardation.— K. Väisänen *et al., Curr. ther. Res.*, 1975, *17*, 202.

Depression. In a single-blind study in 20 patients, sulpiride 0.4 to 1 g daily was shown to be slightly more effective than amitriptyline 75 to 200 mg daily in the treatment of psychotic and neurotic depression.— P. Niskanen *et al., Curr. ther. Res.*, 1975, *17*, 281.

Further references: J. K. Salminen *et al., Curr. ther. Res.*, 1980, *27*, 109.

Gastro-intestinal disorders. Serum-gastrin concentrations following protein stimulation were reduced in 8 of 10 patients with duodenal ulcers after receiving sulpiride 300 mg daily by mouth for 8 days.— C. A. Dinelli *et al., Arzneimittel-Forsch.*, 1976, *26*, 421. See also R. Caldara *et al., Gastroenterology* 1978, *74*, 221.

Further references: G. Albot and J. Boisson, *Sem. Hôp. Paris*, 1970, *46* (*Suppl.* June), 7; J. Felix, *ibid.*, 15; H. Geoffroy *et al., ibid.*, 23; J. B. Dureux and B. Kiffer, *ibid.*, 30; L. Lareng and B. Cathala, *ibid.*, 34; J. Toulet and J. Rousselet, *ibid.*, 41; S. K. Lam *et al., Gastroenterology*, 1979, *76*, 315; W. A. Wiles, *Cent. Afr. J. Med.*, 1979, *25*, 154; J. G. Edwards *et al., Br. J. Psychiat.*, 1980, *137*, 522.

Migraine. References to the use of sulpiride in migraine.— R. Pluvinage, *Thérapie*, 1969, *24*, 703; Y. Barré, *Sem. Hôp. Paris*, 1970, *46* (*Suppl.* June), 80.

Schizophrenia. Similar results with sulpiride in doses of up to 1.8 g daily and chlorpromazine in doses of up to 675 mg daily in schizophrenic patients. No sunrashes occurred in those receiving sulpiride.— O. Bratfos and J. O. Haug, *Acta psychiat. scand.*, 1979, *60*, 1.

Further references: R. Ropert *et al., Sem. Hôp. Paris*, 1970, *46* (*Suppl.* June), 109; M. Toru *et al., J. clin. Pharmac.*, 1972, *12*, 221; D. Cucinotta *et al., Gaz. med. It.*, 1973, *132*, 630; E. Schneider *et al., Arzneimittel-Forsch.*, 1974, *24*, 990; F. Eckmann, *ibid.*, 993; G. B. Cassano *et al., Curr. ther. Res.*, 1975, *17*, 189; A. Elizur and S. Davidson, *Curr. ther. Res.*, 1975, *18*, 578.

Vertigo. References to the use of sulpiride in vestibular disturbances.— W. J. Oosterveld *et al., Thérapie*, 1973, *28*, 35; G. A. Molinari and M. Cenzi, *Curr. ther. Res.*, 1974, *16*, 812.

Proprietary Names
Abilit *(Jap.)*; Championyl *(Vita, Ital.)*; Coolspan *(Jap.)*; Co-Sulpir *(Smaller, Spain)*; Digton *(Areu, Spain)*; Dixibon *(Spain)*; Dobren *(Ravizza, Ital.)*; Dogmatil *(Delagrange, Belg.; Delagrange, Fr.; Schürholz, Ger.; Delagrange, Neth.; Delagrange, Spain; Delagrange, Switz.)*; Drominetas *(Medidroga, Spain)*; Eglonyl *(Noristan, S.Afr.)*; Equilid *(Richter, Ital.)*; Eusulpid *(CT, Ital.)*; Guastil *(Uriach, Spain)*; Isnamide *(Isnardi, Ital.)*; Kapiride *(Kappa, Spain)*; Lavodina *(Turro, Spain)*; Lebopride *(Spyfarma, Spain)*; Lusedan *(Bryan, Spain)*; Miradol *(Jap.)*; Mirbanil *(Boehringer Sohn, Spain)*; Misulvan *(Bernabó, Arg.)*; Neuromyfar *(Emyfar, Spain)*; Normum *(Serpero, Ital.)*; Omperan *(Jap.)*; Psicocen *(Centrum, Spain)*; Quiridil *(Zoja, Ital.)*; Sato *(Scharper, Ital.)*; Sernevin *(Jap.)*; Sicofrenol *(Basileos, Spain)*; Sulpisedan *(Llano, Spain)*; Suprium *(IBYS, Spain)*; Sursumid *(Labif, Ital.)*; Tepavil *(Prodes, Spain)*; Tonofit *(Spain)*; Ulpir *(Lesvi, Spain)*; Vipral *(Roemmers, Arg.)*.

7108-y

Sultopride. LIN-1418. *N*-(1-Ethylpyrrolidin-2-ylmethyl)-5-ethylsulphonyl-2-methoxybenzamide.
$C_{17}H_{26}N_2O_4S$=354.5.

CAS — 53583-79-2.

Sultopride has general properties similar to those of chlorpromazine (p.1509). It has been used in the emergency management of acute psychoses in doses of 0.4 to 1.2 g daily by mouth or intramuscularly; up to 1.6 to 1.8 g daily may be given intramuscularly, and up to 2.4 g daily by mouth. On control of the acute symptoms alternate antipsychotic therapy may be introduced for maintenance, or, in chronically aggressive patients, maintenance doses of sultopride 0.4 to 0.6 g daily may be given.

A study in *animals* suggesting that the central pharmacological activity of sulpiride and sultopride resides in the (−)-enantiomers and that this activity occurs at central dopamine receptors not dependent on adenylate cyclase for functional activity.— P. Jenner *et al., J. Pharm. Pharmac.*, 1980, *32*, 39.

Proprietary Names
Barnetil *(Delagrange, Belg.; Delagrange, Fr.)*.

7109-j

Tetrabenazine. Ro 1-9569; TBZ. 1,3,4,6,7,11b-Hexahydro-3-isobutyl-9,10-dimethoxy-2*H*-benzo[*a*]quinolizin-2-one.
$C_{19}H_{27}NO_3$=317.4.

CAS — 58-46-8.

A white crystalline powder. M.p. 126° to 131°. **Soluble** in hot water; soluble in alcohol and chloroform. **Protect** from light.

Adverse Effects. Drowsiness is the most frequent side-effect of tetrabenazine. Postural hypotension, symptoms of extrapyramidal dysfunction, and depression may also occur. Other side-effects reported include confusion, hallucinations, excess sweating, photophobia, and amenorrhoea. Overdosage has produced sedation, sweating, hypotension, and hypothermia.

Postural hypotension and dysphagia are the serious side-effects of tetrabenazine, which require careful supervision. Depression is common in Huntington's chorea and it is difficult to know whether it is caused by tetrabenazine; parkinsonism was not noted in a series of patients studied.— C. Y. Huang and C. Elliott (letter), *Br. med. J.*, 1977, *2*, 1416. See also C. Y. Huang *et al., Med. J. Aust.*, 1976, *1*, 583.

Extrapyramidal effects. Dysphagia and choking were associated with tetrabenazine in the treatment of Huntington's chorea.— R. P. Snaith and H. de B. Warren (letter), *Lancet*, 1974, *1*, 413.

Overdosage. A patient being treated for involuntary movements who swallowed approximately 1 g (40 tablets) of tetrabenazine during a period of depression became drowsy 2 hours later and marked sweating occurred. Her state of consciousness improved after 24 hours and she talked rationally and gained full control of micturition after 72 hours. Her involuntary movements were reduced when she was somnolent but returned when full consciousness was restored.— D. W. Kidd and D. L. McLellan, *Br. J. clin. Pract.*, 1972, *26*, 179.

Treatment of Adverse Effects. There is no specific treatment. In severe overdosage the stomach should be emptied by aspiration and lavage. For general guidelines to the symptomatic therapy of overdosage with central nervous system depressants, see Phenobarbitone, p.812.

Precautions. Tetrabenazine has been reported to block the action of reserpine. It may also diminish the effects of levodopa and exacerbate the symptoms of parkinsonism.

Interactions. *Monoamine oxidase inhibitors.* Discussion of possible exacerbation of adverse mental effects on concomitant administration of psychotropic agents such as tetrabenazine and monoamine oxidase inhibitors such as iproniazid.— A. Voelkel, *Ann. N.Y. Acad. Sci.*, 1959, *80*, 680. In 2 patients with Huntington's chorea, there was a marked diminution of involuntary movements following treatment with tetrabenazine, up to 50 mg thrice daily. Depression which subsequently developed was successfully treated with isocarboxazid, 10 mg thrice daily.— C. A. Soutar (letter), *Br. med. J.*, 1970, *4*, 55.

Uses. Tetrabenazine is used in the management of movement disorders including chorea and similar symptoms of central nervous system dysfunction. It was formerly tried in the management of psychoses and psychoneuroses.

The usual initial dose is 25 mg thrice daily increased if required by 25 mg every 3 or 4 days to a maximum daily dose of 200 mg. If the patient does not respond within 7 days of receiving the maximum dose further treatment with tetrabenazine will have no effect.

Chorea. Tetrabenazine was given to 30 patients with extrapyramidal movement disorders in doses of 75 to 225 mg daily. At least 80 to 90% reduction in abnormal movements occurred in 18 patients and a complete cessation in 10. Patients with choreiform motor activity showed a gradual diminution in involuntary movement after 2 or 3 days' treatment with doses of 150 to 220 mg. Higher dosage produced sedation. Two of 3 patients with hemiballismus of arteriosclerotic aetiology showed marked improvement after 2 days' treatment with 300 mg the first day and 200 mg for the following day. Tetrabenazine was of no benefit in patients with cerebellar parkinsonian tremors; these conditions could be aggravated. Side-effects occurred in 8 patients, and included fatigue in 3, excessive sweating in 2, and confusion, photophobia, and amenorrhoea in 1 each. Side-effects disappeared on reducing the dose by 25 to 50 mg daily.— M. A. Dalby, *Br. med. J.*, 1969, *2*, 422.

In a double-blind controlled study of 10 patients with chorea there was greater improvement with tetrabenazine 200 mg daily than thiopropazate 30 mg daily, as assessed by observing films of the patients at different stages of treatment.— D. L. McLellan *et al.*, *Lancet*, 1974, *1*, 104. Of 26 patients with chorea given 50 to 150 mg of tetrabenazine daily, choreiform movements were abolished in 10, were improved in 14, and remained unchanged in 2. Treatment was stopped because of hallucinations in 1 and depression in 2 patients.— K. J. Astin and E. W. J. Gumpert (letter), *ibid.*, 512.

A 10-year-old girl and a 12-year-old boy with Sydenham's chorea responded rapidly to treatment with tetrabenazine 25 mg twice or thrice daily.— C. H. Hawkes and C. H. Nourse, *Br. med. J.*, 1977, *1*, 1391.

Following administration of tetrabenazine in doses of up to 200 mg daily to 5 patients with Huntington's chorea and a positive family history, one showed excellent response with complete cessation of involuntary movements, 3 showed moderate improvement, and one showed no improvement. Of 2 patients with Huntington's chorea and no positive family history, one showed moderate improvement and one no improvement. No improvement was noted in a further 7 patients with miscellaneous hyperkinetic movement disorders.— J. U. Toglia *et al.*, *J. clin. Psychiat.*, 1978, *39*, 81.

Further references: J. Pearce (letter), *J. Am. med. Ass.*, 1972, *219*, 1345; D. L. McLellan, *Scott. med. J.*, 1972, *17*, 367; R. Schneider *et al.* (letter), *Br. med. J.*, 1976, *1*, 1212.

Tardive dyskinesia. Tetrabenazine, 50 to 100 mg daily for 1 week, corrected abnormal movements in 3 patients and reduced them in a further 2 when given to 6 patients with persistent dyskinesia associated with phenothiazine treatment. The response was no different from that achieved with diazepam 2 or 4 mg daily for the same period.— R. B. Godwin-Austen and T. Clark, *Br. med. J.*, 1971, *4*, 25.

In a controlled double-blind trial involving 27 patients with extrapyramidal dyskinesias, tetrabenazine 150 mg daily was considered to have caused reduction of involuntary movements in 11 of the 18 patients who completed the trial. Improvement was moderate in 3, and slight in 8 patients.— B. S. Gilligan *et al.*, *Med. J. Aust.*, 1972, *2*, 1054.

Further references: H. Kazamatsuri *et al.*, *Archs gen. Psychiat.*, 1972, *27*, 95; C. P. Chen *et al.*, *Am. J. Psychiat.*, 1973, *130*, 479; H. Pakkenberg, *Archs Neurol.*, 1974, *31*, 352; S. W. Asher and M. J. Aminoff, *Neurology*, 1981, *31*, 1051.

Proprietary Preparations

Nitoman *(Roche, UK).* Tetrabenazine, available as scored tablets of 25 mg. (Also available as Nitoman in *Austral.*).

7110-q

Thiethylperazine Malate *(U.S.P.).* 2-Ethylthio-10-[3-(4-methylpiperazin-1-yl)propyl]phenothiazine di(hydrogen malate).

$C_{22}H_{29}N_3S_2,2C_4H_6O_5$=667.8.

CAS — 1420-55-9 (thiethylperazine); 52239-63-1 (malate).

Pharmacopoeias. In *U.S.*

A white to faintly yellow crystalline powder with not more than a slight odour. **Soluble** 1 in 40 of water, 1 in 90 of alcohol, 1 in 525 of chloroform, and 1 in 3400 of ether. A freshly prepared 1% solution in water has a pH of 2.8 to 3.8. **Store** in airtight containers.

7111-p

Thiethylperazine Maleate *(U.S.P.).* GS 95.

$C_{22}H_{29}N_3S_2,2C_4H_4O_4$=631.8.

CAS — 1179-69-7.

Pharmacopoeias. In *U.S.*

A yellowish granular powder, odourless or with not more than a slight odour and with a bitter taste. M.p. about 183° with decomposition.

Soluble 1 in 1700 of water and 1 in 530 of alcohol; slightly soluble in methyl alcohol; practically insoluble in chloroform and ether. A 0.1% solution in water has a pH of 2.8 to 3.8. **Store** in airtight containers. Protect from light.

Adverse Effects, Treatment, and Precautions. As for Chlorpromazine, p.1509.

Extrapyramidal symptoms may be more common than the other side-effects.

Extrapyramidal effects. Administration of thiethylperazine to a 14-year-old boy resulted in oculogyric crises after only 20 mg; these effects stopped within an hour of discontinuing the drug.— J. McIvor (letter), *Br. med. J.*, 1967, *3*, 438.

Extrapyramidal symptoms were reported in a woman within 60 hours of taking thiethylperazine 10 mg thrice daily.— K. L. De Silva *et al.*, *Practitioner*, 1973, *21*, 316. Extrapyramidal reactions occurred in 40 patients, including children, who had received thiethylperazine, usually as a single intramuscular injection. Akathisia was seen in 4 patients and dyskinesia in 36.— A. R. Ahmad *et al.*, *J. Pakistan med. Ass.*, 1975, *25*, 129. See also P. G. Lacouture *et al.*, *Pediatrics*, 1979, *64*, 954.

Tardive dyskinesia. Tardive dyskinesia associated with long-term administration of thiethylperazine.— H. K. Kief, *Ned. Tijdschr. Geneesk.*, 1979, *123*, 1460.

Absorption and Fate. For an account of the absorption and fate of a phenothiazine, see Chlorpromazine, p.1513.

Uses. Thiethylperazine is a phenothiazine with general properties similar to those of chlorpromazine (see p.1513). It has a piperazine side-chain. Thiethylperazine is used for the control of nausea, vomiting, and vertigo. It has been used for the treatment of motion sickness but is not generally considered effective.

Thiethylperazine is administered by mouth or rectally as the maleate or by injection as the malate. The usual dose is 10 mg of thiethylperazine maleate by mouth twice or thrice daily or 10 mg rectally as suppositories night and morning. Where oral administration is impractical 10 mg of thiethylperazine malate may be given by deep intramuscular injection.

Elderly patients should be given reduced doses. Thiethylperazine is not recommended for use in children.

Nausea and vomiting. A study in 250 out-patients showed that thiethylperazine 10 mg, chlorprothixene 50 mg, and thiopropazate 10 mg, given before meals, were equally effective in countering nausea and vomiting during treatment with fluorouracil.— C. G. Moertel and R. J. Reitemeier, *Gastroenterology*, 1969, *57*, 262.

Thiethylperazine was effective in the prophylaxis and treatment of seasickness in a double-blind study of 300 passengers.— G. Rubensohn, *Läkartidningen*, 1970, *67*, 619.

Further references: A. Kotásek and M. Gráf, *Čslká Gynek.*, 1967, *32*, 486; J. L. Rae, *Med. J. Aust.*, 1967, *1*, 1130; E. J. Messer and J. A. Rensch, *J. oral Surg.*, 1971, *31*, 184; *Clin. Med.*, 1972, *79* (May), 32.

Preparations

Thiethylperazine Malate Injection *(U.S.P.).* A sterile solution in Water for Injections. pH 3 to 4. Protect from light.

Thiethylperazine Maleate Suppositories *(U.S.P.).* Suppositories containing thiethylperazine maleate. Store below 25° in airtight containers. Protect unwrapped suppositories from exposure to sunlight.

Thiethylperazine Maleate Tablets *(U.S.P.).* Tablets containing thiethylperazine maleate. Store in airtight containers. Protect from light.

Proprietary Preparations

Torecan *(Sandoz, UK).* **Injection** containing thiethylperazine *malate* 10.86 mg per ml (equivalent to thiethylperazine 6.5 mg), in ampoules of 1 ml; **Suppositories** each containing thiethylperazine *maleate* 10.28 mg (equivalent to thiethylperazine 6.5 mg); and **Tablets** containing thiethylperazine *maleate* 10 mg (equivalent to thiethylperazine 6.33 mg). (Also available as Torecan in *Arg., Austral., Belg., Canad., Denm., Fr., Ger., Ital., Neth., Norw., Spain, Switz., USA*).

7112-s

Thiopropazate Hydrochloride *(B.P.).* 2-{4-[3-(2-Chlorophenothiazin-10-yl)propyl]piperazin-1-yl}ethyl acetate dihydrochloride.

$C_{23}H_{28}ClN_3O_2S,2HCl$=518.9.

CAS — 84-06-0 (thiopropazate); 146-28-1 (hydrochloride).

Pharmacopoeias. In *Br.*

A white or pale yellow crystalline powder with a faint odour and a bitter taste. M.p. 228° to 232°.

Soluble 1 in 4 of water, 1 in 130 of alcohol, and 1 in 65 of chloroform; very slightly soluble in acetone; practically insoluble in ether. A 10% solution in water has a pH of 1.4 to 1.7. **Protect** from light.

CAUTION. *Thiopropazate may cause severe dermatitis in sensitised persons, and pharmacists, nurses, and others who handle the drug frequently should wear masks and rubber gloves.*

Adverse Effects, Treatment, and Precautions. As for Chlorpromazine, p.1509.

Extrapyramidal symptoms may be more common than the other side-effects.

Absorption and Fate. For an account of the absorption and fate of a phenothiazine, see Chlorpromazine, p.1513.

Uses. Thiopropazate hydrochloride is a phenothiazine with actions and uses similar to those of chlorpromazine (p.1513). It has a piperazine side-chain. The usual initial dose for the treatment of psychoses is 10 mg thrice daily; in severe psychoses up to 100 mg daily has been permitted. Initial doses of 5 to 10 mg thrice daily have been recommended for Huntington's chorea.

Chorea. A study involving thiopropazate in chorea.— D. L. McLellan *et al.*, *Lancet*, 1974, *1*, 104.

Extrapyramidal effects. *Hemiballismus.* A 75-year-old woman with hemiballismus of several months' duration was given thiopropazate hydrochloride 2.5 mg twice daily. Within a week involuntary movements had become only occasional. The effect had been maintained for 5 months.— J. Shafar (letter), *Br. med. J.*, 1972, *1*, 806.

Tardive dyskinesia. Thiopropazate had a beneficial effect on oral dyskinesias compared with placebo but its effect was not significantly greater than that of trifluoperazine.— S. Lal and P. Ettigi, *Curr. ther. Res.*, 1974, *16*, 990.

Administration of thiopropazate hydrochloride 30 mg daily to patients with phenothiazine-induced tardive dyskinesia had no significant effect on the symptoms in 15 patients at 1 and 3 months, but in 10 of the patients who continued for 6 months, significant benefit was noted. Of a total of 11 patients who withdrew from the study 6 had developed a severe exacerbation of their original psychosis which was not controlled by reintroducing their usual antipsychotic medication. In view of the unsatisfactory antipsychotic activity of thiopropazate hydrochloride at these doses and the considerable risk of parkinsonism reported by K. Singer and M.N. Cheng at higher doses, its main value appears to be as an adjunct in patients who need to continue other antipsychotic medication.— J. S. Smith and L. G. Kiloh, *J. Neurol. Neurosurg. Psychiat.*, 1979, *42*, 576. See also K. Singer and M. N. Cheng, *Br. med. J.*, 1971, *4*, 22 and 626.

Further references: R. J. Bullock, *Med. J. Aust.*, 1972, *2*, 314; J. P. Curran, *Am. J. Psychiat.*, 1973, *130*, 925.

Preparations

Thiopropazate Hydrochloride Tablets *(B.P.)*. Thiopropazate Hydrochlor. Tab.; Thiopropazate Tablets. Tablets containing thiopropazate hydrochloride. They are compression-coated.

Dartalan *(Searle, UK)*. Thiopropazate hydrochloride, available as tablets of 5 and 10 mg. (Also available as Dartalan in *Austral., Belg.*).

Other Proprietary Names

Dartal *(Canad., Neth., Switz.)*.

7113-w

Thioproperazine Mesylate.

RP 7843; Thioproperazine Methanesulphonate; Thioproperazine Dimethanesulphonate. *NN*-Dimethyl-10-[3-(4-methylpiperazin-1-yl)propyl]phenothiazine-2-sulphonamide dimethanesulphonate.

$C_{22}H_{30}N_4O_2S_2,2CH_4O_3S=638.8$.

CAS — 316-81-4 (thioproperazine); 2347-80-0 (mesylate).

A fine, white or pale cream, odourless powder which becomes coloured on exposure to light. M.p. about 227°.

Soluble in water; slightly soluble in alcohol; more soluble in boiling alcohol. A 1% solution in water has a pH of about 2.5 which can be adjusted to pH 7 without precipitation of the base. **Protect** from light.

Adverse Effects, Treatment, and Precautions. As for Chlorpromazine, p.1509.

Extrapyramidal symptoms may be more common than the other side-effects.

Absorption and Fate. For an account of the absorption and fate of a phenothiazine, see Chlorpromazine,p.1513.

Uses. Thioproperazine mesylate is a phenothiazine with actions and uses similar to those of chlorpromazine (p.1513). It has a piperazine side-chain. The usual dose for the treatment of psychoses is 5 to 10 mg thrice daily; doses of up to 90 mg daily have been given in severe schizophrenia.

Proprietary Names

Majeptil *(May & Baker, Austral.; Specia, Belg.; Rhône-Poulenc, Canad.; Specia, Fr.; Specia, Neth.; May & Baker, S.Afr.; Specia, Switz.)*; Mayeptil *(Rhodia, Arg.)*.

Thioproperazine mesylate was formerly marketed in Great Britain under the proprietary name Majeptil *(May & Baker)*.

7114-e

Thioridazine *(U.S.P.)*.

10-[2-(1-Methyl-2-piperidyl)ethyl]-2-methylthiophenothiazine.

$C_{21}H_{26}N_2S_2=370.6$.

CAS — 50-52-2.

Pharmacopoeias. In *Nord.* and *U.S.*

A white or slightly yellow crystalline powder, odourless or with a faint odour, which darkens on exposure to light. M.p. 69° to 74°. Thioridazine 100 mg is approximately equivalent to 110 mg of thioridazine hydrochloride. Practically **insoluble** in water; soluble 1 in 6 of alcohol, 1 in 0.8 of chloroform, and 1 in 3 of ether. **Protect** from light.

7115-l

Thioridazine Hydrochloride *(B.P., U.S.P.)*.

$C_{21}H_{26}N_2S_2,HCl=407.0$.

CAS — 130-61-0.

Pharmacopoeias. In *Br., Cz., Jug., Nord.*, and *U.S.*

A white or slightly yellow crystalline powder with a slight odour and a very bitter taste. M.p. 157° to 163° with a range of not more than 3°.

Soluble 1 in 9 of water, 1 in 10 of alcohol, and 1 in 1.5 of chloroform; freely soluble in methyl alcohol; practically insoluble in ether. A 1% solution in water has a pH of 4.2 to 5.2. **Store** in airtight containers. Protect from light.

Adverse Effects. As for Chlorpromazine, p.1509. The incidence of extrapyramidal symptoms is reported to be low.

Pigmentary retinopathy characterised by diminution of visual acuity, brownish colouring of vision, and impairment of night vision has been observed in patients taking large doses. Changes in the T-wave of the electrocardiogram have also occurred. Sexual dysfunction is common with thioridazine but it is reported to have little epileptogenic effect.

Effects on the blood. *Agranulocytosis.* A 73-year-old woman who was taking thioridazine, 25 mg four times daily, developed agranulocytosis which resolved when the treatment was stopped. Thioridazine was stated to have been associated with the development of agranulocytosis in 4 other patients and there appeared to be some evidence that it could have a direct toxic effect on the bone marrow.— D. S. Rosenthal *et al.*, *J. Am. med. Ass.*, 1967, *200*, 81.

Further references: R. L. Ferguson *et al.*, *Sth. med. J.*, 1977, *70*, 110; F. Shabry and J. A. Wolk, *Am. J. Psychiat.*, 1980, *137*, 374.

Haemolytic anaemia. Immune haemolytic anaemia in association with thioridazine.— J. W. Cooper and L. H. Pesnell, *Sth. med. J.*, 1978, *71*, 1443.

Effects on the endocrine system. On 3 occasions a 39-year-old man with chronic schizophrenia developed massive oedema on administration of thioridazine. Prompt diuresis and marked weight loss occurred each time the drug was stopped. On the third occasion the patient suddenly died from multiple pulmonary emboli. Previous authors have suggested that oedema associated with thioridazine may be due to an increase in antidiuretic hormone.— J. Margolis, *J. Am. Geriat. Soc.*, 1972, *20*, 593. Inappropriate secretion of antidiuretic hormone in a woman receiving thioridazine.— F. Matuk and K. Kalyanaraman, *Archs Neurol.*, 1977, *34*, 374.

Conflicting views on the role of thioridazine in inducing water intoxication: K. J. Rao *et al.* (letter), *Ann. intern. Med.*, 1975, *82*, 61; C. M. Fischman (letter), *ibid.*, 852; M. Miller *et al.* (letter), *ibid.*

Effects on the eyes. A description of chorioretinopathy in 3 patients receiving high doses of thioridazine. Progressive changes were noted in 2 of the patients for years after thioridazine was discontinued.— T. A. Meredith *et al.*, *Archs Ophthal., N.Y.*, 1978, *96*, 1172.

Further references: V. Hagopian *et al.*, *Am. J. Psychiat.*, 1966, *123*, 97; M. E. Cameron *et al.*, *Br. J. Ophthal.*, 1972, *56*, 131; F. H. Davidorf, *Archs Ophthal., N.Y.*, 1973, *90*, 251.

Effects on the gastro-intestinal tract. After about 1 month a 68-year-old woman taking thioridazine 150 mg daily developed severe diarrhoea which necessitated withdrawal of the drug. Fluphenazine and trifluoperazine, previously used unsuccessfully, had no effect on bowel function.— A. B. S. Mitchell, *Postgrad. med. J.*, 1975, *51*, 182.

Abdominal distension and aortic obstruction associated with thioridazine treatment.— M. M. Kemeny *et al.*, *J. Am. med. Ass.*, 1980, *243*, 683.

Effects on the heart. In a study of 252 male patients receiving thioridazine, the incidence of T-wave abnormalities only increased with the dose while the severity was related only to age. It was considered that the T-wave abnormalities induced by thioridazine were neither harmful nor cumulative and that they did not necessarily call for a reduction in dose or discontinuation of therapy.— C. C. Thornton and M. H. Wendkos, *Clin. Pharmac. Ther.*, 1971, *12*, 303. See also J. R. Huston and G. E. Bell, *J. Am. med. Ass.*, 1966, *198*, 16.

A 41-year-old man given thioridazine hydrochloride 600 mg daily for alcohol withdrawal developed ventricular ectopic beats, tachycardia, and fibrillation, and died. A 41-year-old woman similarly treated had ventricular tachycardia and frequent episodes of fibrillation, which responded to DC shock. Both patients had acidosis and hypokalaemia.— M. A. Sydney, *Br. med. J.*, 1973, *4*, 467. There was little reason to conclude that thioridazine was responsible for the arrhythmias.— R. W. Newton (letter), *ibid.*, 738.

A 54-year-old woman developed ventricular tachycardia associated with administration of thioridazine 1.3 g daily for manic-depressive psychosis.— T. B. Tri and D. T. Combs, *West. J. Med.*, 1975, *123*, 412.

Abnormal ECG patterns occurring in 4 of 5 schizophrenic patients given thioridazine 4 mg per kg body-weight daily by mouth appeared to be associated with elevated plasma concentrations of the thioridazine ring sulphoxide metabolite.— L. A. Gottschalk *et al.*, *J. pharm. Sci.*, 1978, *67*, 155.

Effects on the liver. Jaundice with increased alkaline phosphatase values and SGPT levels occurred in a patient who was given thioridazine. Altered liver function was also noted in 2 other patients being treated with thioridazine; 1 had increased SGPT levels and the other had increased alkaline phosphatase values and SGPT levels. The third patient continued treatment and the values reverted to normal.— M. J. Reinhart *et al.*, *J. Am. med. Ass.*, 1966, *197*, 767. Criticism.— D. C. H. Sun (letter), *ibid.*, 1967, *199*, 48. A reply.— M. J. Reinhart (letter), *ibid.*, 48.

Further references: M. Barancik *et al.*, *J. Am. med. Ass.*, 1967, *200*, 69; F. J. Kane and L. P. Moore, *Sth. med. J.*, 1971, *64*, 573; P. L. Weiden and C. D. Buckner, *J. Am. med. Ass.*, 1973, *224*, 518.

Effects on sexual function. There was a 60% incidence of sexual dysfunction in 57 male patients taking thioridazine, compared with a 25% incidence in 64 male patients who had taken other neuroleptics. A striking finding in the thioridazine group was the incidence of ejaculatory failures due to retrograde ejaculation; this did not occur in the other group.— J. Kotin *et al.*, *Am. J. Psychiat.*, 1976, *133*, 82. Psychotropic drugs have an adverse effect on male sexual function and thioridazine appears to be the worst offender.— *Br. med. J.*, 1979, *2*, 883.

See also under Uses.

Priapism. A 24-year-old man developed priapism after taking an overdose of thioridazine in a suicide attempt.— R. A. Appell *et al.*, *Br. J. Urol.*, 1977, *49*, 160.

Extrapyramidal effects. The incidence of extrapyramidal effects with thioridazine is low, probably as a result of its high anticholinergic potency; anticholinergic activity, however, has unwanted effects of its own.— *Drug & Ther. Bull.*, 1977, *15*, 57.

Further references: R. J. Miller and D. R. Hiley, *Nature*, 1974, *248*, 596; D. E. Huttenbach (letter), *Am. J. Psychiat.*, 1977, *134*, 820.

Hypotension. Of 48 men who were given up to 800 mg of thioridazine daily, 19 developed hypotension which was severe in 2 patients, 9 experienced tachycardia, and drowsiness occurred in 10. Other side-effects were principally extrapyramidal changes, mainly tremor and rigidity.—Cooperative Study, National Institute of Mental Health, *J. clin. Pharmac.*, 1967, *7*, 287. A further report of hypotension in 1 patient.— B. B. Kumar (letter), *J. Am. med. Ass.*, 1975, *234*, 1321.

Overdosage. Episodic ventricular tachycardia and fibrillation occurred in a patient 36 hours after ingesting 2.5 g of thioridazine. Cardiac monitoring might need to be extended in some patients for at least 48 hours.— D. F. Levine and A. J. Marshall (letter), *Lancet*, 1975, *2*, 990.

Death of 3 patients from overdosage with thioridazine;

in 1 patient the dose was about 2 g, death was apparently due to cardiac arrhythmias. Arrhythmias developed in a further patient who survived after a dose of 500 mg.— P. T. Donlon and J. P. Tupin, *Archs gen. Psychiat.*, 1977, *34*, 955. See also K. R. Burgess *et al.*, *Med. J. Aust.*, 1979, *2*, 177.

See also under Effects on Sexual Function (above).

Treatment of Adverse Effects. As for Chlorpromazine, p.1511.

Four patients with tardive dyskinesia while taking thioridazine were relieved when deanol 600 to 900 mg daily was gradually added to this treatment; it was considered useful for the dyskinesia caused by phenothiazines and butyrophenones.— L. De Silva and C. Y. Huang, *Br. med. J.*, 1975, *3*, 466.

Precautions. As for Chlorpromazine, p.1512.

The influence of antipsychotic therapy on performance of judgement tasks was evaluated in 26 schizophrenic patients. Thioridazine appeared to block use of feedback information, whereas haloperidol and trifluoperazine enhanced use of feedback.— J. S. Gillis, *Curr. ther. Res.*, 1977, *21*, 224.

Interactions. *Adrenaline and other sympathomimetics.* A 27-year-old woman with schizophrenia and T-wave abnormality of the heart, who had responded to thioridazine 100 mg daily with procyclidine 2.5 mg twice daily, died from ventricular fibrillation within 2 hours of taking a single dose of a preparation reported to contain chlorpheniramine maleate 4 mg with phenylpropanolamine hydrochloride 50 mg (Contac. C), concurrently with thioridazine.— G. Chouinard *et al.*, *Can. med. Ass. J.*, 1978, *119*, 729. Critical comment; similar combinations of these drugs have not provoked untoward effects in other patients.— M. H. Wendkos (letter), *ibid.*, 1979, *120*, 1058. Reply, stressing the need for caution in the use of other drugs when large doses of thioridazine are prescribed.— G. Chouinard and B. D. Jones (letter), *ibid.*, 1058.

Antihistamines. For the effect of a preparation containing chlorpheniramine maleate and phenylpropanolamine hydrochloride, on thioridazine, see Adrenaline and Other Sympathomimetics (above).

Phenytoin and other anticonvulsants. Evidence to suggest that concomitant anticonvulsant medication (phenobarbitone and phenytoin) significantly reduces plasma-mesoridazine concentrations in patients given thioridazine; plasma-thioridazine concentration was not significantly different. Plasma concentrations of the anticonvulsants were not affected.— M. Linnoila *et al.*, *Am. J. Psychiat.*, 1980, *137*, 819.

For the effect of thioridazine on phenytoin, see Phenytoin, p.1240.

Tricyclic antidepressants. A woman developed life-threatening ventricular arrhythmias a month after the chlorpromazine in her drug regimen of chlorpromazine 800 mg daily and imipramine 100 mg daily was substituted by thioridazine 800 mg. Another woman, who was taking amitriptyline 300 mg daily, developed ventricular arrhythmias after she reported ingesting about 1.2 g of thioridazine.— E. M. Heiman, *J. nerv. ment. Dis.*, 1977, *165*, 139.

Withdrawal. Thioridazine 125 mg daily, which he had been taking for about 18 months, was abruptly withdrawn from a 9-year-old boy with minimal brain dysfunction characterised by hyperactivity, impulsiveness, and learning disability. Irritability appeared the next day, on the tenth day he complained of stomach aches, dyskinetic movements appeared on the fourteenth day, and nausea and vomiting, which began on the twenty-first day was so severe that he required intravenous fluids from the twenty-third to the twenty-sixth day. The vomiting improved on treatment with trimethobenzamide hydrochloride, but persisted intermittently until the thirty-second day. The extrapyramidal disorder persisted up to 90 days after withdrawal.— L. E. Yepes and B. G. Winsberg, *Am. J. Psychiat.*, 1977, *134*, 574.

Symptoms of nausea and vomiting were noted in a number of patients when long-term use of thioridazine 100 to 800 mg daily was stopped abruptly. The symptoms occurred between 24 and 48 hours after the last dose.— B. B. Kumar (letter), *J. Am. med. Ass.*, 1978, *239*, 25.

Absorption and Fate. For an account of the absorption and fate of a phenothiazine, see Chlorpromazine, p.1513.

The serum half-life of thioridazine has been estimated to range from about 6 to over 40 hours.

In 10 healthy subjects given thioridazine hydrochloride 100 mg, peak serum concentrations of 130 to 520 ng per ml were reached 1¼ to 4 hours after the dose; no correlation was shown between the weight, sex, and serum concentrations. In 3 healthy subjects given thioridazine 200 mg (in divided doses over 7 hours) the serum half-life was about 9 to 10 hours.— E. Mårtensson and B. -E. Roos, *Eur. J. clin. Pharmac.*, 1973, *6*, 181.

A study on the serum concentration and elimination from serum of thioridazine in psychiatric patients. The serum half-life in 38 patients ranged from 6 to 42 hours, with a mean of 16.4 hours in 20 who received only thioridazine and 17.1 hours in those who also received other medication. Elimination was reduced at night and with increasing age.— R. Axelsson and E. Mårtensson, *Curr. ther. Res.*, 1976, *19*, 242.

In 10 psychiatric patients stabilised on thioridazine, therapy was replaced by equipotent doses of the side-chain sulphoxide (mesoridazine) and side-chain sulphone (sulforidazine) metabolites of thioridazine. Both metabolites were shown to have an antipsychotic effect, the dose of each required being about two-thirds that of thioridazine. The serum half-lives were thioridazine 21 hours, mesoridazine 16 hours, and sulforidazine 13 hours. Apathy, depression, and restlessness gradually developed during treatment with the 2 metabolites and they could not be used for any length of time. Extrapyramidal symptoms, hypersalivation, and drowsiness were more common with the metabolites; 2 patients had epileptic seizures, and one receiving sulforidazine developed probable cholestatic jaundice.— R. Axelsson, *Curr. ther. Res.*, 1977, *21*, 587.

A review of the problems encountered in the monitoring of plasma-antipsychotic drug concentrations with specific reference to chlorpromazine, thioridazine, butaperazine, haloperidol, thiothixene, perphenazine, and penfluridol. Owing to wide variations between concentrations and response routine monitoring remained of research interest only.— T. B. Cooper, *Clin. Pharmacokinet.*, 1978, *3*, 14. In 23 patients with acute psychosis treatment with thioridazine increased serum concentrations of prolactin. After normalisation of the data there was a correlation between serum-prolactin concentrations and antipsychotic effect.— R. Öhman and R. Axelsson, *Eur. J. clin. Pharmac.*, 1978, *14*, 111.

Further references: R. Axelsson and E. Mårtensson, *Curr. ther. Res.*, 1977, *21*, 561 (plasma concentrations); G. Nikitopoulou *et al.*, *Clin. Pharmac. Ther.*, 1977, *21*, 422 (plasma-prolactin concentrations); F. A. J. Vanderheeren and R. G. Muusze, *Eur. J. clin. Pharmac.*, 1977, *11*, 135 (plasma concentrations); R. Axelsson and E. Mårtensson, *Curr. ther. Res.*, 1978, *24*, 232 (plasma concentrations).

Metabolism. Gas-chromatographic studies on the serum and urine of psychiatric patients receiving thioridazine identified the main nonconjugated metabolites as side-chain sulphoxide of thioridazine (mesoridazine), side-chain sulphoxide of demethylthioridazine, side-chain sulphone of thioridazine (sulforidazine), thioridazine disulphoxide, and the ring sulphoxide of thioridazine. Other metabolites tentatively identified were demethylthioridazine, the side-chain sulphone and ring sulphoxide of demethylthioridazine, and the ring sulphone of thioridazine.— E. Mårtensson *et al.*, *Curr. ther. Res.*, 1975, *18*, 687.

Plasma protein binding. In 48 patients taking thioridazine the mean amount not bound to serum proteins was 0.15%, that of the side-chain sulphoxide 1.66%, side-chain sulphone 1.17%, and ring sulphoxide 1.7%.— G. Nyberg *et al.*, *Eur. J. clin. Pharmac.*, 1978, *14*, 341.

Uses. Thioridazine is a phenothiazine with actions and uses similar to those of chlorpromazine (p.1513). It has a piperidine side-chain and, unlike chlorpromazine, has little anti-emetic activity.

The usual initial dose for the treatment of psychoses is 50 to 100 mg thrice daily; in severe conditions up to 800 mg daily may be required.

Doses of 30 to 200 mg daily have also been used for non-psychotic emotional disturbances, such as anxiety and tension. In general, however, phenothiazines are only suitable for such purposes in resistant conditions, where more appropriate agents, such as the benzodiazepines (see Diazepam, p.1523) have proved ineffective. If their use is judged to be necessary treatment should be directed at low dosages on a short-term basis.

A suggested dose of thioridazine for children with behaviour disorders is 1 mg per kg body-weight daily, in divided doses. Thioridazine should be given in reduced dosage to elderly patients.

Administration. White plaque formation on the oral mucosa of 3 women receiving thioridazine hydrochloride was attributed to the fact that the patients allowed the tablets to dissolve in the mouth. The symptoms cleared when thioridazine in liquid form was substituted for the tablets.— L. N. Folkerts (letter), *Am. J. Hosp. Pharm.*, 1978, *35*, 384.

In the elderly. Studies involving thioridazine in the elderly: S. E. Goldstein and F. Birnbom, *J. Am. Geriat. Soc.*, 1976, *24*, 355 (organic brain syndrome); M. H. Branchey *et al.*, *J. Am. med. Ass.*, 1978, *239*, 1860 (schizophrenia); L. M. Cowley and R. S. Glen, *J. clin. Psychiat.*, 1979, *40*, 411 (organic brain syndrome).

See also Chlorpromazine, p.1514.

Alcohol and drug withdrawal. Studies of thioridazine in anxiety associated with alcohol withdrawal: W. H. Hague *et al.*, *J. nerv. ment. Dis.*, 1976, *162*, 354; A. Pena-Ramos, *Dis. nerv. Syst.*, 1977, *38*, 144; A. Pena-Ramos and R. Hornberger, *J. clin. Psychiat.*, 1979, *40*, 361.

Anxiety. In a double-blind study in 45 patients with acute neurotic anxiety, thioridazine 25 or 50 mg thrice daily impaired psychomotor skills more than diazepam 5 or 10 mg thrice daily. In subjective studies thioridazine was considered to be less effective than diazepam as an anxiolytic agent.— I. Saario *et al.*, *Br. J. clin. Pharmac.*, 1976, *3*, 843.

Behaviour disorders. Studies on the use of thioridazine for behaviour disorders in children: A. Alexandris and F. W. Lundell, *Can. med. Ass. J.*, 1968, *98*, 92; J. A. Doyle *et al.*, *Curr. ther. Res.*, 1969, *11*, 429; R. Gittelman-Klein *et al.*, *Archs gen. Psychiat.*, 1976, *33*, 1217.

Depression. Thioridazine is the only antipsychotic medication approved by the U.S. Food and Drug Administration for short-term treatment of depression, but there is no good evidence that it has any advantage over other phenothiazines for the treatment of depressed patients.— *Med. Lett.*, 1978, *20*, 49.

Studies on the use of thioridazine in depression or in depression with anxiety: L. Prasad and M. C. Townley, *Curr. ther. Res.*, 1969, *11*, 379. Report No. 172 of the General Practitioner Research Group, *Practitioner*, 1972, *209*, 95; S. H. Rosenthal and C. L. Bowden, *Curr. ther. Res.*, 1973, *15*, 261; J. G. Lofft and J. P. Demars, *Dis. nerv. Syst.*, 1974, *35*, 409.

Effects on sexual function. The use of thioridazine to suppress inappropriate ejaculation.— L. Clein (letter), *Br. med. J.*, 1962, *2*, 548.

Further references: D. Wheatley, *Practitioner*, 1972, *209*, 585.

See also under Adverse Effects.

Extrapyramidal effects. *Tardive dyskinesia.* Criticism of the view that thioridazine may be the phenothiazine of choice for patients with tardive dyskinesia who still require antipsychotic medication. Although anticholinergic agents reduce the frequency of early extrapyramidal side-effects, they may worsen tardive dyskinesia. Hence, thioridazine, with its anticholinergic activity may be relatively contra-indicated.— R. Linden (letter), *New Engl. J. Med.*, 1977, *296*, 1004. Comment.— R. M. Kobayashi (letter), *ibid.*

Pain. Chronic pain was successfully treated with amitriptyline and thioridazine but excessive weight gain occurred when treatment lasted several months.— A. K. Pfister (letter), *J. Am. med. Ass.*, 1978, *239*, 1959. Comment.— J. L. Davis *et al.* (letter), *ibid.*

Psychoses. Thioridazine administered in doses of 100 to 800 mg daily to 47 patients with functional or organic psychoses and 1 with neurotic depression significantly improved their condition at the end of a 5-week trial.— APetrides, *Curr. ther. Res.*, 1973, *15*, 116.

Schizophrenia. Six newly-admitted schizophrenic patients unresponsive to high-dose chlorpromazine or haloperidol were given thioridazine up to 200 mg four times daily. Improvement in 3 patients was associated with a high plasma concentration of the active side-chain sulphoxide (mesoridazine) or sulphone of thioridazine, whereas non-responders had a higher plasma concentration of the inactive ring sulphoxide. Plasma concentrations of thioridazine did not distinguish between the two groups.— G. Sakalis *et al.*, *Curr. ther. Res.*, 1977, *21*, 720.

Further references: J. C. Barker and M. Miller, *Br. J. Psychiat.*, 1969, *115*, 169; J. Walinder *et al.*, *Archs gen. Psychiat.*, 1976, *33*, 501; J. S. Gillis and H. G. Davis, *Curr. ther. Res.*, 1977, *21*, 507; M. Kramer *et al.*, *Curr. ther. Res.*, 1978, *23*, 619.

Preparations

Thioridazine Hydrochloride Oral Solution *(U.S.P.)*. Thioridazine Hydrochloride Solution. A solution containing thioridazine hydrochloride. It contains 2.5 to 4.7% of alcohol. To be diluted before use. Store at 15° to 30° in airtight containers. Protect from light.

Thioridazine Hydrochloride Tablets *(U.S.P.).* Tablets containing thioridazine hydrochloride.

Thioridazine Oral Suspension *(U.S.P.).* A suspension containing thioridazine. pH 8 to 10. Store at a temperature not exceeding 30° in airtight containers. Protect from light.

Thioridazine Tablets *(B.P.).* Tablets containing thioridazine hydrochloride. They are coated.

Proprietary Preparations

Melleril *(Sandoz, UK).* Thioridazine hydrochloride, available as **Tablets** of 10, 25, 50, and 100 mg. **Melleril Suspension** contains thioridazine base 25 and 100 mg in each 5 ml (dilution not recommended). **Melleril Syrup** contains thioridazine base 25 mg in each 5 ml (suggested diluent, syrup free from preservatives). **Melleril Concentrate** is supplied to hospitals for preparing a syrup of the same strength by diluting 1 part to 30 parts with syrup. (Also available as Melleril in *Austral., Belg., Denm., Fr., Ger., Ital., Neth., Norw., S.Afr., Switz.*).

Other Proprietary Names

Arg.— Meleril; *Belg.*— Mellerettes; *Canad.*— Mellaril, Novoridazine, Thioril; *Ger.*— Melleretten; *Ital.*— Mellerette; *Neth.*— Melleretten; *Spain*— Meleril; *Swed.*— Mallorol; *Switz.*— Melleretten; *USA*— Mellaril.

7116-y

Thiothixene *(U.S.P.).* Tiotixene; P 4657B.

(*Z*)-*NN*-Dimethyl-9-[3-(4-methylpiperazin-1-yl)propylidene]thioxanthene-2-sulphonamide.

$C_{23}H_{29}N_3O_2S_2$=443.6.

CAS — 5591-45-7; 3313-26-6 (Z).

Pharmacopoeias. In *U.S.*

A white to tan-coloured almost odourless crystalline powder. M.p. 147° to 152°. Thiothixene 1 mg is approximately equivalent to 1.25 mg of thiothixene hydrochloride (dihydrate). Practically **insoluble** in water; soluble 1 in 110 of dehydrated alcohol, 1 in 2 of chloroform, and 1 in 120 of ether; slightly soluble in acetone and methyl alcohol. **Store** in airtight containers. Protect from light.

7117-j

Thiothixene Hydrochloride *(U.S.P.).*

$C_{23}H_{29}N_3O_2S_2,2HCl,2H_2O$=552.6.

CAS — 58513-59-0 (anhydrous); 49746-04-5 (anhydrous, Z); 22189-31-7 (dihydrate); 49746-09-0 (dihydrate, Z).

Pharmacopoeias. In *U.S.*

A white or almost white crystalline powder with a slight odour. **Soluble** 1 in 8 of water, 1 in 270 of dehydrated alcohol, and 1 in 280 of chloroform; practically insoluble in acetone and ether. **Store** in airtight containers. Protect from light.

Adverse Effects, Treatment, and Precautions. As for Chlorpromazine, p.1509.

Extrapyramidal symptoms are the most common side-effect. Restlessness and insomnia may occur.

Effects on the blood. Leucopenia in a patient associated with thiothixene therapy.— N. R. Cutler and J. F. Heiser, *J. Am. med. Ass.*, 1979, *242*, 2872.

Effects on the endocrine system. A 55-year-old man developed hyponatraemia associated with inappropriate secretion of antidiuretic hormone following administration of thiothixene 30 mg daily for 4 months.— K. Ajlouni *et al.*, *Archs intern. Med.*, 1974, *134*, 1103.

Effects on the mental state. When given to 9 healthy subjects, thiothixene in doses of 5 to 15 mg caused drowsiness while doses of 20 to 40 mg were associated with increasing symptoms of restlessness, difficulty in thinking, and general discomfort.— L. E. Hollister, *J. clin. Pharmac.*, 1968, *8*, 95.

Extrapyramidal effects. *Tardive dyskinesia.* After receiving thiothixene 10 mg daily for a year, a 27-year-old schizophrenic man developed symptoms of tardive dyskinesia.— J. Ananth and A. Costin, *Am. J. Psychiat.*, 1977, *134*, 689.

Withdrawal. Replacement of thiothixene, which he had been taking for 57 days, by thioridazine, was associated with the development of an acute brain syndrome in a 46-year-old man with chronic schizophrenia. Reinstitution of the thiothixene after 7 days controlled the symptoms. The thiothixene was again withdrawn 12 days later, this time without incident; the reason for this was not fully understood.— J. B. Ferholt and W. N. Stone, *J. nerv. ment. Dis.*, 1970, *150*, 400.

Absorption and Fate. For an account of the absorption and fate of a thioxanthene, see Flupenthixol, p.1528.

Plasma concentrations of thiothixene were studied in schizophrenic patients using a method of analysis with a sensitivity equivalent to less than 1 ng per ml of plasma. In 15 adequately controlled patients receiving thiothixene 15 to 60 mg daily in 2, 3, or 4 divided doses by mouth, plasma concentrations were found to be in the relatively narrow range of 10 to 22.5 ng per ml 126 to 150 minutes after the last daily dose despite the fourfold difference in dosage. Investigations in a further 5 patients indicated that peak plasma concentrations were obtained about 1 to 3 hours after a dose, indicating rapid absorption with an absorption half-time of about 30 minutes. There was an early plasma half-life of about 210 minutes and a late half-life of about 34 hours; resurgence of drug concentrations in some subjects might have been due to enterohepatic recycling. Appreciable blood concentrations obtained 24 hours after a single dose indicated that a once-daily dose might be adequate for long-term therapy.— D. C. Hobbs *et al.*, *Clin. Pharmac. Ther.*, 1974, *16*, 473.

In a double-blind study, 40 schizophrenics received either thiothixene or thioridazine hydrochloride, the doses being adjusted for optimal effect. After 3 weeks, plasma concentrations of both drugs were dose-related, but after 8 weeks the plasma concentration of thiothixene had fallen, indicating enzyme induction, whilst the correlation was maintained for thioridazine.— R. Bergling *et al.*, *J. clin. Pharmac.*, 1975, *15*, 178.

Further references: T. Mjorndal and L. Oreland, *Acta pharmac. tox.*, 1971, *29*, 295; T. B. Cooper, *Clin. Pharmacokinet.*, 1978, *3*, 14.

Uses. Thiothixene is a thioxanthene with general properties similar to those of the phenothiazine, chlorpromazine (p.1513). The usual dose of the base or the hydrochloride (expressed in terms of the base) for the treatment of psychoses is 5 mg twice daily gradually increasing to 20 to 30 mg daily; once-daily dosage may be adequate. In severe psychoses doses of up to 60 mg daily may be given. It may also be given intramuscularly as the hydrochloride in doses equivalent to 4 mg of the base two to four times daily increased if necessary to a maximum of 30 mg daily.

Anxiety with depression. In a double-blind trial involving 76 depressed anxious patients, 18 given thiothixene 2 to 12 mg daily achieved moderate to marked improvement compared with 16 patients given a placebo. Side-effects due to thiothixene were stimulation and sedation, but stimulation was also reported by patients receiving the placebo.— B. J. Goldstein and B. Brauzer, *J. clin. Pharmac.*, 1973, *13*, 167.

Psychoses. Thiothixene was used successfully in 2 patients who suffered from pathological jealousy.— N. Herceg, *Med. J. Aust.*, 1976, *1*, 569.

Schizophrenia. Twenty-one of 25 men with chronic schizophrenia benefited from treatment with thiothixene by intramuscular injection for 3 days; the total dose was 26 to 44 mg. Withdrawal of treatment was necessary because of hypotension in 1 patient and extrapyramidal effects in another. Other side-effects observed were dry mouth and facial contracture (5 patients), and sweating and tremor (5 patients).— F. J. M. Belda and T. De Haro, *Curr. ther. Res.*, 1969, *11*, 599.

Further references: L. E. Hollister *et al.*, *Clin. Pharmac. Ther.*, 1971, *12*, 531; A. M. P. Kellam and K. S. Jones, *Acta psychiat. scand.*, 1971, *47*, 174; E. Fischer, *Med. J. Aust.*, 1973, *1*, 436; B. A. Stotsky, *Dis. nerv. Syst.*, 1977, *38*, 967; D. M. Engelhardt *et al.*, *J. clin. Psychiat.*, 1978, *39*, 834; R. G. Knight and A. Harrison, *N.Z. med. J.*, 1979, *89*, 302.

Preparations

Thiothixene Capsules *(U.S.P.).* Capsules containing thiothixene. The *U.S.P.* requires 75% dissolution in 15 minutes. Protect from light.

Thiothixene Hydrochloride Injection *(U.S.P.).* A sterile solution in Water for Injections. Potency is expressed in terms of the equivalent amount of thiothixene. pH 2.5 to 3.5. Protect from light.

Thiothixene Hydrochloride Oral Solution *(U.S.P.).* Thiothixene Hydrochloride Solution. A solution containing thiothixene hydrochloride. Potency is expressed in terms of the equivalent amount of thiothixene. pH 2 to 3. Store in airtight containers. Protect from light.

Proprietary Names

Navane *(Pfizer, Austral.; Roerig, Belg.; Pfizer, Canad.; Pfizer, Denm.; Pfizer, Ital.; Roerig, Neth.; Pfizer, Norw.; Pfizer, S.Afr.; Pfizer, Spain; Roerig, USA)*; Orbinamon *(Pfizer, Ger.)*.

Thiothixene was formerly marketed in Great Britain under the proprietary name Navane *(Pfizer)*.

7118-z

Tofisopam. Tofizopam; Egyt-341. 1-(3,4-Dimethoxyphenyl)-5-ethyl-7,8-dimethoxy-4-methyl-5*H*-2,3-benzodiazepine.

$C_{22}H_{26}N_2O_4$=382.5.

CAS — 22345-47-7.

A white powder. M.p. about 152°. Practically **insoluble** in water; soluble in alcohol and chloroform.

Tofisopam is a benzodiazepine with actions and uses similar to those of diazepam (p.1519). It has been given in doses of 50 mg thrice daily for the treatment of anxiety; in severe conditions doses of up to 300 mg daily have been given.

An introductory comment on tofisopam.— J. Tariska and K. Bolla, *Therapia hung.*, 1975, *23*, 131. The chemistry of tofisopam a 2,3-benzodiazepine.— J. Körösi and T. Láng, *ibid.*, 132. The pharmacology of tofisopam.— L. Petöcz and I. Kosóczky, *ibid.*, 134. A study of the pharmacokinetics of tofisopam in healthy subjects. It was found to have a plasma half-life of about 6 hours.— S. Rónai *et al.*, *ibid.*, 139. The effect of tofisopam on lorry drivers.— J. Gerevich *et al.*, *ibid.*, 143. The use of tofisopam in mild depression.— Z. Böszörményi, *ibid.*, 147. A clinical evaluation of the tranquillising properties of tofisopam in out-patients.— G. Várady *et al.*, *ibid.*, 153. Tofisopam in psychic disorders accompanying myasthenia gravis.— A. Szobor, *ibid.*, 159. Tofisopam for menopausal symptoms.— M. Csillag *et al.*, *ibid.*, 164.

Tofisopam as oral premedication.— A. Pakkanen *et al.*, *Br. J. Anaesth.*, 1980, *52*, 1009.

Proprietary Names

Grandaxine *(L'Ozothine, Fr.)*; Grandaxin *(EGYT, Hung.)*; Sériel *(Fabre, Fr.)*.

7119-c

Triflubazam. ORF-8063; WE 352. 1-Methyl-5-phenyl-7-trifluoromethyl-1*H*-1,5-benzodiazepine-2,4(3*H*,5*H*)-dione.

$C_{17}H_{13}F_3N_2O_2$=334.3.

CAS — 22365-40-8.

Triflubazam is a benzodiazepine with general properties similar to those of diazepam (p.1519). It has been given in doses of 30 to 90 mg daily.

Reviews. Reviews of the actions and uses of triflubazam.— *Drugs Today*, 1975, *11*, 203.

Studies on the metabolism of triflubazam, a 1,5-benzodiazepine.— R. M. Grimes *et al.*, *Pharmacologist*, 1973, *15*, 254; R. E. Huettemann and A. P. Shroff, *J. pharm. Sci.*, 1975, *64*, 1339.

Action. *Animal* studies on the pharmacology of triflubazam.— R. Guerrero-Figueroa and D. M. Gallant, *Curr. ther. Res.*, 1971, *13*, 747; R. D. Heilman *et al.*, *ibid.*, 1974, *16*, 1022.

Alcohol and drug withdrawal. Studies involving triflubazam in alcohol withdrawal.— D. M. Gallant *et al.*, *Curr. ther. Res.*, 1972, *14*, 664; G. Gardos *et al.*, *Curr. ther. Res.*, 1974, *16*, 628.

Anxiety. Studies of triflubazam in anxiety.— G. Sakalis *et al.*, *Curr. ther. Res.*, 1973, *15*, 268; T. M. Itil *et al.*, *Curr. ther. Res.*, 1976, *19*, 307; I. Csanalosi *et al.*, *ibid.*, 1977, *22*, 166.

Hypnotic effect. Triflubazam had no effect on total-sleep time in a double-blind study in 6 healthy subjects who took 20 or 40 mg before retiring. Subjects reported impaired sleep on the night of the single dose and a sense of less wakefulness on the following 2 mornings.—

A. N. Nicholson *et al.*, *Br. J. clin. Pharmac.*, 1977, *4*, 567.

Manufacturers
Boehringer Ingelheim, Ger.

7120-s

Trifluoperazine Hydrochloride *(B.P., U.S.P.)*.

Triphthazinum. 10-[3-(4-Methylpiperazin-1-yl)propyl]-2-trifluoromethylphenothiazine dihydrochloride.
$C_{21}H_{24}F_3N_3S,2HCl=480.4$.

CAS — 117-89-5 (trifluoperazine); 440-17-5 (hydrochloride).

Pharmacopoeias. In *Br.*, *Roum.*, *Rus.*, and *U.S.*

A white to pale yellow, odourless or almost odourless, hygroscopic, crystalline powder with a bitter taste. M.p. 242° with decomposition. Trifluoperazine 1 mg is approximately equivalent to 1.2 mg of trifluoperazine hydrochloride.
Soluble 1 in 2 of water, 1 in 11 of alcohol, and 1 in 100 of chloroform; slightly soluble in isopropyl alcohol; practically insoluble in ether. A 5% solution in water has a pH of 1.7 to 2.6. Solutions are **sterilised** by autoclaving or by filtration; the air in the containers is replaced by nitrogen or other suitable gas. In aqueous solution it is readily oxidised by atmospheric oxygen. **Store** in airtight containers. Protect from light.

Adverse Effects and Treatment. As for Chlorpromazine, p.1509.
Extrapyramidal symptoms may be more common than the other side-effects.

Effects on the blood. *Aplastic anaemia.* Trifluoperazine has been reported to cause aplastic anaemia.— R. H. Girdwood, *Drugs*, 1976, *11*, 394.

Effects on the eyes. Lenticular opacities occurred in 8 out of 31 schizophrenics who were given a succession of phenothiazine derivatives, mainly trifluoperazine, for periods of 3 to 10 years.— L. H. Margolis and J. L. Goble, *J. Am. med. Ass.*, 1965, *193*, 7.

Effects on the heart. A report of a 29-year-old woman with psychosis and congenital heart disease in whom it was considered that trifluoperazine might have precipitated Stokes-Adams attacks.— R. Steinhouse, *Penn. med. J.*, 1972, *75*, 56.

Extrapyramidal effects. Acute dystonia affecting the tongue occurred in 2 patients after a single dose of 10 mg of trifluoperazine.— X. G. Okojie (letter), *Br. med. J.*, 1972, *4*, 796.

Extrapyramidal symptoms were reported in a 17-year-old girl within 60 hours of taking trifluoperazine 1 mg twice daily.— K. L. De Silva *et al.*, *Practitioner*, 1973, *211*, 316.

The Boston Collaborative Drug Surveillance Program monitored consecutively 32 812 medical inpatients. Drug-induced extrapyramidal symptoms occurred in 7 of 73 patients given trifluoperazine hydrochloride. Also 3 patients out of 44 given trifluoperazine with prochlorperazine or chlorpromazine experienced extrapyramidal symptoms.— J. Porter and H. Jick, *Lancet*, 1977, *1*, 587.

Tardive dyskinesia. A placebo-controlled study of phenothiazine-induced tardive dyskinesia in patients given trifluoperazine 16 mg or 80 mg daily. An attempt was made to replicate previous findings with chlorpromazine. The most significant finding was the high incidence of dyskinesia in chronic schizophrenic patients receiving high doses of chlorpromazine or trifluoperazine.— G. E. Crane and C. Chase, *Archs Neurol.*, 1970, *22*, 176.

Overdosage. Seven youths each ingested 60 mg of trifluoperazine. Six had dystonic syndromes which lasted for 24 to 72 hours and were followed by akathisia. One, who had taken chlordiazepoxide 60 mg simultaneously, had an attenuated reaction. Amylobarbitone sodium given intravenously to 2 patients stopped the extrapyramidal attacks instantly, but in 1 patient 3 further severe attacks followed at 8-hourly intervals.— M. X. FitzGerald and O. FitzGerald (letter), *Lancet*, 1969, *1*, 1100.

Further references: P. H. Beighton and D. J. Wilkinson, *Practitioner*, 1967, *199*, 73.

Pregnancy and the neonate. *Early pregnancy.* In 478 pregnant women, known to have been treated with trifluoperazine and preparations containing it, there were 2 abortions and 476 live babies were born who showed no skeletal abnormalities. The statement of the Director of the Canadian Food & Drug Directorate, which implicated Stelazine in producing abnormalities of the foetus, appeared to have no foundation in fact.— I. Schrire, *Smith Kline & French* (letter), *Lancet*, 1963, *1*, 174. See also A. J. Moriarty and M. R. Nance, *Smith Kline & French* (letter), *Can. med. Ass. J.*, 1963, *88*, 375.

Further studies: D. Wheatley (letter), *Br. med. J.*, 1964, *1*, 630 (no association).

Individual reports of malformations in exposed infants: G. Hall, *Med. J. Aust.*, 1963, *1*, 449; D. J. Vince (letter), *Can. med. Ass. J.*, 1969, *100*, 223.

Precautions. As for Chlorpromazine, p.1512.
Severe dystonic reactions have followed the use of trifluoperazine, especially in young people.

Trifluoperazine, given in five 2-mg doses over 36 hours, significantly affected low-speed tests of driving ability; alcohol given concomitantly had little effect. There was no correlation between performance and the objective and subjective effects of medication.— T. A. Betts *et al.*, *Br. med. J.*, 1972, *4*, 580.

Pregnancy and the neonate. For reports and studies on the effects of trifluoperazine in early pregnancy, see Adverse Effects.

Absorption and Fate. For an account of the absorption and fate of a phenothiazine, see Chlorpromazine, p.1513.

Plasma-trifluoperazine concentrations during high-dose therapy.— S. H. Curry *et al.* (letter), *Lancet*, 1981, *1*, 395.

Plasma protein binding. For the comparative protein binding of trifluoperazine and other phenothiazines, see Chlorpromazine, p.1513.

Uses. Trifluoperazine is a phenothiazine with actions and uses similar to those of chlorpromazine (p.1513). It has a piperazine side-chain. Trifluoperazine is given as the hydrochloride but its doses are expressed in terms of the base.
The usual initial dose for the treatment of psychoses is 5 mg twice daily, gradually increased to a usual range of 15 to 20 mg daily in divided doses; in severe psychoses daily doses of 40 mg or more have been given. For the relief of acute psychotic symptoms it may be given by deep intramuscular injection in a dosage of 1 to 3 mg daily in divided doses; up to 6 mg may be given intramuscularly daily in severe psychoses.
For the control of nausea and vomiting the usual dose by mouth is 1 or 2 mg twice daily; up to 6 mg daily may be given in divided doses.
Doses of 1 or 2 mg twice daily have also been used for non-psychotic emotional disturbances, such as anxiety and tension. In general, however, phenothiazines are only suitable for such purposes in resistant conditions, where more appropriate agents, such as the benzodiazepines (see Diazepam, p.1523) have proved ineffective. If their use is judged to be necessary treatment should be directed at low dosages given on a short-term basis.
Trifluoperazine should be given in reduced dosage to elderly patients.

Alcohol and drug withdrawal. Trifluoperazine, 5 mg thrice daily, quickly and effectively suppressed an alcoholic auditory hallucinosis in a 54-year-old woman. She was subsequently maintained on 2 mg thrice daily for 2 months.— D. G. Logan (letter), *J. Am. med. Ass.*, 1967, *202*, 74.

Anxiety. Trifluoperazine was less effective than chlordiazepoxide in the treatment of 126 nonpsychotic patients with anxiety in a placebo-controlled study. Failure of treatment with trifluoperazine was considered to be due to the large number of patients who withdrew from the study because of side-effects which included drowsiness, akathisia, excitement and diarrhoea.— B. L. Weiss *et al.*, *Curr. ther. Res.*, 1977, *22*, 635.

Further references: M. Mirabi *et al.*, *Curr. ther. Res.*, 1978, *23*, 101.

Cholera syndrome. The diarrhoea of a patient with pancreatic cholera syndrome responded dramatically to trifluoperazine.— M. Donowitz *et al.*, *Ann. intern. Med.*, 1980, *93*, 284.

Psychoses. Treatment with trifluoperazine in conjunction with chlorpromazine was given to 620 patients with acute psychotic conditions including delusions and hallucinations. The response occurred quicker than with either drug alone and was good or excellent in 80% of patients after 28 days' treatment.— J. Nemeth and M. Petrovich, *Dis. nerv. Syst.*, 1967, *28*, 812.

Drug-induced psychosis. Trifluoperazine in doses of 2 mg twice daily for 7 days effectively diminished some of the visual disturbances due to lysergide in a 19-year-old man.— W. H. Anderson and J. E. O'Malley (letter), *J. Am. med. Ass.*, 1972, *220*, 1244.

Schizophrenia. A study in 2 matched groups of patients with long-standing schizophrenia showed that treatment for 6 months with trifluoperazine in the usual or in high doses produced no significant improvement when assessed on Lorr's Multidimensional Rating Scale. A dosage increased from 10 to 100 mg daily was unlikely to affect markedly the mental state but would increase the incidence of side-effects.— H. B. Carscallen *et al.*, *Can. psychiat. Ass. J.*, 1968, *13*, 459.

In a double-blind study, the relapse-rate within a year in 12 patients taking a placebo after recovery from an acute episode of schizophrenia was 83%, compared with 33% in 18 similar patients given for maintenance either trifluoperazine 5 to 15 mg (mean 12.3 mg) daily or chlorpromazine 100 to 300 mg (mean 157 mg) daily.— J. P. Leff and J. K. Wing, *Br. med. J.*, 1971, *3*, 599.

Nine schizophrenic patients out of 32 relapsed when treatment mainly with trifluoperazine in a mean dose of 16.1 mg daily for a mean period of 8.8 years was withdrawn. Two patients relapsed out of a matched group of 30 who continued treatment. Of the 23 patients who continued without treatment for a mean period of 16 weeks, motor restlessness worsened or appeared for the first time in 11.— H. I. Hershon *et al.*, *Br. J. Psychiat.*, 1972, *120*, 41.

Preparations

Trifluoperazine Hydrochloride Injection *(U.S.P.)*. A sterile solution in Water for Injections. Potency is expressed in terms of the equivalent amount of trifluoperazine. pH 4 to 5. Protect from light.

Trifluoperazine Hydrochloride Syrup *(U.S.P.)*. A syrup containing trifluoperazine hydrochloride. Potency is expressed in terms of the equivalent amount of trifluoperazine. pH 2 to 3.2. Store in airtight containers. Protect from light.

Trifluoperazine Hydrochloride Tablets *(U.S.P.)*. Tablets containing trifluoperazine hydrochloride. Potency is expressed in terms of the equivalent amount of trifluoperazine. Protect from light.

Trifluoperazine Tablets *(B.P.)*. Tablets containing trifluoperazine hydrochloride. They are sugar-coated. Potency is expressed in terms of the equivalent amount of trifluoperazine.

Proprietary Preparations

Stelabid *(Smith Kline & French, UK)*. **Tablets** each containing trifluoperazine hydrochloride equivalent to trifluoperazine 1 mg and isopropamide iodide equivalent to isopropamide 5 mg and **Forte Tablets** each containing the equivalents of trifluoperazine 2 mg and isopropamide 7.5 mg. For gastro-intestinal spasm and hypersecretion with associated anxiety. *Dose.* 1 tablet 2 or 3 times daily or 1 Forte tablet every 12 hours.

Stelazine *(Smith Kline & French, UK)*. Trifluoperazine hydrochloride, available as an **Injection** containing the equivalent of 1 mg of trifluoperazine per ml, in ampoules of 1 ml; as **Spansule** sustained-release capsules each containing the equivalent of 2, 10, and 15 mg of trifluoperazine; as **Syrup** containing the equivalent of 1 mg of trifluoperazine in each 5 ml (suggested diluent, syrup); as **Concentrate** for hospital use containing the equivalent of 10 mg of trifluoperazine per ml for preparing dilutions convenient for oral administration; and as **Tablets** each containing the equivalent of 1 and 5 mg of trifluoperazine. (Also available as Stelazine in *Austral.*, *Canad.*, *S.Afr.*, *USA*).

Other Proprietary Names

Arg.— Nerolet; *Austral.*— Calmazine, Terfluzin; *Belg.*— Terfluzine; *Canad.*— Clinazine, Novoflurazine, Pentazine, Solazine, Terfluzine, Triflurin, Tripazine; *Denm.*— Terfluzin; *Fr.*— Terfluzine; *Ger.*— Jatroneural; *Ital.*— Modalina; *Neth.*— Terfluzine; *Norw.*— Terfluzin; *Spain*— Eskazine; *Swed.*— Terfluzin; *Switz.*— Eskazinyl, Terfluzine.

A preparation containing trifluoperazine hydrochloride was also formerly marketed in Great Britain under the proprietary name Amylozine (*Smith Kline & French*).

7121-w

Trifluperidol. McN-JR 2498; R 3000. 4′-Fluoro-4-[4-hydroxy-4-(3-trifluoromethylphenyl)piperidino]butyrophenone.
$C_{22}H_{23}F_4NO_2$=409.4.

CAS — 749-13-3.

A white crystalline powder. M.p. 93° to 95°.

7122-e

Trifluperidol Hydrochloride. R 2498.
$C_{22}H_{23}F_4NO_2,HCl$=445.9.

CAS — 2062-77-3.

A white, amorphous or crystalline, flocculent powder. M.p. about 205°. It is stable in air but darkens slowly on exposure to light. Trifluperidol hydrochloride 1.09 mg is approximately equivalent to 1 mg of trifluperidol.
Slightly **soluble** in water; soluble in alcohol; freely soluble in methyl alcohol; slightly soluble in acetone, chloroform, and isopropyl alcohol; practically insoluble in ether and toluene.

Adverse Effects. As for Haloperidol, p.1532.

Treatment of Adverse Effects. As for Chlorpromazine, p.1511.

Precautions. As for Haloperidol, p.1532.

Uses. Trifluperidol is a butyrophenone with general properties similar to those of haloperidol (p.1533), and is used in the treatment of mania and schizophrenia. It is given by mouth as the hydrochloride but doses are stated in terms of the base.
The initial dose is 500 µg daily and the dose is increased at intervals of 3 to 4 days until improvement occurs or a total dose of 6 to 8 mg daily is reached.

Chorea. In 4 patients with Huntington's chorea, treatment with trifluperidol almost abolished involuntary movements in 3 and strikingly reduced them in 1. Side-effects included opisthotonos and hypertonicity and were diminished by reducing the maintenance dose; the average maintenance dose was 1 mg thrice daily.— S. Tarighati and M. F. a'Brook (letter), *Lancet*, 1968, *2*, 458.

Schizophrenia. In a double-blind trial 60 chronic schizophrenics were given trifluperidol or trifluoperazine to a maximum daily dose of 8 mg or 40 mg respectively. Trifluperidol was less effective than trifluoperazine. Side-effects were more frequent in the trifluperidol group and included drowsiness, dizziness, insomnia, over-stimulation, pseudo-parkinsonism, and weakness. It was suggested that trifluperidol was indicated in anergic, withdrawn, and lethargic patients.— W. R. Goodchild *et al.*, *Int. Pharmacopsychiat.*, 1969, *2*, 185.

Trifluperidol in doses of 500 µg thrice daily for 10 weeks was as effective as trifluoperazine 5 mg thrice daily in the treatment of 60 schizophrenic patients.— M. S. Menon and V. Ramachandran, *Curr. ther. Res.*, 1972, *14*, 17.

Further references: M. L. Clark *et al.*, *Psychopharmacologia*, 1968, *12*, 193.

Proprietary Names
Psicoperidol *(Lindeburg & Riemer, Denm.; Lusofarmaco, Ital.; Janssen, S.Afr.; Lindeburg & Riemer, Swed.)*; Triperidol *(Janssen, Belg.; Janssen-Le Brun, Fr.; Janssen, Ger.; Janssen, Neth.; Infal, Spain).*

Trifluperidol hydrochloride was formerly marketed in Great Britain under the proprietary name Triperidol (*Janssen*).

7123-l

Trimetozine. Abbott 22370; PS 2383. 4-(3,4,5-Trimethoxybenzoyl)morpholine.
$C_{14}H_{19}NO_5$=281.3.

CAS — 635-41-6.

Pharmacopoeias. In *Hung.* and *Jug.*

A white crystalline powder. M.p. about 121°. Slightly **soluble** in water and alcohol; freely soluble in chloroform and methyl alcohol.

Trimetozine has been used as a sedative and tranquilliser in usual doses of 0.6 to 1.8 g daily, with a maximum of 3 g daily.

When trimetozine was given in a daily dose of 2.1 g to 10 women with chronic mental illness, no consistent effects were noted to suggest that trimetozine had any useful psychotropic properties. One patient developed hyperglycaemia and glycosuria associated with the treatment.— W. V. Krumholz *et al.*, *J. clin. Pharmac.*, 1967, *7*, 108.

The long-term use of trimetozine.— G. Haits, *Therapia hung.*, 1976, *24*, 145. The use of trimetozine in delirium and other psychotic disorders.— F. Müller and L. Sajtos, *ibid.*, 1977, *25*, 69.

Proprietary Names
Neuristan *(Casasco, Arg.)*; Opalene *(Theraplix, Belg.; Théraplix, Fr.)*; Trioxazine *(EGYT, Hung.; Labatec-Pharma, Switz.).*

7124-y

Tybamate. W713. 2-Methyl-2-propyltrimethylene butylcarbamate carbamate.
$C_{13}H_{26}N_2O_4$=274.4.

CAS — 4268-36-4.

A white crystalline powder or clear viscous liquid, which may congeal to a solid form on standing, with a slight characteristic odour and a bitter taste. M.p. of the powder 49° to 54°.
Very slightly **soluble** in water; very soluble in alcohol and acetone; freely soluble in ether. **Store** in airtight containers.

Adverse Effects, Treatment, and Precautions. As for Meprobamate, p.1546.

Muscular hypotonia. Of 7 patients treated with tybamate, 2 women developed severe muscular hypotonia with marked ataxia on a dose of 1.4 g daily for 2 and 3 weeks respectively. These effects disappeared completely within 10 days of stopping the drug.— J. M. Bachner (letter), *Br. med. J.*, 1967, *1*, 361.

Absorption and Fate. Tybamate is readily absorbed from the gastro-intestinal tract. It is metabolised in the liver and excreted in the urine, mainly as hydroxylated compounds. It has a half-life of about 3 or 4 hours.

Uses. Tybamate is a carbamate with general properties similar to those of meprobamate (p.1546). It has been used in the treatment of anxiety and tension states in usual doses of 250 to 500 mg three or four times daily. The maximum daily dose was 3 g.

References: I. Shapiro, *Curr. ther. Res.*, 1966, *8*, 99; W. B. Spry, *Br. J. clin. Pract.*, 1967, *21*, 175; R. L. Fransway *et al.*, *Curr. ther. Res.*, 1967, *9*, 42; B. J. Goldstein, *Psychosomatics*, 1967, *8*, 334; E. Meshel and H. C. B. Denber, *Dis. nerv. Syst.*, 1968, *29*, 243; F. Veress *et al.*, *J. clin. Pharmac.*, 1969, *9*, 232.

Proprietary Names
Tybatran *(Robins, USA).*

NOTE. The name Nospan has been applied to Tybamate and to Drotaverine Hydrochloride.

7125-j

Valnoctamide. McN-X181. 2-Ethyl-3-methylvaleramide.
$C_8H_{17}NO$=143.2.

CAS — 4171-13-5.

Valnoctamide has been given in doses of 400 to 800 mg daily in 2 or 3 divided doses for anxiety and tension.

References: W. Stephansky, *Curr. ther. Res.*, 1960, *2*, 144.

Proprietary Names
Nirvanil *(Midy, Fr.; Midy, Ital.; Clin-Midy, Neth.; Midy, Switz.).*

Tuberculostatics and Tuberculocides

7550-p

Tuberculosis is caused by *Mycobacterium tuberculosis* or, more rarely, *M. bovis*, and the most usual site of primary infection is the lungs, although extrapulmonary sites may be involved. Tuberculous infection occurs as a result of the inhalation of infected droplets or, in the case of *M. bovis*, by drinking infected milk and may be diagnosed in asymptomatic patients by use of a tuberculin test (p.1611). The term tuberculosis is used when the infected person has a disease process involving one or more parts of the body. In generalised miliary tuberculosis, bacilli are disseminated through the blood and give rise to discrete tubercles scattered throughout the lungs and other tissues.

Compounds used in the treatment or prophylaxis of tuberculosis and described in this chapter include aminosalicylic acid and its salts and derivatives, the antibiotics capreomycin and rifampicin, hydrazides such as isoniazid, thioamines such as ethionamide and prothionamide, and ethambutol, pyrazinamide, and thiacetazone. Other antibiotics used include cycloserine (p.1152), kanamycin (p.1176), and streptomycin (p.1214).

The addition of corticosteroids or corticotrophin to antituberculous therapy may lead to earlier improvement in the patient's condition and in the radiographic clearing of shadows, but generally the slight long-term benefit is not considered to justify their routine use. However, they may be of benefit to seriously ill patients or in the treatment of severe hypersensitivity reactions.

Adverse Effects. Side-effects may be a particular problem when antituberculous agents are given for prolonged periods; chronic toxicity may be reduced with intermittent and short-term treatment schedules. Although adverse effects associated with antituberculous agents are dealt with under the individual monographs it may be difficult to attribute toxicity to specific agents since the treatment of tuberculosis involves the use of 2 or more drugs.

Reviews of the adverse effects of antituberculous agents.— A. Levantine and J. Almeyda, *Br. J. Derm.*, 1972, *86*, 651; G. W. Poole, *Prescribers' J.*, 1975, *15*, 39; D. J. Girling, *Bull. int. Un. Tuberc.*, 1980, *55*, 8.

A controlled study of the adverse effects of drug regimens used in short-term chemotherapy for pulmonary tuberculosis.— M. Zierski and E. Bek, *Tubercle*, 1980, *61*, 41.

Allergy. The testing *in vitro* of hypersensitivity to antituberculous agents.— J. T. Baker *et al.* (letter), *Lancet*, 1974, *2*, 967.

Effects on the liver. The hepatotoxic potential of tuberculostatic drugs.— *Br. med. J.*, 1975, *2*, 522. See also M. Casteels-Van Daele *et al.*, *J. Pediat.*, 1975, *86*, 739.

Effects on mental state. A brief discussion of the role of tuberculostatics in causing depression.— F. A. Whitlock and L. E. J. Evans, *Drugs*, 1978, *15*, 53.

Pregnancy and the neonate. A survey of 1939 reported births to mothers who received isoniazid, ethambutol, rifampicin, and streptomycin, alone or in combination for all or part of their pregnancy. There was no significant increase in congenital abnormalities associated with the use of isoniazid in 1079 births, ethambutol in 369 births, or rifampicin in 101 births. Minor auditory or vestibular disturbances were seen with streptomycin in 24 of 390 births.— D. J. Scheinhorn and V. A. Angelillo, *West. J. Med.*, 1977, *127*, 195. A survey of published reports on 2787 pregnancies in women receiving isoniazid, streptomycin, ethambutol, or rifampicin, and details of 14 women who inadvertently took antituberculous drugs while pregnant. If the disease is not extensive, isoniazid with ethambutol appears to be the most appropriate treatment. If a third drug or a more potent drug is necessary, due to the extensive or serious nature of the disease, rifampicin can be added. Streptomycin should not be used unless these other drugs are contra-indicated. Routine therapeutic abortion for pregnant women taking first-line antituberculous drugs is not medically indicated since, apart from the ototoxicity of streptomycin, the potential teratogenic effect of these drugs has not been established.— D. E. Snider *et al.*, *Am. Rev. resp. Dis.*, 1980, *122*, 65.

A recommendation that pregnancy be avoided in patients taking ethionamide or rifampicin and that the safest combination of antituberculous drugs in pregnant patients is isoniazid with ethambutol.— J. MacVicar, *Practitioner*, 1978, *221*, 885. See also M. de Swiet, *Prescribers' J.*, 1979, *19*, 59.

Further references.— J. C. Marcus, *S. Afr. med. J.*, 1967, *41*, 758; J. Warkany, *Teratology*, 1979, *20*, 133.

Antimicrobial Action. Most of the antituberculous agents are bacteriostatic except for rifampicin and pyrazinamide which are bactericidal. However, ethionamide and isoniazid can also exert a bactericidal effect if high enough concentrations are achieved. Although strains of *Mycobacterium tuberculosis* with primary drug resistance are relatively rare in previously untreated patients in developed countries, resistance develops rapidly to most agents when used alone, so it is necessary to employ 2 or more agents at the same time. Cross-resistance may occur.

The mechanism of action of various tuberculostatic agents.— P. J. McDonald *et al.*, *Med. J. Aust.*, 1974, *2*, 41.

The intracellular growth-rate of tubercle bacilli was found to increase in strains isolated from patients receiving standard antituberculous therapy and despite clinical improvement.— L. B. Hejfec *et al.* (letter), *Lancet*, 1977, *2*, 409.

A report of the bactericidal activity *in vitro* of various antituberculous agents.— J. M. Dickinson *et al.*, *Am. Rev. resp. Dis.*, 1977, *116*, 627.

Sensitivity testing of *Mycobacterium avium* to 14 antimicrobial agents using diffusion through solid media and radioassay.— A. M. Hintz and R. Merkal, *Bull. int. Un. Tuberc.*, 1980, *54*, 347.

Resistance. For reviews and discussions of bacterial resistance to tuberculostatics, see N. W. Horne, *Tubercle*, 1969, *50*, *Suppl.* 2;; D. A. Mitchison, *ibid.*, 44; W. Fox, *ibid.*, 55; J. Crofton, *ibid.*, 65; R. R. Briney and R. G. Cowley, *Am. Rev. resp. Dis.*, 1970, *101*, 700; *Lancet*, 1972, *2*, 412; H. E. Thomas, *Tubercle*, 1972, *53*, 1; C. A. E. G. de Ville de Goyet and H. H. Kleeberg, *ibid.*, 9; G. Canetti *et al.*, *ibid.*, 57; B. G. Guernsey and M. R. Alexander, *Am. J. Hosp. Pharm.*, 1978, *35*, 690.

Variable cross-resistance in 4 mutant strains of *M. tuberculosis* developed to all combinations of capreomycin, kanamycin, and viomycin. There was no cross-resistance between streptomycin and these other injectable antibiotics.— J. K. McClatchy *et al.*, *Tubercle*, 1977, *58*, 29.

Further references.— Y. P. Kataria, *Tubercle*, 1969, *50*, 14.

Incidence of resistance. Of 632 untreated patients with tuberculosis in Kenya, 14.7% had a strain of mycobacterium resistant to 1 or more drugs, 11.1% being resistant to isoniazid and/or streptomycin, 10.3% to isoniazid, 2.2% to streptomycin, and 6% to aminosalicylic acid.—Report of the East African/British MRC Kenya Tuberculosis Survey 1968, *Tubercle*, 1968, *49*, 136. Of 702 untreated patients in Kenya excreting strains of *M. tuberculosis*, 10 (1.4%) had strains resistant to isoniazid and streptomycin and 51 (7.3%) and 10 (1.4%) had strains resistant to isoniazid or streptomycin alone respectively.—Second East African/British MRC Kenya Tuberculosis Survey 1978, *Tubercle*, 1978, *59*, 155.

Of 828 strains of *M. tuberculosis* isolated during 1975-76 in Massachusetts, USA, 163 showed varying degrees of resistance to antituberculous drugs and 41 of these were isolated from untreated patients. This 4.95% incidence of primary drug resistance is not significantly greater than the incidence of 3.1% reported in 1972.— K. D. Stottmeier and S. Baker (letter), *New Engl. J. Med.*, 1977, *296*, 823. The incidence in the Greater Boston area is 2.5 times that of the rest of Massachusetts and had doubled since 1972.— M. A. Khan (letter), *New Engl. J. Med.*, 1977, *297*, 397.

Between 1974 and 1977, 27 of 509 previously untreated Polish patients with pulmonary tuberculosis excreted strains of *M. tuberculosis* resistant to at least one antituberculous agent. Resistance to isoniazid occurred in 22 patients, to streptomycin in 11, and to both drugs in 6. No strains resistant to ethambutol or rifampicin were identified.— M. Janowiec *et al.*, *Tubercle*, 1979, *60*, 233.

In the national survey of tuberculosis notifications in England and Wales for 1978–9, sensitivity tests for streptomycin, isoniazid, rifampicin, and ethambutol were performed on 1070 strains of tubercle bacilli isolated from reported patients. Resistance to streptomycin alone occurred in 12 strains, to isoniazid alone in 12, and to both agents in 7. One further strain was resistant to streptomycin, isoniazid, and rifampicin. Of 801 strains obtained from white patients and 200 strains from patients from the Indian subcontinent, 13 and 15 strains respectively were resistant to one or more agents.—Report from the MRC Tuberculosis and Chest Diseases Unit, *Br. med. J.*, 1980, *281*, 895.

Further references.— Y. E. Chun *et al.*, *Clin. Med.*, 1972, *79* (Dec.), 15; P. L. Schiffman *et al.*, *Am. Rev. resp. Dis.*, 1977, *116*, 821 (California); F. D. Pien *et al.*, *Am. Rev. resp. Dis.*, 1978, *118*, 701 (Hawaii); N. J. Nielsen, *Tubercle*, 1979, *60*, 239 (Eastern Botswana); E. S. Hershfield *et al.*, *Int. J. clin. Pharmac. Biopharm.*, 1979, *17*, 387 (Canada).

Prophylaxis of Tuberculosis. Prophylaxis is intended to prevent the occurrence of acute tuberculosis in susceptible contacts, and to curb its spread through the community. Isoniazid (p.1574) is the antituberculous agent used for this purpose.

A report of the successful use of tuberculosis prophylaxis in Canadian Eskimos using an intermittent regimen of isoniazid 10 mg per kg body-weight, to a maximum of 600 mg, with ethambutol 30 mg per kg, to a maximum of 2000 mg, given thrice weekly for up to 18 months.— S. Grzybowski *et al.*, *Tubercle*, 1976, *57*, 263.

Recommendations for the prophylaxis of tuberculosis. The Joint Tuberculosis Committee of the British Thoracic and Tuberculosis Association considered that chemoprophylaxis against tuberculosis in the UK should be extended and that the following groups should be considered: children with positive tuberculin reactions, adults with positive tuberculin reactions who are either close contacts of infectious cases or who have lesions considered to be inactive, and immigrants, especially those from Asia.— *Tubercle*, 1973, *54*, 309.

Prophylaxis of pulmonary tuberculosis is not considered suitable for mass application in community health. It is considered irrational unless the coinciding treatment programme is widespread, highly organised, and effective. Other disadvantages are the hazards, inconvenience, cost, and difficulty in ensuring adequate patient compliance.— Ninth Report of WHO Expert Committee on Tuberculosis, *Tech. Rep. Ser. Wld Hlth Org. No. 552*, 1974.

Experience with 132 asthmatics did not indicate that prophylaxis is necessary in patients with positive tuberculin reactivity who are receiving prolonged corticosteroid therapy, especially when the toxicity of isoniazid is considered.— M. Schatz *et al.*, *Ann. intern. Med.*, 1976, *84*, 261. The study does not provide an adequate basis for conclusions to be drawn. Corticosteroid therapy can mask symptoms of tuberculosis.— L. B. Reichman *et al.* (letter), *ibid.*, *85*, 538.

Prophylaxis with isoniazid for one year is generally recommended for the following categories of patients who exhibit a positive tuberculin skin test, although the potential toxicity of isoniazid should be borne in mind: 1) household members and other close associates of patients with newly discovered tuberculosis, including children who may still have negative skin tests. These children should be given isoniazid for 3 months and then tested again; if they are positive, treatment should be continued for a total of 1 year, 2) persons with abnormal chest X-rays, 3) newly infected patients whose skin tests have become positive within the past 2 years, 4) compromised patients such as those with leukaemia or diabetes, or receiving immunosuppressive therapy or prolonged treatment with corticosteroids, 5) persons under 35 years who are positive reactors should receive preventative treatment in the absence of additional risk factors. To rule out the possibility of progressive disease all positive skin reactors should be given a chest X-ray.— L. S. Farer, *Center for Disease Control*, *Compr. Ther.*, 1977, *3*, 45.

A double-blind study of isoniazid prophylaxis in 7036 patients with inactive tuberculosis suggested that large-scale prophylaxis in such patients is of no value when they have previously received adequate chemotherapy but is best directed at those individuals with inactive disease who have either been inadequately treated or not previously treated.— A. Falk and G. F. Fuchs, *Chest*, 1978, *73*, 44.

Further references.— J. Noble, *New Engl. J. Med.*, 1971, *285*, 687; W. A. Slagel (letter), *ibid.*, 1972, *286*, 159; W. D. Refshauge, *National Tuberculosis Advisory Council* (letter), *Med. J. Aust.*, 1972, *2*, 570; *Am. Rev. resp. Dis.*, 1974, *110*, 371; *Morb. Mortal.*, 1975, *24*, 71 (joint statement from the American Thoracic Society, American Lung Association, and the Center for Disease Control); L. B. Reichman and R. J. McDonald, *Med. Clins N. Am.*, 1977, *61*, 1185; A. Leff *et al.*, *Am. Rev. resp. Dis.*, 1979, *119*, 161.

For references to the susceptibility of patients on dialysis to tuberculosis, see Administration in Renal Failure, under Treatment of Tuberculosis, below.

Treatment of Tuberculosis. There are differences between developed and developing countries in the choice of antituberculous agents and treatment schedules because of the problems of cost and the supervision of long-term treatment. All treatments of tuberculosis involve the use of 2 or more drugs. Treatment often begins with a schedule of 3 *primary* or 'first-line' agents, to allow for the possibility of bacterial resistance, and after 2 to 3 months is continued with 2 of the drugs. Primary agents available are isoniazid, ethambutol, rifampicin, and streptomycin; the aminosalicylates are still used for primary treatment in some countries but they are poorly tolerated and have often been replaced by other agents such as ethambutol.

In developed countries isoniazid with rifampicin and/or ethambutol is usually the treatment of choice. The availability of the potent bactericidal agent rifampicin has allowed the development of short-term treatment regimens (see below) and these are increasingly important. Some authorities consider that isoniazid with rifampicin for 9 months, supplemented by ethambutol or streptomycin for the first 2 months, is now the standard treatment for tuberculosis. The most common treatment regimen used to be an aminosalicylate, isoniazid, and streptomycin given for up to 3 months and continuation treatment with aminosalicylate and isoniazid for 1 to 2 years.

Pyrazinamide and thiacetazone, 2 antituberculous drugs often considered to be *secondary* agents, are being used successfully in schedules for primary treatment. Other secondary agents, given if resistance or toxicity to primary drugs develops during treatment, include capreomycin, cycloserine, ethionamide, prothionamide, and kanamycin, as well as aminosalicylic acid.

Intermittent and short-term treatment schedules are described below.

For reviews and discussions of the treatment of tuberculosis see Ninth Report of WHO Expert Committee on Tuberculosis, *Tech. Rep. Ser. Wld Hlth Org. No. 552*, 1974; M. Aquinas, *Drugs*, 1975, *9*, 364; A. Rouillon *et al.*, *Tubercle*, 1976, *57*, 275; K. L. Pinsker and S. K. Koerner, *Am. J. Hosp. Pharm.*, 1976, *33*, 275; D. A. Mitchison, *Adv. Med. Topics Ther.*, 1976, *2*, 12 to 25; *Bull. int. Un. Tuberc.*, 1977, *52* (Oct.), 53; E. W. Street, *Scott. med. J.*, 1977, *22*, 279; *Med. Lett.*, 1977, *19*, 97; J. H. Bates, *New Engl. J. Med.*, 1977, *297*, 610; M. Caplin and M. Rehahn, *Topics Ther.*, 1978, *4*, 136; B. G. Guernsey and M. R. Alexander, *Am. J. Hosp. Pharm.*, 1978, *35*, 690; A. Seaton, *Br. med. J.*, 1978, *1*, 701; D. Robinson (letter), *ibid.*, 1053; *Tubercle*, 1978, *59*, 300; J. R. Bignall *et al.*, *Bull. int. Un. Tuberc.*, 1979, *54*, 35; J. M. Grange, *Br. J. Hosp. Med.*, 1979, *22*, 540; J. Glassroth *et al.*, *New Engl. J. Med.*, 1980, *302*, 1441; W. W. Stead and A. K. Dutt, *Ann. intern. Med.*, 1980, *93*, 364.

In a detailed controlled collaborative study of 412 patients with newly-diagnosed sputum-positive tuberculosis, treatment with each of the following 4 schedules was highly effective when assessed at 1 year. (1) Standard treatment with streptomycin, isoniazid with pyridoxine, and aminosalicylic acid (PAS) daily for 3 months then isoniazid and PAS daily; (2) the standard treatment with ethambutol substituted for PAS; (3) as for (1) but with rifampicin substituted for PAS; (4) standard treatment for 3 months followed by isoniazid with pyridoxine and streptomycin twice-weekly. The incidence of side-effects was less in the ethambutol and rifampicin groups than in the other 2 groups.—British MRC Cooperative Study, *Tubercle*, 1973, *54*, 99. See also *ibid.*, 165.

In a study of the role of sensitivity tests in 527 patients with tuberculosis there was no significant difference in response over 3 years between patients who received standard treatment with streptomycin, isoniazid, and sodium aminosalicylate for 3 or 6 months followed by maintenance with isoniazid and sodium aminosalicylate irrespective of pretreatment sensitivity tests and those who received either the standard initial treatment then adjusted according to the sensitivity tests or else treatment based on the result of a relatively rapid slide culture sensitivity test. Even when the incidence of initial resistance was as high as 30%, often to 2 or all 3 of the standard agents, the first standard regimen produced a high bacterial inhibition which was maintained for the 3 years. All 3 groups received initial triple therapy for either 3 or 6 months but there appeared to be little difference in response. Maintenance treatment was continued for 18 to 24 months and again there was no significant difference in response.—Hong Kong Tuberculosis Treatment Services/British MRC, *Tubercle*, 1974, *55*, 169.

A report of bovine tuberculosis in humans.— H. Passes *et al.*, *Morb. Mortal.*, 1978, *27*, 108, per *Int. pharm. Abstr.*, 1978, *15*, 876.

Further references.— M. Tsukamura, *Tubercle*, 1972, *53*, 47.

Administration in renal failure. References to the treatment of tuberculosis in renal transplant patients.— *Tubercle*, 1979, *60*, 193; H. Riska and B. Kuhlback, *Bull. int. Un. Tuberc.*, 1979, *54*, 165.

Comment on the treatment of tuberculosis in patients with renal failure.— *Lancet*, 1980, *1*, 909.

A discussion of the susceptibility of patients on dialysis to tuberculosis and the difficulty of diagnosis.— *Br. med. J.*, 1980, *280*, 349. See also D. A. Mitchison and G. A. Ellard (letter), *ibid.*, 1186 and 1533; A. P. Lundin *et al.*, *Am. J. Med.*, 1979, *67*, 597; O. T. Andrew *et al.*, *ibid.*, 1980, *68*, 59.

Atypical mycobacterial infections. The treatment of atypical mycobacterial infections.— J. J. Van Dyke and K. B. Lake, *J. Am. med. Ass.*, 1975, *233*, 1380 (*Mycobacterium balnei*); G. D. Harris *et al.*, *Am. Rev. resp. Dis.*, 1975, *112*, 31 (*M. kansasii*).

Meningitis, tuberculous. A discussion indicating that isoniazid is still the mainstay of treatment for tuberculous meningitis. In a survey of 52 cases the majority had received isoniazid with streptomycin and aminosalicylic acid and most also received corticosteroids. The mortality-rate was 15% and 69% of the survivors made a complete recovery or had only trivial sequelae. The major factor in producing a poor outcome was a delay in the commencement of treatment. Findings in one patient supported the view that rifampicin and ethambutol do not cross the blood-brain barrier readily and, of themselves, are inadequate therapy. Ethionamide and pyrazinamide penetrate well into the cerebrospinal fluid but are relatively toxic.— R. J. Fallon, *J. antimicrob. Chemother.*, 1978, *4*, 1.

A brief review of the treatment of tuberculous meningitis in infants and children. Treatment has included the 3 major agents, isoniazid, aminosalicylic acid, and streptomycin, and rifampicin in association with isoniazid has been used successfully. Although experience in children is limited and adverse effects difficult to monitor, ethambutol may be added when bacterial resistance is suspected.— G. A. Ahronheim, *Drugs*, 1978, *16*, 136. See also M. S. McKenzie *et al.*, *Clin. Pediat.*, 1979, *18*, 75, 78–79, 82–84.

Tuberculous meningitis in 41 children under 12 years of age was treated with one of the following regimens: (1) isoniazid 20 mg per kg body-weight daily in divided doses for at least 18 months, streptomycin 30 to 50 mg per kg daily for one month, and rifampicin 10 to 15 mg per kg as a single daily dose for 6 months; (2) isoniazid administered as in (1), aminosalicylic acid 200 to 300 mg per kg daily in divided doses for at least 12 months and streptomycin 30 to 50 mg per kg daily for 3 months and in some patients continued 3 times weekly for another 3 months. All patients received corticosteroids at the beginning of treatment. The rate of recovery over 6 months was slightly more rapid in patients who received rifampicin (72.7% compared with 68.4%) and they had fewer neurological sequelae but the differences were not statistically significant. There was little difference between death-rates in the two groups but there was a higher incidence of jaundice amongst children who received rifampicin.— N. N. Rahajoe *et al.*, *Tubercle*, 1979, *60*, 245. See also N. N. Rahajoe *et al.*, *Bull. int. Un. Tuberc.*, 1979, *54*, 297.

A report of 2 women who developed cerebral tuberculomas during the treatment of tuberculous meningitis.— A. J. Lees *et al.*, *Lancet*, 1980, *1*, 1208. Correction.— *ibid.*, 1372. Comments on the role of corticosteroids in the management of cerebral tuberculomas.— J. Lebas *et al.* (letter), *ibid.*, *2*, 84; J. F. Warner (letter), *ibid.*

Further references.— *Lancet*, 1976, *1*, 787.

Pregnancy and the neonate. Isoniazid and ethambutol are considered the safest antituberculous drugs for use during pregnancy.— J. Glassroth *et al.*, *New Engl. J. Med.*, 1980, *302*, 1441.

See also under Adverse Effects, p.1564.

Pulmonary tuberculosis. Reviews of the treatment of pulmonary tuberculosis.— D. J. Girling, *Adv. Med.*, 1977, *13*, 263; W. Fox, *Bull. int. Un. Tuberc.*, 1977, *52* (Oct.), 25; S. Grzybowski and D. A. Enarson, *Bull. int. Un. Tuberc.*, 1978, *53* (June), 70; H. Stott, *Trans. R. Soc. trop. Med. Hyg.*, 1978, *72*, 564; W. W. Addington, *Archs intern. Med.*, 1979, *139*, 1391; G. M. Sterling, *Prescribers' J.*, 1980, *20*, 8.

See also under general reviews, above.

A brief review of the treatment of pulmonary tuberculosis in infants and children.— H. C. Spratt *et al.*, *Drugs*, 1978, *16*, 115. See also J. B. Heycock, *Practitioner*, 1977, *219*, 670.

Except for patients with high-risk factors, the follow-up of patients believed to have taken adequate chemotherapy for pulmonary tuberculosis is no longer considered to be justified. Nevertheless the discharged patient must be encouraged to report any symptoms indicative of relapse.—British Thoracic and Tuberculosis Association Joint Tuberculosis Committee Report, *Br. med. J.*, 1975, *2*, 28.

A favourable report on the use of a regimen consisting of aminosalicylic acid, isoniazid, and streptomycin with or without corticosteroid therapy in the treatment of 113 patients with tuberculous pleural effusion.— B. O. Onadeko, *Tubercle*, 1978, *59*, 269.

A short discussion on the infectivity of patients receiving chemotherapy for pulmonary tuberculosis. The abandonment of routine isolation makes a strict and effective organisation for examining contacts all the more important (see *Tubercle*, 1978, *59*, 245, for a report of standardised contact procedure).— *Br. med. J.*, 1980, *280*, 962. The infectivity of patients with pulmonary tuberculosis is greatest in those with cavities and sputum that is smear-positive for tubercle bacilli but generally falls rapidly after starting chemotherapy. Most patients may return to work quite soon, but if their work includes contact with the public, and especially with children, it is best to wait until treatment has been taken for a month, assuming any cough has ceased.— *Br. med. J.*, 1980, *281*, 434. Criticism.— R. G. Townshend (letter), *ibid.*, 942.

Further references to the treatment of pulmonary tuberculosis.— B. Groth-Petersen, *Scand. J. resp. Dis.*, 1976, *57*, 108 (treatment of relapses); M. Zierski, *Arch. Immunol. & Ther. exp.*, 1976, *24*, 169, per *Abstr. Hyg.*, 1976, *51*, 1069; I. D. Bobrowitz, *Bull. int. Un. Tuberc.*, 1979, *54*, 50 (comparison of ethambutol with rifampicin, given in association with isoniazid); M. W. Long *et al.*, *Am. Rev. resp. Dis.*, 1979, *119*, 879 (US Public Health Service Cooperative Trial of three rifampicin with isoniazid regimens).

Spinal tuberculosis. A series of controlled studies, organised by the British MRC, of different methods of management of patients with spinal tuberculosis, has been carried out in Korea, Rhodesia, Hong Kong, and South Africa. Standard chemotherapy with isoniazid and aminosalicylic acid daily for 18 months, supplemented by streptomycin daily for the first 3 months, has been highly effective in arresting spinal disease in patients fully ambulant from the start of treatment and no extra benefit has been derived from plaster jackets or bed rest in hospital. In countries lacking the resources to perform radical resection of the tuberculous focus, ambulant chemotherapy is the treatment of choice. There was no significant difference between the response obtained in a study of 159 patients with tuberculosis of the spine when 2 different methods of surgical management (radical resection or debridement) were used in addition to standard chemotherapy.—Seventh Report of the MRC Working Party on Tuberculosis of the Spine, *Tubercle*, 1978, *59*, 79.

A discussion of tuberculous paraplegia and its treatment.— *Br. med. J.*, 1979, *1*, 1442.

Further references.— F. A. Waldvogel and H. Vasey, *New Engl. J. Med.*, 1980, *303*, 360.

Tuberculosis of bones and joints. A review of the treatment of tuberculosis of bone and joint showing that favourable results were obtained by the use of tuberculostatic drugs and surgery.— D. L. Griffiths, *Trans. R. Soc. trop. Med. Hyg.*, 1978, *72*, 559.

BCG osteomyelitis was successfully managed in 2 children with standard antituberculous therapy.— M. Pauker *et al.*, *Archs Dis. Childh.*, 1977, *52*, 330.

See also under Spinal Tuberculosis, above.

Tuberculosis of the central nervous system. Five cases of tuberculoma of the central nervous system were treated by surgery and total excision of the tumour followed by intramuscular streptomycin for one month with isoniazid and thiacetazone given daily for one year. Outcome had been good in 4 of the patients.— S. C. Ohaegbulam *et al., Tubercle,* 1979, *60,* 163.

See also under Meningitis, tuberculous, above.

Tuberculosis of the genito-urinary tract. For successful results in the treatment of tuberculosis of the female genital tract in 206 patients given streptomycin, PAS, and isoniazid, see A. M. Sutherland, *Tubercle,* 1976, *57,* 137. See also *idem, Br. J. Obstet. Gynaec.,* 1977, *84,* 881; *idem, Br. J. Hosp. Med.,* 1979, *22,* 569.

The use of rifampicin, isoniazid, and pyrazinamide in short-term chemotherapy of genito-urinary tuberculosis.— J. G. Gow, *Bull. int. Un. Tuberc.,* 1979, *54,* 298. See also *idem, Br. J. Hosp. Med.,* 1979, *22,* 556.

Tuberculosis of the liver. References.— R. D. Rosin, *Tubercle,* 1978, *59,* 47.

Tuberculosis of the lymph nodes. There was no difference between the results obtained in 108 patients with lymph-node tuberculosis who received isoniazid 300 mg and rifampicin 450 or 600 mg daily and those who received isoniazid 300 mg and ethambutol 15 or 25 mg per kg body-weight daily for 18 months. Both groups also received streptomycin 750 mg intramuscularly on 6 days a week for the first 2 months but in 9 patients it had to be withdrawn prematurely.— I. A. Campbell and A. J. Dyson, *Tubercle,* 1977, *58,* 171. No differences have emerged between the 2 regimens in 90 patients followed up to 18 months after the end of chemotherapy. It appears that therapeutic resection is not essential and that chemotherapy alone can achieve good results.— *idem,* 1979, *60,* 95.

Further references.— P. B. Iles and P. A. Emerson, *Br. med. J.,* 1974, *1,* 143; J. B. L. Kabuubi, *Tubercle,* 1978, *59,* 281; J. Newcombe, *Br. J. Hosp. Med.,* 1979, *22,* 553.

Tuberculosis of the skin. A favourable report of the use of streptomycin, isoniazid and rifampicin in the treatment of 4 patients with tuberculosis of the skin.— N. G. Kounis and K. Constantinidis, *Practitioner,* 1979, *222,* 390.

Tuberculosis of the thyroid. A report of a patient with a tuberculous abscess of the thyroid. The patient made a rapid recovery following surgery and was then treated with ethambutol daily and rifampicin and isoniazid twice daily for 3 months followed by rifampicin and isoniazid twice daily for 6 months.— P. Emery, *J. Lar. Otol.,* 1980, *94,* 553.

Intermittent therapy. Intermittent treatment regimens are useful for patients with tuberculosis who cannot be relied on to take their medication unsupervised and may also result in fewer side-effects. After an initial phase of daily treatment for 2 to 3 months, doses are given twice or thrice weekly and occasionally once weekly; in rapid acetylators, once weekly treatment with isoniazid may not be effective and slow-release preparations have been tried in an attempt to overcome this problem. Individual doses used in intermittent regimens are generally higher than the usual daily doses. Regimens usually include isoniazid which has commonly been given twice-weekly by mouth in association with streptomycin by intramuscular injection. Other antituberculous agents used include ethambutol, pyrazinamide, and sodium aminosalicylate. The intermittent administration of rifampicin has been associated with serious adverse effects but, with careful adjustment of dosage, it may be used successfully.

Intermittent schedules may be incorporated into short-term regimens (see below).

A brief review of the intermittent treatment of pulmonary tuberculosis.— D. J. Girling, *Adv. Med.,* 1977, *13,* 263.

A comparison, in patients with newly diagnosed tuberculosis, of the efficacy of twice-weekly supervised doses of sodium aminosalicylate plus isoniazid (with pyridoxine) and daily doses of sodium aminosalicylate plus isoniazid, each regimen being preceded by 2 weeks of daily treatment with streptomycin, sodium aminosalicylate, and isoniazid with pyridoxine. Favourable responses at 1 year were achieved in 79 of 90 on the twice-weekly regimen and in 72 of 83 on the daily regimen. The twice-weekly regimen overcame the problem of failure to take medication and had a lower incidence of hypersensitivity and gastro-intestinal reactions, but the incidence of isoniazid-resistant cultures was higher and response appeared to be more affected by the initial extent of disease.—Tuberculosis Chemotherapy Centre, Madras, *Br. med. J.,* 1973, *2,* 7..

In a study in 404 patients with newly diagnosed pulmonary tuberculosis due to sensitive strains, patients were allocated to daily, thrice-weekly, or twice-weekly treatment with streptomycin (1 g for patients less than 40 years old or 0.75 g for older patients), isoniazid (300 mg daily or 15 mg per kg body-weight twice or thrice weekly), and pyrazinamide (1.5 g daily, 2 g thrice weekly, or 3 g twice weekly in patients under 49.9, 45.5, or 45.5 kg respectively or 2 g, 2.5 g, or 3.5 g respectively in those weighing 49.9, 45.5, and 45.5 kg or more). Treatments were continued for 6 or 9 months and in some on the twice-weekly schedule for 12 months. All treatments were equally effective in eliminating drug-sensitive strains from the sputum but the twice-weekly regimen was marginally less effective in preventing the emergence of isoniazid-resistant strains. Bacteriological relapse-rates after 6 months' chemotherapy were 13, 16, and 18% in patients on daily, thrice-weekly and twice-weekly regimens. Relapse-rates after 9 months' chemotherapy were 3, 4, and 4% respectively. In 110 patients with pretreatment strains resistant to isoniazid and/or streptomycin, the daily regimen was more effective in eliminating streptomycin-resistant strains. After 6 months' chemotherapy 30, 37, and 39% of patients on daily, thrice-weekly, and twice-weekly regimens had an unfavourable bacteriological status. Relapse-rates during follow-up in patients with pretreatment resistant strains were similar to those in patients with initially sensitive strains.—Hong Kong Tuberculosis Treatment Services/British MRC, *Tubercle,* 1975, *56,* 81. See also *Am. Rev. resp. Dis.,* 1977, *115,* 727.

In studies of adverse reactions to a number of drug regimens with isoniazid, streptomycin, rifampicin, and pyrazinamide for the treatment of about 900 patients with pulmonary tuberculosis it was found that the incidence of arthralgia was lower during intermittent than during daily administration of pyrazinamide, and the incidence of hepatic reactions was not apparently increased by the addition of rifampicin.—Hong Kong Tuberculosis Treatment Services/British MRC, *Tubercle,* 1976, *57,* 81. See also G. A. Ellard and R. M. Haslam, *ibid.,* 97.

Assessments at 18 and 36 months in a study involving 280 patients treated for newly-diagnosed pulmonary tuberculosis showed that standard initial triple therapy was as effective given for 6 as 13 weeks when followed by streptomycin with isoniazid given twice weekly for 18 months. Extending the twice-weekly regimen by 6 months offered no advantage. A once-weekly regimen was less effective owing mainly to failures in rapid acetylators.—WHO Collaborating Centre for Tuberculosis Chemotherapy, Prague, *Tubercle,* 1976, *57,* 235; *ibid.,* 1977, *58,* 129.

A report of short-term chemotherapy for tuberculosis with isoniazid and rifampicin given twice weekly.— A. K. Dutt *et al., Chest,* 1979, *75,* 441. See also *Am. Rev. resp. Dis.,* 1977, *116,* 807.

The successful use of twice-weekly regimens of isoniazid with streptomycin or isoniazid with ethambutol in patients with tuberculosis.— J. A. Sbarbaro *et al., Am. Rev. resp. Dis.,* 1980, *121,* 172. See also R. K. Albert *et al., ibid.,* 1976, *114,* 699.

Further references.— *Tubercle,* 1975, *56,* 246; *ibid.,* 1976, *57,* 45 (Third Report of WHO Collaborating Centre for Tuberculosis Chemotherapy, Prague); *ibid.,* 105 (National Research Institute for Tuberculosis, Poland); M. Zierski, *Scand. J. resp. Dis.,* 1978, *102, Suppl.,* 48; *idem, Lung,* 1979, *156,* 17.

Short-term Therapy. The inconvenience of prolonged therapy for tuberculosis has led to the development of effective short intensive courses of treatment for 6 to 9 months with rifampicin and isoniazid, along with other agents including ethambutol, pyrazinamide, streptomycin, and thiacetazone; even shorter treatment regimens are being tried. After an initial intensive phase of treatment, intermittent dosage schedules are sometimes used.

Conclusions and guidelines on the treatment of tuberculosis, with special reference to short-term chemotherapy. The bactericidal combination of isoniazid with rifampicin constitutes the basis of short-term treatment but it is advisable to add one or two supplementary drugs in the initial intensive phase of treatment in order to enhance efficacy and avert the consequences of primary and acquired resistance. From studies carried out around the world over the last 10 years it is agreed that: rifampicin and isoniazid are essential in both the initial and continuation phases of short-term regimens; streptomycin and pyrazinamide contribute to the success of these regimens when used either as supplementary drugs in the initial phase or when rifampicin is not available; for complete effectiveness treatment must continue for a total of 6 to 9 months in patients with bacteriologically-confirmed tuberculosis; and the initial phase of short-term treatment must be intensive with drugs given daily.— *Chronicle Wld Hlth Org.,* 1980, *34,* 101.

Recommendations for the short-term treatment of pulmonary tuberculosis from the American Thoracic Society and the Center for Disease Control. Initial treatment may last from 2 weeks to 2 months and should be with isoniazid 300 mg and rifampicin 600 mg daily; children may be given isoniazid 10 mg per kg body-weight up to 300 mg daily and rifampicin 10 to 20 mg per kg up to 600 mg daily. Ethambutol 15 mg per kg daily should also be given if drug resistance is likely. After the initial phase, isoniazid and rifampicin must be given daily, or twice-weekly if supervised. Treatment should last for a total of at least 9 months and in any event until sputum cultures have been negative for 6 months. After treatment is completed, patients should be followed-up for at least a further 12 months.— M. D. Iseman *et al., Am. Rev. resp. Dis.,* 1980, *121,* 611; *idem, Morb. Mortal.,* 1980, *29,* 97. The British Thoracic Association states that 9 months' chemotherapy with rifampicin and isoniazid, plus ethambutol in the first 2 months, is the preferred treatment for pulmonary tuberculosis in Britain.— *Lancet,* 1980, *1,* 1182; *ibid., 2,* 272.

Short-term regimens are not suitable for patients excreting organisms resistant to isoniazid or rifampicin and cannot yet be recommended for treatment of extrapulmonary tuberculosis or for pulmonary disease in patients with complicating problems such as diabetes or silicosis. Patients should be followed-up for 6 to 12 months after therapy.— J. Glassroth *et al., New Engl. J. Med.,* 1980, *302,* 1441.

Reviews and discussions on the short-term therapy of tuberculosis.— D. J. Girling, *Adv. Med.,* 1977, *13,* 263; *J. Am. med. Ass.,* 1978, *240,* 2526; *Lancet,* 1979, *1,* 1383.

Mention of the bactericidal and sterilising roles of rifampicin and pyrazinamide in short-term therapy of tuberculosis. Isoniazid also has some sterilising activity, that is the ability to kill bacterial persisters; streptomycin has less activity. Bacteriostatic drugs such as ethambutol or thiacetazone do not appear to contribute to short-term therapy in patients with drug sensitive infections although they may prevent the emergence of further drug resistance in patients with an initially resistant strain.— W. Fox, *Bull. int. Un. Tuberc.,* 1978, *53,* 268.

Further reports and references on short-term treatment of tuberculosis.— G. T. Werner and D. K. Sareen (letter), *Lancet,* 1976, *1,* 38; *ibid.,* 162; *Tubercle,* 1977, *58,* 1; S. Pretet *et al., Bull. int. Un. Tuberc.,* 1978, *53,* 244; D. A. Mitchison and J. M. Dickinson, *ibid.,* 254; V. R. Aber and A. J. Nunn, *ibid.,* 260; *ibid.,* 1979, *54,* 9 to 31 (see p. 123 for correction); E. Freerksen and M. Rosenfeld, *ibid.,* 363; J. O. Pearson (letter), *Lancet,* 1979, *2,* 420.

Two-month and three-month treatment regimens. Results of a controlled study of 2- and 3-month chemotherapy regimens in Hong Kong patients indicated that whereas these appeared to be effective for patients who were sputum-culture negative, they were inadequate for those who were sputum-culture positive. One of the following chemotherapy regimens was given to 1072 patients with radiographically active pulmonary tuberculosis: no chemotherapy until confirmation of the activity of the disease; streptomycin, isoniazid, rifampicin, and pyrazinamide daily for 2 months; the same regimen for 3 months; or a standard 12-month control regimen comprising streptomycin, sodium aminosalicylate, and isoniazid. Sputum examination indicated that 691 were initially pretreatment sputum-culture negative, and 381 were pretreatment sputum-culture positive. Of 73 patients with drug-sensitive positive sputum cultures given the 2-month regimen 10 (14%) suffered bacteriological relapse within 12 months, and of 74 given the 3-month regimen 5 (7%) did so, compared with none of 83 in the standard 12-month regimen group. Of 175 and 168 pretreatment sputum-culture negative patients who received these regimens only 1% relapsed. Of 181 sputum-culture negative patients who received no chemotherapy, active disease was confirmed in 61 (34%) within 12 months which indicated that these 2- and 3-month courses had reduced the expected rate of bacteriologically confirmed activity from 34% to 1%.—First Report of the Hong Kong Chest Service, Tuberculosis Research Centre, Madras, India, and British MRC Controlled Trial of 3-Month and 2-Month Regimens of

Chemotherapy, *Lancet,* 1979, *1,* 1361. Comment.—*ibid.,* 1383.

Four-month and six-month treatment regimens. A controlled study on 4-month regimens was carried out initially in 1024 patients, but as a result of high relapse-rates noted on interim analysis the results of only the first 696 patients were taken, the regimen being prolonged to 6 months in the remaining patients. Of the 696 patients, 619 were suitable for analysis and had received the following regimens: streptomycin, isoniazid, rifampicin, and pyrazinamide daily for 8 weeks followed by isoniazid, rifampicin, and pyrazinamide daily for 9 weeks (125 patients); the first 4 drugs for 8 weeks followed by isoniazid plus rifampicin daily for 9 weeks (124 patients); the first 4 drugs for 8 weeks followed by isoniazid plus pyrazinamide daily for 9 weeks (124 patients); the first 4 drugs daily for 8 weeks followed by isoniazid alone daily for 9 weeks (119 patients); isoniazid, rifampicin, and pyrazinamide daily for 8 weeks followed by isoniazid alone daily for 9 weeks (127 patients). In the 2 regimens that included rifampicin throughout the 4 months the rate of bacteriological relapse was 8% in the first 6 months after stopping chemotherapy, but in the 3 where it was only given for the first 2 months it was 24 to 32%. Administration of pyrazinamide in the second 2 months did not appear to reduce the relapse-rate. Administration of streptomycin during the first 2 months appeared to have some beneficial effect, although it did not seem that streptomycin is a major drug for short-course chemotherapy. It was considered that if (as seemed likely with the best regimens in this study) a failure-rate of less than 20% could be achieved with short-term therapy, this would be a major therapeutic advance.—East African/British MRCs, First Report of Fourth Study, *Lancet,* 1978, *2,* 334. A similar study carried out by the Singapore and British MRCs.— S. C. Poh, *Bull. int. Un. Tuberc.,* 1978, *53,* 242. See also *Am. Rev. resp. Dis.,* 1979, *119,* 579.

Six-month treatment regimens. A comparison of 4 regimens involving the daily administration of streptomycin sulphate 1 g intramuscularly and isoniazid 300 mg given alone or with rifampicin 450 or 600 mg, pyrazinamide 2 g, or thiacetazone 150 mg for 6 months, and 1 regimen involving isoniazid and thiacetazone in the above dosages given daily for 18 months, with streptomycin sulphate 1 g intramuscularly daily for the first 8 weeks, in 1137 tuberculous patients. The relapse-rates at 30 months for patients admitted concurrently were 2% of 112 patients in the rifampicin group, 11% of 112 in the pyrazinamide group, 22% of 104 in the thiacetazone group, 29% of 112 in patients given streptomycin only with isoniazid, and 4% for 102 patients on the 18-month course. The rifampicin and pyrazinamide regimens were considered to be superior to the others at 30 months (including the 18-month regimen which had a comparatively high default-rate) when taking both the effectiveness and acceptability of the schedules into account.—East African and British MRCs, *Lancet,* 1972, *1,* 1079; *ibid.,* 1105; *ibid.,* 1973, *1,* 1331; *ibid.,* 1974, *2,* 237.

A second cooperative study was carried out on 953 hospitalised patients with previously untreated pulmonary tuberculosis. After 6 months, analysis was carried out on 734 patients who had been treated as follows: (1) 181 patients received streptomycin sulphate 1 g intramuscularly with isoniazid 300 mg and rifampicin 450 mg for patients under 50 kg body-weight or 600 mg for heavier patients by mouth daily for 6 months; (2) 183 received the same daily dose of isoniazid and rifampicin only for 6 months; (3) 191 received the same doses of streptomycin, isoniazid, and rifampicin as in (1), with pyrazinamide 1.5 g daily for light and 2 g for heavy patients for 2 months followed for the next 4 months by reduced treatment with thiacetazone 150 mg and isoniazid 300 mg daily; (4) 179 patients received the same treatment for the first 2 months as those in group 3, followed for the next 4 months by twice-weekly doses of streptomycin sulphate 1 g intramuscularly, isoniazid 600 mg for light and 900 mg for heavy patients, and pyrazinamide 3 g for light and 4 g for heavy patients. There were only 3 failures in all the groups. However, during the 6 months 61 patients were excluded from the analysis and 4 of these had died of their tuberculosis early in their treatment. A favourable response was achieved with all cultures proving negative in 163 of 181 patients in group 1 (90%), 170 of 183 in group 2 (93%), 170 of 191 in group 3 (89%), and 161 of 179 in group 4 (90%). In the remaining patients responses were doubtful although only 6 resistant strains were obtained. Adverse reactions were evaluated in 943 patients and of these, 22 patients, evenly spread throughout the 4 groups, experienced side-effects. Symptomatic treatment was all that was required in 14 but in the other 8 treatment had to be interrupted or one or more of the drugs withdrawn because of jaundice, rashes, giddiness, paraesthesia, or arthralgia.

Bacteriological follow-up at 12 months, 6 months after treatment had ended, was possible in 677 of the 731 patients who had shown a good or doubtful response and relapses were observed in 31, there being no significant difference between any of the groups. In only 1 patient was the relapse due to a resistant organism. All the schedules were considered to be effective. The use of streptomycin in the triple regimen (group 1) did not appear to add to the effectiveness. However, the initial intensive phases in groups 3 and 4 eliminated sensitive bacilli more quickly than was the case in groups 1 and 2.—East African/British MRCs, *Lancet,* 1974, *2,* 1100. Follow-up of approximately 160 patients in each group showed relapse-rates to be 2, 7, 7, and 4% respectively for the 4 regimens at 18 months (12 months after treatment). Most relapses occurred in the first 6 months with sensitive cultures.— J. F. Heffernan, *Tubercle,* 1975, *56,* 165.

In a 6-month regimen consisting of rifampicin, isoniazid, and ethambutol and reported by M. Zierski it appeared to be unnecessary to give rifampicin and isoniazid daily in the continuation phase after the initial intensive phase in the treatment of tuberculosis. The relapse-rates were similar when rifampicin, isoniazid, and ethambutol were given twice weekly.— J. R. Bignall, *Bull. int. Un. Tuberc.,* 1978, *53* (Mar.), 13.

Bacteriological conversion of sputum cultures occurred in 94% of 56 patients after 2 months' treatment with a regimen containing rifampicin, isoniazid, and pyrazinamide and in 100% after 6 months' treatment. It was considered that pyrazinamide was less well tolerated than ethambutol and ethambutol was a suitable substitute for pyrazinamide in 54 similar patients.— F. J. G. Sanz, *Bull. int. Un. Tuberc.,* 1978, *53* (Mar.), 25.

Excellent results were obtained in tubercular patients given 3 thrice-weekly 6-month treatment regimens (each containing isoniazid and rifampicin, together with: streptomycin, pyrazinamide, and ethambutol, or streptomycin and pyrazinamide, or pyrazinamide and ethambutol) and one daily 6-month regimen (containing isoniazid and rifampicin together with pyrazinamide and ethambutol), all given under supervision. All 4 regimens were highly effective, with bacteriological relapse-rates of 2% or less, as assessed up to 12 months after the end of chemotherapy, even for those with strains initially resistant to isoniazid and streptomycin. A high relapse-rate (8%) occurred in patients given thrice-weekly isoniazid, rifampicin, streptomycin, and ethambutol, confirming the importance of pyrazinamide in short-course chemotherapy, and the very small contribution of ethambutol and streptomycin.—Hong Kong Chest Service/British MRC, *Lancet,* 1981, *1,* 171.

Further references.— J. A. Pilheu, *Chest,* 1977, *71,* 583. Onadeko, B.O.; Sofowora, E.O *Afr. J. Med. med. Sci.,* 1978, *7,* 175.

Six-month and eight-month treatment regimens. Treatment for pulmonary tuberculosis was assessed in 842 of 1056 patients who had not received any previous antituberculous chemotherapy and who were treated with one of the following regimens: (1) streptomycin, isoniazid, and rifampicin given daily for 6 months; (2) streptomycin, isoniazid, rifampicin, and pyrazinamide given daily for 2 months, followed by streptomycin, isoniazid, and pyrazinamide twice a week; (3) the same regimen as (2) but with pyrazinamide replaced by ethambutol throughout; (4) streptomycin, isoniazid, rifampicin, and pyrazinamide given thrice weekly for 4 months, followed by streptomycin, isoniazid, and pyrazinamide twice weekly. The last 3 regimens were given for 6 or 8 months. All except one of 680 patients who had bacilli sensitive to isoniazid, streptomycin, and rifampicin before treatment, had a favourable bacteriological response. Relapse-rates at 24 months were assessed in 639 of these patients and in the ethambutol regimen were 19 of 84 (23%) when given for 6 months and 8 of 84 (10%) when given for 8 months compared with 6 of 87 (7%) and 3 of 87 (3%) in the corresponding pyrazinamide regimen. The relapse rates in regimen (4) were 4 of 71 (6%) and 1 of 83 (1%) and the relapse-rate in regimen (1) was 8 of 143 (6%). Evaluation of the 162 patients with bacilli resistant to isoniazid, streptomycin, or both drugs suggested that short-term regimens used to treat these patients should include rifampicin and another drug other than isoniazid and streptomycin. A course of rifampicin as used in regimens (2) and (4) was considered to be inadequate. Although ethambutol was more effective than pyrazinamide in preventing failure during chemotherapy associated with the emergence of further drug resistance the highest relapse-rates occurred after the ethambutol regimen.—Hong Kong Chest Service/British MRC, *Tubercle,* 1979, *60,* 201.

The final results reported up to 24 months after the end of chemotherapy in a comparative study of 4 treatment regimens, in 932 patients with pulmonary tuberculosis, indicate that 8-month regimens are more effective than 6-month regimens and that thiacetazone with isoniazid is a useful combination in the continuation phase of treatment. An intermittent continuation phase of twice-weekly streptomycin, isoniazid, and pyrazinamide is of value and the place of pyrazinamide in the initial phase of treatment is also confirmed. The 4 regimens, given for 6 or 8 months were: (1) an initial course of streptomycin, isoniazid, rifampicin, and pyrazinamide daily for 2 months followed by a continuation course of thiacetazone and isoniazid given daily; (2) as in (1) but with an initial course of only 1 month; (3) as for (2) but with a continuation course of streptomycin, isoniazid, and pyrazinamide given twice weekly for up to 6 months; followed, in the 8-month regimen by thiacetazone and isoniazid given daily; (4) as for (1) but without pyrazinamide.—Third Study of East African/British MRCs, *Tubercle,* 1980, *61,* 59.

Nine-month treatment regimens. A controlled study was carried out on 696 patients with pulmonary tuberculosis to evaluate the effective duration of treatment. Patients with little or no cavitation (any cavities were less than 2 cm in diameter) were treated with rifampicin 600 mg, or 450 mg where they weighed less than 50 kg, and isoniazid 300 mg both daily for 6 or 12 months. Patients with larger cavitation were treated for 9 or 18 months. In addition all patients under the age of 60 years received either ethambutol 25 mg per kg body-weight by mouth daily or streptomycin 750 mg intramuscularly for 6 days a week for the first 8 weeks of treatment. Patients aged 60 years or more were given ethambutol as the third agent for 8 weeks. Of those with little or no cavitation, 1 out of 174 failed to respond to the 6-month course and during the following year 5 relapsed; this compared with no failures among the 177 treated for 1 year and no relapses during the following 6 months. Of those with larger cavities all 151 responded to 9 months of treatment and no relapses occurred during the next 9 months. The 18-month schedule was equally effective in 155 patients with no failures.—British Thoracic and Tuberculosis Association, *Lancet,* 1975, *1,* 119. See also *idem,* 1976, *2,* 1102.

A report of the final results 54 months from the start of chemotherapy. There was only one further relapse. This was in a patient on the 6-month regimen, bringing the total number of relapses for this group to 9 (7%) of 130 patients still available for analysis. During follow-up ranging from 3 to 4 years after stopping chemotherapy there have been 11 relapses, 10 within 2 years of stopping chemotherapy; in all 11 patients relapse was due to organisms sensitive to streptomycin, rifampicin, ethambutol, and isoniazid. Although follow-up had not been planned beyond 54 months, 2 patients in the 9-month group relapsed 4 to 5 years after stopping chemotherapy, also with organisms sensitive to the drugs used in the study. The research committee of the British Thoracic Association still believes that the 1976 recommendation of 9 months' chemotherapy with rifampicin and isoniazid, plus ethambutol 25 mg per kg body-weight daily in the first 2 months, is the preferred treatment for pulmonary tuberculosis in Britain.—Third Report of a Controlled Trial by the British Thoracic Association, *ibid.,* 1980, *1,* 1182; *ibid.,* *2,* 272.

Further references.— C. O. Anah, *Niger. med. J.,* 1979, *9,* 80; A. W. Lees *et al.* (letter), *Lancet* 1980, *2,* 796.

7551-s

Aminosalicylic Acid *(U.S.P.).*

Para-aminosalicylic Acid; PAS; 4-Aminosalicylic Acid; Aminosalylum; Pasalicylum. 4-Amino-2-hydroxybenzoic acid.

$C_7H_7NO_3$=153.1.

CAS — 65-49-6.

Pharmacopoeias. In *Arg., Aust., Braz., Hung., Pol., Span., Turk.,* and *U.S.*

A white or almost white, bulky powder which darkens on exposure to air and light; it is odourless or has a slight acetous odour and a mild acidic unpleasant taste.

Soluble 1 in about 600 of water, 1 in about 20 of alcohol, 1 in 4000 of chloroform, and 1 in 50 of ether. A saturated solution in water has a pH of 3 to 3.7.

Incompatible with acids, ferric salts, and oxidising agents. Aqueous solutions are unstable. The

U.S.P. directs that a solution must not be used if it is darker in colour than a freshly prepared solution. **Store** at a temperature not exceeding 30° in airtight containers. Protect from light.

Decomposition by heat. On heating a solution of aminosalicylic acid at 100° for 30 minutes, decomposition was negligible at a pH above 7.5, but 15% at pH 6. The decomposition raised the pH, which retarded the decomposition.— V. G. Jensen and E. Jerslev, *J. Pharm. Pharmac.*, 1953, *5*, 328.

Stability. Aqueous solutions of aminosalicylic acid were stable at ordinary temperatures if the pH was not less than 6. At pH 5, 50% decomposed in 10 weeks, at pH 4, in 10 days.— A. Ågren, *J. Pharm. Pharmac.*, 1955, *7*, 549.

The chromogen which discoloured tablets of aminosalicylic acid and the sodium salt was 3,3′-dihydroxyazoxybenzene. This chromogen could be produced by oxidation or sunlight irradiation of *m*-aminophenol, a common impurity of aminosalicylic acid.— I. K. Shih, *J. pharm. Sci.*, 1971, *60*, 1886.

Aminosalicylic acid has the actions described under Sodium Aminosalicylate, p.1582, and has been used in similar doses, with other antituberculous drugs, in the treatment of tuberculosis. It is less well tolerated than the sodium salt.

For references to granules of aminosalicylic acid delaying the absorption of rifampicin, see Rifampicin, p.1578.

Absorption and fate. Aminosalicylic acid crystallised with ascorbic acid (PAS-C) in a single daily dose of 6 g or a divided daily dose of 12 g produced later and higher peak serum concentrations than did equivalent doses of sodium aminosalicylate.— J. M. Schless *et al.*, *Dis. Chest*, 1966, *50*, 595, per *J. Am. med. Ass.*, 1967, *199* (Jan. 30), A140.

Some 58 to 73% of aminosalicylic acid was bound in the body to serum proteins. The half-life in serum was 45 minutes and more than 80% was excreted in urine.— C. M. Kunin, *Ann. intern. Med.*, 1967, *67*, 151.

The biological half-life of aminosalicylic acid was variously reported as 0.75 to 1.9 hours.— W. A. Ritschel, *Drug Intell. & clin. Pharm.*, 1970, *4*, 332.

In 12 healthy subjects the mean peak plasma concentration of aminosalicylic acid was 50 µg per ml following the administration of 4 g by mouth as tablets. The mean half-life was 0.94 hour. About 50% of the drug and metabolites was excreted in 5 to 6 hours, and about 77% of the dose was excreted in 24 hours. About 56% of the dose was metabolised by acetylation.— S. H. Wan *et al.*, *J. pharm. Sci.*, 1974, *63*, 708.

Hyperlipoproteinaemia. A highly purified form of aminosalicylic acid, obtained by recrystallisation with ascorbic acid (PAS-C), was given to 29 patients with type IIa or IIb hyperlipoproteinaemia, in a dose of 6 to 8 g daily in 4 divided doses. A 12-week double-blind crossover study in 14 patients and a similar single-blind crossover study in a further 15 patients both demonstrated a significant decrease in mean serum-cholesterol concentration and a decrease in mean serum-triglyceride concentration. In 13 patients aminosalicylic acid was given for 6 to 12 months and the reduction in serum-cholesterol and triglyceride concentrations was sustained for the duration of the treatment. Changes in body-weight were slight and in general the drug was well tolerated.— P. J. Barter *et al.*, *Ann. intern. Med.*, 1974, *81*, 619. See also R. I. Levy and B. M. Rifkind, *Drugs*, 1973, *6*, 12; *J. Am. med. Ass.*, 1974, *228*, 961; P. T. Kuo *et al.*, *Circulation*, 1976, *53*, 338; B. Vessby *et al.*, *Clin. Pharmac. Ther.*, 1978, *23*, 651.

Preparations

Aminosalicylic Acid Tablets *(U.S.P.)*. Tablets containing aminosalicylic acid. Store at a temperature not exceeding 30° in airtight containers. Protect from light.

Proprietary Names

Gamirpas *(Gamir, Spain)*; Nemasol *(ICN, Canad.)*; Parasal *(Panray, USA)*; Teebacin Acid *(Consolidated Midland, USA)*.

7552-w

Calcium Aminosalicylate *(B.P. 1973)*.

Calc. Aminosal.; Calcii Aminosalicylas; Calcii Para-aminosalicylas; Calcium PAS; Calcium Para-aminosalicylate; Aminosalicylate Calcium *(U.S.P.)*. Calcium 4-amino-2-hydroxybenzoate trihydrate.

$(C_7H_6NO_3)_2Ca,3H_2O=398.4$.

CAS — 133-15-3 (anhydrous).

Pharmacopoeias. In *Arg.* (anhydrous); in *Aust.*, *Braz.*, *Fr.*, *Int.*, *Neth.*, *Swiss* and *U.S.*; in *Ind.* and *Nord.* (½H_2O); in *Port.* (½ or $3H_2O$); and in *Jap.* ($7H_2O$).

A white or slightly yellow, odourless, hygroscopic, crystalline powder with an alkaline bitter-sweet taste. Calcium aminosalicylate trihydrate 1.3 g is approximately equivalent to 1 g of aminosalicylic acid.

Soluble 1 in 7 to 10 of water and slightly soluble in alcohol. A 2% solution in water has a pH of 6 to 8. Aqueous solutions are unstable and darken in colour. The *U.S.P.* directs that solutions should be prepared within 24 hours of administration and that a solution must not be used if it is darker in colour than a freshly prepared solution. **Store** in airtight containers. Protect from light.

Calcium aminosalicylate has the actions described under Sodium Aminosalicylate, p.1582, and has been given in similar doses, with other antituberculous drugs, in the treatment of tuberculosis. It may be more palatable than the sodium salt and can be used in patients on a restricted sodium diet. Calcium aminosalicylate should not be given to patients with hypercalcaemia.

Absorption and fate. In 12 healthy subjects the mean plasma concentration of calcium aminosalicylate was 140 µg per ml following the administration of 4 g by mouth as tablets. The mean half-life was 0.91 hour and about 50% of the drug and its metabolites was excreted in 2 to 3 hours. About 98% of the dose was excreted in 24 hours, about 57% as the acetylated form.— S. H. Wan *et al.*, *J. pharm. Sci.*, 1974, *63*, 708.

Preparations

Aminosalicylate Calcium Capsules *(U.S.P.)*. Calcium Aminosalicylate Capsules. Capsules containing calcium aminosalicylate. Store in airtight containers. Protect from light.

Aminosalicylate Calcium Tablets *(U.S.P.)*. Calcium Aminosalicylate Tablets. Tablets containing calcium aminosalicylate. Store in airtight containers. Protect from light.

Calcium Aminosalicylate Tablets *(B.P.C. 1973)*. Tablets containing calcium aminosalicylate; they are sugar-coated; the coating may be coloured. Store in a cool place in airtight containers.

7553-e

Calcium Benzamidosalicylate. Benzoylpas Calcium *(U.S.P.)*; Bepascum; Calcii Benzamidosalicylas. Calcium 4-benzamido-2-hydroxybenzoate pentahydrate.

$(C_{14}H_{10}NO_4)_2Ca,5H_2O=642.6$.

CAS — 13898-58-3 (4-benzamidosalicylic acid); 528-96-1 (calcium salt, anhydrous); 5631-00-5 (calcium salt, pentahydrate).

Pharmacopoeias. In *Cz.*, *Int.*, *Rus.*, and *U.S.*

A white to cream-coloured odourless almost tasteless powder. Calcium benzamidosalicylate 2.1 g is approximately equivalent to 1 g of aminosalicylic acid.

Soluble 1 in 700 of water; slightly soluble in methyl alcohol; very slightly soluble in alcohol; practically insoluble in chloroform and ether. **Store** in airtight containers at a temperature not exceeding 30°. Protect from light.

Calcium benzamidosalicylate has the actions described under Sodium Aminosalicylate, p.1582, but is absorbed more slowly from the gastro-intestinal tract and is slowly hydrolysed to produce lower though more prolonged plasma concentrations of aminosalicylate. Calcium benzamidosalicylate should not be given to patients with hypercalcaemia but may be used in patients on a restricted sodium diet and is considered to be better tolerated than sodium aminosalicylate. It has been given with other antituberculous drugs in the treatment of tuberculosis in doses of 5 g twice or thrice daily usually after food.

Absorption and fate. The biological half-life of calcium benzamidosalicylate is 2.6 hours.— W. A. Ritschel, *Drug Intell. & clin. Pharm.*, 1970, *4*, 332.

Preparations

Benzoylpas Calcium Tablets *(U.S.P.)*. Tablets containing calcium benzamidosalicylate. Protect from light.

Proprietary Names

B-Pas *(Spain)*.

Calcium benzamidosalicylate was formerly marketed in Great Britain under the proprietary name Therapas *(Smith & Nephew Pharmaceuticals)*.

7554-l

Capreomycin Sulphate *(B.P.)*.

Capromycin Sulphate.

CAS — 11003-38-6 (capreomycin); 1405-37-4 (sulphate).

Pharmacopoeias. In *Br.* *U.S.* includes Sterile Capreomycin Sulfate.

A mixture of the sulphates of the polypeptide antimicrobial substances produced by certain strains of *Streptomyces capreolus* and containing not less than 90% of capreomycin I. It contains not less than 700 units per mg.

Capreomycin I consists of capreomycin IA ($C_{25}H_{44}N_{14}O_8=668.7$) and capreomycin IB ($C_{25}H_{44}N_{14}O_7=652.7$) which predominates. Capreomycin II which makes up about 10% of the mixture consists of capreomycin IIA and capreomycin IIB.

A white or almost white odourless or almost odourless solid. It loses not more than 10% of its weight on drying. One million units of capreomycin is approximately equivalent to 1 g of capreomycin.

Soluble 1 in 1 of water; practically insoluble in alcohol, chloroform, ether, and most other organic solvents. A solution in water is laevorotatory. A 3% solution in water has a pH of 4.5 to 7.5. **Store** at a temperature not exceeding 15° in airtight containers; if intended for parenteral administration, the containers should be sterile and sealed to exclude micro-organisms.

The structure of capreomycin IB. The capreomycins were closely related in structure to viomycin.— B. W. Bycroft *et al.*, *Nature*, 1971, *231*, 301.

Units. One unit of capreomycin is contained in 0.001087 mg of the first International Reference Preparation (1967) of capreomycin sulphate which contains 920 units per mg.

Adverse Effects. The effects of capreomycin on the kidney and eighth cranial nerve are similar to those of streptomycin (p.1213). Nitrogen retention, progressive renal damage, disturbances of calcium and potassium metabolism, and abnormalities in liver function may occur. Vertigo, tinnitus, and occasionally deafness may also occur and are sometimes irreversible. Allergic reactions including skin rashes, fever, and eosinophilia have been reported. The intramuscular injection of capreomycin sometimes causes pain and induration.

Only 14 of 34 patients completed 2 years' treatment with capreomycin. Treatment was withdrawn in 8 due to nitrogen retention or electrolyte disturbances resulting from severe tubular dysfunction, in 3 due to ototoxicity, and in 1 due to a severe allergic reaction. Depression in 3 patients was associated with electrolyte disturbance and 2 other patients developed lethargy and depression. Decreased serum concentrations of calcium, magnesium, and potassium might be detected during treatment.— C. M. Hesling, *Tubercle*, 1969, *50*, *Suppl.*, 39.

Further references: A. M. Holmes *et al.*, *Thorax*, 1970, *25*, 608.

Precautions. Capreomycin should be given with care and in reduced dosage to patients with impaired renal function. Care is also essential in patients with signs of cranial nerve damage or a history of allergy to other drugs. It is advisable to carry out regular checks on renal and auditory function and on blood-potassium concentrations in all patients.

Large doses of capreomycin can produce neuromuscular blockade which is enhanced by ether and may be antagonised by neostigmine or a calcium salt. Capreomycin should not be administered with streptomycin, kanamycin, or viomycin nor with other drugs known to be ototoxic or nephrotoxic.

Antimicrobial Action. Capreomycin is tuberculostatic against various mycobacteria and an MIC of 10 µg per ml has been reported for *Mycobacterium tuberculosis*. Resistance develops readily if capreomycin is used alone. It shows cross-resistance with kanamycin, neomycin, and viomycin, but cross-resistance has not been reported between capreomycin and streptomycin, cycloserine, aminosalicylic acid, ethionamide, isoniazid, ethambutol, or rifampicin.

References: M. Tsukamura, *Am. Rev. resp. Dis.*, 1969, *99*, 780.

Absorption and Fate. Capreomycin is poorly absorbed from the gastro-intestinal tract. A dose of 1 million units of capreomycin (approximately equivalent to 1 g) administered intramuscularly has been reported to give a peak serum concentration of about 30 µg per ml after 1 or 2 hours. Serum concentrations quickly fall and about 50% of a dose is excreted unchanged in the urine within 8 to 12 hours.

Capreomycin is considered to be unable to penetrate to the cavities in fibro-sclerotic lesions in patients with pulmonary tuberculosis.— M. Tsukamura, *Tubercle*, 1972, *53*, 47.

Uses. Capreomycin sulphate is a secondary tuberculostatic. It is less effective than streptomycin or rifampicin and is employed when the patient is unable to tolerate more effective tuberculostatic drugs or when the causative micro-organism has become resistant to them—see Treatment of Tuberculosis, p.1565. It is preferred to kanamycin or viomycin because the incidence of severe side-effects is less. Capreomycin should always be given in conjunction with other antituberculous agents such as ethambutol or rifampicin to prevent the emergence of resistant strains.

Capreomycin sulphate is administered by deep intramuscular injection. The usual dose is 1 million units, equivalent to about 1 g of capreomycin, daily with a maximum of 20 000 units (20 mg) per kg body-weight.

Pulmonary tuberculosis. For early reviews and discussions of the use of capreomycin in the treatment of tuberculosis, see *Tubercle*, 1966, *47*, 234; T. M. Wilson, *Practitioner*, 1967, *199*, 817; *Br. med. J.*, 1969, *3*, 487; *J. Am. med. Ass.*, 1973, *223*, 179.

Preparations

Capreomycin Injection *(B.P.)*. A sterile solution of capreomycin sulphate prepared by dissolving the sterile contents of a sealed container (Capreomycin Sulphate for Injection) in the requisite amount of Water for Injections. If stored at 2° to 8° the solution should be used within 14 days of preparation; at temperatures approaching 20° it should be used within 48 hours.

Sterile Capreomycin Sulfate *(U.S.P.)*. The disulphate of capreomycin; it has a potency equivalent to 700 to 1050 µg of capreomycin per mg.

Capastat *(Dista, UK)*. Capreomycin sulphate, available as powder for preparing injections, in vials each containing 1 million units equivalent to about 1 g of capreomycin. (Also available as Capastat in *Arg., Canad., S.Afr., Spain, Swed., Switz., USA*).

Other Proprietary Names

Caprocin *(Austral.)*; Ogostal *(Ger.)*.

7555-y

Cyacetazide *(B. Vet. C. 1965)*. Cyanoacetohydrazidum; Cyanacetic Acid Hydrazide. Cyanoacetohydrazide.
$C_3H_5N_3O$=99.09.

CAS — 140-87-4.

Pharmacopoeias. In *Nord.*

A white or almost white, almost odourless and tasteless, crystalline powder. M.p. 106° to 108°. **Soluble** 1 in 3.5 of water and 1 in 50 of alcohol; slightly soluble in chloroform and ether. A 10% solution has a pH of 6.5 to 7.5. Aqueous solutions are unstable.

Cyacetazide is a hydrazide derivative and has actions similar to those of isoniazid (p.1571). It was formerly used in the treatment of tuberculosis in conjunction with other tuberculostatic agents.

In veterinary medicine, it has been used as an anthelmintic in the treatment of lungworm infestations.

Proprietary Names

Armazal *(UCB-Pevya, Spain)*; Cianpas (as aminosalicylate) *(Infale, Spain)*.

7556-j

Ethambutol Hydrochloride *(B.P., U.S.P.)*.

(+)-(*R,R*)-*NN'*-Ethylenebis(2-aminobutan-1-ol) dihydrochloride.
$C_{10}H_{24}N_2O_2$,2HCl=277.2.

CAS — 74-55-5 (ethambutol); 1070-11-7 (hydrochloride).

Pharmacopoeias. In *Br., Braz., Jap., Jug., Nord.*, and *U.S.*

A white, odourless or almost odourless crystalline hygroscopic powder with a bitter taste. M.p. 199° to 204°. **Soluble** 1 in 1 of water, 1 in 4 of alcohol, 1 in 850 of chloroform, and 1 in 9 of methyl alcohol; very slightly soluble in ether. A solution in water is dextrorotatory. Solutions are stable when heated at 121° for 10 minutes. **Store** in airtight containers.

Adverse Effects. Ethambutol is generally well tolerated, but may provoke retrobulbar neuritis with a reduction of visual acuity, central scotoma, and green-red colour blindness. The effect on vision depends on the dose, and may be associated with progressive depletion of copper and zinc; it is usually reversible when ethambutol is withdrawn and may affect one or both eyes.

Allergic rashes and gastro-intestinal disturbances have been reported. Jaundice and peripheral neuritis have occurred on rare occasions. Other reactions reported include confusion, disorientation, hallucinations, joint pain, fever, malaise, headache, dizziness, anorexia, and abdominal pain although, since ethambutol is never given alone, other antituberculous drugs may be responsible. Teratogenic effects have been seen in *animals*, but not in man.

Effects on the blood. Neutropenia in a 75-year-old man treated with isoniazid, ethambutol, and rifampicin. Neutropenia was induced, on challenge, by each of the 3 agents.— P. F. Jenkins *et al.*, *Br. med. J.*, 1980, *280*, 1069.

Effects on the eye. Of 59 patients receiving ethambutol in a daily dosage exceeding 35 mg per kg body-weight, 11 developed ocular complications compared with 2 of 59 patients receiving less than 30 mg per kg. The time before onset of toxicity ranged from 69 to 313 days in the high dosage group. Visual acuity took up to 11 months after discontinuation of the drug to return to normal. One patient developed a permanent defect with optic atrophy in 1 eye. Ocular toxicity occurred exclusively in males.— J. E. Leibold, *Ann. N.Y. Acad. Sci.*, 1966, *135*, 904. Abnormal fundi or optic disks and changes in intra-ocular pressure were not seen in 32 patients taking ethambutol about 14 mg per kg body-weight daily for 3 or more months.— P. R. M. Pattisson *et al.*, *Tubercle*, 1978, *59*, 33.

Toxic amblyopia developed in 4 patients given ethambutol in normal doses. Various degrees of recovery occurred over 5 to 12 months when ethambutol was withdrawn.— R. S. Bartholomew, *Br. med. J.*, 1976, *1*, 1535. See also G. J. Barron *et al.*, *Am. J. Ophthal.*, 1974, *77*, 256.

A report of open-angle glaucoma of the hypersecretion type occurring in a study of 17 patients given ethambutol 25 mg per kg body-weight daily for 4 months.— S. S. Bhola and S. D. Purohit, *Ind. J. Chest Dis. Allied Sci.*, 1976, *18*, 189.

Further references: I. Kass, *Tubercle*, 1965, *46*, 166; P. A. Gardiner, *Br. med. J.*, 1979, *1*, 460; B. S. Kuming and L. Braude (letter), *S. Afr. med. J.*, 1979, *55*, 4.

Effects on the kidneys. Ethambutol might have caused renal failure in 2 patients.— J. Collier *et al.*, *Br. med. J.*, 1976, *2*, 1105.

A report of acute diffuse interstitial nephritis in 3 patients attributed to antituberculous therapy and especially isoniazid and/or ethambutol.— W. J. Stone *et al.*, *Antimicrob. Ag. Chemother.*, 1976, *10*, 164.

Effects on the liver. A review indicating that retreatment regimens for tuberculosis based on rifampicin with ethambutol carry a very low risk of hepatitis.— D. J. Girling, *Tubercle*, 1978, *59*, 13.

Effects on the nervous system. Peripheral neuropathy considered to be due to ethambutol was found in 3 tubercular patients who had received ethambutol 13 to 50 mg per kg body-weight, among other drugs. In each case there was improvement and some reversal of damage when ethambutol was discontinued.— P. Tugwell and S. L. James, *Postgrad. med. J.*, 1972, *48*, 667.

Further references: V. S. Nair *et al.*, *Chest*, 1980, *77*, 98.

Effects on the skin. A generalised erythematous macular and papular eruption developed in a 23-year-old woman about 8 days after starting to take ethambutol; challenge confirmed that ethambutol was responsible.— J. S. Pasricha and A. J. Kanwar, *Archs Derm.*, 1977, *113*, 1122.

For a report of the Stevens-Johnson syndrome, associated with rifampicin therapy, possibly being triggered by ethambutol, see Rifampicin, p.1578.

Hyperuricaemia. A report of hyperuricaemia occurring in patients given ethambutol for active tuberculosis.— A. E. Postlethwaite *et al.*, *New Engl. J. Med.*, 1972, *286*, 761.

Acute gouty arthritis considered to be due to ethambutol was reported in 2 tuberculous patients who had received ethambutol 15 mg per kg body-weight daily, among other drugs. Both patients responded to treatment with colchicine. Acute gouty arthritis was also reported in a further patient who had received ethambutol and pyrazinamide; pyrazinamide was considered to be contributory.— T. H. Self *et al.* (letter), *Chest*, 1977, *71*, 561.

Overdosage. Post-mortem findings following a fatal overdose of rifampicin and ethambutol.— D. B. Jack *et al.* (letter), *Lancet*, 1978, *2*, 1107.

Pregnancy and the neonate. Two pregnant patients were treated with ethambutol; 1 delivered a normal infant and in the other, pregnancy was terminated and the foetus was found to be normal. Published reports listed 18 pregnant women who were given ethambutol and no adverse effect was seen on the foetus.— S. Keidan (letter), *Tubercle*, 1973, *54*, 84. See also J. M. Shneerson and R. S. Francis, *Tubercle*, 1979, *60*, 167.

Treatment of Adverse Effects. Overdosage with ethambutol should be treated with gastric lavage. Concentrations in the blood are reduced by haemodialysis or peritoneal dialysis.

Precautions. Ethambutol should be given in reduced dosage to patients with impaired kidney function. It should be given with great care in patients with reduced visual acuity. Ocular examination is recommended before treatment with ethambutol and some authorities consider that regular examinations are necessary during treatment; ethambutol should be withdrawn if vision deteriorates. Serum concentrations of ethambutol should not exceed 5 µg per ml.

Ethambutol may precipitate attacks of gout.

Pregnancy and the neonate. Ethambutol is considered to be one of the safer tuberculostatic drugs in pregnancy.— J. MacVicar, *Practitioner*, 1978, *221*, 885; M. de Swiet, *Prescribers' J.*, 1979, *19*, 59.

See also under Adverse Effects above, and p.1564.

Antimicrobial Action. Ethambutol is bacteriostatic. It is effective against *Mycobacterium tuberculosis* and *M. bovis* with an MIC of 0.5 to 8 µg per ml and also against some atypical mycobacteria including *M. kansasii*. Activity against other micro-organisms has not been reported. It is effective against tubercle bacilli resistant to other tuberculostatics. Cross-resistance has not been reported.

Primary resistance to ethambutol is uncommon but resistant strains of *M. tuberculosis* are readily produced if ethambutol is used alone.

Ethambutol inhibited the transfer of mycolic acids into the cell wall of *Mycobacterium smegmatis in vitro*.— K. Takayama *et al., Antimicrob. Ag. Chemother.*, 1979, *16*, 240.

Absorption and Fate. Ethambutol is readily absorbed after administration by mouth; absorption is not significantly impaired by food. After a single dose of 25 mg per kg body-weight, peak plasma concentrations of up to 5 µg per ml appear within 4 hours, and are less than 1 µg per ml by 24 hours. Most of a dose is excreted unchanged in urine and up to 20% in faeces, within 48 hours. From 8 to 15% of a dose appears in the urine as inactive metabolites.

Ethambutol diffuses readily into red blood cells and into the cerebrospinal fluid when the meninges are inflamed. It has been reported to cross the placenta.

In 6 healthy subjects given a single dose of ethambutol 15 mg per kg body-weight as an aqueous solution and as a commercial tablet preparation mean peak plasma concentrations of 4.45 and 4.01 µg per ml occurred in a mean of 1.91 and 2.83 hours respectively after administration. For plasma concentration measured up to 12 hours after administration the apparent mean elimination half-life was 4.78 and 4.06 hours respectively which increased to about 10 hours for 24 to 72-hour samplings. About 54 to 67% of the dose was excreted unchanged in the urine within 72 hours. The results of studies with pooled human plasma and in 3 subjects indicated that approximately 20 to 30% of ethambutol was bound to plasma proteins.— C. S. Lee *et al., Clin. Pharmac. Ther.*, 1977, *22*, 615. When ethambutol 15 mg per kg was given intravenously or by mouth as tablets or solution a mean of 79.2%, 63.4%, and 61.1% respectively of the administered dose was excreted in the urine unchanged within 72 hours.— C. S. Lee and L. Z. Benet, *J. pharm. Sci.*, 1978, *67*, 470.

Pharmacokinetic studies of ethambutol in elderly patients with tuberculosis.— L. M. O. Omer, *Prax. klin. Pneumol.*, 1978, *32*, 252.

Further references: E. A. Peets *et al., Am. Rev. resp. Dis.*, 1965, *91*, 51; V. Place *et al., Ann. N.Y. Acad. Sci.*, 1966, *135*, 775; T. Lewit *et al.* (letter), *Lancet*, 1970, *2*, 99; T. Dume *et al., Dt. med. Wschr.*, 1971, *96*, 1430.

Absorption. Results suggesting that adequate serum concentrations can be obtained in patients with jejunoileal bypass after a dose of ethambutol of 15 to 25 mg per kg body-weight.— R. E. Polk *et al.* (letter), *Ann. intern. Med.*, 1978, *89*, 430.

Diffusion. *Into cerebrospinal fluid.* In a study of the absorption of ethambutol given in a dose of 25 mg per kg body-weight to 13 healthy subjects and to 21 patients with tuberculous meningitis, mean serum concentrations measured at 3 hours were 4.1 µg per ml (range 2.6 to 6.6) and 4.9 µg per ml (range 3.4 to 8) respectively. A CSF concentration of 0.07 µg per ml was measured at 3 hours in 2 of 5 healthy subjects, no ethambutol being detected in the other 3. The mean CSF concentration at 3 hours was 0.48 µg per ml (0.05 to 1.6) in 4 of 5 patients, no ethambutol being detected in the fifth.— J. A. Pilheu *et al., Tubercle*, 1971, *52*, 117. See also U. Gundert-Remy *et al., Eur. J. clin. Pharmac.*, 1973, *6*, 133.

Into joints. References: D. Mouries *et al., Nouv. Presse méd.*, 1975, *4*, 2734.

Uses. Ethambutol hydrochloride is given with isoniazid (p.1574) and rifampicin (p.1580) in the primary treatment of pulmonary tuberculosis and with rifampicin and sometimes capreomycin (p.1569) in the re-treatment of pulmonary tuberculosis resistant to isoniazid, streptomycin, or aminosalicylic acid. The use of ethambutol with other antituberculous agents is described under Treatment of Tuberculosis, p.1565. Intermittent regimens (p.1566) and short-term treatment (p.1566) including ethambutol are increasingly important.

For initial treatment it is given by mouth in a single daily dose of 15 mg per kg body-weight. In re-treatment it is given in a single daily dose of 25 mg per kg for 60 days then 15 mg per kg daily. A dose of 50 mg per kg has been given twice weekly in intermittent treatment regimens.

Ethambutol has also been administered by injection.

Administration. Plasma concentrations of ethambutol were determined over a period of 8 weeks in patients treated with ethambutol given in divided doses of 5 mg per kg body-weight thrice daily and 8.33 mg per kg thrice daily. Effective concentrations were maintained for 12 hours for the first 3 weeks and for up to 24 hours for the remaining 5 weeks. When ethambutol was given as a single daily dose of 15 or 25 mg per kg, plasma concentrations only remained in the effective range for 4 hours.— H. K. Schwabe *et al., Prax. Pneumol.*, 1973, *27*, 44, per *Int. pharm. Abstr.*, 1974, *11*, 113.

Intravenous use. Reference to the slow intravenous injection of ethambutol.— F. Mandler *et al., Farmaco, Edn prat.*, 1972, *27*, 369.

Administration in renal failure. The dose of ethambutol should be reduced in patients with impaired renal function. Doses of 15 to 25 mg per kg body-weight daily could be given to those with a GFR of 25 to 50 ml per minute; 7.5 to 15 mg per kg to those with a GFR of 10 to 25 ml per minute, and 5 mg per kg for those with a GFR of less than 10 ml per minute or on haemodialysis or peritoneal dialysis.— J. S. Cheigh, *Am. J. Med.*, 1977, *62*, 555.

Data for predicting removal of ethambutol by conventional haemodialysis.— T. P. Gibson and H. A. Nelson, *Clin. Pharmacokinet.*, 1977, *2*, 403. See also C. S. Lee *et al., J. Pharmacokinet. Biopharm.*, 1980, *8*, 69.

The interval between doses of ethambutol should be extended from 24 hours to 24 to 36 hours in those with a glomerular filtration-rate (GFR) of 10 to 50 ml per minute, and to 48 hours in those with a GFR of less than 10 ml per minute. Concentrations of ethambutol were affected by haemodialysis and peritoneal dialysis.— W. M. Bennett *et al., Ann. intern. Med.*, 1980, *93*, 62.

Further references: P. Sharpstone, *Br. med. J.*, 1977, *2*, 36; G. B. Appel and H. C. Neu, *New Engl. J. Med.*, 1977, *296*, 663.

See also under Precautions, above, and in Treatment of Tuberculosis, p.1565.

Leprosy. Ethambutol 800 mg daily was given to 16 patients with lepromatous leprosy for 1 year and to 3 tuberculoid and 1 dimorphic cases for 6 months. There was improvement of the lepromatous lesions after 15 to 30 days and after 1 year 4 were cured, 3 improved, and 5 formerly improved had relapsed showing active lesions again after 9 months. The 3 tuberculoid patients lost all lesions at 6 months and the 1 dimorphic patient appeared cured at 12 months. Resistance might have developed to ethambutol.— A. Saul and R. Barcelata, *Dermatologia, Méx.*, 1969, *13*, 152, per *Lepr. Rev.*, 1971, *42*, 71.

Meningitis, tuberculous. Reports of the use of ethambutol in the treatment of tuberculous meningitis.— I. D. Bobrowitz, *Chest*, 1972, *61*, 629; N. I. Girgis *et al., J. trop. Med. Hyg.*, 1976, *79*, 14.

See also under Treatment of Tuberculosis, p.1565.

Pulmonary tuberculosis. After an initial period of treatment of about 3.5 months with isoniazid, rifampicin, and ethambutol, 63 patients continued treatment with isoniazid 300 mg and rifampicin 600 mg both daily and another 63 with isoniazid 300 mg and ethambutol 15 mg per kg body-weight daily. There were no relapses in either the rifampicin or ethambutol group. Ethambutol was as effective as and cheaper than rifampicin for continuation therapy.— A. W. Lees *et al., Lancet*, 1977, *1*, 1232.

Further reports of ethambutol in the treatment of pulmonary tuberculosis.—US Public Health Service Tuberculosis Program, *Am. Rev. resp. Dis.*, 1968, *98*, 825; G. B. M. Clarke *et al., Br. J. Dis. Chest*, 1972, *66*, 272; B. Doster *et al., Am. Rev. resp. Dis.*, 1973, *107*, 177; G. Daynes, *S. Afr. med. J.*, 1974, *48*, 2352; *Tubercle*, 1981, *62*, 13.

Tuberculosis prophylaxis. For the use of isoniazid with ethambutol in an intermittent regimen for the prophylaxis of tuberculosis, see Prophylaxis of Tuberculosis, p.1564.

Preparations

Ethambutol Hydrochloride Tablets *(U.S.P.)*. Tablets containing ethambutol hydrochloride.

Ethambutol Syrup. The following formula has been recommended by the manufacturers of ethambutol. Ethambutol powder 500 mg, citric acid 100 mg, orange tincture 0.3 ml, syrup 2.5 ml, and double-strength chloroform water to 5 ml. Isoniazid should not be added to this syrup.—Personal Communication, *Lederle*, 1977.

Ethambutol Tablets *(B.P.)*. Tablets containing ethambutol hydrochloride. They may be film-coated.

Proprietary Preparations

Myambutol *(Lederle, UK)*. Ethambutol hydrochloride, available as **Powder** and as **Tablets** of 100 and 400 mg. (Also available as Myambutol in *Arg., Austral., Belg., Canad., Denm., Fr., Ger., Neth., S.Afr., Spain, Swed., Switz., USA*).

Mynah *(Lederle, UK)*. Tablets containing ethambutol hydrochloride and isoniazid. Mynah 200, Mynah 250, Mynah 300, and Mynah 365 contain 200, 250, 300 and 365 mg of ethambutol hydrochloride respectively, with 100 mg of isoniazid.

Other Proprietary Names

Canad.—Etibi; *Fr.*—Dexambutol; *Ger.*—EMB-Fatol; *Ital.*—Etambutyl, Etapiam, Etibi, Miambutol, Mycobutol, Tibutolo; *Spain*—Afimocil, Anvital, Cidanbutol, Etambin, Farmabutol, Fimbutol, Inagen, Tisiobutol.

7557-z

Ethionamide *(B.P., U.S.P.)*. TH 1314; Ethionamidum; Etionamida. 2-Ethylpyridine-4-carbothioamide.

$C_8H_{10}N_2S$ = 166.2.

CAS — 536-33-4.

Pharmacopoeias. In *Br., Braz., Fr., Hung., Int., Jap., Roum.*, and *U.S.*

A bright yellow crystalline powder, darkening on exposure to light, with a slight sulphide-like odour and an unpleasant, sulphurous taste. M.p. 158° to 165°. Practically **insoluble** in water; soluble 1 in 30 of alcohol, 1 in 45 of acetone, 1 in 350 of chloroform, and 1 in 600 of ether; soluble in methyl alcohol; sparingly soluble in propylene glycol. A 1% suspension in water has a pH of 6 to 7. **Store** at 8° to 15° in airtight containers. Protect from light.

The stability of ethionamide in lipophilic suppository bases.— T. Cieszyński, *Acta Pol. pharm.*, 1971, *28*, 59.

Adverse Effects. Ethionamide is more toxic than isoniazid and many patients have to discontinue treatment. The most common side-effect is gastro-intestinal disturbance, with anorexia, excessive salivation, a metallic taste, nausea, vomiting, stomatitis, and diarrhoea.

Other side-effects reported include acne, allergic reactions, alopecia, convulsions, deafness, dermatitis (including photodermatitis), diplopia, dizziness, gynaecomastia, headache, hypotension, impotence, insomnia, liver dysfunction, menstrual disturbances, olfactory disorders, peripheral neuropathy, and rheumatic pains. Mental disturbances, including depression, have been provoked and a tendency towards hypoglycaemia may occur and could be of significance in patients with diabetes mellitus. Racial differences in tolerance may occur; Chinese and Africans are often more tolerant of ethionamide than are Europeans.

Teratogenic effects have been reported in *animals*.

A double-blind study of the incidence and severity of side-effects with individual doses from 0.25 to 1.75 g of ethionamide and from 1.25 to 1.75 g of prothionamide showed that the principal side-effects were gastro-intestinal symptoms, giddiness, and headache. In males, ethionamide had more side-effects than prothionamide while there was no significant difference in females. Females suffered more from the side-effects of either drug than males.— W. Fox *et al., Tubercle*, 1969, *50*, 125.

Effects on the eye. Ethionamide has caused colour vision disturbance especially in the presence of renal failure. Permanent damage is unlikely if the dose is reduced or the drug discontinued.— P. A. MacFaul, *Prescribers' J.*, 1973, *13*, 68.

Ethionamide had been reported to cause optic neuritis and optic atrophy but these rarely occurred when recommended doses were used.— *Med. Lett.*, 1976, *18*, 63.

Effects on the liver. Abnormalities of liver function, but no jaundice, occurred in 12 of 80 patients treated with ethionamide.— J. M. Schless *et al., Am. Rev. resp. Dis.*, 1965, *91*, 728, per *Med. J. Aust.*, 1966, *1*, 229.

A girl developed acute hepatic necrosis and died after treatment with ethionamide, isoniazid, and PAS. Ethionamide was considered to be responsible.— K. Hollinrake, *Br. J. Dis. Chest*, 1968, *62*, 151, per *Abstr. Hyg.*, 1969, *44*, 473.

Effects on mental state. For reports of psychological changes associated with ethionamide, see F. S. Lansdown *et al.*, *Am. Rev. resp. Dis.*, 1967, *95*, 1053; R. K. Narang, *Tubercle*, 1972, *53*, 137; G. S. Sharma *et al.*, *Tubercle*, 1979, *60*, 171.

Effects on the nervous system. A report of encephalopathy with pellagralike symptoms occurring in association with ethionamide in 2 patients and with ethionamide and cycloserine in 1. Treatment was with nicotinamide and compound vitamin preparations.— M. Swash *et al.*, *Tubercle*, 1972, *53*, 132..

Effects on the thyroid. It was suggested that ethionamide had caused a disturbance in the synthesis of thyroid hormone in 2 patients, resulting in hypothyroidism.— T. Moulding and R. Fraser, *Am. Rev. resp. Dis.*, 1970, *101*, 90.

Treatment of Adverse Effects. It is suggested that pyridoxine should be given to patients taking ethionamide who have developed neuropathy on previous isoniazid therapy. Prochlorperazine or trimeprazine tartrate may be of value in the treatment of severe nausea and vomiting.

Precautions. Caution is necessary in administering ethionamide to patients with depression or other psychiatric illness, chronic alcoholism, or epilepsy. Difficulty may be experienced in controlling diabetes when ethionamide is given to diabetics. The side-effects of other tuberculostatic agents may be increased when ethionamide is administered concomitantly. Ethionamide is best avoided during pregnancy. Liver function tests should be carried out before and during treatment with ethionamide.

Interactions. The excretion of ethionamide was reduced by the prior administration of chymotrypsin although serum concentrations were not affected. Chymotrypsin did not affect the half-life or excretion of isoniazid.— M. J. Mattila and H. Tutinen, *Farmaceutiskt Notisbl.*, 1967, *76*, 294, per *Int. pharm. Abstr.*, 1968, *5*, 613.

Antimicrobial Action. Ethionamide is bacteriostatic and, in high concentrations, bactericidal. It is active against various mycobacteria but resistance is reported to develop rapidly. Up to 30% of the organisms that acquire resistance to thiacetazone also develop resistance to ethionamide.

Demonstration of cross-resistance of *Mycobacterium leprae* to thiambutosine, thiacetazone, ethionamide, and prothionamide.— S. R. Pattyn and M. J. Colston (letter), *Lepr. Rev.*, 1978, *49*, 324.

Absorption and Fate. Ethionamide is readily absorbed from the gastro-intestinal tract, and is widely distributed throughout body tissues and fluids, including the cerebrospinal fluid. Peak plasma concentrations occur 2 to 3 hours after a dose. It has a biological half-life of 2 to 4 hours. Ethionamide is extensively metabolised and little appears in the urine as the unchanged drug. One urinary metabolite, ethylisonicotinic acid, appears to be excreted more rapidly than ethionamide.

For references to the pharmacokinetics of ethionamide, see J. P. Johnston *et al.*, *J. Pharm. Pharmac.*, 1967, *19*, 1; M. J. Mattila *et al.*, *Annls Med. intern. Fenn.*, 1968, *57*, 75, per *Abstr. Hyg.*, 1969, *44*, 288; A. Bieder and P. Brunel, *Annls pharm. fr.*, 1971, *29*, 461; J. Pütter, *Arzneimittel-Forsch.*, 1972, *22*, 1027.

Uses. Ethionamide is a thioamide derivative which has been used with other antituberculous agents for the treatment of tuberculosis, generally when resistance to primary agents has developed (see Treatment of Tuberculosis, p.1565). It is less effective than isoniazid. Ethionamide has also been used in the treatment of leprosy.

The usual adult dose is 0.5 to 1 g daily in divided doses with meals. Treatment has been given as a single dose at night.

The usual dose for children is 12 to 15 mg per kg body-weight daily to a maximum of 750 mg daily in divided doses. Some children have received 20 mg per kg daily.

Ethionamide has also been administered as rectal suppositories; the hydrochloride has been given intravenously.

Administration. The maximum dose of ethionamide tolerated in twice-weekly doses over 2 weeks by 10 patients with pulmonary tuberculosis was 1.5 g. The drug was given in conjunction with aminosalicylate and isoniazid. Another 9 patients could not tolerate 1 g. Of 22 patients prescribed their maximum dose for a further 8 weeks, only 2 completed the course at this dose and 2 on a reduced dose.— S. Devadatta *et al.*, *Tubercle*, 1970, *51*, 263.

Studies in *mice* indicated that the efficacy of ethionamide or prothionamide was considerably reduced if they were given less than 3 times a week.— S. R. Pattyn, *Lepr. Rev.*, 1978, *49*, 199.

Atypical mycobacterial infections. Cervical lymphadenitis in a 5-year-old girl, caused by *Mycobacterium fortuitum* only sensitive to ethionamide, gentamicin, or amikacin, was treated with gentamicin and ethionamide 125 mg twice daily for 10 days with ethionamide given thereafter for maintenance.— M. J. Rivron *et al.*, *Archs Dis. Childh.*, 1979, *54*, 312.

Leprosy. Ethionamide 250 mg daily given for 4 to 18 months to 19 patients with leprosy, 13 of them with lepromatous leprosy, brought striking clinical improvement without toxic side-effects.— H. Floch *et al.*, *Bull. Soc. Path. exot.*, 1966, *59*, 715, per *Trop. Dis. Bull.*, 1968, *65*, 133.

Ethionamide was given initially in a dose of 1 g daily then reduced because of side-effects to 500 mg for adults and 250 mg for adolescents in a study of 102 patients, 101 of whom had lepromatous leprosy. There were early signs of improvement at 6 months and after 2 years' treatment 75% of patients had their disease arrested. After 4 years' treatment the bacillary index in most patients had fallen to zero. Ethionamide was considered to have similar activity to dapsone in leprosy.— R. Rollier and M. Rollier, *Maroc. méd.*, 1972, *52*, 148, per *Trop. Dis. Bull.*, 1972, *69*, 917.

Studies in *mice* indicating that ethionamide and prothionamide deserve serious consideration for use in the combined treatment of lepromatous leprosy.— M. J. Colston *et al.*, *Lepr. Rev.*, 1978, *49*, 115.

Pulmonary tuberculosis. Some reports of the use of ethionamide in the treatment of pulmonary tuberculosis.— *Tubercle*, 1966, *47*, 361; A. W. Lees, *Am. Rev. resp. Dis.*, 1967, *95*, 109; *Tubercle*, 1968, *49*, 281; F. J. Chicou *et al.*, *Bull. Wld Hlth Org.*, 1968, *39*, 731.

Preparations

Ethionamide Tablets *(B.P.)*. Tablets containing ethionamide. They may be sugar-coated.

Ethionamide Tablets *(U.S.P.)*. Tablets containing ethionamide. Store at 8° to 15°.

Proprietary Names

Panathide *(Propan, S.Afr.)*; Trecator (also as the hydrochloride) *(Theraplix, Belg.*; *Théraplix, Fr.*; *Ives, USA)*; Trescatyl *(May & Baker, S.Afr.)*; Tubenamide *(Jap.)*.

Ethionamide was formerly marketed in Great Britain under the proprietary name Trescatyl (*May & Baker*).

7558-c

Etocarlide. Aethoxydum; Dialide; Ethoxyd; Etoxid. 4,4'-Diethoxythiocarbanilide 1,3-Bis(4-ethoxyphenyl)thiourea.

$C_{17}H_{20}N_2O_2S = 316.4$.

CAS — 1234-30-6.

Pharmacopoeias. In *Rus.*

A white or almost white crystalline powder with a bitter taste. M.p. 168° to 171°. Practically **insoluble** in water; slightly soluble in alcohol and methyl alcohol; soluble in acetone; freely soluble in chloroform; very slightly soluble in ether. **Store** in airtight containers.

Etocarlide has leprostatic and tuberculostatic properties and has been used in the treatment of leprosy and in conjunction with other tuberculostatics in the treatment of tuberculosis.

Preparations

Tabulettae Aethoxydi *(Rus. P.)*. Tablets each containing 100 or 250 mg of etocarlide.

7559-k

Isoniazid *(B.P., Eur. P., U.S.P.)*. INAH; INH; Isoniaz.; Isoniazidum; Isonicotinic Acid Hydrazide; Isonicotinylhydrazide; Isonicotinylhydrazine; Tubazid. Isonicotinohydrazide.

$C_6H_7N_3O = 137.1$.

CAS — 54-85-3.

Pharmacopoeias. In all pharmacopoeias examined except *Mex.*

Colourless, odourless crystals, or white crystalline powder, with a taste slightly sweet at first and then bitter. M.p. 170° to 174°.

Soluble 1 in 8 of water, 1 in 45 to 50 of alcohol, and 1 in 1000 of chloroform; very slightly soluble in ether. A 5% solution in water has a pH of 6 to 8. A 4.35% solution is iso-osmotic with serum. Solutions are **sterilised** by autoclaving or by filtration.

Incompatible with chloral, sugars, aldehydes and ketones, iodine, hypochlorites, ferric salts, and oxidising agents. Isoniazid absorbs insignificant amounts of moisture at 25° at relative humidities up to about 90%. **Store** in airtight containers. Protect from light.

An aqueous solution of isoniazid iso-osmotic with serum (4.35%) caused 100% haemolysis of erythrocytes cultured in it for 45 minutes.— E. R. Hammarlund and K. Pedersen-Bjergaard, *J. pharm. Sci.*, 1961, *50*, 24.

It was recommended that sugars such as dextrose, laevulose, and sucrose should not be used in isoniazid preparations because the absorption of the drug was impaired by the formation of a condensation product. Sorbitol might be a suitable substitute.— K. V. N. Rao *et al.*, *Bull. Wld Hlth Org.*, 1971, *45*, 625.

Stability. For a report of instability in a mixture containing isoniazid and sodium aminosalicylate, see Sodium Aminosalicylate, p.1582.

Adverse Effects. Patients may experience nausea, vomiting, and other gastro-intestinal effects. Many of the adverse effects of isoniazid are related to hypersensitivity or to the use of large doses; patients who are slow inactivators may experience a greater incidence of toxicity.

Peripheral neuropathy, probably due to pyridoxine deficiency, can occur and the tendency is greater in slow inactivators. Convulsions, optic neuritis, and psychotic reactions have been reported. Liver damage has occurred especially over the age of 35; it may be serious and sometimes fatal with the development of necrosis. Blood disorders that have been reported include haemolytic and aplastic anaemia and agranulocytosis. Various skin reactions, hyperglycaemia, and acidosis have occurred. Pellagra may be related to an isoniazid-induced pyridoxine deficiency which affects the conversion of tryptophan to nicotinic acid. There have been occasional reports of lupus-like reactions, a rheumatic syndrome, and gynaecomastia.

Symptoms of overdosage include slurred speech, acidosis, hyperglycaemia, hallucinations, respiratory and CNS depression, convulsions, and coma. Some patients may experience slight euphoria, and withdrawal symptoms such as headache, irritability, nervousness, insomnia, or excessive dreaming may occasionally occur on cessation of treatment.

During studies of isoniazid prophylaxis in US Public Health Service hospitals, the incidence of adverse effects was 0.4%. Gastro-intestinal disturbances were the commonest complaint. Hypersensitivity reactions, peripheral neuritis, convulsions, and skin reactions were more frequent among older and malnourished persons than among children and adolescents. Peripheral neuritis was commonest in alcoholics who had taken large doses of isoniazid without pyridoxine. Convulsions and other severe reactions generally followed excessive doses. Children with clinical tuberculosis tolerated 20 mg per kg body-weight of isoniazid without ill effects.— F. J. Curry (letter), *New Engl. J. Med.*, 1967, *277*, 1207.

For a brief discussion of the side-effects of isoniazid and methods of testing for slow or rapid inactivation, see N. W. Horne, *Practitioner*, 1972, *208*, 263.

Giddiness characterised by onset at about 12 hours after

dosage, and persisting for about 24 hours was reported among 16% of 75 slow inactivators given a slow-release preparation of isoniazid (matrix isoniazid) 45 mg per kg body-weight. Among rapid inactivators giddiness was reported by 6% of 72 patients given 37.5 to 45 mg per kg and by 25% of 65 patients given 52.5 mg of matrix isoniazid per kg. The incidence was 2% among a total of 101 control patients given isoniazid 15 mg per kg plus matrix base.— R. Parthasarathy *et al.*, *Tubercle*, 1976, *57*, 115. See also T. Santha *et al.*, *ibid.*, 123.

Abuse. Isoniazid in doses of 3 to 5 g has been abused for its hallucinogenic properties. Acute overdoses have been treated with large infusions of pyridoxine.— C. V. Brown (letter), *Lancet*, 1972, *1*, 743.

Allergy. In a retrospective study of 1744 patients treated with various regimens of streptomycin, sodium aminosalicylate, and isoniazid the overall drug intolerance-rate was 12.2%. Intolerance to streptomycin was 10.3%, sodium aminosalicylate 8.8%, and isoniazid 1.3%. The most common reaction to isoniazid was fever. Most patients intolerant to isoniazid and sodium aminosalicylate were successfully desensitised, including those with hepatitis. Reactions appeared to be more frequent when the dose of isoniazid or streptomycin was increased and when streptomycin was added to an existing regimen of isoniazid and sodium aminosalicylate; multiple drug reactions were associated with the number of drugs given rather than dosage.— S. J. Berté *et al.*, *Am. Rev. resp. Dis.*, 1964, *90*, 598.

Reports of febrile reactions in patients receiving isoniazid.— R. S. Davis and B. S. Stoler (letter), *New Engl. J. Med.*, 1977, *297*, 337; N. F. Jacobs and S. E. Thompson, *J. Am. med. Ass.*, 1977, *238*, 1759; J. F. Dasta *et al.*, *Chest*, 1979, *75*, 196.

See also Effects on the Liver, Effects on the Skin, and Lupoid Syndrome, below.

Carcinogenicity. The slight risk of cancer associated with isoniazid prophylaxis outweighs the possible benefits of prevention of active tuberculosis which can usually be treated.— C. T. Miller (letter), *J. Am. med. Ass.*, 1974, *230*, 1254.

In a long-term follow-up (16 to 24 years) of 3842 patients admitted to 2 sanatoria for pulmonary tuberculosis from 1950 to 1957 no evidence of an association between isoniazid treatment and development of malignant neoplasms at any site was found. However, the follow-up is to be continued.— H. Stott *et al.*, *Tubercle*, 1976, *57*, 1.

There was no evidence to support a carcinogenic effect of isoniazid prophylaxis from 2 large prospective studies organised by the US Public Health Service and involving more than 25 000 people who were followed-up for 9 to 14 years.— J. L. Glassroth *et al.*, *Am. Rev. resp. Dis.*, 1977, *116*, 1065.

A study of 11 169 children and 11 169 controls included in a survey of childhood cancers did not support an association between the drugs given during pregnancy, including isoniazid, and the subsequent development of cancer.— B. M. Sanders and G. J. Draper, *Br. med. J.*, 1979, *1*, 717. See also E. C. Hammond *et al.*, *Br. med. J.*, 1967, *2*, 792.

Further references: G. M. Bonser, *Br. med. J.*, 1967, *4*, 129; A. B. Lowenfels and J. Norman (letter), *J. Am. med. Ass.*, 1978, *240*, 434.

Effects on the blood. Bleeding occurred in a patient receiving isoniazid, owing to an acquired inhibitor of fibrin stabilisation associated with isoniazid therapy.— P. T. Otis *et al.*, *Blood*, 1974, *44*, 771, per P. Lechat *et al.*, *Thérapie, 1976* 31, 129.

A report of disseminated intravascular coagulation associated with isoniazid-induced hepatitis in one patient.— J. J. Stuart and H. R. Roberts (letter), *Ann. intern. Med.*, 1976, *84*, 490.

Further reports on the effects of isoniazid on the blood.— G. H. Tomkin, *Practitioner*, 1973, *211*, 773 (sideroblastic anaemia); P. F. Jenkins *et al.*, *Br. med. J.*, 1980, *280*, 1069 (neutropenia).

Haemolytic anaemia. Three episodes of haemolytic anaemia in patients with a deficiency of glucose-6-phosphate dehydrogenase were believed to be precipitated by isoniazid, taken either alone or in conjunction with aminosalicylic acid.— E. R. Burka, *Ann. intern. Med.*, 1966, *64*, 817. Isoniazid did not cause haemolysis in Chinese patients with glucose-6-phosphate dehydrogenase deficiency.— T. K. Chan *et al.*, *Br. med. J.*, 1976, *2*, 1227.

A 3-year-old Negro boy developed haemolytic anaemia and a positive response to the direct Coombs' test after being treated for 1 year with isoniazid 15 mg per kg body-weight daily. The response to the Coombs' test reverted to negative within 18 hours of discontinuing isoniazid. A low concentration of glucose-6-phosphate dehydrogenase was considered coincidental.— M. G. Robinson and M. Foadi, *J. Am. med. Ass.*, 1969, *208*, 656.

Effects on bones and joints. Reports of adverse musculoskeletal effects with isoniazid.— A. E. Good *et al.*, *Ann. intern. Med.*, 1965, *63*, 800 (rheumatic syndrome); J. Y. Doust and F. Moatamed, *Dis. Chest*, 1968, *53*, 62 (arthralgia); P. Periman and T. K. Venkataramani (letter), *Ann. intern. Med.*, 1975, *83*, 667 (arthritis).

Effects on the ear. For the effects of isoniazid on the ear, see D. Dayal and H. Shanta, *Indian J. Tuberc.*, 1970, *17*, 155, per *Abstr. Hyg.*, 1971, *46*, 545.

Effect on the kidney. A report of acute diffuse interstitial nephritis in 3 patients attributed to antituberculous therapy and especially isoniazid and/or ethambutol.— W. J. Stone, *Antimicrob. Ag. Chemother.*, 1976, *10*, 164.

Effects on the liver. In an extensive review of the hepatotoxicity of antituberculosis regimens including isoniazid, especially those used in the controlled studies of the British MRC, D.J. Girling (*Tubercle*, 1978, *59*, 13) stressed that hepatitis occurring during antituberculosis chemotherapy may be attributed to other causes such as the disease itself, alcoholism, cirrhosis, or infectious hepatitis. When treatment is definitely implicated it may not be clear which drug or combination of drugs is responsible. Isoniazid alone is widely used prophylactically in the US and a survey by the US Public Health Service (M. Black *et al.*, *Gastroenterology*, 1975, *69*, 289; D.E. Kopanoff *et al.*, *Am. Rev. resp. Dis.*, 1978, *117*, 991) indicates that there is a definite risk of hepatitis during isoniazid prophylaxis, especially in patients over 35 years of age. M. Black *et al.* (*Gastroenterology*, 1975, *69*, 289) attributed the liver damage to a direct toxic effect of isoniazid metabolites; H.L. Israel (*Gastroenterology*, 1975, *69*, 539) considered it to be a hypersensitivity reaction although many patients have resumed an isoniazid regimen uneventfully after only a short interruption. In Great Britain and many other countries prophylaxis is little used except in children under 6 who have a very low risk of hepatitis. J.R. Mitchell *et al.* (*Ann. intern. Med.*,1976, *84*, 181) and others have suggested that prophylaxis should generally only be used for subjects under 35 years.

Studies of standard first-line treatment regimens based on isoniazid in Great Britain, Africa, and Asia show that the incidence of hepatitis is about 2% or less and this risk is considered acceptable. In Africans many episodes could be attributed to underlying chronic liver disease. Drug-induced hepatitis often appeared to be caused by aminosalicylic acid or thiacetazone rather than by isoniazid. Early reports of a higher incidence of hepatitis with regimens based on isoniazid and rifampicin have not been confirmed in later studies; D.N. Baron and J.L. Bell (*Tubercle*, 1974, *55*, 115) found that transient increases in serum concentrations of liver enzymes were common in the early weeks of antituberculosis therapy but that they rarely implied serious toxicity. J.R. Mitchell *et al.* (*Clin. Pharmac. Ther.*, 1975, *18*, 70) suggested that isoniazid might be more hepatotoxic for rapid rather than slow acetylators; in healthy subjects amounts of acetylisoniazid and isonicotinic acid in the urine were higher in the rapid acetylators. *Animal* work reported by S.D. Nelson *et al.* (*Science*, 1976, *193*, 901) provided evidence that acetylisoniazid can be converted to acetylhydrazine which is further metabolised to a highly reactive compound capable of causing liver necrosis. However, clinical evidence has indicated that the incidence of hepatic damage is no higher among rapid acetylators than among slow acetylators.

In a US Public Health Service Cooperative Surveillance Study probable or possible hepatitis was associated with isoniazid prophylaxis in 174 of 13 838 patients; there were 8 deaths. In the majority of cases hepatitis was seen within the first 6 months of treatment and the incidence was highest in the 50 to 64-year age group; there was no hepatitis in subjects under 20 years. The risk of hepatitis was enhanced by alcohol, especially when consumed daily. Oriental males appeared to be at highest risk of developing isoniazid-associated hepatitis.— D. E. Kopanoff *et al.*, *Am. Rev. resp. Dis.*, 1978, *117*, 991. See also J. E. Thompson, *Med. J. Aust.*, 1978, *1*, 165; R. B. Byrd *et al.*, *J. Am. med. Ass.*, 1979, *241*, 1239; L. A. Dash *et al.*, *Am. Rev. resp. Dis.*, 1980, *121*, 1039.

A view that the benefits of isoniazid chemoprophylaxis outweigh the risks particularly in patients under 50 years of age.— J. E. Thompson, *Med. J. Aust.*, 1978, *1*, 165. Patients receiving isoniazid prophylaxis should receive routine clinical and liver-function evaluation, especially those older than 30 years of age.— R. B. Byrd *et al.*, *J. Am. med. Ass.*, 1979, *241*, 1239. Although an asymptomatic rise in serum-aminotransferase activity occurs in a fifth of patients receiving isoniazid, the risk of developing serious liver disease is considered small and routine liver-function tests seem unnecessary.— *Br. med. J.*, 1980, *280*, 1486.

Further references: R. A. Garibaldi *et al.*, *Am. Rev. resp. Dis.*, 1972, *106*, 357; W. C. Bailey *et al.*, *Am. Rev. resp. Dis.*, 1973, *107*, 523; W. C. Maddrey and J. K. Boitnott, *Ann. intern. Med.*, 1973, *79*, 1; W. W. Stead and E. C. Texter, *ibid.*, 125; R. Rudoy *et al.*, *Am. J. Dis. Child.*, 1973, *125*, 733; W. C. Bailey *et al.*, *Ann. intern. Med.*, 1974, *81*, 200; P. H. Beaudry *et al.*, *Am. Rev. resp. Dis.*, 1974, *110*, 581; A. Austerhoff *et al.*, *Dt. med. Wschr.*, 1974, *99*, 1182; T. Moulding *et al.* (letter), *Ann. intern. Med.*, 1976, *85*, 398; I. F. Litt *et al.*, *J. Pediat.*, 1976, *89*, 133; R. B. Byrd *et al.*, *Archs intern. Med.*, 1977, *137*, 1130; D. Pessayre *et al.*, *Gastroenterology*, 1977, *72*, 284; R. J. Warrington *et al.*, *Clin. exp. Immun.*, 1978, *32*, 97; C. Grönhagen-Riska *et al.*, *Am. Rev. resp. Dis.*, 1978, *118*, 461; G. A. Ellard *et al.*, *ibid.*, 628; P. A. Thomas *et al.*, *Archs Surg., Chicago*, 1979, *114*, 597; W. C. Bailey *et al.*, *Bull. int. Un. Tuberc.*, 1979, *54*, 47; J. A. Pilheu *et al.*, *Bull. int. Un. Tuberc.*, 1979, *54*, 48.

Hepatotoxicity in children. A report of hepatotoxicity in a 2-year-old black boy given isoniazid 200 mg daily.— S. H. Walker and J. O. Park-Hah (letter), *J. Pediat.*, 1977, *91*, 344.

Raised aminotransferase values were recorded in 41 of 239 children receiving isoniazid but only 2 required withdrawal of isoniazid. The remaining 39 continued to take isoniazid under close supervision and values returned to normal within 4 to 8 weeks.— P. Spyridis *et al.*, *Archs Dis. Childh.*, 1979, *54*, 65.

Further references: R. S. Rapp *et al.*, *Am. Rev. resp. Dis.*, 1978, *118*, 794; M. T. Stein, *Pediatrics*, 1979, *64*, 499.

For reports of hepatotoxicity in children receiving rifampicin and isoniazid, see Rifampicin, p.1578.

Malignant neoplasms of the liver. Comment on a theoretical association between hepatic angiosarcoma and substituted hydrazines including isoniazid.— T. K. Daneshmend and J. W. B. Bradfield (letter), *Lancet*, 1979, *2*, 1249.

Effects on mental state. A 16-year-old male with pulmonary tuberculosis developed a psychotic reaction when given isoniazid as part of antituberculous therapy and subsequently developed a similar reaction to treatment with ethionamide. Recovery was complete following withdrawal of each drug and treatment with pyridoxine.— G. S. Sharma *et al.*, *Tubercle*, 1979, *60*, 171.

Effects on metabolism. Reports of metabolic effects associated with the use of isoniazid.— I. Dickson, *Med. J. Aust.*, 1962, *1*, 325 (glycosuria); T. A. Neff, *Chest*, 1971, *59*, 245 (lactic acidosis).

Effects on the nervous system. *Convulsions.* Pyridoxine-responsive convulsions occurred in a 17-day-old infant receiving isoniazid 20 mg twice a day (13 mg per kg body-weight daily) from birth. Doses in excess of 10 mg per kg daily are considered to be dangerous.— S. A. McKenzie *et al.*, *Archs Dis. Childh.*, 1976, *51*, 567; G. Katz (letter), *ibid.*, 1977, *52*, 165.

The Boston Collaborative Drug Surveillance Program monitored consecutively 32 812 medical inpatients. Drug-induced convulsions occurred in 1 of 906 patients given isoniazid.— J. Porter and H. Jick, *Lancet*, 1977, *1*, 587.

Further references to convulsions with isoniazid.— S. Devadatta (letter), *Lancet*, 1965, *2*, 440.

Encephalopathy. Severe aseptic purulent meningoencephalitis in a 27-year-old man resulted from the prophylactic administration of isoniazid for 3 days, and repeated a few months later for 3 days. He rapidly improved after treatment with methylprednisolone sodium succinate 10 mg every 4 hours intramuscularly and ampicillin sodium 1 g intravenously every 2 hours.— V. F. Garagusi *et al.*, *J. Am. med. Ass.*, 1976, *235*, 1141.

A 38-year-old man in chronic renal failure developed encephalopathy when he was mistakenly given isoniazid 300 mg thrice daily. An altered mental status became apparent on the fourth day of treatment. Isoniazid was discontinued and the patient recovered after treatment with pyridoxine and dialysis.— R. L. Gibson and W. J. Stone, *Dialysis Transplant.*, 1979, *8*, 276.

Effects on the skin. Young adults taking isoniazid might develop an acneform syndrome, and pruritus without skin eruption was not unusual. Occasionally urticaria, purpura, and a lupus erythematosus-like syndrome have been reported.— N. Thorne, *Practitioner*, 1973, *211*, 606.

The Stevens–Johnson syndrome developed in a 25-

year-old woman 15 days after starting to take isoniazid. The skin rash and fever reappeared after a test dose of 50 mg.— B. S. Bomb *et al.*, *Tubercle*, 1976, *57*, 229.

Toxic epidermal necrolysis (Lyell's syndrome) occurred in a pregnant patient given isoniazid and streptomycin for the prophylaxis of pulmonary tuberculosis.— J. Kvasnička *et al.*, *Br. J. Derm.*, 1979, *100*, 551.

Further references: L. K. Cohen *et al.*, *Archs Derm.*, 1974, *109*, 377.

Lupoid syndrome. Isoniazid was suspected of causing the induction of antinuclear antibodies after prolonged use in 10 of 55 patients.— A. Cannat and M. Seligmann, *Lancet*, 1966, *1*, 185.

A 39-year-old man developed a lupoid syndrome after the treatment of tuberculosis with isoniazid and PAS. Pericarditis progressing to cardiac tamponade occurred but responded to pericardicentesis. The patient's condition improved considerably after treatment with hydrocortisone and then prednisone. Pericarditis was considered to be a complication of the lupoid syndrome.— J. H. Greenberg and C. L. Lutcher, *J. Am. med. Ass.*, 1972, *222*, 191.

The administration of isoniazid alone or in combination was associated with the development of antinuclear antibodies in 22 of 98 patients with tuberculosis, but no symptoms of lupus-like illness were observed.— N. F. Rothfield *et al.*, *Ann. intern. Med.*, 1978, *88*, 650. See also O. Hübscher *et al.* (letter), *ibid.*, *89*, 1011.

Further references: N. Debeyre *et al.*, *Sem. Hôp. Paris*, 1967, *43*, 3063.

Pellagra. A 31-year-old strict (Vegan) vegetarian Kenyan Asian woman with a low dietary intake of tryptophan and nicotinic acid developed isoniazid-induced pellagra, despite adequate pyridoxine supplementation. Her pellagra rapidly responded to administration of nicotinamide 150 mg daily.— D. A. Bender and R. Russell-Jones (letter), *Lancet*, 1979, *2*, 1125.

Further references: C. I. Harrington, *Practitioner*, 1977, *218*, 716; G. J. Burke and T. Hlangabeza, *S. Afr. med. J.*, 1977, *51*, 719; R. H. M. Thomas *et al.*, *Br. med. J.*, 1981, *283*, 287.

Pregnancy and the neonate. There was no difference between isoniazid and placebo in the frequency of conception, birth-rates, sex ratios, or birthweights in a 5-year controlled study of prophylaxis with isoniazid in 2435 male and female patients.— J. Ludford *et al.*, *Am. Rev. resp. Dis.*, 1973, *108*, 1170.

Results from the Collaborative Perinatal Project suggesting an almost twofold increase in the malformation-rate in children exposed to isoniazid (85) or aminosalicylic acid (43) at some time during the first 4 months of the mothers' pregnancy need independent confirmation before conclusions can be made regarding the possible teratogenicity of these drugs.— O. P. Heinonen *et al.*, *Birth Defects and Drugs in Pregnancy*, Littleton MA, Publishing Sciences Group, 1977, p. 296.

Mesothelioma in a 9-year-old boy might have been caused by administration of isoniazid to his mother during pregnancy.— K. J. Tuman *et al.* (letter), *Lancet*, 1980, *2*, 362.

See also p.1564.

Pyridoxine deficiency. No unequivocal biochemical evidence of pyridoxine deficiency was observed in 6 to 8 weeks in 6 tuberculous patients taking isoniazid 15 mg per kg body-weight, or in 3 taking 300 mg daily. In 2 slow acetylators of isoniazid, a mild increase in pyridoxine excretion was insufficient to account for any deficiency.— L. Levy *et al.*, *Am. Rev. resp. Dis.*, 1967, *96*, 910.

Treatment of Adverse Effects. Peripheral neuritis has been treated with pyridoxine hydrochloride; 50 to 100 mg daily has been recommended for prophylaxis and up to 300 mg daily may be necessary for treatment or for patients at high risk from peripheral neuritis.

Treatment of overdosage consists of gastric lavage following intubation and the control of convulsions by anticonvulsants given intravenously as well as the intravenous injection of large doses of pyridoxine. Any acidosis is corrected with sodium bicarbonate.

Forced diuresis may be tried and haemodialysis or peritoneal dialysis has been used. For a discussion of these active measures for the removal of drugs from the body, see under Treatment of Adverse Effects in Phenobarbitone, p.812.

Paraesthesias arising during isoniazid treatment might be due to peripheral vasoconstriction. Bamethan sulphate, 12.5 mg three or four times daily, suppressed paraesthesias in 9 of 16 adults and brought relief to another 6.— W. Baruffi and J. C. Fadel, *Revta bras. Med.*, 1966, *23*, 853, per *Bull. Hyg., Lond.*, 1967, *42*, 1101.

Pyridoxine is not always effective treatment when peripheral neuropathy has become established.— J. Cawano and L. J. Davis, *Drug Intell. & clin. Pharm.*, 1978, *12*, 112 and 297.

Overdosage. A brief review of dialysis in the management of isoniazid overdosage.— P. Cooper, *Pharm. J.*, 1971, *2*, 507.

A report of the management of 42 patients following isoniazid overdosage. Management consisted of the intravenous infusion of pyridoxine in a dose of 1 g for each gram of isoniazid ingested, correction of acidosis with sodium bicarbonate, and forced diuresis.— C. V. Brown, *Am. Rev. resp. Dis.*, 1972, *105*, 206.

Studies in *rats* and *dogs* suggested that pyridoxine and diazepam act synergistically in antagonising isoniazid-induced convulsions and preventing death due to isoniazid intoxication. Their combined use might be the treatment of choice for isoniazid overdosage.— L. Chin *et al.*, *Toxic. appl. Pharmac.*, 1978, *45*, 713.

Further references: L. Eidus and M. M. Hodgkin (letter), *Can. med. Ass. J.*, 1978, *119*, 692; T. Konigshausen *et al.*, *Vet. hum. Toxicol.*, 1979, *21*, *Suppl.*, 12; J. Miller, *Am. J. Dis. Child.*, 1980, *134*, 290.

Precautions. Isoniazid should not be given to patients who have experienced severe adverse reactions to it including drug-induced liver disease. Care should be taken in giving isoniazid to patients suffering from convulsive disorders, diabetes mellitus, chronic alcoholism, or impaired liver or kidney function or to patients taking other potentially hepatotoxic agents. If symptoms of hepatitis such as malaise, fatigue, anorexia, and nausea develop isoniazid should be discontinued immediately.

When isoniazid is given to patients who inactivate it slowly or to patients receiving PAS concurrently, tissue concentrations may be enhanced, and adverse effects are more likely to appear. There may be an increased risk of liver damage in patients receiving rifampicin and isoniazid but liver enzymes are generally raised only transiently.

Isoniazid enhances the effects of phenytoin and may also inhibit the metabolism of primidone; there may be increased toxicity when used with disulfiram.

Patients may require additional treatment with pyridoxine.

Isoniazid converted the tuberculin response from positive to negative in *rhesus monkeys* despite the presence of gross tuberculous lesions and mycobacteria.— J. P. Gibson *et al.*, *Lab. Anim. Care*, 1971, *21*, 62, per *Int. pharm. Abstr.*, 1972, *9*, 161.

Administration of isoniazid 10 mg per kg body-weight affected skills connected with driving.— M. Linnoila and M. J. Mattila, *J. clin. Pharmac.*, 1973, *13*, 343.

Early deficiencies in pyridoxine status were detected in patients taking isoniazid by measuring red-cell aspartate aminotransferase but not by red-cell alanine aminotransferase. Supplementation with pyridoxine 50 mg daily was adequate even with high doses of isoniazid.— B. R. Standal *et al.*, *Am. J. clin. Nutr.*, 1974, *27*, 479, per *Abstr. Hyg.*, 1974, *49*, 673.

A recommendation that treatment with isoniazid should be stopped when patients develop symptoms of hepatitis, or serum aminotransferase activity rises to three times the normal range, or when any rise in serum aminotransferase activity is accompanied by an increase in serum bilirubin or alkaline phosphatase.— *Med. Lett.*, 1977, *19*, 97.

A review of the clinical consequences of acetylator status in relation to the therapeutic and adverse effects of isoniazid.— D. E. Drayer and M. M. Reidenberg, *Clin. Pharmac. Ther.*, 1977, *22*, 251.

Interactions with drugs. *Alcohol.* A report of isoniazid reducing tolerance to alcohol.— C. -P. Siegers, *Dt. med. Wschr.*, 1977, *102*, 629.

Antacids. Aluminium hydroxide mixture delayed and depressed the absorption of isoniazid. It is recommended that isoniazid be given at least 1 hour before the antacid.— A. Hurwitz and D. L. Schlozman, *Am. Rev. resp. Dis.*, 1974, *109*, 41.

Anticoagulants. For a report of isoniazid enhancing the effect of warfarin, see Warfarin Sodium, p.779.

Anticonvulsants. For the effect of isoniazid on phenytoin, see Phenytoin, p.1240, and for the effect on primidone, see Primidone, p.1254.

Levodopa. Isoniazid might enhance the effects of levodopa.— J. P. Morgan (letter), *Ann. intern. Med.*, 1980, *92*, 434.

Phenelzine. Toxic effects have occurred when isoniazid and phenelzine are used together in slow acetylators.— *Chronicle Wld Hlth Org.*, 1974, *28*, 25.

Rifampicin. For the effect of isoniazid on blood concentrations of rifampicin, see Rifampicin, p.1579.

Sodium salicylate. Although the half-life of isoniazid was shortened by sodium salicylate, possibly by displacement of the isoniazid from plasma proteins, the antimicrobial action *in vitro* was not enhanced and at low isoniazid concentrations it was antagonised.— M. J. Mattila *et al.*, *Arzneimittel-Forsch.*, 1972, *22*, 1769.

Interactions with food. A report of reduced bioavailability when isoniazid was taken with food.— A. Melander *et al.*, *Acta med. scand.*, 1976, *200*, 93.

A 50-year-old Indian patient in Sri Lanka taking isoniazid developed flushing, sweating, giddiness, and a cerebrovascular accident after eating skipjack fish. The reaction was considered due to the inhibition by isoniazid of the histaminase degradation of the high histamine content of the fish, leading to cerebral arterial occlusion during acute hypotension.— N. Senanayake *et al.*, *Br. med. J.*, 1978, *2*, 1127. See also C. G. Uragoda and S. R. Kottegoda, *Tubercle*, 1977, *58*, 83. A similar reaction associated with tuna fish.— C. G. Uragoda, *Am. Rev. resp. Dis.*, 1980, *121*, 157.

A 37-year-old woman who took isoniazid developed symptoms characteristic of those associated with monoamine oxidase inhibitors when she ate cheese.— C. K. Smith and D. T. Durack, *Ann. intern. Med.*, 1978, *88*, 520. See also J. L. Lejonc *et al.* (letter), *Ann. intern. Med.*, 1979, *91*, 793; C. G. Uragoda and S. C. Lodha, *Tubercle*, 1979, *60*, 59.

Pregnancy and the neonate. Isoniazid causes an excessive elimination of pyridoxine and should be avoided during pregnancy.— H. Tuchmann-Duplessis, *Monographs on Drugs, Vol. 2, Drug Effects on the Fetus*, G.S. Avery (Ed.), London, Adis, 1975, p. 35. Isoniazid is considered to be one of the safer tuberculostatic drugs in pregnancy.— J. MacVicar, *Practitioner*, 1978, *221*, 885; M. de Swiet, *Prescribers' J.*, 1979, *19*, 59.

See also under Adverse Effects, above and Absorption and Fate, below.

Antimicrobial Action. Isoniazid is bacteriostatic and, in high concentrations, bactericidal against *Mycobacterium tuberculosis* which it inhibits *in vitro* in concentrations of 0.02 to 0.06 µg per ml. *M. kansasii* may be sensitive to isoniazid but isoniazid has no significant activity against other micro-organisms.

Although the incidence of primary drug resistance is generally low in developed countries mycobacteria rapidly become resistant to isoniazid used alone. For this reason it is usually given in conjunction with other antituberculous drugs, except in prophylaxis.

The MIC of isoniazid for *Mycobacterium tuberculosis* strain H37Rv was greatly diminished when an acridine, such as acriflavine, ethacridine, mepacrine, or proflavine, was added in sub-bacteriostatic concentrations.— V. N. Soloviev and V. S. Zueva (letter), *Lancet*, 1968, *2*, 412.

Further references: M. Steiner and A. Cosio, *New Engl. J. Med.*, 1966, *274*, 755; S. P. Tripathy, *Tubercle*, 1968, *49*, *Suppl.*, 78; R. Narain *et al.*, *Bull. Wld Hlth Org.*, 1968, *39*, 681; C. Allen *et al.*, *Morb. Mortal.*, 1980, *29*, 194.

See also under Antimicrobial Action, p.1564.

Absorption and Fate. Isoniazid is readily absorbed from the gastro-intestinal tract. Peak concentrations appear in blood 1 to 2 hours after a dose by mouth. Isoniazid is not considered to be bound appreciably to plasma proteins and diffuses into all body tissues and fluids, including the cerebrospinal fluid; it appears in foetal blood if given during pregnancy and in the milk of nursing mothers.

Elimination of isoniazid from the body is dependent on the rate of acetylation. In patients with normal renal function at least 50 to 70% of a dose appears in the urine in 24 hours, partly unchanged but mainly as metabolites. The primary metabolic route is the acetylation of isoniazid to acetylisoniazid by *N*-acetyltransferase found in the liver and small intestine. Acetylisoniazid is then hydrolysed to isonicotinic acid and monoacetylhydrazine; isonicotinic acid is conjugated with glycine and monoacetylhydrazine further acetylated to diacetylhydrazine. The metabolites of isoniazid have no tuberculostatic activity and apart possibly from monoacetylhydrazine they are also less toxic. The rate of acetylation of isoniazid and monoacetylhydrazine is genetically determined and there is a bimodal distribution of persons who acetylate them either slowly or rapidly. Various ethnic groups, especially Eskimos, Japanese, and Chinese, are predominantly rapid acetylators whereas in populations of Caucasians, Negroes, and Indians (Madras), proportions of slow and rapid acetylators are similar. Rapid acetylators have been reported to acetylate isoniazid about 5 times more rapidly than slow acetylators.

Slow acetylators of isoniazid have relatively high serum concentrations of free drug and excrete a higher proportion of free isoniazid in the urine than do rapid acetylators, and this may be important in patients on intermittent treatment regimens. Although adverse effects such as hepatitis may be increased in rapid acetylators (but see Adverse Effects) peripheral neuritis occurs more often in slow acetylators. Interactions with other drugs metabolised by acetylation are more likely in slow acetylators.

A review of the clinical pharmacokinetics of isoniazid.— W. W. Weber and D. W. Hein, *Clin. Pharmacokinet.*, 1979, *4*, 401.

A study of the pharmacokinetics of isoniazid in children.— W. A. Olson *et al.*, *Pharmacologist*, 1976, *18*, 153.

Pharmacokinetics of isoniazid in the elderly.— C. Advenier *et al.* (letter), *Br. J. clin. Pharmac.*, 1980, *10*, 167.

Absorption. Results suggesting that adequate serum concentrations can be reliably obtained in patients with jejuno-ileal bypass after a dose of isoniazid of 300 mg.— R. E. Polk *et al.* (letter), *Ann. intern. Med.*, 1978, *89*, 430.

For the effect of food and of aluminium hydroxide mixture on the absorption of isoniazid, see Precautions above.

Bioavailability. Pharmacokinetic studies of slow-release preparations of isoniazid which have been developed in an attempt to compensate for the low blood concentrations achieved in rapid acetylators when once-weekly treatment regimens for tuberculosis are used.— G. A. Ellard *et al.*, *Lancet*, 1972, *1*, 340; G. A. Ellard *et al.*, *Tubercle*, 1973, *54*, 57; L. Eidus *et al.*, *Am. Rev. resp. Dis.*, 1974, *110*, 34; L. Eidus and M. M. Hodgkin, *Arzneimittel-Forsch.*, 1975, *25*, 1077; G. R. Sarma *et al.*, *Tubercle*, 1975, *56*, 314; G. A. Ellard, *Bull. int. Un. Tuberc.*, 1976, *51*, 144; M. M. Hodgkin and B. Eidus, *Bull. int. Un. Tuberc.*, 1979, *54*, 55; M. M. Hodgkin *et al.*, *Res. Commun. chem. Path. Pharmac.*, 1979, *24*, 349.

Diffusion. *Into cerebrospinal fluid.* Mean cerebrospinal fluid concentrations of isoniazid in a patient with tuberculous meningitis were 2 µg per ml 3 to 6 hours after doses of 600 mg by mouth and were about 90% of concentrations found in the serum.— R. Forgan-Smith *et al.* (letter), *Lancet*, 1973, *2*, 374.

Into joints. References: D. Mouries *et al.*, *Nouv. Presse méd.*, 1975, *4*, 2734.

Into saliva. Therapeutic drug monitoring in saliva including details of studies on saliva-isoniazid concentrations.— M. Danhof and D. D. Breimer, *Clin. Pharmacokinet.*, 1978, *3*, 39.

Effects of disease states. Children with Down's syndrome had higher serum concentrations of isoniazid than control children given the same dose. The difference was probably due to a defect in acetylation in children with Down's syndrome.— R. Turpin *et al.* (letter), *Lancet*, 1967, *2*, 1369.

The pharmacokinetics of isoniazid in patients with chronic renal failure.— C. H. Gold *et al.*, *Clin. Nephrol.*, 1976, *6*, 365.

The pharmacokinetics of isoniazid in malnourished children.— Y. Akbani *et al.*, *Acta paediat. scand.*, 1977, *66*, 237; N. Buchanan *et al.*, *S. Afr. med. J.*, 1979, *56*, 299.

Metabolism. Isoniazid is not bound to serum proteins in the body. The biological half-life is 1.1 or 3.6 hours in rapid and slow acetylators respectively and 5 to 27% is excreted in urine.— C. M. Kunin, *Ann. intern. Med.*, 1967, *67*, 151.

The half-life of isoniazid in a slow acetylator given 681 mg by intravenous infusion was 196 minutes, while in a rapid acetylator given 670 mg the half-life was 70.7 minutes. Urinary pH was maintained at 8 in each case. Metabolites found in the urine were acetylisoniazid, isonicotinic acid, and isonicotinuric acid.— H. G. Boxenbaum and S. Riegelman, *J. pharm. Sci.*, 1974, *63*, 1191.

There was no significant difference in the half-life of isoniazid in 23 young people and 27 elderly people; mean half-lives for fast acetylators were 1.4 and 1.5 hours respectively and for slow acetylators they were 3.7 and 4.2 hours respectively.— F. Farah *et al.*, *Br. med. J.*, 1977, *2*, 155.

The following amounts of metabolites, expressed as a percentage of the administered dose, were excreted in the urine by rapid and slow acetylators respectively within 24 hours of a single dose of isoniazid 300 mg: 46.3% and 28.9% as acetylisoniazid, 1.8% and 2.5% as acetylhydrazine, and 23% and 4.9% as diacetylhydrazine.— J. A. Timbrell *et al.*, *Clin. Pharmac. Ther.*, 1977, *22*, 602.

Evidence for a trimodal pattern of acetylation of isoniazid in uraemic patients who were classified as slow, intermediate, or rapid acetylators.— D. J. Chapron *et al.*, *J. pharm. Sci.*, 1978, *67*, 1018.

Determination of acetylator phenotype. Rapid and slow inactivators of isoniazid were detected amongst 124 patients with pulmonary tuberculosis by measuring the ratio of acetylisoniazid to isoniazid in the urine in the first two hours following a dose of 3 mg per kg body-weight given by intramuscular injection. The results obtained by this method correlated with those obtained by measuring blood samples.— P. Venkataraman *et al.*, *Tubercle*, 1972, *53*, 84. Studies in Lapps demonstrated that the phenotype could be determined by measuring the ratio of acetylisoniazid to acid-labile isoniazid in urine within 3 hours of a dose given intravenously.— G. A. Ellard *et al.*, *Tubercle*, 1973, *54*, 201.

Sulphadimidine or matrix isoniazid were used to phenotype over 600 patients with tuberculosis being treated with intermittent regimens including isoniazid. Both methods accurately classified about 99% of the patients as fast or slow acetylators.— G. A. Ellard and P. T. Gammon, *Br. J. clin. Pharmac.*, 1977, *4*, 5. See also G. A. Ellard, *Clin. Pharmac. Ther.*, 1976, *19*, 610.

Further references: P. Venkataraman *et al.*, *Tubercle*, 1968, *49*, 210; D. W. Russell, *Br. med. J.*, 1970, *3*, 324; L. Eidus *et al.*, *Am. Rev. resp. Dis.*, 1971, *104*, 587; W. W. Weber and D. W. Hein, *Clin. Pharmacokinet.*, 1979, *4*, 401.

See also under Sulphadimidine, p.1476.

Distribution of acetylator phenotypes. The incidence of rapid acetylators of isoniazid varies according to the racial and geographic origins of populations and is particularly high in some Far Eastern populations. Reports range from an incidence of about 95% in Canadian Eskimos to 20% or less in Egyptians and certain Jewish groups.— W. W. Weber and D. W. Hein, *Clin. Pharmacokinet.*, 1979, *4*, 401.

Phenotyping by urine test indicated that about 60% of black patients from South Africa and the USA were rapid acetylators of isoniazid compared with about 40% of Canadian and American Caucasians.— L. Eidus *et al.*, *Int. J. clin. Pharmac. Biopharm.*, 1979, *17*, 311.

Further reports of acetylator phenotypes in different populations.— A. Hanngren *et al.*, *Scand. J. resp. Dis.*, 1970, *51*, 61; C. W. L. Jeanes *et al.*, *Can. med. Ass. J.*, 1972, *106*, 331; W. G. L. Allan, *Tubercle*, 1973, *54*, 234; G. A. Ellard, *Clin. Pharmac. Ther.*, 1976, *19*, 610; L. A. Salako and A. F. Aderounmu, *Tubercle*, 1977, *58*, 109.

Pregnancy and the neonate. Isoniazid has been shown to reach the foetus within 15 minutes of administration by mouth. Foetal blood concentrations might exceed maternal blood concentrations of isoniazid. The possibility of adverse effects on the central nervous system from prolonged exposure of the foetus to isoniazid should be considered.— F. Moya and V. Thorndike, *Am. J. Obstet. Gynec.*, 1962, *84*, 1778.

Isoniazid, 5 to 10 mg per kg body-weight, has been reported to give concentrations of 6 to 12 µg per ml in the milk of nursing mothers with a milk to maternal plasma ratio of one.— J. A. Knowles, *J. Pediat.*, 1965, *66*, 1068.

Uses. Isoniazid is a hydrazide derivative which is still one of the best drugs available for the primary treatment of pulmonary tuberculosis and is used with other antituberculous agents as described under Treatment of Tuberculosis, p.1565. Intermittent regimens (p.1566) and short-term treatment (p.1566) including isoniazid are increasingly important. Once-weekly treatment may be less effective in patients who are rapid acetylators of isoniazid. It is also given to selected subjects for the prophylaxis of tuberculosis. Isoniazid also appears to be effective in the treatment of extrapulmonary lesions, including meningitis and genito-urinary disease. Pyridoxine 50 to 100 mg daily is often given in conjunction with isoniazid to avert its neurotoxicity.

The usual dose of isoniazid in tuberculosis is 4 to 5 mg per kg body-weight daily given by mouth in single or divided doses to a maximum of 300 mg daily; up to 10 mg per kg daily may be given particularly during the first 1 or 2 weeks of treatment of tuberculous meningitis. A dose of 15 mg per kg has been given twice weekly in intermittent treatment regimens; slow-release preparations of isoniazid have also been used in such regimens, especially in patients who are rapid acetylators of isoniazid. The usual children's dose is 10 to 20 mg per kg daily in single or divided doses.

Similar doses to those used orally may be given by intramuscular injection when isoniazid cannot be taken by mouth; it may also be given by intravenous injection. Isoniazid has been given intrathecally in doses of 25 to 50 mg daily for adults and 10 to 20 mg daily for children to supplement treatment by mouth. Doses of 50 to 250 mg have been instilled intrapleurally after the removal of pus.

In tuberculosis prophylaxis, daily doses of 300 mg have usually been given for 1 year. The prophylactic dose for children is 10 mg per kg daily to a maximum of 300 mg daily in single or divided doses.

Isoniazid has also been successfully used in the treatment of lupus vulgaris (tuberculosis of the skin). It may be administered in doses of 100 mg or more thrice daily. Treatment must be continued for several months.

The effect of isoniazid on tuberculin sensitivity in 28 children.— A. S. Arneil and B. McMichael, *Can. J. publ. Hlth*, 1974, *65*, 197, per *Abstr. Hyg.*, 1974, *49*, 756.

Administration. A daily dose of 300 mg of isoniazid was adequate even in fast inactivators when given with PAS and streptomycin. The speed of inactivation had little effect on daily regimens, only on weekly schedules.— *Br. med. J.*, 1972, *1*, 305. See also *Drug & Ther. Bull.*, 1974, *12*, 21.

Isoniazid concentrations in fast acetylators receiving isoniazid 30 mg per kg body-weight in a slow-release matrix were comparable to those achieved in slow acetylators receiving 10 mg per kg in ordinary tablets.— C. W. L. Jeanes *et al.*, *Can. med. Ass. J.*, 1973, *109*, 483.

In a study of acetylator phenotyping, the speed of isoniazid inactivation had no effect on the response to twice-weekly regimens of isoniazid with rifampicin given for 12 months to 218 patients with pulmonary tuberculosis. This was not so with once-weekly regimens where 11, all rapid acetylators, of 214 patients so treated did not respond when assessed at 12 months.— G. A. Ellard and P. T. Gammon, *Br. J. clin. Pharmac.*, 1977, *4*, 5. See also WHO Collaborating Centre for Tuberculosis Chemotherapy, Prague, *Tubercle*, 1976, *57*, 235.

For pharmacokinetic studies of slow-release isoniazid preparations and further references to acetylator status, see Absorption and Fate above.

Administration in infants and children. Doses of isoniazid greater than 10 mg per kg body-weight daily are considered dangerous in newborn infants.— S. A. McKenzie *et al.*, *Archs Dis. Childh.*, 1976, *51*, 567; G. Katz (letter), *ibid.*, 1977, *52*, 165. A daily dose for isoniazid of 3 to 5 mg per kg daily has been suggested for the first 2 months of life.— A. Peonides (letter), *Archs Dis. Childh.*, 1977, *52*, 165.

See also under Tuberculosis Prophylaxis, below.

Administration in liver disease. In patients with chronic active liver disease requiring absolutely necessary prophylaxis with isoniazid, serum aspartate aminotransferase concentrations should be monitored weekly and treatment stopped if any rise in concentration persists for longer than 4 weeks or if other signs of toxicity develop.— R. K. Roberts *et al.*, *Drugs*, 1979, *17*, 198.

See also under Precautions, above.

Administration in renal failure. From the results of a controlled study of 10 patients with chronic renal failure, the recommended daily dosage of isoniazid for patients with a serum-creatinine concentration less than 120 µg per ml was 300 mg. Patients with more severe renal failure who were rapid acetylators would need no reduction but in slow acetylators the dose should be reduced so that serum-isoniazid concentrations were less than 1 µg per ml 24 hours after the preceding dose.Doses would seldom need to be reduced to less than 200 mg daily.— D. W. Bowersox *et al.*, *New Engl. J. Med.*, 1973, *289*, 84.

Because of the risk of hepatotoxity the use of prophylactic isoniazid in patients with kidney transplants should be limited to patients at high risk of tuberculosis.— P. A. Thomas *et al.*, *Archs Surg., Chicago*, 1979, *114*, 597.

The normal half-life for isoniazid of 2 to 4 hours (slow acetylators) was increased to 4 hours in end-stage renal failure. Patients with a glomerular filtration-rate of less than 10 ml per minute might require a reduction in the dose to between 66 and 100% of the normal dose. Concentrations of isoniazid were affected by haemodialysis and peritoneal dialysis.— W. M. Bennett *et al.*, *Ann. intern. Med.*, 1980, *93*, 62.

Further references: J. S. Cheigh, *Am. J. Med.*, 1977, *62*, 555; P. Sharpstone, *Br. med. J.*, 1977, *2*, 36; T. P. Gibson and H. A. Nelson, *Clin. Pharmacokinet.*, 1977, *2*, 403; G. B. Appel and H. C. Neu, *New Engl. J. Med.*, 1977, *296*, 663.

See also under Treatment of Tuberculosis, p.1565.

Atypical mycobacterial infections. Lesions in 5 patients aged 6 to 47 years contained *Mycobacterium marinum* sensitive to various tuberculostatic agents. Resolution occurred in a 6-year-old boy following daily treatment with isoniazid and aminosalicylic acid for 5 months.— J. Brown *et al.*, *Can. med. Ass. J.*, 1977, *117*, 912.

Chorea. Slight to marked improvement was seen in 5 of 6 patients with Huntington's chorea when they were given large doses of isoniazid in an attempt to increase brain gamma-aminobutyric acid concentrations. Isoniazid 10 to 21 mg per kg body-weight daily in 3 to 5 divided doses (in association with pyridoxine 100 mg daily) was given for periods of 4 to 25 months; of the 3 patients treated for about 2 years, one showed marked improvement and the other two showed moderate improvement. These preliminary results warrant a double-blind comparison of isoniazid with placebo. Treatment should last for at least 4 months and, since adverse effects are more likely in slow acetylators, phenotype should be determined and the dose adjusted accordingly.— T. L. Perry *et al.*, *Neurology, Minneap.*, 1979, *29*, 370.

Leishmaniasis. For reports of beneficial effects with rifampicin and isoniazid in some patients with leishmaniasis, see Rifampicin, p.1581.

Leprosy. For references to a series of favourable reports on the use of a preparation containing dapsone, isoniazid, and prothionamide (isoprodian) concurrently with rifampicin, see Rifampicin, p.1581.

Meningitis, tuberculous. For reference to isoniazid in the treatment of tuberculous meningitis, see Treatment of Tuberculosis, p.1565.

Pulmonary tuberculosis. Some reports of the use of isoniazid in the treatment of pulmonary tuberculosis.— O. Nazareth *et al.*, *Tubercle*, 1966, *47*, 178; C. V. Ramakrishnan *et al.*, *ibid.*, 1969, *50*, 115; *Bull. Wld Hlth Org.*, 1970, *43*, 143; *Chronicle Wld Hlth Org.*, 1970, *24*, 14; *Br. med. J.*, 1970, *4*, 65; *Tubercle*, 1973, *54*, 23; *J. Am. med. Ass.*, 1974, *227*, 489; K. H. K. Hsu, *ibid.*, *229*, 528; H. Kittel, *Dt. med. Wschr.*, 1979, *104*, 477 (preparation containing dapsone, isoniazid, and prothionamide — Isoprodian).

Spinal tuberculosis. Four reports of various methods of treating spinal tuberculosis in over 700 patients showed that over 80% of patients given isoniazid and aminosalicylic acid for 18 months were alive and well with radiologically healed disease when followed up after a further 18 months. The addition of streptomycin made no significant difference and neither did 6 months in bed, 9 months in a plaster jacket, nor an open debridement operation on the spine. However, there was an average 15-degree increase in kyphosis.— *Br. med. J.*, 1974, *4*, 613.

See also in Treatment of Tuberculosis, p.1565.

Tuberculosis of the skin. Seven patients with tuberculosis verrucosa cutis were cleared of lesions within 6 months by treatment, twice weekly, with streptomycin 1 g intramuscularly and isoniazid 14 mg per kg body-weight with pyridoxine.— V. S. Rajan and Y. S. Goh, *Br. J. Derm.*, 1972, *87*, 270.

Tuberculosis prophylaxis. Following diagnosis of sputum-positive tuberculosis in a member of the medical staff of a paediatric department 82 infants who had been in the baby care unit during the 8 weeks before diagnosis received prophylactic isoniazid therapy in a dosage of 8 mg per kg body-weight daily for 8 weeks. None developed tuberculosis.— C. J. Stewart, *Br. med. J.*, 1976, *1*, 30.

In a 3-month double-blind study about 17% of 60 subjects receiving prophylactic therapy with isoniazid 300 mg daily had abnormal serum aspartate aminotransferase (SGOT) values compared with about 7% of 60 similar patients receiving placebo. Of 10 patients who discontinued isoniazid owing to side-effects these were related to liver dysfunction in 5.— R. B. Byrd *et al.*, *Archs intern. Med.*, 1977, *137*, 1130.

In an international, randomised, double-blind study involving 27 830 patients with fibrotic pulmonary lesions, isoniazid 300 mg or a placebo was administered daily for 12, 24, or 52 weeks. The risk of developing tuberculosis during a 5-year follow up was significantly greater in men than in women and in patients with extensive lung lesions. In general a 12-week regimen of isoniazid reduced the risk by about one quarter and 24 weeks by about two-thirds, but for patients with extensive lung lesions or for patients highly compliant with treatment, 52 weeks of isoniazid was the most effective regimen.— A. Krebs *et al.*, *Bull. int. Un. Tuberc.*, 1979, *54*, 65.

Further references: W. C. Bailey and H. B. Greenberg (letter), *J. Am. med. Ass.*, 1973, *225*, 1121; R. Debre *et al.*, *Int. J. Epidemiol.*, 1973, *2*, 153; *Br. med. J.*, 1974, *4*, 63; O. Horwitz and K. Magnus, *Am. J. Epidem.*, 1974, *99*, 333; *Morb. Mortal.*, 1975, *24*, 71; R. D. Fairshter *et al.*, *Am. Rev. resp. Dis.*, 1975, *112*, 37; S. Grzybowski *et al.*, *Can. med. Ass. J.*, 1976, *114*, 607; G. W. Comstock *et al.*, *Am. Rev. resp. Dis.*, 1979, *119*, 827; A. Horvat *et al.*, *Bull. int. Un. Tuberc.*, 1979, *54*, 69.

For recommendations on the prophylactic use of isoniazid see Prophylaxis of Tuberculosis, p.1564.

See also under Adverse Effects of Isoniazid, p.1571.

Tuberculosis of the vulva. A patient with chronic tuberculous ulceration of the vulva had rapid relief of symptoms and complete healing over a 2-month period when given rifampicin 600 mg and isoniazid 300 mg daily. Treatment was continued for one year.— J. W. Millar *et al.*, *Tubercle*, 1979, *60*, 173.

Preparations

Cachets

Sodium Aminosalicylate and Isoniazid Cachets *(B.P.C. 1973)*. —see under Sodium Aminosalicylate, p.1583.

Elixirs and Syrups

Isoniazid Elixir *(B.P.C. 1973)*. Isoniazid Syrup. Isoniazid 50 mg, citric acid monohydrate 12.5 mg, sodium citrate 60 mg, concentrated anise water 0.05 ml, compound tartrazine solution 0.05 ml, glycerol 1 ml, double-strength chloroform water 2 ml, water to 5 ml. Store at a temperature not exceeding 25° in well-filled airtight containers. Protect from light. Under these conditions it may be expected to retain its potency for 1 year. Not more than a month's supply should be dispensed at a time. When a dose less than 5 ml is prescribed the elixir should be diluted to 5 ml with chloroform water. Such dilutions must be freshly prepared and not used more than 2 weeks after issue. Syrup must not be used as the diluent. *Dose.* Children, twice daily, up to 1 year, 2.5 to 5 ml; 1 to 5 years, 5 to 10 ml.

Isoniazid Syrup *(U.S.P.)*. Contains isoniazid 0.93 to 1.1 g in 100 ml. Store in airtight containers. Protect from light.

Injections

Isoniazid Injection *(B.P.)*. A sterile solution of isoniazid in Water for Injections, the solution being adjusted to pH 5.6 to 6 by the addition of 0.1 M hydrochloric acid. Sterilised by autoclaving.

Isoniazid Injection *(U.S.P.)*. A sterile solution in Water for Injections. pH 6 to 7. Protect from light. If crystals have formed they should be redissolved by warming before use.

Tablets

Isoniazid Tablets *(B.P.)*. Tablets containing isoniazid. The *B.P.* requires 70% dissolution in 45 minutes. Protect from light.

Isoniazid Tablets *(U.S.P.)*. Tablets containing isoniazid. Protect from light.

Proprietary Preparations

Rimifon *(Roche, UK)*. Isoniazid, available as an injection containing 25 mg per ml, in ampoules of 2 ml. (Also available as Rimifon in *Belg., Canad., Fr., Ger., Spain, Switz.*).

Other Proprietary Names

Arg.— Nicotibina; *Austral.*— Isotinyl; *Belg.*— Nicotibine; *Canad.*— Isotamine; *Ger.*— Isozid, Neoteben, Tb-Phlogin, Tebesium-s, Gluronazid *(*as isoniazid glucuronolactone or isoniazid sodium glucuronate*)*; *Ital.*— Cin Vis, Idrazil, Nicazide, Nicizina, Nicozid, Tibizina; *Jap.*— Hydronsan *(*isoniazid sodium glucuronate*)*; *Spain*— Cemidon, Dardex, Fimazid, Hidrafasa, Hidranic, Hidrastol, Hidrazida, Hidrulta, Hiperazida, Iso-Dexter, Kridan Simple, Lefos, Lubacida, Zidafimia, Zideluy; *Swed.*— Tibinide; *Switz.*— Gluronazid *(*isoniazid glucuronolactone*)*; *USA*— Niconyl, Nydrazid, Panazid.

7560-w

Isoniazid Aminosalicylate. GEWO 339; Pasiniazid. Isonicotinohydrazide 4-amino-2-hydroxybenzoate. $C_6H_7N_3O,C_7H_7NO_3=290.3$.

CAS — 2066-89-9.

Yellow crystals. **Soluble** in water and methyl alcohol.

Isoniazid aminosalicylate has the actions and uses of isoniazid (p.1571) and sodium aminosalicylate (p.1582) and has been given in a dose of 10 to 20 mg per kg body-weight daily in divided doses in the treatment of tuberculosis.

Proprietary Names

Dipasic *(Gamaprod, Austral.; Geistlich, Belg.; Gewo, Ger.; Farmerid, Ital.; Geistlich, Neth.; Inibsa, Spain)*; Hidrazida Refor *(Rovi, Spain)*; Paraniazide *(Anphar-Rolland, Fr.)*; Propasal *(Llorente, Spain)*.

7561-e

Metazide. Ro 2-4969; Methazidum. $N^2,N^{2'}$-Methylenebis(isonicotinohydrazide). $C_{13}H_{14}N_6O_2=286.3$.

CAS — 1707-15-9.

Pharmacopoeias. In *Rus.*

A white or creamy-white odourless crystalline powder. M.p. 175° to 181° with decomposition. Practically **insoluble** in water, alcohol, chloroform, and ether; freely soluble in dilute mineral acids. **Store** in airtight containers.

Metazide has been used in the treatment of tuberculosis.

Preparations

Tabulettae Methazidi *(Rus. P.)*. Tablets each containing 100, 300, or 500 mg of metazide.

7562-l

Methaniazide Calcium. Isoniazid Methanesulfonate Calcium. The calcium salt of (2-isonicotinoylhydrazino)methanesulphonic acid. $(C_7H_8N_3O_4S)_2Ca=500.5$.

CAS — 13447-95-5 (methaniazide); 6059-26-3 (calcium salt).

Methaniazide calcium is a tuberculostatic agent related to isoniazid (p.1571).

Proprietary Names

Neo-Tizide *(Carlo Erba, Ital.)*.

7563-y

Morinamide. Morphazinamide. *N*-Morpholinomethylpyrazine-2-carboxamide. $C_{10}H_{14}N_4O_2=222.2$.

CAS — 952-54-5.

Morinamide is a tuberculostatic agent which chemically resembles pyrazinamide (see p.1576); cross-resistance between the 2 drugs has been reported. Morinamide has been given by mouth in a dose of 3 g daily and has also been administered intravenously. Morinamide hydrochloride has also been used.

In 4 subjects given morinamide 3 g by mouth, peak plasma concentrations of about 60 µg per ml were attained after 1 hour. The half-life was about 3.5 hours. The activity of morinamide *in vitro* was not due to the formation of pyrazinamide.— T. C. Bravo *et al.*, *Tubercle*, 1975, *56*, 211.

Further references: D. V. A. Opromolla, *Chemotherapia*, 1966, *11*, 270, per *Int. pharm. Abstr.*, 1967, *4*, 348; M. Alves de Souza, *Schweiz. med. Wschr.*, 1966, *96*, 829, per *Int. pharm. Abstr.*, 1967, *4*, 94; A. Rizzo *et al.*, *Revta bras. Med.*, 1966, *23*, 850, per *Bull. Hyg., Lond.*, 1967, *42*, 1104.

Proprietary Names of Morinamide and Morinamide Hydrochloride
Piazofolina *(Bracco, Ital.)*; Piazolina *(Bracco, S.Afr.*; *Vinas, Spain)*; Piazoline *(Beytout, Fr.)*.

7564-j

Phenyl Aminosalicylate. FR7; Fenamisal; Phenyl PAS. Phenyl 4-amino-2-hydroxybenzoate.
$C_{13}H_{11}NO_3$=229.2.

CAS — 133-11-9.

A white crystalline solid. Phenyl aminosalicylate 1.5 g is approximately equivalent to 1 g of aminosalicylic acid. Practically **insoluble** in water.

Phenyl aminosalicylate has actions and uses similar to those of sodium aminosalicylate (p.1582) and was formerly used with other drugs in the treatment of tuberculosis.

A preparation containing phenyl aminosalicylate was formerly marketed in Great Britain under the proprietary name Dantyl (*Leo Laboratories*).

7565-z

Phthivazid. Phthivazidum; Ftivazidum. 2′-Vanillylideneisonicotinohydrazide monohydrate.
$C_{14}H_{13}N_3O_3,H_2O$=289.3.

CAS — 149-17-7 (anhydrous).

Pharmacopoeias. In *Int.* and *Rus.*

A light yellow tasteless powder with a slightly aromatic odour. Practically **insoluble** in water; soluble in alcohol, mineral acids, and solutions of alkali hydroxides. **Store** in airtight containers.

Phthivazid is a hydrazide derivative with properties and uses similar to those of isoniazid (p.1571). A suggested adult dose in the treatment of tuberculosis has been 0.3 to 1.5 g daily in three divided doses, in association with other antituberculous drugs.

Preparations

Tabulettae Phthivazidi *(Rus. P.)*. Phthivazid Tablets. Tablets of 100, 300, and 500 mg.

7566-c

Potassium Aminosalicylate. Aminosalicylate Potassium *(U.S.P.)*. Potassium 4-amino-2-hydroxybenzoate.
$C_7H_6KNO_3$=191.2.

CAS — 133-09-5.

Pharmacopoeias. In *U.S.*

A white to cream-coloured almost odourless crystalline powder with a saline taste. Potassium aminosalicylate 1.25 g is approximately equivalent to 1 g of aminosalicylic acid. Freely **soluble** in water; sparingly soluble in alcohol; very slightly soluble in chloroform and ether. A 2% solution in water has a pH of 6.5 to 8.5. Aqueous solutions are unstable. The *U.S.P.* directs that solutions should be prepared within 24 hours of administration and that a solution must not be used if it is darker in colour than a freshly prepared solution. **Store** at a temperature not exceeding 40° in airtight containers. Protect from light.

Potassium aminosalicylate has actions and uses similar to those of sodium aminosalicylate (p.1582) and has been given in similar doses. It may be given to patients on a restricted sodium diet.

In 12 healthy subjects the mean peak plasma concentration of potassium aminosalicylate was 121 µg per ml following the administration of 4 g by mouth as tablets. The mean half-life was 0.96 hour and 50% of the drug and metabolites was excreted in 2 to 3 hours. About 99% of the dose was excreted in 24 hours, about 54% as the acetylated form.— S. H. Wan *et al.*, *J. pharm. Sci.*, 1974, *63*, 708.

Preparations

Aminosalicylate Potassium Tablets *(U.S.P.)*. Potassium Aminosalicylate Tablets. Tablets containing potassium aminosalicylate. Store at a temperature not exceeding 40° in airtight containers. Protect from light.

Proprietary Names
Teebacin Kalium *(Consolidated Midland, USA)*.

Potassium aminosalicylate was formerly marketed in Great Britain under the proprietary name Paskalium (*Glenwood*).

7567-k

Prothionamide *(B.P.)*. RP 9778; Th 1321. 2-Propylpyridine-4-carbothioamide.
$C_9H_{12}N_2S$=180.3.

CAS — 14222-60-7.

Pharmacopoeias. In *Br.* and *Jap.*

Odourless or almost odourless, yellow crystals or crystalline powder. M.p. 140° to 143°. Practically **insoluble** in water; soluble 1 in 30 of alcohol, 1 in 200 of chloroform, 1 in 300 of ether, and 1 in 16 of methyl alcohol; soluble in acetone. **Protect** from light.

Adverse Effects, Treatment, and Precautions. As for Ethionamide, p.1570. Prothionamide may be better tolerated.

References: Report of the British Tuberculosis Association 1968, *Tubercle*, 1968, *49*, 125.

Antimicrobial Action. As for Ethionamide, p.1571. There is complete cross-resistance between ethionamide and prothionamide.

Absorption and Fate. Prothionamide is readily absorbed from the gastro-intestinal tract and produces peak plasma concentrations 1 to 2 hours after a dose by mouth. Significant concentrations persist in the blood for about 6 hours. The drug is excreted in urine, mainly as its metabolites.

References: A. Bieder and P. Brunel, *Annls pharm. fr.*, 1971, *29*, 461; J. Pütter, *Arzneimittel-Forsch.*, 1972, *22*, 1027.

Uses. Prothionamide is a thioamide derivative with actions and uses resembling those of ethionamide (p.1571). It appears to be as active an antituberculous agent as ethionamide and to be better tolerated. Strains of *M. tuberculosis* which acquire resistance to ethionamide also become resistant to prothionamide.

The usual dose for adults and children older than 10 years is 0.5 to 1 g daily, taken as single or divided doses with meals. Treatment may be started with lower doses and gradually increased. For children under 10 years of age, an initial dose of 10 mg per kg body-weight daily, gradually increased over 15 days to 20 mg per kg has been recommended.

Prothionamide has also been administered as rectal suppositories; prothionamide hydrochloride has been given intravenously.

Leprosy. Studies in *mice* indicated that the efficacy of ethionamide or prothionamide was considerably reduced if they were given less than 3 times a week. No bacterial multiplication occurred after treatment courses lasting 12 weeks indicating that in paucibacillary leprosy 3- to 6-month treatment courses of prothionamide 500 mg daily should be considered.— S. R. Pattyn, *Lepr. Rev.*, 1978, *49*, 199.

For references to a series of reports on the use of a preparation containing dapsone, isoniazid, and prothionamide (Isoprodian) concurrently with rifampicin, see Rifampicin, p.1581.

Pulmonary tuberculosis. Comparisons of prothionamide and ethionamide in the treatment of pulmonary tuberculosis.— H. Sighart *et al.*, *Prax. Pneumol.*, 1970, *24*, 295; D. K. Gupta *et al.*, *J. Indian med. Ass.*, 1977, *68*, 25.

Further references: J. Miguères *et al.*, *Revue Tuberc. Pneumol.*, 1965, *29*, 1037; A. G. Khomenko and V. I. Tchukanov, *Bull. int. Un. Tuberc.*, 1979, *54*, 49 (comparison of rifampicin and isoniazid with prothionamide or ethambutol); H. Kittel, *Dt. med. Wschr.*, 1979, *104*, 477 (preparation containing dapsone, isoniazid, and prothionamide—Isoprodian).

Preparations

Prothionamide Tablets *(B.P.)*. Tablets containing prothionamide. The tablets may be sugar-coated.

Proprietary Names
Ektebin *(Bayer, Ger.)*; Peteha *(Saarstickstoff-Fatol, Ger.)*; Trevintix *(*also as hydrochloride*) (May & Baker, Austral.*; *Theraplix, Belg.*; *Théraplix, Fr.*; *May & Baker, S.Afr.*; *Rhodia, Spain)*.

Prothionamide was formerly marketed in Great Britain under the proprietary name Trevintix *(May & Baker)*.

7568-a

Pyrazinamide *(B.P., U.S.P.)*. Pyrazinamidum; Pyrazinoic Acid Amide. Pyrazine-2-carboxamide.
$C_5H_5N_3O$=123.1.

CAS — 98-96-4.

Pharmacopoeias. In *Br., Int., Jap., Jug., Nord.*, and *U.S.*

A white or almost white, odourless or almost odourless, crystalline powder with a slightly bitter taste. M.p. 188° to 191°.

Soluble 1 in 60 of water and 1 in 110 of alcohol; soluble in chloroform and ether. A 1.5% solution in water is neutral to litmus. **Store** in airtight containers. Protect from light.

Adverse Effects. Hepatotoxicity is a serious side-effect of pyrazinamide therapy and its frequency appears to be related to dose and duration of treatment. With doses of 3 g daily up to 15% of patients may show signs of liver damage. Other side-effects are anorexia, nausea, vomiting, arthralgia, malaise, fever, sideroblastic anaemia, and difficulty in micturition. Photosensitivity and skin rashes have been reported on rare occasions. Hyperuricaemia commonly occurs and may lead to attacks of gout.

Effects on the liver. A review of the hepatotoxicity of antituberculosis regimens containing pyrazinamide indicates that the risks are much lower than was suggested by early studies, in which large doses were used, often for long periods.— D. J. Girling, *Tubercle*, 1978, *59*, 13. See also J. H. Angel *et al.*, *Bull. int. Un. Tuberc.*, 1979, *54*, 47.

Hyperuricaemia. Studies carried out on one of the authors showed that the urate retention caused by pyrazinamide was mediated by the metabolite pyrazinoic acid. The suppression of urate excretion might be reduced by the intermittent administration of pyrazinamide.— G. A. Ellard and R. M. Haslam, *Tubercle*, 1976, *57*, 97.

Treatment of Adverse Effects. Aminosalicylic acid has been reported to inhibit the hyperuricaemia provoked by pyrazinamide. If hyperuricaemia with acute gouty arthritis occurs pyrazinamide should generally be withdrawn although a uricosuric agent such as probenecid has been given—but see under Precautions below.

Precautions. Pyrazinamide is contra-indicated in patients with liver damage. Liver function should be assessed before and regularly during treatment. Caution should be observed in patients with impaired renal function or a history of gout.

Increased difficulty has been reported in controlling diabetes mellitus when diabetics are given pyrazinamide.

Effect on diagnostic tests. Pyrazinamide could interfere with the Acetest and Ketostix qualitative urine tests for ketones to produce a pink-brown colour.— *Drug & Ther. Bull.*, 1972, *10,* 69.

Interactions. A study of the complex interactions occurring when pyrazinamide and probenecid are given to patients with gout. Urinary excretion of urate depends on the relative size and timing of doses of the two drugs. Probenecid is known to block the excretion of pyrazinamide.— T. F. Yü *et al., Am. J. Med.*, 1977, *63,* 723.

Antimicrobial Action. Pyrazinamide may be bactericidal. It is effective only against *Mycobacterium tuberculosis.* An MIC of 20 µg per ml has been reported *in vitro* at an acid pH; pyrazinamide is inactive at a neutral pH. When used alone resistance may develop within 6 to 8 weeks.

A simple method for detecting pyrazinamide resistance.— E. Brander, *Tubercle,* 1972, *53,* 128.

Absorption and Fate. Pyrazinamide is readily absorbed from the gastro-intestinal tract. Peak serum concentrations occur about 2 hours after a dose by mouth and have been reported to be 33 µg per ml after 1.5 g, and 59 µg per ml after 3 g. Serum concentrations thereafter decline, with a half-life of about 9 to 10 hours. It diffuses into the cerebrospinal fluid. About 30% of the dose is excreted in urine as pyrazinoic acid, and 4% as unchanged pyrazinamide, within 24 hours; 5-hydroxypyrazinoic acid is also an important metabolite.

References: K. D. Stottmeier *et al., Am. Rev. resp. Dis.*, 1968, *98,* 70; G. A. Ellard, *Tubercle,* 1969, *50,* 144; I. M. Weiner and J. P. Tinker, *J. Pharmac. exp. Ther.*, 1972, *180,* 411; G. A. Ellard and R. M. Haslam, *Tubercle,* 1976, *57,* 97.

Diffusion. The average concentrations of pyrazinamide in the cerebrospinal fluid in a patient with tuberculous meningitis were 50 µg per ml, 5 hours after doses of 3 g. Serum concentrations were identical.— R. Forgan-Smith *et al.* (letter), *Lancet,* 1973, *2,* 374.

Uses. Pyrazinamide has not been considered suitable for the primary treatment of pulmonary tuberculosis because of its potential hepatotoxicity. It is however used with other antituberculous drugs in re-treatment regimens, especially in developing countries, see Treatment of Tuberculosis, p.1565, and is now being used more widely in intermittent treatment regimens (p.1566) and short-term treatment regimens (p.1566).

The adult dose of pyrazinamide is 20 to 35 mg per kg body-weight to a maximum of 3 g daily. Children have been given 20 mg per kg daily when there was no satisfactory alternative. It should be given in 3 or 4 equally spaced doses.

A review and criticism of the value of pyrazinamide for assessing urate secretion.— T. H. Steele, *Ann. intern. Med.*, 1973, *79,* 734.

Some reports of the use of pyrazinamide in the treatment of pulmonary tuberculosis.— *Tubercle,* 1969, *50,* 81 (East African/British MRC Pyrazinamide Investigation); *ibid.*, 1970, *51,* 359 (East African/British MRC Pyrazinamide Investigation—Second Report, 1970); J. A. Doyle *et al., ibid.*, 397; *ibid.*, 1971, *52,* 191 (The First Report of the East African/British MRC Retreatment Investigation); *ibid.*, 1973, *54,* 283 (The Second Report of the East African/British MRC Retreatment Investigation).

Preparations

Pyrazinamide Tablets *(B.P., U.S.P.).* Tablets containing pyrazinamide.

Zinamide *(Merck Sharp & Dohme, UK).* Pyrazinamide, available as scored tablets of 500 mg. (Also available as Zinamide in *Austral.*).

Other Proprietary Names

Piraldina *(Ital.)*; Pyrafat *(Ger.)*; Pyrazide *(S.Afr.)*; Tebrazid *(Belg., Canad.)*.

7569-t

Rifampicin *(B.P.).* Rifampin *(U.S.P.)*; Rifaldazine; Rifamycin AMP. 3-(4-Methylpiperazin-1-yliminomethyl)rifamycin SV; (12*Z*,14*E*,24*E*)-(2*S*,16*S*,17*S*,18*R*,19*R*,20*R*,21*S*,22*R*,23*S*)-1,2-Dihydro-5,6,9,17,19-pentahydroxy-23-methoxy-2,4,12,16,18,20,22-heptamethyl-8-(4-methylpiperazin-1-yliminomethyl)-1,11-dioxo-2,7-(epoxypentadeca[1,11,13]trienimino)naphtho-[2,1-*b*]furan-21-yl acetate.

$C_{43}H_{58}N_4O_{12}$=823.0.

CAS — 13292-46-1.

Pharmacopoeias. In *Br., Braz., Roum.*, and *U.S.*

A tasteless brick red to reddish brown crystalline powder. The *U.S.P.* specifies a potency of not less than 900 µg per mg. M.p. about 185° with decomposition. Slightly **soluble** in water, acetone, alcohol, and ether; freely soluble in chloroform; soluble in ethyl acetate and methyl alcohol. Solubility in aqueous solutions is increased at low pH values. A 1% suspension in water has a pH of 4 to 6.5.

The dry powder is stable for more than 5 years at 25°. It loses about 20% of its potency in aqueous solution in 10 hours at room temperature but decomposition is diminished by the addition of a reducing agent such as ascorbic acid. **Store** at a temperature not exceeding 15° in airtight containers in an atmosphere of nitrogen. Protect from light.

At pH 7.5 and a temperature of 25° rifampicin was soluble 1 in 360 of water and desacetylrifampicin was soluble 1 in 135 under the same conditions.— N. Maggi *et al.* , *Lepetit, Arzneimittel-Forsch.*, 1969, *19,* 651.

Adverse Effects. Rifampicin is usually well tolerated. The incidence of side-effects appears to be influenced by the schedule of administration. Gastro-intestinal side-effects have sometimes been severe enough to necessitate withdrawal.

Rifampicin produces abnormalities in liver function. Jaundice may be associated with the concomitant use of other agents, including isoniazid, and fatalities have been reported in patients with pre-existing liver disorders or who had also taken other potentially hepatotoxic agents. Some patients may experience a febrile reaction with influenza-like symptoms. Alterations in kidney function and renal failure have occurred and are considered to be due to hypersensitivity. Skin reactions, eosinophilia, leucopenia, thrombocytopenia, purpura, haemolysis and shock have also occurred.

Other side-effects reported include confusion, drowsiness, weakness, ataxia, dizziness, peripheral neuropathy (which may be due to the concomitant use of isoniazid), blurred vision, transient hearing loss, and menstrual irregularities.

Adverse reactions to daily or intermittent treatment with rifampicin include cutaneous and gastro-intestinal reactions, liver dysfunction, and thrombocytopenic purpura. *Cutaneous reactions* are usually mild and transient and start early in treatment. Typically they consist of flushing of the face and neck sometimes with itching or a rash which may be generalised; up to 5% of patients may be affected. There may be redness and watering of the eyes. Occasionally patients with severe cutaneous reactions may require desensitisation before treatment with rifampicin can be resumed—a dose of 75 mg is given and if there is no reaction it is given twice daily and the dose gradually increased until the original daily dosage is reached. *Gastro-intestinal reactions* are rarely serious and usually consist of anorexia, nausea, and mild abdominal pain; vomiting may occur and, less frequently, diarrhoea. They can often be prevented by giving rifampicin during or immediately after a meal but a few patients seem unable to tolerate rifampicin, in which case it should be withdrawn. There may be transient disturbances of *liver function* during the early weeks of treatment with rifampicin. Hepatitis is uncommon, occurring in up to 1% of patients, and is more likely in alcoholics and patients with pre-existing liver disease. If hepatitis occurs treatment should be stopped, liver-function tests carried out, and supportive treatment given if necessary. Rifampicin may usually be resumed once liver function is normal but should be stopped and alternative chemotherapy used if it becomes abnormal again. A suggestion that patients given rifampicin and isoniazid may be at special risk of liver damage has not been confirmed in later studies. *Thrombocytopenic purpura* is very uncommon but if it occurs rifampicin should be withdrawn immediately and never given again. Some reactions to rifampicin have usually only been reported with intermittent treatment, particularly once-weekly or twice-weekly regimens, and include the 'flu' syndrome, shock, shortness of breath, haemolytic anaemia, and renal failure. They are unlikely to occur when rifampicin is given thrice-weekly or only once a month as in leprosy. The *'flu' syndrome* consists of episodes of fever, chills, and malaise, sometimes with headache, dizziness, and bone pain, starting one to two hours after each dose of rifampicin and lasting for up to 8 hours. The syndrome usually appears after at least 3 months of treatment and may occur in up to 20% of patients receiving once-weekly regimens including rifampicin in a dose of 20 mg or more per kg body-weight. It is more common in women than in men and may be stopped by reducing the dose or changing to daily administration. Circulating rifampicin-dependent antibodies are associated with the occurrence of the 'flu' syndrome which suggests that the symptoms described have an immunological basis. *Shock, shortness of breath, acute haemolytic anaemia,* and *renal failure* have been reported rarely during intermittent therapy but if any of these reactions occur rifampicin should be withdrawn and never given again. When rifampicin is resumed after an interval of several weeks severe reactions have occasionally been experienced by patients who have previously had no reaction or only minor reactions. Treatment should therefore be re-introduced gradually beginning with a daily dose of 75 mg and increasing by 75 mg daily until the required dosage is reached. Despite the potentially dangerous reactions with rifampicin, especially with intermittent regimens, it has been possible to minimise the risks by adjustment of treatment regimens in the light of results from controlled studies.— D. J. Girling, *J. antimicrob. Chemother.*, 1977, *3,* 115; D. J. Girling and K. L. Hitze, *Bull. Wld Hlth Org.*, 1979, *57,* 45.

There is no need to assess the titre of rifampicin-dependent antibodies since no matter how high the titre in patients with reactions, rifampicin can usually be continued without risk by changing to a daily dose. A higher serum-rifampicin concentration was detected in patients experiencing adverse reactions than in patients who did not. Although intermittent treatment can give a higher incidence of side-effects, there is a lower incidence with a twice-weekly than a once-weekly schedule and the incidence with once-weekly rifampicin can be reduced if the schedule is preceded by 2 months of daily treatment.— D. J. Girling *et al.* (letter), *Br. med. J.*, 1974, *3,* 114.

A suggestion that some of the adverse reactions associated with rifampicin may be attributed to its metabolite desacetylrifampicin.— H. Nakagawa *et al., Bull. int. Un. Tuberc.*, 1979, *54,* 171.

Reports of adverse effects in patients receiving intermittent treatment regimens including rifampicin.— G. Poole *et al., Br. med. J.*, 1971, *3,* 343; D. J. Girling and W. Fox (letter), *ibid.*, 1971, *4,* 231; M. Aquinas *et al., Br. med. J.*, 1972, *1,* 765; H. Eule *et al., Tubercle,* 1974, *55,* 81; *ibid.*, 1974, *55,* 193; J. -C. Pujet *et al., Br. med. J.*, 1974, *2,* 415; *Tubercle,* 1975, *56,* 173; J. M. Dickinson *et al., J. antimicrob. Chemother.*, 1977, *3,* 445.

Carcinogenicity. High doses of rifampicin given to *mice* were not carcinogenic.— E. T. Gláz (letter), *Lancet,* 1974, *2,* 404. See also J. Bichel (letter), *Lancet,* 1973, *2,* 1209.

A report of nasopharyngeal lymphoma developing in a 41-year-old man following treatment with isoniazid, ethambutol, and rifampicin for 2 years. It was thought this might be due to the immunosuppressive effects of rifampicin following long-term treatment.— R. Rate *et al.* (letter), *Ann. intern. Med.*, 1979, *90,* 276.

Accelerated growth of lung cancer in association with rifampicin given for tuberculosis.— D. Rodescu *et al.* (letter), *Lancet,* 1981, *2,* 983.

Effects on the blood. *Agranulocytosis.* Mention of a case of fatal aplastic anaemia or agranulocytosis probably due to rifampicin.— W. H. W. Inman, *Br. med. J.*, 1977, *1,* 1500.

Eosinophilia. A case of eosinophilia associated with rifampicin.— I. P. F. Mungall, *Chest,* 1978, *74,* 321. Another case.— M. Lee and H. W. Berger (letter), *ibid.*, 1980, *77,* 579.

Haemolysis. A case of haemolysis associated with rifampicin.— S. Lakshminarayan *et al., Br. med. J.*, 1973, *2,* 282. See also K. Mohring *et al., Dt. med. Wschr.*, 1974,

99, 1458.

Neutropenia. A 75-year-old man treated with isoniazid, ethambutol, and rifampicin developed neutropenia which was re-induced, on challenge, by each of the 3 agents.— P. F. Jenkins *et al.*, *Br. med. J.*, 1980, *280*, 1069.

Thrombocytopenia. Reports of thrombocytopenia associated with rifampicin.— M. A. Blajchman *et al.*, *Br. med. J.*, 1970, *3*, 24; G. C. Ferguson (letter), *Br. med. J.*, 1971, *3*, 638; C. Devred *et al.*, *Nouv. Presse méd.*, 1975, *4*, 2042; J. W. Hadfield, *Postgrad. med. J.*, 1980, *56*, 59.

Effects on bone. Osteomalacia in one patient associated with rifampicin.— S. C. Shah *et al.*, *Tubercle*, 1981, *62*, 207.

Effects on the eye. A study indicated that usual therapeutic doses of rifampicin interfere with colour vision.— J. Laroche and C. Laroche, *Annls pharm. fr.*, 1972, *30*, 433. See also A. W. Lees *et al.*, *Tubercle*, 1971, *52*, 182.

A 34-year-old man suffering from pulmonary tuberculosis developed reversible exudative conjunctivitis as a result of rifampicin therapy.— F. E. Cayley and S. K. Majumdar, *Br. med. J.*, 1976, *1*, 199. Comment.— D. J. Girling (letter), *ibid.*, 585.

Effects on the gastro-intestinal tract. A report of a 59-year-old woman with pseudomembranous colitis probably induced by rifampicin. Underlying hepatic disease may have predisposed her to this.— G. Fournier *et al.* (letter), *Lancet*, 1980, *1*, 101. Criticism.— G. Acocella and V. Arioli, *Lepetit, Ital.* (letter), *ibid.*, 827. Although pseudomembranous colitis may be an exceedingly rare complication of rifampicin, the diagnosis should be considered. Another case of pseudomembranous colitis probably due to rifampicin has occurred (I. Phillips, *Personal Communication*).— R. H. George (letter), *ibid.*, 1304.

A report of pseudomembranous colitis attributed to treatment with rifampicin in association with ethambutol.— H. J. Moriarty and B. A. Scobie, *N.Z. med. J.*, 1980, *91*, 294.

Isolates of *Clostridium difficile* were susceptible to rifampicin (MICs of 0.2 μg or less per ml). However, typical clinical and morphological changes of antibiotic-associated colitis were induced in *hamsters* by rifampicin after the organisms had acquired resistance following frequent exposure.— R. P. O'Connor *et al.* (letter), *Lancet*, 1981, *1*, 499.

Further reports of pseudomembranous colitis associated with the use of rifampicin.— S. P. Borriello *et al.*, *Br. med. J.*, 1980, *281*, 1180; M. Melange *et al.* (letter), *Lancet*, 1980, *2*, 1192; G. Bommelaer *et al.*, *ibid.*

Effects on the kidney. Administration of rifampicin to a 60-year-old man with tuberculosis during a period of fluid restriction induced insidious renal failure with light-chain proteinuria.— R. J. Warrington *et al.*, *Archs intern. Med.*, 1977, *137*, 927.

Other reports of renal failure associated with rifampicin.— V. K. Bansal *et al.*, *Am. Rev. resp. Dis.*, 1977, *116*, 137; W. Y. Qunibi *et al.*, *Sth. med. J.*, 1980, *73*, 791.

Reports of renal failure developing during intermittent treatment with rifampicin and after an interruption in treatment.— D. Cordonnier and J. M. Muller (letter), *Lancet*, 1972, *2*, 1364; D. L. Rothwell and D. E. Richmond, *Br. med. J.*, 1974, *2*, 481; C. T. Flynn *et al.*, *ibid.*, 482; N. Manescu *et al.*, *Münch. med. Wschr.*, 1974, *116*, 2161; K. Mattson *et al.*, *Scand. J. resp. Dis.*, 1974, *55*, 291; M. Cochran *et al.* (letter), *Lancet*, 1975, *1*, 1428; W. C. Chan *et al.*, *Tubercle*, 1975, *56*, 191; P. A. Gabow *et al.*, *J. Am. med. Ass.*, 1976, *235*, 2517; H. Riska *et al.*, *Scand. J. resp. Dis.*, 1976, *57*, 183.

Effects on the liver. A review of the hepatic toxicity of antituberculosis regimens containing isoniazid, rifampicin, or ethambutol.— D. J. Girling, *Tubercle*, 1978, *59*, 13.

In 5 patients with long-standing cirrhosis, jaundice and severe liver failure developed after rifampicin administration; 3 of the patients died.— S. Di Piazza *et al.* (letter), *Lancet*, 1978, *1*, 774.

Predisposing factors in hepatitis induced by isoniazid-rifampicin treatment of tuberculosis.— C. Grönhagen-Riska *et al.*, *Am. Rev. resp. Dis.*, 1978, *118*, 461.

Reports of liver damage in patients receiving rifampicin in association with isoniazid and other drugs.— R. Lesobre *et al.*, *Revue Tuberc. Pneumol.*, 1969, *33*, 393; A. W. Lees *et al.*, *Tubercle*, 1971, *52*, 182; R. Gabriel (letter), *Br. med. J.*, 1971, *3*, 182; S. Lal *et al.*, *Br. med. J.*, 1972, *1*, 148; D. Pessayre *et al.*, *Gastroenterology*, 1977, *72*, 284; J. E. Groopman *et al.* (letter), *New Engl. J. Med.*, 1978, *298*, 1316; A. S. Pier (letter), *ibid.*, 1317.

Hepatotoxicity in children. Reports of severe hepatic reactions in infants and children receiving treatment with rifampicin and isoniazid.— M. Casteels-Van Daele *et al.*, *J. Pediat.*, 1975, *86*, 739; L. Gutman (letter), *J. antimicrob. Chemother.*, 1978, *4*, 283.

Hepatitis occurred in a child treated with rifampicin and ethambutol. Additional symptoms included polyarthritis and the presence of anti-native DNA antibodies.— D. M. Grennan and R. D. Sturrock, *Tubercle*, 1976, *57*, 259.

Effects on mental state. Rifampicin administered daily to a 60-year-old man was associated with the development of an acute organic brain syndrome in which he became confused, disorientated, agitated, and incoherent and suffered hallucinations and delusions.— T. H. Pratt, *J. Am. med. Ass.*, 1979, *241*, 2421.

Further references.— C. W. L. Jeanes *et al.*, *Can. med. Ass. J.*, 1972, *106*, 884.

Effects on muscles. Myopathy in one patient induced by rifampicin.— P. Jenkins and P. A. Emerson, *Br. med. J.*, 1981, *283*, 105.

Effects on the pancreas. Pancreatitis associated with rifampicin therapy might be connected with raised concentrations of the lysosomal enzymes β-glucuronidase and β-*N*-acetyl-glucosaminidase.— W. Perry *et al.* (letter), *Lancet*, 1979, *1*, 492.

Effects on the skin. Chronic papular acneform lesions developed on the face, neck, and shoulders of 8 patients after taking rifampicin, isoniazid, and thiacetazone for about 5 weeks; the lesions disappeared when rifampicin was gradually withdrawn after 12 to 18 weeks of treatment.— U. Nwokolo (letter), *Br. med. J.*, 1974, *3*, 473.

Pemphigus occurring in a 65-year-old woman after about 9 months of treatment with rifampicin, isoniazid, and ethambutol was attributed to rifampicin.— R. W. Gange *et al.*, *Br. J. Derm.*, 1976, *95*, 445.

A 40-year-old African man with tuberculosis given rifampicin, streptomycin, and isoniazid developed the Stevens-Johnson syndrome when ethambutol was added 4 weeks later. All drugs were withdrawn and he responded to treatment with corticosteroids. The condition recurred when rifampicin was again added. Ethambutol had possibly triggered the reaction.— R. Nyirenda and G. V. Gill, *Br. med. J.*, 1977, *2*, 1189.

A report of erythema multiforme bullosum due to rifampicin.— P. Nigam *et al.*, *Lepr. India*, 1979, *51*, 249.

Overdosage. Bright red pigmentation of the skin, orange coloration of sweat, and deep red coloration of plasma and urine were noted in a man who claimed to have taken 40 rifampicin tablets 300 mg. The plasma-rifampicin concentration 12 hours after ingestion was 400 μg per ml but recovery was uneventful and there was only mild liver damage.— R. W. Newton and A. R. W. Forrest, *Scott. med. J.*, 1975, *20*, 55.

Ingestion of about 60 g of rifampicin resulted in death in a 26-year-old man.— R. O. Broadwell *et al.*, *J. Am. med. Ass.*, 1978, *240*, 2283.

Post-mortem findings following a fatal overdose of rifampicin and ethambutol.— D. B. Jack *et al.* (letter), *Lancet*, 1978, *2*, 1107.

Ingestion by a 15-year-old girl of an unknown quantity of rifampicin resulted in marked facial oedema and swelling of the tongue and oropharynx, as well as coloured skin and mucous membranes.— S. Meisel and R. Brower (letter), *Ann. intern. Med.*, 1980, *92*, 262.

Treatment of Adverse Effects. Overdosage with rifampicin should be treated with gastric lavage and intensive supportive measures.

Precautions. Rifampicin is contra-indicated in patients who are hypersensitive to rifamycins. It should not be given to patients with jaundice and should be used with caution in alcoholics and other patients with impaired liver function, especially when given with isoniazid (p.1573) or other hepatotoxic drugs.

Rifampicin accelerates the metabolism of other drugs by inducing microsomal liver enzymes and possibly by interfering with the hepatic uptake of drugs. It has been reported to decrease the effectiveness of corticosteroids, coumarin anticoagulants, digitoxin (and perhaps digoxin), methadone, oral contraceptives, and tolbutamide and may interfere with diagnostic tests. Hypersensitivity reactions including nephrotoxicity appear to be associated with the intermittent use of rifampicin; if treatment with rifampicin is interrupted it should be re-introduced cautiously. Its use is best avoided during pregnancy. Faeces, saliva, sputum, sweat, tears, and urine may be coloured orange-red.

A decline in reactivity to skin tests with tuberculin PPD occurred in 8 of 11 patients and was associated with rifampicin.— P. Mukerjee *et al.*, *Antimicrob. Ag. Chemother.*, 1973, *4*, 607.

A patient's soft contact lenses turned orange after a 2-day course of rifampicin. After the use of a routine cleaning solution one lens continued to have a residual stain.— R. W. Lyons (letter), *New Engl. J. Med.*, 1979, *300*, 372; *idem*, *301*, 224.

Rifampicin produces a shift of peripheral thyroid hormone metabolism towards the activating pathway.— E. E. Ohnhaus and H. Studer, *Br. J. clin. Pharmac.*, 1980, *9*, 285P.

Administration of rifampicin 600 mg daily for 14 days to 8 healthy male subjects reduced plasma concentrations of 25-hydroxycholecalciferol by 56% to 90%. Concentrations of 1,25-dihydroxycholecalciferol were unchanged. The fall in 25-hydroxycholecalciferol may represent the earliest lesion of drug-induced osteomalacia.— M. J. Brodie *et al.*, *Br. J. clin. Pharmac.*, 1980, *9*, 286P; *idem*, *Clin. Pharmac. Ther.*, 1980, *27*, 810.

Effects on laboratory estimations. Studies of the effect of rifampicin on liver function indicated that rifampicin produced competition for the elimination of bilirubin and sulphobromophthalein by the liver. Sulphobromophthalein sodium tests cannot be interpreted until at least 24 hours after rifampicin has been discontinued.— P. Capelle *et al.*, *Gut*, 1972, *13*, 366.

Rifampicin and the assay of folate and vitamin B_{12}.— J. Bate and A. J. Cole, *Med. Lab. Technol.*, 1974, *31*, 199.

Toxic serum concentrations of rifampicin, but not therapeutic concentrations, interfered with the total serum bilirubin assay.— S. Meisel *et al.*, *Antimicrob. Ag. Chemother.*, 1980, *18*, 206.

Interactions with drugs. A review of pharmacokinetic interactions with rifampicin.— W. Zilly *et al.*, *Clin. Pharmacokinet.*, 1977, *2*, 61. See also G. Acocella, *Clin. Pharmacokinet.*, 1978, *3*, 108; G. Acocella and R. Conti, *Tubercle*, 1980, *61*, 171.

A study in 6 healthy subjects demonstrating that rifampicin is a selective inducer of oxidative drug metabolism.— D. D. Breimer *et al.*, *Clin. Pharmac. Ther.*, 1977, *21*, 470.

Further references.— W. C. Buss, *J. antimicrob. Chemother.*, 1979, *5*, 4.

See also under Antimicrobial Action.

Aminosalicylic Acid. Aminosalicylic acid impeded the gastro-intestinal absorption of rifampicin; this could be overcome by administering the drugs separately at an interval of 8 to 12 hours.— G. Boman *et al.* (letter), *Lancet*, 1971, *1*, 800. See also *idem*, *Eur. J. clin. Pharmac.*, 1974, *7*, 217. The decreased absorption of rifampicin was shown to be due to adsorption of rifampicin by bentonite, the main excipient in the granules of aminosalicylic acid.— G. Boman *et al.*, *Eur. J. clin. Pharmac.*, 1975, *8*, 293.

Antidiabetic agents. For a report of increased dose requirements of chlorpropamide in a patient taking rifampicin, see under Chlorpropamide, p.853.

For the effect of rifampicin on tolbutamide, see Tolbutamide, p.860.

Barbiturates. The elimination half-life of hexobarbitone was significantly decreased by treatment with rifampicin in patients with liver disease.— W. Zilly *et al.*, *Eur. J. clin. Pharmac.*, 1977, *11*, 287.

Clofibrate. For the effect of rifampicin in reducing plasma concentrations of clofibric acid, see Clofibrate, p.409.

Corticosteroids. Corticosteroids administered with rifampicin in borderline leprosy exacerbated neuritis in 3 patients with tuberculoid leprosy although in a further patient with lepromatous leprosy neuropathy was alleviated.— G. J. Steenbergen and R. E. Pfaltzgraff, *Lepr. Rev.*, 1975, *46*, 115.

Renal transplant function deteriorated in 3 patients receiving corticosteroids to prevent rejection when they were also given rifampicin.— G. A. Buffington *et al.*, *J. Am. med. Ass.*, 1976, *236*, 1958.

A 6-year-old boy with nephrotic syndrome became unresponsive to prednisolone while receiving rifampicin, evidently the result of hepatic microsomal enzyme induction.— W. Hendrickse *et al.*, *Br. med. J.*, 1979, *1*, 306.

A recommendation that corticosteroid dosage be doubled whenever treatment with rifampicin is initiated.— W. Jubiz and A. W. Meikle, *Drugs*, 1979, *18*, 113.

Dapsone. For references to interactions between dapsone and rifampicin, see Dapsone, p.1490.

Digoxin. For a report of heart failure and reduced serum-digoxin concentrations when rifampicin was given to a woman being treated with digoxin, see under Digoxin, p.534.

Isoniazid. A study in 12 patients with tuberculosis indicated that although isoniazid taken concomitantly with rifampicin had no influence on the metabolic induction of rifampicin it had an unfavourable effect on rifampicin blood concentrations. Isoniazid blood concentrations were unaffected.— R. P. Mouton *et al.*, *J. antimicrob. Chemother.*, 1979, *5*, 447.

Further references.— G. Acocella *et al.*, *Gut*, 1972, *13*, 47; P. Capelle *et al.*, *ibid.*, 366; J. Llorens *et al.*, *Chemotherapy, Basle*, 1978, *24*, 97.

Oral contraceptives. For the effect of rifampicin on oral contraceptives, see Oral Contraceptives, p.1406.

Probenecid. Significant increases in serum-rifampicin concentrations were achieved in 6 subjects given probenecid in association with rifampicin.— S. Kenwright and A. J. Levi, *Lancet*, 1973, *2*, 1401. Probenecid did not significantly increase serum-rifampicin concentrations.— R. J. Fallon *et al.*, *ibid.*, 1975, *2*, 792.

Quinidine. For reports of rifampicin diminishing the effect of quinidine, see Quinidine Sulphate, p.1371.

Porphyria. Although rifampicin has not been implicated as a cause of acute attacks of porphyria, it is a powerful enzyme inducer and should not be given to patients at risk.— *Drug & Ther. Bull.*, 1976, *14*, 72. A study in *rats* indicated that rifampicin would probably not elicit an acute attack in susceptible porphyric individuals.— G. H. Blekkenhorst *et al.* (letter), *Lancet*, 1980, *1*, 1367. Rifampicin is a potent enzyme inducer in man but not in *rats*. It should, therefore, be regarded as contra-indicated for the porphyric patient.— M. J. Brodie (letter), *ibid.*, *2*, 86.

Pregnancy and the neonate. The manufacturers' contra-indication to the use of rifampicin in pregnancy is based on dose-dependent teratogenicity in *rats* and *mice*. In an unpublished report C. Pagani has provided data on 226 women (229 conceptions) who had taken rifampicin during pregnancy. There were 179 babies considered morphologically normal, 9 with malformations, 10 with haemorrhagic tendencies, 4 died in infancy but had no altered morphology, 5 infants died *in utero* (the foetuses showed no abnormalities), and there were 22 abortions, 17 of them induced. The incidence of malformations at birth was 4.3% compared with 1.8% for infants exposed to tuberculosis and 6.5% for infants exposed to other antituberculous regimens. No follow-up was done on the 179 apparently healthy babies and as not all abnormalities could be detected at birth the incidence of 4.3% of malformations can be expected to rise.— J. S. M. Steen and D. M. Stainton-Ellis, *Ciba and Lepetit* (letter), *Lancet*, 1977, *2*, 604.

Although the possibility of rifampicin and isoniazid causing genetic damage seems unlikely it is considered wise for a potential father to refrain from parenthood while receiving these drugs.— D. M. Stainton-Ellis, *Practitioner*, 1977, *219*, 432.

See also under Adverse Effects, p.1564.

Antimicrobial Action. Rifampicin is bactericidal and interferes with the synthesis of nucleic acids in micro-organisms by inhibiting DNA-dependent RNA polymerase. It is active against Gram-positive bacteria, some mycobacteria, especially *Mycobacterium tuberculosis*, *M. bovis*, *M. leprae*, and many strains of *M. kansasii*, and against some Gram-negative bacteria including *Neisseria gonorrhoeae* and *N. meningitidis*. At high concentrations it is active against some viruses. Rifampicin has no effect on fungi but has been reported to enhance the antifungal activity of amphotericin. Minimum inhibitory concentrations tend to vary with the medium used but Gram-positive organisms are usually inhibited by 0.002 to 0.5 µg per ml, mycobacteria by 0.005 to 2 µg per ml, and Gram-negative micro-organisms by 1 to 10 µg per ml. The concomitant use of other antimicrobial agents may enhance the bactericidal activity of rifampicin.

As with other antituberculous compounds resistant mycobacteria rapidly emerge if rifampicin is used alone. Resistant gonococci, meningococci, and staphylococci have been reported. There does not appear to be cross-resistance apart from that between rifampicin and other rifamycins.

Reports of the activity *in vitro* of rifampicin.— L. Verbist and A. Gyselen, *Am. Rev. resp. Dis.*, 1968, *98*, 923 (*M. tuberculosis*); J. H. Subak-Sharpe *et al.*, *Nature*, 1969, *222*, 341 (viruses); Y. Becker and Z. Zakay-Rones, *Nature*, 1969, *222*, 851; Y. Becker *et al.*, *ibid.*, *224*, 33 (*Chlamydia trachomatis*); I. B. Holmes and G. R. Hilson, *J. med. Microbiol.*, 1972, *5*, 251 (*M. leprae*); H. Werner, *Arzneimittel-Forsch.*, 1972, *22*, 1043 (Gram-negative anaerobic bacteria); H. J. Blackman *et al.*, *Antimicrob. Ag. Chemother.*, 1977, *12*, 673 (*Chlamydia trachomatis*).

Phagocytosis was not affected by polymyxin B, rifampicin, or tetracycline.— P. D. Hoeprich *et al.*, *Clin. Pharmac. Ther.*, 1970, *11*, 418. Rifampicin inhibited leucocyte migration (leucotaxis) *in vitro*.— A. Forsgren and D. Schmeling, *Antimicrob. Ag. Chemother.*, 1977, *11*, 580.

Activity against Haemophilus influenzae. Of 98 strains of *H. influenzae* type b, all were inhibited by rifampicin 0.5 µg per ml and 95 by sulphafurazole diethanolamine 10 µg per ml.— R. M. Bannatyne and R. Cheung, *Antimicrob. Ag. Chemother.*, 1978, *13*, 969.

Activity against Legionella pneumophila. Rifampicin was the most active of 22 antimicrobial agents tested *in vitro* against 6 isolates of legionnaires' disease bacterium. The MIC for each isolate was 0.01 µg or less per ml.— C. Thornsberry *et al.*, *Antimicrob. Ag. Chemother.*, 1978, *13*, 78. See also V. J. Lewis *et al.*, *ibid.*, 419.

Activity against meningococci. All of 60 strains of meningococci isolated from 52 patients and 8 carriers were sensitive to rifampicin 0.125 µg per ml. They were all resistant to sulphadiazine sodium 10 µg per ml.— M. Hassan-King *et al.*, *Trans. R. Soc. trop. Med. Hyg.*, 1979, *73*, 567.

Further references.— A. O'Beirne and J. A. Robinson, *Am. J. med. Sci.*, 1971, *262*, 33; W. Brown and R. J. Fallon, *J. antimicrob. Chemother.*, 1980, *6*, 91.

Activity against staphylococci. In a study *in vitro* of the susceptibility of *Staphylococcus aureus* and *Staph. epidermidis* to 65 antimicrobial agents with anti-staphylococcal activity, rifampicin was the most active overall.— L. D. Sabath *et al.*, *Antimicrob. Ag. Chemother.*, 1976, *9*, 962.

Activity with other antimicrobial agents. Reports of enhanced antibacterial activity *in vitro* of rifampicin.— D. C. Shanson and T. Leung, *J. antimicrob. Chemother.*, 1976, *2*, 81 (with novobiocin against *Salmonella typhi*); R. C. Ostenson *et al.*, *Antimicrob. Ag. Chemother.*, 1977, *12*, 655 (with polymyxin B against *Serratia marcescens*); C. U. Tuazon *et al.*, *Antimicrob. Ag. Chemother.*, 1978, *13*, 759 (with nafcillin against *Staph. aureus*); D. Greenwood and J. Andrew, *J. antimicrob. Chemother.*, 1978, *4*, 533 (with nalidixic acid against various Gram-negative bacteria); M. E. Ein *et al.*, *Antimicrob. Ag. Chemother.*, 1979, *16*, 655 (with cephamandole, cephalothin, or vancomycin against methicillin-resistant *Staphyloccus epidermidis*); E. D. Ralph and Y. E. Amatnieks, *ibid.*, 1980, *17*, 379 (with metronidazole against *Bacteroides fragilis*).

Rifampicin did not enhance the bactericidal activity of isoniazid against *M. tuberculosis*, when studied *in vitro* or in infected *guinea-pigs* although it delayed relapse. Rifampicin might have a specific action on a small proportion of the bacterial population which indicated that it might need to be given only for part of a treatment schedule.— J. M. Dickinson and D. A. Mitchison, *Tubercle*, 1976, *57*, 251.

Antagonism occurred against some strains of *Staph. aureus* when the activity of rifampicin was tested *in vitro* with bleomycin and synergism usually occurred when rifampicin was tested with mitomycin. The effect of mitomycin was obtained at concentrations below those usually obtained in serum.— J. Y. Jacobs *et al.*, *Antimicrob. Ag. Chemother.*, 1979, *15*, 580.

Rifampicin used with a penicillin or trimethoprim in experimental infections with staphylococci in *mice* was effective in preventing the development of rifampicin-resistant strains. Enhanced activity was not found.— G. L. Mandell and D. R. Moorman, *Antimicrob. Ag. Chemother.*, 1980, *17*, 658.

With amphotericin. Reports of enhanced activity with rifampicin and amphotericin against various fungi.— M. Kitahara *et al.*, *J. infect. Dis.*, 1976, *133*, 663 (*Histoplasma* and *Blastomyces*); M. Kitahara *et al.*, *Antimicrob. Ag. Chemother.*, 1976, *9*, 915 (*Aspergillus*).

The enhanced activity of rifampicin and amphotericin against *Candida* spp.— W. H. Beggs *et al.*, *J. infect. Dis.*, 1976, *133*, 206. A synergistic effect was observed in only 8 of 51 strains of *Candida albicans*.— R. M. Bannatyne and R. Cheung, *Curr. ther. Res.*, 1979, *25*, 71. In a study *in vitro* of 40 strains of *Candida* spp., all of which were resistant to rifampicin alone, the percentage of strains inhibited by amphotericin 0.4 µg per ml increased from 50 to 90% in the presence of rifampicin 6.25 µg per ml. At the same concentrations 25% of strains were killed with amphotericin and 75% in the presence of rifampicin.— J. E. Edwards *et al.*, *Antimicrob. Ag. Chemother.*, 1980, *17*, 484.

Further references.— L. F. Ayvazian (letter), *Ann. intern. Med.*, 1976, *85*, 539.

With trimethoprim. An enhanced or additive effect *in vitro* was seen against 304 strains of common hospital pathogens when rifampicin and trimethoprim were used together. Enhanced activity was most pronounced against streptococci and *Proteus* spp. and was also noted against other Enterobacteriaceae, *Pseudomonas aeruginosa*, and *Bacteroides fragilis*. Some antagonism was observed against *Staphylococcus aureus* at very low concentrations of rifampicin.— D. W. Kerry *et al.*, *J. antimicrob. Chemother.*, 1975, *1*, 417.

Experimental results indicating that the mutation-rate producing bacteria resistant to the combination of rifampicin and trimethoprim is very low.— V. Arioli *et al.*, *J. antimicrob. Chemother.*, 1977, *3*, 87.

Rifampicin and trimethoprim were antagonistic when used together *in vitro* against *Klebsiella aerogenes* and *Streptococcus faecalis*. The apparent synergism previously reported was shown to be due to trimethoprim suppressing the growth of mutant cells with resistance to low concentrations of rifampicin. It is recommended that if rifampicin is used in association with another antibiotic it should be an inhibitor of protein synthesis such as tetracycline or erythromycin and not trimethoprim.— R. J. Harvey, *J. antimicrob. Chemother.*, 1978, *4*, 315. Criticisms of the study.— V. Arioli and M. Berti (letter), *ibid.*, 1979, *5*, 113; D. L. Steward and J. N. Eble (letter), *ibid.*, 1979, *5*, 114. Reply.— R. J. Harvey (letter), *ibid.*, 1979, *5*, 114. Further criticism and an opinion that antagonism between rifampicin and trimethoprim has not been substantiated.— W. Brumfitt and J. M. T. Hamilton-Miller (letter), *ibid.*, 1979, *5*, 311. Reply.— R. J. Harvey (letter), *ibid.*, 1979, *5*, 312.

Further reports of enhanced activity *in vitro* with rifampicin and trimethoprim.— R. N. Grüneberg and A. M. Emmerson, *J. antimicrob. Chemother.*, 1977, *3*, 453 (urinary pathogens); W. Farrell *et al.*, *ibid.*, 459 (Gram-negative rods); B. P. Goldstein *et al.*, *Antimicrob. Ag. Chemother.*, 1979, *16*, 736 (urinary pathogens); M. Berti *et al.*, *Curr. Microbiol.*, 1979, *2*, 223 (*Haemophilus influenzae*), per *Abstr. Hyg.*, 1980, *55*, 140.

Resistance. A review of resistant patterns of *M. tuberculosis* to rifampicin in countries where its use was restricted to tuberculosis and in countries where it had a wider use did not reveal any change of resistance with the wider use. There was no resistance to rifampicin among 433 strains of Gram-negative bacteria.— G. Acocella *et al.*, *Lancet*, 1977, *1*, 740. See also E. P. Trallero *et al.* (letter), *ibid.*, 956.

A report of resistance *in vitro* of gonococci and meningococci to rifampicin.— H. Schneider *et al.*, *Br. J. vener. Dis.*, 1972, *48*, 500.

The development in one patient of resistance to rifampicin by *M. leprae*.— R. R. Jacobson and R. C. Hastings (letter), *Lancet*, 1976, *2*, 1304.

Rifampicin resistance in strains of *M. kansasii* isolated from 2 infected patients.— P. T. Davidson and R. Waggoner, *Tubercle*, 1976, *57*, 271.

The natural resistance of mycobacteria to rifampicin might be due to permeability barriers.— J. Hui *et al.*, *Antimicrob. Ag. Chemother.*, 1977, *11*, 773.

Further references.— M. Tsukamura, *Tubercle*, 1972, *53*, 111; T. Tanaka *et al.*, *Microbiol. Immunol.*, 1978, *22*, 565.

See also p.1564.

Absorption and Fate. Rifampicin is readily absorbed from the gastro-intestinal tract and peak plasma concentrations of about 9 µg per ml have been reported 2 hours after a dose of 600 mg and 27 µg per ml after a dose of 900 mg. About 75 to 80% of rifampicin in the circulation is bound to plasma proteins. Rifampicin, but not its main metabolite, undergoes enterohepatic circulation. It is widely distributed in body tissues and fluids; it crosses the placenta and diffuses into milk and into the cerebrospinal fluid when the meninges are inflamed. Food may reduce and delay absorption.

Rifampicin is mainly metabolised to active desacetylrifampicin and is excreted in the bile and to a lesser extent in the urine. Up to 30% of a dose of 900 mg may be excreted in the urine, about half of it within 24 hours. The biological half-life of about 3 hours increases with dose and is prolonged in patients with liver disease.

A detailed review of the clinical pharmacokinetics of rifampicin.— G. Acocella, *Clin. Pharmacokinet.*, 1978, *3*, 108.

The main metabolite of rifampicin is the desacetyl derivative, which is active against Gram-positive bacteria and almost unchanged from rifampicin in its activity against Gram-negative bacteria and *Mycobacterium tuberculosis*. Nearly all rifampicin excreted in the bile is in the desacetylated form, the process of desacetylation being almost complete within 5 hours of administration. Of rifampicin excreted in the urine, a small proportion is desacetylated. Following administration of rifampicin and desacetylrifampicin in a dose of 150 mg, serum concentrations after 2, 4, and 8 hours were 2, 1, and 0.4 µg per ml, and 0.1 to 0.2 µg per ml throughout respectively. Four hours after administration of desacetylrifampicin, the concentration in bile was 614 µg per ml.— N. Maggi *et al.*, *Arzneimittel-Forsch.*, 1969, *19*, 651.

Investigation of patients on a prolonged rifampicin regimen indicated that serum concentrations following a dose of rifampicin 450 mg by mouth were lower than those in control subjects or in patients who were receiving alternative antitubercular therapy. Prolonged treatment increased the rate of inactivation or elimination of rifampicin.— S. Virtanen and E. Tala, *Clin. Pharmac. Ther.*, 1974, *16*, 817.

Pharmacokinetic studies on rifampicin with isoniazid.— G. Acocella *et al.*, *Gut*, 1972, *13*, 47.

Pharmacokinetic studies on rifampicin with trimethoprim.— J. M. T. Hamilton-Miller and W. Brumfitt, *J. antimicrob. Chemother.*, 1976, *2*, 181; G. Acocella and R. Scotti, *ibid.*, 271; A. M. Emmerson *et al.*, *ibid.*, 1978, *4*, 523.

A single dose of rifampicin 600 mg intravenously given to 2 patients produced peak serum-rifampicin concentrations of 6.82 and 12.85 µg per ml respectively after 2 hours and in a third patient the peak concentration was 7.72 µg per ml after 4 hours. In 5 patients rifampicin 600 mg daily intravenously for 1 week gave similar concentrations in serum to those reported after oral administration but concentrations in urine were lower.— G. Acocella *et al.*, *Arzneimittel-Forsch.*, 1977, *27*, 1221. See also V. Nitti *et al.*, *Chemotherapy, Basle*, 1977, *23*, 1.

Sex-linked differences in rifampicin kinetics led H. Iwainsky *et al.* (*Scand. J. resp. Dis.*, 1976, *57*, 5) to recommend a reduction in rifampicin dosage of 10% in women relative to that used in men.— J. F. Giudicelli and J. P. Tillement, *Clin. Pharmacokinet.*, 1977, *2*, 157. See also R. Scotti, *Chemotherapy, Basle*, 1973, *18*, 205.

Further references.— K. J. Begg, *Tubercle*, 1967, *48*, 149; H. D. Cohn, *J. clin. Pharmac.*, 1969, *9*, 118; L. F. Devine *et al.*, *J. Am. med. Ass.*, 1970, *214*, 1055; R. V. Makarenkova and I. P. Kopeiko, *Antibiotiki*, 1977, *22*, 259;; I. J. Kiss *et al.*, *Int. J. clin. Pharmac. Biopharm.*, 1978, *16*, 105; I. Pawlowska and T. Pniewski, *Arzneimittel-Forsch.*, 1979, *29*, 1906.

Absorption. Serum-rifampicin concentrations were retarded and reduced when rifampicin was given with food compared with those in the fasting state. However, concentrations achieved when the dose was given with food were still considered to be effective.— D. I. Siegler *et al.*, *Lancet*, 1974, *2*, 197.

The absorption of rifampicin is delayed in patients with coeliac disease.— R. L. Parsons *et al.*, *J. antimicrob. Chemother.*, 1975, *1*, 39.

The absorption of rifampicin in gastrectomised patients.— C. -H. H. Hagelund *et al.*, *Scand. J. resp. Dis.*, 1977, *58*, 241; T. Biehl and K. F. Petersen, *Prax. Pneumol.*, 1978, *32*, 584.

Diffusion. Concentrations of rifampicin in gingival fluid, and minor salivary gland, parotid, and submandibular saliva.— K. W. Stephen *et al.*, *Br. J. clin. Pharmac.*, 1980, *9*, 51.

Into cerebrospinal fluid. Mean concentrations of rifampicin in the cerebrospinal fluid of a patient with tuberculosis meningitis 5 to 6 hours after doses of 900 mg were 400 ng per ml, about 10% of those found in the serum.— R. Forgan-Smith *et al.* (letter), *Lancet*, 1973, *2*, 374..

Further references.— J. J. G. D'Oliveira, *Am. Rev. resp. Dis.*, 1972, *106*, 432; J. E. Sippel *et al.*, *Am. Rev. resp. Dis.*, 1974, *109*, 579.

Into the eye. References.— M. F. Feldman and R. A. Moses, *Am. J. Ophthal.*, 1977, *83*, 862.

Into pleural effusions. References.— G. Boman and A. -S. Malmborg, *Eur. J. clin. Pharmac.*, 1974, *7*, 51.

Excretion. In 20 healthy subjects the percentage of rifampicin plus desacetylrifampicin excreted in the urine increased with the dose of rifampicin. About 4% of a 150-mg dose and 18% of a 900-mg dose was excreted in 24 hours.— S. Brechbühler *et al.*, *Arzneimittel-Forsch.*, 1978, *28*, 480.

Metabolism. Rifampicin is reported to increase its own rate of metabolism.— D. D. Breimer *et al.*, *Clin. Pharmac. Ther.*, 1977, *21*, 470.

The metabolite formylrifampicin accounts for about 10% of the antibacterial activity found in urine after a dose of rifampicin and is thought to form spontaneously in the urine.— G. Acocella, *Clin. Pharmacokinet.*, 1978, *3*, 108.

Further references.— R. A. Ioffe, *Antibiotiki*, 1977, *22*, 177.

Pregnancy and the neonate. Rifampicin 300 mg was taken by a pregnant woman 4 hours before termination. Rifampicin concentrations were assayed in maternal blood, placenta, foetus, and liquor.— I. Rocker (letter), *Lancet*, 1977, *2*, 48.

Protein binding. Studies in tuberculous patients on long-term therapy with rifampicin showed that 84 to 88% was bound to plasma proteins.— G. Boman and V. -A. Ringberger, *Eur. J. clin. Pharmac.*, 1974, *7*, 369.

Further references.— J. J. Vallner, *J. pharm. Sci.*, 1977, *66*, 447.

Uses. Rifampicin belongs to the rifamycin group of antibiotics (p.1085). It may be the most effective drug for administration in association with isoniazid in the primary treatment of pulmonary tuberculosis. It has been used successfully with ethambutol for the re-treatment of pulmonary tuberculosis resistant to the older tuberculostatics; capreomycin has sometimes been given with these two drugs in the initial period of treatment. The use of rifampicin with other antituberculous agents is described under Treatment of Tuberculosis, p.1565. Intermittent regimens (p.1566) and short-term treatment (p.1566) including rifampicin are increasingly important.

Rifampicin has also been used in the treatment of extrapulmonary lesions including tuberculous meningitis as well as in the elimination of meningococci from carriers. It is also given, in association with other antileprotics such as dapsone and clofazimine, in the treatment of leprosy. It has been used in a variety of non-tuberculous conditions caused by susceptible organisms. Rifampicin has been shown to be immunosuppressant.

The usual dose of rifampicin in tuberculosis is 600 mg daily before food as a single dose or 8 to 12 mg per kg body-weight daily; similar doses are used in leprosy. In patients with impaired liver function the dose should generally not exceed 8 mg per kg daily. Intermittent schedules are often employed although this may increase the incidence of side-effects, depending on the schedule adopted; doses of up to 900 mg have been given twice weekly. In the treatment of meningococcal carriers rifampicin is usually given in a dose of 600 mg daily for 4 days. Children may be given 10 to 20 mg per kg to a maximum daily dose of 600 mg.

Rifampicin has also been given intravenously.

Although G. Acocella *et al.* (*Lancet*, 1977, *1*, 740) suggested that the risk of increasing the incidence of rifampicin-resistant strains of *Mycobacterium tuberculosis* is probably small when short courses of the antibiotic were used for non-tuberculous diseases, N.A. Simmons (*J. antimicrob. Chemother.*, 1977, *3*, 109) considered that there was no sound clinical reason to take this risk when alternative antibiotics were available (see also under Gonorrhoea, below). Nevertheless rifampicin has been used in combination with other antibacterial agents in an attempt to achieve enhanced activity and reduce the risk of resistance. W. Brumfitt and J.M.T. Hamilton-Miller have reported (*J. antimicrob. Chemother.*, 1979, *5*, 311) that the combination of rifampicin with trimethoprim is being used in the treatment of urinary-tract infections which have not proved amenable to other commonly used antibiotics (see also under Urinary-tract infections, below).

Reviews of the actions and uses of rifampicin.— I. Phillips, *J. clin. Path.*, 1971, *24*, 410; G. Binda *et al.*, *Arzneimittel-Forsch.*, 1971, *21*, 1907; *Drugs*, 1971, *1*, 354; *Lepr. Rev.*, 1975, *46*, 149.

A review of the use of rifampicin in combination therapy for non-mycobacterial infections.— R. Nessi and G. Fowst, *J. int. med. Res.*, 1979, *7*, 179.

Paediatric experience with rifampicin in non-tuberculous infections.— Y. Naveh, *Curr. ther. Res.*, 1980, *27*, 272.

References to the use of rifampicin in atypical mycobacterial infections.— F. Mandell and P. F. Wright, *Pediatrics*, 1975, *55*, 39.

Reports of the use of rifampicin in non-mycobacterial infections.— P. Lou *et al.*, *Am. J. Ophthal.*, 1977, *83*, 12 (with amphotericin in candidal endophthalmitis); R. C. Ostenson *et al.*, *Antimicrob. Ag. Chemother.*, 1977, *12*, 655 (with polymyxin B in nosocomial infections due to multiple-resistant *Serratia marcescens*).

Administration. A sensitive microbiological test for the detection of rifampicin in urine to monitor dosage compliance.— D. A. Mitchison *et al.*, *Tubercle*, 1974, *55*, 245.

See under Absorption and Fate, above, for reports on the absorption of rifampicin.

Intravenous use. A report of the intravenous use of rifampicin given in a daily dosage of 600 mg for 49 days by infusion in a patient who had undergone massive small bowel resection for jejunoileal tuberculosis.— P. N. Wake *et al.*, *Tubercle*, 1980, *61*, 109.

Topical use. Rifampicin applied topically to vaccination sites of 24 subjects inoculated with vaccinia virus inhibited the vaccination reaction in approximately 50%. There was no inhibition of reaction when rifampicin was given by mouth to 8 subjects.— A. Moshkowitz *et al.* (letter), *Nature*, 1971, *229*, 422.

Administration in infants and children. Pharmacokinetic data indicated that doses of rifampicin higher than 10 mg per kg body-weight need to be given in infants and should possibly be based on body-surface. In newborn infants, a dose of 10 mg per kg should definitely not be exceeded and should probably be reduced.— G. Acocella, *Clin. Pharmacokinet.*, 1978, *3*, 108.

Further references.— N. Kotchabhakdi and C. Junnanond, *J. med. Ass. Thailand*, 1978, *61*, 481.

Administration in liver disease. A recommendation that in chronic liver disease the dose of rifampicin should be less than 10 mg per kg body-weight.— P. Knop *et al.*, *Dt. med. Wschr.*, 1977, *102*, 1913.

Serum concentrations of rifampicin are higher and the biological half-life increased in patients with impaired liver function.— G. Acocella, *Clin. Pharmacokinet.*, 1978, *3*, 108.

Administration in renal failure. Rifampicin can be given to patients with impaired renal function in the usual doses.— P. Sharpstone, *Br. med. J.*, 1977, *2*, 36; J. S. Cheigh, *Am. J. Med.*, 1977, *62*, 555; G. Acocella, *Clin. Pharmacokinet.*, 1978, *3*, 108; W. M. Bennett *et al.*, *Ann. intern. Med.*, 1980, *93*, 62.

Data for predicting removal of rifampicin by conventional haemodialysis.— T. P. Gibson and H. A. Nelson, *Clin. Pharmacokinet.*, 1977, *2*, 403.

A recommendation that in patients with uraemia (creatinine clearance of 10 ml per minute) the dose of rifampicin should be reduced to 300 mg daily.— G. B. Appel and H. C. Neu, *New Engl. J. Med.*, 1977, *296*, 663.

See also p.1565.

Brucellosis. In 23 patients with brucellosis, temperatures returned to normal in a mean of about 6 days (range 1 to 20) after treatment with rifampicin. There were no relapses at 12 months. The usual dose was 900 mg daily, in divided doses of 600 and 300 mg, for an average of 16 days.— P. Agostinelli *et al.*, *G. Mal. infett. parassit.*, 1975, *27*, 22, per *Abstr. Hyg.*, 1975, *50*, 788.

Effective treatment of brucellosis in children with rifampicin or rifampicin with co-trimoxazole; combined treatment is advised.— J. Llorens-Terol and R. M. Busquets, *Archs Dis. Childh.*, 1980, *55*, 486.

Cushing's syndrome. Since rifampicin induced hepatic cortisol-6-hydroxylase as shown by increased urinary excretion of 6-hydroxycortisol, it might be of benefit in Cushing's syndrome.— S. Yamada and K. Iwai (letter), *Lancet*, 1976, *2*, 366.

Endocarditis. For reports of the treatment of endocarditis due to *Staphylococcus aureus* with rifampicin and erythromycin, see M. C. Peard *et al.*, *Br. med. J.*, 1970, *4*, 410; N. D. Burman *et al.*, *Postgrad. med. J.*, 1973, *49*, 920.

Further reports of the treatment of endocarditis with rifampicin.— R. J. Faville *et al.*, *J. Am. med. Ass.*, 1978, *240*, 1963 (*Staph. aureus*); A. G. Jariwalla *et al.*, *Br. med. J.*, 1980, *280*, 155 (*Chlamydia psittaci*).

Enteric infections. In 11 infants with dysentery due to *Shigella flexneri* treatment with furazolidone, co-trimoxazole, chloramphenicol, or ampicillin was ineffective, although tests *in vitro* had indicated sensitivity to these drugs. Subsequent treatment with rifampicin 10 to 12 mg per kg body-weight daily in 2 divided doses for 7 days eradicated the infection; stool cultures remained negative at follow-up 1 month later.— Y. Naveh *et al., Archs Dis. Childh.*, 1977, *52,* 960.

Further references.— Y. Naveh and A. Friedman, *Postgrad. med. J.*, 1974, *50,* 707 (gastro-enteritis in infants due to *Escherichia coli*).

Gonorrhoea. Although gonorrhoea has been treated successfully with rifampicin there are other suitable alternatives to penicillin. Rifampicin should be reserved for the treatment of mycobacterial infections.— *Neisseria gonorrhoea and gonococcal infections, Tech. Rep. Ser. Wld Hlth Org. No. 616,* 1978.

For references to the use of rifampicin in the treatment of gonorrhoea, see Martindale 27th Edn, p. 1599.

Granulomatous disease. Rifampicin was found to penetrate polymorphs from patients with chronic granulomatous disease and to exert its bactericidal activity on bacteria therein. Two patients were given rifampicin 20 mg per kg body-weight daily and 1 improved; the other was eventually thought to be infected with *Aspergillus fumigatus*.— G. Ezer and J. F. Soothill, *Archs Dis. Childh.*, 1974, *49,* 463.

A patient with chronic granulomatous disease responded dramatically to treatment with rifampicin 600 mg twice daily.— B. Lorber (letter), *New Engl. J. Med.*, 1980, *303,* 111.

Histoplasmosis. Two patients with thoracic histoplasmosis were treated with rifampicin 10 mg per kg body-weight daily for 4 and 7 months and other antituberculous drugs. One patient who also received surgery responded satisfactorily.— R. Pieron *et al., Méd. trop. Marseille,* 1973, *33,* 403, per *Abstr. Hyg.*, 1974, *49,* 421.

Immunosuppression. For reports on the immunosuppressant activity of rifampicin, see B. M. Dajani *et al.* (letter), *Lancet,* 1972, *2,* 1094; G. A. W. Rook, *Tubercle,* 1973, *54,* 291; R. Nessi *et al., Arzneimittel-Forsch.*, 1974, *24,* 832; S. Gupta *et al., Ann. intern. Med.*, 1975, *82,* 484; G. Banck and A. Forsgren, *Antimicrob. Ag. Chemother.*, 1979, *16,* 554.

Legionnaires' disease. Erythromycin with or without rifampicin might be effective in the treatment of legionnaires' disease according to a study in infected *guinea-pigs* carried out at the Center for Disease Control.— D. W. Fraser *et al., Lancet,* 1978, *1,* 175.

The association of rifampicin with a tetracycline should be considered for therapy when legionnaires' disease is a possibility in life-threatening pneumonia.— P. L. Meenhorst *et al.* (letter), *Lancet,* 1978, *1,* 711.

A description, based on 16 cases, of distinctive neurological findings associated with legionnaires' disease. Erythromycin is the drug of choice but where response is poor the addition of rifampicin is recommended.— D. H. Kennedy *et al.* (letter), *Lancet,* 1981, *1,* 940.

Leishmaniasis. Successful treatment of cutaneous leishmaniasis with rifampicin in a 19-year-old woman.— F. R. Vásquez (letter), *Archs Derm.*, 1977, *113,* 1610.

A patient with diffuse cutaneous leishmaniasis, which classical antileishmanial drugs had failed to cure, had a remission of the skin lesions when he received antituberculous chemotherapy for an intercurrent mycobacterial infection. Subsequent studies in *mice,* with a strain of *Leishmania mexicana amazonensis* isolated from the patient, showed that when used alone aminosalicylic acid was inactive and rifampicin and isoniazid were only moderately active. However when rifampicin and isoniazid were used together activity was enhanced.— W. Peters *et al., Lancet,* 1981, *1,* 1122.

Limited therapeutic action of rifampicin with isoniazid against *Leishmania aethiopica*.— J. van der Meulen *et al.* (letter), *Lancet,* 1981, *2,* 197. No action of antituberculous drugs against *L. donovani in vivo*.— J. -K. M. E. Schattenkerk *et al.* (letter), *ibid.*, 304.

Further references.— M. M. E. Selim and E. Kandil, *J. Kuwait med. Ass.*, 1972, *6,* 159, per *Trop. Dis. Bull.*, 1973, *70,* 530; I. O. Iskandar, *J. int. med. Res.*, 1978, *6,* 280.

Leprosy. For a short review of the use of rifampicin in the treatment of leprosy, see E. J. Saerens, *Lepr. Rev.*, 1975, *46, Suppl.*, 125.

From a study of 93 previously untreated non-tubercular patients with lepromatous or borderline leprosy it was considered that weekly treatment with rifampicin 15 mg per kg body-weight was as effective as daily treatment with doses of 8 to 10 mg per kg.— S. R. Pattyn *et al., Lepr. Rev.*, 1975, *46, Suppl.*, 129. Rifampicin should not be used alone but in conjunction with other drugs to avoid the emergence of resistant strains of bacilli.— D. V. A. Opromolla and C. J. S. Tonello, *ibid.*, 141.

A series of favourable preliminary reports on the use of rifampicin concurrently with a preparation containing prothionamide, dapsone, and isoniazid (Isoprodian) in the treatment of leprosy.— J. T. de las Aguas, *Lepr. Rev.*, 1975, *46, Suppl.*, 165; S. Innami *et al., ibid.*, 169; M. Aschhoff, *ibid.*, 173; G. Depasquale, *ibid.*, 179; M. Hamzah and A. Kosasih, *ibid.*, 181; H. N. Krenzien, *ibid.*, 189; R. Rohde, *ibid.*, 199; E. Vomstein, *ibid.*, 207. See also Y. Matsuo *et al., Jap. J. Lepr.*, 1978, *47,* 43.

A discussion on the problems of drug resistance in leprosy including mention of rifampicin resistance.— S. G. Browne, *Lepr. Rev.*, 1977, *48,* 79.

Dapsone remains the basis of treatment for leprosy but a combination regimen of long-term dapsone in full dosage with rifampicin (in a tentatively suggested dose of 300 to 600 mg daily for a minimum of 2 weeks) can be given.— Fifth Report of the WHO Expert Committee on Leprosy, *Tech. Rep. Ser. Wld Hlth Org. No. 607,* 1977.

Six months' treatment with dapsone or 3 weeks' treatment with rifampicin rapidly reduces the number of viable bacilli in the nasal discharge of leprosy patients and such patients could virtually be considered as no longer contagious. Patients with lepromatous or borderline leprosy should receive treatment for life even after lesions are no longer active and annual checkups are desirable to check on the development of resistance. Those with tuberculoid or near-tuberculoid leprosy may in most cases stop drug therapy after regular treatment for 2 or 3 years.— S. G. Browne, *Memorandum on Leprosy,* London, HM Stationery Office, 1977.

Studies in 67 patients with lepromatous leprosy (resistant in 65 to dapsone) showed that treatment with rifampicin, usually 600 mg daily, produced a rapid initial clinical improvement but viable bacteria persisted in 7 of 12 patients treated for at least 5 years. Persistence of viable bacteria seemed to be reduced in patients treated with rifampicin plus dapsone 100 mg daily.— M. F. R. Waters *et al., Br. med. J.*, 1978, *1,* 133.

Further reports of rifampicin in the treatment of leprosy.— *Am. J. trop. Med. Hyg.*, 1975, *24,* 475; A. P. León and J. Hernández Silva, *Revta Invest. Salud Publ.*, 1977, *37,* 69; S. Ghosh *et al., Lepr. India,* 1977, *49,* 339; J. P. Digoutte *et al., Bordeaux Méd.*, 1977, *10,* 703, per *Trop. Dis. Bull.*, 1977, *74,* 578; J. Languillon, *Méd. trop. Marseille,* 1977, *37,* 717, per *Trop. Dis. Bull.*, 1979, *76,* 734; B. K. Girdhar *et al., Lepr. India,* 1978, *50,* 363; J. Languillon *et al., Int. J. Lepr.*, 1979, *47,* 37; S. R. Pattyn *et al., Annls Soc. belge Méd. trop.*, 1979, *59,* 79; B. K. Girdhar and K. V. Desikan, *Lepr. India,* 1979, *51,* 475, per *Trop. Dis. Bull.*, 1980, *77,* 742; B. K. Girdhar *et al., Lepr. India,* 1980, *52,* 89, per *Trop. Dis. Bull.*, 1980, *77,* 949.

For further details of the treatment of leprosy, see Dapsone, p.1491.

For earlier reports of rifampicin in the treatment of leprosy, see Martindale 27th Edn, p. 1599.

Liver disease. Findings in patients with liver disease that although hepatic drug metabolism was stimulated by rifampicin there was, unlike phenobarbitone, no improvement in liver function.— W. Zilly *et al., Eur. J. clin. Pharmac.*, 1977, *11,* 287.

Meningitis. *Enterococcal meningitis.* A report of the use of rifampicin in association with vancomycin in the treatment of enterococcal meningitis.— J. L. Ryan *et al., Am. J. Med.*, 1980, *68,* 449.

Meningococcal meningitis. Rifampicin 10 to 25 mg per kg body-weight was given daily in 2 divided doses via a gastric tube to 3 comatose patients with severe meningitis who had not responded to conventional treatment and the 3 improved. Thereafter rifampicin was incorporated into the antibiotic management of patients with meningitis and reduced the mortality-rate over 8 months from between 11 and about 15% to nil.— M. Salour, *Advances in Antimicrobial and Antineoplastic Chemotherapy,* Vol. 1/2, M. Hejzlar *et al.* (Ed.), London, University Park Press, 1972, p. 1203..

Tuberculous meningitis. A survey of 19 patients with tuberculous meningitis seen between 1966 and 1974 indicated that the replacement of aminosalicylic acid or ethambutol with isoniazid therapy, by rifampicin with isoniazid therapy, did not appear to improve the prognosis.— E. J. Haas *et al., Archs intern. Med.*, 1977, *137,* 1518.

Further references.— N. I. Girgis *et al., J. trop. Med. Hyg.*, 1978, *81,* 246.

See also p.1565.

Meningitis prophylaxis. Haemophilus influenzae meningitis prophylaxis. The use of rifampicin to eradicate *H. influenzae* type b from carriers.— J. I. Ward *et al., J. Pediat.*, 1978, *92,* 713; J. I. Ward *et al., New Engl. J. Med.*, 1979, *301,* 122; D. M. Granoff *et al., Pediatrics,* 1979, *63,* 397; R. Yogev *et al., J. Pediat.*, 1979, *94,* 840; D. M. Granoff and R. S. Daum, *J. Pediat.*, 1980, *97,* 854; S. Simasathien *et al., Lancet,* 1980, *2,* 1214; *ibid.*, 1981, *1,* 649.

Meningococcal meningitis prophylaxis. Because of the prevalence of sulphonamide-resistant meningococci and the vestibular side-effects of minocycline, rifampicin is recommended for meningococcal infection prophylaxis. Doses of rifampicin to be given every 12 hours for 4 doses are: adults, 600 mg; children from 1 to 12 years, 10 mg per kg body-weight; and children under 1 year, 5 mg per kg.— J. B. McCormick and J. V. Bennett, *Center for Disease Control, Ann. intern. Med.*, 1975, *83,* 883. See also J. A. Jacobson and D. W. Fraser, *J. Am. med. Ass.*, 1976, *236,* 1053. Children from 4 months to 4 years of age could be given 15 mg per kg, but for infants under 3 months old 5 mg per kg was recommended.— L. Hendeles and B. M. Kagan, *Drug Intell. & clin. Pharm.*, 1978, *12,* 278. Rifampicin is the drug of choice for the prevention of meningococcal disease when the susceptibility of the isolate to sulphadiazine is unknown, or when sulphonamide resistance is documented. For meningococci known to be sensitive to sulphonamides, sulphadiazine is preferred.— *Med. Lett.*, 1981, *23,* 37.

In view of side-effects and the rapid development of rifampicin-resistant meningococci the superiority of rifampicin over minocycline for the prophylactic treatment of meningococcal meningitis contacts was questioned.— R. J. Mangi (letter), *New Engl. J. Med.*, 1976, *294,* 113. Criticism; rifampicin is still the drug of choice.— J. A. Jacobson (letter), *ibid.*, 843.

A comparison of prophylaxis with rifampicin, 600 mg daily for 4 days, or minocycline, in an initial dose of 200 mg then 100 mg every 12 hours for 5 days, in 1540 soldiers during an epidemic caused by sulphonamide-resistant group A *Neisseria meningitidis.* Rates of carriage of *N. meningitidis* were reduced by 78% and 62% respectively but 5 strains highly resistant to rifampicin were found.— A. Sivonen *et al., J. infect. Dis.*, 1978, *137,* 238.

Further references.— W. B. Deal and E. Sanders, *New Engl. J. Med.*, 1969, *281,* 641; W. E. Beam *et al., J. infect. Dis.*, 1971, *124,* 39; C. E. Weidmer *et al., ibid.*, 172; L. F. Devine, *Am. J. med. Sci.*, 1971, *261,* 79; I. S. Blakebrough and H. M. Gilles, *J. Infect.*, 1980, *2,* 137, per *Trop. Dis. Bull.*, 1980, *77,* 1036.

For the use of minocycline to inhibit the emergence of rifampicin-resistant meningococci, see Minocycline Hydrochloride, p.1186.

Mycetoma. For reference to rifampicin being used with streptomycin in the treatment of mycetoma, see E. S. Mahgoub, *Bull. Wld Hlth Org.*, 1976, *54,* 303.

Osteomyelitis. Persistent staphylococcal arthritis attributed to intracellular sequestration, so that the intracellular organisms were protected against bactericidal activity, was successfully cleared with rifampicin which can penetrate leucocyte membranes.— T. R. Beam, *Lancet,* 1979, *2,* 227. See also M. C. Lobo, *Antimicrob. Ag. Chemother.*, 1972, *2,* 195.

Pulmonary tuberculosis. For a brief discussion on treatment regimens for pulmonary tuberculosis based on rifampicin with isoniazid and re-treatment regimens based on rifampicin with ethambutol, see D. J. Girling, *Tubercle,* 1978, *59,* 13.

Some reports of the use of rifampicin in the treatment of pulmonary tuberculosis.— P. Czanik and L. Levendel, *Prax. Pneumol.*, 1970, *24,* 764 (topical use); A. R. Somner *et al., Tubercle,* 1971, *52,* 266; *idem,* 1973, *54,* 141; R. Newman *et al., Am. Rev. resp. Dis.*, 1971, *103,* 461; G. Favez *et al., Chest,* 1972, *61,* 583; M. Aquinas and K. M. Citron, *Tubercle,* 1972, *53,* 153; *ibid.*, 1974, *55,* 1 (Hong Kong Tuberculosis Treatment Services/Brompton Hospital/British MRC Investigation); R. H. Andrews *et al., ibid.*, 105; *ibid.*, 1975, *56,* 1; *Lancet,* 1975, *2,* 1105 (Singapore Tuberculosis Service/British MRC); P. Dubois *et al., Am. Rev. resp. Dis.*, 1977, *115,* 221; M. W. Long *et al., ibid.*, 1979, *119,* 879.

Therapy with rifampicin and a preparation containing dapsone, isoniazid, and prothionamide (Isoprodian) in 40 previously untreated patients with cavernous pulmonary tuberculosis was as effective as therapy with rifampicin, ethambutol, and isoniazid in a similar group of 40 patients.— H. Kittel, *Dt. med. Wschr.*, 1979, *104,* 477.

Trachoma. From a study in 63 patients with paratrachoma (sexually-transmitted trachoma-inclusion conjunctivitis) it appeared that thrice-daily treatment for 6 to 7 weeks with 1% rifampicin eye ointment would clear 90% or more of patients of paratrachoma in London. Treatment for 4 to 6 weeks with 1% chloramphenicol eye ointment reduced the severity of the disease but did not eliminate the infection.— S. Darougar *et al.*, *Br. J. Ophthal.*, 1977, *61*, 255.

Rifampicin or oxytetracycline, each as a 1% eye ointment, had a beneficial effect when applied twice daily for 6 weeks in children with hyperendemic trachoma [trachoma transmitted from eye to eye].— S. Darougar *et al.*, *Br. J. Ophthal.*, 1980, *64*, 37.

Further references.— T. Daghfous *et al.*, *Revue int. Trachome*, 1974, *51*, 71.

Tuberculosis of the skin. Isoniazid 300 mg daily for 3 months was ineffective in treating a localised infection and ulcerative lesion at the site of an accidental BCG inoculation which subsequently responded to rifampicin and ethambutol.— B. Lorber *et al.*, *J. Am. med. Ass.*, 1977, *238*, 55.

Tuberculosis of the vulva. For the successful treatment of vulval tuberculosis with isoniazid and rifampicin, see Isoniazid, p.1575.

Urinary-tract infections. References to the use of rifampicin in urinary-tract infections.— J. M. Murdoch *et al.* (letter), *Lancet*, 1969, *1*, 1094; P. Propaczy, *Wien. med. Wschr.*, 1970, *120*, 743, per *Int. pharm. Abstr.*, 1972, *9*, 618; H. R. Posada *et al.*, *Arzneimittel-Forsch.*, 1972, *22*, 1188.

With trimethoprim. In a controlled study in 40 patients with urinary-tract infections, rifampicin 600 mg with trimethoprim 160 mg (Rifaprim) as a single daily dose was considered to be more effective than co-trimoxazole 960 mg twice daily. Both treatments lasted 10 days.— T. Adachi and T. R. de Almeida, *J. int. med. Res.*, 1979, *7*, 132.

Further references.— R. Palminteri and D. Sassella, *Chemotherapy, Basle*, 1979, *25*, 181.

Preparations

Rifampin Capsules *(U.S.P.)*. Capsules containing rifampicin 300 mg. Store at a temperature not exceeding 40° in airtight containers. Protect from light.

Rifampin and Isoniazid Capsules *(U.S.P.)*. Capsules containing rifampicin 300 mg and isoniazid 150 mg. Store at a temperature not exceeding 40° in airtight containers. Protect from light.

Proprietary Preparations

Rifadin *(Merrell, UK)*. Rifampicin, available as **Capsules** of 150 and 300 mg and as **Syrup** containing 100 mg in each 5 ml. (Also available as Rifadin in *Arg., Austral., Canad., Ital., Neth., Norw., S.Afr., USA*).

Rifinah 150 *(Merrell, UK)*. Tablets each containing rifampicin 150 mg and isoniazid 100 mg. For tuberculosis. **Rifinah 300.** Tablets each containing rifampicin 300 mg and isoniazid 150 mg. *Dose.* Rifinah 150: for patients less than 50 kg body-weight, 3 tablets daily as a single dose; Rifinah 300: for patients over 50 kg body-weight, 2 tablets daily.

Rimactane *(Ciba, UK)*. Rifampicin, available as **Capsules** of 150 and 300 mg, and as **Syrup** containing 100 mg in each 5 ml. (Also available as Rimactane in *Austral., Canad., S.Afr., USA*).

Rimactazid 150 *(Ciba, UK)*. Tablets each containing rifampicin 150 mg and isoniazid 100 mg. For tuberculosis. **Rimactazid 300.** Tablets each containing rifampicin 300 mg and isoniazid 150 mg. *Dose.* Rimactazid 150: for patients less than 50 kg body-weight, 3 tablets daily as a single dose; Rimactazid 300: for patients over 50 kg body-weight, 2 tablets daily.

Other Proprietary Names

Archidyn *(Ital.)*; Fenampicin, Feronia *(both Spain)*; Rifa *(Ger.)*; Rifadine *(Belg., Fr.)*; Rifagen, Rifaldin *(both Spain)*; Rifapiam *(Ital.)*; Rifaprodin *(Spain)*; Rifocina *(Arg.)*; Rifoldin *(Switz.)*; Rifonilo, Riforal *(both Spain)*; Rimactan *(Arg., Belg., Denm., Fr., Ger., Ital., Neth., Norw., Spain, Switz.)*; Rofact *(Canad.)*; Tibirim *(Ind.)*; Tugaldin *(Spain)*.

7570-l

Salinazid. *o*-Hydroxybenzal Isonicotinyl Hydrazone; Salizid. 2′-Salicylideneisonicotinohydrazide.
$C_{13}H_{11}N_3O_2$=241.2.

CAS — 495-84-1.

A pale cream-coloured powder. Very slightly **soluble** in water; soluble in dilute acids and alkalis.

Salinazid is an isoniazid derivative (p.1571) which was formerly used in the treatment of tuberculosis.

7571-y

Sodium Aminosalicylate *(B.P., Eur. P.)*.

Sod. Aminosal.; Natrii Aminosalicylas; Natrii Para-aminosalicylas; Aminosalicylate Sodium *(U.S.P.)*; Aminosalylnatrium; Pasalicylum Solubile; Sodium Para-aminosalicylate; Sodium PAS. Sodium 4-amino-2-hydroxybenzoate dihydrate.
$C_7H_6NNaO_3,2H_2O$=211.1.

CAS — 133-10-8 (anhydrous); 6018-19-5 (dihydrate).

Pharmacopoeias. In *Arg., Aust., Belg., Br., Braz., Chin., Cz., Eur., Fr., Ger., Hung., Ind., Int., It., Jug., Neth., Pol., Port., Roum., Rus., Span., Swiss, Turk.*, and *U.S.*

White or cream-coloured odourless or almost odourless crystals or crystalline powder with a sweet saline taste. Each g of sodium aminosalicylate represents approximately 4.74 mmol (4.74 mEq) of sodium. Sodium aminosalicylate 1.38 g is approximately equivalent to 1 g of aminosalicylic acid.

Soluble 1 in 2 of water; sparingly soluble in alcohol; practically insoluble in chloroform and ether. A 2% solution in water has a pH of 6.5 to 8.5. A 3.27% solution is iso-osmotic with serum. Solutions are **sterilised** by filtration; they should be stored at 4° and must be used within 10 days of preparation. **Incompatible** with acids, ferric salts, and oxidising agents.

Aqueous solutions are unstable and should be freshly prepared. The addition of sodium metabisulphite 0.1% retards oxidation and darkening of the solution. The *U.S.P.* directs that solutions should be prepared within 24 hours of administration and that a solution must not be used if it is darker in colour than a freshly prepared solution. Tablets that have turned brown should not be used. Store at a temperature not exceeding 40° in airtight containers. Protect from light.

Removal of stains. Fabrics contaminated with sodium aminosalicylate should be washed immediately with cold water and rinsed several times. Sodium metabisulphite or other mild bleaching agents may be used for white fabrics if they have been contaminated for a prolonged period. It is not usually possible to remove brown stains in coloured fabrics.

Stability. Deterioration of sodium aminosalicylate solution was caused by an increase of *m*-aminophenol, dependent on pH and temperature.— G. Fischer, *Gyógyszerészet*, 1967, *11*, 146, per *Int. pharm. Abstr.*, 1967, *4*, 890.

The chromogen which discoloured tablets of aminosalicylic acid and the sodium salt was 3,3′-dihydroxyazoxybenzene which could be produced by oxidation or sunlight irradiation of *m*-aminophenol, a common impurity of aminosalicylic acid.— I. K. Shih, *J. pharm. Sci.*, 1971, *60*, 1886.

Solutions of sodium aminosalicylate 5 and 20% containing 25% glycerol were less quickly degraded to *m*-aminophenol than those with syrup or sorbitol but were more quickly discoloured. Solutions with 25% propylene glycol, whilst slightly less stable than those with glycerol, discoloured at a slower rate than any of the solutions.— M. I. Blake *et al.*, *Am. J. Hosp. Pharm.*, 1973, *30*, 441.

A paediatric mixture containing isoniazid 10 g, sodium aminosalicylate 27.5 g, pyridoxine 25 mg, and vehicle for Isoniazid Elixir *B.P.C. 1973* to 100 ml was examined for stability. The pH of the freshly-prepared mixture was 6.2. Overnight storage in a refrigerator resulted in formation of a copious deposit. After storage for 1 week at room temperature the *B.P.C.* limit for 3-aminophenol in isoniazid dry granules (0.3%) was exceeded.— Pharm. Soc. Lab. Rep. P/75/17, 1975.

Adverse Effects. Sodium aminosalicylate may cause the side-effects of salicylates (see p.236) and of the *p*-aminophenyl group which is also formed during the metabolism of such compounds as sulphonamides, phenacetin, and sulphones. Patients hypersensitive to these drugs and to certain hair dyes containing related compounds may also be hypersensitive to sodium aminosalicylate.

Gastro-intestinal side-effects are common and include nausea, vomiting, and diarrhoea; they may be reduced by giving doses with food or in association with an antacid but sodium aminosalicylate may have to be withdrawn. Malabsorption of vitamin B_{12}, folate, and protein, associated with steatorrhoea, has been reported. Hypokalaemia may develop.

Allergic reactions have been reported in over 5% of adults, usually between the second and sixth week of treatment, and include fever, skin rashes, arthralgia, lymphadenopathy, and, more rarely, a syndrome resembling infectious mononucleosis. Other adverse effects which have been attributed to an allergic reaction to aminosalicylate include jaundice, necrosis of the liver, pancreatitis, pulmonary infiltration, encephalitis, nephritis, and renal failure. Blood disorders reported include haemolytic anaemia, agranulocytosis, leucopenia, and thrombocytopenia. Hypoprothrombinaemia and psychosis may occasionally occur. Prolonged treatment with sodium aminosalicylate may induce goitre and hypothyroidism because of interference with the utilisation of iodine.

Allergy. Hypersensitivity reactions to sodium aminosalicylate are often associated with fever and gastro-intestinal symptoms. The rash takes the form of macular or morbilliform exanthema. Findings such as lachrymation, lymphadenopathy, splenomegaly, and leucocytosis might closely simulate infective mononucleosis. Exfoliative dermatitis is a possible complication more common with sodium aminosalicylate than the other tuberculostatics.— N. Thorne, *Practitioner*, 1973, *211*, 606.

Further references: J. M. Smith and V. H. Springett, *Tubercle*, 1966, *47*, 245; T. M. Daniel *et al.*, *J. Lab. clin. Med.*, 1968, *72*, 239; M. Govindaraj and L. J. Grant, *Br. J. Dis. Chest*, 1968, *62*, 27.

See also under Effects on the Blood and Lupoid Syndrome, below.

For reference to the incidence of intolerance to sodium aminosalicylate, see Isoniazid, p.1572.

Effects on the blood. Para-aminosalicylates formed loose associations with red blood cells thus initiating an allergic response, possibly resulting in haemolytic anaemia.— R. R. A. Coombs, *Br. J. Derm.*, 1969, *81*, *Suppl.* 3, 2.

For a report of allergic haemolytic anaemia, see C. Mueller-Eckhardt, *Dt. med. Wschr.*, 1972, *97*, 234.

Aminosalicylic acid was reported to be a haemolytic agent in subjects deficient in glucose-6-phosphate dehydrogenase but only in conjunction with other factors such as infection.— M. E. Pembrey, *Practitioner*, 1974, *213*, 647. Aminosalicylic acid did not cause haemolysis in Chinese patients with glucose-6-phosphate dehydrogenase deficiency.— T. K. Chan *et al.*, *Br. med. J.*, 1976, *2*, 1227.

Effects on the eye. Sodium aminosalicylate could cause optic neuritis.— P. A. MacFaul, *Prescribers' J.*, 1973, *13*, 68.

Effects on the gastro-intestinal tract. For a brief review of aminosalicylic acid-induced malabsorption, see G. F. Longstreth and A. D. Newcomer, *Mayo Clin. Proc.*, 1975, *50*, 284.

Reports of intestinal malabsorption attributed to treatment with aminosalicylic acid or its sodium salt.— A. J. Akhtar *et al.*, *Tubercle*, 1968, *49*, 328; R. A. Levine, *Ann. intern. Med.*, 1968, *68*, 1265; D. J. Coltart, *Br. med. J.*, 1969, *1*, 825.

Effects on the heart. Pericarditis was reported in a patient who took PAS 12 g and isoniazid 300 mg daily for 9 months.— M. D. R. Morris, *Tubercle*, 1970, *51*, 192.

Effects on the liver. Drug-induced hepatitis occurred in 0.32% of 7492 patients receiving antituberculous drugs; aminosalicylic acid was the most common cause among the 38 patients analysed. Patients with aminosalicylate induced hepatitis had lower serum aspartate aminotransferase (SGOT) values than those in whom it was uncertain whether aminosalicylate or isoniazid was responsible.— J. E. Rossouw and S. J. Saunders, *Q.J. Med.*, 1975, *44*, 1. See also *Br. med. J.*, 1975, *2*, 522.

Further references: S. Sochocky, *Br. J. clin. Pract.*, 1971, *25*, 179.

Effects on the metabolism. Two episodes of hypoglycaemic coma occurred in a diabetic patient taking aminosalicylic acid 12 to 18 g daily.— P. Dandona *et al.*, *Postgrad. med. J.*, 1980, *56*, 135.

Lupoid syndrome. A 51-year-old woman with pulmonary tuberculosis developed a lupus-like reaction consisting of arthritis with positive reactions to lupus erythematosus cell tests after 14 months' treatment with aminosalicylate and isoniazid. The effects subsided when therapy was stopped but returned almost immediately when it was restarted.— M. A. Masel, *Med. J. Aust.*, 1967, *2*, 738.

See also under Isoniazid, p.1573.

Pregnancy and the neonate. See under Isoniazid, p.1573.

Treatment of Adverse Effects. If hypersensitivity has occurred the treatment should be stopped and other tuberculostatics such as ethambutol substituted; antihistamines may be tried for symptomatic relief. Desensitisation has been attempted by reducing the dose of sodium aminosalicylate sufficiently to avoid symptoms, and then increasing the amount daily within the limit of toleration till the required daily dose is again being given. Corticosteroids have been given as an adjunct to desensitisation.

If goitre and hypothyroidism occur, thyroxine sodium should be given.

Concentrations of aminosalicylate in the blood are affected by haemodialysis.

Acute liver failure with coma, occurring during treatment with aminosalicylic acid and isoniazid, was successfully treated by exchange transfusion.— R. J. Lederman *et al.*, *Ann. intern. Med.*, 1968, *68*, 830, per *Int. pharm. Abstr.*, 1968, *5*, 661.

Precautions. Great care should be taken in the use of sodium aminosalicylate when renal function is impaired and when sodium restriction is desirable. It should be used with caution in diabetics. The tuberculostatic activity of sodium aminosalicylate is partially inhibited by aminobenzoic acid and by salicylates. The adverse effects of aminosalicylate and salicylates are additive. The urine of patients taking sodium aminosalicylate reduces copper reagents used for testing for glycosuria.

Probenecid can enhance plasma concentrations of aminosalicylate by delaying renal excretion.

Aminosalicylic acid can cause discoloration of the urine.— R. B. Baran and B. Rowles, *J. Am. pharm. Ass.*, 1973, *NS13*, 139.

Effect of disease states. There was an approximate 20% increase in the free fraction of aminosalicylic acid in the serum of patients with kwashiorkor.— N. Buchanan and L. A. Van der Walt, *S. Afr. med. J.*, 1977, *52*, 522.

Effects on laboratory estimations. Aminosalicylic acid can produce a false positive response to Coombs' test and haemolytic anaemia.— A. Huguenin *et al.*, *Algér. méd.*, 1956, *60*, 333, per P. D. Hansten, *Am. J. Hosp. Pharm.*, 1971, *28*, 629.

Sodium aminosalicylate can interfere with qualitative urine estimations for bilirubin by producing a red colour, for ketones by producing a blue-purple colour, and for urobilinogen/porphobilinogen by producing an orange turbidity leading to a yellow solvent extract. It can also interfere technically with chemical estimations for serum aspartate aminotransferase (SGOT) to produce erroneous raised results.— *Drug & Ther. Bull.*, 1972, *10*, 69. See also K. P. Glynn *et al.*, *Ann. intern. Med.*, 1970, *72*, 525.

Interactions. For a report of the effect of diphenhydramine on the absorption of sodium aminosalicylate, see Diphenhydramine Hydrochloride, p.1311.

Antimicrobial Action. Sodium aminosalicylate is bacteriostatic and is active only against mycobacteria. It has a relatively weak action compared with other antituberculous drugs but most strains of *Mycobacterium tuberculosis* have been reported to be inhibited by 1 µg per ml. Resistance emerges slowly over several months.

Absorption and Fate. When given by mouth, sodium aminosalicylate is readily absorbed, and produces peak concentrations in the blood after 1 to 2 hours. Therapeutic concentrations persist for about 4 hours. Sodium aminosalicylate diffuses widely through body tissues and fluids, producing high concentrations in the kidneys, lungs, and liver. Diffusion into the cerebrospinal fluid occurs only if the meninges are inflamed.

Urinary excretion of aminosalicylates is rapid, and about 80% of a dose is excreted within 10 hours. Concentrations of 3 to 5 mg per ml in urine result from therapeutic doses, 50% or more of the dose being excreted in the acetylated form. Though aminosalicylates are acetylated in the body, the rate of the process is not genetically determined as is the case for isoniazid.

In 12 healthy subjects the mean peak plasma concentration of sodium aminosalicylate was 155 µg per ml following administration of 4 g by mouth as tablets. The mean half-life was 0.91 hour and 50% of the drug and metabolites was excreted in 2 to 3 hours. About 93% was excreted in 24 hours, about 56% as the acetylated form.— S. H. Wan *et al.*, *J. pharm. Sci.*, 1974, *63*, 708. For a comparative study of aminosalicylic acid and its calcium, potassium, and sodium salts, see *idem*, *J. Pharmacokinet. Biopharm.*, 1974, *2*, 1.

Uses. Before the introducton of ethambutol and rifampicin, aminosalicylic acid and its salts were widely used with isoniazid and streptomycin in the primary treatment of pulmonary tuberculosis. Because of their low cost aminosalicylates are still used in developing countries and may be valuable when bacterial resistance is a problem—see Treatment of Tuberculosis, p.1565.

The usual daily dosage for adults is 12 g by mouth in divided doses. Doses of up to 20 g daily have been used but may be badly tolerated. If possible it should be given 4-hourly, though for convenience it may be given twice daily; it should be given with or shortly after meals. Children may be given 200 to 300 mg per kg body-weight daily in divided doses. Similar doses have been given twice weekly in intermittent treatment regimens.

Sodium aminosalicylate has been given in tablets, cachets, granules, powders, or as a mixture and has sometimes been given parenterally. Its exceedingly unpleasant taste may make administration difficult; attempts to disguise the taste have not been very successful. Solutions in iced water may be better tolerated, and solutions prepared immediately before use are reported to be less unpleasant. The sodium salt is usually better tolerated than aminosalicylic acid.

Administration in renal failure. Aminosalicylic acid should be avoided in renal failure. Blood-aminosalicylic acid concentrations could be altered by haemodialysis.— P. Sharpstone, *Br. med. J.*, 1977, *2*, 36.

Further references: J. S. Cheigh, *Am. J. Med.*, 1977, *62*, 555; G. B. Appel and H. C. Neu, *New Engl. J. Med.*, 1977, *296*, 663; H. Held and F. Fried, *Chemotherapy, Basle*, 1977, *23*, 405.

Miliary tuberculosis. In 10 of 16 patients with miliary tuberculosis, in whom the usual clinical and radiographic features were absent, treatment with sodium PAS and isoniazid was used diagnostically. A fall of temperature to normal, usually within a week, weight gain, a rise in haemoglobin concentration, and increased well-being were the criteria of improvement.— A. T. Proudfoot *et al.*, *Br. med. J.*, 1969, *2*, 273.

Pulmonary tuberculosis. Some reports of the use of sodium aminosalicylate in the treatment of pulmonary tuberculosis.— *Tubercle*, 1967, *48*, 1; *ibid.*, 1968, *49*, 70; *ibid.*, 1970, *51*, 1; G. Poole and P. Stradling, *Br. med. J.*, 1969, *1*, 82.

Spinal tuberculosis. For reference to the use of aminosalicylic acid with isoniazid in the treatment of spinal tuberculosis, see Treatment of Tuberculosis, p.1565.

Preparations

Cachets

Sodium Aminosalicylate and Isoniazid Cachets *(B.P.C. 1973)*. PAS and Isoniazid Cachets. Cachets containing sodium aminosalicylate and isoniazid. Store in containers which provide adequate protection against moisture, crushing, and light.

Sodium Aminosalicylate Cachets *(B.P.C. 1973)*. PAS Cachets. Cachets containing sodium aminosalicylate. Store in containers which provide adequate protection against moisture, crushing, and light.

Granules

Sodium Aminosalicylate and Isoniazid Granules *(B.P.C. 1973)*. Granules containing sodium aminosalicylate and isoniazid. The granules may be coated and the coating may be coloured. Store in a cool place in airtight containers. Protect from light.

Mixtures

Sodium Aminosalicylate Mixture CF *(A.P.F.)*. PAS Mixture for Children. Sodium aminosalicylate 1 g, sodium metabisulphite 5 mg, orange syrup 2 ml, concentrated chloroform water 0.1 ml, water to 5 ml. *Dose*. 250 to 300 mg of sodium aminosalicylate per kg body-weight daily in 4 divided doses.

Tablets

Aminosalicylate Sodium Tablets *(U.S.P.)*. Sodium Aminosalicylate Tablets. Tablets containing sodium aminosalicylate. Store at a temperature not exceeding 40° in airtight containers. Protect from light.

Sodium Aminosalicylate Tablets *(B.P. 1973)*. Sod. Aminosal. Tab. Sugar-coated tablets containing sodium aminosalicylate.

Proprietary Preparations

Inapasade *(Smith & Nephew Pharmaceuticals, UK)*. Granules of anhydrous sodium aminosalicylate and isoniazid processed with low melting-point waxes, in packets each providing the equivalent of sodium aminosalicylate 6 g and isoniazid 150 mg. **Inapasade Paediatric.** Packets each providing the equivalent of sodium aminosalicylate 2 g and isoniazid 50 mg.

Other Proprietary Names

Apir Pas *(Spain)*; Eupasal Sodico, Italpas Sodico *(both Ital.)*; Parasal Sodium *(USA)*; Parispas *(Spain)*; Pasalba *(Austral.)*; Teebacin *(USA)*.

Sodium aminosalicylate was formerly marketed in Great Britain under the proprietary name Paramisan Sodium (*Smith & Nephew Pharmaceuticals*). A preparation containing sodium aminosalicylate and isoniazid was also formerly marketed under the proprietary name Pasinah-D (*Wander*).

7572-j

Thiacetazone

Thiacetazone *(B.P.C. 1973)*. Amithiozone; Thioacetazonum; TB 1/698; Tebezonum. 4-Acetamidobenzaldehyde thiosemicarbazone.

$C_{10}H_{12}N_4OS$=236.3.

CAS — 104-06-3.

Pharmacopoeias. In *Int.* and *Span.*

Pale yellow odourless or almost odourless crystals or crystalline powder with a bitter taste. Very slightly **soluble** in water; soluble 1 in 500 of alcohol, more soluble in hot alcohol; slightly soluble in methyl alcohol; soluble 1 in 100 of propylene glycol and in other glycols; practically insoluble in chloroform and ether. **Store** in airtight containers. Protect from light.

Adverse Effects. Gastro-intestinal disorders, skin rashes, and vertigo are the side-effects most frequently reported with thiacetazone although the incidence appears to vary from country to country. More serious adverse effects include exfoliative dermatitis, toxic epidermal necrolysis, which has sometimes been fatal, and the Stevens-Johnson syndrome. Agranulocytosis, haemolytic anaemia, cerebral oedema, liver damage, and gynaecomastia have also been reported.

Thiacetazone was administered in a double-blind study in doses of 150 mg increasing by increments of 75 mg to 600 mg for 2589 doses. The incidence of side-effects was 2.3% for thiacetazone and 1.6% for placebo given for 568 doses. All doses of thiacetazone were well tolerated.— W. Fox *et al.*, *Tubercle*, 1974, *55*, 29.

In a 10-year series of 1212 Nigerian patients with tuberculosis who were treated with a regimen of streptomycin, isoniazid, and thiacetazone, 171 (14%) had adverse reactions associated with thiacetazone and in 134 of these aminosalicylic acid had to be substituted for thiacetazone. The most common side-effects were giddiness (10%), occurring mainly in association with streptomycin, and skin rashes (3%) including exfoliation and the Stevens-Johnson syndrome. Despite these adverse effects the advantages of this regimen, in

Nigeria, are considered to outweigh the disadvantages providing adequate precautions are taken.— C. A. Pearson, *J. trop. Med. Hyg.*, 1978, *81*, 238.

Further references: A. B. Miller *et al.*, *Tubercle*, 1966, *47*, 33; *idem*, *Bull. Wld Hlth Org.*, 1970, *43*, 107; S. P. Pamra, *Indian J. med. Res.*, 1971, *59*, 683; A. B. Miller *et al.*, *Bull. Wld Hlth Org.*, 1972, *47*, 211; A. H. Webb, *N.Z. med. J.*, 1973, *78*, 409.

Effects on the blood. In serial haematological studies on 55 patients taking thiacetazone over the previous 4 years, 48.2% showed haematological abnormalities—mainly haemolytic anaemia, but also some neutropenia and thrombocytopenia.— M. A. Masel and N. G. Johnston, *Med. J. Aust.*, 1968, *2*, 840.

Effects on the ear. Auditory and vestibular toxicity was assessed in 469 patients treated with various schedules incorporating isoniazid, thiacetazone, and streptomycin. It was considered that thiacetazone was ototoxic and that it enhanced the ototoxicity of streptomycin.— D. Dayal and H. Shanta, *Indian J. Tuberc.*, 1970, *17*, 155, per *Abstr. Hyg.*, 1971, *46*, 545. The results did not appear to confirm that thiacetazone was more toxic to the ear than isoniazid alone.— D. H. Shennan, *Abstr. Hyg.*, 1971, *46*, 545.

Effects on the skin. Toxic epidermal necrolysis occurred in 2 patients given thiacetazone and was considered to be a hypersensitivity reaction.— F. Handa *et al.*, *Indian J. Tuberc.*, 1974, *21*, 36, per *Abstr. Hyg.*, 1974, *49*, 674.

Further references: G. C. Ferguson *et al.*, *Tubercle*, 1971, *52*, 166.

Precautions. The efficacy and toxicity of a regimen of treatment which includes thiacetazone should be determined in a community before it is used widely since there appears to be a racial or geographical difference in response.

Thiacetazone should not be given to patients with liver impairment and it should generally be discontinued if the patient develops hypersensitivity reactions.

Thiacetazone may displace streptomycin from binding sites on plasma proteins or interfere with its renal excretion, thereby increasing the risk of ototoxicity.

Studies with various regimens of tuberculostatics in 25 patients with tuberculosis suggested that isoniazid enhanced the hepatotoxicity of thiacetazone in British patients.— A. Pines, *Tubercle*, 1964, *45*, 188, per *Abstr. Wld Med.*, 1965, *37*, 163. See also H. L. Gupta *et al.*, *Indian J. med. Res.*, 1977, *65*, 327.

Antimicrobial Action. Thiacetazone is bacteriostatic. It is effective against *Mycobacterium tuberculosis*, *M. bovis*, and *M. leprae* although the sensitivity of strains may vary in different parts of the world. Cross-resistance can develop between thiacetazone and thiocarlide, ethionamide, or prothionamide. When used alone up to 30% of organisms may become resistant in 4 to 6 months.

Sensitivity testing showed that a Kenyan strain of *M. tuberculosis* was more sensitive than a Hong Kong strain; 0.4 µg per ml of thiacetazone could inhibit all the Kenyan strain and most of the Hong Kong strain.— G. A. Ellard *et al.*, *Tubercle*, 1974, *55*, 41.

The sensitivity of *M. tuberculosis* to thiacetazone in Sri Lanka.— M. R. M. Pinto *et al.*, *Tubercle*, 1974, *55*, 129.

Demonstration of cross-resistance of *M. leprae* to thiambutosine, thiacetazone, ethionamide, and prothionamide.— S. R. Pattyn and M. J. Colston (letter), *Lepr. Rev.*, 1978, *49*, 324.

Absorption and Fate. Thiacetazone is absorbed from the gastro-intestinal tract and peak plasma concentrations occur about 4 hours after a dose. Most of the dose is metabolised and excreted mainly in the urine. It is reported to have a biological half-life of 8 to 12 hours.

Peak serum-thiacetazone concentrations occurred about 4 to 5 hours after a dose of 150 mg of thiacetazone and at about 6 hours when the dose was increased to 300 to 600 mg. In Kenyan patients peak concentrations of 1.2 to 1.6 µg per ml were obtained after 150 mg, 2.2 µg per ml after 300 mg, 2.7 µg per ml after 450 mg, and 5 µg per ml after 600 mg. A mean peak concentration of 2.3 µg per ml was measured in 52 patients in Singapore. About 20% of a dose was excreted unchanged by the Kenyans and about 23% by the patients in Singapore irrespective of race.— G. A. Ellard *et al.*, *Tubercle*, 1974, *55*, 41.

Two groups of patients were identified among 114 tuberculous patients and 10 healthy volunteers given 4 mg of thiacetazone per kg body-weight. One group achieved high and the other low blood concentrations of thiacetazone. Treatment was more effective but more toxic in those with high concentrations.— P. K. Sen *et al.*, *Indian J. med. Res.*, 1974, *62*, 557, per *Trop. Dis. Bull.*, 1975, *72*, 197.

Uses. Thiacetazone is a tuberculostatic and antileprotic agent. It is used, in tolerant populations, in the primary treatment of pulmonary tuberculosis with isoniazid and, in the initial phase of treatment, with streptomycin.

The usual adult dose is 2 mg per kg body-weight as a single daily dose but a standard dose of 150 mg daily is often used. It may be preferable to start treatment with 15 mg daily, increasing over 7 to 10 days to the maximum tolerated dose.

In the treatment of leprosy a suggested initial dose of thiacetazone is 50 mg daily, gradually increased over a period of 4 to 8 weeks to a total daily dose of 150 mg.

Leprosy. A study using the *mouse* footpad model indicated that the antileprosy activity of thiambutosine, thiacetazone, and thiocarlide is essentially bacteriostatic. Of the 3 drugs thiacetazone holds the most promise for adjunct use in the combination chemotherapy of leprosy.— M. J. Colston *et al.*, *Lepr. Rev.*, 1978, *49*, 101.

Pulmonary tuberculosis. In a pilot study carried out in East Africa with the collaboration of the East African and British MRCs, a regimen consisting of streptomycin sulphate 1 g with thiacetazone 150 mg and isoniazid 300 mg daily for 4 weeks followed by thiacetazone 450 mg with isoniazid 15 mg per kg body-weight twice weekly for 48 weeks was compared with a second regimen in which the initial intensive phase was continued for 8 weeks and the twice-weekly phase for 44 weeks. After 1 year 20 of 25 (80%) in the first group compared with 22 of 24 (92%) in the second group had responded favourably.— *Tubercle*, 1974, *55*, 211.

Further reports: I. L. Briggs *et al.*, *Tubercle*, 1968, *49*, 48; F. J. Chicou *et al.*, *Chronicle Wld Hlth Org.*, 1969, *23*, 89; *Tubercle*, 1969, *50*, 233 (East African/British MRC Investigation, 1969); *ibid.*, 1970, *51*, 123 and 353 (East African/British MRC Fifth Thiacetazone Investigation, 1970); *idem*, 1973, *54*, 169; *ibid.*, 1971, *52*, 88 (Singapore Tuberculosis Services/Brompton Hospital/British MRC Investigation); *idem*, 1974, *55*, 251 (Second Report).

Preparations

Thiacetazone Tablets *(B.P.C. 1973)*. Tablets containing thiacetazone. Protect from light.

Proprietary Names

Tebewas *(Wassermann, Spain)*; Thetazone *(Propan, S.Afr.)*.

Thiacetazone was formerly marketed in Great Britain under the proprietary name Thioparamizone (*Smith & Nephew Pharmaceuticals*).

7573-z

Thiocarlide. Tiocarlide. 4,4′-Bis(isopentyloxy)thiocarbanilide; 1,3-Bis(4-isopentyloxyphenyl)thiourea.

$C_{23}H_{32}N_2O_2S$=400.6.

CAS — 910-86-1.

A white crystalline powder. Practically **insoluble** in water; soluble in alcohol and macrogol 400. **Protect** from light.

Solutions are decomposed on heating.— L. Eidus and E. J. Hamilton, *Am. Rev. resp. Dis.*, 1964, *90*, 258.

Adverse Effects. Tolerance of thiocarlide has usually been good. Adverse reactions recorded with thiocarlide have included arthralgia, erythema, gastro-intestinal effects, hepatitis, hypoglycaemia, leucopenia, monocytosis, and purpura.

Antimicrobial Action. Thiocarlide is bacteriostatic and inhibits various mycobacteria. Cross-resistance occurs between thiocarlide and thiacetazone.

The MIC of thiocarlide for *Mycobacterium tuberculosis* was about 20 µg per ml. Other mycobacteria examined were equally sensitive.— A. Tacquet *et al.*, *Annls Inst. Pasteur Lille*, 1965, *16*, 31, per *Bull. Hyg., Lond.*, 1967, *42*, 325.

Absorption and Fate. Peak concentrations of thiocarlide exceeding 128 µg per ml have been reported in the blood ½ to 2 hours after a single dose of 6 or 9 g. Some individuals appear to absorb thiocarlide more slowly, and may achieve concentrations of up to 24 µg per ml after 2 to 6 hours. Little unchanged thiocarlide is excreted in urine.

References: O. P. W. Robinson and P. A. Hunter, *Tubercle*, 1966, *47*, 207; H. Eule and E. Werner, *ibid.*, 214.

Uses. Thiocarlide has been used for the treatment of pulmonary tuberculosis in conjunction with other tuberculostatic agents, generally in patients who could not tolerate or who had not responded to other treatments. The usual dose for adults is 6 g daily in divided doses, but up to 10 g daily has been given.

Proprietary Names

Datanil *(Spain)*; Isoxyl *(Fawns & McAllan, Austral.; Continental Pharma, Belg.; Lusofarmaco, Ital.; Continental Pharma, Neth.; Continental Pharma, Switz.)*.

Thiocarlide was formerly marketed in Great Britain under the proprietary name Isoxyl (*Rona*).

7574-c

Viomycin Sulphate *(B.P. 1973)*. Viomycini Sulfas; Tuberactinomycin B.

$C_{25}H_{43}N_{13}O_{10}(+xH_2SO_4)$=685.7.

CAS — 32988-50-4 (viomycin); 37883-00-4 (sulphate).

Pharmacopoeias. In *Int.* and *Jap.* which specifies 1.5 H_2SO_4. *U.S.* includes Sterile Viomycin Sulfate.

The sulphate of an antimicrobial polypeptide base produced by certain strains of *Streptomyces griseus* var. *purpureus* or by any other means.

It is a sterile, white or almost white, odourless or almost odourless, somewhat hygroscopic, crystalline powder with a slightly bitter taste. It contains not less than 700 units per mg of the dried substance.

Very **soluble** in water; slightly soluble in alcohol; practically insoluble in ether. A solution containing 100 000 units per ml in water has a pH of 4.5 to 7. **Incompatible** with novobiocin sodium. Solutions in water are stable at 2° to 10° for 7 days. The dry powder is stable at room temperature for 2 years. **Store** in a cool place in sterile containers sealed to exclude micro-organisms and, as far as possible, moisture.

Incompatibility. A haze developed over 3 hours when viomycin sulphate 4 g per litre was mixed with *amphotericin* 200 mg per litre in dextrose injection, but an immediate precipitate occurred with *heparin* 20 000 units per litre in dextrose injection and sodium chloride injection.— B. B. Riley, *J. Hosp. Pharm.*, 1970, *28*, 228.

Stability. Viomycin sulphate in aqueous solution at pH 6 lost 10% of its potency in 8 hours at 20° when in ampoules filled under air, in 22 days under nitrogen, and 38 days under carbon dioxide. Solutions were less stable at other pH values.— H. Nerlo and S. Umer, *Acta Pol. pharm.*, 1970, *27*, 127, per *Pharm. J.*, 1971, *1*, 228.

Units. One unit of viomycin is contained in 0.0012285 mg of the second International Reference Preparation (1969) of viomycin sulphate which contains 814 units per mg.

Adverse Effects. Viomycin resembles streptomycin (p.1213) and capreomycin (p.1568) in its range of adverse effects but these are considered to be more severe. Renal damage and both auditory and vestibular disturbances have occurred. Other side-effects include allergic reactions, electrolyte disturbances, and electrocardiographic abnormalities. The occurrence and severity of adverse effects are related to dosage.

Precautions. As for Capreomycin Sulphate, p.1568.

Viomycin should not be given to patients with impaired kidney function.

Antimicrobial Action. Viomycin has bacteriostatic activity against *Mycobacterium tuberculosis* and is usually active against strains resistant to streptomycin and isoniazid. The minimum inhibitory concentration of viomycin has been reported to range from 0.6 to 10 µg per ml.

Viomycin also has slight activity against some other organisms, but not sufficient to be of value clinically.

Resistant strains of *M. tuberculosis* readily develop if viomycin is used alone. There is partial cross-resistance between viomycin, kanamycin, and streptomycin and complete cross-resistance with capreomycin.

Absorption and Fate. Little viomycin is absorbed from the gastro-intestinal tract. When given intramuscularly peak plasma concentrations of 22 to 43 μg per ml have been achieved within 1 to 2 hours of a dose of 500 000 units. It does not readily diffuse into cerebrospinal fluid or into peritoneal or pleural effusions. It is mainly excreted by the kidneys.

The biological half-life of viomycin is 3 to 4 hours.—W. A. Ritschel, *Drug Intell. & clin. Pharm.*, 1970, *4*, 332.

Uses. Viomycin sulphate has been used with other agents in the re-treatment of tuberculosis resistant to streptomycin and other antituberculous drugs but has generally been replaced by capreomycin (p.1569).

It is given only by deep intramuscular injection and, for patients with normal renal function, the equivalent of 1 or 2 million units (about 1 to 2 g) of viomycin in 2 equal portions 12 hours apart has been administered twice or thrice weekly. A local anaesthetic has been added to the solution to reduce pain on injection.

Preparations

Sterile Viomycin Sulfate *(U.S.P.)*. Viomycin sulphate suitable for parenteral use. Potency is expressed in terms of the equivalent amount of viomycin. The reconstituted solution should be used within one week if stored at 2° to 8°. pH of a 10% solution 4.5 to 7.

Viomycin Sulphate Injection *(B.P. 1973)*. A sterile solution of viomycin sulphate in Water for Injections, prepared by dissolving the sterile contents of a sealed container in the requisite amount of Water for Injections. pH 4.5 to 7. It should be used within 1 week when stored at room temperature or within 1 month when stored at 2° to 10°.

Proprietary Names

Viocina *(Pfizer, Spain)*; Viocine *(Pfizer, Belg.)*.

Vaccines and other Immunological Products

7930-x

Immunisation is a process of increasing resistance to infection whereby micro-organisms or products of their activity act as *antigens* and stimulate certain body cells to produce *antibodies* with a specific protective capacity.

The process of antibody formation is known as *active immunisation* and may be a natural process following recovery from an infection, or an artificial process following inoculation with a vaccine or toxoid. It is inevitably a slow process dependent on the rate at which the antibody formation can be developed. Immediate protection of short duration may be achieved by *passive immunisation* in which immune serum containing antibodies of the required type, antiserum, or immunoglobulin injection, especially that with a high content of antibodies, is administered.

Vaccines are preparations of antigenic materials which are administered with the object of inducing in the recipient a specific active immunity to specific bacteria or viruses. They may contain living or killed micro-organisms or bacterial toxins or toxoids. Efforts are being made to produce vaccines from particular parts of the bacterium or virus, in order to maintain antigenic activity and reduce reactions to unwanted material. Vaccines may be simple vaccines prepared from a single species or mixed vaccines which are mixtures of 2 or more simple vaccines.

The methods of preparation are designed to ensure that the identity of the specific antigens is maintained and that no microbial contaminants are introduced. The final products are distributed under aseptic conditions into sterile containers which are then sealed to exclude extraneous micro-organisms.

Adverse Effects of Vaccines. Administration of a vaccine by injection may be followed by a local reaction, possibly with inflammation and lymphangitis. At the site of injected vaccine an induration or sterile abscess may develop, particularly with vaccines containing alum administered subcutaneously. The administration of a vaccine may be followed by fever, headache, and malaise starting a few hours after injection and lasting for 1 or 2 days. Vaccines made from viruses grown in eggs and vaccines containing animal serum or antibiotics may cause allergic reactions in hypersensitive persons.

There are very rare reports of infection following the administration of vaccines in which micro-organisms have been inadequately attenuated or inactivated. Very rarely, symptoms of neuritis have been reported about 7 to 10 days after an injection of a vaccine. With some vaccines containing living micro-organisms, local skin lesions are an indication of successful immunisation, but on occasions more general reactions may follow.

Some vaccines, particularly those containing alum, may precipitate paralytic poliomyelitis if administered in communities not immunised against poliomyelitis.

In a group of 77 men, no obvious adverse effects resulted from repeated immunisation for 25 years, although there were abnormal laboratory findings. It was possible that continuing stimulation of immunoreceptor cells by repeated exposure to a single antigen, or closely related group, might initiate immunological abnormalities.— C. S. White *et al., Ann. intern. Med.*, 1974, *81*, 594.

Transient thrombocytopenia had been occasionally reported after immunisation against measles, rubella, measles/mumps/rubella, and rabies using duck-embryo rabies vaccines.— *Br. med. J.*, 1974, *3*, 464.

Transverse myelitis occurred in a 7-month-old girl 6 or 7 days after receiving diphtheria and tetanus vaccine and poliomyelitis vaccine (oral).— E. Whittle and N. R. C. Roberton, *Br. med. J.*, 1977, *1*, 1450.

A 16-year-old girl developed severe vertigo and tinnitus and deafness in the right ear 2 days after revaccination with adsorbed diphtheria and tetanus vaccine and oral poliomyelitis vaccine. Vertigo and tinnitus gradually improved, but the hearing loss persisted.— I. W. S. Mair and H. H. Elverland, *J. Lar. Otol.*, 1977, *91*, 323.

A report of the development of dermatomyositis in children following vaccination against *diphtheria* and *scarlet fever, diphtheria* alone, and *diphtheria, pertussis*, and *tetanus*. There were also reports in the literature of dermatomyositis after vaccination against *diphtheria, pertussis, tetanus*, and *polio*, against *smallpox*, after administration of a *cold* vaccine, and after a second *poliomyelitis* vaccine (*inactivated*). The close temporal relationship between onset of symptoms and vaccinations suggested a causal relationship.— W. Ehrengut (letter), *Lancet*, 1978, *1*, 1040. See also J. A. Cotterill and H. Shapiro (letter), *Lancet*, 1978, *2*, 1158.

Slight ECG changes, without clinical evidence of myocarditis, in 8 of 234 men entering military service, after routine immunisations—usually after smallpox and diphtheria immunisation.— E. -P. J. Helle *et al., Ann. clin. Res.*, 1978, *10*, 280.

The problem of the inadvertent self-injection of oil-emulsion vaccines in veterinary practice.— P. B. Stones, *Glaxo* (letter), *Br. med. J.*, 1979, *1*, 1627.

Precautions for Vaccines. Enquiry regarding previous hypersensitivity should precede the administration of a vaccine and measures to treat reactions should be immediately available. Anaphylactic reactions should be treated with adrenaline, possibly in association with antihistamine and corticosteroid therapy. For detailed recommendations concerning the management of anaphylaxis, see Adrenaline, p.4. Some vaccines contain small amounts of antibiotics and should not be given to patients hypersensitive to them.

The response to some vaccines may be diminished in patients being treated with corticosteroids. Vaccines containing live micro-organisms are contra-indicated in patients with acute febrile illness or intercurrent infection and in those with impaired immune responsiveness whether idiopathic or as a result of radiotherapy or treatment with corticosteroids, cytotoxic drugs, or other immunosuppressants.

While the serum antibody responses to measles vaccine and poliomyelitis vaccine were similar in 20 healthy children and 20 malnourished children the nasopharyngeal secretory antibody response, which in some diseases was more important than the serum response, was impaired in the malnourished children.— R. K. Chandra, *Br. med. J.*, 1975, *2*, 583.

A review of vaccination in the presence of skin diseases.— G. Weber and U. Falk, *Int. J. Derm.*, 1975, *14*, 136, per *Abstr. Hyg.*, 1975, *50*, 657.

Children with eczema should be immunised in the same way as other children; only smallpox vaccination is contra-indicated. The vaccinations are best done when the skin disease is not active.— S. Lingham and R. S. Wells (letter), *Br. med. J.*, 1978, *2*, 355.

A guide to precautions to be taken in vaccination and immunisation.— *Drug & Ther. Bull.*, 1978, *16*, 39.

Discussion of the problem of appropriate storage of vaccines, especially during transport.— H. H. Frankel (letter), *New Engl. J. Med.*, 1979, *301*, 159.

A short discussion on the contra-indications to immunisation in children.— H. B. Valman, *Br. med. J.*, 1980, *280*, 1138. Comments.— J. K. Anand (letter), *Br. med. J.*, 1980, *280*, 1533; S. J. Webb (letter), *ibid.*, 1534; R. H. Hardy (letter), *ibid.*; A. Lloyd-James (letter), *ibid.* Reply.— H. B. Valman (letter), *ibid.* Further comment.— O. G. Brooke (letter), *Br. med. J.*, 1980, *281*, 58; R. Illingworth (letter), *Br. med. J.*, 1980, *281*, 229.

Pregnancy and the neonate. A discussion of the use of vaccines in pregnancy.— M. M. Levine *et al., Lancet*, 1974, *2*, 34. See also *Drug & Ther. Bull.*, 1973, *11*, 13; *Br. med. J.*, 1974, *1*, 511.

Uses of Vaccines. Vaccines are used for active immunisation as a prophylactic measure against some infectious diseases. They provide partial or complete protection for months or years. The first dose generally produces only a slight and rather slow antibody response but, when a second dose is given after a suitable interval, a prompt antibody response follows and high concentrations occur in the blood. Though the antibody concentration may later fall, a further dose of vaccine promptly restores it.

Substances may be added to vaccines to enhance their effectiveness. Adsorbed vaccines should not be given intracutaneously (intradermally). Concomitant administration of vaccines may affect the response to a single vaccine; the effect of diphtheria toxoid is enhanced when administered with pertussis vaccine.

Discussions on immunisation.— M. A. P. S. Downham, *Br. med. J.*, 1976, *1*, 1063; R. B. Heath, *Practitioner*, 1978, *221*, 474; C. Stuart-Harris, *R. Soc. Hlth J.*, 1978, *98*, 99; N. D. Noah, *Br. J. Hosp. Med.*, 1980, *24*, 533; D. D. Rutstein, *New Engl. J. Med.*, 1981, *304*, 1422; A. B. Sabin, *J. Am. med. Ass.*, 1981, *246*, 236.

A review of the effect of vaccines prepared from enteric bacteria and intended to be given by mouth.— Oral Enteric Bacterial Vaccines, *Tech. Rep. Ser. Wld Hlth Org. No. 500*, 1972.

For a discussion of adjuvants, see Immunological Adjuvants, *Tech. Rep. Ser. Wld Hlth Org. No. 595*, 1976.

Discussion of the administration of vaccines by the intranasal route.— D. S. Freestone and A. L. Weinberg, *Br. J. clin. Pharmac.*, 1976, *3*, 827.

Serum antibodies before and after immunisation in haemodialysed children.— C. Kleinknecht *et al., Proc. Eur. Dialysis Transplant Ass.*, 1977, *14*, 209.

A brief report of The International Association of Biological Standardization Congress on the standardisation and use of vaccines in the developing world.— *J. biol. Stand.*, 1978, *6*, 351.

Study of 246 children for whom adequate immunisation histories were available showed the need for reinforcing doses at school entry to maintain adequate titres of diphtheria antitoxin. Tetanus antitoxin titres appeared to be durable but reinforcing doses might prolong immunity through adolescence. With poliomyelitis, reinforcing doses had little effect on titres.— D. Bainton *et al., Br. med. J.*, 1979, *1*, 854.

Recent improvements in the cold chain for vaccine transport and conservation in the tropics.— *Chronicle Wld Hlth Org.*, 1979, *33*, 383.

Pregnancy and the neonate. Breast feeding had a negligible effect on the response to parenteral vaccines; it might prevent some newborn infants from responding to oral poliomyelitis vaccine although in practice this did not appear to have occurred.— *Br. med. J.*, 1972, *4*, 663.

Immunisation Schedules. Protection against several infectious diseases may be provided in early life by active immunisation. In Great Britain, the Department of Health and Social Security has devised immunisation schedules designed to commence immunisation procedures against as many important diseases as possible within the first 2 years of life.

The following schedule of vaccination and immunisation is recommended. During the first year of life, vaccination with Adsorbed Diphtheria, Tetanus, and Pertussis Vaccine and Poliomyelitis Vaccine, Live (Oral). The first doses should preferably be given at the age of 3 months, the second after an interval of 6 to 8 weeks, and the third 4 to 6 months later. If pertussis vaccine is contra-indicated or refused, Adsorbed Diphtheria and Tetanus Vaccine should be given. During the second year of life, vaccination with Measles Vaccine, Live. At school (or nursery school) entry, reinforcing doses of Adsorbed Diphtheria and Tetanus Vaccine and Poliomyelitis Vaccine, Live (Oral) are recommended. Between 11 and 13 years of age BCG Vaccine may be given to tuberculin-negative children. Girls aged 11 to 13 years should receive Rubella Vaccine, Live. On leaving school or before entering employment or further education, reinforcing doses of Adsorbed Tetanus Vaccine and Poliomyelitis Vaccine, either oral or inactivated, are recommended. The schedules are revised from time to time.

Measles, mumps, and rubella vaccines may be given concomitantly and with oral poliomyelitis vaccine. BCG vaccine may be given concomitantly with oral poliomyelitis vaccine. When other live vaccines are given, an interval of at least 3 weeks is generally allowed between the administration of any 2 vaccines containing live micro-organisms. Where this interval is not feasible it is recommended that they be given at the same time but using different sites.

Immunisation of Travellers. An International Certificate of Vaccination in respect of yellow fever is required for travel to countries where the disease is endemic. The Certificate becomes valid 10 days after primary vaccination and immediately on revaccination. It remains valid for 10 years. Certificates in respect of smallpox vaccination are now rarely required; some countries require certificates in respect of cholera vaccination.

A suggested immunisation schedule for travellers who go abroad from time to time: week 1, yellow fever vaccine; week 4, smallpox vaccine, if necessary; weeks 7 and 13, typhoid vaccine and tetanus vaccine; weeks 10, 16, and 22, poliomyelitis vaccine (oral) (or a single reinforcing dose in week 10 for those already immunised); week 39, tetanus vaccine. A suggested alternative schedule which does not provide a satisfactory immunological response but which may be used when there is only brief notice of travel abroad: day 1, cholera vaccine, typhoid vaccine, tetanus vaccine, and poliomyelitis vaccine (oral); day 5, yellow fever vaccine and smallpox vaccine, if necessary (at different sites); day 13, cholera vaccine; day 28, typhoid vaccine, tetanus vaccine, and poliomyelitis vaccine (oral).

For recommendations for immunisation for international travel, see L. Roodyn, *Br. med. J.*, 1974, *4*, 648; A. C. Turner, *Practitioner*, 1978, *220*, 921; *Med. Lett.*, 1981, *25*, 105.

For reviews of immunisation schedules, see J. A. Dudgeon, *Practitioner*, 1975, *215*, 299; M. A. P. S. Downham, *Br. med. J.*, 1976, *1*, 1063; D. Rimland *et al.*, *Ann. intern. Med.*, 1976, *85*, 622; J. M. Mann *et al.*, *ibid.*, 1977, *87*, 380; S. Krugman and S. L. Katz, *J. Am. med. Ass.*, 1977, *237*, 2228; J. C. Delafuente and R. S. Panush, *Drug Intell. & clin. Pharm.*, 1979, *13*, 385.

7931-r

Antisera

Antisera (immunosera) are sterile preparations containing the specific immunoglobulins obtained from the serum of animals by purification. Antisera have the specific power of combining with venins or bacterial toxins, or with the bacterium, virus, or other antigen used for their preparation.

Antisera are obtained from healthy animals immunised by injections of the appropriate toxins or toxoids, venins, or suspensions of micro-organisms or other antigens. The globulins containing the specific immune substances may be obtained from the immune serum by fractional precipitation and enzyme treatment or by other chemical or physical means. A suitable preservative may be added, and is invariably added if the product is issued in multidose containers. The antiserum is distributed aseptically into sterile containers which are sealed so as to exclude micro-organisms. Alternatively they may be supplied as freeze-dried preparations for reconstitution immediately before use.

Immunoglobulins obtained from human blood are described in the chapter on Blood Preparations, p.321. Preparations available include Normal Immunoglobulin Injection, Anti-D (Rh_0) Immunoglobulin Injection, Antihepatitis B Immunoglobulin Injection, Antimeasles Immunoglobulin Injection, Antipertussis Immunoglobulin Injection, Antirabies Immunoglobulin Injection, Antitetanus Immunoglobulin Injection, and Antivaccinia Immunoglobulin Injection.

Antilymphocyte Serum and Antithymocyte Serum are described in the section on Antineoplastic Agents—see pp.188-9.

Adverse Effects of Antisera. Reactions are liable to occur after the injection of any serum of animal origin. Anaphylaxis may occur, with hypotension, dyspnoea, urticaria, and shock. Anaphylactic reactions should be treated with adrenaline, possibly in association with antihistamine and corticosteroid therapy. For detailed recommendations concerning the management of anaphylaxis, see Adrenaline p.4.

Serum sickness may occur frequently 7 to 10 days after the injection of serum of animal origin; symptoms include fever, vomiting, diarrhoea, bronchospasm, and urticaria; there may be nephritis, myocarditis, polyarthritis, neuritis, and uveitis.

Before injecting serum, information should be obtained as to whether previous injections of serum have been received and whether the patient is subject to allergic diseases, such as asthma and infantile eczema. If there is no history of previous serum injection or of allergic reaction, the dose of serum may be given intramuscularly. If the patient is subject to allergic diseases, a trial dose of 0.2 ml of the serum should be given subcutaneously; if no *general* reaction develops during an interval of 30 minutes, the main dose is given intramuscularly.

The patient must be kept under observation for at least 30 minutes after the injection and adrenaline injection kept in readiness for emergency use.

In all urgent cases, the intravenous route is indicated but it should never be used unless a preliminary intramuscular injection, given at least 30 minutes beforehand, has been tolerated. For intravenous use, the serum should be at room temperature, the injection should be given very slowly, and the patient should be recumbent during the injection and for at least an hour afterwards.

The use of convalescent or adult serum of human origin carries the risk of transmitting viral hepatitis type B—see p.321.

Uses of Antisera. Antisera are used for passive immunisation. After injection intravenously, they immediately provide immunity which persists for perhaps 2 or 3 weeks until the antiserum is excreted; other routes of injection have a delayed onset of action.

Immunity may last rather longer after homologous (human) than after heterologous (animal) sera. Sensitisation with previous doses of heterologous sera may result in rapid excretion of the injected antiserum with loss of immunity. It is generally important, therefore, to follow the conferment of passive immunity, which is largely an emergency procedure, by the injection of suitable antigens to produce active immunity.

NOTE. Some antisera and vaccines, including anthrax antiserum, botulinum antitoxin, ovine tetanus antitoxin, and rabies antiserum and vaccines, are not generally available commercially in Great Britain but supplies are kept at designated hospitals and other centres. Changes in distribution arrangements are notified to hospitals from time to time by the Department of Health and Social Security.

7932-f

Adenovirus Vaccine

Vaccines prepared from live or inactivated adenovirus have been given to prevent adenoviral respiratory infections in situations where epidemics are likely to occur, such as military camps, schools, and similar institutions. The vaccines have usually been given as enteric-coated capsules.

Respiratory viruses, including adenoviruses: a review.— *Tech. Rep. Ser. Wld Hlth Org. No. 408*, 1969.

Other references: *Lancet*, 1968, *2*, 721; J. P. Griffin and B. H. Greenberg, *Archs intern. Med.*, 1970, *125*, 981, per *J. Am. med. Ass.*, 1970, *212*, 2138; F. H. Top *et al.*, *J. infect. Dis.*, 1971, *24*, 155, per H. A. Reimann, *Postgrad. med. J.*, 1972, *48*, 363; B. A. Dudding *et al.*, *Am. J. Epidem.*, 1973, *97*, 187.

7933-d

Anthrax Vaccine

A sterile filtrate containing a factor elaborated during the anaerobic growth of *Bacillus anthracis*, precipitated with alum. An adsorbed vaccine is also used. **Store** at 2° to 10° and avoid freezing. Protect from light.

Units. 1 unit of anthrax spore vaccine is contained in approximately 10^8 culturable spores in one ampoule of the first International Reference Preparation (1978).

Adverse Effects and Precautions. As for Vaccines, p.1586.

Moderate local reactions may occur in patients with a past history of anthrax.

Uses. Anthrax Vaccine is used for active immunisation against anthrax. It is recommended for persons exposed to a high risk of infection, such as laboratory workers, veterinary practitioners, and workers handling animal hairs, hides, wool, and bone meal.

It is given in 4 doses, administered by intramuscular injection. The first 3 doses are separated by intervals of 3 weeks and the fourth dose follows after an interval of 6 months. About 90% protection has been reported. Reinforcing doses are required each year.

For brief discussions of the role of a vaccine for the prevention of anthrax, see R. H. Johnson and R. J. Ellis, *Ann. intern. Med.*, 1974, *81*, 61.

NOTE. Preparations of anthrax vaccine are not generally available commercially in Great Britain but supplies are kept at Public Health Laboratories at Cardiff, Leeds, Liverpool, and London, and at hospitals in N. Ireland and Scotland—Belfast, Bridge of Earn, Carluke, and Galashiels.

7934-n

Bacillus Calmette-Guérin Vaccine *(B.P., Eur. P.).*

Vaccinum Tuberculosis (BCG) Cryodesiccatum; Freeze-Dried BCG Vaccine; BCG Vaccine; Dried Tub/Vac/BCG.

NOTE. In Martindale, this vaccine and the vaccine described in the *U.S.P.* (see below) are called BCG vaccine.

A preparation containing live bacteria obtained from a strain derived from the bacillus of Calmette and Guérin and known to protect man against tuberculosis; the strain is maintained so as to preserve its stability, its power of sensitising man to tuberculin, its ability to protect animals against tuberculosis, and its relative non-pathogenicity to man and laboratory animals. It is standardised in relation to its ability to produce, in *guinea-pigs*, a reaction to tuberculin. It is supplied as a dried product, which is reconstituted by the addition of a suitable sterile liquid. The reconstituted vaccine should be used immediately after preparation and any portion not used should be discarded.

Store at 2° to 8°; the liquid vaccine should not be allowed to freeze. Protect from light. Under these conditions the dried product may be expected to retain its potency for at least 1 year from the date of preparation.

A dry BCG vaccine lost 10% of viable organisms per year when stored at 0° to 5°. When stored at temperatures up to 37° there was still sufficient activity after 56 days for vaccination to be carried out successfully in children, and the effects of which were still demonstrated after 14 months.— D. Wright *et al.*, *Tubercle*, 1972, *53*, 92.

Small differences between batches of BCG vaccine detected in some laboratory tests could be associated with marked differences in clinical response. Laboratory tests should be rendered sufficiently precise to detect small differences indicative of inadequate potency.— R. Dobbelaer *et al.*, *J. biol. Stand.*, 1977, *5*, 57.

BCG vaccines prepared from different strains and by different methods varied in protective efficacy. Some vaccines had been associated with lymph-node inflammation and osteitis in the newborn. No recommendations could be made concerning the choice of strain or method of manufacture. The choice of a vaccine for an immunisation programme should be carefully made in the light of all relevant factors including small-scale studies to assess allergenic and reactogenic potential.— *J. biol. Stand.*, 1977, *5*, 83. See also *ibid.*, 85–164.

Comparable stability of BCG vaccine stored under vacuum or under nitrogen in sealed ampoules. Storage under carbon dioxide was also acceptable.— H. Freudenstein, *J. biol. Stand.*, 1978, *6*, 243.

7935-h

BCG Vaccine *(U.S.P.)*.

A dried living culture of the bacillus Calmette-Guérin strain of *Mycobacterium tuberculosis* var. *bovis*; it is grown from a strain that has been maintained to preserve its capacity for conferring immunity. It contains an amount of viable bacteria such that inoculation, in the recommended dose, of tuberculin-negative persons results in an acceptable tuberculin conversion rate. It contains a suitable stabiliser and no antimicrobial agent. The reconstituted vaccine should be used immediately after preparation and any portion not used within 2 hours should be discarded.

Store at 2° to 8° in hermetically-sealed containers. The expiration date is not later than 6 months after issue, or not later than 1 year after issue if stored below 5°.

7936-m

Percutaneous Bacillus Calmette-Guérin Vaccine *(B.P.)*. Percut. BCG Vaccine; Tub/Vac/BCG (Perc).

A suspension of living cells of an authentic strain of the bacillus of Calmette and Guérin with a higher viable bacterial count than Bacillus Calmette-Guérin Vaccine; the strain is maintained so as to preserve its power of sensitising man to tuberculin and its relative non-pathogenicity to man and laboratory animals. A 1 in 25 dilution produces, in *guinea-pigs*, a reaction to tuberculin similar to that produced by Bacillus Calmette-Guérin Vaccine. It is supplied as a dried vaccine and is reconstituted by the addition of a suitable sterile liquid. The reconstituted vaccine should be used immediately after preparation and any portion not used should be discarded. It is given by percutaneous inoculation.

Store at 2° to 8°. Protect from light. Under these conditions the vaccine may be expected to retain its potency for at least 2 years.

Units. The first International Reference Preparation (1965) of BCG vaccine consists of ampoules containing 5.72 mg of dried material derived from 2.5 mg (semi-dry weight) of bacillary mass of BCG and 5 mg of sodium glutamate.

Adverse Effects. As for Vaccines, p.1586.

Side-effects occur rarely with BCG vaccine. They include ulceration of the inoculation site, lymphadenitis, osteitis, and keloid formation. Very rarely, lupus vulgaris has occurred. Generalised reactions, possibly allergic, with a few fatalities have been reported; the fatalities were mostly in patients with peripheral lymphopenia. Disseminated BCG infection may occur.

Tachycardia, liver granulomas, and splenomegaly have occurred after the use of BCG vaccine as adjuvant immunotherapy in neoplastic disease.

Complications induced by BCG vaccination.— A. Lotte *et al.*, *Bull. int. Un. Tuberc.*, 1978, *53* (June), 114. See also *idem*, 1980, *55*, 55.

A report of fatal disseminated BCG infection in an 18-year-old boy 6 years after BCG vaccination. The disease progressed despite antitubercular therapy and 2 courses of transfer factor from Mantoux-positive donors. His macrophage and T lymphocyte function were found to be abnormal.— A. Mackay *et al.*, *Lancet*, 1980, *2*, 1332. See also R. Torriani *et al.*, *Schweiz. med. Wschr.*, 1979, *109*, 708, per *Abstr. Hyg.*, 1979, *54*, 1173.

Allergy and anaphylaxis. An anaphylactic reaction to BCG vaccination occurred in a 6-day-old baby of Middle Eastern parentage.— J. R. Harper (letter), *Lancet*, 1982, *1*, 403.

Effects on bone. Reports of osteomyelitis: M. Pauker *et al.*, *Archs Dis. Childh.*, 1977, *52*, 330; S. Bergdahl *et al.*, *J. Bone Jt Surg.*, 1976, *58-B*, 212; O. Wasz-Hockert *et al.*, *Bull. int. Un. Tuberc.*, 1979, *54*, 325.

Effects on the nervous system. Guillain-Barré syndrome after the use of BCG vaccine.— J. A. M. J. Wils and G. J. M. M. van Gool (letter), *Lancet*, 1975, *1*, 109.

Effects on the skin. A report of 2 boys who developed dermatomyositis subsequent to BCG vaccination.— E. Kåss *et al.* (letter), *Lancet*, 1978, *1*, 772.

Erythema multiforme following BCG vaccination.— M. Dogliotti, *S. Afr. med. J.*, 1980, *57*, 332.

In neoplastic disease. In 13 of 26 patients treated for cancers with BCG vaccine, pyrexia, malaise, vomiting, arthralgia, and headache occurred, requiring hospitalisation in 4 cases. BCG infection followed these symptoms in 2 other patients.— P. W. A. Mansell and E. T. Krementz, *J. Am. med. Ass.*, 1973, *226*, 1570.

Of 25 patients with cancer receiving intratumour injections of BCG vaccine, all developed malaise, 16 had a severe influenza-like syndrome, 6 developed ulcers at the site of injection, and 6 had hepatic dysfunction. It was suggested that to reduce complications in patients previously sensitised to BCG a lower dose should be used and antihistamines given for 24 hours, and aspirin and paracetamol for several days prior to injection. If symptoms still persisted isoniazid 300 mg daily could be given.— F. C. Sparks *et al.*, *New Engl. J. Med.*, 1973, *289*, 827.

Twelve of 21 patients given BCG vaccine for immunotherapy developed hepatic abnormalities; liver biopsy showed 6 had granulomatous reactions and necrosis.— A. Bodurtha *et al.*, *Am. J. clin. Path.*, 1974, *61*, 747, per *J. Am. med. Ass.*, 1974, *229*, 1817. Three further cases.— J. S. Hunt *et al.*, *Lancet*, 1973, *2*, 820.

BCG vaccine 0.1 to 0.6 ml was administered intradermally to more than 300 patients with neoplastic disease, mainly lymphoma and leukaemia. Repeated vaccinations were given to about 100 patients at intervals from 1 week to 1 year. Vaccination was generally well tolerated but in immunocompetent patients repeated vaccinations caused progressively more severe local reactions. After 3 or 4 vaccinations about half of these patients developed systemic reactions with malaise, chills, and fever starting 6 to 10 hours after vaccination and persisting for 5 to 7 days. Two patients developed erythema nodosum and 1 of them pancytopenia with purpura. A further patient had activation of a dormant acid-fast infection. Immunodepressed patients did not respond normally to BCG vaccination (in some cases there was no local reaction) and 2 patients developed persistent disseminated BCG infection. Hypersensitivity reactions could prove a more serious problem than BCG infection which was very sensitive to isoniazid, streptomycin, ethambutol, and rifampicin.— C. W. Aungst *et al.*, *Ann. intern. Med.*, 1975, *82*, 666.

Two patients died following treatment with BCG vaccine given intralesionally for malignant melanoma. Both developed high fever, major coagulation defects, hypotension, and anuria indicating a hypersensitivity reaction.— C. F. McKhann *et al.*, *Cancer*, 1975, *35*, 514, per *Int. pharm. Abstr.*, 1975, *12*, 1019. See also J. W. Proctor *et al.* (letter), *Lancet*, 1978, *2*, 162.

Clinical ascites in 3 patients with malignant melanoma might have been associated with oral BCG immunotherapy.— M. G. Nutting and T. A. McPherson (letter), *New Engl. J. Med.*, 1976, *295*, 395.

Precautions. As for Measles Vaccine, Live, p.1598.

It is suggested that BCG vaccine may be given concomitantly with oral poliomyelitis vaccine, but that killed vaccines or toxoids be not given for 7 days before or 10 days after BCG vaccines and that other live vaccines be not given within 3 weeks.

Of a group of malnourished children who had received BCG vaccine 197 were subsequently retested with tuberculin. A striking difference was noted in skin reactivity: in the kwashiorkor-type of malnutrition sensitivity to tuberculin was greatly depressed whereas in the marasmic type it differed little or not at all from the normal. A clear distinction between different types of nutritional deficiency was relevant in planning mass vaccination programmes.— D. P. Sinha and F. B. Bang, *Lancet*, 1976, *2*, 531. Criticism.— B. Heyworth (letter), *ibid.*, 743.

Impaired response to the tuberculin reaction and BCG in onchocerciasis.— A. Rougemont *et al.* (letter), *Lancet*, 1977, *1*, 309.

Uses. BCG vaccine is used for active immunisation against tuberculosis, principally for the vaccination of selected groups of the population and of persons likely to be exposed to infection. In some countries it is administered only to persons who give a negative tuberculin reaction, but in countries with a high prevalence of tuberculosis, routine vaccination in infancy is recommended. It is generally administered intracutaneously (intradermally) over the insertion of the deltoid muscle. The usual intracutaneous dose is 0.1 ml, or 0.05 ml for infants under 3 months. A reaction, indicated by erythema and papulation, occasionally with superficial ulceration, develops 3 to 6 weeks after administration of the vaccine and subsides during the following 2 to 6 months. Immunity is conferred for about 7 years in up to 80% of those inoculated.

Percutaneous Bacillus Calmette-Guérin Vaccine, a stronger preparation, is administered by multiple puncture (at least 20 punctures).

Because it has been noted that children giving a negative reaction to lepromin gave a positive reaction after BCG vaccine, the vaccine has been used as a prophylactic against leprosy.

Because of its effect on the immune response BCG vaccine has been used in the treatment of various malignant diseases. A methyl-alcohol extraction residue (MER-BCG) has been similarly used; it is reported to cause fewer side-effects.

Arthritis. Of 8 patients with rheumatoid arthritis given BCG vaccine every other day for 1 week, then weekly for 5 months and monthly thereafter, 6 showed some improvement after 3 months. There was no deterioration in any patient during the follow-up period of 12 months.— E. Rewald (letter), *Lancet*, 1974, *2*, 785.

Crohn's disease. Nine patients with Crohn's ileitis or colitis were successfully treated with BCG vaccine. Appetite improved, they gained weight, and diarrhoea diminished. X-rays showed improvement in 4 of 6 patients but no change in 2. Improvement continued after treatment had been withdrawn.— Y. Geffroy *et al.* (letter), *Lancet*, 1970, *2*, 571.

In a double-blind study involving 50 patients with chronic inactive or mildly active Crohn's disease, BCG vaccine taken by mouth for one year had no significant benefit when compared with placebo although there was a slight trend in favour of the vaccine. The need to restrict the concomitant use of corticosteroids, azathioprine, sulphasalazine, or long-term antibacterial agents was a disadvantage.— W. R. Burnham *et al.*, *Gut*, 1979, *20*, 229.

Hepatitis. Immunotherapy with BCG vaccine was effective in 3 of 9 patients with hepatitis B liver disease.— M. F. Bassendine *et al.*, *Gut*, 1980, *21*, A915.

Herpes genitalis. BCG vaccine was given to 15 patients with recurring herpes genitalis infection. Eight had experienced cyclic recurrence with each menstrual period and of these, 3 had no recurrences in 6, 14, and 36 months following vaccination. Of the 7 whose infection did not follow a cyclic pattern 4 reported no recurrences and 3 experienced a decrease in the expected number of infections.— *J. Am. med. Ass.*, 1973, *225*, 466. See also F. D. Anderson *et al.*, *Obstet. Gynec.*, 1974, *43*, 797. Later trials were disappointing.— *Lancet*, 1980, *1*, 26.

Leprosy. In a 9-year trial in 28 220 children in Burma, the incidence of leprosy in children 5 years of age or older was similar in the BCG-vaccinated and unvaccinated groups. In younger children BCG vaccine conferred low protection and then only in early cases.— L. M. Bechelli *et al.*, *Bull. Wld Hlth Org.*, 1974, *51*, 93.

Mass BCG vaccination in an area hyperendemic with leprosy contributed significantly to the decline in the incidence of leprosy by preventing the development of tuberculoid leprosy.— D. L. Leiker and P. Fischer, *Lepr. Rev.*, 1976, *47*, 115.

BCG vaccination should be offered to any child or young adult (not strongly tuberculin-positive) who has been in close contact with a patient suffering from leprosy. BCG vaccine may enhance any existing innate potential resistance to leprosy challenge besides conferring protection against tuberculosis.— S. G. Browne, *Memorandum on Leprosy*, London, HM Stationery Office, 1977.

Comment on the protective effect of BCG vaccination against leprosy and the conflicting results reported from studies in different countries.— *Lancet*, 1982, *1*, 206.

Further references: J. A. K. Brown *et al.*, *Lepr. Rev.*, 1969, *40*, 3; J. Rosenberg and M. C. R. P. Filho, *Revta bras. Leprol.*, 1970, *37*, 51, per *Trop. Dis. Bull.*, 1972, *69*, 755; P. Saint-André *et al.*, *Méd. trop. Marseille*, 1976, *36*, 133; J. P. Digoutte *et al.*, *Bordeaux Méd.*, 1977, *10*, 703.

Leukaemia. Analysis of figures from Quebec and Glasgow where BCG vaccination of infants was commonly carried out did not show that leukaemia mortality-rates were altered.— L. J. Kinlen and M. C. Pike, *Lancet*, 1971, *2*, 398.

In Chicago among 54 414 children who were vaccinated at birth with BCG vaccine there was 1 death from leukaemia compared with 21 deaths among 172 986 children who had not been vaccinated.— S. R. Rosenthal *et al.*, *J. Am. med. Ass.*, 1972, *222*, 1543. A similar report.— F. Ambrosch *et al.*, *Münch. med. Wschr.*, 1978, *120*, 243.

Discussions of the use of immunotherapy, mainly with BCG vaccine, in leukaemia.— *Lancet*, 1974, *1*, 846; R. C. Bast *et al.*, *New Engl. J. Med.*, 1974, *290*, 1458.

Leukaemia, acute lymphoblastic. Patients with acute lymphoblastic leukaemia in whom remission had been obtained by intensive chemotherapy were treated with BCG vaccine. Treatment coincided with long persistence of remission, despite the absence of treatment with pharmacological agents.— Report of a WHO Scientific Group on Immunotherapy of Cancer, *Tech. Rep. Ser. Wld Hlth Org. No. 344*, 1966.

BCG vaccine and irradiated leukaemic cells were used alone and together as active immunotherapy in 20 patients with acute lymphoblastic leukaemia who were in remission after receiving chemotherapy. Eight had not relapsed after periods of 295 to 1150 days. There was no significant difference between the treatments. Ten patients who did not receive immunotherapy relapsed within 130 days.— G. Mathé *et al.*, *Lancet*, 1969, *1*, 697.

In a controlled study BCG vaccine was ineffective in prolonging drug-induced remissions in children with acute lymphocytic leukaemia.— R. M. Heyn *et al.*, *Blood*, 1975, *46*, 431.

Immunotherapy involving BCG in 10 patients with treated acute lymphoblastic leukaemia did not increase survival; all patients relapsed and died within 5 years.— M. A. Baker and R. N. Taub (letter), *Lancet*, 1977, *1*, 1308.

Maintenance of remission of acute lymphocytic leukaemia in children by the use of BCG vaccine.— T. D. Miale *et al.*, *Biomedicine*, 1978, *28*, 96.

Leukaemia, acute myeloid. Discussions on the use of BCG vaccine in acute myelogenous leukaemia.— R. P. Gale, *New Engl. J. Med.*, 1979, *300*, 1189; J. A. Whittaker, *Br. med. J.*, 1980, *281*, 960.

Of 206 newly diagnosed patients over the age of 15 years with acute myeloblastic leukaemia who had completed the Southeastern Cancer Study Group's induction regimen, 45 had completed consolidation treatment for their remission and 41 of these received maintenance with either methotrexate 30 mg per m^2 body-surface twice weekly by mouth (23 patients) or methotrexate with BCG given weekly for 4 weeks. The median duration of remission was 39.4 weeks for the methotrexate/BCG group and 26 weeks for the methotrexate group. When the remission was measured from the onset of the maintenance phase the median duration was 20.4 weeks for methotrexate/BCG and 9.7 weeks for methotrexate alone.— W. R. Vogler and Y. -K. Chan, *Lancet*, 1974, *2*, 128.

Thirty patients in remission from acute myelogenous leukaemia received immunosuppression with BCG and irradiated allogeneic leukaemic cells given at different sites. Half these patients were also given a mixture of BCG and the irradiated leukaemic cells intradermally at 4 sites on 4 occasions at 3-weekly intervals. Four patients in this latter group were still in remission at 92 weeks compared with none of the other 15 patients who had not received the mixture.— R. L. Powles *et al.* (preliminary communication), *Lancet*, 1977, *2*, 1107.

In patients in remission from acute myelogenous leukaemia the duration of remission was comparable in those receiving maintenance therapy or BCG vaccine, but survival was longer in those receiving BCG vaccine and 2nd and 3rd remissions were more common. In patients in remission given maintenance therapy and BCG vaccine or irradiated blast cells, the duration of remission and of survival was similar.— J. A. Whittaker *et al.*, *Br. J. Haemat.*, 1980, *45*, 389.

Further references: J. U. Gutterman *et al.*, *Lancet*, 1974, *2*, 1405; *idem*, 1975, *1*, 454; M. G. Whiteside *et al.*, *Med. J. Aust.*, 1976, *2*, 10.

Lymphoma. References to the use of BCG in lymphoma: J. E. Sokal, *J. surg. Oncol.*, 1973, *5*, 557; P. Gunven *et al.*, *J. natn. Cancer Inst.*, 1973, *51*, 45; J. E. Sokal *et al.*, *New Engl. J. Med.*, 1974, *291*, 1226; *ibid.*, 1255.

Lymphoma, Burkitt's. Absence of benefit with BCG vaccine in Burkitt's lymphoma.— I. T. Magrath and J. L. Ziegler, *Br. med. J.*, 1976, *1*, 615.

Melanoma. Favourable reports of the use of BCG vaccine in malignant melanoma: F. R. Eilber *et al.*, *Am. J. Surg.*, 1976, *132*, 476; A. B. MacGregor *et al.*, *Can. J. Surg.*, 1977, *20*, 25; P. B. McCulloch *et al.*, *Can. med. Ass.J.*, 1977, *117*, 33; W. C. Wood *et al.*, *Surgery, St Louis*, 1978, *83*, 677.

Of 15 patients with malignant melanoma (stage IIB) who were considered to be freed from tumours by wide excision, 8 were treated, 14 days after surgery, with BCG vaccine and autologous irradiated tumour cells. Three vaccinated patients had widespread recurrences at 3 months compared with none of the 7 controls; at 12 months 4 of the vaccinated patients had died compared with none of the controls. Because of these alarming results the study was stopped after 1 year.— M. B. McIllmurray *et al.*, *Br. med. J.*, 1977, *1*, 540. At 2 years of follow-up the higher death-rate in treated patients was less obvious.— M. B. McIllmurray *et al.* (letter), *ibid.*, 1978, *1*, 579.

Further references: F. R. Eilber *et al.*, *New Engl. J. Med.*, 1976, *294*, 237; A. A. El-Domeiri *et al.*, *Archs Surg., Chicago*, 1977, *112*, 257, per *J. Am. med. Ass.*, 1977, *237*, 1508.

For further reports and references on BCG vaccine in malignant melanoma, see Martindale 27th Edn, p. 1610.

Neoplasms. Discussions on the use of BCG vaccine as an antineoplastic agent.— *Med. Lett.*, 1976, *18*, 83; E. M. Hersh *et al.*, *J. Am. med. Ass.*, 1976, *235*, 646; J. L. Fahey *et al.*, *Ann. intern. Med.*, 1976, *84*, 454; A. Coates, *Med. J. Aust.*, 1977, *2*, 143; *Drug & Ther. Bull.*, 1977, *15*, 73; S. P. Richman *et al.*, *Can. med. Ass. J.*, 1979, *120*, 322.

Analysis of the incidence of leukaemia, Hodgkin's disease, and lymphosarcoma in a population of 64 136 subjects who had participated in a study of BCG vaccination did not indicate that BCG vaccine had any influence on these conditions.— G. W. Comstock *et al.*, *Lancet*, 1971, *2*, 1062. See also D. E. Snider *et al.*, *J. natn. Cancer Inst.*, 1978, *60*, 785.

In a clinical trial in 33 patients with localised soft tissue sarcoma 11 of 18 who received adjuvant immunotherapy with BCG vaccine and tumour cell vaccine and 5 of 15 treated by surgery alone were free from recurrences. Immunotherapy had no benefit in patients with osteosarcoma or recurrent or disseminated soft tissue sarcomas.— C. M. Townsend *et al.*, *J. Am. med. Ass.*, 1976, *236*, 2187.

In Sweden, general neonatal BCG vaccination using the same BCG strain was practised for 20 years until May, 1975, when it was stopped because of a high incidence of side-effects, mainly osteitis. Preliminary data on subsequent tumour incidence did not reveal an increase, and therefore did not support the view that its incidence is influenced by BCG vaccination.— B. S. Nilsson and O. Widström (letter), *Lancet*, 1979, *1*, 222.

See also under Leukaemia, Lymphoma, and Melanoma, above.

Bladder. A discussion, generally favourable, of the use of BCG vaccine in the treatment of superficial bladder cancer.— A. Morales, *Can. med. Ass. J.*, 1980, *122*, 1133.

Breast. Prolongation of remission and survival in women with breast cancer treated with chemotherapy and BCG vaccine.— J. U. Gutterman *et al.*, *Br. med. J.*, 1976, *2*, 1222. Criticism.— P. B. Iles *et al.* (letter), *ibid.*, 1560; M. H. Maor (letter), *ibid.*

Gastro-intestinal tract. In 83 patients with colorectal cancer the disease-free interval after surgery and overall survival were significantly increased by treatment with BCG vaccine weekly for 3 months and every other week thereafter and, in 50 patients, fluorouracil 150 mg per m^2 body-surface 4 times daily for 5 days every 4 weeks.— G. M. Mavligit *et al.*, *Lancet*, 1976, *1*, 871. Criticisms: J. T. Evans (letter), *ibid.*, 1248; P. R. M. Thomas *et al.* (letter), *ibid.*, 1349.

The failure of nonspecific immunotherapy in cancer of the large bowel.— R. J. Nicholls, *Br. J. Hosp. Med.*, 1980, *24*, 309.

Further references: S. K. Carter, *Cancer Immunol. & Immunother.*, 1976, *1*, 199, per *Drugs*, 1977, *14*, 463.

Head and neck. Unfavourable reports of the use of BCG vaccine as adjuvant immunotherapy for neoplasms of the head and neck.— J. Y. Suen *et al.*, *Am. J. Surg.*, 1977, *134*, 474, per *J. Am. med. Ass.*, 1978, *239*, 982; R. Papac *et al.*, *Cancer Res.*, 1978, *38*, 3150.

Lung. Favourable reports of the adjuvant use of BCG vaccine in neoplasms of the bronchus and lung.— M. F. McKneally *et al.*, *Lancet*, 1976, *1*, 377; A. Pines, *ibid.*, 380; M. F. McKneally *et al.*, *ibid.*, 1977, *1*, 1003; E. C. Holmes *et al.* (preliminary communication), *ibid.*, 1977, *2*, 586; H. M. Jansen *et al.*, *Thorax*, 1978, *33*, 429; K. Yasumoto *et al.*, *Cancer Res.*, 1979, *39*, 3262.

Unfavourable reports.— P. Roscoe *et al.*, *Cancer Immunol. & Immunother.*, 1977, *3*, 115; A. B. Miller *et al.*, *Can. med. Ass. J.*, 1979, *121*, 45; J. Lowe *et al.*, *Lancet*, 1980, *1*, 11.

A report of severe adverse reactions in patients with resected bronchogenic carcinoma given BCG vaccine intrapleurally.—The Ludwig Lung Cancer Study Group, (letter), *New Engl. J. Med.*, 1981, *305*, 167.

Ovary. Immunotherapy with BCG and irradiated tumour cells in 10 patients with ovarian cancer considered to be in a static state due to conventional chemotherapy was considered to prolong stasis or remission and survival time when compared with a retrospective group of 25 controls. Immunotherapy was probably of no use in progressive disease.— C. N. Hudson *et al.* (preliminary communication), *Lancet*, 1976, *2*, 877.

Skin ulcers. Vaccination with BCG vaccine gave some protection for a few months against chronic necrotising skin ulcers caused by infection with *Mycobacterium ulcerans*, Buruli ulcer, in a refugee settlement in Uganda. The degree of protection from vaccination ranged from 18% in areas with a high incidence of infection to 74% in areas with a low incidence.—First Results by the Uganda Buruli Group, *Lancet*, 1969, *1*, 111.

A study carried out in an endemic area of Uganda showed that BCG vaccination gave short-term protection against Buruli ulcer, caused by *Mycobacterium ulcerans;* vaccination gave no additional protection to persons with previously acquired lesions.— P. G. Smith *et al.*, *Trans. R. Soc. trop. Med. Hyg.*, 1976, *70*, 449.

Tuberculosis immunisation. The BCG Vaccination Sub-Committee of the Department of Health recommended that despite the fall in the risk of infection the use of BCG vaccine should be continued on a community basis in the United Kingdom. Special measures were recommended for immigrants, especially from Africa, Bangladesh, India, and Pakistan in whom the incidence of tuberculosis remained high, and included in these communities the vaccination of children at birth or soon after entry.— *Lancet*, 1975, *2*, 778.

An account of the present knowledge of immunisation against tuberculosis.— H. G. ten Dam *et al.*, *Bull. Wld Hlth Org.*, 1976, *54*, 255.

From an 18-month study of 181 children in The Gambia vaccinated with BCG it was recommended that if children were malnourished vaccination might be repeated to give adequate protection, and that BCG vaccination should not be given when other infections such as measles or malaria were likely to cause immunosuppression.— B. Heyworth, *Trans. R. Soc. trop. Med. Hyg.*, 1977, *71*, 251.

In the final report to the MRC the protective efficacy of BCG vaccine and vole bacillus vaccine was 77% over the 20-year period after vaccination.— P. D' A. Hart and I. Sutherland, *Br. med. J.*, 1977, *2*, 293.

In a study made in Finland in 1961, tuberculous foci were found at autopsy in 35 of 83 BCG-vaccinated subjects and in 61 of 67 non-vaccinated subjects. It appears that BCG vaccination does not prevent the establishment of infection in exposed subjects but does limit the multiplication and dissemination of the bacilli and the development of lesions following infection.— I. Sutherland and I. Lindgren, *Tubercle*, 1979, *60*, 225.

The Tuberculosis Prevention Trial in 260,000 persons in S. India comparing BCG vaccine and placebo (the Madras study) showed that BCG vaccination afforded no protection for the first 7.5 years of follow-up.— *Bull. Wld Hlth Org.*, 1979, *57*, 819. A scientific group, jointly sponsored by the Indian Council of Medical Research and the World Health Organization recognised the high scientific quality of the trial; the absence of protective effect should not be regarded as automatically applying to other parts of the world; epidemiological, environmental, and immunological factors might be involved.— *Tech. Rep. Ser. Wld Hlth Org. No. 651*, 1980. A WHO Study Group reviewed BCG vaccination, including the results of the South Indian trial, where tuberculosis in the trial area showed an unprecedented pattern of behaviour. The effectiveness of BCG vaccination could not be predicted with certainty. Vaccination programmes should continue and should be appropriate to the epidemiological situation in each country.— *Tech. Rep. Ser. Wld Hlth Org. No. 652,* 1980. Further discussions and comment: *Chronicle Wld Hlth Org.*, 1980, *34,* 118; *Lancet,* 1980, *1,* 73; *Lancet,* 1981, *1,* 309; D. B. Travers (letter), *Lancet,* 1981, *1,* 1001; *Tubercle,* 1981, *62,* 219.

It would be wise to use isoniazid-resistant BCG vaccine for an infant taking isoniazid.— *Br. med. J.*, 1979, *2,* 530.

Discussions of the use of BCG vaccine in the newborn.— H. G. ten Dam and K. L. Hitze, *Bull. Wld Hlth Org.*, 1980, *58,* 37. See also *Br. med. J.*, 1980, *281,* 1445; J. D. Cartwright, *S. Afr. med. J.*, 1978, *54,* 65; R. Alloula and D. Larbaoui, *Bull. int. Un. Tuberc.*, 1979, *54,* 328.

Administration. BCG vaccine administered by mouth was as effective as intradermal vaccination in producing tuberculin skin sensitivity.— H. Kahn *et al.*, *Tubercle,* 1970, *51,* 423.

In a study of 1736 children the results of BCG vaccination carried out using a jet injector were similar to those produced by the technique using a syringe and needle.—A Report from the Research Council of the British Thoracic and Tuberculosis Association, *Tubercle,* 1971, *52,* 155. Poorer seroconversion with jet injection than with syringe and needle.— H. D. Wilson, *Lancet,* 1973, *1,* 927. Whereas 19 of 10 800 children who had been vaccinated with BCG vaccine given by a jet injector (Dermojet) had persistent deep discharging abscesses at the site of inoculation, there was only 1 in 27 000 who had been vaccinated with a needle and syringe. However, administration by jet injector was considered to be an adequate method of vaccination if the guns were regularly checked to ensure an accurate dose was given to the correct depth of skin.— J. A. Marston and R. J. Pye, *Practitioner,* 1978, *220,* 625.

Results of a pilot programme indicated that BCG vaccination using a bifurcated needle was significantly inferior to the intradermal technique.— A. M. Darmanger *et al.*, *Bull. Wld Hlth Org.*, 1977, *55,* 49. See also *Bull. int. Un. Tuberc.*, 1978, *53* (Mar.), 30.

Further references: S. Landi *et al.*, *Can. med. Ass. J.*, 1967, *97,* 222 (multiple puncture compared with intradermal injection); *Tubercle,* 1971, *52,* 19 (multiple puncture); W. G. L. Allan and A. Tanaka, *ibid.*, 247 (infants).

Diagnostic use. Tuberculin testing before and after BCG vaccination for detecting the prevalence of infection in areas with a high prevalence of non-specific sensitivity.— H. G. ten Dam and K. L. Hitze, *Bull. Wld Hlth Org.*, 1980, *58,* 475. See also K. V. Krishnaswami *et al.*, *Indian J. Tuberc.*, 1979, *26,* 70, per *Trop. Dis. Bull.*, 1980, *77,* 243.

Proprietary Preparations

BCG Vaccine (Intradermal) *(Evans Medical, UK).* A brand of Bacillus Calmette-Guérin Vaccine, available as powder for preparation before use, in multidose ampoules of 1 and 5 ml; supplied with diluent.

BCG Vaccine (Percutaneous) *(Evans Medical, UK).* A brand of Percutaneous Bacillus Calmette-Guérin Vaccine, available as powder for preparation before use, in multidose ampoules.

Other Proprietary Names

BCG Vaccine *(Lilly, USA).*

7937-b

Blastomycin

CAS — 1362-89-6.

A sterile standardised liquid concentrate of the soluble growth products developed by the fungus *Blastomyces dermatitidis* when grown in the mycelial phase on a synthetic medium; it contains suitable preservatives and an approved red dye. It is a clear reddish-amber liquid, **miscible** with water. **Store** at 2° to 8°, when it may be expected to retain its potency for 2 years from the date of manufacture.

Blastomycin has been used as an aid in the diagnosis of North American blastomycosis in a dose of 0.1 ml of a 1 in 100 dilution, intradermally, but is considered to be unreliable.

7938-v

Botulinum Antitoxin *(B.P., Eur. P.).* Botulinum Antiserum; Immunoserum Antibotulinicum; Bot/Ser.

A sterile preparation containing the specific antitoxic globulins that have the power of neutralising the toxins formed by *Clostridium botulinum,* type A, type B, or type E, or any mixture of types A, B, and E.

It is an almost colourless or very faintly yellow liquid, free from turbidity and almost odourless except for the odour of any added bactericide. It contains not less than 500 units of each of type A and type B and not less than 50 units of type E per ml. pH 6 to 7.

Store at 2° to 8° and avoid freezing. Protect from light. The *B.P.* states that the method of preparation of antisera is such that they lose, at pH 6, not more than 5% of their activity per year at 20° and not more than 20% at 37°.

The label states the animal source.

NOTE. The *B.P.* states that when Mixed Botulinum Antitoxin or Botulinum Antitoxin is prescribed or demanded and the types to be present are not stated, Botulinum Antitoxin prepared from types A, B, and E shall be dispensed or supplied.

7939-g

Botulism Antitoxin *(U.S.P.).*

A sterile solution of the refined and concentrated antibodies, chiefly globulins, obtained from the blood of healthy horses that have been immunised against the toxins produced by type A and type B and/or E strains of *Clostridium botulinum.* It contains a suitable antimicrobial agent and not more than 20% of solids.

An almost colourless, clear or slightly opalescent liquid, almost odourless or with the odour of the antimicrobial agent.

Store at 2° to 8°. The expiration date of antitoxin containing 20% excess potency is not later than 5 years after release from manufacturer's cold storage. The label states the animal source.

Units. 500 units of *Clostridium botulinum* Type A antitoxin, equine are contained in 68.0 mg of dried hyperimmune horse serum in one ampoule of the first International Standard Preparation (1963). 500 units of Type B antitoxin are contained in 87.0 mg of dried hyperimmune horse serum in one ampoule of the first International Standard Preparation (1963). 1000 units of Type E antitoxin are contained in 69.1 mg of dried hyperimmune horse serum in one ampoule of the first International Standard Preparation (1963).

Adverse Effects. As for Antisera, p.1587.

Botulinum antitoxin is prepared from the serum of animals and reactions due to the injection of animal serum may occur.

Uses. Botulinum Antitoxin is used in the treatment of botulism, caused by the ingestion of infected food. It has been found of value in the treatment of intoxications due to toxins of types B and E but is less effective for the more toxic and quicker acting type A toxin. It should be given as early as possible in the course of the disease though late administration may be of value against B and E toxins which remain in the circulation for some time.

Since the type of botulinum toxin is seldom known the polyvalent antitoxin is usually given. Not less than 50 000 units each of types A and B and 5000 units of type E should be injected intramuscularly or intravenously; the dose may need to be repeated. Persons who have consumed suspected food and in whom symptoms have not developed should be given not less than 10 000 units each of types A and B and 1000 units of type E intramuscularly or subcutaneously as a prophylactic measure.

Monovalent (E) and bivalent (A, B) antitoxin is also used.

NOTE. Botulinum antitoxin is available from designated hospitals and other centres.

7940-f

Cholera Vaccine *(B.P., Eur. P.).* Vaccinum Cholerae; Cho/Vac.

A sterile homogeneous suspension of a suitable killed strain or strains of the cholera vibrio, *Vibrio cholerae.* It consists of a mixture of equal parts of vaccines prepared from smooth strains of 2 main serological types, Inaba and Ogawa of the classical biotype with or without the *eltor* biotype. A single strain or several strains of each type may be included. All strains must contain, in addition to their type O antigens, the heat-stable O antigen common to the Inaba and Ogawa types. If more than one strain each of Inaba and Ogawa are used they may be selected to contain other O antigens. It contains not less than 8000 million *V. cholerae* per dose, which does not exceed 1 ml. It contains not more than 0.5% of phenol.

It may also be supplied as a dried vaccine (Dried Cho/Vac) which is reconstituted immediately before use by the addition of a suitable sterile liquid. Phenol may not be used in the preparation of the dried vaccine. *Eur P.* includes the dried vaccine as Freeze-Dried Cholera Vaccine; Vaccinum Cholerae Cryodesiccatum.

Store at 2° to 8° and avoid freezing. Protect from light. Under these conditions the liquid vaccine may be expected to retain its potency for at least 18 months and the dried vaccine for at least 5 years.

7941-d

Cholera Vaccine *(U.S.P.).*

A sterile suspension, in sodium chloride injection or other suitable diluent, of a suitable killed strain or strains of *Vibrio cholerae* selected for high antigenic efficiency. It consists of a mixture of equal parts of suspensions of cholera vibrios of the Inaba and Ogawa strains. It has a potency of not less than 8 units per serotype per ml. It contains a suitable antimicrobial agent.

Store at 2° to 8° and avoid freezing. The expiration date is not later than 18 months after release from manufacturer's cold storage.

The stability of cholera vaccines.— I. Joó and J. Zsidai, *J. biol. Stand.*, 1979, *7,* 341.

Units. The second International Reference Preparations (1971) of cholera vaccine (Inaba) and cholera vaccine (Ogawa) each consist of ampoules of freeze-dried material from monovalent vaccine (4×10^{10} organisms per ampoule).

A report of an international collaborative assay of a sample of cholera vaccine (Inaba) and of a sample of cholera vaccine (Ogawa) proposed for acceptance as the British Reference Preparation of Cholera Vaccine (Inaba) and of Cholera Vaccine (Ogawa). The potency of the Inaba vaccine was 0.89 and that of the Ogawa vaccine 2.39 in terms of the corresponding International Reference Preparations. The vaccines were established as the first British Reference Preparations.— A. Ford and V. Seagroatt, *J. biol. Stand.*, 1977, *5,* 69.

Adverse Effects and Precautions. As for Vaccines, p.1586.

Slight swelling, erythema, and tenderness occasionally occur at the injection site. Fever and malaise have been reported and general reactions, including anaphylaxis and hypersensitivity reactions, have occurred. Neurological and psychiatric reactions have occasionally occurred.

Myocardial infarction occurred in a previously healthy 40-year-old man after active immunisation with cholera vaccine.— K. G. Koutsaimanis and G. H. Rée (letter), *New Engl. J. Med.*, 1978, *299,* 153.

Reactions were reduced if the second and subsequent doses of cholera vaccine were given, in appropriate volume, intradermally.— *Br. med. J.*, 1981, *282*, 201.

For a report of vibriocidal activity being reduced when yellow fever vaccine was given with or within 3 weeks of cholera vaccine, see Yellow Fever Vaccine, p.1613.

Uses. Cholera Vaccine is used for active immunisation but it is not considered to be very effective and the immunity conferred is short-lived. It is given by subcutaneous or intramuscular injection. A primary prophylactic course of 2 injections given at an interval of at least a week and preferably 4 weeks may confer immunity in about 50% of patients for up to 6 months. Further doses should therefore be given at intervals of 6 months. The first dose is usually at least 4000 million *Vibrio cholerae;* the second and subsequent doses usually contain at least 8000 million *V. cholerae.*

Children have been given doses of up to one-half the adult dose; the use of Cholera Vaccine is not recommended for children less than 1 year of age.

Cholera Vaccine has been given intracutaneously (intradermally) especially for second and subsequent doses; doses of 20 to 40% of the subcutaneous dose have been used.

Field trials of cholera vaccines had shown that protection against infection with *Vibrio cholerae*, lasting for 3 to 6 months, was achieved in 30 to 80% of those vaccinated. Protection had been poorest in those under 10 years of age.— *Tech. Rep. Ser. Wld Hlth Org. No. 414*, 1969.

A controlled study in 101 healthy Africans, aged 14 to 20 years, showed that the antibody response 2 weeks after vaccination with a single dose of monovalent Inaba or Ogawa cholera vaccine was appreciably greater in those given 1 ml subcutaneously than in those given 0.2 ml intracutaneously.— A. M. McBean, *Lancet*, 1972, *1*, 527.

Cholera vaccine given annually for 3 years just before the start of the cholera season to children aged up to 14 years gave increased protection. One dose produced 43% protection, 2 doses 64%, 3 doses 81%, and 4 doses 76%. This level of effectiveness and the need for annual immunisation indicated that cholera treatment centres using oral maintenance therapy were more effective and cheaper than the use of cholera vaccine.— W. H. Mosley *et al.*, *Bull. Wld Hlth Org.*, 1972, *47*, 229.

In a field trial in the Philippines, tests with a monovalent cholera vaccine prepared from *V. cholerae* Ogawa strain showed that it reduced the incidence of cholera from about 23% in a control group to 11.5% in persons receiving 0.2 ml vaccine intradermally and to 6.1% in those given 0.5 ml by subcutaneous injection. Intradermal administration protected for 4 months and subcutaneous injection for 6 months.—Report of Philippines Cholera Committee, WHO Cholera Research Project, *Bull. Wld Hlth Org.*, 1973, *49*, 389.

Study of a cholera vaccine adsorbed on aluminium hydroxide.— J. S. Saroso *et al.*, *Bull. Wld Hlth Org.*, 1978, *56*, 619.

There was no justification for mass vaccination for the control of cholera.— *Chronicle Wld Hlth Org.*, 1978, *32*, 369.

P and V plasmids in *Cholera vibrio*; possible use for oral immunisation.— V. B. Sinha and B. S. Srivastava, *Bull. Wld Hlth Org.*, 1979, *57*, 643. See also B. S. Srivastava *et al.*, *ibid.*, 649.

Studies on the effects of purified cholera toxoid given either subcutaneously or by direct instillation into the jejunum to healthy subjects.— M. M. Levine *et al.*, *Trans. R. Soc. trop. Med. Hyg.*, 1979, *73*, 3.

Discussion of developments in cholera vaccination, including reference to adjuvant vaccines, single-strain vaccines, toxoids (detoxified with formaldehyde and glutaraldehyde), live vaccines, and oral vaccines.— *Bull. Wld Hlth Org.*, 1979, *57*, 719. See also J. A. Green, *Bull. Hattkine Inst.*, 1978, *6*, 51; *Bull. Wld Hlth Org.*, 1980, *58*, 353.

Proprietary Preparations

Cholera Vaccine *(Wellcome, UK)*. A brand of Cholera Vaccine containing not less than 8000 million *V. cholerae* per ml, in vials of 1.5 and 10 ml.

Other Proprietary Names

Cholera Vaccine (India Strains)*(Lederle, USA)*; Cholera Vaccine *(Sclavo, USA)*; Cholera Vaccine *(Wyeth, USA)*.

Cholera vaccine was also formerly marketed in Great Britain under the proprietary name Vibriomune (*Duncan, Flockhart*).

7942-n

Coccidioidin *(U.S.P.)*.

CAS — 12622-73-0.

A sterile solution containing the antigens obtained from the byproducts of mycelial growth or from the spherules of the fungus *Coccidioides immitis*; it contains a suitable antimicrobial agent. It is a clear almost colourless or amber-coloured liquid. **Store** at 2° to 8°. Dilutions should be stored at 2° to 8° and used within 24 hours. The expiration date is not later than 3 years (mycelial product) or 18 months (spherule-derived product) after release from manufacturer's cold storage.

Coccidioidin is used in the diagnosis of coccidioidomycosis in doses of 0.1 ml of a 1 in 10 000 to 1 in 10 dilution, intracutaneously (intradermally).

Negative reactions in serious forms of the disease can pose a problem; there may be cross-reactions with histoplasmin and in patients with other fungal infections.— *FDA Drug Bull.*, 1978, *8*, 15.

Proprietary Names

Spherulin *(Berkeley, USA)*.

In Great Britain supplies of coccidioidin are available on a named-patient basis from *Cutter*.

7943-h

Cold Vaccines

These are usually mixtures of suspensions of various species of bacteria.

Mixed vaccines containing some of the micro-organisms commonly found in infections of the respiratory tract have been used for prophylaxis and treatment of the common cold, bronchitis, etc., though controlled trials have failed to establish any definite prophylactic properties. Bacterial vaccines have been used to reduce secondary infections occurring during a common cold.

In Great Britain a Catarrh Vaccine is available on a named-patient basis from *Swiss Serum and Vaccine Institute, UK* and *Lilly, USA*.

7944-m

Oral Cold Vaccines

It has been suggested that when cold vaccines are given by mouth the soluble antigenic substances penetrate the intestinal mucosa and give rise to antibody formation. Though there is little evidence that the vaccines have prophylactic value they have been widely used.

Oral bacterial vaccines and colds.— *Lancet*, 1974, *2*, 1552. See also C. H. Drake and J. E. Smith (letter), *ibid.*, 1975, *2*, 614.

Proprietary Preparations

Lantigen B (known in *S.Afr.* as Coldvac and Imuvac) *(Ashe, UK)*. A liquid stated to contain in each ml the antigenic extracts of *Neisseria catarrhalis, Haemophilus influenzae, Staphylococcus aureus*, pneumococci, and streptococci, of each 1000 million, and *Klebsiella pneumoniae* 500 million, with chlorhexidine acetate 50 µg and thiomersal 100 µg. For the prevention of some bacterial infections of the upper respiratory tract. *Dose.* 1 metered dose, under the tongue, twice daily.

References: H. C. Price and G. Henley, *Practitioner*, 1974, *213*, 720.

Oral cold vaccines containing mixed organisms were also formerly marketed in Great Britain under the proprietary names Buccaline Berna (*Swiss Serum and Vaccine Institute*) and Esobactulin (*Southon-Horton*).

7945-b

Diphtheria and Tetanus Vaccine *(B.P.)*.

Diphtheria-Tetanus Prophylactic; DT/Vac/FT.

A sterile mixture of diphtheria formol toxoid and tetanus formol toxoid. It conforms with the test for potency for Diphtheria Vaccine in its ability to prevent a positive Schick reaction in animals and with the test for potency for Tetanus Vaccine.

Store at 2° to 8° and avoid freezing. Protect from light.

7946-v

Adsorbed Diphtheria and Tetanus Vaccine *(B.P., Eur. P.)*.

Adsorbed Diphtheria-Tetanus Prophylactic; Vaccinum Diphthericum et Tetanicum Adsorbatum; Diphtheria and Tetanus Vaccine (Adsorbed); DT/Vac/Ads.

It is prepared from diphtheria formol toxoid containing not less than 1500 Limes flocculationis (Lf) per mg of protein nitrogen, tetanus formol toxoid containing not less than 500 Lf per mg of protein nitrogen, and a mineral carrier, which may be hydrated aluminium hydroxide, aluminium phosphate, or calcium phosphate in a saline solution or other appropriate solution iso-osmotic with blood. The name of the mineral carrier is stated on the label. The antigenic properties are adversely affected by certain bactericides such as phenol or cresol. It complies with the tests for potency for Adsorbed Diphtheria Vaccine and for Adsorbed Tetanus Vaccine. The *Eur. P.* requires the potency of each component to be expressed in terms of international units.

Store at 2° to 8° and avoid freezing. Protect from light. Under these conditions it may be expected to retain its potency for at least 3 years.

7947-g

Diphtheria and Tetanus Toxoids *(U.S.P.)*.

A sterile solution prepared by mixing suitable quantities of diphtheria toxoid and tetanus toxoid. The antigenicity or potency and the proportions of the toxoids are such as to provide an immunising dose of each toxoid in the labelled dose.

A colourless to brownish-yellow clear or very slightly turbid liquid free from evident clumps and particles and with a slight characteristic odour.

Store at 2° to 8° and avoid freezing. The expiration date is not later than 2 years after release from manufacturer's cold storage.

7948-q

Diphtheria and Tetanus Toxoids Adsorbed *(U.S.P.)*.

A sterile suspension prepared by mixing suitable quantities of plain or adsorbed diphtheria toxoid and plain or adsorbed tetanus toxoid and, if plain toxoids are used, an aluminium adsorbing agent. The antigenicity or potency and the proportions of the toxoids are such as to provide an immunising dose of each toxoid in the labelled dose.

Store at 2° to 8° and avoid freezing. The expiration date is not later than 2 years after release from manufacturer's cold storage.

7949-p

Tetanus and Diphtheria Toxoids Adsorbed for Adult Use *(U.S.P.)*.

A sterile suspension prepared by mixing suitable quantities of adsorbed diphtheria toxoid and adsorbed tetanus toxoid using the same precipitating or adsorbing agent for both toxoids. The antigenicity or potency and the proportions of the toxoids are such as to provide, in the labelled dose, an immunising dose of adsorbed tetanus

toxoid and one-tenth of the immunising dose of adsorbed diphtheria toxoid specified for children and not more than 2 Lf of diphtheria toxoid.
Store at 2° to 8° and avoid freezing. The expiration date is not later than 2 years after release from manufacturer's cold storage.

Adverse Effects and Precautions. As for Vaccines, p.1586.
Local reactions occur occasionally but are generally not severe; the frequency of reactions is reported to be less in children under 5 years of age than in older children.

Side-effects in adults.— J. P. Middaugh, *Am. J. publ. Hlth*, 1979, *69*, 246.

Uses. Adsorbed Diphtheria and Tetanus Vaccine is used for active immunisation against diphtheria and tetanus, particularly in those for whom the pertussis component of Diphtheria, Tetanus, and Pertussis Vaccine is contra-indicated or the subject of parental objection. It is given in usual doses of 0.5 ml by deep subcutaneous or intramuscular injection, the first dose being given at the age of 3 to 6 months, preferably 3 months, followed after 6 to 8 weeks by the second dose, and after a further 4 to 6 months by the third dose. Some authorities recommend 2 doses, with a third dose of Adsorbed Tetanus Vaccine after 6 to 12 months.
It is also used as a reinforcing dose at school entry in children who have previously been immunised against diphtheria and tetanus, or against diphtheria, tetanus, and pertussis and in whom the pertussis component is no longer needed.
Diphtheria and Tetanus Vaccine (formol toxoid) is used only for reinforcing doses.
Adsorbed Diphtheria and Tetanus Vaccine may be given in a reduced dose of 0.2 ml to children over 10 years and adults in whom a Schick test has shown susceptibility to diphtheria.
Diphtheria and Tetanus Vaccine (but not the adsorbed vaccine) may be given in a dose of 0.1 ml intradermally to those who have shown reactions to an earlier dose of adsorbed vaccine.

An adsorbed vaccine containing only 1.5 Lf of diphtheria toxoid and 7.5 Lf of tetanus toxoid was given to about 120 adults; one dose was often sufficient to provide immunity and side-effects were slight. For those adequately protected against tetanus an adsorbed vaccine containing only the diphtheria toxoid was desirable.— F. W. Sheffield *et al.*, *Br. med. J.*, 1978, *2*, 249.

Proprietary Preparations

Adsorbed Diphtheria and Tetanus Vaccine (PTAH) *(Duncan, Flockhart, UK)*. A brand of Adsorbed Diphtheria and Tetanus Vaccine, with aluminium hydroxide as the mineral carrier, each 0.5-ml dose containing 30 international units of diphtheria toxoid and 40 international units of tetanus toxoid, in ampoules of 0.5 ml and vials of 5 ml.

Diphtheria and Tetanus Vaccine *(Wellcome, UK)*. A brand of Diphtheria and Tetanus Vaccine, each 0.5-ml dose containing 25 Lf of diphtheria toxoid and 3.5 Lf of tetanus toxoid, available in vials of 5 ml. **Adsorbed Diphtheria and Tetanus Vaccine.** A brand of Adsorbed Diphtheria and Tetanus Vaccine, with aluminium hydroxide as the mineral carrier, each 0.5-ml dose containing 30 international units of diphtheria toxoid and 40 international units of tetanus toxoid, available in ampoules of 0.5 ml and vials of 5 ml.

Other Proprietary Names

Diphtheria and Tetanus Toxoids, Combined, Purogenated *(Lederle, USA)*; Diphtheria and Tetanus Toxoids, Adsorbed *(Sclavo, USA)*; Diphtheria and Tetanus Toxoids, Adsorbed (Pediatric), Aluminium Phosphate Adsorbed (Ultrafined)*(Wyeth, USA)*; Tetanus and Diphtheria Toxoids Adsorbed *(Connaught, USA)*.

7950-n

Diphtheria Antitoxin *(B.P., Eur. P.)*. Immunoserum Diphthericum; Dip/Ser.

A sterile preparation containing the specific antitoxic globulins that have the power of neutralising the toxin formed by *Corynebacterium diphtheriae*.
It is an almost colourless or very faintly yellow liquid free from turbidity and almost odourless except for the odour of any added bactericide. It has a potency of not less than 1000 units per ml when obtained from horse serum and not less than 500 units per ml when obtained from other species. pH 6 to 7.
Storage. As for Botulinum Antitoxin, p.1590.
The label states the animal source.

7951-h

Diphtheria Antitoxin *(U.S.P.)*.

A sterile solution of the refined and concentrated proteins, chiefly globulins, containing antitoxic antibodies obtained from the serum or plasma of healthy horses that have been immunised against diphtheria toxin or toxoid. It contains not less than 500 units per ml and not more than 20% of solids.
An almost colourless, clear or slightly opalescent liquid, almost odourless or with the odour of the preservatives.
Store at 2° to 8°. The expiration date of antitoxin containing 20% excess potency is not later than 5 years after release from manufacturer's cold storage.
The label states the animal source.

Units. One unit of diphtheria antitoxin, equine, is contained in 0.0628 mg of the first International Standard Preparation (1934).

Adverse Effects. As for Antisera, p.1587.
Diphtheria antitoxin is prepared from the serum of animals and reactions due to injection of animal serum may occur.

Uses. Diphtheria antitoxin neutralises the toxin produced by *Corynebacterium diphtheriae* locally at the site of infection and in the circulation but it does not affect the pathological changes already induced by the toxin.
Diphtheria is usually treated by the concomitant administration of an antibiotic such as erythromycin or penicillin.
When the attack is mild or of moderate severity doses of 10 000 to 30 000 units of diphtheria antitoxin may be given intramuscularly, after a test dose to eliminate hypersensitivity; doses of 40 000 to 100 000 units or even more may be given in the severe cases. Doses of more than 40 000 units may be given intravenously.
The prophylactic dose is 500 to 2000 units, usually injected intramuscularly. The passive immunity thus conferred usually lasts about 2 weeks. Passive immunisation may be combined with active immunisation with Diphtheria Vaccine.

Preparations

Diphtheria Antitoxin is available from *Regent Laboratories*.

Proprietary Names

Diphtheria Antitoxin *(Connaught, USA)*; Diphtheria Antitoxin *(Sclavo, USA)*.

7952-m

Diphtheria, Tetanus, and Pertussis Vaccine *(B.P.)*. Diphtheria-Tetanus-Whooping-cough Prophylactic; Triple Vaccine; DTPer/Vac.

NOTE. In USA the title Triple Vaccine has been applied to typhoid-paratyphoid A and B vaccines.

A sterile mixture of diphtheria formol toxoid, tetanus formol toxoid, and a suspension of killed *Bordetella pertussis*. It complies with the test for potency for Diphtheria Vaccine in its ability to prevent a positive Schick reaction in animals, and with the test for potency for Tetanus Vaccine, and the volume stated on the label as the dose contains not less than 4 pertussis units, calculated with reference to the second British Reference Preparation (1968).
Store at 2° 8° and avoid freezing. Protect from light.

7953-b

Adsorbed Diphtheria, Tetanus, and Pertussis Vaccine *(B.P., Eur. P.)*. Adsorbed Diphtheria-Tetanus-Whooping-cough Prophylactic; Vaccinum Diphthericum Tetanicum et Pertussis Adsorbatum; Diphtheria, Tetanus and Pertussis Vaccine (Adsorbed); DTPer/Vac/Ads.

It is prepared from diphtheria formol toxoid containing not less than 1500 Lf per mg of protein nitrogen, tetanus formol toxoid containing not less than 500 Lf per mg of protein nitrogen, a suspension of killed *Bordetella pertussis* (not more than 20×10^9 per dose), and a mineral carrier, which may be hydrated aluminium hydroxide, aluminium phosphate, or calcium phosphate in a saline solution or other appropriate solution iso-osmotic with blood. The name of the mineral carrier is stated on the label. The antigenic properties are adversely affected by certain bactericides such as phenol or cresol. It complies with the tests for potency for Adsorbed Diphtheria Vaccine, for Adsorbed Tetanus Vaccine, and for Pertussis Vaccine.
Store at 2° to 8° and avoid freezing. Protect from light. Under these conditions it may be expected to retain its potency for at least 3 years.

7954-v

Diphtheria and Tetanus Toxoids and Pertussis Vaccine *(U.S.P.)*.

A sterile suspension prepared by mixing suitable quantities of pertussis vaccine component of killed *Bordetella pertussis*, or a fraction of this organism, diphtheria toxoid, and tetanus toxoid. The antigenicity or potency and the proportions of the components are such that the labelled dose provides an immunising dose of each component.
A whitish or light yellowish or brownish, more or less turbid liquid, free from evident clumps after shaking, with a faint odour.
Store at 2° to 8° and avoid freezing. The expiration date is not later than 18 months after release from manufacturer's cold storage.

7955-g

Diphtheria and Tetanus Toxoids and Pertussis Vaccine Adsorbed *(U.S.P.)*.

A sterile suspension prepared by mixing suitable quantities of plain or adsorbed diphtheria toxoid, plain or adsorbed tetanus vaccine, plain or adsorbed pertussis vaccine, and, if plain antigen components are used, an aluminium adsorbing agent. The antigenicity or potency and the proportions of the components are such that the labelled dose provides an immunising dose of each component.
A whitish markedly turbid liquid, free from evident clumps after shaking, nearly odourless or with a faint odour of the preservative.
Store at 2° to 8° and avoid freezing. The expiration date is not later than 18 months after release from manufacturer's cold storage.

Adverse Effects and Precautions. As for Pertussis Vaccine, p.1600.
An interval of at least 3 to 4 weeks is generally allowed between the administration of Diphtheria, Tetanus, and Pertussis Vaccine and any

vaccine containing live micro-organisms other than oral poliomyelitis vaccine.

Of 516 276 children in Sweden vaccinated with triple vaccine, neurological reactions occurred in 167—destructive encephalopathy 3, convulsions 80, hypsarrhythmia 4, shock 54, uncontrollable screaming 24, and serous meningitis 2.— J. Ström, *Br. med. J.*, 1967, *4*, 320.

Amongst children aged 5 to 6 months or more who received primary courses of diphtheria, tetanus, and pertussis vaccine, 2 per 1000 suffered moderate reactions and 0.6 per 1000 suffered severe reactions.— J. B. O'Regan, *Br. med. J.*, 1970, *2*, 783.

A report of postvaccination granuloma in 2 patients after immunisation with [Adsorbed] Diphtheria, Tetanus, and Pertussis Vaccine. The tumours measured 17×11×6 mm and 16×9 mm respectively and were considered due to the aluminium hydroxide component of the vaccine.— M. Erdohazi and R. L. Newman, *Br. med. J.*, 1971, *3*, 621.

Severe progressive proliferative glomerulonephritis in a woman aged about 35 years was attributed to the repeated injection over 4 years of Diphtheria, Tetanus, and Pertussis Vaccine.— J. M. Boulton-Jones *et al.*, *Br. med. J.*, 1974, *3*, 387.

Uses. Diphtheria, Tetanus, and Pertussis Vaccine or Adsorbed Diphtheria, Tetanus, and Pertussis Vaccine is used for active immunisation against diphtheria, tetanus, and whooping cough. The antigenicity of the diphtheria vaccine is enhanced by the pertussis vaccine.

The vaccines are given in 3 doses during the first year of life and followed by a reinforcing dose of Diphtheria and Tetanus Vaccine at the age of 5 years or at school entry. The first dose may be given at the age of 3 to 6 months, but preferably at the age of 3 months. The second dose should be given 6 to 8 weeks later and the third dose to follow after 4 to 6 months. The injections are given by deep subcutaneous or intramuscular injection.

When the primary immunisation course is completed by the age of 6 to 8 months (e.g. because of a pertussis epidemic) a further injection of Diphtheria, Tetanus, and Pertussis Vaccine, or of Diphtheria and Tetanus Vaccine, is sometimes given 12 months later.

Though local and systemic reactions occurred in a proportion of children vaccinated with diphtheria, tetanus, and pertussis vaccine together with typhoid vaccine, the use of this quadruple vaccine was still recommended in areas where typhoid fever was present.— B. Cvjetanovic *et al.*, *Bull. Wld Hlth Org.*, 1972, *46*, 47.

The successful use, in the Philippines, of a 2-dose, 6-month schedule of vaccination using an adsorbed diphtheria, tetanus, and pertussis vaccine with an increased content of aluminium phosphate.— A. Mangay-Angara *et al.*, *J. biol. Stand.*, 1980, *8*, 87. See also J. M. Mahieu *et al.*, *Bull. Wld Hlth Org.*, 1978, *56*, 773.

Intradermal administration. A study in Uganda in which diphtheria, tetanus, and pertussis vaccine was given by intradermal jet injector and in which antibody titres were comparable with those produced after standard intramuscular injection, suggested that the technique might become the method of choice. The dose consisted of 3 jet injections each of 0.05 to 0.08 ml.— J. P. Stanfield *et al.*, *Br. med. J.*, 1972, *2*, 197.

Proprietary Preparations

Adsorbed Diphtheria, Tetanus and Pertussis Vaccine (PTAH) *(Duncan, Flockhart, UK)*. A brand of Adsorbed Diphtheria, Tetanus, and Pertussis Vaccine, with aluminium hydroxide as the mineral carrier, containing in each 0.5-ml dose not less than 30 international units of diphtheria toxoid, 60 international units of tetanus toxoid, and 4 international units of killed *B. pertussis*, in ampoules of 0.5 ml and vials of 5 ml.

Trivax *(Wellcome, UK)*. A brand of Diphtheria, Tetanus, and Pertussis Vaccine, containing in each 0.5-ml dose 25 Lf of diphtheria toxoid, 3.5 Lf of tetanus toxoid, and not more than 20 000 million killed *B. pertussis*, available in ampoules of 0.5 ml and in vials of 5 ml. **Trivax-AD.** A brand of Adsorbed Diphtheria, Tetanus, and Pertussis Vaccine, with the same antigens and aluminium hydroxide as the mineral carrier, available in ampoules of 0.5 ml and in vials of 5 ml.

Other Proprietary Names

Diphtheria and Tetanus Toxoids and Pertussis Vaccine Adsorbed *(Connaught, USA)*; Diphtheria and Tetanus Toxoids and Pertussis Vaccine Adsorbed, Ultrafined, Triple Antigen *(Wyeth, USA)*; Tri-Immunol *(Lederle, USA)*.

7956-q

Diphtheria, Tetanus, and Poliomyelitis Vaccine. *(B.P.)*. DTPol/Vac.

A sterile mixture of diphtheria formol toxoid, tetanus formol toxoid, and Poliomyelitis Vaccine (Inactivated). It conforms with the test for potency for Diphtheria Vaccine in its ability to prevent a positive Schick reaction in animals and with the tests for potency for Tetanus Vaccine and for Inactivated Poliomyelitis Vaccine.

Store at 2° to 8° and avoid freezing. Protect from light. Under these conditions it may be expected to retain its potency for at least a year.

Adverse Effects and Precautions. As for Vaccines, p.1586.

Uses. Diphtheria, Tetanus, and Poliomyelitis Vaccine is used to reinforce the immunity of children who have previously been immunised against diphtheria, tetanus, and poliomyelitis, particularly at the age of 5 years or at school entry. The volume indicated on the label as the dose is given by deep subcutaneous or intramuscular injection.

Manufacturers

Connaught, Canad.

In Great Britain, diphtheria, tetanus, and poliomyelitis vaccine is available on a named-patient basis from *Connaught, Canad.*

7957-p

Diphtheria, Tetanus, Pertussis, and Poliomyelitis Vaccine *(B.P. 1973)*. Diphtheria-Tetanus-Whooping-cough-Poliomyelitis Prophylactic; DTPerPol/Vac.

A mixture of diphtheria formol toxoid, tetanus formol toxoid, a suspension of killed *Bordetella pertussis*, and Poliomyelitis Vaccine (Inactivated). It conforms with the test for potency for Diphtheria Vaccine in its ability to prevent a positive Schick reaction in animals and with the tests for potency for Tetanus Vaccine, Pertussis Vaccine, and Inactivated Poliomyelitis Vaccine.

Store at 2° to 10° and avoid freezing. Protect from light. Under these conditions it may be expected to retain its potency for at least 12 months.

Adverse Effects and Precautions. As for Pertussis Vaccine, p.1600.

Uses. Diphtheria, Tetanus, Pertussis, and Poliomyelitis Vaccine has been used for active immunisation of infants against diphtheria, tetanus, pertussis, and poliomyelitis. The volume indicated on the label as the dose is given by deep subcutaneous or intramuscular injection in a schedule similar to that for Diphtheria, Tetanus, and Pertussis Vaccine.

Manufacturers

Connaught, Canad.

In Great Britain, diphtheria, tetanus, pertussis, and poliomyelitis vaccine is available on a named-patient basis from *Connaught, Canad.* and *Swiss Serum and Vaccine Institute, UK.*

7958-s

Diphtheria Vaccine *(B.P.)*. Diphtheria Prophylactic; Diphtheria Formol Toxoid; Dip/Vac/FT.

It is prepared from diphtheria toxin produced by the growth of *Corynebacterium diphtheriae*. The toxin is converted to diphtheria formol toxoid by treatment with formaldehyde solution. Diphtheria Vaccine is standardised in terms of its ability to prevent a positive Schick reaction in animals and in terms of Lf equivalents (see below under Units); it contains not less than 25 Lf in the dose stated on the label.

Store at 2° to 8° and avoid freezing. Protect from light.

7959-w

Adsorbed Diphtheria Vaccine *(B.P., Eur. P.)*. Adsorbed Diphtheria Prophylactic; Vaccinum Diphthericum Adsorbatum; Diphtheria Vaccine (Adsorbed); Dip/Vac/Ads.

It is prepared from diphtheria formol toxoid containing not less than 1500 Lf (see under Units) per mg of protein nitrogen and a mineral carrier which may be hydrated aluminium hydroxide, aluminium phosphate, or calcium phosphate in a saline solution or other appropriate solution iso-osmotic with blood. The name of the mineral carrier is stated on the label. The antigenic properties are adversely affected by certain bactericides such as phenol or cresol. Adsorbed Diphtheria Vaccine is standardised in terms of its ability to protect *guinea-pigs* from the erythrogenic effects of diphtheria toxin; it contains not less than 30 units per dose. Potency may also be assessed on the basis of its ability to protect *guinea-pigs* from the lethal effects of diphtheria toxin. The *Eur. P.* requires the potency to be expressed in terms of international units.

Store at 2° to 8° and avoid freezing. Protect from light.

7960-m

Diphtheria Toxoid *(U.S.P.)*.

A sterile solution of the formaldehyde-treated products of growth of the diphtheria bacillus *Corynebacterium diphtheriae*.It contains a non-phenolic preservative.

A brownish-yellow clear or slightly turbid liquid free from evident clumps or particles and with a slight characteristic odour.

Store at 2° to 8° and avoid freezing. The expiration date is not later than 2 years after release from manufacturer's cold storage.

7961-b

Diphtheria Toxoid Adsorbed *(U.S.P.)*.

A sterile preparation of diphtheria toxoid precipitated or adsorbed by alum, aluminium hydroxide, or aluminium phosphate adjuvants.

A white, faintly grey, or faintly pink suspension, free from evident clumps after shaking.

Store at 2° to 8° and avoid freezing. The expiration date is not later than 2 years after release from manufacturer's cold storage.

Units. 200 units of diphtheria toxoid, plain, are contained in 21 mg of formalin-treated diphtheria toxoid, freeze-dried, in one ampoule of the second International Standard Preparation (1975).

132 units of diphtheria toxoid, adsorbed, are contained in 75 mg of diphtheria toxoid adsorbed on aluminium hydroxide 1 mg (with polygeline 26 mg) in one ampoule of the second International Standard Preparation (1978).

The Limes flocculationis (Lf) of diphtheria toxin, diphtheria toxoid, or diphtheria vaccine is determined by incubation with a standard preparation of diphtheria antitoxin for flocculation test; when the concentration of antitoxin is varied in mixtures of constant volume, the mixture flocculating first is that which contains the most nearly equivalent quantities of toxin, or toxoid, and antitoxin.

There is no simple correlation between international units and Lf equivalents.

Adverse Effects. As for Vaccines, p.1586.

Local reactions occur occasionally but are generally not severe; the frequency of reactions is reported to be less in children under 5 years of age than in older children.

Precautions. As for Vaccines, p.1586.

Diphtheria vaccines, especially alum-precipitated diphtheria/pertussis vaccine, have precipitated paralytic poliomyelitis; immunisation should therefore be delayed during outbreaks of poliomyelitis.

A family history of allergy was not a contra-indication to diphtheria, tetanus, and poliomyelitis vaccination, but diphtheria and tetanus vaccine should be given with care to patients with a history of convulsions.— *Br. med. J.*, 1978, *2*, 944.

Uses. Diphtheria vaccines are used for active immunisation against diphtheria. Diphtheria formol toxoid has weak immunological properties and its effects are usually enhanced by administration as adsorbed toxoid or with pertussis vaccine. Diphtheria Vaccine is therefore unsuitable for primary immunisation.

Active immunisation against diphtheria should preferably be started when the infant is 3 months old. Primary immunisation may be achieved by the use of Adsorbed Diphtheria Vaccine given by deep subcutaneous or by intramuscular injection in usual doses of 0.5 ml. The first dose is followed 6 to 8 weeks later by the second dose and the third dose follows after a further interval of 4 to 6 months. Some authorities recommend 2 doses. A reinforcing dose may be given at the age of 5 or at school entry; for this purpose Diphtheria Vaccine or Adsorbed Diphtheria Vaccine may be used.

Primary immunisation against diphtheria is commonly associated with immunisation against tetanus, pertussis, and poliomyelitis. For this purpose Adsorbed Diphtheria and Tetanus Vaccine, Diphtheria, Tetanus, and Pertussis Vaccine, or Adsorbed Diphtheria, Tetanus, and Pertussis Vaccine may be used; immunisation against poliomyelitis is generally provided by giving Poliomyelitis Vaccine, Live (Oral).

If it is necessary to provide primary immunisation in children above the age of 10 or in adults a schedule of 2 doses, each of 0.2 ml, has been suggested after a Schick test has shown susceptibility to diphtheria. The Schick test is also used to identify those patients likely to suffer reactions.

A short discussion of the use of diphtheria vaccine.— J. W. G. Smith, *Practitioner*, 1978, *220*, 929.

Diphtheria toxoid made up into lozenges which were allowed to dissolve slowly in the mouth had been found to stimulate an antibody response in previously immunised children.— J. W. G. Smith, *Br. med. Bull.*, 1969, *25*, 177.

The use of diphtheria toxoid for assessing cellular immunity.— M. John *et al.*, *Dte GesundhWes.*, 1978, *33*, 463, per *Int. pharm. Abstr.*, 1978, *15*, 1123.

Regardless of age, all persons require protection from diphtheria.— R. H. Bernier, *J. Am. med. Ass.*, 1980, *243*, 2525.

Proprietary Preparations

Adsorbed Diphtheria Vaccine Wellcome *(Wellcome, UK)*. A brand of Adsorbed Diphtheria Vaccine, each 0.5-ml dose containing not less than 30 international units of diphtheria toxoid, with aluminium phosphate as the mineral carrier, in vials of 5 ml.

Diphtheria Vaccine TAF *(Wellcome, UK)*. A suspension of the floccules formed by the interaction between diphtheria toxoid and its antitoxin, each 0.5-ml dose containing not less than 100 Lf of the original diphtheria toxoid, available in vials of 5 ml. For active immunisation against diphtheria in patients for whom other vaccines are unsuitable. *Dose*. 3 doses of 0.5 ml at intervals of not less than 4 weeks. Contra-indicated in patients allergic to horse serum.

7962-v

Gas-gangrene Antitoxin (Oedematiens)

(B.P., Eur. P.). Immunoserum Anticlostridium Oedematiens; Oed/Ser.

A sterile preparation containing the specific antitoxic globulins that have the power of neutralising the alpha toxin formed by *Clostridium oedematiens*.

It is an almost colourless or very faintly yellow liquid, free from turbidity, and almost odourless except for the odour of any added bactericide. It has a potency of not less than 3750 units per ml. pH 6 to 7.

Storage . As for Botulinum Antitoxin, p.1590.

The label states the animal source.

Units. 1100 units of gas-gangrene antitoxin (oedematiens) are contained in 91 mg in one ampoule of the third International Standard Preparation (1966).

Adverse Effects. As for Antisera, p.1587.

Gas-gangrene antitoxin is prepared from the serum of animals and reactions due to the injection of animal serum may occur.

Uses. Gas-gangrene Antitoxin (Oedematiens) is used mainly in conjunction with other gas-gangrene antitoxins, as in Mixed Gas-gangrene Antitoxin. The monovalent antitoxin is not much used in practice owing to the difficulty of rapidly identifying the infecting organism.

The usual initial therapeutic dose is not less than 30 000 units intravenously. Further injections may be given every 4 to 6 hours.

Doses of 10 000 units intramuscularly or intravenously have been given for prophylaxis.

7963-g

Gas-gangrene Antitoxin (Perfringens).

(B.P., Eur. P.). Gas-gangrene Antitoxin (Welchii); Immunoserum Anticlostridium Perfringens; Perf/Ser.

A sterile preparation containing the specific antitoxic globulins that have the power of neutralising the alpha toxin formed by *Clostridium perfringens* (*C. welchii*, type A).

It is an almost colourless or very faintly yellow liquid, free from turbidity and almost odourless except for the odour of any added bactericide. It has a potency of not less than 1500 units per ml. pH 6 to 7.

Storage .As for Botulinum Antitoxin, p.1590.

The label states the animal source.

The development and testing of a *Clostridium welchii* type C vaccine.— P. D. Walker *et al.*, *J. biol. Stand.*, 1979, *7*, 315. See also P. A. Knight *et al.*, *ibid.*, 373.

Units. 270 units of gas-gangrene antitoxin (perfringens) (type A antitoxin) are contained in 90.35 mg in one ampoule of the fifth International Standard Preparation (1963).

The collaborative assay of material now established as the International Reference Preparations of *Clostridium welchii (C. perfringens)* Beta and Epsilon Toxoids.— I. Davidson *et al.*, *Bull. Wld Hlth Org.*, 1978, *56*, 641.

Adverse Effects. As for Antisera, p.1587.

Gas-gangrene antitoxin is prepared from the serum of animals and reactions due to the injection of animal serum may occur.

Uses. Gas-gangrene Antitoxin (Perfringens) is used mainly in conjunction with other gas-gangrene antitoxins, as in Mixed Gas-gangrene Antitoxin. The monovalent antitoxin is not much used in practice owing to the difficulty of rapidly identifying the infecting organism.

The usual initial therapeutic dose is not less than 30 000 units intravenously. Further injections may be given every 4 to 6 hours.

Doses of 10 000 units intramuscularly or intravenously have been given for prophylaxis.

7964-q

Gas-gangrene Antitoxin (Septicum) *(B.P., Eur. P.)*.

Gas-gangrene Antitoxin (Vibrion septique); Immunoserum Anticlostridium Septicum; Sep/Ser.

A sterile preparation containing the specific antitoxic globulins that have the power of neutralising the alpha toxin formed by *Clostridium septicum*,also known as *Vibrion septique*.

It is an almost colourless or very faintly yellow liquid, free from turbidity and almost odourless except for the odour of any added bactericide. It has a potency of not less than 1500 units per ml. pH 6 to 7.

Storage. As for Botulinum Antitoxin, p.1590.

The label states the animal source.

Units. 500 units of gas-gangrene antitoxin (septicum) are contained in 59 mg in one ampoule of the third International Standard Preparation (1957).

Adverse Effects. As for Antisera, p.1587.

Gas-gangrene antitoxin is prepared from the serum of animals and reactions due to the injection of animal serum may occur.

Uses. Gas-gangrene Antitoxin (Septicum) is used mainly in conjunction with other gas-gangrene antitoxins, as in Mixed Gas-gangrene Antitoxin. The monovalent antitoxin is not much used in practice owing to the difficulty of rapidly identifying the infecting organisms. The usual initial therapeutic dose is not less than 15 000 units intravenously. Further injections may be given every 4 to 6 hours.

Doses of 5000 units intramuscularly or intravenously have been given for prophylaxis.

8039-n

Mixed Gas-gangrene Antitoxin *(B.P., Eur. P.)*.

Immunoserum Anticlostridium Mixtum; Gas/Ser.

Prepared by mixing Gas-gangrene Antitoxin (Oedematiens), Gas-gangrene Antitoxin (Perfringens), and Gas-gangrene Antitoxin (Septicum) in appropriate quantities.

It is an almost colourless or very faintly yellow liquid, free from turbidity, and almost odourless except for the odour of any added bactericide. It has a potency of not less than 1000 units of Gas-gangrene Antitoxin (Oedematiens), not less than 1000 units of Gas-gangrene Antitoxin (Perfringens) and not less than 500 units of Gas-gangrene Antitoxin (Septicum) in 1 ml. pH 6 to 7.

Storage. As for Botulinum Antitoxin, p.1590.

The label states the animal source.

Adverse Effects. As for Antisera, p.1587.

Gas-gangrene antitoxin is prepared from the serum of animals and reactions due to the injection of animal serum may occur.

Uses. Mixed Gas-gangrene Antitoxin should be given, as soon as possible after infliction of a wound, when infection is suspected, as a prophylactic measure against the development of gas-gangrene. The usual dose is 25 000 units. Intravenous injection ensures rapid distribution of the antitoxin, but if this route is impracticable the injection may be given intramuscularly into healthy tissue. The dose may be doubled, or repeated if the clinical condition of the patient deteriorates or if an operation is necessary. It may be given with Tetanus Antitoxin.

The therapeutic dose is at least 75 000 units and is administered intravenously in order to neutralise the toxaemia with a minimum of delay. Repeated administration may be required every 4 to 6 hours according to the response of the patient.

As soon as the infecting micro-organism has been

identified, monovalent antitoxin may be substituted, if available, for polyvalent antitoxin, though this course is seldom possible in practice.

Preparations

Mixed Gas-gangrene Antitoxin is available from *Servier*

8040-k

Histoplasmin *(U.S.P.).*

CAS — 9008-05-3.

A sterile solution containing standardised culture filtrates of the fungus *Histoplasma capsulatum* grown on a synthetic liquid medium; it may contain a suitable antimicrobial agent. It is a clear liquid which is **miscible** with water. **Store** at 2° to 8°. The expiration date is not later than 2 years after release from manufacturer's cold storage.

Histoplasmin, in an intracutaneous (intradermal) dose of 0.1 ml of a 1 in 100 dilution, is used as an aid to the diagnosis of histoplasmosis.

The histoplasmin skin test is relatively effective; lack of specificity is due to extensive cross-reactions in individuals sensitised to other fungi.— *FDA Drug Bull.*, 1978, *8,* 15.

Manufacturers

Parke, Davis, USA.

7965-p

Inactivated Influenza Vaccine *(B.P., Eur. P.).*

Influenza Vaccine; Influenza Vaccine (Inactivated); Vaccinum Influenzae Inactivatum; Flu/Vac.

A sterile aqueous suspension of a suitable strain or strains of influenza virus types A and B, either individually or mixed, grown in the allantoic cavity of fertile incubated chick embryos, inactivated so that they are non-infective but retain their antigenic properties, purified by centrifugation or other suitable means, and suspended in a neutral buffered saline solution containing a suitable bactericide. Not more than 2 strains of the same sub-type may be included. Formaldehyde solution may be used to inactivate the virus. Suitable strains of influenza virus are those currently recommended by the World Influenza Centre of the World Health Organization. It is a slightly opalescent liquid which contains not less than 600 units per dose.

It may also be supplied as an adsorbed vaccine (Adsorbed Influenza Vaccine; Flu/Vac/Ads) prepared with the addition of aluminium hydroxide, aluminium phosphate, or calcium phosphate. *Eur. P.* includes the adsorbed vaccine as Influenza Vaccine (Adsorbed); Vaccinum Influenzae Adsorbatum. The name of the mineral carrier is stated on the label.

Store at 2° to 8° and avoid freezing. Protect from light. Under these conditions it may be expected to retain its potency for at least 18 months.

CAUTION. *The vaccine should not be brought into contact with alcohol or other disinfectant and care is needed when sterilising syringes and skin before immunisation.*

NOTE. When Inactivated Influenza Vaccine is prescribed or demanded, Inactivated Influenza Vaccine or Inactivated Influenza Vaccine (Surface Antigen) or the adsorbed versions may be dispensed or supplied.

7966-s

Influenza Virus Vaccine *(U.S.P.).*

A sterile aqueous suspension of suitably inactivated influenza virus types A and B, either individually or combined, or virus sub-units prepared from the extra-embryonic fluid of virus-infected chick embryos. It may contain a suitable antimicrobial agent.

A slightly turbid liquid or suspension, which may have a slight yellow or reddish tinge and an odour of the preservative.

Store at 2° to 8° and avoid freezing. The expiration date is not later than 18 months after release from manufacturer's cold storage.

7967-w

Inactivated Influenza Vaccine (Surface Antigen) *(B.P.).*

Flu/Vac/SA; Flu/Vac/SA/Ads.

A sterile aqueous suspension of the immunologically active haemagglutinin and neuraminidase surface antigens, of a suitable strain or strains of inactivated influenza virus types A and B either individually or mixed. The virus may be grown as for Inactivated Influenza Vaccine; after purification by centrifugation or other suitable means the virus particles are disrupted by treatment with suitable agents and the surface antigens are separated and suspended in a buffered solution containing a suitable preservative. The vaccine contains an approved quantity of haemagglutinin antigen which represents at least 25% of the total protein and not more than traces of viral protein other than haemagglutinin and neuraminidase. The vaccine may be plain or adsorbed and thus may contain a suitable adjuvant or mineral carrier. Potency is expressed in terms of micrograms of haemagglutinin per virus strain. For adsorbed vaccine the name of the mineral carrier is stated on the label.

Store at 2° to 8° and avoid freezing. Protect from light. Under these conditions it may be expected to retain its potency for not less than one year.

The antigenic composition of the influenza virus.— G. C. Schild, *Postgrad. med. J.*, 1979, *55,* 87.

Nomenclature of strains. Influenza virus strains were formerly classified into types A, B, and C on the basis of their ribonucleoprotein antigens. It was now established that the surface of the virus contained an additional virus-coded antigen, the neuraminidase, which was morphologically and immunologically distinct from the haemagglutinin and which underwent independent antigenic variation. A revised system of nomenclature, designed to be used from the beginning of 1972, was therefore proposed.— *Bull. Wld Hlth Org.*, 1971, *45,* 119. A revised system of nomenclature, based on double immunodiffusion reactions, should be used from the date of publication. The strain designation for influenza virus types A, B, and C contains: a description of the antigenic specificity of the nucleoprotein antigen (types A, B, or C) (an internal antigen, the matrix antigen, has also been described); the host of origin (if not man, including, if appropriate, the inanimate source); the geographical origin; the strain number; and the year of isolation; e.g. A/lake water/Wisconsin/1/79. For type A viruses the antigenic description follows (in parenthesis) including the antigenic character of the haemagglutinin (H1 up to H12) and the antigenic character of the neuraminidase (N1 up to N9). There is no provision for describing subtypes of B and C viruses. Recombination between viruses within a type is readily accomplished; the letter R should be added after the strain description to indicate the recombinant nature of the virus, e.g. A/Hong Kong/1/68(H3N2)R. In addition the strain of origin of the H and N antigens of antigenic hybrid recombinant A and B viruses should be given, e.g. A/BEL/42(H1)—Singapore/1/57(N2)R.— *Bull. Wld Hlth Org.*, 1980, *58,* 585.

Units. One unit of influenza virus haemagglutinin (type A) was contained in 0.093661 mg of the first International Reference Preparation (1967) (now discontinued).

It was possible to express CCA (chick-cell agglutination) units in terms of international units, the factor being 1.74, i.e. 500 CCA units ≡ 870 international units.— P. Krag and M. W. Bentzon, *Bull. Wld Hlth Org.*, 1971, *45,* 473.

The bacterial endotoxin content of 12 influenza vaccines varied widely but did not correlate with the incidence of adverse reactions.— F. A. Ennis, *J. biol. Stand.*, 1977, *5,* 165.

Haemagglutinin activity, as measured by haemagglutination or chick-cell agglutination techniques, does not provide a reliable measure of the haemagglutinin content of influenza vaccines. The International Reference Preparation (1967) was discontinued and should not be used. A reference material would be made available annually containing the haemagglutinin and neuraminidase components of viruses causing prevalent infections and would be known as WHO Influenza Virus Reference Haemagglutinin, with the year of production in brackets. Potency should be expressed as the quantity of haemagglutinin expressed in mg per dose.— WHO Expert Committee on Biological Standardization, *Tech. Rep. Ser. Wld Hlth Org. No. 626,* 1978.

Adverse Effects. As for Vaccines, p.1586.

Local and general reactions may occur but are usually mild. Fever and malaise sometimes occur and severe febrile reactions have been reported. Severe allergic reactions have occurred in persons hypersensitive to egg protein or any antibiotic present in the vaccine.

A 23-year-old nurse developed thrombotic thrombocytopenic purpura 2 to 3 weeks after receiving influenza vaccine (Flenzavax).— R. C. Brown *et al.* (letter), *Br. med. J.*, 1973, *2,* 303.

Acute polyarteritis leading to generalised muscle wasting and ultimate death was attributed to influenza vaccine.— C. F. P. Wharton and R. Pietroni (letter), *Br. med. J.*, 1974, *2,* 331.

Reports of a relatively high incidence of adverse effects in children.— W. M. Marine and C. Stuart-Harris, *J. Pediat.*, 1976, *88,* 26, per *Int. pharm. Abstr.*, 1976, *13,* 988; P. F. Wright *et al.*, *J. Pediat.*, 1976, *88,* 31; T. W. Hoskins (letter), *Br. med. J.*, 1976, *2,* 1131; T. W. Hoskins, *Practitioner,* 1977, *219,* 400; S. Schevill and M. I. Marks, *Can. med. Ass. J.*, 1977, *116,* 271.

A report of pericarditis following influenza vaccination.— J. J. Streifler *et al.*, *Br. med. J.*, 1981, *283,* 526.

Allergic reactions. Reports of allergic reactions.— U. N. Kumbar and B. Varkey (letter), *Can. med. Ass. J.*, 1977, *116,* 724; D. A. Moneret-Vautrin and J. P. Grilliat (letter), *Lancet,* 1977, *2,* 666; K. E. L. McColl *et al.* (letter), *Lancet,* 1978, *2,* 434.

Neurological disorders. Brief details of 9 patients who developed neuropathy after administration of influenza vaccine; symptoms included encephalopathy (3), polyneuropathy, transverse myelopathy, radiculopathy, paraparesis, blurred vision due to occlusion of the central retinal vein, and paraesthesia and pain.— C. E. C. Wells, *Br. med. J.*, 1971, *3,* 755.

One patient developed paraesthesia of the arm and another vague annoying sensations in the arm following influenza vaccination.— T. W. Furlow (letter), *Lancet,* 1977, *1,* 253. Bilateral hand and forearm pain with paraesthesia developed in a patient 3 weeks after vaccination. Investigations led to a diagnosis of carpal-tunnel syndrome.— P. Hasselbacher (letter), *ibid.*, 551.

Four cases of meningo-encephalitis occurring after inoculation with influenza vaccine.— R. D. Gens and H. J. Beecham (letter), *New Engl. J. Med.*, 1978, *299,* 721. These 4 cases had been included in 38 reports of CNS inflammation received as a result of national surveillance following the vaccination of over 45 million people in the USA between October and December 1976.— I. C. Guerrero *et al.* (letter), *ibid.*, 1979, *300,* 565.

Bilateral optic neuritis associated with influenza vaccine.— H. D. Perry *et al.*, *Ann. Ophthal.*, 1979, *11,* 545.

Severe progressive polyneuropathy after trivalent influenza vaccination.— H. Fowler *et al.* (letter), *Lancet,* 1979, *2,* 1193.

Analysis of the data relating to more than 40 million adults in the USA who received swine influenza vaccine, and of more than 500 cases of the Guillain-Barré syndrome, with 25 fatalities.— A. D. Langmuir, *J. R. Soc. Med.*, 1979, *72,* 660. See also J. S. Marks and T. J. Halpin, *J. Am. med. Ass.*, 1980, *243,* 2490. Further references to the Guillain-Barré syndrome and influenza vaccination: *Br. med. J.*, 1977, *1,* 1373; W. Ehrengut (letter), *Br. med. J.*, 1977, *1,* 1662; P. M. Boffey, *Science,* 1977, *195,* 155; L. B. Schonberger *et al.*, *Am. J. Epidem.*, 1979, *110,* 105.

In about 12.5 million persons vaccinated with influenza vaccine in the 1978–79 season the risk factor in respect of Guillain-Barré syndrome was 1.4 (not significant)—significantly less than the risk factor of 6.2 for 1976–77.— E. S. Hurwitz *et al.*, *New Engl. J. Med.*, 1981, *304,* 1557.

See also under Precautions.

Pregnancy and the neonate. There were reports, though not unanimous, of congenital malformations and leukaemia in children born to mothers who had influenza during pregnancy; there was no evidence that influenza vaccination posed any special risk.— *Ann. intern. Med.*,

1978, *89*, 373.

Possible teratogenic effect of influenza vaccine.— H. B. Sarnat *et al.*, *Teratology*, 1979, *20*, 93.

Precautions. As for Vaccines, p.1586.

Influenza Vaccine should not be used in persons hypersensitive to egg protein. Care is necessary in administering the vaccine to persons with allergic conditions, such as asthma or dermatitis.

A patient who had recovered from a single attack of retrobulbar neuritis received an injection of influenza vaccine 7 years later and soon afterwards became blind and quadriplegic. It was suggested that patients who had had a demyelinating disease should not receive vaccines.— J. Rabin (letter), *J. Am. med. Ass.*, 1973, *225*, 63.

Progression of renal disease in Henoch-Schönlein purpura after influenza vaccination.— I. Damjanov and J. A. Amato (letter), *J. Am. med. Ass.*, 1979, *242*, 2555.

From results of a double-blind, placebo-controlled study involving a total of 88 patients it did not appear that swine-influenza vaccination posed a serious risk to patients with multiple sclerosis.— L. W. Myers *et al.* (letter), *New Engl. J. Med.*, 1976, *295*, 1204. Influenza vaccine was well tolerated by 93 patients with multiple sclerosis who received a total of 209 doses of vaccine.— W. A. Sibley *et al.*, *J. Am. med. Ass.*, 1976, *236*, 1965. Comment on 5 cases of multiple sclerosis with onsets 2 weeks to 4 months after swine influenza vaccination.— J. A. Morris and B. G. Young (letter), *Lancet*, 1978, *2*, 636.

Use in systemic lupus erythematosus. A number of studies demonstrated that influenza vaccination did not cause undue exacerbations of systemic lupus erythematosus, although patients with the severe form were not studied. G.W. Williams *et al.* (*Ann. intern. Med.*, 1978, *88*, 729) recorded low antibody titres after immunisation and suggested that protection might be poor but double immunisation carried out by R. Brodman *et al.* (*Ann. intern. Med.*, 1978, *88*, 735) produced similar antibody responses in 37 patients as in 42 controls. Other studies found no overall difference in antibody response in vaccinated patients and controls (S.C. Ristow *et al.*, *Ann. intern. Med.*, 1978, *88*, 786; J.S. Louie *et al.*, *ibid.*, 790). Immunosuppressant therapy did not appear to affect the response.— E. V. Hess and B. Hahn, *Ann. intern. Med.*, 1978, *88*, 833. Criticism.— L. F. Ayvazian (letter), *ibid.*, 1979, *90*, 127.

Uses. Inactivated Influenza Vaccine is used for active immunisation against epidemic influenza. Protection develops in 2 to 3 weeks in about 70% of those immunised, but lasts only for a few months. The surface antigen vaccine or split-product vaccine (also known as SPV, subunit, or subvirion vaccine, may be better tolerated than the whole virus vaccine.

Influenza vaccination is recommended for persons considered to be under special risk, such as patients with chronic cardiac disease, chronic pulmonary disease, chronic renal disease, or diabetes, and for medical and nursing personnel, key workers, and residents in closed institutions.

Influenza vaccine is administered by deep subcutaneous injection or intramuscular injection. It is generally given in the autumn as a single dose, but a second dose after 4 to 6 weeks is suggested for young adults, who will not have been exposed naturally to prevalent strains.

Surface antigen vaccine should be used in children.

A series of papers on influenza.— *Br. med. Bull.*, 1979, *35*, 3–91.

Reviews and discussions of vaccination against influenza.— D. Hobson, *Postgrad. med. J.*, 1973, *49*, 180; *Br. med. J.*, 1976, *1*, 730; *ibid.*, 1977, *2*, 1435; P. A. Gross and F. A. Ennis, *New Engl. J. Med.*, 1977, *296*, 567 (split-virus vaccines); *Drug & Ther. Bull.*, 1978, *16*, 85; N. J. McCarthy, *Med. J. Aust.*, 1978, *1*, 314; B. J. Feery, *Med. J. Aust.*, 1978, *1*, 321; S. C. Schoenbaum, *New Engl. J. Med.*, 1978, *298*, 621; D. A. J. Tyrrell and J. W. G. Smith, *Br. med. Bull.*, 1979, *35*, 77; J. Stevenson, *Practitioner*, 1979, *223*, 759; *Ann. intern. Med.*, 1980, *93*, 466 (Recommendations of the Public Health Service Immunization Practices Advisory Committee); *Br. med. J.*, 1980, *281*, 527; *Med. Lett.*, 1980, *22*, 91; *Med. Lett.*, 1981, *23*, 99; *Ann. intern. Med.*, 1981, *95*, 461 and 512 (Recommendations of the Public Health Service Immunization Practices Advisory Committee).

Studies in the UK had shown that 40 to 80% protection against infection was obtained with influenza vaccine. In the USA, trials extending over 17 years had indicated a high degree of protection against infection, ranging from about 70 to 90% except for 2 intervening years. The difference between the results obtained in the studies was attributed to differences in the vaccines used, the populations observed, and the methods used to estimate vaccine efficacy.— Report of a WHO Scientific Group on Respiratory Viruses. *Tech. Rep. Ser. Wld Hlth Org. No. 408*, 1969.

Seroconversion only after the second dose of influenza vaccine in some patients and increased antibody titres in others after the second dose justified a 2-dose immunisation schedule for high-risk patients.— J. S. MacKenzie, *Br. med. J.*, 1977, *1*, 200.

In 121 healthy volunteers given varying doses of a bivalent subunit influenza vaccine the haemagglutination-inhibition antibody response to the A/Victoria/3/75 component was independent of the dosage given but the response to the B/Hong Kong/8/73 component was dose related. There was no appreciable increase in the HI titre to the strains after a second dose.— B. J. Feery *et al.*, *Med. J. Aust.*, 1977, *2*, 324.

The use of chemically disrupted (split-virus) influenza vaccine was reported to have fewer side-effects than whole-virus vaccines; only split-virus vaccines were recommended for the vaccination of children under 13 years of age.— *Can. med. Ass. J.*, 1978, *119*, 821.

In a double-blind clinical study involving 225 patients 116 received a bivalent subunit influenza vaccine about 1 to 2 months before the expected onset of an influenza epidemic and 109 acted as controls. Of the patients in these 2 groups 1 and 14 respectively contracted influenza indicating that vaccination afforded about an 80% protection rate.— M. L. Hammond *et al.*, *Med. J. Aust.*, 1978, *1*, 301.

A study of influenza vaccine in schoolboys was started in 1970 and outbreaks of influenza A occurred in 1972 and 1974; a third outbreak occurred in 1976, caused by an A/Victoria strain. The cumulative confirmed-case reports in 375 evaluable boys indicated that boys vaccinated for the first time were partially protected against the strain causing the next outbreak; revaccination with updated strains did not produce the anticipated protection, and, in the long term, boys who received appropriate vaccination before each outbreak had a similar total experience to boys who never received influenza-A vaccine. These observations suggest that annual revaccination with influenza-A vaccine confers no long-term advantage. The practice of offering annual revaccination to adults appears to be open to question.— T. W. Hoskins *et al.*, *Lancet*, 1979, *1*, 33. Similar findings had been obtained in *animal* studies. Yearly vaccination of those most likely to suffer harm from influenza might leave them most at risk when the next pandemic strikes.— J. Lindenmann (letter), *ibid.*, 269. Similar findings at another boys' school.— J. P. Sparks (letter), *ibid.*, 317.

Influenza vaccination of the elderly.— W. H. Barker and J. P. Mullooly, *J. Am. med. Ass.*, 1980, *244*, 2547.

Further references to influenza vaccination.— J. H. D. Briscoe, *J. R. Coll. gen. Pract.*, 1977, *27*, 28; R. Jennings *et al.*, *J. infect. Dis.*, 1978, *138*, 577; L. M. Eastwood *et al.*, *J. clin. Path.*, 1979, *32*, 534; B. J. Feery *et al.*, *J. infect. Dis.*, 1979, *139*, 237; T. Luthardt *et al.*, *Dt. med. Wschr.*, 1979, *104*, 56; G. R. Hodges *et al.*, *Sth. med. J.*, 1979, *72*, 29; S. J. Lerman *et al.*, *J. Pediat.*, 1980, *96*, 271; P. A. Gross *et al.*, *J. Pediat.*, 1980, *97*, 56; H. M. Foy *et al.*, *J. Am. med. Ass.*, 1981, *245*, 1736; T. F. Nolan, *ibid.*, 1762.

Administration. Patients given influenza vaccines by aerosol derived significantly better protection than those given subcutaneous injections.— R. H. Waldman and W. J. Coggins, *J. infect. Dis.*, 1972, *126*, 242, per *J. Am. med. Ass.*, 1972, *222*, 1084.

Influenza vaccine (Admune) had been given intradermally to 2000 schoolchildren and teachers; reactions had been slight. In 32 patients studied antibody-titre responses had been disappointing.— D. K. Payler (letter), *Br. med. J.*, 1977, *2*, 1152.

A favourable report of the intradermal use of influenza vaccine.— W. Halperin *et al.*, *Am. J. publ. Hlth*, 1979, *69*, 1247.

Herpes. Of 61 patients with herpes infections 54 were reported to show response to subcutaneous injection of small doses (assessed by intracutaneous testing) of influenza vaccine. The duration of lesions was reported to be reduced.— J. B. Miller, *Ann. Allergy*, 1979, *42*, 295. See also D. G. Mayne (letter), *Br. med. J.*, 1979, *2*, 1368.

Use in malignant disease. It was recommended that patients with malignant disease should receive influenza immunisation. There was a greater antibody response in 14 patients immunised between courses of cancer chemotherapy than in 22 immunised at the time of administration of chemotherapy.— D. W. Ortbals *et al.*, *Ann. intern. Med.*, 1977, *87*, 552. See also B. J. Feery *et al.*, *Med. J. Aust.*, 1977, *1*, 292; *idem* (letter), 640; P. A. Gross *et al.*, *J. Pediat.*, 1978, *92*, 30.

Use in renal failure. References, generally favourable, to the use of influenza vaccination in renal failure and dialysis.— M. C. Jordan *et al.*, *Ann. intern. Med.*, 1973, *79*, 790; R. N. P. Carroll *et al.*, *Br. med. J.*, 1974, *2*, 701; R. C. Pabico *et al.*, *Ann. intern. Med.*, 1976, *85*, 431; K. J. Sheth *et al.*, *J. Am. med. Ass.*, 1978, *239*, 2559; D. W. Ortbals *et al.*, *ibid.*, 2562; G. R. Noble, *ibid.*, 2592; S. S. Kumar *et al.*, *J. Am. med. Ass.*, 1978, *239*, 840; B. Haldimann and C. Descoeudres, *Schweiz. med. Wschr.*, 1978, *108*, 52; W. A. Briggs *et al.*, *Ann. intern. Med.*, 1980, *92*, 471.

Proprietary Preparations

Fluvirin *(Duncan, Flockhart, UK)*. A brand of Inactivated Influenza Vaccine (Surface Antigen), available in disposable syringes of 0.5 ml and vials of 5 and 25 ml. *Dose*. 0.5 ml; children, 4 to 9 years, 0.5 ml, repeated 4 weeks later.

Influvac *(Duphar, UK)*. A brand of Inactivated Influenza Vaccine inactivated with propiolactone, available in ampoules and disposable syringes of 0.5 ml and vials of 5 and 25 ml. It contains traces of neomycin and polymyxin. *Dose*. 0.5 ml; persons, 9 to 26 years, 0.5 ml, repeated after 4 weeks.

MFV-Ject *(Mérieux, Fr.: Servier, UK)*. A brand of Inactivated Influenza Vaccine, available in syringes of 0.5 ml and vials of 5 and 25 ml. *Dose*. Adults and children over 13 years, 0.5 ml.

Other Proprietary Names

Fluax, Fluogen, Fluzone *(all USA)*.

An inactivated influenza vaccine was also formerly marketed in Great Britain under the proprietary name Admune *(Duncan, Flockhart)*.

7968-e

Influenza Vaccine, Live (Intranasal) *(B.P.)*. Influenza Vaccine (Live Attenuated); Influenza Vaccine (Live); Flu/Vac(Live)/Nas.

An aqueous suspension of a suitable live attenuated strain of influenza virus of either type A or type B, grown in embryonated eggs. It is supplied as a freeze-dried vaccine which is reconstituted, immediately before use, by the addition of a suitable sterile liquid. Potency is assessed in terms of virus titre.

Store at 2° to 8° *in vacuo* or in an atmosphere of nitrogen. Protect from light. Under these conditions it may be expected to retain its potency for at least 1 year.

Adverse Effects and Precautions. As for Vaccines, p.1586.

Uses. Influenza Vaccine, Live (Intranasal) has been used for active immunisation against influenza in selected populations.

It has been given by intranasal administration, 5 drops of the reconstituted vaccine being instilled into each nostril while the patient is supine; the dose is repeated after 1 to 2 weeks. It is not recommended for use in children.

References.— G. M. Schiff *et al.*, *Infect. & Immunity*, 1975, *11*, 754; J. M. Prevost *et al.*, *Scand. J. resp. Dis.*, 1975, *56*, 58; C. A. Morris *et al.*, *Lancet*, 1975, *2*, 196; K. G. Nicholson *et al.*, *Lancet*, 1976, *1*, 1309; C. A. Morris *et al.*, *Lancet*, 1976, *1*, 1118; W. W. Storms *et al.*, *J. Allergy & clin. Immunol.*, 1976, *58*, 284; R. J. Rubin *et al.*, *J. infect. Dis.*, 1976, *133*, 613; J. S. Mackenzie, *Aust. N.Z. J. Med.*, 1977, *7*, 431; J. D. Lee *et al.*, *J. infect. Dis.*, 1977, *135*, 824; I. G. Winson *et al.*, *Thorax*, 1977, *32*, 726; P. J. Fell *et al.*, *Lancet*, 1977, *1*, 1282; D. D. Richman, *New Engl. J. Med.*, 1979, *300*, 137; H. Kessler (letter), *Lancet*, 1980, *2*, 431.

Influenza Vaccine, Live (Attenuated) was formerly marketed in Great Britain under the proprietary name Nasoflu *(Smith Kline & French)*.

7969-l

Leptospira Antiserum *(B.P.C. 1973).* Leptospira Icterohaemorrhagiae Antiserum; Lep/Ser.

Native serum, or a preparation from native serum, containing the antibodies that give a specific protection against strains of *Leptospira icterohaemorrhagiae.*
It is an almost colourless to yellow or yellow-brown liquid, clear but which may become turbid with age, and almost odourless except for the odour of any added bactericide. pH 6 to 8.5.
Store at 2° to 10° and avoid freezing. Protect from light. At 5° it may be expected to lose not more than 5% of its activity in a year; at 20° the loss may approach 20%.

Adverse Effects. As for Antisera, p.1587.
Leptospira antiserum is prepared from the serum of the horse and reactions due to the injection of animal serum may occur.

Uses. Leptospira Antiserum has occasionally been used in the treatment of leptospirosis icterohaemorrhagica (spirochaetal jaundice, Weil's disease), mainly as an adjuvant to chemotherapy. Intravenous administration is preferable in severe cases.
The usual dose is 20 to 40 ml intramuscularly or intravenously.

7970-v

Lymphogranuloma Venereum Antigen *(U.S.P.).* Frei Antigen.

A sterile suspension of the inactivated agent of *Miyagawanella lymphogranulomatis*, prepared by growing the virus in chick-embryo cells. It is a slightly turbid whitish liquid. It contains an antimicrobial agent. **Store** at 2° to 8°. The expiration date is not later than one year after release from manufacturer's cold storage.

Lymphogranuloma venereum antigen has been used in the diagnosis of lymphogranuloma venereum. A control injection should give no reaction. The usual dose was 0.1 ml intracutaneously (intradermally).

Lymphogranuloma venereum antigen was not reactive in many patients with previous *Chlamydia trachomatis* infection and the test might be negative in confirmed cases of the disease. Removal from the market was recommended; it was so removed.— *FDA Drug Bull.*, 1978, *8*, 15.

7971-g

Measles and Mumps Virus Vaccine Live *(U.S.P.).*

A bacterially sterile preparation of a suitable live strain of measles virus (see Measles Virus Vaccine Live, p.1597) and a suitable live strain of mumps virus (see Mumps Virus Vaccine Live, p.1598). It may contain suitable antimicrobial agents. Each labelled dose provides an immunising dose of each component. It is supplied as a freeze-dried vaccine which is reconstituted, just prior to use, by the addition of a suitable sterile liquid.
Store at 2° to 8°. Protect from light. The expiration date is about 1 year after manufacture.

Uses. Measles and Mumps Virus Vaccine Live is used for simultaneous vaccination against measles and mumps.

7972-q

Measles and Rubella Virus Vaccine Live *(U.S.P.).*

A bacterially sterile preparation of suitable live strains of measles virus (see Measles Virus Vaccine Live, p.1597) and live rubella virus (see Rubella Virus Vaccine Live, p.1605). It may contain suitable antimicrobial agents. Each labelled dose provides an immunising dose of each component. It is supplied as a freeze-dried vaccine which is reconstituted, immediately before use, by the addition of a suitable sterile liquid.
Store at 2° to 8°. Protect from light. The expiration date is about 1 year after manufacture.

Adverse Effects and Precautions. As for Measles Vaccine, Live, below and Rubella Vaccine, Live, p.1605.
It must not be given to pregnant women.

Uses. Measles and Rubella Virus Vaccine Live is used for the concomitant active immunisation of children against measles and rubella—see Measles Vaccine, Live, p.1598 and Rubella Vaccine, Live, p.1606.

In 375 seronegative children given measles and rubella vaccine the measles antibody response was 98.9% and the rubella response 95.5%. Fever was comparable to that developing after measles vaccine alone.— V. M. Villarejos *et al.*, *J. Pediat.*, 1971, *79*, 599, per *Int. pharm. Abstr.*, 1973, *10*, 25.

A discussion on the value of measles and rubella vaccines, recommending that their use should be more widespread in childhood.— J. A. Dudgeon, *Archs Dis. Childh.*, 1977, *52*, 907.

See also S. Krugman, *J. Pediat.*, 1977, *90*, 1.

Proprietary Names
M-R-Vax *(Merck Sharp & Dohme, USA).*

In Great Britain supplies are available on a named-patient basis from *Merck Sharp & Dohme.*

7973-p

Measles, Mumps, and Rubella Virus Vaccine Live *(U.S.P.).*

A bacterially sterile preparation of suitable live strains of measles virus (see Measles Virus Vaccine Live, p.1597), mumps virus (see Mumps Virus Vaccine Live, p.1598), and rubella virus (see Rubella Virus Vaccine Live, p.1605). It may contain suitable antimicrobial agents. Each labelled dose provides an immunising dose of each component. It is supplied as a freeze-dried vaccine which is reconstituted, immediately before use, by the addition of a suitable sterile liquid.
Store at 2° to 8°. Protect from light. The expiration date is about 1 year after manufacture.

The stability of measles, mumps, and rubella virus vaccine, stabilised in a buffered sorbitol/gelatin medium.— W. J. McAleer *et al.*, *J. biol. Stand.*, 1980, *8*, 281.

Adverse Effects and Precautions. As for Measles Vaccine, Live, below and Rubella Vaccine, Live, p.1605.
It must not be given to pregnant women.

Bilateral optic neuritis in a 6-year-old boy about 3 weeks after measles, mumps, and rubella immunisation.— E. L. Kazarian and W. E. Gager, *Am. J. Ophthal.*, 1978, *86*, 544.

Uses. Measles, Mumps, and Rubella Virus Vaccine Live is used for the concomitant active immunisation of children against measles, mumps, and rubella—see Measles Vaccine, Live, p.1598, Mumps Virus Vaccine Live, p.1598, and Rubella Vaccine, Live, p.1606.

A trivalent vaccine which consisted of measles, mumps, and rubella vaccines was administered subcutaneously to 715 children aged 7 months to 7 years. Antibodies to measles were developed in 96% of the children, to mumps in 95%, and to rubella in 94%. Slight fever developed in many children in the 5- to 12-day period after vaccination.— J. Stokes *et al.*, *J. Am. med. Ass.*, 1971, *218*, 57. See also E. B. Buynak *et al.*, *J. Am. med. Ass.*, 1969, *207*, 2259.

Further references.— N. J. Ehrenkranz *et al.*, *Bull. Wld Hlth Org.*, 1975, *52*, 81.

Proprietary Names
M-M-R *(Merck Sharp & Dohme, USA).*

In Great Britain supplies are available on a named-patient basis from *Merck Sharp & Dohme.*

7974-s

Inactivated Measles Vaccine. Measles Vaccine (Inactivated) *(B.P. 1968)*; Measles Vaccine (Killed); Meas/Vac (Inactivated).

An aqueous suspension of a suitable measles virus grown in cultures of monkey kidney tissue or chick-embryo cells and inactivated by a suitable method; it may contain aluminium hydroxide or aluminium phosphate, a suitable pH indicator such as phenol red, and antibiotics in the minimum effective concentration. Formaldehyde solution may be used to inactivate the virus.
It is a clear or opalescent liquid; if phenol red has been used in its production, it has a reddish tinge.
Store at 2° to 10° and avoid freezing. Protect from light. Under these conditions it may be expected to retain its potency for at least 1 year.

Adverse Effects and Precautions. As for Vaccines, p.1586.
For reports of atypical measles in patients previously given inactivated measles vaccines, see Measles Vaccine, Live, p.1598.

Uses. Inactivated Measles Vaccine was formerly used for active immunisation against measles but immunisation with Measles Vaccine, Live is now used. It was also given prior to inoculation with Measles Vaccine, Live to reduce side-effects.

7975-w

Measles Vaccine, Live *(B.P., Eur. P.).*

Measles Vaccine (Live Attenuated); Vaccinum Morbillorum; Meas/Vac (Live).

An aqueous suspension of a suitable live modified (attenuated) strain of measles virus grown in cultures of chick-embryo cells. It is supplied as a freeze-dried vaccine which is reconstituted, immediately before use, with Water for Injections; bactericides must not be added. If phenol red has been used in its production, it may have a reddish tinge. It contains a suitable stabiliser. Potency is expressed in terms of virus titre.
Store at 2° to 8°. Protect from light. Under these conditions it may be expected to retain its potency for at least 1 year.

CAUTION. *The vaccine is readily inactivated by chemical disinfectants and antiseptics and care is needed to avoid contact with these substances when sterilising syringes and skin before immunisation.*

7976-e

Measles Virus Vaccine Live *(U.S.P.).*

A bacterially sterile freeze-dried preparation of a suitable live strain of measles virus grown in cultures of chick-embryo cells. It contains not less than the equivalent of 1000 TCID50 in each immunising dose, and may contain suitable antimicrobial agents.
Store at 2° to 8°. Protect from light. The reconstituted vaccine should be used within 8 hours of preparation.

Discussion of the problem of appropriate storage of measles vaccine, especially during transport.— M. D. Coulter and B. M. Jones (letter), *Br. med. J.*, 1977, *2*, 120.

The successful use of a heat-stable measles vaccine in Cameroon. There was a negligible loss of titre after storage for 7 days at about 25°.— D. L. Heymann *et al.*, *Br. med. J.*, 1979, *2*, 99.

Adverse Effects. As for Vaccines, p.1586.
Fever and skin rashes occur frequently following the administration of Measles Vaccine, Live. The fever generally starts 5 to 10 days after the injection and lasts for about 1 or 2 days. Conjunctivitis, coryza, pharyngitis, and bronchitis may also occur. More serious effects reported to be associated with the use of the vaccine include convulsions, encephalitis, and thrombocytopenic purpura.

General reactions occurred in 32%, and were severe in 6%, of 50 children vaccinated with live measles vaccine, but there were no serious complications.— J. E. Miller and B. Harding-Cox, *Practitioner*, 1969, *203*, 352.

All 8 children given a live measles vaccine developed some symptoms 7 to 8 days after vaccination. Temporary EEG changes were noted in 6 and were similar to those seen in the prodromal phase of measles. Measles antibodies were not detected in the serum until the 28th to 31st day.— G. Pampiglione *et al.*, *Lancet*, 1971, *2*, 5.

Three patients developed the nephrotic syndrome after receiving measles vaccine.— J. A. Kuzemko (letter), *Br. med. J.*, 1972, *4*, 665.

Atypical measles. Comment on the cause of the atypical-measles syndrome. Although this is generally associated with the killed vaccine, reports that it has been described as arising in people who have had the live vaccine, if confirmed, are disturbing. Atypical measles seems unlikely to arise very often after the attenuated vaccine but as the years pass and immunity begins to wane the possibility must be kept in mind.— *Lancet*, 1979, *1*, 962.

Further references.— J. W. St. Geme *et al.*, *Pediatrics*, 1976, *57*, 148; M. Chatterji and V. Mankad, *J. Am. med. Ass.*, 1977, *238*, 2635; E. M. Nichols, *Am. J. publ. Hlth*, 1979, *69*, 160; V. A. Fulginiti and R. E. Helfer, *J. Am. med. Ass.*, 1980, *244*, 804.

Leucopenia. Inoculation of children with live measles vaccine was constantly followed by leucopenia, which usually started 4 days after the injection and lasted for about 9 days.— F. L. Black and S. R. Sheridan, *Am. J. Dis. Childh.*, 1967, *113*, 301, per *Abstr. Wld Med.*, 1967, *41*, 755.

Lymphadenopathy. An 11-month-old Negro girl developed inguinal lymphoid hyperplasia a few days after being given an injection of live measles virus vaccine into a gluteal muscle. Other reports had previously indicated that regional lymphadenopathy could develop as an occasional complication up to 2 weeks after administration of attenuated measles vaccine.— R. F. Dorfman and J. C. Herweg, *J. Am. med. Ass.*, 1966, *198*, 320.

Neurological complications. In 50.9 million doses of measles vaccine distributed in USA between 1963 and 1971 there were 84 cases of neurological disorders occurring less than 30 days after vaccination. Of these, encephalitis or encephalopathy in 45 occurred 6 to 15 days after vaccination suggesting that measles vaccine was the cause.— P. J. Landrigan and J. J. Witte, *J. Am. med. Ass.*, 1973, *223*, 1459.

A 19-month-old girl developed Guillain-Barré syndrome 5 days after being given live measles and rubella vaccine; after 4 days of progressive weakness motor function returned to normal over the following 8 weeks; a second 10-month-old child became similarly ill after receiving live measles vaccine as well as vaccination against polio, diphtheria, pertussis and tetanus, and she too recovered.— C. Grose and I. Spigland, *Am. J. Med.*, 1976, *60*, 441.

A review of 375 cases of subacute sclerosing panencephalitis occurring in the USA suggested that live measles vaccine might be implicated in this condition. However, the risk from vaccination appeared less than the risk from measles and since the introduction of measles vaccination there had been a decline in the incidence of subacute sclerosing panencephalitis.— J. F. Modlin *et al.*, *Pediatrics*, 1977, *59*, 505.

In a boy with subacute sclerosing panencephalitis rapid deterioration and death followed immunisation with a measles vaccine.— W. E. Dodson *et al.* (letter), *Lancet*, 1978, *1*, 767. The national registry of subacute sclerosing panencephalitis showed 9 patients who had received live and/or inactivated measles vaccine after the onset of SSPE. There was no evidence that measles vaccine accelerated the disease process.— N. A. Halsey *et al.* (letter), *ibid.*, 1978, *2*, 783.

Precautions. As for Vaccines, p.1586.

Measles Vaccine, Live should not be given to persons with hypogammaglobulinaemia, leukaemia or other malignant conditions, acute illness or active tuberculosis, or to those being treated with corticosteroids or immunosuppressive drugs. It should not be given to persons hypersensitive to egg protein.

Care is necessary in administering the vaccine to persons with allergic conditions, such as asthma or dermatitis, or a family history of convulsions, to the undernourished, or to children with chronic heart or lung disorders. It should not be given during pregnancy.

It should generally not be administered within 3 weeks of another vaccine containing live micro-organisms.

Measles vaccination may temporarily reduce the reaction to tuberculin and other skin tests.

In about 11% of children previously immunised against diphtheria, the reaction to a Schick test became positive 4 to 6 weeks after vaccination with live measles vaccine. The occurrence of diphtheria in children apparently adequately immunised had been attributed to this effect.— M. P. Bondarenko and K. M. Celyseva, *Zh. Mikrobiol. Épidem. Immunobiol.*, 1967, *44*, 26, per *Abstr. Wld Med.*, 1968, *42*, 323.

Inoculation with live measles vaccine suppressed the reaction to a histoplasmin skin test for about 1 to 4 weeks.— W. T. Hughes *et al.*, *Am. J. Dis. Child.*, 1968, *116*, 402, per *J. Am. med. Ass.*, 1968, *206*, 1101.

Inoculation with a vaccine of live measles virus suppressed for 1 to 4 weeks a delayed hypersensitivity reaction to antigens of *Candida*, diphtheria toxoid, poison ivy, smallpox, and tuberculin purified protein derivative. Administration of the vaccine did not affect existing titres of antibodies to diphtheria or poliomyelitis or immediate wheal and flare reactions.— P. Fireman *et al.*, *Pediatrics*, 1969, *43*, 264, per *J. Am. med. Ass.*, 1969, *208*, 193.

Measles vaccine temporarily suppressed the response to a tuberculin skin test in some tuberculin-positive persons.— *J. Am. med. Ass.*, 1969, *208*, 783. A case report.— M. J. Wilmers (letter), *Br. med. J.*, 1972, *4*, 665.

Uses. Measles Vaccine, Live is used for active immunisation against measles. Immunity to measles develops in about 90% of children given a single dose, antibody being detectable in the serum about the twelfth day after injection. Protection is considered to last for at least 15 years.

In the newborn, maternally transmitted antibodies prevent the development of immunity following administration of Measles Vaccine, Live, and generally the vaccine should not be given to infants before the age of 9 months. Measles Vaccine, Live should preferably be given during the second year of life; because the incidence of side-effects is lower in children aged 3 or over, some authorities would defer immunisation until that age; it may also be given to susceptible children up to the age of 15 years. In the USA it is generally given from the age of 15 months, and it is recommended that those receiving it before 12 months of age should be revaccinated at 15 months.

Reactions may be reduced by giving a small dose of Normal Immunoglobulin Injection with a known content of measles antibodies at the same time as the vaccine, but at a different site.

Measles Vaccine, Live is given by subcutaneous or intramuscular injection. The usual dose is 0.5 ml.

Discussions of measles and measles vaccination.— *Lancet*, 1977, *2*, 387; *Lancet*, 1979, *2*, 834; *Med. Lett.*, 1979, *21*, 102; *Lancet*, 1981, *2*, 236.

Discussion of measles and a suggestion for selective immunisation.— H. Smith, *Br. med. J.*, 1980, *280*, 766. Criticism and comment.— J. A. Frank *et al.* (letter), *Br. med. J.*, 1980, *280*, 1185; J. Desmyter and S. Krugman (letter), *ibid;* G. Dick (letter), *ibid.*, 1186; C. Miller (letter), *Br. med. J.*, 1980, *280*, 1451.

In a controlled trial, 19 972 children, aged 10 months to 2 years, were given either inactivated measles vaccine followed 1 month later by live vaccine or a single dose of live vaccine; 16 239 children acted as controls. Up to 6 months after inoculation substantial protection against measles was provided by both vaccination schedules but the incidence of side-effects, particularly serious side-effects, was higher in those who received the single dose of live vaccine than in those given the 2 vaccines. When the degrees of protection were compared up to 33 months after inoculation, the single dose of live vaccine generally was superior; it provided protection in about 90% of those inoculated children remaining in the trial. Evaluation after 57 months yielded similar results and follow-up over a 12-year period of 11 516 vaccinated children showed no evidence of declining protection. In the last 5 years of the study there was no difference in protection between the single dose of the live vaccine and the schedule of the killed followed by the live vaccine.—Reports to the MRC by the Measles Vaccines Committee and the Measles Sub-Committee of the Committee on Development of Vaccines and Immunisation Procedures, *Br. med. J.*, 1966, *1*, 441; *ibid.*, 1968, *2*, 449; *Practitioner*, 1971, *206*, 458; *Lancet*, 1977, *2*, 571.

A study in Nigerian children indicated that dose reduction would not be a satisfactory economy measure in measles vaccine campaigns.— R. B. Wallace *et al.*, *Bull. Wld Hlth Org.*, 1976, *53*, 361.

Results of a collaborative study by the Ministry of Health of Kenya and the World Health Organization suggested that in countries with conditions similar to those in Kenya the optimum age for measles vaccination was 7½ months. At this age seroconversion would occur and protection should last for at least 2 to 3 years thus covering a high proportion of children when they were most vulnerable to malnutrition.— *Bull. Wld Hlth Org.*, 1977, *55*, 21.

References generally supporting immunisation at 14 to 15 months rather than at 12 months.— D. M. Shasby *et al.*, *New Engl. J. Med.*, 1977, *296*, 585; A. S. Yeager *et al.*, *J. Am. med. Ass.*, 1977, *237*, 347; J. S. Marks *et al.*, *Pediatrics*, 1978, *62*, 955; J. D. Shelton, *ibid.*, 961.

A recommendation for immunisation from 12 months.— J. Wilkins and P. F. Wehrle, *Am. J. Dis. Child.*, 1978, *132*, 164.

The possible role of measles vaccination after exposure.— *Lancet*, 1978, *2*, 930.

A 12.2% incidence of measles complications in 147 patients previously vaccinated compared with 9.8% in 348 not vaccinated.— G. A. Jackson (letter), *Br. med. J.*, 1979, *2*, 332.

Serological screening programmes should be carried out to identify and vaccinate susceptible adult subjects, rather than widespread vaccination of all subjects.— P. J. Krause *et al.*, *Ann. intern. Med.*, 1979, *90*, 873.

The limited usefulness of intradermal injection.— P. B. Wood *et al.*, *Trans. R. Soc. trop. Med. Hyg.*, 1980, *74*, 381.

Further references.— J. B. McCormick *et al.*, *J. Pediat.*, 1977, *90*, 13; R. D. Krugman *et al.*, *J. Pediat.*, 1977, *91*, 766; J. Celers, *Bull. Inst. Pasteur, Paris*, 1977, *75*, 327, per *Abstr. Hyg.*, 1978, *53*, 845; J. Deseda-Tous *et al.*, *Am. J. Dis. Child.*, 1978, *132*, 287; The Kasongo Project Team, *Lancet*, 1981, *1*, 764.

Hodgkin's disease. Regression of Hodgkin's disease after measles and a proposal for a trial of attenuated live measles vaccine as an adjunct to chemotherapy in the treatment of Hodgkin's disease in children.— A. M. Taqi *et al.* (letter), *Lancet*, 1981, *1*, 1112.

Multiple sclerosis. A brief discussion of the possible role of measles and measles vaccination in multiple sclerosis.— *Br. med. J.*, 1979, *1*, 937.

Proprietary Preparations

Attenuvax *(Morson, UK).* A brand of Measles Vaccine, Live (Enders' attenuated Edmonston strain), supplied in single-dose vials with ampoules of diluent. It contains traces of neomycin. (Also available as Attenuvax in *USA*).

Mevilin-L *(Duncan, Flockhart, UK).* A brand of Measles Vaccine, Live (Schwarz strain), supplied in single-dose vials with 0.5-ml ampoules of Water for Injections. It may contain traces of neomycin and polymyxin.

Rimevax *(Smith Kline & French, UK).* A brand of Measles Vaccine, Live (Schwarz strain), supplied in single-dose vials with ampoules of diluent. It contains traces of neomycin sulphate.

7977-l

Meningococcal Polysaccharide Vaccine Group A *(U.S.P.).*

A sterile preparation of the group-specific polysaccharide antigen from *Neisseria meningitidis* group A, consisting of a polymer of *N*-acetyl mannosamine phosphate. It is supplied as a dried vaccine which is reconstituted before use with Bacteriostatic Sodium Chloride Injection containing thiomersal. When reconstituted each 0.5-ml dose contains 50 µg of the antigen with 2.5 to 5 mg of lactose as a stabiliser. The potency is such that the serum antibody titre is increased at least 4-fold in not less than 90% of 25 healthy subjects.

Store at 2° to 8°. The expiration date is not

later than 18 months after release from manufacturer's cold storage. The reconstituted vaccine should be used immediately after preparation, or within 8 hours if stored at 2° to 8°.

7978-y

Meningococcal Polysaccharide Vaccine Group C *(U.S.P.).*

A sterile preparation of the group-specific polysaccharide antigen from *Neisseria meningitidis* group C, consisting of a polymer of sialic acid. It is supplied as a dried vaccine which is reconstituted before use with Bacteriostatic Sodium Chloride Injection containing thiomersal. When reconstituted each 0.5-ml dose contains 50 µg of the antigen with 2.5 to 5 mg of lactose as a stabiliser. The potency is such that the serum antibody titre is increased at least 4-fold in not less than 90% of 25 healthy subjects.
Store at 2° to 8°. The expiration date is not later than 18 months after release from manufacturer's cold storage. The reconstituted vaccine should be used immediately after preparation, or within 8 hours if stored at 2° to 8°.

7979-j

Meningococcal Polysaccharide Vaccine Groups A and C Combined *(U.S.P.).*

A sterile preparation of meningococcal polysaccharide group A and C specific antigens (see above). It is supplied as a dried vaccine which is reconstituted before use with Bacteriostatic Sodium Chloride Injection containing thiomersal. When reconstituted each 0.5-ml dose contains 50 µg of each antigen with 2.5 to 5 mg of lactose as a stabiliser. The antigenicity or potency is such that the dose provides an immunising dose of each component.
Store at 2° to 8°. The expiration date is not later than 18 months after release from manufacturer's cold storage. The reconstituted vaccine should be used immediately after preparation, or within 8 hours if stored at 2° to 8°.

Recommended requirements for meningococcal polysaccharide vaccine, including the name *Vaccinum meningitidis cerebrospinalis*.— WHO Expert Committee on Biological Standardization, *Tech. Rep. Ser. Wld Hlth Org. No. 594,* 1976.

The standardisation and control of meningococcal vaccines.— K. H. Wong *et al., J. biol. Stand.,* 1977, *5,* 197.

The enhancement of stability of meningococcal polysaccharide vaccines by using lactose instead of mannitol as a menstruum for lyophilisation.— R. H. Tiesjema *et al., Bull. Wld Hlth Org.,* 1977, *55,* 43.

The biological and physicochemical characteristics of meningococcus polysaccharide group C prepared by 2 different methods of purification.— M. Porro *et al., J. biol. Stand.,* 1980, *8,* 7.

Adverse Effects. As for Vaccines, p.1586.
Localised erythema lasting 1 or 2 days has been reported.

Precautions. As for Vaccines, p.1586.

Impairment of response to meningococcal vaccine in acute malaria.— W. A. Williamson and B. M. Greenwood, *Lancet,* 1978, *1,* 1328.

Uses. Meningococcal polysaccharide monovalent or bivalent vaccines are used to control outbreaks of meningococcal disease caused by *Neisseria meningitidis* serogroup A and/or C. Vaccination may also be of value to travellers to countries where the disease is endemic, and as an adjunct to antibiotic prophylaxis for household contacts of persons with the disease.
An antibody response to group A antigen is considered likely to develop in children from the age of 3 months, and to group C antigen from the age of 2 years. An antibody response develops within about 5 days in about 90% of subjects (of appropriate age) vaccinated. The duration of immunity remains to be established.

Discussions of the use of meningococcal polysaccharide vaccine.— Cerebrospinal Meningitis Control, *Tech. Rep. Ser. Wld Hlth Org. No. 588,* 1976; M. L. Lepow and R. Gold, *New Engl. J. Med.,* 1977, *297,* 721; *Lancet,* 1978, *2,* 1185.

The American Public Health Service Advisory Committee on Immunization Practices recommendations for the use of meningococcal polysaccharide vaccines.— *Ann. intern. Med.,* 1978, *89,* 949.

In a double-blind study, during an epidemic in Finland, Group A capsular polysaccharide (meningococcal) vaccine was administered to 49 295 children aged 3 months to 5 years and a further 48 977 children received a control *H. influenzae* type b polysaccharide vaccine; 31 906 remained unvaccinated. No children in the meningococcal vaccine group suffered meningitis or sepsis, whereas 6 cases occurred in those vaccinated with the *H. influenzae* vaccine and 13 in the unvaccinated group. In a second study none of 21 007 vaccinated children suffered disease caused by Group A meningococci whereas 5 to 7 cases would have been expected.— H. Peltola *et al., New Engl. J. Med.,* 1977, *297,* 686.

In a double-blind study in Egypt 1 of more than 88 000 children aged 6 to 15 years vaccinated with a single dose of meningococcal polysaccharide (50 µg in 0.5 ml) prepared from *N. meningitidis* serogroup A, developed cerebrospinal meningitis due to this serogroup during the following 12 months, compared with 9 in a similar control group given tetanus toxoid. In the second year there was no evidence of a protective effect. The difference in the duration of protection from another reported series was possibly related to the difference in molecular weight of the polysaccharide. During the first year the vaccine reduced the incidence of new carriers among vaccinees and shortened the duration of carriage.— M. H. Wahden *et al., Bull. Wld Hlth Org.,* 1977, *55,* 645.

In an epidemic of cerebrospinal meningitis 65 000 children were immunised in 1974/5 with meningococcal vaccine of serogroup A. Morbidity in non-immunised children was 12 times higher than in the immunised group.— G. Jamba *et al., Bull. Wld Hlth Org.,* 1979, *57,* 943.

Selective vaccination of the inhabitants of African villages, using 50 µg of combined group-A and group-C meningococcal vaccine, reduced the incidence of meningococcal disease compared with control villages. Subsequent analysis of the data indicated that the vaccination policy would have been more effective had it been given as soon as a single case of meningococcal disease had been identified.— B. M. Greenwood and S. S. Wali, *Lancet,* 1980, *1,* 729. See also B. M. Greenwood *et al., Br. med. J.,* 1978, *1,* 1317.

The control of epidemic meningococcal meningitis in Nigeria by mass vaccination with meningococcal vaccine containing groups A and C polysaccharide antigen.— I. Mohammed and K. Zaruba, *Lancet,* 1981, *2,* 80.

Further references.— H. H. Erwa *et al., Bull. Wld Hlth Org.,* 1973, *49,* 301; P. H. Makela *et al., Lancet,* 1975, *2,* 883; M. L. Lepow *et al., Pediatrics,* 1977, *60,* 673; E. C. Gotschlich, *Am. J. Med.,* 1978, *65,* 719; A. E. Taunay *et al., Revta Instil. Adolfo Lutz,* 1978, *38,* 77, per *Trop. Dis. Bull.,* 1980, *77,* 433; J. Wilkins and P. F. Wehrle, *J. Pediat.,* 1979, *94,* 828.

Pregnancy and the neonate. A mixed meningococcal vaccine (A and C) was evaluated in pregnant women and infants during an epidemic of meningitis in Brazil. Antibodies were detected in the women and there was some placental transfer of antibody although this was irregular. Vaccination of children in the first 6 months of life was unsuccessful.— A. de A. Carvalho *et al., Lancet,* 1977, *2,* 809.

Proprietary Names
Meningovax-AC *(Merck Sharp & Dohme, USA)*; Menomune (group A, group C, or groups A and C) *(Connaught, USA).*

In Great Britain supplies of group A and group C vaccine are available on a named-patient basis from *Elkins-Sinn, USA* and the combined vaccine is available similarly from *Servier* and *Smith Kline & French.*

7980-q

Mumps Skin Test Antigen *(U.S.P.).*

A sterile aqueous suspension of formaldehyde-inactivated mumps virus prepared from the extra-embryonic fluid of virus-infected chick embryos, concentrated and purified by differential centrifugation, and suspended in iso-osmotic sodium chloride solution containing glycine as a preservative. Each ml contains not less than 20 complement-fixing units.
Store at 2° to 8°. The expiration date is not later than 18 months after manufacture or release from manufacturer's cold storage.

Recovery from mumps produces skin hypersensitivity to mumps virus. A positive reaction to Mumps Skin Test Antigen, 0.1 ml intracutaneously (intradermally), may indicate previous infection with mumps virus but it is not considered to be very reliable. It should not be given to patients hypersensitive to egg protein.

Mumps Skin Test Antigen is unreliable for identifying susceptible persons because of poor sensitivity and specificity and variable potency. It is now used as one of a number of tests to evaluate immunological (T-cell) competence.— *FDA Drug Bull.,* 1978, *8,* 15.

A 2-year-old child with recurrence of laryngeal papillomas had a beneficial response to local injection of 0.1 ml of mumps skin test antigen into the base of 2 polyps. The injections were subsequently repeated twice and it was felt that the rate and extent of recurrence had been markedly suppressed. The child had been immunised with live mumps virus vaccine at about 16 months of age, which was a prerequisite of the treatment protocol.— A. Greensher (letter), *Lancet,* 1980, *2,* 920.

Manufacturers
Lilly, USA.

7981-p

Inactivated Mumps Vaccine. Mumps Vaccine (Inactivated); Inactivated Mumps Virus Vaccine.

A sterile aqueous suspension of killed mumps virus prepared from the extra-embryonic fluid of virus-infected chick embryos, concentrated and purified by centrifugation, inactivated with formaldehyde solution, and suspended in iso-osmotic sodium chloride solution containing glycine and thiomersal. It is a turbid white suspension.
Store at 2° to 8°, when it may be expected to retain its potency for 18 months.

Inactivated mumps vaccine has been used for active immunisation against mumps.

7982-s

Mumps Virus Vaccine Live *(U.S.P.).*

A bacterially sterile freeze-dried preparation of a suitable strain of mumps virus grown in cultures of chick-embryo cells. It is reconstituted with a suitable diluent immediately before use. It contains not less than 5000 TCID50 in each immunising dose. It may contain suitable antimicrobial agents. **Store** at 2° to 8°. Protect from light. The expiration date is about 1 year after manufacture.

CAUTION. *The vaccine should not be brought into contact with alcohol or other disinfectants and care is needed when sterilising syringes and skin before immunisation.*

Adverse Effects. As for Vaccines,p.1586.
Unilateral nerve deafness and encephalitis have occured rarely.

Precautions. As for Measles Vaccine, Live, above.

Parotid swelling occurred in 20 children who had received live attenuated mumps vaccine 3 to 39 months earlier. The diagnosis of mumps was confirmed in 8 of 17 studied serologically; in the remainder the cause of the swelling was not identified.— P. A. Brunell *et al., Pediatrics,* 1972, *50,* 441, per *Int. pharm. Abstr.,* 1973, *10,* 287.

Uses. Mumps Virus Vaccine Live is used for active immunisation against mumps. An antibody response in over 90% of susceptible persons inoculated has been reported, persisting for at least 12 years. In the USA vaccination is recommended for infants 12 months and over, and for susceptible children, adolescents, and adults. The vaccine is given subcutaneously as a single dose.
It is not recommended for children below the age of 1 year in whom maternal antibodies might

prevent a response.
It can be given concomitantly with live measles, rubella, and poliomyelitis vaccines.

A brief review of mumps vaccine.— J. A. Dudgeon, *Archs Dis. Childh.*, 1980, *55*, 3.

The complications of mumps justified attempts to prevent the disease; it could be considered especially for postpubertal boys likely to be exposed to infection.— *Drug & Ther. Bull.*, 1975, *13*, 23.

There was no place for the uncontrolled use of mumps vaccine; it could however be offered to adolescents and adults shown by a radial haemolysis test to be susceptible.— P. P. Mortimer, *Br. med. J.*, 1978, *2*, 1523. A similar conclusion.— J. W. G. Smith, *Practitioner*, 1978, *220*, 929.

While mumps vaccination might be an advantage for the individual it might have the reverse effect for the general population, by altering the pattern of natural infection which led to 95% of adults being immune.— *Br. med. J.*, 1980, *281*, 1231. A differing view.— J. Desmyter (letter), *ibid.*, 1637.

Recommendations of the Immunization Practice Advisory Committee of the Center for Disease Control. Susceptible children over 12 months of age, adolescents, and nonpregnant adults should be vaccinated against mumps unless vaccination is contra-indicated. Subjects born before 1957 are likely to have been infected naturally and generally may be considered to be immune. Testing for susceptibility is unnecessary before vaccination since nonsusceptible subjects are not considered to be at enhanced risk from vaccination and since tests are unreliable or nonspecific or, if reliable, difficult to obtain.— *Ann. intern. Med.*, 1980, *92*, 803.

Proprietary Preparations

Mumpsvax *(Morson, UK)*. Mumps virus vaccine, live attenuated, (Jeryl-Lynn strain) in single-dose vials each containing not less than 5000 TCID50, supplied with disposable syringes of diluent, for reconstitution immediately before use. (Also available as Mumpsvax in *USA*).

7983-w

Pertussis Vaccine *(B.P., Eur. P.)*.

Whooping-cough Vaccine; Vaccinum Pertussis; Per/Vac.

A sterile suspension, in a saline or other appropriate solution iso-osmotic with blood, of a suitable killed strain or strains of *Bordetella pertussis*. The estimated potency of the volume stated on the label as the dose, which does not exceed 1 ml, is not less than 4 units with relation to the second British Reference Preparation (1968) which contains 1 unit in 1.5 mg of dried vaccine. It may contain a suitable bactericide.
It may also be supplied as an adsorbed vaccine (Per/Vac/Ads) adsorbed on aluminium hydroxide, aluminium phosphate, or calcium phosphate, containing not more than 20×10^9 bacilli per dose. *Eur. P.* includes the adsorbed vaccine as Pertussis Vaccine (Adsorbed); Vaccinum Pertussis Adsorbatum. The label states the name of the mineral carrier.
Store at 2° to 8° and avoid freezing. Protect from light. Under these conditions it may be expected to retain its potency for at least 2 years.

NOTE. When Pertussis Vaccine is prescribed or demanded the plain or the adsorbed vaccine may be dispensed or supplied.

7984-e

Pertussis Vaccine *(U.S.P.)*.

A sterile bacterial fraction or suspension of killed *Bordetella pertussis* of a strain or strains selected for high antigenicity. It contains a preservative. It contains 12 protective units per immunising dose.
Store at 2° to 8° and avoid freezing. The expiration date is not later than 18 months after release from manufacturer's cold storage.

7985-l

Pertussis Vaccine Adsorbed *(U.S.P.)*.

A sterile bacterial fraction or suspension of killed *Bordetella pertussis* of a strain or strains selected for high antigenicity, precipitated or adsorbed by the addition of aluminium hydroxide or aluminium phosphate. It contains a preservative. It contains not less than 12 protective units per immunising dose.
Store at 2° to 8° and avoid freezing. The expiration date is not later than 18 months after release from manufacturer's cold storage.

Potency measurement of pertussis vaccines and consistency in production.— J. D. van Ramshorst *et al.*, *J. biol. Stand.*, 1979, *7*, 307. See also *Bull. Wld Hlth Org.*, 1978, *56*, 220.

Discussion of the varying US and WHO standards for pertussis vaccines.— J. Cameron (letter), *New Engl. J. Med.*, 1980, *303*, 157.

Research prospects for the development of better pertussis vaccines.— C. R. Manclark, *Bull. Wld Hlth Org.*, 1981, *59*, 9.

Units. 34.7 units are contained in 52 mg in one ampoule of the first International Standard Preparation (1957).

Adverse Effects. As for Vaccines, p.1586.
Reactions are common following the administration of pertussis vaccine or of vaccines in which it is a component. The more severe general effects include anorexia, fever, vomiting, malaise, uncontrollable screaming, collapse, and convulsions leading, rarely, to chronic epilepsy, encephalopathy, infantile spasms, and mental retardation. In some cases these reactions have followed after reactions to a previous dose. Fatalities have been reported.

A 45-year-old man developed fever, lymphadenopathy, haemoptysis, renal failure, diffuse vasculitis, and died after receiving 8 intramuscular injections of pertussis vaccine at frequent intervals for the development of specific immunoglobulin.— W. B. Bishop *et al.*, *New Engl. J. Med.*, 1966, *274*, 616.

Neurological complications. The role of pertussis vaccine in causing convulsions and permanent cerebral damage is controversial; few detailed case reports have been published, many cases are not reported, and accurate assessment is difficult. However, it does appear that there is some causal relationship between pertussis vaccine and neurological complications although the incidence is such that pertussis vaccination is generally recommended as part of the basic course of immunisation of childhood except in certain susceptible groups (see Precautions).
This is discussed in detail in Reports from the Committee on Safety of Medicines and the Joint Committee on Vaccination and Immunisation in *Whooping Cough*, Department of Health and Social Security, London, HM Stationery Office, 1981. See also *Lancet*, 1981, *1*, 1113.

Other reviews and discussions of the complications of pertussis vaccination.— *Drug & Ther. Bull.*, 1976, *14*, 1; *Br. med. J.*, 1977, *2*, 5; *Lancet*, 1977, *1*, 918; *Lancet*, 1977, *2*, 71; W. Ehrengut, *ibid.*, 1978, *1*, 370; R. A. Ouvrier, *Med. J. Aust.*, 1978, *2*, 300; G. F. Grady and L. H. Wetterlow, *New Engl. J. Med.*, 1978, *298*, 966; M. Eastman, *Am. Pharm.*, 1979, *NS19* (Jan.), 16; J. P. Koplan *et al.*, *New Engl. J. Med.*, 1979, *301*, 906; *Br. med. J.*, 1981, *282*, 1563; *Lancet*, 1981, *1*, 1138; R. J. Robinson, *Archs Dis. Childh.*, 1981, *56*, 577.

Fifty children were seen in an 11-year period with neurological illness believed to be due to the pertussis component of diphtheria, tetanus, and pertussis vaccine; adequate data were available for 36 whose illness occurred within 14 days of inoculation; in 24, reactions occurred within 24 hours. Of the 36, 32 had convulsions, 23 within 24 hours and 7 within 7 days. Of the 36, 22 became mentally retarded with epilepsy, 4 were retarded without epilepsy, and 3 had epilepsy without retardation. Possible contributory factors in 12 included previous convulsions, infection, family history of epilepsy in a first-degree relative, a perinatal problem, and previous reactions to the vaccine.— M. Kulenkampff *et al.*, *Archs Dis. Childh.*, 1974, *49* 46.

A study of 160 cases of neurotoxicity possibly associated with pertussis vaccine and the features of a pertussis reaction syndrome. It was impossible to estimate the prevalence of the syndrome or of subsequent brain damage. The incidence was unlikely to be lower than 1 in 60 000 and might be as high as 1 in 10 000. If it were 1 in 20 000 then 30 children each year would suffer brain damage in the UK.— G. T. Stewart, *Lancet*, 1977, *1*, 234. See also G. T. Stewart, *J. Epidem. Community Health*, 1979, *33*, 150. Criticism.— J. S. Robertson (letter), *Br. med. J.*, 1979, *2*, 735; J. B. P. Stephenson (letter), *ibid.*, 1979, *2*, 933.

One serious neurological complication possibly related to pertussis vaccine in 450 000 doses given in an area of the USA.— M. Bader (letter), *New Engl. J. Med.*, 1978, *299*, 492.

A report on the first 1000 cases notified to the National Childhood Encephalopathy Study; 3.5% of the notified children had been immunised with diphtheria, tetanus, and pertussis vaccine within 7 days before the onset of disease, compared with 1.7% in controls. The estimated attributable risk of serious neurological disorders within 7 days of immunisation in previously normal children was 1 in 110 000 (regardless of outcome) or 1 in 310 000 (neurological sequelae persisting one year later).— D. L. Miller *et al.*, *Br. med. J.*, 1981, *282*, 1595. See also *idem*, in *Whooping Cough*, Department of Health and Social Security, London, HM Stationery Office, 1981, p. 79.

Discussion of some of the problems in evaluating the safety of pertussis vaccination.— T. W. Meade (letter), *Br. med. J.*, 1981, *283*, 59.

Further references.— C. L. Miller *et al.*, *Lancet*, 1974, *2*, 510; J. C. Melchior, *Archs Dis. Childh.*, 1977, *52*, 134; A. H. Griffith, *Wellcome*, *Br. med. J.*, 1978, *1*, 809; L. H. Collier, *Lister* (letter), *ibid.*, 985; J. B. P. Stephenson (letter), *Lancet*, 1979, *2*, 416.

See also under Diphtheria, Tetanus, and Pertussis Vaccine, p.1593.

Precautions. As for Vaccines, p.1586.
It is considered that pertussis vaccine should not be given to children with a history of seizures, convulsions, or cerebral irritation in the neonatal period, with developmental neurological defects, with a febrile illness, especially respiratory, until fully recovered, or with a personal or family history of epilepsy or other diseases of the central nervous system. It should not be given to patients who have shown a severe local or general reaction to a previous dose. Opinion is divided as to whether a personal or family history of allergy is a contra-indication. If used in such patients adrenaline and appropriate resuscitative facilities should be available.
If a reaction follows the first dose of diphtheria, tetanus, and pertussis vaccine, further immunisation with diphtheria and tetanus vaccine may be considered.

The recommended contra-indications to pertussis vaccination were felt to be too ambiguous. Parents may be advised against immunisation only if: the baby has already had a convulsion or displayed evidence of severe brain damage; or a parent or sibling has established epilepsy or severe neurological disorder; or the baby is in the acute phase of a febrile illness—that is, *not* an ordinary cold or the convalescent phase of a febrile illness.— *Br. med. J.*, 1980, *280*, 307. The contra-indications should be strictly observed.— R. J. Robinson, *Archs Dis. Childh.*, 1981, *56*, 577. Uncertainty as to how the contra-indications should be interpreted.— D. Hull, *Br. med. J.*, 1981, *283*, 1231.

Uses. Pertussis Vaccine and Adsorbed Pertussis Vaccine are used for active immunisation of infants against whooping cough.
Whooping cough is most dangerous in early life, and immunisation should be started when the infant is 3 months old.
Pertussis Vaccine is given in 3 doses by deep subcutaneous or intramuscular injection; the second dose is given after 6 to 8 weeks, and the third dose 4 to 6 months later. It is generally administered as Diphtheria, Tetanus, and Pertussis Vaccine.
In Great Britain, the Joint Committee on Vaccination and Immunisation re-affirmed in 1977, and again in 1981, its support for immunisation

against whooping cough (see under Adverse Effects).

Immunisation with adsorbed pertussis vaccine produced higher titres of agglutinins than did plain vaccine; there was no obvious difference in response between those who received the 3 doses at intervals of 1 to 2 months, starting at 3 to 4 months of age, and those in whom the third dose followed 6 months after the second.— N. W. Preston *et al.*, *J. Hyg., Camb.*, 1974, *73*, 119, per *J. Am. med. Ass.*, 1974, *230*, 1469.

The use of pertussis vaccine, in reduced dosage, in adults during a hospital epidemic of whooping cough. Of 286 volunteers 77% showed a fourfold rise in pertussis agglutinins. Reactions to the vaccine were common.— C. C. Linnemann *et al.*, *Lancet*, 1975, *2*, 540. See also T. L. Kurt and A. S. Yeager (letter), *New Engl. J. Med.*, 1978, *299*, 492.

A report of 119 patients with whooping cough; 66% of those over 3 months of age had incomplete immunisation and 41% had no immunisation. There was complete immunisation in 34% of the patients. Pertussis vaccine was considered to be effective although not completely so.— T. T. Salmi *et al.* (letter), *Lancet*, 1975, *2*, 811.

During an outbreak of whooping cough in rural Shetland the incidence of the disease was similar in those who had been immunised and in those, aged under 3 years 3 months, who had not been immunised.— R. K. Ditchburn, *Br. med. J.*, 1979, *1*, 1601.

Evidence from the 1978 whooping-cough epidemic in Hertfordshire indicated that immunisation provides more than 90% protection.— M. A. Church, *Lancet*, 1979, *2*, 188. A similar report.— N. W. Preston, *Lancet*, 1976, *1*, 1065.

In a study of 658 children, pertussis vaccination reduced the incidence of whooping cough and the severity and duration of the disease.— P. R. Grob *et al.*, *Br. med. J.*, 1981, *282*, 1925.

An epidemic of whooping cough associated with a low acceptance of pertussis vaccine.— Report from the Swansea Research Unit of the Royal College of General Practitioners, *Br. med. J.*, 1981, *282*, 23. See also E. Miller *et al.* (letter), *Lancet*, 1980, *1*, 718; R. Pollard, *Lancet*, 1980, *1*, 1180.

Proprietary Preparations

Pertussis Vaccine Wellcome *(Wellcome, UK)*. A brand of Pertussis Vaccine containing not less than 4 units and not more than 20 000 million organisms in each 0.5-ml dose, with thiomersal 0.01%.

7986-y

Plague Vaccine *(B.P. 1973)*. Plague/Vac.

A sterile suspension of suitable killed strains of the capsulated form of *Pasteurella pestis* (=*Yersinia pestis*). It contains 3000 million bacteria (*P. pestis*) in 1 ml and 0.5% of phenol. Formaldehyde solution may be used to inactivate the bacteria.
Store at 2° to 10° and avoid freezing. Protect from light.

7987-j

Plague Vaccine *(U.S.P.)*.

A sterile suspension of formaldehyde-killed *Yersinia pestis*. Potency is assessed by comparison with a reference substance.
A whitish turbid liquid, almost odourless or with a slight odour of the preservative.
Store at 2° to 8° and avoid freezing. The expiration date is not later than 18 months after release from manufacturer's cold storage.

Adverse Effects and Precautions. As for Vaccines, p.1586.
Local and general reactions of moderate severity sometimes occur, but usually subside after 1 or 2 days.

Uses. Plague Vaccine is used for active immunisation against plague in those occupationally exposed to the organism and in workers in infected areas when normal precautionary measures are not possible.
Plague Vaccine is administered by intramuscular injection; the initial dose is usually 0.5 ml, and is followed 4 weeks later by a second dose, with a third dose (40% of the original dose) 4 to 12 weeks later. Three doses at weekly intervals afford some protection. Two booster doses may be given at 6-monthly intervals, with further doses every 1 to 2 years.

The effectiveness of live or inactivated plague vaccines was not well established. They might reduce morbidity and mortality in bubonic plague but not in pneumonic plague. Vaccines conferred immunity which lasted not longer than 6 months; revaccination was necessary to maintain immunisation.— *Tech. Rep. Ser. Wld Hlth Org. No. 447*, 1970.

Plague surveillance and control.— *Chronicle Wld Hlth Org.*, 1980, *34*, 139.

Manufacturers
Cutter, USA.

In Great Britain supplies are available on a named-patient basis from *Cutter.*

7988-z

Pneumococcal Vaccine

A sterile preparation of the polysaccharide capsular antigens from 14 serotypes of *Streptococcus pneumoniae*. It contains in each dose (usually 0.5 ml) 50 μg of the polysaccharide from each of the 14 serotypes. **Store** at 2° to 8°.

Adverse Effects. As for Vaccines, p.1586.
Erythema, soreness, and possibly induration may occur at the injection site. Fever and, rarely, allergic reactions have occurred.

Pneumococcal vaccine, polyvalent (Pneumovax), was administered to over 13 000 elderly individuals. Mild reactions at the injection site were reported by about 5% of patients and mild febrile reactions occurred in less than 1%.— N. J. Fiumara and G. E. Waterman, *Curr. ther. Res.*, 1979, *25*, 185.

Reports of acute febrile reactions.— G. Uhl *et al.* (letter), *New Engl. J. Med.*, 1978, *299*, 1318; E. P. Gabor and M. Seeman, *J. Am. med. Ass.*, 1979, *242*, 2208.

Hypersensitivity in 2 patients.— K. Nelson *et al.*, *Sth. med. J.*, 1980, *73*, 264.

Precautions. As for Vaccines, p.1586.
Pneumococcal vaccine should not be given to patients with febrile illness, or to patients with Hodgkin's disease after chemotherapy or irradiation.
Care should be exercised if it is given to patients with severe cardiac or pulmonary impairment, or to those who have suffered pneumonia during the past 3 years.
Its use is not recommended during pregnancy.

Pneumococcal vaccine failed to protect a 46-year-old man with defective immunoglobulin synthesis associated with chemotherapy for chronic lymphocytic leukaemia.— M. Rytel (letter), *Lancet*, 1978, *2*, 1317.

Two patients with angioimmunoblastic lymphadenopathy in a quiescent phase both had sudden reactivation of their disease after immunisation with polyvalent pneumococcal vaccine.— P. Schulman *et al.* (letter), *Lancet*, 1979, *2*, 1141.

Relapse of 2 patients with thrombocytopenia after pneumococcal or influenza vaccination.— J. G. Kelton, *J. Am. med. Ass.*, 1981, *245*, 369.

Uses. Of the many serotypes of *Streptococcus pneumoniae* the 14 from which antigens are obtained for pneumococcal vaccine are considered to cause about 80% of pneumococcal disease.
The use of pneumococcal vaccine may be considered in those at increased risk from infection with *Streptococcus pneumoniae*—those who have undergone splenectomy, those with splenic dysfunction such as sickle-cell anaemia, those, especially the elderly, with cardiac, pulmonary, hepatic, or renal impairment or diabetes, and those in closed communities.
An antibody response develops by the third week, and probably lasts some years.
A single dose is given by subcutaneous or intramuscular injection, and should not be repeated within 3 years.

Reviews and discussions of the use of pneumococcal vaccine.— *Morb. Mortal.*, 1978, *27*, 25 (The American Public Health Service Advisory Committee on Immunization Practice); *Med. Lett.*, 1978, *20*, 13; K. Hales and S. L. Barriere, *Am. J. Hosp. Pharm.*, 1979, *36*, 773; *Lancet*, 1980, *1*, 240; *Drug & Ther. Bull.*, 1980, *18*, 23; *Med. Lett.*, 1980, *22*, 114; A. M. Emmerson, *J. antimicrob. Chemother.*, 1980, *6*, 301; *Lancet*, 1981, *1*, 251.

Antibody production was satisfactory in 92% of persons given a 14-valent pneumococcal vaccine; the incidence of pneumonia was reduced by 76 to 92%. Children under 2 years of age might not respond satisfactorily to some of the capsular types. The duration of immunity was not yet known; booster injections at 1 year (not considered necessary) caused increased erythema and induration at the injection site.— M. R. Hilleman *et al.*, *Bull. Wld Hlth Org.*, 1978, *56*, 371.

Discussion on the limited acceptance of pneumococcal vaccine.— R. H. Pantell and T. J. Stewart, *J. Am. med. Ass.*, 1979, *241*, 2272. See also R. Austrian, *Am. J. Med.*, 1979, *67*, 547. A review of the use of pneumococcal vaccine concluded that there was currently no evidence to support widespread pneumococcal vaccination in the USA.— J. V. Hirschmann and B. A. Lipsky, *J. Am. med. Ass.*, 1981, *246*, 1428.

A discussion on the need for uniformity in the capsular polysaccharides and for a single polyvalent pneumococcal vaccine.— Austrian R. *et al.* (letter), *Lancet*, 1980, *1*, 1354.

Findings which suggest that immunisation of mothers with pneumococcal vaccine in an attempt to increase maternal antibody to type III group B streptococcus is unlikely to prevent neonatal infection caused by this organism.— C. J. Baker *et al.*,, *New Engl. J. Med.*, 1980, *303*, 173.

Findings in the high-risk groups of patients for which pneumococcal vaccine is recommended suggest that the efficacy of the vaccine may be considerably less in children and in patients with underlying disease than in the generally healthy adults previously studied.— C. V. Broome *et al.*, *New Engl. J. Med.*, 1980, *303*, 549. Comments.— R. Austrian, *ibid.*, 578; N. A. Halsey and F. J. Mather (letter), *ibid.*, 1981, *304*, 116; A. J. Ammann (letter), *ibid.* Reply.— C. V. Broome *et al.* (letter), *ibid.*

Second injections of pneumococcal vaccine had been given to several hundred children whose antibody responses were smaller than those of adults; only mild reactions were seen. This could be expected to apply to older patients with impaired responses.— P. H. Makela (letter), *Lancet*, 1981, *1*, 496.

Further references.— P. Smit *et al.*, *J. Am. med. Ass.*, 1977, *238*, 2613; J. O. Klein and E. A. Mortimer, *Pediatrics*, 1978, *61*, 321; M. J. Cowan *et al.*, *Pediatrics*, 1978, *62*, 721; M. R. Jacobs *et al.*, *New Engl. J. Med.*, 1978, *299*, 735; G. W. Fischer *et al.*, *Lancet*, 1979, *1*, 75; I. D. Riley *et al.*, *Archs Dis. Childh.*, 1981, *56*, 354.

Asplenic patients. Polyvalent pneumococcal vaccine should be given to all patients with impaired splenic function. In addition, continuous antibiotic prophylaxis should be used after splenectomy up to the age of 5 years.— A. J. Ammann and L. K. Diamond (letter), *New Engl. J. Med.*, 1978, *299*, 778.

A report of vaccine-type pneumococcal pneumonia developing in an asplenic patient 20 months after vaccination with polyvalent pneumococcal vaccine.— G. S. Giebink *et al.*, *J. Am. med. Ass.*, 1979, *241*, 2736.

A proposal for a multicentre trial of pneumococcal vaccine in asplenic patients.— P. M. Emerson *et al.* (letter), *Lancet*, 1979, *2*, 1191.

Reduced antibody response to 8 pneumococcal polysaccharides of a 9-valent vaccine in splenectomised patients, when assessed by enzyme-linked immunoabsorbent assay.— S. W. Hosea *et al.*, *Lancet*, 1981, *1*, 804.

Hodgkin's disease. Significant antibody response was obtained in all of 27 patients with Hodgkin's disease given polyvalent pneumococcal vaccine before radiotherapy and/or chemotherapy regardless of whether the vaccine was given before or after splenectomy, and only one of the 27 patients has had a serious pneumococcal infection since the project started in February 1978. Administration of a polyvalent pneumococcal vaccine (14 types) is therefore recommended for all patients with Hodgkin's disease, to be given before or after splenectomy, but before specific immunosuppressive therapy is started.— J. E. Addiego *et al.* (preliminary communication), *Lancet*, 1980, *2*, 450.

Reports showing an absence of antibody response after radiotherapy and/or chemotherapy.— G. R. Siber *et al.*, *New Engl. J. Med.*, 1978, *299*, 442; E. Cadman *et al.* (letter), *New Engl. J. Med.*, 1978, *299*, 1317; D. R. Minor *et al.*, *Ann. intern. Med.*, 1979, *90*, 887. See also A. M. Levine *et al.*, *Blood*, 1979, *54*, 1171.

Diabetes. Adequate antibody response to pneumococcal vaccine in diabetic patients.— E. A. Friedman *et al.*, *J. Am. med. Ass.*, 1980, *244*, 2310; T. R. Beam *et al.*, *ibid.*, 2621. See also J. M. Moss, *ibid.*, *243*, 2301.

Lupus erythematosus. In a double-blind study in 40 patients with systemic lupus erythematosus there was a significant increase in antibody concentrations after polyvalent pneumococcal vaccine though the concentrations were lower in treated patients than in controls.— J. H. Klippel *et al.*, *Arthritis Rheum.*, 1979, *22*, 1321. See also M. P. Jarrett *et al.*, *ibid.*, 1980, *23*, 1287.

Myeloma. The possible value of pneumococcal vaccine in patients with multiple myeloma.— H. M. Lazarus *et al.*, *Am. J. Med.*, 1980, *69*, 419.

Otitis media. A controlled study of the efficacy of 14-valent pneumococcal vaccine in children aged 3 months to 6 years who had had one or more attacks of otitis media. The pneumococcal vaccine was given to 500 children while another 327 received a control vaccine (*Haemophilus influenzae* type b capsular polysaccharide). The pneumococcal vaccine provided no protection to infants aged less than 6 months but in those over 6 months of age protection of the order of 50 to 60% was obtained. It was somewhat better in those aged over 2 years than in the younger group.— P. H. Mäkelä *et al.*, *Lancet*, 1980, *2*, 547. Comment.— G. A. Filice (letter), *ibid.*, 1248. Reply.— P. H. Mäkelä and P. Karma (letter), *ibid.*, 1981, *1*, 152.

Renal failure. Adequate antibody response to pneumococcal vaccine in patients with azotaemia and those on dialysis.— E. A. Friedman *et al.*, *J. Am. med. Ass.*, 1980, *244*, 2310.

A report of the failure of pneumococcal vaccine to prevent *Streptococcus pneumoniae* sepsis in two 4-year-old children with the nephrotic syndrome.— W. A. Primack *et al.* (letter), *Lancet*, 1979, *2*, 1192.

Sickle-cell anaemia. During a 2-year period following immunisation with octavalent pneumococcal-polysaccharide vaccine none of 77 children with sickle-cell disease developed *Streptococcus pneumoniae* infection whereas 8 of 106 similar control patients did.— A. J. Ammann, *New Engl. J. Med.*, 1977, *297*, 897.

A 3-year-old boy with sickle-cell disease died from pneumococcal septicaemia despite immunisation with 14-valent pneumococcal vaccine (Pneumovax) about 2½ months earlier.— G. D. Overturf *et al.* (letter), *New Engl. J. Med.*, 1979, *300*, 143. Failure in 2 further patients.— V. I. Ahonkhai *et al.*, *New Engl. J. Med.*, 1979, *301*, 26.

Eight children, all except 1 under 2 years of age, with sickle-cell anaemia, were given a single dose of pneumococcal vaccine. Antibody responses were measured for 12 of the 14 serotypes; a twofold or greater response was achieved in 60 of the 96 concentrations.— G. R. Buchanan and G. Schiffman, *J. Pediat.*, 1980, *96*, 264.

Sjögren's syndrome. A controlled study against placebo in 32 patients with Sjögren's syndrome indicated that pneumococcal vaccine elevated antibody concentrations against the 12 capsular serotypes measured. Concentrations fell but generally remained above baseline values at 6 months. The disease was not exacerbated.— J. Karsh *et al.*, *Arthritis Rheum.*, 1980, *23*, 1294.

Proprietary Preparations

Pneumovax *(Morson, UK).* Pneumococcal vaccine, containing in each 0.5-ml syringe 50 µg of each polysaccharide type derived from the capsules of 14 strains of pneumococci, with phenol 0.25%. (Also available as Pneumovax in *USA*).

Other Proprietary Names

Pnu-imune *(USA).*

7989-c

Inactivated Poliomyelitis Vaccine *(B.P., Eur. P.).*

Poliomyelitis Vaccine (Inactivated); Poliomyelitis Vaccine (Killed); Vaccinum Poliomyelitidis Inactivatum; Pol/Vac (Inact).

NOTE. This vaccine is sometimes called Salk vaccine.

A sterile aqueous suspension of suitable strains of poliomyelitis virus, types 1, 2, and 3, grown in cultures of monkey kidney tissue and inactivated by a suitable method. It may contain minimal amounts of permitted antibiotics and preservatives.

It is a clear liquid; if phenol red has been used in its production, it has a reddish tinge. It is assayed with respect to its ability to promote the production of neutralising antibodies to each of the 3 types of virus.

Store at 2° to 8° and avoid freezing. Protect from light. Under these conditions it may be expected to retain its potency for at least 18 months.

7990-s

Poliovirus Vaccine Inactivated *(U.S.P.).*

A sterile aqueous suspension of poliomyelitis virus, types 1, 2, and 3, grown in cultures of monkey kidney tissue and inactivated. It may contain suitable antimicrobial agents. It is standardised with respect to its ability to promote the production of neutralising antibodies to each of the 3 types of virus.

A clear yellowish or reddish liquid which may have the odour of the preservative.

Store at 2° to 8°. The expiration date is not later than 1 year after release from manufacturer's cold storage.

Adverse Effects. As for Vaccines, p.1586.

Local reactions are generally infrequent. Thrombocytopenia, convulsions, and encephalopathy have been reported.

The increased incidence of subacute sclerosing panencephalitis in New Zealand between 1956–66 might have been associated with the poliomyelitis vaccination programme.— D. M. Baguley and G. L. Glasgow, *Lancet*, 1973, *2*, 763. Comment.— *ibid.*, 772. A report of over 60 patients with subacute sclerosing panencephalitis who had been reimmunised with poliomyelitis vaccine.— O. Kolar (letter), *ibid.*, 1082. There was no association in South Africa where the Sabin vaccine rather than the Salk vaccine was used.— A. Kipps *et al.* (letter), *ibid.*, 1388.

Pregnancy and the neonate. Two women who were vaccinated against poliomyelitis during pregnancy gave birth to infants with flaccid paralysis and other birth defects.— H. E. Thelander (letter), *J. Am. med. Ass.*, 1966, *198*, 791.

Data derived from a cohort of 50 897 pregnancies showed that the rate of stillbirth among women who received killed polio vaccine during the first 4 months of pregnancy was 20% greater than the rate among other women.— D. Slone *et al.*, *Clin. Pharmac. Ther.*, 1973, *14*, 648.

Of 50 282 children born to mothers monitored by the Collaborative Perinatal Project 9222 were found to have been exposed to vaccines, and possibly other drugs, at some time during the first 4 months of the pregnancy. Although no association between malformations and exposure to vaccines in general was found a slight suggestion of association between poliomyelitis vaccine (inactivated) and malignant tumours and between poliomyelitis vaccine (oral) and gastro-intestinal malformations especially malrotation of the intestine was noted.— O. P. Heinonen *et al.*, *Birth Defects and Drugs in Pregnancy*, Littleton MA, Publishing Sciences Group, 1977, p. 314.

Precautions. As for Vaccines, p.1586.

Uses. Inactivated Poliomyelitis Vaccine is used for active immunisation against poliomyelitis, though the live oral vaccine is generally preferred. It is given in 3 doses administered by subcutaneous or intramuscular injection. The first dose is followed 4 to 6 weeks later by the second dose and the third dose follows after an interval of 6 or more months. Some regimens consist of 4 injections, the first 3 at 4 to 6 week intervals and the fourth 6 to 12 months later.

It may be given to patients with immune deficiency diseases and those undergoing immunosuppressive therapy, for whom the use of oral poliomyelitis vaccine is contra-indicated.

It is a component of Diphtheria, Tetanus, and Poliomyelitis Vaccine and of Diphtheria, Tetanus, Pertussis, and Poliomyelitis Vaccine.

Two doses of poliomyelitis vaccine, adsorbed on calcium phosphate, given at the age of 5 and 6 months, conferred protection on 86 to 92% of 167 children, with protection against the 3 types of virus in 81%; protection was reinforced by a third dose at the age of 17 months. The procedure offered advantages for mass vaccination in the tropics.— P. Sureau *et al.*, *Bull. Wld Hlth Org.*, 1977, *55*, 739.

For references to the respective advantages and disadvantages of inactivated poliomyelitis vaccine, see Poliomyelitis Vaccine, Live (Oral), p.1603.

Further references.— J. Salk and D. Salk, *Science*, 1977, *195*, 834; O. Ruuskanen *et al.*, *Acta paediat. scand.*, 1980, *69*, 397.

Preparations

Supplies are available in England, Wales, and Northern Ireland through the Department of Health and Social Security, and in Scotland through the Scottish Health Service.

Proprietary Names

Poliomyelitis Vaccine (Purified)*(Connaught, USA).*

7991-w

Poliomyelitis Vaccine, Live (Oral) *(B.P., Eur. P.).*

Poliomyelitis Vaccine (Live); Vaccinum Poliomyelitidis Perorale; Pol/Vac (Oral).

NOTE. This vaccine is sometimes called Sabin vaccine.

An aqueous suspension of suitable live attenuated strains of poliomyelitis virus, types 1, 2, or 3, grown in suitable tissue cultures; it may contain any one of the 3 virus types or combinations of them. It may contain a stabilising agent.

It is a clear liquid which, if phenol red has been used in its production, has a reddish tinge. It is standardised for virus titre which is not less than 3×10^5 CCID50 for types 1 and 3 and not less than 1×10^5 CCID50 for type 2.

Store at a temperature not exceeding −20°. Protect from light. When thawed and stored at 0° to 4°, it should be used within 3 months; when exposed to higher temperatures it should be used within a few hours. When a stabiliser such as magnesium chloride or sucrose is present the periods of storage may be extended to 6 months at 0° to 4° and to 2 weeks at temperatures up to 25°.

7992-e

Poliovirus Vaccine Live Oral *(U.S.P.).*

A preparation of one or a combination of the 3 types of suitable live attenuated polioviruses, grown in cultures of monkey kidney tissue or of suitable human tissue. Monovalent vaccine contains not less than $10^{5.3}$ to 10^6 TCID50 per dose Trivalent vaccine contains not less than $10^{5.4}$ to $10^{6.4}$ TCID50 for type 1, not less than $10^{4.5}$ to $10^{5.5}$ for type 2, and not less than $10^{5.2}$ to $10^{6.2}$ for type 3.

A clear colourless yellowish or red-tinged liquid or a frozen solid.

Store at 2° to 8° or in the frozen state. The expiration date is not later than 30 days (liquid vaccine) or 1 year (frozen vaccine) after release from manufacturer's cold storage. Liquid vaccine should be used within 7 days of first opening the container.

Adverse Effects. As for Vaccines, p.1586.

Side-effects occur very rarely and include diarrhoea and skin rashes of an allergic type. Neurological disorders have been reported following the administration of oral poliomyelitis vaccine. Paralytic poliomyelitis has been attributed to the vaccine.

Following mass vaccination of children in Japan with Sabin vaccine in 1961 the incidence of poliomyelitis fell dramatically. Between 1962 and 1968 among over 11 million newborn infants vaccinated, 36 developed vaccine-related poliomyelitis.— T. Takatsu *et al.*, *Bull. Wld Hlth Org.*, 1973, *49*, 129.

The findings in a WHO Consultative Study in 8 countries at the end of the first 5 years of an international investigation into the relation between acute persisting spinal paralysis and oral polio vaccine. Marked differences were noted between countries and a single cause could not be identified although the quality of the vaccine played an important role. It was confirmed that oral poliomyelitis vaccines made from the Sabin attenuated strains are among the safest vaccines in use.— F. A. Assaad *et al.*, *Bull. Wld Hlth Org.*, 1976, *53*, 319.

About 242 million doses of oral poliomyelitis vaccine

were distributed in the years 1969–78; 76 cases of paralysis were reported—18 in healthy recipients, 47 in healthy close contacts, and 11 in persons with immune deficiencies.— *Morbid. Mortal.*, 1979, *28*, 510.

Pregnancy and the neonate. See under Inactivated Poliomyelitis Vaccine, p.1602.

Precautions. As for Vaccines, p.1586.

Poliomyelitis Vaccine, Live (Oral) should not generally be administered during periods of illness or indifferent health and it should not be given to patients with diarrhoea or gastro-intestinal dysfunction. It should not be given to patients with immune deficiency diseases such as hypogammaglobulinaemia, or those with leukaemia, lymphoma, or generalised malignancy, or to patients receiving corticosteroids, immunosuppressants, or radiation. It use is generally considered to be contra-indicated during the first trimester of pregnancy. It should not generally be administered within 3 or 4 weeks of another vaccine containing live micro-organisms.

The slight risk of poliomyelitis being induced by the oral vaccine could not be ruled out, but was too small to warrant a restriction of the vaccination programme in Great Britain.— *Immunisation Against Infectious Disease*, London, Department of Health and Social Security, 1972.

A report of chronic poliomyelitis in an immunodeficient child secondary to vaccination with trivalent oral poliomyelitis vaccine. Immunodeficiency should be diagnosed as early as possible so that live-virus vaccines could be avoided.— L. E. Davis *et al.*, *New Engl. J. Med.*, 1977, *297*, 241.

Infection from vaccinated contacts. Because of the occasional occurrence of vaccine-related poliomyelitis, the whole family should be treated together, for primary or reinforcing doses.— *Br. med. J.*, 1978, *2*, 764.

Pregnancy and the breast-feeding infant. A pregnant woman travelling to a developing area should be immunised against poliomyelitis; the risk of the disease was far greater than any risk to the foetus.— M. M. Levine *et al.*, *Lancet*, 1974, *2*, 34.

There is no reason to restrict breast-feeding in infants given oral poliomyelitis vaccine.— *Br. med. J.*, 1979, *1*, 27.

Use in hypogammaglobulinaemia. About a third of 176 patients with primary hypogammaglobulinaemia were given live vaccines, including poliomyelitis vaccine, while being treated with normal immunoglobulin injection. There were no apparent ill-effects. It was recommended that immunisation should only be started after careful consideration and after ensuring that normal circulating lymphocytes and normal delayed skin hypersensitivity were present.— Report of an MRC Working-party, *Lancet*, 1969, *1*, 163.

Use in systemic lupus erythematosus. Vaccination and immunisation against poliomyelitis could be carried out if necessary in patients with systemic lupus erythematosus which was controlled, but should be withheld in those with active disease and those on large doses of steroids.— N. R. Rowell, *Br. med. J.*, 1969, *2*, 427.

Uses. Poliomyelitis Vaccine, Live (Oral) is used for active immunisation against poliomyelitis. It stimulates the formation of antibodies in the blood and also produces a local resistance in the intestinal tissues to infection with virulent poliomyelitis viruses. It is commonly given as a trivalent single vaccine containing the 3 virus types. The efficacy of Poliomyelitis Vaccine, Live (Oral) is reported to be reduced in some tropical countries, possibly because of the interference of other enteroviruses.

When trivalent vaccine is used, 3 doses are administered. In infants the first dose may be given at the age of 3 months, the second dose 6 to 8 weeks later, and the third dose after an interval of 4 to 6 months. Unvaccinated parents should be offered vaccination at the same time as their infants.

Reinforcing doses of Poliomyelitis Vaccine, Live (Oral) are recommended at school entry and at 15 to 19 years of age. Further reinforcing doses are necessary only in adults exposed to infection.

On the occurrence of a single case of paralytic poliomyelitis, a dose of Poliomyelitis Vaccine, Live (Oral) is recommended for all persons in the neighbourhood, regardless of whether they have previously been immunised.

The incidence of paralytic poliomyelitis in Italy was not reduced after 4 years in which a mass vaccination programme was carried out using inactivated poliomyelitis vaccine. A programme of vaccination was then carried out with oral poliomyelitis vaccine, initially using types 1, 2, and 3 Sabin vaccines, and later a trivalent Sabin vaccine, and 67.3% of the child population of ages 4 months to 6 years were vaccinated. The incidence of paralytic poliomyelitis, which before vaccination had been about 6 per 100 000 total population, fell to 0.16 per 100 000, and to 0.04 per 100 000 in those areas where the percentage of children vaccinated was highest.— A. Giovanardi, *J. Am. med. Ass.*, 1969, *209*, 525.

Six of 39 nursery schoolchildren who had been given oral poliomyelitis vaccine usually in 3 doses had antibodies to only 1 poliomyelitis virus type, 15 had antibodies to 2 types, and 18 to all 3 types.— D. Reid *et al.*, *Lancet*, 1973, *2*, 899. See also C. M. Rasmussen *et al.*, *Am. J. Dis. Child.*, 1973, *126*, 465, per *J. Am. med. Ass.*, 1973, *226*, 579.

Following a study of 78 infants it was concluded that owing to poor seroconversion rates the primary course of immunisation with oral polio vaccine for infants in developing countries, especially those in the tropics, should consist of at least 5 doses of oral polio vaccine given at intervals of 4 weeks or more.— T. J. John, *Br. med. J.*, 1976, *1*, 812. See also T. J. John *et al.*, *Bull. Wld Hlth Org.*, 1976, *54*, 115. Conversion-rates of 71 to 96% (despite low-potency vaccine) in children in India given 3 doses of oral poliomyelitis vaccine at approximately monthly intervals.— T. J. John *et al.*, *Br. med. J.*, 1980, *281*, 542. A study indicating that diphtheria, tetanus, pertussis, and poliomyelitis vaccine may be used in the routine immunisation of infants in developing countries. The immune response to injectable poliomyelitis vaccine was better than that achieved with oral vaccine.— R. Krishnan *et al.*, *ibid.*, 1982, *284*, 164.

The Institute of Medicine Committee for the Study of Poliomyelitis Vaccines unanimously recommend the continued use of oral poliomyelitis vaccine as the principal vaccine. Inactivated vaccine should be available for persons with heightened susceptibility to infection, including immunodeficient children and their siblings and immunodepressed persons, adults undergoing initial vaccination (if time permits) and travelling to areas with a high incidence of disease, and for those preferring the inactivated vaccine.— E. O. Nightingale, *New Engl. J. Med.*, 1977, *297*, 249. Comment.— D. T. Karzon, *ibid.*, 275. Further references supporting the use of oral poliomyelitis vaccine.— *Lancet*, 1977, *2*, 21; D. M. McLean, *Can. med. Ass. J.*, 1977, *116*, 7.

Discussions of the choice between inactivated or live poliomyelitis vaccine.— *Br. med. J.*, 1978, *2*, 845; J. L. Melnick, *Bull. Wld Hlth Org.*, 1978, *56*, 21.

Further references to poliomyelitis vaccination.— R. D. Krugman *et al.*, *Pediatrics*, 1977, *60*, 80; D. Metselaar *et al.*, *Bull. Wld Hlth Org.*, 1977, *55*, 747; D. Metselaar *et al.*, *ibid.*, 755; Y. E. Cossart, *Br. med. J.*, 1977, *1*, 1621. See also *ibid.*, 1617; *Lancet*, 1978, *2*, 1030; *Br. med. J.*, 1980, *280*, 1555.

Herpes. Of 23 patients with recurrent herpes simplex 74% were completely relieved of attacks, without relapse for 1 to 4 years, after receiving oral poliomyelitis vaccine 4 drops per month for 3 months.— A. Tager, *Harefuah*, 1974, *86*, 363, per *J. Am. med. Ass.*, 1974, *228*, 1729.

Beneficial results with oral poliomyelitis vaccine in patients with recurrent herpes infections.— J. Garrel *et al.*, *Nouv. Presse méd.*, 1979, *8*, 47.

Proprietary Preparations

Merieux Poliomyelitis Vaccine (Oral) *(Mérieux, Fr.: Servier, UK).* Poliomyelitis Vaccine, Live (Oral), containing virus types 1, 2, and 3, grown in monkey kidney-cell cultures; stabilised with magnesium chloride and albumin. It may contain traces of neomycin and penicillin. *Dose.* 0.5 ml from a single-dose ampoule or 2 drops (0.1 ml) from a multidose vial.

Poliomyelitis Vaccine (Oral) *(Smith Kline & French, UK).* Poliomyelitis Vaccine, Live (Oral), grown in monkey kidney-cell cultures; stabilised with magnesium chloride. It contains traces of neomycin sulphate. *Dose.* 3 drops.

Poliomyelitis Vaccine (Oral) Wellcome *(Wellcome, UK).* Poliomyelitis Vaccine, Live (Oral), containing virus types 1, 2, and 3, grown in monkey kidney-cell cultures. It may contain traces of polymyxin, neomycin, kanamycin, penicillin, and streptomycin. *Dose.* 3 drops.

Other Proprietary Names

Orimune *(Lederle, USA).*

7993-l

Pseudomonas Vaccine

Vaccines prepared from *Pseudomonas* spp. have been given to patients suffering from burns to prevent the development of overwhelming pseudomonal infections. A 16-component vaccine (PEV-01) prepared from 16 serotypes of *Pseudomonas aeruginosa* is under study.

Pseudomonas vaccine given to 176 patients with various neoplasms reduced the fatality-rate from pseudomonas infections when compared with a control group of 185.— L. S. Young, *Ann. intern. Med.*, 1973, *79*, 518. See also G. N. Hortobagyi *et al.*, *Cancer Immunol. & Immunother.*, 1978, *4*, 201 (heptavalent vaccine).

The preparation and characterisation of a 16-component *Pseudomonas* vaccine.— J. M. Miler *et al.*, *J. med. Microbiol.*, 1977, *10*, 19.

Results of 2 controlled studies at Birmingham Accident Hospital, England, and one at Safdarjang Hospital, New Delhi, India, indicated that a polyvalent pseudomonas vaccine had a beneficial effect in protecting patients with extensive burns, from infection with *Pseudomonas aeruginosa*. *Ps. aeruginosa* was not found in the blood cultures of any of the vaccinated patients in the trial; only one of 31 blood cultures from vaccinated patients grew a Gram-negative bacterium (*Klebsiella aerogenes*), compared with 20 of 42 blood cultures from unvaccinated patients which grew Gram-negative bacteria. *Ps. aeruginosa* and *Kleb. aerogenes* were the 2 main species of bacteria found in blood cultures of unvaccinated patients, suggesting that the pseudomonas vaccine had also reduced the likelihood of *Kleb. aerogenes* septicaemia. Death from *Ps. aeruginosa* is uncommon in the Birmingham Unit, but in the New Delhi Unit, where it is common, the mortality in adults was reduced from 13 of 32 (40.6%) to 2 of 30 (6.6%) in the vaccinated group; in children it was reduced from 5 of 24 (20.8%) in the unvaccinated group to 1 of 21 (4.8%) in the vaccinated group.— R. J. Jones *et al.*, *Lancet*, 1979, *2*, 977.

Results of a controlled study at Safdarjang Hospital, New Delhi, involving 106 extensively burned children, indicated that passive immunisation with pseudomonas immunoglobulin (obtained from the plasma of healthy subjects vaccinated with the polyvalent pseudonomas vaccine, PEV-01) was superior in preventing death to pseudomonas vaccine and to combined immunoglobulin and vaccine. In the 173 adults in the study, however, vaccination seemed slightly more effective than passive immunisation, in preventing death. Deaths were 5 of 60 (8.3%) in vaccinated adults compared with 22 of 61 (36%) in unvaccinated controls.— R. J. Jones *et al.*, *Lancet*, 1980, *2*, 1263. Criticism.— B. Bose (letter), *ibid.*, 1981, *1*, 435.

Further references: J. E. Pennington, *J. infect. Dis.*, 1974, *130*, *Suppl.*, S159.

Manufacturers

Wellcome, UK.

7994-y

Rabies Antiserum *(B.P., Eur. P.).* Antirabies Serum; Immunoserum Antirabicum; Rab/Ser.

A sterile preparation containing the specific antiviral globulins that have the power of neutralising the virus of rabies. The strain of rabies virus used for the immunisation of the animals is a suitable 'fixed' strain prepared in animals of a different species from that which is used for the preparation of rabies vaccine.

It is an almost colourless or very faintly yellow liquid, free from turbidity, and almost odourless except for the odour of any added bactericide. It contains not less than 80 units per ml. pH 6 to 7.

Storage. As for Botulinum Antitoxin, p.1590.

The label states the animal source.

7995-j

Antirabies Serum *(U.S.P.).*

A sterile solution containing antiviral substances obtained from the blood or plasma of a healthy animal, usually the horse, that has been immunised by vaccine against rabies. It contains a suitable antimicrobial agent.

A faintly brownish, yellowish, or greenish clear

or slightly opalescent liquid, almost odourless or with a slight odour of the antimicrobial agent.

Store at 2° to 8°. The expiration date is not later than 2 years after release from manufacturer's cold storage.

The label states the animal source.

Units. 86.6 units of rabies antiserum, equine, are contained in approximately 86.6 mg in one ampoule of the first International Standard Preparation (1955).

Adverse Effects. As for Antisera, p.1587.

Rabies Antiserum is prepared from the serum of animals and reactions due to the injection of animal serum may occur.

Uses. Rabies Antiserum is given in a single dose of 40 units per kg body-weight with Rabies Vaccine (see p.1604) for the prevention of rabies in patients who have received bites from rabid animals or animals suspected of being rabid. Antirabies immunoglobulin injection is preferred.

For a brief discussion of the treatment of rabies with antiserum and vaccines, see A. D. Macrae, *Br. med. J.*, 1973, *1*, 604.

Proprietary Names

Antirabies Serum *(Sclavo, USA)*; Rabies Antiserum *(Lederle, USA)*.

In Great Britain supplies are available on a named-patient basis from the *Swiss Serum and Vaccine Institute, UK.*

7996-z

Rabies Vaccine *(B.P.)*. Antirabic Vaccine; Rab/Vac.

A sterile aqueous suspension of inactivated rabies virus; a suitable strain is grown in an approved cell culture. The vaccine may be issued as a liquid or as a freeze-dried solid which is reconstituted, immediately before use, by the addition of a suitable sterile liquid. The estimated potency is not less than 2.5 times that of the second International Reference Preparation (the assay is imprecise).

A clear liquid which may have a reddish colour if phenol red has been used in the preparation, or friable solid.

Store the liquid vaccine at 2° to 8° and avoid freezing. The dried vaccine is stored *in vacuo* or under nitrogen at 2° to 8°. Protect from light. Under these conditions the dried vaccine may be expected to retain its potency for at least 18 months.

7997-c

Rabies Vaccine *(U.S.P.)*.

A sterile preparation, in dried form, of killed fixed rabies virus obtained from infected duck embryos.

Store at 2° to 8°. The expiration date is not later than 18 months after release from manufacturer's cold storage.

By removing much non-essential protein the potency of duck-embryo rabies vaccine was increased 90-fold. Limited studies suggested antigenicity comparable with that of human diploid-cell vaccine.— K. R. Schell *et al.*, *J. biol. Stand.*, 1980, *8*, 97.

Units. 10 units are contained in approximately 49.45 mg of human diploid-cell rabies vaccine in one ampoule of the third International Reference Preparation (1978).

Adverse Effects. As for Vaccines, p.1586.

Most patients experience pain, erythema, and induration at the injection site after the use of duck-embryo vaccine; pruritus may occur. Fever, malaise, or myalgia may occur in about one-third of patients, usually after 5 to 8 doses. Anaphylactic reactions and lymphadenopathy may occur. Neuroparalytic reactions (transverse myelitis, neuropathy, or encephalopathy) have been reported.

Side-effects after human diploid-cell vaccine are considerably less common—erythema and induration may occur in about 10 to 25% of patients and fever in 1%; headache, nausea, abdominal pain, muscle aches, and dizziness may occur; neuroparalytic reactions do not appear to be a problem.

Neuroparalytic complications after the earlier brain-tissue vaccine were much more frequent than after duck-embryo vaccine.

Vaccinations against rabies provoked the onset of multiple sclerosis in a patient.— H. Miller *et al.*, *Br. med. J.*, 1967, *2*, 210.

In an estimated 424 000 patients receiving duck-embryo rabies vaccine in the USA from 1958 to 1971 there were 22 reports of anaphylaxis, 137 of minor transient neurological reactions, and 4 of transverse myelitis, 5 of neuropathy, and 4 of encephalopathy (2 fatal). In a prospective study in 116 patients receiving the vaccine after exposure local reactions were a constant feature; other reactions included regional adenopathy (18%), generalised adenopathy (3%), malaise, myalgia, fever, chills, and anaphylaxis (0.9%).— R. H. Rubin *et al.*, *Ann. intern. Med.*, 1973, *78*, 643.

Permanent and progressive neurological damage occurred in 2 veterinary surgeons following postexposure treatment with a brain-based rabies vaccine (Hempt vaccine).— H. D. Schoop and P. Rohrbach, *Dt. med. Wschr.*, 1974, *99*, 1923, per *Abstr. Hyg.*, 1975, *50*, 697.

Acute renal failure after rabies vaccine.— P. Stosiek *et al.*, *Dte GesundhWes.*, 1976, *31*, 262, per *Int. pharm. Abstr.*, 1976, *13*, 826.

Guillain-Barré syndrome after rabies vaccine produced on suckling mouse brain.— I. Vergara *et al.* (letter), *Archs Neurol., Chicago*, 1979, *36*, 254. After human diploid-cell vaccine.— E. Bøe and H. Nyland, *Scand. J. infect. Dis.*, 1980, *12*, 231.

Precautions. As for Vaccines, p.1586.

Corticosteroids and immunosuppressants may interfere with the development of antibodies; when their use is essential the serum should be tested for antibody response.

Uses. Rabies Vaccine is used, as part of postexposure treatment, for the prevention of rabies in patients who have been bitten by rabid animals or animals suspected of being rabid. Infection does not take place through unbroken skin but it is possible through uninjured mucous membranes and has been reported after the inhalation of virus in the laboratory.

Major bites (multiple bites or bites on the face, head, neck, or finger) or licks of the mucosa by an animal rabid or suspected of being rabid require immediate local attention to the wounds, a single dose of Rabies Antiserum (see p.1604) 40 units per kg body-weight or antirabies immunoglobulin injection 20 units per kg body-weight, followed by rabies vaccine. Treatment with vaccine should commence immediately, but at a different site. Treatment may be stopped if the animal remains healthy for 5 days or if laboratory examination of the killed animal proves negative.

Minor bites (covered areas of the arms, legs, or trunk) or licks of the skin, scratches, or abrasions by a rabid animal require treatment as for major bites. If the animal is suspected of being rabid the wound should receive local attention and a course of vaccine should be commenced and completed unless the animal proves to be healthy.

Various dose schedules for Rabies Vaccine are used. Human diploid-cell vaccine is now available and is the vaccine of choice—it produces a better immunological response and causes fewer side-effects—six injections are given intramuscularly or subcutaneously on days 0, 3, 7, 14, 30, and 90. For brain-tissue vaccine 14 daily doses are commonly given. For duck-embryo vaccine 14 or more daily doses may be given subcutaneously into the abdomen, lower back, or lateral aspect of the thigh. Some countries have adopted 7- to 10-day courses; such courses should only be used if studies have demonstrated adequate antibody concentrations. Reinforcing doses are recommended 10, 20, and 90 days after the completion of the initial course with brain-tissue or duck-embryo vaccine.

Persons exposed to a high risk of infection may be given two 1-ml intramuscular injections of diploid-cell vaccine 4 weeks apart, followed by a reinforcing dose 12 months later, and further doses every 2 to 3 years. An immunological response occurs in substantially all of those vaccinated. A schedule of 3 doses at days 0, 7, and 21 or 28 also affords immunity in practically all immunised subjects. Alternative regimens that have been used involve the use of two 1-ml subcutaneous injections of duck-embryo vaccine 6 weeks apart, followed by a reinforcing dose 6 months later, to provide active immunisation. Further reinforcing doses should be given every year. An immunological response usually occurs in about 80% of those vaccinated but if a suitable antibody response has not occurred within 1 month of the third dose, further reinforcing doses should be given. Schedules of 3 doses at 5- to 7-day intervals with a fourth dose one month later have also been used. Vaccines cultured on brain tissue are not recommended for this purpose.

Exposure to rabies following successful immunisation should be treated by a single dose of vaccine. Persons who have previously been immunised but whose antibody status is not known may be given a single dose on exposure with further doses 10, 20, and 90 days later; some authorities recommend the full immunisation programme in such patients.

Reviews and discussions of rabies and of the use of rabies vaccine before and after exposure.— C. Kaplan, *Br. J. clin. Pract.*, 1976, *30*, 208; *Br. med. J.*, 1976, *2*, 197; *Med. Lett.*, 1977, *19*, 43; M. Goulon and P. Gajdos, Neuromuscular diseases, in *Recent Advances in Intensive Therapy*, No. 1, I.M. Ledingham (Ed.), London, Churchill Livingstone, 1977, p. 159; S. D. Gardner, *Hlth Trends*, 1977, *9*, 35; K. G. Ferguson and V. A. Callcott-Stevens, *Can. med. Ass. J.*, 1977, *117*, 12; *Can. med. Ass. J.*, 1979, *120*, 1044; G. Dempster *et al.*, *Can. med. Ass. J.*, 1979, *120*, 1069; *Med. Lett.*, 1980, *22*, 93; *Morb. Mortal.*, 1980, *29*, 265 (Recommendations of the Immunization Practices Advisory Committee of the Center for Disease Control).

Rabies developed in a child 20 days after being bitten by a rabid bat and 2 days after completing a 14-day course of duck-embryo rabies vaccine. The child recovered after aggressive symptomatic treatment.— M. A. W. Hattwick *et al.*, *Ann. intern. Med.*, 1972, *76*, 931.

A discussion of the development of rabies vaccines, including: Fermi vaccine, partially inactivated, the use of which was now declining; Semple vaccine, from mammalian brain tissue, inactivated, and associated with a risk of encephalitis—modified Semple vaccines were being evaluated; vaccines produced in the brains of suckling animals, the brains of very young animals being low in myelin content and therefore in encephalitic potential—vaccines purified by centrifugation and chromatography had been used experimentally; Flury live vaccines developed in avian tissue and generally limited to use in animals; duck-embryo vaccine of comparatively low antigenic potency, but widely recommended and used; hamster kidney cell cultures used in animals; and a vaccine grown in human diploid cells highly antigenic with a reduced dose frequency, but difficult to produce in adequate potency on a large scale.— J. Crick, *Postgrad. med. J.*, 1973, *49*, 551.

The recommended treatment of all wounds involving possible exposure to rabies was to wash and flush the site of infection with soap and water, detergent, or water alone then to apply alcohol 40% to 70%, tincture or aqueous solutions of iodine, or, making sure that all soap had been removed, 0.1% solutions of quaternary ammonium compounds. Rabies antiserum should be injected in and around the wound. Rabies vaccine should be given daily for 14 consecutive days. It was recommended that booster doses of vaccine should be given to all patients 10, 20, and 90 days after the last daily dose of brain-tissue or duck-embryo vaccine to ensure the production and maintenance of high concentrations of serum-neutralising antibodies. The combined use of antiserum and vaccine was considered to be the best specific treatment for the postexposure prophylaxis of rabies in man.— Sixth Report of a WHO Expert Committee on Rabies, *Tech. Rep. Ser. Wld Hlth Org. No. 523*, 1973. These recommendations were endorsed.

Human diploid cell vaccine was the vaccine of choice and for postexposure prophylaxis 1 ml should be given intramuscularly on days 0, 3, 7, 14, 30 and 90.— *Memorandum on Rabies*, London, HM Stationery Office, 1977.

In a study of 177 persons receiving postexposure rabies prophylaxis 23% of those who received rabies antiserum plus a duck embryo vaccine failed to develop an adequate neutralising antibody response. Additional doses of the vaccine did not increase the percentage of persons who responded adequately to antiserum plus vaccine although they did improve the percentage of responders who received the vaccine alone. A dose of antiserum greater than that recommended (40 units per kg) was also associated with low antibody response as was the administration of corticosteroids during therapy. Persons under 15 years responded with better antibody titre to the combined therapy than did those over 15 despite the higher doses of antiserum used.— L. Corey *et al.*, *Ann. intern. Med.*, 1976, *85*, 170.

Comment on dumb rabies (paralytic rabies with absence of hydrophobia).— *Lancet*, 1978, *2*, 1031. See also R. P. Mills *et al.*, *Cent. Afr. J. Med.*, 1978, *24*, 115.

Because of the theoretical risk of person-to-person transmission, the Center for Disease Control will continue to recommend prophylaxis for persons exposed to human rabies.— L. J. Anderson *et al.* (letter), *New Engl. J. Med.*, 1980, *302*, 967.

Human diploid-cell vaccine. A human diploid cell vaccine was used in 45 patients bitten by rabid dogs and wolves. Rabies antiserum was also given to 44 patients initially and vaccine was given on days 0, 3, 7, 14, 30, and 90. No patient developed rabies.— M. Bahmanyar *et al.*, *J. Am. med. Ass.*, 1976, *236*, 2751.

In 8 volunteers given human diploid-cell rabies vaccine 1 ml intramuscularly on days 0, 3, 7, 14, 30, and 90 an antibody response was present in each by day 14. In 8 further volunteers and 3 patients given the vaccine similarly, and rabies immunoglobulin 20 units per kg body-weight intramuscularly on day 0, a response was evident by day 7 in the volunteers and in 2 of the patients. Combined treatment was recommended for patients at high risk.— E. K. Kuwert *et al.*, *J. biol. Stand.*, 1978, *6*, 211.

Neutralising antibody persisted one year later in persons given 3 doses of diploid-cell rabies vaccine, compared with half the persons originally given duck-embryo vaccine. All responded to a single booster dose of diploid-cell vaccine, with much higher antibody concentrations in those initially given diploid-cell vaccine.— E. I. Rosanoff and H. Tint, *Am. J. Epidem.*, 1979, *110*, 322.

Human diploid-cell rabies vaccine was given to 255 patients (132 with allergy to duck-embryo vaccine, 86 with inadequate response to duck-embryo vaccine, and 37 prior to exposure). Of 185 without antibody titres of 1:16 (considered adequate) all achieved titres of 1:16 after diploid-cell vaccine and most achieved titres of 1:50. Local reactions occurred at the injection site (28%); other reactions included headache, nausea, dizziness, and fever. No neuroparalytic reactions occurred and none had been confirmed after use of diploid-cell vaccine in more than 5000 patients.— L. J. Anderson *et al.*, *J. Am. med. Ass.*, 1980, *244*, 781.

References to the intradermal use of rabies vaccine.— F. Y. Aoki *et al.*, *Lancet*, 1975, *1*, 660 (high incidence of local reactions); P. Morgan *et al.*, *Bull. Pan Am. Hlth Org.*, 1978, *12*, 257; N. Ajjan *et al.*, *J. Am. med. Ass.*, 1980, *244*, 2528; J. Furlong and G. Lea (letter), *Lancet*, 1981, *1*, 1311; K. G. Nicholson *et al.*, *Lancet*, 1981, *2*, 915.

Further references mainly to human diploid-cell rabies vaccine: U. Shah *et al.*, *Br. med. J.*, 1976, *1*, 997; G. S. Turner *et al.*, *Lancet*, 1976, *1*, 1379; K. E. Nelson *et al.*, *J. Am. med. Ass.*, 1977, *238*, 218; K. G. Nicholson *et al.*, *J. infect. Dis.*, 1978, *137*, 783; S. A. Plotkin and T. Wiktor, *Pediatrics*, 1979, *63*, 219; K. G. Nicholson *et al.*, *J. infect. Dis.*, 1979, *140*, 176; *Lancet*, 1981, *1*, 1036.

Proprietary Preparations

Merieux Rabies Vaccine *(Mérieux, Fr.: Servier, UK)*. An inactivated rabies vaccine prepared from the Wistar PM/WI 38 1503-3M virus strain propagated in human diploid cells, and inactivated with propiolactone; supplied as powder for preparation before use in single-dose vials, with 1 ml of diluent. *Dose.* 1 ml.

Other Proprietary Names

Rabies Vaccine (duck-embryo)*(Lilly, USA)*.

7998-k

Rocky Mountain Spotted Fever Vaccine *(U.S.P.)*.

A sterile aqueous suspension of inactivated *Rickettsia rickettsii* prepared by growing the virus in the infected yolk sac and chorioallantoic membranes of embryonated chick eggs. It may be purified by chemical treatment and contains an antimicrobial agent. It is a slightly turbid white or slightly reddish liquid. **Store** at 2° to 8°. The expiration date is not later than 18 months after release from manufacturer's cold storage.

For active immunisation against Rocky Mountain spotted fever three 1-ml doses of vaccine have been administered subcutaneously at intervals of 7 to 10 days. Children under 12 years of age have been given 3 doses of 0.5 ml.

Comment on the ineffectiveness of an established Rocky Mountain spotted fever vaccine and development of a new vaccine.— T. H. Maugh, *Science*, 1978, *201*, 604. See also M. S. Ascher *et al.*, *J. infect. Dis.*, 1978, *138*, 217.

7999-a

Rubella and Mumps Virus Vaccine Live *(U.S.P.)*.

A bacterially sterile preparation of a suitable live strain of rubella virus (see Rubella Virus Vaccine Live, p.1605) and a suitable live strain of mumps virus (see Mumps Virus Vaccine Live, p.1599). It may contain suitable antimicrobial agents. Each labelled dose provides an immunising dose of each component. It is supplied as a freeze-dried vaccine which is reconstituted, immediately before use, by the addition of a suitable sterile liquid.

Store at 2° to 8°. Protect from light. The expiration date is about 1 year after manufacture.

Adverse Effects and Precautions. As for Rubella Vaccine, p.1605.

It must not be given to pregnant women and its use is not recommended in children aged less than 1 year.

A 20-month-old boy developed the Guillain-Barré syndrome, with ascending flaccid paralysis, 10 days after receiving mumps and rubella vaccine.— J. R. Gunderman, *Am. J. Dis. Child.*, 1973, *125*, 834, per *Int. pharm. Abstr.*, 1973, *10*, 892.

Uses. Rubella and Mumps Virus Vaccine Live is used for the concomitant active immunisation of children against mumps and rubella—see Mumps Virus Vaccine Live, p.1598, and Rubella Vaccine, Live, below.

In a study in 415 seronegative children given mumps and rubella vaccine, antibodies to mumps developed in 96% and to rubella in 94% of the patients.— R. E. Weibel *et al.*, *J. Am. med. Ass.*, 1971, *216*, 983.

Proprietary Names

Biavax *(Merck Sharp & Dohme, USA)*.

In Great Britain supplies are available on a named-patient basis from *Merck Sharp & Dohme*.

8000-s

Rubella Vaccine, Live *(B.P.)*. Rubella Vaccine (Live Attenuated); Rub/Vac (Live);

An aqueous suspension of a suitable live attenuated strain of rubella virus grown in suitable cell cultures. Potency is expressed in terms of virus titre.

It is supplied as a freeze-dried vaccine, which is reconstituted, immediately before use, by the addition of a suitable sterile liquid. Bactericides must not be added; it contains a suitable stabiliser.

Store at 2° to 8° *in vacuo* or in an atmosphere of nitrogen. Protect from light. Under these conditions it may be expected to retain its potency for at least 12 months.

CAUTION. *The vaccine is readily inactivated by chemical disinfectants and antiseptics and care is needed to avoid contact with these substances when sterilising syringes and skin before immunisation.*

8001-w

Rubella Virus Vaccine Live *(U.S.P.)*.

A bacterially sterile freeze-dried preparation of a suitable live strain of rubella virus grown in cultures of duck-embryo tissue, rabbit kidney-cell tissue, or human tissue. It contains the equivalent of not less than 1000 TCID50 in each immunising dose.

Store at 2° to 8°. Protect from light.

A comparison of methods for testing the potency of rubella vaccine.— M. Rapicetta *et al.*, *J. biol. Stand.*, 1977, *5*, 231.

Adverse Effects. As for Vaccines, p.1586.

Generally, side-effects have not been severe. Those occurring most commonly are skin rashes and arthralgia. Coryza, pharyngitis, bronchitis, fever, arthritis, lymphatic adenitis, neuropathy, and paraesthesia have also been reported.

The incidence of joint and muscular pains was acceptably low with Cendehill and DE-5 rubella vaccines but was higher and the effects more prolonged with DK-12 vaccine in a survey of children aged 1 to 12 years.— M. G. Grand *et al.*, *J. Am. med. Ass.*, 1972, *220*, 1569.

HPV-77 duck-cell attenuated rubella vaccine was given to 653 susceptible females aged 8 months to 41 years. After vaccination arthritis and/or arthralgia was not seen in children under 12 years, but was seen in 7.5% of females aged 12 to 25 years, and in 58.3% of women aged 26 to 41 years. These joint reactions were generally mild and transient.— R. E. Weibel *et al.*, *J. Am. med. Ass.*, 1972, *222*, 805.

A follow-up study was conducted in 1964 women who were given rubella vaccine. The vaccine was given within 3 months of conception in 27 instances and pregnancy was terminated in 10 women. In 17 pregnancies continued to term all infants appeared normal at birth and at subsequent follow-up. Side-effects reported were painful or stiff joints (664), swollen joints (190), rash (227), enlarged glands (212), sore throat (207), headache (106), and fever (78). Side-effects were more frequent after HPV-77-DE-5 than Cendehill strain virus and in those over 25. The stage of menstrual cycle and method of contraception also affected the frequency of side-effects. In 776 previously seronegative women followed up the conversion rate was 88.4%. It was suggested that many vaccine failures could be attributed to pre-existing low-level immunity.— J. P. Fox *et al.*, *J. Am. med. Ass.*, 1976, *236*, 837.

Other references to arthralgia.— S. L. Spruance *et al.*, *J. Pediat.*, 1972, *80*, 413; R. B. Wallace *et al.*, *Am. J. publ. Hlth*, 1972, *62*, 658; G. R. Thompson *et al.*, *Am. J. Dis. Child.*, 1973, *125*, 526; *Br. med. J.*, 1973, *4*, 186; A. J. Tingle *et al.*, *Ann. intern. Med.*, 1979, *90*, 203; D. Vergani *et al.* (letter), *Lancet*, 1980, *2*, 321.

Neurological complications. A myeloradiculoneuritic syndrome occurred in 36 children after a mass rubella vaccination programme; it occurred equally after each of 3 vaccines, and developed in an average of 6 weeks after vaccination. Some children had daily recurrences of neuritic pain while others had leg pain and a distinctive limp.— R. C. Gilmartin *et al.*, *J. Pediat.*, 1972, *80*, 406, per *Drugs*, 1972, *4*, 112.

Of 32 children with neuropathy after rubella vaccine 2 had major recurrences involving the leg syndrome and a crouching gait.— W. Schaffner *et al.*, *Am. J. Dis. Child.*, 1974, *127*, 684, per *J. Am. med. Ass.*, 1974, *228*, 1177. See also C. Grose *et al.* (letter), *J. Am. med. Ass.*, 1973, *223*, 799.

Two patients developed diffuse myelitis, with persistent motor impairment of the legs, after receiving rubella vaccine.— S. Holt *et al.*, *Br. med. J.*, 1976, *2*, 1037. A 27-year-old woman had paraesthesia of both legs and mild paraparesis 8 days after receiving rubella vaccine; a similar attack occurred 14 months later after exposure to rubella.— P. O. Behan (letter), *Br. med. J.*, 1977, *1*, 166.

Precautions. As for Vaccines, p.1586.

Rubella vaccines should not be given to persons with hypogammaglobulinaemia, leukaemia or other malignant conditions, or febrile illness, or to those being treated with corticosteroids or immunosuppressive drugs. Care is necessary in administering the vaccine to persons with allergic conditions.

Generally, it should not be administered within 3 or 4 weeks of another vaccine containing live micro-organisms.

It must not be given during pregnancy or within 3 months of conception.

Rubella virus has been recovered from the decidua, placenta, and foetus from some patients inadvertently given rubella vaccine during pregnancy and from some patients given rubella vaccine prior to therapeutic abortion. However, healthy infants have been delivered after the inadvertent use of rubella vaccine during pregnancy.

There was a significantly greater incidence of mild thrombocytopenia in 25 seronegative women given live rubella vaccine than in matched controls. Since the reaction occurred before seroconversion it might have been due to an infective rather than an immunological mechanism.— J. M. Forrest *et al.*, *Aust. N.Z. J. Med.*, 1974, *4*, 352, per *Int. pharm. Abstr.*, 1975, *12*, 824.

A study among small groups of children and young adults showed that 4 to 5 years after vaccination with rubella vaccine there were detectable amounts of antibody in the blood of the children but 19 of 25 examined had no cell-mediated immunity; in contrast 22 of 25 of the young adults who had been naturally infected with rubella virus had both types of immunity. Since cell-mediated immunity was normally depressed during pregnancy, there was a risk that foetuses of women who had been vaccinated might not be protected against rubella.— E. Rossier *et al.*, *Can. med. Ass. J.*, 1977, *116*, 481. See also A. J. Rhodes, *ibid.*, 463.

Failure of rubella vaccination evidently due to antibodies in a recent blood transfusion.— R. W. Watt and R. B. McGucken, *Br. med. J.*, 1980, *281*, 977.

Pregnancy and the neonate. A report from the Center for Disease Control. Rubella vaccine is not suitable for pregnant women because of the possible risk of foetal abnormality; the vaccine virus could cross the placenta. The risk of teratogenicity should be much lower from the vaccine virus than from the wild virus. Infants born to more than 60 susceptible women inadvertently immunised during early pregnancy and continued to term did not have any recognisable malformations attributable to rubella.— *Ann. intern. Med.*, 1978, *88*, 543.

There is no reason to withhold rubella vaccination if someone else in the household is pregnant.— *Br. med. J.*, 1979, *1*, 1696.

Further references: J. F. Modlin *et al.*, *New Engl. J. Med.*, 1976, *294*, 972; J. P. Fox *et al.*, *J. Am. med. Ass.*, 1976, *236*, 837; J. M. Forrest and M. A. Menser (letter), *Med. J. Aust.*, 1977, *1*, 77; S. R. Preblud *et al.* (letter), *Br. med. J.*, 1978, *2*, 960; C. Peckham and W. C. Marshall, *J. antimicrob. Chemother.*, 1979, *5*, *Suppl.* A, 71; E. Broadbent *et al.*, *J. clin. Path.*, 1980, *33*, 24; J. E. Banatvala *et al.* (letter), *Lancet*, 1981, *1*, 392.

For earlier references, see Martindale 27th Edn, p. 1627.

Uses. Rubella Vaccine, Live is used for active immunisation against German measles. It appears to induce an antibody response in over 90% of susceptible persons inoculated. It is given as a single dose by subcutaneous injection. Protection has been maintained for 8 years and is expected to be prolonged. The virus may be present in nasopharyngeal secretions during the 2nd and 3rd weeks after inoculation, but the risk of infection appears to be remote.

In Great Britain it is recommended that vaccination should be offered to all girls between their 11th and 14th birthdays. Vaccination may be given to women of childbearing age if they are seronegative. Women who are found to be seronegative during pregnancy should be offered vaccination in the early postpartum period. Seronegative women with an occupational risk of acquiring or transmitting rubella should also be offered vaccination. Effective precautions against pregnancy must be observed for at least 3 months following vaccination.

In the USA vaccination is recommended for children from the age of 12 months.

Discussions of rubella vaccination.— C. S. Peckham *et al.*, *Br. med. J.*, 1976, *1*, 760; J. W. G. Smith, *Practitioner*, 1978, *220*, 929; *Ann. intern. Med.*, 1978, *88*, 543 (Center for Disease Control); *Lancet*, 1979, *1*, 989; *Med. Lett.*, 1979, *21*, 53.

Of 142 seronegative women 36 received Cendehill rubella vaccine, 35 received HPV-77 DE-5 vaccine, 36 received RA 27/3 vaccine, and 35 received To-336 vaccine. Geometric mean antibody titres were 39.3, 63.1, 61.9, and 65.7 respectively. The incidence of joint symptoms was lowest with the Japanese To-336 vaccine. The possible nonteratogenicity of the To-336 vaccine needed to be confirmed.— J. M. Best *et al.*, *Br. med. J.*, 1974, *3*, 221.

A comparative study of Almevax and Cendevax rubella vaccines.— M. A. Menser *et al.*, *Med. J. Aust.*, 1978, *2*, 85.

Discussions and controversy regarding the respective merits of Cendehill and RA 27/3 rubella vaccines: T. H. Ingalls (letter), *Lancet*, 1979, *1*, 831 (favouring RA 27/3); F. E. André *et al.* , *Smith Kline-RIT* (letter), *Lancet*, 1979, *2*, 417 (defence of Cendehill); J. M. Best *et al.* (letter), *Lancet*, 1979, *2*, 690 (criticism of Cendehill); T. H. Ingalls (letter), *ibid.*, 791; D. S. Freestone, *Wellcome* (letter), *ibid.*, 858; F. E. André *et al.* (letter), *ibid.*, 1980, *1*, 657.

Lack of effect of rubella vaccine in the USA especially in children vaccinated when less than 15 months of age.— H. H. Balfour and D. P. Amren (letter,), *Lancet*, 1977, *2*, 1130.

A suggestion that women vaccinated against rubella should have follow-up serological screening to determine whether immunity had been established.— P. Curzen (letter), *Br. med. J.*, 1977, *2*, 186. See also *Lancet*, 1979, *1*, 1329; G. E. D. Urquhart and N. Fernando (letter), *ibid.*, 1981, *2*, 47; D. Gilmore *et al.*, *Br. med. J.*, 1982, *284*, 628.

Four of 12 hospital staff given rubella vaccine failed to show immunity when tested 3 to 6 weeks later.— W. J. C. Roberts (letter), *Br. med. J.*, 1978, *2*, 433.

Of 82 women given rubella vaccine 4 failed to produce haemagglutination-inhibiting antibodies.— E. D. Pereira *et al.* (letter), *Br. med. J.*, 1978, *2*, 773.

Results of the 1979 survey on rubella antibody status of young adults in the UK suggest that the effect of the rubella vaccine campaign on the immunological status of young females is being maintained.— M. Clarke *et al.*, *Lancet*, 1980, *1*, 537.

A long-term follow-up study of girls given RA 27/3 or Cendehill rubella vaccine in their 13th to 14th year and a group of girls found to be naturally immune at that age. A high proportion of subjects in all groups had persistent rubella antibody 6 to 7 years later. Some, who were seronegative using standard screening methods, were found to be immune when retested using more sensitive assays.— H. Zealley and E. Edmond, *Br. med. J.*, 1982, *284*, 382.

Further references: M. A. Menser *et al.*, *Med. J. Aust.*, 1978, *2*, 83; G. M. Schiff *et al.*, *J. Am. med. Ass.*, 1978, *240*, 2635; P. N. Goldwater *et al.*, *Lancet*, 1978, *2*, 1298.

Intranasal administration. References to the use of rubella vaccine, given intranasally.— F. Buser and A. Nicolas, *Am. J. Dis. Child.*, 1971, *122*, 53; T. A. Ingalls and H. W. Horne, *Lancet*, 1971, *1*, 830; C. F. W. Fairfax *et al.*, *Community Med.*, 1972, *128*, 213; E. E. Petersen *et al.*, *Dt. med. Wschr.*, 1973, *98*, 1842; H. Zealley *et al.*, *J. biol. Stand.*, 1974, *2*, 111; J. E. Banatvala *et al.* (letter), *Lancet*, 1979, *1*, 970; T. H. Ingalls (letter), *ibid.*, 1290; C. H. Taylor-Robinson and H. Mallinson (letter), *Lancet*, 1979, *2*, 1128; F. R. Philbrook and T. H. Ingalls (letter), *ibid.*, 1980, *1*, 147.

Postpartum use. The conversion-rate was 97% in 589 seronegative women given rubella vaccine within 4 days post partum, 100% in 58 who also received anti-D immunoglobulin, but 50% (4 of 8) in those who had received blood transfusions.— L. Grillner and L. Forssman (letter), *Br. med. J.*, 1974, *4*, 47.

Rubella antibody titres in 15 women given anti-D immunoglobulin injection 250 μg within 48 hours of delivery followed 3 days later by 0.5 ml of rubella vaccine were comparable with those in 10 patients given rubella vaccine on the fifth postpartum day. Rubella antibodies in the anti-D preparation did not prevent the development of active immunity.— E. Maroni and J. Munzinger, *Br. med. J.*, 1975, *2*, 541.

Proprietary Preparations

Almevax *(Wellcome, UK)*. A live rubella vaccine prepared from the Wistar RA 27/3 virus propagated in WI-38 human diploid cells, and containing in each 0.5 ml not less than 1000 TCID50; supplied as powder for preparation before use, with diluent. It contains traces of neomycin sulphate and polymyxin B sulphate. *Dose.* 0.5 ml.

Cendevax (known in some countries as Ervevax) *(Smith Kline & French, UK)*. A live rubella vaccine, prepared from the Cendehill strain of virus cultured in rabbit kidney cells, and containing in each 0.5 ml not less than 1000 TCID50; supplied as powder for preparation before use, with diluent. It contains traces of neomycin sulphate. *Dose.* 0.5 ml.

Other Proprietary Names

Meruvax II *(*Wistar RA 27/3*) (USA)*.

A live rubella vaccine prepared from the HPV-77 strain of virus (and propagated in duck-embryo cells) was formerly available in Great Britain under the proprietary name Meruvax (*Morson*). It is anticipated that *Morson* will market in Great Britain a live vaccine prepared from the RA 27/3 strain (and propagated in human diploid cells) under the proprietary name Meruvax II.

8002-e

Schick Control *(B.P., Eur. P.)*.

Schick Test Toxin which has been heated at 70° to 85° for not less than 5 minutes in order to destroy the specific toxin. It must be prepared from the same batch of Schick Test Toxin as that with which it is issued for use.

8003-l

Schick Test Control *(U.S.P.)*.

Diphtheria Toxin for Schick Test that has been inactivated by heat.

Store at 2° to 8°. The expiration date is not later than 1 year after release from manufacturer's cold storage.

Uses. Schick Control is used in conjunction with Schick Test Toxin in the Schick test to distinguish between the true Schick-positive reaction, due to the absence of diphtheria antitoxin in the blood, and a pseudo-reaction, due to susceptibility to non-specific substances.

A dose of 0.1 to 0.2 ml is administered intracutaneously (intradermally) into the flexor surface of the forearm.

8004-y

Schick Test Toxin *(B.P., Eur. P.)*. Toxinum Diphthericum Diagnosticum.

A preparation from sterile filtrate from a culture in a liquid medium of a toxigenic strain (a well-characterised PW-8 subculture is satisfactory) of *Corynebacterium diphtheriae*; the toxin may be purified; it is then diluted so that 0.1 or 0.2 ml contains the test dose. The diluent may be a sterile aqueous solution containing 1.5% of a mixture of 57 g of borax, 85 g of boric acid, and 99 g of sodium chloride, or some other buffer solution of pH 7.2 to 7.4 which will equally well render the mixture iso-osmotic with blood. It contains a suitable bactericide. It is a clear colourless or very pale straw-coloured liquid. It is standardised in terms of the amount necessary to produce a local reaction in *guinea-pigs* or *rabbits*, and of its ability to combine with antitoxin.

Store at 2° to 8° when Schick Test Toxin prepared with borax-boric acid buffer solution in saline may be expected to retain its potency for 6 months when packed in containers of not more than 0.25 ml and for 2 years in containers of not less than 1.5 ml. When Schick Test Toxin is stored at 25° it retains its potency for 2 months.

8005-j

Diphtheria Toxin for Schick Test. *(U.S.P.)*.

A sterile solution of the diluted standardised toxic products of growth of *Corynebacterium diphtheriae* prepared from toxin of specified

minimum potency.
Store at 2° to 8°. The expiration date is not later than 1 year after release from manufacturer's cold storage.

Uses. Schick Test Toxin is used in the Schick test for the diagnosis of susceptibility to diphtheria and to detect patients aged 8 to 10 years or over who are immune (*negative-and-pseudo reaction*) who might experience a reaction to diphtheria toxoid.
A dose of 0.1 or 0.2 ml is administered intracutaneously (intradermally) into the flexor surface of the forearm. A similar dose of Schick Control is injected into the other forearm. The reaction to the injections may be read after 24 to 48 hours, though 5 to 7 days may be necessary for late reactors and to confirm a reading taken earlier.
A *negative reaction*, indicating that the patient is immune to diphtheria, occurs when there is no redness at either injection site. A *negative-and-pseudo reaction* or *pseudo-reaction*, also indicating immunity, is shown by a flush which develops rapidly at each injection site within about 24 hours. This reaction fades more rapidly than a positive reaction. A *positive reaction*, indicating susceptibility to diphtheria, occurs as a red flush about 10 mm or more in diameter at the site of injection of the test dose with no reaction to the control injection.
A *combined* or *positive-and-pseudo reaction*, also indicating susceptibility, is shown by a flush which develops rapidly at each injection site, but as it fades a positive reaction develops at the site of the test dose.

In 3205 children previously vaccinated against diphtheria, a high incidence of positive reactions to Schick test was found, particularly in children who had recently had various infections or who had other vaccines within 2 months of being vaccinated for diphtheria.— M. A. Zhogova *et al.*, *Zh. Mikrobiol. Épidem. Immunobiol.*, 1966, *43*, 44, per *J. Am. med. Ass.*, 1966, *196* (Apr. 25), A209.

Proprietary Preparations

Schick Test Toxin Wellcome *(Wellcome, UK)*. A brand of Schick Test Toxin, with control, in packs of 1 ml.

8006-z

Scorpion Venom Antiserum *(B.P.)*. Anti-scorpion Serum.

A sterile preparation containing the specific antitoxic globulins that have the power of neutralising the venom of one or more species of scorpion. The species of scorpion against whose venom or venoms the antiserum is intended to be used varies according to the geographical region and for any particular region should include those species prevalent in the region. The potency should be such that the dose stated on the label will completely neutralise the maximum amount of venom likely to be delivered by a single sting.
It is an almost colourless or very faintly yellow liquid, free from turbidity, and almost odourless except for the odour of any added bactericide. pH 6 to 7.
Storage. As for Botulinum Antitoxin, p.1590.
The label states the species of scorpion against whose venom or venoms the antiserum is effective.

Adverse Effects. As for Antisera, p.1587.
Scorpion venom antiserum is prepared from the serum of animals and reactions due to the injection of animal serum may occur.

Uses. A scorpion sting is not usually fatal to healthy adults in the African and Middle East areas but the sting of South and Central American scorpions frequently results in death.
The injection of antiserum suitable for the species of scorpion can prevent symptoms and reduce pain provided it is done with the least possible delay. The volume stated on the label as the dose should preferably be made directly into the site of the sting but, if this cannot be done, as much as possible should be injected into the site and the remainder intramuscularly into a convenient proximal position.

A brief report of a WHO meeting emphasising the fragmentary knowledge of the epidemiology on snake bites, spider bites, and scorpion stings and the need for a manual on treatment.— *Bull. Wld Hlth Org.*, 1980, *58*, 576.

Preparations

Scorpion venom antiserum is available from the Lister Institute of Preventive Medicine.

8007-c

Smallpox Vaccine *(B.P., Eur. P.)*. Liquid Smallpox Vaccine (Dermal); Vaccine Lymph; Vaccinum Vacciniae; Vaccinum Variolae Fluidum Dermicum; Var/Vac.

A suspension of a suitable strain of the living virus of vaccinia prepared from material obtained from the lesions produced by the inoculation of vaccinia virus in the skin of healthy animals, in a solution having stabilising properties; it contains no antibiotics. Smallpox vaccine contains not less than 1×10^8 pock-forming units per ml, when compared with the first International Reference Preparation (1962). Smallpox Vaccine is a viscid colourless or straw-coloured liquid.
It may also be supplied as a dried vaccine (Dried Var/Vac) which is reconstituted before use by the addition of a suitable sterile liquid. *Eur. P.* includes the dried vaccine as Freeze-Dried Smallpox Vaccine (Dermal); Vaccinum Variolae Cryodesiccatum Dermicum.
Store as specified on the label at a temperature above its freezing point. Protect from light. Under these conditions it will retain its potency for at least 1 year. When stored at 2° to 5°, it may be expected to retain its potency for only 4 weeks. The dried vaccine should be stored *in vacuo* or in an atmosphere of an inert gas below 5° when it may be expected to retain its potency for 3 years. The reconstituted vaccine may be expected to retain its potency for 7 days at 2° to 8°.

CAUTION. *The vaccine should not be brought into contact with acetone, alcohol, ether, or other chemical disinfectants and care is necessary to avoid contact with these substances when preparing the skin before immunisation.*

8008-k

Smallpox Vaccine *(U.S.P.)*.

A suspension or solid containing a suitable strain of the living virus of vaccinia grown in the skin of bovine calves; it may contain a suitable preservative.
Its potency is compared with a reference vaccine (when intended for multiple-puncture administration) or with a 1 : 30 dilution of the reference vaccine (when intended for jet injection). If it is intended for jet injection the label so states; it also states the animal source.
Store below 0° (liquid vaccine) or at 2° to 8° (dried vaccine). The expiration date is not later than 3 months and 18 months respectively after release from manufacturer's cold storage.

Unused reconstituted smallpox vaccine can be destroyed by autoclaving or boiling for 5 minutes. Alternatively the opened ampoule can be totally immersed in Strong Sodium Hypochlorite Solution (10% 'available chlorine') for at least 12 hours.— *Br. med. J.*, 1979, *2*, 509.

Units. The first International Reference Preparation (1962) of smallpox vaccine consists of ampoules containing 14 mg of freeze-dried smallpox vaccine.

Uses. Smallpox Vaccine, when inoculated by multiple pressure or by scarification, stimulates the formation of antibodies, and the resulting immunity persists for a number of years.
Following the global eradication of smallpox, vaccination is recommended by the World Health Organization only for investigators at special risk. Very few countries demand certificates of vaccination, and the number of those countries is falling.
The World Health Organization has recommended that stocks of virus be destroyed or transferred to not more than 4 collaborating centres for research.

A brief discussion of accidental smallpox in a laboratory worker.— *Lancet*, 1979, *1*, 83.

A discussion of the need to retain smallpox viruses in laboratories, with reference to other pox viruses.— W. H. Foege, *New Engl. J. Med.*, 1979, *300*, 670.

Formal declaration of the global eradication of smallpox. Smallpox vaccination (except for investigators at special risk) and requirements for international certificates of vaccination should be terminated.— *Chronicle Wld Hlth Org.*, 1980, *34*, 258.

Sufficient vaccine to vaccinate 200 million people will be maintained by WHO as an 'insurance against the unknown' for an indefinite period.—. Chronicle Wld Hlth Org., 1980, *34*, 81.

Suspected smallpox in 139 patients, since eradication, was not confirmed. Vaccination continued to be offered to military personnel in British services and NATO armies, evidently because of the risk of smallpox being used in biological warfare. Vaccinia reactions were reported in contacts of vaccinated persons.— *Br. med. J.*, 1981, *282*, 1880.

Further references: J. G. Breman and I. Arita, *New Engl. J. Med.*, 1980, *303*, 1263.

For the adverse effects, precautions, and uses of smallpox vaccine, see Martindale 27th Edn, p. 1629–31.

Preparations

In the UK freeze-dried smallpox vaccine is available from Public Health Laboratories and from *Vestric* .

Proprietary Names

Dryvax *(Wyeth, USA)*.

8009-a

Snake Venom Antiserum *(B.P.C. 1973)*. Antivenene; Antivenin; Antivenom; Antivenom Serum; Venom Antitoxin; Antisnakebite Serum.

Native serum, or a preparation from native serum, containing the antitoxic globulins, or their derivatives, that have the power of neutralising the venom of one or more kinds of snake.
Snake venom antiserum (native serum) is a yellow or yellow-brown liquid, pH 7 to 8.5; if a preparation from native serum it is usually almost colourless but may be yellowish-brown or greenish-yellow, pH 6 to 7. At 5° it may be expected to lose not more than 5% of its activity in a year; at 20° the loss may approach 20%.
Store at 2° to 10° and avoid freezing. Protect from light.

8010-e

Antivenin (Crotalidae) Polyvalent *(U.S.P.)*. Polyvalent Crotaline Antivenin.

A sterile freeze-dried preparation of specific venom-neutralising globulins obtained from the serum of healthy horses immunised against 4 species of pit vipers, *Crotalus atrox* (Western diamondback), *Crotalus adamanteus* (Eastern diamondback), *Crotalus durissus terrificus* (South American rattlesnake), and *Bothrops atrox* (South American fer de lance). One dose neutralises the venoms in not less than 180 mouse LD50 of *C. atrox*, 1320 of *C. durissus terrificus*, and 780 of *B. atrox*. It may contain a suitable preservative. When reconstituted as specified it contains not more than 20% of solids.
Store at a temperature not exceeding 40°. The

expiration date of antivenin containing 10% excess potency is not more than 5 years after release from manufacturer's cold storage.
The label states the species of pit viper against which the antivenin is to be used and the animal source.

8011-l

Antivenin (Micrurus Fulvius) *(U.S.P.)*.

A sterile freeze-dried preparation of specific venom-neutralising globulins obtained from the serum of healthy horses immunised against venom of *Micrurus fulvius* (Eastern Coral snake). One dose neutralises the venom in not less than 250 mouse LD50 of *M. fulvius*. It may contain a suitable preservative. When reconstituted as specified it contains not more than 20% of solids.
Store at a temperature not exceeding 40°. The expiration date of antivenin containing 10% excess potency is not more than 5 years after release from manufacturer's cold storage.
The label states the animal source.

Units. 300 units of *Naja* antivenin, equine, are contained in 807 mg of purified, dried, polyvalent (*Naja* and *Hemachatus* spp.) horse serum in one ampoule of the first International Standard Preparation (1964).

Adverse Effects. As for Antisera, p.1587.
Snake venom antiserum is prepared from animal serum and reactions due to the injection of animal serum may occur.
Serum sickness is not uncommon and anaphylactic reactions may occur.

References to adverse effects: S. K. Sutherland, *Med. J. Aust.*, 1977, *1*, 613 (role of anticomplement); S. K. Sutherland and K. E. Lovering, *Med. J. Aust.*, 1979, *2*, 671; H. A. Reid, *WHO Collaborative Centre for the Control of Antivenoms* (letter), *Lancet*, 1980, *1*, 1024. Comment.— *ibid.*, 1009.

Uses. Venomous snakes comprise the Crotalidae (rattlesnakes and pit vipers), Viperidae (true vipers), Elapidae (cobras, kraits, and mambas), and the Hydrophidae (sea snakes).
The venom of snakes is a complex mixture chiefly of proteins, many of which have enzymatic activity, and may also provoke local inflammatory reactions. The venom may have profound effects on tissue, blood vessels and other organs, blood cells, coagulation, and neurotoxic effects with sensory, motor, cardiac, and respiratory involvement.
In Great Britain the only poisonous snake is the adder, *Viperus berus*. Zagreb antivenin may be used as part of the overall treatment, if hypotension exists or recurs, though opinion on its use is divided.
In the USA a polyvalent crotaline antivenin and an antivenin against the Eastern Coral snake are available. In Australia a polyvalent antivenin and a number of monovalent antivenins are available. In many other countries a wide variety of antivenins are available.
The use of antivenim is an essential part of the treatment of bites from highly venomous snakes.
Antivenin is generally given cautiously by intravenous infusion, after dilution with sodium chloride injection or dextrose injection. Resuscitative facilities should be available; preliminary test doses are not considered reliable. Some authorities recommended the use of antihistamine cover.

Reviews and discussions of the treatment of snake bite: F. E. Russell *et al.*, *J. Am. med. Ass.*, 1975, *233*, 341; S. K. Sutherland (letter), *Med. J. Aust.*, 1977, *2*, 841; *Med. J. Aust.*, 1978, *1*, 137; *Med. Lett.*, 1978, *20*, 101; D. A. Warrell, *Prescribers' J.*, 1979, *19*, 190; *ibid.*, *20* (Apr.).

In 4 patients with massive local swelling after being bitten by the puff-adder (*Bitis arietans*) antivenom probably prevented the development of local necrosis. Antivenom and intravenous fluids restored the blood pressure in a further 2 patients with hypotension. Victims of *B. arietans* with swelling of more than half of the bitten limb or with signs of systemic envenoming should be given at least 80 ml of specific polyvalent antivenom.— D. A. Warrell *et al.*, *Br. med. J.*, 1975, *4*, 697.

A review of adder bites and their management. It was recommended that Zagreb antivenom should be given if hypotension persisted or recurred unless there was a history of allergy. Antivenom might also be indicated if there was leucocytosis, evidence of acidosis, ECG changes or raised serum creatine phosphokinase concentrations. Extensive swelling seen within 2 hours of a bite was also a possible indication in adults to minimise morbidity. Serum sensitivity tests were not recommended as they had been found to be misleading and adrenaline was always effective when given promptly to treat reactions. The contents of 2 ampoules of Zagreb antivenom was a suitable dose for all ages; this was diluted in 100 ml of sodium chloride injection and infused at an initial rate of 15 drops a minute increased to complete the dose within an hour. Further antivenom might be considered if there was no improvement. Should a reaction occur the drip should be stopped temporarily and 0.5 ml of a 1 in 1000 solution of adrenaline given intramuscularly. Once the reaction was controlled the infusion of antivenom could be restarted.— H. A. Reid, *Br. med. J.*, 1976, *2*, 153.

Venom of the small-scaled snake (*Parademansia microlepidotus*), Australia's potentially most venomous snake, is neutralised by either taipan antivenom or the Australian polyvalent antivenom. Brown snake and tiger snake antivenoms are not effective.— S. K. Sutherland *et al.*, *Med. J. Aust.*, 1978, *1*, 288.

A case report of severe envenomation after a bite from *Rhabdophis subminiatus* (red-neck keel-back snake), commonly considered harmless.— H. M. Mather *et al.*, *Br. med. J.*, 1978, *1*, 1324.

A report of the treatment, in 8 years, of 32 bites by foreign venomous snakes in Britain. Antiserum was given to 9 patients and might have been helpful in a further 2. Antiserum should be given if there was potentially serious systemic poisoning or if the bite was from a snake whose venom caused local necrosis; intravenous infusion was essential; large doses were needed after elapid bites; after viper bites producing defibrination, clot quality might be useful in assessing whether dosage was adequate.— H. A. Reid, *Br. med. J.*, 1978, *1*, 1598.

An account of the treatment of 60 patients who had been bitten by the carpet or saw-scaled viper, *Echis carinatus*. Thirteen patients had no evidence of poisoning and 15 had local swelling but normal clotting, the whole limb being swollen in 4. The remaining 32 had local swelling and non-clotting blood. Administration of either Behringwerke North and West African polyvalent (*Bitis, Echis, Naja*) antivenom, or South African Institute for Medical Research (SAIMR) *Echis* antivenom, intravenously through an infusion of iso-osmotic sodium chloride solution, once only in 24 patients, twice in 2 patients, and thrice in 1 patient, restored normal clotting. The remaining 5 patients received treatment elsewhere owing to shortage of antivenom supplies. The hazards of *E. carinatus* and the value of effective therapy with antivenom are emphasised.— R. N. H. Pugh *et al.*, *Lancet*, 1979, *2*, 625. A comparison of 2 antivenoms for the treatment of bites by the carpet viper (*Echis carinatus*) in Nigeria.— D. A. Warrell *et al.*, *Br. med. J.*, 1980, *280*, 607.

The bacteriology of rattlesnake serum.— E. J. C. Goldstein *et al.*, *J. infect. Dis.*, 1979, *140*, 818.

The treatment of unidentified viper bites.— K. A. Markwalder, *Br. med. J.*, 1980, *281*, 648.

NOTE. Zagreb antivenom is available from *Regent Laboratories*; stocks are also held at Guy's Hospital Poisons Centre. Small stocks of antivenin against American, Australian, and other exotic snakes are held at Guy's Hospital and some other centres.

8012-y

Staphylococcus Antitoxin *(B.P. 1968)*. Sta/Ser.

A preparation from native serum containing the antitoxic globulins or their derivatives that have the specific power of neutralising the lethal, skin-necrosing, and haemolytic properties of the alpha toxin formed by *Staphylococcus aureus*. It is an almost colourless or very faintly yellow liquid, free from turbidity, and almost odourless except for the odour of any added bactericide. It has a potency of not less than 1000 units per ml. pH 6 to 7.
Store at 2° to 10° and avoid freezing. Protect from light.

Staphylococcus Antitoxin was employed in the treatment of acute staphylococcal infections where toxaemia was a marked feature but this form of treatment has been superseded by antibiotic therapy.

8013-j

Staphylococcus Toxoid *(B.P. 1968)*. Sta/Tox.

Prepared by treating staphylococcus alpha toxin produced by the growth of *Staphylococcus aureus* with formaldehyde solution until its specific toxicity has been completely removed or reduced to a low level.
Store at 2° to 10° and avoid freezing. Protect from light. Under these conditions it may be expected to retain its potency for at least 2 years after the date of manufacture; a 1 in 10 dilution will retain its potency for 3 months.

Staphylococcus Toxoid has been given intramuscularly in a combined method of prophylaxis and treatment of chronic infections such as recurring boils, carbuncles, and infected acne.

Manufacturers
Connaught, Canad.; Lederle, USA.

8014-z

Tetanus and Pertussis Vaccine *(B.P. 1973)*.
Tetanus-Whooping-cough Prophylactic; TPer/Vac.

A mixture of tetanus formol toxoid and a suspension of killed *Bordetella pertussis*. It conforms with the test for potency for Tetanus Vaccine, and the volume stated on the label as the dose contains not less than 4 pertussis units, calculated with reference to the second British Reference Preparation (1968).
Store at 2° to 10° and avoid freezing. Protect from light.

Adverse Effects and Precautions. As for Pertussis Vaccine, p.1600.

Uses. Tetanus and Pertussis Vaccine has been used for active immunisation against tetanus and whooping cough but simultaneous immunisation against diphtheria, tetanus, and whooping cough is generally preferred. The volume stated on the label as the dose has been given by deep subcutaneous or intramuscular injection in a schedule similar to that for Diphtheria, Tetanus, and Pertussis Vaccine.

8015-c

Tetanus Antitoxin *(B.P., Eur. P.)*. Immunoserum Antitetanicum; Tet/Ser.

A sterile preparation containing the specific antitoxic globulins that have the power of neutralising the toxin formed by *Clostridium tetani*.
It is an almost colourless or very faintly yellow liquid, free from turbidity, and almost odourless except for the odour of any added bactericide.
For prophylactic use, it has a potency of not less than 1000 units per ml, and for therapeutic use not less than 3000 units per ml. pH 6 to 7.
Storage. As for Botulinum Antitoxin, p.1590.
The label states the animal source and whether the preparation is intended for prophylactic or therapeutic use.

8016-k

Tetanus Antitoxin *(U.S.P.)*.

A sterile solution of the refined and concentrated proteins, chiefly globulins, containing antitoxic antibodies obtained from the serum or plasma of healthy horses that have been immunised against tetanus toxin or toxoid. It contains not less than 400 units per ml.
A faintly brownish, yellowish, or greenish clear or slightly opalescent liquid, odourless or with

odour of the antimicrobial agent.
Store at 2° to 8°. The expiration date of antitoxin containing 20% excess potency is not later than 5 years after release from manufacturer's cold storage.
The label states the animal source.

Units. 1400 units (1000 Lf-equivalents for flocculation) of tetanus antitoxin, equine are contained in 47 mg in one ampoule of the second International Standard Preparation (1969).

The estabishment of the British Reference preparation for tetanus antitoxin for the flocculation test.— F. Sheffield *et al.*, *J. biol. Stand.*, 1979, *7*, 301.

Adverse Effects. As for Antisera, p.1587.
Tetanus Antitoxin is prepared from the serum of animals and reactions due to the injection of animal serum may occur.

Severe and irreversible perceptive deafness followed the administration of antitoxin for tetanus prophylaxis.— P. E. Pantazopoulos, *Laryngoscope, St Louis*, 1965, *75*, 1836, per *Med. J. Aust.*, 1966, *2*, 327.

Uses. Tetanus Antitoxin neutralises the toxin produced by *Clostridium tetani*; the toxin has a high affinity for nerve cells and antitoxin is unlikely to have an effect on toxin that is no longer circulating.
Tetanus Antitoxin has been used to provide temporary passive immunity but Antitetanus Immunoglobulin Injection (see p.333) is preferred. For prophylaxis after injury non-immune or partially immune persons may be given, as early as possible, 1500 units of Tetanus Antitoxin subcutaneously or intramuscularly. Doses of not less than 10 000 units intramuscularly or intravenously have been given as part of the regimen of treatment of established tetanus.
Whenever a non-immune patient is seen because of injury opportunity should be taken to institute a course of active immunisation.

Tetanus antitoxin given intrathecally as an adjunct to systemic antitoxin therapy (750 units given thrice over 50 hours) in a single-blind study of 295 patients with adult-type tetanus reduced the overall mortality; 13 of 184 (7%) dying in the intrathecal group compared with 16 of 111 (14%) in the control group. A dose of 200 units intrathecally was more effective than one of 1500 units. Additional treatment consisted of sedation, betamethasone, procaine penicillin, and wound toilet.— R. K. M. Sanders *et al.*, *Lancet*, 1977, *1*, 974.

The use of tetanus antitoxin injected around the umbilicus in neonatal tetanus.— A. H. Rathore and A. E. M. Vreebrug, *J. Pakistan med. Ass.*, 1978, *28*, 3, per *Trop. Dis. Bull.*, 1979, *76*, 901.

In a study of 60 infants with tetanus neonatorum, treatment with human antitetanus immunoglobulin 150 units intrathecally, with equine tetanus antitoxin 20 000 units intravenously and 20 000 units intramuscularly, was no more effective in reducing the mortality rate, days in hospital, and days of sedation than the same doses of tetanus antitoxin given alone.— M. R. Sedaghatian, *Archs Dis. Childh.*, 1979, *54*, 623.

In a study in 107 patients with neonatal tetanus mortality was 37% in those given tetanus antitoxin 50 or 100 units intrathecally, with steroids, compared with 68% in controls.— A. K. Singh *et al.*, *Archs Dis. Childh.*, 1980, *55*, 527. See also S. Singhi and P. Singhi (letter), *ibid.*, 1979, *54*, 650.

Proprietary Names
Tetanus Antitoxin *(Sclavo, USA)*.

In Great Britain supplies are available on a named-patient basis from *Swiss Serum and Vaccine Institute, UK*.

8017-a

Tetanus Vaccine *(B.P.)*.

Tetanus Toxoid; Tetanus Formol Toxoid; Tet/Vac/FT.

It is prepared from tetanus toxin produced by the growth of *Clostridium tetani*. The toxin is converted to tetanus formol toxoid by treatment with Formaldehyde Solution. The potency of the vaccine is determined by its ability to promote the development of antibodies in guinea-pigs.
Store at 2° to 8° and avoid freezing. Protect from light.
NOTE. When Tetanus Vaccine is prescribed or demanded and the form is not stated, Adsorbed Tetanus Vaccine may be dispensed or supplied.

8018-t

Adsorbed Tetanus Vaccine *(B.P., Eur. P.)*.

Adsorbed Tetanus Toxoid; Tetanus Vaccine (Adsorbed); Vaccinum Tetanicum Adsorbatum; Tet/Vac/Ads.

It is prepared from tetanus formol toxoid containing not less than 500 Lf per mg of protein nitrogen and a mineral carrier which may be hydrated aluminium hydroxide, aluminium phosphate, or calcium phosphate in a saline solution or other appropriate solution iso-osmotic with blood. The name of the mineral carrier is stated on the label. The antigenic properties are adversely affected by certain bactericides such as phenol or cresol. It contains not less than 40 units per dose.
Store at 2° to 8° and avoid freezing. Protect from light. Under these conditions it may be expected to retain its potency for at least 3 years.
NOTE. When Tetanus Vaccine is prescribed or demanded and the form is not stated, Adsorbed Tetanus Vaccine may be dispensed or supplied.

8019-x

Tetanus Toxoid *(U.S.P.)*.

A sterile solution of the formaldehyde-treated products of growth of *Clostridium tetani*. It contains a non-phenolic preservative.
Store at 2° to 8° and avoid freezing. The expiration date is not later than 2 years after release from manufacturer's cold storage.

8020-y

Tetanus Toxoid Adsorbed *(U.S.P.)*.

A sterile preparation of tetanus toxoid precipitated or adsorbed by alum, aluminium hydroxide, or aluminium phosphate adjuvants.
Store at 2° to 8° and avoid freezing. The expiration date is not later than 2 years after release from manufacturer's cold storage.

Units. 833 units of tetanus toxoid, plain, are contained in 25 mg of alcohol-purified tetanus toxoid, plain, with glycine, in one ampoule of the first International Standard Preparation (1951).
120 units of tetanus toxoid, adsorbed, are contained in 80 mg of a dried mixture of tetanus toxoid adsorbed to aluminium hydroxide, and an equal part of guinea-pig serum, in one ampoule of the first International Standard Preparation (1965).
Potency has also been expressed in terms of Limes flocculationis (Lf); there is no simple correlation between international units and Lf equivalents.

Adverse Effects. As for Vaccines, p.1586.
Local reactions occur occasionally, usually following the usc of adsorbed vaccines. The incidence of reactions increases with the second and third injections but the reactions are generally not severe. Reactions are more common in adults that in children and an incidence in adults of 1 to 2% has been reported. Hypersensitivity reactions, possibly associated with skin rashes, have been reported.

A discussion of toxic reactions, particularly local reactions, to tetanus vaccine.— *Br. med. J.*, 1974, *1*, 48.

Intramuscular injection of tetanus toxoid into the gluteal region produced fewer side-effects than intramuscular deltoid injections or subcutaneous injections into the arm. The incidence and severity of side-effects did not vary between persons receiving primary vaccination and those with a history of vaccination.— D. David and B. Zehntner, *Schweiz. med. Wschr.*, 1971, *101*, 1055, per *Clin. Med.*, 1973, *80* (Jan.), 43.

A woman who inadvertently received 3.8 ml of tetanus vaccine was given diphenhydramine 50 mg four times a day. A local reaction with mild erythema, heat, induration, and slight tenderness developed at the injection sites in the buttocks. This reaction had disappeared after 5 days.— S. Lerner (letter), *J. Am. med. Ass.*, 1974, *228*, 159.

Allergic reactions. Local allergic reactions to tetanus toxoid were fairly common and systemic reactions were not rare.— P. E. Klein (letter), *J. Am. med. Ass.*, 1967, *199*, 282. Intradermal inoculations gave adequate protection, and reactions were mild or local.— S. Fisher (letter), *ibid.*, 947.

A 24-year-old woman developed anaphylactic shock and died 30 minutes after an injection of tetanus vaccine. Previous injections with the vaccine had been well tolerated.— M. Staak and E. Wirth, *Dt. med. Wschr.*, 1973, *98*, 110.

There was a high incidence of cutaneous hypersensitivity reactions to tetanus toxoid in 70 patients previously immunised without untoward effect.— M. A. Facktor *et al.*, *J. Allergy & clin. Immunol.*, 1973, *52*, 1, per *J. Am. med. Ass.*, 1973, *226*, 492.

Further references: D. F. Fardon, *J. Am. med. Ass.*, 1967, *199*, 125.

Aspirin (for its effect on prostaglandins) and an antihistamine could be given 1 hour before a test dose of tetanus vaccine in a patient suspected of being hypersensitive; if there was no reaction within 20 minutes the full dose of vaccine could be given.— H. R. C. Riches, *Practitioner*, 1979, *223*, 601.

Epidermal necrolysis. A fatal case of toxic epidermal necrolysis in a patient given tetanus vaccine. Swelling, shock, and epidermal necrolysis occurred after the 3rd injection of vaccine and the patient died after 4 days.— M. Halm *et al.*, *Dte GesundhWes.*, 1974, *29*, 1430, per *Int. pharm. Abstr.*, 1975, *12*, 194.

Neuropathy. Peripheral neuropathy with paralysis of the right radial nerve developed in a medical student a few hours after he had been given tetanus vaccine.— G. I. Blumstein and H. Kreithen, *J. Am. med. Ass.*, 1966, *198*, 1030.

Precautions. As for Vaccines, p.1586.

It was advisable not to administer tetanus vaccine within 48 hours of giving corticotrophin.— M. L. Brandon, *J. Am. med. Ass.*, 1969, *207*, 1724.

Use in systemic lupus erythematosus. Vaccination and immunisation against tetanus with tetanus toxoid could be carried out if necessary in patients with systemic lupus erythematosus which was controlled but should be withheld in those with active disease and those on large doses of steroids.— N. R. Rowell, *Br. med. J.*, 1969, *2*, 427.

Uses. Tetanus vaccines are used for active immunisation against tetanus. Tetanus Vaccine is less potent as an antigen than Adsorbed Tetanus Vaccine when given as a first dose; subsequent doses may be either Tetanus Vaccine or Adsorbed Tetanus Vaccine. A high degree of protection is provided for about 5 years after an immunisation course. A reinforcing dose given several years after the primary immunisation will rapidly stimulate the production of antibodies.
Tetanus Vaccine and Adsorbed Tetanus Vaccine are administered by deep subcutaneous or intramuscular injection in 3 doses, usually of 0.5 ml; the first dose is followed 6 to 12 weeks later by the second dose, and the third dose follows after an interval of 6 to 12 months. A reinforcing dose is desirable 5 years later with a further dose after a further 5 to 15 years. In the event of injury an additional reinforcing dose may be given, to promote an immediate antibody response, provided such a dose has not been given in the preceding 12 months.
Active immunisation against tetanus should be started in infants aged 3 months and the vaccine is generally given as Diphtheria, Tetanus, and Pertussis Vaccine (see p.1593). For a reinforcing dose at the age of 5 years or at school entry, when immunisation against whooping cough is no longer necessary, Diphtheria and Tetanus Vaccine may be given.
In the event of injury in non-immunised persons opportunity is usually taken to initiate a course of primary immunisation. This provides no immediate protection; prophylactic treatment with Antitetanus Immunoglobulin Injection, possibly

with antibiotics, may be needed. The first dose of Adsorbed Tetanus Vaccine may be given concomitantly, but not into the same limb.

Tetanus Vaccine, but not Adsorbed Tetanus Vaccine, is sometimes given intracutaneously (intradermally) in doses of 0.1 ml, for the second and subsequent doses.

Serum-tetanus antitoxin concentrations were significantly lower in 41 children who had been given tetanus vaccine more than 2 years before the study compared with the concentrations in 58 children who had been vaccinated within 2 years. Vaccination might need to be repeated every 2 to 3 years.— A. R. Meira, *Lancet*, 1973, *2*, 659.

A single dose of Adsorbed Tetanus Vaccine, given at the age of 5 months, conferred protection on 257 of 260 children; protection was reinforced by a second dose 12 months later. The procedure offered advantages for mass vaccination in the tropics.— P. Sureau *et al.*, *Bull. Wld Hlth Org.*, 1977, *55*, 739.

A recommendation that travellers abroad should receive booster doses of tetanus vaccine every 3 to 5 years.— A. C. Turner, *Practitioner*, 1979, *222*, 16.

The use of tetanus toxoid by mouth.— R. Veronesi *et al.*, *Revta bras. med.*, 1979, *36*, 26, per *Trop. Dis. Bull.*, 1979, *76*, 1096.

Discussions of the need for vaccination against tetanus in elderly patients in institutions.— F. T. Sherman (letter), *J. Am. med. Ass.*, 1980, *244*, 2159; P. Irvine and K. Crossley (letter), *ibid.*

Reduced incidence of pain, tenderness, swelling, and erythema in children aged 15 to 16 given reinforcing doses of Tetanus Vaccine, compared with those given Adsorbed Tetanus Vaccine.— L. H. Collier *et al.*, *Lancet*, 1979, *1*, 1364. From extensive experience with plain and adsorbed vaccines in thousands of employees at a motor car factory the wisdom of perpetuating the use of plain vaccine is doubted. The only advantage it appears to have over the adsorbed vaccine is its suitability for intradermal administration in the occasional patient who has had a severe reaction to previous inoculations of adsorbed vaccine, aluminium-containing preparations being unsuitable for intradermal inoculation. Alternatively 2 Lf doses of adsorbed tetanus vaccine intramuscularly have proved virtually non-toxic and have provided adequate antitoxin response.— W. G. White (letter), *ibid.*, 1980, *1*, 42.

In a study in India, 80% of 410 patients who had not been immunised had measurable tetanus antitoxin concentrations which were protective in 3%. Adsorbed tetanus toxoid in a single dose of 100 Lf was given to 131 adults with naturally acquired antitoxin and single doses of 250 Lf were given to 38 similar children. Protective concentrations of antibody were produced in all patients with an average 10-fold rise after the 100 Lf dose and a 20-fold rise after the 250 Lf dose at one month. Antibody concentrations remained protective for 3 years after the 100 Lf dose and protection in excess of 5 years was expected for the 250 Lf dose. The results suggested that single-dose vaccination may be better than the conventional 3-dose scheme for a population with poor compliance and in whom naturally acquired antitoxin is associated with partial tolerance to tetanus toxoid.— F. D. Dastur *et al.*, *Lancet*, 1981, *2*, 219.

Pregnancy and the neonate. Tetanus toxoid was effective in preventing tetanus in the newborn. No tetanus developed in 341 babies born to women who had received 2 or 3 spaced injections of adsorbed toxoid during pregnancy or up to 5 years previously compared with 27 occurrences amongst 347 babies born to women who had not received toxoid.— J. W. G. Smith, *Br. med. Bull.*, 1969, *25*, 177. See also K. W. Newell *et al.*, *Bull. Wld Hlth Org.*, 1971, *45*, 773; J. P. Stanfield *et al.*, *Lancet*, 1973, *1*, 215.

Proprietary Preparations

Adsorbed Tetanus Vaccine Wellcome *(Wellcome, UK)*. A brand of Adsorbed Tetanus Vaccine, with aluminium hydroxide as the mineral carrier, each 0.5-ml dose containing not less than 40 international units of tetanus toxoid, in ampoules of 0.5 ml and vials of 5 ml.

Adsorbed Tetanus Vaccine (PTAH) *(Duncan, Flockhart, UK)*. A brand of Adsorbed Tetanus Vaccine, with aluminium hydroxide as the mineral carrier, each 0.5-ml dose containing not less than 40 international units of tetanus toxoid, in ampoules of 0.5 ml and vials of 5 ml.

Tetanus Vaccine in Simple Solution Welcome *(Wellcome, UK)*. A brand of Tetanus Vaccine, each 0.5-ml dose containing 14 Lf of tetanus toxoid, in ampoules of 0.5 ml and vials of 5 ml.

Other Proprietary Names

Tetanus Toxoid *(Connaught, USA)*; Tetanus Toxoid Adsorbed *(Connaught, USA)*; Tetanus Toxoid Purogenated *(Lederle, USA)*; Tetanus Toxoid Adsorbed *(Lederle, USA)*; Tetanus Toxoid Adsorbed *(Parke, Davis, USA)*; Tetanus Toxoid, Adsorbed *(Sclavo, USA)*; Tetanus Toxoid, Fluid, Purified *(Wyeth, USA)*; Tetanus Toxoid Adsorbed, Aluminium Phosphate *(Wyeth, USA)*.

8021-j

Trichinella Extract

CAS — 8016-91-9.

An aqueous extract of the killed, washed, defatted, and powdered larvae of *Trichinella spiralis*, usually obtained from inoculated rodents. It consists of the water-soluble antigens of the larvae in a buffered saline solution containing 0.4% of phenol as a preservative. **Store** at 2° to 8°.

It was formerly used for making intradermal diagnostic tests in the diagnosis of trichiniasis.

Trichinella extract was ineffective as a diagnostic agent because of poor sensitivity and inadequate standardisation. It has been largely supplanted by serological tests. Removal from the market was recommended; it had been so removed.— *FDA Drug Bull.*, 1978, *8*, 15.

8022-z

Old Tuberculin *(B.P., Eur. P.)*.

Tuberculinum Crudum; OT. The sterile heat-concentrated filtrate from a fluid medium on which *Mycobacterium tuberculosis* or *M. bovis* has been grown. It contains a suitable preservative.

It is a clear, yellow to brown, viscous fluid containing not less than 100 000 units per ml. It is distributed under aseptic conditions into sterile containers which are then sealed to exclude micro-organisms.

Store at 2° to 8° and avoid freezing. Protect from light. Under these conditions it may be expected to retain its potency for at least 8 years. Diluted solutions are less stable depending on the degree of dilution and the nature of the diluent. Diluted solutions should be kept in full containers and used as soon as possible after preparation; once a container is opened any unused portion should be discarded.

8023-c

Tuberculin Purified Protein Derivative *(B.P., Eur. P.)*.

Tuberculini Derivatum Proteinosum Purificatum; Tuberculin PPD.

A sterile preparation made from the heat-treated products of growth and lysis of the appropriate species of mycobacterium which reveal delayed hypersensitivity in animals sensitised by micro-organisms of the same species. The active fraction, predominantly protein, is isolated by precipitation.

It is a colourless to pale straw-coloured liquid, or a freeze-dried cream-coloured powder or tablets. It is distributed under aseptic conditions into sterile containers which are then sealed to exclude micro-organisms. The liquid contains 100 000 units per ml. pH 6.5 to 7.5. The dry powder contains 30 000 units per mg.

Store at 2° to 8° and avoid freezing. Protect from light. In dried form it retains its potency indefinitely. Concentrated solutions containing 0.5% of phenol may be expected to retain their potency for at least 8 years. Diluted solutions are less stable depending on the mode of preparation and the nature of the diluent. Diluted solutions should be kept in full containers and used as soon as possible after preparation; once a container is opened any unused portion should be discarded.

CAUTION. *As traces of tuberculin are liable to adhere to glassware, syringes used for tuberculin tests should not be used for other purposes. Tuberculin Purified Protein Derivative may produce toxic effects if inhaled and care must be taken when handling the powder.*

8024-k

Tuberculin *(U.S.P.)*.

A sterile solution derived from the concentrated soluble products of growth of *Mycobacterium tuberculosis* or *M. bovis*, prepared in a suitable medium. It is supplied as Old Tuberculin, a standardised culture filtrate or as Purified Protein Derivative (PPD), a further standardised purified protein fraction.

Old Tuberculin is a clear brownish liquid with a characteristic odour. Purified Protein Derivative (PPD) of Tuberculin is a slightly opalescent colourless solution.

Store at 2° to 8°. Multiple-puncture devices may be stored at a temperature not exceeding 30°.

The expiration date of concentrated Old Tuberculin containing 50% of glycerol is not later than 5 years (dilutions 1 year) after release from manufacturer's cold storage; the expiration date of PPD containing 50% of glycerol is not later than 2 years (dilutions 1 year) after release from manufacturer's cold storage. Multiple-puncture devices may be stored for not more than 2 years after release.

Commercially available and standard tuberculin PPD gave a high proportion of false negative results in tuberculous patients, probably as a result of loss of potency of the preparation by adsorption on glass. Preparations stabilised with polysorbate 80 gave more consistent results.— M. Holden *et al.*, *New Engl. J. Med.*, 1971, *285*, 1506. See also P. Q. Edwards, *ibid.*, 1972, *286*, 374; O. P. Sharma and P. A. Evans (letter), *ibid.*, 375.

In a group of 121 patients exposed to tuberculosis, a tuberculin purified protein derivative stabilised with polysorbate 80 gave fewer negative or doubtful results than non-stabilised purified protein derivatives.— F. J. Erdtmann *et al.*, *J. Am. med. Ass.*, 1974, *228*, 479.

Agreement between PPD and PPD-polysorbate 80 tuberculin reactions was 91% among lepromatous patients and 94% for other patients.— T. H. Rea *et al.* (letter), *J. Am. med. Ass.*, 1974, *229*, 1165.

The biological reactivity of 2 commercially available tuberculin preparations was measured in 168 subjects. Differences between the tuberculins were more evident when an induration of 10 mm or more was considered positive. Using a criterion of 5 mm or more the differences were smaller, but the frequency of non-tuberculous responders was increased.— S. Landi *et al.*, *Tubercle*, 1975, *56*, 55.

Stability. The biological potency of 15 commercially available tuberculin solutions was measured at 4, 24, and 37° when diluted to 1, 5, and 250 units per dose with a diluent containing 0.0005% of Tween 80 and phenol 0.3%. Preparations at all 3 strengths were stable for at least 3 years at 4°, 2 years at 24°, and 1 year at 37°.— S. Landi and H. R. Held, *Tubercle*, 1978, *59*, 121. The activity of skin tests containing mycobacterial purified protein derivatives was not adversely affected by the addition of Tween 80. However, Tween 80 appeared to enhance the reaction of a given dose of antigen to a greater degree than would be expected if the sole effect were to prevent adsorption of protein to glass.— R. C. Good and M. J. Selin, *Bull. int. Un. Tuberc.*, 1979, *54*, 163.

Units. 500 000 units of mammalian tuberculin purified protein derivative are contained in 10 mg with 4 mg of salts in one ampoule of the first International Standard Preparation (1951).

500 000 units of avian tuberculin purified protein derivative are contained in 10 mg with 26.3 mg of salts in one ampoule of the first International Standard Preparation (1954).

The third International Standard Preparation (1965) of Old Tuberculin contains 90 000 units per ml.

Adverse Effects. Pain and pruritus may occur at the injection site, occasionally with vesiculation, ulceration, or necrosis in highly sensitive persons. If given to patients with tuberculosis a severe reaction, with cough, dyspnoea, limb pain, vomiting, fever, rigor, and lymphopenia, may occur.

Granuloma has been reported after Heaf tests.
Allergic reactions to tuberculin tine tests have been reported rarely and measures to deal with them should be available. For detailed recommendations concerning the management of anaphylaxis, see Adrenaline, p.4.

A 19-year-old youth collapsed and died shortly after receiving a Tuberculin Tine Test (old tuberculin intradermal test). He had also been given an oral poliomyelitis vaccine before the tine test. Death was considered probably to be due to an anaphylactic reaction to the tine test. No abnormality was found at autopsy.— V. J. M. DiMaio and R. C. Froede (letter), *J. Am. med. Ass.*, 1975, *233*, 769.

Application of 1% hydrocortisone ointment would prevent severe reactions to PPD: application of an occlusive dressing enhanced absorption.— T. F. Plaut (letter), *New Engl. J. Med.*, 1976, *295*, 1263. In a large, controlled, double-blind, prospective study by M.L. Hanson and G.W. Comstock (*Am. Rev. resp. Dis.*, 1968, *97*, 472) hydrocortisone ointment 1% was no more effective than a placebo.— L. B. Reichman (letter), *ibid.*, 1977, *296*, 175.

Precautions. Sensitivity to tuberculin is diminished in the undernourished. It may also be diminished during measles or other virus infections, after ultraviolet light treatment, during corticosteroid therapy, and after virus vaccines.

Reduced response with corticosteroids.— M. Schatz *et al.*, *Ann. intern. Med.*, 1976, *84*, 261.

Impaired response to the tuberculin reaction and BCG in onchocerciasis.— A. Rougemont *et al.* (letter), *Lancet*, 1977, *1*, 309.

During periodic mass testings of inmates of Arkansas prisons, local skin sensitisation was shown not to be responsible for the 'booster' effects of repeated tuberculin PPD tests which could cause apparent conversion from negative to positive tests in about 10% of individuals.— W. W. Stead (letter), *New Engl. J. Med.*, 1977, *297*, 225.

The tuberculin reactions of 725 school children in Brisbane following BCG vaccinations were larger in those tested with purified protein derivatives of *Mycobacterium avium* than those with purified protein derivatives of BCG vaccine, *M. bovis* or *M. tuberculosis*. It was suggested that the vaccination was enhancing a pre-existing latent hypersensitivity to *M. avium* even in children with a previous negative tuberculin reaction. These findings would be of importance in BCG studies where, though a tuberculin test had been used to exclude infected individuals, some of the vaccinated and unvaccinated persons would have latent tuberculin hypersensitivity.— E. W. Abrahams, *Tubercle*, 1979, *60*, 109.

For a report of false positive reactions due to the inclusion of thiomersal in Old Tuberculin, see Thiomersal, p.576.

Uses. Tuberculin is used as a diagnostic agent for tuberculosis. A person showing a specific sensitivity to tuberculin is considered to have been infected with tubercle bacillus, though the infection may be inactive.

Sensitivity tests to tuberculin can be performed in different ways. In the intracutaneous (intradermal) test of Mantoux, the diagnostic dose varies with the circumstances because of the great variation in sensitivity to tuberculin. In a full-scale test, the initial dose injected is 1 unit of either Old Tuberculin or Tuberculin Purified Protein Derivative in 0.1 ml. The test is read at 72 hours. A positive reaction is characterised by an area of palpable infiltration of not less than 5 or 6 mm in diameter, which may or may not be surrounded by erythema. Necrosis may occur in hypersensitive people. If the reaction is negative, the test is repeated with 10 units of tuberculin in 0.1 ml. If the second test is negative, a final test may be made with 100 units in 0.1 ml before regarding the person as 'Mantoux-negative'. In the USA induration of 10 mm is considered positive.

Frequently, where the sensitivity of the person is not expected to be unduly high, the initial test is with 5 or 10 units, followed, if negative, by the test with 100 units. It is also common practice in epidemiological surveys to use a single test with 5 or 10 units.

To avoid injections, a multiple-puncture (Heaf) method, with an undiluted tuberculin, is frequently employed. The test is read at 3 days. Absence of induration represents a negative response; a positive response involves induration of at least 2 mm diameter at 4 or more of the puncture points or a greater response which may include coalescence of papules to form a ring, formation of a plaque, or vesicle formation with erythema.

Disposable tine tests, coated with dried old tuberculin or moistened before use from an attached reservoir of tuberculin purified protein derivative are also used.

Tuberculin PPD has been used in healthy persons to measure the anti-inflammatory effects of drugs such as flufenamic acid and mefenamic acid used in the treatment of rheumatoid arthritis.— P. A. Bacon and P. A. Dieppe, *J. clin. Pharmac.*, 1972, *12*, 249.

A differential skin test for opportunist mycobacterial infections in children using a composite antigen from *M. avium*, *M. intracellulare*, and *M. scrofulaceum* with tuberculin PPD.— J. Marks *et al.*, *Tubercle*, 1977, *58*, 19.

A review on tuberculosis, including the diagnosis of tuberculous infection.— J. Glassroth *et al.*, *New Engl. J. Med.*, 1980, *302*, 1441. Comment that it is not unusual for the tuberculin test to be positive and to remain so throughout adulthood in persons who have been immunised with BCG vaccine in infancy.— I. Feferman (letter), *ibid.*, *303*, 940. Reply. The recommendation of the US Public Health Service to disregard a history of BCG vaccination in evaluating a positive tuberculin reaction is believed to be a reasonable approach.— J. Glassroth *et al.* (letter), *ibid.*

A comparison of the effects of PPD-S (the standard tuberculin) and of PPD-T (with Tween), and of 3 atypical antigens used in dual skin testing—PPD-B (Battey), PPD-Y (*M. kansasii*), and PPD-X (*M. xenopi*).— W. F. Larrabee and R. Talavera, *Tubercle*, 1980, *61*, 239.

Comparison of Mantoux and tine tests. Discussion of Mantoux, Heaf, and tine tests.— *Br. med. J.*, 1979, *1*, 1300.

Of 307 subjects 59% were positive as judged by the Mantoux test; when assessed by the tine test performed at the same time in the opposite arm only 3.9% were judged positive, with 15.5% in the doubtful category. The tine test could not be recommended.— *Br. med. J.*, 1978, *1*, 1451 (Report of the Tuberculin Subcommittee of the Research Committee of the British Thoracic Association).

In a study in 190 subjects there was an 87% correlation between the results of the Mantoux test (10 units) and those of the tine test, when the latter was applied for 2 seconds and induration of 2 to 4 mm was considered positive. While the Mantoux test remained the most suitable for hospital use the tine test was valuable.— D. J. M. Sinclair and R. N. Johnston, *Br. med. J.*, 1979, *1*, 1325.

Simultaneous tests for tuberculosis using the Mantoux test (10 units) and the tuberculin tine test were performed on 393 patients. The overall agreement between the tests was 78%, this rose to 90% if all doubtful tests were reclassified as positive or 82% if reclassified as negative. It was suggested that the doubtful category should be abandoned and readings in this range classified as positive.— N. J. C. Snell, *Tubercle*, 1979, *60*, 99.

A purified protein derivative tine test compared favourably with the Mantoux test and old tuberculin tine test with respect to accuracy in diagnosing tuberculin hypersensitivity in patients with *Mycobacterium tuberculosis* infection.— E. L. Stull and S. A. Szumski, *Curr. ther. Res.*, 1979, *26*, 89.

Variations in response to the tuberculin tine test appeared to depend on the coating of the tines; some tines were uniformly coated at the tip while in others the coating had formed a globule at the base. Of 144 smooth-coated tines 2 produced no visible reaction, while of 144 globular-coated tines 37 produced no visible reaction.— J. A. Lunn, *Br. med. J.*, 1980, *280*, 223.

A favourable comparison of multiple puncture liquid tuberculin test (Imotest) with the Mantoux test.— J. A. Lunn *et al.*, *Lancet*, 1981, *1*, 695. Criticism.— S. A. Szumski, *Lederle* (letter), *ibid.*, 1363. Reply.— J. A. Lunn (letter), *ibid.*, *2*, 93. Evidence confirming Lunn's findings (*Br. med. J.*, 1980, *280*, 223) of the variable tuberculin coating of tines.— C. Herzog (letter), *ibid.*, 417.

References criticising the dry tine test: H. Welke *et al.*, *S. Afr. med. J.*, 1976, *50*, 2073; J. Houghton (letter), *Br. med. J.*, 1978, *2*, 54; C. K. Connolly *et al.* (letter), *ibid.*, 1367; J. M. Platts (letter), *ibid.*, 1979, *1*, 823; P. K. Wilson (letter), *ibid.*, 1979, *2*, 53.

References defending the dry tine test: M. Caplin *et al.* (letter), *Br. med. J.*, 1978, *2*, 54; V. M. Hawthorne (letter), *ibid.*, 280; A. A. Cunningham (letter), *ibid.*, 503; K. Sauer and O. Brändli (letter), *ibid.*, 1367; P. R. Bull *et al.* (letter), *ibid.*, 1979, *1*, 1712; E. L. Stull, *Curr. ther. Res.*, 1979, *25*, 657.

Heaf test. In 213 children aged 12 to 14 years who had shown grade 1 positive reactions to the Heaf test, only 25 who showed positive reactions to subsequent Mantoux testing were considered likely to have been infected with *M. tuberculosis*, and none had evidence of active tuberculosis 12 months later. It was recommended that all children who showed negative or grade 1 reactions to the Heaf test be given the benefit of BCG vaccination. The criteria used for evaluating the Heaf test were: grade 1, four or more discrete palpable papules at least 1 mm in diameter; grade 2, papules forming a ring with normal skin in the middle; grade 3, a plateau of induration; grade 4, vesiculation or ulceration.— N. S. Galbraith *et al.*, *Br. med. J.*, 1972, *1*, 647.

For a review of the grading of the Heaf test, see *Lancet*, 1972, *1*, 240. See also *Br. med. J.*, 1974, *2*, 49; *ibid.*, 1974, *3*, 622.

Proprietary Preparations

Imotest-tuberculin *(Servier, UK)*. A disposable plastic unit bearing 9 tines which are wetted before application by 0.05 ml of tuberculin purified protein derivative contained in an attached removable reservoir; the amount of tuberculin injected is stated to be equivalent to at least 5 units. For intradermal tuberculin testing.

Tuberculin, Old, Tine Test (Rosenthal) *(Lederle, UK)*. A disposable plastic unit with a stainless steel disk bearing 4 tines coated with old tuberculin; the amount of old tuberculin on the tines is equivalent to 5 units. For intradermal tuberculin testing. (Also available as Tuberculin, Old, Tine Test in *USA*).

Tuberculin PPD is also manufactured in Great Britain by *Evans Medical* .

Other Proprietary Names

*(*Old Tuberculin or Tuberculin Purified Protein Derivative, including diluted solutions and tine tests*)*: Aplisol, Aplitest, Tuberculin Purified Protein Derivative Tine Test, Tubersol *(*all *USA)*.

8025-a

Typhoid and Tetanus Vaccine *(B.P.)*.

Typhoid/Tet/Vac.

A sterile mixture of a suspension of killed *Salmonella typhi* and tetanus formol toxoid, containing 1000 or 2000 million typhoid bacteria per ml. It conforms with the test for potency for Tetanus Vaccine.

The suspension is prepared from a strain or strains of *S. typhi* that are smooth and have a full complement of H, O, and Vi antigens. The bacteria are killed by heat or by a suitable bactericide such as formaldehyde or phenol.

Store at 2° to 8° and avoid freezing. Protect from light.

Adverse Effects and Precautions. As for Tetanus Vaccine, p.1609 and Typhoid Vaccine, p.1612.

Uses. Typhoid and Tetanus Vaccine may be used for primary immunisation against typhoid fever and tetanus. The volume stated on the label as the dose is followed after 4 to 6 weeks by a second dose. To provide adequate protection against tetanus a third dose, of Tetanus Vaccine or Adsorbed Tetanus Vaccine, is needed 4 to 6 months later.

Typhoid and Tetanus Vaccine may also be used as a reinforcing dose in persons already immunised; for this purpose a single intramuscular dose is adequate.

8026-t

Typhoid Vaccine *(B.P., Eur. P.)*. Vaccinum Typhoidi; Typhoid/Vac.

It is a sterile suspension of killed *Salmonella typhi* containing not less than 500 million and not more than 1000 million bacteria in the volume, which does not exceed 1 ml, indicated on the label as the dose.

It is prepared from a strain or strains of *S. typhi* that are smooth and have a full complement of H, O, and Vi antigens. The bacteria are killed by heat or by a suitable bactericide such as formaldehyde or phenol.

It may also be supplied as a dried vaccine (Dried Typhoid/Vac) which is reconstituted immediately before use by the addition of suitable sterile liquid. Phenol may not be used in the preparation of the dried vaccine. *Eur. P.* includes the dried vaccine as Freeze-Dried Typhoid Vaccine; Vaccinum Typhoidi Cryodesiccatum.

Store at 2° to 8° and avoid freezing. Protect from light. Under these conditions the liquid vaccine may be expected to retains its potency for at least 2 years and the dried vaccine for at least 5 years.

8027-x

Typhoid Vaccine *(U.S.P.)*.

A sterile suspension or solid containing killed typhoid bacilli (*Salmonella typhosa*) of the Ty 2 strain. It has a potency of 8 units per ml. Dried vaccine contains no preservative; aqueous vaccine and reconstituting fluid contain a preservative. The *U.S.P.* specifies a nitrogen content for acetone-extracted and non-extracted preparations.

Store at 2° to 8° and avoid freezing. The expiration date is not later than 18 months after release from manufacturer's cold storage.

The stability of typhoid vaccines.— I. Joó and J. Zsidai, *J. biol. Stand.*, 1979, *7*, 341.

Units. The first International Reference Preparation (1962) of acetone-inactivated typhoid vaccine consists of ampoules containing 11 mg of dried vaccine.

The first International Reference Preparation (1962) of heat-phenol-inactivated typhoid vaccine consists of ampoules containing 34 mg of freeze-dried vaccine.

Adverse Effects. As for Vaccines, p.1586.

Adverse effects may be more marked in patients over 35 years of age, and are less marked after intracutaneous (intradermal) injection.

In a double-blind study in which subjects were injected with either saline or a monovalent acetone-inactivated typhoid vaccine, it was found that local reactions to the vaccine occurred in about 85% of subjects vaccinated by jet injection and in about 24% of those vaccinated by a conventional syringe. No increase in local reactions occurred when a second jet injection was given 5 weeks after the first. This vaccine was not significantly immunogenic to antigens O and Vi, but induced a high seroconversion rate to typhoid H antigen.— E. A. Edwards *et al.*, *Bull. Wld Hlth Org.*, 1974, *51*, 501.

Precautions. As for Vaccines, p.1586.

Typhoid vaccine is not recommended for patients with acute infections or chronic illness, or for children less than 1-year-old.

Vaccinations against typhoid provoked the onset of multiple sclerosis in a patient and in 3 it produced an exacerbation of established multiple sclerosis.— H. Miller *et al.*, *Br. med. J.*, 1967, *2*, 210.

In patients with rheumatoid arthritis typhoid vaccine might provoke activity; intradermal doses were therefore preferable.— *Br. med. J.*, 1977, *1*, 39.

Use in systemic lupus erythematosus. Vaccination and immunisation against typhoid could be carried out if necessary in patients with systemic lupus erythematosus which was controlled, but should be withheld in those with active disease and those on large doses of corticosteroids.— N. R. Rowell, *Br. med. J.*, 1969, *2*, 427.

Uses. Typhoid Vaccine is used for active immunisation against typhoid fever. Protection is adequate in about 70% of those inoculated and immunity lasts for at least 2 years.

For primary immunisation of adults, 2 doses, usually of 0.5 ml, are given by deep subcutaneous or by intramuscular injection, preferably 4 to 6 weeks apart; reinforcing doses may be given every 3 years, or annually if the risk of exposure is high. Children are given one-half the adult dose.

The second dose may be given intracutaneously (intradermally) in a dose of 0.1 ml for adults and children.

The status of available agents for immunisation against typhoid and prospects for development.— *Bull. Wld Hlth Org.*, 1979, *57*, 719.

One batch of acetone-killed typhoid vaccine had given 79 to 94% protection in 3 trials; heat-killed vaccines had protected 51 to 86% in 6 trials; formalin-killed vaccine had protected 90% in 1 trial; alcohol-killed vaccines protected 39 to 75% in 4 trials; and antigenic extracts or miscellaneous preparations had protected 11 to 77% in 8 trials.— G. Edsall (letter), *New Engl. J. Med.*, 1968, *278*, 795.

Single doses of typhoid vaccine afforded significant protection against infection. Doses of 0.4 to 0.5 ml of an acetone-killed vaccine (K-66) or of a heat-killed vaccine (G-66) were administered in Russia to about 104 000 children aged 7 to 20 years; about 52 000 further children served as controls. The incidence of typhoid during the following 10 months was significantly lower in the vaccinated groups than in controls. The incidence of infection in a further 11 months was low, but the number of cases did not permit conclusions to be drawn.— L. B. Hejfec *et al.*, *Bull. Wld Hlth Org.*, 1969, *40*, 903.

An oral typhoid vaccine (Ty 58) gave no protection against typhoid.— C. S. Chuttani *et al.*, *Bull. Wld Hlth Org.*, 1973, *48*, 754. A favourable report of the use of live oral typhoid vaccine (Ty 21a) in children.— M. H. Wahdan, *Bull. Wld Hlth Org.*, 1980, *58*, 469.

Proprietary Preparations

Typhoid Vaccine (Monovalent) Wellcome *(Wellcome, UK)*. Contains 1000 million *Salmonella typhi* (heat-killed) per ml, in vials of 1.5 ml. *Dose*. 0.5 ml.

Other Proprietary Names

Typhoid Vaccine *(Wyeth, USA)*.

8028-r

Typhoid-paratyphoid A and B Vaccine *(B.P. 1973)*. TAB Vaccine; TAB/Vac.

A sterile mixed suspension of *Salmonella typhi*, *S. paratyphi A*, and *S. paratyphi B*. It contains 1000 million *S. typhi*, 500 or 750 million *S. paratyphi A*, and 500 or 750 million *S. paratyphi B* in 1 ml.

It consists of vaccines prepared from strains of the bacteria that are smooth and have the full complement of O and H antigens and, in the case of *S. typhi*, contain also the Vi antigen. Either a single strain or several strains of each species may be included. The bacteria are killed by heat or by a bactericide.

Store at 2° to 10° and avoid freezing. Protect from light. Under these conditions it may be expected to retain its potency for 18 months from the date of manufacture.

8029-f

Intracutaneous Typhoid-paratyphoid A and B Vaccine *(B.P. 1973)*. Intracut. TAB Vaccine; Intradermal Typhoid-paratyphoid A and B Vaccine; TAB/Vac (Intracut).

A sterile mixed suspension of *Salmonella typhi*, *S. paratyphi A*, and *S. paratyphi B*. It contains *either* 2500 million *S. typhi*, 1250 million *S. paratyphi A*, and 1250 million *S. paratyphi B*, *or* 2000 million *S. typhi*, 1500 million *S. paratyphi A*, and 1500 million *S. paratyphi B* in 1 ml.

It is prepared from strains of the bacteria that are smooth and have the full complement of O and H antigens and, in the case of *S. typhi*, contain also the Vi antigens. Either a single strain or several strains of each species may be included. The bacteria are killed by heat or by a bactericide.

Store at 2° to 10° and avoid freezing. Protect from light.

Adverse Effects and Precautions. As for Typhoid Vaccines, p.1612.

Local reactions are common. Serious side-effects which have occurred rarely include cardiovascular reactions, arthropathies, encephalitis, and nephritis. Use of the vaccine has activated latent infections with herpes, poliomyelitis, and tuberculosis.

Uses. Typhoid-paratyphoid A and B Vaccine has been used for active immunisation against typhoid and paratyphoid fevers, but the value of the paratyphoid component has not been established. Vaccination against paratyphoid fever is no longer recommended.

The use of typhoid-paratyphoid vaccines should be discontinued because (1) of the low incidence of paratyphoid A and B disease, (2) the immunogenicity of paratyphoid A vaccine has never been proved, and (3) the immunogenicity of *S. paratyphi B* was low—an adequate content would make the vaccine unacceptable.— *Bull. Wld Hlth Org.*, 1979, *57*, 719.

8030-z

Typhoid-paratyphoid A and B and Cholera Vaccine *(B.P. 1973)*. TAB and Cholera Vaccine; TAB-Cho/Vac.

NOTE. TABC Vaccine is a synonym for Typhoid-paratyphoid A, B, and C Vaccine; no such abbreviation should be made in respect of Typhoid-paratyphoid A and B and Cholera Vaccine. .

A sterile mixed suspension of *Salmonella typhi*, *S. paratyphi A*, *S. paratyphi B*, and *Vibrio cholerae*. It contains 1000 million *S. typhi*, 500 or 750 million *S. paratyphi A*, 500 or 750 million *S. paratyphi B*, and 8000 million *V. cholerae* in 1 ml. The bacteria are described under Typhoid-paratyphoid A and B Vaccine, and Cholera Vaccine.

Store at 2° to 10° and avoid freezing. Protect from light. Under these conditions it may be expected to retain its potency for 18 months from the date of manufacture.

Adverse Effects and Precautions. As for Typhoid Vaccine, p.1612.

In 1 patient vitreous haemorrhage occurred in both eyes shortly after receiving a typhoid cholera inoculation.— P. J. Lewis and B. L. Jones (letter), *Med. J. Aust.*, 1974, *2*, 914.

A report of anuria and hepatitis apparently related to a reaction to revaccination with typhoid-paratyphoid A and B and cholera vaccine.— A. J. Eisinger and J. G. Smith, *Br. med. J.*, 1979, *1*, 381.

Uses. Typhoid-paratyphoid A and B and Cholera Vaccine was formerly used instead of the constituent vaccines for active immunisation against typhoid and paratyphoid fevers and cholera. Vaccination against paratyphoid fever is no longer recommended.

8031-c

Typhoid-paratyphoid A and B and Tetanus Vaccine *(B.P. 1973)*. Typhoid-paratyphoid A and B Vaccine-Tetanus Toxoid; TAB and Tetanus Vaccine; TABT/Vac.

A sterile mixed suspension of *Salmonella typhi*, *S. paratyphi A*, and *S. paratyphi B*, with tetanus formol toxoid. It contains 500 or 1000 million *S. typhi*, 250 or 500 million *S. paratyphi A*, and 250 or 500 million *S. paratyphi B* in 1 ml. The potency of the tetanus component is comparable to that of Tetanus Vaccine.

Store at 2° to 10° and avoid freezing. Protect from light. Under these conditions it may be expected to retain its potency for 18 months from the date of manufacture.

Adverse Effects and Precautions. As for Typhoid Vaccine, p.1612.

Uses. Typhoid-paratyphoid A and B and Tetanus Vaccine was formerly used for active immunisation against typhoid and paratyphoid fevers and tetanus but vaccination against paratyphoid fever is no longer recommended.

8032-k

Typhoid-paratyphoid A, B, and C Vaccine *(B.P. 1968).* TABC Vaccine; TABC/Vac.

A sterile mixed suspension of *Salmonella typhi, S. paratyphi A, S. paratyphi B,* and *S. paratyphi C.* It contains 1000 million *S. typhi,* 500 or 750 million *S. paratyphi A,* 500 or 750 million *S. paratyphi B,* and 500 or 750 million *S. paratyphi C* in 1 ml.

It consists of vaccines prepared from strains of the bacteria that are smooth and have the full complement of O and H antigens and, in the case of *S. typhi* and *S. paratyphi C,* contain also the Vi antigen. Either a single strain or several strains of each species may be included. The bacteria are killed by heat or by a bactericide.

Store at 2° to 10° and avoid freezing. Protect from light.

Uses. Typhoid-paratyphoid A, B, and C Vaccine was formerly used to provide immunity against typhoid and paratyphoid fevers.

8033-a

Typhus Vaccine *(B.P.).* Typhus/Vac.

A sterile suspension of killed epidemic typhus rickettsiae prepared in the yolk sacs of fertile eggs, rodent lungs, or the peritoneal cavity of gerbils. Potency is assessed on the basis of the production, in *guinea-pigs,* of serum which protects *mice* against the toxin.

The label states the material from which the vaccine has been obtained, and whether the vaccine has been purified.

It is a slightly turbid liquid which deposits on standing; the deposit is readily redistributed by shaking.

Store at 2° to 8° and avoid freezing. Protect from light. Under these conditions it may be expected to retain its potency for at least 1 year.

8034-t

Typhus Vaccine *(U.S.P.).*

A sterile suspension of killed rickettsiae of a strain or strains of epidemic typhus rickettsiae (*Rickettsia prowazeki*) selected for antigenicity; it consists of the refined material derived from a suspension of the yolk sacs of infected chick embryos; the rickettsiae are killed chemically; it may contain a suitable preservative.

Store at 2° to 8°. The expiration date is not later than 18 months after release from manufacturer's cold storage.

Adverse Effects and Precautions. As for Vaccines, p.1586.

Local reactions are usually mild, but reactions of moderate severity may occur.

Care is necessary in persons hypersensitive to egg protein.

Uses. Typhus Vaccine is used for active immunisation against louse-borne typhus. Its use may be considered for those living in or visiting the few endemic areas, for medical workers, and laboratory workers. It does not provide complete protection, but lessens the severity of the disease and the incidence of serious complications. It does not provide protection against scrub typhus.

The primary course is 2 doses given subcutaneously at intervals of 7 to 10 days, with a third dose several months later. Reinforcing doses should be given annually.

Manufacturers
Commonwealth Serum Laboratories, Austral.

8035-x

Widow Spider Species Antivenin (Latrodectus mactans) *(U.S.P.).*

A sterile freeze-dried preparation of specific venom-neutralising globulins obtained from the serum of healthy horses immunised against venom of black widow spiders (*Latrodectus mactans*) or related species. One dose neutralises the venom in not less than 6000 *mouse* LD50 of *L. mactans.* When reconstituted as specified it contains not more than 20% of solids. It contains thiomersal 0.01%.

Store at a temperature not exceeding 40°. The expiration date of antivenin containing 10% excess potency is not more than 5 years after release from manufacturer's cold storage.

The label states the animal source.

Adverse Effects. As for Antisera, p.1587.

Black widow spider antivenin is prepared from the serum of animals and reactions to the injection of animal serum may occur.

Uses. Black widow spider antivenin is used as part of the treatment of bites by the black widow spider.

A single dose may be given intramuscularly into the thigh and repeated if necessary. In severe cases the dose is diluted with 10 to 50 ml of sodium chloride injection and given intravenously over 15 minutes.

Proprietary Names
Antivenin (Black Widow Spider)*(Merck Sharp & Dohme, USA).*

8037-f

Yellow Fever Vaccine, Live *(B.P.).* Yel/Vac.

An aqueous suspension of chick-embryo tissue infected with the strain of yellow fever virus known as 17D, which is virulent for mice, but, though avirulent for man, has retained its immunising efficiency. It is supplied as a freeze-dried product which is reconstituted before use with a saline or other appropriate solution so that the reconstituted vaccine is iso-osmotic with blood.

The potency of the vaccine is such that it contains plaque-forming units equivalent to not less than 1000 mouse LD50 in each dose.

Store *in vacuo* or in an atmosphere of nitrogen at 2° to 8°. Protect from light. Under these conditions it may be expected to retain its potency for at least 1 year; at lower temperatures it retains its potency for longer periods. At 20° it loses its potency within a few days.

8038-d

Yellow Fever Vaccine *(U.S.P.).*

A freeze-dried preparation of a selected attenuated strain of live yellow fever virus cultured in chick embryos. Potency is expressed in terms of mouse LD50. It contains no human serum and no antimicrobial agent. It is reconstituted, just prior to use, by the addition of sodium chloride injection.

Store under nitrogen preferably below 0° but not above 5°. The expiration date is not later than 1 year after release from manufacturer's cold storage.

Three of 8 yellow fever vaccines from different manufacturing laboratories retained their potency for 2 weeks at 37° and all the vaccines could be kept for 2 weeks at 22°.— Y. Robin *et al., Bull. Wld Hlth Org.,* 1971, *44,* 729.

A stabilised yellow fever vaccine (Arilvax-stabilised) had a half-life of more than 2 years when stored at −20° or 4°; of about 292 days at about 20°; of 10.1 days at 37°; and 2.4 days at 46°. After reconstitution the half-life was at least 90 minutes at 37°.— C. Burfoot *et al., J. biol. Stand.,* 1977, *5,* 173.

Yellow fever vaccine of high initial potency, reconstituted with water, or diluted 1 : 10 with sodium chloride injection and ready for use, could be kept, protected as far as possible from light, for up to a day at 22°. Vaccines of minimum allowable initial potency might fall below strength. The study was based on vaccine from one manufacturer and might not be universally applicable.— C. Lucasse and C. Visser, *J. biol. Stand.,* 1978, *6,* 1.

The development of an improved experimental yellow fever vaccine.— G. A. Tannock *et al., J. biol. Stand.,* 1980, *8,* 23.

Adverse Effects. As for Vaccines, p.1586.

Local and general reactions are not common after vaccination for yellow fever. Hypersensitivity reactions have occurred in persons allergic to egg protein and, very rarely, encephalitis has followed vaccination, generally in infants under 9 months of age.

Side-effects following the use of 17D vaccine in about 120 000 instances during an epidemic in Senegal were transient bleeding at the injection site and haematomas. Meningoencephalitic complications, including 25 fatalities, occurred in 240 patients following about 1 850 000 vaccinations using Dakar yellow fever vaccine.— L. Chambon *et al., Bull. Wld Hlth Org.,* 1967, *36,* 113.

Encephalitis occurred in 248 patients in Dakar after vaccination for yellow fever, but only 2 of them had been given vaccine made from the 17D virus.— I. D. Mar *et al., Annls Pédiat., Paris,* 1967, *43,* 689, per *J. Am. med. Ass.,* 1967, *200* (May 22), A191.

Precautions. As for Vaccines, p.1586.

Yellow Fever Vaccine, Live should be given with care to persons hypersensitive to egg protein. It should not generally be given to infants less than 9 months of age.

The vibriocidal activity and the yellow fever neutralising antibody titres were reduced in subjects vaccinated with yellow fever vaccine given with or within 3 weeks of cholera vaccine.— O. Felsenfeld *et al., Lancet,* 1973, *1,* 457.

Yellow fever vaccine could be given with little added risk to a patient receiving steroid therapy.— *Br. med. J.,* 1977, *1,* 39. But see Precautions for Vaccines, p.1586.

Pregnancy and the neonate. Pregnant women might be vaccinated in an epidemic or if travel to an endemic area could not be delayed; otherwise vaccination should be delayed until after the first trimester.— M. M. Levine *et al., Lancet,* 1974, *2,* 34.

Uses. Yellow Fever Vaccine, Live produces an active immunity which is usually established within 10 days of administration and persists for many years. Only 1 dose is required for immunisation but re-inoculation every 10 years is desirable, and probably more frequently during an epidemic. Yellow Fever Vaccine, Live is given by subcutaneous injection; the dose is the volume containing at least 1000 mouse LD50 doses.

An International Certificate of Vaccination against yellow fever is valid only if the vaccine used has been approved by WHO and administered at a designated vaccinating centre. Lists of designated centres are published periodically.

Eleven women with recurrent labial herpes simplex eruptions reported that yellow fever vaccine had a delaying effect on herpes providing them with long periods without eruptions.— H. H. Neumann (letter), *Lancet,* 1977, *2,* 250.

Proprietary Preparations
Arilvax *(Wellcome, UK).* A brand of Yellow Fever Vaccine, Live, available as dried powder for preparation before use, in ampoules of 1, 5, and 10 doses, with diluent. It contains traces of neomycin sulphate and polymyxin B sulphate.

Vasodilators

9200-h

The vasodilators described in this section are mainly those used for angina pectoris or for cerebral or peripheral vascular disorders.

Vasodilators used in the management of angina pectoris were formerly termed *coronary* vasodilators, but their mode of action is now considered to be a reduction of oxygen demand. For further details, see Glyceryl Trinitrate, p.1621.

Cerebral and *peripheral* vasodilators fall primarily into 3 main groups: (1) alpha-adrenoceptor blocking agents; (2) smooth muscle relaxants; and (3) those that act by simulating the effects of beta-adrenoceptor stimulation.

Other drugs with a peripheral vasodilator effect include co-dergocrine mesylate (see p.663), histamine (see p.518), acetylcholine (see p.1037), and nicotinic acid (see p.1649). Many anti-hypertensive agents have powerful peripheral vasodilator effects and are described under Anti-hypertensive Agents, p.135.

Cerebrovascular disease. A review of the use of vasodilators in senile dementia. The difficulties in mounting clinical trials in dementia are many, and it will be some time before any firm conclusions about the efficacy of cerebral vasodilators are reached. On present evidence, it appears that simple vasodilators have no place in the treatment of vascular dementia.— *Br. med. J.*, 1979, *2*, 511.

A review summarising the pathophysiology of cerebrovascular disease and dementia and the pharmacology of cerebral vasodilators, including their use in these disorders. Cerebral vasodilators must be regarded as contra-indicated in all patients with acute stroke and may sometimes be harmful in chronic cerebrovascular disease. Co-dergocrine mesylate and naftidrofuryl have shown some promise in senile dementia but can only be cautiously recommended. Cyclandelate and vincamine have not been clearly shown to be of value and there is insufficient evidence to justify the use of other cerebral vasodilators for senile dementia.— P. Cook and I. James, *New Engl. J. Med.*, 1981, *305*, 1508 and 1560.

Further reviews: J. A. Yesavage *et al.*, *Archs gen. Psychiat.*, 1979, *36*, 220.

Cardiac disorders. *Angina pectoris.* Reviews of the use of vasodilators in angina pectoris: *Br. med. J.*, 1978, *2*, 462; L. H. Opie, *Lancet*, 1980, *1*, 966; *Drug & Ther. Bull.*, 1981, *19*, 37.

Heart failure. Reviews of the use of vasodilators in heart failure: J. N. Cohn and J. A. Franciosa, *New Engl. J. Med.*, 1977, *297*, 27 and 254; *Med. Lett.*, 1978, *20*, 89; M. Packer and J. Meller, *Am. J. Cardiol.*, 1978, *42*, 686; *Lancet*, 1979, *2*, 777.

Peripheral vascular disorders. A review of the non-surgical management of peripheral vascular disease. There is little evidence that vasodilators have much to offer.— C. A. C. Clyne, *Br. med. J.*, 1980, *281*, 794. Peripheral vasodilators are of no benefit in intermittent claudication and may do harm by reducing flow where it is needed.— *Lancet*, 1980, *1*, 404. See also *Med. Lett.*, 1978, *20*, 11.

9201-m

Adenosine Phosphate. AMP; Adenosine 5′-Monophosphate; Adenosine-5′-phosphoric Acid; 5′-Adenylic Acid; Muscle Adenylic Acid; Monophosadénine. 6-Amino-9-β-D-ribofuranosylpurine 5′-(dihydrogen phosphate).
$C_{10}H_{14}N_5O_7P$=347.2.

CAS — 61-19-8.

A crystalline solid, readily **soluble** in boiling water; the sodium salt is soluble in cold water. It is a nucleotide constituent of animal cells, being concerned with the storage and release of energy.

Adverse Effects. Adverse effects associated with adenosine phosphate include flushing, dizziness, dyspnoea, and palpitations after injection, particularly with large doses in aqueous solution. Anaphylactic reactions have been reported.

Uses. Adenosine phosphate has vasodilator properties and has been used in the treatment of complications of varicose ulcers. It has been given in usual doses of 20 to 140 mg daily sublingually or orally or up to 100 mg daily by intramuscular injections as the sodium salt. It has also been given for pruritus, porphyria, multiple sclerosis, hepatic disorders, and rheumatism.

Adenosine phosphate 160 to 200 mg daily for at least 4 weeks was effective in controlling all the symptoms of porphyria cutanea tarda, apart from the hypersensitivity of the skin to slight injuries, in 19 of 21 patients. The improvement lasted for several years in about half the group. Relapses responded to further treatment.— A. Gajdos (letter), *Lancet*, 1974, *1*, 163.

Proprietary Names

Adenyl *(Auclair, Fr.; Auclair, Switz.)*; My-B-Den *(Dome, USA)*.

Adenosine phosphate was formerly marketed in Great Britain under the proprietary name Adenyl (*Rona*).

9202-b

Cyclic Adenosine Phosphate. Cyclic AMP; cAMP. Adenosine 3′,5′-(hydrogen phosphate).
$C_{10}H_{12}N_5O_6P$=329.2.

CAS — 60-92-4.

Pharmacopoeias. In *Chin.* which specifies the monohydrate.

Cyclic adenosine phosphate is of considerable pharmacological interest in that it appears to function as 'second messenger' in the mediation of hormone action. It is considered that a hormone, such as adrenaline or glucagon, is bound to a receptor site on the target cell membrane and that it there activates adenyl cyclase under the influence of which, in the presence of magnesium, adenosine triphosphate is converted to cyclic adenosine phosphate which evokes the characteristic hormone response in the cell before being converted, under the influence of phosphodiesterase, to adenosine phosphate. Hormones whose action may be mediated by cyclic adenosine phosphate include catecholamines with predominantly beta-adrenoceptor activity, calcitonin, parathyroid, corticotrophin, glucagon, follicle-stimulating hormone, luteinising hormone, protirelin, and vasopressin. The action of histamine and prostaglandins may be similarly mediated.

The role of cyclic adenosine phosphate in the aetiology of disease is as yet little understood.

The cardiovascular effects of exogenous cyclic adenosine phosphate.— R. A. Levine *et al.*, *Clin. Pharmac. Ther.*, 1968, *9*, 168. The effect on glucose metabolism.— R. A. Levine, *Metabolism*, 1968, *17*, 34. The antidiuretic effect.— *idem*, *Clin. Sci.*, 1968, *34*, 253. The effect of the dibutyryl derivative.— *idem*, *Clin. Pharmac. Ther.*, 1970, *11*, 238.

Discussions of the role of cyclic adenosine phosphate as a mediator of hormone action.— *Lancet*, 1970, *2*, 1119; G. W. Liddle and J. G. Hardman, *New Engl. J. Med.*, 1971, *285*, 560. Role in the regulation of lymphocyte function.— C. W. Parker, *New Engl. J. Med.*, 1976, *295*, 1180. Potential role in therapeutics.— B. Weiss and W. N. Hait, *A. Rev. Pharmac. & Toxic.*, 1977, *17*, 441.

Despite positive findings *in vitro*, dibutyryl cyclic adenosine phosphate had no effect on induced inflammation in 6 subjects, nor had cyclic adenosine phosphate inducers, theophylline and salbutamol, given in conjunction to 9 patients with chronic urticaria.— J. L. Burton and M. W. Greaves (letter), *Lancet*, 1972, *2*, 1151.

In 7 patients with psoriasis, dibutyryl cyclic adenosine phosphate 200 ng per ml in acetone followed by papaverine 1% was applied thrice daily to psoriatic areas cleaned of scale. After 4 weeks the treated areas were unchanged or worse.— R. Auerbach (letter), *J. Am. med. Ass.*, 1974, *227*, 326. Comment on results observed.— A. E. Warren (letter), *ibid.*, *228*, 695.

9203-v

Adenosine Triphosphate. ATP; Adenosine 5′-Triphosphate; 5′-Adenyldiphosphoric Acid; Adenylpyrophosphoric Acid; Triphosadénine. Adenosine 5′-(tetrahydrogen triphosphate).
$C_{10}H_{16}N_5O_{13}P_3$=507.2.

CAS — 56-65-5.

Pharmacopoeias. Cz. includes the disodium salt under the title Natrium Adenosintriphosphoricum ($C_{10}H_{14}N_5Na_2O_{13}P_3$=551.1).

A white amorphous odourless powder with a faint sour taste. Very **soluble** in water; practically insoluble in alcohol, ether, and other organic solvents. A 1% aqueous solution has a pH of about 2. Unstable in alkaline solution.

Adenosine triphosphate is a nucleotide constituent of animal cells with a fundamental role in biological energy transformations, being concerned with the storage and release of energy; it is converted to cyclic adenosine monophosphate, release of energy occurring during the process. It has been postulated that adenosine triphosphate might be involved in neurotransmission in the central nervous system and also in the gastro-intestinal tract and urinary bladder. Its administration has been claimed to improve circulation and muscular power. It has been given in the treatment of a variety of rheumatic conditions and has been used in the treatment of coronary insufficiency and supraventricular tachycardia.

Muscular dystrophy. A mixture of nucleotides and nucleosides including adenosine triphosphate has been suggested for the treatment of the Duchenne type of muscular dystrophy. Controlled trials have not shown it to produce any observable benefits (J.M.S. Pearce *et al.*, *Br. med. J.*,1964, *2*, 915 and J.N. Walton *et al.*, *ibid.*, 1965, *2*, 533), though improvement has been noted in an uncontrolled trial (J.K. Wilkie, *ibid.*, 821).

Radiological protection. Adenosine triphosphate given with deoxyribonucleic acid decreased the rate of cells with structural chromosome aberrations in 3 radiologists chronically exposed to X-rays.— V. Goyanes-Villaescusa (letter), *Lancet*, 1973, *2*, 575.

Proprietary Preparations

Adenotriphos *(Rona, UK)*. **Ampoules** of 2 ml of an injection containing the neutral sodium salt of adenosine triphosphoric acid equivalent to 10 mg of adenosine triphosphoric acid per ml and **Tablets** each containing 3 mg of the disodium salt of adenosine triphosphoric acid. *Dose.* By mouth, initial, 2 tablets thrice daily for 1 week; maintenance, 4 to 8 tablets daily; by intramuscular injection, initial, the contents of 1 or 2 ampoules daily for 2 to 4 days; maintenance, the same or half dosage every other day to a total of 10 to 20 ampoules. (Also available as Adenotriphos in *Austral.*).

Other Proprietary Names

Atepodin *(Spain)*; Atriphos (sodium salt) *(Hung.)*; Estriadin *(Spain)*; Nucleocardyl *(Spain)*; Striadyne *(Belg., Fr.)*; Striadyne forte *(Switz.)*; Triadenyl ATP (calcium and sodium salts) *(Ger.)*; Triadesin-A, Trinosin (both *Jap.*).

9204-g

Ammi Visnaga Fruit. Khella; Khellah; Picktooth Fruit; Visnaga.

Pharmacopoeias. In *Fr.*, *Ger.*, and *Pol.*

The dried ripe fruits of *Ammi visnaga* (Umbelliferae). Ammi visnaga fruit usually contains about 1% of khellin (p.1625), 0.3% of khelloside ($C_{19}H_{20}O_{10}$,$2H_2O$=444.4), and about 0.1% of visnagin.

Ammi visnaga fruit has been used as a liquid extract containing 0.5% w/v of khellin (*max. dose:* 0.5 ml) and a tincture containing 0.05% w/v of khellin (*max. dose:* 4 ml) as an antispasmodic in renal colic and ureteric spasm.

'Visnagan', the oil remaining after the extraction of the principal crystalline constituents of ammi visnaga fruit, has been investigated by a number of workers and several crystalline components have been isolated, at least 3 of which, samidine ($C_{21}H_{22}O_7$), dihydrosamidine, and visnadine (p.1634), have been reported to be strongly vasodilatory; the last 2 are isomers with the formula $C_{21}H_{24}O_7$.

References: G. V. Anrep *et al.*, *J. Pharm. Pharmac.*, 1949, *1*, 164; M. M. Bagouri, *ibid.*, 177; S. Collett, *Mfg Chem.*, 1952, *23*, 235; E. Smith *et al.*, *J. Am. chem. Soc.*, 1957, *79*, 3534.

Proprietary Names

Visnacorin ('visnagan') *(Infale, Spain)*.

9205-q

Amyl Nitrite *(B.P.C. 1973).* Amylis Nitris; Isoamyl Nitrite; Amylium Nitrosum; Isopentyl Nitrite; Pentanoli Nitris; Azotito de Amilo; Nitrito de Amilo.

Pharmacopoeias. In *Arg., Aust., Belg., Cz., Hung., Ind., Int., It., Jap., Jug., Mex., Nord., Pol., Port., Rus., Span., Swiss, Turk.,* and *U.S.*

A clear, yellow, volatile, inflammable liquid with a fragrant odour and pungent aromatic taste. Wt per ml 0.868 to 0.878 g. B.p. 96°. Flash-point 10° (closed-cup test). It consists of the nitrites of 3-methylbutan-1-ol, $(CH_3)_2CH.CH_2.CH_2OH$, and 2-methylbutan-1-ol, $CH_3.CH_2.CH(CH_3).CH_2OH$, with other nitrites of the homologous series, and contains not less than 90% w/w of nitrites calculated as $C_5H_{11}NO_2$. The *U.S.P.* specifies a mixture of the nitrite esters of 3-methylbutan-1-ol and 2-methylbutan-1-ol, with not less than 85% of $C_5H_{11}NO_2$.

Practically **insoluble** in water; miscible with alcohol, chloroform, ether, and light petroleum. **Incompatible** with alcohol, alkaline carbonates, caustic alkalis, bromides, iodides, ferrous salts, and phenazone. It is volatile even at low temperatures and is liable to decompose with evolution of nitrogen, particularly if it has become acid in reaction. **Store** in a cool place in airtight containers. Protect from light.

CAUTION. *Amyl nitrite forms an explosive mixture with air or oxygen. It is very inflammable and must not be used where it may be ignited.*

Adverse Effects, Treatment, and Precautions. As for Glyceryl Trinitrate, p.1620.

Abuse. Comment on the abuse of volatile nitrites, in the belief that they expand creativity, stimulate music appreciation, promote a sense of abandon in dancing, and intensify sexual experience.— L. T. Sigell *et al., Am. J. Psychiat.,* 1978, *135,* 1216. A brief report on the widespread use of inhaled nitrites ('poppers') by homosexual men.— T. J. McManus *et al.* (letter), *Lancet,* 1982, *1,* 503. See also under Butyl Nitrite, p.1687.

Results suggesting that nitrites may be immunosuppressive in the setting of repeated viral antigenic stimulation and may contribute to the high frequency of Kaposi's sarcoma and opportunistic infections in homosexual men.— J. J. Goedert *et al., Lancet,* 1982, *1,* 412.

Absorption and Fate. Amyl nitrite is absorbed into the circulation from mucous membranes, the rate of absorption being most rapid from the lungs. It is rapidly inactivated by hydrolysis. Amyl nitrite is rapidly hydrolysed in the gastro-intestinal tract; it is inactive by mouth.

Uses. When inhaled, amyl nitrite has an action similar to that of glyceryl trinitrate (p.1621). It is the most rapid in action of the nitrites, the effect being evident within 10 seconds. The vessels of the head and neck are most affected, and within 30 to 40 seconds after inhalation the face flushes, the head and neck perspire, and the heart-rate increases. The action is of short duration and usually lasts only about 5 minutes.

Amyl nitrite has been used in doses of 0.12 to 0.3 ml by inhalation as a short-acting vasodilator in the treatment of attacks of angina pectoris, in which it brings almost instant relief. It has also been used for the relief of renal and biliary colic.

It is employed by repeated inhalations in the immediate treatment of cyanide poisoning to induce the formation of methaemoglobin which combines with the cyanide to form non-toxic cyanmethaemoglobin; for further details see under Stronger Hydrocyanic Acid (Treatment of Adverse Effects), p.790.

Diagnostic use. References to the use of amyl nitrite in the diagnosis of some cardiac disorders: K. E. Cohn *et al., Am. J. Cardiol.,* 1968, *21,* 681; T. Sawayama *et al., Am. Heart J.,* 1968, *76,* 746; *idem, Circulation,* 1969, *40,* 327.

Poisoning. For reference to the use of amyl nitrite in the management of hydrogen sulphide poisoning, see Hydrogen Sulphide, p.1718.

Preparations

Amyl Nitrite Inhalant *(U.S.P.).* Crushable glass capsules containing amyl nitrite *U.S.P.*; they contain a suitable stabiliser. Store in a cool place. Protect from light.

Amyl Nitrite Vitrellae *(B.P.C. 1973).* Vitrell. Amyl. Nitrit. Amyl nitrite in crushable glass capsules. To be crushed between finger and thumb, and the vapour inhaled. Store in a cool place, as decomposition may occur at higher temperatures with loss of activity and development of high pressure.

Proprietary Names

Nitrit *(DAK, Denm.).*

9206-p

Azapetine Phosphate. Azepine Phosphate; Ro 2-3248. 6-Allyl-6,7-dihydro-5*H*-dibenz[*c,e*]azepine dihydrogen phosphate.

$C_{17}H_{17}N,H_3PO_4=333.3.$

CAS — 146-36-1 (azapetine); 130-83-6 (phosphate).

Azapetine phosphate 35 mg is approximately equivalent to 25 mg of azapetine.

Adverse Effects. Adverse effects associated with azapetine include dry mouth, nausea, vomiting, dizziness, anorexia, fever, headache, nasal congestion, palpitations, tachycardia, and orthostatic hypotension.

Uses. Azapetine is an alpha-adrenoceptor blocking agent which has also a direct dilator effect on peripheral blood vessels.

It has been used in doses equivalent to 25 to 75 mg of azapetine 3 times daily in the treatment of peripheral vascular disorders due to arterial spasm.

Proprietary Names

Ilidar *(Roche, Belg.; Roche, Ger.; Roche, Swed.; Roche, Switz.).*

9207-s

Bamethan Sulphate. 2-Butylamino-1-(4-hydroxyphenyl)ethanol sulphate.

$(C_{12}H_{19}NO_2)_2,H_2SO_4=516.6.$

CAS — 3703-79-5 (bamethan); 5716-20-1 (sulphate).

Adverse Effects. Bamethan sulphate may cause dizziness and other signs of hypotension, facial flushing, and tachycardia.

Treatment of Adverse Effects. In severe overdosage the stomach should be emptied by inducing emesis or by aspiration and lavage. If necessary the circulation should be maintained with infusions of suitable electrolytes.

Precautions. Bamethan sulphate should be given with caution to patients with angina pectoris and is contra-indicated in recent cardiac infarction.

Uses. Bamethan sulphate is a peripheral vasodilator which acts directly on vascular smooth muscle. It is used in the treatment of peripheral vascular disorders in usual doses of 25 mg four times daily.

Proprietary Preparations

Vasculit *(Boehringer Ingelheim, UK).* Bamethan sulphate, available as tablets of 12.5 mg.

Other Proprietary Names

Angiolast (as nicotinate) *(Ital.)*; Patol *(Jap.)*; Rotesar *(Arg.)*; Simpelate *(Jap.)*; Vasculat *(Arg., Belg., Fr., Ger., Ital., Neth., S.Afr., Spain, Switz.).*

9208-w

Bencyclane Fumarate. Bencyclane Hydrogen Fumarate. 3-(1-Benzylcycloheptyloxy)-*NN*-dimethylpropylamine hydrogen fumarate.

$C_{19}H_{31}NO,C_4H_4O_4=405.5.$

CAS — 2179-37-5 (bencyclane); 14286-84-1 (fumarate).

A crystalline substance. M.p. about 132°. **Soluble** about 1 in 100 of water and 1 in 50 of hot water; readily soluble in alcohol.

Bencyclane fumarate is a vasodilator which has been given in the treatment of peripheral and cerebral vascular disorders.

References to the inhibition of platelet aggregation by bencyclane fumarate: H. J. Klose *et al., Arzneimittel-Forsch.,* 1975, *25,* 1064; W. Jäger *et al., ibid.,* 1938; J. Bédi and A. L. Pálos, *Therapia hung.,* 1976, *24,* 50.

Effects on the nervous system. Details of adverse effects of bencyclane fumarate on the nervous system, additional to the previously reported headache and dizziness. The following adverse reactions were noted in a total of 21 patients: hallucination (6), insomnia (5), tremor (5), walking difficulty (5), excitement (3), aggravation of tremor (3), light-headed feeling (3), talkativeness (2), incontinence (2), speech disorder (1), convulsion (1), aggravation of right hemiplegia (1), numbness of lower limbs (1), micturition disorder (1), discomfort in occipital area (1), malaise (1), increase in blood pressure (1), decrease in blood pressure (1).— *Japan med. Gaz.,* 1979, *16* (Apr. 20), 11.

Proprietary Names

Angiociclan *(Ravasini, Ital.)*; Bioarterol *(Unifa, Arg.)*; Desoblit *(Elmu, Spain)*; Dilangio (cyclamate or fumarate) *(Montpellier, Arg.; Andreu, Spain)*; Fludilat *(Organon, Arg.; Organon, Fr.; Thiemann, Ger.; Thiemann, Switz.)*; Flussema *(Italfarmaco, Switz.)*; Fluxema *(Italfarmaco, Ital.)*; Halidor *(EGYT, Hung.; Jap.)*; Inphos *(Landó, Arg.)*; Vasodarkey *(Cuatrecasas-Darkey, Spain).*

9209-e

Bendazol Hydrochloride. Dibazol. 2-Benzylbenzimidazole hydrochloride.

$C_{14}H_{12}N_2,HCl=244.7.$

CAS — 621-72-7 (bendazol); 1212-48-2 (hydrochloride).

Pharmacopoeias. In *Rus.*

A white or slightly greyish- or yellowish-white hygroscopic crystalline powder with a bitter saline taste. Sparingly **soluble** in water and chloroform; very soluble in hot water; freely soluble in alcohol; slightly soluble in acetone; practically insoluble in ether. Solutions in water are acid to litmus. **Store** in airtight containers.

Bendazol hydrochloride has been stated to have vasodilating, antispasmodic, and antihypertensive properties. Doses in the *Rus. P.* are: max. single, 50 mg by mouth; max. in 24 hours, 150 mg.

9210-b

Benfurodil Hemisuccinate. CB 4091. 1-[5-(2,5-Dihydro-5-oxo-3-furyl)-3-methylbenzofuran-2-yl]ethyl hydrogen succinate.

$C_{19}H_{18}O_7=358.3.$

CAS — 3447-95-8.

Crystals. M.p. 144°.

Benfurodil hemisuccinate is stated to be a vasodilator used in the treatment of vascular disease. It is given in doses of about 150 mg twice or thrice daily by mouth or 200 to 300 mg daily by intramuscular or intravenous injection.

Proprietary Names

Clinodilat *(Liade, Spain)*; Eucilat *(Clin-Comar-Byla, Fr.).*

9211-v

Benziodarone. L 2329. 2-Ethylbenzofuran-3-yl 4-hydroxy-3,5-di-iodophenyl ketone.

$C_{17}H_{12}I_2O_3=518.1.$

CAS — 68-90-6.

Adverse Effects. Gastro-intestinal disturbances, hypothyroidism and hyperthyroidism, and jaundice have been reported.

Hyperthyroidism. Two cases of thyrotoxicosis were noted during administration of benziodarone for gout. Recovery occurred on discontinuation of the medicament but it was suggested that benziodarone should not be used in gouty patients with thyroid irregularities.— J. P. Camus *et al.*, *Revue Rhum. Mal. ostéo-articulaires*, 1973, *40*, 148, per *Thérapie*, 1974, *29*, 15.

Jaundice. The Committee on Safety of Drugs had received reports of 11 cases of jaundice occurring in patients being treated with benziodarone (Cardivix).— D. A. Cahal (letter), *Br. med. J.*, 1964, *2*, 882. Scrutiny of individual case histories and clinical data of the 11 cases of jaundice reported above did not confirm that benziodarone was responsible. Two cases had features which suggested there might be a connection and another case proved to be a carcinoma of the head of the pancreas. As the specific cause was in doubt, Cardivix could not be cleared and the manufacturers had withdrawn the drug from the market pending further information.— J. Valentine *et al.*, *Fisons* (letter), *ibid.*, 882.

Precautions. Benziodarone should be given only with caution to patients with iodine sensitivity and to patients taking anticoagulants.

Interactions. For the effects of benziodarone on anticoagulants, see Ethyl Biscoumacetate, p.771, Phenprocoumon, p.774, and Warfarin Sodium, p.778.

Absorption and Fate. Benziodarone is absorbed from the gastro-intestinal tract. It has been reported that maximum concentrations in plasma occur about 6 hours after a dose; benziodarone is concentrated in the liver. Excretion is mainly in the faeces and may be delayed by reabsorption.

Uses. Benziodarone is a vasodilator which has been used in the prophylaxis of angina pectoris and after myocardial infarction.
Benziodarone has also been given to diminish uricaemia in gout.

Cardiac disorders. References to the use of benziodarone in angina pectoris: P. Dailheu-Geoffroy and J. Nataf, *Presse méd.*, 1961, *69*, 971; P. Davies *et al.*, *Br. med. J.*, 1963, *2*, 359; S. Blake and D. Keelan, *J. Irish med. Ass.*, 1964, *54*, 42.

Hyperuricaemia. In 59 patients with gout (without renal calculi and with a blood-urea concentration not exceeding 1 mg per ml) serum-uric acid concentrations were reduced, in all except one, to less than 70 µg per ml after treatment with benziodarone 300 mg daily, though the effects on blood concentrations and clearance of urea were variable. Side-effects included weakness (11 patients), restless legs (2), dizziness (1), and impotence (2).— A. Ryckewaert *et al.*, *Thérapeutique*, 1971, *47*, 371, per *Abstr. Wld Med.*, 1971, *45*, 772.

In 40 patients with hypertension and normal renal function mean initial serum-uric acid concentrations of 62 µg per ml rose rapidly after commencing treatment with diuretics—usually thiazides—reaching a mean of 88 µg per ml; the concentration fell to normal in all but 1 patient within a week of being given benziodarone 100 to 200 mg daily, the mean value after 4.5 months being 53 µg per ml. Most of 11 patients with impaired renal function also received benefit.— G. Lagrue *et al.*, *Presse méd.*, 1971, *79*, 849, per *Abstr. Wld Med.*, 1971, *45*, 750.

Proprietary Names
Ampliacor *(RBS Pharma, Ital.)*; Amplivix *(Labaz, Belg.; Labaz, Fr.; Sigmatau, Ital.; Labaz, Neth.; Labaz, Switz.)*; Becumaron *(Riedel, Arg.)*; Coronal *(Crinos, Ital.)*; Dilacoron *(Sierochimica, Ital.)*; Dilafurane *(Labaz, Spain)*; Plexocardio *(Benvegna, Ital.)*; Uricor *(Ravizza, Ital.)*.

9212-g

Benzyl Nicotinate.
$C_{13}H_{11}NO_2$=213.2.

CAS — 94-44-0.

Benzyl nicotinate is a topical vasodilator used, in a concentration of 2.5%, in rubefacient creams and ointments.

Proprietary Preparations
See under Methyl Nicotinate, p.1626.

9213-q

Betahistine Hydrochloride.
PT 9. *N*-Methyl-2-(2-pyridyl)ethylamine dihydrochloride.
$C_8H_{12}N_2,2HCl$=209.1.

CAS — 5638-76-6 (betahistine); 5579-84-0 (hydrochloride).

A white or creamy-white, odourless, hygroscopic, crystalline powder with a bitter taste. M.p. about 152°. Freely **soluble** in water; soluble in alcohol; practically insoluble in chloroform and ether. **Store** in airtight containers. Protect from light.

Adverse Effects. Nausea, headache, and exacerbation of peptic ulcer have been reported.

Treatment of Adverse Effects. In the case of severe overdosage the stomach should be emptied by aspiration and lavage. If necessary the circulation should be maintained by infusion of suitable electrolyte solutions. The vasodilator effect of betahistine is stated to be inhibited by antihistamines.

Precautions. Betahistine hydrochloride should be given with care to patients with asthma, peptic ulcer or a history of peptic ulcer. It should not be given to patients with phaeochromocytoma. It has been suggested that it should not be given concomitantly with antihistamines.

Absorption and Fate. Betahistine hydrochloride is readily absorbed from the gastro-intestinal tract. It is converted to 2 metabolites and peak concentrations in blood of the 2 metabolites are achieved within 3 to 5 hours. Most of a dose is excreted in the urine, in the form of the metabolites, in about 3 days.

Uses. Betahistine hydrochloride is an analogue of histamine and is claimed to improve the microcirculation. It is used to reduce the frequency of episodes of dizziness in some patients with Ménière's disease. The usual dose is 8 mg thrice daily taken preferably with meals; not more than 48 mg should be taken in any one day. Betahistine has also been used in the treatment of histamine headache.

Bedsores. In a study in 18 elderly patients with decubitus ulcers, 9 treated for about 3 months with betahistine 2 tablets [each 4 mg] 4 times daily received significantly greater benefit than those treated with placebo.— C. Pecora *et al.*, *Clin. Med.*, 1971, *78* (July), 26. Comment that similar results might follow the application of local heat alone or combined with hydrotherapy.— M. R. Sather *et al.*, *Drug Intell. & clin. Pharm.*, 1977, *11*, 162.

Dementia. Studies into the role of betahistine in arteriosclerosis and dementia: J. H. Seipel and J. E. Floam, *J. clin. Pharmac.*, 1975, *15*, 144; J. H. Seipel *et al.*, *ibid.*, 155; J. S. Meyer *et al.*, *ibid.*, 1974, *14*, 280; J. H. Seipel *et al.*, *ibid.*, 1977, *17*, 140.

Headache. Ninety-three of 160 patients, most of whom suffered from headache of varied cause, were improved after treatment with betahistine hydrochloride, 2 to 25 mg daily.— B. T. Horton and H. von Leden, *Proc. Staff Meet. Mayo Clin.*, 1962, *37*, 692. Of 184 patients with histamine headache, 105 obtained relief after treatment with betahistine hydrochloride, 2 to 25 mg daily.— B. T. Horton, *ibid.*, 713.

Ménière's disease. Reports and studies on betahistine hydrochloride in Ménière's disease: J. C. Elia, *J. Am. med. Ass.*, 1966, *196*, 187; D. M. Le Pere, *Clin. Med.*, 1967, *74* (Apr.), 63; A. Burkin, *ibid.*, *74* (Oct.), 41; J. J. Hicks *et al.*, *Archs Otolar.*, 1967, *86*, 610; *Drug & Ther. Bull.*, 1971, *9*, 42; R. A. Bertrand, *Laryngoscope, St Louis*, 1971, *80*, 889; I. J. C. Frew and G. N. Menon, *Postgrad. med. J.*, 1976, *52*, 501; T. J. Wilmot and G. N. Menon, *J. Lar. Otol.*, 1976, *90*, 833; *Drug & Ther. Bull.*, 1981, *19*, 17.

Proprietary Preparations
Serc *(Duphar, UK)*. Betahistine hydrochloride, available as scored tablets of 8 mg. (Also available as Serc in *Austral., Canad., Fr., S.Afr.*).

Other Proprietary Names
Aequamen *(mesylate)* *(Ger.)*; Betaserc *(Belg., Cyp., Denm., Egypt, Fin., Greece, Neth., Switz.)*; Deanosart, Hainimeru, Medan, Meginalisk, Meniace, Menietol, Merislon, Menitazine *(all mesylate)* *(all Jap.)*; Meotels *(Jap.)*; Microser *(Ital.)*; Pyritylulon, Remark, Riptonin *(all mesylate)* *(all Jap.)*; Sinmenier *(Spain)*; Suzotolon, Tenyl-D *(both mesylate)* *(both Jap.)*; Vasomotal *(Ger.)*; Urutal *(Jug.)*.

9214-p

Buphenine Hydrochloride.
Nylidrin Hydrochloride *(U.S.P.)*; Nylidrinium Chloride. 1-(4-Hydroxyphenyl)-2-(1-methyl-3-phenylpropylamino)propan-1-ol hydrochloride.
$C_{19}H_{25}NO_2,HCl$=335.9.

CAS — 447-41-6 (buphenine); 849-55-8 (hydrochloride).

Pharmacopoeias. In *U.S.*

An odourless, white, crystalline powder. **Soluble** 1 in 65 of water and 1 in 40 of alcohol; slightly soluble in chloroform and ether. A 1% solution in water has a pH of 4.5 to 6.5. **Store** in airtight containers.

Adverse Effects. Buphenine hydrochloride may cause nausea and vomiting, trembling, nervousness, weakness, dizziness, and palpitations.

Treatment of Adverse Effects. In severe overdosage the stomach should be emptied by aspiration and lavage. If necessary, the circulation should be maintained with infusions of suitable electrolytes.

Precautions. Buphenine hydrochloride is contra-indicated in patients with myocardial infarction, hyperthyroidism, paroxysmal tachycardia, or severe angina pectoris.

Absorption and Fate. Buphenine hydrochloride is readily absorbed from the gastro-intestinal tract; its effect begins in about 10 minutes, reaches a maximum in about 30 minutes, and lasts for about 2 hours.

Investigations in *dogs* indicated that buphenine is excreted in the urine as the free base and its glucuronide.— H. Li and P. Cervoni, *J. pharm. Sci.*, 1976, *65*, 1352.

Uses. Buphenine produces the effects of beta-adrenoceptor stimulation. It is reported to increase peripheral blood flow mainly by direct action on the arteries and arterioles of the skeletal muscles. It has little effect on the vessels of the skin.
Buphenine has been used in the treatment of peripheral vascular disease.
It has also been used in the treatment of Ménière's disease and other disorders of the internal ear.
The usual initial dose of buphenine hydrochloride is 6 mg by mouth thrice daily, which may be increased to 36 or 48 mg daily in divided doses, if necessary. It has also been given by subcutaneous or intramuscular injection.

Deafness. For the use of buphenine hydrochloride in perceptive deafness, see T. J. Wilmot and J. C. Seymour, *Lancet*, 1960, *1*, 1098.

Dementia. A study of buphenine in elderly patients with cognitive, emotional, and physical impairment.— S. E. Goldstein and F. Birnbom, *J. clin. Psychiat.*, 1979, *40*, 520.

Peripheral vascular disease. On the basis of studies by F.S. Caliva *et al.* (*Am. J. med. Sci.*, 1959, *238*, 174), S. Zetterquist (*Acta med. scand.*, 1968, *183*, 487), and H.L. Karpman and R. Okun (*Geriatrics*, 1972, *27*, 101) there is no indication for the use of buphenine in peripheral vascular diseases.— J. D. Coffman, *New Engl. J. Med.*, 1979, *300*, 713.

Premature labour. Studies of buphenine in the prevention of premature labour: O. Castrén *et al.*, *Acta obstet. gynec. scand.*, 1975, *54*, 95; K. S. Koh, *Can. med. Ass. J.*, 1976, *114*, 700; R. Richter, *Am. J. Obstet. Gynec.*, 1977, *127*, 482.

Preparations
Nylidrin Hydrochloride Injection *(U.S.P.)*. A sterile solution of buphenine hydrochloride in Water for Injections.

Nylidrin Hydrochloride Tablets *(U.S.P.)*. Tablets containing buphenine hydrochloride. Store in airtight containers.

Proprietary Names
Arlibide *(US Vitamin, Arg.)*; Arlidin *(USV, Canad.; USV Pharmaceutical Corp., USA)*; Bufedon *(Cedona, Neth.)*; Dilatol *(Tropon, Ger.)*; Dilydrin *(Medichemie, Switz.)*; Opino *(Bayropharm, Ital.)*; Penitardon *(Woelm, Ger.)*; Pervadil *(ICN, Canad.)*; Tocodrin *(Medichemie, Switz.)*.

Buphenine hydrochloride was formerly marketed in Great Britain under the proprietary name Perdilatal Forte (*Smith & Nephew Pharmaceuticals*).

9215-s

Butalamine Hydrochloride. LA 1221. *NN*-Dibutyl-*N'*-(3-phenyl-1,2,4-oxadiazol-5-yl)ethylenediamine hydrochloride.
$C_{18}H_{28}N_4O,HCl=352.9$.

CAS — 22131-35-7 (butalamine); 56974-46-0 (hydrochloride).

A white crystalline powder. M.p. 135° to 141°. **Soluble** 1 in 7 of water, 1 in 10 of alcohol, and 1 in 2.5 of chloroform.

Butalamine hydrochloride is a vasodilator which has been given in the treatment of peripheral vascular disorders.

Proprietary Names
Adrevil *(Zyma, Ger.)*; Hemotrope *(Andromaco, Arg.)*; Surem *(CEPA, Spain)*; Surheme *(Aron, Fr.; Spemsa, Ital.)*.

9216-w

Butoxyethyl Nicotinate. 2-Butoxyethyl nicotinate.
$C_{12}H_{17}NO_3=223.3$.

CAS — 13912-80-6.

Butoxyethyl nicotinate is a topical vasodilator used, in a concentration of 2.5%, in rubefacient ointments.

Proprietary Preparations

See under Methyl Nicotinate, p.1626..

9217-e

Cetiedil Citrate. 2-(Perhydroazepin-1-yl)ethyl α-cyclohexyl-α-(3-thienyl)acetate dihydrogen citrate monohydrate.
$C_{20}H_{31}NO_2S,C_6H_8O_7,H_2O=559.7$.

CAS — 14176-10-4 (cetiedil); 16286-69-4 (citrate, anhydrous).

Cetiedil citrate is a vasodilator which has been given in the treatment of peripheral vascular disorders.

After intravenous injection of radioactively labelled cetiedil, 50% of the dose was metabolised within 5 minutes, and after 1 hour only labelled metabolites were recovered from the urine. Cetiedil was also shown to be rapidly metabolised after administration by mouth, and after first pass through the liver only metabolites would enter the general circulation. It was concluded that the metabolites of cetiedil were active as inhibition of saliva secretion persisted when cetiedil could no longer be detected in plasma.— A. M. Soeterboek *et al.*, *Eur. J. clin. Pharmac.*, 1977, *12*, 205.

Asthma. References to bronchodilator activity of cetiedil citrate: J. Orehek *et al.*, *Nouv. Presse méd.*, 1976, *5*, 1577; Y. W. Cho *et al.*, *Int. J. clin. Pharmac. Biopharm.*, 1978, *16*, 402.

Peripheral vascular disorders. An evaluation of cetiedil, administered intravenously, intramuscularly, or by mouth, in the treatment of peripheral vascular disorders.— R. Barbe *et al.*, *Clin. Trials J.*, 1980, *17*, 20.

Proprietary Names
Stratene *(Innothéra, Fr.; Sigmatau, Ital.)*.

9218-l

Chromonar Hydrochloride. Carbocromen Hydrochloride; A27053; AG 3; Cassella 4489. Ethyl 3-(2-diethylaminoethyl)-4-methylcoumarin-7-yloxyacetate hydrochloride.
$C_{20}H_{27}NO_5,HCl=397.9$.

CAS — 804-10-4 (chromonar); 655-35-6 (hydrochloride).

A white crystalline powder with a bitter taste. M.p. about 159°. **Soluble** in water, alcohol, and chloroform.

Chromonar hydrochloride is a vasodilator which has been used in the prophylaxis of angina pectoris.

For reports of pharmacological studies, see R. E. Nitz and E. Potzsch, *Arzneimittel-Forsch.*, 1963, *13*, 243; W. Lochner and H. Hirche, *ibid.*, 251; H. J. Bretschneider *et al.*, *ibid.*, 255.

Absorption, blood concentrations, and excretion of chromonar.— Y. C. Martin and R. -G. Wiegand, *J. pharm. Sci.*, 1970, *59*, 1313.

Cardiac disorders. A multicentre double-blind crossover study of 187 patients with angina pectoris who received chromonar for 8 weeks (79 patients) or 12 weeks (108 patients) at a dosage of 150 mg thrice daily (73 patients) or 225 mg thrice daily (114 patients) demonstrated significant prevention of anginal attacks by the lower dose, and improvement in attack-rate and glyceryl trinitrate requirement by the higher dose although the higher dose failed to show any advantage over placebo when the glyceryl trinitrate requirement was considered alone.— R. J. Bing *et al.*, *Clin. Pharmac. Ther.*, 1974, *16*, 4. See also H. Bell *et al.*, *ibid.*, 1968, *9*, 40.

Further references: G. Faucon *et al.*, *Thérapie*, 1975, *30*, 185; E. Schraven, *Arzneimittel-Forsch.*, 1976, *26*, 197; E. Schraven *et al.*, *ibid.*, 200; R. Sirbulescu *et al.*, *ibid.*, 204; N. N. Kipsidze and G. M. Kikava, *ibid.*, 1976, *26*, 882.

Proprietary Names
Antiangor *(ISM, Ital.)*; Cardiocap *(Fidia, Ital.)*; Cromene *(Scharper, Ital.)*; Intensain *(Cassella-Riedel, Belg.; Diamant, Fr.; Cassella-Riedel, Ger.; Pierrel, Ital.; Jap.;Boehringer Mannheim, S.Afr.; Albert-Farma, Spain; Cassella-Riedel, Switz.)*; Intensacrom *(Albert-Farma, Spain)*.

9219-y

Cinepazet Maleate. Cinepazic Acid Ethyl Ester Maleate. Ethyl 4-(3,4,5-trimethoxycinnamoyl)piperazin-1-ylacetate hydrogen maleate.
$C_{20}H_{28}N_2O_6,C_4H_4O_4=508.5$.

CAS — 23887-41-4 (cinepazet); 50679-07-7 (maleate).

A white powder. M.p. 130°.

Cinepazet maleate is a vasodilator which has been used in the treatment of angina pectoris.

Absorption and fate of cinepazet in man. Most of a dose given by mouth was eliminated within 24 hours, 60% being excreted in the urine. The major metabolite was cinepazic acid.— L. F. Chasseaud *et al.*, *Arzneimittel-Forsch.*, 1972, *22*, 2003.

Proprietary Names
Vascoril *(Delalande, Belg.; Delalande, Fr.; Delalande, Ital.; Delalande, Switz.)*.

9220-g

Cinepazide Maleate. 1-(Pyrrolidin-1-ylcarbonylmethyl)-4-(3,4,5-trimethoxycinnamoyl)piperazine hydrogen maleate.
$C_{22}H_{31}N_3O_5,C_4H_4O_4=533.6$.

CAS — 23887-46-9 (cinepazide); 26328-04-1 (maleate).

Cinepazide maleate is a vasodilator which has been given in peripheral and cerebral vascular disorders and in coronary insufficiency.

Pharmacology in *animals*.— B. Pourrias *et al.*, *Thérapie*, 1974, *29*, 29 and 43.

Proprietary Names
Vasodistal *(Delalande, Fr.; Delalande, Ital.; Delalande, Switz.)*.

9221-q

Cloridarol. Clobenfurol. α-(Benzofuran-2-yl)-α-(4-chlorophenyl)methanol.
$C_{15}H_{11}ClO_2=258.7$.

CAS — 3611-72-1.

A white odourless crystalline powder. M.p. about 48°.

Cloridarol has been given in the prevention and treatment of coronary insufficiency.

Proprietary Names
Cordium *(Massone, Arg.)*; Menacor *(Menarini, Ital.)*; Menoxicor *(Menarini, Spain)*.

9222-p

Cyclandelate.
BS 572. 3,3,5-Trimethylcyclohexyl mandelate.
$C_{17}H_{24}O_3=276.4$.

CAS — 456-59-7.

A white to off-white amorphous powder with a slight menthol-like odour and a bitter taste. M.p. below 60°. On storage it may sublime into a crystalline form resembling cotton wool.

Practically **insoluble** in water; soluble 1 in about 1 of alcohol and 1 in about 2 of light petroleum; very soluble in ether and other common organic solvents. **Store** in a cool place in airtight containers. Protect from light.

Adverse Effects. Nausea, gastro-intestinal distress, or flushing may follow high doses of cyclandelate.

Other adverse effects reported include tingling and headache.

Toxicity of cyclandelate was low, though with large doses there might be flushing, tingling, nausea, or headache.— T. Winsor and C. Hyman, *Clin. Pharmac. Ther.*, 1961, *2*, 652.

Treatment of Adverse Effects. In severe overdosage the stomach should be emptied by aspiration and lavage. If necessary the circulation should be maintained with infusions of suitable electrolytes, and if necessary by vasopressors.

Precautions. Cyclandelate is contra-indicated in the acute phase of a cerebrovascular accident.

Uses. Cyclandelate is a vasodilator used in the treatment of cerebrovascular and peripheral vascular disorders. It is given in a dosage of 1.6 g daily in divided doses.

Action. *Animal* studies into the mode of action of cyclandelate: A. B. H. Funcke *et al.*, *Curr. med. Res. Opinion*, 1974, *2*, 37 (brain glucose uptake); G. van Hell, *Curr. med. Res. Opinion*, 1974, *2*, 211 (collateral vessel formation).

Cerebrovascular disease. Several double-blind studies of cyclandelate have shown improvement in orientation, disturbed behaviour, and vocabulary without improvement in self-care, recent memory, or mood. Nevertheless, the overall results are inconsistent, and improvements in clinical and psychological tests are not always matched by useful changes in the activities of daily living.— *Br. med. J.*, 1978, *2*, 348. See also *Drug & Ther. Bull.*, 1975, *13*, 85. Further reviews: *Med. Lett.*, 1976, *18*, 38; P. Cook and I. James, *New Engl. J. Med.*, 1981, *305*, 1508 and 1560.

Individual reports and studies on the role of cyclandelate in cerebrovascular disease: J. Young *et al.*, *Br. J. Psychiat.*, 1974, *124*, 177; P. Hall, *J. Am. Geriat. Soc.*, 1976, *24*, 41; G. Davies *et al.*, *Age and Ageing*, 1977, *6*, 156; D. B. Rao *et al.*, *J. Am. Geriat. Soc.*, 1977, *25*, 548; R. Brasseur, *Angiology*, 1978, *29*, 121; B. Capote and N. Parikh, *J. Am. Geriat. Soc.*, 1978, *26*, 360; G. F. A. Harding *et al.*, *Angiology*, 1978, *29*, 139; L. Sourander and C. B. Blakemore, *ibid.*, 133.

Diabetic retinopathy. In a double-blind randomised study deterioration of the blood-retinal barrier was assessed in 22 diabetic patients, without retinal involvement, by vitreous fluorophotometry after the injection of fluorescein. It was considered that deterioration of the blood-retinal barrier, an early sign of diabetic retinopathy, was delayed in the third month in those patients given cyclandelate 400 mg four times daily for 3 months. Long-term studies were considered to be indicated.— J. G. Cunha-Vaz *et al.*, *Br. J. Ophthal.*, 1977,

61, 399.

Dysmenorrhoea. Over a period of 15 years, 60 women with spasmodic dysmenorrhoea had been treated with cyclandelate with consistently good results; 800 mg daily in divided doses was given for 3 days before the expected date of menstruation and for the first 2 days of menstruation.— D. Kerslake (letter), *Br. med. J.*, 1973, *2*, 614.

Peripheral vascular disease. A review of drugs used in the management of peripheral vascular disease, including cyclandelate. There is no substantial evidence to recommend the use of cyclandelate in peripheral vascular diseases.— J. D. Coffman, *New Engl. J. Med.*, 1979, *300*, 713. Further references: R. E. Fremont, *Am. J. med. Sci.*, 1964, *247*, 182; T. Reich, *J. Am. Geriat. Soc.*, 1977, *25*, 202.

Proprietary Preparations

Cyclobral *(Norgine, UK)*. Cyclandelate, available as capsules of 400 mg.

Cyclospasmol *(Brocades, UK)*. Cyclandelate, available as **Capsules** of 400 mg; as **Suspension** containing 400 mg in each 5 ml; and as **Tablets** of 400 mg. (Also available as Cyclospasmol in *Austral., Belg., Canad., Denm., Fr., Neth., Norw., S.Afr., Switz., USA*).

Other Proprietary Names

Arto-Espasmol *(Spain)*; Ciclospasmol *(Ital.)*; Cyclomandol *(Swed.)*; Spasmocyclon *(Ger.)*; Vasodyl *(Spain)*.

9223-s

Di-isopropylammonium Dichloroacetate. DIPA; Di-isopropylamine Dichloroethanoate; Di-isopropylamine Dichloroacetate.
$C_8H_{17}Cl_2NO_2$=230.1.

CAS — 660-27-5.

Crystals with an odour of chlorine and a slightly bitter taste. M.p. 119° to 121°. **Soluble** 1 in less than 2 of water; very soluble in alcohol and chloroform.

Di-isopropylammonium dichloroacetate is a vasodilator which has been given in the treatment of peripheral and cerebral vascular disorders.

A review of the pharmacology and therapeutic effects of di-isopropylammonium dichloroacetate.— P. W. Stacpoole, *J. clin. Pharmac.*, 1969, *9*, 282.

Proprietary Names

Cubisol *(Piam, Ital.)*; Dedyl *(Difrex, Austral.; Houdé I.S.H., Fr.)*; Diedi *(Atem, Belg.; ISF, Ital.; Seber, Spain)*; Kalodil *(Fidia, Ital.)*; Neovascoril *(Saita, Ital.)*; Nutricor *(Llorens, Spain)*; Vasculene *(Von Boch, Ital.)*.

9224-w

Dilazep Hydrochloride. Asta C 4898. Perhydro-1,4-diazepin-1,4-diylbis(trimethylene 3,4,5-trimethoxybenzoate) dihydrochloride.
$C_{31}H_{44}N_2O_{10}$,2HCl=677.6.

CAS — 35898-87-4 (dilazep); 20153-98-4 (hydrochloride).

Dilazep hydrochloride is a vasodilator which has been given in the treatment of coronary insufficiency and angina pectoris.

Pharmacology in *animals*.— D. Leuke *et al.*, *Arzneimittel-Forsch.*, 1972, *22*, 639. Toxicity studies in *animals*.— H. H. Able *et al.*, *ibid.*, 667; H. Schriewer and H. M. Rauen, *ibid.*, 1455.

The myocardial blood flow was measured in 5 patients with catheterised hearts given dilazep and found to be increased after doses of 160 to 310 μg per kg body-weight.— I. Hensel *et al.*, *Arzneimittel-Forsch.*, 1972, *22*, 652. Evidence of coronary vascularisation induced by dilazep in *animals*.— G. Schmidt *et al.*, *ibid.*, 663.

Metabolism.— E. Schaumlöffel and R. Prignitz, *Arzneimittel-Forsch.*, 1972, *22*, 1651.

For a series of papers on the pharmacology and use of dilazep in ischaemic heart disease, see *Arzneimittel-Forsch.*, 1974, *24*, 1851 to 1926.

The effects of dilazep on blood platelet aggregation.— F. Kuzuya, *Arzneimittel-Forsch.*, 1979, *29*, 539.

Proprietary Names

Cormelian *(Asta, Ger.; Schering, Ital.)*; Komerian *(Jap.)*.

9225-e

Diltiazem Hydrochloride. Latiazem Hydrochloride; CRD-401. *cis*-(+)-3-Acetoxy-5-(2-dimethylaminoethyl)-2,3-dihydro-2-(4-methoxyphenyl)-1,5-benzothiazepin-4(5*H*)-one hydrochloride.
$C_{22}H_{26}N_2O_4S$,HCl=451.0.

CAS — 42399-41-7 (diltiazem); 33286-22-5 (hydrochloride).

A white odourless crystalline powder with a bitter taste. M.p. about 212° with decomposition. Freely **soluble** in water, chloroform, and methyl alcohol; slightly soluble in dehydrated alcohol. **Protect** from light.

Diltiazem hydrochloride exists in 2 crystalline forms; prisms and plates.— K. Kohno *et al.*, *Arzneimittel-Forsch.*, 1977, *27*, 1424.

Diltiazem hydrochloride is a vasodilator which has been used in the management of angina pectoris.

Animal pharmacology studies of diltiazem: D. Saito *et al.*, *Arzneimittel-Forsch.*, 1977, *27*, 1669; Y. Ito *et al.*, *Br. J. Pharmac.*, 1978, *64*, 503.

Cardiac disorders. *Angina pectoris.* References: R. Kusukawa *et al.*, *Arzneimittel-Forsch.*, 1977, *27*, 878; I. Nakayama, *Int. J. clin. Pharmac. Biopharm.*, 1979, *17*, 410.

Heart failure. The effect of diltiazem hydrochloride on sodium diuresis and renal function in chronic congestive heart failure.— M. Kinoshita *et al.*, *Arzneimittel-Forsch.*, 1979, *29*, 676.

Hypoglycaemia. Diltiazem hydrochloride 44 mg given intravenously over 2 hours to a woman with hypoglycaemic attacks due to an insulinoma reduced insulin secretion for the first 10 minutes but also reduced the blood-glucose concentration. A dose of 180 mg daily by mouth for 15 days reduced the frequency of attacks.— H. Taniguchi *et al.* (letter), *Lancet*, 1977, *2*, 501.

Proprietary Names

Herbesser *(Jap.)*; Masdil *(Esteve, Spain)*.

9226-l

Dipyridamole.

RA 8. 2,2′,2″,2‴-[(4,8-Dipiperidinopyrimido[5,4-*d*]pyrimidine-2,6-diyl)dinittrilo]tetraethanol.
$C_{24}H_{40}N_8O_4$=504.6.

CAS — 58-32-2.

An odourless, intensely yellow, crystalline powder with a bitter taste. Solutions have a yellowish-blue fluorescence. M.p. about 163°.

Very slightly **soluble** in water; soluble in chloroform, methyl alcohol, and dilute acids; slightly soluble in acetone; practically insoluble in ether and light petroleum.

Adverse Effects. Gastric disturbances, diarrhoea, headache, dizziness, faintness, and skin rash may occur after administration of dipyridamole. Some patients experience facial flushing and a bitter taste after intravenous injection. Rapid intravenous injection of dipyridamole may cause a lowering of blood pressure, especially in patients with hypertension. Dipyridamole can also induce angina in some patients.

Alopecia. A 38-year-old woman with the haemolytic-uraemic syndrome initially treated with streptokinase and heparin, was subsequently treated with aspirin 3 g daily and dipyridamole 300 mg daily. Alopecia during treatment might have been due to dipyridamole.— J. A. Utting and D. R. Shreeve, *Br. med. J.*, 1973, *2*, 591.

Effects on the heart. Comment on the role of dipyridamole in myocardial scintigraphy, including mention that a rather unexpected effect of distal coronary vasodilators is angina, which may be reversed by glyceryl trinitrate or, in severe cases, aminophylline.— *Lancet*, 1980, *2*, 1346.

Precautions. Dipyridamole should be given only with care to patients with hypotension and should not be given to patients with hypotension following myocardial infarction.

Interactions. In 24 patients with glomerulonephritis who were stabilised on either warfarin or phenindione, dipyridamole in doses up to 400 mg daily did not affect prothrombin activity. It was recommended that when dipyridamole was used the prothrombin activity should be maintained at the upper end of the therapeutic range in order to avoid possible bleeding complications due to the slight anticoagulant activity of dipyridamole.— S. Kalowski and P. Kincaid-Smith, *Med. J. Aust.*, 1973, *2*, 164.

Interference with diagnostic tests. Serum from a patient taking dipyridamole gave very high readings when lipoproteins were being measured by nephelometry. Dipyridamole imparts a yellowish-blue fluorescence to solutions and could interfere in other laboratory tests involving fluorescence or nephelometry measurements.— K. Wiener (letter), *Lancet*, 1981, *2*, 634.

Pregnancy and the neonate. A young woman with a prosthetic heart valve was successfully managed throughout pregnancy with the aid of dipyridamole and delivered a healthy infant.— R. Ahmad *et al.* (letter), *Lancet*, 1976, *2*, 1414. See also Y. Biale *et al.* (letter), *Lancet*, 1977, *1*, 907.

Absorption and Fate. Dipyridamole is readily absorbed from the gastro-intestinal tract. It is concentrated in the liver and is mainly excreted in the faeces. Excretion may be delayed by reabsorption. A small amount is excreted in the urine as glucuronide.

For a study suggesting that blood-dipyridamole concentrations below 3.5 μmol per litre may not be effective in suppressing platelet function, see under Cardiac Disorders, below.

Uses. Dipyridamole has antithrombotic activity and is used in conditions where modification of platelet function may be beneficial. For this purpose the usual dose is 100 mg four times daily before food increased if necessary, to 600 mg daily.

It has also been used as a vasodilator in the long-term management of chronic angina pectoris in usual doses of 50 mg thrice daily. It has also been given by slow intravenous injection in a dose of 10 to 20 mg twice or thrice daily.

Action. Evidence to suggest that the antithrombotic activity of phosphodiesterase inhibitors, such as dipyridamole, depend upon the activation of platelet adenylcyclase by potentiation of endogenous prostacyclin.— S. Moncada and R. Korbut, *Lancet*, 1978, *1*, 1286. Comments.— D. F. Horrobin *et al.* (letter), *ibid.*, *2*, 270; A. K. Pedersen (letter), *ibid. In vitro* studies pointing to an effect of dipyridamole on prostaglandin metabolism in platelets, which might provide an additional explanation of its activity as an inhibitor of platelet function.— L. C. Best *et al.* (letter), *ibid.*, 846. *In vitro* tests indicating that inhibition of thromboxane synthetase cannot explain the antithrombotic effects of dipyridamole.— S. Moncada *et al.* (letter), *ibid.*, 1257. Findings indicating that dipyridamole has an inhibitory effect on platelet aggregation, dependent on albumin but independent of prostacyclin and thromboxane.— K. A. Jørgensen and E. Stoffersen (letter), *ibid.*, 1258. Data suggesting that the most important mechanism of action of dipyridamole might be enhancement of the effects of prostacyclin.— G. Di Minno *et al.* (letter), *ibid.*

In a study involving 10 healthy subjects dipyridamole 8 μg per kg body-weight per minute, infused for 2 hours, induced an increase of prostacyclin release, probably by a direct effect on the metabolic pathways of arachidonic acid.— G. Masotti *et al.* (letter), *Lancet*, 1979, *1*, 1412. A study in 4 healthy subjects indicating that dipyridamole ingestion appeared to diminish rather than enhance the effect of prostacyclin (and other prostaglandins) as platelet-aggregate inhibitors in human platelet-rich plasma. These findings do not support the hypothesis that the antithrombotic action of dipyridamole is caused by enhancement of platelet aggregate inhibition by 'circulating' prostacyclin.— G. Di Minno *et al.* (letter), *ibid.*, 1979, *2*, 701. In 10 juvenile-onset, insulin-dependent diabetics, dipyridamole significantly decreased their raised plasma concentrations of β-thromboglobulin without affecting metabolic control. This might be based on enhancement or release of prostacyclin.— G. Schernthaner *et al.* (letter), *ibid.*, 748.

Cardiac disorders. For the role of dipyridamole in the prevention of myocardial infarction, see Aspirin, p.242.

Cardiac surgery. Dipyridamole was considered to reduce the incidence of thrombo-embolic episodes during the year following heart-valve replacement. In a study in 70 patients, 27 were given dipyridamole 400 mg daily and 36 a placebo, starting 10 to 14 days after operation. All patients received warfarin sodium. There were 11 thrombo-embolic episodes among the patients receiving placebos but none among those continuously taking dipyridamole. Two of 7 patients who discontinued dipyridamole after 3 and 4 months respectively because of side-effects suffered single cerebral embolisms.— J. M. Sullivan *et al.*, *New Engl. J. Med.*, 1968, *279*, 576.

Platelet function was significantly decreased in 11 patients who had undergone mitral valve replacement when dipyridamole was given in doses sufficient to produce blood concentrations above 3.5 μmol per litre. The usual dose was 100 mg four times daily.— S. M. Rajah *et al.*, *Br. J. clin. Pharmac.*, 1977, *4*, 129.

The treatment of cardiac transplantation patients with dipyridamole and warfarin, together with the reduction of plasma-lipid concentrations associated with a low-fat dietary regimen, may be responsible for the reduction of graft atherosclerosis.— S. W. Jamieson *et al.*, *Br. med. J.*, 1979, *1*, 93.

Results of a controlled study in 50 patients who had undergone coronary-artery bypass surgery indicated that anticoagulant treatment with warfarin or antiplatelet treatment with aspirin and dipyridamole, starting on the third postoperative day and continuing for 6 months, failed to improve the patency of the grafts.— G. A. Pantely *et al.*, *New Engl. J. Med.*, 1979, *301*, 962. A suggestion that treatment should be started earlier.— I. D. Goldberg and M. B. Stemerman (letter), *ibid.*, 1980, *302*, 865. The dosage of aspirin was inappropriate.— L. Klotz (letter), *ibid.*, 866. Comment on an earlier study on the effects of aspirin and dipyridamole in similar patients.— S. J. Phillips *et al.* (letter), *ibid.* Criticism of the study.— H. B. Barner (letter), *ibid.* Reply.— G. A. Pantely *et al.* (letter), *ibid.*

Cerebrovascular disease. Dipyridamole 100 mg four times daily was an effective treatment for vertebrobasilar insufficiency in a 50-year-old male.— L. Simons (letter), *Med. J. Aust.*, 1977, *1*, 229.

Dengue fever. Addition of dipyridamole and aspirin to the standard treatment, which included heparin, of children with dengue haemorrhagic fever did not significantly reduce mortality-rate but it was considered that the additional treatment prevented progression of the disease.— L. K. Kho *et al.*, *S.E. Asian J. trop. med. publ. Hlth*, 1979, *10*, 385.

Diagnostic use. Comment on the British Nuclear Medicine Society's 1980 autumn regional meeting discussion of dipyridamole administration as a possible alternative to exercise stress for thallium-201 myocardial scintigraphy in suspected coronary heart disease. The message from the meeting was that dipyridamole, alone or in association with isometric handgrip, is a useful alternative to exercise, and is the method of choice when exercise is impractical or contra-indicated.— *Lancet*, 1980, *2*, 1346.

A crossover study in 12 patients comparing dipyridamole 300 mg by mouth with 40 mg intravenously in thallium-201 myocardial imaging. It was concluded that oral dipyridamole is at least as effective as intravenous dipyridamole in thallium-201 myocardial imaging, and that the technique is safe, easy to perform, and suitable for out-patient use. One patient developed angina and ST-segment depression after oral dipyridamole, which was abolished by aminophylline 50 mg intravenously.— P. Walker *et al.*, *Clin. Sci.*, 1980, *59*, 5P.

Headache. A double-blind study of dipyridamole in migraine was abandoned when it was found to exacerbate the migraine.— C. H. Hawkes (letter), *Lancet*, 1978, *2*, 153. Beneficial results had been obtained in the prevention of migraine using dipyridamole in a dosage of 150 or 200 mg daily.— H. Damasio (letter), *ibid.*, 478.

Further references: B. E. Masel *et al.*, *Neurology, Minneap.*, 1978, *28*, 371; *idem*, *Headache*, 1980, *20*, 13.

Necrobiosis lipoidica. For reports of the use of dipyridamole in association with aspirin in necrobiosis lipoidica, see Aspirin, p.240.

Peripheral vascular disorders. In patients in whom stenosis or segmental occlusion of a large artery of the lower limb had been successfully removed by surgery 84% of the arteries remained open in 51 given dipyridamole 75 mg and aspirin 330 mg thrice daily for 14 days, compared with 70% remaining open in 50 given only aspirin.— H. Hess *et al.*, *Dt. med. Wschr.*, 1978, *103*, 1994.

Thrombocythaemia. A study of the relationship between platelet hyperaggregability and thrombosis in patients with thrombocythaemia.— K. K. -Y. Wu, *Ann. intern. Med.*, 1978, *88*, 7. Comment.— C. Y. Thomas (letter), *ibid.*, 845. Reply, emphasising that antiplatelet drugs are indicated only for thrombocythaemic patients with acute thrombotic complications and possibly also for those who exhibit platelet hyperaggregability. They should be avoided in patients with bleeding complications or poor platelet function, otherwise serious bleeding will occur.— K. K. Wu (letter), *ibid.*

Comment on the excellent clinical response of patients with essential thrombocythaemia, to antiplatelet drugs, and the view that in its milder forms the diagnosis may often be overlooked. In 19 of 35 patients given enteric-coated aspirin 325 mg and dipyridamole 100 mg, both thrice daily, there was complete disappearance of pain and gangrene with healing of previous gangrenous changes within 4 to 6 weeks of starting therapy. Five patients relapsed on withdrawal of aspirin and dipyridamole, but again responded when therapy was reintroduced.— W. Morris-Jones and F. E. Preston (letter), *Br. med. J.*, 1981, *282*, 317.

Pulmonary disorders. Administration of dipyridamole 100 mg four times daily to 7 patients with chronic obstructive lung disease caused no significant changes in cardiorespiratory function after 10 days, but raised plasma concentrations of β-thromboglobulin (an indicator of *in vivo* platelet-release reaction) were reduced.— G. G. Nenci *et al.* (letter), *New Engl. J. Med.*, 1981, *304*, 1044.

Renal disorders. The use of therapy with prednisolone, azathioprine or cyclophosphamide, dipyridamole, and heparin followed by warfarin in the treatment of 15 patients with rapidly progressing glomerulonephritis.— C. B. Brown *et al.*, *Lancet*, 1974, *2*, 1166.

Further references: K. Kan *et al.*, *J. Am. med. Ass.*, 1974, *229*, 557 (proliferative glomerulonephritis); E. B. Arenson and C. S. August, *J. Pediat.*, 1975, *86*, 957 (haemolytic-uraemic syndrome, with aspirin and heparin); H. Hasegawa *et al.*, *Curr. ther. Res.*, 1977, *22*, 413 (chronic renal failure); G. H. Neild *et al.*, *Br. med. J.*, 1978, *1*, 743 (relapsing polychondritis, with prednisolone, azathioprine, and anticoagulants); S. Okada *et al.* (letter), *Lancet*, 1981, *1*, 719 (lupus nephritis).

Renal transplants. In a controlled study of 54 patients who had received primary renal allografts, the use of dipyridamole 100 to 400 mg daily with phenindione or warfarin sodium was associated with a significant improvement in the histological appearance of the glomeruli and blood vessels.— T. H. Mathew *et al.*, *Lancet*, 1974, *1*, 1307. See also P. Kincaid-Smith, *Lancet*, 1969, *2*, 920; H. S. Carlin *et al.*, *Hosp. Top.*, 1972, *50*, 41, per *Int. pharm. Abstr.*, 1973, *10*, 375.

Thrombocytopenic purpura. For reference to dipyridamole in the management of thrombocytopenic purpura, see Aspirin, p.241.

Thrombo-embolic disorders. By itself, dipyridamole has been shown to have no clinical value in the prevention of stroke or venous thrombo-embolism. In association with aspirin it prevents embolisation from prosthetic heart valves, but this combination does not appear to be as effective in venous thrombo-embolism.— J. R. A. Mitchell, *Prescribers' J.*, 1979, *19*, 74. See also J. R. A. Mitchell, *Practitioner*, 1979, *223*, 668.

Results of a double-blind placebo-controlled study involving 38 patients with recurrent deep-vein thrombosis and shortened platelet survival time demonstrated a reduced incidence of new venous thrombosis in those given dipyridamole 25 mg in association with aspirin 300 mg, four times daily, compared with those given placebo (one of 19 compared with 7 of 19 respectively).— P. Steele, *Lancet*, 1980, *2*, 1328.

Homocystinaemia. It was reported by L.A. Harker *et al.* (*New Engl. J. Med.*, 1974, *291*, 537) that 4 patients with homocystinaemia due to cystathionine synthase deficiency manifested a shortened platelet survival *in vivo*, and that this platelet survival could be increased to normal by treatment with dipyridamole and aspirin. Treatment with dipyridamole 100 mg and aspirin 1 g daily appeared to be associated with an abolition of subsequent vascular occlusive or thrombo-embolic events in their patients. The shortening of platelet survival was not confirmed by E.R. Uhlemann *et al.* (*New Engl. J. Med.*, 1976, *295*, 1283) in 6 patients, but nevertheless they elected to prescribe long-term dipyridamole and aspirin for patients with homocystinaemia in the hope that the regimen might be of benefit. Experience with a 13-year-old boy who developed bilateral pulmonary emboli following appendicectomy, despite treatment with dipyridamole and aspirin from the third postoperative day, however, has prompted these workers to raise the need for a controlled clinical study (see J.D. Schulman *et al.* (letter), *New Engl. J. Med.*, 1978, *299*, 661).

Use in surgery. The incidence of postoperative deep-vein thrombosis was reduced to 14% among 85 patients given dipyridamole 100 mg together with calcium aspirin 1 g, by mouth or as a suppository on the evening before the operation and for 7 days postoperatively, compared with an incidence of 32% among a control group of 75 patients. None of these patients had leg or thyroid surgery and significant differences in incidences were noted when the results of the study were classified according to the type of operation performed.— J. T. G. Renney *et al.*, *Br. med. J.*, 1976, *1*, 992. See also under Aspirin, p.243.

See also under Cardiac Disorders (Cardiac Surgery), above.

For the absence of effect of dipyridamole or dipyridamole and aspirin in the prophylaxis of deep-vein thrombosis after fracture of the femoral neck, see Heparin, p.768.

For a regimen incorporating dipyridamole for patients with homozygous hypercholesterolaemia undergoing surgery, see Dextran 70 Intravenous Infusion, p.513.

Transient brain ischaemia. The best drug for occasional transient ischaemic attacks is still aspirin (enteric-coated) 300 mg daily. There may be advantage in combining this with dipyridamole 100 mg thrice daily.— *Br. med. J.*, 1980, *280*, 1004.

Further references: G. Fassio *et al.*, *J. int. med. Res.*, 1979, *7*, 492 (aspirin with dipyridamole).

Proprietary Preparations

Persantin *(Boehringer Ingelheim, UK)*. Dipyridamole, available in 2-ml **Ampoules** of an injection containing 5 mg per ml, and as **Tablets** of 25 and 100 mg. (Also available as Persantin in *Arg.*, *Austral.*, *Denm.*, *Ger.*, *Ital.*, *Neth.*, *Norw.*, *S.Afr.*, *Spain*, *Switz.*).

Other Proprietary Names

Belg.—Persantine; *Canad.*—Persantine; *Fr.*—Coronarine, Natyl, Péridamol, Persantine, Prandiol; *Ger.*—Dipyrida, Functiocardon; *Ital.*—Coribon, Corosan, Coroxin, Novodil, Stenocardil, Stenocor, Stimolcardio, Trancocard, Viscor; *Jap.*— Anginal; *USA*—Persantine.

9227-y

Efloxate. Rec 1/0185; Efloxatum; 7-Ethyloxyacetate Flavone; Ethyl Flavone-7-oxyacetate; Flavone-7-ethyloxyacetate; 7-(Carbethoxymethoxy)flavone. Ethyl 4-oxo-2-phenyl-4*H*-chromen-7-yloxyacetate.

$C_{19}H_{16}O_5$=324.3.

CAS — 119-41-5.

Crystals. M.p. 123° to 124°. Slightly **soluble** in water; soluble in most organic solvents.

Efloxate is a vasodilator which has been given in the treatment of angina pectoris.

Proprietary Names

Dilatan Kore *(Lenza, Ital.)*; Recordil *(Recordati, Belg.; Recordati, Ital.)*; Recordil LA *(Méram, Fr.; Recordati, Switz.)*.

9228-j

Erythrityl Tetranitrate.

Erythritol Tetranitrate; Erythrol Nitrate or Tetranitrate; Nitroerythrite; Nitroerythrol; Tetranitrol. Butane-1,2,3,4-tetrol tetranitrate.

$C_4H_6(O.NO_2)_4$=302.1.

CAS — 7297-25-8.

White tasteless crystals. M.p. about 61°. It explodes on percussion. Practically **insoluble** in water; soluble in alcohol, acetone, acetonitrile, chloroform, ether, and glycerol.

9229-z

Diluted Erythrityl Tetranitrate *(U.S.P.)*.

Pharmacopoeias. In *Aust.* (25% in lactose), *Nord.* (10% in lactose), and *U.S.* (in lactose or other suitable inert excipient; the strength is not specified).

A mixture of erythrityl tetranitrate and lactose, the latter being added to minimise the risk of explosion.

It is a white powder with a slight odour of nitric oxides and a slightly sweet taste. Partly **soluble** in cold water and alcohol. **Store** at a temperature not exceeding 40° in airtight containers. Protect from light.

Adverse Effects, Treatment, and Precautions. As for Glyceryl Trinitrate, p.1620.

Absorption and Fate. Erythrityl tetranitrate is readily absorbed from the oral mucosa and probably less effectively absorbed from the gastro-intestinal tract.

Uses. Erythrityl tetranitrate is a vasodilator with general properties similar to glyceryl trinitrate (p.1621). When administered sublingually its effects are evident in 5 to 10 minutes and when swallowed in 20 to 30 minutes.

Erythrityl tetranitrate is of less value for the treatment of an acute attack than for the prophylaxis of angina pectoris. The usual dose is 5 to 10 mg sublingually or by mouth thrice daily, increased after 2 or 3 days to up to 3 or more times these amounts.

Cardiac disorders. Erythrityl tetranitrate in valvular heart disease.— S. Goldberg *et al.*, *Am. J. Med.*, 1978, *65*, 161.

Preparations

Erythrityl Tetranitrate Tablets *(U.S.P.).* Tablets containing diluted erythrityl tetranitrate *U.S.P.* Store at a temperature not exceeding 40° in airtight containers.

Proprietary Names

Cardilate *(Wellcome, Austral.; Calmic, Canad.; Wellcome, Ital.; Wellcome, USA)*; Cardiwell *(Wellcome, Fr.)*.

9230-p

Etafenone Hydrochloride. LG-11457. 2′-(2-Diethylaminoethoxy)-3-phenylpropiophenone hydrochloride.
$C_{21}H_{27}NO_2,HCl=361.9$.

CAS — 90-54-0 (etafenone); 2192-21-4 (hydrochloride).

Etafenone hydrochloride is a vasodilator which has been used in the treatment of angina pectoris.

References: W. R. Kukovetz and G. Pöch, *Arzneimittel-Forsch.*, 1975, *25*, 31; H. Flohr and W. Breull, *Arzneimittel-Forsch.*, 1975, *25*, 1400.

Proprietary Names

Baxacor *(Mack, Illert., Ger.)*; Dialicor *(Guidotti, Ital.)*; Relicor *(Davur, Spain)*; Asamedel, Cardilicor, Corodilan, Corofenon, Coronabason, Dialicor, Esanthin-S, Etafenarin, Hypochit *(all Jap.)*.

9231-s

Ethyl Nicotinate.
$C_8H_9NO_2=151.2$.

CAS — 614-18-6.

A liquid; very **soluble** in water, alcohol, and ether.

Ethyl nicotinate is a topical vasodilator used, in a concentration of 1 to 2%, in rubefacient creams and ointments.

Proprietary Preparations

See under Methyl Nicotinate, p.1626..

9232-w

Fenalcomine Hydrochloride. 1-{4-[2-(α-Methylphenethylamino)ethoxy]phenyl}propan-1-ol hydrochloride.
$C_{20}H_{27}NO_2,HCl=349.9$.

CAS — 34616-39-2 (fenalcomine); 34535-83-6 (hydrochloride).

Fenalcomine hydrochloride is a vasodilator which has been given in the treatment of angina pectoris.

Proprietary Names

Cordoxène *(Laroche Navarron, Fr.)*.

9233-e

Fendiline Hydrochloride. *N*-(2-Benzhydrylethyl)-α-methylbenzylamine hydrochloride.
$C_{23}H_{25}N,HCl=351.9$.

CAS — 13042-18-7 (fendiline); 13636-18-5 (hydrochloride).

Fendiline hydrochloride is a vasodilator which has been used in the treatment of angina pectoris and coronary insufficiency.

Proprietary Names

Sensit *(Thiemann, Ger.; Thiemann, Switz.)*.

9234-l

Gapicomine Citrate. 4,4′-(Iminodimethylene)dipyridine dihydrogen citrate.
$C_{12}H_{13}N_3,C_6H_8O_7=391.4$.

CAS — 1539-39-5 (gapicomine); 24631-38-7 (citrate).

A crystalline solid. M.p. about 191°. **Soluble** in water. **Protect** from light.

Gapicomine citrate is a vasodilator which has been used in coronary disorders.

Proprietary Names

Bicordin *(Polfa, Pol.)*.

9235-y

Glyceryl Trinitrate.

Trinitroglycerin; Glonoin; Trinitrin; Nitroglycerin; Nitroglycerol. Propane-1,2,3-triol trinitrate.
$C_3H_5(O.NO_2)_3=227.1$.

CAS — 55-63-0.

A colourless, slightly volatile, odourless, oily liquid, with a sweet, aromatic, and pungent taste. It explodes on rapid heating or on percussion. Wt per ml about 1.6 g.

Soluble 1 in 800 of water, 1 in 4 of alcohol, 1 in 120 of carbon disulphide, and 1 in 6 of almond oil; miscible with acetone, chloroform, ether, and glacial acetic acid; sparingly soluble in glycerol and light petroleum.

CAUTION. *In fatty or oily solution it is perfectly safe and stable but in alcoholic solution the substance must be handled with the utmost caution.*

9236-j

Glyceryl Trinitrate Solution *(B.P.C. 1973).*

Glyc. Trinit. Soln.; Glyceryl Trinitrate Spirit; Nitroglycerin Solution; Trinitrin Solution; Guttae Glycerylі Nitratis; Liquor Glycerylis Trinitratis; Solutio Nitroglycerini Spirituosa.

Pharmacopoeias. In *Arg., Aust., Belg., Chin., Cz., Hung., Jug., Mex., Nord., Pol., Port., Rus., Span.,* and *Swiss.*

A 1% w/v solution of glyceryl trinitrate in alcohol (90%). It is a clear colourless liquid, neutral to litmus. Mixed with an equal volume of water the solution keeps clear, but diluted with twice its volume a turbid mixture is produced and glyceryl trinitrate, which explodes on percussion, deposits on standing. Wt per ml 0.829 to 0.838 g. The name 'Liquor Glonoini' is sometimes used for solutions of various strengths.

Incompatibility. Glyceryl trinitrate is precipitated when the solution is diluted with about 2 to 8 volumes of water. Glyceryl trinitrate is decomposed by caustic alkalis. **Store** in a cool place in airtight containers. Protect from light.

CAUTION. *Glass-stoppered bottles containing the solution should be opened with caution. It is dangerous if spilled and allowed to evaporate; it may be rendered harmless by potassium or sodium hydroxide solution.*

9237-z

Concentrated Glyceryl Trinitrate Solution *(B.P.).*

Pharmacopoeias. In *Br.* and *Nord.*

A 9 to 11% w/v solution of glyceryl trinitrate in alcohol (96%). It is a clear, colourless or pale yellow liquid. Wt per ml 0.83 to 0.85 g.

Miscible with acetone and ether. **Store** in a cool place in airtight containers. Protect from light.

CAUTION. *Glass-stoppered bottles containing the solution should be opened with caution. It is dangerous if spilled and allowed to evaporate; it may be rendered harmless by potassium or sodium hydroxide solution.*

Stability. Many studies have demonstrated that glyceryl trinitrate tablets are very unstable and subject to considerable loss of potency in contact with packaging components such as adhesive labels, cotton and rayon fillers, and plastic bottles and caps, but V.A. Russell *et al.* (*Pharm. J.*, 1973, *2*, 466) found that tablets stored at 25° in glass containers sealed with foil-lined screw caps and opened 4 times daily to simulate use still had 90.9% of their activity after 35 days. For further reports and studies on the instability and deterioration of glyceryl trinitrate tablets, see D. Banes (letter), *J. pharm. Sci.*, 1968, *57*, 893; R. F. Shangraw and A. M. Contractor, *J. Am. pharm. Ass.*, 1972, *NS12*, 633; S. A. Fusari, *J. pharm. Sci.*, 1973, *62*, 122 and 2012; G. A. Mayer, *Can. med. Ass. J.*, 1974, *110*, 788; D. P. Page *et al.*, *J. pharm. Sci.*, 1975, *64*, 140.

The Council of the Pharmaceutical Society of Great Britain recommends that glyceryl trinitrate tablets should be labelled with an indication that they should be discarded after eight weeks in use. The recommendation applies both to dispensed tablets and to tablets sold over the counter. Pharmacists are reminded that glyceryl trinitrate tablets should be dispensed only in glass containers sealed with a foil lined cap and containing no cotton wool wadding.— *Pharm. J.*, 1980, *2*, 405. See also *ibid.*, 1973, *1*, 56.

Stability studies on glyceryl trinitrate solutions intended for intravenous use.— J. K. Sturek *et al.*, *Am. J. Hosp. Pharm.*, 1978, *35*, 537; D. J. Ludwig and C. T. Ueda, *ibid.*, 541; J. C. Boylan *et al.* (letter), *ibid.*, 1031.

Accelerated stability studies indicated a loss of potency of glyceryl trinitrate from an aqueous solution containing macrogol 400. Dehydrated alcohol, glycerol, propylene glycol, and povidone had no deleterious effect on stability.— P. Suphajettra *et al.*, *J. pharm. Sci.*, 1978, *67*, 1394.

An almost 50% loss of potency occurred in 2 hours from glyceryl trinitrate intravenous infusion solutions in plastic bags (Travenol Viaflex). This loss was considered to be due to adsorption or absorption by the plastic and it was recommended that only glass bottles should be used together with the shortest length of giving set possible.— W. G. Crouthamel *et al.* (letter), *New Engl. J. Med.*, 1978, *299*, 262. Flow-related loss of potency of glyceryl trinitrate infusion solutions was prevented by replacing the plastic giving-set. Much reduction in potency loss was obtained when glyceryl trinitrate was infused from glass syringes attached to high-density polyethylene tubing .— P. A. Cossum *et al.*, *Lancet*, 1978, *2*, 349.

Further reports, studies, and comments on the stability of glyceryl trinitrate in solution for injection: H. Christiansen *et al.*, *J. clin. Hosp. Pharm.*, 1980, *5*, 209; M. S. Roberts *et al.*, *J. Pharm. Pharmac.*, 1980, *32*, 237.

Adverse Effects. Glyceryl trinitrate may cause flushing of the face, dizziness, tachycardia, and throbbing headache. Large doses cause vomiting, restlessness, hypotension, syncope, cyanosis, and methaemoglobinaemia; coldness of the skin, impairment of respiration, and bradycardia may ensue.

Chronic nitroglycerin poisoning may occur in industry but tolerance develops when nitroglycerin is regularly handled and severe withdrawal symptoms occur in subjects abruptly removed from chronic exposure. Loss of such tolerance is rapid and may cause poisoning on re-exposure. Prolonged contact on the skin produces eruptions.

Maximum permissible atmospheric concentration 0.2 ppm.

Comment on glyceryl trinitrate and nitrosamine formation.— *Br. med. J.*, 1980, *280*, 163.

Abuse. For comment on the abuse of volatile nitrites, see under Amyl Nitrite, p.1615.

Allergy. Allergic reactions to glyceryl trinitrate ointment occurred in 5 male patients. It was suggested that sublingual glyceryl trinitrate should be instituted prior to discontinuation of the ointment to prevent possible glyceryl trinitrate withdrawal reactions.— P. A. N. Chandraratna and R. E. O'Dell, *Curr. ther. Res.*, 1979, *25*, 481. See also W. F. Sausker and F. D. Frederick (letter), *J. Am. med. Ass.*, 1978, *239*, 1743; A. A. Hendricks and G. W. Dec, *Archs Derm.*, 1979, *115*, 853.

Cardiovascular effects. Reports of adverse cardiovascular effects associated with glyceryl trinitrate therapy: R. L. Feldman *et al.*, *Am. J. Cardiol.*, 1978, *42*, 517 (coronary artery narrowing); C. A. Hales, *Am. J. Med.*, 1978, *65*, 911 (hypoxaemia); E. A. Kopman *et al.*, *Am. Heart J.*, 1978, *96*, 444 (hypoxaemia); G. T. St Lee, *Am. Heart J.*, 1978, *95*, 273 (leg oedema); P. A. N. Chandraratna *et al.*, *Br. Heart J.*, 1979, *41*, 354 (acute deterioration of left ventricular function in an alcoholic); E. A. Ong and S. Bassn, *Chest*, 1980, *77*, 244 (bradycardia and hypotension); A. A. Bove and R. E. Vlietstra (letter), *New Engl. J. Med.*, 1982, *306*, 484 (paradoxical angina after injection into the left coronary artery).

Effects on the skin. For a report of extensive erythroderma due to pentaerythritol tetranitrate and glyceryl trinitrate, see Pentaerythritol Tetranitrate, p.1630.

Overdosage. Methaemoglobinaemia in an 80-year-old man was believed to have been induced by an overdose of glyceryl trinitrate. He had taken 100 tablets of glyceryl trinitrate 400 µg during the 36 hours before admission to hospital.— J. B. Marshall and R. E. Ecklund (letter), *J. Am. med. Ass.*, 1980, *244*, 330.

Treatment of Adverse Effects. Syncope should be treated by keeping the patient in a recumbent position with the head lowered. Severe poisoning should be treated with gastric aspiration and lavage and the administration of oxygen, with assisted respiration if necessary. If methaemoglobinaemia occurs give methylene blue 1 to 4 mg per kg body-weight by intravenous injection. The circulation may be maintained with infusions of plasma or suitable electrolyte solutions.

Precautions. Glyceryl trinitrate should not be used in patients with marked anaemia or with head trauma or cerebral haemorrhage, and should be used with caution in patients who are predisposed to closed-angle glaucoma. Some effects of glyceryl trinitrate are enhanced by alcohol.

Glaucoma. No increase in intra-ocular pressure occurred after a single dose of glyceryl trinitrate or pentaerythritol tetranitrate in 34 patients, including some with open-angle glaucoma, threatened closed-angle glaucoma, or in remission from closed-angle glaucoma. In some patients the intra-ocular pressure was reduced slightly. When the findings were examined in conjunction with other published reports it was considered that nitrite and nitrate vasodilators were not contra-indicated in patients with open-angle glaucoma and it seemed unlikely that they would induce angle closure.— C. G. Whitworth and W. M. Grant, *Archs Ophthal., N.Y.*, 1964, *71*, 492. See also *Br. med. J.*, 1979, *1*, 1473.

Interference with diagnostic tests. In laboratory tests for catecholamines, glyceryl trinitrate could cause increased readings or false positives.— *Med. Lett.*, 1971, *13*, 82.

Withdrawal and tolerance. A diminished response to glyceryl trinitrate was found in 10 patients after treatment for 1 week with pentaerythritol tetranitrate.— J. -L. Schelling and L. Lasagna, *Clin. Pharmac. Ther.*, 1967, *8*, 256. A double-blind crossover study of isosorbide dinitrate and placebo in 17 male patients indicated that long-acting nitrates (which the authors considered to be no more effective than placebo) did not reduce the efficacy of glyceryl trinitrate given sublingually for the relief of angina pectoris.— W. S. Aronow and H. M. Chesluk, *Circulation*, 1970, *42*, 61.

Myocardial ischaemia accompanied by wide oscillations in arterial pressure after coronary bypass surgery in a 59-year-old woman may have been secondary to coronary vasospasm after abrupt withdrawal of high doses of glyceryl trinitrate; she had received glyceryl trinitrate intravenously over the previous 10 days in doses gradually increased to 1.32 g daily.— C. J. Wilkinson and J. H. Sanders, *Anesth. Analg.*, 1980, *59*, 707.

Serious adverse effects on withdrawal from occupational exposure: R. P. Lund *et al.*, *Br. J. ind. Med.*, 1968, *25*, 136; J. C. Klock, *Am. Heart J.*, 1975, *89*, 510.

Absorption and Fate. Glyceryl trinitrate is readily absorbed from the oral mucosa, but rapidly metabolised so that it only has a fleeting duration of action.

Glyceryl trinitrate is also readily absorbed from the gastro-intestinal tract, but owing to extensive first-pass metabolism in the liver its bioavailability is reduced. In view of its short plasma half-life various long-acting formulations are available for oral administration.

Glyceryl trinitrate is also absorbed through the skin from an ointment basis.

Glyceryl trinitrate is metabolised by hydrolysis to dinitrates and the mononitrate, which is the main urinary metabolite.

Bioavailability. Application of glyceryl trinitrate ointment 2% to the chest or flank in amounts containing 12.5 to 25 mg to 9 patients and 50 mg to 5 patients with congestive heart failure produced mean plasma concentrations of glyceryl trinitrate 1 hour after application of 3.1 ng per ml and 8.9 ng per ml respectively and these concentrations were maintained for a further 3 hours. The patients in the low-dose group (12.5 to 25 mg) who were characterised as sensitive to glyceryl trinitrate by prior intravenous infusion studies demonstrated haemodynamic benefit concomitant with plasma concentrations of about 3 ng per ml but those in the high-dose group (50 mg) who had shown a prior attenuated response to intravenous infusion demonstrated a minimal response despite plasma concentrations of 9 ng per ml. An unexpected finding was that although plasma concentrations decreased substantially following removal of the ointment, glyceryl trinitrate was still detectable in the plasma 30 minutes thereafter suggesting that a depot for glyceryl trinitrate exists in the skin after percutaneous application. It was concluded that glyceryl trinitrate ointment provides therapeutic concentrations that are associated with substantial haemodynamic benefit in selected patients with heart failure but in those in whom an attenuated response is found during intravenous infusion large doses of ointment are unlikely to be beneficial.— P. W. Armstrong *et al.*, *Am. J. Cardiol.*, 1980, *46*, 670.

Further references: H. P. Blumenthal *et al.* (letter), *Br. clin. Pharmac.*, 1977, *4*, 242.

Metabolism and pharmacokinetics. Peak plasma concentrations of glyceryl trinitrate given sublingually to patients appeared within 4 minutes and at least half of the intact glyceryl trinitrate was cleared from the blood in 1 to 3 minutes.— M. G. Bogaert *et al.*, *J. Pharm. Pharmac.*, 1972, *24*, 737. See also P. W. Armstrong *et al.*, *Circulation*, 1979, *59*, 585.

In 10 healthy volunteers given glyceryl trinitrate 560 µg sublingually mean peak blood concentrations of glyceryl dinitrate 25 ng per ml and glyceryl mononitrate 36 ng per ml occurred after 10 minutes and 2 hours respectively. About 22% of the administered dose was excreted in the urine after 24 hours, mainly as the mononitrate.— G. B. Neurath and M. Dünger, *Arzneimittel-Forsch.*, 1977, *27*, 416.

Uses. Glyceryl trinitrate relaxes smooth muscle, including vascular muscle, and reduces systolic blood pressure. It is believed that its anti-anginal effect mainly depends on reducing myocardial oxygen demand by means of peripheral vasodilatation which causes decreased venous return, permitting a reduction in left ventricular volume and energy expenditure. The effect of glyceryl trinitrate in relaxing coronary vessels is not considered appreciably to increase coronary blood flow.

The effect of glyceryl trinitrate sublingually occurs in about 2 to 3 minutes and its action lasts for about 30 to 60 minutes. Tolerance may develop with daily use but withdrawal for a week re-establishes the original sensitivity.

Glyceryl trinitrate solution is used as a vasodilator in the prophylaxis and treatment of angina pectoris. It has also been used for the relief of renal and gall-bladder colic.

Glyceryl trinitrate solution is usually administered as tablets which should be allowed to dissolve in the mouth. The usual dose is the equivalent of 0.5 to 1 mg of glyceryl trinitrate. Sustained-action tablets, which should be swallowed, are also available for prophylaxis; tablets of 2.6, 6.4, or 10 mg may be taken thrice daily depending on the severity of the angina pectoris. It is also applied in the form of an ointment.

Glyceryl trinitrate may also be given by intravenous infusion as a solution containing 400 µg or less per ml in sodium chloride injection or dextrose injection. For the control of hypertension during cardiac surgery the recommended starting dose is 25 µg per minute increasing in steps of 25 µg per minute at 5-minute intervals until the desired fall in blood pressure is achieved; although most patients respond to doses between 10 and 200 µg per minute during some surgical procedures doses of up to 400 µg per minute have been required. In the treatment of perioperative myocardial ischaemia the recommended starting dose is 15 to 20 µg per minute increasing in steps of 10 to 15 µg per minute until the desired effect is achieved. For unresponsive congestive cardiac failure secondary to acute myocardial infarction an initial dose of 20 to 25 µg per minute is recommended which may be decreased to 10 µg per minute or increased in steps of 20 to 25 µg per minute at intervals of 15 to 30 minutes until the desired effect occurs. In unstable angina refractory to treatment with standard therapy a recommended starting dose is 10 µg per minute increasing in steps of 5 to 10 µg per minute at approximately 30-minute intervals.

Administration. Symptoms of cerebral ischaemia, characterised by syncope, weakness, or mild paralysis, occurred in 3 elderly anginal patients after taking glyceryl trinitrate while in a standing position. It was suggested that the standing position should be avoided and that the initial dose should be 250 µg instead of the usual therapeutic dose of 0.5 to 1 mg.— V. Rønnov-Jessen, *Acta med. scand.*, 1963, *174*, 523.

For psychological reasons glyceryl trinitrate ointment is usually applied to the chest wall, but the same effect can be achieved when it is applied to any other part of the skin.— U. Elkayam and W. S. Aronow, *Drugs*, 1982, *23*, 165.

Cardiac disorders. Comment on the beneficial role of long-acting nitrates in cardiovascular disease, with special reference to oral sustained-action glyceryl trinitrate, glyceryl trinitrate ointment, and isosorbide dinitrate. The prevailing concept of the action of glyceryl trinitrate in angina is that it works predominantly by reducing myocardial oxygen demands by a reduction in both afterload and preload of the left ventricle. Thus, the peripheral actions of glyceryl trinitrate to decrease venous return and lower systemic arterial resistance appear to be critical in effecting the balance between myocardial oxygen supply and demand in coronary atherosclerosis. Since decreases in afterload and preload have been documented in patients with coronary disease or heart failure given long-acting nitrates, it is logical to assume that these same physiological actions will be effective in protecting anginal patients for prolonged periods. It must be recognised that long-acting nitrates have a wide and poorly understood dose-response spectrum, so that individualisation of therapy is imperative for each patient. Although the side-effects, including dizziness, syncope, and severe headache, may sometimes preclude the clinical use of these drugs, there is ample evidence that they can play a useful role in the treatment of patients with both angina pectoris and congestive heart failure.— J. Abrams, *Am. J. Med.*, 1978, *64*, 183.

Comment on nitrates which are primarily reducers of preload or left-ventricular filling pressure which is raised in left-heart failure. Drugs such as nitrates dilate the systemic veins and by reducing venous return ultimately reduce the filling pressure on the left heart. The filling pressure should not be allowed to fall below optimum for the diseased heart.— L. H. Opie, *Lancet*, 1980, *1*, 966. See also *idem*, 750.

A review on glyceryl trinitrate ointment.— U. Elkayam and W. S. Aronow, *Drugs*, 1982, *23*, 165.

Further reviews and comments: *Lancet*, 1976, *2*, 1287; *ibid.*, 1979, *2*, 1340; J. R. Parratt, *J. Pharm. Pharmac.*, 1979, *31*, 801; J. Abrams, *New Engl. J. Med.*, 1980, *302*, 1234; *idem*, *J. Am. med. Ass.*, 1981, *246*, 1557.

Angina pectoris. Glyceryl trinitrate is often believed to have failed because it is not used in the best manner, or because of headaches. While it is usually employed to relieve the pain of an anginal attack, it is also of great value when used prophylactically, for example before a walk or before sexual intercourse. Patients require reassurance that this prophylactic use will not cause the drug to lose its effect or mask the pain rather than prevent an attack. Patients should be warned that a throbbing headache is a common adverse effect. Headaches are more severe in younger patients and those with migraine; they may be reduced by using the smaller dose tablet of 300 µg or by spitting out the standard 500 µg tablet after about half has dissolved. If headaches are a problem it is usually better to change to isosorbide.— P. J. B. Hubener, *Prescribers' J.*, 1979, *19*, 143.

An interim report of a prospective randomised study of coronary bypass surgery compared with treatment with propranolol and vasodilators in 100 patients suffering from chronic stable disabling angina pectoris. So far there was no overall difference in major cardiac morbidity or mortality between the two groups although greater symptomatic improvement and a lower incidence of unstable angina pectoris had occurred in the surgical group.— F. E. Kloster *et al.*, *New Engl. J. Med.*, 1979, *300*, 149.

In 17 patients with angina pectoris exercise tolerance (mean 2.83 minutes) was not affected by placebo ointment (mean 2.9 minutes 30 minutes after application) but was improved by the application of 2% glyceryl trinitrate ointment (mean 6.8 minutes). Five patients were free from pain after 15 minutes' exercise. In some patients benefit lasted for 3 hours.— H. H. Salem and S. P. Singh, *Postgrad. med. J.*, 1979, *55*, 874. For a brief discussion on glyceryl trinitrate ointment for the prophylaxis of angina pectoris, see *Med. Lett.*, 1981, *23*, 82.

Further reports and studies on the role of glyceryl trinitrate in angina pectoris: E. M. Krantz *et al.*, *Br. J. Anaesth.*, 1980, *52*, 945; H. S. Loeb, *Chest*, 1980, *77*, 374; J. R. Mikolich *et al.*, *ibid.*, 375; M. E. Davidov, *Angiology*, 1981, *32*, 16.

Arrhythmias. Intravenous administration of glyceryl trinitrate at a rate of 40 µg per minute resulted in rapid and complete control of severe ventricular arrhythmias associated with angina at rest in a 63-year-old man. Previous treatment with lignocaine intravenously, isosorbide dinitrate sublingually, and propranolol orally had been unsuccessful.— R. M. Gagnon *et al.*, *Can. med. Ass. J.*, 1980, *123*, 1131. A similar report.— E. Antman *et al.*, *Br. Heart J.*, 1980, *43*, 88.

Further references to the use of glyceryl trinitrate in cardiac arrhythmias: D. Pitcher *et al.*, *Br. J. clin. Pract.*, 1979, *33*, 326.

Cardiac surgery. During pedicle operation for coronary insufficiency any change in the T-wave or S-T segment was considered an indication for glyceryl trinitrate, given intramuscularly or intravenously. The treatment reversed the changes within 10 minutes in almost all cases.— W. H. Sewell *et al.*, *J. thorac. cardiovasc. Surg.*, 1965, *49*, 317.

In 20 acutely hypertensive patients undergoing coronary-artery surgery glyceryl trinitrate infused during surgery, in a mean dose of 960 ng per kg body-weight per minute, reduced systolic, diastolic, and mean arterial blood-pressure; it appeared to reduce myocardial oxygen demand and relieve myocardial ischaemia.— J. A. Kaplan *et al.*, *Anesthesiology*, 1976, *45*, 14.

Evidence from a study involving 8 patients with coronary heart disease who underwent aortocoronary bypass surgery that combined treatment with dopamine and glyceryl trinitrate intravenously may be of value in patients with pre-existing high left-ventricular filling pressure or with pulmonary hypertension.— W. Hess *et al.*, *Br. J. Anaesth.*, 1979, *51*, 1063.

Heart failure. Nitrate preparations have lately been assessed for the therapy of both acute left-ventricular failure and chronic heart failure. As the major effect of nitrates is venodilatation rather than arteriolar dilatation they are most suited to patients with raised pulmonary wedge pressure and clinical features of pulmonary congestion. In the control of severe chronic congestive heart failure nitrates are less effective than prazosin or hydralazine but may be very useful in combination with these agents to achieve the greatest possible preload reduction, especially in patients with severe pulmonary congestion.— L. H. Opie, *Lancet*, 1980, *1*, 966.

Reports and studies on the role of glyceryl trinitrate in heart failure: J. A. Franciosa *et al.*, *Curr. ther. Res.*, 1977, *22*, 231; N. A. Cagin *et al.*, *N.Y. St. J. Med.*, 1978, *78*, 888; P. A. N. Chandraratna *et al.*, *Cardiology*, 1978, *63*, 337; J. Mehta *et al.*, *Br. Heart J.*, 1978, *40*, 845.

Myocardial infarction. Comment on the role of glyceryl trinitrate in myocardial infarction. Although glyceryl trinitrate was formerly shunned in acute myocardial infarction, it may indeed be beneficial. Since the hazard of hypotension induced by glyceryl trinitrate cannot be dismissed the possibility of counteracting a fall in blood pressure with phenylephrine or, in selected patients, avoiding it by direct intracoronary administration of glyceryl trinitrate should be considered.— E. Braunwald, *New Engl. J. Med.*, 1978, *299*, 1301. Comment on the potential hazard of injecting commercial preparations of glyceryl trinitrate containing propylene glycol directly into coronary arteries.— M. L. S. Cuddy *et al.* (letter), *New Engl. J. Med.*, 1981, *305*, 1651.

Ten patients with acute myocardial infarction were given glyceryl trinitrate by intravenous infusion sufficient to reduce the arterial pressure by about 20 mmHg for 60 minutes. Left ventricular filling pressure was reduced and the magnitude of the ST-segment elevation decreased when compared with 7 controls. However the subsequent infusion of phenylephrine caused an increase in the magnitude of the ST-segment elevation and in left ventricular filling pressure. It was considered that the addition of phenylephrine to glyceryl trinitrate therapy was not beneficial to patients with acute myocardial infarction.— P. C. Come *et al.*, *New Engl. J. Med.*, 1975, *293*, 1003. A similar study indicating an additional benefit with phenylephrine only in patients without left-ventricular failure.— J. S. Borer *et al.*, *ibid.*, 1008.

Initial favourable results on the extent of necrosis had been obtained following infusion of glyceryl trinitrate in patients with acute myocardial infarction.— J. P. Derrida *et al.* (letter), *New Engl. J. Med.*, 1977, *297*, 336. See also *idem*, *Am. Heart J.*, 1978, *96*, 833.

Further reports of the use of glyceryl trinitrate in myocardial infarction: P. W. Armstrong *et al.*, *Am. J. Cardiol.*, 1976, *38*, 474; N. A. Awan *et al.*, *Circulation*, 1976, *54*, 761; M. Chiariello *et al.*, *ibid.*, 766; P. C. Come and B. Pitt, *ibid.*, 624; K. B. Ramanathan *et al.*, *ibid.*, 1979, *60*, 1230.

Hypertension of pregnancy. A report of the use of glyceryl trinitrate by intravenous infusion to control severe hypertension of pregnancy during caesarean section in a severely obese patient.— S. W. Snyder *et al.*, *Anesthesiology*, 1979, *51*, 563.

Impotence. Impotence in a 56-year-old man with a history of depression and hypochondriacal neurosis was alleviated on taking glyceryl trinitrate tablets for chest pains.— J. W. Mudd, *Am. J. Psychiat.*, 1977, *134*, 922.

For comments on the abuse of volatile nitrites for purposes of sexual gratification, see under Amyl Nitrite, p.1615.

Oesophageal spasm and achalasia. Administration of glyceryl trinitrate 400 µg sublingually during attacks gave rapid and complete relief to a man with diffuse oesophageal spasm and permitted him to continue eating without further difficulty.— R. C. Orlando and E. M. Bozymski, *New Engl. J. Med.*, 1973, *289*, 23. See also N. Swamy, *Gastroenterology*, 1977, *72*, 23.

Clinical improvement in vigorous achalasia in a woman following therapy with propantheline bromide 15 mg and a long-acting preparation of glyceryl trinitrate 2.5 mg both thrice daily.— F. V. Ona and L. S. Polintan, *Archs intern. Med.*, 1980, *140*, 1118.

Peripheral vascular disorders. A recommendation for the topical use of glyceryl trinitrate as a 2% ointment in the treatment of peripheral vascular diseases.— W. N. Beaucher (letter), *New Engl. J. Med.*, 1979, *301*, 159. Comment.— J. D. Coffman (letter), *New Engl. J. Med.*, 1979, *301*, 159.

A 75-year-old man with intermittent claudication, who was unable to renounce his life-long habit of cigarette smoking, obtained a therapeutic response to smoking a cigarette impregnated with glyceryl trinitrate. In a subsequent study, 13 patients with various forms of vasospasm had a beneficial response to smoking cigarettes impregnated with glyceryl trinitrate 400 µg, six to twenty times daily for periods of up to 2 years.— W. T. Foley, *J. clin. Pharmac.*, 1979, *19*, 75.

A dramatic and immediate response to glyceryl trinitrate sublingually in a woman with peripheral vascular insufficiency associated with oxalosis.— A. J. Dennis *et al.*, *Ann. intern. Med.*, 1980, *92*, 799.

Proctalgia fugax. Some patients with proctalgia fugax (an obscure type of rectal pain in adults) respond to inhalation of amyl nitrite and others find relief from a soluble tablet of glyceryl trinitrate 300 µg placed beneath the tongue.— *Br. med. J.*, 1979, *2*, 32.

Pulmonary disorders. Failure of glyceryl trinitrate in conventional doses to produce effective bronchodilatation in 10 asthmatic patients.— W. C. Miller and T. F. Shultz (letter), *Am. Rev. resp. Dis.*, 1979, *120*, 471.

The use of glyceryl trinitrate in patients with chronic obstructive pulmonary disease.— B. Niehues *et al.*, *Dt. med. Wschr.*, 1979, *104*, 691.

Pulmonary oedema. Beneficial effects of glyceryl trinitrate sublingually in the emergency treatment of severe pulmonary oedema.— W. -D. Bussmann and D. Schupp, *Am. J. Cardiol.*, 1978, *41*, 931.

Preparations

Glyceryl Trinitrate Aerosol. Glyceryl trinitrate 1%, propylene glycol 3%, dehydrated alcohol 15%, dichlorodifluoromethane 16%, dichlorotetrafluoroethane 65%, all by wt. The metered valve provided about 500 µg of glyceryl trinitrate.—A.M. Contractor *et al.*, *J. pharm. Sci.*, 1974, *63*, 907.

Glyceryl Trinitrate Ointment. A 2% ointment of glyceryl trinitrate in hydrous wool fat for the treatment of cardiovascular disease might be prepared using a 10% adsorbate of glyceryl trinitrate in lactose. A glass mortar was coated with the hydrous wool fat and the adsorbate gradually incorporated. Careful handling of the adsorbate was necessary and the mixing should be carried out near to an open window. The operator should take care not to breathe the vapour or allow the material to come in contact with the skin.—*J. Am. pharm. Ass., pract. Pharm. Edn*, 1950, *11*, 619.

Glyceryl Trinitrate Tablets *(B.P.)*. Glyc. Trinit. Tab.; Trinitrin Tablets; Nitroglycerin Tablets. Tablets containing glyceryl trinitrate in a basis of mannitol. They should be protected from light and stored at a temperature not exceeding 25° in a glass container closed by means of a screw closure lined with aluminium or tin foil; additional packing that absorbs glyceryl trinitrate should be avoided. Glyceryl trinitrate tablets should be issued for patients in containers of not more than 100 tablets. The tablets should be allowed to dissolve slowly in the mouth.

Nitroglycerin Tablets *(U.S.P.)*. Tablets containing glyceryl trinitrate. Store at 15° to 30° in airtight containers, preferably of glass, containing not more than 100 tablets. For sublingual use.

Proprietary Preparations

Cardiac Dellipsoids D 18 *(Pilsworth, UK)*. Tablets each containing glyceryl trinitrate 600 µg, caffeine hydrobromide 60 mg, and the equivalent of digitalis tincture 0.12 ml and a strophanthus tincture 0.06 ml.

Natirose *(Wilcox, UK: Lewis, UK)*. Tablets each containing glyceryl trinitrate 750 µg, ethylmorphine hydrochloride 3 mg, and hyoscyamine hydrobromide 50 µg. For the prevention and treatment of attacks of angina pectoris. *Dose.* Prophylactic, 1 tablet chewed once or twice daily; treatment, 1 crushed and chewed for 1 or 2 minutes before swallowing: not more than 5 tablets in 24 hours.

Nitrocontin (formerly known as Nitrolan) *(Napp, UK)*. Sustained-release tablets each containing glyceryl trinitrate 2.6 or 6.4 mg. *Dose.* 1 tablet, swallowed whole, morning and night.

Nitrolingual *(Rona, UK)*. A pressurised spray for application to the oral mucosa, providing glyceryl trinitrate for buccal absorption 400 µg in each metered dose.

Percutol *(Reckitt & Colman Pharmaceuticals, UK)*. Glyceryl trinitrate, available as ointment containing 2% in a basis containing hydrous wool fat and soft paraffin. One inch of ointment is stated to contain glyceryl trinitrate 16.64 mg. *Administration.* ½ to 2 inches at each application; not to be rubbed in.

Sustac *(Pharmax, UK)*. Glyceryl trinitrate, available as sustained-release tablets of 2.6, 6.4, and 10 mg. These tablets must be swallowed whole. *Dose.* 1 tablet twice or thrice daily. (Also available as Sustac in *Austral.*, *Denm.*, *Neth.*).

NOTE. The name Sustac is also applied to Carbenoxolone Sodium, see p.78..

Tridil *(American Hospital Supply, UK)*. Glyceryl trinitrate, available as solutions for preparing intravenous infusions; **Tridil 5 mg** contains 500 µg per ml, in ampoules of 10 ml, with alcohol 10%, monobasic potassium phosphate, and lactose; **Tridil 50 mg** contains 5 mg per ml, in ampoules of 10 ml, with alcohol 30% and propylene glycol 30% in Water for Injections. A loss of potency may occur if Tridil is administered via PVC infusion bags.

Other Proprietary Names

Arg.—Nitrolingual, Nitroprontan; *Austral.*—Anginine, Nitrolate; *Belg.*—A 12, Nitrobaat, Nitrolingual, Nitrong, Nitroprol, Nysconitrine Forte, Trinalgon; *Canad.*—Nitrol, Nitrong, Nitrostabilin, Nitrostat; *Denm.*—Nitrolingual, Nitrong; *Fr.*—Lénitral; *Ger.*—Gilucor nitro, Klavikordal, Nitrangin, Nitrogesanit retard, Nitrolingual, Nitro Mack, Nitrorectal, Nitrozell-retard, Sustac-Retard, Trinitrosan; *Ital.*—Lentonitrina, Nitroglyn, Nitrong, Nitro Retard, Venitrin; *Neth.*—Nitrobaat, Nitrolingual, Nitrong, Nitrozell; *Norw.*—Nitrong, Nitroretard; *S.Afr.*—Angised, Nitrong; *Spain*—Lentonitrina, Nitro Mack Retard, Nitrozel LP; *Swed.*—Nitroglyn, Nitrong, Nitroretard; *Switz.*—Niong retard, Nitracut, Nitrochron Retard, Nitro-lent, Nitrolingual, Nitro Mack retard, Nitromint, Nitroran; *USA*—Cardabid, Nitora, Nitro-Bid, Nitroglyn, Nitrol, Nitrong, Nitro-SA, Nitrospan, Nitrostat, Nitrovas, Trates.

9238-c

Hepronicate. Heptylidynetris(methylene nicotinate).
$C_{28}H_{31}N_3O_6$=505.6.

CAS — 7237-81-2.

Hepronicate is a vasodilator which has been given in the treatment of peripheral vascular disorders.

Proprietary Names
Megrin *(Jap.)*.

9239-k

Hexobendine Hydrochloride. ST 7090. *NN'*-Ethylenebis(3-methylaminopropyl 3,4,5-trimethoxybenzoate) dihydrochloride.
$C_{30}H_{44}N_2O_{10}$,2HCl=665.6.

CAS — 54-03-5 (hexobendine); 50-62-4 (hydrochloride).

A white crystalline powder. **Soluble** in water and chloroform; slightly soluble in alcohol; practically insoluble in ether.

Hexobendine hydrochloride is a vasodilator which has been given in the treatment of coronary insufficiency and angina pectoris.

References: H. W. Kirchhoff *et al.*, *Arzneimittel-Forsch.*, 1969, *19*, 64; L. McInnes and J. R. Parratt, *Br. J. Pharmac.*, 1969, *37*, 272; J. S. Meyer *et al.*, *Neurology, Minneap.*, 1971, *21*, 691, per *Abstr. Wld Med.*, 1971, *45*, 866; C. E. Hansing *et al.*, *Arzneimittel-Forsch.*, 1972, *22*, 398; H. Herrschaft, *ibid.*, 1976, *26*, 1240.

Proprietary Names
Flussicor *(Farmalabor, Ital.)*; Reoxyl *(Hormonchemie, Ger.)*; Ustimon *(Chemie-Linz, Aust.*; *Merck-Clévenot, Fr.*; *Petersen, S.Afr.*; *Lacer, Spain*; *Chemie-Linz, Switz.)*.

9240-w

Hexyl Nicotinate. *n*-Hexyl nicotinate.
$C_{12}H_{17}NO_2$=207.3.

CAS — 23597-82-2.

Hexyl nicotinate is a topical vasodilator used, in a concentration of 2%, in rubefacient creams.

Proprietary Preparations

See under Methyl Nicotinate, p.1626..

9241-e

Ifenprodil Tartrate. RC 61-91. (±)-2-(4-Benzylpiperidino)-1-(4-hydroxyphenyl)propan-1-ol tartrate.
$(C_{21}H_{27}NO_2)_2$,$C_4H_6O_6$=801.0.

CAS — 23210-56-2 (ifenprodil); 23210-58-4 (tartrate).

A white amorphous powder. M.p. 180°. **Soluble** 1 in 50 of water; soluble in alcohol; very slightly soluble in acetone and chloroform; practically insoluble in ether.

Ifenprodil tartrate is a vasodilator, with alpha-adrenoceptor blocking properties, which has been given in peripheral and cerebral vascular disorders.

Prior administration of ifenprodil protected *rats, guinea-pigs, rabbits* and *mice* against the effects of cyanide. The protective action was also observed *in vitro*.— T. Furukawa *et al.*, *Toxic. appl. Pharmac.*, 1976, *37*, 289.

A beneficial effect on some parameters following intravenous administration of ifenprodil tartrate to patients with intermittent claudication.— M. O. Spach and J. Schwartz, *Thérapie*, 1977, *32*, 301.

Proprietary Names
Dilvax *(Promeco, Arg.)*; Vadilex *(Robert et Carrière, Fr.)*; Serocral *(Jap.)*.

9242-l

Imolamine Hydrochloride. LA 1211. 2-(5-Imino-3-phenyl-1,2,4-oxadiazolin-4-yl)triethylamine hydrochloride.
$C_{14}H_{20}N_4O$,HCl=296.8.

CAS — 318-23-0 (imolamine); 15823-89-9 (hydrochloride).

A white odourless powder with a bitter taste. **Soluble** 1 in 1 of water, 1 in 500 of alcohol; slightly soluble in chloroform.

Imolamine hydrochloride is a vasodilator which has been used in the treatment of angina pectoris.

Proprietary Names
Coremax *(Ciba, Arg.)*; Irrigor *(Aron, Fr.*; *Karlspharma, Ger.*; *Spemsa, Ital.)*; Irrigor 3 *(Heineking, Switz.)*.

9243-y

Inositol Nicotinate.

meso-Inositol Hexanicotinate; Inositol Niacinate; Win 9154. *meso*-Inositol hexanicotinate.
$C_{42}H_{30}N_6O_{12}$=810.7.

CAS — 6556-11-2.

A crystalline solid. Practically **insoluble** in water and most organic solvents; soluble in dilute acids.

Uses. Inositol nicotinate is a vasodilator and is believed to be slowly hydrolysed to nicotinic acid. It is given in the treatment of peripheral vascular disorders and has been suggested for cerebral vascular disease.

Treatment is usually started with 1.5 g daily and increased, if necessary, to 3 to 4 g daily in divided doses. Initial doses of 1 g thrice daily have been used in cerebral vascular disease.

Inositol nicotinate is claimed to have a fibrinolytic effect and to reduce hypercholesterolaemia.

Hyperlipoproteinaemia. Reports and studies on inositol nicotinate in hyperlipoproteinaemia: H. Pristautz, *Arzneimittel-Forsch.*, 1977, *27*, 152; K. Bolzano *et al.*, *ibid.*, 1979, *29*, 1621.

Necrobiosis lipoidica. Preliminary observations showed that treatment for up to 2½ years with inositol nicotinate 1 g thrice daily used alone or following treatment with stanozolol caused improvement in 16 patients with necrobiosis lipoidica and cleared 2 other patients; of 3 further patients given stanozolol alone, 1 found no effect and 2 some improvement.— E. L. Rhodes, *Br. J. Derm.*, 1976, *95*, 673.

Peripheral vascular disorders. Reports and studies on inositol nicotinate in peripheral vascular disorders: E. F. J. Ring and P. A. Bacon, *J. int. med. Res.*, 1977, *5*, 217; V. C. H. Tyson, *Practitioner*, 1979, *223*, 121.

Proprietary Preparations

Hexopal *(Winthrop, UK)*. Inositol nicotinate, available as **Suspension** containing 1 g in each 5 ml and as **Tablets** of 500 mg. **Hexopal Forte.** Inositol nicotinate, available as scored tablets of 750 mg.

Other Proprietary Names
Dilcit *(Denm., Swed.)*; Dilexpal *(Fr.)*; Esantene *(Ital.)*; Evicyl *(Arg.)*; Hämovannad *(Ger.)*; Hexanicit *(Denm., Ger., Norw., Swed., Switz.)*; Linodil *(Canad.)*; Palohex *(Belg., Neth.)*; Vasodil *(Austral.)*.

9244-j

Isosorbide Dinitrate.

Sorbide Nitrate. 1,4:3,6-Dianhydro-D-glucitol 2,5-dinitrate.
$C_6H_8N_2O_8$=236.1.

CAS — 87-33-2.

Pharmacopoeias. In *Chin.* and *Jap.*

A white crystalline powder. Very slightly **soluble** in water; sparingly soluble in alcohol; very soluble in acetone; freely soluble in chloroform; soluble in methyl alcohol.

CAUTION. Isosorbide dinitrate may explode if subjected to percussion or excessive heat.

9245-z

Diluted Isosorbide Dinitrate *(B.P., U.S.P.)*.

Diluted Sorbide Nitrate.

Pharmacopoeias. In *Br. Braz.* and *U.S.* specify about 25% of isosorbide dinitrate.

A mixture of isosorbide dinitrate (usually 20 to 50%) with lactose, mannitol, or other suitable inert excipients, the latter being added to minimise the risk of explosion. It may contain up to 1% of a suitable stabiliser such as ammonium phosphate.

A fine white to ivory-white odourless crystalline powder. Very slightly **soluble** in water; sparingly soluble in alcohol; very soluble in acetone; freely soluble in chloroform. **Store** in airtight containers; the *B.P.* specifies a cool place; the *U.S.P.* specifies a temperature not exceeding 40°. Protect from light.

Adverse Effects, Treatment, and Precautions. As for Glyceryl Trinitrate, p.1620.

Halitosis had occurred in several patients taking isosorbide dinitrate sublingually.— D. Bauman (letter), *J. Am. med. Ass.*, 1975, *234*, 482.

Cardiovascular effects. Reports of ankle oedema associated with isosorbide dinitrate therapy.— J. C. Rodger, *Br. med. J.*, 1981, *283*, 1365.

Effects on the eyes. There was no increase in intra-ocular pressure in 12 normal subjects, 3 with raised intra-ocular pressure, and 3 with glaucoma up to 60 minutes after the administration of isosorbide dinitrate 5 mg sublingually.— D. Robertson and R. M. Stevens (letter), *J. Am. med. Ass.*, 1977, *237*, 117.

Withdrawal and tolerance. In 19 patients taking isosorbide dinitrate 10 to 50 (mean 27.4) mg usually 4 times daily for 3.5 to 10 months a smaller reduction in blood pressure and a smaller increase in heart-rate compared with pretreatment values indicated the development of tolerance, but exercise tolerance was not adversely affected. Because of the possibility of dependence withdrawal should be gradual and continuous prophylaxis was not recommended for patients controlled by less intensive therapy.— D. T. Danahy and W. S. Aronow, *Circulation*, 1977, *56*, 205.

Lack of tolerance to isosorbide dinitrate after 3 months of therapy.— J. A. Franciosa and J. N. Cohn, *Am. J. Cardiol.*, 1980, *45*, 648.

Absorption and Fate. Like glyceryl trinitrate, isosorbide dinitrate is readily absorbed from the oral mucosa and has a fairly fleeting duration of action. Isosorbide dinitrate is also readily absorbed following administration by mouth. In view of its short plasma half-life various long-acting formulations are available for oral administration.

Isosorbide dinitrate is also absorbed through the skin from an ointment basis.

In 2 healthy male volunteers isosorbide dinitrate 5 mg by mouth was rapidly and almost completely absorbed from the gastro-intestinal tract. Up to 25% was excreted in the urine in 6 hours, 49% in 12 hours, and 78% in 24 hours. After 5 days up to 99% had been excreted in the urine and 0.8% in the faeces. Isosorbide dinitrate was excreted in the urine, mainly as polar metabolites, with a half-life of about 10 hours.— W. H. Down *et al.*, *J. pharm. Sci.*, 1974, *63*, 1147.

Following administration of isosorbide dinitrate 10 mg sublingually to 2 subjects, significant plasma concentrations of isosorbide dinitrate were detected at 10 minutes and up to 1 hour after dosage. Two metabolites isosorbide 2-mononitrate and 5-mononitrate reached a maximum concentration in plasma 30 minutes after administration of the isosorbide dinitrate.— D. A. Chin *et al.*, *J. pharm. Sci.*, 1977, *66*, 1143.

In a comparative crossover study of different tablet formulations administration of isosorbide dinitrate 5 mg as standard tablets sublingually and by mouth gave mean peak plasma concentrations of about 9 ng per ml fifteen minutes after sublingual administration and 3 ng per ml thirty minutes after oral administration respectively, these concentrations subsequently declining rapidly, to below the limits of detection (0.5 ng per ml) after 4 hours; the mean half-lives were not significantly different being calculated as 0.5 and 0.67 hours respectively (overall range 0.47 to 1.05 hours). An initial peak of about 1.4 ng per ml was obtained 40 minutes after administration of the sustained-release tablets, remaining at this level for a further 5 hours and declining to the limits of detection after about 12 hours.— D. F. Assinder *et al.*, *J. pharm. Sci.*, 1977, *66*, 775.

In 10 healthy male volunteers isosorbide dinitrate 5 mg (Cedocard) by mouth gave a mean peak plasma concentration of 5.8 ng per ml after 30 minutes and a half-life of 48 minutes. A sustained-release preparation containing 20 mg (Iso Mack Retard, *Mack, Ger.*) gave a peak plasma concentration of 3.2 ng per ml after 2 to 4 hours and declined slowly over 12 hours.— D. F. Assinder *et al.*, *Arzneimittel-Forsch.*, 1977, *27*, 156.

Isosorbide dinitrate 10 mg four times daily initially, increased gradually to 360 to 720 mg daily in divided doses for about 1 to 8 weeks was well-tolerated in 7 patients with angina pectoris. Prolonged high plasma concentrations of isosorbide dinitrate and higher concentrations of its metabolites isosorbide 2-mononitrate (up to 5-fold higher) and isosorbide 5-mononitrate (up to 30-fold higher) were achieved although there was considerable individual variation. It was considered that high plasma concentrations were attained because the high chronic doses of isosorbide dinitrate had saturated the intrahepatic biotransformation process.— S. J. Shane *et al.*, *Br. J. clin. Pharmac.*, 1978, *6*, 37.

Further references: D. Mansel-Jones *et al.*, *J. clin. Pharmac.*, 1978, *18*, 544 (cutaneous and sublingual); A. Schinz *et al.*, *Int. J. clin. Pharmac. Biopharm.*, 1978, *16*, 297 (ointment); T. Taylor *et al.*, *Arzneimittel-Forsch.*, 1978, *28*, 1426 (sustained-release formulation).

Uses. Isosorbide dinitrate is a vasodilator with general properties similar to those of glyceryl trinitrate (p.1621). Isosorbide dinitrate is suitable for oral as well as sublingual administration. In view of its brief plasma half-life preparations of isosorbide dinitrate for oral administration are available in sustained-release form. When administered sublingually its effects begin within about 5 minutes and last for about 2 hours; when swallowed its effects are evident after about 30 minutes and last for about 5 hours.

It is used prophylactically in the treatment of angina pectoris in oral doses of 5 to 20 mg twice or thrice daily according to the patient's needs. Increases in dosage should be gradual to avoid side-effects. Up to 120 mg daily in divided doses may be necessary. For acute attacks the usual dose is 5 to 10 mg sublingually. Isosorbide dinitrate may also be used in similar doses as adjunctive therapy in congestive heart failure.

Isosorbide dinitrate may also be given by intravenous infusion as a solution usually containing about 75 to 100 µg per ml in sodium chloride injection or dextrose injection. For unresponsive congestive cardiac failure or unstable angina a recommended starting dose is 2 mg per hour increased if necessary to 7 mg per hour; doses of up to 10 mg per hour may be necessary in some patients.

Isosorbide dinitrate has also been applied topically.

A review of the pharmacological properties and therapeutic use of isosorbide dinitrate.— U. Elkayam and W. S. Aronow, *Drugs*, 1982, *23*, 165.

Administration. A preliminary report of experience with isosorbide dinitrate cream.— B. Cheadle *et al.* (letter), *Br. med. J.*, 1981, *283*, 1549.

Cardiac disorders. For detailed comments on the role of long-acting nitrates in cardiovascular disease, see Glyceryl Trinitrate, p.1621.

Angina pectoris. Reports and studies on the role of isosorbide dinitrate in angina pectoris: H. Kasparian *et al.*, *Am. Heart J.*, 1975, *90*, 68; D. J. Battock *et al.*, *Am. Heart J.*, 1976, *92*, 455; D. T. Danahy *et al.*, *Circulation*, 1977, *55*, 381; D. L. Glancy *et al.*, *Am. J. Med.*, 1977, *62*, 39; G. Lee *et al.*, *Chest*, 1978, *73*, 327; B. Pugh *et al.*, *Am. J. Cardiol.*, 1978, *41*, 1291; A. A. Kattus *et al.*, *Chest*, 1979, *75*, 17; J. E. Markis *et al.*, *Am. J. Cardiol.*, 1979, *43*, 265; J. Whittington and E. B. Raftery, *Br. J. clin. Pharmac.*, 1980, *10*, 211.

Heart failure. Reports and studies on the role of isosorbide dinitrate in heart failure: R. Gray *et al.*, *Am. Heart J.*, 1975, *90*, 346; R. H. Baxter *et al.*, *Br. Heart J.*, 1977, *39*, 1067; W. D. Bussmann *et al.*, *Am. J. Cardiol.*, 1977, *39*, 91; T. Hardarson *et al.*, *Am. J. Cardiol.*, 1977, *40*, 90; D. O. Williams *et al.*, *Am. J. Cardiol.*, 1977, *39*, 84; J. A. Gomes *et al.*, *Am. J. Med.*, 1978, *65*, 794; G. L. Pierpont *et al.*, *Chest*, 1978, *73*, 8; K. P. Schüren and H. N. Macha, *Dt. med. Wschr.*, 1978, *103*, 777; J. Stephens *et al.*, *Br. Heart J.*, 1978, *40*, 832 and 838; J. Figueras *et al.*, *Br. Heart J.*, 1979, *41*, 317; J. A. Franciosa and J. N. Cohn, *Am. J. Cardiol.*, 1979, *43*, 1009; K. Venkataraman *et al.*, *Clin. Pharmac. Ther.*, 1979, *25*, 43; J. A. Franciosa *et al.*, *Am. J. Med.*, 1980, *69*, 559; J. D. Stephens *et al.*, *Br. Heart J.*, 1980, *43*, 220.

Pulmonary hypertension. Isosorbide dinitrate, in doses of 25 to 40 mg, may be useful in reducing pulmonary hypertension in patients with chronic obstructive pulmonary disease.— D. T. Danahy *et al.*, *Clin. Pharmac. Ther.*, 1979, *25*, 541.

Preparations

Isosorbide Dinitrate Tablets *(B.P.)*. Sorbide Nitrate Tablets. Tablets containing isosorbide dinitrate. The label states whether they are to be swallowed, chewed before swallowing, or allowed to dissolve in the mouth.

Isosorbide Dinitrate Tablets *(U.S.P.)*. Tablets containing isosorbide dinitrate. Store at a temperature not exceeding 40°. For sublingual use.

Proprietary Preparations

Cedocard *(Cedona, Neth.: Tillotts, UK)*. Isosorbide dinitrate, available as scored tablets of 5 and 10 mg for oral or sublingual administration. **Cedocard Retard**. Scored sustained-release tablets each containing isosorbide dinitrate 20 mg. *Dose*. 1 tablet of Cedocard Retard morning and evening. (Also available as Cedocard in *Belg., Neth., S.Afr., Switz.*).

Cedocard-20 *(Cedona, Neth.: Tillotts, UK)*. Isosorbide dinitrate, available as scored tablets of 20 mg. For oral administration.

Cedocard I.V *(Cedona, Neth.: Tillotts, UK)*. Isosorbide dinitrate, available as solution for preparing intravenous infusions, containing 1 mg per ml, in ampoules of 10 ml. A 15 to 30% loss of potency may occur if Cedocard I.V. is administered via PVC infusion bags.

Isoket Ampoules *(Sanol Schwarz, UK)*. Isosorbide dinitrate, available as solution for preparing intravenous infusions, containing 1 mg per ml, in ampoules of 10 ml. A loss of potency of up to 40% may occur if Isoket is administered via PVC infusion bags.

Isoket Retard *(Sanol Schwarz, UK)*. Isosorbide dinitrate, available as sustained-release scored tablets of 20 mg. *Dose*. 1 tablet every 12 hours. (Also availabe as Isoket in *Ger., Spain, Switz.*, and as Isoket-10 in *Arg.*).

Isordil *(Ayerst, UK)*. Isosorbide dinitrate, available as sublingual tablets of 5 mg and as scored oral tablets of 10 and 30 mg. (Also available as Isordil in *Arg., Austral., Belg., Canad., S.Afr., Switz., USA*).

Isordil Tembids *(Ayerst, UK)*. Isosorbide dinitrate, available as sustained-release capsules of 40 mg. *Dose*. 1 capsule twice or thrice daily.

Soni-Slo *(Rona, UK)*. Isosorbide dinitrate, available as sustained-release capsules of 20 mg. *Dose*. 1 capsule twice or thrice daily.

Sorbichew (formerly known as Sorbitrate Chewable) *(Stuart, UK)*. Isosorbide dinitrate, available as scored chewable tablets of 5 mg.

Sorbid SA *(Stuart, UK)*. Tablets each containing 40 mg of isosorbide dinitrate, 10 mg for immediate release and 30 mg for sustained release. *Dose*. Prophylactic, 1 or 2 tablets twice daily.

Sorbitrate Tablets *(Stuart, UK)*. Isosorbide dinitrate, available as scored tablets of 10 and 20 mg. For oral administration. (Also available as Sorbitrate in *USA*).

Vascardin *(Nicholas, UK)*. Isosorbide dinitrate, available as scored tablets of 10 mg for oral or sublingual administration.

Other Proprietary Names

Arg.— Conducil, Corosorbide, Maycor, Sigillum, Surantol, Vasodilat; *Austral.*— Carvasin, Isotrate; *Belg.*— Sorbidilat; *Canad.*— Coronex; *Fr.*— Risordan; *Ger.*— Cardio, Corovliss, Iso Mack, Maycor, Nitro, Nitrosorbon, Sorbidilat, Vermicet; *Ital.*— Carvasin, Nitrosorbide; *Jap.*— Directan, Nitrol; *Mex.*— Isorbid; *Norw.*— Sorbangil; *Swed.*— Sorbangil; *Switz.*— Iso Mack, Myorexon, Sorbidilat; *USA*— Dilatrate-SR, Iso-Bid, Iso-D, Isotrate, Sorbide, Sorquad, Vasotrate.

9246-c

Isoxsuprine Hydrochloride *(B.P., U.S.P.)*.

Caa 40; Phenoxyisopropylnorsuprifen. 1-(4-Hydroxyphenyl)-2-(1-methyl-2-phenoxyethylamino)propan-1-ol hydrochloride.

$C_{18}H_{23}NO_3,HCl=337.8$.

CAS — 395-28-8 (isoxsuprine); 579-56-6 (hydrochloride).

Pharmacopoeias. In *Br.* and *U.S.*

A white or almost white odourless crystalline powder with a bitter taste. M.p. about 200° with decomposition. **Soluble** 1 in 500 of water, 1 in 100 of alcohol and dilute sodium hydroxide solution, and 1 in 2500 of dilute hydrochloric acid; practically insoluble in chloroform and ether. A 1% solution in water has a pH of 4.5 to 6. **Store** in airtight containers.

Adverse Effects and Treatment. As for Buphenine Hydrochloride, p.1616.

Transient flushing may occur. Larger doses cause tachycardia and hypotension, particularly in hypertensive patients. A slight increase in the rate of the foetal heart-beat has been noted when isoxsuprine has been given by intravenous infusion during the late stages of pregnancy. Rarely, severe skin rashes have been associated with its administration.

Allergy. A report of allergic dermatitis in 2 women given isoxsuprine for premature labour. The eruption was pruritic and papular in both women.— J. J. Horowitz and R. K. Creesy, *Am. J. Obstet. Gynec.*, 1978, *131*, 225.

Pregnancy and the neonate. In a retrospective study of 26 premature infants whose mothers had received isoxsuprine during labour, no infant had any symptoms of the respiratory distress syndrome to which they were considered to be susceptible. A further 12 mothers were given isoxsuprine 80 to 160 mg intravenously over 1 to 2 days up to the end of labour and none of the premature infants (gestational age 28 to 35 weeks) developed the respiratory distress syndrome.— P. Kero *et al.* (letter), *Lancet*, 1973, *2*, 198.

In a study involving 40 neonates whose mothers had received isoxsuprine within 24 hours of delivery and 40 matched controls, ileus was found to be more common in the isoxsuprine group than in the controls. The isoxsuprine group was subdivided according to concentrations found in the cord blood and the incidence of respiratory distress syndrome was minimal in the group with absent or low drug values but rose to surpass the control group as the isoxsuprine concentration exceeded 10 ng per ml; likewise the incidence of hypocalcaemia and hypotension rose progressively with increasing concentrations. The cord concentrations correlated inversely with the drug-free interval before delivery and it was suggested that with frequent assessment of uterine response it should be possible to avoid delivering infants at a time when they have high plasma-isoxsuprine concentrations.— J. E. Brazy *et al.*, *J. Pediat.*, 1981, *98*, 146.

Bowel distension occurred in 2 patients given orciprenaline for premature labour. The patients were also taking isoxsuprine.— G. V. Nair *et al.* (letter), *Lancet*, 1976, *1*, 907.

Further references: R. W. Stander *et al.*, *Am. J. Obstet. Gynec.*, 1964, *89*, 792 (foetal tachycardia).

Precautions. Isoxsuprine is reported to be contra-indicated following recent arterial haemorrhage, in patients with known heart disease, or in severe anaemia. It should not be administered parenterally to patients with hypotension or tachycardia.

It should not be given where there is premature detachment of the placenta or immediately post partum.

In premature labour patients should be maintained in the lateral position during infusion.

Absorption and Fate. Isoxsuprine hydrochloride is absorbed from the gastro-intestinal tract. The maximum concentration in the circulation occurs about 1 hour after administration by mouth or intramuscular or subcutaneous injection, and is maintained for about 3 hours. Isoxsuprine is in part conjugated in the blood and is excreted in the urine. Faecal excretion is insignificant.

Pregnancy and the neonate. See above under Adverse Effects.

Uses. Isoxsuprine produces the effects of beta-adrenoceptor stimulation and alpha-adrenoceptor antagonism, the former effect predominating. Its dilating action is greater on the arteries supplying skeletal muscles than on those supplying skin.

Isoxsuprine hydrochloride is used in the treatment of cerebral and peripheral vascular disease. It may be given by mouth in doses of up to 20 mg four times daily, or by intramuscular or intra-arterial injection in doses of up to 10 mg four times daily. Isoxsuprine hydrochloride may also be given by intravenous infusion as a solution containing 100 mg in 500 ml of sodium chloride infusion. A recommended schedule for a maximum infusion time of 1 hour twice daily is 0.5 ml per minute (100 μg per minute) for 10 minutes, 1 ml per minute (200 μg per minute) for the next 10 minutes, 1.5 ml per minute (300 μg per minute) for the following 10 minutes, and 2 ml per minute (400 μg per minute) for the remaining 30 minutes; if after a rate of 2 ml per minute for 10 minutes there have been no side-effects 2.5 ml per minute (500 μg per minute) may be given for the last 20 minutes.

Isoxsuprine hydrochloride inhibits contractions of the uterus and is used by intravenous injection to arrest premature labour. It is given initially by intravenous infusion; a solution containing 100 mg in 500 ml of sodium chloride injection is infused at the rate of 1 to 1.5 ml per minute (200 to 300 μg per minute) increased, according to the patient's response, to 2.5 ml per minute (500 μg per minute) with regular monitoring of blood pressure and maternal and foetal heart-rates, and continued until control is established. Subsequent treatment consists of intramuscular injections of 10 mg every 3 hours for 24 hours, every 4 to 6 hours for a further 48 hours, and then 20 mg by mouth 4 times daily.

Cerebrovascular disease. Cerebral vasodilators have proved disappointing for senile dementia in clinical practice. None of the few studies on isoxsuprine has shown it to be of any practical value.— *Br. med. J.*, 1979, *2*, 511. Criticism.— A. J. Martin, *Duphar* (letter), *ibid.*, 866. Reply.— *ibid.* See also P. Cook and I. James, *New Engl. J. Med.*, 1981, *305*, 1560.

Reports and studies on the use of isoxsuprine in cerebrovascular disease: A. D. Dhrymiotis and J. R. Whittier, *Curr. ther. Res.*, 1962, *4*, 124; J. F. Fazekas and R. W. Alman, *Am. J. med. Sci.*, 1964, *248*, 16; S. M. A. Hussain *et al.*, *Practitioner*, 1976, *216*, 222; B. M. Guyer, *Clin. Trials J.*, 1977, *14*, 159.

Dysmenorrhoea. In doses of 10 to 20 mg three or four times daily, starting prior to menstruation, isoxsuprine gave relief to 44 of 53 women subject to severe pelvic cramp.— D. M. Voulgaris, *Obstet. Gynec.*, 1960, *15*, 220.

Eye disorders. A 65-year-old man with central retinal artery occlusion recovered his vision within 10 minutes of the intravenous administration of isoxsuprine hydrochloride 20 mg in 20 ml of sodium chloride injection. Treatment was started within 10 minutes of the onset of blindness and was continued intramuscularly and by mouth, for 4 weeks.— T. G. Judge, *Br. J. clin. Pract.*, 1968, *22*, 223.

Peripheral vascular disorders. Results of studies do not support the use of isoxsuprine in obstructive arterial disease; since it is not a cutaneous vasodilator, it should not be used in vasospastic disease.— J. D. Coffman, *New Engl. J. Med.*, 1979, *300*, 713.

Reports and studies of the use of isoxsuprine in peripheral vascular disorders: S. B. Samuels and H. E. Shaftal, *J. Am. med. Ass.*, 1959, *171*, 142; T. T. Zsostér and R. J. Baird, *Can. med. Ass. J.*, 1974, *110*, 1260; T. Di Perri *et al.*, *Br. J. clin. Pharmac.*, 1978, *5*, 255.

Premature labour. A review of drugs, including isoxsuprine, used for the arrest of premature labour.— *Drug & Ther. Bull.*, 1980, *18*, 34.

See also under Salbutamol, p.31.

Reports and studies on isoxsuprine in premature labour: E. H. Bishop and T. B. Woutersz, *J. Am. med. Ass.*, 1961, *178*, 812,; C. C. Briscoe, *Am. J. Obstet. Gynec.*, 1966, *95*, 885; A. I. Csapo and J. Herczeg, *Am. J. Obstet. Gynec.*, 1977, *129*, 482.

Sickle-cell crisis. Experience with isoxsuprine in the relief of pain in sickle-cell crisis.— C. Psomadakis *et al.*, *Angiology*, 1981, *32*, 249.

Preparations

Isoxsuprine Hydrochloride Injection *(B.P.).* Isoxsuprine Hydrochlor. Inj.; Isoxsuprine Injection. A sterile solution in Water for Injections. Sterilised by autoclaving.

Isoxsuprine Hydrochloride Injection *(U.S.P.).* A sterile solution in Water for Injections. pH 4.9 to 6.0.

Isoxsuprine Hydrochloride Tablets *(B.P.).* Isoxsuprine Hydrochlor. Tab. Tablets containing isoxsuprine hydrochloride.

Isoxsuprine Hydrochloride Tablets *(U.S.P.).* Tablets containing isoxsuprine hydrochloride. Store in airtight containers.

Proprietary Preparations

Defencin CP *(Bristol-Myers Pharmaceuticals, UK).* Isoxsuprine resinate, available as sustained-release capsules each containing the equivalent of 40 mg of isoxsuprine hydrochloride. *Dose.* 1 capsule every 12 hours.

Duvadilan *(Duphar, UK).* Isoxsuprine hydrochloride, available as **Injection** containing 5 mg per ml, in ampoules of 2 and 10 ml, and as scored **Tablets** of 20 mg. **Duvadilan Retard.** Sustained-release capsules of isoxsuprine resinate, each containing the equivalent of isoxsuprine hydrochloride 40 mg. *Dose.* 1 sustained-release capsule morning and evening. (Also available as Duvadilan in *Arg.*, *Austral.*, *Belg.*, *Fr.*, *Ger.*, *Ital.*, *Neth.*, *S.Afr.*, *Spain*, *Swed.*, *Switz.*).

Other Proprietary Names

Aust.— Xuprin; *Canad.*— Vasodilan; *Ger.*—Vasoplex; *Ital.*—Fenam, Largiven, Vascuprin, Vasodilene, Vasosuprina; *Jap.*—Isokulin, Synzedrin, Vahodilan; *Norw.*—Cardilan; *Switz.*—Suprilent; *USA*—Isolait, Vasodilan.

Isoxsuprine hydrochloride was also formerly marketed in Great Britain under the proprietary name Vasotran (*Bristol Laboratories*).

9247-k

Itramin Tosylate. 2-Aminoethyl nitrate toluene-4-sulphonate.

$C_2H_6N_2O_3,C_7H_8O_3S=278.3.$

CAS — 646-02-6 (itramin); 13445-63-1 (tosylate).

Itramin tosylate is a vasodilator formerly used in the treatment of angina pectoris.

9248-a

Kallidinogenase. Kallikrein; Callicrein; Kalléone.

CAS — 9001-01-8.

A vasodilator substance isolated from the pancreas and urine of mammals.

Readily **soluble** in water and alcohol (50%); practically insoluble in alcohol (95%) and the common organic solvents.

The properties and assay methods of kallidinogenase.— Kallikrein, in *Pharmaceutical Enzymes*, R. Ruyssen and A. Lauwers (Ed.), Gent, E. Story-Scientia, 1978, p. 145.

Adverse Effects. Side-effects reported include flushing, dizziness, and palpitations; rarely, allergic reactions have occurred. Large doses given by intravenous injection produce hypotension which may persist for several hours.

For a report of pre-kallidinogenase activator being identified as Hageman-factor (factor XII) fragments and being responsible for severe transient hypotension in patients given infusions of albumin fraction, see Plasma Protein Fraction, p.335.

Precautions. Kallidinogenase should be used with caution after recent cerebral vascular episodes. It should not be given in the presence of increased intracranial pressure or cardiac failure.

Uses. Kallidinogenase has vasodilating properties and has been used in the treatment of peripheral vascular disorders.

Studies *in vitro* showed that human urinary kallidinogenase activated inactive renin and it was considered that it might be a part of a control system for the release of renin.— J. E. Sealey *et al.*, *Nature*, 1978, *275*, 144.

Comment on the possible role of kallidinogenase as an activator of inactive renin.— D. H. Osmond *et al.* (letter), *Lancet*, 1978, *2*, 1375; J. A. Millar *et al.* (letter), *ibid.*, 1376.

The pharmacology of bradykinin and related kinins.— D. Regoli and J. Barabé, *Pharmac. Rev.*, 1980, *32*, 1. See also M. Schachter, *ibid.*, 1979, *31*, 1.

Proprietary Names

Depot-Padutin *(Bayer, Denm.*; *Bayropharm, Ger.)*; Padutin *(Bayer, Denm.*; *Bayropharm, Ger.)*; Padutina Depot *(Bayer, Spain)*; Padutine-Dépot *(Bayer, Belg.)*; Bioactin, Onokrein-P, Prokrein *(all Jap.)*.

Kallidinogenase was formerly marketed in Great Britain under the proprietary name Glumorin (*Bayer*).

9249-t

Khellin. Khellinum; Khelline; Visammin. 4,9-Dimethoxy-7-methyl-5*H*-furo[3,2-*g*]chromen-5-one.

$C_{14}H_{12}O_5=260.2.$

CAS — 82-02-0.

Pharmacopoeias. In *Aust.* and *Rus.*

White odourless crystals, sometimes with a slight yellowish tinge, and with a bitter taste. M.p. about 153°. Obtained by extraction from ammi visnaga fruit (p.1614) or by synthesis.

Very slightly **soluble** in cold water; sparingly soluble in boiling water; soluble in acetone, alcohol, chloroform, and glacial acetic acid; less soluble in ether and light petroleum; readily soluble in dilute mineral acids.

Uses. Khellin relaxes smooth muscle and has been employed in the treatment of angina pectoris, and in the treatment of asthma.

Cardiac disorders. A discussion on abandoned treatments for angina pectoris, including khellin, which is now believed to have no specific physiological efficacy yet was formerly found to be effective and was used extensively.— H. Benson and D. P. McCallie, *New Engl. J. Med.*, 1979, *300*, 1424.

Preparations

Tabulettae Khellini *(Rus. P.).* Tablets each containing khellin 20 mg.

Proprietary Names

Aspas *(Zanardi, Ital.)*; Kellina *(UCB, Ital.)*; Kellosal *(Biosint, Ital.)*; Kelicorin *(Infale, Spain)*.

9250-l

Lidoflazine. McN-JR-7904; R 7904; Ordiflazine. 4-[3-(4,4′-Difluorobenzhydryl)propyl]piperazin-1-ylaceto-2′,6′-xylidide.

$C_{30}H_{35}F_2N_3O=491.6.$

CAS — 3416-26-0.

A white or slightly yellow amorphous powder. Practically **insoluble** in water; very soluble in chloroform.

Adverse Effects. Side-effects associated with lidoflazine include gastro-intestinal upset, transient dizziness, tinnitus and headache.

Treatment of Adverse Effects. In overdosage by mouth, the stomach should be emptied by aspiration and lavage.

Uses. Lidoflazine is used for the long-term management of angina pectoris. It has calcium-antagonist properties. A recommended dosage schedule is 120 mg daily initially for the first week, increased to 120 mg twice daily for the second week, subsequently increased to 120 mg thrice daily thereafter.

It should not be used for the primary treatment of cardiac arrhythmias.

Action. Comment on the different action of drugs given the general description of calcium antagonists, and the view that they should be subdivided into 4 or more classes according to their principal therapeutic effects; lidoflazine inhibits excess ingress of calcium into cells deprived of oxygen without affecting calcium homoeostasis in the well-oxygenated cell.— A. L. Macnair and H. A. Waldron, *Janssen* (letter), *Br. med. J.*, 1981, *282*, 400.

For further comments on the mode of action of calcium antagonists, see under Nifedipine, p.1628.

Cardiac disorders. Angina pectoris. In a double-blind crossover study on 31 patients with angina pectoris, lidoflazine 60 mg thrice daily was compared with placebo for 6-week periods. In more severe cases, lidoflazine reduced both number of attacks and glyceryl trinitrate consumption, but had less effect in milder cases. There was a carry-over effect of lidoflazine into the placebo period.— B. Brantmark *et al., Eur. J. clin. Pharmac.*, 1973, *6*, 156.

Further reports and studies of the role of lidoflazine in angina pectoris: L. K. Verhaeghe, *Arzneimittel.Forsch.*, 1969, *19*, 1842; J. Piessens and H. De Geest, *Cardiology*, 1972, *57*, 135; V. Bernstein and D. I. Peretz, *Curr. ther. Res.*, 1972, *14*, 483; C. Aravanis *et al., ibid.*, 1973, *15*, 285; L. A. Nordstrom and F. L. Gobel, *Chest*, 1978, *74*, 50.

Cardiac arrhythmias. Ectopic multifocal beats occurred in 15 of 30 patients with atrial fibrillation (29) or atrial flutter (1) who were given lidoflazine 60 mg thrice daily. Although conversion to sinus rhythm occurred in 19 of the 31 episodes of arrhythmia treated, atrial fibrillation was felt to be a contra-indication to the use of lidoflazine.— M. Schlepper and R. Derro, *Arzneimittel-Forsch.*, 1972, *22*, 923. Six hyperthyroid patients with chronic atrial fibrillation were given lidoflazine by mouth at a dose increased weekly from 60 mg up to 180 mg daily. Sinus rhythm was achieved in all patients within 12 hours to 6 weeks and maintained for at least 5 to 14 months, independently of thyroid function. Lidoflazine was continued at the cardioversion dose or less. Antithyroid treatment with methimazole was started before or after cardioversion with lidoflazine.— K. Bruyneel *et al., Postgrad. med. J.*, 1975, *51*, 4.

Further reports and studies of lidoflazine in cardiac arrhythmias: O. A. Beck *et al., Dt. med. Wschr.*, 1978, *103*, 1068 (chronic atrial fibrillation and flutter).

Proprietary Preparations

Clinium *(Janssen, UK).* Lidoflazine, available as tablets of 120 mg. (Also available as Clinium in *Arg., Belg., Fr., Ger., Ital., Neth., S.Afr.*).

Other Proprietary Names

Clavidene *(Ital.)*; Corflazine *(Fr.)*; Klinium *(Spain)*.

9251-y

Mannityl Hexanitrate. Mannitol Hexanitrate; Nitromannite; Nitromannitol.
$C_6H_8(O.NO_2)_6$=452.2.

CAS — 15825-70-4.

Pharmacopoeias. Swiss P. has Mannitylium Hexanitricum Trituratum 10% (in lactose).

A white crystalline powder with a faint odour. Practically **insoluble** in water; soluble in warm alcohol and in chloroform, ether, and glacial acetic acid. For medicinal purposes it is supplied diluted with an inert substance such as lactose (usually 1 part of mannityl hexanitrate to 9 or more parts of lactose), since the undiluted compound is explosive. **Store** in airtight containers. Protect from light.

Mannityl hexanitrate has general properties similar to those of glyceryl trinitrate (p.1620) and has been used in the prophylaxis of angina pectoris.

Proprietary Names

Moloid *(Südmedica, Ger.)*.

9252-j

Medibazine Hydrochloride. 4105S. 1-Benzhydryl-4-piperonylpiperazine dihydrochloride.
$C_{25}H_{26}N_2O_2$,2HCl=459.4.

CAS — 53-31-6 (medibazine); 22193-78-8 (hydrochloride).

Medibazine hydrochloride is a vasodilator which has been used in the treatment of coronary insufficiency.

Proprietary Names

Vialibran *(Servier, Fr.; Servier, Spain)*.

9253-z

Methyl Nicotinate *(B.P.)*.
$C_7H_7NO_2$=137.1.

CAS — 93-60-7.

Pharmacopoeias. In *Br.*

White or almost white crystals or crystalline powder with a characteristic odour; it darkens in colour on keeping, becoming reddish; m.p. 40° to 42°. **Soluble** 1 in 0.7 of water and alcohol, 1 in 0.4 of chloroform, and 1 in 1 of ether.

Methyl nicotinate, usually in a concentration of 1%, is used in ointments and creams for topical application as a rubefacient for the relief of pain in muscular rheumatism, lumbago, and fibrositis.
Other nicotinates are used in a similar way.

A report of an investigation of the rate of diffusion of methyl nicotinate in water, macrogol 300, propylene glycol, and tetrahydrofurfuryl alcohol; of the volatility, viscosity, and surface tension of these bases; and of the effect upon vasodilatation of preparations of methyl nicotinate formulated in these bases.— B. S. Baker *et al., Br. J. Derm.*, 1969, *81*, 60.

A report of an investigation into the rate of absorption and duration of action of solutions of methyl nicotinate in water, macrogol 300, propylene glycol, and tetrahydrofurfuryl alcohol.— R. B. Fountain *et al., Br. J. Derm.*, 1969, *81*, 202.

The effect of glycerol on the percutaneous absorption of methyl nicotinate from aqueous solutions.— J. Hadgraft *et al., Br. J. Derm.*, 1972, *87*, 30. See also W. J. Albery and J. Hadgraft, *J. Pharm. Pharmac.*, 1979, *31*, 140.

Proprietary Preparations containing Nicotinates

Algipan Balm *(Wyeth, UK).* A non-greasy cream containing methyl nicotinate 1%, histamine hydrochloride 0.1%, glycol salicylate 10%, and capsicum oleoresin 0.1%. For non-articular rheumatism, sprains, and other affections of the muscles.

Bayolin *(Bayer, UK).* A cream containing in each 100 g benzyl nicotinate 2.5 g, glycol salicylate 10 g, and a heparinoid (obtained by sulphation of polysaccharides from the cell walls of certain *Penicillium* strains) equivalent to 5000 units of heparin. For muscular pains and rheumatic conditions.

Cremalgex *(Norton, UK: Vestric, UK).* A non-greasy cream containing methyl nicotinate 1%, glycol salicylate 10%, capsicum oleoresin 0.15%, and histamine hydrochloride 0.1%. For rheumatic pain, fibrositis, and sciatica.

Cremalgin *(Berk Pharmaceuticals, UK).* A cream containing methyl nicotinate 1%, glycol salicylate 10%, histamine hydrochloride 0.1%, and capsicum oleoresin 0.1%. For rheumatism, fibrositis, and similar conditions.

Cremathurm *(Sinclair, UK).* A cream containing ethyl nicotinate 1%, methyl salicylate 10%, histamine acid phosphate 0.1%, and capsicum oleoresin 0.1%. For rheumatic conditions.

Finalgon *(Boehringer Ingelheim, UK).* Ointment containing butoxyethyl nicotinate 2.5% and nonivamide 0.4%. For fibrositis, sprains, and other painful musculoskeletal conditions.

Transvasin *(Lloyd-Hamol, Reckitt & Colman Pharm., UK).* A cream containing ethyl nicotinate 2%, hexyl nicotinate 2%, thurfyl salicylate 14%, and benzocaine 2%, in a water-miscible basis. For rheumatic disorders, and for use as an adjuvant in the treatment of sprains and strains.

Other Proprietary Names of Nicotinates

Rubriment (benzyl nicotinate) *(Ger.)*; Trafuril (thurfyl nicotinate) *(Fr., Switz.)*.

Thurfyl nicotinate was formerly marketed in Great Britain under the proprietary name Trafuril (*Ciba*). Preparations containing nicotinates were also formerly marketed in Great Britain under the proprietary names Dubalm (*Norma*), No-Del (*Rybar*), and Thoracin (*Lloyd-Hamol*).

9254-c

Methylchromone. 3-Methyl-4*H*-chromen-4-one.
$C_{10}H_8O_2$=160.2.

CAS — 85-90-5.

A white crystalline powder. Sparingly **soluble** in water; soluble in alcohol and ether.

Methylchromone is a vasodilator which has been given in the treatment of angina pectoris and coronary insufficiency. It has also been used as an antispasmodic for the relief of biliary, hepatic, or renal spasm.

Overdosage. Reversible renal failure in a 3-year-old boy after the ingestion of methylchromone 3.5 g.— J. Otten and H. L. Vis, *J. Pediat.*, 1968, *73*, 422, per *J. Am. med. Ass.*, 1968, *206*, 944.

Proprietary Names

Cromonalgina *(Ceccarelli, Ital.)*; Diacromone *(Millot-Solac, Fr.)*.

9255-k

Methylpropylpropanediol Dinitrate. 2-Methyl-2-propylpropane-1,3-diol dinitrate.
$C_7H_{14}N_2O_6$=222.2.

Methylpropylpropanediol dinitrate is a vasodilator that has been used in the prophylaxis of angina pectoris.

9256-a

Naftidrofuryl Oxalate. Nafronyl Oxalate; EU-1806; LS-121. 2-Diethylaminoethyl 3-(1-naphthyl)-2-tetrahydrofurfurylpropionate hydrogen oxalate.
$C_{24}H_{33}NO_3,C_2H_2O_4$=473.6.

CAS — 31329-57-4 (naftidrofuryl); 3200-06-4 (oxalate).

A white odourless powder. M.p. about 108°. Readily **soluble** in water.

Adverse Effects. Naftidrofuryl oxalate may cause nausea, epigastric pain, and insomnia.

Acute and chronic administration of naftidrofuryl did not affect serum-creatinine concentration and aminohippurate/inulin clearance in patients with occlusive arterial disease.— H. Heidrich *et al., Arzneimittel-Forsch.*, 1975, *25*, 429.

Thrombophlebitis occurred at 10 of 13 naftidrofuryl infusion sites in 7 consecutive patients, often after about 2 hours of infusion. The aetiology was multifactorial; the low pH (3.4) of the infusion in dextrose-saline (200 mg in 200 ml) might be involved; other possible factors were being studied.— C. R. J. Woodhouse and D. G. A. Eadie, *Br. med. J.*, 1977, *1*, 1320. Thrombophlebitis was common when naftidrofuryl was given as a continuous drip, but no trouble was experienced when it was given as an infusion (200 mg in 500 ml of dextrose-saline) over 2 hours, the line being kept open with saline until the second infusion was due.— M. Gann (letter), *ibid.*, 1598. See also D. Charlesworth (letter), *ibid.*, 1537; J. Chamberlain (letter), *ibid.*, *2*, 121; W. Morris-Jones (letter), *ibid.*; D. G. MacLellan (letter), *ibid.*, 267; V. F. Standing *et al.* (letter), *ibid.*, 895; H. Heidrich, *ibid.*, 1978, *1*, 618.

Oesophageal ulceration in a patient attributed to the taking of naftidrofuryl capsules without an adequate accompanying amount of fluid.— E. C. McCloy and S. Kane (letter), *Br. med. J.*, 1981, *282*, 1703.

Absorption and Fate. Naftidrofuryl oxalate is absorbed from the gastro-intestinal tract. Its effects appear to last for some hours.

For a study of the metabolism of naftidrofuryl in *mice* and *rats*, see A. -G. Rico *et al., Thérapie*, 1974, *29*, 281.

Uses. Naftidrofuryl oxalate is used in the treatment of peripheral and cerebral vascular disorders. It is claimed to enhance cellular oxidative capacity, to antagonise bradykinin, and to be an antispasmodic.
The usual dose is 100 mg thrice daily by mouth. Initial therapy may also be given by intramuscular or intravenous injection for 7 to 14 days in doses of 40 mg once or twice daily, together with 100 mg thrice daily by mouth. Rest pain, gross ischaemia, and incipient gangrene may initially be treated for 7 to 10 days with 200 mg twice daily by intravenous or intra-arterial infusion over a period of 90 to 120 minutes in 250 to 500 ml of sodium chloride injection, dextrose injection, or Dextran 40 Intravenous Infusion, together with oral therapy.

Reduced postoperative nitrogen loss in patients given naftidrofuryl by infusion twice daily.— H. J. G. Burns *et al.*, *Br. med. J.*, 1981, *283*, 7.

Cerebrovascular disease. A review of drugs used in senile dementia. Several well-conducted studies have suggested that naftidrofuryl improves memory and behaviour, but further studies are needed to establish whether it improves activities of daily living.— *Br. med. J.*, 1979, *2*, 511. A similar view and the warning that all cerebral vasodilator therapy must be regarded as contra-indicated in patients with acute stroke and may sometimes be harmful in patients with chronic cerebrovascular disease.— P. Cook and I. James, *New Engl. J. Med.*, 1981, *305*, 1508 and 1560.

Reports and studies on the use of naftidrofuryl oxalate in cerebrovascular disease: T. G. Judge and A. Urquhart, *Curr. med. Res. Opinion*, 1972, *1*, 166; J. Gerin, *Br. J. clin. Pract.*, 1974, *28*, 177; N. H. Brodie, *Practitioner*, 1977, *218*, 274; I. M. James *et al.* (letter), *Br. J. clin. Pharmac.*, 1978, *6*, 545; A. K. Admami, *Br. med. J.*, 1978, *2*, 1678; T. Steiner *et al.* (letter), *ibid.*, 1979, *1*, 412.

Topical application of naftidrofuryl (as Praxilene Forte 200 mg in 10 ml) on the superficial temporal artery when performing extracranial/intracranial anastomosis for cerebral revascularisation has been found to be a useful means of increasing the diameter of the vessel and increasing the blood flow.— C. M. Bannister (letter), *Lancet*, 1980, *2*, 372.

Ménière's disease. Mention of increased hearing in patients with Ménière's disorder during intravenous infusion of naftidrofuryl and a reduction in vertiginous symptoms when subsequently given therapy by mouth.— W. P. R. Gibson *et al.*, *J. Lar. Otol.*, 1977, *91*, 679.

Peripheral vascular disorders. A brief discussion on the actions and uses of naftidrofuryl oxalate in peripheral vascular disorders.— *Drug & Ther. Bull.*, 1979, *17*, 83.

Reports on studies of the use of naftidrofuryl oxalate in peripheral vascular disorders: M. B. Clyne and A. Lask, *Br. J. clin. Pract.*, 1978, *32*, 169; C. V. Ruckley *et al.*, *Br. med. J.*, 1978, *1*, 622 (no benefit in intermittent claudication); K. H. Nilsen, *ibid.*, 1979, *1*, 20 (increase in low basal skin blood flow in patients with Raynaud's phenomenon); P. M. Gaylarde *et al.*, *Br. J. Derm.*, 1980, *102*, 7 (blood flow changes in systemic sclerosis and Raynaud's phenomenon).

Proprietary Preparations

Praxilene *(Lipha, UK)*. Naftidrofuryl oxalate, available as capsules of 100 mg. **Praxilene Forte**. Ampoules of 10 ml for the preparation of intravenous infusion solutions, each containing naftidrofuryl oxalate 200 mg. (Also available as Praxilene in *Belg., Fr., Ital., Spain, Switz.*).

Other Proprietary Names

Citoxid *(Arg.)*; Dusodril *(Ger.)*; Iridus *(Arg.)*.

9257-t

Nicametate Citrate. Nicametate Dihydrogen Citrate; Diethylaminoethyl Nicotinate Citrate. 2-Diethylaminoethyl nicotinate dihydrogen citrate.
$C_{12}H_{18}N_2O_2,C_6H_8O_7=414.4$.

CAS — 3099-52-3 (nicametate); 1641-74-3 (citrate).

Nicametate citrate is a vasodilator with general properties similar to those of nicotinic acid (see p.1648), to which it is slowly hydrolysed. It is given for the treatment of peripheral vascular disorders in a usual dosage of 300 mg daily for 20 days a month. It has also been given by intramuscular injection or intravenous or intra-arterial infusion.

Proprietary Names
Euclidan *(Millot-Solac, Fr.; Crinos, Ital.; Solac, Switz.)*; Nicopile *(Jap.)*.

9258-x

Niceritrol. PETN. Pentaerythritol tetranicotinate; 2,2-Bis(hydroxymethyl)propane-1,3-diol tetranicotinate.
$C_{29}H_{24}N_4O_8=556.5$.

CAS — 5868-05-3.

NOTE. The synonym PETN is also applied to pentaerythritol tetranitrate.

Very slightly **soluble** in water; more soluble in dilute acids.

Niceritrol, an ester of pentaerythritol and nicotinic acid, is a vasodilator with general properties similar to those of nicotinic acid (see p.1648), to which it is slowly hydrolysed. It is given in the treatment of peripheral vascular disorders and angina pectoris in a usual dosage of 250 to 500 mg twice to thrice daily. Doses of up to 1 g thrice daily have been used to reduce blood-cholesterol concentrations.

Absorption and fate.— L. Harthon and K. Sigroth, *Arzneimittel-Forsch.*, 1974, *24*, 1688.

A brief discussion of niceritrol alone and in conjunction with clofibrate in the treatment of type IIa and IIb hyperlipoproteinaemia.— L. Orö *et al.*, *Postgrad. med. J.*, 1975, *51*, *Suppl.* 8, 76.

Proprietary Names
Bufor *(Astra, Denm.)*; Perycit *(Tosi, Ital.; Inibsa, Spain; Astra, Swed.; Bofors, Switz.)*.

9259-r

Nicofuranose. ES 304; Tetranicotinoylfructofuranose; Tetranicotinoylfructose. β-D-Fructofuranose 1,3,4,6-tetranicotinate.
$C_{30}H_{24}N_4O_{10}=600.5$.

CAS — 15351-13-0.

A creamy-white crystalline powder. M.p. 132° to 143°. Practically **insoluble** in water, soluble 1 in 4 of chloroform; sparingly soluble in dilute solutions of hydrochloric acid and sodium hydroxide.

Nicofuranose is a vasodilator with general properties similar to those of nicotinic acid (see p.1648), to which it is slowly hydrolysed. It is given in the treatment of peripheral vascular disorders in a usual dosage of 500 mg thrice daily but doses of 0.75 to 1 g thrice daily may be given.

Similar doses have been given to lower blood-cholesterol concentrations.

In 27 healthy young men given, while fasting, a single dose of 500 mg of nicofuranose, mean plasma concentrations of nicotinic acid (with wide individual variations) were 0.51, 0.72, 0.47, and 0.19 μg per ml at 1.5, 3, 4, and 6 hours respectively. The corresponding values in 14 given the same dose as an enteric-coated tablet were 0.28, 0.41, 0.5, and 0.31 μg per ml.— H. A. Salmi and H. Frey, *Curr. ther. Res.*, 1974, *16*, 669.

Necrobiosis lipoidica. Preliminary observations showed that long-term treatment with nicofuranose 500 mg thrice daily improved the condition of 5 patients and had no effect in 1 patient with necrobiosis lipoidica; when nicofuranose was given to 3 patients already treated with stanozolol, 1 patient showed improvement.— E. L. Rhodes, *Br. J. Derm.*, 1976, *95*, 673.

Peripheral vascular disorders. References to nicofuranose in peripheral vascular disorders: G. Holti *et al.*, *Practitioner*, 1971, *207*, 654; G. Andrews *et al.*, *ibid.*, 1973, *211*, 83.

Proprietary Preparations
Bradilan *(Napp, UK)*. Nicofuranose, available as enteric-coated tablets of 250 mg. (Also available as Bradilan in *Ger., Ital., S.Afr.*).

Other Proprietary Names
Buclidan *(Spain)*; Vasperdil *(Switz.)*.

9260-j

Nicomethanol Nicotinate. 3-Pyridylmethyl nicotinate.
$C_{12}H_{10}N_2O_2=214.2$.

CAS — 49673-77-0.

Nicomethanol nicotinate is a vasodilator given in the treatment of peripheral and cerebral vascular disorders in a usual dosage of 300 to 600 mg daily.

Proprietary Names
Nicodue *(SIT, Ital.)*.

9261-z

Nicotinyl Alcohol. Nicotinic Alcohol; 3-Hydroxymethylpyridine; NU 2121; 3-Pyridinemethanol; β-Pyridylcarbinol. 3-Pyridylmethanol.
$C_6H_7NO=109.1$.

CAS — 100-55-0.

A very hygroscopic liquid; very **soluble** in water and ether; sparingly soluble in light petroleum. **Store** in airtight containers.

Nicotinyl alcohol is a vasodilator with general properties similar to those of nicotinic acid (see p.1648), to which it is partly hydrolysed. It was formerly given parenterally in peripheral vascular disorders when a rapid effect was required in a usual dosage of 100 to 200 mg by subcutaneous or intramuscular injection, or 100 mg by slow intravenous injection, repeated several times a day as required.

9262-c

Nicotinyl Tartrate. 3-Pyridylmethanol hydrogen tartrate.
$C_6H_7NO,C_4H_6O_6=259.2$.

CAS — 6164-87-0.

A white crystalline powder with a bitter taste. M.p. 146° to 149°. Nicotinyl tartrate 2.4 g is approximately equivalent to 1 g of nicotinyl alcohol. **Soluble** in water, alcohol, and ether.

Adverse Effects. Flushing of the skin of the face and neck, dizziness, and a feeling of faintness may occur. These symptoms usually abate on reduction of the dosage. Slight swelling of the face, nausea and vomiting, and hypotension have also been reported.

Treatment of Adverse Effects. In severe overdosage the stomach should be emptied by inducing emesis or by aspiration and lavage. If necessary the circulation should be maintained with infusions of suitable electrolytes.

Precautions. Nicotinyl tartrate should be given with care to patients with diabetic or prediabetic disorders.

Absorption and Fate. Nicotinyl tartrate is absorbed from the gastro-intestinal tract and is in part metabolised to nicotinic acid. It is excreted in the urine.

Uses. Nicotinyl tartrate is a vasodilator with general properties similar to those of nicotinic acid (see p.1649), to which it is partly hydrolysed.

It is given by mouth in the treatment of peripheral vascular disorders in usual doses equivalent to 25 to 50 mg of nicotinyl alcohol 4 times daily. A sustained-release preparation containing the equivalent of 150 mg of nicotinyl alcohol may be given in a dose of 1 or 2 tablets twice daily.

Nicotinyl tartrate has also been given to lower blood-cholesterol concentrations.

Reports and studies of the use of nicotinyl alcohol and nicotinyl tartrate to reduce blood-cholesterol concentrations: E. Böhle *et al.*, *Dte Arzt*, 1967, *64*, 504, per *J. Am. med. Ass.*, 1967, *200* (Apr. 10), A241; S. Heyden-Stucky, *Schweiz. med. Wschr.*, 1967, *97*, 451; Z. N. Gaut and W. J. R. Taylor, *J. clin. Pharmac.*, 1968, *8*, 370; F. A. Nelemans, *Arzneimittel-Forsch.*, 1972, *22*, 1410; C. A. Dujovne *et al.*, *Am. J. med. Sci.*, 1979, *277*, 255.

Proprietary Preparations

Ronicol *(Roche, UK)*. Nicotinyl tartrate, available as scored tablets each containing the equivalent of 25 mg of nicotinyl alcohol. **Ronicol Timespan.** Sustained-release tablets each containing the equivalent of 150 mg of nicotinyl alcohol. *Dose.* 1 or 2 sustained-release tablets night and morning. (Also available as Ronicol in *Austral., Denm., Fr., Ger., Ital., Neth., Norw., S.Afr., Spain, Switz.*).

Other Proprietary Names

Roniacol *(Arg., Canad., USA)*; Selcarbinol *(Ital.)*; Tebarcon *(Ger.)*.

9263-k

Nifedipine. BAY a 1040; Nifedipinum. Dimethyl 1,4-dihydro-2,6-dimethyl-4-(2-nitrophenyl)pyridine-3,5-dicarboxylate.
$C_{17}H_{18}N_2O_6$=346.3.

CAS — 21829-25-4.

A yellow odourless tasteless crystalline powder. Practically **insoluble** in water; slightly soluble in alcohol; soluble in acetone and chloroform. **Protect** from light.

Adverse Effects. Nifedipine may cause transient headache, flushing, and lethargy. Other side-effects reported include dizziness, allergic reactions, hypotension, palpitations, and sometimes precipitation of anginal pain.

Overdosage with nifedipine may be associated with bradycardia and hypotension.

Allergy. Two women developed erythematous oedema of the legs while taking nifedipine 10 mg thrice daily; the condition regressed when nifedipine was withdrawn and recurred in 1 patient given a challenge.— J. F. Bridgman (letter), *Br. med. J.*, 1978, *1*, 578.

See also under Effects on the Liver, below.

Cerebral ischaemia. A report of cerebral ischaemia in 2 elderly patients given nifedipine.— E. Nobile-Orazio and R. Sterzi, *Br. med. J.*, 1981, *283*, 948.

Diabetogenic effect. Significantly increased plasma-glucose concentrations after a glucose-tolerance test in 6 healthy subjects who had received nifedipine 20 mg every 8 hours for 3 days.— S. Charles *et al.*, *Br. med. J.*, 1981, *283*, 19. A lack of effect on glucose or insulin secretion in diabetics and non-diabetics after a single 10-mg dose of nifedipine or after 30 mg daily for one month.— A. D. B. Harrower and T. Donnelly (letter), *ibid.*, 796. A lack of effect in 6 healthy men given nifedipine 40 mg daily for 7 days and the view that changes in carbohydrate tolerance, if any, are small when nifedipine is given at usual doses of 30 to 40 mg daily.— R. H. Greenwood (letter), *ibid.*, 1982, *284*, 501.

Effects on the heart. Three patients experienced precordial pain, simulating angina pectoris or myocardial infarction and lasting 0.5 to 2 hours, after taking nifedipine.— A. G. Jariwalla and E. G. Anderson, *Br. med. J.*, 1978, *1*, 1181.

Effects on the liver. Hepatitis developed in a 69-year-old man after 10 days' therapy with nifedipine 40 mg daily for severe stable angina. The clinical features, immunological studies, and a later positive challenge test indicated a hypersensitive mechanism.— H. H. Rotmensch *et al.*, *Br. med. J.*, 1980, *281*, 976. See also A. R. Davidson (letter), *ibid.*, 1364.

Hypotension. Severe hypotension in 2 patients with severe chronic heart failure given nifedipine 20 or 30 mg.— N. Brooks *et al.*, *Br. med. J.*, 1980, *281*, 1324.

See also under Interactions, below.

Pulmonary oedema. A report of nifedipine precipitating acute pulmonary oedema in a 71-year-old man with symptoms of severe angina pectoris and a clinical diagnosis of moderate aortic valve stenosis and probable coronary artery disease. The patient had taken two 10-mg doses.— D. J. Gillmer and P. Kirk, *Br. med. J.*, 1980, *280*, 1420.

For the use of nifedipine in the management of pulmonary oedema, see under Cardiac Disorders, below.

Tremor. A 46-year-old man experienced fine tremor, particularly of the upper limbs, while taking nifedipine 30 mg daily. When the dose was increased to 60 mg daily he experienced chest pain after most doses; the pain ceased when nifedipine was withdrawn.— C. Rodger and A. Stewart (letter), *Br. med. J.*, 1978, *1*, 1620.

Treatment of Adverse Effects. In overdosage by mouth the stomach should be emptied by aspiration and lavage. Hypotension may be treated by placing the patient in the supine position with the feet raised; standard measures, such as atropine for bradycardia and noradrenaline for hypotension, have been suggested if necessary. It also has been suggested that calcium gluconate may be of benefit.

Precautions. Nifedipine should be used with caution in patients whose cardiac reserve is poor.

Nifedipine may enhance the antihypertensive effects of beta-adrenoceptor blocking agents. The use of nifedipine in diabetic patients may require adjustment of their control.

In patients who experience ischaemic pain following administration of nifedipine, therapy should be discontinued.

Interactions. *Beta-blockers.* Two patients developed heart failure when nifedipine was given in addition to beta-blockers.— C. J. Anastassiades, *Br. med. J.*, 1980, *281*, 1251. See also R. H. Robson and M. C. Vishwanath, *Br. med. J.*, 1982, *284*, 104; C. Anastassiades (letter), *ibid.*, 506.

A report of severe hypotension in a patient with hypertension and angina taking atenolol when nifedipine was added to his treatment. When atenolol was withdrawn he developed unstable angina. In such situations the nifedipine should be withdrawn.— L. H. Opie and D. A. White, *Br. med. J.*, 1980, *281*, 1462. See also J. S. Staffurth and P. Emery (letter), *ibid.*, *282*, 225.

For the use of nifedipine in association with beta-adrenoceptor blocking agents, see under Hypertension, below.

Cardiac glycosides. For the effect of nifedipine on digoxin, see Digoxin, p.534.

Absorption and Fate. Nifedipine is readily and almost completely absorbed from the gastro-intestinal tract. Following administration by mouth peak blood concentrations are reported to occur after 20 to 45 minutes with a half-life of about 4 to 5 hours and an elimination half-life from serum of 3 to 4 days. Its duration of action is about 8 to 12 hours.

Nifedipine is mainly excreted in the urine as an inactive metabolite.

Following administration of labelled nifedipine 10 mg by mouth or sublingually to 25 persons 90% of the administered activity was absorbed. About 70 to 80% of the administered activity was excreted in the urine with more than 90% of this quantity appearing in the first day indicating a half-life of 4 to 5 hours. Up to 15% of the administered activity was detected in the faeces after 4 days. The elimination from the serum corresponded to a half-life of 3 to 4 days.— F. A. Horster *et al.*, *Arzneimittel-Forsch.*, 1972, *22*, 330.

Protein binding. Studies indicating that nifedipine is very strongly bound (91 to 98%) to serum proteins.— H. Rosenkranz *et al.*, *Arzneimittel-Forsch.*, 1974, *24*, 455.

Uses. Nifedipine is used in the treatment and prophylaxis of angina pectoris and in the treatment of hypertension. Although nifedipine has calcium-antagonist properties it has not been found to have any therapeutic anti-arrhythmic effect; it is also a vasodilator. Nifedipine is reported to act by reducing cardiac work and myocardial oxygen demand, and by reducing peripheral resistance and heart load.

The usual oral dose is 10 mg thrice daily taken during or after meals increased, if necessary, to 20 mg thrice daily. A recommended dose for elderly patients or those on concomitant medication is 5 mg thrice daily.

It may also be taken sublingually.

Action. A review of calcium-antagonists, including nifedipine. Nifedipine has verapamil-like effects on the conduction system of *animals* but not in man; hence, in association with beta-adrenoceptor blocking agents it should theoretically be less hazardous than verapamil. The action of nifedipine on coronary smooth muscle is ten to twelve times more powerful than that of verapamil. Clinically, it is used against coronary artery spasm but not against supraventricular arrhythmias; it should, however, be indirectly effective against ventricular arrhythmias resulting from coronary spasm. Nifedipine is a promising agent, with few side-effects and useful in various disorders, especially angina (whether induced by spasm or by effort) and hypertension. It may eventually emerge as the agent of choice in patients with angina or hypertension together with bronchospasm, left-ventricular failure, or other specific contra-indications to beta-adrenoceptor blockade.— L. H. Opie, *Lancet*, 1980, *1*, 806.

Comment on calcium antagonists, including nifedipine. Nifedipine has been shown to relieve symptoms in many patients with variant angina (Prinzmetal's angina) whose symptoms are often attributed to coronary artery spasm. Nifedipine is also effective in classic angina of effort where it probably acts by peripheral dilatation rather than a local effect on the coronary vessels. In angina, nifedipine may usefully be combined with a beta-blocker, but care must be taken about the possibility of heart failure. Nifedipine has also been shown to have an antihypertensive effect which is rapid in onset and of prolonged duration. The reflex increase in sympathetic activity manifest by a rise in pulse-rate and plasma-renin concentration suggests that associated treatment with beta-blockade may be appropriate in hypertension.— *Br. med. J.*, 1981, *282*, 89. Comment on the different actions of drugs given the general description of calcium antagonist, and the view that they should be subdivided into 4 or more classes according to their principal therapeutic effects.— A. L. Macnair and H. A. Waldron, *Janssen* (letter), *ibid.*, 400.

Comment on the mode of action of calcium antagonists. The description of this group of drugs as 'calcium antagonists' can be misleading. A more accurate name is 'slow channel inhibitors'.— P. A. Poole-Wilson (letter), *Lancet*, 1981, *1*, 219.

Further reviews and comments: *Drug & Ther. Bull.*, 1979, *17*, 22; E. M. Antman *et al.*, *Ann. intern. Med.*, 1980, *93*, 875; P. H. Stone *et al.*, *ibid.*, 886; *Lancet*, 1980, *2*, 352.

Asthma. Studies involving 20 patients with asthma indicated that nifedipine premedication prevents exercise-induced asthma but does not modify the basal bronchial tone of such patients.— J. Cerrina *et al.*, *Am. Rev. resp. Dis.*, 1981, *123*, 156.

In a study of 10 patients with chronic stable asthma nifedipine 20 mg had no significant bronchodilator activity but provided protection against histamine-induced bronchoconstriction when compared with placebo. It was concluded that nifedipine would not be therapeutically useful in asthma but could be given safely and was preferred to beta-blockers in the treatment of angina in patients with asthma.— D. O. Williams *et al.*, *Br. med. J.*, 1981, *283*, 348.

Further references: S. S. Jaiprakash *et al.*, *Postgrad. med. J.*, 1980, *56*, 624 (angina pectoris and chronic airways obstruction).

Cardiac disorders. *Angina pectoris.* Nifedipine produced a significant reduction in the frequency of anginal attacks and requirements for glyceryl trinitrate in an uncontrolled study of 127 patients with coronary-artery spasm and *variant angina* not controlled by conventional therapy. Daily doses of nifedipine ranged from 40 to 160 mg, average 64 mg daily, and were given for a mean duration of 9 months. Only 7 patients were considered to be true treatment failures. Side-effects severe enough to stop treatment occurred in 6 patients and included dizziness, flushing, and headache. Pedal oedema, postural hypotension, a generalised rash (1 patient), and muscle cramps (2 patients) were also reported.— E. Antman *et al.*, *New Engl. J. Med.*, 1980, *302*, 1269. Criticism of the uncontrolled nature of the study and the lack of relevant detail about symptomatic relief.— A. Ippoliti (letter), *ibid.*, *303*, 939. Reply.— E. Antman *et al.* (letter), *ibid.*

In a double-blind study involving 16 patients with severe *exertional angina pectoris* the incidence of pain and consumption of glyceryl trinitrate were significantly decreased by nifedipine 30 or 60 mg daily compared with placebo, but a significantly greater reduction was produced by propranolol 240 or 480 mg daily. Although the higher dose of propranolol had no additional benefit over the lower dose, the higher dose of nifedipine was significantly more effective than the lower. Combination of the 2 drugs in the higher doses produced further significant improvement.— P. Lynch *et al.*, *Br. med. J.*, 1980, *281*, 184. See also G. D. G. Oakley *et al.*, *ibid.*, 1979, *1*, 1540.

Further references to nifedipine and angina pectoris: J. E. Müller and S. J. Gunther, *Circulation*, 1978, *57*, 137 (variant angina); A. C. F. Kenmure and J. H. Scruton, *Br. J. clin. Pract.*, 1979, *33*, 49; R. Battye and C. M. Ordille, *J. int. med. Res.*, 1979, *7*, 360 (variant angina); M. Previtali *et al.*, *Am. J. Cardiol.*, 1980, *45*, 825 (variant angina); J. W. Moses *et al.*, *Ann. intern. Med.*, 1981, *94*, 425 (variant angina); A. C. Tweddel *et al.*, *Br. J. clin. Pharmac.*, 1981, *12*, 229 (with propranolol).

Arrhythmias. Resistance of ventricular arrhythmias to nifedipine.— A. L. Gutovitz *et al.*, *Circulation*, 1977, *56*, *Suppl.* 3, 179.

Cardiomyopathy. Nifedipine improved diastolic compliance and systolic performance, and relieved dyspnoea and chest pain in a 54-year-old woman with severe hypertrophic cardiomyopathy.— B. H. Lorell *et al.*, *New Engl. J. Med.*, 1980, *303*, 801.

Heart failure. Nifedipine 10 mg sublingually relieved acute pulmonary oedema in 7 patients with hypertensive heart disease, 7 with primary heart disease, and 10 with rheumatic heart disease. Its beneficial effect in acute heart failure seems to result from simultaneous reduction in preload and afterload and, possibly, improved myocardial contractility.— A. Polese *et al.*, *Am. J. Med.*, 1979, *66*, 825.

Evidence that nifedipine may be beneficial for vasodilatation in patients with congestive heart failure.— S. Matsumoto *et al.*, *Am. J. Cardiol.*, 1980, *46*, 476. See also S. Klugmann *et al.*, *Br. Heart J.*, 1980, *43*, 440.

Dysmenorrhoea. In 10 women with severe primary dysmenorrhoea given nifedipine 20 to 40 mg by mouth on the first menstrual day pain relief occurred within 10 to 30 minutes of administration.— K. -E. Andersson and U. Ulmsten, *Br. J. Obstet. Gynaec.*, 1978, *85*, 142.

Hypertension. Nifedipine 10 mg by mouth or sublingually in 17 and 9 patients respectively with severe primary hypertension produced peak hypotensive effects 20 to 30 and 5 to 15 minutes respectively after administration. In a further 3 patients with hypertensive encephalopathy and acute left ventricular failure nifedipine 10 mg sublingually also effectively reduced systemic and pulmonary arterial pressure.— M. Guazzi *et al.*, *Clin. Pharmac. Ther.*, 1977, *22*, 528.

In 17 patients with arterial hypertension sublingual doses of 10 or 20 mg of nifedipine caused a rapid and significant reduction in blood pressure; heart-rate increased; forearm blood flow increased; vascular resistance decreased. There was considerable individual variation in plasma concentrations of nifedipine which did not correlate with reduction in blood pressure. In 10 patients treated for 6 weeks with 10 to 20 mg thrice daily mean supine blood pressure fell from 175/115 to 151/96 mmHg. Some patients experienced sensations of heat 20 to 40 minutes after taking nifedipine and mean serum-potassium concentrations were reduced. Concomitant treatment with a beta blocker to control the heart-rate was suggested.— O. L. Pedersen and E. Mikkelsen, *Eur. J. clin. Pharmac.*, 1978, *14*, 375.

Substitution of nifedipine 10 to 30 mg thrice daily for hydralazine or prazosin reduced blood pressure in 10 patients whose blood pressure control was unsatisfactory despite adequate doses of a beta-blocker (metoprolol, acebutolol, or nadolol), a diuretic, and hydralazine or prazosin. No cases of hypotension occurred and the only side-effect noted was diuretic-resistant oedema in 1 patient. These results confirmed previous suggestions that nifedipine and beta-blockers are a potentially useful combination.— S. Dean and M. J. Kendall (letter), *Br. med. J.*, 1981, *282*, 1322.

Further references to the use of nifedipine in hypertension: M. T. Olivari *et al.*, *Circulation*, 1979, *59*, 1056; M. D. Guazzi *et al.*, *Circulation*, 1980, *61*, 913; M. Thibonnier *et al.*, *Eur. J. clin. Pharmac.*, 1980, *17*, 161.

Oesophageal disorders. In clinical studies involving 29 patients with achalasia given nifedipine 10 to 20 mg sublingually 15 to 30 minutes before each meal and up to a maximum of 60 mg daily, responses were classified as excellent or good in 21, moderate in 5, and poor in 3.— M. Bortolotti and G. Labo, *Gastroenterology*, 1981, *80*, 39.

Further references: J. N. Blackwell *et al.*, *Gut*, 1979, *20*, A919.

Peripheral vascular disorders. Beneficial results with nifedipine in Raynaud's phenomenon.— A. Kahan *et al.* (letter), *Ann. intern. Med.*, 1981, *94*, 546.

Pulmonary hypertension. Results from studies involving 13 patients with acute respiratory failure given nifedipine 20 mg sublingually indicated that nifedipine vasodilates pulmonary vessels constricted by hypoxia, without deleterious effects on arterial oxygenation. However the potential benefit of long-term administration of nifedipine in such patients remains entirely conjectural.— G. Simmonneau *et al.*, *New Engl. J. Med.*, 1981, *304*, 1582.

Urinary incontinence. Administration of a single dose of nifedipine 10 to 30 mg by mouth had an inhibiting effect on the detrusor contractions in 10 women with urge incontinence; following treatment with nifedipine 10 to 20 mg twice daily for 1 week all patients reported subjective improvement.— T. Rud *et al.*, *Urol. int.*, 1979, *34*, 421.

Proprietary Preparations

Adalat *(Bayer, UK)*. Nifedipine, available as capsules of 10 mg. **Adalat 5.** Nifedipine, available as capsules of 5 mg. For oral or sublingual administration; for sublingual use the capsules should first be bitten open. (Also available as Adalat in *Arg., Belg., Denm., Ger., Ital., Jap., Norw., S.Afr., Spain, Switz.*).

Other Proprietary Names

Adalate *(Fr.)*; Nifelat *(Arg.)*.

9264-a

Nitrous Ether Spirit *(B.P.C. 1959)*. Sp. Aether. Nitros.; Sweet Nitre Spirit; Ethyl Nitrite Spirit.

CAS — 109-95-5 (nitrous ether).

A clear, faintly yellow, volatile liquid with a characteristic penetrating apple-like odour and a characteristic taste, consisting of an alcoholic solution of ethyl nitrite, $C_2H_5NO_2$, 1.25 to 2.5% w/v, together with acetaldehyde and other related substances. Wt per ml 0.827 to 0.836 g.

Incompatible with salicylates and ferrous sulphate, and with phenazone and potassium iodide unless previously neutralised with sodium bicarbonate. **Store** in a cool place in small well-filled airtight containers. Protect from light.

Adverse Effects. Methaemoglobinaemia has been reported in infants.

Methaemoglobinaemia occurred in 2 infants given a folk remedy containing nitrous ether spirit. Despite treatment with methylene blue one infant died.— R. R. Chilcote *et al.*, *Pediatrics*, 1977, *59*, 280.

Uses. Nitrous ether spirit has the vasodilator effects of the other nitrites but has been mainly used as a diaphoretic. It also has been reported to have a slight diuretic action.

Preparations

Concentrated Ethyl Nitrite Solution *(B.P. 1932)*. Concentrated Nitrous Ether Solution; Liq. Aethyl. Nitrit. Conc. A solution of ethyl nitrite in alcohol. It contains 17 to 20% w/v of ethyl nitrite when freshly prepared. After storage and when the container has been opened occasionally, it contains not less than 10% w/v. When diluted 1 to 8 with water it yields a solution which is equivalent in content of ethyl nitrite to Nitrous Ether Spirit. Store in a cool place in small well-filled airtight containers. Protect from light.

9265-t

Nonivamide. *N*-Vanillylnonamide.
$C_{17}H_{27}NO_3$=293.4.

CAS — 2444-46-4.

Nonivamide is a topical vasodilator structurally related to capsaicin. It is used, in a concentration of 0.4%, in rubefacient ointments.

Proprietary Preparations

See under Methyl Nicotinate, p.1626..

Other Proprietary Names

Rheumaplast *(Ger.)*.

9266-x

Octyl Nitrite *(B.P.C. 1968)*. Octylis Nitris. 2-Ethylhexyl nitrite.
$C_8H_{17}NO_2$=159.2.

Pharmacopoeias. In *Ind.*

A clear yellow liquid with a characteristic aromatic and pungent odour. B.p. about 169°. Wt per ml 0.88 to 0.886 g. Practically **insoluble** in water; miscible with alcohol and ether. It is liable to decompose with evolution of nitrogen, particularly if it has become acid in reaction. **Store** in a cool place in airtight containers. Protect from light.

Adverse Effects, Treatment, and Precautions. As for Glyceryl Trinitrate, p.1620.

Octyl nitrite is less toxic than amyl nitrite and has a reduced tendency to cause methaemoglobinaemia.

For references to the abuse of inhaled nitrites, see Amyl Nitrite, p.1615.

Absorption and Fate. Octyl nitrite is absorbed into the circulation from mucous membranes, the rate of absorption being most rapid from the lungs. It is rapidly inactivated, though less rapidly than amyl nitrite.

Uses. When inhaled, octyl nitrite has an action similar to that of glyceryl trinitrate (p.1621). Its effects are evident within 30 seconds of inhalation and its vasodilator effect is of longer duration than that of amyl nitrite, the fall in blood pressure reaching its maximum in 2 or 3 minutes and lasting for about 6 minutes.

It has been used in doses of 0.2 to 0.4 ml by inhalation as a short-acting vasodilator in the treatment of angina pectoris. It has also been used in the treatment of cardiospasm, to produce relaxation of involuntary muscle in the bronchi and gastro-intestinal tract, and to relax spasm of the cardiac and pyloric sphincters during radiological examination of the gastro-intestinal tract.

Inhalation of octyl nitrite could give temporary relief from achalasia of the cardia.— A. J. Moon, *Practitioner*, 1974, *212*, 346.

Preparations

Octyl Nitrite Vitrellae *(B.P.C. 1968)*. Vitrell. Octyl. Nitrit. Octyl nitrite in crushable glass capsules. To be crushed between finger and thumb, and the vapour inhaled. Store in a cool place.

9267-r

Oxpentifylline. Pentoxifylline; BL 191. 3,7-Dimethyl-1-(5-oxohexyl)xanthine.
$C_{13}H_{18}N_4O_3$=278.3.

CAS — 6493-05-6.

A white odourless crystalline powder. M.p. 102° to 105°. **Soluble** in water.

Adverse Effects. Nausea, gastro-intestinal disturbances, dizziness, and flushing may occur.

Side-effects of nausea and vomiting caused 4 of 10 healthy subjects given oxpentifylline 200 mg thrice daily to withdraw from a double-blind study.— P. E. M. Jarrett *et al.*, *Curr. med. Res. Opinion*, 1977, *4*, 492.

Absorption and Fate. Oxpentifylline is readily absorbed from the gastro-intestinal tract. It is extensively metabolised and numerous metabolites have been identified. Elimination appears to be biphasic; half-lives of 8.3 minutes and 1.8 hours have been reported after intravenous injection. Elimination is virtually complete in 12 hours; in 24 hours about 94% of a dose is recovered in the urine and 4% in the faeces.

References.— H. -J. Hinze *et al.*, *Arzneimittel-Forsch.*, 1972, *22*, 1144; H. -J. Hinze, *ibid.*, 1492.

Uses. Oxpentifylline is a vasodilator used in the treatment of peripheral vascular disorders. The usual initial dose is 200 mg by mouth thrice daily reduced, when improvement is seen, to a maintenance dose of 100 mg thrice daily. Sustained-release tablets are also available.

Oxpentifylline may also be given by intravenous or intra-arterial infusion or by intravenous injection. A recommended initial dosage for intravenous infusion is 100 mg in 250 to 500 ml of sodium chloride injection, dextrose injection, or laevulose 5% given over 90 to 180 minutes; this dosage may be increased by 50 mg daily to a maximum of 400 mg daily. For intra-arterial infusion a recommended dose is 100 to 300 mg daily given in 20 to 50 ml of sodium chloride injection over 10 to 30 minutes. A recommended dose for intravenous injection is 100 mg given slowly with the patient lying down; it is suggested that a course of intravenous injections should be started with a preliminary dose of 50 to 100 mg diluted in 5 ml of sodium chloride injection given over several minutes.

Cerebrovascular disease. Reports and comments on the use of oxpentifylline in cerebrovascular disease: K. Koppenhagen *et al.*, *Curr. med. Res. Opinion*, 1977, *4*, 521; K. Koppenhagen *et al.*, *ibid.*, 681; D. Harwart, *ibid.*, 1979, *6*, 73; P. Martin and P. Vives, *ibid.*, 1980, *6*, 518; S. Janaki, *J. int. med. Res.*, 1980, *8*, 56 and 180; E. Herskovits *et al.*, *Lancet*, 1981, *1*, 966; C. Warlow and R. Peto (letter), *ibid.*, 1103; M. J. Gawel *et al.* (letter), *ibid.*, 1266.

Peripheral vascular disorders. References to the use of oxpentifylline in peripheral vascular disorders: J. C. Baumann and H. -W. Muth, *Medsche Welt, Stuttg.*, 1971, *22*, 1288; O. Hammer and A. Neuner, *Medsche Mschr., Stuttg.*, 1972, *26*, 127; R. Herger, *Fortschr. Med.*, 1972, *90*, 865; W. Bossong, *Z. Haut- u. GeschlKrankh.*, 1972, *47*, 711; M. O. Spach and J. Schwartz, *Thérapie*, 1977, *32*, 301; A. M. Ehrly, *Curr. med. Res. Opinion*, 1978, *5*, 608; B. Angelkort *et al.*, *ibid.*, 1979, *6*, 255.

Proprietary Preparations

Trental *(Hoechst, UK)*. Oxpentifylline, available as

Injection containing 20 mg per ml, in ampoules of 5 ml, and as **Tablets** of 100 mg. **Trental 400.** Oxpentifylline, available as sustained-release tablets of 400 mg. *Dose.* 1 sustained-release tablet thrice daily; maintenance, 1 twice daily. (Also available as Trental in *Arg., Ger., Ital., Jap., Switz.*).

Other Proprietary Names
Elorgan *(Spain)*; Tarontal *(Greece)*; Terental *(Mex.)*; Torental *(Fr., Mor., Tun.)*.

9268-f

Oxyfedrine Hydrochloride.
D 563; Oxifedrini Chloridum. L-3-(β-Hydroxy-α-methylphenethylamino)-3′-methoxypropiophenone hydrochloride.
$C_{19}H_{23}NO_3,HCl=349.9$.

CAS — 15687-41-9 (oxyfedrine); 16777-42-7 (hydrochloride).

Pharmacopoeias. In *Nord.*

A white tasteless almost odourless crystalline powder. M.p. about 195°. **Soluble** 1 in 200 of water, 1 in 80 of alcohol, and 1 in 1200 of chloroform; practically insoluble in ether.

Adverse Effects. Oxyfedrine administration has been associated with reversible loss of taste sensation.

A study indicating that usual therapeutic doses of oxyfedrine strongly interfere with colour vision.— J. Laroche and C. Laroche, *Annls pharm. Fr.*, 1977, *35*, 173.

Absorption and Fate. Oxyfedrine hydrochloride is absorbed from the gastro-intestinal tract. It is reported to be metabolised to phenylpropanolamine.

Results indicating that oxyfedrine when given by mouth in doses of up to 16 mg is almost completely metabolised to phenylpropanolamine.— E. Appel *et al.*, *Eur. J. clin. Pharmac.*, 1975, *8*, 161.

Uses. Oxyfedrine hydrochloride is used in the treatment of angina pectoris. It is given in usual doses of 8 to 16 mg thrice daily. It may also be given by slow intravenous injection in a usual dosage of 4 mg thrice daily.

Action. Comment on the anti-anginal properties of oxyfedrine despite properties which could be classified as those of a beta-adrenoceptor agonist.— *Lancet*, 1981, *1*, 25. Oxyfedrine is not simply a beta-adrenoceptor agonist; it is a partial agonist at these receptors and could be accurately described as a beta-adrenoceptor blocking drug with marked intrinsic sympathomimetic activity. Other properties, however, including a combination of myocardial stimulation with peripheral venodilatation may adequately explain its beneficial effects.— J. R. Parratt (letter), *ibid.*, 441.

Cardiac disorders. Indication that oxyfedrine has a beneficial effect in angina pectoris comparable to that of propranolol.— J. Whittington and E. B. Raftery, *Br. J. clin. Pharmac.*, 1980, *10*, 439.

Proprietary Names
Ildamen *(Homburg, Belg.; Pharmacia, Denm.; Homburg, Ger.; Farmades, Ital.; Homburg, Neth.; Lacer, Spain; Treupha, Switz.)*; Modacor *(Houdé-I.S.H., Fr.)*.

9269-d

Pentaerythritol Tetranitrate.
Pentaerythrityl Tetranitrate; Erynite; Nitropentaerythrol; Nitropenthrite; Pentaerythritolum Tetranitricum; Pentanitrol. 2,2-Bis(hydroxymethyl)propane-1,3-diol tetranitrate.
$C_5H_8N_4O_{12}=316.1$.

CAS — 78-11-5.

Pharmacopoeias. In *Cz.*

A white crystalline powder. Practically **insoluble** in water; slightly soluble in alcohol; soluble in acetone. For medicinal purposes it is supplied diluted with an inert substance such as lactose, since the undiluted compound may explode upon percussion or on exposure to heat. **Store** in a cool place in airtight containers. Protect from light.

9270-c

Diluted Pentaerythritol Tetranitrate *(B.P.C. 1973).*
Dil. Pentaerythr. Tetranit.; Diluted Pentaerythrityl Tetranitrate; Pentaerythritol Tetranitrate *(20 per cent)*.

Pharmacopoeias. In *Aust.* (25% in lactose), *Swiss* (10% in lactose), and *Braz.* and *U.S.* (in lactose, mannitol, or other suitable inert excipient; strength not specified).

A mixture of pentaerythritol tetranitrate with lactose, or with a mixture of 3 parts of lactose and 1 part of starch. It is a white odourless or almost odourless crystalline powder and contains 20% of pentaerythritol tetranitrate. **Store** in a cool place in airtight containers. Protect from light.

Adverse Effects, Treatment, and Precautions. As for Glyceryl Trinitrate, p.1620.

Effects on the skin. A 63-year-old man who had taken pentaerythritol tetranitrate and glyceryl trinitrate for 8 years developed extensive erythroderma due to the drugs. The condition regressed when the drugs were withdrawn but re-appeared after separate challenge doses of each drug.— F. P. Ryan, *Br. J. Derm.*, 1972, *87*, 498. See also J. K. Wilkin, *Archs Derm.*, 1980, *116*, 598.

Absorption and Fate. Pentaerythritol tetranitrate is absorbed from the gastro-intestinal tract, and to some extent from the oral mucosa. It has been reported to be absorbed through intact skin.

In 15 healthy men given 20 or 40 mg of radioactive pentaerythritol tetranitrate, radioactivity was detected in the blood within 15 minutes, with peak concentrations 4 to 8 hours after the dose. The tetranitrate and trinitrate were not detected in the blood; pentaerythritol and pentaerythritol mononitrate were the principal metabolites, with traces of the dinitrate. Of the 20-mg and 40-mg doses 32 and 41% respectively were eliminated in the faeces, partly as unchanged tetranitrate. About 60% of the 20-mg dose and 50% of the 40-mg dose were recovered in the urine in 48 hours, chiefly as pentaerythritol and the mononitrate. The proportion of pentaerythritol to mononitrate after the 20-mg dose was 1:1 compared with 1:3 after the 40-mg dose, possibly indicating a limiting rate of de-esterification of the mononitrate.— I. W. F. Davidson *et al.*, *J. pharm. Sci.*, 1971, *60*, 274.

Variation in absorption. Ten healthy volunteers given a dose of a sustained-release capsule of pentaerythritol tetranitrate 80 mg showed marked variations in individual blood-nitrate concentrations for up to 12 hours. The mean concentration remained within the therapeutic range of 6 to 9 µg per ml, except in 1 subject, who demonstrated malabsorption of the drug.— A. K. Sim *et al.*, *Br. J. clin. Pract.*, 1969, *23*, 293.

Further references: I. W. F. Davidson *et al.*, *J. Pharmac. exp. Ther.*, 1970, *175*, 42.

Uses. Pentaerythritol tetranitrate is a vasodilator with general properties similar to those of glyceryl trinitrate (p.1621) but its duration of action is more prolonged. Its effect begins in about 1 hour and lasts about 5 hours.

It is used prophylactically in the treatment of angina pectoris, usually in doses of 10 to 30 mg three or four times daily before meals; doses of 60 mg three or four times daily are also used. It is also given as sustained-release preparations.

Cardiac disorders. Data indicating that in congestive heart failure pentaerythritol tetranitrate may have a beneficial effect on preload and afterload lasting 5 hours or more.— F. G. Shellock *et al.*, *Clin. Pharmac. Ther.*, 1980, *28*, 436.

For detailed comments on the role of long-acting nitrates in cardiovascular disease, see Glyceryl Trinitrate, p.1621.

Preparations

Pentaerythritol Tablets *(B.P.).* Tablets containing pentaerythritol tetranitrate. Store at a temperature not exceeding 25°. Protect from light.

Pentaerythritol Tetranitrate Tablets *(U.S.P.).* Tablets containing diluted pentaerythritol tetranitrate *U.S.P.* Store in airtight containers.

Tabulettae Eryniti *(Rus. P.).* Tablets containing pentaerythritol tetranitrate 10 or 20 mg. Protect from light.

Proprietary Preparations

Cardiacap *(Consolidated Chemicals, UK).* Sustained-release capsules each containing pentaerythritol tetranitrate 30 mg. *Dose.* 1 capsule every 12 hours.

Mycardol (known in some countries as Mycartal) *(Winthrop, UK).* Pentaerythritol tetranitrate, available as scored tablets of 30 mg. (Also available as Mycardol in *Austral.*).

Peritrate *(Warner, UK).* Pentaerythritol tetranitrate, available as tablets of 10 mg. **Peritrate SA.** Sustained-release tablets each containing pentaerythritol tetranitrate 80 mg. *Dose.* 1 sustained-release tablet before breakfast and 1 before the evening meal. (Also available as Peritrate in *Arg., Austral., Belg., Canad., Fr., Ital., Neth., S.Afr., Spain, USA*).

An elderly man developed sudden severe dysphagia due to oesophageal obstruction caused by a tablet of Peritrate SA. The wax base layer of the tablet remained undissolved and had to be removed. Three years previously he had undergone a subtotal gastrectomy and gastro-jejunostomy.— A. J. Cummins (letter), *J. Am. med. Ass.*, 1966, *196*, 917.

Other Proprietary Names
Austral.—Penritol; *Fr.*—Nitrodex, Pentanitrine; *Ger.*—Dilcoran; *Neth.*—Pentrit; *S.Afr.*—Cordilate, Pentral 80; *Swed.*—Nitropent; *Switz.*—Dilcoran, Lentrat, Nitrodex, Pentrit; *USA*—Antime, Duotrate, El-Petn, Metranil, Pentafin, Pentritol, Pentryate, Quintrate, Terpate, Tranite, Vasolate.

Pentaerythritol tetranitrate was also formerly marketed in Great Britain under the proprietary name Pentral 80 Tempules (*Concept Pharmaceuticals*). A preparation containing pentaerythritol tetranitrate was also formerly marketed under the proprietary name Pentrium (*Roche*).

639-q

Pentifylline.
SK7; 1-Hexyltheobromine. 1-Hexyl-3,7-dimethylxanthine.
$C_{13}H_{20}N_4O_2=264.3$.

CAS — 1028-33-7.

A crystalline solid. M.p. about 82°. **Store** in a cool place. Protect from light.

Uses. Pentifylline is structurally related to caffeine (see p.340) and was formerly used in conjunction with nicotinic acid in the treatment of peripheral vascular insufficiency.

Reference: *Drug & Ther. Bull.*, 1972, *10*, 66.

A preparation containing pentifylline was formerly marketed in Great Britain under the proprietary name Cosaldon (*Hoechst*).

9271-k

Pentrinitrol.
Pentaerythritol Trinitrate; W 2197. 2,2-Bis(hydroxymethyl)propane-1,3-diol trinitrate.
$C_5H_9N_3O_{10}=271.1$.

CAS — 1607-17-6.

Pentrinitrol is a vasodilator with general properties similar to those of glyceryl trinitrate (p.1620).

The metabolism of pentrinitrol.— I. W. F. Davidson *et al.*, *Clin. Pharmac. Ther.*, 1971, *12*, 972.

Persistent plasma concentrations of pentaerythritol dinitrate and mononitrate metabolites were unlikely to be responsible for the sustained action of pentrinitrol in man, since they had almost no vasodilator activity in *dogs*.— J. C. Parker *et al.*, *Eur. J. Pharmac.*, 1975, *31*, 29.

Following sublingual administration of radioactively labelled pentrinitrol 10 mg as tablets to 4 healthy subjects the mean 72-hour urinary recovery of the dose was about 91% (range 85 to 96%) indicating that excretion is almost entirely renal. A mean of only about 0.08% was present as unchanged drug, with a mean of about 0.9% as the dinitrate, 53% as the mononitrate, 14% as pentaerythritol, 8.4% as the trinitrate glucuronide, 12.6% as the dinitrate glucuronide, and 1.7% as the mononitrate glucuronide. Concentration of the unchanged drug was also found to be low in the pooled plasma (becoming undetectable an hour after ingestion), and the same 6 metabolites were found. The trinitrate glucuronide metabolite was of major interest because its ability to reconvert to the active trinitrate, possibly coupled with enterohepatic recycling, might explain the duration of the drug's action, particularly since the trinitrate was detected in urine for up to 48 hours although it had disappeared from plasma after only 1 hour.— F. J. Di Carlo *et al.*, *Clin. Pharmac. Ther.*, 1977, *22*, 309.

Proprietary Names

Petrin *(Parke, Davis, USA)*.

9272-a

Perhexiline Maleate. WSM 3978G. 2-(2,2-Dicyclohexylethyl)piperidine hydrogen maleate.

$C_{19}H_{35}N,C_4H_4O_4$=393.6.

CAS — 6621-47-2 (perhexiline); 6724-53-4 (maleate).

A white crystalline powder. M.p. about 189°. Slightly **soluble** in water; soluble in chloroform and methyl alcohol. **Protect** from light.

Adverse Effects. Some adverse effects associated with perhexiline therapy are dizziness, headache, nausea, vomiting, and other gastro-intestinal disturbances, ataxia, moderate hypoglycaemia, alterations in the electrocardiogram, and liver enzyme abnormalities. Weakness, anxiety, tremors, syncope, changes in libido, paraesthesias, genito-urinary symptoms, flushing and sweating, and skin rash and urticaria have also been reported. Other adverse effects reported include diplopia, abdominal pain, extrapyramidal syndromes and convulsions. Severe adverse effects associated with perhexiline include severe hypoglycaemia, severe hepatic toxicity, marked weight loss, and severe peripheral neuropathy affecting all 4 limbs sometimes with associated papilloedema.

Details on the adverse-reactions warning about perhexiline maleate, circulated by the Committee on Safety of Medicines. The Committee on Safety of Medicines has received reports of peripheral neuropathy, abnormalities of liver function, hypoglycaemia, and weight loss in patients on the drug. The patient usually recovers if the drug is promptly withdrawn at the onset of symptoms or signs.— *Lancet*, 1977, *2*, 260.

Comment on peripheral neuropathy associated with perhexiline therapy. Symptomatic neuropathy occurs in about 0.1% of treated patients, but subclinical disorders have been found in as many as two-thirds of patients studied electrophysiologically. Sensory symptoms, including muscle pain and tenderness, are usually prominent, appearing as early as three weeks after treatment begins, and may be followed by severe weakness of distal and even of proximal muscle groups. In most cases symptoms have occurred only after several months of treatment with daily doses of 200 to 300 mg of the drug. Papilloedema, dysgeusia, deafness, cerebellar signs, autonomic disorders, and raised concentrations of protein in cerebrospinal fluid have been reported. Histological studies of peripheral-nerve biopsy specimens have shown prominent segmental demyelination with associated axonal degeneration, and membranous and paracrystalline inclusions in Schwann cells and endothelial cells. Biochemical studies have shown an increased ganglioside content in peripheral nerve. Complete recovery usually occurs within several months of stopping treatment.— Z. Argov and F. L. Mastaglia, *Br. med. J.*, 1979, *1*, 663.

A study indicating that the development of neuropathy in patients receiving perhexiline may be linked with impaired oxidative metabolism. Routine determination of drug oxidation phenotype using debrisoquine might be of predictive value in determining perhexiline dosage and controlling its neurotoxicity.— R. R. Shah *et al.*, *Br. med. J.*, 1982, *284*, 295.

Some individual references to adverse reactions associated with perhexiline maleate: G. Feldman, *Nouv. Presse méd.*, 1974, *3*, 2580 (hypoglycaemia); D. J. Howard and J. R. Rees, *Br. med. J.*, 1976, *1*, 133 (liver toxicity, impotence, reversible dysuria); F. Lhermitte *et al.*, *Br. med. J.*, 1976, *1*, 1256 (peripheral neuropathy); D. M. Fraser *et al.*, *Br. med. J.*, 1977, *2*, 675 (peripheral and autonomic neuropathy); P. Kopelman and P. G. M. Morgan (letter), *Lancet*, 1977, *1*, 705 (liver toxicity); A. Lageron *et al.* (letter), *Lancet*, 1977, *1*, 483 (liver toxicity); J. Laroche and C. Laroche, *Annls pharm. Fr.*, 1977, *35*, 173 (interference with colour vision); G. S. A. MacDonald (letter), *Lancet*, 1977, *1*, 1056 (liver toxicity); S. Pollet *et al.*, *Lancet*, 1977, *1*, 1258 (peripheral neuropathy); I. W. Tomlinson and F. D. Rosenthal., *Br. med. J.*, 1977, *1*, 1319 (muscle weakness and skin rash); K. D. Dawkins and E. O'Connor (letter), *Lancet*, 1978, *1*, 831 (symptoms mimicking bronchial carcinoma); D. M. Fraser and H. C. Miller (letter), *Br. med. J.*, 1978, *1*, 858 (peripheral and autonomic neuropathy); W. Murray *et al.*, *Practitioner*, 1978, *221*, 757 (dizziness, vomiting, and ataxia); J. B. Myers and M. Ronthal, *Med. J. Aust.*, 1978, *2*, 465 (weight loss and neuropathy); P. Paliard *et al.*, *Digestion*, 1978, *17*, 419 (liver toxicity, peripheral neuropathy, hypoglycaemia, and renal failure); E. Singlas *et al.*, *Eur. J. clin. Pharmac.*, 1978, *14*, 195 (peripheral neuropathy); W. P. Stephens *et al.*, *Br. med. J.*, 1978, *1*, 21 (raised intracranial pressure with headache, papilloedema, and ataxia); D. Lewis *et al.*, *Gut*, 1979, *20*, 186 (liver toxicity); D. Pessayre *et al.*, *Gastroenterology*, 1979, *76*, 170 (liver toxicity); J. C. Wijesekera *et al.*, *J. neurol. Scis*, 1980, *46*, 303 (peripheral neuropathy); K. W. G. Heathfield and F. Carabott (letter), *Lancet*, 1982, *1*, 507 (peripheral neuropathy and cirrhosis of the liver).

Treatment of Adverse Effects. In overdosage by mouth the stomach should be emptied by aspiration and lavage.

Precautions. In view of severe toxicity associated with perhexiline it should only be used in patients who have not responded to other anti-anginal agents.

It is contra-indicated in patients with impaired hepatic or renal function and in the acute stage of myocardial infarction. Perhexiline should be administered with caution to diabetic patients.

During treatment with perhexiline it is recommended that the patient should be examined for the signs and symptoms of peripheral neuropathy, hepatic toxicity, hypoglycaemia, and loss of weight and that treatment should be discontinued should any of these occur.

Perhexiline may produce or exacerbate ventricular conduction disorders.

Absorption and Fate. Perhexiline is absorbed from the gastro-intestinal tract. It is slowly excreted as metabolites in the urine and faeces with a half-life ranging from 3 to 12 days. Elimination is dependent primarily upon ability to metabolise perhexiline oxidatively.

The absorption, excretion, and metabolism of perhexiline maleate.— G. J. Wright *et al.*, *Postgrad. med. J.*, 1973, *49* (Apr.), *Suppl.*, 8.

Uses. Perhexiline maleate may be used in the prophylaxis of angina pectoris in patients who have not responded to other anti-anginal agents. It may be considered to be a calcium antagonist. The usual initial dose is 100 to 200 mg daily in 2 divided doses adjusted at intervals of 2 to 4 weeks according to the response of the patient; it is generally recommended not to administer more than 300 mg daily although doses of 400 mg daily have been necessary in some patients.

Perhexiline has also been used to control some forms of cardiac arrhythmias, such as ventricular extrasystoles.

Cardiac disorders. A review of drugs and the heart, including perhexiline, which has complex actions, with both anti-anginal and anti-arrhythmic activities. Although perhexiline has been designated as a calcium antagonist, additional quinidine-like and mild diuretic properties make the true classification difficult; it also differs from other calcium antagonists in lacking an acute effect against Prinzmetal's angina. Experimentally, there is a nitrate-like effect with redistribution of blood flow to the endocardial zones. Perhexiline has been used as an anti-anginal agent when beta-blockade and nitrates fail, but in view of the very serious side-effects now recognised, other calcium antagonists should be tried first.— L. H. Opie, *Lancet*, 1980, *1*, 806.

Anti-arrhythmic action and The Puzzle of Perhexiline, E.M. Vaughan Williams, London, Academic Press, 1980.

For further comments on the mode of action of calcium antagonists, see Nifedipine, p.1628.

Proprietary Preparations

Pexid *(Merrell, UK)*. Perhexiline maleate, available as scored tablets of 100 mg. (Also available as Pexid in *Austral., Belg., Fr., Ger., Ital., S.Afr., Spain, Switz.*).

Other Proprietary Names

Corzepin *(Spain)*; Daprin *(Arg.)*.

9273-t

Phenethyl Nicotinate.

$C_{14}H_{13}NO_2$=227.3.

Phenethyl nicotinate is a topical vasodilator which has been used, in a concentration of 2%, in rubefacient creams.

9274-x

Pipratecol. 1-(3,4-Dihydroxyphenyl)-2-[4-(2-methoxyphenyl)piperazin-1-yl]ethanol.

$C_{19}H_{24}N_2O_4$=344.4.

CAS — 15534-05-1.

Pipratecol is a vasodilator which has been given in conjunction with raubasine (p.1632) in the treatment of peripheral vascular disorders.

9275-r

Prenylamine Lactate *(B.P.)*. B 436 (prenylamine); Hoechst 12512; Prenylamini Lactas. *N*-(2-Benzhydrylethyl)-α-methylphenethylamine lactate.

$C_{24}H_{27}N,C_3H_6O_3$=419.6.

CAS — 69-43-2.

Pharmacopoeias. In *Br., Chin., Cz., Jap.,* and *Roum.*

A white, odourless or almost odourless, crystalline powder with a bitter numbing taste. M.p. 137° to 140°. Prenylamine lactate 76.4 mg is approximately equivalent to 60 mg of prenylamine. **Soluble** about 1 in 200 of water, 1 in 5 of alcohol, and 1 in 2 of chloroform; very soluble in glacial acetic acid. **Protect** from light.

Adverse Effects. Prenylamine may cause sedation and lassitude, gastro-intestinal disturbances including nausea, vomiting, and diarrhoea, headache, flushing of the skin, and dizziness. Skin reactions, extrapyramidal symptoms, and intention tremor have been reported. Ventricular arrhythmias have also been reported. Overdosage may cause hypotension, tachycardia, acute myocardial depression, and possibly convulsions.

Effects on the heart. Ventricular tachycardia associated with syncope and prolongation of the Q-T interval occurred in 2 elderly women taking prenylamine. The ECG should be checked every 3 months in patients taking prenylamine.— R. Puritz *et al.*, *Br. med. J.*, 1977, *2*, 608. Comment.— W. Bogie, *Hoechst* (letter), *ibid.*, 829. See also P. F. Fazzini *et al.*, *Am. Heart J.*, 1975, *90*, 805.

A study indicating significant prolongation of the Q-T interval in patients with angina pectoris given prenylamine. The Q-T interval returned to normal on withdrawal of prenylamine and no serious problems were encountered.— D. Oakley *et al.*, *Postgrad. med. J.*, 1980, *56*, 753.

A case of prenylamine toxicity possibly showing the *torsade de pointes* phenomenon in sinus rhythm.— C. I. Meanock and M. I. M. Noble, *Postgrad. med. J.*, 1981, *57*, 381.

Effects on the liver. A patient taking prenylamine 240 mg daily developed nausea and raised SGOT values which returned to normal when the dose was reduced to 180 mg daily.— N. Cardoe, *Br. J. clin. Pract.*, 1968, *22*, 299.

Treatment of Adverse Effects. In severe poisoning the stomach should be emptied by aspiration and lavage. Treatment is symptomatic, but it has been recommended that adrenaline, noradrenaline, or isoprenaline should not be given because of the possibility of ventricular fibrillation. Diazepam may be given intravenously if convulsions are present.

Precautions. Prenylamine should not be given to patients with severe uncompensated heart failure, defects of cardiac conduction, or with severe hepatic or renal impairment.

Prenylamine should not be administered concurrently with beta-adrenoceptor blocking agents or with cardiac depressants. It should be given only with care to patients taking antihypertensive agents, the dose of which may need to be reduced, or to patients receiving drugs liable to produce hypokalaemia.

Absorption and Fate. Prenylamine lactate is readily absorbed from the gastro-intestinal tract. An initial half-life of about 7 hours after administration by mouth has been reported. Prenylamine is extensively bound to plasma proteins. Numerous metabolites, including traces of amphetamine, have been detected in the urine; some prenylamine is also excreted in the faeces, even after intravenous administration.

Uses. Prenylamine is used prophylactically in the treatment of angina pectoris. It may be considered to be a calcium antagonist. The usual initial dosage of prenylamine lactate is the equivalent of 180 mg of prenylamine daily in 3 divided doses, increased to 300 mg daily if necessary, and reduced after a few weeks to the lowest effective maintenance dose.

Cardiac disorders. A review of drugs and the heart, including prenylamine lactate. Prenylamine has an anti-anginal effect which has so far eluded satisfactory explanation, but its properties include calcium antagonism and a general attenuating effect on the adrenergic system.— L. H. Opie, *Lancet*, 1980, *1*, 806.

Reports and studies on prenylamine lactate in angina pectoris: T. Winsor *et al.*, *Am. Heart J.*, 1971, *82*, 43; H. Tucker *et al.*, *Br. Heart J.*, 1974, *36*, 1001; W. P. Leary *et al.*, *Curr. ther. Res.*, 1976, *19*, 180.

For further comments on the mode of action of calcium antagonists, see Nifedipine, p.1628.

Preparations

Prenylamine Lactate Tablets *(B.P.)*. Tablets containing prenylamine lactate; they are sugar-coated. Potency is expressed in terms of the equivalent amount of prenylamine.

Synadrin *(Hoechst, UK)*. Prenylamine lactate, available as tablets each containing the equivalent of 60 mg of prenylamine. (Also available as Synadrin in *Neth., Norw., Spain*).

Other Proprietary Names

Angormin *(Arg.)*; Angorsan *(Ital.)*; Bismetin *(Jap.)*; Carditin *(Ital.)*; Crepasin, Epocol *(both Jap.)*; Eucardion *(Ital.)*; Herzcon *(Jap.)*; Hostaginan *(Arg., Belg.)*; Incoran *(Ital.)*; Lactamine *(Jap.)*; NP 30, Nyuple, Onlemin *(all Jap.)*; Piboril *(Arg.)*; Reocorin *(Ital.)*; Sedolatan *(Swed.)*; Segontin *(Austral., Canad., Denm., Ger., Ital., S.Afr., Switz.)*; Ségontine *(Fr.)*; Wasangor *(Ital.)*.

9276-f

Propatylnitrate. Ettriol Trinitrate; Propatyl Nitrate; Trinettriol; ETTN; Win 9317. 2-Ethyl-2-hydroxymethylpropane-1,3-diol trinitrate.

$C_6H_{11}N_3O_9$=269.2.

CAS — 2921-92-8.

A white, odourless, tasteless, crystalline powder. M.p. about 52°. Explosive, but only slightly sensitive to shock.

Practically **insoluble** in water; readily soluble in acetone and dehydrated alcohol.

Adverse Effects, Treatment, and Precautions. As for Glyceryl Trinitrate, p.1620.

Absorption and Fate. Propatylnitrate is absorbed from the oral mucosa and from the gastro-intestinal tract. It is probably slowly hydrolysed in the body to nitrite

Uses. Propatylnitrate is a vasodilator with general properties similar to those of glyceryl trinitrate (p.1621). It has been given sublingually in usual doses of 5 to 10 mg thrice daily for the prophylaxis of angina pectoris and in doses of 10 mg for acute attacks.

Proprietary Names

Etrynit *(Astra, Denm.; Astra, Swed.)*; Vasangor *(Winthrop, Belg.)*.

Propatylnitrate was formerly marketed in Great Britain under the proprietary name Gina (*Winthrop*).

9277-d

Raubasine. Ajmalicine; Alkaloid F; δ-Yohimbine. Methyl 16,17-didehydro-19α-methyl-18-oxayohimban-16-carboxylate.

$C_{21}H_{24}N_2O_3$=352.4.

CAS — 483-04-5.

Raubasine is an alkaloid obtained from *Vinca rosea* (= *Catharanthus roseus* (Apocynaceae).

It is related chemically to reserpine (see p.163) but has less antihypertensive activity. It has been given in peripheral and cerebral vascular disorders.

Absorption and excretion of raubasine in healthy subjects.— A. Marzo *et al.*, *Arzneimittel-Forsch.*, 1977, *27*, 2343.

Proprietary Names

Circolene *(Inverni della Beffa, Ital.)*; Hydrosarpan *(Servier, Canad.)*; Hydrosarpan Fort *(Eutherapie, Belg.; Servier, Canad.; Servier, Fr.; Servier, Switz.)*; Isoarteril *(Isola-Ibi, Ital.)*; Lamuran *(Boehringer, Arg.; Galenus Mannheim, Ger.; Boehringer Biochemia, Ital.; Boehringer Mannheim, Switz.)*; Loparol *(Boehringer Mannheim, Spain)*; Melanex *(Boehringer Mannheim, S.Afr.)*; Raubasil *(Zanardi, Ital.)*; Rauvasil *(SAM, Ital.)*; Sarpan *(Farge, Ital.)*.

9278-n

Suloctidil. CP 556 S. 1-(4-Isopropylthiophenyl)-2-octylaminopropan-1-ol.

$C_{20}H_{35}NOS$=337.6.

CAS — 54767-75-8.

Suloctidil is a vasodilator used in the treatment of peripheral and cerebral vascular disorders in a usual dosage of 100 mg twice or thrice daily.

Peripheral vascular disorders. Reports and studies on suloctidil in peripheral vascular disorders: H. Adriaensen, *Curr. med. Res. Opinion*, 1976, *4*, 395; P. Gillot, *Curr. ther. Res.*, 1978, *23*, 724.

Proprietary Names

Locton *(Lepetit, Ital.)*; Sulocton *(Continental Pharma, Belg.; Continental Pharma, Switz.)*.

9279-h

Thurfyl Nicotinate. Nicotafuryl. Tetrahydrofurfuryl nicotinate.

$C_{11}H_{13}NO_3$=207.2.

CAS — 70-19-9.

Thurfyl nicotinate is a topical vasodilator used, in a concentration of 5%, in rubefacient creams.

Proprietary Names

See under Methyl Nicotinate, p.1626.

9280-a

Thymoxamine Hydrochloride *(B.P.)*.

Moxisylyte Hydrochloride. 4-(2-Dimethylaminoethoxy)-5-isopropyl-2-methylphenyl acetate hydrochloride.

$C_{16}H_{25}NO_3,HCl$=315.8.

CAS — 54-32-0 (thymoxamine); 964-52-3 (hydrochloride).

Pharmacopoeias. In *Br.*

A white odourless crystalline powder with a bitter taste. M.p. about 212°. Thymoxamine hydrochloride 45.2 mg is approximately equivalent to 40 mg of thymoxamine. **Soluble** 1 in 2.5 of water, 1 in 11 of alcohol, and 1 in 3 of chloroform; practically insoluble in ether and light petroleum. A 5% solution in water has a pH of 4.5 to 5.5. **Protect** from light.

Adverse Effects. Thymoxamine hydrochloride may cause nausea, diarrhoea, headache, vertigo, and flushing of the skin. Overdosage may cause hypotension.

Drowsiness, nasal stuffiness, palpitations, and postural hypotension have been reported after intravenous injection.

Treatment of Adverse Effects. As for Tolazoline Hydrochloride, p.1633.

Precautions. Thymoxamine hydrochloride should be given with care to patients with coronary artery disease or diabetes mellitus.

Thymoxamine may enhance the effects of antihypertensive agents and the hypotensive effect of thymoxamine may be enhanced by tricyclic antidepressants.

Absorption and Fate. Thymoxamine is poorly absorbed from the gastro-intestinal tract. It is active when given by inhalation.

Following intravenous infusion of thymoxamine at a mean rate of 210 µg per minute for 30 minutes the plasma half-life was 2.4 minutes; a steady plasma concentration of 300 ng per ml was achieved and fell to zero within 10 minutes of stopping the infusion.— J. P. Griffin *et al.* (letter), *Lancet*, 1972, *1*, 1288.

Further references: A. G. Arbab and P. Turner, *Br. J. Pharmac.*, 1971, *43*, 479P; *idem* (letter), *J. Pharm. Pharmac.*, 1971, *23*, 719.

Uses. Thymoxamine is an alpha-adrenoceptor blocking agent which is used for the treatment of peripheral vascular disorders.

The usual dose is the equivalent of 40 mg of thymoxamine four times daily. It is also given intravenously in a dose of 100 µg per kg bodyweight, which may be given 4 times daily. A single dose of 5 mg may be given intra-arterially into a distal artery to reduce spasm after arterial surgery or before the withdrawal of a cardiac catheter.

Action. Thymoxamine is a specific and reversible alpha-adrenoceptor blocking agent. It has a weak antihistaminic action.— G. Brownlee, *Angiology*, 1966, *17*, 186.

Asthma. It has been suggested (H. Herxheimer (letter), *Lancet*, 1972, *2*, 491) that an antihistaminic effect of thymoxamine (A.T. Birmingham and J. Szolcsányi, *J. Pharm. Pharmac.*, 1965, *17*, 449) might be responsible for any bronchodilating properties, but this has been challengcd (J. Gaddie *et al.* (letter), *Lancet*, 1972, *2*, 657).

Experience in 10 patients with bronchial asthma demonstrated an increase in respiratory function when thymoxamine or phentolamine was combined with isoprenaline.— K. R. Patel and J. W. Kerr (letter), *Lancet*, 1975, *1*, 348. See also K. R. Patel, *Br. J. clin. Pharmac.*, 1976, *3*, 601. Inhibition of post-exercise bronchoconstriction following thymoxamine inhalation.— K. R. Patel *et al.*, *J. Allergy clin. Immunol.*, 1976, *57*, 285.

In a study in 7 patients with bronchial asthma only 1 claimed benefit (not supported by FEV_1) from the inhalation 4-hourly of 0.3 ml of thymoxamine 1.5% in addition to their salbutamol and sodium cromoglycate.— E. N. Wardle (letter), *Br. med. J.*, 1977, *1*, 1085.

Further references: J. P. Griffin *et al.* (letter), *Lancet*, 1972, *1*, 1288; K. N. V. Palmer *et al.* (letter), *Br. med. J.*, 1974, *4*, 409; A. M. Haddock *et al.*, *ibid.*, 1975, *2*, 357.

Ménière's syndrome. References to thymoxamine in Ménière's syndrome: N. W. Gill, *J. Lar. Otol.*, 1968, *82*, 231; *Drug & Ther. Bull.*, 1969, *7*, 99; J. R. Young, *J. int. med. Res.*, 1978, *6*, 166; L. Naftalin and K. J. H. Mallett, *J. Lar. Otol.*, 1980, *94*, 311 (possible hormonal vertigo in one patient).

Peripheral vascular disorders. Reports and studies on the use of thymoxamine in peripheral vascular disorders: K. A. Myers *et al.*, *Cardiovasc. Res.*, 1968, *4*, 360; P. Turner *et al.*, *Lancet*, 1969, *1*, 1238; C. Ramsay, *J. clin. Pharmac.*, 1969, *9*, 239; S. P. Kane, *Br. J. Surg.*, 1970, *57*, 921; J. G. Collier *et al.*, *Br. J. Pharmac.*, 1972, *44*, 294; M. Thomas *et al.*, *Br. J. Surg.*, 1973, *60*, 545; S. S. Rose, *Br. J. clin. Pract.*, 1979, *33*, 223; D. M. Williamson and M. Gatecliff, *Curr. med. Res. Opinion*,

1980, *6*, 500; G. V. Jaffe and J. J. Grimshaw, *Br. J. clin. Pract.*, 1980, *34*, 343.

Shock, septic. For reference to the use of thymoxamine as part of a therapeutic regimen for the treatment of septic shock, see Isoprenaline Sulphate, p.17.

Spasticity. Thymoxamine 40 mg four times daily increased to 80 mg six times daily by mouth was ineffective in reducing spasticity in 12 patients.— G. M. Yuill and D. Neary (letter), *Lancet*, 1973, *2*, 1504.

In a double-blind study of 6 patients with severe spasticity due to lesions at spinal or supraspinal sites, thymoxamine 100 µg per kg body-weight by intravenous injection reduced spasticity measured electromyographically.— C. de B. White and A. Richens (letter), *Lancet*, 1974, *1*, 686.

Further references: S. J. Phillips *et al.*, *Br. J. Pharmac.*, 1973, *47*, 595; J. Mai, *Acta neurol. scand.*, 1978, *57*, 65.

Use in ophthalmology. Thymoxamine eye-drops (0.1% solution buffered to pH 7 with borax 0.3% and boric acid 1.5%) when instilled into eyes produced miosis lasting up to 2 hours. Pretreatment with thymoxamine eye-drops prevented the production of mydriasis by phenylephrine 10% or ephedrine 2%. Thymoxamine also reversed the mydriasis produced by hydroxyamphetamine 1%.— P. Turner and J. M. Sneddon, *Clin. Pharmac. Ther.*, 1968, *9*, 45. See also J. H. Stewart-Jones, *Pharm. J.*, 1974, *1*, 335.

Of a group of 6 patients, 4 treated with thymoxamine eye-drops 0.5% had a change in the pupillary response to dark adaptation and 3 of 4 recovered pupillary reflexes to light.— V. J. Marmion (letter), *Br. med. J.*, 1969, *2*, 450.

In 12 healthy students thymoxamine eye-drops 0.1% completely reversed the mydriasis produced by ephedrine 5% but incompletely reversed that caused by homatropine 0.5% or by ephedrine and homatropine. A small reduction in accommodation produced by ephedrine was reversed by thymoxamine but the greater reduction in accommodation produced by homatropine was only partially reversed.— S. Small *et al.*, *Br. J. Ophthal.*, 1976, *60*, 132.

Thymoxamine caused incomplete reversal of mydriasis produced by tropicamide; 0.2% solutions of thymoxamine were tolerated in the eye but did not appear to be more effective than 0.1% solutions.— G. L. Mayer *et al.*, *Curr. med. Res. Opinion*, 1977, *4*, 660.

Further references: A. H. Halasa and P. C. Rutkowski, *Archs Ophthal., N.Y.*, 1973, *90*, 177; R. S. Dixon *et al.*, *Archs Ophthal., N.Y.*, 1979, *97*, 2147.

Preparations

Thymoxamine Tablets *(B.P.)*. Tablets containing thymoxamine hydrochloride. Protect from light.

Opilon *(Warner, UK)*. Thymoxamine hydrochloride, available as an injection containing the equivalent of 5 mg of thymoxamine per ml, in ampoules of 1 ml. **Opilon-Forte.** An injection containing the equivalent of 15 mg of thymoxamine per ml, in ampoules of 2 ml. **Opilon Tablets.** Scored tablets each containing the equivalent of 40 mg of thymoxamine. (Also available as Opilon in *Ital., S.Afr.*).

NOTE. The code THY is permitted in Great Britain for single-dose eye-drops of thymoxamine.

Other Proprietary Names

Apifor *(Spain)*; Arlitene *(Ital.)*; Carlytène Fort *(Fr.)*; Valyten *(Spain)*; Vasoklin *(Ger.)*.

9281-t

Tolazoline Hydrochloride *(B.P., U.S.P.)*.

Tolazol. Hydrochlor.; Benzazoline Hydrochloride; Tolazolinium Chloratum. 2-Benzyl-2-imidazoline hydrochloride.

$C_{10}H_{12}N_2,HCl=196.7$.

CAS — 59-98-3 (tolazoline); 59-97-2 (hydrochloride).

Pharmacopoeias. In *Arg., Aust., Br., Braz., Cz., Hung., Ind., It., Jug., Nord., Pol., Roum.,* and *U.S.*

A white or creamy-white, odourless, or almost odourless crystalline powder with a bitter taste. M.p. 172° to 176°.

Soluble 1 in 0.5 of water, 1 in 2 of alcohol, and 1 in 2.5 to 3 of chloroform; practically insoluble in ether. A 1% solution in water has a pH of 5 to 7. A 3.05% solution is iso-osmotic with serum. Solutions are **sterilised** by autoclaving or by filtration. **Store** in airtight containers. Protect from light.

A 3.05% solution of tolazoline hydrochloride in water, iso-osmotic with serum, caused 93% haemolysis of erythrocytes cultured in it for 45 mintues.— E. R. Hammarlund and K. Pedersen-Bjergaard, *J. pharm. Sci.*, 1961, *50*, 24.

Incompatibility. There were changes in the u.v. spectra indicating chemical change and possible incompatibility when ethacrynate sodium was added to sodium chloride injection containing tolazoline hydrochloride.— P. N. Catania and J. C. King, *Am. J. Hosp. Pharm.*, 1972, *29*, 141.

Adverse Effects. Minor side-effects of tolazoline hydrochloride include pilo-erection and flushing, but these may subside with continued use of the drug. Severe tachycardia, cardiac arrhythmias, apprehension, tingling, chilliness, shivering, sweating, nausea, vomiting, diarrhoea, and epigastric pain may also occur. Orthostatic hypotension may occur, especially with large doses.

Anginal pain or marked hypertension may also occur, particularly after parenteral administration; tolazoline has been implicated as a precipitating factor in myocardial infarction. Intra-arterial injection may be followed by a burning sensation in the limb. Administration of tolazoline has been associated with exacerbation of peptic ulcer.

Pregnancy and the neonate. Hypochloraemic metabolic alkalosis in an infant with respiratory distress was apparently related to gastric hypersecretion following infusion of tolazoline.— J. M. Adams *et al.*, *Pediatrics*, 1980, *65*, 298.

Studies in young *animals* have indicated that the combination of severe hypoxaemia and the use of tolazoline in the newborn infant whose systemic arterial blood pressure is inadequately controlled, may predispose to hypotension and acute renal failure. Two infants in whom this combination of circumstances occurred required peritoneal dialysis before return of renal function.— R. S. Trompeter *et al.*, *Lancet*, 1981, *1*, 1219.

Treatment of Adverse Effects. In severe overdosage by mouth the stomach should be emptied by aspiration and lavage. Hypotension is probably best treated by keeping the patient recumbent with the head lowered. If necessary the circulation may be maintained by infusion of suitable electrolyte solutions. Adrenaline is not suitable for the reversal of hypotension induced by alpha-adrenoceptor blocking agents since it may exacerbate the hypotension by stimulating beta-receptors.

Precautions. Tolazoline hydrochloride should be given with care to patients with coronary artery disease. Since tolazoline hydrochloride stimulates gastric secretion of hydrochloric acid, it should not be used in the presence of peptic ulceration.

For the effect of tolazoline on dopamine, see Dopamine Hydrochloride, p.9.

Absorption and Fate. Tolazoline hydrochloride is absorbed from the gastro-intestinal tract and its maximum effects are produced after 45 to 100 minutes. It is more rapidly absorbed after intramuscular injection, producing the maximum effects after 30 to 60 minutes. The effects last for several hours. Tolazoline hydrochloride is rapidly excreted in the urine, largely unchanged.

Uses. Tolazoline hydrochloride is an alpha-adrenoceptor blocking agent which also has a direct dilator action on the peripheral blood vessels, especially the arterioles and capillaries, and increases the peripheral blood flow.

Tolazoline is mainly used in the treatment of peripheral vascular disorders. Tolazoline hydrochloride is generally given by mouth. It is usual to commence with a small dose, such as 12.5 mg once or twice daily, increased, according to the response obtained, to 25 to 50 mg four times daily.

Tolazoline hydrochloride has been given in doses of up to 50 mg by subcutancous, intramuscular, intravenous, or slow intra-arterial injection.

Tolazoline has also been used in the form of a 10% ointment or solution for local application and as a 5 or 10% solution as eye-drops in the treatment of ophthalmic conditions such as iritis, keratitis, and iridocyclitis.

Action. Work in *animals* showed tolazoline to be a histaminergic agonist acting at H_2 receptors in addition to its alpha-adrenoceptor blocking activity.— T. O. Yellin *et al.* (letter), *Nature*, 1975, *253*, 561.

Animal studies suggesting a partial α- agonist action of tolazoline.— S. Naujoks and J. -P. Guignard (letter), *Lancet*, 1979, *2*, 1075.

Adjunct to X-ray examination. The infusion of 35 mg of tolazoline prior to arteriography facilitated the diagnosis of polyarteritis nodosa in 2 patients.— K. Bron *et al.*, *Radiology*, 1971, *99*, 295, per *Int. pharm. Abstr.*, 1973, *10*, 595.

In 64 consecutive bone and soft tissue arteriographies tolazoline 25 to 50 mg diluted to 10 ml with iso-osmotic saline solution was given intra-arterially to improve the visualisation of normal vascular anatomy and tumour vascularity.— I. Hawkings and T. Hudson, *Radiology*, 1974, *110*, 541, per *Int. pharm. Abstr.*, 1975, *12*, 205.

Preference for angiotensin over tolazoline for angiographic enhancement.— L. Ekelund *et al.*, *Radiology*, 1977, *122*, 95, per *Int. pharm. Abstr.*, 1977, *14*, 737.

Further references: H. M. Goldstein *et al.*, *Radiology*, 1976, *119*, 275.

Hypertension, pulmonary. A patient with primary pulmonary hypertension obtained a beneficial response to tolazoline hydrochloride 50 mg but the therapy could not be tolerated owing to nausea and vomiting.— U. R. Shettigar *et al.*, *New Engl. J. Med.*, 1976, *295*, 1414.

Cystic fibrosis. Improvement in vital capacity was seen in 10 patients with cystic fibrosis who received tolazoline 2 mg per kg body-weight on alternate days for 1 month for the treatment of pulmonary involvement unresponsive to conventional therapy. Thoracic gas volume decreased and arterial oxygen tensions increased during tolazoline therapy; temporary cessation of treatment caused deterioration of these factors. Only minimal radiologic changes indicating improvement in lung function were evident in some patients at the end of the trial.— *J. Am. med. Ass.*, 1968, *204* (Apr. 1), A25. See also L. L. Kelminson *et al.*, *Pediatrics*, 1967, *39*, 24.

Diaphragmatic hernia. Tolazoline in the treatment of congenital diaphragmatic hernias.— E. Sumner and J. D. Frank, *Archs Dis. Childh.*, 1981, *56*, 350.

Respiratory distress syndrome. Of 36 neonates with hypoxaemia and evidence of pulmonary disease, 21 responded to an intravenous infusion of tolazoline 1 to 2 mg per kg body-weight over 10 minutes followed by a continuous intravenous infusion of 1 to 2 mg per kg per hour for a mean of 36 hours. There were 13 survivors from the infants who had responded, whereas only 3 of those infants who had little or no response survived. In a group of 10 neonates with hypoxaemia but without pulmonary disease, 8 improved after a similar infusion of tolazoline but one died later. Both infants who did not respond died. Side-effects occurred in 14 infants and included gastro-intestinal or pulmonary haemorrhage, abdominal distension, oliguria, haematuria, renal failure and thrombocytopenia. It was recommended that blood pressure should be carefully monitored during administration of tolazoline to neonates.— B. W. Goetzman *et al.*, *J. Pediat.*, 1976, *89*, 617.

Tolazoline hydrochloride 1 to 2 mg per kg body-weight injected intravenously or via the umbilical artery produced clinical improvement in 10 of 20 preterm infants with severe hyaline membrane disease. Renal failure occurred in one infant and 2 suffered irritability associated with blood-stained cerebrospinal fluid.— N. McIntosh and R. O. Walters, *Archs Dis. Childh.*, 1979, *54*, 105.

Further references: D. K. Stevenson *et al.*, *J. Pediat.*, 1979, *95*, 595.

See also under Adverse Effects (Pregnancy and the Neonate).

Peripheral vascular disorders. A review of drugs, including tolazoline, used in the management of peripheral vascular disease. In the author's clinical experience, tolazoline has not been of benefit in obstructive vascular disease, but in association with other agents, is occasionally useful in patients with Raynaud's phenomenon.— J. D. Coffman, *New Engl. J. Med.*, 1979, *300*, 713. See also J. D. Coffman and A. S. Cohen, *ibid.*, 1971, *285*, 259.

Individual reports and studies of tolazoline in peripheral vascular disorders: A. G. Prandoni and M. Moser,

Circulation, 1954, *9,* 73; W. G. Guntheroth *et al., Circulation,* 1967, *36,* 724; M. Thomas *et al., Br. J. Surg.,* 1973, *60,* 545.

Leprosy. Twenty-five patients with leprosy ulcers of the hand or foot were treated with perineural injections of tolazoline hydrochloride, 25 mg in 1 ml being injected twice weekly near the ulnar nerve in patients with ulcers of the hand and round the popliteal nerve in patients with ulcers of the foot. Smaller ulcers healed after 2 to 6 weeks' treatment; trophic ulcers of the sole healed with prolonged treatment. All the treated ulcers except 1 either healed or were reduced in size.— J. S. Mathur *et al., Lepr. Rev.,* 1966, *37,* 249.

Marked improvement of leprotic lagophthalmos in a patient given 2 courses of 6 weekly local injections of 25 mg (1 ml) of tolazoline hydrochloride in the neighbourhood of the main facial nerve.— H. V. Nema and J. S. Mathur, *Lepr. Rev.,* 1967, *38,* 159.

Preparations

Tolazoline Hydrochloride Injection *(U.S.P.).* A sterile solution in Water for Injections. pH 3 to 4.

Tolazoline Hydrochloride Tablets *(U.S.P.).* Tablets containing tolazoline hydrochloride.

Tolazoline Tablets *(B.P.).* Tablets containing tolazoline hydrochloride. Protect from light.

Unguentum Tolazolini *(Nord. P.).* Tolazoline Ointment. Tolazoline hydrochloride 10 g, water 5 g, wool fat 17 g, and white soft paraffin 68 g.

Proprietary Preparations

Priscol *(Ciba, UK).* Tolazoline hydrochloride, available as scored tablets of 25 mg. (Also available as Priscol in *Austral., Ger., Spain, Switz.*).

Other Proprietary Names

Dilazol *(Switz.)*; Priscoline *(Canad., USA)*; Zoline *(Austral.).*

9282-x

Trimetazidine Hydrochloride. Trimetazine Hydrochloride. 1-(2,3,4-Trimethoxybenzyl)piperazine dihydrochloride.
$C_{14}H_{22}N_2O_3,2HCl=339.3.$

CAS — 5011-34-7 (trimetazidine); 13171-25-0 (hydrochloride).

A white crystalline powder. **Soluble** in water.

Trimetazidine hydrochloride is a vasodilator which has been used prophylactically in the treatment of angina pectoris.

Cardiac disorders. References to the use of trimetazidine in angina pectoris: P. Brodbin and C. A. O'Connor, *Br. J. clin. Pract.,* 1968, *22,* 395; T. N. Mehrotra and E. T. Bassadone, *ibid.,* 1967, *21,* 553.

Proprietary Names

Vastarel *(Servier, Fr.)*; Cartoma, Vastazin *(both Jap.).*

Trimetazidine hydrochloride was formerly marketed in Great Britain under the proprietary name Vastarel *(Servier).*

9283-r

Trolnitrate Phosphate. Aminotrate Phosphate; Nitranolum; Trinitrotriethanolamine Diphosphate. Nitrilotrisethylene trinitrate diphosphate.
$C_6H_{12}N_4O_9,2H_3PO_4=480.2.$

CAS — 7077-34-1 (trolnitrate); 588-42-1 (phosphate).

Pharmacopoeias. In *Rus. Cz.* includes Trolnitratium Diphosphoricum cum Saccharo Lactis, containing trolnitrate phosphate 25% in lactose.

A fine, white, odourless or almost odourless, crystalline powder. Decomposes at 106° to 110°. Sparingly **soluble** in water with hydrolysis; freely soluble in alcohol and dilute mineral acids; practically insoluble in chloroform and ether.

Trolnitrate phosphate is a vasodilator with general properties similar to those of glyceryl trinitrate (see p.1620). It has been used for the prophylaxis of angina pectoris in usual doses of 2 to 4 mg three or four times daily. Doses of up to 40 mg daily have been employed.

Proprietary Names

Angitrit *(Leo, Belg.; Leo, Denm.; Nordmark-Werke, Ger.; Leo, Neth.)*; Nitroduran *(Lövens, Swed.)*; Praenitron *(Pfizer, Austral.).*

9284-f

Visnadine. 10-Acetoxy-9,10-dihydro-8,8-dimethyl-2-oxo-2*H*,8*H*-pyrano[2,3-*f*]chromen-9-yl 2-methylbutyrate.
$C_{21}H_{24}O_7=388.4.$

CAS — 477-32-7.

Visnadine is a vasodilator obtained from ammi visnaga fruit (see p.1614) which has been used in the treatment of circulatory deficiencies.

Proprietary Names

Carduben *(Madaus, Ger.)*; Vibeline *(Bellon, Fr.; Promesa, Spain)*; Visnamine *(Chinoin, Ital.).*

9285-d

Xanthinol Nicotinate.

Xanthinol Niacinate; SK 331A. 7-{2-Hydroxy-3-[(2-hydroxyethyl)methylamino]propyl}theophylline nicotinate.
$C_{13}H_{21}N_5O_4,C_6H_5NO_2=434.5.$

CAS — 2530-97-4 (xanthinol); 437-74-1 (nicotinate).

Pharmacopoeias. In *Cz.*

Colourless crystals. **Soluble** in water.

Adverse Effects. Flushing of the skin, abdominal pain, skin rash, and hypotension have been reported following the administration of xanthinol nicotinate.

Precautions. Care is necessary in giving xanthinol nicotinate by mouth to patients with peptic ulceration, and it should probably not be given to patients with mitral stenosis or myocardial or cerebral infarction, or concomitantly with sympatholytic agents.

Uses. Xanthinol nicotinate has been given in the treatment of peripheral and cerebral vascular disorders.

A suggested dosage by mouth is to start treatment with 150 mg thrice daily, gradually increasing, if necessary, up to 900 mg or more daily. It has also been given by intramuscular or slow intravenous injection in doses of 900 mg or more daily.

Xanthinol nicotinate has a transient fibrinolytic action.

Studies of xanthinol nicotinate in healthy subjects showed it to produce a brisk but transient fibrinolytic activity when injected or infused intravenously. A refractory state soon appeared, in which subjects did not respond to further therapy. It appeared that resistance to repeated injections was not due to exhaustion of the body's fibrinolytic potential. Side-effects included flushing of the skin, adbominal pain, and hypotension. Because of the transient nature of the fibrinolytic response and the danger of hypotension, xanthinol nicotinate did not appear to have a place in the treatment of thrombo-embolic occlusive vascular disease.— G. P. McNicol and A. S. Douglas, *Br. med. J.,* 1965, *1,* 1149.

The main action of xanthinol nicotinate was considered to be an improvement in peripheral blood flow, with the transient fibrinolytic effect of secondary importance. Intravenous injections of 150 mg of xanthinol nicotinate caused a distinct flush but, in general, pulse and blood pressure were little affected. This was in contrast to the fall in blood pressure reported by McNicol and Douglas.— A. Hedbom (letter), *Br. med. J.,* 1965, *1,* 1554.

Eclampsia. Evidence that xanthinol nicotinate 5 mg four times daily for 7 days corrected insufficient placental circulation and improved placental function in women with pre-eclampsia.— N. A. M. Bergstein and H. I. J. M. v. Kessel (letter), *Lancet,* 1968, *2,* 111.

Peripheral vascular disorders. Reports and studies of the use of xanthinol nicotinate in peripheral vascular disorders: V. R. Witek, *Arzneimittel-Forsch.,* 1968, *18,* 156; E. Davis and H. Rozov, *Practitioner,* 1975, *215,* 793.

Proprietary Names

Angioamin *(Dompè, Ital.)*; Complamin *(Wulfing, Belg.; Nordic, Canad.; Tika, Denm.; Beecham-Wülfing, Ger.; Italchimici, Ital.; Bencard, Neth.; Tika, Norw.; Adcock Ingram, S.Afr.; Tika, Swed.; Wülfing, Switz.)*; Complamina *(Raffo, Arg.)*; Complamine *(Latéma, Fr.)*; Emodinamin *(Sigurtà, Ital.)*; Landrina *(Landerlan, Spain)*; Vasoprin *(Alfa Farmaceutici, Ital.)*; Vedrin *(Polifarma, Ital.).*

Xanthinol nicotinate was formerly marketed in Great Britain under the proprietary name Complamex *(Gemini).*

Vitamins

7820-j

Vitamins are constituents of the diet other than carbohydrate, fat, protein, and inorganic salts and are necessary for the normal metabolic function of the body. Some compounds with vitamin activity, such as the active metabolites of vitamin D, have hormonal activity.

Minimum daily requirements have been recommended for the principal vitamins and these are noted in the respective monographs. In assessing dietary intakes account should also be taken of those substances which are not vitamins but which can be converted to vitamins in the body.

Deficiencies may occur in persons on restricted or deficient diets, in persons with malabsorption syndromes, and when requirements are increased, such as during periods of growth, in pregnancy and during lactation, and in increased metabolic states such as hyperthyroidism, fever, and wasting diseases. It is the treatment of these deficiency states which represents the main clinical application for vitamins or their synthetic analogues. There is little justification in the use of vitamins as 'tonics'.

Large doses of vitamins (megavitamin therapy) have been proposed for the treatment of a wide variety of disorders including arthritis, asthma, nephritis, rheumatic fever, schizophrenia, and vascular disorders but adequate evidence of their value is lacking.

The vitamins and principal substances with vitamin activity described in this section may be classified as follows:

Compounds with **vitamin A** activity include vitamin A, p.1635; betacarotene, p.1638; halibut-liver oil, p.1638.

Compounds with **vitamin B_1** activity include thiamine hydrochloride, p.1639; thiamine mononitrate, p.1640.

Compounds with **vitamin B_2** activity include riboflavine, p.1641; riboflavine sodium phosphate, p.1642.

Compounds with **vitamin B_6** activity include pyridoxine hydrochloride, p.1642.

Compounds with **vitamin B_{12}** activity include cobalamins, p.1643; cyanocobalamin, p.1644; hydroxocobalamin, p.1645; liver extracts, p.1646.

Other vitamins of the B group include biotin, p.1646; folic acid, p.1647; folinic acid, p.1648; calcium folinate, p.1648; nicotinic acid, p.1648; nicotinamide, p.1650; pantothenic acid, p.1650; calcium pantothenate, p.1650; dexpanthenol, p.1650.

Other compounds traditionally considered as part of the B group include aminobenzoic acid, p.1651; choline, p.1651; inositol, p.1652.

Compounds with **vitamin C** activity include ascorbic acid, p.1653; sodium ascorbate, p.1657; black currant, p.1657; rose fruit, p.1657.

Compounds with **vitamin D** activity include vitamin D, p.1657; alfacalcidol, p.1659; calcifediol, p.1660; calcitriol, p.1660; cholecalciferol, p.1661; cod-liver oil, p.1661; dihydrotachysterol, p.1662; ergocalciferol, p.1662.

Compounds with **vitamin E** activity include vitamin E, p.1662; alpha tocopheryl acetate, p.1664; wheat germ oil, p.1665.

Compounds with **vitamin K** activity include vitamin K, p.1665; acetomenaphthone, p.1666; menadiol sodium diphosphate, p.1666; menadione, p.1666; menadione sodium bisulphite, p.1667; phytomenadione, p.1665.

These compounds are discussed in this section in the above order.

Recommendations on vitamin requirements:. Requirements of Vitamin A, Thiamine, Riboflavine and Niacin, Report of a Joint FAO/WHO Expert Group, *Tech. Rep. Ser. Wld Hlth Org. No. 362,* 1967; Requirements of Ascorbic Acid, Vitamin D, Vitamin B_{12}, and Iron, Report of a Joint FAO/WHO Expert Group, *Tech. Rep. Ser. Wld Hlth Org. No. 452,* 1970; *Manual of Nutrition*, Ministry of Agriculture, Fisheries and Food, London, HM Stationery Office, 1970; Requirements of Folate, Report of a WHO Group of Experts on Nutritional Anaemias, *Tech. Rep. Ser. Wld Hlth Org. No. 503,* 1972; T. H. Jukes, *J. Am. med. Ass.,* 1975, *233,* 550; Recommended Daily Amounts of Food Energy and Nutrients for Groups of People in the United Kingdom, Report by the Committee on Medical Aspects of Food Policy, *Report on Health and Social Subjects No. 15,* London, HM Stationery Office, 1979; Present Day Practice in Infant Feeding: 1980, Report of a Working Party of the Panel on Child Nutrition Committee on Medical Aspects of Food Policy, *Report on Health and Social Subjects, 20,* London, HM Stationery Office, 1980; Artificial Feeds for the Young Infant: 1980, Report of the Working Party on the Composition of Foods for Infants and Young Children, Committee on Medical Aspects of Food Policy, *Report on Health and Social Subjects, 18,* London, HM Stationery Office, 1980; *Recommended Dietary Allowances,* 9th Edn, Washington, The National Research Council, 1980.

Adverse effects. A review of vitamin toxicity.— J. R. DiPalma and D. M. Ritchie, *A. Rev. Pharmac. & Toxic.,* 1977, *17,* 133 to 148. See also J. G. Lewis, *Adverse Drug React. Bull.,* 1980, June, 296.

Deficiency states. Deficiences of vitamins during parenteral nutrition.— *Br. med. J.,* 1978, *2,* 913.

In the elderly. A review of nutritional deficiency in the elderly.— A. C. M. Windsor, *Practitioner,* 1979, *222,* 625.

In a nutrition survey of 879 elderly subjects aged 65 or over, the measurement of haemoglobin concentrations, where carried out, indicated a 7.3% incidence of anaemia. Mean serum concentrations of iron, folate, cyanocobalamin, and pyridoxine were lower in these subjects than in the younger population but there was not a corresponding incidence of anaemia.— Report by the Panel on Nutrition of the Elderly, A Nutrition Survey of the Elderly, London, HM Stationery Office, 1972.

There was no valid evidence that medical treatment, including the use of vitamins, was of value in senile cataract.— *Br. med. J.,* 1978, *1,* 908.

Intramuscular vitamin supplementation in the elderly.— H. Baker *et al., J. Am. Geriat. Soc.,* 1980, *28,* 42.

Interactions. A review of vitamin deficiencies which could be caused by various drugs.— F. Clark, *Adverse Drug React. Bull.,* 1976, Apr., 196.

A review of drugs known to cause vitamin deficiency, symptoms of deficiency, and the mechanisms involved in the development of such deficiency states.— L. Ovesen, *Drugs,* 1979, *18,* 278.

The effects of oral contraceptives on vitamin status.— V. Wynn, *Lancet,* 1975, *1,* 561.

The increased need for vitamins in smokers.— *FDA Drug Bull.,* 1979, *9,* 4.

Pregnancy and the neonate. A report of the possible prevention of neural-tube defects by periconceptional vitamin supplementation. Only 1 of 178 infants or foetuses of fully supplemented mothers at risk had a neural-tube defect (a provisional recurrence rate of 0.6%), compared with 13 of 260 infants or foetuses of similar control mothers (a provisional recurrence rate of 5%). The supplemented women were given one tablet of Pregnavite Forte F thrice daily for not less than 28 days before conception and continuing until at least the date of the second missed period (i.e., until well after the time of neural-tube closure).— R. W. Smithells *et al.* (preliminary communication), *Lancet,* 1980, *1,* 339. Addition of interim results of a second cohort of mothers, demonstrated 3 recurrences among 397 offspring of fully supplemented mothers and 23 recurrences among 493 offspring of unsupplemented mothers.— *idem* (letter), 1981, *2,* 1425. See also M. Holmes-Siedle *et al.* (letter), *ibid.,* 1982, *1,* 276. Criticism, including comments on the need for confirmation and for identification of the vitamin involved: G. M. Stirrat (letter), *ibid.,* 625; J. H. Renwick (letter), *ibid.,* 748; P. Meier (letter), *ibid.,* 859.

See also below under Megavitamin Therapy.

Further references and comments.— D. H. Stone (letter), *Lancet,* 1980, *1,* 647; R. W. Smithells and S. Sheppard (letter), *ibid.;* P. M. Fernhoff (letter), *ibid.,* 648; J. H. Elwood (letter), *ibid.;* C. J. Schorah *et al.* (letter), *ibid.,* 880; P. N. Kirke (letter), *ibid.,* 1300; D. L. J. Freed (letter), *ibid.,* 1301; G. M. Raab and S. M. Gore (letter), *ibid.;* R. Sharpe (letter), *ibid.;* N. C. Nevin (letter), *ibid.;* J. A. Davis (letter), *ibid.,* 1302; J. H. Edwards (letter), *ibid.,* 1982, *1,* 275.

See also under Folic Acid, p.1648.

Megavitamin therapy. A committee set up to evaluate megavitamin therapy agreed that such treatment was experimental and largely unproven, but recommended wide-ranging controlled research.— A. Imlac, *Can. med. Ass. J.,* 1977, *116,* 557.

A discussion on the hazards of megavitamin therapy. Vitamins generally functioned as coenzymes which bound to apoenzymes. Apoenzymes were generally saturated at levels approximating the recommended daily allowances of vitamins, and the production of apoenzymes was limited. In megadoses vitamins functioned therefore as chemicals.— V. D. Herbert, *J. Am. pharm. Ass.,* 1977, *NS17,* 764. See also M. Eastman, *Am. Pharm.,* 1978, *NS18* (Feb.), 16.

An account of vitamin homoeostasis in the brain, with a critical view of the use of megavitamin therapy. Homoeostatic processes provide an ultrastable environment for the brain, and they break down only in extreme nutritional deficiency or when they are disrupted by diseases such as meningitis.— R. Spector, *New Engl. J. Med.,* 1977, *296,* 1393.

Pregnancy and the neonate. An anencephalic foetus was detected at 17 weeks of pregnancy in a healthy normal 28-year-old mother who had taken large doses of ascorbic acid, thiamine, folic acid, pyridoxine, and yeast during psychiatric treatment in the first 10 weeks of pregnancy. Large doses of vitamins were taken for 6 months before conception.— P. Averback (letter), *Can. med. Ass. J.,* 1976, *114,* 995.

See also above under Deficiency States.

7821-z

Vitamin A *(Eur. P., U.S.P.).*

Vitaminum A; Retinol; Anti-infective Vitamin; Anti-xerophthalmic Vitamin; Axerophthol; Axerophthylium. 15-Apo-β-caroten-15-ol; 3,7-Dimethyl-9-(2,6,6-trimethylcyclohex-1-enyl)nona-2,4,6,8-*all-trans*-tetraen-1-ol.

$C_{20}H_{30}O = 286.5$.

CAS — 68-26-8.

Pharmacopoeias. In *Arg., Braz., Eur., Fr., Ger., It., Neth., Pol., Port., Swiss, Turk.,* and *U.S.*

The name vitamin A is applied to a number of substances of very similar structure found in animal tissues and possessing similar activity. The principal and most active substance is all-*trans* retinol which may be prepared by synthesis while material derived from natural sources (fish or marine mammalian liver oils and natural concentrates) is accompanied by several isomers. Retinal is vitamin A aldehyde, and retinoic acid is vitamin A acid—see Tretinoin, p.508 and Isotretinoin, p.496. The term 'provitamin A' is used to refer to all carotenoids and related compounds such as the β-apo-carotenals that are converted into vitamin A. Retinol is generally used in the form of esters such as the acetate, palmitate, or propionate.

All-*trans* retinol occurs as pale yellow crystals, practically **insoluble** in water, and freely soluble in alcohol, ether, light petroleum, and in fixed oils.

Vitamin A is very sensitive to the action of air, oxidising agents, light, and acids. Vitamin A and its precursors are stable to heat in the absence of oxidising agents, and the ordinary cooking processes do not destroy the vitamin A activity of vegetables. Frozen foods may lose 5 to 10% of their vitamin A activity during storage for 12 months at −23°. Vitamin A is stable in vegetable oils containing antioxidants, but not during heating; rancid fats have a catalytic effect on vitamin A destruction.

The foods which may serve as sources of vitamin A, either directly or through carotene, are butter, cream, margarine, egg yolk, liver, fish-liver oils, spinach, watercress, and carrots; of less value are

milk, nuts, fruit, and tomatoes.
Vitamin A of the *U.S.P.* contains a suitable form of retinol which may consist of retinol or its esters formed from edible fatty acids, principally acetic and palmitic acids. It is a light yellow to red oil which may solidify upon refrigeration; practically odourless or with a mild fishy odour but no rancid odour or taste. It may be diluted with edible oils or be incorporated in solid edible carriers or excipients, and may contain suitable antoxidants, dispersants, and antimicrobial agents.
Store in a cool place, in well-filled airtight containers, preferably under an atmosphere of inert gas. Protect from light.

7822-c

Vitamin A Acetate. Retinol Acetate; Retinyl Acetate; Axerophtholum Aceticum; Axerophthylium Aceticum.
$C_{22}H_{32}O_2$=328.5.
CAS — 127-47-9.

Pharmacopoeias. In *Chin., Cz., Jap., Jug., Pol., Roum.,* and *Rus.*

White to yellow crystals with a faint characteristic odour, containing about 2.9 million units per g. Vitamin A acetate 1.15 g is approximately equivalent to 1 g of retinol. M.p. about 57°. Practically **insoluble** in water; soluble in alcohol, chloroform, ether, light petroleum, and fats and fixed oils. **Store** at a temperature of 15° in airtight containers under an atmosphere of nitrogen. Protect from light.

7823-k

Vitamin A Palmitate. Retinol Palmitate; Retinyl Palmitate; Axerophthylium Palmiticum.
$C_{36}H_{60}O_2$=524.9.
CAS — 79-81-2.

Pharmacopoeias. In *Cz., Jap.,* and *Pol. It.* has Retinolo Palmitato in Microsfere, which contains not less than 485 000 units of vitamin A per g.

Yellow crystals or a yellow oily substance with a faint characteristic odour, containing about 1.8 million units per g. Vitamin A palmitate 1.83 g is approximately equivalent to 1 g of retinol. M.p. 28° to 30°. Practically **insoluble** in water; soluble in chloroform, ether, and vegetable oils. **Store** at a temperature of 15° in airtight containers under an atmosphere of nitrogen. Protect from light.

Sorption of vitamin A by glass and plastic. When an aqueous solution of vitamin A acetate 3 μg per ml solubilised in 0.01% polysorbate 80 was stored in the dark in a plastic intravenous fluid bag for 24 hours at 25° a considerable amount of vitamin A was adsorbed onto the bag. Further increases in adsorption occurred when vitamin A was in normal saline solution or dextrose solution 5%.— W. L. Chiou and P. Moorhatch (letter), *J. Am. med. Ass.,* 1973, *223,* 328.

The amounts of vitamin A delivered to the patient from glass and polyvinyl chloride containers were 77% and 71% respectively when protected from light and 61% and 49% when exposed to light. These differences were not considered medically significant.— R. L. Nedich (letter), *J. Am. med. Ass.,* 1973, *224,* 1531.

Absorption of vitamin A acetate increased with temperature and time when solutions in water were exposed to polyvinyl chloride. Absorption into the plastic was greater when dextrose injection or sodium chloride injection were the diluents.— P. Moorhatch and W. L. Chiou, *Am. J. Hosp. Pharm.,* 1974, *31,* 72.

Stability. Oxidation of vitamin A was catalysed by traces of metals, notably copper and iron, but this could be inhibited appreciably by the addition of antioxidants such as propyl gallate, hydroquinone, α-tocopherol, and especially by combinations of these antoxidants. Vitamin A dissolved in vegetable oil could be destroyed when the oil became rancid owing to formation of peroxides.— T. J. Macek, *Am. J. Pharm.,* 1960, *132,* 433.

dl-α-Tocopherol did not stabilise aqueous dispersions of vitamin A unless the concentration exceeded 0.5%. The best stabiliser was a combination of *dl-α*-tocopherol 3%, ascorbic acid 0.1%, nordihydroguaiaretic acid 0.01%, and disodium edetate 0.2%.— L. Klotz *et al., Pharmazie,* 1964, *19,* 606.

A study of the stability of vitamin A acetate in aqueous cetomacrogol solutions.— E. Azaz and R. Segal, *J. Pharm. Pharmac.,* 1977, *29,* 322.

The stability of microencapsulated vitamin A acetate.— R. Cadorniga *et al., Boll. chim.-farm.,* 1979, *118,* 380, per *Int. pharm. Abstr.,* 1980, *17,* 836.

In tablets. The stability of vitamin A esters in protected beadlet form in tablets was severely reduced by increases in moisture content from 0 to 2%, particularly in the absence of antoxidants.— J. T. Carstensen *et al., J. pharm. Sci.,* 1966, *55,* 561.

Units. The International Standards for vitamin A and for provitamin A were discontinued in 1954 and 1956 respectively but the International units for these substances have continued to be widely used. In 1960–1, the WHO Expert Committee on Biological Standardization redefined the International unit for vitamin A as the activity of 0.000344 mg of pure all-*trans* vitamin A acetate and the International unit for provitamin A as the activity of 0.0006 mg of pure all-*trans* β-carotene.
The activity of one International unit is contained in 0.0003 mg of all-*trans* retinol, in 0.00055 mg of all-*trans* retinol palmitate, and in 0.000359 mg of all-*trans* retinol propionate.
The *U.S.P.* unit is defined as the specific biologic activity of 0.0003 mg of the all-*trans* isomer of retinol, and is equivalent to the International unit.
In England and Wales, the Labelling of Food Regulations 1970 (SI 1970: No. 400) as amended (SI 1972: No. 1510) require that in any food labelled as containing vitamin A the vitamin must be calculated as micrograms of retinol.

Adverse Effects and Precautions. Hypervitaminosis A is usually caused by the administration of excessive amounts of vitamin A over long periods. It is characterised by fatigue, irritability, anorexia and loss of weight, vomiting and other gastro-intestinal disturbances, low-grade fever, polyuria, hepatosplenomegaly, pruritus, loss of hair, cracking and bleeding lips, and dry skin with desquamation, hyperkeratosis, and yellow pigmentation. Anaemia, headache, and visual disturbances have also been reported. These symptoms usually clear rapidly on withdrawal of vitamin A. Subcutaneous swelling, pains in bones and joints, and tenderness over the long bones commonly occur; in children, premature closure of the epiphyses of the long bones may result in arrested bone growth. Intracranial hypertension and papilloedema, mimicking brain tumours, have been reported, usually in children.
Acute vitamin A intoxication may occur with very high doses and is characterised by sedation, headache, irritability, papilloedema, and generalised peeling of the skin.
Toxic effects may result from the acute ingestion of more than 500 mg or the chronic ingestion of 50 mg daily, or lower doses in children.
In *animals,* teratogenic effects and decalcification of bones have occurred.

In a statement by the Drugs and Nutrition Committees of the American Academy of Pediatrics, the free sale and misuse of high potency vitamin A preparations was condemned. Ingestion of as little as 8 to 16 mg (25 000 to 50 000 units) daily for as little as 30 days could induce signs of increased intracranial pressure. The incidence of hypervitaminosis A was increasing and might be increased by the use of bizarre, highly fortified health foods. The use of large amounts of vitamin A for acne in adolescents was not of proven value.— S. J. Yaffe and L. J. Filer, *Pediatrics,* 1971, *48,* 655.

Hypervitaminosis A occurred in patients with advanced chronic renal failure and in those undergoing dialysis, but not in patients with acute renal failure.— H. Yatzidis *et al., Br. med. J.,* 1975, *3,* 352.

Further references to hypervitaminosis A: *Bulletin of the National Clearinghouse for Poison Control Centers,* 1972, 4; H. I. Silverman, *Am. J. Optom.,* 1972, *49,* 335; S. T. Teo *et al., Med. J. Aust.,* 1973, *2,* 324; E. Foldi *et al., Dt. med. Wschr.,* 1976, *101,* 205; M. L. Eaton, *Am. J. Hosp. Pharm.,* 1978, *35,* 1099; B. A. Shaywitz *et al., J. Am. med. Ass.,* 1977, *238,* 1749; *Med. Lett.,* 1980, *22,* 19.

Allergy. Allergy to vitamin A and its precursors in the diet in a young child was confirmed by challenge tests.— J. Greenbaum, *Ann. Allergy,* 1979, *43,* 98.

Effects on the eye. Reports of papilloedema associated with vitamin A.— M. H. Feldman and N. S. Schlezinger, *Archs Neurol., Chicago,* 1970, *22,* 1; C. Edmunds *et al.* (letter), *J. Am. med. Ass.,* 1973, *226,* 674.

Effects on the liver. Nodular liver cirrhosis and portal hypertension occurred in a 36-year-old man 3.5 years after receiving vitamin A 70 million units by mouth over 7 weeks for psoriasis vulgaris.— R. Fleischmann *et al., Dt. med. Wschr.,* 1977, *102,* 1637.

Further references: B. P. Lane, *Am. J. Path.,* 1968, *53,* 591; E. Rubin *et al., Am. J. Dis. Child.,* 1970, *119,* 132; M. D. Muenter *et al., Am. J. Med.,* 1971, *50,* 129; E. A. Jacques *et al., Gastroenterology,* 1979, *76,* 599.

Effects on the nervous system. Peripheral neuritis and pain developed in 2 leprotic patients treated with thiambutosine when vitamin A 15 000 and 120 000 units daily respectively were taken. The nerve pains stopped when the excess vitamin A was withdrawn.— A. G. Warren (letter), *Lepr. Rev.,* 1973, *44,* 220.

Effects on serum calcium. Hypercalcaemia and skeletal changes occurred in 3 patients who had taken excessive amounts of vitamin A.— B. Frame *et al., Ann. intern. Med.,* 1974, *80,* 44.

Hypervitaminosis A and hypercalcaemia occurred in a woman who had taken 150 000 units of vitamin A daily for 3 years and a further 2500 units of vitamin A plus 400 units of vitamin D daily for 1 year. Vitamin A was discontinued and the hypercalcaemia was treated by frusemide 80 to 120 mg daily and intravenous infusion of sodium chloride.— G. Fisher and P. G. Skillern, *J. Am. med. Ass.,* 1974, *227,* 1413.

A further report of hypercalcaemia.— K. J. Hofman *et al., S. Afr. med. J.,* 1978, *54,* 579.

Effects on serum cholesterol. Excessive serum concentrations of vitamin A were found in 10 of 50 patients with chronic laryngitis. Six of these patients and a further 10 patients had high serum-cholesterol concentrations.— P. M. Stell and M. P. McLoughlin (letter), *Lancet,* 1972, *1,* 147. See also J. M. Kordylas (letter), *Lancet,* 1972, *2,* 606.

Pregnancy and the neonate. For the absence of a correlation between high serum concentrations of vitamin A and congenital malformation, see J. Wild *et al., Br. med. J.,* 1974, *1,* 57. Criticism of the analytical procedure and hence also of the conclusions.— F. A. Bubb (letter), *ibid.,* 391. The increase in serum concentrations of vitamin A in women taking oral contraceptives was due to an increase in bound retinol and not to free retinol. The teratogenic effects of vitamin A in *animals* occurred with doses of vitamin A which greatly exceeded the binding capacity of retinol-binding protein in the serum.— M. H. Briggs (letter), *ibid.,* 1974, *3,* 170.

The birth of 2 malformed children to mothers who had taken an excess of vitamin A during pregnancy and the birth of 2 malformed children associated with deficiency of vitamin A suggested an association.— J. L. Schardein, *Drugs as Teratogens,* Cleveland, CRC, 1976, p. 237.

Further references: L. Stange *et al., Acta obstet. gynec. scand.,* 1978, *57,* 298.

Absorption and Fate. Vitamin A is usually readily absorbed from the diet but absorption may be diminished when liver function is impaired. Large doses of vitamin A are somewhat less effectively absorbed. If ingested as an ester this is largely hydrolysed to retinol which is emulsified by bile salts and phospholipids and absorbed in a micellar form. Part is conjugated with glucuronic acid in the liver and part is metabolised in the liver and kidney, leaving 30 to 50% of the dose for storage in the liver. It is bound to a globulin (retinol-binding protein) in the blood. It does not readily diffuse across the placenta but is present in the milk of nursing mothers. Metabolites of vitamin A are excreted in the faeces and in the urine.

There was no difference between plasma concentrations of vitamin A and its precursor, beta-carotene, in 39 patients with genetically-determined retinitis pigmentosa and 84 controls.— W. H. Massoud *et al., Br. J. Ophthal.,* 1975, *59,* 200.

Human Requirements. An optimum daily dietary intake of about 750 μg of vitamin A is recommended for healthy adults. An alternative source of vitamin A is provided by the carotenoid pigments of plants but they are less effectively utilised by the body.

The average daily recommended intake of vitamin A for adults was 750 μg of retinol (vitamin A alcohol). For infants, children, and young people, recommended daily intakes ranged from 300 μg at 6 to 12 months to 725 μg at 13 to 15 years.— Report of a Joint FAO/WHO Expert Group, *Tech. Rep. Ser. Wld Hlth Org. No. 362,* 1967.

Recommended daily intake of vitamin A or its equivalent: boys and girls up to 1 year, 450 μg; 1 to 6 years, 300 μg; 7 to 8 years, 400 μg; boys and girls 9 to 17 years, 575 to 750 μg; men and women 18 years or over, 750 μg; during pregnancy, 750 μg; during lactation, 1.2 mg. One μg of retinol was considered equivalent to 6 μg of β-carotene or 12 μg of other biologically active carotenoids.— *Report on Health and Social Subjects No. 15,* London, HM Stationery Office, 1979.

The recommendation that any infant formula should contain not less than 0.4 μg and not more than 1.5 μg retinol equivalent per ml reconstituted feed.— Artificial Feeds for the Young Infant: 1980, Report of the Working Party on the Composition of Foods for Infants and Young Children, Committee on Medical Aspects of Food Policy, *Report on Health and Social Subjects, 18,* London, HM Stationery Office, 1980.

Recommended daily dietary allowance of vitamin A: up to 6 months, 420 retinol equivalents (RE); 6 months to 3 years, 400 RE; 4 to 6 years, 500 RE; 7 to 10 years, 700 RE; males 11 years and over, 1000 RE; females 11 years and over, 800 RE; in pregnancy, 1000 RE; in lactation, 1200 RE. One retinol equivalent represents 1 μg of retinol, 6 μg of β-carotene, or 12 μg of other provitamin A carotenoids.— *Recommended Dietary Allowances,* 9th Edn, Washington, The National Research Council, 1980.

Uses. Vitamin A is essential for normal vision in dim light. Vitamin A interacts with various opsins of the retina to form visual pigments. One of the earliest symptoms of the deficiency is night-blindness. A later and more serious manifestation is xerophthalmia, a condition more commonly met with in the Far East and parts of Africa than in Europe.

Night-blindness due to vitamin-A deficiency is successfully treated by administration of vitamin A, but xerophthalmia, except in the early stages, is not amenable to treatment.

Vitamin A is believed to be involved in differentiation of epithelial tissues, though its exact role is obscure; deficiency of vitamin A may therefore give rise to skin changes, causing a dry rough skin, with a lowered resistance to minor skin infections. Some skin disorders have responded to topical treatment with vitamin A usually applied in the form of tretinoin (see p.508). The change in the epithelial cells of the periodontal tissues leads to inflammation of the gums and eventually to pyorrhoea. In the less severe types of deficiency the administration of vitamin A in adequate amounts rapidly leads to revitalisation of the affected tissues, usually within 2 or 3 weeks.

Deficiency of vitamin A, usually accompanied by protein-energy malnutrition, is linked with an increased frequency of infection and with defective immunological defence mechanisms. Deficient absorption of the precursors of vitamin A occurs in certain conditions such as coeliac disease and sprue, and excessive use of liquid paraffin as a laxative may reduce the utilisation of the provitamin by carrying away large amounts in the faeces.

Vitamin A is released very slowly, if at all, after intramuscular injection of oily solutions; water-miscible preparations should therefore be used. Oily solutions may be used orally.

In areas where vitamin A deficiency is common, foods such as sugar and milk have been fortified with vitamin A.

In the treatment of xerophthalmia an initial dose of vitamin A palmitate 55 mg (100 000 units), as a water-miscible preparation, is given initially by intramuscular injection, with a similar dose by mouth on the following day. A further dose of 110 mg (200 000 units) is given before discharge from hospital (55 mg; 100 000 units for children under 1 year). Single doses are given every 3 to 6 months to prevent recurrence.

In other severe deficiency states doses of 100 000 units by mouth have been given daily for 3 days, followed by 50 000 units daily for 14 days and 10 000 to 20 000 units daily for 2 months.

For the recommended daily dietary allowances to prevent deficiency, see under Human Requirements.

Acne and psoriasis. For the use of derivatives of vitamin A in various skin disorders, including acne and psoriasis, see under Tretinoin, p.508.

Administration in renal failure. For reference to vitamin A in renal failure see under Deficiency States (Dialysis), below.

Crohn's disease. Response of one patient with Crohn's disease to vitamin A.— M. Skogh *et al.* (letter), *Lancet,* 1980, *1,* 766. Comment.— A. M. Dvorak (letter), *Lancet,* 1980, *1,* 1303.

Deficiency states. A review of vitamin A deficiency, xerophthalmia, and its prevention and treatment. The preferred treatment of xerophthalmia was an immediate intramuscular injection of 100 000 units of retinyl palmitate in a water-miscible form then 100 000 units by mouth as an oily solution of the acetate or palmitate with vitamin E on the next day. A further oral dose of 100 000 units should be given to children under 1 year of age before discharge, or 200 000 units for patients over 1 year. For control and prevention in areas with a xerophthalmia problem similar oral doses of oily solution should be given to children aged 1 to 6 years every 6 months.— Vitamin A Deficiency and Xerophthalmia, Report of a Joint WHO/USAID Meeting, *Tech. Rep. Ser. Wld Hlth Org. No. 590,* 1976. See also *Chronicle Wld Hlth Org.,* 1978, *32,* 306, 310, and 322; B. A. Underwood, *Bull. Wld Hlth Org.,* 1978, *56,* 525; R. A. Thoft, *New Engl. J. Med.,* 1978, *298,* 1239.

Vitamin A deficiency did not affect colour vision.— V. Reddy and Vijayalaxmi, *Br. med. J.,* 1977, *1,* 81.

In a comparative study 69 children with corneal xerophthalmia were given oil-miscible vitamin A 200 000 units by mouth while 45 similar children were given water-miscible vitamin A 100 000 units intramuscularly. Both groups were given an additional dose by mouth the following day, consisting of the contents of a standard UNICEF capsule containing oil-miscible vitamin A palmitate 200 000 units and vitamin E 40 units, expressed into the child's mouth. Results indicated that corneal xerophthalmia responds just as rapidly to double-dose oral therapy as to parenteral. Fears that oral therapy alone would delay healing, especially in children with diarrhoea or protein-energy malnutrition, appear to have been unfounded and treatment, which is a medical emergency, need not be delayed in order to give it parenterally. No evidence of toxicity was encountered except for occasional asymptomatic papilloedema. It is considered that a third dose of oil-miscible vitamin A given one or two weeks later would probably improve liver stores even further and delay or reduce the risk of clinical relapse.— A. Sommer *et al., Lancet,* 1980, *1,* 557. Vitamin A absorption is markedly suppressed after acute watery diarrhoea.— D. R. Nalin and R. Russell (letter), *ibid.,* 1411. Nevertheless, enough is absorbed after a large dose to prevent xerophthalmia.— A. Sommer (letter), *ibid.*

Other reports of vitamin A deficiency and its treatment.— G. Venkataswamy, *Br. J. Ophthal.,* 1967, *51,* 854; B. S. Kuming and W. M. Politzer, *Br. J. Ophthal.,* 1967, *51,* 649; S. M. Pereira *et al., Am. J. clin. Nutr.,* 1967, *20,* 297, per *Abstr. Wld Med.,* 1967, *41,* 759; S. M. Pereira and A. Begum, *Am. J. clin. Nutr.,* 1969, *22,* 858, per *J. Am. med. Ass.,* 1969, *209,* 1558; F. Bors and P. Fells, *Br. J. Ophthal.,* 1971, *55,* 210; R. M. Russell *et al., Ann. intern. Med.,* 1978, *88,* 622.

Dialysis. Although the inter-patient variation was large there was no significant change in mean plasma concentrations of β-carotenoid measured in 6 patients and only a small decrease in the mean plasma concentrations of vitamin A following 8 hours of haemodialysis in 10 patients with chronic uraemia who were receiving maintenance haemodialysis.— L. Gotloib *et al., J. Am. med. Ass.,* 1978, *239,* 751.

Studies on the raised plasma concentrations of vitamin A in patients on maintenance haemodialysis, and advice that supplements of vitamin A should be avoided: K. Farrington *et al., Br. med. J.,* 1981, *282,* 1999; M. O'Fearghail *et al.* (letter), *ibid., 283,* 919; W. K. Stewart and L. W. Fleming (letter), *ibid.,* 1187.

Night blindness. In a study of 13 patients with treated chronic small-intestinal disease but without signs of malnutrition, all 13 had visual alterations in dark adaption despite 10 of them taking 3 500 to 10 000 units of vitamin A daily. There was a significant decrease in adaption threshold in 2 of 4 patients given 50 000 units intramuscularly and in 6 of 8 patients given 50 000 units daily by mouth for 30 days.— R. M. Russell *et al., Lancet,* 1973, *2,* 1161.

Malignant neoplasms. Reports and discussions of a possible connection between low concentrations of vitamin A and the development of cancer.— C. Mettlin *et al., J. natn. Cancer Inst.,* 1979, *62,* 1435; *Lancet,* 1980, *1,* 575; *Br. med. J.,* 1980, *281,* 957; N. Wald *et al., Lancet,* 1980, *2,* 813; A. Sakula (letter), *ibid.,* 1029; Z. A. Leitner *et al.* (letter), *ibid.,* 1030; N. Wald (letter), *ibid.,* 1144; D. S. McLaren (letter), *ibid.;* M. Briggs (letter), *ibid.,* 1145; R. B. Shekelle *et al., Lancet,* 1981, *2,* 1185; J. D. Kark *et al., Br. med. J.,* 1982, *284,* 152; H. B. Stähelin (letter), *Lancet,* 1982, *1,* 394; J. Gouveia *et al., ibid.,* 710 (use of the retinoid, *[etretinate]*).

For a reference to vitamin A enhancing the effect of cyclophosphamide in tumours, see Cyclophosphamide, p.201.

Sunburn. A preparation containing vitamin A and calcium carbonate (Sylvasun) taken the night before and 1 hour before exposure to u.v. radiation was no more effective than a placebo in providing protection from sunlight or from u.v. radiation from an artificial source when used in 2 double-blind trials involving 74 people.— F. E. Anderson, *Med. J. Aust.,* 1968, *1,* 802.

A study in 24 boys aged about 17 years showed that vitamin A 75 000 units (22.5 mg) at night and 50 000 units (15 mg) the next morning significantly increased the serum concentration of vitamin A, but had no significant effect on sunburning on subsequent exposure.— F. E. Anderson, *Aust. J. Derm.,* 1969, *10,* 26, per *Abstr. Wld Med.,* 1969, *43,* 877.

There was no convincing evidence that vitamin A 25 000 units with calcium carbonate 115 mg (Sylvasun) gave any protection against sunburn and there was strong evidence that it did not.— *Drug & Ther. Bull.,* 1975, *13,* 64. Comment.— *Pharm. J.,* 1975, *2,* 142.

Preparations

Concentrated Vitamin A Solution *(B.P.C. 1973).* Conc. Vit. A Soln.; Liquor Vitamini A Concentratus; Liq. Vitamin. A Conc. A solution of vitamin A containing 50 000 units in 1 g. It consists either of a suitable fish-liver oil or a blend of such oils, or a solution of a source of vitamin A in a suitable vegetable oil such as arachis oil. Any suitable source of vitamin A may be used, such as fish-liver oil rich in vitamin or a concentrate prepared therefrom; synthetic vitamin A or its esters may also be used. It contains not more than 500 units of vitamin D per g. A pale yellow or yellow oily liquid with a faint but not rancid odour and a bland or slightly fishy taste. Store in a cool place in well-filled airtight containers. Protect from light.

A similar preparation, containing 30 000 to 1 million units per g, is included in several pharmacopoeias.

Synthetic Vitamin A Concentrate (Oily Form) *(B.P., Eur. P.).* Synthetic Retinol Concentrate (Oily Form). A synthetic ester or a mixture of synthetic esters of retinol (usually the acetate, palmitate, or propionate); it may be diluted with a suitable vegetable oil. It contains not less than 500 000 units of vitamin A activity in 1 g and not less than 95% and not more than 110% of the number of units stated on the label. It may contain suitable stabilising agents such as antoxidants. It is a yellow to brownish-yellow oily liquid with a faint characteristic odour. Partial crystallisation may occur in highly concentrated solutions. Store in a cool place in an atmosphere of nitrogen or other suitable gas in hermetically sealed containers. Any part of the contents of a container not used at once should be protected by an atmosphere of an inert gas. Protect from light. A similar preparation is included in some pharmacopoeias.

Vitamin A Capsules *(U.S.P.).* Capsules containing vitamin A. Store in airtight containers. Protect from light.

Vitamin A Ester Concentrate (Natural) *(B.P.).* Retinol Ester Concentrate. A natural ester or a mixture of natural esters of retinol or a solution of the ester or mixture of esters in arachis oil or other suitable vegetable oil. It contains not less than 485 000 units of vitamin A activity in 1 g and not less than 97% of the number of units stated on the label. It may contain a suitable antoxidant or mixture of antoxidants. It is a yellow oil or a mixture of oil and crystalline material which when warmed yields a homogeneous yellow oil. It has a faint odour and bland taste. Store in a cool place in an atmosphere of nitrogen or other suitable gas in hermetically sealed containers. Any part of the contents of a container not used at once should be protected by an atmosphere of an inert gas. Protect from light. A similar preparation is included in *It. P.*

Proprietary Preparations

Ro-A-Vit Ampoules *(Roche, UK)*. Each 1-ml ampoule contains vitamin A palmitate (synthetic) equivalent to 300 000 units of vitamin A, in an oily vehicle.

Ro-A-Vit Tablets *(Roche, UK)*. Each contains vitamin A acetate (synthetic) equivalent to 50 000 units of vitamin A. (Also available as Ro-A-Vit in *Arg., Austral.*).

Other Proprietary Names of Vitamin A and its Esters

Arg.—Aquasol-A, Atunol, Bagoderm A, Bagovit-A, Vit-A-Plos; *Belg.*—Acaren, Anol Standard, Arovit, Dagravit A Forte, Neo-Dohyfral A; *Canad.*—Afaxin, Aquasol A; *Denm.*—Ariovit, Avimin; *Fr.*—A313, Arovit, Avibon; *Ger.*—A-Mulsin, Arovit, A-Vicotrat, Oculotect, Ophtosan, Vogan; *Ital.*—Alfa Monovit, Alfatar, Amirale, Arovit, Avitina, Euvit A, Euvitol, Farmobion A, Idrurto A, Primavit; *Neth.*—Arovit, Dagravit A, Davitamon A, Dohyfral A; *S.Afr.*—Arovit, Avita, Fabavit; *Spain*—A-Om, Amplex-A, Arovit, Auxina A Masiva, Avitam Masivo, Biominol A, Dolce-A, Evitex A, Fiviton-A, Ido-A50, Mulsal-A Megadosis, Neominas A, Perlaminas A Masivas, Vitaendil A; *Swed.*—Arovit, Ido-A; *Switz.*—Arovit, Axerol, Oculotect; *USA*—Aquasol A, Vi-Dom A.

A preparation containing vitamin A and tocopheryl acetate was formerly marketed in Great Britain under the proprietary name Rovigon (*Roche*).

7824-a

Betacarotene. all-*trans*-β-Carotene. β,β-Carotene.
$C_{40}H_{56}$=536.9.

CAS — 7235-40-7.

Purple or red crystals. M.p. about 181°. Practically **insoluble** in water, acid, or alkalis; very sparingly soluble in alcohol and methyl alcohol; soluble in chloroform and carbon disulphide; moderately soluble in ether, petroleum ether, and oils. **Store** at −20° in airtight containers. Protect from light.

Carotene exists in 3 isomeric forms, all of which are converted to some extent into vitamin A in the livers of man and animals. Of the 3 isomers of carotene, the *beta* compound is more active than the *alpha*- or *gamma*-isomers. The vitamin A activity of plants is due to the presence of *alpha*-, *beta*-, and *gamma*-carotenes and to kryptoxanthine; that of animal tissues is due to both vitamin A and carotene, while fish-liver oils contain vitamin A but no carotene.

Units. See under Vitamin A, p.1636.

Uses. Betacarotene is a precursor of vitamin A. It has been tried, in doses of 30 to 300 mg daily, in erythropoietic protoporphyria. Betacarotene and other carotenoids are used as colouring agents for foods.

An increase in serum carotene of less than 350 ng per ml after the administration of carotene 15 000 units thrice daily with meals for 3 days indicated steatorrhoea.— G. R. Onstad and L. Zieve, *J. Am. med. Ass.*, 1972, *221*, 677.

Lupus erythematosus. Complete cures of chronic discoid lupus erythematosus of from 12 to 23 years duration, and previously controlled by chloroquine or topical corticosteroid treatment, occurred within 3 weeks in 3 patients given betacarotene 50 mg thrice daily, for up to 2 months.— P. C. H. Newbold, *Br. J. Derm.*, 1976, *95*, 100. A contrary report.— E. L. Dubois and C. Patterson (letter), *J. Am. med. Ass.*, 1976, *236*, 138.

Photosensitivity. In 2 patients with actinic reticuloid and 3 with idiopathic solar urticaria, treatment with betacarotene afforded no consistent photoprotection.— A. Kobza *et al.*, *Br. J. Derm.*, 1973, *88*, 157.

A patient with polymorphous light eruption, photosensitive in the range 290 to 500 nm, was successfully treated with betacarotene 180 mg daily plus frequent topical applications of sulisobenzone. However neither medicament alone gave adequate protection.— J. J. Nordlund *et al.*, *Archs Derm.*, 1973, *108*, 710.

In a study comparing PUVA and betacarotene in 29 patients with polymorphous light eruption, 9 of 10 treated with PUVA and 6 of 19 treated with betacarotene showed complete remission. All 6 patients treated with both in consecutive years had remissions with betacarotene.— J. A. Parrish *et al.*, *Br. J. Derm.*, 1979, *100*, 187.

Protection of 5 American Indians from hereditary polymorphous light eruption by the use of betacarotene.— R. M. Fusaro and J. A. Johnson (letter), *J. Am. med. Ass.*, 1980, *243*, 231.

Porphyria. In 53 patients with erythropoietic protoporphyria who were given betacarotene by mouth in doses of 30 to 180 mg, 46 experienced a fourfold or more increase in the time they could tolerate exposure to sunlight, and 3 doubled their exposure time. There was no evidence of hypervitaminosis A or of leucopenia.— M. M. Mathews-Roth *et al.*, *J. Am. med. Ass.*, 1974, *228*, 1004.

From the results of a controlled crossover study, lasting several months, of 13 patients with erythropoietic protoporphyria, betacarotene 25 mg four times daily had no more influence than a placebo on signs and symptoms of photosensitivity in these patients.— M. F. Corbett *et al.*, *Br. J. Derm.*, 1977, *97*, 655.

The administration of betacarotene 75 to 200 mg daily to adults or 50 mg daily to children 12 years of age or under appeared to be associated with some improvement in tolerance to bright sunlight among the 16 patients with erythropoietic protoporphyria studied, but the results did not correlate with the concentration of porphyrin in the blood and faeces of these patients.— S. T. Zaynoun *et al.*, *Br. J. Derm.*, 1977, *97*, 663.

Carotenoids (betacarotene alone or combined with canthaxanthin) 50 to 150 mg daily by mouth were given to 23 patients with porphyria and 16 with various other photodermatoses. In 19 of 20 with erythropoietic protoporphyria good results were obtained but no improvement occurred in the other types of porphyria. Of the 16 with various photodermatoses only 6 responded to therapy. The only side-effect was a yellow discoloration of the skin.— G. Goerz and H. Ippen, *Dt. med. Wschr.*, 1977, *102*, 1051.

Further reports of protection: M. M. Mathews-Roth *et al.*, *New Engl. J. Med.*, 1970, *282*, 1231; T. B. Fitzpatrick *et al.*, *Proc. R. Soc. Med.*, 1971, *64*, 861; E. G. Jung, *Dt. med. Wschr.*, 1977, *102*, 279.

Sunburn. Betacarotene 180 mg by mouth daily for 10 weeks had a small but significant effect in increasing the minimal erythema dose of sunburn radiation compared with placebo in 30 male subjects. The effect was too small to be useful.— M. M. Mathews-Roth *et al.*, *J. invest. Derm.*, 1972, *59*, 349, per *J. Am. med. Ass.*, 1972, *222*, 1580.

Proprietary Names

Carotin *(Prosana, Austral.)*; Solatene *(Roche, Austral.; Roche, USA)*.

7825-t

Halibut-liver Oil *(B.P.)*. Oleum Jecoris Hippoglossi; Oleum Hippoglossi; Ol. Hippogloss.; Heilbuttleberöl; Aceite de Higado de Hipogloso.

CAS — 8001-46-5.

Pharmacopoeias. In *Aust., Br., Ger., Int., Mex.*, and *Swiss.* Some pharmacopoeias specify higher minima than the *B.P.* for vitamin A.

The refined fixed oil extracted from the fresh or suitably preserved liver of the halibut species belonging to the genus *Hippoglossus* (Pleuronectidae). It contains not less than 30 000 units of vitamin A activity per g. Halibut-liver oil may contain up to about 3000 units of vitamin D activity per g. Halibut-liver oil containing 30 000 units of vitamin A in 1 g contains approximately 5000 units in 0.2 ml.

A pale to golden-yellow liquid with a fishy but not rancid odour and taste. Wt per ml 0.915 to 0.925 g. Practically **insoluble** in alcohol; miscible with chloroform, ether, carbon disulphide, ethyl acetate, and light petroleum. **Store** in a cool place in well-filled airtight containers. Protect from light.

Halibut-liver oil is used as a means of administering vitamins A and D; the proportion of vitamin A to vitamin D is usually greater in halibut-liver oil than in cod-liver oil. It is usually given in capsules. Doses of about 0.2 ml daily are employed.

Eleven fishermen developed symptoms of vitamin A poisoning, characterised especially by generalised desquamation of the skin, after eating from 20 to 300 g of fried halibut-liver—an intake of about 2 to 30 million units of vitamin A.— J. P. Nater and H. M. G. Doeglas, *Acta derm.-vener., Stockh.*, 1970, *50*, 109, per *Trop. Dis. Bull.*, 1970, *67*, 1368.

Preparations

Halibut-liver Oil Capsules *(B.P.)*. Capsulae Olei Hippoglossi; Caps. Ol. Hippogloss. Flexible capsules containing halibut-liver oil diluted, if necessary, with a suitable fixed oil to a volume of 0.12 to 0.18 ml. Each capsule contains halibut-liver oil equivalent to about 4000 units of vitamin A activity. Vitamin D activity is also present. If stored at a temperature not exceeding 20° and protected from light, they may be expected to retain their potency for at least 3 years. *Dose.* 1 daily.

Halibut Oil Capsules *(Crookes Products, UK)*. Each contains vitamin A 4000 units and vitamin D 450 units.

Proprietary Names

Viton *(Asche, Ger.)*.

7826-x

Shark-liver Oil. The fixed oil extracted from the liver of various species of shark.

Pharmacopoeias. In *Chin.* and *Ind.*

The content of vitamin A is usually high while the content of vitamin D is low; shark-liver oil has therefore been used as a source of vitamin A.

7827-r

Preparations of Vitamins A and D

Concentrated Vitamins A and D Solution *(B.P.C. 1973)*. Conc. Vit. A and D Soln.; Liquor Vitaminorum A et D Concentratus; Liq. Vitamin. A et D Conc. A fish-liver oil or blend of fish-liver oils, or a solution of sources of vitamins A and D in a vegetable oil such as arachis oil, containing vitamin A 50 000 units and vitamin D 5000 units in 1 g.

A pale yellow or yellow oily liquid with a faint but not rancid odour and a bland or slightly fishy taste. Very slightly **soluble** in alcohol; miscible with chloroform, ether, and light petroleum. **Store** in a cool place in well-filled airtight containers. Protect from light. *Dose.* 0.05 to 0.5 g or 0.06 to 0.6 ml. A similar preparation is contained in some pharmacopoeias.

Oleovitamin A and D *(U.S.P.)*. A solution of vitamin A and vitamin D in fish-liver oil or in an edible vegetable oil; the vitamin D is present as ergocalciferol or cholecalciferol, or from natural sources. Store in a dry place, preferably under an atmosphere of an inert gas, in airtight containers. Protect from light.

Oleovitamin A and D Capsules *(U.S.P.)*. Capsules containing oleovitamin A and D. Store in airtight containers in a dry place. Protect from light.

Vitamins A and D Capsules *(B.P.C. 1973)*. Each contains vitamin A 4000 units and vitamin D 400 units. The capsule shells may be coloured. Store in a cool place. Protect from light. *Dose.* prophylactic, 1 capsule daily; therapeutic, 2 capsules daily.

See also Cod-liver Oil, p.1661 and Halibut-liver Oil, p.1638.

Proprietary Preparations

Halycitrol Vitamin Emulsion *(Laboratories for Applied Biology, UK)*. Contains in each 5 ml vitamin A 4600 units and vitamin D 460 units. *Dose.* 5 ml daily.

Minadex *(Farley, UK)*. An orange-flavoured syrup containing in each 5 ml vitamin A 650 units, ergocalciferol 65 units, iron (as ferric ammonium citrate) 12 mg, calcium glycerophosphate 11.25 mg, potassium glycerophosphate 1.125 mg, manganese sulphate 500 μg, and copper sulphate 500 μg (suggested diluent, syrup). *Dose.* 10 ml thrice daily after meals; children, 5 ml twice or thrice daily.

Tonivitan A & D Syrup *(Medo Chemicals, UK)*. Contains in each 5 ml vitamin A 700 units, ergocalciferol 70 units, green ferric ammonium citrate 150 mg, calcium glycerophosphate 25 mg, manganese glycerophosphate 400 μg, and copper sulphate 400 μg. *Dose.* 10 ml thrice daily; children, 2.5 to 10 ml.

Vitlipid Adult *(KabiVitrum, UK)*. Emulsion containing in each ml vitamin A palmitate equivalent to vitamin A 250 units, ergocalciferol 12 units, and phytomenadione 15 μg, with fractionated soya oil, fractionated ovolecithin, and glycerol, available in ampoules of 10 ml. **Vitlipid Infant** is a similar emulsion containing in each ml vitamin A palmitate equivalent to vitamin A 333 units, ergocalciferol 100 units, and phytomenadione 50 μg, available in ampoules of 4 ml. For addition to Intralipid as a supplement in parenteral nutrition.

7828-f

Vitamin B_1

Thiamine is vitamin B_1 and is described below, together with a number of related compounds with similar activity.

7829-d

Thiamine Hydrochloride *(B.P., B.P. Vet., Eur. P., U.S.P.)*.

Aneurine Hydrochloride; Thiaminii Chloridum; Thiamini Hydrochloridum; Vitamin B_1; Aneurine Chloride Hydrochloride; Thiaminium Chloride. 3-(4-Amino-2-methylpyrimidin-5-ylmethyl)-5-(2-hydroxyethyl)-4-methylthiazolium chloride hydrochloride.
$C_{12}H_{17}ClN_4OS,HCl=337.3$.

CAS — 59-43-8 (thiamine); 67-03-8 (hydrochloride).

Pharmacopoeias. In all pharmacopoeias examined. ***Rus.*** also has the bromide (Thiamini Bromidum), $C_{12}H_{17}BrN_4OS,HBr,½H_2O = 435.2$. Some pharmacopoeias specify the monohydrate.

Thiamine is present in rice-polishings, liver, yeast, and pork; it is synthesised by intestinal bacteria, but it is not known whether it is absorbed from this site. It is also prepared synthetically.

Colourless crystals or white or almost white crystalline powder with a characteristic somewhat meat-like odour and a bitter taste. M.p. about 248° with decomposition.

Soluble 1 in 1 of water, 1 in 100 of alcohol, and 1 in 20 of glycerol; soluble in methyl alcohol; practically insoluble in acetone, dehydrated alcohol, and ether. A 2.5% solution in water has a pH of 2.7 to 3.3. A 4.24% w/v solution is iso-osmotic with serum. Solutions are **sterilised** by filtration; chlorbutol 0.5% w/v is a suitable bacteriostat. **Store** in airtight nonmetallic containers. Protect from light.

Sterile solutions of pH 4 or less lose activity only very slowly but neutral or alkaline solutions deteriorate rapidly, especially in contact with air. When exposed to air, the anhydrous material rapidly absorbs about 4% of water.

Incompatible with oxidising and reducing substances, mercuric chloride, iodides, carbonates, acetates, and ferric sulphate. Tannic acid, ferric ammonium citrate, and iodine produce brown precipitates. Destruction of thiamine hydrochloride in solution is accelerated by copper ions.

Preparations containing thiamine hydrochloride are usually incompatible with phenobarbitone sodium. Precipitation of phenobarbitone depends on the strength of the solution and of any alcohol present. Phenobarbitone sodium, being alkaline, may raise the pH of a thiamine solution and cause it to deteriorate rapidly.

The loss of thiamine from food during cooking is variable but may reach 50%.

An aqueous solution of thiamine hydrochloride iso-osmotic with serum (4.24%) caused 87% haemolysis of erythrocytes cultured in it for 45 minutes. The solution and the erythrocytes darkened in colour.— E. R. Hammarlund and K. Pedersen-Bjergaard, *J. pharm. Sci.*, 1961, *50*, 24.

Incompatibility. Thiamine was incompatible with riboflavine in aqueous solutions; trace precipitation of thiochrome or chloroflavin occurred.— T. J. Macek, *Am. J. Pharm.*, 1960, *132*, 433.

Thiamine was incompatible with benzylpenicillin.— M. A. Schwartz and F. H. Buckwalter, *Australas. J. Pharm.*, 1963, *44*, S86.

Thiamine or vitamin-B complex injections were incompatible with dextrose injections or additives containing metabisulphite. Loss of potency of thiamine increased with the concentration of metabisulphite and increased in pH above 3.— E. A. Parker *et al.*, *Abbott, Bull. parent. Drug Ass.*, 1967, *21*, 197.

Radiosensitivity. Multivitamin preparations of vitamins of the B group were relatively stable to ionising radiations. However, individual vitamins in solution were relatively radiosensitive.— P. A. Wills, *Australas. J. Pharm.*, 1963, *44*, S50.

Stability in preparations. Sodium sulphite, potassium metabisulphite, and sodium hydrosulphite accelerated the degradation of thiamine in solution.— S. Rigamonti, *Boll. chim.-farm.*, 1964, *103*, 358.

A further reference.— J. C. Sanders, *Pharm. Weekbl. Ned.*, 1968, *103*, 853.

Adverse Effects and Precautions. No untoward effects occur when thiamine is administered by mouth in amounts many times greater than the therapeutic dose. Anaphylactic reactions have occasionally been produced by injections of thiamine, given alone, and sudden death has been reported; this risk of anaphylactic shock increases with repeated administration by the parenteral route.

The main symptom of overdosage (more than 400 mg intravenously) was acute mental alertness without pressure of ideas; this lasted for a few hours. After several days of injections, subacute symptoms were lethargy, somnolence, mild ataxia, heaviness in the limbs, and diminution of gut tone; relief was obtained in 48 hours if thiamine hydrochloride was withheld. Chronic symptoms were milder versions of the subacute ones with nausea and lack of appetite and an obvious smell of thiamine in newly washed skin and in the excreta. Relief occurred within 72 hours by omitting the vitamin.— J. Gould, *Proc. R. Soc. Med.*, 1954, *47*, 217.

For the effect of large doses of thiamine on some estimations of blood-theophylline concentrations, see Aminophylline, p.343.

Allergy. Thiamine hydrochloride given on its own by intravenous injection was liable to induce allergic reactions. This risk was negligible if the injection was given with other vitamins of the B group, even when doses as large as 100 mg of thiamine hydrochloride were given.— N. T. Pollitt (letter), *J. Am. med. Ass.*, 1968, *203*, 153.

Death from anaphylactic shock in a woman aged about 30 years after receiving thiamine 125 mg by intramuscular injection.— E. S. K. Assem, *Practitioner*, 1973, *211*, 565.

Absorption and Fate. Thiamine is absorbed from the gastro-intestinal tract and is widely distributed to most body tissues. It is not stored to any appreciable extent in the body and amounts in excess of the body's requirements are excreted in the urine as unchanged thiamine or as metabolites. About 1 mg of thiamine is metabolised in the body daily.

Human Requirements. Since thiamine is not stored in the body and is rapidly lost from the tissues during short periods of deficiency, normal health cannot be maintained unless the diet regularly contains an adequate amount of the vitamin. The requirement is directly related to the carbohydrate intake and the metabolic-rate. A daily intake of 400 µg per 4200 kJ (1000 kcal) is recommended. The total requirement is increased during periods of active growth or heavy muscular work, during pregnancy and lactation, in pathological conditions such as fevers and hyperthyroidism, and in other conditions causing increased metabolism or diuresis.

Thiamine deficiency commonly occurs in association with deficiency of other vitamins, especially in severe malnutrition.

The basic recommended intake of thiamine was 400 µg per 4200 kJ (1000 kcal) of diet, so that men required 1.3 mg of thiamine and women required 900 µg daily.— Report of a Joint FAO/WHO Expert Group, *Tech. Rep. Ser. Wld Hlth Org. No. 362*, 1967.

Recommended daily intake of thiamine: boys and girls up to 8 years of age, 300 to 800 µg; boys 9 to 17 years, 0.9 to 1.2 mg; girls 9 to 17 years, 800 to 900 µg; men 18 to 64 years, 1 to 1.3 mg; over 65 years, 0.9 to 1 mg; women over 18 years, 0.7 to 1 mg; during pregnancy, 1 mg; during lactation, 1.1 mg.— Recommended Daily Amounts of Food Energy and Nutrients for Groups of People in the United Kingdom, Report by the Committee on Medical Aspects of Food Policy, *Report on Health and Social Subjects No. 15*, London, HM Stationery Office, 1979.

Recommended daily dietary allowance of thiamine: up to 6 months, 0.3 mg; 6 to 12 months, 0.5 mg; 1 to 3 years, 0.7 mg; 4 to 6 years, 0.9 mg; 7 to 10 years and males 51 years and over, 1.2 mg; males 11 to 18 years, and 23 to 50 years, 1.4 mg; males 19 to 22 years, 1.5 mg; females 11 to 22 years, 1.1 mg; females 23 years and over, 1 mg; in pregnancy, an additional 0.4 mg; in lactation, an additional 0.5 mg.— *Recommended Dietary Allowances*, 9th Edn, Washington, The National Research Council, 1980.

The recommendation that foods for the young infant should contain thiamine in amounts not less than 130 ng per ml (based on the lower limit of the range in pooled samples of human milk).— Artificial Feeds for the Young Infant: Report of the Working Party on the Composition of Foods for Infants and Young Children, Committee on Medical Aspects of Food Policy, *Report on Health and Social Subjects, 18*, London, HM Stationery Office, 1980.

Pregnancy and the neonate. Brief discussion of a possible association between Down's syndrome and maternal thiamine deficiency.— C. Reading (letter), *Med. J. Aust.*, 1976, *1*, 505.

Uses. Thiamine is fundamentally associated with carbohydrate metabolism. By combining with the pyrophosphoric acid in nucleated cells, particularly in the liver, kidneys, and white blood-cells, it is converted in the body to its pyrophosphate (cocarboxylase) which acts as a coenzyme in such reactions as the decarboxylation of α-keto acids, particularly of pyruvate and α-ketoglutarate. In the presence of thiamine deficiency pyruvic and lactic acids accumulate in the tissues. Thiamine pyrophosphate also acts as a coenzyme in the direct oxidative pathway of glucose metabolism.

The use of thiamine hydrochloride is indicated only in conditions in which there is a known, or assumed, deficiency. The outstanding example of its effective use is in the treatment of beri-beri, in which there is a gross deficiency not only of thiamine but of other factors of the vitamin-B group.

Deficiency of thiamine results in fatigue, anorexia, gastro-intestinal disturbances, tachycardia, irritability, and neurological symptoms, and where there is reason to assume that this syndrome may be of dietary origin thiamine may be usefully employed. It may also be employed with benefit as a supplement to the diet in conditions in which thiamine deficiency may be caused by interference with its ingestion, absorption, and utilisation, or by increasing its destruction or excretion.

Wernicke's encephalopathy associated with beri-beri or alcoholism responds to treatment with thiamine.

There is some evidence that neuritis associated with pregnancy and the neuritis of pellagra are attributable to thiamine deficiency and will therefore benefit from thiamine hydrochloride added to the diet. Claims for its value in the treatment of other types of neuritis not associated with a vitamin-B deficiency in the diet are unfounded.

Thiamine hydrochloride is usually given by mouth; parenteral administration is unnecessary except in patients with impaired absorption or cardiac failure in beri-beri. The usual therapeutic dose is 10 to 100 mg daily by mouth or, if necessary, by intramuscular injection. In severe deficiency states up to 600 mg has been given daily. The usual prophylactic dose is 2 to 5 mg daily.

Deficiency states. A patient with lactic acidosis in alcoholic beri-beri responded to treatment with thiamine.— C. L. H. Majoor, *J.R. Coll. Physns*, 1978, *12*, 143. See also K. Thirunavukkarasu, *Med. J. Aust.*, 1979, *2*, 583.

Dialysis. A depletion syndrome could appear during long-term dialysis.— *Br. med. J.*, 1969, *2*, 778.

Treatment of dialysis dementia with thiamine.— J. L. James *et al.*, *Neurology, Minneap.*, 1976, *26*, 391.

Wernicke's encephalopathy. This was usually associated with chronic malnutrition and was secondary to alcoholism, gastro-intestinal disorders, or pernicious vomiting of pregnancy. Most of the clinical features (nystagmus, ophthalmoplegia, ataxia, and mental confusion) could be reversed by thiamine.— J. Yudkin, *Practitioner*, 1959, *182*, 30.

All chronic alcoholics should receive maintenance thiamine. Thiamine was urgently needed by patients with

Wernicke's encephalopathy.— *Drug & Ther. Bull.*, 1973, *11*, 85. Wernicke's encephalopathy is treatable, and preventable, with high doses of thiamine.— *Lancet*, 1979, *1*, 1122.

Reports of Wernicke's encephalopathy in 6 patients receiving adequate amounts of thiamine during parenteral nutrition.— D. Lonsdale (letter), *J. Am. med. Ass.*, 1978, *239*, 1133.

A suggestion for the fortification of alcoholic drinks with thiamine to prevent the development of the Wernicke-Korsakoff syndrome in alcoholics. Studies into safety, stability, and effect on flavour of such additions were necessary.— B. S. Centerwall and M. H. Criqui, *New Engl. J. Med.*, 1978, *299*, 285. Studies suggested no problems of stability, safety, or adverse effect on flavour.— J. Price and M. T. Theodoros (letter), *Med. J. Aust.*, 1979, *1*, 285.

Insect repellent. More than 70% of 100 insect-sensitive patients, when taking thiamine hydrochloride 75 to 150 mg daily, reported that insects bothered them little or not at all.— *Med. Lett.*, 1968, *10*, 55. Two reported studies had not demonstrated any protective effect.— D. E. Weidhaas (letter), *J. Am. med. Ass.*, 1977, *237*, 2114.

Metabolic disorders. Thiamine hydrochloride 10 mg daily corrected hyperaminoacidaemia in a new form of maple-syrup-urine disease. This was an example of vitamin-responsive hereditary metabolic disease.— C. R. Scriver *et al.*, *Lancet*, 1971, *1*, 310.

Preparations

Blockley Cocktail. An injection, 'Blockley cocktail', containing 50 ml of dextrose 50%, 5 units of soluble insulin, and 2 ml of vitamin B complex or thiamine 100 mg was mixed in a large syringe and administered by slow intravenous injection in the treatment of the acute alcoholic.—P.E. Farrell, *J. Am. med. Ass.*, 1968, *204*, 641.

Thiamine Hydrochloride Injection *(B.P.)*. Thiamine Hydrochlor. Inj.; Thiamine Injection; Aneurine Hydrochloride Injection; Vitamin B_1 Injection. A sterile solution in Water for Injections. Sterilised by filtration. pH 2.8 to 3.4. Protect from light.

Thiamine Hydrochloride Injection *(U.S.P.)*. A sterile solution of thiamine hydrochloride in Water for Injections. pH 2.5 to 4.5. Protect from light.

Thiamine Hydrochloride Tablets *(B.P.)*. Thiamine Hydrochlor. Tab.; Vitamin B_1 Tablets. Tablets containing thiamine hydrochloride. Avoid contact with metals. Protect from light.

Thiamine Hydrochloride Tablets *(U.S.P.)*. Tablets containing thiamine hydrochloride. Store in airtight containers. Protect from light.

Proprietary Preparations

Aneurone *(Philip Harris, UK)*. Mixture containing in each 10 ml thiamine hydrochloride 1 mg, strychnine hydrochloride 500 µg, caffeine 30 mg, sodium acid phosphate 60 mg, and compound gentian infusion 2.5 ml (suggested diluent, syrup). *Dose.* 5 to 10 ml thrice daily before meals; children, 2.5 to 5 ml.

Benerva *(Roche, UK)*. Thiamine hydrochloride, available as 1-ml **Ampoules** of injection containing 25 or 100 mg per ml and as **Tablets** of 3, 10, 25, 50, 100, and 300 mg. (Also available as Benerva in *Arg., Belg., Denm., Fr., Ger., Ital., Spain, Swed., Switz.*).

Other Proprietary Names

Austral.—Betamin, Beta-Sol, Bewon, Invite B_1, Juvabe '300' (see also under Thiamine Mononitrate); *Belg.*—Aneurol, Benavit, Beneurol 300, Benol, Betamine; *Canad.*—Betaxin, Bewon, Megamin; *Fr.*—Bévitine; *Ger.*—Betabion; *Ital.*—Aberil, Betabion, Betar, Bisolvit, Farmobion B_1; *Spain*—Bemarr Fortisimo, Betabion, Dextamina B_1, Extraneurina (as monophosphate), Lifaton B_1, Trifosfaneurina (phosphoric esters), Vitantial; *Switz.*—Vitaneurin; *USA*—Betalin S.

7830-c

Thiamine Mononitrate *(U.S.P.)*. Aneurine Mononitrate; Thiamine Nitrate; Vitamin B_1 Mononitrate. 3-(4-Amino-2-methylpyrimidin-5-ylmethyl)-5-(2-hydroxyethyl)-4-methylthiazolium nitrate.
$C_{12}H_{17}N_5O_4S$=327.4.

CAS — 532-43-4.

Pharmacopoeias. In *Braz., Ger., Ind., Jap.*, and *U.S.*

White crystals or crystalline powder with a slight characteristic odour. M.p. about 193° with decomposition. **Soluble** 1 in 44 of water; slightly soluble in alcohol and chloroform. A 2% solution in water has a pH of 6 to 7.5. **Store** in airtight containers. Protect from light.

Uses. Thiamine mononitrate has actions and uses similar to those of thiamine hydrochloride.

Proprietary Names
B_1-Vicotrat *(Heyl, Ger.)*; Dagravit B_1 Retard *(Dagra, Belg.; Medinsa, Spain)*; Juvabe '300' (see also under Thiamine Hydrochloride) *(Cambridge Laboratories, Austral.)*.

7831-k

Benfotiamine. *S*-Benzoylthiamine *O*-Monophosphate. *N*-(4-Amino-2-methylpyrimidin-5-ylmethyl)-*N*-(2-benzoylthio-4-dihydroxyphosphinyloxy-1-methylbut-1-enyl)formamide.
$C_{19}H_{23}N_4O_6PS$=466.6.

CAS — 22457-89-2.

A white odourless crystalline powder with a slightly bitter taste. M.p. about 200° with decomposition. Slightly **soluble** in water, alcohol, and chloroform; soluble in solutions of sodium hydroxide, sodium carbonate, and hydrochloric acid.

Uses. Benfotiamine has the actions and uses of thiamine hydrochloride (see p.1639). It has been given in doses of up to 600 mg daily.

Proprietary Names
Berdi *(Elea, Arg.)*; Neuroluy Retard *(Miluy, Spain)*; Neurostop *(Lacer, Spain)*; Tabiomyl *(Roussel, Belg.)*; Vitanévril *(Porcher-Lavril, Fr.)*.

7832-a

Bisbentiamine. *O*-Benzoylthiamine Disulphide. *NN'*-{Dithiobis[2-(2-benzoyloxyethyl)-1-methylvinylene]}bis-[*N*-(4-amino-2-methylpyrimidin-5-ylmethyl)formamide].
$C_{38}H_{42}N_8O_6S_2$=771.0.

CAS — 2667-89-2.

Uses. Bisbentiamine has the actions and uses of thiamine hydrochloride (see p.1639). It has been given in doses of up to 150 mg daily.

Short review.— *Japan med. Gaz.*, 1975, *12* (Feb. 20), 18.

Proprietary Names
Beston (see also under Bisbutiamine) *(Triosol, Belg.; Jap.)*; Bithiamin *(Jap.)*; Supra B_1 *(Esteve, Spain)*.

7833-t

Bisbutiamine. *O*-Butyrylthiamine Disulphide. *NN'*-{Dithiobis[2-(2-butyryloxyethyl)-1-methylvinylene]}bis-[*N*-(4-amino-2-methylpyrimidin-5-ylmethyl)formamide].
$C_{32}H_{46}N_8O_6S_2$=702.9.

CAS — 18481-23-7.

Uses. Bisbutiamine has the actions and uses of thiamine hydrochloride (see p.1639). It has been given in doses of up to 100 mg daily, by subcutaneous, intramuscular, or intravenous injection.

Proprietary Names
Beston (see also under Bisbentiamine)*(Jap.)*.

7834-x

Bisibutiamine. *O*-Isobutyrylthiamine Disulphide. *NN'*-{Dithiobis[2-(2-isobutyryloxyethyl)-1-methylvinylene]}bis[*N*-(4-amino-2-methylpyrimidin-5-ylmethyl)formamide].
$C_{32}H_{46}N_8O_6S_2$=702.9.

CAS — 3286-46-2.

Uses. Bisibutiamine has the actions and uses of thiamine hydrochloride (see p.1639). It has been given in doses of up to 100 mg daily.

Proprietary Names
Arcalion *(Servier, Spain)*; Neodaian *(Jap.)*; Vitaberin *(Jap.)*.

7835-r

Cetotiamine Hydrochloride. DCET; Dicethiam Hydrochloride; *O,S*-Bis(ethoxycarbonyl)thiamine Hydrochloride. *N*-(4-Amino-2-methylpyrimidin-5-ylmethyl)-*N*-[4-(ethoxycarbonyloxy)-2-(ethoxycarbonylthio)-1-methylbut-1-enyl]formamide hydrochloride.
$C_{18}H_{26}N_4O_6S,HCl$=562.9.

CAS — 137-76-8 (cetotiamine); 616-96-6 (hydrochloride).

Colourless odourless crystals. M.p. about 120°. Freely **soluble** in water, chloroform, and methyl alcohol; practically insoluble in ether.

Uses. Cetotiamine has the actions and uses of thiamine hydrochloride (see p.1639). It has been given in doses of up to 100 mg daily.

Proprietary Names
Dicetamin *(Jap.)*.

7836-f

Cocarboxylase. Diphosphothiamine; Thiamine Pyrophosphate. 3-(4-Amino-2-methylpyrimidin-5-ylmethyl)-5-{2-[dihydroxyphosphinyloxy(hydroxy)phosphinyloxy]-ethyl}-4-methylthiazolium hydroxide.
$C_{12}H_{20}N_4O_8P_2S$ (hydroxide form)=442.3.

CAS — 154-87-0 (chloride form).

A form of thiamine found in the body.

Proprietary Names
B-Carbossilasi *(Cif, Ital.)*; Berolase *(Roche, Belg.; Roche, Ger.; Roche, Ital.; Roche, Switz.)*; Bester *(Salvat, Spain)*; Bioxilasi *(Zyma, Ital.)*; Bivitasi *(ISI, Ital.)*; Co-B_1 *(Bruco, Ital.)*; Cocarbasi *(Zarri, Ital.)*; Cocarbil *(UCB-Pevya, Spain)*; Co-Carbox *(Wassermann, Spain)*; Cocarvit *(CT, Ital.)*; Co-Enzyme B *(Inwood, USA)*; Coneurina *(SIRT-BBP, Ital.)*; Magnesiocarbina (as magnesium salt) *(FIRMA, Ital.)*; Pirofosfasi *(Mitim, Ital.)*; Vitaendil Cocarboxilasa 500 *(Boizot, Spain)*; Bicholase, Cocalose, Cocarbose, Paraboramin, Proffit (all *Jap.)*.

7837-d

Cycotiamine. Cyclocarbothiamine. *N*-(4-Amino-2-methylpyrimidin-5-ylmethyl)-*N*-[1-(2-oxo-1,3-oxathian-4-ylidene)ethyl]formamide.
$C_{13}H_{16}N_4O_3S$=308.4.

CAS — 6092-18-8.

White to yellowish-white, almost odourless, crystalline powder. Slightly **soluble** in water and alcohol. The hydrochloride is very soluble in water and soluble in alcohol.

Uses. Cycotiamine has the actions and uses of thiamine hydrochloride (see p.1639). It has been given in doses of up to 100 mg daily or up to 100 mg of the hydrochloride daily by subcutaneous, intramuscular, or intravenous injection.

Proprietary Names
Cometamin *(Jap.)*.

7838-n

Fursultiamine. Thiamine Tetrahydrofurfuryl Disulphide; TTFD. *N*-(4-Amino-2-methylpyrimidin-5-ylmethyl)-*N*-[4-hydroxy-1-methyl-2-(tetrahydrofurfuryldithio)but-1-enyl]formamide.
$C_{17}H_{26}N_4O_3S_2$=398.5.

CAS — 804-30-8.

A white or pale yellow crystalline powder. M.p. about 130° with decomposition. Slightly **soluble** in water; soluble in acetone and alcohol.

Uses. Fursultiamine has the actions and uses of thiamine hydrochloride (see p.1639). It has been given in doses of up to 100 mg daily, by mouth, or by subcutaneous, intramuscular, or intravenous injection.

It has also been used in the treatment of children with subacute necrotising encephalopathy (Leigh's disease).

Use in the Wernicke-Korsakoff syndrome.— J. P. Blass and G. E. Gibson, *New Engl. J. Med.*, 1977, *297*, 1367.

Proprietary Names
Alinamin-F *(Jap.)*; Judolor *(Woelm, Ger.; Woelm, Switz.)*.

7839-h

Octotiamine. Thioctothiamine. *N*-[2-(3-Acetylthio-7-methoxycarbonylheptyldithio)-4-hydroxy-1-methylbut-1-enyl]-*N*-(4-amino-2-methylpyrimidin-5-ylmethyl)formamide.

$C_{23}H_{36}N_4O_5S_3$=544.7.

CAS — 137-86-0.

A white crystalline solid with a slightly bitter taste.

Uses. Octotiamine has the actions and uses of thiamine hydrochloride (see p.1639).

Proprietary Names

Neuvita *(Jap.)*.

7840-a

Dried Yeast *(B.P.C. 1973)*.

Cerevisiae Fermentum Siccatum; Faex Siccata; Saccharomyces Siccum; Levure de Bière; Trockenhefe; Levedura Sêca; Fermento de Cerveja.

Pharmacopoeias. In *Aust., Braz., Chin., Cz., Jap., Mex., Port., Spain,* and *Swiss.*

Unicellular fungi belonging to the family Saccharomycetaceae, dried by a process which avoids decomposition of the vitamins present. The chief species are *Saccharomyces cerevisiae, S. carlsbergensis,* and *S. monacensis.* Yeast is obtained as a by-product in the manufacture of spirits, or as the sole product of yeast factories.

It is a buff or brownish-buff, somewhat granular powder with a characteristic odour and not excessively bitter characteristic taste. It contains in 1 g not less than 100 µg of thiamine, calculated as the hydrochloride, not less than 300 µg of nicotinic acid, and not less than 40 µg of riboflavine; it also contains pyridoxine, pantothenic acid, biotin, folic acid, vitamin B_{12}, aminobenzoic acid, and inositol. It contains about 46% of proteins, some of which are combined with nucleic acid to form nucleins and nucleoproteins, about 36% of carbohydrates, and a number of enzymes, including zymase, invertase, and maltase. **Store** in airtight containers.

Uses. Dried yeast is used for the prevention and treatment of vitamin-B deficiency. As a dietary supplement it has been given in the following doses: infants, 1 to 2.5 g daily in milk; children, 4 to 6 g; and adults, 6 to 8 g. In conditions of severe vitamin-B deficiency, such as beri-beri, pellagra, or ariboflavinosis, adults may be given doses up to 30 g daily. It may be administered as tablets or as powder; proprietary yeast extracts are also available.

There was no evidence that yeast was of value in multiple sclerosis.— *Br. med. J.*, 1979, *1,* 666.

Preparations

Yeast Tablets *(B.P.C. 1973).* Tabellae Cerevisiae Fermenti; Dried Yeast Tablets. Tablets containing dried yeast. Store in airtight containers.

Proprietary Preparations

DCL Vitamin B_1 Yeast *(Distillers Co., UK).* A pure-culture yeast containing in each g thiamine hydrochloride 1 mg, riboflavine 40 µg, and nicotinic acid 300 µg, available as tablets of 300 mg. *Dose.* 6 to 12 tablets daily.

Grandilase *(Keimdiät, Ger.: Thomson & Joseph, UK).* A vitamin-B concentrate prepared from yeast and rice bran. It contains 150 mg of thiamine hydrochloride per 100 g, with riboflavine, pyridoxine hydrochloride, and nicotinic acid. For use as a pharmaceutical and dietary additive.

Marmite *(Bovril, UK).* A concentrated yeast extract prepared by autolysis with salt and flavoured with vegetables and spices; it contains sodium 46.4 mg (2 mmol), riboflavine 53 µg, and nicotinic acid 581 µg per g.

Proper-Myl Injection *(Consolidated Chemicals, UK).* Ampoules each stated to contain 10 million irradiated lyophilised yeast cells, prepared from selected yeast strains, together with 5 ml of solvent.

Other Proprietary Names

Perenterol *(Ger.)*; Ultra-Levure *(Switz.)*.

A preparation containing dried yeast was also formerly marketed in Great Britain under the proprietary name Mycolactine (*Wilcox*).

7841-t

Vitamin B_2

Riboflavine is vitamin B_2 and is described below together with riboflavine derivatives.

7842-x

Riboflavine *(B.P., B.P. Vet., Eur. P.)*.

Riboflav.; Lactoflavin; Riboflavin *(U.S.P.)*; Riboflavinum; Vitamin B_2; Vitamin G. 7,8-Dimethyl-10-(1-D-ribityl)isoalloxazine; 3,10-Dihydro-7,8-dimethyl-10-(D-*ribo*-2,3,4,5-tetrahydroxypentyl)benzopteridine-2,4-dione.

$C_{17}H_{20}N_4O_6$=376.4.

CAS — 83-88-5.

Pharmacopoeias. In all pharmacopoeias examined.

A yellow or orange-yellow crystalline powder with a slight odour and a persistent bitter taste, obtained from yeast or other natural sources or prepared synthetically. M.p. about 280° with decomposition.

Soluble 1 in 3000 to 1 in 20 000 of water, the variation in solubility being due to the variation in the internal crystalline structure; more soluble in physiological saline and in 10% urea solution; practically insoluble in alcohol, acetone, chloroform, and ether; very soluble in dilute solutions of alkali hydroxides. A solution in hydrochloric acid is dextrorotatory. A saturated solution in water has a pH of 5.5 to 7.2. Solutions are **sterilised** by autoclaving or by filtration.

Incompatible with alkalis and salts of heavy metals. **Store** in airtight containers. Protect from light. When dry it is not appreciably affected by diffused light, but in solution, especially in the presence of alkali, it deteriorates rapidly, the decomposition being accelerated by light.

Liver, kidney, eggs, milk, yeast, and green vegetables are considered the richest dietary sources. There is little loss of riboflavine from these foods during cooking. It is also synthesised by bacteria in the large intestine but it is unlikely to be absorbed from this site.

Inactivation of antibiotics. Riboflavine reduced the antibacterial activity of solutions of streptomycin, erythromycin, tyrothricin, carbomycin, and tetracyclines. At least in the case of tetracycline the reaction was a photochemical oxidation. No inactivation occurred with chloramphenicol, penicillin, or neomycin.— J. Dony-Crotteux, *J. Pharm. Belg.*, 1957, *12,* 179, per *Can. pharm. J.*, 1958, *91,* 224. See also L. J. Leeson and J. F. Weidenheimer, *J. pharm. Sci.*, 1969, *58,* 355 (tetracycline); J. Dony and M. J. Devleeschouwer, *J. Pharm. Belg.*, 1976, *31,* 479 (macrolides).

Absorption and Fate. Riboflavine is absorbed from the gastro-intestinal tract, and in the circulation it is bound to plasma proteins. Although riboflavine is widely distributed little is stored in the body, and amounts in excess of the body's requirements are excreted in the urine. Riboflavine in the faeces is probably the product of intestinal micro-organisms.

Riboflavine is converted in the body to flavine mononucleotide (FMN) and then to flavine adenine dinucleotide (FAD).

Patients with hepatitis and cirrhosis of the liver, and those given probenecid, had reduced absorption of riboflavine.— P. S. Rivlin, *New Engl. J. Med.*, 1970, *283,* 463.

Renal clearance of riboflavine involved renal tubular secretion and exceeded endogenous creatinine clearance by up to 3 times. Clearance was reduced at low serum concentrations of riboflavine. Riboflavine was 60% bound to serum protein. Prior administration of probenecid decreased the renal clearance of riboflavine but did not affect its protein binding.— W. J. Jusko *et al., J. pharm. Sci.*, 1970, *59,* 473.

Riboflavine caused discoloration of the urine.— R. B. Baran and B. Rowles, *J. Am. pharm. Ass.*, 1973, *NS13,* 139.

A review, chiefly from *animal* studies, of the effects of hormones and drugs on riboflavine. Thyroid hormones, corticotrophin, and aldosterone enhanced the formation of FMN and FAD, while phenothiazines and possibly tricyclic antidepressants inhibited FAD formation. Boric acid increased the excretion of riboflavine.— R. S. Rivlin, *Nutr. Rev.*, 1979, *37,* 241.

Human Requirements. The riboflavine requirement is often related to the energy intake but it appears to be more closely related to resting metabolic requirements. The normal adult requires about 1.3 to 1.8 mg daily. Requirements are increased during pregnancy and lactation.

The basic recommended intake of riboflavine was 550 µg per 4200 kJ (1000 kcal) of diet, so that men required 1.8 mg of riboflavine and women required 1.3 mg of riboflavine.— Report of a Joint FAO/WHO Expert Group, *Tech. Rep. Ser. Wld Hlth Org. No. 362,* 1967.

In a nutrition survey of elderly subjects aged 65 or over, 57 of 778 had angular stomatitis and cheilosis and a riboflavine intake of 1.2 mg a day compared with 1.3 mg for those without lip lesions; 4 of 23 subjects with a riboflavine intake of less than 700 µg daily for men or less than 550 µg daily for women had lip lesions.— Report by the Panel on Nutrition of the Elderly, *A Nutrition Survey of the Elderly,* London, HM Stationery Office, 1972.

Recommended daily intake of riboflavine calculated on resting metabolism: boys and girls up to 8 years of age, 0.4 to 1 mg; boys and girls 9 to 17 years, 1.2 to 1.7 mg; men over 17 years, 1.6 mg; women over 17 years, 1.3 mg; during pregnancy, 1.6 mg; during lactation 1.8 mg.— Recommended Daily Amounts of Food Energy and Nutrients for Groups of People in the United Kingdom, Report by the Committee on Medical Aspects of Food Policy, *Report on Health and Social Subjects No. 15,* London, HM Stationery Office, 1979.

Recommended daily dietary allowance for riboflavine: up to 6 months, 0.4 mg; 6 to 12 months, 0.6 mg; 1 to 3 years, 0.8 mg; 4 to 6 years, 1 mg; 7 to 10 years, 1.4 mg; males 11 to 14 years and 23 to 50 years, 1.6 mg; males 15 to 22 years, 1.7 mg; males 51 years and over, 1.4 mg; females 11 to 22 years, 1.3 mg; 23 years and over, 1.2 mg; in pregnancy, an additional 0.3 mg; in lactation, an additional 0.5 mg.— *Recommended Dietary Allowances,* 9th Edn, Washington, The National Research Council, 1980.

The recommendation that foods for the young infant should contain riboflavine in amounts not less than 300 ng per ml (based on the lower limit of the range in pooled samples of human milk).— Artificial Feeds for the Young Infant: Report of the Working Party on the Composition of Foods for Infants and Young Children, Committee on Medical Aspects of Food Policy, *Report on Health and Social Subjects, 18,* London, HM Stationery Office, 1980.

Uses. Riboflavine is inactive until phosphorylated; flavine mononucleotide and flavine adenine dinucleotide are its active forms and these are involved as coenzymes in the respiratory chain and in oxidative phosphorylation.

Riboflavine deficiency in man is characterised by a well-defined syndrome, the features of which are angular stomatitis, glossitis, reddened, shiny, and denuded lips, seborrhoeic follicular keratosis of the nasolabial folds, nose, and forehead, dermatitis of the ano-genital region, and 'burning feet'. Certain ocular manifestations, such as itching and burning of the eyes, photophobia, and corneal vascularisation, are seen in a large proportion but not in all cases. There is little evidence that riboflavine is of therapeutic value except in the treatment of ariboflavinosis, for which doses of 2 to 10 mg daily are given according to the severity of the condition. It is usually administered by mouth but it may be injected if for any reason it cannot be absorbed or utilised by the oral route.

See also Riboflavine Sodium Phosphate.

Riboflavine is a permitted colouring agent for food.

Since riboflavine could be easily detected in the urine by fluorescence in a narrow beam of light, incorporation of riboflavine 2.5 mg within a tablet could enable detection of patients who took medications irregularly.— I. H. Jones, *Med. J. Aust.*, 1967, *1*, 202.

Estimated acceptable daily intake of riboflavine: up to 500 µg per kg body-weight.— Thirteenth Report of FAO/WHO Expert Committee on Food Additives, *Tech. Rep. Ser. Wld Hlth Org. No. 445*, 1971.

Riboflavine might have a beneficial effect in patients with transfusion-dependent β-thalassaemia who had a reduced red-cell conversion-rate of pyridoxine to pyridoxal.— B. B. Anderson *et al.*, *Nature*, 1976, *264*, 574.

In view of the possible association between prolonged ascorbic acid administration and hyperoxaluria, a 33-year-old man and a 4-month-old infant with recessive congenital methaemoglobinaemia, were both successfully transferred from ascorbic acid therapy to riboflavine therapy. The maintenance doses of riboflavine of 30 mg daily and 20 mg daily respectively, depressed methaemoglobin concentrations to about 5%.— J. C. Kaplan and M. Chirouze (letter), *Lancet*, 1978, *2*, 1043.

Deficiency states. Details of ocular manifestations caused by deficiency of B-complex vitamins, particularly riboflavine, which included blepharo-conjunctivitis, epithelial keratitis, nutritional amblyopia, and possibly corneal vascularisation, night-blindness and general blindness.— G. Venkataswamy, *Br. J. Ophthal.*, 1967, *51*, 749.

Eight of 22 patients with cataracts had riboflavine deficiency. It was suggested that riboflavine might be of value in the prevention or regression of cataract.— J. T. Prchal *et al.*, *Lancet*, 1978, *1*, 12.

There was no valid evidence that medical treatment, including the use of vitamins, was of value in senile cataract.— *Br. med. J.*, 1978, *1*, 908.

Riboflavine deficiency in infants exposed to phototherapy did not appear to be harmful and attempts to provide supplementary riboflavine would probably be unwise.— *Lancet*, 1978, *1*, 1191.

Preparations

Riboflavin Injection *(U.S.P.)*. A sterile solution of riboflavine in Water for Injections. It may contain nicotinamide or other suitable solubilising agents. pH 4.5 to 7. Protect from light.

Riboflavin Tablets *(U.S.P.)*. Tablets containing riboflavine. Store in airtight containers. Protect from light.

Riboflavine Tablets *(B.P.C. 1973)*. They may be coated and coloured. Store in airtight containers. Protect from light.

Proprietary Names

Beflavin *(Roche, Ger.)*; Beflavina *(Roche, Ital.)*; Beflavine *(Roche, Belg.*; *Roche, Fr.)*; Berivine *(Meuse, Belg.)*.

Riboflavine was formerly marketed in Great Britain under the proprietary name Beflavit (*Roche*).

7843-r

Riboflavine Sodium Phosphate *(B.P.)*. Riboflavine Phosphate (Sodium Salt); Natrii Riboflavinophosphas; Riboflavine Phosphate; Vitamin B_2 Phosphate; Riboflavine 5′-Phosphate Sodium. The dihydrate of the sodium salt of riboflavine 5′-phosphate.
$C_{17}H_{20}N_4NaO_9P,2H_2O=514.4$.

CAS — 130-40-5 (anhydrous).

Pharmacopoeias. In *Br.* and *Nord. Jap.* specifies the anhydrous salt.

A yellow to orange-yellow, odourless or almost odourless, crystalline hygroscopic powder with a slightly bitter taste. Riboflavine sodium phosphate 1.37 g is approximately equivalent to 1 g of riboflavine. **Soluble** 1 in 20 of water; very slightly soluble in alcohol; practically insoluble in chloroform and ether. A solution in 5 M hydrochloric acid is dextrorotatory. A 2% solution in water has a pH of 4 to 6.3. Solutions are **sterilised** by autoclaving at a pH not above 6, by heating with a bactericide at 98° to 100° for 30 minutes, or by filtration. **Store** in airtight containers. Protect from light.

Uses. Riboflavine sodium phosphate has actions similar to those of riboflavine and is used for the preparation of injections as solutions are readily prepared. It is a permitted food colour in Great Britain.

Riboflavine sodium phosphate had the same absorption and excretion characteristics as riboflavine. Administration after a meal enhanced absorption due to prolonged retention at the gastro-intestinal absorption sites. The phosphate was excreted in the urine as riboflavine. Enterohepatic cycling occurred.— W. J. Jusko and G. Levy, *J. pharm. Sci.*, 1967, *56*, 58.

Preparations

Injectabile Riboflavini *(Nord. P.)*. Riboflavine Injection. Riboflavine sodium phosphate (anhydrous) 640 mg (equivalent to 500 mg of riboflavine), citric acid monohydrate 60 mg, sodium chloride 850 mg, Water for Injections to 100 ml. Sterilised by autoclaving. Phenylmercuric nitrate 0.001% is a suitable preservative; *Dan. Disp.* specifies 0.1% methyl hydroxybenzoate.
Jap. P. also includes a similar injection.

Proprietary Names

Bisulase *(Jap.)*.

7844-f

Riboflavine Tetrabutyrate. Riboflavine Butyrate.
$C_{33}H_{44}N_4O_{10}=656.7$.

CAS — 752-56-7.

Orange-yellow crystals or crystalline powder. M.p. about 146°. Practically **insoluble** in water; soluble in acetone, alcohol, and chloroform, and in natural oils and fats.

Uses. Riboflavine tetrabutyrate has the properties of riboflavine (see p.1641). It is also claimed to facilitate the elimination of lipid peroxides and has been tried as a hypolipidaemic agent. For riboflavine deficiency the usual dose is up to 20 mg daily; in hyperlipidaemia it is 60 to 120 mg daily in 2 or 3 divided doses.

Proprietary Names

Liperox *(Byk Liprandi, Arg.)*; Multiscleran *(Boehringer Mannheim, Spain)*; Bisanorin, Bituvitan, Bonabon B_2, Butirid, Eyekas, Hibon, Ribobis, Ribobutin, Riboract, Wakaflavin-L *(all Jap.)*.

7845-d

Flavine Adenine Dinucleotide. FAD. Riboflavine 5′-(adenosine diphosphate).
$C_{27}H_{33}N_9O_{15}P_2=785.6$.

CAS — 146-14-5.

A yellow powder. Readily **soluble** in water; practically insoluble in alcohol.

Uses. Flavine adenine dinucleotide is an active form of riboflavine. It has been given by mouth in doses of 5 to 15 mg thrice daily, and has also been given by subcutaneous, intramuscular, and intravenous injection.

Proprietary Names

Adeflavin, B2-Elite-10, Fademin, Fladd, Flamitajin-B, Flanin F, Flavinin, Flavitan, Flaziren D, Hokurabin, Mohaflan, Wakedenin *(all Jap.)*.

7846-n

Vitamin B_6

Pyridoxine is vitamin B_6 and is described below together with pyridoxine derivatives.

7847-h

Pyridoxine Hydrochloride *(B.P., Eur. P., U.S.P.)*. Pyridox. Hydrochlor.; Pyridoxinii Chloridum; Pyridoxini Hydrochloridum; Pyridoxinium Chloride; Pyridoxol Hydrochloride; Vitamin B_6; Adermine Hydrochloride; Piridossina Cloridrato. 3-Hydroxy-4,5-bis(hydroxymethyl)-2-methylpyridine hydrochloride.
$C_8H_{11}NO_3,HCl=205.6$.

CAS — 65-23-6 (pyridoxine); 58-56-0 (hydrochloride).

NOTE. Pyridoxine is only one of 3 similar compounds that may be referred to as vitamin B_6; the other two are pyridoxal and pyridoxamine.

Pharmacopoeias. In *Arg., Aust., Belg., Br., Braz., Chin., Cz., Eur., Fr., Ger., Hung., Ind., Int., It., Jap., Jug., Neth., Nord., Port., Roum., Rus., Swiss, Turk.*, and *U.S.*

A white or almost white odourless crystalline powder, or crystals, with a slightly bitter saline taste. M.p. 202° to 206° with decomposition. **Soluble** 1 in 5 of water and 1 in 100 to 115 of alcohol; practically insoluble in acetone, chloroform, and ether. A 5% solution in water has a pH of 2.3 to 3.5. A 3.04% solution is iso-osmotic with serum. Solutions are **sterilised** by autoclaving or by filtration. **Store** in airtight containers. Protect from light.

Pyridoxine occurs in yeast, liver, cereals, meat, and many other foodstuffs, and is prepared synthetically.

Effect of gamma-irradiation. With irradiation of 30 000 Gy or less, pyridoxine and folic acid in aqueous solution were partially or totally destroyed depending on the irradiation dose and the pH of the solution. In the solid state, pyridoxine and folic acid lost hydrogen atoms on irradiation, but these were replaced when the irradiated samples were dissolved in acid solutions.— I. Galatzeanu and F. Antoni, *Radiosterilization of Medical Products*, Vienna, International Atomic Energy Agency, 1967, p. 33.

Incompatibility. Pyridoxine hydrochloride was stated to be incompatible with alkaline solutions, iron salts, and oxidising solutions.— W. Kramer *et al.*, *Drug Intell. & clin. Pharm.*, 1971, *5*, 211.

Precautions. Pyridoxine reduces the effects of levodopa (see p.884).

Deterioration in acne vulgaris or an acneform eruption was associated with pyridoxine or cyanocobalamin therapy in a study of 14 patients.— O. Braun-Falco and H. Lincke, *Münch. med. Wschr.*, 1976, *118*, 155, per *J. Am. med. Ass.*, 1976, *235*, 1387.

Pregnancy and the neonate. A recommendation that, since there was evidence that pyridoxine inhibits lactation, it should not be given to nursing mothers.— L. B. Greentree (letter), *New Engl. J. Med.*, 1979, *300*, 141. Criticism.— N. I. Lande (letter), *ibid.*, 926; R. S. Rivlin (letter), *ibid.*, 927; B. A. Underwood (letter), *ibid.*, *301*, 107. Pyridoxine failed to suppress lactation when 300 mg was given twice daily to 11 postpartum women, nor could prolactin-inhibitory properties be demonstrated in normal volunteers.— E. del Pozo and R. Brun del Re (letter), *ibid.*, 107. Similar negative reports.— H. N. MacDonald *et al.*, *Br. J. Obstet. Gynaec.*, 1976, *83*, 54; N. Husami *et al.*, *Fert. Steril.*, 1978, *30*, 393.

Absorption and Fate. Pyridoxine is absorbed from the gastro-intestinal tract and is converted to the active form pyridoxal phosphate. Pyridoxal and pyridoxamine are also absorbed and converted. It is excreted in the urine as 4-pyridoxic acid.

Pyridoxine was not bound to plasma proteins but its metabolites pyridoxal phosphate and pyridoxal were totally bound and partially bound respectively.— B. B. Anderson *et al.* (letter), *Nature*, 1974, *250*, 502.

Human Requirements. For adults, the daily requirement of pyridoxine is probably about 2 mg and this amount is present in most normal diets. Convulsions and hypochromic anaemia have occurred in infants deficient in pyridoxine and in adults deprived of the vitamin. Lesions of the skin and mouth resembling those of ariboflavinosis and nicotinic acid deficiency have been observed in adults deprived of pyridoxine. Peripheral neuritis has also occurred and the neuritis associated with isoniazid therapy may be due to pyridoxine deficiency, for further details, see Isoniazid (Treatment of Adverse Effects), p.1573.

Recommendations for allowances for vitamin B_6 are difficult to make since requirements increase as the protein content of the diet increases. A daily dietary allowance of 2.2 mg should be suitable for men and 2 mg for women; 300 µg daily should be suitable for infants up to 6 months and 600 µg for children from 6 months to 1 year. Older children can be given up to 2 mg daily. Pregnant women should generally take 2.6 mg daily and lactating women 2.5 mg. Supplementation with vitamin B_6 did not appear to be necessary in women taking oral contraceptives.— *Recommended Dietary Allowances*, 9th Edn, Washington, The National Research Council, 1980, p. 96.

The recommendation that foods for the young infant should contain pyridoxine hydrochloride in amounts not less than 50 ng per ml (based on the lower limit of the range in pooled samples of human milk).— Artificial Feeds for the Young Infant: Report of the Working Party on the Composition of Foods for Infants and Young Children, Committee on Medical Aspects of

Food Policy, *Report on Health and Social Subjects, 18*, London, HM Stationery Office, 1980.

Uses. Pyridoxine, pyridoxal, and pyridoxamine, which occur in foodstuffs, are collectively known as vitamin B_6. In the body they are converted to pyridoxal phosphate which is the coenzyme for a variety of metabolic transformations. Though, owing to the wide distribution of vitamin B_6 in nature, clinical deficiency symptoms are seldom observed, pyridoxine is essential in human nutrition. As a nutritional supplement it is usually employed in conjunction with other vitamins of the B group.

Pyridoxine hydrochloride is administered by mouth as tablets or by injection. For convulsions caused by pyridoxine deficiency in infants, the dosage is 4 mg per kg body-weight daily for short periods. For the treatment of anaemia induced by pyridoxine deficiency in an adult, the dosage is 50 to 150 mg daily in divided doses. Some types of megaloblastic anaemia possibly caused by pyridoxine deficiency have been treated with 100 to 200 mg daily. Large doses of pyridoxine are also given in the management of homocystinuria. A daily dose of 150 mg may be given as a prophylactic against peripheral neuritis in patients on isoniazid therapy; children may be given 25 to 50 mg daily. Pyridoxine hydrochloride has been used in doses ranging from 20 to 200 mg daily for the treatment of the nausea and vomiting of pregnancy and irradiation sickness but the evidence of its value in these conditions is not impressive.

Administration in renal failure. In chronic renal failure patients on low-protein diets were usually given pyridoxine 50 mg daily to ensure adequate protein metabolism.— *Drug & Ther. Bull.*, 1978, *16*, 61.

Deficiency states. Pyridoxine dependency, an uncommon and, probably, hereditary disorder of neonates, produced a typical clinical syndrome of meconium staining and respiratory distress at birth, followed 3 to 7 hours later by hyperirritability, rolling eyes, grimacing, intermittent apnoea, and generalised tonic-clonic convulsions. After treatment with pyridoxine hydrochloride 10 to 100 mg intramuscularly or intravenously the convulsions ceased within seconds. The maintenance dose was 4 to 10 mg daily by mouth. All neonates with convulsions should be given pyridoxine parenterally as a diagnostic test.— M. M. Robins, *J. Am. med. Ass.*, 1966, *195*, 491. See also M. Bejšovec *et al.*, *Archs Dis. Childh.*, 1967, *42*, 201, per *J. Am. med. Ass.*, 1967, *200* (June 26), A186.

Homocystinuria. References to pyridoxine in homocystinuria: C. Hooft *et al.* (letter), *Lancet*, 1967, *1*, 1384; B. Turner (letter), *ibid.*, 1967, *2*, 1151; G. E. Gaull *et al.* (letter), *ibid.*, 1968, *2*, 1302; N. A. J. Carson and I. J. Carre, *Archs Dis. Childh.*, 1969, *44*, 387.

Hyperoxaluria. In about one-third of patients with primary hyperoxaluria the urinary oxalate excretion was reduced by pyridoxine in high doses of 1 g daily in divided doses.— R. W. E. Watts, *Postgrad. med. J.*, 1977, *53*, *Suppl.* 2, 7. See also A. R. Harrison *et al.*, *Br. med. J.*, 1981, *282*, 2097.

Mental disorders. Prolonged improvement occurred over a period of 8 to 10 weeks in 8 schizophrenic patients in a pilot study of 15 who were given pyridoxine 50 mg thrice daily in addition to normal treatment.— L. Bucci (letter), *Br. J. Psychiat.*, 1973, *122*, 240.

The effect of high doses of pyridoxine on autistic children.— B. Rimland *et al.*, *Am. J. Psychiat.*, 1978, *135*, 472.

For a critical view of vitamin therapy for mental disorders, see in the general section under Megavitamin Therapy, p.1635.

Depression. Pyridoxine 50 mg daily for 5 days relieved symptoms of depression and irritability in a woman in the fourth month of pregnancy. Similarly, pyridoxine relieved the irritability of a woman in the second half of the menstrual cycle.— F. Winston (letter), *Lancet*, 1969, *1*, 1209.

Initial experience with pyridoxine hydrochloride in 3 patients prompted a controlled crossover study in 13 women with premenstrual tension and depression where only 1 patient improved significantly when given pyridoxine.— J. Stokes and J. Mendels (letter), *Lancet*, 1972, *1*, 1177.

In a study of 39 depressed patients receiving oral contraceptives, 19 had absolute pyridoxine deficiency and these patients achieved improvement in their mood when treated with pyridoxine.— P. W. Adams *et al.* (letter), *Lancet*, 1974, *2*, 516.

There was no justification for the routine use of pyridoxine in depressed women who were taking oral contraceptives. In those few women with very troublesome symptoms with no psychosocial cause, pyridoxine 50 mg daily could be given for a trial period of 4 weeks after which it should be stopped if there was no definite improvement.— *Drug & Ther. Bull.*, 1978, *16*, 86.

Further references: M. J. Baumblatt and F. Winston (letter), *Lancet*, 1970, *1*, 832; S. A. Price and P. A. Toseland (letter), *ibid.*, 1969, *2*, 158; F. Winston (letter), *ibid.*, 377; *idem*, *Am. J. Psychiat.*, 1973, *130*, 1217, per *Int. pharm. Abstr.*, 1974, *11*, 570.

Neuropathies. A discussion of the use of pyridoxine hydrochloride for the treatment of peripheral neuropathies induced by hydralazine or isoniazid; pyridoxine was not always effective when the neuropathy had become established.— J. Cawano and L. J. Davis, *Drug Intell. & clin. Pharm.*, 1978, *12*, 112 and 297.

Hydrazine poisoning. Fourteen hours after sustaining a thermal burn in an industrial hydrazine explosion a 36-year-old man became comatose and remained so for 60 hours. He then received pyridoxine 600 mg intramuscularly and 1 g as an intravenous infusion over 3 hours. Four hours after the start of therapy he demonstrated spontaneous purposeful activity and could follow simple commands; 12 hours later he was alert and conversant. Subsequent neurological examinations revealed no discernible deficit; an EEG was normal.— J. K. Kirklin *et al.*, *New Engl. J. Med.*, 1976, *294*, 938.

Ocular disorders. Encouraging preliminary findings had been obtained following administration of pyridoxine to 4 patients with gyrate atrophy of the choroid and retina, a progressive genetic disorder which leads to blindness by the age of 40 or 50 years.— R. G. Weleber *et al.* (letter), *Lancet*, 1978, *2*, 1213.

Pregnancy and the neonate. All of 14 women with gestational diabetes had low-normal or subnormal blood-pyridoxine concentrations. After treatment with pyridoxine these concentrations rose and on repeat oral glucose-tolerance tests only 2 were considered to have diabetes. Pyridoxine possibly reduced abnormal xanthurenic acid synthesis by restoring tryptophan metabolism.— H. J. T. C. Bennink and W. H. P. Schreurs, *Br. med. J.*, 1975, *3*, 13.

See also under Tryptophan Metabolism.

In 13 women, at least 26 weeks pregnant, abnormal glucose tolerance was reduced (to normal values in 5) after treatment for 2 weeks with pyridoxine 25 mg four times daily.— W. N. Spellacy *et al.*, *Am. J. Obstet. Gynec.*, 1977, *127*, 599.

Further references: M. D. Gillmer and D. Mazibuko, *Am. J. Obstet. Gynec.*, 1979, *133*, 499.

Tardive dyskinesia. In 4 of 5 patients tardive dyskinesia following earlier neuroleptic medication was reduced by pyridoxine 1 to 1.4 g daily in 4 divided doses; the most severe conditions responded most readily. Dyskinesia returned when pyridoxine was withdrawn. Treatment was well tolerated.— J. DeVeaugh-Geiss and L. Manion, *J. clin. Psychiat.*, 1978, *39*, 573.

Thrombosis. The role of pyridoxine as a possible antithrombotic agent.— M. A. Packham *et al.* (letter), *Lancet*, 1981, *2*, 809.

Tryptophan metabolism. Long-term treatment with pyridoxine 200 mg daily benefited 76 asthmatic children with a metabolic block in tryptophan metabolism.— P. J. Collipp *et al.*, *Ann. Allergy*, 1975, *35*, 93, per *Int. pharm. Abstr.*, 1976, *13*, 837.

Preparations

Pyridoxine Hydrochloride Injection *(U.S.P.)*. A sterile solution of pyridoxine hydrochloride in Water for Injections. pH 2 to 3.8. Protect from light.

Rus. P. specifies 1, 2.5, and 5%, in ampoules of 1 ml. Protect from light.

Pyridoxine Hydrochloride Tablets *(B.P.)*. Pyridoxine Hydrochlor. Tab.; Pyridoxine Tablets; Vitamin B_6 Tablets. Tablets containing pyridoxine hydrochloride. Store at a temperature not exceeding 30°. Protect from light.

Pyridoxine Hydrochloride Tablets *(U.S.P.)*. Tablets containing pyridoxine hydrochloride. Protect from light.

Pyridoxine Injection *(B.P.C. 1973)*. Pyridoxine Hydrochloride Injection. A sterile solution of pyridoxine hydrochloride in Water for Injections. Protect from light.

Proprietary Preparations

Benadon *(Roche, UK)*. Pyridoxine hydrochloride, available as tablets of 20 mg and scored tablets of 50 mg. (Also available as Benadon in *Arg., Belg., Ger., Ital., Spain, Swed., Switz.*).

Comploment *(Napp, UK)*. Pyridoxine hydrochloride, available as sustained-release tablets of 100 mg.

Other Proprietary Names

Austral.— Pydox, Pyroxin; *Belg.*— Bedoxine; *Canad.*— Hexa-Betalin, Hexavibex; *Fr.*—Bécilan, Dermo 6, Pyricamphre *(camsylate)*; *Ger.*—B_6-Vicotrat, Hexobion; *Ital.*—Bivit-6, Farmobion B_6, Seibion, Xanturenasi; *S.Afr.*—Lactosec 200; *Spain*—Dextamina B6, Godabion B6, Hexobion, Sibevit B6, Vitanoxi B6; *Swed.*—Hexapyral; *USA*—Hexa-Betalin.

7848-m

Pyridoxal Phosphate. Pyridoxal 5-Phosphate; Codecarboxylase. 3-Hydroxy-5-hydroxymethyl-2-methylpyridine-4-carboxaldehyde 5′-phosphate.
$C_8H_{10}NO_6P$=247.1.

CAS — 54-47-7.

Yellow crystals; **soluble** in water.

Uses. Pyridoxal phosphate is the active form of vitamin B_6 (see Pyridoxine Hydrochloride, p.1642). It may be given by mouth or by subcutaneous, intramuscular, or intravenous injection, in doses of up to 60 mg daily.

A patient with sideroblastic anaemia unresponsive to pyridoxine responded dramatically to pyridoxal phosphate.— D. Y. Mason and P. M. Emerson, *Br. med. J.*, 1973, *1*, 389.

Proprietary Names

Himitan, Hysix, Pidopidon, Sechvitan *(all Jap.)*.

7849-b

Vitamin B_{12}

Strictly, vitamin B_{12} is cyanocobalamin. The name is sometimes used for the group of cobalamin compounds having biological activity.

7850-x

Cobalamins

Vitamin B_{12} is present in the body mainly as methylcobalamin (mecobalamin) and as adenosylcobalamin (cobamamide) and hydroxocobalamin. Both mecobalamin and cobamamide act as coenzymes; the first is involved in the transmethylation of homocysteine to methionine and the second in the isomerisation of methylmalonyl coenzyme to succinyl coenzyme. Mecobalamin is closely involved with folate in several important metabolic pathways.

Reports and discussions of the problems associated with the measurement of cobalamin concentrations in serum and of their use in diagnosis.— J. F. Kolhouse *et al.*, *New Engl. J. Med.*, 1978, *299*, 785; B. A. Cooper and V. M. Whitehead, *ibid.*, 816; R. M. Donaldson, *ibid.*, 827; E. Hippe (letter), *ibid.*, 1979, *300*, 141; J. M. England and J. C. Linnell, *Lancet*, 1980, *2*, 1072; I. C. Balfour and D. W. Lane (letter), *ibid.*, 1246; A. M. Streeter *et al.* (letter), *ibid.*, 1981, *1*, 39; H. Baker *et al.* (letter), *ibid.*, 154.

Absorption and Fate. The cobalamins are extensively bound to specific plasma proteins called transcobalamins; transcobalamin II appears to be involved in the rapid transport of the cobalamins to tissues.

Cobalamins are absorbed from the gastro-intestinal tract, but may be irregularly absorbed when given in large therapeutic doses and absorption is impaired in patients with an absence of intrinsic factor, with a malabsorption syndrome or with disease or abnormality of the gut, or after gastrectomy.

Cobalamins are stored in the liver, excreted in the bile, and undergo some enterohepatic recycling; part of a dose is excreted in the urine, most of it in the first 8 hours.

Cobalamins diffuse across the placenta.

Reduced absorption of vitamin B_{12} in bile acid deficiency.— N. H. Teo *et al.*, *Gut*, 1980, *21*, A908.

Human Requirements. Body stores of vitamin B_{12} range from 1 to 5 mg. About 0.1 to 0.2% of the body's stores are lost daily. In most developed countries daily requirements will be adequately met by a balanced diet but in under-developed countries this may not be so; persons on strict vegetarian diets that exclude dairy products also require supplements. To replace losses and to provide for biological variations in individuals, a daily intake of 2 to 3 µg is required.

The following daily intakes of vitamin B_{12} were recommended: up to 1 year of age, 0.3 µg; 1 to 3 years, 0.9 µg; 4 to 9 years, 1.5 µg; 10 years and over, 2 µg; in pregnancy, 3 µg; during lactation, 2.5 µg.— Report of a Joint FAO/WHO Expert Group, *Tech. Rep. Ser. Wld Hlth Org. No. 452*, 1970.

The recommended daily dietary allowance of vitamin B_{12} for adults is 3 µg; for breast-fed infants, 0.5 µg daily; for infants fed on milk formulas and for children up to adolescence, 0.15 µg per 418 kJ; for pregnant or lactating women, 4 µg.— *Recommended Dietary Allowances*, 9th Edn, Washington, The National Research Council, 1980, p. 117.

The recommendation that foods for the young infant should contain vitamin B_{12} in amounts not less than 0.1 ng per ml (based on the lower limit of the range in pooled samples of human milk).— Artificial Feeds for the Young Infant: Report of the Working Party on the Composition of Foods for Infants and Young Children, Committee on Medical Aspects of Food Policy, *Report on Health and Social Subjects, 18*, London, HM Stationery Office, 1980.

Uses. Deficiency of vitamin B_{12} interferes with haemopoiesis and produces megaloblastic anaemia. There may also be irreversible damage to the nervous system.

Treatment of deficiency is generally with hydroxocobalamin. Cobamamide and mecobalamin have also been used. Cyanocobalamin is not suitable as optic neuropathies may deteriorate.

Treatment produces prompt haematological improvement and a striking clinical response, the patients feeling stronger and their appetites improving. Subacute combined degeneration of the spinal cord, responds more slowly and remission may not be complete. Treatment must be continued indefinitely.

Preparations

Cobalamin Concentrate *(U.S.P.)*. Vitamin B_{12} Activity Concentrate. The dried partially purified product resulting from the growth of selected *Streptomyces* cultures or other cobalamin-producing micro-organisms. It contains not less than 500 µg of cobalamin (measured as cyanocobalamin) per g, and it may contain harmless diluents and stabilising agents. A 0.5% solution in water has a pH of 4 to 8. Store in airtight containers. Protect from light.

A less purified form of vitamin B_{12} suitable for use in oral preparations.

7851-r

B_{12}TAM. A suspension of a cyanocobalamin-tannin complex in a sesame oil/aluminium monostearate gel.

Uses. B_{12}TAM is a long-acting cyanocobalamin preparation which has been used in the treatment of vitamin-B_{12} deficiency and pernicious anaemia.

References: P. Bastrup-Madsen *et al.*, *Lancet*, 1966, *1*, 739.

Proprietary Names

Betolvex *(Dumex, Denm.; Dumex, Neth.; Dumex, Norw.; Dumex, Swed.; Dumex, Switz.)*; Depinar (zinc tannate complex) *(Petersen, S.Afr.)*.

7852-f

Cobamamide. Coenzyme B_{12}; Dibencozide; Dibenzcozamide; Dimebenzcozamide. (5′-Deoxy-5′-adenosyl)cobalamin; *Coα*-[α-(5,6-Dimethylbenzimidazolyl)]-*Coβ*-(5′-deoxy-5′-adenosyl)cobamide.

$C_{72}H_{100}CoN_{18}O_{17}P$=1579.6.

CAS — 13870-90-1.

A form of vitamin B_{12} found in the body (see p.1643). It is unstable to light.

Cobamamide has been used in doses of about 1 to 5 mg daily, by mouth or injection. Larger doses have been used.

References: L. W. Sullivan and V. Herbert, *New Engl. J. Med.*, 1965, *272*, 240; K. Boddy *et al.*, *Lancet*, 1968, *2*, 710.

Proprietary Names

Arg.—Activanat, Cobafor; *Belg.*—Heraclene; *Fr.*—Cobalion, Cobanzyme, Dibencozan, Héraclène, Indusil T, Névrizide; *Ger.*—Xobaline; *Ital.*—Aima, Anabasi, Anazym, Betarin, Ciclozim, Cobaforte, Cobalin, Cobazina, Coben B_{12}, Coezim B_{12}, Conzibi 12, Cromazim, Dimazin, Dodecozim B_{12}, Extrabolin, Fisiocobal, Fortezim, Glade, Indusil, Marvizim, Maximal, Medozim, Neocobal, Nutricon, Paidozim, Radiozima, Rubenzim Forte, Trillovit, Trofozim, Unifort, Zervital, Zidovit; *Jap.*—Cobaltamin-S, Cobamyde, Hycobal; *Spain*—Ambritan, Anabolizante, Anabozima, Be-Livita, Benydiol soluble, Gradalin Co-B_{12}, Indusil, Panhor, Protemi, Sartoenzim, Thencel, Vitosit, Xobaline; *Switz.*—Cobazymase.

7853-d

Cyanocobalamin *(B.P., Eur. P., U.S.P.)*.

Cyanocobal.; Cyanocobalaminum; Cobamin; Cycobemin; Vitamin B_{12}. *Coα*-[α-(5,6-Dimethylbenzimidazolyl)]-*Coβ*-cyanocobamide.

$C_{63}H_{88}CoN_{14}O_{14}P$=1355.4.

CAS — 68-19-9.

Pharmacopoeias. In all pharmacopoeias examined except *Span.*

A cobalt-containing substance obtained from liver or separated from the products of metabolism of various micro-organisms. It occurs as dark red, odourless, tasteless, hygroscopic crystals or crystalline or amorphous powder; it loses not more than 12% of its weight on drying.

Soluble 1 in 80 of water and 1 in 180 of alcohol (90%); practically insoluble in acetone, chloroform, and ether. Solutions are **sterilised** by autoclaving or by filtration. **Incompatible** with oxidising and reducing agents and with salts of heavy metals. It is stable in neutral aqueous solutions but is slowly decomposed in alkaline solutions and in strongly acid solutions. Benzyl alcohol 2% and phenylmercuric nitrate 0.001% are suitable preservatives for solutions of cyanocobalamin. **Store** in airtight containers. Protect from light.

It is present in liver, kidney, milk, eggs, and muscle tissue; it is produced by bacterial synthesis in the colon but is not absorbed from this site. About 30% of vitamin B_{12} in food is destroyed by cooking.

Effect of gamma-irradiation. Solutions of cyanocobalamin at 25 000 Gy became turbid and reddish-brown and at 250 000 Gy turbid and yellow. Potency was reduced to 10% at 25 000 Gy and to about 1% at 250 000 Gy.— *The Use of Gamma Radiation Sources for the Sterilisation of Pharmaceutical Products*, London, ABPI, 1960.

Incompatibility. Cyanocobalamin 10 µg was 'physically incompatible' with warfarin sodium 10 mg in 100 ml of dextrose injection.— R. D. Dunworth and F. R. Kenna, *Am. J. Hosp. Pharm.*, 1965, *22*, 190.

There was loss of clarity when intravenous solutions of cyanocobalamin were mixed with those of ascorbic acid, dextrose, phytomenadione, or (in dextrose injection) warfarin sodium.— J. A. Patel and G. L. Phillips, *Am. J. Hosp. Pharm.*, 1966, *23*, 409.

A number of incompatibilities which had been quoted in the literature for cyanocobalamin injection were due to hydroxocobalamin which was formerly present in considerable quantities as a contaminant. Cyanocobalamin could be stored for 24 hours, protected from light at room temperature, in the presence of ascorbic acid without loss of activity and was stable for the life of an extemporaneously prepared intravenous infusion solution in the presence of many iron salts administered parenterally including iron-dextran complex. Cyanocobalamin was compatible with other vitamins of the B complex for short-term storage.— C. L. J. Coles and K. A. Lees, *Glaxo* (letter), *Pharm. J.*, 1971, *1*, 153.

Stability. In solutions containing thiamine hydrochloride, cyanocobalamin, and other factors of the vitamin-B complex, breakdown products of thiamine hydrochloride caused rapid destruction of cyanocobalamin. Low concentrations of ferric ions could protect cyanocobalamin against the effects of thiamine breakdown products without appreciably affecting the stability of the thiamine.— J. Heathcote and B. A. Wills, *J. Pharm. Pharmac.*, 1962, *14*, 232. See also D. A. Zuck and J. W. Conine, *J. pharm. Sci.*, 1963, *52*, 59.

Whilst cyanocobalamin alone was stable in solution when exposed to light, a destructive effect occurred in the presence of riboflavine. This photolysis of cyanocobalamin was accelerated by nicotinamide and inhibited by the antoxidants ethyl hydrocaffeate and thiourea.— R. P. Patel and V. K. Soni, *Indian J. Pharm.*, 1964, *26*, 35.

For a review on the stability and stabilisation of cyanocobalamin in vitamin-B complex injections containing thiamine and nicotinamide, see S. K. Baveja, *Australas. J. Pharm.* , 1966, *47*, S108.

Adverse Effects. Cyanocobalamin is usually well tolerated. Rarely, allergic reactions have been reported after injection.

Reports of allergic reactions.— G. Høvding, *Br. med. J.*, 1968, *3*, 102; J. James and R. P. Warin, *Br. med. J.*, 1971, *2*, 262; A. A. Fisher (letter), *J. Am. med. Ass.*, 1975, *233*, 21. Further references: I. Pevny *et al.*, *Hautzart*, 1977, *28*, 600.

Rapid maturation of cells following vitamin B_{12} administration increased degradation of nucleic acid and increased uric acid, resulting in gout.— *Drug & Ther. Bull.*, 1975, *13*, 73.

For a report of deterioration in acne and acneform eruption associated with cyanocobalamin, see Pyridoxine Hydrochloride, p.1642.

Precautions. Cyanocobalamin should not be given before a diagnosis has been fully established because of the possibility of masking symptoms of subacute degeneration of the spinal cord. Cyanocobalamin is not a suitable form of vitamin B_{12} for the treatment of optic neuropathies associated with raised plasma concentrations of cyanocobalamin (for further details see below).

Interactions. A review of the compounds which inhibit cyanocobalamin.— S. Waxman *et al.*, *Am. J. Med.*, 1970, *48*, 599.

Metformin reduced intestinal absorption of cyanocobalamin.— V. Herbert, *Ann. intern. Med.*, 1972, *76*, 140.

Impaired absorption of vitamin B_{12} was observed in 30% of a group of 50 patients receiving potassium citrate and/or calcium gluconate.— I. P. Palva *et al.*, *Acta. med. scand.*, 1974, *196*, 525, per *Drug Intell. & clin. Pharm.*, 1975, *9*, 466.

Ascorbic acid destroyed cyanocobalamin *in vitro*. The destructive effect was affected by the concentration of both and the food source of cyanocobalamin.— V. Herbert and E. Jacob, *J. Am. med. Ass.*, 1974, *230*, 241.

In 3 subjects who had taken a minimum of 1 g of ascorbic acid with each meal for more than 3 years, serum-cyanocobalamin concentrations ranged from 65 to 100 picograms per ml. Two had hypersegmented neutrophils and occasional ovalomacrocytes but none was anaemic. In 1 subject cessation of high-dose ascorbic acid therapy was followed by an increase in the serum-cyanocobalamin concentration from 100 to 180 picograms per ml.— J. D. Hines (letter), *J. Am. med. Ass.*, 1975, *234*, 24. Further references: H. L. Newmark *et al.*, *J. Am. med. Ass.*, 1979, *242*, 2319.

Impairment of absorption by eggs.— A. Doscherholmen (letter), *J. Am. med. Ass.*, 1978, *240*, 2045.

Absorption and Fate. See under Cobalamins, above.

After an oral dose of labelled vitamin B_{12} had been administered to a healthy subject, the vitamin was quickly taken up by the intestinal mucosa and held there for at least 2 to 3 hours. Labelled vitamin B_{12} did not appear in the blood or tissues for 2 to 3 hours and peak concentrations did not occur until 8 to 12 hours after the dose. It accumulated and reached maximum concentrations in the liver within 24 hours. By 5 to 6 days, 60 to 70% of the dose was in the liver.— D. L. Mollin and A. H. Waters, *The Study of Vitamin B_{12} Absorption Using Labelled Cobalamins*, Amersham, The Radiochemical Centre, 1968, p. 5.

The rate of absorption of cyanocobalamin, hydroxocobalamin, and cyanocobalamin-zinc-tannate complex from injection sites was such that 50% of the dose had left the site in 40 minutes, 2½ hours, and 2 days respectively. After injection of 1 mg, the amounts excreted in the urine in 72 hours were 75, 30, and 10% respectively. Serum concentrations in excess of 0.1 ng per ml were maintained for an average of 2.1, 7.1, and 6.3 months respectively.— A. Killander and I. Werner, *Acta haemat.*, 1969, *40*, 305, per *J. Am. med. Ass.*, 1969, *207*, 1950.

In 2 volunteers given ^{57}Co-labelled cyanocobalamin by mouth no radioactivity was detected in the blood for 2 hours but it was detected at 3 hours and persisted for 48 hours. Cyanocobalamin was shown by chromatography to be bound to plasma proteins transcobalamin I and II and also to a third carrier which might be a polymer of transcobalamin II.— I. Chanarin *et al.*, *Br. med. J.*, 1972, *2*, 441. See also A. Doscherholmen *et al.* (letter), *J. Am. med. Ass.*, 1974, *227*, 800.

Absorption of cyanocobalamin was impaired in 8 of 14 patients who had undergone radiotherapy for carcinoma of the bladder. The mucosa of the terminal ileum had probably been damaged.— M. P. McBrien, *Br. med. J.*, 1973, *1*, 648.

Pancreatic extract 2 g increased the absorption and urinary excretion of vitamin B_{12} in 7 patients with pancreatic exocrine insufficiency; it had no effect in patients with vitamin B_{12} malabsorption associated with pernicious anaemia or drug-induced disease.— P. P. Toskes *et al.*, *Gastroenterology*, 1973, *65*, 199, per *J. Am. med. Ass.*, 1973, *226*, 584.

Study in 5 subjects showed that cyanocobalamin was absorbed from the gut as a complex with transcobalamin II; the complex had a reported plasma half-life of about 5 minutes.— I. Chanarin *et al.*, *Br. med. J.*, 1978, *1*, 1453.

Pregnancy and the neonate. Reports of vitamin-B_{12} deficiency in infants born to and breast-fed by mothers who were vegetarian or had pernicious anaemia.— M. C. Higginbottom *et al.*, *New Engl. J. Med.*, 1978, *299*, 317; J. Frader *et al.* (letter), *ibid.*, 1319; D. Heaton (letter), *ibid.*, 1979, *300*, 202.

Uses. Cyanocobalamin has been used in the treatment of cobalamin deficiency but hydroxocobalamin is now preferred (see below and under Cobalamins, p.1644).

The usual initial dose is 0.25 to 1 mg intramuscularly on alternate days for 1 to 2 weeks, followed by 250 µg weekly until the blood count is normal, then a maintenance dose of 1 mg monthly. If there are neurological complications the initial dose is 1 mg on alternate days while improvement is occurring followed by a maintenance dose of 1 mg monthly.

Cyanocobalamin is sometimes given by mouth, when injections are impracticable, but it is much less reliable by this route than by intramuscular injection; doses of 50 to 150 µg or more daily have been given; in pernicious anaemia doses of at least 300 µg daily have been given.

An account of the different forms of vitamin B_{12} and of some of the inborn errors of cobalamin metabolism, including a detailed explanation of why hydroxocobalamin, and not cyanocobalamin, is the form of vitamin B_{12} most suitable for therapeutic use. The 3 main cobalamins in man and *animals* are hydroxocobalamin (and/or closely related compounds), adenosylcobalamin, and methylcobalamin; cyanocobalamin is present only in traces and is often undetectable, its biochemical significance, if any, being uncertain. Conditions in which plasma-cyanocobalamin concentrations are raised include *tobacco amblyopia, Leber's optic atrophy*, and *dominantly inherited optic atrophy*; some of the optic neuropathies appear to respond to massive doses of hydroxocobalamin and have been claimed to be adversely affected by administration of cyanocobalamin; common sense suggests the undesirability of raising a plasma-cyanocobalamin concentration that is already abnormally high. Comment is also made on the serious discrepancies between the results of microbiological and radioisotopic assays for total cobalamins, together with the recommendation that every laboratory should specify the assay method used, and that the term 'vitamin B_{12}' should be abandoned and replaced by 'the cobalamins'.— D. M. Matthews and J. C. Linnell, *Br. med. J.*, 1979, *2*, 533.

A plea for the withdrawal of cyanocobalamin in favour of hydroxocobalamin.— A. G. Freeman (letter), *Lancet*, 1978, *1*, 777.

Mental disorders. Comparison of a group of 40 mentally disturbed geriatric patients with a matched control group of 40 mentally normal patients showed no marked difference in serum concentrations of vitamin B_{12}, which suggested that deficiency was unlikely to be a common cause of mental disturbance in geriatric patients.— P. K. Buxton *et al.*, *Geront. clin.*, 1969, *11*, 22. A similar report in 1004 patients.— F. Murphy *et al.*, *Br. med. J.*, 1969, *3*, 559. See also R. Shulman, *ibid.*, 1967, *3*, 266.

See also under Hydroxocobalamin, below.

For a critical view of vitamin therapy for mental disorders, see in the general section under Megavitamin Therapy, p.1635.

Methylmalonicaciduria. References to cyanocobalamin in the treatment of methylmalonicaciduria: G. W. Frimpter, *New Engl. J. Med.*, 1973, *289*, 895; M. G. Ampola *et al.*, *New Engl. J. Med.*, 1975, *293*, 313; B. A. Gordon *et al.*, *Can. med. Ass. J.*, 1976, *115*, 233; D. T. Whelan *et al.*, *Can. med. Ass. J.*, 1979, *120*, 1230; I. Auchterlonie *et al.*, *Archs Dis. Childh.*, 1979, *54*, 802.

Preparations

Cyanocobalamin Injection *(B.P.)*. Vitamin B_{12} Injection. A sterile solution of cyanocobalamin in Water for Injections containing sufficient acetic acid or hydrochloric acid to adjust the pH to about 4 (limits 3.8 to 5.5); it may contain a suitable buffering agent. Sterilised by autoclaving. Potency is expressed in terms of the equivalent amount of anhydrous cyanocobalamin. Protect from light.

Cyanocobalamin Injection *(U.S.P.)*. A sterile solution of cyanocobalamin in Water for Injections, or in Water for Injections rendered iso-osmotic by the addition of sodium chloride. pH 4.5 to 7. Potency is expressed in terms of the equivalent amount of anhydrous cyanocobalamin. Protect from light.

NOTE. Some Liver Preparations are standardised for cyanocobalamin content—see p.1646.

Ce-Cobalin Syrup *(Paines & Byrne, UK)*. Contains in each ml cyanocobalamin 6 µg and ascorbic acid 2 mg. *Dose.* Infants, 2.5 ml daily; children, 5 ml thrice daily; adults, 5 to 10 ml thrice daily.

Cytacon *(Glaxo, UK)*. Cyanocobalamin, available as **Liquid** containing 35 µg in each 5 ml (suggested diluent, syrup) and as **Tablets** of 50 µg. (Also available as Cytacon in *Austral.*).

Cytamen *(Glaxo, UK)*. Cyanocobalamin, available as injection containing 250 or 1000 µg per ml, in ampoules of 1 ml. (Also available as Cytamen in *Arg., Austral., S.Afr.*).

Hepacon-B12 *(Consolidated Chemicals, UK)*. Cyanocobalamin, available as injection containing 100 or 1000 µg per ml, in ampoules of 1 ml.

Hepanorm Tablets *(Wallace Mfg Chem., UK: Farillon, UK)*. Each contains cyanocobalamin 7.5 mg, intrinsic factor concentrate 25 mg, folic acid 2.5 mg, and liver fraction 150 mg. *Dose.* 2 tablets daily for 14 days, then 1 tablet daily.

Other Proprietary Names

Arg.—Reedvit; *Austral.*—Panalamine; *Belg.*— Cytaman; *Canad.*—Anacobin, Bedoz, Bio-12, Cyanabin, Neo-Rubex, Redisol, Rubramin, Rubion; *Denm.*—Behepan; *Fr.*—Docémine; *Ger.*—Berubi, Cobalparen, Cytobion, Docivit, Millevit, Pharmatovit B_{12}, Vicapan B_{12}; *Ital.*—Bimil, Dobetin, Docigram 1000, Dodevitina, Eritrovit B_{12}, Neurobaltina, Robelvit B_{12}, Rotamin, Sorbigen B_{12}, Viemin 12; *S.Afr.*—Balamin forte, Depinar, Norivite-12, Nubee 12; *Spain*—Bedocefarm, Cincomil Bedoce, Co-Vitam B12, Docetasan, Eocill B12, Fiviton B12, Lifaton B12, Milbedoce, Neuro Liser B12, Noventabedoce, Optovite B12, Plentasal, Retidex B12, Rubraluy, Sorbevit B12, Surgevit; *Swed.*—Behepan (see also under Hydroxocobalamin), Cykobemin; *Switz.*—Lagavit B_{12}, Mepharubin, Pharmatovit B_{12}, Rubrovit 1000, Vitarubin; *USA*—Berubigen, Betalin 12, Dodex, Redisol, Rubesol, Rubramin PC, Ruvite, Sytobex.

Cyanocobalamin was also formerly marketed in Great Britain under the proprietary name Cobalin (*Paines & Byrne*).

7854-n

Hydroxocobalamin *(B.P., B.P. Vet.)*. Hydroxocobal.; Idrossocobalamina; Vitamin B_{12a}; Vitamin B_{12b}. *Coα*-[α-(5,6-Dimethylbenzimidazolyl)]-*Coβ*-hydroxocobamide.

$C_{62}H_{89}CoN_{13}O_{15}P$=1346.4.

CAS — 13422-51-0.

Pharmacopoeias. In *Br.*, *Fr.*, *It.*, and *U.S.*
Fr. also includes Hydroxocobalamin Acetate and Chloride. *Jap. P.* has Hydroxocobalamin Acetate.

Hydroxocobalamin occurs either as aquocobalamin chloride [α-(5,6-dimethylbenzimidazol-1-yl)aquocobamide chloride], which when dried contains not less than 96% of $C_{62}H_{90}ClCoN_{13}O_{15}P$, or as aquocobalamin sulphate, which when dried contains not less than 96% of $C_{124}H_{180}Co_2N_{26}O_{34}P_2S$. It is in the form of dark red, almost odourless and tasteless crystals or crystalline powder. The chloride loses 8 to 12% of its weight and the sulphate 8 to 16% on drying. Some decomposition may occur on drying.

Soluble 1 in 50 of water and 1 in 100 of alcohol; sparingly soluble in methyl alcohol; practically insoluble in acetone, chloroform, and ether. A 2% solution in water has a pH of 8 to 10. Solutions are **sterilised** by filtration. **Store** in a cool place in airtight containers. Protect from light.

Aquocobalamin. In acid solutions, hydroxocobalamin took up a hydrogen ion which converted the hydroxyl to a coordinated water molecule. In this form the molecule (aquocobalamin) was basic and formed salts with acids. Thus, in solution it existed as an equilibrium mixture with hydroxocobalamin and, since it was more stable at acid pH values, commercial products were likely to be mainly in the aquocobalamin form. Therefore 'aquocobalamin' would be a more appropriate designation. However, the term 'hydroxocobalamin' had become established in the medical literature.— E. L. Smith *et al.*, *Analyst, Lond.*, 1962, *87*, 183.

Adverse Effects and Precautions. As for Cyanocobalamin, p.1644.

Patients receiving hydroxocobalamin 1 mg at 3-day intervals for the treatment of pernicious anaemia might have an attack of gout on the 4th to 6th day of treatment.— A. V. Hoffbrand, *Prescribers' J.*, 1972, *12*, 118.

Absorption and Fate. See under Cobalamins, above.

Uses. Hydroxocobalamin has the actions and uses described under Cobalamins (see p.1644). It is administered by intramuscular injection.

The usual dose for pernicious anaemia is 0.25 to 1 mg on alternate days for 1 or 2 weeks, then 0.25 mg weekly till the blood count is normal, with maintenance doses of 1 mg every 2 or 3 months. In the presence of neurological involvement doses of 1 mg are given on alternate days while improvement continues.

For prophylaxis in subjects taking diets deficient in vitamin B_{12}, doses of 1 mg are given every 2 or 3 months.

In tobacco amblyopia and Leber's optic atrophy doses of 1 mg are given daily for 2 weeks, then twice weekly while improvement continues, with maintenance doses of 1 mg monthly.

For explanation why hydroxocobalamin, and not cyanocobalamin, should be used when vitamin B_{12} is required, see under Cyanocobalamin, p.1645.

Deficiency states. Of 130 consecutive patients with recurrent aphthous stomatitis, 23 had deficiencies of vitamin B_{12}, folic acid, or iron; 15 showed complete remission after treatment with hydroxocobalamin 1 mg intramuscularly every 2 months, folic acid 5 mg thrice daily, or iron by mouth for at least 6 months. Local treatment was considered unlikely to have produced lasting clinical improvement.— D. Wray *et al.*, *Br. med. J.*, 1975, *2*, 490.

Mental disorders. In 39 elderly subjects with low serum concentrations of vitamin B_{12} but without macrocytic anaemia or neuropathy, intramuscular injection of hydroxocobalamin 1 mg twice in the first week and then weekly for 4 weeks was no more effective than placebo in effecting an improvement in the psychiatric state or general well-being.— D. Hughes *et al.*, *Br. med. J.*, 1970, *2*, 458.

For a critical view of vitamin therapy for mental disorders, see in the general section under Megavitamin Therapy, p.1635.

Treatment of cyanide poisoning. Due to its cyanide-binding capacity hydroxocobalamin could be used to treat cyanide poisoning.— L. M. Dalderup (letter), *Lancet*, 1973, *2*, 625.

Although it had been suggested that hydroxocobalamin could be of benefit in cyanide poisoning, existing preparations were unsuitable, about 10 litres of the available injections (0.1%) being required to neutralise a fatal dose of about 200 mg of cyanide.— *Lancet*, 1977, *2*, 1167.

For reference to the use of hydroxocobalamin in the prevention of nitroprusside-induced cyanide poisoning, see Sodium Nitroprusside, p.166.

Preparations

Hydroxocobalamin Injection *(B.P.)*. A sterile solution of hydroxocobalamin in Water for Injections containing sufficient acetic acid or hydrochloric acid to adjust the pH to about 4 (range: pH 3.8 to 5.5); it may also contain a suitable buffering agent. Sterilised by filtration. Potency is expressed in terms of the equivalent amount of anhydrous hydroxocobalamin. Protect from light.

Hydroxocobalamin Injection *(U.S.P.)*. A sterile solution of hydroxocobalamin in Water for Injections. Potency is expressed in terms of the equivalent amount of anhydrous hydroxocobalamin. pH 3.5 to 5. Protect from light.

Proprietary Preparations

Cobalin-H *(Paines & Byrne, UK)*. Hydroxocobalamin, available as injection containing 250 and 1000 µg per ml, in ampoules of 1 ml.

Neo-Cytamen *(Glaxo, UK)*. Hydroxocobalamin, available as injection containing 250 and 1000 µg per ml, in ampoules of 1 ml. (Also available as Neo-Cytamen in *Arg., Austral., Ital., S.Afr.*).

Other Proprietary Names

Arg.—Dosixbe, Droxodoce 10 000, Droxofor; *Belg.*—Forta-B12, Mega-B12 *(acetate)*, Novobedouze; *Denm.*—Vibeden; *Fr.*—Dodécavit, Hydroxo, Novobédouze; *Ger.*—Aquo-Cytobion, Axlon, Berubi-long, Depogamma *(acetate)*, Docivit Depot *(acetate)*, Novidroxin *(acetate)*; *Ind.*—Macrabin H; *Ital.*—Biocobal VCA, Bradirubra, Cobalidrina 1000, Cobalvit, Fravit B_{12}, Idro Apavit, Idrobamina, Idrocobalamin, Idrospes B_{12}, Idrozima, Longicobal, Natur B_{12}, Red 1000, Rossobivit 1000, Rubitard B_{12}; *Neth.*—Hydrocobamine; *Spain*—Acuo-Godabion B12 *(acetate)*, Aquodavur, Docevita, Hidroxuber *(acetate)*, Megamilbedoce, Milbedoce Depot; *Swed.*—Behepan *(see also under Cyanocobalamin)*; *Switz.*—Acimexan, Hydroxo, Liodozal, Novobédouze, Vitarubin Depot; *USA*—Alpha Redisol, Alpha-Ruvite, Hydroxo B_{12}, Neo-Betalin 12, Rubesol-LA, Sytobex-H.

7855-h

Liver Extracts

CAS — 8002-47-9.

Liver extracts were formerly widely used in the treatment of pernicious anaemia but they have now been almost entirely replaced by hydroxocobalamin and are no longer recommended for routine treatment. They contain variable but usually small amounts of cyanocobalamin, some folic acid, and possibly other haemopoietic factors.

Proprietary Liver Preparations for Injection

Hemoplex *(Paines & Byrne, UK)*. A crude liver extract for injection with thiamine hydrochloride 10 mg, riboflavine 500 µg, pyridoxine hydrochloride 2.5 mg, and nicotinamide 10 mg per ml; in vials of 10 ml.

Hepacon *(Consolidated Chemicals, UK)*. Liver extract for intramuscular injection, standardised to contain 100 or 1000 µg of cyanocobalamin per ml, in ampoules of 2 ml. **Hepacon-B Forte.** Liver extract for injection, containing in each 2-ml ampoule cyanocobalamin 15 µg, cocarboxylase 50 mg, and folic acid 2.5 mg.

Hepanorm Fortissimum *(Wallace Mfg Chem., UK: Farillon, UK)*. Injection containing crude liver extract equivalent to not less than 15 µg vitamin B_{12} activity per ml; in ampoules of 2 ml.

Parenamps *(Paines & Byrne, UK)*. An extract of whole liver for intramuscular injection containing not less than 2 µg of cyanocobalamin per ml, in ampoules of 2 ml.

Ripason *(Robapharm, Switz.: Welbeck, UK)*. An albumin-free total liver extract, available as an **Injection** in vials of 10 ml and as **Tablets**. *Dose.* Injection, initial, a test-dose of 2 deep intramuscular injections each of 1 ml into the buttocks; maintenance, 2 to 3 ml intramuscularly or 2 to 4 ml by slow intravenous injection daily; tablets, 1 or 2 thrice daily. (Also available as Ripason in *Spain*).

A critical reference.— P. J. Toghill *et al.*, *Gut*, 1969, *10*, 882.

Proprietary Liver Preparations for Oral Use

Ironorm Tonic with Iron *(Wallace Mfg Chem., UK: Farillon, UK)*. Contains in each 5 ml proteolysed liver extract equivalent to fresh liver 2 g, ferric ammonium citrate 250 mg, calcium glycerophosphate 10.75 mg, manganese glycerophosphate 1 mg, potassium glycerophosphate 1.75 mg, sodium glycerophosphate 21.25 mg, calcium pantothenate 125 µg, cyanocobalamin 2.5 µg, nicotinamide 3.75 mg, pyridoxine hydrochloride 125 µg, riboflavine 250 µg, and thiamine hydrochloride 500 µg. *Dose.* 10 to 20 ml thrice daily; children, 5 to 10 ml.

Minamino Compound *(Consolidated Chemicals, UK)*. A syrup containing in each 100 ml extracts from fresh liver 70 g, fresh spleen 15 g, and fresh gastric mucosa 7 g, with cyanocobalamin 100 µg, nicotinamide 400 mg, pyridoxine hydrochloride 35 mg, riboflavine 40 mg, thiamine hydrochloride 300 mg, ferric ammonium citrate 410 mg, manganese sulphate 1.7 mg, copper sulphate 2.8 mg, and mixed amino acids 2 g. *Dose.* 20 ml thrice daily; children, 10 ml with water.

Valonorm Tonic Elixir *(Wallace Mfg Chem., UK: Farillon, UK)*. Contains in each 5 ml proteolysed liver equivalent to fresh liver 2 g, calcium glycerophosphate 10.75 mg, sodium glycerophosphate 21.25 mg, potassium glycerophosphate 1.75 mg, manganese glycerophosphate 1 mg, calcium pantothenate 125 µg, cyanocobalamin 2.5 µg, nicotinamide 3.75 mg, pyridoxine hydrochloride 125 µg, riboflavine 250 µg, and thiamine hydrochloride 500 µg. *Dose.* 10 to 20 ml thrice daily.

Other Proprietary Names of Liver Preparations for Injection or Oral Use

Austral.—Hepasol; *Belg.*—Campolon Forte; *Fr.*—Ficarmore, Hépatrol, Hépatophal, Hormantoxone; *Ital.*—Disintox, Emazian, Eparmone, Epatomaster, Epatormon, Eupakriton; *Spain*—Lipohepal.

Liver extract was also formerly marketed in Great Britain under the proprietary name Anahaemin *(Duncan, Flockhart)*.

7856-m

Mecobalamin. Methylcobalamin. *Coα*-[α-(5,6-Dimethylbenzimidazolyl)]-*Coβ*-methylcobamide.
$C_{63}H_{91}CoN_{13}O_{14}P$=1344.4.

CAS — 13422-55-4.

A red crystalline powder. Sparingly **soluble** in water; practically insoluble in acetone and ether.

Uses. Mecobalamin is a form of vitamin B_{12} found in the body (see p.1643). It has been used in doses of 500 µg intramuscularly.

Proprietary Names

Algobaz *(Labaz, Fr.)*; Asimil B12 *(Torlan, Spain)*; Cobaldocemetil *(Clariana, Spain)*; Cobimetil-B12 *(Sastre, Spain)*; Dunyl *(Exa, Arg.)*; Methylcobaz*(Labaz, Fr.)*; Metil-Vitelix *(Emyfar, Spain)*; Calomide-ME, Cobamain, Cobametin 500, Hitocobamin-M, Methycobal, Vancomin-S *(all Jap.)*.

7857-b

Desiccated Stomach *(B.P.C. 1949)*. Ventriculus Desiccatus; Dried Stomach; Powdered Stomach.

A coarse granular powder with a faint odour and a slight taste, prepared from the fresh stomach of the pig, *Sus scrofa* (Suidae), freed from extraneous fat, ground, and dried *in vacuo* below 45°; the dried material is defatted, dried without heat, and ground to a coarse powder.

Desiccated stomach was formerly used in the treatment of pernicious anaemia.

Proprietary Preparations of a Stomach and Intestinal Extract

Robaden (known in some countries as Robuden) *(Robapharm, Switz.: Welbeck, UK)*. A combination of extracts of the stomach and duodenum of animals. Available as **Tablets** containing equal parts of the water-insoluble and water-soluble fractions of stomach and duodenum; as injections in **Ampoules (gastric)** containing the water-soluble protein-free extractives from stomach 70% and duodenum 30%; and in **Ampoules (duodenal)** containing the water-soluble protein-free extractives from stomach 30% and duodenum 70%. For gastric and duodenal ulcers, gastritis, and duodenitis.

7858-v

Other Vitamins of the B Group

Described below are biotin, folic acid, folinic acid, nicotinic acid, and pantothenic acid and their related compounds.

7859-g

Biotin. Vitamin H; Coenzyme R. *cis*-5-(Hexahydro-2-oxo-1*H*-thieno[3,4-*d*]imidazol-4-yl)valeric acid.
$C_{10}H_{16}N_2O_3S$=244.3.

CAS — 58-85-5.

Pharmacopoeias. In *Swiss.*

Odourless, tasteless, colourless crystals or a white crystalline powder. M.p. 227° to 231°. Slightly **soluble** in water, alcohol, and other organic solvents; soluble in dilute alkaline solutions. A 0.1% solution in water has a pH of 3.0 to 3.6. **Protect** from light.

Biotin is widely distributed in plants and animals, the richest sources being liver, kidney, pancreas, yeast, milk, and egg-yolk. It is a coenzyme for carboxylation during the metabolism of proteins and carbohydrates. Biotin combines with a glycoprotein, avidin, present in raw egg-white, to form a complex from which biotin cannot be absorbed from the intestine and which is excreted in the faeces. Deficiency states have been induced both in **animals** and man by administering a diet containing large amounts of raw egg-white or of avidin. In *animals*, the deficiency syndrome includes dermatitis, depilation, and loss of muscular control; deficiency symptoms in man resemble those of any type of B-group deficiency—seborrhoeic dermatitis, lassitude, anorexia, and paraesthesia.

The daily human requirement is unknown but 100 to 300 µg is considered adequate; this amount is provided by the diet and intestinal flora and there is no evidence of the spontaneous occurrence of biotin deficiency in adults. An intake of 50 µg per 4.18 MJ daily is considered suitable for infants and children.

A recommended dietary allowance could not be established for biotin. Conventional dietary intake of 100 to 300 µg daily appeared satisfactory for adults. Infants and children should be adequately provided for with 50 µg per 4.18 MJ; human milk provides 10 µg per 4.18 MJ, milk formulas provide 15 µg per 4.18 MJ.— *Recommended Dietary Allowances*, 9th Edn, Washington, The National Research Council, 1980, p. 120.

The recommendation that foods for the young infant should contain biotin in amounts not less than 5 ng per ml (based on the lower limit of the range in pooled samples of human milk).— Artificial Feeds for the Young Infant: Report of the Working Party on the Composition of Foods for Infants and Young Children, Committee on Medical Aspects of Food Policy, *Report on Health and Social Subjects, 18*, London, HM Stationery Office, 1980.

Deficiency states. Discussions on biotin deficiency and carboxylase deficiency.— K. Tanaka, *New Engl. J. Med.*, 1981, *304*, 839; *Lancet*, 1981, *1*, 1195.

A child of 2 years 9 months with the juvenile form of biotin-responsive multiple carboxylase deficiency responded dramatically to treatment with biotin 10 mg daily by mouth.— J. Thoene *et al.*, *New Engl. J. Med.*, 1981, *304*, 817. See also D. M. Mock *et al.*, *ibid.*, 820.

Further case reports of response to biotin in deficiency states.— M. J. Cowan *et al.*, *Lancet*, 1979, *2*, 115; B. M. Charles *et al.*, *ibid.*, 118; A. Munnich *et al.* (letter), *ibid.*, 1980, *1*, 1080.

Skin disorders. In a double-blind crossover trial in 19 infants with seborrhoeic dermatitis, biotin 4 mg daily by mouth was no more effective than placebo. All patients were also treated with betamethasone valerate cream 0.02%.— J. A. Keipert, *Med. J. Aust.*, 1976, *1*, 584.

A preliminary study suggesting that biotin incorporated in a cream or shampoo could be used to control excessive hair loss.— E. Settel, *Drug Cosmet. Ind.*, 1977, *121* (Oct.), 34.

Proprietary Names
Biodermatin *(Lafare, Ital.)*; Medebiotin *(Medea, Spain)*.

7860-f

Folic Acid *(B.P., U.S.P.)*. Acidum Folicum; Folacin; Pteroylglutamic Acid; Pteroylmonoglutamic Acid; Folinsyre. *N*-[4-(2-Amino-4-hydroxypteridin-6-ylmethylamino)benzoyl]-L(+)-glutamic acid.
$C_{19}H_{19}N_7O_6$=441.4.
CAS — 59-30-3.

Pharmacopoeias. In *Arg., Aust., Br., Braz., Chin., Cz., Ger., Ind., Int., It., Jap., Jug., Mex., Nord., Pol., Port., Rus., Swiss, Turk.*, and *U.S.*

Folic Acid is present, chiefly combined with several L(+)-glutamic acid moieties in peptide linkages, in liver, yeast, leafy vegetables, and certain other natural products, and it may be prepared synthetically. It is a yellow to orange, odourless or almost odourless and tasteless, microcrystalline powder containing 5 to 8.5% of water.

Practically **insoluble** in water, alcohol, acetone, chloroform, and ether; soluble in dilute solutions of alkali hydroxides and carbonates, yielding a clear orange-brown solution; soluble in hydrochloric acid and in sulphuric acid, yielding very pale yellow solutions. A solution in 0.1 M sodium hydroxide is dextrorotatory. Solutions of the sodium salt are **sterilised** by filtration.

Incompatible with oxidising and reducing agents and with ions of heavy metals. Acid solutions of folic acid are sensitive to heat but towards neutrality stability progressively increases; solutions are inactivated by ultraviolet light and alkaline solutions are sensitive to oxidation. Fifty to 90% of folic acid may be destroyed during cooking. **Store** in airtight containers. Protect from light.

Effect of gamma-irradiation. For the effect of gamma-irradiation on folic acid, see Pyridoxine Hydrochloride, p.1642.

Stability. A solution of folic acid 1 mg per ml, in a vehicle of purified water preserved with hydroxybenzoates and adjusted to pH 8 to 8.5 with sodium hydroxide, had little loss of potency when stored at 25° for 8 weeks.— S. G. Smith, *Pharm. J.*, 1976, *1*, 108.

Adverse Effects. Folic acid is usually well tolerated.

Of 3 patients with a history suggesting allergy to folic acid, 1 gave marked reactions to intradermal skin tests with folic acid, folinic acid, and aminopterin, but not methotrexate.— H. J. Woodliff and R. E. Davis, *Med. J. Aust.*, 1966, *1*, 351.

In 14 healthy adults of mean age 36 years, folic acid 15 mg daily caused anorexia, nausea, abdominal distension, and flatulence in 4 within 1 week, and in 4 within 4 weeks; 6 reported a simultaneous bitter taste, and 3 women each lost about 3 kg in weight. Nine suffered altered sleep and dream patterns. Eight complained of malaise and irritability which became more pronounced with time and 5 became over-active.— R. Hunter *et al.* (preliminary communication), *Lancet*, 1970, *1*, 61. Comments.— R. E. Davis and H. J. Woodliff (letter), *ibid.*, 308; J. A. Blair (letter), *ibid.*, 360.

Folic acid, 15 mg daily for up to 1 year, produced no unwanted side-effects in 30 epileptic patients who were also given phenytoin.— F. B. Gibberd *et al.* (letter), *Lancet*, 1970, *1*, 360. Folic acid 15 mg daily given for one month to 20 healthy subjects caused no toxicity in a double-blind study.— L. Hellström, *ibid.*, 1971, *1*, 59.

No adverse effects were observed in a physician who had taken folic acid 60 mg daily for 3 years.— T. W. Sheehy (letter), *Lancet*, 1973, *1*, 37.

Folic acid hypersensitivity and fever in a 36-year-old anephric man.— G. P. Sesin and H. Krischenbaum, *Am. J. Hosp. Pharm.*, 1979, *36*, 1565.

Precautions. Folic acid should never be given alone or in conjunction with inadequate amounts of hydroxocobalamin for the treatment of megaloblastic or pernicious anaemia. Though folic acid produces a haemopoietic response, it fails to prevent the onset of subacute combined degeneration of the cord. Folic acid should not be given before a diagnosis has been fully established. The inclusion of folic acid in multivitamin preparations may be dangerous.

Large and continuous doses of folic acid may lower the blood concentration of vitamin B_{12}.

Folic acid has been given to correct the folate deficiency associated with the use of anticonvulsants (for further details see Phenytoin, p.1236).

Absorption studies carried out in 6 subjects with a systemic bacterial infection and 6 without demonstrated impairment of folic acid absorption in the patients with infection.— G. C. Cook *et al.*, *Lancet*, 1974, *2*, 1416.

Interactions. A review of compounds which reduce the effectiveness of folic acid and cyanocobalamin.— S. Waxman *et al.*, *Am. J. Med.*, 1970, *48*, 599.

Metformin reduced intestinal absorption of folic acid.— V. Herbert, *Ann. intern. Med.*, 1972, *76*, 140.

Absorption studies using folate compounds indicated that the availability of folates from the diet appeared to be inhibited by gastric acidity and the presence of ascorbate in the gastro-intestinal tract.— K. Ratanasthien *et al.*, *J. clin. Path.*, 1977, *30*, 438.

Phenytoin. For the interaction between folic acid and phenytoin, see Phenytoin, p.1240.

Absorption and Fate. Folic acid is absorbed mainly from the proximal part of the small intestine. Folate polyglutamates are considered to be deconjugated to monoglutamates during absorption. Folic acid rapidly appears in the blood, where it is extensively bound to plasma proteins. The amounts of folic acid absorbed from normal diets are rapidly distributed in body tissues and about 4 to 5 µg is excreted in the urine daily. When larger amounts are absorbed a high proportion is metabolised in the liver to other active forms of folate and a proportion is stored as reduced and methylated folate. Larger amounts of folate are rapidly excreted in the urine.

Folic acid administered by mouth appeared in the portal blood unaltered and was converted to 5-methyltetrahydrofolate, mainly in the liver.— V. Melikian *et al.*, *Lancet*, 1971, *2*, 955. Comment.— V. M. Whitehead *et al.* (letter), *ibid.*, 1972, *1*, 326.

Human Requirements. Body stores of folate in healthy persons have been reported as being between 5 to 10 mg, however, body stores may be much higher. A considerable proportion of folate is stored in the liver. About 400 µg of folate a day is considered a suitable average intake.

The recommended daily intakes of total folate were: infants up to 6 months, 40 to 50 µg; 7 to 12 months, 120 µg; children 1 to 12 years, 200 µg; persons 13 years and over, 400 µg; pregnant women, 800 µg; lactating women, 600 µg. All pregnant women needed daily supplements of about 500 µg of folic acid.— Report of a WHO Group of Experts on Nutritional Anaemias, *Tech. Rep. Ser. Wld Hlth Org. No. 503*, 1972.

Recommended daily intake of total folate: infants under 1 year, 50 µg; children 1 to 4 years, 100 µg; boys 5 to 11 years 200 µg; girls 5 to 8 years, 200 µg; older persons 300 µg; during pregnancy 500 µg; during lactation, 400 µg.— Recommended Daily Amounts of Food Energy and Nutrients for Groups of People in the United Kingdom, Report by the Committee on Medical Aspects of Food Policy, *Report on Health and Social Subjects No. 15*, London, HM Stationery Office, 1979.

The recommended daily dietary allowance of folate is 400 µg for adults and adolescents; for infants 5 µg per kg body-weight; for children 8 to 10 µg per kg; for pregnant women 800 µg; for lactating women 500 µg.— *Recommended Dietary Allowances*, 9th Edn, Washington, The National Research Council, 1980, p. 109.

The recommendation that foods for the young infant should contain folic acid in amounts not less than 30 ng per ml (based on the lower limit of the range in pooled samples of human milk).— Artificial Feeds for the Young Infant: Report of the Working Party on the Composition of Foods for Infants and Young Children, Committee on Medical Aspects of Food Policy, *Report on Health and Social Subjects, 18*, London, HM Stationery Office, 1980.

For further comments on folate requirements during pregnancy, see under Deficiency States, in Uses.

Uses. Folic acid is a member of the vitamin-B group. Folic acid is reduced in the body to tetrahydrofolate, which is a coenzyme for various metabolic processes including the synthesis of purine and pyrimidine nucleotides, and hence in the synthesis of DNA; it is also involved in some amino-acid conversion, and in the formation and utilisation of formate.

Deficiency of folic acid leads to megaloblastic anaemia. Deficiency may result from a diminished intake, as in malnutrition, from malabsorption, or from the concomitant use of anticonvulsants or dihydrofolate reductase inhibitors such as pyrimethamine, trimethoprim, or methotrexate. Folic acid does not correct folate deficiency due to dihydrofolate reductase inhibitors; calcium folinate (p.1648) is used for this purpose.

In the treatment of megaloblastic anaemia, folic acid may be given by mouth in an initial dosage of 10 to 20 mg daily for 14 days, or until a haemopoietic response has been obtained; the daily maintenance dose is 2.5 to 10 mg. Children may be given 5 to 15 mg daily according to the severity of the deficiency state. It may also be administered by intramuscular injection as the sodium salt.

In the prophylaxis of megaloblastic anaemia of pregnancy, the usual dose is 200 to 500 µg daily.

Reviews of the sources, absorption and fate, and actions of folic acid.— N. K. Shinton, *Br. med. J.*, 1972, *1*, 556; V. Herbert, *New Engl. J. Med.*, 1972, *286*, 214.

A report of the use of folic acid as a possible xanthine oxidase inhibitor.— K. A. Oster (letter), *Ann. intern. Med.*, 1977, *86*, 367. A criticism.— J. Plachetka (letter), *ibid.*, *87*, 252.

Discussion on the use of folic acid to reverse cervical dysplasia in women taking oral contraceptives.— *J. Am. med. Ass.*, 1980, *244*, 633.

Administration in renal failure. For reference to folic acid in renal failure see under Deficiency States (Dialysis), below.

Deficiency states. The role of malabsorption in folate deficiency, and its treatment.— A. V. Hoffbrand, *Clin. Med.*, 1972, *79* (Jan.), 19.

The role of folate deficiency in neurological disorders.— *Br. med. J.*, 1976, *2*, 71; *Lancet*, 1976, *2*, 836.

In 24 patients with severe folate deficiency (mean 1.6 ng per ml of serum), the incidence of neurological disease (organic brain syndrome, neuropathy, or positive Babinski response) was higher than in 21 patients with normal serum-folate concentrations (mean 12.7 ng per ml).— E. H. Reynolds *et al.*, *Br. med. J.*, 1973, *2*, 398.

Reports and comment on folate deficiency occurring during intensive care or parenteral nutrition.— D. Steinberg (letter), *J. Am. med. Ass.*, 1972, *222*, 490; R. M. Ibbotson *et al.*, *Br. med. J.*, 1975, *4*, 145; C. A. J. Wardrop *et al.* (letter), *ibid.*, 344; R. M. Ibbotson *et al.* (letter), *ibid.*, 522; M. E. J. Beard *et al.*, *Br. med. J.*, 1978, *1*, 624.

Dialysis. Following studies in 6 stable anephric patients it was recommended that the administration of folic acid 1 mg after each haemodialysis could provide adequate dosage.— V. A. Skoutakis *et al.*, *Clin. Pharmac. Ther.*, 1975, *18*, 200.

There was no need for folic acid supplements in adequately nourished patients undergoing haemodialysis.— J. Cunningham *et al.*, *Br. med. J.*, 1981, *282*, 1582.

In children. A discussion of folate deficiency in children.— *Lancet*, 1973, *1*, 813.

In a double-blind controlled study of 62 infants with low birth-weight folic acid 50 µg daily from the age of 2 weeks to 6 months produced no greater benefit than placebo.— A. C. Kendall *et al.*, *Archs Dis. Childh.*, 1974, *49*, 736.

Folic-acid deficiency may be the cause of reduced birth-weight and growth in erythroblastic infants. Folic-acid supplementation in 17 such infants improved weight gain although when folic acid was stopped some regressed.— G. Gandy and W. Jacobson, *Archs Dis. Childh.*, 1977, *52*, 1, 7, and 16.

Folic acid treatment of megaloblastosis in preterm infants and warning to avoid excess.— M. K. Strelling *et al.*, *Archs Dis. Childh.*, 1979, *54*, 699; D. Stevens *et al.*, *Pediatrics*, 1979, *64*, 333.

In the elderly. In a survey of serum-folate concentrations, no significant difference was found in elderly persons living at home and younger controls, but the levels were lower in patients in geriatric hospitals. There was little evidence of folate deficiency and no evidence of vitamin-B_{12} deficiency due to malnutrition.— R. H. Girdwood *et al.*, *Br. med. J.*, 1967, *2*, 670. See also *ibid.*, 652.

Neuropathic disorder clinically similar to subacute combined degeneration of the spinal cord occurred in 10 elderly patients with folate deficiency and normal serum concentrations of cyanocobalamin in 9 patients. Following treatment with folic acid 30 mg daily by mouth, neuropathy was reversed in 3 patients, and some improvement in reflex and sensory abnormalities occurred in all but 2 patients.— M. Manzoor and J. Runcie, *Br. med. J.*, 1976, *1*, 1176. Comments.— A. C. Young (letter), *ibid.*, 1406; M. C. Bateson (letter), *ibid.*, 1528.

Pregnancy and the neonate. Megaloblastic anaemia occurred in up to 4% of pregnancies when folate was not given; it was particularly likely in twin pregnancies. Elemental iron 100 mg plus folic acid 350 µg daily was adequate in areas where dietary intake was poor and had almost eliminated haematinic deficiency.— M. C. Macnaughton, *Prescribers' J.*, 1979, *19*, 52.

In a comparative study 11 pregnant women received a preparation containing ferrous fumarate, cyanocobalamin, and folic acid, and 10 received the same preparation without folic acid. In the first group only 1 suffered the restless leg syndrome whereas it occurred in 9 of the second group.— M. I. Botez and B. Lambert (letter), *New Engl. J. Med.*, 1977, *297*, 670.

Folic acid 4 mg daily taken before and during early pregnancy appeared to protect against recurrence of neural tube defects in the infants, in women who had already borne such an infant.— K. M. Laurence *et al.*, *Br. med. J.*, 1981, *282*, 1509. Criticism.— R. Mamtani and S. J. Watkins (letter), *ibid.*, 2056.

For studies on the role of vitamin supplementation in the prevention of neural-tube defects see in the general section, p.1635.

Mental disorders. A discussion of folate-responsive schizophrenia.— *Lancet*, 1975, *1*, 1283. See also E. H. Reynolds (letter), *ibid.*, 1975, *2*, 189.

For a critical view of vitamin therapy for mental disorders, see in the general section under Megavitamin Therapy, p.1635.

Preparations

Folic Acid Injection *(U.S.P.)*. A sterile solution of folic acid in Water for Injections prepared with the aid of sodium hydroxide or sodium carbonate. pH 8 to 11.

Folic Acid Tablets *(B.P.)*. Tablets containing folic acid. Protect from light.

Folic Acid Tablets *(U.S.P.)*. Tablets containing folic acid.

Proprietary Preparations

Lexpec Folic Acid *(R.P. Drugs, UK)*. Syrup containing folic acid 2.5 mg in each 5 ml (recommended diluent, Sorbitol Solution or Sorbitol Solution and water, equal parts).

Other Proprietary Names

Acfol *(Spain)*; Folacid *(Neth.)*; Folacin *(Norw., Swed.)*; Folaemin *(Neth.)*; Folasic *(Austral.)*; Foldine *(Fr.)*; Folettes *(Austral.)*; Folico, Folina (both *Ital.)*; Folsan *(Ger.)*; Folvite *(Canad., Switz., USA)*; Nifolin *(Denm.)*; Novofolacid *(Canad.)*.

7861-d

Sodium Folate. Sodium Pteroylglutamate.
$C_{19}H_{18}N_7NaO_6$=463.4.

CAS — 6484-89-5.

Available as a solution in water, prepared from sodium hydroxide or sodium carbonate and folic acid. Sodium folate solution is a clear, mobile, yellow to orange-yellow liquid. A solution in water has a pH of 8 to 11. Solutions are **sterilised** by filtration.

Uses. Sodium folate has the actions and uses of folic acid and it is used for parenteral folic acid therapy.

Preparations

See under Folic Acid, p.1648..

7862-n

Folinic Acid. Citrovorum Factor; Leucovorin; Formyl Tetrahydropteroylglutamic Acid. 5-Formyltetrahydropteroylglutamate trihydrate; *N*-[4-(2-Amino-5-formyl-5,6,7,8-tetrahydro-4-hydroxypteridin-6-ylmethylamino)benzoyl]-L(+)-glutamic acid trihydrate.
$C_{20}H_{23}N_7O_7,3H_2O$=527.5.

CAS — 58-05-9 (anhydrous).

A crystalline substance. Sparingly **soluble** in water. A saturated solution in water has a pH of about 3.

Uses. Folinic acid is used therapeutically in the form of its calcium salt, see Calcium Folinate, p.1648.

7863-h

Calcium Folinate.

Calcium Leucovorin; Calcium Folinate-SF; Leucovorin Calcium *(U.S.P.)*; NSC-3590. Calcium 5-formyltetrahydropteroylglutamate pentahydrate; Calcium *N*-[4-(2-amino-5-formyl-5,6,7,8-tetrahydro-4-hydroxypteridin-6-ylmethylamino)benzoyl]-L(+)glutamate pentahydrate.
$C_{20}H_{21}CaN_7O_7,5H_2O$=601.6.

CAS — 1492-18-8 (anhydrous); 41927-89-3 (pentahydrate).

Pharmacopoeias. In *Braz.* and *U.S.*

A yellowish-white or yellow, odourless, microcrystalline powder. Very **soluble** in water; practically insoluble in alcohol. **Protect** from light.

The manufacturers reported that calcium folinate injections diluted in dextrose, dextrose/saline, Ringer's injection, and lactated Ringer's injection were stable (90% potency, and maintenance of pH, clarity, and colour) for 24 hours. The *U.S.P.* injection could be diluted with milk or alkaline solutions for oral use within 24 hours.— R. D. Lauper (letter), *Am. J. Hosp. Pharm.*, 1978, *35*, 377.

Adverse Effects. Occasional allergic reactions have been reported; pyrexia has occurred after injections.

Precautions. As with folic acid, folinic acid should never be given alone or in conjunction with inadequate amounts of hydroxocobalamin for the treatment of pernicious anaemia.

Uses. Folinic acid is the 5-formyl derivative of tetrahydrofolic acid, the active form of folic acid. Folinic acid is used principally as an antidote to folic acid antagonists, such as methotrexate, which block the conversion of folic acid to tetrahydrofolate by binding the enzyme dihydrofolate reductase.

In cases of inadvertent overdosage of a folic acid antagonist, folinic acid should be administered as soon as possible; if a period of more than 4 hours intervenes, the treatment may not be effective. Where large doses of methotrexate have been given calcium folinate may be given, by intravenous infusion in a dose equivalent to 75 mg of folinic acid within 12 hours, followed by 12 mg intramuscularly every 6 hours for 4 doses. Doses equal to or greater than the dose of methotrexate have been recommended. In less severe overdosage 6 to 12 mg of folinic acid intramuscularly every 6 hours for 4 doses may be adequate.

Folinic acid is used in conjunction with methotrexate to reduce the toxicity of the methotrexate ('folinic acid rescue'; 'calcium leucovorin rescue'). Folinic acid is given after an appropriate interval, usually of up to 24 hours, has elapsed for methotrexate to exert its antineoplastic effect. Doses of up to 120 mg have been given over 12 to 24 hours, by intramuscular injection or intravenous injection or infusion, followed by 12 to 15 mg intramuscularly, or 15 mg by mouth, every 6 hours for the next 48 hours. With lower doses of methotrexate folinic acid 15 mg by mouth every 6 hours for 48 to 72 hours may suffice. For further details see under Methotrexate, p.217.

Folinic acid, like folic acid, is effective in the treatment of megaloblastic anaemia. The dosage suggested in the treatment of megaloblastic anaemia varies from 15 mg daily down to 1 mg daily.

Folinic acid was effectively absorbed when given by mouth and produced peak concentrations of folate in the serum after about 1 hour.— P. F. Nixon and J. R. Bertino, *New Engl. J. Med.*, 1972, *286*, 175.

Deficiency states. Severe folate deficiency considered to be potentially fatal developed in 2 patients receiving intravenous nutrition. Both patients developed jaundice. Calcium folinate 9 mg daily by intravenous injection produced haematological recovery.— P. J. Green (letter), *Lancet*, 1977, *1*, 814.

Associated with dihydrofolate reductase inhibitors. The administration of folinic acid 10 mg daily had been recommended for the prevention of haematological toxicity due to pyrimethamine.— *Med. Lett.*, 1975, *17*, 32.

Among 194 patients with *Pneumocystis carinii* pneumonia, 35.5% had acute leukaemia. It was suggested that folinic acid should not be administered to reduce the side-effects of pyrimethamine in the treatment of *Pneumocystis carinii* pneumonia associated with leukaemia because folic acid could produce haematological relapse in patients with leukaemia.— R. E. Helmer (letter), *Ann. intern. Med.*, 1975, *82*, 124.

Methotrexate. A discussion of the use of folinic acid to prevent the toxicity of some folic acid antagonists, particularly methotrexate ('folinic acid rescue therapy'). Much research is still needed to determine the optimum dose and frequency of administration, and to define the ideal interval between the end of methotrexate therapy and the start of folinic acid.— *Drug & Ther. Bull.*, 1978, *16*, 11.

In 10 patients with methotrexate toxicity after high doses, and resistant to standard doses of calcium folinate, skin and mucosal toxicity was arrested within 24 hours and was recovering usually within 48 hours after massive doses of calcium folinate—1 to 5 g in a day or 4 to 8 g in 2 days by infusion. Bone-marrow depression occurred in all the patients but there were no methotrexate-related deaths. Further study was needed to assess the minimum dose of calcium folinate.— I. Djerassi, *Cancer Treat. Rep.*, 1977, *61*, 749.

For the use of folinic acid in vincristine overdosage, see p.231.

Preparations

Leucovorin Calcium Injection *(U.S.P.)*. A sterile solution of calcium folinate in Water for Injections. Sodium hydroxide or hydrochloric acid may be added to adjust the pH (range: 6.5 to 8.5); it may contain suitable preservatives. Potency is expressed in terms of the equivalent amount of folinic acid. Protect from light.

Calcium Leucovorin *(Lederle, UK)*. Calcium folinate, available as **Injection** containing the equivalent of folinic acid 3 mg per ml, in ampoules of 1 and 10 ml, and as scored **Tablets** each containing the equivalent of folinic acid 15 mg. (Also available as Calcium Leucovorin in *Canad.*).

Other Proprietary Names

Lederfoline *(Fr.)*; Ledervorin *(Neth.)*; Ledervorin Calcium *(Belg.)*; Leucovorin *(Austral., Denm., Ger., Ital., S.Afr.)*.

7864-m

Nicotinic Acid *(B.P., B.P. Vet., Eur. P.)*.

Nicotin. Acid; Acidum Nicotinicum; Niacin *(U.S.P.)*; Nikotinsäure. Pyridine-3-carboxylic acid.
$C_6H_5NO_2$=123.1.

CAS — 59-67-6.

Pharmacopoeias. In *Aust., Belg., Br., Braz., Chin., Eur., Fr., Ger., Hung., Ind., Int., It., Jap., Mex., Neth., Nord., Port., Roum., Rus., Span., Swiss, Turk.*, and *U.S.*

It is prepared synthetically and occurs in rice-polishings, yeast, liver, lean meats, and to a lesser extent in potatoes and vegetables.

White or creamy-white, odourless or almost odourless, crystals or crystalline powder with a feebly acid taste. M.p. 234° to 237°.

Soluble 1 in 55 to 60 of water and 1 in 100 of alcohol; soluble in boiling water and boiling alcohol and in solutions of alkali hydroxides and carbonates; very slightly soluble in chloroform; practically insoluble in ether. A 1.3% solution in water has a pH of 3 to 3.5. Solutions of the sodium salt are **sterilised** by autoclaving or by filtration. **Incompatible** with oxidising agents. There is little loss of nicotinic acid from foods during cooking. **Protect** from light.

Adverse Effects. Nicotinic acid has a vasodilator action and when given by mouth or by injection in therapeutic doses it may cause flushing of the face, a sensation of heat, and a pounding in the head. These symptoms are transient and may be avoided by substituting nicotinamide.

Other adverse effects which have been reported, especially following high doses of nicotinic acid, include flushing and dryness of the skin, urticaria, pruritus, furunculosis, other skin lesions, abdominal cramps, diarrhoea, nausea and vomiting, malaise, anorexia, activation of peptic ulcer, amblyopia, jaundice and impairment of liver function, decrease in glucose tolerance, mild diabetes, and hyperuricaemia. Most of these effects subside on withdrawal of the drug.

Effects on the eye. Three patients receiving nicotinic acid 3 to 5 g daily for hypercholesterolaemia developed blurring of vision due to cystoid macular oedema. Vision deteriorated further with time but improved on stopping nicotinic acid.— J. D. M. Gass, *Am. J. Ophthal.*, 1973, *76*, 500.

Effects on liver function. Studies of liver function in 8 patients with hypercholesterolaemia who had been treated with nicotinic acid, 1.5 to 6 g daily for up to 9 years, showed slight retention of sulphobromophthalein and grade 3 cephalin flocculation in 1. Three untreated patients with hypercholesterolaemia acted as controls and an abnormal serum aspartate aminotransferase (SGOT) value was found in 1 of them. Histological changes were evident in the treated patients but were not severe enough to affect clinical and laboratory assessments of hepatic impairment. The changes were not considered a contra-indication for the use of nicotinic acid in carefully supervised patients with hypercholesterolaemia.— A. H. Baggenstoss *et al.*, *Mayo Clin. Proc.*, 1967, *42*, 385.

Jaundice occurring in a 69-year-old man was attributed to nicotinic acid which he had taken in doses of 750 mg daily for less than 3 months. The jaundice became more severe in the 3 weeks following discontinuation of the drug but began to recede within a month.— A. A. Sugerman and C. G. Clark, *J. Am. med. Ass.*, 1974, *228*, 202.

Hepatitis in a young woman was possibly due to nicotinic acid. She had taken 3 g daily with several other vitamins for 2½ years, but her condition did not improve until the nicotinic acid was withdrawn.— N. Einstein *et al.*, *Am. J. dig. Dis.*, 1975, *20*, 282.

Effects on mental state. In 2 patients the ingestion of nicotinic acid 1.5 and 3 g, respectively, appeared to enhance psychotic symptoms. The patients had previously experienced mainly pleasant effects after marijuana or lysergide, but these turned to frightening psychotic experiences after nicotinic acid.— G. R. Heninger and M. B. Bowers (letter), *J. Am. med. Ass.*, 1968, *204*, 1010. Since 1952, over 1000 patients had been treated with nicotinic acid, and other agents, in doses of 3 to 30 g daily with no evidence of exacerbation of psychotic symptoms. Nicotinic acid was less toxic than tranquillisers and antidepressants.— A. Hoffer (letter), *J. Am. med. Ass.*, 1969, *207*, 1355.

Precautions. Nicotinic acid should be given cautiously to patients with a history of peptic ulceration.

Effect on diagnostic tests. In laboratory tests for blood bilirubin, nicotinic acid could cause increased blood levels or give false positives.— *Med. Lett.*, 1971, *13*, 82.

Nicotinic acid could cause chemical interference in laboratory tests for catecholamines.— *Med. Lett.*, 1971, *13*, 82.

Absorption and Fate. Nicotinic acid is readily absorbed from the gastro-intestinal tract and is widely distributed in the body tissues. It has a short half-life. The principal metabolites after low doses are *N*-methylnicotinamide and the 2-pyridone and 4-pyridone derivatives; after large doses the principal metabolites are nicotinuric acid, *N*-methylnicotinamide, and the 2-pyridone derivative.

A review of the clinical pharmacokinetics of nicotinic acid.— R. Gugler, *Clin. Pharmacokinet.*, 1978, *3*, 425.

Further references: M. Weiner, *Drug Metab. Rev.*, 1979, *9*, 99.

Human Requirements. The normal daily human requirement, though not definitely known, is probably about 15 to 20 mg, depending on the protein intake. Primary dietary deficiency is rare. Secondary deficiency may be caused by an inadequate intake as a result of oropharyngeal lesions, gastro-intestinal disorders, or alcoholism.

To allow for the metabolic conversion of tryptophan into nicotinic acid, the recommended intake of the vitamin should be expressed as 'niacin equivalents' per 1000 kcal; 6.6 niacin equivalents were required for every 1000 kcal. One such equivalent was equal to 1 mg of nicotinic acid or 60 mg of tryptophan.— Report of a Joint FAO/WHO Expert Group, *Tech. Rep. Ser. Wld Hlth Org. No. 362*, 1967.

Recommended daily intake of nicotinic acid, calculated on resting metabolism: boys and girls up to 8 years, 5 to 11 mg; 9 to 17 years, 14 to 19 mg; men 18 years and over, 18 mg; women 18 years and over, 15 mg; during pregnancy, 18 mg; during lactation, 21 mg. One mg of available nicotinic acid was considered equivalent to 60 mg of tryptophan.— Recommended Daily Amounts of Food Energy and Nutrients for Groups of People in the United Kingdom, Report by The Committee on Medical Aspects of Food Policy, *Report on Health and Social Subjects No. 15*, London, HM Stationery Office, 1979.

Recommended daily dietary allowances of nicotinic acid: up to 6 months, 6 mg; 6 to 12 months, 8 mg; 1 to 3 years, 9 mg; 4 to 6 years, 11 mg; 7 to 10 years, 16 mg; males 11 to 18 years and 23 to 50 years, 18 mg; males 19 to 22 years, 19 mg; males 51 years and over, 16 mg; females 11 to 14 years, 15 mg; 15 to 22 years, 14 mg; 23 years and over, 13 mg; in pregnancy, an additional 2 mg; in lactation, an additional 5 mg. The allowances are calculated as nicotinic acid equivalents; one nicotinic acid equivalent equals 1 mg of nicotinic acid or 60 mg of dietary tryptophan.— *Recommended Dietary Allowances*, 9th Edn, Washington, The National Research Council, 1980.

The recommendation that foods for the young infant should contain nicotinic acid/nicotinamide in amounts not less than 2.3 µg per ml (based on the lower limit of the range in pooled samples of human milk).— Artificial Feeds for the Young Infant: Report of the Working Party on the Composition of Foods for Infants and Young Children, Committee on Medical Aspects of Food Policy, *Report on Health and Social Subjects, 18*, London, HM Stationery Office, 1980.

Uses. Nicotinic acid is converted in the body to nicotinamide adenine dinucleotide (NAD) and nicotinamide adenine dinucleotide phosphate (NADP) which are involved in electron transfer reactions in the respiratory chain.

Deficiency of nicotinic acid produces pellagra, which is characterised by loss of appetite, lethargy, weakness, diarrhoea, skin lesions, and mental and neurological changes. In the treatment of pellagra up to 500 mg is given by mouth daily in divided doses.

Nicotinic acid or nicotinamide produce improvement in the mental, dermal, and alimentary manifestations of pellagra but neurological symptoms may need prolonged treatment and the concomitant use of other vitamins of the B group.

Nicotinic acid has been employed for its vasodilator action in the treatment of a variety of disorders; its value is not considered to be established.

Nicotinic acid in high doses lowers plasma concentrations of very low-density and low-density lipoproteins. It has therefore been used, often in association with other lipid-regulating agents, in type II, III, IV, and V hyperlipoproteinaemias. Doses of 3 g or more daily have been given; side-effects may be a limiting factor.

The addition of any of the following substances to raw and unprocessed meat intended for human consumption is prohibited in Great Britain by the Meat (Treatment) Regulations, 1964: ascorbic acid, isoascorbic acid, nicotinic acid, nicotinamide, and any derivative of these substances. The ban on the addition of nicotinic acid to raw and unprocessed meat should be extended to include uncooked processed meat and meat products.— *Food Additivies and Contaminants Committee Report on Further Classes of Food Additives*, London, HM Stationery Office, 1968.

Administration in renal failure. The dose of nicotinic acid should be reduced to 50% in patients with a glomerular filtration-rate (GFR) of 10 to 50 ml per minute, and should be titrated to the needs of the patient in those with a GFR of less than 10 ml per minute.— W. M. Bennett *et al.*, *Ann. intern. Med.*, 1980, *93*, 286.

Diagnosis of Gilbert's syndrome. The mean increase in plasma bilirubin 180 minutes after the slow intravenous injection of nicotinic acid 50 mg was 23.3 µmol per litre in 16 patients with Gilbert's syndrome compared with 6.5 µmol per litre in 6 controls. The nicotinic acid test was more reliable than the reduced energy intake test.— A. R. Davidson *et al.*, *Br. med. J.*, 1975, *2*, 480. See also V. L. Fromke and D. Miller, *Medicine, Baltimore*, 1972, *51*, 451, per *Gut*, 1973, *14*, 820; W. Röllinghoff *et al.*, *ibid.*, 1981, *22*, 663.

Effects on serum lipids. Reviews and discussions of the effect of nicotinic acid on plasma lipids.— R. I. Levy and B. M. Rifkind, *Drugs*, 1973, *6*, 12; *Med. Lett.*, 1975, *17*, 49; W. R. Fisher and D. H. Truitt, *Ann. intern. Med.*, 1976, *85*, 497; R. I. Levy, *A. Rev. Pharmac. & Toxic.*, 1977, *17*, 499; S. Margolis, *J. Am. med. Ass.*, 1978, *239*, 2696; *Med. Lett.*, 1980, *22*, 65; *Drug & Ther. Bull.*, 1980, *18*, 25; P. Samuel, *Am. Heart J.*, 1980, *100*, 573; H. Keen *et al.* (letter), *Lancet*, 1980, *2*, 1241.

The mechanism of the hypolipidaemic action of nicotinic acid.— B. J. Kudchodkar *et al.*, *Clin. Pharmac. Ther.*, 1978, *24*, 354. See also J. Shepherd *et al.*, *J. clin. Invest.*, 1979, *63*, 858.

Nicotinic acid was considered an acceptable alternative to cholestyramine in the treatment of hyperlipoproteinaemia type IIa. In a controlled crossover study of 8 patients, nicotinic acid 1 g thrice daily reduced plasma-cholesterol concentrations by 21%, and plasma-triglyceride concentrations by 23%, which might indicate potential benefit in type IIb hyperlipoproteinaemia. Cholestyramine 4 g four times daily reduced cholesterol concentrations by 27% but had no effect on triglyceride concentration. Two patients withdrew from the study because of flushing due to nicotinic acid.— J. I. Mann *et al.*, *Br. J. clin. Pharmac.*, 1977, *4*, 305.

Three patients with type IIb and three with type IV hyperlipidaemia on chronic dialysis were treated with a sustained-release preparation of nicotinic acid 1 to 2 g daily for 6 weeks. Concentrations of cholesterol and triglycerides were reduced but persistent flushing caused 2 patients to cease treatment; 2 others continued to have flushing and gastro-intestinal symptoms. Treatment by diet was preferable.— R. Gokal *et al.*, *Br. med. J.*, 1978, *1*, 82.

For discussions of the use of nicotinic acid in the treatment of hyperlipoproteinaemia, and for classifications of hyperlipoproteinaemia, see Clofibrate, p.408.

For the use of nicotinic acid with colestipol, see p.412.

Myocardial infarction. In a 5-year double-blind trial on the efficacy and safety of nicotinic acid and other lipid-influencing drugs in long-term therapy of coronary heart disease, 1119 males, aged initially between 30 and 64 years and who had experienced 1 or more episodes of myocardial infarction, were allocated to treatment with nicotinic acid 3 g daily. Nicotinic acid was no more effective than placebo in reducing overall or cause-specific mortality; there was a statistically significant lower incidence of non-fatal cardiac infarction in the nicotinic acid group, but a statistically significant higher incidence of atrial fibrillation and other cardiac arrhythmias. There was also an increased incidence of gastro-intestinal problems, and elevated levels of serum enzymes, serum uric acid, and plasma glucose in men taking nicotinic acid.— The Coronary Drug Project Research Group, *J. Am. med. Ass.*, 1975, *231*, 360. Comment.— *Br. med. J.*, 1975, *2*, 103; *Lancet*, 1975, *1*, 501.

Mental disorders. A critical review of the use of nicotinic acid in the treatment of schizophrenia; there was no clear evidence that nicotinic acid or nicotinamide were of value in acute or chronic schizophrenia.— *Med. Lett.*, 1973, *15*, 107.

For another critical view of vitamin therapy for mental disorders, see in the general section under Megavitamin Therapy, p.1635.

Peripheral vascular disorders. There was no basis for the use of nicotinic acid in peripheral vascular diseases.— J. D. Coffman, *New Engl. J. Med.*, 1979, *300*, 713.

Limited value of nicotinic acid in 6 patients with stasis dermatitis.— J. K. Wilkin *et al.*, *Br. J. Derm.*, 1979, *100*, 471.

Vasculitis. Nicotinic acid 300 to 500 mg daily produced remissions of livedoid vasculitis in 9 of 12 patients; 2 were not changed, and 1 became worse.— R. K. Winkelmann *et al.*, *Mayo Clin. Proc.*, 1974, *49*, 746.

Preparations

Injectabile Acidi Nicotinici *(Nord. P.).* Nicotinic acid 5 g, sodium bicarbonate 3 g, Water for Injections to 100 ml. Sterilised by autoclaving. A suitable preservative is 0.001% phenylmercuric nitrate; *Dan. Disp.* specifies 1% benzyl alcohol.

Niacin Injection *(U.S.P.).* Nicotinic Acid Injection. A sterile solution of nicotinic acid and sodium nicotinate in Water for Injections, made with the aid of sodium carbonate or sodium hydroxide. pH 4 to 6. Potency is expressed in terms of nicotinic acid.

Niacin Tablets *(U.S.P.).* Tablets containing nicotinic acid.

Nicotinic Acid Tablets *(B.P.).* Tablets containing nicotinic acid.

Proprietary Names

Akotin 250 *(Glaxo, Arg.)*; Nicangin *(Astra, Swed.)*; Nico-400 *(Marion Laboratories, USA)*; Nicobid *(Armour, USA)*; Nicolar *(Armour, USA)*; Niconacid *(Wander, Ger.)*; Nicorol *(Paramed, Switz.)*; Nico-Span *(Key, USA)*; Nicotinex *(Fleming, USA)*; Nicyl *(Astra, Fr.)*; SK-Niacin *(Smith Kline & French, USA)*; Vasotherm *(Nutrition Control Products, USA)*.

NOTE. For proprietary preparations containing nicotinic acid and acetomenaphthone for chilblains, see under Acetomenaphthone, p.1666.

7865-b

Nicotinamide *(B.P., B.P. Vet., Eur. P.).* Nicotinamidum; Niacinamide *(U.S.P.)*; Nicotinic Acid Amide; Nicotylamide; Vitamin PP. Pyridine-3-carboxamide.

$C_6H_6N_2O$=122.1.

CAS — 98-92-0.

Pharmacopoeias. In all pharmacopoeias examined.

A white crystalline powder or colourless crystals, odourless or with a faint characteristic odour and a salty and bitter taste. M.p. 128° to 131°. It absorbs insignificant amounts of moisture at relative humidities up to about 90% at 25°.

Soluble 1 in 1 of water and 1 in 10 of boiling water, 1 in 1.5 of alcohol, and 1 in 10 of glycerol; slightly soluble in chloroform and ether. A 5% solution in water has a pH of 6 to 7.5. A 4.49% solution is iso-osmotic with serum. Solutions are **sterilised** by autoclaving or by filtration. **Incompatible** with alkalis and mineral acids. **Store** in airtight containers.

An aqueous solution of nicotinamide iso-osmotic with serum (4.49%) caused 100% haemolysis of erythrocytes cultured in it for 45 minutes.— E. R. Hammarlund and K. Pedersen-Bjergaard, *J. pharm. Sci.*, 1961, *50*, 24.

Addition compound with ascorbic acid. A canary-yellow addition compound was formed when equimolecular amounts of ascorbic acid and nicotinamide were mixed. The reaction product maintained essentially the full potency of each constituent but had a melting point different from either component.— T. J. Macek, *Am. J. Pharm.*, 1960, *132*, 433.

Adverse Effects. Nicotinamide does not cause vasodilatation like nicotinic acid.

A patient with schizophrenia receiving nicotinamide, fluphenazine, and thiothixene was admitted repeatedly to hospital for nausea and vomiting. He was found to have abnormal liver function on each occasion which returned to normal during his stay in hospital. It was discovered that for several days before each attack he had increased the dose of nicotinamide from 3 g to 9 g daily. Liver dysfunction returned with challenge doses of nicotinamide.— S. L. Winter and J. L. Boyer, *New Engl. J. Med.*, 1973, *289*, 1180.

Uses. Nicotinamide has the actions described under Nicotinic Acid (above), but it has no vasodilator action. It is used as an alternative to nicotinic acid for the prevention and treatment of pellagra in daily doses of up to 250 mg.

Mention of the use of nicotinamide 25 mg daily or weekly in 6 children with Hartnup disease.— B. Wilcken *et al.*, *Archs Dis. Childh.*, 1977, *52*, 38.

Preparations

Niacinamide Injection *(U.S.P.).* A sterile solution of nicotinamide in Water for Injections. pH 5 to 7.

Niacinamide Tablets *(U.S.P.).* Tablets containing nicotinamide. Store in airtight containers.

Nicotinamide Tablets *(B.P.).* Nicotinic Acid Amide Tablets; Niacinamide Tablets. Tablets containing nicotinamide. Store in airtight containers. Protect from light.

Proprietary Names

Farmobion PP *(Farmochimica Italiana, Ital.)*; Nicobion *(Astra, Fr.*; *E. Merck, Ger.*; *Lematte & Boinot, Switz.)*; Nicotilamida *(Igoda, Spain)*.

7866-v

Pantothenic Acid. (+)-(*R*)-3-(2,4-Dihydroxy-3,3-dimethylbutyramido)propionic acid.

$C_9H_{17}NO_5$=219.2.

CAS — 79-83-4.

An unstable, extremely hygroscopic, viscous oil. Freely **soluble** in water, ethyl acetate, dioxan, and glacial acetic acid; soluble in ether and amyl alcohol; practically insoluble in chloroform. **Store** in airtight containers.

It is found in meat, fresh vegetables, yeast, egg-yolk, and milk and it may be prepared synthetically.

Absorption and Fate. Pantothenic acid is readily absorbed from the gastro-intestinal tract and is widely distributed in the body tissues. About 70% of pantothenic acid is excreted unchanged in the urine and about 30% in the faeces.

Human Requirements.

The recommendation that foods for the young infant should contain pantothenic acid in amounts not less than 2 µg per ml (based on the lower limit of the range in pooled samples of human milk).— Artificial Feeds for the Young Infant: Report of the Working Party on the Composition of Foods for Infants and Young Children, Committee on Medical Aspects of Food Policy, *Report on Health and Social Subjects, 18*, London, HM Stationery Office, 1980.

Uses. Pantothenic acid is present in living tissues and is commonly considered a member of the vitamin-B group. It is a component of coenzyme A which is concerned with the transfer of two-carbon groups.

Little is known about the significance of pantothenic acid in human nutrition and no specific symptoms in man have been correlated with a deficiency of the vitamin, though a syndrome has been described involving fatigue, headache, sleep disturbances, epigastric pain, paraesthesias, muscle cramps, and incoordination. On the basis of animal requirements the daily human requirement is probably 5 to 10 mg. A normal diet usually provides 10 to 20 mg daily. Pantothenic acid is relatively stable in foodstuffs during long periods of storage and little is destroyed during cooking.

Pantothenic acid has no accepted therapeutic uses in human medicine, though it has been used, particularly in the form of its calcium salt, with variable results, in a variety of conditions including streptomycin intoxication, postoperative ileus, and rheumatoid conditions. It is usually administered as the calcium salt (see p.1650) and it is employed, usually in conjunction with other vitamins of the B group, as a nutritional supplement.

See also Dexpanthenol, p.1650.

7867-g

Calcium Pantothenate *(Eur. P., U.S.P.).* Calcii Pantothenas; Dextro Calcium Pantothenate. The calcium salt of (+)-pantothenic acid.

$(C_9H_{16}NO_5)_2Ca$=476.5.

CAS — 137-08-6.

Pharmacopoeias. In *Arg., Belg., Braz., Chin., Cz., Eur., Fr., Ger., It., Jap., Jug., Neth., Pol., Port., Swiss,* and *U.S.*

A white, odourless, slightly hygroscopic powder with a bitter taste. M.p. 197° to 204°. **Soluble** 1 in 3 of water; soluble in glycerol; practically insoluble in alcohol, chloroform, and ether. A 5% solution in water is dextrorotatory and has a pH of 7 to 9. A 5.5% solution is iso-osmotic with serum. Solutions are not stable to autoclaving and are **sterilised** by filtration. Solutions are most stable between pH 5 and 7; in more strongly acid or in alkaline solution hydrolysis is fairly rapid. **Incompatible** with sulphates, phosphates, and carbonates. **Store** in airtight containers.

Uses. See Pantothenic Acid, p.1650.

Calcium pantothenate given initially in a dose of 500 mg daily increasing to 2 g daily in patients with arthritic conditions.—Report No. 199 of the General Practitioner Research Group, *Practitioner*, 1980, *224*, 208.

Preparations

Calcium Pantothenate Tablets *(U.S.P.).* Tablets containing calcium pantothenate. Store in airtight containers.

Cantopal Compound Capsules (KW55) *(Koch-Light, UK: Cantassium Co., UK).* Each contains calcium pantothenate 125 mg, calcium phosphate 62.5 mg, cysteine hydrochloride 75 mg, sebacic acid ($C_{10}H_{18}O_4$ = 202.3) 25 mg, and ethyl n-heptyloxyacetate ($C_{11}H_{22}O_3$ = 202.3) 25 mg. For rheumatoid arthritis. *Dose.* 4 capsules 30 minutes before breakfast.

Cantothen Injection (KW21/2) *(Koch-Light, UK: Cantassium Co., UK).* Vials each containing calcium pantothenate 200 mg and cysteine hydrochloride 30 mg, for preparing injections. For osteoarthritis and osteoporosis. *Dose.* By intragluteal injection, the contents of 1 vial thrice weekly for 2 weeks, reduced thereafter according to the needs of the patient.

Other Proprietary Names

Cal-Pan *(Canad.)*; Galamila *(Ger.)*; Megapantho *(Canad.)*; Pantenil *(Spain)*; Pantholin *(USA)*; Pantogen *(Austral.)*; Sili-met-san *(Belg.)*.

7868-q

Racemic Calcium Pantothenate *(U.S.P.).*

$(C_9H_{16}NO_5)_2Ca$=476.5.

CAS — 599-54-2 [(±)-pantothenic acid]; 6381-63-1 (calcium salt).

Pharmacopoeias. In *U.S.*

A white slightly hygroscopic powder with a faint characteristic odour and a bitter taste. It is a mixture of the calcium salts of the dextrorotatory and laevorotatory isomers of pantothenic acid and contains not less than 42.5% of dextrorotatory calcium pantothenate, calculated on the dried basis. Potency is expressed in terms of the equivalent amount of calcium pantothenate (dextrorotatory).

Freely **soluble** in water; soluble in glycerol; practically insoluble in alcohol, chloroform, and ether. A solution in water is neutral or alkaline to litmus. Solutions are **sterilised** by filtration. **Store** in airtight containers.

Uses. As for Pantothenic Acid, p.1650. It has been used in doses of up to 200 mg.

7869-p

Dexpanthenol. Pantothenol; Dextro-Pantothenyl Alcohol. (*R*)-2,4-Dihydroxy-*N*-(3-hydroxypropyl)-3,3-dimethylbutyramide.

$C_9H_{19}NO_4$=205.3.

CAS — 81-13-0.

Pharmacopoeias. In *Aust.* and *Nord.*

A clear, colourless or slightly yellow, odourless, hygroscopic, viscous liquid with a bitter taste.

Miscible with water and alcohol; soluble 1 in 70 of chloroform and 1 in 200 of ether; practically insoluble in fats and oils. A 5.6% solution in water is iso-osmotic with serum. Solutions may be **sterilised** by maintaining at 98° to 100° for 30 minutes with a bactericide or by filtration, the pH being adjusted to between 4 and 7. **Store** in airtight containers.

Precautions. Dexpanthenol is contra-indicated in haemophiliacs and in patients with ileus due to mechanical obstruction. It should be given cautiously with or immediately after parasympathomimetic drugs or suxamethonium.

Uses. Dexpanthenol is the alcoholic analogue of pantothenic acid (see p.1650); it is readily converted to the acid when administered internally. It has been given intramuscularly in doses of 250 to 500 mg to prevent or control gastro-intestinal atony but its value has not been established.

Dexpanthenol has been used topically as an ointment, cream, or solution, usually in a strength of 2%, for the

treatment of various minor skin disorders. It has been used in various cosmetic preparations.
Dexpanthenol has also been given with the aim of reducing the adverse effects of streptomycin and salicylates.
The actions and use of dexpanthenol and panthenol in cosmetics.— B. Idson, *Drug Cosmet. Ind.*, 1974, *114*, (May), 36.

Proprietary Names
Bepanten *(Roche, Ital.)*; Bepanthen *(Roche, Austral.; Roche, Denm.; Roche, Ger.; Roche, Neth.; Roche, Switz.)*; Bepanthene *(Roche, Belg.; Roche, Fr.; Roche, Spain)*; Bepantol *(Roche, S.Afr.)*; Ilopan *(Adria, USA)*; Motilyn *(Abbott, Canad.)*; Panthoderm *(US Vitamin, Arg.; USV, Canad.; USV Pharmaceutical Corp., USA)*; Thenalton *(Fulton, Ital.)*.

7870-n

Other Compounds Traditionally Considered as Part of the B Group

Described below are aminobenzoic acid, choline, and inositol and their related compounds.

7871-h

Aminobenzoic Acid *(B.P., U.S.P.)*. Amben; PAB; PABA; Pabacidum; Para-aminobenzoic Acid; Vitamin H′; Acidum Paraminobenzoicum. 4-Aminobenzoic acid.
$C_7H_7NO_2$=137.1.

CAS — 150-13-0.

Pharmacopoeias. In *Aust., Br., Braz., Cz., Pol., Roum., Span., Swiss,* and *U.S.*

White or slightly yellow odourless or almost odourless crystals or crystalline powder. M.p. 186° to 189°. It gradually darkens on exposure to air and light.
Soluble 1 in 200 of water, 1 in 10 of boiling water, 1 in 8 of alcohol, and 1 in 50 of ether; slightly soluble in chloroform; freely soluble in solutions of alkali hydroxides and carbonates. **Incompatible** with ferric salts and oxidising agents. **Store** in airtight containers. Protect from light.

Adverse Effects. Contact and photocontact dermatitis has been reported.

From patch tests carried out in 413 patients with contact dermatoses, 1 was found to be allergic to aminobenzoic acid.— E. Epstein, *J. Am. med. Ass.*, 1966, *198*, 517.

Precautions. Aminobenzoic acid lotion may stain clothing.

Uses. Aminobenzoic acid has sometimes been included as a member of the vitamin-B group. It is involved in the synthesis by micro-organisms of folic acid and is therefore of importance in the mode of action of sulphonamides and of dihydrofolate reductase inhibitors, such as methotrexate. A deficiency of aminobenzoic acid in man or animals has not been demonstrated.
Aminobenzoic acid and its esters are used by topical application in alcoholic lotions or creams as sunscreen agents; a 5% solution is commonly used. In some countries their use in cosmetics is prohibited.
See also under Potassium Aminobenzoate (p.1651).

Aminobenzoic acid has no useful role in human nutrition.— V. Herbert, *J. Am. med. Ass.*, 1980, *243*, 1092.

The efficacy of aminobenzoic acid as a sunscreen agent was much greater than that of its esters, padimate (amyl dimethylaminobenzoate) and glyceryl aminobenzoate, both immediately after application and after 30 minutes of profuse sweating. Immersion in water caused a serious loss of protection, particularly in the first 30 minutes after application. Aminobenzoic acid appeared to diffuse into the horny layer of the skin and significant protection remained for 3 days after a single application of a 5% preparation. Alcohol 50% or 60% was more effective than a number of other bases. Application of 5% alcoholic solutions once daily for 10 days did not give rise to toxic symptoms. Aminobenzoic acid had no protective effect when given by mouth.— I. Willis and A. Kligman, *Archs Derm.*, 1970, *102*, 405, per *J. Am. med. Ass.*, 1970, *214*, 613. See also M. A. Pathak *et al.*, *New Engl. J. Med.*, 1969, *280*, 1459; *Drug & Ther. Bull.*, 1971, *9*, 95.

Studies with aminobenzoic acid 5% in alcohol (55%) showed that application of 60 µl per cm² usually gave protection against 30 minimal erythemal doses. Daily application enhanced the amount and duration of protection. The amount of residual protection after 10 minutes of water immersion was greatest 2 hours after application.— A. Langner and A. M. Kligman, *Archs Derm.*, 1972, *105*, 851. See also *idem*, *106*, 338, per *J. Am. med. Ass.*, 1972, *221*, 1423; R. L. Garcia and C. M. Davis, *Milit. Med.*, 1973, *138*, 331, per *Int. pharm. Abstr.*, 1974, *11*, 95.

Solutions of aminobenzoic acid 5% in 50 to 70% alcohol were considered to be the most effective non-opaque sunscreens.— *Med. Lett.*, 1974, *16*, 60.

For other reports of aminobenzoic acid as a sunscreen agent, see Sunscreen Agents, p.1495.

Preparations

Aminobenzoic Acid Lotion *(B.P., A.P.F.)*. Aminobenzoic acid 5 g, glycerol 20 ml, alcohol (or industrial methylated spirit) 60 ml, freshly boiled and cooled water to 100 ml. Protect from light. It discolours slightly on storage.

Aminobenzoic Acid Lotion. Aminobenzoic acid 5 g, chocolate brown FB, food grade of commerce, 2 mg, industrial methylated spirit 80 ml, water to 100 ml.—Pharm. Soc. Lab. Rep., P/71/2, 1971.

Aminobenzoic Acid Topical Solution *(U.S.P.)*. Aminobenzoic Acid Solution. Contains aminobenzoic acid 4.5 to 5.5% and alcohol 65 to 75%. Store in airtight containers. Protect from light.
Used topically as a sunscreening agent; to be re-applied every 2 hours and after bathing.

Proprietary Names
Hachemina *(Medea, Spain)*; Hill-Shade *(Hill, USA)*; Pabagel *(Owen, Canad.)*; Pabanol *(Elder, Canad.)*; Pabina *(SCS, S.Afr.)*; Paraminan *(Gallier, Fr.)*; Presun 8 *(Westwood, Canad.; Westwood, USA)*; RV Paba *(Elder, USA)*.

A preparation containing aminobenzoic acid was formerly marketed in Great Britain under the proprietary name Pabamin (*Medo-Chemicals*).

7872-m

Potassium Aminobenzoate. Potassium 4-aminobenzoate.
$C_7H_6KNO_2$=175.2.

CAS — 138-84-1.

A crystalline powder with a saline taste. Very **soluble** in water; less soluble in alcohol; practically insoluble in ether. A 1% solution has a pH of about 7.

Adverse Effects and Precautions. Anorexia, nausea, fever, and skin rash have been reported.
Potassium aminobenzoate should not be given concomitantly with sulphonamides.

After 6 weeks' treatment with potassium aminobenzoate 20 g daily a 48-year-old woman with systemic sclerosis developed a generalised macular rash and became jaundiced. Her condition steadily improved when she was treated with prednisone. Later, when potassium aminobenzoate 1 g thrice daily was given as a provocative test the patient experienced tingling in the extremities, felt sick after each dose, and her temperature rose. The reaction was considered to be of the hypersensitivity type.— D. M. Davies and J. Cavanagh (letter), *Lancet*, 1967, *1*, 896.

Uses. Potassium aminobenzoate has been used in the treatment of various disorders associated with excessive fibrosis, such as scleroderma. The usual dose is 12 g daily in divided doses.

A group of 14 patients with localised scleroderma showed softening of the sclerotic lesions when treated with potassium aminobenzoate. Adults were given a daily dose of 12 g, as capsules or as a 10% aqueous solution. The daily dose for children was 220 mg per kg body-weight.— C. J. D. Zarafonetis, *Am. J. med. Sci.*, 1962, *243*, 147. See also *idem*, *Ann. intern. Med.*, 1959, *50*, 343.

A controlled trial had not confirmed the value of potassium aminobenzoate in scleroderma.— W. Silber and N. Gitlin, *S. Afr. med. J.*, 1973, *44*, 1001, per *Br. med. J.*, 1975, *4*, 397.

Relief of symptoms, healing of ulcers, and increased skin and joint motility occurred in a 55-year-old woman with scleroderma who was treated with potassium aminobenzoate 12 g daily together with reserpine 250 µg twice daily. After 5 months potassium aminobenzoate was reduced to 8 g daily and further improvement occurred.— D. Meyers, *Med. J. Aust.*, 1977, *1*, 887. Criticism.— A. J. Barnett (letter), *Med. J. Aust.*, 1977, *2*, 105.

Objective evaluation of the value of potassium aminobenzoate in Peyronie's disease was not possible.— *Br. med. J.*, 1978, *2*, 330.

Proprietary Preparations

Potaba *(Glenwood, UK)*. Potassium aminobenzoate, available as **Capsules** of 500 mg, as **Envules** (sachets) of 3 g, and as **Tablets** of 500 mg. (Also available as Potaba in *Austral., Switz., USA*).

Potaba+6 *(Glenwood, UK)*. Tablets each containing potassium aminobenzoate 500 mg and pyridoxine hydrochloride 1 mg. For disorders associated with excessive fibrosis. *Dose.* 24 tablets daily in divided doses.

7873-b

Choline. 2-Hydroxyethyltrimethylammonium hydroxide.
$C_5H_{15}NO_2$=121.2.

CAS — 62-49-7 (cation).

A colourless, viscid, hygroscopic, strongly alkaline liquid. It is the basic constituent of lecithin.
Very **soluble** in water and alcohol; practically insoluble in ether. **Store** in airtight containers.

Adverse Effects. Nausea, vomiting, gastro-intestinal discomfort, and diarrhoea have been reported after large doses. Other side-effects reported include incontinence or exacerbation of incontinence, depression or exacerbation of depression, and an unpleasant fishy odour.

Uses. Though choline is an essential factor in animal and human nutrition it cannot strictly be classified as a vitamin. Choline deficiency can only be produced as the result of a combined deficiency of choline and methyl donors, e.g. methionine; that is, by limiting the intake of both choline and protein. The daily requirement has not been established.
Choline functions as a methyl donor in metabolic processes.
In *animals* choline is capable of preventing or curing fatty infiltration of the liver, and has therefore been described as a lipotropic agent. There is, however, no valid evidence that the supplementation of a normally adequate diet with choline or other lipotropic agents is likely to effect a speedier or more complete recovery in cirrhosis of the liver or other conditions than might be attained by the diet alone.
Choline has been given in disorders believed to be associated with cholinergic activity in the brain e.g. ataxia, Huntington's chorea, Alzheimer's disease, and tardive dyskinesia. Some encouraging results have been reported and study continues.
Choline is used as its acid tartrate, chloride, and acid citrate. It is also given as lecithin (see p.55).

A short review of the use of tryptophan and choline in the treatment of brain diseases characterised respectively by decreased concentrations of serotonin and acetylcholine.— J. H. Growdon *et al.*, *Ann. intern. Med.*, 1977, *86*, 337.

It was not universally accepted that raising brain concentrations of acetylcholine increased central cholinergic activity; some investigators believed there was an inverse relationship; the mechanisms were not simple.— I. Hanin (letter), *New Engl. J. Med.*, 1979, *300*, 1113.

Further references: *Lancet*, 1980, *1*, 293; M. K. Schneck *et al.*, *Int. Drug Ther. Newslett.*, 1981, *16*, 5.

Alzheimer's disease. Pilot study of 7 patients with senile dementia of the Alzheimer type indicated that choline chloride 5 g daily might provide some improvement. There were no significant changes in symptoms but behaviour appeared to improve in 2 patients in the first 24 hours of the study. A dose of 10 g daily produced nausea, diarrhoea, and a small reduction in blood pressure.— W. D. Boyd *et al.* (letter), *Lancet*, 1977, *2*, 711.

Choline bitartrate had no beneficial effect in 3 elderly patients with Alzheimer's disease. One patient became incontinent with foul odour.— P. Etienne *et al.* (letter), *Lancet*, 1978, *1*, 508.

In a double-blind placebo-controlled crossover study, 3 of 10 patients with Alzheimer's disease seemed less confused following administration of choline 9 g daily (as the bitartrate) for 2 weeks. Exacerbation of pre-existing urinary incontinence occurred in 3 patients, and some patients suffered gastro-intestinal discomfort; an additional patient, whose diagnosis was changed to depression, felt more depressed. Although the results were not encouraging, possible benefit from choline therapy could not be ruled out; it was considered that the dose used was too high.— C. M. Smith *et al.* (letter), *Lancet*, 1978, *2*, 318. Initial encouraging results had been obtained following administration of choline dihydrogen citrate 9 g daily for 21 days to younger patients (under 65 years) with early Alzheimer's disease.— J. L. Signoret *et al.* (letter), *ibid.*, 1978, *2*, 837.

The pathogenesis of Alzheimer's disease.— D. M. Bowen *et al.*, *Lancet*, 1979, *1*, 11; I. Grundke-Iqbal *et al.*, *Lancet*, 1979, *1*, 578.

In a double-blind study of 18 women with Alzheimer's disease there was no beneficial effect when choline chloride 15 g daily was taken for 2 months.— E. B. Renvoize and T. Jerram (letter), *New Engl. J. Med.*, 1979, *301*, 330.

Concomitant use of piracetam and choline in patients with senile dementia of the Alzheimer's type.— E. Friedman *et al.* (letter), *New Engl. J. Med.*, 1981, *304*, 1490.

See also under Lecithins, p.55.

Ataxia. A 56-year-old man with cerebellar ataxia improved dramatically while taking choline 4 or 5 g daily.— N. J. Legg, *Br. med. J.*, 1978, *2*, 1403. An earlier report of improvement in cerebellar ataxia in a patient treated with choline chloride had not been confirmed in a further 13 patients; they had not benefited.— N. Legg (letter), *Br. med. J.*, 1979, *2*, 133.

None of 6 patients with hereditary ataxia benefited from treatment with choline chloride 1 g four times daily for a week followed, after a 2-week rest, by treatment for a month.— D. V. Philcox and B. Kies (letter), *Br. med. J.*, 1979, *2*, 613.

Preliminary results of a double-blind crossover study in 8 patients with Friedreich's ataxia, 6 with sporadic cerebellar degeneration, and 6 with atypical spinocerebellar degeneration with cerebellar ataxia and spasticity of the lower limbs showed some improvement in upper limb coordination after treatment with choline 6 or 12 g daily but only 2 patients had improvement in gait.— I. R. Livingstone and F. L. Mastaglia (letter), *Br. med. J.*, 1979, *2*, 939.

Blepharospasm. Possible benefit of choline in blepharospasm.— B. Skarf and J. A. Sharpe (letter), *New Engl. J. Med.*, 1981, *305*, 957.

Deficiency states. Evidence of choline deficiency in 15 patients receiving total parenteral nutrition.— M. E. Burt *et al.* (letter), *Lancet*, 1980, *2*, 638.

Gilles de la Tourette's syndrome. For choline therapy in Gilles de la Tourette's syndrome see under Lecithins, p.55.

Huntington's chorea. In 5 patients with Huntington's chorea choline chloride 3 to 15 g daily produced dose-dependent elevation of free choline in plasma but had little or no effect on symptoms.— S. -M. Aquilonius and S. -A. Eckernas, *Neurology, Minneap.*, 1977, *27*, 887.

Tardive dyskinesia. In a double-blind placebo-controlled study of 20 patients with tardive dyskinesia choline chloride 150 mg per kg body-weight daily (in 3 divided doses) for 1 week increased to 200 mg per kg daily for a second week, decreased choreic movements in 9, increased them in 1, and had no effect in 10. Plasma concentrations of choline increased from a range of 8.6 to 20.5 nmol per ml before treatment to 18.2 to 60.1 nmol per ml 1 hour after a dose in the second week.— J. H. Growdon *et al.*, *New Engl. J. Med.*, 1977, *297*, 524.

In 5 patients with tardive dyskinesia choline chloride 150 to 200 mg per kg body-weight daily in divided doses, or lecithin 21 to 105 g daily, reduced abnormal movements. The bitter taste of choline, the development of a fishy odour, and gastro-intestinal effects made lecithin preferable.— A. J. Gelenberg *et al.*, *Am. J. Psychiat.*, 1979, *136*, 772.

Further references: *Med. Lett.*, 1979, *21*, 34.

Trimethylaminuria. Adjustment of the diet to lower the intake of choline to a minimal safety concentration was effective within 3 weeks in controlling the production of trimethylamine in a 13-year-old boy who had been suffering from a fishy odour for about 7 years. While trimethylamine was still excreted in the urine it was barely detectable in the sweat and breath.— R. Marks *et al.*, *Br. J. Derm.*, 1976, *95*, *Suppl.* 14, 11.

Choline bitartrate 5 g given in 3 doses at 8-hourly intervals had been found useful as a diagnostic aid for patients with trimethylaminuria.— R. Marks *et al.*, *Br. J. Derm.*, 1977, *96*, 399.

Proprietary Names

Neurotropan *(Itting, Ger.)*.

7874-v

Choline Bitartrate.

Choline Acid Tartrate; Bitartarato de Colina. 2-Hydroxyethyltrimethylammonium hydrogen tartrate.

$C_9H_{19}NO_7$=253.3.

CAS — 87-67-2.

Pharmacopoeias. In *Braz.*, *Ger.*, *Nord.*, and *Port.*

A white, hygroscopic, crystalline powder with an acid taste and a faint amine-like odour. Very **soluble** in water; slightly soluble in alcohol; very slightly soluble in acetone and light petroleum; practically insoluble in chloroform and ether. Solutions are **sterilised** by autoclaving or by filtration. **Store** in airtight containers.

Uses. Choline bitartrate has the same actions as choline, p.1651.

Proprietary Names

Colyne (see also under Choline Chloride) *(Saita, Ital.)*.

7875-g

Choline Chloride.

Cholinii Chloridum. 2-Hydroxyethyltrimethylammonium chloride.

$C_5H_{14}ClNO$=139.6.

CAS — 67-48-1.

Pharmacopoeias. In *Aust.*, *Belg.*, *Cz.*, *Ger.*, *Hung.*, and *It.*

White, odourless, tasteless, very hygroscopic crystals. Very **soluble** in water and alcohol; very slightly soluble in acetone and light petroleum; practically insoluble in chloroform and ether. A 10% solution in water has a pH of 5 to 6. Solutions may be **sterilised** by filtration. **Store** in airtight containers.

Uses. Choline chloride has the same actions as choline, p.1651.

Proprietary Names

Becholine *(Medical Research, Austral.)*; Becholine D *(Medical Research, Austral.)*; Colyne (see also under Choline Bitartrate) *(Saita, Ital.)*.

7876-q

Choline Dihydrogen Citrate.

Choline Citrate; Cholinum Citricum; Citrato de Colina. 2-Hydroxyethyltrimethylammonium dihydrogen citrate.

$C_{11}H_{21}NO_8$=295.3.

CAS — 77-91-8.

Pharmacopoeias. In *Belg.* and *Pol.*

Colourless translucent hygroscopic crystals or white crystalline powder with an acid taste; it is odourless or has a faint amine-like odour. **Soluble** 1 in 1 of water and 1 in 45 of alcohol; very slightly soluble in chloroform and ether. A 25% solution in water has a pH of 3.5 to 4.5. **Store** in airtight containers.

Uses. Choline dihydrogen citrate has the same actions and uses as choline, p.1651.

Cystinuria. For a report of choline dihydrogen citrate being given to facilitate enzymic remethylation of homocystine to methionine in the treatment of homocystinuria, see Cystine, p.50.

Proprietary Preparations

Wallachol *(Wallace Mfg Chem., UK: Farillon, UK)*. **Syrup** containing in each 100 ml choline dihydrogen citrate 4.5 g, the antitoxic principle from 7.5 g of fresh liver, proteolysed liver equivalent to fresh liver 50 g, racemethionine 375 mg, inositol 500 mg, thiamine hydrochloride 20 mg, riboflavine 5 mg, pyridoxine hydrochloride 5 mg, cyanocobalamin 50 µg, and nicotinamide 100 mg. **Tablets** each containing choline dihydrogen citrate 224 mg, the antitoxic principle from 250 mg of fresh liver, dried liver 50 mg, racemethionine 112 mg, inositol 56 mg, thiamine hydrochloride 1 mg, riboflavine 1 mg, pyridoxine hydrochloride 250 µg, cyanocobalamin 1 µg, and nicotinamide 5 mg. For liver dysfunction and impaired fat metabolism. *Dose.* 10 to 15 ml of syrup, or 2 or 3 tablets, thrice daily.

7877-p

Inositol.

i-Inositol; *meso*-Inositol. *myo*-Inositol.

$C_6H_{12}O_6$=180.2.

CAS — 87-89-8.

Pharmacopoeias. In *Aust.*, *Belg.*, and *Chin.*

Odourless fine white crystals or white crystalline powder with a sweet taste. M.p. about 224°. It is optically inactive. **Soluble** 1 in 6 of water; slightly soluble in alcohol; practically insoluble in chloroform and ether. Solutions in water are neutral to litmus.

Inositol is present in animal tissues and in plants, especially in seeds and cereal brans.

Apart from its presence in organic matter in various forms, little is known about the specific function of inositol, though it is stated to be curative of *mouse* alopecia and to be capable of preventing fatty liver in *rats*. It is an essential nutrient for some micro-organisms. Deficiency symptoms in *mice* have been cured by feeding 10 mg of inositol in 100 g of food. Most purified rations used for experimental purposes contain this level of inositol. Its role in human nutrition is unknown. The consumption of inositol by man is about 1 g daily.

Preliminary findings following administration of inositol 500 mg twice daily to 7 diabetic subjects for 2 weeks, suggested that it might be beneficial in the treatment of diabetic neuropathy.— J. G. Salway *et al.*, *Lancet*, 1978, *2*, 1282.

Tablet excipient. Inositol was considered suitable as an excipient for chewable tablets because it was non-hygroscopic, inert, non-toxic, and physically stable.— S. S. Nasir and L. O. Wilken, *J. pharm. Sci.*, 1966, *55*, 794.

Proprietary Preparations

Inositol Capsules *(Bioglan, UK)*. Each contains 500 mg.

Other Proprietary Names

Inosital, Inositina (both *Ital.*); Inosit-Zyma *(Ger.)*.

7878-s

Compound Preparations of Vitamins of the B Group

Compound Vitamin B Tablets *(B.P.C. 1973)*. Compound Thiamine Tablets; Compound Aneurine Tablets; Vitamin B Compound Tablets. Each contains nicotinamide 15 mg, riboflavine 1 mg, and thiamine hydrochloride 1 mg. Store in airtight containers and avoid contact with metal. Protect from light. *Dose.* Prophylactic, 1 or 2 tablets daily.

Strong Compound Vitamin B Tablets *(B.P.C. 1973)*. Strong Compound Thiamine Tablets; Strong Compound Aneurine Tablets; Strong Vitamin B Compound Tablets. Each contains nicotinamide 20 mg, pyridoxine hydrochloride 2 mg, riboflavine 2 mg, and thiamine hydrochloride 5 mg. They may be coated. Store in airtight containers and avoid contact with metal. Protect from light. *Dose.* Therapeutic, 1 or 2 tablets thrice daily.

Vitamins B and C Injection *(B.P.C. 1973)*. A sterile solution of vitamins B and C in Water for Injections prepared, immediately before use, by mixing the contents of a pair of ampoules. Sterilised by autoclaving, by maintaining at 98° to 100° for 30 minutes with a bactericide, or by filtration. Store in a cool place. Protect from light. The air in ampoules containing ascorbic acid is replaced with nitrogen or other suitable gas. The strength and route of administration must be stated on the prescription or order. When *Strong Vitamins B and C Injection for intravenous use* is prescribed, a pair of ampoules is supplied, one containing a solution of pyridoxine hydrochloride 50 mg, riboflavine or the equivalent amount of riboflavine sodium phosphate 4 mg, and thiamine hydrochloride 250 mg in 5 ml, and the other containing a solution of ascorbic acid (as sodium salt)

500 mg and anhydrous dextrose 1 g in 5 ml and either of the 2 ampoules containing nicotinamide 160 mg. When *Weak Vitamins B and C Injection for intravenous use* is prescribed, a pair of ampoules is supplied, one containing a solution of pyridoxine hydrochloride 50 mg, riboflavine or the equivalent amount of riboflavine sodium phosphate 4 mg, and thiamine hydrochloride 100 mg in 5 ml, and the other ascorbic acid (as sodium salt) 500 mg in 5 ml. Either of the 2 ampoules contains nicotinamide 160 mg. When *Strong Vitamins B and C Injection for intramuscular use* is prescribed, a pair of ampoules is supplied, one containing a solution of pyridoxine hydrochloride 50 mg, riboflavine or the equivalent amount of riboflavine sodium phosphate 4 mg, thiamine hydrochloride 250 mg, and benzyl alcohol 0.14 ml in 5 ml, and the other ascorbic acid (as sodium salt) 500 mg in 2 ml. Either of the 2 ampoules contains nicotinamide 160 mg. When *Weak Vitamins B and C Injection for intramuscular use* is prescribed, a pair of ampoules is supplied, one containing a solution of pyridoxine hydrochloride 50 mg, riboflavine or the equivalent amount of riboflavine sodium phosphate 4 mg, thiamine hydrochloride 100 mg, and benzyl alcohol 0.08 ml in 2 ml, and the other ascorbic acid (as sodium salt) 500 mg in 2 ml. Either of the 2 ampoules contains nicotinamide 160 mg.

Incompatibility. An immediate precipitate occurred when Strong Vitamins B and C Injection for intravenous use, 4-pairs per litre, was mixed with amphotericin 200 mg per litre, and a crystalline precipitate occurred with methohexitone sodium 2 g per litre in dextrose injection. A crystalline precipitate occurred when the vitamin injection was mixed with sulphadiazine sodium 4 g per litre in dextrose injection and sodium chloride injection.— B. B. Riley, *J. Hosp. Pharm.*, 1970, *28*, 228.

Proprietary Compound Preparations of Vitamins of the B Group

Allbee with C *(Robins, UK).* **Capsules** each containing calcium pantothenate 10 mg, nicotinamide 50 mg, pyridoxine hydrochloride 5 mg, riboflavine 10 mg, thiamine mononitrate 15 mg, and ascorbic acid 300 mg; **Elixir** containing in each 5 ml nicotinamide 20 mg, pyridoxine hydrochloride 2 mg, riboflavine sodium phosphate 4 mg, thiamine mononitrate 6 mg, and ascorbic acid 120 mg. *Dose.* 1 to 3 capsules daily or 5 to 10 ml of elixir 2 or 3 times daily; children, 1 capsule or 5 to 10 ml daily.

BC 500 (known in some countries as Beminal 500 or Todobe) *(Ayerst, UK).* Tablets each containing calcium pantothenate 20 mg, cyanocobalamin 5 µg, nicotinamide 100 mg, pyridoxine hydrochloride 10 mg, riboflavine 12.5 mg, thiamine mononitrate 25 mg, and sodium ascorbate equivalent to ascorbic acid 500 mg. **BC 500 with Iron.** Tablets each containing calcium pantothenate 20 mg, nicotinamide 100 mg, pyridoxine hydrochloride 10 mg, riboflavine 12.5 mg, sodium ascorbate equivalent to ascorbic acid 500 mg, thiamine mononitrate 25 mg, and ferrous fumarate 200 mg. *Dose.* 1 tablet of BC 500 or BC 500 with Iron daily.

Becosym *(Roche, UK).* **Syrup** containing in each 5 ml nicotinamide 20 mg, pyridoxine hydrochloride 2 mg, riboflavine 2 mg, and thiamine hydrochloride 5 mg (suggested diluent, syrup). **Tablets** are a brand of Strong Compound Vitamin B Tablets. **Forte Tablets** each containing nicotinamide 50 mg, pyridoxine hydrochloride 10 mg, riboflavine 15 mg, and thiamine hydrochloride 15 mg. *Dose.* 5 to 15 ml of syrup or 1 to 3 tablets daily.

Benerva Compound Tablets *(Roche, UK).* A brand of Compound Vitamin B Tablets.

Bravit *(Galen, UK).* Tablets each containing nicotinamide 200 mg, pyridoxine hydrochloride 5 mg, riboflavine 5 mg, thiamine hydrochloride 50 mg, and ascorbic acid 100 mg. *Dose.* 1 to 3 tablets daily.

Effico *(Pharmax, UK).* Mixture containing in each 5 ml nicotinamide 2.1 mg, thiamine hydrochloride 180 µg, caffeine 20.2 mg, compound gentian infusion 0.31 ml (suggested diluent, syrup). *Dose.* 10 ml thrice daily.

Hepacon-Plex *(Consolidated Chemicals, UK).* Ampoules of 2 ml each containing calcium pantothenate 10 mg, cyanocobalamin 8 µg, nicotinamide 150 mg, pyridoxine hydrochloride 5 mg, riboflavine 2 mg, and thiamine hydrochloride 100 mg. *Dose.* 2 to 4 ml by intramuscular injection.

Lance B+C Tablets *(Kirby-Warrick, UK).* Each contains thiamine hydrochloride 50 mg, riboflavine 5 mg, pyridoxine hydrochloride 5 mg, nicotinamide 200 mg, and ascorbic acid 100 mg. *Dose.* 1 tablet thrice daily.

Lederplex *(Lederle, UK).* Contains in each 5 ml nicotinamide 10 mg, pyridoxine hydrochloride 200 µg, riboflavine 2 mg, thiamine hydrochloride 2 mg, pantothenic acid 2 mg, choline 20 mg, inositol 10 mg, soluble liver fraction 470 mg, and cyanocobalamin 5 µg. *Dose.* 10 ml daily.

Lipoflavonoid Capsules *(Lewis, UK).* Each contains dexpanthenol 330 µg, nicotinamide 3.33 mg, pyridoxine hydrochloride 330 µg, riboflavine 330 µg, thiamine hydrochloride 330 µg, hydroxocobalamin 1.66 µg, choline bitartrate 233 mg, inositol 111 mg, racemethionine 28 mg, ascorbic acid 100 mg, and lemon bioflavonoid complex 100 mg. For migraine, vertigo, and neurosensory deafness associated with Ménière's syndrome. *Dose.* Initial, 3 capsules thrice daily for 6 to 8 weeks; maintenance, 2 capsules thrice daily.

Lipotriad *(Lewis, UK).* **Capsules** containing in each dose of 3, dexpanthenol 1 mg, nicotinamide 10 mg, pyridoxine hydrochloride 1 mg, riboflavine 1 mg, thiamine hydrochloride 1 mg, hydroxocobalamin 5 µg, choline bitartrate 700 mg, inositol 334 mg, and racemethionine 84 mg; **Liquid** containing the equivalent of 3 capsules in each 5 ml. For senile macular degeneration, arteriosclerotic retinopathy, and diabetic retinopathy. *Dose.* 3 capsules or 5 ml of liquid thrice daily, preferably after meals.

N.29 Tablets *(Norton, UK: Vestric, UK).* Each contains nicotinamide 200 mg, pyridoxine hydrochloride 5 mg, riboflavine 5 mg, thiamine hydrochloride 50 mg, and ascorbic acid 100 mg. *Dose.* 1 to 3 tablets daily.

Noravita Syrup *(Wallace Mfg Chem., UK: Farillon, UK).* Contains in each 5 ml nicotinamide 80 mg, pyridoxine hydrochloride 2 mg, riboflavine 2 mg, thiamine hydrochloride 20 mg, and ascorbic acid 40 mg. *Dose.* 5 to 15 ml thrice daily.

Norvits Syrup *(R.P. Drugs, UK).* Contains in each 5 ml thiamine hydrochloride 5 mg, riboflavine sodium phosphate 2 mg, nicotinamide 20 mg, and pyridoxine hydrochloride 2 mg. *Dose.* Adults and children: prophylactic, 5 to 15 ml daily; therapeutic, 15 to 45 ml daily in divided doses; infants: prophylactic only, 5 ml daily.

Orovite *(Bencard, UK).* **Elixir** containing in each 5 ml nicotinamide 80 mg, pyridoxine hydrochloride 2 mg, riboflavine 2 mg, thiamine hydrochloride 20 mg, and ascorbic acid 40 mg, in syrup (suggested diluent, syrup). **Tablets** each containing nicotinamide 200 mg, pyridoxine hydrochloride 5 mg, riboflavine 5 mg, thiamine hydrochloride 50 mg, and ascorbic acid 100 mg. *Dose.* 10 ml of elixir or 1 tablet thrice daily; children, 5 ml.
For Orovite 7, see p.1668.

Pabrinex *(Paines & Byrne, UK).* Concentrated injections of the vitamin-B complex and ascorbic acid. **High Potency Injection.** Each pair of ampoules contains thiamine hydrochloride 250 mg, riboflavine sodium phosphate equivalent to riboflavine 4 mg, pyridoxine hydrochloride 50 mg, nicotinamide 160 mg, ascorbic acid 500 mg, with anhydrous dextrose 1 g (for intravenous injection) or benzyl alcohol 140 mg (for intramuscular injection). **Intramuscular Maintenance Injection.** Each pair of ampoules contains thiamine hydrochloride 100 mg, riboflavine sodium phosphate equivalent to riboflavine 4 mg, pyridoxine hydrochloride 50 mg, nicotinamide 160 mg, ascorbic acid 500 mg, and benzyl alcohol 80 mg.

Parentrovite *(Bencard, UK).* Concentrated injections of the vitamin-B complex and ascorbic acid. **High Potency Injection.** Each pair of ampoules containing nicotinamide 160 mg, pyridoxine hydrochloride 50 mg, riboflavine 4 mg, thiamine hydrochloride 250 mg, and sodium ascorbate equivalent to ascorbic acid 500 mg, with anhydrous dextrose 1 g (for intravenous injection) or benzyl alcohol 140 mg and chlorocresol 0.2% (for intramuscular injection). **Maintenance Injection.** Each pair of ampoules containing nicotinamide 160 mg, pyridoxine hydrochloride 50 mg, riboflavine 4 mg, thiamine hydrochloride 100 mg, and sodium ascorbate equivalent to ascorbic acid 500 mg with benzyl alcohol 80 mg and chlorocresol 0.2% (for intramuscular injection).

Ventricular fibrillation in a 67-year-old woman developed immediately after an intravenous bolus injection of Parentrovite High Potency Injection; this was possibly due to the thiamine component.— R. H. Falk and D. E. Protheroe, *Postgrad. med. J.*, 1979, *55*, 201.

Solivito *(KabiVitrum, UK).* Vials each containing biotin 300 µg, cyanocobalamin 2 µg, folic acid 200 µg, nicotinamide 10 mg, pyridoxine hydrochloride 2.43 mg, riboflavine sodium phosphate 2.47 mg, sodium ascorbate 34 mg, sodium pantothenate 11 mg, and thiamine mononitrate 1.24 mg, with glycine 100 mg, sodium edetate, and methyl hydroxybenzoate. For use as a supplement in parenteral nutrition. For infusion in dextrose injection after reconstitution with dextrose injection or Water for Injections.

Surbex T *(Abbott, UK).* Tablets each containing thiamine mononitrate 15 mg, riboflavine 10 mg, nicotinamide 100 mg, pyridoxine hydrochloride 5 mg, and sodium ascorbate equivalent to ascorbic acid 500 mg. *Dose.* 1 or more tablets daily.

Tonivitan B Syrup *(Medo Chemicals, UK).* An elixir containing in each 5 ml nicotinamide 2.5 mg, pyridoxine hydrochloride 16.5 µg, riboflavine 400 µg, thiamine hydrochloride 500 µg, calcium glycerophosphate 20 mg, and manganese glycerophosphate 5 mg. *Dose.* 5 to 10 ml thrice daily.

Vigranon B *(Wallace Mfg Chem., UK: Farillon, UK).* **Syrup** containing in each 5 ml dexpanthenol 3 mg, nicotinamide 20 mg, pyridoxine hydrochloride 2 mg, riboflavine 2 mg, and thiamine hydrochloride 5 mg and as **Tablets** each containing calcium pantothenate 500 µg, nicotinamide 10 mg, pyridoxine hydrochloride 100 µg, riboflavine 2 mg, thiamine hydrochloride 3 mg, and dried yeast 125 mg. *Dose.* 5 to 15 ml of syrup or 1 to 3 tablets thrice daily.

7879-w

Vitamin C

Ascorbic acid is vitamin C and is described below with other compounds with similar activity.

7880-m

Ascorbic Acid *(B.P., B.P. Vet., Eur. P., U.S.P.).*

Ascorb. Acid; Acidum Ascorbicum; Vitamin C; L-Ascorbic Acid; Cevitamic Acid. The enolic form of 3-oxo-L-gulofuranolactone; 2,3-Didehydro-L-*threo*-hexono-1,4-lactone.
$C_6H_8O_6$=176.1.

CAS — 50-81-7.

Pharmacopoeias. In all pharmacopoeias examined.

Odourless or almost odourless, colourless crystals or white or very pale yellow crystalline powder with an acid taste. It may be extracted from the ripe fruit of *Capsicum annuum* or from other vegetable sources, such as rose hips, black currants, and the juice of citrus fruits, or it may be prepared synthetically. M.p. about 190° with decomposition.

Soluble 1 in 3 to 3.5 of water, 1 in 25 of alcohol, and 1 in 10 of methyl alcohol; soluble in acetone; practically insoluble in chloroform, ether, and light petroleum. A solution in water is dextrorotatory. A 5% solution in water has a pH of 2.2 to 2.5. A 5.04% solution is iso-osmotic with serum.

Solutions are **sterilised** by heating at 98° to 100° for 30 minutes with a bactericide or by filtration, the air in the final containers being replaced by nitrogen or other suitable gas; chlorocresol is a suitable bactericide. Solutions, especially when made alkaline, deteriorate rapidly in air, the change being accelerated by heat and light; the optimum pH is 5.4. The first stage in the oxidation, the formation of dehydroascorbic acid, is reversible.

Ascorbic acid is readily destroyed during cooking. The loss is generally about 50% but appropriate precautions such as reducing access to oxygen, using the minimum of water, and not stirring cooked food in heated conditions may reduce the loss of ascorbic acid to about 30%.

Incompatible with ferric salts, oxidising agents, and salts of heavy metals, particularly copper.

Store in airtight non-metallic containers. Protect from light.

An aqueous solution of ascorbic acid iso-osmotic with serum (5.04%) caused 100% haemolysis of erythrocytes cultured in it for 45 minutes. The solution turned dark brown.— E. R. Hammarlund and K. Pedersen-Bjergaard, *J. pharm. Sci.*, 1961, *50*, 24.

Samples of fresh orange juice contained considerably more biologically active ascorbic acid (L-ascorbic acid and dehydro-L-ascorbic acid) than pasteurised orange juice which contained more of the biologically inactive oxidation product 2,3-diketo-L-gulonic acid. Frozen concentrates contained intermediate concentrations of active and inactive ascorbic acid. Total ascorbic acid concentrations were similar for all 3 products.— I. Horowitz *et al.*, *J. Am. med. Ass.*, 1976, *235*, 2624.

Effects of gamma-irradiation. Ascorbic acid did not appear to be adversely affected by gamma-irradiation. In solution, irradiation caused a slight deepening in colour and in the more dilute solutions (i.e. 20 mg per ml) the assays showed some reduction in strength.— *The Use of Gamma Radiation Sources for the Sterilisation of Pharmaceutical Products,* London, ABPI, 1960.

Incompatibility. Injections of ascorbic acid have been reported to be incompatible with aminophylline, bleomycin sulphate, erythromycin lactobionate, nafcillin sodium, nitrofurantoin sodium, conjugated oestrogens, sodium bicarbonate, and sulphafurazole diethanolamine. Occasional incompatibility, depending on pH or concentration, has occurred with chloramphenicol sodium succinate, chlorothiazide sodium, and hydrocortisone sodium succinate.

Stability in solution. Ascorbic acid was most stable at pH 6 to 6.5 and sodium bicarbonate was preferable to triethanolamine for adjusting the pH. Propylene glycol had a stabilising effect. Solutions should be protected from light.— M. A. Kassem *et al., Pharm. Acta Helv.,* 1969, *44,* 611. Heavy metal ions such as Cu^{2+}, Fe^{3+}, Zn^{2+}, and Mn^{2+} decreased the stability of ascorbic acid, but Fe^{2+} and Mg^{2+} had little effect. Carbon dioxide was more effective than nitrogen for replacing dissolved oxygen in the water.— *idem,* 667. A similar report.— P. Finholt *et al., J. pharm. Sci.,* 1966, *55,* 1435. The degradation of ascorbic acid solution in aerobic conditions at pH 3.5 to 7.2.— S. M. Blaug and B. Hajratwala, *J. pharm. Sci.,* 1972, *61,* 556.

The stability of ascorbic acid solutions during autoclaving was markedly increased by the addition of *N*-hydroxyethylethylene-diaminetriacetic acid or diethylenetriaminepenta-acetic acid (pentetic acid). Stability was also improved by sodium diethyldithiocarbamate, disodium edetate, and dimercaprol and, to a lesser extent, by hydroxyquinoline and propyl gallate. The increase in stability resulted from chelation from solution of the heavy metal ions which cause decomposition of ascorbic acid. There was an optimum concentration of chelating agent for maximum stability, which depended on the amounts of metal ions present and which should be determined experimentally for each formulation. On storage, precipitates appeared in solutions containing hydroxyquinoline and higher concentrations of dimercaprol, and hydrogen sulphide was detected in the sodium diethyldithiocarbamate solutions.— M. A. Kassem *et al., Pharm. Acta Helv.,* 1972, *47,* 89.

In very dilute solutions (0.01% of critical micelle concentrations) the nonionic surfactants polysorbate 80 and poloxamer increased the rate of oxidation of ascorbic acid. At surfactant concentrations equal to 0.1% of critical micelle concentration the rate was the same as that obtained in surfactant-free water. Above this concentration the oxidation-rate decreased, while polysorbate did not affect oxidation.— S. M. Blaug and B. Hajratwala, *J. pharm. Sci.,* 1974, *63,* 1240.

Tablet formulation. Colour stability and formulation of ascorbic acid tablets.— R. B. Wortz, *J. pharm. Sci.,* 1967, *56,* 1169.

The stability of ascorbic acid tablets.— S. H. Rubin *et al., J. pharm. Sci.,* 1976, *65,* 963.

Adverse Effects and Precautions. Ascorbic acid is usually well tolerated. Large doses may cause diarrhoea and the formation of renal calcium oxalate calculi. Doses of 600 mg or more daily have a diuretic action. Ascorbic acid should be given with care to patients with hyperoxaluria. Tolerance may be induced in patients taking high doses.

A discussion on the effects and hazards of ascorbic acid.— *Lancet,* 1979, *1,* 308.

Caries developed in infants given fruit juice preparations.—First Report of the Panel of Cariogenic Foods, Committee on Medical Aspects of Food Policy,, per *Br. dent. J.,* 1969, *126,* 273. Comments.— E. B. D. Jones, *National Rose Hip Products Association* (letter), *ibid.,* 299.

Acute reactions in 3 cancer patients appeared to be associated with large doses of ascorbic acid (up to 20 g daily) given intravenously.— A. Campbell and T. Jack, *Scott. med. J.,* 1979, *24,* 151.

A man ingested ascorbic acid 15 g daily for more than 4 months without adverse effects.— J. D. White (letter), *New Engl. J. Med.,* 1981, *304,* 1491.

Allergy. A report of an allergic response to ascorbic acid in 3 patients, presenting as eczema, urticaria, or asthma.— P. Vassal, *Revue fr. Allerg.,* 1976, *16,* 103.

Anaemia. Ascorbic acid 1.5 g daily had been reported to cause haemolytic anaemia in certain individuals with a deficiency of glucose-6-phosphate dehydrogenase. The reaction was not considered clinically significant under normal circumstances (e.g. in the absence of infection).— E. Beutler, *Pharmac. Rev.,* 1969, *21,* 73.

Dependence. When daily ascorbic acid intake significantly exceeded 250 mg for prolonged periods, the rate of clearance from the body increased so that blood concentrations did not increase with larger doses. Dependence on larger than normal maintenance doses could occur and deficiency might occur if treatment was withdrawn.— W. J. Rhead and G. N. Schrauzer (letter), *Nutr. Rev.,* 1971, *29,* 262.

A 32-year-old man with migraine apparently became dependent on ascorbic acid which he had substituted for methysergide and codeine. Interrupting an intake of ascorbic acid 6 g daily resulted in acute onset of headache.— LBali and E. Callaway (letter), *New Engl. J. Med.,* 1978, *299,* 364.

Effects on fertility. The mucolytic effect of ascorbic acid might render the cervical mucus less permeable to spermatozoa.— M. H. Briggs (letter), *Lancet,* 1973, *2,* 677. Of 15 women taking ascorbic acid, 9 who took doses of up to 1 g conceived readily, 1 who took 1 to 5 g daily had a spontaneous abortion and failed to conceive again, and the other 5 who took 2 to 4 g daily either alone or with other vitamins failed to conceive although 2 did conceive 3 months after stopping the vitamin. To prevent any alteration in fertility the daily dose of ascorbic acid should not exceed 500 mg.— *idem,* 1083. Ascorbic acid did not appear to have any effect on fertility. Four patients taking 2 to 3 g daily became pregnant.— A. Hoffer (letter), *ibid.,* 1146.

Effect on the eye. At usual therapeutic doses rutin improved colour vision whereas rutin in association with ascorbic acid caused a slight deterioration. This confirmed previous findings of an adverse effect of ascorbic acid on colour vision.— J. Laroche and C. Laroche, *Annls pharm. Fr.,* 1977, *35,* 173.

Effects on iron overload. Cardiac deterioration in 8 of 11 patients with iron overload treated with desferrioxamine and ascorbic acid.— W. L. Henry and A. W. Nienhuis, *Circulation,* 1977, *56, Suppl.* 3, 218. A conference considered 7 deaths which had occurred in patients treated with desferrioxamine and ascorbic acid. Six had cardiac disease before receiving chelation therapy. Cardiac disease was common in patients with transfusion-dependent anaemia and survival beyond 25 years of age was rare. It was not possible to determine whether either drug had precipitated or aggravated cardiac dysfunction.— A. W. Nienhuis (letter), *New Engl. J. Med.,* 1977, *296,* 114.

For further comment on the hazards of ascorbic acid in the iron-overloaded patient, see Desferrioxamine, p.381.

Effects on the kidney. An abrupt loss of renal function in an infant with congenital nephrotic syndrome was associated with the administration of high doses of ascorbic acid.— V. M. Reznik *et al.* (letter), *New Engl. J. Med.,* 1980, *302,* 1418.

Hyperoxaluria. Ascorbic acid could be partly metabolised to oxalic acid. Average reported production-rates were 1 mg oxalate from 1 g ascorbate, 12 mg from 4 g, and 68 mg from 9 g, but with wide individual variations. Some patients would have a high risk of renal calcification during treatment with high doses of ascorbic acid.— M. H. Briggs *et al.* (letter), *Med. J. Aust.,* 1973, *2,* 48.

A report of hyperoxaluria associated with ascorbic acid.— M. Briggs (letter), *Lancet,* 1976, *1,* 154.

A calcium oxalate stone was recovered from the urine of a 21-year-old man who had taken ascorbic acid 1 g daily for many months. Urinary oxalate concentrations were raised but concentrations decreased after discontinuing ascorbic acid.— D. A. Roth and R. V. Breitenfield (letter), *J. Am. med. Ass.,* 1977, *237,* 768.

Five patients with a history of calcium oxalate urolithiasis developed new stones 1 to 3 years after starting to take ascorbic acid 4 g or more daily. The stone formation of patients with a history of calcium oxalate urolithiasis might be activated by high doses of ascorbic acid.— L. H. Smith (letter), *New Engl. J. Med.,* 1978, *298,* 856.

Interactions. In 14 elderly men without clinical signs of hypovitaminosis, the administration of tetracycline 250 mg four times daily for 5 days resulted in a reduction of ascorbic acid concentration in leucocytes to less than half initial values. In 2 further subjects the urinary excretion of ascorbic acid was increased.— A. C. M. Windsor *et al., Br. med. J.,* 1972, *1,* 214.

Concomitant administration of aspirin 600 mg and ascorbic acid 500 mg prevented the normal elevation of leucocyte ascorbic acid after 4 hours and caused a significantly higher increase of plasma ascorbic acid than occurred when ascorbic acid only was administered.— M. Greene and C. W. M. Wilson, *Br. J. clin. Pharmac.,* 1975, *2,* 369P.

Drugs which induced tissue desaturation of ascorbic acid included aspirin, nicotine from cigarettes, alcohol, several appetite suppressants, iron, phenytoin, some convulsant drugs, the oestrogen component of oral contraceptives, and tetracycline.— G. Coffey and C. W. M. Wilson (letter), *Br. med. J.,* 1975, *1,* 208.

Deficiency of vitamin C caused a small but demonstrable impairment in drug metabolism and could account for the reduction in drug-metabolising ability in the elderly.— D. J. Smithard and M. J. S. Langman (letter), *Br. med. J.,* 1977, *1,* 1029.

Following findings by E.M. Baker *et al.* (*Science,* 1971, *173,* 826) that ascorbic acid was converted partly to ascorbic acid sulphate in man, a study in 5 healthy subjects demonstrated that high doses of ascorbic acid increased the apparent half-life of paracetamol, this effect being prevented by concurrent administration of sodium sulphate. This interaction was unlikely to be of much clinical significance at therapeutic doses, but similar interactions might occur between ascorbic acid and steroids or other compounds that conjugated with sulphate. The possibility of interaction with drugs subject to pronounced first-pass metabolism, such as isoprenaline, was of particular concern.— J. B. Houston and G. Levy, *J. pharm. Sci.,* 1976, *65,* 1218.

For the effect of ascorbic acid on ethinyloestradiol, and the possible implications for women taking oral contraceptives, see Ethinyloestradiol, p.1412.

For reports of the interaction of ascorbic acid with warfarin, see Warfarin Sodium, p.777.

For the effect of ascorbic acid on fluphenazine, see Fluphenazine, p.1530.

Interference with biochemical laboratory tests. Ascorbic acid could cause chemical interference in laboratory tests for blood or urine creatinine, glucose, and uric acid.— *Med. Lett.,* 1971, *13,* 82; J. Millhouse, *Adverse Drug React. Bull.,* 1974, Dec., 164.

Ascorbic acid in large doses could interfere technically with chemical estimations for glucose in the blood and urine to produce erroneous lowered results.— *Drug & Ther. Bull.,* 1972, *10,* 69.

False-negative results for glycosuria could be obtained if the glucose-oxidase method were used with urine containing ascorbic acid.—, per J. S. Mayson *et al.* (letter), *Lancet,* 1973, *1,* 780.

The effect of ascorbic acid on laboratory estimation of liver enzymes and bilirubin.— M. H. Briggs *et al.* (letter), *Med. J. Aust.,* 1973, *2,* 48; H. E. Spiegel and E. Pinili (letter), *ibid.,* 1974, *2,* 265. Patients who had received 10 to 80 g of ascorbic acid intravenously could be expected to have blood concentrations which would interfere with bilirubin estimations.— M. H. Briggs (letter), *ibid.,* 542.

A patient who took 1 g of ascorbic acid daily for 2 years developed a vivid yellow coloration of the urine, which also caused a reduction of Benedict's solution.— L. Martin and J. G. Lines (letter), *Lancet,* 1974, *2,* 103.

False-negative occult blood tests occurred in a woman who took ascorbic acid 2 g daily as a dietary supplement. Faecal excretion of 55 mg daily of ascorbic acid could inhibit aqueous occult blood tests and ascorbic acid should not be taken for 2 to 3 days before such tests.— R. M. Jaffe *et al., Ann. intern. Med.,* 1975, *83,* 824.

A study in 9 healthy subjects indicated that ascorbic acid in doses of 3 and 9 g both given in dosage regimens of once and thrice daily did not interfere with the determination of urinary glucose by the 2-drop Clinitest method.— D. Smith and W. W. Young, *Am. J. Hosp. Pharm.,* 1977, *34,* 1347.

Ascorbic acid produced false negative results for paracetamol in an indophenol method of detection of paracetamol in the urine.— J. Swale (letter), *Lancet,* 1977, *2,* 981.

Pregnancy and the neonate. Ascorbic acid in doses greater than 1 g daily should not be taken during pregnancy since the effect of large doses on the foetus was unknown.— *Med. Lett.,* 1973, *15,* 67.

There were no significant differences in plasma concentrations of ascorbic acid between women with uneventful pregnancies and those ending in abortion, stillbirth, or the birth of a congenitally malformed infant in a study of 1500 pregnant women.— J. S. Vobecky *et al.* (letter), *Lancet,* 1974, *1,* 630.

A brief discussion of rebound scurvy in infants born to mothers taking high doses of ascorbic acid.— V. D. Herbert, *J. Am. pharm. Ass.,* 1977, *NS17,* 764.

Uricosuria. Significant uricosuria occurred after the administration of ascorbic acid 4 g but not after 0.5 or

2 g in a study involving 14 subjects. Chronic administration of ascorbic acid 2 g four times daily for 3 to 7 days resulted in sustained uricosuria and decrease in serum concentrations of uric acid. Ascorbic acid in large doses might obscure the diagnosis of gout or in some patients it might precipitate acute gouty arthritis.— H. B. Stein *et al.*, *Ann. intern. Med.*, 1976, *84*, 385.

Absence of effect of ascorbic acid 4 or 12 g on serum concentrations or excretion of uric acid.— W. E. Mitch *et al.*, *Clin. Pharmac. Ther.*, 1981, *29*, 318.

Further references: L. Berger *et al.*, *Am. J. Med.*, 1977, *62*, 71, per *Int. pharm. Abstr.*, 1977, *14*, 495.

Absorption and Fate. Ascorbic acid is readily absorbed from the gastro-intestinal tract and is widely distributed in the body tissues. The amount present in the body in health is in excess of 1.5 g. The concentration is higher in leucocytes and platelets than in erythrocytes and plasma. In deficiency states the concentration in leucocytes declines later and at a slower rate, and has been considered to be a better criterion for the evaluation of deficiency than the concentration in plasma.

Ascorbic acid in excess of the body's needs is rapidly eliminated in the urine and its elimination is usually accompanied by a mild diuresis.

A report of the differing rates of excretion of ascorbic acid in smokers and non-smokers.— *J. Am. med. Ass.*, 1969, *208*, 626.

Ascorbate-3-sulphate, a metabolite of ascorbic acid, was found in the urine of patients with scurvy.— E. M. Baker *et al.*, *Science*, 1971, *173*, 826.

Leucocyte and plasma concentrations of ascorbic acid and their role in estimating body stores.— H. S. Loh and C. W. M. Wilson, *Br. med. J.*, 1971, *3*, 733.

Reports of the behavioural and clinical changes observed in ascorbic acid deficiency, and of the metabolism of ascorbic acid in deficiency states.— R. E. Hodges *et al.*, *Am. J. clin. Nutr.*, 1971, *24*, 432. See also E. M. Baker *et al.*, *ibid.*, 444; R. A. Kinsman and J. Hood, *ibid.*, 455.

In a study in 25 healthy subjects given ascorbic acid 1 or 2 g daily for 12 weeks resting blood concentrations of ascorbic acid rose initially but returned to pretreatment values in about 10 days. Similar adaptation occurred when ascorbic acid was withdrawn.— L. M. Spero and T. W. Anderson (letter), *Br. med. J.*, 1973, *4*, 354.

Plasma concentrations of ascorbic acid fell with increasing age and without any alteration of intake in a study of 34 women aged 19 to 89 years.— M. L. Burr *et al.* (letter), *Lancet*, 1974, *1*, 163.

Ascorbic acid was partly metabolised to the sulphate and could modify the biotransformation of drugs similarly metabolised. Concomitant administration of ascorbic acid and salicylamide caused a significant decrease in the excretion of salicylamide as sulphate in 8 of 10 volunteers. This was compensated by a rise in glucuronide excretion.— J. B. Houston; G. Levy (letter), *Nature*, 1975, *255*, 78.

Most young women excreted less than 20% of a dose of ascorbic acid in 24 hours; by the second day plasma and urine concentrations were comparable with those in controls. Excretion appeared to be in some form other than ascorbic acid; oxalate and dehydroascorbic acid were possibilities.— A. B. Harris (letter), *Lancet*, 1976, *1*, 366.

A study on the metabolism of supplementary ascorbic acid during the common cold.— C. W. M. Wilson *et al.*, *J. clin. Pharmac.*, 1976, *16*, 19.

Of 14 healthy subjects who took ascorbic acid 500 mg, 5 were defined as high and 9 as low excretors of ascorbic acid.— A. Mullen and C. W. M. Wilson, *Br. J. clin. Pharmac.*, 1977, *4*, 731P.

In 5 healthy subjects, previously saturated with ascorbic acid, the mean half-life of ascorbic acid after a 1-g dose intravenously was 3.37 hours. About 83% of the dose was recovered in the urine, chiefly (84%) as ascorbic acid.— S. Yung *et al.* (letter), *J. pharm. Sci.*, 1978, *67*, 1491.

Further references: H. S. Loh *et al.*, *Clin. Pharmac. Ther.*, 1974, *14*, 390; E. W. Nelson *et al.*, *J. clin. Pharmac.*, 1978, *18*, 325.

Human Requirements. The minimum protective dose of ascorbic acid against clinical scurvy is 10 mg daily, but this does not provide a satisfactory vitamin allowance which for adults ranges between 30 and 60 mg daily.

These quantities are normally supplied in the diet, but individuals vary greatly in their requirements, and the higher the metabolic-rate the greater the need; more is required in pregnancy and lactation, thyrotoxicosis, postoperative states, and possibly infections.

The recommended daily intake of ascorbic acid was: from birth to 12 years, 20 mg; 13 years and over, 30 mg; in the second and third trimesters of pregnancy and during lactation, 50 mg.— Report of a Joint FAO/WHO Expert Group, *Tech. Rep. Ser. Wld Hlth Org. No. 452*, 1970.

White blood-cell concentrations of ascorbic acid in 305 elderly subjects aged 65 or over correlated with their recorded ascorbic acid intake.— Report by the Panel on Nutrition of the Elderly, *A Nutrition Survey of the Elderly*, London, HM Stationery Office, 1972.

Low white-cell concentrations of ascorbic acid were found in 6 of 12 patients with multiple injuries requiring artificial ventilation. Variations in these values were noted during the following 2 weeks but in 2 patients with the severest injury ascorbic acid concentrations continued to fall.— E. L. Lloyd and W. G. Edge (letter), *Br. J. Anaesth.*, 1973, *45*, 532.

Recommended daily intake of ascorbic acid: boys and girls, up to 8 years, 20 mg; 9 to 17 years, 25 to 30 mg; men and women 18 years and over, 30 mg; during pregnancy and lactation, 60 mg.— Recommended Daily Amounts of Food Energy and Nutrients for Groups of People in the United Kingdom, Report by the Committee on Medical Aspects of Food Policy, *Report on Health and Social Subjects, No. 15*, London, HM Stationery Office, 1979.

The recommendation that infant feeds should provide a minimum of 30 μg ascorbic acid per ml reconstituted feed.— Artificial Feeds for the Young Infant: 1980, Report of the Working Party on the Composition of Foods for Infants and Young Children, Committee on Medical Aspects of Food Policy, *Report on Health and Social Subjects, 18*, London, HM Stationery Office, 1980.

The recommended daily dietary allowance of ascorbic acid for adults is 60 mg; for infants in the first week of life 100 mg; for older breast- or bottle-fed infants 35 mg; for children up to 11 years of age 45 mg; for pregnant women 80 mg; for lactating women 100 mg.— *Recommended Dietary Allowances*, 9th Edn, Washington, The National Research Council, 1980, p. 75.

Uses. Ascorbic acid is essential for the synthesis of collagen and intercellular material. It is involved in the conversion of folic acid to folinic acid, in electron transport processes, and in the healing of wounds, and is believed to be involved in the metabolism of tyrosine.

Clinical scurvy, which is the outcome of severe ascorbic acid deficiency, is seldom seen now in adults but is still occasionally found in infants, and an ample intake of ascorbic acid is therefore important during pregnancy and lactation. For the prevention of infantile scurvy, at least 20 mg of ascorbic acid daily should be provided as a supplement for bottle-fed infants.

Ascorbic acid is used in the treatment of idiopathic methaemoglobinaemia. It has been used empirically in a wide variety of other disorders but there is little evidence that it has any beneficial effect. Controversy continues as to its value in large doses in the prophylaxis of the common cold.

Ascorbic acid is usually administered orally as tablets or fruit juice, but in the presence of persistent vomiting, diarrhoea, or other conditions preventing its adequate utilisation by mouth, it may be administered by injection as sodium ascorbate. Typical doses are 1 g twice or thrice daily to promote wound healing; 0.5 to 1 g twice or thrice daily for scurvy; and 200 to 500 mg daily for other purposes.

Ascorbic acid has been used as an antoxidant in emulsions of fats and oils, in iron mixtures, in certain injections and eye-drops, and as a browning inhibitor in unprocessed cut fruits, fruit pulps, and juices.

The addition of any of the following substances to raw and unprocessed meat intended for human consumption is prohibited in Great Britain by the Meat (Treatment) Regulations, 1964: ascorbic acid, isoascorbic acid, nicotinic acid, nicotinamide, and any derivative of these substances.

The ban on the addition of ascorbic acid to raw and unprocessed meat should be extended to include uncooked processed meat and meat products.— *Food Additives and Contaminants Committee Report on Further Classes of Food Additives*, London, HM Stationery Office, 1968.

Ascorbic acid was a good preservative of red blood cells because it maintained the concentrations of 2,3-diphosphoglycerate in the cells.— L. Wood and E. Beutler, *J. Am. med. Ass.*, 1972, *222*, 260.

Ascorbic acid was reported to prevent the formation of nitrosamines and nitrosamides *in vitro* and *in vivo*.— J. H. Weisburger (letter), *Lancet*, 1977, *2*, 607. See also H. Marquardt *et al.*, *Science*, 1977, *196*, 1000.

Use as an antoxidant. A review of the uses and efficacy in food of ascorbic acid as an antoxidant and synergist.— *Fd Add. Ser. Wld Hlth Org. No. 3*, 1972.

Estimated acceptable daily intake as antoxidant in food: up to 15 mg per kg body-weight in addition to that naturally present in food.— Seventeenth Report of FAO/WHO Expert Committee on Food Additives, *Tech. Rep. Ser. Wld Hlth Org. No. 539*, 1974. For background toxicological information, see *Fd Add. Ser. Wld Hlth Org. No. 5*, 1974.

Acidification of urine. A study in 10 healthy subjects given 4 regimens of ascorbic acid 4 and 6 g daily (divided into 4 or 6 daily doses) did not demonstrate any clinically significant effect on the pH of 24-hour urine samples compared with controls.— D. C. McLeod and M. C. Nahata (letter), *New Engl. J. Med.*, 1977, *296*, 1413.

From a study in 16 healthy subjects it was concluded that ascorbic acid in doses of 2 to 4 g daily did not consistently and reliably lower the pH of urine, and was not of value for this purpose.— V. E. Muiznieks, *Can. J. Hosp. Pharm.*, 1978, *31*, 18.

Administration in renal failure. For reference to ascorbic acid in renal failure see under Deficiency States (Dialysis), below.

Antimicrobial action. Ascorbic acid inhibited *in vitro* 16 strains of *Pseudomonas aeruginosa*. Minimum inhibitory concentrations ranged from 3.3 to 217 mg per ml. Ascorbic acid enhanced the antibacterial activity *in vitro* of ampicillin, erythromycin, chloramphenicol, colistin, and sulphamethoxazole and trimethoprim separately and together against *Ps. aeruginosa*. In 5 patients with cystic fibrosis whose sputum contained viable *Ps. aeruginosa*, co-trimoxazole 960 mg and ascorbic acid 2 g were given twice daily for 4 weeks. The number of viable *Ps. aeruginosa* diminished by 10- to 100-fold during treatment.— B. D. Rawal *et al.*, *Med. J. Aust.*, 1974, *1*, 169.

Leprosy. Studies of the metabolism of *Mycobacterium leprae* had shown that it required the enzyme β-glucuronidase, which was inhibited by ascorbic acid, for the utilisation of nutrients. In 1 patient with lepromatous leprosy treatment with ascorbic acid 1.5 g daily was found to fragment leprosy bacilli.— O. K. Skinsnes, *J. Am. med. Ass.*, 1975, *233*, 188.

Bronchospasm. Absence of effect of ascorbic acid on antigen-induced bronchospasm.— D. Kordansky *et al.*, *J. Allergy clin. Immunol.*, 1979, *63*, 61, per *Int. pharm. Abstr.*, 1980, *17*, 319.

Collagen disorders. Ten patients, aged 5 to 27 years, with osteogenesis imperfecta and 4 healthy persons were given a low hydroxyproline diet and after an initial 4-day period 1 g of ascorbic acid daily. Retention of ascorbic acid ranged from 255 to 612 mg after 3 months in the patients and younger healthy persons, but was lower in the elderly who were healthy. Decreased urinary excretion of hydroxyproline occurred after 3 months in 6 of the 10 patients and there was a substantially decreased incidence of broken bones.— E. A. Winterfeldt *et al.* (letter), *Lancet*, 1970, *1*, 1347.

There was a decreased tendency to fracture and a feeling of energy which increased physical activity in 13 infants and children with osteogenesis imperfecta whilst receiving ascorbic acid. The older children received 1 to 2 g daily and the infants 250 to 600 mg. Ten of 11 patients who had serum-zinc determinations showed a decrease in serum zinc, most marked during the first months of therapy whilst 8 controls receiving ascorbic acid showed an increase in serum zinc.— D. Kurz and E. J. Eyring, *Pediatrics*, 1974, *54*, 56.

In a study of 7 healthy children and 8 children being given prednisolone 2 mg per kg body-weight daily for at least 15 days, ascorbic acid 500 mg every 8 hours for 4 days had no effect on hydroxyproline excretion in the first group but induced a rise in the second group. Since reduced hydroxyproline excretion is an indication of decreased collagen formation large doses of ascorbic acid might counteract the adverse effect of corticosteroids on collagen formation.— D. Liakakos *et al.*, *Archs*

Dis. Childh., 1974, *49*, 400. Only 1 of 5 patients with juvenile rheumatoid arthritis experienced a rise in hydroxyproline excretion. Ascorbic acid was not considered to improve collagen synthesis.— P. Saphyakhajon *et al.* (letter), *Archs Dis. Childh.*, 1977, *52*, 82.

Common cold. Discussions of the status of ascorbic acid in relation to the common cold.— *Br. med. J.*, 1972, *4*, 786; *ibid.*, 1973, *3*, 311; C. W. M. Wilson and H. S. Loh (letter), *ibid.*, 1973, *4*, 166; *Med. Lett.*, 1974, *16*, 85; M. H. M. Dykes and P. Meier, *J. Am. med. Ass.*, 1975, *231*, 1073; C. W. M. Wilson, *Practitioner*, 1975, *215*, 343; *Br. med. J.*, 1976, *1*, 606; *Lancet*, 1979, *1*, 308.

In a double-blind trial lasting less than 4 months, 131 of 407 persons who took 1 g ascorbic acid daily in divided doses, increased to 4 g daily for the first 3 days of illness, did not experience any nose or throat symptoms and 105 were free from illness. This compared with 101 having no nose and throat symptoms and 76 with no illness out of 411 who took a placebo for the same period. The mean duration of illness per episode and incidence of work days lost was lower among persons who received ascorbic acid. There was no difference in sense of well-being experienced by the 2 groups; of 182 others who did not complete the trial 15 of 93 taking ascorbic acid and 13 of 89 taking the placebo complained of side-effects.— T. W. Anderson *et al.*, *Can. med. Ass. J.*, 1972, *107*, 503.

In a controlled study of the effects of ascorbic acid on colds in schoolboys and girls, the complexities of cold symptoms were reduced in the girls and the severity and intensity of colds considered to be catarrhal were also reduced in girls.— C. W. M. Wilson and H. S. Loh (preliminary communication), *Lancet*, 1973, *1*, 638. Criticism.— L. Kinlen and R. Peto (letter), *ibid.*, 944.

In a double-blind study ascorbic acid, 1 or 2 g depending on age, or a placebo was administered daily to 641 schoolchildren over a period of 14 weeks. Although the incidences of respiratory illness were similar in both groups, the length of illness was shorter in the treated group. The less severe symptoms of cold (cough and nasal discharge) were less frequent in the ascorbic acid group although other symptoms (sore throat, headache and fever) were similar in frequency, suggesting a local mucosal action of ascorbic acid. Measurement of blood-ascorbic acid in 100 children showed that those with higher blood concentrations had fewer sick days than those with the lower concentrations.— J. L. Coulehan *et al.*, *New Engl. J. Med.*, 1974, *290*, 6. Statistical criticism.— R. I. Shader, *Curr. ther. Res.*, 1974, *16*, 655.

Illnesses were less severe and shorter duration in volunteers taking ascorbic acid than in those taking a placebo. In this double-blind study the vitamin group received 500 mg once a week either as a tablet or sustained-release capsule and 1500 mg on the first day of illness plus 1000 mg on the next four days.— T. W. Anderson *et al.*, *Can. med. Ass. J.*, 1975, *112*, 823.

In a study in 1524 volunteers there was no evidence that ascorbic acid 10 g in 2.5 days relieved respiratory or general constitutional symptoms of the common cold. Men taking ascorbic acid had fewer recurrences of cold; the effect was not seen in women. Ascorbic acid was not considered of value.— D. A. J. Tyrrell *et al.*, *Br. J. prev. soc. Med.*, 1977, *31*, 189, per *Abstr. Hyg.*, 1977, *52*, 1242. See also P. C. Elwood *et al.*, *Practitioner*, 1977, *218*, 133.

In a 5-month double-blind study in 42 pairs of twins aged 6 to 15 years, ascorbic acid 0.5 to 1 g daily had no significant overall effect on cold symptoms compared with placebo. In girls receiving ascorbic acid in the 2 youngest groups cold symptoms were less severe and significantly shorter in duration. The severity of symptoms was diminished in the youngest group of treated boys.— J. Z. Miller *et al.*, *J. Am. med. Ass.*, 1977, *237*, 248.

Further references suggesting possible benefit: S. S. Charleston and K. M. Clegg (letter), *Lancet*, 1972, *1*, 1401; A. B. Carr *et al.*, *Med. J. Aust.*, 1981, *2*, 411.

Negative reports: G. H. Walker *et al.*, *Br. med. J.*, 1967, *1*, 603. Report No. 117 of the General Practitioner Research Group, *Practitioner*, 1968, *200*, 442; T. W. Anderson *et al.*, *Can. med. Ass. J.*, 1974, *111*, 31; M. Carson *et al.* (letter), *Br. med. J.*, 1974, *1*, 577; M. H. Briggs (letter), *Lancet*, 1974, *2*, 1211; J. L. Coulehan *et al.*, *New Engl. J. Med.*, 1976, *295*, 973.

Cot death. There is no evidence that large doses of ascorbic acid prevent sudden infant deaths.— P. Phelan (letter), *Med. J. Aust.*, 1979, *2*, 696.

Cystinosis. In a double-blind study involving 64 children with nephropathic cystinosis, ascorbic acid 200 mg per kg body-weight daily for up to about 2 years had no beneficial effect when compared with placebo and might be harmful.— J. A. Schneider *et al.*, *New Engl. J. Med.*, 1979, *300*, 756.

Deficiency states. From a study of 109 patients with duodenal ulceration it was concluded that depletion of ascorbic acid was common in patients with duodenal ulcer, duodenal stenosis, and the postgastrectomy syndrome.— I. W. Dymock *et al.* (letter), *Br. med. J.*, 1968, *1*, 179. In 33 patients undergoing surgery for peptic ulcer, both dietary intake and leucocyte concentrations of ascorbic acid were lower than those accepted as normal. After vagotomy the dietary intake was increased by the rise in leucocyte concentrations of ascorbic acid was small, possibly because of the hypochlorhydria induced by vagotomy. Patients who had undergone vagotomy might need routine supplements before any subsequent surgery.— J. A. E. MacDonald and M. M. Cohen, *Br. med. J.*, 1972, *2*, 738.

Persistent oral ulceration due to ascorbic acid deficiency responded to treatment with ascorbic acid 150 mg daily. Dietary advice was also given.— M. M. Ferguson and J. H. Dagg (letter), *Lancet*, 1974, *1*, 164.

A discussion of the need for supplements of ascorbic acid in patients with liver disease.— *Br. med. J.*, 1977, *1*, 735.

Scurvy in 1 patient with Crohn's disease and low leucocyte-ascorbic acid concentrations in a further 9 suggested that patients with Crohn's disease should receive regular treatment with ascorbic acid at a dose of 50 to 100 mg daily.— B. D. Linaker, *Postgrad. med. J.*, 1979, *55*, 26.

Dialysis. Patients on long-term haemodialysis showed a lowering of ascorbic acid concentrations which could be rectified by the addition of 1 g of ascorbic acid to the dialysate both at the beginning and at the midpoint of dialysis.— J. F. Sullivan and A. B. Eisenstein, *J. Am. med. Ass.*, 1972, *220*, 1697.

In the elderly. Administration of ascorbic acid 1 g daily for 28 days to long-stay geriatric in-patients led to slight but significant clinical improvement, compared with administration of placebo to similar patients. Of those who had been thought unlikely to improve, 7 of 23 in the ascorbic acid group did so whereas only 1 of 24 in the placebo group did so.— C. J. Schorah *et al.*, *Lancet*, 1979, *1*, 403.

In children. Administration of ascorbic acid 200 mg daily to a 9-month-old girl with Chediak-Higashi syndrome corrected the functional defects of her polymorphonuclear leucocytes.— L. A. Boxer *et al.*, *New Engl. J. Med.*, 1976, *295*, 1041.

Benefit following administration of ascorbic acid 0.5 to 1 g daily to an infant with hawkinsinuria (a defect of tyrosine metabolism).— B. Wilcken *et al.*, *New Engl. J. Med.*, 1981, *305*, 865.

Effects on serum cholesterol. A correlation in elderly men but not women between ascorbic acid status and the high-density lipoprotein fraction of cholesterol.— C. J. Bates *et al.* (letter), *Lancet*, 1977, *2*, 611.

Although ascorbic acid did not effectively lower serum-cholesterol concentrations in healthy subjects with initial values under 2 mg per ml, the effect was clear in hypercholesterolaemic subjects with a low intake of ascorbic acid. A daily ascorbic acid intake of about 500 mg represented a simple method of managing secondary hypercholesterolaemia.— E. Ginter (letter), *Lancet*, 1979, *2*, 958. Criticism and comment.— J. McMichael (letter), *ibid.*, 1182; R. J. Jarrett (letter), *ibid.*, 1375; A. E. Hugh (letter), *ibid.*; R. J. Farrell (letter), *ibid.*, 1376.

Further references: C. R. Spittle, *Lancet*, 1971, *2*, 1280; T. W. Anderson *et al.* (letter), *ibid.*, 1972, *2*, 876; H. S. Loh (letter), *Lancet*, 1973, *2*, 153; E. H. Derrick (letter), *Med. J. Aust.*, 1974, *2*, 577.

Thrombo-embolism. Ascorbic acid given to 271 geriatric subjects appeared to be no more effective than placebo given to 267 in preventing vascular thrombosis.— C. T. Andrews and T. S. Wilson (letter), *Lancet*, 1973, *2*, 39. The dose of ascorbic acid was too low to influence white-cell concentrations.— H. S. Loh and C. W. M. Wilson (letter), *ibid.*, 317.

Ascorbic acid 1 g daily or placebo was given from the time of admission to hospital for 2 weeks or until 2 weeks after surgery to 63 patients who were considered to be at risk from venous thrombo-embolisms. Scanning with iodinated (^{125}I) human fibrinogen injection identified thrombo-embolisms in 10 of the 30 patients given ascorbic acid compared with 20 of 33 given placebo.— C. R. Spittle (letter), *Lancet*, 1973, *2*, 199.

Growth. A study of the effect of ascorbic acid on growth.— J. Z. Miller *et al.*, *J. Am. med. Ass.*, 1977, *237*, 248. Criticism.— T. H. Jukes (letter), *ibid.*, *238*, 937.

Hyperhidrosis. Excessive sweating in thalidomide victims with reduction deformities of the limbs might respond to administration of ascorbic acid. One girl had achieved complete control with a dose of 50 mg daily.— R. W. Smithells (letter), *Lancet*, 1978, *1*, 1042.

The effects of ascorbic acid on heat acclimatisation.— H. F. Kotze *et al.*, *J. appl. Physiol.*, 1977, *42*, 711.

Intracardiac tests. Ascorbic acid was successfully used as an indicator for detecting and localising cardiac defects, particularly right-left shunts, by the dilution method. Doses of 50 to 200 mg of ascorbic acid were introduced through a cardiac catheter into the heart and the catheter was rinsed with either a further 100 mg of ascorbic acid or with sodium chloride injection. Doses of up to 800 mg of ascorbic acid was injected without complications occurring. Changes in electrical potential produced by the strong reducing properties of ascorbic acid were used to measure the dilution of ascorbic acid in the brachial artery.— A. M. Levy *et al.*, *Br. Heart J.*, 1967, *29*, 22.

Malignant neoplasms. Concentrations of potentially carcinogenic N-nitroso compounds decreased in the faeces of 20 healthy men after administration of ascorbic acid 250 mg four times daily.— *J. Am. med. Ass.*, 1977, *238*, 19.

A discussion of the role of ascorbic acid in neoplasms.— E. Cameron *et al.*, *Cancer Res.*, 1979, *39*, 663.

The results of a randomised double-blind study in 123 patients with advanced cancer indicated that ascorbic acid 10 g daily was of no benefit when compared with placebo. All but 9 of the patients had previously received radiotherapy or chemotherapy.— E. T. Creagan *et al.*, *New Engl. J. Med.*, 1979, *301*, 687. Critical comments.— M. L. Rossman and W. S. Brostoff (letter), *ibid.*, 1980, *302*, 298; E. Cameron (letter), *ibid.*, 299; C. H. Zaeslein (letter), *ibid.*; D. Small and E. S. Geringer (letter), *ibid.* A reply.— E. T. Creagan and C. G. Moertel (letter), *ibid.*

Mental disorders. Relief of depression in 4 patients treated with ascorbic acid 50 mg per kg body-weight intravenously per day for 2 weeks.— P. Cocchi *et al.*, *Pediatrics*, 1980, *65*, 862.

For a critical view of vitamin therapy for mental disorders, see in the general section under Megavitamin Therapy, p.1635.

Paraquat poisoning. The possible use of massive doses of ascorbic acid in paraquat poisoning.— B. Halliwell (letter), *Lancet*, 1976, *2*, 854.

Prickly heat. In a double-blind trial 30 children who had suffered from prickly heat for 8 weeks were given either ascorbic acid 15 mg per kg body-weight daily or a placebo for 2 weeks. Fourteen of the 15 treated with ascorbic acid improved or were free from lesions after completing the course compared with only 4 of 15 given placebo.— T. C. Hindson, *Lancet*, 1968, *1*, 1347. Comments.— F. P. Ellis (letter), *ibid.*, 1968, *2*, 173.

See also under Hyperhidrosis, above.

Thalassaemia. For the use of ascorbic acid in the management of iron overload in patients with thalassaemia, see Desferrioxamine, p.381.

See also under Adverse Effects, above.

Wound healing. The role of ascorbic acid in wound healing.— *Br. med. J.*, 1979, *1*, 437.

In a double-blind study of 20 patients with pressure-sores, ascorbic acid 500 mg twice daily given to 10 produced a mean white blood-cell concentration of 65.5 μg per 10^8 white blood cells compared with 25.8 per 10^8 in the 10 control patients. There was a mean reduction in area of the pressure-sore of 84% in the treated patients and 43% in the control patients.— T. V. Taylor *et al.*, *Lancet*, 1974, *2*, 544. Doses as high as 1 g might not be necessary.— C. R. Lee (letter), *ibid.*, 775. See also *Br. med. J.*, 1971, *2*, 604.

In a double-blind crossover pilot study of 8 patients with thalassaemia who had multiple leg ulcers, the administration of ascorbic acid 3 g daily resulted in a high rate of total or partial healing.— A. M. Afifi *et al.*, *Br. J. Derm.*, 1975, *92*, 339.

For the hazards of ascorbic acid in the iron-overloaded patient see under Adverse Effects, above.

Preparations

Ascorbic Acid Injection *(B.P.C. 1973).* Inj. Acid. Ascorb. Ascorbic acid 10% and sodium bicarbonate 4.8% in Water for Injections. Sterilise by filtration. Supplied, under nitrogen or other suitable gas, in single-dose ampoules. Protect from light. *Dose.* Therapeutic, 2 to 6 ml daily. A similar injection is included in several pharmacopoeias.

Ascorbic Acid Injection *(U.S.P.).* A sterile solution, in Water for Injections, of ascorbic acid prepared with the aid of sodium hydroxide, sodium carbonate, or sodium bicarbonate. pH 5.5 to 7. Protect from light.

Ascorbic Acid Tablets *(B.P.).* Ascorb. Acid Tab.; Vitamin C Tablets. Tablets containing ascorbic acid. Store in airtight containers. Protect from light and avoid contact with metal. Tablets containing 500 mg should be chewed then swallowed.

Ascorbic Acid Tablets *(U.S.P.).* Tablets containing ascorbic acid. Store in airtight containers. Protect from light.

Potassium Ascorbate Eye-drops *(Moorfields Eye Hosp.).* Ascorbic acid 10 g, potassium bicarbonate 5.7 g, disodium edetate 200 mg, sodium metabisulphite 300 mg, benzalkonium chloride 10 mg, water to 100 ml. pH 6.5. Sterilise by filtration. For glaucoma and lime burns.

Proprietary Preparations

Ascorbef *(Cox Continental, UK).* Ascorbic acid available as effervescent tablets of 1 g.

Roscorbic *(Roche, UK).* Ascorbic acid, available as tablets of 25, 50, 200, and 500 mg. **Roscorbic Effervescent Tablets.** Each contains ascorbic acid 1 g.

NOTE. This preparation is also known as Redoxon and is marketed as Roscorbic for prescription use.

Other Proprietary Names of Ascorbic Acid or Sodium Ascorbate

Arg.—Agruvit, Cewin; *Aust.*—Cebion; *Austral.*—Ascorb, Cecon, Cetamin, Citrets, Citrion, Flavettes, Juva-C, Invite-C, Multi-C, Vitascorb, Vitoran; *Belg.*—Abbo-C, Cebion, Cenol, Cevitan, Cevitine, Cevitol 500, C-Will, Orantine, Viascor, Vio-C, Vitascorbol 500; *Canad.*—Adenex, Ce-Vi-Sol, Megascorb; *Fr.*—Abriscor, Laroscorbine, Vitascorbol; *Ger.*—Cebion, Cedoxon, Ce-Fortin, Ceglycon, C-Vicotrat-forte, Taxofit, Xitix; *Greece*—Cebion; *Ital.*—Acidylina, Agrumina, Agruvit, Aran C, Asco C, Ascomed, Ascor, Ascorbivit, Aster C, Bio-ci,Cebion, Cecon, Cevigen, Cevit, Ci-Agro, Cidalma, Cith, Citran, Citrovitamina, Clisa, C-Tard, Duo-C, Esurvit, Euvit C, Farmobion C, Idro-C, Kosmo-C, Lacivit, Lemonvit, Orange, Pasta Al Cebion, Pronto C, Vicisin, Vicitina; *Jap.*—Hicee; *Neth.*—Cebion; *S.Afr.*—Cebion; *Spain*—Abboce, Amplex-C, C-Vit, Cantil (see also under Mepenzolate Bromide), Cebion, Cecrisina, Cetasan, Cetin, Cevitasi Fuerte, Citrovit, Dextamina C, Dif-Vitamin C, Godabion C, Gradalin C, Iskia C, Kronoletas C Lenta, Ledovit-C, Lifaton-C Normal, Pancervo-C, Sergovit-C, Vicomin-C, Vitaceland, Vitafardi-C, Viterra C, Yoguis-C; *Swed.*—Cebion, C-vimin, Cevitil, Hybrin, Ido-C; *Switz.*—Ascorbin, Cebion, C-Tron, Frubiose 500, Mephacevin, Vitascorbal, Vicemex, Vita Cé; *USA*—Alba-Ce, CC-Kaps, Cemill, Cenolate, Cetane, Cevalin, Cevi-Bid, Ce-vi-sol, Duoscorb, Viterra C.

7881-b

Sodium Ascorbate *(U.S.P.).* 3-Oxo-L-gulofuranolactone sodium enolate.

$C_6H_7NaO_6$=198.1.

CAS — 134-03-2.

Pharmacopoeias. In *U.S.*

White or very faintly yellow, odourless or almost odourless, crystals or crystalline powder. It gradually darkens on exposure to light.

Soluble 1 in 1.3 of water; very slightly soluble in alcohol; practically insoluble in chloroform and ether. A 10% solution in water is dextrorotatory and has a pH of 7 to 8. A 3% solution is iso-osmotic with serum. **Store** in airtight containers. Protect from light.

Uses. Sodium ascorbate has properties similar to those of ascorbic acid and is suitable for the preparation of solutions for injection.

It is used as an antoxidant in the food industry.

A review of the uses and efficacy of sodium ascorbate as an antoxidant and synergist.— *Fd Add. Ser. Wld Hlth Org. No. 3,* 1972.

Estimated acceptable daily intake: up to 15 mg per kg body-weight in addition to that naturally present in food.— Seventeenth Report of FAO/WHO Expert Committee on Food Additives, *Tech. Rep. Ser. Wld Hlth Org. No. 539,* 1974.

For proprietary names of preparations containing sodium ascorbate see under Ascorbic Acid, above.

7882-v

Black Currant *(B.P.).* Ribes Nigrum; Rib. Nig.

Pharmacopoeias. In *Br.*

The fresh ripe fruit of *Ribes nigrum* (Grossulariaceae) together with their pedicels and rachides. Black currant contains invert sugar 6 to 8%; citric, malic, and ascorbic acids together equivalent to about 3% of citric acid; and pectin and colouring matter. The ascorbic acid content of the fruit varies between about 100 to 300 mg per 100 g.

Uses. Black currant is rich in ascorbic acid and is used in the form of a syrup as a dietary supplement, particularly for children. The syrup is also used as a flavouring agent.

Preparations

Black Currant Syrup *(B.P.).* Syrupus Ribis Nigri; Syr. Rib. Nig. Prepared by dissolving sucrose 70 g in 56 ml of clarified juice from fresh black currants, previously diluted to a weight per ml of 1.045 g, or in 56 ml of a similarly diluted solution of concentrated black currant juice of commerce; benzoic acid (equivalent to not more than 800 ppm), or sodium metabisulphite or other suitable sulphite (equivalent to not more than 350 ppm of SO_2) is added. Permitted food-grade colours may be added. Wt per ml 1.27 to 1.3 g. It contains not less than 0.055% w/w of ascorbic acid (about 7.5 mg in 10 ml) but this standard does not apply to syrup used for pharmaceutical purposes as a flavouring agent. Store at a temperature not exceeding 25° in well-filled containers. Protect from light.

7883-g

Rose Fruit *(B.P.C. 1954).* Rosae Fructus; Dog Rose Fruits; Brier Fruit; Hips; Cynosbati Fructus; Hypanthium Rosae.

Pharmacopoeias. In *Hung., Jap., Pol., Rus.,* and *Swiss.*

The fresh ripe fruits of various species of *Rosa* (Rosaceae), containing 0.1 to 1% of ascorbic acid together with vitamin A, thiamine, riboflavine, and nicotinic acid.

Uses. Rose fruit is a rich source of ascorbic acid, containing from 3 to 4 times as much as black currant and about 10 times as much as orange juice. It is used in the form of a syrup as a dietary supplement, particularly for children.

7884-q

Vitamin D

The term vitamin D is used for a range of compounds which possess the property of preventing or curing rickets; they include: ergocalciferol (vitamin D_2), cholecalciferol (D_3), 25-hydroxycholecalciferol or calcifediol, 1,25-dihydroxycholecalciferol or calcitriol, 1α-hydroxycholecalciferol or alfacalcidol, and dihydrotachysterol.

The vitamin-D content of food appears to be relatively unaffected by cooking.

Comment on the variable potency of some intramuscular preparations of vitamin D.— M. P. Whyte *et al.* (letter), *New Engl. J. Med.,* 1979, *300,* 142.

Units. The Second International Standard Preparation (1949) of vitamin D consists of bottles containing approximately 6 g of a solution of cholecalciferol in vegetable oil (1000 units per g). NOTE. One unit of vitamin D is contained in 0.000025 mg of cholecalciferol.

In England and Wales, the Labelling of Food Regulations 1970 (SI 1970: No. 400) as amended (SI 1972: 1510) require that in any food labelled as containing vitamins D, D_2 or D_3 the vitamin must be calculated as micrograms of cholecalciferol.

The eventual discontinuation of the International Standard for Vitamin D (and International Unit) was recommended by the WHO Expert Committee on Biological Standardization.— *Chronicle Wld Hlth Org.,* 1973, *27,* 31.

Adverse Effects. Symptoms of vitamin-D overdosage are anorexia, lassitude, nausea, vomiting, diarrhoea, loss of weight, polyuria, profuse sweating, headache, extreme thirst, and vertigo; the calcium and phosphorus concentrations of serum and urine are increased and calcium may be deposited in many tissues including the arteries and kidneys, which may lead to hypertension and renal failure; the cholesterol concentration of plasma may be increased. Patients intentionally on high doses of the vitamin should be kept under close observation.

Myocardial infarction. In 118 patients who had suffered myocardial infarction the estimated daily consumption of vitamin D was significantly higher than in 118 controls; a daily intake of 30 μg might be the critical level. There was no correlation between the intake of vitamin D and the incidence of angina pectoris or degenerative joint disease.— V. Lindén, *Br. med. J.,* 1974, *3,* 647. Criticism.— O. Lindahl and L. Lindwall (letter), *ibid.,* 1975, *2,* 560.

A study of the content in serum of 25-hydroxy vitamin D in 30 patients who had suffered myocardial infarction and in 60 controls afforded no support for the suggestion that the intake of vitamin D was related to the higher risk of myocardial infarction in northern Norway.— T. Vik *et al., Br. med. J.,* 1979, *2,* 176.

Overdose. A report of 8 patients who were suffering from vitamin-D intoxication, in 6 of whom the vitamin-D therapy was unnecessary.— M. Davies and P. H. Adams, *Lancet,* 1978, *2,* 621. An account of hypercalcaemia in 21 patients due to vitamin-D poisoning. Five had been inappropriately prescribed milligram doses. Milligram doses were appropriate for the other 16 but control of therapy was inadequate. Constant vigilance is essential for patients taking large doses of vitamin D.— C. R. Paterson, *Lancet,* 1980, *1,* 1164.

Deafness after long-term treatment with ergocalciferol 2.5 mg daily.— H. N. Cohen *et al.* (letter), *Lancet,* 1979, *1,* 985.

Massive acute vitamin-D intoxication in a family after eating food cooked in an oil with a high cholecalciferol content and intended as a supplement for animal feeding.— P. F. Down *et al., Postgrad. med. J.,* 1979, *55,* 897.

Pregnancy and the neonate. In 1964 R.E. Garcia *et al.* (*New Engl. J. Med.,* 1964, *271,* 117) suggested an association between idiopathic hypercalcaemia and a syndrome characterised by mental subnormality, a peculiar facies, and supraventricular aortic stenosis. Attention was called to the similarity between the cardiovascular lesion seen in experimental vitamin-D intoxication and idiopathic hypercalcaemia. An association between the syndrome and excessive maternal ingestion of vitamin D was demonstrated in *rabbits* by W.F. Friedman and W.C. Roberts (*Circulation,* 1966, *34,* 77). Further references: W. F. Friedman and L. F. Mills, *Pediatrics,* 1969, *43,* 12.

Reproduction studies with calcitriol in *animals*.— R. M. McClain *et al., Toxic. appl. Pharmac.,* 1980, *52,* 89.

Treatment of Adverse Effects. The treatment of hypercalcaemia is described in the section on calcium salts, p.619. Excessive exposure to sunlight should be avoided.

Precautions. The effects of hypercalcaemia should be borne in mind when giving vitamin D as should the role of the liver and kidney on the different forms of vitamin D. Special care should be taken to ensure correct dosage in infants.

The effects of vitamin D may be reduced in patients taking barbiturates or anticonvulsants.

Evidence that isoniazid interferes with vitamin-D metabolism, although in a manner different to the vitamin-D-wasting effect of rifampicin. Patients on long-term treatment with isoniazid and rifampicin may be at risk of developing metabolic bone disease.— M. J. Brodie *et al., Br. J. clin. Pharmac.,* 1981, *11,* 422P.

Resistance. Resistance to vitamin D in one patient might have been due to absence of parathyroid hormone and high plasma concentrations of calcitonin.— C. R. Paterson, *Br. med. J.,* 1977, *1,* 952.

Further references: L. C. Aschinberg *et al., J. Pediat.,* 1977, *91,* 56.

Absorption and Fate. Vitamin D in man is derived from 2 main sources. During exposure to sunlight cholecalciferol (vitamin D_3) is formed in the skin from 7-dehydrocholesterol; vitamin D is also ingested in the diet as ergocalciferol (vitamin D_2) or as cholecalciferol.

Cholecalciferol in the circulation is hydroxylated

in the liver to 25-hydroxycholecalciferol (calcifediol is 25-hydroxycholecalciferol), the most abundant form in the circulation; it is subject to enterohepatic circulation, and is further hydroxylated to 1,25-dihydroxycholecalciferol (calcitriol is 1,25-dihydroxycholecalciferol) in the renal tubule cells, production being regulated by the concentrations of 1,25-dihydroxycholecalciferol, parathyroid hormone, calcium, phosphate, and probably prolactin in the circulation. There are believed to be other possible pathways for the metabolism of 25-hydroxycholecalciferol, and small amounts of 24,25-dihydroxycholecalciferol and possibly other metabolites are produced in the kidney; their significance is not clear. 1,25-Dihydroxycholecalciferol is reported to be metabolised to 1,24,25-trihydroxycholecalciferol and to another unidentified metabolite. The metabolism of ergocalciferol has been less extensively studied than that of cholecalciferol but is believed to be similar. Vitamin-D metabolites are bound to specific plasma proteins.

1,25-Dihydroxycholecalciferol is considered to be the active metabolite of vitamin D and is considered to be hormonal. 1α-Hydroxycholecalciferol (alfacalcidol is 1α-hydroxycholecalciferol), a synthetic analogue of 1,25-dihydroxycholecalciferol, is considered to be hydroxylated in the liver to 1,25-dihydroxycholecalciferol.

The various forms of vitamin D are absorbed from the gastro-intestinal tract. The roles of the liver and kidney should be considered when giving vitamin D.

Reviews and discussions of the metabolism of vitamin D.— H. F. DeLuca, *Ann. intern. Med.*, 1976, *85*, 367; *Lancet*, 1977, *1*, 840; R. Larkins, *Med. J. Aust.*, 1977, *2*, 175; M. R. Haussler and T. A. McCain, *New Engl. J. Med.*, 1977, *297*, 974 and 1041; S. Tomlinson and J. L. H. O'Riordan, *Br. J. Hosp. Med.*, 1978, *19*, 40; R. G. Long and M. R. Wills, *Br. J. Hosp. Med.*, 1978, *20*, 312; J. Reeve, *Br. med. J.*, 1979, *2*, 888; *Lancet*, 1979, *2*, 292.

The absorption and fate of calcitriol given by mouth and by intravenous injection. Although doses of 1 µg by mouth seldom produced serum concentrations above 20 ng per litre they did increase serum-calcium concentrations possibly by a direct action on the intestinal mucosal-cell nucleus. Since the half-life of calcitriol was shorter than that of cholecalciferol and 25-hydroxycholecalciferol any hypercalcaemia due to inadvertent overdosage would be of a shorter duration.— E. B. Mawer *et al.*, *Lancet*, 1976, *1*, 1203.

Plasma concentrations of 25-hydroxy vitamin D in patients treated with high doses of ergocalciferol or cholecalciferol for metabolic bone disease or hypoparathyroidism. High priming doses were necessary for a rapid response.— J. M. Gertner and M. Domenech, *J. clin. Path.*, 1977, *30*, 144.

Most vitamin D was normally transported on a specific binding globulin; in a 9-month-old boy who had received large doses of ergocalciferol, binding to globulin was reduced and binding to lipoprotein and albumin increased.— J. Silver *et al.*, *Br. med. J.*, 1978, *2*, 93.

The role of pituitary hormones in regulating renal vitamin-D metabolism in man.— D. J. Brown *et al.*, *Br. med. J.*, 1980, *280*, 277.

In 4 healthy subjects given calcitriol 4 µg, peak concentrations were achieved at 4 hours and had returned to normal 27 hours after administration. In 3 subjects given 24,25-dihydroxycholecalciferol 250 µg peak concentrations were achieved at 6 hours and were still considerably raised at 48 hours. In 1 subject studied the concentration returned to the normal range in 9 days but not to the pre-treatment value by 21 days.— R. S. Mason *et al.*, *Br. med. J.*, 1980, *280*, 449.

Synthesis and metabolism of vitamin D after ultraviolet irradiation of normal and vitamin-D-deficient subjects.— J. S. Adams *et al.*, *New Engl. J. Med.*, 1982, *306*, 722.

Further references: S. W. Stanbury and E. B. Mawer, *Clin. Sci.*, 1980, *58*, 523.

Human Requirements. The daily requirements of vitamin D in adults are small and are met in part by exposure to sunlight. An intake of about 100 to 200 units (2.5 to 5 µg) is generally considered adequate in adults. The requirements are greater in infancy and during pregnancy and lactation.

The following daily intakes of vitamin D were recommended: from birth to 6 years of age, 400 units (10 µg); 7 years and over, 100 units (2.5 µg); during the second and third trimesters of pregnancy, and during lactation, 400 units (10 µg).— Report of a Joint FAO/WHO Expert Group, *Tech. Rep. Ser. Wld Hlth Org. No. 452*, 1970.

Studies indicated that babies received substantial amounts of vitamin D during the first 6 to 12 months of life, though there was considerable variation. In some older children the amount of vitamin D received was well below the allowance of 400 units suggested by most countries. It seemed that the use of unfortified cow's milk for young babies should be discouraged. As the main source of vitamin D in older children was margarine, and its consumption was variable, further research was required to indicate whether deficiency of vitamin D necessitated a revision of the scheme for fortifying foods.— *Interim Report on Vitamin D by the Panel on Child Nutrition*, London, HM Stationery Office, 1970.

In a nutrition survey of 879 elderly subjects aged 65 or over the average content of vitamin D in the diet was 104 units and was considered to match recommended intake. However, it was felt that the elderly might be less able to obtain vitamin D from sunlight and that those who were housefast might be at special risk.— Report by the Panel on Nutrition of the Elderly, *A Nutrition Survey of the Elderly*, London, HM Stationery Office, 1972.

Human milk contained more vitamin D than had hitherto been considered. This was accounted for by the presence of a water-soluble sulphate complex of vitamin D that would not previously have been considered as earlier measurements were based on the fat-soluble form. The mean concentration of this sulphate form in samples taken on days 3 to 5 was 1.78 µg per 100 ml, on days 6 to 8, 1.00 µg per 100 ml, and during established lactation 0.91 µg per 100 ml. The biological activity of the sulphate form was under study while the effect of these findings on maternal vitamin-D requirements still remained to be studied.— D. R. Lakdawala and E. M. Widdowson, *Lancet*, 1977, *1*, 167.

The following daily intakes of vitamin D (as cholecalciferol) were recommended: infants under 1 year, 7.5 µg; children 1 to 4 years, 10 µg; in pregnancy and lactation, 10 µg; dietary sources might not be necessary for children and adults sufficiently exposed to sunlight; adults insufficiently exposed to sunlight might need 10 µg daily; children and adolescents should receive that amount during winter.— Daily Amounts of Food and Energy and Nutrients for Groups of People in the United Kingdom, Report by the Committee on Medical Aspect of Food Policy, *Report on Health and Social Subjects No. 15*, London, HM Stationery Office, 1979.

The recommendation that any infant feed should provide about 10 ng vitamin D (0.4 i.u.) per ml reconstituted feed and acceptance of the range 7 to 13 ng vitamin D per ml feed. The recommendation that the vitamin be added as ergocalciferol (vitamin D_2) or cholecalciferol (vitamin D_3).— Artificial Feeds for the Young Infant: 1980, Report of the Working Party on the Composition of Foods for Infants and Young Children, Committee on Medical Aspects of Food Policy, *Report on Health and Social Subjects, 18*, London, HM Stationery Office 1980.

Recommended daily dietary allowance of vitamin D (as cholecalciferol) for infants, children, and adolescents is 10 µg (400 units); for adults aged 19 to 22 years 7.5 µg (300 units); for adults more than 22 years of age 5 µg (200 units); pregnant or lactating women require an additional 5 µg (200 units).— *Recommended Dietary Allowances*, 9th Edn, Washington, The National Research Council, 1980, p. 61.

A study of ergocalciferol supplements in Asian women during pregnancy; such supplements should be given to all pregnant Asian women, for at least the last trimester, in the UK.— O. G. Brooke *et al.*, *Br. med. J.*, 1980, *280*, 751 and 1168.

Uses. Vitamin D is necessary for the absorption of calcium and phosphate from the gastro-intestinal tract and for their transport. Deficiency of vitamin D is associated with the occurrence of rickets in children and osteomalacia in adults and is a factor in the production of tetany.

Poor absorption may occur in persistent diarrhoea, steatorrhoea, and biliary obstruction and intake of vitamin D may need to be increased in these conditions. It is advisable to monitor serum-calcium concentrations during treatment with vitamin D.

Vitamin D is administered clinically as alfacalcidol (p.1660), calcifediol (p.1660), calcitriol (p.1660), cholecalciferol (p.1661), dihydrotachysterol (p.1662), and ergocalciferol (p.1662).

The use of vitamin D_2 and D_3 as additives in animal feeding stuffs is controlled in Great Britain by The Fertilisers and Feeding Stuffs Regulations 1973 (SI 1973: No. 1521) as amended (SI 1976: No. 840; SI 1977: No. 115).

Details of the different forms of vitamin D.— *Drug & Ther. Bull.*, 1981, *19*, 103.

Reviews of vitamin D and its function and uses.— P. H. Stern, *Pharmac. Rev.*, 1980, *32*, 47; A. M. Pierides, *Drugs*, 1981, *21*, 241; D. R. Fraser, *Br. med. Bull.*, 1981, *37*, 37.

Cirrhosis. A study involving 39 patients with symptomatic primary biliary cirrhosis demonstrated that the condition was associated with reduced serum concentrations of hydroxy vitamin D. A single dose of ergocalciferol given intramuscularly had no effect but regular monthly injections could produce normal serum concentrations. Such patients could therefore hydroxylate ergocalciferol if given in adequate amounts.— R. K. Skinner *et al.*, *Lancet*, 1977, *1*, 720. A single dose of 10 µg of calcifediol per kg body-weight by mouth had no effect on the plasma concentrations of hydroxy vitamin D in 11 similar patients when compared with 15 controls. Osteomalacia in 4 of the patients was associated with the use of cholestyramine.— J. E. Compston and R. P. H. Thompson, *ibid.*, 721.

A discussion on osteomalacia in primary biliary cirrhosis and the need to give ergocalciferol parenterally, sometimes in doses of 150 000 units monthly.— *Lancet*, 1978, *1*, 1138.

Treatment for 5 to 13 months with calcifediol 50 µg daily by mouth in 2 patients or ergocalciferol 3.75 mg (150 000 units) once a week by intramuscular injection in 2 similar patients effectively healed osteomalacia associated with primary biliary cirrhosis. Low plasma concentrations of 25-hydroxy vitamin D became normal in all 4 patients which suggested that the doses used were in the therapeutic range. Liver function continued to deteriorate in 3 patients and 2 had since died.— J. E. Compston *et al.*, *Gut*, 1979, *20*, 133.

Administration of ergocalciferol did not prevent development of bone disease in patients with chronic cholestatic or alcoholic liver disease.— R. G. Long *et al.*, *Gut*, 1978, *19*, 85.

Further references: D. B. Posner *et al.*, *Gastroenterology*, 1978, *74*, 866; J. E. Compston *et al.*, *Br. med. J.*, 1979, *2*, 309; J. S. Reed *et al.*, *Gastroenterology*, 1980, *78*, 512.

Deficiency states. A review of vitamin-D deficiency and bone disease.— J. C. Gallagher and B. L. Riggs, *New Engl. J. Med.*, 1978, *298*, 193.

Reports of vitamin-D deficiency: In Asians.— S. P. Hunt *et al.*, *Br. med. J.*, 1976, *2*, 1351; J. A. Ford *et al.*, *Archs Dis. Childh.*, 1976, *51*, 939; J. Pietrek *et al.*, *Lancet*, 1976, *1*, 1145.

A working party has advised against the fortification of food with vitamin D as a means of combating deficiencies in Asians.— *Lancet*, 1981, *1*, 229. Annual prophylaxis with ergocalciferol 2.5 mg by mouth each autumn.— W. P. Stephens *et al.*, *ibid.*, *2*, 1199.

Advice that not only children but also young adults (aged 13 to 18 years) of Asian origin living in Great Britain should be given supplements of vitamin D. A particular target should be pregnant Asian women.— K. M. Goel *et al.*, *Lancet*, 1981, *2*, 405.

Vitamin-D deficiency in gastro-intestinal disease.— J. G. Haddad, *Ann. intern. Med.*, 1977, *87*, 629.

Vitamin-D deficiency associated with fracture of the femur.— Y. Weisman *et al.*, *Br. med. J.*, 1978, *2*, 1196; M. R. Baker *et al.*, *Br. med. J.*, 1979, *1*, 589.

In the elderly. In 11 patients in a long-stay geriatric unit with plasma concentrations of 25-hydroxy vitamin D (25-OHD) of 2 to 22.8 ng per ml given ergocalciferol 500 units daily, concentrations of plasma 25-OHD rose significantly by the second month of treatment compared with 12 controls; the effect was greater in those with low initial 25-OHD values. A four-fold increase in dose produced only a marginally greater improvement in 25-OHD. A daily dose of 500 units of vitamin D was adequate in most old people.— W. J. MacLennan and J. C. Hamilton, *Br. med. J.*, 1977, *2*, 859. A similar report.— J. Conely *et al.* (letter), *Br. med. J.*, 1977, *2*, 1668.

Rickets. In 81 children, some of whom had rickets, with alkaline phosphatase values of 30 KA units or more and treated with ergocalciferol 1.25 mg daily, growth in a year was significantly greater than in controls.— W. T. Cooke *et al.*, *Br. med. J.*, 1974, *2*, 293.

A survey of the vitamin-D status of 256 schoolboys from Asian, West Indian, and European homes in Birmingham during 1976. It was considered that 1 mg of cholecalciferol given as one tablet each school term during adolescence would prevent rickets in schoolboys from such communities.— G. Ellis *et al.*, *Lancet*, 1977, *1*, 825.

Alfacalcidol 100 ng per kg body-weight was given daily by mouth for 3 weeks in the treatment of nutritional rickets in a premature baby. The hypocalcaemia was reversed, skeletal mineralisation improved, reactive hyperparathyroidism halted, and rickets healed.— J. F. T. Glasgow and M. Reid (letter), *Lancet*, 1977, *2*, 302. See also Y. Seino *et al.*, *Archs Dis. Childh.*, 1981, *56*, 628.

A report of the successful treatment with alfacalcidol of 2 children with cystinotic rickets.— S. I. Beer *et al.* (letter), *Archs Dis. Childh.*, 1978, *53*, 761.

Hypocalcaemia and secondary hyperparathyroidism were corrected in a 22-year-old black woman with osteomalacia when she was given cholecalciferol 100 μg daily for 4 weeks but the very high serum concentration of 1,25-dihydroxyvitamin D was elevated still further. The disorder was attributed to impaired responsiveness of target organs to 1,25-dihydroxyvitamin D and was designated vitamin-D-dependent rickets Type II.— M. H. Brooks *et al.*, *New Engl. J. Med.*, 1978, *298*, 996.

Epilepsy. Of 21 patients with epilepsy given ergocalciferol 2000, 10 000, or 50 000 units daily for up to 1 year, minor seizures were reduced in 11 and increased in 7 while major seizures were reduced in 6 and increased in 8. These results were not considered sufficiently promising to proceed to a controlled trial.— A. Richens and D. J. F. Rowe (letter), *Br. med. J.*, 1974, *3*, 251.

In 23 patients with epilepsy taking anticonvulsants the number of seizures was significantly reduced when ergocalciferol 4000 to 16 000 units daily was added to their treatment. The reduction in seizures was not correlated with changes in serum concentrations of calcium or magnesium.— C. Christiansen *et al.* (preliminary communication), *Br. med. J.*, 1974, *2*, 258.

Hyperparathyroidism. In 6 patients with primary hyperparathyroidism treated with alfacalcidol prior to surgery the postoperative course was comparable with that in 6 patients not given alfacalcidol. Alfacalcidol might increase hypercalcaemia and could not be recommended for routine pre-operative use in such patients.— D. A. Heath *et al.*, *Br. med. J.*, 1979, *1*, 450.

Calcitriol 250 to 500 ng daily arrested or improved the radiological features of hyperparathyroidism in a study in 57 patients undergoing regular dialysis.— D. E. Memmos *et al.*, *Br. med. J.*, 1981, *282*, 1919.

See also under Hypoparathyroidism (below).

Hypocalcaemia. The use of alfacalcidol in hypocalcaemic psychosis.— J. M. Gertner *et al.*, *Clin. Endocr.*, 1976, *5*, 539.

Convulsions ceased in a 40-year-old man with hypocalcaemia secondary to hypoparathyroidism after treatment with ergocalciferol; anticonvulsant-induced hypocalcaemia in a young man was slowly reversed, with cessation of convulsions, when he was given ergocalciferol intramuscularly; a third patient with convulsions secondary to hypocalcaemia and osteomalacia died despite treatment with calcium gluconate and ergocalciferol.— M. M. Gupta and D. N. Grover, *Postgrad. med. J.*, 1977, *53*, 330.

Symptoms of neonatal hypocalcaemia in 48 infants were initially alleviated by brief intravenous infusion of calcium gluconate. Subsequent treatment of 24 infants with alfacalcidol 330 ng in arachis oil by mouth twice daily for 5 days was more rapidly effective in correcting hypocalcaemia than intravenous infusion of calcium 20 mg per kg body-weight daily, as calcium gluconate injection 10%, used to treat the other 24 infants.— Y. Barak *et al.*, *Archs Dis. Childh.*, 1979, *54*, 642.

Hypoparathyroidism. Calcitriol given by mouth to 8 patients with proven hypoparathyroidism increased serum-calcium concentration within 6 to 8 days. Normal serum-calcium concentrations were achieved within 10 to 57 days (mean 26 days); 4 or 5 patients were also taking calcium supplements. The increase in serum-calcium concentration was associated with a reduction in serum-phosphorus concentration although high phosphorus values persisted in 3 patients. There were 3 episodes of hypercalcaemia in 2 patients and these responded quickly to withdrawal of therapy. Treatment had continued for between 4 and 24 months (mean 15 months) and the minimum effective dose varied from 0.25 to 1 μg daily.— M. Davies *et al.*, *Lancet*, 1977, *1*, 55.

Further references: R. G. G. Russell *et al.*, *Lancet*, 1974, *2*, 14; H. P. Kind *et al.* (letter), *Lancet*, 1975, *1*, 1145; S. W. Kooh *et al.*, *New Engl. J. Med.*, 1975, *293*, 840; L. D. Lambert and A. J. Johanson, *J. Pediat.*, 1977, *90*, 654.

See also Hyperparathyroidism, above.

Hypophosphataemia. In the treatment of familial and non-familial hypophosphataemia, administration of vitamin D 40 000 to 140 000 units daily had a beneficial effect on the intestinal transport of phosphate, though it did not completely correct defective absorption. The response to treatment with vitamin D could be assessed by an oral test of phosphate tolerance, in which venous blood and urine samples were collected and analysed for inorganic phosphate at intervals after the administration of sodium phosphate 6.9 g (equivalent to 1.5 g of phosphorus).— J. R. Condon *et al.*, *Br. med. J.*, 1970, *3*, 138.

Osteitis deformans. Brief discussions of the role of vitamin D in Paget's disease.— E. D. Williams *et al.* (letter), *Lancet*, 1981, *1*, 384; C. Nagant de Deuxchaisnes *et al.* (letter), *ibid.*, 833.

Osteomalacia. Reviews and discussions of the treatment of osteomalacia with vitamin D: S. J. Darke and J. M. L. Stephen, *Topics of our Time No. 1*, Department of Health and Social Security, London, HM Stationery Office, 1976; B. Frame and A. M. Parfitt, *Ann. intern. Med.*, 1978, *89*, 966.

Vitamin-D requirements in anticonvulsant osteomalacia.— *Br. med. J.*, 1976, *2*, 1340. See also under Phenytoin, p.1236.

The successful use of alfacalcidol 2 to 8 μg daily in a 51-year-old woman with anticonvulsant osteomalacia.— J. R. Juttmann *et al.*, *Br. med. J.*, 1977, *1*, 551 and 846. See also J. E. Compston *et al.*, *ibid.*, 1977, *2*, 612; *idem*, *Lancet*, 1978, *1*, 9.

Nutritional osteomalacia responded to vitamin D 3000 units daily, with added calcium. In the presence of malabsorption vitamin D was best given by injection—20 000 to 50 000 units weekly until the bone was healing.— G. L. Chalmers, *Practitioner*, 1978, *220*, 711.

The beneficial use of calcifediol in a patient with osteomalacia after ileal resection and cholestyramine treatment.— J. E. Compston and L. W. L. Horton, *Gastroenterology*, 1978, *74*, 900.

In 4 patients with hepatic cirrhosis and osteomalacia (3 with myopathy) the intramuscular injection of calcitriol 15 μg in arachis oil every 4 weeks relieved bone pain and myopathy and reduced the amount of osteoid tissue; serum and urinary biochemical changes were not pronounced.— R. G. Long *et al.*, *Br. med. J.*, 1978, *1*, 75. Critical comment.— T. C. B. Stamp (letter), *ibid.*, 511.

Patients with osteomalacia due to vitamin-D deficiency responded within weeks to treatment with ergocalciferol 1.25 mg by mouth twice weekly. Larger doses might be necessary in patients with malabsorption and renal failure.— S. Posen *et al.*, *Drugs*, 1979, *17*, 297.

Evidence that 1,25-dihydroxycholecalciferol is the most important factor for the healing of vitamin-D deficient osteomalacia, and that other hydroxy metabolites are unimportant.— S. E. Papapoulos *et al.*, *Lancet*, 1980, *2*, 612.

Osteoporosis. A discussion on the management of osteoporosis.— *Br. med. J.*, 1975, *4*, 307.

A discussion on the management of postmenopausal osteoporosis.— B. E. C. Nordin, *Drugs*, 1979, *18*, 484. For details of the hormone therapy of postmenopausal osteoporosis see Oestradiol, p.1426 and Mestranol, p.1418.

Alfacalcidol was given by mouth in a daily dose of 2 μg with 1 g of calcium to 7 patients with osteoporosis of old age and 6 improved clinically after about 5 weeks' treatment. There was an improvement in fitness and mobility and increased bone formation and mineralisation. Severe reversible hypercalcaemia occurred in 1 patient.— B. Lund *et al.*, *Lancet*, 1975, *2*, 1168.

Decrease of back pain in 11 of 15 patients with osteoporosis and increased mobility in 7 after treatment with alfacalcidol or calcitriol.— I. Wandless *et al.* (letter), *Br. med. J.*, 1980, *280*, 1320. Correction to dose *ibid.*, *281*, 65.

Further references: O. H. Sorensen *et al.*, *Israel J. med. Scis*, 1977, *13*, 253.

For an unfavourable report of the use of vitamin D 10 000 to 50 000 units daily in the treatment of postmenopausal osteoporosis, and the recommended use of alfacalcidol with hormones, see Calcium Salts, p.621.

Renal Osteodystrophy. In 12 patients with stable non-terminal renal failure who complained of skeletal pain, ergocalciferol 50 000 to 100 000 units daily for periods of 3 to 24 months resulted in symptomatic improvement in 9.— J. P. Ingham *et al.*, *Med. J. Aust.*, 1974, *1*, 873.

Two patients with advanced chronic renal failure and extensive vascular calcification of pelvis and extremities were treated for renal osteodystrophy. Maintenance haemodialysis was performed twice weekly and cholecalciferol 15 mg given 2 or 3 times weekly with aluminium hydroxide (about 4 g daily in 1 patient), treatment being continued for about 7 months. Serum calcium and phosphorous concentrations were carefully controlled. In both patients there was a marked regression of renal osteodystrophy and vascular calcifications of hands and feet almost disappeared.— R. Verberckmoes *et al.*, *Ann. intern. Med.*, 1975, *82*, 529.

Cholecalciferol or ergocalciferol in high doses of 1.5 mg (600 000 units) a week for 6 months was given to 8 patients with severe bone disease undergoing haemodialysis. The renal bone disease improved in 6 patients.— D. Brancaccio *et al.* (letter), *Lancet*, 1977, *1*, 199.

Rheumatoid arthritis. The role of deficiency of vitamin D in spontaneous fractures in patients with rheumatoid arthritis.— P. J. Maddison and P. A. Bacon, *Br. med. J.*, 1974, *4*, 433.

Preparations

Concentrated Vitamin D Solution *(B.P.C. 1973, Ind. P.)*. Conc. Vit. D Soln.; Liquor Vitamini D Concentratus; Liq. Vitamin. D Conc. A solution of vitamin D containing 10 000 units in 1 g. It consists either of a suitable fish-liver oil or blend of such oils or of a solution of a source of vitamin D in a vegetable oil such as arachis oil. Any suitable source of vitamin D may be used, such as ergocalciferol, a fish-liver oil rich in vitamin D, a concentrate prepared from such oils, or any other source of the antirachitic substance found in fish livers. It contains not more than 5000 units of vitamin A per g.

See also Halibut-liver Oil, p.1638.
See also under Preparations of Vitamins A and D.

7885-p

Alfacalcidol. 1α-Hydroxycholecalciferol; 1α-Hydroxy-vitamin D_3; 1α-OHD_3; EB 644. (5*Z*,7*E*)-9,10-Secocholesta-5,7,10(19)-triene-1α,3β-diol.
$C_{27}H_{44}O_2$=400.6.
CAS — 41294-56-8.

A crystalline substance. M.p. 132° to 133°.

Adverse Effects and Treatment. As for Vitamin D (p.1657).

Four of 16 patients on dialysis treated with alfacalcidol 1 to 2 μg daily developed varying degrees of conjunctival injection and dilatation of blood vessels.— R. Ahmad and B. Large (letter), *Br. med. J.*, 1977, *2*, 1027.

Severe peri-articular calcification (tumoral calcinosis) developed in 2 patients on regular dialysis treated with alfacalcidol. Pruritus might be a useful warning sign of calcification.— G. S. Walker *et al.*, *Postgrad. med. J.*, 1977, *53*, 570.

Effects on the kidneys. A study in 12 patients with bone disease after jejuno-ileal bypass for obesity suggested that alfacalcidol might produce small increases in serum-creatinine concentrations in people with normal renal function.— J. E. Compston *et al.* (letter), *Lancet*, 1979, *1*, 386.

Accelerated deterioration in renal function associated with alfacalcidol administration. The need for careful supervision was emphasised.— L. R. Solomon and N. P. Mallick (letter), *Lancet*, 1980, *2*, 261. See also under Calcitriol, p.1660.

Although 2 brothers with vitamin-D-dependent rickets and normal glomerular filtration-rates had received alfacalcidol for 24 months with no complications, administration to 4 children with chronic renal failure and renal osteodystrophy had accelerated the decline in glomerular filtration-rate.— M. H. Winterborn *et al.* (letter), *Lancet*, 1978, *2*, 150. Of 8 patients only 1 had a rapid acceleration of renal failure after starting treatment with alfacalcidol.— T. G. Feest *et al.* (letter), *ibid.*, 427. Of 14 children with bone disease, not on dialysis, 2 with hypophosphataemic rickets had taken alfacalcidol for 15 months with maintenance of normal renal function; 2 patients showed decreased rate of fall in creatinine clearance, 2 increased, and 4 no change; in 4 data were inadequate.— R. J. Postlethwaite and I. B. Houston (letter), *ibid.*, 428. Discussion of the problems of assessing the effects of drugs on renal function in patients with progressive renal failure. In 14 patients treated with alfacalcidol or calcitriol 9 had an unaltered rate of decline of renal function, in 3 it accelerated, and in 2 it slowed.— J. A. Kanis *et al.* (letter), *ibid.*, 316. In 9 patients with chronic renal failure, not on dialysis, creatinine clearance fell by 5.4% in the 6 months before treatment with alfacalcidol and by 21.6% during 6 months' treatment with alfacalcidol.— H. E. Nielsen *et al.* (letter), *ibid.*, 1259.

Precautions. As for Vitamin D (p.1657).

A 43-year-old woman with chronic renal failure who was subsequently discovered to have been regularly taking a magnesium-containing antacid powder developed serious magnesium intoxication on administration of alfacalcidol. There was a special risk of magnesium intoxication in patients with chronic renal failure treated with alfacalcidol.— E. Sörensen *et al.*, *Br. med. J.*, 1976, *2*, 215.

Studies in 15 patients, some on haemodialysis, showed that the long-term administration of alfacalcidol had little effect on magnesium absorption in chronic renal failure. Increases in magnesium concentrations might reflect dietary changes.— J. A. Kanis, *Br. med. J.*, 1977, *1*, 211.

Absorption and Fate. See under Vitamin D (p.1657).

Alfacalcidol is considered to be converted in the liver to 1,25-dihydroxycholecalciferol.

Uses. Alfacalcidol is an analogue of calcitriol which, as 1,25-dihydroxycholecalciferol, is considered to be the active metabolite of vitamin D. It has activity similar to that of calcitriol (p.1660) and is used in the treatment of hypoparathyroidism, pseudohypoparathyroidism, renal osteodystrophy associated with secondary hyperparathyroidism, vitamin-D-dependent rickets, and in malabsorption rickets.

The usual initial dose is 1 μg daily (0.05 μg per kg body-weight for children under 20 kg) adjusted according to the biochemical response; most patients respond to 1 to 3 μg daily. Maintenance doses may be 0.25 to 1 μg daily.

See also Vitamin D (p.1658).

Discussions of the uses of alfacalcidol.— *Clin. Endocr.*, 1977, *7*, *Suppl.* (Dec.);; *Lancet*, 1978, *1*, 973; *Br. med. J.*, 1978, *1*, 1571; *Drug & Ther. Bull.*, 1979, *17*, 25.

An elderly woman with long-standing malabsorption of calcium and severe hypocalcaemia unresponsive to cholecalciferol responded promptly to very-high-dose treatment with alfacalcidol 5 μg daily increased to 12 μg daily; the maintenance dose was 9 μg daily.— E. Hylander and S. Madsen, *Acta med. scand.*, 1979, *205*, 603.

Renal osteodystrophy. Ten patients with uraemia and undergoing regular haemodialysis were treated with alfacalcidol 0.5 to 2 μg daily for a minimum of 5 months. Response was good among 5 patients with secondary hyperparathyroidism, osteitis fibrosa and raised serum alkaline phosphatase concentration. Bone mineralisation improved in the 4 of these patients with osteomalacia; their serum phosphatase returned to normal and hypercalcaemia was not troublesome. Intestinal calcium absorption improved in all 10 patients treated. The 5 patients who did not improve did not have osteitis or increased serum alkaline phosphate concentration; they all had moderately severe osteomalacia with myopathy. Hypercalcaemia developed during treatment in this group, causing troublesome irritation and requiring treatment to be interrupted; and hypophosphataemia was also noted in these 5 patients.— A. M. Pierides *et al.*, *Lancet*, 1976, *1*, 1092.

The use of alfacalcidol 40 to 80 ng per kg body-weight daily, in 10 children with renal osteodystrophy.— R. J. Postlethwaite and I. B. Houston, *Archs Dis. Childh.*, 1977, *52*, 420.

In 14 patients with renal osteodystrophy undergoing dialysis treated with alfacalcidol 1 μg daily initially adjusted to a range of 1 μg a week to 3 μg daily for 12 to 18 months, mean plasma-calcium concentrations rose from 94 to 107 μg per ml at 1 year and inorganic phosphate from 40 to 53 μg per ml; plasma alkaline phosphatase, initially increased in 12 patients, fell in 11 (often after a transient rise) and became normal in 7; the mean serum concentration of parathyroid hormone fell from 4.74 to 1.74 ng per ml at 1 year. Episodes of severe hypercalcaemia occurred; careful monitoring was therefore essential.— A. M. Brownjohn *et al.*, *Br. med. J.*, 1977, *2*, 721.

Experience with 27 patients on dialysis given alfacalcidol 1 or 2 μg daily and 9 given calcitriol 1 or 1.5 μg daily confirmed that alfacalcidol and calcitriol enhanced calcium absorption in such patients.— A. M. Pierides *et al.*, *Nephron*, 1978, *20*, 203.

The essential point in the pathogenesis and therapy of the complex bone disease of uraemic patients was the hepatic 25-hydroxylation of vitamin D rather than the renal 1α-hydroxylation.— D. Brancaccio *et al.* (letter), *Lancet*, 1978, *1*, 1314. A study in 8 patients with chronic renal failure and 7 healthy subjects indicated that the hepatic metabolism of vitamin D in chronic renal failure is probably normal.— K. Farrington *et al.* (letter), *ibid.*, 1979, *1*, 321.

In 6 patients with chronic renal failure alfacalcidol 1 μg daily increased calcium absorption in the proximal small intestine and raised serum concentrations and urinary excretion of calcium. 24*R*,25-Dihydroxycholecalciferol had no consistent effect in 6 further patients.— J. Szymendera and K. Galus, *Br. med. J.*, 1978, *2*, 1465. Comment.— J. A. Kanis *et al.* (letter), *ibid.*, 1979, *1*, 822. A reply.— J. Szymendera (letter), *ibid.*

Further references: G. R. D. Catto *et al.*, *Br. med. J.*, 1975, *1*, 12; J. C. M. Chan *et al.*, *J. Am. med. Ass.*, 1975, *234*, 47; L. Tougaard *et al.*, *Lancet*, 1976, *1*, 1044; G. R. D. Catto and M. Macleod, *Am. J. Med.*, 1976, *61*, 64; S. Castells *et al.*, *Curr. ther. Res.*, 1976, *19*, 410; M. W. J. Davie *et al.*, *Ann. intern. Med.*, 1976, *84*, 281; J. C. M. Chan and H. F. DeLuca, *J. Am. med. Ass.*, 1977, *238*, 2053; R. B. Naik *et al.*, *Proc. Eur. Dialysis Transplant Ass.*, 1977, *14*, 425; B. Krolner *et al.*, *Ugeskr. Laeg.*, 1977, *139*, 880; J. C. M. Chan *et al.*, *J. Pediat.*, 1977, *90*, 820; J. A. Kanis *et al.*, *Archs Dis. Childh.*, 1977, *52*, 473; P. Bordier *et al.*, *Am. J. Med.*, 1978, *64*, 101.

For accelerated deterioration in renal function associated with alfacalcidol, see under Adverse Effects, above.

Proprietary Preparations

One-Alpha *(Leo, UK)*. Alfacalcidol, available as **Capsules** of 0.25 and 1 μg and as **Drops** containing 5 μg per ml (250 ng per drop). (Also available as One-Alpha in *Canad., Eire*).

Other Proprietary Names

Delakmin, EinsAlpha *(both Ger.)*; Etalpha *(Denm., Neth., Norw., Swed.)*; Un-alfa *(Fr.)*.

7886-s

Calcifediol.

U-32070E; 25-Hydroxycholecalciferol; 25-Hydroxyvitamin D_3; 25-$(OH)D_3$. (5*Z*,7*E*)-9,10-Secocholesta-5,7,10(19)-triene-3β,25-diol monohydrate.

$C_{27}H_{44}O_2,H_2O = 418.7$.

CAS — 19356-17-3 (anhydrous); 63283-36-3 (monohydrate).

A white powder. M.p. about 105°.

Practically **insoluble** in water; soluble in organic solvents.

Adverse Effects and Treatment. As for Vitamin D (p.1657).

Precautions. As for Vitamin D (p.1657).

An idiosyncratic reaction with headache, nausea, vomiting, diarrhoea, and fever occurred in a woman given calcifediol. The reaction did not occur when the patient was given alfacalcidol.— C. G. Gegick *et al.* (letter), *Ann. intern. Med.*, 1974, *80*, 416.

Absorption and Fate. See under Vitamin D (p.1657).

Calcifediol was given by mouth in a dose of 10 μg per kg body-weight to 12 healthy subjects and produced a mean maximum rise in plasma concentration of 109 ng per ml. Absorption was also studied in 10 patients with disturbed calcium metabolism and/or gastro-intestinal function and demonstrated their abnormalities in vitamin-D absorption. Calcifediol could be used as a tolerance test for such patients.— T. C. B. Stamp, *Lancet*, 1974, *2*, 121.

Uses. Calcifediol is 25-hydroxycholecalciferol which is a metabolite of ergocalciferol and cholecalciferol and is used similarly.

Typical doses are 50 to 125 μg daily.

See also under vitamin D (p.1658).

A patient with fractures which failed to heal after treatment with vitamin D and phosphates responded to treatment with calcifediol.— J. Manis and A. Norman, *Br. med. J.*, 1975, *2*, 478.

Doses of ergocalciferol and cholecalciferol needed to be 10 times as high as those of calcifediol to produce similar values for hydroxyvitamin-D-plasma concentrations in a study of over 200 subjects.— T. C. B. Stamp *et al.*, *Lancet*, 1977, *1*, 1341.

Cirrhosis. A study in 8 female patients indicated that the 25-hydroxy derivative given by mouth might be the preferred form of vitamin-D therapy in primary biliary cirrhosis.— J. B. Wagonfeld *et al.*, *Lancet*, 1976, *2*, 391.

Rickets. An account of the long-term therapy of vitamin D-resistant rickets with calcifediol in 2 children.— J. B. Puschett *et al.*, *Clin. Pharmac. Ther.*, 1975, *17*, 202.

Further references: J. B. Puschett *et al.*, *Lancet*, 1974, *2*, 920; A. Frederich *et al.*, *Thérapie*, 1974, *29*, 681; F. Daum *et al.*, *J. Pediat.*, 1976, *88*, 1041.

Hypoparathyroidism. Trial of calcifediol in vitamin D-resistant hypoparathyroidism.— C. Y. C. Pak *et al.*, *Archs intern. Med.*, 1970, *126*, 239.

Osteomalacia. The treatment of vitamin-D-resistant osteomalacia (of hepatic origin) with calcifediol in 2 patients.— J. C. Renier *et al.*, *Revue Rhum. Mal. osteo-artic.*, 1978, *45*, 7.

Renal osteodystrophy. In 5 patients undergoing long-term haemodialysis, treatment with calcifediol 100 or 40 μg daily resulted in increased absorption of calcium, a decrease in circulating immunoreactive parathyroid hormone and alkaline phosphatase, and a striking improvement in bone lesions.— S. L. Teitelbaum *et al.*, *J. Am. med. Ass.*, 1976, *235*, 164.

One haemodialysis patient with renal bone disease who did not respond to high doses of cholecalciferol or ergocalciferol was considered to have an impaired ability for hepatic 25-hydroxylation. Treatment with calcifediol produced a beneficial response. Calcifediol was recommended for the treatment of uraemic osteodystrophy in patients with this impairment.— D. Brancaccio *et al.* (letter), *Lancet*, 1977, *1*, 199.

Further references: R. Dumas *et al.*, *Archs Dis. Childh.*, 1979, *54*, 322.

Proprietary Names

Calderol *(Upjohn, USA)*; Dédrogyl *(Roussel, Fr.)*; Hidroferol *(Juventus, Spain)*.

7887-w

Calcitriol.

1,25-Dihydroxycholecalciferol; 1α,25-Dihydroxycholecalciferol; 1α,25-Dihydroxyvitamin D_3; 1α,25$(OH_2)D_3$; Ro 21-5535. (5*Z*,7*E*)-9,10-Secocholesta-5,7,10(19)-triene-1α,3β,25-triol.

$C_{27}H_{44}O_3 = 416.6$.

CAS — 32222-06-3.

A colourless crystalline substance. Relatively **insoluble** in water; soluble in organic solvents.

Adverse Effects, Treatment, and Precautions. As for Vitamin D (p.1657).

In a controlled study, deterioration in renal function was noted after 6 months in all of 8 patients who received calcitriol to correct abnormal mineral metabolism, and in 7 of 9 who received cholecalciferol, although it had remained stable for the previous 6 months. Decreased formation of 1,25-dihydroxycholecalciferol might protect renal function in chronic renal failure and treatment should be restricted to patients with severe symptomatic renal osteodystrophy.— C. Christiansen *et al.*, *Lancet*, 1978, *2*, 700. See also B. Lund *et al.* (letter), *ibid.*, 731. Criticism.— K. Farrington *et al.* (letter), *ibid.*, 941. A reply.— C. Christiansen *et al.* (letter), *ibid.*, 1979, *1*, 50.

Further references: S. G. Massry and D. A. Goldstein, *J. Am. med. Ass.*, 1979, *242*, 1875.

See also under Alfacalcidol, p.1659.

Uses. Calcitriol is 1α,25-dihydroxycholecalciferol, which is considered to be the most active form of vitamin D.

It exerts a rapid effect, and hypercalcaemia, if it occurs, can be rapidly reversed.

Because it is not dependent on 1α-hydroxylation in the kidney it is effective in conditions in which this metabolic process is impaired, including renal disease, and in anephric patients.

It has been used in the treatment of neonatal hypocalcaemia, in hypoparathyroidism, in pseudohypoparathyroidism, in renal osteodystrophy associated with secondary hyperparathyroidism, and in vitamin-D-dependent rickets.

Doses have generally been in the range of 0.5 to

2 μg daily.

Calcitriol is also used in the treatment of hypocalcaemia in patients undergoing chronic dialysis; an adequate intake of calcium is essential. The initial dose is 250 ng daily which may be increased at 2- to 4-week intervals by 250 ng daily until a satisfactory biochemical and clinical response is obtained; most patients are controlled on a daily dose of 0.5 to 1 μg daily.

See also under Vitamin D (p.1658).

A reproducible diuretic response to calcitriol in 1 patient.— M. Andrae *et al.* (letter), *Lancet*, 1977, *2*, 1080.

Preliminary studies in 6 healthy subjects appear to indicate that 1α,25-dihydroxyprevitamin D_3, formed in the skin after topical application of 1α,25-dihydroxy-7-dehydrocholesterol and ultraviolet irradiation, thermally isomerises to 1α,25-dihydroxyvitamin D_3. Although the amount of 1α,25-dihydroxyvitamin D_3 reaching the target tissues is much smaller for topical application than for oral therapy the biological response appears to be markedly prolonged. Similarly, cutaneous absorption of 1α,25-dihydroxyvitamin D_3 has been found to provide sustained and relatively constant blood concentrations when compared with those achieved after oral doses.— M. F. Holick *et al.*, *New Engl. J. Med.*, 1980, *303*, 349.

Cirrhosis. Improvement in both calcium and phosphate absorption was found in 10 patients with primary biliary cirrhosis receiving calcitriol 500 ng daily.— K. Farrington *et al.*, *Gut*, 1979, *20*, 616.

Deficiency states. Rickets. Results in 11 children indicating that a regimen of calcitriol and phosphate is beneficial in the treatment of vitamin D-resistant rickets. Long-term administration of phosphate, as Joulie's solution, alone or in association with ergocalciferol, induced mineralisation of the epiphyseal plate but not of the endosteal bone surface, whereas phosphate in association with calcitriol 0.25 to 1 μg daily greatly improved the mineralisation of trabecular bone. Further studies are needed to determine whether, as patients reach the end of their growth period, it will be possible to maintain the results achieved with small doses of calcitriol without the burden of aggressive phosphate supplementation.— F. H. Glorieux *et al.*, *New Engl. J. Med.*, 1980, *303*, 1023.

Renal osteodystrophy. Discussions of the use of calcitriol and alfacalcidol in renal osteodystrophy.— M. Peacock, *Practitioner*, 1978, *220*, 913; *Lancet*, 1979, *2*, 1339; S. L. Teitelbaum, *Ann. intern. Med.*, 1981, *94*, 404.

In a double-blind study involving 31 patients who were undergoing regular haemodialysis, calcitriol 0.5 to 1.5 μg daily was effective in raising mean serum-calcium concentrations and reducing circulating parathyroid-hormone concentrations whereas cholecalciferol 10 to 30 μg daily was not. Calcitriol was associated with a histologic improvement of bone disease. Five of the 15 patients who received calcitriol developed hypercalcaemia but this was rapidly reversible on reduction of dosage. Calcitriol was considered of value in renal osteodystrophy.— T. Berl *et al.*, *Ann. intern. Med.*, 1978, *88*, 774.

Five patients with renal failure (2 of whom were undergoing haemodialysis) and renal osteodystrophy received calcitriol 500 ng and calcium carbonate 4 g daily for 4 to 16 months. The intestinal absorption of calcium was increased with increases in plasma concentrations, and plasma values for alkaline phosphatase and hydroxyproline fell. Serum concentrations of parathyroid hormone were also reduced and bone mineralisation improved.— K. Y. Ahmed *et al.*, *Lancet*, 1978, *1*, 629.

Administration of calcitriol for periods of 4 to 26 months promoted growth in 6 children aged 3 months to 14 years with renal osteodystrophy.— R. W. Chesney *et al.*, *New Engl. J. Med.*, 1978, *298*, 238. Comment.— B. S. Roof and C. F. Piel (letter), *ibid.*, 1424. A reply.— R. W. Chesney *et al.* (letter), *ibid.*, 1425.

Further references: A. S. Brickman *et al.*, *Archs intern. Med.*, 1974, *134*, 883; A. S. Brickman *et al.*, *Am. J. Med.*, 1974, *57*, 28; R. G. Henderson *et al.*, *Lancet*, 1974, *1*, 379; A. M. Pierides *et al.*, *Archs Dis. Childh.*, 1977, *52*, 464; P. Bordier *et al.*, *Am. J. Med.*, 1978, *64*, 101; D. R. Maxwell *et al.*, *Clin. Pharmac. Ther.*, 1978, *23*, 515; J. C. Prior *et al.*, *Am. J. Med.*, 1979, *67*, 583.

For accelerated deterioration in renal function associated with calcitriol, see under Adverse Effects, above.

Proprietary Preparations

Rocaltrol *(Roche, UK)*. Calcitriol, available as capsules of 250 and 500 ng. (Also available as Rocaltrol in *Aust., Austral., Belg., Canad., Ger., Switz., USA*).

7888-e

Cholecalciferol *(B.P., B.P. Vet., U.S.P.).*

Colecalciferol; Activated 7-Dehydrocholesterol; Vitamin D_3. (5*Z*,7*E*)-9,10-Secocholesta-5,7,10(19)-trien-3β-ol.

$C_{27}H_{44}O = 384.6$.

CAS — 67-97-0.

Pharmacopoeias. In *Arg., Aust., Br., Chin., Cz., Hung., Jap., Pol., Roum., Swiss,* and *U.S.*

White or almost white, odourless or almost odourless crystals which are affected by air and light. M.p. about 84°.

Practically **insoluble** in water; freely soluble in alcohol, acetone, chloroform, and ether; soluble in fixed oils. A solution in alcohol is dextrorotatory. Solutions in volatile solvents are unstable and should be used immediately. **Store** in a cool place in hermetically sealed containers in which the air has been replaced by an inert gas. The contents of an opened container should be used immediately. Protect from light.

Cholecalciferol contains 40 000 units of antirachitic activity (vitamin D) in 1 mg.

In England and Wales, the Labelling of Food Regulations 1970 (SI 1970: No. 400) as amended (SI 1972: No. 1510) require that in any food labelled as containing vitamins D, D_2, or D_3 the vitamin must be calculated as micrograms of cholecalciferol.

Isomerisation. For a report of isomerisation of cholecalciferol and its effect on vitamin-D activity, see Ergocalciferol, p.1662.

Adverse Effects and Treatment. As for Vitamin D (p.1657).

Precautions. As for Vitamin D (p.1657).

For a report of decreased renal function in patients taking cholecalciferol, see Calcitriol, p.1660.

Cirrhosis. Malabsorption of cholecalciferol given by mouth occurred in 4 of 6 patients with primary biliary cirrhosis; there was also increased urinary excretion.— E. L. Krawitt *et al.*, *Lancet*, 1977, *2*, 1246.

Vitamin D metabolism was studied, in winter, in 10 patients with cirrhosis (8 alcoholic, 2 cryptogenic) and 12 controls. Plasma concentration of 25-hydroxycholecalciferol was not significantly lower in the cirrhotics, and 3 of 4 patients re-investigated in late summer had a considerable rise in concentration compared with the winter value. The half-life of tritium-labelled cholecalciferol given intravenously was short in the cirrhotics and did not correlate with plasma concentration of 25-hydroxycholecalciferol; 4 hours after injection there was also a reduction in the appearance of tritium-labelled 25-hydroxycholecalciferol when compared with the controls. An increased rate of metabolism of cholecalciferol but reduced production of the hydroxylated metabolite appeared to contribute to vitamin-D deficiency in liver disease.— R. T. Jung *et al.*, *Gut*, 1978, *19*, 290.

Absorption and Fate. See under Vitamin D (p.1657).

After an intravenous injection of cholecalciferol, serum concentrations of cholecalciferol and its metabolites showed the same biphasic exponential decay. In the initial phase the half-life in serum was usually less than 2 days and in the following phase the half-life was in excess of 18 days.— E. B. Mawer *et al.* (letter), *Nature*, 1969, *222*, 482.

Uses. Cholecalciferol is formed in the skin from 7-dehydrocholesterol during exposure to sunlight. It is also present in fish-liver oils and in some articles of diet. Cholecalciferol may be used for the same purposes as ergocalciferol (p.1662).

See also Vitamin D (p.1658).

Preparations

Cholecalciferol Capsules *(Univ. Coll. Hosp.)*. Contain cholecalciferol 0.25 or 1 mg in arachis oil of low peroxide value containing 0.1% of hydroquinone.

Cholecalciferol Injection. Crystalline cholecalciferol 100 mg, dehydrated alcohol 10 ml, propylene glycol to 100 ml. The solution was filtered into 1-ml ampoules, the air in which was replaced by nitrogen, and sterilised by autoclaving. The solution was refrigerated [to reverse isomerisation] before use. *Dose.* As a test of vitamin-D deficiency, 1 ml intravenously. It was mixed with venous blood immediately prior to injection.— H. Whittle, *et al.*, *Lancet*, 1969, *1*, 747.

Proprietary Names

Actifral D3 *(Duphar, Spain)*; Aqua-Sterogyl D3 *(Roussel, Belg.)*; D-cure *(SMB, Belg.)*; Detin D3 *(Efeyn, Spain)*; D-Mulsin *(Mucos, Ger.)*; D_3-Vicotrat forte *(Heyl, Ger.)*; Iper D_3 *(Zambon, Ital.)*; Neo-Dohyfral D_3 *(Philips-Duphar, Belg.; Duphar, Neth.)*; Tridelta *(Ceccarelli, Ital.)*; Vi-De-3 *(Sandoz, S.Afr.; Wander, Switz.)*; Vitaendil D-3 *(Boizot, Spain)*.

7889-l

Cholecalciferol-Cholesterin.

Colecalciferol-Cholesterin; Cholecalciferol-Cholesterol; Vitamin-D_3-Cholesterol. An equimolecular compound of cholecalciferol and cholesterol.

$C_{27}H_{44}O,C_{27}H_{46}O = 771.3$.

Pharmacopoeias. In *Ger.*

Colourless crystals or a white crystalline powder. Practically **insoluble** in water; sparingly soluble in alcohol and fixed oils; freely soluble in acetone, chloroform, ether, and methyl alcohol. **Store** as for Ergocalciferol, p.1662.

Uses. Cholecalciferol-cholesterin may be used similarly to cholecalciferol. It contains about 20 000 units of antirachitic activity (vitamin D) in 1 mg.

Proprietary Names

D-Tracetten *(Albert-Roussel, Ger.)*; Vigorsan *(Albert-Roussel, Ger.)*; D_3-Vicotrat *(Heyl, Ger.)*; Vigantol *(E. Merck, Ger.)*; Vigantoletten *(E. Merck, Ger.)*.

7890-v

Cod-liver Oil *(B.P., B.P. Vet.).*

Oleum Jecoris Aselli; Oleum Morrhuae; Ol. Morrh.; Cod Liver Oil *(U.S.P.)*; Huile de Foie de Morue; Lebertran; Aceite de Hígado de Bacalao; Óleo de Bacalhau; Olio di Fegato di Merluzzo.

CAS — 8001-69-2.

Pharmacopoeias. In *Arg., Aust., Belg., Br., Cz., Hung., Int., Jap., Mex., Nord., Pol., Port., Roum., Rus., Span., Swiss, Turk.,* and *U.S.*

Some pharmacopoeias permit oil from other species of the family Gadidae and several specify higher minima than the *B.P.* for vitamin A and vitamin D.

The oil obtained from the fresh liver of the cod, *Gadus callarias* (=*G. morhua*) and other species of *Gadus* (Gadidae), refined, and clarified by filtration at about 0°. The *B.P.* specifies not less than 600 units of vitamin A activity per g and not less than 85 units of antirachitic activity (vitamin D) per g and may contain up to 100 ppm of dodecyl gallate, octyl gallate, or propyl gallate, or any mixture of these as an antoxidant. The *U.S.P.* specifies not less than 850 units of vitamin A and not less than 85 units of vitamin D per g, and permits up to 1% of a suitable flavour or flavours.

A pale yellow oil with a slightly fishy but not rancid odour and taste. Wt per ml 0.917 to 0.924 g.

Practically **insoluble** in alcohol; miscible with chloroform, ether, carbon disulphide, ethyl acetate, and light petroleum. **Store** in a cool place in well-filled airtight containers. Protect from light.

On exposure to sunlight the vitamin A is rapidly destroyed. On exposure to air the oil absorbs oxygen and becomes thicker but does not dry to a hard varnish. Inferior or old oils are liable to be dark in colour, acrid or bitter, unduly acid, and somewhat rancid. But if properly stored, cod-liver oil retains its potency and characters for many years.

Uses. Cod-liver oil is a source of vitamins A and D; because of its high content of vitamin D it is used as a supplement to the diet of infants for the prevention of rickets. Doses of up to 10 ml daily are employed. It also contains several unsaturated fatty acids which are essential food factors and do not occur in vitamin A and D concentrates.

The antirachitic activity of cod-liver oil is due principally to the presence of vitamin D_3 (cholecalciferol).

Cod-liver oil dressings or ointment have been advocated to accelerate healing in burns, ulcers, and superficial wounds, but controlled observations have failed to substantiate claims of their value.

A suggestion that cod-liver oil may be a convenient source of eicosapentaenoic acid with possible protective value against thrombosis.— S. A. Reed (letter), *Lancet*, 1979, *2*, 739.

See also under Eicosapentaenoic Acid, p.1706.

Preparations

Cod-liver Oil Emulsion *(B.P.C. 1959)*. Emuls. Ol. Morrh. Cod-liver oil 50 ml, acacia 12.5 g, tragacanth 700 mg, volatile bitter almond oil 0.1 ml, saccharin sodium 10 mg, chloroform 0.2 ml, water to 100 ml. *Dose.* 8 to 30 ml daily.

Proprietary Preparations

M & M Tulle *(Malam, UK: Vestric, UK)*. A sterilised gauze dressing impregnated with cod-liver oil 23%, purified honey 23%, and hexachlorophane 0.5%. For bedsores, varicose ulcers, and burns.

Morhulin *(Priory Laboratories, UK)*. Ointment containing cod-liver oil 11.4%, a diluted sodium hypochlorite solution 1%, and zinc oxide 38% in a wool fat and soft paraffin basis. For wounds, varicose ulcers, and bedsores.

Morsep *(Priory Laboratories, UK)*. A cream containing cetrimide 0.5%, a diluted sodium hypochlorite solution 1%, vitamin A 70 units per g, and ergocalciferol 10 units per g in a non-greasy basis. For napkin rash.

Ung. Morrhuae Co *(Philip Harris, UK)*. An ointment containing cod-liver oil 12.5% and zinc oxide 12.5% in a perfumed wool fat basis. For varicose ulcers and napkin rash.

Other Proprietary Names

Dermovitamina *(Ital.)*; Gelosellan *(Ger.)*; Jecovitol *(Neth.)*; Swansolan-Lebertransalbe *(Ger.)*; Ung-Morrhuol-Lohr *(Austral.)*; Unguentolan *(Ger.)*.

7891-g

Dihydrotachysterol *(B.P., U.S.P.)*.

Dichysterol. (5*E*,7*E*,22*E*)-10α-9,10-Secoergosta-5,7,22-trien-3β-ol.

$C_{28}H_{46}O = 398.7$.

CAS — 67-96-9.

Pharmacopoeias. In *Br.*, *Jug.*, and *U.S.*

Odourless colourless crystals or white crystalline powder. M.p. 123.5° to 129°. May also occur in a form melting at about 113°. Practically **insoluble** in water; soluble 1 in 20 of alcohol, 1 in 0.7 of chloroform, 1 in 3 of ether, and 1 in 50 of arachis oil. **Store** in a cool place in sealed glass containers in which the air has been replaced by nitrogen or other inert gas. Protect from light.

Preparation of capsules. Flexible gelatin capsules were prepared with a solution of dihydrotachysterol in a low peroxide arachis oil containing 0.1% of hydroquinone as an antioxidant. The requisite dose of dihydrotachysterol (0.1, 0.25, or 1 mg) was dissolved in 165 mg of solvent with the aid of *gentle* heat. The capsules showed no loss of activity after storage for 2 years.— C. E. Dent and M. Friedman, *Lancet*, 1964, *2*, 164.

Adverse Effects and Treatment. As for Vitamin D (p.1657).

Precautions. As for Vitamin D (p.1657).

For a suggestion that dihydrotachysterol might accelerate bone loss in patients with renal osteodystrophy on dialysis, see *J. Am. med. Ass.*, 1977, *237*, 752.

Interactions. Three patients receiving dihydrotachysterol and calcium for postoperative hypoparathyroidism, following thyroidectomy, developed hypercalcaemia when their concomitant thyroxine therapy was discontinued before a radio-iodine scan. The dose of dihydrotachysterol should be reduced and serum-calcium concentrations should be monitored when thyroid treatment is interrupted, since elimination of dihydrotachysterol may be delayed in hypothyroidism.— B. -A. Lamberg and M. J. Tikkanen, *Br. med. J.*, 1981, *283*, 461.

Absorption and Fate. Dihydrotachysterol is 25-hydroxylated in the liver.

Uses. Dihydrotachysterol is closely related chemically to calcitriol (see p.1660). While it requires 25-hydroxylation, it does not require 1α-hydroxylation. It acts more rapidly and has a shorter duration of action than ergocalciferol so dosage is more readily controlled, but the effect may persist for up to a month.

Dihydrotachysterol is used in the treatment of the hypocalcaemia of hypoparathyroidism, in the treatment of vitamin-D-resistant rickets, in osteomalacia, and in renal osteodystrophy.

Dosage must be controlled by regular blood-calcium estimations. Typical doses for the treatment of acute hypocalcaemic tetany are 0.75 to 2.5 mg daily initially for about 3 days. Less acute conditions may respond to 0.25 to 0.5 mg daily. Maintenance doses may vary from 0.25 mg a week to 1 mg daily.

See also Vitamin D (p.1658).

Renal osteodystrophy. Beneficial responses to dihydrotachysterol in 4 patients on dialysis with persistent hypophosphataemia and osteomalacia and who had not taken phosphate-binders for at least 2 years.— K. Y. Ahmed *et al.*, *Lancet*, 1976, *2*, 439. See also *J. Am. med. Ass.*, 1970, *212*, 1797.

Bone diseases which developed in 9 of 24 patients on long-term haemodialysis were treated in 8 with dihydrotachysterol 250 to 375 μg daily; for 4 patients higher doses were required and the dose was increased progressively at 2-monthly intervals up to 1 mg daily. The incidence of corneal calcification did not increase, and there were no new fractures after treatment started. In some patients the dose of dihydrotachysterol could be reduced when the bones were healed.— P. E. Cordy, *Can. med. Ass. J.*, 1977, *117*, 766.

Preparations

Dihydrotachysterol Capsules *(Univ. Coll. Hosp.)*. Contain dihydrotachysterol 0.25 or 1 mg in arachis oil of low peroxide value containing 0.1% of hydroquinone.

Dihydrotachysterol Tablets *(U.S.P.)*. Tablets containing dihydrotachysterol. Protect from light.

Proprietary Preparations

AT 10 *(Sterling Research, UK)*. Dihydrotachysterol, available as an oily solution containing 250 μg in each ml (dilution not recommended). (Also available as AT 10 in *Austral., Belg., Ger., Ital., Neth., S.Afr., Switz.*).

Tachyrol *(Duphar, UK)*. Dihydrotachysterol, available as scored tablets of 200 μg.

Other Proprietary Names

Atecen *(Swed.)*; Calcamine *(Fr.)*; Dihydral *(see also under Diphenhydramine Hydrochloride) (Belg., Iraq, Neth., Spain)*; Dygratyl *(Denm., Swed.)*; Hytakerol *(Canad., USA)*.

7892-q

Ergocalciferol *(B.P., Eur. P., U.S.P.)*.

Ergocalciferolum; Calciferol *(B.P. Vet.)*; Calcif.; Vitamin D_2; Irradiated Ergosterol; Viosterol. (5*Z*,7*E*,22*E*)-9,10-Secoergosta-5,7,10(19),22-tetraen-3β-ol.

$C_{28}H_{44}O = 396.7$.

CAS — 50-14-6.

Pharmacopoeias. In *Arg., Aust., Belg., Br., Braz., Chin., Cz., Eur., Fr., Ger., Hung., Ind., Int., It., Jap., Jug., Neth., Nord., Port., Roum., Swiss., Turk.*, and *U.S.*

An antirachitic substance obtained from ergosterol by ultraviolet irradiation. Odourless or almost odourless, tasteless, colourless or slightly yellow crystals or white or slightly yellow crystalline powder. It contains 40 000 units of antirachitic activity (vitamin D) in 1 mg. M.p. 113° to 119°. Practically **insoluble** in water; soluble 1 in 2 of alcohol, 1 in 10 of acetone, 1 in 0.7 of chloroform, 1 in 2 of ether, and 1 in 50 to 100 of fixed oils. A solution in alcohol is dextrorotatory. Solutions are **sterilised** by filtration. **Store** in a cool place in hermetically sealed containers in which the air has been replaced by an inert gas. Protect from light.

In England and Wales, the Labelling of Food Regulations 1970 (SI 1970: No. 400) as amended (SI 1972: No. 1510) require that in any food labelled as containing vitamins D, D_2, or D_3 the vitamins must be calculated as micrograms of cholecalciferol.

Isomerisation. Ergocalciferol and cholecalciferol were reversibly isomerised to precalciferols and precholecalciferols. The equilibrium fractions of precalciferol and ergocalciferol depended on the storage temperature. Isomerisation proceeded until equilibrium was reached. The relative activity of precalciferol had been reported as 40, 56, or 34% of ergocalciferol, and that of precholecalciferol as 35%. The potential vitamin-D content was the important quantity for standardisation purposes: standardisation on ergocalciferol alone could lead to overdosage by 40%. Assay samples and standard solutions should be equilibrated under the same conditions before assay.— J. A. K. Buisman *et al.*, *J. pharm. Sci.*, 1968, *57*, 1326.

Adverse Effects, Treatment, and Precautions. As for Vitamin D (p.1657).

Absorption and Fate. See under Vitamin D (p.1657).

Uses. Ergocalciferol takes slightly longer to act than dihydrotachysterol and its effects last rather longer. It has a cumulative action and dosage must be carefully controlled. The effects of changes in dosage may not be apparent for about 6 weeks.

In the treatment of rickets the minimum daily dose is 25 μg (1000 units), but usually doses of 75 to 100 μg (3000 to 4000 units) are prescribed for rapid healing; in vitamin-D-dependent rickets doses of 0.25 to 1.25 mg (10 000 to 50 000 units) or more daily may be required; very high doses were formerly given to resistant patients.

In hypoparathyroidism doses of 1.25 to 2.5 mg (50 000 to 100 000 units) daily may be required.

In vitamin-D-dependent rickets, hypoparathyroidism, and renal osteodystrophy, calcitriol (see p.1660) or alfacalcidol (see p.1660) may be preferable.

In the treatment of hypocalcaemic tetany daily doses of 50 000 to 400 000 units (1.25 to 10 mg) have been given.

Ergocalciferol is also used for the prevention of anticonvulsant-induced osteomalacia.

Ergocalciferol has been promoted for use in the treatment of chilblains; there appears to be no rationale for such use.

See also Vitamin D (p.1658).

Rodenticide. Ergocalciferol as a rodenticide.— J. H. Greaves *et al.*, *J. Hyg., Camb.*, 1974, *73*, 341, per *Abstr. Hyg.*, 1975, *50*, 26; F. P. Rowe *et al.*, *J. Hyg., Camb.*, 1974, *73*, 353, per *Abstr. Hyg.*, 1975, *50*, 26; B. D. Rennison, *J. Hyg., Camb.*, 1974, *73*, 361, per *Abstr. Hyg.*, 1975, *50*, 26; *Br. med. J.*, 1975, *2*, 105.

Preparations

Calciferol Capsules *(Univ. Coll. Hosp.)*. Contain ergocalciferol 0.25 or 1 mg in arachis oil of low peroxide value containing 0.1% of hydroquinone.

Calciferol Injection *(B.P.)*. Inj. Calciferol.; Vitamin D_2 Injection. A sterile solution of ergocalciferol or cholecalciferol in ethyl oleate, containing 7.5 mg (300 000 units) in each ml. Sterilised by filtration. Store at a temperature not exceeding 25° in ampoules in which the air has been replaced by nitrogen or other suitable gas. Protect from light. For intramuscular use only.

Calciferol Solution *(B.P.)*. Calcif. Soln.; Liquor Calciferoli; Vitamin D_2 Solution. A solution of ergocalciferol or cholecalciferol in a suitable vegetable oil, such as arachis oil, containing 63.5 to 90 μg (about 3000 units) in 1 ml. It is a pale yellow oily liquid with a slight but not rancid odour. Store at a temperature not exceeding 25° in well-filled containers. Protect from light.

Many pharmacopoeias include solutions of ergocalciferol in vegetable oils, the strengths varying from 3000 to 650 000 units per g.

Ergocalciferol Capsules *(U.S.P.)*. Calciferol Capsules. Usually an edible vegetable oil solution of ergocalciferol, encapsulated with gelatin. Store in airtight containers. Protect from light.

Ergocalciferol Oral Solution *(U.S.P.)*. Ergocalciferol Solution. A solution of ergocalciferol in an edible vegetable oil, in polysorbate 80, or in propylene glycol. Store in airtight containers. Protect from light.

Ergocalciferol Tablets *(U.S.P.)*. Tablets containing ergocalciferol. Store in airtight containers. Protect from light.

High-Strength Calciferol Tablets *(B.P.)*. Sugar-coated tablets containing ergocalciferol or cholecalciferol 225 to 312.5 μg (about 10 000 units). Store at a temperature not exceeding 25°.

NOTE. These tablets are approximately one-fifth the strength of Strong Calciferol Tablets *B.P. 1973*.

When calciferol tablets are prescribed or demanded, high-strength calciferol tablets should *not* be dispensed or supplied unless it is confirmed that the high-strength tablets are intended. For the treatment of rickets, see Calcium with Vitamin D Tablets, p.624.

Proprietary Preparations Containing Vitamin D

Sterogyl-15 *(Roussel, UK)*. Ergocalciferol, available as alcoholic solution in ampoules each containing 600 000 units in 1.5 ml for oral use. (Also available as Sterogyl-15 in *Austral., Belg., Fr., S.Afr., Spain, Switz.*).

For proprietary preparations containing calcium and vitamin D, see p.625..

Other Proprietary Names

Deltar, Endo D (both *Ital.)*; Drisdol *(Canad.)*; Esterosol *(Spain)*; Farmobion D_2 *(Ital.)*; Fiviton D *(Spain)*; Genevis D_2 *(Switz.)*; Ostelin *(Austral., Ital.)*; Radiosterina *(Ital.)*; Radiostol *(Canad.)*; Raquiferol *(Arg.)*; Vidue, Vigantolo (both *Ital.)*; Vigantol, Vitanoxi D-2, Vitavera D (all *Spain)*.

7893-p

Vitamin E. Alpha Tocopherols.

Pharmacopoeias. U.S. specifies *d* or *dl* alpha tocopherols or their acetates or acid succinates. *It.* has Tocoferoli Misti Concentrati containing not less than 34% total tocopherols.

Vitamin E occurs in the oil from the soya bean, wheat germ, rice germ, cottonseed, and maize, and in green leaves. The concentrates are clear yellow viscous oils. Vitamin E does not appear to be destroyed by cooking.

Store in airtight containers; *d* or *dl* alpha tocopherol should be stored in an atmosphere of inert gas. Protect from light.

Units. Though the potency of preparations of vitamin E is still sometimes expressed in units, the International standard for vitamin E was discontinued in 1956. The International unit was the activity contained in 1 mg of a standard preparation *dl*-α-tocopheryl acetate.

The *U.S.P.* states that in expressing vitamin E activity of tocopherol products, the following equivalents of 1 mg are employed:

dl-alpha tocopheryl acetate, 1 unit;
dl-alpha tocopheryl acid succinate, 0.89 unit;
dl-alpha tocopherol, 1.1 units;
d-alpha tocopheryl acetate, 1.36 units;
d-alpha tocopherol, 1.49 units;
d-alpha tocopheryl acid succinate, 1.21 units.

Adverse Effects. Vitamin E is usually well tolerated. Large doses have occasionally caused gastro-intestinal disturbances, fatigue, and weakness. Contact dermatitis has occurred following topical application.

A brief review of adverse effects associated with vitamin E, including mention of severe weakness with creatinuria and raised serum-creatine-kinase activity, in 2 male volunteers, after taking 800 units daily for 3 weeks.— M. H. Briggs (letter), *Lancet*, 1974, *1*, 220. See also V. D. Herbert, *J. Am. pharm. Ass.*, 1977, *NS17*, 764.

In 52 patients given tocopherol 300 mg daily, the serum-cholesterol value rose by a mean of 74 mg per 100 ml.— S. Dahl (letter), *Lancet*, 1974, *1*, 465.

A review of the use of large doses of vitamin E in the treatment or prevention of heart disease. The likelihood of serious adverse effects appears to be very low.— *Med. Lett.*, 1975, *17*, 69.

Over a period of 10 years thrombophlebitis had occurred in 46 patients taking vitamin E; pulmonary embolism was considered to have occurred in 26 of the patients.— H. J. Roberts (letter), *Lancet*, 1978, *1*, 49.

Fifty patients had been seen with thrombophlebitis associated with the ingestion of vitamin E, usually 400 units or more daily. In some the phlebitis improved when vitamin E was withdrawn or the dose reduced. The suggested association urgently required confirmation.— H. J. Roberts, *Angiology*, 1979, *30*, 169.

A description of the function of vitamin E as an antoxidant, including the comment that large doses appear to be tolerated with relative impunity, although megavitamin therapy may have side-effects, including enhancement of the anticoagulant effect of warfarin and impairment *in vitro* of the bactericidal capacity of leucocytes.— F. A. Oski, *New Engl. J. Med.*, 1980, *303*, 454.

Interactions. In a 55-year-old man taking warfarin sodium, clofibrate, digoxin, and procainamide, vitamin E up to 1200 units daily caused a prolongation of the prothrombin time and ecchymoses. Concentrations of vitamin K-dependent coagulation factors were reduced during a test period of vitamin E ingestion, and returned to normal after the patient stopped taking vitamin E.— J. J. Corrigan and F. I. Marcus, *J. Am. med. Ass.*, 1974, *230*, 1300.

Malignant hyperpyrexia. A suggestion (P. James, letter, *Br. med. J.*, 1978, *1*, 1345) of an association between the ingestion of vitamin E and fatal malignant hyperpyrexia was later withdrawn (*idem*, 1979, *1*, 200) in view of familial susceptibility.

Absorption and Fate. Vitamin E is absorbed from the gastro-intestinal tract. Most of the vitamin appears in the lymph and is then widely distributed to all tissues. Most of a dose is slowly excreted in the bile and the remainder is eliminated in the urine as glucuronides of tocopheronic acid or other metabolites.

α-Tocopherol was the naturally-occurring active form of vitamin E but the acetate and succinate were used because of their greater stability to oxidation. Both esters underwent hydrolysis in the gastro-intestinal tract to release the active free form when given by mouth. Injection of a micellar aqueous dispersion of alpha tocopheryl acetate did not correct a rapid decline in blood-tocopherol concentration in a stress situation. Intramuscular or intravenous injection of an aqueous dispersion of *dl*-alpha tocopherol in *dogs* produced a relatively rapid and substantial rise in blood-tocopherol concentrations when compared with injection of a similar aqueous dispersion of the acetate.— H. L. Newmark *et al.*, *J. pharm. Sci.*, 1975, *64*, 655.

Human Requirements. The minimum daily requirements of vitamin E have not been clearly defined. There appears to be no evidence that supplements are required in subjects on balanced diets. Requirements increase with increased dietary amounts of polyunsaturated fatty acids.

The recommendation that the amount of α-tocopherol should be such as to ensure that the ratio of α-tocopherol (mg) to polyunsaturated fatty acids (g) is at least 0.4 : 1.0. The recommendation that an infant feed should contain not less than 3 μg α-tocopherol per ml of reconstituted feed, i.e., the amount found on average in mature human milk.— Artificial Feeds for the Young Infant: 1980, Report of the Working Party on the Composition of Foods for Infants and Young Children, Committee on Medical Aspects of Food Policy, *Report on Health and Social Subjects, 18*, London, HM Stationery Office, 1980.

Human milk contains 2 to 5 units of vitamin E per litre and provides an adequate intake for nursing infants. Milk formulas used for feeding low-birth-weight infants should provide 0.7 units for 0.42 MJ and at least 1 unit per g of linoleic acid. An oral supplement of 5 units of water-soluble vitamin E is also recommended. For children an intake of 5 units daily at 9 kg body-weight increasing to 12 units at 40 kg should be satisfactory in diets providing 4 to 7% of calories as linoleic acid. Most adult diets in the USA provide adequate amounts of vitamin E; balanced diets providing about 10 to 20 units and high-fat diets about 25 units. The increased calorie intake in pregnancy should normally be accompanied by sufficient additional vitamin E.— *Recommended Dietary Allowances*, 9th Edn, Washington, The National Research Council, 1980, p. 63.

Uses. Vitamin E has been advocated for a variety of disorders largely on the basis of deficiency states in *animals*, but evidence for any clinical benefit has generally been inconclusive. Deficiency of vitamin E has, however, been identified in disorders, such as cystic fibrosis, where fat absorption is impaired, and the benefit of supplements has been demonstrated.

Use has also been made of the antoxidant properties of vitamin E in attempts to combat oxygen toxicity in preterm infants and thereby reduce the severity of retrolental fibroplasia.

Vitamin E may be given as *d* or *dl* alpha tocopherol or as the respective acetates or acid succinates. The racemate has also been given as the calcium succinate. Other compounds with vitamin-E activity include other tocopherols and tocotrienols.

Vitamin E may also be administered in the form of preparations such as wheat-germ oil.

An account of superoxide radicals produced within cells and the body's mechanisms to deal with their potentially damaging effects, with special reference to the antoxidant properties of vitamin E and studies describing its therapeutic benefits.— F. A. Oski, *New Engl. J. Med.*, 1980, *303*, 454.

Further reviews and discussions of the use of vitamin E.— *Drug & Ther. Bull.*, 1976, *14*, 69; *Lancet*, 1977, *2*, 1268; *Br. med. J.*, 1978, *1*, 1201; *ibid.*, 1980, *280*, 697.

Use as an antoxidant. A review of the uses and efficacy of tocopherols as antoxidants and synergists in food.— *Fd Add. Ser. Wld Hlth Org. No. 3*, 1972.

Estimated acceptable daily intake as an antoxidant: up to 2 mg per kg body-weight of α-tocopherol or mixed tocopherol concentrate (as α-tocopherol).— Seventeenth Report of FAO/WHO Expert Committee on Food Additives, *Tech. Rep. Ser. Wld Hlth Org. No. 539*, 1974. For background toxicological information, see *Fd Add. Ser. Wld Hlth Org. No. 5*, 1974.

Cardiac disorders. In a double-blind study of 22 patients with ischaemic heart disease 11 received α-tocopherol succinate 1600 units daily and 11 a placebo. All patients were placed on a strict diet and exercise programme. Three patients in each group were able to reduce the number of glyceryl trinitrate tablets needed each month, whilst 4 of the vitamin group almost eliminated their tablets by reducing average monthly intake from 150 to 1 or 2 tablets.— W. M. Toone (letter), *New Engl. J. Med.*, 1973, *289*, 979.

In a double-blind study of the effect of vitamin E 3200 units daily on the symptoms of angina pectoris in 51 patients, vitamin E did not appear to be more beneficial than a placebo.— T. W. Anderson, *Can. med. Ass. J.*, 1974, *110*, 401.

In a double-blind study in 48 patients with angina pectoris given vitamin E 1600 units daily for 6 months and a placebo for 6 months, vitamin E afforded no benefit.— R. E. Gillilan *et al.*, *Am. Heart J.*, 1977, *93*, 444.

A discussion on abandoned treatments for angina pectoris, including vitamin E.— H. Benson and D. P. McCallie, *New Engl. J. Med.*, 1979, *300*, 1424.

Deficiency states. Excess platelet aggregation in 2 children with vitamin-E deficiency was reversed by vitamin E.— A. M. Lake *et al.*, *J. Pediat.*, 1977, *90*, 722.

The management of 8 patients with abetalipoproteinaemia by diet and supplements of vitamins A, E, and K. Vitamin E might have had a beneficial effect, when given early, in delaying or preventing neurological and retinal symptoms.— D. P. R. Muller *et al.*, *Archs Dis. Childh.*, 1977, *52*, 209.

A progressive neurological syndrome in 6 children with chronic liver disease and low serum concentrations of vitamin E, possibly the result of defective absorption.— J. L. Rosenblum *et al.*, *New Engl. J. Med.*, 1981, *304*, 503.

Epidermolysis bullosa dystrophica. In a double-blind crossover study in 2 sisters with epidermolysis bullosa dystrophica, vitamin E 400 units four times daily produced a marked reduction in blister formation.— E. B. Smith and W. M. Michener, *Archs Derm.*, 1973, *108*, 254. See also J. D. Michaelson *et al.*, *ibid.*, 1974, *109*, 67.

Negative reports.— W. P. Unger and J. R. Nethercott, *Can. med. Ass. J.*, 1973, *108*, 1136; R. H. Adams *et al.*, *Br. J. Derm.*, 1975, *93*, *Suppl.* 11, 10.

Haemolysis. Vitamin E 400 or 800 units by mouth daily was used in the treatment of haemolytic anaemia due to abnormalities of glutathione metabolism in 2 children. Erythrocyte survival was increased, reticulocytosis was decreased, and, in 1 patient, the haematocrit was improved.— S. P. Spielberg *et al.*, *Ann. intern. Med.*, 1979, *90*, 53. See also L. A. Boxer *et al.*, *New Engl. J. Med.*, 1979, *301*, 901; J. D. Schulman *et al.*, *Ann. intern. Med.*, 1980, *93*, 330.

High doses of vitamin E by mouth had a beneficial effect on chronic haemolysis in 23 patients with Mediterranean-type glucose-6-phosphate dehydrogenase deficiency.— L. Corash *et al.*, *New Engl. J. Med.*, 1980, *303*, 416.

Further references: S. S. Lo *et al.*, *Archs Dis. Childh.*, 1973, *48*, 360; *Br. med. J.*, 1974, *2*, 625; C. B. Modell *et al.* (letter), *ibid.*, 1974, *3*, 259; *Med. J. Aust.*, 1976, *1*, 685.

Cystic fibrosis. Liability to lipid peroxidation in membranes is a function of the polyunsaturated fatty acid content of the phospholipids. Cystic fibrosis is invariably associated with vitamin E deficiency where there is pancreatogenic steatorrhoea. It has been shown by P.M. Farrell *et al.* (*J. clin. Invest.*, 1977, *1*, 904) that most non-supplemented cystic fibrosis patients are so deficient that their erythrocytes are inadequately protected against the oxidative stress of exposure to peroxide.— *Lancet*, 1977, *2*, 1268. See also E. Elias *et al.*, *ibid.*, 1981, *2*, 1319 (neurological symptoms requiring intramuscular vitamin E).

In the neonate. Reductions in carboxyhaemoglobin in 10 premature infants given a total dose of vitamin E 125 mg per kg body-weight over 4 days compared with 10 control infants suggested that vitamin E might reduce the accelerated destruction of red blood cells seen in premature infants.— S. J. Gross *et al.*, *Pediatrics*, 1977, *59*, *Suppl.*, 995.

In a study in 35 premature infants vitamin E in a total dose of 125 to 150 mg per kg body-weight intramuscularly in the first 8 days of life protected against haemolysis, even when iron was given intramuscularly concomitantly.— J. E. Graeber *et al.*, *J. Pediat.*, 1977, *90*, 282.

Thirty-five infants weighing 2 kg or less were sequentially given either tocopheryl acetate (a total of 125 mg per kg body-weight intramuscularly over the first week of life) or no vitamin E therapy. The severity of complications did not vary significantly between the 2 groups and the study provided no evidence to support the contention that vitamin E reduced the fall of haemoglobin in premature infants; nor did it affect the rate of growth of preterm infants. Its routine use, either by mouth or by intramuscular injection, could not be recommended.— M. I. Levene (letter), *Lancet*, 1979, *2*, 1186.

Herpes. Favourable results with topical vitamin E in an uncontrolled survey of 50 patients with herpes simplex.— M. Fink and J. Fink (letter), *Br. dent. J.*, 1980, *148*, 246.

Huntington's chorea. In a double-blind 24-week crossover study deterioration in 9 patients with Huntington's chorea was similar while taking tocopheryl acetate 400 mg thrice daily or a placebo. The claimed benefit of vitamin E in Huntington's chorea should be discounted.— A. J. Caro and S. Caro, *Br. med. J.*, 1978, *1*, 153.

Intermittent claudication. Vitamin E was not proven to be of value in the treatment of intermittent claudication.— E. Housley and I. J. McFadyen (letter), *Lancet*, 1974, *1*, 458.

A significant difference in walking distance and lower-leg arterial pressure was found between patients treated with α-tocopherol for 4 to 7 years and controls.— K. Haeger (letter), *Lancet*, 1974, *1*, 1352.

Neurological disorders. Absence of benefit in 12 patients with amyotrophic lateral sclerosis.— J. D. Dorman *et al.*, *J. Am. med. Ass.*, 1969, *209*, 257.

Neuralgia. Favourable results with topical vitamin E in post-herpetic neuralgia.— S. Ayres and R. Mihan, *Archs Derm.*, 1973, *108*, 855.

Porphyria. In 4 patients with porphyria, urinary excretion of porphyrins decreased to normal levels following treatment with vitamin E.— P. P. Nair *et al.*, *Archs intern. Med.*, 1971, *128*, 411.

Vitamin E in doses ranging from 100 to 400 mg daily was of no benefit to 5 patients with porphyria.— P. Mustajoki (letter), *J. Am. med. Ass.*, 1972, *221*, 714.

Respiratory distress syndrome. In a controlled study of neonates with the respiratory distress syndrome who required increased concentrations of oxygen (greater than 40%), 20 received vitamin E 20 mg per kg body-weight daily by intramuscular injection during the acute phase of the syndrome and a further 20 acted as controls. Over the first 2 months of treatment, in infants surviving for more than about 10 days and still requiring supplemental oxygen, 6 of 13 controls had X-ray changes indicative of bronchopulmonary dysplasia and 4 died whilst none of the 9 vitamin-treated infants had abnormal chest X-rays and all survived. Administration of vitamin E during the acute phase might have diminished the toxic effects of oxygen, one of the causal factors of bronchopulmonary dysplasia.— R. A. Ehrenkranz *et al.*, *New Engl. J. Med.*, 1978, *299*, 564. Comment, including the features of bronchopulmonary dysplasia and concern about the design of the study: further study was certainly warranted.— W. H. Northway, *ibid.*, 599.

Retrolental fibroplasia. Evidence that vitamin E in high doses of 100 mg per kg body-weight daily by mouth can reduce the severity of retrolental fibroplasia in preterm infants requiring oxygen.— H. M. Hittner *et al.*, *New Engl. J. Med.*, 1981, *305*, 1365. A warning on the possible association between vitamin E and necrotising enterocolitis.— S. Sobel *et al.* (letter), *ibid.*, 1982, *306*, 867.

Sickle-cell anaemia. A decrease in irreversibly sickled erythrocytes in sickle-cell anaemia patients given vitamin E.— C. L. Natta *et al.*, *Am. J. clin. Nutr.*, 1980, *33*, 968.

Sunscreening. A discussion on the use of tocopherols as sunscreen agents.— *Mfg Chem.*, 1979, *50* (July), 57.

Use by athletes. In brief reviews of the use of vitamin E by athletes there was no convincing evidence of improved performance.— *Br. med. J.*, 1971, *4*, 251; J. Thomas, *Aust. J. Pharm.*, 1972, *53*, 280. See also I. M. Sharman *et al.*, *Br. J. Nutr.*, 1971, *26*, 265.

Vitamin E 1200 units daily for 50 days had no effect on oxygen consumption in 10 subjects when compared with placebo in 10 similar subjects.— T. Watt *et al.* (letter), *Lancet*, 1974, *2*, 354.

Vitamin E 300 mg daily controlled muscular cramps in an uncontrolled series of about 50 patients.— L. Lotzof (letter), *Med. J. Aust.*, 1977, *1*, 904.

Preparations

Vitamin E Capsules *(U.S.P.)*. Capsules containing Vitamin E or Vitamin E preparation. Store in airtight containers. Protect from light.

Vitamin E Preparation *(U.S.P.)*. A combination of a single form of vitamin E with one or more inert substances; it may be in liquid or solid form. Preparations containing the *dl*-form may contain also a small amount of the *d*-form occurring as a minor constituent of an added substance. Store in airtight containers. Preparations containing *d*- or *dl*-alpha tocopherol should be stored in an atmosphere of inert gas. Protect from light.

Proprietary Names

Aquasol E *(USV Pharmaceutical Corp., USA)*; Dextamina-E Fuerte *(Dexter, Spain)*; Dif-Vitamin E *(Andreu, Spain)*; E Sir *(Farmades, Ital.)*; E-ferol *(O'Neal, USA)*; Egermol *(UPB, Belg.)*; Eprolin *(Lilly, Switz.)*; Eta-Monovit *(Libra, Ital.)*; Everol *(Kin, Spain)*; Evion *(Igoda, Spain)*; Fertilvit *(Lafare, Ital.)*; Godabion E *(Igoda, Spain)*; Ilitia *(Biologici Italia, Ital.)*; Invite E *(Nelson, Austral.)*; Lethopherol *(Nutrition Control Products, USA)*; Na-To-Caps *(Jamco, Ital.)*; Pheryl E *(Miller, USA)*; Propan E *(Propan, S.Afr.)*; Solucap E *(Jamieson-McKames, USA)*; Tocerol *(Prosana, Austral.)*; Tocovite *(Akarana, Austral.)*; Viteril *(Panthox & Burck, Ital.)*.

7894-s

d-Alpha Tocopherol. *RRR*-α-Tocopherol. (+)-2,5,7,8-Tetramethyl-2-(4,8,12-trimethyltridecyl)chroman-6-ol.
$C_{29}H_{50}O_2$=430.7.

CAS — 59-02-9.

A clear yellow or greenish-yellow viscous oil. Practically **insoluble** in water; soluble in alcohol; miscible with acetone, chloroform, ether, and vegetable oils. It is oxidised on exposure to air and light, particularly in alkaline solutions. **Store** in an atmosphere of inert gas. Protect from light.

d-Alpha tocopherol is considered to be the form of vitamin E found in nature.

7895-w

***dl*-Alpha Tocopherol.** Tocoferol; *dl*-α-Tocoferolo. (±)-2,5,7,8-Tetramethyl-2-(4,8,12-trimethyltridecyl)chroman-6-ol.
$C_{29}H_{50}O_2$=430.7.

CAS — 10191-41-0.

Pharmacopoeias. In *Braz.*, *It.*, and *Jap.* The nomenclature of *Arg.* is confused.

A clear yellow or greenish-yellow, almost odourless, viscous oil. Wt per ml about 0.95 g. Practically **insoluble** in water; very soluble in alcohol; miscible with chloroform, ether, acetone, and vegetable oils. It is oxidised on exposure to air and light, particularly in alkaline solutions, darkening in colour. **Store** in an atmosphere of inert gas. Protect from light.

Uses. *dl*-Alpha tocopherol is given for its vitamin-E activity. It is a permitted antoxidant for foods.

Proprietary Names

Fravit E *(Francia Farm., Ital.)*.

7896-e

Alpha Tocopheryl Acetate *(B.P., B.P. Vet., Eur. P.)*. α-Tocopheryl Acetate; α-Tocopherol Acetate; α-Tocopheroli Acetas; *dl*-α-Tocopherol Acetate; Vitamin E Acetate. (±)-α-Tocopherol acetate.
$C_{31}H_{52}O_3$=472.8.

CAS — 7695-91-2.

Pharmacopoeias. In *Aust.*, *Br.*, *Braz.*, *Chin.*, *Cz.*, *Eur.*, *Fr.*, *Ger.*, *Hung.*, *It.*, *Jap.*, *Neth.*, *Nord.*, *Pol.*, and *Swiss. It.* also includes *d*-alpha tocopheryl acetate. *Jug.*, *Roum.*, and *Rus.* include tocopheryl acetate without specification of the structure.

A clear, odourless or almost odourless, slightly greenish-yellow, viscous oily liquid. Relative density 0.952 to 0.966. Practically **insoluble** in water; freely soluble in acetone, dehydrated alcohol, chloroform, ether, and fixed oils; soluble in alcohol. Unstable in alkaline solutions. **Protect** from light.

Uses. Alpha tocopheryl acetate is given for its vitamin E activity.

Proprietary Preparations

Ephynal *(Roche, UK)*. Tocopheryl acetate (synthetic), available as tablets of 3 and 10 mg, and as scored tablets of 50 and 200 mg. (Also available as Ephynal in *Arg.*, *Austral.*, *Belg.*, *Denm.*, *Fr.*, *Ger.*, *Ital.*, *S.Afr.*, *Spain*, *Swed.*, *Switz.*).

Vita-E *(Bioglan, UK)*. *d*-Alpha tocopheryl acetate, available as **Gels** (capsules) of 75, 200, and 400 units; as **Gelucaps** (tablets) of 75 units; and as **Ointment** containing 30 units per g. (Also available as Vita-E Gelucaps in *Austral.*).

Other Proprietary Names of Alpha Tocopheryl Acetates

Canad.—Aquasol E; *Denm.*— Fertilan; *Fr.*—Tocomine; *Ger.*—E-Mulsin, E-Vicotrat, Evion; *Ital.*—Evion Forte, E-Vit, Evitina, Farmobion E, Tocogen, Tocopherex; *Jap.*—Juvela (see also under Dietary and Nutritive Preparations, p.64); *Neth.*—Davitamon E; *Norw.*—Ido-E; *Spain*—Auxina E; *Swed.*—E-vimin, Ido-E; *USA*—Tokols.

7897-l

***d*-Alpha Tocopheryl Acid Succinate.** Dextocoferyli Succinas. (+)-α-Tocopherol hydrogen succinate.
$C_{33}H_{54}O_5$=530.8.

CAS — 4345-03-3.

Pharmacopoeias. In *Nord.*

Colourless or almost colourless crystals or white or yellowish crystalline powder, almost odourless and tasteless. M.p. 75°. Practically **insoluble** in water; soluble 1 in 5 of alcohol, 1 in 0.8 of chloroform, and 1 in 1 of ether; soluble in vegetable oils. **Incompatible** with alkalis and oxidising agents. **Protect** from light.

Uses. *d*-Alpha tocopheryl acid succinate is given for its vitamin-E activity.

Preparations

Vita-E Succinate *(Bioglan, UK)*. *d*-Alpha tocopheryl acid succinate, available as scored tablets of 200 units.

Other Proprietary Names

Daltose *(Canad.)*.

7898-y

***dl*-Alpha Tocopheryl Calcium Succinate.** Tocopheroli Calcii Succinas; Vitamin E Calcium Succinate. The calcium salt of (±)-α-tocopherol succinate.
$(C_{33}H_{53}O_5)_2Ca$=1099.6.

CAS — 14638-18-7.

Pharmacopoeias. In *Jap.*

A white to yellowish-white, odourless powder. Practically **insoluble** in water, alcohol, and acetone; freely soluble in chloroform and ether. **Store** in airtight containers. Protect from light.

Uses. *dl*-Alpha tocopheryl calcium succinate is used for its vitamin-E activity.

Proprietary Names
E-Tap-S *(Jap.)*.

7899-j

Tocopheryl Nicotinate. Vitamin E Nicotinate. (±)-α-Tocopherol nicotinate.
$C_{35}H_{53}NO_3$=535.8.

CAS — 51898-34-1.

A yellow oily substance. M.p. about 38°. Practically **insoluble** in cold water; soluble in most organic solvents.

Uses. Tocopheryl nicotinate has been given in doses of up to 900 mg initially to patients with hyperlipidaemia.

Proprietary Names
Disclar *(Casen-Roncales, Spain)*; Renascin *(Mack, Illert., Ger.)*; Juvela Nicotinate, Nicobita-E, Nicoferol *(all Jap.)*.

7900-j

Tocopherylquinone. α-Tocopherylquinone; α-Tocoquinone; Tocoferylchinonum. 2-(3-Hydroxy-3,7,11,15-tetramethylhexadecyl)-3,5,6-trimethyl-1,4-benzoquinone.
$C_{29}H_{50}O_3$=446.7.

CAS — 7559-04-8.

A yellow oil. Practically **insoluble** in water; soluble in alcohol.

Uses. Tocopherylquinone has been used in a variety of conditions including hypertension and disorders of muscle and skin. Daily doses have ranged from 100 to 600 mg.

Proprietary Names
Eutrophyl *(Riker, Fr.)*; Ipotensil *(Tosi-Novara, Ital.)*; Tensiopress *(Biosint, Ital.)*; Trimina *(Iti, Ital.)*; Vitapressina *(Coli, Ital.)*.

7901-z

Wheat-germ Oil *(B.P.C. 1954)*. Oleum Tritici Germinis.

CAS — 8006-95-9.

A bland yellow oil with a nutty odour and taste, obtained by expression or solvent extraction of the embryos of wheat, *Triticum aestivum* (Gramineae).
Slightly **soluble** in alcohol; miscible with chloroform, ether, and light petroleum. Wt per ml about 0.93 g. It contains α-tocopherol accompanied by other tocopherols. **Store** in a cool place in well-filled airtight containers. Protect from light.

Uses. Wheat-germ oil has been given as a source of vitamin E. Doses of up to 5 ml have been employed.

Proprietary Preparations
Atlagran-D *(Keimdiät, Ger.: Thomson & Joseph, UK)*. An oil prepared from wheat-germ oil 15% and other vegetable oils, containing about 41% of phosphatides. For use in pharmaceutical and dietary preparations. **Atlagran K 70** is similar; for use in cosmetics.

Auxigran *(Keimdiät, Ger.: Thomson & Joseph, UK)*. An alcohol extract of the oil-soluble and water-soluble constituents of wheat embryos. For use as an ingredient of pharmaceutical, dermatological, and cosmetic preparations. **Auxigran Forte.** A similar preparation, concentrated, and standardised for vitamin content.

Crookes Wheat-germ Oil Capsules *(Crookes Products, UK)*. Each 0.18-ml capsule provides 3 mg of combined tocopherols.

E-Grandelan 8470 *(Keimdiät, Ger.: Thomson & Joseph, UK)*. Wheat-germ oil with a low content of free fatty acids. A source of vitamin E for use in pharmaceutical, cosmetic, and dietary preparations.

Redoxogran *(Keimdiät, Ger.: Thomson & Joseph, UK)*. An oil prepared from wheat embryos and specific moulds. For use, in a concentration of 0.05 to 0.1%, as an antoxidant for oils and fats.

Other Proprietary Names
E-Grandelat *(Ger.)*.

7902-c

Vitamin K

Vitamin K is present, as phytomenadione (vitamin K_1), in fresh green vegetables, fruit, and egg-yolk, and vitamin K_2 (menaquinone) is synthesised in the intestine by normal bacterial action. In normal adults, requirements of vitamin K are adequately met from the diet, together with that formed by bacterial action in the intestine. There is little loss of vitamin K from food during cooking.
Naturally occurring vitamin K is fat-soluble and depends on the presence of adequate quantities of bile salts for its satisfactory absorption from the intestine. There are also several synthetic naphthaquinone derivatives with vitamin K activity and some of these are water-soluble.

Absorption and Fate. Phytomenadione is absorbed from the gastro-intestinal tract in the presence of bile. Vitamin K_2 is also synthesised by intestinal bacteria. Vitamin K is rapidly metabolised and excreted; it is not significantly stored by the body.

The pharmacokinetics of phytomenadione in young and in elderly subjects.— A. M. M. Shepherd *et al.*, *Clin. Pharmac. Ther.*, 1977, *21*, 117.

Human Requirements. The minimum daily requirements of vitamin K are not clearly defined but an intake of about 2 µg per kg body-weight daily appears to be adequate and can be supplied in the average diet and by synthesis within the intestine.

A study of a patient with obstructive jaundice suggested that the daily requirement of vitamin K_1 was about 100 to 500 ng per kg body-weight.— P. Barkhan and M. J. Shearer, *Proc. R. Soc. Med.*, 1977, *70*, 93.

No specific recommended dietary allowance could be made for vitamin K. A daily intake of 2 µg per kg body-weight appeared satisfactory. Even if intestinal synthesis contributed little to the intake, most diets could still provide adequate amounts and this included both breast- and bottle-bed infants; current artificial feeds contain 4 µg per 0.42 MJ and breast milk 15 µg per litre.— *Recommended Dietary Allowances*, 9th Edn, Washington, The National Research Council, 1980, p. 69.

The suggestion that an infant feed should contain not less than 15 ng per ml vitamin K.— Artificial Feeds for the Young Infant: 1980, Report of the Working Party on the Composition of Foods for Infants and Young Children, Committee on Medical Aspects of Food Policy, *Report on Health and Social Subjects, 18*, London, HM Stationery Office, 1980.

Uses. Vitamin K is essential for the formation of prothrombin (factor II) and other clotting factors (factors VII, IX, and X) in the liver. Deficiency of vitamin K produces hypoprothrombinaemia, in which the clotting time of the blood is prolonged and spontaneous haemorrhage may occur.
Deficiency of vitamin K may result from poor intestinal absorption of the vitamin, from obstructive jaundice or severe liver disease, or from the administration of coumarin or indanedione anticoagulants which interfere with vitamin K metabolism. It is possible that the prolonged administration of antibiotics may interfere with the bacterial synthesis of vitamin K in the intestine and lead to a deficiency of the vitamin.
In newborn infants, hypoprothrombinaemia may result from a vitamin-K deficiency which is thought to be due primarily to lack of bacterial synthesis of the vitamin in the intestine.

A report of a symposium on vitamin K.— *Mayo Clin. Proc.*, 1974, *49*, 911–944.

A discussion on carboxylated calcium-binding proteins and vitamin K.— P. M. Gallop *et al.*, *New Engl. J. Med.*, 1980, *302*, 1460.

A severe coagulation defect due to a dietary deficiency of vitamin K occurred in one patient while being treated with antibiotics. She responded to phytomenadione 10 mg intravenously daily for 3 days followed by oral treatment.— B. T. Colvin and M. J. Lloyd, *J. clin. Path.*, 1977, *30*, 1147.

When treating warfarin overdosage account must be taken of the rapid turnover of phytomenadione compared with the slow elimination of warfarin.— T. D. Bjornsson and T. F. Blaschke (letter), *Lancet*, 1978, *2*, 846.

Mention of the use of vitamin K parenterally after liver biopsy.— J. R. F. Walters and A. Paton, *Br. med. J.*, 1980, *280*, 777.

Neonatal haemorrhage. A study of plasma from 43 healthy neonates indicated that healthy babies did not have vitamin-K deficiency and that the practice of giving vitamin-K prophylaxis to such infants was of no value.— J. M. van Doorm *et al.* (letter), *Lancet*, 1977, *1*, 852. See also U. Göbel *et al.* (letter), *ibid.*, 1977, *2*, 187; P. G. Mori *et al.* (letter), *ibid.*, 188. Criticism. The pattern of feeding may affect the vitamin-K status in the first few days of life. It would be inadvertent to discontinue the custom of prophylaxis with vitamin K.— J. R. Edson (letter), *ibid.*, 187.

A discussion of the use of vitamin K in the newborn, including the view that human milk is deficient in vitamin K. While the need for prophylaxis had been challenged the effectiveness of vitamin K in vitamin-K-dependent coagulation factor deficiency was beyond dispute. Selective prophylaxis was recommended for preterm and low birth weight infants, those who had difficult births, those due for early discharge or to be wholly breast-fed, those with inadequate intakes or taking antibiotics, those with evidence of bruising or bleeding, and those needing surgery.— *Lancet*, 1978, *1*, 755.

Intravenous administration of phytomenadione 2 mg corrected hypoprothrombinaemia following lumbar puncture and venepuncture in a 6-week-old breast-fed infant. It was considered advisable to investigate prothrombin time before undertaking invasive procedures in breast-fed infants of this age.— A. M. B. Minford and O. B. Eden, *Archs Dis. Childh.*, 1979, *54*, 310.

7903-k

Phytomenadione *(B.P., B.P. Vet.)*. Phytomenad.; Phytonadione *(U.S.P.)*; Phylloquinone; Vitamin K_1; Methylphytylnaphthochinonum. 2-Methyl-3-phytyl-1,4-naphthoquinone.
$C_{31}H_{46}O_2$=450.7.

CAS — 84-80-0.

Pharmacopoeias. In *Arg.*, *Br.*, *Braz.*, *Chin.*, *Cz.*, *Jap.*, *Turk.*, and *U.S.*

A clear, deep yellow, very viscous, odourless or almost odourless oil which is stable in air but decomposes on exposure to light. Specific gravity about 0.967.
Practically **insoluble** in water; soluble 1 in 70 of alcohol; more soluble in dehydrated alcohol; freely soluble in chloroform, ether, and fixed oils. A 5% solution in dehydrated alcohol is neutral to litmus. Aqueous dispersons for injection may be **sterilised** by autoclaving. **Store** in airtight containers. Protect from light.

Incompatibility. Particulate matter was observed within 2 hours when 1 ml of commercial phytomenadione injection was mixed with 5 ml of sterile water and 1 ml of commercial phenytoin sodium injection solution.— R. Misgen, *Am. J. Hosp. Pharm.*, 1965, *22*, 92.

There was a loss of clarity when intravenous solutions of phytomenadione were mixed with those of ascorbic acid, cyanocobalamin, dextran, or phenytoin sodium.— J. A. Patel and G. L. Phillips, *Am. J. Hosp. Pharm.*, 1966, *23*, 409.

Stability. As phytomenadione was unstable to light it should not be added to intravenous infusions.— R. L. Longe (letter), *Am. J. Hosp. Pharm.*, 1974, *31*, 1039.

Adverse Effects and Precautions. Intravenous administration of phytomenadione has caused reactions, including altered sensations of taste, flushing of the face, sweating, bronchospasm and cyanosis, tachycardia, and hypotension. It has been suggested that these reactions may have been caused by the vehicle. Fatalities have occurred. Pain and swelling may occur at the injection site. Intravenous injections should be given very slowly.

Cerebral arterial thrombosis developed in 2 patients with malabsorption syndromes due to coeliac disease during treatment with vitamin K for severe deficiency of vitamin-K-dependent coagulation factors.— J. Florholmen *et al.*, *Br. med. J.*, 1980, *281*, 541.

Allergy. Erythematous rashes around the injection site developed in 6 patients with chronic liver disease 7 to 16 days after they were given phytomenadione in a total dose of 270 to 440 mg (Konakion) by injection. Reactions resolved within 22 days.— A. W. Bullen *et al.*, *Br. J. Derm.*, 1978, *98*, 561. See also H. M. Barnes and I. Sarkany, *Br. J. Derm.*, 1976, *95*, 653; J. W. Robison and R. B. Odom, *Archs Derm.*, 1978, *114*, 1790.

Absorption and Fate. See under Vitamin K, p.1665.

Uses. Phytomenadione is a naturally occurring vitamin K which causes a rise in the plasma prothrombin concentration and reduction in the clotting time.

Phytomenadione is used in the treatment of hypoprothrombinaemia and haemorrhage caused by anticoagulant therapy. It is not effective in overdosage with heparin. If treatment with anticoagulants is to be continued, the smallest effective dose of phytomenadione should be employed. Dosage should be controlled by prothrombin-time estimations.

Initial doses of phytomenadione are usually in the range 2.5 to 25 mg (exceptionally 50 mg) by subcutaneous or intramuscular injection, the dose being repeated after 6 to 8 hours if necessary. It may also be given by mouth in doses of 5 to 20 mg, repeated after 8 to 12 hours if necessary. In severe bleeding it may be given intravenously at a rate not greater than 1 mg per minute; a recommended dose for severe bleeding is 10 to 20 mg by slow intravenous injection, followed by estimation of the prothrombin level 3 hours later; if the dose has been inadequate it should be repeated; not more than 40 mg should be given intravenously in 24 hours. In some countries not all commercial injections are suitable for intravenous use.

In the treatment of haemorrhagic disease of the newborn it may be given in a dose of 1 mg intramuscularly and, if necessary, further doses may be given 8-hourly. As a prophylactic measure, 0.5 to 1 mg may be given intramuscularly or it may be given to the mother in a dose of 1 to 5 mg by intramuscular injection 12 to 24 hours before delivery.

Preparations

Phytomenadione Capsules *(B.P. 1968)*. Phytomenad. Caps.; Vitamin K_1 Capsules. Flexible capsules containing an emulsion of phytomenadione with suitable dispersing and stabilising agents; the shells are coloured brown. Store in a cool place; avoid freezing.

Phytomenadione Injection *(B.P.)*. Phytomenad. Inj.; Vitamin K_1 Injection. A sterile preparation of phytomenadione in Water for Injections containing suitable dispersing and stabilising agents. Sterilised by autoclaving. pH 5 to 7.5. Protect from light and avoid freezing. If oil droplets have appeared or separation has occurred, it should not be used.

Phytomenadione Tablets *(B.P.)*. Vitamin K_1 Tablets. Tablets containing phytomenadione; they may be sugar-coated. They should be chewed or allowed to dissolve slowly in the mouth.

Phytonadione Injection *(U.S.P.)*. A sterile aqueous dispersion of phytomenadione; it contains suitable solubilising and/or dispersing agents. pH 5 to 7. Protect from light.

Phytonadione Tablets *(U.S.P.)*. Tablets containing phytomenadione. Protect from light.

Proprietary Preparations

Konakion *(Roche, UK)*. Phytomenadione, available as **Injection** containing 2 mg per ml in ampoules of 0.5 ml, and 10 mg per ml in ampoules of 1 ml, and as **Tablets** of 10 mg. (Also available as Konakion in *Arg., Austral., Belg., Canad., Ger., Ital., Neth., Norw., S.Afr., Spain, Switz., USA*).

Other Proprietary Names

Aquamephyton *(Austral., Canad., Neth., USA)*; Kaywan, Vita-K1 *(both Jap.)*; Mephyton *(Canad., USA)*.

Phytomenadione was also formerly marketed in Great Britain under the proprietary name Aquamephyton *(Merck Sharp & Dohme)*.

7904-a

Acetomenaphthone *(B.P. 1973)*. Acetomenaph.; Acetomenadione; Menadiol Diacetate. 2-Methylnaphthalene-1,4-diyl diacetate.

$C_{15}H_{14}O_4$=258.3.

CAS — 573-20-6.

Pharmacopoeias. In *Ind.* and *Jug.*

A white crystalline powder with a bitter taste. It is odourless or has a slight odour of acetic acid. M.p. 112° to 115°.

Practically **insoluble** in water; soluble in acetic acid, slightly soluble in cold alcohol; soluble 1 in 3.3 of boiling alcohol.

Uses. Acetomenaphthone has actions and uses similar to those of phytomenadione (see p.1665) but it exerts its effects more slowly and phytomenadione is therefore generally preferred. It has been administered by mouth in doses of 5 to 20 mg daily.

Traditionally acetomenaphthone has been used in conjunction with nicotinic acid or nicotinamide for the prevention and treatment of chilblains; the role of acetomenaphthone is obscure.

Preparations

Acetomenaphthone Tablets *(B.P. 1973)*. Acetomenaph. Tab. Tablets containing acetomenaphthone. They may be sugar-coated.

Proprietary Preparations

Chilblain Treatment Dellipsoids D 27 *(Pilsworth, UK)*. Tablets each containing acetomenaphthone 7 mg and nicotinic acid 25 mg. *Dose.* 1 tablet night and morning.

Pernivit *(Duncan, Flockhart, UK)*. Tablets each containing acetomenaphthone 7 mg and nicotinic acid 25 mg. For chilblains. *Dose.* 6 to 9 tablets daily; prophylactic, half the recommended dose.

A preparation containing acetomenaphthone was also formerly marketed in Great Britain under the proprietary name Amisyn Tablets (*Armour*).

7905-t

Menadiol Sodium Diphosphate. U.S.P.;

Menadiolum Solubile. 2-Methylnaphthalene-1,4-diyl bis(disodium phosphate) hexahydrate.

$C_{11}H_8Na_4O_8P_2,6H_2O$=530.2.

CAS — 481-85-6 (menadiol); 84-98-0 (menadiol diphosphate); 131-13-5 (tetrasodium salt, anhydrous); 6700-42-1 (tetrasodium salt, hexahydrate).

Pharmacopoeias. In *Arg., Cz.,* and *U.S.*

A white to pink hygroscopic powder with a characteristic odour. Very **soluble** in water; practically insoluble in alcohol. A solution in water has a pH of about 8. **Store** at a temperature not exceeding 8° in airtight containers. Protect from light.

Adverse Effects. Gastric discomfort may occasionally occur. Allergic reactions have been reported.

For comments on hyperbilirubinaemia associated with water-soluble derivatives of menadione, see Menadione, p.1666.

Uses. Menadiol sodium diphosphate is a water-soluble derivative of menaphthone. For the treatment of severe hypoprothrombinaemia caused by anticoagulants it has largely been superseded by phytomenadione (see p.1666), but it may be employed for less severe conditions. It is administered either by mouth or by subcutaneous, intramuscular, or intravenous injection.

For the prevention of haemorrhagic disorders in conditions such as obstructive jaundice or steatorrhoea or during prolonged courses of treatment with salicylates, doses of 5 to 10 mg may be given daily.

For the prevention of haemorrhagic disease of the newborn 10 mg daily has been given by mouth to the mother for 3 to 4 days before delivery or 5 mg given by injection to the mother during delivery. For administration to the infant, phytomenadione is preferred.

Menadiol sodium diphosphate may be used in doses of 100 mg by injection as a radiosensitiser in the treatment of cancer.

Malignant neoplasms. A brief review of the radiosensitising action of menadiol sodium diphosphate.— *Lancet*, 1972, *2*, 638. Comment.— G. E. Adams (letter), *ibid.*, 921.

A short review of the use of radioactive vitamin K for the treatment of malignant diseases.— N. M. Bleehen, *Br. med. Bull.*, 1973, *29*, 54.

Preparations

Menadiol Sodium Diphosphate Injection *(U.S.P.)*. A sterile solution in Water for Injections. pH 7.5 to 8.5. Protect from light.

Menadiol Sodium Diphosphate Tablets *(U.S.P.)*. Tablets containing menadiol sodium diphosphate. Protect from light.

Synkavit *(Roche, UK)*. Anhydrous menadiol sodium diphosphate, available as scored **Tablets** of 12.63 mg (equivalent to 10 mg of the anhydrous free ester) and as **Injection** in 1-ml ampoules of 12.63 mg and 2-ml ampoules of 126.3 mg (equivalent to 10 mg and 100 mg respectively of the anhydrous free ester). (Also available as Synkavit in *Arg., Austral., Belg., S.Afr., Switz.*).

Other Proprietary Names

Kappadione *(USA)*; Synkavite *(Canad.)*; Synkayvite *(USA)*.

7906-x

Menadione *(Eur. P., U.S.P.)*. Menaphthone *(B.P. 1963)*; Menaph.; Menaphthene; Menadionum; Methylnaphthochinonum; Vitamin K_3. 2-Methyl-1,4-naphthoquinone.

$C_{11}H_8O_2$=172.2.

CAS — 58-27-5.

Pharmacopoeias. In *Arg., Aust., Belg., Braz., Eur., Fr., Ger., Ind., Int., It., Mex., Neth., Swiss, Turk.,* and *U.S.*

A bright yellow crystalline powder with a faint characteristic odour. M.p. 105° to 107°. On exposure to light it decomposes and darkens to light brown.

Practically **insoluble** in water; soluble 1 in 60 of alcohol, and 1 in 50 of fixed oils; freely soluble in chloroform; soluble in ether and carbon disulphide. Solutions in oils are **sterilised** by maintaining at 150° for 1 hour. **Incompatible** with alkalis and reducing agents. **Protect** from light.

CAUTION. *The powder is irritating to the respiratory tract and to the skin. The alcoholic solution has vesicant properties.*

Stability. Menadione formed complexes in aqueous solution with electron donors such as caffeine, nicotinamide, salicyclic acid and theobromine. These complexes could reduce photodecomposition of menadione.— S. Hata *et al.*, *Chem. pharm. Bull., Tokyo*, 1967, *15*, 1791. Stability of menadione increased with increase in concentration of electron donor.— *idem*, 1796.

A solution of menadione in dimethicone 20 was more stable than in maize oil at room temperature. There was a 10% loss of potency in about 230 days in dimethicone 20 or in about 40 days in maize oil.— R. T. Turnbull and K. E. Avis, *J. pharm. Sci.*, 1968, *57*, 1409.

Adverse Effects. Menadione and its water-soluble derivatives have been reported to compete with bilirubin during their metabolism and thereby to induce hyperbilirubinaemia in neonates. They have also been reported to induce haemolysis in subjects deficient in glucose-6-phosphate dehydrogenase, which can exacerbate the hyperbilirubinaemia. These adverse effects are not considered to be a hazard of phytomenadione.

Water-soluble derivatives of menadione such as the phosphate (Synkavit) and the sulphate (Hykinone) have been accused of causing excessive jaundice and also haemolysis in glucose-6-phosphate dehydrogenase deficient infants and are no longer used in the neonatal period, although these adverse effects were almost certainly due to excessive dosage.— *Lancet*, 1978, *1*, 755.

Absorption and Fate. Unlike phytomenadione, menadione and its water-soluble derivatives can be absorbed from the gastro-intestinal tract in the absence of bile.

Uses. Menadione is a provitamin; following activation it exerts vitamin K effects. It has been largely replaced by phytomenadione (see p.1666).
Menadione is usually administered by intramuscular injection as a 0.5% solution in oil.
For references to the use of menadione in multiple sclerosis and muscular dystrophy, see Martindale 27th Edn, p. 1690.

Preparations

Menadione Injection *(U.S.P.)*. A sterile solution of menadione in oil.

Menadione Tablets *(U.S.P.)*. Tablets containing menadione.

Proprietary Names

Bilkaby *(Bailly, Fr.)*; Kaergona Hidrosoluble *(IBYS, Spain)*; Karanum *(Igoda, Spain)*; Katerap Hidrosoluble *(Sintyal, Arg.)*; Vita-Noxi K *(Therapia, Spain)*; Zimema-K *(Saet, Spain)*.

7907-r

Menadione Sodium Bisulphite. Menaphthone Sodium Bisulphite *(B.P. 1963)*; Menaph. Sod. Bisulphite; Menadione Sodium Bisulfite *(U.S.P.)*; Methylnaphthochinonumnatrium Bisulfurosum; Kavitanum; Vikasolum; Vitamin K_3 Sodium Bisulphite. Sodium 1,2,3,4-tetrahydro-2-methyl-1,4-dioxonaphthalene-2-sulphonate trihydrate.
$C_{11}H_8O_2NaHSO_3,3H_2O=330.3$.

CAS — 130-37-0 (anhydrous); 6147-37-1 (trihydrate).

Pharmacopoeias. In *Arg., Belg., Braz., Hung., Ind., Jug., Nord., Pol., Port., Rus., Swiss,* and *U.S. Braz.* and *U.S.* specify a mixture containing 63 to 75% menadione sodium bisulphite and 30 to 38% sodium bisulphite. *Nord.* and *Swiss* specify $2H_2O$.

A white, odourless, hygroscopic, crystalline powder. **Soluble** 1 in 3 of water; very slightly soluble in alcohol, chloroform, and ether. A solution in water is neutral to litmus. A 5.07% solution is iso-osmotic with serum. Solutions are **sterilised** by filtration. **Store** in airtight containers. Protect from light.

Incompatibility. Particulate matter was observed within 2 hours when 1 ml of commercial injection of menadione sodium bisulphite was mixed with 5 ml of sterile water and 1 ml of commercial injection solutions of phenytoin sodium or promazine hydrochloride.— R. Misgen, *Am. J. Hosp. Pharm.*, 1965, *22*, 92.

Stability. On prolonged storage, solutions of menadione sodium bisulphite became yellow and a precipitate was formed, decomposition being accelerated by heat and light; solutions were most stable below pH 2.5. The addition of sodium chloride improved the stability of the injection; the breakdown to menadione and sodium bisulphite was prevented by adding 0.2% of sodium metabisulphite. When solutions containing added sodium metabisulphite were stored under an inert gas, the yellow colour and precipitate did not appear unless the ampoules were stored in sunlight; under these conditions, however, the rate of conversion to inactive 2-methyl-1,4-naphthoquinone-3-sulphonate was increased. Solutions which contained 0.2% of sodium metabisulphite and 0.7% of sodium chloride, sterilised by filtration and filled into ampoules under air, were shown to have a shelf-life of 2½ years at 20° or 1½ years at 30°.— Shu-yuan Yeh and G. A. Wiese, *Drug Stand.*, 1958, *26*, 22.

Adverse Effects. Hyperbilirubinaemia has been reported in infants given menadione sodium bisulphite, for further details see under Menadione, p.1666.
Menadione sodium bisulphite did not cause haemolysis in Chinese patients with glucose-6-phosphate dehydrogenase deficiency.— T. K. Chan *et al.*, *Br. med. J.*, 1976, *2*, 1227.

Uses. Menadione sodium bisulphite is a water-soluble derivative of menaphthone. It has been mainly replaced by phytomenadione (see p.1666).
Doses of 1 to 2 mg have been given subcutaneously or intramuscularly, with larger doses if necessary. It has also been given by mouth.

Preparations

Menadione Sodium Bisulfite Injection *(U.S.P.)*. A sterile solution of menadione sodium bisulfite *U.S.P.* in Water for Injections. pH 2 to 4. The label indicates the content of $C_{11}H_9NaO_5S,3H_2O$ and of $NaHSO_3$.

Menaphthone Sodium Bisulphite Injection *(B.P. 1963)*. Menaph. Sod. Bisulphite Inj. A sterile solution of menadione sodium bisulphite in Water for Injections containing 0.2% of sodium metabisulphite. Protect from light.

Proprietary Names

K Thrombin *(Fawns & McAllan, Austral.)*; Nuvit *(Propan, S.Afr.)*.

7908-f

Menatetrenone. Menatetren. 2-Methyl-3-(3,7,11,15-tetramethylhexadeca-2,6,10,14-tetraenyl)-1,4-naphthoquinone.
$C_{31}H_{40}O_2=444.7$.

CAS — 863-61-6.

Yellow crystals or oily liquid. Practically **insoluble** in water.

Uses. Menatetrenone has the typical properties of phytomenadione (see p.1665) and is used for the same purposes. It has been given in doses of 10 to 20 mg by intramuscular or slow intravenous injection.

Proprietary Names

Kaytwo, Kephton-Two (both *Jap.*).

7909-d

Vitamin K_5 Hydrochloride. 4-Amino-2-methyl-1-naphthol hydrochloride.
$C_{11}H_{11}NO,HCl=209.7$.

CAS — 130-24-5.

Vitamin K_5 hydrochloride has the general properties of vitamin K and has been given in doses equivalent to 1 to 5 mg of vitamin K_5 by subcutaneous, intramuscular, or intravenous injection.

7910-c

Vitamin P

The name vitamin P was formerly applied to a substance claimed to increase the resistance of the capillaries and reduce their permeability to red blood cells. This name has since been abandoned because all substances having vitamin P activity are flavone derivatives, generally described as bioflavonoids.
Compounds claimed to possess such activity include hesperidin (see p.1717), rutin (see p.1752), and troxerutin (see p.1767).
The source, actions, and uses of compounds with bioflavonoid activity.— *Br. med. J.*, 1969, *1*, 235.

7911-k

Multivitamin Preparations

WARNING. Excessive dosage of vitamin A and D can lead to hypervitaminosis: see under Adverse Effects of Vitamin D, p.1657, and Adverse Effects of Vitamin A, p.1636. When multivitamin preparations are prescribed, allowance should be made for vitamins obtained from other sources.

Decavitamin Capsules *(U.S.P.)*. Each capsule contains not less than the labelled amounts of vitamin A (as retinol), vitamin D (as ergocalciferol or cholecalciferol), ascorbic acid or its equivalent as sodium ascorbate, calcium pantothenate or its equivalent as racemic calcium pantothenate, dexpanthenol, or racemic panthenol, cyanocobalamin, folic acid, nicotinamide, pyridoxine hydrochloride, riboflavine, thiamine hydrochloride or its equivalent as thiamine mononitrate, and a suitable form of alpha tocopherol. Store in airtight containers. Protect from light. **Decavitamin Tablets** (*U.S.P.*) contain the same ingredients. Protect from light.

Hexavitamin Capsules *(U.S.P.)*. Each capsule contains not less than 5000 units of vitamin A (as retinol), 400 units of vitamin D (as ergocalciferol, cholecalciferol, or from natural sources), 75 mg of ascorbic acid or the equivalent amount of sodium ascorbate, 2 mg of thiamine hydrochloride or an equivalent amount of thiamine mononitrate, 3 mg of riboflavine, and 20 mg of nicotinamide. Store in airtight containers. Protect from light. **Hexavitamin Tablets** (*U.S.P.*) contain the same ingredients. Store in airtight containers.

Vitamins Capsules *(B.P.C. 1973)*. Capsulae Vitaminorum. Each contains vitamin A 2500 units, thiamine hydrochloride 1 mg, riboflavine 500 µg, nicotinamide 7.5 mg, ascorbic acid 15 mg, and vitamin D 300 units. The shells may be coloured. Store in a cool place. Protect from light. *Dose.* 1 or 2 capsules daily.

Proprietary Multivitamin Preparations

Abidec Drops *(Parke, Davis, UK)*. A solution containing in each 0.6 ml vitamin A 4000 units, vitamin D 400 units, thiamine hydrochloride 1 mg, riboflavine 400 µg, nicotinamide 5 mg, ascorbic acid 50 mg, and pyridoxine hydrochloride 500 µg. *Dose.* Infants under 1 year 0.3 ml, children 0.6 ml daily.

Abidec Capsules *(Parke, Davis, UK)*. Each contains vitamin A 4000 units, vitamin D 400 units, thiamine hydrochloride 1 mg, riboflavine 1 mg, pyridoxine hydrochloride 500 µg, nicotinamide 10 mg, and ascorbic acid 25 mg. *Dose.* 1 capsule daily.

Adexolin Vitamin Drops *(Farley, UK)*. A sugar-free water-miscible solution containing in 1 ml vitamin A (as palmitate) 5250 units, vitamin D (as ergocalciferol) 1400 units, and ascorbic acid 105 mg; and on the basis of 35 drops per ml, 150 units, 40 units, and 3 mg respectively per drop. *Dose.* Children, 0 to 5 years, 10 drops daily; over 5 years, 5 drops daily.

Calavite *(Carlton Laboratories, UK)*. Tablets each containing vitamin A 4000 units, thiamine hydrochloride 500 µg, riboflavine 100 µg, nicotinamide 20 mg, ascorbic acid 15 mg, and ergocalciferol 12.5 µg.

Calcimax *(Wallace Mfg Chem., UK: Farillon, UK)*. Syrup containing in each 5 ml thiamine hydrochloride 500 µg, riboflavine 125 µg, pyridoxine hydrochloride 125 µg, cyanocobalamin 0.125 µg, ascorbic acid 5 mg, ergocalciferol 400 units, nicotinamide 2 mg, calcium pantothenate 125 µg, and calcium glycine hydrochloride 500 mg. Calcium and vitamin supplement. *Dose.* 20 ml in water twice daily; children, 5 to 10 ml thrice daily.

Children's Vitamin Drops *(Hough, Hoseason, UK)*. A solution containing in 1 ml (equivalent to 35 drops) vitamin A 5000 units, vitamin D (as ergocalciferol) 2000 units, and ascorbic acid 150 mg. *Dose.* 5 drops daily.

Concavit *(Wallace Mfg Chem., UK: Farillon, UK)*. **Capsules** each containing vitamin A 5000 units, thiamine hydrochloride 2.5 mg, riboflavine 2.5 mg, pyridoxine hydrochloride 1 mg, ascorbic acid 40 mg, cyanocobalamin 5 µg, ergocalciferol 500 units, vitamin E 2 units, calcium pantothenate 5 mg, and nicotinamide 20 mg. **Drops** containing in each 0.5 ml and **Syrup** containing in each 5 ml vitamin A 5000 units, thiamine hydrochloride 2 mg, riboflavine 1 mg, pyridoxine hydrochloride 1 mg, ascorbic acid 50 mg, cyanocobalamin 5 µg, ergocalciferol 500 units, dexpanthenol 2 mg, and nicotinamide 12.5 mg. *Dose.* 1 or 2 capsules, 1 ml of drops, or 10 ml of syrup daily; children, 5 ml of syrup daily.

Dalivit *(Paines & Byrne, UK)*. **Capsules** each containing vitamin A 10 000 units, vitamin D 1000 units, thiamine mononitrate 3 mg, riboflavine 3 mg, pyridoxine hydrochloride 1 mg, ascorbic acid 75 mg, nicotinamide 25 mg, and calcium pantothenate 5 mg. **Drops** containing in each 0.6 ml vitamin A 5000 units, vitamin D 400 units, thiamine hydrochloride 1 mg, riboflavine 400 µg, pyridoxine hydrochloride 500 µg, ascorbic acid 50 mg, and nicotinamide 5 mg. **Syrup** containing in each 5 ml vitamin A 5000 units, vitamin D 1000 units, thiamine hydrochloride 2.5 mg, riboflavine 1 mg, pyridoxine hydrochloride 1 mg, ascorbic acid 25 mg, nicotinamide 10 mg, and calcium pantothenate 5 mg. *Dose.* 1 capsule or 15 ml of syrup daily; children up to 1 year, 0.3 ml of drops, over 1 year, 0.6 ml.

Eso-Tabs *(Southon-Horton, UK)*. Tablets each containing vitamin A 6000 units, thiamine hydrochloride 1 mg, riboflavine 500 µg, nicotinamide 10 mg, biotin 10 µg, pyridoxine hydrochloride 100 µg, ascorbic acid 20 mg, vitamin D 400 units, dried ferrous sulphate 500 µg, anhydrous manganese sulphate 500 µg, and anhydrous copper sulphate 100 µg. *Dose.* 1 tablet daily.

Esotone Tablets *(Southon-Horton, UK)*. Each contains vitamin A 4500 units, vitamin D 450 units, and ascorbic acid 30 mg. *Dose.* 1 tablet daily.

Forceval *(Unigreg, UK: Vestric, UK)*. Capsules each containing vitamin A (as retinol) 5000 units, vitamin D (as cholecalciferol) 600 units, tocopheryl acetate 10 mg, thiamine mononitrate 10 mg, riboflavine 5 mg, pyridoxine hydrochloride 500 µg, cyanocobalamin 2 µg, ascorbic acid 50 mg, nicotinamide 20 mg, calcium pantothenate 2 mg, calcium 70 mg, L-lysine hydrochloride 60 mg, inositol 60 mg, choline bitartrate 40 mg, iron 10 mg, copper 500 µg, phosphorus 55 mg, magnesium 2 mg, potassium 3 mg, zinc 500 μg, iodine 100 μg, and manganese 500 μg. *Dose.* 1 capsule daily.

Gevral Capsules *(Lederle, UK).* Each contains vitamin A acetate 5000 units, vitamin D 500 units, cyanocobalamin 1 μg, thiamine mononitrate 5 mg, riboflavine 5 mg, nicotinamide 15 mg, pyridoxine hydrochloride 500 μg, calcium pantothenate 5 mg, choline bitartrate 50 mg, inositol 50 mg, ascorbic acid 50 mg, vitamin E (as *d*-alpha tocopheryl acetate) 10 units, L-lysine monohydrochloride 25 mg, iron (as ferrous fumarate) 10 mg, iodine (as potassium iodide) 100 μg, calcium (as calcium hydrogen phosphate) 145 mg, phosphorus (as calcium hydrogen phosphate) 110 mg, copper (as oxide) 1 mg, manganese (as dioxide) 1 mg, magnesium (as oxide) 1 mg, potassium (as sulphate) 5 mg, and zinc (as oxide) 500 μg. *Dose.* 1 daily.

Juvel *(Bencard, UK).* **Tablets** each containing vitamin A 5000 units, vitamin D 500 units, thiamine hydrochloride 2.5 mg, riboflavine 2.5 mg, pyridoxine hydrochloride 2.5 mg, nicotinamide 50 mg, and ascorbic acid 50 mg. **Elixir** containing four-fifths of the above amounts in each 5 ml (suggested diluent, syrup). *Dose.* 1 tablet or 5 ml of elixir daily; children under 2 years, 2.5 ml.

Ketovite *(Paines & Byrne, UK).* **Tablets** each containing thiamine hydrochloride 1 mg, riboflavine 1 mg, pyridoxine hydrochloride 330 μg, nicotinamide 3.3 mg, calcium pantothenate 1.16 mg, ascorbic acid 16.6 mg, alpha tocopheryl acetate 5 mg, acetomenaphthone 500 μg, inositol 50 mg, biotin 170 μg, and folic acid 250 μg; and **Supplement Liquid** containing in each 5 ml vitamin A 2500 units, vitamin D 400 units, choline chloride 150 mg, and cyanocobalamin 12.5 μg. For use in phenylketonuria and other disorders of amino-acid or disaccharide metabolism. *Dose.* 1 tablet thrice daily and 5 ml of supplement liquid daily.

Multibionta *(E. Merck, UK).* Ampoules of 10 ml each containing vitamin A 10 000 units, ascorbic acid 500 mg, dexpanthenol 25 mg, nicotinamide 100 mg, pyridoxine hydrochloride 15 mg, riboflavine sodium phosphate 10 mg, thiamine hydrochloride 50 mg, and tocopheryl acetate 5 mg. *Dose.* 10 ml daily in an intravenous infusion.

Multivite *(Duncan, Flockhart, UK).* Pellets each containing vitamin A 2500 units, vitamin D 250 units, thiamine hydrochloride 500 μg, and ascorbic acid 12.5 mg. *Dose.* 2 pellets daily; children, 1 pellet.

Orovite 7 *(Bencard, UK).* Granules containing in each sachet vitamin A palmitate 2500 units, ascorbic acid 60 mg, ergocalciferol 100 units, nicotinamide 18 mg, pyridoxine hydrochloride 2 mg, riboflavine sodium phosphate 1.7 mg, and thiamine mononitrate 1.4 mg. *Dose.* The contents of 1 sachet, dispersed in water, daily.

For other Orovite Preparations, see p.1653.

Polyvite Capsules *(Medo Chemicals, UK).* Each contains vitamin A 4500 units, ergocalciferol 11 μg, thiamine hydrochloride 2.5 mg, riboflavine 1.5 mg, pyridoxine hydrochloride 1.5 mg, calcium pantothenate 2 mg, nicotinamide 15 mg, and ascorbic acid 30 mg. *Dose.* 1 or 2 capsules daily.

Supplementary Vitamin Tablets *(Cow & Gate, UK).* Each contains most of the vitamins and minerals normally present in human milk and cows' milk, and sucrose; vitamins A and D are omitted to allow flexibility of dosage of these vitamins, and sodium, calcium, lactose, and galactose are not present in significant amounts. For supplementing specialised infant foods of a synthetic character lacking vitamins and trace elements, particularly Edosol, Galactomin, and Locasol. *Dose.* Up to 4 months, 1 tablet per feed; 4 to 8 months, 2 tablets per feed; over 8 months, 3 tablets per feed.

Tonivitan Capsules *(Medo Chemicals, UK).* Each contains vitamin A 4500 units, thiamine hydrochloride 1 mg, nicotinic acid 15 mg, ascorbic acid 15 mg, ergocalciferol 600 units, and dried yeast 50 mg. *Dose.* 1 to 3 capsules thrice daily.

Tri-Vitamin Dellipsoids D 21A *(Pilsworth, UK).* Tablets each containing thiamine hydrochloride 150 units, ascorbic acid 250 units, and vitamin D 500 units.

Vi-Daylin *(Abbott, UK).* Contains in each 5 ml vitamin A palmitate 3000 units, ergocalciferol 400 units, thiamine hydrochloride 1.5 mg, riboflavine 1.2 mg, ascorbic acid 50 mg, nicotinamide 10 mg, and pyridoxine hydrochloride 1 mg. *Dose.* Children 5 to 10 ml daily; infants, 2.5 to 5 ml.

Vitavel Syrup *(Bencard, UK).* A syrup containing in each 5 ml vitamin A 4000 units, vitamin D 300 units, thiamine hydrochloride 800 μg, and ascorbic acid 16 mg, with purified dextrose 25% w/v, in a flavoured basis containing sucrose (suggested diluent, syrup). *Dose.* 5 to 10 ml daily; infants, 2.5 to 5 ml in water.

A multivitamin preparation was also formerly marketed in Great Britain under the proprietary name Vita-Six (*Paines & Byrne*).

Water

7700-g

Water. Aqua; Aqua Communis; Aqua Fontana; Aqua Potabilis; Eau Potable; Wasser. H_2O=18.015.

CAS — 7732-18-5.

In *Martindale,* as in the *B.P.* and *Eur. P.,* the term 'water' refers to Purified Water (see p.1670). In the *B.P.C. 1973* the term 'water' refers to suitable potable water or, if this is not available, freshly boiled and cooled Purified Water; this may be called Water for Preparations.

Potable water is derived mainly from surface sources such as lakes, rivers, and streams, and from underground sources such as wells and springs. In emergencies it may be obtained directly from the sea either by distillation or by demineralisation with ion-exchange materials. All statutory water undertakings are required to provide a supply of water which is both palatable and safe to drink; it must be clear, colourless, odourless, and tasteless, and it must be free from toxic substances, pathogenic organisms, and excessive amounts of substances in solution not normally detectable by the unaided senses.

The chemical composition of potable water is variable and the nature and concentration of the impurities in it depend upon the source from which it is drawn. In any water obtained from a surface source, traces of organic matter are present. Algae, bacteria, viruses, and pyrogens may occasionally be present. In addition, ammonia, residual chlorine, and traces of metals may be detected.

There are international standards for the quality of water intended for human consumption. Toxic substances such as arsenic, barium, cadmium, chromium, copper, cyanide, lead, and selenium may constitute a danger to health if present in drinking water in excess of the recommended concentrations.

Fluoride is regarded as an essential constituent of drinking water but may endanger health if present in excess—see Sodium Fluoride, p.700.

Ingestion of water containing 45 mg or more per litre of nitrates may cause methaemoglobinaemia in infants.

The use of tap water containing metal ions (such as aluminium, copper, and lead), fluoride, or chloramine, for dialysis may be hazardous.

A hard water contains soluble calcium and magnesium salts, which cause the precipitation of soap and prevent its lathering and form scale and sludge in boilers, water pipes, and autoclaves. Temporary hardness in water is due to the presence of bicarbonates which are converted to insoluble carbonates on heating. Permanent hardness is due to dissolved chlorides, nitrates, and sulphates, which do not form a precipitate on heating.

Without further purification, potable water may be unsuitable for certain pharmaceutical purposes. For example, the concentration of calcium present in water affects the sol viscosities and gel strengths of alginate and pectin dispersions, the colour of some mixtures may be affected by the pH of the water employed, and precipitates may be formed when hard water is used. In such instances, purified water should always be used.

Adverse effects associated with potable water. Analysis of the infant mortality-rates in 61 county boroughs demonstrated an association between high infant mortality and low calcium content of drinking water.— M. D. Crawford *et al., Lancet,* 1972, *1,* 988.

In a study in the USA the incidence of urolithiasis was greater in soft water areas.— D. Churchill *et al., Ann. intern. Med.,* 1978, *88,* 513.

A report of 2 patients who developed angio-oedema and urticaria after drinking tap water.— D. J. Rapp (letter), *J. Am. med. Ass.,* 1972, *221,* 305.

A report of allergic reactions caused by endotoxin in tap water obtained from a small lake heavily contaminated with Gram-negative bacteria.— A. Muittari *et al.* (letter), *Lancet,* 1980, *2,* 89.

A report of aquagenic pruritus in 3 patients; the condition was probably common.— M. W. Greaves *et al., Br. med. J.,* 1981, *282,* 2008.

Carcinogenicity. A discussion on whether chlorinated water is associated with an increased cancer risk.— *Lancet,* 1981, *1,* 1142.

Effects associated with haemodialysis. During haemodialysis solutes are transferred from the water solution into the blood at the same time as impurities are removed from the blood. Since excessive amounts of solute may be absorbed from the large volume of water used each week, some units deionise tap water to remove the very small amounts of iron, calcium, magnesium, and other natural or added solutes, such as fluoride, before it is used in dialysis.— *Br. dent. J.,* 1979, *147,* 246.

Both plasma and red blood cells readily took up lead from potable water during haemodialysis. Dialysis with 200 to 500 litres of fluid containing 100 µg per litre of lead twice or thrice weekly could expose the patient to over 6 mg of lead daily.— J. Blomfield (letter), *Lancet,* 1973, *2,* 666.

References to bone disease associated with haemodialysis.— A. Rashid *et al., Med. Instrumn,* 1974, *8,* 204 (attributed to the presence of fluoride and other elements); M. K. Ward *et al., Lancet,* 1978, *1,* 841 (osteomalacia possibly associated with the aluminium content of water supplies).

See also under Aluminium, p.926.

For reports of haemolysis occurring in patients undergoing haemodialysis with potable water containing chloramine, see Chloramine, p.554.

Effects of fluoride in potable water. Analysis of the standardised mortality-rates in 34 areas did not reveal any significant correlation between mortality and the natural fluoride content of the water supplies.— J. M. Nixon and R. G. Carpenter, *Lancet,* 1974, *2,* 1068.

See also under Sodium Fluoride, p.700.

Effects of lead in potable water. A comprehensive survey of lead in drinking water in Great Britain, 1975–76.— Report of an Interdepartmental Working Group, *Pollution Paper No. 12,* London, HM Stationery Office, 1977.

A proposed maximum limit for lead in running drinking water was 50 µg per litre.— *Chronicle Wld Hlth Org.,* 1978, *32,* 42 and 132.

Reports of excessive lead concentrations in water, attributed to lead water pipes and storage tanks, and the correlation between lead concentrations in water and blood: A. D. Beattie *et al., Br. med. J.,* 1972, *2,* 488 (blood-lead concentrations above 400 µg per litre); D. Malcolm (letter), *ibid.,* 1972, *4,* 366 (criticism); A. D. Beattie *et al., Br. med. J.,* 1972, *2,* 491 (lead concentrations in water of 108 µg per litre); P. C. Elwood *et al.* (letter), *Lancet,* 1976, *1,* 1295 (a slight relationship between blood-lead concentrations and high water-lead concentrations); H. F. Thomas and P. C. Elwood (letter), *Lancet,* 1978, *2,* 109 (flushing a domestic tap for 1 minute substantially reduced lead concentrations in water in homes with lead piping).

An association between the lead content of water and mental retardation in a comparison of 77 retarded children and 77 controls.— A. D. Beattie *et al., Lancet,* 1975, *1,* 589. See also M. R. Moore *et al., ibid.,* 1977, *1,* 717. The lead content of domestic water in homes where 41 educationally subnormal children had been born was not significantly different from that in 82 control homes.— P. C. Elwood *et al.* (letter), *ibid.,* 1976, *1,* 590.

Further references to lead in the water supply: M. D. Crawford and D. G. Clayton, *Br. med. J.,* 1973, *2,* 21 (correlation with lead in rib bone); B. C. Campbell *et al., Br. med. J.,* 1977, *1,* 482 (elevated serum-urea concentrations and hyperuricaemia associated with excessive lead in the domestic water supply).

See also under Effects on the Cardiovascular System.

Effects on the cardiovascular system. Comment on epidemiological studies linking mortality from cardiovascular disease with the quality of drinking water. Studies in the USA and Great Britain have shown an inverse relationship between water hardness and mortality with soft water areas having higher death-rates from heart disease, although findings in other countries have varied. Hard and soft water differ in the concentration of many trace elements as well as of calcium and it has been suggested that the factor involved may be one or more of these elements.— *Br. med. J.,* 1978, *1,* 264. See also *Chronicle Wld Hlth Org.,* 1973, *27,* 534; *Lancet,* 1980, *1,* 555.

Studies on the relationship between cardiovascular disease and the softness of water: M. D. Crawford *et al., Lancet,* 1971, *2,* 327 (positive correlation between cardiovascular deaths and decreasing water hardness); F. W. Stitt *et al., ibid.,* 1973, *1,* 122 (higher mean heart-rates, plasma-cholesterol concentrations, and mean blood pressure, in the 56 to 65 years age-group, in men living in soft water areas); E. G. Knox, *ibid.,* 1465 (an inverse relationship between deaths due to ischaemic heart disease and calcium intake, and a positive correlation with fat and vitamin-D intake); S. P. A. Allwright *et al., ibid.,* 1974, *2,* 860 (no association); P. C. Elwood *et al., ibid.,* 1470 (an apparent association between calcium and mortality); M. L. Bierenbaum *et al., ibid.,* 1975, *1,* 1008 (a higher incidence of cardiovascular deaths and increased hypertension in a hard water area, possibly related to increased serum-cadmium concentrations); B. Chipperfield *et al., ibid.,* 1976, *1,* 121 (a lower magnesium/potassium ratio in normal heart muscle in soft water areas); I. Gyárfás *et al., Népegészségügy,* 1976, *57,* 342, per *Abstr. Hyg.,* 1977, *52,* 386; P. C. Elwood *et al., Br. J. prev. soc. Med.,* 1977, *31,* 178; Arterial Hypertension, Report of a WHO Expert Committee, *Tech. Rep. Ser. Wld Hlth Org. No. 628,* 1978, p. 19 (evidence of an association between high blood pressure and soft demineralised water); B. Chipperfield and J. R. Chipperfield, *Lancet,* 1979, *2,* 709 (metal and water content of normal heart muscle in hard water and soft water districts); E. A. Cameron and R. B. Singh (letter), *ibid.,* 1084; R. Masironi *et al., Bull. Wld Hlth Org.,* 1979, *57,* 291 (a negative correlation between water hardness and the incidence of myocardial infarction); S. J. Pocock *et al., Br. med. J.,* 1980, *280,* 1243 (British Regional Heart Study: a significant negative association between water hardness and cardiovascular mortality); C. G. Caro and M. J. Lever (letter), *Lancet,* 1981, *1,* 50.

An epidemiological study in north-west Wales failed to support an association between lead in water and death from cardiovascular disease or cancer.— P. C. Elwood *et al.* (letter), *Lancet,* 1976, *1,* 748. A positive correlation between blood-lead concentrations, tap-water lead concentration, and hypertension in men in the west of Scotland but not in women who had no correlation between lead and hypertension.— D. G. Beevers *et al., ibid.,* *2,* 1.

Methaemoglobinaemia. Cyanosis in an infant was possibly due to the preparation of feeds with water which had been subjected to prolonged boiling. The concentration of nitrate in tap water was increased by 30% by boiling for 5 minutes; nitrate could be reduced by bacteria to nitrite with consequent methaemoglobinaemia.— *Community Med.,* 1972, *127,* 133.

Water intoxication. A discussion on water intoxication induced deliberately. Symptoms are due to intracellular overhydration; headache and vomiting may be followed by confusion, disorientation, and restlessness progressing to convulsions and coma. The excess water is distributed throughout the total body water (about 42 litres in a 70-kg man) and the plasma-sodium concentration needs to fall below 120 mmol (120 mEq) per litre before symptoms are likely. Mild symptoms are best treated by withdrawing water. More severe symptoms, especially the onset of stupor, are treated with hypertonic saline, a 5% solution of sodium chloride being given at a rate of 1 ml per minute until there is improvement; more than 250 ml is rarely necessary. The substantial increase in plasma volume resulting from this treatment may precipitate heart failure and pulmonary oedema in susceptible patients and frusemide in association with a slow infusion of hypertonic saline may be preferable in such patients.— *Br. med. J.,* 1979, *1,* 913.

Treatment with an aerosol of water was commonly used in the treatment of croup, asthma, and respiratory distress syndrome in infants and children. Water intoxication could occur in small infants due to water absorbed during the nebulisation process. In 24 hours a gain in body water of 200 to 400 ml could occur using an ultrasonic nebuliser.— R. L. Harris and H. D. Riley,

J. Am. med. Ass., 1967, *201*, 953.

Acute water intoxication in a 10-month-old girl following the consumption of about 1 litre of water in 2½ hours. Convulsions were not controlled by diazepam but she recovered within a few hours of the intravenous infusion of 300 ml of 2% sodium chloride injection.— A. Etzioni *et al.*, *Archs Dis. Childh.*, 1979, *54*, 551.

Further reports of water intoxication: T. H. Bewley, *Br. med. J.*, 1964, *2*, 864; S. Dugan and M. A. Holliday, *Pediatrics*, 1967, *39*, 418; E. R. Alexander *et al.*, *Br. med. J.*, 1973, *1*, 89; D. Maclean *et al.*, *Postgrad. med. J.*, 1976, *52*, 532; J. G. Mortimer, *Archs Dis. Childh.*, 1980, *55*, 401 (acute water intoxication as a manifestation of child abuse).

Water-borne infections. An assessment of the public health importance of human viruses in water, waste water, and soil, including sources of infection and methods for the monitoring and removal of viruses. It was concluded that the contamination of water and soil by waste water and human faeces containing enteric viruses may pose real public health problems. There have been reports of water-borne viral hepatitis A and gastroenteritis and the constant exposure of large population groups to even relatively small numbers of enteric viruses may lead to an endemic state of viral dissemination in the community which can and should be prevented. Enteric viruses may be present in water despite conventional water treatment considered adequate for protection against bacterial pathogens. It is recommended that wherever possible drinking water should be free from human enteric viruses and when derived from virus-contaminated sources should be treated by methods of proven high efficiency for removing or inactivating viruses and not only bacteria. Coastal bathing and shellfish growing areas should be protected from contamination by waste water and sludge and control procedures should be instituted when waste water or sludge is used for irrigation or fertilisation.— Report of a WHO Scientific Group on Human Viruses in Water, Wastewater and Soil, *Tech. Rep. Ser. Wld Hlth Org. No. 639*, 1979. Criticism.— D. R. Gamble, *Lancet*, 1979, *1*, 425. Reports and discussions on the viral contamination of water: J. L. Melnick *et al.*, *Bull. Wld Hlth Org.*, 1978, *56*, 499; *Br. med. J.*, 1978, *2*, 1662; D. M. Morens *et al.*, *Lancet*, 1979, *1*, 964 (gastro-enteritis); T. F. Smith, *Ann. intern. Med.*, 1979, *91*, 119.

Further reports on the contamination of potable water and water-borne infections: *Lancet*, 1980, *1*, 1176 (giardiasis); J. O'H. Tobin *et al.*, *Lancet*, 1980, *2*, 118 (legionnaires' disease); R. Feachem (letter), *Lancet*, 1980, *2*, 255 (faecal bacteria); P. J. Redding and P. W. McWalter, *Br. med. J.*, 1980, *281*, 275 (*Pseudomonas fluorescens* in distilled water used for humidifiers); S. P. Fisher-Hoch *et al.*, *Lancet*, 1981, *1*, 932 (legionnaires' disease).

Cold urticaria. Although 12 of 19 patients with disabling cold urticaria were successfully rendered cold-tolerant with a regimen of 5-minute cold baths in hospital, subsequent experience in out-patients argued against its use as a routine treatment.— A. K. Black *et al.* (letter), *Lancet*, 1979, *2*, 964.

Heat stroke. The treatment of heat stroke by immersing the patient in ice cold water or by cold sprays induces vasoconstriction which reduces heat transport from body core to skin, induces shivering which raises temperature, and is distressing to the conscious patient. A technique of keeping the whole of the skin surface wet by atomised spraying of ordinary tap water while holding the skin temperature above 32°, and so maintaining an active circulation from core to skin surface is considered superior. This is achieved by blowing dry warm air over the body at the same time as the skin is sprayed. Studies in volunteers have indicated that a 2° fall in core temperature can be achieved at a steady rate in less than 7 minutes.— J. S. Weiner and M. Khogali (letter), *Lancet*, 1979, *1*, 1135. The effectiveness of the warm air spray method in which there is good air circulation and air temperature at the body surface is 30° to 35° during spraying was confirmed in patients suffering from heat stroke during the Mecca pilgrimages in 1978 and 1979.— *idem*, 1980, *1*, 507. Rapid cooling was achieved in 18 hyperpyrexial patients; 16 recovered and 2, who were diabetic, died.— M. Khogali and J. S. Weiner, *ibid.*, *2*, 276.

References to the use of ice packs in the treatment of heat stroke or heat exhaustion: *Lancet*, 1979, *2*, 1344 (heat exhaustion); C. L. Sprung and M. J. Hauser (letter), *Lancet*, 1980, *2*, 642 (heat stroke).

Herpes. Application of ice-cubes to treat recurrent herpes labialis had provided beneficial results in 14 patients. Treatment involved continuous application for 90 to 120 minutes within 24 hours of the prodrome.— S. Danziger (letter), *Lancet*, 1978, *1*, 103. See also D. R. Zimmerman (letter), *ibid.*, *2*, 1260; A. S. Russell (letter), *ibid.*, 1979, *1*, 325; I. J. Wilson (letter), *ibid.*, 613.

Muscle damage. Muscles damaged by crush injury and unresponsive to electrical stimulation were stroked with ice. There was slight contraction in the affected leg muscles.— M. Swaby, *Physiotherapy*, 1975, *61*, 191.

7701-q

Purified Water *(B.P., Eur. P.)*. Aqua Purificata.

Pharmacopoeias. In *Br.*, *Eur.*, *Fr.*, *Ger.*, *Ind.*, *It.*, *Jug.*, *Nord.*, *Pol.*, and *U.S. Fr.* also includes distilled water. *Arg.*, *Aust.*, *Mex.*, *Port.*, *Rus.*, and *Span.* include only distilled water; *Cz.*, *Hung.*, *Int.*, *Jap.*, *Neth.*, *Roum.*, *Swiss*, and *Turk.* include demineralised water and distilled water; *Cz.*, *Jap.*, and *Nord.* include sterile purified water.

A clear, colourless, odourless, and tasteless liquid prepared from suitable potable water either by distillation or by treatment with ion-exchange materials or any other suitable method. *U.S.P.* specifies pH 5 to 7. **Store** in airtight containers which do not alter the properties of the water.

The *B.P.* directs that when Distilled Water is prescribed or demanded Purified Water be dispensed or supplied.

Purified Water is unsuitable for preparing injections; for this purpose Water for Injections must be used.

PREPARATION BY DEIONISATION. By passing potable water through columns of anionic and cationic ion-exchange resins, ionisable substances can be removed, producing a water of high specific resistance. Colloidal and non-ionisable impurities such as pyrogens may not be removed by this process. For further information see under Ion-exchange Resins: Purification of Water, p.869.

PREPARATION BY DISTILLATION. In this process water is separated as vapour from non-volatile impurities and is subsequently condensed. In practice, non-volatile impurities may be carried into the distillate by entrainment unless a suitable baffle is fitted to the still.

Odour, frothing, adsorption in ultraviolet light, and low surface tension in samples of distilled water were frequently associated with the use of plastics in the distillation apparatus.— A. D. Bangham and M. W. Hill (letter), *Nature*, 1972, *237*, 408.

For reviews of the use of deionised water in haemodialysis solutions, see *Recent Developments in Haemodialysis*, Report of a Conference at London, 1973, Romford, Macarthys Laboratories Ltd and Elga Products Ltd, 1973.

A discussion of energy-conserving methods for the production and distribution of purified water.— J. D. Benedictus, *Merrell-National, USA*, *J. parent. Drug Ass.*, 1978, *32*, 26. See also A. L. Kunz, *Bull. parent. Drug Ass.*, 1973, *27*, 266 (reverse osmosis); *ibid.*, 1974, *28*, 64–87 (distillation; filtration; ozonisation; reverse osmosis).

7702-p

Water for Injections *(B.P., Eur. P.)*. Aqua pro Injectionibus; Aq. pro Inj.; Water for Injection *(U.S.P.)*; Aqua ad Iniectabilia; Aqua ad Injectionem; Aqua Injectabilis; Aqua pro Injectione; Eau pour Préparations Injectables; Wasser für Injektionszwecke.

Pharmacopoeias. In all pharmacopoeias examined except *Braz.* and *Roum.*

U.S.P. also includes Sterile Water for Injection, Sterile Water for Inhalation, Sterile Water for Irrigation, and Bacteriostatic Water for Injection.

Water for Injections (*B.P.*) is sterilised distilled water free from pyrogens; it is prepared by distillation of potable water, purified water, or distilled water from a neutral glass, quartz, or suitable metal still fitted with an efficient device for preventing the entrainment of droplets; the first portion of the distillate is rejected, and the remainder collected in a suitable container and sterilised by autoclaving. The reaction of distilled water is often acidic but the titratable acidity is very low; the *B.P.* and *Eur. P.* specify a limit for acidity and alkalinity.

Water for Injection (*U.S.P.*) is water purified by distillation or by reverse osmosis, pyrogen-free, and containing no added substance. It is intended for use as a solvent in parenteral solutions which are to be sterilised after preparation. Sterile Water for Injection (*U.S.P.*) is the subject of a separate monograph.

When Water for Injections free from carbon dioxide or dissolved air is required for a preparation, the distillate, freshly prepared as above, is boiled for at least 10 minutes with as little exposure to air as possible, cooled, distributed into the final containers, and sterilised by autoclaving. It is used for the preparation of solutions of the soluble salts of weakly acidic substances, since the slight acidity due to dissolved carbon dioxide might cause the formation of a precipitate.

All aqueous injections should be prepared with Water for Injections. For those aqueous injections which are sterilised by heat or by filtration, freshly distilled water collected under the same conditions as given for Water for Injections may be used provided that the final preparation is immediately sterilised.

The preparation of Water for Injection (*U.S.P.*) by reverse osmosis.— C. F. Frith *et al.*, *Bull. parent. Drug Ass.*, 1976, *30*, 118. See also D. L. Juberg *et al.*, *ibid.*, 1977, *31*, 70.

7703-s

Pyrogens

Pyrogens are of bacterial origin and consist of lipids associated with a polysaccharide or protein, or both. They may be found on occasion in tap water and they may be detected in potable or distilled water which has been allowed to stand for some time.

Many pyrogens may not be inactivated by sterilisation processes and it is therefore important that solutions for injection should be prepared with ingredients free from pyrogens and that they should be sterilised as soon as possible after preparation.

The Proceedings of an International Symposium on Pyrogens, London, Pharmaceutical Society of Great Britain, 1975.

A study of the stability, under different conditions, of the International Pyrogen Reference Preparation showed that steaming for 30 minutes caused a loss of at least 52% of activity and autoclaving at 115° for 30 minutes caused almost complete destruction. Refrigeration for 16 weeks at 4° also caused loss, and pyrogens could be removed from solution by a strongly basic anion-exchange resin but were unaffected by a strongly acid cation-exchange resin.— C. H. R. Palmer and T. D. Whittet, *J. Pharm. Pharmac.*, 1961, *13*, 62T.

Heating at 100° for 30 minutes destroyed 92% of a lipopolysaccharide pyrogen from *Staphylococcus aureus*, whilst autoclaving at 115° for 30 minutes destroyed 97%. Passage through columns of 2 ion-exchange resins resulted in absorption of 82 and 84% respectively of pyrogen, whilst storage at 15° to 22° for 10 weeks resulted in 57% loss.— C. H. R. Palmer and T. D. Whittet, *J. Hosp. Pharm.*, 1968, *25*, 7.

Glass or plastic syringes sterilised by gamma irradiation were unlikely to cause pyrogenic responses as a result of pre-sterilisation bacterial contamination.— *Pharm. J.*, 1972, *2*, 368.

Discussions on the preparation of pyrogen-free water.— J. C. Holcombe, *Bull. parent. Drug Ass.*, 1975, *29*, 153; R. Saari *et al.*, *ibid.*, 1977, *31*, 248.

For the use of the Limulus test for pyrogens, see Limulus Test, p.520.

Solutions containing pyrogens cause a febrile reaction if injected.

Bacterial pyrogen has been given by intravenous injection as a test for pituitary-adrenal function.

Pituitary-adrenal function. In 7 healthy subjects plasma concentrations of corticotrophin were in the range 24 to 111 pg per ml, and of corticosteroids 63 to 242 ng per ml. The intravenous injection of pyrogen (*Organon*) 5 ng per kg body-weight substantially increased the plasma concentration of corticotrophin to a mean of 643 pg per ml (range 209 to 1725) and of corticosteroids to a mean of 372 ng per ml (range 223 to 514). After the intravenous injection of insulin 0.15 unit per kg body-weight (to produce a blood-sugar concentration of less than 400 µg per ml) the corresponding values were 256 pg per ml (range 114 to 364) and 267 ng per ml (range 189 to 353). After the intramuscular injection of lypressin 10 pressor units the corresponding values were 95 pg per ml (range 49 to 141) and 235 ng per ml (range 169 to 287). The pituitary-adrenal response to lypressin was best judged by the corticosteroid response, but for insulin and pyrogen the corticotrophin response was a more sensitive indicator.— J. J. Staub *et al.*, *Br. med. J.*, 1973, *1*, 267. See also J. S. Jenkins and W. Else, *Lancet*, 1968, *2*, 940; J. A. Wider *et al.*, *J. Am. med. Ass.*, 1969, *209*, 669.

Part 2

Supplementary Drugs and Other Substances

12300-l

A-124. 3,5-Dibromo-2-methoxybenzyl Alcohol β-Diethylaminoethyl Ether Hydrochloride. 2-(3,5-Dibromo-2-methoxybenzyloxy)triethylamine hydrochloride.
$C_{14}H_{21}Br_2NO_2,HCl=431.6$.

Crystals. M.p. 124° to 127°.

A-124 has a spasmolytic effect on smooth muscle.

12301-y

A-73025. SSHA-73025.

CAS — 64082-61-7.

A semi-synthetic heparin analogue; it is a glycosaminoglycan polysulphate of bovine origin with a molecular weight about half that of heparin. It is suggested that it has a specific action on antithrombin III with less effect than heparin on clotting parameters.

References: D. P. Thomas *et al.* (preliminary communication), *Lancet*, 1977, *1*, 120; D. A. Lane *et al.*, *Br. J. Haemat.*, 1977, *37*, 239; R. Michalski *et al.*, *ibid.*, 247; V. V. Kakkar *et al.* (letter), *Lancet*, 1981, *1*, 1167.

Manufacturers
Luitpold, Ger.

Glycosaminoglycan polysulphate (Arteparon, *Luitpold, Ger.*) is a similar compound which has been used by intra-articular injection in arthritic joints.

References: G. L. Bach *et al.*, *Z. Rheumatol.*, 1977, *36*, 260; E. Rau *et al.*, *ibid.*, 265; S. Santavirta *et al.* (letter), *Br. med. J.*, 1978, *1*, 1140; M. Zbojanová, *Clin. Trials J.*, 1979, *16*, 183.

12303-z

Abrus *(B.P.C. 1934).* Abrus Seed; Indian Liquorice; Jequirity Bean; Jumble Beads; Prayer Beads; Rosary Beans.

CAS — 1393-62-0 (abrin).

The seeds of *Abrus precatorius* (Leguminosae), which contain *N*-methyltryptophan, abric acid, glycyrrhizin, a lipolytic enzyme, and the toxic albumin, abrin.

Abrin is considered responsible for the toxic effects of abrus seeds. Deaths of children have occurred from eating one or more seeds. Toxic effects include gastro-enteritis, haemorrhages, inflammation, necrosis of the liver and kidneys, agglutination and haemolysis of the red blood cells, and convulsions. Treatment is symptomatic.

A report of cases of poisoning with abrus seeds.— M. Hart, *New Engl. J. Med.*, 1963, *268*, 885.

A patient became critically ill after drinking tea in which 1 seed of *Abrus precatorius* had been soaked for 15 minutes.— *J. Am. med. Ass.*, 1969, *207*, 1159.

Inhibition of tumour growth in *animals* by abrin, a protein isolated from *Abrus precatorius*.— J. Lin *et al.* (letter), *Nature*, 1970, *227*, 292.

12304-c

Acarbose. Bay g-5421. *O*-{4-Amino-4,6-dideoxy-*N*-[(1*S*,4*R*,5*S*,6*S*)-4,5,6-trihydroxy-3-hydroxymethylcyclohex-2-enyl]-α-D-glucopyranosyl}-(1→4)-*O*-α-D-glucopyranosyl-(1→4)-D-glucopyranose.
$C_{25}H_{43}NO_{18}=645.6$.

CAS — 56180-94-0.

Acarbose is an inhibitor of glucoside hydrolase which reduces the increase in blood-sugar concentrations after a carbohydrate load. Its possible use in diabetes mellitus is under study.

References: W. F. Caspary, *Lancet*, 1978, *1*, 1231; H. Vierhapper *et al.* (letter), *ibid.*, 1978, *2*, 1386; R. H. Taylor *et al.*, *Gut*, 1978, *19*, A969; J. C. McLoughlin *et al.*, *Lancet*, 1979, *2*, 603 and 808; D. J. A. Jenkins *et al.*, *ibid.*, 924; R. J. Walton *et al.*, *Br. med. J.*, 1979, *1*, 220; D. Sailer and G. Röder, *Arzneimittel-Forsch.*, 1980, *30*, 2182; H. Vierhapper, *Diabetologia*, 1981, *20*, 586.

Manufacturers
Bayer, UK.

12305-k

Aceglatone. 2,5-Di-*O*-acetyl-D-glucaro-1,4:6,3-dilactone.
$C_{10}H_{10}O_8=258.2$.

CAS — 642-83-1.

A white or almost white, odourless, tasteless powder or crystals. M.p. about 192° with decomposition. Practically **insoluble** in water; sparingly soluble in acetone; slightly soluble in alcohol and methyl alcohol; soluble in dimethylformamide.

Aceglatone inhibits the activity of β-glucuronidase and has an anti-inflammatory action. It has been given by mouth to prevent the recurrence of carcinoma of the bladder after surgery. Adverse effects have included anorexia, gastric discomfort, dry skin, and pigmentation.

Proprietary Names
Glucaron *(Chugai, Jap.).*

12306-a

Aceglutamide. N^2-Acetyl-L-glutamine; 2-Acetylamino-L-glutaramic acid.
$C_7H_{12}N_2O_4=188.2$.

CAS — 2490-97-3.

Aceglutamide has been given in an attempt to improve memory and concentration.

Proprietary Names
Acutil-S Italseber *(ISF, Ital.).*

12307-t

Aceglutamide Aluminium. KW-110. A complex of aceglutamide with aluminium hydroxide.

Aceglutamide aluminium is used in the treatment of gastric ulcer.

Proprietary Names
Glumal *(Kyowa, Jap.).*

12308-x

Acemetacin. Bay f-4975; TVX-1322. *O*-[(1-*p*-Chlorobenzoyl-5-methoxy-2-methylindol-3-yl)acetyl]glycolic acid.
$C_{21}H_{18}ClNO_6=415.8$.

CAS — 53164-05-9.

A derivative of indomethacin (see p.257) used in inflammatory and rheumatic disorders.

Proprietary Names
Rantudil *(Tropon, Ger.).*

12302-j

Aceprometazine. 16-64 CB. 10-(2-Dimethylaminopropyl)phenothiazin-2-yl methyl ketone.
$C_{19}H_{22}N_2OS=326.5$.

CAS — 13461-01-3.

Aceprometazine is a phenothiazine compound which has been used as a sedative, usually in conjunction with other tranquillisers such as clorazepate dipotassium or meprobamate. It has been given by mouth or rectally.

14035-b

Acesulfame Potassium. The potassium salt of 6-methyl-1,2,3-oxothiazin-4-(3H)-one 2,2-dioxide.
$C_4H_4KNO_4S=201.2$.

CAS — 33665-90-6 (acesulfame).

White odourless crystalline powder or granules with an intensely sweet taste. A 1% solution in water has a pH of 6.5 to 7.5.

The Food Additives and Contaminants Committee on the review of sweetners in food has recommended that acesulfame potassium be permitted for use as a sweetner in food, other than food manufactured specifically for babies and young children.

12309-r

Acethiamine Hydrochloride. Acetiamine Hydrochloride; Diacethiamine Hydrochloride. *N*-(5-Acetoxy-3-acetylthiopent-2-en-2-yl)-*N*-(4-amino-2-methylpyrimidin-5-ylmethyl)formamide hydrochloride monohydrate.
$C_{16}H_{22}N_4O_4S,HCl,H_2O=420.9$.

CAS — 299-89-8 (acethiamine).

Acethiamine has the general properties of thiamine.

Proprietary Names
Névriton *(Spret-Mauchant, Fr.)*; Thianeuron *(Badische, Ger.).*

12310-j

Acetohydroxamic Acid. AHA.
$C_2H_5NO_2=75.07$.

CAS — 546-88-3.

Acetohydroxamic acid is a specific inhibitor of urease. Its use has been suggested in the treatment of hyperammonaemia and hepatic coma.

References: T. Aoyagi and W. H. J. Summerskill, *Lancet*, 1966, *1*, 296; W. H. J. Summerskill *et al.*, *Gastroenterology*, 1968, *54*, 20; M. Peacock and W. G. Robertson, *Drugs*, 1980, *20*, 225 (use in infected stone disease to prevent the formation of ammonia and alkali from urea).

12311-z

Acetyldihydrocodeine Hydrochloride. 4,5-Epoxy-3-methoxy-9a-methylmorphinan-6-yl acetate hydrochloride.
$C_{20}H_{25}NO_4,HCl=379.9$.

CAS — 3861-72-1 (acetyldihydrocodeine).

Acetyldihydrocodeine hydrochloride has been used for the relief of cough.

Proprietary Names
Acetylcodone *(Bios-Coutelier, Belg.).*

12312-c

Acetylectylurea. *N*-Acetyl-*N'*-(2-ethylisocrotonoyl)urea.
$C_9H_{14}N_2O_3$=198.2.

Acetylectylurea has been used as a sedative.

12313-k

Acetylleucine. Acetyl-DL-leucine; RP-7542. *N*-Acetyl-DL-leucine.
$C_8H_{15}NO_3$=173.2.

Acetylleucine has been tried in the treatment of vertigo. The ethanolamine derivative has been given by injection.

Proprietary Names
Tanganil *(Specia, Fr.).*

12314-a

Acetylphenylhydrazine. Pyrodin; Hydracetin. *N*-Acetyl-*N'*-phenylhydrazine.
$C_8H_{10}N_2O$=150.2.

CAS — 114-83-0.

Colourless odourless crystals. **Soluble** 1 in 50 of water; readily soluble in alcohol.

Acetylphenylhydrazine has similar actions to those of phenylhydrazine (p.1740).

12315-t

Acexamic Acid. CY-153; Acide Acéxamique; Acidum Acexamicum; Epsilon Acetamidocaproic Acid. 6-Acetamidohexanoic acid.
$C_8H_{15}NO_3$=173.2.

CAS — 57-08-9.

Crystals. M.p. about 108°.

Acexamic acid is related structurally to the antifibrinolytic agent aminocaproic acid (p.733) and is used as the sodium or calcium salt. It has been administered topically and by mouth to promote the healing of ulcers and various other lesions.

Proprietary Names
Plastenan (as calcium or sodium salt) *(Armstrong, Arg.; de Bournonville, Belg.; Choay, Fr.; Italfarmaco, Ital.; Boizot, Spain).*

12316-x

Acipimox. K-9321. 5-Methylpyrazine-2-carboxylic acid 4-oxide.
$C_6H_6N_2O_3$=154.1.

CAS — 51037-30-0.

Acipimox has been reported to reduce cholesterol and triglyceride concentrations.

References: L. M. Fuccella *et al.*, *Clin. Pharmac. Ther.*, 1980, *28*, 790.

Manufacturers
Carlo Erba, Ital.

12317-r

Acivicin. AT-125; NSC-163501; U-42126. (αS,5*S*)-α-Amino-3-chloro-2-isoxazolin-5-ylacetic acid.
$C_5H_7ClN_2O_3$=178.6.

CAS — 42228-92-2.

Acivicin is reported to have antineoplastic activity.

Manufacturers
Upjohn, USA.

12318-f

Aclarubicin. Aclacinomycin A; NSC-208734.
$C_{42}H_{53}NO_{15}$=811.9.

CAS — 57576-44-0.

An anthracycline antineoplastic antibiotic derived from *Streptomyces galilaeus.*

References: H. Suzuki *et al.* (letter), *Lancet*, 1979, *1*, 870; G. Mathé *et al.* (letter), *ibid.*, *2*, 310.

Manufacturers
Bristol, USA.

12319-d

Aclatonium Napadisylate. Celatonium Napadisilate; Choline Naphthalene-1,5-Disulphonate (2:1) Dilactate Diacetate. 2-(2-Acetoxypropionyloxy)ethyltrimethylammonium naphthalene-1,5-disulphonate (2:1).
$2C_{10}H_{20}NO_4,C_{10}H_6O_6S_2$=722.8.

CAS — 55077-30-0.

An antispasmodic agent that has been tried in gastro-intestinal disorders.

Manufacturers
Toyama, Jap.

12320-c

Aconite *(B.P.C. 1973).* Aconit.; Aconit Napel; Aconite Root; Monkshood Root; Wolfsbane Root; Aconiti Tuber; Eisenhutknollen.

CAS — 8063-12-5.

Pharmacopoeias. In *Arg., Belg., Braz., Chin., Fr., Ind., Mex., Port., Roum., Span.,* and *Swiss. Chin.* specifies *A. carmichaeli.*

The dried root of *Aconitum napellus* agg. (Ranunculaceae), containing from 0.2 to 1.5% of total alkaloids. The ether-soluble alkaloids (chiefly aconitine) vary in amount, usually between 0.2 and 0.6%. The *B.P.C. 1973* specifies not less than 0.5% of alkaloids, calculated as aconitine, and the minimum content specified by pharmacopoeias varies between 0.15 and 0.8%.

Adverse Effects. Aconite affects both the heart and the central nervous system; the heart is first slowed through the vagus centre but it is also affected directly, its excitability is increased, and its coordination disturbed. Eventually the heart stops, often suddenly. Respiration is depressed progressively. With large doses death is almost instantaneous.

With moderately toxic doses there is a tingling of the tongue, mouth, stomach, and skin (this is the most important diagnostic feature) followed by numbness and anaesthesia. Other symptoms are nausea, vomiting, and diarrhoea; excessive salivation; irregular, weak, and slow pulse, later becoming rapid; difficult respiration; cold, clammy, and livid skin; muscular weakness, incoordination, and vertigo. Death may occur from paralysis of the heart or the respiratory centre.

Symptoms of aconite poisoning may appear almost immediately and are rarely delayed beyond an hour; in fatal poisoning death usually occurs with 6 hours. As little as 5 to 10 ml of aconite tincture may prove fatal.

Treatment of Adverse Effects. After the ingestion of aconite, empty the stomach by aspiration and lavage; give atropine sulphate; assisted respiration may be necessary if there are signs of respiratory depression. The patient should be kept warm and lying down with the head rather low.

Uses. Internally, aconite acts as a mild diaphoretic and diminishes the force and rate of the heart but owing to the closeness of its therapeutic and toxic doses and the variability of its potency it is a dangerous therapeutic agent and should not be used.

When applied to the skin it produces tingling followed by numbness, and aconite liniments were formerly used extensively in the treatment of neuralgia, sciatica, and rheumatism. However, sufficient aconitine may be absorbed through the skin to cause serious poisoning; liniments should never be applied to wounds or abraded surfaces.

A preparation of aconite is used in homoeopathic medicine.

Preparations

For preparations containing aconite, see Martindale 27th Edn, p. 1716.

12321-k

Aconitine *(B.P.C. 1934).* Acetylbenzoylaconine. 8-Acetoxy-3,11,18-trihydroxy-16-ethyl-1,6,19-trimethoxy-4-methoxymethylaconitan-10-yl benzoate.
$C_{34}H_{47}NO_{11}$=645.7.

CAS — 302-27-2.

Pharmacopoeias. In *Arg., Aust., Port., Span.,* and *Swiss.*

An alkaloid obtained from aconite. Colourless crystals or white crystalline powder. A drop of dilute solution placed on the tongue produces a characteristic tingling sensation. **Soluble** 1 in 4500 of water, 1 in 40 of alcohol (90%), 1 in 3 of chloroform, 1 in 70 of ether, and 1 in 2800 of light petroleum. **Incompatible** with iodine and tannic acid. **Protect** from light.

Aconitine has the actions described for aconite (above). It is one of the most potent and quick-acting of poisons; as little as 2 mg may prove fatal.

Accidental poisoning of 2 medical students by aconitine, the amount taken by each student being between 5 and 10 mg. Both recovered without treatment.— F. S. Fiddes, *Br. med. J.*, 1958, *2*, 779.

12322-a

Acrolein. Acrylic Aldehyde; Acraldehyde; Acrylaldehyde. Prop-2-enal.
C_3H_4O=56.1.

CAS — 107-02-8.

An inflammable liquid with a pungent odour.

Acrolein is irritant to the skin and may cause vesiculation. The vapour causes lachrymation and nasal irritation. Inhalation may cause pulmonary oedema. It has various industrial uses.

A review.— C. Izard and C. Libermann, *Mutat. Res.*, 1978, *47*, 115.

12323-t

Acrosoxacin. Rosoxacin; Win-35213. 1-Ethyl-1,4-dihydro-4-oxo-7-(4-pyridyl)quinoline-3-carboxylic acid.
$C_{17}H_{14}N_2O_3$=294.3.

CAS — 40034-42-2.

Adverse Effects and Precautions. Headaches and gastro-intestinal disturbances have been reported occasionally with acrosoxacin. Dizziness and drowsiness may occur and patients should be advised not to drive or operate machinery if affected. Acrosoxacin should be given with caution to patients with impaired renal or hepatic function.

In experimental studies acrosoxacin has induced lesions in weight-bearing joints in young *animals* and frequent doses in patients under 18 years are not recommended.

Uses. Acrosoxacin is an antibacterial agent with activity against *Neisseria gonorrhoeae.* It is given by mouth in the treatment of gonorrhoea as a single dose of 300 mg, preferably on an empty stomach.

A brief review of acrosoxacin.— *Drug & Ther. Bull.*, 1982, *20*, 10.

An evaluation of acrosoxacin in male gonorrhoea.— B. M. Limson *et al.*, *Curr. ther. Res.*, 1979, *26*, 842.

Acrosoxacin resistance in *Neisseria gonorrhoeae*.— M. E. Macaulay (letter), *Lancet*, 1982, *1*, 171; C. Jones and L. Cohen (letter), *ibid.*, 855.

Proprietary Preparations

Eradacin *(Sterling Research, UK)*. Acrosoxacin, available as capsules of 150 mg.

12324-x

Acrylamide. Propenamide.
$C_3H_5NO=71.1$.

CAS — 79-06-1.

Acrylamide is highly toxic and irritant; it can be absorbed through unbroken skin. Symptoms of poisoning include increased sweating and neuropathy which may be persistent. Poisoning has occurred from the accidental ingestion of water contaminated with low concentrations of acrylamide. It has industrial applications, including use as a plasticiser and a waterproof 'chemical grout'.

References: R. B. Auld and S. F. Bedwell, *Can. med. Ass. J.*, 1967, *96*, 652; H. Igisu, *J. Neurol. Neurosurg. Psychiat.*, 1975, *38*, 581, per *Pharm. J.*, 1976, *1*, 466; *Br. med. J.*, 1976, *2*, 960; C. M. Kesson *et al.*, *Postgrad. med. J.*, 1977, *53*, 16.

12325-r

Adenine. Vitamin B_4. 6-Aminopurine.
$C_5H_5N_5=135.1$.

CAS — 73-24-5.

Adenine is a constituent of coenzymes and nucleic acids.

Adenine has been used to extend the storage life of Whole Blood (see p.322).

Striking improvement in megaloblastic anaemia in a 9-year-old boy with Lesch-Nyhan syndrome followed treatment with adenine in divided doses of up to 1.5 g daily. Hyperuricaemia resulting from degradation of adenine was corrected by allopurinol.— S. P. M. van der Zee *et al.* (letter), *Lancet*, 1968, *1*, 1427.

A review of toxicological and pharmacological aspects, in *animals* and man, of the use of adenine to improve preservation of red blood cells. The only toxic effect of purified adenine appears to result from deposition of the metabolite 2,8-dioxyadenine in the kidney tubules, although this does not lead to chronic disease and tubular function is re-established after discontinuation of the drug. The amount of drug which produces functional changes in man is great enough to permit extensive use of blood containing the small quantities of adenine needed for enhanced preservation. J.S. Falk *et al.* (*Transfusion*, 1972, *12*, 376) concluded that human tolerance (maximum dosage of adenine with no crystal deposition in the kidney tubules) is at least 15 mg per kg body-weight. The toxicity of adenine in patients with chronic liver and kidney dysfunction has not been studied and the effects, if any, of the 8-oxyadenine intermediate are not known.— W. L. Warner, *Transfusion*, 1977, *17*, 326.

Proprietary Names

B4 Hemosan *(Pons, Spain)*; Biadenina *(Biagini, Ital.)*; Leuco-4 *(Villette, Fr.)*.

12326-f

***S*-Adenosyl-L-methionine.** 5′-[(3-Amino-3-carboxypropyl)methylsulphonio]-5′-deoxyadenosine hydroxide, inner salt.
$C_{15}H_{22}N_6O_5S=398.4$.

CAS — 29908-03-0.

S-Adenosyl-L-methionine, the active derivative of methionine, has been studied for the treatment of hepatic disorders.

References: G. Ideo, *Minerva med., Roma*, 1975, *66*, 1571; F. Consolo *et al.*, *Curr. ther. Res.*, 1977, *22*, 751; R. Mazzanti *et al.*, *Curr. ther. Res.*, 1979, *25*, 25; P. Cavallo-Perin *et al.*, *Curr. ther. Res.*, 1979, *26*, 982; V. Pecoraro *et al.*, *G. Mal. infett. parassit.*, 1979, *31*, 390, per *Abstr. Hyg.*, 1980, *55*, 626.

Proprietary Names

Samyr (disulphate ditosylate) *(Bioresearch, Ital.)*.

12327-d

Adinazolam. U-41123. 8-Chloro-1-(dimethylaminomethyl)-6-phenyl-4*H*-1,2,4-triazolo[4,3-*a*]-[1,4]benzodiazepine.
$C_{19}H_{18}ClN_5=351.8$.

CAS — 37115-32-5.

A benzodiazepine tranquilliser structurally related to diazepam.

Manufacturers

Upjohn, USA.

12328-n

Adipic Acid. Hexanedioic Acid.
$C_6H_{10}O_4=146.1$.

CAS — 124-04-9.

White crystals or crystalline powder. M.p. 151.5° to 154°. Slightly **soluble** in water; freely soluble in alcohol; soluble in acetone.

Adipic acid is used as an acidulating agent in foods.

Estimated acceptable daily intake of free acid, potassium, sodium, and ammonium salts: up to 5 mg per kg body-weight.— Twenty-first Report of the Joint FAO/WHO Expert Committee on Food Additives, *Tech. Rep. Ser. Wld Hlth Org. No. 617*, 1978.

12329-h

Aesculus. Horse-chestnut; Semen Hippocastani; Marron d'Inde; Castaño de Indias; Rosskastaniensamen.

CAS — 6805-41-0 (aescin).

Pharmacopoeias. In *Ger.*, *Port.*, and *Span.*

The seeds of the horse-chestnut, *Aesculus hippocastanum* (Hippocastanaceae) containing aescin (escin) and other saponins. **Protect** from light.

Aescin has been used in the prevention and treatment of various peripheral vascular disorders, including traumatic swellings and post-operative oedema, but is of doubtful value. It has been reported to cause acute renal failure. Aescin has been given by mouth and has been applied topically. Sodium aescinate has been administered by intravenous injection.
See also Esculoside, p.1496.

A pseudolupus syndrome which occurred in 15 patients was associated with the use of a preparation containing Venocuran—an aesculus extract, phenopyrazone (a pyrazolone derivative), and various cardiac glycosides.— P. J. Grob *et al.*, *Lancet*, 1975, *2*, 144.

Proprietary Names

Femirosine *(Jap.)*; Feparil *(Madaus Cerafarm, Spain)*; Reparil *(Bellon, Fr.*; *Madaus, Ger.*; *Ibi, Ital.*; *Madaus, S.Afr.*; *Madaus, Switz.)*; Tochief *(Jap.)*; Venostasin *(Klinge, Switz.)*.

12330-a

Aflatoxins

CAS — 1162-65-8 (aflatoxin B_1); 7220-81-7 (aflatoxin B_2); 1165-39-5 (aflatoxin G_1); 7241-98-7 (aflatoxin G_2).

Aflatoxins are toxic metabolites produced by many strains of *Aspergillus flavus*, growing on many vegetable foods, notably peanuts. Aflatoxin B_1, B_2, G_1, and G_2 have been identified.

Aflatoxin B_1 causes hepatic damage and is a potent hepatocarcinogen in *animals* and there is considerable suggestive evidence for a link in humans.

A review and discussion on naturally occurring toxic substances in foods, including aflatoxins.— R. L. Gross and P. M. Newberne, *Clin. Pharmac. Ther.*, 1977, *22*, 680.

Aflatoxin B_1 was found in the blood of 2 children with Reye's syndrome (characterised by acute encephalopathy and fatty degeneration of the viscera) during the acute phase of the disease.— G. R. Hogan *et al.* (letter), *Lancet*, 1978, *1*, 561.

A report of a woman who remained well 14 years after taking aflatoxin 1.5 mg per kg body-weight over a period of approximately 2 weeks in an attempt at suicide. Additional factors, such as malnutrition and hepatitis virus, may be necessary for aflatoxin carcinogenesis in man, or the latent period for tumour formation may exceed 14 years.— R. M. Willis *et al.* (letter), *Lancet*, 1980, *1*, 1198.

12331-t

Afloqualone. HQ-495. 6-Amino-2-fluoromethyl-3-*o*-tolylquinazolin-4(3*H*)-one.
$C_{16}H_{14}FN_3O=283.3$.

CAS — 56287-74-2.

A muscle relaxant used in conditions associated with muscle spasm.

12332-x

Aklomide. 2-Chloro-4-nitrobenzamide.
$C_7H_5ClN_2O_3=200.6$.

CAS — 3011-89-0.

Aklomide is a coccidiostat used in veterinary practice.

Manufacturers

Salsbury, UK.

12333-r

AL-1612. 3-Ethyl-5-(4,4-ethylenedioxypiperidinomethyl)-4,5,6,7-tetrahydro-2-methyl-1*H*-indol-4-one.
$C_{19}H_{28}N_2O_3=332.4$.

CAS — 25331-92-4.

A white crystalline substance with low **solubility** in water.

AL-1612 has been used in the treatment of schizophrenia.

References: A. A. Sugerman, *Curr. ther. Res.*, 1971, *13*, 743; A. Elizur and S. Gershon, *ibid.*, 584; C. H. Chen *et al.*, *ibid.*, 1972, *14*, 303; S. W. Holmes and J. A. Gylys, *Arzneimittel-Forsch.*, 1973, *23*, 1314 (anti-emetic effects in *animals*).

Manufacturers

Bristol, USA.

12334-f

Alafosfalin. Alaphosphin; Ro-03-7008.
(1*R*)-1-(L-Alaninamido)ethylphosphonic acid.
$C_5H_{13}N_2O_4P=196.1$.

CAS — 60668-24-8.

Alafosfalin has antibacterial activity against many Gram-negative and some Gram-positive organisms; it has no significant activity against *Pseudomonas* and *Proteus* spp. It appears to enhance the activity of some beta-lactam antibiotics.

References: *Lancet*, 1978, *1*, 314; R. Wise, *J. antimicrob. Chemother.*, 1979, *5*, 121; J. G. Allen *et al.*, *Antimicrob. Ag. Chemother.*, 1979, *15*, 684; F. R. Atherton *et al.*, *ibid.*, 696; J. G. Allen *et al.*, *ibid.*, *16*, 306; H. B. Maruyama *et al.*, *ibid.*, 444; J. G. Allen and L. J. Lees, *ibid.*, 1980, *17*, 973; P. G. Welling *et al.*, *J. antimicrob. Chemother.*, 1980, *6*, 373.

Manufacturers

Roche, UK.

12335-d

Alanosine. L-Alanosine. L-3-(Hydroxynitrosoamino)alanine; L-2-Amino-3-(hydroxynitrosoamino)propionic acid.
$C_3H_7N_3O_4=149.1$.

CAS — 5854-93-3.

Alanosine is reported to have antineoplastic activity.

References: G. Powis *et al.*, *Clin. Pharmac. Ther.*, 1980, *27*, 279.

12336-n

Alaproclate. GEA-654. 4-Chloro-αα-dimethylphenethyl DL-alaninate; 2-(4-Chlorobenzyl)prop-2-yl 2-aminopropionate.
$C_{13}H_{18}ClNO_2$=255.7.

CAS — 60719-82-6.

Alaproclate is reported to be an antidepressant.

Manufacturers
Astra, USA.

12337-h

Albumen *(B.P.C. 1934).* Egg Albumen; White of Egg; Albumen Ovi Recens.

CAS — 9006-50-2.

The liquid white of the egg of *Gallus bankiva* var. *domesticus* (Phasianidae). A nearly colourless or pale yellow fluid. Wt per ml about 1.045 g. It is coagulated on heating to about 70°, or by adding alcohol. It is precipitated by most mineral acids and some organic acids. It is **soluble** in caustic alkalis but forms precipitates with the salts of most heavy metals. It is also precipitated by volatile oils, camphor, phenol, and tannic acid.

Albumen may be used in the treatment of poisoning by salts of heavy metals and as a demulcent after the ingestion of corrosive substances such as hydrochloric acid. It is also used as a clarifying agent.

12338-m

Alclometasone Dipropionate. Sch-22219. 7α-Chloro-11β,17α,21-trihydroxy-16α-methylpregna-1,4-diene-3,20-dione 17,21-dipropionate.
$C_{28}H_{37}ClO_7$=521.0.

CAS — 67452-97-5 (alclometasone); 66734-13-2 (dipropionate).

Alclometasone dipropionate is a topical corticosteroid.

Manufacturers
Schering, UK.

12339-b

Alfentanil Hydrochloride. R-39209. *N*-{1-[2-(4-Ethyl-5-oxo-2-tetrazolin-1-yl)ethyl]-4-(methoxymethyl)-4-piperidyl}propionanilide hydrochloride monohydrate.
$C_{21}H_{32}N_6O_3,HCl,H_2O$=471.0.

CAS — 71195-58-9 (alfentanil); 69049-06-5 (hydrochloride, anhydrous); 70879-28-6 (hydrochloride, monohydrate).

Alfentanil hydrochloride is a short-acting narcotic analgesic.

References: J. H. Brown *et al.*, *Br. J. Anaesth.*, 1980, *52*, 1101; B. Kay and B. Pleuvry, *ibid.*, 631P; B. Kay and B. Pleuvry, *Anaesthesia*, 1980, *35*, 952; B. Kay and D. K. Stephenson, *ibid.*, 1197.

Manufacturers
Janssen, Belg.

12340-x

Algeldrate. W-4600. A hydrated aluminium hydroxide of the general formula
$Al(OH)_3,xH_2O$ = 78.0.

CAS — 1330-44-5.

Algeldrate is an antacid.

Proprietary Names
Alucol *(Sandoz, Ital.)*; Pepsamar *(Winthrop, Arg.)*.

12341-r

Alginic Acid *(B.P.C. 1973, U.S.N.F.).* Acide Alginique; Acidum Alginicum. A polyuronic acid composed of residues of D-mannuronic and L-guluronic acids extracted from algae belonging to the Phaeophyceae, mainly species of *Laminaria*, which grow in large quantities off the west coasts of Scotland and Ireland. Equivalent wt about 200.

CAS — 9005-32-7.

Pharmacopoeias. In *Fr.* and *Nord.* Also in *U.S.N.F.*

A white to pale yellowish-brown, odourless or almost odourless, tasteless powder. The *B.P.C. 1973* allows a small proportion of the acid groups of alginic acid to be neutralised with sodium carbonate to produce a more granular and less bulky material. It loses not more than 18% of its weight on drying; *U.S.N.F.* specifies not more than 15% loss on drying.
Practically **insoluble** in water and organic solvents; soluble in solutions of alkali hydroxides. A 3% dispersion in water has a pH of 1.5 to 3.5. Alginic acid may be **sterilised** by autoclaving; solutions of soluble alginates may be similarly sterilised. Some loss of viscosity usually occurs in solutions prepared from sterilised alginic acid and in sterilised alginate solutions to an extent which depends on the other substances present. **Store** in airtight containers.

Alginic acid is a tablet disintegrant and binder; it is preferably incorporated by a dry-mixing process. See also Sodium Alginate, p.960. Alginates are used as haemostatics—see Calcium Alginate, p.735. Alginic acid is also an ingredient of antacid preparations.

For the use of alginic acid in tablet manufacture by direct compression, see E. J. Mendell, *Mfg Chem.*, 1972, *43* (June), 31.

Estimated acceptable daily intake of alginic acid and its ammonium, calcium, potassium, and sodium salts: up to 25 mg per kg body-weight.— Seventeenth Report of the FAO/WHO Expert Committee on Food Additives, *Tech. Rep. Ser. Wld Hlth Org. No. 539*, 1974.

12342-f

Almitrine Dimesylate. S-2620(almitrine). *NN'*-Diallyl-6-[4-(4,4'-difluorobenzhydryl)piperazin-1-yl]-1,3,5-triazine-2,4-diyldiamine bis(methanesulphonate).
$C_{26}H_{29}F_2N_7,2CH_4SO_3$=669.8.

CAS — 27469-53-0 (almitrine).

Almitrine dimesylate is used as a respiratory stimulant.

Proprietary Names
Vectarion *(Servier, Fr.)*.

12343-d

Aloglutamol. 2-Amino-2-hydroxymethylpropane-1,3-diol gluconate dihydroxyaluminate.
$C_{10}H_{24}AlNO_{12}$=377.3.

Aloglutamol is an antacid.

Proprietary Names
Altris *(Chemil, Ital.)*; Tasto *(Scharper, Ital.)*.

12344-n

Alpha Fetoprotein. α-Fetoprotein.

Units. 100 000 units of human alpha fetoprotein are contained in 139.91 mg of freeze-dried alpha fetoprotein in one ampoule of the first International Standard Preparation (1975).

Alpha fetoprotein (AFP) is an alpha globulin of similar molecular weight to albumin. The concentration in foetal serum exceeds that of maternal serum and amniotic fluid. In the second trimester of pregnancy AFP concentrations in maternal serum are elevated in relation to non-pregnant concentrations.
Screening of AFP concentrations in maternal serum and amniotic fluid has been used for the diagnosis of neural tube defects associated with anencephaly and spina bifida.

Some references: *Lancet*, 1977, *1*, 1323 (Report of UK Collaborative Study on Alpha-fetoprotein in Relation to Neural Tube Defects); C. J. Smith *et al.*, *Br. med. J.*, 1979, *1*, 920; D. J. H. Brock, *ibid.*, 1979, *2*, 1402; R. Harris, *ibid.*, 1980, *280*, 1199; N. J. Wald and H. S. Cuckle, *Br. J. Hosp. Med.*, 1980, *23*, 473; S. J. Standing *et al.*, *Br. med. J.*, 1981, *283*, 705.

Recommendations and discussions of alpha fetoprotein and chorionic gonadotrophin as tumour markers in patients with testicular tumours.— B. Nørgaard-Pedersen *et al.* (letter), *Lancet*, 1978, *2*, 1042; E. E. Fraley *et al.*, *New Engl. J. Med.*, 1979, *301*, 1370.

Detection of hydatidiform mole.— D. H. Smith *et al.*, *Br. med. J.*, 1980, *280*, 1213.

Localisation of malignant germ cell tumours by external scanning after injection of radioactive anti alphafetoprotein.— A. K. Halsall *et al.*, *Br. med. J.*, 1981, *283*, 942.

12345-h

Althiazide. Altizide; P-1779. 3-Allylthiomethyl-6-chloro-3,4-dihydro-2*H*-1,2,4-benzothiadiazine-7-sulphonamide 1,1-dioxide.
$C_{11}H_{14}ClN_3O_4S_3$=383.9.

CAS — 5588-16-9.

Althiazide is a thiazide diuretic (see p.581) that has been used in the treatment of hypertension.

References: D. Levitt, *Curr. med. Res. Opinion*, 1979, *6*, 136; E. N. Mngola, *J. int. med. Res.*, 1980, *8*, 199.

Manufacturers
Pfizer, USA.

12346-m

Altrenogest. A-35957; A-41300; RH-2267; RU-2267. 17α-Allyl-17β-hydroxy-19-norandrosta-4,9,11-trien-3-one; 17β-Hydroxy-19,21,24-trinorchola-4,9,11,22-tetraen-3-one.
$C_{21}H_{26}O_2$=310.4.

CAS — 850-52-2.

Altrenogest is reported to have progestational activity.

Manufacturers
Hoechst, UK; Roussel-UCLAF, USA.

12347-b

Aluminium Lactate. Tris(lactato)aluminium.
$C_9H_{15}AlO_9$=294.2.

CAS — 537-02-0; 18917-91-4.

Aluminium lactate is used in the local treatment of various disorders of the mouth.

Proprietary Names
Aluctyl *(Roussel, Arg.; Beytout, Fr.; Brocades, Ital.; Tió, Spain; Beytout, Switz.)*.

12348-v

Aluminium Oxide.
Al_2O_3=102.0.

CAS — 1344-28-1.

Fused synthetic aluminium oxide, of graded particle size, is used as an abrasive paste as an adjunct in the treatment of acne.

Proprietary Preparations
Brasivol *(Stiefel, UK)*. Cleansing pastes containing graded particles of fused synthetic aluminium oxide in a detergent basis; supplied in three grades: No. 1 (fine), No. 2 (medium), and No. 3 (coarse). (Also available as Brasivol in *Austral., S.Afr.*).

Other Proprietary Names
Brasivil *(Ger.)*.

Other Proprietary Abrasive Preparations
Ionax Scrub *(Alcon, UK: Farillon, UK)*. Gel containing polyethylene granules in an alcoholic detergent basis,

with benzalkonium chloride 0.25%. For the abrasive treatment of acne.

12349-g

AM-715. 1-Ethyl-6-fluoro-1,4-dihydro-4-oxo-7-(piperazin-1-yl)quinoline-3-carboxylic acid.
$C_{16}H_{18}FN_3O_3$=319.3.

CAS — 70458-96-7.

AM-715 is an antimicrobial agent that has been tried in urinary-tract infections.

References: A. Ito *et al.*, *Antimicrob. Ag. Chemother.*, 1980, *17*, 103.

Manufacturers
Kyorin, Jap.

12350-f

Amanita phalloides

CAS — 17466-45-4 (phalloidin); 28227-92-1 (phalloin); 23109-05-9 (α-amanitin); 21150-22-1 (β-amanitin); 21150-23-2 (γ-amanitin).

Amanita phalloides 'death cap' is the most toxic of the poisonous mushrooms and is reported to be responsible for about 90% of fatal mushroom poisoning.

The toxic principles are heat-stable cyclic polypeptides including phallotoxins (phalloidin, phalloin) and amatoxins (α-, β-, γ-amanitin), of which α-amanitin is the most significant. A single mushroom weighing 20 to 25 g may be lethal. Symptoms occur 6 to 12 or more hours after ingestion and initially consist of severe gastro-intestinal symptoms including pain, nausea, vomiting, and diarrhoea sometimes simulating cholera. Dehydration and cardiovascular collapse may follow. This initial phase is followed by a phase of apparent improvement. Two or three days later the more serious phase supervenes representing the toxic effects of amanitin on the liver; jaundice occurs, and there may be renal, cardiac, and CNS involvement. The mortality-rate is 30 to 50% despite treatment.

There is no specific antidote and treatment consists primarily of symptomatic and supportive measures. Expert identification of the ingested material is desirable. Procedures recommended include: empty the stomach by inducing emesis or by aspiration and lavage (though because of the delay in appearance of symptoms this may not be productive); use activated charcoal to adsorb the toxin; a radioimmunoassay is available in some countries for the detection of amatoxins; some authorities leave *in situ* a duodenal tube for regular aspiration of the products of enterohepatic circulation. Correct fluid and electrolyte imbalance.

Some authorities recommend a saline purgative such as sodium sulphate and high colonic enemas to promote peristalsis.

Haemodialysis, haemoperfusion over charcoal, and exchange transfusion have been used; the toxins are bound to plasma proteins; the use of high doses of penicillin to displace the toxins has been suggested. Forced diuresis has been advocated.

Various drug therapy has been advocated in an attempt to protect the liver. Cytochrome C has been suggested; there is no evidence that it is of value. Silymarin is used in hepatic disorders and has protected *mice* from the effects of *Amanita phalloides*, but evidence of its clinical usefulness is sparse. The use of thioctic acid is controversial; the more recent *animal* studies do not, in general, support a protective effect, but some authorities consider it worth a trial. The intravenous use of insulin and growth hormone has been advocated in an attempt to promote hepatic regeneration.

Some other *Amanita* spp. have similar activity; they include *A. verna* ('deadly agaric', 'fool's mushroom', sometimes called 'destroying angel'), *A. virosa* (sometimes also called 'destroying angel'), and *A. bisporigera*. Some *Galerina* spp. have similar activity.

Some *Amanita* spp. such as *A. muscaria* ('fly agaric') and *A. pantherina* have muscarinic and/or hallucinatory effects. If the effects are muscarinic atropine is indicated for treatment.

Coprinus atramentarius ('ink cap') has disulfiram-like activity. Numerous other toxic mushrooms occur, some with hallucinatory activity.

Wild mushrooms should be eaten only if positively identified as being edible.

Recovery of 16 patients with mushroom (not *A. phalloides*) poisoning.— D. J. McCormick *et al.*, *Ann. intern. Med.*, 1979, *90*, 332.

Reviews and discussions of *Amanita phalloides* poisoning and its treatment: *Drug & Ther. Bull.*, 1976, *14*, 91; K. F. Lampe, *Paediatrician*, 1977, *6*, 289; K. H. Usadel *et al.* (letter), *New Engl. J. Med.*, 1979, *300*, 1223; *Lancet*, 1980, *2*, 351; T. Weber (letter), *ibid.*, 640; H. Faulstich (letter), *ibid.*, 794.

A plea for the use of forced diuresis.— S. Vesconi *et al.* (letter), *Lancet*, 1980, *2*, 854.

Comment on favourable results in 3 patients with *Amanita phalloides* poisoning treated with Bastien's emergency therapy, and emphasis that the regimen must be started as soon as possible. Bastien's therapy consists of oral therapy with nifuroxazide 1.2 g daily and dihydrostreptomycin 1.5 g daily and intravenous therapy with ascorbic acid 3 g daily, the 3 drugs being given for 3 days. During this treatment a carrot soup broth is the sole source of nutrition.— A. -M. Dumont *et al.* (letter), *Lancet*, 1981, *1*, 722.

12351-d

Amcinonide. CL-34699. 16α,17α-Cyclopentylidenedioxy-9α-fluoro-11β,21-dihydroxypregna-1,4-diene-3,20-dione 21-acetate.
$C_{28}H_{35}FO_7$=502.6.

CAS — 51022-69-6.

NOTE. The name amcinopol was formerly applied to amcinonide.

Amcinonide is a fluorinated corticosteroid applied topically, usually used in a concentration of 0.1%.

References: G. L. Rocha *et al.*, *Curr. ther. Res.*, 1976, *19*, 538; O. Binet *et al.*, *ibid.*, 1979, *25*, 500; R. Woodford and J. M. Haigh, *ibid.*, *26*, 301; *Med. Lett.*, 1980, *22*, 51.

Proprietary Names
Amicla *(Lederle, Neth.)*; Cyclocort *(Lederle, Canad.; Lederle, USA)*.

12352-n

Ametantrone Acetate. Cl-881. 1,4-Bis[2-(2-hydroxyethylamino)ethylamino]anthraquinone acetate.
$C_{22}H_{28}N_4O_4,xC_2H_4O_2$=412.5 (ametantrone).

CAS — 64862-96-0 (ametantrone); 73334-06-2 (acetate).

Ametantrone acetate is a potential antineoplastic agent.

Manufacturers
Parke, Davis, USA.

12353-h

Amezinium Methylsulphate. Amezinium Metilsulfate. 4-Amino-6-methoxy-1-phenylpyridazinium methylsulphate.
$C_{12}H_{15}N_3O_5S$=313.3.

CAS — 30578-37-1.

Amezinium methylsulphate has been used in the treatment of hypotension.

Proprietary Names
Regulton *(Ger.)*.

12354-m

Amfenac Sodium. AHR-5850; AHR-5850D. Sodium (2-amino-3-benzoylphenyl)acetate monohydrate.
$C_{15}H_{12}NNaO_3,H_2O$=295.3.

CAS — 51579-82-9 (amfenac); 61618-27-7 (sodium salt).

Amfenac sodium is a phenylalkanoic acid derivative (see p.234) with anti-inflammatory and analgesic activity.

References: A. K. Jain *et al.*, *Clin. Pharmac. Ther.*, 1980, *27*, 260.

Manufacturers
Robins, UK.

12355-b

Amicarbalide Isethionate *(B.P. Vet.)*. M & B 5062A. 3,3′-Diamidinocarbanilide isethionate; 1,3-Bis(3-amidinophenyl)urea bis(2-hydroxyethanesulphonate).
$C_{19}H_{28}N_6O_9S_2$=548.6.

CAS — 3459-96-9 (amicarbalide); 3671-72-5 (isethionate).

A white or slightly cream-coloured, odourless or almost odourless powder. M.p. 200° to 204°. **Soluble** 1 in less than 1 of water and 1 in 250 of alcohol; practically insoluble in chloroform and ether. A 50% solution in water has a pH of 5 to 7. Solutions are **sterilised** by filtration.

Amicarbalide isethionate is an antiprotozoal agent used in veterinary medicine in the treatment of bovine babesiasis.

A comparison of the pharmacological effects of amicarbalide and quinuronium.— P. Eyre, *J. Pharm. Pharmac.*, 1967, *19*, 509.

Proprietary Names
Diampron *(May & Baker, UK)*.

12356-v

Amikhelline Hydrochloride. 9-(2-Diethylaminoethoxy)-4-hydroxy-7-methyl-5*H*-furo[3,2-g][1]benzopyran-5-one hydrochloride.
$C_{18}H_{21}NO_5,HCl$=367.8.

CAS — 4439-67-2 (amikhelline); 40709-23-7 (hydrochloride).

Amikhelline has antispasmodic properties and is used in disorders of the gastro-intestinal tract.

Proprietary Names
Nokhel *(Promesa, Spain)*.

12357-g

Aminaphtone. Aminaftone. 2-Hydroxy-3-methylnaphtho-1,4-hydroquinone 2-(4-aminobenzoate); 3-Methylnaphthalene-1,2,4-triol 2-(4-aminobenzoate).
$C_{18}H_{15}NO_4$=309.3.

CAS — 14748-94-8.

Aminaphtone has been used as an oral haemostatic agent.

Proprietary Names
Capillarema *(Baldacci, Ital.)*.

12358-q

Amineptine Hydrochloride. S-1694. 7-(10,11-Dihydro-5*H*-dibenzo[*a,d*]cyclohepten-5-ylamino)heptanoic acid hydrochloride.
$C_{22}H_{27}NO_2,HCl$=373.9.

CAS — 57574-09-1 (amineptine); 30272-08-3 (hydrochloride).

NOTE. The name amineptic has been applied to amineptine.

Amineptine hydrochloride is an antidepressant.

References: P. van Amerongen, *Curr. med. Res. Opinion*, 1979, *6*, 93; C. Vauterin and M. Bazot, *ibid.*, 101; S. Bornstein, *ibid.*, 107.

Proprietary Names
Survector *(Euthérapie, Fr.)*.

12359-p

Aminobutyric Acid.
Gamma-aminobutyric Acid; GABA. 4-Aminobutyric acid.
$C_4H_9NO_2$=103.1.

CAS — 56-12-2.

White crystals with a bitter taste. Freely **soluble** in water; slightly soluble in hot alcohol; practically insoluble in other organic solvents.

Aminobutyric acid is believed to act as an inhibitory neurotransmitter in the CNS. It has been claimed to be of value in cerebral disorders and coma and to have an antihypertensive effect. Adverse effects have included gastro-intestinal disorders, insomnia, headache, and pyrexia.

Over a period of 2 months 7 patients with Huntington's chorea were treated with aminobutyric acid starting at a dose of 1 g and increasing to 12 to 32 g daily. Two patients gained improvement of function and a decrease in choreiform movements and a third patient showed moderate improvement.— R. Fisher *et al.* (letter), *Lancet*, 1974, *1*, 506.

Severe peripheral vascular collapse occurred in one of the authors 90 minutes after taking 8 g of chromatographically pure aminobutyric acid.— T. L. Perry *et al.* (letter), *Lancet*, 1974, *1*, 995. Doses of 1 to 2 g daily and 40 g given over 48 hours had produced no serious side-effects.— R. Fisher *et al.* (letter), *ibid.*, 1347.

γ-Vinyl aminobutyric acid, an irreversible inhibitor of aminobutyric acid transaminase, had a beneficial effect in 7 of 9 patients with tardive dyskinesia when given by mouth in doses ranging from 2 to 6 g daily. Dyskinesia was aggravated in the other 2 patients. Sedation was the most prominent side-effect.— G. P. Tell *et al.* (letter), *New Engl. J. Med.*, 1981, *305*, 581. See also J. Grove *et al.* (letter), *Lancet*, 1980, *2*, 647.

Proprietary Names
Gamarex *(Causyth, Ital.)*; Gammalon *(Daiichi, Jap.)*; Mielogen *(Made, Spain)*.

12360-n

Aminohydroxybutyric Acid.
4-Amino-3-hydroxybutyric acid.
$C_4H_9NO_3$=119.1.

CAS — 352-21-6.

Odourless white crystals or crystalline powder with a slight characteristic taste. Very **soluble** in water; very slightly soluble in alcohol, chloroform, and other organic solvents.

Aminohydroxybutyric acid has been claimed to be of value in neurological disorders and to have an antihypertensive effect. Adverse effects have included dizziness and anorexia.

Proprietary Names
Aminoxan *(Kaken, Jap.)*; Bogil *(Llorente, Spain)*; Gabimex *(Gramon, Arg.)*; Gabob *(Jap.)*; Gamibetal *(ISF, Ital.*; *Ono, Jap.*; *Ibsa, Switz.)*; Gabomade *(Made, Spain)*; Gaboril *(Seber, Spain)*.

12361-h

Aminomethiazole Tartrate.
2-Amino-4-methylthiazole hydrogen tartrate.
$C_4H_6N_2S,C_4H_6O_6$=264.3.

Aminomethiazole tartrate is an antithyroid agent.

Proprietary Names
Normotiroide *(Vita, Ital.)*.

12362-m

Aminonitrothiazole
(B. Vet. C. 1965). Aminonitrothiazolum. 2-Amino-5-nitrothiazole.
$C_3H_3N_3O_2S$=145.1.

CAS — 1320-42-9.

Pharmacopoeias. In *Nord.*

A greenish-yellow to orange-yellow light odourless powder with a slightly bitter taste. Slightly **soluble** in water; soluble 1 in 250 of alcohol and of ether; practically insoluble in chloroform.

Aminonitrothiazole has been used in veterinary medicine in the prevention and treatment of blackhead (histomoniasis) in turkeys and chickens, and in the treatment of canker (trichomoniasis) in pigeons.

12363-b

Aminopicoline Camsylate.
2-Amino-4-methylpyridine camphor-10-sulphonate.
$C_6H_8N_2,C_{10}H_{16}O_4S$=340.4.

Aminopicoline camsylate has been used for its reputed beneficial effect on the circulation.

Proprietary Names
Piricardio *(Nagel, Ital.)*.

12364-v

4-Aminopyridine.
$C_5H_6N_2$=94.1.

CAS — 504-24-5.

4-Aminopyridine is reported to reverse the effects of non-depolarising muscle relaxants and to have analeptic effects. Improvement of myasthenia gravis has been reported. Aminopyridine hydrochloride and aminopyridine sulphate have been used.

References: W. C. Bowman *et al.*, *J. Pharm. Pharmac.*, 1977, *29*, 616; H. Lundh *et al.*, *J. Neurol. Neurosurg. Psychiat.*, 1977, *40*, 1109; S. Agoston *et al.*, *Br. J. Anaesth.*, 1978, *50*, 383; H. Lundh *et al.*, *J. Neurol. Neurosurg. Psychiat.*, 1979, *42*, 171; S. Agoston *et al.*, *Br. J. Anaesth.*, 1980, *52*, 367; J. Evenhuis *et al.*, *ibid.*, 1981, *53*, 567.

Proprietary Names
Pymadin.

12365-g

Aminorex.
Aminoxaphen; McN-742. 2-Amino-5-phenyl-2-oxazoline.
$C_9H_{10}N_2O$=162.2.

CAS — 2207-50-3.

Aminorex is an anorectic agent which was withdrawn from use because of its association with pulmonary hypertension which sometimes proved fatal.

12366-q

Ammonium Benzoate
(B.P.C. 1949). Ammonii Benzoas; Ammonium Benzoicum.
$C_6H_5.CO_2NH_4$=139.2.

CAS — 1863-63-4.

White almost odourless scaly crystals. **Soluble** 1 in 6 of water, 1 in 30 of alcohol, and 1 in 8 of glycerol. **Incompatible** with acids, fruit syrups, ferric salts, and alkali hydroxides and carbonates.

Ammonium benzoate has been used for increasing the acidity of the urine and as an expectorant in chronic bronchitis.

12367-p

Ammonium Citrate
(B.P.C. 1949). Ammon. Cit.
$C_6H_5O_7(NH_4)_3$=243.2.

CAS — 3458-72-8.

A white or almost white, very deliquescent, crystalline powder with a saline taste. It tends to lose ammonia and to be partly converted to an acid salt. Very **soluble** in water. **Store** in airtight containers.

Ammonium citrate has been used as a mild expectorant and diuretic. After absorption it is converted into carbonate and urea and increases the alkalinity of the urine only slightly.

12368-s

Ammonium Persulphate
(B.P.C. 1934).
$(NH_4)_2S_2O_8$=228.2.

CAS — 7727-54-0.

Colourless odourless crystals or white granules or crystalline powder, containing about 7% of available oxygen. **Soluble** 1 in 2 of water; practically insoluble in dehydrated alcohol. It is stable under normal conditions of storage but it decomposes rapidly at about 95°. It decomposes in the presence of moisture and of traces of certain metallic impurities. **Store** in a cool place in airtight containers. Protect from light.

Ammonium persulphate is a powerful oxidising agent which has been used in photography and various industrial processes. Strong solutions are irritant to the skin.

Severe reactions, including loss of consciousness, occurred after using hair bleach containing ammonium persulphate.— C. D. Calnan and S. Shuster, *Archs Derm.*, 1963, *88*, 812, per *J. Soc. cosmet. Chem.*, 1967, *18*, 681.

12369-w

Ammonium Phosphate
(U.S.N.F., B.P.C. 1949). Diammonium Hydrogen Phosphate. Diammonium hydrogen orthophosphate.
$(NH_4)_2HPO_4$=132.1.

CAS — 7783-28-0.

Pharmacopoeias. In *U.S.N.F.*

Colourless crystals or granules with a slight odour and a saline taste. Loses ammonia on exposure to air, forming some ammonium dihydrogen orthophosphate, $NH_4H_2PO_4$. **Soluble** 1 in 2 of water; practically insoluble in alcohol. A 1% solution in water has a pH of 7.6 to 8.2. A 1.76% solution is iso-osmotic with serum. **Incompatible** with alkalis, ferric salts, and salts of heavy metals. **Store** in airtight containers.

Ammonium phosphate was formerly used as a diuretic. It may be used as a buffering agent in pharmaceutical preparations.

12370-m

Ammonium Salicylate.
$C_7H_9NO_3$=155.2.

CAS — 528-94-9.

Ammonium salicylate has been used topically in skin disorders.

Proprietary Names
Salicyl-Vasogen *(Pearson, Ger.)*.

12371-b

Amoscanate.
GO-9333; C-9333-Go/CGP-4540. 4-*p*-Nitroanilinophenyl isothiocyanate.
$C_{13}H_9N_3O_2S$=271.3.

CAS — 26328-53-0.

A tasteless yellow substance. M.p. 204° to 206°. Practically **insoluble** in water.

Amoscanate is an anthelmintic structurally related to bitoscanate (see p.89). It is effective against hookworm, *Ancylostoma duodenale* and *Necator americanus*, and against *Schistosoma mansoni* and *S. japonicum*; it has limited value against *S. haematobium*.
Adverse effects reported include gastro-intestinal effects, skin rash, and giddiness.

References: B. J. Vakil *et al.*, *Trans. R. Soc. trop. Med. Hyg.*, 1977, *71*, 247; B. V. Ashok *et al.*, *Br. J. clin. Pharmac.*, 1977, *4*, 463; J. C. Doshi *et al.*, *Am. J. trop. Med. Hyg.*, 1977, *26*, 636; P. S. Gupta *et al.*, *J. trop. Med. Hyg.*, 1979, *82*, 117, per *Trop. Dis. Bull.*, 1980, *77*, 391; Tech. Rep. Ser. Wld Hlth Org. No. 643, 1980.

Manufacturers
Ciba-Geigy, Switz.

12372-v

Amprolium Hydrochloride *(B.P. Vet.).* 1-(4-Amino-2-propylpyrimidin-5-ylmethyl)-2-methylpyridinium chloride hydrochloride.
$C_{14}H_{19}ClN_4,HCl$=315.2.

CAS — 121-25-5 (amprolium); 137-88-2 (hydrochloride).

A white or almost white, odourless or almost odourless powder. **Soluble** 1 in 2 of water and 1 in 170 of alcohol; very slightly soluble in ether; practically insoluble in chloroform.

Amprolium hydrochloride is an antiprotozoal agent used in veterinary practice for the prevention of coccidiosis in poultry.

12373-g

Amrinone. Win-40680. 5-Amino-3,4′-bipyridyl-6(1*H*)-one.
$C_{10}H_9N_3O$=187.2.

CAS — 60719-84-8.

Amrinone is an inotropic agent under study for the treatment of heart failure. It has been given by injection and by mouth.

References: J. R. Benotti *et al.*, *New Engl. J. Med.*, 1978, *299*, 1373; A. M. Katz, *ibid.*, 1409; T. H. Le Jemtel *et al.*, *Circulation*, 1979, *59*, 1098; T. H. Le Jemtel *et al.*, *Am. J. Cardiol.*, 1980, *45*, 123; J. Wynne *et al.*, *ibid.*, 1245; M. P. Kullberg *et al.*, *Clin. Pharmac. Ther.*, 1981, *29*, 394; J. Edelson *et al.*, *ibid.*, 723.

A report of thrombocytopenia and fever.— S. A. Rubin *et al.* (letter), *New Engl. J. Med.*, 1979, *301*, 1185.

Proprietary Names
Inocor *(Winthrop, USA).*

12374-q

Amsacrine. *m*-AMSA; CI-880; NSC-156303; NSC-249992. 4′-(Acridin-9-ylamino)methanesulphon-*m*-anisidide.
$C_{21}H_{19}N_3O_3S$=393.5.

CAS — 51264-14-3.

Amsacrine is an antineoplastic agent which has been tried in the treatment of acute leukaemia and other neoplastic diseases.

References: S. S. Legha *et al.*, *Ann. intern. Med.*, 1980, *93*, 17 (leukaemia); G. Rivera *et al.*, *Clin. Pharmac. Ther.*, 1980, *27*, 280 (leukaemia and solid tumours); Z. A. Arlin, *Cancer Res.*, 1980, *40*, 3304 (leukaemia); M. A. Goldsmith *et al.*, *Cancer clin. Trials*, 1980, *3*, 197 (leukaemia and solid tumours); R. B. Weiss *et al.*, *ibid.*, 203.

Manufacturers
Bristol, USA; Parke, Davis, USA.

12375-p

Anagrelide Hydrochloride. BL-4162A. 6,7-Dichloro-1,5-dihydroimidazo[2,1-*b*]quinazolin-2(3*H*)-one hydrochloride.
$C_{10}H_7Cl_2N_3O,HCl$=292.6.

CAS — 68475-42-3 (anagrelide); 58579-51-4 (hydrochloride).

Anagrelide is reported to be an inhibitor of platelet aggregation.

References: R. C. Gaver *et al.*, *Clin. Pharmac. Ther.*, 1981, *29*, 381 (disposition and metabolism).

Manufacturers
Bristol, USA.

12376-s

Androisoxazole. 17α-Methyl-5α-androstano-[3,2-*c*]isoxazol-17β-ol.
$C_{21}H_{31}NO_2$=329.5.

CAS — 360-66-7.

Androisoxazole is used as an anabolic agent.

Proprietary Names
Neo-Ponden *(Serono, Ital.)*; Neo-Pondus *(Farma-Lepori, Spain).*

12377-w

Androstenediol Dipropionate. Androst-5-ene-3β,17β-diol dipropionate.
$C_{25}H_{38}O_4$=402.6.

CAS — 521-17-5 (androstenediol); 2297-30-5 (dipropionate).

Androstenediol is reported to have androgenic and oestrogenic activity and has been used in menopausal and other disorders and in prostatic carcinoma.

Proprietary Names
Bisexovis *(Vister, Ital.).*

12378-e

Aniline Mustard. NSC-18429. *NN*-Bis(2-chloroethyl)aniline.
$C_{10}H_{13}Cl_2N$=218.1.

CAS — 553-27-5.

Aniline mustard is an antineoplastic agent.

References: *Br. med. J.*, 1973, *2*, 566; R. A. Kyle *et al.*, *Cancer Res.*, 1973, *33*, 956, per *J. Am. med. Ass.*, 1973, *225*, 329.

12379-l

Anitrazafen. LY-122512. 5,6-Bis(4-methoxyphenyl)-3-methyl-1,2,4-triazine.
$C_{18}H_{17}N_3O_2$=307.4.

CAS — 63119-27-7.

Anitrazafen is reported to be a topical anti-inflammatory agent.

Manufacturers
Lilly, USA.

12380-v

Antigastrin. SC-15396. 2-Phenyl-2-(2-pyridyl)thioacetamide.
$C_{13}H_{12}N_2S$=228.3.

CAS — 10400-14-3.

Practically **insoluble** in water; slightly soluble in alcohol and light petroleum; readily soluble in acetone and chloroform.

Antigastrin is an antagonist of gastric secretion, particularly gastrin-stimulated gastric secretion.

12381-g

Antimony Barium Tartrate *(B. Vet. C. 1965).* Barium Antimonyltartrate. A salt of varying composition corresponding approximately to the formula $(C_4H_4O_7Sb)_2Ba$.

CAS — 12655-04-8.

A white or creamy-white, odourless, tasteless powder. Very slightly **soluble** in water and alcohol; soluble, with decomposition, in aqueous solutions of mineral acids and alkalis.

Antimony barium tartrate has the adverse effects described under Antimony Sodium Tartrate, p.87. It has been used in veterinary medicine in the treatment of gapeworm infestation in poultry and game; it has been administered by inhalation as a fine dust.
Maximum permissible atmospheric concentration of antimony 500 μg per m^3.

12382-q

Antimony Trichloride *(B. Vet. C. 1965).*
$SbCl_3$=228.1.

CAS — 10025-91-9.

Pharmacopoeias. In *Port.*

Colourless very deliquescent crystals, fuming in moist air. **Soluble** in dilute hydrochloric acid, giving a clear solution; almost entirely soluble in dehydrated alcohol and in chloroform, giving solutions which are not more than slightly turbid. It is hydrolysed by water to basic antimony oxychloride. **Store** in a cool place in airtight containers. Protect from light.

Antimony trichloride is an escharotic and is used in veterinary medicine in dishorning solutions, such as Antimony Trichloride Collodion, for dishorning calves. It has the adverse effects described under Antimony Sodium Tartrate, p.87.
Maximum permissible atmospheric concentration of antimony 500 μg per m^3.

Case histories of 7 men accidentally exposed to antimony trichloride fumes.— P. J. Taylor, *Br. J. ind. Med.*, 1966, *23*, 318, per *Abstr. Wld Med.*, 1967, *41*, 153.

Preparations

Antimony Trichloride Collodion *(B. Vet. C. 1965).* Antimony trichloride 28 g, salicylic acid 7 g, pyroxylin 2.6 g, castor oil 2 g, camphor 1.3 g, solvent ether 63 ml, and dehydrated alcohol 21 ml. Store in a cool place in well-filled airtight containers. The container should be labelled 'Caution. Flammable: keep away from an open flame'.

12383-p

Antimony Trisulphide. Black Antimony Sulphide; Antimonious Sulphide; Antimonous Sulphide; Trisulfure d'Antimoine; Spiessglanz; Stibnite.
Sb_2S_3=339.7.

CAS — 1345-04-6.

Pharmacopoeias. In *Port.* and *Span.*

Greyish-black powder or masses. Practically **insoluble** in water and alcohol; soluble in warm solutions of alkali hydroxides.

Antimony trisulphide has the adverse effects described under Antimony Sodium Tartrate, p.87. Its use as a medicinal antimonial has been abandoned.
Maximum permissible atmospheric concentration of antimony 500 μg per m^3.

For a reference to the topical use of antimony trisulphide together with zinc chloride in the treatment of breast carcinoma, see Zinc Chloride, p.945.

12384-s

Antrafenine. 2-[4-(ααα-Trifluoro-*m*-tolyl)piperazin-1-yl]ethyl *N*-(7-trifluoromethyl-4-quinolyl)anthranilate.
$C_{30}H_{26}F_6N_4O_2$=588.6.

CAS — 55300-29-3.

Antrafenine is an analgesic used in rheumatic and other disorders.

Proprietary Names
Stakane *(Dausse, Fr.).*

15329-m

Apalcillin. PC-904 (sodium salt). (6*R*)-6-[(*R*)-2-(4-Hydroxy-1,5-naphthyridin-3-ylcarboxamido)-2-phenylacetamido]penicillanic acid.
$C_{25}H_{23}N_5O_6S$=521.5.

CAS — 63469-19-2 (apalcillin); 58795-03-2 (sodium salt).

Apalcillin is a semi-synthetic penicillin derivative.

References: G. P. Bodey *et al.*, *Antimicrob. Ag. Chemother.*, 1978, *13*, 14; H. Noguchi *et al.*, *ibid.*, 745; G. P. Bodey and B. Le Blanc, *ibid.*, *14*, 78.

Manufacturers
Sumitomo, Jap.

12385-w

Apholate. 2,2,4,4,6,6-Hexakis(aziridin-1-yl)-1,3,5,2,4,6-triazatriphosphorine.
$C_{12}H_{24}N_9P_3$=387.3.

CAS — 52-46-0.

Apholate is a chemosterilant which has been used in the control of the mosquito.

References: D. E. Weidhaas, *Nature*, 1962, *195*, 786; D. A. Dame and H. R. Ford, *ibid.*, 1964, *201*, 733; E. F. Knippling *et al.*, *Bull. Wld Hlth Org.*, 1968, *38*, 421; M. K. K. Pillai and K. K. Grover, *ibid.*, 1969, *40*, 229.

12386-e

Apis mellifera. The honey bee.

A preparation containing the venom of *Apis mellifera* is used in homoeopathic medicine where it is known as Apis mellifica or Apis mel.

12387-l

Apramycin. Nebramycin Factor 2; Lilly 47657; EL-857/820. 4-*O*-[3-Amino-6-(4-amino-4-deoxy-α-D-glucopyranosyloxy)-8-hydroxy-7-methylaminoperhydropyrano[3,2-*b*]pyran-2-yl]-2-deoxystreptamine.
$C_{21}H_{41}N_5O_{11}$=539.6.

CAS — 37321-09-8.

An antibiotic produced by *Streptomyces tenebrarius*.

Apramycin is an aminocyclitol antibiotic used as the sulphate for bacterial intestinal disorders in veterinary practice.

References: R. Ryden and B. J. Moore, *J. antimicrob. Chemother.*, 1977, *3*, 609; J. R. Walton, *ibid.*, 1978, *4*, 309.

Proprietary Names
Apralan (sulphate)*(Elanco, UK)*.

12388-y

Arginine Glucose-1-phosphate. L-Arginine α-D-glucopyranose-1-phosphate.
$(C_6H_{14}N_4O_2)_2,C_6H_{13}O_9P$=608.5.

CAS — 18822-82-7.

Arginine glucose-1-phosphate has been used in hepatic disorders.

Proprietary Names
Arginil *(SPA, Ital.)*; Fosfarginil *(Wassermann, Spain)*.

12389-j

Arginine Oxoglutarate. Arginine Oxoglurate. L-Arginine 2-oxoglutarate.
$C_6H_{14}N_4O_2,C_5H_6O_5$=320.3.

CAS — 16856-18-1.

Arginine oxoglutarate has been used in the treatment of hepatic disorders. Di(arginine) oxoglutarate has been similarly used.

Proprietary Names
Eucol *(Lefrancq, Fr.)*; Leberam *(Chephasaar, Ger.)*.

12390-q

Arginine Tidiacicate. The L-arginine salt of thiazolidine-2,4-dicarboxylic acid.
$C_6H_{14}N_4O_2,C_5H_7NO_4S$=351.4.

Arginine tidiacicate has been used in hepatic disorders.

Proprietary Names
Tiadilon *(Crinex, Fr.)*.

12391-p

Aristolochia Sodium. Sodium 8-methoxy-6-nitrophenanthro[3,4-*d*]-1,3-dioxole-5-carboxylate.
$C_{17}H_{10}NNaO_7$=363.3.

CAS — 313-67-7 (aristolochic acid); 52232-70-9 (sodium salt).

Aristolochia is an aromatic bitter obtained from *Aristolochia* spp. (Aristolochiaceae).

The sodium salt of aristolochic acid has been given by mouth in various inflammatory conditions. Aristolochic acid is carcinogenic in *animals*.

Proprietary Names
Tardolyt *(Madaus, Ger.)*.

12392-s

AR-L-115-BS. 2-(2-Methoxy-4-methylsulphinylphenyl)-1*H*-imidazo[4,5-*b*]pyridine.
$C_{14}H_{13}N_3O_2S$=287.3.

AR-L-115-BS is reported to have inotropic effects on the heart.

For a series of papers, including *animal* and human studies, see *Arzneimittel-Forsch.*, 1981, *31*, 129–278.

Proprietary Names
Vardax *(Thomae, Ger.)*.

12393-w

Arrowroot *(B.P.C. 1973)*. Maranta; Amylum Marantae; Araruta.

Pharmacopoeias. In *Belg.*, *Port.*, and *Span.*

The starch granules of the rhizomes of *Maranta arundinacea* (Marantaceae). A white odourless tasteless powder, much of which may cohere in small irregular masses. It loses not more than 16% of its weight on drying. When 1 g is boiled with 15 ml of water and cooled, a translucent whitish gelatinous mass is formed.

Arrowroot has the general properties of starch and is used as a gruel in the treatment of diarrhoea. One tablespoonful to 500 ml of boiling water produces a demulcent mucilage. It has been used as a suspending agent in the preparation of barium meals and is sometimes used in place of starch in tablet making.

12394-e

Arsanilic Acid *(B.P. Vet.)*. AS-101; Aminarsonic Acid. 4-Aminophenylarsonic acid.
$C_6H_8AsNO_3$=217.1.

CAS — 98-50-0.

A white or creamy-white almost odourless granular powder. **Soluble** 1 in 200 of water and 1 in 40 of alcohol; practically insoluble in chloroform and ether; soluble in solutions of alkali hydroxides.

In veterinary medicine, arsanilic acid is used in pigs and poultry for the prophylaxis and treatment of enteric infections due to *Escherichia coli* and *Vibrio coli*; it has also been administered in low concentrations as a growth-promoting agent.

12395-l

Arsenic Triiodide *(B.P.C. 1949)*. Arsen. Triiod.; Arsenous Iodide; Arsenious Iodide; Arsenium Iodatum; Arsenicum Triioduratum; Arsenii Iodetum.
AsI_3=455.6.

CAS — 7784-45-4.

Pharmacopoeias. In *Port.*

An almost odourless orange-red crystalline powder. **Soluble** partly or almost entirely 1 in 18 of water forming a slightly cloudy acid solution, and 1 in 42 of alcohol; soluble in chloroform and ether. **Incompatible** with alkaloids and many other substances. **Store** in airtight containers. Protect from light.

Arsenic triiodide has the adverse effects described under Arsenic Trioxide, p.1680. It was formerly used internally, usually in the form of Donovan's Solution, in the treatment of syphilitic skin conditions and was employed externally, as an ointment, in lupus and other skin conditions.

Preparations

Donovan's Solution. Liq. Arsen. et Hydrarg. Iod. *(B.P.C. 1949)*; Solution of Arsenous and Mercuric Iodides. Arsenic triiodide 1 g, red mercuric iodide 1 g, water to 100 ml. Protect from light in well-filled containers. *Dose.* 0.3 to 1 ml.

12396-y

Arsenic Trioxide *(B.P.C. 1963)*. Arsen. Trioxid.; Arseni Trioxydum; Arsenous Oxide; Arsenious Oxide; Arsenic; White Arsenic; Arsenious Anhydride; Arsenious Acid; Acidum Arsenicosum (Anhydricum); Anhydridum Arsenicosum.
As_2O_3=197.8.

CAS — 1327-53-3.

Pharmacopoeias. In *Arg.*, *Aust.*, *Belg.*, *Hung.*, *Int.*, *Jap.*, *Jug.*, *Mex.*, *Pol.*, *Port.*, *Rus.*, *Span.*, *Swiss*, and *Turk.*

A heavy white powder or irregular lumps with a vitreous fracture and often containing both transparent and opaque varieties. Very slowly **soluble** 1 in about 60 of water, the rate of solution depending on the relative proportions of the two varieties present, and on the degree of subdivision; more soluble in water acidified with hydrochloric acid and in alkali hydroxide and carbonate solutions; slightly soluble in alcohol and ether; very slowly soluble, at 20°, in glycerol but readily soluble in hot glycerol. **Incompatible** with calcium and magnesium salts, salts of heavy metals, iodine, and tannins.

Legislation in Great Britain controls the amount of arsenic in certain foods and beverages.

The tentative maximum acceptable daily load of arsenic in the diet was 50 µg per kg body-weight.— Tenth Report of Joint FAO/WHO Expert Committee on Food Additives, *Tech. Rep. Ser. Wld Hlth Org. No. 373*, 1967.

The standards of the WHO for drinking water stated that the concentration of arsenic in communal drinking water supplies should not exceed 0.05 ppm. The standards of the US Public Health Services for drinking water stated that if a communal water supply contained 0.01 to 0.05 ppm, alternative supplies should be used.— *Br. med. J.*, 1969, *3*, 70.

In a review of drinking water standards in April 1972 the WHO decided the present limit of 0.05 ppm for arsenic should remain.— S. Hernberg, *Chronicle Wld Hlth Org.*, 1973, *27*, 192.

Adverse Effects. Overdosage with arsenic is indicated by severe gastric pain, vomiting, profuse watery diarrhoea, proteinuria, numbness and tingling of the extremities, particularly the feet, followed by intense thirst and muscular cramps. From 100 to 300 mg of arsenic trioxide may be lethal if absorption is rapid and if adequate treatment is not given. Neuropathy, nephritis, and encephalopathy may follow acute arsenical poisoning.

Chronic arsenical poisoning is characterised by oedema of the face and eyelids, pruritus, soreness of the mouth, inflammation of the conjunctiva and nasal mucosa, loss of appetite, nausea, vomiting, and diarrhoea. The continued administration of small doses for long periods may lead to dryness of the skin, dermatitis, pigmentation, and keratinisation. Loss of hair and nails may follow. Among late symptoms and signs of chronic arsenical poisoning are anaemia, cirrhosis of the liver, jaundice, and peripheral neuritis. An association between the chronic administration of inorganic arsenic and neoplasms of the skin and lungs has long been suspected.

Maximum permissible atmospheric concentration of arsenic 200 µg per m^3.

Reviews and discussions on the toxicity and hazards associated with arsenic and arsenical compounds: M. M. Black, *Pharm. J.*, 1967, *2*, 593 (chronic ingestion); *Br. med. J.*, 1974, *3*, 487 (used as herbicides and animal feeding supplements); L. M. Klevay, *Pharmac. Ther.*, 1976, *1*, 189 (pharmacology and toxicology); W. L. Schoolmeester and D. R. White, *Sth. med. J.*, 1980, *73*,

198.

Chronic arsenical poisoning of the American Ambassador in Rome was believed to be due to her ingesting in her food over 2 or 3 years arsenate dust which had fallen from the paint on her bedroom ceiling. Symptoms developed slowly.— *Lancet*, 1956, *2*, 182.

A report of 11 cases of acute and subacute arsenical poisoning from drinking well-water contaminated with grasshopper bait buried in the area.— E. J. Feinglass, *New Engl. J. Med.*, 1973, *288*, 828.

A report of 74 cases of arsenic poisoning in Singapore resulting from the use of herbal preparations intended for the treatment of asthma and other illnesses.— C. -H. Tay and C. -S. Seah, *Med. J. Aust.*, 1975, *2*, 424.

References to industrial exposure to arsenic and mortality: O. Axelson *et al.*, *Br. J. ind. Med.*, 1978, *35*, 8, per *J. Am. med. Ass.*, 1978, *240*, 882; S. S. Pinto *et al.*, *Archs environ. Hlth*, 1978, *33*, 325.

Effects on blood. Thrombocytopenia had been associated with treatment with arsenic.— M. G. Wilson, *Am. J. Obstet. Gynec.*, 1962, *83*, 818.

A woman aged 18, treated for over 2 years with Fowler's solution for psoriasis, developed chronic arsenical poisoning which was associated with megaloblastic anaemia and folic acid deficiency.— J. H. M. van Tongeren *et al.*, *Lancet*, 1965, *1*, 784.

Aplastic anaemia and eventually acute myelogenous leukaemia developed in a 67-year-old man in association with the extensive use of arsenical pesticides.— C. R. Kjeldsberg and H. P. Ward, *Ann. intern. Med.*, 1972, *77*, 935.

Further references: J. R. Feussner *et al.*, *Blood*, 1979, *53*, 820.

Effects on the gastro-intestinal tract. A report of a massive haemorrhage from the upper gastro-intestinal tract of a previously healthy 64-year-old man who had taken a proprietary asthma relief preparation containing arsenic trioxide and potassium iodide daily for 55 years.— I. M. Szuler *et al.*, *Can. med. Ass. J.*, 1979, *120*, 168.

Effects on the heart. A report of severe arsenic poisoning complicated by atypical life-threatening ventricular tachycardia, with marked prolongation of the Q-T interval, in a 57-year-old man. ECG monitoring is considered mandatory during the initial phase in patients poisoned with arsenic. Ventricular tachycardia associated with a prolonged Q-T interval may be worsened by agents such as procainamide, quinidine, or disopyramide and in the short term isoprenaline is the treatment of choice.— S. Goldsmith and A. H. L. From, *New Engl. J. Med.*, 1980, *303*, 1096. Comments.— F. H. Meyers (letter), *ibid.*, 1981, *304*, 607; T. L. Kurt (letter), *ibid.* Reply.— S. Goldsmith and A. H. L. From (letter), *ibid.*

Effects on the liver. Non-cirrhotic portal hypertension occurred in 2 men as a result of chronic treatment with Fowler's solution; it was suggested that arsenic damaged the intrahepatic portal veins. Other side-effects included skin pigmentation and tumours in both and carcinoma of the larynx and bronchus in 1.— J. S. Morris *et al.*, *Gut*, 1973, *14*, 821.

See also under Malignant Neoplasms, below.

Effects on the nervous system. Of 57 patients in North Carolina who had been acutely poisoned by inorganic arsenicals, 37 developed neuropathy and 5 encephalopathy, 7 to 14 days after the incident. Unless dimercaprol was administered within the first 18 hours of the illness, it failed to prevent the development of neuropathies.— R. B. Jenkins, *Brain*, 1966, *89*, 479.

A 59-year-old man developed arsenical peripheral neuropathy, acute respiratory involvement, and chronic bronchitis, and died following the application to the face of an arsenical paste as a quack cancer cure.— T. J. Robinson, *Br. med. J.*, 1975, *3*, 139.

Further references: L. G. Garb and C. H. Hine, *J. occup. Med.*, 1977, *19*, 567, per *Abstr. Hyg.*, 1978, *53*, 6.

Effects on the respiratory system. A report of acute respiratory failure following severe arsenic poisoning.— C. Greenberg *et al.*, *Chest*, 1979, *76*, 596.

See also under Malignant Neoplasms, below.

Effects on the skin. An illustrated description of cutaneous and other symptoms of arsenical poisoning.— F. A. J. Kingery, *J. Am. med. Ass.*, 1966, *196*, 173.

Arsenicals might cause bullous eruptions and exfoliative dermatitis.— R. L. Baer and H. Harris, *J. Am. med. Ass.*, 1967, *202*, 710.

The administration of arsenic compounds might cause photosensitivity.— J. Kalivas, *J. Am. med. Ass.*, 1969, *209*, 1706.

See also under Malignant Neoplasms, below.

Effects on the vascular system. Polyarteritis had been reported following the administration of arsenicals.— P. D. B. Davies, *Br. J. Dis. Chest*, 1969, *63*, 57.

Characteristic vascular lesions were found on postmortem examination of 5 infants who had suffered chronic arsenic poisoning.— H. G. Rosenberg, *Archs Path.*, 1974, *97*, 360, per *J. Am. med. Ass.*, 1974, *228*, 1323.

Malignant neoplasms. Retrospective studies showed the presence of malignant tumours in 12% and of premalignant keratoses in 44% of 144 subjects, 21 to 47 years after they had received medical treatment with arsenic.— S. Evans, *Br. J. Derm.*, 1977, *97*, *Suppl.* 15, 13.

A retrospective study of data of patients who had received arsenic for various skin diseases, obtained from the Danish Cancer Registry for the years 1930 to 1939, indicated that there was an increased incidence of internal malignant neoplasms associated with those patients who had arsenic keratoses.— F. R. Reymann *et al.*, *Archs Derm.*, 1978, *114*, 378.

Kidney. Adenocarcinoma of the kidney developed in a 45-year-old man 17 years after receiving inorganic arsenic therapy for 5 years for psoriasis.— D. S. Nurse (letter), *Med. J. Aust.*, 1978, *1*, 102.

Liver. Angiosarcoma of the liver occurred in a patient and was associated with chronic ingestion of Fowler's solution; angiosarcoma of the skin developed subsequently.— J. J. Lander *et al.*, *Gastroenterology*, 1975, *68*, 166, per *J. Am. med. Ass.*, 1975, *233*, 1327.

Further references: H. Falk *et al.*, *Lancet*, 1979, *2*, 1120.

Lung. Of 173 deceased subjects exposed primarily to lead and calcium arsenate a definite increase in respiratory cancer was found in comparison with 1809 who had not been exposed. Among the more heavily exposed an excess of respiratory cancer was observed more than 35 years after the initial exposure.— M. G. Ott *et al.*, *Archs environ. Hlth*, 1974, *29*, 250, per *J. Am. med. Ass.*, 1974, *230*, 769. See also A. M. Lee and J. F. Fraumeni, *J. natn. Cancer Inst.*, 1969, *42*, 1045, per *J. Am. med. Ass.*, 1969, *209*, 1121.

There was no association between arsenical air pollution arising from a copper smelter and lung cancer.— J. L. Lyon *et al.* (letter), *Lancet*, 1977, *2*, 869.

Nasopharynx. Nasopharyngeal carcinoma developed in a 41-year-old woman who had been treated with an arsenical solution for psoriasis for at least 20 years. Palmar and plantar keratoses were also present.— S. D. Prystowsky *et al.*, *Archs Derm.*, 1978, *114*, 602.

Skin. The causal relationship of arsenic to skin cancer was well established. In 6 patients (4 female and 2 male) arsenic was prescribed for psoriasis, rheumatic fever, convulsions, or as a general tonic. The average latent period before the clinical onset of lung cancer was 32 years and all tumours were poorly differentiated carcinomas. All patients had skin manifestations of chronic ingestion of arsenic. The period of administration varied from 3 to 15 years.— A. O. Robson and A. M. Jelliffe, *Br. med. J.*, 1963, *2*, 207.

Further references: S. L. Wagner *et al.*, *Archs Derm.*, 1979, *115*, 1205; *Br. med. J.*, 1979, *1*, 44.

Pregnancy and the neonate. A 17-year-old mother with depression took about 30 ml of a preparation containing 1.32% of elemental arsenic during the third trimester of pregnancy. Four days later, she gave birth to a premature infant who died from hyaline membrane disease 11 hours later. High concentrations of arsenic were found in the liver, brain, and kidneys.— G. Lugo *et al.*, *Am. J. Dis. Child.*, 1969, *117*, 328.

Treatment of Adverse Effects. Acute poisoning due to the ingestion of arsenic compounds should be treated by immediate gastric aspiration and lavage, followed by a saline purgative, such as sodium sulphate 30 g in 250 ml of water, to promote peristalsis. Dimercaprol is specific, and treatment should be started immediately the cause of poisoning is suspected—see Dimercaprol, p.383 for details of dosage. Morphine may be given to control severe abdominal pain. Water and electrolytes lost by vomiting and diarrhoea should be replaced.

Peritoneal dialysis or haemodialysis may be required for renal failure and exchange blood transfusion for severe liver damage.

Arsenic Antidote (see *Martindale 27th Edn*, p. 1723), which consisted principally of freshly precipitated ferric hydroxide, has been administered in the past in the early stages of the treatment of acute poisoning by inorganic arsenical compounds, but its efficacy was never proved, and it should no longer be used, especially since a specific treatment is available.

For the symptoms and treatment of poisoning with arsenic compounds, see *Poisonous Chemicals used on Farms and Gardens*, London, Department of Health and Social Security, 1969.

References to the use of penicillamine in the treatment of arsenic poisoning: A. Kuruvilla *et al.*, *Clin. Toxicol.*, 1975, *8*, 535; R. G. Peterson and B. H. Rumack, *J. Pediat.*, 1977, *91*, 661.

Absorption and Fate.

Studies on the absorption and fate of arsenic in man.— G. K. H. Tam *et al.*, *Toxic. appl. Pharmac.*, 1979, *50*, 319; C. Pomroy *et al.*, *ibid.*, 1980, *53*, 550.

Uses. The therapeutic use of inorganic arsenical preparations is no longer recommended. Arsenical Solution (Fowler's Solution) was formerly used in the treatment of some types of skin disease, especially dermatitis herpetiformis and eczema, and in leukaemia.

Externally, arsenic trioxide has a caustic action.

Arsenic trioxide has been widely employed as a constituent of weedkillers and sheepdips and for the destruction of rats and mice.

Arsenic trioxide is used in homoeopathic medicine.

Arsenic trioxide known locally as *Bhasma* was used in India as an aphrodisiac additive to opium.— D. V. Datta (letters), *Lancet*, 1977, *1*, 484 and 903. An Ayurvedic medicine (*Bhasam*), which contains arsenic, is commonly taken during pregnancy by women in some parts of India, in the hope of producing a male child.— D. V. Datta *et al.* (letter), *ibid.*, 1979, *2*, 641.

Preparations

For preparations containing arsenic trioxide, see Martindale 27th Edn, p. 1723.

12397-j

Arsine. Arsenic Trihydride; Hydrogen Arsenide.

AsH_3=77.9.

CAS — 7784-42-1.

A colourless gas with a disagreeable garlic-like odour.

Arsine is highly toxic. It causes severe haemolysis which may result in acute renal failure. Exposure to as little as 3 ppm may cause symptoms, after a latent period of 2 to 24 hours, including headache, fever, dyspnoea, tachycardia, abdominal pain, nausea, vomiting, jaundice, haemolytic anaemia, haematuria, oliguria, and anuria. Treatment involves exchange transfusions and haemodialysis; dimercaprol has been used but may not be effective. See also under Arsenic Trioxide, above.

Maximum permissible atmospheric concentration 0.05 ppm.

A review of arsine poisoning.— B. A. Fowler and J. B. Weissberg, *New Engl. J. Med.*, 1974, *291*, 1171.

Reports of arsine poisoning.— S. P. Wilkinson *et al.*, *Br. med. J.*, 1975, *3*, 559; S. S. Pinto, *J. occup. Med.*, 1976, *18*, 633; R. V. Rosvoll *et al.*, *Morb. Mortal.*, 1978, *27*, 165, per *Int. pharm. Abstr.*, 1979, *16*, 428; E. Rathus *et al.*, *Med. J. Aust.*, 1979, *1*, 163.

12398-z

Arsphenamine. Arsenobenzene; Arsenobenzol; Arsenophenolamine; Salvarsan; '606'. 4,4'-Arsenobis(2-aminophenol) dihydrochloride dihydrate.

$C_{12}H_{12}As_2N_2O_2,2HCl,2H_2O$=475.0.

CAS — 139-93-5 (anhydrous); 5794-20-7 (dihydrate).

A light yellow, odourless or almost odourless, hygroscopic powder containing about 32% of As. **Soluble** 1 in 5 of water, forming a thick syrupy liquid, and 1 in 12 of alcohol; very slightly soluble in chloroform and ether. Unstable in air. **Store** below 15° in sealed containers from which the air has been removed or replaced by an inert gas. Protect from light. If discoloured (either grey or brownish) arsphenamine must not be used.

Arsphenamine was formerly used similarly to neoarsphenamine (p.1731) in the treatment of syphilis.

12399-c

Artificial Saliva

Artificial saliva is used in conditions in which the normal secretion of saliva is reduced or absent.

An 'ideal' formula would be slightly viscous, have lubricating properties and a neutral reaction, not contain sucrose or inorganic elements other than buffers, be acceptably flavoured, be stable, and be harmless when swallowed. A preparation based on carmellose sodium, with phosphate buffer, hydroxybenzoates as preservatives, and flavoured with saccharin sodium and peppermint, chloroform, cinnamon, or anise may prove acceptable.

For formulas in *Martindale*, see Carmellose Sodium, p.951; Hypromellose, p.956; and Methylcellulose, p.948.

12400-c

Artificial Tears

Artificial tears are used in conditions in which the normal lachrymal secretion is reduced or absent.

Preparations should be lubricant, non-irritant, and sterile.

For formulas in *Martindale*, see Hypromellose, p.956; Methylcellulose, p.948; and Povidone, p.958.

12401-k

Asarabacca. Hazelwort; Wild Nard; Rhizoma Asari.

Pharmacopoeias. In *Swiss.*

The dried rhizome, roots, and leaves of *Asarum europaeum* (Aristolochiaceae).

Asarabacca is an ingredient of snuffs. It is also an irritant emetic and has been used in rodent poisons.

12402-a

Asbestos

The name asbestos is applied to several naturally occurring and widely distributed fibrous mineral silicates. They include amosite (brown asbestos), anthophyllite, chrysotile (white asbestos), and crocidolite (blue asbestos).

Asbestos has properties of heat resistance, insulation, and reinforcement and has been used extensively for heat or electrical insulation, fire protection, in friction materials, and in the construction industry in a wide variety of materials including cement, pipes, and tiles.

When inhaled asbestos fibres can cause asbestosis (pulmonary fibrosis), lung cancer, and mesothelioma of the pleura and peritoneum. Mesothelioma has been reported in persons exposed to relatively small amounts of asbestos after a latent period of more than 20 years. Occupational exposure has sometimes been associated with an increased incidence of gastro-intestinal and laryngeal cancers. Some types of asbestos are more hazardous than others; crocidolite is considered to be the most dangerous and is no longer imported into Great Britain. Occupational exposure to asbestos dust is now rigorously controlled.

Reviews and comments on asbestos and the hazards of exposure to asbestos dust: K. Constantinidis, *Br. J. clin. Pract.*, 1977, *31*, 89; *Lancet*, 1977, *2*, 1211; W. R. Lee, *Practitioner*, 1978, *221*, 581; *Br. med. J.*, 1978, *1*, 1164; C. M. Spooner, *New Engl. J. Med.*, 1979, *301*, 782; J. C. Wagner, *Practitioner*, 1979, *223*, 28; *Lancet*, 1979, *2*, 887; D. Gloag, *Br. med. J.*, 1981, *282*, 551; *idem*, 623 and 978; C. P. de Fonseka (letter), *ibid.*, 1707.

Asbestos and cancer.— *Chronicle Wld Hlth Org.*, 1977, *31*, 114.

Ingested asbestos fibres may penetrate the gastro-intestinal wall but there is insufficient evidence that ingested fibre can produce cancer. Inhalation of fibres can produce cancer.— Twenty-second Report of Joint FAO/WHO Expert Committee on Food Additives, *Tech. Rep. Ser. Wld Hlth Org. No. 631*, 1978.

An examination of asbestos in relation to food and drink. Although there is no clear evidence of an increased incidence of carcinoma of the gastro-intestinal tract attributable to asbestos in non-occupationally exposed populations, asbestos by inhalation is known to be carcinogenic. It would be prudent to ensure that contamination of drinking water, beverages, and food is reduced to a minimum and all possible action should be taken to achieve this.— Food Additives and Contaminants Committee, FAC/REP/30, London, HM Stationery Office, 1979. The hazards of asbestos in water.— *Lancet*, 1981, *2*, 132. Comment.— R. Murray and K. Browne (letter), *ibid.*, 415.

Comment on the epidemiology of mesothelioma and the role of asbestos.— K. H. Antman, *New Engl. J. Med.*, 1980, *303*, 200.

Reports of mesothelioma associated with asbestos: K. J. Arul and P. F. Holt, *Int. Archs occup. environ. Hlth*, 1977, *40*, 141, per *Abstr. Hyg.*, 1977, *52*, 1393; J. R. Edge and S. L. Choudhury, *Thorax*, 1978, *33*, 26, per *Abstr. Hyg.*, 1978, *53*, 316; D. B. Jefferys and J. A. Vale, *Br. med. J.*, 1978, *2*, 607; F. P. Li *et al.*, *J. Am. med. Ass.*, 1978, *240*, 467; N. J. Vianna and A. K. Polan, *Lancet*, 1978, *1*, 1061; V. L. Roggli (letter), *New Engl. J. Med.*, 1981, *304*, 1045.

12403-t

Astemizole. R-43512. 1-(4-Fluorobenzyl)-2-{[1-(4-methoxyphenethyl)-4-piperidyl]amino}benzimidazole.

$C_{28}H_{31}FN_4O$=458.6.

CAS — 68844-77-9.

Astemizole is an antihistamine.

References: J. Callier *et al.*, *Curr. ther. Res.*, 1981, *29*, 24.

Manufacturers

Janssen, Belg.

12404-x

Astromicin Sulphate. Astromicin Sulfate; Fortimicin A; Abbott-44747; KW-1070. 4-Amino-1-(2-amino-*N*-methylacetamido)-1,4-dideoxy-3-*O*-(2,6-diamino-2,3,4,6,7-pentadeoxy-β-L-*lyxo*-heptopyranosyl)-6-*O*-methyl-L-*chiro*-inositol sulphate.

$C_{17}H_{35}N_5O_6,2H_2SO_4$=601.6.

CAS — 55779-06-1 (astromicin); 72275-67-3 (sulphate); 66768-12-5 (xH_2SO_4).

An antibiotic produced by *Micromonospora* spp.

Astromicin sulphate is an antibiotic with a spectrum of activity broadly similar to that of gentamicin.

References: R. N. Jones *et al.*, *Antimicrob. Ag. Chemother.*, 1979, *16*, 823 (antimicrobial activity); Y. Ohashi *et al.*, *ibid.*, 1980, *17*, 138 (antimicrobial activity); E. T. Kimura *et al.*, *Toxic. appl. Pharmac.*, 1980, *53*, 399 (toxicity studies in *animals*).

Manufacturers

Abbott, USA; Kyowa, Jap.

12405-r

Atracurium Besylate. 33A74. 2,2′-(3,11-Dioxo-4,10-dioxatridecamethylene)bis(1,2,3,4-tetrahydro-6,7-dimethoxy-2-methyl-1-veratrylisoquinolinium) di(benzenesulphonate).

$C_{53}H_{72}N_2O_{12},2C_6H_5O_3S$=1243.5.

CAS — 64228-81-5.

Atracurium besylate is a non-depolarising muscle relaxant.

References: R. Hughes and D. J. Chapple, *Br. J. Anaesth.*, 1980, *52*, 238P (*animal* studies); T. M. Hunt *et al.*, *ibid.*, (preliminary studies in 28 patients); R. Hughes *et al.*, *ibid.*, 634P (recovery); R. Hughes *et al.*, *ibid.*, 956P (clinical studies); R. Hughes and D. J. Chapple, *ibid.*, 1981, *53*, 31 (pharmacology).

Manufacturers

Wellcome, UK.

12406-f

Atromepine. Tropine (−)-α-methyltropate; (1*R*,3*r*,5*S*)-Tropan-3-yl (−)-α-methyltropate.

$C_{18}H_{25}NO_3$=303.4.

CAS — 428-07-9.

Atromepine is an anticholinergic agent.

Proprietary Names

Analgispan *(Lepetit, Spain).*

12407-d

Aurotioprol. Sodium 3-aurothio-2-hydroxypropane-1-sulphonate.

$C_3H_6AuNaO_4S_2$=390.2.

CAS — 27279-43-2.

Aurotioprol is a gold compound used in the treatment of arthritic disorders.

Proprietary Names

Allochrysine *(Sarbach, Fr.).*

12408-n

Avena. Aven; Cultivated White Oats; Oats; Oatmeal.

The grain of *Avena sativa* (Gramineae).

Avena is reputed to have antidepressant activity and has been administered as a liquid extract or tincture. It has been claimed to counteract dependence on nicotine and morphine.

Avenin, a protein present in oats, might be harmful to patients with coeliac disease.

Variable reports of the effects of avena on nicotine and morphine dependence: C. L. Anand (letter), *Nature*, 1971, *233*, 496; *idem* (letter), *Br. med. J.*, 1971, *3*, 640; C. G. Le Fevre (letter), *Med. J. Aust.*, 1972, *1*, 140; C. Bye *et al.* (letter), *Nature*, 1974, *252*, 580; J. W. Gabrynowicz (letter), *Med. J. Aust.*, 1974, *2*, 306; J. Connor *et al.*, *J. Pharm. Pharmac.*, 1975, *27*, 92.

Proprietary Preparations

Aveeno Colloidal *(Cooper, UK).* A bath additive containing colloidal oat fraction. **Aveeno Oilated.** A bath additive containing colloidal oat fraction 40% and liquid paraffin 37%. **Aveenobar.** A skin cleanser containing colloidal oat fraction 52.6%, isopropyl myristate 3%, and a lanolin derivative 0.9%, in a soapless basis. **Aveenobar Oilated.** A skin cleanser containing colloidal oat fraction 30%, vegetable oils 23%, and a lanolin derivative 1%, in a soapless basis.

12409-h

Azaclorzine Hydrochloride. AY-25329; Nonachlazine; Nonakhlazine. 2-Chloro-10-[3-(perhydropyrrolo[1,2-*a*]pyrazin-2-yl)propionyl]-phenothiazine dihydrochloride.

$C_{22}H_{24}ClN_3OS,2HCl$=486.9.

CAS — 49864-70-2 (azaclorzine); 49780-10-1 (hydrochloride).

A creamish or yellow-greenish crystalline powder. M.p. 218° to 228°. Freely **soluble** in water; sparingly soluble in alcohol.

Azaclorzine hydrochloride is a phenothiazine derivative used in the USSR as a coronary vasodilator.

Manufacturers

Ayerst, USA.

12410-a

Azalomycin. A mixture of related antibiotics produced by *Streptomyces hygroscopicus* var. *azalomyceticus*. Azalomycins B, F, and M have been identified.

CAS — 54182-65-9; 11003-23-9 (azalomycin B); 11003-24-0 (azalomycin F); 28380-24-7 (azalomycin M).

Azalomycin F, containing at least 5 components, is a white to light yellow amorphous or crystalline powder. Practically **insoluble** in water; sparingly soluble in dimethylformamide and methyl alcohol.

Azalomycin has been used in the treatment of vaginitis due to *Trichomonas* spp. or *Candida albicans*.

The properties of azalomycin F.— M. Arai, *Arzneimittel-Forsch.*, 1968, *18*, 1396.

Manufacturers
Sankyo, Jap.

12411-t

Azanidazole. F-4. 4-[(*E*)-2-(1-Methyl-5-nitroimidazol-2-yl)vinyl]pyrimidin-2-ylamine.
$C_{10}H_{10}N_6O_2$=246.2.

CAS — 62973-76-6.

NOTE. The name Nitromidine has been suggested for azanidazole.

Azanidazole has been used for the treatment of vaginal trichomonal infections.

Proprietary Names
Triclose *(Ist. Chem. Ital., Ital.).*

NOTE. Triclos is a proprietary name for triclofos sodium.

12412-x

Azaperone *(B.P. Vet.).* R-1929. 4′-Fluoro-4-[4-(2-pyridyl)piperazin-1-yl]butyrophenone.
$C_{19}H_{22}FN_3O$=327.4.

CAS — 1649-18-9.

A white to yellowish-white microcrystalline powder. M.p. 90° to 95°. Practically **insoluble** in water; soluble 1 in 29 of alcohol, 1 in 4 of chloroform, and 1 in 31 of ether. Solutions are **sterilised** by filtration. **Protect** from light.

Azaperone is a tranquilliser used in veterinary practice.

References: C. J. E. Niemegeers *et al.*, *Arzneimittel-Forsch.*, 1974, *24*, 1798; A. G. Rauws *et al.*, *Toxic. appl. Pharmac.*, 1976, *35*, 333.

Proprietary Names
Suicalm (Janssen)*(Crown, UK).*

14036-v

Azelaic Acid. Nonanedioic acid; Heptane-1,7-dicarboxylic acid.
$C_9H_{16}O_4$=188.2.

CAS — 123-99-9.

Azelaic acid has been applied as a 15% cream to the lesions of malignant melanoma; it has also been given by mouth. A cytotoxic effect on the malignant melanocyte has been reported.

References: M. Nazzaro-Porro *et al.* (preliminary communication), *Lancet*, 1980, *1*, 1109.

12413-r

Azelastine. A-5610. 4-(4-Chlorobenzyl)-2-(perhydro-1-methylazepin-4-yl)phthalazin-1-one.
$C_{22}H_{24}ClN_3O$=381.9.

CAS — 58581-89-8.

Azelastine has antihistamine activity.

For a series of studies in *animals*, see *Arzneimittel-Forsch.*, 1981, *31*, 1184–1230.

12414-f

Azolimine. CL-90748. 2-Imino-3-methyl-1-phenylimidazolidin-4-one.
$C_{10}H_{11}N_3O$=189.2.

CAS — 40828-45-3.

A crystalline solid. M.p. about 169°.

Azolimine is a potassium-sparing diuretic.

Pharmacology in *animals*.— R. Z. Gussin *et al.*, *J. Pharmac. exp. Ther.*, 1975, *195*, 8.

Manufacturers
Lederle, USA.

12415-d

Azosemide. BM-02001; Ple-1053. 2-Chloro-5-(1*H*-tetrazol-5-yl)-4-(2-thenylamino)benzenesulphonamide.
$C_{12}H_{11}ClN_6O_2S_2$=370.8.

CAS — 27589-33-9.

Azosemide is a diuretic with actions similar to those of frusemide.

References: F. Krück *et al.*, *Eur. J. clin. Pharmac.*, 1978, *14*, 153; D. C. Brater, *Clin. Pharmac. Ther.*, 1979, *25*, 428; D. C. Brater *et al.*, *ibid.*, 435; C. Brater *et al.*, *ibid.*, 1979, *26*, 437; R. Seiwell and C. Brater, *ibid.*, 1980, *27*, 285; K. Horky *et al.*, *Eur. J. Pharmac.*, 1981, *69*, 439.

Manufacturers
Boehringer Mannheim, Ger.

12416-n

Bambermycin. Bambermycins; Flavophospholipol. An antibiotic complex containing mainly moenomycin A and moenomycin C and which may be obtained from cultures of *Streptomyces bambergiensis*.

CAS — 11015-37-5.

Bambermycin is used in feedstuffs for pigs and poultry and in veterinary supplements—see under Antibiotic Supplements for Animal Feeds, p.1082.

Proprietary Names
Flavomycin *(Hoechst, USA).*

12417-h

Barbetonium Iodide. Diethyl[2-(5-ethylperhydro-2,4,6-trioxo-5-phenylpyrimidin-1-yl)ethyl]methylammonium iodide.
$C_{19}H_{28}IN_3O_3$=473.4.

CAS — 6191-48-6.

Barbetonium iodide is an anticholinergic agent which has been used for its spasmolytic effects on the gastro-intestinal tract.

Proprietary Names
Defenale *(IBIS, Ital.).*

12418-m

Barbexaclone. (−)-2-Cyclohexyl-*N*,1-dimethylethylamine 5-ethyl-5-phenylbarbiturate.
$C_{12}H_{12}N_2O_3,C_{10}H_{21}N$=387.5.

CAS — 4388-82-3.

Barbexaclone is a compound of (−)-propylhexedrine and phenobarbitone. It has been used in the treatment of epilepsy.

Proprietary Names
Maliasin *(Knoll, Arg.; Knoll AG, Austral.; Knoll, Ger.; Knoll, Switz.).*

12419-b

Batroxobin. A thrombin-like enzyme obtained from the venom of the viper *Bothrops atrox*.

CAS — 9039-61-6; 54182-64-8.

NOTE. The name Hemocoagulase has also been used for preparations of batroxobin. The names batroxobin and hemocoagulase have also been used for preparations from the venom of *Bothrops jararaca*.

Batroxobin has been used as a haemostat in haemorrhagic disorders. Some authorities consider that its action depends on the production of a low-grade disseminated intravascular coagulation and that it cannot therefore be recommended.

The effect of prophylactic administration of a coagulant fraction from *Bothrops jararaca* on blood loss in vaginal operations.— P. Godts and R. Dewitte, *Acta ther.*, 1978, *4*, 63.

Proprietary Names
Reptilase *(Stago, Fr.; Knoll, Ger.; Richter, Ital.; Kramer, Switz.).*

Proprietary Names of Preparations from *Bothrops jararaca*
Botropase *(Ravizza, Belg.; Ravizza, Ital.).*

12420-x

Bearberry. Uva Ursi; Bearberry Leaves; Busserole; Bärentraubenblätter; Ptarmiganberry Leaves.

Pharmacopoeias. In *Aust., Belg., Cz., Ger., Hung., Jap., Jug., Pol., Port., Rus.,* and *Swiss.*

The dried leaves of the bearberry, *Arctostaphylos uva-ursi* (Ericaceae).

Bearberry has been reported to be a diuretic and astringent. It has been given as an infusion or liquid extract in the treatment of urethritis and cystitis.

12421-r

Beclobrate. Sgd-24774. Ethyl (±)-2-(4-*p*-chlorobenzylphenoxy)-2-methylbutyrate.
$C_{20}H_{23}ClO_3$=346.9.

CAS — 55937-99-0.

Beclobrate is reported to lower blood concentrations of cholesterol.

References: K. Thiele *et al.*, *Arzneimittel-Forsch.*, 1979, *29*, 711.

Manufacturers
Siegfried, Ger.

12422-f

Befuraline Hydrochloride. DIV-154. Benzofuran-2-yl 4-benzylpiperazin-1-yl ketone hydrochloride.
$C_{20}H_{20}N_2O_2$,HCl=356.9.

CAS — 41717-30-0 (befuraline); 41716-84-1 (hydrochloride).

Befuraline hydrochloride has antidepressant properties.

References: J. Komarek and F. J. Neumann, *Arzneimittel-Forsch.*, 1977, *27*, 2066; R. Clemens and U. Clemens, *ibid.*, 2416; I. J. E. Boksay *et al.*, *ibid.*, 1979, *29*, 193.

Manufacturers
Hoechst, Ger.

12423-d

Bemetizide. Diu-60. 6-Chloro-3,4-dihydro-3-(α-methylbenzyl)-2*H*-1,2,4-benzothiadiazine-7-sulphonamide 1,1-dioxide.
$C_{15}H_{16}ClN_3O_4S_2$=401.9.

CAS — 1824-52-8.

Bemetizide is a thiazide diuretic which has been used with guabenxan in the treatment of hypertension.

12424-n

Benfluorex Hydrochloride. JP-992; 780-SE. 2-[α-Methyl-3-(trifluoromethyl)phenethylamino]ethyl benzoate hydrochloride. $C_{19}H_{20}F_3NO_2,HCl=387.8$.

CAS — 23602-78-0 (benfluorex); 35976-51-3 (benfluorex, ±); 23642-66-2 (hydrochloride).

Benfluorex hydrochloride has been used in the treatment of hypertriglyceridaemia and hypercholesterolaemia. It has been reported to have anorectic and hypoglycaemic activity.

Absence of interaction with phenprocoumon.— P. De Witte and H. M. Brems, *Curr. med. Res. Opinion*, 1980, *6*, 478.

Proprietary Names
Médiator *(Servier, Fr.)*.

12425-h

Benorterone. SKF-7690. 17β-Hydroxy-17α-methyl-*B*-norandrost-4-en-3-one. $C_{19}H_{28}O_2=288.4$.

CAS — 3570-10-3.

Benorterone is an anti-androgen. It has been tried in acne and idiopathic hirsutism.

Twenty of 23 women with acne benefited from treatment with benorterone, for 2 to 17 months, as did 20 of 28 women with idiopathic hirsutism who received benorterone for 5 to 17 months. Two of 62 patients treated with benorterone developed a 50% decrease in prothrombin time after treatment for 1 month, with a return to normal on discontinuing therapy.— A. Zarate *et al.* (letter), *J. clin. Endocr. Metab.*, 1966, *26*, 1394.

Benorterone was beneficial in patients with acne and idiopathic hirsutism but after withdrawal of the drug symptoms recurred in all patients with acne and in most of those with hirsutism.— S. D. Pria *et al.*, *J. invest. Derm.*, 1969, *52*, 348, per *J. Am. med. Ass.*, 1969, *208*, 1053.

Manufacturers
Smith Kline & French, USA.

12426-m

Benperazine Bromide. LBC-132. (Piperazine-1,4-diyldiethylene)bis(benzyldiethylammonium bromide). $C_{30}H_{50}Br_2N_2=598.5$.

CAS — 17172-31-5.

Benperazine bromide is a muscle relaxant which has been used in spastic disorders.

Proprietary Names
Isocurine *(Du Bled, Belg.)*.

12427-b

Benproperine. 1-[2-(2-Benzylphenoxy)-1-methylethyl]piperidine. $C_{21}H_{27}NO=309.5$.

CAS — 2156-27-6.

Benproperine has been used for the relief of cough. The embonate and phosphate have been used.

Proprietary Names of Benproperine Salts
Blascorid *(Guidotti, Ital.)*; Pirexil *(Astra, Arg.)*; Pirexyl *(Pharmacia, Swed.)*; Tussafug *(Robugen, Ger.; Robugen, Switz.)*; Cofrel.

12428-v

Bensuldazic Acid. (5-Benzylperhydro-6-thioxo-1,3,5-thiadiazin-3-yl)acetic acid. $C_{12}H_{14}N_2O_2S_2=282.4$.

CAS — 1219-77-8.

A fungicide; the sodium salt of bensuldazic acid is used in veterinary medicine for the external treatment of ringworm.

Proprietary Names
Defungit *(sodium salt) (Hoechst, UK)*.

12429-g

Bentazepam. Thiadipone; CI-718; QM-6008. 1,3,6,7,8,9-Hexahydro-5-phenyl-2*H*-[1]benzothieno[2,3-*e*]-1,4-diazepin-2-one. $C_{17}H_{16}N_2OS=296.4$.

CAS — 29462-18-8.

A crystalline solid. M.p. about 242°.

Bentazepam is a substituted benzodiazepine tranquilliser.

Pharmacology in *animals*.— M. P. Fernández-Tomé *et al.*, *Arzneimittel-Forsch.*, 1975, *25*, 926.

Manufacturers
Parke, Davis, USA.

12431-d

Benzalamide. 3-Methyl-4-phenylbut-3-enamide. $C_{11}H_{13}NO=175.2$.

CAS — 7236-47-7.

Benzalamide has been used in the treatment of lipid disorders.

Proprietary Names
Kata-Lipid *(Ibi, Ital.; IBE, Spain)*.

12432-n

Benzarone. L-2197. 2-Ethylbenzofuran-3-yl 4-hydroxyphenyl ketone. $C_{17}H_{14}O_3=266.3$.

CAS — 1477-19-6.

Benzarone has been given by mouth and applied topically in the treatment of various peripheral vascular disorders.

Pharmacology of benzarone in *cats*.— E. Betz and W. Eitel, *Arzneimittel-Forsch.*, 1978, *28*, 626.

Proprietary Names
Fragivix *(Labaz, Belg.; Labaz, Fr.; Sanol, Ger.; Sigmatau, Ital.; Labaz, Spain; Labaz, Switz.)*; Venagil *(Cristalfarma, Ital.)*.

12433-h

Benzpiperylone. KB-95. 4-Benzyl-2-(1-methyl-4-piperidyl)-5-phenyl-4-pyrazolin-3-one. $C_{22}H_{25}N_3O=347.5$.

CAS — 53-89-4.

Benzpiperylone is a pyrazole derivative which has been used in the treatment of rheumatic disorders.

Proprietary Names
Benzometan *(Castejon, Spain)*; Humedil *(Bio-Mar, Spain)*.

12434-m

Benzyl Isothiocyanate. Benzyl Mustard Oil; Benzylsenföl; Oleum Tropaeoli. $C_8H_7NS=149.2$.

CAS — 622-78-6.

An oil obtained from Capuchin cress, *Tropaeolum majus* (Tropaeolaceae). B.p. 243°. Practically **insoluble** in water; soluble in alcohol.

Benzyl isothiocyanate has been given as an antibacterial agent.

Proprietary Names
Tromacaps *(Madaus, Ger.; Madaus, Switz.)*.

12435-b

Bepridil Hydrochloride. CERM-1978. *N*-(3-Isobutoxy-2-pyrrolidin-1-ylpropyl)-*N*-phenylbenzylamine hydrochloride monohydrate. $C_{24}H_{34}N_2O,HCl,H_2O=421.0$.

CAS — 64706-54-3 (bepridil); 64616-81-5 (hydrochloride, anhydrous); 74764-40-2 (hydrochloride, monohydrate).

Bepridil hydrochloride is reported to be a vasodilator.

Manufacturers
Wallace, USA.

12436-v

Betaine Nicotinate. (Carboxymethyl)trimethylammonium nicotinate. $C_{11}H_{16}N_2O_4=240.3$.

Betaine nicotinate has been used as a hypolipidaemic agent.

Proprietary Names
Nibet *(Zoja, Ital.)*.

12437-g

Betamethasone Adamantoate. 9α-Fluoro-11β,17α,21-trihydroxy-16β-methylpregna-1,4-diene-3,20-dione 21-adamantoate. $C_{33}H_{43}FO_6=554.7$.

Betamethasone adamantoate is a long-acting corticosteroid with the general properties of betamethasone (p.461). It is used systemically in veterinary practice.

12438-q

Betanaphthyl Benzoate. Benzonaphthol; Naphthol Benzoate. 2-Naphthyl benzoate. $C_{17}H_{12}O_2=248.3$.

CAS — 93-44-7.

Pharmacopoeias. In *Belg., Pol., Port.,* and *Span.*

A white, crystalline, odourless, tasteless powder. Practically **insoluble** in water; very slightly soluble in cold alcohol but soluble in hot alcohol; soluble in chloroform, ether, and glacial acetic acid. **Incompatible** with alkaline substances, iron salts, salol, and thymol. **Protect** from light.

Betanaphthyl benzoate has been used for the treatment of intestinal infections and has been employed as an ointment in parasitic infections of the skin.

12439-p

Betaxolol Hydrochloride. SL-75212. 1-{4-[2-(Cyclopropylmethoxy)ethyl]phenoxy}-3-isopropylaminopropan-2-ol hydrochloride. $C_{18}H_{29}NO_3,HCl=343.9$.

CAS — 63659-18-7 (betaxolol); 63659-19-8 (hydrochloride).

Betaxolol hydrochloride is a beta-adrenoceptor blocking agent.

References: G. Bianchetti *et al.*, *Br. J. clin. Pharmac.*, 1979, *8*, 403P; *idem*, 403P; R. Gomeni *et al.*, *ibid.*, 404P; B. J. Davis and P. Turner, *ibid.*, 405P; G. Bianchetti *et al.*, *ibid.*, 407P; *idem*, 408P; J. R. Kilborn *et al.*, *ibid.*, 409P; K. Balnave *et al.*, *ibid.*, 1980, *9*, 297P; G. Bianchetti *et al.*, *ibid.*, 299P; P. J. Cadigan *et al.*, *ibid.*, 569; J. F. Giudicelli *et al.*, *ibid.*, *10*, 41; B. M. Assael *et al.*, *Clin. Pharmac. Ther.*, 1981, *29*, 232; K. Balnave *et al.*, *Br. J. clin. Pharmac.*, 1981, *11*, 171.

Manufacturers
Synthelabo, Fr.

12440-n

Bevantolol Hydrochloride. Cl-775. (±)-1-(3,4-Dimethoxyphenethylamino)-3-*m*-tolyloxypropan-2-ol hydrochloride.
$C_{20}H_{27}NO_4,HCl=381.9$.

CAS — 59170-23-9 (bevantolol); 42864-78-8 (hydrochloride).

Bevantolol hydrochloride is a beta-adrenoceptor blocking agent.

References: A. D. Mackay *et al., Clin. Pharmac. Ther.*, 1981, *29*, 1.

Manufacturers
Parke, Davis, USA.

12441-h

Bezafibrate. BM-15075; LO-44. 2-[4-(2-*p*-Chlorobenzamidoethyl)phenoxy]-2-methylpropionic acid.
$C_{19}H_{20}ClNO_4=361.8$.

CAS — 41859-67-0.

Bezafibrate is used in the treatment of hypertriglyceridaemia and hypercholesterolaemia. The usual dose is 600 mg daily; 400 mg daily may be adequate for maintenance.

Enhancement of the effect of phenprocoumon by bezafibrate.— R. Zimmerman *et al., Dt. med. Wschr.*, 1977, *102*, 509.

In a 12-week study in 13 well-controlled diabetic patients with hyperlipidaemia, bezafibrate 600 mg daily significantly reduced serum concentrations of cholesterol and triglycerides. During the study no change in antidiabetic medication was necessary.— P. Wahl *et al., Dt. med. Wschr.*, 1978, *103*, 1233. See also R. Fellin *et al., Curr. ther. Res.*, 1981, *29*, 657.

Disposition pharmacokinetics of bezafibrate in man.— U. Abshagen *et al., Eur. J. clin. Pharmac.*, 1979, *16*, 31. See also U. Abshagen *et al., ibid.*, 1980, *17*, 305.

Proprietary Preparations
Bezalip *(MCP Pharmaceuticals, UK).* Bezafibrate, available as tablets of 200 mg.

Other Proprietary Names
Cedur *(Ger.).*

12442-m

Bicyclomycin. 6-Hydroxy-5-methylene-1-(1,2,3-trihydroxy-2-methylpropyl)-2-oxa-7,9-diazabicyclo[4.2.2]deca-8,10-dione.
$C_{12}H_{18}N_2O_7=302.3$.

CAS — 38129-37-2.

An antibiotic obtained from strains of *Streptomyces sapporonensis* and *S. aizunensis.*
Freely **soluble** in water; sparingly soluble in alcohol; soluble in methyl alcohol; slightly soluble in acetone; practically insoluble in chloroform and ethyl acetate.

Bicyclomycin is an antibiotic reported to be effective *in vitro* against *Escherichia coli, Neisseria gonorrhoeae, Shigella* spp., and *Salmonella* spp. It has been given intramuscularly.

References: M. Nishida *et al., J. Antibiot., Tokyo*, 1972, *25*, 582; *idem*, 594.

Manufacturers
Fujisawa, Jap.

12443-b

Bietaserpine. DL-152; S-1210; 1-(2-Diethylaminoethyl)reserpine. Methyl 1-(2-diethylaminoethyl)-18-*O*-(3,4,5-trimethoxybenzoyl)reserpate.
$C_{39}H_{53}N_3O_9=707.9$.

CAS — 53-18-9.

Bietaserpine is an antihypertensive agent. It is used as the tartrate.

Proprietary Names
Pleiatensin Simplex (tartrate) *(Guidotti, Ital.)*; Tensibar (tartrate) *(Lefrancq, Fr.).*

12444-v

Bifonazole. Bay h-4502. 1-(α-Biphenyl-4-ylbenzyl)imidazole.
$C_{22}H_{18}N_2=310.4$.

CAS — 60628-96-8.

Bifonazole is reported to be a topical antifungal agent.

Manufacturers
Bayer, UK.

12445-g

Bismuth Dipropylacetate. Bismuth Valproate. Bismuth tris(2-propylvalerate).
$C_{24}H_{45}BiO_6=638.6$.

Bismuth dipropylacetate has been given rectally for the treatment of infections of the mouth and throat. The potential toxicity of the bismuth ion should be considered.

Proprietary Names
Birectal *(Labaz, Fr.)*; Maribis *(Gazzini, Ital.)*; Neo-Laryngobis *(Bio-Chemical Laboratory, Canad.)*; Suppangin *(Südmedica, Ger.).*

12446-q

Bisoxatin Acetate. Bisoxatin Diacetate; Wy-8138. 2,2-Bis(4-hydroxyphenyl)-1,4-benzoxazin-3(2*H*,4*H*)-one diacetate.
$C_{24}H_{19}NO_6=417.4$.

CAS — 17692-24-9 (bisoxatin); 14008-48-1 (acetate).

Bisoxatin acetate is used as a purgative.

Proprietary Names
Kritel *(Gramon, Arg.)*; Laxonalin *(Fher, Spain)*; Maratan *(Ravizza, Ital.)*; Wylaxine *(Wyeth, Belg.; Wyeth, Neth.).*

12447-p

Bitolterol Mesylate. Win-32784. 4-[2-(*tert*-Butylamino)-1-hydroxyethyl]-*o*-phenylene di(*p*-toluate) methanesulphonate.
$C_{28}H_{31}NO_5,CH_4O_3S=557.7$.

CAS — 30392-40-6 (bitolterol); 30392-41-7 (mesylate).

Bitolterol mesylate has bronchodilator properties.

References: I. Kass and T. S. Mingo, *Chest*, 1980, *78*, 283.

Manufacturers
Winthrop, USA.

12448-s

BL-3459. 1,2,3,5-Tetrahydro-6-methylimidazo[2,1-*b*]quinazolin-2-one hydrochloride monohydrate.
$C_{11}H_{11}N_3O,HCl,H_2O=255.7$.

CAS — 50608-63-4 (anhydrous).

BL-3459 is an inhibitor of platelet aggregation, potentially useful as an antithrombotic agent.

Pharmacology of BL-3459 in *animals.*— J. S. Fleming *et al., J. Pharmac. exp. Ther.*, 1975, *194*, 435; M. V. Griffiths *et al., Archs Otolar.*, 1977, *103*, 318.

Manufacturers
Bristol, USA.

12449-w

Black Nightshade. Morelle Noire.

Pharmacopoeias. In *Chin.*

The leaves and flowering tops of the black or garden nightshade, *Solanum nigrum* (Solanaceae). It contains solanine and its allied alkaloids.

Black nightshade is distributed throughout most of the world as a weed of cultivation. It appears to have little medicinal value but has been used in liniments, poultices, and decoctions for external application. The treatment of adverse effects is as described under Atropine, p.290.

12450-m

Boldenone Undecenoate. Ba-29038; Boldenone Undecylenate. 17β-Hydroxyandrosta-1,4-dien-3-one 17-(undec-10-enoate).
$C_{30}H_{44}O_3=452.7$.

CAS — 846-48-0 (boldenone); 13103-34-9 (undecenoate).

Boldenone undecenoate is an anabolic steroid used in veterinary practice.

Proprietary Names
Vebonol *(Ciba-Geigy Agrochemicals, UK).*

12451-b

Bradykinin. Kallidin-9.

CAS — 58-82-2.

Bradykinin is a potent vasoactive nonapeptide described by M. Rocha e Silva *et al., Am. J. Physiol.*, 1949, *156*, 261. They showed that it is formed by the action of certain enzymes (such as trypsin or those in some snake venoms, e.g. *Bothrops jararaca*) on plasma globulins. It has since been synthesised. [R.A. Boissonnas *et al., Experientia*, 1960, *16*, 26]. Physiologically, it is formed by the action of proteolytic enzymes (kallikreins) on a plasma globulin (kininogen). It is rapidly inactivated by peptidases. Its main pharmacological effects are smooth muscle stimulation, vasodilatation, increase in capillary permeability, production of oedema, and production of pain.

The pharmacology of bradykinin and related polypeptides.— A. P. Somlyo and A. V. Somlyo, *Pharmac. Rev.*, 1970, *22*, 249; H. P. J. Bennett and C. McMartin, *ibid.*, 1978, *30*, 247; D. Regoli and J. Barabe, *ibid.*, 1980, *32*, 1.

Further references: G. Bertaccini, *Pharmac. Rev.*, 1976, *28*, 127 (non-mammalian); *Am. Pharm.*, 1979, *NS19* (Feb.), 40 (possible significance in contraception).

12452-v

Brocresine. CL-54998; NSD-1055. α-Amino-oxy-6-bromo-*m*-cresol.
$C_7H_8BrNO_2=218.0$.

CAS — 555-65-7.

Brocresine is claimed to be a histidine decarboxylase inhibitor although this has been disputed. It has been used in pruritus, chronic urticaria, and parkinsonism.

References: *J. Am. med. Ass.*, 1968, *205* (Aug. 26), A27 (pruritus); H. Zachariae *et al., J. invest. Derm.*, 1969, *53*, 341 (urticaria), per *J. Am. med. Ass.*, 1969, *210*, 1789; M. W. Greaves, *Br. J. Derm.*, 1971, *85*, 467 (urticaria); P. M. Howse and W. B. Matthews, *J. Neurol. Neurosurg. Psychiat.*, 1973, *36*, 27 (parkinsonism).

12453-g

Bromophenylpropenal. 2-Bromo-3-phenylprop-2-enal.
$C_9H_7BrO=211.1$.

CAS — 5443-49-2.

Bromophenylpropenal is reported to have antifungal activity.

Proprietary Names
Amplimykol *(Fides, Spain).*

12454-q

Bromopride. CM-8252; VAL-13081. 4-Amino-5-bromo-*N*-(2-diethylaminoethyl)-*o*-anisamide.
$C_{14}H_{22}BrN_3O_2$=344.3.

CAS — 4093-35-0.

Bromopride has been used in a variety of gastro-intestinal disorders, including the relief of nausea and vomiting.

Use in radiology.— V. S. Benakis *et al.*, *Pharmatherapeutica*, 1978, *2*, 53.

Proprietary Names
Cascapride *(Cascan, Ger.)*; Emoril *(Roemmers, Arg.)*; Plesium *(Chiesi, Ital.)*; Praiden *(Italchemi, Ital.)*; Valopride *(Vita, Ital.)*; Viaben *(Schürholz, Ger.)*.

12455-p

Bromovinyldeoxyuridine. (*E*)-5-(2-Bromovinyl)-2′-deoxyuridine.
$C_{11}H_{13}BrN_2O_5$=333.1.

Bromovinyldeoxyuridine is reported to have antiviral activity.

Studies in *animals*.— J. Descamps *et al.*, *Antimicrob. Ag. Chemother.*, 1979, *16*, 680; P. C. Maudgal *et al.*, *Antimicrob. Ag. Chemother.*, 1980, *17*, 8.

Use in 4 patients with herpes zoster.— E. de Clercq *et al.*, *Br. med. J.*, 1980, *281*, 1178.

12456-s

Broparestrol. α-Bromo-β-(4-ethylphenyl)stilbene.
$C_{22}H_{19}Br$=363.3.

CAS — 479-68-5.

Broparestrol is a synthetic compound with oestrogenic activity. It has been given for the suppression of lactation and in neoplastic disease. It has been used topically in acne and similar skin disorders.

Proprietary Names
Acnestrol *(Scharper, Ital.)*; Longestrol *(Laroche Navarron, Fr.; Landerlan, Spain)*.

12457-w

Brotianide. Bay-4059Va; FBA-4059. 2-Bromo-6-(4-bromophenylthiocarbamoyl)-4-chlorophenyl acetate; 2-Acetoxy-3,4′-dibromo-5-chlorothiobenzanilide.
$C_{15}H_{10}Br_2ClNO_2S$=463.6.

CAS — 23233-88-7.

Brotianide is a veterinary anthelmintic used in the treatment of liver-fluke infestation.

12458-e

Brotizolam. We-941; We-941-BS. 2-Bromo-4-(2-chlorophenyl)-9-methyl-6*H*-thieno[3,2-*f*]-[1,2,4]triazolo[4,3-*a*][1,4]diazepine.
$C_{15}H_{10}BrClN_4S$=393.7.

CAS — 57801-81-7.

Brotizolam is a hypnotic.

References: J. Grünberger *et al.*, *Curr. ther. Res.*, 1978, *24*, 427; B. Saletu *et al.*, *Arzneimittel-Forsch.*, 1979, *29*, 700; A. N. Nicholson *et al.*, *Br. J. clin. Pharmac.*, 1980, *10*, 75; M. Fink and P. Irwin, *Clin. Pharmac. Ther.*, 1981, *30*, 336.

Manufacturers
Boehringer Ingelheim, Ger.

12459-l

Brucellin

CAS — 11028-17-4.

Pharmacopoeias. In *Chin.* and *Rus.*

A sterile filtrate of a broth culture of *Brucella* organisms.

Brucellin has been used in an intradermal skin test for the diagnosis of brucellosis but results are unreliable.

Results indicating that the brucellin skin test should not be used for the diagnosis of brucellosis.—Report by a Working-party to the Director of the Public Health Laboratory Service, *Lancet*, 1972, *1*, 676.

See also Fifth Report of the Joint FAO/WHO Expert Committee on Brucellosis, *Tech. Rep. Ser. Wld Hlth Org. No. 464*, 1971, p. 34.

12460-v

Bryonia. The root of *Bryonia alba* (Cucurbitaceae).

Bryonia is used in homoeopathic medicine.

12461-g

Buchu *(B.P.C. 1963)*. Buchu Leaves; Bucco; Folia Bucco.

CAS — 68650-46-4 (buchu oil).

Pharmacopoeias. In *Cz.*

The dried leaves of 'short' or 'round' buchu, *Agathosma betulina* (=*Barosma betulina*) (Rutaceae) containing not less than 1.8% v/w of volatile oil. **Store** in a cool dry place. Protect from light.

Buchu is a weak diuretic and urinary antiseptic and was formerly administered as an infusion in mixtures for urinary-tract infections.

12462-q

Bucindolol Hydrochloride. MJ-13105-1. 2-[2-Hydroxy-3-(2-indol-3-yl-1,1-dimethylethylamino)propoxy]benzonitrile hydrochloride.
$C_{22}H_{25}N_3O_2$,HCl=399.9.

CAS — 71119-11-4 (bucindolol); 70369-47-0 (hydrochloride).

Bucindolol hydrochloride is a beta-adrenoceptor blocking agent.

Manufacturers
Bristol-Myers, UK; Mead Johnson, USA.

12463-p

Budesonide. S-1320. An epimeric mixture of the α- and β-propyl forms of 16α,17α-butylidenedioxy-11β,21-dihydroxypregna-1,4-diene-3,20-dione.
$C_{25}H_{34}O_6$=430.5.

CAS — 51333-22-3 (11β,16α); 51372-29-3 [11β,16α(R)]; 51372-28-2 [11β,16α(S)].

Budesonide is a topical corticosteroid.

References: H. Schmidt *et al.*, *J. int. med. Res.*, 1981, *9*, 236 (comparison with betamethasone valerate); H. Degreef and L. Salde, *Curr. ther. Res.*, 1981, *29*, 880 (comparison with betamethasone dipropionate).

Proprietary Names
Preferid *(Tika, Denm.)*.

12464-s

Bufeniode. HF-241; Di-iodobuphenine. 4-Hydroxy-3,5-di-iodo-α-{1-[(1-methyl-3-phenylpropyl)amino]ethyl}benzyl alcohol.
$C_{19}H_{23}I_2NO_2$=551.2.

CAS — 22103-14-6.

Bufeniode is an antihypertensive agent.

Proprietary Names
Proclival *(Roussel, Arg.; Houdé-I.S.H., Fr.)*.

12465-w

Buflomedil Hydrochloride. LL-1656. 2′,4′,6′-Trimethoxy-4-(pyrrolidin-1-yl)butyrophenone hydrochloride.
$C_{17}H_{25}NO_4$,HCl=343.8.

CAS — 55837-25-7 (buflomedil).

Buflomedil hydrochloride is reported to have vasodilator properties.

References: G. Rosas *et al.*, *Angiology*, 1981, *32*, 291.

Proprietary Names
Fonzylane *(Lafon, Fr.)*; Lofton; Loftyl.

12466-e

Bunamidine Hydrochloride *(B.P. Vet.)*. N^1,N^1-Dibutyl-4-hexyloxy-1-naphthamidine hydrochloride.
$C_{25}H_{38}N_2O$,HCl=419.0.

CAS — 3748-77-4 (bunamidine); 1055-55-6 (hydrochloride).

A white, odourless or almost odourless, crystalline powder. M.p. about 210°. **Soluble** 1 in 200 of water, 1 in 2 of alcohol, and 1 in 2 of chloroform; practically insoluble in ether.

Bunamidine is a veterinary anthelmintic, administered as tablets in the treatment of tapeworm infestations in dogs and cats.

Proprietary Names
Scolaban *(Wellcome, UK)*.

12467-l

Bunamidine Hydroxynaphthoate *(B. Vet. C. 1965)*. N^1,N^1-Dibutyl-4-hexyloxy-1-naphthamidine 3-hydroxy-2-naphthoate.
$C_{36}H_{46}N_2O_4$=570.8.

CAS — 13501-04-7.

A pale yellow, almost odourless, crystalline powder. M.p. 170° to 175°. Practically **insoluble** in water; soluble 1 in 35 of alcohol, 1 in 3 of chloroform, and 1 in 300 of ether.

Bunamidine hydroxynaphthoate is a veterinary anthelmintic active against 2 species of tapeworm, *Moniezia expansa* and *M. benedeni*, in sheep and goats.

12468-y

Bupicomide. Sch-10595. 5-Butylpyridine-2-carboxamide.
$C_{10}H_{14}N_2O$=178.2.

CAS — 22632-06-0.

Bupicomide is an antihypertensive agent.

Inhibition of dopamine-β-hydroxylase by bupicomide in *animals*.— C. A. Korduba *et al.*, *J. Pharmac. exp. Ther.*, 1973, *184*, 671.

In 6 patients with mild or moderate hypertension bupicomide 0.9 to 2 g daily reduced blood pressure to a similar extent as hydralazine 300 to 600 mg daily.— M. Velasco *et al.*, *Clin. Pharmac. Ther.*, 1975, *18*, 145. See also M. Velasco and J. L. McNay, *Mayo Clin. Proc.*, 1977, *52*, 430.

12469-j

Bupropion Hydrochloride. Amfebutamone Hydrochloride; BW-323. (±)-2-(*tert*-Butylamino)-3′-chloropropiophenone hydrochloride.
$C_{13}H_{18}ClNO$,HCl=276.2.

CAS — 34911-55-2 (bupropion); 31677-93-7 (hydrochloride).

Bupropion hydrochloride is an antidepressant.

References: L. F. Fabre *et al.*, *Clin. Pharmac. Ther.*, 1977, *21*, 102; W. E. Fann *et al.*, *Curr. ther. Res.*, 1978, *23*, 222; L. F. Fabre and D. M. McLendon, *ibid.*, 393; A. W. Peck *et al.*, *Br. J. clin. Pharmac.*, 1979, *7*, 469; H. Canning *et al.*, *Br. J. Pharmac.*, 1979, *66*, 104P; W. C. Stern and N. Harto-Truax, *Psychopharmac. Bull.*, 1980, *16*, 43; W. E. Fann *et al.*, *Clin. Pharmac. Ther.*, 1981, *29*, 244.

Manufacturers
Wellcome, UK.

12470-q

Buquineran. UK-14275. 1-Butyl-3-[1-(6,7-dimethoxyquinazolin-4-yl)-4-piperidyl]urea.
$C_{20}H_{29}N_5O_3$=387.5.

CAS — 59184-78-0.

Buquineran is a phosphodiesterase inhibitor with inotropic effects on the heart.

References: F. Follath *et al.*, *Br. J. clin. Pharmac.*, 1975, *2*, 372P; F. Follath *et al.*, *Clin. Pharmac. Ther.*, 1976, *20*, 24; I. Hutton *et al.*, *Br. J. clin. Pharmac.*, 1977, *4*, 513; C. T. Alabaster *et al.*, *Br. J. Pharmac.*, 1977, *60*, 284P; P. G. Jackson *et al.*, *Br. J. clin. Pharmac.*, 1978, *5*, 7; K. Jennings *et al.*, *ibid.*, 13.

Possible adverse effects due to prolongation of the QT interval.— *Lancet*, 1979, *2*, 777.

Manufacturers
Pfizer, UK.

14039-p

Buserelin Acetate. HOE-766; S74 6766 (buserelin). (6-*O*-*tert*-Butyl-D-serine)-des-10-glycinamidegonadorelin ethylamide acetate.
$C_{60}H_{86}N_{16}O_{13},C_2H_4O_2$=1299.5.

CAS — 57982-77-1 (buserelin); 68630-75-1 (acetate).

Buserelin is a nonapeptide, an analogue of gonadorelin (see p.1267). It has been used experimentally for the inhibition of ovulation, and in premenopausal women with metastatic breast cancer.

Effect on ovulation.— R. Baumann *et al.*, *Contraception*, 1980, *21*, 191.

See also p.1267.

Luteolytic effect.— A. Lemay *et al.*, *Fert. Steril.*, 1979, *32*, 646.

Use in metastatic breast cancer.— J. G. M. Klijn and F. H. de Jong, *Lancet*, 1982, *1*, 1213.

Manufacturers
Hoechst, Ger.

12471-p

Buspirone Hydrochloride. MJ-9022-1. 1-[4-(4-Pyrimidin-2-ylpiperazin-1-yl)butyl]piperidine-4-spirocyclopentane-2,6-dione hydrochloride.
$C_{21}H_{31}N_5O_2$,HCl=422.0.

CAS — 36505-84-7 (buspirone); 33386-08-2 (hydrochloride).

Buspirone hydrochloride is a tranquilliser.

References: H. L. Goldberg, *Psychopharmac. Bull.*, 1979, *15*, 90; H. L. Goldberg and R. J. Finnerty, *Am. J. Psychiat.*, 1979, *136*, 1184.

Manufacturers
Bristol-Myers, UK; Mead Johnson, USA.

12472-s

Butaclamol Hydrochloride. AY-23028. (±)-3α-*tert*-Butyl-2,3,4,4aβ,8,9,13bα,14-octahydro-1*H*-benzo[6,7]cyclohepta[1,2,3-*de*]pyrido-[2,1-*a*]isoquinolin-3-ol hydrochloride.
$C_{25}H_{31}NO$,HCl=398.0.

CAS — 36504-93-5 (butaclamol); 36504-94-6 (hydrochloride).

Butaclamol is a tranquilliser which has been tried in schizophrenia.

Butaclamol was compared to chlorpromazine in a double-blind placebo-controlled study in 27 chronic schizophrenics. Initial doses of butaclamol 5 mg and chlorpromazine 100 mg daily were gradually increased to a maximum of 50 mg or 1 g daily, respectively. After 12 weeks, improvement was seen in both groups receiving active drug, compared to the placebo group. However, extrapyramidal side-effects were much more pronounced with butaclamol and it was suggested that the maintenance dose of butaclamol might be in the range 5 to 20 mg daily.— M. L. Clark *et al.*, *J. clin. Pharmac.*, 1977, *17*, 529.

Further references: T. A. Pugsley and W. Lippmann, *J. Pharm. Pharmac.*, 1977, *29*, 135 (mode of action); J. N. Nestoros, *Int. Pharmacopsychiat.*, 1978, *13*, 138 (comparison with fluphenazine).

Manufacturers
Ayerst, USA.

12473-w

Butaverine Hydrochloride. Butyl 3-phenyl-3-piperidinopropionate hydrochloride.
$C_{18}H_{27}NO_2$,HCl=325.9.

CAS — 55837-14-4 (butaverine).

Butaverine hydrochloride has been used for its antispasmodic effects on the gastro-intestinal tract.

Proprietary Names
Espasmo Gemora *(Prodes, Spain).*

12474-e

Butazopyridine. 2,6-Diamino-6′-butoxy-3,3′-azopyridine.
$C_{14}H_{18}N_6O$=286.3.

Butazopyridine has been used in the treatment of biliary and urinary disorders.

Proprietary Names
Neotropina *(Schering, Ital.).*

12475-l

Butibufen. FF-106. 2-(4-Isobutylphenyl)butyric acid.
$C_{14}H_{20}O_2$=220.3.

CAS — 55837-18-8.

Butibufen is a phenylalkanoic acid derivative (see p.234) with analgesic and anti-inflammatory activity.

Proprietary Names
Butilopan *(Juste, Spain).*

12476-y

Butidrine Hydrochloride. CO-405 (butidrine). 2-*sec*-Butylamino-1-(5,6,7,8-tetrahydro-2-naphthyl)ethanol hydrochloride.
$C_{16}H_{25}NO$,HCl=283.8.

CAS — 7433-10-5 (butidrine); 1506-12-3 (hydrochloride).

Butidrine hydrochloride is a beta-adrenoceptor blocking agent.

Proprietary Names
Betabloc *(Farmasimes, Spain).*

15310-z

Butikacin. UK-18892. 6-*O*-(3-Amino-3-deoxy-α-D-glucopyranosyl)-4-*O*-(6-amino-6-deoxy-α-D-glucopyranosyl)-N^1-[(2*S*)-4-amino-2-hydroxybutyl]-2-deoxy-D-streptamine.
$C_{22}H_{45}N_5O_{12}$=571.6.

CAS — 59733-86-7.

Butikacin is an aminoglycoside antibiotic with activity similar to that of amikacin.

References: R. Wise and J. M. Andrews, *Antimicrob. Ag. Chemother.*, 1978, *14*, 228; S. Jevons *et al.*, *ibid.*, 277; R. J. Andrews *et al.*, *ibid.*, 846; M. J. Kendall *et al.*, *J. antimicrob. Chemother.*, 1978, *4*, 459; A. J. Carter, *Antimicrob. Ag. Chemother.*, 1979, *16*, 362; B. Trollfors *et al.* (letter), *J. antimicrob. Chemother.*, 1980, *6*, 685.

Manufacturers
Pfizer, UK.

12477-j

Butinoline. Butinolinum; Dibutidin. 1,1-Diphenyl-4-(pyrrolidin-1-yl)but-2-yn-1-ol.
$C_{20}H_{21}NO$=291.4.

CAS — 968-63-8.

Butinoline has antispasmodic properties and has been used in the treatment of various gastro-intestinal disorders. Butinoline phosphate has also been used.

Manufacturers
Heumann, Ger.

12478-z

Butixirate. MG-5771. The *trans*-4-phenylcyclohexylamine salt of 2-(biphenyl-4-yl)butyric acid.
$C_{16}H_{16}O_2,C_{12}H_{17}N$=415.6.

CAS — 19992-80-4.

Butixirate has been applied topically in a variety of inflammatory and oedematous disorders.

Proprietary Names
Flectar *(Maggioni, Ital.).*

12479-c

Butofilolol. CM-6805a. (±)-2′-(3-*tert*-Butylamino-2-hydroxypropoxy)-5′-fluorobutyrophenone.
$C_{17}H_{26}FNO_3$=311.4.

CAS — 64552-17-6.

Butofilolol is a beta-adrenoceptor blocking agent.

12480-s

Butopamine. LY-131126. (*R*)-4-Hydroxy-α-{[(*R*)-3-(4-hydroxyphenyl)-1-methylpropyl]aminomethyl}benzyl alcohol.
$C_{18}H_{23}NO_3$=301.4.

CAS — 66734-12-1.

Butopamine is structurally related to dobutamine and is reported to have inotropic effects on the heart.

References: M. J. Thompson *et al.*, *Clin. Pharmac. Ther.*, 1980, *28*, 324.

Manufacturers
Lilly, USA.

12481-w

Butopiprine Hydrobromide. 2-Butoxyethyl 2-phenyl-2-(2-piperidyl)acetate hydrobromide.
$C_{19}H_{29}NO_3$,HBr=400.4.

CAS — 55837-15-5 (butopiprine); 60595-56-4 (hydrobromide).

Butopiprine hydrobromide has been used for the relief of cough.

Proprietary Names
Laucalon *(Castejon, Spain)*; Rutacel *(Promeco, Arg.).*

12482-e

Butyl Acetate. *n*-Butyl acetate.
$C_6H_{12}O_2$=116.2.

CAS — 123-86-4.

A colourless flammable liquid with a strong fruity odour. Wt per ml about 0.88 g.

Butyl acetate is used as a solvent.

12483-l

Butyl Nitrite.
$C_4H_9NO_2$=103.1.

Commercial butyl nitrite or isobutyl nitrite, sometimes with other additives, is not used medicinally. It is used as a drug of abuse and has effects similar to those of amyl nitrite.

A discussion of the abuse of nitrites including butyl nitrite.— C. W. Sharp and R. C. Stillman, *Ann. intern.*

Med., 1980, *92*, 700.

Reports of methaemoglobinaemia: M. K. Horne *et al.*, *Ann. intern. Med.*, 1979, *91*, 417; R. Shesser *et al.* (letter), *ibid.*, 1980, *92*, 131; R. W. Steiner and A. S. Manoguerra (letter), *ibid.*, 570; S. Wason *et al.*, *ibid.*, 637; M. Smith *et al.* (letter), *ibid.*, 719.

12484-y

Butylamine. *n*-Butylamine.
$C_4H_{11}N$=73.2.

CAS — 109-73-9.

A colourless liquid with an ammoniacal odour. Wt per ml about 0.744 g; b.p. about 78°.

Butylamine is used as a solvent.

15308-r

Cafaminol. 7-Methyl-8-(2-hydroxy-*N*-methylethylamino)theophylline.
$C_{11}H_{17}N_5O_3$=267.3.

CAS — 30924-31-3.

Cafaminol has been used by mouth to relieve nasal congestion.

Proprietary Names
Rhinoptil *(Promonta, Ger.).*

15309-f

Cafcycline. A salt of chloramphenicol succinate and tetracycline.
$C_{37}H_{40}Cl_2N_4O_{16}$=867.6.

Cafcycline has been used for the treatment of infections susceptible to chloramphenicol and tetracycline.

Proprietary Names
Complessomicina *(Medosan, Ital.).*

12500-x

Cafedrine Hydrochloride. H-8351; Kafedrin Hydrochloride. 7-[2-(β-Hydroxy-α-methylphenethylamino)ethyl]theophylline hydrochloride.
$C_{18}H_{23}N_5O_3,HCl$=393.9.

CAS — 58166-83-9 (cafedrine).

Cafedrine hydrochloride is a theophylline derivative which has been used in the treatment of hypotension.

12501-r

Cafrolicycline. A salt of chloramphenicol succinate and rolitetracycline.
$C_{42}H_{49}Cl_2N_5O_{16}$=950.8.

Cafrolicycline is an antibiotic which has the activity of chloramphenicol and the tetracyclines.

Proprietary Names
Ciclincaf *(Medici, Ital.)*; Clorociclin *(Panthox & Burck, Ital.)*; Metilcaf *(Ital Suisse, Ital.)*; Reicaf *(San Carlo, Ital.)*; Tecaf *(Farmochimica Italiana, Ital.)*; Tetrafenicol *(Medici Domus, Ital.).*

12502-f

Calcined Magnesite *(B.P. Vet.).* Consists mainly of magnesium oxide and is usually prepared by igniting naturally occurring magnesite (magnesium carbonate).

A white or sand-coloured powder or granules. Very slightly **soluble** in water; incompletely soluble in dilute mineral acids.

Calcined magnesite is used as a source of magnesium in the prevention of hypomagnesaemia in calves, adult cattle, and sheep.

12503-d

Calcium Borogluconate *(B. Vet. C. 1965).* Calcii Borogluconas; Calcium Borogluconicum.

CAS — 5743-34-0.

Pharmacopoeias. In *Aust.*

A mixture of 83 parts of calcium gluconate with 17 parts of boric acid. It occurs as an odourless white powder, white granules, or colourless transparent scales. Slowly **soluble** 1 in 5 of cold water and readily soluble in boiling water, forming a clear or slightly opalescent solution. Solutions are usually **sterilised** by filtration but they may be sterilised by autoclaving or by maintaining at 98° to 100° for 30 minutes with a bactericide, provided that precautions are taken to ensure that a precipitate does not form during sterilisation or storage.

Calcium borogluconate has been given in veterinary medicine for hypocalcaemia, by subcutaneous or intravenous injection.

12504-n

Calcium Bromolactobionate. Calcium Bromobionate. Calcium bromide lactobionate hexahydrate.
$Ca(C_{12}H_{21}O_{12})_2,CaBr_2,6H_2O$=1062.6.

CAS — 33659-28-8 (anhydrous).

Calcium bromolactobionate is used as a source of calcium and of bromide. The use of bromides is generally deprecated.

Proprietary Names
Calcibronat *(Sandoz, Arg.; Sandoz-Wander, Belg.; Sandoz, Fr.; Sandoz, Ger.; Sandoz, Ital.; Sandoz, Spain; Sandoz, Switz.)*; Calcibromin *(Astra, Arg.).*

12505-h

Calcium Copperedetate *(B.P. Vet.).* The dihydrate of the copper chelate of the calcium salt of ethylenediamine-*NNN'N'*-tetra-acetic acid.
$C_{10}H_{12}CaCuN_2O_8,2H_2O$=427.9.

CAS — 66317-91-7 (anhydrous).

A blue, almost odourless, crystalline powder. It contains 9.1 to 9.7% of Ca and 14.4 to 15.3% of Cu. **Soluble** 1 in 7 of water, the solution gradually precipitating the insoluble tetrahydrate; practically insoluble in alcohol.

Calcium copperedetate is used by subcutaneous injection in the prevention and treatment of copper deficiency in cattle and sheep.

Proprietary Names
Coprin *(Glaxovet, UK).*

12506-m

Calcium Dobesilate. 205E; Calcii Dobesilas; Calcium Doxybenzylate. Calcium 2,5-dihydroxybenzenesulphonate.
$C_{12}H_{10}CaO_{10}S_2$=418.4.

CAS — 88-46-0 (dobesilic acid); 20123-80-2 (calcium salt).

Calcium dobesilate is claimed to reduce capillary permeability and has been used in diabetic retinopathy and other vascular disorders. Gastro-intestinal disturbances have occurred occasionally.

The action of calcium dobesilate on the pathological permeability of the capillary walls in diabetics indicated its use in the treatment of simple diabetic retinopathy.— R. Sevin and J. -F. Cuedet, *Ophthalmologica, Basel,* 1971, *162*, 33, per *J. Am. med. Ass.*, 1971, *215*, 1536.

In a double-blind study, calcium dobesilate had a very slight inhibitory effect on the deterioration of diabetic retinopathy.— P. G. Binkhorst and O. P. Van Bijsterveld, *Curr. ther. Res.*, 1976, *20*, 283.

The metabolism and pharmacokinetics of calcium dobesilate in man.— A. Benakis *et al.*, *Thérapie*, 1974, *29*, 211.

Proprietary Names
Dexium *(Delalande, Ger.)*; Dobesifar *(Farmila, Ital.)*; Doxium *(Alcon, Arg.; Delalande, Belg.; Carrion, Fr.; Biogal, Hung.; Delalande, Ital.; Ethnor, S.Afr.; Esteve, Spain; Om, Switz.).*

12507-b

Calcium Fluoride.
CaF_2=78.1.

CAS — 7789-75-5.

Calcium fluoride is used similarly to sodium fluoride for the prevention of dental caries.

Native calcium fluoride (Calcarea Fluorica; Calc. Fluor) is used in homoeopathic medicine.

Proprietary Names
Fluor Monal *(Monal, Fr.).*

12508-v

Calcium Glycolate. The calcium salt of α-hydroxyacetic acid.
$(CH_2OH.CO_2)_2Ca$=190.2.

CAS — 26257-13-6.

A white solid.

Calcium glycolate has been used for its diuretic effect.

Proprietary Names
Glycuril *(Laphal, Fr.).*

12509-g

Calcium Hopantenate. Calcium Homopantothenate. The hemihydrate of the calcium salt of D(+)-4-(2,4-dihydroxy-3,3-dimethylbutyramido)butyric acid.
$Ca(C_{10}H_{18}NO_5)_2,½H_2O$=513.6.

CAS — 17097-76-6 (anhydrous).

Calcium hopantenate is a homologue of pantothenic acid and has been used in the treatment of various behavioural disorders including hyperkinesis.

Proprietary Names
Hopate *(Tanabe, Jap.).*

12510-f

Calcium Oxide *(B.P.C. 1934).* Calc. Oxid.; Lime *(U.S.P.)*; Quicklime; Calcium Oxydatum; Calx; Calx Usta; Chaux Vive; Gebrannter Kalk.
CaO=56.08.

CAS — 1305-78-8.

Pharmacopoeias. In *Arg., Belg., Hung., Jap., Jug., Nord., Pol., Port., Span., Swiss,* and *U.S.*

Hard, odourless, white or greyish-white masses, granules, or powder. It readily absorbs moisture and carbon dioxide from the atmosphere. When it is moistened with water a reaction occurs, heat being evolved and calcium hydroxide formed. **Soluble** 1 in 840 of water, 1 in 1740 of boiling water; soluble in glycerol and syrup; practically insoluble in alcohol. **Store** in airtight containers.

Calcium oxide is used in the preparation of Sulfurated Lime Topical Solution (*U.S.P.*), p.505. It has been used in the preparation of caustic pastes such as London Paste.

Maximum permissible atmospheric concentration 2 mg per m^3.

The antidote for lime burns in the eye was a saturated solution of glucose.— P. A. Gardiner, *Br. med. J.*, 1978, *2*, 1347.

For the use of disodium edetate in treatment of lime burns of the eye, see p.383.

Preparations

London Paste. Pasta Londinensis. Equal parts of calcium oxide and sodium hydroxide, reduced to a fine powder and kept in a well-stoppered bottle. To be made into a paste with water when required. An escharotic. Similar to Vienna Paste, p.44.

12511-d

Calcium Pidolate. The calcium salt of 5-oxopyrrolidine-2-carboxylic acid.
$Ca(C_5H_6NO_3)_2$=296.3.

Calcium pidolate is used as a source of calcium.

Proprietary Names
Efical *(Millot-Solac, Fr.)*.

12512-n

Calcium Sucrose Phosphate. A mixture having the approximate empirical formula of the calcium salt of a monophosphate ester of sucrose.
$C_{12}H_{21}CaO_{14}P,2H_2O$=496.4.

CAS — 12676-30-1; 25584-76-3 (both anhydrous).

Calcium sucrose phosphate has been used in the prevention of dental caries.

For reviews of its use in preventing dental caries, see *Br. med. J.*, 1968, *1*, 267; *Lancet*, 1968, *1*, 1187; G. G. Craig, *Br. dent. J.*, 1975, *138*, 25.

12513-h

Calcium Sulfexanoate. The calcium salt of 2,2′-dithiodi(hexanoic acid).
$C_{12}H_{20}CaO_4S_2$=332.5.

CAS — 22414-93-3.

Calcium sulfexanoate has been used in the treatment of hepatic disorders.

Proprietary Names
Lepexal *(Berna, Ital.)*; Lipexal *(Berna, Spain)*.

12514-m

Camphoscapine. Noscapine Camsylate. Noscapine camphor-10-sulphonate.
$C_{22}H_{23}NO_7,C_{10}H_{16}O_4S$=645.7.

CAS — 25333-79-3.

Camphoscapine is used for the relief of cough.

Proprietary Names
Tulisan *(Logeais, Fr.)*.

NOTE. The name Tulisan has also been used for thiram..

12515-b

Camptothecin.
$C_{20}H_{16}N_2O_4$=348.4.

CAS — 7689-03-4.

An alkaloid from *Camptotheca acuminata* (Nyssaceae). Pale yellow crystals. M.p. 264° to 267° with decomposition.

Camptothecin has antineoplastic activity.

A review of the biogenesis, synthesis, and pharmacology of camptothecin.— M. Shamma and V. St. Georgiev, *J. pharm. Sci.*, 1974, *63*, 163.

A brief review of the antileukaemic properties of camptothecin.— M. E. Wall and M. C. Wani, *A. Rev. Pharmac. & Toxic.*, 1977, *17*, 117.

12516-v

Canella *(B.P.C. 1934)*. White Cinnamon; Wild Cinnamon Bark.

CAS — 8022-43-3 (canella oil).

The bark of *Canella alba* (= *C. winterana*) (Canellaceae), containing a bitter principle and about 1% of a volatile oil.

Canella is a mild aromatic bitter. A mixture of the powdered bark with aloes is known as Hiera Picra and has been used as an emmenagogue.

12517-g

Cantharides *(B.P.C. 1949)*. Cantharis; Blistering Beetle; Lytta; Russian Flies; Spanish Fly; Insectes Coléoptères Hétéromères; Méloides.

Pharmacopoeias. In *Aust., Hung., Nord., Port.,* and *Swiss.*

The dried beetle *Cantharis vesicatoria* (=*Lytta vesicatoria*) (Meloidae) or other spp., containing not less than 0.6% of cantharidin. **Store** in airtight containers. Protect from light. Cantharides having an ammoniacal odour should not be used.

Adverse Effects. Following ingestion of cantharides there is burning pain in the throat and stomach, with difficulty in swallowing; nausea, vomiting, colic, bloody diarrhoea, and tenesmus; renal pain, frequent micturition, haematuria; chill, syncope, and circulatory failure. Toxic effects have been produced by 600 mg, and death by 1.5 to 3 g, though recovery has occurred from much larger doses.

Acute cantharides intoxication in a 20-year-old man.— A. J. Presto and E. C. Muecke, *J. Am. med. Ass.*, 1970, *214*, 591.

Treatment of Adverse Effects. Empty the stomach by inducing emesis or by aspiration and lavage; activated charcoal and sodium sulphate have been recommended; give demulcent drinks freely (but *not* oils or fats) and morphine for pain; hot applications to the abdomen may relieve the pain. The circulation should be maintained by the intravenous infusion of plasma or of suitable electrolyte solutions.

Uses. Preparations of cantharides have been employed externally as rubefacients, counter-irritants, and vesicants. They should not be taken internally or applied over large surfaces owing to the risk of absorption.
Cantharides is used in homoeopathic medicine.

12518-q

Cantharidin *(B.P.C. 1949, B. Vet. C. 1965)*. Hexahydro-3aα,7aα-dimethyl-4β,7β-epoxyisobenzofuran-1,3-dione.
$C_{10}H_{12}O_4$=196.2.

CAS — 56-25-7.

Pharmacopoeias. In *Span.*

Cantharidin is obtained from cantharides (see above) or mylabris (see p.1730). It occurs as colourless, odourless, glistening crystals which sublime at about 120°. M.p. 216° to 218°.
Very slightly **soluble** in water; soluble 1 in about 1100 of alcohol, 1 in 40 of acetone, 1 in 55 of chloroform, 1 in 700 of ether, and 1 in 150 of ethyl acetate; soluble in fixed oils.

Cantharidin was formerly used as a counter-irritant and vesicant and was usually preferred to cantharides since the strength of preparations could be more readily controlled. Preparations of cantharidin were used in hair lotions for their rubefacient action. Cantharidin in flexible collodion has been applied for the removal of warts. It has also been used in veterinary medicine. Owing to the high toxicity of cantharidin it is recommended that preparations containing it should not be used medicinally. Adverse effects and treatment are those described for Cantharides (see above). The fatal dose is less than 60 mg.

For reports of fatalities after accidental poisoning with cantharidin, see *Pharm. J.*, 1953, *2*, 467; L. C. Nickolls and D. Teare, *Br. med. J.*, 1954, *2*, 1384; J. D. Craven and A. Polak, *ibid.*, 1386; M. A. Lécutier, *ibid.*, 1399.

A 42-year-old man took a teaspoonful of a preparation containing approximately 20 mg of cantharidin. He developed symptoms of renal damage which responded to treatment including a magnesium sulphate enema and high fluid intake of milk. Hydrocortisone pellets were effective against mouth ulcers.— R. D. Rosin, *Br. med. J.*, 1967, *4*, 33.

An 18-year-old woman who swallowed about 2 ml of a preparation containing cantharidin (Cantharone) developed electrocardiographic changes indicative of myocardial damage, in addition to local effects in the mouth, throat, and pharynx, which responded to treatment with hydrocortisone sodium succinate and with ampicillin, given parenterally.— W. B. Ewart *et al.* (letter), *Can. med. Ass. J.*, 1978, *118*, 1199.

Proprietary Names
Cantharone *(Seres, USA)*.

12519-p

Caoutchouc. Cautchuc; Elastica; Kautschak; Gummi Elasticum; Resina Elastica; Rubber *(B.P.C. 1934)*; India-Rubber.

CAS — 9006-04-6.

The principal constituent of the coagulated latex obtained chiefly from the trunks of *Hevea brasiliensis* (Euphorbiaceae).
A yellowish-white to brown elastic material with a characteristic odour. Almost completely **soluble** in chloroform; partially soluble in petroleum ether.

Caoutchouc is used pharmaceutically in the manufacture of adhesive plasters.

Allergic contact sensitivity to thiuram compounds (present in rubber) in patients in a haemodialysis unit.— N. S. Penneys *et al.*, *Archs Derm.*, 1976, *112*, 811.

Contact urticaria to rubber.— A. F. Nutter, *Br. J. Derm.*, 1979, *101*, 597.

12520-n

Capobenic Acid. C-3. 6-(3,4,5-Trimethoxybenzamido)hexanoic acid.
$C_{16}H_{23}NO_6$=325.4.

CAS — 21434-91-3.

Capobenic acid is a vasodilator which has been used in the prevention and treatment of myocardial infarction and other cardiac disorders.

Proprietary Names
Cardiobiol *(Lifepharma, Spain)*; Cardiobiomar *(Bio-Mar, Spain)*; C-Tre *(sodium salt) (Ist. Chem. Ital., Ital.)*; Kelevitol *(Migra, Arg.)*; Pectoris *(Llorens, Spain)*; Trifartine *(Phoenix, Arg.)*.

12521-h

Carazolol. BM-51052. 1-(Carbazol-4-yloxy)-3-isopropylaminopropan-2-ol.
$C_{18}H_{22}N_2O_2$=298.4.

CAS — 57775-29-8.

Carazolol is a beta-adrenoceptor blocking agent.

Pharmacology of carazolol in *animals*.— W. Bartsch *et al.*, *Arzneimittel-Forsch.*, 1977, *27*, 1022.

Proprietary Names
Conducton *(Klinge, Ger.)*.

12522-m

Carbadox. GS-6244. Methyl 3-(quinoxalin-2-ylmethylene)carbazate N^1N^4-dioxide.
$C_{11}H_{10}N_4O_4$=262.2.

CAS — 6804-07-5.

A yellow crystalline powder. M.p. about 245°. Practically **insoluble** in water.

Carbadox is an antibacterial agent used in veterinary practice for treating swine dysentery and enteritis and for promoting growth.

Manufacturers
Pfizer, UK.

12523-b

Carbamylglutamic Acid. *N*-Carbamoyl-L-glutamic acid.
$C_6H_{10}N_2O_5$=190.2.

CAS — 1188-38-1.

Carbamylglutamate has been used in the treatment of hyperammonaemia.

References to the use of carbamylglutamate with arginine in the treatment of hyperammonaemia.— C. Bachmann *et al.* (letter), *New Engl. J. Med.*, 1981, *304*, 543.

12524-v

Carbazeran. UK-31557. 1-(6,7-Dimethoxyphthalazin-1-yl)-4-piperidyl ethylcarbamate.
$C_{18}H_{24}N_4O_4$=360.4.

CAS — 70724-25-3.

Carbazeran is reported to have inotropic effects on the heart.

Manufacturers
Pfizer, USA.

12525-g

Carbon Monoxide.
CO=28.01.

CAS — 630-08-0.

A colourless, odourless, tasteless, highly inflammable gas.
Carbon monoxide is a constituent of coal gas and illuminating gas and of some fuel gases used in industrial processes; the exhaust fumes from internal combustion engines and some waste gases produced in industrial processes contain a high proportion of carbon monoxide; carbon monoxide is formed during the incomplete combustion of natural gas and other fuels. Small amounts are inhaled during the smoking of tobacco.

Adverse Effects. Carbon monoxide is highly toxic when inhaled and it is the cause of many deaths, both accidental and suicidal; infants, small children, and elderly people are particularly susceptible to carbon monoxide. When inhaled, carbon monoxide combines with haemoglobin in the blood to form carboxyhaemoglobin which is useless as a carrier of oxygen; the symptoms of carbon monoxide poisoning are due to anoxia.
Unconsciousness may occur suddenly or may be preceded by dizziness, weakness, nausea, vomiting, headache, skin lesions, excessive sweating, pyrexia, and mental dullness and confusion; there may be involuntary defaecation and urination and loss of muscular control, followed by circulatory failure. Death results from respiratory or cardiac failure, pulmonary oedema, bronchopneumonia, or cerebral damage. The lethal concentration of carboxyhaemoglobin in the blood is about 50% or more. Concentrations over 1000 ppm of carbon monoxide in inspired air may be fatal in 1 hour. Lower concentrations may have subtle effects on brain function.
The maximum permissible concentration in the atmosphere in occupations in which carbon monoxide is a hazard is 50 ppm for continuous exposure 8 hours a day, or 400 ppm for short exposure.

For the hazard of exposure to carbon monoxide from gases used in industry, and the diagnosis, treatment, and prevention of carbon monoxide poisoning, see F. J. Wagner, *Z. ges. Hyg.*, 1964, *10,* 621. A symposium on carbon monoxide poisoning.— *Rass. Med. ind.*, 1964, *33,* 243, per *Bull. Hyg., Lond.*, 1965, *40,* 806. See also P. M. Winter and J. N. Miller, *J. Am. med. Ass.*, 1976, *236,* 1502.

Exposure to carbon monoxide poisoning: review of the literature and 567 post mortems.— P. A. Finck, *Milit. Med.*, 1966, *131,* 1513.

Carbon monoxide poisoning: causes and prevention, Department of Employment, London, HM Stationery Office, 1971.

For studies of the effects of carbon monoxide on time perception, lung function, driving skills, and driving performance, see R. D. Stewart *et al.*, *Archs environ. Hlth*, 1973, *27,* 155; S. M. Ayres *et al.*, *ibid.*, 168; G. Wright *et al.*, *ibid.*, 349; R. A. McFarland, *ibid.*, 355.

A discussion on environmental carbon monoxide from cigarette smoking.— H. R. R. Wakeham, *Prev. Med.*, 1977, *6,* 526. See also *Drug & Ther. Bull.*, 1978, *16,* 17.

Computerised tomography as an indication of long-term outcome after acute carbon monoxide poisoning.— Y. Sawada *et al.*, *Lancet*, 1980, *1,* 783.

Comment on the reduced incidence of carbon monoxide poisoning in Great Britain.— *Lancet*, 1981, *2,* 75.

Effects on the blood. An association between the raised blood-carboxyhaemoglobin concentrations associated with cigarette smoking, and polycythaemia.— J. R. Smith and S. A. Landaw, *New Engl. J. Med.*, 1978, *298,* 6.

Effects on the cardiovascular system. A review of carbon monoxide poisoning and coronary heart disease.— J. R. Goldsmith and W. S. Aronow, *Environ. Res.*, 1975, *10,* 236.

The relationship between carbon monoxide (bound to haemoglobin) from tobacco smoke and atherosclerotic diseases.— M. Heliövaara *et al.*, *Br. med. J.*, 1978, *1,* 268.

Effects on the gastro-intestinal tract. A report of carbon monoxide poisoning mimicking gastroenteritis.— J. M. Hopkinson *et al.*, *Br. med. J.*, 1980, *281,* 214.

Effects on the liver. In 18 patients who had suffered severe occupational carbon monoxide poisoning an early rise in serum aspartate aminotransferase (SGOT) and in malate and sorbitol dehydrogenase was followed fairly rapidly by a fall towards normal. Similar changes occurred in serum immunoglobulins.— L. Gramer and H. Ruof, *Dt. med. Wschr.*, 1968, *93,* 2275, per *J. Am. med. Ass.*, 1968, *206,* 2773.

Effects on the muscles. Myonecrosis may develop as a complication of carbon monoxide poisoning.— *J. Am. med. Ass.*, 1976, *236,* 2589.

Effects on the skin. Chronic carbon monoxide poisoning was associated in 2 patients with blisters and bullous lesions; 1 of these patients also had erythema and oedema of the scalp, progressing to alopecia.— P. I. Long, *J. Am. med. Ass.*, 1968, *205,* 50. The location of lesions corresponded with pressure areas; the lesions were the result of hypoxia due to prolonged compression.— H. Ippen and G. Goerz (letter), *ibid.*, 1969, *207,* 1718.

Neurological complications. A discussion of the neurological complications of carbon monoxide poisoning.— *Lancet*, 1968, *1,* 77. See also *Br. med. J.*, 1968, *1,* 398; R. D. Snyder, *Neurology, Minneap.*, 1970, *20,* 177.

Of 74 patients who had suffered acute carbon monoxide poisoning and who were followed for an average of 3 years after exposure, 8 had gross neuropsychiatric damage (cognitive change, personality change, or frank abnormality) attributable to carbon monoxide, 8 had favourable personality changes, 21 had unfavourable personality changes, and 27 had memory defects. Many had received treatment only in a casualty department and many had not been followed up. The importance of adequate oxygenation, reduction of cerebral oedema, and follow-up was emphasised.— J. S. Smith and S. Brandon, *Br. med. J.*, 1973, *1,* 318.

A report of sensorineural hearing loss from acute carbon monoxide poisoning.— S. R. Baker and D. J. Lilly, *Ann. Otol. Rhinol. Lar.*, 1977, *86,* 323.

Retrobulbar neuritis with neuroretinal oedema as a delayed effect of carbon monoxide poisoning.— N. C. Reynolds and I. Shapiro, *Milit. Med.*, 1979, *144,* 472.

Pregnancy and the neonate. A review of the biological effects of carbon monoxide on the pregnant woman, the foetus, and the newborn infant.— L. D. Longo, *Am. J. Obstet. Gynec.*, 1977, *129,* 69. See also E. F. Rose and M. Rose, *Clin. Med.*, 1971, *78* (Aug.), 12.

Treatment of Adverse Effects. Remove the patient from the contaminated atmosphere; if necessary, apply suction to remove obstruction (vomitus) from the airway and assist the respiration; give oxygen (under pressure if available) for at least 1 hour (a mixture of 95% oxygen and 5% carbon dioxide may be of value when the patient is breathing spontaneously but the respiratory centre is still depressed); after a long period of unconsciousness, if dehydrated, give dextrose injection intravenously; and maintain the circulation with infusions of plasma or suitable electrolyte solutions. If cerebral oedema is suspected 500 ml of 20% mannitol solution should be given intravenously over a period of 15 minutes, followed by 500 ml of 5% dextrose injection over the next 4 hours.
Absolute rest should be maintained for 3 days while possible cardiac damage is assessed.

Only 1 death had occurred in 100 patients with acute carbon monoxide poisoning who had been treated with mannitol intravenously. No side-effects had occurred.— H. Matthew (letter), *Lancet*, 1970, *1,* 518.

It was exceptional for the skin to be pink in the living patient poisoned by carbon monoxide; such patients were commonly cyanosed and pale. The breathing was not usually depressed unless the patient was moribund; it was usually more than adequate although the arterial pCO_2 was usually low and hypoxia had induced such a fall in standard bicarbonate that the arterial pH was below normal. The addition of carbon dioxide in any concentration to the oxygen being administered was clearly irrational as it would tend to reduce arterial pH even further. Similarly blood transfusion in a condition characterised by myocardial damage could be extremely dangerous.— H. Matthew, *Br. med. J.*, 1971, *1,* 519.

An 8-year-old boy exposed to carbon monoxide in a house fire was apnoeic on arrival at hospital and had a carboxyhaemoglobin concentration of more than 80% two hours after admission. He recovered with minimal spastic diplegia and dyskinesia after treatment which included intubation, 100% oxygen, correction of acidosis, bronchial lavage, hydrocortisone intravenously, 10% mannitol to reverse any cerebral oedema, and dexamethasone subsequently to alleviate neurological symptoms.— J. A. Sills *et al.*, *Postgrad. med. J.*, 1974, *50,* 519.

The treatment of carbon monoxide poisoning with hyperbaric oxygen.— G. K. Anderson, *Milit. Med.*, 1978, *143,* 538.

A reminder that carbon monoxide is a leading cause of fire-associated deaths and the view that hyperbaric oxygen therapy is mandatory in confirmed cases of carbon monoxide exposure with evidence of CNS dysfunction.— R. M. Roberts (letter), *Lancet*, 1981, *2,* 816.

Detection of Carbon Monoxide. The standard method for the detection of carbon monoxide in industry is described in Booklet No. 7 (1955) (Carbon Monoxide) issued by HM Factories Inspectorate, Ministry of Labour.

Uses.
A report on a technique using carbon monoxide for the detection of intrapulmonary haemorrhage in patients with Goodpasture's syndrome.— P. W. Ewan *et al.*, *New Engl. J. Med.*, 1976, *295,* 1391. Comments.— A. P. Fishman, *ibid.*, 1430; P. W. Ewan and A. J. Rees (letter), *ibid.*, 1977, *296,* 574; A. P. Fishman (letter), *ibid.*, 575.

12526-q

Carcainium Chloride. QX-572. Dimethylbis(phenylcarbamoylmethyl)ammonium chloride.
$C_{18}H_{22}ClN_3O_2$=347.8.

CAS — 1042-42-8.

Carcainium chloride is a quaternary ammonium anti-arrhythmic agent which has been given by intravenous infusion in the treatment of ventricular arrhythmias.

References: M. L. Schwartz *et al.*, *J. clin. Pharmac.*, 1967, *7,* 278; L. Rydén *et al.*, *Br. Heart J.*, 1974, *36,* 811; L. Rydén *et al.*, *Eur. J. clin. Pharmac.*, 1975, *8,* 277 (metabolism); L. Rydén *et al.*, *Br. Heart J.*, 1975, *37,* 65 (haemodynamics); B. Bergdahl *et al.*, *Acta med. scand.*, 1978, *204,* 311.

Manufacturers
Astra, Swed.

12527-p

Carnauba Wax *(U.S.N.F.).* Caranda Wax; Cera Coperniciae.

Pharmacopoeias. In *U.S.N.F.*

It is obtained from the leaves of the Brazilian wax palm, *Copernicia cerifera* (Palmae).
Light brown to pale yellow moderately coarse powder or flakes with a characteristic bland odour free from rancidity. Sp. gr. about 0.99. M.p. 81° to 86°. Practically **insoluble** in water; slightly soluble in boiling alcohol; soluble in warm chloroform and in toluene.

Carnauba wax is used in pharmacy as a tablet-coating and tablet-polishing agent. Various types and grades are used industrially in the manufacture of polishes. Its use is also permitted in certain foods.

Specifications for carnauba wax set by American Wax Importers and Refiners Association.— *Soap chem. Spec.*, 1966, *42* (4A, Apr.), 260.

Use in food. The use of carnauba wax is permitted in chocolate confectionery, chocolate products, and sugar confectionery under the Miscellaneous Additives in Food Regulations 1980 (SI 1980: No. 1834) for England and Wales and the Miscellaneous Additives in Food (Scotland) Regulations 1980 [SI 1980: No. 1889 (S. 176)].

12528-s

Carnitine. Vitamin B_T. (3-Carboxy-2-hydroxypropyl)trimethylammonium hydroxide, inner salt.
$C_7H_{15}NO_3$=161.2.

CAS — 461-06-3; 541-14-0 (D); 541-15-1 (L); 406-76-8 (DL).

L-Carnitine is a constituent of living tissues, especially striated muscle and is involved in the metabolism of fatty acids. It has also been claimed to stimulate gastric and pancreatic secretions. Carnitine has been given as the DL- or L-isomer in deficiency states, in the treatment of hyperlipidaemia, especially in patients undergoing haemodialysis, and in coronary heart disease. It has also been given as carnitine orotate ($C_7H_{15}NO_3,C_5H_4N_2O_4$=317.3) for its supposed protective effect on liver cells.

The pharmacokinetics of L-carnitine following intravenous infusion of DL-carnitine.— P. G. Welling *et al.*, *Int. J. clin. Pharmac. Biopharm.*, 1979, *17*, 56.

Action. Carnitine acts as a carrier in fatty-acid transport into mitochondria of skeletal and cardiac muscle, where β-oxidation occurs, with the production of energy. Carnitine is synthesised in the liver from the amino acid lysine. A deficiency of carnitine may arise from either a failure of hepatic synthesis or a failure of transport from liver into muscle and results in lipid-storage disorders with cellular accumulation of neutral fat, the common triglyceride.— *Lancet*, 1978, *1*, 757. If carnitine deficiency is limited to muscle the syndrome is called myopathic; if several tissues and plasma are involved the illness is termed systemic.— J. D. McGarry and D. W. Foster, *New Engl. J. Med.*, 1980, *303*, 1413.

Serum concentrations of carnitine were significantly reduced in pregnant women and an increased demand for carnitine by the growing foetus was suggested.— H. R. Scholte *et al.* (letter), *New Engl. J. Med.*, 1978, *299*, 1079.

Further references: S. G. Gilgore and S. L. De Felice, *J. new Drugs*, 1966, *6*, 124, 349, and 351 (antagonism of thyroid hormones); H. Brooks *et al.*, *J. clin. Pharmac.*, 1977, *17*, 561; S. Bongrani *et al.*, *Farmaco, Edn prat.*, 1980, *35*, 239 (vasodilatation and inotropic effect in *animals*).

Deficiency states. A 3½-year-old boy with systemic carnitine deficiency improved dramatically when he was given L-carnitine 2 g daily (100 to 120 mg per kg body-weight daily in 3 divided doses; (DL-carnitine 4 g daily was used until L-carnitine became available). Two episodes of diarrhoea improved when the dose was temporarily halved. Carnitine has been given for nearly a year and has been shown to be well absorbed. High doses have not caused serious gastro-intestinal symptoms and there appears to be no need to give the drug intravenously.— P. R. Chapoy *et al.*, *New Engl. J. Med.*, 1980, *303*, 1389. Comment.— J. D. McGarry and D. W. Foster, *ibid.*, 1413.

Further references: C. Angelini (letter), *Lancet*, 1975, *2*, 554; G. P. Hosking *et al.* (letter), *ibid.*, 1977, *1*, 853; M. E. Tripp *et al.*, *New Engl. J. Med.*, 1981, *305*, 385.

Haemodialysis. Addition of L-carnitine to the dialysate of 4 patients completely prevented the fall in plasma-carnitine noted during haemodialysis.— A. Bizzi *et al.* (letter), *Lancet*, 1979, *1*, 882.

Administration of carnitine to 3 patients on long-term dialysis was associated with development of severe weakness and myasthenia-like symptoms.— G. Bazzato *et al.* (letter), *Lancet*, 1979, *1*, 1041. A myasthenia-like syndrome occurred after DL- but not L-carnitine.— G. Bazzato *et al.* (letter), *ibid.*, 1981, *1*, 1209.

In a study of 51 patients undergoing chronic haemodialysis administration of DL-carnitine 2.4 g daily in 3 divided doses reduced raised fasting serum-triglyceride concentrations and increased serum high-density lipoprotein to or towards normal. The correction of these lipid abnormalities by carnitine supplementation may reduce the incidence of atherosclerosis and other complications in such patients.— B. Lacour *et al.*, *Lancet*, 1980, *2*, 763. Less promising results with L-carnitine 1.5 g daily in 10 patients.— J. Aubia *et al.* (letter), *ibid.*, 1028. Comment on the treatment of 10 hypertriglyceridaemic haemodialysis patients and, in particular, the practical problems involved. Severe neuromuscular transmission problems were encountered in 2 patients given DL-carnitine 1.2 g daily.— M. K. Chan *et al.* (letter), *ibid.* Comment.— B. Lacour *et al.* (letter), *ibid.*, 1981, *1*, 212.

Preliminary results in 7 dialysis patients suggesting that L-carnitine can significantly improve the lipoprotein pattern in patients on haemodialysis and unaffected by hypertriglyceridaemia.— C. U. Casciani *et al.* (letter), *Lancet*, 1980, *2*, 1309.

Hyperlipoproteinaemia. Administration of DL-carnitine chloride 900 mg daily in 3 divided doses daily for 8 weeks significantly reduced serum-triglyceride concentrations in 14 patients with type IV hyperlipoproteinaemia. On stopping the carnitine the concentrations gradually increased, reaching pretreatment concentrations after 4 weeks. A slight lowering effect on total cholesterol concentrations was also noted but this was not statistically significant. Intravenous infusion of carnitine in 4 healthy subjects was found to have the same effect. No side-effects were observed.— M. Maebashi *et al.*, *Lancet*, 1978, *2*, 805.

Further references: P. F. Bougneres *et al.* (letter), *Lancet*, 1979, *1*, 1401; P. Pola *et al.*, *Curr. ther. Res.*, 1980, *27*, 208.

Proprietary Names of Carnitine Hydrochloride
Bicarnésine *(Labaz, Fr.)*; Bicarnesine *(Petersen, S.Afr.)*; Biomux *(Chiesi, Ital.)*; Carn *(Benvegna, Ital.)*; Carnetina *(Sigmatau, Ital.)*; Carnitolo *(SIRT-BBP, Ital.)*; Flatistine (chloride) *(Sauba, Fr.)*; Framil (bicarnitine chloride) *(Francia Farm., Ital.)*; Metina *(Francia Farm., Ital.)*; Monocamin *(Jap.)*.

12529-w

Caroverine Hydrochloride. 1-(2-Diethylaminoethyl)-1,2-dihydro-3-(4-methoxybenzyl)quinoxalin-2-one hydrochloride.
$C_{22}H_{27}N_3O_2,HCl$=401.9.

CAS — 23465-76-1 (caroverine).

Caroverine hydrochloride is used for its spasmolytic properties.

Proprietary Names
Espasmofibra *(Faes, Spain)*; Spasmium *(Medichemie, Switz.)*.

12530-m

Carperone. AL-1021. 4′-Fluoro-4-(4-isopropylcarbamoyloxypiperidino)butyrophenone; 1-[3-(4-Fluorobenzoyl)propyl]-4-piperidyl isopropylcarbamate.
$C_{19}H_{27}FN_2O_3$=350.4.

CAS — 20977-50-8.

Carperone is a derivative of butyrophenone which has been tried in the treatment of schizophrenia.

References: R. Guerrero-Figueroa *et al.*, *Curr. ther. Res.*, 1969, *11*, 121; D. M. Gallant *et al.*, *ibid.*, 456; A. A. Sugerman, *ibid.*, 775; J. W. S. Angus *et al.*, *ibid.*, 779; J. L. Gendron and B. C. Shiele, *ibid.*, 1971, *13*, 169; J. L. Gendron *et al.*, *ibid.*, 1973, *15*, 333.

Manufacturers
Bristol, USA.

12531-b

Carprofen. C-5720; Ro-20-5700/000. (±)-2-(6-Chlorocarbazol-2-yl)propionic acid.
$C_{15}H_{12}ClNO_2$=273.7.

CAS — 53716-49-7.

Carprofen is an analgesic with anti-inflammatory and antipyretic activity.

Pharmacokinetics.— J. E. Ray *et al.*, *J. clin. Pharmac.*, 1979, *19*, 635; F. Rubio *et al.*, *J. pharm. Sci.*, 1980, *69*, 1245; J. F. Kelly *et al.*, *Clin. Pharmac. Ther.*, 1981, *29*, 257.

Comparison with indomethacin.— B. Kirchheiner *et al.*, *Curr. ther. Res.*, 1980, *28*, 875.

Use as an analgesic for dental pain.— S. A. Cooper *et al.*, *Clin. Pharmac. Ther.*, 1981, *29*, 237.

Proprietary Names
Imadyl *(Roche, Switz.)*.

12532-v

Cartazolate. SQ-65396. Ethyl 4-butylamino-1-ethyl-1*H*-pyrazolo[3,4-*b*]pyridine-5-carboxylate.
$C_{15}H_{22}N_4O_2$=290.4.

CAS — 34966-41-1.

Cartazolate has been tried in the treatment of anxiety and depression.

References: G. Sakalis *et al.*, *Curr. ther. Res.*, 1974, *16*, 861; G. Sathananthan *et al.*, *ibid.*, 1976, *19*, 475; P. Collins *et al.*, *ibid.*, 512.

Manufacturers
Squibb, USA.

12533-g

Carteolol Hydrochloride. Abbott 43326; OPC-1085. 1,2,3,4-Tetrahydro-5-(2-hydroxy-3-*tert*-butylaminopropoxy)quinolin-2-one hydrochloride.
$C_{16}H_{24}N_2O_3,HCl$=328.8.

CAS — 51781-06-7 (carteolol); 51781-21-6 (hydrochloride).

Carteolol hydrochloride is a beta-adrenoceptor blocking agent.

References: S. Morita *et al.*, *Arzneimittel-Forsch.*, 1977, *27*, 2380; A. Tarkiainen *et al.*, *Eur. J. clin. Pharmac.*, 1981, *19*, 239.

Proprietary Names
Mikelan *(Otsuka, Jap.)*.

12534-q

Carubicin Hydrochloride. Carminomycin Hydrochloride; NSC-180024. 10-*O*-Demethyldaunorubicin; (1*S*,3*S*)-3-Acetyl-1,2,3,4,6,11-hexahydro-3,5,10,12-tetrahydroxy-6,11-dioxonaphthacen-1-yl 3-amino-2,3,6-trideoxy-α-L-lyxopyranoside hydrochloride.
$C_{26}H_{27}NO_{10},HCl$=550.0.

CAS — 39472-31-6; 50935-04-1 (both carubicin); 52794-97-5 (hydrochloride).

Carubicin hydrochloride is an antineoplastic agent related to doxorubicin.

References: S. T. Crooke, *J. Med.*, 1977, *8*, 295; H. M. Olson and C. C. Capen, *Toxic. appl. Pharmac.*, 1978, *44*, 605; S. K. Carter, *Drugs*, 1980, *20*, 375; R. C. Young *et al.*, *New Engl. J. Med.*, 1981, *305*, 139.

Manufacturers
Bristol, USA.

12535-p

Casoni-test Antigen. An antigen solution prepared from hydatid-cyst fluid obtained from man or sheep under sterile conditions.

It is used in the Casoni test, an intradermal test for the diagnosis of hydatid disease. Complement-fixation tests are more reliable. An injection of 0.25 ml of the solution is made into the skin on the outer half of the upper arm and a control injection of sterile saline is made 3 to 4 cm above this. A wheal may appear after 10 minutes reaching maximum size in 30 minutes; if the diameter of the wheal is at least 2 cm, the reaction is positive. A delayed response consisting of infiltration or oedema may occur after about 6 hours lasting for 18 to 24 hours; if the diameter of swelling is at least 4 cm, the reaction is positive.

The Casoni test for the diagnosis of hydatid disease was compared with a complement-fixation test in 1081 patients over the period 1957 to 1967 in Great Britain. The complement-fixation test gave more reliable results than the Casoni test but the latter was useful for diagnosing past or present infection in a community.— C. M. P. Bradstreet, *J. med. Microbiol.*, 1969, *2*, 419.

A bentonite flocculation test which used antigen-coated particles mixed with the patient's serum, and an indirect haemagglutination test for the presence of hydatid disease were both considered more sensitive and specific than the Casoni test during studies of 44 patients and

50 healthy subjects.— R. C. Mahajan and N. L. Chitkara, in Tropical Diseases II, *Progress in Drug Research*, Vol. 19, E. Jucker (Ed.), Basle, Birkhäuser Verlag, 1975, p. 75.

12536-s

Castor *(B.P.C. 1934)*. Castoreum.

Pharmacopoeias. In *Port.*

The dried preputial follicles of the beaver, *Castor fiber* (Castoridae). Dark brown or grey pear-shaped masses with an empyreumatic odour.

The chief use of castor is as a fixative in perfumery.

12537-w

Catha. Kat; Kath; Khat; Miraa; Abyssinian, African, or Arabian Tea.

CAS — 71031-15-7 (cathinone).

The fresh or dried leaves of *Catha edulis* (Celastraceae), containing cathine (see p.1692), cathinone ($C_9H_{11}NO$ = 149.2), celastrin, choline, tannins, and inorganic salts.

Catha is an excitant of the central nervous system and is used in northern and eastern Africa as a stimulant, the leaves either being chewed or used as an infusion. Dependence on catha has been reported.

Preparations of the catha type were dependence-producing.— Nineteenth Report of WHO Expert Committee on Drug Dependence, *Tech. Rep. Ser. Wld Hlth Org. No. 526*, 1973.

Further references: Z. Marešová, *Vnitř. Lék.*, 1967, *13*, 753; W. Luqman and T. S. Danowski, *Ann. intern. Med.*, 1976, *85*, 246; P. Kalix, *J. Pharm. Pharmac.*, 1980, *32*, 662 ((−)-cathinone).

12538-e

Cathine. (+)-Norpseudoephedrine. *threo*-2-Amino-1-phenylpropan-1-ol.
$C_9H_{13}NO$=151.2.

CAS — 492-39-7; 36393-56-3.

Cathine is a constituent of catha (p.1692) and has been used as an anorectic agent.

The chemistry and pharmacology of cathine.— R. A. Heacock and J. E. Forrest, *Can. J. pharm. Sci.*, 1974, *9*, 64.

Cathine was excreted unchanged in the urine 30 to 50 minutes after ingestion of the synthetic drug, about 40% being recovered in the urine within 6 hours. Trace amounts were detected 24 hours later.— C. K. Maitai and G. M. Mugera, *J. pharm. Sci.*, 1975, *64*, 702. Cathine 60 mg by mouth produced a mean peak plasma concentration in 6 healthy subjects of 200 ng per ml after 1.3 hours. Cathine could not be detected in the plasma after 24 hours.— F. Frosch, *Arzneimittel-Forsch.*, 1977, *27*, 665. The bioavailability of cathine from capsules or sustained-release dragees.— *idem*, 1076.

Proprietary Names of Cathine and Cathine Hydrochloride

Adiposetten N *(Reiss, Ger.)*; Amorphan Depot *(Heumann, Ger.)*; Miniscap M.D. *(Cooper, Switz.)*; Minusin Depot *(Otto Jann, Switz.)*; Mirapront N *(polystyrol-divinylbenzol-sulphonic acid derivative) (Mack, Illert., Ger.)*; Neo-Soldana *(Girol, Switz.)*; Nobese *(Restan, S.Afr.)*; Reduform *(Para-Pharma, Switz.)*.

12539-l

CEA. Carcinoembryonic Antigen; TAA; Tumour-associated Antigen.

A number of studies have suggested that CEA concentrations in plasma are elevated in malignant disease and that estimations, by radioimmunoassay, of CEA concentrations may be of value in the diagnosis of such disease and of relapse.

A summary of an NIH Consensus Statement on the role of CEA as a marker in the management of cancer. It was concluded that: a) the plasma CEA assay is not sufficiently sensitive or specific for routine cancer screening, b) CEA values cannot be used independently to establish a diagnosis of cancer, c) CEA values should be obtained in patients with either colorectal or bronchial carcinomas and used as an adjunct to staging methods, d) regular and sequential assay of plasma CEA is the best non-invasive method available for postoperative surveillance of patients with colorectal cancer. The role of CEA monitoring in other types of cancer is less convincing.— *Br. med. J.*, 1981, *282*, 373. Precautions to be followed when testing for CEA in patients with cancer. Tests for CEA are to be used only for managing cancer and assessing prognosis; they are not intended for screening or diagnosis.— W. C. Dierksheide, *FDA* (letter), *New Engl. J. Med.*, 1981, *304*, 174.

Earlier discussions on CEA.— *Br. med. J.*, 1977, *2*, 535; *Lancet*, 1978, *2*, 461.

An account of CEA titres in effusion fluid, and their potential use for diagnosis.— J. S. Nystrom *et al.*, *Archs intern. Med.*, 1977, *137*, 875. See also R. A. Rittgers *et al.*, *Ann. intern. Med.*, 1978, *88*, 631; M. S. Loewenstein *et al.*, *ibid.*, 635.

Localisation of tumour deposits by external scanning after injection of radiolabelled antibody to CEA.— P. W. Dykes *et al.*, *Br. med. J.*, 1980, *280*, 220. See also J. -P. Mach *et al.*, *New Engl. J. Med.*, 1980, *303*, 5.

15311-c

Cefazedone. EMD-30087 *(sodium salt)*. (7*R*)-7-[2-(3,5-Dichloro-4-oxo-1-pyridyl)acetamido]-3-(5-methyl-1,3,4-thiadiazol-2-ylthiomethyl)-3-cephem-4-carboxylic acid.
$C_{18}H_{15}Cl_2N_5O_5S_3$=548.4.

CAS — 56187-47-4 (cefazedone); 63521-15-3 (sodium salt).

Cefazedone is a cephalosporin antibiotic.

For a series of papers on cefazedone, see *Arzneimittel-Forsch.*, 1979, *29*, 361–462.

Further references: D. von Kobyletzki *et al.*, *Arzneimittel-Forsch.*, 1979, *29*, 1763; D. Adam *et al.*, *ibid.*, 1901; A. D. Russell and D. T. Rogers (letter), *J. antimicrob. Chemother.*, 1980, *6*, 288.

Manufacturers
E. Merck, Ger.

15312-k

Cefmenoxime Hydrochloride. Abbott-50912; SCE-1365 (cefmenoxime). (*Z*)-(7*R*)-7-[2-(2-Aminothiazol-4-yl)-2-methoxyiminoacetamido]-3-[(1-methyl-1*H*-tetrazol-5-yl)thiomethyl]-3-cephem-4-carboxylic acid hydrochloride.
$(C_{16}H_{17}N_9O_5S_3)_2,HCl$=1059.6.

CAS — 65085-01-0 (cefmenoxime); 75738-58-8 (hydrochloride).

Cefmenoxime hydrochloride is a cephalosporin antibiotic.

Manufacturers
Abbott, USA; Takeda, Jap.

12540-v

Cefmetazole. CS-1170; SKF-83088. (7*S*)-7-[2-(Cyanomethylthio)acetamido]-7-methoxy-3-(1-methyl-1*H*-tetrazol-5-ylthiomethyl)-3-cephem-4-carboxylic acid.
$C_{15}H_{17}N_7O_5S_3$=471.5.

CAS — 56796-20-4.

Cefmetazole is a cephamycin antibiotic.

References: *Chemotherapy, Tokyo*, 1978, *26*, *Suppl.* 5;; S. Ohya *et al.*, *Antimicrob. Ag. Chemother.*, 1978, *14*, 780; K. Dornbusch *et al.*, *J. antimicrob. Chemother.*, 1980, *6*, 207; K. Sato *et al.*, *Antimicrob. Ag. Chemother.*, 1980, *17*, 736.

See also a series of papers in *Jap. J. Antibiot.*, 1979, *32*..

Manufacturers
Sankyo, Jap.

12541-g

Ceforanide. BL-S786. (7*R*)-7-[2-(α-Amino-*o*-tolyl)acetamido]-3-(1-carboxymethyl-1*H*-tetrazol-5-ylthiomethyl)-3-cephem-4-carboxylic acid.
$C_{20}H_{21}N_7O_6S_2$=519.5.

CAS — 60925-61-3.

Ceforanide is a cephalosporin antibiotic.

Antimicrobial activity.— F. Leitner *et al.*, *Antimicrob. Ag. Chemother.*, 1976, *10*, 426; R. D. Meyer, *J. Antibiot., Tokyo*, 1977, *30*, 326; S. Shadomy *et al.*, *Antimicrob. Ag. Chemother.*, 1978, *13*, 412; M. Laverdiere *et al.*, *ibid.*, 669; N. Aswapokee *et al.*, *ibid.*, *14*, 1; K. H. Burch *et al.*, *ibid.*, 1979, *16*, 386; K. Dombusch *et al.*, *J. antimicrob. Chemother.*, 1980, *6*, 207.

Pharmacokinetics.— R. D. Smyth *et al.*, *Antimicrob. Ag. Chemother.*, 1979, *16*, 615; F. H. Lee *et al.*, *ibid.*, 1980, *17*, 188; J. R. Hess *et al.*, *ibid.*, 251; E. H. Estey *et al.*, *Clin. Pharmac. Ther.*, 1981, *30*, 398; S. S. Hawkins *et al.*, *ibid.*, 468.

Pharmacokinetics of the lysine salt.— M. Pfeffer *et al.*, *J. pharm. Sci.*, 1980, *69*, 398.

Clinical studies.— R. J. Wallace *et al.*, *Infection*, 1979, *7*, 176; K. H. Burch *et al.*, *Antimicrob. Ag. Chemother.*, 1979, *16*, 386; D. M. Musher *et al.*, *ibid.*, 1980, *17*, 254.

Manufacturers
Bristol, USA.

15313-a

Cefotetan. YM-09330. (7*S*)-7-[(4-Carbamoylcarboxymethylene-1,3-dithietan-2-yl)carboxamido]-7-methoxy-3-[(1-methyl-1*H*-tetrazol-5-yl)thiomethyl]-3-cephem-4-carboxylic acid.
$C_{17}H_{17}N_7O_8S_4$=575.6.

CAS — 69712-56-7.

Cefotetan is a cephamycin antibiotic.

Manufacturers
Yamanouchi, Jap.

12542-q

Cefotiam Hydrochloride. Abbott-48999; CGP-14221/E; SCE-963 *(cefotiam)*. (7*R*)-7-[2-(2-Aminothiazol-4-yl)acetamido]-3-[1-(2-dimethylaminoethyl)-1*H*-tetrazol-5-ylthiomethyl]-3-cephem-4-carboxylic acid dihydrochloride.
$C_{18}H_{23}N_9O_4S_3,2HCl$=598.5.

CAS — 61622-34-2 (cefotiam); 66309-69-1 (hydrochloride).

Cefotiam hydrochloride is a cephalosporin antibiotic.

Antimicrobial activity.— K. Tsuchiya *et al.*, *Antimicrob. Ag. Chemother.*, 1978, *14*, 557; M. Ogawa *et al.*, *J. antimicrob. Chemother.*, 1979, *5*, 681; Y. Nozaki *et al.*, *Antimicrob. Ag. Chemother.*, 1979, *15*, 20; K. Sato *et al.*, *ibid.*, 1980, *17*, 736.

Manufacturers
Abbott, USA; Ciba-Geigy, USA; Takeda, Jap.

12543-p

Cefroxadine. CGP-9000. (7*R*)-[D-2-Amino-2-(cyclohexa-1,4-dienyl)acetamido]-3-methoxy-3-cephem-4-carboxylic acid.
$C_{16}H_{19}N_3O_5S$=365.4.

CAS — 51762-05-1.

Cefroxadine is a cephalosporin antibiotic.

References: H. Lode *et al.*, *Antimicrob. Ag. Chemother.*, 1979, *16*, 1; K. Yasuda *et al.*, *ibid.*, 1980, *18*, 105; T. Bergan, *Chemotherapy, Basle*, 1980, *26*, 225; M. Ohkawa *et al.*, *ibid.*, 1981, *27*, 149.

Manufacturers
Ciba-Geigy, Switz.

12544-s

Cefsulodin Sodium. Sulcephalosporin Sodium; Abbott-46811; CGP-7174E; SCE-129. The monosodium salt of (7*R*)-3-(4-carbamoylpyridiniomethyl)-7-[(2*R*)-2-phenyl-2-sul-

phoacetamido]-3-cephem-4-carboxylate.
$C_{22}H_{19}N_4NaO_8S_2$=554.5.

CAS — 62587-73-9 (cefsulodin); 52152-93-9 (sodium salt).

Cefsulodin sodium is a cephalosporin antibiotic with activity against *Pseudomonas aeruginosa.* The usual dose in respiratory and urinary-tract infections is 1 to 4 g daily in divided doses. It may be given by intramuscular or intravenous injection or by intravenous infusion.

Antimicrobial activity.— K. Tsuchiya *et al., Antimicrob. Ag. Chemother.,* 1978, *13,* 137; K. Tsuchiya and M. Kondo, *ibid.,* 536; M. Kondo and K. Tsuchiya, *ibid., 14,* 151; H. C. Neu and K. P. Fu, *ibid.,* 1979, *15,* 646; G. A. Jacoby and L. Sutton, *ibid., 16,* 243; R. Wise *et al., ibid.,* 341; U. Ullmann, *J. antimicrob. Chemother.,* 1979, *5,* 563; M. P. E. Slack *et al., ibid.,* 687; M. V. Borobio *et al., Antimicrob. Ag. Chemother.,* 1980, *17,* 129; A. King *et al., ibid.,* 165; R. R. Bulger and J. A. Washington, *ibid.,* 393; K. Sato *et al., ibid.,* 736.

Pharmacokinetics.— G. R. Granneman *et al., Clin. Pharmac. Ther.,* 1982, *31,* 95.

Proprietary Preparations

Monaspor *(Ciba, UK).* Cefsulodin sodium, available as powder for preparing injections, in vials of 0.5 and 1 g; supplied with 3-ml ampoules of lignocaine hydrochloride 0.5% solution for the preparation of a solution when intramuscular injection is intended.

Other Proprietary Names

Pseudocef *(Ger.)*; Takesulin, Tilmapor *(both Jap.).*

12545-w

Ceftazidime. GR-20263. (*Z*)-(7*R*)-7-[2-(2-Aminothiazol-4-yl)-2-(1-carboxy-1-methylethoxyimino)acetamido]-3-(1-pyridiniomethyl)-3-cephem-4-carboxylate.
$C_{22}H_{22}N_6O_7S_2$=546.6.

CAS — 72558-82-8.

Ceftazidime is a cephalosporin antibiotic.

Comparative susceptibility of *Pseudomonas aeruginosa* to ceftazidime and 4 other cephalosporin antibiotics.— B. Van Klingeren *et al.* (letter), *J. antimicrob. Chemother.,* 1980, *6,* 674.

For the proceedings of a symposium, see *J. antimicrob. Chemother.,* 1981, *8, Suppl.* B, 1–358.

Manufacturers

Glaxo, UK.

12546-e

Ceftizoxime Sodium. FK-749; FR-13749; SKF-88373-Z. Sodium (*Z*)-(7*R*)-7-[2-(2-aminothiazol-4-yl)-2-methoxyiminoacetamido]-3-cephem-4-carboxylate.
$C_{13}H_{12}N_5NaO_5S_2$=405.4.

CAS — 68401-81-0 (ceftizoxime); 68401-82-1 (sodium salt).

Ceftizoxime sodium is a cephalosporin antibiotic.

Antimicrobial activity.— T. Kamimura *et al., Antimicrob. Ag. Chemother.,* 1979, *16,* 540; H. Kojo *et al., ibid.,* 549; D. Greenwood *et al., ibid.,* 1980, *17,* 397; K. P. Fu and H. C. Neu, *ibid.,* 583; K. Sato *et al., ibid.,* 736.

Pharmacokinetics.— H. C. Neu and S. Srinivasan, *Antimicrob. Ag. Chemother.,* 1981, *20,* 366.

Manufacturers

Fujisawa, Jap.; Smith Kline & French, USA.

12547-l

Ceftriaxone Sodium. Cefatriaxon Sodium; Ro-13-9904. (*Z*)-(7*R*)-7-[2-(2-Aminothiazol-4-yl)-2-methoxyiminoacetamido]-3-[(2,5-dihydro-6-hydroxy-2-methyl-5-oxo-1,2,4-triazin-3-yl)thiomethyl]-3-cephem-4-carboxylic acid, disodium salt.
$C_{18}H_{16}N_8Na_2O_7S_3$=598.5.

CAS — 73384-59-5 (ceftriaxone); 74578-69-1 (disodium salt).

Ceftriaxone sodium is a cephalosporin antibiotic, reported to have a long half-life.

Antimicrobial activity.— R. Wise *et al., J. antimicrob. Chemother.,* 1980, *6,* 595.

Pharmacokinetics.— K. Stoeckel *et al., Clin. Pharmac. Ther.,* 1981, *29,* 284; *idem,* 650.

Manufacturers

Roche, Switz.

12548-y

Cefuracetime. 640/1. (*Z*)-(7*R*)-7-[2-(2-Furyl)-2-methoxyiminoacetamido]cephalosporanic acid.
$C_{17}H_{17}N_3O_8S$=423.4.

CAS — 39685-31-9.

Cefuracetime is a cephalosporin antibiotic.

Manufacturers

Glaxo, UK.

12549-j

Cerium Oxalate *(B.P.C. 1949).*

CAS — 139-42-4 (cerous oxalate, anhydrous).

Pharmacopoeias. In *Aust.*

A white or pinkish, granular, odourless, tasteless powder consisting of about 50% of cerous oxalate, $(C_2O_4)_3Ce_2,10H_2O$=724.5, with the oxalates of numerous other rare earths, especially lanthanum, praseodymium, and neodymium. Practically **insoluble** in water; soluble in warm dilute acids.

Cerium oxalate was formerly used as an anti-emetic.

12550-q

Cerous Nitrate. Cerium Nitrate.
$Ce(NO_3)_3$=326.1.

CAS — 10108-73-3.

Cerous nitrate has been used topically in the treatment of burns.

References: W. W. Monafo *et al., Archs Surg., Chicago,* 1978, *113,* 397.

The antibacterial activity of cerous nitrate *in vitro.*— R. M. E. Richards and V. Magan, *J. Pharm. Pharmac.,* 1979, *31, Suppl.,* 33P.

15314-t

Cetraxate Hydrochloride. DV-1006. 4-(2-Carboxyethyl)phenyl tranexamate hydrochloride; 4-(2-Carboxyethyl)phenyl *trans*-4-aminomethylcyclohexanecarboxylate hydrochloride.
$C_{17}H_{23}NO_4$,HCl=341.8.

CAS — 34675-84-8 (cetraxate); 27724-96-5 (hydrochloride).

Cetraxate hydrochloride has been used in the treatment of peptic ulcer.

Comparison with gefarnate.— A. Ishimori *et al., Arzneimittel-Forsch.,* 1979, *29,* 1625.

Manufacturers

Daiichi, Jap.

12551-p

Cetylamine Hydrofluoride. Amine Fluoride 242. Hexadecylamine hydrofluoride.
$C_{16}H_{35}N$,HF=261.5.

CAS — 143-27-1 (cetylamine); 3151-59-5 (hydrofluoride).

Cetylamine hydrofluoride has been used as an additive to toothpaste for the prevention of caries.

References: T. M. Marthaler, *Br. dent. J.,* 1968, *124,* 510.

12552-s

Chlordesmethyldiazepam. Clordesmethyldiazepam. 7-Chloro-5-(2-chlorophenyl)-1,3-dihydro-2*H*-1,4-benzodiazepin-2-one.
$C_{15}H_{10}Cl_2N_2O$=305.2.

CAS — 2894-67-9.

Chlordesmethyldiazepam is a derivative of diazepam and has hypnotic and tranquillising properties.

References: C. Zimmermann-Tansella *et al., J. clin. Pharmac.,* 1976, *16,* 481; G. Cesco *et al., Arzneimittel-Forsch.,* 1977, *27,* 146; V. Andreoli *et al., ibid.,* 436; A. Castellani *et al., Acta ther.,* 1978, *4,* 77; A. Castellani *et al., Clin. Ther.,* 1978, *2,* 68, per *Int. pharm. Abstr.,* 1980, *17,* 511; A. Castellani *et al., Clin. Ther.,* 1979, *2,* 343, per *Int. pharm. Abstr.,* 1980, *17,* 511; L. De Angelis *et al., Curr. ther. Res.,* 1979, *26,* 920.

Proprietary Names

En *(Ravizza, Ital.).*

12553-w

Chloroacetophenone. CN; Phenacyl Chloride. 2-Chloroacetophenone.
C_8H_7ClO=154.6.

CAS — 532-27-4.

NOTE. The name mace is applied to solutions of chloroacetophenone.

Chloroacetophenone is a lachrymatory which is irritant to the skin and eyes. It has been used in a riot-control gas.
Maximum permissible atmospheric concentration 0.05 ppm.

Recommended treatment of exposure to chloroacetophenone included neutralisation by washing the skin with sodium bicarbonate solution and the instillation of boric acid solution into the eyes.— H. W. Jolly and C. L. Carpenter (letter), *J. Am. med. Ass.,* 1968, *203,* 808.

In a comparative study of chloroacetophenone and CS gas applied under a 4-cm diameter watch glass for a period of 1 hour to the skin of healthy subjects, chloroacetophenone was shown to present a far greater cutaneous hazard than CS gas. The reactions were more severe when it was applied moist. Treatment was not considered necessary in the subjects studied, but in the case of extreme irritation, the use of calamine cream with antihistamine therapy at night to aid sleep was recommended. The blisters would resolve spontaneously.— P. Holland and R. G. White, *Br. J. Derm.,* 1972, *86,* 150.

12554-e

Chloropicrin. Nitrochloroform. Trichloronitromethane.
CCl_3NO_2=164.4.

CAS — 76-06-2.

A slightly oily liquid with an intense odour. B.p. about 112°. **Soluble** 1 in about 600 of water; miscible with dehydrated alcohol, acetone, carbon disulphide, carbon tetrachloride, ether, and methyl alcohol.

Chloropicrin is a lachrymatory agent and is intensely irritating to the skin and mucous membranes. It is an insecticide and is used for fumigating stored grain and soil. Chloropicrin is also added to other fumigants as a warning gas.
Maximum permissible atmospheric concentration 0.1 ppm.

12555-l

Chloroplatinic Acid. Kloroplatinasyra. Hexachloroplatinic acid hexahydrate.
$H_2PtCl_6,6H_2O$=517.9.

CAS — 16941-12-1 (anhydrous); 18497-13-7 (hexahydrate).

Pharmacopoeias. In *Nord.*

Yellowish-brown to red-brown odourless deliquescent crystals with a warming bitter taste. Very **soluble** in water; freely soluble in alcohol. **Store** in airtight containers.

Aqueous solutions of platinic chloride ($PtCl_4$=336.9) are used in corneal tattooing solutions.

A review of sensitivity to platinum compounds.— G. M. Levene, *Br. J. Derm.*, 1971, *85*, 590.

Platinum nephrotoxicity.— N. E. Madias and J. T. Harrington, *Am. J. Med.*, 1978, *65*, 307.

Occupational inhalation allergy in workers in the platinum- associated industry.— G. Schultze-Werninghaus *et al.*, *Dt. med. Wschr.*, 1978, *103*, 972.

Preparations

Platinum Chloride Solution *(Addenbrooke's Hosp.)*. Platinic chloride 2 g in water to 100 ml. It is applied to a small area denuded of superficial epithelium and allowed to dry; a freshly prepared solution of hydrazine hydrate 2 g in water to 100 ml is then applied and allowed to dry; the area is stained black. The solutions should be sterile. For corneal tattooing.

12556-y

Chloroquine Gentisate.
Chloroquine 2,5-dihydroxybenzoate.
$C_{18}H_{26}ClN_3,C_7H_6O_4$=474.0.

CAS — 16510-14-8.

Chloroquine gentisate is used in the treatment of rheumatic and similar disorders.

Proprietary Names
Quinercyl *(Robert et Carrière, Fr.)*.

12557-j

Cholesteryl Benzoate.
Cholesterol Benzoate. Cholest-5-en-3β-yl benzoate.
$C_{34}H_{50}O_2$=490.8.

CAS — 604-32-0.

Crystals. M.p. 150°

Cholesteryl benzoate is a dermatological agent used as a 1% ointment with bismuth subnitrate.

12558-z

Chondroitin Sulphate A.
CSA.

CAS — 24967-93-9.

An acid mucopolysaccharide which is a constituent of most mammalian cartilaginous tissues.

Chondroitin sulphate A has been given to patients with ischaemic heart disease and has also been used in osteoporosis and related disorders.

In a study of 46 elderly patients with atherosclerosis, 60 mg per kg body-weight daily of chondroitin sulphate A or placebo were given by mouth for 6 to 64 months. Serum cholesterol and triglyceride concentrations were reduced and clotting time was prolonged in the treated group although there was evidence of tolerance developing on long-term treatment in some patients.— K. Nakazawa and K. Murata, *J. int. med. Res.*, 1978, *6*, 217.

Further references: L. M. Morrison, *J. Am. Geriat. Soc.*, 1968, *16*, 779; *idem*, *J. Am. Geriat. Soc.*, 1969, *17*, 913; L. M. Morrison *et al.*, *J. Am. med. Ass.*, 1969, *208*, 1474; *ibid.*, *209*, 352.

Proprietary Names
Structum (sodium salt) *(Grémy-Longuet, Fr.; Grémy-Longuet, Switz.)*.

12559-c

Chrome Alum *(B.P.C. 1934)*.
Chromium Potassium Sulphate.
$KCr(SO_4)_2,12H_2O$=499.4.

CAS — 10141-00-1 (anhydrous).

Large violet crystals. **Soluble** 1 in 7 of water forming a violet solution which becomes green on heating to 60° to 80°; on prolonged standing the solution returns to the original colour.

Chrome alum is used in tanning, as a mordant in dyeing, and for hardening gelatin in photographic materials. It has been used as a sclerosant in medicine.

Proprietary Names
Sclérémo *(Bouteille, Fr.)*.

12560-s

Chromium Trichloride.
Chromic Chloride.
$CrCl_3$=158.4.

CAS — 10025-73-7.

Chromium is an essential trace element and chromium trichloride has been given as a chromium supplement.

For a comprehensive review of chromium deficiency, metabolism, human requirements, and toxicity, see Report of a WHO Expert Group on Trace Elements in Human Nutrition, *Tech. Rep. Ser. Wld Hlth Org. No. 532*, 1973, 20. See also A. S. Prasad, *Trace Elements and Iron in Human Metabolism*, Chichester, John Wiley, 1978.

The administration of supplementary chromium (as trichloride) 150 µg daily for 2 months resulted in the normalisation of impaired glucose tolerance in 4 of 8 nondiabetic subjects and some benefit in most of the others.— *J. Am. med. Ass.*, 1968, *206*, 36. Criticisms of the use of chromium trichloride in diabetes.— A. Wise (letter), *ibid.*, 1978, *240*, 2045.

Further references: W. H. Glinsmann and W. Mertz, *Metabolism*, 1966, *15*, 510; W. H. Glinsmann *et al.*, *Science*, 1966, *152*, 1243; R. A. Levine *et al.*, *Metabolism*, 1968, *17*, 114.

12561-w

Chromocarb Diethylamine.
The diethylamine salt of 4-oxo-4*H*-1-benzopyran-2-carboxylic acid.
$C_{14}H_{17}O_4N$=263.3.

CAS — 4940-39-0 (chromocarb).

Chromocarb diethylamine is used for its reputed effect on capillary fragility.

Proprietary Names
Fludarène *(Egic, Fr.)*.

12562-e

Chrysoidine Hydrochloride Citrate.
4-Phenylazobenzene-1,3-diamine hydrochloride citrate; Azobenzene-2,4-diamine hydrochloride citrate.
$C_{12}H_{12}N_4,HCl,C_6H_8O_7$=440.8.

CAS — 532-82-1 (hydrochloride); 5909-04-6 (xHCl, citrate).

Soluble 1 in 25 of water; soluble in alcohol.

Chrysoidine hydrochloride citrate is an antimicrobial agent which has been used in the treatment of urinary-tract and other infections.

Proprietary Names
Azoangin *(Permicutan, Ger.)*; Azohel *(Permicutan, Ger.)*.

12563-l

Cianidanol.
(+)-Cyanidanol-3; Dexcyanidanol; (+)-Catechol. *trans*-2-(3,4-Dihydroxyphenyl)-3,4-dihydro-2*H*-1-benzopyran-3,5,7-triol.
$C_{15}H_{14}O_6$=290.3.

CAS — 154-23-4.

NOTE. The name cianidol has been used for this compound.

Cianidanol has been used in the treatment of viral hepatic disorders.

Cianidanol in a dose of 2 g daily for 4 weeks was more effective than placebo in a double-blind controlled study of 100 patients with acute viral hepatitis. Active treatment was associated with greater elimination of hepatitis-B surface antigen, a reduction in serum-bilirubin concentration, and alleviation of anorexia, nausea, pruritus, and possibly abdominal discomfort. Follow-up for 6 months in 96 revealed no relapse.— A. L. Blum *et al.*, *Lancet*, 1977, *2*, 1153. Further encouraging results with cianidanol in 50 consecutive adults with acute viral hepatitis.— F. Di Nola (letter), *ibid.*, 1980, *2*, 1379.

Further references: L. Balant *et al.*, *Arzneimittel-Forsch.*, 1979, *29*, 1758 (pharmacokinetics); I. Vido *et al.*, *Dt. med. Wschr.*, 1980, *105*, 330 (hepatitis); *Lancet*, 1982, *1*, 549 (brief review and report of conference); K. H. Kimbel (letter), *ibid.*, 737 (mention of haemolysis and fever); M. J. World *et al.* (letter), *ibid* (possible use of higher doses).

Proprietary Names
Ausoliver *(Ausonia, Ital.)*; Catergen *(Zyma, Ger.; Zyma, Ital.; Zyma, Switz.)*.

15315-x

Cibenzoline.
Ro-22-7796. (±)-2-(2,2-Diphenylcyclopropyl)-2-imidazoline.
$C_{18}H_{18}N_2$=262.4.

CAS — 53267-01-9.

Cibenzoline is reported to have anti-arrhythmic activity.

Manufacturers
Roche, Switz.

12564-y

Ciclazindol Hydrochloride.
Wy-23409. 10-(3-Chlorophenyl)-2,3,4,10-tetrahydropyrimido[1,2-*a*]indol-10-ol hydrochloride.
$C_{17}H_{15}ClN_2O,HCl$=335.2.

CAS — 37751-39-6 (ciclazindol); 37647-52-2 (hydrochloride).

Ciclazindol hydrochloride is reported to have antidepressant and anorectic properties.

References: A. J. Swaisland *et al.*, *Br. J. clin. Pharmac.*, 1977, *4*, 61; K. Ghose *et al.*, *Psychopharmacology*, 1978, *57*, 109; V. M. S. Oh *et al.*, *ibid.*, 1979, *60*, 177; F. A. Kerr and E. Szabadi, *Br. J. clin. Pharmac.*, 1979, *8*, 396P; S. Levine, *J. int. med. Res.*, 1979, *7*, 1.

Manufacturers
Wyeth, UK.

12565-j

Ciclobendazole.
Cyclobendazole; R-17147. Methyl 5-(cyclopropylcarbonyl)benzimidazol-2-ylcarbamate.
$C_{13}H_{13}N_3O_3$=259.3.

CAS — 31431-43-3.

Ciclobendazole is an anthelmintic which has been tried in roundworm (*Ascaris*), hookworm, and *Trichuris* infection.

References: A. Degrémont and E. Stahel, *Schweiz. med. Wschr.*, 1978, *108*, 1430; R. Guggenmoos *et al.*, *Tropenmed. Parasit.*, 1978, *29*, 423.

Manufacturers
Cilag-Chemie, Switz.; Janssen, Belg.

12566-z

Ciclonicate.
Cyclonicate. *trans*-3,3,5-Trimethylcyclohexyl nicotinate.
$C_{15}H_{21}NO_2$=247.3.

CAS — 53449-58-4.

Ciclonicate is a vasodilator and is used in circulatory disorders.

Proprietary Names
Cortofludan *(Knoll, Switz.)*.

12567-c

Ciclosidomine Hydrochloride.
PR-G-138-CL. *N*-(Cyclohexylcarbonyl)-3-morpholinosydnone imine hydrochloride.
$C_{13}H_{20}N_4O_3,HCl$=316.8.

CAS — 66564-16-7 (ciclosidomine).

Ciclosidomine hydrochloride is reported to be an antihypertensive.

Manufacturers
Boehringer Ingelheim, UK.

12568-k

Ciclotizolam. We-973-BS. 2-Bromo-4-(2-chlorophenyl)-9-cyclohexyl-6*H*-thieno[3,2-*f*][1,2,4]triazolo[4,3-*a*][1,4]diazepine.
$C_{20}H_{18}BrClN_4S=461.8$.

CAS — 58765-21-2.

Ciclotizolam is reported to be a tranquilliser.

Manufacturers
Boehringer Ingelheim, UK.

12569-a

Cicloxilic Acid. *cis*-2-Hydroxy-2-phenylcyclohexanecarboxylic acid.
$C_{13}H_{16}O_3=220.3$.

CAS — 57808-63-6.

Cicloxilic acid has been used in the treatment of hepatic disorders.

Studies, including *animal* studies, on cicloxilic acid.— *Arzneimittel-Forsch.*, 1978, *28*, 1205–52.

Reduction of cholesterol supersaturation of gall-bladder bile.— M. Zuin *et al.*, *Arzneimittel-Forsch.*, 1979, *29*, 837.

Use in chronic alcoholics.— S. Geminiani *et al.*, *Farmaco, Edn prat.*, 1979, *34*, 449.

Proprietary Names
Plecton *(Guidotti, Ital.).*

12580-y

Cilobamine Mesylate. Clobamine Mesylate; RMI-81182EF. *cis*-2-(3,4-Dichlorophenyl)-3-isopropylaminobicyclo[2.2.2]octan-2-ol methanesulphonate.
$C_{17}H_{23}Cl_2NO,CH_4O_3S=424.4$.

CAS — 69429-85-2.

Cilobamine mesylate is reported to be an antidepressant.

Manufacturers
Merrell-National, USA.

12570-e

Cimicifuga. The roots of *Cimicifuga racemosa* (Ranunculaceae).

Pharmacopoeias. Jap. includes the rhizome of *C. simplex* (=*C. foetida*) and other spp. *B.P.C. 1934* included the dried rhizome and roots of *C. racemosa.*

Cimicifuga is used in homoeopathic medicine where it is known as Actaea racemosa or Actaea rac.

12571-l

Cinanserin Hydrochloride. NSC-125717; SQ-10643. 2′-(3-Dimethylaminopropylthio)cinnamanilide hydrochloride.
$C_{20}H_{24}N_2OS,HCl=376.9$.

CAS — 1166-34-3 (cinanserin); 54-84-2 (hydrochloride).

Cinanserin hydrochloride is a serotonin antagonist which has been tried in the treatment of mania and schizophrenia. Adverse effects reported include nausea, lethargy, paranoid ideation, and extrapyramidal symptoms; liver tumours have occurred in *animals.*

References: F. J. Kane, *Am. J. Psychiat.*, 1970, *126*, 1020; J. M. C. Holden *et al.*, *J. clin. Pharmac.*, 1971, *11*, 220; T. M. Itil, *Dis. nerv. Syst.*, 1971, *32*, 193.

Manufacturers
Squibb, USA.

12572-y

Cinmetacin. (1-Cinnamoyl-5-methoxy-2-methylindol-3-yl)acetic acid.
$C_{21}H_{19}NO_4=349.4$.

CAS — 20168-99-4.

Cinmetacin has anti-inflammatory activity and has been used in the treatment of rheumatic disorders.

References: T. Komatsu *et al.*, *Arzneimittel-Forsch.*, 1973, *23*, 1690.

Proprietary Names
Cindomet *(Chiesi, Ital.).*

12573-j

Cinpropazide. *N*-Isopropyl-2-[4-(3,4,5-trimethoxycinnamoyl)piperazin-1-yl]acetamide.
$C_{21}H_{31}N_3O_5=405.5$.

CAS — 23887-47-0.

Cinpropazide is reported to be a coronary vasodilator.

Pharmacology in *animals.*— B. Pourrias *et al.*, *Thérapie*, 1974, *29*, 233.

Manufacturers
Delalande, Fr.

15316-r

Ciprofibrate. Win-35833. 2-[4-(2,2-Dichlorocyclopropyl)phenoxy]-2-methylpropionic acid.
$C_{13}H_{14}Cl_2O_3=289.2$.

CAS — 52214-84-3.

Ciprofibrate is reported to have hypolipidaemic activity.

Manufacturers
Winthrop, USA.

12574-z

Ciramadol. WY-15705. (−)-2-(α-Dimethylamino-3-hydroxybenzyl)cyclohexanol.
$C_{15}H_{23}NO_2=249.4$.

CAS — 63269-31-8.

Ciramadol is an analgesic.

References: A. D. Cochrane *et al.*, *Med. J. Aust.*, 1979, *2*, 501; M. J. Staquet, *Curr. med. Res. Opinion*, 1980, *6*, 475; F. Camu, *Eur. J. clin. Pharmac.*, 1981, *19*, 259.

Manufacturers
Wyeth, USA.

12575-c

Citalopram Hydrobromide. Nitalapram Hydrobromide; Lu-10-171. 1-(3-Dimethylaminopropyl)-1-(4-fluorophenyl)-1,3-dihydroisobenzofuran-5-carbonitrile hydrobromide.
$C_{20}H_{21}FN_2O,HBr=405.3$.

CAS — 59729-33-8 (citalopram); 59729-32-7 (hydrobromide).

Citalopram hydrobromide is reported to inhibit serotonin uptake and has been tried in the treatment of depression.

References: K. F. Overø, *Eur. J. clin. Pharmac.*, 1978, *14*, 69.

Manufacturers
Lundbeck, UK.

12576-k

Citicoline. Citidoline; CDP-Choline; Cytidine Diphosphate Choline. Choline cytidine-5′-pyrophosphate.
$C_{14}H_{26}N_4O_{11}P_2=488.3$.

CAS — 987-78-0.

A hygroscopic white powder. Freely **soluble** in water; practically insoluble in alcohol, acetone, and chloroform. **Store** in airtight containers.

Citicoline is a derivative of choline and cytidine involved in the biosynthesis of lecithin. It is claimed to increase blood flow and oxygen consumption in the brain and has been given by injection in the treatment of cerebrovascular disorders.

References: F. Salvadorini *et al.*, *Curr. ther. Res.*, 1975, *18*, 513 (use in depression); F. Boismare *et al.*, *Thérapie*, 1977, *32*, 345 (*animal* study); G. Palma *et al.*, *Curr. ther. Res.*, 1979, *26*, 1 (use in cardiac arrhythmias).

Proprietary Names
Brassel *(Schiapparelli, Ital.)*; Cidifos *(Neopharmed, Ital.)*; Cidilin *(Errekappa, Ital.)*; Nicholin *(Cyanamid, Ital.)*; Rexort *(Cassenne-Takeda, Fr.)*; Sauran *(Abello, Spain)*; Somazina *(Ferrer, Spain)*; Cereb, Colite, Corenalin, Cyscholin, Ensign, Haocolin, Hornkest, Neucolis, Nicholin, Recognan, Suncholin *(all Jap.).*

12577-a

Citiolone. BO-714. *N*-(Perhydro-2-oxo-3-thienyl)acetamide.
$C_6H_9NO_2S=159.2$.

CAS — 1195-16-0.

Citiolone has been used in the treatment of hepatic disorders.

Proprietary Names
Citiolase *(Roussel Maestretti, Ital.)*; Mucorex *(Berenguer-Beneyto, Spain)*; Sitilon *(Roussel, Arg.)*; Thioxidrène *(Bottu, Fr.).*

12578-t

Clidanac. TAI-284. 6-Chloro-5-cyclohexylindan-1-carboxylic acid.
$C_{16}H_{19}ClO_2=278.8$.

CAS — 28968-07-2; 34148-01-1.

Clidanac is reported to have anti-inflammatory and antipyretic activity.

References: *Curr. ther. Res.*, 1981, *30*, 71.

Manufacturers
Takeda, Jap.

12579-x

Clioxanide. CI-633; SYD-230. 2-(4-Chlorophenylcarbamoyl)-4,6-di-iodophenyl acetate.
$C_{15}H_{10}ClI_2NO_3=541.5$.

CAS — 14437-41-3.

A white crystalline powder. M.p. 215° to 216°. Sparingly **soluble** in water; moderately soluble in alcohol, acetone, dimethylformamide, and ethyl acetate; soluble in chloroform.

Clioxanide has been used as a veterinary anthelmintic.

15317-f

Clobuzarit. ICI-55897. 2-(4′-Chlorobiphenyl-4-ylmethoxy)-2-methylpropionic acid.
$C_{17}H_{17}ClO_3=304.8$.

CAS — 22494-47-9.

Clobuzarit has been studied for its anti-rheumatic activity.

References: B. McConkey *et al.*, *Ann. rheum. Dis.*, 1980, *39*, 18.

12581-j

Clocanfamide. 4-Chloro-*N*-(2-hydroxyethyl)-*N*-(3-methyl-8,9,10-trinorborn-2-ylmethyl)benzamide.
$C_{18}H_{24}ClNO_2$=321.8.

CAS — 18966-32-0.

Clocanfamide has been used in the treatment of peptic ulcer.

Proprietary Names
Clamiren *(Zilliken, Ital.)*.

12582-z

Clocapramine Hydrochloride. Y-4153.
1′-[3-(3-Chloro-10,11-dihydro-5*H*-dibenz[*b,f*]azepin-5-yl)propyl][1,4′-bipiperidine]-4′-carboxamide dihydrochloride monohydrate.
$C_{28}H_{37}ClN_4O,2HCl,H_2O$=572.0.

CAS — 47739-98-0 (clocapramine).

An odourless white crystalline powder with a bitter taste. Sparingly **soluble** in water; slightly soluble in alcohol and chloroform; practically insoluble in acetone and ether; freely soluble in glacial acetic acid. M.p. about 260° with decomposition. **Protect** from light.

Clocapramine is a chlorinated derivative of carpipramine (p.1506) and has been used in the treatment of schizophrenia. Clocapramine is teratogenic in *mice*.

Pharmacology of clocapramine in *animals*.— M. Nakanishi *et al.*, *Arzneimittel-Forsch.*, 1971, *21*, 391; M. Nakanishi and M. Setoguchi, *ibid.*, 1973, *23*, 806.

Proprietary Names
Clofekton *(Yoshitomi, Jap.)*.

12583-c

Clocinizine Hydrochloride. Chlorcinnazine Dihydrochloride. 1-(4-Chlorobenzhydryl)-4-cinnamylpiperazine dihydrochloride.
$C_{26}H_{27}ClN_2,2HCl$=475.9.

CAS — 298-55-5 (clocinizine).

Clocinizine hydrochloride is an antihistamine and has been given in the treatment of rhinitis.

12584-k

Clocortolone Pivalate. SH-863. 9α-Chloro-6α-fluoro-11β,21-dihydroxy-16α-methylpregna-1,4-diene-3,20-dione 21-pivalate.
$C_{27}H_{36}ClFO_5$=495.0.

CAS — 4828-27-7 (clocortolone); 34097-16-0 (pivalate).

Clocortolone pivalate is a fluorinated corticosteroid for topical use, usually at a concentration of 0.1%.

References: R. H. Binder, *Curr. ther. Res.*, 1977, *21*, 796; K. H. Kolb *et al.*, *Arzneimittel-Forsch.*, 1978, *28*, 1648.

Proprietary Names
Cloderm *(Ortho, USA)*; Purantix *(Schering, Ital.; Sandoz, Spain; Wander, Switz.)*.

12585-a

Clofexamide. ANP-246. 2-(4-Chlorophenoxy)-*N*-(2-diethylaminoethyl)acetamide.
$C_{14}H_{21}ClN_2O_2$=284.8.

CAS — 1223-36-5.

Clofexamide has been used with dipyrone or phenylbutazone in analgesic anti-inflammatory preparations.

12586-t

Clofoctol. 2-(2,4-Dichlorobenzyl)-4-(1,1,3,3-tetramethylbutyl)phenol.
$C_{21}H_{26}Cl_2O$=365.3.

CAS — 37693-01-9.

Clofoctol is an antimicrobial compound administered as suppositories for respiratory infections.

Proprietary Names
Octofène *(Debat, Fr.)*.

12587-x

Cloforex. D-237. Ethyl (*p*-chloro-α,α-dimethylphenethyl)carbamate.
$C_{13}H_{18}ClNO_2$=255.7.

CAS — 14261-75-7.

Cloforex is an anorectic agent.

Proprietary Names
Lipociden *(Lesvi, Spain)*.

12588-r

Clomestrone. Chloro-oestrone Methyl Ether; 16α-Chloro-oestrone 3-Methyl Ether; SC-8246. 16α-Chloro-3-methoxyestra-1,3,5(10)-trien-17-one.
$C_{19}H_{23}ClO_2$=318.8.

CAS — 4091-75-2.

Clomestrone is a synthetic oestrogen which has been used in lipid disorders.

Proprietary Names
Arterolo *(Nuovo, Ital.)*; Athéran-N *(Sobio, Switz.)*; Iposclerone *(ION, Ital.)*.

12589-f

Clopidol. Clopindol; Meticlorpindol. 3,5-Dichloro-2,6-dimethylpyridin-4-ol.
$C_7H_7Cl_2NO$=192.0.

CAS — 2971-90-6.

A white crystalline powder. M.p. greater than 320°. Practically **insoluble** in water; slightly soluble in alcohol, soluble in methyl alcohol.

Clopidol is a coccidiostat and is added to chicken feeding stuffs for fattening.
Maximum permissible atmospheric concentration 10 mg per m³.

12590-z

Clopirac. BRL-13856; CP-172 AP. [1-(4-Chlorophenyl)-2,5-dimethylpyrrol-3-yl]acetic acid.
$C_{14}H_{14}ClNO_2$=263.7.

CAS — 42779-82-8.

Clopirac is a phenylalkanoic acid derivative (see p.234) with anti-inflammatory, analgesic, and antipyretic properties.

Proprietary Names
Clopiran *(Continental Pharma, Belg.)*.

12591-c

Cloranolol. GYKI-41099. 1-(*tert*-Butylamino)-3-(2,5-dichlorophenoxy)propan-2-ol.
$C_{13}H_{19}Cl_2NO_2$=292.2.

CAS — 39563-28-5 (cloranolol); 52427-25-5 (hydrochloride).

Cloranolol is a beta-adrenoceptor blocking agent.

Proprietary Names
Tobanum *(Gedeon Richter, Hung.)*.

12592-k

Clotiazepam. Y-6047. 5-(2-Chlorophenyl)-7-ethyl-1,3-dihydro-1-methyl-2*H*-thieno[2,3-*e*]-1,4-diazepin-2-one.
$C_{16}H_{15}ClN_2OS$=318.8.

CAS — 33671-46-4.

Clotiazepam is a benzodiazepine tranquilliser with properties similar to those of diazepam.

Proprietary Names
Trecalmo *(Tropon, Ger.)*; Rize *(Jap.)*.

12593-a

Clovoxamine. DU-13811. 4′-Chloro-5-methoxyvalerophenone (*E*)-*O*-(2-aminoethyl)oxime.
$C_{14}H_{21}ClN_2O_2$=284.8.

CAS — 54739-19-4.

Clovoxamine has been tried as an antidepressant.

References: V. Claassen *et al.*, *Arzneimittel-Forsch.*, 1978, *28*, 1756 (*animal* pharmacology); J. H. Wright *et al.*, *Curr. ther. Res.*, 1981, *29*, 148 (depression).

Manufacturers
Duphar, Neth.

12594-t

Cloxacillin Benzathine *(B.P. Vet.)*. The *NN*′-dibenzylethylenediamine salt of cloxacillin.
$C_{16}H_{20}N_2,(C_{19}H_{18}ClN_3O_5S)_2$=1112.1.

CAS — 23736-58-5; 32222-55-2.

A white or almost white, almost odourless powder. Slightly **soluble** in water; soluble 1 in 110 of alcohol, 1 in 80 of acetone, 1 in 18 of chloroform, 1 in 170 of isopropyl alcohol, and 1 in 3 of methyl alcohol. **Store** at a temperature not exceeding 25° in airtight containers. If it is intended for injection, the containers should be sterile and sealed to exclude micro-organisms.

Cloxacillin benzathine has the actions and uses of cloxacillin sodium (see p.1148) and is used in veterinary medicine as an intramammary injection in the treatment of bovine mastitis.

Proprietary Names
Embaclox DC *(May & Baker, UK)*; Orbenin Dry Cow *(Beecham Animal Health, UK)*.

15330-t

Cloxyquin. Cloxiquine. 5-Chloroquinolin-8-ol.
C_9H_6ClNO=179.6.

CAS — 130-16-5.

Cloxyquin is an antimicrobial agent which has been used topically in mycotic infections. It is a component of halquinol, p.980.

12595-x

Clozapine. HF-1854. 8-Chloro-11-(4-methylpiperazin-1-yl)-5*H*-dibenzo[*b,e*][1,4]diazepine.
$C_{18}H_{19}ClN_4$=326.8.

CAS — 5786-21-0.

Yellow crystals. M.p. about 183°.

Adverse Effects. Agranulocytosis has been reported during treatment with clozapine. Sedation and hypotension have also occurred.

Clozapine caused hyperthermia associated with influenza-like symptoms in 4 of 16 patients.— E. Guirguis *et al.*, *Curr. ther. Res.*, 1977, *21*, 707.

Effects on blood. During a 2-month period in Finland there were 18 reports of severe blood disorders (9 fatal) associated with clozapine. Agranulocytosis accounted for 8 of the deaths and leukaemia probably for the ninth. The sale and use of clozapine was stopped in Finland until further notice.— J. Idänpään-Heikkilä *et al.* (letter), *Lancet*, 1975, *2*, 611. See also *idem*, *Eur. J. clin. Pharmac.*, 1977, *11*, 193. Experience in 22 other countries outside Finland where clozapine had been marketed indicated an incidence of agranulocytosis of 0.3 per 1000 compared with an incidence almost 20 times as high in Finland and with 0.1 to 0.8 per 1000 for other tricyclic neuroleptics. A local factor or factors were possibly responsible for the higher incidence in Finland.— R. W. Griffith and K. Saameli, *Sandoz, Switz.* (letter), *Lancet*, 1975, *2*, 657. It was suggested that the frequency of agranulocytosis associated with clozapine was no higher than with phenothiazines. Weekly blood counts during the first 4 months of treatment would detect incipient granulocytopenia, and so reduce the mortality rate.— B. Anderman and R. W. Griffith, *Sandoz, Switz., Eur. J. clin. Pharmac.*, 1977, *11*, 199.

Further references: H. -J. Senn *et al.* (letter), *Lancet*, 1977, *1*, 547; A. Kirkegaard and A. Jensen, *Arzneimittel-Forsch.*, 1979, *29*, 851.

Effects on the nervous system. The reversal of clozapine-induced delirium by physostigmine.— P. Schuster *et al.* (letter), *Lancet*, 1976, *1*, 37. See also P. Schuster *et al.*, *Clin. Toxicol.*, 1977, *10*, 437.

Absorption and Fate.

Studies on the relationship between plasma concentrations of clozapine and its effects.— M. Ackenheil *et al.*, *Arzneimittel-Forsch.*, 1976, *26*, 1156; M. Thorup and R. Fog, *Acta psychiat. scand.*, 1977, *55*, 123; H. Bräu *et al.*, *Arzneimittel-Forsch.*, 1978, *28*, 1300; G. M. Simpson and T. A. Cooper, *Am. J. Psychiat.*, 1978, *135*, 99.

The metabolism of clozapine.— B. Stock *et al.*, *Arzneimittel-Forsch.*, 1977, *27*, 982.

Uses. Clozapine is a tranquilliser which has been given by mouth and by intramuscular injection in the treatment of schizophrenia. Extrapyramidal effects are usually absent but clozapine has been withdrawn from use in several countries because of reports of agranulocytosis.

References to the use of clozapine in schizophrenia: G. M. Simpson and E. Varga, *Curr. ther. Res.*, 1974, *16*, 679; R. Matz *et al.*, *ibid.*, 687; B. Ekblom and J. E. Haggstrom, *ibid.*, 945; M. Ackenheil *et al.*, *Arzneimittel-Forsch.*, 1974, *24*, 984; H. Gross *et al.*, *ibid.*, 987; G. Chouinard and L. Annable, *J. clin. Pharmac.*, 1976, *16*, 289; A. J. Gelenberg and J. C. Doller, *J. clin. Psychiat.*, 1979, *40*, 238; B. Shopsin *et al.*, *Archs gen. Psychiat.*, 1979, *36*, 657; Y. D. Lapierre *et al.*, *Curr. ther. Res.*, 1980, *27*, 391.

References to the effect of clozapine in dyskinesias: K. J. Zander and E. Rüther, *Arzneimittel-Forsch.*, 1978, *28*, 1495; G. M. Simpson *et al.*, *Psychopharmacology*, 1979, *136*, 317; E. D. Caine *et al.*, *Am. J. Psychiat.*, 1979, *136*, 317.

Proprietary Names

Leponex *(Sandoz, S.Afr.; Sandoz, Spain; Wander, Switz.)*.

12596-r

Clupadonic Acid.

Docosa-7,10,13,16,19-pentaenoic acid.

$C_{22}H_{34}O_2$=330.5.

CAS — 2234-74-4.

An active principle of cod-liver oil.

Proprietary Names

Clupadene *(SAIS, Ital.)*; Clupanina *(Arnaldi, Ital.)*.

12597-f

Cobalt Chloride *(B. Vet. C. 1965)*.

Cobaltous Chloride.

$CoCl_2,6H_2O$=237.9.

CAS — 7646-79-9 (anhydrous).

Pharmacopoeias. In *Aust.*, *Fr.*, and *Nord.*

Deep red, slightly deliquescent, monoclinic crystals. **Soluble** 1 in 2 of water and 1 in 2.5 of alcohol; soluble in acetone, ether, and glycerol. A solution in water is pink but becomes blue on heating to about 50°; a solution in alcohol is blue. Solutions are **sterilised** by autoclaving or by filtration. **Store** in airtight containers.

Adverse Effects. Reactions to cobalt have included anorexia, nausea and vomiting, diarrhoea, precordial pain, cardiomyopathy, flushing of the face and extremities, skin rashes, temporary nerve deafness, renal injury, diffuse thyroid enlargement, and hypothyroidism. Cobalt induces severe nausea and vomiting in patients with pernicious anaemia.

Maximum permissible atmospheric concentration, as cobalt, 0.1 mg per m^3.

A report of increased concentrations of cobalt in the blood and urine of patients with cobalt-containing metallic hip replacements.— R. F. Coleman *et al.*, *Br. med. J.*, 1973, *1*, 527.

Allergy. Of 1205 persons with dermatitis or eczema submitted to patch testing with 2% aqueous solution of cobalt chloride, 12.3% gave a positive reaction.— E. Rudzki and D. Kleniewska, *Br. J. Derm.*, 1970, *83*, 543.

Of 4000 patients subjected to patch testing in 5 European clinics 7.4% of males and 6.6% of females showed positive reactions to cobalt chloride 2% in soft paraffin.— H. Bandmann *et al.*, *Archs Derm.*, 1972, *106*, 335.

For reports and comments on cobalt sensitivity in patients with cobalt-containing hip prostheses, see M. W. Elves *et al.*, *Br. med. J.*, 1975, *4*, 376; G. K. McKee (letter), *ibid.*, 646; D. A. Jones and K. Lucas (letter), *ibid.*, 647; D. A. Jones *et al.*, *J. Bone Jt Surg.*, 1975, *57B*, 289.

Further references: N. K. Veien and K. Kaaber, *Contact Dermatitis*, 1979, *5*, 371.

Effects on the heart. Autopsy on 4 patients with renal failure indicated that cobalt might be a prime cause of uraemic cardiomyopathy.— K. Pehrsson and L. -E. Lins (letter), *Lancet*, 1978, *2*, 51.

A report of cobalt cardiomyopathy in a 17-year-old girl on maintenance haemodialysis, who had been given cobalt chloride 25 mg twice daily for about 9 months.— I. H. Manifold *et al.*, *Br. med. J.*, 1978, *2*, 1609.

Fatal myocardial disease associated with industrial exposure to powdered cobalt.— A. Kennedy *et al.*, *Lancet*, 1981, *1*, 412.

Uses. Cobalt chloride, when administered to both normal and anaemic subjects, produces reticulocytosis and a rise in the erythrocyte count. This property suggested its use in the treatment of certain types of anaemia, but its general therapeutic use is, however, unjustified and not without danger.

In veterinary medicine, cobalt chloride has been given as a dietary supplement to ruminants.

For a review of cobalt deficiency and toxic effects, see Report of a WHO Expert Group on Trace Elements in Human Nutrition, *Tech. Rep. Ser. Wld Hlth Org. No. 532*, 1973, 29. See also E. J. Underwood, *Nutr. Rev.*, 1975, *33*, 65.

References to the use of cobalt chloride: M. S. Edwards and J. R. Curtis, *Lancet*, 1971, *2*, 582; L. S. Valberg (letter), *ibid.*, 1092; E. A. Bowie and P. J. Hurley, *Aust. N.Z. J. Med.*, 1975, *5*, 306, per *J. Am. med. Ass.*, 1975, *234*, 662; J. M. Duckham and H. A. Lee (letter), *Lancet*, 1976, *1*, 1350; *idem*, *Q. J. Med.*, 1976, *45*, 277; *Lancet*, 1976, *2*, 26.

12598-d

Cobalt Oxide *(B.P. Vet.)*.

Tricobalt Tetroxide. It consists of cobalt (II, III) oxide (tricobalt tetroxide) with a small proportion of cobalt (III) oxide (dicobalt trioxide).

Co_3O_4=240.8.

CAS — 1308-06-1.

A black odourless hygroscopic powder. Practically **insoluble** in water; soluble in mineral acids and in solutions of the alkali hydroxides. **Store** in airtight containers.

Cobalt oxide is used in veterinary practice for the prevention of cobalt deficiency in ruminants.

12599-n

Cobalt Protoporphyrin.

A complex of cobalt and protoporphyrin.

Cobalt protoporphyrin has been given intravenously in the treatment of malignant disease.

Proprietary Names

Copp *(Green Cross Corp., Jap.)*.

12600-n

Cobalt Sulphate *(B. Vet. C. 1965)*.

Cobaltous Sulphate.

$CoSO_4,7H_2O$=281.1.

CAS — 10124-43-3 (anhydrous); 65492-00-4 (hydrate).

Pharmacopoeias. In *Fr.*

Red or orange-red monoclinic crystals. **Soluble** 1 in 2 of water; slightly soluble in alcohol.

Cobalt sulphate has been used in veterinary medicine in the prevention and treatment of cobalt-deficiency diseases in ruminants.

For a review of reports of cardiac toxicity after the addition of cobalt suphate to improve the 'head' of beer, see *Lancet*, 1967, *2*, 928.

12601-h

Cobaltous Besylate.

Cobalt di(benzenesulphonate).

$C_{12}H_{10}CoO_6S_2$=373.3.

CAS — 23384-69-2.

Cobaltous besylate has been used in hypertension. The potential toxicity of the cobalt ion should be considered.

Proprietary Names

Ipertensan *(Ceccarelli, Ital.)*.

12602-m

Coconut Water.

The clear liquid obtained from young coconuts, the fruit of *Cocos nucifera* (Palmae).

Coconut water has been given as an intravenous infusion for electrolyte replacement in patients with severe dehydration. It has been reported to be sterile and pyrogen-free.

References: S. Hinderaker, *Lancet*, 1966, *2*, 57; K. Rajasuriya, *ibid.*, 166; Q. M. Iqbal, *ibid.*, 346; D. B. Jelliffe, *ibid.*, 968; J. M. Garvan and B. W. Gunner, *ibid.*, 1967, *1*, 1278; H. Nurasid *et al.*, *Paediatrica Indones.*, 1979, *19*, 219.

For the use of coconut water to replace potassium loss during cholera, see Potassium Citrate, p.631.

12604-v

Coenzyme A.

CoA; CoASH. 5′-*O*-{3-Hydroxy-3-[2-(2-mercaptoethylcarbamoyl)ethylcarbamoyl]-2,2-dimethylpropyl}adenosine-3′-dihydrogenphosphate-5′-trihydrogendiphosphate.

$C_{21}H_{36}N_7O_{16}P_3S$=767.5.

CAS — 85-61-0.

A colourless powder. **Soluble** in water.

Formed from adenosine triphosphate, cysteine, and pantothenic acid, coenzyme A is involved in the body in many physiological roles, including the formation of citrate, the oxidation of pyruvate, the oxidation and synthesis of fatty acids, the synthesis of triglycerides, cholesterol, and phospholipids, and the acetylation of amines, choline, and glucosamine. It has been given by injection in a variety of metabolic disorders and for protection against irradiation. Coenzyme A is contra-indicated in acute myocardial infarction.

The administration of coenzyme A was associated with a delay in the progression of muscular dystrophy.— H. Radu (letter), *Lancet*, 1973, *2*, 576.

Proprietary Names

Aluzime *(Alter, Spain)*; Co-A *(Robilliart, Fr.)*; Coalip *(ISF, Ital.)*.

12605-g

Cogalactoisomerase Sodium.

Uridine-5′-diphosphoglucose Sodium; UDPG.

$C_{15}H_{22}N_2Na_2O_{17}P_2,3H_2O$=664.3.

CAS — 133-89-1 (cogalactoisomerase).

Cogalactoisomerase is used in various hepatic disorders. It is used as the disodium salt.

Proprietary Names
Anatox, Antitoxicum, Atoxepan, Bivitox, Detoxasi, Encrevar, Eparasi, Epatoxil, Evident, Gilasi, Glucodin, Glucoepasi, Glucuril, Liotoxid, Liverasi, Netox, Toxalen, Toxizim, Udepasi, Udetox, Udicit, Udifos, Urepasina, Uridasi *(all Ital.)*; Toxepasi *(Ital., Spain)*.

NOTE. The name Glucodin is also applied to a preparation of dextrose..

12606-q

Collagenase.
Clostridiopeptidase A.

CAS — 9001-12-1.

An enzyme derived from the fermentation of *Clostridium histolyticum* with the ability to digest native and denatured collagen. Potency is expressed in terms of its ability to digest undenatured bovine collagen *in vitro.*

Preparations containing collagenase are used for the debridement of dermal ulcers and burns, and possibly other necrotic lesions, to facilitate granulation and epithelialisation. Optimal activity is at pH 6 to 8; enzyme activity is reduced in the presence of detergents, hexachlorophane, and heavy metal ions. Infections may require additional treatment.

A report of a symposium on collagenase.— *J. Am. med. Ass.*, 1970, *212*, 560.

A review of the properties and role of collagen and collagenase.— G. S. Lazarus, *Br. J. Derm.*, 1972, *86*, 193. See also M. R. Sather *et al.*, *Drug Intell. & clin. Pharm.*, 1977, *11*, 161.

A report of contact allergy associated with the use of collagenase.— W. P. H. Braun, *Contact Dermatitis*, 1975, *1*, 241.

Collagenase had been suggested for the treatment of pressure sores.— *Drug & Ther. Bull.*, 1977, *15*, 69.

Proprietary Names
Santyl (ointment) *(Pentagone, Canad.; Knoll, USA)*.

12607-p

Comfrey
(B.P.C. 1934). Symphytum; Comfrey Root. The dried root and rhizome of *Symphytum officinale* (Boraginaceae). It contains about 0.7% of allantoin, large quantities of mucilage, and some tannin.

Pharmacopoeias. In *Pol.*

Comfrey was formerly used as an application to wounds and ulcers to stimulate healing and was also given internally for gastric ulcers. The healing action of comfrey has been attributed to the presence of allantoin (see p.490).

Results indicating that contrary to some claims comfrey leaves are not a source of vitamin B_{12}.— R. W. Payne and B. F. Savage (letter), *Br. med. J.*, 1977, *2*, 458.

Comment on the potential carcinogenicity of comfrey. Liver tumours have been reported in *rats* fed on diets containing high doses of comfrey.— *Br. med. J.*, 1979, *1*, 598.

Work carried out by the Toxicology Unit of the MRC Laboratories has demonstrated toxic pyrrolizidine alkaloids in comfrey. The alkaloid concentrations are highest in small, young leaves, especially early in the season; large, mature leaves carry the lowest concentrations of toxic alkaloids. Moreover, protein extracted from comfrey should not be harmful. The external use of comfrey preparations should not be hazardous since the alkaloids are converted to toxic metabolites by liver enzymes.— A. R. Mattocks (letter), *Lancet*, 1980, *2*, 1136. Comment on comfrey and liver damage, and the recommendation that its use should be discouraged.— J. N. Roitman (letter), *ibid.*, 1981, *1*, 944. Comfrey toxicity in perspective.— C. Anderson (letter), *ibid.*, 1424.

12603-b

Conorphone Hydrochloride.
Codorphone Hydrochloride; TR-5109. 9a-Cyclopropylmethyl-4,5α-epoxy-8β-ethyl-3-methoxymorphinan-6-one hydrochloride.
$C_{23}H_{29}NO_3,HCl=403.9.$

CAS — 72060-05-0 (conorphone); 70865-14-4 (hydrochloride).

Conorphone hydrochloride is reported to be an analgesic.

Manufacturers
Miles, USA.

12608-s

Copper Oleate.
$Cu(C_{18}H_{33}O_2)_2=626.5.$

CAS — 1120-44-1.

Copper oleate has been used in a concentration of 0.03% for the treatment of pediculosis.

Proprietary Names
Cuprex *(Merck, Arg.)*.

12609-w

Corynebacterium parvum.
C. parvum; *Propionibacterium acnes*; NSC-220537. A species of Gram-positive bacteria.

Corynebacterium parvum is available as a preparation containing inactivated freeze-dried organisms.

Adverse Effects and Precautions. Inactivated *Corynebacterium parvum* is claimed to be better tolerated than most other treatments for malignant effusions but fever has been reported in 10 to 40% of patients following intracavitary injection and abdominal pain or discomfort in 20% following intraperitoneal injection. Nausea and vomiting may occur and leakage into tissues may result in local discomfort.
The incidence and severity of side-effects may be enhanced if it is given intrapleurally within 10 days of thoracic surgery.

The toxicity of *Corynebacterium parvum* given intravenously to patients with solid tumours. Side-effects included fever, shaking chills, and nausea and vomiting; these diminished with continued treatment. Three of 9 patients showed increased serum-alkaline-phosphatase values.— R. C. Ossorio *et al.* (letter), *Lancet*, 1975, *2*, 1090.

Side-effects arising from *Corynbacterium parvum* have included hypotension, fever, and malaise. Premedication with hydrocortisone, chlorpromazine and promethazine has reduced the hypotension and malaise. Dyspnoea, hyperaesthesia, and transient hemiparesis have occurred causing infusions of *C. parvum* to be stopped.— I. H. McIntosh *et al.* (letter), *Lancet*, 1976, *2*, 803.

Three of 87 patients receiving antineoplastic regimens involving intravenous administration of *Corynebacterium parvum* developed a syndrome of nephrotoxicity with renal failure which resolved on withdrawal of *Corynebacterium parvum.* A fourth patient with *Corynebacterium parvum*-induced renal failure was identified in another hospital.— G. M. Dosik *et al.*, *Ann. intern. Med.*, 1978, *89*, 41.

Uses. Inactivated *Corynebacterium parvum* is used in the treatment of malignant effusions. Usual doses of 7 to 14 mg of inactivated freeze-dried *Corynebacterium parvum* in 10 to 20 ml of sodium chloride injection are injected into the pleural or peritoneal cavity immediately after the effusion has been aspirated. If necessary injections may be repeated every 1 to 4 weeks.
Corynebacterium parvum has immunostimulant activity and has been tried as an adjuvant to cancer chemotherapy. It has been injected subcutaneously, intramuscularly, intravenously, and into tumours.

Malignant effusions. In 6 patients with malignant ascitic or pleural effusions there was a reduction in effusions and a decrease in the number of malignant cells after treatment with *Corynebacterium parvum*, given as a suspension (7 mg dry weight of formalin-killed organisms per ml in 0.01% thiomersalate); the dose was 0.5 to 2 ml intraperitoneally, intrapleurally, or occasionally intramuscularly.— H. E. Webb *et al.*, *Br. med. J.*, 1978, *1*, 338.

In a comparative study of 21 patients with recurrent malignant pleural effusions treatment with *Corynebacterium parvum* was better tolerated and more effective than with mustine. The relative contributions of chemical irritation and immunological reaction to the mode of action of *Corynebacterium parvum* were not clear.— J. W. Millar *et al.*, *Thorax*, 1980, *35*, 856. See also *idem* (letter), *Lancet*, 1981, *1*, 726.

Malignant neoplasms. Discussions and reports on the use of *Corynebacterium parvum* in cancer immunotherapy: *Lancet*, 1975, *1*, 502; L. Israel and R. Edelstein (letter), *ibid.*, 979; J. L. Fahey *et al.*, *Ann. intern. Med.*, 1976, *84*, 454; B. Rao *et al.*, *Cancer*, 1977, *39*, 514; I. R. Gough and C. M. Furnival (letter), *Lancet*, 1978, *2*, 999; I. R. Gough *et al.*, *Aust. N.Z. J. Surg.*, 1978, *48*, 296.

Proprietary Preparations
Coparvax *(Calmic, UK). Corynebacterium parvum*, available as vials containing 7 mg of inactivated freeze-dried organisms with thiomersal. Store at 2° to 8°. Protect from light.

12610-m

Cosmetics
In Great Britain The Cosmetic Products Regulations 1978 (SI 1978: No. 1354) define a 'cosmetic product' as 'any substance or preparation intended to be applied to any part of the external surfaces of the human body (that is to say, the epidermis, hair system, nails, lips and external genital organs) or to the teeth or buccal mucosa wholly or mainly for the purpose of cleaning, perfuming or protecting them or keeping them in good condition or changing their appearance or combating body odour or perspiration except where such cleaning, perfuming, protecting, keeping, changing, or combating is wholly for the purpose of treating or preventing disease'. A 'cosmetic product intended to come into contact with the mucous membranes' means 'a cosmetic product intended to be applied in the vicinity of the eyes, on the lips, in the oral cavity or to the external genital organs, and does not include any cosmetic product which is intended to come into only brief contact with the skin'.
The use of a large number of substances or groups of substances (generally with potent pharmacological activity or recognised toxicity) is prohibited in cosmetics.
The use of colouring agents for cosmetics is controlled. Some substances or groups of substances may be used only for specified purposes, with specified maximum concentrations, and subject to labelling and other requirements. In Great Britain these substances include ammonia, boric acid, chlorates of the alkali metals, chlorbutol, chloroform, formaldehyde, fluorides, fluorophosphates, fluorosilicates, hexachlorophane, hydrogen peroxide, hydroquinone, methyl alcohol, oxalic acid, its esters and alkaline salts, phenol, phenylmercuric compounds, potassium or sodium hydroxide, pyrogallol, quinine and its salts, resorcinol, sodium nitrite, zinc chloride, and zinc sulphate. Cosmetic products containing lanolin should be labelled 'contains lanolin'.

A discussion of dermatitis caused by perfumes in cosmetics.— *Br. med. J.*, 1977, *2*, 782.

12611-b

Cotarnine Chloride
(B.P.C. 1934). Cotarnine Hydrochloride; Cotarninium Chloratum; Stypticine. 7,8-Dihydro-4-methoxy-6-methyl-1,3-dioxolo[4,5-*g*]isoquinolinium chloride dihydrate.
$C_{12}H_{14}ClNO_3,2H_2O=291.7.$

CAS — 82-54-2 (cotarnine); 10018-19-6 (chloride).

Pharmacopoeias. In *Aust., Jug., Rus.*, and *Span.*

The chloride of cotarnine, an alkaloid obtained by oxidising noscapine with nitric acid. A pale yellow deliquescent powder. **Soluble** in water, alcohol, and chloroform; practically insoluble in ether. Solutions are **sterilised** by filtration. **Store** in airtight containers. Protect from light.

Cotarnine chloride has been used locally and systemically to arrest bleeding, especially in menstrual disorders, but is of doubtful value.

12612-v

Co-tetroxazine.

A mixture of tetroxoprim and sulphadiazine in the proportion of 1:2.5.

CAS — 73173-12-3.

Co-tetroxazine has the general properties of co-trimoxazole (see p.1460) and is used in the treatment of infections of the respiratory and urinary tracts.

Proprietary Names

Sterinor *(Heumann, Ger.)*; Tibirox *(Roche, Ger.)*.

12614-q

Covering Creams

Covering creams usually contain opacifying agents and pigments in a suitable basis. They are used for the concealment of birth marks, scars, and disfiguring skin disease.

Proprietary Preparations

Boots Covering Cream *(Boots, UK)*. An opaque, pigmented cream.

Covermark *(Medexport, UK)*. An opaque cream based on beeswax and mineral oil, available in a variety of tints. A range of other covering and tinting products is also available.

Keromask *(Sterling Industrial, UK)*. 'Base' cream and 'toning' cream, containing titanium dioxide and pigments.

12615-p

CR Gas.

EA-3547. Dibenz[*b,f*][1,4]oxazepine.
$C_{13}H_9NO$=195.2.

CAS — 257-07-8.

A riot-control gas with properties similar to those of CS gas (see below). CR gas is reported not to be hydrolysed by water and therefore to be capable of use in water cannons.

References: *Lancet*, 1973, *1*, 1370; *ibid.*, 1973, *2*, 1184; *Br. med. J.*, 1973, *3*, 5; D. G. Upshall, *Toxic. appl. Pharmac.*, 1974, *29*, 301; R. W. Foster and A. G. Ramage, *Br. J. Pharmac.*, 1975, *53*, 436; J. L. Pinkus (letter), *New Engl. J. Med.*, 1978, *299*, 901.

Effect on skin.— P. Holland, *Br. J. Derm.*, 1974, *90*, 657.

12616-s

Creatinolfosfate Sodium.

The sodium salt of 1-(2-hydroxyethyl)-1-methylguanidine *O*-phosphate.
$C_4H_{11}N_3NaO_4P$=219.1.

CAS — 6903-79-3 (creatinolfosfate).

Creatinolfosfate is used as an adjuvant in the treatment of cardiac disorders.

For a series of papers, see *Arzneimittel-Forsch.*, 1979, *29*, 1445–94.

Proprietary Names

Aplodan *(Simes, Ital.)*; Dragosil *(Farmasimes, Spain)*; Gipron *(Serpero, Ital.)*.

12617-w

Crotarbital.

Crotylbarbital. 5-(But-2-enyl)-5-ethylbarbituric acid.
$C_{10}H_{14}N_2O_3$=210.2.

CAS — 1952-67-6.

Crotarbital is a barbiturate used as a sedative.

Proprietary Names

Chavotan *(Taranto, Arg.)*.

12618-e

CS Gas.

α-(*o*-Chlorobenzylidene)malononitrile.
$C_{10}H_5ClN_2$=188.6.

CAS — 2698-41-1.

CS gas has been used as a riot-control gas.

Its toxic effects include irritation of the eyes and nose, with copious lachrymation and rhinorrhoea; a burning sensation of the mouth and throat; pain in the chest, with difficulty in breathing; coughing; an increase in salivation; and retching and vomiting. These effects usually disappear a few minutes after exposure ends. The effects of pre-existing disease of the chest may be exacerbated. Erythema and blistering of the skin may occur.

Exposed persons should be removed from the contaminated area. Treatment is symptomatic. Contaminated skin should be washed with soap and water. If contamination of the eyes has been severe they should be irrigated with physiological saline or water and amethocaine instilled to relieve pain.

Application of CS gas 20 to 30 mg under a watch glass on the skin of healthy men for a period of 1 hour produced faint erythema and transient irritation. The erythema faded over a period of 1 to 2 days leaving no residual pigmentation or blanching of the skin; there was no irritation or pruritus during the stage of erythema, and no vesication occurred. When the material was moistened the reactions were slightly more severe and occurred with quantities of 10 mg.— P. Holland and R. G. White, *Br. J. Derm.*, 1972, *86*, 150.

A discussion of the possible carcinogenicity of CS gas.— *Br. med. J.*, 1973, *1*, 129.

CS gas, administered by inhalation to *rats* and *rabbits*, and by intraperitoneal injection to *rats*, was not teratogenic.— D. E. Upshall, *Toxic. appl. Pharmac.*, 1973, *24*, 45.

Further references: *Report of the Enquiry into the Medical and Toxicological aspects of CS*, Part 1, London, HM Staionery Office, 1969; *ibid.*, Part 2, London, HM Stationery Office, 1971; G. R. N. Jones, *Nature*, 1972, *235*, 257; S. Park and S. T. Giammona, *Am. J. Dis. Child.*, 1972, *123*, 245, per *Int. pharm. Abstr.*, 1972, *9*, 878; L. Leadbeater, *Toxic. appl. Pharmac.*, 1973, *25*, 101.

15331-x

Cuproxoline.

Copper(II) bis(5,7-disulpho-8-quinolyl oxide)—diethylamine (1:4).
$C_{34}H_{56}CuN_6O_{14}S_4$=964.6.

CAS — 13007-93-7.

Cuproxoline is used in veterinary medicine for the prevention and treatment of copper deficiency.

Proprietary Names

Cujec *(Tasman, UK)*.

12619-l

Cyanoacrylate Adhesives

CAS — 1069-55-2 (bucrylate); 6606-65-1 (enbucrilate); 137-05-3 (mecrylate).

A number of cyanoacrylate compounds have been used as surgical tissue adhesives. They include bucrylate (isobutyl 2-cyanoacrylate, $C_8H_{11}NO_2$=153.2), enbucrilate (butyl 2-cyanoacrylate,$C_8H_{11}NO_2$=153.2), and mecrylate (methyl 2-cyanoacrylate, $C_5H_5NO_2$=111.1).

Bucrylate has been tried in occlusive therapy.

The manufacturers of a cyanoacrylate adhesive have stated that accidental spilling of cyanoacrylates on skin, mucous membranes, or eyes causes no permanent damage and surgery should never be necessary to separate accidentally bonded skin. In the event of accidental skin adhesion they recommend that the bonded surfaces should be immersed in warm soapy water, the surfaces peeled or rolled apart with the aid of a spatula, and the adhesive removed from the skin with soap and water; attempts should not be made to pull the surfaces apart. Eyelids stuck together or bonded to the eyeball should be washed thoroughly with warm water and a gauze patch applied; the eye will open without further action in 1 to 4 days. Manipulative attempts to open the eyes should not be made. Although cyanoacrylate introduced into the eyes may cause double vision and lachrymation they state that there is no residual damage. If lips are accidentally stuck together plenty of warm water should be applied and maximum wetting and pressure from saliva inside the mouth encouraged. Lips should be peeled or rolled apart and not pulled. Adhesive introduced into the mouth solidifies and adheres, but saliva will lift the adhesive in ½ to 2 days. Care should be taken to avoid choking.

Heat is evolved on solidification of cyanoacrylate and in rare cases may cause burns.

The use of enbucrilate as an adjunct in some types of retinal detachment surgery.— L. Regenbogen *et al.*, *Br. J. Ophthal.*, 1976, *60*, 561.

The successful removal of a stone from the oesophagus using Loctite Super Glue 3.— D. S. Macpherson and R. Wyatt, *Br. med. J.*, 1978, *2*, 476.

Complete pain relief was obtained in 3 of 6 patients with chronic alcoholic pancreatitis, following ductal obstruction by low-pressure injection of a rapid-setting cyanoacrylate glue into the pancreatic duct. The patients were given pancreatic supplements by mouth.— J. M. Little *et al.* (preliminary communication), *Lancet*, 1979, *2*, 557. Encouraging results with similar glues.— W. Rosch and C. Gebhardt (letter), *ibid.*, 1131; W. Land and H. Weitz (letter), *ibid.*

Proprietary Names

Histoacryl Blue *(Davis & Geck, UK)*.

12620-v

Cycloheximide.

U-4527. 3-{(*R*)-2-[(1*S*,3*S*,5*S*)-3,5-Dimethyl-2-oxocyclohexyl]-2-hydroxyethyl}glutarimide.
$C_{15}H_{23}NO_4$=281.4.

CAS — 66-81-9.

An antimicrobial substance produced by strains of *Streptomyces griseus*.

Cycloheximide has antifungal properties and has been used for the treatment and control of certain mycotic plant diseases. It may be added to bacteriological media to facilitate the isolation or counting of bacteria in the presence of yeasts or moulds; similarly, it has been used in the detection and isolation of *Chlamydia trachomatis*. It is a potent skin irritant and if spilled on the skin should be washed off immediately with soap and water. Cycloheximide is claimed to be of value in the treatment of psoriasis.

Intravenous infusion of cycloheximide, which was known to inhibit protein synthesis, reliably caused lysis of fever in 15 chronically febrile patients with Hodgkin's disease and no detectable bacterial, fungal, or viral infection. Antipyretic effects were also noted in other neoplastic diseases but it had no effect in 4 patients with normal granulocyte reserves who were febrile as a result of bacterial infection.— C. W. Young and M. D. Dowling, *Cancer Res.*, 1975, *35*, 1218, per *J. Am. med. Ass.*, 1975, *233*, 1326.

Proprietary Names

Acti-dione *(Upjohn, USA)*.

15318-d

Cyhalothrin.

PP-563. (*RS*)-α-Cyano-3-phenoxybenzyl (*Z*)-(1*RS*,3*RS*)-3-(2-chloro-3,3,3-trifluoropropenyl)-2,2-dimethylcyclopropane-carboxylate.
$C_{23}H_{19}ClF_3NO_3$=449.9.

Cyhalothrin is an insecticide for veterinary use.

Manufacturers

ICI Pharmaceuticals, UK.

12621-g

Cytisine. Baptitoxine; Laburnine; Sophorine; Ulexine. 1,2,3,4,5,6-Hexahydro-1,5-methano-8*H*-pyrido[1,2-*a*][1,5]diazocin-8-one.
$C_{11}H_{14}N_2O$=190.2.

CAS — 485-35-8.

Pharmacopoeias. In *Rus.* which also includes Cytitone, a solution of cytisine.

A white or slightly yellowish crystalline powder. M.p. 154° to 157°. Freely **soluble** in water, alcohol, and chloroform.

Cytisine is a highly toxic alkaloid found in laburnum and some other leguminous plants. It resembles nicotine in its actions. Adverse effects include nausea and vomiting, dilatation of the pupils, and tachycardia, followed by dizziness, mental confusion, muscular incoordination and weakness, and convulsions; respiratory paralysis may occur leading to death by asphyxia. Treatment of adverse effects is as described under Nicotine, p.1732.

12622-q

Cytochrome C. A haemoprotein occurring in the body and involved in electron and hydrogen transport in biological oxidation processes.

CAS — 9007-43-6.

Pharmacopoeias. Chin. includes Cytochrome C Solution and preparations for injection.

Cytochrome C has been given intravenously in various hypoxic conditions.

Earlier encouraging results with cytochrome C have not been substantiated in subsequent *animal* studies on the treatment of poisoning with *Amanita phalloides* (see p.1677).

Proprietary Names
Biocytmet *(Biosedra, Arg.)*; Cytochrom C-Uvocal *(Mulli, Ger.)*; Cyto-Mack *(Szama, Arg.; Mack, Switz.)*.

12623-p

Danitracen. WA-335; WA-335BS. 9,10-Dihydro-10-(1-methyl-4-piperidylidene)-9-anthrol.
$C_{20}H_{21}NO$=291.4.

CAS — 31232-26-5.

Danitracen, structurally related to cyproheptadine, has antihistamine and antiserotonin properties. It also has antidepressant and sedative effects.

Pharmacology of danitracen in *animals*.— G. Engelhardt, *Arzneimittel-Forsch.*, 1975, *25*, 1723; J. Kähling *et al.*, *ibid.*, 1737.

Comparable effects of danitracen 3 mg daily and amitriptyline 150 mg daily in 116 patients with depression.— N. Matussek *et al.*, *Arzneimittel-Forsch.*, 1976, *26*, 1160. See also S. Kaumeier *et al.*, *Curr. ther. Res.*, 1977, *21*, 108.

Further references: B. Saletu *et al.*, *Curr. ther. Res.*, 1976, *20*, 810 (psychoactivity and cerebral bioavailability); F. G. Sulman *et al.*, *Headache*, 1977, *17*, 203 (use in migraine).

Manufacturers
Thomae, Ger.

12624-s

Deanol. Démanol. 2-Dimethylaminoethanol.
$C_4H_{11}NO$=89.12.

CAS — 108-01-0.

Adverse Effects and Precautions. Headache, constipation, muscle tension, insomnia, pruritus, transient skin rash, and postural hypotension may occur with deanol. Extreme changes of mood have been reported.

Deanol should not be given to patients with grand mal epilepsy.

Severe cholinergic effects (rhinorrhoea, sialorrhoea, and dyspnoea) in a 37-year-old woman were associated with the administration of deanol.— R. Nesse and B. J. Carroll (letter), *Lancet*, 1976, *2*, 50.

Further references: D. E. Casey, *Psychopharmacology*, 1979, *62*, 187 (mood disorders).

Uses. Deanol may be a precursor of acetylcholine and has been claimed to enhance cholinergic activity. It has been employed as a central stimulant in behavioural disorders of children and has been used in the treatment of dyskinesias, with variable success in both indications.

It has been used as deanol hydrogen *N*-acetylglutamate (deanol aceglumate), deanol acetamidobenzoate, deanol cyclohexylpropionate (cyprodenate; cyprodémanol), deanol hydrogen succinate (deanol hemisuccinate), deanol dihydrogen phosphate, deanol pyroglutamate (=deanol pidolate), and deanol hydrogen tartrate. Meclofenoxate (see p.365) is a similar derivative.

A brief review of the clinical efficacy and postulated mechanism of action of deanol acetamidobenzoate.— O. Ré, *Curr. ther. Res.*, 1974, *16*, 1238.

The use of cyprodenate in geriatric patients.— M. Bergener and H. Frestein, *Arzneimittel-Forsch.*, 1972, *22*, 2058.

Two patients with blepharospasm were successfully treated with deanol, in doses of 600 mg and 1 g daily.— E. Miller (letter), *New Engl. J. Med.*, 1973, *289*, 697.

Behavioural disorders. In a double-blind study of 64 children with learning and behavioural disorders, including many with hyperactivity, daily maintenance doses of deanol 500 mg (as the acetamidobenzoate) or methylphenidate 40 mg both improved performance when compared with placebo. Although deanol has been postulated to be an acetylcholine precursor its mechanism of action remains speculative.— J. A. Lewis and R. Young, *Clin. Pharmac. Ther.*, 1975, *17*, 534.

Dyskinesias. In 8 of 11 patients levodopa-induced dyskinesias were relieved by deanol 600 to 900 mg daily; one further patient was improved. Dyskinesias recurred when placebo was substituted.— E. Miller, *Neurology, Minneap.*, 1974, *24*, 116, per *J. Am. med. Ass.*, 1974, *228*, 783. The beneficial results achieved by others with deanol 300 to 900 mg daily in various dyskinesias were not confirmed in 25 patients given 225 or 450 to 900 mg daily.— E. C. Laterre and E. Fortemps (letter), *Lancet*, 1975, *1*, 1301. Response of tardive dyskinesia was variable following deanol administration; there might be different subtypes.— D. E. Casey (letter), *New Engl. J. Med.*, 1976, *295*, 1078. In a double-blind study involving 14 patients with tardive dyskinesia treatment with deanol acetamidobenzoate 2 g daily for 4 weeks resulted in no more improvement than occurred with placebo.— P. Penovich *et al.*, *J. Am. med. Ass.*, 1978, *239*, 1997.

Further references: D. Mehta *et al.* (letter), *Am. J. Psychiat.*, 1976, *133*, 1467; I. Ray (letter), *Can. med. Ass. J.*, 1977, *117*, 129; I. V. Jackson, *Curr. ther. Res.*, 1978, *24*, 725; J. Amsterdam and J. Mendels, *Am. J. Psychiat.*, 1979, *136*, 1197.

Proprietary Names
Actébral *(maleic acid derivative of cyprodenate) (Laboratoires Biologiques de l'Île-de-France, Fr.; Boizot, Spain)*; Clérégil *(aceglumate) (Merck-Clévenot, Fr.; Merck-Clévenot, Switz.)*; Cervoxan *(acetamidobenzoate) (see also under Vinburnine) (SMB, Belg.)*; Deaner *(acetamidobenzoate) (Riker, Arg.; Riker, Austral.; Riker, Canad.; Riker, USA)*; Diforène *(Choay, Fr.)*; Endocaina *(acetamidobenzoate hydrochloride) (Lafage, Arg.)*; Pabenol *(acetamidobenzoate) (Gentili, Ital.)*; Panclar *(phosphate) (Astra, Arg.; Astra, Fr.; Made, Spain)*; Plenium *(cyprodenate) (Millet, Arg.)*; Risatarun *(aceglumate) (Ravensberg, Ger.)*; Rischiaril *(aceglumate) (Piam, Ital.)*; Tonibral *(hemisuccinate) (Sobio, Fr.)*.

12625-w

Deanol Benzilate. Benzacine; Deanol Diphenylglycolate; Dimethylaminoethyl Diphenylglycolate; 2-Dimethylaminoethyl Benzilate. 2-Dimethylaminoethyl αα-diphenyl-α-hydroxyacetate.
$C_{18}H_{21}NO_3$=299.4.

CAS — 968-46-7; 71-79-4 (hydrochloride).

Deanol benzilate has been given to relieve the symptoms of rhinitis and as an antispasmodic agent. The hydrochloride and benzilic acid salt have been used.

Proprietary Names
Arinol *(hydrochloride)(Macchia, Ital.)*; Asaletten *(benzilic acid salt and hydrochloride)(Thilo, Ger.)*; Labotropin *(hydrochloride)(Labopharma, Ger.)*.

12626-e

Decoquinate *(B.P. Vet.)*. M & B-15497; HC-1528. Ethyl 6-decyloxy-7-ethoxy-4-hydroxyquinoline-3-carboxylate.
$C_{24}H_{35}NO_5$=417.5.

CAS — 18507-89-6.

A cream to buff-coloured, odourless or almost odourless, microcrystalline powder. M.p. about 242°. Practically **insoluble** in water and alcohol; very slightly soluble in chloroform and ether.

Decoquinate is a coccidiostat used in poultry and is also added to feeding stuffs for the fattening of chickens.

Proprietary Names
Deccox Premix *(May & Baker, UK)*.

12627-l

Deflazacort. L-5458; Azacort. 11β,21-Dihydroxy-2′-methyl-5′βH-pregna-1,4-dieno[17,16-*d*]-oxazole-3,20-dione 21-acetate.
$C_{25}H_{31}NO_6$=441.5.

CAS — 14484-47-0.

NOTE. The name oxazacort has been suggested for this compound.

Deflazacort is a corticosteroid under study for systemic use.

References: A. Caniggia *et al.*, *Int. J. clin. Pharmac. Biopharm.*, 1977, *15*, 126; G. Buniva *et al.*, *Curr. ther. Res.*, 1979, *26*, 69; M. G. Mazzucconi *et al.*, *Int. J. clin. Pharmac. Biopharm.*, 1980, *18*, 538.

Manufacturers
Lepetit, Ital.

12628-y

Delmadinone Acetate. RS-1301. 6-Chloro-3,20-dioxopregna-1,4,6-trien-17α-yl acetate.
$C_{23}H_{27}ClO_4$=402.9.

CAS — 15262-77-8 (delmadinone); 13698-49-2 (acetate).

A white crystalline powder. M.p. about 169°.

Delmadinone acetate is a progestogen with anti-androgen and anti-oestrogen activity. It has been used as an anti-androgen in veterinary practice.

Proprietary Names
Tardak *(Syntex, UK)*.

12629-j

Demegestone. R-2453. 17α-Methyl-19-norpregna-4,9-diene-3,20-dione.
$C_{21}H_{28}O_2$=312.5.

CAS — 10116-22-0.

Demegestone is a progestogen and has been used in menstrual disorders.

Proprietary Names
Lutionex *(Roussel, Fr.)*.

12630-q

Demoxytocin. ODA-914; Desamino-oxytocin. [1-(3-Mercaptopropionic acid)]-oxytocin.
$C_{43}H_{65}N_{11}O_{12}S_2$=992.2.

CAS — 113-78-0.

Demoxytocin has been used by mouth, as buccal tablets, for the induction of labour.

References: G. Lykkesfeldt and M. Osler, *Acta obstet. gynec. scand.*, 1979, *58*, 321.

Proprietary Names
Sandopart *(Sandoz-Wander, Belg.; Sandoz, Ital.; Sandoz, S.Afr.; Sandoz, Switz.)*.

12631-p

2-Deoxy-D-glucose.
$C_6H_{12}O_5$=164.2.

CAS — 154-17-6.

2-Deoxy-D-glucose has been tried topically as an antiviral agent.

References: D. R. Woodman and J. C. Williams, *Antimicrob. Ag. Chemother.*, 1977, *11*, 475; H. A. Blough and R. L. Giuntoli, *J. Am. med. Ass.*, 1979, *241*, 2798; L. Corey and K. K. Holmes (letter), *ibid.*, *243*, 29; *ibid.*, 1980, *244*, 2022.

12632-s

Deoxyribonucleic Acid. Desoxypentose Nucleic Acid; Desoxyribose Nucleic Acid; Desoxyribonucleic Acid; DNA; ADN; Thymus Nucleic Acid; Animal Nucleic Acid.

Pharmacopoeias. In *Fr.*

A nucleotide polymer, and 1 of the 2 distinct varieties of nucleic acid (see p.1735). It is found in the cell nuclei of living tissues. It occurs as a white or pale cream-coloured powder. Practically **insoluble** in water and most organic solvents. Freely soluble in alkaline solutions.

Several proprietary preparations of deoxyribonucleic acid are marketed in some countries and are advocated for a variety of asthenic and convalescent conditions.

For the use of deoxyribonucleic acid by intradermal injection in the diagnosis of systemic lupus erythematosus, see R. O. Ores and E. H. Mandel, *Br. J. Derm.*, 1971, *84*, 217.

A review of the use of deoxyribonucleic acid as a carrier for antineoplastic agents.— A. Trouet *et al.*, Desoxyribonucleic Acid as Carrier of Antitumour Drugs, in *Drug Carriers in Biology and Medicine*, G. Gregoriadis (Ed.), London, Academic Press, 1979, pp. 87–105.

For a report of deoxyribonucleic acid in conjunction with adenosine triphosphate inducing radioprotection, see Adenosine Triphosphate, p.1614.

Recombinant DNA research. A discussion on the merits and risks of work on recombinant DNA.— L. Thomas, *New Engl. J. Med.*, 1977, *296*, 324. See also C. Cohen, *ibid.*, 1203; R. Goldstein, *ibid.*, 1226; *Lancet*, 1979, *1*, 1123.

Proprietary Names
Desoxiribon *(Craveri, Arg.)*; Eucytol *(Mayoly-Spindler, Fr.*; *Mayoly-Spindler, Switz.)*; Nuclifort *(Mayoly-Spindler, Fr.)*.

12633-w

Desogestrel. Org-2969. 13β-Ethyl-11-methylene-18,19-dinor-17α-pregn-4-en-20-yn-17β-ol.
$C_{22}H_{30}O$=310.5.

CAS — 54024-22-5.

Adverse Effects and Precautions. As for Progesterone, p.1431.
See also under Oral Contraceptives, p.1402.

Uses. Desogestrel is a progestogen used in oral contraceptive preparations.

References: S. O. Skouby, *Contraception*, 1976, *14*, 529; L. Viinikka *et al.*, *Contraception*, 1977, *16*, 51, per *Int. pharm. Abstr.*, 1978, *15*, 315; L. Viinikka *et al.*, *Eur. J. clin. Pharmac.*, 1979, *15*, 349.

Proprietary Preparations of Desogestrel with Ethinyloestradiol

Marvelon *(Organon, UK)*. Tablets each containing desogestrel 150 µg and ethinyloestradiol 30 µg. For use as an oral contraceptive. *Dose.* One tablet daily for 21 days starting on the first day of the first treated cycle and after 7 tablet-free days for succeeding cycles. (Also available as Marvelon in *Ger.*).

12634-e

Detaxtran Hydrochloride. The hydrochloride of a water-soluble cationic substance, of high molecular weight, obtained from dextran.

Detaxtran hydrochloride is reported to reduce the absorption of lipids and has been used in hyperlipidaemia.

Proprietary Names
Dexide *(Fargal-Pharmasint, Ital.)*; Pulsar *(Medosan, Ital.)*.

12635-l

Detorubicin. {(2*S*,4*S*)-4-[(3-Amino-2,3,6-trideoxy-α-L-*lyxo*-hexopyranosyl)oxy]-1,2,3,4,6,11-hexahydro-2,5,12-trihydroxy-7-methoxy-6,11-dioxonaphthacen-2-yl}carbonylmethyl glyoxylate 2-(diethyl acetal).
$C_{33}H_{39}NO_{14}$=673.7.

CAS — 66211-92-5.

Detorubicin is an analogue of doxorubicin under study as an antineoplastic agent.

References: C. Jacquillat *et al.*, *Cancer Treat. Rep.*, 1979, *63*, 889; S. K. Carter, *Drugs*, 1980, *20*, 375.

Manufacturers
Rhône-Poulenc, Fr.

12636-y

Deximafen Hydrochloride. R-26333; R-25540 *(racemic)*. (+)-2,3,5,6-Tetrahydro-5-(or 3-)-phenyl-1*H*-imidazo[1,2-*a*]imidazole hydrochloride.
$C_{11}H_{13}N_3$,HCl=223.7.

CAS — 42116-77-8 (deximafen).

Deximafen hydrochloride has been studied as a potential antidepressant agent.

Manufacturers
Janssen, Belg.

12637-j

Dezocine. Wy-16225. (−)-13β-Amino-5,6,7,8,9,10,11α,12-octahydro-5α-methyl-5,11-methanobenzocyclodecen-3-ol.
$C_{16}H_{23}NO$=245.4.

CAS — 53648-55-8.

Dezocine is an analgesic and narcotic antagonist which has been given by injection for the relief of severe pain.

A study in 5 healthy subjects indicated that dezocine is 8.6 times as potent as pentazocine in terms of its respiratory depressant effect. The clinical significance of these findings remains to be determined.— H. P. Wuest and J. W. Bellville, *J. clin. Pharmac.*, 1979, *19*, 205.

After a single intravenous injection of dezocine 20 mg, 21 of 25 patients with severe pain remained free of pain for a mean of 3.5 hours. Doses of 10 or 15 mg were less effective. Pronounced dizziness occurred in 23 of the 25 patients. Other side-effects included nausea, vomiting, aching of the nose (each in 1 patient), and sweating (2 patients).— W. Oosterlinck and A. Verbaeys, *Curr. med. Res. Opinion*, 1980, *6*, 472.

In a double-blind controlled study of 20 cancer patients suffering continuous pain, dezocine 10 mg by intramuscular injection was significantly more effective than placebo in relieving pain. Side-effects reported included nausea, slight perspiration, and sensation of heat.— M. Staquet, *Curr. med. Res. Opinion*, 1980, *6*, 634.

A double-blind study in 160 patients indicated that dezocine was efficient and safe for the relief of moderate pain after lower abdominal obstetric or gynaecological surgery. Dezocine 10 mg was equipotent with morphine 10 mg, both given by intramuscular injection.— J. W. Downing *et al.*, *Br. J. Anaesth.*, 1981, *53*, 59.

Further references: R. J. Fragen and N. Caldwell, *Anesth. Analg. curr. Res.*, 1978, *57*, 563.

Manufacturers
Wyeth, USA.

12638-z

Diacetolol Hydrochloride. EU-4891; M & B-16942A. (±)-3′-Acetyl-4′-(2-hydroxy-3-isopropylaminopropoxy)acetanilide hydrochloride.
$C_{16}H_{24}N_2O_4$,HCl=344.8.

CAS — 28197-69-5 (diacetolol); 69796-04-9 (hydrochloride).

Diacetolol is an active metabolite of acebutolol and has beta-adrenoceptor blocking activity.

References: A. Gulaid *et al.* (letter), *Br. J. clin. Pharmac.*, 1978, *5*, 261; B. Flouvat *et al.*, *Eur. J. clin. Pharmac.*, 1981, *19*, 287.

Manufacturers
May & Baker, UK; Norwich-Eaton, USA.

12639-c

Diamphenethide *(B.P. Vet.)*. Diamfenetide. β,β′-Oxybis(aceto-*p*-phenetidide).
$C_{20}H_{24}N_2O_5$=372.4.

CAS — 36141-82-9.

A white to pale buff-coloured powder. Practically **insoluble** in water and in ether; soluble 1 in 160 of alcohol, 1 in 500 of chloroform, and 1 in 150 of methyl alcohol.

Diamphenethide is used for the control of liver fluke in sheep.

Proprietary Names
Coriban *(Wellcome, UK)*.

12640-s

Dianhydrogalactitol. Dianhydrodulcitol; DAG; NSC-132313. 1,2:5,6-Dianhydrogalactitol; 1,2:5,6-Diepoxyhexane-3,4-diol.
$C_6H_{10}O_4$=146.1.

CAS — 23261-20-3.

Dianhydrogalactitol is reported to have antineoplastic activity.

References: B. Hoogstraten and C. Haas, *Clin. Pharmac. Ther.*, 1976, *19*, 108; S. Eckhardt *et al.*, *Cancer Treat. Rep.*, 1977, *61*, 841; R. T. Eagan *et al.*, *J. Am. med. Ass.*, 1979, *241*, 2046.

Manufacturers
Chinoin, Hung.

12641-w

Diaveridine *(B.P. Vet.)*. BW-49-210. 5-Veratrylpyrimidine-2,4-diyldiamine.
$C_{13}H_{16}N_4O_2$=260.3.

CAS — 5355-16-8.

A white or creamy-white, odourless, tasteless powder. M.p. about 233°. Very slightly **soluble** in water and alcohol; soluble 1 in 600 of chloroform.

Diaveridine has been used in veterinary medicine as a coccidiostat in poultry. It also has bacteriostatic properties.

Manufacturers
May & Baker, UK.

12642-e

Dibromochloropropane. 1,2-Dibromo-3-chloropropane.
$C_3H_5Br_2Cl$=236.3.

CAS — 96-12-8.

Dibromochloropropane is a pesticide. Concern has been expressed at low sperm counts in workers exposed to dibromochloropropane.

References: D. Whorton *et al.* (preliminary communication), *Lancet*, 1977, *2*, 1259; *ibid.*, 1978, *2*, 79; R. I. Glass *et al.*, *Am. J. Epidem.*, 1979, *109*, 346; D. Whorton *et al.*, *J. occup. Med.*, 1979, *21*, 161; G. Potashnik *et al.*, *Israel J. med. Scis*, 1979, *15*, 438, per *J. Am. med. Ass.*, 1979, *242*, 1210.

12643-l

Dibromotyrosine. 3,5-Dibromo-L-tyrosine.
$C_9H_9Br_2NO_3$=339.0.

CAS — 300-38-9.

Dibromotyrosine is reported to have antithyroid activity.

Proprietary Names
Biotiren *(Benvegna, Ital.)*; Bromotiren *(Baldacci, Ital.; Saet, Spain)*.

12644-y

Dichlofenthion *(B.P. Vet.)*. V-C-13. *O*-2,4-Dichlorophenyl *O,O*-diethyl phosphorothioate.
$C_{10}H_{13}Cl_2O_3PS$=315.2.

CAS — 97-17-6.

A colourless or pale yellow oily liquid. Wt per ml 1.296 to 1.316 g. **Immiscible** with water; miscible with alcohol and chloroform.

Dichlofenthion is an organophosphorus compound (see p.832), used as an insecticide in veterinary practice.

12645-j

Dichlorisone Acetate. Diclorisone Acetate. 9α,11β-Dichloro-17α,21-dihydroxypregna-1,4-diene-3,20-dione 21-acetate.
$C_{23}H_{28}Cl_2O_5$=455.4.

CAS — 7008-26-6 (dichlorisone); 79-61-8 (acetate).

Dichlorisone acetate is a topical corticosteroid.

Proprietary Names
Astroderm *(Aristochimica, Ital.)*; Dermaren *(Areu, Spain)*; Diclasone *(Liberman, Spain)*.

12646-z

Dichlorophenarsine Hydrochloride. Chlorarsenum Hydrochloricum. (3-Amino-4-hydroxyphenyl)dichloroarsine hydrochloride.
$C_6H_6AsCl_2NO,HCl$=290.4.

CAS — 455-83-4 (dichlorophenarsine); 536-29-8 (hydrochloride).

Pharmacopoeias. In *Belg.*, *Braz.*, *Mex.*, and *Pol.*

A white odourless powder containing 25.3 to 27% of As; it is usually mixed with buffering agents and other suitable substances to make its solution physiologically compatible with blood. **Soluble** in water, alcohol, acetone, solutions of alkali hydroxides and carbonates, and dilute mineral acids. **Store** below 25°, in sealed glass containers from which the air has been removed or replaced by an inert gas.

In clinical efficacy and toxicity dichlorophenarsine resembles oxophenarsine, and was formerly used in the treatment of syphilis.

12647-c

Diclofensine Hydrochloride. Moxifensine Hydrochloride; Ro-8-4650. (±)-4-(3,4-Dichlorophenyl)-1,2,3,4-tetrahydro-7-methoxy-2-methylisoquinoline hydrochloride.
$C_{17}H_{17}Cl_2NO,HCl$=358.7.

CAS — 67165-56-4 (diclofensine); 34041-84-4 (hydrochloride).

Diclofensine hydrochloride has been tried in parkinsonism and depression.

References: E. Birket-Smith *et al.*, *Acta neurol. scand.*, 1978, *58*, 74 (parkinsonism); J. Presthus *et al.*, *ibid.*, 77 (parkinsonism); G. Heinze and L. M. O. Omer, *Curr. ther. Res.*, 1981, *29*, 567 (depression).

Manufacturers
Roche, Switz.

12648-k

Diethylaminoethanol. 2-Diethylaminoethanol.
$C_6H_{15}NO$=117.2.

CAS — 100-37-8.

Diethylaminoethanol is an analogue of deanol (see p.1700) and has been similarly used.

Proprietary Names
Cérébrol (malate) *(Laboratoires Français de Thérapeutique, Fr.)*.

12649-a

Diethylthiambutene Hydrochloride *(B.P. Vet.)*. *NN*-Diethyl-1-methyl-3,3-di-(2-thienyl)prop-2-enylamine hydrochloride.
$C_{16}H_{21}NS_2,HCl$=327.9.

CAS — 86-14-6 (diethylthiambutene); 132-19-4 (hydrochloride).

A white, odourless or almost odourless, crystalline powder. M.p. 151° to 154°. **Soluble** 1 in 2 of water and 1 in 1 of alcohol; practically insoluble in ether.

Diethylthiambutene hydrochloride is a narcotic analgesic which has been used in veterinary medicine.

12650-e

Difenpiramide. Diphenpyramide; Z-876. *N*-(2-Pyridyl)-2-(biphenyl-4-yl)acetamide.
$C_{19}H_{16}N_2O$=288.3.

CAS — 51484-40-3.

Difenpiramide has anti-inflammatory, analgesic, and antipyretic activity and has been used in the treatment of rheumatic and other disorders.

Proprietary Names
Difenax *(Zambeletti, Ital.)*.

12651-l

Diflorasone Diacetate. U-34865. 6α,9α-Difluoro-11β,17α,21-trihydroxy-16β-methylpregna-1,4-diene-3,20-dione 17,21-diacetate.
$C_{26}H_{32}F_2O_7$=494.5.

CAS — 2557-49-5 (diflorasone); 33564-31-7 (diacetate).

Diflorasone diacetate is a fluorinated corticosteroid for topical application, usually in a concentration of 0.05%.

References: S. M. Bluefarb *et al.*, *J. int. med. Res.*, 1976, *4*, 454; M. M. Cahn *et al.*, *Curr. ther. Res.*, 1977, *22*, 297; S. Hammarström *et al.*, *Science*, 1977, *197*, 994; J. F. Lawless and S. S. Stubbs, *Curr. ther. Res.*, 1978, *23*, 159; *Med. Lett.*, 1978, *20*, 112; D. J. P. Squires and E. L. Masson, *J. int. med. Res.*, 1981, *9*, 79.

Proprietary Names
Florone *(Upjohn, Canad.; Upjohn, Neth.; Upjohn, USA)*.

12652-y

Difluprednate. CM-9155; W-6309. 6α,9α-Difluoro-11β,17α,21-trihydroxypregna-1,4-diene-3,20-dione 21-acetate 17-butyrate.
$C_{27}H_{34}F_2O_7$=508.6.

CAS — 23674-86-4.

Difluprednate is a fluorinated corticosteroid for topical application.

Proprietary Names
Epitopic *(Porcher-Lavril, Fr.)*.

12653-j

Dihexazine. The 3-hydroxy-5-hydroxymethyl-2-methylisonicotinaldehyde 5-phosphate salt of 4-(5*H*-dibenzo[*a,d*]cyclohepten-5-ylidene)-1-methylpiperidine.
$C_{21}H_{21}N,C_8H_{10}NO_6P$=534.5.

Dihexazine is the pyridoxal phosphate salt of cyproheptadine and has been used as an appetite stimulant.

Proprietary Names
Viternum *(Argentia, Arg.; Juste, Spain)*.

12654-z

Dihydroxydibutylether. Hydroxybutyloxide. 4,4′-Oxybis(butan-2-ol).
$C_8H_{18}O_3$=162.2.

CAS — 821-33-0.

Dihydroxydibutylether is a choleretic agent.

Biliary secretion was increased by dihydroxydibutylether 300 to 750 mg by mouth.— F. Fici *et al.*, *Curr. ther. Res.*, 1976, *20*, 772.

Proprietary Names
Boutybil *(Bouty, Ital.)*; Cistoquine *(Casasco, Arg.)*; Colenormol *(Beta, Ital.)*; Dis-Cinil *(Lusofarmaco, Ital.)*; Diskin *(Benedetti, Ital.)*; Dyskinebyl *(CCP, Belg.)*; Dyskinébyl *(Laphal, Fr.)*; Kinepar *(Lusofarmaco, Spain)*; Liver-Chol *(Radiumfarma, Ital.)*.

12655-c

Diiodhydrin. Iodazone; Iothion. 1,3-Di-iodopropan-2-ol.
$C_3H_6I_2O$=311.9.

CAS — 534-08-7.

NOTE. Distinguish iodazone from iodazine.

Diiodhydrin is an organic iodine-containing material for topical use; it is reported to have antibacterial properties.

Proprietary Names
Glico-Iodazol *(Zambeletti, Ital.)*; Iodazol *(Zambeletti, Ital.)*.

9005-f

Diiodotyrosine. Diiodothyrosinum; Iodogorgoic Acid. 3,5-Di-iodo-L-tyrosine dihydrate.
$C_9H_9I_2NO_3,2H_2O$=469.0.

CAS — 66-02-4 (anhydrous); 300-39-0 (L, anhydrous).

Pharmacopoeias. In *Aust.*, *Cz.*, and *Rus.*

A white to slightly yellowish-brown powder, containing about 58% of organically combined iodine. Slightly **soluble** in water and alcohol; practically insoluble in chloroform and ether; soluble in solutions of alkali hydroxides and strong acids. **Protect** from light.

Uses. Diiodotyrosine is a precursor of both tri-iodothyronine and thyroxine in the thyroid gland. It has been advocated for hyperthyroidism and some types of goitre.

Proprietary Names
Itir *(Boniscontro & Gazzone, Ital.)*; Normotiroides Fuerte *(Inexfa, Spain)*.

12656-k

Dimelazine Hydrochloride. 10-(1,3-Dimethylpyrrolidin-3-ylmethyl)phenothiazine hydrochloride.
$C_{19}H_{22}N_2S,HCl$=346.9.

CAS — 15302-12-2 (dimelazine).

Dimelazine hydrochloride has antihistaminic and sedative properties.

Proprietary Names
Centrophène *(Biosédra, Fr.)*.

12657-a

Dimethylaminoethyl Reserpilinate Hydrochloride. 2-Dimethylaminoethyl (3β,19α,20α)-16,17-didehydro-10,11-dimethoxy-19-methyloxayohimban-16-carboxylate hydrochloride.
$C_{26}H_{35}N_3O_5,2HCl=542.5$.

CAS — 5585-67-1 (dimethylaminoethyl reserpilinate).

A derivative of reserpiline, an alkaloid obtained from *Rauwolfia vomitoria*. It has been used in the treatment of hypertension.

Proprietary Names
Paratensiol *(Latéma, Fr.)*; Belnalin, Dimeserpin, Hypertenin, Moderyl, Morandamin, Parenin, Perserin, Pilinate, Pullsmalin R, Resporisan, Shinnabrein *(all Jap.)*.

12658-t

4-Dimethylaminophenol Hydrochloride.

$C_8H_{11}NO,HCl=173.6$.

CAS — 619-60-3 (4-dimethylaminophenol).

4-Dimethylaminophenol hydrochloride is used as an adjunct in the treatment of cyanide poisoning. It is reported to oxidise haemoglobin to ferrihaemoglobin (methaemoglobin) which has an affinity with cyanide ions. Sodium thiosulphate is then given to produce thiocyanate. Few clinical reports are available.
See also Hydrocyanic Acid, p.790.

Proprietary Names
4-DMAP *(Köhler, Ger.)*.

12659-x

3,5-Dimethyl-3′-isopropyl-L-thyronine. L-2-Amino-3-[4-(4-hydroxy-3-isopropylphenoxy)-3,5-dimethylphenyl]propionic acid.
$C_{20}H_{25}NO_4=343.4$.

3,5-Dimethyl-3′-isopropyl-L-thyronine is a thyroid hormone analogue.

A study in *rats* on the possible role of the thyroid hormone analogues 3,5-dimethyl-3′-isopropyl-L-thyronine (DIMIT), 3,5-di-iodo-3′-isopropyl-L-thyronine (DIIIT), and 3,5-di-iodo-3′-*sec*-butyl-L-thyronine (DISBT) in the prevention of foetal goitre *in utero*.— F. Comite *et al., Endocrinology*, 1978, *102*, 1670.

Further references: I. J. Chopra, *New Engl. J. Med.*, 1976, *295*, 335.

12660-y

Dimethylphenyliminothiazolidine Hydrorhodanide. (−)-2-Imino-3,4-dimethyl-5-phenylthiazolidine thiocyanate.
$C_{11}H_{14}N_2S,HCNS=265.4$.

CAS — 14007-67-1 (dimethylphenyliminothiazolidine).

Dimethylphenyliminothiazolidine hydrorhodanide has been used in the treatment of various respiratory disorders. The hydrochloride and theophylline-7-acetate have also been used.

12662-z

Dimetridazole *(B.P. Vet.)*. 1,2-Dimethyl-5-nitroimidazole.
$C_5H_7N_3O_2=141.1$.

CAS — 551-92-8.

An almost white to brownish-yellow, odourless or almost odourless powder which darkens on exposure to light. M.p. 138° to 141°. Slightly **soluble** in water; soluble 1 in 30 of alcohol, 1 in 5 of chloroform, and 1 in 170 of ether; soluble in mineral acids. **Protect** from light.

Dimetridazole is used in veterinary medicine in the prevention and treatment of blackhead (histomoniasis) in turkeys and chickens and for the control of swine dysentery and trichomoniasis in pigeons. It is also used as a growth promoter in pigs and poultry.

Proprietary Names
Emtryl *(May & Baker, UK)*.

12663-c

Dimophebumine Hydrochloride. Sp-281. 1-(3,4-Dimethoxyphenyl)-*NN*-dimethyl-4-phenylbutylamine hydrochloride.
$C_{20}H_{27}NO_2,HCl=349.9$.

CAS — 3735-45-3 (dimophebumine).

A white crystalline powder. M.p. 137° to 148°. **Soluble** 1 in 3 of water, alcohol, and methyl alcohol; slightly soluble in acetone and ether.

Dimophebumine hydrochloride is a uterine relaxant which has been used to facilitate parturition.

Proprietary Names
Monzal *(Thomae, Ger.)*; Monzaldon (veterinary) *(Boehringer Ingelheim, UK)*.

12664-k

Dimorpholamine. *NN*′-Ethylenebis(*N*-butylmorpholine-4-carboxamide).
$C_{20}H_{38}N_4O_4=398.5$.

CAS — 119-48-2.

Pharmacopoeias. In *Jap.* which also includes an injection.

Dimorpholamine is reported to stimulate the circulation and the respiration.

Proprietary Names
Theraplina Théraplix *(Vaillant, Ital.)*.

12665-a

Dinitolmide *(B.P. Vet.)*. Dinitrotoluamide; Methyldinitrobenzamide. 3,5-Dinitro-*o*-toluamide.
$C_8H_7N_3O_5=225.2$.

CAS — 148-01-6.

Pharmacopoeias. In *Fr.*

A cream-coloured to light tan-coloured odourless powder. M.p. 177° to 181°. Practically **insoluble** in water; soluble 1 in 100 of alcohol, 1 in 15 of acetone, 1 in 650 of chloroform, and 1 in 850 of ether.

Dinitolmide is a coccidiostat used in poultry.

Proprietary Names
Salcostat *(Salsbury, UK)*.

12666-t

2,4-Dinitrochlorobenzene. DNCB. 1-Chloro-2,4-dinitrobenzene.
$C_6H_3ClN_2O_4=202.6$.

CAS — 97-00-7.

Yellow crystals. M.p. 50° to 52°. Practically **insoluble** in water; slightly soluble in alcohol; soluble in ether and carbon disulphide.

Solubilisation. An aqueous solution of 2,4-dinitrochlorobenzene could be prepared by solubilisation with dimethyl sulphoxide.— G. Scherbel and G. Weidemann, *Arzneimittel-Forsch.*, 1975, *25*, 678.

Adverse Effects. Skin contact with 2,4-dinitrochlorobenzene usually produces hypersensitivity which becomes evident on subsequent exposure.

Four workers developed contact dermatitis following exposure to 2,4-dinitrochlorobenzene which had been used as an algicide in cooling water.— R. M. Adams *et al., Archs Derm.*, 1971, *103*, 183, per *J. Am. med. Ass.*, 1971, *215*, 1342.

Not only was 2,4-dinitrochlorobenzene a potent sensitiser but it had been shown to cross-react with chloramphenicol.— R. J. Pye and J. L. Burton (letter), *Br. med. J.*, 1976, *2*, 1130. Further comment on the hazards of sensitisation, especially in laboratory workers.— T. Green *et al.* (letter), *Chem. in Br.*, 1977, *13*, 163.

Uses. 2,4-Dinitrochlorobenzene is a potent sensitiser and the modification or absence of a hypersensitivity response to the topical application of 2,4-dinitrochlorobenzene has been used diagnostically in certain diseases. It has also been used as an immunostimulant in leprosy and some forms of cancer and in the treatment of alopecia and warts.

A discussion on the use of immunotherapy with 2,4-dinitrochlorobenzene.— E. C. Holmes *et al., J. Am. med. Ass.*, 1975, *232*, 1052.

Sensitivity to 2,4-dinitrochlorobenzene could be used to monitor changes in cell-mediated immunity in patients during immunosuppression.— D. N. H. Hamilton *et al., Lancet*, 1976, *2*, 1170.

From studies with 46 Caucasian subjects it was concluded that histological differentiation between an allergic and a toxic reaction to 2,4-dinitrochlorobenzene was not possible and to avoid incorrect interpretations challenge patch tests should be made with doses within the range 3 to 10 μg per cm^2.— A. Hartman *et al., Br. J. Derm.*, 1976, *94*, 407.

A technique for measuring 2,4-dinitrochlorobenzene skin sensitivity.— H. F. Pabst and R. C. Urtasun (letter), *Lancet*, 1977, *1*, 433.

For earlier references to the diagnostic and investigative use of 2,4-dinitrochlorobenzene and its use in the treatment of cancer, see Martindale 27th Edn, p. 1751.

Alopecia. The mild contact dermatitis arising from application of a solution of 2,4-dinitrochlorobenzene in acetone was assessed in the treatment of alopecia areata. Sensitisation was induced by a 2% solution in 43 patients then a 0.1% solution was applied weekly to half the head until a skin reaction was obtained when the concentration was further adjusted; 33 patients showed a significant difference in hair growth between the treated and the untreated sides.— R. Happle and K. Echternacht, *Lancet*, 1977, *2*, 1002.

Acquired tolerance to 2,4-dinitrochlorobenzene being used for the treatment of alopecia was reversed by 2 days' treatment with cimetidine 300 mg four times daily.— L. A. Daman and E. W. Rosenberg (letter), *Lancet*, 1977, *2*, 1087. Of 30 patients being treated with 2,4-dinitrochlorobenzene for alopecia, 15 acquired tolerance and were treated with cimetidine 400 mg to 1 g daily. In 7 of the 15 patients hypersensitivity was restored within the first week; cimetidine was ineffective in 4 patients and was stopped after 2 weeks, and in 5 treatment was stopped after 1 to 3 weeks owing to adverse effects.— F. Breuillard and E. Szapiro (letter), *ibid.*, 1978, *1*, 726.

All of 8 patients with long-standing alopecia totalis or very extensive alopecia areata became sensitised to 2,4-dinitrochlorobenzene but none had a cosmetically acceptable regrowth of hair and all continue to wear a wig. Moreover, a marked eczematous reaction is necessary to achieve even moderate regrowth, with itching and even weeping of the scalp for 24 to 48 hours after each treatment. 2,4-Dinitrochlorobenzene does not appear from this study to be a useful therapy for alopecia areata, although it may have a role in alopecia areata of very short duration, to accelerate the growth that usually occurs without treatment.— A. P. Warin (letter), *Lancet*, 1979, *1*, 927. See also P. S. Friedmann (letter), *ibid.*, 1412.

Further reports and comments on 2,4-dinitrochlorobenzene in the treatment of alopecia: F. Breuillard and E. Szapiro (letter), *Lancet*, 1978, *2*, 1304; L. A. Daman *et al., Archs Derm.*, 1978, *114*, 1036; *Br. med. J.*, 1979, *1*, 505; I. Ralfs (letter), *ibid.*, 820; C. I. Harrington (letter), *ibid.*, 1017; P. S. Friedmann, *Br. J. Derm.*, 1981, *105*, 285.

Leprosy. Reduced reactivity to 2,4-dinitrochlorobenzene in leprosy patients and controls in Kenya.— A. Hartman, *Lepr. Rev.*, 1976, *47*, 193.

References to the use of 2,4-dinitrochlorobenzene as an immunostimulant in leprosy: Le Kinh Due, *Bull. int. Un. Tuberc.*, 1979, *54*, 366; T. H. Rea and N. E. Levan, *Int. J. Lepr.*, 1980, *48*, 120.

Warts. A discussion of immunotherapy with 2,4-dinitrochlorobenzene, from an uncontrolled study completed by 35 patients with recalcitrant warts. Patients were sensitised by epicutaneous application of 0.15 ml of a 2% solution of 2,4-dinitrochlorobenzene in acetone to the upper arm and after patch testing for sensitivity they were treated with daily or twice daily applications of 2,4-dinitrochlorobenzene in acetone in concentrations ranging from 0.05 to 1%, the usual concentration being 0.1%. A moderate degree of localised pruritus, oedema, and erythema was regarded as a normal reaction. Localised contact dermatitis occurred in 7 patients and widespread contact dermatitis or autosensitisation in 3; these patients required treatment with systemic corticosteroids. The study indicated that treatment with 2,4-dinitrochlorobenzene may result in the resolution of 66% of recalcitrant warts.— D. Buckner and N. M. Price, *Br. J. Derm.*, 1978, *98*, 451. See also D. L. J. Freed and K. E. Eyres, *Br. J. Derm.*, 1979, *100*, 731.

Reports of beneficial results with 2,4-dinitrochlorobenzene in the treatment of warts: M. Goihman-Yahr *et al.* (letter), *Lancet*, 1978, *1*, 447; P. S. Bekhor *et al.*, *Aust. J. Derm.*, 1978, *19*, 28; B. B. Sanders and K. W. Smith, *Cutis*, 1981, *27*, 389.

12667-x

Diosmine. 5-Hydroxy-2-(3-hydroxy-4-methoxyphenyl)-7-rutinosyloxy-4*H*-chromen-4-one.
$C_{28}H_{32}O_{15}$=608.6.

CAS — 520-27-4.

An odourless yellow powder. M.p. about 281°. Practically **insoluble** in water and most organic solvents.

Diosmine is a bioflavonoid isolated from citrus fruits or prepared synthetically. It has been used similarly to rutin (see p.1752) in the treatment of venous disorders.

Excellent or good results were achieved in 36 of 43 patients with vascular disorders, menorrhagia, or metrorrhagia associated with the use of oral contraceptives or intra-uterine contraceptive devices, when given diosmine 300 mg twice daily for 1 to 2 months.— M. Monrozies and D. Rodriguez, *Revue fr. Gynéc. Obstét.*, 1976, *71*, 301.

Proprietary Names
Daflon *(Servier, Fr.; Servier, Ital.; Servier, Switz.)*; Diovenor *(Innothéra, Fr.)*; Flebotropin *(Bagó, Arg.)*; Ven-Detrex *(Hommel, Switz.)*; Venosmine *(Geymonat Sud, Ital.)*.

12668-r

Dipenine Bromide. Diponium Bromide; HL-267; Sa-267. 2-(Dicyclopentylacetoxy)ethyltriethylammonium bromide.
$C_{20}H_{38}BrNO_2$=404.4.

CAS — 2001-81-2.

Dipenine bromide is an antispasmodic agent. It has been tried with indifferent results in the treatment of renal colic.

Proprietary Names
Unospaston *(Wolfs, Belg.)*.

12669-f

Diphenhydramine Di(acefyllinate). Bietanautine. Diphenhydramine bis(theophyllin-7-ylacetate).
$C_{17}H_{21}NO,2C_9H_{10}N_4O_4$=731.8.

CAS — 6888-11-5.

NOTE. The name Etanautine was formerly applied to diphenhydramine monoacefyllinate; it is now applied to ethylbenzhydramine, see p.1707.

Diphenhydramine di(acefyllinate) has been used as an anti-emetic.

Proprietary Names
Nautamine *(Delagrange, Fr.)*.

12670-z

Dipivefrin. Dipivefrine; Dipivalyl Adrenaline; Dipivalyl Epinephrine; DPE. (±)-4-(1-Hydroxy-2-methylaminoethyl)-1,2-phenylene dipivalate.
$C_{19}H_{29}NO_5$=351.4.

CAS — 52365-63-6.

Dipivefrin is an ester and prodrug of adrenaline. A 0.1% solution applied to the eye in the treatment of glaucoma is reported to be as effective as 2% adrenaline.

References: M. E. Yablonski *et al.*, *Archs Ophthal., N.Y.*, 1977, *95*, 2157; M. A. Kass *et al.*, *ibid.*, 1979, *97*, 1865; A. N. Kohn *et al.*, *Am. J. Ophthal.*, 1979, *87*, 196; J. Theodore and H. M. Leibowitz, *ibid.*, *88*, 1013; J. A. Anderson, *Archs Ophthal., N.Y.*, 1980, *98*, 350.

Proprietary Names
Glaucothil (hydrochloride) *(Thilo, Ger.)*.

12671-c

Disobutamide. SC-31828. 2-(2-Chlorophenyl)-2-[2-(di-isopropylamino)ethyl]-4-piperidinobutyramide.
$C_{23}H_{38}ClN_3O$=408.0.

CAS — 68284-69-5.

Disobutamide is reported to have anti-arrhythmic properties.

Manufacturers
Searle, USA.

12672-k

Disodium Aminohydroxypropylidenediphosphonate. APD; Aminohydroxypropylidenebisphosphonate Disodium. Disodium 3-amino-1-hydroxy-propylidenediphosphonate.
$C_3H_9NNa_2O_7P_2$=279.0.

CAS — 40391-99-9 (aminohydroxypropylidenediphosphonic acid); 57248-88-1 (disodium salt).

Disodium aminohydroxypropylidenediphosphonate has been used similarly to disodium etidronate (p.1704) in the treatment of osteitis deformans (Paget's disease of bone). Unlike disodium etidronate it is claimed selectively to inhibit osteoclast activity and bone resorption without disturbing mineralisation.

Disodium aminohydroxypropylidenediphosphonate, shown by *animal* studies to reduce bone turnover at a dose 500 times less than that which causes osteomalacia, was given in gelatin capsules thrice daily half-an-hour before meals to 18 patients with moderately severe Paget's disease. Five patients received 30 µmol per kg body-weight daily for 10 days subsequently reduced to 15 µmol per kg, and 9 received the initial dose for 30 days, subsequently similarly reduced; one received an initial dose of 60 µmol per kg for 20 days, and 3 started with 15 µmol per kg. In most patients remission was achieved within 4 months and with a maintenance dose of 15 µmol per kg body-weight daily. Bone resorption generally became normal within a few days but return to normal bone formation required a few months, this difference creating a positive calcium balance associated with transient secondary hyperparathyroidism. No fractures or recrudescence of pain similar to that encountered with disodium etidronate occurred.— W. B. Frijlink *et al.*, *Lancet*, 1979, *1*, 799. Similar encouraging preliminary results in 14 patients with osteolytic bone disease due to breast cancer or myeloma. The drug was well tolerated in most respects: some patients had slight gastric discomfort; a transient rise of body temperature of 1 or 2° never lasted more than 72 hours.— F. J. M. van Breukelen *et al.*, *ibid.*, 803.

A report of beneficial results in Paget's disease with aminohydroxypropylidenediphosphonate (APD). All but 4 of 67 patients given APD 250 to 500 mg daily obtained complete biochemical remission with histological improvement within 6 months; 4 slow responders are still improving. Treatment, always continued until 6 months after the beginning of biochemical remission, has been stopped in 49. Of these, 28 have stayed in remission for up to 12 months, 8 for up to 24 months, and 2 for up to 30 months. The 11 patients with recurrences were completely sensitive to retreatment. Clinical and histological improvement was evident, and radiology of long bones gave evidence of improvement, consisting of disappearance of osteolytic lesions and return towards normal cortical architecture of long bones.— O. L. M. Bijvoet *et al.* (letter), *Lancet*, 1980, *1*, 1416.

Manufacturers
Henkel, Ger.

12673-a

Disodium Clodronate. Clodronate Disodium; Clodronate Sodium; Dichloromethane Diphosphonate Disodium; Dichloromethylene Diphosphonate Disodium; Sodium Clodronate; Cl_2MDP. Disodium (dichloromethylene)diphosphonate.
$CH_2Cl_2Na_2O_6P_2$=288.9.

CAS — 10596-23-3 (clodronic acid).

Disodium clodronate is a diphosphonate with properties similar to those of disodium etidronate (p.1704) but is reported to be more effective in decreasing bone resorption while having less effect on mineralisation. It has been used in the treatment of osteitis deformans (Paget's disease of bone) and in hypercalcaemia.

Ten patients with Paget's disease of bone received disodium clodronate 1.6 g daily and 9 received 400 mg daily, both doses being given for 6 months. Clinical improvement occurred with both doses and was striking with the higher dose. The higher dose significantly reduced urine hydroxyproline, serum alkaline phosphatase, urine calcium, and the number of pagetic bone osteoclasts. Unlike disodium etidronate which induces bone demineralisation at doses above 5 mg per kg body-weight daily, no mineralisation defect was induced. A transient increase occurred in serum concentrations of parathyroid hormone in 13 of the 19 patients during treatment.— P. J. Meunier *et al.*, *Lancet*, 1979, *2*, 489.

Administration of disodium clodronate 1.6 g daily, usually in a single dose half-an-hour before breakfast, had a beneficial effect in 13 patients with Paget's disease of bone. Pain, which was the main symptom in 9 of the 13 patients, was reduced in all but one, and in all patients the biochemical values returned to normal or near-normal within 3 to 7 months. Beneficial effects were also obtained in 17 patients with hypercalcaemia due to primary hyperparathyroidism or secondary to malignant disease given doses ranging from 0.8 to 3.2 g daily.— D. L. Douglas *et al.*, *Lancet*, 1980, *1*, 1043.

Results of a double-blind crossover study indicate that disodium clodronate may be a useful inhibitor of the skeletal mobilisation of calcium in multiple myeloma. Patients with multiple myeloma and hypercalcaemia or sustained hypercalciuria took clodronate 1.6 g twice daily for 8 weeks and placebo for 8 weeks. Five of 10 patients completed the study and 4 of them showed evidence of an effect within 7 days of starting treatment with clodronate; they had sustained and highly significant decreases in urinary excretion of calcium compared with the pre-study or placebo periods. The fifth patient had recurrent hypercalciuria and hypercalcaemia while receiving clodronate. The remaining 5 patients died before completion of the study. Clodronate was well tolerated apart from transient mild diarrhoea in most of the patients.— E. S. Siris *et al.*, *New Engl. J. Med.*, 1980, *302*, 310. Comment.— L. G. Raisz, *ibid.*, 347.

Further references: K. A. Conrad and S. M. Lee, *Clin. Pharmac. Ther.*, 1981, *30*, 114 (pharmacokinetics); T. P. Jacobs *et al.*, *Ann. intern. Med.*, 1981, *94*, 312 (hypercalcaemia of malignancy); E. Shane *et al.*, *ibid.*, *95*, 23 (hyperparathyroidism).

Manufacturers
Procter & Gamble, USA.

12674-t

Disodium Etidronate. Etidronate Disodium; EHDP; Na_2EHDP. Disodium 1-hydroxyethylidenediphosphonate.
$C_2H_6Na_2O_7P_2$=250.0.

CAS — 2809-21-4 (etidronic acid); 7414-83-7 (disodium salt).

The name sodium etidronate is used for a variable mixture of sodium salts which may be monosodium, trisodium, or tetrasodium.

A white powder. Very **soluble** in water.

Adverse Effects. Nausea and diarrhoea have been reported. With high doses of disodium etidronate impaired mineralisation of bone has been associated with increased bone pain, osteomalacia, and fractures. Hyperphosphataemia may occur.

Disodium etidronate should be given with great care to patients with impaired renal function.

A report of gastric ulceration associated with the use of disodium etidronate.— R. L. Saunders, *Sth. med. J.*, 1977, *70*, 1327.

Absorption and Fate. From 1 to 6% of a dose of disodium etidronate is absorbed from the gastro-intestinal tract. It is not metabolised. The majority of absorbed drug disappears from the blood within 6 hours. About 50% is excreted in the urine within 24 hours, the remainder being chemically adsorbed on bone and slowly eliminated. Unabsorbed disodium etidronate is excreted in the faeces.

In 4 adults given disodium etidronate 5 mg per kg body-weight, mean absorption varied from 1.49 to 3.35% (depending upon assessment) and 1.8% of the dose was recovered in the urine in 24 hours. In 5 adults given 30 mg per kg, mean absorption varied from 3.99 to 10.2% and 3.1% was recovered in the urine in 48 hours.— R. R. Recker and P. D. Saville, *Toxic. appl. Pharmac.*, 1973, *24*, 580.

Uses. Disodium etidronate is a diphosphonate which inhibits the growth and dissolution of hydroxyapatite crystals in bone and may also directly impair osteoclast activity. It diminishes bone resorption and bone formation.

Disodium etidronate is used in the treatment of osteitis deformans (Paget's disease of bone). It reduces accelerated bone turnover and decreases elevated serum concentrations of alkaline phosphatase and urinary excretion of hydroxyproline. Bone pain is generally relieved but has occasionally been exacerbated, especially with high doses. It has also been tried in other disorders of calcium metabolism including ectopic calcification, renal calculi, hypercalcaemia, and osteoporosis. Radioactively labelled etidronate has been used as a bone scanning agent.

In the treatment of osteitis deformans, disodium etidronate is given by mouth in doses of 5 to 20 mg per kg body-weight daily. The usual dose is 5 mg per kg daily for not more than 6 months. Retreatment should only be given after a drug-free interval of at least 3 months, after evidence of relapse, and should not be continued for more than 6 months. Doses above 10 mg per kg daily should not be given for more than 3 months. Disodium etidronate is usually administered as a single dose 2 hours before a meal and food should be avoided for 2 hours before and after the meal, especially milk and other products with a high calcium content.

The diphosphonates disodium clodronate (p.1704) and disodium aminohydroxypropylidenediphosphonate (p.1704) have also been used in the treatment of osteitis deformans and hypercalcaemia. Other diphosphonates include disodium medronate (disodium methylene diphosphonate; MDP; $CH_4Na_2O_6P_2$=220.0) and oxidronic acid ($CH_6O_7P_2$=192.0).

Reviews of diphosphonates.— R. G. G. Russell, *Br. J. Hosp. Med.*, 1975, *14*, 297; *Lancet*, 1981, *2*, 1326.

Comment on the use of newer diphosphonates to block bone resorption.— L. G. Raisz, *New Engl. J. Med.*, 1980, *302*, 347.

Ectopic calcification. A 6-year-old boy with progressive fibrodysplasia ossificans was given disodium etidronate 100 mg twice daily increased to thrice daily after 4 weeks. Nail growth which had ceased started again. Swellings on the head, neck, and back, which at first continued to grow, regressed without leaving indurations. At follow-up 9 months later no further calcifications and ossifications were observed.— K. von Schnakenburg *et al.*, *Dt. med. Wschr.*, 1972, *97*, 1873, per *Int. pharm. Abstr.*, 1973, *10*, 410. Lack of benefit.— J. G. Hall *et al.*, *J. Pediat.*, 1979, *94*, 679.

Disodium etidronate was not effective in the management of calcification in a study of 6 patients with dermatomyositis or scleroderma.— A. L. Metzger *et al.*, *New Engl. J. Med.*, 1974, *291*, 1294.

Disodium etidronate 10 mg per kg body-weight per day (raised to 20 mg per kg in 1 case) was given to 3 children with diseases involving ectopic calcification. Therapy had continued for at least 2 years and calcium balance was reduced in all 3 children due to increased faecal excretion. Clinical improvement, with a marked decrease in calcification and general improvement in mobility, occurred in only 1 child.— W. S. Uttley *et al.*, *Archs Dis. Childh.*, 1975, *50*, 187.

Further references: R. G. G. Russell *et al.*, *Lancet*, 1972, *1*, 10.

Hypercalcaemia. Six patients with primary hyperparathyroidism and 1 patient with hyperparathyroidism secondary to carcinoma of the oesophagus were given disodium etidronate 20 mg per kg body-weight daily. Initially all patients were hypercalcaemic; after 5 weeks' treatment 2 patients had a small decrease in serum-calcium concentration, and there was no significant decrease in the others. There was a significant decrease in urinary calcium excretion in 4 patients, and a smaller decrease in the other 3. These decreases were not maintained during 6 months of treatment. Serum phosphorus increased in all patients after 5 weeks' treatment, and was maintained for 6 months in 4 patients. The results suggest that disodium etidronate decreases bone resorption, but the consistent increase in serum phosphorus in the presence of elevated calcium concentrations might predispose to soft-tissue calcification.— R. A. Kaplan *et al.*, *J. clin. Pharmac.*, 1977, *17*, 410.

While receiving disodium etidronate 600 mg daily, serum concentrations of calcium returned to normal in a patient with breast cancer who had extensive bone metastases, intractable excruciating bone pain, and hypercalcaemia.— J. I. Zweig and N. Shafer (letter), *J. Am. med. Ass.*, 1980, *244*, 437.

Osteitis deformans. Reviews and comments on osteitis deformans and its treatment with diphosphonates.— R. Smith, *Br. med. J.*, 1977, *1*, 365; *Med. Lett.*, 1978, *20*, 78; *Lancet*, 1978, *1*, 914; H. K. Ibbertson *et al.*, *Drugs*, 1979, *18*, 33; R. G. G. Russell, *Clins rheum. Dis.*, 1979, *5*, 673; E. S. Siris *et al.*, *Bull. N.Y. Acad. Med.*, 1980, *56*, 285; D. J. Hosking, *Br. med. J.*, 1981, *283*, 686.

Three of 5 patients with Paget's disease of bone and deafness had improved hearing after treatment for 180 days with disodium etidronate 1.2 g daily.— C. Gennari and I. Sensini (letter), *Br. med. J.*, 1975, *1*, 331.

In 9 patients with Paget's disease concomitant treatment with disodium etidronate 7.5 mg per kg body-weight daily and synthetic human calcitonin 500 µg daily subcutaneously resulted in normal values for serum alkaline phosphatase and urinary hydroxyproline excretion in 6 to 12 months without the complications associated with conventional doses of either agent used alone.— D. J. Hosking *et al.*, *Lancet*, 1976, *1*, 615. In a report of 30 patients with Paget's disease treated with disodium etidronate 7.5 mg per kg body-weight daily and calcitonin, 25 were in complete biochemical remission after 6 to 12 months. Seven had a recurrence within 3 months of withdrawal and 7 between 3 and 50 months; recurrences were normally sensitive to disodium aminohydroxypropylidenediphosphonate. Maintained remission has been observed in 11 patients for up to 5 years.— O. L. M. Bijvoet *et al.* (letter), *Lancet*, 1980, *1*, 1416.

Of 109 patients with Paget's disease of bone, 67 showed clinical improvement after taking disodium etidronate 5, 10, or 20 mg per kg body-weight daily for periods between 6 and 24 months. Maximum clinical improvement occurred after 6 months' therapy, there being no significant further improvement when treatment was longer and no significant difference between the improvement produced by 5, 10, or 20 mg per kg. Side-effects, which generally occurred in those patients taking 10 or 20 mg per kg, included diarrhoea in 12, pseudomembranous colitis in 1, increasing bone pain in 13, and bone fractures in 18. There was also mineralisation delay in those patients receiving 10 or 20 mg per kg but not in those receiving 5 mg per kg. Forty-two patients who received a second course of treatment responded as well as they did to the first course. It was recommended that intermittent courses of disodium etidronate were preferable to continuous therapy and a dose of 5 mg per kg would have the best therapeutic ratio.— M. R. A. Khairi *et al.*, *Ann. intern. Med.*, 1977, *87*, 656.

Comment on the role of disodium etidronate as the only practical alternative to calcitonin in the treatment of Paget's disease of bone.— C. N. de Deuxchaisnes *et al.* (letter), *Lancet*, 1980, *1*, 374. A reminder of the merits of mithramycin.— A. S. Russell (letter), *ibid.*, 884.

Osteoporosis. Disodium etidronate 20 mg per kg body-weight daily administered to 5 osteoporotic patients for 6 months and to 5 for 12 months produced a small positive balance shift in bone calcium although the effect was too small to be of much potential therapeutic benefit in osteoporosis. No chemical, or haematological, or urinary changes were associated with the therapy apart from a clear rise in serum-phosphorus concentrations in 9 of 10 patients and a small significant increase in serum-calcium concentrations in most patients.— R. P. Heaney and P. D. Saville, *Clin. Pharmac. Ther.*, 1976, *20*, 593.

Proprietary Preparations

Didronel Tablets *(Brocades, UK)*. Each contains disodium etidronate 200 mg. (Also available as Didronel in *Canad.*, *USA*).

Other Proprietary Names

Calcimux *(Arg.)*; Etidron *(Ital.)*.

12675-x

Disodium Guanylate.

Sodium 5′-Guanylate; Disodium Guanosine-5′-monophosphate. Guanosine 5′-(disodium phosphate).

$C_{10}H_{12}N_5Na_2O_8P,xH_2O$=407.2.

CAS — 5550-12-9 (anhydrous).

Colourless or white crystals or a white crystalline powder with a characteristic taste. It loses not more than 25% of its weight on drying. **Soluble** in water; sparingly soluble in alcohol; practically insoluble in ether. A 5% solution in water has a pH of 7 to 8.5.

Disodium guanylate is a flavour enhancer.

12676-r

Disodium Inosinate.

Sodium 5′-Inosinate; Disodium Inosine-5′-monophosphate. Inosine 5′-(disodium phosphate).

$C_{10}H_{11}N_4Na_2O_8P,xH_2O$=392.2.

CAS — 4691-65-0 (anhydrous).

Colourless or white crystals or a white crystalline powder with a characteristic taste. It contains not more than 28.5% of water. **Soluble** in water; sparingly soluble in alcohol; practically insoluble in ether. A 5% solution in water has a pH of 7 to 8.5.

Disodium inosinate is a flavour enhancer.

12677-f

Disoprofol.

ICI-35868. 2,6-Di-isopropylphenol.

$C_{12}H_{18}O$=178.3.

CAS — 2078-54-8.

Disoprofol is an intravenous anaesthetic agent.

Studies in *animals* J. W. Dundee, *Br. J. Anaesth.*, 1979, *51*, 641; J. B. Glen, *ibid.*, 1980, *52*, 230P; *idem*, 731; H. K. Adam *et al.*, *ibid.*, 743.

Clinical studies.— K. M. Rogers, *Br. J. Anaesth.*, 1980, *52*, 230P; K. M. Rogers *et al.*, *ibid.*, 807; B. Kay and D. K. Stephenson, *Anaesthesia*, 1980, *35*, 1182; D. V. Rutter *et al.*, *ibid.*, 1188; E. Major *et al.*, *Br. J. Anaesth.*, 1981, *53*, 267.

Manufacturers

ICI Pharmaceuticals, UK.

12678-d

Domiodol.

MG-13608. 2-Iodomethyl-1,3-dioxolan-4-ylmethanol.

$C_5H_9IO_3$=244.0.

CAS — 61869-07-6.

Domiodol has been used for the relief of respiratory disorders.

Proprietary Names

Mucolitico *(Maggioni, Ital.)*.

12679-n

Doxpicomine Hydrochloride.

Doxpicodin Hydrochloride; LY-108380. (−)-α-1,3-Dioxan-5-yl-*NN*-dimethyl-3-pyridylmethylamine hydrochloride.

$C_{12}H_{18}N_2O_2,HCl$=258.7.

CAS — 62904-71-6 (doxpicomine); 69494-04-8 (hydrochloride).

Doxpicomine hydrochloride is a potent analgesic which has been given by injection in doses of up to 400 mg.

References: M. S. Mok *et al.*, *Clin. Pharmac. Ther.*, 1981, *29*, 266 (comparison with pethidine); R. I. H. Wang and N. Robinson, *ibid.*, 771 (comparison with morphine).

Manufacturers

Lilly, USA.

12680-k

Dropropizine. UCB-1967. 3-(4-Phenylpiperazin-1-yl)propane-1,2-diol.
$C_{13}H_{20}N_2O_2$=236.3.

CAS — 17692-31-8.

Dropropizine has been used for the relief of cough.

Proprietary Names
Catabex *(Sarva, Belg.)*; Ribex *(Formenti, Ital.)*.

12681-a

Drosera. Sundew; Droserae Herba; Herba Rorellae; Rorela; Ros Solis.

Pharmacopoeias. In *Belg.* and *Span.*

The air-dried entire plant *Drosera rotundifolia* (Droseraceae).

Drosera has been used for its reputed value in chronic bronchitis, asthma, and whooping cough, usually as a tincture or liquid extract, but is of doubtful value.
It is used in homoeopathic medicine.

12682-t

Drotaverine. 1-(3,4-Diethoxybenzylidene)-6,7-diethoxy-1,2,3,4-tetrahydroisoquinoline.
$C_{24}H_{31}NO_4$=397.5.

CAS — 14009-24-6.

Drotaverine has been used for its spasmolytic properties.

Proprietary Names
Deprolen *(Lostaló, Arg.)*; No-Spa *(Chinoin, Hung.)*; Nospasin *(Phoenix, Arg.)*.

12683-x

Duazomycin. Duazomycin A; NSC-51097. L-2-Acetamido-6-diazo-5-oxohexanoic acid.
$C_8H_{11}N_3O_4$=213.2.

CAS — 1403-47-0.

A pale yellow powder.

Duazomycin is an antibiotic with antineoplastic activity isolated from cultures of *Streptomyces ambofaciens*.

References: J. Colsky *et al.*, *Clin. Pharmac. Ther.*, 1966, *7*, 352; H. T. Foley *et al.*, *J. new Drugs*, 1966, *6*, 105.

12684-r

Dulcamara *(B.P.C. 1934)*. Bittersweet; Woody Nightshade; Dulcamarae Caulis; Douce-Amère.

The dried stems and branches of *Solanum dulcamara* (Solanaceae).

Dulcamara was formerly a popular remedy for chronic rheumatism and skin eruptions and was administered as an infusion.
All parts of the plant are poisonous due to the presence of solanine ($C_{45}H_{73}NO_{15}$=868.1) and its allied alkaloids. The berries have caused poisoning in children. Adverse effects are treated as described under Atropine, p.290.

It was recommended that dulcamara be prohibited for use in foods as a flavouring agent.— *Food Standards Committee Report on Flavouring Agents*, London, HM Stationery Office, 1965.

12685-f

Eicosapentaenoic Acid. Eicosa-5,8,11,14,17-pentaenoic acid.
$C_{20}H_{30}O_2$=302.5.

CAS — 25378-27-2.

Eicosapentaenoic acid is a precursor of some prostaglandins (see p.1353).
Because some populations with a diet rich in eicosapentaenoic acid have a low incidence of myocardial infarction it has been suggested that supplementing the diet by foods with a high content of eicosapentaenoic acid (such as mackerel or fish-liver oils) might reduce the incidence of myocardial infarction.

References: J. Dyerberg *et al.*, *Lancet*, 1978, *2*, 117; J. Dyerberg and H. O. Bang, *ibid.*, 1979, *2*, 433; S. A. Reed (letter), *ibid.*, 739; T. G. Taylor *et al.* (letter), *ibid.*, 1378; C. M. van Gent *et al.* (letter), *ibid.*, 1249; *idem*, 1980, *1*, 108; W. Siess *et al.*, *ibid.*, 441; *ibid.*, 464; T. A. B. Sanders *et al.* (letter), *ibid.*, 1189; A. Hirai *et al.* (letter), *ibid.*, *2*, 1132; E. J. Goetzl, *New Engl. J. Med.*, 1980, *303*, 822; S. Kobayashi *et al.* (letter), *Lancet*, 1981, *2*, 197; M. Thorngren and A. Gustafson, *ibid.*, 1190.

12686-d

Elantrine. EX-10-029. 3-(5,6-Dihydro-5-methyldibenz[*b,e*]azepin-11-ylidene)-*NN*-dimethylpropylamine.
$C_{20}H_{24}N_2$=292.4.

CAS — 1232-85-5.

Elantrine is structurally related to the tricyclic antidepressants (see p.110) and has been used similarly to benzhexol (see p.295) in the treatment of drug-induced extrapyramidal symptoms. The dicyclamate salt has been tried.

References: H. Freeman and I. S. Mehta, *Curr. ther. Res.*, 1972, *14*, 470; E. R. Blonsky *et al.*, *Clin. Pharmac. Ther.*, 1974, *15*, 46.

Manufacturers
Merrell-National, USA.

12687-n

Embutramide. *N*-(*β*,*β*-Diethyl-*m*-methoxyphenethyl)-4-hydroxybutyramide.
$C_{17}H_{27}NO_3$=293.4.

CAS — 15687-14-6.

Embutramide is a narcotic analgesic.

12969-e

Enalapril. MK-421. *N*-(1-Ethoxycarbonyl-3-phenylpropyl)-L-alanyl-L-proline hydrogen maleate.
$C_{20}H_{28}N_2O_5,C_4H_4O_4$=492.5.

Enalapril maleate is an angiotensin-converting-enzyme inhibitor, under study as an antihypertensive agent.

References: A. A. Patchett *et al.*, *Nature*, 1980, *288*, 280; D. B. Brunner *et al.*, *Br. J. clin. Pharmac.*, 1981, *11*, 461; J. Biollaz *et al.*, *Clin. Pharmac. Ther.*, 1981, *29*, 665; H. Gavras *et al.*, *Lancet*, 1981, *2*, 543; G. A. MacGregor *et al.*, *Br. med. J.*, 1981, *283*, 401.

Manufacturers
Merck Sharp & Dohme, UK.

12688-h

Endralazine. BQ-22-708. 6-Benzoyl-5,6,7,8-tetrahydropyrido[4,3-*c*]pyridazin-3-ylhydrazine.
$C_{14}H_{15}N_5O$=269.3.

CAS — 39715-02-1 (endralazine); 65322-72-7 (mesylate).

Endralazine is reported to be a vasodilator and has been tried in the treatment of hypertension.

References: H. -U. Lehmann *et al.*, *Med. Klin.*, 1977, *72*, 1203.

Manufacturers
Sandoz, UK.

12689-m

Endrysone. Endrisone. 11*β*-Hydroxy-6*α*-methylpregna-1,4-diene-3,20-dione.
$C_{22}H_{30}O_3$=342.5.

CAS — 35100-44-8.

Endrysone is a corticosteroid for topical use.

Proprietary Names
Aldrisone *(SIFI, Ital.)*.

12690-t

Enilconazole. R-23979. (±)-1-(*β*-Allyloxy-2,4-dichlorophenethyl)imidazole.
$C_{14}H_{14}Cl_2N_2O$=297.2.

CAS — 35554-44-0.

Enilconazole is reported to have antifungal activity.

Manufacturers
Janssen, Belg.

12691-x

Enviomycin. Tuberactinomycin N. Stereoisomer of 9,12-bis(hydroxymethyl)-15-(3,6-diamino-4-hydroxyhexanamido)-3-(hexahydro-2-iminopyrimidin-4-yl)-2,5,8,11,14-pentaoxo-1,4,7,10,13-pentaazacyclohexadec-6-ylidenemethylurea.
$C_{25}H_{43}N_{13}O_{10}$=685.7.

CAS — 33103-22-9.

An antibiotic produced by *Streptomyces griseoverticillatus* var. *tuberacticus*.

Enviomycin is an antibiotic which has been used, as the sulphate, in the treatment of pulmonary tuberculosis.

Proprietary Names
Tuberactin (sulphate) *(Jap.)*.

12692-r

Enviroxime. LY-122772. (*E*)-2-Amino-6-benzoyl-1-(isopropylsulphonyl)-1*H*-benzimidazole oxime.
$C_{17}H_{18}N_4O_3S$=358.4.

CAS — 72301-79-2.

Enviroxime has antiviral activity against rhinoviruses.

References: R. J. Phillpotts *et al.*, *Lancet*, 1981, *1*, 1342.

Manufacturers
Lilly, UK.

12693-f

Epimestrol. NSC-55975; Org-817. 3-Methoxyestra-1,3,5(10)-triene-16*α*,17*α*-diol.
$C_{19}H_{26}O_3$=302.4.

CAS — 7004-98-0.

Epimestrol is an oestrogen which has been used in the treatment of infertility and amenorrhoea and other disturbances of the menstrual cycle.

Proprietary Names
Stimovul *(Organon, Ger.; Ravasini, Ital.; Organon, Neth.)*.

12694-d

Epitiostanol. 10275-S. 2*α*,3*α*-Epithio-5*α*-androstan-17*β*-ol.
$C_{19}H_{30}OS$=306.5.

CAS — 2363-58-8.

Epitiostanol is reported to have anabolic activity. It has been used in various breast disorders including neoplasms of the breast.

Proprietary Names
Thiodrol *(Jap.)*.

12695-n

Epomediol. 1,8-Epoxy-4-isopropyl-1-methylcylcohexane-2,6-diol.
$C_{10}H_{18}O_3$=186.3.

Epomediol is used in the treatment of hepatic disorders.

Proprietary Names
Clesidren *(Corvi, Ital.)*.

12696-h

Eprazinone Hydrochloride. CG-B6K (eprazinone); CE-746 (eprazinone). 3-[4-(β-Ethoxyphenethyl)piperazin-1-yl]-2-methylpropiophenone dihydrochloride.
$C_{24}H_{32}N_2O_2,2HCl=453.5$.

CAS — 10402-90-1 (eprazinone); 10402-53-6 (hydrochloride).

Eprazinone hydrochloride is an antitussive and expectorant and has been used in the treatment of respiratory disorders.

Proprietary Names
Eftapan *(Merckle, Ger.)*; Mucitux *(Sanders-Probel, Belg.; Riom, Fr.; Liade, Spain)*; Resplene *(Chugai, Jap.)*.

12697-m

Eprozinol Hydrochloride. 3-[4-(β-Methoxyphenethyl)piperazin-1-yl]-1-phenylpropan-1-ol dihydrochloride.
$C_{22}H_{30}N_2O_2,2HCl=427.4$.

CAS — 32665-36-4 (eprozinol).

A white crystalline powder. **Soluble** in water, alcohol, and chloroform.

Eprozinol hydrochloride inhibits bronchoconstriction and has been used in the treatment of asthmatic and bronchitic disorders. It also has a sedative action.

Proprietary Names
Alecor *(Andromaco, Arg.)*; Brovel *(Lepetit, Ital.)*; Eupnéron *(Lyocentre, Fr.)*.

12698-b

Eptazocine. ST-2121. (−)-(1*S*,6*S*)-2,3,4,5,6,7-Hexahydro-1,4-dimethyl-1,6-methano-1*H*-4-benzazonin-10-ol.
$C_{15}H_{21}NO=231.3$.

CAS — 72522-13-5.

Eptazocine is reported to be a narcotic analgesic.

Proprietary Names
Sedapain *(Jap.)*.

12699-v

Equisetum. Horsetail; Herba Equiseti; Schachtelhalmkraut.

Pharmacopoeias. In *Aust., Ger., Hung., Pol., Roum.,* and *Swiss. Arg.* specifies *E. giganteum.*

The dried sterile green stems of the common horsetail, *Equisetum arvense* (Equisetaceae).

Equisetum has weak diuretic properties. It has been used in the treatment of respiratory disorders.

Alkaloids present in equisetum of British origin included nicotine and palustrine.— J. D. Phillipson and C. Melville, *J. Pharm. Pharmac.*, 1960, *12*, 506.

12700-v

Erythromycin Thiocyanate *(B. Vet. C. 1965).*
$C_{37}H_{67}NO_{13},HSCN=793.0$.

CAS — 7704-67-8.

A white or almost white powder with a faint characteristic odour. Erythromycin thiocyanate 1.1 g is approximately equivalent to 1 g of erythromycin. **Soluble** 1 in 250 of water, 1 in 25 of alcohol, and 1 in 250 of chloroform. **Store** in airtight containers. Protect from light.

Erythromycin thiocyanate has the actions and uses of erythromycin (see p.1158) and has been used in veterinary medicine.

12701-g

Etamiphylline Heparinate

CAS — 314-35-2 (etamiphylline); 59547-58-9 (heparinate).

A complex of etamiphylline and heparin.

Etamiphylline heparinate is promoted for the treatment of hyperlipidaemia and associated disorders.

Proprietary Names
Milhéparine *(Millot-Solac, Fr.)*.

12702-q

Etamocycline. Etamicycline. *NN'*-[Ethylenebis(methyliminomethylene)]bis(4-dimethylamino-1,4,4a,5,5a,6,11,12a-octahydro-3,6,10,12,12a-pentahydroxy-6-methyl-1,11-dioxonaphthacene-2-carboxamide).
$C_{50}H_{60}N_6O_{16}=1001.1$.

CAS — 15590-00-8.

Etamocycline is an antibiotic derived from tetracycline.

12703-p

Ethomoxane Hydrochloride. *N*-Butyl-8-ethoxy-1,4-benzodioxan-2-ylmethylamine hydrochloride.
$C_{15}H_{23}NO_3,HCl=301.8$.

CAS — 3570-46-5 (ethomoxane); 6038-78-4 (hydrochloride).

Ethomoxane hydrochloride has been claimed to allay nervousness.

12704-s

Ethonam Nitrate. Ethonamidate; Etonam Nitrate; R-10100. Ethyl 1-(1,2,3,4-tetrahydro-1-naphthyl)imidazole-5-carboxylate nitrate.
$C_{16}H_{18}N_2O_2,HNO_3=333.3$.

CAS — 15037-44-2 (ethonam); 15037-55-5 (nitrate).

Ethonam nitrate is an antifungal agent reported to be active against dermatophytes but inactive against yeasts. It has been used as lotion and powder both containing 2%.

References: R. Vanbreuseghem *et al.*, *Chemotherapia*, 1967, *12*, 107; J. Brugmans and J. van Cutsem, *Dermatologica*, 1969, *138*, 403, per *Abstr. Wld Med.*, 1969, *43*, 697.

Manufacturers
Janssen, Belg.

12705-w

Ethopabate *(B.P. Vet.).* Methyl 4-acetamido-2-ethoxybenzoate.
$C_{12}H_{15}NO_4=237.3$.

CAS — 59-06-3.

A white or pinkish-white, odourless or almost odourless powder. M.p. about 148°. **Soluble** 1 in 2000 of water, 1 in 30 of alcohol, 1 in 10 of chloroform, 1 in 600 of ether, and 1 in 15 of methyl alcohol.

Ethopabate is used, usually in conjunction with other agents such as amprolium, pyrimethamine, or sulphaquinoxaline, in the prevention of coccidiosis in poultry.

Manufacturers
Merck Sharp & Dohme, UK.

12706-e

Ethyl Deoxyuridine. 5-Ethyl-2′-deoxyuridine.
$C_{11}H_{16}N_2O_5=256.3$.

CAS — 15176-29-1.

Ethyl deoxyuridine has been used in herpes infection of the eye.

Proprietary Names
Aedurid *(Robugen, Ger.)*; Edurid *(Robugen, Switz.)*.

15319-n

Ethyl Loflazepate. Ethyl 7-chloro-5-(2-fluorophenyl)-1,3-dihydro-2-oxo-2*H*-1,4-benzodiazepine-3-carboxylate.
$C_{18}H_{14}ClFN_2O_3=360.8$.

CAS — 29177-84-2.

Ethyl loflazepate in a benzodiazepine compound (see Diazepam p.1519), with anxiolytic activity.

Manufacturers
Clin Midy, Fr.

12707-l

Ethyl Salicylate. Ethyl 2-hydroxybenzoate.
$C_9H_{10}O_3=166.2$.

CAS — 118-61-6.

A very refractive colourless liquid with an odour similar to that of methyl salicylate. It becomes yellowish-brown on long exposure to light and air. B.p. about 232°. Slightly **soluble** in water; miscible with alcohol and ether. **Protect** from light.

Ethyl salicylate has properties similar to those of methyl salicylate (see p.263). It is used in perfumery.

12708-y

Ethylamphetamine Hydrochloride. Etilamfetamine Hydrochloride. *N*-Ethyl-α-methylphenethylamine hydrochloride.
$C_{11}H_{17}N,HCl=199.7$.

CAS — 457-87-4 (ethylamphetamine); 1858-47-5 (hydrochloride).

Ethylamphetamine hydrochloride has been used as an anorectic agent.

Proprietary Names
Apetinil *(Medial, Neth.)*; Apetinil-Depo *(Will-Pharma, Belg.; Syntex, Switz.)*.

12709-j

Ethylbenzhydramine Hydrochloride. Etanautine Hydrochloride; Diethylaminoethoxydiphenylmethane Hydrochloride; β-Diethylaminoethylbenzhydryl Ether Hydrochloride. 2-(Benzhydryloxy)triethylamine hydrochloride.
$C_{19}H_{25}NO,HCl=319.9$.

CAS — 642-58-0 (ethylbenzhydramine); 86-24-8 (hydrochloride).

NOTE. The name Etanautine was formerly applied to diphenhydramine monoacefyllinate.

Crystals with a bitter taste. M.p. 140°. Freely **soluble** in water; soluble in acetone, alcohol, and chloroform; very slightly soluble in ether. A 1% solution in water has a pH of about 5.5.

Ethylbenzhydramine hydrochloride has been used in the treatment of spastic conditions such as parkinsonism.

Proprietary Names
PKM *(Montavit, Switz.)*.

12710-q

Ethylene Dibromide. EDB. 1,2-Dibromoethane.
$C_2H_4Br_2$=187.9.
CAS — 106-93-4.

A heavy colourless liquid. **Soluble** 1 in about 250 of water at 30°; soluble in alcohol, ether, and most organic solvents.

Ethylene dibromide is used as an insecticide by fumigation and as a lead scavenger in the petroleum industry. It is more toxic than carbon tetrachloride or ethylene dichloride. It is irritant to the eyes, skin, and mucous membranes. Inhalation leads to drowsiness, CNS depression, and possibly pulmonary oedema. Contact with the skin causes blistering. Kidney and liver damage may occur.
Ethylene dibromide is reported to be carcinogenic in experimental *animals*.

A study in *rats* showed an increased incidence of morbidity and mortality in animals exposed to a combination of ethylene dibromide and disulfiram. The clinical significance was not known but the advisability of continued occupational exposure to ethylene dibromide by patients receiving disulfiram was uncertain.— H. B. Plotnick (letter), *J. Am. med. Ass.*, 1978, *239*, 1609. See also R. E. Yodaiken, *ibid.*, 2783.

Ethylene dibromide is recognised as a potential carcinogen in man. Industrial workers should be properly equipped to ensure virtually no contact with it.— *Threshold Limit Values 1980*, Guidance Note EH 15/80, London, Health and Safety Executive, 1980.

12711-p

Ethylene Dichloride. Dutch Liquid; Brocide. 1,2-Dichloroethane.
$C_2H_4Cl_2$=98.96.
CAS — 107-06-2.

A colourless inflammable liquid with a chloroform-like odour. **Soluble** 1 in about 250 of water; soluble in most organic solvents.

Ethylene dichloride is used as an industrial solvent and, usually in conjunction with carbon tetrachloride, as an insecticide by fumigation. Exposure to the vapour may cause lachrymation and corneal clouding, nasal irritation, and vertigo due to the depressant effect on the CNS. Contact with the skin may cause dermatitis. Kidney and liver damage may follow ingestion.
Maximum permissible atmospheric concentration 10 ppm.
Ethylene dichloride has been reported to be carcinogenic in experimental *animals*.

The maximum acceptable concentration of ethylene dichloride in cereals after fumigation.— Report of the 1971 Joint FAO/WHO Meeting on Pesticide Residues in Food, *Tech. Rep. Ser. Wld Hlth Org. No. 502*, 1972. The Food Additives and Contaminants Committee recommended that ethylene dichloride be temporarily permitted for use as a solvent in food and recommended a maximum concentration for use in food as consumed of 5 ppm. Further toxicity studies were required.— *Report on the Review of Solvents in Food*, FAC/REP/25, Ministry of Agriculture, Fisheries and Food, London, HM Stationery Office, 1978. Ethylene dichloride is not suitable for use as a food additive.— Twenty-third Report of Joint FAO/WHO Expert Committee on Food Additives, *Tech. Rep. Ser. Wld Hlth Org. No. 648*, 1980.

12712-s

Etifelmine. 2-Diphenylmethylenebutylamine.
$C_{17}H_{19}N$=237.3.
CAS — 341-00-4.

Etifelmine hydrochloride has been used for the treatment of hypotension. A mixture of the hydrochloride and nicotinate is similarly used.

Proprietary Names
Gilutensin (hydrochloride and nicotinate) *(Giulini, Ger.)*; Tensinase-D (hydrochloride) *(Jap.)*.

12713-w

Etintidine Hydrochloride. BL-5641A. 2-Cyano-1-[2-(5-methyl-1*H*-imidazol-4-ylmethylthio)ethyl]-3-(prop-2-ynyl)guanidine hydrochloride.
$C_{12}H_{16}N_6S,HCl$=312.8.
CAS — 69539-53-3 (etintidine); 71807-56-2 (hydrochloride).

Etintidine hydrochloride is reported to be a histamine H_2 blocking agent.

Manufacturers
Bristol, USA.

12714-e

Etiocholanolone. 3α-Hydroxy-5β-androstan-17-one.
$C_{19}H_{30}O_2$=290.4.
CAS — 53-42-9.

A white crystalline powder. **Soluble** in propylene glycol.

Etiocholanolone is one of the 17-ketosteroids produced by the metabolism of steroid hormones and excreted in the urine. The rise in the number of blood granulocytes which follows an intramuscular injection of etiocholanolone has been used to assess bone-marrow granulocyte reserves in patients receiving cytotoxic drugs. It has pyrogenic properties and has been used to study the mechanisms of fever.
In addition to fever and granulocytosis etiocholanolone has been reported to cause muscle and joint pain, anorexia, malaise, and inflammation at the site of injection.

Nine of 10 patients with severe bone-marrow failure improved when treated with etiocholanolone 300 μg per kg body-weight daily for 2 to 4 weeks in propylene glycol at a concentration of 20 mg per ml, and thereafter on alternate days. Treatment was by intramuscular injection with prednisolone acetate 400 μg per kg in a concentration of 50 mg per ml being given in the same syringe to reduce any inflammation.— E. C. Besa, *Lancet*, 1977, *1*, 728.

Preparations
Etiocholanolone Injection *(Queen Eliz. Hosp., S. Australia)*. Etiocholanolone 10 mg and propylene glycol 1 ml. Sterilised by filtration. Store at 2° to 8°. Shelf-life 3 months. *Dose.* 100 μg per kg body-weight intramuscularly for the estimation of bone-marrow reserves.

Proprietary Names
Etiolone *(Vister, Ital.)*.

12715-l

Etiroxate Hydrochloride. CG-635. Ethyl DL-2-amino-3-[4-(4-hydroxy-3,5-di-iodophenoxy)-3,5-di-iodophenyl]-2-methylpropionate hydrochloride.
$C_{18}H_{17}I_4NO_4,HCl$=855.4.
CAS — 17365-01-4 (etiroxate); 55327-22-5 (hydrochloride).

Etiroxate is the racemic ethyl ester of the methyl derivative of thyroxine, and has been used in the treatment of hyperlipoproteinaemia type II.

References: W. Schwartzkopff and E. Russ, *Münch. med. Wschr.*, 1975, *117*, 827, per *J. Am. med. Ass.*, 1975, *233*, 834.

Proprietary Names
Skleronorm *(Grünenthal, Ger.; Grünenthal, Switz.)*.

12716-y

Etisazole Hydrochloride. Bay VA-9387 (etisazole). *N*-Ethyl-1,2-benzisothiazol-3-ylamine hydrochloride.
$C_9H_{10}N_2S,HCl$=214.7.
CAS — 7716-60-1 (etisazole).

Etisazole hydrochloride is an antifungal agent used in veterinary practice.

Proprietary Names
Netrosylla *(Bayer Agrochem, UK)*.

12717-j

Etodolac. Etodolic Acid; AY-24236. 1,8-Diethyl-1,3,4,9-tetrahydropyrano[3,4-*b*]indol-1-ylacetic acid.
$C_{17}H_{21}NO_3$=287.4.
CAS — 41340-25-4.

Etodolac is reported to have anti-inflammatory activity.

Manufacturers
Ayerst, USA.

12718-z

Etodroxizine Dimaleate. 2-{2-[2-(4-*p*-Chlorobenzhydrylpiperazin-1-yl)ethoxy]ethoxy} ethanol dimaleate.
$C_{23}H_{31}ClN_2O_3,2C_4H_4O_4$=651.1.
CAS — 17692-34-1 (etodroxizine).

Etodroxizine dimaleate has been used as a hypnotic.

Proprietary Names
Indunox *(UCB, Belg.; UCB, Neth.; UCB, S.Afr.)*.

12719-c

Etofibrate. 2-Nicotinoyloxyethyl 2-(4-chlorophenoxy)-2-methylpropionate.
$C_{18}H_{18}ClNO_5$=363.8.
CAS — 31637-97-5.

The molecule of etofibrate comprises the molecules of clofibrate and nicotinic acid.

Etofibrate has been used in the treatment of hyperlipidaemias.

References: A. Gustafson, *Int. J. clin. Pharmac. Biopharm.*, 1979, *17*, 498.

Proprietary Names
Lipo-Merz *(Merz, Ger.)*.

12720-s

Etofylline Clofibrate. ML-1024. 2-(Theophyllin-7-yl)ethyl 2-(4-chlorophenoxy)-2-methylpropionate.
$C_{19}H_{21}ClN_4O_5$=420.9.
CAS — 54504-70-0.

Etofylline clofibrate is an ester of etofylline and clofibric acid and has been used in the treatment of hyperlipidaemias.

For a series of papers, see *Arzneimittel-Forsch.*, 1980, *30*, 2013–74.

Proprietary Names
Duolip *(Merckle, Ger.)*.

12721-w

Etoperidone Hydrochloride. Clopradone Hydrochloride; ST-1191 (etoperidone). 2-{3-[4-(3-Chlorophenyl)piperazin-1-yl]propyl}-4,5-diethyl-2,4-dihydro-1,2,4-triazol-3-one hydrochloride.
$C_{19}H_{28}ClN_5O,HCl$=414.4.
CAS — 52942-31-1 (etoperidone); 57775-22-1 (hydrochloride).

Etoperidone hydrochloride is reported to have antidepressant activity.

Proprietary Names
Staff *(Sigmatau, Ital.)*.

12722-e

Etozolin. Gö-687; W-2900A. Ethyl (3-methyl-4-oxo-5-piperidinothiazolidin-2-ylidene)acetate.
$C_{13}H_{20}N_2O_3S$=284.4.
CAS — 73-09-6.

Etozolin is a diuretic.

For a series of papers on etozolin, see *Arzneimittel-Forsch.*, 1977, *27*, 1742–1817.

Proprietary Names
Elkapin *(Gödecke, Ger.)*.

12723-l

Etymemazine Hydrochloride. RP-6484 *(etymemazine)*. 3-(2-Ethylphenothiazin-10-yl)-2,*N*,*N*-trimethylpropylamine hydrochloride.
$C_{20}H_{26}N_2S,HCl=363.0$.

CAS — 523-54-6 (etymemazine); 13994-15-5 (hydrochloride).

Etymemazine hydrochloride is a phenothiazine compound with sedative and tranquillising properties.

Proprietary Names
Nuital *(Vaillant-Defresne, Fr.)*; Sergetyl *(Vaillant-Defresne, Fr.; Vaillant-Defresne, Switz.)*.

12724-y

Euphrasia. The whole plant of *Euphrasia officinalis* (Scrophulariaceae).

Euphrasia is used in homoeopathic medicine.

12725-j

Examestrone. Hexoxymestrone. 3-Hexyloxy-17α-methylandrosta-3,5-dien-17β-ol.
$C_{26}H_{42}O_2=386.6$.

Examestrone is a derivative of testosterone, with anabolic and androgenic activity.

Proprietary Names
Enoltestovis *(Vister, Ital.)*.

12726-z

Exiproben Sodium. DCH-21. Sodium 2-(3-hexyloxy-2-hydroxypropoxy)benzoate.
$C_{16}H_{23}NaO_5=318.3$.

CAS — 26281-69-6 (exiproben); 3478-44-2 (sodium salt).

Exiproben sodium has been used in the treatment of hepatic disorders.

Proprietary Names
Droctil *(Geigy, Ital.)*; Etopalin *(Geigy, Arg.)*.

12727-c

Famotine Hydrochloride. UK-2054. 1-[(4-Chlorophenoxy)methyl]-3,4-dihydroisoquinoline hydrochloride.
$C_{16}H_{14}ClNO,HCl=308.2$.

CAS — 18429-78-2 (famotine); 10500-82-0 (hydrochloride).

Famotine is claimed to be an antiviral agent but was of no benefit in influenza and respiratory syncytial virus infections.

Manufacturers
Pfizer, USA.

12729-a

Febantel. Bay h 5757; BAY Vh 5757. Dimethyl 2-[2-(2-methoxyacetamido)-4-(phenylthio)phenyl] guanidine-1,3-dicarboxylate.
$C_{20}H_{22}N_4O_6S=446.5$.

CAS — 58306-30-2.

Febantel is an anthelmintic with possible application in veterinary practice.

Manufacturers
Bayer, UK.

12728-k

Febarbamate. Phenobamate; Go-560. 1-(3-Butoxy-2-carbamoyloxypropyl)-5-ethyl-5-phenylbarbituric acid.
$C_{20}H_{27}N_3O_6=405.4$.

CAS — 13246-02-1.

Febarbamate is reported to have sedative and tranquillising properties.

Proprietary Names
G-Tril *(Sapos, Neth.; Vinas, Spain)*; Solium *(Lirca, Ital.)*.

12730-e

Fenaftic Acid. 1-Diethylcarbamoyl-1,2,3,4,5,6,7,8-octahydro-6,6-dimethyl-8-oxo-3-phenyl-2-naphthoic acid.
$C_{24}H_{31}NO_4=397.5$.

CAS — 27736-80-7.

Fenaftic acid has been claimed to increase bile secretion and to improve its composition. It has been given in illness involving hepatobiliary insufficiency or dysfunction.

12731-l

Fenalamide. Ethyl *N*-(2-diethylaminoethyl)-2-ethyl-2-phenylmalonamate.
$C_{19}H_{30}N_2O_3=334.5$.

CAS — 4551-59-1.

Fenalamide has antispasmodic activity.

Proprietary Names
Spasmamide Semplice *(Schering, Ital.)*.

12732-y

Fenbutamidol. An equimolecular combination of phenyramidol and oxyphenbutazone.
$C_{32}H_{34}N_4O_4=538.6$.

CAS — 25146-18-3.

Fenbutamidol has been used for the reduction of inflammation.

Proprietary Names
Febutolo *(ISM, Ital.)*.

12733-j

Fenbutyramide. Fenbutiramide. 2-Phenylbutyramide.
$C_{10}H_{13}NO=163.2$.

Fenbutyramide has been used in the treatment of hypercholesterolaemia.

Proprietary Names
Hyposterol *(Vaillant, Ital.)*; Liosterin *(Medici Domus, Ital.)*; Normosterolo *(Salfa, Ital.)*.

12734-z

Fencamine Hydrochloride. ST-374. 8-[2-(*N*,α-Dimethylphenethylamino)ethylamino]-7-methyltheophylline hydrochloride.
$C_{20}H_{28}N_6O_2,HCl=420.9$.

CAS — 28947-50-4 (fencamine); 24356-67-0 (hydrochloride).

Fencamine hydrochloride is reported to be a CNS stimulant and has been used in depression.

Proprietary Names
Sicoclor *(Gramon, Arg.)*.

12735-c

Fencibutirol. 2-(1-Hydroxy-4-phenylcyclohexyl)butyric acid.
$C_{16}H_{22}O_3=262.3$.

CAS — 5977-10-6.

Fencibutirol has been used in the treatment of hepatic disorders.

Proprietary Names
Verecolene *(Maggioni, Ital.)*.

12736-k

Fenclonine. CP-10118; DL-*p*-Chlorophenylalanine; Parachlorophenylalanine. 2-Amino-3-(4-chlorophenyl)propionic acid.
$C_9H_{10}ClNO_2=199.6$.

CAS — 7424-00-2.

Fenclonine is an inhibitor of the biosynthesis of serotonin. It has been given to patients with carcinoid syndrome and some relief of symptoms, especially of diarrhoea, has been reported. Hypothermia has been reported during treatment with fenclonine. Doses of 2 to 4 g daily have been used; higher doses have been reported to produce psychic side-effects.

References: K. Engelman *et al.*, *New Engl. J. Med.*, 1967, *277*, 1103; M. Shani and C. Sheba, *Br. med. J.*, 1970, *4*, 784; A. B. Vaidya and R. J. Levine, *New Engl. J. Med.*, 1971, *284*, 255.

Manufacturers
Pfizer, USA.

12737-a

Fenclozic Acid. ICI-54450. [2-(4-Chlorophenyl)thiazol-4-yl]acetic acid.
$C_{11}H_8ClNO_2S=253.7$.

CAS — 17969-20-9.

A white crystalline powder. M.p. about 155°. Sparingly **soluble** in water; soluble in most organic solvents.

Fenclozic acid is an analgesic and anti-inflammatory agent which was withdrawn from study because of hepatotoxicity.

12738-t

Fenethylline Hydrochloride. H-814; R-720-11; Fenetylline Hydrochloride; Amfetyline Hydrochloride; 7-Ethyltheophylline Amphetamine Hydrochloride. 7-[2-(α-Methylphenethylamino)ethyl]theophylline hydrochloride.
$C_{18}H_{23}N_5O_2,HCl=377.9$.

CAS — 3736-08-1 (fenethylline); 1892-80-4 (hydrochloride).

A white crystalline powder. **Soluble** in water.

Fenethylline is a theophylline derivative of amphetamine which has been used for its central stimulant effect.

Proprietary Names
Captagon *(de Bournonville, Belg.; Gerda, Fr.; Homburg, Ger.)*.

12739-x

Fenmetozole Hydrochloride. DH-524. 2-(3,4-Dichlorophenoxymethyl)-2-imidazoline hydrochloride.
$C_{10}H_{10}Cl_2N_2O,HCl=281.6$.

CAS — 41473-09-0 (fenmetozole); 23712-05-2 (hydrochloride).

Fenmetozole is a compound with central nervous system activity which has been tried in the treatment of depression with equivocal results. Its suggested potential as an alcohol antagonist has not been confirmed.

References: C. -P. Chien and R. M. Kaplan, *Curr. ther. Res.*, 1969, *11*, 471; *idem*, 1971, *13*, 350; H. B. McNamee *et al.*, *Clin. Pharmac. Ther.*, 1975, *17*, 735; M. Fink and P. Irwin, *Curr. ther. Res.*, 1975, *18*, 590; L. C. Griffis *et al.*, *Clin. Pharmac. Ther.*, 1978, *24*, 350.

Manufacturers
Dow, USA.

12740-y

Fenobam. McN-3377-98. 1-(3-Chlorophenyl)-3-(1-methyl-4-oxo-2-imidazolin-2-yl)urea monohydrate.
$C_{11}H_{11}ClN_4O_2,H_2O=284.7$.

CAS — 57653-26-6 (anhydrous); 63540-28-3 (monohydrate).

Fenobam is reported to have tranquillising properties.

References: T. M. Itil *et al.*, *Curr. ther. Res.*, 1978, *24*, 708; J. C. Pecknold *et al.*, *ibid.*, 1980, *27*, 119; C. T. H. Friedmann *et al.*, *ibid.*, 144.

Manufacturers
McNeil, USA.

12741-j

Fenozolone. LD-3394; Phenozolone. 2-Ethylamino-5-phenyl-2-oxazolin-4-one.
$C_{11}H_{12}N_2O_2=204.2$.

CAS — 15302-16-6.

Fenozolone is a psychostimulant which has been used in the treatment of nervous disorders.

Proprietary Names
Ordinator *(Sintyal, Arg.; Dausse, Fr.).*

12742-z

Fenpentadiol. Rd-292. 2-(4-Chlorophenyl)-4-methylpentane-2,4-diol.
$C_{12}H_{17}ClO_2=228.7$.

CAS — 15687-18-0.

Fenpentadiol has been used in depression and psychosomatic disorders.

Proprietary Names
Trédum *(Anphar-Rolland, Fr.).*

12743-c

Fenpiprane Hydrochloride. 1-(3,3-Diphenylpropyl)piperidine hydrochloride.
$C_{20}H_{25}N,HCl=315.9$.

CAS — 3540-95-2 (fenpiprane); 3329-14-4 (hydrochloride).

Fenpiprane hydrochloride is used in veterinary practice, in association with fenpipramide hydrochloride ($C_{21}H_{26}N_2O,HCl,H_2O=376.9$), for arresting cervical spasm and hastening normal labour.

Proprietary Names
Efosin *(Hoechst, UK).*

12744-k

Fenpyramine Hydrochloride. 3,3-Diphenyl-*N*-(4-pyridyl)propylamine hydrochloride.
$C_{20}H_{20}N_2,HCl=324.9$.

CAS — 29769-70-8.

Fenpyramine hydrochloride has been used for its spasmolytic effects, especially on the gastro-intestinal tract.

Proprietary Names
Fenprin *(RBS Pharma, Ital.).*

12745-a

Fenquizone Potassium. MG-13054. The potassium salt of 7-chloro-1,2,3,4-tetrahydro-4-oxo-2-phenylquinazoline-6-sulphonamide.
$C_{14}H_{11}ClKN_3O_3S=375.9$.

CAS — 20287-37-0 (fenquizone).

Fenquizone potassium is a diuretic.

Proprietary Names
Idrolone *(Maggioni, Ital.).*

12746-t

Fenspiride Hydrochloride. JP-428; NAT-333; NDR-5998A; Decaspiride. 8-Phenethyl-1-oxa-3,8-diazaspiro[4.5]decan-2-one hydrochloride.
$C_{15}H_{20}N_2O_2,HCl=296.8$.

CAS — 5053-06-5 (fenspiride); 5053-08-7 (hydrochloride).

Fenspiride is reported to have bronchodilator and anti-inflammatory properties. It has been given in asthma and other respiratory disorders.

References: *J. Am. med. Ass.*, 1969, *209*, 1615.

Proprietary Names
Abronquil *(S. Chobet, Arg.)*; Espiràn *(Farnex, Ital.)*; Fendel *(Sidus, Arg.)*; Pneumorel *(Dumas, Belg.; Biopharma, Fr.)*; Respiride *(Schiapparelli, Ital.)*; Tegencia *(Elmu, Spain)*; Viarespan *(Norka, Spain).*

12747-x

Fentiazac. BR-700; Wy-21894. [4-(4-Chlorophenyl)-2-phenylthiazol-5-yl]acetic acid.
$C_{17}H_{12}ClNO_2S=329.8$.

CAS — 18046-21-4.

Fentiazac is reported to have analgesic, anti-inflammatory, and antipyretic activity.

References: F. Natale and G. Perna, *J. int. med. Res.*, 1977, *5*, 96.

A series of 7 papers on fentiazac in rheumatic conditions.— *Curr. med. Res. Opinion*, 1979, *6*, *Suppl.* 2, 53–100.

Proprietary Names
Flogene *(Polifarma, Ital.)*; Norvedan *(LPB, Ital.)*; Ragilon *(Szabó, Arg.).*

12748-r

Fenugreek *(B.P.C. 1949).* Faenum-Graecum; Semen Foenugraeci; Semen Trigonellae; Bockshornsame.

Pharmacopoeias. In *Aust.*, *Chin.*, *Pol.*, and *Swiss.*

The dried seeds of *Trigonella foenumgraecum* (Leguminosae), containing not less than 30% of water-soluble extractive.

Fenugreek has been used chiefly in veterinary medicine as an aromatic.

Studies of the steroidal sapogenin yield of fenugreek.— R. Hardman and F. R. Y. Fazli, *Planta med.*, 1972, *21*, 322.

A report of 'maple-syrup' urine odour due to the ingestion of fenugreek.— G. B. Bartley *et al.* (letter), *New Engl. J. Med.*, 1981, *305*, 467.

Metabolic effects. An infusion prepared from fenugreek seeds and an aqueous solution of trigonelline, an alkaloid present in the seeds to the extent of 0.13%, had both been shown to have hypoglycaemic effects in *animals*. A transient hypoglycaemic effect was noted in 5 of 10 diabetic patients who were given 500 mg of trigonelline while fasting but treatment with 1.5 to 3 g of trigonelline daily for 5 days did not decrease the diurnal blood-glucose concentration.— J. Mishkinsky *et al.* (letter), *Lancet*, 1967, *2*, 1311.

Proprietary Names
Fénugrène *(Lemoine, Fr.).*

12749-f

Ferrous Ascorbate.
$C_{12}H_{14}FeO_{12}=406.1$.

CAS — 24808-52-4.

Ferrous ascorbate has been used as a source of iron in the treatment of iron-deficiency anaemias.

Proprietary Names
Ascofer *(Desbergers, Canad.; Roland-Marie, Fr.; Roland-Marie, Switz.)*; Cefer *(Phoenix, Arg.)*; Nedifer *(Servier, Neth.).*

12750-z

Fibracillin. Amidacilina; AL-70-35. (6*R*)-6-{D-2-[2-(4-Chlorophenoxy)-2-methylpropionamido]-2-phenylacetamido}penicillanic acid.
$C_{26}H_{28}ClN_3O_6S=546.0$.

CAS — 51154-48-4.

Fibracillin is reported to have an antimicrobial spectrum similar to that of ampicillin.

Proprietary Names
Alongapen *(Lafarquim, Spain).*

12751-c

Fipexide Hydrochloride. BP-662. 1-(4-Chlorophenoxyacetyl)-4-piperonylpiperazine hydrochloride.
$C_{20}H_{21}ClN_2O_4,HCl=425.3$.

CAS — 34161-24-5 (fipexide); 34161-23-4 (hydrochloride).

Fipexide hydrochloride is a stimulant of the central nervous system and has been used in the treatment of depression and memory defects.

Proprietary Names
Vigilor *(Bouchard, Fr.).*

12752-k

Flavodate Sodium. Flavodate Disodium. Disodium (4-oxo-2-phenyl-4*H*-chromene-5,7-diyldioxy)diacetate.
$C_{19}H_{12}Na_2O_8=414.3$.

CAS — 37470-13-6 (flavodic acid); 13358-62-8 (disodium salt).

Flavodate sodium is stated to increase the resistance of capillaries and to reduce their permeability. It has been given in vascular disorders.

Proprietary Names
Comparison *(Casasco, Arg.)*; Intercyton *(Roland-Marie, Fr.; Semar, Spain)*; Pericel *(Lirca, Ital.).*

12753-a

Flecainide Acetate. R-818. *N*-(2-Piperidylmethyl)-2,5-bis(2,2,2-trifluoroethoxy)benzamide acetate.
$C_{17}H_{20}F_6N_2O_3,C_2H_4O_2=474.4$.

CAS — 54143-55-4 (flecainide); 54143-56-5 (acetate).

Flecainide acetate is reported to have anti-arrhythmic activity, and to be effective when given by mouth.

References: P. Somani, *Clin. Pharmac. Ther.*, 1980, *27*, 464; J. B. Schwartz *et al.*, *Drugs*, 1981, *21*, 23; M. Hodges *et al.*, *Clin. Pharmac. Ther.*, 1981, *29*, 251; J. L. Anderson *et al.*, *New Engl. J. Med.*, 1981, *305*, 473.

Manufacturers
Riker, USA.

12755-x

Fluazacort. L-6400. 9α-Fluoro-11β,21-dihydroxy-2′-methyl-5′β*H*-pregna-1,4-dieno[17,16-*d*]-oxazole-3,20-dione 21-acetate.
$C_{25}H_{30}FNO_6=459.5$.

CAS — 19888-56-3.

Fluazacort is a fluorinated corticosteroid for topical use.

Proprietary Names
Azacortid *(Richter, Ital.).*

12756-r

Flubendazole. Fluoromebendazole; R-17889. Methyl 5-(4-fluorobenzoyl)-1*H*-benzimidazole-2-ylcarbamate.
$C_{16}H_{12}FN_3O_3=313.3$.

CAS — 31430-15-6.

Flubendazole is an anthelmintic.

The activity of flubendazole against nematode and cestode infections in *animals*.— D. Thienpont *et al.*, *Janssen, Belg.*, *Arzneimittel-Forsch.*, 1978, *28*, 605.

Clinical reports of use in various helminth infections.— H. Schenone *et al.*, *Boln chil. Parasit.*, 1977, *32*, 85, per *Trop. Dis. Bull.*, 1978, *75*, 670; A. Canese *et al.*, *Revta Paraguaya Microbiol.*, 1978, *13*, 31, per *Trop. Dis. Bull.*, 1978, *75*, 983; J. P. Nozais, *Méd. Afr. noire*, 1978, *25*, 473, per *Trop. Dis. Bull.*, 1978, *75*, 1211; C. Penot *et al.*, *Bull. Soc. Path. exot.*, 1978, *71*, 370, per *Trop. Dis. Bull.*, 1979, *76*, 927.

Mention of the use of flubendazole in hydatid cyst disease (echinococcosis).— P. Bouree and R. Molinard (letter), *Br. med. J.*, 1978, *1*, 301.

Manufacturers
Janssen, Belg.

12757-f

Flumequine. R-802. 9-Fluoro-6,7-dihydro-5-methyl-1-oxo-1*H*,5*H*-benzo[*ij*]quinolizine-2-carboxylic acid.
$C_{14}H_{12}FNO_3=261.3$.

CAS — 42835-25-6.

Flumequine is an antibacterial agent used in the treatment of urinary-tract infections.

References: S. R. Rohlfing *et al.*, *Antimicrob. Ag. Chemother.*, 1976, *10*, 20; S. R. Rohlfing *et al.*, *J. antimicrob. Chemother.*, 1977, *3*, 615; D. Greenwood, *Antimicrob. Ag. Chemother.*, 1978, *13*, 479.

Proprietary Names
Apurone *(Riker, Fr.)*.

15320-k

Flumeridone. R-45486. 5-Chloro-1-{1-[3-(5-fluoro-2-oxobenzimidazolin-1-yl)propyl]-4-piperidyl}benzimidazolin-2-one.
$C_{22}H_{23}ClFN_5O_2=443.9$.

CAS — 75444-64-3.

Flumeridone is reported to have anti-emetic activity.

Manufacturers
Janssen, Belg.

15321-a

Flumethrin. Bay Vl-6045. α-Cyano-4-fluoro-3-phenoxybenzyl 3-(β,4-dichlorostyryl)-2,2-dimethylcyclopropanecarboxylate.
$C_{28}H_{22}Cl_2FNO_3=510.4$.

CAS — 69770-45-2.

Flumethrin is an insecticide for veterinary use.

Manufacturers
Bayer Agrochem, UK.

12758-d

Flumizole. CP-22665. 4,5-Bis(4-methoxyphenyl)-2-(trifluoromethyl)imidazole.
$C_{18}H_{15}F_3N_2O_2=348.3$.

CAS — 36740-73-5.

Flumizole is an anti-inflammatory agent.

References: E. H. Wiseman *et al.*, *J. pharm. Sci.*, 1975, *64*, 1469.

Manufacturers
Pfizer, USA.

12759-n

Flunarizine Hydrochloride. R-14950. *trans*-1-Cinnamyl-4-(4,4′-difluorobenzhydryl)piperazine dihydrochloride.
$C_{26}H_{26}F_2N_2,2HCl=477.4$.

CAS — 52468-60-7 (flunarizine); 30484-77-6 (hydrochloride).

Flunarizine is the difluorinated derivative of cinnarizine. Flunarizine hydrochloride has vasodilator properties.

References: R. Boniver, *Arzneimittel-Forsch.*, 1978, *28*, 1800 (vertigo); J. Schetz *et al.*, *Curr. ther. Res.*, 1978, *23*, 121 (intermittent claudication); F. Roekaerts *et al.*, *Curr. ther. Res.*, 1979, *26*, 363 (venous insufficiency); J. Heykants *et al.*, *Arzneimittel-Forsch.*, 1979, *29*, 1168 (plasma concentrations); J. H. Palmer *et al.*, *Lancet*, 1981, *2*, 279 (urinary incontinence); N. P. Zissis *et al.*, *Curr. ther. Res.*, 1981, *29*, 395.

Proprietary Names
Sibelium *(Janssen, Ger.)*.

12760-k

Flunixin. Sch-14714. 2-(2-Methyl-3-trifluoromethylanilino)nicotinic acid; 2-(α^3,α^3,α^3-Trifluoro-2,3-xylidino)nicotinic acid.
$C_{14}H_{11}F_3N_2O_2=296.2$.

CAS — 38677-85-9.

Flunixin is reported to have analgesic activity.

References: J. -E. Gjöres *et al.*, *Clin. Trials J.*, 1976, *13*, 105; B. Zederfeldt *et al.*, *Br. J. Anaesth.*, 1977, *49*, 467.

Manufacturers
Schering, UK.

12761-a

Fluocortin Butyl. SH K-203. Butyl 6α-fluoro-11β-hydroxy-16α-methyl-3,20-dioxopregna-1,4-dien-21-oate.
$C_{26}H_{35}FO_5=446.6$.

CAS — 33124-50-4 (fluocortin); 41767-29-7 (butyl ester).

Fluocortin butyl is a fluorinated corticosteroid for topical use.

For a series of papers on fluocortin butyl, see *Arzneimittel-Forsch.*, 1977, *27*, 2185–2246.

Further references: P. H. Vlasses *et al.*, *Clin. Pharmac. Ther.*, 1981, *29*, 643.

Proprietary Names
Vaspit *(Schering, Ger.; Schering, Switz.)*.

12762-t

Fluotracen Hydrochloride. SK&F-28175. (±)-*cis*-3-(9,10-Dihydro-10-methyl-2-trifluoromethylanthracen-9-yl)-*NN*-dimethylpropylamine hydrochloride.
$C_{21}H_{24}F_3N,HCl=383.9$.

CAS — 35764-73-9 (fluotracen); 57363-14-1 (hydrochloride).

Fluotracen hydrochloride is reported to have antidepressant activity.

References: P. J. Fowler *et al.*, *Arzneimittel-Forsch.*, 1977, *27*, 1589.

Clinical studies: T. M. Itil *et al.*, *Curr. ther. Res.*, 1977, *21*, 343.

Manufacturers
Smith Kline & French, USA.

12763-x

Fluoxetine. Lilly-103472; Lilly-110140. (±)-*N*-Methyl-3-phenyl-3-(4-trifluoromethylphenoxy)propylamine.
$C_{17}H_{18}F_3NO=309.3$.

CAS — 54910-89-3.

Fluoxetine is reported to be an inhibitor of serotonin uptake.

References: L. Lemberger *et al.*, *Clin. Pharmac. Ther.*, 1978, *23*, 421; L. Lemberger *et al.*, *Science*, 1978, *199*, 436; H. Y. Meltzer *et al.*, *J. neural Transmission*, 1979, *45*, 165; *J. Am. med. Ass.*, 1980, *243*, 1705.

Manufacturers
Lilly, USA.

12764-r

Flupamesone. UR-105. Bis(9α-fluoro-11β,21-dihydroxy-16α,17α-isopropylidenedioxypregna-1,4-diene-3,20-dione) 21,21′-[4,4′-methylenebis(3-methoxy-2-naphthoate)].
$C_{73}H_{78}F_2O_{16}=1249.4$.

CAS — 55461-42-2.

Flupamesone is a fluorinated corticosteroid for topical use.

References: V. Rimbau and F. Lleonart, *Arzneimittel-Forsch.*, 1975, *25*, 1040; T. R. Moreno *et al.*, *Curr. ther. Res.*, 1977, *21*, 183.

Proprietary Names
Flutenal *(Uriach, Spain)*.

12765-f

Fluproquazone. 46-790; RF-46-790; RF-46-790-n. 4-(4-Fluorophenyl)-1-isopropyl-7-methylquinazolin-2(1*H*)-one.
$C_{18}H_{17}FN_2O=296.3$.

CAS — 40507-23-1.

Fluproquazone is reported to have analgesic and anti-inflammatory activity.

For a series of papers on fluproquazone, see *Arzneimittel-Forsch.*, 1981, *31*, 871–940.

Further references: B. Von Graffenried and E. Nüesch, *Curr. ther. Res.*, 1979, *26*, 275; B. Maeglin *et al.*, *ibid.*, 284; U. Herrmann *et al.*, *Clin. Pharmac. Ther.*, 1980, *27*, 379.

Proprietary Names
Tormosyl *(Sandoz, Switz.)*.

12766-d

Flutiorex. SL-72340. (±)-*N*-Ethyl-α-methyl-*m*-(trifluoromethylthio)phenethylamine.
$C_{12}H_{16}F_3NS=263.3$.

CAS — 59173-25-0 (flutiorex); 53993-67-2 (tiflorex).

Tiflorex is the (+)-isomer.

Flutiorex is an anorectic agent similar to fenfluramine (p.66).

In 6 healthy subjects flutiorex 20 mg had an anorectic effect similar to that of fenfluramine 40 mg; its α-adrenergic sympathomimetic effect and its stimulant effect on the CNS were more pronounced.— J. F. Giudicelli *et al.*, *Br. J. clin. Pharmac.*, 1976, *3*, 113. A study with flutiorex in which men experienced more marked CNS stimulation than women. Flutiorex and its metabolite norflutiorex were detected in the blood of 4 of the 5 men and in 1 of the 5 women. The basis of the differences of blood concentrations was not understood.— *idem*, *Eur. J. clin. Pharmac.*, 1976, *10*, 325.

An evaluation of the anorectic activity of a sustained-release formulation of flutiorex was carried out in 6 healthy female subjects. Significant reduction in hunger occurred after 5 to 7 hours. Flutiorex produced no effect on pulse-rate or blood pressure and there was no evidence of CNS stimulation, but mydriasis did occur. Headache was also reported.— T. Silverstone *et al.*, *Br. J. clin. Pharmac.*, 1979, *7*, 353.

Manufacturers
Synthelabo, Fr.

12767-n

Flutroline. CP-36584. (±)-8-Fluoro-α,5-bis(4-fluorophenyl)-1,3,4,5-tetrahydro-2*H*-pyrido-[4,3-*b*]indol-2-ylbutan-1-ol.
$C_{27}H_{25}F_3N_2O=450.5$.

CAS — 70801-02-4.

Flutroline is reported to have tranquillising activity.

Manufacturers
Pfizer, USA.

12768-h

Fluvoxamine.

DU-23000 (maleate). 5-Methoxy-4′-trifluoromethylvalerophenone (*E*)-*O*-(2-aminoethyl)oxime.
$C_{15}H_{21}F_3N_2O_2$=318.3.

CAS — 54739-18-3 (fluvoxamine); 61718-82-9 (maleate).

Fluvoxamine is reported to have antidepressant activity.

References: T. M. Itil *et al.*, *Prog. Neuro-Psychopharm.*, 1977, *1*, 309; J. H. Wright and H. C. B. Denber, *Curr. ther. Res.*, 1978, *23*, 83; M. Schachter and J. D. Parkes, *J. Neurol. Neurosurg. Psychiat.*, 1980, *43*, 171.

Manufacturers
Duphar, Neth.

12769-m

Folescutol Hydrochloride.

LD-2988. 6,7-Dihydroxy-4-(morpholinomethyl)coumarin hydrochloride.
$C_{14}H_{15}NO_5$,HCl=313.7.

CAS — 15687-22-6 (folescutol).

Folescutol is stated to increase venous circulation and to reduce capillary permeability and has been used in a wide range of circulatory disorders.

Proprietary Names
Covalan *(Dausse, Fr.).*

12770-t

Fosazepam.

48390; HR-930. 7-Chloro-1-dimethylphosphinylmethyl-1,3-dihydro-5-phenyl-2*H*-1,4-benzodiazepin-2-one.
$C_{18}H_{18}ClN_2O_2P$=360.8.

CAS — 35322-07-7.

Fosazepam is a benzodiazepine compound with the general properties of diazepam (see p.1519). It has been tried as a hypnotic.

A possible hypnotic dose for fosazepam might be 40 to 60 mg.— A. N. Nicholson *et al.*, *Br. J. clin. Pharmac.*, 1976, *3*, 533.

Further references: S. Allen and I. Oswald, *Br. J. clin. Pharmac.*, 1976, *3*, 165; A. -M. Risberg *et al.*, *Eur. J. clin. Pharmac.*, 1977, *12*, 105.

Manufacturers
Hoechst, UK.

12771-x

Fosforylcholine.

Phosphorylcholine. (2-Hydroxyethyl)trimethylammonium chloride dihydrogen phosphate.
$C_5H_{15}ClNO_4P$=219.6.

CAS — 107-73-3.

Fosforylcholine has been used in the treatment of hepatic disorders. The calcium salt has been used as a source of calcium and phosphorus.

Proprietary Names of the Calcium Salt
Arenzil *(San Carlo, Ital.)*; Bifos *(Sidus, Ital.)*; Colincalcium *(Farmacologico Milanese, Ital.)*; Colinef *(Brocchieri, Ital.)*; Contrasthen *(Müller/Göppingen, Ger.)*; Epafosforil *(Coli, Ital.)*; Epaspes *(Nuovo, Ital.)*; Fisiocolina *(IBIS, Ital.)*; Fosfocolina *(Azienda Farm. Ital., Ital.)*; Isocolin *(Isola-Ibi, Ital.)*; Tonepar *(Molteni, Ital.).*

Proprietary Names of the Magnesium Salt
Héparexine *(Astra, Fr.).*

15322-t

Fosfosal.

UR-1521. 2-Phosphono-oxybenzoic acid.
$C_7H_7O_6P$=218.1.

CAS — 6064-83-1.

Fosfosal has analgesic, antipyretic, and anti-inflammatory activity.

Manufacturers
Uriach, Spain.

12772-r

Frentizole.

Lilly 53616. 1-(6-Methoxybenzothiazol-2-yl)-3-phenylurea.
$C_{15}H_{13}N_3O_2S$=299.3.

CAS — 26130-02-9.

Frentizole has immunosuppressant activity and has been tried in systemic lupus erythematosus; toxicity, especially liver damage, appears to be a problem. It has also been tried in idiopathic thrombocytopenic purpura.

References: J. D. O'Duffy *et al.*, *Mayo Clin. Proc.*, 1980, *55*, 601.

Manufacturers
Lilly, USA.

12773-f

FST-Sawada Antigen

FST-Sawada antigen has been used in a skin test for filariasis. Tests in proven cases of infection with *Wuchereria bancrofti, Loa loa,* and *Onchocerca volvulus* have given positive results.

FST-Sawada antigen is obtainable from Division of Malaria and Other Parasitic Diseases, World Health Organization, Geneva.— *Br. med. J.*, 1977, *2*, 170.

Further references: Second Report of the WHO Expert Committee on Filariasis, *Tech. Rep. Ser. Wld Hlth Org. No. 359*, 1967.

12775-n

Furaltadone.

Furmethonol; Nitrofurmethonum. (±)-5-Morpholinomethyl-3-(5-nitrofurfurylideneamino)oxazolidin-2-one.
$C_{13}H_{16}N_4O_6$=324.3.

CAS — 139-91-3; 59302-14-6 (±).

An odourless yellow crystalline powder with a bitter taste. M.p. about 205°. **Soluble** 1 in 2000 of water, 1 in 1000 of alcohol, 1 in 300 of chloroform; practically insoluble in ether.

Furaltadone was formerly administered by mouth as an antibacterial agent but was later withdrawn owing to its toxic effects. It has been used in veterinary medicine.

Manufacturers
Norwich-Eaton, USA.

12776-h

Furonazide.

2′-(α-Methylfurfurylidene)isonicotinohydrazide.
$C_{12}H_{11}N_3O_2$=229.2.

CAS — 3460-67-1.

Furonazide has been used in the treatment of tuberculosis.

Proprietary Names
Clitizina *(Menarini, Belg.)*; Menazone *(Menarini, Ital.).*

12777-m

Gabexate Mesylate.

Ethyl 4-(6-guanidinohexanoyloxy)benzoate methanesulphonate.
$C_{16}H_{23}N_3O_4$,CH_4SO_3=417.5.

CAS — 39492-01-8 (gabexate); 56974-61-9 (mesylate).

Gabexate mesylate is a proteolytic enzyme inhibitor used in the treatment of pancreatitis.

Proprietary Names
Foy *(Ono, Jap.).*

12778-b

Galactose.

D-Galactose.
$C_6H_{12}O_6$=180.2.

CAS — 59-23-4.

Pharmacopoeias. In *Neth.* and *Swiss.*

A white odourless crystalline or fine granular powder with a slightly sweet taste. M.p. about 168°. **Soluble** 1 in 1.7 of water and 1 in 600 of alcohol. A 4.92% solution in water is iso-osmotic with serum. Solutions are **sterilised** by autoclaving.

Galactose has been used in liver-function tests.

Galactosaemia. Hereditary galactosaemia and its treatment by a diet free from lactose and galactose.— R. G. Hansen, *J. Am. med. Ass.*, 1969, *208*, 2077.

Galactose elimination capacity. After an 8-hour fast, galactose was given by intravenous injection over a period of 3 minutes as a 25 or 30% solution in a dose of 350 mg per kg body-weight. The galactose concentrations in blood samples taken at 10-minute intervals were determined and the half-life of galactose in the blood stream calculated. Although galactose was not entirely metabolised or eliminated by the liver the results correlated with the liver's elimination capacity. The half-life was about 12 minutes in patients without liver disease.— B. Tengström, *Scand. J. clin. Lab. Invest.*, 1966, *18*, *Suppl.* 92, 132.

In 25 patients with fulminant liver failure, the galactose elimination capacity after a dose of 25 g intravenously over 5 minutes was significantly higher in 5 patients who survived (17.6 µmol per minute per kg body-weight) than in 20 who died (12.2 µmol per minute per kg). Capillary blood samples were taken every 5 minutes from 25 to 60 minutes after the start of injection and analysed enzymatically. Other routine liver tests showed no difference between the patients.— L. Ranek *et al.*, *Gut*, 1976, *17*, 959.

Influence on insulin secretion. Stimulation of pancreatic insulin secretion followed the administration of galactose by mouth and intravenously. The effect was attributed to the conversion of galactose to glucose.— K. Rommel *et al.*, *Diabetologia*, 1969, *5*, 309, per *J. Am. med. Ass.*, 1969, *210*, 1796.

12779-v

β-Galactosidase.

Lactase.

CAS — 9031-11-2.

β-Galactosidase is the enzyme involved in the hydrolysis of lactose. Deficiency of the enzyme may result in alactasia or lactose intolerance.

A discussion of lactose intolerance.— *Med. Lett.*, 1981, *23*, 67.

Proprietary Names
LactAid *(USA)*; Lactozyma, Lysolac *(both Ital.)*; Lactyme, Lamitase, Organase *(all Jap.).*

12780-r

Gallium Nitrate.

NSC-15200; WR-135675.
$Ga(NO_3)_3$,$9H_2O$=417.9.

CAS — 13494-90-1 (anhydrous).

Gallium nitrate has antineoplastic activity.

References: K. E. Kinnamon *et al.*, *Antimicrob. Ag. Chemother.*, 1979, *15*, 157; S. W. Hall *et al.*, *Clin. Pharmac. Ther.*, 1979, *25*, 82.

12781-f

Gelsemium

(B.P.C. 1973). Gelsemium Root; Jessamine; Yellow Jasmine Root. The dried rhizome and roots of *Gelsemium sempervirens* (Loganiaceae) containing not less than 0.32% of total alkaloids, calculated as gelsemine ($C_{20}H_{22}N_2O_2$ = 322.4).

CAS — 509-15-9 (gelsemine).

Adverse Effects. These include giddiness, ptosis, double vision, dilated pupils, weakness, and respiratory depression. They may be delayed for some hours and may result from quite small doses of gelsemium. Fatal doses cause slowing and arrest of the respiration.

Treatment of Adverse Effects. After ingestion of gelsemium, empty the stomach by inducing emesis or by aspiration and lavage; give atropine by subcutaneous injection; assisted respiration may be necessary.

Uses. Gelsemium depresses the central nervous system and has been used mainly in neuralgic conditions, particularly trigeminal neuralgia and migraine. It has usually been employed as the tincture given in mixtures with bromides or other sedatives.

Gelsemium is used in homoeopathic medicine.

Preparations

Compound Gelsemium and Hyoscyamus Mixture *(B.P.C. 1973).* Gelsemium tincture 0.3 ml, potassium bromide 500 mg, hyoscyamus tincture 1 ml, double-strength chloroform water 5 ml, water to 10 ml. It should be recently prepared. *Dose.* 10 to 20 ml.

Gelsemium Tincture *(B.P.C. 1973).* Tinct. Gelsem. Prepared from gelsemium by percolation with alcohol (60%) and adjusted to contain 0.03 to 0.034% w/v of total alkaloids, calculated as gelsemine. *Dose.* 0.3 to 1 ml.

Gowers' Mixture. A mixture containing gelsemium and used in the treatment of migraine. Various formulas have been used. They usually contained a bromide and strychnine as well as gelsemium tincture.

12782-d

Gestrinone. A-46745; R-2323; RU-2323.

13β-Ethyl-17β-hydroxy-18,19-dinor-17α-pregna-4,9,11-trien-20-yn-3-one.

$C_{21}H_{24}O_2$=308.4.

CAS — 16320-04-0; 40542-65-2.

Gestrinone is a progestogen which has been tried as a contraceptive. It has been given by mouth once weekly, or used as subdermal implants or as vaginal rings. It has also been tried in males for the suppression of spermatogenesis.

References: O. Akinla *et al.*, *Contraception*, 1976, *14*, 671 (vaginal rings), per *Int. pharm. Abstr.*, 1978, *15*, 315; G. Azadian-Boulanger *et al.*, *Am. J. Obstet. Gynec.*, 1976, *125*, 1049 (mid-cycle administration), per *Int. pharm. Abstr.*, 1977, *14*, 123; S. Diaz *et al.*, *Contraception*, 1977, *16*, 155 (subdermal implants), per *Int. pharm. Abstr.*, 1978, *15*, 314; W. N. Spellacy *et al.*, *Contraception*, 1978, *18*, 121 (metabolic effects during once-weekly administration), per *Int. pharm. Abstr.*, 1979, *16*, 107; R. Alvarez *et al.*, *Contraception*, 1978, *18*, 151 (subdermal implants), per *Int. pharm. Abstr.*, 1979, *16*, 107; W. N. Spellacy, *Fert. Steril.*, 1978, *30*, 289 (metabolic effects during once-weekly administration), per *Int. pharm. Abstr.*, 1979, *16*, 170; S. S. David *et al.*, *Fert. Steril.*, 1979, *31*, 278 (once-weekly administration), per *Int. pharm. Abstr.*, 1979, *16*, 1113.

12783-n

Gibberellic Acid. GA; Gibberellin A_3.

$C_{19}H_{22}O_6$=346.4.

CAS — 77-06-5.

Gibberellins are plant growth stimulators obtained from culture filtrates of the fungus *Gibberella fujikuroi*. Gibberellic acid is **soluble** 1 in 170 of water and soluble in alcohol, acetone, and methyl alcohol. Aqueous solutions lose potency when stored and should be freshly prepared.

Gibberellic acid is the most important of the gibberellins and is has been used for promoting the growth of plants.

12784-h

Ginseng. Ginseng Radix; Ninjin; Panax; Pannag. The dried root of *Panax ginseng* (= *P. schinseng*) (Araliaceae). Other varieties of ginseng include *Panax quinquefolium* (North America) and *P. pseudoginseng*.

Pharmacopoeias. In *Chin.*, *Jap.*, and *Rus. Chin.* also includes Radix Notoginseng from *P. notoginseng*. Red Gingseng (*Jap. P.*) is the dried root of *P. ginseng* which has been steamed. Panax Rhizome (*Jap. P.*) is the rhizome of *P. japonicum*.

Ginseng contains a mixture of several saponin glycosides termed ginsenosides. The main ones are based on the aglycones oleanolic acid, (20*S*)-protopanaxadiol, and (20*S*)-protopanaxtriol. The sugars glucose, rhamnose, arabinose, and xylose are present in varying amounts.

Studies in *animals* have demonstrated that ginseng has a wide range of pharmacological activities but their possible clinical significance has not been elucidated by controlled studies in man. Ginseng has been claimed to enhance the natural resistance and recuperative power of the body and to have both stimulant and sedative activity. Its toxicity appears to be low. It is used as a decoction, liquid extract, or as a powder.

For reviews of ginseng, see W. E. Court, *Pharm. J.*, 1975, *1*, 180; E. J. Shellard, *Chemist Drugg.*, 1978, *210*, 370; L. Cartwright, *Aust. J. Pharm.*, 1979, *60*, 346; *Med. Lett.*, 1980, *22*, 72.

Ginseng was used in Chinese medicine in the People's Republic of China for weakness after vomiting of blood, for menorrhagia, and for vomiting. It was also used with other herbal remedies for rectocele, fever, gasping, excessive sweating, and thirst.— *Herbal Pharmacology in the People's Republic of China: A Trip Report of the American Herbal Pharmacology Delegation*, Washington D.C., National Academy of Sciences, 1975.

A 2-year study of ginseng in 133 subjects who had used a wide variety of commercial preparations including roots, capsules, tablets, teas, extracts, cigarettes, chewing gum, and candies. The majority of preparations were taken by mouth but a few subjects had experimented with intranasal or parenteral routes and topical preparations had also been used. The stimulant effects of ginseng were confirmed but there was also a high incidence of side-effects including morning diarrhoea (47 subjects), skin eruptions (33), sleeplessness (26), nervousness (25), hypertension (22), euphoria (18), and oedema (14). The 'ginseng abuse syndrome' defined as hypertension together with nervousness, sleeplessness, skin eruptions, and morning diarrhoea was experienced by 14 subjects who took ginseng by mouth in an average daily dose of 3 g. Abrupt withdrawal precipitated hypotension, weakness, and tremor in one user. About 50% of the subjects had discontinued the use of ginseng within 2 years.— R. K. Siegel, *J. Am. med. Ass.*, 1979, *241*, 1614. Comment.— R. K. Siegel (letter), *ibid.*, 1980, *243*, 32.

The analytical, pharmacological, and clinical aspects of ginseng were considered at an international symposium at Lugano, 1975, sponsored by the World Health Organization and *Pharmaton, Switz.* and a similar symposium at Singapore, 1977, sponsored by *Pharmaton, Switz.*

Oestrogenic effects. A 70-year-old woman developed swollen tender breasts with diffuse nodularity on 3 occasions after taking ginseng.— B. V. Palmer (letter), *Br. med. J.*, 1978, *1*, 1284. See also *ibid.*, 1556; M. N. G. Dukes (letter), *ibid.*, 1621.

A report of an oestrogen-like effect on the vaginal epithelium in a 62-year-old woman taking ginseng.— R. Punnonen and R. Lukola, *Br. med. J.*, 1980, *281*, 1110.

12785-m

Glaziovine. (±)-1,2,2a,3,4,5-Hexahydro-8-hydroxy-7-methoxy-3-methylcyclopent[*ij*]isoquinoline-1-spiro-1′-cyclohexa-2′,5′-dien-4′-one.

$C_{18}H_{19}NO_3$=297.4.

CAS — 6808-72-6; 17127-48-9 (±).

Glaziovine is an alkaloid obtained from *Ocotea glaziovii* or prepared synthetically.

Glaziovine is reported to have tranquillising and antidepressant properties.

References: B. Buffa *et al.*, *Curr. ther. Res.*, 1974, *16*, 621; D. Sardini and A. Marzo, *Farmaco, Edn prat.*, 1977, *32*, 503; A. Marzo *et al.*, *Eur. J. clin. Pharmac.*, 1978, *13*, 219.

Proprietary Names

Suavedol *(Simes, Ital.)*.

12786-b

Glipentide. Glypentide; UR-661. 1-Cyclopentyl-3-[*p*-(2-*o*-anisamidoethyl)benzenesulphonyl]urea.

$C_{22}H_{27}N_3O_5S$=445.5.

CAS — 32797-92-5.

Glipentide is a sulphonylurea hypoglycaemic agent.

In a study on 22 patients with maturity-onset diabetes uncontrolled by diet, glipentide was shown to have similar hypoglycaemic potency to glibenclamide. The daily requirement of glipentide ranged from 2.5 to 10 mg, and could be given as a single dose at breakfast.— E. M. Lorenzo *et al.*, *Curr. ther. Res.*, 1977, *21*, 50.

Proprietary Names

Staticum *(Uriach, Spain)*.

12787-v

Glisolamide. 1-Cyclohexyl-3-{[*p*-[2-(5-methylisoxazole-3-carboxamido)ethyl]benzene]sulphonyl}urea.

$C_{20}H_{26}N_4O_5S$=434.5.

CAS — 24477-37-0.

Glisolamide is a sulphonylurea used in the treatment of diabetes mellitus.

Proprietary Names

Diabenor *(IFI, Ital.)*.

12788-g

Gloxazone. BW-356-C-61. 3-Ethoxy-2-oxobutyraldehyde bis(thiosemicarbazone).

$C_8H_{16}N_6OS_2$=276.4.

CAS — 2507-91-7.

Gloxazone has been tried in the treatment of anaplasmosis in cattle.

Proprietary Names

Contrapar *(Wellcome, UK)*.

12789-q

Gluconiazide. D-Glucuronic acid γ-lactone 1-(isonicotinoylhydrazone).

$C_{12}H_{13}N_3O_6$=295.3.

CAS — 3691-74-5.

Gluconiazide has been used in the treatment of tuberculosis.

Proprietary Names

Glucazide *(Stholl, Ital.)*; Guidazide *(Guidotti, Ital.)*.

12790-d

Glucosamine. NSC-758; Chitosamine. 2-Amino-2-deoxy-β-D-glucopyranose.

$C_6H_{13}NO_5$=179.2.

CAS — 3416-24-8.

Glucosamine is found in chitin, mucoproteins, and mucopolysaccharides; it is isolated from chitin or prepared synthetically.

Needle crystals. M.p. 110° with decomposition. Very **soluble** in water; soluble 1 in 38 of boiling methyl alcohol; sparingly soluble in cold methyl alcohol and alcohol; practically insoluble in chloroform and ether.

Glucosamine sulphate and hydriodide have been given in the treatment of rheumatic disorders. The hydrochloride has also been used.

References: A. Drovanti *et al.*, *Clin. Ther.*, 1980, *3*, 260; G. Crolle and E. D'Este, *Curr. med. Res. Opinion*, 1980, *7*, 104; J. M. Pujalte *et al.*, *ibid.*, 110; E. D'Ambrosio *et al.*, *Pharmatherapeutica*, 1981, *2*, 504; Y. Vajaradul, *Clin. Ther.*, 1981, *3*, 336.

Proprietary Names of Glucosamine Sulphate

Adaxil *(with the hydriodide) (Spedrog-Caillon, Arg.)*; Anartril *(with the hydriodide) (Farma-Lepori, Spain)*; Arthryl *(with the hydriodide) (Synlab, Fr.)*; Dona *(Opfermann, Ger.)*; Viartril *(with the hydriodide) (Rotta, Ital.)*.

12791-n

Glutaminase

CAS — 9001-47-2.

An enzyme obtained from *Achromobacter* spp. which hydrolyses glutamine and asparagine.

Glutaminase has been tried, similarly to colaspase (p.198), in the treatment of acute leukaemia. It depletes blood glutamine for about 12 hours.

References: A. S. D. Spiers and H. E. Wade, *Br. med. J.*, 1976, *1*, 1317.

12792-h

Gluten. A mixture of 2 proteins, gliadin and glutenin, present in wheat flour and to a lesser extent in barley, oats, and rye. Gliadin is a prolamine, one of the 2 chief groups of plant proteins, and glutenin belongs to the other main group termed glutelins.

CAS — 8002-80-0.

Gluten is of medicinal and pharmaceutical interest in that patients with coeliac disease (non-tropical sprue; primary malabsorption syndrome; idiopathic steatorrhoea; gluten-induced enteropathy) are sensitive to the gliadin fraction of gluten contained in the normal diet. Claims that only the α-gliadin fraction is toxic have not been substantiated. Treatment consists of the use of gluten-free diets; wheat products are particularly to be avoided. Rye, which contains a small amount of gluten, and barley and oats, which contain the prolamines hordein and avenin respectively, should also be excluded from the diet of patients with coeliac disease.

A warning that some prescription medicines contained gluten and should be avoided by patients on a gluten-free diet. They included Dimotane LA, Dimotapp LA, Donnatal LA, Fybranta, Nardil, Natirose, Nulacin, Saroten, and Veracolate.— *Br. med. J.*, 1976, *2*, 185.

A discussion on transient gluten intolerance.— J. A. Walker-Smith, *Practitioner*, 1978, *220*, 562.

A report of a child who was sensitive to wheat and who responded to a gluten-free dietary regimen yet who did not suffer from coeliac disease. She was considered to have a hereditary genetic disposition.— A. Jonas (letter), *Lancet*, 1978, *2*, 1047.

Mention of the use of prolamine (a rapidly solidifying aminoacid solution) to occlude the pancreatic duct to exclude any still present excretory pancreatic function in the residual pancreatic tissue during partial duodenopancreatectomy.— F. P. Gall and C. Gebhardt, *Dt. med. Wschr.*, 1979, *104*, 1003.

Coeliac disease. Reviews, reports, and comments on gluten and coeliac disease: *Br. med. J.*, 1973, *2*, 130; P. G. Baker *et al.*, *ibid.*, 1975, *1*, 486; C. Edwards and P. Stillman, *Pharm. J.*, 1979, *1*, 463; J. A. Dodge, *Archs Dis. Childh.*, 1980, *55*, 143; J. M. Littlewood *et al.* (letter), *Lancet*, 1980, *2*, 1359; D. N. Challacombe and J. M. Baylis (letter), *ibid.*, 1360; T. Lindberg (letter), *ibid.*, 1981, *1*, 449.

References to α-gliadin and mechanisms of gluten toxicity in coeliac disease: A. S. Dissanayake *et al.*, *Lancet*, 1973, *2*, 709; D. A. Hudson *et al.*, *ibid.*, 1976, *1*, 339; M. M. Weiser and A. P. Douglas, *ibid.*, 567; *Br. med. J.*, 1978, *1*, 3; P. J. Ciclitira *et al.*, *Lancet*, 1980, *2*, 234; A. L. Patey (letter), *ibid.*, 427.

For data on the protein content of cereals, see P. G. Baker (letter), *Lancet*, 1975, *2*, 1307; P. G. Baker and A. E. Read, *Postgrad. med. J.*, 1976, *52*, 264.

In a series of 202 patients with coeliac disease, 37 of the 97 deaths between 1941 and 1975 had been caused by malignant disease, particularly reticulum cell sarcoma and gastro-intestinal cancer. A gluten-free diet did not appear to protect against malignant complications but a longer follow-up would be needed.— G. K. T. Holmes *et al.*, *Gut*, 1976, *17*, 612.

Advice that children with coeliac disease must adhere to a gluten-free diet indefinitely.— A. S. McNeish, *Archs Dis. Childh.*, 1980, *55*, 110. Suggestions for the flavouring of gluten, acceptable to children.— G. Lloyd (letter), *Pharm. J.*, 1977, *2*, 113.

Diagnosis. Comment on coeliac disease and its diagnosis.— *Lancet*, 1981, *1*, 593.

A protocol for gluten challenge to diagnose coeliac disease.— C. J. Rolles and A. S. McNeish, *Br. med. J.*, 1976, *1*, 1309. Comment on the variable response to gluten challenge.— *Lancet*, 1979, *2*, 1169.

References to a skin test for coeliac disease using a subfraction of gluten: B. S. Anand *et al.*, *Lancet*, 1977, *1*, 118; *ibid.*, 130; R. F. A. Logan and A. Ferguson (letter), *ibid.*, 1978, *2*, 1042; R. E. Offord *et al.* (letter), *ibid.*, 1043; S. Auricchio *et al.* (letter), *ibid.*, 1979, *1*, 611.

An immunological assay for coeliac disease.— A. Ashkenazi *et al.*, *Lancet*, 1981, *1*, 914.

Dermatitis herpetiformis. Comment on dermatitis herpetiformis and its association with gluten-sensitive enteropathy (coeliac disease).— *Lancet*, 1978, *2*, 458.

Reports on the beneficial effect of a gluten-free diet in some patients with dermatitis herpetiformis.— L. Fry *et al.*, *Lancet*, 1973, *1*, 288; T. Reunala *et al.*, *Br. J. Derm.*, 1977, *97*, 473; C. I. Harrington and N. W. Read, *Br. med. J.*, 1977, *1*, 872; K. Ljunghall and U. M. Tjernlund (letter), *Lancet*, 1978, *2*, 1003.

Multiple sclerosis. Comparison of jejunal biopsy samples from 11 patients with multiple sclerosis and 11 control subjects demonstrated no evidence that gluten sensitivity has any role in the aetiology of multiple sclerosis.— M. C. Bateson *et al.*, *Lancet*, 1979, *1*, 1108.

Schizophrenia. In a double-blind study in 14 patients with schizophrenia on constant antipsychotic therapy, there was deterioration of their condition when challenged with wheat gluten.— M. M. Singh and S. R. Kay, *Science*, 1976, *191*, 401. Comment.— *Lancet*, 1976, *1*, 844.

A study indicating that 7 autistic children and one child believed to have childhood schizophrenia, were not benefiting from gluten-free dietary regimens.— D. M. McCarthy and M. Coleman, *Lancet*, 1979, *2*, 877.

Preparations

For some gluten-free dietary preparations, see p.63.

12794-b

Glyceryl Mono-octanoate. Mono-octanoin. $C_{11}H_{22}O_4=218.3$.

CAS — 26402-26-6.

A preparation containing glyceryl mono-octanoate 70% has been used, by perfusion, for the dissolution of gall-stones.

References: U. Leuschner *et al.* (letter), *Lancet*, 1979, *2*, 103; B. Schmack *et al.* (letter), *ibid.*, 1979, *2*, 423; J. L. Thistle *et al.*, *Gastroenterology*, 1980, *78*, 1016; L. Witzel *et al.* (letter), *New Engl. J. Med.*, 1980, *303*, 465; L. N. Jarrett *et al.*, *Lancet*, 1981, *1*, 68; U. Leuschner and H. Baumgärtel (letter), *ibid.*, 336; J. C. K. Lojenga and A. A. van Sorge (letter), *ibid.*; P. B. Cotton *et al.* (letter), *ibid.*, 436; E. Mack *et al.*, *Archs Surg.*, 1981, *116*, 341; T. R. Gadacz, *Surgery, St Louis*, 1981, *89*, 527.

Proprietary Names

Capmul 8210.

12795-v

Glyguetol. Guaietolin; Glycerylguethol. 3-(2-Ethoxyphenoxy)propane-1,2-diol. $C_{11}H_{16}O_4=212.2$.

CAS — 63834-83-3.

The ethoxy analogue of guaiphenesin. It has been used as a mucolytic agent.

Proprietary Names

Guéthural *(Élerté, Fr.)*.

12796-g

Glypressin. Triglycyl-lysine-vasopressin; Terlipressin. *N*-[*N*-(*N*-Glycylglycyl)glycyl]lypressin.

$C_{52}H_{74}N_{16}O_{15}S_2=1227.4$.

CAS — 14636-12-5.

Glypressin is a synthetic analogue of vasopressin. It has been given for the arrest of uterine bleeding.

References: J. Vosmík *et al.*, *Gastroenterology*, 1977, *72*, 605; M. Akerlund and T. Laudánski, *Br. J. Obstet. Gynaec.*, 1978, *85*, 525; V. Pavlín *et al.*, *ibid.*, 801; J. C. Douglas *et al.*, *Gut*, 1979, *20*, 565; C. V. Prowse *et al.*, *Eur. J. clin. Invest.*, 1980, *10*, 49.

Proprietary Names

Glycylpressin (acetate) *(Ferring, Ger.)*.

12797-q

Gold Keratinate. Aurothiopolypeptide.

CAS — 9078-78-8.

A gold compound stated to contain 13% of Au.

It has been used in the treatment of arthritic disorders.

Proprietary Names

Auro-Detoxin *(Beecham-Wülfing, Ger.)*.

12798-p

Gossypol. 2,2′-Bis(1,6,7-trihydroxy-3-methyl-5-isopropylnaphthalene-8-carboxaldehyde). $C_{30}H_{30}O_8=518.6$.

CAS — 303-45-7.

Gossypol is an ingredient extracted from cottonseed oil.

Gossypol is being studied, especially in China, as a male contraceptive.

Side-effects have included weakness, changes in appetite, gastro-intestinal effects, and some loss of libido. Hypokalaemia has occurred.

Gossypol acetate and gossypol formate have been used.

Brief discussions: *Lancet*, 1979, *1*, 395; A. de Peyster and Y. Y. Wang (letter), *New Engl. J. Med.*, 1979, *301*, 275; *Med. J. Aust.*, 1979, *2*, 121; *Practitioner*, 1979, *223*, 428; H. Pösö *et al.* (letter), *Lancet*, 1980, *1*, 885.

Further references: *Chin. med. J.*, 1978, *4*, 417; *Gynec. obstet. Invest.*, 1979, *10*, 163; K. -F. Cheng *et al.*, *Am. J. Obstet. Gynec.*, 1980, *138*, 1227; *Chin. med. J.*, 1980, *93*, 477.

12799-s

Graphites. A mineral form of carbon, containing a small amount of iron.

CAS — 7782-42-5.

Graphites is used in homoeopathic medicine.

12800-s

Guabenxan. 1-(1,4-Benzodioxan-6-ylmethyl)guanidine. $C_{10}H_{13}N_3O_3=223.2$.

CAS — 19889-45-3.

Guabenxan is used, as the sulphate, as an antihypertensive agent.

Proprietary Names

Tensigradyl (with a thiazide diuretic) *(Oberval, Fr.)*.

12801-w

Guacetisal. Acetylsalicylic Acid Guaiacol Ester. 2-Methoxyphenyl 2-acetoxybenzoate. $C_{16}H_{14}O_5=286.3$.

CAS — 55482-89-8.

Guacetisal has been given by mouth and as suppositories for painful respiratory disorders.

Proprietary Names

Broncaspin *(Bayer, Ital.)*.

12802-e

Guaiacol Phenylacetate. 2-Methoxyphenyl phenylacetate. $C_{15}H_{14}O_3=242.3$.

CAS — 4112-89-4.

Guaiacol phenylacetate is used for its reputed mucolytic and expectorant properties.

Proprietary Names

Gujaphenyl *(Galactina, Ger.)*; Gunyl *(Galactina, Switz.)*.

12803-l

Guaiapate. MG-5454. 1-{2-[2-(2-*o*-Methoxyphenoxyethoxy)ethoxy]ethyl}piperidine.
$C_{18}H_{29}NO_4$=323.4.

CAS — 852-42-6.

Guaiapate has been used for the relief of cough.

Proprietary Names
Klamar *(Maggioni, Ital.).*

12804-y

Guamecycline Dihydrochloride. *N*[2]-(4-Guanidinoformimidoylpiperazin-1-ylmethyl)tetracycline dihydrochloride.
$C_{29}H_{38}N_8O_8$,2HCl=699.6.

CAS — 16545-11-2 (guamecycline); 19115-46-9 (xHCl).

An antibiotic with the general properties of tetracycline.

Proprietary Names
Bronco-Was *(Wassermann, Spain)*; Guanamycine *(Prospa, Belg.)*; Xantociclina *(SPA, Ital.).*

12805-j

Guanazodine Sulphate. Egyt-739. 1-(Octahydroazocin-2-ylmethyl)guanidine sulphate monohydrate.
$C_9H_{20}N_4$,H_2SO_4,H_2O=300.4.

CAS — 32059-15-7 (guanazodine); 42839-36-1 (sulphate, anhydrous).

Guanazodine sulphate is an antihypertensive agent.

References: W. Reiterer and H. Czitober, *Arzneimittel-Forsch.*, 1977, *27*, 2163; B. Síró *et al.*, *Therapia hung.*, 1977, *25*, 134.

Proprietary Names
Sanegyt *(EGYT, Hung.).*

12806-z

Guanfacine Hydrochloride. BS-100-141; LON-798. *N*-Amidino-2-(2,6-dichlorophenyl)acetamide hydrochloride.
$C_9H_9Cl_2N_3O$,HCl=282.6.

CAS — 29110-47-2 (guanfacine); 29110-48-3 (hydrochloride).

Guanfacine hydrochloride 1.15 mg is approximately equivalent to 1 mg of guanfacine.

Adverse Effects. Guanfacine has adverse effects similar to those of clonidine (p.139). Dryness of the mouth and sedation are the effects most frequently reported especially in the initial stages of treatment.

A report on side-effects and withdrawal symptoms encountered in 580 hypertensive patients treated with guanfacine for 1 year and 169 patients who continued treatment for a second year. The most frequent side-effect was dryness of the mouth but the overall incidence of 60% during the first year had fallen to 15% by the end of the year. Sedation occurred in 33% of patients and had fallen to 5.7% by the end of the first year. Other side-effects reported during the first and second years respectively included orthostatic disturbances (15 and 6.5%), constipation (14 and 4.1%), male sexual dysfunction (4.6 and 0.6%), insomnia (5.5 and 2.2%), gastro-intestinal discomfort (4.1 and 2.2%), and sweating (5.3 and 1.7%). Sinus bradycardia was seen in only 12 patients and was transient in 9. The frequency and severity of adverse effects was dose-related and doses of 2 mg or less caused virtually no dry mouth. A withdrawal syndrome occurred in 2 to 4% of patients 2 to 7 days after discontinuation of guanfacine. No signs of tachyphylaxis or tolerance were seen.— P. Jerie, *Sandoz, Switz., Br. J. clin. Pharmac.*, 1980, *10, Suppl.* 1, 157S.

Absorption and Fate. Guanfacine is absorbed from the gastro-intestinal tract. It is reported to enter the brain more slowly than clonidine.

A review of the pharmacokinetics and metabolism of guanfacine. Absorption from the gastro-intestinal tract is rapid and complete with no evidence of any first-pass effect and distribution is characterised by low blood concentrations, low plasma protein binding, and a relatively high affinity for tissues. After single doses the mean elimination half-life was 17.7 hours after intravenous and 21.4 hours after oral administration respectively with 85 and 82% of a dose excreted in the urine in 4 days. Major metabolites were the glucuronide and sulphate of 3-hydroxy guanfacine, which represented about 50% of the amounts excreted in the urine in 48 hours.— J. R. Kiechel, *Br. J. clin. Pharmac.*, 1980, *10, Suppl.* 1, 25S.

In 5 healthy subjects given the equivalent of 3 mg of guanfacine by mouth, peak plasma concentrations occurred at 1.5 to 4 hours and ranged from 9.2 to 11.7 ng per ml in 4 subjects, while the fifth subject had a much lower peak concentration of 4.5 ng per ml. The mean plasma half-life was 12.1 hours (range 9.4 to 15.3 hours) and plasma concentrations 24 hours after the dose were about 3 ng per ml. At 24 hours about 37% of the guanfacine had been excreted unchanged in the urine.— C. T. Dollery and D. S. Davies, *Br. J. clin. Pharmac.*, 1980, *10, Suppl.* 1, 5S.

Results in patients with normal and impaired renal function suggested that non-renal elimination of guanfacine plays an important role in patients with renal failure.— W. Kirch *et al.*, *Br. J. clin. Pharmac.*, 1980, *10, Suppl.* 1, 33S.

Further references: M. Guerret *et al.*, *J. pharm. Sci.*, 1979, *68*, 219; Y. A. Weiss *et al.*, *Clin. Pharmac. Ther.*, 1979, *25*, 283; W. Kirch *et al.*, *Clin. Pharmacokinet.*, 1980, *5*, 476.

Uses. Guanfacine is a centrally acting antihypertensive agent with actions and uses similar to those of clonidine (p.140). Guanfacine hydrochloride has been given by mouth in the treatment of hypertension in usual doses equivalent to 2 mg of guanfacine daily, with a range of 0.5 to 6 mg daily.

A symposium on guanfacine hydrochloride.— *Br. J. clin. Pharmac.*, 1980, *10, Suppl.* 1, 1–208S.

An evaluation of guanfacine in 580 hypertensive patients treated for 1 year and in 169 who continued for a second year. Initial doses of 0.5 mg twice daily were increased gradually according to response and a diuretic, beta-blocker, or vasodilator added if necessary. Mean daily doses of guanfacine after 1 year were the equivalent of 3.4 mg for monotherapy and 6 mg for combined therapy; after 2 years mean doses were 3.2 and 5 mg respectively. In general guanfacine was found to be an effective antihypertensive agent. Once daily or twice daily dosage regimens were recommended.— P. Jerie, *Sandoz, Switz., Br. J. clin. Pharmac.*, 1980, *10, Suppl.* 1, 37S.

Guanfacine in relatively high single doses of 3 or 4 mg cuased a substantial fall in supine and standing blood pressure within 6 hours; the effect was maximal by 10 to 12 hours and lasted for more than 36 hours. A recommended initial dose in routine practice was the equivalent of 0.5 to 1 mg. Maintenance doses ranged rom 2 to 6 mg daily.— C. Zamboulis and J. L. Reid, *Clin. Pharmac. Ther.*, 1980, *28*, 715.

In a study of 5 healthy subjects guanfacine 3 mg by mouth had a similar antihypertensive effect to that of clonidine 0.3 mg but its onset of action was slower, beginning about 2 hours after a dose and reaching a maximum at 6 hours, and the duration of action was longer.— C. T. Dollery and D. S. Davies, *Br. J. clin. Pharmac.*, 1980, *10, Suppl.* 1, 5S.

Further references: A. Jäättelä, *Eur. J. clin. Pharmac.*, 1976, *10*, 69; *idem*, 73; U. C. Dubach *et al.*, *Arzneimittel-Forsch.*, 1977, *27*, 674; I. Lancranjan and P. Marbach, *Sandoz* (letter), *Br. med. J.*, 1977, *1*, 1472; *idem, Metabolism*, 1977, *26*, 1225; W. Kirch and A. Distler, *Int. J. clin. Pharmac. Biopharm.*, 1978, *16*, 132; P. MacCarthy *et al.*, *Clin. exp. Pharmac. Physiol.*, 1978, *5*, 187; Y. K. Seedat, *Curr. ther. Res.*, 1978, *24*, 288; S. Lochaya *et al.*, *Am. Heart J.*, 1980, *99*, 58; C. J. van der Merwe and S. A. Kruger, *S. Afr. med. J.*, 1980, *57*, 400; A. J. Bune *et al.*, *Eur. J. clin. Pharmac.*, 1981, *19*, 309; M. Karesoja and H. Takkunen, *Curr. ther. Res.*, 1981, *29*, 60; C. Zamboulis and J. L. Reid, *Eur. J. clin. Pharmac.*, 1981, *19*, 19.

Proprietary Names
Estulic *(Wander, Belg.; Sandoz, Eire; Sandoz, Fr.; Wander, Ger.; Sandoz, Greece; Sandoz, Neth.; Sandoz, Switz.).*

12807-c

Guanidine Hydrochloride. Carbamidine Hydrochloride; Iminourea Hydrochloride.
CH_5N_3,HCl=95.53.

CAS — 113-00-8 (guanidine); 50-01-1 (hydrochloride).

A white crystalline powder. Very **soluble** in water and alcohol. A 1.47% solution in water is iso-osmotic with serum.

Adverse Effects. The most serious side-effect of guanidine is suppression of the bone marrow; this may be dose-related.

Guanidine in a dose of 21 mg per kg body-weight caused diarrhoea, salivation, hypotension, and atrial fibrillation in a 70-year-old patient with carcinoma of the lung. When given a second time in the same dose, guanidine caused the same arrhythmia.— K. K. Nakano and H. R. Tyler (letter), *Ann. intern. Med.*, 1972, *77*, 658.

Adverse reactions to guanidine were more varied and more serious than was generally recognised. Minor side-effects included mild gastro-intestinal disturbances (which could be controlled with atropine) and paraesthesias of the lips, face, hands, and feet. More disturbing neurological symptoms were hyperirritability, tremor, ataxia, and rare seizures; administration of calcium had been shown to control the neurological symptoms. Unusual side-effects included atrial fibrillation and hypotension, skin reactions, hypoglycaemia, and raised blood-creatinine concentrations. Suppression of bone marrow was the most serious side-effect recorded.— S. J. Oh and K. W. Kim, *Neurology, Minneap.*, 1973, *23*, 1084.

Guanidine hydrochloride was associated with markedly increased weakness in 2 Chinese patients with motor neurone disease. This effect appeared to be dose-related and Oriental men might be more sensitive to the postulated guanidine-induced depletion of axonal acetylcholine.— F. H. Norris *et al.*, *Neurology, Minneap.*, 1974, *24*, 135, per *J. Am. med. Ass.*, 1974, *228*, 783.

Bone-marrow depression. Guanidine caused bone-marrow depression in 3 of 150 patients treated for amyotrophic lateral sclerosis.— F. H. Norris *et al.*, *Archs Neurol., Chicago*, 1974, *30*, 184, per *J. Am. med. Ass.*, 1974, *227*, 688.

Effects on the kidney. Severe fibrosing interstitial nephritis in an elderly man was possibly due to guanidine which he had taken, in a dose of 250 mg four times daily, for about 7 years for the control of the Eaton-Lambert syndrome.— L. D. Blumhardt *et al.*, *Br. med. J.*, 1977, *1*, 946.

Uses. Guanidine hydrochloride has been used in the Eaton-Lambert syndrome; it has been tried in myasthenia gravis and other neurological disorders with less satisfactory results. It has also been tried in the treatment of botulism.

A review of guanidine hydrochloride.— S. Gerrard, *J. Hosp. Pharm.*, 1975, *33*, 15.

The pharmacodynamics of guanidine hydrochloride in healthy subjects.— W. Mayer and A. Komarek, *Arzneimittel-Forsch.*, 1978, *28*, 680.

Amyotrophic lateral sclerosis. Twenty-four patients with amyotrophic lateral sclerosis were randomly assigned to guanidine 2 or 25 mg per kg body-weight daily. At 10 months 6 of 13 patients in the lower dose group had died compared with 2 of 11 in the higher dose group; no patient improved although the higher dose group had had significantly more stable cases up to 6 months. It was considered that although administration of guanidine might confer short-term benefit the risk of major side-effects including acute paralysis and bone-marrow depression should be balanced against the possiblity of the disease taking a relatively benign course.— F. H. Norris *et al.*, *Neurology, Minneap.*, 1974, *24*, 721, per *J. Am. med. Ass.*, 1974, *230*, 1344.

Botulism. Improvement in limb and eye muscle weakness but not in respiratory muscle weakness was reported within 48 hours in 2 patients with botulism who received 35 mg per kg body-weight daily of guanidine hydrochloride.— M. Puggiari and M. Cherington, *J. Am. med. Ass.*, 1978, *240*, 2276.

Further references: M. Cherington, *Archs Neurol., Chicago*, 1974, *30*, 432; M. Cherington and D. Schultz, *Clin. Toxicol.*, 1977, *11*, 19.

Eaton-Lambert syndrome. Administration of guanidine in doses of 12 to 58.3 mg per kg body-weight daily brought about clinical and electrophysiological improvement in 3 patients with the Eaton-Lambert syndrome.

Guanidine was the drug of choice in the Eaton-Lambert syndrome and could reverse the basic defect of neuromuscular transmission in this condition.— S. J. Oh and K. W. Kim, *Neurology, Minneap.*, 1973, *23*, 1084.

Myasthenia gravis. A report of increased neuromuscular block and clinical worsening in 3 patients with severe myasthenia gravis who received guanidine.— J. C. Brown and R. J. Johns, *Johns Hopkins med. J.*, 1969, *124*, 1, per *J. Am. med. Ass.*, 1969, *207*, 1551.

12808-k

Guanoxabenz Hydrochloride.

43-663 *(guanoxabenz)*. 1-(2,6-Dichlorobenzylideneamino)-3-hydroxyguanidine hydrochloride.
$C_8H_8Cl_2N_4O,HCl=283.5$.

CAS — 24047-25-4 (guanoxabenz).

Guanoxabenz hydrochloride has been used as an antihypertensive agent.

Proprietary Names
Benzérial *(Houdé-I.S.H., Fr.)*.

12809-a

Gutta Percha *(U.S.P., B.P.C. 1949)*.

Gutt. Perch.; Gummi Plasticum.

Pharmacopoeias. In *Span.* and *U.S.*

The coagulated, dried, purified latex of trees of the genera *Palaquium* and *Payena* and most commonly *Palaquium gutta* (Sapotaceae).
It occurs in lumps or blocks with a slight characteristic odour and is of a brown or greyish-brown or greyish-white colour externally and reddish-yellow or reddish-grey internally with a laminated or fibrous appearance; it is flexible, but only slightly elastic. Practically **insoluble** in water; partly soluble in carbon disulphide and turpentine oil; almost entirely soluble in chloroform.

Gutta percha has been used in various dressings. In dentistry, gutta percha has been used as a filling material and as the basis of compounds for taking dental impressions.

12810-e

Haematin.

Hematin; Ferriheme Hydroxide; Ferriprotoporphyrin Hydroxide.
$C_{34}H_{32}N_4O_4,FeOH=633.5$.

CAS — 15489-90-4.

Haematin is the ferric iron complex of protoporphyrin IX and is formed from haemoglobin. It has been used in the treatment of acute porphyria.

A method for the preparation of haematin injection.— J. R. B. J. Brouwers, *Pharm. Weekbl. Ned. scient. Edn*, 1979, *1*, 33, per *Int. pharm. Abstr.*, 1980, *17*, 102.

Porphyria. Administration of haematin should be as early as possible in an attack of porphyria not only to correct the biochemical abnormalities but also to prevent chronic porphyric neuropathy.— C. A. Pierach and C. J. Watson (letter), *Lancet*, 1978, *1*, 1361.

A 33-year-old woman who suffered regular monthly attacks of porphyria with her menstrual periods, which were not alleviated by hormone therapy, obtained complete relief on weekly intravenous administration of haematin 200 mg for 6 months. Her symptoms recurred on stopping the prophylactic haematin therapy.— J. M. Lamon *et al.*, *Lancet*, 1978, *2*, 492.

A prolonged attack of porphyria in a 29-year-old woman was terminated by a 3-day course of haematin 4 mg per kg body-weight daily administered over 20 minutes into a slow-running intravenous infusion of sodium chloride injection. A further course of 4 mg per kg every 12 hours for 3 days was again dramatically successful 7 weeks later. Since previous infusions of laevulose had damaged her veins, the infusions had to be given into small peripheral veins which caused mild temporary irritation, but haematin appears to be less destructive of veins than laevulose.— K. E. L. McColl *et al.*, *Lancet*, 1979, *1*, 133.

Further references: G. J. Dhar *et al.*, *Ann. intern. Med.*, 1975, *83*, 20; A. Peterson *et al.*, *J. Am. med. Ass.*, 1976, *235*, 520; K. E. L. McColl *et al.*, *Gut*, 1980, *21*, A898.

12811-l

Haematoporphyrin.

A red pigment free from iron obtained from haematin.
$C_{34}H_{38}N_4O_6=598.7$.

CAS — 14459-29-1.

Haematoporphyrin has been used in the treatment of anaemia, debility, and depressive states.

A complex of haematoporphyrin with deanol (Hematodeanol) reduced the CNS depression induced by pentobarbitone and delayed hypothermia induced by reserpine in animals.— A. Brucato *et al.*, *Arzneimittel-Forsch.*, 1977, *27*, 1015.

Photosensitisation in 2 patients after the intravenous use of haematoporphyrin.— G. L. Zalar *et al.*, *Archs Derm.*, 1977, *113*, 1392.

Discussion on the use of a haematoporphyrin derivative, activated by light energy, as a treatment for tumours.— G. McBride, *J. Am. med. Ass.*, 1979, *242*, 403.

Proprietary Names
Ematodyn *(dihydrochloride) (Cifa, Ital.)*; Hémédonine *(Laboratoires de l'Hémédonine, Fr.)*; Porfidyna *(Spain)*.

12812-y

Haemoglobin.

The red pigment of red blood cells. It is a tetrameric compound, each of the 4 subunits consisting of an iron-protoporphyrin complex containing 1 atom of ferrous iron (haem), in association with a polypeptide (globin).

Haemoglobin has the property of reversible oxygenation and is the respiratory pigment of blood. It contains about 0.34% of iron and it has been used in iron-deficiency anaemias as a substitute for iron salts but it is much less effective.

Manufacturers
Harimex-Ligos, Neth.

12813-j

Halofuginone.

(±)-*trans*-7-Bromo-6-chloro-3-[3-(3-hydroxy-2-piperidyl)acetonyl]quinazolin-4(3*H*)-one.
$C_{16}H_{17}BrClN_3O_3=414.7$.

CAS — 55837-20-2.

Halofuginone is used for the prevention of coccidiosis in poultry.

Proprietary Names
Stenorol *(Hoechst, UK)*.

12814-z

Halopredone Acetate.

2-Bromo-6β,9α-difluoro-11β,17α,21-trihydroxypregna-1,4-diene-3,20-dione 17,21-diacetate.
$C_{25}H_{29}BrF_2O_7=559.4$.

CAS — 57781-15-4 (halopredone); 57781-14-3 (acetate).

Halopredone acetate is a halogenated corticosteroid for topical use.

References: L. Toscano *et al.*, *Arzneimittel-Forsch.*, 1977, *27*, 1636; Rampini E. *et al.*, *ibid.*, 2396; E. Rampini *et al.*, *ibid.*, 2399; B. Palmerio and P. Magnani, *ibid.*, 2404; E. Rampini *et al.*, *Eur. J. clin. Pharmac.*, 1978, *14*, 325.

Manufacturers
Pierrel, Ital.

12815-c

Haloxon *(B.P. Vet.)*.

Bis(2-chloroethyl) 3-chloro-4-methylcoumarin-7-yl phosphate.
$C_{14}H_{14}Cl_3O_6P=415.6$.

CAS — 321-55-1.

A white or almost white, odourless or almost odourless powder. M.p. 88° to 93°. Practically **insoluble** in water; soluble 1 in 9 of alcohol, 1 in 4 of acetone, and 1 in 2 of chloroform.

Haloxon is an anthelmintic used in veterinary medicine.

Proprietary Names
Equilox *(Crown, UK)*.

12817-a

Henna *(B.P.C. 1934)*.

Henna Leaf; Lawsonia.

The dried leaves of *Lawsonia inermis* (= *L. alba*) (Lythraceae), containing lawsone (see p.1497).

Powdered henna is used for dyeing the hair and skin.

Henna is used in India by both men and women as a cooling and decorative cosmetic on the palms and soles.— Sadgopal (letter), *Soap Perfum. Cosm.*, 1966, *39*, 389.

12818-t

Hepatitis B Vaccine

A suspension of 20-nm particles of hepatitis B surface antigen derived from chronic carriers, purified to remove whole virus, treated with formalin to inactivate any residual live virus, and adsorbed on alum.

When hepatitis B vaccine is given to populations at high risk (homosexuals, dialysis patients, medical personnel) usually in a course of 3 injections at monthly intervals with a re-inforcing dose about 6 months after the first injection, a protective effect has been demonstrated. Its value in other populations and in areas where hepatitis is endemic remains to be established.

Discussions of the development and potential value of hepatitis B vaccines.— C. S. Marwick, *Am. Pharm.*, 1979, *NS19* (May), 13; *Br. med. J.*, 1980, *280*, 203; *ibid.*, *281*, 1585; *Lancet*, 1980, *2*, 1229; J. L. Dienstag, *New Engl. J. Med.*, 1980, *303*, 874.

Minimum requirements for hepatitis B vaccine.— Report of the WHO Expert Committee on Viral Hepatitis, *Tech. Rep. Ser. Wld Hlth Org. No. 602*, 1977.

A good response to hepatitis B vaccine (*Merck*) among 79 dialysis patients. Forty of the patients received 2 initial intramuscular injections of 40 µg in 1 ml and 39 received 3 similar initial injections, at intervals of one month; all participants were then given a booster dose 6 months after their first injection. Within 6 months of the first injection 79.7% of the 79 study patients had detectable anti-HBs, and an additional 8.9% became antibody-positive after the 6-month booster dose, making a total of 89%.— C. E. Stevens *et al.*, *Lancet*, 1980, *2*, 1211.

Demonstration of the efficacy of hepatitis B vaccine in a placebo-controlled randomised double-blind study in 1083 homosexual men. The vaccine was given intramuscularly as a 40-µg (1-ml) dose (*Merck*), and the dose repeated one month and 6 months later if blood specimens were negative for HBsAg, anti-HBs (antibody to hepatitis B surface antigen), and anti-HBc (antibody to hepatitis B core antigen). The placebo consisted of alum alone in the vaccine diluent. Hepatitis B vaccine induced high concentrations of anti-HBs but not antibodies directed against core or 'e' antigens. Within one month of the first injection of vaccine, 31.4% had acquired antibody; within 2 months, 77%; within 3 months, 87%; and within 6 months, 90%. After the third injection the antibody response-rate increased to 96% and then remained essentially unchanged for the rest of the 18-month follow-up period. This antibody response was associated with a dramatic reduction in the incidence of heptatitis B virus events when compared with the placebo group.— W. Szmuness *et al.*, *New Engl. J. Med.*, 1980, *303*, 833.

Seroconversion in 96% of 50 health care workers after 3 doses of hepatitis B vaccine (*Merck*) at monthly intervals. The response in children with thalassaemia was similar.— N. Matsaniotis *et al.* (letter), *Lancet*, 1981, *1*, 210.

An antibody response in 94% of 298 children in an area where hepatitis B is endemic, after 3 injections at monthly intervals of hepatitis B vaccine (10 µg per dose) (*Pasteur*).— P. Maupas *et al.*, *Lancet*, 1981, *1*, 289.

Hepatitis in 3.6% of 164 personnel of dialysis, transplant, or nephrology units given 3 injections of hepatitis B vaccine (*Pasteur*) at monthly intervals compared with 12.3% in 154 controls.— J. Crosnier *et al.*, *Lancet*, 1981, *1*, 455.

Comparable antibody responses in medical personnel given antihepatitis B immunoglobulin followed by hepatitis B vaccine (*Merck*) in 20-µg doses, immunoglobulin with vaccine followed by vaccine, or vaccine only.— W. Szmuness *et al.*, *Lancet*, 1981, *1*, 575.

Hepatitis occurred in 10 of 48 haemodialysis patients who generally received 3 injections of hepatitis B vaccine (*Pasteur*) compared with 21 of 47 patients receiving placebo—a significant reduction.— J. Crosnier *et al.*, *Lancet*, 1981, *1*, 797.

Manufacturers
Merck Sharp & Dohme, USA; Institut Pasteur, Fr.; Green Cross Corp., Jap.

12819-x

Heptaminol Hydrochloride. RP-2831. 6-Amino-2-methylheptan-2-ol hydrochloride.

$C_8H_{19}NO,HCl=181.7$.

CAS — 372-66-7 (heptaminol); 543-15-7 (hydrochloride).

Heptaminol hydrochloride is a cardiac stimulant and vasodilator and has been given in the treatment of cardiovascular disorders.

Proprietary Names
Altocor *(Coop. Farm., Ital.)*; Arcor *(Manetti Roberts, Ital.)*; Coreptil *(Delalande, Ital.)*; Cortensor *(Wander, Switz.)*; Delmiton *(Rhodia, Arg.)*; Eoden *(Woelm, Ger.; ICN, Spain)*; Hept-a-myl *(Delalande, Belg.; Delalande, Fr.; Delalande, Switz.)*; Heptylon *(Delalande, Ger.)*.

12820-y

Herniaria. Bruchkraut; Herba Herniariae; Herniary; Rupture-wort.

Pharmacopoeias. In *Aust., Cz., Hung., Jug.,* and *Pol.*

The dried leaves and flowering tops of various species of rupture-wort, chiefly *Herniaria glabra* and *H. hirsuta* (Caryophyllaceae).

Herniaria has astringent and diuretic properties and has been given by mouth, usually as an infusion, in bladder affections.

Eight saponins were isolated and identified in *Herniaria glabra*. Hydrolysis produced sugars and 7 aglycones.— T. Kartnig and O. Wegschaider, *Planta med.*, 1972, *21*, 144, per *Int. pharm. Abstr.*, 1973, *10*, 164.

12821-j

Hesperidin. 5-Hydroxy-2-(3-hydroxy-4-methoxyphenyl)-4-oxo-4*H*-chromen-7-yl rutinoside.

$C_{28}H_{34}O_{15}=610.6$.

CAS — 520-26-3.

A colourless or yellowish crystalline glycoside isolated from the rind of certain citrus fruits. Very slightly **soluble** in water.

Hesperidin has the same actions and has been used for the same purposes as rutin (see p.1752).

12822-z

Hesperidin Methyl Chalcone

CAS — 24292-52-2.

Hesperidin methyl chalcone is a flavonoid which has been used similarly to rutin (p.1752) in the treatment of capillary fragility.

12823-c

Hexachlorobenzene.

$C_6Cl_6=284.8$.

CAS — 118-74-1.

A white crystalline solid. Practically **insoluble** in water; slightly soluble in alcohol; soluble in chloroform and ether.

NOTE. Hexachlorobenzene should not be confused with Benzene Hexachloride.

Hexachlorobenzene has been used as an agricultural fungicide. It is not biodegradable to any significant extent and hexachlorobenzene residues in food have arisen as a result of its occurrence in industrial wastes as well as its use as a fungicide.

Hexachlorobenzene is reported to be excreted in breast milk.

Porphyria cutanea tarda in 348 patients was traced to consumption of wheat for planting which had been treated with a fungicide containing 10% of hexachlorobenzene. The patients had probably ingested 50 to 200 mg daily. Acute manifestations disappeared without specific therapy 20 to 30 days after consumption had ceased.— C. Cam and G. Nigogosyan, *J. Am. med. Ass.*, 1963, *183*, 88.

Report on 8 patients with porphyria induced by ingestion of seed grain treated with hexachlorobenzene. Disodium edetate appeared to be effective in reversing the symptoms.— H. A. Peters *et al.*, *Am. J. med. Sci.*, 1966, *251*, 314, per *J. Am. med. Ass.*, 1966, *195* (Mar. 28), A229.

Samples of perirenal fat taken during postmortem examinations of 75 bodies of varying ages in Sydney were all found to contain hexachlorobenzene in amounts up to 8.2 ppm. Since hexachlorobenzene was also found in samples of eggs and animal fats the human contamination was considered to be due to the illegal feeding of treated seed wheat to livestock.— M. N. Brady and D. S. Siyali, *Med. J. Aust.*, 1972, *1*, 158.

A value of 600 ng per kg body-weight should be used as a provisional guide for setting upper limits of hexachlorobenzene residues until it was possible to establish an acceptable daily intake based on the results of comprehensive toxicological studies.— 1973 Evaluations of some Pesticide Residues in Food, *Pestic. Residue Ser. Wld Hlth Org. No. 3*, 1974. See also Pesticide Residues in Food, *Tech. Rep. Ser. Wld Hlth Org. No. 574*, 1975.

For toxicological studies in animals, see E. J. Gralla *et al.*, *Toxic. appl. Pharmac.*, 1977, *40*, 227; T. Kuiper-Goodman *et al.*, *ibid.*, 529; J. R. P. Cabral *et al.*, *ibid.*, *41*, 155.

Further references: J. E. Burns *et al.*, *Archs envir. Hlth*, 1974, *29*, 192, per *J. Am. med. Ass.*, 1974, *230*, 157; J. E. Burns and F. M. Miller, *Archs envir. Hlth*, 1975, *30*, 44, per *J. Am. med. Ass.*, 1975, *231*, 426; K. D. Courtney, *Environ. Res.*, 1979, *20*, 225 (review); G. Koss *et al.*, *Arch. Tox.*, 1979, *42*, 19.

12824-k

Hexacyprone Calcium. Calcium 3-(1-benzyl-2-oxocyclohexyl)propionate.

$(C_{16}H_{19}O_3)_2Ca=558.7$.

CAS — 892-01-3 (hexacyprone); 3837-23-8 (calcium salt).

Hexacyprone calcium has been used in the treatment of hepatic disorders.

Proprietary Names
Epadren *(Vister, Ital.)*.

12825-a

Histamine-Azoprotein. A synthetic complex of histamine and horse serum globulin.

Histamine-azoprotein has been used as a desensitising agent in the treatment of allergic conditions.

Manufacturers
Parke, Davis, USA.

12826-t

Homidium Bromide *(B.P. Vet.)*. RD-1572; Ethidium Bromide. 3,8-Diamino-5-ethyl-6-phenylphenanthridinium bromide.

$C_{21}H_{20}BrN_3=394.3$.

CAS — 1239-45-8.

A dark purple, odourless or almost odourless, crystalline or amorphous powder with a persistent bitter taste. It loses not more than 10% of its weight on drying. **Soluble** 1 in 20 of water and 1 in 750 of chloroform. A 2% solution in water has a pH of 4 to 7.

Homidium bromide is a trypanocide used in veterinary medicine.

12827-x

Homonicotinic Acid. 3-Pyridylacetic acid.

$C_7H_7NO_2=137.1$.

CAS — 501-81-5.

Homonicotinic acid is used in the treatment of hypercholesterolaemia.

Proprietary Names
Minedil *(Formenti, Ital.)*; Piridil *(Nagel, Ital.)*; Piristerol *(Janus, Ital.)*.

12828-r

Hydrastine Hydrochloride *(B.P.C. 1949)*.

6,7-Dimethoxy-3-(5,6,7,8-tetrahydro-6-methyl-1,3-dioxolo[4,5-*g*]isoquinolin-5-yl)isobenzofuran-1(3*H*)-one hydrochloride.

$C_{21}H_{21}NO_6,HCl=419.9$.

CAS — 118-08-1 (hydrastine); 5936-28-7 (hydrochloride).

Pharmacopoeias. In *Span.*

The hydrochloride of an alkaloid obtained from hydrastis.

A white or creamy-white, odourless, hygroscopic powder with a very bitter and pungent taste. **Soluble** in water and alcohol; slightly soluble in chloroform. Solutions in water are acid to litmus. **Store** in airtight containers. Protect from light.

Hydrastine hydrochloride constricts peripheral vessels and has been reputed to cause uterine contractions and arrest uterine haemorrhage but it is of doubtful value.

12829-f

Hydrastinine Hydrochloride *(B.P.C. 1934)*.

Idrastinina Cloruro. 5,6,7,8-Tetrahydro-6-methyl-1,3-dioxolo[4,5-*g*]isoquinolin-5-ol hydrochloride.

$C_{11}H_{11}NO_2,HCl=225.7$.

CAS — 6592-85-4 (hydrastinine); 4884-68-8 (hydrochloride).

Pharmacopoeias. In *It.*

The hydrochloride of an alkaloid produced by oxidation of hydrastine.

Pale yellow odourless crystals or crystalline powder with a very bitter taste. M.p. 212° with decomposition. Very **soluble** in water and alcohol; sparingly soluble in chloroform and ether. Solutions in water are neutral and show a blue fluorescence. **Store** in a cool place. Protect from light.

Hydrastinine hydrochloride appears to stimulate involuntary muscle and was formerly employed in various forms of uterine haemorrhage.

12830-z

Hydrastis *(B.P.C. 1949)*. Hydrast.; Golden Seal; Yellow Root; Hidraste; Idraste.

Pharmacopoeias. In *Arg., Belg., Braz., Fr., It., Mex., Port., Roum.,* and *Span.*

The dried rhizome and roots of golden seal, *Hydrastis canadensis* (Ranunculaceae), containing not less than 1.5% of hydrastine; it also contains the alkaloids berberine and canadine.

The content of hydrastine specified in pharmacopoeias varies from 1.5% to not less than 2.5%.

Hydrastis was formerly used to check excessive uterine haemorrhage.

12831-c

Hydrazine Sulphate.

$H_6N_2O_4S$=130.1.

CAS — 302-01-2 (hydrazine); 10034-93-2 (sulphate).

Crystals. **Soluble** 1 in about 33 of water, freely soluble in hot water; practically **insoluble** in alcohol. A 0.2M solution in water has a pH of 1.3.

Hydrazine sulphate is employed in various industrial processes. It is used in the preparation of hydrazine hydrate which is applied after a solution of platinic chloride for corneal tattooing (see Chloroplatinic Acid, p.1693).

An account of the successful treatment of industrial hydrazine poisoning with pyridoxine.— J. K. Kirklin *et al.*, *New Engl. J. Med.*, 1976, *294*, 938.

A report of fatal choroidal melanoma in a worker who had been exposed to hydrazine for 6 years.— D. M. Albert and C. A. Puliafito (letter), *New Engl. J. Med.*, 1977, *296*, 634.

The use of hydrazine sulphate by a laboratory worker was associated with the development of a syndrome similar to systemic lupus erythematosus.— P. J. Durant and R. A. Harris (letter), *New Engl. J. Med.*, 1980, *303*, 584.

A discussion of hydrazine sulphate as an antineoplastic agent.— W. Regelson, *J. Am. med. Ass.*, 1980, *243*, 337.

12832-k

Hydrogen Sulphide. Sulphuretted Hydrogen.

H_2S=34.08.

CAS — 7783-06-4.

A colourless inflammable gas with a characteristic odour; the intensity of the smell gives no indication of concentration.

Adverse Effects. Hydrogen sulphide poisoning is a common industrial hazard and is encountered in such places as chemical works, mines, sewage works, and stores of decomposing protein; concentrations of 0.1 to 0.2% in the atmosphere may be fatal in a few minutes. Pulmonary irritation, oedema, and respiratory failure usually occur after acute poisoning; prolonged exposure to low concentrations may give rise to severe conjunctivitis with photophobia and corneal opacity, irritation of the respiratory tract, rhinitis, bronchitis, stomatitis, pharyngitis, digestive disturbances, headache, lassitude, and skin rashes. There are some similarities to poisoning with cyanides.

A discussion of poisoning by hydrogen sulphide.— *Lancet*, 1978, *1*, 28. Comments.— A. Downie (letter), *ibid.*, 219; C. H. B. Binns (letter), *ibid.*, 501; A. Downie (letter), *ibid.*

Concentrations of about 200 ppm caused irritation of the respiratory tract and, on prolonged exposure, pulmonary oedema. Toxicity to the CNS could occur suddenly at concentrations in excess of 500 ppm and immediate death might follow concentrations in excess of 1000 ppm. Irritation to the eyes occurred at concentrations of less than 50 ppm.— *Methods for the Detection of Toxic Substances in Air, Hydrogen Sulphide*, London, HM Stationery Office, 1969.

Further references: W. W. Burnett *et al.*, *Can. med. Ass. J.*, 1977, *117*, 1277; R. P. Smith (letter), *ibid.*, 1978, *118*, 775; W. W. Burnett and E. G. King (letter), *ibid.*, 776; *J. Am. med. Ass.*, 1978, *239*, 1374.

Treatment of Adverse Effects. After exposure to hydrogen sulphide place the patient in fresh air, give inhalations of oxygen and, if necessary, assist the respiration. Antibiotics may be necessary if pulmonary infection occurs. The conjunctival sacs should be carefully washed out if eye irritation is severe.

In severe poisoning, amyl nitrite inhalation and sodium nitrite by intravenous injection have been suggested.

A brief review of the management of sulphide poisoning.— R. P. Smith and R. E. Gosselin, *A. Rev. Pharmac. & Toxic.*, 1976, *16*, 189.

The successful treatment of a 47-year-old man with severe hydrogen sulphide poisoning using oxygen, amyl nitrite inhalations for 30 seconds out of each minute for 5 minutes, and then sodium nitrite 300 mg intravenously for 3 minutes. Treatment was aimed at producing methaemoglobinaemia to inactivate the sulphide. In addition he received sodium thiosulphate 12.5 g by intravenous injection.— R. J. Stine *et al.*, *Ann. intern. Med.*, 1976, *85*, 756.

Further references: R. P. Smith and R. E. Gosselin, *J. occup. Med.*, 1979, *21*, 93.

Uses. Hydrogen sulphide is widely employed in many industrial processes.

12833-a

Hydroxyestrone Diacetate. 16α-Hydroxyoestrone Diacetate. 3,16α-Dihydroxyestra-1,3,5(10)-trien-17-one diacetate.

$C_{22}H_{26}O_5$=370.4.

CAS — 566-76-7 (hydroxyestrone); 1247-71-8 (diacetate).

Hydroxyestrone diacetate is a derivative of oestrone. It is claimed to have minimal systemic oestrogenic effects when given by mouth but to retain effects on the vaginal mucosa. It is used in the treatment of vaginitis and associated disorders.

Proprietary Names

Colpoginon *(Boizot, Spain)*; Colpogynon *(Laboratories de l'Hepatrol, Switz.)*; Colpormon *(Millet, Arg.; Anphar-Rolland, Fr.)*.

12834-t

Hydroxyethylpromethazine Chloride.

(2-Hydroxyethyl)dimethyl[1-methyl-2-(phenothiazin-10-yl)ethyl]ammonium chloride.

$C_{19}H_{25}ClN_2OS$=364.9.

CAS — 7647-63-4 (hydroxyethylpromethazine); 2090-54-2 (chloride).

Hydroxyethylpromethazine chloride is an antihistamine.

Proprietary Names

Aprobit *(Recip, Swed.)*.

12835-x

Hydroxymethylnicotinamide. Nicotinylmethylamide; *N*-Hydroxymethylnicotinamide. *N*-Hydroxymethylpyridine-3-carboxamide.

$C_7H_8N_2O_2$=152.2.

CAS — 3569-99-1.

Crystals. M.p. 141° to 142°. Sparingly **soluble** in water and alcohol; freely soluble in hot water and alcohol.

Hydroxymethylnicotinamide is a choleretic and has been used in the treatment of various disorders of the gall-bladder.

Proprietary Names

Bilamid *(Cilag, Ger.; Bracco, Ital.; Cilag-Chemie, Switz.)*; Bilamide *(Cilag-Chemie, Belg.)*; Biloide *(Labatec-Pharma, Switz.)*.

12836-r

5-Hydroxytryptophan. 5-HTP; Ro-0783/B. 2-Amino-3-(5-hydroxy-1*H*-indol-3-yl)propionic acid.

$C_{11}H_{12}N_2O_3$=220.2.

CAS — 56-69-9.

NOTE. The form of 5-hydroxytryptophan used clinically is generally the L-form.

5-Hydroxytryptophan is a precursor of serotonin (see p.1753) and has been used clinically in attempts to treat disorders believed to be associated with serotonin deficiency.

Changes in mood, mostly elevation, were observed in 7 neurological patients without affective disorders and 1 healthy subject given L-5-hydroxytryptophan 100 to 300 mg by intravenous infusion in sodium chloride injection. Carbidopa was also given to reduce the severity of vomiting which always occurred 30 to 90 minutes after infusion and to increase the amount of L-5-hydroxytryptophan entering the brain. Neurotoxicity occurred with doses of 200 mg and above and included dilatation of the pupil, hyperreflexia, ataxia, and dysarthria. There was some similarity to the effects of alcohol.— M. Trimble *et al.* (letter), *Lancet*, 1975, *1*, 583. See also M. H. Greenwood *et al.*, *Br. J. clin. Pharmac.*, 1975, *2*, 165.

Severe insomnia in a 33-year-old woman following a road accident responded to 4 consecutive nightly doses of L-5-hydroxytryptophan totalling 3 g.— M. Webb and J. G. Kirker (letter), *Lancet*, 1981, *1*, 1365.

Manganese poisoning. A beneficial response to DL-5-hydroxytryptophan, up to 3 g daily, was achieved in a patient in whom the symptoms of manganese poisoning failed to respond to levodopa.— I. Mena *et al.*, *New Engl. J. Med.*, 1970, *282*, 5.

Mental disorders. Of 107 patients with endogenous depression given L-5-hydroxytryptophan daily in divided doses by mouth for at least 5 weeks, the majority rapidly obtained a beneficial response.— I. Sano, *Münch. med. Wschr.*, 1972, *114*, 1713, per *J. Am. med. Ass.*, 1972, *222*, 1085. Further studies in depression: N. S. Kline *et al.*, *Am. J. Psychiat.*, 1964, *121*, 379, per *Int. pharm. Abstr.*, 1965, *2*, 918; T. Persson and B. -E. Roos (letter), *Lancet*, 1967, *2*, 987; G. d'Elia *et al.*, *Acta psychiat. scand.*, 1978, *57*, 239; L. J. van Hiele, *Neuropsychobiology*, 1980, *6*, 230.

After oral administration of L-5-hydroxytryptophan with a peripheral decarboxylase inhibitor, mild to moderate improvement was obtained in 6 of 7 chronic undifferentiated schizophrenic patients who were resistant to phenothiazines. Of 4 chronic paranoid schizophrenic patients who were resistant to phenothiazines 2 became worse after treatment with 5-hydroxytryptophan and 1 improved. Some schizophrenic patients might have an abnormality in serotonin metabolism.— R. J. Wyatt *et al.*, *Science*, 1972, *177*, 1124.

Further studies in schizophrenia: V. Zarcone *et al.*, *Archs gen. Psychiat.*, 1973, *28*, 843; R. J. Wyatt *et al.*, *ibid.*, *29*, 597.

Myoclonus. Comment on the use of the investigational drug L-5-hydroxytryptophan in the treatment of myoclonus and the view that in general its use should be discouraged. L-5-Hydroxytryptophan is usually effective in posthypoxic intention myoclonus, a rare condition, but may exacerbate some other myoclonic syndromes. Significant adverse effects, especially gastro-intestinal disturbances, are almost universal, even when given with a peripheral decarboxylase inhibitor such as carbidopa.— R. R. Young, *J. Am. med. Ass.*, 1980, *243*, 1569.

L-5-Hydroxytryptophan with carbidopa was administered to 23 patients with myoclonus and 16 patients with other neurological disorders. Following administration by mouth of maximum doses of 0.4 to 2 g daily with carbidopa 100 to 300 mg daily more than 50% improvement was obtained in 11 of 18 patients with intention myoclonus due to anoxia or other brain damage; only 1 patient obtained no improvement and in 3 it was 90% or more; some patients derived sustained benefit for more than 3 years. No benefit was obtained by 2 patients with athetotic cerebral palsy, 2 with multiple sclerosis, 2 with essential tremor, 4 with cerebellar intention tremor, 1 with infantile spasms, 2 with dystonia musculorum deformans, 2 with central pain syndromes, or 3 with idiopathic epilepsy; some benefit was obtained in 1 patient with myoclonus epilepsy and in 1 of 2 patients with familial essential myoclonus. Side-effects included anorexia, nausea, diarrhoea, and occasional vomiting and were reduced by prochlorperazine or trimethobenzamide, and diphenoxylate; prior administration of carbidopa for 1 or 2 days before therapy also reduced the gastro-intestinal side-effects. During the first week of therapy 3 patients developed dyspnoea followed by hyperventilation and lightheadedness, with fainting in 1; pulmonary function tests remained normal. Varying degrees of mental stimulation occurred in 10 patients; these were reversible on dosage reduction and frequently disappeared or diminished after 4 to 6 weeks without reduction, but 2 patients required concurrent administration of perphenazine to maintain their antimyoclonic dosage. Other side-effects included mydriasis, blurring of vision, abdominal pain, and bradycardia.— M. H. Van Woert *et al.*, *New Engl. J. Med.*, 1977, *296*, 70. Comment.— T. L. Munsat, *ibid.*, 101.

Studies suggesting that the treatment of intention myoclonus with L-5-hydroxytryptophan and carbidopa in a 70-year-old man unmasked an abnormality in his ability to metabolise kynurenine and resulted in the development of a scleroderma-like illness.— E. M. Sternberg *et al.*, *New Engl. J. Med.*, 1980, *303*, 782.

Further references: D. Chadwick *et al.*, *Lancet*, 1975, *2*, 434; J. DeLéan and J. C. Richardson (letter), *ibid.*, 870; J. H. Growdon *et al.*, *Neurology, Minneap.*, 1976, *26*, 1135; W. M. Carroll and P. J. Walsh, *Br. med. J.*,

1978, *2,* 1612.

Parkinsonism. Following administration of L-5-hydroxytryptophan and a peripheral decarboxylase inhibitor to 7 parkinsonian patients significant increase in bradykinesia and rigidity occurred together with an exacerbation of functional disability.— T. N. Chase *et al., Neurology, Minneap.,* 1972, *22,* 479, per *J. Am. med. Ass.,* 1972, *221,* 429. See also T. N. Chase (letter), *Lancet,* 1970, *2,* 1029.

An antidepressant and tremor-decreasing effect was noted in the majority of 13 patients with Parkinson's disease after administration of L-5-hydroxytryptophan by mouth. Any effect on muscle rigidity was difficult to evaluate.— I. Sano and K. Taniguchi, *Münch. med. Wschr.,* 1972, *114,* 1717, per *J. Am. med. Ass.,* 1972, *222,* 1085.

Self-mutilation. The self-mutilation associated with the Lesch-Nyhan syndrome, an inborn error of purine metabolism, was abolished by L-5-hydroxytryptophan in 4 patients.— T. -I. Mizuno and Y. Yugari (letter), *Lancet,* 1974, *1,* 761.

Administration of L-5-hydroxytryptophan 1.6 g daily in divided doses with carbidopa 75 mg four times daily controlled the tics, vocalisations and self-mutilation in a 15-year-old boy with Gilles de la Tourette syndrome. Lip and buccal ulcers healed and it was possible to reduce major and minor tranquilliser therapy. Symptoms recurred during 3 periods of placebo therapy.— M. H. Van Woert *et al., New Engl. J. Med.,* 1977, *296,* 210.

Further references: C. D. Frith *et al., J. Neurol. Neurosurg. Psychiat.,* 1976, *39,* 656.

Proprietary Names

Prétonine *(Arkodex, Fr.)*; Quiétim *(Nativelle, Fr.)*; Telesol *(Lasa, Spain).*

12837-f

Hypoglycin A.
L-2-Amino-3-(2-methylenecyclopropyl)propionic acid.
$C_7H_{11}NO_2$=141.2.

CAS — 156-56-9.

A toxic substance present in the arillus of unripe akee, the fruit of *Blighia sapida* (Sapindaceae).

Hypoglycin A is responsible for Jamaican vomiting sickness, with symptoms of acute and severe vomiting, hypoglycaemia, CNS depression, convulsions, and coma, frequently fatal.

Glycine might be useful in the treatment of poisoning by the unripe fruits of the Jamaican ackee [akee].— H. S. A. Sherratt and S. S. Al-Bassam (letter), *Lancet,* 1976, *2,* 1243. See also K. Tanaka (letter), *ibid.,* 1977, *1,* 370; H. S. A. Sherratt and S. S. Al-Bassam (letter), *ibid.,* 604.

Further references: R. Haeckel, *Germ. Med.,* 1972, *2,* 69; K. Tanaka *et al., New Engl. J. Med.,* 1976, *295,* 461; R. Bressler, *ibid.,* 500; D. Billington *et al., ibid.,* 1482.

12838-d

Ibopamine Hydrochloride.
SB-7505. 4-(2-Methylaminoethyl)-*o*-phenylene di-isobutyrate hydrochloride.
$C_{17}H_{25}NO_4,HCl$=343.8.

CAS — 66195-31-1 (ibopamine).

Ibopamine hydrochloride is reported to be a dopamine agonist with inotropic effects which increases renal blood flow and thereby induces diuresis.

References: G. F. Melloni *et al., Curr. ther. Res.,* 1979, *25,* 406; G. F. Melloni *et al., ibid., 26,* 466; F. Gicchetti *et al., ibid.,* 1980, *27,* 741; L. Verga *et al., Clin. Trials J.,* 1980, *17,* 15; G. F. Melloni *et al., Eur. J. clin. Pharmac.,* 1981, *19,* 177; S. Stefoni *et al., Br. J. clin. Pharmac.,* 1981, *11,* 69.

Manufacturers

Simes, Ital.

12839-n

Ibufenac.
(4-Isobutylphenyl)acetic acid.
$C_{12}H_{16}O_2$=192.3.

CAS — 1553-60-2.

Colourless crystals. M.p. 85° to 87°. Practically **insoluble** in water; soluble in organic solvents.

Ibufenac has anti-inflammatory, analgesic, and antipyretic properties. It was formerly used in the treatment of rheumatic conditions but was found to cause jaundice.

Proprietary Preparations

Ibufenac was formerly marketed in Great Britain under the proprietary name Dytransin (*Boots*).

12840-k

Ibuprofen Lysine.
Soluphene. Lysine 2-(4-isobutylphenyl)propionate.
$C_{19}H_{32}N_2O_4$=352.5.

CAS — 57469-77-9.

Ibuprofen lysine has anti-inflammatory, analgesic, and antipyretic activity.

References: R. Latini *et al., Int. J. clin. Pharmac. Biopharm.,* 1977, *15,* 492, per *Int. pharm. Abstr.,* 1978, *15,* 482.

Proprietary Names

Saren *(Bracco, Ital.).*

12841-a

Ibuproxam.
4-Isobutylhydratropohydroxamic acid.
$C_{13}H_{19}NO_2$=221.3.

CAS — 53648-05-8.

Ibuproxam has anti-inflammatory, analgesic, and antipyretic activity.

References: G. Orzalesi *et al., Arzneimittel-Forsch.,* 1977, *27,* 1006 (pharmacology in *rats*); *idem,* 1012 (metabolism to ibuprofen in *rats*); S. Chimichi *et al., J. pharm. Sci.,* 1980, *69,* 521.

Proprietary Names

Ibudros *(Manetti Roberts, Ital.).*

12842-t

Idrocilamide.
LCB-29. *N*-(2-Hydroxyethyl)cinnamamide.
$C_{11}H_{13}NO_2$=191.2.

CAS — 6961-46-2.

Idrocilamide has been used for the relief of muscle spasm in disorders such as hemiplegia or paraplegia.

References: K. Fasshauer and G. Huffmann, *Arzneimittel-Forsch.,* 1977, *27,* 1612.

A critical reference: G. D. Perkin and M. J. Aminoff, *Br. J. clin. Pharmac.,* 1976, *3,* 879.

Inhibition by idrocilamide of the disposition of caffeine.— J. L. Brazier *et al., Eur. J. clin. Pharmac.,* 1980, *17,* 37.

Proprietary Names

Brolitène *(Médicia, Fr.).*

15323-x

Imcarbofos.
CL-217658. Tetraethyl {(2-methoxy-*p*-phenylene)bis[imino(thiocarbonyl)]}diphosphoramidate.
$C_{17}H_{30}N_4O_7P_2S_2$=528.5.

CAS — 66608-32-0.

Imcarbofos is an organophosphorus compound (see p.832) for use as a veterinary anthelmintic.

Manufacturers

American Cyanamid, USA.

12843-x

Imexon.
BM-06002. 4-Imino-1,3-diazabicyclo-[3.1.0]hexan-2-one.
$C_4H_5N_3O$=111.1.

CAS — 59643-91-3.

Imexon is reported to have immunostimulant properties with possible use in neoplastic disease.

Manufacturers

Boehringer Mannheim, Ger.

12844-r

Imidocarb Hydrochloride.
4A65. 3,3′-Di(2-imidazolin-2-yl)carbanilide dihydrochloride; 1,3-Bis[3-(2-imidazolin-2-yl)phenyl]urea dihydrochloride.
$C_{19}H_{20}N_6O,2HCl$=421.3.

CAS — 27885-92-3 (imidocarb); 5318-76-3 (hydrochloride).

Imidocarb hydrochloride is a babesicide used in veterinary medicine.

Manufacturers

Wellcome, USA.

12845-f

Impromidine Hydrochloride.
SK&F-92676-A_3. 1-(3-Imidazol-4-ylpropyl)-3-[2-(5-methylimidazol-4-ylmethylthio)ethyl]guanidine trihydrochloride.
$C_{14}H_{23}N_7S,3HCl$=430.8.

CAS — 55273-05-7 (impromidine); 65573-02-6 (hydrochloride).

Impromidine hydrochloride is a histamine H_2 agonist, with potential use in the study of gastric secretion.

References:. W. L. Burland *et al., Br. J. clin. Pharmac.,* 1979, *7,* 421P; U. Bangerter *et al., Gut,* 1979, *20,* A938; R. H. Hunt *et al., Gastroenterology,* 1980, *78,* 505; R. H. McIsaac *et al., Gut,* 1981, *22,* 529.

Manufacturers

Smith Kline & French, UK.

12846-d

Improsulfan Tosylate.
Iminodipropyl dimethanesulphonate 4-toluenesulphonate.
$C_8H_{19}NO_6S_2,C_7H_8O_3S$=461.6.

CAS — 13425-98-4 (improsulfan); 32784-82-0 (tosylate).

Improsulfan tosylate is reported to have antineoplastic activity in leukaemia.

Proprietary Names

Protecton *(Jap.).*

NOTE. The name Protecton has also been applied to a topical contraceptive preparation.

12847-n

Indacrinone.
Indacrinic Acid; MK-196. (±)-[(6,7-Dichloro-2-methyl-1-oxo-2-phenylindan-5-yl)oxy]acetic acid.
$C_{18}H_{14}Cl_2O_4$=365.2.

CAS — 57296-63-6.

Indacrinone is a loop diuretic.

Comparison with hydrochlorothiazide.— C. E. Wilhelmsson *et al., Br. J. clin. Pharmac.,* 1979, *8,* 261.

The response to indacrinone, and to indacrinone plus amiloride, in healthy subjects.— P. J. Ravenscroft *et al., Clin. Pharmac. Ther.,* 1980, *28,* 45.

Comparison with frusemide.— J. D. Irvin *et al., Clin. Pharmac. Ther.,* 1980, *28,* 376.

The effects of different enantiomers.— J. D. Irvin *et al., Clin. Pharmac. Ther.,* 1980, *27,* 260; J. A. Tobert *et al., ibid.,* 1981, *29,* 344; P. H. Vlasses *et al., ibid.,* 798.

Further references: K. F. Tempero *et al., Clin. Pharmac. Ther.,* 1976, *19,* 116; K. F. Tempero *et al., ibid.,* 1977, *21,* 119; *Nephron,* 1979, *23, Suppl.* 1, 1–66; B. A. Brooks *et al., Br. J. clin. Pharmac.,* 1980, *10,* 249.

Manufacturers
Merck Sharp & Dohme, USA.

12848-h

Indanazoline.
2-(Indan-4-ylamino)-2-imidazoline.
$C_{12}H_{15}N_3$=201.3.

CAS — 40507-78-6.

Indanazoline has been used as a spray for the relief of nasal catarrh.

Proprietary Names
Farial *(Nordmark-Werke, Ger.).*

15324-r

Indeloxazine Hydrochloride.
CI-874. (±)-2-(Inden-7-yloxymethyl)morpholine hydrochloride.
$C_{14}H_{17}NO_2$,HCl=267.8.

CAS — 60929-23-9 (indeloxazine); 65043-22-3 (hydrochloride).

Indeloxazine hydrochloride is reported to have antidepressant activity.

Manufacturers
Parke, Davis, USA.

12849-m

Indenolol Hydrochloride.
Sch-28316Z *(indenolol)*; YB-2. A 2:1 tautomeric mixture of 1-(inden-7-yloxy)-3-isopropylaminopropan-2-ol hydrochloride and 1-(inden-4-yloxy)-3-isopropylaminopropan-2-ol hydrochloride.
$C_{15}H_{21}NO_2$,HCl=283.8.

CAS — 60607-68-3 (indenolol); 68906-88-7 (hydrochloride).

Indenolol hydrochloride is a beta-adrenoceptor blocking agent.

References: F. E. Okupa *et al., Clin. Pharmac. Ther.*, 1981, *29*, 434.

Proprietary Names
Pulsan *(Jap.).*

12850-t

Indobufen.
K-3920. (±)-2-[4-(1-Oxo-isoindolin-2-yl)phenyl]butyric acid.
$C_{18}H_{17}NO_3$=295.3.

CAS — 63610-08-2.

Indobufen is an inhibitor of platelet aggregation.

Pharmacokinetics: L. M. Fuccella *et al., Eur. J. clin. Pharmac.*, 1979, *15*, 323; V. Tamassia *et al., ibid.*, 329.

Effects on platelet aggregation: T. D. Perri *et al., Arzneimittel-Forsch.*, 1979, *29*, 104; N. Ciavarella *et al., Curr. ther. Res.*, 1981, *29*, 503; A. Vittoria *et al., J. int. med. Res.*, 1981, *9*, 12.

Manufacturers
Farmitalia, Ital.

12851-x

Indorenate Hydrochloride.
TR-3369. Methyl (±)-3-amino-2-(5-methoxyindol-3-yl)propionate hydrochloride.
$C_{13}H_{16}N_2O_3$,HCl=284.7.

CAS — 73758-06-2 (indorenate); 72318-55-9; 73523-17-8 (both hydrochloride).

Indorenate hydrochloride is reported to have antihypertensive properties.

Manufacturers
Miles, USA.

12852-r

Inosine.
Hypoxanthine Riboside. 6,9-Dihydro-9-β-D-ribofuranosyl-1*H*-purin-6-one.
$C_{10}H_{12}N_4O_5$=268.2.

CAS — 58-63-9.

Inosine has been used in the treatment of cardiac insufficiency and other cardiac disorders.

The successful use of inosine for perfusing the kidney during conservative renal surgery in 5 patients.— J. E. A. Wickham *et al., Br. med. J.*, 1978, *2*, 173.

Proprietary Names
Inosipsina *(Zilliken, Ital.)*; Oxiamin *(Made, Spain)*; Tebertin *(Berenguer-Beneyto, Spain)*; Trophicardyl *(Innothéra, Fr.).*

12853-f

Iodazine.
Iodazine M; Dimethylenediethylenediamine Di-iodomethylate. 1,1,4,4-Tetramethylpiperazinium di-iodide.
$C_8H_{20}I_2N_2$=398.1.

NOTE. Distinguish iodazine from iodazone.

Iodazine is used in the treatment of rheumatic disorders. It may be administered orally, parenterally, or rectally.

12854-d

Iododesoxycytidine.
2′-Deoxy-5-iodocytidine.
$C_9H_{12}IN_3O_4$=353.1.

CAS — 611-53-0.

Iododesoxycytidine is reported to be an antiviral agent.

Proprietary Names
Cébé-Viran *(Chauvin-Blache, Fr.; Chauvin-Blache, Switz.)*; Cuterpès *(Chauvin-Blache, Fr.).*

12855-n

Ioglicic Acid.
SH-H-200-AB. 5-Acetamido-2,4,6-tri-iodo-*N*-(methylcarbamoylmethyl)isophthalamic acid.
$C_{13}H_{12}I_3N_3O_5$=671.0.

CAS — 49755-67-1.

Ioglicic acid is an iodinated contrast medium used, as the meglumine and sodium salts, for a variety of angiographic and related procedures.

Proprietary Names
Rayvist *(Schering, Ger.).*

12856-h

Iohexol.
Win-39424. *NN′*-Bis(2,3-dihydroxypropyl)-5-[*N*-(2,3-dihydroxypropyl)acetamido]-2,4,6-tri-iodoisophthalamide.
$C_{19}H_{26}I_3N_3O_9$=821.1.

CAS — 66108-95-0.

Iohexol is an iodinated contrast medium.

Manufacturers
Nyco, Norw.; Winthrop, USA.

14037-g

Iopamidol.
B-15000; SQ-13396. NN′-Bis[2-hydroxy-1-(hydroxymethyl)ethyl]-2,4,6-tri-iodo-5-lactamidoisophthalamide.
$C_{17}H_{22}I_3N_3O_8$=777.1.

CAS — 60166-93-0; 62883-00-5.

Iopamidol is a contrast medium used for a variety of angiographic procedures; it is also used in myelography.

Proprietary Preparations
Niopam 200 *(E. Merck, UK).* Contains iopamidol 40.8%, equivalent to 20% of iodine, in ampoules of 10 ml. **Niopam 300.** Contains iopamidol 61.2%, equivalent to 30% of iodine, in ampoules of 10 ml and bottles of 50 ml. **Niopam 370.** Contains iopamidol 75.5%, equivalent to 37% of iodine, in ampoules of 10 ml and bottles of 50 ml.

12857-m

Ioprocemic Acid.
SH-H-332; ZK-10720. 3-[3-(*N*-ethylacetamido)-2,4,6-tri-iodophenyl]propionic acid.
$C_{13}H_{14}I_3NO_3$=613.0.

CAS — 1456-52-6.

Ioprocemic acid is an iodinated contrast medium.

Manufacturers
Schering, Ger.

12858-b

Iotasul.
ZK-79112. 5,5′-[Thiobis(ethylenecarboxamido)]bis[*NN′*-bis(2,3-dihydroxypropyl)-2,4,6-tri-iodo-*NN′*-dimethylisophthalamide.
$C_{38}H_{50}I_6N_6O_{14}S$=1608.3.

CAS — 71767-13-0.

Iotasul is an iodinated contrast medium.

Manufacturers
Schering, Ger.

12859-v

Iotroxic Acid.
SH-213AB. 3,3′-(3,6,9-Trioxaundecanedioyldi-imino)bis(2,4,6-tri-iodobenzoic acid).
$C_{22}H_{18}I_6N_2O_9$=1215.8.

CAS — 51022-74-3.

12860-r

Meglumine Iotroxate.
Meglumine Iotroxinate; Iotroxamide; SH.H-273. The *N*-methylglucamine salt of iotroxic acid.
$C_{22}H_{18}I_6N_2O_9$,$2C_7H_{17}NO_5$=1606.2.

Iotroxic acid is a contrast medium used, as the meglumine salt, intravenously for visualisation of the biliary tract.

References: J. Doran *et al., Br. J. clin. Pharmac.*, 1978, *6*, 311.

Proprietary Preparations
Biliscopin *(Schering, UK).* Meglumine iotroxate, available as a 38% sterile solution in ampoules of 30 ml. It contains the equivalent of 180 mg of iodine per ml. **Biliscopin for infusion.** Meglumine iotroxate, available as a 10.5% sterile solution in bottles of 100 ml. It contains the equivalent of 50 mg of iodine per ml.

12861-f

Ioxaglic Acid.
N-(2-Hydroxyethyl)-2,4,6-tri-iodo-5-[2′,4′,6′-tri-iodo-3′-(*N*-methylacetamido)-5′-methylcarbamoylhippuramido]isophthalamic acid.
$C_{24}H_{21}I_6N_5O_8$=1268.9.

CAS — 59017-64-0.

Ioxaglic acid is an iodinated contrast medium. The meglumine and sodium salts are under study.

Manufacturers
May & Baker, UK.

12862-d

Ipexidine Mesylate.
CK-0569 *(ipexidine)*. 1,1′-[Piperazine-1,4-diylbis(trimethyleneiminocarbonimidoyl)]bis(3-hexylurea) dimethanesulphonate.
$C_{26}H_{54}N_{10}O_2$,$2CH_4O_3S$=731.0.

CAS — 69017-89-6 (ipexidine); 69017-90-9 (mesylate).

Ipexidine mesylate is reported to reduce dental plaque and gingivitis.

Manufacturers
Cooper, USA.

12863-n

Ipronidazole. M&B-16905; Ro-7-1554. 2-Isopropyl-1-methyl-5-nitroimidazole.
$C_7H_{11}N_3O_2$=169.2.

CAS — 14885-29-1.

Ipronidazole is used in veterinary practice in the management of blackhead (histomoniasis) in turkeys.

Proprietary Names
Iproprán *(Roche, Ger.).*

12864-h

Iron Polymaltose. Ferromaltose; Ferrum Polyisomaltose. A complex of ferric hydroxide and isomaltose.

NOTE. The precise structure is rarely defined accurately. There may therefore be differences between preparations similarly described.

Iron polymaltose is used as a source of iron, usually for intramuscular injection.

Proprietary Names
Fer Lucien *(Lucien, Fr.)*; Ferrum H *(Sigma, Austral.)*; Ferrum Hausmann IM *(see also under Dextriferron, Ferrous Fumarate, Saccharated Iron Oxide) (Biothera-Asperal, Belg.; Spain)*; Intrafer *(Manzoni, Ital.).*

12865-m

ISF-2123. 1-[*N*-(3-Hydrazinopyridazin-6-yl)-*N*-methylamino]propan-2-ol dihydrochloride.
$C_8H_{15}N_5O,2HCl$=270.2.

CAS — 56393-22-7.

ISF-2123 has antihypertensive properties.

References: C. Carpi and L. Dorigotti, *Br. J. Pharmac.*, 1974, *52*, 459P.

Manufacturers
ISF, Ital.

12866-b

Isobromindione. 5-Bromo-2-phenyl-indan-1,3-dione.
$C_{15}H_9BrO_2$=301.1.

CAS — 1470-35-5.

Isobromindione has been used in the treatment of hyperuricaemia. It appears to lack the anticoagulant activity of bromindione.

Proprietary Names
Uridion *(Gentili, Ital.).*

12867-v

Isobutiacilic Acid. 2-(4-Hydroxy-6-methylpyrimidin-2-yl)-2-(methyl)thiopropionic acid.
$C_9H_{12}N_2O_2S$=212.3.

Isobutiacilic acid has been used as an antithyroid agent.

Proprietary Names
Isotiran *(Zilliken, Ital.).*

12868-g

Isoconazole Nitrate. FF-149 *(isoconazole)*; R-15454. 1-[2,4-Dichloro-β-(2,6-dichlorobenzyloxy)phenethyl]imidazole nitrate.
$C_{18}H_{14}Cl_4N_2O,xHNO_3$=416.1 (isoconazole).

CAS — 27523-40-6 (isoconazole); 24168-96-5 (mononitrate); 40036-10-0 (xHNO₃).

Isoconazole nitrate is used topically for the treatment of fungal infections. Vaginal fungal infections are treated by the insertion of 600 mg of isoconazole nitrate.

References: H. Wendt and J. Kessler, *Arzneimittel-Forsch.*, 1979, *29*, 846.

Proprietary Preparations
Travogyn Vaginal Tablets *(Keymer, UK)*. Each contains isoconazole nitrate 300 mg.

Other Proprietary Names
Fazol *(Fr.).*

12869-q

Isoflupredone Acetate. 9α-Fluoroprednisolone Acetate; U-6013. 9α-Fluoro-11β,17α,21-trihydroxypregna-1,4-diene-3,20-dione 21-acetate.
$C_{23}H_{29}FO_6$=420.5.

CAS — 338-95-4 (isoflupredone); 338-98-7 (acetate).

Isoflupredone is a fluorinated corticosteroid for topical use.

Proprietary Names
Menaderm Simplex *(Menarini, Ital.).*

14038-q

Isomalt. BAY i-3930. An approximately equimolar mixture of 6-*O*-(α-D-glucopyranosyl)-D-glucitol ($C_{12}H_{24}O_{11}$ = 344.3) and 1-*O*-(α-D-glucopyranosyl)-D-mannitol ($C_{12}H_{24}O_{11},2H_2O$ = 380.3).

A white, odourless, crystalline, slightly hygroscopic solid with a sweet taste.

The Food Additives and Contaminants Committee on the review of sweeteners in food has recommended that isomalt be permitted temporarily for use as a sweetener in food, other than food manufactured specifically for babies and young children.

12870-d

Isonixin. 2-Hydroxy-*N*-(2,6-dimethylphenyl)nicotinamide.
$C_{14}H_{14}N_2O_2$=242.3.

CAS — 57021-61-1.

Isonixin has analgesic and anti-inflammatory activity.

Studies in *animals*.— R. Cadena *et al.*, *Arzneimittel-Forsch.*, 1977, *27*, 1457 (anti-inflammatory activity); M. T. Mitjavila *et al.*, *ibid.*, 1460 (toxicology).

Proprietary Names
Nixyn Oral *(Hermes, Spain).*

12872-h

Isoxepac. HP-549; P-720549. 6,11-Dihydro-11-oxodibenz[*b,e*]oxepin-2-ylacetic acid.
$C_{16}H_{12}O_4$=268.3.

CAS — 55453-87-7.

Isoxepac has anti-inflammatory activity.

Use in rheumatoid arthritis.— L. S. Gerlis and J. M. Gumpel, *Rheumatol. Rehab.*, 1981, *20*, 50.

Manufacturers
Hoechst, UK.

12873-m

Isoxicam. W-8495. 4-Hydroxy-2-methyl-*N*-(5-methylisoxazol-3-yl)-2*H*-1,2-benzothiazine-3-carboxamide 1,1-dioxide.
$C_{14}H_{13}N_3O_5S$=335.3.

CAS — 34552-84-6.

Isoxicam is an anti-inflammatory agent under study.

Manufacturers
Parke, Davis, USA.

12874-b

Ivermectin. A mixture of ivermectin component B_{1a} (5-*O*-demethyl-22,23-dihydroavermectin A_{1a}) and ivermectin component B_{1b} (5-*O*-demethyl-25-de(1-methylpropyl)-22,23-dihydro-25-(1-methylethyl)avermectin A_{1a}).

CAS — 70161-11-4 (component B_{1a}); 70209-81-3 (component B_{1b}); 70288-86-7 (mixture).

Ivermectin is a veterinary parasiticide used for a variety of infections in cattle.

Proprietary Names
Ivomec *(Merck Sharp & Dohme, UK).*

12875-v

Jojoba Oil. An oil derived from the desert plant *Simmondsia californica.*

CAS — 61789-91-1.

It is proposed as a substitute for sperm whale oil.

References: *Drug Cosmet. Ind.*, 1980, *127* (Aug.), 14; *ibid.*, (Sept.), 60.

12876-g

Kasugamycin.
$C_{14}H_{25}N_3O_9$=379.4.

CAS — 6980-18-3.

An antimicrobial substance produced by the growth of *Streptomyces kasugaensis.* **Soluble** in water; practically insoluble in most organic solvents.

Kasugamycin is an aminoglycoside antibiotic with antifungal activity and generally weak antibacterial properties apart from activity against mycobacteria, *Pseudomonas* spp., and leptospira.

12877-q

Katemfe. The fruit of *Thaumatococcus daniellii* (Scitamineae).

Katemfe contains a water-soluble proteinaceous sweet principle which has been characterised as thaumatin I and thaumatin II, many times sweeter than sucrose, but labile to heat.

References: H. van der Wel, in *Symposium: Sweeteners*, G.E. Inglett (Ed.), Westport, AVI, 1974, p. 194; K. J. Parker, *Nature*, 1978, *271*, 493.

12878-p

Kava *(B.P.C. 1934).* Kava-Kava.

CAS — 500-64-1 (kawain); 495-85-2 (methysticin); 500-62-9 (yangonin).

The rhizome of *Piper methysticum* (Piperaceae), a shrub indigenous to islands of the South Pacific. It contains pyrones including kawain, methysticin, and yangonin.

Kava is reported to have mild hallucinogenic properties and has been used in a beverage to allay anxiety and reduce fatigue. It was formerly used as an antiseptic and diuretic in inflammatory conditions of the genito-urinary tract in the form of a liquid extract.

A patient who drank a tea made from kava 5 to 6 times daily for 6 months experienced a chronic intoxicated feeling, ataxia, loss of appetite, diarrhoea, and skin reactions. Also his skin was yellow which might have been due to deposition of kava pyrones in the keratin. Use of the tea was discontinued and most symptoms had disappeared when he was examined 12 months later.— R. K. Siegel, *J. Am. med. Ass.*, 1976, *236*, 473.

Proprietary Names
Neuronika *(kawain) (Klinge, Ger.).*

12879-s

Keracyanin. 3-[6-*O*-(α-L-Rhamnopyranosyl)-β-D-glucopyranosyloxy]-3′,4′,5,7-tetrahydroxyflavylium chloride.
$C_{27}H_{31}ClO_{15}$=631.0.

CAS — 18719-76-1.

Keracyanin is claimed to improve visual adaptation to darkness.

Proprietary Names
Meralop *(ISF, Ital.).*

12880-h

Keratin *(B.P.C. 1934).* A name applied to a group of proteins which form the main constituents of horns, hoofs, feathers, quills, etc.

CAS — 68238-35-7.

Pharmacopoeias. In *Span.*

Keratin occurs as an odourless tasteless brownish-yellow powder or transparent, white, or greyish-white scales. Practically **insoluble** in water, alcohol, ether, and dilute acids; soluble in solutions of ammonia and in glacial acetic acid.

Keratin was formerly employed as an 'enteric' coating for pills and tablets.

12881-m

Ketanserin. R-41468; R-49945 *(tartrate).* 3-{2-[4-(4-Fluorobenzoyl)piperidino]ethyl-}quinazoline-2,4(1*H*,3*H*)-dione.
$C_{22}H_{22}FN_3O_3$=395.4.

CAS — 74050-98-9.

Ketanserin blocks serotonin receptors, and is being studied for its effects in hypertension.

References: J. M. Van Neuten *et al.*, *J. Pharmac. exp. Ther.*, 1981, *218,* 217; J. De Cree *et al.* (letter), *Lancet*, 1981, *1,* 1161; J. -C. Demoulin *et al.*, *ibid.*, 1186; J. De Cree *et al.*, *Angiology*, 1981, *32,* 137.

Manufacturers
Janssen, Belg.

12882-b

Ketocaine Hydrochloride. Chetocaina Cloridrata. 2′-(2-Di-isopropylaminoethoxy)butyrophenone hydrochloride.
$C_{18}H_{29}NO_2$,HCl=327.9.

CAS — 1092-46-2 (ketocaine); 1092-47-3 (hydrochloride).

Ketocaine hydrochloride is an injectable local anaesthetic.

Topical application of ketocaine (base) 10% in skin grafting.— L. Ohlsén and S. Englesson, *Br. J. Anaesth.*, 1980, *52,* 413.

Further references: A. Berlin-Wahlén *et al.*, *Acta pharm. suec.*, 1977, *14,* 425; G. Haegerstam *et al.*, *Arzneimittel-Forsch.*, 1979, *29,* 1177.

Proprietary Names
Vericaina *(Recordati, Ital.).*

12883-v

Kinkéliba. Combreti Folium. The dried leaves of *Combretum micranthum* (=*C. altum; C. raimbaultii*) (Combretaceae), a shrub indigenous to West Africa.

Pharmacopoeias. In *Fr.* and *Span.*

Kinkéliba has been used as a liquid extract or tincture and is reputed to be of value in blackwater and other fevers.

A decoction of *Combretum mucronatum* root was apparently successful in the treatment of guinea-worm infection.— *Chronicle Wld Hlth Org.*, 1977, *31,* 428.

12884-g

Krebiozen

CAS — 9008-19-9.

Krebiozen is the name of a preparation that received much publicity, particularly in the USA, as a 'cancer cure'. It was stated to be obtained from the blood of horses previously injected with an extract of *Actinomyces bovis.*
The claims made for Krebiozen were never scientifically substantiated and, in 1966, the US Food and Drugs Administration pronounced it to be totally discredited.

12885-q

Kveim Antigen. A fine suspension in physiological saline of material from granulomatous lymph nodes taken from patients with active sarcoidosis.

Kveim antigen is used as an intradermal injection of 0.15 ml of a 10% suspension in the Kveim test (also known as the Kveim-Siltzbach test) for the diagnosis of sarcoidosis. A positive reaction consists of a papule at the site of injection, 1 to 3 weeks or longer after the injection is given, which remains palpable for at least 42 days from the time of its appearance. A biopsy should be taken at the site of the injection about 4 to 6 weeks after administration of the antigen to confirm the result of the test histologically.
Kveim antigen is available in Great Britain from the Central Public Health Laboratory.

For reviews of the Kveim test, see *Br. med. J.*, 1971, *2,* 604; *Med. Lett.*, 1972, *14,* 71.

A vindication of the Kveim-Siltzbach test.— *Lancet*, 1972, *1,* 188. Criticism.— H. L. Israel (letter), *ibid.*, 486.

Kveim tests were carried out with 3 batches of material in 81 patients with various diseases and positive results were obtained in tuberculosis, lymphomas, inflammatory bowel diseases, and rheumatoid arthritis as well as sarcoidosis.— T. H. Hurley *et al.*, *Lancet*, 1975, *1,* 494.

12886-p

Laburnum. Golden Chain; Golden Rain. *Laburnum anagyroides* (= *L. vulgare; Cytisus laburnum*) (Leguminosae).

All parts of laburnum are toxic. The toxic principle is cytisine (see p.1700).

A report of laburnum poisoning in 10 children.— R. G. Mitchell, *Lancet*, 1951, *2,* 57.

Comments on the incidence of laburnum poisoning in children and the suggestion that in general it is not as dangerous as has been thought.— R. M. Forrester, *Lancet*, 1979, *1,* 1073; J. M. Morfitt (letter), *ibid.*, 1195; K. C. Chin and T. J. Beattie (letter), *ibid.*, 1299; A. Bramley and R. Goulding, *Br. med. J.*, 1981, *283,* 1220.

12887-s

Laetrile. Laetrile consists chiefly of amygdalin (*O*-[6-*O*-β-D-glucopyranosyl-β-D-glucopyranosyl]-D-mandelonitrile, $C_{20}H_{27}NO_{11}$ = 457.4), a cyanogenic glycoside derived from apricot stones.

CAS — 29883-15-6 (amygdalin).

Laetrile is a controversial 'cancer' treatment; it has been postulated that amygdalin is preferentially hydrolysed in cancer cells by the enzyme β-glucosidase to yield benzaldehyde and hydrogen cyanide in sufficient quantities to kill malignant cells. More recently laetrile has been claimed to be 'vitamin B_{17}', also referred to as nitriloside, the deficiency of which is said to result in cancer; there is no evidence for accepting this view and laetrile is of no known value in human nutrition.
Laetrile has been used, usually in association with a special diet, by many cancer patients in the USA and elsewhere. However it is not licensed by the FDA and acceptable evidence of an antitumour effect is lacking. A recent clinical study conducted by the National Cancer Institute has indicated that laetrile is of no benefit in the treatment of cancer.
Despite claims for its lack of toxicity there have been several reports of cyanide poisoning and other adverse reactions associated with the use of laetrile, especially when taken by mouth.

Reviews and discussions on laetrile in the treatment of cancer: C. Holden, *Science*, 1976, *193,* 982; *FDA Drug Bull.*, 1977, *7,* 2; F. J. Ingelfinger, *New Engl. J. Med.*, 1977, *296,* 1167; A. S. Relman, *ibid.*, 1978, *298,* 215; G. R. Newell, *ibid.*, 216; C. G. Moertel, *ibid.*, 218; R. T. Dorr and J. Paxinos, *Ann. intern. Med.*, 1978, *89,* 389; B. J. Culliton and W. K. Waterfall, *Br. med. J.*, 1979, *1,* 802.

A report of chemically subpotent and microbially contaminated preparations of laetrile.— J. P. Davignon (letter), *New Engl. J. Med.*, 1977, *297,* 1355.

A brief description of the 'nutritional and metabolic antineoplastic diet' of laetrile proponents which includes: no meat, fish, or fowl; no dairy products; no animal protein; increased ingestion of fruit and vegetables; large doses of ascorbic acid (which may increase the probability of cyanide poisoning) and vitamin E; oral pancreatic enzymes; pangamic acid ('vitamin B_{15}'); and laetrile.— V. Herbert (letter), *J. Am. med. Ass.*, 1978, *240,* 1139.

In a retrospective analysis by the National Cancer Institute of cancer patients who were thought to have shown objective benefit from laetrile, 6 of 67 evaluable patients were judged to have complete or partial responses.— N. M. Ellison *et al.*, *New Engl. J. Med.*, 1978, *299,* 549.

One hundred and seventy-eight patients with advanced cancer, but in good general condition, were given laetrile in doses typical of those which had been promoted, in association with vitamins, pancreatic enzymes, and a 'metabolic diet'. Of the 175 evaluable patients 79% had progression of disease at 2 months and 91% had progression at 3 months; only one patient had a transient partial response. Of the 178 patients 152 had died; the median survival for all patients was 4.8 months. Laetrile is of no substantive value in cancer; further investigation or clinical use is not justified.— C. G. Moertel *et al.*, *New Engl. J. Med.*, 1982, *306,* 201. See also A. S. Relman, *ibid.*, 236.

Toxicity. A review of cyanide poisoning and other adverse reactions associated with laetrile. Some 37 poisonings and 17 deaths, mostly from the ingestion of apricot or other fruit kernels, have now been recorded. Cyanide release from amygdalin is known to occur in the presence of hydrolysing β-glucosidase enzymes which are present in some raw fruits and vegetables including lettuce, mushrooms, certain fresh fruits, green peppers, celery, and sweet almonds; ingestion of any of these uncooked foods with amygdalin can produce cyanide poisoning. Other adverse reactions reported with laetrile include hypotension, haemoglobinuria, gastro-intestinal haemorrhage, vomiting, headache, diarrhoea, fever, rash, and muscular weakness. It is advised that physicians with patients using laetrile should watch for signs and symptoms of acute and chronic cyanide intoxication and be prepared to administer emergency treatment. Patients who use laetrile should be warned against taking the parenteral preparation by mouth since the high concentration can be rapidly fatal.— *FDA Drug Bull.*, 1977, *7,* 26.

An 11-month-old baby died from cyanide poisoning after accidentally swallowing between one and 5 laetrile tablets each containing amygdalin 500 mg and yielding 12 to 26 mg of cyanide on hydrolysis. The potential toxicity of this preparation had not been realised, which contributed to a delay in the start of treatment with amyl nitrite by inhalation followed by 1.5 ml of a 3% sodium nitrite solution intravenously and 6 ml of 25% sodium thiosulphate solution.— K. T. Braico *et al.*, *New Engl. J. Med.*, 1979, *300,* 238. See also J. R. Humbert *et al.* (letter), *J. Am. med. Ass.*, 1977, *238,* 482.

Individual reports of adverse reactions and cyanide poisoning in patients using laetrile: F. P. Smith *et al.* (letter), *J. Am. med. Ass.*, 1977, *238,* 1361; *idem*, *Cancer Treat. Rep.*, 1978, *62,* 169; L. Sadoff *et al.*, *J. Am. med. Ass.*, 1978, *239,* 1532; J. A. Ortega and J. E. Creek, *J. Pediat.*, 1978, *93,* 1059; J. H. Carter and P. Goldman (letter), *ibid.*, *94,* 1018; D. L. Morse *et al.* (letter), *New Engl. J. Med.*, 1979, *301,* 892; M. J. Rubino and F. Davidoff (letter), *J. Am. med. Ass.*, 1979, *241,* 359; C. G. Moertel *et al.*, *ibid.*, 1981, *245,* 591.

12888-w

Laminaria Stalks. Stipites Laminariae; Styli Laminariae.

Pharmacopoeias. In *Arg.*, *Port.*, and *Span.*

The dried stalks of the seaweeds *Laminaria cloustoni*, *L. digitata*, and possibly other species of *Laminaria*.

Laminaria stalks swell in water to about 6 times their volume and have been used surgically to dilate cavities. For this purpose they are usually made into either solid or hollow cylinders ('laminaria tents') from 50 to 75 mm long and 8 to 12 mm wide. They have been supplied singly in sealed tubes after being sterilised by alcohol vapour in an autoclave at 120° for 50 minutes.

References to the use of laminaria for the induction of abortion: J. H. Duenhoelter *et al.*, *Obstet. Gynec.*, 1976, *47*, 469; J. H. Strauss *et al.*, *Am. J. Obstet. Gynec.*, 1979, *134*, 260; M. Hachamovitch *et al.*, *ibid.*, *135*, 327; K. Edström, *Bull. Wld Hlth Org.*, 1979, *57*, 481.

12889-e

Lappa. Burdock; Burdock Root; Bardane (Grande); Bardanae Radix.

Pharmacopoeias. In *Fr.* and *Span. Fr. P.* also describes the leaves.

The dried root of the great burdock, *Arctium lappa* (= *A. majus*), and other species of *Arctium* (Compositae).

Lappa was formerly used in the form of a decoction as a diuretic and diaphoretic.

A report of symptoms of anticholinergic poisoning in a 26-year-old woman who had taken burdock root tea contaminated with atropine.— P. D. Bryson *et al.*, *J. Am. med. Ass.*, 1978, *239*, 2157. See also *idem* (letter), *240*, 1586; F. F. Hyde (letter), *Pharm. J.*, 1978, *2*, 204.

12890-b

Lasalocid. Ro-02-2985. 6-[(3*R*,4*S*,5*S*,7*R*)-7-{(2*S*,3*S*,5*S*)-5-Ethyl-5-[(2*R*,5*R*,6*S*)-5-ethyl-tetrahydro-5-hydroxy-6-methyl-2*H*-pyran-2-yl]-tetrahydro-3-methyl-2-furyl}-4-hydroxy-3,5-dimethyl-6-oxononyl]-2-hydroxy-*m*-toluic acid.
$C_{34}H_{54}O_8$=590.8.

CAS — 11054-70-9; 25999-31-9.

Lasalocid is used in veterinary practice as a coccidiostat for poultry. The sodium salt has also been used.

12891-v

Lead Arsenate *(B. Vet. C. 1965).* Plumbi Arsenas.
$PbHAsO_4$=347.1.

CAS — 7645-25-2 (xPb).

Pharmacopoeias. In *Arg.*

A white or nearly white powder, free from lumps or grit. Practically **insoluble** in cold water; soluble in nitric acid and solutions of alkali hydroxides.

Lead arsenate has been used in veterinary medicine for the control of tapeworm infection in ruminants. It has been used in horticulture as a spray for controlling some pests.
Maximum permissible atmospheric concentration, as lead, 150 μg per m^3.

12892-g

Lepromin. A suspension of killed *Mycobacterium leprae* prepared from the skin of heavily infected patients suffering from lepromatous leprosy or from armadillo tissue infected with *M. leprae*. .

CAS — 63163-81-5.

Lepromin is used in an intradermal skin test for the classification of leprosy and the assessment of immune responsiveness to *M. leprae*. The test is not diagnostic for leprosy and reactions may be found in persons who have not been exposed to leprosy. An intradermal injection of suspension is made; an early reaction may occur after 48 hours and consists of oedema and erythema around the site of injection; a late reaction may occur after about 4 weeks and takes the form of a definite nodule which may be ulcerating.
Supplies of lepromin are available in Great Britain from Laboratories for Leprosy and Mycobacterial Research, National Institute for Medical Research, Mill Hill, London, NW7 1AA.

An account of the lepromin reaction. The original lepromin (of Mitsuda and Hayashi), a suspension of the whole autoclaved homogenised leproma including some tissue elements, was sometimes called integral lepromin, whereas purified bacillary suspensions were sometimes called bacillary lepromins. Leprolins were the soluble proteins of the bacilli with or without proteins of the lepra, not coagulated by heating, and did not elicit the early reaction. The Dharmendra antigen was neither a lepromin nor a leprolin and was used especially for testing the early reactions; it gave only a weak late reaction.— M. Abe *et al.*, *Lepr. Rev.*, 1974, *45*, 244.

A WHO memorandum on recommendations for the preparation of standard integral (Mitsuda-type) lepromin and its testing. The source material should be *M. leprae* from biopsy specimens of skin obtained from heavily infected patients suffering from lepromatous leprosy or from armadillo tissues infected with *M. leprae*.— *Bull. Wld Hlth Org.*, 1979, *57*, 921.

Further references: E. P. Elliston and C. E. Taylor, *Int. J. Lepr.*, 1976, *44*, 319; J. Walter *et al.*, *Lepr. Rev.*, 1977, *48*, 169; U. Sengupta *et al.*, *Lepr. India*, 1978, *50*, 599; G. Ramu *et al.*, *Lepr. Rev.*, 1980, *51*, 207.

12893-q

Letosteine. 2-[2-(Ethoxycarbonylmethylthio)ethyl]thiazolidine-4-carboxylic acid.
$C_{10}H_{17}NO_4S_2$=279.4.

CAS — 53943-88-7.

Letosteine has been used as a mucolytic agent in respiratory disorders.

Proprietary Names
Viscotiol *(Farmitalia Carlo Erba, Fr.)*.

12894-p

Leucocianidol. 2-(3,4-Dihydroxyphenyl)chroman-3,4,5,7-tetrol.
$C_{15}H_{14}O_7$=306.3.

CAS — 480-17-1.

Leucocianidol has been used for its reputed beneficial effects on capillary circulation.

Proprietary Names
Flavan *(Millot-Solac, Fr.)*; Okavena *(Pan Química Farmac., Spain)*; Résivit *(Oberlin, Fr.)*.

12895-s

Leuprolide Acetate. Abbott-43818; TAP-144. 5-OxoPro-His-Trp-Ser-Tyr-D-Leu-Leu-Arg-*N*-ethyl-L-prolinamide acetate.
$C_{59}H_{84}N_{16}O_{12},C_2H_4O_2$=1269.5.

CAS — 74381-53-6.

A polypeptide reported to have antineoplastic activity.

Manufacturers
Abbott, USA; Takeda, Jap.

12896-w

Levonantradol Hydrochloride. CP-50556-1. (−)-(6*S*,6a*R*,9*R*,10a*R*)-5,6,6a,7,8,9,10,10a-Octahydro-9-hydroxy-6-methyl-3-[(1*R*)-1-methyl-4-phenylbutoxy]phenanthridin-1-yl acetate hydrochloride.
$C_{27}H_{35}NO_4,HCl$=474.0.

CAS — 71048-87-8 (levonantradol); 70222-86-5 (hydrochloride).

Levonantradol is a synthetic cannabinoid with analgesic and anti-emetic activity.

References: A. K. Jain *et al.*, *Clin. Pharmac. Ther.*, 1981, *29*, 255.

Manufacturers
Pfizer, UK.

12897-e

Lignin. A polymer occurring in plant fibrous tissue.

CAS — 9005-53-2.

Lignin has been reported to adsorb bile salts and acids and has been used in the treatment of diarrhoea.

For references to the use of lignin, see Martindale 27th Edn, p. 1774.

12899-y

Lodoxamide. *NN'*-(2-Chloro-5-cyano-*m*-phenylene)dioxamic acid.
$C_{11}H_6ClN_3O_6$=311.6.

CAS — 53882-12-5 (lodoxamide); 53882-13-6 (lodoxamide ethyl); 63610-09-3 (lodoxamide trometamol).

Lodoxamide and its ethyl derivative (lodoxamide ethyl; U-42718) and its trometamol derivative (lodoxamide trometamol; lodoxamide tromethamine; U-42585E) have potential anti-asthmatic and anti-allergic activity.

References: M. L. Katcher and C. E. Reed, *J. Allergy & clin. Immunol.*, 1980, *66*, 223.

Manufacturers
Upjohn, USA.

12900-y

Lofentanil Oxalate. R-34995. (−)-Methyl *t*-3-methyl-1-phenethyl-4-(*N*-phenyl-propionamido)piperidine-*r*-4-carboxylate oxalate.
$C_{25}H_{32}N_2O_3,C_2H_2O_4$=498.6.

CAS — 61380-40-3 (lofentanil); 61380-41-4 (oxalate).

Lofentanil oxalate is reported to be a narcotic analgesic.

Manufacturers
Janssen, Belg.

12901-j

Lofexidine. Ba-168; RMI-14042A. 2-[1-(2,6-Dichlorophenoxy)ethyl]-2-imidazoline.
$C_{11}H_{12}Cl_2N_2O$=259.1.

CAS — 31036-80-3.

Lofexidine is structurally related to clonidine (p.139) and has been studied in the treatment of hypertension.

Effects on blood pressure and haemodynamics: F. M. Fouad *et al.*, *Clin. Pharmac. Ther.*, 1980, *27*, 254; W. St. J. LaCorte *et al.*, *ibid.*, 1981, *29*, 259; F. M. Fouad *et al.*, *ibid.*, 498; H. S. Schultz *et al.*, *J. clin. Pharmac.*, 1981, *21*, 65; B. N. Garrett and N. M. Kaplan, *ibid.*, 173.

Lofexidine in opiate withdrawal.— A. M. Washton *et al.* (letter), *Lancet*, 1981, *1*, 991; M. S. Gold *et al.* (letter), *ibid.*, 992.

Manufacturers
Richardson-Vicks, UK; Nattermann, Ger.

12902-z

Lonazolac. 3-(4-Chlorophenyl)-1-phenyl-pyrazol-4-ylacetic acid.
$C_{17}H_{13}ClN_2O_2$=312.8.

CAS — 53808-88-1.

Lonazolac has analgesic and anti-inflammatory activity.

Manufacturers
Byk Gulden, Ger.

12903-c

Loprazolam. 6-(2-Chlorophenyl)-2,4-dihydro-2-(4-methylpiperazin-1-ylmethylene)-8-nitro-1*H*-imidazo[1,2-*a*][1,4]benzodiazepin-1-one. $C_{23}H_{21}ClN_6O_3$=464.9.

CAS — 61197-73-7.

Loprazolam is a benzodiazepine reported to have hypnotic properties.

Manufacturers
Roussel, UK.

12904-k

Lucimycin. Lucensomycin. An antifungal substance produced by the growth of *Streptomyces lucensis* and closely related to natamycin. $C_{36}H_{53}NO_{13}$=707.8.

CAS — 11035-14-6; 13058-67-8.

It is a white crystalline powder. Practically **insoluble** in water and alcohol.

Lucimycin has been used in mycotic skin infections.

12905-a

Luténurine. Lutenurin. The hydrochloride of an alkaloid extracted from the rhizomes of the yellow water lily, *Nuphar lutea* (Nymphaeaceae).

CAS — 12698-70-3.

Luténurine is an antibacterial, antifungal, and antitrichomonal agent which has been used in the treatment of vaginitis.

Proprietary Names
Situcidine *(UCB, Fr.).*

12906-t

Lysidine. Methylglyoxalidine. 2-Methyl-2-imidazoline.
$C_4H_8N_2$=84.12.

CAS — 534-26-9.

Crystals. M.p. 105°. **Soluble** in water, alcohol, and chloroform; less soluble in carbon tetrachloride and petroleum ether; practically insoluble in ether. **Incompatible** with acids, metal salts, and alkaloids.

Lysidine bitartrate has been used in the treatment of rheumatism.

12907-x

Magnesium Ascorbate.
$(C_6H_7O_6)_2Mg$=374.5.

CAS — 15431-40-0.

Magnesium ascorbate has been used as a source of magnesium.

Proprietary Names
Magnorbin *(E. Merck, Ger.; Bracco, Ital.).*

12908-r

Magnesium Ferulate. Magnesium 4-hydroxy-3-methoxycinnamate.
$(C_{10}H_9O_4)_2Mg$=410.7.

CAS — 32179-46-7.

Magnesium ferulate has been used as a choleretic agent.

Proprietary Names
Fruchol *(Laboratoires Français de Thérapeutique, Fr.).*

12909-f

Magnesium Gluceptate. Magnesium glucoheptonate.
$C_{14}H_{26}MgO_{16}$=474.7.

Magnesium gluceptate has been used as a source of magnesium.

Proprietary Names
Magnesium-Rougier *(Rougier, Canad.).*

12910-z

Magnesium Glutamate Hydrobromide. Magnesium Bromoglutamate; Magnesium α-Aminoglutarate Hydrobromide.
$(C_5H_8NO_4)_2Mg,HBr$=397.5.

Magnesium glutamate hydrobromide has been used as a sedative and hypnotic in the treatment of insomnia, neuroses, and behavioural disorders.

Proprietary Names
Bromolate *(Roner, Austral.)*; Hyposed *(Nelson, Austral.)*; Psicosoma *(Trommsdorff, Ger.)*; Psycho-Soma *(Roner, Austral.; Boots-Dacour, Fr.)*; Psychoverlan *(Verla, Ger.).*

12911-c

Magnesium Lactate.
$C_6H_{10}MgO_6$=202.4.

CAS — 18917-93-6.

Magnesium lactate has been used as a source of magnesium.

Proprietary Names
Magnespasmyl *(CCP, Belg.; Millot-Solac, Fr.; Laboromand, Switz.).*

12912-k

Magnesium Pidolate. Magnesium Pyroglutamate. Magnesium 5-oxopyrrolidine-2-carboxylate.
$(C_5H_6NO_3)_2Mg$=280.5.

CAS — 62003-27-4.

Magnesium pidolate has been used as a source of magnesium.

Proprietary Names
MAG 2 *(Méram, Fr.).*

12913-a

Mammalian Tissue Extracts

Many medicinal preparations with definite pharmacological activity and valid clinical uses are of mammalian or similar origin and are described under their appropriate monographs—for example, calcitonin, corticotrophin, hydrocortisone (cortisol), some enzymes, heparin, insulin, parathyroid, pituitary hormones, some sex hormones, thyroid.
Traditionally many other preparations of similar origin have been promoted for a wide variety of disorders. Evidence of pharmacological activity is often lacking, and many have fallen into disuse.

Some Proprietary Preparations

H. 11 Extract *(Standard Laboratories, UK).* A solution prepared from human urine by alcohol extraction and dialysis containing a polypeptide, with amino acids; stated to inhibit the growth of tumours. For subcutaneous injection. Also available as **Ointment, Oral Liquid, Suppositories,** and **Tablets.**

Raveron *(Robapharm, Switz.: Welbeck, UK).* An extract of the prostate of healthy mature animals, available as an injection in ampoules of 1 ml. For the initial stage of prostatic hypertrophy, chronic prostatitis, and urinary incontinence. *Dose.* 1 ml daily or 2 ml every other day by deep intramuscular injection, for 4 to 6 weeks.

Recosen *(Robapharm, Switz.: Welbeck, UK).* An extract from the whole hearts of freshly killed animals. The water-soluble protein-free fractions are available in **Ampoules** of 1 ml, and the insoluble fractions are available as **Tablets**. For diseases of the heart. *Dose.* 1 ml by intramuscular injection daily or 1 to 2 ml on alternate days up to a total of 15 to 25 injections; 1 tablet thrice daily before meals concurrently and for several weeks afterwards.

12914-t

Mazaticol Hydrochloride. KAO-264; PG-501. 6,6,9-Trimethyl-9-azabicyclo[3.3.1]-non-3β-yl di(2-thienyl)glycolate hydrochloride monohydrate.
$C_{21}H_{27}NO_3S_2,HCl,H_2O$=460.0.

CAS — 42024-98-6 (mazaticol).

Mazaticol hydrochloride has been used in the treatment of drug-induced parkinsonism.

Proprietary Names
Pentona *(Tanabe, Jap.).*

12915-x

Mebolazine. 3,3′-Azinobis(2α,17α-dimethyl-5α-androstan-17β-ol).
$C_{42}H_{68}N_2O_2$=633.0.

CAS — 3625-07-8.

Mebolazine has been used as an anabolic agent.

Proprietary Names
Roxilon *(Lepetit, Spain).*

12916-r

Mecinarone. 1-[6-(2-Dimethylaminoethoxy)-4,7-dimethoxybenzofuran-5-yl]-3-(4-methoxyphenyl)prop-2-en-1-one.
$C_{24}H_{27}NO_6$=425.5.

CAS — 26225-59-2.

Mecinarone is reported to be a vasodilator.

Pharmacology in *animals.*— B. Pourrias *et al., Arzneimittel-Forsch.*, 1975, *25*, 782; B. Pourrias and F. Friedrich, *Eur. J. Pharmac.*, 1978, *49*, 203.

The stability of mecinarone maleate.— R. Gimet and J. Rabiant, *Farmaco, Edn prat.*, 1977, *32*, 214.

Manufacturers
Delalande, Fr.

12917-f

Mecloralurea. 75-25-C. 1-Methyl-3-(2,2,2-trichloro-1-hydroxyethyl)urea.
$C_4H_7Cl_3N_2O_2$=221.5.

CAS — 1954-79-6.

Mecloralurea has been used for the relief of anxiety.

Proprietary Names
Héraldium *(Millot-Solac, Fr.).*

12918-d

Meclorisone Dibutyrate. Sch-11572. 9,11β-Dichloro-17α,21-dihydroxy-16α-methylpregna-1,4-diene-3,20-dione dibutyrate.
$C_{30}H_{40}Cl_2O_6$=567.5.

CAS — 4732-48-3 (meclorisone); 10549-91-4 (dibutyrate).

Meclorisone dibutyrate is reported to be a topical corticosteroid.

Manufacturers
Schering, UK.

12919-n

Mecrifurone Hydrochloride. 9-[(2-Diethylamino)ethoxy]-7-methyl-5-oxo-5*H*-furo[3,2-*g*][1]-benzopyran-4-yl 3-(3-pyridyl)prop-2-enoate hydrochloride.
$C_{26}H_{26}N_2O_6,HCl$=499.0.

CAS — 23845-79-6 (mecrifurone); 23829-65-4 (hydrochloride).

Mecrifurone has been used for the prevention and treatment of angina pectoris and related disorders.

Proprietary Names
Coronplat *(Intersint, Ital.).*

12920-k

Medifoxamine Fumarate. *NN*-Dimethyl-2,2-diphenoxyethylamine fumarate.
$C_{16}H_{19}NO_2,C_4H_4O_4$=373.4.

CAS — 32359-34-5 (medifoxamine); 16604-45-8 (fumarate).

Medifoxamine fumarate has been used for the relief of anxiety.

Proprietary Names
Gerdaxyl *(Sidus, Arg.; Gerda, Fr.; Promesa, Spain).*

12921-a

Medroxalol Hydrochloride. RMI-81968A. 5-{1-Hydroxy-2-[1-methyl-3-(3,4-methylenedioxyphenyl)propylamino]ethyl-}salicylamide hydrochloride.
$C_{20}H_{24}N_2O_5,HCl$=408.9.

CAS — 56290-94-9 (medroxalol); 70161-10-3 (hydrochloride).

Medroxalol hydrochloride is reported to have alpha- and beta-adrenoceptor blocking activity.

References: P. Jaillon *et al., Clin. Pharmac. Ther.*, 1981, *29*, 254.

Manufacturers
Merrell-National, USA.

12922-t

Mefexamide. ANP-297; NP-297. *N*-(2-Diethylaminoethyl)-2-(4-methoxyphenoxy)acetamide.
$C_{15}H_{24}N_2O_3$=280.4.

CAS — 1227-61-8.

Mefexamide is a central nervous system stimulant which has been used in the treatment of fatigue and depression. Mefexamide hydrochloride has also been used.

Proprietary Names
Méfexadyne *(Anphar-Rolland, Fr.)*; Perneuron *(Crinos, Ital.)*; Timodyne *(Montpellier, Arg.; Anphar-Rolland, Fr.; Max Ritter, Switz.).*

NOTE. Timodine is a preparation containing nystatin and hydrocortisone.

12923-x

Meladrazine. Ba-13155; Hydramitrazine. NNN'N'-Tetraethyl-6-hydrazinotriazin-2,4-diyldiamine.
$C_{11}H_{23}N_7$=253.3.

CAS — 13957-36-3.

Meladrazine has muscle-relaxant properties. It has been used as the tartrate.

References: E. Pedersen and V. Grynderup, *Br. med. J.*, 1966, *2*, 271.

Proprietary Names
Lisidonil *(Ciba, Denm.; Ciba, Norw.).*

12924-r

Melatonin. *N*-Acetyl-5-methoxytryptamine. Melatonin is a hormone produced in the pineal gland. *N*-[2-(5-Methoxyindol-3-yl)ethyl]acetamide.
$C_{13}H_{16}N_2O_2$=232.3.

CAS — 73-31-4.

Results mainly from *animal* studies indicate that melatonin increases the concentration of aminobutyric acid and serotonin in the midbrain and hypothalamus and enhances the activity of pyridoxal-kinase, an enzyme involved in the synthesis of aminobutyric acid, dopamine, and serotonin. Melatonin is involved in the inhibition of gonadal development and in the control of oestrus; there appears to be a diurnal rhythm of melatonin secretion. It has been used in parkinsonism with disappointing results.

A discussion on the actions of melatonin.— *Lancet*, 1974, *2*, 1235. See also *The Pineal Gland*, G.E.W. Wolstenholme and J. Knight (Ed.), Edinburgh, Churchill Livingstone, 1971; K. P. Minneman and R. J. Wurtman, *A. Rev. Pharmac. Toxic.*, 1976, *16*, 33; K. M. Shaw, *Adv. Drug Res.*, 1977, *11*, 75.

The effect on melatonin on sleep and growth-hormone secretion.— H. Cramer *et al., Arzneimittel-Forsch.*, 1976, *26*, 1076.

A hypothesis that the pineal gland may play a role in the aetiology of breast cancer and that melatonin might suppress induction of breast cancer.— M. Cohen *et al., Lancet*, 1978, *2*, 814. Comment and disagreement.— E. Tapp (letter), *ibid.*, 1001; R. A. Karmali *et al.* (letter), *ibid.*, 1002; H. -O. Adami *et al.* (letter), *ibid.*, 1312; M. Cohen *et al.* (letter), *ibid.*, 1381.

12925-f

Melengestrol Acetate. BDH-1921; NSC-70968. 6-Methyl-16-methylene-3,20-dioxopregna-4,6-dien-17α-yl acetate.
$C_{25}H_{32}O_4$=396.5.

CAS — 5633-18-1 (melengestrol); 2919-66-6 (acetate).

Melengestrol acetate is a progestational agent. It is also reported to have glucocorticoid activity.

12926-d

Memotine Hydrochloride. UK-2371. 3,4-Dihydro-1-[(4-methoxyphenoxy)methyl]isoquinoline hydrochloride.
$C_{17}H_{17}NO_2,HCl$=303.8.

CAS — 18429-69-1 (memotine); 10540-97-3 (hydrochloride).

Memotine is an antiviral agent which has been tried in the prophylaxis of influenza.

References: A. S. Beare *et al., Lancet*, 1968, *1*, 843; K. W. Brammer *et al.* (letter), *Nature*, 1968, *219*, 515; G. M. Williamson and D. Jackson, *Bull. Wld Hlth Org.*, 1969, *41*, 665; J. E. Stark *et al., Thorax*, 1970, *25*, 649, per *Abstr. Wld Med.*, 1971, *45*, 241.

Manufacturers
Pfizer, USA.

12927-n

Menbutone. 4-(4-Methoxy-1-naphthyl)-4-oxobutyric acid.
$C_{15}H_{14}O_4$=258.3.

CAS — 3562-99-0.

Menbutone has been used as a choleretic agent. The magnesium salt has been similarly used.

Proprietary Names
Hepalande (magnesium salt) *(Delalande, Ger.)*; Icteryl (magnesium salt) *(Delalande, Belg.; Delalande, Fr.)*; Sintobilina *(Azienda Farm. Ital., Ital.).*

12928-h

Mepindolol. LF-17895; SHE-222 (sulphate). 1-Isopropylamino-3-(2-methylindol-4-yloxy)propan-2-ol.
$C_{15}H_{22}N_2O_2$=262.4.

CAS — 23694-81-7 (mepindolol); 56396-94-2 (sulphate).

Mepindolol is a beta-adrenoceptor blocking agent.

References: J. Bonelli, *Int. J. clin. Pharmac. Biopharm.*, 1977, *15*, 325; H. M. Beumer *et al., ibid.*, 1978, *16*, 249; J. Bonelli, *J. int. med. Res.*, 1978, *6*, 317; M. Sukerman *et al., Curr. ther. Res.*, 1979, *25*, 384; M. Sukerman *et al., ibid.*, 1980, *27*, 178; J. Bonelli *et al., Int. J. clin. Pharmac. Biopharm.*, 1980, *18*, 169.

Proprietary Names
Corindolan (sulphate)*(Schering, Ger.).*

12929-m

Mepiprazole. H-4007 (dihydrochloride). 1-(3-Chlorophenyl)-4-[2-(5-methylpyrazol-3-yl)ethyl]piperazine.
$C_{16}H_{21}ClN_4$=304.8.

CAS — 20326-12-9 (mepiprazole); 20344-15-4 (dihydrochloride).

Mepiprazole is reported to have psychotropic activity.

In a double-blind crossover study in 19 patients with the irritable bowel syndrome treatment for 4 weeks with mepiprazole 5 mg thrice daily was significantly more effective than treatment with a placebo. Side-effects included headache, vertigo, nausea, and increased irritability.— G. Dotevall and E. Groll, *Br. med. J.*, 1974, *4*, 16.

Proprietary Names
Psigodal *(Igoda, Spain).*

12930-t

Mepitiostane. S-10364. 17β-(1-Methoxycyclopentyloxy)-2α,3α-epithio-5α-androstane.
$C_{25}H_{40}O_2S$=404.6.

CAS — 21362-69-6.

Mepitiostane has been used in the treatment of breast cancer.

References: K. Inoue *et al., Cancer Treat. Rep.*, 1978, *62*, 743.

Proprietary Names
Thioderon *(Jap.).*

12931-x

Mepixantone. 3-Methoxy-4-piperidinomethyl-9*H*-xanthen-9-one.
$C_{20}H_{21}NO_3$=323.4.

CAS — 17854-59-0.

Mepixantone has been used as a respiratory stimulant.

Proprietary Names
Pimexone *(Formenti, Ital.).*

12932-r

Meptazinol Hydrochloride. Wy-22811. 3-(3-Ethyl-1-methylperhydroazepin-3-yl)phenol hydrochloride.
$C_{15}H_{23}NO,HCl$=269.8.

CAS — 54340-58-8 (meptazinol); 59263-76-2 (hydrochloride); 34154-59-1 (hydrochloride, ±).

Meptazinol hydrochloride is an analgesic with narcotic antagonist activity. It has been given intramuscularly as well as by mouth and rectally.

When 11 healthy fasting subjects were given meptazinol hydrochloride 50, 100, or 200 mg by mouth the drug was rapidly and almost completely absorbed, less than 10% appearing in the faeces. The drug was rapidly excreted and more than 60% appeared in the urine in the first 24 hours. Plasma concentrations of unchanged meptazinol remained below a detectable value of 20 ng per ml following administration by mouth. Intravenous administration of 20 mg to 2 subjects produced peak plasma concentrations of 53 and 60 ng per ml with an elimination half-life of about 2 hours. Meptazinol was considered to undergo extensive first-pass metabolism, its main metabolite being the glucuronide.— R. A. Franklin *et al., Br. J. clin. Pharmac.*, 1976, *3*, 497. Meptazinol hydrochloride 50 or 75 mg was rapidly absorbed and produced peak plasma concentrations of 39 to 190 ng per ml 30 minutes after rectal administration. The elimination half-life was approximately 2 hours. No obvious dose and concentration relationship was evident. Gastric emptying is seriously slowed by meptazinol. It is metabolised in the liver. In a study on 2 subjects given 50 mg by mouth peak plasma concentrations remained below 10 ng per ml.— *idem*, 1977, *4*, 163.

Intramuscular injections of meptazinol 100 mg, pethidine 100 mg, or pentazocine 60 mg all produced significant postoperative analgesia when they were compared in a double-blind study in 75 patients. Analgesia was at a maximum 30 to 60 minutes after injection and was still appreciable after 2 hours. There was no significant difference in the frequency of side-effects although meptazinol appeared to produce less sedation.— N. J. Paymaster, *Br. J. Anaesth.*, 1977, *49*, 1139.

Meptazinol 100 mg per 70 kg body-weight intramuscularly caused substantially less respiratory depression than morphine 10 mg per 70 kg or pentazocine 60 mg per 70 kg in 7 healthy subjects. Nausea and vomiting occurred in 5 subjects after meptazinol but euphoria or dysphoria did not.— C. Jordan *et al.*, *Br. J. Anaesth.*, 1979, *51*, 497.

Meptazinol 100 mg by mouth produced significantly better relief of moderate to severe pain than pentazocine 25 mg in a double-blind placebo-controlled crossover study in 30 elderly patients. Meptazinol also caused less mental confusion than pentazocine.— V. Pearce and P. J. Robson, *Postgrad. med. J.*, 1980, *56*, 474.

In a study of 13 women given an intramuscular injection of 100 to 150 mg during labour, meptazinol was found to cross the placenta readily but was rapidly eliminated from the neonate. This contrasted with pethidine which was known to be excreted very slowly from neonates.— R. A. Franklin *et al.* (letter), *Br. J. clin. Pharmac.*, 1981, *12*, 88.

Further references to the use of meptazinol: W. Oosterlinck and W. De Sy, *Curr. med. Res. Opinion*, 1975, *3*, 187; *idem*, 1976, *3*, 716; M. Staquet, *J. clin. Pharmac.*, 1978, *18*, 76; D. G. Moyes *et al.*, *S. Afr. med. J.*, 1979, *55*, 865; S. G. Flavell-Matts and P. J. Ward, *Br. J. clin. Pract.*, 1980, *34*, 286; A. Hedges *et al.*, *Br. J. Anaesth.*, 1980, *52*, 295; M. B. A. Jackson and P. J. Robson, *Br. J. Obstet. Gynaec.*, 1980, *87*, 296; C. P. Nel *et al.*, *S. Afr. med. J.*, 1981, *59*, 908; A. G. Wade and P. J. Ward, *J. int. med. Res.*, 1981, *9*, 74.

Manufacturers
Wyeth, UK.

12933-f

Metamivan. 3-Ethoxy-*NN*-diethyl-4-hydroxybenzamide.
$C_{13}H_{19}NO_3$=237.3.

Metamivan is an analogue of ethamivan and has been used as a cardiac and respiratory stimulant.

Proprietary Names
Anacardiol *(Ibi, Ital.)*.

12934-d

Metescufylline. 7-(2-Diethylaminoethyl)theophylline (7-hydroxy-4-methylcoumarin-6-yloxy)acetate.
$C_{25}H_{31}N_5O_8$=529.5.

CAS — 15518-82-8.

Metescufylline has been used for its reputed effect on capillary circulation.

Proprietary Names
Veinartan *(Millot-Solac, Fr.)*; Venarterin *(Boi, Spain)*.

12935-n

Methallibure *(B. Vet. C. 1965)*. AY-61122; ICI-33828; Metallibure. 1-Methyl-6-(1-methylallyl)-2,5-dithiobiurea.
$C_7H_{14}N_4S_2$=218.3.

CAS — 926-93-2.

CAUTION. *Protective gloves should be worn when handling methallibure.*

A white powder with a faintly garlic-like odour. M.p. about 187°. Practically **insoluble** in water and chloroform; soluble 1 in 100 of acetone and 1 in 200 of methyl alcohol; soluble in pyridine.

Methallibure has the property of reversibly inhibiting certain hypothalamic and anterior pituitary functions. It has been used in veterinary medicine to control the time of oestrus in pigs and has been administered to poultry to delay ovulation and for force moulting in laying hens.

Precocious puberty. Methallibure suppressed ovarian activity and ovulation in a 9-year-old girl with precocious puberty.— J. A. Loraine *et al.*, *Br. med. J.*, 1965, *1*, 98.

Teratogenicity. A report of the anti-gestation and teratogenic effects of methallibure in *gilts*.— J. U. Akpokodje and C. A. V. Barker, *Can. vet. J.*, 1971, *12*, 121, per *Int. pharm. Abstr.*, 1972, *9*, 344.

12936-h

Methetoin. N-3. 5-Ethyl-1-methyl-5-phenylhydantoin.
$C_{12}H_{14}N_2O_2$=218.3.

CAS — 5696-06-0.

Methetoin is an anticonvulsant which has been tried in the treatment of epilepsy. It has actions similar to those of phenytoin (see p.1235).

References: L. Oettinger and R. Simonds, *Dis. nerv. Syst.*, 1962, *23*, 403; W. Z. Baro, *ibid.*, 1964, *25*, 38; G. Selby and I. T. Lorentz, *Med. J. Aust.*, 1966, *2*, 940; J. Logothetis, *Dis. nerv. Syst.*, 1967, *28*, 515, per *Abstr. Wld Med.*, 1968, *42*, 239.

12937-m

Methicotinium Iodide. 3-Methoxycarbonyl-1-methylpyridinium iodide.
$C_8H_{10}INO_2$=279.1.

CAS — 4685-10-3.

Methicotinium iodide has been used in the treatment of hypertension and atherosclerosis.

Proprietary Names
Iodonicot *(Farmacosmici, Ital.)*.

12938-b

Methindizate Hydrochloride. Metindizate Hydrochloride. 2-(1-Methylperhydroindol-3-yl)ethyl benzilate hydrochloride.
$C_{25}H_{31}NO_3,HCl$=430.0.

CAS — 15687-33-9 (methindizate).

Methindizate hydrochloride is an antispasmodic used in veterinary medicine.

Manufacturers
Bayer Agrochem, UK.

12939-v

Methiosulfonium Chloride. Methylmethionine Sulfonium Chloride. (3-Amino-3-carboxypropyl)dimethylsulphonium chloride.
$C_6H_{14}ClNO_2S$=199.7.

CAS — 1115-84-0.

Methiosulfonium chloride has been used for its reputed protective effect on the liver and gastro-intestinal mucosa.

Proprietary Names
Epadyn-U *(Archifar, Ital.)*; Cabagin-U *(Jap.)*.

12940-r

Methiosulfonium Iodide. Methylmethionine Sulfonium Iodide. (3-Amino-3-carboxypropyl)dimethylsulphonium iodide.
$C_6H_{14}INO_2S$=291.1.

CAS — 3493-11-6.

Methiosulfonium iodide has been used in rheumatic and other disorders.

Proprietary Names
Lobarthrose *(Opodex, Fr.)*.

12941-f

Methisoprinol. NPT-10381; Inosiplex; Isoprinosine. A 1:3 molar complex of inosine and 1-dimethylaminopropan-2-ol 4-acetamidobenzoate.

CAS — 36703-88-5.

Methisoprinol is an antiviral agent and has been used in the treatment of subacute sclerosing panencephalitis. It has also been tried in other viral infections.

Methisoprinol 2.5 g twice daily for 10 days by mouth was no more effective than a placebo in a double-blind study in 30 subjects infected, 48 hours after starting treatment, with an intranasal instillation of Hong Kong influenza virus.— S. Longley *et al.*, *Antimicrob. Ag. Chemother.*, 1973, *3*, 506. Methisoprinol 4 g daily, taken by mouth in divided doses, reduced symptoms when compared with placebo in a double-blind study of healthy subjects infected experimentally with influenza A virus.— R. A. Khakoo *et al.*, *J. antimicrob. Chemother.*, 1981, *7*, 389.

Recovery started within a month of treatment with methisoprinol 5 g daily in a 10-year-old girl with subacute sclerosing panencephalitis. Steady improvement was noted over the next 2½ years.— R. H. Mattson, *Neurology, Minneap.*, 1974, *24*, 383. A study of methisoprinol in 2 patients with subacute sclerosing panencephalitis, one of whom may have obtained some benefit.— L. J. Streletz and J. Cracco, *Ann. Neurol.*, 1977, *1*, 183. Twenty-three of 27 patients with acute viral encephalitis treated with methisoprinol recovered; 19 of these did so without sequelae. The usual dose of methisoprinol was 100 mg per kg body-weight daily by mouth or intravenously, in courses of 8 to 10 days, with 8 days between courses; 1 to 3 courses were given for benign forms, and 2 to 6 or 9 courses for severe forms. In general, therapy was well tolerated; vomiting sometimes occurred at the beginning of oral therapy. Discontinuous therapy at moderate doses yields the best results for all forms of the disorder. Immunostimulants given continuously or in high doses may enhance proliferation of suppressor T lymphocytes yielding results opposite to those sought.— A. Buge *et al.* (letter), *Lancet*, 1979, *2*, 691.

A report of no benefit with methisoprinol in patients with acute viral hepatitis.— K. C. Lam *et al.*, *Am. J. dig. Dis.*, 1978, *23*, 893.

Lymphocytes from 6 children with cancer and herpes zoster, who had received methisoprinol in a dose of 1.8 to 2.7 g per m^2 body-surface daily for at least 5 days, were no more responsive to varicella-zoster antigen than those from 7 similar patients who received a placebo. Methisoprinol had been reputed to be a stimulator of virus-sensitised lymphocytes.— S. Feldman *et al.*, *Antimicrob. Ag. Chemother.*, 1978, *14*, 495.

Further references: T. E. Lynes, *Pharmacologist*, 1970, *12* (2), 271; L. A. Glasgow and G. J. Galasso, *J. infect. Dis.*, 1972, *126*, 162, per *Int. pharm. Abstr.*, 1973, *10*, 262; T. W. Chang and L. Weinstein, *Am. J. med. Sci.*, 1973, *265*, 143, per *Abstr. Hyg.*, 1973, *48*, 1050; P. Gordon *et al.*, *Antimicrob. Ag. Chemother.*, 1974, *5*, 153; P. R. Huttenlocher, *Neurology, Minneap.*, 1976, *26*, 364; P. R. Huttenlocher and R. H. Mattson, *ibid.*, 1979, *29*, 763; J. S. Wolinsky *et al.*, *Clin. exp. Immun.*, 1979, *35*, 397.

Proprietary Names
Delimmun *(Delalande, Ger.)*; Viruxan *(Gramon, Arg.; Sigmatau, Ital.)*.

12942-d

Methocidin. Hydroxymethyl Gramicidin.

CAS — 1407-05-2.

Methocidin is an antimicrobial agent with the actions and uses of gramicidin (see p.1173) from which it is derived.

Proprietary Names
Argicilline *(Aron, Fr.)*.

12943-n

2-Methoxyethanol. Ethylene Glycol Monomethyl Ether.
$C_3H_8O_2$=76.1.

CAS — 109-86-4.

A colourless liquid. Wt per ml about 0.96 g; b.p. about 125°.

2-Methoxyethanol is used as a solvent.

12944-h

5-Methoxypsoralen. Bergapten. 5-Methoxypsoralen is an ingredient of bergamot oil. 4-Methoxyfuro[3,2-*g*]chromen-7-one.
$C_{12}H_8O_4$=216.2.

CAS — 484-20-8.

5-Methoxypsoralen has been used similarly to methoxsalen (p.497) in the PUVA treatment of psoriasis.

Concern has been expressed at the possible risk of cancer, and the widespread use of 5-methoxypsoralen in cosmetic suntan preparations is considered unwise by some authorities.

A discussion of the possible risk of cancer from sunlight, from the use of psoralens in the PUVA treatment of psoriasis, and from the use of 5-methoxypsoralen in suntan preparations.— *Br. med. J.*, 1981, *283*, 335.

References to the use of 5-methoxypsoralen in the treatment of psoriasis.— H. Hönigsmann *et al.*, *Br. J. Derm.*, 1979, *101*, 369.

Warning against the use of 5-methoxypsoralen in suntan preparations.— M. J. Ashwood-Smith (letter), *Br. med. J.*, 1979, *2*, 1144; P. Kersey (letter), *ibid.*, 1980, *280*, 940.

Defence of the use of 5-methoxypsoralen.— P. Forlot (letter), *Br. med. J.*, 1980, *280*, 648; C. Grupper and B. Beretti (letter), *ibid.*, 940.

12945-m

Methscopolamine Methylsulphate. *N*-Methyl Hyoscine Methylsulphate. (−)-(1*S*,3*s*,5*R*,6*R*,7*S*)-6,7-Epoxy-8-methyl-3-[(*S*)-tropoyloxy]tropanium methyl sulphate.
$C_{18}H_{24}NO_4,CH_3O_4S$=429.5.

CAS — 13265-10-6 (methscopolamine); 18067-13-5 (methylsulphate).

Methscopolamine methylsulphate has the general properties of hyoscine methobromide and has been used for its antispasmodic effects.

Proprietary Names
Daipin *(Jap.)*; Sandrix *(Sanders-Probel, Belg.)*; Ulix *(Substantia, Fr.)*.

12946-b

Methyl Benzoquate *(B.P. Vet.)*. AY-20385; ICI-55052; Nequinate. Methyl 7-benzyloxy-6-butyl-1,4-dihydro-4-oxoquinoline-3-carboxylate.
$C_{22}H_{23}NO_4$=365.4.

CAS — 13997-19-8.

A white or creamy-white, odourless or almost odourless, amorphous powder. Practically **insoluble** in water; very slightly soluble in alcohol, chloroform, and methyl alcohol.

Methyl benzoquate is used in veterinary medicine as a coccidiostat in poultry.

12947-v

Methyl Butetisalicylate. Methyl Diethylacetylsalicylate. Methyl *O*-(2-ethylbutyryl)salicylate.
$C_{14}H_{18}O_4$=250.3.

Methyl butetisalicylate has been applied topically in rheumatic and similar disorders.

Proprietary Names
Doloderm *(Montedison, Arg.; Bellon, Fr.; RBS Pharma, Ital.)*.

12951-n

Methyl Fluorosulphate. Methyl Fluorosulphonate.
$CH_3O.SO_2F$=114.1.

Methyl fluorosulphate is a laboratory methylating agent. Pulmonary oedema has occurred after inhalation, and concern expressed concerning carcinogenicity.

References: J. Admiral (letter), *Lancet*, 1976, *2*, 854 (fatal pulmonary oedema); J. E. Cummings and J. F. King (letter), *Chem. in. Br.*, 1979, *15*, 329 (possible carcinogenicity).

12948-g

Methylheptaminol Hydrochloride. 2-Methyl-6-methylaminoheptan-2-ol hydrochloride.
$C_9H_{21}NO,HCl$=195.7.

Methylheptaminol hydrochloride has been used in the treatment of cardiac insufficiency.

Proprietary Names
Corsanil *(SIT, Ital.)*; Eptaminal *(Washington, Ital.)*.

12949-q

Methylhydroxyquinoline Methylsulphate. 1-Methyl-8-hydroxyquinolinium methyl sulphate.
$C_{10}H_{10}NO,CH_3O_4S$=271.3.

Methylhydroxyquinoline methylsulphate has been used as eye-drops in a variety of conditions.

Proprietary Names
Chibro-Uvélina *(Davur, Spain)*; Chibro-Uveline *(UPB, Belg.)*; Uveline *(Merck Sharp & Dohme-Chibret, Fr.)*.

12950-d

Methylmethacrylate. Methyl 2-methylacrylate.
$C_5H_8O_2$=100.1.

CAS — 80-62-6.

A liquid. Wt per ml about 0.94 g. **Soluble** in methyl ethyl ketone and in aromatic and chlorinated hydrocarbons.

Methylmethacrylate forms the basis of acrylic bone cements used in orthopaedic surgery. A liquid consisting chiefly of methylmethacrylate monomer with a polymerisation initiator is mixed with a powder consisting of polymethylmethacrylate (PMMA) or polymethylmethacrylate and methylmethacrylate-styrene copolymer. Barium sulphate or zirconium dioxide may be added as a contrast medium. The reaction is exothermic. The liquid is sterilised by filtration and the powder by irradiation. Beads of polymethylmethacrylate containing gentamicin have been implanted in the prophylaxis and treatment of bone infections. A bone cement containing gentamicin is also available.

Copolymers of methacrylate esters, including substances based on dimethylaminoethylmethacrylate, have been used in the film-coating of tablets and in sustained-release preparations.

A multiplicity of factors may be involved in adverse reactions to the use of bone cement, including direct effects or the results of insufficient fixation.

Maximum permissible atmospheric concentration of methylmethacrylate 100 ppm.

A discussion of the use of methylmethacrylate in pathological fractures including those resulting from metastatic cancer.— *Br. med. J.*, 1977, *2*, 4.

Based on experience of 7000 arthroplasties, involving the use of acrylic cement, performed over 10 years, the following considerations emerged: hypotension occurred in about 80% of cases; it rarely exceeded 15 mmHg after insertion of cement into the reamed acetabulum; it rarely exceeded 30 mmHg after insertion into the reamed femoral shaft; cardiac arrest had not occurred; hypotension appeared to be related to the absorption of free monomer into the circulation; hypotension was not affected by the anaesthetic technique.— G. J. C. Brittain and D. J. Ryan (letter), *Br. med. J.*, 1972, *4*, 667.

The use of methylmethacrylate cement in total hip replacement in arthritic patients appeared to carry no greater risk of cardiac arrest than might be expected in patients of similar age undergoing major surgery. The use of the cement in elderly patients with transcervical fracture of the femoral head undergoing Thompson's prosthetic replacement and in patients with rheumatoid arthritis undergoing total knee replacement with intra-medullary stems might carry an increased risk of cardiac arrest. Cardiac arrest and hypotension in association with the cement in orthopaedic surgery might be multifactorial. The risk of carcinogenicity in older patients need not be a practical consideration but long-term studies in *animals* were needed before its use in young people could be recommended. The use of the cement was not considered a factor in late deep infection. The possibility of hypersensitivity should be borne in mind. Disposable syringes made of polystyrene or polymethylmethacrylate should not be used in preparing the cement; syringes of polypropylene or glass and utensils of polypropylene or stainless steel were suitable.— Working Party on Acrylic Cement in Orthopaedic Surgery, Report to Department of Health and Social Security, London 1974.

Dizziness, dyspnoea, nausea, and vomiting were experienced by operating room personnel during and after operations for total hip replacement using methylmethacrylate. Adequate ventilation was necessary when using methylmethacrylate. A concentration of 100 ppm had been recommended as a time-weighted average concentration for industrial inhalation exposure for a 40-hour week by the American Conference on Governmental Industrial Hygienists.— *J. Am. med. Ass.*, 1976, *235*, 2652. See also N. L. Schenck (letter), *ibid.*, *236*, 1694.

A study of the adverse cardiovascular effects of methylmethacrylate during total hip replacement in 10 subjects aged 55 to 82 years, and observations on its effects on the isolated *rabbit* heart.— K. C. Wong *et al.*, *Clin. Pharmac. Ther.*, 1977, *21*, 709.

Seven patients with contact dermatitis due to acrylic monomers present in some u.v. printing inks showed no cross-reactivity to methylmethacrylate.— J. R. Nethercott, *Br. J. Derm.*, 1978, *98*, 541.

Bowen's resin, prepared from glycidyl methacrylate and bisphenol A (=4,4′-isopropylidenediphenol) had replaced silicate cement and acrylic resin for the dental filling of anterior teeth, with advantage in colour matching and mechanical properties. Methylmethacrylate was successfully used for making dentures despite disadvantages which included low impact strength, high shrinkage, poor abrasion and fatigue resistance, and inhibition of taste.— E. A. Mason, *Chem. in Br.*, 1980, *16*, 190.

Further references to adverse effects: J. H. Adams *et al.*, *Br. med. J.*, 1972, *3*, 740 (fatal fat embolism and cerebral infarction); R. Routledge (letter), *ibid.*, 1973, *1*, 487 (cystitis, granuloma, and carcinoma in industrial workers); R. D. Wines (letter), *ibid.*, *3*, 409 (bladder carcinoma); E. D. Dorofeeva, *Gig. Truda prof. Zabol.*, 1974, *10*, 23 (industrial poisoning), per *J. Am. med. Ass.*, 1975, *232*, 314; I. B. Fries *et al.*, *J. Bone Jt Surg.*, 1975, *57*, 547 (contact dermatitis), per *J. Am. med. Ass.*, 1975, *234*, 116; T. Kallos, *Anesthesiology*, 1975, *42*, 210 (impaired arterial oxygenation); G. E. Foster and J. B. Bourke (letter), *Lancet*, 1978, *2*, 267 (intestinal obstruction).

Proprietary Preparations

CMW Orthopaedic Bone Cement *(CMW Laboratories, UK)*. A sterile powder containing polymethylmethacrylate, supplied together with a sterile liquid containing monomethylmethacrylate. The powder and liquid are mixed together before use.

Garamycin Chains *(Kirby-Warrick, UK)*. Sterile polymethylmethacrylate-methylacrylate copolymer beads each containing gentamicin sulphate equivalent to gentamicin 4.5 mg together with zirconium dioxide 20 mg as an X-ray contrast medium. Each chain consists of 30 beads threaded on multiple-thread surgical wire. For the prophylaxis and treatment of bone infections.

Palacos R *(Kirby-Warrick, UK)*. A sterile bone cement consisting of a powder containing polymethylmethacrylate with zirconium dioxide (as an X-ray contrast medium), supplied together with a liquid containing monomethylmethacrylate. The powder and liquid are mixed together before use. **Palacos R with Gentamicin.** The powder component contains in addition gentamicin sulphate equivalent to gentamicin 500 mg in each 40-g pack. **Palacos R-20 with Gentamicin** is a half-size pack.

Septopal Chains *(E. Merck, UK)*. Sterile polymethylmethacrylate-methylacrylate copolymer beads each containing gentamicin sulphate equivalent to gentamicin 4.5 mg together with zirconium dioxide 20 mg as an X-ray contrast medium. Each chain consists of 30 beads threaded on multiple-thread surgical wire. For the prophylaxis and treatment of bone infections.

Surgical Simplex Plain Bone Cement *(Howmedica, UK)*. A sterile powder containing methylmethacrylate-styrene copolymer and polymethylmethacrylate, supplied together with a sterile liquid containing monomethylmethacrylate. The powder and liquid are mixed together before use. **Surgical Simplex Radiopaque Bone Cement.** The powder contains in addition barium sulphate 10%.

12952-h

Methyridine *(B. Vet. C. 1965)*. Metyridine. 2-(2-Methoxyethyl)pyridine.
$C_8H_{11}NO$=137.2.

CAS — 114-91-0.

A clear colourless or pale yellow to pale brown

liquid with a faint odour. Wt per ml 0.996 to 1 g. **Miscible** with water, alcohol, and most organic solvents. **Store** in airtight containers. Protect from light.

Methyridine is an anthelmintic which has been used in veterinary medicine for the treatment of roundworm infections.

12953-m

Meticrane. 6-Methylthiochroman-7-sulphonamide 1,1-dioxide.
$C_{10}H_{13}NO_4S_2$=275.3.

CAS — 1084-65-7.

Meticrane is a diuretic. There have been reports of thrombocytopenia associated with its use.

Proprietary Names
Arresten *(Jap.)*; Fontilix *(Diamant, Fr.)*.

12954-b

Metioprim. 5-(3,5-Dimethoxy-4-methylthiobenzyl)pyrimidine-2,4-diyldiamine.
$C_{14}H_{18}N_4O_2S$=306.4.

CAS — 68902-57-8.

Metioprim is closely related structurally to trimethoprim (see p.1484), and has antibacterial activity.

Manufacturers
Heumann, Ger.

15325-f

Metirosine. Metyrosine; L-588357-0. (−)-α-Methyl-L-tyrosine.
$C_{10}H_{13}NO_3$=195.2.

CAS — 672-87-7; 620-30-4 (racemetirosine).

NOTE. The term α-methyltyrosine (α-MPT; α-MT; α-methyl-*p*-tyrosine) is used below since although metirosine, the (−)-isomer, is the active form the manufacturers state that some racemate (racemetirosine; (±)-α-methyl-DL-tyrosine) is produced during synthesis but that the material supplied contains mainly (−)-isomer with a small amount of (+)-isomer.
The code name MK 781, applied to earlier investigational material, may have described a racemate or a preparation containing a smaller proportion of (−)-isomer than the product now available commercially.
Potency of the proprietary preparation (Demser) is expressed in terms of metirosine.

Adverse Effects. Sedation occurs in the majority of patients receiving α-methyltyrosine. Extrapyramidal symptoms; anxiety and psychic disturbances including depression, hallucinations, disorientation, and confusion; and diarrhoea have also been reported. Crystalluria, transient dysuria, and haematuria have been seen in a few patients. Other adverse effects reported occasionally include slight swelling of the breast, galactorrhoea, nasal stuffiness, decreased salivation, gastro-intestinal disturbances, headache, impotence or failure of ejaculation, and allergic reactions.
Hypotension and cardiac arrhythmias may occur during surgery for phaeochromocytoma, when α-methyltyrosine is used pre-operatively.

Precautions. To minimise the risk of crystalluria, patients receiving α-methyltyrosine should have a fluid intake sufficient to maintain a urine volume of at least 2 litres daily and their urine should be examined regularly for the presence of crystals.
α-Methyltyrosine has sedative effects and patients should be warned of the hazards of driving a motor vehicle or operating machinery while receiving the drug. It may have additive effects with alcohol and other CNS depressants. The extrapyramidal effects of phenothiazines or haloperidol may be exacerbated. Symptoms of psychic stimulation and insomnia may occur when α-methyltyrosine is withdrawn.
When α-methyltyrosine is used pre-operatively in patients with phaeochromocytoma, blood pressure and the ECG should be monitored continuously during surgery.
α-Methyltyrosine may cause spurious increases in urinary catecholamines because of the presence of metabolites of the drug.

Absorption and Fate. α-Methyltyrosine is well absorbed from the gastro-intestinal tract and is excreted mainly unchanged by the kidneys. Less than 0.5% of a dose may be excreted as the metabolites α-methyldopa, α-methyldopamine, and α-methylnoradrenaline.

Uses. α-Methyltyrosine is an inhibitor of the enzyme tyrosine hydroxylase, and consequently of the synthesis of catecholamines. It is used to control hypertension and symptoms of excessive sympathetic stimulation in patients with phaeochromocytoma and may be given for pre-operative preparation, to those patients for whom surgery is contra-indicated, or to those with malignant phaeochromocytoma.
α-Methyltyrosine is given by mouth in a dose of 250 mg four times daily, increased daily by 250 mg or 500 mg to a maximum of 4 g daily in divided doses. The optimum dose, achieved by monitoring clinical symptoms and catecholamine excretion, is usually in the range of 2 to 3 g daily and when used pre-operatively it should be given for at least 5 to 7 days before surgery.
The concomitant use of alpha-adrenoceptor blocking agents may be necessary.

A review of the pharmacology and clinical use of α-methyltyrosine.— R. N. Brogden *et al., Drugs,* 1981, *21,* 81.

The suppression of craving and the withdrawal syndrome by α-methyltyrosine in subjects addicted to narcotics or amphetamines.— J. Pozuelo, *Cleveland Clin. Q.,* 1976, *43,* 89. See also L. -E. Jönsson *et al., Clin. Pharmac. Ther.,* 1971, *12,* 889; J. Pozuelo and F. W. L. Kerr, *Mayo Clin. Proc.,* 1972, *47,* 621.

Further references: K. Engelman *et al., J. clin. Invest.,* 1968, *47,* 577.

Phaeochromocytoma. Reviews of the use of α-methyltyrosine in phaeochromocytoma.— *Lancet,* 1968, *2,* 1130; *Med. Lett.,* 1980, *22,* 28.

Experience in a 31-year-old woman with bilateral phaeochromocytoma suggested that α-methyltyrosine was best used in conjunction with an alpha and a beta blocker such as phenoxybenzamine and propranolol.— W. E. Bagnall *et al., Postgrad. med. J.,* 1976, *52,* 653.

Further references: A. Sjoerdsma *et al., Lancet,* 1965, *2,* 1092; N. F. Jones *et al., ibid.,* 1968, *2,* 1105; R. G. Robinson *et al., J. Pediat.,* 1977, *91,* 143.

Schizophrenia. In a study of 10 patients with psychotic diseases given α-methyltyrosine up to 4 g daily, 5 of 7 of the patients with mania improved significantly and in 3 this continued after treatment was stopped. The 3 patients with depression became worse and improved when treatment was discontinued. Hypotension, lethargy, and day-time sedation occurred in patients given doses of over 2 g daily.— H. K. H. Brodie *et al., Clin. Pharmac. Ther.,* 1971, *12,* 218.

The antipsychotic action of phenothiazine drugs was enhanced in 5 patients with chronic schizophrenia when α-methyltyrosine 2 g daily was given concomitantly.— A. Carlsson *et al., J. neural Transmission,* 1972, *33,* 83, per *Br. med. J.,* 1973, *1,* 551. A double-blind study in 10 chronic schizophrenics did not confirm that α-methyltyrosine up to 3 g daily enhanced the effect of their existing phenothiazine medication, possibly because of differences from the study populations in which such effect had been reported.— H. A. Nasrallah *et al., Archs gen. Psychiat.,* 1977, *34,* 649.

Further references: W. E. Bunney *et al., Am. J. Psychiat.,* 1971, *127,* 872; J. Walinder *et al., Archs gen. Psychiat.,* 1976, *33,* 501.

Proprietary Preparations

Demser *(Merck Sharp & Dohme, UK).* α-Methyltyrosine, mainly as the (−)-isomer (metirosine), available as capsules containing the equivalent of 250 mg of metirosine. (Also available as Demser in *Neth.* and *USA*).

12955-v

Metofenazate Fumarate. Methophenazine Fumarate. 2-{4-[3-(2-Chlorophenothiazin-10-yl)propyl]piperazin-1-yl}ethyl 3,4,5-trimethoxybenzoate difumarate.
$C_{31}H_{36}ClN_3O_5S,2C_4H_4O_4$=830.3.

CAS — 388-51-2 (metofenazate); 522-23-6 (fumarate).

Metofenazate fumarate is a phenothiazine which has been used in the treatment of psychotic disorders. The diesylate is also used.

Proprietary Names
Frenolon *(EGYT, Hung.; Labatec-Pharma, Switz.)*.

12956-g

Metomidate Hydrochloride. R-7315. Methyl 1-(α-methylbenzyl)imidazole-5-carboxylate hydrochloride.
$C_{13}H_{14}N_2O_2,HCl$=266.7.

CAS — 5377-20-8 (metomidate); 35944-74-2 (hydrochloride).

An off-white crystalline powder. M.p. about 172°. Very **soluble** in water.

Metomidate is the methyl analogue of etomidate (p.749). Metomidate hydrochloride is used in veterinary practice as a sedative and, in conjunction with azaperone, to produce surgical anaesthesia.

Proprietary Names
Hypnodil *(Janssen)(Crown, UK)*.

12957-q

Mibolerone. NSC-72260; U-10997. 17β-Hydroxy-7α,17α-dimethylestr-4-en-3-one.
$C_{20}H_{30}O_2$=302.5.

CAS — 3704-09-4.

Mibolerone is an anabolic and androgenic agent used in veterinary practice as a contraceptive for bitches.

12958-p

Midazolam Maleate. Ro-21-3981/001. 8-Chloro-6-(2-fluorophenyl)-1-methyl-4*H*-imidazo-[1,5-*a*][1,4]benzodiazepine maleate.
$C_{18}H_{13}ClFN_3,C_4H_4O_4$=441.8.

CAS — 59467-70-8 (midazolam); 59467-94-6 (maleate).

Midazolam maleate is a benzodiazepine used for the induction of anaesthesia.

A brief review.— J. W. Dundee, *Br. J. Anaesth.,* 1979, *51,* 641.

Further references: R. J. Fragen *et al., Anesthesiology,* 1978, *49,* 41 (comparison with diazepam); J. G. Reves *et al., Can. Anaesth. Soc. J.,* 1979, *26,* 42 (comparison with thiopentone); C. R. Brown *et al., Anesthesiology,* 1979, *50,* 467 (clinical pharmacology and pharmacokinetics); F. H. Sarnquist *et al., Clin. Pharmac. Ther.,* 1980, *27,* 283 (pharmacokinetics); J. W. Dundee *et al., Br. J. clin. Pharmac.,* 1980, *9,* 305P (comparison with diazepam); A. Forster *et al., Br. J. Anaesth.,* 1980, *52,* 907 (effect on CNS and cardiovascular system); J. A. S. Gamble *et al., ibid.,* 951P (induction of anaesthesia); J. W. Dundee *et al., Anaesthesia,* 1980, *35,* 454 (pharmacokinetics); J. W. Dundee and D. B. Wilson, *ibid.,* 459 (induction of anaesthesia); M. T. Smith *et al., Eur. J. clin. Pharmac.,* 1981, *19,* 271 (clinical pharmacology and pharmacokinetics); I. Gath *et al., Clin. Pharmac. Ther.,* 1981, *29,* 533 (clinical pharmacology).

Manufacturers
Roche, UK.

12959-s

Midodrine Hydrochloride. ST-1085. 2-Amino-*N*-(β-hydroxy-2,5-dimethoxyphenethyl)acetamide hydrochloride.
$C_{12}H_{18}N_2O_4,HCl$=290.7.

CAS — 42794-76-3 (midodrine); 3092-17-9 (hydrochloride).

Midodrine hydrochloride is a sympathomimetic agent which has been used in the treatment of hypotension.

Use in incontinence.— D. Jonas, *J. Urol.*, 1977, *118*, 980.

Vasoconstrictor effects.— O. Thulesius *et al.*, *Eur. J. clin. Pharmac.*, 1979, *16*, 423.

Use in idiopathic orthostatic hypotension and Shy-Drager syndrome.— A. Schirger *et al.*, *Mayo Clin. Proc.*, 1981, *56*, 429.

Proprietary Names
Gutron *(Chemie-Linz, Aust.; Hormonchemie, Ger.).*

12960-h

Mikamycin. Antimicrobial substances produced by *Streptomyces mitakaensis.*

CAS — 11006-76-1.

Mikamycin is an antibiotic used topically in conjunction with hydrocortisone.

12961-m

Milenperone. R-34009. 5-Chloro-1-{3-[4-(4-fluorobenzoyl)piperidino]propyl}-1,3-dihydro-2*H*-benzimidazol-2-one.
$C_{22}H_{23}ClFN_3O_2$=415.9.

CAS — 59831-64-0.

Milenperone is reported to have neuroleptic activity.

Manufacturers
Janssen, Belg.

12962-b

Miloxacin. AB-206. 1,4-Dihydro-6,7-methylenedioxy-1-methoxy-4-oxoquinoline-3-carboxylic acid.
$C_{12}H_9NO_6$=263.2.

CAS — 37065-29-5.

Miloxacin is a urinary antimicrobial agent.

References A. Izawa *et al.*, *Antimicrob. Ag. Chemother.*, 1980, *18*, 37 (antimicrobial activity); *idem*, 41 (pharmacokinetics); A. Yoshitake *et al.*, *ibid.*, 45 (pharmacokinetics).

Manufacturers
Sumitomo, Jap.

12963-v

Minaprine. Agr-1240; CB-30038. *N*-(4-Methyl-6-phenylpyridazin-3-yl)-2-morpholinoethylamine.
$C_{17}H_{22}N_4O$=298.4.

CAS — 25905-77-5.

Minaprine is used in a variety of psychiatric disorders.

Proprietary Names
Cantor *(Clin-Comar-Byla, Fr.).*

12964-g

Minaxolone. CCI-12923. Minaxolone, as the citrate, is a water-soluble compound structurally related to alphaxalone. 11α-Dimethylamino-2β-ethoxy-3α-hydroxy-5α-pregnan-20-one.
$C_{25}H_{43}NO_3$=405.6.

CAS — 62571-87-3.

Minaxolone has been studied as an intravenous anaesthetic agent but clinical study has ceased pending long-term toxicity studies in *animals.*

References: J. W. Dundee, *Br. J. Anaesth.*, 1979, *51*, 641; W. Aveling *et al.*, *Lancet*, 1979, *2*, 71; H. G. McNeill *et al.*, *ibid.*, 73; W. Aveling *et al.*, *Br. J. Anaesth.*, 1979, *51*, 564P; G. L. Dunn *et al.*, *Can. Anaesth. Soc. J.*, 1980, *27*, 140; J. W. Sear *et al.*, *Anaesthesia*, 1980, *35*, 169; L. E. Mather *et al.* (letter), *Br. J. Anaesth.*, 1980, *52*, 241; G. G. Harrison and D. F. Morrell (letter), *ibid.*, 706; G. H. Blekkenhorst *et al.*, *ibid.*, 759; C. J. Hull, *ibid.*, 1981, *53*, 323; J. W. Sear *et al.*, *ibid.*, 339.

Manufacturers
Glaxo, UK.

12965-q

Miracle Fruit. The fruit of *Synsepalum dulcificum* (Sapotaceae).

Miracle fruit contains a glycoprotein 'miraculin' with no apparent taste of its own but able to make sour substances taste sweet and to improve the flavour of foods. Its activity is reduced by heating.

References: H. van der Wel, in *Symposium: Sweeteners*, G.E. Inglett (Ed.), Westport, AVI, 1974, p. 194; F. R. Dastoli and R. J. Harvey, *ibid.*, p. 204.

12966-p

Misonidazole. Ro-7-0582. 1-Methoxy-3-(2-nitroimidazol-1-yl)propan-2-ol.
$C_7H_{11}N_3O_4$=201.2.

CAS — 13551-87-6.

Misonidazole has been given to sensitise neoplastic cells to the effects of irradiation. Peripheral neuropathy may be a dose-limiting factor.

Discussions of the use of misonidazole as a radiosensitiser: *Lancet*, 1978, *2*, 617; J. D. Chapman, *New Engl. J. Med.*, 1979, *301*, 1429; *Br. med. J.*, 1980, *281*, 1089.

Further references: A. B. M. F. Karim (letter), *Lancet*, 1978, *2*, 891; P. Workman *et al.*, *Br. J. Cancer*, 1978, *38*, 709; J. Partington *et al.*, *Cancer Treat. Rep.*, 1979, *63*, 123; A. V. Reynolds, *J. Pharm. Pharmac.*, 1979, *31*, *Suppl.*, 29P; M. D. Walker and T. A. Strike, *Cancer clin. Trials*, 1980, *3*, 105; G. E. Adams (letter), *Br. med. J.*, 1981, *282*, 906.

Study of the effect of phenytoin on the metabolism of misonidazole in 6 patients showed a shortening of the half-life without lowering the concentration 4 hours after a dose. The effect might reduce neurotoxicity associated with misonidazole.— P. Workman *et al.*, *Br. J. Cancer*, 1980, *41*, 302.

Manufacturers
Roche, UK.

12967-s

Mitoxantrone Hydrochloride. CL-232315; NSC-301739. 1,4-Dihydroxy-5,8-bis[2-(2-hydroxyethylamino)ethylamino]anthraquinone dihydrochloride.
$C_{22}H_{28}N_4O_6,2HCl$=517.4.

CAS — 65271-80-9 (mitoxantrone); 70476-82-3 (hydrochloride).

Mitoxantrone is reported to have antineoplastic activity.

References: D. S. Alberts *et al.*, *Cancer Chemother. Pharmac.*, 1980, *5*, 11.

Manufacturers
Lederle, USA.

12968-w

MK-251. αα-Dimethyl-4-(ααββ-tetrafluorophenethyl)benzylamine.
$C_{17}H_{17}F_4N$=311.3.

CAS — 40396-83-6 (isethionate).

MK-251 has anti-arrhythmic properties. It has been studied as the isethionate and hydrochloride.

Pharmacology in *animals.*— M. L. Torchiana *et al.*, *J. Pharmac. exp. Ther.*, 1975, *194*, 415; A. G. Zacchei and L. Weidner, *J. pharm. Sci.*, 1975, *64*, 814.

Manufacturers
Merck Sharp & Dohme, USA.

12970-b

Mocimycin. MYC-8003. An antibiotic obtained from *Streptomyces ramocissimus.*
$C_{43}H_{60}N_2O_{12}$=797.0.

CAS — 50935-71-2; 52212-85-8.

Mocimycin has been added to animal feeding stuffs for promoting growth.

12971-v

Molsidomine. Morsydomine; CAS-276; SIN-10. *N*-Ethoxycarbonyl-3-morpholinosydnonimine.
$C_9H_{14}N_4O_4$=242.2.

CAS — 25717-80-0.

Molsidomine is a vasodilator which has been used in the treatment of angina pectoris.

References: G. Blazek *et al.*, *Dt. med. Wschr.*, 1977, *102*, 81; N. Grewe and M. Stauch, *ibid.*, 1758; A. Takeshita *et al.*, *Circulation*, 1977, *55*, 401; D. Dell *et al.*, *Hoechst*, *Br. J. clin. Pharmac.*, 1978, *5*, 359P; K. R. Karsch *et al.*, *Eur. J. clin. Pharmac.*, 1978, *13*, 241; S. Guerchicoff *et al.*, *ibid.*, 247; B. Niehues *et al.*, *Dt. med. Wschr.*, 1978, *103*, 853; P. A. Majid *et al.*, *New Engl. J. Med.*, 1980, *302*, 1; M. Aptecar *et al.*, *Am. Heart J.*, 1981, *101*, 369.

Proprietary Names
Corvaton *(Cassella-Riedel, Ger.)*; Molsidolat *(Hoechst, Ital.)*; Morial *(Jap.).*

12972-g

Monalazone Disodium. Disodium 4-(*N*-chlorosulphamoyl)benzoate.
$C_7H_4ClNNa_2O_4S$=279.6.

CAS — 61477-95-0.

Monalazone disodium is closely related structurally to halazone and is used as a vaginal disinfectant and spermicide.

Proprietary Names
Speton *(Temmler, Ger.).*

12973-q

Monensin Sodium. Lilly-67314 (monensin). An antibiotic isolated from *Streptomyces cinnamonensis.* Sodium 4-{2-[2-ethyl-3′-methyl-5′-(tetrahydro-6-hydroxy-6-hydroxymethyl-3,5-dimethyl-2*H*-pyran-2-yl)perhydro-2,2′-bifuran-5-yl]-9-hydroxy-2,8-dimethyl-1,6-dioxaspiro[4.5]dec-7-yl}-3-methoxy-2-methylvalerate.
$C_{36}H_{61}NaO_{11}$=692.9.

CAS — 17090-79-8 (monensin); 22373-78-0 (sodium salt).

Monensin sodium is used in veterinary practice for the prevention of coccidiosis in chickens and as a growth promoter for cattle.

Proprietary Names
Elancoban *(Elanco, UK)*; Romensin *(Elanco, UK).*

12974-p

Monoacetin. Acetin; Monacetin. Glyceryl monoacetate.
$C_5H_{10}O_4$=134.1.

CAS — 26446-35-5.

A colourless hygroscopic liquid with a characteristic odour. Wt per ml about 1.21 g. **Soluble** in water and alcohol; slightly soluble in ether. **Store** in airtight containers.

Monoacetin is a solvent. It has been suggested for use in the treatment of sodium fluoroacetate poisoning (see p.702).

The Food Additives and Contaminants Committee recommended that the mono-, di-, and tri-acetates of glycerol be temporarily permitted for use as solvents in food. Further studies on hydrolysis and toxicity were required.— *Report on the Review of Solvents in Food*, FAC/REP/25, Ministry of Agriculture, Fisheries and Food, London, HM Stationery Office, 1978.

12975-s

Mopidamol. Ra-233. 2,2′,2″,2‴-(4-Piperidinopyrimido[5,4-*d*]pyrimidine-2,6-diyldinitrilo)tetraethanol.
$C_{19}H_{31}N_7O_4$=421.5.

CAS — 13665-88-8.

Mopidamol is reported to inhibit platelet aggregation. It also has antineoplastic activity.

Proprietary Names
Rapenton *(Thomae, Ger.).*

12976-w

Moprolol Hydrochloride. SD-1601. 1-Isopropylamino-3-(2-methoxyphenoxy)propan-2-ol hydrochloride.
$C_{13}H_{21}NO_3$,HCl=275.8.

CAS — 5741-22-0 (moprolol); 27058-84-0 (hydrochloride).

Moprolol hydrochloride is a beta-adrenoceptor blocking agent. The activity resides in the (−)-enantiomer.

Studies with the active (−)-enantiomer.— P. Ghirardi and F. Grosso, *J. cardiovasc. Pharmac.*, 1980, *2*, 471; G. Catenazzo *et al.*, *Curr. ther. Res.*, 1981, *29*, 651; G. Vrebos *et al.*, *ibid.*, 655; H. Höffkes, *ibid.*, *30*, 88; J. Nicaise *et al.*, *ibid.*, 93.

Proprietary Names
Omeral *(Simes, Ital.).*

12977-e

Morantel Tartrate. CP-12009-18; UK-2964-18. (*E*)-1,4,5,6-Tetrahydro-1-methyl-2-[2-(3-methyl-2-thienyl)vinyl]pyrimidine hydrogen tartrate.
$C_{12}H_{16}N_2S,C_4H_6O_6$=370.4.

CAS — 20574-50-9 (morantel); 26155-31-7 (tartrate).

Pale yellow to greenish-yellow crystals. M.p. 167° to 170°. Readily **soluble** in water; practically insoluble in ethyl acetate.

Morantel tartrate is a veterinary anthelmintic.

Manufacturers
Pfizer, UK.

12978-l

Moricizine. Moracizine; Ethmosine; Ethmozine; Etmozin; EN-313. Ethyl [10-(3-morpholinopropionyl)phenothiazin-2-yl]carbamate.
$C_{22}H_{25}N_3O_4S$=427.5.

CAS — 31883-05-3.

Moricizine is a phenothiazine compound with anti-arrhythmic activity.

A brief review.— J. B. Schwartz *et al.*, *Drugs*, 1981, *21*, 23.

Further references: J. Morganroth *et al.*, *Circulation*, 1977, *56*, *Suppl.* 3, 180; D. P. Zipes and P. J. Troup, *Am. J. Cardiol.*, 1978, *41*, 1005; J. Morganroth *et al.*, *Am. Heart J.*, 1979, *98*, 621; P. J. Podrid *et al.*, *Circulation*, 1980, *61*, 450.

Manufacturers
Endo, USA.

12979-y

Moroxydine Hydrochloride. ABOB. 1-(Morpholinoformimidoyl)guanidine hydrochloride.
$C_6H_{13}N_5O$,HCl=207.7.

CAS — 3731-59-7 (moroxydine); 3160-91-6 (hydrochloride).

Moroxydine hydrochloride has been reported to have some beneficial influence in the prophylaxis and treatment of various viral infections, but several studies failed to substantiate early reports of its value.

A study indicating that usual therapeutic doses of moroxydine strongly interfere with colour vision.— J. Laroche and C. Laroche, *Annls pharm. fr.*, 1977, *35*, 173.

Proprietary Names
Biguan *(Septa, Spain)*; Flumadon *(Globopharm, Switz.)*; Flumidin *(Kabi, Ger.)*; Virustat *(Delagrange, Belg.; Delagrange, Fr.).*

12980-g

Motretinide. Ro-11-1430. (*all-trans*)-*N*-Ethyl-9-(4-methoxy-2,3,6-trimethylphenyl)-3,7-dimethylnona-2,4,6,8-tetraenamide.
$C_{23}H_{31}NO_2$=353.5.

CAS — 56281-36-8.

Motretinide has been used topically, similarly to tretinoin, in the treatment of acne.

References: J. Christiansen *et al.*, *Dermatologica*, 1977, *154*, 219; J. Christiansen *et al.*, *ibid.*, 1979, *159*, 466.

Proprietary Names
Tasmaderm *(Roche, Switz.).*

12981-q

Moxestrol. R-2858. 11β-Methoxy-19-nor-17α-pregna-1,3,5(10)-trien-20-yne-3,17-diol.
$C_{21}H_{26}O_3$=326.4.

CAS — 34816-55-2.

Moxestrol is a synthetic oestrogen.

References: C. Robyn *et al.*, *J. clin. Pharmac.*, 1978, *18*, 29.

Proprietary Names
Surestryl *(Roussel, Fr.).*

12982-p

Musk. Moschus; Mosc.; Deer Musk; Almíscar. The dried secretions from the preputial follicles of the musk deer, *Moschus moschiferus* (Cervidae).

CAS — 8001-04-5 (musk); 541-91-3 (muskone).

Pharmacopoeias. In *Jap.* and *Port.*

It has a powerful penetrating and persistent odour which is due to the presence of the ketone muskone, $C_{16}H_{30}O$. **Store** in airtight containers.

Musk is used as a fixative in perfumery. It was formerly regarded as a powerful medullary stimulant.

A series of nitrated tertiary butyl toluenes or xylenes, or related compounds, are used as artificial musks.

12983-s

Green-lipped Mussel

An extract from the green-lipped mussel *Perna canaliculata* (Mytilidae), stated to contain amino acids, fats, carbohydrates, and minerals, is promoted for the treatment of rheumatic disorders.

In a double-blind crossover study completed by 26 patients treatment of rheumatoid arthritis for 4 weeks with Seatone was no more effective than a placebo.— E. C. Huskisson *et al.*, *Br. med. J.*, 1981, *282*, 1358.

Other adverse comment: *Br. med. J.*, 1978, *2*, 49; M. J. Ahern *et al.*, *Med. J. Aust.*, 1980, *2*, 151; P. M. Brooks (letter), *ibid.*, 158; *Lancet*, 1981, *1*, 85.

A favourable report from a homoeopathic hospital.— R. G. Gibson and S. L. M. Gibson (letter), *Lancet*, 1981, *1*, 439.

Proprietary Names
Seatex *(English Grains, UK)*; Seatone *(McFarlane, UK).*

12984-w

Mycophenolic Acid. Lilly-68618; NSC-129185. An antimicrobial substance produced by the growth of *Penicillium stoloniferum*. (*E*)-6-(1,3-Dihydro-4-hydroxy-6-methoxy-7-methyl-3-oxoisobenzofuran-5-yl)-4-methylhex-4-enoic acid.
$C_{17}H_{20}O_6$=320.3.

CAS — 24280-93-1.

Mycophenolic acid is an antimetabolite which interferes with the synthesis of nucleic acids. It has been used in the treatment of psoriasis. Antitumour activity in *animals* has not generally been substantiated in clinical studies.

Mycophenolic acid has been used in the treatment of psoriasis. Side-effects included nausea, vomiting, and diarrhoea. Mycophenolic acid reacted only in tissue which contained the enzyme beta-glucuronide hydrolase, which was found in the skin.— *J. Am. med. Ass.*, 1974, *227*, 606. Mycophenolic acid, administered by mouth, was converted to an inactive glucuronide by the liver; glucuronidase in the skin reconverted the glucuronide to the active form. It has been shown to clear psoriasis lesions.— E. J. Van Scott, *ibid.*, 1976, *235*, 197.

Of 35 patients with psoriasis resistant to conventional treatment given mycophenolic acid 2.4 to 7.2 g daily for up to 2 years, 20 were cleared of lesions and 13 definitely improved. Side-effects included soft stools, diarrhoea, and anal tenderness; weakness; insomnia; and influenza-like syndrome; herpes simplex; herpes zoster; and dysuria. There was a reduction in haemoglobin concentrations in 13 patients, leucopenia in 1, thrombocytopenia in 2, and a mild increase in alkaline phosphatase in 4.— R. Marinari *et al.*, *Archs Derm.*, 1977, *113*, 930. See also S. Spatz *et al.*, *Br. J. Derm.*, 1978, *98*, 429.

For references to the properties of mycophenolic acid and its use as an antineoplastic agent, see Martindale 27th Edn, p. 1783.

Manufacturers
ICI Pharmaceuticals, UK; Leo, Denm.; Lilly, USA.

15302-z

Mylabris *(B.P.C. 1949).* Mylab.; Chinese Blistering Beetle; Chinese Cantharides; Indian Blistering Beetle. The dried beetles *Mylabris sidae (=M. phalerata), M. cichorii*, and *M. pustulata* (Meloidae), containing not less than 1% of cantharidin.

Pharmacopoeias. In *Chin.*

Mylabris has been used as a source of cantharidin and as a substitute for cantharides in the East.

12986-l

Myrtecaine. Nopoxamine. 2-[2-(10-Norpin-2-en-2-yl)ethoxy]triethylamine.
$C_{17}H_{31}NO$=265.4.

CAS — 7712-50-7.

A liquid. B.p. 135° to 140° at 2 to 3 mmHg.

Myrtecaine is a local anaesthetic which has been used topically. Myrtecaine lauryl sulphate has also been used.

12987-y

Myrtillus. Bilberry; Blaeberry; Heidelbeere; Huckleberry; Hurtleberry; Whortleberry; Myrtilli Fructus; Baccae Myrtilli. The dried fruits of *Vaccinium myrtillus* (Ericaceae).

Pharmacopoeias. In *Aust.*, *Cz.*, *Pol.*, and *Swiss.*

Myrtillus has diuretic and astringent properties. It has also been used for degenerative retinal conditions.

Proprietary Names
Antocin *(Tubi Lux, Ital.)*; Purpuralin *(Alcon, Arg.).*

12988-j

N-5′. *N*-(3′,4′-Dimethoxycinnamoyl)anthranilic acid.
$C_{18}H_{17}NO_5$=327.3.

CAS — 53902-12-8.

N-5′ has been studied as an anti-allergic agent in the control of asthma.

References: A. Koda *et al.*, *J. Allergy & clin. Immunol.*, 1976, *57*, 396; H. Azuma *et al.*, *Br. J. Pharmac.*, 1976, *58*, 483; H. Shioda *et al.*, *Allergy*, 1979, *34*, 213.

Manufacturers
Kissei, Jap.

12989-z

Naboctate Hydrochloride. SP-325. (±)-7,8,9,10-Tetrahydro-6,6,9-trimethyl-3-(1-methyloctyl)-6*H*-dibenzo[*b,d*]pyran-1-yl 4-diethylaminobutyrate hydrochloride.
$C_{33}H_{53}NO_3,HCl$=548.2.

CAS — 74912-19-9 (naboctate); 73747-21-4 (hydrochloride).

Naboctate hydrochloride is reported to have anti-emetic activity.

12990-p

Nabumetone. BRL-14777. 4-(6-Methoxy-2-naphthyl)butan-2-one.
$C_{15}H_{16}O_2$=228.3.

CAS — 42924-53-8.

Nabumetone is reported to have anti-inflammatory activity.

Manufacturers
Beecham Research, UK.

12991-s

Nadide. CO-1; Codehydrogenase I; Coenzyme I; DPN; Diphosphopyridine Nucleotide; NAD; Nicotinamide Adenine Dinucleotide. Nadide is a naturally occurring coenzyme substance. 1-(3-Carbamoylpyridinio)-β-D-ribofuranoside 5-(adenosine-5′-pyrophosphate).
$C_{21}H_{27}N_7O_{14}P_2$=663.4.

CAS — 53-84-9.

Nadide has been tried without success in the treatment of schizophrenia and is claimed to be of value in the treatment of alcohol and drug addiction.

Proprietary Names
Nad-Medical *(Medical, Spain)*; Nicodrasi *(Bruco, Ital.)*.

12992-w

Nadoxolol Hydrochloride. LL-1530. 3-Hydroxy-4-(1-naphthyloxy)butyramide oxime hydrochloride.
$C_{14}H_{16}N_2O_3,HCl$=296.8.

CAS — 54063-51-3 (nadoxolol); 35991-93-6 (hydrochloride).

Nadoxolol hydrochloride is a beta-adrenoceptor blocking agent.

Proprietary Names
Bradyl 250 *(Lafon, Fr.)*.

12993-e

Nafazatrom. Bay g-6575. 3-Methyl-1-[2-(2-naphthyloxy)ethyl]-5-pyrazolone.
$C_{16}H_{16}N_2O_2$=268.3.

CAS — 59040-30-1.

Nafazatrom has been claimed to inhibit platelet aggregation and to have an antithrombotic effect.

References: J. Vermylen *et al.*, *Lancet*, 1979, *1*, 518; F. Seuter *et al.*, *Arzneimittel-Forsch.*, 1979, *29*, 54.

Manufacturers
Bayer, UK.

12994-l

Nafiverine Hydrochloride. *NN*′-Bis{2-[2-(1-naphthyl)propionyloxy]ethyl}piperazine dihydrochloride.
$C_{34}H_{38}N_2O_4,2HCl$=611.6.

CAS — 5061-22-3 (nafiverine).

Nafiverine hydrochloride has been used for its antispasmodic effects. The dimesylate has also been used.

Proprietary Names
Naftidan *(De Angeli, Ital.)*.

12995-y

Naftifine. SN-105-843. (*E*)-*N*-Cinnamyl-*N*-methyl(1-naphthylmethyl)amine.
$C_{21}H_{21}N$=287.4.

CAS — 65472-88-0.

NOTE. The name naftifungine was formerly applied to this compound.

Naftifine is reported to have antifungal activity.

Manufacturers
Sandoz, UK.

12996-j

Naftypramide. DA-992; Naphthipramide. 4-Dimethylamino-2-isopropyl-2-(1-naphthyl)butyramide.
$C_{19}H_{26}N_2O$=298.4.

CAS — 1505-95-9.

Naftypramide is an anti-inflammatory agent.

References: E. Camarri *et al.*, *Curr. ther. Res.*, 1970, *12*, 1.

Manufacturers
De Angeli, Ital.

12997-z

Nandrolone Hemisuccinate. 3-Oxoestr-4-en-17β-yl hydrogen succinate.
$C_{22}H_{30}O_5$=374.5.

CAS — 6785-62-2.

Nandrolone hemisuccinate is a soluble derivative of nandrolone used as an anabolic agent. Nandrolone sodium sulphate has also been used.

Proprietary Names
Menidrabol *(Menarini, Ital.)*; Kératyl (nandrolone sodium sulphate) *(Chauvin-Blache, Fr.)*.

12998-c

Nandrolone Laurate *(B.P. Vet.)*. Nandrolone Dodecanoate. 3-Oxoestr-4-en-17β-yl dodecanoate.
$C_{30}H_{48}O_3$=456.7.

CAS — 26490-31-3.

A white to creamy-white crystalline powder with a faint characteristic odour. M.p. about 47°. Practically **insoluble** in water; soluble 1 in 1 of alcohol; readily soluble in chloroform, ether, fixed oils, and esters of fatty acids. Solutions in oil are **sterilised** by maintaining at 150° for 1 hour. **Store** at 2° to 8°. Protect from light.

Nandrolone laurate is a long-acting anabolic agent used in veterinary practice.

Proprietary Names
Laurabolin *(Intervet, UK)*.

12999-k

Napactadine Hydrochloride. DL-588. *NN*′-Dimethylnaphthalene-2-acetamidine hydrochloride.
$C_{14}H_{16}N_2,HCl$=248.8.

CAS — 76631-45-3 (napactadine); 57166-13-9 (hydrochloride).

Napactadine hydrochloride is reported to have antidepressant activity.

Manufacturers
Dow, USA.

13000-p

Naphthalophos. Bay-9002; Naftalofos; Phthalophos. Diethyl naphthalimido-oxyphosphonate.
$C_{16}H_{16}NO_6P$=349.3.

CAS — 1491-41-4.

Naphthalophos is a veterinary anthelmintic.

15301-j

Neoarsphenamine *(B.P.C. 1963)*. Neoarsphenaminum; Novarsenobenzene; Neoarsaminol; Neoarsenobenzol; Neoarsphenolamine; Neosalvarsan; Novarsenol; NAB; '914'.

CAS — 457-60-3.

Pharmacopoeias. In *Aust.*, *Belg.*, *Fr.*, *Int.*, *It.*, *Mex.*, *Pol.*, *Port.*, *Rus.*, and *Span. Jap.* includes Neoarsphenamine Sodium for Injection.

A yellow dry powder with no odour except that due to traces of ether or alcohol. It consists mainly of sodium 3-amino-4,4′-dihydroxy-3′-sulphinomethylaminoarsenobenzene ($C_{13}H_{13}As_2N_2NaO_4S$ = 466.1) and contains 18 to 21% of As. Very **soluble** in water; slightly soluble in alcohol (90%); soluble in glycerol; practically insoluble in dehydrated alcohol, chloroform, and ether. A 6% solution in water has a pH of 7 to 9. A 2.32% solution is iso-osmotic with serum. It is unstable in air, and is distributed in sealed containers from which the air has been removed or replaced by an inert gas. Solutions for injection should not be shaken during preparation and must be used immediately. **Store** at a temperature not exceeding 15°; it should not be used if it has become darker in colour.

An aqueous solution of neoarsphenamine iso-osmotic with serum (2.32%) caused 17% haemolysis of erythrocytes cultured in it for 45 minutes.— E. R. Hammarlund and K. Pedersen-Bjergaard, *J. pharm. Sci.*, 1961, *50*, 24.

Neoarsphenamine was formerly used in the treatment of syphilis, yaws, relapsing fever, and rat-bite fever and has been used topically in Vincent's angina. For details of the adverse effects of neoarsphenamine and precautions to be taken in its use, see *Martindale 27th Edn*, p. 1785.

Preparations

Neoarsphenamine Injection *(B.P.C. 1963)*. Inj. Neoarsphenamin. A sterile solution of neoarsphenamine prepared by dissolving, immediately before use, the sterile contents of a sealed container in the requisite amount of Water for Injections. The injection must be used within 5 minutes of preparation as it rapidly decomposes, with increase of toxicity.

Neoarsphenamine Sodium for Injection *(Jap. P.)*. It contains suitable stabilisers and is dissolved in Water for Injections before use.

Proprietary Names
Collunovar *(Dexo, Fr.)*.

13002-w

Neodymium Sulfisonicotinate. Neodymium 3-sulphoisonicotinate octahydrate. $C_{18}H_9N_3Nd_2O_{15}S_3,8H_2O=1036.1$.

CAS — 13957-51-2 (anhydrous).

Neodymium sulfisonicotinate has been used for the prophylaxis and treatment of thrombo-embolic disorders.

Proprietary Names
Isothrodym *(Mulli, Ger.).*

13003-e

Neohesperidin Dihydrochalcone. 3,5-Dihydroxy-4-[3-(3-hydroxy-4-methoxyphenyl)propionyl]phenyl 2-*O*-(6-deoxy-α-L-mannopyranosyl)-β-D-glucopyranoside. $C_{28}H_{36}O_{15}=612.6$.

CAS — 20702-77-6 (neohesperidin dihydrochalcone); 18916-17-1 (naringin dihydrochalcone); 65520-51-6 (neoeriocitrin dihydrochalcone).

Neohesperidin dihydrochalcone is a sweetening agent derived from naringin present in citrus peel. Other dihydrochalcone sweeteners that have been studied include hesperetin dihydrochalcone glucoside ($C_{22}H_{26}O_{11}$ = 466.4), naringin dihydrochalcone ($C_{27}H_{34}O_{14}$ = 582.6), neoeriocitrin dihydrochalcone ($C_{27}H_{34}O_{15}$ = 598.6), and poncirin dihydrochalcone ($C_{28}H_{36}O_{14}$ = 596.6).

References to neohesperidin dihydrochalcone (Neo-DHC): *Mfg Chem.*, 1976, *47* (Aug.), 10; *Chemist Drugg.*, 1977, *208*, 114; R. P. Batzinger *et al.*, *Science*, 1977, *198*, 944. See also R. M. Horowitz and B. Gentili, in *Symposium: Sweeteners*, G.E. Inglett (Ed.), Westport, AVI, 1974, p.182.

13004-l

Neuraminidase. Neuraminidase is an enzyme widely distributed in nature.

CAS — 9001-67-6.

Neuraminidase derived from *Vibrio cholerae* (VCN) has been shown experimentally to increase the immunogenicity of tumour cells. VCN-treated cells injected into *animals* have prevented or impaired the growth of tumour grafts and have caused the regression of small tumours.

It is being used experimentally in the immunological treatment of leukaemia.

References: *Lancet*, 1972, *1*, 523; F. E. Rosato *et al.*, *Surgery Gynec. Obstet.*, 1974, *139*, 675, per *J. Am. med. Ass.*, 1975, *232*, 876; *J. Am. med. Ass.*, 1975, *234*, 371; R. P. Gale, *New Engl. J. Med.*, 1979, *300*, 1189.

Manufacturers
Hoechst, UK.

13005-y

Neutral Red. CI Basic Red 5; Colour Index No. 50040; Neutral Red Chloride; Nuclear Fast Red; Toluylene Red. 3-Amino-7-dimethylamino-2-methylphenazine hydrochloride. $C_{15}H_{16}N_4,HCl=288.8$.

CAS — 553-24-2.

A dark green powder. **Soluble** 1 in 25 of water; 1 in 55 of alcohol; and 1 in 33 of ethylene glycol.

Neutral red is a photoactive dye that has been tried in the treatment of recurrent herpes simplex infections. Some viruses can incorporate such dyes which attach to viral guanosine and subsequent exposure to light in the presence of oxygen causes breakage of DNA and RNA strands. Photodynamic inactivation by application of a 0.1% solution of neutral red followed by exposure to light has met with limited success; there is some evidence for the potential carcinogenicity of inactivated herpes simplex viruses. Allergic contact dermatitis has also been reported.

References: T. D. Felber *et al.*, *J. Am. med. Ass.*, 1973, *223*, 289; *Med. Lett.*, 1974, *16*, 112; T. D. Felber, *J. Am. med. Ass.*, 1975, *231*, 79; M. G. Myers *et al.*, *New Engl. J. Med.*, 1975, *293*, 945; A. P. C. H. Roome *et al.*, *Br. J. vener. Dis.*, 1975, *51*, 130, per *Abstr. Hyg.*, 1975, *50*, 798; E. G. Friedrich *et al.*, *Obstet. Gynec.*, 1976, *48*, 564, per *Int. pharm. Abstr.*, 1977, *14*, 470; R. S. Berger and C. M. Papa, *J. Am. med. Ass.*, 1977, *238*, 133; A. W. Kopf *et al.* (letter), *ibid.*, 1978, *239*, 615; B. E. Juel-Jensen, *Practitioner*, 1979, *222*, 745.

13006-j

Niaprazine. *N*-[3-(4-*p*-Fluorophenylpiperazin-1-yl)-1-methylpropyl]nicotinamide. $C_{20}H_{25}FN_4O=356.4$.

CAS — 27367-90-4.

Niaprazine is an antihistamine which has been used for its sedative and hypnotic properties.

Proprietary Names
Nopron *(Carrion, Fr.).*

13007-z

Nicarbazin *(B. Vet. C. 1965).* An equimolecular complex of 1,3-bis(4-nitrophenyl)urea ($C_{13}H_{10}N_4O_5$) and 4,6-dimethylpyrimidin-2-ol ($C_6H_8N_2O$). $C_{19}H_{18}N_6O_6=426.4$.

CAS — 330-95-0.

A pale yellow odourless or almost odourless powder. Very slightly **soluble** in water, alcohol, chloroform, and ether; soluble 1 in 700 of dimethylformamide.

Nicarbazin is used in veterinary medicine for the prevention of coccidiosis in poultry.

Proprietary Names
Nicrazin *(Merck Sharp & Dohme, UK).*

13008-c

Nicardipine Hydrochloride. RS-69216; RS-69216-XX-07-0; YC-93. 2-(*N*-Methylbenzylamino)ethyl methyl 1,4-dihydro-2,6-dimethyl-4-(3-nitrophenyl)pyridine-3,5-dicarboxylate hydrochloride. $C_{26}H_{29}N_3O_6,HCl=516.0$.

CAS — 55985-32-5 (nicardipine); 54527-84-3 (hydrochloride).

Nicardipine hydrochloride is a vasodilator which is claimed to improve cerebral circulation.

References: T. Seki and T. Takenaka, *Int. J. clin. Pharmac. Biopharm.*, 1977, *15*, 267; T. Takenaka and J. Handa, *ibid.*, 1979, *17*, 1.

Manufacturers
Syntex, UK; Yamanouchi, Jap.

13009-k

Niclofolan. Bayer-9015; Menichlopholan. 5,5′-Dichloro-3,3′-dinitrobiphenyl-2,2′-diol. $C_{12}H_6Cl_2N_2O_6=345.1$.

CAS — 10331-57-4.

Niclofolan is a fasciolacide.

Promising results have been reported with niclofolan in doses of 1 to 2 mg per kg body-weight [daily] for 2 to 3 days in the treatment of liver-fluke disease caused by *Clonorchis* and *Opisthorchis* spp.— Parasitic Zoonoses, Report of a WHO Expert Committee with the participation of FAO, *Tech. Rep. Ser. Wld Hlth Org. No. 637*, 1979, p. 70.

Further references: C. Nwokolo and K. J. Volkmer, *Am. J. trop. Med. Hyg.*, 1977, *26*, 688 (paragonimiasis), per *Trop. Dis. Bull.*, 1977, *74*, 1139.

13010-w

Nicofurate. 1-(4-Methoxycarbonyl-5-methyl-2-furyl)butane-1,2,3,4-tetrayl tetranicotinate. $C_{35}H_{28}N_4O_{11}=680.6$.

CAS — 4397-91-5.

Nicofurate has the general properties of nicotinic acid (see p.1648) and has been used as a vasodilator and in lipid disorders.

Proprietary Names
Arteriolase *(Marxer, Arg.).*

13011-e

Nicomol. (2-Hydroxycyclohexane-1,3-diylidene)tetrakis(methylene nicotinate). $C_{34}H_{32}N_4O_9=640.6$.

CAS — 27959-26-8.

A white, odourless, tasteless, crystalline powder. M.p. about 178°. Practically **insoluble** in water and ether; soluble in chloroform and hydrochloric acid.

Nicomol is a nicotinic acid derivative with a hypocholesterolaemic action and has been used in the treatment of abnormal lipid metabolism.

Proprietary Names
Cholexamin *(Kyorin, Jap.).*

13012-l

Nicomorphine Hydrochloride. 3,6-Di-*O*-nicotinoylmorphine hydrochloride; (−)-(5*R*,6*S*)-4,5-Epoxy-9a-methylmorphin-7-en-3,6-diyl dinicotinate hydrochloride. $C_{29}H_{25}N_3O_5,HCl=532.0$.

CAS — 639-48-5 (nicomorphine); 12040-41-4 (hydrochloride); 35055-78-8 (xHCl).

Nicomorphine hydrochloride is a narcotic analgesic.

Proprietary Names
Vilan *(Nourypharma, Neth.; Synmedic, Switz.).*

15303-c

Nicotine *(B.P.C. 1934).* 3-(1-Methylpyrrolidin-2-yl)pyridine. $C_{10}H_{14}N_2=162.2$.

CAS — 54-11-5.

A liquid alkaloid obtained from the dried leaves of the tobacco plant, *Nicotiana tabacum* (Solanaceae). Tobacco leaves contain 2 to 8% of nicotine combined as malate or citrate. Nicotine is a colourless to pale yellow, very hygroscopic, oily liquid with an unpleasant pungent odour and a sharp burning persistent taste. Wt per ml about 1.01 g. It gradually becomes brown on exposure to air or light.

Soluble in water, alcohol, chloroform, ether, kerosene, light petroleum, and fixed oils. **Store** in airtight containers. Protect from light.

Adverse Effects. Nicotine is a highly toxic substance and in acute poisoning death may occur within a few minutes due to respiratory failure arising from paralysis of the muscles of respiration. The fatal dose of nicotine for an adult is from 40 to 60 mg.

Less severe poisoning causes nausea and salivation, abdominal pain, vomiting, diarrhoea, dizziness, mental confusion, disturbed hearing and vision, faintness, convulsions, sweating, and prostration. Chronic poisoning, usually arising from continued excessive smoking, causes local irritation of the respiratory tract, digestive and nutritional disturbances, peripheral vasoconstriction and a rise in blood pressure, and, more rarely, amblyopia.

Nicotine is rapidly absorbed through the skin or by inhalation and most cases of nicotine poisoning are due to careless handling when it is employed as a horticultural insecticide.

The effects of nicotine in relation to the smoking of tobacco and the tar and nicotine content of cigarettes: *Br. med. J.*, 1968, *1*, 73; R. Kumar *et al.*, *Clin. Pharmac. Ther.*, 1977, *21*, 520; *Drug & Ther. Bull.*, 1978, *16*, 17; M. Lader, *Br. J. clin. Pharmac.*, 1978, *5*, 289; J. C. Robinson *et al.*, *Can. med. Ass. J.*, 1980, *123*, 889; L. T. Kozlowski, *J. Am. med. Ass.*, 1981, *245*, 158.

A report of nicotine poisoning in tobacco pickers.— S. H. Gehlbach *et al.*, *J. Am. med. Ass.*, 1974, *229*, 1880.

A study of the absorption and metabolism of nicotine from cigarettes by 8 healthy men, 3 of whom were non-smokers. All the smokers who inhaled had an increase in their heart-rate proportional to the blood-concentrations of nicotine; blood pressure also rose but the correlation was not so clear. The results of the study supported the view that many smokers smoke to dose themselves with nicotine.— A. K. Armitage *et al.*, *Br. med. J.*, 1975, *4*, 313. Estimation of urinary excretion of cotinine (a major metabolite of nicotine) may provide a useful index of smoking habits.— S. Matsukura *et al.*, *Clin. Pharmac. Ther.*, 1979, *25*, 555. For further pharmacokinetic studies of nicotine, see K. J. Ivey and E. J. Triggs, *Am. J. dig. Dis.*, 1978, *23*, 809 (absorption by the stomach); A. E. Klein and J. W. Gorrod, *Eur. J. Drug Metab. Pharmacokinet.*, 1978, *3*, 51 (metabolism); S. Matsukura *et al.*, *Clin. Pharmac. Ther.*, 1979, *25*, 549 (renal excretion); J. Rosenberg *et al.*, *ibid.*, 1980, *28*, 517 (intravenous administration); E. R. Gritz *et al.*, *ibid.*, 1981, *30*, 201 (plasma nicotine and cotinine concentrations in smokeless tobacco users).

Pharmacological effects of nicotine and smoking: P. E. Cryer *et al.*, *New Engl. J. Med.*, 1976, *295*, 573; R. J. Lefkowitz, *ibid.*, 615 (noradrenaline release); D. K. Chattopadhyay *et al.*, *Gut*, 1977, *18*, 833 (reduced lower oesophageal sphincter pressure); Å. Wennmalm, *Br. J. Pharmac.*, 1977, *59*, 95 (stimulation of prostaglandin synthesis); W. W. Winternitz and D. Quillen, *J. clin. Pharmac.*, 1977, *17*, 389 (plasma cortisol and growth hormone concentrations); Å. Wennmalm, *Br. J. Pharmac.*, 1978, *64*, 559 (prostaglandins).

Reports on mortality and cigarette smoking.— R. Doll and R. Peto, *Br. med. J.*, 1976, *2*, 1525; G. D. Friedman *et al.*, *New Engl. J. Med.*, 1979, *300*, 213; C. C. Seltzer (letter), *ibid.*, 1162; G. D. Friedman (letter), *ibid.*; G. D. Friedman *et al.*, *ibid.*, 1981, *304*, 1407.

Results of the Walnut Creek Contraceptive Drug Study involving 17 939 women enrolled between 1969 and 1971 and during which 16 759 women were followed for an average of 6.5 years, indicated that the risk of subarachnoid haemorrhage in smokers was 5.7 times that of non-smokers, and of current oral contraceptive users 6.5 times that of non-users. The relative risk estimate for the association of smoking and current oral contraceptive use was 21.9.— D. B. Petitti and J. Wingerd, *Lancet*, 1978, *2*, 234.

Prinzmetal's variant angina and diffuse oesophageal spasm developed one week after a 41-year-old women gave up cigarettes after years of heavy smoking. Nitrates were only partially effective and her pain was only controlled when verapamil was given.— S. A. Lipton *et al.* (letter), *New Engl. J. Med.*, 1978, *299*, 775.

References to the effects of passive smoking (the breathing of air containing cigarette smoke): W. S. Aronow, *New Engl. J. Med.*, 1978, *299*, 21; H. Wakeham (letter), *ibid.*, 896; B. F. Robinson (letter), *ibid.*; C. L. Waite (letter), *ibid.*, 897; A. Coodley (letter), *ibid.*; W. S. Aronow (letter), *ibid.*; J. R. White and H. F. Froeb, *ibid.*, 1980, *302*, 720; C. Lenfant and B. M. Liu, *ibid.*, 742; F. Adlkofer *et al.* (letter), *ibid.*, *303*, 392; G. L. Huber (letter), *ibid.*; A. P. Freedman (letter), *ibid.*, 393; D. M. Aviado (letter), *ibid.*; R. E. Shor and D. C. Williams (letter), *ibid.*; F. Kauffman (letter), *ibid.*; J. R. White and H. F. Froeb (letter), *ibid.*; T. S. Bocanegra and L. R. Espinoza (letter), *ibid.*, 1419; S. L. Stock (letter), *Lancet*, 1981, *2*, 1044.

A study indicating that snuff can provide enough nicotine to satisfy the nicotine-dependent cigarette smoker. Snuff may be a satisfactory and acceptable substitute for cigarette smoking, with considerable health benefits.— M. A. H. Russell *et al.*, *Lancet*, 1980, *1*, 474. Comment.— J. J. Pindborg and N. H. Axelsen (letter), *ibid.*, 775. Snuff may be a factor in the aetiology of buccal and gingival carcinoma.— D. F. Goldsmith and D. M. Winn (letter), *ibid.*, 825. See also A. G. Christen (letter), *New Engl. J. Med.*, 1980, *302*, 818; D. M. Winn *et al.*, *ibid.*, 1981, *304*, 745; D. Schottenfeld, *ibid.*, 778.

Effects on the cardiovascular system. Reports on the association between cigarette smoking and coronary heart disease.— C. Bain *et al.*, *Lancet*, 1978, *1*, 1087; A. C. Arntzenius *et al.*, *ibid.*, 1221; D. Slone *et al.*, *New Engl. J. Med.*, 1978, *298*, 1273; F. Gyntelberg *et al.*, *Lancet*, 1981, *1*, 987; W. P. Castelli *et al.*, *ibid.*, *2*, 109; P. N. Lee (letter), *ibid.*, 642; W. P. Castelli (letter), *ibid.*

Evidence against nicotine as a cause of coronary heart disease.— N. J. Wald *et al.*, *Lancet*, 1981, *2*, 775.

Effects on the lungs. A study of matched pairs of men who had died in the periods 1955–60 and 1970–77 compared changes in the bronchial epithelium of smokers and non-smokers. The drop in tar and nicotine content of cigarettes over the last 25 years was reflected in less extensive histological changes in the 1970–77 group but in both groups all smokers had more abnormalities than non-smokers.— O. Auerbach *et al.*, *New Engl. J. Med.*, 1979, *300*, 381. Comments.— A. P. Fishman, *ibid.*, 428; T. L. Kurt (letter), *ibid.*, 1394; D. G. Haack (letter), *ibid.*; G. H. Miller *et al.* (letter), *ibid.*, 1395; P. Bernfeld (letter), *ibid.*; O. Auerbach *et al.* (letter), *ibid.*

Further references: *Br. med. J.*, 1975, *4*, 247; T. Higenbottam *et al.*, *Lancet*, 1980, *1*, 409; R. V. Ebert, *New Engl. J. Med.*, 1981, *304*, 1486.

Effects on sexual function. References to sperm abnormalities and cigarette smoking: H. J. Evans *et al.*, *Lancet*, 1981, *1*, 627; E. M. Berry (letter), *ibid.*, 1159.

Interactions. The effect of tobacco smoking on drug metabolism.— A. P. Alvares, *Clin. Pharmacokinet.*, 1978, *3*, 462.

Further references: W. J. Jusko, *J. Pharmacokinet. Biopharm.*, 1978, *6*, 7.

Pregnancy and the neonate. A discussion on the retarding effects of smoking on intra-uterine growth and the resulting association with an increased risk of spontaneous abortion, pre-term delivery, perinatal death, and possible long-term harmful effects on the infant's development.— *Lancet*, 1979, *1*, 536.

Concentrations of nicotine in the milk of lactating women who smoke.— B. B. Ferguson *et al.*, *Am. J. Dis. Child.*, 1976, *130*, 837.

Further references: H. Van Vunakis *et al.*, *Am. J. Obstet. Gynec.*, 1974, *120*, 64, per *Int. pharm. Abstr.*, 1975, *12*, 415; T. G. B. Dow *et al.*, *Br. med. J.*, 1975, *4*, 253; R. W. Payne (letter), *ibid.*, 521; J. Kline *et al.*, *New Engl. J. Med.*, 1977, *297*, 793; *Br. med. J.*, 1978, *1*, 259; R. L. Naeye, *J. Am. med. Ass.*, 1979, *241*, 867; R. L. Naeye (letter), *Lancet*, 1980, *1*, 765; S. M. Garn *et al.* (letter), *ibid.*, *2*, 912.

Treatment of Adverse Effects. Prompt treatment of nicotine poisoning is essential. If contact was with the skin, remove contaminated clothing and wash the skin thoroughly with cold water without rubbing. If the patient has swallowed nicotine, induce emesis if there are no convulsions and the respiration is normal. Wash out the stomach with water or with a 1 in 5000 solution of potassium permanganate (very pale pink); it may be followed by a suspension of activated charcoal. Diazepam, or if necessary a short-acting barbiturate such as thiopentone sodium, should be given intravenously to control convulsions. Assisted respiration may be required.

Uses. Nicotine has no therapeutic uses but is of considerable pharmacological interest. The main physiological action is paralysis of all autonomic ganglia, preceded by stimulation. Centrally, small doses cause respiratory stimulation, while larger doses produce convulsions of the medullary type and cause arrest of respiration. The effects on skeletal muscle are similar to those on ganglia.

Nicotine is mainly used as a horticultural insecticide either as a vapour or as a spray.

Precautions should be taken when using these sprays to avoid inhalation or contact with the skin.

A chewing gum containing nicotine has been used as an aid to giving up smoking.

Reviews of the clinical use of nicotine chewing gum as an aid to giving up smoking.— M. A. H. Russell *et al.*, *Br. med. J.*, 1980, *280*, 1599; *Drug & Ther. Bull.*, 1980, *18*, 83; *ibid.*, 1981, *19*, 4.

The abuse and intoxication potential of nicotine chewing gum intended to help smokers to stop smoking.— J. Hartelius and L. Tibbling (letter), *Br. med. J.*, 1976, *2*, 812.

In 8 healthy subjects the daily consumption of about 8 pieces of nicotine chewing gum (each 2 mg) significantly increased the mean blood-nicotine concentration from 26.3 to 35.3 ng per ml but did not reduce cigarette smoking.— J. A. M. Turner *et al.*, *Postgrad. med. J.*, 1977, *53*, 683.

Of 69 dependent smokers treated with nicotine chewing gum 26 were abstinent at one-year follow-up. These results compared favourably with those of an earlier study involving 49 patients who received psychological therapy where only 7 were abstinent at one-year follow-up. Side-effects reported by the patients receiving the nicotine gum were aching of the jaw (3), mouth ulcers (3), slight nausea (2), and palpitations (1). Only 2 patients became addicted to the gum.— M. Raw *et al.*, *Br. med. J.*, 1980, *281*, 481.

Proprietary Preparations

Nicorette *(Lundbeck, UK: Farillon, UK)*. Nicotine, available as chewing gum containing 2 or 4 mg. (Also available as Nicorette in *Switz.*).

13014-j

Nifuroxazide. 2′-(5-Nitrofurfurylidene)-4-hydroxybenzohydrazide.

$C_{12}H_9N_3O_5$=275.2.

CAS — 965-52-6.

Nifuroxazide has been used in the treatment of colitis and diarrhoea.

For the possible use of nifuroxazide in the treatment of amanita poisoning, see *Amanita phalloides*, p.1677. See also G. L. Floersheim, *Toxic. appl. Pharmac.*, 1975, *34*, 499.

Proprietary Names

Ercefuryl *(Robert & Carriere, Belg.; Robert et Carrière, Fr.)*; Pentofuryl *(Karlspharma, Ger.)*.

13015-z

Nifursol. 3,5-Dinitro-2′-(5-nitrofurfurylidene)salicylohydrazide.

$C_{12}H_7N_5O_9$=365.2.

CAS — 16915-70-1.

Nifursol is used in veterinary practice for the management of blackhead (histomoniasis) in turkeys.

Proprietary Names

Salfuride *(Salsbury, UK)*.

13016-c

Nifurtoinol. Hydroxymethylnitrofurantoin. 3-Hydroxymethyl-1-(5-nitrofurfurylideneamino)hydantoin.

$C_9H_8N_4O_6$=268.2.

CAS — 1088-92-2.

Nifurtoinol has been used similarly to nitrofurantoin in urinary-tract infections.

References: A. J. Beysens and H. C. L. V. Kock, *Pharm. Weekbl. Ned.*, 1973, *108*, 149; R. H. A. Sorel and H. Roseboom, *Int. J. Pharmaceut.*, 1979, *3*, 93.

Proprietary Names

Urfadyn *(Inpharzam, Belg.; Arsac, Fr.; Zambon, Ital.; Inpharzam, Neth.)*; Urfadyne *(Inpharzam, Ger.; Inpharzam, Switz.)*.

13017-k

Nimesulide. R-805. 4′-Nitro-2′-phenoxymethanesulphonanilide.

$C_{13}H_{12}N_2O_5S$=308.3.

CAS — 51803-78-2.

Nimesulide is reported to have anti-inflammatory activity.

References: R. L. Vigdahl and R. H. Tukey, *Biochem. Pharmac.*, 1977, *26*, 307; R. Weissenbach, *J. int. med. Res.*, 1981, *9*, 349.

Manufacturers

Riker, UK.

13018-a

Nimetazepam. Menifazepam; S-1530. 1,3-Dihydro-1-methyl-7-nitro-5-phenyl-2*H*-1,4-benzodiazepin-2-one.

$C_{16}H_{13}N_3O_3$=295.3.

CAS — 2011-67-8.

Nimetazepam is a benzodiazepine (see Diazepam, p.1519) with sedative and hypnotic properties.

Proprietary Names
Erimin *(Sumitomo, Jap.).*

13019-t

Nimustine. Pimustine; ACNU; NSC-245382. 1-(4-Amino-2-methylpyrimidin-5-ylmethyl)-3-(2-chloroethyl)-3-nitrosourea.
$C_9H_{13}ClN_6O_2$=272.7.

CAS — 42471-28-3.

Nimustine is a nitrosourea compound reported to have antineoplastic activity.

References: N. Saijo and H. Niitani, *Cancer Chemother. Pharmac.*, 1980, *4*, 165.

Proprietary Names
Nidran *(Sankyo, Jap.).*

13020-l

Niprofazone. *N*-[(2,3-Dimethyl-5-oxo-1-phenyl-3-pyrazolin-4-yl)isopropylaminomethyl]-nicotinamide.
$C_{21}H_{25}N_5O_2$=379.5.

CAS — 15387-10-7.

Niprofazone is reported to have analgesic, anti-inflammatory, and antipyretic activity.

Proprietary Names
Ravalgene *(Ravasini, Ital.).*

13021-y

Nisin. An antimicrobial substance produced by the growth of *Streptococcus lactis.*

CAS — 1414-45-5.

It is a crystalline substance consisting of a number of closely related polypeptides. **Soluble** in water; slightly soluble in alcohol; very soluble in chloroform. Stable to boiling in acid solution.

Units. One unit of nisin is contained in 0.001 mg of the first International Reference Preparation (1969) of nisin which contains 1000 units per mg.

Uses. Nisin is used as a preservative for cheese, clotted cream, and canned foods—see under Antibiotics as Food Preservatives, p.1083.

The use of nisin for the preservation of foods. A discussion and review of the literature.— G. Vanini and S. Moro, *G. Batt. Virol. Immun.*, 1966, *59*, 220, per *Bull. Hyg., Lond.*, 1967, *42*, 382.

13022-j

Nisoldipine. Bay k-5552. Isobutyl methyl 1,4-dihydro-2,6-dimethyl-4-(2-nitrophenyl)pyridine-3,5-dicarboxylate.
$C_{20}H_{24}N_2O_6$=388.4.

CAS — 63675-72-9.

Nisoldipine has vasodilator properties.

Pharmacology in *animals*.— S. Kazda *et al.*, *Arzneimittel-Forsch.*, 1980, *30*, 2144. Haemodynamic effects in man.— A. Vogt *et al.*, *ibid.*, 2162.

Manufacturers
Bayer, UK.

13023-z

Nitrefazole. EMD-15700. 2-Methyl-4-nitro-1-(4-nitrophenyl)imidazole.
$C_{10}H_8N_4O_4$=248.2.

CAS — 21721-92-6.

Nitrefazole has possible application in the treatment of alcoholism.

Manufacturers
E. Merck, UK.

13024-c

Nitro Blue Tetrazolium. Nitroblue Tetrazolium; Nitro BT; Nitro NBT. 3,3′-(3,3′-Dimethoxy-4,4′-biphenylylene)bis[2-(4-nitrophenyl)-5-phenyl-2*H*-tetrazolium chloride].
$C_{40}H_{30}Cl_2N_{10}O_6$=817.6.

CAS — 298-83-9.

A yellow dye. **Soluble** in water.

Nitro blue tetrazolium is converted by reduction by neutrophils to dark blue water-insoluble formazan, the reduction being enhanced by phagocytosis. This reaction forms the basis of nitro blue tetrazolium tests in which blood is incubated with a solution of nitro blue tetrazolium, under standard conditions, and the presence of formazan is assessed microscopically. Such tests have been used, with variable success, for the detection of bacterial infections, as a measure of the circulating concentration of functional neutrophils, and for the detection of chronic granulomatous disease. There have been many reports of factors yielding false results.

Discussions of the nitro blue tetrazolium test.— *Lancet*, 1971, *2*, 909; A. W. Segal *et al.*, *ibid.*, 1973, *2*, 879; *ibid.*, 1974, *1*, 664; A. W. Segal, *ibid.*, *2*, 1248.

13025-k

Nitrobenzene *(B.P.C. 1934).* Nitrobenzol; Oil of Mirbane.
$C_6H_5NO_2$=123.1.

CAS — 98-95-3.

A pale yellow liquid with a benzaldehyde-like odour. B.p. 210° to 212°. Wt per ml about 1.203 g. Practically **insoluble** in water; miscible with alcohol and ether.

Adverse Effects. Nitrobenzene is highly toxic and the ingestion of 1 g may be fatal. Toxic effects from ingestion are usually delayed for several hours and may include nausea, prostration, burning headache, methaemoglobinaemia with cyanosis, haemolytic anaemia, vomiting (with characteristic odour), convulsions, and coma, ending in death after a few hours. Poisoning may also occur from absorption through the skin, or by inhalation.

Maximum permissible atmospheric concentration 1 ppm.

Treatment of Adverse Effects. After ingestion of nitrobenzene the stomach should be emptied by aspiration and lavage; alcohol or oils must not be given. Methaemoglobinaemia may be treated with methylene blue. Blood transfusions may be necessary. Oxygen should be given if cyanosis is severe.

If the skin or eyes are splashed with nitrobenzene contaminated clothing should be removed immediately and the affected areas washed with running water for at least 15 minutes.

Uses. Nitrobenzene is used in the manufacture of aniline, as a preservative in polishes, in perfumery and soaps, and as an insect repellent.

It was recommended that nitrobenzene be prohibited for use in foods as a flavouring agent.— *Food Standards Committee Report on Flavouring Agents*, London, HM Stationery Office, 1965.

13026-a

***p*-Nitrophenol.**
$C_6H_5NO_3$=139.1.

CAS — 100-02-7.

p-Nitrophenol is reported to have antifungal activity.

Proprietary Preparations
Phortinea Liquid *(Philip Harris, UK).* Contains *p*-nitrophenol 2%. For fungal infections of the skin, especially tinea. To be applied twice daily.

13027-t

Nitroscanate. CGA-23654; GS-23654. 4-(4-Nitrophenoxy)phenyl isothiocyanate.
$C_{13}H_8N_2O_3S$=272.3.

CAS — 19881-18-6.

An almost odourless beige-coloured crystalline powder. M.p. about 122°. Practically **insoluble** in water; soluble in organic solvents.

Nitroscanate is an anthelmintic for *dogs*.

Proprietary Names
Lopatol *(Ciba-Geigy Agrochemicals, UK).*

13028-x

Nitrovin Hydrochloride. CL-48401. Bis-[2-(5-nitro-2-furyl)vinyl]methylenehydrazinoformamidine hydrochloride; 1,5-Bis(5-nitro-2-furyl)penta-1,4-dien-3-one amidinohydrazone hydrochloride.
$C_{14}H_{12}N_6O_6$,HCl=396.7.

CAS — 804-36-4 (nitrovin); 2315-20-0 (hydrochloride).

Nitrovin hydrochloride is used as a food additive in veterinary practice to promote growth.

Proprietary Names
Payzone *(Cyanamid, UK).*

13029-r

Nitroxynil *(B.P. Vet.).* Nitroxinil. 4-Hydroxy-3-iodo-5-nitrobenzonitrile.
$C_7H_3IN_2O_3$=290.0.

CAS — 1689-89-0 (nitroxynil); 27917-82-4 (eglumine salt).

A yellow odourless or almost odourless powder. M.p. 136° to 139°. Practically **insoluble** in water; soluble 1 in 120 of alcohol and 1 in 60 of ether; soluble in solutions of alkali hydroxides. Solutions of the eglumine salt of nitroxynil are **sterilised** by autoclaving or by filtration. **Protect** from light.

Nitroxynil is a veterinary anthelmintic used in the treatment of liver-fluke infestations in cattle and sheep. It is administered by subcutaneous injection as the eglumine salt.

Proprietary Names
Trodax (eglumine salt) *(May & Baker, UK).*

13030-j

Norclostebol Acetate. 4-Chloro-3-oxoestr-4-en-17β-yl acetate.
$C_{20}H_{27}ClO_3$=350.9.

CAS — 13583-21-6 (norclostebol).

Norclostebol acetate has been used as an anabolic agent.

Proprietary Names
Anabol 4-19 *(Piam, Ital.).*

13031-z

Norgestimate. D-138; ORF-10131. (+)-13-Ethyl-3-hydroxyimino-18,19-dinor-17α-pregn-4-en-20-yn-17β-yl acetate.
$C_{23}H_{31}NO_3$=369.5.

CAS — 35189-28-7.

NOTE. The name dexnorgestrel acetime was formerly applied to this compound.

Norgestimate is a progestogen which has been used with ethinyloestradiol as an oral contraceptive.

References: H. S. Weintraub *et al.*, *J. pharm. Sci.*, 1978, *67*, 1406; J. S. Lawson *et al.*, *Am. J. Obstet. Gynec.*, 1979, *134*, 315, per *J. Am. med. Ass.*, 1979, *242*, 1802.

Manufacturers
Ortho, USA.

13032-c

Norgestrienone. 17β-Hydroxy-19-nor-17α-pregna-4,9,11-trien-20-yn-3-one.
$C_{20}H_{22}O_2$=294.4.

CAS — 848-21-5.

Norgestrienone is a progestogen which has been used, as subdermal implants, and orally with ethinyloestradiol as a contraceptive.

References: E. Coutinho *et al.*, *Contraception*, 1978, *18*, 315, per *Int. pharm. Abstr.*, 1979, *16*, 305; E. Coutinho *et al.*, *Contraception*, 1978, *18*, 335, per *Int. pharm. Abstr.*, 1979, *16*, 311; A. Faundes *et al.*, *Contraception*, 1978, *18*, 355, per *Int. pharm. Abstr.*, 1979, *16*, 305; S. Diaz *et al.*, *Contraception*, 1978, *18*, 429, per *Int. pharm. Abstr.*, 1979, *16*, 459; J. Toivonen, *Contraception*, 1979, *20*, 511, per *Int. pharm. Abstr.*, 1980, *17*, 779.

Proprietary Names of Norgestrienone with Ethinyloestradiol
Planor *(Roussel, Fr.)*.

13033-k

Normethadone Hydrochloride. Desmethylmethadone Hydrochloride; Phenyldimazone Hydrochloride. 6-Dimethylamino-4,4-diphenylhexan-3-one hydrochloride.
$C_{20}H_{25}NO,HCl$=331.9.

CAS — 467-85-6 (normethadone); 847-84-7 (hydrochloride).

Crystals. M.p. 174° to 177°. **Soluble** in water and alcohol. A 1% solution in water has a pH of about 5.

Normethadone is closely related to methadone (p.1015). The hydrochloride has been used as a cough suppressant.

13034-a

Nosiheptide. RP-9671. A peptide antibiotic obtained from cultures of *Streptomyces actuosus* or by any other means.
$C_{51}H_{43}N_{13}O_{12}S_6$=1222.3.

CAS — 56377-79-8.

Nosiheptide is used as a food additive in veterinary practice to promote growth.

15306-t

Nucleic Acid *(B.P.C. 1934)*. Nucleinic Acid; Acide Zymonucléique; Acidum Nucleicum.

Pharmacopoeias. In *Port.* and *Span.*

A complex mixture of phosphorus-containing organic acids present in living cells. Commercially, nucleic acid is obtained from yeast; other sources include wheat embryo, fish sperm, and thymus gland. It occurs as a white or off-white amorphous powder. Practically **insoluble** in water, alcohol, and ether; soluble in dilute alkalis.

Nucleic acids are of 2 types, ribonucleic acids (RNA) (see p.1751) and deoxyribonucleic acids (DNA) (see p.1701). They are composed of chains of nucleotides (phosphate esters of purine or pyrimidine bases and pentose sugars).

Since the administration of nucleic acid gives rise to a marked temporary leucocytosis (usually preceded by a short period of leucopenia) it was formerly given in the treatment of a variety of bacterial infections in the hope of enhancing the natural defence mechanisms. Its therapeutic value, however, was never established.

13036-x

Octacaine Hydrochloride. 3-Diethylaminobutyranilide hydrochloride.
$C_{14}H_{22}N_2O,HCl$=270.8.

CAS — 13912-77-1 (octacaine); 59727-70-7 (hydrochloride).

Octacaine hydrochloride has been used as a local anaesthetic.

Proprietary Names
Amplicain *(Geistlich, Switz.)*.

13037-r

Octaverine Hydrochloride. 6,7-Dimethoxy-1-(3,4,5-triethoxyphenyl)isoquinoline hydrochloride.
$C_{23}H_{27}NO_5,HCl$=433.9.

CAS — 549-68-8 (octaverine); 6775-26-4 (hydrochloride).

Octaverine hydrochloride has antispasmodic properties and has been used in the treatment of various gastro-intestinal disorders.

13038-f

Octostanol. 3-Octyloxy-5α-androst-3-en-17β-ol.
$C_{27}H_{46}O_2$=402.7.

Octostanol has been used in the palliative treatment of breast cancer.

Proprietary Names
Ectovis *(Vister, Ital.)*.

13039-d

Oestradiol Hexahydrobenzoate. Estra-1,3,5(10)-triene-3,17β-diol 17-cyclohexanecarboxylate.
$C_{25}H_{34}O_3$=382.5.

CAS — 15140-27-9.

Oestradiol hexahydrobenzoate is a long-acting ester of oestradiol.

Proprietary Names
Benzo-Gynoestryl Retard *(Roussel, Fr.)*.

13040-c

Onion. The bulb of *Allium cepa* (Liliaceae).

Onion has been reported to reduce platelet aggregation and to enhance fibrinolysis.

References: I. S. Menon (letter), *Br. med. J.*, 1969, *1*, 845; I. S. Menon (letter), *Br. med. J.*, 1970, *2*, 421; H. J. Goldsmith *et al.*, *Lancet*, 1971, *2*, 738; K. I. Baghurst *et al.* (letter), *Lancet*, 1977, *1*, 101; C. Phillips and N. L. Poyser (letter), *Lancet*, 1978, *1*, 1051.

Hypoglycaemic effect in *animals*.— R. C. Jain *et al.* (letter), *Lancet*, 1973, *2*, 1491; R. C. Jain and C. R. Vyas (letter), *Br. med. J.*, 1974, *2*, 730.

The antihypertensive action of onions was associated with the presence of prostaglandin A_1, 1 ppm.— T. H. Maugh, *Science*, 1979, *204*, 293.

13041-k

Ononis. Restharrow Root; Radix Ononidis; Racine de Bugrane; Arrête-Boeuf; Hauhechelwurzel. The dried roots of *Ononis spinosa* (Leguminosae), containing saponins.

Pharmacopoeias. In *Aust.*, *Cz.*, *Hung.*, and *Pol.*

Ononis has been used as a diuretic.

13042-a

Orazamide. Oroxamide; Aica Orotate. 5-Aminoimidazole-4-carboxamide orotate dihydrate.
$C_9H_{10}N_6O_5,2H_2O$=318.2.

CAS — 2574-78-9 (anhydrous); 60104-30-5 (dihydrate).

A white odourless almost tasteless crystalline powder. M.p. about 280° with decomposition. Slightly **soluble** in water; practically insoluble in most organic solvents.

Orazamide is claimed to correct abnormal metabolism of protein, lipids, and glucose, and has been used in the treatment of liver disorders.

Proprietary Names
Aica-Hepat *(Montpellier, Arg.)*; Aicamin *(Labaz, Belg.; Crinos, Ital.; Fujisawa, Jap.; Made, Spain)*; Aïcamine *(Labaz, Fr.)*; Aicorat *(Mack, Illert., Ger.)*.

13043-t

Orgotein. Ormetein; Bovine Superoxide Dismutase. A group of water-soluble protein congeners isolated from liver, red blood cells, and other tissues; mol. wt about 33 000 with a compact formation maintained by about 4 gram-atoms of chelated divalent metals. It is produced from beef liver as Cu-Zn mixed chelate having superoxide dismutase activity.

CAS — 9016-01-7.

Orgotein has anti-inflammatory properties. It has been given by intra-articular injection in degenerative joint disease, and for bladder disorders and the amelioration of side-effects of radiotherapy. It is also used in veterinary practice.

A report on the use of orgotein in the successful treatment of a child with paraquat poisoning.— *Nature*, 1973, *245*, 64.

For a series of reports on the actions and uses of orgotein, see *Eur. J. Rheumatol. Inflamm.*, 1981, *4*, 151–270.

Joint disorders. Twenty-two patients with degenerative joint disease were treated with intra-articular injections of orgotein; of 19 adequately followed 16 derived benefit in terms of pain or joint size or motion. Orgotein was given in sodium chloride injection in concentrations of 0.5 to 2 mg per ml; the usual dose was 2 to 3 mg and patients received from 1 to 15 injections. Benefit lasted from 14 to more than 450 days after the last injection.— K. Lund-Olesen and K. B. Menander, *Curr. ther. Res.*, 1974, *16*, 706.

A report of beneficial results with orgotein in a double-blind study of 30 patients with active classical rheumatoid arthritis affecting the knee. Orgotein 4 mg or aspirin 4 mg was given in physiological saline at pH 7 as a weekly intra-articular injection for 6 weeks. Follow-up continued for a further 6 weeks. Patients given orgotein had a significantly better rheumatoid activity index than those who had received aspirin. No serious side-effects were noted but 9 of 15 patients given orgotein had local painful subcutaneous reactions.— K. -M. Goebel *et al.*, *Lancet*, 1981, *1*, 1015.

Further references: M. Walravens and J. Dequeker, *Curr. ther. Res.*, 1976, *20*, 62; P. H. Proctor *et al.* (letter), *Lancet*, 1978, *2*, 95.

Radiotherapy. A double-blind study in 38 patients given orgotein 4 mg or placebo intramuscularly for 8 weeks after each session of irradiation for bladder tumours indicated that orgotein had a significant effect in ameliorating the side-effects of irradiation.— F. Edsmyr *et al.*, *Curr. ther. Res.*, 1976, *19*, 198.

Further references: H. Marberger *et al.*, *Curr. ther. Res.*, 1975, *18*, 466.

Proprietary Names
Ontosein *(Leo, Aust.)*.

13044-x

Ornicarbase. Ornithine Carbamoyl-transferase.

CAS — 9001-69-8.

Ornicarbase has been used in hepatic disorders.

Proprietary Names
Ociter *(Bracco, Ital.)*; Préortan *(Leurquin, Fr.)*.

13045-r

Orotic Acid. Animal Galactose Factor; Whey Factor; Uracil-6-carboxylic Acid. 1,2,3,6-Tetrahydro-2,6-dioxopyrimidine-4-carboxylic acid monohydrate.
$C_5H_4N_2O_4,H_2O$=174.1.

CAS — 65-86-1 (anhydrous); 50887-69-9 (monohydrate).

A white crystalline powder. Slightly **soluble** in water; practically insoluble in ether.

Orotic acid occurs naturally in the body; it is found in milk. It is an intermediate in the biosynthesis of pyrimidine nucleotides which in turn are involved in the synthesis of DNA and RNA. Orotic acid and its lysine, magnesium, and potassium salts have been used in the treatment of hyperuricaemia and hypercholesterolaemia and in liver disorders. Calcium and magnesium orotate have been used as a mineral source.

Four patients with gout were given 4 g of orotic acid daily for 6 days. Plasma-uric acid concentrations fell by 20 µg per ml and a marked increase in urinary oxypurines was noted.— G. D. Kersley, *Ann. rheum. Dis.*, 1966, *25*, 353.

Orotic acid had been given to premature and full-term infants to lower concentrations of bilirubin. Results were conflicting.— *Br. med. J.*, 1972, *2*, 62.

Proprietary Names

Calora *(calcium orotate) (Miller, USA)*; Crataron *(lysine orotate) (Rether, Spain)*; Dioron *(potassium orotate) (Lepetit, Belg.)*; Lactinium *(Roland, Ger.)*; Lysortine *(lysine orotate) (Théraplix, Fr.)*; Magora *(magnesium orotate) (Miller, USA)*; Oroturic *(Grémy-Longuet, Fr.)*.

13046-f

Oryzanol. γ-Oryzanol; Gamma Oryzanol; γ-OZ. A substance extracted from rice bran oil and rice embryo bud oil. Triacontanyl 3-(4-hydroxy-3-methoxyphenyl)prop-2-enoate.
$C_{40}H_{58}O_4$=602.9.

CAS — 11042-64-1.

Pharmacopoeias. In *Chin.*

Oryzanol has been used in autonomic and endocrine disturbances.

Proprietary Names

Caclate, Gammariza, Gammatsul, Guntrin, Hi-Z, Maintenan, Oliver, Thiaminogen *(all Jap.)*.

13047-d

Osmium Tetroxide. Osmic Acid.
OsO_4=254.2.

CAS — 20816-12-0.

CAUTION. *Osmium tetroxide solution and its fumes are corrosive to the eyes, mucous membranes, and skin .*

A white or cream-coloured very deliquescent crystalline powder or yellow crystals, with an unpleasant pungent odour. **Soluble** in water, alcohol, and ether. **Store** in airtight containers. Protect from light.

Osmium tetroxide is an oxidising agent. It has been given by intra-articular injection in rheumatic disorders of the knee.

Maximum permissible atmospheric concentration, as osmium, 0.0002 ppm.

References: A. Kajander and A. Ruotsi, *Annls Med. intern. Fenn.*, 1967, *57*, 87, per *Abstr. Wld Med.*, 1968, *42*, 636; J. W. Brooke, *Clin. Med.*, 1968, *75* (June), 37; H. Ott *et al.*, *Schweiz. med. Wschr.*, 1977, *107*, 1165, per *J. Am. med. Ass.*, 1978, *239*, 453; M. Nissilä *et al.*, *Scand. J. Rheumatol.*, 1978, *7*, 79; M. Nissilä, *ibid.*, 1979, *Suppl.* 29;; H. Sheppeard and D. J. Ward, *Rheumatol. Rehabil.*, 1980, *19*, 25.

13048-n

Otilonium Bromide. Diethylmethyl{2-[4-(2-octyloxybenzamido)benzoyloxy]ethyl-}ammonium bromide.
$C_{29}H_{43}BrN_2O_4$=563.6.

CAS — 26095-59-0.

Otilonium bromide has been used for its antispasmodic effects on the gastro-intestinal tract.

Proprietary Names

Spasmomen *(Menarini, Ital.)*.

13049-h

Ouricury Wax. Ouricuri Wax; Licuri Wax.

A hard, brittle, light tan to dark brown wax obtained from the leaves of a native Brazilian palm tree, *Syagrus coronata* (= *Cocos coronata*) (Palmae). M.p. 81.5° to 84°.

Ouricury wax resembles carnauba wax (see p.1690) and is used in polishes.

Specifications for ouricury wax set by American Wax Importers and Refiners Association.— *Soap chem. Spec.*, 1966, *42* (4A, Apr.), 261.

13050-a

Oxabolone Cypionate. Oxabolone Cipionate. 4,17β-Dihydroxyestr-4-en-3-one 17-(β-cyclopentylpropionate).
$C_{26}H_{38}O_4$=414.6.

CAS — 1254-35-9.

Oxabolone cypionate has been used as an anabolic agent and in osteoporosis.

Proprietary Names

Steranabol Depot *(Farmitalia, Ger.)*; Steranabol Ritardo *(Farmitalia, Ital.)*.

NOTE. Steranabol is used as a proprietary name for clostebol acetate.

13051-t

Oxaceprol. Acetylhydroxyproline. (−)-1-Acetyl-4-hydroxy-L-proline.
$C_7H_{11}NO_4$=173.2.

CAS — 33996-33-7.

A white powder with a slightly acid taste. M.p. 135°. **Soluble** in water and alcohol; practically insoluble in chloroform and ether.

Oxaceprol is reported to affect connective-tissue metabolism and has been used in dermatology, to promote wound healing, and in rheumatic disorders.

Proprietary Names

Jonctum *(Merrell Toraude, Fr.; Merrell, Ital.; Inibsa, Spain)*; Tejuntivo *(Valderrama, Spain)*.

13052-x

Oxametacin. Oxamethacin. 1-(4-Chlorobenzoyl)-5-methoxy-2-methylindole-3-acetohydroxamic acid.
$C_{19}H_{17}ClN_2O_4$=372.8.

CAS — 27035-30-9.

Oxametacin is closely related structurally to indomethacin and has analgesic and anti-inflammatory activity.

Comparison with indomethacin.— J. Polderman and M. Colon, *J. int. med. Res.*, 1979, *7*, 83; *idem*, 1980, *8*, 156.

Proprietary Names

Flogar *(UCB, Belg.; ABC, Ital.)*.

13053-r

Oxapium Iodide. Cyclonium Iodide; SH-100. 1-(2-Cyclohexyl-2-phenyl-1,3-dioxolan-4-ylmethyl)-1-methylpiperidinium iodide.
$C_{22}H_{34}INO_2$=471.4.

CAS — 6577-41-9.

A white odourless crystalline powder with a bitter taste. M.p. about 200°. Very slightly **soluble** in water; soluble in alcohol; freely soluble in chloroform and methyl alcohol.

Oxapium iodide has anticholinergic properties and has been used for the relief of smooth-muscle spasm. Oxapium bromide has also been used.

Proprietary Names

Esperan *(Toyama, Jap.)*.

13054-f

Oxaprotiline Hydrochloride. C-49802B-Ba. (±)-1-(9,10-Dihydro-9,10-ethanoanthracen-9-yl)-3-methylaminopropan-2-ol hydrochloride.
$C_{20}H_{23}NO,HCl$=329.9.

CAS — 56433-44-4 (oxaprotiline); 39022-39-4 (hydrochloride).

Oxaprotiline hydrochloride is a tetracyclic antidepressant.

References: J. P. Feighner *et al.*, *Curr. ther. Res.*, 1981, *29*, 363.

Manufacturers

Ciba-Geigy, USA.

13055-d

Oxaprozin. Wy-21743. 3-(4,5-Diphenyloxazol-2-yl)propionic acid.
$C_{18}H_{15}NO_3$=293.3.

CAS — 21256-18-8.

Oxaprozin has analgesic and anti-inflammatory activity and has been tried in patients with rheumatic disorders.

References: R. Jamar and J. Dequeker, *Curr. med. Res. Opinion*, 1978, *5*, 433; W. J. Reynolds *et al.*, *J. Rheumatol.*, 1979, *6*, 345; J. A. Hubsher *et al.*, *J. int. med. Res.*, 1979, *7*, 69; F. W. Janssen *et al.*, *Clin. Pharmac. Ther.*, 1980, *27*, 352; P. D. Mitnick *et al.*, *Clin. Pharmac. Ther.*, 1980, *28*, 680; F. L. Lanza *et al.*, *J. clin. Pharmac.*, 1981, *21*, 157.

Manufacturers

Wyeth, UK.

13056-n

Oxatomide. R-35443. 1-[3-(4-Benzhydrylpiperazin-1-yl)propyl]benzimidazolin-2-one.
$C_{27}H_{30}N_4O$=426.6.

CAS — 60607-34-3.

NOTE. The name oxatimide was suggested for this compound.

Oxatomide is an antihistamine; it has been suggested that it has mast-cell stabilising properties. The usual dose is 30 to 60 mg twice daily.

References: R. De Beule *et al.*, *Acta Allerg.*, 1977, *32*, 278; A. Ahonen *et al.*, *Curr. ther. Res.*, 1979, *26*, 82; C. Möller and B. Björkstén, *Allergy*, 1980, *35*, 319; J. De Cree *et al.*, *Clin. Trials J.*, 1980, *17*, 84; J. De Cree *et al.*, *Curr. med. Res. Opinion*, 1980, *6*, 380; I. S. Petheram *et al.*, *Br. J. Dis. Chest*, 1980, *74*, 319; S. Gatti *et al.*, *Br. J. Derm.*, 1980, *103*, 671; J. Blockeel and O. Leuridan, *Ophthalmologica, Basel*, 1980, *181*, 133; P. Dockx *et al.*, *Curr. ther. Res.*, 1981, *29*, 510; E. F. Juniper *et al.*, *Clin. Allergy*, 1981, *11*, 61; S. F. Wood and J. H. Barber, *ibid.*, 491; W. Peremans *et al.*, *Dermatologica*, 1981, *162*, 42.

Proprietary Preparations

Tinset *(Janssen, UK)*. Oxatomide, available as scored tablets of 30 mg.

13057-h

Oxdralazine. L-6150 *(dihydrochloride)*. *N*-(6-Hydrazinopyridazin-3-yl)-2,2′-iminodiethanol.
$C_8H_{15}N_5O_2$=213.2.

CAS — 17259-75-5 (oxdralazine); 27464-23-9 (dihydrochloride).

Oxdralazine is reported to have vasodilator and antihypertensive properties.

References: A. Maseri *et al.*, *J. int. med. Res.*, 1976, *4*, 402; A. Salvadeo *et al.*, *Arzneimittel-Forsch.*, 1979, *29*, 1753; E. Bartoli *et al.*, *J. clin. Pharmac.*, 1979, *19*, 751; R. M. Moskowitz and J. N. Cohn, *Clin. Pharmac. Ther.*, 1980, *27*, 773.

Manufacturers

Lepetit, Ital.

13058-m

Oxepinac. 6,11-Dihydro-11-oxodibenz[*b,e*]oxepin-3-ylacetic acid.
$C_{16}H_{12}O_4$=268.3.

CAS — 55689-65-1.

Oxepinac is reported to have analgesic activity and has been tried in arthritic disorders.

For a series of papers on oxepinac, including *animal* studies, see *Arzneimittel-Forsch.*, 1978, *28*, 428–468.

Manufacturers
Daiichi, Jap.

13059-b

Oxetorone Fumarate. L-6257. 3-(6,12-Dihydrobenzofuro[3,2-*c*][1]benzoxepin-6-ylidene)-*NN*-dimethylpropylamine hydrogen fumarate.
$C_{21}H_{21}NO_2,C_4H_4O_4$=435.5.

CAS — 26020-55-3 (oxetorone); 34522-46-8 (fumarate).

Oxetorone fumarate has been used in the treatment of migraine.

Proprietary Names
Nocertone *(Armstrong, Arg.; Labaz, Belg.; Labaz, Fr.; Labaz, Ger.; Labaz, Spain; Labaz, Switz.).*

13060-x

Oxfendazole. RS-8858. Methyl 5-phenylsulphinyl-1*H*-benzimidazol-2-ylcarbamate.
$C_{15}H_{13}N_3O_3S$=315.3.

CAS — 53716-50-0.

Oxfendazole is a veterinary anthelmintic.

Proprietary Names
Synanthic *(Syntex, UK)*; Systamex *(Wellcome, UK).*

13061-r

Oxfenicine. UK-25842. L-2-(4-Hydroxyphenyl)glycine.
$C_8H_9NO_3$=167.2.

CAS — 32462-30-9.

Oxfenicine is reported to have potential application in the treatment of ischaemic heart disease.

Manufacturers
Pfizer, UK.

13062-f

Oxibendazole. SKF-30310. Methyl 5-propoxy-1*H*-benzimidazol-2-ylcarbamate.
$C_{12}H_{15}N_3O_3$=249.3.

CAS — 20559-55-1.

Oxibendazole is a veterinary anthelmintic.

Manufacturers
Smith Kline & French, UK.

13063-d

Oxidopamine. 6-Hydroxydopamine. 5-(2-Aminoethyl)benzene-1,2,4-triol.
$C_8H_{11}NO_3$=169.2.

CAS — 1199-18-4.

An off-white unstable powder. **Store** at 5° in a desiccator.

Oxidopamine has been used by subconjunctival injection to produce reversible chemical sympathectomy in glaucoma.

Oxidopamine 1 to 5 mg in 0.5 ml of 0.005M ascorbic acid solution, buffered to pH 6 with sodium ascorbate, injected subconjunctivally lowered intra-ocular pressure within 3 hours in 9 of 11 glaucomatous eyes resistant to other medication. Topical application of adrenaline 1% eye-drops four times daily maintained the reduction in intra-ocular pressure for up to 3 months. A further injection of oxidopamine produced a similar response.—J. G. Diamond, *Archs Ophthal., N.Y.*, 1976, *94*, 41.

Further references: H. Watanabe *et al.*, *Trans. Am. Acad. Ophthal. Oto-lar.*, 1977, *83*, 69.

Manufacturers
Cooper, USA.

13064-n

Oxiperomide. Foxamide; Peromide; R-4714. 1-[1-(2-Phenoxyethyl)-4-piperidyl]benzimidazolin-2-one.
$C_{20}H_{23}N_3O_2$=337.4.

CAS — 5322-53-2.

Oxiperomide has been tried for the control of dyskinesias.

References: P. Bédard *et al.*, *Br. med. J.*, 1978, *1*, 954; *Lancet*, 1980, *1*, 1119; D. E. Casey and J. Gerlach, *J. Neurol. Neurosurg. Psychiat.*, 1980, *43*, 264.

Manufacturers
Janssen, Belg.

13065-h

Oxitropium Bromide. Ba-253-HR. 6,7-Epoxy-8-ethyl-3-[(*S*)-tropoyloxy]tropanium bromide.
$C_{19}H_{26}BrNO_4$=412.3.

CAS — 30286-75-0.

Oxitropium bromide is structurally related to ipratropium bromide. It is reported to have anticholinergic and bronchodilator activity.

References: D. Nolte, *Respiration*, 1978, *36*, 32; E. Flohr and K. O. Bischoff, *ibid.*, 1979, *38*, 98.

Manufacturers
Boehringer Ingelheim, Ger.

13066-m

Oxmetidine Hydrochloride. SKF-92994-A_2. 2-[2-(5-Methylimidazol-4-ylmethylthio)ethylamino]-5-piperonylpyrimidin-4(1*H*)-one dihydrochloride.
$C_{19}H_{21}N_5O_3S,2HCl$=472.4.

CAS — 72830-39-8 (oxmetidine); 63204-23-9 (hydrochloride).

Oxmetidine is reported to have histamine H_2 receptor blocking activity.

Manufacturers
Smith Kline & French, UK.

13067-b

Oxolamine Citrate. AF-438; 683M; SKF-9976; Quoxolamine Citrate. 2-(3-Phenyl-1,2,4-oxadiazol-5-yl)triethylamine citrate.
$C_{14}H_{19}N_3O,C_6H_8O_7$=437.4.

CAS — 959-14-8 (oxolamine); 1949-20-8 (citrate).

Crystals. Slightly **soluble** in water and alcohol.

Oxolamine citrate is an antitussive agent with analgesic and anti-inflammatory properties. It has been used in the treatment of inflammatory respiratory conditions. Oxolamine phosphate has also been used.

Proprietary Names
Bentox *(Falorni, Ital.)*; Bredon *(Organon, Austral.; Organon, Belg.; Organon, Denm.; Organon, Neth.)*; Broncatar *(Pulitzer, Ital.)*; Encelad *(Italchemi, Ital.)*; Flogobron *(Intersint, Ital.)*; Oxolev *(Barlocco, Ital.)*; Perebron *(Angelini, Ital.; Farma-Lepori, Spain)*; Tussibron *(Sella, Ital.).*

15307-x

Oxophenarsine Hydrochloride *(B.P.C. 1963).* Oxophenarseni Hydrochloridum; Arsphenoxidi Hydrochloridum; Phenarsoxydum Hydrochloricum. 2-Amino-4-arsenosophenol hydrochloride.
$C_6H_6AsNO_2,HCl$=235.5.

CAS — 306-12-7 (oxophenarsine); 538-03-4 (hydrochloride).

Pharmacopoeias. In *Int.* and *Mex.*

A white, or nearly white, odourless, deliquescent, amorphous powder containing 30 to 32% of As. **Soluble** in water, solutions of alkali hydroxides and carbonates, and mineral acids; sparingly soluble in alcohol; practically insoluble in acetone, chloroform, and ether. A solution in water is acid to litmus but alkaline to congo red. A 3.67% solution is iso-osmotic with serum. When sodium carbonate or bicarbonate is added to the aqueous solution, carbon dioxide is evolved and the base precipitated, but the precipitate dissolves on shaking.
It is distributed in sealed containers, usually mixed with alkali carbonates and buffering agents to increase the pH and make it physiologically compatible with human blood. It is very stable when anhydrous but the stability decreases with increase in water content. **Store** at a temperature not exceeding 20° in hermetically sealed containers.

Oxophenarsine was formerly used similarly to neoarsphenamine (p.1731) in the treatment of syphilis. Oxophenarsine tartrate was also used.

13069-g

Oxybromonaftoic Acid. 4-Bromo-3-hydroxy-2-naphthoic acid.
$C_{11}H_7BrO_3$=267.1.

CAS — 2208-15-3.

Oxybromonaftoic acid has been used in hepatic disorders.

Proprietary Names
Naftocol *(Panthox & Burck, Ital.).*

13070-f

Oxychlorpromazine Hydrochloride. 3-(2-Chlorophenothiazin-10-yl)-*NN*-dimethylpropylamine 5-oxide hydrochloride.
$C_{17}H_{19}ClN_2OS,HCl$=371.3.

CAS — 969-99-3 (oxychlorpromazine); 316-07-4 (hydrochloride).

Oxychlorpromazine hydrochloride has been used similarly to chlorpromazine hydrochloride.

Proprietary Names
Transedon *(Sintetica, Switz.).*

13071-d

Oxyclozanide *(B.P. Vet.).* ICI-46683. 3,3′,5,5′,6-Pentachloro-2′-hydroxysalicylanilide.
$C_{13}H_6Cl_5NO_3$=401.5.

CAS — 2277-92-1.

Pharmacopoeias. In *Nord.*

A cream-coloured, odourless, tasteless powder. M.p. about 208°. Very slightly **soluble** in water; soluble 1 in 20 of alcohol, 1 in 5 of acetone, and 1 in 600 of chloroform; soluble in solutions of alkali hydroxides and carbonates.

Oxyclozanide is a veterinary anthelmintic used in the control of liver-fluke infestations in cattle and sheep.

Proprietary Names
Zanil *(ICI Pharmaceuticals, UK).*

13073-h

Pamabrom. 2-Amino-2-methylpropan-1-ol 8-bromotheophyllinate.
$C_4H_{11}NO,C_7H_7BrN_4O_2$=348.2.

CAS — 606-04-2.

A fine white powder. M.p. 300° with decomposition. **Soluble** in water. A saturated aqueous solution has a pH of 8 to 8.5.

Pamabrom is a mild diuretic which has been used for the relief of premenstrual tension.

13074-m

Pangamic Acid

A substance isolated from apricot kernels and rice bran was termed pangamic acid and has also been described as 'vitamin B_{15}'. Although pangamic acid has been identified by some sources as gluconic acid 6-bis(*N*-di-isopropylamino)acetate, there is much uncertainty about the identity of products sold in health food stores as 'vitamin B_{15}', pangamic acid, or calcium pangamate and different brands have been reported to have completely different compositions.

Claims for the activity of pangamic acid as a promoter of tissue oxygenation and its alleged value in numerous disorders have not been substantiated. There is no evidence that pangamic acid is a vitamin.

References: *Med. Lett.*, 1978, *20*, 44; *J. Am. med. Ass.*, 1980, *243*, 2473.

13075-b

Pantethine. (+)-(*R*)-*NN'*-[Dithiobis(ethyleneiminocarbonylethylene)]bis(2,4-dihydroxy-3,3-dimethylbutyramide).
$C_{22}H_{42}N_4O_8S_2$=554.7.

CAS — 16816-67-4.

Pantethine has activity similar to that of pantothenic acid.

Proprietary Names
Pantetina *(Maggioni, Ital.).*

13076-v

Papaverine Monophosadenine. Papaverine Adenylate; 3209 CERM. Papaverine adenosine 5'-monophosphate.
$C_{30}H_{35}N_6O_{11}P$=686.6.

CAS — 39024-96-9.

Papaverine monophosadenine has been used for its reputed effects on the cerebral circulation.

Proprietary Names
Dicertan *(Sarget, Fr.).*

13077-g

Papaveroline Meglumine. The *N*-methylglucamine salt of 1-(3,4-dihydroxybenzyl)isoquinoline-6,7-diol.
$C_{16}H_{13}NO_4,C_7H_{17}NO_5$=478.5.

CAS — 574-77-6 (papaveroline).

Papaveroline meglumine has been used in the treatment of circulatory disorders. The sulphonate has also been used.

Proprietary Names
Modus *(Scharper, Ital.).*

13078-q

Paraphenylenediamine.
$C_6H_4(NH_2)_2$=108.1.

CAS — 106-50-3.

Commonly known in the hairdressing trade as '*para*'.

White or reddish crystals; **soluble** 1 in 100 of water; soluble in alcohol and chloroform.

Adverse Effects. It is estimated that about 4% of apparently normal subjects are sensitive to 'para', and 1% acutely sensitive.
The local effects consist of oedema and severe dermatitis of the scalp, sometimes spreading to the face and even the upper part of the thorax.
The systemic effects which have been reported include cardiovascular damage, vertigo, gastritis, asthenia, diplopia, chemosis, exophthalmos, asthma, and exfoliative dermatitis.
Some studies have linked hair dyes with mutagenicity and carcinogenicity.
Maximum permissible atmospheric concentration 100 μg per m^3.

Of 1205 persons with dermatitis or eczema submitted to patch testing with paraphenylenediamine 2% in yellow soft paraffin, 15.2% gave a positive reaction.— E. Rudzki and D. Kleniewska, *Br. J. Derm.*, 1970, *83*, 543.

Carcinogenicity. In a study of chromosomal damage and hair dyes no excess of chromosomal damage was noted in 60 professional hair tinters compared with 36 control subjects, possibly owing to the protective effect of gloves and poor percutaneous absorption through the hands. A significant excess of chromosomal damage (mainly chromatid breaks), was, however, noted in women with dyed hair compared with matched controls. This latter finding warranted further study in view of the known mutagenicity and carcinogenicity of some hair-dye constitutents.— D. J. Kirkland *et al.*, *Lancet*, 1978, *2*, 124. Severe criticisms and comments.— N. J. Van Abbé (letter), *ibid.*, 271; D. J. Kirkland *et al.* (letter), *ibid.*, 272; N. J. Van Abbé (letter), *ibid.*, 368; D. J. Price (letter), *ibid.;* A. R. Feinstein (letter), *ibid.*, 627; D. J. Kirkland *et al.* (letter), *ibid.*, 628; C. Burnett (letter), *ibid.*, 685.

Analysis of data from 120 557 married, female, registered US nurses did not indicate evidence of any material carcinogenic risk occurring during the initial 20 years following first use of permanent hair dyes.— C. H. Hennekens *et al.*, *Lancet*, 1979, *1*, 1390. Criticisms.— A. K. Bahn (letter), *ibid.*, *2*, 475; J. M. Davies (letter), *ibid.*, 536.

For references to the mutagenic activity in bacteria of paraphenylenediamine derivatives used as hair dyes and its relevance to carcinogenicity, see C. E. Searle *et al.*, *Nature*, 1975, *255*, 506; D. J. Kirkland and S. Venitt, *Mutation Res.*, 1976, *40*, 37; C. Burnett (letter), *Lancet*, 1976, *1*, 482; S. Venitt *et al.* (letter), *ibid.*, 641.

Further references: D. G. MacPhee and D. M. Podger (letter), *Med. J. Aust.*, 1975, *2*, 32; M. Jain *et al.* (letter), *Can. med. Ass. J.*, 1977, *117*, 1132; K. M. Stavraky *et al.*, *J. natn. Cancer Inst.*, 1979, *63*, 941.

Uses. Paraphenylenediamine is used as a hair dye and for dyeing furs.
When used as hair dyes, concentrations of the ortho, meta, and para isomers of phenylenediamine and their *N*-substituted derivatives are restricted in Great Britain by the Cosmetic Products Regulations 1978 (SI 1978: No. 1354).

13079-p

Pararosaniline Embonate. Pararosaniline Pamoate; Tris-(aminophenyl)carbonium Pamoate; TAC Pamoate; CI-403A. 4-[(4-Aminophenyl)(4-iminocyclohexa-2,5-dien-1-ylidene)methyl]aniline 4,4'-methylenebis(3-hydroxy-2-naphthoate) (2:1) dihydrate.
$(C_{19}H_{18}N_3)_2,C_{23}H_{14}O_6,2H_2O$=999.1.

CAS — 569-61-9 (pararosaniline); 7232-51-1 (embonate, dihydrate).

Pararosaniline embonate is a schistosomicide with activity against *Schistosoma mansoni*, *S. haematobium* , and *S. japonicum*.

A study in 166 patients with *Schistosoma japonicum* infection treated with pararosaniline embonate indicated that of 4 dosage schedules the following was the most effective: the equivalent of 35 to 40 mg of pararosaniline per kg body-weight daily in 3 divided doses for 14 days, the course being repeated after 7 days' rest. In a further study in 323 patients improved control was achieved when the above course was modified and followed by a single daily dose once a week for 16 to 24 weeks. Negative stools were achieved in up to 98% of patients. Side-effects (nausea, vomiting, body weakness, skin eruptions, dizziness, anorexia) were generally mild and transient.— T. P. Pesigan *et al.*, *Bull. Wld Hlth Org.*, 1967, *36*, 263.

Further references: T. P. Pesigan *et al.*, *J. Philipp. med. Ass.*, 1966, *42*, 653, per *Trop. Dis. Bull.*, 1968, *65*, 904; *Chronicle Wld Hlth Org.*, 1966, *20*, 92.

Manufacturers
Parke, Davis, USA.

13080-n

Paratoluenediamine. 2-Methyl-1,4-phenylenediamine.
$C_7H_{10}N_2$=122.2.

CAS — 95-70-5.

Paratoluenediamine is used as a hair dye.

Of 612 persons with dermatitis or eczema submitted to patch testing with paratoluenediamine 2% in yellow soft paraffin, 4.2% gave a positive reaction.— E. Rudzki and D. Kleniewska, *Br. J. Derm.*, 1970, *83*, 543.

A report of aplastic anaemia in a woman who used a hair dye containing paratoluenediamine.— P. J. Toghill and R. G. Wilcox, *Br. med. J.*, 1976, *1*, 502. For comments suggesting that the aplastic anaemia might be attributed to antibiotics taken by the patient, see A. J. Jouhar, *Bristol-Myers* (letter), *ibid.*, 1074.

For references to the potential mutagenicity and carcinogenicity of hair dyes, see Paraphenylenediamine (above).

13081-h

Parbendazole *(B.P. Vet.).* SKF-29044. Methyl 5-butylbenzimidazol-2-ylcarbamate.
$C_{13}H_{17}N_3O_2$=247.3.

CAS — 14255-87-9.

A white or almost white, odourless or almost odourless, crystalline powder. Practically **insoluble** in water; soluble 1 in 900 of alcohol and 1 in 300 of chloroform; very slightly soluble in ether; soluble in dilute mineral acids.

Parbendazole is a veterinary anthelmintic used in the treatment of nematode infestations.

In the usual veterinary doses parbendazole had a marked teratogenic effect in *rats*, a slight teratogenic effect in *mice*, and no teratogenic effect in *rabbits*.— L. Mercier-Parot, *Thérapie*, 1976, *31*, 491. A study of the embryotoxic and antimitotic effect of drugs of the benzimidazole series.— P. Delatour and Y. Richard, *ibid.*, 505.

Proprietary Names
Helmatac*(Smith Kline & French, UK).*

13082-m

Parethoxycaine Hydrochloride. 2-Diethylaminoethyl 4-ethoxybenzoate hydrochloride.
$C_{15}H_{23}NO_3,HCl$=301.8.

CAS — 94-23-5 (parethoxycaine); 136-46-9 (hydrochloride).

Parethoxycaine hydrochloride has been used as a local anaesthetic for topical use in the mouth.

Proprietary Names
Maxicaïne *(Fumouze, Fr.).*

13083-b

Paroxypropione. 4'-Hydroxypropiophenone.
$C_9H_{10}O_2$=150.2.

CAS — 70-70-2.

A crystalline solid. M.p. 149°. **Soluble** 1 in 3000 of cold water and 1 in 30 of boiling water; soluble in alcohol and ether.

Paroxypropione is a pituitary gonadotrophic hormone inhibitor which has been used for the control of pituitary hyperactivity.

Proprietary Names
Frenantol *(UPB, Belg.)*; Frénantol *(Anglo-French Laboratories, Canad.*; *Laroche Navarron, Fr.)*; Frenantole *(Landerlan, Spain)*; Frenormon Fuerte *(Medea, Spain)*; Possipione *(Recordati, Ital.).*

13084-v

Parsalmide. 54106-CB; MY-41-6. 5-Amino-*N*-butyl-*O*-(prop-2-ynyl)salicylamide; 5-Amino-*N*-butyl-2-(prop-2-ynyloxy)benzamide.
$C_{14}H_{18}N_2O_2$=246.3.

CAS — 30653-83-9.

Parsalmide is reported to have analgesic and anti-inflammatory activity and has been used in the treatment of rheumatic and other disorders.

For a series of papers on parsalmide, see *Minerva med., Roma*, 1976, *67*, 3361–3417.

Further references: A. Pedrazzoli *et al., Boll. chim.-farm.*, 1976, *115*, 125, per *Int. pharm. Abstr.*, 1976, *13*, 1144; G. Maffi *et al., Boll. chim.-farm.*, 1976, *115*, 135, per *Int. pharm. Abstr.*, 1976, *13*, 1144; L. Fleischmann and A. Pedrazzoli, *Arzneimittel-Forsch.*, 1977, *27*, 1199.

Proprietary Names
Parsal *(Midy, Ital.)*.

13085-g

Pashydrazide. 4-Aminosalicylohydrazide.
$C_7H_9N_3O_2$=167.2.

CAS — 6946-29-8.

Pashydrazide has been used in the treatment of tuberculosis.

Proprietary Names
Pasdrazide *(Bruco, Ital.)*.

13086-q

Passion Flower. Passiflora; May-pop; Grenadille; Pasionaria.

CAS — 486-84-0 (harman).

Pharmacopoeias. In *Belg., Fr., Span.*, and *Swiss. Braz.* includes the leaves of *P. alata*, (Maracujá).

The dried flowering and fruiting tops of *Passiflora incarnata* (Passifloraceae). *Swiss P.* specifies not less than 0.01% of alkaloids calculated as harman ($C_{12}H_{10}N_2$).

Passion flower is reputed to have antispasmodic and sedative properties. It has been used as a liquid extract and as a tincture.

13088-s

Peganum *(B.P.C. 1934).* Harmal; Armel; Hurmal; Syrian Rue; Wild Rue. The dried seeds of *Peganum harmala* (Zygophyllaceae), containing 2.5 to 4% of total alkaloids. The principal alkaloid is harmaline, $C_{13}H_{14}N_2O$ (about 60%), in association with harmine, $C_{13}H_{12}N_2O$, harmalol, $C_{12}H_{12}N_2O$, and peganine (= vasicine, see Adhatoda, p.686.

CAS — 304-21-2 (harmaline); 442-51-3 (harmine); 525-57-5 (harmalol); 6159-55-3 (peganine).

Peganum has been used in India for various medicinal purposes, particularly as an anthelmintic and narcotic, in the form of an infusion and tincture. Harmaline and harmine have been reported to have hallucinogenic properties—see p.925.

13089-w

Pendecamaine. Dimethyl(3-palmitamidopropyl)ammonioacetate.
$C_{23}H_{46}N_2O_3$=398.6.

CAS — 32954-43-1.

Pendecamaine is an ampholytic surfactant (see p.1443) which has been used in surgical scrubs and in cosmetic and toilet preparations.

Proprietary Names of Related Preparations
Tego Betain L7 *(Goldschmidt, UK)* (also known as Tego Betain C) (based on C_{11} to C_{17} fatty acids).

13090-m

Pentaerythritol. 2,2-Bis(hydroxymethyl)propane-1,3-diol.
$C_5H_{12}O_4$=136.1.

CAS — 115-77-5.

Pentaerythritol has been used in the treatment of constipation.

Proprietary Names
Auxinutril *(Gallier, Fr.)*.

13091-b

Pentamustine. NCNU. 1-(2-Chloroethyl)-3-neopentyl-1-nitrosourea.
$C_8H_{16}ClN_3O_2$=221.7.

CAS — 73105-03-0.

Pentamustine is a nitrosourea compound reported to have antineoplastic activity.

13092-v

Peplomycin. Pepleomycin; NK-631 (sulphate 1:1). N^1-{3-[(*S*)-(α-Methylbenzyl)amino]propyl-}bleomycinamide.
$C_{61}H_{88}N_{18}O_{21}S_2$=1473.6.

CAS — 68247-85-8 (peplomycin); 70384-29-1 (sulphate).

Peplomycin is a derivative of bleomycin with antineoplastic activity.

Proprietary Names
Pepleo (sulphate) *(Nippon Kayaku, Jap.)*.

13093-g

Pepstatin. Pepstatin A. It is obtained from several species of *Streptomyces* . *N*-[Isovaleryl-L-valyl-L-valyl-4-amino-3-hydroxy-6-methylheptanoyl-L-alanyl]-4-amino-3-hydroxy-6-methylheptanoic acid.
$C_{34}H_{63}N_5O_9$=685.9.

CAS — 26305-03-3.

Pepstatin inhibits the effect of pepsin probably by binding to form a pepsin-pepstatin complex. It has been tried in patients with duodenal or gastric ulcers. Other pepstatins, with differing radicals substituted at four places in the molecule, have been identified.

Pepstatin and the inhibition of leukokinins and formation of ascitic fluid.— L. M. Greenbaum *et al., Cancer Res.*, 1975, *35*, 706, per *Int. pharm. Abstr.*, 1975, *12*, 1123.

In a double-blind randomised clinical study in 54 patients with duodenal ulcer pepstatin 100 mg seven times a day for 6 weeks had no significant advantage over placebo in ulcer healing.— O. Bonnevie *et al., Gut*, 1979, *20*, 624.

Manufacturers
Bristol, USA.

13094-q

Peracetic Acid. Acetyl Hydroperoxide; Peroxyacetic Acid.
$C_2H_4O_3$=76.05.

CAS — 79-21-0.

A liquid with an acrid odour. **Soluble** in water, alcohol, and ether.

Peracetic acid is a strong oxidising agent which is corrosive to the skin. It has been used as a spray for sterilisation of the air and interior of germ-free animal laboratories.

References: V. Kestnerová and F. Volná, *Čslká Epidem. Mikrobiol. Imunol.*, 1966, *15*, 275, per *Int. pharm. Abstr.*, 1967, *4*, 337; A. Pazdiora and V. Kubiček, *Vojen. zdrav. Listy*, 1967, *36*, 116, per *Int. pharm. Abstr.*, 1967, *4*, 1188; R. D. Barnes *et al., Lancet*, 1969, *1*, 168; V. Kubiček, *Čslká Farm.*, 1970, *19*, 67, per *Int. pharm. Abstr.*, 1972, *9*, 546; D. Dworschak and J. Linde, *Dte GesundhWes.*, 1976, *31*, 1622, per *Int. pharm. Abstr.*, 1977, *14*, 217; P. Schiller, *Čslká Epidem. Mikrobiol. Imunol.*, 1979, *28*, 116, per *Abstr. Hyg.*, 1979, *54*, 1084.

13095-p

Pergolide Mesylate. LY-127809. 8β-Methylthiomethyl-6-propylergoline methanesulphonate.
$C_{19}H_{26}N_2S,CH_4O_3S$=410.6.

CAS — 66104-22-1 (pergolide); 66104-23-2 (mesylate).

Pergolide mesylate is a dopamine receptor agonist which reduces plasma concentrations of prolactin. It has been tried, usually with levodopa, in the treatment of parkinsonism.

References: A. N. Lieberman *et al.* (letter), *Lancet*, 1979, *2*, 1129; D. L. Kleinberg *et al., J. clin. Endocr. Metab.*, 1980, *51*, 152; L. Lemberger *et al., Clin. Pharmac. Ther.*, 1980, *27*, 265; *idem*, 642; A. Lieberman *et al., Neurology, Minneap.*, 1981, *31*, 675; E. R. González, *J. Am. med. Ass.*, 1981, *246*, 11; A. Rubin *et al., Clin. Pharmac. Ther.*, 1981, *30*, 258; A. J. Lees and G. M. Stern (letter), *Lancet*, 1981, *2*, 577; S. Franks *et al., ibid.*, 659.

Manufacturers
Lilly, UK.

13096-s

Perisoxal. Perixazole; 31252-S (citrate). 1-(5-Phenylisoxazol-3-yl)-2-piperidinoethanol.
$C_{16}H_{20}N_2O_2$=272.3.

CAS — 2055-44-9.

Perisoxal is reported to have analgesic and anti-inflammatory activity.

Proprietary Names
Isoxal (citrate) *(Jap.)*.

13097-w

Permethrin. 3-Phenoxybenzyl 3-(2,2-dichlorovinyl)-2,2-dimethylcyclopropanecarboxylate.
$C_{21}H_{20}Cl_2O_3$=391.3.

CAS — 52645-53-1.

Permethrin is a pyrethroid insecticide for veterinary use.

References: J. M. B. Harley, *Trans. R. Soc. trop. Med. Hyg.*, 1978, *72*, 112.

13098-e

Peruvoside. A glycoside obtained from *Thevetia neriifolia* (Apocynaceae), related to thevetin A.
$C_{30}H_{44}O_9$=548.7.

CAS — 1182-87-2.

Peruvoside has been used in congestive heart failure.

Slow injection of peruvoside 600 to 900 µg into the pulmonary artery in 6 patients with congestive heart failure had an immediate and marked positive inotropic and negative chronotropic effect. Peruvoside was also effective in 22 patients with congestive heart failure who received peruvoside by mouth in an average dose of 2.4 mg, followed by an average maintenance dose of 600 µg.— M. L. Bhatia *et al., Br. med. J.*, 1970, *3*, 740.

Further references: G. Lohmöller and H. Lydtin, *Arzneimittel-Forsch.*, 1971, *21*, 1567.

Proprietary Names
Encordin *(E. Merck, Ger.)*; Largitor *(Inverni della Beffa, Ital.)*; Nerial *(Simes, Ital.)*; Perusid *(Malesci, Ital.)*.

13099-l

Phenamidine Isethionate *(B. Vet. C. 1965).* 4,4′-Oxydibenzamidine bis(2-hydroxyethanesulphonate).
$C_{18}H_{26}N_4O_9S_2$=506.5.

CAS — 101-62-2 (phenamidine); 620-90-6 (isethionate).

White or nearly white, odourless crystals or powder, with a bitter taste. **Soluble** 1 in 1.4 of water and 1 in 300 of alcohol; practically insoluble in chloroform and ether. A 5% solution in water has a pH of 5 to 7. Solutions are **sterilised** by filtration or by maintaining at 98° to 100° for 30 minutes with a bactericide.

Phenamidine isethionate has bactericidal properties but has mainly been used in veterinary medicine in the treatment of babesiasis in cattle, horses, and dogs.

13100-l

Phencyclidine Hydrochloride *(B. Vet. C. 1965).* CI-395; PCP. 1-(1-Phenylcyclohexyl)piperidine hydrochloride.

$C_{17}H_{25}N,HCl=279.9$.

CAS — 77-10-1 (phencyclidine); 956-90-1 (hydrochloride).

A white odourless crystalline powder. M.p. about 228°. **Soluble** 1 in 6 of water, 1 in 7 of alcohol, and 1 in 2 of chloroform; very slightly soluble in ether. A 10% solution in water has a pH of 2 to 5. Solutions are **sterilised** by filtration.

Adverse Effects. Phencyclidine can induce a psychosis clinically indistinguishable from schizophrenia. Several deaths have resulted from its illicit use. Adverse effects reported include respiratory depression, hallucinations, agitation, catatonic rigidity, disorientation, incoordination, nystagmus, hypersalivation, vomiting, convulsions, numbness, and maculopapular skin rash.

For a short review of the toxic effects of phencyclidine hydrochloride, see R. E. Lister, *J. Pharm. Pharmac.*, 1966, *18,* 364 (Symposium on the Toxicity of Analgesic Substances).

The pharmacology and toxicology of phencyclidine.— J. C. Munch, *Bull. Narcot.*, 1974, *26* (Oct.–Dec.), 9; J. P. Morgan and J. L. Solomon, *N.Y. St. J. Med.*, 1978, *78,* 2035.

Abuse. Street names for phencyclidine used illicitly have included: angel dust, angel hair, angel mist, crystal, cyclone, dust, elephant tranquilliser, embalming fluid, goon, hog, horse tranquilliser, killer weed, KW, mint weed, mist, monkey dust, peace pills, peace weed, rocket fuel, scuffle, sheets, super weed, surfer, and T.

Reviews on the abuse of phencyclidine.— *Med. Lett.*, 1977, *19,* 70; S. Cohen, *J. Am. med. Ass.*, 1977, *238,* 515; M. Dolan, *Am. Pharm.*, 1978, *NS18* (Feb.), 22; R. C. Petersen and R. C. Stillman, *Phencyclidine: A Review*, Rockville, Maryland, National Institute on Drug Abuse, 1978; L. J. Sioris and E. P. Krenzelok, *Am. J. Hosp. Pharm.*, 1978, *35,* 1362; E. J. Khantzian and G. J. McKenna, *Ann. intern. Med.*, 1979, *90,* 361; M. L. Richards *et al.*, *Drug Intell. & clin. Pharm.*, 1979, *13,* 336; R. Stillman and R. C. Petersen, *Ann. intern. Med.*, 1979, *90,* 428; *Br. med. J.*, 1980, *281,* 1511.

A review of the causes of phencyclidine-related deaths.— R. S. Burns and S. E. Lerner, *Clin. Toxicol.*, 1978, *12,* 463.

Phencyclidine was a major component of street drug preparations. In liquid form it was sprayed on marihuana, parsley, oregano, or other plant leaves and sold as 'angel dust'. In powder form it was marketed as phencyclidine or 'peace pills'. It was frequently sold as lysergide, mescaline, psilocybin, cocaine, 3,4-methylenedioxyamphetamine (MDA), tetrahydrocannabinol and other drugs, or it might be mixed with these agents. Many unrecognised toxic reactions secondary to sympathomimetic anaesthetic abuse were occurring and phencyclidine, a major drug of abuse, was a member of this group.— J. M. Rainey and M. K. Crowder, *J. Am. med. Ass.*, 1974, *230,* 824. When used illicitly phencyclidine has been sniffed, injected, eaten, or smoked. Many analogues have been synthesised and at least 6 are sold illicitly in the U.S.— *Br. med. J.*, 1980, *281,* 1511.

A series of papers on the abuse of phencyclidine.— *Clin. Toxicol.*, 1976, *9,* 473–600, per *Abstr. Hyg.*, 1977, *52,* 382.

A report of near death in a 3-year-old child who had ingested 3 tablets of phencyclidine and a less serious response in a 17-year-old who had also ingested 3 tablets. Recommended treatment included hydration to ensure adequate urinary output for excretion of the drug, avoidance of sympathomimetic agents, respiratory support, barbiturates to control seizures, and diazepam, or phenothiazines for control of spasticity and oculogyric crisis.— C. B. Liden *et al.*, *J. Pediat.*, 1973, *83,* 844.

Fatal status epilepticus occurred in a 17-year-old girl found to have 7 µg of phencyclidine per ml in blood and 30 µg per ml in urine. Phenobarbitone was also detected in the blood in a concentration of 21 µg per ml.— G. F. Kessler *et al.* (letter), *New Engl. J. Med.*, 1974, *291,* 979.

A 13-year-old boy with phencyclidine poisoning developed acute hypertension on the third day and became comatose. He died on the seventh day.— J. W. Eastman and S. N. Cohen, *J. Am. med. Ass.*, 1975, *231,* 1270. Comment.— R. H. Libman (letter), *ibid.*, *233,* 1257. Hypertension during recovery from phencyclidine intoxication.— B. McMahon *et al.*, *Clin. Toxicol.*, 1978, *12,* 37.

The plasma half-life of phencyclidine in subjects suffering from overdosage was found to be about 11 hours which explains the slow clinical improvement of such patients. In 3 patients with a history of multiple-drug abuse, suffering from phencyclidine overdosage, symptoms included coma, excessive salivation and bronchial secretions, excessive lachrymation, conjunctival hyperaemia, muscular spasms with tonic-extensor spasms most pronounced in the neck and back, increased tendon reflexes, nystagmus, and paranoid psychosis.— J. A. Marshman *et al.*, *Toxic. appl. Pharmac.*, 1976, *35,* 129.

Irregular burst-like nystagmus was noted in 2 boys who had ingested phencyclidine. These strikingly abnormal eye movements might aid the diagnosis of phencyclidine poisoning.— J. Herskowitz and E. Y. Oppenheimer (letter), *New Engl. J. Med.*, 1977, *297,* 1405.

Phencyclidine abuse in 2 patients was associated with depression of the central nervous system and acute rhabdomyolysis. It was recommended that all patients with, or suspected of, phencyclidine poisoning should be screened for acute rhabdomyolysis so that prompt treatment to forestall myoglobinuric renal failure could be started.— F. C. Cogen *et al.*, *Ann. intern. Med.*, 1978, *88,* 210. Further reports of rhabdomyolysis and acute renal failure associated with phencyclidine abuse: B. Hoogwerf *et al.*, *Clin. Toxicol.*, 1979, *14,* 47; C. H. Barton *et al.*, *Archs intern. Med.*, 1980, *140,* 568.

A radioimmunoassay screening test for the detection and management of phencyclidine intoxication.— B. Kaul and B. Davidow, *J. clin. Pharmac.*, 1980, *20,* 500.

Individual reports of adverse effects resulting from phencyclidine abuse: J. I. Stein, *Milit. Med.*, 1973, *138,* 590 (psychosis), per *Int. pharm. Abstr.*, 1974, *11,* 618; R. M. Allen and S. J. Young, *Am. J. Psychiat.*, 1978, *135,* 1081 (psychosis); R. G. Fariello and J. A. Black, *J. clin. Psychiat.*, 1978, *39,* 579 (EEG abnormalities); K. -M. Jan *et al.* (letter), *New Engl. J. Med.*, 1978, *299,* 722 (malignant hyperthermia); C. J. Crosley and E. F. Binet, *J. Pediat.*, 1979, *94,* 316 (cerebrovascular complications); V. E. Grove, *J. Am. med. Ass.*, 1979, *242,* 655 (painless self-injury); A. Rosen, *Am. J. Psychiat.*, 1979, *136,* 118 (mania); R. L. Corales *et al.*, *J. Am. med. Ass.*, 1980, *243,* 2323 (effects mimicking head injury); N. L. Golden *et al.*, *Pediatrics*, 1980, *65,* 18 (effects on the foetus).

References to the increasing importance of phencyclidine as a drug of abuse in the USA: N. C. Jain *et al.* (letter), *New Engl. J. Med.*, 1977, *297,* 673; R. D. Budd (letter), *ibid.*, 1980, *303,* 588.

Treatment of overdosage. Until more is known about interactions, other drugs should be used with caution in the treatment of phencyclidine poisoning. If diazepam is used to decrease excitement, agitation, and possibly seizures, small intravenous doses of 2 to 5 mg should be used. If antipsychotic medication is needed butyrophenones such as haloperidol are preferred to phenothiazines. Additional treatment measures include isolation with minimal sensory input and adequate hydration to promote urinary excretion of phencyclidine and its metabolites. Severe respiratory depression and coma requires endotracheal intubation, continuous gastric suctioning, acidification of the urine with ammonium chloride, and careful fluid management.— E. J. Khantzian and G. J. McKenna, *Ann. intern. Med.*, 1979, *90,* 361.

The diagnosis and management of phencyclidine overdosage.— R. Aronow and A. K. Done, *J. Am. Coll. emergency Physns*, 1978, *7,* 56.

Comment on *animal* studies suggesting the possible beneficial effect of tacrine in phencyclidine intoxication.— M. S. Albin (letter), *J. Am. med. Ass.*, 1978, *240,* 529. Lack of benefit with tacrine or physostigmine in *dogs*.— E. F. Domino (letter), *ibid.*, *241,* 2505.

Studies in *animals* suggested that charcoal would inhibit gastro-intestinal absorption of phencyclidine when given soon after an overdose and would reduce the prolonged systemic toxicity by inhibiting reabsorption.— A. L. Picchioni and P. F. Consroe (letter), *New Engl. J. Med.*, 1979, *300,* 202.

The possible value of desipramine in phencyclidine withdrawal.— F. S. Tennant *et al.*, *Am. J. Psychiat.*, 1981, *138,* 845.

Further references to the treatment of phencyclidine toxicity: T. G. Tong *et al.*, *J. Am. med. Ass.*, 1975, *234,* 512; C. B. Liden *et al.*, *ibid.*, 513; P. V. Lvisada and B. I. Brown, *Clin. Toxicol.*, 1976, *9,* 539, per *Int. pharm. Abstr.*, 1977, *14,* 420; A. Chari-Bitron, *J. Pharm. Pharmac.*, 1977, *29,* 55; R. T. Rappolt *et al.*, *J. Am. Coll. emergency Physns*, 1979, *8,* 68.

See also reviews on abuse (above).

Uses. Phencyclidine is related chemically to ketamine (p.750) and is a potent analgesic and anaesthetic. It was formerly given intravenously to produce an amnesic trance-like state, with analgesia, but severe adverse effects, especially postoperative psychoses, precluded its use. It was formerly used in veterinary medicine as an immobilising agent and is widely used in the USA as a hallucinogenic drug of abuse (see above).

13101-y

Phenolphthalol. 2-(4,4′-Dihydroxybenzhydryl)benzyl alcohol.

$C_{20}H_{18}O_3=306.4$.

CAS — 81-92-5.

Phenolphthalol has been used as a purgative.

Proprietary Names

Gentiapol *(Pohl, Ger.)*; Normolax *(Biagini, Ital.)*; Regolax *(Corvi, Ital.)*.

15300-y

Phenylhydrazine Hydrochloride *(B.P.C. 1949).*

$C_6H_5.NH.NH_2,HCl=144.6$.

CAS — 100-63-0 (phenylhydrazine); 59-88-1 (hydrochloride).

A white or slightly coloured crystalline powder, becoming brown on keeping, particularly if exposed to bright light. **Soluble** 1 in 5 of water; soluble in alcohol. **Protect** from light.

Phenylhydrazine has a specific effect in destroying erythrocytes and was formerly used in the treatment of polycythaemia vera but it has been replaced by more effective and less toxic medicaments. Phenylhydrazine may be absorbed from the skin.

Maximum permissible atmospheric concentration of phenylhydrazine 5 ppm.

13103-z

Phenylthiourea. Phenylthiocarbamide; PTC. 1-Phenylthiourea.

$C_7H_8N_2S=152.2$.

CAS — 103-85-5.

NOTE. The abbreviation PTC has also been applied to Factor IX, a blood-clotting factor.

Sensitivity to the bitter taste of phenylthiourea has been found to be genetically determined; weak solutions (about 1 in 100 000) usually taste bitter to 3 of 4 persons in the population. The possibility that some individuals or groups are predisposed genetically to certain diseases has been investigated by correlation of the occurrence of disease with taste sensitivity to phenylthiourea.

For a review of taste sensitivity with reference to the role of phenylthiourea, see *Chemist Drugg.*, 1972, *197,* 390.

References: H. Harris and H. Kalmus, *Ann. Eugen.*, 1949, *15,* 24; G. R. Fraser, *Lancet*, 1961, *1,* 964; N. Freire-Maia *et al.* (letter), *ibid.*, 1967, *1,* 576; F. W. Clements *et al.*, *Bull. Wld Hlth Org.*, 1968, *38,* 297; K. T. Veselý *et al.*, *Gut*, 1968, *9,* 57; H. J. McDonald (letter), *New Engl. J. Med.*, 1979, *300,* 1224.

13104-c

Phloroglucinol. Phloroglucin. Benzene-1,3,5-triol.
$C_6H_6O_3$=126.1.

CAS — 108-73-6.

White crystals with a sweet taste. M.p. about 218°. **Soluble** 1 in 100 of water and 1 in 10 of alcohol; soluble in ether. **Protect** from light.

Phloroglucinol is an antispasmodic and has been given for the relief of smooth muscle spasm. Trimethylphloroglucinol has also been used.

Proprietary Names
Dilospan S *(Nippon Roussel, Jap.)*; Spasfon-Lyoc *(Lafon, Fr.)*.

13105-k

Phosgene. Carbonyl Chloride; Chloroformyl Chloride.
$COCl_2$=98.92.

CAS — 75-44-5.

A colourless volatile liquid or a colourless gas with a slight odour of new-mown hay. B.p. about 8°. The gas is heavier than air.

Adverse Effects. Poisoning may occur from industrial use or from the generation of phosgene from chlorinated compounds such as chloroform or carbon tetrachloride in the presence of heat. Symptoms of poisoning, which may be delayed for up to 24 hours, include burning of the eyes and throat, cough, dyspnoea, cyanosis, and pulmonary congestion and oedema. Exposure to 50 ppm may be rapidly fatal. Massive exposure may cause intravascular haemolysis, thrombus formation, and immediate death. Maximum permissible atmospheric concentration 0.1 ppm.

Treatment of Adverse Effects. After inhalation of phosgene or absorption from the skin, treatment consists of complete rest and the administration of oxygen. The mouth, eyes, nose, and skin should be irrigated with water; a 1% solution of sodium bicarbonate has also been advocated. Corticosteroids may reduce tissue damage. Further treatment is symptomatic.

Uses. Phosgene is used in the chemical industry. It was formerly used as a war gas.

13106-a

Phosphorus. Yellow Phosphorus; Fósforo.
P=30.97376.

CAS — 7723-14-0.

Pharmacopoeias. In *Port.* and *Span.*

Translucent, colourless or pale yellow, wax-like sticks. M.p. 44°, igniting at a slightly higher temperature. Practically **insoluble** in water; soluble 1 in 320 of dehydrated alcohol, 1 in 25 of chloroform, 1 in 80 of ether, 1 in 100 each of oleic acid, suet, and oils of almond, olive, castor, and theobroma, and 1 in 0.5 of carbon disulphide. It is unstable in air and should be **stored** under water.

WARNING. *The Council of the Pharmaceutical Society of Great Britain advises pharmacists not to supply materials likely to be used for making fireworks, including phosphorus, to children under any circumstances, and recommends that it should be sold only to persons who are, or appear to be, 18 years of age or over.*

Adverse Effects. Symptoms of acute poisoning by phosphorus, a general protoplasmic poison, may include an odour of garlic in the breath, burning pain in the abdomen, intense thirst, nausea, vomiting, profuse diarrhoea, renal disorders, hypoprothrombinaemia and haemorrhage, delirium, convulsions, and coma. After a period usually of between 1 and 2 days there may be a remission of symptoms followed by jaundice, hepatic failure, peripheral circulatory collapse, prostration, coma, and death.

The fatal dose is about 100 mg, though it may be as low as 50 mg; a dose of 15 mg may be severely toxic.

Symptoms of chronic poisoning are very slow in onset and are associated with lowered resistance to infection and defective tissue repair. They include periostitis and necrosis of the upper and lower jaw ('phossy jaw').

Externally, phosphorus causes severe burns to the skin.

Maximum permissible atmospheric concentration 100 µg per m^3.

Three cases of acute phosphorus poisoning in children after accidental ingestion of unknown amounts of rat poisons. Two children (aged 2 and 3 years) died 5 hours after ingestion; both had a cardiopulmonary arrest and passed 'smoking' stools. One child aged 7 years recovered within 3 days. Gastric lavage (using physiological saline and liquid paraffin or potassium permanganate) was performed in 2 children including 1 who died.— F. A. Simon and L. K. Pickering, *J. Am. med. Ass.*, 1976, *235*, 1343.

Haemolytic anaemia. For a reference to 3 cases of haemolytic anaemia following phosphorus burn injuries, see J. V. Dacie and S. M. Worrledge, *Prog. Hemat.*, 1969, *6*, 82, per M. Swanson, *Drug Intell. & clin. Pharm.*, 1973, *7*, 6.

Treatment of Adverse Effects. After ingestion of phosphorus the stomach should be washed out with copious amounts of water; a 1 in 5000 solution of potassium permanganate (very pale pink) or a 1 in 1000 solution of copper sulphate have also been advocated.

Give alkaline drinks and dextrose, but *not* animal or vegetable oils and fats or white of egg. Solutions of dextrose should be given intravenously to correct dehydration and the circulation should be maintained by intravenous infusions of plasma or of suitable electrolyte solutions.

Treat for liver damage with a high-carbohydrate diet. Phytomenadione should be given intravenously and repeated according to the prothrombin time. Injections of hydrocortisone have been suggested for severe liver failure; exchange blood transfusions have also been suggested. Peritoneal dialysis or haemodialysis may be required for renal failure. Treat burns by irrigation with water and then large quantities of a 1% copper sulphate solution; sodium bicarbonate solution has also been used.

Phosphorus particles from flares and rockets in Vietnam were removed from wounds as soon as possible. Copper sulphate solution was applied to the burning phosphorus, washed away with saline, and sodium perborate was then applied to prevent copper poisoning.— E. J. Jones *et al.*, *Archs Surg., Chicago*, 1968, *97*, 1, per *Can. med. Ass. J.*, 1968, *99* (Nov. 23), 10.

Uses. Phosphorus is no longer used in medicine. Inorganic phosphates are given in deficiency states and bone diseases. Phosphorus has been used in the manufacture of rat poisons.

It is used in homoeopathic medicine.

Phosphorus in a 1 to 2% paste had been used as a cockroach poison and rodenticide. Because of the risk of fire, phosphorus should never be mixed with bait but should be mixed with substances containing liquids, such as molasses, fat, or water. However, it was recommended that phosphorus should no longer be used on account of its toxicity; 15 mg could be severely toxic and 50 mg fatal. Other more effective rodenticides were available.— Safe Use of Pesticides, Twentieth Report of the WHO Expert Committee on Insecticides, *Tech. Rep. Ser. Wld Hlth Org. No. 513*, 1973.

13107-t

***o*-Phthaldialdehyde.** Phthalaldehyde.
$C_8H_6O_2$=134.1.

CAS — 643-79-8.

A 5% solution of *o*-phthaldialdehyde in xylene has been used to locate functioning sweat glands. It is applied to the skin and after 10 minutes functioning sweat-gland orifices appear as black dots.

References: L. Juhlin and H. Hansson, *Archs Derm.*, 1968, *97*, 327.

13108-x

Phthalofyne. Methylpentynol Phthalate; Methylparafynol Phthalate; Methylpentynyl Phthalate. 3-Methylpent-1-yn-3-yl hydrogen phthalate.
$C_{14}H_{14}O_4$=246.3.

CAS — 131-67-9.

Phthalofyne is a veterinary anthelmintic used in whipworm infection.

13109-r

Physalis. Alkekengi; Bladder Cherry; Chinese Lantern; Ground Cherry; Strawberry Tomato; Winter Cherry.

The berries of *Physalis alkekengi* (Solanaceae), reputed to have diuretic properties.

Cape gooseberry is the edible fruit of *P. peruviana.*

13110-j

Phytohaemagglutinin. Phytohemagglutin; PHA.

CAS — 9008-97-3.

Phytohaemagglutinin is one of a group of proteins termed lectins that are reported to agglutinate cells by binding to specific carbohydrate residues. It is a complex mucoprotein extract from the seeds of the bean, *Phaseolus vulgaris*, and certain other plants. It consists of at least 3 factors which, respectively, cause haemagglutination, serum-protein precipitation, and the stimulation of mitosis in white blood cells and has been found to stimulate the production of an interferon-like substance by human leucocytes *in vitro.* The blastogenic response of lymphocytes to phytohaemagglutinin has been used extensively as a measure of immunocompetence and may be of value in detecting and monitoring malignant disease.

It has been tried in the treatment of aplastic anaemia but results have been equivocal.

Intradermal tests with 1 and 10 µg of phytohaemagglutinin in physiological saline produced strong positive reactions with erythema, induration, and local heat in 11 patients with defective immune mechanisms due to chronic lymphocytic leukaemia, and in 38 healthy controls.— R. Ariò *et al.*, *Lancet*, 1967, *1*, 899. A finding of cancer-specific changes in lymphocytes after stimulation with phytohaemagglutinin.— J. A. V. Pritchard *et al.*, *ibid.*, 1978, *2*, 1275.

In an evaluation of phytohaemagglutinin as a diagnostic agent for sarcoidosis both the 6 control subjects and the 16 patients with sarcoidosis developed local reactions within 48 hours of an intradermal injection of 2 or 10 µg. However, the *in vitro* lymphocyte response to phytohaemagglutinin was lower in the patients with sarcoidosis than in the control subjects.— R. J. Bonforte *et al.* (letter), *Lancet*, 1972, *1*, 958.

Detection of toxic phytohaemagglutinins in immature legume seeds and their effect on *rats*.— F. I. Ikegwuonu and O. Bassir, *Toxic. appl. Pharmac.*, 1977, *40*, 217.

Further references: W. J. Byrd *et al.*, *Lancet*, 1964, *2*, 420; E. F. Wheelock, *Science*, 1965, *149*, 310; R. Edelman and E. F. Wheelock, *ibid.*, 1966, *154*, 1053; M. W. Elves *et al.*, *Acta haemat.*, 1967, *37*, 100, per *Abstr. Wld Med.*, 1967, *41*, 491; J. W. Thomas *et al.*, *Can. med. Ass. J.*, 1967, *97*, 832 and 836; G. Astaldi *et al.* (letter), *Lancet*, 1968, *2*, 172; M. J. Simons *et al.*, *Nature*, 1968, *219*, 1021; I. Scherwenke, *Planta med.*, 1971, *20*, 320, per *Int. pharm. Abstr.*, 1973, *10*, 299; R. J. Bonforte *et al.*, *J. Pediat.*, 1972, *81*, 775, per *Int. pharm. Abstr.*, 1973, *10*, 285; W. H. Marshall *et al.*, *Can. med. Ass. J.*, 1977, *116*, 1257; P. Rouge *et al.*, *Annls pharm. fr.*, 1978, *36*, 143.

13111-z

Phytolacca *(B.P.C. 1934)*. Poke Root.

Pharmacopoeias. In *Chin.*

The dried root of the poke plant, *Phytolacca americana* (= *P. decandra*) (Phytolaccaceae).

Phytolacca has emetic, purgative, and mildly narcotic properties. It is sometimes found as an adulterant of belladonna root. The powdered drug is powerfully sternutatory.

Children and adults who had ingested berries of *P. americana* (poke-berries) or brought them into contact with skin abrasions developed plasmacytosis and mitotic changes in peripheral blood cells.— B. E. Barker *et al.* (letter), *New Engl. J. Med.*, 1966, *275*, 965.

Report of haematological abnormalities in 9 patients after exposure to poke berries.— B. E. Barker *et al.* (letter), *Lancet*, 1967, *1*, 437.

A report of poisoning in a 43-year-old woman who drank a cup of herbal tea made from powdered phytolacca.— W. H. Lewis and P. R. Smith (letter), *J. Am. med. Ass.*, 1979, *242*, 2759.

13112-c

Picadex *(B. Vet. C. 1965)*. Piperazine Carbon Disulphide Complex. A polymer of the equimolecular complex of piperazine and carbon disulphide.

$(C_5H_{10}N_2S_2)_n$=162.3×*n*.

CAS — 99-00-3 ($C_5H_{10}N_2S_2$).

A pale yellow almost odourless crystalline powder. Very slightly **soluble** in water and organic solvents. **Protect** from light.

Picadex is an anthelmintic which has been used in veterinary medicine.

13113-k

Picobenzide. M-14012-4. 3,5-Dimethyl-*N*-(4-pyridylmethyl)benzamide.

$C_{15}H_{16}N_2O$=240.3.

CAS — 51832-87-2.

Picobenzide is reported to have neuroleptic activity.

Pharmacokinetics in *animals*.— P. D. García de Jalón *et al.*, *Arzneimittel-Forsch.*, 1979, *29*, 1704.

Manufacturers

Made, Spain.

13114-a

Picodralazine. Picodralazinum. [4-(4-Pyridylmethyl)phthalazin-1-yl]hydrazine.

$C_{14}H_{13}N_5$=251.3.

CAS — 17692-43-2.

Picodralazine is a peripheral vasodilator which has been used in the treatment of hypertension.

13115-t

Pifarnine. U-27. 1-Piperonyl-4-(3,7,11-trimethyldodeca-2,6,10-trienyl)piperazine.

$C_{27}H_{40}N_2O_2$=424.6.

CAS — 56208-01-6.

Pifarnine has been used in the treatment of peptic ulcer.

References: A. Bianchetti *et al.*, *Arzneimittel-Forsch.*, 1975, *25*, 580; A. Porro *et al.*, *Farmaco, Edn prat.*, 1979, *34*, 85; M. Petrillo *et al.*, *Curr. ther. Res.*, 1979, *25*, 457.

Proprietary Names

Pifazin *(Pierrel, Ital.)*.

13116-x

Pimeclone Hydrochloride. Spiractin. 2-Piperidinomethylcyclohexanone hydrochloride.

$C_{12}H_{21}NO,HCl$=231.8.

CAS — 534-84-9 (pimeclone); 6966-09-2 (hydrochloride).

Pimeclone has respiratory stimulant properties similar to those of lobeline.

References: H. Barrie *et al.*, *Lancet*, 1962, *2*, 742.

13117-r

Pimefylline Nicotinate. 7-[2-(3-Pyridylmethylamino)ethyl]theophylline pyridine-3-carboxylate.

$C_{15}H_{18}N_6O_2$=314.3.

CAS — 10001-43-1 (pimefylline); 10058-07-8 (nicotinate).

Pimefylline nicotinate has been used in the treatment of cardiovascular disorders.

Proprietary Names

Teonicon *(Neopharmed, Ital.)*.

13118-f

Pimethixene. BP-400. 9-(1-Methyl-4-piperidylidene)thioxanthene.

$C_{19}H_{19}NS$=293.4.

CAS — 314-03-4.

Pimethixene is reported to have antihistaminic and sedative properties and to be an inhibitor of serotonin. It has been used in the treatment of respiratory disorders in children.

References: F. Grover, *Ann. Allergy*, 1963, *21*, 233, per *Am. J. Hosp. Pharm.*, 1963, *20*, 592.

Proprietary Names

Calmixène *(Sandoz, Fr.)*; Muricalm *(Wander, Belg.)*; Sedosil *(Cooper, Switz.)*.

13119-d

Pinaverium Bromide. 4-(6-Bromoveratryl)-4-{2-[2-(10-norpinan-2-yl)ethoxy]ethyl}morpholinium bromide.

$C_{26}H_{41}Br_2NO_4$=591.4.

CAS — 59995-65-2 (pinaverium); 53251-94-8 (bromide).

Pinaverium bromide is used as an antispasmodic agent in the treatment of gastro-intestinal disorders.

Proprietary Names

Dicetel *(Charton, Canad.; Latéma, Fr.)*.

13120-c

Pipacycline. N^2-[4-(2-Hydroxyethyl)piperazin-1-ylmethyl]tetracycline.

$C_{29}H_{38}N_4O_9$=586.6.

CAS — 1110-80-1.

Pipacycline is an antibiotic with a spectrum of activity similar to that of tetracycline.

Proprietary Names

Boniciclina *(Boniscontro & Gazzone, Ital.)*; Sieromicin *(Sierochimica, Ital.)*; Valtomicina (guaiacolglycolate) *(Midy, Ital.)*.

13121-k

Piperazine Camsylate. Piperazine di(camphor-10-sulphonate).

$C_4H_{10}N_2,(C_{10}H_{16}O_4S)_2$=550.7.

CAS — 27016-31-5.

Piperazine camsylate has been used for its reputed stimulant effect on the cardiovascular and respiratory systems.

Proprietary Names

Solucamphre *(Delalande, Fr.; Delalande, Switz.)*.

13122-a

Piperazinedione. 593A; NSC-135758. 3,6-Bis(5-chloro-2-piperidyl)piperazine-2,5-dione dihydrochloride.

$C_{14}H_{22}Cl_2N_4O_2,2HCl$=422.2.

CAS — 41109-80-2.

Piperazinedione is reported to have antineoplastic activity

References: C. A. Presant and C. Klahr, *Cancer*, 1977, *40*, 1386; M. W. Pasmantier *et al.*, *Cancer Treat. Rep.*, 1977, *61*, 1731; V. Currie *et al.*, *ibid.*, 1979, *63*, 73; K. A. Dicke *et al.*, *Lancet*, 1979, *1*, 514.

Manufacturers

Merck Sharp & Dohme, USA.

13123-t

Pipethanate Ethobromide. Ethylpipethanate Bromide. 1-(2-Benziloyloxyethyl)-1-ethylpiperidinium bromide.

$C_{23}H_{30}BrNO_3$=448.4.

CAS — 4546-39-8 (pipethanate); 23182-46-9 (ethobromide).

A crystalline powder with a bitter taste. M.p. about 219°. Slightly **soluble** in water and alcohol; soluble in methyl alcohol; practically insoluble in ether.

Pipethanate ethobromide is an anticholinergic agent which has been used for relieving spasm of the gastro intestinal and urinary tracts.

Proprietary Names

Panpurol *(Nippon Shinyaku, Jap.)*.

13124-x

Piracetam. CI-871; UCB-6215; Pyrrolidone Acetamide. 2-(2-Oxopyrrolidin-1-yl)acetamide.

$C_6H_{10}N_2O_2$=142.2.

CAS — 7491-74-9.

A white almost odourless crystalline powder with a slightly bitter taste. M.p. about 152°. **Soluble** 1 in 4 of water; slightly soluble in alcohol; practically insoluble in acetone.

Piracetam acts on the central nervous system and has been described as a cerebral stimulant although its mode of action is not certain. It is said to protect the cerebral cortex against hypoxia and has been used following trauma or surgery and in a variety of disorders including alcoholism, vertigo, senile dementia, cerebrovascular accidents, and behavioural disorders in children. Piracetam has been given by mouth in doses of 800 mg thrice daily. In severe disorders it has been given by intramuscular or intravenous injection.

Piracetam has also been tried in the treatment of sickle-cell anaemia.

A report of basic toxicological studies on piracetam.— M. Giurgea, *Farmaco, Edn prat.*, 1977, *32*, 47.

After administration by mouth to 6 fasting subjects, piracetam 800 mg gave peak plasma concentrations of about 15 to 19 µg per ml in about 30 minutes and declined with a half-life of about 5 to 6 hours. Elimination after intravenous injection was similar. Piracetam was mainly excreted unchanged in the urine.— J. G. Gobert and E. L. Baltès, *Farmaco, Edn prat.*, 1977, *32*, 83.

Effects on the blood. *Sickle-cell anaemia.* A report of piracetam inhibiting and reversing sickling *in vitro* and producing beneficial effects in 12 patients. The dose in a crisis was 80 mg per kg body-weight in 300 ml of dextrose injection infused every 8 hours for 3 days. Maintenance was with 1 g intramuscularly daily for 6 months then 1.2 g every 8 hours by mouth. Maintenance in children was with 600 mg thrice daily by mouth.— J. T. de Araujo and G. S. Nero (letter), *Lancet*, 1977, *2*, 411. A report of *animal* studies casting doubt on any beneficial effect of piracetam in sickle-cell anaemia.— F. F. Costa *et al.* (letter), *ibid.*, 1979, *2*, 1302. Studies *in vitro* suggesting that piracetam has a non-specific antisickling effect.— I. M. Franklin (letter), *ibid.*, 1980, *1*, 767.

Further references: G. O. S. de Melo, *Lancet*, 1976, *2*,

1139; R. M. Nalbandian *et al.* (letter), *ibid.*, 1978, *2*, 570.

Thrombosis. A study in 10 healthy subjects suggests that piracetam is an effective antiplatelet agent, and deserves clinical study as an antithrombotic (platelet-inhibiting) agent.— R. L. Bick (letter), *Lancet*, 1979, *2*, 752.

Neurological disorders. The general mental condition of 40 of 98 elderly patients with psycho-organic symptoms given piracetam 800 mg thrice daily for 8 weeks was improved compared with 24 of 98 patients given placebo.— A. J. Stegink, *Arzneimittel-Forsch.*, 1972, *22*, 975. In patients with reversible encephalopathic psychosyndromes combined with depression or paranoid syndrome piracetam aided restoration of memory, vigilance, lucidity, and differentiation. In latent psychotic conditions it provoked reactions and thus aided diagnosis.— A. Voelkel, *ibid.*, 1974, *24*, 1127. In 78 elderly patients with psycho-organic symptoms treatment with piracetam 4.8 g daily by mouth for 6 weeks was significantly more effective than a placebo whereas there was no significant difference between piracetam 2.4 g daily and a placebo.— J. H. Kretschmar and C. Kretschmar, *ibid.*, 1976, *26*, 1158. A report of the use of piracetam in association with choline in the treatment of patients with senile dementia of the Alzheimer's type.— E. Friedman *et al.* (letter), *New Engl. J. Med.*, 1981, *304*, 1490.

Piracetam 10 g daily was well accepted in a controlled study of 100 patients and was considered to improve the level of consciousness postoperatively.— A. E. Richardson and F. J. Bereen (preliminary communication), *Lancet*, 1977, *2*, 1110. Findings suggesting that piracetam appears to exert a beneficial effect on recovery of consciousness in patients with brain impairment following trauma or neurosurgery.— R. B. Carrington da Costa *et al.*, *Acta ther.*, 1978, *4*, 109.

In a double-blind study in 60 chronic alcoholic patients piracetam 1.6 g thrice daily was as effective as chlormethiazole, 2.7 g daily initially reducing to 0.6 g daily after 1 week, in the relief of withdrawal symptoms. The incidence of side-effects was similar for both drugs.— S. J. Dencker *et al.*, *J. int. med. Res.*, 1978, *6*, 395. See also N. S. Marks, *Acta ther.*, 1977, *3*, 181; J. G. Meyer *et al.*, *Dt. med. Wschr.*, 1979, *104*, 911.

In a double-blind crossover study of 16 epileptic patients with learning difficulties, aged between 8 and 20 years, treatment with piracetam 1.2 to 2.4 g daily in divided doses, depending on body-weight, resulted in significant improvements in alertness, some aspects of visual perception, and achievement at school. The patients recovered more rapidly and were less confused following seizures.— P. S. Kunneke and G. M. Malan, *Br. J. clin. Pract.*, 1979, *33*, 266.

Further references: J. Pogady *et al.*, *Acta ther.*, 1977, *3*, 217 (nocturnal enuresis); D. Bente *et al.*, *Arzneimittel-Forsch.*, 1978, *28*, 1529 (elderly psychiatric patients); L. Gustafson *et al.*, *Psychopharmacology*, 1978, *56*, 115 (dementia); N. G. Maritz *et al.*, *S. Afr. med. J.*, 1978, *53*, 889 (cerebral palsy); S. Lloyd-Evans *et al.*, *Curr. med. Res. Opinion*, 1979, *6*, 351 (chronic brain failure).

Proprietary Names
Cerebropan *(ISM, Ital.)*; Ciclocetam *(Callol, Spain)*; Ciclofalina *(Almirall, Spain)*; Encefalux *(Geve, Spain)*; Genogris *(Vita, Spain)*; Gericetam *(Level, Spain)*; Huberdasen *(Hubber, Spain)*; Idéaxan *(Millot-Solac, Fr.)*; Merapiran *(Finadiet, Arg.)*; Noostan *(Rhodia, Arg.)*; Nootrop *(UCB, Ger.)*; Noo-Tropicon *(Sidus, Arg.)*; Nootropil *(UCB, Belg.; UCB, Ital.; UCB, Neth.; UCB, S.Afr.; UCB-Pevya, Spain; UCB, Switz.)*; Nootropyl *(UCB, Fr.)*; Normabrain *(Cassella-Riedel, Ger.)*; Pirroxil *(SIT, Ital.)*; Stimucortex *(Kali-Farma, Spain)*; Tonibral *(Bagó, Arg.)*.

13125-r

Pirandamine Hydrochloride.
AY-23713. *NN*-Dimethyl-2-(1,3,4,9-tetrahydro-1-methylindeno[2,1-*c*]pyran-1-yl)ethylamine hydrochloride.
$C_{17}H_{23}NO,HCl=293.8$.

CAS — 42408-79-7 (pirandamine); 42408-78-6 (hydrochloride).

Pirandamine hydrochloride is a tricyclic antidepressant.

Manufacturers
Ayerst, USA.

13126-f

Pirazolac.
ZK-76604. 4-(4-Chlorophenyl)-1-(4-fluorophenyl)pyrazol-3-ylacetic acid.
$C_{17}H_{12}ClFN_2O_2=330.7$.

CAS — 71002-09-0.

Pirazolac is reported to have antirheumatic activity.

Manufacturers
Schering, Ger.

13127-d

Pirbuterol Hydrochloride.
Pyrbuterol Hydrochloride; CP-24314-1. 2-*tert*-Butylamino-1-(5-hydroxy-6-hydroxymethyl-2-pyridyl)ethanol dihydrochloride.
$C_{12}H_{20}N_2O_3,2HCl=313.2$.

CAS — 38677-81-5 (pirbuterol); 38029-10-6 (hydrochloride).

Pirbuterol hydrochloride is a sympathomimetic compound being studied for its effects as a bronchodilator in asthma. Pirbuterol acetate has also been studied.

Studies of the effects of pirbuterol given by mouth.— S. N. Steen *et al.*, *Curr. ther. Res.*, 1974, *16*, 1077; R. F. Willey *et al.*, *Br. J. clin. Pharmac.*, 1976, *3*, 595; I. C. Paterson *et al.* (letter), *ibid.*, 1977, *4*, 376; N. K. Burk and L. Diamond, *Clin. Pharmac. Ther.*, 1978, *24*, 84; T. J. Ence *et al.*, *Ann. Allergy*, 1979, *43*, 229; B. A. Votteri and L. Melcher, *ibid.*, 348; H. Poppius *et al.*, *Eur. J. clin. Pharmac.*, 1979, *15*, 389; H. M. Beumer, *Int. J. clin. Pharmac. Biopharm.*, 1979, *17*, 18; M. L. Brandon, *Ann. Allergy*, 1980, *45*, 8; A. J. Dyson and A. D. MacKay, *Br. J. Dis. Chest*, 1980, *74*, 70.

Use of pirbuterol by inhalation.— H. M. Beumer, *Int. J. clin. Pharmac. Biopharm.*, 1979, *17*, 237.

Studies of the haemodynamic effects of pirbuterol in patients with heart failure.— N. A. Awan *et al.*, *Am. J. Cardiol.*, 1981, *47*, 665; J. R. Dawson *et al.*, *Br. med. J.*, 1981, *282*, 1423; W. S. Colucci *et al.*, *New Engl. J. Med.*, 1981, *305*, 185.

Manufacturers
Pfizer, USA.

13128-n

Pirenperone.
R-47465. 3-{2-[4-(4-Fluorobenzoyl)piperidino]ethyl}-2-methyl-4*H*-pyrido[1,2-*a*]-pyrimidin-4-one.
$C_{23}H_{24}FN_3O_2=393.5$.

CAS — 75444-65-4.

Pirenperone is reported to have psychotropic activity.

Manufacturers
Janssen, Belg.

13129-h

Pirenzepine Hydrochloride.
LS-519 (pirenzepine); LS-519-CL-2 (hydrochloride). 5,11-Dihydro-11-(4-methylpiperazin-1-ylacetyl)pyrido-[2,3-*b*][1,4]benzodiazepin-6-one dihydrochloride.
$C_{19}H_{21}N_5O_2,2HCl=424.3$.

CAS — 28797-61-7 (pirenzepine); 29868-97-1 (hydrochloride).

Pirenzepine hydrochloride is reported to inhibit gastric secretion with minimal systemic anticholinergic effects. It has been used in the treatment of hyperacidity and peptic ulcer.

For a series of papers on pirenzepine, see *Scand. J. Gastroenterol.*, 1979, *14*, *Suppl.* 57.

Further references: M. Giger *et al.*, *Schweiz. med. Wschr.*, 1979, *109*, 617; G. Stacher *et al.*, *Int. J. clin. Pharmac. Biopharm.*, 1979, *17*, 442; R. Stockbrügger *et al.*, *Scand. J. Gastroenterol.*, 1979, *14*, 615; B. H. Jaup *et al.*, *ibid.*, 621; W. Londong *et al.*, *Gut*, 1980, *21*, A451; M. Guslandi *et al.*, *Curr. ther. Res.*, 1980, *27*, 714; S. Čerlek *et al.*, *J. int. med. Res.*, 1981, *9*, 148; W. Londong *et al.*, *Gut*, 1981, *22*, 542.

Proprietary Names
Gastrozepin *(Bender, Aust.; Thomae, Ger.; Boehringer Ingelheim, Ital.; Boehringer Sohn, Switz.)*; Leblon *(De Angeli, Ital.)*; Ulcosan *(Dompè, Ital.)*; Gastrozepina.

13130-a

Piretanide.
Hoe-118; S-734118. 4-Phenoxy-3-(pyrrolidin-1-yl)-5-sulphamoylbenzoic acid.
$C_{17}H_{18}N_2O_5S=362.4$.

CAS — 55837-27-9.

Piretanide is a loop diuretic with effects generally comparable with those of frusemide.

Comparison with frusemide.— C. J. C. Roberts *et al.*, *Br. J. clin. Pharmac.*, 1978, *6*, 129; J. R. Lawrence *et al.*, *Clin. Pharmac. Ther.*, 1978, *23*, 558; H. Valette *et al.* (letter), *Br. J. clin. Pharmac.*, 1979, *7*, 219; C. Marone and F. C. Reubi, *Eur. J. clin. Pharmac.*, 1980, *17*, 165; W. P. Leary *et al.*, *Curr. ther. Res.*, 1981, *29*, 249; A. J. Reyes *et al.*, *ibid.*, 253.

Comparison with bumetanide.— M. Homeida *et al.*, *Br. J. clin. Pharmac.*, 1979, *8*, 173.

Use in cirrhosis with ascites.— V. Arroyo *et al.*, *Gut*, 1980, *21*, 855.

Use of high doses of piretanide in renal failure.— A. Hadj Aissa *et al.*, *Br. J. clin. Pharmac.*, 1981, *11*, 63.

Further references: H. Valette and E. Apoil (letter), *Br. J. clin. Pharmac.*, 1979, *8*, 592; P. Teredesai and J. B. Puschett, *Clin. Pharmac. Ther.*, 1979, *25*, 331; A. Alvestrand and J. Bergström, *Curr. ther. Res.*, 1979, *25*, 786; N. Pozet *et al.*, *Br. J. clin. Pharmac.*, 1980, *9*, 577.

Proprietary Names
Arelix *(Hoechst, Ital.)*.

13131-t

Pirfenoxone Sodium.
Catalin Sodium. Sodium 1-hydroxy-5-oxo-5*H*-pyrido[3,2-*a*]phenoxazine-3-carboxylate.
$C_{16}H_7N_2NaO_5=330.2$.

CAS — 1043-21-6 (pirfenoxone); 51410-30-1 (sodium salt).

Pirfenoxone sodium has been used in the treatment of cataracts, usually as eye-drops.

References: M. Nakagaki and H. Tereda, *J. pharm. Soc. Japan*, 1967, *87*, 817; A. Pirie and R. van Heyningen (letter), *Lancet*, 1974, *2*, 169; H. Maclean *et al.* (letter), *ibid.*, 895.

Proprietary Names
Clarvisan *(Tubi Lux, Ital.; Abello, Spain)*.

13132-x

Pirglutargine.
Arginine Pyroglutamate; Arginine Pidolate. L-Arginine DL-pyroglutamate.
$C_{11}H_{21}N_5O_5=303.3$.

CAS — 64855-91-0.

Pirglutargine has been used for its reputed cerebral stimulant effect.

Proprietary Names
Adiuvant *(Manetti Roberts, Ital.)*.

13133-r

Piridoxilate.
Pyridoxylate; Pyridoxine α_5-Hemiacetal Glyoxylate. The reciprocal salt of 2-(5-hydroxy-4-hydroxymethyl-6-methyl-3-pyridylmethoxy)glycolic acid with 2-[4,5-bis(hydroxymethyl)-2-methyl-3-pyridyloxy]glycolic acid (1:1).
$C_{10}H_{13}NO_6,C_{10}H_{13}NO_6=486.4$.

CAS — 24340-35-0.

An odourless white or slightly yellow crystalline powder. M.p. about 166°. **Soluble** in water; practically insoluble in alcohol, chloroform, and ether.

Piridoxilate is claimed to increase tissue oxygenation. It has been used in the treatment of circulatory insufficiency, including peripheral, cerebral, and coronary disorders.

Proprietary Names
Glyo-6 *(Houdé-I.S.H., Fr.; Dieckmann, Ger.; Roussel Maestretti, Ital.)*.

13134-f

Pirifibrate. EL-466. 6-Hydroxymethyl-2-pyridylmethyl 2-(4-chlorophenoxy)-2-methylpropionate.
$C_{17}H_{18}ClNO_4$=335.8.

CAS — 55285-45-5.

Pirifibrate has been used to lower cholesterol and triglyceride concentrations in lipid disorders.

References: A. J. Domingo *et al.*, *Clin. Ther.*, 1980, *3*, 219.

Proprietary Names
Bratenol *(Elmu, Spain).*

13135-d

Pirlindole Hydrochloride. 2,3,3a,4,5,6-Hexahydro-8-methyl-1*H*-pyrazino[3,2,1-*jk*]carbazole hydrochloride.
$C_{15}H_{18}N_2$,HCl=262.8.

CAS — 60762-57-4 (pirlindole); 16154-78-2 (hydrochloride).

Pirlindole hydrochloride is reported to have antidepressant activity.

Pharmacology in *animals*.— P. A. Martorana and R. -E. Nitz, *Arzneimittel-Forsch.*, 1979, *29*, 946. See also P. A. Martorana *et al.*, *ibid.*, 950.

Further reference including brief summary of clinical use.— M. D. Mashkovsky and N. I. Andrejeva, *Arzneimittel-Forsch.*, 1981, *31*, 75.

13136-n

Piroheptine Hydrochloride. 3-(10,11-Dihydro-5*H*-dibenzo[*a,d*]cyclohepten-5-ylidene)-1-ethyl-2-methylpyrrolidine hydrochloride.
$C_{22}H_{25}N$,HCl=339.9.

CAS — 16378-21-5 (piroheptine); 16378-22-6 (hydrochloride).

Odourless white or yellowish-white crystals or crystalline powder with a bitter numbing taste. M.p. about 253° with decomposition. Sparingly **soluble** in water; freely soluble in alcohol, chloroform, methyl alcohol, and glacial acetic acid; slightly soluble in acetone; practically insoluble in ether. **Protect** from light.

Piroheptine is structurally related to the tricyclic antidepressants (seep.110) and has been used in the treatment of parkinsonism and drug-induced extrapyramidal symptoms.

Pharmacological studies in *animals*.— M. Hitomi *et al.*, *Arzneimittel-Forsch.*, 1972, *22*, 953; *ibid.*, 961; T. Ohashi, *ibid.*, 966.

Proprietary Names
Trimol *(Fujisawa, Jap.).*

13137-h

Pirquinozol. SQ-13847. 2-(Hydroxymethyl)pyrazolo[1,5-*c*]quinazolin-5(6*H*)-one.
$C_{11}H_9N_3O_2$=215.2.

CAS — 65950-99-4.

Pirquinozol is reported to have anti-allergic activity.

Manufacturers
Squibb, UK.

13138-m

Pivcephalexin Hydrochloride. Pivcefalexin Hydrochloride; ST-21. Pivaloyloxymethyl (7*R*)-3-methyl-7-(α-D-phenylglycylamino)-3-cephem-4-carboxylate hydrochloride.
$C_{22}H_{27}N_3O_6S$,HCl=498.0.

CAS — 27726-31-4.

Pivcephalexin hydrochloride has the general properties of cephalexin, see p.1123.

Proprietary Names
Sigmacef *(Sigmatau, Ital.).*

13139-b

Plafibride. ITA-104. 1-[2-(4-Chlorophenoxy)-2-methylpropionyl]-3-morpholinomethylurea.
$C_{16}H_{22}ClN_3O_4$=355.8.

CAS — 63394-05-8.

Plafibride is reported to inhibit platelet aggregation and to reduce plasma concentrations of lipids.

Proprietary Names
Idonor, Perifunal, Plafibrinol *(all Spain).*

13140-x

Plasminogen

CAS — 9001-91-6.

Plasminogen is the specific substance derived from plasma which, when activated to plasmin by streptokinase, has the property of lysing fibrinogen, fibrin, and some other proteins.

In a double-blind study involving 500 premature infants of birth-weight 1 to 2.5 kg and at risk from hyaline membrane disease, 251 were treated with plasminogen shortly after birth and 249 received placebo. Mild respiratory distress, severe respiratory distress, and deaths occurred in 35, 19, and 6, and 22, 31, and 20 patients in each group respectively. Eleven deaths in the placebo group and 2 deaths in the treated group were attributed to hyaline membrane disease.— C. L. Ambrus *et al.*, *J. Am. med. Ass.*, 1977, *237*, 1837.

For the use of plasminogen with streptokinase in the treatment of deep-vein thrombosis, see Streptokinase, p.657.

13141-r

Plastics

Pharmacopoeias. Fr. includes several monographs on plastics including Polystyrene, Styrene-Butadiene Copolymer, Polyvinyl Chloride (PVC), Polyethylene, and Polypropylene.

Plastic materials used in medicine and pharmacy may give rise to various adverse effects, either by direct contact of the plastic with tissues or by indirect contact as when a solution stored in a plastic container, such as a disposable syringe, is injected. Adverse effects may also arise among workers through handling the materials during manufacture.

Pure plastics appear to be of low toxicity, but some substances added during manufacture to impart specific physical properties are toxic. These additives include plasticisers added to reduce brittleness, ultraviolet-ray absorbers to prevent degradation by light, and antoxidants and lubricants which are sometimes needed for satisfactory processing. These additives leach out from the finished plastic materials and have been the main cause of the adverse effects that have been reported though carcinogenic effects have been produced by prolonged implantation of some pure plastics. The adverse effects produced are diverse, depending upon the nature of the plastic and the toxicity of the additives as well as upon the site and duration of contact; they include haemolysis of blood cells, thrombosis, sensitisation reactions, precancerous changes, and local tissue necrosis.

See also under Vinyl Chloride, p.1769.

The hazards of various additives to plastics.— *Lancet*, 1977, *2*, 19.

An evaluation of the safety of plastics used in medicine, including pure polymers and polymers with additives. At present there was no evidence of toxicity from the use of polvinyl chloride (PVC) plasticised plastics.— W. L. Guess, *Clin. Toxicol.*, 1978, *12*, 77.

Apparatus and containers. Reviews, comments, and studies on plastic containers for pharmaceuticals: J. B. Murray and G. Smith, *Pharm. J.*, 1968, *1*, 88; J. Autian, *Bull. parent. Drug Ass.*, 1968, *22*, 276; *Pharm. J.*, 1971, *2*, 374 (British Pharmacopoeia Commission Committee Report); B. Mueller-Dieckmann, *Pharm. J.*, 1971, *2*, 564; A. M. Beyerlein *et al.*, *J. pharm. Sci.*, 1971, *60*, 1317; WHO Expert Committee on Specifications for Pharmaceutical Preparations, *Tech. Rep. Ser. Wld Hlth Org. No. 614*, 1977; R. C. Shah *et al.*, *Pharm. J.*, 1978, *2*, 58; W. Lund (letter), *ibid.*, 105; *Med. Lett.*, 1980, *22*, 43.

Loss of antibacterial preservatives from contact lens solutions stored in plastic containers.— N. E. Richardson *et al.*, *J. Pharm. Pharmac.*, 1977, *29*, 717. Comment.— H. D. Blackburn *et al.* (letter), *ibid.*, 1978, *30*, 666. For further references to the sorption of preservatives by plastics, see Preservatives, p.1281.

Silicone particles from haemodialysis tubing.— A. S. -Y. Leong *et al.* (letter), *Lancet*, 1981, *2*, 210; J. Bommer and E. Ritz (letter), *ibid.*, 420; A. S. -Y. Leong *et al.*, *New Engl. J. Med.*, 1982, *306*, 135; E. A. Friedman and A. P. Lundin, *ibid.*, 167.

Plasticisers. References to the leaching of the plasticiser bis(2-ethylhexyl) phthalate [di(2-ethylhexyl) phthalate] from polyvinyl chloride containers and apparatus, including blood bags and haemodialysis tubing: T. E. Needham and L. A. Luzzi (letter), *New Engl. J. Med.*, 1973, *289*, 1256; T. D. Darby and R. K. Ausman (letter), *ibid.*, 1974, *290*, 579; T. E. Needham and J. H. Corley (letter), *ibid.*, 1976, *294*, 398; K. Ono *et al.*, *J. Am. med. Ass.*, 1975, *234*, 948; *Lancet*, 1975, *1*, 1172; *Br. med. J.*, 1975, *3*, 262; S. W. Kim *et al.*, *J. pharm. Sci.*, 1976, *65*, 670; M. A. Stenchever *et al.*, *ibid.*, 1648; S. Fayz *et al.*, *J. Pharm. Pharmac.*, 1977, *29*, 407; A. R. Nissenson (letter), *Ann. intern. Med.*, 1977, *87*, 245; T. E. Needham and R. D. Jones (letter), *New Engl. J. Med.*, 1978, *299*, 1472.

See also under Whole Blood, p.322.

Pulmonary haemorrhage and haemolytic anaemia in 2 young men exposed to trimellitic anhydride (TMA), which is used in the manufacture of plasticisers, as a constituent of alkyl resins, and as a curing agent for epoxy resins.— D. Ahmad *et al.*, *Lancet*, 1979, *2*, 328. See also *J. Am. med. Ass.*, 1980, *244*, 1667.

Carcinogenicity. Plastic implants and neoplasms.— R. H. Rigdon, *Sth. med. J.*, 1974, *67*, 1459, per *Int. pharm. Abstr.*, 1976, *13*, 21.

Squamous cell carcinoma of the buccal mucosa associated with chronic exposure to polyvinyl chloride.— C. L. Casterline *et al.*, *Cancer*, 1977, *39*, 1686.

Effects on the respiratory system. A patient suffered more than 40 attacks of polymer-fume fever in 9 months after smoking cigarettes contaminated with the pyrolysis products of polytef (polytetrafluoroethylene; PTFE).— N. Williams and F. K. Smith, *J. Am. med. Ass.*, 1972, *219*, 1587.

Respiratory symptoms, wheezing, shortness of breath, tightness of chest, and coughing occurred in 3 patients after inhalation of fumes generated by cutting polyvinyl chloride plastic film with a hot wire.— W. N. Sokol *et al.*, *J. Am. med. Ass.*, 1973, *226*, 639. Two women engaged in thermocutting polyvinyl chloride paper suffered from similar symptoms.— J. J. Stevens (letter), *J. Am. med. Ass.*, 1974, *227*, 1005. Comments: J. J. Trautlein (letter), *ibid.*; W. B. Buckingham (letter), *ibid.*; W. B. Triplett (letter), *ibid.*; P. M. Papoff (letter), *ibid.*

Symptoms of asthma in a 51-year-old woman with no history of atopy or lung disease were caused by exposure to thermal degradation products of polyethylene (Polythene). The source of exposure was a crimp-film wrapping machine for tins, which cut and crimped Polythene film, using hot metal. Two further patients have been seen with bronchospasm induced by Polythene fumes, and a third with bronchospasm induced by polypropylene, but all 3 had pre-existing bronchospastic disease.— S. Skerfving *et al.* (letter), *Lancet*, 1980, *1*, 211.

Further references: H. Falk and B. Portnoy, *J. Am. med. Ass.*, 1976, *235*, 915; R. H. Andrasch and E. J. Bardana, *ibid.*, 937; R. E. Brubaker, *J. occup. Med.*, 1977, *19*, 693, per *Abstr. Hyg.*, 1978, *53*, 428; D. P. Schlueter *et al.*, *J. occup. Med.*, 1978, *20*, 183, per *Abstr. Hyg.*, 1978, *53*, 597.

See also Plasticisers (above).

Pregnancy and the neonate. Eight phthalate esters, commonly used as plasticisers in containers for blood and parenteral solutions, were injected into pregnant *rats*. Although fertility was unaffected, resorption or death of the foetus, gross foetal abnormalities, skeletal malformation, and decrease in foetal size were observed in some or all of the animals.— A. R. Singh *et al.*, *J. pharm. Sci.*, 1972, *61*, 51.

Prostheses. References to the use of plastic prostheses: R. Bagnall, *Chem. in Br.*, 1978, *14*, 598; C. H. Bamford and A. Ledwith, *ibid.*, *15*, 19.

See also under Polytef, p.1745.

Soft contact lenses. A brief review of contact lenses

manufactured from hydrophilic plastic polymer materials.— *Br. med. J.*, 1976, *1*, 608.

Proprietary Preparations of Some Plastic Support Materials

Baycast *(Bayer, UK)*. A bandage consisting of a cotton fabric coated with a polyurethane polymer which, when wetted by immersion in water, hardens into a rigid cast.

Crystona *(Smith & Hill, UK)*. A splinting material containing a water-soluble polymer and a glass which, when wetted by immersion in water, becomes rigid.

Glassona Bandage *(Smith & Nephew, UK)*. A mixture of glass and cellulose acetate fibres knitted into a stockingette type of material to form a bandage which, when wetted by immersion in acetone, hardens into a rigid cast.

Lightcast II *(3M United Kingdom, UK)*. A range of open-weave fibreglass tapes, impregnated with a photosensitive resin, which become rigid when exposed to u.v. light.

Neofract *(Johnson & Johnson Orthopaedic, UK)*. A two-component splinting material, based on polyurethane, which expands to a foam and then sets hard when the 2 components are mixed together.

Orthoplast *(Johnson & Johnson Orthopaedic, UK)*. A thermoplastic isoprene rubber splinting material; it is warmed by hot water or hot air before being moulded to the patient's requirements.

Plastazote *(Smith & Nephew, UK)*. A polyethylene foam material for preparing orthopaedic supports. It is softened by heating at 140° in a hot air oven and is then moulded, while still warm, to the patient's requirements.

Scotchcast *(3M United Kingdom, UK)*. A knitted fibreglass fabric impregnated with a polyurethane polymer which, when wetted by immersion in water, hardens into a rigid cast.

13143-d

Poly A.poly U

CAS — 24936-38-7.

Poly A.poly U is a double-stranded polyribonucleotide comprising polyadenylic and polyuridylic acids, and is believed to be a stimulant of the immune system. It has been studied in patients with breast cancer who have undergone surgery with or without radiotherapy. Improved survival has been reported.

References: J. Lacour *et al.*, *Lancet*, 1980, *2*, 161.

13144-n

Poly I.poly C. Polyinosinic-polycytidylic Acid.

CAS — 24939-03-5.

Poly I.poly C is a synthetic helical double-stranded polyribonucleotide complex of equimolar concentrations of polyinosinic and polycytidylic acids.

It has been found to induce the production of interferon.

A review of interferons and their inducers.— S. E. Grossberg, *New Engl. J. Med.*, 1972, *287*, 13, 79, and 122.

Unlike interferon, interferon inducers were toxic, producing effects rather like endotoxin, and damaging the *mouse* thymus. They could be used locally because they were apparently little absorbed.— *Lancet*, 1974, *2*, 761. Since a modified poly I.poly C complex [poly I.poly C and poly L-lysine; poly(ICLC)] produced metabolic changes when injected into *rats* it was suggested that treatment with trace metals and nitrogen supplementation may be required during prolonged therapy.— M. C. Powanda *et al.*, *Antimicrob. Ag. Chemother.*, 1977, *12*, 602.

Clinical studies of poly I.poly C or poly(ICLC) in cancer patients: R. A. Robinson *et al.*, *J. natn. Cancer Inst.*, 1976, *57*, 599, per *Int. pharm. Abstr.*, 1977, *14*, 223; A. S. Levine *et al.*, *Cancer Res.*, 1979, *39*, 1645.

The production *in vitro* of interferon through induction by poly I.poly C or by a complex of poly I.poly C and a dextran was enhanced from 10 to 100 times by pretreatment of cells with amphotericin or other polyene macrolides.— E. C. Borden *et al.*, *Antimicrob. Ag. Chemother.*, 1978, *13*, 159. See also *idem*, 1979, *16*, 203.

References to *animal* studies: M. Absher and W. R. Stinebring, *Nature*, 1969, *223*, 715; H. L. Lindsay *et al.*, *ibid.*, 717; R. H. Adamson and S. Fabro, *ibid.*, 718; M. R. Hilleman, *Bull. Wld Hlth Org.*, 1969, *41*, 696; P. Fenje and B. Postic, *J. infect. Dis.*, 1971, *123*, 426, per *Trop. Dis. Bull.*, 1971, *68*, 946; L. Levy and T. C. Merigan, *Antimicrob. Ag. Chemother.*, 1977, *11*, 122; D. A. Stringfellow and S. D. Weed, *ibid.*, 1980, *17*, 988.

Viral infections. An evaluation of poly I.poly C as an interferon inducer in viral respiratory diseases. A small but definite reduction in symptoms of upper respiratory tract illness had been associated with intranasal administration of poly I.poly C.— D. A. Hill *et al.*, *J. Am. med. Ass.*, 1972, *219*, 1179.

In a double-blind study of 24 children with cancer and herpes zoster the topical application to the herpes lesions of poly I.poly C in varying strengths was of no benefit.— S. Feldman *et al.*, *Antimicrob. Ag. Chemother.*, 1975, *8*, 289. See also *idem*, *J. Am. med. Ass.*, 1972, *222*, 624.

A stabilised derivative of poly I.poly C, poly(ICLC), has antiviral activity against hepatitis B virus infection in *chimpanzees*.— R. H. Purcell *et al.*, *Lancet*, 1976, *2*, 757.

Poly I.poly C inhibited strains of herpes simplex virus isolated from patients with herpetic keratitis. Of 50 strains, 44 were inhibited by 0.1 µg or less per ml; the remaining 6 were inhibited by up to 2 µg per ml.— O. Smetana *et al.*, *Antimicrob. Ag. Chemother.*, 1977, *11*, 797.

The successful use of poly I.poly C with a single dose of human diploid rabies vaccine for the protection of rhesus *monkeys* from lethal doses of rabies virus.— G. M. Baer *et al.*, *Bull. Wld Hlth Org.*, 1979, *57*, 807.

13145-h

Polydextrose. CP-31081.

CAS — 68424-04-4.

A randomly bonded glucose polymer, of average molecular weight 1500, with some sorbitol end-groups, and with citric acid residues attached to the polymer by mono- or di-ester bonds.

Polydextrose has potential as a low-energy replacement for sugar and fats in foods.

Manufacturers

Pfizer, USA.

13146-m

Polyhexanide. ICI-9073. Poly(1-hexamethylenebiguanide hydrochloride). $(C_8H_{17}N_5,HCl)_n$=219.7×*n*.

CAS — 28757-48-4.

Polyhexanide is an antibacterial agent which has been used in contact lens solutions and in veterinary preparations.

13147-b

Polyphloretin Phosphate. PPP. A mixture of phosphorylated phloretin polymers.

CAS — 9014-72-6.

Polyphloretin phosphate is an inhibitor of alkaline phosphatase, hyaluronidase, and prostaglandins. It is also reported to reduce the permeability of serous membranes and to diminish serous exudates.

In 15 subjects 3 intradermal injections of 100 µg of polyphloretin phosphate at hourly intervals reduced the erythema produced by 1 µg of alprostadil given intradermally 1 hour after the last dose, but had no effect on the size of the wheal, nor on the erythema or wheal produced by histamine or bradykinin. Polyphloretin phosphate 100 mg intravenously did not affect the erythema or wheal produced by alprostadil, histamine, or bradykinin.— J. Søndergaard and H. P. Jørgensen, *Br. J. Derm.*, 1973, *88*, 51.

Further references to *animal* or in vitro studies: E. Diczfalusy *et al.*, *Acta chem. scand.*, 1953, *7*, 913; B. R. Beitch and K. E. Eakins, *Br. J. Pharmac.*, 1969, *37*, 158; K. E. Eakins *et al.*, *ibid.*, 1970, *39*, 556; A. A. Mathé *et al.* (letter), *Nature New Biol.*, 1971, *230*, 215; R. Villanueva *et al.*, *Fedn Proc.*, 1971, *30*, 626; R. A. Bethel and K. E. Eakins, *ibid.*; A. A. Mathé *et al.*, *J. Pharm. Pharmac.*, 1972, *24*, 378.

13148-v

Polyphloroglucinol Phosphate. Poly[benzene-1,3,5-triol mono(dihydrogen phosphate)]. $(C_6H_7O_6P)_n$=206.1×*n*.

CAS — 68922-92-9 (polyphloroglucinol); 9014-68-0 (phosphate).

Polyphloroglucinol phosphate has an inhibitory effect on hyaluronidase and phosphatases and has been used as a 1% cream in the treatment of eczema.

Proprietary Names

Dealyd B *(Leo, Swed.)*.

13149-g

Polyricinate *(B. Vet. C. 1965)*. A condensate of castor oil fatty acids and ethylene oxide.

A golden-brown to reddish-brown, clear, moderately viscous liquid with a faint odour. It readily forms emulsions on dilution with water. Slightly **soluble** in water; miscible with alcohol and other organic solvents.

Polyricinate is an antifrothing agent which has been used in veterinary medicine for the treatment of frothy bloat in ruminants.

13150-f

Polytef. Politef. Poly(tetrafluoroethylene). $(C_2F_4)_n$.

CAS — 9002-84-0.

Polytef has numerous industrial applications. As 'Teflon' it is used on 'non-stick' cooking utensils.

A paste of polytef has been used in the treatment of aphonia.

References to use in aphonia: *Br. med. J.*, 1980, *281*, 1615.

Prostheses. Polytetrafluoroethylene (PTFE) for replacement grafts in vascular surgery: H. C. Stansel *et al.*, *Archs Surg.*, 1979, *114*, 1291; G. D. Vaughan *et al.*, *J. Trauma*, 1979, *19*, 403.

See also under Plastics, p.1744.

Proprietary Preparations

Polytef Paste for Injection *(Ethicon, UK)*. A sterile paste containing 50% of modified poly(tetrafluoroethylene) in glycerol and polysorbate 20. For injection into the vocal cords in aphonia.

13151-d

Porcine Skin

Sterile denatured lyophilised skin, of porcine origin, consisting of the dermal and/or epidermal layers.

Porcine skin is used as a temporary dressing in burns, ulcers, and other injuries associated with skin loss. The rationale is to prevent fluid and heat loss, to reduce infection, to protect exposed structures, to reduce pain, and to prepare the site for grafting.

The material is reconstituted by immersion in sterile water or suitable saline solution and applied, dermal side to the wound, using strict aseptic technique, and changed as required. Bovine skin is similarly used.

References: *Drug & Ther. Bull.*, 1976, *14*, 71; J. S. H. Rundle *et al.*, *Br. med. J.*, 1976, *2*, 216; A. V. Kaisary, *Postgrad. med. J.*, 1977, *53*, 672; D. N. Bremner *et al.*, *Practitioner*, 1977, *218*, 708; D. S. Chatterjee, *Curr. med. Res. Opinion*, 1978, *5*, 726; A. M. Yiacoumettis, *Br. J. clin. Pract.*, 1979, *33*, 99.

Proprietary Preparations

Armoderm *(Armour, UK)*. A temporary biological dressing consisting of sterilised freeze-dried porcine skin. For topical application to burns and varicose ulcers, after reconstitution in a sterile, balanced electrolyte solution.

Corethium 1 *(Johnson & Johnson, UK)*. A temporary biological dressing consisting of sterilised freeze-dried porcine skin. For topical application to burns, after reconstitution in sodium chloride injection or Ringer's solution. Also available glutaraldehyde-treated for use in oral surgery. **Corethium 2.** A similar temporary dressing consisting of porcine dermis. For application to varicose ulcers and similar skin conditions. **Corethium 3.** A similar temporary dressing consisting of bovine dermis. For application to burns and skin donor sites.

Fascia Lata *(Ethicon, UK)*. Sterilised strips of bovine connective tissue obtained from below the hide. A substitute for human fascia lata for use in surgery.

Zenoderm Corium Implant *(Ethicon, UK)*. A sterile material prepared from porcine dermis by enzyme treatment and glutaraldehyde-crosslinking. For use by surgical implantation as a supporting tissue.

Proprietary Preparations of Similar Material

Synthaderm *(Armour, UK)*. A temporary dressing consisting of a sterile plastic film with a hydrophobic outer layer and a hydrophilic inner layer. Stated to be permeable to gases but impermeable to bacteria and fluids.

13152-n

Potassium Borotartrate.

Potassium Sodium Borotartrate; Soluble Cream of Tartar.

A white odourless powder. It may be prepared by evaporating a solution of borax 2 parts and potassium bitartrate 5 parts. Freely **soluble** in water.

Potassium borotartrate has been used in nervous disorders and is used in photography as a retarder for alkaline developers. The toxic effects of chronic boron poisoning have been reported following the use of potassium borotartrate internally (see under Boric Acid, p.337).

Proprietary Names

Neurobore *(Bouteille, Fr.)*.

13153-h

Potassium Bromate.

$KBrO_3$=167.0.

CAS — 7758-01-2.

A white, odourless, tasteless, crystalline powder or granules. **Soluble** 1 in 12.5 of water and 1 in 2 of boiling water; practically insoluble in alcohol. A 5% solution is neutral to litmus.

Adverse Effects. Ingestion of potassium bromate is followed by nausea, vomiting, severe abdominal pain, and diarrhoea. The patient becomes apathetic but very irritable; loss of consciousness, central nervous depression, and loss of tendon reflexes ensue, but convulsions may occur. Methaemoglobinaemia may occur. Kidney damage, with albuminuria and oliguria or anuria may arise. Respiration becomes shallow and rapid, the heart-rate increases, and the blood pressure falls. Body temperature is lowered. Hepatitis, pulmonary oedema, and toxic myocarditis have been reported. Death from renal failure may occur within 1 to 2 weeks.

An account of potassium bromate poisoning in 55 patients due to the ingestion of contaminated sugar.— A. H. Paul, *N.Z. med. J.*, 1966, *65*, 33, per *Bull. Hyg., Lond.*, 1966, *41*, 864.

Report of potassium bromate poisoning in 816 persons who had eaten bread prepared from dough containing an excessive amount of potassium bromate which had been added as a flour improver. The bread contained 1.1% w/w instead of a permitted 40 ppm.— T. H. Stewart *et al.*, *S. Afr. med. J.*, 1969, *43*, 200, per *Abstr. Wld Med.*, 1969, *43*, 709.

An account of deafness and renal failure due to potassium bromate poisoning.— C. A. Quick *et al.*, *Archs Otolar.*, 1975, *101*, 494, per *J. Am. med. Ass.*, 1975, *233*, 568.

Treatment of Adverse Effects.. After the ingestion of potassium bromate the stomach should be emptied by aspiration and lavage and demulcent drinks such as milk given. Pain is relieved by the injection of pethidine. An intravenous infusion of 100 to 500 ml of a 1% sodium thiosulphate solution or intravenous injection of 10 to 50 ml of a 10% solution has been recommended; it must *not* be given by mouth. If vomiting is protracted, fluid intake should be maintained with copious drinks or the intravenous infusion of dextrose injection. Oxygen may be indicated and if methaemoglobinaemia is severe exchange transfusion with whole blood may be necessary; the use of methylene blue should be avoided since it may enhance the toxicity of bromate.

The prompt use of haemodialysis or peritoneal dialysis has been suggested.

Uses. Potassium bromate is an oxidising agent. It has no therapeutic uses but it has been widely used in home permanent-wave sets as the 'neutraliser' of thioglycollate hair-waving lotions (see p.1761). It is also used as a flour-maturing agent.

13154-m

Potassium Iodate *(B. Vet. C. 1965)*.

KIO_3=214.0.

CAS — 7758-05-6.

A white crystalline odourless powder. **Soluble** 1 in 12 of water; practically insoluble in alcohol. A 5% solution in water is neutral to litmus.

Potassium iodate has been used as a source of iodine in mineral supplements for animal feeds. It has also been used prophylactically in areas where there is endemic goitre.

Potassium iodate was considered unsafe for use in food.— Ninth Report of the Joint FAO/WHO Expert Committee on Food Additives, *Tech. Rep. Ser. Wld Hlth Org. No. 339*, 1966.

Potassium iodate 169 mg (equivalent to about 100 mg of iodine) has been used to prevent uptake of radioactive iodine by the thyroid.— A. Cronquist *et al.*, *Hlth Phys.*, 1971, *21*, 393. A comment that in the UK tablets of potassium iodate are kept in readiness for distribution to the exposed population on a one-off basis in the event of radiation exposure due to a nuclear power plant disaster.— J. A. Bonnell and G. C. Dale (letter), *Lancet*, 1981, *2*, 207. See also J. A. Bonnell (letter), *Br. med. J.*, 1980, *281*, 1278.

Goitre. The incorporation of 2 parts per million of potassium iodate in bread was an effective prophylactic against endemic goitre in Tasmania in comparison with the distribution of tablets containing 10 mg of potassium iodide to schoolchildren.— F. W. Clements *et al.*, *Lancet*, 1970, *1*, 489. The addition gave a mean daily iodine intake of between 80 and 270 µg and resulted within a few months in increased incidence of thyrotoxicosis, mainly in patients over 50 years old.— R. J. Connolly *et al.*, *ibid.*, 500. Comments.— S. Whittingham and I. R. Mackay (letter), *ibid.*, 520.

The addition of potassium iodate 1 part to 40 000 parts of salt given to children in an area of the Himalayan foothills reduced the prevalence of thyroid enlargement from 40.3% in 1962 to 17.1% in 1968. In areas where salt with either potassium iodide or potassium iodate had been distributed continuously since 1956 the incidence of goitre was nil in children under 5, and negligible in children under 10 years of age. Concentrations of protein-bound serum iodine among individuals in these areas were however lower than those found in nonendemic areas of India.— S. S. Sooch *et al.*, *Bull. Wld Hlth Org.*, 1973, *49*, 307.

13155-b

Potassium Nitrate *(B.P.)*.

Pot. Nit.; Nitre; Saltpetre; Kalii Nitras; Kalium Nitricum; Azotato de Potássio.

KNO_3=101.1.

CAS — 7757-79-1.

Pharmacopoeias. In *Arg.*, *Belg.*, *Br.*, *Braz.*, *Cz.*, *Fr.*, *Hung.*, *Int.*, *Jap.*, *Nord.*, *Pol.*, *Port.*, *Span.*, and *Swiss.*

Odourless colourless crystals or white crystalline powder with a cooling saline taste. **Soluble** 1 in 3.3 of cold water, 1 in 0.5 of boiling water, and 1 in 620 of alcohol. Solutions in water are neutral to litmus. A 1.62% solution in water is iso-osmotic with serum.

When heated to about 350° potassium nitrate melts and forms, on cooling, a solid mass known as 'sal prunella' which is usually supplied in small balls.

WARNING. *The Council of the Pharmaceutical Society of Great Britain advises pharmacists not to supply materials likely to be used for making fireworks, including potassium nitrate, to children under any circumstances, and recommends that it should be sold only to persons who are, or appear to be, 18 years of age or over.*

Adverse Effects. After ingestion of potassium nitrate gastro-enteritis, with severe abdominal pain, vomiting, vertigo, muscular weakness, irregular pulse, cyanosis, convulsions, and collapse may occur. The toxic dose varies greatly; from 15 to 30 g may prove fatal but much larger doses have been taken without serious effects. Symptoms of chronic poisoning from prolonged therapeutic use resemble those of bromism or iodism.

Potassium nitrate may be reduced to nitrite in the gastro-intestinal tract by the action of bacteria and ingestion can therefore cause methaemoglobinaemia. Poisoning has frequently been reported in infants given water from wells contaminated with nitrates. For reference to nitrites as precursors of nitrosamines and the potential role of nitrosamines as carcinogens, see p.392.

Toxicological information on potassium and sodium nitrates in food. The safe upper limit for nitrate in the drinking water of infants was probably 10 to 20 ppm.— *Fd Add. Ser. Wld Hlth Org. No. 5*, 1974.

Nitrates might be found in water and they were present in high concentrations in foods such as beets, spinach, carrots, and cabbages; conversion of nitrates to nitrites (which could cause methaemoglobinaemia) was enhanced when nitrate-containing foods spoiled. The lower stomach acidity of infants under 4 months of age might permit growth of bacteria capable of reducing nitrates to nitrites; deaths had occurred as a result of giving infants water with a high nitrate content and toxicity had also occurred in infants after nitrate was reduced to nitrite when jars of baby food were left open or cooked vegetables were kept at room temperature for some time. Although nitrates and nitrites were effective food preservatives they could lead to the formation of nitrosamines which were carcinogenic in *animals* and might act similarly in man.— *Med. Lett.*, 1974, *16*, 75.

Allergy. A patient who suffered attacks of palindromic rheumatism after ingesting a wide range of foods was found to be sensitive to sodium nitrate. Test doses of sodium nitrite only elicited minor joint discomfort.— S. Epstein, *Ann. Allergy*, 1969, *27*, 343.

Effects on the blood. A report of severe methaemoglobinaemia in 3 workers (fatal in one) following absorption of sodium and potassium nitrate through burnt skin areas after an industrial accident.— J. C. Harris *et al.*, *J. Am. med. Ass.*, 1979, *242*, 2869.

Treatment of Adverse Effects. Acute overdosage with potassium nitrate may be treated by administering large quantities of water by mouth, and by gastric lavage and aspiration. Demulcents such as milk and egg-white may delay absorption. Methaemoglobinaemia should be treated with methylene blue (see p.384). Oxygen and assisted respiration may be necessary and blood transfusions have been suggested.

Following ingestion of 50 g of potassium nitrate over a period of 12 days a 22-year-old woman developed methaemoglobinaemia which was successfully treated with methylene blue, 5 ml of 1% solution by slow intravenous injection (1 mg per kg body-weight). Supportive therapy included ascorbic acid by intravenous injection.— J. Paccalin *et al.*, *Thérapie*, 1973, *28*, 1143.

Absorption and Fate. Nitrates are readily absorbed from the gastro-intestinal tract and are rapidly excreted almost entirely unchanged in the urine; a small amount may be reduced to nitrite (but see Adverse Effects, above). Their excretion is similar to that of chloride ions.

Uses. Potassium nitrate, when taken by mouth in dilute solution, acts as a diuretic and it was formerly used for this purpose. It is an ingredient of Mitigated Silver Nitrate (*B.P.C. 1968*) and Toughened Silver Nitrate (*B.P.*). It has been included in 'asthma powders' to assist combustion. It is used as a preservative in foods (see p.1282).

Estimated acceptable daily intake of nitrates: up to 500 µg per kg body-weight. No change was made from the Seventeenth Report [however, in that report an intake of up to *5 mg* per kg was given].— Twenty-third Report of Joint FAO/WHO Expert Committee on Food Additives, *Tech. Rep. Ser. Wld Hlth Org. No. 648*, 1980. Nitrate should on no account be added to baby foods.— *Fd Add. Ser. Wld Hlth Org. No. 5*, 1974.

13156-v

Potassium Nitrite.
KNO_2=85.10.

CAS — 7758-09-0.

A white crystalline deliquescent powder. **Soluble** in water; practically insoluble in alcohol. A 5% solution has a pH of 6 to 9. **Store** in airtight containers.

Potassium nitrite has the pharmacological effects of the other nitrites (see Sodium Nitrite, p.392). It is used as a preservative in foods (see p.1282).

Food for babies less than 6 months of age should not contain added nitrites.— Twentieth Report of the Joint FAO/WHO Expert Committee on Food Additives, *Tech. Rep. Ser. Wld Hlth Org. No. 599*, 1976. Estimated acceptable daily intake of nitrites: up to 20 µg per kg body-weight. No change was made from the acceptable daily intake provided in the Seventeenth Report [however, in that report an intake of up to *200 µg* per kg was given].— Twenty-third Report of Joint FAO/WHO Expert Committee on Food Additives, *Tech. Rep. Ser. Wld Hlth Org. No. 648*, 1980.

13157-g

Potassium Polystyrene Sulphonate.
The potassium form of a cation-exchange resin.

CAS — 9011-99-8.

Potassium polystyrene sulphonate has the general properties of the ion-exchange resins (see p.869) and is used in the treatment of hypercalcaemia.

Proprietary Names
Campanyl *(Temmler, Ger.).*

13158-q

Potassium Quadroxalate *(B.P.C. 1934).*
Potassium Tetroxalate; Salt of Sorrel; Salts of Lemon; Sal Acetosella.
$KHC_2O_4,H_2C_2O_4,2H_2O$=254.2.

CAS — 127-96-8 (anhydrous).

Colourless transparent crystals with an acid taste. **Soluble** 1 in 30 of water and 1 in 2 of boiling water.

Potassium quadroxalate has been used for removing ink stains and iron mould from clothing and table-linen and for bleaching straw. It has the adverse effects of Oxalic Acid, p.787.
The names 'Salts of Lemon' and 'Salt of Sorrel' have also been applied to Potassium Binoxalate, KHC_2O_4,H_2O = 146.1.

13159-p

Potassium Selenate *(B.P. Vet.).*
K_2SeO_4=221.2.

CAS — 7790-59-2.

Colourless odourless crystals or a white crystalline powder. **Soluble** 1 in 1 of water.

Potassium selenate is used in veterinary practice in conjunction with vitamin E in the prevention and treatment of deficiency syndrome, including nutritional muscular dystrophy (white muscle disease, stiff lamb disease) in calves and lambs.

13160-n

Pranosal.
3-(2,5-Dimethylpyrrolidin-1-yl)propyl salicylate.
$C_{16}H_{23}NO_3$=277.4.

CAS — 17716-89-1.

Pranosal has been used as the salicylate as a topical analgesic in rheumatic and other disorders.

Proprietary Names
Pyradol (salicylate) *(Sarbach, Fr.).*

13161-h

Praziquantel.
EMBAY-8440. 2-Cyclohexylcarbonyl-1,2,3,6,7,11b-hexahydropyrazino-[2,1-*a*]isoquinolin-4-one.
$C_{19}H_{24}N_2O_2$=312.4.

CAS — 55268-74-1.

Praziquantel is an anthelmintic effective against tapeworm infections and against *Schistosoma* (*S. haematobium, S. mansoni*, and *S. japonicum*).

Pharmacokinetics.— G. Leopold *et al., Eur. J. clin. Pharmac.*, 1978, *14*, 281; K. U. Bühring *et al., Eur. J. Drug Metab. Pharmacokinet.*, 1978, *3*, 179; K. Patzschke *et al., ibid.*, 1979, *4*, 149.

Schistosomiasis. A favourable review of the use of praziquantel in schistosomiasis.— *Lancet*, 1980, *1*, 635.

Favourable reports:. A. Davis *et al., Bull. Wld Hlth Org.*, 1979, *57*, 773 (*S. haematobium*); N. Katz *et al., ibid.*, 781 (*S. mansoni*); T. Ishizaki *et al., ibid.*, 787 (*S. japonicum*); A. T. Santos *et al., ibid.*, 793 (*S. japonicum*); J. E. McMahon and N. Kolstrup, *Br. med. J.*, 1979, *2*, 1396 (*S. haematobium*); *Chin. med. J.*, 1980, *93*, 375.

Tapeworm infection. References: H. Schenone *et al., Boln chil. Parasit.*, 1977, *32*, 11 (77.3% to 100% cure in *Hymenolepis nana* infection), per *Trop. Dis. Bull.*, 1978, *75* 378; M. C. Baranski, *Boln chil. Parasit.*, 1977, *32*, 37, per *Trop. Dis. Bull.*, 1978, *75* 380; C. J. Canzonieri *et al., Boln chil. Parasit.*, 1977, *32*, 41 (100% cure in *Taenia saginata* and generally 80.8 to 93.3% in *Hymenolepis nana* infections), per *Trop. Dis. Bull.*, 1978, *75*, 379; H. -J. Rim *et al., Korean J. Parasit.*, 1979, *17*, 67 (cure in 52 of 53 patients with *T. solium* infection), per *Trop. Dis. Bull.*, 1980, *77*, 687; H. Schenone, *Am. J. trop. Med. Hyg.*, 1980, *29*, 320 (76 to 98.5% cure in *Hymenolepis nana* infection), per *Trop. Dis. Bull.*, 1980, *77*, 687.

Proprietary Names
Cesol *(E. Merck, Ger.)*; Biltricide *(Bayer, Ger.)*; Droncit (veterinary).

15332-r

Prednazoline.
Prednisolone-fenoxazoline Compound. 11β,17α,21-Trihydroxypregna-1,4-diene-3,20-dione 21-(dihydrogen phosphate) compound with 2-(2-isopropylphenoxymethyl)-2-imidazoline.
$C_{21}H_{29}O_8P,C_{13}H_{18}N_2O$=658.7.

CAS — 6693-90-9.

Prednazoline has the general properties of prednisolone (see p.479) and of fenoxazoline (see p.13) and has been used locally in the treatment of pharyngitis, rhinitis, and sinusitis.

Proprietary Names
Déturgylone *(Dausse, Fr.).*

13162-m

Prednisolone Valeroacetate.
11β,17α,21-Trihydroxypregna-1,4-diene-3,20-dione 17-valerate 21-acetate.
$C_{28}H_{38}O_7$=486.6.

CAS — 72064-79-0.

Prednisolone valeroacetate is a corticosteroid for topical use.

Proprietary Names
Acepreval *(Parke, Davis, Ital.).*

13163-b

Pregnenolone Succinate.
3β-Hydroxypregn-5-en-20-one hydrogen succinate.
$C_{25}H_{36}O_5$=416.6.

CAS — 145-13-1 (pregnenolone); 4598-67-8 (succinate).

Pregnenolone is a synthetic corticosteroid. The succinate is applied topically. Pregnenolone acetate has also been used.

Proprietary Names
C.S. (acetate) *(Armstrong, Arg.).*

13164-v

Prenalterol Hydrochloride.
CGP-7760-B; H133/22; H-80/62 (racemate); C-50005/A-Ba (racemate). (−)-(*S*)-1-(4-Hydroxyphenoxy)-3-isopropylaminopropan-2-ol hydrochloride.
$C_{12}H_{19}NO_3,HCl$=261.7.

CAS — 57526-81-5 (prenalterol); 61260-05-7 (hydrochloride).

Adverse Effects and Precautions. Palpitations and nervousness may occur with prenalterol hydrochloride. Isolated ventricular ectopic beats have been reported. The incidence of anginal attacks may be increased in patients with angina pectoris.

Uses. Prenalterol hydrochloride is a sympathomimetic agent with stimulant effects on $beta_1$-adrenoceptors. It has an inotropic action on the heart with relatively little chronotropic effect. Prenalterol hydrochloride is used in the treatment of heart failure associated with myocardial infarction or open-heart surgery or shock. A suggested dose is 0.5 mg per minute by slow intravenous infusion to a total of not more than 20 mg.
It is also promoted for the reversal of beta-blockade.

Reversal of metoprolol-induced haemodynamic changes in 10 patients by prenalterol.— R. Ariniego *et al., Br. Heart J.*, 1979, *42*, 139. See also O. Rönn *et al., Eur. J. clin. Pharmac.*, 1979, *15*, 9.

Haemodynamic effects of prenalterol in healthy subjects.— D. H. T. Scott *et al., Br. J. clin. Pharmac.*, 1979, *7*, 365; O. Rönn *et al., Eur. J. clin. Pharmac.*, 1980, *17*, 81.

Haemodynamic effects of prenalterol in patients with ischaemic heart disease or heart failure.— I. Hutton *et al., Br. Heart J.*, 1980, *43*, 134; P. C. Kirlin and B. Pitt, *Am. J. Cardiol.*, 1981, *47*, 670; A. L. Muir *et al., Br. J. clin. Pharmac.*, 1981, *12*, 475; N. A. Awan *et al., Am. Heart J.*, 1981, *101*, 158.

Use of prenalterol in 21 patients with heart failure or hypotension.— S. Reiz *et al., Clin. Cardiol.*, 1980, *3*, 96.

Proprietary Preparations

Hyprenan *(Astra, UK).* Prenalterol hydrochloride, available as solution for intravenous use containing 1 mg per ml, in ampoules of 5 ml.

Varbian *(Ciba, UK).* Prenalterol hydrochloride, available as solution for intravenous use containing 1 mg per ml, in ampoules of 5 ml.

13165-g

Pretamazium Iodide.
66-269. 4-(Biphenyl-4-yl)-3-ethyl-2-[4-(pyrrolidin-1-yl)styryl]thiazolium iodide.
$C_{29}H_{29}IN_2S$=564.5.

CAS — 24840-59-3.

An anthelmintic for threadworm infection.

13166-q

Primaperone.
Flufenone. 4′-Fluoro-4-piperidinobutyrophenone.
$C_{15}H_{20}FNO$=249.3.

CAS — 1219-35-8.

Primaperone has been reported to be a vasodilator and antihypertensive agent. It has been claimed to exert a central effect on the vasomotor centre and to decrease peripheral vascular resistance.

13167-p

Primidolol.
UK-11443. 1-[2-(2-Hydroxy-3-*o*-tolyloxypropylamino)ethyl]-5-methyluracil.
$C_{17}H_{23}N_3O_4$=333.4.

CAS — 67227-55-8.

Primidolol is reported to be a beta-adrenoceptor blocking agent.

References: P. Fauchald, *Curr. med. Res. Opinion*, 1980, *6*, 528; A. Lehtonen, *Int. J. clin. Pharmac. Biopharm.*, 1981, *19*, 228.

Manufacturers
Pfizer, UK.

13168-s

Prizidilol Hydrochloride. SKF-92657-A. 1-*tert*-Butylamino-3-[2-(6-hydrazinopyridazin-3-yl)phenoxy]propan-2-ol dihydrochloride monohydrate.
$C_{17}H_{25}N_5O_2,2HCl,H_2O=422.4$.

CAS — 59010-44-5 (prizidilol); 63642-19-3 (hydrochloride, anhydrous); 73398-12-6 (hydrochloride, monohydrate).

Prizidilol hydrochloride is reported to have vasodilator and antihypertensive properties.

References: A. Bell *et al.*, *Br. J. clin. Pharmac.*, 1980, *9*, 299P; D. W. Pitcher *et al.*, *ibid.*, 300P; J. G. Collier and D. W. Pitcher, *ibid.*, 301P; R. Larsson *et al.*, *Clin. Pharmac. Ther.*, 1981, *29*, 588; A. Clancy *et al.*, *Br. J. clin. Pharmac.*, 1981, *11*, 428P.

Manufacturers
Smith Kline & French, UK.

13169-w

Proadifen Hydrochloride. Propyladiphenine Hydrochloride; SKF-525A. 2-Diethylaminoethyl 2,2-diphenylvalerate hydrochloride.
$C_{23}H_{31}NO_2,HCl=390.0$.

CAS — 302-33-0 (proadifen); 62-68-0 (hydrochloride).

Proadifen has been found to enhance the effects of a large number of drugs. It may act by inhibiting drug metabolism.

References: G. V. Rossi, *J. pharm. Sci.*, 1963, *52*, 819; W. R. Ravis and S. Feldman, *ibid.*, 1979, *68*, 945.

Manufacturers
Smith Kline & French, USA.

13170-m

Probicromil. 4,6-Dioxo-10-propyl-4*H*,6*H*-pyrano[3,2-g]chromene-2,8-dicarboxylic acid.
$C_{17}H_{12}O_8=344.3$.

CAS — 58805-38-2.

Probicromil has possible anti-allergic activity.

Manufacturers
Fisons, UK.

13171-b

Procaterol Hydrochloride. CI-888; OPC-2009. (±)-*erythro*-8-Hydroxy-5-(1-hydroxy-2-isopropylaminobutyl)quinolin-2(1*H*)-one hydrochloride.
$C_{16}H_{22}N_2O_3,HCl=326.8$.

CAS — 72332-33-3 (procaterol); 62929-91-3 (hydrochloride).

Procaterol hydrochloride is reported to be a sympathomimetic agent with possible application as a bronchodilator.

Pharmacology.— N. Himori and N. Taira, *Br. J. Pharmac.*, 1977, *61*, 9; Y. Yabuuchi, *ibid.*, 513; I. Takayanagi *et al.*, *J. Pharm. Pharmac.*, 1977, *29*, 187; S. Yamashita *et al.*, *ibid.*, 1978, *30*, 273.

Manufacturers
Otsuka, Jap.; Parke, Davis, USA.

13172-v

Procodazole. 3-(Benzimidazol-2-yl)propionic acid.
$C_{10}H_{10}N_2O_2=190.2$.

CAS — 23249-97-0.

Procodazole is reported to have immunostimulant properties.

Proprietary Names
Estimulocel *(Lafarquim, Spain).*

13173-g

Profadol Hydrochloride. A-2205; CI-572. 3-(1-Methyl-3-propylpyrrolidin-3-yl)phenol hydrochloride.
$C_{14}H_{21}NO,HCl=255.8$.

CAS — 428-37-5 (profadol); 2324-94-9 (hydrochloride).

A white solid. M.p. 145° to 146°. **Soluble** in water.

Profadol hydrochloride is a narcotic analgesic reported to be about one-quarter to one-half as potent as morphine. Side-effects are typical of narcotic analgesics.

For references to profadol, see Martindale 27th Edn, p. 1802.

13174-q

Proglumetacin Maleate. Protacine Maleate; CR-604. 3-{4-[2-(1-*p*-Chlorobenzoyl-5-methoxy-2-methylindol-3-ylacetoxy)ethyl]piperazin-1-yl}propyl 4-benzamido-*NN*-dipropylglutaramate dimaleate.
$C_{46}H_{58}ClN_5O_8,2C_4H_4O_4=1076.6$.

CAS — 57132-53-3 (proglumetacin); 59209-40-4 (maleate).

Proglumetacin maleate is reported to have analgesic and anti-inflammatory activity and has been used in the treatment of rheumatic and similar disorders.

Comparison with indomethacin.— V. Pipitone *et al.*, *Curr. med. Res. Opinion*, 1979, *6*, 287.

Bioavailability.— A. A. Bignamini and P. L. Casula, *Curr. med. Res. Opinion*, 1979, *6*, 299.

Comparisons with oxyphenbutazone.— V. Pietrogrande *et al.*, *Clin. Ther.*, 1979, *2*, 368; J. Munzenberg and S. Tachibana, *Pharmatherapeutica*, 1980, *2*, 279; P. Loizzi *et al.*, *ibid.*, 285.

Proprietary Names
Afloxan *(Rotta, Ital.)*; Proxil *(Rorer, Ital.).*

13175-p

Prolonium Iodide. *NN*-(2-Hydroxytrimethylene)bis(trimethylammonium) di-iodide.
$C_9H_{24}I_2N_2O=430.1$.

CAS — 123-47-7.

Prolonium iodide has been given in a variety of disorders in which iodine has traditionally been used.

Proprietary Names
Endo-Iodo *(Cozzolino, Ital.)*; Endojodin *(Bayer, Ger.)*; Intrajodina *(Gentili, Ital.)*; Iodopropano *(Farmochimica Italiana, Ital.)*; Iorganisan *(Santos, Spain)*; Soluyodina *(Luyma, Spain)*; Yodofasa *(Lifasa, Spain).*

13176-s

Promestriene. 17β-Methoxy-3-propoxyestra-1,3,5(10)-triene.
$C_{22}H_{32}O_2=328.5$.

CAS — 39219-28-8.

Promestriene has been used topically in vaginitis and seborrhoea.

Proprietary Names
Colpotrophine *(Théramex, Fr.)*; Délipoderm *(Théramex, Fr.).*

13177-w

Propafenone Hydrochloride. SA-79; WZ-884642; WZ-884643; Fenopraine *(propafenone)*. 2′-(2-Hydroxy-3-propylaminopropoxy)-3-phenylpropiophenone hydrochloride.
$C_{21}H_{27}NO_3,HCl=377.9$.

CAS — 54063-53-5 (propafenone).

Propafenone hydrochloride has been used in the treatment of cardiac arrhythmias.

References: E. Aldor and H. Heeger, *Dt. med. Wschr.*, 1976, *101*, 1318; O. A. Beck *et al.*, *ibid.*, 1978, *103*, 1068; O. A. Beck and H. Hochrein, *ibid.*, 1261; H. Blanke *et al.*, *ibid.*, 1979, *104*, 587.

Proprietary Names
Rytmonorm *(Knoll, Ger.).*

13178-e

Propizepine Hydrochloride. UP-106 *(propizepine)*. 6-(2-Dimethylaminopropyl)-6,11-dihydro-5*H*-pyrido[2,3-*b*][1,5]benzodiazepin-5-one hydrochloride.
$C_{17}H_{20}N_4O,HCl=332.8$.

CAS — 10321-12-7 (propizepine); 14559-79-6 (hydrochloride).

Propizepine hydrochloride is a tricyclic antidepressant.

Proprietary Names
Vagran 50 *(UPSA, Fr.).*

13179-l

Proquamezine Fumarate. Aminopromazine Fumarate; Tetrameprozine Fumarate; Bayer-A-124; RP-3828. *NNN′N′*-Tetramethyl-3-(phenothiazin-10-yl)propane-1,2-diamine fumarate.
$(C_{19}H_{25}N_3S)_2,C_4H_4O_4=771.0$.

CAS — 58-37-7 (proquamezine); 3688-62-8 (fumarate).

A white powder. M.p. about 168° with decomposition. Proquamezine fumarate 118 mg is approximately equivalent to 100 mg of proquamezine. **Soluble** 1 in 11 of water, 1 in 200 of alcohol, and 1 in 20 of methyl alcohol; practically insoluble in ether.

Proquamezine fumarate is a phenothiazine derivative with antispasmodic properties and is used in veterinary medicine.

Proprietary Names
Myspamol *(May & Baker, UK).*

13180-v

Proquazone. 43-715; RU-43-715-n. 1-Isopropyl-7-methyl-4-phenylquinazolin-2(1*H*)-one.
$C_{18}H_{18}N_2O=278.4$.

CAS — 22760-18-5.

Proquazone has analgesic and anti-inflammatory activity and has been used in the treatment of rheumatic and related disorders.

Comparisons with indomethacin.— M. Karakaya, *Curr. ther. Res.*, 1977, *22*, 127; R. Allan and M. Bleicher, *J. int. med. Res.*, 1977, *5*, 253; H. Broll *et al.*, *Curr. ther. Res.*, 1978, *23*, 27; M. Schattenkirchner and Z. Fryda-Kaurimsky, *ibid.*, *24*, 905; B. Skrifvars and M. Nissilä, *Scand. J. Rheumatol.*, 1980, *9*, 33.

Comparison with naproxen.— J. T. Vainio and P. V. Lepistö, *Scand. J. Rheumatol.*, 1978, *Suppl.* 21, 25.

A comparison with aspirin.— J. A. Forbes *et al.*, *J. clin. Pharmac.*, 1980, *20*, 465.

Absence of effect on coagulation parameters.— H. Vinazzer, *Int. J. clin. Pharmac. Biopharm.*, 1977, *15*, 214.

Further references: *Scand. J. Rheumatol.*, 1978, *Suppl.* 21, 1–42.

Proprietary Names
Biarison *(Sandoz, Ger.; Wander, Neth.; Wander, Switz.).*

13181-g

Prospidium Chloride. 3,12-Bis(3-chloro-2-hydroxypropyl)-3,12-diaza-6,9-diazoniadispiro-[5.2.5.2]hexadecane dichloride monohydrate. $C_{18}H_{36}Cl_4N_4O_2,H_2O$=500.3.

CAS — 23476-83-7 (anhydrous).

Prospidium chloride is reported to have antineoplastic activity.

Proprietary Names
Prospidin *(Casen-Roncales, Spain).*

13182-q

Prosultiamine. Thiamine Propyl Disulphide. *N*-(4-Amino-2-methylpyrimidin-5-ylmethyl)-*N*-(4-hydroxy-1-methyl-2-propyldithiobut-1-enyl)formamide.
$C_{15}H_{24}N_4O_2S_2$=356.5.

CAS — 59-58-5.

Prosultiamine has the general properties of thiamine hydrochloride.

Proprietary Names
Binova *(Gentili, Ital.)*; Jubedel Fuerte *(Septa, Spain)*; Taketron *(Takeda, Neth.)*; Trofotiamin *(IBP, Ital.).*

13183-p

Protheobromine. 3,7-Dihydro-1-(2-hydroxypropyl)-3,7-dimethylpurine-2,6(1*H*)-dione.
$C_{10}H_{14}N_4O_3$=238.2.

CAS — 50-39-5.

Protheobromine is a derivative of theobromine and has been used similarly.

Proprietary Names
Idromin *(Arnaldi, Ital.)*; Tebe *(Simes, Ital.)*; Tebesimes *(Farmasimes, Spain)*; Teocorin *(Cif, Ital.)*; Thebes *(Sintesa, Belg.).*

13184-s

Proxicromil. FPL-57787. 6,7,8,9-Tetrahydro-5-hydroxy-4-oxo-10-propyl-4*H*-benzo[*g*]-chromene-2-carboxylic acid.
$C_{17}H_{18}O_5$=302.3.

CAS — 60400-92-2.

Proxicromil was under study as a prophylactic anti-allergic agent but study has ceased because of toxicity in *animals.*

References: N. C. Thomson *et al., Clin. Allergy,* 1980, *10,* 43; J. P. Girard and T. J. Sullivan, *ibid.,* 271.

Manufacturers
Fisons, UK.

13185-w

Proxorphan Tartrate. BL-5572 (proxorphan); BL-5572M. 9a-Cyclopropylmethyl-6-oxamorphinan-3-ol tartrate.
$(C_{19}H_{25}NO_2)_2,C_4H_6O_6$=748.9.

CAS — 69815-38-9 (proxorphan); 69815-39-0 (tartrate).

Proxorphan tartrate is reported to have analgesic and antitussive activity.

Manufacturers
Bristol, USA.

13186-e

Prussian Blue

NOTE. The name Prussian Blue (Berlin Blue; CI Pigment Blue 27; CI No. 77520; Potassium Ferric Cyanoferrate(II)) is applied to potassium ferric hexacyanoferrate(II), $KFe[Fe(CN)_6]$ = 306.9. The name Prussian Blue (CI Pigment Blue 27; CI No. 77510) is also applied to ferric ferrocyanide, $Fe_4[Fe(CN)_6]_3$ = 859.2.
The name Turnbull's Blue (CI No. 77525) is applied to ferrous ferricyanide, $FeFe_2[Fe(CN)_6]_2,H_2O$ = 609.5, prepared by treating prussian blue (CI No. 77510) with oxalic acid.

A deep blue pigment.

Prussian blue has been given by mouth in the treatment of thallium poisoning. Thallium is exchanged for potassium in the lattice and is excreted in the faeces. For reports, see Thallium Acetate, p.1760.
It has been used similarly for the removal of radiocaesium from the body.

For reports of the removal of radiocaesium (^{137}Cs) from the body using Prussian blue, see V. Nigrović, *Physics Med. Biol.,* 1965, *10,* 81; K. Madshus *et al.* (letter), *Int. J. Radiat. Biol.,* 1966, *10,* 519; V. Nigrović *et al., Strahlentherapie,* 1966, *130,* 413; K. Madshus and A. Strömme, *Z. Naturforsch.,* 1968, *23b,* 391.

Proprietary Names
Antidotum Thallii Heyl *(Heyl, Ger.)*; Radiogardase-Cs *(Heyl, Ger.).*

13187-l

Pulsatilla. The whole plant of *Pulsatilla nigricans* (Ranunculaceae).

CAS — 62887-80-3.

Pulsatilla is used in homoeopathic medicine.

13188-y

Punarnava. Punarnaba.

Pharmacopoeias. In *Ind.*

The fresh or dried plant *Boerhaavia diffusa* (= *B. repens*) (Nyctaginaceae), containing an alkaloid, punarnavine.

Punarnava has been used in India as a diuretic, usually in the form of a liquid extract.

13189-j

Pyran Copolymer. NSC-46015C; DIVEMA. An anionic copolymer of divinyl ether and maleic anhydride, with an average molecular weight of 17 000.

CAS — 27100-68-1.

Pyran copolymer is an antiviral agent which has been reported to induce the production of interferon in man.

References: T. C. Merigan and W. Regelson, *New Engl. J. Med.,* 1967, *277,* 1283; T. J. Leavitt *et al., Am. J. Dis. Child.,* 1971, *121,* 43; R. S. McCord *et al., Antimicrob. Ag. Chemother.,* 1976, *10,* 28.

13190-q

Pyrantel Tartrate *(B. Vet. C. 1965).* CP-10423-18; UK-2500. 1,4,5,6-Tetrahydro-1-methyl-2-[(*E*)-2-(2-thienyl)vinyl]pyrimidine hydrogen tartrate.
$C_{15}H_{20}N_2O_6S$=356.4.

CAS — 15686-83-6 (pyrantel); 33401-94-4 (tartrate).

Pharmacopoeias. In *Nord.*

A white to pale greenish-yellow crystalline powder with a faint odour. M.p. 147° to 151°. **Soluble** 1 in 5 of water and 1 in 9 of methyl alcohol; slightly soluble in chloroform and isopropyl alcohol; practically insoluble in ether. A 1% solution in water has a pH of 3.3 to 3.7. **Store** in airtight containers. Protect from light.

Pyrantel tartrate is a veterinary anthelmintic which has been used in the treatment of roundworm infections.

13191-p

Pyridinolcarbamate. Pyridine-2,6-diylbis(methylene *N*-methylcarbamate).
$C_{11}H_{15}N_3O_4$=253.3.

CAS — 1882-26-4.

A white odourless crystalline powder. M.p. 135° to 138°. Slightly **soluble** in water; soluble in alcohol and chloroform.

Pyridinolcarbamate has been reported to be a bradykinin antagonist and has been claimed to have beneficial effects in the treatment of the complications of atherosclerosis. Adverse effects have included gastro-intestinal disturbances and liver damage.

Reports on the use of pyridinolcarbamate in atherosclerosis and related disorders: T. Shimamoto *et al., Am. Heart J.,* 1966, *71,* 297; D. T. Nash, *J. clin. Pharmac.,* 1968, *8,* 259; T. Shimamoto *et al., Am. Heart J.,* 1970, *79,* 5; H. Yamazaki *et al., ibid.,* 640; A. Zelikovsky *et al., Jap. Heart J.,* 1973, *14,* 12; T. G. Judge, *Practitioner,* 1974, *213,* 10; A. Gulyás and I. Szám, *Therapia hung.,* 1976, *24,* 63; L. Hunyi, *ibid.,* 67; J. Bédi *et al., ibid.,* 91.

Pharmacokinetic studies of pyridinolcarbamate: R. Mallein *et al., Thérapie,* 1973, *28,* 115; R. Mallein *et al., ibid.,* 129; J. Sassard *et al., J. pharm. Sci.,* 1979, *68,* 1190.

Platelet hyper-aggregation was reduced in patients with damaged blood vessel walls receiving pyridinolcarbamate.— R. J. Prost-Djovakovic *et al., Thérapie,* 1975, *30,* 429. See also A. Girolami *et al., Arzneimittel-Forsch.,* 1977, *27,* 1202.

Reports of liver damage associated with the use of pyridinolcarbamate.— *Japan med. Gaz.,* 1976, *13* (Sept. 20), 8; Y. Litvin *et al.* (letter), *Lancet,* 1977, *1,* 1257.

Proprietary Names
Anginin *(Banyu, Jap.; Teva, Israel)*; Angioxil *(FIRMA, Ital.)*; Angioxine *(Roussel, Fr.)*; Aterofal *(Nativelle, Ital.)*; Aterosan *(Lancet, Ital.)*; Atrombogen *(Migra, Arg.)*; Cicloven *(AGIPS, Ital.)*; Colesterinex *(Prodes, Spain; Galenica, Switz.)*; Duaxol *(Argentia, Arg.)*; Exibral *(Marxer, Arg.)*; Movecil *(Carlo Erba, Ital.)*; Prodectin *(Gedeon Richter, Hung.)*; Ravenil *(Caber, Ital.)*; Tripsix *(Landó, Arg.)*; Vasagin *(Sidus, Ital.)*; Vasapril *(Cifa, Ital.)*; Vasocil *(Magis, Ital.)*; Vasoverin *(Banyu, Switz.)*; Acesterol, Angio-Reder, Aterograso, Aterollano, Ateronova, Carbatona, Dual-Xol, Duvaline, Gasparol, Idobernal, Katrombin, Plavolex, Veranterol *(all Spain).*

13192-s

Pyrisuccideanol Maleate. 2-Dimethylaminoethyl 5-hydroxy-4-hydroxymethyl-6-methyl-3-pyridylmethyl succinate maleate.
$C_{16}H_{24}N_2O_6,(C_4H_4O_4)_2$=572.5.

CAS — 33605-94-6 (pyrisuccideanol); 53659-00-0 (maleate).

Pyrisuccideanol is the succinic acid ester of pyridoxine (see p.1642) and of deanol (see p.1700).

Pyrisuccideanol has been used as the maleate in the treatment of cerebrovascular and similar disorders.

Proprietary Names
Mentis *(Menarini, Ital.)*; Stivane *(Beaufour, Fr.; IBYS, Spain).*

13193-w

Pyrithidium Bromide *(B.P. Vet.).* RD-2801; Pyritidium Bromide. 3-Amino-8-(2-amino-1,6-dimethylpyrimidinium-4-ylamino)-6-(4-aminophenyl)-5-methylphenanthridinium dibromide.
$C_{26}H_{27}Br_2N_7$=597.4.

CAS — 3616-05-5 (pyrithidium); 14222-46-9 (bromide).

A brick-red to reddish-purple, odourless or almost odourless, hygroscopic powder. It loses not more than 10% of its weight on drying. **Soluble** 1 in 40 of water and 1 in 1900 of alcohol. A 2% suspension in water has a pH of 4 to 7. **Store** in airtight containers.

Pyrithidium bromide is used in veterinary medicine as a trypanocide in cattle.

13194-e

Pyritinol Hydrochloride. Pyrithioxine Hydrochloride. 3,3′-Dithiodimethylenebis(5-hydroxy-6-methyl-4-pyridylmethanol) dihydrochloride monohydrate.
$C_{16}H_{20}N_2O_4S_2,2HCl,H_2O = 459.4$.

CAS — 1098-97-1 (pyritinol); 10049-83-9 (hydrochloride, anhydrous).

Pyritinol hydrochloride is claimed to promote the uptake of glucose by the brain and has been used in the treatment of various cerebrovascular disorders. It has been given by mouth in doses of 300 to 600 mg daily; it has also been given by intravenous infusion in doses of 200 to 400 mg daily.

A review of the treatment of senile dementia with various drugs, including pyritinol.— J. A. Yesavage *et al.*, *Archs gen. Psychiat.*, 1979, *36*, 220.

Patients with organic brain disorders based on disturbed cerebral glucose metabolism improved after treatment with pyritinol hydrochloride 900 mg by mouth or 1 g by intravenous infusion daily for an average of 3 weeks.— S. Hoyer *et al.*, *Arzneimittel-Forsch.*, 1977, *27*, 671.

References to the cerebral effects of pyritinol hydrochloride and it use in various cerebral vascular disorders: E. Stoica *et al.*, *Eur. Neurol.*, 1972, *7*, 348 (cerebral infarct); C. Fehling-Joss, *Clin. Trials J.*, 1974, *11*, 123 (dyslexia); G. Logue *et al.*, *S. Afr. med. J.*, 1974, *48*, 2245 (behavioural disorders in children); D. J. L. O'Kelly, *J. int. med. Res.*, 1975, *3*, 323 (chronic alcoholism); J. Glatzel, *Medsche Klin.*, 1976, *71*, 1958 (various psychopathological syndromes); Z. Bystřický *et al.*, *Medsche Welt, Stuttg.*, 1977, *28*, 643 (brain contusion); W. Hamouz, *Pharmatherapeutica*, 1977, *1*, 398 (senile dementia); H. Herrschaft, *Münch. med. Wschr.*, 1978, *120*, 1263 (acute cerebral ischaemia); Y. Tazaki *et al.*, *J. int. med. Res.*, 1980, *8*, 118 (various cerebrovascular disorders).

Further references: L. Davies, *S. Afr. pharm. J.*, 1964, *31* (Dec.), 26; K. Becker and S. Hoyer, *Dt. Z. Nerv-Heilk.*, 1966, *188*, 200, per *Abstr. Wld Med.*, 1966, *40*, 209; W. Darge *et al.*, *Arzneimittel-Forsch.*, 1969, *19*, 9.

Pyritinol was associated with hepatitis in 1 patient.— S. Imoto *et al.* (letter), *Ann. intern. Med.*, 1979, *91*, 129.

Proprietary Names
Biocefalin, Cefalogen, Cerebropirina, Cerebrotrofina, Cervitalin, Encebrovit, Encefabol, Encefort, Encerebron, Fulneurina, Leonar, Life, Maind, Musa, Scintidin, Tonobrein, Tonomentis *(all Ital.)*; Bonifen *(Igoda, Spain)*; Divalvon-D, Enbol, Neuroxin, Piritiomin *(all Jap.)*; Encephabol *(Merck, Aust.; E. Merck, Austral.; Merck, Belg.; E. Merck, Ger.; E. Merck, Neth.; Merck, S.Afr.; E. Merck, Switz.)*; Encéphabol *(Merck-Clévenot, Fr.)*; Epocan *(Merck, Arg.)*.

13195-l

Pyrovalerone. F-1983 (hydrochloride). 4′-Methyl-2-(pyrrolidin-1-yl)valerophenone.
$C_{16}H_{23}NO = 245.4$.

CAS — 3563-49-3 (pyrovalerone); 1147-62-2 (hydrochloride).

Pyrovalerone is a central stimulant which has been used in asthenia, reactive depression, and for the relief of drug-induced lethargy.

A report of the abuse of pyrovalerone.— E. Fournier *et al.*, *Thérapie*, 1976, *31*, 557.

Further references: G. Gardos and J. O. Cole, *Curr. ther. Res.*, 1971, *13*, 631.

13196-y

Quazepam. Sch-16134. 7-Chloro-5-(2-fluorophenyl)-1,3-dihydro-1-(2,2,2-trifluoroethyl)-2*H*-1,4-benzodiazepine-2-thione.
$C_{17}H_{11}ClF_4N_2S = 386.8$.

CAS — 36735-22-5.

Quazepam is a benzodiazepine (see Diazepam, p.1519), used as a hypnotic.

References: F. R. Freemon *et al.*, *J. clin. Pharmac.*, 1977, *17*, 398; E. I. Tietz *et al.*, *Curr. ther. Res.*, 1979, *26*, 894; T. Roth *et al.*, *J. int. med. Res.*, 1979, *7*, 583; A. Kales *et al.*, *J. clin. Pharmac.*, 1980, *20*, 184; M. Mamelak *et al.*, *Curr. ther. Res.*, 1981, *29*, 135; A. Kales *et al.*, *Clin. Pharmac. Ther.*, 1981, *30*, 194; H. K. Uhthoff *et al.*, *J. int. med. Res.*, 1981, *9*, 288.

Manufacturers
Schering, UK.

13197-j

Quinalbital. Chinalbital.
$C_{20}H_{26}N_2O_2,C_{11}H_{18}N_2O_3 = 552.7$.

Quinalbital is the hydroquinidine salt of amylobarbitone and has been used in the treatment of cardiac disorders.

Proprietary Names
Amoquine *(Houde, Belg.)*; Amosedil *(Roussel Maestretti, Ital.)*.

13198-z

Quinbolone. 17β-(Cyclopent-1-enyloxy)androsta-1,4-dien-3-one.
$C_{24}H_{32}O_2 = 352.5$.

CAS — 2487-63-0.

Quinbolone is an anabolic agent.

Proprietary Names
Anabolicum *(Vister, Ital.)*.

13199-c

Quincarbate. DU-23187. Ethyl 10-chloro-3-ethoxymethyl-2,3,6,9-tetrahydro-9-oxo-*p*-dioxino-[2,3-*g*]quinoline-8-carboxylate.
$C_{17}H_{18}ClNO_6 = 367.8$.

CAS — 54340-59-9.

Quincarbate is a diuretic with natriuretic properties.

References: J. van Dijk *et al.*, *J. med. Chem.*, 1976, *19*, 982.

Manufacturers
Duphar, Neth.

13200-c

Quindoxin. ICI-8173. Quinoxaline 1,4-dioxide.
$C_8H_6N_2O_2 = 162.1$.

CAS — 2423-66-7.

Quindoxin is a growth promoter formerly used in pigs and poultry.

Five patients developed contact eczema after handling animal meals containing quindoxin. All gave strong reactions to patch tests.— T. A. J. Dawson and K. W. Scott (letter), *Br. med. J.*, 1972, *3*, 469.

As a result of the development of tumours of the nose and liver in *animals* fed with quindoxin (Grofas) at a level of intake far higher than would be absorbed by humans or farm animals, *ICI Pharmaceuticals* had withdrawn the product in order to protect subjects who handled the product in concentrated form.— *Pharm. J.*, 1973, *2*, 237.

13201-k

Quinine and Urea Hydrochloride *(B.P.C. 1949)*. Carbamidated Quinine Dihydrochloride; Chininum Dihydrochloricum Carbamidatum; Urea-Quinine.
$C_{20}H_{24}N_2O_2,CH_4N_2O,2HCl,5H_2O = 547.5$.

CAS — 549-52-0 (anhydrous).

Pharmacopoeias. In *Arg.*, *Mex.*, and *Port.*

White odourless crystals or powder with a bitter taste. **Soluble** 1 in 1 of water and 1 in 3 of alcohol. A solution in water is acid to litmus; a 4.5% solution in water is iso-osmotic with serum. Solutions are **sterilised** by autoclaving or by filtration. **Protect** from light.

Quinine and urea hydrochloride was formerly used as a local anaesthetic, especially following rectal operations. It has also been administered intramuscularly for the therapeutic actions of quinine.

13202-a

Quinine Ascorbate. Quinine Biascorbate. A compound (2 : 1) of ascorbic acid with quinine.
$C_{20}H_{24}N_2O_2,2C_6H_8O_6 = 673.7$.

CAS — 146-40-7.

Quinine ascorbate has been used as a smoking deterrent.

13203-t

Quinizarin-2,6-disulphonic Acid. 9,10-Dihydro-1,4-dihydroxy-9,10-dioxoanthracene-2,6-disulphonic acid.
$C_{14}H_8O_{10}S_2 = 400.3$.

CAS — 81-64-1 (quinizarin); 1337-62-8 (disulphonic acid).

Quinizarin-2,6-disulphonic acid is the active constituent of Quinizarin Compound, which also contains anhydrous sodium carbonate as a desiccant and maize starch as a diluent. The usual proportions are quinizarin-2,6-disulphonic acid 28%, anhydrous sodium carbonate 24%, maize starch 48%. The resulting mixture is a reddish-grey fine powder which may become blue-grey after storage.

When moistened, Quinizarin Compound powder has a dark violet colour and this reaction is used to determine the pattern of sweat secretion as a diagnostic aid in nerve damage, and in dermatological and endocrinological investigations. The powder is applied to the skin but in special investigations it may first be mixed with olive oil or liquid paraffin. The powder should not be allowed to enter the eyes or nose. Quinizarin Compound can be removed with soap and warm water and, if necessary, weak acetic acid solution or vinegar.

Quinizarin Compound applied on cellulose tape as a test of sudomotor function in leprosy.— A. B. A. Karat *et al.*, *Lancet*, 1969, *1*, 651.

13204-x

Quinupramine. LM-208. 10,11-Dihydro-5-(quinuclidin-3-yl)-5*H*-dibenz[*b,f*]azepine.
$C_{21}H_{24}N_2 = 304.4$.

CAS — 31721-17-2.

Quinupramine is a tricyclic antidepressant.

Proprietary Names
Kevopril *(Pharmuka, Belg.)*; Kinupril *(Fournier Frères, Fr.)*.

13205-r

Quinuronium Sulphate *(B. Vet. C. 1965)*. Quinolyl Urea. 6,6′-Ureylenebis(1-methylquinolinium) bis(methyl sulphate).
$C_{23}H_{26}N_4O_9S_2 = 566.6$.

CAS — 135-14-8.

A creamy-white to canary-yellow odourless crystalline powder with a bitter taste. Very **soluble** in water; very slightly soluble in organic solvents. A 5% solution in water has a pH of 2 to 3.5. On heating, aqueous solutions darken and some decomposition may occur.

Quinuronium sulphate is used in veterinary medicine for the treatment of babesiasis.

A review of the pharmacological effects of quinuronium and a comparison with amicarbalide.— P. Eyre, *J. Pharm. Pharmac.*, 1967, *19*, 509.

Proprietary Names
Ludobal *(Bayer Agrochem, UK)*; Pirevan V *(Evans Medical, UK)*.

13206-f

Rafoxanide *(B.P. Vet.)*. MK-990. 3′-Chloro-4′-(4-chlorophenoxy)-3,5-di-iodosalicylanilide.
$C_{19}H_{11}Cl_2I_2NO_3$=626.0.

CAS — 22662-39-1.

A greyish-white to brown powder. M.p. about 175°. Practically **insoluble** in water; soluble 1 in 25 of acetone, 1 in 40 of chloroform, 1 in 35 of ethyl acetate, and 1 in 200 of methyl alcohol. **Protect** from light.

Rafoxanide is used for the treatment and control of liver fluke in sheep and cattle.

Proprietary Names
Flukanide *(Merck Sharp & Dohme, UK)*.

13207-d

Raspberry Leaf *(B.P.C. 1949)*. Rubi Idaei Folium. The dried leaflets of *Rubus idaeus* (Rosaceae).

Raspberry leaf contains a principle, readily extracted with hot water, which relaxes the smooth muscle of the uterus and intestine of some *animals*.
Raspberry 'tea' has been a traditional remedy for painful and profuse menstruation and for use before and during confinement. The infusion has also been used as an astringent gargle.

13208-n

Relaxin. A polypeptide hormone extracted from the corpus luteum of the ovaries of pregnant sows. It is reported to be related structurally to insulin and has a molecular weight of about 6000.

CAS — 9002-69-1.

Relaxin acts on connective tissue, including collagen, and causes relaxation of the pubic symphysis and softening of the uterine cervix. In many *animal* species it appears to play a major part in cervical ripening before parturition. Relaxin is secreted by the human corpus luteum during pregnancy although its role has not been established. Early clinical studies with impure extracts given parenterally or orally produced conflicting results. More recently a purified porcine relaxin preparation, used intravaginally in obstetric patients, induced cervical changes in the majority of patients.
Relaxin was formerly tried in the treatment of collagen diseases.

In a double-blind study 30 women were given 2 mg of intravaginal purified porcine relaxin in a viscous gel on the evening before surgical induction of labour, while 30 similar women received the gel alone. Ten of the 30 women given relaxin went into labour before the proposed induction whereas none of the 30 control women did so. Twenty-five of the 30 women treated with relaxin had improved cervical scores after treatment and significantly fewer required intravenous oxytocin than those in the control group. No side-effects were experienced by the patients receiving relaxin and no neonatal complications were recorded. Relaxin 2 mg intravaginally appears to be at least as safe and effective as dinoprost 25 mg intravaginally and, in this study, labour was significantly shorter than in the control group.— A. H. MacLennan *et al.*, *Lancet*, 1980, *1*, 220.

Further references: G. Weiss *et al.*, *Science*, 1976, *194*, 948; R. James *et al.*, *Nature*, 1977, *267*, 544; S. Bedarkar *et al.*, *ibid.*, *270*, 449.

For earlier reports on the use of relaxin, see Martindale 27th Edn, p. 1807.

13209-h

Reserpiline Hydrochloride. Methyl 16,17-didehydro-10,11-dimethoxy-19α-methyl-3β,20α-oxayohimban-16-carboxylate hydrochloride.
$C_{23}H_{28}N_2O_5$,HCl=448.9.

CAS — 131-02-2 (reserpiline); 63647-55-2 (hydrochloride).

Reserpiline is an alkaloid derived from *Rauwolfia serpentina*. The hydrochloride has been used as an antihypertensive agent.

Proprietary Names
Grona *(Llorens, Spain)*; Redouline *(Roterpharma, Belg.)*.

13210-a

Rhus *(B.P.C. 1934)*. Sumach Berries. The dried fruits of the smooth or Pennsylvanian sumach, *Rhus glabra* (Anacardiaceae).

Rhus has astringent and reputed diuretic properties. Poison ivy (*Rhus radicans*) and poison oak (*R. toxicodendron*), species growing in the USA, are irritant poisons producing severe contact dermatitis. Extracts of poison ivy and poison oak have been used for the prophylaxis of poison ivy dermatitis but their effectiveness has not been proved.
Poison oak is used in homoeopathic medicine.

Five patients who were exquisitely sensitive to *Rhus* antigen developed a generalised eczematous dermatitis after eating large amounts of unroasted cashew nuts. Raw cashew nuts sold in organic food stores contained appreciable amounts of cashew-nut shell oil on their surfaces; this oil was antigenically similar to *Rhus* oleoresin and would cause a generalised eruption when ingested in large quantities by subjects highly sensitive to *Rhus* antigen.— J. H. Ratner *et al.*, *Archs Derm.*, 1974, *110*, 921, per *J. Am. med. Ass.*, 1974, *230*, 1744.

13211-t

Ribonuclease. RNAase.

CAS — 9001-99-4.

An enzyme present in most mammalian tissue, with optimum activity at pH 7 to 8; mol. wt about 13 000. It has been synthesised.

Ribonuclease is involved in the catalytic cleavage of ribonucleic acid. It has been used in ointments in the treatment of traumatic and articular pain.

A favourable report of the use of ribonuclease in tick-borne encephalitis.— B. M. Gluchov *et al.*, *Zh. Nevropat. Psikhiat.*, 1968, *68*, 361, per *Abstr. Wld Med.*, 1968, *42*, 838.

15326-d

Ribonucleic Acid. Ribose Nucleic Acid; RNA; ARN; Yeast Nucleic Acid; Plant Nucleic Acid.

Pharmacopoeias. In *Fr.*

A nucleotide polymer, and 1 of the 2 distinct varieties of nucleic acid (see p.1735). It is found in the cytoplasm and in small amounts in the cell nuclei of living tissues. It can be extracted from beer or bread yeast.
A white or slightly cream powder containing not less than 14.5% of nitrogen and 9% of phosphorus calculated with reference to the dried substance.
Practically **insoluble** in water and organic solvents; freely soluble in alkaline solutions.

Ribonucleic acid has been tried in the treatment of mental retardation and to improve memory and proprietary preparations containing various salts of ribonucleic acid have been advocated for a variety of asthenic and convalescent conditions.

References: S. Zimányi *et al.* (letter), *Lancet*, 1962, *2*, 1283; S. DeCarvalho, *Nature*, 1963, *197*, 1077; W. Dingman and M. B. Sporn, *Science*, 1964, *144*, 26; K. Wolff, *J. Am. Geriat. Soc.*, 1964, *12*, 226; B. F. Brown, *Sci. Horiz.*, 1967, (May), 13.

13213-r

Ricin. A highly toxic albuminoid protein present in castor seeds, the seeds of *Ricinus communis* (Euphorbiaceae) from which castor oil (see p.695) is obtained.

CAS — 9009-86-3.

NOTE. The title ricin is used for the castor seed in *Fr. P.*

Ricin is extremely toxic and the fatal dose by intravenous injection in experimental *animals* has been reported to be as low as 300 ng per kg body-weight. It has been used in chemical warfare.
Ingestion of castor seeds has proved fatal and signs and symptoms of poisoning are similar to those described for Abrus seeds (p.1673). After expression of the oil from castor seed, the ricin remains in the seed cake or 'pomace', which is subjected to steam treatment to destroy the ricin. The detoxified pomace is used as a fertiliser.

A review of the literature on ricin poisoning and a report of an extensive investigation of ricin poisoning in port workers while handling cargoes of castor pomace that had not been subjected to heat treatment.— W. C. Cooper *et al.*, *Am. ind. Hyg. Ass. J.*, 1964, *25*, 431, per *Bull. Hyg., Lond.*, 1965, *40*, 457.

Inhibition of tumour growth in *animals* by ricin.— J. Lin *et al.*, *Nature*, 1970, *227*, 292.

A 57-year-old man suffered acute ricin intoxication after chewing a single castor bean. For a brief period he felt a sensation of burning in the mouth and throat, then collapsed and was in shock when admitted to hospital. He recovered in 2½ hours after symptomatic treatment with adrenaline, calcium, metaraminol, and infusions of electrolyte solutions and dextran 40.— J. Kingma, *Ned. Tijdschr. Geneesk.*, 1971, *115*, (July 10), per *Int. pharm. Abstr.*, 1972, *9*, 43.

A discussion of the toxic effects of ricin and of its use for political assassination.— B. Knight, *Br. med. J.*, 1979, *1*, 350.

13214-f

Rimazolium Methylsulphate. Rimazolium Metilsulfate; MZ-144. 3-Ethoxycarbonyl-6,7,8,9-tetrahydro-1,6-dimethyl-4-oxo-4*H*-pyrido-[1,2-*a*]pyrimidinium methyl sulphate.
$C_{14}H_{22}N_2O_7S$=362.4.

CAS — 35615-72-6 (rimazolium); 28610-84-6 (methylsulphate).

Rimazolium methylsulphate is reported to have analgesic properties.

References: M. Haataja *et al.*, *Curr. ther. Res.*, 1977, *22*, 784; M. Haataja and H. Saarimaa, *ibid.*, 1978, *23*, 277; M. Haataja *et al.*, *ibid.*, *24*, 284; S. Fink and K. O. Nielsen, *ibid.*, 900; E. Ihasz, *Therapia hung.*, 1980, *28*, 22.

Proprietary Names
Dolcuran *(Szabó, Arg.)*; Probon *(Chinoin, Hung.)*; Rimagin *(Fin.)*.

13215-d

Ro-15-1788. Ethyl 8-fluoro-5,6-dihydro-5-methyl-6-oxo-4*H*-imidazo[1,5-*a*][1,4]benzodiazepine-3-carboxylate.
$C_{15}H_{14}FN_3O_3$=303.3.

Ro-15-1788 is reported to antagonise the CNS effects of benzodiazepines.

References: W. Hunkeler *et al.*, *Nature*, 1981, *290*, 514; A. Darragh *et al.*, *Lancet*, 1981, *2*, 8; *idem*, 1042.

Manufacturers
Roche, Switz.

13216-n

Robenidine Hydrochloride. Robenzidene Hydrochloride; CL-78116. 1,3-Bis(4-chlorobenzylideneamino)guanidine hydrochloride.
$C_{15}H_{13}Cl_2N_5,HCl=370.7$.

CAS — 25875-51-8 (robenidine); 25875-50-7 (hydrochloride).

A white crystalline powder. M.p. about 289°

Robenidine hydrochloride is used in veterinary practice as a coccidiostat for poultry.

Proprietary Names
Robenz *(American Cyanamid, USA).*

13217-h

Rociverine. LG-30158. 2-Diethylamino-1-methylethyl *cis*-1-hydroxy(bicyclohexyl)-2-carboxylate.
$C_{20}H_{37}NO_3=339.5$.

CAS — 53716-44-2.

Rociverine has been used in spastic disorders of the gastro-intestinal and urinary tracts, and as an aid to endoscopy.

References: M. Laudi and G. Fontana, *Farmaco, Edn prat.*, 1979, *34*, 553; A. Manganelli, *Farmaco, Edn prat.*, 1979, *34*, 384.

Proprietary Names
Rilaten *(Guidotti, Ital.).*

13218-m

Rolipram. ZK-62711. 4-(3-Cyclopentyloxy-4-methoxyphenyl)pyrrolidin-2-one.
$C_{16}H_{21}NO_3=275.3$.

CAS — 61413-54-5.

Rolipram is reported to have neuroleptic activity.

Manufacturers
Schering, Ger.

13219-b

Ronidazole. (1-Methyl-5-nitroimidazol-2-yl)methyl carbamate.
$C_6H_8N_4O_4=200.2$.

CAS — 7681-76-7.

Ronidazole is an antiprotozoal agent used in veterinary medicine for the treatment of swine dysentery. It has also been added to turkey feeding stuffs.

Experimental comparison with metronidazole.— A. C. Cuckler *et al.*, *Am. J. trop. Med. Hyg.*, 1970, *19*, 916, per *Trop. Dis. Bull.*, 1971, *68*, 816.

Proprietary Names
Ridzol *(Merck Sharp & Dohme, UK).*

13220-x

Roxarsone. NSC-2101. 4-Hydroxy-3-nitrophenylarsonic acid.
$C_6H_6AsNO_6=263.0$.

CAS — 121-19-7.

Roxarsone is used as a growth promoter in animal feeds. The monosodium salt has also been used for the control of swine dysentery.

Manufacturers
Salsbury, UK.

13221-r

Royal Jelly. Queen Bee Jelly. A milky-white viscid secretion from the salivary glands of the worker hive bee, *Apis mellifera* (Apidae); it is essential for the development of queen bees.

It is a complex mixture of proteins, amino acids, lipids, carbohydrates, fatty acids, and vitamins (particularly pantothenic acid). One constituent is 10-hydroxydec-2-enoic acid, which has antimicrobial properties.

Royal jelly has been used as a general 'tonic', to ward off the effects of old age, and to ease sufferers from chronic degenerative diseases, but of the many and diverse claims made for the therapeutic value of the jelly, none has been substantiated.

Royal jelly is also incorporated in some cosmetic preparations for its supposed beneficial effect on skin tissue.

References: *Br. med. J.*, 1957, *1*, 1136; *Drug Cosmet. Ind.*, 1957, *81*, 452; M. S. Blum *et al.*, *Science*, 1959, *130*, 452; A. H. Dayan, *J. Pharm. Pharmac.*, 1960, *12*, 377.

15304-k

Rutin. Rutoside. 2-(3,4-Dihydroxyphenyl)-3,5,7-trihydroxy-4-oxo-4*H*-chromen-3-yl rutinoside trihydrate.
$C_{27}H_{30}O_{16},3H_2O=664.6$.

CAS — 153-18-4 (anhydrous).

Pharmacopoeias. In *Aust.*, *Belg.*, *Braz.*, *Ger.*, *Hung.*, *Pol.*, *Roum.*, *Rus.*, and *Swiss.*

A greenish-yellow, tasteless, microcrystalline powder obtained from buckwheat, *Fagopyrum esculentum* (Polygonaceae), or from other sources which include the flower buds of the Chinese pagoda-tree, *Sophora japonica*, and the leaves of several species of *Eucalyptus*. **Soluble** 1 in 10 000 of water and 1 in 650 of alcohol; soluble in isopropyl alcohol, methyl alcohol, pyridine, and solutions of alkali hydroxides; practically insoluble in chloroform and ether. **Incompatible** with acids and salts of heavy metals. **Protect** from light.

The stability of rutin in alkaline solutions was very limited; decomposition occurred within a few days. Stabilised solutions should not be used after 1 year.— E. Winde, *Dt. ApothZtg.*, 1977, *117*, 2138. See also R. Reingraber, *ibid.*, 1978, *118*, 1279.

Rutin or rutin-like moieties were possibly contained in a tobacco glycoprotein, with allergenic and thrombogenic potential, present in cured tobacco leaves or cigarette smoke condensates.— *J. Am. med. Ass.*, 1978, *239*, 1476.

Rutin has been used in the treatment of disease states characterised by capillary bleeding associated with increased capillary fragility but evidence of its value is inconclusive.

At usual therapeutic doses rutin improved colour vision.— J. Laroche and C. Laroche, *Annls pharm. fr.*, 1977, *35*, 173.

Preparations

Tabulettae Rutini *(Rus. P.).* Rutin Tablets. Each contains rutin 20 mg.

Proprietary Names
Birutan *(E. Merck, Ger.)*; Lifaton-P *(Lifasa, Spain)*; Neorutin *(Neomed, Switz.)*; Pecitrol *(Ferran, Spain)*; Permol *(UCB-Pevya, Spain)*; Rutinion *(Rhein-Pharma, Ger.).*

13223-d

Saramycetin. X-5079C; Ro-2-7758. An antimicrobial polypeptide produced by the growth of a species of *Streptomyces*.

CAS — 11130-70-4.

Saramycetin has antifungal properties and was formerly tried in various systemic fungal infections.

13224-n

Scoparium *(B.P.C. 1949).* Broom Tops; Scoparii Cacumina; Planta Genista; Genêt; Genêt à Balai. The dried tops of broom, *Sarothamnus scoparius* (=*Cytisus scoparius*) (Leguminosae).

Pharmacopoeias. In *Fr.*

Scoparium is a mild diuretic and has been administered as a decoction or infusion.

13225-h

Sebacic Acid. Decanedioic acid; Octane-1,8-dicarboxylic acid.
$C_{10}H_{18}O_4=202.2$.

CAS — 111-20-6.

Leaflets or a white powder with a mild fatty-acid odour. M.p. 133° to 135°. **Soluble** 1 in 1000 of water and of ether; freely soluble in alcohol; sparingly soluble in hydrocarbons.

Sebacic acid is an emollient included in preparations used to protect damaged skin.

Diisopropyl sebacate ($C_{16}H_{30}O_4$ = 286.4) is used as a skin moisturising agent.

13226-m

Seclazone. W-2354. 7-Chloro-3,3a-dihydro-2*H*,9*H*-isoxazolo[3,2-*b*][1,3]benzoxazin-9-one.
$C_{10}H_8ClNO_3=225.6$.

CAS — 29050-11-1.

Seclazone is an anti-inflammatory compound with uricosuric properties.

References: A. Jain and H. Hoyt, *Clin. Pharmac. Ther.*, 1972, *13*, 141; J. Edelson *et al.*, *J. pharm. Sci.*, 1973, *62*, 229; N. B. Banerjee *et al.*, *Toxic. appl. Pharmac.*, 1973, *25*, 444.

13227-b

Secnidazole. PM-185184; RP-14539. 1-(2-Methyl-5-nitroimidazol-1-yl)propan-2-ol.
$C_7H_{11}N_3O_3=185.2$.

CAS — 3366-95-8.

Secnidazole is closely related structurally to metronidazole, but is reported to have a longer half-life. It has been used in amoebiasis and trichomoniasis.

Use in amoebiasis.— L. J. Andre and G. Charmot, *Méd. trop. Marseille*, 1973, *33*, 311, per *Trop. Dis. Bull.*, 1974, *71*, 150.

Use in trichomoniasis.— D. Videau *et al.*, *Br. J. vener. Dis.*, 1978, *54*, 77.

Activity *in vitro* against *Bacteroides fragilis*.— J. Symonds (letter), *J. antimicrob. Chemother.*, 1979, *5*, 484.

Proprietary Names
Flagentyl.

13228-v

Selegiline Hydrochloride. (−)-(*R*)-*N*,α-Dimethyl-*N*-(prop-2-ynyl)phenethylamine hydrochloride.
$C_{13}H_{17}N,HCl=223.7$.

CAS — 14611-51-9 (selegiline); 14611-52-0 (hydrochloride).

NOTE. Synonyms used in the literature are confusing and include (−)-Deprenil, L-Deprenil, Deprenyl, (−)-Deprenyl, L-Deprenyl, L-Deprenaline, E-250. It is the (−)-isomer which is active.

Selegiline is an inhibitor of monoamine oxidase type B. It has been given with levodopa and decarboxylase inhibitors in the treatment of parkinsonism and has been tried in depression. It is reported not to interact with tyramine in food.

Use with levodopa, and sometimes a decarboxylase inhibitor, in parkinsonism.— L. Ambrozi *et al.*, *Br. J. Pharmac.*, 1976, *58*, 423P; W. Birkmayer *et al.*, *Lancet*, 1977, *1*, 439; A. J. Lees *et al.*, *ibid.*, *2*, 791; W. Birkmayer, *J. neural Transmission*, 1978, *43*, 239; M.

Streifler *et al.*, *Curr. ther. Res.*, 1980, *27*, 643; M. Schachter *et al.*, *J. Neurol. Neurosurg. Psychiat.*, 1980, *43*, 1016; P. Reiderer and G. P. Reynolds (letter), *Br. J. clin. Pharmac.*, 1980, *9*, 98; T. Eisler *et al.*, *Neurology, Minneap.*, 1981, *31*, 19.

Use in depression.— J. Mendlewicz and M. B. H. Youdim, *J. Affect. Dis.*, 1980, *2*, 137; N. Mendis *et al.*, *Psychopharmacology*, 1981, *73*, 87.

Further references: J. Mendlewicz and M. B. H. Youdim (letter), *Lancet*, 1977, *2*, 507; J. D. Elsworth *et al.*, *Psychopharmacology*, 1978, *57*, 33; G. P. Reynolds *et al.* (letter), *Br. J. clin. Pharmac.*, 1978, *6*, 542; M. Schachter *et al.* (letter), *Lancet*, 1979, *1*, 831.

Proprietary Names
Jumex *(Chinoin, Hung.)*.

13229-g

Senecio

Many species of the genus *Senecio* (Compositae), which includes the ragworts and groundsels, are poisonous and have been found to contain pyrrolizidine alkaloids which produce hepatic necrosis. The ragwort, *S. jacobaea*, which is abundant throughout the British Isles, is poisonous to livestock when eaten in quantity.

The ragwort and, in the USA, the golden ragwort, *Senecio aureus*, in the form of extracts have been used as emmenagogues but are of doubtful value. Ragwort, in the form of a decoction or ointment, has also been applied externally to aid wound healing.

Two alkaloids, senecionine and senecionine *N*-oxide were isolated from *Senecio triangularis*, growing in Colorado, USA. They inhibited growth of a carcinosarcoma in *mice* and this could be an explanation for the ancient use of *Senecio* spp. in the treatment of cancer.— S. M. Kupchan and M. I. Suffness (letter), *J. pharm. Sci.*, 1967, *56*, 541.

Toxicity. An extensive review of the toxicity of pyrrolizidine alkaloids present in *Senecio* spp. and other plants.— E. K. McLean, *Pharmac. Rev.*, 1970, *22*, 429.

The oral administration of ragwort, which contained 6 pyrrolizidine alkaloids, to *rats* produced hypertensive pulmonary vascular disease.— J. M. Kay *et al.*, *Thorax*, 1971, *26*, 262, per *Drugs*, 1972, *4*, 301.

A report of liver damage and death associated with a herbal tea (Gordolobos) prepared from *Senecio longilobus* in Arizona, USA.— R. Huxtable, *J. Am. med. Ass.*, 1977, *238*, 1233. See also A. E. Stillman *et al.*, *Gastroenterology*, 1977, *73*, 349; A. E. Stillman *et al.* (letter), *Br. J. clin. Pharmac.*, 1977, *26*, 257, per *Int. pharm. Abstr.*, 1978, *15*, 260.

Further references: D. W. Fox *et al.*, *J. Pediat.*, 1978, *93*, 980.

13230-f

Sepia. The dried inky secretion of the cuttle fish.

Sepia is used in homoeopathic medicine.

13231-d

Serendipity Berry. The fruit of *Dioscoreophyllum cumminsii* (Menispermaceae).

Serendipity berries contain a water-soluble proteinaceous sweet principle, many times sweeter than sucrose, but labile to heat.

References: H. van der Wel, *Symposium: Sweeteners*, G.E. Inglett (Ed.), Westport, IVA, 1974, p. 194.

15305-a

Serotonin. Enteramine; 5-Hydroxytryptamine; 5-HT. 3-(2-Aminoethyl)-1*H*-indol-5-ol.
$C_{10}H_{12}N_2O$=176.2.

CAS — 50-67-9.

Serotonin is widely distributed in the body; it also occurs in stinging nettles (*Urtica dioica*), bananas, and other fruit.

Serotonin is released by tryptaminergic neurones in the central nervous system, where it is believed to act as a neurotransmitter, and to be involved in the transmission of nervous impulses and in the control of the tone of the viscera. Serotonin is stored and synthesised mainly in enterochromaffin cells and in neurones and is also stored in blood platelets. It is considered to be implicated in causing the vascular headache of migraine; support for this view has been gained by the relief often obtained from the use of serotonin antagonists, such as methysergide and cyproheptadine. Serotonin has been suggested for use in the treatment of depression but as it does not pass the blood-brain barrier adequately, its precursor 5-hydroxytryptophan (see p.1718) has been used.

Cardiac lesions have been found in patients with carcinoid tumours producing excessive amounts of serotonin, and endomyocardial fibrosis has been reported prevalent amongst Nigerians eating large quantities of serotonin-rich matoke bananas. Teratogenic effects have been found in *animals* given large amounts of serotonin.

A review of the origin, distribution in the body, physiological effects, and clinical and pharmacological aspects of serotonin.— A. Sirek and O. V. Sirek, *Can. med. Ass. J.*, 1970, *102*, 846. See also G. Bignami, *A. Rev. Pharmac. & Toxic.*, 1976, *16*, 329; A. R. Green and D. G. Grahame-Smith, *Nature*, 1976, *260*, 487.

A discussion on serotonin and psychiatric illness.— *Lancet*, 1981, *2*, 788.

Biochemical studies of serotonin: H. M. van Praag and J. Korf, *Psychopharmacologia*, 1971, *19*, 148 (in depression), per *Abstr. Wld Med.*, 1971, *45*, 616; M. Coleman, *J. Pediat.*, 1971, *78*, 985 (in hyperactive children), per *Abstr. Wld Med.*, 1971, *45*, 880; Y. A. Habib *et al.*, *Acta allerg.*, 1971, *26*, 39 (in nasal allergy), per *Abstr. Wld Med.*, 1971, *45*, 581; D. L. Murphy *et al.*, *Archs Neurol., Chicago*, 1973, *28*, 239 (in muscular dystrophy), per *J. Am. med.Ass.*, 1973, *224*, 261; R. K. Winkelmann *et al.*, *Br. J. Derm.*, 1976, *95*, 51 (in scleroderma and Raynaud's phenomenon); N. C. Tye *et al.*, *Nature*, 1977, *268*, 741 (in conflict behaviour); *Br. med. J.*, 1978, *1*, 1651 (in autism).

Serotonin competitively inhibited cholinesterase *in vitro*.— Y. S. Mohammed *et al.*, *Arzneimittel-Forsch.*, 1975, *25*, 1714.

Serotonin creatinine sulphate was the form of serotonin available for research and clinical use. Vertigo and tachycardia had followed rapid intravenous injection. There was no evidence that it was effective as a haemostatic.— M. Verstraete, *Haemostatic Drugs*, The Hague, Martinus Nijhoff, 1977, p. 68.

13233-h

Serrapeptase. A proteolytic enzyme derived from *Serratia* spp.

Serrapeptase has been used in the treatment of inflammatory disorders.

Proprietary Names
Danzen *(Cyanamid, Ital.)*.

13234-m

Sevoflurane. BAX-3084. Fluoromethyl 2,2,2-trifluoro-1-(trifluoromethyl)ethyl ether.
$C_4H_3F_7O$=200.1.

CAS — 28523-86-6.

Sevoflurane is an inhalation anaesthetic.

Manufacturers
Travenol, USA.

13235-b

Shea Butter. A natural fat obtained from the shea tree *Butyrospermum parkii* (Sapotaceae) indigenous to W. Africa.

It may be purified by hot filtration and decolorisation with activated charcoal. After filtration it yields a yellowish-cream mass, and after decolorisation a white granular mass. M.p. about 38°.

Shea butter is used as an ointment and cream basis.

Physico-chemical properties of shea butter.— H. C. Mital and F. R. Dove, *Planta med.*, 1971, *20*, 283.

References to the properties of creams and ointments prepared with shea butter: H. C. Mital and F. R. Dove, *Drug Cosmet. Ind.*, 1973, *113* (Oct.), 46 (physical properties); H. C. Mital *et al.*, *Pharm. Acta Helv.*, 1974, *49*, 28 (antoxidants; release of medicaments); G. H. Konning and H. C. Mital, *ibid.*, 192 (stability of medicaments); D. O. Gyane, *Drug Cosmet. Ind.*, 1976, *118* (May), 36 (lemon grass oil as a preservative); G. H. Konning and L. B. Acheampong, *ibid.*, 1979, *125* (Dec.), 42 (release of medicaments).

Pharmaceutical and cosmetic applications of creams and ointments prepared from shea butter.— H. C. Mital, *Drug Cosmet. Ind.*, 1977, *120* (May), 30.

Salicylic acid and benzoic acid were released from an ointment basis prepared from shea butter 75%, arachis oil 25%, and hard paraffin 10% at a faster rate than from white soft paraffin *B.P.* or simple ointment *B.P.*— G. H. Konning and H. C. Mital, *J. pharm. Sci.*, 1978, *67*, 374.

Nasal decongestion. Shea butter was an effective nasal decongestant when applied to the nostrils of 21 subjects suffering from allergic rhinitis. The airways cleared within 0.5 to 1.5 minutes of application and remained clear for 5 to 8.5 hours. Xylometazoline 0.1% cleared the nasal airways within 1 minute of application and the effect lasted for 2 to 4.5 hours in 7 similar patients. Shea butter did not irritate the nasal mucosa or cause rebound congestion.— A. Tella, *Br. J. clin. Pharmac.*, 1979, *7*, 495.

13236-v

Silymarin. The active principle from the fruit of *Silybum marianum (=Carduus marianus)* (Compositae). The principal component is the flavonoid silybin.
$C_{25}H_{22}O_{10}$=482.4.

CAS — 65666-07-1 (silymarin); 22888-70-6 (silybin).

Pharmacopoeias. Ger. includes Milk Thistle Fruit, the ripe liberated fruit of *Silybum marianum* containing not less than 1% of silymarin calculated as silybin.

Silymarin has been used for the treatment of hepatic disorders. *Animal* studies have suggested a possible protective role in *Amanita phalloides* poisoning, but clinical evidence is sparse.

Liver function in patients with chronic hepatitis and cholangitis improved after 3 months' therapy with silymarin.— G. Poser, *Arzneimittel-Forsch.*, 1971, *21*, 1209.

Silymarin 420 mg daily was given to 375 patients with cirrhosis. Of 20 followed up for 6 to 36 months 10 were definitely improved and 4 had deteriorated.— I. Benda and W. Zenz, *Wien. med. Wschr.*, 1973, *123*, 512, per *Int. pharm. Abstr.*, 1975, *12*, 58.

The chemistry and active constituents of *Silybum marianum*.— H. Wagner *et al.*, *Arzneimittel-Forsch.*, 1974, *24*, 466; G. Halbach and W. Trost, *ibid.*, 866; I. Morelli, *Boll. chim.-farm.*, 1978, *117*, 258.

A dimer of silybin had 10 times the activity of silybin.— G. Vogel and W. Trost, *Arzneimittel-Forsch.*, 1975, *25*, 392.

Animal studies suggesting a protective effect against *Amanita phalloides* poisoning.— G. L. Floersheim, *Toxic. appl. Pharmac.*, 1975, *34*, 499; G. L. Floersheim *et al.*, *ibid.*, 1978, *46*, 455; B. Tuchweber *et al.*, *ibid.*, 1979, *51*, 265.

A commercial preparation of silymarin (Legalon) enhanced the activity of the mixed function oxidation system in *rats* but did not prevent carbon tetrachloride-induced depression of the system. In human subjects the half-life of phenazone and phenylbutazone was not altered by silymarin and it was doubtful whether silymarin had a hepatic protective role in man.— H. W. Leber and S. Knauff, *Arzneimittel-Forsch.*, 1976, *26*, 1603.

Further references: G. Vogel *et al.*, *Arzneimittel-Forsch.*, 1975, *25*, 82; A. Desplaces *et al.*, *ibid.*, 89; G. Vogel *et al.*, *ibid.*, 179; H. Schriewer *et al.*, *ibid.*, 188.

Proprietary Names
Ciscolex *(Lemonier, Arg.)*; DuraSilymarin *(Durachemie, Ger.)*; Enterohepat *(Dexter, Arg.)*; Epacardo *(Savio, Ital.)*; Hepadestal *(Krugmann, Ger.)*; Laragon *(Roemmers, Arg.)*; Legalon *(Bellon, Fr.; Madaus, Ger.; Ibi, Ital.; Madaus Cerafarm, Spain; Madaus, Switz.)*; Silirex *(Lampugnani, Ital.)*; Silliver *(Abbott, Ital.)*; Cordomarin, Cronol, Emil, Eparfit, Escarmine, Halodren, Hepagerina, Hepalar, Hepallolina, Hepato-Framan, Lecemin, Pluropon, Sematron, Silarine, Silgen, Silibancol, Silimazu *(all Spain)*.

13237-g

Sitofibrate. Stigmast-5-en-3β-ol 2-(4-chlorophenoxy)-2-methylpropionate.
$C_{39}H_{59}ClO_3$=611.3.

CAS — 55902-94-8.

Sitofibrate has been used in the treatment of hyperlipidaemia. It is claimed to have a dual effect due to its clofibrate-like activity and its sitosterol-like activity.

Proprietary Names
Longeril *(Ferrer, Spain).*

13238-q

Sitogluside. AW-10; BSSG; EU-4906; WA-184. 3β-(β-D-Glucopyranosyloxy)stigmast-5-ene.
$C_{35}H_{60}O_6$=576.9.

CAS — 474-58-8.

Sitogluside is reported to have activity against prostatic hypertrophy.

Manufacturers
Norwich-Eaton, USA.

13239-p

Sobrerol. *p*-Menth-6-ene-2,8-diol.
$C_{10}H_{18}O_2$=170.3.

CAS — 498-71-5.

Sobrerol is claimed to have expectorant and mucolytic activity and is used in respiratory disorders.

References: V. Dalla Valle, *Boll. chim.-farm.*, 1970, *109*, 761, per *Int. pharm. Abstr.*, 1972, *9*, 714.

Proprietary Names
Sobrepin *(Unifa, Arg.; Corvi, Ital.; Zambeletti, Spain).*

13240-n

Sodium Apolate. Sodium Lyapolate.
Poly(sodium ethylenesulphonate).
$(C_2H_3NaO_3S)_n$.

CAS — 25053-27-4.

Sodium apolate is a synthetic heparinoid anticoagulant. It has been used in ointments for the resolution of haematomas and for the relief of sprains and contusions.

Proprietary Names
Pergagel *(Albert-Roussel, Ger.).*

13241-h

Sodium Arsanilate *(B.P. Vet.).* Anhydrous Sodium Aminarsonate. Sodium hydrogen 4-aminophenylarsonate.
$C_6H_7AsNNaO_3$=239.0.

CAS — 127-85-5.

A white or creamy-white, almost odourless, hygroscopic, granular powder. **Soluble** 1 in 3 of water and 1 in 150 of alcohol; practically insoluble in chloroform and ether. **Store** in airtight containers.

Sodium arsanilate is used in veterinary medicine for similar purposes to arsanilic acid (p.1680).

13242-m

Sodium Arsenate. Sodium Arseniate; Natrium Arsenicicum.
$Na_2HAsO_4,7H_2O$=312.0.

CAS — 7778-43-0 (anhydrous); 10048-95-0 (heptahydrate).

Pharmacopoeias. In *Belg., Fr., Pol., Port., Rus.,* and *Swiss.*

Odourless colourless transparent crystals which are efflorescent in dry air and somewhat deliquescent in moist air. **Soluble** 1 in 1.5 of water and 1 in 2 of glycerol; slightly soluble in alcohol. A solution in water is alkaline to litmus. A 3.83% solution is iso-osmotic with serum. Solutions are **sterilised** by autoclaving or by filtration. **Incompatible** with calcium and magnesium salts, alkaloidal salts, and salts of heavy metals. **Store** in airtight containers.

Sodium arsenate was formerly used in the treatment of chronic skin diseases, in parasitic diseases of the blood, and in some forms of anaemia. It has the adverse effects of Arsenic Trioxide, p.1680.

13243-b

Sodium Bromebrate. MBBA; NSC-104801; WR-149912. The sodium salt of (*E*)-3-*p*-anisoyl-3-bromoacrylate.
$C_{11}H_8BrNaO_4$=307.1.

CAS — 5711-40-0 (bromebric acid); 21739-91-3 (sodium salt).

Pharmacopoeias. In *Cz.*

Sodium bromebrate is an antineoplastic agent which has been administered intravenously.

Discovered in Czechoslovakia and introduced as a folate inhibitor, research in Britain suggested bromebric acid might also possess an alkylating action.— J. Q. Matthias, *Practitioner*, 1973, *211*, 465.

Further references: S. Frytak *et al.*, *Cancer*, 1976, *37*, 1248; J. H. Edmonson *et al.*, *J. natn. Cancer Inst.*, 1977, *59*, 1619 (ovarian carcinoma); D. D. Von Hoff *et al.*, *Biomedicine*, 1977, *26*, 388.

Proprietary Names
Cytembena *(Cz.).*

13244-v

Sodium Buniodyl. Buniodyl Sodium; Sodium Bunamiodyl. Sodium 3-butyramido-α-ethyl-2,4,6-tri-iodocinnamate.
$C_{15}H_{15}I_3NNaO_3$=661.0.

CAS — 1233-53-0 (buniodyl); 1923-76-8 (sodium salt).

A white odourless slightly hygroscopic powder. Slightly **soluble** in water and alcohol. **Store** in airtight containers. Protect from light.

Sodium buniodyl is a contrast medium administered by mouth for the examination of the biliary tract. It has been associated with acute renal failure and death and has been withdrawn from the market in several countries.

Proprietary Names
Orabilix *(Codali, Belg.; Guerbet, Fr.; Hefa-Frenon, Ger.; Guerbet, Switz.).*

13245-g

Sodium Cacodylate *(B.P.C. 1949).* Sod. Cacodyl.; Sodium Dimethylarsonate. Sodium dimethylarsinate trihydrate.
$C_2H_6AsNaO_2,3H_2O$=214.0.

CAS — 75-60-5 (cacodylic acid); 124-65-2 (sodium salt, anhydrous); 6131-99-3 (sodium salt, trihydrate); 5968-84-3 (ferric salt).

Pharmacopoeias. In *Aust., It., Mex., Port.,* and *Span. Span.* also includes ferric cacodylate.

A white, odourless, very deliquescent, crystalline or granular powder. **Soluble** 1 in 0.5 of water and 1 in 2.5 of alcohol. A 3.3% solution in water is iso-osmotic with serum. Solutions are **sterilised** by autoclaving or by filtration. **Incompatible** with alkaloidal salts. **Store** in airtight containers.

The effects of sodium cacodylate are essentially those of the inorganic arsenic to which it is partly reduced in the body. It was formerly used, usually by subcutaneous injection, for the same purposes as arsenic trioxide. It has the adverse effects of Arsenic Trioxide, p.1680. Sodium cacodylate is more toxic when given by mouth than when injected because of the rapid release of inorganic arsenic; it imparts a strong garlic-like odour to the breath, urine, and perspiration, particularly when taken by mouth, due to the release of cacodylic oxide.

Ferric cacodylate (iron cacodylate; ferric dimethylarsinate), strychnine cacodylate, and sodium cacodylate were once popular ingredients of proprietary injections advocated for their stimulant effects in debilitated conditions.

13246-q

Sodium Cyanate.
NaCNO=65.01.

CAS — 917-61-3.

White crystals. Solutions in water have a pH of 9.2 to 9.8.

A method was described for purification of sodium cyanate from the technical grade available. The dried purified product was stable to heat at 200° for 2 hours. In aqueous solutions it was unstable to heat, dependent on concentration and temperature. Stability was impaired at low pH.— R. F. Labbe, *J. pharm. Sci.*, 1973, *62*, 1727.

Adverse Effects. Peripheral neuropathies, gastro-intestinal effects, fatigue, and drowsiness have been reported with sodium cyanate.

Polyneuropathy occurred in 2 patients given sodium cyanate for sickle-cell anaemia.— C. M. Peterson *et al.*, *Ann. intern. Med.*, 1974, *81*, 152.

Two patients with sickle-cell disease who had been taking sodium cyanate up to 41 or 44 mg per kg body-weight daily for 440 to 600 days developed motor and sensory neuropathy.— A. Ohnishi *et al.*, *Archs Neurol., Chicago*, 1975, *32*, 530, per *J. Am. med. Ass.*, 1975, *233*, 568.

Of 6 patients with sickle-cell anaemia given sodium cyanate 30 mg per kg body-weight daily for 3 to 6 months, 4 developed toxicity, including peripheral neuropathy, nerve conduction abnormalities, psychiatric disturbances, and weight loss.— S. Charache *et al.*, *Archs intern. Med.*, 1975, *135*, 1043, per *Trop. Dis. Bull.*, 1976, *73*, 17.

Bilateral cataracts occurred in 2 patients receiving sodium cyanate. There was spontaneous regression in 1 patient when sodium cyanate was withdrawn.— D. H. Nicholson *et al.*, *Archs Ophthal., N.Y.*, 1976, *94*, 927, per *J. Am. med. Ass.*, 1976, *235*, 2667.

Uses. Sodium cyanate is an antisickling agent which causes carbamoylation of the terminal valine residues of haemoglobin and increases its oxygen affinity.

Preliminary clinical studies were encouraging when sodium cyanate was given by mouth to patients with sickle-cell disease but a subsequent controlled study demonstrated no beneficial effect and increasing evidence of unacceptable toxicity.

There have been some encouraging results using extracorporeal treatment in which cyanate is added to blood previously withdrawn from the patient and then returned to the body.

Discussions on the use of cyanate in the treatment of sickle-cell disease.— A. May and E. R. Huehns, *Trans. R. Soc. trop. Med. Hyg.*, 1974, *68*, 85; *idem, Br. med. Bull.*, 1976, *32*, 223; J. Dean and A. N. Schechter, *New Engl. J. Med.*, 1978, *299*, 804.

Carbamoylation did not directly inhibit sickling, but the increased oxygen affinity decreased the proportion of deoxyhaemoglobin at any particular partial pressure of oxygen, thereby reducing the tendency to sickle and increasing red-cell survival.— A. May *et al.*, *Lancet*, 1972, *1*, 658.

References to extracorporeal treatment with sodium cyanate in sickle-cell disease.— D. A. Diederich *et al.*, *J. clin. Invest.*, 1976, *58*, 642, per *J. Am. med. Ass.*, 1977, *237*, 76; E. E. Langer *et al.*, *J. Lab. clin. Med.*, 1976, *87*, 462.

For earlier reports on the use of sodium cyanate in patients with sickle-cell disease, see Martindale 27th Edn, p. 1812.

13247-p

Sodium Dichloroacetate. DCA.
$C_2HCl_2NaO_2$=150.9.

CAS — 2156-56-1.

Sodium dichloroacetate activates pyruvate dehydrogenase. It has been tried in the treatment of lactic acidosis, including that caused by phenformin, but its use has been suspended by some workers because of toxicity in *animals* and a report of polyneuropathy in clinical studies.

After initial results in 7 diabetic subjects, more detailed studies in 4 diabetic subjects with fasting hyperglycaemia and hyperlipoproteinaemia indicated that sodium dichloroacetate 3 or 4 g once daily for 6 or 7 days significantly decreased the following values: fasting blood-sugar concentrations, plasma-lactate concentrations, plasma-alanine concentrations, plasma-cholesterol concentrations (in 3 of the patients), and plasma-triglyceride concentrations (the very low-density lipoprotein fraction being most affected); the following values were significantly increased: plasma-ketone-body concentrations and serum-uric acid concentrations (with falls in both urate excretion and clearance); plasma-insulin, free fatty acid and glycerol concentrations were unaffected. No other laboratory indexes were affected and no adverse clinical effects were noted except mild sedation in about half the patients in both phases of the study. Further studies were indicated to elucidate the efficacy and safety of sodium dichloroacetate, its mode of action, and its clinical significance.— P. W. Stacpoole *et al.*, *New Engl. J. Med.*, 1978, *298*, 526. Comment.— A. S. Relman, *ibid.*, 564. It was not proved that dichloroacetate offered any advantage over bicarbonate in the treatment of lactic acidosis.— R. D. Cohen and R. A. Iles (letter), *ibid.*, 1364. Comments on the metabolic effects of dichloroacetate in *rats*.— D. W. Crabb and R. A. Harris (letter), *ibid.*, *299*, 255; D. Stansbie and R. J. Sherriff (letter), *ibid.*, 256. Blood concentrations of lactate and pyruvate were decreased in an 18-month-old child with congenital lactic acidosis when sodium dichloroacetate was given. Lactate concentrations at the upper limit of normal were maintained when a dose of 150 mg per kg body-weight daily was given for 6 months but there was no clinical improvement, and growth and psychomotor retardation remained unchanged.— F. X. Coude *et al.* (letter), *ibid.*, 1365. The chronic oral administration of dichloroacetate has been suspended because of adverse effects in *animals* and a polyneuropathy which developed in a patient given dichloroacetate for 16 weeks.— P. W. Stacpoole *et al.* (letter), *ibid.*, 1979, *300*, 372. Mention of the mutagenicity of dichloroacetate.— V. Herbert *et al.* (letter), *ibid.*, 625.

A suggestion that 2-chloropropionate may be preferable to dichloroacetate in metabolic studies with pyruvate dehydrogenase activators.— D. W. Crabb and R. A. Harris (letter), *New Engl. J. Med.*, 1978, *299*, 255.

The biological disposition of sodium dichloroacetate after intravenous administration.— G. Lukas *et al.*, *J. pharm. Sci.*, 1980, *69*, 419.

Further references to sodium dichloroacetate in the treatment of lactic acidosis: K. G. M. M. Alberti and M. Nattrass, *Lancet*, 1977, *2*, 25; K. Irsigler *et al.*, *ibid.*, 1027; K. G. M. M. Alberti *et al.* (letter), *ibid.*, 1136; E. Standl *et al.*, *Klin. Wschr.*, 1977, *55*, 969; K. Irsigler *et al.*, *Arzneimittel-Forsch.*, 1979, *29*, 555; P. G. Wells *et al.*, *Diabetologia*, 1980, *19*, 109.

13248-s

Sodium Dithionite.
Sodium Hydrosulphite; Sodium Sulphoxylate.
$Na_2S_2O_4$=174.1, or $Na_2S_2O_4,2H_2O$ = 210.1.

CAS — 7775-14-6 (anhydrous).

NOTE. The name sodium hydrosulfite is also applied to $NaHSO_2$ = 88.06.

A white or slightly grey crystalline powder with a slight characteristic odour. **Soluble** in water yielding a solution which rapidly absorbs oxygen and becomes turbid.

A 0.25% solution of sodium dithionite is used to remove phenazopyridine stains.

13249-w

Sodium 2-Ethylmercurithiobenzoxazole-5-carboxylate.

$C_{10}H_8HgNNaO_3S$=445.8.

CAS — 16509-11-8.

An almost white powder. **Soluble** in water and methyl alcohol; less soluble in alcohol.

Sodium 2-ethylmercurithiobenzoxazole-5-carboxylate has bacteriostatic and antifungal properties. A 0.02% solution is used for the storage of bone for transplantation.

References: P. Van den Broek and W. Kuijpers, *Acta oto-lar.*, 1974, *77*, 335; E. Eitschberger *et al.*, *Archs Otorhinolar.*, 1978, *220*, 141.

Proprietary Preparations

Cialit *(Hoechst, UK)*. A brand of sodium 2-ethylmercurithiobenzoxazole-5-carboxylate.

13250-m

Sodium Glycarsamate *(B. Vet. C. 1965)*.
Sodium Glycollylarsanilate. Sodium *N*-glycoloylarsanilate; Sodium [4-(2-hydroxyacetamido)phenyl]arsonate.
$C_8H_9AsNNaO_5$=297.1.

CAS — 140-45-4.

A white or creamy-white, odourless, almost tasteless, crystalline powder. **Soluble** 1 in 6 of water and 1 in 280 of alcohol. **Store** in a cool place in small airtight containers. Protect from light.

Sodium glycarsamate is an anthelmintic used in veterinary medicine for the treatment of equine strongyloidosis.

Proprietary Names

Astryl *(May & Baker, UK)*.

13251-b

Sodium Hyaluronate.
The sodium salt of a high-viscosity mucopolysaccharide of high molecular weight.

CAS — 9004-61-9 (hyaluronic acid); 9067-32-7 (sodium salt).

Hyaluronic acid is widely distributed in body tissues and intracellular fluids.

Sodium hyaluronate is used as an adjuvant to promote tissue repair.

Proprietary Preparations

Healonid *(Pharmacia, UK)*. Solution containing in each ml sodium hyaluronate 10 mg (obtained from avian tissue), sodium chloride 8.5 mg, sodium phosphate dihydrate 280 µg, and sodium acid phosphate monohydrate 40µg in Water for Injections, available in single-use syringes of 0.4 ml. Store at 2° to 8°. For intra-ocular injecttion during eye surgery.

Other Proprietary Names

Connettivina *(Kreussler, Ger.; Fidia, Ital.)*.

13252-v

Sodium Hydrogen Sulphate.
Sodium Acid Sulphate; Sodium Bisulphate.
$NaHSO_4,H_2O$=138.1.

CAS — 7681-38-1 (anhydrous); 10034-88-5 (monohydrate).

Colourless odourless crystals or fused masses. **Soluble** 1 in less than 1 of water, yielding an acid solution. It is decomposed by alcohol.

Sodium hydrogen sulphate is used for preparing effervescing baths.

13253-g

Sodium Methylarsinate.
Sodium Metharsinite; Natrium Methylarsonicum. Disodium methylarsonate hexahydrate.
$CH_3AsNa_2O_3,6H_2O$=292.0.

CAS — 5967-62-4.

Pharmacopoeias. In *Fr.*, *It.*, *Port.*, and *Span.*

A white crystalline powder containing 25.65% of As. **Soluble** 1 in about 1 of water; slightly soluble in alcohol; practically insoluble in ether. **Incompatible** with alkaloids and iron salts.

Sodium methylarsinate has the actions and uses of sodium cacodylate but was stated not to impart the garlic odour to the breath characteristic of the cacodylates.

Proprietary Names

Arsozon *(Takeda, Jap.)*; Disomear *(Nakataki, Jap.)*.

13254-q

Sodium Nitrate.
Natrii Nitras; Natrium Nitricum.
$NaNO_3$=84.99.

CAS — 7631-99-4.

NOTE. Crude sodium nitrate is known as Chile Saltpetre.

Pharmacopoeias. In *Fr.*

Colourless, odourless, hygroscopic crystals with a cooling saline taste. **Soluble** 1 in 1 of water, 1 in 0.6 of boiling water, and 1 in 125 of alcohol. A 1.36% solution in water is iso-osmotic with serum. **Store** in airtight containers.

WARNING. *The Council of the Pharmaceutical Society of Great Britain advises pharmacists not to supply materials likely to be used for making fireworks, including sodium nitrate, to children under any circumstances, and recommends that it should be sold only to persons who are, or appear to be, 18 years of age or over.*

Adverse Effects and Treatment. As for Potassium Nitrate, p.1746.

Uses. Sodium nitrate has similar properties to potassium nitrate.

The Preservatives in Food Regulations 1979 (SI 1979: No. 752) as amended (SI 1982: No. 15) and The Preservatives in Food (Scotland) Regulations 1979 [SI 1979: No. 1073 (S.96)] as amended permit as a preservative not more than 50 ppm of sodium nitrate and sodium nitrite (both expressed as sodium nitrite) in certain types of cheese and limits of not more than 150 to 500 ppm of sodium nitrate and sodium nitrite (both expressed as sodium nitrite) in cured meats including cured meat products. The Regulations also prohibit the sale of any food specially prepared for babies or young children if it has in it or on it any added sodium nitrate or sodium nitrite.

Crude sodium nitrate is used as a fertiliser.

Estimated acceptable daily intake of nitrates: up to 500 µg per kg body-weight. No change was made from the Seventeenth Report [however, in that report an intake of up to 5 mg per kg was given].— Twenty-third Report of Joint FAO/WHO Expert Committee on Food Additives, *Tech. Rep. Ser. Wld Hlth Org. No. 648*, 1980. Nitrate should on no account be added to baby foods.— *Fd Add. Ser. Wld Hlth Org. No. 5*, 1974.

13255-p

Sodium Perchlorate.
$NaClO_4,H_2O$=140.5.

CAS — 7601-89-0 (anhydrous); 7791-07-3 (monohydrate).

Colourless crystals or white crystalline powder. **Soluble** in water.

WARNING. *The Council of the Pharmaceutical Society of Great Britain advises pharmacists not to supply materials likely to be used for making fireworks, including chlorates, to children under any circumstances, and recommends that they should be sold only to persons who are, or appear to be, 18 years of age or over.*

Sodium perchlorate has properties similar to those of potassium perchlorate (p.358) and has also been used to protect the thyroid gland during treatment with radioisotopes. It has been given by intravenous injection in doses of 75 mg. Sodium perchlorate has also been used in the preparation of patients for brain scanning.

The use of sodium perchlorate in the differentation of patients with Hashimoto's disease from those with goitre.— H. W. Gray, *Lancet*, 1974, *1*, 335.

Proprietary Names

Irenat *(Tropon, Ger.; Medichemie, Switz.)*.

13256-s

Sodium Pidolate. Sodium Pyroglutamate; Sodium Pyrrolidone Carboxylate; NaPCA. Sodium 5-oxopyrrolidine-2-carboxylate.
$C_5H_6NNaO_3$=151.1.

CAS — 28874-51-3.

White odourless hygroscopic crystals with an acid taste. **Soluble** in water; slightly soluble in organic solvents. **Store** in airtight containers.

Sodium pidolate is used as a humectant.

Proprietary Preparations

Ajidew A-100 *(Ajinomoto, Jap.: K & K-Greeff, UK).* Consists of pidolic acid ($C_5H_7NO_3$ = 129.1). **Ajidew N-50** is a 50% solution of the sodium salt. They are used as humectants.

Lacticare *(Stiefel, UK).* A lotion containing sodium pidolate 2.5% and lactic acid 5% in an oil-in-water basis. For hyperkeratotic and other dry skin conditions.

13257-w

Sodium Pteroyl Triglutamate. PteGlu3. Sodium *N*-{*N*-[*N*-*p*-(2-amino-4-hydroxypteridin-6-ylmethylamino)benzoyl-L-γ-glutamyl]-L-γ-glutamyl}-L-glutamate.
$C_{29}H_{32}N_9NaO_{12}$=721.6.

CAS — 89-38-3 (pteroyltriglutamic acid).

Sodium pteroyl triglutamate is a folate compound with weak folic acid activity obtained from microbial fermentation. It was formerly used as a palliative in the treatment of malignant disease.

13258-e

Sodium 5′-Ribonucleotide. A mixture, in approximately equal proportions, of disodium guanylate and disodium inosinate.

A flavour enhancer.

13259-l

Sodium Salamidacetate. Sodium (2-carbamoylphenoxy)acetate.
$C_9H_8NNaO_4$=217.2.

CAS — 25395-22-6 (salamidacetic acid); 3785-32-8 (sodium salt).

Sodium salamidacetate is reported to have analgesic, anti-inflammatory, and antipyretic activity.

Proprietary Names

Neosalid *(Bruco, Ital.).*

13260-v

Sodium Silicate. Soluble Glass; Water Glass.

CAS — 1344-09-8.

Concentrated aqueous solutions of sodium silicate are commercially available and have many industrial uses. The solutions vary in composition, viscosity, and density; the greater the ratio of Na_2O to SiO_2 the more tacky and alkaline the solution. A solution has been used, similarly to Plaster of Paris, for making fixed dressings for fractures. One of the most commonly used solutions, which is employed for egg preserving contains about 40% $Na_2Si_3O_7$.

13261-g

Sodium Succinate.
$C_4H_4Na_2O_4,6H_2O$=270.1.

CAS — 150-90-3 (anhydrous); 6106-21-4 (hexahydrate).

A crystalline powder. **Soluble** 1 in 5 of water; practically insoluble in alcohol. An aqueous solution is neutral or slightly alkaline.

Sodium succinate has been used experimentally in the treatment of various psychotic disorders. Succinic dinitrile ($C_4H_4N_2$ = 80.09) has been used in the treatment of exhaustion and depression.

13262-q

Sorbinicate. D-Glucitol hexanicotinate.
$C_{42}H_{32}N_6O_{12}$=812.7.

CAS — 6184-06-1.

Sorbinicate has been used in the treatment of lipid disorders.

Hypolipidaemic effects.— G. Magnati *et al., Farmaco, Edn prat.*, 1978, *33,* 162.

Reduction of platelet aggregation.— G. Avellone *et al., Farmaco, Edn prat.*, 1980, *35,* 147.

Fibrinolytic activity.— S. Novo *et al., Farmaco, Edn prat.*, 1980, *35,* 155.

Proprietary Names

Nicosterolo *(Guidotti, Ital.).*

13263-p

Soterenol Hydrochloride. MJ-1992. 2′-Hydroxy-5′-(1-hydroxy-2-isopropylaminoethyl)methanesulphonanilide hydrochloride.
$C_{12}H_{20}N_2O_4S,HCl$=324.8.

CAS — 13642-52-9 (soterenol); 14816-67-2 (hydrochloride).

Soterenol is a sympathomimetic agent but was reported to cause benign tumours in *rats.*

References: B. M. Cohen, *Curr. ther. Res.*, 1969, *11,* 713; D. Poynter *et al.* (letter), *Br. med. J.*, 1978, *1,* 46.

13264-s

Sparteine Sulphate *(B.P.C. 1949).* Spart. Sulph.; (−)-Sparteine Sulphate; *l*-Sparteine Sulphate; Sparteinum Sulfuricum; Sulfato de Esparteina. Dodecahydro-7,14-methano-2*H*,6*H*-dipyrido[1,2-*a*:1′,2′-*e*][1,5]diazocine sulphate pentahydrate.
$C_{15}H_{26}N_2,H_2SO_4,5H_2O$=422.5.

CAS — 90-39-1 (sparteine); 299-39-8 (sulphate, anhydrous); 6160-12-9 (sulphate, pentahydrate).

Pharmacopoeias. In *Arg., Belg., It., Port., Roum.,* and *Span.*

Sparteine sulphate is a salt of the dibasic alkaloid, sparteine, obtained from scoparium, *Sarothamnus scoparius (=Cytisus scoparius)* (Leguminosae). It occurs as odourless colourless crystals or white crystalline granules or powder with a bitter saline taste. **Soluble** 1 in 2 of water and 1 in 5 of alcohol; practically insoluble in chloroform and ether. Solutions are **sterilised** by autoclaving or by filtration. **Incompatible** with alkalis, iodides, and tannic acid. **Protect** from light.

Sparteine sulphate has been reported to lessen the irritability and conductivity of cardiac muscle and has been used in the treatment of cardiac arrhythmias. Small doses stimulate and large doses paralyse the autonomic ganglia. Peripherally, it has a fairly strong curare-like action, arresting respiration by paralysing the phrenic endings.

Sparteine sulphate has also been used as an oxytocic agent to induce labour at term but its action is unpredictable. Several hours should be allowed to elapse before giving oxytocin after the administration of sparteine sulphate.

Sparteine camsylate has also been used.

Proprietary Names

Depasan *(Giulini, Ger.)*; Spartopan (adenylate) *(Bouchard, Fr.).*

13265-w

Spirogermanium Hydrochloride. NSC-192965. 3-(8,8-Diethyl-2-aza-8-germaspiro[4.5]-dec-2-yl)-*NN*-dimethylpropylamine dihydrochloride.
$C_{17}H_{36}GeN_2,2HCl$=414.0.

CAS — 41992-23-8 (spirogermanium); 41992-22-7 (hydrochloride).

Spirogermanium hydrochloride is reported to have antineoplastic activity.

Manufacturers

Boehringer Ingelheim, UK; Unimed, USA.

13266-e

SQ-26776

SQ-26776 belongs to a new class of monocyclic beta-lactam antibiotics (monobactams) produced by bacteria. It is reported to be highly active against Gram-negative bacteria including beta-lactamase-producing strains.

References: *Lancet,* 1981, *2,* 620; R. B. Sykes *et al., Nature,* 1981, *291,* 489.

Manufacturers

Squibb, USA.

13267-l

Statolon. Vistatolon; NSC-71901. An antiviral substance derived from *Penicillium stoloniferum.* The active constituent is a polyanionic polysaccharide.

CAS — 11006-77-2.

Statolon has been shown to induce the production of interferon by *animal* cells.

References: W. J. Kleinschmidt and G. W. Probst, *Antibiotics Chemother.*, 1962, *12,* 298; W. J. Kleinschmidt and E. B. Murphy, *Virology,* 1965, *27,* 484, per *J. Am. med. Ass.*, 1966, *195* (Feb. 7), A257.

Manufacturers

Lilly, USA.

13268-y

Stenbolone Acetate. 2-Methyl-3-oxo-5α-androst-1-en-17β-yl acetate.
$C_{22}H_{32}O_3$=344.5.

CAS — 5197-58-0 (stenbolone); 1242-56-4 (acetate).

Stenbolone acetate has been used as an anabolic agent.

Proprietary Names

Stenobolone *(Infal, Spain).*

13269-j

Stibamine Glucoside. The *N*-glucoside of sodium *p*-aminophenylstibonate.
$C_{36}H_{49}N_3NaO_{22}Sb_3$=1264.0.

CAS — 6543-62-0 (stibamine); 1344-34-9 (glucoside).

An odourless, pale cream-coloured to light buff, amorphous powder. Readily **soluble** in water. A 6% solution in water has a pH of 8.5 to 9.

Stibamine glucoside is a pentavalent antimony compound which was formerly used in the treatment of leishmaniasis.

13270-q

Strontium Chloride.
$SrCl_2,6H_2O$=266.6.

CAS — 10476-85-4 (anhydrous).

Colourless odourless crystals or white granules. Readily **soluble** in water; soluble 1 in 8 of alcohol.

Strontium chloride is used as a 10% toothpaste for the relief of dental hypersensitivity.

Strontium was rachitogenic in *chicks;* it inhibited the intestinal absorption of calcium and the synthesis of 1,25-dihydroxycholecalciferol.— J. L. Omdahl and H. F. DeLuca, *J. biol. Chem.*, 1972, *247*, 5520.

The Council on Dental Therapeutics of the American Dental Association had not seen adequate evidence to justify claims for dentifrices promoted to provide relief from hypersensitive teeth.— A.D.T. 1975.

Brief comment on the potential use of strontium in the prevention of dental decay, in the treatment of osteoporosis, and as an adjunct to cancer chemotherapy.— *Am. Pharm.*, 1979, *NS19* (Aug.), 38.

13271-p

Succinimide.

Butanimide. Pyrrolidine-2,5-dione.
$C_4H_5NO_2$=99.09.

CAS — 123-56-8.

A crystalline substance. M.p. about 126°. **Soluble** 1 in about 3 of water and 1 in 24 of alcohol; practically insoluble in ether and chloroform.

Succinimide has been claimed to inhibit the formation of oxalic acid calculi in the kidney and to reduce hyperoxaluria.

References: K. E. Schulte and G. Henke, *Eur. J. Drug Metab. Pharmacokinet.*, 1978, *3*, 161.

Proprietary Names
Succinimide-Sauba *(Sauba, Fr.)*.

13272-s

Succisulfone.

1500F; Fourneau-1500; Succinylsulphone. 4′-Sulphanilylsuccinanilic acid; 4-Amino-4′-(3-carboxypropionamido)diphenyl sulphone.
$C_{16}H_{16}N_2O_5S$=348.4.

CAS — 5934-14-5.

Crystals. M.p. 157°. **Soluble** in ammonia.

Succisulfone is a bacteriostatic agent applied topically as a 10% powder. It has also been used as a mouth-wash containing 5% and an eye lotion containing 25%.

Proprietary Names
Exosulfonyl *(Vaillant-Defresne, Fr.)*.

13273-w

Sucrose Octa-acetate *(U.S.N.F.)*.

$C_{28}H_{38}O_{19}$=678.6.

CAS — 126-14-7.

Pharmacopoeias. In *U.S.N.F.*

A white, almost odourless, hygroscopic powder with an intensely bitter taste. M.p. not less than 78°. **Soluble** 1 in 1100 of water, 1 in 11 of alcohol, 1 in 0.3 of acetone, and 1 in 0.5 of toluene; soluble in ether; very soluble in chloroform and methyl alcohol. **Store** in airtight containers.

Sucrose octa-acetate is used as an alcohol denaturant.

13274-e

Sufentanil.

R-30730; R-33800 *(citrate)*. *N*-{4-(Methoxymethyl)-1-[2-(2-thienyl)ethyl]-4-piperidyl}propionanilide.
$C_{22}H_{30}N_2O_2S$=386.6.

CAS — 56030-54-7 (sufentanil); 60561-17-3 (citrate).

Sufentanil is a narcotic analgesic.

Animal pharmacology.— W. F. M. Van Bever *et al.*, *Arzneimittel-Forsch.*, 1976, *26*, 1548; C. J. E. Niemegeers *et al.*, *ibid.*, 1551.

Further references: J. Kugler *et al.*, *Anaesthesist*, 1977, *26*, 343.

Manufacturers
Janssen, Belg.

13275-l

Sulbactam.

CP-45899. Penicillanic acid 1,1-dioxide; (2*S*,5*R*)-3,3-Dimethyl-7-oxo-4-thia-1-azabicyclo[3.2.0]heptane-2-carboxylic acid 4,4-dioxide.
$C_8H_{11}NO_5S$=233.2.

CAS — 68373-14-8 (sulbactam); 69388-79-0 (pivsulbactam).

Sulbactam is reported to inhibit beta-lactamase and thereby to increase the antibacterial activity of penicillins and cephalosporins against beta-lactamase-producing organisms. Pivsulbactam (sulbactam pivoxil; CP-47904) is reported to have similar activity.

References: A. R. English *et al.*, *Antimicrob. Ag. Chemother.*, 1978, *14*, 414; K. P. Fu and H. C. Neu, *ibid.*, 1979, *15*, 171; B. Olsson *et al.*, *ibid.*, 263; K. P. Fu and H. C. Neu, *ibid.*, *16*, 561; J. A. Retsema *et al.*, *ibid.*, 1980, *17*, 615; R. Wise *et al.*, *J. antimicrob. Chemother.*, 1980, *6*, 197; I. Braveny and K. Machka (letter), *Lancet*, 1980, *2*, 752.

Manufacturers
Pfizer, UK.

13276-y

Sulfachrysoidine Sodium.

Sodium 4,6-diamino-4′-sulphamoylazobenzene-2-carboxylate.
$C_{13}H_{12}N_5NaO_4S$=357.3.

CAS — 485-41-6 (sulfachrysoidine).

Sulfachrysoidine sodium is a sulphonamide which has been used topically.

Proprietary Names
Collubiazol *(Roussel, Arg.*; *Roussel, Belg.)*; Rubiazol *(Roussel Maestretti, Ital.)*.

13277-j

Sulfadicramide.

3-Methyl-*N*-sulphanilylcrotonamide.
$C_{11}H_{14}N_2O_3S$=254.3.

CAS — 115-68-4.

Sulfadicramide is a sulphonamide used by topical application to the eye.

Proprietary Names
Irgamid *(Zyma-Galen, Belg.*; *Dispersa, Ger.*; *Zyma, Neth.*; *Zyma, Switz.)*.

13278-z

Sulfametomidine.

N[1]-(6-Methoxy-2-methylpyrimidin-4-yl)sulphanilamide.
$C_{12}H_{14}N_4O_3S$=294.3.

CAS — 3772-76-7.

Sulfametomidine has the typical properties of the sulphonamides. It is given in once-daily dosage.

Proprietary Names
Télémid *(Nativelle, Fr.)*.

13279-c

Sulfanitran.

Sulphanitran. 4′-(4-Nitrophenylsulphamoyl)acetanilide.
$C_{14}H_{13}N_3O_5S$=335.3.

CAS — 122-16-7.

Sulfanitran is a sulphonamide coccidiostatic agent. It is used as an additive to veterinary feedstuffs—see under Antibiotic Supplements for Animal Feeds, p.1082.

Manufacturers
Salsbury, UK.

13280-s

Sulfaperin.

BT-325. *N*[1]-(5-Methylpyrimidin-2-yl)sulphanilamide.
$C_{11}H_{12}N_4O_2S$=264.3.

599-88-2

Sulfaperin is a sulphonamide used in the treatment of susceptible infections.

Proprietary Names
Grosulan *(Grossmann, Switz.)*; Pallidin *(E. Merck, Ger.)*; Retardon *(Chassot, Switz.)*; Ultrasulfon *(Streuli, Switz.)*; Ipersulfidin, Palidin, Retardsulf, Rexulfa, Sintosulfa, Sulfalast, Sulfapenta, Sulfatreis, Sulfixone, Sulfopiran, Sulfopirimidina *(all Ital.)*.

13281-w

Sulfonaphtine Glucoside.

Naphthionine Glucoside. 4-(β-D-Glucopyranosylamino)naphthalene-1-sulphonic acid.
$C_{16}H_{19}NO_8S$=385.4.

CAS — 1328-93-4 (glucoside, sodium salt).

Sulfonaphtine glucoside has been used, as the sodium salt, as a haemostatic agent.

Proprietary Names
Emostane *(*sodium salt*) (Jamco, Ital.)*.

13282-e

Sulglycotide.

Sulglicotide. The sulphuric polyester of a glycopeptide isolated from pig duodenum.

CAS — 54182-59-1.

Sulglycotide has been used in the treatment of gastric and duodenal ulcer and gastritis.

In a double-blind multicentre study in 77 patients with proven duodenal ulcer the effect of sulglycotide 100 mg thrice daily and 200 mg at night for 30 days was not significantly different from that of cimetidine 200 mg thrice daily and 400 mg at night. The effect of cimetidine was more rapid. Ulcers larger than 1 cm in diameter healed better with cimetidine.— G. B. Porro *et al.*, *Br. med. J.*, 1979, *2*, 17.

Pharmacological studies in 75 healthy subjects indicated that the salt obtained from *N*-methyl-octatropinium and sulglycotide may be suitable for the treatment of gastric ulcer.— G. C. Allegra *et al.*, *Curr. ther. Res.*, 1979, *25*, 485.

Proprietary Names
Gliptid *(Merck, Arg.)*; Gliptide *(Crinos, Ital.)*; Ulcodavur *(Davur, Spain)*.

13283-l

Sulisatin Sodium.

The disodium salt of 3,3-bis(4-hydroxyphenyl)-7-methylindolin-2-one bis(hydrogen sulphate) (ester).
$C_{21}H_{15}NNa_2O_9S_2$=535.5.

CAS — 54935-03-4 (sulisatin); 54935-04-5 (sodium salt).

Sulisatin sodium has been used as a purgative.

References: F. Cantal *et al.*, *Clin. Ther.*, 1977, *1*, 216, per *Int. pharm. Abstr.*, 1978, *15*, 1071.

Proprietary Names
Laxitex *(Andreu, Spain)*.

13284-y

Sulmarin.

MG-143. 4-Methylcoumarin-6,7-diyl bis(hydrogen sulphate).
$C_{10}H_8O_{10}S_2$=352.3.

CAS — 29334-07-4.

Sulmarin is reported to have a protective effect on capillary fragility.

Manufacturers
Maggioni, Ital.

13285-j

Sulodexide. Glucurono-2-amino-2-deoxyglucoglucan sulphate.

CAS — 57821-29-1.

Sulodexide has been used as a hypolipidaemic agent.

Proprietary Names
Provenal *(Pulitzer, Ital.)*; Vessel *(Alfa Farmaceutici, Ital.)*.

13286-z

Sulphaproxyline. Sulfaproxyline. N^1-(4-Isopropoxybenzoyl)sulphanilamide; *p*-Isopropoxy-*N*-sulphanilylbenzamide.
$C_{16}H_{18}N_2O_4S$=334.4.

CAS — 116-42-7.

Sulphaproxyline is a sulphonamide used, usually with sulfamerazine, in the treatment of susceptible infections.

Proprietary Names of Sulphaproxyline with Sulfamerazine
Dosulfin *(Geigy, Ger.)*; Dosulfine *(Gomenol, Fr.)*.

A preparation containing sulphaproxyline and sulfamerazine was formerly marketed in Great Britain under the proprietary name Dosulfin (*Geigy*).

13287-c

Sulpharsphenamine *(B.P. 1953)*. Sulpharsenobenzene; Myarsenol; Myoarsenobenzol; Thioarsphenamine.

CAS — 618-82-6.

Pharmacopoeias. In *Belg., Mex., Port., Rus.,* and *Span.*

A yellow powder consisting mainly of disodium 4,4′-dihydroxy-3,3′-di(sulphomethylamino)arsenobenzene, $C_{14}H_{14}As_2N_2Na_2O_8S_2$ = 598.2, and containing 18 to 21% of As. **Soluble** 1 in 0.5 of water (pH not less than 3); practically insoluble in alcohol and ether. Unstable in air. **Store** below 15° in sealed containers from which the air has been removed or replaced by an inert gas. Injections must be used immediately after preparation.

Sulpharsphenamine was formerly used similarly to neoarsphenamine (p.1731) in the treatment of syphilis.

13288-k

Sulphatolamide. Sulfatolamide. The *N*-sulphanilylthiourea salt of α-amino-*p*-toluenesulphonamide.
$C_{14}H_{19}N_5O_4S_3$=417.5.

CAS — 1161-88-2.

Sulphatolamide is a sulphonamide which has been used in local infections of the mouth.

Proprietary Names
Marbaletten *(Bayer, Switz.)*.

13289-a

Surfomer. AOMA. Poly(1,2-dicarboxy-3-hexadecyltetramethylene).
$(C_{22}H_{40}O_4)_n$.

CAS — 71251-04-2.

Surfomer is reported to have hypolipidaemic activity.

Manufacturers
Monsanto, USA.

13290-e

Surgibone. Sterile heterogeneous bone and cartilage for surgical use, obtained from young calves and bovine embryos and subjected to special processing which reduces the antigenicity.

Surgibone has been used for grafting procedures in orthopaedic and reconstructive surgery.

Surgibone had little or no value in encouraging new bone growth or preventing ingrowth of fibrous tissue into bone defects. An intense inflammatory response had also attended its use.— *J. Am. med. Ass.*, 1967, *199* (Feb. 6), A35.

Further references: *J. Am. med. Ass.*, 1966, *195*, 951.

Proprietary Preparations of Related Products
Kiel Bone Graft *(Braun Melsungen, Ger.: Davis & Geck, UK)*. Sterile bone obtained from calves, processed to reduce its antigenicity, for use in surgery.

References to the use of Kiel Bone Graft: G. Fuchs and J. Schlachetzki, *Chirurg.*, 1966, *37*, 174, per *J. Am. med. Ass.*, 1966, *196* (June 13), A253; W. A. W. Maney, *Br. J. clin. Pract.*, 1967, *21*, 519; D. Churchill-Davidson *et al.*, *Proc. R. Soc. Med.*, 1967, *60*, 1077; P. S. Ramani *et al.*, *Br. J. Surg.*, 1975, *62*, 147.

13291-l

Suriclone. 31264-RP. (±)-6-(7-Chloro-1,8-naphthyridin-2-yl)-2,3,6,7-tetrahydro-7-oxo-5*H*-[1,4]dithi-ino[2,3-*c*]pyrrol-5-yl 4-methylpiperazine-1-carboxylate.
$C_{20}H_{20}ClN_5O_3S_2$=478.0.

CAS — 53813-83-5.

Suriclone is reported to have tranquillising and hypnotic activity.

Manufacturers
May & Baker, UK.

13292-y

Sutoprofen. Suprofen; R-25061. 2-[4-(2-Thenoyl)phenyl]propionic acid.
$C_{14}H_{12}O_3S$=260.3.

CAS — 40828-46-4.

Sutoprofen is an anti-inflammatory analgesic.

For a series of papers reporting *animal* pharmacology, see *Arzneimittel-Forsch.*, 1975, *25*, 1495–1542.

Proprietary Names
Surfrex *(Janssen, Belg.)*.

13293-j

Suxamidofylline. 7-[2-(3-Diethylcarbamoylpropionyloxy)ethyl]theophylline.
$C_{17}H_{25}N_5O_5$=379.4.

CAS — 12712-75-3.

Suxamidofylline, a derivative of theophylline, has been used in conditions similar to those in which aminophylline is used.

Proprietary Names.
Argecor *(Farge, Ital.)*; Cardiodest *(Biotrading, Ital.)*.

13294-z

Talmetacin. BA-7605-06. (±)-1,3-Dihydro-3-oxoisobenzofuran-1-yl [1-(4-chlorobenzoyl)-5-methoxy-2-methyl-1*H*-indol-3-yl]acetate.
$C_{27}H_{20}ClNO_6$=489.9.

CAS — 67489-39-8.

Talmetacin is structurally related to indomethacin and is reported to have analgesic, antipyretic, and anti-inflammatory activity.

Manufacturers
Bagó, Arg.; Resfar, Ital.

13295-c

Tametraline Hydrochloride. CP-24441-1. (1*R*,4*S*)-1,2,3,4-Tetrahydro-*N*-methyl-4-phenyl-1-naphthylamine hydrochloride.
$C_{17}H_{19}N,HCl$=273.8.

CAS — 52795-02-5 (tametraline); 52760-47-1 (hydrochloride).

Tametraline hydrochloride is reported to have antidepressant activity.

Manufacturers
Pfizer, USA.

13296-k

Tamitinol. 4-(Ethylaminomethyl)-2-methyl-5-(methylthiomethyl)pyridin-3-ol.
$C_{11}H_{18}N_2OS$=226.3.

CAS — 59429-50-4.

Tamitinol is reported to be of possible value in cerebral disease.

Manufacturers
E. Merck, UK.

13297-a

Tandamine Hydrochloride. AY-23946. 2-(9-Ethyl-1,3,4,9-tetrahydro-1-methylthiopyrano-[3,4-*b*]indol-1-yl)-*NN*-dimethylethylamine hydrochloride.
$C_{18}H_{26}N_2S,HCl$=338.9.

CAS — 42408-80-0 (tandamine); 58167-78-5 (hydrochloride).

Tandamine hydrochloride has antidepressant properties.

References: R. S. B. Ehsanullah *et al.*, *Br. J. clin. Pharmac.*, 1976, *3*, 950P; *idem*, *Psychopharmacology*, 1977, *52*, 73; I. Jirkovsky *et al.*, *Arzneimittel-Forsch.*, 1977, *27*, 1642; B. Saletu *et al.*, *Int. Pharmacopsychiat.*, 1977, *12*, 137.

Manufacturers
Ayerst, USA.

13298-t

Tantalum.
Ta=180.9479.

CAS — 7440-25-7.

Finely powdered tantalum has been used as an X-ray contrast medium.

Maximum permissible atmospheric concentration 5 mg per m^3.

Use of tantalum in bronchography.— *J. Am. med. Ass.*, 1969, *210*, 1382; N. Zamel *et al.*, *Radiology*, 1970, *94*, 547, per *J. Am. med. Ass.*, 1970, *212*, 512; R. B. Dilley and J. A. Nadel, *Ann. Otol. Rhinol. Lar.*, 1970, *79*, 945, per *Int. pharm. Abstr.*, 1972, *9*, 46.

Use of tantalum in X-ray examination of the oesophagus.— J. A. Nadel *et al.*, *Invest. Radiol.*, 1969, *4*, 57, per *J. Am. med. Ass.*, 1969, *208*, 1219.

Use of tantalum in tracheography.— F. P. Stitik *et al.*, *Am. J. Roentg.*, 1978, *130*, 35.

13299-x

Taurine. 2-Aminoethanesulphonic acid.
$C_2H_7NO_3S$=125.1.

CAS — 107-35-7.

Bile acids are conjugated in the body with glycine or with taurine. Taurine has been tried as an adjunct in the treatment of hypercholesterolaemia and in cardiovascular disorders.

Taurine 1 g thrice daily for 7 days effectively reduced or prevented alcohol-withdrawal symptoms. Psychotic and convulsive symptoms occurred in 3 of 22 patients so treated compared with 17 of 38 control patients. There was also a significant reduction in the incidence of these symptoms when present before withdrawal.— H. Ikeda (letter), *Lancet*, 1977, *2*, 509.

Other references: N. A. Soter and T. B. Fitzpatrick, *Practitioner*, 1969, *202*, 102; N. E. Miller *et al.*, *Med. J. Aust.*, 1973, *1*, 1223; R. G. Fariello and R. Mutani (letter), *Lancet*, 1974, *2*, 1201; S. W. Schaffer and J. J. Kocsis, *Am. Pharm.*, 1979, *NS19* (Nov.), 36.

Proprietary Names
O-Due *(Falorni, Ital.)*.

13300-x

Tazolol Hydrochloride. RS-6245; ITP. (±)-1-Isopropylamino-3-(thiazol-2-yloxy)propan-2-ol hydrochloride.
$C_9H_{16}N_2O_2S,HCl=252.8$.

CAS — 39832-48-9 (tazolol); 38241-39-3 (hydrochloride).

Although originally described as a selective β_1-adrenoceptor agonist, further experimental work suggested that tazolol was a non-specific beta-blocking agent.

References: G. Vanquelin *et al.*, *Biochem. Pharmac.*, 1976, *25*, 2605; S. J. Clark and R. H. Poyser, *J. Pharm. Pharmac.*, 1977, *29*, 630.

13301-r

TCDD. 2,3,7,8-Tetrachlorodibenzo-*p*-dioxin.
$C_{12}H_4Cl_4O_2=322.0$.

CAS — 1746-01-6.

NOTE. The name Dioxin is often used for TCDD, and has also been applied to dimethoxane.

TCDD is a by-product in the manufacture of trichlorophenol and a contaminant of the herbicide trichlorophenoxyacetic acid (see p.842). It has been incriminated as causing chloracne (a severe and persistent acne caused by chlorinated compounds), liver and kidney damage, hirsutism, and personality changes. It is a potent teratogen. It is an inducer of the enzyme aryl hydrocarbon hydroxylase which is implicated in carcinogenesis. Other chlorinated dibenzodioxins, sometimes called dioxins, have similar but lower toxicity.

References: *Dioxin, Toxicological and Chemical Aspects*, F. Cattabeni *et al.* (Ed.), London, John Wiley, 1978.

13302-f

Teasuprine. Isoxsuprine Theophylline-7-acetate; TI-72. 1-(4-Hydroxyphenyl)-2-(1-methyl-2-phenoxyethylamino)propan-1-ol theophyllin-7-ylacetate.
$C_{27}H_{33}N_5O_7=539.6$.

CAS — 60640-79-1.

Teasuprine is reported to be a peripheral vasodilator.

Proprietary Names
Angiclan *(Juste, Spain).*

13303-d

Tefazoline Nitrate. Tenaphtoxaline Nitrate. 2-(5,6,7,8-Tetrahydro-1-naphthylmethyl)-2-imidazoline nitrate.
$C_{14}H_{18}N_2,HNO_3=277.3$.

CAS — 1082-56-0 (tefazoline).

Tefazoline nitrate has been used as a nasal decongestant.

Proprietary Names
Tenaphto *(UPB, Belg.).*

13304-n

Tenitramine. *NNN'N'*-Tetrakis(2-hydroxyethyl)ethylenediamine tetranitrate (ester).
$C_{10}H_{20}N_6O_{12}=416.3$.

CAS — 21946-79-2.

Tenitramine has been used for the prophylaxis and treatment of angina pectoris and as an adjunct in other cardiac disorders.

Proprietary Names
Tenitran *(Elea, Arg.; Bioindustria, Ital.; Roger, Spain).*

13305-h

Tenoxicam. Ro-12-0068. 4-Hydroxy-2-methyl-*N*-(2-pyridyl)-2*H*-thieno[2,3-*e*][1,2]thiazine-3-carboxamide 1,1-dioxide.
$C_{13}H_{11}N_3O_4S_2=337.4$.

CAS — 59804-37-4.

Tenoxicam is reported to have analgesic and anti-inflammatory activity.

Manufacturers
Roche, Switz.

13306-m

Terazosin Hydrochloride. Abbott-45975. 1-(4-Amino-6,7-dimethoxyquinazolin-2-yl)-4-(tetrahydro-2-furoyl)piperazine hydrochloride dihydrate.
$C_{19}H_{25}N_5O_4,HCl,2H_2O=459.9$.

CAS — 63590-64-7 (terazosin); 63074-08-8 (hydrochloride, anhydrous); 70024-40-7 (hydrochloride, dihydrate).

Terazosin hydrochloride is reported to have antihypertensive activity.

Manufacturers
Abbott, USA.

13307-b

Terconazole. Triaconazole; R-42470. 1-{4-[-[2-(2,4-Dichlorophenyl)-*r*-2-(1*H*-1,2,4-triazol-1-ylmethyl)-1,3-dioxolan-*c*-4-yl]methoxy]phenyl}-4-isopropylpiperazine.
$C_{26}H_{31}Cl_2N_5O_3=532.5$.

CAS — 67915-31-5.

Terconazole is reported to have antifungal activity.

Manufacturers
Janssen, Belg.

13308-v

Terfenadine. RMI-9918. 1-(4-*tert*-Butylphenyl)-4-[4-(α-hydroxybenzhydryl)piperidino]-butan-1-ol.
$C_{32}H_{41}NO_2=471.7$.

CAS — 50679-08-8.

Terfenadine is an antihistamine; it is reported to have low sedative potential.

References: K. J. Hüther *et al.*, *Eur. J. clin. Pharmac.*, 1977, *12*, 195; V. K. Kulshrestha *et al.*, *Br. J. clin. Pharmac.*, 1978, *6*, 25; C. H. Clarke and A. N. Nicholson, *ibid.*, 31; A. Reinberg *et al.*, *Eur. J. clin. Pharmac.*, 1978, *14*, 245; L. Moser *et al.*, *ibid.*, 417; M. L. Brandon *et al.*, *Ann. Allergy*, 1980, *44*, 71; V. H. Van Landeghem *et al.*, *Clin. Pharmac. Ther.*, 1980, *27*, 290.

Proprietary Preparations
Triludan *(Merrell, UK).* Terfenadine, available as scored tablets of 60 mg.

Other Proprietary Names
Teldane *(Fr.).*

13309-g

Terizidone. B-2360. 4,4'-[*p*-Phenylenebis(methyleneamino)]bis(isoxazolidin-3-one).
$C_{14}H_{14}N_4O_4=302.3$.

CAS — 25683-71-0.

Terizidone has been used in the treatment of tuberculosis and infections of the urinary tract.

Proprietary Names
Terivalidin *(SCS, S.Afr.; Vinas, Spain)*; Urovalidin *(Bracco, Ital.).*

13310-f

Terodiline Hydrochloride. *N-tert*-Butyl-1-methyl-3,3-diphenylpropylamine hydrochloride.
$C_{20}H_{27}N,HCl=317.9$.

CAS — 15793-40-5 (terodiline); 7082-21-5 (hydrochloride).

A white crystalline powder. **Soluble** in water and chloroform.

Terodiline has been used in the treatment of angina pectoris. The mode of action is not entirely clear.

Terodiline blocked the bronchoconstrictor actions of acetylcholine but not of serotonin and bradykinin.— J. Iravani and G. N. Melville, *Arzneimittel-Forsch.*, 1975, *25*, 415.

Terodiline hydrochloride 150 mg daily was given to 10 patients with obstructive pulmonary disease. Two patients developed severe anticholinergic side-effects, and discontinued treatment; 2 patients dropped out for other reasons. The remaining 6 showed some bronchodilatation. During the study, the dose was reduced to 75 mg daily, and this was considered to be the maximum daily dose.— H. Castenfors *et al.* (preliminary study), *Eur. J. clin. Pharmac.*, 1975, *8*, 197.

Proprietary Names
Bicor *(Recip, Swed.).*

13311-d

Tetragastrin. The C-terminal tetrapeptide of gastrin.

CAS — 1947-37-1.

Tetragastrin has been used similarly to pentagastrin to test the secretory action of the stomach.

Tetragastrin in a dose of 2.5 µg per kg body-weight by subcutaneous injection produced a lower gastric-acid response than 40 µg of histamine per kg, but a comparable response followed a dose of 5 µg per kg. No side-effects were reported.— P. Rødbro and K. H. Køster (letter), *Lancet*, 1967, *2*, 1092. For a similar report, see Histamine Acid Phosphate, p.518.

13312-n

Tetrahydrobiopterin. 2-Amino-5,6,7,8-tetrahydro-6-(1,2-dihydroxypropyl)pteridin-4(3*H*)-one.
$C_9H_{15}N_5O_3=241.2$.

CAS — 17528-72-2.

An atypical phenylketonuria has been described, attributed to deficiency of tetrahydrobiopterin; there have been reports of response to tetrahydrobiopterin.

References: D. M. Danks *et al.* (letter), *Lancet*, 1975, *2*, 1043; D. M. Danks *et al.* (letter), *ibid.*, 1976, *1*, 1236; J. Schaub *et al.*, *Archs Dis. Childh.*, 1978, *53*, 674; S. D. Cederbaum (letter), *New Engl. J. Med.*, 1979, *301*, 441; F. A. Firgaira *et al.*, *Lancet*, 1979, *2*, 1260.

13313-h

Tetramethylammonium Iodide.
$C_4H_{12}IN=201.0$.

CAS — 75-58-1.

Pale yellow crystals. M.p. 230° with decomposition. Sparingly **soluble** in water; freely soluble in dehydrated alcohol; practically insoluble in chloroform and ether.

Tetramethylammonium iodide is a quaternary ammonium ganglion-blocking agent which has been used as an antihypertensive and antispasmodic agent. It has also been used as a disinfectant.

Proprietary Names
Artilacer *(Lacer, Spain)*; Banikol *(Techni-Pharma, Mon.).*

13314-m

Tetrazepam. CB-4261. 7-Chloro-5-(cyclohex-1-enyl)-1,3-dihydro-1-methyl-2*H*-1,4-benzodiazepin-2-one.
$C_{16}H_{17}ClN_2O$=288.8.

CAS — 10379-14-3.

Tetrazepam is a benzodiazepine derivative (see Diazepam, p.1519) which has been used for its muscle relaxant properties.

Proprietary Names
Myolastan *(Clin-Comar-Byla, Fr.).*

13315-b

Tetroxoprim. 5-[3,5-Dimethoxy-4-(2-methoxyethoxy)benzyl]pyrimidine-2,4-diyldiamine.
$C_{16}H_{22}N_4O_4$=334.4.

CAS — 53808-87-0.

Tetroxoprim is closely related chemically to trimethoprim (see p.1484). It is a dihydrofolate reductase inhibitor. It has been used in conjunction with sulphonamides similarly to co-trimoxazole.

For a report of a symposium on antibacterial folate inhibitors, see *J. antimicrob. Chemother.*, 1979, *5, Suppl.* B, 1–239.

Manufacturers
Heumann, Ger.

13316-v

Thalidomide. K-17. 2-Phthalimidoglutarimide.
$C_{13}H_{10}N_2O_4$=258.2.

CAS — 50-35-1.

Adverse Effects. Thalidomide, a non-barbiturate hypnotic, was synthesised in Germany in 1953 and became generally available in West Germany in 1957 and in Great Britain in 1958. In November 1961 it was reported that thalidomide apparently had teratogenic effects when administered to women early in pregnancy and this was soon followed by further reports which implicated thalidomide beyond doubt. Thalidomide was withdrawn from the British market in December 1961.

Other toxic effects due to thalidomide include paraesthesias and peripheral neuropathy.

Deformities caused by thalidomide. For the pharmacology of thalidomide, its clinical aspects, and a detailed survey of deformed children born alive in England and Wales between 1st January 1960 and 31st August 1962, see Deformities Caused by Thalidomide, *Report on Public Health and Medical Subjects No. 112*, London, HM Stationery Office, 1964.

An analysis of the defects caused by thalidomide in 154 children.— R. W. Smithells, *Br. med. J.*, 1973, *1*, 269. See also T. Kajii *et al.*, *Teratology*, 1973, *8*, 163, per *J. Am. med. Ass.*, 1974, *227*, 356.

A discussion of the possible aetiology of thalidomide embryopathy.— E. Gardner and R. O'Rahilly (letter), *Lancet*, 1976, *1*, 635. See also J. McCredie, *Lancet*, 1973, *2*, 1058; W. G. McBride, *Teratology*, 1977, *16*, 79.

Comment on the young men and women affected by thalidomide.— *Lancet*, 1981, *2*, 510.

References to thalidomide and cranial nerve abnormalities: R. Murphy and P. Mohr, *Br. med. J.*, 1977, *2*, 1191; P. D. Phelps and P. E. Roland (letter), *ibid.*, 1672; G. C. Gordon (letter), *ibid.*, 1978, *1*, 237.

Further abnormalities: D. N. Bremner and G. Mooney (letter), *Lancet*, 1978, *1*, 826 (agenesis of appendix); R. W. Smithells (letter), *ibid.*, 1042 (absent appendix and sweating).

For other references to reviews and clinical and pharmacological reports of the teratogenic effects of thalidomide, see Extra Pharmacopoeia 25th Edn, pp. 310 and 311.

Neuropathy. A review of reports on the progress of patients who had suffered from peripheral neuropathy after treatment with thalidomide.— *Lancet*, 1969, *1*, 713.

Toxic metabolites. Thalidomide metabolites were derived from D-glutamic acid instead of the natural L-form. One metabolite, *N*-(*O*-carbobenzoxyl)glutamic acid, was similar to folic acid; thalidomide metabolites might act as folic acid antagonists and could be used as antineoplastics.— A. U. De and D. Pal, *J. pharm. Sci.*, 1975, *64*, 262.

Uses. Thalidomide has been shown to have immunosuppressive activity. It has been found beneficial in the treatment of lepra reactions in doses ranging from 50 to 400 mg daily, depending on the severity of the symptoms. It should not be used in women of child-bearing potential.

Leprosy. In a double-blind crossover study of thalidomide in the treatment of severe chronic erythema nodosum leprosum, the dose of prednisolone necessary to suppress symptoms was considerably reduced in 9 of 10 patients while they were receiving thalidomide 300 mg daily. Seven patients subsequently relapsed. Two developed mild allergic dermatitis during thalidomide treatment.— M. F. R. Waters, *Lepr. Rev.*, 1971, *42*, 26. For a comment that prednisolone should not be given with thalidomide see *Lepr. Rev.*, 1979, *50*, 326.

Of 50 patients with lepromatous leprosy who were treated with thalidomide for 7 days, 52% did not have further lepra reactions over 9 months.— C. G. S. Iyer *et al.*, *Bull. Wld Hlth Org.*, 1971, *45*, 719.

Thalidomide usually in a dose of 100 mg at bedtime relieved the symptoms of erythema nodosum leprosum in 20 of 22 patients.— L. Levy *et al.* (letter), *Lancet*, 1973, *2*, 324. Due to the risk of peripheral neuritis thalidomide should not be used.— C. L. Crawford (letter), *ibid.*, 567. No evidence of neurotoxicity had been seen during the use of thalidomide to control erythema nodosum leprosum (ENL) and indeed thalidomide seemed particularly valuable in ENL neuritis.— M. F. R. Waters, *Lepr. Rev.*, 1974, *45*, 337.

A preliminary report of a study of 61 adult male dapsone-sensitive patients with lepromatous leprosy and recurrent lepra reactions showed that thalidomide acted more rapidly than clofazimine, but it was not better in controlling the reactions or in increasing tolerance of dapsone, and its beneficial effect ceased when dosage with thalidomide stopped, while clofazimine continued to exert its effect.— K. Ramanujam *et al.*, *Lepr. Rev.*, 1975, *46*, *Suppl.*, 117.

A reminder that rifampicin impairs the effectiveness of oral contraceptives. The consequences of this could be disastrous in a lepromatous woman of child-bearing age receiving thalidomide to control a prolonged and severe lepra reaction.— W. H. Jopling and J. H. S. Pettit (letter), *Lepr. Rev.*, 1979, *50*, 331.

Other reports of the use of thalidomide in lepra reactions: R. C. Hastings *et al.*, *Clin. Pharmac. Ther.*, 1970, *11*, 481; J. Sheskin, *Medna Cutánea*, 1970, *4*, 379, per *Trop. Dis. Bull.*, 1972, *69*, 213; M. B. Marques and D. V. A. Opromolla, *Revta bras. Leprol.*, 1970, *37*, 41, per *Trop. Dis. Bull.*, 1972, *69*, 754; A. Magora *et al.*, *Int. J. Lepr.*, 1971, *39*, 863, per *Trop. Dis. Bull.*, 1973, *70*, 247; M. Goihman-Yahr *et al.*, *Int. Archs Allergy appl. Immun.*, 1978, *57*, 317, per *Trop. Dis. Bull.*, 1978, *75*, 950; J. Sheskin, *Int. J. Derm.*, 1978, *17*, 82, per *Trop. Dis. Bull.*, 1978, *75*, 506.

Skin disorders. A 12-year-old boy with a polymorphous light eruption was successfully treated with thalidomide 25 mg daily.— P. F. Geraghty (letter), *Med. J. Aust.*, 1977, *2*, 785.

Further references: H. van den Broek, *Archs Derm.*, 1980, *116*, 571 (prurigo nodularis).

Ulcerative colitis. Subjective and objective improvement occurred in a 28-year-old woman with ulcerative colitis, not adequately controlled by corticosteroids and sulphasalazine, when she was given thalidomide 400 mg daily. Other medication was withdrawn and the dose of thalidomide reduced to 200 mg daily, without relapse.— M. F. R. Waters *et al.*, *Br. med. J.*, 1979, *1*, 792.

Weber-Christian disease. A patient with Weber-Christian disease (relapsing, non-suppurative panniculitis) not controlled by fluocortolone responded rapidly to thalidomide 300 mg daily in 2 divided doses reduced after 3 weeks to 200 mg daily and after 10 weeks to 100 mg daily. There was no expected relapse when thalidomide was withdrawn at 13 weeks and the patient followed up for 13 months.— J. Eravelly and M. F. R. Waters (letter), *Lancet*, 1977, *1*, 251.

15328-h

Thallium Acetate. Thallous Acetate.
$C_2H_3O_2Tl$=263.4.

CAS — 563-68-8.

White odourless deliquescent crystals or crystalline powder. **Soluble** in water and alcohol.

Adverse Effects. Thallium salts are toxic when inhaled, ingested, or absorbed through the skin. Symptoms of poisoning appear within 12 to 24 hours of a single toxic dose and include severe abdominal pain, vomiting, diarrhoea, gastro-intestinal haemorrhage, and in severe cases tremors, delirium, convulsions, paralysis, and coma, leading to death in 1 to 2 days. However, the acute reaction may subside to be followed within about 10 days by the development of polyneuritis; psychosis, delirium, convulsions, and other signs of encephalopathy; tachycardia, hypertension, and arrhythmias; skin eruptions; and hepatorenal injury. Alopecia occurs within 15 to 20 days. Death may result from respiratory failure.

Smaller repeated doses are also toxic, with symptoms appearing over several weeks.

Maximum permissible atmospheric concentration of soluble thallium compounds, as thallium, 100 μg per m^3.

A brief review of the toxicity of thallium.— *Br. med J.*, 1972, *3*, 717. See also *Lancet*, 1974, *2*, 564; F. Barbier (letter), *ibid.*, 965.

Further reviews: C. H. Henning, *Dt. ApothZtg*, 1979, *119*, 1782; L. P. Shabalina and V. S. Spiridonova, *J. Hyg. Epidem. Microbiol. Immun.*, 1979, *23*, 247.

The *minimum lethal dose* in an adult was about 800 mg of thallium sulphate, i.e. 12 mg per kg body-weight. Accidental poisoning by thallium showed 3% fatality, mostly in children; suicidal poisoning showed 10% fatality and homicidal 100%.— R. Hausman and W. J. Wilson, *J. forens. Sci.*, 1964, *9*, 72.

In view of the toxicity of thallium sulphate to man and other animals, its lack of unpleasant odour or taste or irritant effects on the skin, its ready absorption through the skin and gastro-intestinal tract, and its slow elimination, it was recommended that it should not be used as a rodenticide.— Safe Use of Pesticides, Twentieth Report of the WHO Expert Committee on Insecticides, *Tech. Rep. Ser. Wld Hlth Org. No. 513*, 1973.

The pigment deposition in the hair of patients suffering from thallium poisoning could be easily recognised by the microscopic examination of some head hair in a 10% solution of sodium hydroxide.— E. Gerdts (letter), *Lancet*, 1974, *2*, 1268.

Treatment of Adverse Effects. After the acute ingestion of thallium the stomach should be emptied by emesis or lavage and a saline purgative such as sodium sulphate may be given. Intensive supportive therapy is necessary and suitable electrolyte solutions should be administered intravenously to correct dehydration and maintain a good urine flow.

Various methods have been employed in an attempt to increase the faecal and urinary excretion of thallium. A suspension of activated charcoal has been given to reduce intestinal absorption but is less successful than Prussian blue administered by duodenal tube. Chelating agents have been tried but are of doubtful value and potentially dangerous. The administration of potassium chloride by mouth may mobilise thallium from the tissues but is also hazardous.

The value of haemodialysis has not been established.

Chelating agents. Loss of consciousness had been noted during infusions of sodium diethyldithiocarbamate in patients undergoing treatment for thallium poisoning and EEG disturbances were noted which lasted for several weeks. These did not correlate with the initial high blood-thallium concentrations and it was suspected that they were due to the chelate. From experiments in *rats* the chelate was found to be lipophilic and it easily crossed the blood-brain barrier, thereby probably causing the coma. Thallium released in the brain by the chelate would then account for the long-term neurological disturbances.— H. H. Kamerbeek *et al.*, *Acta med. scand.*, 1971, *189*, 149.

Haemodialysis. A report of the use of haemodialysis in the treatment of thallium poisoning.— P. Piazolo *et al.*, *Dt. med. Wschr.*, 1971, *96*, 1215, per *Pharm. J.*, 1972, *1*, 177.

Thallium was still present in the urine after haemodialysis and forced diuresis.— A. Klöppel and G. Weiler, *Dt. med. Wschr.*, 1978, *103*, 75.

Potassium chloride. Although potassium chloride administered by mouth released tissue thallium, the symptoms were then aggravated by the increased plasma-thallium concentrations.— W. J. Bank *et al.*, *Archs Neurol., Chicago*, 1972, *26*, 456, per *J. Am. med. Ass.*, 1972, *220*, 877.

Prussian blue. Thallium was found to be more strongly bound *in vitro* to Prussian blue than to activated charcoal. In *rats* the thallium concentration in the brain in the treated group was less than half and in muscle one-quarter that of the control group after 4 days' therapy with Prussian blue. Three patients suffering from thallium poisoning, one of whom had ingested 2 g of thallium 14 days previously and was seriously ill, were given Prussian blue 10 g twice daily for 10 to 14 days by duodenal tube. All patients recovered, although the one who had taken 2 g had some residual neurological disturbances.— H. H. Kamerbeek *et al.*, *Acta med. scand.*, 1971, *189*, 321. See also P. Dvořák, *Z. Naturforsch.*, 1971, *26*, 277.

Two patients who had intentionally ingested about 700 mg of thallium sulphate were given Prussian blue 250 mg per kg body-weight daily in 4 divided doses through a duodenal tube. Mannitol 15% was also given via the tube to aid defaecation. Treatment was discontinued when the urinary-thallium excretion fell below 500 µg per 24 hours. Both patients recovered.— C. F. Van der Merwe, *S.Afr. med. J.*, 1972, *46*, 960.

The successful use of Prussian blue in the treatment of thallium poisoning in 11 patients, with a review of older methods of treatment.— W. Stevens *et al.*, *Int. J. clin. Pharmac. Biopharm.*, 1974, *10*, 1.

Uses. Thallium acetate was formerly used for depilation in ringworm and in depilatory creams but owing to numerous fatalities following both systemic and local treatments it is now very rarely used for such purposes. However, it is used in industry and as a rodenticide and pesticide and is therefore still a hazard.

13318-q

Thenitrazole.

TC-109. *N*-(5-Nitrothiazol-2-yl)thiophene-2-carboxamide.
$C_8H_5N_3O_3S_2$=255.3.

CAS — 3810-35-3.

Thenitrazole has been used in the treatment of vaginal trichomoniasis.

Proprietary Names
Atrican *(Innothéra, Fr.; Bouty, Ital.).*

13319-p

Thenoic Acid.

α-Thiophenic Acid. Thiophene-2-carboxylic acid.
$C_5H_4O_2S$=128.1.

CAS — 527-72-0.

Needles. M.p. about 128°. Very **soluble** in hot water, alcohol, and ether; moderately soluble in chloroform; slightly soluble in light petroleum.

Thenoic acid is an antimicrobial agent which has been administered by mouth, rectally, or as nasal drops as the sodium salt ($C_5H_3NaO_2S$ = 150.1) and by mouth as the lithium salt ($C_5H_3LiO_2S$ = 134.1), in the treatment of respiratory-tract infections.

Proprietary Names
Soufrane (sodium salt) *(Roland-Marie, Fr.)*; Thiophéol (lithium salt) *(Inava, Fr.).*

13320-n

Theobromine Magnesium Oleate.

Magnesium 3,7-dimethylxanthine oleate. The magnesium double salt of theobromine ($C_7H_8N_4O_2$) and oleic acid ($C_{18}H_{34}O_2$).

CAS — 6767-73-3.

Theobromine magnesium oleate has been given by mouth in the treatment of arteriosclerosis and peripheral vascular disease in doses of 200 or 400 mg thrice daily. Transient flushing and pruritus have been reported. It is contra-indicated in patients with renal disease.

Proprietary Names
Athemol *(Glaxo, USA).*

13321-h

Theodrenaline Hydrochloride.

H-8352. 7-[2-(3,4,β-Trihydroxyphenethylamino)ethyl]theophylline hydrochloride.
$C_{17}H_{21}N_5O_5$,HCl=411.8.

CAS — 13460-98-5 (theodrenaline); 2572-61-4 (hydrochloride).

Theodrenaline is an analeptic which has been used with cafedrine hydrochloride (see p.1688) in the treatment of hypotension.

13322-m

Thiamine Disulphide Hydrochloride.

NN'-[2,2'-Dithiobis(4-hydroxy-1-methylbut-1-enyl)]bis[*N*-(4-amino-2-methylpyrimidin-5-ylmethyl)]formamide hydrochloride.
$C_{24}H_{34}N_8O_4S_2$,HCl=559.2.

CAS — 67-16-3 (thiamine disulphide); 18642-10-9 (hydrochloride).

Thiamine disulphide hydrochloride has the general properties of thiamine hydrochloride.

Proprietary Names
Algoneurina *(IBIS, Ital.).*

13323-b

Thiobutabarbital Sodium.

Sodium 5-*sec*-butyl-5-ethyl-2-thiobarbiturate.
$C_{10}H_{15}N_2NaO_2S$=250.3.

CAS — 2095-57-0 (thiobutabarbital); 947-08-0 (sodium salt).

Thiobutabarbital sodium has been used for the induction of anaesthesia.

Proprietary Names
Inactin *(Byk Gulden, Ger.).*

13324-v

Thiocolchicoside.

3,10-Di(demethoxy)-3-glucopyranosyloxy-10-methylthiocolchicine.
$C_{27}H_{33}NO_{10}S$=563.6.

CAS — 602-41-5.

Pharmacopoeias. In *Fr.*

A yellow crystalline powder. **Soluble** in water and alcohol; practically insoluble in acetone and ether.

Thiocolchicoside is a muscle relaxant which has been used in rheumatic, traumatic, and gynaecological disorders.

Proprietary Names
Coltramyl *(Roussel, Belg.; Roussel, Fr.)*; Liviane *(Made, Spain)*; Musco-Ril *(Inverni della Beffa, Ital.).*

13325-g

Thioctic Acid.

Lipoic Acid. 5-(1,2-Dithiolan-3-yl)valeric acid.
$C_8H_{14}O_2S_2$=206.3.

CAS — 62-46-4.

Thioctic acid, its sodium salt, and its amide have been used in the treatment of liver dysfunction; it has also been tried in subacute necrotising encephalopathy. Beneficial results have been claimed in amanitin poisoning following ingestion of the mushroom *Amanita phalloides*, but its use is controversial; some authorities consider it worth a trial.

Thioctic acid, given to 36 children with epidemic hepatitis in doses of 3 mg per kg body-weight for 2 to 3 weeks in infants and 1 mg per kg for older children, produced improvement in those in the acute or subchronic stage after 10 to 21 days' treatment. The best route was intravenously as higher doses were required intramuscularly and the effect was delayed.— W. Kitlak, *Arch. Kinderheilk.*, 1963, *168*, 166, per *J. Am. med. Ass.*, 1963, *185* (Sept. 14), A209.

Use in Leigh's subacute necrotising encephalopathy.— B. E. Clayton *et al.*, *Archs Dis. Childh.*, 1967, *42*, 467.

Amanita poisoning. A report of 12 patients treated successfully for mushroom [*Amanita phalloides*] poisoning by gastric lavage, dextrose injection, prednisone 100 mg given intravenously and, where the transaminase concentrations were greater than 100 units per 100 ml, thioctic acid 100 mg intravenously twice daily for 9 to 12 days.— R. Zulik *et al.* (letter), *Lancet*, 1972, *2*, 228.

Thioctic acid as an antidote to *Amanita phalloides* poisoning.— B. J. Culliton, *Science*, 1974, *185*, 600. Criticism. Experimental results with thioctic acid in both *mice* and *dogs* had been negative.— F. R. Alleva (letter), *ibid.*, 1975, *187*, 216. Criticism of the study in *dogs*. Although amanitin poisoning and thioctic acid could both produce hypoglycaemia this had not been adequately corrected. In human subjects thioctic acid should be given with a sustained intravenous infusion of dextrose solution to provide a total dose of at least 100 g of dextrose daily. With this regimen no subject had been reported to show hypoglycaemia.— F. C. Bartter, *ibid.*

Animal studies failing to show benefit in *Amanita phalloides* poisoning.— F. R. Alleva *et al.*, *Toxic. appl. Pharmac.*, 1975, *33*, 184; G. L. Floersheim, *ibid.*, *34*, 499.

Thioctic acid was successfully used to treat 6 patients suffering from the hepatotoxic effects of mushroom poisoning.— B. M. Berkson (letter), *New Engl. J. Med.*, 1979, *300*, 371.

Further references: C. E. Becker *et al.*, *West. J. Med.*, 1976, *125*, 100.

Proprietary Names
Biletan *(Gador, Arg.)*; Lipoamid (amide) *(Fuso, Jap.)*; Lipoamin (amide) *(Sawai, Jap.)*; Thioami (amide) *(Hokuriku, Jap.)*; Thioctacid *(Homburg, Ger.)*; Thioctan *(Katwijk, Neth.)*; Tioctidasi (sodium salt) *(ISI, Ital.).*

15327-n

Thioglycollic Acid.

Mercaptoacetic acid.
HS.CH_2.CO_2H=92.11.

CAS — 68-11-1.

A colourless or nearly colourless liquid with a strong unpleasant odour. It is readily oxidised in air. **Miscible** with water, alcohol, ether, and many other organic solvents.

Ammonium, monoethanolamine, and sodium thioglycollates are used in home permanent-wave sets in the 'waving lotion', which is subsequently neutralised with potassium bromate (see p.1746) or other less toxic substances. A sensitivity dermatitis to thioglycollates may occur, with symptoms of oedema, erythema, itching, and a papular rash; these disappear on discontinuing the use of the solution.

Thioglycollates are also used in depilatory preparations.

Report of 5 cases of dermatitis associated with thioglycollate hair-waving.— L. H. Cotter, *J. Am. med. Ass.*, 1946, *131*, 592.

Thioglycollic acid was found to be a potential skin irritant in 146 women. The following precautions were recommended: (1) no solution to be left on the skin of the neck or forehead not covered by hair; (2) the scalp to be thoroughly rinsed as soon as possible; (3) any areas giving a burning sensation to be washed clean immediately; (4) if erythema occurred any further contact with thioglycollate to be avoided; (5) the hairdresser or operator should handle thioglycollate as infrequently as possible, should use protective gloves whenever giving cold wave treatment and not use barrier creams, and should avoid any further contact with thioglycollate wave lotions and detergents when the skin was inflamed.— L. Goldman *et al.*, *J. Am. med. Ass.*, 1948, *137*, 354.

Details of 2 depilatory creams containing thioglycollic acid or calcium thioglycollate. The pH value for optimum activity was 12 to 12.5 for 4% of thioglycollic acid or 5 to 10% of calcium thioglycollate; increased concentration of thioglycollate did not further accelerate activity. An excess of calcium hydroxide was required to assure the optimum pH values.— B. N. Bloch, *Soap Perfum. Cosm.*, 1972, *45*, 283.

13328-s

Thiophanate.
4,4′-*o*-Phenylenebis(ethyl 3-thioallophanate).

$C_{14}H_{18}N_4O_4S_2$=370.4.

CAS — 23564-06-9.

Thiophanate is used as a veterinary anthelmintic.

Proprietary Names

Nemafax *(May & Baker, UK).*

13329-w

Thiophene.
Thiofuran; Thiole; Thiotetrole; Divinylene Sulphide.

C_4H_4S=84.14.

CAS — 110-02-1.

A colourless liquid with a benzene-like odour. B.p. about 84°. Practically **insoluble** in water; miscible with alcohol and other organic solvents.

Thiophene is an antimicrobial agent which has been administered in suppositories.

13330-m

Thiram.
TMT; TMTD; SQ-1489; NSC-1771. Tetramethylthiuram disulphide.

$C_6H_{12}N_2S_4$=240.4.

CAS — 137-26-8.

A white crystalline powder. Practically **insoluble** in water; slightly soluble in alcohol and ether; more soluble in chloroform.

Thiram is the methyl analogue of disulfiram (p.579) and has antibacterial and antifungal activity. It has been used as a fungicide in agriculture, and in industry as a rubber accelerator. Thiram is irritant to mucous membranes and skin.

Of 1205 persons with dermatitis or eczema submitted to patch testing with thiram 2% in yellow soft paraffin, 4.8% gave a positive reaction.— E. Rudzki and D. Kleniewska, *Br. J. Derm.*, 1970, *83*, 543. See also A. M. Kligman, *J. invest. Derm.*, 1966, *47*, 393; H. T. H. Wilson, *Br. J. Derm.*, 1969, *81*, 175.

Temporary maximum acceptable daily intake of thiram 5 µg per kg body-weight.— Report of the 1974 Joint FAO/WHO Meeting on Pesticide Residues in Food, *Tech. Rep. Ser. Wld Hlth Org. No. 574*, 1975.

13331-b

Thonzonium Bromide.
NC-1264; Tonzonium Bromide. Hexadecyl[2-(*N*-*p*-methoxybenzyl-*N*-pyrimidin-2-ylamino)ethyl]dimethylammonium bromide.

$C_{32}H_{55}BrN_4O$=591.7.

CAS — 553-08-2.

Thonzonium bromide is a cationic detergent. As an additive in ear-drops and aerosol sprays it has been claimed to lower surface tension and facilitate the penetration of mucus by the active ingredients.

References: R. H. L. Wilson and N. L. Wilson, *Clin. Pharmac. Ther.*, 1966, *7*, 189.

Proprietary Names

Thonzide *(Parke, Davis, USA).*

13332-v

Thorium Dioxide.
Thorium Oxide.

ThO_2=264.0.

CAS — 1314-20-1.

A heavy white powder; practically **insoluble** in water.

Colloidal solutions of thorium dioxide have been used as X-ray contrast media for examination of the liver and spleen, for arteriography, and occasionally for outlining the cerebral ventricles. Its elimination is very slow and incomplete. It accumulates in the reticulo-endothelial system, especially in the liver and spleen. As it is radioactive (half-life: 1.41 × 10^{10} years), this accumulation is dangerous and there is strong evidence that the ensuing prolonged exposure to its radiation is a contributing factor in the development of malignant diseases and blood disorders often 20 to 30 years after its administration.

Discussion of the toxicity of thorium dioxide.— *Lancet*, 1977, *1*, 1297.

Of 1107 patients given thorium dioxide between 1930 and 1952 primarily for the radiological visualisation of blood vessels, 699 had died and 408 were alive up to the end of 1963. The long-term sequelae were shown, statistically, to include local granulomas in 81, cirrhosis of the liver in 42, fatal blood disorders in 16, and haemangioendotheliomas occurring in 22 and virtually thorium-dioxide specific. It was considered that the use of thorium dioxide was never justified in patients with a life expectation of more than 2 years.— J. da Silva Horta *et al.*, *Lancet*, 1965, *2*, 201.

Brief case histories of 6 patients seen between 1967 and 1975, who had received thorium dioxide many years earlier. Complications included leukaemia, aplastic anaemia, tumours, and, in all patients, hyposplenism. The literature was reviewed and included 61 cases of leukaemia and 40 cases of marrow failure, almost all of which were attributed to thorium dioxide; liver cirrhosis or fibrosis and splenic atrophy were common. The re-introduction of the contrast medium for the visualisation of brain-stem abscesses had recently been proposed.— S. A. N. Johnson *et al.*, *Q. J. Med.*, 1977, *46*, 259.

Other reports of long-term sequelae following the use of thorium dioxide: R. H. Kyle *et al.*, *New Engl. J. Med.*, 1963, *268*, 80; *Minerva med., Roma*, 1963, *54*, 122; P. Germon *et al.*, *J. Am. med. Ass.*, 1963, *186*, 437; G. L. Maltby, *New Engl. J. Med.*, 1964, *270*, 490; K. Schlager, *Radiol. Aust.*, 1963, *14*, 285, per *Int. pharm. Abstr.*, 1965, *2*, 553; G. Blümel *et al.*, *Wien. med. Wschr.*, 1964, *114*, 345, per *Int. pharm. Abstr.*, 1965, *2*, 554; J. S. MacKay and R. C. Ross, *Can. med. Ass. J.*, 1966, *94*, 1298; A. O. Langlands and E. R. D. Williamson, *Br. med. J.*, 1967, *3*, 206; T. Mori *et al.*, *Strahlentherapie*, 1967, *134*, 229; J. T. Boyd *et al.*, *Br. med. J.*, 1968, *2*, 517; M. L. Janower *et al.*, *New Engl. J. Med.*, 1968, *279*, 186; K. G. McNeill *et al.*, *Br. J. Radiol.*, 1968, *41*, 755; H. von Leden, *Archs Otolar.*, 1970, *91*, 520; H. J. Woodliff *et al.*, *Med. J. Aust.*, 1972, *2*, 768; G. L. Smoron and H. A. Battifora, *Cancer*, 1972, *30*, 1252, per *Int. pharm. Abstr.*, 1974, *11*, 536; J. M. Kiely *et al.*, *Cancer*, 1973, *31*, 1312, per *Int. pharm. Abstr.*, 1974, *11*, 536; P. K. Johnson and R. B. Babb, *Am. J. dig. Dis.*, 1975, *20*, 384; A. I. Gotlieb *et al.*, *Can. med. Ass. J.*, 1976, *115*, 433; C. C. Waddell *et al.*, *J. Am. med. Ass.*, 1977, *238*, 423; J. M. Isner *et al.*, *Am. J. Med.*, 1978, *64*, 1069; A. Ødegaard *et al.*, *J. clin. Path.*, 1978, *31*, 893; W. F. Sindelar *et al.*, *Cancer*, 1978, *42*, 2604; J. C. E. Underwood and P. Huck, *ibid.*, 2610; A. G. Arnold and M. H. Oelbaum, *Postgrad. med. J.*, 1980, *56*, 124.

Thorium dioxide was formerly marketed under the proprietary name Thorotrast.

13333-g

Thuja.
The fresh leaves and twigs of *Thuja occidentalis* (Coniferae).

Thuja is used in homoeopathic medicine.

13334-q

Thymidine.
Thymine 2-Deoxyriboside. 1-(2-Deoxy-β-D-ribofuranosyl)-5-methyluracil; 1-(2-Deoxy-β-D-ribofuranosyl)-1,2,3,4-tetrahydro-5-methylpyrimidine-2,4-dione.

$C_{10}H_{14}N_2O_5$=242.2.

CAS — 50-89-5.

Soluble in water and hot alcohol, sparingly soluble in hot chloroform.

Thymidine is a nucleoside constituent of cells. It has been suggested that an intravenous injection of a solution containing thymidine may reverse, at least partially, the systemic effects of idoxuridine (see p.820). Thymidine has also been used to modulate the toxicity of methotrexate and fluorouracil. An anti-tumour effect has been demonstrated in *animals*.

A review of thymidine.— D. S. Martin *et al.*, *Cancer*, 1980, *45, Suppl.* (Mar. 15), 1117.

A study indicating that acute lymphoblastic leukaemic cells are highly sensitive to growth inhibition by thymidine. Thymidine may have a role in the management of certain acute lymphoblastic leukaemias or lymphomas.— R. M. Fox *et al.* (preliminary communication), *Lancet*, 1979, *2*, 391.

References to the use of thymidine in preventing methotrexate toxicity: W. D. Ensminger and E. Frei, *Cancer Res.*, 1977, *37*, 1857; S. B. Howell *et al.*, *ibid.*, 1978, *38*, 325.

Further references: W. D. Ensminger and E. Frei, *Clin. Pharmac. Ther.*, 1978, *24*, 610 (pharmacokinetic study); D. F. Chiuten *et al.*, *Cancer Res.*, 1980, *40*, 818 (clinical and pharmacokinetic study in cancer patients).

For a report of the enhancement of the effect of vinblastine by thymidine, see Vinblastine Sulphate, p.231.

13335-p

Thymus Hormones

CAS — 69521-94-4 (thymosin α_1); 60529-76-2 (thymopoietin); 63340-72-7 (thymic humoral factor).

The thymus gland controls the development of T-lymphocytes and thereby plays a central role in cell-mediated immunity and the regulation of immune responses. It secretes hormones although the multiplicity of factors isolated has led to some confusion. Several polypeptides characterised in the thymus or serum are able to induce lymphocyte differentiation *in vitro* and *in vivo*. They include: thymosin fraction 5, a crude thymus gland extract; thymosin α_1, a component of fraction 5 which has been synthesised; thymopoietin, a polypeptide of known amino-acid sequence; thymic humoral factor (THF), isolated from crude thymic extract dialysate; and serum thymic factor (Facteur Thymique Serique, FTS), a nonapeptide which has been synthesised.

Various preparations, including crude extracts from calf thymus gland, thymosin fraction 5, and thymosin α_1 have been tried as immunostimulants in immunodeficiency disorders and as an adjunct in the treatment of malignant disease.

Reviews on thymus hormones: *Br. med. J.*, 1977, *1*, 1559; *J. Am. med. Ass.*, 1977, *237*, 429; J. -F. Bach, *A. Rev. Pharmac. & Toxic.*, 1977, *17*, 281; *J. Am. med. Ass.*, 1981, *246*, 205.

Reviews on lymphocyte function and immunodeficiency diseases: W. Pruzanski and E. C. Keystone, *Can. med. Ass. J.*, 1977, *117*, 114; A. M. Denman, *Br. med. J.*, 1978, *2*, 980; *idem*, 1980, *281*, 1376.

Reviews on thymus hormones in cancer therapy: *J. Am. med. Ass.*, 1978, *239*, 1945; S. P. Richman *et al.*, *Can. med. Ass. J.*, 1979, *120*, 322.

Seven children with various primary immune deficiency diseases had low proportions of T-cell rosettes, which increased after incubation with thymosin. Clinical improvement occurred in a 5½-year-old girl with thymic hypoplasia and abnormal immunoglobulin synthesis during treatment with thymosin derived from calf thymus 1 mg per kg body-weight daily by intramuscular injection. Improvement was maintained by weekly injections of 1 mg per kg.— D. W. Wara *et al.*, *New Engl. J. Med.*, 1975, *292*, 70. See also R. Hong and S. Horowitz, *ibid.*, 104.

Thymosin prepared from calf thymus was given in doses of 10 to 250 mg per m^2 body-surface intramuscularly daily for 7 days for immunostimulation to 10 patients with various tumours and immunoincompetence. Immunocompetence was partially restored and 1 patient achieved an objective clinical response. Three of the patients also received a further 5 weekly injections of 75 mg per m^2. The only side-effects were mild urticaria in 1 patient, low-grade fever in 2 patients, and pain on injection in 1 patient.— J. J. Costanzi *et al.*, *Cancer*, 1977, *40*, 14.

Of 2 siblings with adenosine deaminase deficiency one child responded to enzyme replacement therapy with transfusions of red blood cells alone. The other child required supplementation with thymosin injections as well as red blood cells before there was improvement of immunological function.— A. Rubinstein *et al.*, *New Engl. J. Med.*, 1979, *300*, 387.

Ten of 17 patients with histiocytosis-X responded to treatment with thymic extract. This was at least as good as results with a historical control group given chemotherapy. Positive responses were associated with the correction of immunological abnormalities. After a test dose, extract of calf thymus gland was given daily by intramuscular injection in a dose of 1 mg of protein per kg body-weight. The average number of injections required to achieve initial remission was 27. Three of the patients who responded have not required further treatment with extract; the other 7 relapsed and received further courses but all 10 patients are currently in remission. Most patients experienced localised tenderness at the injection site and allergic reactions occurred in 2.— M. E. Osband *et al.*, *New Engl. J. Med.*, 1981, *304*, 146.

Further references: M. A. Scheinberg *et al.*, *Lancet*, 1975, *1*, 424 (role of thymosin in systemic lupus erythematosus); M. C. Dalakas *et al.* (letter), *New Engl. J. Med.*, 1980, *302*, 1092 (role of thymosin α_1 in myasthenia gravis).

13336-s

Tiamenidine Hydrochloride. HOE-440; HOE-42-440. *N*-(2-Chloro-4-methyl-3-thienyl)-2-imidazolin-2-ylamine hydrochloride.
$C_8H_{10}ClN_3S,HCl=252.2$.

CAS — 31428-61-2 (tiamenidine); 51274-83-0 (hydrochloride).

Tiamenidine hydrochloride has antihypertensive activity.

References: D. Findlay and J. R. Lawrence, *Eur. J. clin. Pharmac.*, 1978, *14*, 231; C. Zamboulis *et al.*, *Br. J. clin. Pharmac.*, 1979, *8*, 390P; L. S. Gerlis and N. Wright, *Pharmatherapeutica*, 1980, *2*, 408; B. C. Campbell *et al.*, *Eur. J. clin. Pharmac.*, 1980, *18*, 449; B. E. Hansson and B. Hökfelt, *Br. J. clin. Pharmac.*, 1981, *11*, 73.

Manufacturers
Hoechst, UK.

13337-w

Tiamulin Fumarate. 81723-hfu; SQ-22947; SQ-14055. 11-Hydroxy-6,7,10,12-tetramethyl-1-oxo-10-vinylperhydro-3a,7-pentanoinden-8-yl (2-diethylaminoethylthio)acetate hydrogen fumarate.
$C_{28}H_{47}NO_4S,C_4H_4O_4=609.8$.

CAS — 55297-95-5 (tiamulin); 555297-96-6 (fumarate).

Tiamulin fumarate is used in the treatment of dysentery in *pigs*.

Proprietary Names
Dynamutilin *(Squibb, UK).*

13338-e

Tiapamil. Ditian Tetraoxide; Verocainine; Ro-11-1781. *N*-(3,4-Dimethoxyphenethyl)-3-[2-(3,4-dimethoxyphenyl)-1,3-dithian-2-yl]-*N*-methylpropylamine 1,1,3,3-tetraoxide.
$C_{26}H_{37}NO_8S_2=555.7$.

CAS — 57010-31-8.

Tiapamil is a calcium antagonist with potential use in cardiac arrhythmias.

References: G. Cocco and C. Strozzi, *Boll. chim.-Farm.*, 1978, *117*, 660; R. Gmeiner *et al.*, *Eur. J. clin. Pharmac.*, 1979, *16*, 155.

Manufacturers
Roche, UK.

13339-l

Tiapride. FLO-1347 *(hydrochloride)*. *N*-(2-Diethylaminoethyl)-2-methoxy-5-methylsulphonylbenzamide.
$C_{15}H_{24}N_2O_4S=328.4$.

CAS — 51012-32-9 (tiapride); 51012-33-0 (hydrochloride).

Tiapride is a neuroleptic drug with anti-emetic actions. It has been tried in the treatment of various psychiatric disorders and dyskinesias. Tiapride hydrochloride has also been used.

References: M. Strolin-Benedetti *et al.*, *Annls pharm. fr.*, 1978, *36*, 279 (absorption and fate); P. Price *et al.* (letter), *Lancet*, 1978, *2*, 1106 (levodopa-induced dyskinesia); A. J. Lees *et al.*, *J. Neurol. Neurosurg. Psychiat.*, 1979, *42*, 380 (levodopa-induced dyskinesia).

Proprietary Names of Tiapride and Tiapride Hydrochloride
Sereprile *(Vita, Ital.)*; Tiapridal *(Millet, Arg.; Delagrange, Belg.; Delagrange, Fr.)*; Tiapridex *(Schürholz, Ger.).*

13341-g

Tibezonium Iodide. Rec-15/0691. Diethylmethyl{2-[4-(4-phenylthiophenyl)-3*H*-1,5-benzodiazepin-2-ylthio]ethyl}ammonium iodide.
$C_{28}H_{32}IN_3S_2=601.6$.

CAS — 54663-47-7.

Tibezonium iodide has been used in the treatment of infections of the mouth and throat.

Physicochemical profile.— F. Fontani *et al.*, *Boll. chim.-Farm.*, 1977, *116*, 705.

Antibacterial activity.— M. Veronese *et al.*, *Chemotherapy, Basle*, 1977, *23*, 90.

Proprietary Names
Antoral *(Recordati, Ital.).*

13342-q

Tibolone. Org-OD-14. 17β-Hydroxy-7α-methyl-19-nor-17α-pregn-5(10)-en-20-yn-3-one.
$C_{21}H_{28}O_2=312.5$.

CAS — 5630-53-5.

Tibolone is an anabolic agent. It has been tried for the prevention of osteoporosis.

References: R. Lindsay *et al.*, *Br. med. J.*, 1980, *280*, 1207. Comment.— J. Coope (letter), *ibid.*, *281*, 456. A reply.— R. Lindsay and D. M. Hart (letter), *ibid.*

13343-p

Ticlopidine Hydrochloride. 5-(2-Chlorobenzyl)-4,5,6,7-tetrahydrothieno[3,2-*c*]pyridine hydrochloride.
$C_{14}H_{14}ClNS,HCl=300.2$.

CAS — 55142-85-3 (ticlopidine); 53885-35-1 (hydrochloride).

Ticlopidine is an inhibitor of platelet aggregation.

Pharmacology in *animals*.— A. Akashi *et al.*, *Arzneimittel-Forsch.*, 1980, *30*, 409; *idem*, 415.

In a double-blind study 15 patients with cerebral disorders received ticlopidine 750 mg daily for 7 days and 15 received placebo. Notable prolongation of bleeding time was observed in the patients who received ticlopidine with no change in platelet count; ADP-induced aggregation was reduced and disaggregation enhanced; collagen and adrenaline-induced aggregation was unaffected.— C. Lecrubier *et al.*, *Thérapie*, 1977, *32*, 189.

Further references: J. J. Thebault *et al.*, *Clin. Pharmac. Ther.*, 1975, *18*, 485; J. -J. Thebault *et al.*, *J. int. med. Res.*, 1977, *5*, 405; J. -J. Thebault *et al.* (letter), *Br. J. clin. Pharmac.*, 1980, *10*, 311; E. J. P. Brommer, *J. int. med. Res.*, 1981, *9*, 203; D. J. Ellis *et al.*, *Clin. Pharmac. Ther.*, 1981, *29*, 243.

Proprietary Names
Ticlid *(Millot-Solac, Fr.; Labaz, Neth.)*; Tiklid *(Labaz, Ger.; Labaz, Spain).*

13344-s

Tiletamine Hydrochloride. CI-634. 2-Ethylamino-2-(2-thienyl)cyclohexanone hydrochloride.
$C_{12}H_{17}NOS,HCl=259.8$.

CAS — 14176-49-9 (tiletamine); 14176-50-2 (hydrochloride).

Tiletamine has been reported to have anaesthetic and anticonvulsant properties.

Manufacturers
Parke, Davis, USA.

13345-w

Tilorone Hydrochloride. 2,7-Bis(2-diethylaminoethoxy)fluoren-9-one dihydrochloride.
$C_{25}H_{34}N_2O_3,2HCl=483.5$.

CAS — 27591-97-5 (tilorone); 27591-69-1 (hydrochloride).

Tilorone hydrochloride is an antiviral agent active by mouth. It has been reported to induce interferon production in *mice*.

Tilorone was reported to be toxic and unlikely to be studied in man.— *Lancet*, 1974, *2*, 761.

Lack of benefit with tilorone in amyotrophic lateral sclerosis.— W. H. Olson *et al.*, *Neurology, Minneap.*, 1978, *28*, 1293.

References to *animal* studies of tilorone: R. F. Krueger and G. D. Mayer, *Science*, 1970, *169*, 1213 and 1214 (antiviral activity); R. F. Kruegar *et al.*, *Antimicrob. Ag. Chemother.*, 1970, 486 (antiviral activity); R. H. Adamson (letter), *Lancet*, 1971, *1*, 398 (antitumour activity); A. W. Ford-Hutchinson *et al.*, *J. Pharm. Pharmac.*, 1976, *28*, 790 (anti-inflammatory activity); R. W. Kuehne *et al.*, *Antimicrob. Ag. Chemother.*, 1977, *11*, 92 (antiviral activity); W. G. Clark and J. A. Robins, *Br. J. Pharmac.*, 1978, *62*, 281 (antipyretic activity); L. Levy *et al.*, *Lepr. Rev.*, 1978, *49*, 215 (antileprotic activity).

Manufacturers
Merrell-National, USA.

13346-e

Timepidium Bromide. SA-504. 3-[Di-(2-thienyl)methylene]-5-methoxy-1,1-dimethylpiperidinium bromide monohydrate.
$C_{17}H_{22}BrNOS_2,H_2O=418.4$.

CAS — 35035-05-3 (anhydrous).

Timepidium bromide is an anticholinergic agent which has been used for the relief of spasm of the gastro-intestinal tract.

Comparison with hyoscine butylbromide.— N. Tohei *et al.*, *Arzneimittel-Forsch.*, 1975, *25*, 1813.

Proprietary Names
Sesden *(Tanabe, Jap.).*

13347-l

Tioclomarol. LM-550. 3-[5-Chloro-α-(4-chloro-β-hydroxyphenethyl)-2-thenyl]-4-hydroxycoumarin.
$C_{22}H_{16}Cl_2O_4S=447.3$.

CAS — 22619-35-8.

Tioclomarol is a coumarin anticoagulant.

Proprietary Names
Apegmone *(Oberval, Fr.).*

13348-y

Tioconazole. UK-20349. 1-[2,4-Dichloro-β-(2-chloro-3-thenyloxy)phenethyl]imidazole.
$C_{16}H_{13}Cl_3N_2OS=387.7$.

CAS — 65899-73-2.

Tioconazole has antifungal activity.

References: S. Jevons *et al.*, *Pfizer*, *Antimicrob. Ag. Chemother.*, 1979, *15*, 597.

Manufacturers
Pfizer, UK.

13349-j

Tiopronin. Tioprotide. *N*-(2-Mercaptopropionyl)glycine.
$C_5H_9NO_3S=163.2$.

CAS — 1953-02-2.

A white crystalline powder with a characteristic sulphurous odour. **Soluble** in water.

Tiopronin is a sulphydryl compound with properties similar to those of glutathione (p.53) and penicillamine (p.385). It has been used in the treatment of hepatic and skin disorders and in cystinuria.

Beneficial results were obtained in 15 patients with cystinuria treated with tiopronin in doses gradually increased to 2 g daily for periods of up to several months. In all patients the urine was kept free of cystine and in 5 patients partial or total dissolution of urinary calculi was noted. Tolerance was good with no signs of haematological, renal, or hepatic toxicity.— J. Thomas *et al.*, *Thérapie*, 1976, *31*, 623.

Parenteral administration of tiopronin (30 g over a period of 10 days) to 27 men with symptoms of chronic lead poisoning had a beneficial effect on the biochemical indices of lead poisoning. The mechanism of action is not clear.— F. Candura *et al.* (letter), *Lancet*, 1979, *1*, 330.

Proprietary Names
Capen *(Phoenix, Arg.)*; Epatiol *(Medici, Ital.)*; Mucolysin *(Proter, Ital.)*; Sutilan *(Cusi, Spain)*; Thiola *(Sidus, Arg.*; *Coop. Farm., Ital.*; *Jap.*; *Multipharmax, Switz.)*; Thiosol *(Coop. Farm., Ital.)*; Vincol *(Reig Jofré, Spain)*.

13350-q

Tiopropamine Hydrochloride. 3,3-Diphenyl-3′-(phenylthio)dipropylamine hydrochloride.
$C_{24}H_{27}NS,HCl=398.0$.

CAS — 39516-21-7 (tiopropamine).

Tiopropamine hydrochloride is used in the treatment of peptic ulcer.

Proprietary Names
Redden *(Alfa Farmaceutici, Ital.)*.

13351-p

Tiotidine. ICI-125211. 2-Cyano-1-{2-[2-(diaminomethyleneamino)thiazol-4-ylmethylthio]-ethyl}-3-methylguanidine.
$C_{10}H_{16}N_8S_2=312.4$.

CAS — 69014-14-8.

Tiotidine has histamine H_2-receptor blocking activity. Development of the compound has ceased because of tumours in *animals*.

Manufacturers
ICI Pharmaceuticals, UK.

13352-s

Tipepidine Hybenzate. Tipepidine Hibenzate. 3-[Di(2-thienyl)methylene]-1-methylpiperidine 2-(4-hydroxybenzoyl)benzoate.
$C_{15}H_{17}NS_2,C_{14}H_{10}O_4=517.7$.

CAS — 5169-78-8 (tipepidine); 31139-87-4 (hybenzate).

Pale yellow odourless tasteless crystals. Very slightly **soluble** in water; slightly soluble in alcohol; freely soluble in glacial acetic acid.

Tipepidine hybenzate is a cough suppressant which is claimed also to have an expectorant action.

Proprietary Names
Asvelik *(tipepidine) (Andromaco, Spain)*; Asverin *(ISF, Ital.*; *Tanabe, Jap.)*; Sotal *(Gramon, Arg.)*.

13353-w

Tipropidil Hydrochloride. MJ-12880-1. 1-[4-(Isopropylthio)phenoxy]-3-octylaminopropan-2-ol hydrochloride.
$C_{20}H_{35}NO_2S,HCl=390.0$.

CAS — 70895-45-3 (tipropidil); 70895-39-5 (hydrochloride).

Tipropidil hydrochloride is reported to have vasodilator activity.

Manufacturers
Bristol, USA; Mead Johnson, USA.

13354-e

Tiquinamide. Wy-24081. 5,6,7,8-Tetrahydro-3-methylquinoline-8-carbothioamide.
$C_{11}H_{14}N_2S=206.3$.

CAS — 53400-67-2.

Tiquinamide is reported to have weak histamine H_2-receptor blocking activity, but significant activity in blocking gastric acid secretion.

References: D. M. Pierce *et al.* (letter), *Br. J. clin. Pharmac.*, 1976, *3*, 943; D. E. Beattie *et al.*, *Arzneimittel-Forsch.*, 1979, *29*, 1564; A. Johnston *et al.* (letter), *Lancet*, 1979, *2*, 1191.

Manufacturers
Wyeth, UK.

13355-l

Titanium.
Ti=47.90.

CAS — 7440-32-6.

Titanium plate has been used in the repair of skull damage.

For the use of titanium in cranioplasty, see D. S. Gordon and G. A. S. Blair, *Br. med. J.*, 1974, *2*, 478; G. A. S. Blair *et al.*, *ibid.*, 1976, *2*, 907.

An evaluation of titanium cones for use as a root filling material.— J. J. Messing, *Br. dent. J.*, 1980, *148*, 41.

Preparations used in Cranioplasty
Anodising Solution *(Roy. Victoria Hosp.)*. Phosphoric acid 80, sulphuric acid 10, water to 100.
Pickling Solution *(Roy. Victoria Hosp.)*. Nitric acid 8, hydrofluoric acid 1.5, water to 100.

13356-y

Tixocortol Pivalate. JO-1016. 11β,17α-Dihydroxy-21-mercaptopregn-4-ene-3,20-dione 21-pivalate.
$C_{26}H_{38}O_5S=462.6$.

CAS — 61951-99-3 (tixocortol).

Tixocortol pivalate is a topical corticosteroid. Preparations are available for use in the nose, mouth, and ear.

For a series of *animal* and *in vitro* studies, see *Arzneimittel-Forsch.*, 1981, *31*, 453–469.

Proprietary Names
Pivalone *(Jouveinal, Fr.)*.

13357-j

Tizanidine. DS-103-282. 5-Chloro-*N*-(2-imidazolin-2-yl)-2,1,3-benzothiadiazol-4-ylamine.
$C_9H_8ClN_5S=253.7$.

CAS — 51322-75-9.

Tizanidine has been used in the treatment of disorders associated with muscle spasticity.

References: A. Bragstad and G. Blikra, *Curr. ther. Res.*, 1979, *26*, 39 (comparison with chlorzoxazone); P. Lepistö, *Curr. ther. Res.*, 1979, *26*, 454 (placebo); U. K. Rinne, *Curr. ther. Res.*, 1980, *28*, 827 (placebo, diazepam, baclofen); O. L. Hennies, *J. int. med. Res.*, 1981, *9*, 62 (diazepam); C. Smolenski *et al.*, *Curr. med. Res. Opinion*, 1981, *7*, 374 (baclofen).

Manufacturers
Sandoz, UK.

13358-z

Todralazine Hydrochloride. Todrazoline Hydrochloride; Ecarazine Hydrochloride; BT-621; CEPH. Ethyl 3-(phthalazin-1-yl)carbazate hydrochloride monohydrate.
$C_{11}H_{12}N_4O_2,HCl,H_2O=286.7$.

CAS — 14679-73-3 (todralazine); 3778-76-5 (hydrochloride, anhydrous).

Todralazine hydrochloride is an antihypertensive agent structurally related to hydralazine.

References: W. Reiterer and H. Czitober, *Arzneimittel-Forsch.*, 1977, *27*, 2163.

Proprietary Names
Aperdor, Apiracohl, Apride, Atapren, Deprezid, Dypirecohl, Ecahain, Ecara, Hydrapron, Illcut, Marukunan, Propat, Prorazin, Seirof *(all Jap.)*; Binazin *(Biosedra, Arg.)*; Binazine *(Polfa, Pol.)*.

13359-c

Toldimfos. (4-Dimethylamino-*o*-tolyl)phosphinic acid.
$C_9H_{14}NO_2P=199.2$.

CAS — 57808-64-7.

Toldimfos is a phosphorus source used in veterinary medicine.

Proprietary Names
Foston *(sodium salt) (Hoechst, UK)*.

13360-s

Tolmesoxide. RX-71107. 4,5-Dimethoxy-*o*-tolyl methyl sulphoxide.
$C_{10}H_{14}O_3S=214.3$.

CAS — 38452-29-8.

Tolmesoxide is reported to have vasodilator activity.

References: J. A. Buylla *et al.*, *Br. J. clin. Pharmac.*, 1979, *8*, 402P; B. C. Campbell *et al.*, *ibid.*, 1981, *11*, 431P.

For a comparison with diazoxide, see p.144.

Manufacturers
Reckitt & Colman Pharmaceuticals, UK.

13361-w

Toloconium Methylsulphate. Toloconium Metilsulfate. Trimethyl[1-(*p*-tolyl)dodecyl]ammonium methylsulphate.
$C_{23}H_{43}NO_4S=429.7$.

CAS — 552-92-1.

Toloconium methylsulphate is a quaternary ammonium compound which has been used in infections of the mouth.

Proprietary Names
Albert Crème *(Fessenmayer, Switz.)*; Desogen *(Geigy, Neth.*; *Ciba-Geigy, Switz.)*; Stomatosan *(Medital, Ital.)*.

NOTE. The name Desogen has also been used for preparations containing dofamium chloride.

13362-e

Tolynol. 1-(*p*-Tolyl)ethanol; *p*,α-Dimethylbenzyl alcohol.
$C_9H_{12}O=136.2$.

CAS — 536-50-5.

Tolynol has been used as a choleretic in the treatment of hepatic disorders.

Proprietary Names
Curcumyl *(SMB, Belg.)*; Norbilan *(Face, Ital.)*.

13363-l

Tonazocine Mesylate. Win-42156-2. (±)-1-[(2R*,6S*,11S*)-1,2,3,4,5,6-Hexahydro-8-hydroxy-3,6,11-trimethyl-2,6-methano-3-benzazocin-11-yl]octan-3-one methanesulphonate.
$C_{23}H_{35}NO_2,CH_4O_3S$=453.6.

CAS — 71461-18-2 (tonazocine); 73789-00-1 (mesylate).

Tonazocine mesylate is reported to have analgesic properties.

Manufacturers
Winthrop, USA.

13364-y

Tracazolate. ICI-136753. Ethyl 4-butylamino-1-ethyl-6-methyl-1*H*-pyrazolo[3,4-*b*]pyridine-5-carboxylate.
$C_{16}H_{24}N_4O_2$=304.4.

CAS — 41094-88-6.

Tracazolate is reported to have tranquillising activity.

Manufacturers
ICI Pharmaceuticals, UK.

13365-j

Transfer Factor. A non-immunogenic small peptide which is a constituent of thymus-derived lymphocytes.

Transfer factor can passively transfer cell-mediated immunity from a sensitised donor to a non-sensitised recipient. It is prepared from the lymphocytes of the donor, whose sensitivity may have been demonstrated by skin tests. Crude dialysates of disrupted lymphoid cells have been used. It has also been prepared by gel filtration.
Transfer factor has been suggested for use in infections due to bacteria, fungi, and viruses, inflammatory disorders, immunodeficiency diseases, leprosy, and malignancies. Its ultimate place in therapeutics remains to be established.

Discussions of transfer factor including its potential use as a therapeutic agent.— *Lancet*, 1973, *2*, 79; L. E. Spitler, *Int. J. Derm.*, 1978, *17*, 445; C. H. Kirkpatrick, *New Engl. J. Med.*, 1980, *303*, 390.

A report of a fatal lymphoproliferative disorder and concomitant polyclonal gammopathy 3 weeks after the administration of transfer factor to a 10-month-old child.— E. W. Gelfand *et al.*, *New Engl. J. Med.*, 1973, *289*, 1385.

A crude dialysate of buffy-coat leucocytes was concentrated and subjected to gel filtration. Three fractions A, B, and C were identified of which only fraction B conferred delayed reactivity to *Candida* antigen. Fraction B appeared to have a molecular weight of 2000 to 4000; in conjunction with the observed density this indicated a molecule of 12 amino acids and 3 or 4 RNA bases.— A. A. Gottlieb *et al.* (preliminary communication), *Lancet*, 1973, *2*, 822. Criticism.— L. E. Spitler (letter), *ibid.*, 1492.

A fraction of a preparation of transfer factor with biological activity contained a high proportion of hypoxanthine; it was not known if the hypoxanthine was responsible for biological activity.— R. H. Tomar *et al.*, *J. Allergy & clin. Immunol.*, 1976, *58*, 190, per *J. Am. med. Ass.*, 1976, *236*, 1518.

The use of *animal* transfer factor in man.— C. Boucheix *et al.* (letter), *Lancet*, 1977, *1*, 198.

Some references to the use of transfer factor: *J. Am. med. Ass.*, 1974, *227*, 131 (with BCG vaccine in Hodgkin's disease); I. -L. Strannegård *et al.* (letter), *Lancet*, 1975, *2*, 702 (severe atopic disease); A. Alonso (letter), *ibid.*, 1976, *1*, 1352 (severe atopic disease); D. G. Jose *et al.*, *ibid.*, 1976, *1*, 263 (protein-energy malnutrition and infections); J. E. Montie *et al.*, *J. Urol.*, 1977, *117*, 553 (immunotherapy of disseminated renal cell carcinoma), per *J. Am. med. Ass.*, 1977, *238*, 1690; R. E. Wolf *et al.*, *J. Am. med. Ass.*, 1977, *238*, 869 (Behçet's syndrome); C. H. Kirkpatrick, *ibid.*, 891 (Behçet's syndrome); R. S. Freedman *et al.*, *Am. J. Obstet. Gynec.*, 1978, *130*, 572 (gynaecology); H. M. Høyeraal *et al.*, *Ann. rheum. Dis.*, 1978, *37*, 175 (lack of benefit in juvenile rheumatoid arthritis); W. R. Faber *et al.*, *Clin. exp. Immun.*, 1979, *35*, 45 (lack of benefit in lepromatous leprosy).

Fungal infections. References to the use of transfer factor in candidiasis: H. F. Pabst and R. Swanson, *Br. med. J.*, 1972, *2*, 442; R. D. Feigin *et al.*, *Pediatrics*, 1974, *53*, 63; C. H. Kirkpatrick and T. K. Smith, *Ann. intern. Med.*, 1974, *80*, 310; M. de Sousa *et al.*, *Br. J. Derm.*, 1976, *94*, 79; R. M. MacKie, *ibid.*, 107; C. C. Benz *et al.*, *ibid.*, 1977, *97*, 87; J. E. Edwards *et al.*, *Ann. intern. Med.*, 1978, *89*, 91; M. Horsmanheimo *et al.*, *Archs Derm.*, 1979, *115*, 180; R. H. Tomar *et al.*, *Ann. Allergy*, 1979, *42*, 241; H. Mobacken *et al.*, *Acta derm.-vener., Stockh.*, 1980, *60*, 51.

References to the use of transfer factor in coccidioidomycosis: R. W. Steele *et al.*, *Am. J. Med.*, 1976, *61*, 283, per *Abstr. Hyg.*, 1976, *51*, 1228.

Multiple sclerosis. Absence of effect in patients with multiple sclerosis given transfer factor or placebo.— P. O. Behan *et al.*, *Lancet*, 1976, *1*, 988; T. Fog *et al.*, *ibid.*, 1978, *1*, 851.

In a double-blind placebo-controlled study the clinical state of 29 patients with multiple sclerosis of varying severity given transfer factor was compared with that of 29 carefully matched patients given placebo. The transfer factor was obtained from a pool of 20 spouses sharing the same house as an affected patient. Although the transfer factor did not significantly improve the clinical state of multiple sclerosis patients, the rate of progression in those with mild to moderate disease activity was slowed. The benefit of treatment with transfer factor was not apparent until 18 months to 2 years after its commencement. The findings justify long-term studies with transfer factor and comparison of transfer factor with other immunopotentiating agents, such as interferon.— A. Basten *et al.*, *Lancet*, 1980, *2*, 931. Comment.— *ibid.*, 953. A very important difference between the immunosuppressant approach to multiple sclerosis and attempts to stimulate the immune system with transfer factor is that immunosuppression is hazardous whereas transfer factor is at least safe.— H. Valdimarsson (letter), *ibid.*, 1191. Criticisms of the designation double-blind to the immunosuppressant regimen.— E. H. Jellinek (letter), *ibid.*, 1192; G. S. Plaut (letter), *ibid.*

Skin disorders. References to the use of transfer factor in various skin disorders: P. Gröhn *et al.*, *Acta derm.-vener., Stockh.*, 1978, *58*, 153 (severe cystic acne); M. K. Sharma *et al.*, *Clin. Immunol. Immunopath.*, 1979, *12*, 183 (cutaneous leishmania infection).

Viral infections. The failure of therapy with transfer factor in a patient with chronic active hepatitis type B.— M. J. Tong *et al.*, *New Engl. J. Med.*, 1976, *295*, 209. In a double-blind study 5 of 6 patients with active chronic aggressive hepatitis who received transfer factor and 2 of 6 who received saline showed at least moderate improvement.— S. T. Shulman *et al.* (letter), *ibid.*, 898. Reply.— M. J. Tong *et al.* (letter), *ibid.*

In a preliminary study, one injection of transfer factor 2 units given every 2 weeks for 3 months appeared to have a beneficial effect in 7 of 9 patients with chronic active hepatitis and HbsAg in their serum and liver. Two patients received a second series of injections 6 months after completion of the first course. Transfer factor might have both immunological and antiviral activities.— G. Pizza *et al.* (letter), *New Engl. J. Med.*, 1979, *300*, 1332.

Further references: S. Shulman *et al.* (letter), *Lancet*, 1974, *2*, 650; S. Jain *et al.*, *Clin. exp. Immun.*, 1977, *30*, 10, per *Abstr. Hyg.*, 1978, *53*, 724.

A report of the effective use of transfer factor to treat 1 patient with varicella pneumonia.— J. Lankford *et al.* (letter), *J. Am. med. Ass.*, 1979, *241*, 2598.

The results of a randomised double-blind placebo-controlled study in 61 children with acute lymphocytic leukaemia confirmed those of previous studies and demonstrated the efficacy of transfer factor in preventing varicella-zoster infection in susceptible subjects. Patients were given dialysable transfer factor by subcutaneous injection in doses of 1×10^8 lymphocyte equivalents per 7 kg of body-weight or placebo and have been followed-up for 12 to 30 months so far. Of the 31 children exposed to chicken-pox during the study, 14 became clinically infected and all but one of these were in the placebo group. Long-term follow-up is necessary before protection can be considered absolute.— R. W. Steele *et al.*, *New Engl. J. Med.*, 1980, *303*, 355. Comments.— C. H. Kirkpatrick, *ibid.*, 390.

After treatment with bovine transfer factor by mouth, clinical symptoms and viruria disappeared in a 4-year-old boy with combined Epstein-Barr virus and cytomegalovirus infection and specific immunity to cytomegalovirus developed.— J. F. Jones *et al.*, *Lancet*, 1981, *2*, 122. See also I. T. Thomas *et al.*, *ibid.*, 1977, *2*, 1056 (congenital cytomegalovirus infection).

13366-z

Trapidil. AR-12008. 7-Diethylamino-5-methyl-1,2,4-triazolo[1,5-*a*]pyrimidine.
$C_{10}H_{15}N_5$=205.3.

CAS — 15421-84-8.

Trapidil is reported to be a coronary vasodilator.

Mention of the use of trapidil in angina pectoris.— K. Hasegawa *et al.*, *Br. med. J.*, 1980, *281*, 27.

Proprietary Names
Locorunal; Rocornal.

13367-c

Trengestone. Ro-4-8347. 6-Chloro-9β,10α-pregna-1,4,6-triene-3,20-dione.
$C_{21}H_{25}ClO_2$=344.9.

CAS — 5192-84-7.

Trengestone is a progestogen which has been used in menstrual disorders.

Proprietary Names
Retroid *(Roche, Switz.).*

13368-k

Treoxytocin. [4-L-Threonine]-oxytocin.
$C_{42}H_{65}N_{11}O_{12}S_2$=980.2.

CAS — 26995-91-5.

A synthetic analogue of oxytocin with similar properties.

Proprietary Names
Metrodin *(Serono, Ital.).*

13369-a

Trepibutone. Trepionate; AA-149. 3-(2,4,5-Triethoxybenzoyl)propionic acid.
$C_{16}H_{22}O_6$=310.3.

CAS — 41826-92-0.

Trepibutone is reported to have spasmolytic and choleretic activity.

Proprietary Names
Supacal *(Jap.).*

13370-e

Trepipam Maleate. Trimopam Maleate; Sch-12679. (+)-2,3,4,5-Tetrahydro-7,8-dimethoxy-3-methyl-1-phenyl-1*H*-3-benzazepine hydrogen maleate.
$C_{19}H_{23}NO_2,C_4H_4O_4$=413.5.

CAS — 56030-50-3 (trepipam); 39624-66-3 (maleate).

Trepipam maleate has been tried in the treatment of psychotic disorders.

References: A. Keskiner *et al.*, *Curr. ther. Res.*, 1971, *13*, 714; T. M. Itil *et al.*, *ibid.*, 1972, *14*, 136; S. Park *et al.*, *ibid.*, 298; I. Huston *et al.*, *ibid.*, 1977, *21*, 70; J. -M. Albert *et al.*, *ibid.*, 786; Y. D. Lapierre, *ibid.*, 1978, *24*, 204.

Manufacturers
Schering, USA.

13371-l

Triamcinolone Aminobenzal Benzamidoisobutyrate. 16α,17α-(4-Dimethylaminobenzylidenedioxy)-9α-fluoro-11β,21-dihydroxypregna-1,4-diene-3,20-dione 21-(3-benzamido-2-methylpropionate).
$C_{41}H_{47}FN_2O_8$=714.8.

Triamcinolone aminobenzal benzamidoisobutyrate is a corticosteroid for topical use.

Proprietary Names
Taucorten *(Sigmatau, Ital.).*

13372-y

Triamcinolone Benetonide. Triamcinolone Acetonide Benzamidoisobutyrate. 9α-Fluoro-11β,21-dihydroxy-16α,17α-isopropylidenedioxypregna-1,4-diene-3,20-dione 21-(3-benzamido-2-methylpropionate).
$C_{35}H_{42}FNO_8$=623.7.

CAS — 31002-79-6.

Triamcinolone benetonide is a corticosteroid for topical use.

References: F. E. Roessel, *J. int. med. Res.*, 1977, *5*, 207; H. V. N. vd Kroon and L. M. J. van Driel, *ibid.*, 213; D. J. Tazelaar, *ibid.*, 338.

Proprietary Names
Tibicorten *(Sigmatau, Ital.)*.

13373-j

Triazinate. Baker's Antifol; BAF; NSC-139105; WR-219427. 3-[2-Chloro-4-(4,6-diamino-2,2-dimethyl-1,3,5-triazin-1(2*H*)-yl)phenoxymethyl]-*NN*-dimethylbenzamide.
$C_{21}H_{25}ClN_6O_2$=428.9.

CAS — 48223-06-9 (triazinate); 41191-04-2 (esylate).

Triazinate is a folate antagonist which has been tried in neoplastic disease. It is used as the esylate.

References: R. T. Skeel *et al.*, *Cancer Res.*, 1976, *36*, 48; R. H. McCreary *et al.*, *Cancer*, 1977, *40*, 9; V. Rodriguez *et al.*, *Cancer Res.*, 1977, *37*, 980; T. L. Loo *et al.*, *Drug Metab. Rev.*, 1978, *8*, 137.

13374-z

Tribenoside. Ba-21401. Ethyl 3,5,6-tri-*O*-benzyl-D-glucofuranoside.
$C_{29}H_{34}O_6$=478.6.

CAS — 10310-32-4.

Tribenoside has been used in inflammatory and varicose disorders of the veins.

References: A. Casagrande and R. S. Lodovici, *Gazz. int. Med. Chir.*, *Roma*, 1968, *73*, 714, per *Abstr. Wld Med.*, 1969, *43*, 90; W. C. Dick *et al.*, *Ann. rheum. Dis.*, 1969, *28*, 187, per *Abstr. Wld Med.*, 1969, *43*, 690; A. Sioufi and F. Pommier, *J. pharm. Sci.*, 1980, *69*, 167.

Proprietary Names
Alven *(FIRMA, Ital.)*; Flebosan *(Dukron, Ital.)*; Glyvenol *(Ciba, Arg.; Ciba, Belg.; Ciba, Fr.; Ciba, Ger.; Ciba, Ital.; Ciba, Spain; Ciba-Geigy, Switz.)*; Hemocuron *(Takeda, Jap.)*; Venalisin *(AGIPS, Ital.)*; Venodin *(Tosi-Novara, Ital.)*.

13375-c

Tricaprylin. Caprylic Acid Triglyceride; Glycerin Tricaprylate. Glyceryl trioctanoate; Propane-1,2,3-triyl trioctanoate.
$C_{27}H_{50}O_6$=470.7.

CAS — 538-23-8.

Tricaprylin has the general properties of the medium-chain triglycerides (see under Fractionated Coconut Oil, p.696) and has been similarly used.

Proprietary Names
Mac-Eight *(Ono, Jap.)*.

13376-k

Tricarbaurinium. Aluminon. The triammonium salt of 3-(3,3′-dicarboxy-4,4′-dihydroxybenzhydrylidene)-6-oxocyclohexa-1,4-diene-1-carboxylic acid.
$C_{22}H_{23}N_3O_9$=473.4.

CAS — 569-58-4.

Tricarbaurinium is claimed to inhibit the action of hyaluronidase and has been used topically in the treatment of mouth disorders.

Proprietary Names
Lysofon *(Lafon, Fr.)*.

13377-a

Trientine Dihydrochloride. Trien; Triethylenetetramine Dihydrochloride. 2,2′-Ethylenedi-iminobis(ethylamine) dihydrochloride.
$C_6H_{18}N_4$,2HCl=219.2.

CAS — 112-24-3 (trientine); 38260-01-4 (dihydrochloride).

Trientine dihydrochloride is a copper chelating agent which has been used as an alternative to penicillamine in patients with Wilson's disease. It has been given in usual doses of 1.2 to 2.1 g daily.

Trientine intended for use as a laboratory reagent should not be included in pharmaceutical preparations without purification.— J. M. Walshe (letter), *Lancet*, 1970, *2*, 154. A method for purifying trientine.— H. B. F. Dixon *et al.* (letter), *ibid.*, 1972, *1*, 853. A modified method of preparation.— I. Bucur and K. H. Hasselgren (letter), *ibid.*, 1975, *2*, 1218.

References to the use of trientine in Wilson's disease: J. M. Walshe, *Lancet*, 1969, *2*, 1401; R. S. Dubois *et al.* (letter), *ibid.*, 1970, *2*, 775; H. Harders and E. Cohnen, *Proc. R. Soc. Med.*, 1977, *70*, *Suppl.* 3, 10, per *Int. pharm. Abstr.*, 1978, *15*, 514; J. M. Walshe, *Lancet*, 1982, *1*, 643.

Further references: O. Epstein and S. Sherlock, *Gastroenterology*, 1980, *78*, 1442 (toxicity of trientine dihydrochloride when used in primary biliary cirrhosis).

Manufacturers
K & K-Greeff, UK.

13378-t

Trifluomeprazine Maleate *(B.P. Vet.)*. Triflutrimeprazine Maleate; SKF-5354A; SKF-5354I. 2,*N*,*N*-Trimethyl-3-(2-trifluoromethylphenothiazin-10-yl)propylamine hydrogen maleate.
$C_{19}H_{21}F_3N_2S$,$C_4H_4O_4$=482.5.

CAS — 2622-37-9 (trifluomeprazine).

A white or almost white, odourless or almost odourless, crystalline powder. M.p. about 178°. Very slightly **soluble** in water; soluble 1 in 25 of alcohol and 1 in 25 of chloroform; practically insoluble in ether. **Protect** from light.

Trifluomeprazine maleate is a tranquilliser used in veterinary medicine.

13379-x

Triflusal. UR-1501. 2-Acetoxy-4-trifluoromethylbenzoic acid.
$C_{10}H_7F_3O_4$=248.2.

CAS — 322-79-2.

Triflusal is a fluorinated analogue of aspirin and is reported to inhibit platelet aggregation.

References: J. Garcia-Rafanell and J. Morell, *Thérapie*, 1977, *32*, 337; -M. L. Rutllant *et al.*, *Curr. ther. Res.*, 1977, *22*, 510; R. M. Masso *et al.*, *ibid.*, 1979, *25*, 791.

Manufacturers
Uriach, Spain.

13380-y

Trilostane. Win-24540. 4α,5α-Epoxy-17β-hydroxy-3-oxoandrostane-2α-carbonitrile.
$C_{20}H_{27}NO_3$=329.4.

CAS — 13647-35-3.

Adverse Effects. Side-effects reported with high doses of trilostane have included flushing, nausea, vomiting, rhinorrhoea, and oedema of the palate.

Precautions. Trilostane is contra-indicated in pregnancy and should be used with caution in patients with renal or hepatic dysfunction. It may interfere with the activity of oral contraceptives.

A preliminary report of trilostane interference with fluorimetric steroid assays.— D. Mattingly and C. Tyler (letter), *Lancet*, 1981, *1*, 561. Comment.— G. H. Beastall *et al.* (letter), *ibid.*, 727.

Marked depression of plasma-testosterone concentrations in a man given trilostane for recurrent Cushing's syndrome.— P. E. Belchetz *et al.* (letter), *Lancet*, 1981, *1*, 897.

Uses. Trilostane is an adrenocortical suppressant which inhibits the enzyme system essential for the production of glucocorticoids and mineralocorticoids. It has been used in the treatment of Cushing's syndrome and primary aldosteronism.

The usual dose is 60 mg by mouth four times daily for at least 3 days and then adjusted, according to the patient's response, within the range of 120 to 480 mg daily. Doses of 960 mg daily have been given.

An evaluation of trilostane.— *Drug & Ther. Bull.*, 1982, *20*, 7.

Proprietary Preparations
Modrenal Capsules *(Sterling Research, UK)*. Each contains trilostane 60 mg.

13381-j

Trimebutine Maleate. 2-Dimethylamino-2-phenylbutyl 3,4,5-trimethoxybenzoate hydrogen maleate.
$C_{22}H_{29}NO_5$,$C_4H_4O_4$=503.5.

CAS — 39133-31-8 (trimebutine); 34140-59-5 (maleate).

Trimebutine maleate has antispasmodic properties and has been used in the treatment of gastro-intestinal disorders.

In an 8-week double-blind study in 20 patients with irritable bowel syndrome, trimebutine 200 mg thrice daily was more effective than placebo in relieving symptoms.— M. G. Moshal and M. Herron, *J. int. med. Res.*, 1979, *7*, 231.

Further references: K. Lüttecke, *J. int. med. Res.*, 1978, *6*, 86; *idem*, *Curr. med. Res. Opinion*, 1980, *6*, 437.

Proprietary Names
Debridat *(Armstrong, Arg.; Jouveinal, Fr.; Sigmatau, Ital.)*; Foldox *(Sidus, Arg.)*; Miopropan *(Bernabó, Arg.)*; Polibutin *(Juste, Spain)*.

13382-z

Trimetrexate. CI-898. 5-Methyl-6-(3,4,5-trimethoxyanilinomethyl)quinazoline-2,4-diyldiamine.
$C_{19}H_{23}N_5O_3$=369.4.

CAS — 52128-35-5.

Trimetrexate is reported to have antineoplastic activity.

Manufacturers
Parke, Davis, USA.

13383-c

Tritiozine. Trithiozine; ISF-2001. 4-(3,4,5-Trimethoxythiobenzoyl)morpholine.
$C_{14}H_{19}NO_4S$=297.4.

CAS — 35619-65-9.

Crystalline powder. M.p. 140° to 141°. **Soluble** 1 in 5000 of water, 1 in 12 of acetone, 1 in 7 of benzyl alcohol, 1 in 2 of chloroform, and 1 in 200 of propylene glycol. A saturated solution in water has a pH of 7. **Stable** on exposure to air, moisture, and light.

Tritiozine is reported to reduce gastric secretion and has been given in the treatment of gastric and duodenal ulcers.

A short review of tritiozine.— R. Pellegrini, *J. int. med. Res.*, 1979, *7*, 452.

A favourable report of the use of tritiozine for the treatment of 658 patients with peptic ulcers or other hypersecretory disorders. Reported side-effects, occurring in under 2% of patients, included drowsiness, nausea, headache, myalgia, paraesthesia, and pyrosis. The mechanism of action was not yet understood.— R. Pellegrini and A. Albrici, *ISF* (letter), *Farmaco, Edn prat.*, 1979, *34*, 138.

In a comparative study in 49 patients with duodenal ulcers similar healing-rates were achieved with tritiozine

1.2 g daily or cimetidine 1 g daily.— P. Tomassetti *et al.*, *Curr. ther. Res.*, 1981, *29*, 517.

Further references: R. Corinaldesi *et al.*, *Farmaco, Edn prat.*, 1977, *32*, 25; G. Dobrilla *et al.*, *Acta ther.*, 1977, *3*, 247; J. A. Frias *et al.*, *Clin. Ther.*, 1978, *1*, 251; R. Cheli *et al.*, *Curr. ther. Res.*, 1979, *26*, 62; R. Corinaldesi *et al.*, *Farmaco, Edn prat.*, 1979, *34*, 121; K. Gibiński *et al.*, *Int. J. clin. Pharmac. Biopharm.*, 1979, *17*, 48.

Proprietary Names
Tresanil *(ISF, Ital.)*.

13384-k

Tritoqualine. L-554. 7-Amino-4,5,6-triethoxy-3-(5,6,7,8-tetrahydro-4-methoxy-6-methyl-1,3-dioxolo[4,5-*g*]isoquinolin-5-yl)phthalide.
$C_{26}H_{32}N_2O_8$=500.5.
CAS — 14504-73-5.

Tritoqualine is stated to inhibit histidine decarboxylase which catalyses the conversion of histidine to histamine. It has the typical uses of the antihistamines (see p.1294).

References: R. Petry and G. Trenkner (letter), *Lancet*, 1967, *1*, 1111.

Proprietary Names
Hypostamine *(Promedica, Fr.)*; Inhibostamin *(Swiss-Pharma, Ger.)*.

13385-a

Tropatepine Hydrochloride. SD-1248-17. 3-(Dibenzo[*b,e*]thiepin-11(6*H*)-ylidene)tropane hydrochloride.
$C_{22}H_{23}NS,HCl$=370.0.
CAS — 27574-24-9 (tropatepine); 27574-25-0 (hydrochloride).

Tropatepine hydrochloride is an anticholinergic agent which has been used in the treatment of parkinsonism and drug-induced dyskinesias.

Proprietary Names
Lepticur *(Diamant, Fr.)*.

13386-t

Troxerutin. Trioxyethylrutin. 3′,4′,7-Tris[*O*-(2-hydroxyethyl)]rutin; 2-[3,4-Bis(2-hydroxyethoxy)phenyl]-5-hydroxy-7-(2-hydroxyethoxy)-4-oxo-4*H*-chromen-3-yl rutinoside.
$C_{33}H_{42}O_{19}$=742.7.
CAS — 7085-55-4.

The principal component of a mixture, commonly called trihydroxyethylrutoside, which contains also the mono-, di-, and tetra-derivatives. The term oxerutins is applied to a mixture of 5 different hydroxyethylrutosides, not less than 45% of which is troxerutin. The mixture is a fine, slightly hygroscopic, yellow to brownish-yellow powder with a faint odour and a faint slightly saline taste. It is **soluble** in water, methyl alcohol, glycerol, and propylene glycol; slightly soluble in alcohol; and practically insoluble in chloroform and ether. A 10% solution has a pH of 4.4 to 5.

Adverse Effects. Side-effects reported include gastro-intestinal disturbances, flushing, and headache.

Absorption and Fate. Troxerutin is absorbed from the gastro-intestinal tract. The principal route of excretion appears to be in the bile.

In 3 healthy subjects given radioactive hydroxyethylrutosides (Paroven) 300 mg by mouth peak plasma concentrations occurred 2 to 9 hours after administration and 27 to 29% of the radioactivity was protein-bound. Urinary excretion accounted for about 3 to 6% of the administered dose and was almost complete after 48 hours.— A. M. Hackett *et al.*, *Arzneimittel-Forsch.*, 1976, *26*, 925.

Following administration of troxerutin 500 mg by mouth to a healthy subject only trace amounts of unchanged drug were detected in the urine. However after β-glucuronidase treatment of the urine a cumulative urinary excretion corresponding to 5.3% of the administered dose was found after 78.6 hours.— H. S. I. Tan *et al.*, *J. pharm. Sci.*, 1978, *67*, 1142.

Uses. Troxerutin is a flavonoid derivative which is claimed to reduce capillary fragility and permeability. It has been used in the treatment of haemorrhoids and venous disorders of the lower limbs.

The usual dose is 250 mg of a mixture of hydroxyethylrutosides, containing not less than 45% of troxerutin, 3 or 4 times daily for 3 or 4 weeks, followed by a maintenance dose of 250 to 500 mg daily.

Evaluations of troxerutin: *Br. med. J.*, 1969, *1*, 235; *Drug & Ther. Bull.*, 1970, *8*, 91.

Complete healing within 6 weeks followed the administration of troxerutin (Paroven) 250 mg four times daily and local application of Sofra-Tulle dressings in a man with a gangrenous left fourth toe due to thrombosis of the fourth digital artery. Local treatment with crystal violet and systemic treatment with ampicillin had been unsuccessful.— E. D. M. Tod (letter), *Br. med. J.*, 1969, *1*, 642.

The use of troxerutin in lymphangiography.— P. D. Broks, *Am. J. Roentg.*, 1977, *128*, 263, per *Int. pharm. Abstr.*, 1977, *14*, 1040.

Diabetic retinopathy. In a double-blind study in 20 patients with diabetic retinopathy, troxerutin caused a significant reduction in the retinal vascular permeability to fluorescein.— M. Tschopp *et al.*, *Diabetologia*, 1970, *102*, 475, per *J. Am. med. Ass.*, 1970, *214*, 1598.

Haemorrhoids. In 91 patients with haemorrhoids, treatment with troxerutin in a dose of two 100-mg capsules thrice daily for 3 weeks resulted in significant improvement related to severe pain, bleeding, pruritus, inflammation, and serous oozing. The treatment was of most value in second- and third-degree haemorrhoids.— M. B. Clyne *et al.*, *Practitioner*, 1967, *198*, 420. A further report.— Report No. 125 of the General Practitioner Research Group 1968, 378.

In a double-blind trial 34 patients with haemorrhoids treated with hydroxyethylrutosides 200 mg thrice daily for a week then 100 mg thrice daily for 2 weeks achieved significantly greater relief in respect of bleeding, pruritus, anal discharge, and objective reduction of haemorrhoids than did 30 similar patients given a placebo. Of 24 of the patients with second- or third-degree haemorrhoids 19 obtained objective reduction with hydroxyethylrutosides compared with none of 19 given placebo. Of a further 14 patients with thrombosed internal haemorrhoids and given also 500 mg of hydroxyethylrutosides intravenously daily for 3 days, 9 were relieved more quickly than was usual with conventional treatment.— C. S. Sinnatamby, *Clin. Trials J.*, 1973, *10* (2), 45.

Raynaud's syndrome. Clear clinical improvement occurred in 7 patients with severe Raynaud's syndrome given troxerutin 2 to 3 g daily (in 2 doses) intravenously for 2 to 4 weeks, followed by 3 to 6 g daily (in 3 or 4 doses) by mouth. Similar results had been achieved in patients with chronic ischaemic legs.— F. Lund *et al.* (letter), *Br. med. J.*, 1980, *280*, 334.

Further references: A. H. Sorensen and H. Hansen (letter), *Br. med. J.*, 1969, *3*, 532.

Varicose veins. Cramps and burning and restless legs in 80 patients with chronic venous disorders of the leg were greatly reduced after treatment with troxerutin, 250 mg thrice daily for 4 weeks. The larger wet ulcers of the legs improved more quickly than did those which were smaller and dry.— S. Allen, *Practitioner*, 1970, *205*, 221.

Blood was examined from the legs of 6 healthy subjects and 14 patients with varicose veins, 9 of whom received hydroxyethylrutosides (Paroven) in a dose of 250 mg four times daily for 4 weeks. Treatment with hydroxyethylrutosides significantly altered the oxygen tension, saturation, and content of varicose vein blood. The treatment seemed significantly to improve tissue perfusion and oxygenation, with amelioration of symptoms attributed to venous insufficiency. Side-effects were negligible.— A. J. McEwan and C. S. McArdle, *Br. med. J.*, 1971, *2*, 138. A further report.— D. E. Fitzgerald, *Practitioner*, 1967, *198*, 406.

In a double-blind multicentre study completed by 90 patients with varicose veins, hydroxyethylrutosides (Paroven) 250 mg or a placebo were administered 4 times daily and patients assessed after 4 and 8 weeks. Treatment with hydroxyethylrutosides was significantly more effective than placebo in reducing pitting oedema and relieving symptoms of tired and heavy legs and nocturnal muscle cramps.— T. B. Pulvertaft, *Zyma, Practitioner*, 1979, *223*, 838.

Proprietary Preparations

Paroven *(Zyma, UK)*. Hydroxyethylrutosides, containing not less than 45% of troxerutin, available as capsules of 250 mg. (Also available as Paroven in *Austral.*).

Other Proprietary Names
Pherarutin *(Ger.)*; Pur-Rutin 20% *(Switz.)*; Relvène, Rutilémone *(both Fr.)*; Varemoid *(Austral.)*; Venamitol *(Fr.)*; Venoruton *(Arg., Belg., Ger., Ital., Neth., Spain, Switz.)*.

13387-x

Tyformin. Augmentin; Tiformin; HL-523. 4-Guanidinobutyramide.
$C_5H_{12}N_4O$=144.2.
CAS — 4210-97-3.

NOTE. A preparation containing amoxycillin and potassium clavulanate is marketed under the name Augmentin (see p.1144).

Tyformin has been found to lower the blood concentration of urea when given to patients with uraemic diabetes.

References: W. J. H. Butterfield *et al.* (letter), *Lancet*, 1969, *2*, 381; G. L. Schless *et al.* (letter), *ibid.*, 1970, *1*, 780; K. Brown *et al.* (letter), *ibid.*, 1971, *1*, 141.

13388-r

Tylosin *(B. Vet. C. 1965)*. An antimicrobial substance with a macrolide structure, produced by a strain of *Streptomyces fradiae*.
CAS — 1401-69-0.

An almost white to buff-coloured powder with a characteristic odour. **Soluble** 1 in 400 of water, 1 in 15 of alcohol, 1 in 30 of chloroform, and 1 in 6 of methyl alcohol; soluble in dilute mineral acids. A 2.5% suspension in water has a pH of 8.5 to 10.5. **Store** in airtight containers.

One unit of tylosin is contained in 0.001 mg of the first International Standard Preparation (1966) of tylosin base which contains 1000 units per mg.

Tylosin has similar antimicrobial activity to erythromycin (p.1158). It is used in veterinary medicine in the treatment of vibrionic scour in pigs and in the treatment of respiratory infections in animals, including the prevention of respiratory mycoplasmosis in chickens and infectious sinusitis and air sacculitis in turkeys.

Tylosin phosphate is added to animal feeding stuffs as a growth promoter for pigs.

A report of 2 cases of contact dermatitis due to tylosin contained in animal feed supplements. The second patient was also allergic to feed supplements containing nitrofurazone.— K. H. Neldner, *Archs Derm.*, 1972, *106*, 722.

Proprietary Names of Tylosin and its Salts
Tylamix *(Elanco, UK)*; Tylan *(Elanco, UK)*.

13389-f

Tylosin Tartrate *(B. Vet. C. 1965)*.
CAS — 1405-54-5.

A white to buff-coloured odourless powder. **Soluble** 1 in 10 of water; slightly soluble in alcohol; very slightly soluble in chloroform; practically insoluble in ether. A 2.5% solution in water has a pH of 5 to 7.5. **Store** in airtight containers.

Tylosin tartrate is used in veterinary medicine for the purposes described above under tylosin; 1.2 g of tylosin tartrate is approximately equivalent to 1 g of tylosin.

14000-c

Ubidecarenone. Ubiquinone-10; Coenzyme Q10. 2-Deca(3-methylbut-2-enylene)-5,6-dimethoxy-3-methyl-*p*-benzoquinone.
$C_{59}H_{90}O_4$=863.4.
CAS — 303-98-0.

A yellow to yellowish-orange, odourless, tasteless, crystalline powder. M.p. about 48°. Practically **insoluble** in water and methyl alcohol; very slightly soluble in alcohol; freely soluble in acetone and ether; very soluble in chloroform. **Protect** from light.

Ubidecarenone is a naturally occurring coenzyme involved in electron transport in the mitochondria. It is claimed to be involved in the metabolism of cardiac muscle and in high doses has protected *animals* from isoprenaline-induced myocardial damage. It has been used, in conjunction with standard treatment, in mild or moderate congestive heart failure.

Ubidecarenone has also been tried in conditions associated with coenzyme deficiency.

References to clinical studies: E. G. Wilkinson *et al.*, *Res. Commun. chem. Path. Pharmac.*, 1975, *12*, 111 (periodontal disease); E. G. Wilkinson *et al.*, *ibid.*, 1976, *14*, 715 (periodontal disease); T. Yamagami *et al.*, *ibid.*, 721 (essential hypertension); I. L. Hansen *et al.*, *ibid.*, 729 (periodontal disease).

Proprietary Names

Inokiten, Neuquinone, Ube-Q (all *Jap.*).

14001-k

Urapidil Hydrochloride.

B-66256 (*urapidil*). 6-[3-(4-*o*-Methoxyphenylpiperazin-1-yl)propylamino]-1,3-dimethylpyrimidine-2,4(1*H*,3*H*)-dione hydrochloride.

$C_{20}H_{29}N_5O_3,HCl=423.9$.

CAS — 34661-75-1 (urapidil); 64887-14-5 (hydrochloride).

Urapidil hydrochloride has been used in the treatment of hypertensive crises and severe hypertension.

For a series of papers on the pharmacology of urapidil in *animals*, see *Arzneimittel-Forsch.*, 1977, *27*, 1895–1932. See also W. R. Kukovetz *et al.*, *ibid.*, 2406 (pharmacokinetics in man); E. G. Bruckschen *et al.*, *ibid.*, 1978, *28*, 1176 (pharmacology and use in man).

Proprietary Names

Ebrantil (*Byk Gulden, Ger.*).

14002-a

Urate Oxidase.

Uricase; CB-8129. An enzyme obtained from *Aspergillus flavus*.

CAS — 9002-12-4.

It has been used in the treatment of hyperuricaemia.

The use of urate oxidase to treat hyperuricaemia in patients being treated for malignant disorders.— P. Kissel *et al.* (letter), *Lancet*, 1975, *1*, 229.

The use of urate oxidase derived from *Candida utilis* and bound to polyethylene glycol to treat hyperuricaemia in 5 men with neoplastic disease, without producing antibodies.— S. Davis *et al.*, *Lancet*, 1981, *2*, 281.

Proprietary Names

Uricozyme (*Clin-Comar-Byla, Fr.*).

14003-t

Urazamide.

5-Aminoimidazole-4-carboxamide ureidosuccinate.

$C_9H_{14}N_6O_6=302.2$.

Urazamide has been used in the treatment of hepatic disorders.

Proprietary Names

Carbaica (*Selvi, Ital.*); Colahepat Plus (*Ima, Arg.*).

14004-x

Uridine.

Uracil Riboside. 1-β-D-Ribofuranosyluracil; 1-β-D-Ribofuranosylpyrimidine-2,4(1*H*,3*H*)-dione.

$C_9H_{12}N_2O_6=244.2$.

CAS — 58-96-8.

Needle crystals; **soluble** in water.

Uridine is one of the four nucleosides present in ribonucleic acid.

Haematological remission was induced when uridine was given to a 17-month-old boy with refractory megaloblastic anaemia associated with hereditary orotic aciduria.— D. M. O. Becroft and L. I. Phillips, *Br. med. J.*, 1965, *1*, 547.

For studies indicating that addition of uridine rendered media containing thymine suitable for trimethoprim sensitivity testing, see S. G. B. Amyes and J. T. Smith, *J. antimicrob. Chemother.*, 1978, *4*, 415 and 421.

14005-r

Uridine Triphosphate.

UTP; Uridine Triphosphoric Acid. Uridine 5′-(tetrahydrogen triphosphate).

$C_9H_{15}N_2O_{15}P_3=484.1$.

CAS — 63-39-8.

Uridine triphosphate has been claimed to be of value in muscular atrophy and muscular weakness.

Proprietary Names of the Sodium Salt of Uridine Triphosphate

Fosforudin (*Francia Farm., Ital.*); Miosprint (*Biosint, Ital.*); Uteplex (*Ayerst, Belg.*; *Auclair, Fr.*; *Auclair, Switz.*); Utipina (*Dexter, Arg.*).

Uridine triphosphate was formerly marketed in Great Britain under the proprietary name Uteplex (*Rona*).

14006-f

Usnea barbata.

Usnea barbata is a lichen.

CAS — 125-46-2 (usnic acid).

Usnea barbata contains usnic acid which is reported to have antimicrobial activity.

Proprietary Preparations

Omnigran (*Keimdiät, Ger.: Thomson & Joseph, UK*). Ground lichen, *Usnea barbata*. For use in pharmaceutical and cosmetic preparations.

Usnagran-A (*Keimdiät, Ger.: Thomson & Joseph, UK*). An alcoholic extract of lichen, *Usnea barbata*. For use in pharmaceutical and cosmetic preparations. **Usnagran-T**. Contains the fat-soluble and water-soluble constituents of lichen. For use in pharmaceutical and cosmetic preparations. **Usnagran-TP**. A 1% solution of Usnagran-T in propylene glycol.

Other Proprietary Names

Granobil (*Ger.*).

14007-d

Vadrine.

S-131. 5-(4-Pyridyl)-1,3,4-oxadiazol-2(3*H*)-one 4-aminosalicylate.

$C_{14}H_{12}N_4O_5=316.3$.

CAS — 3547-60-2.

Vadrine was formerly used in the treatment of lepromatous leprosy and tuberculosis.

14008-n

Valepotriates.

Epoxy-iridoid esters, isolated from valerian.

CAS — 18296-45-2 (didrovaltrate); 18296-44-1 (valtrate); 25161-41-5 (acevaltrate).

They include *didrovaltrate* (6-acetoxy-1,4a,5,6,7,7a-hexahydro-1-isovaleryloxy-4-isovaleryloxymethylcyclopenta[*c*]pyran-7-spiro-2′-oxiran, $C_{22}H_{32}O_8=424.5$), *valtrate* (4-acetoxymethyl-1,6-di-isovaleryloxy-1,6,7,7a-tetrahydrocyclopenta[*c*]pyran-7-spiro-2′-oxiran, $C_{22}H_{30}O_8=422.5$), and *acevaltrate* (4-acetoxymethyl-(1 or 6)-3-acetoxy-3-methylbutyryloxy)-1,6,7,7a-tetrahydro-(6 or 1)-isovaleryloxycyclopenta[*c*]pyran-7-spiro-2′-oxiran, $C_{24}H_{32}O_{10}=480.5$). On prolonged storage and drying they are hydrolysed to yield isovaleric acid.

A mixture stated to contain didrovaltrate, valtrate, and acevaltrate has been used as a sedative.

Proprietary Names

Valmane (*Kali-Chemie, Ger.*; *Kali-Chemie, Neth.*; *Kali-Farma, Spain*).

14009-h

Valerian

(*B.P., Eur. P.*). Baldrianwurzel; Valerianae Radix; Valer; Valerian Rhizome; Valerian Root.

CAS — 8057-49-6 (valerian extract).

Pharmacopoeias. In *Arg., Aust., Belg., Br., Cz., Eur., Fr., Ger., Hung., It., Jug., Neth., Nord., Pol., Port., Roum., Rus., Span.,* and *Swiss. Br.* also describes Powdered Valerian.

Ind. P. has valerian from *V. wallichii* (Indian Valerian). *Jap. P.* has Japanese Valerian from *V. fauriei* or allied plants; it also describes Powdered Japanese Valerian.

The subterranean organs, including the rhizome, root, and stolon of *Valeriana officinalis* (Valerianaceae), dried below 40°, and containing not less than 15% of alcohol (60%)-soluble extractive. It has a characteristic odour resembling that of valeric acid and camphor, and a sweet taste with a spicy bitter after-taste. It contains an odourless crystalline principle (methyl 2-pyrrolyl ketone), alkaloids, valepotriates (see above), and about 1% of volatile oil. **Store** in a cool place. Protect from light.

Valerian has been used as an extract, infusion, or tincture, often in conjunction with bromides, chloral hydrate, and phenobarbitone, in the treatment of hysteria and other nervous conditions. It has also been used as a carminative.

NOTE. The odour of valerian may be removed from a scale pan or from the hands by rubbing with sodium bicarbonate.

Preparations

Valerian Extract (*B.P.C. 1954*). Ext. Valerian. A soft alcoholic extract. Store in a cool place in airtight containers. *Dose.* 60 to 300 mg.

Valerian Liquid Extract (*B.P.C. 1963*). Ext. Valerian. Liq. 1 in 1; prepared by percolation with alcohol (60%). *Dose.* 0.3 to 1 ml. *Belg. P.* includes a similar liquid extract, prepared with alcohol (80%).

For other preparations containing valerian, see Martindale 27th Edn, p. 1828.

Proprietary Preparations

Nerve Dellipsoids D16 (*Pilsworth, UK*). Tablets each containing valerian extract 125 mg, potassium bromide 200 mg, calcium phosphate 125 mg, and strychnine hydrochloride 200 μg.

Sedative Tonic Dellipsoids D14 (*Pilsworth, UK*). Tablets each containing valerian extract 125 mg, phenobarbitone 12.5 mg, nux vomica dry extract equivalent to nux vomica tincture 0.3 ml, and calcium phosphate 125 mg.

Other Proprietary Names

Baldrisedon (*Ger., Switz.*); Recvalysat (*Ger.*); Valdispert (*Ger., Neth.*).

14010-a

Valeric Acid.

Valerianic Acid; Baldriansäure; Acido Focénico; Acido Delfinico.

$C_5H_{10}O_2=102.1$.

CAS — 109-52-4.

Pharmacopoeias. In *Port.* and *Span. Span. P.* specifies a mixture of 2 isomers of valeric acid.

A colourless oily liquid with a characteristic disagreeable odour and a pungent sour taste. Wt per ml about 0.93 g. **Soluble** 1 in 30 of water from which it separates on the addition of calcium chloride or other soluble salts; miscible with alcohol and ether.

Valeric acid was formerly used in the treatment of hysteria and other nervous conditions.

Various salts of valeric acid have been used similarly to valerian and to valeric acid.

14011-t

Varicella Vaccine

A live attenuated varicella vaccine has been produced and has prevented the development of varicella (chicken-pox) in small groups of contacts, in patients with leukaemia, and in immunosuppressed patients.

Discussions and the prospects for development.— A. B. Sabin, *J. Am. med. Ass.*, 1977, *238*, 1731; J. A. Dudgeon, *Archs Dis. Childh.*, 1980, *55*, 3.

Protection of contacts: M. Takahashi *et al.* (preliminary communication), *Lancet*, 1974, *2*, 1288; Y. Asano *et al.* (letter), *Lancet*, 1976, *1*, 965; Y. Asano *et al.*, *Pediatrics*, 1977, *59*, 3 and 8.

Protection in leukaemia: H. Nakagawa and N. Katsushima, *Tohoku J. exp. Med.*, 1978, *126*, 393, per *Abstr. Hyg.*, 1979, *54*, 576; K. Ha *et al.*, *Pediatrics*, 1980, *65*, 346, per *Int. pharm. Abstr.*, 1980, *17*, 512.

14012-x

Vecuronium Bromide.

Org-NC-45. 1-(3α,17β-Diacetoxy-2β-piperidino-5α-androstan-16β-yl)-1-methylpiperidinium bromide.
$C_{34}H_{57}BrN_2O_4$=637.7.

CAS — 50700-72-6.

Vecuronium bromide is a non-depolarising neuromuscular blocking agent.

References: R. J. Marshall and J. A. O. Ojewole, *Br. J. Pharmac.*, 1979, *66*, 77P; N. N. Durant *et al.*, *Br. J. Anaesth.*, 1980, *52*, 723; N. Krieg *et al.*, *Br. J. Anaesth.*, 1980, *52*, 783; J. Norman *et al.*, *Br. J. Anaesth.*, 1980, *52*, 956P; *Br. J. Anaesth.*, 1980, *52*, *Suppl.* 1, 1–72S; N. Krieg *et al.*, *Br. J. Anaesth.*, 1981, *53*, 259; J. J. Savarese, *Anesthesiology*, 1981, *55*, 1; M. R. Fahey *et al.*, *Anesthesiology*, 1981, *55*, 6.

Manufacturers
Organon, UK.

14013-r

Veratrine *(B.P.C. 1934).*

CAS — 8051-02-3 (mixture).

NOTE. Veratrine should be distinguished from protoveratrines obtained from veratrum.

Pharmacopoeias. In *Aust.*, *Pol.*, *Port.*, and *Span.*

A mixture of alkaloids from sabadilla (see p.842). It is a white or greyish-white powder with an intensely acrid and numbing taste. Practically **insoluble** in water; soluble 1 in 3 of alcohol, 1 in 3 of chloroform, 1 in 6 of ether, and in other organic solvents. **Store** in airtight containers. Protect from light.

Adverse Effects and Treatment. Veratrine resembles aconite (p.1674) in its action on the peripheral nerve endings and poisoning should be treated similarly. It is an intense local irritant and has a powerful direct stimulating action on all muscle tissues. *It has a violent irritant action on mucous membranes, even in minute doses, and must be handled with great care.* Internally, it causes violent vomiting, purging, an intense burning sensation in the mouth and throat, and general muscular weakness.

Uses. Veratrine should not be used internally. It was formerly applied externally for its analgesic properties and as a parasiticide, especially for head lice, but even when used in this way there is danger of systemic poisoning from absorption.

14014-f

Vinburnine.

Vincamone; CH-846; (−)-Eburnamonine; 3α,16α-Eburnamonine. (3α,16α)-Eburnamenin-14(15*H*)-one.
$C_{19}H_{22}N_2O$=294.4.

CAS — 4880-88-0.

Vinburnine is used in conditions associated with cerebral circulatory insufficiency.

Proprietary Names
Cervoxan [see also under Deanol (acetamidobenzoate)]-*(Sobio, Fr.)*; Eburnal *(Chiesi, Ital.)*.

14015-d

Vincamine.

An alkaloid obtained from *Vinca minor* (Apocynaceae). Methyl (3α,16α)-14,15-dihydro-14β-hydroxyeburnamenine-14-carboxylate.
$C_{21}H_{26}N_2O_3$=354.4.

CAS — 1617-90-9.

Vincamine is claimed to increase cerebral circulation and utilisation of oxygen and has been used in a variety of cerebral disorders. It has been given by mouth in doses of 40 to 80 mg daily and has also been administered intramuscularly and by intravenous infusion.

Vincamine hydrochloride and vincamine tartrate have also been used.

For a series of papers on vincamine, see *Arzneimittel-Forsch.*, 1977, *27*, 1238–98.

References to pharmacokinetic studies of vincamine: K. Ventouras *et al.*, *Pharm. Acta Helv.*, 1977, *52*, 97; P. W. Lücker *et al.*, *Arzneimittel-Forsch.*, 1978, *28*, 79; W. Erking *et al.*, *ibid.*, 2332.

References to clinical studies of vincamine: P. Foltyn, *Arzneimittel-Forsch.*, 1978, *28*, 90 (psychiatric disturbances in the elderly); W. J. Dekoninck *et al.*, *ibid.*, 1654 (acute stroke); P. Mikus, *ibid.*, 2165 (cerebrovascular insufficiency); E. Thiery *et al.*, *ibid.*, 1979, *29*, 571 (acute stroke).

Proprietary Names
Arg.—Atervit, Sostenil, Vincalex, Vincapan, Vinodrel; *Belg.*—Cerebroxine, Pervincamine, Vinca, Vincamed *(also hydrochloride)*; *Fr.*—Perphal, Pervincamine, Tripervan, Vasculogène, Vinca *(also hydrochloride)*, Vincabrain, Vincafor Retard, Vincasaunier, Vincimax; *Ger.*—Cetal *(also hydrochloride)*, Equipur, Esberidin *(hydrochloride)*, Novicet, Pervincamin *(also hydrogen tartrate)*, VincaHexal, Vincapront; *Hung.*—Devincan; *Ital.*—Anasclerol *(hydrochloride)*, Ausomina, Cerebramina, Gibivi, Pervincamina, Teproside *(teprosilate)*, Vasonett, Vinca, Vincadar, Vinca-Dil, Vincafolina, Vincamidol; *Spain*—Artensen, Arteriovinca, Asnai, Centractiva, Cetovinca *(ketoglutarate)*, Horusvin, Oxicebral, Tefavinca, Vadicate, Vincabiomar, Vincacen, Vincadar, Vincagalup, Vincane, Vincavix; *Switz.*— Aethroma, Cetal Retard, Oxygeron, Pervincamine, Pervone, Tonifor, Vinca, Vincabrain, Vincapront.

14016-n

Vinpocetine.

Ethyl Apovincaminate; Ethyl Apovincaminoate; RGH-4405. Ethyl (3α,16α)-eburnamenine-14-carboxylate.
$C_{22}H_{26}N_2O_2$=350.5.

CAS — 42971-09-5.

Vinpocetine has been used in cerebral circulatory disorders.

For a series of papers on *animal* and clinical studies with vinpocetine, see *Arzneimittel-Forsch.*, 1976, *26*, 1907–1989.

Pharmacokinetics.— L. Vereczkey *et al.*, *Arzneimittel-Forsch.*, 1979, *29*, 957.

Proprietary Names
Cavinton *(Gedeon Richter, Hung.)*.

14017-h

Vinyl Chloride.

Vinyl Chloride Monomer; VCM. Chloroethylene.
C_2H_3Cl=62.50.

CAS — 75-01-4.

A colourless gas with a characteristic odour. It liquefies on cooling. B.p. −13.9°. It is inflammable and forms explosive mixtures with air in the range 4 to 22% v/v. **Soluble** in alcohol.

Vinyl chloride is used in the manufacture of polyvinyl chloride (PVC) and other vinyl polymers. Occupational exposure to vinyl chloride in polymerisation plants has been associated with acro-osteolysis, especially in the terminal phalanges of the fingers, a condition resembling Raynaud's phenomenon, and sclerodermatous skin changes; liver damage and hepatic angiosarcoma; splenomegaly; thrombocytopenia; impaired respiratory function; and chromosomal abnormalities.

As a result of these toxic effects the use of vinyl chloride as an aerosol propellent and in cosmetics has been banned in many countries and efforts are being made to limit the amount of vinyl chloride present in food packaging materials.

Maximum permissible atmospheric concentration 5 ppm.

See also under Plastics, p.1744.

A detailed review of the chemistry, biotransformation, toxicology, and carcinogenicity of vinyl chloride. An increase in reported cases of vinyl chloride-induced liver malfunction, angiosarcoma, Raynaud's syndrome, scleroderma, and acro-osteolysis should be expected in the near future due to past exposures; the exposure of the general population to vinyl chloride-propelled aerosols and household products might contribute to these disease states. Occupational exposures would probably decrease as vinyl chloride-polyvinyl chloride plants met the new exposure limit of 1 ppm.— T. J. Haley, *J. Toxic. envir. Hlth*, 1975, *1*, 47, per *Abstr. Hyg.*, 1976, *51*, 7.

A symposium reviewing the British experience of the environmental, epidemiological, and pathological effects of exposure to vinyl chloride arising during the course of polymerisation to polyvinyl chloride.— *Proc. R. Soc. Med.*, 1976, *69*, 275–310.

The FDA proposed to ban certain food packaging material made from vinyl chloride since it was found that residual vinyl chloride gas trapped in polyvinyl chloride could migrate into food.— *FDA Consumer*, 1976, (Dec.–Jan.), 5.

Pregnancy and the neonate. The incidence of foetal deaths was significantly increased in wives whose husbands were occupationally exposed to vinyl chloride.— P. F. Infante *et al.*, *Lancet*, 1976, *1*, 734.

Following exposure to vinyl chloride no teratogenic response was noted in *mice*, *rats*, or *rabbits*.— J. A. John *et al.*, *Toxic. appl. Pharmac.*, 1977, *39*, 497.

14018-m

Vinzolidine Sulphate.

Vinzolidine Sulfate; LY-104208.
$C_{48}H_{58}ClN_5O_9,H_2SO_4$=982.5.

CAS — 67699-40-5 (vinzolidine); 67699-41-6 (sulphate).

Vinzolidine sulphate is structurally related to vinblastine sulphate and is reported to have antineoplastic activity.

Manufacturers
Lilly, USA.

14019-b

Viquidil Hydrochloride.

Quinicine Hydrochloride; Mequiverine Hydrochloride; LM-192. 1-(6-Methoxy-4-quinolyl)-3-(3-vinyl-4-piperidyl)propan-1-one hydrochloride.
$C_{20}H_{24}N_2O_2,HCl$=360.9.

CAS — 84-55-9 (viquidil); 52211-63-9 (hydrochloride).

A yellow odourless powder with a bitter taste. M.p. about 184°. Sparingly **soluble** in water; soluble in alcohol; practically insoluble in acetone.

Viquidil has been claimed to reduce arterial spasm, to increase cerebral blood flow, and to facilitate oxygen utilisation. It has been used in various cerebral disorders.

Effect on blood platelets *in vitro*.— C. Lecrubier *et al.*, *Arzneimittel-Forsch.*, 1972, *22*, 1334.

Effect on cerebral circulation.— B. Hünermann *et al.*, *Arzneimittel-Forsch.*, 1973, *23*, 1074.

Proprietary Names
Desclidium *(Ima, Arg.; Pharmuka, Belg.; Spret-Mauchant, Fr.; Badische, Ger.; Rorer, Ital.; Sideta, Spain; Spret, Switz.)*; Vasexten *(Bernabó, Arg.)*.

14020-x

Xantofyl Palmitate.
Xanthophyl Dipalmitate; Heleniene. β,ε-Carotene-3,3′-diyl dipalmitate.

$C_{72}H_{116}O_4$=1045.7.

CAS — 547-17-1.

Xantofyl palmitate has been used by mouth in the treatment of some visual disturbances.

Proprietary Names
Adaptinol *(Bayer, Fr.; Bayropharm, Ital.)*.

14021-r

Xenbucin.
2-(Biphenyl-4-yl)butyric acid.

$C_{16}H_{16}O_2$=240.3.

CAS — 959-10-4.

Xenbucin has been used in the treatment of lipid disorders

Proprietary Names
Liposana *(Farmaroma, Ital.)*.

14022-f

Xibornol.
CP-3H; IBX; IHP. 6-(Isoborn-2-yl)-3,4-xylenol; 6-[(1*R*,2*S*,4*S*)-Born-2-yl]-3,4-xylenol.

$C_{18}H_{26}O$=258.4.

CAS — 38237-68-2.

Xibornol is an antimicrobial agent which has been used in the treatment of infections of the respiratory tract.

Proprietary Names
Nanbacine *(Fournier Frères, Fr.)*.

14023-d

Xylazine.
N-(5,6-Dihydro-4*H*-1,3-thiazin-2-yl)-2,6-xylidine.

$C_{12}H_{16}N_2S$=220.3.

CAS — 7361-61-7 (xylazine); 23076-35-9 (hydrochloride).

Xylazine is a sedative, analgesic, and muscle relaxant used in veterinary medicine.

The varying pharmacological effects of xylazine in *animals*.— P. Simon *et al.*, *Thérapie*, 1973, *28*, 735.

A report of an overdosage with xylazine in man.— S. G. Carruthers *et al.*, *Clin. Toxicol.*, 1979, *15*, 281.

Proprietary Names
Rompun *(Bayer Agrochem, UK)*.

14024-n

Yohimbine Hydrochloride *(B.P.C. 1949)*.
Aphrodine Hydrochloride; Corynine Hydrochloride; Chlorhydrate de Québrachine. The hydrochloride of the principal alkaloid of the bark of the yohimbe tree, *Pausinystalia yohimbe* (= *Corynanthe yohimbi*) (Rubiaceae). Methyl 17α-hydroxy-yohimban-16α-carboxylate hydrochloride.

$C_{21}H_{26}N_2O_3,HCl$=390.9.

CAS — 146-48-5 (yohimbine); 65-19-0 (hydrochloride).

Pharmacopoeias. In *Aust., Cz., Fr., Span.,* and *Swiss.*

A white odourless crystalline powder with a bitter taste. **Soluble** 1 in 100 of water; more soluble in hot water and alcohol. Solutions are **sterilised** by maintaining at 98° to 100° for 30 minutes with a bactericide or by filtration. **Incompatible** with alkalis, bromides, and iodides.

Yohimbine produces an α-adrenoceptor block of short duration. It has been reported to have an antidiuretic action. It has been used for its alleged aphrodisiac properties but convincing evidence of such an effect is lacking. It is contra-indicated in renal or hepatic disease.

Yohimbine is an α_2-selective adrenoceptor antagonist that enhances noradrenaline efflux without blocking postsynaptic vascular α_1 receptors.— B. B. Hoffman and R. J. Lefkowitz, *New Engl. J. Med.*, 1980, *302*, 1390.

Four of 6 impotent diabetics with incapacitating paraesthesia of the lower limbs noted prompt relief of paraesthesia after taking yohimbine 6 mg thrice daily by mouth. Paraesthesia recurred when treatment was interrupted.— A. Morales *et al.* (letter), *New Engl. J. Med.*, 1981, *305*, 1221.

A report of favourable effects with yohimbine in a double-blind placebo-controlled study of patients with clomipramine-induced orthostatic hypotension.— Y. Lecrubier *et al.* (letter), *Br. J. clin. Pharmac.*, 1981, *12*, 90.

Interactions. For the effect of yohimbine on clonidine, see Clonidine Hydrochloride, p.139.

Proprietary Preparations
Vikonon *(Savoy Laboratories, UK: Farillon, UK)*. Tablets each containing yohimbine hydrochloride 5 mg, caffeine 65 mg, calcium glycerophosphate 130 mg, ergocalciferol 240 units, cyanocobalamin 20 µg, thiamine hydrochloride 3 mg, and tocopheryl succinate 10 mg. *Dose.* 1 tablet morning and evening as required.

Preparations containing yohimbine hydrochloride were also formerly marketed in Great Britain under the proprietary names Potensan and Potensan Forte (*Medo-Chemicals*).

14025-h

Zanthoxylum Fruit.
Prickly Ash Berries. The pericarp of the ripe fruit of *Zanthoxylum piperitum (= Xanthoxylum piperitum)* (Rutaceae) or other species of *Zanthoxylum*.

Pharmacopoeias. In *Jap.* which also includes Powdered Zanthoxylum Fruit.

It contains about 3.3% v/w of essential oil. It is an ingredient of Bitter Tincture (*Jap. P.*).

Zanthoxylum *B.P.C. 1934* Toothache Bark; Xanthoxylum) is the dried bark of the northern prickly ash, *Z. americanum*, or the southern prickly ash, *Z. clavaherculis*.

Zanthoxylum fruit has carminative properties.

14026-m

Zaprinast.
1,4-Dihydro-5-(2-propoxyphenyl)-7*H*-1,2,3-triazolo[4,5-*d*]pyrimidin-7-one.

$C_{13}H_{13}N_5O_2$=271.3.

CAS — 37762-06-4.

Zaprinast is reported to have anti-allergic activity.

References: B. J. Broughton *et al.* (letter), *Nature*, 1974, *251*, 650.

Manufacturers
May & Baker, UK.

14027-b

Zeranol.
Zearalanol; MK-188; P-1496; THFES(HM). (3*S*,7*R*)-3,4,5,6,7,8,9,10,11,12-Decahydro-7,14,16-trihydroxy-3-methyl-1*H*-2-benzoxacyclotetradecin-1-one.

$C_{18}H_{26}O_5$=322.4.

CAS — 26538-44-3.

Zeranol is an oestrogenic agent. It has also been used as a growth promoter in veterinary practice.

In a study in women who had undergone hysterectomy and ovariectomy 15 were given zeranol 75 mg daily, 15 were given conjugated oestrogens 1.25 mg daily, and 15 were given a placebo. Zeranol had oestrogenic properties similar to those of conjugated oestrogens, reducing the incidence of hot flushes and promoting the maturation of vaginal epithelial cells, without significant side-effects.— W. H. Utian, *Br. med. J.*, 1973, *1*, 579.

Proprietary Names
Frideron *(Sandoz, Ital.)*; Ralone *(Ist. Chem. Ital., Ital.; Llorens, Spain)*.

14028-v

Zimelidine Hydrochloride.
H-102/09. (*Z*)-4-Bromo-*NN*-dimethyl-γ-(3-pyridyl)cinnamylamine dihydrochloride monohydrate.

$C_{16}H_{17}BrN_2,2HCl,H_2O$=408.2.

CAS — 56775-88-3 (zimelidine); 60525-15-7 (hydrochloride, anhydrous); 61129-30-4 (hydrochloride, monohydrate).

Zimelidine hydrochloride is an inhibitor of serotonin uptake and has been used in the treatment of depression. The usual dose is 200 to 300 mg daily, and 100 to 200 mg daily for elderly patients. It should not be given with monoamine oxidase inhibitors.

Reports of the use of zimelidine in depression.— O. Benkert *et al.*, *Arzneimittel-Forsch.*, 1977, *27*, 2421; B. Siwers *et al.*, *Clin. Pharmac. Ther.*, 1977, *21*, 194; J. Cox *et al.*, *Prog. Neuro-Psychopharmac.*, 1978, *2*, 379; A. Aberg and G. Holmberg, *Acta psychiat. scand.*, 1979, *59*, 45.

Use in migraine.— E. Syvälahti *et al.*, *Curr. ther. Res.*, 1979, *25*, 299.

Further references: C. D. Burgess *et al.*, *Postgrad. med. J.*, 1979, *55*, 704; W. Z. Potter *et al.*, *Clin. Pharmac. Ther.*, 1980, *27*, 278; D. Brown *et al.*, *Eur. J. Clin. Pharmac.*, 1980, *17*, 111; R. J. Simpson *et al.*, *Br. med. J.*, 1980, *280*, 1133; R. J. Simpson *et al.*, *Br. J. clin. Pharmac.*, 1981, *11*, 96; *Acta psychiat scand.*, 1981, *63*, *Suppl.* 290, 1–477.

Proprietary Preparations
Zelmid *(Astra, UK)*. Zimelidine hydrochloride, available as tablets of 100 and 200 mg.

14029-g

Zinc Bromide.

$ZnBr_2$=225.2.

CAS — 7699-45-8.

A very hygroscopic granular powder with a sharp metallic taste. **Soluble** 1 in 0.25 of water and 2 in 1 of alcohol (90%); soluble in ether and in solutions of alkali hydroxides. A solution in water is acid to litmus (pH about 4). **Store** in airtight containers.

Zinc bromide in concentrated aqueous solutions has been used as a biological shielding material against gamma-rays and X-rays.

Proprietary Preparations
Zinc Bromide Optical Grade Solution *(Steetley Mfg, UK)*. A 77% aqueous solution. Wt per ml 2.45 to 2.55 g. A transparent solution which is employed as a biological shield in viewing-windows used for the viewing of radioactive materials.

14030-f

Zinviroxime.
LY-122771. (*Z*)-2-Amino-6-benzoyl-1-(isopropylsulphonyl)-1*H*-benzimidazole oxime.

$C_{17}H_{18}N_4O_3S$=358.4.

CAS — 72301-78-1.

Zinviroxime is an isomer of enviroxime and is reported to have antiviral activity.

Manufacturers
Lilly, USA.

14031-d

Zopiclone. RP-27267. 6-(5-Chloro-2-pyridyl)-6,7-dihydro-7-oxo-5*H*-pyrrolo[3,4-*b*]-pyrazin-5-yl 4-methylpiperazine-1-carboxylate. $C_{17}H_{17}ClN_6O_3$=388.8.

CAS — 43200-80-2.

Zopiclone, though differing structurally, is reported to have hypnotic and sedative activity similar to that of the benzodiazepines (see Diazepam, p.1519).

References: E. Wickstrøm and K. -E. Giercksky, *Eur. J. clin. Pharmac.*, 1980, *17*, 93; K. -E. Giercksky and E. Wickstrøm, *Clin. Ther.*, 1980, *3*, 21.

Manufacturers
May & Baker, UK.

14032-n

Zorubicin. Rubidazone; NSC-164011 (hydrochloride); RP-22050. Benzoic acid (2*S*,4*S*)-{1-[4-(3-amino-2,3,6-trideoxy-α-L-lyxopyranosyloxy)-1,2,3,4,6,11-hexahydro-2,5,12-trihydroxy-7-methoxy-6,11-dioxonaphthacen-2-yl]ethylidene}hydrazide. $C_{34}H_{35}N_3O_{10}$=645.7.

CAS — 54083-22-6 (zorubicin); 36508-71-1 (hydrochloride).

Zorubicin is a derivative of daunorubicin and has antineoplastic activity.

References: C. Jacquillat *et al.*, *Br. med. J.*, 1972, *4*, 468; C. Jacquillat *et al.*, *Cancer*, 1976, *37*, 653; R. S. Benjamin *et al.*, *Cancer Res.*, 1977, *37*, 4623.

Manufacturers
Rhône-Poulenc, Fr.

Part 3

Formulas of British Proprietary Medicines

Proprietary medicines that are primarily intended for supply against prescriptions written by medical practitioners for individual patients are described in Parts 1 and 2 of Martindale.

'Counter' Proprietaries

The formulas given in the following list are for proprietary medicines licensed in Great Britain (excluding herbal products) and advertised for over-the-counter sale to the public in the press, by broadcasting, or by display. These proprietary medicines may be for general sale or for sale only through a pharmacy. No sharp distinction can be drawn between proprietary medicines in this list and those described in Parts 1 and 2 of this volume, as some of the medicines in this list may be prescribed, just as some of the medicines in Parts 1 and 2 of *Martindale* may lawfully be supplied to the public without a prescription.

Many of these preparations have a 'licence of right' and remain to be examined by the Committee on the Review of Medicines. Inclusion of a proprietary medicine in this list does not necessarily signify that the ingredients are innocuous or efficacious and reference should be made to the monographs in Parts 1 and 2 for information on the possible adverse effects, abuse potential, contra-indications, and hypersensitivity to the ingredients. It should also be noted that the contents of these preparations are as described by the manufacturers.

Over a period of years the Council of the Pharmaceutical Society of Great Britain has advised its members not to supply the following over the counter:

(a) preparations for slimming purposes, other than foods, unless to be taken on medical advice,
(b) preparations claimed to counteract the undesirable effects of alcoholic beverages,
(c) mixtures containing morphine for administration to infants as carminatives and sedatives,
(d) teething powders containing mercury compounds, and
(e) glycerin of borax and honey of borax.

10 Hour Capsules *(Cupal, UK).* Each capsule contains paracetamol 150 mg, noscapine 10 mg, terpin hydrate 30 mg, and phenylephrine hydrochloride 5 mg.

Abdine *(Abdine, UK).* Each **Single Strength** powder contains sodium and potassium tartrate 2.75 g, sodium bicarbonate 2.75 g, and tartaric acid 2.5 g; each **Double Strength** powder contains sodium and potassium tartrate 7 g, sodium bicarbonate 3 g, and tartaric acid 2.5 g.

Acnaid Lotion *(Cupal, UK).* Contains cetrimide 1%, salicylic acid 0.05% and alcohol (90%) 30%.

Acne-Aid Soap *(Stiefel, UK).* Active ingredient: sulphated surfactant blend 6.3%.

Acriflex *(Farley, UK).* A cream containing chlorhexidine gluconate solution 5%.

Actron *(Miles, UK).* Tablets each containing aspirin 267 mg, paracetamol 133 mg, caffeine 40 mg, sodium bicarbonate 1.606 g, and citric acid 954 mg.

Adrifax Spray Dressing *(Industrial Pharmaceutical, UK).* Benzocaine 5% and cetrimide 0.5%.

Adult Cough Balsam *(Cupal, UK).* Contains morphine hydrochloride 0.0165%, ammonium acetate 3.5%, squill vinegar 12%, acetic acid 3.33%, glycerol 10%, and sucrose 40%.

Aerocol Pain-relieving Spray *(Thornton & Ross, UK).* Trichloromonofluoromethane 85% and dichlorodifluoromethane 15%.

Afrazine Nasal Spray *(Kirby-Warrick, UK).* Contains oxymetazoline hydrochloride 0.05%.

Aidex Cream *(Cuxson, Gerrard, UK).* Aminacrine hydrochloride 0.1% and benzocaine 0.1%.

Airball Breathe Easy *(Temana, UK).* Active constituents: eucalyptus oil 11.4%, menthol 0.57%, and thymol 0.47%.

Alcovite *(Booker Health, UK).* Each tablet contains ascorbic acid 500 mg, cysteine 10 mg, pyridoxine hydrochloride 5 mg, thiamine hydrochloride 20 mg, and zinc (as amino acid chelate) 2 mg.

Algispray *(Kirby-Warrick, UK: Sangers Agencies, UK).* Glycol salicylate 5%, diethylamine salicylate 5%, methyl nicotinate 1%, vehicle to 100%.

Alka-Mints *(Miles, UK).* Flavoured tablets each containing calcium carbonate 450 mg and aluminium hydroxide-magnesium carbonate co-dried gel 50 mg.

Alka-Seltzer Tablets *(Miles, UK).* Each contains aspirin 324 mg, citric acid, anhydrous, 965 mg, and sodium bicarbonate 1.625 g.

All Clear Shampoo *(Elida Gibbs, UK).* Active constituent: pyrithione zinc 1%.

Aluzyme *(Phillips Yeast, UK).* Tablets each containing thiamine 160 µg, riboflavine 210 µg, niacin 2.5 mg, folic acid 14 µg, with other vitamins of the B complex natural to brewers' yeast.

Amm-i-dent *(Stafford-Miller, UK).* Active ingredient: carbamide [urea] 13%.

Amovon Corn Caps *(Amovon, UK).* Plasters spread with an ointment containing salicylic acid 40%.

Anadin Maximum Strength Capsules *(International Chemical, UK).* Each contains aspirin 500 mg and caffeine 32 mg.

Anadin Soluble Tablets *(International Chemical, UK).* Effervescent tablets each containing aspirin 325 mg and caffeine citrate 30 mg.

Anadin Tablets *(International Chemical, UK).* Each contains aspirin 325 mg, caffeine 15 mg, and quinine sulphate 1 mg.

Anbesol *(International Chemical, UK).* Active ingredients: lignocaine hydrochloride 0.9%, chlorocresol 0.1%, and cetylpyridinium chloride 0.02%.

Andrews Liver Salt *(Sterling Health).* Contains anhydrous citric acid 19.5%, sodium bicarbonate 22.6%, magnesium sulphate (dihydrate) 17.4%, and sucrose 40.5%.

Andrews Liver Salt for Diabetics *(Sterling Health).* Contains tartaric acid 40%, sodium bicarbonate 42.33%, magnesium sulphate (dihydrate) 17.63%, and saccharin sodium 0.05%.

Anestan Tablets *(Crookes Products, UK).* Each contains ephedrine hydrochloride 15 mg, theophylline hydrate 60 mg, and salicylamide 130 mg.

Angiers Junior Aspirin *(Bristol-Myers, UK).* Tablets each containing aspirin 75 mg.

Anodesyn *(Crookes Products, UK).* **Ointment** containing ephedrine hydrochloride 0.25%, lignocaine hydrochloride 0.5%, and allantoin 0.5%. **Suppositories** contain in addition bronopol 0.2%.

Anorm Ointment *(Norma, UK).* Aldioxa 0.5%, bismuth subgallate 3%, boric acid 5%, zinc oxide 10%, Peru balsam 2%, and lauromacrogol '400' 3%.

An-Skels Pastilles *(Smith Kendon, UK).* Cetylpyridinium chloride 1 mg.

Anthical Cream *(May & Baker, UK).* Contains mepyramine maleate 1.5% and zinc oxide 15% in a vanishing cream basis.

Antipeol *(Medico-Biological Laboratories, UK: Sestri, UK).* Ointment containing zinc oxide 20%, ichthammol 2.8%, urea 0.1%, and salicylic acid 0.1%.

Antussin Cough Syrup *(Sterling Health).* Each 5 ml contains dextromethorphan hydrobromide 5.28 mg, phenylephrine hydrochloride 3.52 mg, ammonium chloride 44 mg, and ipecacuanha liquid extract 0.005 ml.

Aphagel *(Savory & Moore, UK).* Contains benzocaine 1% and cetylpyridinium chloride 0.01% in a protective basis.

Aqua-Ban Tablets *(Thompson Medical, UK).* Each contains ammonium chloride 325 mg and caffeine 100 mg.

Askit Powders *(Askit, UK).* Each contains microfined aspirin 530 mg, aloxiprin 140 mg, caffeine citrate 110 mg, and aluminium glycinate 30 mg. **Hot Lemon Askit** contains the same active ingredients.

Askit Tablets *(Askit, UK).* Each contains aspirin 230 mg, aloxiprin 110 mg, caffeine 20 mg, and aluminium glycinate 10 mg.

Aspergum *(Plough, UK).* Chewing gum tablets each containing aspirin 227 mg.

Aspro *(Nicholas, UK).* Each tablet contains microfined aspirin 320 mg. **Effervescent Aspro.** Each tablet contains aspirin 300 mg. **Aspro Clear.** Each soluble tablet contains aspirin 300 mg, in an effervescent basis.

Atkinson & Barker's Infants' Gripe Mixture *(Strenol, UK).* Each 5 ml contains light magnesium carbonate 250 mg, sodium bicarbonate 75 mg, sucrose 487.5 mg, alcohol 0.356 ml, fennel oil 0.004 ml, and dill oil 0.004 ml.

Atrixo Hand Cream *(Smith & Nephew Toiletries, UK).* An emulsion containing a silicone oil and fatty alcohols with parabens.

Avrogel *(Vincent, UK: De Witt, UK).* Contains salicylic acid 1.5%, resorcinol monoacetate 1%, and hexachlorophane 0.2%.

Ayrtons Antiseptic Cream *(Ayrton, Saunders, UK).* Contains zinc oxide 5%, boric acid 1%, phenol 1%, methyl salicylate 0.5%, anhydrous lanolin 20%, paraffin ointment to 100%.

Ayrtons Bronchial Emulsion *(Ayrton, Saunders, UK).* Contains liquid paraffin 25%, glycerol 5%, sodium hypophosphite 1%, calcium hypophosphite 1%, compound benzoin tincture 2.5%, squill vinegar 5%, acetic acid 1%, and capsicum tincture 0.25%.

Ayrtons Burn Cream *(Ayrton, Saunders, UK).* Aminacrine hydrochloride 0.1% in a non-greasy basis.

Ayrtons Childrens Cough Syrup *(Ayrton, Saunders, UK).* Each 5 ml contains blackcurrant syrup 0.75 ml, wild cherry syrup 0.5 ml, tolu syrup 0.835 ml, glycerol 0.25 ml, and ipecacuanha liquid extract 0.00625 ml.

Ayrtons Cold Sore Lotion *(Ayrton, Saunders, UK).* Contains camphor 1.5%, eucalyptus oil 1.5%, flexible collodion 25%, and benzoin tincture to 100%.

Ayrtons Corn and Wart Paint *(Ayrton, Saunders, UK).* Contains salicylic acid 12.5%, zinc chloride 2%, hypophosphorous acid 0.1%, and collodion basis to 100%.

Ayrtons Heart Shaped Indigestion Tablets *(Ayrton, Saunders, UK).* Each contains sodium bicarbonate 55 mg, heavy magnesium carbonate 80 mg, calcium carbonate 475 mg, pepsin 1 mg, pancreatin 1 mg, and oleoresin capsicum 5 µg.

Ayrtons Insect Bite Cream *(Ayrton, Saunders, UK).* Contains antazoline hydrochloride 2%, benzocaine 3%, and cetrimide 0.5%.

Ayrtons IVY Tablets *(Ayrton, Saunders, UK).* Each contains ferrous gluconate 98 mg, dried yeast 195 mg, vitamin B_1 170 µg, and ascorbic acid 4 mg.

Babelix Baby Cough Syrup *(Cupal, UK).* Each 5 ml contains dilute acetic acid 0.4165 ml, tolu solution 0.0625 ml, and sucrose 2.225 g.

Baby Chest Rub *(Cupal, UK).* Contains camphor 5%, turpentine oil 5%, menthol 2%, eucalyptus oil 2%, cedar wood oil 0.5%, nutmeg oil 0.1%, and thyme oil 0.1%.

Baby Gripe Mixture *(Cupal, UK).* Each 5 ml contains dill oil 0.0017 ml, caraway oil 0.0017 ml, and sodium bicarbonate 124 mg.

Baby Gum Lotion *(Cupal, UK).* Contains cetylpyridinium chloride 0.01%.

Bactrian Antiseptic Cream *(Loveridge, UK).* Contains cetrimide 1%.

Bakese 1 Tablets *(Fulford Williams, UK).* Pink tablets each containing paracetamol 500 mg and codeine phosphate 8 mg. **Bakese 2 Tablets.** Yellow tablets each containing paracetamol 500 mg.

Banish *(Max Factor, UK).* Active ingredients: benzethonium chloride 0.064%, *N*-(trichloromethylthio)cyclohex-4-ene-1,2-dicarboximide[captan] 0.108%, and sp. meth. indust. 16.7% by wt.

Banish Shampoo *(Max Factor, UK).* Active ingredients: sodium *o*-phenylphenate tetrahydrate 0.3% and *para*-chloro-*meta*-xylenol 0.2%.

Bankof *(Parkinsons, UK).* Contains oxymel 2%, tolu tincture 0.5%, benzoin tincture 0.5%, capsicum tincture 0.75%, ipecacuanha liquid extract 0.45%, camphor 0.03%, and sucrose 22%.

Bansor Mouth and Throat Antiseptic *(Thornton & Ross, UK).* Active ingredient: cetrimide 0.01%.

Beecham's Catarrh Capsules *(Beecham Proprietaries, UK).* Aluminium-guaiphenesin complex 127 mg and phenylpropanolamine hydrochloride 25 mg.

Beecham's Pills *(Beecham Proprietaries, UK).* Each contains ginger 20.3 mg, coriander 4.4 mg, hard soap 9.7 mg, aloes 42 mg, rosemary oil 700 µg, juniper oil 700 µg, anise oil 200 µg, capsicum oleoresin 100 µg, ginger oleoresin 400 µg, and light magnesium carbonate 2.5 mg.

Beecham's Powders *(Beecham Proprietaries, UK).* Each contains aspirin 600 mg and caffeine 50 mg, in a basis containing cinnamon oil.

Beecham's Powders + Hot Lemon *(Beecham Proprietaries, UK).* Each contains aspirin 600 mg, caffeine 50 mg, and ascorbic acid 40 mg, in a basis containing lemon juice and cinnamon.

Beecham's Powders Mentholated *(Beecham Proprietaries, UK).* Each contains aspirin 600 mg and caffeine 50 mg with menthol and flavourings.

Beecham's Powders (Tablet Form) *(Beecham Proprietaries, UK).* Each contains aspirin 300 mg and caffeine 25 mg, in a basis containing cinnamon oil.

Bemax *(Beecham Foods, UK).* Stabilised wheat germ containing in each oz carbohydrate 10.1 g, protein 7.2 g, vitamin B_1 400 µg, vitamin B_2 160 µg, niacin 1.5 mg, vitamin B_6 270 µg, vitamin E 6.3 mg, manganese 3.6 mg, iron 1.9 mg, and copper 180 µg.

Bengers *(Fisons, UK).* Ingredients: partially dextrinished wheaten flour, sodium bicarbonate, and the pancreatic enzymes amylase and trypsin.

Biactol *(Richardson-Vicks, UK).* Active ingredients: sodium lauryl ether sulphate 2.6% and propylene phenoxetol 2%.

Bidex Spray *(Optrex, UK).* Contains chlorhexidine hydrochloride 0.1%.

Bidex Towelettes *(Optrex, UK).* Contain chlorhexidine gluconate 0.1% and cetrimide 0.3%.

Bile Beans *(Fisons, UK).* Each contains cascara dry extract 17.8 mg, jalap resin 3.09 mg, peppermint oil 890 µg, ginger oleoresin 1.57 mg, powdered ginger 12.59 mg, capsicum oleoresin 790 µg, simple aqueous extract of colocynth (1–4) 4.97 mg, powdered aloes 23.4 mg, cardamom fruit 1.82 mg, ipmoea resin 4.38 mg, sodium tauroglycocholate 11.24 mg, powdered gentian 5.11 mg, liquorice 14.81 mg, and aqueous extract of gentian (1–1) 10.37 mg.

Bio-Strath Elixir *(Vessen, UK).* Contains 84% candida, 7% extract of malt, 4.5% honey (natural), 4.5% orange juice. **Bio-Strath Drops.** A similar preparation without malt, honey, or orange juice.

Biovital Liquid *(Radiol, UK).* Each 20 ml contains vitamin B_1 hydrochloride 600 µg, riboflavine (as riboflavine 5′-phosphate sodium) 2.6 mg, vitamin B_6 hydrochloride 1 mg, nicotinamide 10 mg, cyanocobalamin 2 µg, vitamin C 20 mg, iron (as sodium ferric citrate) 12 mg, manganese (as manganese citrate) 60 µg, and alcohol 2.341 g.

Biovital Tablets *(Radiol, UK).* Each contains vitamin B_1 600 µg, vitamin B_2 600 µg, vitamin B_6 1 mg, nicotinamide 10 mg, vitamin B_{12} 2 µg, vitamin C 20 mg, iron 32.5 mg, and manganese 150 µg.

Birley's Antacid Powder *(Strenol, UK).* Contains dried aluminium hydroxide gel 1%, magnesium trisilicate 11.1%, and light magnesium carbonate 87.9%.

Bisma-Calna Cream *(Charnwood, UK).* Active constituents: bismuth carbonate 82.5 mg, light magnesium carbonate 262.5 mg, chalk 250 mg, and sodium bicarbonate 187.5 mg.

Bismag Powder *(International Chemical, UK).* Contains light magnesium carbonate 47.6%, heavy magnesium carbonate 3%, sodium bicarbonate 48.15%, and bismuth carbonate 1.25%.

Bismag Tablets *(International Chemical, UK).* Each contains sodium bicarbonate 149 mg, heavy magnesium carbonate 130 mg, and light magnesium carbonate 26 mg.

Bisma-Rex Antacid Powder *(Minnesota, UK).* Sodium bicarbonate 65%, calcium carbonate 15%, heavy magnesium carbonate 5%, light kaolin 4%, bismuth carbonate 1%, light magnesium carbonate 10%, peppermint oil 0.125%.

Bisma-Rex Antacid Tablets *(Minnesota, UK).* Each contains bismuth carbonate 13 mg, magnesium trisilicate 90 mg, calcium carbonate 460 mg, magnesium carbonate 160 mg, and peppermint oil 2 mg.

Bismuthated Magnesia Ovals *(Cupal, UK).* Tablets each containing bismuth carbonate 3.9 mg, sodium bicarbonate 15.6 mg, heavy kaolin 62.5 mg, heavy magnesium carbonate 220 mg, and calcium carbonate 220 mg with peppermint flavour.

BiSoDoL Powder *(International Chemical, UK).* Contains light magnesium carbonate 37.58%, heavy magnesium carbonate 2%, sodium bicarbonate 57.88%, and diastase 1.4%.

BiSoDoL Tablets *(International Chemical, UK).* Each contains calcium carbonate 518 mg, light magnesium carbonate 66.7 mg, sodium bicarbonate 63.3 mg, diastase 9.2 mg, and sucrose 538 mg.

Bis-Peps Tablets *(Guest, UK).* Pepsin 1.563 mg, sodium bicarbonate 25 mg, heavy magnesium carbonate 200 mg, bismuth carbonate 25 mg, with peppermint oil.

Blake's Witch Hazel Cream *(Blake, UK).* Active ingredients: olive oil 29%, distilled witch hazel 40%, lanolin 5%, calamine 5%.

Blisteze *(DDD, UK: Dendron, UK).* Cream containing strong ammonia solution 0.2%, aromatic ammonia solution 6.04%, camphor 0.9%, and liquefied phenol 0.49%.

Blistik Medicated Lip Balm *(DDD, UK: Dendron, UK).* Active constituents: padimate O, camphor, and thymol.

BN Liniment *(Minnesota, UK).* Turpentine oil 12%, ammonium carbonate 4%, ammonium chloride 2% and strong ammonia solution 2%.

Boldolaxine *(Dales, UK: Farillon, UK)*. Each tablet contains boldo 70 mg, phenolphthalein 75 mg, belladonna dry extract 3 mg, and Iceland moss 10 mg.

Bon Voyage *(Cupal, UK)*. Each tablet contains cyclizine hydrochloride 50 mg.

Bonomint Laxative Chewing Gum *(Westminster, Reckitt & Colman Pharmaceuticals, UK)*. Tablets each containing yellow phenolphthalein 97 mg, with sucrose, liquid glucose, starch, and peppermint oil in a chewing gum basis.

Boots Adrenaline Cream *(Boots, UK)*. Contains adrenaline acid tartrate equivalent to adrenaline 0.02%.

Boots Antiseptic Cream *(Boots, UK)*. Contains dybenal (2,4-dichlorobenzyl alcohol) 0.5%, cetrimide 0.5%, and allantoin 0.2%.

Boots Antiseptic Lozenges *(Boots, UK)*. Each contains tyrothricin 1 mg and benzocaine 5 mg.

Boots Antiseptic Mouthwash & Gargle (Strepsol) *(Boots, UK)*. Contains dybenal (2,4-dichlorobenzyl alcohol) 0.5% and amylmetacresol 0.125%.

Boots Antiseptic Throat Drops *(Boots, UK)*. Each contains amylmetacresol 0.023% with menthol and eucalyptus, cherry menthol, or lemon flavour.

Boots Bronchial Cough Mixture *(Boots, UK)*. Contains in each 5 ml ammonium chloride 150 mg, ammonium carbonate 100 mg, and guaiphenesin 32.5 mg.

Boots Bronchial Lozenges *(Boots, UK)*. Balsam of tolu 0.7%, menthol 0.2%, anise oil 0.24%, alcoholic extract from 0.06% of capsicum, aqueous extracts from 0.1% of coltsfoot leaf and 0.15% of horehound, liquorice juice 6.3%, basis to 100%.

Boots Catarrh Cough Syrup *(Boots, UK)*. Each 10 ml contains codeine phosphate 3 mg, creosote 0.015 ml, and sucrose 7.8 g.

Boots Catarrh Pastilles *(Boots, UK)*. Contain menthol 1%, creosote 0.2%, and pine oil 0.45%.

Boots Chilblain Cream *(Boots, UK)*. Contains benzyl alcohol 7.5% and eucalyptus oil 1%.

Boots Chilblain Tablets *(Boots, UK)*. Each contains acetomenaphthone 7 mg, nicotinic acid 25 mg, and calcium hydrogen phosphate 320 mg.

Boots Children's Cough Linctus *(Boots, UK)*. Contains in each 5 ml ephedrine hydrochloride 3 mg, ipecacuanha liquid extract 0.00625 ml, tolu syrup 1.4 ml, citric acid 50 mg, sodium benzoate 10 mg, and sucrose 2.78 g.

Boots Children's Cough Pastilles *(Boots, UK)*. Contain honey 4.5%, glycerol 6.2%, ipecacuanha liquid extract 0.04%, and squill liquid extract 0.05%.

Boots Children's Soluble Aspirin *(Boots, UK)*. Each tablet contains aspirin 75 mg, calcium carbonate 25 mg, and anhydrous citric acid 7.5 mg.

Boots Children's Vitamin Syrup *(Boots, UK)*. Contains in each 5 ml vitamin A 2500 units, thiamine hydrochloride 500 µg, riboflavine 600 µg, nicotinamide 5 mg, ascorbic acid 15 mg, and ergocalciferol 250 units.

Boots Cold and Influenza Mixture *(Boots, UK)*. Contains in each 10 ml camphor 0.015 g, ether spirit 0.062 ml, squill vinegar 0.35 ml, strong ammonium acetate solution 0.16 ml, benzoic acid 0.02 g, anise oil 0.003 ml, and rectified spirit 0.56 ml.

Boots Cold Relief *(Boots, UK)*. Sachets each containing paracetamol 650 mg, sodium citrate 500 mg, and ascorbic acid 50 mg, in a blackcurrant-flavoured basis.

Boots Cold Sore Lotion *(Boots, UK)*. Camphor 3%, menthol 0.2%, dybenal (2,4-dichlorobenzyl alcohol) 0.25%, basis to 100%.

Boots Compound Laxative Syrup of Figs *(Boots, UK)*. Contains in each 5 ml: 45% alcoholic extract from 750 mg of senna fruit, aqueous extract from 550 mg of fig, malt extract 1.87 g, clove oil 0.001 ml, peppermint oil 0.00025 ml, and benzoic acid 10 mg.

Boots Corn Paint *(Boots, UK)*. Salicylic acid 14.3%, lactic acid 3%, ether solvent 10.4%, chlorophyll 0.3%, flexible collodion to 100%.

Boots Cough Relief for Adults *(Boots, UK)*. Each 10 ml contains pholcodine 7.5 mg, diphenhydramine hydrochloride 25 mg, and dehydrated alcohol 0.48 ml.

Boots Cough Relief for Children *(Boots, UK)*. Each 5 ml contains pholcodine 1.5 mg, diphenhydramine hydrochloride 12.5 mg, and dehydrated alcohol 0.24 ml.

Boots Cream of Magnesia Tablets *(Boots, UK)*. Each contains magnesium hydroxide 300 mg.

Boots Day Cold Comfort *(Boots, UK)*. Linctus containing in each 30 ml pholcodine 10 mg, pseudoephedrine hydrochloride 40 mg, and paracetamol 600 mg.

Boots Decongestant Nasal Spray *(Boots, UK)*. Xylometazoline hydrochloride 0.1%.

Boots Deep Skin Cleanser *(Boots, UK)*. Active ingredients: dichlorobenzyl alcohol 0.2%, salicylic acid 0.25%, glycerol 0.5%, and industrial methylated spirit 44%.

Boots Diarrhoea Mixture *(Boots, UK)*. Each 20 ml contains activated attapulgite 3 g.

Boots Diarrhoea Tablets *(Boots, UK)*. Each white tablet contains codeine phosphate 10 mg and each brown tablet contains activated attapulgite 600 mg.

Boots Dusting Powder *(Boots, UK)*. Contains allantoin 0.5%.

Boots Dyspepsia Tablets *(Boots, UK)*. Each contains magnesium trisilicate 100 mg, ginger 5 mg, and sodium bicarbonate 150 mg.

Boots Effervescent Vitamin C Tablets *(Boots, UK)*. Each contains ascorbic acid 1 g.

Boots Embrocation *(Boots, UK)*. Active ingredients: acetic acid (80%) 6.27%, camphor 0.8%, and turpentine oil 40%.

Boots Eye Drops *(Boots, UK)*. Contain boric acid 2.5%, sodium borate 0.5%, hamamelis water 5%, and cetrimide 0.01%.

Boots Family Antiseptic *(Boots, UK)*. Contains chloroxylenol 3%, terpineol 5%, and aromatic pine oil 1%.

Boots Feeding Bottle Steriliser Tablets *(Boots, UK)*. Contain sodium hypochlorite equivalent to 1% available chlorine.

Boots Foot Cream *(Boots, UK)*. Contains menthol 1%, cetrimide 0.5%, and distearyldimethylammonium chloride 3.75%.

Boots Foot Powder *(Boots, UK)*. Dichlorophen 0.2%, sodium polymetaphosphate 4%, light kaolin 20%, basis to 100%.

Boots Glycerin Honey and Lemon Linctus *(Boots, UK)*. Contains in each 5 ml glycerol 0.75 ml, honey 1.11 g, citric acid monohydrate 50 mg, lemon oil 0.006 ml, and sucrose 1.96 g. **Boots Glycerin Honey and Lemon Linctus with Ipecacuanha** contains, in addition, ipecacuanha liquid extract 0.015 ml.

Boots Glycerin of Thymol Pastilles with AMC *(Boots, UK)*. Contain sodium benzoate 0.49%, sodium salicylate 0.3%, sodium carbonate 1%, glycerol 3.8%, menthol 0.02%, thymol 0.03%, pumilio pine oil 0.03%, cineole 0.08%, methyl salicylate 0.02%, and amylmetacresol 0.036%.

Boots Gripe Mixture *(Boots, UK)*. Each 5 ml contains sodium bicarbonate 50 mg, weak ginger tincture 0.025 ml, concentrated caraway water 0.075 ml, concentrated spearmint water (*B.P.C. 1959*) 0.005 ml, concentrated peppermint water 0.0005 ml, and rectified spirit 0.15 ml.

Boots Indigestion Mixture *(Boots, UK)*. Contains in each 5 ml light magnesium carbonate 225 mg, sodium bicarbonate 225 mg, calcium carbonate 175 mg, peppermint oil 0.005 ml, and chloroform water to 5 ml.

Boots Indigestion Powder *(Boots, UK)*. Each teaspoonful (approximately 2.5 g) contains heavy magnesium carbonate 937.5 mg, sodium bicarbonate 312.5 mg, magnesium trisilicate 234.4 mg, light kaolin 78.1 mg, and prepared chalk 937.5 mg.

Boots Insect Repellent *(Boots, UK)*. **Gel** contains diethyltoluamide; **Liquid** contains diethyltoluamide, dimethyl phthalate, and dibutyl phthalate; and **Spray** contains diethyltoluamide.

Boots Iodized Throat Tablets *(Boots, UK)*. Each tablet contains iodophenol 0.4 mg, potassium iodide 0.4 mg, phenol 1.5 mg, and menthol 2 mg.

Boots Iron Tonic Tablets *(Boots, UK)*. Each contains ferrous fumarate 25 mg, dried yeast 300 mg, and thiamine hydrochloride 3 mg.

Boots Medicated Foot Spray *(Boots, UK)*. Chlorhexidine acetate 0.1% and dichlorophen 0.25%.

Boots Medicated Skin Treatment Gel *(Boots, UK)*. Active ingredients: glycerol 3%, allantoin 0.2%, industrial methylated spirit 50%, menthol 0.08%, and dichlorobenzyl alcohol 0.5%.

Boots Medicated Skin Wash *(Boots, UK)*. Active ingredients: cetrimide 0.5% and benzalkonium chloride solution 0.5%.

Boots Medicated Soap *(Boots, UK)*. Contains triclocarban 2%.

Boots Menthol and Wintergreen Embrocation *(Boots, UK)*. Active constituents: menthol 2.4%, cineole 2%, cajuput oil 0.5%, eucalyptus oil 1.5%, methyl salicylate 14.2%.

Boots Nappy Rash Cream *(Boots, UK)*. Contains dimethicone 10% and cetrimide 0.5%.

Boots Night Cold Comfort *(Boots, UK)*. Linctus containing in each 30 ml pseudoephedrine hydrochloride 40 mg, pholcodine 10 mg, diphenhydramine hydrochloride 10 mg, paracetamol 600 mg, and alcohol 6 ml.

Boots Ointment for Haemorrhoids *(Boots, UK)*. Contains boric acid 2.1%, zinc oxide 4.2%, methyl salicylate 0.05%, belladonna liquid extract 0.72%, tannic acid 0.6% and heavy kaolin 16.8%.

Boots Original Indigestion Tablets *(Boots, UK)*. Each contains calcium carbonate 200 mg, magnesium trisilicate 60 mg, heavy magnesium carbonate 60 mg, sodium bicarbonate 60 mg, and ginger 10 mg.

Boots Pain Relieving Balm *(Boots, UK)*. Contains glycol monosalicylate 7.5%, ethyl nicotinate 1%, and vanillylnonamide 0.015%.

Boots Pink Healing Ointment *(Boots, UK)*. Zinc oxide 8%, methyl salicylate 3.6%, liquefied phenol 2%, menthol 0.01%, basis to 100%.

Boots Senna Laxative Tablets *(Boots, UK)*. Each contains standardised senna equivalent to 7.5 mg of total sennosides.

Boots Sore Mouth Gel *(Boots, UK)*. Lignocaine 0.6% and cetylpyridinium chloride 0.02%.

Boots Sore Mouth Pastilles *(Boots, UK)*. 2,4-Dichlorobenzyl alcohol 0.1%, alcoholic (90%) extractive from 0.1% of myrrh, glycerol 4.5%, menthol 0.02%.

Boots Sparkling Health Salt *(Boots, UK)*. Sucrose 38.9%, sodium bicarbonate 22.5%, tartaric acid 6.9%, citric acid 13.8%, dried magnesium sulphate 17.3%, and sodium chloride 0.6%.

Boots Sting Relief *(Boots, UK)*. Zinc oxide 2%, benzyl alcohol 1.5%, chloroxylenol 1.5%, eucalyptus oil 1%, borax 1%, menthol 0.5%, camphor 0.25%, basis to 100%.

Boots Suppositories for Haemorrhoids *(Boots, UK)*. Each contains zinc oxide 230 mg, glycol monosalicylate 104 mg, benzyl alcohol 52 mg, and methyl salicylate 10 mg.

Boots Tooth Tincture *(Boots, UK)*. Contains menthol 5%, camphor 3.5%, clove oil 0.1%, and rectified spirit 64%.

Boots Vapour Rub *(Boots, UK)*. Contains eucalyptus oil 1.5%, camphor 6%, turpentine oil 4%, menthol 1%, thymol 0.1%, and pumilio pine oil 0.4%.

Boots Vegetable Laxative Tablets *(Boots, UK)*. Each tablet contains compound colocynth extract 60 mg, hyoscyamus dry extract 15 mg, jalap resin 15 mg, and peppermint oil 0.006 ml.

Boots Vitamin and Iron Tonic *(Boots, UK)*. Contains in each 10 ml ferrous gluconate 225 mg, calcium gluconate 200 mg, manganese glycerophosphate 6 mg, caffeine 32 mg, thiamine hydrochloride 700 µg, riboflavine 400 µg, and nicotinamide 6 mg.

Boots Vitamin E Tablets *(Boots, UK)*. Each contains vitamin E 100 mg.

Boots Vitamin Yeast Tablets *(Boots, UK)*. Each contains dried yeast 300 mg, thiamine 0.192 mg, riboflavine 0.215 mg, and nicotinic acid 2.144 mg.

Box's Herbal Ointment *(Box, UK)*. Contains slippery elm 10.5%, althaea 10.5%, and yellow soft paraffin to 100%.

Box's Indigestion Pills *(Box, UK)*. Each contains myrrh 25 mg, gentian extract 7.5 mg, ginger 25 mg, capsicum 25 mg, aloes 27.5 mg, and cajuput oil 0.0045 ml.

Box's Multivitamin Capsules *(Box, UK)*. DL-Alpha tocopheryl acetate 2.2 mg, ergocalciferol 0.625 µg, vitamin A palmitate 5.5 mg, thiamine mononitrate 3.125 mg, riboflavine 2.75 mg, sodium ascorbate 19.52 mg, ascorbic acid 31.73 mg, nicotinamide 22 mg, pyridoxine 0.55 mg, calcium pantothenate 8.75 mg, cyanocobalamin 1.25 µg, and folic acid 0.55 mg.

Bragg's Charcoal Biscuits *(Bragg, UK)*. Contain carbo ligni (*B.P.C. 1934*) 12.5%.

Bragg's Charcoal Tablets *(Bragg, UK)*. Contain carbo ligni (*B.P.C. 1934*) 90%.

Brentan *(Janssen, UK)*. Cream containing miconazole nitrate 2%.

Bronal Cough and Catarrh Elixir *(Cupal, UK)*. Contains in each 5 ml dextromethorphan hydrobromide 10 mg, ephedrine hydrochloride 10 mg, tolu solution 156.25 mg, menthol 0.5 mg, glycerol 0.25 ml, and alcohol (90%) 1 ml. **Diabetic Bronal** contains the same active ingredients.

Bronalin *(Cupal, UK)*. Each 5 ml contains ammonium chloride 135 mg, diphenhydramine hydrochloride 14 mg, and sodium citrate 57 mg.

Bronalin Paediatric *(Cupal, UK)*. Each 5 ml contains diphenhydramine hydrochloride 7 mg and sodium citrate 28.5 mg.

Bronchipax *(Ashe, UK)*. Extended-action tablets each containing ephedrine resinate equivalent to ephedrine hydrochloride 30 mg, theophylline 40 mg, and salicylamide 250 mg.

Bronskels Pastilles *(Smith Kendon, UK)*. Each pastille contains pholcodine 2 mg.

Brontussin *(Sandersons, UK)*. Each 5 ml contains dextromethorphan hydrobromide 5.7 mg, ephedrine hydrochloride 14.25 mg, ammonium chloride 47.5 mg, ipecacuanha liquid extract 0.0052 ml, glycerol 0.75 ml, and menthol 1.1 mg, in a basis free from sugar.

Brooklax Chocolate Laxative *(Westminster, Reckitt & Colman Pharmaceuticals, UK)*. Tablets containing chocolate 90% and yellow phenolphthalein 10%.

Buf Acne Lotion *(Minnesota, UK)*. Contains benzoyl peroxide 5%.

Burgess' Lion Ointment *(Burgess, UK)*. Contains yellow soft petroleum jelly 65%, anhydrous lanolin 15%, zinc oleostearate 5%, yellow beeswax 5%, rosin 5%, and methylated spirit 5%.

Burn Aid Cream *(Cupal, UK)*. Aminacrine hydrochloride 0.1% and antazoline hydrochloride 1%.

Burneze *(Potter & Clarke, UK: De Witt, UK)*. An aerosol containing mepyramine maleate 0.5% and benzocaine 1%.

Buttercup Baby Cough Linctus *(LRC Products, UK)*. Each 5 ml contains squill liquid extract 0.0015 ml, ipecacuanha liquid extract 0.01 ml, chloroform spirit 0.225 ml, tolu solution 0.04 ml, and glycerol 1 ml.

Buttercup Medicated Sweets *(LRC Products, UK)*. Honey 1%, lemon oil 0.68%, menthol 0.15%, and eucalyptus 0.15%.

Buttercup Syrup *(LRC Products, UK)*. Each 5 ml contains squill liquid extract 0.0031 ml, stronger capsicum tincture 0.0025 ml, strong ginger tincture 0.005 ml, acetic acid 0.19 ml, and chloroform 0.025 ml.

Buxton Rubbing Bottle *(Buxton Chemical Products, UK)*. Contains capsicum oleoresin 2.19%, turpentine oil 12.69%, camphor 2.3%, methyl salicylate 2.3%, and soft paraffin to 100%.

C & M Lotion *(Wigglesworth, UK)*. Contains calamine 15%, mepyramine maleate 1%, and glycerol 10%.

Cabdrivers Adult Linctus *(De Witt, UK)*. Each 5 ml contains dextromethorphan hydrobromide 11.5 mg, terpin hydrate 11.5 mg, menthol 7 mg, pumilio pine oil 0.0015 ml, eucalyptus oil 0.0025 ml, glycerol 0.825 ml, glucose syrup 2.83 ml, and alcohol (90%) 0.79 ml.

Cabdrivers Diabetic Linctus *(De Witt, UK)*. Contains in 5 ml ephedrine hydrochloride 6 mg and dextromethorphan hydrobromide 15 mg.

Cabdrivers Junior Glucose Linctus *(De Witt, UK)*. Ephedrine hydrochloride 0.12%, vinegar of ipecacuanha 4.17%, red-poppy syrup 8.33%, anise syrup 4.17%, and glucose syrup 26%.

Caffexen *(Charnwood, UK)*. Contains caffeine 2.74%, sodium iodide 9%, liquorice liquid extract 8.33%, chloroform 0.21%, and ephedrine hydrochloride 0.3%.

Calamousse *(Kirby-Warrick, UK)*. Foam spray containing calamine 4% and witch hazel extract 5%.

Calazean Cream *(Cox, UK)*. Contains antazoline hydrochloride 1%, calamine 8%, camphor 0.1%, and cetrimide 0.5%.

California Syrup of Figs *(Sterling Health)*. Contains aqueous extract of senna leaf (1–1) 27.8%.

Calsalettes *(Torbet Laboratories, UK)*. Tablets containing aloin 38 mg, starch 16 mg, lactose 3 mg, and stearic acid 3 mg.

Cantab-17 *(Cantassium Co., UK)*. Consists of apricot kernel powder.

Cantaba *(Cantassium Co., UK)*. Each tablet contains aminobenzoic acid 100 mg.

Cantapollen Naturtabs *(Cantassium Co., UK)*. Each tablet contains bee pollen 250 mg and dolomite 350 mg.

Cantarna *(Cantassium Co., UK)*. Each tablet contains ribonucleic acids 450 mg.

Cantassium Discs *(Cantassium Co., UK)*. Each contains ferrous fumarate 2 mg, potassium sulphate 4 mg, potassium iodide 2 mg, and potassium bicarbonate 296 mg.

Carmil *(Ex-Lax, UK)*. Each 5 ml contains pectin 40 mg, light kaolin 500 mg, morphine hydrochloride 350 µg, and atropine methonitrate 100 µg.

Carnation Callous Caps *(Cuxson, Gerrard, UK)*. Plasters bearing an ointment containing salicylic acid 40%.

Carnation Corn Caps *(Cuxson, Gerrard, UK)*. Plasters bearing an ointment containing salicylic acid 40%.

Carters Infurno Embrocation *(Herbal Laboratories, UK)*. Contains methyl salicylate 17%, capsicin 1.25%, eucalyptus oil 4.25%, rectified camphor oil 4.25%, and menthol 0.8%.

Carter's Little Pills *(Carter-Wallace, UK)*. Each contains phenolphthalein 16 mg and aloin 8 mg.

Carters Varicose Ointment *(Herbal Laboratories, UK)*. Contains ichthammol 2.95%, liquefied phenol 0.92%, hamamelis water 5.9%, and zinc oxide 10.3%.

Castellan No. 10 Bronchial Pastilles *(Ayrton, Saunders, UK)*. Contain liquorice extract 5.7%, menthol 0.5%, peppermint oil 0.025%, anise oil 0.3%, capsicin 0.001%, benzoin tincture 0.5%, and clove oil 0.05%.

Castellan No. 10 Cough Mixture *(Ayrton, Saunders, UK)*. Contains morphine hydrochloride 0.025%, liquorice liquid extract 1%, squill liquid extract 1.5%, acetic acid 0.48%, ether 0.375%, chloroform 0.5%, anise oil 0.094%, and peppermint oil 0.094%.

Celaton CH3 Plus *(Celaton, UK)*. Each contains riboflavine 0.6 mg, pyridoxine hydrochloride 0.7 mg, nicotinamide 6 mg, ascorbic acid 25 mg, vitamin E acetate 1.4 mg, rutin 1 mg, methionine 1 mg, calcium pantothenate 2.5 mg, thiamine hydrochloride 0.6 mg, cyanocobalamin 1 µg, biotin 1 µg, vitamin A acetate 2 mg, procaine hydrochloride 15 mg, ginseng powder 2 mg, and ergocalciferol 5 µg.

Celaton CH3 Strong and Calm Tablets *(Celaton, UK)*. Tablets each containing para-aminobenzoic acid 7.5 mg, biotin 1 µg, vitamin A acetate 0.5 mg, vitamin B_1 0.6 mg, vitamin B_2 0.6 mg, vitamin B_6 0.7 mg, nicotinamide 6 mg, calcium pantothenate 2.5 mg, cyanocobalamin 1 µg, ascorbic acid 25 mg, vitamin D_2 2.5 µg, vitamin E acetate 10.5 mg, sucrose 141 mg, acacia 3 mg, povidone 6.25 mg, methyl *p*-hydroxybenzoate 0.22 mg, and sodium propyl-*p*-hydroxybenzoate 0.11 mg.

Celaton CH3 Tri-Plus Tablets *(Celaton, UK)*. Each contains vitamin A acetate 0.5 mg, vitamin B_2 0.6 mg, vitamin B_1 0.6 mg, vitamin B_6 0.7 mg, nicotinamide 6 mg, biotin 1 µg, calcium pantothenate 2.5 mg, cyanocobalamin 2.5 µg, ascorbic acid 25 mg, vitamin D 2.5 µg, vitamin E 10.5 mg, para-aminobenzoic acid 7.5 mg, ginseng root 2 mg, heart powder 30 mg, brain powder 30 mg, and intrinsic factor 20 mg.

Cephos Powders *(Beecham Proprietaries, UK)*. Each contains aspirin 570 mg, caffeine 20 mg, and salicylamide 40 mg.

Cephos Tablets *(Beecham Proprietaries, UK)*. Each tablet contains aspirin 285 mg, salicylamide 20 mg, and caffeine 10 mg.

Cepton Cleansing Milk *(Care, UK)*. Contains chlorhexidine gluconate solution 2.5%.

Cepton Medicated Clear Gel *(Care, UK)*. Contains chlorhexidine gluconate solution 2.5%.

Cetrimax Antiseptic Cream *(Thornton & Ross, UK)*. Contains cetrimide 0.5%.

Chap Stick *(Robins Consumer Products, UK)*. Ointment containing wool fat 1%, padimate 0.4%, and camphor 1.6% in a wax basis.

Cheb's Bruise Easer *(Halas, UK)*. Contains heparin 50 units per g, glycol salicylate 10%, and cetrimide 0.1%.

Chilblain Cream *(Pickles, UK)*. Contains histamine acid phosphate 0.1% and methyl nicotinate 1%.

Child's Pain Elixir *(Cupal, UK)*. Each 5 ml contains paracetamol 120 mg.

Chilvax Tablets *(British Chemotheutic, UK)*. Each contains paracetamol 400 mg, thiamine hydrochloride 0.5 mg, caffeine 15 mg, and nicotinamide 5 mg.

Christy's Skin Emulsion *(Christy, UK)*. Contains wool fat 4.8%, glyceryl monostearate 4.8%, white beeswax 0.7%, spermaceti 0.7%, propyl hydroxybenzoate 0.04%, methyl hydroxybenzoate 0.08%, glycerol 2.16%, industrial methylated spirit 7.5%, parachlorometaxylenol 0.05%, and aminacrine hydrochloride 0.00035%.

Cidal *(Albion, UK)*. Soap containing Irgasan 0.75%.

Citramins *(Minnesota, UK)*. Chewable tablets each containing retinol 750 µg, ascorbic acid 25 mg, and cholecalciferol 5 µg.

Clarke's Blood Mixture *(Halas, UK)*. Potassium iodide 1.15%, sodium salicylate 1.85%, potassium bicarbonate 1.85%, ammonium chloride 0.7%, concentrated compound gentian infusion 0.75%, and concentrated compound sarsaparilla decoction 0.75%.

Clean & Clear *(Beecham Proprietaries, UK)*. Contains triclosan 0.5%, ethoxylated lauryl alcohol 40%, nonyl phenol ethylene oxide condensate 10%, with sodium salts of alkyl ether sulphate and sulphosuccinates.

Clearasil Clearguard Cleansing Lotion *(Richardson-Vicks, UK)*. Contains allantoin 0.1%, salicylic acid 0.25%, IMS 38.27%.

Clearasil Clearguard Cream *(Richardson-Vicks, UK)*. Contains sulphur 8% and triclosan 0.1%.

Clearasil Clearguard Soap *(Richardson-Vicks, UK)*. Contains colloidal sulphur 2%.

Clearine Eye Drops *(Optrex, UK)*. Hamamelis water 12.5% and naphazoline hydrochloride 0.01%.

Clinic Shampoo *(Elida Gibbs, UK)*. **Cream Beauty** contains 2,4,4′-trichloro-2-hydroxy diphenyl ether [triclosan] 0.03% and **Deep Health** contains 0.05%.

Codanin *(International Chemical, UK)*. Tablets each containing paracetamol 500 mg and codeine phosphate 10 mg.

Codella *(Napp, UK)*. Hand cream containing povidone-iodine 0.2%.

Codural Period Pain Tablets *(Minnesota, UK)*. Each contains caffeine 50 mg, paracetamol 250 mg, and homatropine methylbromide 750 µg.

Cojene *(Fisons, UK)*. Each tablet contains aspirin 300 mg, caffeine citrate 105 mg, and codeine phosphate 8 mg.

Cold and Influenza Capsules *(Regent Laboratories, UK)*. Paracetamol 240 mg, ascorbic acid 66 mg, caffeine 10 mg, quinine sulphate 6 mg.

Cold Discs *(Cox, UK)*. Tablets each containing ascorbic acid 50 mg, paracetamol 400 mg, phenylephrine hydrochloride 5 mg, terpin hydrate 25 mg, and noscapine 15 mg.

Coldrex Antiseptic Throat Lozenges *(Sterling Health)*. Menthol 3 mg and amylmetacresol 0.6 mg.

Coldrex Cold & Flu Treatment *(Sterling Health)*. Tablets containing paracetamol 500 mg, phenylephrine hydrochloride 5 mg, caffeine 25 mg, terpin hydrate 20 mg, and ascorbic acid 30 mg.

Coldrex Nasal Spray *(Sterling Health)*. Contains phenylephrine hydrochloride 0.5%.

Coldrex Powders *(Sterling Health)*. Sachets each containing paracetamol 1 g, phenylephrine hydrochloride 10 mg, and ascorbic acid 60 mg.

Coldrex Tablets *(Sterling Health)*. Each contains paracetamol 500 mg, phenylephrine hydrochloride 5 mg, caffeine 25 mg, terpin hydrate 20 mg, and vitamin C 30 mg.

Collins Elixir *(Collins of Norwich, UK)*. Contains ethylmorphine hydrochloride 0.03%, chloroform 0.4%, tartaric acid 1.87%, and lemon oil 0.31%.

Collins Elixir Pastilles *(Collins of Norwich, UK)*. Each contains chloroform 0.34%, citric acid 1.65%, lemon oil 0.26%, squill vinegar 0.42%, and glycerol 0.21%.

Collis Browne's (J.) Mixture *(International Laboratories, UK)*. Each 5-ml dose contains: opium liquid extract equivalent to morphine 1 mg, peppermint oil 0.0015 ml, and capsicum tincture 0.0012 ml, in a vehicle containing chloroform water.

Colsor Cream *(Pickles, UK)*. Tannic acid 5%, camphor 5%, menthol 0.5%, phenol 1%, lanolin basis to 100%.

Colsor Lotion *(Pickles, UK)*. Contains tannic acid 5%, camphor 5%, phenol 0.5%, and menthol 0.5%.

Coltex Cream *(Thornton & Ross, UK)*. Contains diphenhydramine hydrochloride 2%.

Compound W *(International Chemical, UK)*. A wart remover containing salicylic acid 14.2%, menthol 1.9%, glacial acetic acid 11%, and camphor 1.5%.

Congreve's Balsamic Elixir *(Fennings, UK)*. Contains aqueous extracts of horehound 0.5%, coltsfoot leaf 0.5%, hyssop 0.25%, and rosemary 0.375%, alcoholic (48%) extracts of tolu balsam 2%, catechu 2%, guaiacum resin 1%, cochineal 0.2%, and squill 0.5%, turpentine oil 0.0625%, and alcohol 27.5%.

Contac 400 *(Menley & James, UK)*. Sustained-release capsules each containing phenylpropanolamine hydrochloride 50 mg and belladonna alkaloids (calculated as hyoscyamine sulphate) 250 µg.

Correctol Tablets *(Plough, UK)*. Docusate sodium 100 mg, yellow phenolphthalein 65 mg, sodium benzoate 18 mg, and calcium gluconate 59 mg.

Covonia Mentholated Bronchial Balsam *(Thornton & Ross, UK)*. Active ingredients: dextromethorphan hydrobromide 0.075%, guaiphenesin 0.5%, menthol 0.05%, and eucalyptol 0.03%.

Cox's Bronchial Mixture *(Cox, UK)*. Contains in each 10 ml squill liquid extract 0.095 ml, senega liquid extract 0.0475 ml, ipecacuanha tincture 0.15 ml, tolu solution 0.12 ml, capsicum tincture 0.125 ml, camphor 2 mg, benzoic acid 12 mg, anise oil 0.002 ml, ammonium bicarbonate 235 mg, and glycerol 0.01 ml.

Cox's Catarrh and Bronchial Syrup *(Cox, UK)*. Contains in each 10 ml codeine phosphate 2.125 mg, chloroform 0.006 ml, creosote 0.011 ml, alcoholic (68%) extract of aconite (0.05% aconitine) 0.0125 ml, calcium lactate 8 mg, calcium tetrahydrogen phosphate 10 mg, and cinnamon oil 0.00083 ml.

Cox's Cetrimide Cream *(Cox, UK)*. Contains cetrimide 0.5%.

Cox's Children's Cherry Cough Syrup *(Cox, UK)*. Contains in each 5 ml tolu solution 0.067 ml, red-poppy syrup 0.535 ml, wild cherry syrup 0.535 ml, ipecacuanha tincture 0.1 ml, squill vinegar 0.33 ml, and glycerol 0.75 ml.

Cox's Digestive Mints *(Cox, UK)*. Each contains dihydroxyaluminium sodium carbonate 300 mg.

Cox's Junior Soluble Aspirin *(Cox, UK)*. Each tablet contains aspirin 75 mg.

Cox's Nasal Spray *(Cox, UK)*. Contains phenylephrine hydrochloride 0.5%.

Cox's Pain Relief Tablets *(Cox, UK)*. Each contains paracetamol 450 mg, codeine phosphate 8.1 mg, caffeine citrate 15 mg, and nicotinamide 15 mg.

Cradocap *(Napp, UK)*. A shampoo containing cetrimide 10%, cetyl alcohol 15%, and lanolin 1%.

Crampex Tablets *(International Laboratories, UK)*. Each contains guaiphenesin 60 mg, nicotinic acid 20 mg, calcium gluconate 200 mg, and ergocalciferol 20 µg.

Cream E45 *(Crookes Products, UK)*. An emollient basis containing white soft paraffin 14.5%, light liquid paraffin 11.6%, and wool fat 1% with self-emulsifying glyceryl monostearate, stearic acid, triethanolamine, and methyl hydroxybenzoate.

Creds *(Ernest Jackson, UK)*. Contain menthol 0.5%, peppermint oil 0.025%, aniseed oil 0.3%, benzoin tincture 0.5%, capsicin 0.001%, and clove oil 0.05%.

Cremaffin *(Boots, UK)*. A brand of Liquid Paraffin and Magnesium Hydroxide Emulsion.

Cremathurm *(Sinclair, UK)*. Cream containing methyl salicylate 10%, ethyl nicotinate 1%, histamine acid phosphate 0.1%, and capsicum oleoresin 0.1%.

Cremosan *(Ayrton, Saunders, UK)*. Contains zinc oxide 5.3%, beeswax 10.7%, resin 10.7%, wool fat 22.2%, cresol 2.3%, formaldehyde solution 0.2%, thymol 0.2%, and paraffin basis to 100%.

Crest Plus *(Proctor & Gamble, UK)*. Toothpaste containing sodium fluoride 0.24%.

Crookes Multivitamins *(Crookes Products, UK)*. Each tablet contains vitamin A 5000 units, vitamin B_1 2 mg, vitamin B_2 2 mg, vitamin B_6 1 mg, vitamin B_{12} 2 µg, vitamin C 50 mg, vitamin D 400 units, nicotinamide 20 mg, iron 15 mg, and copper 0.75 mg.

Croupline Cough Syrup *(Waterhouse, UK)*. Contains the water-soluble constituents of lobelia 3.62%, grindelia 0.36%, anise 0.9%, coltsfoot leaf 1.06%, and wild cherry bark (free from hydrocyanic acid) 1.25%, together with guaiphenesin 0.25%, anise oil 0.1%, acetic acid 0.24%, and sucrose 75.93%.

Cupal Burn Aid *(Cupal, UK)*. Cream containing aminacrine hydrochloride 0.1% and antazoline hydrochloride 1%.

Cupal Child's Pain Elixir *(Cupal, UK)*. Each 5 ml contains paracetamol 120 mg.

Cupal Cold Sore Lotion *(Cupal, UK)*. Contains tannic acid 5%, salicylic acid 1%, and myrrh 10%.

Cupal Cold Sore Ointment *(Cupal, UK)*. Contains allantoin 1%, diperodon hydrochloride 1%, camphor 1%, and zinc oxide 5%.

Cupal Insect Bite Cream *(Cupal, UK)*. Contains antazoline hydrochloride 2%.

Cupal Nail Bite Lotion *(Cupal, UK)*. Contains denatonium benzoate.

Cupal Verruca Ointment *(Cupal, UK)*. Contains salicylic acid 50%.

Cupal Wart Solvent *(Cupal, UK)*. Contains glacial acetic acid 86.25%.

Cupal Worm Elixir *(Cupal, UK)*. Consists of Piperazine Citrate Elixir.

Cuticura Ointment *(Cuticura, UK)*. Mineral oil 28.5%, yellow soft paraffin 50.43%, beeswax 18.17%, pine oil 0.04%, rose geranium oil 0.17%, chlorophyll 0.04%, oxyquinoline 0.05%, sulphur praecip. 0.5%, and phenol 0.16%.

Cymex *(De Witt, UK).* Contains urea 1%, cetrimide 0.5%, dimethicone 9%, and chlorocresol 0.1%.

Day Nurse *(Beecham Proprietaries, UK).* Each 20-ml dose contains: paracetamol 500 mg, vitamin C 60 mg, phenylpropanolamine hydrochloride 25 mg, dextromethorphan hydrobromide 15 mg, and alcohol 3.08 ml.

DDD Medicated Cream *(DDD, UK: Dendron, UK).* Contains thymol 0.09%, menthol 0.15%, methyl salicylate 1.15%, chlorbutol 1.11%, resorcin 0.25%, liquefied phenol 0.98%, and titanium dioxide 0.5%.

DDD Lotion (Extra Strength) *(DDD, UK: Dendron, UK).* Contains thymol 0.09%, menthol 0.14%, salicylic acid 1.84%, resorcinol 0.74%, chlorbutol 1.1%, methyl salicylate 0.92%, glycerol 7.72%, liquefied phenol 0.98%, and alcohol 34.74%.

DDD Lotion (Ordinary Strength) *(DDD, UK: Dendron, UK).* Contains thymol 0.09%, menthol 0.14%, salicylic acid 0.75%, resorcinol 0.75%, chlorbutol 1.13%, methyl salicylate 0.94%, glycerol 7.93%, liquefied phenol 0.98%, and alcohol 34.11%.

De Witt's Analgesic Pills *(De Witt, UK).* Each contains paracetamol 330 mg and caffeine 30 mg.

De Witt's Antacid Powder *(De Witt, UK).* Contains magnesium trisilicate 12%, light magnesium carbonate 10%, calcium carbonate 20%, sodium bicarbonate 48.5%, light kaolin 9% and peppermint oil 0.5%.

De Witt's Antacid Tablets *(De Witt, UK).* Each contains calcium carbonate 324 mg, heavy magnesium carbonate 194.4 mg, magnesium trisilicate 64.8 mg, peppermint oil 3.6 mg, and lactose 129.6 mg.

De Witt's Kidney and Bladder Pills *(De Witt, UK).* Each contains potassium nitrate 50 mg, juniper oil 2 mg, alcoholic (60%) extract of buchu (1–4) 10 mg, methylene blue 10 mg, aqueous extract of uva ursi (2–7) 20 mg, cascara dry extract 15 mg.

De Witt's Throat Lozenges *(De Witt, UK).* Each contains tyrothricin 1.25 mg, benzocaine 8 mg, and cetylpyridinium chloride 2 mg.

Deakin's Cough and Cold Healer *(Deakin & Hughes, UK).* Contains camphor 0.05%, liquefied phenol 0.42%, anise oil 0.04%, benzoic acid 0.025%, glacial acetic acid 0.5%, aqueous extract (1 in 1) of coltsfoot flower 0.5%, senega liquid extract 0.25%, liquorice liquid extract 2.08%, squill liquid extract 0.25%, concentrated chloroform water 1.25%, and syrup 10%.

Deakin's Fever and Inflammation Remedy *(Deakin & Hughes, UK).* Contains sodium salicylate 2.8%, sodium citrate 2.8%, concentrated quassia infusion 2%, alcoholic (25%) extract of bearberry (2 in 5) 2%, alcoholic (25%) extract of caryophyllum (1 in 5) 3%, taraxacum juice 5%, strong ginger tincture 0.5%, camphor 0.05%, peppermint oil 0.04%, liquefied phenol 0.41%, cinnamon oil 0.04%, and anise oil 0.04%.

Delax *(Boots, UK).* An emulsion containing in each 5 ml liquid paraffin 2.5 ml, phenolphthalein 45 mg, and benzoic acid 5.5 mg.

Delrosa Blackcurrant and Rose Hip Syrup *(Sterling Health).* A sucrose-free syrup containing not less than 110 mg of ascorbic acid per fl oz.

Delrosa Real Orange Juice and Rose Hip Syrup *(Sterling Health).* A sucrose-free syrup containing not less than 110 mg of ascorbic acid per fl oz.

Delrosa Rose Hip Syrup *(Sterling Health).* A sucrose-free syrup containing ascorbic acid not less than 110 mg per fl oz.

Dentinox Colic Drops *(DDD, UK: Dendron, UK).* Active ingredient: dimethicone 42 mg per ml.

Dentinox Teething Liquid *(DDD, UK: Dendron, UK).* Contains lignocaine hydrochloride 0.33%, myrrh tincture 0.8%, alcoholic (60%) chamomile extract (1–5) 15%, honey 17%, cetylpyridinium chloride 0.1%, and alcohol 3%. **Dentinox Teething Gel** contains the same active ingredients.

Dentosine *(Cuxson, Gerrard, UK).* Mouthwash containing tannic acid 2.2%, phenol 2.2%, glycerol 11%, isopropyl alcohol 18%, tincture of krameria 7%, witch hazel (distilled extract) 10%.

Dermidex Lotion *(International Laboratories, UK).* Lignocaine 1.2%, aldioxa 0.25%, chlorbutol 1%, and cetrimide 0.5%.

Diamond Corn Treatment *(Cupal, UK).* Contains salicylic acid 13%, amyl acetate 2%, pyroxylin 1.625%, acetone to 100%.

Diamond Foot & Body Powder *(Cupal, UK).* Active ingredients: chlorphenesin 1.5%, zinc oxide 10%, and boric acid 10%.

Diarrhoea & Sickness Mixture *(Savory & Moore, UK).* Each 5 ml contains kaolin 1.83 g, pectin 50 mg, and belladonna tincture 0.1 ml.

Digespirin Antacid *(Spencer, UK).* Tablets each containing dihydroxyaluminium sodium carbonate 300 mg.

Dijex Liquid *(Crookes Products, UK).* Contains aluminium hydroxide gel 98%, and magnesium hydroxide 1.7%.

Dijex Tablets *(Crookes Products, UK).* Each contains aluminium hydroxide-magnesium carbonate co-dried gel 400 mg.

Dinneford's Magnesia Gripe Mixture *(Beecham Proprietaries, UK).* Contains heavy magnesium carbonate 1.57%, citric acid monohydrate 3.54%, sodium bicarbonate 2.13%, sucrose 25%, and rectified spirit 5.28%.

Diocalm Tablets *(Beecham Proprietaries, UK).* Each contains morphine hydrochloride 230 µg and activated attapulgite 280 mg.

Disprin *(Reckitt & Colman Pharmaceuticals, UK).* Tablets each containing aspirin 300 mg, calcium carbonate 90 mg, and anhydrous citric acid 30 mg.

Disprin, Junior *(Reckitt & Colman Pharmaceuticals, UK).* Tablets each containing aspirin 75 mg, calcium carbonate 24 mg, and anhydrous citric acid 8 mg.

Diversey Divocream *(Diversey, UK).* Benzalkonium chloride solution (50%) 0.5%.

Doan's Backache Pills *(Fulford Williams, UK).* Each contains paracetamol 97.2 mg, sodium salicylate 48.6 mg, and aloin 650 µg.

Doctor's Catarrh Pastilles (Sure Shield) *(Guest, UK: English Grains, UK).* Contain menthol 0.36%, creosote 0.18%, and pine oil 0.36%.

Do-Do *(International Laboratories, UK).* Tablets each containing ephedrine hydrochloride 22 mg, anhydrous caffeine 30 mg, and theophylline sodium glycinate 50 mg.

Dolomite Tablets *(Booker Health, UK).* Each provides calcium 90 mg and magnesium 55 mg.

Dols Rub Cream *(Smith & Walker, UK).* Camphor 0.4%, methyl salicylate 9.5%, capsicum extract 0.075%, sodium iodide 0.45%, and chlorocresol 0.09%.

Doom Insect Bite Repellent with Sunscreen *(Napa, UK).* Active ingredients: diethyltoluamide 10% and cinoxate 2.5%.

Dorant Mouthwash *(Laboratories for Applied Biology, UK).* Active ingredients per 100 ml: parahydroxybenzoic acid esters: ethyl 250 mg, propyl 500 mg, and benzyl 250 mg; chloroform 4.9 ml.

Dristan Decongestant Tablets with Antihistamine *(International Chemical, UK).* Each contains phenylephrine hydrochloride 5 mg, chlorpheniramine maleate 2 mg, aspirin 325 mg, and caffeine 16.2 mg.

Dristan Nasal Mist with Oxymetazoline *(International Chemical, UK).* Active ingredient: oxymetazoline hydrochloride 0.05%.

Dry-Clear Acne Lotion *(International Chemical, UK).* Active ingredient: benzoyl peroxide 5%.

Dusk *(Cupal, UK).* Active ingredients: diethyltoluamide 20%.

Duttons Cough Mixture *(Spencer, UK).* Each 5 ml contains liquorice liquid extract 0.133 ml, acetic acid (80%) 0.133 ml, honey 0.267 ml, chloroform 0.025 ml, glycerol 0.2 ml, capsicum tincture 0.025 ml, treacle 2.275 ml.

Earache Drops *(Ayrton, Saunders, UK).* Camphor liniment 12.5, cajuput oil 3.12, rosemary oil 3.12, safrol 3.12, arachis oil to 100.

Earex *(International Laboratories, UK).* Ear-drops containing arachis oil 33.3%, almond oil 33.3% and rectified camphor oil 33.3%.

Ecdilyn Expectorant Syrup *(De Witt, UK).* Each 5 ml contains diphenhydramine hydrochloride 14 mg, ammonium chloride 135 mg, sodium citrate 57 mg, and menthol 1.1 mg.

Ectodyne Worm Syrup *(Wigglesworth, UK).* Contains piperazine citrate 12.6%.

Efavite *(Agricultural Holdings, UK: Britannia Health, UK).* Tablets each containing ascorbic acid 125 mg, pyridoxine hydrochloride 25 mg, nicotinamide 7.5 mg, and zinc sulphate 2.5 mg.

Effer-C *(Cox, UK).* Effervescent tablets each containing ascorbic acid 1 g.

Eftab Effervescent Mouth Wash Tablets *(Thornton & Ross, UK).* Contain peppermint oil 0.56%, clove oil 0.33%, spearmint oil 0.03%, menthol 0.62%, thymol 0.23%, methyl salicylate 0.02%, effervescent basis to 100%.

Elastoplast Antiseptic Cream *(Smith & Nephew Pharmaceuticals, UK).* Contains chloroxylenol 0.3%, triclosan 0.3%, and edetic acid 0.2%.

Elastoplast Antiseptic Liquid *(Smith & Nephew Pharmaceuticals, UK).* Contains cetrimide 3% and chlorhexidine gluconate solution 1.5%.

Elastoplast Antiseptic Wipes *(Smith & Nephew Pharmaceuticals, UK).* Active constituent of impregnating fluid: cetrimide 1%.

Elastoplast Insect Repel Wipes *(Smith & Nephew Pharmaceuticals, UK).* Active constituents of impregnating fluid: diethyltoluamide 20% and dimethyl phthalate 10%.

Elliman's Embrocation *(Beecham Proprietaries, UK).* Contains turpentine oil 35.41% and acetic acid 10.37%.

Emlab Brewers' Yeast Tablets *(Minnesota, UK).* Each contains dried yeast 300 mg.

Emlab Iron and Brewers' Yeast Tablets *(Minnesota, UK).* Each contains dried yeast 300 mg and ferrous fumarate 15 mg.

Eno *(Beecham Proprietaries, UK).* Each 5-g dose is prepared from sodium bicarbonate 2.99 g, tartaric acid 1.43 g, and citric acid 870 mg.

Enterosan *(Mayfair Chemicals, UK).* Each tablet contains kaolin 700 mg, morphine hydrochloride 275 µg, and belladonna dry extract 1.8 mg.

Envoy Pastilles *(Ernest Jackson, UK).* Benzalkonium chloride solution (50%) 0.00108 ml and hexylresorcinol 0.54 mg.

EP Tablets *(Strenol, UK: Farillon, UK).* Each contains paracetamol 300 mg, caffeine 50 mg, and codeine phosphate 8 mg.

Erytex Acute Eczema Ointment *(Charnwood, UK)*. Active constituents: calamine 12.5%, zinc oxide 10%, salicylic acid 1.25%.

Eso-Dex Indigestion Tablets *(Southon-Horton, UK)*. Each contains dried aluminium hydroxide 130 mg, magnesium trisilicate 130 mg, magnesium carbonate 65 mg, and calcium carbonate 195 mg.

Eso-Pax Capsules *(Southon-Horton, UK)*. Each contains paracetamol 240 mg, ascorbic acid 60 mg, caffeine 10 mg, and quinine sulphate 6 mg.

Esopyn Inhalant Capsules *(Regent Laboratories, UK)*. Camphor 8.15 mg, menthol 16.3 mg, eucalyptol 16.3 mg, pumilio pine oil 8.15 mg, thymol 3.26 mg.

Esotérica *(Norcliff Thayer, UK)*. **Facial** and **Fortified** contain hydroquinone 2%, padimate O 3.3%, and oxybenzone 2.5%; **Regular** contains hydroquinone 2%.

Etsonal Stomach Treatment *(Mawson & Proctor, UK)*. Contains bismuth and ammonium citrate solution 14.4%, sodium citrate 1.16%, chloroform and morphine tincture 1.08% chloroform emulsion 0.58%, and sodium bicarbonate 4.02%.

Eucarbon *(Trenka, Aust.: Farillon, UK)*. Each tablet contains charcoal 180 mg, sublimed sulphur 50 mg, senna leaf 105 mg, rhubarb extract 25 mg, peppermint oil and fennel oil.

Exa-mol Antiseptic Ointment *(Wigglesworth, UK)*. Contains yellow soft paraffin 73.1%, wool fat 4.8%, phenol 3.5%, zinc oxide 6%, ammoniated mercury 1%, coal tar solution 2.4%, and starch 10%.

Ex-Lax, Junior *(Ex-Lax, UK)*. Each tablet contains yellow phenolphthalein 48 mg in a chocolate basis.

Ex-Lax Pills *(Ex-Lax, UK)*. Each contains phenolphthalein 95 mg.

Ex-Lax Tablets *(Ex-Lax, UK)*. Each tablet contains yellow phenolphthalein 98 mg in a chocolate basis.

Extra Energy Tablets *(Kirby-Warrick, UK: Sangers Agencies, UK)*. Each contains caffeine 50 mg, ascorbic acid 5 mg, thiamine hydrochloride 1 mg, riboflavine 1 mg, nicotinic acid 5 mg, dextrose 150 mg.

Face-Savers Cream Medication *(Sterling Health)*. Colloidal sulphur 6.4% and resorcinol 1.5%.

Famel Catarrh & Throat Pastilles *(Optrex, UK)*. Active ingredients: creosote 0.29%, cassia oil 0.21%, lemon oil 0.08%, and menthol 0.34%.

Famel Expectorant *(Optrex, UK)*. Linctus containing guaiphenesin 50 mg in each 5 ml.

Famel Honey and Lemon Cough Linctus *(Optrex, UK)*. Contains in each 5 ml guaiphenesin 50 mg, purified honey 250 mg, lemon juice 0.5 ml, and liquid glucose 4.68 g.

Famel Honey and Lemon Cough Pastilles *(Optrex, UK)*. Each contains guaiphenesin 20 mg.

Famel Inhalant Capsules *(Optrex, UK)*. Each contains pumilio pine oil 58.4 mg, chlorbutol 53.1 mg, menthol 47.8 mg, rectified camphor oil 21.3 mg, creosote 21.3 mg, and lavandin oil 10.6 mg.

Famel Linctus *(Optrex, UK)*. Each 5 ml contains pholcodine 5 mg and papaverine hydrochloride 0.5 mg.

Famel Nasal Inhaler *(Optrex, UK)*. Contains eucalyptol 10%, pumilio pine oil 10%, rectified camphor oil 7.5%, cinnamon oil 5%, menthol 50%, and creosote 17.5%.

Famel Syrup (Original) *(Optrex, UK)*. Contains creosote 0.335%, calcium lactate 0.051%, calcium hydrogen phosphate 0.01%, codeine 0.03%, and liquid glucose 94%

Family Antiseptic Cream *(Cupal, UK)*. Active ingredients: cetrimide 0.35% and benzalkonium chloride solution 0.3%.

Family Cherry Linctus *(Cupal, UK)*. Each 5 ml contains dilute acetic acid 0.782 ml, ipecacuanha liquid extract 0.01 ml, glycerol 0.25 ml, and sucrose 2.1 g.

Fam-Lax Laxative Tablets *(Cussons, UK)*. Each contains phenolphthalein 125 mg and powdered rhubarb 27.5 mg.

Febrilix *(Boots, UK)*. A brand of Paediatric Paracetamol Elixir.

Febs Cold Relief Tablets with Vitamin C *(Boots, UK)*. Each contains paracetamol 400 mg, ascorbic acid 50 mg, caffeine 30 mg, and phenylephrine hydrochloride 5 mg.

Feen-a-mint *(Plough, UK)*. Chewing gum tablets each containing phenolphthalein 97.2 mg.

Female Hormone Cream 1934 *(Blakoe, UK)*. Contains oestrone 330 units per g.

Femfresh Intimate Deodorant Spray *(Crookes Products, UK)*. Contains chlorhexidine hydrochloride 0.075%, talc, perfume, and propellents.

Feminax *(Nicholas, UK)*. Tablets each containing paracetamol 250 mg, salicylamide 250 mg, codeine phosphate 8 mg, caffeine 50 mg, and hyoscine hydrobromide 100 µg.

Fennings' Adult Cooling Powders *(Fennings, UK)*. Each 300-mg powder contains anhydrous caffeine 30 mg, paracetamol 180 mg, heavy magnesium carbonate 30 mg, liquorice 24 mg, and light kaolin 26.67 mg.

Fennings' Children's Cooling Powders *(Fennings, UK)*. Each 200-mg powder contains paracetamol 50 mg.

Fennings' Gripe Mixture *(Fennings, UK)*. Each 5 ml contains sodium bicarbonate 50 mg, ginger tincture 0.025 ml, peppermint oil 0.000625 ml, dill oil 0.00125 ml, and caraway oil 0.00125 ml.

Fennings' Little Healers *(Fennings, UK)*. Each tablet contains prepared ipecacuanha 20 mg.

Fennings' Mixture, Lemon Flavoured *(Fennings, UK)*. Sodium salicylate 5%, sodium metabisulphite 0.1%, oil of lemon (terpeneless) 0.1%, spirit of chloroform 2.5%, and extract of quassia liq. (1–1) 0.5%.

Fennings' Original Mixture *(Fennings, UK)*. Each 15 ml contains nitric acid 0.2 ml, peppermint oil 0.001 ml, and sanguis draconis 150 µg.

Fennings' Soluble Junior Aspirin *(Fennings, UK)*. Each tablet contains aspirin 75 mg.

Fenox *(Crookes Products, UK)*. Phenylephrine hydrochloride, available as **Nasal Drops** and as **Nasal Spray** each containing 0.5%.

Fibrosine Balm *(International Chemical, UK)*. Active ingredients: methyl nicotinate 1%, glycol salicylate 5%, histamine dihydrochloride 0.05%, and capsicum oleoresin 0.12%.

Fiery Jack Ointment *(Fylde, UK)*. Contains iodine 0.28%, capsicum oleoresin 0.7%, arachis oil 0.72%, capsicum 20%, lard 8%, hard paraffin 8%, and yellow soft paraffin to 100%.

Fiery Jack Rubbing Cream *(Fylde, UK)*. Capsicin 1.25%, histamine dihydrochloride 0.1%, methyl nicotinate 1%, glycol salicylate 5%, diethylamine salicylate 5%, water-miscible basis to 100%.

Fisherman's Friend Aniseed Flavoured Cold and Flu Lozenges *(Lofthouse of Fleetwood, UK)*. Active ingredients: liquorice powder 7.6%, menthol 0.5%, and anise oil 0.17%.

Fisherman's Friend Extra Strong Throat & Chest Lozenges *(Lofthouse of Fleetwood, UK)*. Contain eucalyptus oil 0.153%, cubeb oil 0.305%, capsicum tincture 0.02%, liquorice extract 7.317%, and menthol 0.9%.

Fisherman's Friend Honey Cough Syrup *(Lofthouse of Fleetwood, UK)*. Honey 1.25 ml, squill vinegar 0.9 ml, citric acid 50 mg, saccharin solution 0.05 ml, anise oil 0.005 ml, benzoic acid 5 mg, peppermint oil 0.0025 ml, menthol 2.5 mg, and eucalyptol 0.001 ml.

Fisherman's Friend Rubbing Ointment *(Lofthouse of Fleetwood, UK)*. Active ingredients: capsicum oleoresin 2%, menthol 10%, chlorbutol 10%, and camphor 10%.

Flucaps Capsules *(Industrial Pharmaceutical, UK)*. Each contains codeine phosphate 8 mg and paracetamol 500 mg.

Flu-rex *(Cupal, UK)*. Each tablet contains paracetamol 400 mg, caffeine 30 mg, phenylephrine hydrochloride 5 mg, and noscapine 7.5 mg.

Frador *(Fassett & Johnson, UK)*. Active constituents: menthol 0.1%, chlorbutol 1%, prep. storax 2%, and the alcohol-soluble matter of 15% of benzoin, in alcoholic solution.

Franolyn Expect *(WinPharm, UK)*. Each 10 ml contains guaiphenesin 50 mg, ephedrine 9.5 mg, and theophylline 120 mg.

Freezone *(International Chemical, UK)*. Active constituents: salicylic acid 14.41% and zinc chloride 2.36%.

Fynnon Calcium Aspirin *(Beecham Proprietaries, UK)*. Each tablet contains aspirin 500 mg, calcium carbonate 150 mg, and citric acid 50 mg.

Fynnon Salt *(Beecham Proprietaries, UK)*. Sodium sulphate 95.96%, sodium bicarbonate 1.95%, potassium sulphate 2.05%, lithium sulphate 0.033%, and traces of iron and sodium chloride.

Galloways Baby Cough Linctus *(LRC Products, UK)*. Each 5 ml contains squill liquid extract 0.0015 ml, ipecacuanha liquid extract 0.01 ml, chloroform spirit 0.225 ml, tolu solution 0.04 ml, and glycerol 1 ml.

Galloways Bronchial Expectorant *(LRC Products, UK)*. Contains ether spirit 0.357%, ipecacuanha liquid extract 0.067%, squill vinegar 0.535%, acetic acid 4.2%, chloroform 0.2%, and syrup 78.6%.

Galloways Cough Syrup *(LRC Products, UK)*. Each 5 ml contains ipecacuanha liquid extract 0.0045 ml, chloroform 0.01 ml, acetic acid 0.21 ml, squill vinegar 0.0267 ml, and ether 0.0028 ml.

Galloways Honey and Lemon Cough Syrup *(LRC Products, UK)*. Contains ether spirit 0.00842 ml, acetic acid 0.21 ml, ipecacuanha tincture 0.045 ml, squill vinegar 0.0268 ml, honey 0.25 ml, syrup to 5 ml.

Galloways Junior Cough Linctus *(LRC Products, UK)*. Contains squill liquid extract 0.3%, ipecacuanha liquid extract 0.2%, chloroform spirit 4.5%, tolu solution 0.8%, glycerol 20%, and syrup.

Gamma Formula *(Booker Health, UK)*. Capsules containing evening primrose oil.

GEB6 *(Booker Health, UK)*. Each capsule contains ginseng root 400 mg, pyridoxine hydrochloride 50 mg, and vitamin E 400 units.

Genasprin *(Fisons, UK)*. Tablets each containing aspirin 300 mg.

George's American Marvel Liniment *(Thomas, UK)*. Contains alcoholic (45%) extract of arnica flower (10–1) 3.7%, alcoholic (60%) capsicum extract (5–1)3.7%, turpentine oil 5%, water 6%, camphor 2%, eucalyptus oil 2%, rosemary oil 0.3%, soft soap 8%, and industrial methylated spirit to 100%.

Germ Ointment *(Parkinsons, UK).* Zinc oxide 8, starch 5, phenol 0.5, methyl salicylate 3, chloroxylenol 0.25, basis to 100.

Germolene *(Beecham Proprietaries, UK).* **Tin** contains lanolin 35%, yellow soft paraffin 40%, liquid paraffin 3.9%, starch 10%, zinc oxide 6.55%, methyl salicylate 3%, octaphonium chloride 0.3%, chloroxylenol 0.05%, phenol 1.19%, and menthol 0.01%; **Tube** contains anhydrous lanolin 35%, yellow soft paraffin 36%, liquid paraffin 7.9%, starch 10%, phenol 1.19%, zinc oxide 6.55% methyl salicylate 3%, octaphonium chloride 0.3%, and menthol 0.01%.

Germolene Footspray *(Beecham Proprietaries, UK).* Contains triclosan 0.03% and dichlorophen 0.1%.

Germolene Medicated Plasters *(Beecham Proprietaries, UK).* Adhesive plasters with a medicated pad containing domiphen bromide 0.15%.

Germolene New-Skin *(Beecham Proprietaries, UK).* Contains ethyl acetate 57.3%, alcohol 25.1%, pyroxylin 6.9%, butyl alcohol 5%, castor oil 3%, amyl acetate 2%, and camphor 0.6%.

Germoloids *(Beecham Proprietaries, UK).* **Ointment** contains yellow soft paraffin 84.5%, zinc oxide 6.6%, wool fat 3.5%, methyl salicylate 3.05%, bismuth oxychloride 1.1%, phenol 1%, menthol 0.2%, and chloroxylenol 0.05%. **Suppositories** each contain lignocaine hydrochloride 13.2 mg and zinc oxide 284 mg.

Germoloids Moist Toilet Tissues *(Beecham Proprietaries, UK).* Active constituents of impregnating fluid: benzalkonium chloride 0.133%, chlorhexidine gluconate 0.2%, and menthol 0.04%.

Gerovital H3 Face Cream *(Tudor, UK).* Active constituent: procaine hydrochloride 100 mg in each 27-g pack.

Gerovital H3 Tablets *(Tudor, UK).* Each contains procaine hydrochloride 100 mg, benzoic acid 6 mg, potassium metabisulphite 5 mg, and disodium phosphate 500 µg.

Gibbs SR *(Elida Gibbs, UK).* Toothpaste containing sodium monofluorophosphate 0.8% and zinc citrate trihydrate 0.5%.

Gill's Medicated Dandruff Remover Shampoo *(Beautisales, UK).* Active ingredients: methyl salicylate 1.5% and rosemary oil 0.5%.

Glacier Cream *(Farillon, UK).* **Green tube:** a non-greasy cream containing ethylparadimethylaminobenzoate 1% and titanium dioxide 1%. **Red tube:** a greasy cream containing ethylparadimethylaminobenzoate 1%, titanium dioxide 1%, and zinc oxide 1%.

Glacier Cream Lip Salve *(Farillon, UK).* Contains ethylparadimethylaminobenzoate 1%.

Glempec *(Parkinsons, UK).* Contains glycerol 5%, citric acid 0.6%, acetic acid 1.2%, ipecacuanha liquid extract 0.13%, camphor 0.04%, liquid glucose 3.7%, and lemon juice 5%.

Glinteel Lotion *(Wigglesworth, UK).* Contains tannic acid 5.25%, Peru balsam 6.25%, cinnamon oil 0.5%, water 8.6%, and industrial methylated spirit to 100%.

Goddard's White Oil Embrocation *(LRC Products, UK).* Active ingredients: turpentine oil 22%, dilute acetic acid 30%, and dilute ammonia solution 14%.

Gold Label *(Thomson & Joseph, UK).* Tablets each containing Korean ginseng 200 mg.

Gon *(Medico-Biological Laboratories, UK).* Tablets each containing acetomenaphthone 10 mg and nicotinamide 50 mg.

Grapefruit Health Salts *(Cupal, UK).* Contains tartaric acid 40%, sodium bicarbonate 42.04%, dried magnesium sulphate 17.66%, saccharin sodium 0.05%, and grapefruit oil 0.25%.

Grasshopper Ear Drops *(Spencer, UK).* Docusate sodium 5%.

Grasshopper Ointment *(Spencer, UK).* Contains colophony 31.68%, yellow beeswax 7.94%, larch oleoresin 23.74%, arachis oil 15.84%, white soft paraffin 19.81%, and copper acetate 0.99%.

Gum-eze *(De Witt, UK).* Contains myrrh tincture 10%, krameria tincture 2.5%, thymol 0.1%, oil of cloves 0.1%, propylene glycol 50%, glycerol 37.0875%, sodium benzoate 0.1%, cetylpyridinium chloride 0.1%, and saccharin 0.0125%.

H_3 Plus *(Eucomark, UK).* Each capsule contains vitamin A 2850 units, vitamin D 250 units, vitamin B_{12} 0.5 µg, vitamin C 40 mg, aminobenzoic acid 25 mg, thiamine hydrochloride 5 mg, riboflavine 5 mg, nicotinamide 12 mg, pyridoxine hydrochloride 500 µg, calcium pantothenate 3 mg, inositol 30 mg, choline dihydrogen citrate 42 mg, tocopherol acid succinate 10 units, biotin 0.5 µg, folic acid 25 µg, L-lysine monohydrochloride 24 mg, iron 10 mg, iodine 150 µg, calcium 46.5 mg, phosphorus 37 mg, copper 1 mg, manganese 1 mg, potassium 5 mg, zinc 500 µg, and magnesium 1 mg.

Hacks *(Barker Dobson, UK).* Active ingredients: menthol 0.1%, eucalyptus oil 0.06%, anise oil 0.11%, tolu liquid 0.02%, coltsfoot extract equivalent to coltsfoot 0.008%, horehound extract equivalent to horehound 0.03%, compound benzoin tincture 0.02%, sucrose 63.7%, and liquid glucose 31.9%.

Hactos Chest & Cough Mixture *(Thomas, UK).* Contains chloroform 0.5%, capsicum extract 0.01%, peppermint oil 0.01%, anise oil 0.01%, clove oil 0.01%, and sucrose 10%.

Haemorex *(Cupal, UK).* Ointment containing zinc oxide 7.5, diperodon hydrochloride 1, allantoin 1, and basis to 100.

Haemorrhoidal Spray *(International Chemical, UK).* Contains lignocaine 0.08% and chlorhexidine hydrochloride 0.1%.

Haemostatic Dressing Strip *(Wallace, Cameron, UK).* Sodium alginate, calcium alginate, domiphen bromide 0.15%.

Haliborange Tablets *(Farley, UK).* Each contains vitamin A 2500 units, cholecalciferol 200 units, and ascorbic acid 25 mg.

Halls Cherry Flavour Cough Drops *(Warner-Lambert, UK).* Active ingredients: menthol 1.5 mg and eucalyptus oil 1 mg.

Head & Shoulders *(Proctor & Gamble, UK).* Shampoo containing zinc pyrithione 1%.

Healthy Feet Cream *(Pickles, UK).* Contains glycerol 5%, menthol 1.5%, undecylenic acid 2.5%, and dibromopropamidine isethionate 0.15%.

Hedex *(Sterling Health).* Tablets each containing paracetamol 500 mg.

Hedex Seltzer *(Sterling Health).* Sachets each containing paracetamol 1 g, caffeine 60 mg, sodium bicarbonate 1.54 g, and anhydrous citric acid 1.25 g.

Hewlett's Antiseptic Cream *(Astra, UK).* Active ingredients: zinc oxide 80 mg, boric acid 25 mg, lanolin 40 mg, in each g of cream.

Hill's Bronchial Balsam *(Hill's Pharmaceuticals, UK).* Each 5 ml contains morphine hydrochloride 900 µg, ammonium acetate 180 mg, capsicum tincture 0.0105 ml, compound benzoin tincture 0.3125 ml, ipecacuanha liquid extract 0.025 ml, acetic acid 0.11 ml, and simple lobelia tincture 0.125 ml.

Hill's Bronchial Balsam Pastilles *(Hill's Pharmaceuticals, UK).* Contain compound benzoin tincture 0.793%, capsicum oleoresin 0.001%, peppermint oil 0.04%, ipecacuanha liquid extract 0.5%, simple lobelia tincture 2.5%, and menthol 0.11%.

Hill's Junior Balsam *(Hill's Pharmaceuticals, UK).* Contains compound benzoin tincture 3.125%, ipecacuanha liquid extract 0.2%, simple lobelia tincture 1.25%, acetic acid (80%) 1.13%, capsicum tincture 0.1%, ammonium acetate 1.8%, and squill vinegar 3.12%.

Hip-C *(Paines & Byrne, UK).* Rose hip syrup containing vitamin C not less than 3 mg per ml.

Homocea Ointment *(Mawson & Proctor, UK).* Contains coconut oil 20%, lard 2%, white beeswax 7.5%, hard paraffin 20%, soft white paraffin 30%, camphor 2%, eucalyptus oil 0.5%, rosemary oil 0.5%, cajuput oil 2.5%, turpentine oil 10%, strong ammonia solution 3%, and water 2%.

Honey Kof Syrup *(Parkinsons, UK).* Contains honey 13.5%, glycerol 8%, lemon tincture 0.2%, chloroform 0.1%, benzoic acid 0.025%, lemon juice 7%, ipecacuanha liquid extract 0.25%, dilute sulphuric acid 0.56%, acetic acid 1.5%, and sucrose 52%.

Hot Measure (Solution) *(Reckitt & Colman Pharmaceuticals, UK).* Each liquid dose contains paracetamol 600 mg, dextromethorphan hydrobromide 15 mg, chlorpheniramine maleate 4 mg, phenylpropanolamine hydrochloride 25 mg, and alcohol 5.7 ml.

Iglodine *(Ayrton, Saunders, UK).* An antiseptic solution containing the equivalent of phenol 0.089% and combined iodine 0.04%.

Iglodine Ointment *(Ayrton, Saunders, UK).* Combined iodine 0.14%, zinc oxide 1.43%, phenol 0.32%, bismuth oxychloride 2.86%.

Iloderm *(Ilon Laboratories, UK).* Contains zinc oxide 19.8%, talc 3.3%, kaolin 2.5%, wool fat 2.5%, and cod-liver oil 1.5%.

Ilonium *(Ilon Laboratories, UK).* Ointment containing colophony 15.6%, larch turpentine 8.1%, turpentine oil 8%, phenol 0.1%, and thymol 0.03%.

Indi-Go *(Lofthouse of Fleetwood, UK).* Lozenges containing bismuth carbonate 2.5%, dried aluminium hydroxide 5%, sodium bicarbonate 5%, calcium carbonate 10%, and magnesium trisilicate 5%.

Interlene *(WinPharm, UK).* A medicated shampoo containing loramine 2%.

Iron Blood Tonic Number 20 *(Cupal, UK).* Active ingredients: concentrated compound sarsaparilla decoction 0.08%, potassium iodide 0.5%, ferric ammonium citrate 2.5%, sassafras oil 0.05%.

Iron Jelloids *(Beecham Proprietaries, UK).* Each contains dried ferrous sulphate 65 mg, copper carbonate 170 µg, dried yeast 138 mg, thiamine hydrochloride 170 µg, riboflavine 290 µg, nicotinamide 1.67 mg, and ascorbic acid 4.17 mg.

Ironplan *(Menley & James, UK).* Sustained-release capsules each containing exsiccated ferrous sulphate 150 mg and vitamin B_1 3 mg.

Jackson's All Fours Cough Mixture *(Waterhouse, UK).* Contains in each 5 ml anise oil 0.00325 ml, peppermint oil 0.0006 ml, chloroform spirit 0.0125 ml, chloroform 0.01185 ml, anaesthetic ether 0.003 ml, capsicum extract 0.02375 ml, and liquorice extract 0.125 ml.

Jackson's Antiseptic Throat Pastilles *(Ernest Jackson, UK).* Contain liquorice extract 5.7%, acetic acid 0.9%, menthol 0.12%, camphor 0.03%, terebene 0.49%, benzoic acid 0.01%, thymol 0.003%, methyl salicylate 0.005%, cineole 0.005%, capsicum oleoresin 0.00001%, and pumilio pine oil 0.2%.

Jackson's Bronchial Catarrh Pastilles *(Ernest Jackson, UK).* Contain creosote 0.15%, chloroform 1.5%, menthol 0.6%, anise oil 0.02%, peppermint oil 0.02%, capsicin 0.001%, and benzoin tincture 0.5%.

Jackson's Catarrh Pastilles *(Ernest Jackson, UK)*. Contain menthol 0.6%, sylvestris pine oil 0.3%, siberian fir oil 0.3%, and creosote 0.2%.

Jackson's Children's Cough Pastilles *(Ernest Jackson, UK)*. Honey 12%, ipecacuanha liquid extract 0.36%, squill liquid extract 0.73%, and citric acid 0.9%.

Jackson's Eucalyptus & Menthol Pastilles *(Ernest Jackson, UK)*. Contain eucalyptus oil 0.6% and menthol 0.8%.

Jackson's Febrifuge *(Waterhouse, UK)*. Contains sucrose 4.19%, sodium sulphate 4.19%, potassium nitrate 0.76%, chloroform 0.13%, ammonium chloride 0.76%, liquorice liquid extract 2%, rhubarb liquid extract 0.19%, taraxacum extract 0.66%, burnt sugar 0.66%, strong ginger tincture 0.47%, potassium iodide 0.04%, iodine 0.04%, capsicum tincture 0.1%, camphor 0.02%, alcohol 1.4%, anise oil 0.02%, and clove oil 0.04%.

Jackson's Glycerin Thymol Pastilles *(Ernest Jackson, UK)*. Contain sodium benzoate 0.3%, thymol 0.04%, menthol 0.03%, cineole 0.06%, siberian fir oil 0.02%, methyl salicylate 0.01%, and glycerol 3%.

Jackson's Iodised Throat Lozenges *(Ernest Jackson, UK)*. Citric acid 10.27 mg, phenol 6.5 mg, menthol 2.86 mg, aqueous iodine solution 0.0039 ml, and methyl salicylate 0.920 mg.

Jackson's Night-Cough Pastilles *(Ernest Jackson, UK)*. Contain cinnamic acid 0.009%, benzoic acid 0.002%, aqueous extract of wild cherry bark (1–1) 3.2%, and codeine phosphate 0.178%.

Jackson's Pholcodine Pastilles *(Ernest Jackson, UK)*. Each contains pholcodine 2.2 mg, menthol 1.1 mg, aniseed oil 540 μg, peppermint oil 120 μg, and eucalyptus oil 120 μg.

Jenners Antacid Suspension *(Savory & Moore, UK)*. Each 5 ml contains magnesium hydroxide mixture 1.29 g, aluminium hydroxide gel 2.56 g, polydimethylsiloxane 7.5 mg, in a flavoured basis.

Jenners Tablets *(Savory & Moore, UK)*. Each contains aluminium hydroxide/magnesium carbonate co-dried gel 500 mg in a flavoured basis.

Johnson's Celebrated Liniment *(Amovon, UK)*. Eucalyptus oil 27% and dipentene 73%.

Johnson's XX Oils *(Amovon, UK)*. Castor oil 88%, dipentene 9%, and eucalyptus oil 3%.

Joy-rides *(Stafford-Miller, UK)*. Each tablet contains hyoscine hydrobromide 150 μg.

Junior Kil Kof *(Parkinsons, UK)*. Contains honey 13.5%, glycerol 8%, chloroform spirit 1%, ipecacuanha liquid extract 0.25%, benzoic acid 0.025%, lemon juice 7%, acetic acid 1.5%, dilute sulphuric acid 0.56%, lemon tincture 0.2%, chloroform 0.1%, and sucrose 52%.

Juno Junipah Salts *(Cox, UK)*. Contain anhydrous sodium sulphate 88%, anhydrous sodium phosphate 0.8%, sodium bicarbonate 11%, saccharin 0.04%, and juniper oil 0.1%.

Juno Junipah Tablets *(Cox, UK)*. Contain anhydrous sodium sulphate 450 mg, anhydrous sodium phosphate 60 mg, phenolphthalein 25 mg, and juniper oil 0.00025 ml, with sodium chloride and terpeneless lime oil.

Kao-C Adults Diarrhoea Mixture *(Cupal, UK)*. Light kaolin 10% and calcium carbonate 5%.

Kao-C Junior Diarrhoea Mixture *(Cupal, UK)*. Contains light kaolin 10% and calcium carbonate 5%.

Kemazoid Throat Lozenges *(British Chemotheutic, UK)*. Each contains benzalkonium chloride 1 mg. **Kemazoid Throat Lozenges with Benzocaine**. Each contains cetrimide 1 mg and benzocaine 5 mg.

Keroderm *(Sterling Industrial, UK)*. An ointment containing titanium dioxide 2%, zinc oxide 10%, bismuth oxyquinolinate 0.25%, in a water-in-oil emulsion basis.

Kest *(Berk Pharmaceuticals, UK)*. Each tablet contains magnesium sulphate 300 mg and phenolphthalein 50 mg.

KH3 Geriatricum *(Schwarzhaupt, Ger.: Farillon, UK)*. Capsules each containing procaine hydrochloride 50 mg and haematoporphyrin base 200 μg.

Kil Kof *(Parkinsons, UK)*. Contains liquorice liquid extract 0.5%, ipecacuanha liquid extract 0.05%, benzoin tincture 1.67%, tolu tincture 1.67%, capsicum tincture 0.4%, anaesthetic ether 0.2%, anise oil 0.16%, oxymel 5%, cetylpyridinium chloride 0.05%, chloroform 0.6%, liquid glucose 8%, and treacle 25%.

Kilpain Menthol & Wintergreen Cream with Mustard *(Wigglesworth, UK)*. Contains eucalyptus oil 1.3%, menthol 0.23%, methyl salicylate 11.22%, thymol 0.75%, phenol 0.38%, camphor 0.38%, and volatile mustard oil 0.07%.

Kilpain Toothache Tincture *(Wigglesworth, UK)*. Contains camphor 7.6%, clove oil 3.4%, solvent ether 32.7%, phenol 13%, and IMS to 100%.

Koladex Tablets *(Laboratories for Applied Biology, UK)*. Each contains caffeine 21 mg, stabilised kola extract 4.5 mg (equivalent to 80 mg dry kola nuts), and glucose 700 mg.

Kompo *(J.F. White, UK)*. Contains black catechu 6%, clove oil 0.065%, cassia oil 0.09%, and capsicum oleoresin 0.019%.

Kruschen Salts *(Ashe, UK)*. Sodium chloride 10%, anhydrous sodium sulphate 2%, potassium chloride 1%, potassium sulphate 5.5%, citric acid 1.5%, potassium iodide 0.001%, magnesium sulphate, exsiccated ($MgSO_4,2.75H_2O$) to 100%.

Laboprin *(Laboratories for Applied Biology, UK)*. Tablets containing aspirin 300 mg and lysine 245 mg.

Ladybird *(Booker Health, UK)*. Each capsule contains ascorbic acid 200 mg, cyanocobalamin 5 μg, folic acid 25 μg, pyridoxine hydrochloride 20 mg, riboflavine 5 mg, and zinc (as amino acid chelate) 4 mg.

Lanacane *(Combe, UK: Nicholas, UK)*. Cream containing benzocaine 3%, resorcinol 2%, and chlorothymol 0.0325%.

Lang's Bruise Relief Spray *(DHL Products, UK)*. Non-metered aerosol containing heparin and cetrimide 0.02%.

Langdale's Cinnamon Essence *(Langdale, UK)*. Contains cinnamon oil 2.72%, alcohol (60%) 54.35%, ipecacuanha tincture 0.85%, squill tincture 0.85%, and senega tincture 0.47%.

Langdale's Tablets *(Langdale, UK)*. Contain cinnamon oil 1%, squill liquid extract 0.006%, senega liquid extract 0.001%, and ipecacuanha liquid extract 0.001%.

Lantex Moist Toilet Tissues *(Sterling Health)*. Active constituent of the impregnating fluid: methylbenzethonium chloride 0.25%.

Lecigran *(Lane, UK)*. Consists of vegetable (soya) lecithin.

Lemeze Cough Syrup *(Guest, UK: English Grains, UK)*. Contains in each 5 ml cetylpyridinium chloride 2 mg, ipecacuanha liquid extract 0.003 ml, lemon oil 0.006 ml, purified honey 500 mg, ammonium chloride 30 mg, glycerol 500 mg, and citric acid monohydrate 125 mg.

Lemon Flu Cold Syrup *(Cupal, UK)*. Contains in each 5 ml codeine phosphate 5 mg, ephedrine hydrochloride 7.5 mg, and diphenhydramine hydrochloride 5 mg, in a basis containing terpeneless lemon oil 0.01 ml.

Lem-Plus Cough Linctus with Honey and Lemon *(Clark Proprietaries, UK)*. Each 5 ml contains ipecacuanha liquid extract 0.015 ml, honey 1.12 g, glycerol 0.75 ml, citric acid 50 mg, terpeneless lemon oil 0.00006 ml, lemon oil 0.006 ml, lime oil 0.00125 ml, and sucrose 1.96 g.

Lem-Plus Instant Hot Lemon Drink *(Clark Proprietaries, UK)*. Granules for solution containing paracetamol 650 mg, sodium citrate 500 mg, and ascorbic acid 50 mg.

LemSip *(Reckitt & Colman Pharmaceuticals, UK)*. Each sachet contains paracetamol 650 mg, phenylephrine hydrochloride 5 mg, ascorbic acid 10 mg, and sodium citrate 500 mg, in a flavoured basis.

LemSip, Junior *(Reckitt & Colman Pharmaceuticals, UK)*. Each sachet contains paracetamol 217 mg, phenylephrine hydrochloride 1.7 mg, ascorbic acid 3.3 mg, and sodium citrate 167 mg, in a blackcurrant-flavoured basis.

Limb-Ease Tablets *(Sterling Health)*. Each contains inositol nicotinate 200 mg.

Linctoid C *(Loveridge, UK)*. Contains oxymel 6%, chloroform spirit 3%, tolu syrup 30%, horehound syrup 12%, ipecacuanha tincture 2%, and black currant syrup 20%.

Linus Brand Vitamin C Powder *(Chatfield Laboratories, UK)*. Consists of ascorbic acid.

Lipgarde *(Pickles, UK)*. Contains lanolin, modified wheat-germ oil, and Nipastat in an emollient basis.

Lipsavers *(Carter-Wallace, UK)*. Active ingredients: 2-ethylhexyl salicylate 4%, sorbic acid 0.5%, and allantoin 0.25%.

Liptrex *(Pickles, UK)*. Contains lanolin, modified wheat-germ oil, and Nipastat in a vegetable-oil basis.

Liqufruta Honey *(LRC Products, UK)*. Each 5 ml contains chondrus 20 mg, liquorice extract 37 mg, linseed 33 mg, chamomile 6.25 mg, peppermint oil 0.005 ml, anise oil 0.002 ml, ipecacuanha liquid extract 0.008 ml, and honey 840 mg.

Liqufruta Lemon *(LRC Products, UK)*. Contains the water-soluble constituents of linseed 0.66%, and chamomile 0.125%, with noscapine 0.08%, ipecacuanha liquid extract 0.15%, tolu solution 2%, and lemon basis to 100%.

Liqufruta Medica *(LRC Products, UK)*. The water-soluble constituents of linseed 0.66%, chondrus 0.4%, and chamomile 0.125%, together with garlic oil 0.0195%, peppermint oil 0.104%, anise oil 0.052%, ipecacuanha liquid extract 0.165%, liquorice juice 0.75%, burnt sugar 1.25%, and sucrose 1.25%.

Liqufruta Standard *(LRC Products, UK)*. The water-soluble constituents of linseed 0.66%, chondrus 0.4%, and chamomile 0.125%, together with garlic oil 0.013%, perppermint oil 0.104%, anise oil 0.052%, ipecacuanha liquid extract 0.165%, liquorice juice 0.75%, burnt sugar 1.25%, and sucrose 1.25%.

Listerine Antiseptic *(Warner-Lambert, UK)*. Alcohol (95%) 28.4%, benzoic acid 0.12%, eucalyptol 0.09%, menthol 0.04%, methyl salicylate 0.05%, thymol 0.06%, water to 100%.

Lloyd's Cream *(Reckitt & Colman Pharmaceuticals, UK)*. Contains diethylamine salicylate 10%.

Lockets Lozenges *(Mars, UK)*. Eucalyptol 0.25%, menthol 0.27%, honey 14.7%, and glycerol 2.4%.

Lotil *(Fassett & Johnson, UK)*. Active constituents: wool alcohols 6%, self-emulsifying glyceryl monostearate 10%, glycerol 6%, benzyl alcohol 5%, cetostearyl alcohol 3%, chlorocresol 0.2%.

Loveridge Adults Cough Mixture *(Loveridge, UK)*. Euphorbia extract 0.21 ml, cocillana liquid extract 0.021 ml, squill liquid extract 0.021 ml, senega liquid extract 0.021 ml, menthol 1.1 mg, anise oil 0.0105 ml, in each 5 ml.

Loveridge Children's Cherry Bark Cough Syrup *(Loveridge, UK)*. Wild cherry syrup 0.175 ml, acetic acid 0.075 ml, ipecacuanha liquid extract 0.0025 ml, camphor 2.5 mg, anise oil 0.0004 ml, in each 5 ml.

Loveridge Children's Cough Mixture *(Loveridge, UK)*. Cocillana extract 0.008 ml, squill liquid extract 0.02 ml, vinegar of ipecacuanha 0.16 ml, in each 5 ml.

Loveridge Cold and Influenza Mixture *(Loveridge, UK)*. Sodium citrate 0.345 g, strong ammonium acetate solution 0.473 ml, camphor 2.5 mg, in each 5 ml.

Loveridge Cold Sore Lotion *(Loveridge, UK)*. Cetrimide 0.5%, camphor 5%, menthol 1%, tolu balsam 2%.

Loveridge Corn and Wart Solvent *(Loveridge, UK)*. Salicylic acid 12%.

Loveridge Creosote Bronchial Mixture *(Loveridge, UK)*. Creosote 0.04 ml, potassium iodide 0.11 g, liquorice liquid extract 0.4 ml, tolu solution 0.125 ml, anise oil 0.0015 ml, in each 5 ml.

Loveridge Indigestion Mixture No. 2 *(Loveridge, UK)*. Magnesium carbonate, light 0.275 g, bismuth carbonate 0.075 g, bismuth salicylate 0.075 g, peppermint oil 0.004 ml, in each 5 ml.

Loveridge Mentholated Balsam *(Loveridge, UK)*. Squill oxymel 1.4 ml, liquorice liquid extract 0.185 ml, menthol 3.5 mg, in each 5 ml.

Lucozade *(Beecham Foods, UK)*. Contains glucose syrup 22.4%, lactic acid 0.11%, caffeine 0.018%, and vitamin C 0.0082%, with flavouring and preservative.

Luma Bath Salts *(Sestri, UK)*. Contain methyl salicylate, capsicum oleoresin, potassium iodide, and sodium carbonate.

Mac Blackcurrant Lozenges *(Beecham Proprietaries, UK)*. Each contains amylmetacresol 600 μg, with sucrose and glucose syrup solids.

Mac Lozenges Honey-Lem *(Beecham Proprietaries, UK)*. Each lozenge contains amylmetacresol 600 μg, sucrose and glucose syrup solids 2.4 g.

Mac Lozenges Medicated *(Beecham Proprietaries, UK)*. Each lozenge contains amylmetacresol 600μg, menthol 4 mg, glucose syrup solids 2.7 g.

Mackenzie Decongestant Tablets *(Cox, UK)*. Each contains paracetamol 250 mg, guaiphenesin 50 mg, methylephedrine hydrochloride 15 mg, chlorpheniramine maleate 2 mg, and menthol 1 mg.

Mackenzies Smelling Salts *(Cox, UK)*. Active constituents: ammonia 15% and eucalyptus oil 3%.

Macleans Indigestion Powder *(Beecham Proprietaries, UK)*. Contains heavy magnesium carbonate 15.5%, calcium carbonate 37.2%, and stabilised aluminium hydroxide equivalent to 17.4% of dried aluminium hydroxide.

Macleans Indigestion Tablets *(Beecham Proprietaries, UK)*. Each contains light magnesium carbonate 150 mg, calcium carbonate 400 mg, and stabilised aluminium hydroxide equivalent to 183 mg of dried aluminium hydroxide.

Matthews' Fullers Earth Cream *(Ashe, UK)*. Contains Matthews' fullers earth 5.3%, zinc oxide 2.9%, calcium carbonate 2.9%, and lanolin 3.4% in an emollient basis.

Maw's Baby Lotion *(Ashe, UK)*. Contains chlorhexidine gluconate 0.01%.

Maw's Cold Sore Ointment *(Ashe, UK)*. Contains tannic acid 5%.

Maw's Orange Halibut Tablets *(Ashe, UK)*. Each tablet contains vitamin A 2500 units, ergocalciferol 250 units, and ascorbic acid 25 mg.

Medacalm Tablets *(British Chemotheutic, UK)*. Activated magnesium aluminium trisilicate 225 mg and pectin 50 mg.

Medex Elixir *(Savory & Moore, UK)*. Each 5 ml contains diphenhydramine hydrochloride 14 mg, ammonium chloride 100 mg, and sodium citrate 44 mg.

Medicaid *(Newton, UK: Farillon, UK)*. Cream containing cetrimide 0.5% in a hydrophilic basis.

Medicalm *(Savory & Moore, UK)*. Each 5 ml contains light kaolin 1.83 g and belladonna tincture 0.1 ml, in an aqueous pectin suspending vehicle.

Medicol Liquid Antiseptic *(Jeyes, UK)*. Dichloroxylenol 2.5%, terpineol 5%, and isopropyl alcohol 13.5%.

Medijel *(DDD, UK: Dendron, UK)*. Contains glycerol 5%, lignocaine hydrochloride 0.66%, and aminacrine hydrochloride 0.05%.

Medijel Soft Pastilles *(DDD, UK: Dendron, UK)*. Contain lignocaine hydrochloride 0.25% and aminacrine hydrochloride 0.025%.

Medipain *(Savory & Moore, UK)*. Tablets each containing paracetamol 500 mg, codeine phosphate 8 mg, and casein 30 mg.

Meditus Pastilles *(Savory & Moore, UK)*. Contain calcium lactophosphate 0.4%, codeine phosphate 0.03%, creosote 0.35%, aconite tincture 0.25%, cinnamon oil 0.275%, peppermint oil 0.35%, and lemon oil 0.1%.

Meditus Syrup *(Savory & Moore, UK)*. Each 5 ml contains calcium lactate 50 mg, calcium phosphate 20 mg, lactic acid 0.0165 ml, phosphoric acid 0.044 ml, tinct. aconite (*B.P.C. 1949*) 0.0415 ml, codeine phosphate 900 μg, creosote 12.5 mg.

Meggezones *(Plough, UK)*. Pastilles each containing menthol 16 mg, benzoin 5.5 mg, peppermint oil 3.1 mg, liquorice liquid extract 17.5 mg and myrrh 0.09 mg.

Melissin *(Surf Ski International, UK)*. Contains in each 5 ml guaiphenesin 100 mg, menthol 1 mg, glycerol 1.66 ml, melissa, dried 125 mg, benzoic acid 5 mg, citric acid 50 mg, and aromatic oils.

Meloids *(Boots, UK)*. Lozenges each containing liquorice juice 93.3%, menthol 1.5%, cinnamon oil 0.37%, and stronger capsicum tincture 0.12%.

Melrose *(Roberts & Sheppey, UK)*. Contains hard paraffin 27.9%, yellow soft paraffin 67.3%, wool fat 1.9%, isopropyl linoleate 1.5%, and chloroxylenol 0.1%.

Meltus Adult Cough & Catarrh Linctus *(Cupal, UK)*. Contains in each 5 ml guaiphenesin 25 mg, cetylpyridinium chloride 2.5 mg, sucrose 1.75 g, and purified honey 500 mg.

Meltus Junior Cough & Catarrh Linctus *(Cupal, UK)*. Contains in each 5 ml guaiphenesin 12.5 mg, cetylpyridinium chloride 2.5 mg, sucrose 2 g, and purified honey 500 mg.

Mentho Lyptus Extra Strong *(Warner-Lambert, UK)*. Active ingredients: menthol 0.39% and eucalyptus oil 0.14%.

Mentho Lyptus Original *(Warner-Lambert, UK)*. Active ingredients: menthol 0.1% and eucalyptus oil 0.08%.

Mentho Lyptus Spearmint Lozenges *(Warner-Lambert, UK)*. Menthol 0.04% and eucalyptus oil 0.1%.

Menthol and Wintergreen Cream *(Cupal, UK)*. Contains eucalyptus oil 1.25%, methyl salicylate 11.2%, menthol 0.22%, camphor 0.34%, and volatile mustard oil 0.1%.

Mentholated Balsam *(Savory & Moore, UK)*. Ipecacuanha tincture 2%, chloroform and morphine tincture 5%, liquorice liquid extract 5%, squill oxymel 25%, menthol 0.05%, camphor spirit 2%.

Mentholatum Antiseptic Lozenges *(Mentholatum, UK)*. Each contains menthol 16 mg, eucalyptus oil 12 mg, and amylmetacresol 600 μg.

Mentholatum Balm *(Mentholatum, UK)*. Contains menthol 1.66%, camphor 10%, eucalyptus oil 0.66%, pumilio pine oil 0.66%, and methyl salicylate 0.66%.

Mentholatum Deep Heat Lotion *(Mentholatum, UK)*. Contains menthol 1.58%, methyl salicylate 18.94%, and liquid lanolin 1.9%.

Mentholatum Deep Heat Rub *(Mentholatum, UK)*. Contains menthol 5.91%, eucalyptus oil 1.97%, methyl salicylate 12.8% and turpentine oil 1.47%.

Mentholatum Deep Heat Spray *(Mentholatum, UK)*. Non-metered aerosol containing glycol salicylate 5%, methyl salicylate 1%, methyl nicotinate 1.6%, and ethyl salicylate 5%.

Mentholatum Nasal Inhaler *(Mentholatum, UK)*. Contains menthol 40%, camphor 40%, methyl salicylate 11%, eucalyptus oil 5%, and pine oil 4%.

Merocaine Lozenges *(Merrell, UK)*. Each contains benzocaine 10 mg and cetylpyridinium chloride 1.4 mg.

Mijex *(Pickles, UK)*. Contains diethyltoluamide and citronella oil.

Milk of Magnesia *(Sterling Health)*. Each 5 ml contains magnesium hydroxide 415 mg.

Milk of Magnesia Tablets *(Sterling Health)*. Each contains magnesium hydroxide 300 mg.

Mil-Par *(Sterling Health)*. Contains approx. 6% magnesium hydroxide and 25% liquid paraffin.

Minalka *(Concept Pharmaceuticals, UK)*. Each tablet contains calcium gluconate 243 mg, potssium citrate 132 mg, disodium phosphate 19 mg, magnesium phosphate 4 mg, ferrous gluconate 540 μg, manganese sulphate 540 μg, copper sulphate 270 μg, zinc sulphate 270 μg, cobalt sulphate 270 μg, potassium iodide 3 μg, and vitamin D_3 1.25 μg, with excipients.

Mist Nerve Sedative *(Industrial Pharmaceutical, UK)*. Potassium bromide mixture (*B.P.C. 1963*) 100%.

Modantis *(Surf Ski International, UK)*. Cream containing antazoline hydrochloride 1%, cetrimide 0.5%, titanium dioxide 2%, and allantoin 0.5%, with cetostearyl alcohol, liquid paraffin, and water.

Moncler Derma Gel *(Roche, UK)*. Active ingredients: *N*-ethyl-9-(4-methoxy-2,3,6-trimethylphenyl)-3,7-dimethyl-2,4,6,8-nonatetraenamide (Vibenoid) and D-panthenol. **Moncler Derma Lotion**. Active ingredients: allantoin, salicylic acid, phenoxyethanol, and D-panthenol ethyl ether.

Moorland Indigestion Tablets *(Crookes Products, UK)*. Each contains bismuth aluminate 5.4 mg, magnesium trisilicate 29 mg, dried aluminium hydroxide 11.6 mg, heavy magnesium carbonate 94 mg, light kaolin 27 mg, and calcium carbonate 464 mg.

Mothereze Tablets *(Herbal Laboratories, UK)*. Each contains dry extracts of raspberry leaf 27.7% and of senna leaf 11.1%.

Mrs. Cullen's Cuts 'n' Grazes Antiseptic Cream *(Cullen & Davison, UK)*. Contains chlorhexidine gluconate solution 0.5%.

Mrs. Cullen's Lem-Clear *(Cullen & Davison, UK)*. Each single-dose sachet contains aspirin 585 mg, salicylamide 95 mg, caffeine 60 mg, and ascorbic acid 80 mg.

Mrs. Cullen's Powders *(Cullen & Davison, UK)*. Contain aspirin 600 mg, caffeine 62 mg, calcium phosphate 34.08 mg, saccharin sodium 3.84 mg, and sodium lauryl sulphate 80 µg.

Mu-Cron Liquid for Children *(International Laboratories, UK)*. Contains phenylpropanolamine hydrochloride 0.2% and guaiphenesin 0.5%.

Mu-Cron Tablets *(International Laboratories, UK)*. Each contains guaiphenesin 32 mg, phenylpropanolamine hydrochloride 25 mg, prepared ipecacuanha 11 mg, and paracetamol 250 mg.

Mulcets Mouth Ulcer Tablets *(Minnesota, UK)*. Each contains ascorbic acid 25 mg and cetylpyridinium chloride 1 mg.

Multone Iron Vitamin Tonic *(Cupal, UK)*. Tablets each containing ferrous gluconate 150 mg, ascorbic acid 5 mg, nicotinamide 3 mg, thiamine hydrochloride 0.5 mg, and riboflavine 0.3 mg.

Murine *(Abbott, UK)*. Eye-drops containing naphazoline hydrochloride 0.012%.

'N' for Burns *(Tidebrook, UK)*. Sodium salts of dihydroxy diaryl methane sulphonic acid polymers 15% in a water-soluble jelly basis.

N Tonic *(Cupal, UK)*. Each 5 ml contains calcium hypophosphite 7.5 mg, potassium hypophosphite 7.5 mg, manganese hypophosphite 2.5 mg, ferric hypophosphite 1.25 mg, thiamine hydrochloride 0.53 mg, potassium citrate 2.2 mg, phosphoric acid 0.0009 ml, and quassia extract 2.5 mg.

Napisan *(Richardson-Vicks, UK)*. A preparation for cleansing and disinfecting babies' napkins, based on potassium monopersulphate and sodium chloride.

Nasciodine *(Strenol, UK: Farillon, UK)*. Active ingredients: iodine 1.26%, menthol 0.59%, methyl salicylate 3.87%, essential oil of camphor 3.87%, and turpentine oil 3.87%.

Natusan Baby Cream *(Benzon, UK)*. Contains boric acid 2.85%, borax 0.15%, and glycerol in an emollient basis.

Natusan Baby Lotion *(Benzon, UK)*. Contains polyoxyethylene alcohol 0.55%, polyoxyethylene derivative of wool fat 0.87%, carboxypolymethylene 0.78%, and glycerol 2.73%, in an emollient basis.

Nazex Nasal Spray *(Cupal, UK)*. Phenylephrine hydrochloride 0.5% in an iso-osmotic basis.

Nella Red Oil *(Nella, UK: Pharmagen, UK)*. Contains methyl nicotinate 1 g, mustard oil 25 ml, clove oil 1.5 ml, red tax. oil 10 mg, and arachis oil to 100 ml.

Neo Baby Cream *(Neo Laboratories, UK: Farillon, UK)*. Contains cetrimide 0.2%, benzalkonium chloride solution 0.1%, in a silicone/lanolin basis.

Neo Baby Mixture *(Neo Laboratories, UK)*. Each 5 ml contains sodium bicarbonate 50 mg, ginger tincture, strong 0.01 ml, and dill oil 0.005 ml.

Neovita Capsules *(Savoy Laboratories, UK: Farillon, UK)*. Each contains vitamin A 2400 units, vitamin B_1 2.5 mg, vitamin B_2 2.5 mg, vitamin B_6 1 mg, vitamin B_{12} 4.9 µg, vitamin C 40 mg, vitamin D 240 units, vitamin E 2 mg, nicotinamide 20 mg, calcium phosphate 100 mg, ginseng 100 mg, magnesium oxide 10 mg, copper sulphate 2 mg, zinc oxide 5 mg, manganese sulphate 2 mg, dried ferrous sulphate 33 mg, calcium pantothenate 10 mg, and lecithin 9.5 mg.

Nicobrevin Anti-Smoking Capsules *(Miller of Golden Square, UK)*. Each contains menthyl valerianate 100 mg, quinine 15 mg, camphor 10 mg, and eucalyptus oil 10 mg.

Night Nurse *(Beecham Proprietaries, UK)*. Each 20 ml contains promethazine hydrochloride 20 mg, dextromethorphan hydrobromide 15 mg, paracetamol 500 mg, and alcohol 3.08 ml.

Nigroids *(Arcadian Confections, UK)*. Pellets containing liquorice extract 68.6% and menthol 2.06%.

Nirolex Expectorant Linctus *(Boots, UK)*. Contains in each 5 ml guaiphenesin 50 mg, ephedrine hydrochloride 15 mg, menthol 1 mg, glycerol 1 ml, and sucrose 2.5 g.

Nivea Creme *(Smith & Nephew Toiletries, UK)*. A water-in-oil emulsion prepared from solid alcohols of the cholesterol series and neutral hydrocarbons.

Nostroline *(Kirby-Warrick, UK: Sangers Agencies, UK)*. Contains eucalyptol 0.2%, menthol 0.3%, phenol 1.6%, and geranium oil 0.2%.

Novasil Antacid Suspension *(Cupal, UK)*. Contains in each 10 ml sodium bicarbonate 445 mg, light magnesium carbonate 333 mg, and peppermint oil 0.01 ml.

Novasil Antacid Tablets *(Cupal, UK)*. Each contains sodium bicarbonate 15.6 mg, heavy kaolin 62.5 mg, calcium carbonate 220 mg, heavy magnesium carbonate 220 mg, and peppermint flavour 3.9 mg.

Noxacorn Antiseptic Corn Remover *(Cox, UK)*. Contains benzocaine 2.2%, camphor 2.2%, salicylic acid 10.6%, iodine 0.11%, castor oil 2.6%, phenol 0.31%, and collodion to 100%.

Noxzema Skin Cream *(Noxell, UK: Ever Ready Razor Blade, UK)*. Contains camphor 0.37%, eucalyptus oil 0.12%, menthol 0.075%, clove oil 0.12%, and phenol 0.32%.

Nurodol *(Beecham Proprietaries, UK)*. Each tablet contains paracetamol 500 mg and caffeine 50 mg.

Nurse Harvey's Gripe Mixture *(Harvey-Scruton, UK)*. Contains dill oil 0.069%, caraway oil 0.069%, weak ginger tincture 5.2%, sodium bicarbonate 1.33%, and syrup 15%.

Nurse Sykes Bronchial Balsam *(Waterhouse, UK)*. Contains compound benzoin tincture 3.1%, capsicum tincture 0.26%, camphor 0.02%, acetic acid 1.5%, glycerol 6.25%, tolu syrup 25%, syrup 25%, alpha-glyceryl-guaiacol ether [guaiphenesin] 0.175%, and chloroform q.s.

Nurse Sykes Powders *(Waterhouse, UK)*. Contain aspirin 41.33%, paracetamol 30%, caffeine 15%, and excipient to 100%.

Nylax Laxative Tablets *(British Chemotheutic, UK)*. Each contains vitamin B_1 3 mg, phenolphthalein 60 mg, cascara dry extract 30 mg, aloin 2 mg, senna leaf 15 mg, and bisacodyl 2 mg.

Olbas Oil *(Lane, UK)*. Contains cajuput oil 18.5%, clove oil 0.1%, eucalyptus oil 35.45%, juniper berry oil 2.7%, menthol 4.1%, peppermint oil 35.45%, and wintergreen oil 3.7%.

Olbas Pastilles *(Lane, UK)*. Contain eucalyptus oil 1.16%, peppermint oil 1.12%, menthol 0.1%, juniper berry oil 0.067%, wintergreen oil 0.047%, and clove oil 0.0025%.

Omega-H3 *(Vitabiotics, UK)*. Each capsule contains aminobenzoic acid 50 mg, wheat-germ oil 100 mg, vegetable lecithin 20 mg, choline 100 mg, inositol 100 mg, rutin 10 mg, thiamine hydrochloride 15 mg, riboflavine 3 mg, pantothenic acid 3 mg, pyridoxine hydrochloride 1 mg, cyanocobalamin 20 µg, biotin 3 µg, folic acid 0.5 mg, ascorbic acid 60 mg, nicotinamide 15 mg, vitamin A 2000 units, ergocalciferol 200 units, vitamin E 25 mg, ferrous sulphate 13.25 mg, ferrous fumarate 32 mg, calcium hydrogen phosphate 180 mg, magnesium sulphate 3.32 mg, zinc oxide 1.26 mg, copper sulphate 2.84 mg, and manganese sulphate 3.32 mg.

On and Off Hair Removing Cream *(Innoxa, UK)*. Active ingredient: calcium thioglycollate.

One-a-day Tablets *(Crookes Laboratories, UK)*. Each contains vitamin A palmitate 5000 units, vitamin B_1 2 mg, vitamin B_2 2 mg, vitamin B_6 1 mg, vitamin B_{12} 2 µg, nicotinamide 20 mg, sodium ascorbate 50 mg, vitamin D 400 units, ferrous carbonate 15 mg, copper carbonate 0.75 µg.

Opas Indigestion Powder *(Wigglesworth, UK)*. Contains sodium bicarbonate 20% calcium carbonate 40%, and heavy magnesium carbonate 40%.

Opas Indigestion Tablets *(Wigglesworth, UK)*. Each contains sodium bicarbonate 68 mg, calcium carbonate 136 mg, and heavy magnesium carbonate 136 mg.

Opazimes *(Wigglesworth, UK)*. Each tablet contains dried aluminium hydroxide 160 mg, light kaolin 700 mg, morphine hydrochloride 250 µg, and belladonna dry extract 3 mg.

Optabs Eye Lotion Tablets *(British Chemotheutic, UK)*. Tablets containing phenylephrine hydrochloride 0.05%, adrenaline 0.6%, and acriflavine 0.005%.

Optrex Eye Drops *(Optrex, UK)*. Hamamelis water 12.5%, allantoin 0.08%, and chlorbutol 0.06%.

Optrex Eye Lotion *(Optrex, UK)*. Contains in 100 ml distilled witch hazel 12.95 g, allantoin 50 mg, salicylic acid 25 mg, chlorbutol 20 mg, and zinc sulphate 4 mg.

Optrex Eye Ointment *(Optrex, UK)*. Contains gramicidin 0.02% and aminacrine hydrochloride 0.02%.

Optrose Rose Hip Syrup *(Optrex, UK)*. Contains ascorbic acid not less than 110 mg per fl oz.

Orajel *(Pickles, UK)*. Contains benzocaine 7.5%.

Orange & Halibut Vitamins *(Kirby-Warrick, UK: Sangers Agencies, UK)*. Each tablet contains vitamin A 2500 units, vitamin D_2 200 units, and vitamin C 25 mg.

Orobronze *(De Witt, UK)*. Each capsule contains canthaxanthin 30 mg.

Ortracin Chewing Gum Pastilles *(Industrial Pharmaceutical, UK)*. Tyrothricin 0.5 mg in each tablet.

Over-Nite *(Cupal, UK)*. Contains in each 20 ml paracetamol 500 mg, diphenhydramine hydrochloride 10 mg, ephedrine hydrochloride 15 mg, and codeine phosphate 10 mg.

Owbridge's *(Chefaro, UK)*. Each 5 ml contains cetylpyridinium chloride 1.25 mg, anise oil 0.0025 ml, clove oil 0.0025 ml, acetic acid 0.06 ml, capsicum tincture 0.025 ml, strong ammonium acetate solution 0.16 ml.

Owbridge's Cold Control *(Chefaro, UK)*. Each liquid dose provides paracetamol 500 mg, phenylpropanolamine hydrochloride 25 mg, and ammonium chloride 300 mg.

Oxy5 *(Norcliff Thayer, UK)*. Lotion containing benzoyl peroxide 5%. **Oxy10.** Lotion containing benzoyl peroxide 10%. **Oxy Wash.** Contains benzoyl peroxide 10%.

P.M.T. Tablets *(English Grains, UK)*. Each contains pyridoxine hydrochloride 20 mg.

Pan-A-Gel *(Ursula-Ruth, UK)*. Capsules containing royal jelly. **Pan-B-Gel.** Capsules containing royal jelly.

Panaleve Elixir *(Wigglesworth, UK)*. Contains paracetamol 120 mg in each 5 ml.

Panaleve Tablets *(Wigglesworth, UK)*. Each contains paracetamol 500 mg.

Panets *(Optrex, UK)*. Each tablet contains paracetamol 500 mg.

Panets Baby Syrup *(Optrex, UK)*. Each 5 ml contains paracetamol 120 mg in an orange-flavoured basis.

Papaya Enzyme *(Booker Health, UK)*. Each tablet contains papain 22.5 mg, prolase 8.1 mg, mylase 2.1 mg, papaya leaves 5 mg, and papaya fruit 2.5 mg.

Parkilax *(Parkinsons, UK)*. Contains fig aqueous extract (1–4) 5%, prune aqueous extract (1–4) 5%, senna liquid extract 12%, cascara liquid extract (free from bitterness) 3.5%, and chloroform 0.2%.

Parkinsons Children's Aspirin Tablets *(Parkinsons, UK)*. Each contains aspirin 75 mg.

Parkinsons Glycerin, Lemon, Ipec Cough Mixture *(Parkinsons, UK)*. Contains lemon juice 10%, glycerol 7%, ipecacuanha tincture 1%, dilute sulphuric acid 1.1%, ether 0.1%, chloroform 0.1%, camphor 0.03%, phosphoric acid 0.04%, benzoic acid 0.03%, and sucrose 50%.

Parkinsons Indian Brandee *(Parkinsons, UK)*. Contains nitrous ether spirit 5%, capsicum tincture 2%, compound gentian tincture 0.04%, compound cardamom tincture 5%, glycerol 0.6%, sodium citrate 1.5%, and sucrose 35.6%.

Parkinsons Toothache Tincture *(Parkinsons, UK)*. Contains camphor 18.8%, chloroform 0.4%, phenol 0.8%, clove oil 11.4%, benzalkonium chloride solution 0.2%, and industrial methylated spirit to 100%.

Parkinsons White Embrocation *(Parkinsons, UK)*. Contains turpentine oil 15.5%, camphor 3.5%, industrial methylated spirit 9%, and acetic acid 7.5%.

Parlice *(De Witt, UK)*. Active ingredients: bioallethrin 0.66% and piperonyl butoxide 2.64%.

Pastilaid Indigestion Pastilles *(Arcadian Confections, UK)*. Each contains aluminium hydroxide-magnesium carbonate co-dried gel 200 mg and magnesium trisilicate 200 mg.

Paton's Mouth Treatment *(Paton, UK)*. Contains wool fat 48.95%, yellow soft paraffin 48.95%, iodoform 0.05%, tannic acid 2%, and saccharin 0.05%.

Pediclex Shampoo *(Ansun, UK)*. Contains malathion 0.5%.

Pediclex Sprinkle 'n Comb Lotion *(Ansun, UK)*. Contains malathion 0.75%.

Penetrol Catarrh Lozenges *(Crookes Products, UK)*. Each contains menthol 7.3 mg, ammonium chloride 26.25 mg, phenylephrine hydrochloride 5.5 mg, and creosote 1.8 mg.

Penetrol Inhalant *(Crookes Products, UK)*. Contains menthol 17.5%, cajuput oil 2.5%, lavender oil 8%, eucalyptus oil 7.5%, otto lavender 4%, peppermint oil 0.2%, and industrial methylated spirit 60%.

Pennine Eye Drops *(Thornton & Ross, UK)*. Contain zinc sulphate 0.05%, boric acid 1.6%, borax 0.16%, sodium potassium tartrate 0.2%, hamamelis water 5%, and phenylmercuric acetate 0.002%.

Peplax *(Cupal, UK)*. Peppermint flavoured tablets each containing phenolphthalein 130 mg.

Pepto-Bismol *(Norwich-Eaton, UK: Farillon, UK)*. Liquid containing bismuth subsalicylate 1.752%, veegum, and methyl salicylate 0.09%.

Persomnia *(Ashe, UK)*. Tablets each containing paracetamol 500 mg and codeine phosphate 8 mg.

Pharmacin *(Optrex, UK)*. Capsules each containing aspirin 325 mg.

Pharmaton *(Pharmaton, Switz.: Pharmagen, UK)*. Capsules each containing dimethylaminoethanol bitartrate 26 mg, ginseng complex 200 mg, vitamin A 4000 units, vitamin B_1 2 mg, vitamin B_2 2 mg, vitamin B_6 1 mg, vitamin B_{12} 1 µg, vitamin C 60 mg, vitamin D 400 units, vitamin E 10 mg, nicotinamide 15 mg, calcium pantothenate 10 mg, rutin 20 mg, iron 10 mg, calcium 90.3 mg, phosphorus 70 mg, fluorine 200 µg, copper 1 mg, potassium 8 mg, manganese 1 mg, magnesium 10 mg, zinc 1 mg, with choline, inositol, linoleic acid and linolenic acid.

Pharmaton Ginseng Extract Capsules *(Pharmaton, Switz.: Pharmagen, UK)*. Each contains 100 mg of standardised extract from Korean panax ginseng 500 mg.

Phensic *(Beecham Proprietaries, UK)*. Each tablet contains aspirin 325 mg and caffeine 50 mg.

Phensic Soluble *(Beecham Proprietaries, UK)*. Tablets each containing aspirin 325 mg and calcium carbonate 97.5 mg.

Phillips Iron Tonic *(Phillips Yeast, UK)*. Tablets each containing iron (as saccharated ferrous carbonate) 20 mg, dried yeast 170 mg, vitamin C 10 mg, vitamin B_1 160 µg, vitamin B_2 300 µg, and nicotinic acid 2 mg.

Phillips Tonic Yeast *(Phillips Yeast, UK)*. Each tablet of brewers' yeast contains thiamine hydrochloride 110 µg, riboflavine 200 µg, nicotinic acid 1.4 mg, pyridoxine 9 µg, calcium pantothenate 12 µg, and other vitamins natural to brewers' yeast.

pHiso-Ac *(WinPharm, UK)*. Cream containing colloidal sulphur 6.4% and resorcinol 1.5%.

pHiso-Clear *(WinPharm, UK)*. Contains salicylic acid 0.5%, IMS 25.4%.

pHisoderm *(WinPharm, UK)*. Contains sodium octylphenoxyethoxyethyl ether sulphonate, lanolin derivatives, and petrolatum.

pHisohex *(WinPharm, UK)*. Active ingredient: chlorhexidine gluconate 1%.

Pholtussa Mixture *(Philip Harris, UK)*. Pholcodine 0.08%, ipecacuanha extract 1.5%, and blackcurrant syrup 50%.

Phosferine Liquid *(Beecham Proprietaries, UK)*. Contains cinchonidine sulphate 0.06% and quinine sulphate 0.47%.

Phosferine Tablets *(Beecham Proprietaries, UK)*. Each contains cinchonidine sulphate 151 µg and quinine sulphate 703 µg.

Phyllosan *(Beecham Proprietaries, UK)*. Each tablet contains ferrous fumarate 35 mg, nicotinic acid 8.5 mg, thiamine hydrochloride 166 µg, riboflavine 333 µg, and ascorbic acid 5 mg.

Pickles Foot Ointment *(Pickles, UK)*. Contains salicylic acid 50%.

Pickles SCR *(Pickles, UK)*. Contains salicylic acid 1.5%.

Pickles Smelling Salts *(Pickles, UK)*. Strong ammonia solution 28.5%, pumilio pine oil 14.25%, and eucalyptus oil 14.25%.

Pickles Toothache Tincture *(Pickles, UK)*. Lignocaine hydrochloride 0.7% and clove oil 10%.

Pilease *(Ayrton, Saunders, UK)*. Contains ethyl aminobenzoate 6%, zinc oxide 5%, hexachlorophane 0.5%, starch 5%, wool fat 10%, and paraffin basis to 100%.

Pilogene Compound *(Hanson, UK)*. Contains hamamelis 1.05%, almond oil 1.35%, and zinc oxide 0.9% in a saponaceous basis.

Placidex *(De Witt, UK)*. Contains paracetamol 240 mg in each 10 ml.

Plurivite M Tablets *(Boots, UK)*. Tablets each containing vitamin A palmitate 5000 units, thiamine hydrochloride 2 mg, riboflavine 2 mg, pyridoxine hydrochloride 1 mg, cyanocobalamin 2 µg, nicotinamide 20 mg, vitamin C (as sodium ascorbate) 50 mg, calciferol solution 400 units, iron (as ferrous carbonate) 15 mg, and copper (as copper carbonate) 0.75 mg.

Plurivite Tablets *(Boots, UK)*. Each contains vitamin A palmitate 4000 units, thiamine hydrochloride 2 mg, riboflavine 2 mg, pyridoxine hydrochloride 1 mg, cyanocobalamin 2 µg, nicotinamide 20 mg, ascorbic acid 50 mg, calciferol solution 400 units, vitamin E 5 mg, and calcium pantothenate 5 mg.

Pollen-B *(Wassen, UK: Fassett & Johnson, UK)*. Tablets each containing bee-collected pollen 150 mg.

Potter's Asthma Cigarettes *(Potter & Clarke, UK: De Witt, UK)*. Active constituents: the active principles of stramonium leaves equivalent to 0.15% of alkaloids calculated as hyoscyamine.

Potter's Asthma Remedy *(Potter & Clarke, UK: De Witt, UK)*. Active constituents: the active principles of stramonium leaves equivalent to 0.12% of alkaloids calculated as hyoscyamine.

Potter's Catarrh Pastilles *(Potter & Clarke, UK: De Witt, UK)*. Contain sylvestris pine oil 0.41%, pumilio pine oil 0.41%, eucalyptus oil 0.02%, creosote 0.2%, menthol 0.83%, thymol 0.02%, and aqueous extractive from althaea 0.5%.

Potter's Childrens Cough Pastilles *(Potter & Clarke, UK: De Witt, UK)*. Honey 90 mg, glycerol 22 mg, menthol 430 µg, and creosote 120 µg.

Potter's Dermacreme Ointment *(Potter's Herbal Supplies, UK)*. Menthol 0.015%, methyl salicylate 3%, liquefied phenol 1%, starch 8%, zinc oxide 8%, hard paraffin 5%, wool fat 3.25%, and yellow soft paraffin to 100%.

Potter's Psoriasis Ointment *(Potter's Herbal Supplies, UK)*. Starch 5%, sublimed sulphur 7%, zinc oxide 7%, phytolacca 0.5%, butamyrate citrate 0.18%, hydrous wool fat 28%, and yellow soft paraffin to 100%.

Potter's Skin Clear Ointment *(Potter's Herbal Supplies, UK)*. Phenols 0.33%, starch 17%, sulphur sublimed 5%, zinc oxide 23%, and yellow soft paraffin to 100%.

Potter's Varicose Vein Ointment *(Potter's Herbal Supplies, UK)*. Boric acid 3.7%, cade oil 2.3%, emulsifying wax 2.4%, hamamelis liquid extract 7.4%, hard paraffin 1.85%, wool alcohols 1.48%, zinc oxide 3.57%, and yellow soft paraffin to 100%.

Potter's Walk Easy Ointment *(Potter's Herbal Supplies, UK)*. Contains salicylic acid 12.5%.

Powerin *(International Chemical, UK)*. Tablets each containing paracetamol 200 mg, caffeine 45 mg, and aspirin 300 mg.

PP Tablets *(Lane, UK)*. Each contains gentian extract 6 mg, valerian liquid extract 12 mg, passion flower extract (1 in 1) 6 mg, theobromine 15 mg, paracetamol 150 mg, caffeine 7.5 mg, and kola liquid extract 12 mg.

PR Pain Relief Tablets *(Boots, UK)*. Each tablet contains aspirin 250 mg, paracetamol 125 mg, and caffeine 25 mg.

PR Spray *(Crookes Products, UK)*. A refrigerant skin spray containing dichlorodifluoromethane 15% and trichlorofluoromethane 85%.

Preparation H *(International Chemical, UK)*. **Ointment** containing the alcohol-soluble extract of 2 g of live yeast cells per g (Bio-Dyne), shark-liver oil 3%, and phenylmercuric nitrate 0.01% and **Suppositories** each containing the alcohol-soluble extract of 72 mg of live yeast cells, shark-liver oil 72 mg, and phenylmercuric nitrate 0.24%.

Primes Premiums *(Newton, UK: Farillon, UK)*. Each tablet contains magnesium trisilicate 40 mg, dried aluminium hydroxide 125 mg, magnesium carbonate 150 mg, calcium carbonate 250 mg, and peppermint oil.

Procol *(Menley & James, UK)*. Sustained-action capsules each containing isopropamide iodide 3.4 mg and phenylpropanolamine hydrochloride 50 mg.

Proctors' Pinelyptus Pastilles *(Ernest Jackson, UK)*. Contain menthol 0.548%, eucalyptus oil 0.842%, abietis oil 0.12%, and sylvestris pine oil 0.12%.

Pro-Hyd 50 *(E.C.M. Laboratories, UK)*. Capsules each containing procaine hydrochloride 50 mg and haematoporphyrin hydrochloride 200 μg.

Pronel *(Bioglan, UK)*. Capsules each containing gelatin 320 mg.

Propa PH *(Optrex, UK)*. Active constituents: cetrimide 0.1%, menthol 0.034%, thymol 0.017%, thyme oil 0.0085%, benzoic acid 0.185%, chlorthymol 0.017%, eucalyptol 0.017%, methyl salicylate 0.0085%, and cineole 0.017%.

Pro-Plus Tablets *(Ashe, UK)*. Each contains caffeine 50 mg.

Pro-Ven Gel *(Stiefel, UK)*. Contains benzoyl peroxide 2.5%.

Pru-Sen *(Herbal Laboratories, UK)*. Contains senna leaf 5%, figs 10%, prunes 1.67%, raisins 3.33%, and dates 80%.

Pruven *(Stiefel, UK)*. Gel containing benzoyl peroxide 2.5%.

Pulmo Bailly *(Bengué, UK)*. Each 5 ml contains guaiacol 75 mg, codeine 7 mg, and phosphoric acid 75 mg.

Pylatum Regulators *(Laboratory Facilities, UK: Dendron, UK)*. Active ingredients: senna leaf 5%, cascara dry extract 56%, aloin 16%, colocynth 6%, ginger oleoresin 4%, peppermint oil 4%, and hard soap 1.5%.

Pyorex *(Bengué, UK)*. Toothpaste containing acetarsol lithium equivalent to acetarsol 0.45%, aminacrine hydrochloride 0.006%, and sodium ricinoleate 0.76%.

Q-Panol Elixir *(Cupal, UK)*. Contains in each 5 ml paracetamol 120 mg.

Quatoral Lozenges *(Guest, UK)*. Each contains tyrothricin 1 mg, benzocaine 5 mg, and cetylpyridinium chloride 1.5 mg.

Quick Action Cough Cure *(Spencer, UK)*. Each dose provides dextromethorphan hydrobromide 3.75 mg and guaiphenesin 25 mg.

Quick Kwells *(Nicholas, UK)*. Tablets each containing hyoscine hydrobromide 300 μg.

Radian Massage Cream *(Radiol, UK)*. Contains menthol 2.54%, camphor 1.43%, methyl salicylate 0.42%, and water-soluble capsicin 0.042%.

Radian Warm-up Sports Rub *(Radiol, UK)*. Contains capsicin and methyl salicylate in a lotion basis.

Radian-B Spirit Liniment *(Radiol, UK)*. Manufactured from menthol 1.4%, aspirin 1.2%, camphor 0.6%, and methyl salicylate 0.6%, in alcohol. **Radian-B Spray** is prepared from the same ingredients but contains no alcohol.

Radox *(Nicholas, UK)*. Bath salts containing extracts of herbs with witch hazel, horse-chestnut, rosemary, hops, and camomile; sea salt with salts of calcium, magnesium, and sodium; a mixture of sodium carbonate and sodium bicarbonate; and soapless cleansing agents.

Ralgex Balm *(Beecham Proprietaries, UK)*. Contains methyl nicotinate 1%, histamine dihydrochloride 0.05%, and capsicin 0.12%.

Ralgex Embrocation *(Beecham Proprietaries, UK)*. Turpentine oil 22%, dilute acetic acid 30%, and dilute ammonia solution 14%.

Ralgex Embrocation Stick *(Beecham Proprietaries, UK)*. Active ingredients: glycol salicylate 3.01%, ethyl salicylate 3.01%, methyl salicylate 0.6%, capsicin 1.67%, and menthol 6.19%.

Ralgex Spray *(Beecham Proprietaries, UK)*. Active ingredients: glycol salicylate 4.8%, ethyl salicylate 4.8%, methyl salicylate 0.96%, and methyl nicotinate 1.6%.

Rayglo BKB *(Cupal, UK)*. Each tablet contains buchu extract 10 mg and methylene blue 4 mg.

Rayglo Chest Rub *(Cupal, UK)*. Contains camphor 6.1%, menthol 2.03%, cedar wood oil 0.5%, eucalyptus oil 2%, nutmeg oil 0.1%, thyme oil 0.1%, guaiacol 0.0011%, turpentine oil 6.1%, pine oil 3%, Peru balsam 0.05%, and white soft paraffin to 100%.

Rayglo Laxative Tablets *(Cupal, UK)*. Each contains phenolphthalein 125 mg.

Rayglo Toothache Tincture *(Cupal, UK)*. Contains camphor 10%, sandarac substitute 10%, and clove 5%.

Red Kooga *(English Grains, UK)*. A range of preparations containing Korean panax ginseng.

Redelan Effervescent tablets *(Roche, UK)*. Each contains vitamin A 5500 units, thiamine mononitrate 1.2 mg, riboflavine sodium phosphate 1.8 mg, pyridoxine hydrochloride 1.6 mg, cyanocobalamin 1.4 μg, nicotinamide 15 mg, calcium pantothenate 13 mg, ascorbic acid 75 mg, ergocalciferol 400 units, and DL-alpha-tocopheryl acetate 10 mg.

Redoxon *(Roche, UK)*. Tablets each containing ascorbic acid 25, 50, 200, or 500 mg. **Redoxon Effervescent.** Tablets each containing ascorbic acid 1 g; in standard, blackcurrant, lemon, or orange flavours.

Reguletts *(Cupal, UK)*. Tablets each containing phenolphthalein 120 mg in a chocolate basis.

Relcol Tablets *(Industrial Pharmaceutical, UK)*. Paracetamol 240 mg, quinine bisulphite 1 mg, ephedrine 7.5 mg.

Rennie Tablets *(Nicholas, UK)*. Each contains chalk 680 mg and light magnesium carbonate 80 mg.

Ress-Q Pastilles *(Ernest Jackson, UK)*. Each contains benzalkonium chloride 600 μg, tinct. benzoin co. 10 mg, and menthol 2 mg.

Revive *(Ethical Research Products, UK)*. Fructose 20 g, dextrose 18 g, and sucrose 2 g in 100 ml, with lime juice, and citric acid.

Revlon ZP11 Formula *(Revlon, UK)*. **Medicated Hair Dressing** containing zinc pyrithione 0.5% and **Medicated Shampoo** containing zinc pyrithione 1%.

Rheumaban Cream *(Pickles, UK)*. Active ingredients: histamine acid phosphate 0.1%, eucalyptus oil 3%, methyl nicotinate 1.5%, camphor oil 2%, glycol salicylate 7.5%, and pumilio pine oil 3%.

Rinstead Gel *(Plough, UK)*. Contains benzocaine 2%, sodium ricinoleate 0.1%, chloroxylenol 0.1%, clove oil 0.1%, myrrh 0.1%, glycerol 10%, CMC 2%, and SVR 30%.

Rinstead Pastilles *(Plough, UK)*. Each contains menthol 0.37 mg, myrrh 1.25 mg, sodium ricinoleate 0.62 mg, chloroxylenol 0.75 mg, phenolphthalein 0.75 mg, and tartaric acid 3.25 mg.

Ruban *(Evans Medical, UK)*. Active constituents: glycol salicylate 2%, methyl nicotinate 0.75%, capsicum oleoresin 0.2%, in a non-greasy basis.

Rutivite Tablets *(Rutin Products, UK)*. Each contains dried buckwheat (leaf and flower) equivalent to 30 mg of rutin.

Sainsbury's Cold Powders *(Sainsbury, UK)*. Each contains paracetamol 1 g, phenylephrine hydrochloride 10 mg, and vitamin C 60 mg.

St. James' Balm *(Medico-Biological Laboratories, UK: Sestri, UK)*. Contains zinc oxide 20%, ichthammol 2.8%, urea 0.1%, and salicylic acid 0.1%.

Saltair Lotion *(Salt, UK)*. Magnesium trisilicate 2.05%, bismuth carbonate 0.25%, aldioxa 0.5%, hexachlorophane 0.1%, starch 11%, kaolin, light 0.7%, zinc oxide 27.5%, and silicon dioxide 0.35%.

Samaritan Anti-midge Cream *(Thornton & Ross, UK)*. Contains dimethyl phthalate 1% and diethyltoluamide 15%.

Samaritan Chilblain Cream *(Thornton & Ross, UK)*. Active ingredients: methyl nicotinate 1.5%, phenol 0.5%, camphor 1.5%, and benzocaine 4%.

Samaritan Menthol and Wintergreen Cream *(Thornton & Ross, UK)*. Methyl salicylate 12.5% and menthol 1% in a water-miscible basis.

Sanatogen *(Fisons, UK)*. Consists of casein 94.5%, sodium glycerophosphate 5%, and glyceryl mono-oleate 0.5%.

Sanatogen High C *(Fisons, UK)*. Each tablet contains ascorbic acid 1.020 g and riboflavine 300 μg, with tartaric acid and adipic acid.

Sanatogen Junior Vitamins *(Fisons, UK)*. Tablets each containing vitamin A acetate 2500 units, vitamin C 50 mg, and vitamin D_2 200 units.

Sanatogen Multivitamins *(Fisons, UK)*. Tablets each containing vitamin A 4000 units, vitamin B_1 1.2 mg, vitamin B_2 1.8 mg, vitamin C 30 mg, vitamin D_2 400 units, vitamin E 2 mg, nicotinamide 12 mg, potassium iodide 130 μg.

Sanatogen Multivitamins Plus Iron *(Fisons, UK)*. Vitamin A acetate 4000 units, vitamin B_1 1.2 mg, vitamin B_2 1.8 mg, nicotinamide 12 mg, coated ascorbic acid 30 mg, vitamin D_2 400 units, vitamin E 0.5 mg, potassium iodide 130 μg, and ferrous fumarate 45.6 mg.

Sanatogen Vitamin C Tablets *(Fisons, UK)*. Each contains ascorbic acid 75 mg.

Sanatogen Vitamin E *(Fisons, UK)*. Each tablet contains vitamin E 100 mg.

Sanderson's Cough Linctus *(Sandersons, UK: Vestric, UK)*. Contains in each 5 ml compound cardamom tincture 0.2 ml and citric acid 1.4 mg.

Sanderson's Throat Specific *(Sandersons, UK: Vestric, UK)*. **Mixture** contains in each 5 ml squill extract 0.025 ml, capsicum liquid extract 0.025 ml, quassia extract 0.008 ml, and acetic acid 0.113 ml. **Pastilles** each contain honey 145 mg, squill vinegar 96 mg, capsicum oleoresin 19 μg, tolu tincture 3 mg, menthol 1.5 mg, benzoic acid 0.966 mg, eucalyptus oil 0.376 mg, and cinnamic acid 37.5 μg.

Savlon Antiseptic Cream *(Care, UK)*. Contains cetrimide 0.5% and chlorhexidine gluconate 0.1%.

Savlon Antiseptic Liquid *(Care, UK)*. Contains chlorhexidine gluconate 0.3% and cetrimide 3%.

Savlon Babycare Cream *(Care, UK)*. Contains cetrimide 0.5%.

Savlon Dry First Aid Spray *(Care, UK)*. Aerosol containing povidone-iodine 0.5%.

Scholl Antiseptic Foot Balm *(Scholl, UK)*. Active ingredients: halquinol 0.4%, menthol 0.5%, methyl salicylate 0.1%, and basis to 100%.

Scholl Athlete's Foot Powder *(Scholl, UK)*. Contains chlorphenesin 1%, zinc oxide 20%, and talc 79%.

Scholl Athlete's Foot Treatment (S1) *(Scholl, UK)*. Contains borotannic complex 9.9% and methyl salicylate 0.76%.

Scholl Bunion Lotion *(Scholl, UK)*. Contains weak iodine solution 10.8%, capsicum oleoresin 0.014%, and menthol 2.7%.

Scholl Corn and Callous Salve *(Scholl, UK)*. Contains salicylic acid 39%, eucalyptus oil 1%, and anhydrous lanolin to 100%.

Scholl Corn Removing Liquid *(Scholl, UK).* Active ingredients: salicylic acid 11.25% and camphor 2.8%.

Scholl Fixo Corn Plasters *(Scholl, UK).* The spread material contains salicylic acid 40%.

Scholl Foot Powder *(Scholl, UK).* Contains salicylic acid 3% and aluminium chlorhydroxide 10%.

Scholl Ingrown Toenail Treatment *(Scholl, UK).* Active constituents: potassium acetate 3%, triethanolamine 10%, and urea 10%.

Scholl Zino Corn, Callous, and Bunion Pads *(Scholl, UK).* Plasters with medicated disks impregnated with salicylic acid 40%.

Scott's Cod Liver Oil Capsules *(Beecham Proprietaries, UK).* Each contains vitamin A 625 units and vitamin D 62.5 units in 315 mg of cod-liver oil.

Scott's Emulsion *(Beecham Proprietaries, UK).* Each 5 ml contains cod-liver oil 1.68 g, calcium hypophosphite 48 mg, sodium hypophosphite 24 mg.

Sea-legs *(Farley, UK).* Tablets each containing meclozine hydrochloride 12.5 mg.

Seba Med *(Sebamat Chemie, Ger.: Pharmagen, UK).* Soap-free **Liquid Cleanser** contains amino acids, nicotinic acid, nicotinamide, lactic acid, vitamin B_6, vitamin H, and vitamin F. Soap-free **Cleansing Bar** contains amino acids, cholesterol, lecithin, phosphatides, glycerides, and vitamins.

Sebbix Shampoo *(Ashe, UK).* Contains purified coal fraction 0.25% stated to be therapeutically equivalent to crude coal tar 2%, with sodium sulphosuccinated undecylenic monoalkylolamide 1%.

Secaderm Salve *(Rorer, UK).* Active ingredients: phenol 2.4%, terebene 5.25%, melaleuca oil 5.6%, rectified oil of turpentine 6%, and resin 26%.

Secron *(De Witt, UK).* Each 5 ml contains phenylpropanolamine hydrochloride 7.5 mg and guaiphenesin 30 mg.

Sek Ointment *(International Chemical, UK).* Active constituents: sodium propionate 12.1%, propionic acid 1.5%, sodium octoate 9.8%, zinc octoate 4.9%, and docusate sodium 0.15%.

Selenium-ACE *(Christy, UK).* Each tablet contains vitamin C 100 mg, selenium yeast 80 mg (50 µg Se), vitamin A 500 units, and vitamin E (natural) 50 units.

Sensodyne Toothpaste *(Stafford-Miller, UK).* Active ingredient: strontium chloride 10%.

Sereen *(Boots, UK).* Tablets each containing hyoscine hydrobromide 300 µg.

Setlers *(Beecham Proprietaries, UK).* Tablets each containing calcium carbonate 534 mg and light magnesium carbonate 72 mg.

Seven Rubbing Oils *(Parkinsons, UK).* Contains rectified camphor oil 0.9%, clove oil 0.18%, cajuput oil 0.18%, sweet birch oil 0.18%, amber oil 0.36%, eucalyptus oil 0.36%, expressed mustard oil 16.2%, methyl salicylate 0.9%, and camphor 1.08%.

Seven Seas *(British Cod Liver Oils, UK).* Consists of cod-liver oil.

Seven Seas Capsules *(British Cod Liver Oils, UK).* Each contains 0.3 ml of cod-liver oil, providing vitamin A 600 units, vitamin D 60 units, and vitamin E 0.3 units.

Seven Seas Cherry Flavour *(British Cod Liver Oils, UK).* Consists of cod-liver oil with cherry flavouring.

Seven Seas Orange Syrup *(British Cod Liver Oils, UK).* Active ingredients per 10 ml: cod liver oil 2.8 g, vitamin A 4000 units, vitamin B_6 0.7 mg, vitamin C 35 mg, vitamin D 400 units, and vitamin E 3 mg, with concentrated orange juice and polyunsaturates.

Si-Ko *(Ever Ready Razor Blade, UK).* Toothpaste containing silica-hydro-glycero-gel 67.8%, emulsifying agent 1.2%, essential oils 0.5%, sodium fluoride 0.2%, cream of tartar 29.8%, and buffers 0.5%.

Simpkins Antiseptic Throat Lozenges *(Simpkin, UK).* Contain weak iodine solution 1.13%, menthol 0.04%, and phenol 0.02%.

Simpkins Bronchial Catarrh Lozenges *(Simpkin, UK).* Contain cinnamon oil 0.02%, menthol 0.12%, and compound benzoin tincture 1.1%.

Simpkins Children's Cough Lozenges *(Simpkin, UK).* Contain ipecacuanha extract 0.0026 ml, squill extract 0.0026 ml, menthol 1.3 mg, chloroform spirit 0.0013 ml, glycerol 0.021 ml, anise oil 0.0026 ml, and tolu extract.

Simpkins Menthol & Eucalyptus Drops *(Simpkin, UK).* Contain menthol 0.25% and eucalyptus oil 0.215%.

Simpkins Menthol & Eucalyptus Mini-Tabs *(Simpkin, UK).* Contain eucalyptus oil 0.95% and menthol 0.52%.

Simpkins Teddy Cough Lozenges *(Simpkin, UK).* Contain anise oil 0.0013 ml, peppermint oil 0.0013 ml, coltsfoot extract 0.00054 ml, menthol 0.48 mg, ipecacuanha extract 0.00036 ml, and squill extract 0.00036 ml, and chloroform spirit 0.00048 µl.

Simpson's Foot Ointment *(Dendron, UK).* Active ingredients: potassium iodide 0.25%, sublimed sulphur 3%, salicylic acid 0.187%, camphor 2%, menthol 0.2%, pine oil 0.25%, zinc oxide 0.25%, zinc stearate 1.67%.

Sine-Off *(Menley & James, UK).* Each tablet contains aspirin 325 mg, phenylpropanolamine hydrochloride 18.75 mg, and chlorpheniramine maleate 2 mg.

Skintex Medicinal Cream *(Lloyd, Aimee, UK).* Chloroxylenol 0.25%, glycerol 18%, castor oil 10%, and camphor 0.5%.

Slim-Line *(Thompson Medical, UK).* Chewing gum containing benzocaine 6 mg in each tablet.

Sloan's Liniment *(Warner-Lambert, UK).* Contains methyl salicylate 2.65%, camphor 0.63%, pine oil 6.77%, turpentine oil 48.9%, and capsicum oleoresin 0.72%.

Smokers Supplement *(Booker Health, UK).* Each tablet contains ascorbic acid 500 mg, cysteine 10 mg, pyridoxine hydrochloride 5 mg, and thiamine hydrochloride 20 mg.

Snef Nasal Drops *(Thornton & Ross, UK).* Active constituent: phenylephrine hydrochloride 0.25% in an iso-osmotic basis.

Snowfire Healing Tablet *(Pickles, UK).* Contains benzoin 0.02%, citronella oil 0.06%, thyme oil 0.01%, clove oil 0.04%, cade oil 0.04%, lemon oil 0.01%, in a soft paraffin basis.

Snufflebabe *(Pickles, UK).* Contains camphor 3.5%, menthol 1.5%, pine oil 0.5%, cedar oil 0.25%, thyme oil 0.5%, and cajuput oil 1%.

Solarcaine Cream *(Plough, UK).* Benzocaine 1% and triclosan 0.2%. **Solarcaine Lotion**. Benzocaine 0.5% and triclosan 0.2%. **Solarcaine Spray**. Benzocaine 5% and triclosan 0.1%.

Solasil *(Cuticura, UK).* Contains hamamelis liquid extract 1.5%, almond oil 1.35%, zinc oxide 0.9%, camphor 0.1%, and menthol 0.1%.

Soleze *(Pickles, UK).* Contains dibromopropamidine isethionate 0.15% in an emollient basis.

Solution 41 *(Innoxa, UK).* Contains salicylic acid 0.07% and triclosan 0.05%.

Soothadent *(Ashe, UK).* Contains lignocaine hydrochloride 2%.

Soothake *(Paton, UK).* Benzyl alcohol 5%, clove oil 5%, benzocaine 7.5%, wool fat 12.5%, and basis to 100%.

Sovol Liquid *(Carter-Wallace, UK).* Each 5 ml contains aluminium hydroxide 200 mg, magnesium hydroxide 200 mg, and dimethylpolysiloxane 25 mg.

Sovol Tablets *(Carter-Wallace, UK).* Each contains aluminium hydroxide-magnesium carbonate co-dried gel 300 mg, magnesium hydroxide 100 mg, and dimethylpolysiloxane 25 mg.

Spotoway Antiseptic Cream *(Pure Plant Products, UK).* Extrapone No. 4 Special 0.5% and chlorhexidine gluconate solution 1%.

Spotoway Lotion *(Pure Plant Products, UK).* Chlorhexidine gluconate solution 0.5%, cetrimide 0.04%, and industrial methylated spirit 10%.

Steedman's Teething Jelly *(Beecham Proprietaries, UK).* Active constituents: cetylpyridinium chloride 0.02% and ethyl nicotinate 0.0025%.

Steiner Treatment Shampoo *(Steiner, UK: Richards & Appleby, UK).* Contains zinc omadine 1%.

Sterotabs *(Boots, UK).* Tablets each containing halazone 4 mg.

Stingo *(Potter & Clarke, UK).* Aerosol containing trichlorofluoromethane 85% and dichlorodifluoromethane 15%.

Stings Cream *(Savory & Moore, UK).* Contains diphenhydramine hydrochloride 2% and menthol 1%.

Stomosol Liquid Concentrate *(Thackray, UK).* Chlorhexidine gluconate solution 5%, benzalkonium chloride solution (50%) 20%, and cetomacrogol '1000' 10%.

Stop 'n Grow *(Mentholatum, UK).* Active ingredients: denatonium benzoate 0.14%, sucrose octa-acetate 7.69%.

Strepsils *(Crookes Products, UK).* Lozenges each containing amylmetacresol 600 µg and dichlorobenzyl alcohol 1.2 mg. **Strepsils Honey and Lemon**. Contain the same active ingredients in a flavoured basis.

Sublamin *(Wyngood, UK).* Liquid containing benzoic acid 4.85%, salicylic acid 3%, benzalkonium chloride solution 0.1%, and cetylpyridinium chloride 0.05%.

Sucrets *(Beecham Proprietaries, UK).* Throat lozenges each containing hexylresorcinol 2.4 mg.

Sunnimax *(Warne, UK).* Tablets each containing vitamin A 4500 units, vitamin D 450 units, and vitamin C 40 mg.

Sunspot Healing Paint *(Surf Ski International, UK).* Camphor 8%, benzoin 2%, ethylene glycol 0.02%, benzalkonium chloride 0.1%, allantoin 0.4%, isopropyl alcohol (90%) to 100%.

Super Plenamins *(Minnesota, UK).* Tablets each containing vitamin A 5000 units, vitamin B_1 2.25 mg, vitamin B_2 2.25 mg, vitamin B_3 500 µg, vitamin B_6 100 µg, vitamin B_{12} 2 µg, vitamin C 40 mg, vitamin D 300 units, vitamin E 2 mg, nicotinamide 20 mg, dried ferrous sulphate 51 mg, calcium 75 mg, phosphorus 58 mg, magnesium 10 mg, iodine 150 µg, copper 750 µg, manganese 1.25 mg, potassium 3 mg, and zinc 1 mg.

Surama Medicated Cigarettes *(Vines Biocrin, UK).* Contain cascarilla bark 1.5%, cubeb fruit 1.5%, benzoin 1.5%, stramonium leaf 92.5%, eucalyptus oil 1.5%, menthol 0.5%, and pumilio pine oil 1%.

Sure Shield Adult Travel Tablets *(Guest, UK: English Grains, UK).* Each contains chlorbutol 150 mg.

Sure Shield Antibactic Throat Lozenges *(Guest, UK: English Grains, UK).* Each contains tyrothricin 1 mg and cetylpyridinium chloride 1.5 mg.

Sure Shield Bronchial Mixture *(Guest, UK: English Grains, UK).* Each 5 ml contains ammonium bicarbonate 50 mg, squill liquid extract 0.021 ml, ipecacuanha liquid extract 0.0085 ml, senega liquid extract 0.0145 ml, liquorice extract 0.425 ml, glycerol 310 mg, tolu syrup 0.245 ml, capsicin 0.000125 ml, and treacle 1.75 g.

Sure Shield Children's Travel Tablets *(Guest, UK: English Grains, UK)*. Each contains chlorbutol 75 mg.

Sure Shield Diarrhoea Mixture *(Guest, UK: English Grains, UK)*. Each 5 ml contains sodium bicarbonate 125 mg, light kaolin 470 mg, compound rhubarb tincture 0.0625 ml, catechu tincture 0.125 ml, chalk 32 mg, and aromatic ammonia solution 0.195 ml.

Sure Shield Dyspepsia Tablets *(Guest, UK: English Grains, UK)*. Each contains bismuth carbonate 11.25 mg, heavy magnesium carbonate 62.5 mg, sodium bicarbonate 43.75 mg, calcium carbonate 400 mg, pepsin 870 µg, pancreatin 625 µg, capsicin 50 µg.

Sure Shield Footballer's Linctus *(Guest, UK: English Grains, UK)*. Each 5 ml contains menthol 12.5 mg, anise oil 0.0125 ml, tolu syrup 0.5 ml, capsicum tincture 0.167 ml, euphorbia liquid extract 0.05 ml, coltsfoot liquid extract 0.05 ml, and treacle 2.75 g.

Sure Shield Iodised Throat Tablets *(Guest, UK: English Grains, UK)*. Active constituents: iodine (free and combined) 0.0478%, methyl salicylate 0.0617%, phenol (free and combined) 0.379%, menthol 0.228%, citric acid 0.446%, and cetylpyridinium chloride 0.044%.

Sure Shield Mouth Ulcer Tablets *(Guest, UK: English Grains, UK)*. Each contains amylmetacresol 500 µg, ascorbic acid 25 mg, and cetylpyridinium chloride 1.5 mg.

Sure Shield Sure-Lax Tablets *(Guest, UK: English Grains, UK)*. Tablets each containing phenolphthalein 90 mg and natural raspberry juice.

Sure Shield Rum Cough Elixir *(Guest, UK: English Grains, UK)*. Contains in each 5 ml cocillana liquid extract 0.02 ml, squill liquid extract 0.01 ml, senega liquid extract 0.01 ml, cascara liquid extract 0.125 ml, ipecacuanha tincture 0.125 ml, menthol 460 µg, and Jamaica rum 2.5 ml.

Surgolene Liquid *(Thomas, UK)*. Liquefied phenol 0.63%, hydrochloric acid 0.4%, salicylic acid 0.045%, and iodine 0.11%.

Swarm *(Pickles, UK)*. Cream containing dibromopropamidine isethionate 0.15%, mepyramine maleate 1.5%, and calamine 10%.

Sweet Relief Liniment *(Dalton Supplies, UK)*. Menthol 0.6%, methyl salicylate 0.1%, sodium chloride 0.5%, and isopropyl alcohol 60%.

Sylphen Tablets *(Industrial Pharmaceutical, UK)*. Contain paracetamol 300 mg, ephedrine hydrochloride 5 mg, and caffeine 30 mg.

Tabasan *(Ayrton, Saunders, UK)*. Tablets each containing ephedrine hydrochloride 15 mg, theobromine 30 mg, and salicylamide 60 mg.

Tabmint *(Radiol, UK)*. Chewing gum containing silver acetate 6 mg, ammonium acetate 14.5 mg, sodium chloride 11 mg, and co-carboxylase 25 µg in each tablet.

Tangeroil Worm Syrup *(English Grains, UK)*. Each 5 ml contains piperazine citrate 800 mg.

TCP First Aid Gel *(Unicliffe, UK)*. Contains TCP Liquid Antiseptic 80% in a gel basis.

TCP Liquid Antiseptic *(Unicliffe, UK)*. An aqueous solution containing halogenated phenols and salicylic acid made from chlorine 0.4%, iodine 0.005%, phenol 0.63%, and sodium salicylate 0.052%, with the partial elimination of ionisable halides.

TCP Ointment *(Unicliffe, UK)*. TCP Liquid Antiseptic 6.4%, iodine 0.2%, methyl salicylate 1.3%, precip. sulphur 1.5%, kaolin 8.5%, with camphor 1.3%, tannic acid 0.4%, salicylic acid 0.4%, and glycerol 2.4%.

TCP Throat Pastilles *(Unicliffe, UK)*. Active ingredients: TCP Liquid Antiseptic 10% (1.74 mg); available in black currant and lemon flavours.

Tellodont *(Tell, UK)*. Gargle and mouthwash tablets each containing sodium benzoate 5%, peppermint oil 0.9%, thymol 0.3%, menthol 1.2%, cinnamon oil 0.3%, methyl salicylate 0.3%, and saccharin 0.1%, in an effervescent basis.

Tellora *(Tell, UK)*. Powder for preparing mouthwash containing menthol, thymol, sodium benzoate, cetrimide, clove oil, aniseed oil, saccharin, sodium bicarbonate, tartaric acid, and empicol.

Terperoin Elixir *(Savory & Moore, UK)*. Each 5 ml contains codeine phosphate 10.4 mg, menthol 5 mg, terpin hydrate 20 mg, in a flavoured syrup basis.

Terperoin Pastilles *(Savory & Moore, UK)*. Contain pine oil 0.05%, cineole 0.028%, ipecacuanha liquid extract 0.014%, terpin hydrate 0.64%, codeine phosphate 0.097%, and menthol 0.14%.

Test Sixty *(Ashe, UK)*. Packs of 8 tablets each containing lobeline hydrochloride 2 mg, and 30 lozenges each containing methylcellulose 187 mg, oil of bitter orange 2 mg, peppermint oil 6 mg, and bergamot oil 2 mg.

Thornton & Ross Diarrhoea Mixture *(Thornton & Ross, UK)*. Contains in each 5 ml aromatic chalk powder 250 mg and catechu 40 mg.

Thornton & Ross Indian Brandee *(Thornton & Ross, UK)*. Contains in each 5 ml potassium nitrate 25 mg, ether 0.05 ml, compound rhubarb tincture 0.75 ml, capsicum tincture 0.125 ml, and compound cardamom tincture 0.05 ml.

Thornton & Ross Indigestion Mixture *(Thornton & Ross, UK)*. Each 5 ml contains aluminium oxide 150 mg, light magnesium oxide 118 mg, aromatic cardamom tincture 0.05 ml, and peppermint oil 0.0004 ml.

Thornton & Ross Vapour Rub *(Thornton & Ross, UK)*. Menthol 2.5%, Camphor 2.5%, methyl salicylate 2.75%, eucalyptus oil 2.5%, turpentine oil 5%, pine oil 1%, thyme oil 0.2%, and creosote 0.025%.

Three Flasks Bronchial Emulsion *(Thornton & Ross, UK)*. Contains liquid paraffin 25%, anise oil 0.2%, pumilio pine oil 0.05%, cinnamon oil 0.05%, calcium hypophosphite 1.2%, sodium hypophosphite 1.2%, glycerol 5%, and compound benzoin tincture 1%.

Three Flasks Cold Sore Lotion *(Thornton & Ross, UK)*. Contains camphor 1.1%, menthol 1.1%, diethyl phthalate 0.825%, and benzoin tincture (meth.) 84.475%.

Three Flasks Corn & Wart Solvent *(Thornton & Ross, UK)*. Active ingredients: pyroxylin 1.27%, Canada balsam 4.7%, zinc chloride 1.7%, salicylic acid 12%, castor oil 2.85%, and colophony 2.4%.

Three Flasks Juniper Pills *(Thornton & Ross, UK)*. Each contains bearberry extract (aqueous 5–2) 16.2 mg, buchu extract (aqueous 8–3) 16.2 mg, capsicum 16.2 mg, squill 16.2 mg, potassium nitrate 65 mg, aloin 9.7 mg, juniper oil 4 mg, and methylene blue 4 mg.

Three Flasks Nail Bite Lotion *(Thornton & Ross, UK)*. Soap spirit 50%, capsicum oleoresin 0.1%, and quassia extract 0.2%.

Three Flasks Proflavine Cream *(Thornton & Ross, UK)*. Contains proflavine hemisulphate 0.1%.

Three Flasks Tooth-Ache Solution *(Thornton & Ross, UK)*. Contains menthol 2%, phenol 0.9%, clove oil 6%, camphor 4%, chloroform 0.95%, colour q.s., and IMS to 100%.

Three Noughts Cough Syrup *(Carter Bond, UK)*. Active constituents when manufactured: anise oil 0.04%, clove oil 0.01%, cassia oil 0.02%, spearmint oil 0.01%, ether 0.1%, chloroform 0.65%, chloroform spirit 0.66%, alcoholic (90%) tincture of capsicum (1–5) 0.08%, ipecacuanha liquid extract 0.19%, cetylpyridinium chloride 0.018%, acetic acid 0.9%, and benzoic acid 0.05%.

Throat Chest and Lung Drops *(Simpkin, UK)*. Lozenges each containing clove oil 0.0014 ml, eucalyptus oil 0.0021 ml, anise oil 0.0028 ml, peppermint oil 0.0028 ml, ginger extract 0.0014 ml, menthol 0.14 mg, with citric acid, benzoic acid, and chloroform spirit.

Throaties Original Flavour *(Arcadian Confections, UK)*. Active ingredients: benzoin tincture 0.5%, menthol 0.45%, aniseed oil 0.1%, peppermint oil 0.025%, and capsicin 0.001%. **Throaties Catarrh Pastilles.** Active ingredients: menthol 0.6%, abietis pine oil 0.3%, sylvestris pine oil 0.3%, and creosote 0.2%. **Throaties, Lemon Honey & Menthol.** Active ingredients: honey 2.4%, lemon oil 0.3%, and menthol 0.09%.

Tiger Balm *(Vessen, UK)*. Contains menthol, camphor, clove oil, and cajuput oil.

Tilloderm White Tar Ointment *(Tillotts, UK)*. Lanolin 39.3%, soft paraffin 46.7%, zinc oxide 10%, resorcin 4%, cresol 0.002%.

Tinoxid Tablets *(Ayrton, Saunders, UK)*. Tin powder 110 mg and stannic oxide 19.5 mg.

Topex *(Richardson-Vicks, UK)*. Lotion containing benzoyl peroxide 5%.

Topex Acne Cream *(Richardson-Vicks, UK)*. Contains benzoyl peroxide 5%.

Torbetol *(Torbet Laboratories, UK)*. Contains cetrimide 0.7%, benzalkonium bromide 0.05%, and hexachlorophane 0.75%.

Torbetol Shampoo *(Torbet Laboratories, UK)*. Contains cetrimide 17.5% and benzalkonium bromide 2.5%.

Totavit Capsules *(Cupal, UK)*. Each contains vitamin A 5000 units, ergocalciferol 400 units, thiamine hydrochloride 1.5 mg, riboflavine 1.2 mg, pyridoxine hydrochlroride 0.5 mg, nicotinamide 10 mg, ascorbic acid 30 mg, tocopheryl acetate 1 unit, copper (as copper sulphate) 0.1 mg, iron (as ferrous sulphate) 15 mg, calcium 24 mg, phosphorus 18.5 mg, and DL-methionine 30 mg.

Touch and Go Toothache Tincture *(Ayrton, Saunders, UK)*. Contains camphor 10%, menthol 1.25%, chloroform 7.5%, ether 7.5%, cajuput oil 2.5%, clove oil 3.12%, and tolu balsam 1.25%.

Trinity Ointment *(Thornton & Ross, UK)*. Contains eucalyptus oil 8.33%, zinc ointment 25%, hydrous wool fat 25%, soft paraffin to 100%.

Trisonovin *(Menley & James, UK)*. Cream containing resorcinol 2% and sulphur 8%.

Tums *(Norcliff Thayer, UK: Pharmagen, UK)*. Each tablet contains calcium carbonate 500 mg and peppermint oil 1.1 mg.

Tunes, Cherry Menthol *(Mars, UK)*. Tolu balsam 0.036%, menthol 0.162%, thyme oil 0.0025%, and camphor 0.0086%.

Tunes, Honey Menthol *(Mars, UK)*. Contain menthol 0.135%, anethole 0.114%, cinnamon oil 0.018%, peppermint oil 0.015%, eucalyptol 0.015%, with sugar, glucose syrup, and honey.

Tusana Cough Linctus *(Boots, UK)*. Contains in each 5 ml dextromethorphan hydrobromide 5 mg, ipecacuanha liquid extract 0.025 ml, and tolu syrup 3.71 ml.

Tussils Cough Lozenges *(Boots, UK)*. Each contains dextromethorphan hydrobromide 2.5 mg and phenylephrine hydrochloride 500 µg.

Tussobron Cough Suppressant Syrup *(Wigglesworth, UK)*. Contains in each 5 ml dextromethorphan hydrobromide 5 mg, ephedrine hydrochloride 10 mg, and ammonium chloride 37.5 mg.

Tyrocane Paediatric *(Cupal, UK)*. Lozenges each containing cetylpyridinium chloride 2.5 mg.

Tyrocane Throat Lozenges *(Cupal, UK)*. Tyrothricin 500 µg, cetylpyridinium chloride 2.5 mg, and benzocaine 5 mg.

Tyroco Throat Lozenges *(Cox, UK)*. Each contains tyrothricin 1 mg, benzocaine 5 mg, cetylpyridinium chloride 4 mg.

Tyromycin Lozenges *(Industrial Pharmaceutical, UK)*. Tyrothricin 1 mg, benzocaine 5 mg, cetylpyridinium chloride 1 mg.

T-Zone Decongestant Tablets *(Newton, UK: Farillon, UK)*. Each contains salicylamide 324 mg, caffeine 16.2 mg, ephedrine sulphate 4 mg, atropine sulphate 120 µg, magnesium hydroxide 65 mg, sodium citrate 16.2 mg, and dried aluminium hydroxide 16.2 mg.

Ulcaid Tablets *(Cupal, UK)*. Benzocaine 5 mg, cetylpyridinium chloride 2.5 mg, and tyrothricin 0.5 mg.

Ultra Cleancut Spray Solution *(Wallace, Cameron, UK)*. Benzalkonium chloride solution (50%) 2%, lignocaine hydrochloride 0.5%.

Ultra Plastron Spray Dressing *(Wallace, Cameron, UK)*. Benzocaine 1%, cetrimide 0.1%, polyvinylpyrrolidone co-polymer 3%.

Ultra Steriflow Eye Wash *(Wallace, Cameron, UK)*. Sodium acid phosphate 0.52%, sodium phosphate 1.19%, sodium chloride 0.48%.

Ultra Throat Lozenges *(Wallace, Cameron, UK)*. Each contains benzalkonium chloride solution (50%) 0.0006 ml.

Ultracach Analgesic Capsules *(Wallace, Cameron, UK)*. Paracetamol 300 mg, caffeine 30 mg.

Ultradal Antacid Stomach Tablets *(Wallace, Cameron, UK)*. Light magnesium carbonate 60 mg, magnesium trisilicate 150 mg, dried aluminium hydroxide gel 90 mg, calcium carbonate 105 mg.

Ultrakool Aerosol Spray *(Wallace, Cameron, UK)*. Trichlorofluoromethane 85%, dichlorodifluoromethane 15%.

Ultralief Tablets *(Wallace, Cameron, UK)*. Salicylamide 200 mg, paracetamol 200 mg, caffeine 25 mg.

Unichem Throat & Catarrh Pastilles *(Unichem, UK)*. Menthol 0.62%, sylvestris pine oil 0.31%, peppermint oil 0.31%, and thymol 0.073%.

Uvicool *(WB Pharmaceuticals, UK: Boehringer Ingelheim, UK)*. Active ingredient: para-aminobenzoic acid.

Vadarex Nasal Inhaler *(Parkinsons, UK)*. Each contains menthol 225 mg, rectified camphor oil 0.01 ml, cedar wood oil 0.05 ml, pine oil 0.05 ml, camphor 25 mg, creosote 0.02 ml, and methyl salicylate 0.02 ml.

Vadarex Wintergreen Ointment *(Parkinsons, UK)*. Contains sweet birch oil 0.12%, cajuput oil 0.12%, eucalyptus oil 1%, menthol 0.5%, and methyl salicylate 9%.

Valderma Antiseptic Cream *(Reckitt & Colman Pharmaceuticals, UK)*. Active constituent: di-8-hydroxyquinoline *p*-aminosalicylate 0.3% in a water-miscible basis.

Valomel Hand Lotion *(Hough, Hoseason, UK)*. Contains hydrogen peroxide solution 2.5%, chlorocresol 0.25%, benzoin tincture 1%, and glycerol 14%.

Valpeda Foot Balm *(Reckitt & Colman Pharmaceuticals, UK)*. Contains halquinol 0.3%.

Vanamil *(Richardson-Vicks, UK)*. Tablets each containing dried aluminium hydroxide 200 mg, magnesium hydroxide 200 mg, and activated dimethicone 20 mg.

Vanispot *(Cox, UK)*. Cream containing resorcinol 2%, precipitated sulphur 8%, hexachlorophane 0.25%, and titanium dioxide 3%.

Vapex Inhalant *(Kerfoot, UK: Fisons, UK)*. Menthol 17.5, linalyl acetate 0.468, eucalyptus oil 4.687, lavender oil 4.687, bornyl acetate 0.416, essential oil of camphor 1.5, and alcohol (IMS) 70.742.

Varemoid *(Zyma, UK)*. Each tablet contains hydroxyethylrutosides 100 mg.

Vaseline *(Chesebrough-Pond's, UK)*. Brands of white and yellow petroleum jelly.

Vaseline Medicated Shampoo *(Chesebrough-Pond's, UK)*. Contains triclosan 0.2%.

Vaydar Vapour-Rub *(Parkinsons, UK)*. Contains menthol 2.7%, camphor 5.7%, turpentine oil 5%, eucalyptus oil 2.5%, cedar wood oil 0.5%, pine oil 1%, and chloroxylenol 0.1%.

VeetO *(Reckitt & Colman Pharmaceuticals, UK)*. **Cream** and **Lotion** contain calcium and potassium thioglycollates, in an oil-in-water basis.

Veno's Adult Formula Cough Mixture *(Beecham Proprietaries, UK)*. Each 5 ml contains noscapine hydrochloride 8.5 mg and liquid glucose 4.25 g.

Veno's Honey and Lemon Cough Mixture *(Beecham Proprietaries, UK)*. Contains in each 5 ml lemon juice 1 ml, honey 250 mg, ammonium chloride 30 mg, and ipecacuanha liquid extract 0.003 ml.

Veno's Original Cough Mixture *(Beecham Proprietaries, UK)*. Contains camphor 0.02%, aniseed oil 0.03%, capsicum tincture 0.12%, liquid glucose 63.5%, and molasses 34%.

Verrugon *(Pickles, UK)*. Contains salicylic acid 50% and glycerol 7%.

Vick VapoRub *(Richardson-Vicks, UK)*. Menthol 2.82%, camphor 5.25%, turpentine oil 4.77%, eucalyptus oil 1.35%, nutmeg oil 0.48%, cedar wood oil 0.45%, thymol 0.1%.

Vicks Cough Calmers *(Richardson-Vicks, UK)*. Lozenges each containing dextromethorphan 4.05 mg and benzocaine 2.4 mg.

Vicks Double-Action Medicated Lozenges *(Richardson-Vicks, UK)*. Each contains menthol 7.04 mg, camphor 0.24 mg, and eucalyptus oil 2.35 mg.

Vicks Expectorant Cough Syrup *(Richardson-Vicks, UK)*. Each 5 ml contains guaiphenesin 50 mg, sodium citrate 200 mg, and cetylpyridinium chloride 1.25 mg.

Vicks Inhaler *(Richardson-Vicks, UK)*. Menthol 125 mg, camphor 50 mg, methyl salicylate 5 mg, and oil of pine needles 10 mg.

Vicks Lozenges *(Richardson-Vicks, UK)*. Each contains menthol 1.74 mg and vitamin C 3.9 mg; available in menthol, lemon, blackcurrant, and wild cherry flavours.

Vicks Lozenges, Lemon Plus *(Richardson-Vicks, UK)*. Each contains menthol 2.75 mg and vitamin C 100 mg.

Vicks Medinite *(Richardson-Vicks, UK)*. Each 30-ml dose contains ephedrine sulphate 8 mg, doxylamine succinate 7.5 mg, paracetamol 600 mg, dextromethorphan hydrobromide 15 mg, and alcohol 19%.

Vicks Sinex Nasal Spray *(Richardson-Vicks, UK)*. Contains oxymetazoline hydrochloride 0.05%, menthol 0.025%, camphor 0.015%, and eucalyptol 0.0075% in a buffered aqueous solution. **Sinex Nose Drops** contain the same active ingredients.

Vine's Anti-Scurf Hair Dressing *(Vines Biocrin, UK)*. Active ingredients: *p*-chloro-*m*-cresol 0.25%, sodium alkyl sulphates 0.25%, alkyl aliphatic esters 8.7%, aliphatic alcohols 4.9%, cholesterol 0.37%, lanosterol 0.3%, sulphur 1.97%, and carbamide 0.98%.

Visine Eye Drops *(Unicliffe, UK)*. Tetrahydrozoline hydrochloride 0.05% and benzalkonium chloride solution (50%) 0.02%.

Vita-Glucose Tablets *(Simpkin, UK)*. Contain dextrose with not less than 40 mg ascorbic acid in each 28 g.

Vitaplus Multivitamins *(Farley, UK)*. Tablets each containing vitamin A 2500 units, B_1 1.1 mg, B_2 1.5 mg, B_6 1.0 mg, B_{12} 4.0 µg, nicotinamide 17 mg, folic acid 25 µg, vitamin C 30 mg, vitamin D 100 units, vitamin E 5 mg.

Vitaplus Multivitamins with Iron *(Farley, UK)*. Tablets each containing vitamin A 2500 units, B_1 1.1 mg, B_2 1.5 mg, B_6 1.0 mg, B_{12} 4.0 µg, nicotinamide 17 mg, folic acid 25 µg, vitamin C 30 mg, vitamin D 100 units, vitamin E 5 mg, iron, as ferrous fumarate, 15 mg.

Vitathone Chilblain Cream *(Cupal, UK)*. Contains methyl nicotinate 1.25%, azulene 0.05%, and dimethicone 3%.

Vitathone Chilblain Tablets *(Cupal, UK)*. Each contains acetomenaphthone 7 mg and nicotinic acid 25 mg.

Vitocee Tablets *(Boots, UK)*. Each contains vitamin A 750 µg, vitamin C 25 mg, and cholecalciferol 5 µg.

Vitrite Multi-Vitamin Syrup *(British Cod Liver Oils, UK)*. Each 5 ml contains vitamin A 2000 units, cholecalciferol 200 units, vitamin E 1.5 mg, nicotinamide 9 mg, thiamine hydrochloride 0.7 mg, riboflavine 0.85 mg, pyridoxine hydrochloride 0.35 mg, and ascorbic acid 17.5 mg.

Vocalzone Pastilles *(Guest, UK: English Grains, UK)*. Menthol 1%, peppermint oil 0.5%, myrrh 0.25%, and liquorice extract 1.1%.

Vosene *(Beecham Proprietaries, UK)*. Active constituents (%): thymol 0.1, resorcinol 0.03, coal tar solution 3.3, rosemary oil 0.1, and biomin (sulphosuccinated undecylenic monoalkylolamide) 2.5.

Vykmin E *(Beecham Proprietaries, UK)*. Each capsule contains retinol 2000 units, cholecalciferol 200 units, vitamin E 100 mg, vitamin B_1 1.2 mg, vitamin B_2 1.8 mg, vitamin B_6 100 µg, vitamin B_{12} 1 µg, vitamin C 40 mg, nicotinamide 12 mg, calcium pantothenate 1 mg, manganese 500 µg, potassium 3 mg, zinc 1 mg, iodine 150 µg, molybdenum 100 µg, iron 15 mg, and calcium phosphate 92.34 mg.

Vykmin Fortified *(Beecham Proprietaries, UK)*. Capsules each containing retinol 5000 units, ergocalciferol 350 units, vitamin B_1 1.2 mg, riboflavine 1.8 mg, vitamin B_6 100 µg, vitamin B_{12} 1 µg, vitamin C 40 mg, vitamin E 2 mg, nicotinamide 12 mg, calcium pantothenate 1 mg, dried ferrous sulphate 51 mg, potassium molybdate 340 µg, manganese sulphate 2.2 mg, potassium sulphate 6.68 mg, potassium iodide 200 µg, zinc sulphate 4.4 mg, and calcium phosphate 92.34 mg.

Wartex Ointment *(Pickles, UK)*. Contains salicylic acid 50% and glycerol 7%.

Wasp-Eze *(Potter & Clarke, UK: De Witt, UK)*. An aerosol for insect-bite relief containing mepyramine maleate 0.5% and benzocaine 1%.

Waxaid Ear drops *(Cupal, UK)*. Paradichlorobenzene 2%, chlorbutol 5%, turpentine oil 10%, arachis oil to 100%.

Waxwane Ear Drops *(Thornton & Ross, UK)*. Turpentine oil 15%, terpineol 5%, and chloroxylenol 0.2%, in arachis oil.

Wigglesworth Acne Cream *(Wigglesworth, UK)*. Contains resorcinol 0.5%, precipitated sulphur 1%, cetylpyridinium chloride 0.5%, and isopropyl myristate 2%.

Wigglesworth Rapid Energy Release Tablets *(Wigglesworth, UK)*. Each contains caffeine 50 mg, nicotinic acid 5 mg, riboflavine 1 mg, and thiamine hydrochloride 1 mg.

Wigglesworth Syrup of Honey Glycerin & Blackcurrant with Ipecac *(Wigglesworth, UK)*. Contains purified honey 14%, glycerol 5%, black currant syrup 5%, ipecacuanha liquid extract 0.2%, tolu syrup 7.6%, citric acid 0.75%, glacial acetic acid 0.25%, and sucrose 50%.

Wigglesworth Vitamin ACD Tablets *(Wigglesworth, UK)*. Each contains vitamin A 4000 units, vitamin D 550 units, vitamin C 25 mg.

Willocare Adults Bronchial Balsam *(Wigglesworth, UK)*. Contains potassium citrate 9.06%, potassium iodide 0.47%, ipecacuanha liquid extract 0.3%, camphorated opium tincture 4.05%, liquorice liquid extract 2.5%, and cetylpyridinium chloride 0.03%.

Willocare Chilblain Ointment *(Wigglesworth, UK)*. Contains phenol 1%, camphor 6%, and Peru balsam 2%.

Willocare Children's Cherry Cough Linctus *(Wigglesworth, UK)*. Contains in each 5 ml squill liquid extract 0.02 ml, ipecacuanha liquid extract 0.003 ml, wild cherry syrup 0.08 ml, camphor 2 mg, glycerol 0.12 ml, and honey 350 mg.

Willocare Children's Cough Balsam *(Wigglesworth, UK)*. Contains potassium citrate 3%, ipecacuanha liquid extract 0.1%, and liquorice liquid extract 2.5%.

Willocare Glycerin Lemon & Honey with Ipecac *(Wigglesworth, UK)*. Contains glycerol 12.5%, purified honey 30%, ipecacuanha liquid extract 0.42%, and lemon oil 0.04%.

Willocare Golden Ear Drops *(Wigglesworth, UK)*. Contain rectified camphor oil 15%, cineole 7.5%, nutmeg oil 0.4%, terpineol 2%, and arachis oil to 100%.

Willocare Infants Nasal Drops *(Wigglesworth, UK)*. Contain ephedrine hydrochloride 0.5%.

Willocare Junior Expectorant *(Wigglesworth, UK)*. Contains in each 5 ml dextromethorphan hydrobromide 3.75 mg, ephedrine hydrochloride 2.5 mg, phenylephrine hydrochloride 2.5 mg, ipecacuanha liquid extract 0.0037 ml, and sucrose 4.25 g.

Willocare Mentholated Balsam *(Wigglesworth, UK)*. Contains purified honey 5.17%, glacial acetic acid 0.86%, liquorice liquid extract 1.29%, formaldehyde solution 0.02%, menthol 0.005%, and syrup 25.86%.

Wintogeno *(Cox, UK)*. Active constituents: capsicin 0.3%, thymol 0.11%, eucalyptol 0.11%, menthol 2.6%, methyl salicylate 12.2%.

Witch Doctor *(Ethichem, UK: Farillon, UK)*. Gel containing witch hazel liquid extract 81.5%, propylene glycol 7%, and alkoyl diethanolamide 0.75%.

Witch Stik *(Ethichem, UK: Farillon, UK)*. Witch hazel extract containing not less than 65% alcohol.

Woodward's Gripe Water *(LRC Products, UK)*. Dill water, concentrated 3.6%, sodium bicarbonate 1%, ginger tincture 1.25%, rectified spirit 3.67%, and syrup 15%.

X.89 Geriomar *(Pan-American Pharmaceuticals, UK)*. Capsules each containing para-aminobenzoic acid 25 mg, haematoporphyrin hydrochloride 250 µg, 2-dimethylaminoethanol hydrogen tartrate 15 mg, with traces of minerals and excipients.

Yeast Pac Medicated *(De Witt, UK)*. Contains coal tar solution 0.6%, bentonite 2.3%, precipitated sulphur 3%, zinc oxide 13%, kaolin 36.2%, and dried yeast 1.9%.

Yeast-Vite *(Beecham Proprietaries, UK)*. Each tablet contains salicylamide 162 mg, caffeine 50 mg, thiamine hydrochloride 167 µg, riboflavine 167 µg, and nicotinamide 1.5 mg.

Zam-Buk *(Fisons, UK)*. Active ingredients: eucalyptus oil 5%, camphor 1.8%, thyme oil 0.5%, colophony 2.5%, and sassafras oil 0.65%.

Zanthine Tablets *(Approved Prescription Services, UK)*. Each contains caffeine 30 mg and dextrose 150 mg.

Zefringe Sachets *(British Chemotheutic, UK)*. Each contains paracetamol 800 mg and caffeine 60 mg in an effervescent basis.

Zincast Baby Cream *(Parkinsons, UK)*. Contains zinc oxide 7.5%, wool fat 4%, and castor oil 4.5%.

Zubes Lemon and Honey Cough Lozenges *(Cussons, UK)*. Contain menthol 0.1%, lemon oil 0.22%, citric acid 1.5%, and honey 5%. **Zubes Original**. Contain anise oil 0.2%, peppermint oil 0.13%, clove oil 0.02%, menthol 0.3%, camphor 0.01%, tolu balsam 0.07%, benzoin 0.07%, capsicum tincture 0.02%, gingerin 0.02%, aqueous extract of horehound (1 in 15), quassia (1 in 48), and coltsfoot leaf (1 in 60) 0.015%, with sucrose and liquid glucose.

Directory of Manufacturers

The names and addresses of the manufacturers (or distributors) of the products and proprietary medicines mentioned in Martindale are listed below in alphabetical order of the abbreviated names used in the text.

3M United Kingdom, UK. 3M United Kingdom Ltd, 3M House, P.O. Box 1, Bracknell, Berks RG12 1JU, England.

Abbott, Arg. Abbott Laboratories Arg., Sarmiento 1113-8° piso, 1041 Buenos Aires, Argentina.

Abbott, Austral. Abbott Laboratories Pty Ltd, Captain Cook Drive, Kurnell NSW 2231, Australia.

Abbott, Belg. Abbott S.A., rue du Bosquet 2, 1340 Ottignies, Belgium.

Abbott, Canad. Abbott Laboratories Ltd, 5400 Côte de Liesse Rd, Montreal, Quebec H4P 1A5, Canada.

Abbott, Denm. Abbott Laboratories A/S, Bygstubben 15, Trørød, 2950 Vedbaek, Denmark.

Abbott, Fr. Societé Française des Laboratoires Abbott, 28380 Saint-Rémy-sur-Avre, France.

Abbott, Ger. Deutsche Abbott GmbH, Binger Strasse 173, Postfach: 200, 6507 Ingelheim am Rhein, W. Germany.

Abbott, Ital. Abbott s.p.a., 04010 Campoverde, Italy.

Abbott, Norw. Abbott Norge, Hofstadgt. 60, Postboks 78, 1375 Høn, Norway.

Abbott, NZ. Abbott Laboratories (NZ) Ltd, P.O. Box 35-078, Naenae, New Zealand.

Abbott, S.Afr. Abbott Laboratories SA (Pty) Ltd, P.O. Box 1616, Johannesburg 2000, S. Africa.

Abbott, Spain. Abbott Laboratories SA, Josefa Valcarcel 48, Madrid 27, Spain.

Abbott, Swed. Abbott Scandinavia AB, Box 1074, 163 11 Spånga, Sweden.

Abbott, Switz. Abbott AG, Loretostrasse 1, 6300 Zug, Switzerland.

Abbott, UK. Abbott Laboratories Ltd, Queenborough, Kent ME11 5EL, England.

Abbott, USA. Abbott Laboratories, Pharmaceutical Products Division, 14th & Sheridan Rd, North Chicago IL 60064, USA.

ABC, Ital. Istituto Biologico Chemioterapico ABC s.p.a., Viale Thovez 26, 10131 Torino, Italy.

Abdine, UK. Abdine Ltd, 2 Woodhead Rd, Darnley Industrial Estate, Glasgow G53 7NU, Scotland.

Abello, Spain. Laboratorios Abello SA, Julian Camarillo 8, Madrid 17, Spain.

ABM Chemicals, UK. A.B.M. Chemicals Ltd, Woodley, Stockport, Cheshire SK6 1PQ, England.

Acbel, Switz. Lab. Acbel S.A., rue Coulouvrenière 20, 1204 Geneva, Switzerland.

Accepted Foods, UK. Accepted Foods Ltd, 49 Kingston Rd, Leatherhead, Surrey, England.

ACF, Neth. ACF Chemiefarma N.V., Straatweg 2, 3604 BB Maarssen, Netherlands.

ACO, Denm. See *KabiVitrum, Denm.*

ACO, Norw. See *KabiVitrum, Norw.*

ACO, Swed. ACO Läkemedel AB, Box 3026, 171 03 Solna, Sweden.

Actipharm, Switz. Actipharm S.àr.l., rue Prévost-Martin 42-44, 1205 Geneva, Switzerland.

Adam, Austral. Adam Drug Co., 41 Barry Ave, Mortdale NSW 2223, Australia.

Adcock Ingram, S.Afr. Adcock Ingram Laboratories Ltd, 50 Commando Rd, Industria West, Johannesburg, S. Africa.

Adima, Switz. Adima S.A., Case postale 540, 1211 Geneva 3, Switzerland.

Adipharm, Switz. Adipharm AG, alte Winterthurerstr. 42, 8304 Wallisellen, Switzerland.

Adria, Canad. Adria Laboratories of Canada Ltd, 4500 Dixie Rd, Mississauga, Ontario L4W 1V7, Canada.

Adria, USA. Adria Laboratories Inc., P.O. Box 16529, Columbus OH 43216, USA.

Adrian-Marinier, Fr. Laboratoires Adrian-Marinier (Adrim), 22 cours Albert-1er, B.P. 753.08, 75360 Paris Cedex 08, France.

Adroka, Switz. Adroka AG, Hegenheimermattweg, 4123 Allschwil, Switzerland.

Adrosanol, Switz. Adrosanol Pharma AG, Dufourstrasse 11, 4052 Basel, Switzerland.

Aesculapius, Ital. Aesculapius, Laboratorio Chimico Farmaceutico s.p.a., St. Padana Superiore 290, 20090 Vimodrone, Italy.

Affeltranger, Switz. H. Affeltranger, Zürcherstrasse 153, 8500 Frauenfeld, Switzerland.

AFI, Norw. A/S Farmaceutisk Industri, Lillogt. 3, Postboks 4284 Torshov, Oslo 4, Norway.

AFOM, Ital. AFOM Laboratorio Farmacogeno s.a.s. di dott. Bianco & C., Via Basilica 5, 10122 Torino, Italy.

AGIPS, Ital. Azienda Generale Italiana Prodotti Specializzati, Via Amendola 4, 16035 Rapallo, Italy.

AGM, Ger. Aktiengesellschaft für medizinische Produkte (Schwarzhaupt-Gruppe), Sachsenring 37-47, 5000 Cologne 1, W. Germany.

Agol, Switz. Agol Chemie O. Luginbühl AG, Freiburgstrasse 618, 3172 Niederwangen, Switzerland.

Agpharm, Switz. Agpharm AG, Reussinsel, 6003 Luzern, Switzerland.

Agricultural Holdings, UK. Agricultural Holdings Co. Ltd, 40 Warton Rd, London E15 2JU, England.

Aguettant, Fr. Laboratoires Aguettant, 1 ave J.-Carteret, 69007 Lyon, France.

Aicardi, Ital. Aicardi Farmaceutici s.r.l., Via del Faggiolo 42 A/B, 40132 Bologna, Italy.

Aima, Ital. Aima Plasmaderivati s.p.a., 55020 Castelvecchio Pascoli, Italy.

Airkem, USA. Airkem, Division of Airwick Industries Inc., 380 North St, Teterboro NJ 07608, USA.

Airwick, Switz. Airwick AG, Technische Produkte, 4002 Basel, Switzerland.

Ajinomoto, Jap. Ajinomoto Co. Inc., 5-8 Kyobashi 1-chome, Chuo-ku, Tokyo 104, Japan.

Akarana, Austral. Akarana, Australia.

Akzo, UK. Akzo Chemie UK Ltd, 12 St Ann's Crescent, London SW18 2LS, England.

A.L., Denm. See *Apothekernes Laboratorium, Denm.*

A.L., Norw. See *Apothekernes Laboratorium, Norw.*

A.L.-Pharma, Denm. A.L.-Pharma a/s, Emdrupvej 28 B, 2100 Copenhagen Ø, Denmark.

A.L., Swed. See *Apothekernes Laboratorium, Swed.*

Albert-Farma, Ital. Albert-Farma s.p.a., Strada Statale 17 Km. 22, 67019 Scoppito, Italy.

Albert-Farma, Spain. Albert-Farma, Spain.

Albert-Roussel, Ger. Albert-Roussel Pharma GmbH, Abraham-Lincoln-Strasse 38-42, Postfach: 1160, 6200 Wiesbaden, W. Germany.

Albion, UK. Albion Soap Co. Ltd, 113 Station Rd, Hampton, Middx TW12 2DY, England.

Albright & Wilson, Eire. Albright & Wilson (Ireland) Ltd, Sandyford Industrial Estate, Fox Rock, Dublin 18, Eire.

Albright & Wilson, Marchon Division, UK. Albright & Wilson Ltd, Detergents Division, Marchon Works, Whitehaven, Cumbria CA28 9QQ, England.

Albright & Wilson, Medical Division, UK. Albright & Wilson Ltd, Oldbury Medical Dept, P.O. Box 80, Oldbury, Warley, West Midlands B69 4LN, England.

Alcina, Switz. Alcina Labor, Zimmerwaldstr. 49, 3122 Kehrsatz, Switzerland.

Alcon, Arg. Alcon Laboratorio Arg. S.R.L., Estados Unidos 1852, 1227 Buenos Aires, Argentina.

Alcon, Canad. Alcon Laboratories Ltd, 6500 Kitimat Rd, Mississauga, Ontario L5N 2B8, Canada.

Alcon-Couvreur, Belg. Ets A. Couvreur S.A., rue Vanderlinden 46, 1030 Brussels, Belgium.

Alcon, Denm. See *Meda, Denm.*

Alcon, Norw. See *Meda, Norw.*

Alcon, S.Afr. See *Adcock Ingram, S.Afr.*

Alcon, UK. Alcon Laboratories (UK) Ltd, Imperial Way, Watford, Herts WD2 4YR, England.

Alcon, USA. Alcon Laboratories Inc., 6201 South Freeway, P.O. Box 1959, Fort Worth TX 76101, USA.

Alcor, Spain. Alcor, Spain.

Aldepha, Switz. Aldepha AG, Witikonerstr. 37, 8032 Zurich, Switzerland.

Aldon, Spain. Aldon, Spain.

Alembic Products, UK. Alembic Products Ltd, Oaklands House, Oaklands Drive, Sale, Manchester M33 1WS, England.

Alet, Arg. Laboratorio Alet S.A., Cramer 2968, 1429 Buenos Aires, Argentina.

Alfa Farmaceutici, Ital. Alfa Farmaceutici s.p.a., Via Ragazzi del 99 n.5, 40133 Bologna, Italy.

Alfa, UK. Alfa Chemicals Ltd, Shirley Lodge, 470 London Rd, Slough, Berks SL3 8QY, England.

Alfar, Spain. Alfar, Spain.

Alginate Industries, UK. Alginate Industries Ltd, 22 Henrietta St, London WC2E 8NB, England.

Alimedic, Switz. Alimedic S.A., av. de Provence 16, 1007 Lausanne, Switzerland.

Alkaloida Chemical Factory, Hung. Alkaloida Vegyészeti Gyár, Tiszavasvári, Hungary.

Allard, Fr. Laboratoires Allard, 10 ave de Messine, 75008 Paris, France.

Allcock, Norw. See *Collett, Norw.*

Allemann, Switz. John Allemann, Prod. pharmaceutiques, 1095 Lutry, Switzerland.

Allen & Hanburys, Austral. Allen & Hanburys, 1061 Mountain Highway, Boronia Vic. 3155, Australia.

Allen & Hanburys, Canad. Allen & Hanburys, 1025 The Queensway, Toronto, Ontario M8Z 5S6, Canada.

Allen & Hanburys, UK. Allen & Hanburys Ltd, Horsenden House, Oldfield Lane North, Greenford, Middx UB6 0HB, England.

Allergan, Arg. Allergan S.A.I.C.yF., Independencia 766, 1099 Buenos Aires, Argentina.

Allergan, Austral. Allergan Pharmaceuticals Pty Ltd, 32 Punch St, Artarmon NSW 2064, Australia.

Allergan, Belg. See *Roterpharma, Belg.*

Allergan, Canad. Allergan Inc., 263 Labrosse Ave, Pointe Claire, Quebec H9R 1A3, Canada.

Allergan, Denm. See *Biofarma, Denm.*

Allergan, Ger. Pharm-Allergan Vertrieb GmbH, Liststr. 24, Postfach: 5180, 7500 Karlsruhe 21, W. Germany.

Allergan, Neth. See *Bournonville, Neth.*

Allergan, S.Afr. Allergan International, P.O. Box 6747, Johannesburg, S. Africa.

Allergan, UK. Allergan Ltd, Fennels Lodge, St Peter's Close, Loudwater, High Wycombe, Bucks HP11 1JT, England.

Allergan, USA. Allergan Pharmaceuticals Inc., 2525 Dupont Dr., P.O. Box DP, Irvine CA 92713, USA.

Almed, Switz. Almed AG, Ankerstr. 53, 8004 Zurich, Switzerland.

Almedica, Switz. Almedica, Laufenstrasse 12, 4018 Basel, Switzerland.

Almirall, Spain. Laboratorios Almirall SA, Cardoner 68-74, Barcelona, Spain.

Alpes, Arg. Alpes Aem S.A.I.C., Nazca 366, 1406 Buenos Aires, Argentina.

Alphar, Switz. Alphar S.A., rue Tour de l'Ile, 1200 Geneva, Switzerland.

Alpinapharm, Switz. Alpinapharm AG, Gsteigstr. 52, 8049 Zurich, Switzerland.

Also, Ital. Also Lab. s.a.s., Via Settembrini 26/A, 20124 Milan, Italy.

Alter, Spain. Alter SA, Mateo Inurria 30, Madrid 16, Spain.

Alther, Switz. Dr R. Alther, Burggraben 28, 9000 St Gallen, Switzerland.

Alvarez Gómez, Spain. Alvarez Gómez, Spain.

Alza, Neth. See *Pharbil, Neth.*

Alza, Norw. See *Astra, Norw.*

Alza, USA. Alza Corporation, 950 Page Mill Rd, Palo Alto CA 94304, USA.

Amerchol, USA. Amerchol Corporation, A Unit of CPC International Inc., P.O. Box 351, Talmadge Rd, Edison NJ 08817, USA.

American Chicle, USA. American Chicle Sales Division, Warner-Lambert Co., 201 Tabor Rd, Morris Plains NJ 07950, USA.

American Critical Care, USA. American Critical Care, Division of American Hospital Supply Corp., 1600 Waukegan Rd, McGaw Park IL 60085, USA.

American Cyanamid, USA. American Cyanamid Co., P.O. Box 400, Princeton NJ 08540, USA.

American Hospital Supply, UK. American Hospital Supply (UK) Ltd, 53 Church Rd, Ashford, Middx TW15 2TY, England.

Amersham International, UK. Amersham International Ltd, White Lion Rd, Amersham, Bucks HP7 9LL, England.

Ames, Arg. Ames Division de Lab. Miles de Argentina S.R.L., C. Correo N° 46, 1651 San Andres (Bs.As.), Argentina.

Ames, UK. Ames Company, Division of Miles Laboratories Ltd, P.O. Box 37, Stoke Court, Stoke Poges, Slough SL2 4LY, England.

Amfre-Grant, USA. Amfre-Grant Inc., 16600 NW 54th Ave, Miami FL 33014, USA.

Amid, USA. Amid Laboratories Inc., 611 Moore St, P.O. Box 299, Marion AL 36756, USA.

Amido, Fr. Laboratoires Amido, 65 r. du Dr-Jenner, 59010 Lille Cedex, France.

Amino, Switz. Amino AG, 5430 Wettingen 1, Switzerland.

Amovon, UK. Amovon Ltd, Tree Tops, 208 Seabridge Lane, Newcastle, Staffs ST5 3LS, England.

Amrein, Switz. St. Th. Amrein, 9053 Teufen, Switzerland.

AMSA, Ital. Ascaridolo Mancini s.n.c., P.za Cavour 19, 50031 Barberino di Mugello, Italy.

Ana, Fr. Laboratoires Ana, 171 av. Charles-de-Gaulle, 92200 Neuilly, France.

Anca, Canad. Anca Laboratories, 111 Consumers Dr., Whitby, Ontario L1N 5Z5, Canada.

Andard-Mount, UK. Andard-Mount (London) Ltd, 24 London Rd, Wembley, Middx HA9 7HD, England.

Andersen, Norw. Jan F. Andersen, Postboks 1132 Flattum, 3501 Hønefoss, Norway.

Andreu, Arg. Laboratorio Andreu S.A., Constitucion 4234, 1254 Buenos Aires, Argentina.

Andreu, Spain. Dr Andreu SA, Moragas 15, Barcelona, Spain.

Andromaco, Arg. Laboratorio Andromaco S.A.I.C.I., Ing. Huergo 1145, 1107 Buenos Aires, Argentina.

Andromaco, Spain. Laboratorios Andromaco SA, Solana 22, Torrejon de Ardoz (Madrid), Spain.

Angelini, Ital. Aziende Chimiche Riunite Angelini Francesco s.p.a., Viale Amelia 70, 00181 Rome, Italy.

Anglo-French Laboratories, Canad. Anglo-French Laboratories, 582 rue Orly, Dorval, Quebec H9P 1E9, Canada.

Anlikerhaus, Switz. Anlikerhaus AG, Postfach 114, 8820 Wädenswil, Switzerland.

Anphar-Rolland, Fr. Laboratoires Anphar-Rolland, 2 rue de la Division-Leclerc, 91380 Chilly-Mazarin, France.

Anstead, UK. D.F. Anstead Ltd, Victoria House, Radford Way, Billericay, Essex CM12 0DE, England.

Ansun, UK. Ansun Proprietaries Ltd, 3 Chester Crescent, Newcastle, Staffs ST5 3RT, England.

Antibioticos, Spain. Antibioticos SA, Bravo Murillo 38, Madrid 3, Spain.

Antogen, Switz. Antogen AG, Arbonerstrasse 145, 9302 Kronbühl, Switzerland.

Antonetto, Ital. Marco Antonetto, Via Arsenale 29/31, 10121 Torino, Italy.

Antonioli, Switz. Dr M. Antonioli, Postfach 6, 4006 Basel, Switzerland.

Aplin & Barrett, UK. Aplin & Barrett Ltd, Bythesea Rd, Trowbridge, Wilts BA14 8TR, England.

Apothekernes Laboratorium, Denm. See *A.L.-Pharma, Denm.*

Apothekernes Laboratorium, Norw. A/S Apothekernes Laboratorium for Specialpraeparater, Skøyen, Oslo 2, Norway.

Apothekernes Laboratorium, Swed. See *Kemi-Intressen, Swed.*

Appleford, UK. Appleford Ltd, 14 Villiers Rd, Kingston-on-Thames, Surrey KT1 3AS, England.

Approved Prescription Services, UK. Approved Prescription Services Ltd, P.O. Box 15, Whitcliffe Rd, Cleckheaton, West Yorkshire BD19 3BZ, England.

Arcadian Confections, UK. Arcadian Confections Ltd, Crediton, Devon EX17 3AP, England.

Archifar, Ital. Archifar Laboratori Chimico Farmacologici s.p.a., Via R. Lepetit 8, 20124 Milan, Italy.

Archifar, Switz. See *Allemann, Switz.*

Arco, Switz. Arco S.A., via Besso 44, 6900 Lugano, Switzerland.

Arden, UK. Elizabeth Arden Ltd, 13 Hanover Sq., London W1R 0PA, England.

Arduin, Ital. Lab. Chim. Farm. Arduin s.n.c., Stradone S.Agostino 26/1, 16123 Genoa, Italy.

Areu, Spain. Areu, Spain.

Argentia, Arg. Quimica Argentia S.A.C.I.F.I., Larrea 790, 1030 Buenos Aires, Argentina.

Aristegui, Spain. Laboratorios del Dr Aristegui, Alameda de Urquijo 18-24, Bilbao 8, Spain.

Aristochimica, Ital. Aristochimica s.p.a., Via Doberdò 16, 20126 Milan, Italy.

Ariston, Arg. Quimica Ariston S.A., O'Connor 555/59, 1704 Ramos Mejia, Argentina.

Aristopharm, Switz. Aristopharm AG, Mattenstr. 16, 4002 Basel, Switzerland.

Arkodex, Fr. Laboratoires Arkodex, 58 rue de la Glacière, 75013 Paris, France.

Armedic, Denm. Armedic A/S Laegemidler, Søndermarksvej 16, 2500 Valby, Denmark.

Armour, Austral. Armour Pharmaceutical Co., Division of USV Australia Pty Ltd, 172 Princes Highway, Arncliffe NSW 2205, Australia.

Armour, Denm. See *Johnson, Denm.*

Armour, Ital. Armour Medicamenta s.p.a., Viale Europa, 21040 Origgio (Varese), Italy.

Armour-Montagu, Fr. Laboratoires Armour-Montagu, 4 rue de la Gare, 92300 Levallois, France.

Armour, Norw. See *Andersen, Norw.*

Armour, S.Afr. See *Berk, S.Afr.*

Armour, UK. Armour Pharmaceutical Co. Ltd, St Leonard's House, St Leonard's Rd, Eastbourne, East Sussex BN21 3YG, England.

Armour, USA. Armour Pharmaceutical Co., P.O. Box 1849, Scottsdale AZ 85252, USA.

Armstrong, Arg. Lab. Armstrong S.A., Joaquín V. Gonzales 653, 1407 Buenos Aires, Argentina.

Arnaldi, Ital. Arnaldi Emilio, Via Oldoini 55, 19100 La Spezia, Italy.

Arnaldi-Uscio, Ital. Colonia della Salute Carlo Arnaldi s.p.a., 16030 Uscio, Italy.

Arnold, Switz. Dr E. & J. Arnold, Alpenstrasse 8, 6000 Luzern, Switzerland.

Aron, Fr. S.N.E. des Laboratoires Aron, 116 rue Carnot, 92152 Suresnes Cedex, France.

Arsac, Fr. Laboratoires Arsac, 177 ave Victor-Hugo, 26007 Valence, France.

Artesan, Ger. Artesan GmbH, Fabrik chem.-pharm. Präparate, Wendlandstrasse 1, Postfach: 52, 3130 Lüchow, W. Germany.

Arthromedica, Switz. Arthromedica S.A., Via Molinazzo 14, 6900 Lugano-Cassarate, Switzerland.

Arznei Müller-Rorer, Ger. Arznei Müller-Rorer GmbH, Stieghorster Strasse 86, Postfach: 520, 4800 Bielefeld 1, W. Germany.

Asba, Switz. Lab. Asba S.A., 9 rue Bellot, 1206 Geneva, Switzerland.

Asche, Ger. Asche AG, Fischersallee 49, Postfach: 50 0132, 2000 Hamburg 50, W. Germany.

Ascher, USA. B.F. Ascher & Co. Inc., 5100 East 59th St, Kansas City MO 64130, USA.

Asco, Switz. Asco Pharmaceutica AG, Seefeldstr. 81, 8008 Zurich, Switzerland.

Ascot, Austral. Ascot Pharmaceuticals Pty Ltd, 33 Myrtle St, North Sydney NSW 2060, Australia.

Ash Dental, UK. Ash Dental, Summit House, Moon Lane, Barnet, Herts EN5 5UA, England.

Ashe, UK. Ashe Laboratories Ltd, Ashetree Works, Kingston Rd, Leatherhead, Surrey KT22 7JZ, England.

Askit, UK. Askit Laboratories Ltd, 93 Saracen St, Glasgow G22 5HX, Scotland.

Asla, Spain. Asla, Spain.

Associated Hospital Supply, UK. Associated Hospital Supply, P.O. Box 4, Pershore, Worcs, England.

Asta, Aust. See *Laevosan, Aust.*

Asta, Belg. See *de Bournonville, Belg.*

Asta, Denm. See *Schering Kemi, Denm.*

Asta, Ger. Asta-Werke AG, Chemische Fabrik, Artur-Ladebeck-Strasse 128, Postfach: 14 01 29, 4800 Bielefeld 14, W. Germany.

Asta, Neth. See *Multi-Pharma, Neth.*

Asta, Switz. See *Adroka, Switz.* and *Max Ritter, Switz.*

Astor, UK. Astor Chemical Ltd, Tavistock Rd, West Drayton, Middx UB7 7RA, England.

Astra, Arg. Astra S.A. Prod. Farm. y Quim., Argerich 536, 1706 Haedo, Argentina.

Astra, Austral. Astra Chemicals Pty Ltd, 10 Khartoum Rd, North Ryde NSW 2113, Australia.

Astra, Belg. Astra Chemicals S.A., Chaussée d'Alsemberg 1001, 1180 Brussels, Belgium.

Astra, Denm. Astra-Gruppen A/S, Roskildevej 22, 2620 Albertslund, Denmark.

Astra, Fr. Laboratoires Astra France, Groupe pharmaceutique Astra Suède, 64 rue du 8 Mai 1945, 92025 Nanterre Cedex, France.

Astra, Ger. Astra Chemicals GmbH, Tinsdaler Weg 183, Postfach: 249, 2000 Wedel (Holstein), W. Germany.

Astra Meditec, Denm. Astra Meditec A/S, Roskildevej 22, 2620 Albertslund, Denmark.

Astra Meditec, Norw. Astra Meditec A/S, Skårervn. 116, Postboks 1, 1473 Skårer, Norway.

Astra, Neth. Astra Pharmaceutica B.V., Treubstraat 16, 2288 EJ Rijswijk, Netherlands.

Astra, Norw. Astra Farmasøytiske A/S, Skårervn. 116, Postboks 1, 1473 Skårer, Norway.

Astra, Swed. Astra Läkemedel AB, Strängnäsvägen 44, 151 85 Södertälje, Sweden.

Astra, Switz. See *Globopharm, Switz.* and *Pharmac-Service, Switz.*

Astra-Syntex, Denm. Astra-Syntex Terapeutika ApS, C.F. Richsvej 103, 2000 Copenhagen F, Denmark.

Astra-Syntex, Norw. Astra-Syntex A/S, Strømsveien 66 C, Postboks 44, 2011 Strømmen, Norway.

Astra, UK. Astra Pharmaceuticals Ltd, St Peter's House, 2 Bricket Rd, St Albans, Herts AL1 3JW, England.

Astra, USA. Astra Pharmaceutical Products Inc., 7 Neponset St, Worcester MA 01606, USA.

Atem, Belg. Applications Therapeutiques et Medicales, Chaussée d'Alsemberg 1001, 1180 Brussels, Belgium.

Athenstaedt, Ger. Athenstaedt & Redeker KG, Hemelinger Bahnhofstrasse 13, Postfach: 448660, 2800 Bremen 44, W. Germany.

Athrodax, UK. Athrodax Ltd, Athrodax House, Telford Rd, Bicester, Oxon OX6 0TX, England.

Atlas, UK. Atlas Chemical Industries (UK) Ltd, Cleeve Rd, Leatherhead, Surrey KT22 7SW, England.

Auclair, Fr. Laboratoires Auclair, 4 rue Guillot, B.P. 390, 92541 Montrouge Cedex, France.

Auclair, Switz. See *Opopharma, Switz.*

Auriema, UK. Auriema Ltd, 442 Bath Rd, Slough, Berks, England.

Ausonia, Ital. Ausonia Farmaceutici s.r.l., Via Laurentina Km. 24.730, 00040 Pomezia (Roma), Italy.

Ausonia, Spain. Ausonia, Spain.

Avon, UK. Avon Medicals Ltd, Moons Moat Drive, Redditch, Worcs B98 9HA, England.

Ayerst, Arg. Ayerst Laboratorio Inc., Wenceslao Villafañe 1236, 1295 Buenos Aires, Argentina.

Ayerst, Austral. Ayerst Laboratories Pty Ltd, Gregory Place, Parramatta NSW 2150, Australia.

Ayerst, Belg. Ayerst Benelux S.A., rue Royale 247, 1030 Brussels, Belgium.

Ayerst, Canad. Ayerst Laboratories, PO Box 6115, Montreal, Quebec H3C 3J1, Canada.

Ayerst, Denm. See *Ferring, Denm.*

Ayerst, Ital. Ayerst Italiana s.p.a., Via dei M. Lepini Km. 53, 04100 Latina, Italy.

Ayerst, Neth. Ayerst Benelux N.V., Pilotenstraat 35, 1059 CH Amsterdam, Netherlands.

Ayerst, Norw. See *AFI, Norw.*

Ayerst, S.Afr. Ayerst Laboratories (Pty) Ltd, P.O. Box 573, Halfway House 1685, S. Africa.

Ayerst, Switz. See *Doetsch, Grether, Switz.* and *Sodip, Switz.*

Ayerst, UK. Ayerst Laboratories Ltd, South Way, Andover, Hants SP10 5LT, England.

Ayerst, USA. Ayerst Laboratories, 685 Third Ave, New York NY 10017, USA.

Ayrton, Saunders, UK. Ayrton, Saunders & Co. Ltd, 34 Hanover St, Liverpool L69 1BL, England.

Azienda Farm. Ital., Ital. A.F.I.-Azienda Farmaceutica Italian, Via A. de Gasperi 47, 21040 Sumirago, Italy.

Bachmann, Switz. Dr W. Bachmann & Co., Zürcherstrasse 89, 8805 Richterswil, Switzerland.
Badische, Ger. Badische Arzneimittel GmbH, Rheinstrasse 93-95, Postfach: 1406, 7570 Baden-Baden, W. Germany.
Badrial, Fr. Laboratoires Badrial, B.P. 292, 51060 Reims Cedex, France.
Baer, Ger. Chemisch-pharmazeutische Fabrik Dr Baer KG GmbH & Co., Ehrwalder Strasse 21, Südmedica-Haus, Postfach:70 16 69, Munich 70, W. Germany.
Baer, Switz. Paul Baer AG, Oberhusstrasse 6, 8134 Adliswil, Switzerland.
Bagó, Arg. Lab. Bagó S.A.C.I.F.A.M.S., Bdo. de Irigoyen 248, 1072 Buenos Aires, Argentina.
Bailly, Fr. Laboratoires A. Bailly (S.P.E.A.B.), 6 rue du Rocher, 75008 Paris, France.
Bajer, Arg. Lab. Felipe Bajer S.A.I.C., Alfredo R. Bufano 1265, 1416 Buenos Aires, Argentina.
Baker, Neth. J.T. Baker Chemicals B.V., P.O. Box 1, 7400 AA Deventer, Netherlands.
Baldacci, Ital. Laboratori Baldacci s.p.a., Via S. Michele Scalzi 73, 56100 Pisa, Italy.
Baliarda, Arg. Lab. Baliarda S.R.L., Saavedra 1260/2, 1247 Buenos Aires, Argentina.
Bama, Spain. Bama SA, Bailen 95-97, Barcelona, Spain.
Banyu, Jap. Banyu Pharmaceutical Co. Ltd, 7 Nihonbashi Honcho 2-chome, Chuo-ku, Tokyo 103, Japan.
Banyu, Switz. See *Biochimica, Switz.*
Barbezat, Switz. Barbezat & Cie S.A., 5a ruelle Rousseau, 2114 Fleurier, Switzerland.
Barker Dobson, UK. Barker Dobson Ltd, Everton, Liverpool L6 5DF, England.
Barlocco, Ital. Lab. Farm. Barlocco E. s.r.l., Via Giovanni Santolini 10, 16132 Genoa, Italy.
Barlowe Cote, Canad. Barlowe Cote Laboratories of Canada, 2400 Finch Ave West, Weston, Ontario M9M 2C8, Canada.
Barnes-Hind, Canad. Barnes-Hind Canada, 1821 Albion Rd, Rexdale, Ontario M9W 5S8, Canada.
Barnes-Hind, UK. Barnes-Hind Ltd, Isis Trading Estate, Stratton Rd, Swindon, Wilts SN1 2PQ, England.
BASF, Ger. BASF AG, Carl-Bosch-Strasse 38, 6700 Ludwigshafen, W. Germany.
BASF, UK. BASF (UK) Ltd, Earl Rd, Cheadle Hulme, Cheadle, Cheshire, England.
BASF Wyandotte, USA. BASF Wyandotte Corporation, 100 Cherry Hill Rd, Parsippany NJ 07054, USA.
Basileos, Spain. Basileos, Spain.
Basotherm, Ger. Basotherm GmbH Präparate gegen Erkrankungen von Haut und Schleimhaut, Leipzigstrasse 26, Postfach:130, 7950 Biberach an der Riss 1, W. Germany.
Bateman-Jackson, UK. Bateman-Jackson, Tubiton House, Medlock St, Oldham, Lancs, England.
Baumann, Switz. Walter Baumann & Co., Postfach 336, 8034 Zurich, Switzerland.
Baungaard, Denm. R. Baungaard & Co., Naerumgårdsvej 10, 2850 Naerum, Denmark.
Baxter, Ital. Laboratori Don Baxter s.p.a., Via Flavia 124, 34147 Trieste, Italy.
Bayer Agrochem, UK. Bayer UK Ltd, Agrochem Division, Eastern Way, Bury St Edmunds, Suffolk IP32 7AH, England.
Bayer, Arg. Bayer Argentina S.A.C.I.F.I.y, de M. Empedrado 2435, 1417 Buenos Aires, Argentina.
Bayer, Aust. Bayer-Pharma GmbH, Biberstrasse 15, 1011 Vienna 1, Austria.
Bayer, Austral. Bayer Pharmaceutical Co., 47 Wilson St, Botany NSW 2019, Australia.
Bayer, Belg. Bayer Belgium S.A., Ave Louise 143, 1050 Brussels, Belgium.
Bayer, Denm. Bayer Kemi A/S, Christian IX's gade 2, 1111 Copenhagen K, Denmark.
Bayer, Fr. Bayer-Pharma, rue Bellocier, 89104 Sens Cedex, France.
Bayer, Ger. Bayer AG, 5090 Leverkusen, W. Germany.
Bayer, Ital. Bayer Italia s.p.a., Viale Certosa 126, 20156 Milan, Italy.
Bayer, Neth. Bayer Nederland B.V., divisie Bayer Farma, Nijverheidsweg 26, 3641 RR Mijdrecht, Netherlands.
Bayer, Norw. Bayer Kjemi A/S, Haakon VII's gt. 2, Postboks 1615 Vika, Oslo 1, Norway.
Bayer, S.Afr. Bayer Pharmaceuticals (SA) (Pty) Ltd, P.O. Box 10233, Johannesburg, S. Africa.
Bayer, Spain. Química Farmacéutica Bayer SA, Calabria 268, Barcelona, Spain.
Bayer, Swed. Bayer (Sverige) AB, Div. Farma, Box 5148, 102 43 Stockholm, Sweden.
Bayer, Switz. Bayer Pharma AG, 8036 Zurich, Switzerland.
Bayer, UK. Bayer UK Ltd, Pharmaceutical Division, Haywards Heath, West Sussex RH16 1TP, England.
Baylor, USA. Baylor Laboratories Inc., P.O. Drawer 277, Hurst TX 76053, USA.
Bayropharm, Ger. Bayropharm GmbH, Wiener Platz 4, Postfach: 800146, 5000 Cologne 80, W. Germany.
Bayropharm, Ital. Bayropharm Italiana s.p.a., Via dei Cignoli 9, 20151 Milan, Italy.
BDH Chemicals, UK. BDH Chemicals Ltd, Broom Rd, Poole, Dorset BH12 4NN, England.
Beaufour, Belg. See *de Bournonville, Belg.*
Beaufour, Fr. Laboratoires Beaufour, 18 place Doguereau, 28104 Dreux, France.
Beautisales, UK. Beautisales Ltd, 65 Loveridge Rd & Mews, London NW6 2DR, England.
Beecham Animal Health, UK. Beecham Animal Health, Veterinary Dept, Beecham House, Brentford, Middx TW8 9BD, England.
Beecham, Arg. Prod. Beecham S.A., Florida 378-3[er] piso, Galeria Central, 1005 Buenos Aires, Argentina.
Beecham, Austral. Pharmaceutical Division of Beecham (Australia) Pty Ltd, 212 Chesterville Rd, Moorabbin Vic. 3189, Australia.
Beecham, Canad. Beecham Laboratories Inc., 115 Brunswick Blvd, Pointe Claire, Quebec H9R 1A4, Canada.
Beecham, Denm. See *Møller, Denm.*
Beecham Foods, UK. Beecham Products, Research and Development (Foods), 11 Stoke Poges Lane, Slough, Berks SL1 3NW, England.
Beecham, Ital. Beecham Italia s.p.a., Via Pirelli 19, 20124 Milan, Italy.
Beecham, Neth. Beecham Research Lab., Afd. van Beecham Farma B.V., Sportlaan 198, 1185 TH Amstelveen, Netherlands.
Beecham Proprietaries, UK. Beecham Proprietaries, Beecham House, Great West Rd, Brentford, Middx TW8 9BD, England.
Beecham Research, UK. Beecham Research Laboratories, Beecham House, Great West Rd, Brentford, Middx TW8 9BD, England.
Beecham, Switz. Beecham AG, Weltpoststr. 4, 3015 Bern, Switzerland.
Beecham, USA. Beecham Laboratories, Division of Beecham Inc., 501 Fifth St, Bristol TN 37620, USA.
Beecham-Wülfing, Ger. Beecham-Wülfing GmbH & Co. KG, Stresemannallee 6, Postfach: 25, 4040 Neuss 1, W. Germany.
Behring, Norw. See *Hoechst, Norw.*
Behringer, Switz. Behringer Pharma, 42 rue du Lac, 1400 Yverdon, Switzerland.
Behringwerke, Denm. See *Hoechst, Denm.*
Behringwerke, Ger. Behringwerke AG, Postfach: 1130, 3550 Marburg (Lahn), W. Germany.
Beiersdorf, Ger. Beiersdorf AG, Unnastrasse 48, 2000 Hamburg 20, W. Germany.
Beiersdorf, Ital. Beiersdorf s.p.a., Via Eraclito 30, 20128 Milan, Italy.
Belgana, Belg. Laboratoires Belgana S.A., rue Saint-Ghislain 41, 1000 Brussels, Belgium.
Bellon, Belg. See *Wellcome, Belg.*
Bellon, Fr. Laboratoires Roger Bellon, B.P. 105, 159 ave du Roule, 92201 Neuilly-sur-Seine Cedex, France.
Bellon, Neth. See *Rhône-Poulenc, Neth.*
Bellon, Switz. See *Rhodia-Pharm, Switz.*
Bencard, Neth. See *Beecham, Neth.*
Bencard, UK. Bencard, Great West Rd, Brentford, Middx TW8 9BE, England.
Bender, Aust. Bender & Co. GmbH, Dr Boehringer-Gasse 5-11, 1121 Vienna XII, Austria.
Bene-Chemie, Ger. Bene-Chemie GmbH, Herterichstrasse 1, Postfach: 710269, 8000 Munich 71, W. Germany.
Benedetti, Ital. Labor. Chim. Biol. Benedetti Oreste, Via Donizetti 52, 50018 Scandicci, Italy.
Bengué, UK. Bengué & Co. Ltd, St Ives House, St Ives Rd, Maidenhead, Berks SL6 1RD, England.
Benitol, Arg. Lab. Benitol S.A.C.I., Av. del Libertador 7748, 1429 Buenos Aires, Argentina.
Benvegna, Ital. Neoterapici Benvegna s.r.l., Via Liborio Giuffrè 52/B, 90127 Palermo, Italy.
Benzon, Denm. A/S Alfred Benzon, Halmtorvet 29, 1700 Copenhagen V. Denmark.
Benzon, Swed. Benzons Farmaceutiska AB, Box 1423, 251 02 Helsingborg, Sweden.
Benzon, UK. Alfred Benzon (UK) Ltd, 26 Heathlands Rd, Boldmere, Sutton Coldfield, West Midlands B73 5DZ, England.
Berenguer-Beneyto, Spain. Laboratorios Berenguer-Beneyto SA, Marques de Ahumada 5, Madrid 28, Spain.
Bergamon, Ital. Bergamon s.r.l., Via di Cancelliera 34, 00040 Ariccia (Roma), Italy.
Berk Pharmaceuticals, UK. Berk Pharmaceuticals Ltd, St Leonard's House, St Leonard's Rd, Eastbourne, East Sussex BN21 3YG, England.
Berk, S.Afr. Berk Pharmaceuticals (SA) (Pty) Ltd, P.O. Box 301, Isando 1600, S. Africa.
Berkeley, USA. Berkeley Biologicals, 1831 Second St, Berkeley CA 94710, USA.
Berlex, USA. Berlex Laboratories Inc., 110 East Hanover Ave, Cedar Knolls NJ 07927, USA.
Berlimed, S.Afr. Berlimed (Pty) Ltd, P.O. Box 10259, Johannesburg 2000, S. Africa.
Berna, Ital. Istituto Sieroterapico Berna s.r.l., Via Bellinzona 39, 22100 Como, Italy.
Berna, Spain. Instituto Berna de España SA, Av. Generalisimo 71, Madrid 16, Spain.
Bernabó, Arg. Lab. Bernabó & Cía. S.A.I.yC., Terrada 2346/48, 1416 Buenos Aires, Argentina.
Bernauer, Switz. A. Bernauer & Co., Rosenweg 1, 6052 Hergiswil, Switzerland.
Berol Kemi, UK. Berol Kemi (UK) Ltd, 55 Clarendon Rd, Watford, Herts WD1 1SP, England.
Berset, Switz. P. Berset, Lab. pharmaceutique, 1723 Marly-le-Grand, Switzerland.
Berta, Ital. Berta Michele s.a.s. Farmaceutici, Piazza Martelli 7, 20162 Milan, Italy.
Berthet, Switz. R. Berthet, 16 bd des philosophes, 1205 Geneva, Switzerland.
Besins-Iscovesco, Fr. Laboratoires Besins-Iscovesco, 5 rue du Bourg-l'Abbé, 75003 Paris, France.
Besse, Switz. R. Besse, 1933 Sembrancher, Switzerland.
Beta, Arg. Lab. Beta S.A.I.C.A., San Juan 2266/74, 1232 Buenos Aires, Argentina.
Beta, Ital. Laboratorio Biologico Chemioterapico Beta s.r.l., Via G. Uberti 8, 25100 Brescia, Italy.
Beta Medical Products, UK. Beta Medical Products Ltd, 33 Arkwright Rd, Astmoor, Runcorn, Cheshire, England.
Bettschart, Switz. Dr A. Bettschart, 8840 Einsiedeln, Switzerland.
Beutlich, USA. Beutlich Inc., 7006 North Western Ave, Chicago IL 60645, USA.
Beytout, Fr. Laboratoires Beytout, 10 rue Guynemer, 94160 Saint-Mandé, France.
Beytout, Switz. See *Pharmacal, Switz.* and *Uhlmann-Eyraud, Switz.*
Biagini, Ital. Farmaceutici Biagini s.p.a., 55020 Castelvecchio Pascoli, Italy.
Bichsel, Switz. Dr G. Bichsel, Postfach 29, 3800 Interlaken, Switzerland.
Bichsel-Werder, Switz. Dr E. Bichsel-Werder, 3001 Bern, Switzerland.
Bicsa, Spain. Bicsa, Spain.
Bieder, Switz. Bieder & Cie, Tribschenstrasse 66, 6005 Luzern, Switzerland.
Bier, Ital. Bier, Lab. Chim. Farm. Partenopeo di Rosa Frattolillo, Via S. Gregorio Armeno 21, 80138 Napoli, Italy.
Billerud-Uddeholm, Swed. Billerud-Uddeholm AB, 663 00 Skoghall, Sweden.
Bio-Chemical Laboratory, Canad. Bio-Chemical Laboratory Inc., 2323 Montée St.-Aubin, Ville De Laval, Quebec H7S 1Z7, Canada.
Bio-Mar, Spain. Bio-Mar, Spain.
Bio-Oil Research, UK. Bio-Oil Research Ltd, Royal Oak Building, High St, Crewe, Cheshire CW2 7BL, England.
Biobasal, Switz. Biobasal AG, Münzgasse 3, 4051 Basel, Switzerland.
Biochimica, Switz. Biochimica AG, Schäppistr. 12, Postfach 203, 8033 Zurich, Switzerland.
Biocodex, Fr. Laboratoires Biocodex, 19 rue Barbès, 92126 Montrouge Cedex, France.
Biodica, Fr. Laboratoires Biodica, 10 ave du Général-de-Gaulle, 92160 Antony, France.

Biofarma, Denm. Biofarma A/S, Nyvej 16, 1851 Copenhagen V, Denmark.

Bioforce, Switz. Bioforce AG, 9325 Roggwil, Switzerland.

Biogal, Hung. Biogal Gyógyszergyár, Debrecen, Hungary.

Bioglan, UK. Bioglan Laboratories Ltd, Spirella Building, Bridge Rd, Letchworth, Herts SG6 4ET, England.

Bioindustria, Ital. Bioindustria Farmaceutici s.p.a., Via De Ambrosiis 2, 15067 Novi Ligure, Italy.

Biokema, Switz. Biokema S.A., 39-41 rue de Lausanne, 1020 Renens, Switzerland.

Biokosma, Switz. Biokosma AG, 9642 Ebnat-Kappel, Switzerland.

Biol, Arg. Inst. Biológico Arg. S.A.I.C., J.E. Uriburu 153, 1027 Buenos Aires, Argentina.

Biolabor, Switz. Biolabor AG, Seestrasse 26, 8702 Zollikon, Switzerland.

Biologici Italia, Ital. Laboratori Biologici Italia Petrucci Dr G. & C. s.r.l., Via Sarzanese 160/A, 55100 Lucca, Italy.

Biologische Arbeitsgemeinschaft, Ger. Biologische Arbeitsgemeinschaft GmbH, Pharmazeutische Fabrik, Amtsgerichtsstrasse 1-3, Postfach: 28, 6302 Lich 1, W. Germany.

Biomed, Switz. Biomed AG, Stauffacherstr. 45, 8004 Zurich, Switzerland.

Biomedica Foscama, Ital. Biomedica Foscama Industria Chimico Farmaceutica s.p.a., Via Tiburtina Km. 14.5, 00131 Rome, Italy.

Biopect-H, Denm. Damino A/S, Staushedevej 10, 6621 Gesten, Denmark.

Biopharm, S.Afr. Biopharm (Pty) Ltd, Access City, 32 Stalb St, New Doornfontein, Johannesburg, S. Africa.

Biopharma, Fr. Laboratoires Biopharmaceutiques de France, 27 rue du Pont, 92201 Neuilly, France.

Bioq. Aplicada, Arg. Lab. Bioq. Aplicada (Dr Rafael Quesada), Saavedra 363/77, 1704 Ramos Mejia, Argentina.

Bioresearch, Ital. Bioresearch s.r.l., 20060 Liscate (Milano), Italy.

Biorex, Switz. Biorex AG, 9642 Ebnat-Kappel, Switzerland.

Biorex, UK. Biorex Laboratories Ltd, Biorex House, Canonbury Villas, London N1 2HB, England.

Bios-Coutelier, Belg. Bios-Coutelier S.A., rue de Potter 37, 1030 Brussels, Belgium.

Biosa, Switz. Biosa S.A., 28 ch. du Grand-Puits, 1217 Meyrin, Switzerland.

Biosedra, Arg. Lab. Biosedra S.A.C.I.E.I., Manuela Pedraza 3345, 1429 Buenos Aires, Argentina.

Biosédra, Fr. Laboratoires Biosédra, 42 ave Augustin-Dumont, 92240 Malakoff, France.

Biosedra, Switz. See *Actipharm, Switz.*

Biosint, Ital. Biosint, Laboratori Farmaco Biologici s.r.l., Via Zorutti 54, 33030 Campoformido, Italy.

Biostabilex, Fr. Laboratoires Biostabilex, 121 ave de Wagram, 75017 Paris, France.

Biotest, Ger. Biotest-Serum-Institut GmbH, Flughafenstrasse 4, Postfach: 730 260, 6000 Frankfurt 73, W. Germany.

Biothera-Asperal, Belg. See *CCP, Belg.*

Biothérax, Denm. See *Tjellesen, Denm.*

Biothérax, Fr. Laboratoires Biothérax, 58 rue du Landy, 93211 La Plaine Saint-Denis Cedex, France.

Biothérax, Norw. See *Remifarm, Norw.*

Biotrading, Ital. Biotrading Co. s.r.l., Via L. Pogliaghi 1, 20146 Milan, Italy.

Biphar, Fr. Laboratoires Biphar, 27 rue de la Procession, 75737 Paris Cedex 15, France.

Biphar, Switz. Biphar S.A., 12-14 chemin Rieu, 1208 Geneva, Switzerland.

Bipharma, Neth. Bipharma B.V., Pilotenstraat 35, 1059 CH Amsterdam, Netherlands.

Birnstiel, Switz. Dr W. Birnstiel's Erben, Hauptstrasse, 3780 Gstaad, Switzerland.

Bismag, Norw. See *Kobro, Norw.*

Black, UK. S. Black (Import & Export) Ltd, 30 Islington Green, London N1 8DU, England.

Blagden, UK. Blagden Campbell Chemicals Ltd, AMP House, Dingwall Rd, Croydon, Surrey CR9 3QU, England.

Blair, USA. Blair Laboratories Inc., 50 Washington St, Norwalk CT 06856, USA.

Blake, UK. Thomas Blake & Co., 20 Blatchford Close, Horsham, West Sussex RH13 5RQ, England.

Blakoe, UK. Blakoe Ltd, 225 Putney Bridge Rd, London SW15, England.

Blend-a-med, Ger. Blendax-Werke R. Schneider GmbH & Co., Blend-a-med-Forschung, Rheinallee 88, Postfach: 1580, 6500 Mainz 1, W. Germany.

BOC Medishield, UK. BOC Medishield, Elizabeth Way, Harlow, Essex CM19 5AB, England.

Bode, Ger. Bacillofabrik Dr Bode & Co., Melanchthonstrasse 27, Postfach: 540709, 2000 Hamburg 54, W. Germany.

Bode, Switz. See *Pharmacolor, Switz.*

Boehringer, Arg. Boehringer Argentina S.A., Viamonte 2213/15, 1056 Buenos Aires, Argentina.

Boehringer Biochemia, Ital. Boehringer Biochemia Robin s.p.a., Via S. Uguzzone 5, 20126 Milan, Italy.

Boehringer Corp., UK. The Boehringer Corporation (London) Ltd, Bell Lane, Lewes, East Sussex BN7 1LG, England.

Boehringer Ingelheim, Austral. Boehringer Ingelheim Pty Ltd, 50 Broughton Rd, Artarmon NSW 2064, Australia.

Boehringer Ingelheim, Belg. Boehringer Ingelheim S.A., rue du Collège St-Michel 17, 1150 Brussels, Belgium.

Boehringer Ingelheim, Denm. Boehringer Ingelheim A/S, Hanebred 2, 2720 Vanløse, Denmark.

Boehringer Ingelheim, Fr. Laboratoires Boehringer Ingelheim, B.P. 292, 51060 Reims Cedex, France.

Boehringer Ingelheim, Ger. Boehringer Ingelheim KG, Binger Strasse, Postfach: 200, 6507 Ingelheim am Rhein, W. Germany.

Boehringer Ingelheim, Ital. Boehringer Ingelheim s.p.a., 50100 Firenze, Italy.

Boehringer Ingelheim, Neth. Boehringer Ingelheim B.V., Stephensonstraat 38, 2014 KD Haarlem, Netherlands.

Boehringer Ingelheim, Norw. See *Collett, Norw.*

Boehringer Ingelheim, S.Afr. Boehringer Ingelheim (Pty) Ltd, Private Bag X3032, Randburg 2125, S. Africa.

Boehringer Ingelheim, Swed. Boehringer Ingelheim AB, Box 44, 127 21 Skärholmen, Sweden.

Boehringer Ingelheim, UK. Boehringer Ingelheim Ltd, Southern Industrial Estate, Bracknell, Berks, England.

Boehringer Ingelheim, USA. Boehringer Ingelheim Ltd, 90 East Ridge, P.O. Box 368, Ridgefield CT 06877, USA.

Boehringer Mannheim, Belg. See *Boehringer Pharma, Belg.*

Boehringer Mannheim, Ger. Boehringer Mannheim GmbH, Sandhofer Strasse 116, Postfach: 310 120, 6800 Mannheim 31, W. Germany.

Boehringer Mannheim, S.Afr. Boehringer Mannheim (SA) (Pty) Ltd, 192 Hendrik Verwoerd Drive, Randburg, Johannesburg, S. Africa.

Boehringer Mannheim, Spain. Boehringer Mannheim SA, Copernico 61-63, Barcelona, Spain.

Boehringer Mannheim, Swed. Boehringer Mannheim Scandinavia AB, Box 147, 161 26 Bromma 1, Sweden.

Boehringer Mannheim, Switz. Boehringer Mannheim (Schweiz) AG, Riedstr., 6330 Cham, Switzerland.

Boehringer Pharma, Belg. Boehringer Pharma S.A., Ave des Croix de Guerre 90, 1120 Brussels, Belgium.

Boehringer Sohn, Arg. C.H. Boehringer Sohn, Chile 80 6° 7° 8°piso, 1098 Buenos Aires, Argentina.

Boehringer Sohn, Spain. C.H. Boehringer Sohn Ingelheim SA, Pablo Alcover 33, Barcelona, Spain.

Boehringer Sohn, Switz. C.H. Boehringer Sohn GmbH, Peter-Merian-Strasse 19, Basel, Switzerland.

Boffi, Ital. Boffi Antonio, Via M. di Lando 88, 00162 Rome, Italy.

Bofors, Norw. See *Playtex-Wallco, Norw.*

Bofors, Switz. See *Globopharm, Switz.*

Boi, Spain. Boi Laboratorios, Padilla 370, Barcelona, Spain.

Boizot, Spain. Laboratorio E. Boizot, Luis Cabrera 63, Madrid 2, Spain.

Bonal, Switz. Bonal S.A., 3 place de la Riponne, 1005 Lausanne, Switzerland.

Bonfield, Eire. Bonfield Ltd, Ballymore Eustace, Co. Kildare, Eire.

Boniscontro & Gazzone, Ital. Lab. Prod. Farm. Boniscontro & Gazzone del Dr M. Pensa & C., Corso Racconigi 23, 10139 Torino, Italy.

Bonmati, Spain. Bonmati, Spain.

Bonomelli-Hommel, Ital. Bonomelli Hommel Farmaceutici, Divisione della Bonomelli s.p.a., Via Montecuccoli 1, 22042 Dolzago, Italy.

Bonru Perel, Arg. Lab. Bonru Perel, Rafaela 4831, 1407 Buenos Aires, Argentina.

Booker Health, UK. Booker Health Foods Ltd, Healthways House, 45 Station Approach, West Byfleet, Surrey, England.

Boots-Dacour, Fr. Laboratoires Boots-Dacour, 49 rue de Bitche, B.P. 66, 92404 Courbevoie Cedex, France.

Boots, Denm. See *A.L.-Pharma, Denm.*

Boots-Formenti, Ital. Boots Formenti s.p.a., Via Correggio 28, 20149 Milan, Italy.

Boots, Norw. See *Apothekernes Laboratorium, Norw.*

Boots, UK. The Boots Company Ltd, Nottingham NG2 3AA, England.

Boots, USA. Boots Pharmaceuticals Inc., 6540 Line Ave, P.O. Box 6750, Shreveport LA 71106, USA.

Borromeo, Ital. Borromeo Laboratori Farmaco-biologici s.r.l., Via Mac Mahon 45, 20155 Milan, Italy.

Bottasso, Ital. Farmaceutici Bottasso s.a.s., Via Dal Lino 23, 40134 Bologna, Italy.

Bottu, Belg. Laboratoire Bottu c/o Roussel S.A., Ave Adolphe Lacomblé 59-61, 1040 Brussels, Belgium.

Bottu, Fr. Bottu, 52 ave du Maréchal-Joffre, 92024 Nanterre Cedex, France.

Bottu, Switz. See *Siegfried, Switz.*

Bouchara, Fr. Laboratoires du Dr E. Bouchara, 8 rue Pastourelle, 75003 Paris, France.

Bouchard, Fr. Laboratoires Bouchard, 6 rue Anna-Jacquin, 92102 Boulogne-sur-Seine, France.

Bournonville, Neth. Bournonville-Pharma B.V., De Steiger 196, 1351 AV Almere, Netherlands.

Bouteille, Fr. Laboratoires Bouteille, 7 rue des Belges, 87000 Limoges, France.

Bouty, Ital. Laboratori Bouty s.p.a. it., Via Teodosio 17, 20131 Milan, Italy.

Bovril, UK. Bovril Ltd, Southbury Rd, Enfield, Middx EN1 1YP, England.

Box, UK. W.H. Box, 47 Mayflower St, Plymouth, England.

BP Chemicals, UK. BP Chemicals Ltd, Belgrave House, 76 Buckingham Palace Rd, London SW1W 0SU, England.

Bracco, Ital. Bracco Industria Chimica s.p.a., Via E. Folli 50, 20134 Milan, Italy.

Bracco, S.Afr. See *SCS, S.Afr.*

Bragg, UK. J.L. Bragg (Ipswich) Ltd, Tower St, Ipswich, Suffolk IP1 3BE, England.

Brassovora, Arg. Brassovora S.R.L., Cerrito 836-8°Piso, 1010 Buenos Aires, Argentina.

Braun, Denm. See *Ottosen, Denm.*

Braun Melsungen, Ger. B. Braun Melsungen AG, Carl-Braun-Strasse 1, Postfach: 110+120, 3508 Melsungen, W. Germany.

Braun, Norw. See *KSL, Norw.*

Brentchem, UK. Brentchem Ltd, International Way, Southall Lane, Heston, Middx TW5 9NJ, England.

Breon, USA. Breon Laboratories Inc., 90 Park Ave, New York NY 10016, USA.

Bristol, Austral. Bristol Laboratories, 345 Pacific Highway, Crows Nest NSW 2065, Australia.

Bristol, Belg. S.A. Bristol Benelux, chaussée de la Hulpe 185, 1170 Brussels, Belgium.

Bristol, Canad. Bristol Laboratories of Canada, Bristol-Myers Canada Inc., 100 Industrial Blvd, Candiac, Quebec J5R 1J1, Canada.

Bristol Europe, Ital. Bristol Europe s.p.a., Mead Johnson Divisione Farmaceutici, Via A. Bargoni 8/78, 00153 Rome, Italy.

Bristol, Fr. Laboratoires Bristol, 32 rue de l'Arcade, 75008 Paris, France.

Bristol, Ger. Bristol-Arzneimittel, Niederlassung Bensberg der Bristol-Myers GmbH, Rosenstrasse 10, Postfach: 209, 5060 Bergisch Gladbach 1, W. Germany.

Bristol Italiana Sud, Ital. Bristol Italiana (Sud) s.p.a., Via A. Bargoni 8, 00153 Rome, Italy.

Bristol-Myers Pharmaceuticals, UK. Bristol-Myers Pharmaceuticals, A division of Bristol-Myers Co. Ltd, Station Rd, Langley, Slough SL3 6EB, England.

Bristol-Myers, Spain. Bristol-Myers SA, Isla de Java 1, Madrid 34, Spain.

Bristol-Myers, UK. Bristol-Myers Co. Ltd, Station Rd, Langley, Slough SL3 6EB, England.

Bristol, Neth. Bristol-Myers B.V., Slochterenlaan 12, 1405 AM Bussum, Netherlands.

Bristol, Norw. See *Apothekernes Laboratorium, Norw.*

Bristol, NZ. Bristol Laboratories, P.O. Box 37-117, Parnell, Auckland 1, New Zealand.

Bristol, Swed. Bristol Laboratorier AB, Box 4100, 171 04 Solna, Sweden.

Bristol, Switz. Bristol-Myers S.A., Riedstrasse 3, 6330 Cham, Switzerland.

Bristol, USA. Bristol Laboratories, Division of Bristol-Myers Co., Thompson Rd, P.O. Box 657, Syracuse NY 13201, USA.

Britannia Health, UK. Britannia Health Products Ltd, 7 High St, Reigate, Surrey, England.

British Celanese, UK. British Celanese Ltd, P.O. Box 5, Spondon, Derby DE2 7BP, England.

British Chemotheutic, UK. British Chemotheutic Products Ltd, Kemtheutic House, Grant St, Bradford, West Yorkshire BD3 9HF, England.

British Cod Liver Oils, UK. British Cod Liver Oils Ltd, Marfleet, Hull, North Humberside HU9 5NJ, England.

British Traders & Shippers, UK. British Traders & Shippers Ltd, 6 Merrielands Crescent, Dagenham, Essex, England.

Brocades, Ital. Brocades s.p.a., Viale Spagna 45, 20093 Cologno Monzese, Italy.

Brocades, UK. Brocades (Great Britain) Ltd, Brocades House, Pyrford Rd, West Byfleet, Weybridge, Surrey KT14 6RA, England.

Brocchieri, Ital. Stabilimento Chimico Farmaceutico Brocchieri dr. L. s.r.l., Via Tiburtina Km. 14.4, 00131 Rome, Italy.

Brothier, Fr. Laboratoires Brothier, 41 rue de Neuilly, 92000 Nanterre, France.

Brown, Austral. J.L. Brown, Australia.

Bruco, Ital. Farmaceutici Bruco s.r.l., Via E. Bazzano 12, 16019 Ronco Scrivia, Italy.

Bruneau, Belg. See *Du Bled, Belg.*

Bruneau, Fr. Laboratoires Bruneau, 204 ave du Maréchal-Juin, 92107 Boulogne Cedex, France.

Brunnengräber, Ger. Dr Christian Brunnengräber Chemische Fabrik GmbH Lübeck, Ratzeburger Allee 106, Postfach: 2052, 2400 Lübeck, W. Germany.

Bruschettini, Ital. Bruschettini s.r.l., Via Isonzo 6, 16147 Genova Sturla, Italy.

Bryan, Spain. Bryan, Spain.

BTP Cocker Chemicals, UK. BTP Cocker Chemicals Ltd, Nook Lane, Oswaldtwistle, Lancs BB5 3PQ, England.

Bucaneve, Ital. Bucaneve di Nerci Alessandro, Via Sercognani 15, 20156 Milan, Italy.

Budin, Ital. Dr Budin & C., Via Ombrone 1/A, 00198 Rome, Italy.

Burgess, UK. Edwin Burgess Ltd, Longwick Rd, Princes Risborough, Aylesbury, Bucks HP17 9RR, England.

Burton, Parsons, USA. Burton, Parsons & Co. Inc., 120 Westhampton Ave, Washington DC 20027, USA.

Bush Boake Allen, UK. Bush Boake Allen, A division of Albright & Wilson Ltd, Blackhorse Lane, London E17 5QP, England.

Buxton Chemical Products, UK. Buxton Chemical Products, 6 Channing Rd, Lytham St Annes, Lancs FY8 1BJ, England.

Byk, Belg. Byk Belga S.A., rue Anatole France 115-121/Bte 5, 1030 Brussels, Belgium.

Byk Essex, Ger. Byk-Essex Pharmazeutische GmbH, Sonnenstrasse 33 a, 8000 Munich 2, W. Germany.

Byk Gulden, Denm. See *Nordisk Droge, Denm.*

Byk Gulden, Ger. Byk Gulden Lomberg Chemische Fabrik GmbH, Byk-Gulden-Strasse 2, Postfach: 6500, 7750 Konstanz, W. Germany.

Byk Gulden, Ital. Byk Gulden Italia s.p.a., Via Giotto 1, 20032 Cormano, Italy.

Byk Gulden, Norw. See *Collett, Norw.*

Byk Gulden, S.Afr. Byk-Gulden, P.O. Box 51476, Randburg 2125, S. Africa.

Byk Gulden, Spain. Byk Gulden, Spain.

Byk Gulden, Swed. Byk Gulden Scandinavian Office, Skiljevägen 4A, 191 49 Sollentuna, Sweden.

Byk Gulden, Switz. See *Iromedica, Switz.*

Byk Liprandi, Arg. Byk Liprandi S.A.C.E.I., Delgado 1565, 1426 Buenos Aires, Argentina.

Byk-Mallinckrodt, UK. Byk-Mallinckrodt (UK) Ltd, 129G, Building 521, Southampton Rd, Heathrow Airport, Hounslow, Middx TW6 3JX, England.

Byk, Neth. Byk Nederland B.V., Weerenweg 29, 1161 AG Zwanenburg, Netherlands.

Caber, Ital. Caber Farmaceutici s.a.s., Via Trieste 41, 48100 Ravenna, Italy.

Calbiochem, USA. Calbiochem Co., P.O. Box 12087, San Diego CA 92119, USA.

Callol, Spain. Callol, Spain.

Calmic, Canad. Calmic Medical Division, Burroughs Wellcome Inc., 60 Riverview Ave, LaSalle, Quebec H8R 3S1, Canada.

Calmic, UK. Calmic Medical Division, The Wellcome Foundation Ltd, Crewe Hall, Crewe, Cheshire CW1 1UB, England.

Calor, UK. Calor Group Ltd, Key West, Windsor Rd, Slough, England.

Cambridge Laboratories, Austral. Cambridge Laboratories Pty Ltd, 397 Little Lonsdale St, Melbourne Vic. 3000, Australia.

Camlab, UK. Camlab Ltd, Nuffield Rd, Cambridge CB4 1TH, England.

Canderm, Canad. Canderm Pharmacal Ltd, 3300 Sartelow, St Laurent, Quebec H4R 1E3, Canada.

Candioli, Ital. Istituto Candioli Profilattico & Farmaceutico s.p.a., Via Manzoni 2, 10092 Torino Beinasco, Italy.

Cantassium Co., UK. The Cantassium Company, 225 Putney Bridge Rd, London SW15, England.

Capitol, Spain. Capitol, Spain.

Caranza, Ital. Laboratori Farmaceutici Caranza, Via Carrea 12, 16149 Genoa, Italy.

Care, UK. Care Laboratories Ltd, Badminton Court, Amersham, Bucks, England.

Carlo Erba & Deutsche Farmitalia, Switz. See *Essex, Switz.*

Carlo Erba, Ital. Farmitalia Carlo Erba s.p.a., Gruppo Montedison, Via Imbonati 24, 20159 Milan, Italy.

Carlton Laboratories, UK. Carlton Laboratories (UK) Ltd, 4 Manor Parade, Salvington Rd, Durrington, Worthing, West Sussex BN13 2JP, England.

Carnation Foods, UK. Carnation Foods Co. Ltd, Danesfield House, Medmenham, Marlow, Bucks SL7 2ES, England.

Carnegie, UK. Carnegie Medical, 1 Morley St, Loughborough, Leics LE11 1EP, England.

Carnrick, UK. Carnrick Laboratories, 52 The Parade, Oadby, Leicester LE2 5BB, England.

Carnrick, USA. Carnrick Laboratories Inc., 65 Horse Hill Rd, Cedar Knolls NJ 07927, USA.

Carrion, Fr. Laboratoires Carrion, 30 rue Henri-Régnault, 92400 Courbevoie, France.

Carter Bond, UK. Carter Bond Ltd, Attercliffe Rd, Sheffield S4 7XG, England.

Carter-Wallace, UK. Carter-Wallace Ltd, Wear Bay Rd, Folkestone, Kent, England.

Carulla Vekar, Spain. Carulla Vekar SA, Av. de Madrid 110, Barcelona, Spain.

Casasco, Arg. Lab. Casasco S.A., Boyacá 237/41, 1406 Buenos Aires, Argentina.

Cascan, Ger. Cascan GmbH, Hüttenstrasse 10, Postfach: 1907, 6200 Wiesbaden-Schierstein, W. Germany.

Casen-Roncales, Spain. Laboratorios Casen-Roncales SA, Tenor Fleta 5, Zaragoza, Spain.

Casgrain & Charbonneau, Canad. Casgrain & Charbonneau Ltée, 445 St Lawrence Blvd, Montreal, Quebec H2Y 2Y8, Canada.

Cassella-med, Ger. Cassella-med GmbH, ein Unternehmen der Hoechst-Gruppe, Gereonstrasse 50, Postfach: 101104, 5000 Cologne 1, W. Germany.

Cassella-Riedel, Belg. See *CCP, Belg.*

Cassella-Riedel, Ger. Cassella-Riedel Pharma GmbH, Hanauer Landstrasse 521, 6000 Frankfurt (Main) 61, W. Germany.

Cassella-Riedel, Switz. See *Hoechst, Switz.* and *Opopharma, Switz.*

Cassenne, Fr. Laboratoires Cassenne, 3 square Desaix, 75015 Paris, France.

Cassenne-Takeda, Fr. Laboratoires Cassenne-Takeda, 3 square Desaix, 75015 Paris, France.

Cassenne, UK. Cassenne Ltd, Roussel House, Wembley Park, Middx HA9 0NF, England.

Castejon, Spain. Laboratorio Castejon SA, Edificio Europharma, Autopista de Barajas Km 12, Madrid 22, Spain.

Castillon, Spain. Laboratorios Castillon SA, Breton de los Herreros 69, Madrid, Spain.

Causyth, Ital. Causyth s.p.a., Via Serio 6, 20139 Milan, Italy.

CAVF, Spain. CAVF, Spain.

CCP, Belg. Comptoir Chimico Pharmaceutique, chaussée d'Alsemberg 1001, 1180 Brussels, Belgium.

Ceccarelli, Ital. Ceccarelli A. & C. dei F.lli dr. Tanganelli, Via G. Caponsacchi 31, 50126 Firenze, Italy.

Cecef, Spain. Cecef, Spain.

Cedona, Neth. Cedona Haarl. Pharm. Fabriek B.V., Oudeweg 147, 2031 CC Haarlem, Netherlands.

Celaton, UK. Celaton Laboratory Research Ltd, 201 Headstone Lane, Harrow, Middx HA2 6ND, England.

Celtia, Arg. Lab. Celtia S.R.L., B. Mitre 4284, 1201 Buenos Aires, Argentina.

Central Pharmacal, USA. The Central Pharmacal Co., 110-128 East Third St, Seymour IN 47274, USA.

Centrallab., Denm. Central Laboratoriet, Kirkevejen 20, Teestrup, 4690 Haslev, Denmark.

Centrum, Spain. Centrum SA, Sagitario 12, Llano del Espartal (Alicante), Spain.

CEPA, Spain. Compania Española de la Penicilina Antibioticos, Avda. Generalisimo 15-17, Madrid 16, Spain.

Ceresium, Switz. Ceresium S.A., Corso Elvezia, 6900 Lugano, Switzerland.

Cétrane, Fr. Laboratoire Cétrane, 92 rue Baudin, 92307 Levallois, France.

Cetus, Arg. Laboratorio Cetus, Querandíes 4275, 1183 Buenos Aires, Argentina.

Cevep, Switz. Cevep S.A., 5 rue M.A.-Calame, 2400 Le Locle, Switzerland.

Chamberlains, S.Afr. See *Warner, S.Afr.*

Charnwood, UK. Charnwood Pharmaceuticals Ltd, 69 Abbey Lane, Leicester LE4 5QT, England.

Charton, Canad. Charton Laboratories, 9393 Louis-H. Lafontaine, Montreal, Quebec H1J 1Y8, Canada.

Chassot, Switz. Chassot & Cie AG, Sägestrasse 73, 3098 Köniz, Switzerland.

Chatfield Laboratories, UK. Chatfield Laboratories, Rear of 208 York Rd, London SW11, England.

Chauvin-Blache, Fr. Laboratoires Chauvin-Blache, S.A., 104 rue de la Galera, B.P. 1174, 34009 Montpellier Cedex, France.

Chauvin-Blache, Switz. See *Novopharma, Switz.*

Chefaro, Ger. Deutsche Chefaro Pharma GmbH, Bäkkerstrasse 3, Postfach: 1330, 4670 Lünen (Westf.), W. Germany.

Chefaro, Neth. Chefaro International B.V., Keileweg 8, 3029 BS Rotterdam, Netherlands.

Chefaro, UK. Chefaro Proprietaries Ltd, Crown House, London Rd, Morden, Surrey, England.

Chelsea Drug & Chemical, UK. Chelsea Drug & Chemical Co. Ltd, 310 Old Brompton Rd, London SW5 9JQ, England.

Chemfarma, S.Afr. See *Restan, S.Afr.*

Chemical & Insulating Co., UK. The Chemical & Insulating Co. Ltd, West Auckland Rd, Darlington, Co Durham DL3 0UR, England.

Chemie-Linz, Aust. Chemie-Linz AG, St-Peter-Strasse 25, 4021 Linz, Austria.

Chemie-Linz, Denm. See *Astra, Denm.*

Chemie-Linz, Switz. See *Globopharm, Switz.* and *Max Ritter, Switz.*

Chemil, Ital. Chemil, Chemioterapici Milano s.r.l., Via Cavour 41/43, 20026 Novate Milanese, Italy.

Cheminova, Spain. Cheminova Española SA, Emilio Muñoz 15, Madrid 17, Spain.

Chemipharm, Ger. Chemipharm GmbH & Co., Chemisch-pharmazeutische Fabrik KG, Sachsenring 37-47, 5000 Cologne 1, W. Germany.

Chemipharm, Switz. See *Rutara, Switz.*

Chephasaar, Ger. Chephasaar, Chemisch-Pharmazeutische Fabrik GmbH, Mühlstrasse 50, Postfach: 120, 6670 St Ingbert, W. Germany.

Chesebrough-Pond's, UK. Chesebrough-Pond's Ltd, P.O. Box 242, Consort House, Victoria St, Windsor, Berks SL4 1EX, England.

Chibret, Belg. See *UPB, Belg.*

Chibret, Neth. Chibret, divisie van Merck, Sharp & Dohme B.V., Waarderweg 39, 2031 BN Haarlem, Netherlands.

Chiesi, Ital. Chiesi Farmaceutici s.p.a., Via Palermo 30, 43100 Parma, Italy.

Chimimportexport, Switz. See *Grosclaude, Switz.*

Chinoin, Hung. Chinoin Gyógyszer-és Vegyészeti Termékek Gyára, 26 Rottenbiller V., 1077 Budapest, Hungary.

Chinoin, Ital. Chinoin s.p.a., Via Zanella 3/5, 20133 Milan, Italy.

Chinosol, Denm. See *Baungaard, Denm.*

Chinosolfabrik, Ger. Chinosolfabrik Zweigniederlassung der Riedel-de Haën Aktiengesellschaft, 3016 Seelze 1 (Hannover), W. Germany.

Chipman, UK. Chipman Ltd, Goods Yard, Station, Horsham, West Sussex, England.

Chlor-Chem, UK. Chlor-Chem Ltd, Hauxton, Cambridge CB2 5HU, England.

Choay, Fr. Laboratoire Choay, 46 ave Théophile-Gautier, 75782 Paris Cedex 16, France.

Christiaens, Belg. A. Christiaens S.A., rue de l'Etuve 60, 1000 Brussels, Belgium.

Christiaens, Neth. See *Lamepro, Neth.*

Christiaens, Switz. See *Biomed, Switz.* and *Laboromand, Switz.*

Christy, UK. Thomas Christy Ltd, North Lane, Aldershot, Hants, England.

Chugai, Jap. Chugai Pharmaceutical Co. Ltd, TMM Bldg, 10-6 Iwamotocho 1-chome, Chiyoda-ku, Tokyo 101, Japan.

Ciba, Arg. Ciba-Geigy S.A.I.C.yF., Arias 1851, 1429 Buenos Aires, Argentina.

Ciba, Austral. Ciba Pharmaceuticals, 14 Orion Rd, Lane Cove NSW 2066, Australia.

Ciba, Belg. Ciba-Geigy, Noordkustlaan 18, 1720 Groot-Bijgaarden, Belgium.

Ciba, Canad. Ciba Pharmaceuticals, Division of Ciba-Geigy Canada Ltd, 205 Bouchard Blvd, Dorval, Quebec H9S 1B1, Canada.

Ciba, Denm. Ciba-Geigy A/S, Lyngbyvej 172, 2100 Copenhagen Ø, Denmark.

Ciba, Fr. Laboratoires Ciba-Geigy, Dépt. Ciba, 2 et 4 rue Lionel-Terray, 92506 Rueil-Malmaison, France.

Ciba-Geigy Agrochemicals, UK. Ciba-Geigy Agrochemicals, Whittlesford, Cambridge CB2 4QT, England.

Ciba-Geigy, Switz. Ciba-Geigy AG, Schwarzwaldallee 215, 4058 Basel, Switzerland.

Ciba-Geigy, UK. Ciba-Geigy (UK) Ltd, Industrial Chemicals Division, Tenax Rd, Trafford Park, Manchester M17 1WT, England.

Ciba-Geigy, USA. Ciba-Geigy Corporation, 556 Morris Ave, Summit NJ 07901, USA.

Ciba, Ger. Ciba Pharmazeutika, Ciba-Geigy GmbH, Öflinger Strasse, Postfach: 1160/1180, 7867 Wehr (Baden), W. Germany.

Ciba, Ital. Ciba Geigy s.p.a., 21040 Origgio, Italy.

Ciba, Neth. Ciba Farmaca, Raapopseweg 1, 6824 DP Arnhem, Netherlands.

Ciba, Norw. Ciba-Geigy Pharma A/S, Strømsvn. 49-53, Postboks 124, 2011 Strømmen, Norway.

Ciba, NZ. Ciba Pharmaceuticals, P.O. Box 19, 109 Avondale, Auckland, New Zealand.

Ciba, S.Afr. Ciba (Pharmaceutical Division), P.O. Box 92, Isando 1600, S. Africa.

Ciba, Spain. Ciba-Geigy SA, Paseo Carlos I 206, Barcelona, Spain.

Ciba, Swed. Ciba-Geigy Läkemedel AB, Box 605, 421 26 V Frölunda, Sweden.

Ciba, Switz. See *Ciba-Geigy, Switz.*

Ciba, UK. Ciba Laboratories, Wimblehurst Rd, Horsham, West Sussex RH12 4AB, England.

Ciba, USA. Ciba Pharmaceutical Co., Division of Ciba-Geigy Corporation, 556 Morris Ave, Summit NJ 07901, USA.

Ciccarelli, Ital. Farmaceutici dott. Ciccarelli s.p.a., Via Clemente Prudenzio 13, 20138 Milan, Italy.

Cidan, Spain. Cidan SA, Ulldecona 77, Benicarlo (Castellon), Spain.

Cif, Ital. Cif Prodotti Medicinali s.r.l., Via Roccagiovine 253/255, 00156 Rome, Italy.

Cifa, Ital. Cifa Farmaceutici s.p.a., Corso Venezia 10, 10155 Torino, Italy.

Cilag-Chemie, Aust. Cilag-Chemie GmbH, Inzersdorfer Strasse 64, 1102 Vienna X, Austria.

Cilag-Chemie, Belg. Cilag-Chemie S.A., Stationstraat 82, 2300 Turnhout, Belgium.

Cilag-Chemie, Denm. See *Mecobenzon, Denm.*

Cilag-Chemie, Ital. Cilag Chemie Italiana s.p.a., Via Palmanova 67, 20132 Milan, Italy.

Cilag-Chemie, Neth. See *ACF, Neth.*

Cilag-Chemie, Norw. Cilag-Chemie Informasjonskontor, Boks 166, 1312 Slependen, Norway.

Cilag-Chemie, Swed. Cilag-Chemie AB, Box 7073, 191 07 Sollentuna, Sweden.

Cilag-Chemie, Switz. Cilag-Chemie AG, Hochstrasse 205-209, 8200 Schaffhausen, Switzerland.

Cilag, Ger. Cilag GmbH, Neue Bergstrasse 9, Postfach: 32, 6146 Alsbach, W. Germany.

Cinfa, Spain. Cinfa, Spain.

City Chemical Corp., USA. City Chemical Corporation, 132 West 22nd St, New York NY 10011, USA.

Clarben, Spain. Clarben, Spain.

Clariana, Spain. Clariana-Pico SA, Carr Carlet-Valencia km 0.500, Apart 4, Carlet (Valencia), Spain.

Clark Proprietaries, UK. Clark Proprietary Medicines (UK) Ltd, P.O. Box 3, Pangbourne, Berks, England.

Climax, Arg. Climax Argentina S.R.L., San Nicolas 674/78, 1407 Buenos Aires, Argentina.

Clin-Comar-Byla, Fr. Laboratoires Clin Midy, Dépt. Clin-Comar-Byla, 20 rue des Fossés-St-Jacques, 75240 Paris Cedex 05, France.

Clin-Midy, Belg. Clin-Midy S.A., ave Jean Jaures 50, 1030 Brussels, Belgium.

Clin Midy, Fr. Laboratoires Clin Midy, 20 rue des Fossés-St-Jacques, 75240 Paris Cedex 05, France.

Clin-Midy, Neth. Clin-Midy B.V., Verrijn Stuartlaan 27, 2288 EK Rijswijk, Netherlands.

Clin-Midy, Spain. Clin-Midy SA, Ecuador 6, Barcelona, Spain.

Clin-Midy, Switz. Clin-Midy S.A., rte de la Galaise 32, 1228 Plan-les-Ouates, Switzerland.

CMW Laboratories, UK. CMW Laboratories Ltd, Bone Cement Division, Cornford Rd, Blackpool, England.

Co-Caps, UK. Co-Caps (Coded Capsules), 361 Lillie Rd, London SW6 7PA, England.

Coates & Cooper, UK. Coates & Cooper Ltd, Hill Farm Ave, Watford WD2 7RA, England.

Cochard, Belg. Lab. Cochard S.A., rue Charles Parenté 5-7, 1070 Brussels, Belgium.

Codali, Belg. Codali S.A., square Ambiorix 10, 1040 Brussels, Belgium.

Coirre, Belg. See *Pharmethic, Belg.*

Coles, Belg. R. Coles S.A., Mommaertslaan 14, 1920 Diegem, Belgium.

Colgate-Palmolive, UK. Colgate-Palmolive Ltd, 76 Oxford St, London W1A 1EN, England.

Coli, Ital. Farmaceutici Coli s.r.l., Via Giacinto Carini 23, 00152 Rome, Italy.

Collett, Denm. See *Nordisk Droge, Denm.*

Collett, Norw. Collett-Marwell Hauge A/S, Drammensvn. 852, Postboks 204, 1371 Asker, Norway.

Collins of Norwich, UK. Collins of Norwich, 25 Gentleman's Walk, Norwich NR2 1NA, England.

Collins, UK. L.D. Collins & Co. Ltd, Sunray House, 9 Plantagenet Rd, New Barnet, Herts EN5 5JG, England.

Coloplast, UK. Coloplast Ltd, Bridge House, Orchard Lane, Huntingdon, Cambs PE17 4LN, England.

Colson & Kay, UK. Colson & Kay Ltd, Shentonfield Rd, Manchester M22 4RW, England.

Combe, UK. Combe UK Ltd, AMP House, Dingwall Rd, Croydon, Surrey, England.

Combustinwerk, Ger. Combustinwerk Eulitz & Co., Griesberg 2, Postfach: 1116, 8031 Seefeld/Obb., W. Germany.

Commonwealth Serum Laboratories, Austral. Commonwealth Serum Laboratories, 45 Poplar Rd, Parkville Vic. 3052, Australia.

Comprehensive Pharmaceuticals, UK. Comprehensive Pharmaceuticals Ltd, 95 Frampton St, London NW8 8NA, England.

Concept Pharmaceuticals, UK. Concept Pharmaceuticals Ltd, 59 High St, Rickmansworth, Herts WD3 2DA, England.

Connaught, Canad. Connaught Laboratories Ltd, 1755 Steeles Ave West, Willowdale, Ontario M2N 5T8, Canada.

Connaught, USA. Connaught Laboratories Inc., Swiftwater PA 18370, USA.

Consolidated Chemicals, UK. Consolidated Chemicals Ltd, The Industrial Estate, Wrexham, Clwyd LL13 9PS, Wales.

Consolidated Midland, USA. Consolidated Midland Corporation, 195 East Main St, P.O. Box 74, Brewster NY 10509, USA.

Contactasol, UK. Contactasol Ltd, Unit 2, Leigh Close, 161 Kingston Rd, New Malden, Surrey KT3 3NW, England.

Conti, Ital. Laboratorio Chimico Carlo Conti s.a.s., Via L. Gereschi 32, 56100 Pisa, Italy.

Continental Ethicals, S.Afr. Continental Ethicals (Pty) Ltd, P.O. Box 55307, Northlands 2116, S. Africa.

Continental Pharma, Belg. Continental Pharma S.A., ave Louise 135, 1050 Brussels, Belgium.

Continental Pharma, Neth. Continental Pharma Holland, Gerritsenweg 5, 7202 BP Zutphen, Netherlands.

Continental Pharma, Switz. See *Pharmos, Switz.*

Coop. Farm., Ital. Cooperativa Farmaceutica Società Cooperativa, Via Passione 8, 20122 Milan, Italy.

Cooper, Canad. Cooper Laboratories Ltd, 670 Curé Boivin Blvd, Boisbriand, Quebec J7G 2A7, Canada.

Cooper, Ger. Cooper Laboratories (Deutschland) GmbH, Pehmertanger Weg 3, Postfach: 1220, 2908 Friesoythe (Oldb.), W. Germany.

Cooper, Switz. Cooper S.A., 1701 Fribourg-Moncor, Switzerland.

Cooper, UK. Cooper Health Products Ltd, Gatehouse Rd, Aylesbury, Bucks HP19 3ED, England.

Cooper, USA. Cooper Laboratories Inc., 305 Fairfield Ave, Fairfield NJ 07006, USA.

CooperVision, UK. CooperVision Ltd, 21 The Avenue, Southampton SO9 1NP, England.

Coopervision, USA. Coopervision Pharmaceuticals Inc., P.O. Box 367, San German PR 00753, USA.

Cophar, Switz. Cophar S.A., 1701 Fribourg-Moncor, Switzerland.

Cortec, Norw. Cortec medisiner A/S, Drammensvn. 10, Oslo 2, Norway.

Cortec, Swed. Cortec Aktiebolag, Box 5073, 200 71 Malmo, Sweden.

Corvi, Ital. Camillo Corvi s.p.a., Viale dei Mille 3, 29100 Piacenza, Italy.

Cosmopharm, Switz. Cosmopharm AG, Zimmerlistrasse 6, 8004 Zurich, Switzerland.

Costantino, Ital. Costantino A. & C. s.p.a., Via F. Romana 11, 10083 Favria Canavese, Italy.

Cottrell, UK. Cottrell & Co., 15 Charlotte St, London W1P 2AA, England.

Courtois, Ital. Courtois Laboratori Farmaco Biologici s.r.l., Corso Chieri 13, 10132 Torino, Italy.

Covor, Belg. Laboratoires Covor S.A., rue Hobbema 41, 1040 Brussels, Belgium.

Cow & Gate, UK. Cow & Gate Ltd, Cow & Gate House, Trowbridge, Wilts BA14 8YX, England.

Cox Continental, UK. Cox Continental Ltd, Whiddon Valley, Barnstaple, Devon EX32 8NS, England.

Cox, UK. Arthur H. Cox & Co. Ltd, Whiddon Valley, Barnstaple, Devon EX32 8NS, England.

Cozzolino, Ital. Laboratori Cozzolino e Vecchione Cove s.n.c., Via delle Brecce 145, 80146 Naples, Italy.

Craveri, Arg. Craveri S.A.I.C., Arangreen 830, 1405 Buenos Aires, Argentina.

Creighton, Austral. R.M. Creighton Pty Ltd, Australia.

Crinex, Fr. Laboratoires Crinex, 1 ave du Dr-Lannelongue, 92120 Montrouge, France.

Crinos, Ital. Industria Farmacobiologica Crinos s.p.a., Piazza XX Settembre 2, 22079 Como Villaguardia, Italy.

Crippa e Berger, Ital. Crippa e Berger s.p.a., Corso Italia 22, 20122 Milan, Italy.

Cristalfarma, Ital. Cristalfarma s.r.l., Via L. da Vinci 168, 20090 Trezzano S.N., Italy.

Criston, Ital. Laboratorio del Criston di Vettorazzo Giovanni, Via Gaia da Camino 7, 31100 Treviso, Italy.

Croda, UK. Croda (Goole) Ltd, Rawcliffe Bridge, Goole, North Humberside DN14 8PN, England.

Croklaan, Neth. Croklaan B.V., Postbus 4, Wormerveer, Netherlands.

Crookes Laboratories, UK. Crookes Laboratories Ltd, P.O. Box 94, 1 Thane Rd West, Nottingham NG2 3AA, England.

Crookes Products, UK. Crookes Products Ltd, P.O. Box 94, 1 Thane Rd West, Nottingham NG2 3AA, England.

Crosara, Ital. Lab. Farmaco Biologico Crosara s.r.l., Via G. Carini 23, 00152 Rome, Italy.

Crown, UK. Crown Chemical Co. Ltd, Lamberhurst, Kent TN3 8DJ, England.

CT, Ital. C.T., Laboratorio Farmaceutico s.r.l., Via D. Alighieri 49-51, 18038 Sanremo, Italy.

Cuatrecasas-Darkey, Spain. Cuatrecasas-Darkey SA, Iradier 12, Barcelona, Spain.

Cullen & Davison, UK. Cullen & Davison Ltd, Portadown, Craigavon, Co Armagh, Northern Ireland.

Cupal, UK. Cupal Ltd, King St, Blackburn, Lancs BB2 2DX, England.

Cusi, Spain. Laboratorios Cusi SA, Carretera de Francia, Masnou (Barcelona), Spain.

Cussons, UK. Cussons (UK) Ltd, Kersal Vale, Manchester M7 0GL, England.

Cuticura, UK. Cuticura Laboratories Ltd, Clivemont Rd, Cordwallis Trading Estate, Maidenhead, Berks, England.

Cutter, Canad. Cutter Ltd, 8241 30th St SE, Calgary, Alberta T2C 1H7, Canada.

Cutter, UK. Cutter Laboratories Inc., 10 Quarry St, Guildford, Surrey GU1 3UZ, England.

Cutter, USA. Cutter Laboratories Inc., 4th & Parker Sts, Berkeley CA 94710, USA.

Cuxson, Gerrard, UK. Cuxson, Gerrard & Co. (Dressings) Ltd, 26 Fountain Lane, Oldbury, Warley, West Midlands B69 3BB, England.

Cyanamid, Belg. Cyanamid Benelux S.A. (Lederle), rue de Hennin 79, 1050 Brussels, Belgium.

Cyanamid, Ital. Cyanamid Italia s.p.a., Zona Ind. XV Strada, 95030 Catania, Italy.

Cyanamid-Lederle, Ger. Cyanamid GmbH, Abt. Lederle Arzneimittel, Pfaffenrieder Strasse 7, 8190 Wolfratshausen, W. Germany.

Cyanamid, Spain. Cyanamid Iberica SA, Apartado 471, Madrid, Spain.

Cyanamid, Swed. Cyanamid Nordiska AB, Archimedesvägen 4, 161 70 Bromma, Sweden.

Cyanamid, UK. Cyanamid of Great Britain Ltd, Chemicals Division, Fareham Rd, Gosport, Hants PO13 0AS, England.

Dagra, Belg. Dagra S.A., rue St-Ghislain 41, 1000 Brussels, Belgium.

Dagra, Neth. Dagra N.V., Verrijn Stuartweg 60, 1112 AX Diemen, Netherlands.

Daiichi, Jap. Daiichi Seiyaku Co. Ltd, 14-10 Nihonbashi 3-chome, Chuo-ku, Tokyo 103, Japan.

Dainippon, Jap. Dainippon Pharmaceutical Co. Ltd, 25 Doshomachi 3-chome, Higashi-ku, Osaka 541, Japan.

DAK, Denm. Danmarks Apotekerforening, Hammerichsgade 14, 1611 Copenhagen V, Denmark.

Dalcross, Austral. Dalcross, Australia.

Dales, UK. Dales Pharmaceuticals Ltd, Snaygill Industrial Estate, Keighley Rd, Skipton, North Yorkshire BD23 2RW, England.

Dallas, Arg. Dallas S.R.L., Perú 1236, 1141 Buenos Aires, Argentina.

Dalton Supplies, UK. Dalton Supplies Ltd, Nettlebed, Henley-on-Thames, Oxon RG9 5AB, England.

Daniel-Brunet, Fr. Laboratoires Daniel-Brunet, 112 rue de Silly, 92100 Boulogne-sur-Seine, France.

Danning, UK. P.A. Danning, 44 Morley Rd, Twickenham, Middx, England.

Dansk Dental Depot, Denm. Dansk Dental Depot A/S, Adelgade 5-7, 1304 Copenhagen K, Denmark.

Daro, Neth. Daro B.V., Lutmastraat 181-183, 1073 GX Amsterdam, Netherlands.

Daufresne, Switz. See *Pharmac-Service, Switz.*

Dausse, Fr. Laboratoires Dausse, 60 rue de la Glacière, 75621 Paris Cedex 13, France.

Dausse, Switz. See *Pharmac-Service, Switz.*

Davenport, UK. J.T. Davenport Ltd, 83 Union St, London SE1, England.

Davis & Geck, UK. Davis & Geck, A division of Cyanamid of Great Britain Ltd, Fareham Rd, Gosport, Hants PO13 0AS, England.

Davur, Spain. Davur SA, Pantoja 14, Madrid 2, Spain.

DDD, UK. DDD Ltd, 94 Rickmansworth Rd, Watford, Herts WD1 7JJ, England.

DDSA Pharmaceuticals, UK. DDSA Pharmaceuticals Ltd, 310 Old Brompton Rd, London SW5 9JQ, England.

De Angeli, Ital. Istituto De Angeli s.p.a., Via Serio 15, 20139 Milan, Italy.

De Angeli, S.Afr. See *Restan, S.Afr.*

de Angeli, Switz. See *Boehringer Sohn, Switz.* and *Unipharma, Switz.*

de Bournonville, Belg. Ets A. de Bournonville et Fils S.A., rue aux Fleurs 30-38, 1000 Brussels, Belgium.

De-No-Fa Lilleborg, Norw. A/S Denofa og Lilleborg Fabriker, Sandakervn. 56, Postboks 4236 Torshov, Oslo 4, Norway.

De-Nol, S.Afr. De-Nol Laboratories (SA) (Pty) Ltd, 112 Pritchard St, Johannesburg 2001, S. Africa.

De Witt, UK. De Witt International Ltd, Seymour Rd, London E10 7LX, England.

Deakin & Hughes, UK. G. Deakin & Hughes Ltd, 31 Somerset St, Abertillery, Gwent, Wales.

Debat, Belg. See *Dumas, Belg.*

Debat, Fr. Laboratoires Debat, 60 rue de Monceau, 75008 Paris, France.

Debat, Neth. See *Roussel, Neth.*

Debat, Switz. See *Pharmacal, Switz.*

Decon Laboratories, UK. Decon Laboratories Ltd, Conway St, Hove, Sussex BN3 3LY, England.

Degesch, Ger. Degesch GmbH, Frankfurt Main, W. Germany.

Degussa, UK. Degussa Ltd, 175 Tottenham Court Rd, London W1P 0BJ, England.

Deiters, Spain. Deiters, Spain.

Delagrange, Belg. See *Dumas, Belg.*

Delagrange, Fr. Laboratoires Delagrange, 39 blvd de Latour-Maubourg, 75340 Paris Cedex 07, France.

Delagrange, Neth. See *Pharmexport, Neth.*

Delagrange, Spain. Laboratorios Delagrange SA, Apartado 101, Alcobendas (Madrid), Spain.

Delagrange, Switz. See *Pharmos, Switz.*

Delalande, Belg. Lab. Delalande S.A., rue du Méridien 22, 1030 Brussels, Belgium.

Delalande, Fr. Laboratoires Delalande, 16 rue Henri-Regnault, 92402 Courbevoie, France.

Delalande, Ger. Delalande Arzneimittel GmbH, Aachener Strasse 201-209, Postfach: 410320, 5000 Cologne 41, W. Germany.

Delalande, Ital. Laboratori Delalande s.p.a., Via Torino 19, 10044 Pianezza Torino, Italy.

Delalande, Switz. Lab. Delalande S.A., Case postale 252, 1211 Geneva, Switzerland.

Delandale, UK. Delandale Laboratories Ltd, Delandale House, 37 Old Dover Rd, Canterbury, Kent CT1 3JB, England.

Delta Laboratories, Eire. Delta Laboratories Ltd, Fairdale Works, Artane, Dublin 5, Eire.

Dendron, UK. Dendron Distributors, 94 Rickmansworth Rd, Watford, Herts WD1 7JJ, England.

Dental Health Promotion, UK. Dental Health Promotion Ltd, 130 Finchley Rd, London NW3 5HS, England.

Dentinox, Ger. Dentinox Gesellschaft für Pharmazeutische Präparate Lenk & Schuppan, Nunsdorfer Ring 19, 1000 Berlin 48, W. Germany.

Denver, Austral. Denver Laboratories (Australia) Pty Ltd, 10 Clarke St, Crows Nest NSW 2065, Australia.

Dergo, Belg. Ets Dergo S.A., rue Franz Gailliard 2A, 1060 Brussels, Belgium.

Dermal Laboratories, UK. Dermal Laboratories Ltd, Tatmore Place, Gosmore, Hitchin, Herts SG4 7QR, England.

Dermalex, UK. Dermalex Co. Ltd, 146 Kilburn High Rd, London NW6 4JD, England.

Dermik, USA. Dermik Laboratories Inc., 500 Virginia Dr., Fort Washington PA 19034, USA.

Desbergers, Canad. Desbergers Ltd, 8480 St Lawrence Blvd, Montreal, Quebec H2P 2M6, Canada.

Desitin, Ger. Desitin-Werk Carl Klinke GmbH, Weg beim Jäger 214, Postfach: 63 01 20, 2000 Hamburg 63, W. Germany.

Dessy, Ital. Istituto Biologico Dessy s.p.a., Via S. Domenico 107-109, 50133 Firenze, Italy.

Deutsche Hydrierwerke, Ger. Deutsche Hydrierwerke, W. Germany.

Dexo, Fr. Laboratoires Dexo, 31 rue d'Arras, 92000 Nanterre, France.

Dexter, Arg. Dexter S.A.I.C., Corrientes 617-3°piso, 1043 Buenos Aires, Argentina.

Dexter, Spain. Dexter, Spain.

DHL Products, UK. DHL Products Ltd, New Mill, New St, Idle, Bradford, West Yorkshire, England.

Diabetylin, Ger. Diabetylingesellschaft, Nachf. Apotheker Hans Meixner, Dr-Georg-Spohn-Strasse 7, Postfach: 1161, 7902 Blaubeuren, W. Germany.

Diamant, Fr. Laboratoires Diamant, ave du Général-de-Gaulle, 92800 Puteaux, France.

Diamed, UK. Diamed Diagnostics Ltd, Mast House, Derby Rd, Bootle, Merseyside, England.

Diasan, Switz. Diasan AG, Stampfenbachstrasse 59, 8006 Zurich, Switzerland.

Dieckmann, Ger. Dieckmann Arzneimittel GmbH, Klasingstrasse 1-11, Postfach 2125 u. 2320, 4800 Bielefeld 1, W. Germany.

Dietary Foods, UK. Dietary Foods (Bletchley) Ltd, Cumberland House, Regal Drive, Soham, Ely, Cambs, England.

Dietary Specialities, UK. Dietary Specialities Ltd, London House, 42 Upper Richmond Rd West, London SW14 8DD, England.

Diethelm, Switz. Diethelm & Co. AG, Eggbühlerstrasse 14, 8050 Zurich, Switzerland.

Dietisa, Spain. Dietisa SA, Buenaventura Plaja 9, Barcelona, Spain.

Difa, Ital. Difa s.p.a., Gruppo Cooper Laboratories Inc., Via Monterosso 273, 21042 Caronno Pertusella, Italy.

Difrex, Austral. Difrex (Aust.) Laboratories, 13-19 Glebe St, Glebe NSW 2037, Australia.

Dismedic, Arg. Dismedic Arg. S.R.L., Thames 1144/46, 1414 Buenos Aires, Argentina.

Dispersa, Denm. See *Erco, Denm.*

Dispersa, Ger. Dispersa Baeschlin GmbH, Dornierstrasse 4, Postfach: 145, 8034 Germering, W. Germany.

Dispersa, Norw. See *Andersen, Norw.*

Dispersa, Switz. Dispersa Labor, Dr E. Baeschlin AG, Postfach 1086, 8401 Winterthur, Switzerland.

Dispert, Arg. Dispert S.A.I.C.A.I.yF., Ituzaingó 1010, 1272 Buenos Aires, Argentina.

Disprovent, Arg. Disprovent S.A. Esp. Med., Cervantes 2950, 1417 Buenos Aires, Argentina.

Dista, Denm. See *Lilly, Denm.*

Dista, Spain. Dista SA, Apartado 585, Madrid, Spain.

Dista, UK. Dista Products Ltd, Fleming Rd, Speke, Liverpool L24 9LN, England.

Dista, USA. Dista Products Company, Division of Eli Lilly & Co., P.O. Box 1407, Indianapolis IN 46206, USA.

Distillers Co., UK. The Distillers Co. (Malt Products) Ltd, Kirkliston, West Lothian EH29 9DN, Scotland.

Diversey, UK. Diversey Ltd, Weston Favell Centre, Northampton NN3 4PD, England.

Doak, Canad. See *Trans-Canada Dermapeutics, Canad.*

Doak, USA. Doak Pharmacal Co. Inc., 700 Shames Dr., Westbury, Long Island NY 11590, USA.

Doetsch, Grether, Switz. Doetsch, Grether & Cie AG, Steinentorstr. 23, 4051 Basel, Switzerland.

Dolorgiet, Ger. Dolorgiet Arzneimittelfabrik, Peter Doll KG, Koblenzer Strasse 112, Postfach: 2007 44, 5300 Bonn 2, W. Germany.

Dome, Austral. Dome Laboratories, Wellington Rd, Mulgrave Vic. 3170, Australia.

Dome, Denm. See *Baungaard, Denm.*

Dome/Hollister-Stier, UK. Dome/Hollister Stier, Division of Miles Laboratories Ltd, Stoke Court, Stoke Poges, Slough SL2 4LY, England.

Dome, Norw. See *Meda, Norw.*

Dome, USA. Dome Division, Miles Laboratories Inc., 400 Morgan Lane, West Haven CT 06516, USA.

Dominguez, Arg. Lab. Dominguez S.R.L., Av. La Plata 2552, 1437 Buenos Aires, Argentina.

Dompè, Ital. Dompè Farmaceutici s.p.a., Via S. Martino 12, 20122 Milan, Italy.

Doms, Fr. Laboratoires Doms, 4 rue Ficatier, 92400 Courbevoie, France.

Dorsey, USA. Dorsey Laboratories, Division of Sandoz Inc., P.O. Box 83288, Lincoln NE 68501, USA.

Dow, Canad. Dow Pharmaceuticals, Dow Chemical of Canada Ltd, 380 Elgin Mills Road East, Richmond Hill, Ontario L4C 5H2, Canada.

Dow Corning, UK. Dow Corning Ltd, Reading Bridge House, Reading, Berks RG1 8PW, England.

Dow Corning, USA. Dow Corning Corporation, Midland MI 48640, USA.

Dow, USA. Dow Pharmaceuticals, The Dow Chemical Co., P.O. Box 68511, Indianapolis IN 46268, USA.

Downs, UK. Downs Surgical Ltd, Church Path, Mitcham, Surrey CR4 3UE, England.

Draco, Denm. See *Astra, Denm.*

Draco, Norw. See *Astra, Norw.*

Draco, Swed. AB Draco, Box 1707, 221 01 Lund, Sweden.

Dreikehl, Spain. Dreikehl, Spain.

Dreluso, Ger. Dreluso Pharmazeutika, Dr Elten & Sohn, Market 5, Postfach: 140, 3253 Hessisch Oldendorf 1, W. Germany.

Drobena, Ger. Drobena Arzneimittel GmbH, Motzener Strasse 17, 1000 Berlin 48, W. Germany.

Du Bled, Belg. Du Bled, avenue Jean Jaurès 46/48, 1030 Brussels, Belgium.

Du Pont Pharmaceuticals, UK. Du Pont Pharmaceuticals, Du Pont (UK) Ltd, Wedgwood Way, Stevenage, Herts SG1 4QN, England.

Dubernard, Fr. Dubernard Hospital S.A., Laboratoire Pharmaceutique (Groupe Sanofi), 22 quai de Bacalan, 33075 Bordeaux Cedex, France.

Dukron, Ital. Dukron Italiana s.p.a., 04010 Campoverde, Italy.

Dulcis, Neth. See *Bournonville, Neth.*

Dumas, Belg. Labo. Dumas S.A., rue F. Debelder 15-17, 1200 Brussels, Belgium.

Dumas, UK. Dumas Chemicals (Tunbridge Wells) Ltd, Pantiles House, Neville St, Tunbridge Wells, Kent, England.

Dumex, Denm. A/S Dumex (Dumex Ltd), Prags Boulevard 37, 2300 Copenhagen S, Denmark.

Dumex, Neth. Dumex B.V., Min. Hartsenlaan 11, 1217 LR Hilversum, Netherlands.

Dumex, Norw. A/S Dumex, Postboks 53, Gml. Drammensv. 107, 1322 Høvik, Norway.

Dumex, S.Afr. Dumex, S. Africa.

Dumex, Swed. Dumex Läkemedel AB, Box 3501, 250 03 Helsingborg 3, Sweden.

Dumex, Switz. Dumex S.A., Baarerstrasse 10, 6300 Zug, Switzerland.

Dumont, Arg. Química Dumont Freres, Charcas 5013/15, 1425 Buenos Aires, Argentina.

Duncan, Flockhart, UK. Duncan, Flockhart & Co. Ltd, 700 Oldfield Lane North, Greenford, Middx UB6 0HD, England.

Dunhall, USA. Dunhall Pharmaceuticals Inc., Highway 59N, P.O. Box 100, Gravette AR 72736, USA.

Duphar, Belg. Duphar, Division de Philips, Place de Brouckère 2, 1000 Brussels, Belgium.

Duphar, Neth. Duphar Nederland B.V., Drentestraat 11, 1083 HK Amsterdam, Netherlands.

Duphar, Spain. Duphar SA, Martinez Villergas 2, Madrid 27, Spain.

Duphar, UK. Duphar Laboratories Ltd, Gaters Hill, West End, Southampton SO3 3JD, England.

Dupomar, Arg. Dupomar S.A.C.I.F., Av. Juan B. Justo 4840, 1416 Buenos Aires, Argentina.

DuPont de Nemours, USA. E.I. DuPont de Nemours & Co. Inc., Pharmaceutical Division, 1007 Market St, Wilmington DE 19898, USA.

Durachemie, Ger. Durachemie GmbH & Co. KG, Riedersteinstrasse 30, 8180 Tegernsee, W. Germany.

Dymond, Canad. Dymond Drugs Ltd, P.O. Box 697, 46 Spalding Drive, Brantford, Ontario N3T 5P9, Canada.

Dynamit Nobel, UK. Dynamit Nobel (UK) Ltd, Chemicals Division, Gateway House, 302 High St, Slough, Berks SL1 1HF, England.

E. Merck, Austral. E. Merck Pty Ltd, Australia.

E. Merck, Denm. See *Nordisk Droge, Denm.*

E. Merck, Ger. E. Merck, Frankfurter Strasse 250, Postfach: 4119, 6100 Darmstadt 1, W. Germany.

E. Merck, Neth. E. Merck Nederland B.V., Basisweg 34, 1043 AP Amsterdam, Netherlands.

E. Merck, Norw. Merck A/S, Platousgt. 2, Oslo 1, Norway.

E. Merck, Swed. E. Merck Aktiebolag, Sturegatan 8, 114 35 Stockholm, Sweden.

E. Merck, Switz. See *Oscar Brandenberger, Switz.*

E. Merck, UK. E. Merck Ltd, Four Marks, Alton, Hants GU34 5HG, England.

Eastman, UK. Eastman Chemical International AG, P.O. Box 66, Kodak House, Station Rd, Hemel Hempstead, Herts HP1 1JU, England.

E.C.M. Laboratories, UK. E.C.M. Laboratories, Jedburgh House, Jedburgh Rd, London E13 9LQ, England.

Ecobi, Ital. Farmaceutici Ecobi s.p.a., Via E. Bazzano, 16019 Ronco Scrivia, Italy.

Econo Med, USA. Econo Med Pharmaceuticals Inc., P.O. Box 3303, Burlington NC 27215, USA.

Eddé, Canad. J. Eddé Ltd, 202 Laurier Ave E, Montreal, Quebec H2T 1G1, Canada.

Efesal, Spain. Efesal, Spain.

Efeyn, Spain. Laboratorios Efeyn SA, Bravo Murillo 81, Madrid 3, Spain.

Eggochemia, Aust. Eggochemia, Fabrik chemischer u. pharmazeutischer Präparate, Dr Rigobert Plass, Heiligenstädter Strasse Nr. 158, 1195 Vienna XIX, Austria.

Egic, Belg. See *Atem, Belg.*

Egic, Fr. Egic, 45-Amilly, B.P. 172, 45203 Montargis Cedex, France.

Egic, Neth. See *Multi-Pharma, Neth.*

Egic, S.Afr. See *Remedia, S.Afr.*

Egic, Switz. See *Panpharma, Switz.*

Ego, Austral. Ego Pharmaceuticals Pty Ltd, 71-73 Taunton Drive, Cheltenham Vic. 3192, Australia.

EGYT, Hung. EGYT Gyógyszervegyészeti Gyár, 30 Kereszturi ut, 1106 Budapest, Hungary.

Eifelfango, Ger. Eifelfango, chemisch pharmazeutische Werke, J. Graf Metternich GmbH & Co. KG, Ringener Strasse 45, Postfach: 265, 5483 Bad Neuenahr-Ahrweiler, W. Germany.

Eisai, Jap. Eisai Co. Ltd, 6-10 Koishikawa 4-chome, Bunkyo-ku, Tokyo 112, Japan.

Elanco, UK. Elanco Products Ltd, Kingsclere Rd, Basingstoke, Hants RG21 2XA, England.

Elder, Belg. See *Wolfs, Belg.*

Elder, Canad. See *Canderm, Canad.*

Elder, S.Afr. See *Propan, S.Afr.*

Elder, Switz. See *Medicina, Switz.* and *Panpharma, Switz.*

Elder, USA. Paul B. Elder Co., 705 East Mulberry St, P.O. Box 31, Bryan OH 43506, USA.

Elea, Arg. Lab. Elea S.A.C.I.F.yA., Saladillo 2452, 1440 Buenos Aires, Argentina.

Electrolactil, Spain. Electrolactil, Spain.

Élerté, Fr. Laboratoires des Réalisations Thérapeutiques Élerté, 181 rue de la Goutte-d'Or, 93303 Aubervilliers Cedex, France.

Elida Gibbs, UK. Elida Gibbs Ltd, P.O. Box 1DY, Portman Square, London W1A 1DY, England.

Eliovit, Ital. Laboratori Eliovit, Via Marsala 31/C, 25100 Brescia, Italy.

Elkins-Sinn, USA. Elkins-Sinn Inc., A subsidiary of A.H. Robins Co., 2 Esterbrook Lane, P.O. Box 5483, Cherry Hill NJ 08034, USA.

Ellem, Ital. Laboratori Farmaco Biologici Ellem s.p.a., Corso Ticinese 89, 20123 Milan, Italy.

Elmu, Spain. Elmu SA, Emilio Vargas 2, Madrid 27, Spain.

Emyfar, Spain. Laboratorio Emyfar SA, Unificación 22-24, Hospitalet de Llobregat (Barcelona), Spain.

Endo, Austral. Endo Laboratories (Australia) Pty Ltd, 448 Pacific Highway, Artarmon NSW 2064, Australia.

Endo, Canad. Endo Laboratories, Subsidiary of E. I. du Pont de Nemours & Co. (Inc.), P.O. Box 550, Town of Mount Royal, Quebec H3P 3C7, Canada.

Endo, Denm. See *Winthrop, Denm.*

Endo, S.Afr. See *Berk, S.Afr.*

Endo, USA. Endo Laboratories Inc., 1000 Stewart Ave, Garden City NY 11530, USA.

Endopharm, Ger. Endopharm Arzneimittelfabrik GmbH, Philipp-Reis-Strasse 14, Postfach: 10 20 48, 6072 Dreieich-Sprendlingen, W. Germany.

Engelhard, Ger. Karl Engelhard, Fabrik pharmazeutischer Präparate, Sandweg 94, Postfach: 2764, 6000 Frankfurt am Main 1, W. Germany.

English Grains, UK. English Grains Ltd, Swains Park, Park Rd, Overseal, Burton-on-Trent, Staffs, England.

Enzypharm, UK. Enzypharm Biochemicals Ltd, P.O. Box 69, Harrogate, North Yorkshire HG1 4BB, England.

Epsilon, Arg. Laboratorio Epsilon S.A., Calle 118 (Ex. Martin Fierro), San Martin, Argentina.

Erba, Denm. See *Montedison, Denm.*

Erba, Norw. See *Montedison, Norw.*

Erco, Denm. Ercopharm A/S, Skelstedet 13-15, 2950 Vedbaek, Denmark.

Erco, Norw. See *Organon, Norw.*

Erco, Swed. Erco Läkemedel AB, Grevgatan 34, 114 53 Stockholm, Sweden.

Ern, Spain. Ern SA, Pedro IV 499, Barcelona, Spain.

Ernest Jackson, UK. Ernest Jackson & Co. Ltd, Crediton, Devon EX17 3AP, England.

Errekappa, Ital. Errekappa Euroterapici (Divisione della Bioresearch), Via Marcona 37, 20129 Milan, Italy.

Essex, Arg. Essex Arg. S.A.I.C., Maipu 1300 6°piso, 1006 Buenos Aires, Argentina.

Essex, Austral. Essex Laboratories Pty Ltd, Australian Subsidiary of Schering Corporation USA, 11 Gibbon Rd, Baulkham Hills NSW 2153, Australia.

Essex, Belg. N.V. Essex (Belgium) S.A., Subsidiary of Schering Corporation USA, ave de la Couronne 163, 1050 Brussels, Belgium.

Essex, Denm. Essex Pharma A/S, Hvedemarken 12, 3520 Farum, Denmark.

Essex, Ital. Essex Italia s.p.a., Via Ripamonti 89, 20139 Milan, Italy.

Essex, Neth. Essex (Nederland) B.V., Bankrashof 3, 1183 NP Amstelveen, Netherlands.

Essex, NZ. Essex Laboratories (NZ) Ltd, P.O. Box 22-074, Otahuhu, Auckland 6, New Zealand.

Essex, Spain. Essex (España) SA, Apartado 36220, Madrid 16, Spain.

Essex, Swed. Essex Läkemedel AB, Box 27190, 102 52 Stockholm, Sweden.

Essex, Switz. Essex Chemie AG, Postfach 834, 6002 Luzern, Switzerland.

Estedi, Spain. Estedi, Spain.

Ester, Spain. Laboratorio Farmacéutico Ester SA, Antonio Cabezon 17, Madrid 34, Spain.

Esterfarm, Ital. Esterfarm Laboratori Farmaceutici, Via del Tritone 66, 00187 Rome, Italy.

Esteve, Spain. Laboratorios del Dr Esteve SA, Avda. Virgen de Montserrat 221, Barcelona, Spain.

Ethical Research Products, UK. Ethical Research Products, Tunbridge Wells, England.

Ethichem, UK. Ethichem Ltd, 2 Mansfield Rd, South Croydon, Surrey CR2 6HN, England.

Ethicon, UK. Ethicon Ltd, P.O. Box 408, Bankhead Ave, Edinburgh EH11 4HE, Scotland.

Ethimed, S.Afr. Ethimed (Pty) Ltd, Waltloo, Pretoria, S. Africa.

Ethnor, Austral. Ethnor Pty Ltd, 1 Khartoum Rd, North Ryde NSW 2113, Australia.

Ethnor, S.Afr. Ethnor (Pty) Ltd, P.O. Box 273, Halfway House 1685, S. Africa.

Etris, Fr. Etris S.A.R.L., 14 rue de la Comète, 75007 Paris, France.

Eucomark, UK. Eucomark Distributors Ltd, Jedburgh House, Jedburgh Rd, London E13 9LQ, England.

Eufarma, Ital. Eufarma Cosmetici s.r.l., Via delle Panche 44, 50141 Firenze, Italy.

Eutherapie, Belg. Eutherapie Benelux, rue François Debelder 15-17, 1200 Brussels, Belgium.

Euthérapie, Fr. Euthérapie, 27 rue du Pont, B.P. 126, 92201 Neuilly-sur-Seine Cedex, France.

Evans Medical, UK. Evans Medical Ltd, 891 Greenford Rd, Greenford, Middx UB6 0HE, England.

Evans Vanodine, UK. Evans Vanodine International Ltd, Brierley Rd, Walton Summit Centre, Bamber Bridge, Preston PR5 8AH, England.

Evening Primrose Oil Co., UK. Evening Primrose Oil Co. Ltd, 17 Royal Crescent, Cheltenham, Glos GL50 3DA, England.

Ever Ready Razor Blade, UK. Ever Ready Razor Blade Co. Ltd, Quadrant Works, Manor Park Crescent, Edgware, Middx HA8 7LY, England.

Evident Dental Co., UK. Evident Dental Co. Ltd, 57 Wellington Court, Wellington Rd, London NW8 9TD, England.

Ex-Lax, UK. Ex-Lax Ltd, Fishponds Rd, Wokingham, Berks RG11 2QD, England.

Exa, Arg. Impex Ltda. S.A.C.I.F.I.A., Pedro Echague 2437, 1261 Buenos Aires, Argentina.

Fabo, Ital. Fabo Farmindustria s.a.s., Via del Borghetto 3 B, 40122 Bologna, Italy.

Fabre, Fr. Laboratoires Pierre Fabre, Départment médical de Fimex S.A., 125 rue de la Faisanderie, 75116 Paris, France.

Face, Ital. Face di Sergio Cavasotto & C., Laboratori Farmaceutici s.r.l., Via D. Menini 129, 16137 Genoa, Italy.

Faes, Spain. Fabrica Española de Productos Químicos y Farmacéuticos SA, Apartado 555, Bilbao, Spain.

FAIR Laboratories, UK. FAIR Laboratories Ltd, Squibb House, 141 Staines Rd, Hounslow, Middx TW3 3JB, England.

Falk, Neth. See *Tramedico, Neth.*

Falorni, Ital. Istituto Farmochimico Falorni s.p.a., Via Vasco De Gama 207, 50127 Firenze, Italy.

Famaco, Swed. Famaco AB, Box 9007, 102 71 Stockholm, Sweden.

Family Planning Sales, UK. Family Planning Sales Ltd, 28 Kelburne Rd, Cowley, Oxford OX4 3SZ, England.

Farber-Ref, Ital. Farber Ref s.p.a., Via Imperia 35, 20142 Milan, Italy.

Farco-Pharma, Ger. Farco-Pharma GmbH Pharmazeutische Präparate, Bergisch Gladbacher Strasse 180, Postfach: 800326, 5000 Cologne 80, W. Germany.

Fargal-Pharmasint, Ital. Laboratori Biochimici Fargal Pharmasint s.r.l., Via P. Cavallini 24, 00192 Rome, Italy.

Farge, Ital. Farge, Via Tortona 12, 16139 Genoa, Italy.

Farillon, UK. Farillon Ltd, Bryant Ave, Romford, Essex RM3 0PJ, England.

Farlabo, Spain. Farlabo, Spain.

Farley, UK. Farley Health Products Ltd, Torr Lane, Plymouth PL3 5UA, England.

Farma-Lepori, Spain. Farma-Lepori SA, Osio 7-9, Barcelona, Spain.

Farmabion, Spain. Farmabion SA, Carretera de Alcobendas Km 6.400, Madrid 16, Spain.

Farmacologico Milanese, Ital. Lab. Farmacologico Milanese s.n.c., Via Monterosso 273, 21042 Caronno Pertusella, Italy.

Farmacosmici, Ital. Farmacosmici s.r.l., Via A. Volta 24, 22100 Como, Italy.

Farmades, Ital. Farmades s.p.a. Farmaceutici Degussa & Schering, Via di Tor Cervara 282, 00155 Rome, Italy.

Farmalabor, Ital. Farmitalia Carlo Erba s.p.a., Gruppo Montedison, Via Imbonati 24, 20159 Milan, Italy.
Farmaroma, Ital. Farmaroma s.r.l., Laboratori Farmacobiologici, Via Prenestina 707, 00171 Rome, Italy.
Farmasimes, Spain. Simes Farmasimes SA, Zamora 46-48, Barcelona, Spain.
Farmer Hill, Austral. Farmer Hill, Australia.
Farmerid, Ital. Farmerid s.r.l., Via E. Nicolardi 254/B, 80151 Naples, Italy.
Farmigea, Ital. Farmigea s.p.a., Industria Chimico Farmaceutica, Via Carmignani 2, 56100 Pisa, Italy.
Farmila, Ital. Farmila-Farmaceutici Milano s.p.a., Via E. Fermi 50, 20019 Settimo Milanese, Italy.
Farmitalia Carlo Erba, Fr. Laboratoires Farmitalia Carlo Erba S.A., Tour Franklin, Cedex 11, 92081 Paris-La-Défense, France.
Farmitalia Carlo Erba, UK. Farmitalia Carlo Erba Ltd, Kingmaker House, Station Rd, Barnet, Herts EN5 1NU, England.
Farmitalia, Ger. Farmitalia Carlo Erba GmbH, Merzhauser Strasse 112, Postfach: 480, 7800 Freiburg, W. Germany.
Farmitalia, Ital. Farmitalia Carlo Erba s.p.a., Gruppo Montedison, Via Imbonati 24, 20159 Milan, Italy.
Farmitalia, Neth. See *ICN, Neth.*
Farmochimica Italiana, Ital. La Farmochimica Italiana s.p.a., Via N. d'Apulia 8, 20125 Milan, Italy.
Farmos, Denm. See *Nordisk Droge, Denm.*
Farnex, Ital. Farnex Laboratori s.p.a., Via Borsa 11, 20073 Codogno, Italy.
Fassett & Johnson, UK. Fassett & Johnson Ltd, New Rd, Winsford, Cheshire CW7 2NX, England.
Faulding, Austral. F.H. Faulding & Co. Ltd, 48 Beans Rd, Thebarton SA 5031, Australia.
Faure, Fr. Laboratoires H. Faure (Les Vitacollyres), 07104 Annonay Cedex, France.
Fawns & McAllan, Austral. Fawns & McAllan Pty Ltd, 432 Mount Dandenong Rd, Croydon Vic. 3136, Australia.
Fecofar, Arg. Fed. Arg. Coop. Farmac., John F. Kenedy 2742, 1754 San Justo (Pcia. de Bs. As.), Argentina.
Fedal, Spain. Fedal, Spain.
Federico Bonet, Spain. Federico Bonet SA, P. General Primo de Rivera 13, Madrid 5, Spain.
Fellows, USA. Fellows-Testagar, Subsidiary of Chromalloy Pharmaceuticals Inc., 12741 Capital Ave, Oak Park MI 48237, USA.
Fennings, UK. Fennings Pharmaceuticals, 46 London Rd, Horsham, West Sussex RH12 2DT, England.
Ferndale, USA. Ferndale Laboratories Inc., 780 West Eight Mile Rd, Ferndale MI 48220, USA.
Ferran, Spain. Instituto Ferran, Garcilaso 206-232, Barcelona, Spain.
Ferraton, Denm. Ferraton, Kirkevejen 20, 4690 Haslev, Denmark.
Ferrer, Spain. Ferrer Internacional SA, Gran Via Carlos III 94, Barcelona, Spain.
Ferring, Denm. Ferring A/S, Indertoften 5, 2720 Vanløse, Denmark.
Ferring, Ger. Ferring Arzneimittel GmbH, Wittland 11, Postfach: 2145 Fearz, 2300 Kiel, W. Germany.
Ferring, Norw. See *AFI, Norw.*
Ferring, Swed. Ferring AB, Box 305 61, 200 62 Malmo, Sweden.
Ferring, UK. Ferring Pharmaceuticals Ltd, 11 Mount Rd, Feltham, Middx TW13 6JG, England.
Ferrosan, Denm. A/S Ferrosan, Sydmarken 1-5, 2860 Søborg, Denmark.
Ferrosan, Norw. A/S Ferrosan, Treschowsgt. 2 b, Oslo 4, Norway.
Ferrosan, Swed. AB Ferrosan, Box 839, 201 80 Malmo, Sweden.
Fessenmayer, Switz. C. Fessenmayer, Postfach 52, 4011 Basel, Switzerland.
Feversham, UK. Feversham Products Ltd, 11 Lamb St, London E1, England.
Fher, Spain. Laboratorios Fher SA, Avda. Generalisimo Franco 635, Barcelona, Spain.
Fides, Spain. Laboratorio Fides, Vizcaya 417, Barcelona, Spain.
Fidia, Ital. Fidia, Farmaceutici Italiani Derivati Industriali e Affini s.p.a., Via Ponte d/ Fabbrica 3/A, 35031 Abano Terme, Italy.
Finadiet, Arg. Finadiet S.A.C.I.F.I., Hipólito Yrigoyen 3771, 1208 Buenos Aires, Argentina.
Fine Organics, USA. Fine Organics Inc., 205 Main St, Lodi NJ 07644, USA.
Fink, Ger. Johann Georg Fink GmbH & Co., Daimlerstrasse 3, Postfach: 1160, 7033 Herrenberg, W. Germany.
FIRMA, Ital. Fabbr. Ital. Ritrov. Medic. Aff. s.p.a., Via di Scandicci 37, 50143 Firenze, Italy.
Fisher, USA. Fisher Scientific Co., 52 Fadem Rd, Springfield NJ 07081, USA.
Fisons, Canad. Fisons Corporation Ltd, 80 Melford Dr., Scarborough, Ontario M1B 2G3, Canada.
Fisons, Denm. Fisons A/S, Rosenkaeret 22 A, 2860 Søborg, Denmark.
Fisons, Norw. Fisons, Vaekerøvn. 213, Oslo 7, Norway.
Fisons, S.Afr. Fisons Pharmaceuticals (Pty) Ltd, P.O. Box 5788, Johannesburg 2000, S. Africa.
Fisons, UK. Fisons Ltd, Pharmaceutical Division, Derby Rd, Loughborough, Leics LE11 0BB, England.
Fisons, USA. Fisons Corporation, Pharmaceutical Division, Two Preston Court, Bedford MA 01730, USA.
Fleming, USA. Fleming & Co., 1600 Fenpark Dr., Fenton MO 63026, USA.
Flint, USA. Flint Laboratories, Division of Travenol Laboratories Inc., One Baxter Parkway, Deerfield IL 60015, USA.
FMC Corp., USA. FMC Corporation, 1105 Coleman Ave, San Jose CA 95110, USA.
Ford, Austral. Ford, Australia.
Ford, Jackson, UK. Ford, Jackson & Co. (Sales) Ltd, Church St, Castleford, West Yorkshire, England.
Forest, Denm. See *Nordisk Droge, Denm.*
Formenti, Ital. Prodotti Formenti s.r.l., Via Correggio 43, 20149 Milan, Italy.
Forrest, Austral. Forrest Pharmaceutical Co. Pty Ltd, 7 Willis St, Arncliffe NSW 2205, Australia.
Fortbenton, Arg. Fortbenton Co. Laboratories S.R.L., Escalada 133, 1407 Buenos Aires, Argentina.
Fortuny, Spain. Fortuny SA, Pablo Piferrer 23, Palma de Mallorca, Spain.
Fougera, USA. E. Fougera & Co., Division of Byk-Gulden Inc., Cantiague Rd, Hicksville, Long Island NY 11802, USA.
Fournier Frères, Belg. See *Christiaens, Belg.*
Fournier Frères, Fr. Laboratoires Fournier Frères, 35 quai du Moulin-de-Cage, 92231 Gennevilliers, France.
Fournier S.A., Fr. Laboratoires Fournier S.A., 9 rue Petitot, 21100 Dijon, France.
Fournier, Switz. See *Galenica, Switz.* and *Vögelin, Switz.*
Francia Farm., Ital. Francia Farmaceutici s.r.l., Via dei Pestagalli 7, 20138 Milan, Italy.
Franklin Medical, UK. Franklin Medical, Division of Virgocrest Ltd, P.O. Box 138, Turnpike Rd, Cressex Industrial Estate, High Wycombe, Bucks HP12 3NB, England.
Fresenius, Ger. Dr E. Fresenius Chem.-Pharm. Industrie KG, Borkenberg 14, Postfach: 1809, 6370 Oberursel/Ts. 1, W. Germany.
Friis, Denm. Christian Friis & Co., Maltegårdsvej 18, 2820 Gentofte, Denmark.
Frosst, Canad. Charles E. Frosst & Co., P.O. Box 1005, Pointe Claire-Dorval, Quebec H9R 4P8, Canada.
Frumtost, Spain. Productos Frumtost SA, Suiza 9-11, Barcelona, Spain.
Fuchs, Switz. Dr med. H. Fuchs, Kurhaus, 6936 Cademario, Switzerland.
Fujisawa, Jap. Fujisawa Pharmaceutical Co. Ltd, 3 Doshomachi 4-chome, Higashi-ku, Osaka 541, Japan.
Fujisawa, S.Afr. See *Intal, S.Afr.*
Fujizoki, Jap. Fujizoki Pharmaceutical Co. Ltd, 6-7 Shimoochiai 4-chome, Shinjuku-ku, Tokyo 161, Japan.
Fulford Williams, UK. Fulford Williams (International) Ltd, Cornwall Rd, Hatch End, Pinner, Middx, England.
Fulton, Ital. Fulton Company s.a.s., Via M. Gonzaga 5, 20123 Milan, Italy.
Fumouze, Fr. Laboratoires Fumouze S.A., 1 rue Méchin, 93450 Ile-Saint-Denis, France.
Funk, Spain. Laboratorios Funk SA, Mallorca 288, Barcelona, Spain.
Furt, Fr. Laboratoires Furt, 2 rue de Rivière, 33074 Bordeaux Cedex, France.
Fushimi, Denm. See *Astra Meditec, Denm.*
Fuso, Jap. Fuso Pharmaceutical Industries Ltd, 3-11 Morinomiya 2-chome, Joto-ku, Osaka 536, Japan.
Fylde, UK. Fylde Laboratories, Kent St, Preston, Lancs PR1 1RR, England.
Gador, Arg. Lab. Dr Gador & Cía S.A.C.I., Florida 868, 1006 Buenos Aires, Argentina.
GAF, UK. GAF (Great Britain) Ltd, Tilson Rd, Roundthorn, Wythenshawe, Manchester M23 9PH, England.
Galactina, Ger. Galactina GmbH, Hans-Böckler-Strasse 22, Postfach: 301, 6078 Neu-Isenberg, W. Germany.
Galactina, Switz. Galactina AG, Birkenweg 2-8, 3123 Belp, Switzerland.
Galen, UK. Galen Ltd, 19 Lower Seagoe Industrial Estate, Craigavon, Co. Armagh BT63 5QD, Northern Ireland.
Galenica, Switz. Galenica Vertretungen AG, Untermattweg 8, 3001 Bern, Switzerland.
Galenus Mannheim, Ger. Galenus Mannheim GmbH, Geheimrat-Haas-Platz 50, Postfach: 310105, 6800 Mannheim 31, W. Germany.
Galepharma, Spain. Galepharma Ibérica SA, Via Augusta 173, Barcelona, Spain.
Gallier, Fr. Laboratoires Gallier S.A., 1 bis place du Président-Mithouard, 75007 Paris, France.
Galter, Ital. Farmaceutici Galter s.a.s., Via Tiburtina 1010, 00156 Rome, Italy.
Galup, Spain. Galup, Spain.
Gamaprod, Austral. Gamaprod Pty Ltd, Australia.
Gamir, Spain. Gamir SA Aurelio, Carr Barcelona 2, Almacera (Valencia), Spain.
Ganassini, Ital. Istituto Ganassini s.p.a. di Ricerche Biochimiche, Via Gaggia 16, 20139 Milan, Italy.
Garlisol, UK. The Garlisol Co. Ltd, 36 Cambridge Rd, Hastings, East Sussex, England.
Gattefossé, Fr. Ets Gattefossé, 36 chemin de Genas, 69800 St Priest, France.
Gayoso Wellcome, Spain. Gayoso Wellcome SA (Burroughs Wellcome), Carretera de Barcelona Km 26.300, Alcala de Henares (Madrid), Spain.
Gazzini, Ital. Farmaceutici Gazzini, Effegi, Via Francesco Cilea 4, 50144 Firenze, Italy.
GEA, Denm. Aktieselskabet GEA, Holger Danskesvej 89, 2000 Copenhagen F, Denmark.
GEA, Switz. See *Heineking, Switz.*, *Max Ritter, Switz.*, and *Revit, Switz.*
Gedeon Richter, Hung. Chemical Works of Gedeon Richter Ltd, 21 Gyomrol ut, 1475 Budapest 10, Hungary.
Gee Lawson, UK. Gee Lawson Chemicals Ltd, 404 Finchley Rd, London NW2 2HR, England.
Geigy, Arg. Ciba Geigy S.A.I.C.yF., Arias 1851, 1429 Buenos Aires, Argentina.
Geigy, Austral. Geigy Pharmaceuticals, 14 Orion Rd, Lane Cove NSW 2066, Australia.
Geigy, Belg. Ciba-Geigy, Noordkustlaan 18, 1720 Groot-Bijgaarden, Belgium.
Geigy, Denm. Ciba-Geigy A/S, Lyngbyvej 172, 2100 Copenhagen Ø, Denmark.
Geigy, Eire. Geigy Pharmaceuticals, 70 Northumberland Rd, Dublin 4, Eire.
Geigy, Fr. Laboratoires Ciba-Geigy, Dépt. Geigy, 2 et 4 rue Lionel-Terray, 92506 Rueil-Malmaison, France.
Geigy, Ger. Geigy Pharmazeutika, Ciba-Geigy GmbH, Öflinger Strasse, Postfach: 1160/1180, 7867 Wehr (Baden), W. Germany.
Geigy, Ital. Ciba-Geigy s.p.a., 21040 Origgio (Varese), Italy.
Geigy, Neth. Geigy farmaca, Raapopseweg 1, 6824 DP Arnhem, Netherlands.
Geigy, Norw. Ciba-Geigy Pharma A/S, Strømsvn. 49-53, Postboks 124, 2011 Strømmen, Norway.
Geigy, S.Afr. Geigy (Pharmaceutical Division), P.O. Box 92, Isando 1600, S. Africa.
Geigy, Spain. Ciba-Geigy SA, Paseo Carlos I 206, Barcelona, Spain.
Geigy, Swed. Ciba-Geigy Läkemedel AB, Box 605, 421 26 V Frölunda, Sweden.
Geigy, Switz. See *Ciba-Geigy, Switz.*
Geigy, UK. Geigy Pharmaceuticals, Wimblehurst Rd, Horsham, West Sussex RH12 4AB, England.
Geigy, USA. Geigy Pharmaceuticals, Division of Ciba-Geigy Corporation, Saw Mill River Rd, Ardsley NY 10502, USA.
Geistlich, Belg. See *Pharma-Produits, Belg.*
Geistlich, Denm. See *Meda, Denm.*
Geistlich, Neth. See *ICN, Neth.*
Geistlich, Switz. Ed. Geistlich Söhne AG, 6110 Wolhusen, Switzerland.
Geistlich, UK. Geistlich Sons Ltd, Newton Bank, Long Lane, Chester CH2 3QZ, England.
Gemini, UK. Gemini Pharmaceutical Products Ltd, Rawlings House, Rawlings St, London SW3, England.

General Diagnostics, UK. General Diagnostics, Warner-Lambert (UK) Ltd, Chestnut Ave, Eastleigh, Hants SO5 3ZQ, England.

General Pharm. Prods, USA. General Pharmaceutical Products Inc., 3205 Johnson Rd, Steubenville OH 43952, USA.

Génévrier, Fr. Laboratoires Génévrier, 45 rue Madeleine-Michelis, B.P. 149, 92202 Neuilly-sur-Seine, France.

Gentili, Ital. Istituto Gentili s.p.a., Via Mazzini 112, 56100 Pisa, Italy.

Gerda, Fr. Laboratoires Gerda, 6 rue Pierre-Basset, 69160 Tassin-la-Demi-Lune, France.

Gerot, Belg. See *Byk, Belg.*

Gerot, Switz. Gerot Pharmaceutica AG, 6280 Hochdorf, Switzerland.

Geve, Spain. Laboratorio Geve, Ciudad 3, Tortosa (Tarragona), Spain.

Gewo, Ger. Gewo Chemie GmbH, Schneidweg 5, Postfach: 110172, 7570 Baden-Baden 11, W. Germany.

Geyfarm, Ital. Geyfarm Industria Chimico-Farmaceutica s.p.a., Via Filatoio 12, 10066 Torre Pellice (Torino), Italy.

Geymonat Sud, Ital. Geymonat Sud s.p.a., Via S. Anna 2, 03012 Anagni, Italy.

G.F. Dietary Supplies, UK. G.F. Dietary Supplies Ltd, Lowther Rd, Stanmore, Middx HA7 1EL, England.

Ghimas, Ital. Ghimas s.p.a., Via R. Fucini 2, 40033 Casalecchio di Reno, Italy.

Gibipharma, Ital. Gibipharma s.p.a., Via Carlo Pisacane 10, 20016 Pero (Milano), Italy.

Girod, Switz. Ets. Henri Girod S.A., Ch. du Grand-Puits 28, 1217 Genève-Meyrin, Switzerland.

Girol, Switz. Girol AG, Helenastrasse 4, 8008 Zurich, Switzerland.

Gist-Brocades/Brocatrade, Neth. Gist-Brocades N.V., afd. Brocatrade, Wateringseweg 1, 2611 XT Delft, Netherlands.

Gist-Brocades, Denm. See *Nordisk Droge, Denm.*

Gist-Brocades, Neth. Gist-Brocades Farmaca Nederland B.V., Frijdastraat 7-9, 2288 EX Rijswijk, Netherlands.

Gist-Brocades, Norw. See *Collett, Norw.*

Giulini, Denm. See *Meda, Denm.*

Giulini, Ger. Giulini Pharma GmbH, Hans-Böckler-Allee 20, Postfach:220, 3000 Hannover 1, W. Germany.

Giulini, Neth. See *Schmidt, Neth.*

Giulini, Swed. See *Famaco, Swed.*

Giulini, Switz. See *Hausmann, Switz.*

Givaudan, USA. Givaudan Corporation, 100 Delawanna Ave, Clifton NJ 07014, USA.

Glaxo, Arg. Laboratorio Glaxo (Arg.) S.A.C.eI., J.J. Castelli 6701, 1605 Munro (Bs.As.), Argentina.

Glaxo, Denm. Glaxo Laegemidler A/S, Vermlandsgade 67, 2300 Copenhagen S, Denmark.

Glaxo, Ind. Glaxo Laboratories (India) Ltd, Dr Annie Besant Rd, Worli, Bombay-400 018, India.

Glaxo, Neth. Glaxo B.V., Parklaan 6-8, 2132 BN Hoofddorp, Netherlands.

Glaxo, Norw. See *Nyco, Norw.*

Glaxo, NZ. Glaxo Laboratories (NZ) Ltd, P.O. Box 1543, Palmerston North, New Zealand.

Glaxo, S.Afr. Glaxo, P.O. Box 485, Germiston 1400, S. Africa.

Glaxo, UK. Glaxo Laboratories Ltd, Greenford, Middx UB6 0HE, England.

Glaxo, USA. Glaxo Inc., 1900 West Commercial Blvd, Fort Lauderdale FL 33309, USA.

Glaxovet, UK. Glaxovet Ltd, Greenford, Middx UB6 0HE, England.

Glenden, Switz. See *Imal, Switz.*

Glenwood, UK. Glenwood Laboratories Ltd, 19 Wincheap, Canterbury, Kent CT1 3TB, England.

Globopharm, Arg. Globopharm Argentina S.A.C.I.F.I., B. Mitre 4284, 1201 Buenos Aires, Argentina.

Globopharm, Switz. Globopharm AG, Seestrasse 200, 8700 Küsnacht, Switzerland.

Gobbi-Novag, Arg. Laboratorio Gobbi-Novag S.A.I.C., F. Onsari 498 (Ex. Gral. Cadorna), 1875 Wilde, Argentina.

Gödecke, Ger. Gödecke Aktiengesellschaft, Salzufer 16, Postfach:10 02 50, 1000 Berlin 10, W. Germany.

Gödecke, Switz. See *Cosmopharm, Switz.*

Goldschmidt, UK. Th. Goldschmidt Ltd, Initial House, 150 Field End Rd, Eastcote, Middx HA5 1SA, England.

Goldschmidt, USA. Goldschmidt Chemical Corporation, P.O. Box 1299, Hopewell VA 23860, USA.

Gomenol, Fr. Laboratoires du Gomenol, 48 rue des Petites-Écuries, 75010 Paris, France.

Gonnon, Fr. Laboratoires Gonnon, 16 rue François-Dauphin, 69002 Lyon, France.

Goodrich, UK. B F Goodrich Chemical (UK) Ltd, Wellington House, 6 Upper St Martin's Lane, London WC2H 9DL, England.

Goupil, Fr. Laboratoires Goupil S.A., 30 ave du Président-Wilson, 94230 Cachan, France.

G.P. Laboratories, Austral. G.P. Laboratories, Division of Pfizer Pty Ltd, Wharf Rd, West Ryde NSW 2114, Australia.

Grace, UK. W.R. Grace Ltd, Northdale House, North Circular Rd, London NW10 7UH, England.

Graham Chemical Corp., USA. Graham Chemical Corporation Inc., P.O. Box 9434, Greensboro NC 27408, USA.

Gramon, Arg. Gerardo Ramón y Cía. S.A.I.yC., Cangallo 2683, 1040 Buenos Aires, Argentina.

Granata, Ital. Laboratori Chimico Biologici Granata s.p.a., Strada Padana Superiore 32, 20063 Cernusco (Milano), Italy.

Greeff, USA. Greeff, USA.

Green Cross Corp., Jap. The Green Cross Corporation, 1-47 Chuo 1-chome, Joto-ku, Osaka 536, Japan.

Greiter, Switz. Greiter Distribution AG, Bahnhofstrasse 51, 9450 Alstätten, Switzerland.

Grémy-Longuet, Fr. Laboratoires Grémy-Longuet, 15 rue Jean-Jaurès, 92807 Puteaux Cedex, France.

Grémy-Longuet, Switz. See *Uhlmann-Eyraud, Switz.*

Grimault, Fr. Laboratoires Grimault, 41 rue Camille-Pelletan, 92305 Levallois-Perret, France.

Grosclaude, Switz. Grosclaude S.A., Case postale 478, 1211 Geneva, Switzerland.

Grossmann, Switz. Dr Grossmann AG, Pharmaca, Binningerstrasse 95, 4123 Allschwil, Switzerland.

Grünenthal, Belg. See *Bios-Coutelier, Belg.*

Grünenthal, Ger. Grünenthal GmbH, Steinfeldstrasse 2, Postfach:129, 5190 Stolberg, W. Germany.

Grünenthal, S.Afr. Grünenthal (SA) Pty Ltd, P.O. Box 41298, Craighall 2024, S. Africa.

Grünenthal, Switz. See *Pharmacolor, Switz.*

Guadalupe, Spain. Guadalupe, Spain.

Guardian, USA. Guardian Chemical Corporation, 230 Marcus Blvd, Hauppauge, Long Island NY 11787, USA.

Guerbet, Belg. See *Codali, Belg.*

Guerbet, Denm. See *Lindeburg, Denm.*

Guerbet, Fr. Laboratoires Guerbet, 16 rue Jean-Chaptal, B.P. 15, F 93601 Aulnay-sous-Bois Cedex, France.

Guerbet, Neth. See *Byk, Neth.*

Guerbet, Switz. See *Max Ritter, Switz.*

Guest, UK. Thos Guest & Co. Ltd, Carruthers St, Ancoats, Manchester M4 7HX, England.

Guidi, Ital. Laboratorio Biochimico dr Guidi di P. Barone e C. s.n.c., Via Osoppo 7, 20148 Milan, Italy.

Guidotti, Ital. Laboratorio Guidotti & C. s.p.a., Via Trieste 40, 56100 Pisa, Italy.

Gunnar Kjems, Denm. See *Meda, Denm.*

Gønget, Denm. F.F. Gønget & Co., Englandsvej 382 A, 2770 Kastrup, Denmark.

Halas, UK. Halas Laboratories Ltd, Thorp Arch Trading Estate, Wetherby, West Yorkshire LS23 7BJ, England.

Hall Bros, UK. Hall Bros (Whitefield) Ltd, Dumers Lane, Radcliffe, Manchester, England.

Hall Forster, UK. Hall Forster & Co. Ltd, P.O. Box 1DB, Pooley Close, Newcastle upon Tyne NE99 1DB, England.

Halocarbon, Denm. See *Friis, Denm.*

Halty, Fr. Laboratoires Halty, 1 ave Foch, 64200 Biarritz, France.

Hamilton, Austral. Hamilton Laboratories Pty Ltd, 217 Flinders St, Adelaide SA 5000, Australia.

Hanson, UK. A.C. Hanson, Bon Acord, Athol Park, Port Erin, Isle of Man.

Harimex-Ligos, Neth. Harimex-Ligos B.V., Kieveen 20, 7371 GD Loenen, Netherlands.

Harris, Canad. Harris Laboratories, 1050 Chemin du Golf, Ile des Soeurs, Montreal, Quebec H3E 1H4, Canada.

Harvard, S.Afr. See *Restan, S.Afr.*

Harvey-Scruton, UK. Harvey-Scruton Ltd, 4 Baker Lane, York, England.

Harvey, Switz. See *Mundipharma, Switz.*

Harvey, USA. Harvey Laboratories Inc., 113 West Wyoming Ave, Philadelphia PA 19140, USA.

Hässle, Denm. See *Astra, Denm.*

Hässle, Norw. See *Astra, Norw.*

Hässle, Swed. AB Hässle, Kärragatan 5, 431 83 Mölndal, Sweden.

Hauck, USA. W.E. Hauck Inc., P.O. Box 1065, Roswell GA 30075, USA.

Hauser, Denm. See *Tjellesen, Denm.*

Hausmann, Denm. See *Meda, Denm.*

Hausmann, Norw. See *Andersen, Norw.*

Hausmann, Switz. Laboratorien Hausmann AG, 9001 St Gallen, Switzerland.

Health & Diet Food Co., UK. Health & Diet Food Co. Ltd, Seymour House, 79 High St, Godalming, Surrey GU7 1AW, England.

Heath & Heather, UK. Heath & Heather Ltd, Division of Associated Health Foods, Station Approach, West Byfleet, Surrey, England.

Hefa-Frenon, Ger. Hefa-Frenon Arzneimittel GmbH & Co. KG, Am Bahnhof 1-3, Postfach:220, 4712 Werne an der Lippe, W. Germany.

Hefti, Switz. Hefti AG, 8048 Zurich, Switzerland.

Heilit, Ger. Heilit Arzneimittel GmbH, Danziger Strasse 5, Postfach:1248, 2057 Reinbek, W. Germany.

Heineking, Switz. L. Heineking & Cie, alte Landstrasse 32, 8800 Thalwil, Switzerland.

Helge Kjelstrup, Denm. Helge Kjelstrup ApS, Emdrupvej 28 B, 2100 Copenhagen Ø, Denmark.

Helvepharm, Switz. Helvepharm AG, Bahnhofstr., 3185 Schmitten, Switzerland.

Henkel, Ger. Henkel KGaA, Henkelstrasse 67, Postfach:1100, 4000 Düsseldorf 13, W. Germany.

Henleys, UK. Henleys Medical Supplies Ltd, Alexandra Works, Clarendon Rd, London N8 0DL, England.

Henning Berlin, Ger. Henning Berlin GmbH, Chemie- und Pharmawerk, Komturstrasse 19/20, 1000 Berlin 42, W. Germany.

Henning, Denm. See *Gønget, Denm.*

Henry Christenson, Norw. Henry Christenson & Co., Vibesgt. 2, Oslo 3, Norway.

Herbal Laboratories, UK. Herbal Laboratories, Kilbane St, Copse Rd, Fleetwood, Lancs FY7 7PF, England.

Herbrand, Ger. Dr Herbrand KG, chem.-pharm. Werk, Nollenstrasse 54, Postfach:1107, 7614 Gengenbach, W. Germany.

Herbrand, Switz. See *Adima, Switz.*

Hercules, UK. Hercules Ltd, 20 Red Lion St, London WC1R 4PB, England.

Hermal, Ger. Hermal-Chemie Kurt Herrmann, Danziger Strasse 5, Postfach:1228/9, 2057 Reinbek, W. Germany.

Hermal, Neth. See *Bipharma, Neth.*

Hermal, Swed. See *E. Merck, Swed.*

Hermal, Switz. See *Lubapharm, Switz.*

Hermes, Spain. Laboratorios Hermes SA, Pl. Duque Medinaceli 4, Barcelona, Spain.

Hetty, Arg. Laboratorio Hetty, Cabrera 3156, 1186 Buenos Aires, Argentina.

Heumann, Ger. Ludwig Heumann & Co. GmbH, Heideloffstrasse 18, Postfach:2260, 8500 Nürnberg 1, W. Germany.

Hexcel, USA. Hexcel, USA.

Heyden, Denm. See *Meda, Denm.*

Heyden, Ger. von Heyden GmbH, Volkartstrasse 83, 8000 Munich 19, W. Germany.

Heyden, Norw. See *Kobro, Norw.*

Heyden, Swed. See *Meda, Swed.*

Heyl, Ger. Heyl & Co., chem.-pharm. Fabrik, Goerzallee 253, 1000 Berlin 37, W. Germany.

Hill, USA. Hill Dermaceuticals Inc., 3102 Corrine Dr., P.O. Box 19283, Orlando FL 32814, USA.

Hill's Pharmaceuticals, UK. Hill's Pharmaceuticals Ltd, Talbot St, Briercliffe, Burnley, Lancs BB10 2JY, England.

Hindustan Antibiotics, Ind. Hindustan Antibiotics Ltd, Pimpri, Pune-411 008, India.

Hishiyama, Jap. Hishiyama Pharmaceutical Co. Ltd, 37 Doshomachi 2-chome, Higashi-ku, Osaka 541, Japan.

Hispano-Medial, Spain. Laboratorios Hispano-Medial, Muntaner 468, Barcelona, Spain.

Hispano Quimica, Spain. Hispano Quimica Farmacéutica SA, Carretera Del Medio S/N Hospitallet, Spain.

Hobein, Ger. Dr Hobein & Co. Nachf. GmbH, Grenzstrasse 2, 5309 Meckenheim-Merl, W. Germany.

Hoechst, Arg. Química Hoechst S.A., Corrientes 222, 1043 Buenos Aires, Argentina.

Hoechst, Austral. Hoechst Australia Ltd, 606 St Kilda Rd, Melbourne Vic. 3000, Australia.

Hoechst, Belg. Hoechst Belgium S.A., chaussée de Charleroi 111, 1060 Brussels, Belgium.

Hoechst, Braz. Hoechst do Brasil Quimica e Farmaceutica S.A., Rua Basilio da Gama 77, Sao Paulo, Brazil.

Hoechst, Canad. Hoechst Canada Inc., Pharmaceutical Division, 4045 Côte Vertu Blvd, Montreal, Quebec H4R 1R6, Canada.

Hoechst, Denm. Hoechst Danmark A/S, Islevdalvej 110, 2610 Rødovre, Denmark.

Hoechst, Fr. Laboratoires Hoechst, 3 ave Général-de-Gaulle, 92800 Puteaux, France.

Hoechst, Ger. Hoechst Aktiengesellschaft, Brüningstrasse 45, Postfach:800320, 6230 Frankfurt (Main) 80, W. Germany.

Hoechst, Ital. Hoechst AG, Strada Statale 17 Km. 22, 67019 Scoppito, Italy.

Hoechst, Jap. Hoechst Japan Ltd, New Hoechst Bldg, 10-16 Akasaka 8-chome, Minato-ku, Tokyo 107, Japan.

Hoechst, Neth. Hoechst Holland N.V., Verkoop (divisie Pharma), Sara Burgerhartstraat 25, 1055 KV Amsterdam, Netherlands.

Hoechst, Norw. Norske Hoechst A/S, Økernvn. 145, Postboks 177 Økern, Oslo 5, Norway.

Hoechst, S.Afr. Hoechst Pharmaceuticals (Pty) Ltd, P.O. Box 8692, Johannesburg 2000, S. Africa.

Hoechst, Spain. Hoechst Ibérica SA, Travesera de Gracia 47, Barcelona, Spain.

Hoechst, Swed. Svenska Hoechst AB, Avd. Läkemedel, Box 42026, 126 12 Stockholm 42, Sweden.

Hoechst, Switz. Hoechst-Pharma AG, Bernerstrasse/Herostrasse 7, 8048 Zurich, Switzerland.

Hoechst, UK. Hoechst UK Ltd, Pharmaceutical Division, Hoechst House, Salisbury Rd, Hounslow, Middx TW4 6JH, England.

Hoechst, USA. Hoechst-Roussel Pharmaceuticals Inc., Route 202-206 North, Somerville NJ 08876, USA.

Hokuriku, Jap. Hokuriku Seiyaku Co. Ltd, 3-14 Tatekawacho 1-chome, Katsuyama-shi, Fukuiken 911, Japan.

Holland-Rantos, USA. Holland-Rantos Co. Inc., 865 Centennial Ave, P.O. Box 385, Piscataway NJ 08854, USA.

Holphar, Ger. Holphar Pharmazeutische Präparate GmbH, Albert-Weisgerber-Allee 67, Postfach: 1760, 6670 St Ingbert, W. Germany.

Holpro, S.Afr. Holpro Pharmaceuticals (Pty) Ltd, P.O. Box 7856, Johannesburg 2000, S. Africa.

Homburg, Belg. See *de Bournonville, Belg.*

Homburg, Ger. Chemiewerk Homburg, Zweigniederlassung der Degussa AG, Daimlerstrasse 25, Postfach: 2514, 6000 Frankfurt am Main 1, W. Germany.

Homburg, Neth. See *Multi-Pharma, Neth.*

Homburg, S.Afr. See *Remedia, S.Afr.*

Hommel, Belg. See *CCP, Belg.*

Hommel, Ger. Chemische Werke Hommel GmbH, Postfach: 1263, 7840 Müllheim/Baden 1, W. Germany.

Hommel, Neth. See *Reckitt & Colman, Neth.*

Hommel, Switz. Hommel AG, Industriering 34, 8134 Adliswil, Switzerland.

Honeywill & Stein, UK. Honeywill & Stein Ltd, Greenfield House, 69 Manor Rd, Wallington, Surrey SM6 0BP, England.

Hopkin & Williams, UK. Hopkin & Williams, P.O. Box 1, Romford RM1 1HA, England.

Hormonchemie, Ger. Hormon-Chemie München GmbH, Freisinger Landstrassc 74, Postfach: 45 03 61, 8000 Munich 45, W. Germany.

Horner, Canad. Frank W. Horner Inc., 5485 Ferrier St, Town of Mount Royal, Quebec H4P 1M6, Canada.

Hortel, Spain. Hortel, Av. Cieza 58, Abaran (Murcia), Spain.

Horus, Spain. Horus, Spain.

Horwell, UK. Arnold R. Horwell Ltd, 2 Grangeway, Kilburn High Rd, London NW6 2BP, England.

Hosbon, Spain. Hosbon SA, Avda. José Antonio 512, Barcelona, Spain.

Houde, Belg. Laboratoires Houde, avenue Adolphe Lacomblé 69-71, 1040 Brussels, Belgium.

Houdé-I.S.H., Fr. Laboratoires Houdé-I.S.H., 15 rue Olivier-Métra, 75980 Paris Cedex 20, France.

Hough, Hoseason, UK. Hough, Hoseason & Co. Ltd, Levenshulme, Manchester M19 3PT, England.

Howard Lloyd, UK. Howard Lloyd & Co. Ltd, Clerk Green, Batley, West Yorkshire WF17 5RU, England.

Howmedica, UK. Howmedica (UK) Ltd, 622 Western Ave, London W3 0TF, England.

Hoyer, Ger. Hoyer GmbH & Co., Pharmazeutische Präparate, Siemensstrasse 14, Postfach: 1240, 4040 Neuss 21, W. Germany.

Hoyt, UK. Hoyt Laboratories, Division of Colgate-Palmolive Ltd, 76 Oxford St, London W1A 1EN, England.

Hubber, Spain. Laboratorios Hubber SA, Berlin 38-48, Barcelona, Spain.

Hughes & Hughes, UK. Hughes & Hughes Ltd, Elms Industrial Estate, Church Rd, Harold Wood, Romford, Essex RM3 0HR, England.

Hynson, Austral. Hynson, Australia.

Hynson, Westcott & Dunning, Canad. See *Lloyd Wood, Canad.*

Hynson, Westcott & Dunning, USA. Hynson, Westcott & Dunning Inc., Charles & Chase Sts, Baltimore MD 21201, USA.

Hyrex, USA. Hyrex Pharmaceuticals, 3494 Democrat Rd, P.O. Box 18385, Memphis TN 38118, USA.

Hythe, UK. Hythe Chemicals Ltd, Hythe, Southampton, Hants SO4 6ZG, England.

I. Bioq., Arg. Instituto Bio-Químico Arg. S.A., Rocamora 4047, 1184 Buenos Aires, Argentina.

IBE, Spain. IBE, Spain.

Ibi, Ital. Ibi, Istituto Biochimico Italiano Giovanni Lorenzini s.p.a., Via G. Lorenzini 2-4, 20139 Milan, Italy.

Ibirn, Ital. Istituto Bioterapico Nazionale s.r.l., Via A. Vertunni 40 A/B, 00155 Rome (Tor Sapienza), Italy.

IBIS, Ital. IBIS, Istituto Biochimico Sperimentale s.p.a., Viale Machiavelli 29, 50125 Firenze, Italy.

IBP, Ital. Istituto Biochimico Pavese s.p.a., Viale Alzaia 29, 27100 Pavia, Italy.

Ibsa, Switz. Ibsa S.A., Via al Ponte 13, 6900 Massagno/Lugano, Switzerland.

Ibse, Spain. Ibse SA, Pedro IV 499, Barcelona, Spain.

IBYS, Spain. Instituto de Biológica y Sueroterapia SA, Bravo Murillo 53, Madrid 3, Spain.

ICB, Ital. Industria Chimica Biologica s.p.a., Via Tanini 37-D, 16133 Genoa, Italy.

Ichthyol, Ger. Ichthyol-Gesellschaft Cordes, Hermanni & Co., Sportallee 85, Postfach: 630380, 2000 Hamburg 63, W. Germany.

Ichthyol, Switz. See *Opopharma, Switz.*

ICI, Austral. ICI Australia Ltd, ICI House, 1 Nicholson St, Melbourne Vic. 3001, Australia.

ICI, Denm. ICI-Pharma AS, Islands Brygge 41, 2300 Copenhagen S, Denmark.

ICI-Farma, Arg. División de Duperial S.A.I.C. (Dist. Lepetit), Paseo Colón 285, 1330 Buenos Aires, Argentina.

ICI Mond, UK. Imperial Chemical Industries Ltd, Mond Division, P.O. Box 13, The Heath, Runcorn, Cheshire WA7 4QF, England.

ICI, Norw. A/S ICI-Pharma, Drammensvn. 126A, Postboks 173 Skøyen, Oslo 2, Norway.

ICI Organics, UK. Imperial Chemical Industries Ltd, Organics Division, P.O. Box 42, Hexagon House, Blackley, Manchester M9 3DA, England.

ICI Petrochemicals, UK. Imperial Chemical Industries Ltd, Petrochemicals Division, P.O. Box 90, Wilton, Middlesbrough, Cleveland, England.

ICI Pharmaceuticals, UK. Imperial Chemical Industries Ltd, Pharmaceuticals Division, Mereside, Alderley Park, Macclesfield, Cheshire SK10 4TG, England.

ICI Plant Protection, UK. Imperial Chemical Industries Ltd, Plant Protection Division, Fernhurst, Haslemere, Surrey GU27 3JE, England.

ICI, S.Afr. ICI SA (Pharmaceuticals) Ltd, 1 Leyds St, Braamfontein, Johannesburg, S. Africa.

ICI, Spain. ICI-Farma SA, Conde de Penalver 45, Madrid 6, Spain.

ICI, Swed. ICI-Pharma AB, Stora Badhusgatan 20, 411 21 Göteborg, Sweden.

ICN Arco, Norw. See *Remed, Norw.*

ICN, Canad. ICN Canada Ltd, 1956 Bourdon St, St Laurent, Montreal, Quebec H4M 1V1, Canada.

ICN, Neth. ICN Pharmaceuticals Holland B.V., Stephensonstraat 1, 2723 RM Zoetermeer, Netherlands.

ICN, Spain. ICN Pharmaceuticals España SA, Apartado de Correos 63, Angana del Rey, Madrid, Spain.

ICN, USA. ICN Pharmaceuticals Inc., 222 North Vincent Ave, Covina CA 91722, USA.

IFI, Ital. Istituto Farmacoterapico Italiano s.p.a., Via Archimede 124, 00197 Rome, Italy.

Igoda, Spain. Igoda, Spain.

Ilon Laboratories, UK. Ilon Laboratories (Hamilton) Ltd, Lorne St, Hamilton, Lanarkshire ML3 9AB, Scotland.

Ima, Arg. Laboratorio Ima S.A.I.C., Cramer 1030, 1426 Buenos Aires, Argentina.

Imal, Switz. Imal Pharmaceutica AG, Witikonerstrasse 15, 8032 Zurich, Switzerland.

Imba, Spain. Imba, Spain.

Immuno, Arg. Immuno S.A.C.I.F.I.A., 25 de Mayo 362, 1002 Buenos Aires, Argentina.

Immuno, Ger. Immuno GmbH, Slevogtstrasse 3, Postfach: 103080, 6900 Heidelberg, W. Germany.

Immuno, UK. Immuno Ltd, Arctic House, Rye Lane, Dunton Green, Nr Sevenoaks, Kent TN14 5HB, England.

IMS, UK. International Medication Systems (UK) Ltd, 11 Royal Oakway South, Daventry, Northants NN11 5PJ, England.

Inava, Fr. Laboratoires Inava, département médical de Fimex S.A., 125 rue de la Faisanderie, 75116 Paris, France.

Inca, Arg. Inca Laboratorios de Especialidades Medicinales, Cramer 4130, Buenos Aires, Argentina.

Incasa-Wolff, Spain. Incasa-Wolff, Spain.

Independent Chemists Marketing, UK. Independent Chemists Marketing Ltd, 51 Boreham Rd, Warminster, Wilts BA12 9JU, England.

Industrial Pharmaceutical, UK. Industrial Pharmaceutical Services Ltd, Bridgewater Rd, Broadheath, Altrincham, Cheshire, England.

Inexfa, Spain. Inexfa, Spain.

Infal, Spain. Instituto Farmacológico Latino SA, Rios Rosas 57, Madrid 3, Spain.

Infale, Spain. Industrial Farmacéutica de Levante SA, Mallorca 216, Barcelona, Spain.

Ingasetter, UK. Ingasetter Ltd, Banchory, Grampian, Scotland.

Ingeborg Vidnes, Norw. Ingeborg Vidnes, Sandbuktvn. 3, 1420 Svartskog., Norway.

Ingram & Bell, Canad. Ingram & Bell Ltd, 20 Bond Ave, Don Mills, Ontario M3B 1L9, Canada.

Ingram, USA. Ingram Pharmaceutical Co., 202 Green St, San Francisco CA 94111, USA.

Inibsa, Spain. Industrial Iberica Químico Farmaceutica SA, Aribau 200-210, Barcelona, Spain.

Innothéra, Fr. Laboratoires Innothéra (Chantereau), 10 ave P.-Vaillant-Couturier, 94117 Arcueil Cedex, France.

Innoxa, UK. Innoxa (England) Ltd, 202 Terminus Rd, Eastbourne, East Sussex BN21 3DF, England.

Inolex, USA. Inolex Pharm., Division of Inolex Corporation, 3 Science Rd, Glenwood IL 60425, USA.

Inpharzam, Belg. Inpharzam S.A., ave Roger Vandendriessche 18, 1150 Brussels, Belgium.

Inpharzam, Ger. Inpharzam GmbH, Alfred-Schmidt-Strasse 5, Postfach: 701009/701026, 8000 Munich 70, W. Germany.

Inpharzam, Neth. Inpharzam Nederland N.V., De Paal 41, 1351 JH Almere, Netherlands.

Inpharzam, Switz. Inpharzam S.A., 6814 Lamone, Switzerland.

Institut Pasteur, Fr. Institut Pasteur Production, 3 bd Raymond-Poincaré, 92430 Marnes La Coquette, France.

Intal, S.Afr. Intal Ethical Promotions (Pty) Ltd, P.O. Box 10534, Johannesburg, S. Africa.

International Chemical, UK. International Chemical Co. Ltd, Chenies St, London WC1E 7ET, England.

International Laboratories, UK. International Laboratories Ltd, Charwell House, Wilsom Rd, Alton, Hants GU34 2TJ, England.

International Pharmaceutical, USA. International Pharmaceutical Corporation, Subsidiary of Marion Laboratories Inc., 10236 Bunker Ridge Rd, Kansas City MO 64137, USA.

Interox, UK. Interox Chemicals Ltd, P.O. Box 6, Kingsway, Luton LU4 8HL, England.

Intersint, Ital. Intersint Italiana s.r.l., Industria Terapeutici di Sintesi, Via Laurentina Km. 26.500, 00040 Pomezia (Roma), Italy.

Intervet, UK. Intervet Laboratories Ltd, Science Park, Milton Rd, Cambridge CB4 4BH, England.

Inverni della Beffa, Ital. Inverni della Beffa s.p.a., Via Ripamonti 99, 20141 Milan, Italy.

Inwood, USA. Inwood Laboratories Inc., Division of Forest Laboratories Inc., Prospect St, Inwood NY 11696, USA.

ION, Ital. ION, Istituto Opoterapico Nazionale Pisa s.p.a., Via Contessa Matilde 66, 56100 Pisa, Italy.

IPC, Canad. See *Marion Laboratories, USA.*

IPSEN, Fr. Institut de Produits de Synthèse et d'Extraction Naturelle, 51-53 rue du Dr-Blanche, 75016 Paris, France.

IRBI, Ital. Istituto Ricerche Biochimiche Italiane A.A. Neri s.a.s., S.S. Pontina 28, 00040 Pomezia (Roma), Italy.

Iromedica, Switz. Iromedica AG, Haggenstrasse 45, 9014 St Gallen, Switzerland.

Irving, Austral. F.H. Irving (Medical Products) Pty Ltd, 6th Floor, 363 George St, Sydney NSW 2000, Australia.

ISA, Arg. Inst. Seroterápico Arg. S.A.I.C., Larrazabal 1848/50, 1440 Buenos Aires, Argentina.

ISC Chemicals, UK. ISC Chemicals Ltd, St Andrew's Rd, Avonmouth, Bristol BS11 9HP, England.

Isdin, Spain. Isdin SA, Diagonal 520, Barcelona, Spain.

ISF, Ital. ISF s.p.a., Via Leonardo da Vinci 1, 20090 Trezzano S/N, Italy.

ISI, Ital. Istituto Sieroterapico Italiano s.p.a., 80029 S. Antimo, Italy.

Iskia, Spain. Iskia, Spain.

ISM, Ital. Ist. Sieroterapico Mil. S. Belfanti (Ente Morale aggregato all'Università di Milano), Via Darwin 20, 20143 Milan, Italy.

Isnardi, Ital. Pietro Isnardi & C. s.p.a., Via XXV Aprile 69, 18100 Imperia Oneglia, Italy.

Isola-Ibi, Ital. Isola Ibi, Istituto Bioterapico Internazionale, Viale Pio VII 50, 16148 Genova Quarto, Italy.

ISOM, Ital. I.S.O.M., Medicinali s.p.a., Via Solari 19, 20144 Milan, Italy.

Ist. Chem. Ital., Ital. Istituto Chemioterapico Italiano s.p.a., Via Crocefisso 12, 20122 Milan, Italy.

Ist. Chim. Inter., Ital. Istituto Chimico Internazionale di Rende dr. Giuseppe s.n.c., Via Salaria 1240, 00138 Rome, Italy.

Ital Suisse, Ital. Ital Suisse Co. s.a.s. di Giancarlo Ceroni & C., Via Binasco 54, 20080 Casarile, Italy.

Italchemi, Ital. Italchemi Pharma s.p.a., St. Asolana Km. 11.2, 43056 S.Polo di Torrile, Italy.

Italchimici, Ital. Italchimici s.p.a., Viale Tiziano 25, 00196 Rome, Italy.

Italfarmaco, Ital. Italfarmaco s.p.a., Viale F. Testi 330, 20126 Milan, Italy.

Italfarmaco, Switz. See *Pharnova, Switz.*

Italquimica, Spain. Italquimica, Spain.

Iti, Ital. Iti s.p.a. Istituto Terapeutico Internazionale, Via Principe Eugenio 23, 20155 Milan, Italy.

Itting, Ger. Franz Itting KG, Lauensteiner Strasse 41/42, Postfach: 40, 8642 Ludwigsstadt, W. Germany.

Ives, USA. Ives Laboratories Inc., 685 Third Ave, New York NY 10017, USA.

J. Martin, Spain. Juan Martin, Spain.

Jamco, Ital. Jamco Laboratori Farmaceutici s.r.l., Via Luzzatti 13-A/13-B, 00185 Rome, Italy.

Jamieson-McKames, USA. Jamieson-McKames Inc., 3227 Morganford Rd, St Louis MO 63116, USA.

Janovich, Spain. Janovich, Spain.

Janssen, Aust. See *Cilag-Chemie, Aust.*

Janssen, Belg. Janssen Pharmaceutica, Turnhoutsebaan 30, 2340 Beerse, Belgium.

Janssen, Denm. Janssenpharma A/S, Hammerbakken 21, 3460 Birkerød, Denmark.

Janssen, Ger. Janssen GmbH, Raiffeisenstrasse 8, Postfach: 1168, 4040 Neuss 21, W. Germany.

Janssen, Ital. Janssen Farmaceutici s.p.a., Viale Caravaggio 107, 00147 Rome, Italy.

Janssen-Le Brun, Fr. Janssen-Le Brun, 5 rue de Lübeck, 75116 Paris, France.

Janssen, Neth. See *ACF, Neth.*

Janssen, S.Afr. Janssen Pharmaceutica, Private Bag X3014, Randburg 2125, S. Africa.

Janssen, Switz. See *Cilag-Chemie, Switz.*

Janssen, UK. Janssen Pharmaceutical Ltd, Janssen House, Marlow, Bucks SL7 1ET, England.

Janus, Ital. Janus s.r.l., Industrie Chimiche Riunite, Via Torino 8, 67050 Paterno di Avezzano, Italy.

Jeyes, UK. Jeyes Group Ltd, Brunel Way, Thetford, Norfolk IP24 1HF, England.

J.F. White, UK. J.F. White & Co. Ltd, Lovington Laboratory, Benson St, Leeds 7, England.

Johnson & Johnson Orthopaedic, UK. Johnson & Johnson Orthopaedic Division, 260 Bath Rd, Slough, Berks SL1 4EA, England.

Johnson & Johnson, UK. Johnson & Johnson Ltd, 260 Bath Rd, Slough, Berks SL1 4EA, England.

Johnson & Johnson, USA. Johnson & Johnson, 501 George St, New Brunswick NJ 08903, USA.

Johnson, Arg. Johnson & Johnson de Arg. S.A.C.eI., Darwin 471, 1414 Buenos Aires, Argentina.

Johnson, Denm. A. Johnson & Co. A/S, Jaegersborg alle 14-16, 2920 Charlottenlund, Denmark.

Johnson, Swed. A. Johnson & Co. Läkemedels AB, Box 57, 201 20 Malmo, Sweden.

Jorba, Spain. Laboratorios Jorba SA, Josefa Valcarcel 30, Madrid, Spain.

Joullié, Fr. Laboratoires Joullié S.A., 20 bis place Boieldieu, 92803 Puteaux, France.

Jouveinal, Fr. Jouveinal Laboratoires, 1 rue des Moissons, 94260 Fresnes, France.

Juste, Spain. Juste SA Químico Farmaceutica, Madrid, Spain.

Juventus, Spain. Juventus SA, Valentin Beato 44, Madrid, Spain.

K. & G., Norw. Koren & Gedde A/S, Nycovn. 2, Postboks 4220 Torshov, Oslo 4, Norway.

K & K-Greeff, UK. K & K-Greeff Chemicals Ltd, Suffolk House, George St, Croydon CR9 3QL, England.

K/L Pharmaceutical, UK. K/L Pharmaceutical Ltd, 25 Macadam Place, South Newmoor Industrial Estate, Irvine KA11 4HP, Scotland.

Kabi, Denm. See *KabiVitrum, Denm.*

Kabi Diagnostica, Swed. AB Kabi Diagnostica, Lindhagensgatan 133, 112 87 Stockholm, Sweden.

Kabi, Ger. Deutsche KabiVitrum GmbH, Levelingstrasse 18, Postfach: 800468, 8000 Munich 80, W. Germany.

Kabi, Neth. See *KabiVitrum, Neth.*

Kabi, Norw. See *KabiVitrum, Norw.*

Kabi, Swed. Kabi AB, Lindhagensgatan 133, 112 87 Stockholm, Sweden.

KabiVitrum, Denm. KabiVitrum A/S, Halmtorvet 29, 1700 Copenhagen V, Denmark.

Kabivitrum, Fr. Kabivitrum S.A., 71 ave Victor-Hugo, 75116 Paris, France.

KabiVitrum, Neth. KabiVitrum B.V., Ingelandenweg 1, 1069 WE Amsterdam, Netherlands.

KabiVitrum, Norw. A/S KabiVitrum, Nesbruvn. 33, Postboks 22, 1362 Billingstad, Norway.

KabiVitrum, UK. KabiVitrum Ltd, KabiVitrum House, Riverside Way, Uxbridge, Middx UB8 2YF, England.

Kade, Ger. Dr Kade Pharmazeutische Fabrik GmbH, Erkelenzdamm 3, 1000 Berlin 36, W. Germany.

Kaigai, Jap. Kaigai Koeki Co. Ltd, 2-2 Marunouchi 2-chome, Chiyoda-ku, Tokyo 100, Japan.

Kairon, Spain. Kairon, Spain.

Kaken, Jap. Kaken Chemical Co. Ltd, 28-8 Honkomagome 2-chome, Bunkyo-ku, Tokyo 113, Japan.

Kali-Chemie, Denm. See *Meda, Denm.*

Kali-Chemie, Ger. Kali-Chemie Pharma GmbH, Hans-Böckler-Allee 20, Postfach: 220, 3000 Hannover 1, W. Germany.

Kali-Chemie, Neth. See *Schmidt, Neth.*

Kali-Chemie, Norw. See *Meda, Norw.*

Kali-Chemie, Switz. See *Hausmann, Switz.* and *Pharmacolor, Switz.*

Kali-Farma, Spain. Kali-Farma SA, Avda. Generalisimo Franco 618, Barcelona, Spain.

Kalopharma, Ital. Kalopharma s.p.a., Via Montanara 2, 20019 Settimo Milanese (Milano), Italy.

Kanoldt, Ger. Kanoldt Arzneimittel GmbH, Oberer Weberberg 11, Postfach: 1160, 8884 Höchstädt (Donau), W. Germany.

Kappa, Spain. Kappa, Spain.

Karlspharma, Ger. Karlspharma Pharmazeutische Produkte GmbH, Benzstrasse 4, Postfach: 1154, 8011 Kirchheim b. München, W. Germany.

Kasdorf, Arg. Kasdorf & Cía. S.A., Gentenera 649, 1686 Hurlingham, Argentina.

Katwijk, Neth. Katwijk B.V., Chemische Industrie Katwijk, Prins Hendrikkade 11, 2225 TZ Katwijk aan Zee, Netherlands.

Kayaku, Jap. Kayaku Antibiotics Research Co. Ltd, 16-23 Mejiro 2-chome, Toshima-ku, Tokyo 171, Japan.

Keene, USA. Keene Pharmaceuticals Inc., 333 S. Mockingbird, P.O. Box 7, Keene TX 76059, USA.

Keimdiät, Ger. Keimdiät GmbH - Vertrieb Synpharma GmbH, Pfladergasse 7, Postfach: 111 649, 8900 Augsburg, W. Germany.

Kela, Belg. Kela Laboratoria N.V., Industriezone de Kluis, Postbus 4, 2320 Hoogstraten, Belgium.

Kelco, USA. Kelco, Division of Merck & Co. Inc., 8355 Aero Dr., San Diego CA 92123, USA.

Keller, Switz. E. Keller Erben AG, 6901 Lugano, Switzerland.

Kemi-Intressen, Swed. Kemi-Intressen AB, Box 6018, 172 06 Sundbyberg, Sweden.

Kenwood, USA. Kenwood Laboratories Inc., 490-A Main St, New Rochelle NY 10801, USA.

Kerfoot, UK. Thomas Kerfoot & Co. Ltd, Vale of Bardsley, Ashton-under-Lyne, Lancs OL7 9RR, England.

Kessler, Spain. Kessler, Spain.

Kettelhack Riker, Ger. Kettelhack Riker Pharma GmbH, Wilbecke 12-14, Postfach: 1340, 4280 Borken, W. Germany.

Key, USA. Key Pharmaceuticals Inc., 50 NW 176th St, P.O. Box 3670, Miami FL 33169, USA.

Keymer, UK. Keymer Pharmaceuticals Ltd, The Brow, Burgess Hill, West Sussex RH15 9NE, England.

Kin, Spain. Kin SA, San Mario 53-55, Barcelona, Spain.

Kinney, USA. Kinney & Co. Inc., 1307 12th St, Columbus IN 47201, USA.

Kirby-Warrick, UK. Kirby-Warrick Pharmaceuticals Ltd, Mildenhall, Bury St Edmunds, Suffolk IP28 7AX, England.

Kissei, Jap. Kissei Pharmaceutical Co. Ltd, 105 Nomizo, Yoshikawa-ku, Matsumoto-shi, Nagano 399-65, Japan.

Klein, Ger. Dr Gustav Klein, Am Bach 1, Postfach: 7, 7615 Zell-Harmersbach, W. Germany.

Klinge, Ger. Klinge Pharma GmbH & Co., Leopoldstrasse 16, Postfach: 40 04 20, 8000 Munich 40, W. Germany.

Klinge, Switz. See *Galenica, Switz.*

Kneipp, Ger. Kneipp-Werke Kneipp.Mittel-Zentrale Leusser & Oberhäusser, Steinbachtal 43, Postfach: 5960, 8700 Würzburg, W. Germany.

Knoll AG, Austral. See *Schering Pty, Austral.*

Knoll, Arg. Knoll Arg. S.A., Guemes 3475, 1425 Buenos Aires, Argentina.

Knoll, Austral. Knoll Laboratories Division USV Australia Pty Ltd, 172 Princes Highway, Arncliffe NSW 2205, Australia.

Knoll, Belg. See *Coles, Belg.*

Knoll, Denm. See *Meda, Denm.*

Knoll, Ger. Knoll AG, Knollstrasse (Eingang Sudermannstrasse), Postfach: 210805, 6700 Ludwigshafen, W. Germany.

Knoll, Ital. Knoll s.p.a., Via Soperga 37, 20127 Milan, Italy.

Knoll, Neth. Knoll AG Afd. Specialité's Nederland, Donker Curtiusstraat 7-IVB, 1051 JL Amsterdam, Netherlands.

Knoll, Norw. See *Meda, Norw.*

Knoll, S.Afr. See *Holpro, S.Afr.*

Knoll, Swed. See *Meda, Swed.*

Knoll, Switz. Knoll & Cie AG, Postfach 172, 4410 Liestal, Switzerland.

Knoll, USA. Knoll Pharmaceutical Co., 30 North Jefferson Rd, Whippany NJ 07981, USA.

Kobro, Norw. Kobro & Co. A/S, Sørkedalsvn. 10 A, Postboks 5295, Oslo 3, Norway.

Koch-Light, UK. Koch-Light Laboratories Ltd, 2 Willow Rd, Colnbrook, Slough SL3 0BZ, England.

Kohjin, Jap. Kohjin Co. Ltd, 1-1 Shinbashi 1-chome, Minato-ku, Tokyo 105, Japan.

Köhler, Ger. Dr Franz Köhler Chemie GmbH, Neue Bergstrasse 3-7, Postfach: 17, 6146 Alsbach-Hähnlein 1, W. Germany.

Kowa, Jap. Kowa Co. Ltd, 6-29 Nishiki 3-chome, Naka-ku, Nagoya 460, Japan.

Kramer, Switz. Paul Kramer S.A., 42 rue de Genève, 1003 Lausanne, Switzerland.

Kremers-Urban, USA. Kremers-Urban Co., 5600 West County Line Rd, P.O. Box 2038, Milwaukee WI 53201, USA.

Kreussler, Denm. See *Ferraton, Denm.*

Kreussler, Ger. Chemische Fabrik Kreussler & Co. GmbH, Rheingaustrasse 87-95, Postfach: 129105, 6200 Wiesbaden 12, W. Germany.

Kreussler, Neth. See *Multi-Pharma, Neth.*

Krugmann, Ger. Krugmann GmbH, Mundipharma Strasse 4, Postfach: 350, 6250 Limburg (Lahn), W. Germany.

KSL, Norw. Knut Spaerens Laboratorier A/S, Lardalgt. 46, Postboks 610, 3101 Tønsberg, Norway.

Kyorin, Jap. Kyorin Pharmaceutical Co. Ltd, 5 Kanda Surugadai 2-chome, Chiyoda-ku, Tokyo 101, Japan.

Kyowa Hakko Kogyo, S.Afr. See *Pharmafrica, S.Afr.*

Kyowa, Jap. Kyowa Hakko Kogyo Co. Ltd, 6-1 Ohtemachi 1-chome, Chiyoda-ku, Tokyo 100, Japan.

L'Ozothine, Fr. Laboratoires de l'Ozothine S.A., 18 rue d'Arras, 92003 Nanterre Cedex, France.

Labatec-Pharma, Switz. Labatec-Pharma S.A., 36 rue du 31-Décembre, 1217 Meyrin, Switzerland.

Labaz, Belg. Labaz, ave de Béjart 1, 1120 Brussels, Belgium.

Labaz, Fr. Laboratoires Labaz, B.P. 599, 33003 Bordeaux Cedex, France.

Labaz, Ger. Labaz GmbH, Pharmaz. Präparate, Heinrich-Hertz-Strasse 44, 4006 Erkrath 1, W. Germany.

Labaz, Neth. Labaz B.V., Govert van Wijnkade 48, 3140 AB Maassluis, Netherlands.

Labaz-Pisagara, Spain. Labaz-Pisagra, Spain.

Labaz, S.Afr. See *Reckitt & Colman, S.Afr.*

Labaz Sanofi, UK. Labaz Sanofi UK Ltd, Regent House, Heaton Lane, Stockport SK4 1AG, England.

Labaz, Spain. Labaz, Spain.

Labaz, Switz. Labaz AG, Spiegelgasse 1, 4051 Basel, Switzerland.

Labcatal, Fr. Laboratoires Labcatal, 7 rue Roger-Salengro, 92120 Montrouge, France.

Labif, Ital. Labif Medicinali Zatta s.r.l., Via S. Slataper 10, 50134 Firenze, Italy.

Labinca, Arg. Labinca S.A., Cramer 4130, 1429 Buenos Aires, Argentina.

Labohain, Belg. Laboratoire Pharmaceutique d'Ohain, chemin du Catty 2, 1328 Ohain, Belgium.

Labopharma, Ger. Labopharma, Chemische-pharmazeutische Fabrik GmbH, Nordhauser Strasse 30, 1000 Berlin 10 10, W. Germany.

Laboratoire Européen du Médicament, Fr. Laboratoire Européen du Médicament, 125 rue de la Faisanderie, 75116 Paris, France.

Laboratoires Biologiques de l'Île-de-France, Fr. Laboratoires Biologiques de l'Île-de-France S.A., 45 rue de Clichy, 75009 Paris, France.

Laboratoires de l'Hémédonine, Fr. Laboratoires de l'Hémédonine, 117 rue Félix-Faure, 59110 La Madeleine, France.

Laboratoires de l'Opocalcium, Fr. Laboratoires de l'Opocalcium, 7 rue de l'Industrie, 95310 St-Ouen l'Aumone, France.

Laboratoires Français de Thérapeutique, Fr. Laboratoires Français de Thérapeutique S.A., 41 rue de Tauzia, 33800 Bordeaux, France.

Laboratories de l'Hepatrol, Switz. See *Pharmos, Switz.*

Laboratories for Applied Biology, UK. Laboratories for Applied Biology Ltd, 91 Amhurst Park, London N16 5DR, England.

Laboratory Facilities, UK. Laboratory Facilities Ltd, 24 Britwell Rd, Burnham, Slough, Berks SL1 8AG, England.

Laboromand, Switz. Laboromand S.A., 1 rue Madeleine, 1204 Geneva, Switzerland.

Lacefa, Arg. Laboratorio Lacefa S.A.I.C.A., Av. de Mayo 666-Piso 1°, 1084 Buenos Aires, Argentina.

Lacer, Spain. Lacer SA, Cerdena 350, Barcelona, Spain.

Lacroix, Fr. Laboratoires Lacroix, 37 rue Pajol, 75018 Paris, France.

Laevosan, Aust. Laevosan GmbH & Co. KG, Estermannstrasse 17, 4020 Linz, Austria.

Laevosan, Switz. See *Boehringer Mannheim, Switz.* and *Wander, Switz.*

Lafage, Arg. Laboratorio Lafage S.R.L., José E. Uriburu 61, 1027 Buenos Aires, Argentina.

Lafare, Ital. Laboratorio Farmaceutico Reggiano s.n.c., Via S.B. Cozzolino 67, 80056 Ercolano Resina, Italy.

Lafarge, Fr. Laboratoires Lafarge, 62 rue de la Brauderie, 36000 Chateauroux, France.

Lafarquim, Spain. Laboratorios Lafarquim (Alonga) SA, Rufino Gonzalez 4, Madrid 17, Spain.

Lafon, Fr. Laboratoires Lafon, B.P. 22, 94701 Maisons-Alfort Cedex, France.

Lagap, Switz. Lagap S.A., P.O. Box 7, 6943 Vezia, Switzerland.

Lainco, Spain. Lainco, Spain.

Laing-National, UK. Laing-National Ltd, Ashburton Rd, Trafford Park, Manchester M17, England.

Lambda Pharmacal, USA. Lambda Pharmacal Corporation, Plainview NY 11803, USA.

Lamepro, Neth. Lamepro B.V., Lissenveld 49, 4941 VL Raamsdonksveer, Netherlands.

Lampugnani, Ital. Lampugnani Farmaceutici s.p.a., Via Gramsci 4, 20014 Nerviano (Milano), Italy.

Lancet, Ital. Lancet s.r.l., Passeggiata di Ripetta 19, 00136 Rome, Italy.

Landerlan, Spain. Laboratorios Landerlan SA, Agastia 67, Madrid, Spain.

Landó, Arg. Laboratorio Landó S.A., Allende 2186, 1407 Buenos Aires, Argentina.

Lane, UK. G.R. Lane Health Products Ltd, Sisson Rd, Gloucester GL1 3QB, England.

Langdale, UK. E.F. Langdale Ltd, Vulcan Way, New Addington, Surrey CR9 0BS, England.

Langley, Austral. Langley Laboratories Pty Ltd, 116 Cabramatta Rd, Cremorne NSW 2090, Australia.

Lannacher, Denm. See *Ringsted & Semler, Denm.*

Laphal, Fr. Laboratoires Laphal, 13190 Allauch, France.

Laporte, UK. Laporte Industries Ltd, P.O. Box 2, Moorfield Rd, Widnes, Cheshire WA8 0JU, England.

Lappe, Ger. Lappe Arzneimittel, Niederlassung Bensberg der Bristol-Myers GmbH, Rosenstrasse 10-20, Postfach: 209, 5060 Bergisch Gladbach 1, W. Germany.

Larco, Arg. See *Disprovent, Arg.*

Larkhall Laboratories, UK. Larkhall Laboratories, 225 Putney Bridge Rd, London SW15 2PY, England.

Larma, Spain. Laboratorios Larma SA, Avda. de los Madronos 33, Madrid, Spain.

Laroche Navarron, Belg. See *UPB, Belg.*

Laroche Navarron, Fr. Laboratoires Laroche Navarron, 20 rue Jean-Jaurès, 92800 Puteaux, France.

Lasa, Spain. Lasa Laboratorios SA, Plaza Centenario 5, San Sebastian, Spain.

Laser, USA. Lasser Inc., 2000 N. Main St, Crown Point IN 46307, USA.

Latema, Belg. See *Triosol, Belg.*

Latéma, Fr. Laboratoires de Thérapeutique Moderne, Latéma, 42 rue Rouget de Lisle, 92151 Suresnes Cedex, France.

Latéma, Switz. See *Pharmacolor, Switz.*

Laves, Ger. Laves-Arzneimittel GmbH, Hildesheimer Strasse 111 A, Postfach: 810340, 3000 Hannover, W. Germany.

Lawrence Industries, UK. Lawrence Industries, Mitcham Industrial Estate, Streatham Rd, Mitcham, Surrey CR4 2AP, England.

Lazar, Arg. Laboratorio Lazar & Cía S.A., Av. Vélez Sarfield 5855, 1605 Munro, Argentina.

Le-Han, Canad. Le-Han, 123 Edward St, Suite A-15, Toronto, Ontario H5G 1E2, Canada.

Lederle, Arg. Cyanamid de Arg. S.A., Charcas 5051/63, 1425 Buenos Aires, Argentina.

Lederle, Austral. Lederle Laboratories, 88 Christie St, St. Leonards NSW 2065, Australia.

Lederle, Belg. See *Cyanamid, Belg.*

Lederle, Canad. Lederle Products Dept, Cyanamid Canada Inc., 2255 Sheppard Ave East, Willowdale, Ontario M2J 4Y5, Canada.

Lederle, Denm. Cyanamid Danmark Lederle Informationsafdeling, St. Kongensgade 68, 1264 Copenhagen K, Denmark.

Lederle, Neth. Lederle Nederland B.V., Waarderweg 45, 2031 BN Haarlem, Netherlands.

Lederle, S.Afr. Lederle Laboratories (Pty) Ltd, P.O. Box 7552, Johannesburg 2000, S. Africa.

Lederle, Swed. See *Cyanamid, Swed.*

Lederle, Switz. See *Opopharma, Switz.*

Lederle, UK. Lederle Laboratories, Division of Cyanamid of Great Britain Ltd, Fareham Rd, Gosport, Hants PO13 0AS, England.

Lederle, USA. Lederle Laboratories, Division of American Cyanamid Co., Pearl River NY 10965, USA.

Leeming, USA. Leeming/Pacquin Divisions, Pfizer Inc., 235 East 42nd St, New York NY 10017, USA.

LEFA, Spain. Laboratorios Españoles de Farmacologia Aplicada, Luis Cabrera 9, Madrid 2, Spain.

Lefrancq, Fr. Laboratoires Lefrancq, 36 ave de Metz, 93230 Romainville, France.

Legere, USA. R.J. Legere & Co. Inc., 7326 E. Evans Rd, Scottsdale AZ 85260, USA.

Leiras, Denm. See *Nordisk Droge, Denm.*

Leiras, Norw. See *Remifarm, Norw.*

Lelong, Fr. Laboratoires Lelong, 45200 Amilly, France.

Lema, Arg. Lema S.A., Constitución 4234, 1254 Buenos Aires, Argentina.

Lematte & Boinot, Switz. See *Labatec-Pharma, Switz.* and *Pharmac-Service, Switz.*

Lemmon, USA. Lemmon Co., P.O. Box 30, Sellersville PA 18960, USA.

Lemoine, Fr. Laboratoires Lemoine, 36 rue du Magasin, 59000 Lille, France.

Lemonier, Arg. Lemonier & Cía S.R.L., Misiones 159/61, 1083 Buenos Aires, Argentina.

Lemos, Arg. Laboratorio Lemos S.R.L., Sgo. del Estero 1162, 1075 Buenos Aires, Argentina.

Len-Tag, USA. Len-Tag Co., 5101 E. Davison Ave, Detroit MI 48212, USA.

Lensa, Spain. Lensa, Spain.

Lenza, Ital. Farmaceutici Lenza s.r.l., Via Padula (Racc. Autos), 80026 Casoria (Napoli), Italy.

Leo, Aust. Leo-Arzneimittel GmbH, Brigittagasse 22-26, Postfach: 201, 1201 Vienna, Austria.

Leo, Belg. Leo, ave de la Porte de Hal 38/39, 1060 Brussels, Belgium.

Leo, Denm. Løvens kemiske Fabrik, Industriparken 55, 2750 Ballerup, Denmark.

Leo, Fr. Laboratoires Leo, 38 ave Hoche, 75008 Paris, France.

Leo, Neth. See *Leo Pharm., Neth.* and *UCB, Neth.*

Leo, Norw. Løvens kemiske Fabrik, Hegdehaugsvn. 36, Postboks 7186 Homansbyen, Oslo 3, Norway.

Leo Pharm., Neth. Leo Pharm. Producte B.V., Jules Verne-weg 31, 7821 AD Emmen, Netherlands.

Leo Rhodia, Swed. AB Leo Rhodia, Box 945, 251 09 Helsingborg, Sweden.

Leo, Spain. Laboratorios Leo SA, Avda. Pio XII 99, Madrid 16, Spain.

Leo, Swed. AB Leo, Box 941, 251 09 Helsingborg, Sweden.

Leo, Switz. Leo AG, Dübendorfstr. 2, 8051 Zurich, Switzerland.

Leo, UK. Leo Laboratories Ltd, Longwick Rd, Princes Risborough, Aylesbury, Bucks HP17 9RR, England.

Lepetit, Arg. Lepetit S.A.Q.I.yC., L.N. Alem 896, 1001 Buenos Aires, Argentina.

Lepetit, Austral. Lepetit (Pharmaceuticals) Pty Ltd, 105 Miller St, North Sydney NSW 2060, Australia.

Lepetit, Belg. Lepetit Belgica, ave de Tervuren 35, 1040 Brussels, Belgium.

Lepetit, Fr. Laboratoires Lepetit S.A., 64 rue du Ranelagh, 75016 Paris, France.

Lepetit, Ital. Gruppo Lepetit s.p.a., Via Roberto Lepetit 8, 20124 Milan, Italy.

Lepetit, Neth. Lepetit B.V., Aert van Nesstraat 45, 3012 CA Rotterdam, Netherlands.

Lepetit, Spain. Laboratorios Lepetit SA, Madrid, Spain.

Lepetit, Switz. See *Biochimica, Switz.* and *Tettamanti, Switz.*

Lepetit, UK. See *Merrell, UK.*

Lesvi, Spain. Lesvi SA, Gossol 9-13, Barcelona, Spain.

Leurquin, Fr. Laboratoires Leurquin, 22 rue du Capitaine-Ferber, 75020 Paris, France.

Level, Spain. Level SA, Pedro IV 499, Barcelona, Spain.

Lewis, UK. Lewis Laboratories Ltd, Lavender Walk, Leeds LS9 8JG, England.

Lexalabs, USA. Lexalabs Inc., Lenexa KS 66215, USA.

Liade, Spain. Laboratorios Liade SA, Joaquín Costa 26, Madrid 6, Spain.

Liberman, Spain. Liberman SL, Pedro IV 84, Barcelona, Spain.

Libra, Ital. Chemical Lab. Libra s.r.l., Via Schiaparelli 1, 20125 Milan, Italy.

Lifasa, Spain. Lifasa, Los Centelles 7, Valencia 6, Spain.

Lifepharma, Spain. Laboratorios Lifepharma de España SA, Ruiz Parello 15, Madrid, Spain.

Lilly, Arg. Eli Lilly Argentina S.A., Suipacha 664-4°Piso, 1008 Buenos Aires, Argentina.

Lilly, Austral. Eli Lilly (Australia) & Co., Wharf Rd, West Ryde NSW 2114, Australia.

Lilly, Canad. Eli Lilly & Co. (Canada) Ltd, 3650 Danforth Ave, Scarborough, Ontario M1N 2E8, Canada.

Lilly, Denm. Eli Lilly and Company Denmark ApS, Tømmerup Stationsvej 10, 2770 Kastrup, Denmark.

Lilly, Ger. Eli Lilly GmbH, Marienbader Platz, Postfach: 1420, 6380 Bad Homburg v.d.H., W. Germany.

Lilly, Ital. Eli Lilly Italia s.p.a., Via Gramsci 733, 50019 Sesto Fiorentino, Italy.

Lilly, Neth. Lilly Nederland, Stationsplein 97, 3511 ED Utrecht, Netherlands.

Lilly, Norw. Eli Lilly S.A. Informasjonsavdeling Norge, Brynsengvn. 1, Postboks 122 Bryn, Oslo 6, Norway.

Lilly, NZ. Eli Lilly (NZ) & Co., P.O. Box 76205, Manukau City, New Zealand.

Lilly, S.Afr. Lilly Laboratories (SA) (Pty) Ltd, P.O. Box 98, Short St, Isando, Transvaal, S. Africa.

Lilly, Spain. Lilly Indiana de España SA, Apartado 585, Madrid, Spain.

Lilly, Switz. See *Schweiz. Serum & Impfinstitut, Switz.*

Lilly, UK. Lilly Industries Ltd, Kingsclere Rd, Basingstoke, Hants RG21 2XA, England.

Lilly, USA. Eli Lilly & Co., P.O. Box 618, Indianapolis IN 46206, USA.

Limas, Ital. c/o Aesculapius Laboratorio Chimico Farmaceutico s.p.a., Strada Padana Sup. 290, 20090 Vimodrone, Italy.

Lindeburg & Riemer, Denm. Lindeburg & Riemer, c/o A. Johnson & Co. A/S, hospitalsafd., Jaegersborg alle 14-16, 2920 Charlottenlund, Denmark.

Lindeburg & Riemer, Swed. See *Johnson, Swed.*

Lindeburg, Denm. Lindeburg Farma, Naerum Hovedgade 2, 2850 Naerum, Denmark.

Lindopharm, Ger. Lindopharm, Fabrik chemisch-pharmazeutischer Erzeugnisse v.d. Linde KG, Neustrasse 82, Postfach: 560, 4010 Hilden, W. Germany.

Lingner & Fischer, Ger. Lingner & Fischer GmbH, Hermannstrasse 7, Postfach: 1440, 7580 Bühl (Baden), W. Germany.

Linton, UK. G.H. Linton & Co. Ltd, 4 Herbert St, Hemel Hempstead, Herts, England.

Lipha, Belg. See *Sopar, Belg.*

Lipha, Ger. Lipha Arzneimittel GmbH, Annastrasse 38, Postfach: 10 23 65, 4300 Essen, W. Germany.

Lipha, UK. Lipha Pharmaceuticals Ltd, Old Farm Rd, West Drayton, Middx UB7 7LD, England.

Liqufruta, UK. Liqufruta Ltd, Sanitas House, 15 Stockwell Green, London SW9 9JJ, England.

Lirca, Ital. Lirca Farmaceutici s.p.a., Via Rivoltana 35, 20090 Limito, Italy.

Lisapharma, Ital. Lisapharma s.p.a., Via Licinio 11, 22036 Erba (Como), Italy.

Lister, UK. Lister Institute of Preventive Medicine, Elstree, Herts, England.

Llano, Spain. Laboratorios Farmacéuticos Dr Llano, Madrid, Spain.

Llorens, Spain. Llorens, Spain.

Llorente, Spain. Instituto Llorente SA, General Rodrigo 6, Madrid 3, Spain.

Lloyd, Aimee, UK. Lloyd, Aimee & Co. Ltd, 145a High St, Tenterden, Kent TN30 6JS, England.

Lloyd, Austral. See *Muir & Neil, Austral.*

Lloyd-Hamol, Reckitt & Colman Pharm., UK. Lloyd-Hamol Ltd, Reckitt & Colman Pharmaceutical Division, Dansom Lane, Kingston-upon-Hull HU8 7DS, England.

Lloyd Wood, Canad. W. Lloyd Wood Co. Ltd, 833 Oxford St, Toronto, Ontario M8Z 5X4, Canada.

Lloyds Pharmaceuticals, Reckitt & Colman Pharm., UK. Lloyds Pharmaceuticals Ltd, Reckitt & Colman Pharmaceutical Division, Dansom Lane, Kingston-upon-Hull HU8 7DS, England.

LOA, Arg. Laboratorio Oftalmol Arg. S.A.I.C.I.F., Dr J.F. Aranguren 344, 1405 Buenos Aires, Argentina.

Loders & Nucoline, UK. Loders & Nucoline Ltd, Sussex House, Burgess Hill, West Sussex RH15 9AW, England.

Lofthouse of Fleetwood, UK. Lofthouse of Fleetwood Ltd, Maritime St, Fleetwood, Lancs FY7 7LP, England.

Logeais, Belg. See *Dumas, Belg.*

Logeais, Fr. Laboratoires Jacques Logeais, 71 ave du Général-de-Gaulle, 92130 Issy-les-Moulineaux, France.

Logeais, Switz. See *Biphar, Switz.* and *Pharmos, Switz.*

Lohmann, Ger. Dr Paul Lohmann GmbH KG, Hauptstrasse 2, Postfach: 1220, 2354 Emmerthal-Kirchohsen, W. Germany.

Longuet, Belg. See *Du Bled, Belg.*

Lopez-Brea, Spain. Lopez-Brea, Spain.

Lostaló, Arg. Laboratorio R.A. Lostaló S.A.I.C.I.F.A.M., Quintino Bocayuva 1786, 1257 Buenos Aires, Argentina.

Lövens, Swed. Lövens Läkemedel, Box 404, 201 24 Malmo, Sweden.

Loveridge, UK. J.M. Loveridge Ltd, 6 Millbrook Rd, Southampton, England.

Loxley, UK. Loxley Medical, Bessingby Estate, Bridlington, North Humberside YO16 4SU, England.

LPB, Ital. LPB Istituto Farmaceutico s.p.a., Via dei Lavoratori 54, 20092 Cinisello Balsamo, Italy.

LRC Products, UK. LRC Products Ltd, North Circular Rd, London E4 8QA, England.

Lubapharm, Switz. Lubapharm AG, Drosselstrasse 47, 4059 Basel, Switzerland.

Lucchini, Switz. Lab. Lucchini S.A., 20 rue Coulouvrenière, 1204 Geneva, Switzerland.

Lucien, Fr. Laboratoires Lucien, 3 rue des Écoles, 92704 Colombes Cedex, France.

Luitpold, Denm. See *Helge Kjelstrup, Denm.*

Luitpold, Ger. Luitpold-Werk, Chemisch-pharmazeutische Fabrik, Zielstattstrasse 9, Postfach: 70 12 09, 8000 Munich 70, W. Germany.

Luitpold, Norw. See *AFI, Norw.*

Luitpold, Switz. See *Medichemie, Switz.*

Luitpold-Werk, UK. Luitpold-Werk Munich, Hayes Gate House, 27 Uxbridge Rd, Hayes, Middx UB4 0JN, England.

Lundbeck, Belg. Lundbeck S.A., blvd de Smet de Naeyer 410a, 1090 Brussels, Belgium.

Lundbeck, Denm. H. Lundbeck & Co. A/S, Ottiliavej 7, 2500 Valby, Denmark.

Lundbeck, Neth. Lundbeck B.V., Kabelweg 55, 1014 BA Amsterdam, Netherlands.

Lundbeck, Norw. H. Lundbeck & Co. A/S, Drammensvn. 342, Postboks 188, 1324 Lysaker, Norway.

Lundbeck, S.Afr. See *SCS, S.Afr.*

Lundbeck, Swed. AB H. Lundbeck & Co., Djäknegatan 21, 211 35 Malmo, Sweden.

Lundbeck, Switz. Lundbeck AG, Dübendorfstrasse 2, 8051 Zurich, Switzerland.

Lundbeck, UK. Lundbeck Ltd, Lundbeck House, Hastings St, Luton, Beds LU1 5BE, England.

Lusofarmaco, Ital. Istituto Luso Farmaco D'Italia s.p.a., Via Carnia 26, 20132 Milan, Italy.

Lusofarmaco, Spain. Lusofarmaco SAE, Federico Salmon 9, Madrid, Spain.

Lusty, UK. Lusty's Natural Products Ltd, Sisson Rd, Gloucester GL1 3OB, England.

Luyma, Spain. Luyma, Spain.

Lyocentre, Fr. Laboratoires Lyocentre, 63203 Riom Cedex, France.

MacAndrews & Forbes, UK. MacAndrews & Forbes Ltd, Pembroke House, 44 Wellesley Rd, Croydon CR9 3QE, England.

Macarthys, UK. Macarthys Laboratories Ltd, Chesham House, Chesham Close, Romford RM1 4JX, England.

Macchia, Ital. Macchia Lab. Chim. Farm., Via Bartoli 1, Cascina, 56026 S. Frediano a Settimo, Italy.

Macfarlan Smith, UK. Macfarlan Smith Ltd, Wheatfield Rd, Edinburgh EH11 2QA, Scotland.

Mack, Illert., Ger. Heinrich Mack Nachf., Chemisch-Pharmazeutische Fabrik, Heinrich-Mack-Strasse 35, Postfach: 140, 7918 Illertissen/Bayern, W. Germany.

Mack, Reichenhall, Ger. Josef Mack KG, Natürliche Heil- und Kurmittel, Innsbrucker Strasse 37, Postfach: 467, 8230 Bad Reichenhall, W. Germany.

Mack, Switz. See *Opopharma, Switz.*

Madariaga, Spain. Madariaga, Bocangel 21, Madrid, Spain.

Madaus Cerafarm, Spain. Laboratorios Madaus Cerafarm SA, Calle Fuego s/n, Barcelona, Spain.

Madaus, Ger. Dr Madaus & Co., Ostmerheimer Strasse 198, Postfach: 932 001, 5000 Cologne 91, W. Germany.

Madaus, S.Afr. Madaus Pharmaceuticals (Pty) Ltd, P.O. Box 76246, Wendywood 2144, S. Africa.

Madaus, Switz. See *Biomed, Switz.*

Made, Ital. Made Italiana s.r.l., Via Tiburtina 1310, 00131 Rome, Italy.

Made, Spain. Laboratorios Made SA, Avda de Burgos, Madrid, Spain.

Maggioni, Ital. Maggioni Farmaceutici s.p.a., Via G. Colombo 40, 20133 Milan, Italy.

Maggioni, Switz. See *Ceresium, Switz.*

Magis, Ital. Laboratorio Magis Farmaceutici, Viale Europa 36, 25100 Brescia, Italy.

Maipe, Spain. Maipe, Spain.

Maizena-Compagniet, Denm. Maizena-Compagniet A/S, Hanne Nielsensvej 14, 2840 Holte, Denmark.

Malam, UK. Malam Laboratories Ltd, Highbank House, Marshdale Rd, Bolton BL1 5AQ, England.

Malco, Austral. Malco Agency, Australia.

Malesci, Ital. Malesci s.p.a. Istituto Farmacobiologico, Via Porpora 22, 50144 Firenze, Italy.

Mallard, USA. Mallard Inc., 3021 Wabash Ave, Detroit MI 48216, USA.

Mallinckrodt, USA. Mallinckrodt Pharmaceuticals, Division Mallinckrodt Inc., 675 Brown Rd, St Louis MO 63134, USA.

Maltown, UK. Maltown Ltd, P.O. Box 53, Harrogate, North Yorkshire HG2 0NH, England.

Manceau, Denm. See *Tjellesen, Denm.*

Manchem, UK. Manchem Ltd, Ashton New Rd, Manchester M11 4AT, England.

Manetti Roberts, Ital. Manetti L. & Roberts H. s.p.a., Via Antonio da Noli 4, 50127 Firenze, Italy.

Mann, Ger. Dr Gerhard Mann, Chemisch-pharmazeutische Fabrik GmbH, Brunsbütteler Damm 165-173, 1000 Berlin 20, W. Germany.

Mann, Neth. See *Tramedico, Neth.*

Manzoni, Ital. Lab. Manzoni Giulio & C. s.p.a., Via V. Vela 5, 20133 Milan, Italy.

Marion Laboratories, USA. Marion Laboratories Inc., 10236 Bunker Ridge Rd, Kansas City MO 64137, USA.

Mars, UK. Mars Ltd, Dundee Rd, Slough, England.

Marshall's Pharmaceuticals, UK. Marshall's Pharmaceuticals Ltd, 38 Greenhill, Hampstead High St, London, England.

Martin Santos, Spain. Dr Martin Santos SA, Av Gijon 64, Valladolid, Spain.

Martindale Pharmaceuticals, UK. Martindale Pharmaceuticals Ltd, Chesham House, Chesham Close, Romford, Essex RM1 4JX, England.

Martindale Samoore, UK. Martindale Samoore Ltd, Chesham House, Chesham Close, Romford, Essex RM1 4JX, England.

Martinet, Fr. Laboratoires Martinet, 222 blvd Pereire, 75848 Paris Cedex 17, France.

Marupi-Merck Sharp & Dohme, Jap. Marupi-Merck Sharp & Dohme K.K., Takeda Bldg, 17-1 Junkeimachidori 4-chome, Minami-ku, Osaka 542, Japan.

Marxer, Arg. Productos Marxer, Bdo. de Irigoyen 248, 1072 Buenos Aires, Argentina.

Massone, Arg. Inst. Massone S.A. Prod. Químicos Biológicos, Arias 4431, 1430 Buenos Aires, Argentina.

Matthews & Wilson, UK. Matthews & Wilson Ltd, 225 Putney Bridge Rd, London SW15 2PY, England.

Mawson & Proctor, UK. Mawson & Proctor Pharmaceuticals Ltd, Kingsway South, Gateshead NE8 1YX, England.

Max Factor, UK. Max Factor Ltd, P.O. Box 7, Wallisdown Rd, Bournemouth BH11 8PL, England.

Max Jenne, Denm. A/S Max Jenne, Skolevej 1, 6200 Åbenrå, Denmark.

Max Ritter, Switz. Max Ritter, Postfach Selnau, 8039 Zurich, Switzerland.

May & Baker, Austral. May & Baker Australia Pty Ltd, 19 Paramount Rd, West Footscray Vic. 3012, Australia.

May & Baker, S.Afr. Maybaker (SA) (Pty) Ltd, P.O. Box 1130, Port Elizabeth 6000, S. Africa.

May & Baker, UK. May & Baker Ltd, Dagenham, Essex RM10 7XS, England.

Mayfair Chemicals, UK. Mayfair Chemicals Ltd, Eastfield House, Eastfield Lane, Whitchurch, Nr Pangbourne, Berks RG8 7EJ, England.

Mayoly-Spindler, Fr. Laboratoires Mayoly-Spindler, B.P. 206, 92502 Rueil-Malmaison, France.

Mayoly-Spindler, Switz. See *Uhlmann-Eyraud, Switz.*

Mayrand, USA. Mayrand Inc., 1026 E. Lindsay St, P.O. Box 20246, Greensboro NC 27420, USA.

Mazuelos, Spain. Mazuelos SA, Medina y Galnares 52, Sevilla, Spain.

McFarlane, UK. McFarlane Laboratories Ltd, 11th Floor, New Zealand House, Haymarket, London SW1Y 4TE, England.

McGaw, USA. McGaw, USA.

McNeil, Canad. McNeil Laboratories (Canada) Ltd, 600 Main St West, Stouffville, Ontario L0H 1L0, Canada.

McNeil, USA. McNeil, Camp Hill Rd, Fort Washington PA 19034, USA.

MCP Pharmaceuticals, UK. MCP Pharmaceuticals Ltd, Simpson Parkway, Kirkton Campus, Livingston, West Lothian, Scotland.

Mead Johnson, Arg. Mead Johnson Inter, Ltda., Av. Belgrano 1248/50, 1093 Buenos Aires, Argentina.

Mead Johnson, Austral. Mead Johnson, 345 Pacific Highway, Crows Nest NSW 2065, Australia.

Mead Johnson, Belg. Mead Johnson, chaussée de la Hulpe 185/187, 1170 Brussels, Belgium.

Mead Johnson, USA. Mead Johnson & Co., 2404 Pennsylvania St, Evansville IN 47721, USA.

Mecobenzon, Denm. Mecobenzon A/S, Halmtorvet 29, 1700 Copenhagen V, Denmark.

Med-Kjemi, Norw. Med-Kjemi A/S, Hofstadgt. 60, 1375 Høn, Norway.

Med. y Prod. Quím., Spain. Med. y Prod. Quím, Spain.

Meda, Denm. Meda AS, Dynamovej 11, 2730 Herlev, Denmark.

Meda, Norw. Meda A/S, Billingstadsletta 14, Postboks 70, 1312 Slependen, Norway.

Meda, Swed. Meda AB, Box 138, 401 22 Göteborg 1, Sweden.

Medea, Spain. Medea SA, Sta Carolina 53-59, Barcelona, Spain.

Medex, Arg. Medex Omicron S.A.I.C., 23 esq. 66, 1615 Villa Zagala Pdo. San Martín Pcia Bs. As., Argentina.

Medexport, UK. Medexport Ltd, P.O. Box 25, Arundel, West Sussex BN18 0SW, England.

Medexport, USSR. Medexport, 31 Kakhovka, Building 2, 113461 Moscow, USSR.

Medial, Neth. See *Will-Pharma, Neth.*

Medica, Fin. Lääketehdas-Medica Oy, Teollisuuskatu 23-25, Helsinki, Finland.

Medical & Industrial, UK. Medical & Industrial Equipment Ltd, Falcon Rd, Sowton Industrial Estate, Sowton, Exeter, Devon, England.

Medical Research, Austral. Medical Research (Marketing) Pty Ltd, Cnr. Talavera and Khartoum Rds, North Ryde NSW 2113, Australia.

Medical, Spain. Medical SA, Virgen de las Angustias 2, Cordoba, Spain.

Medical Wire, UK. Medical Wire & Equipment Co. (Bath) Ltd, Potley, Corsham, Wilts, England.

Medichem, Austral. Medichem Pharmaceuticals Pty Ltd, 30 Thorby Ave, Leichardt NSW 2040, Australia.

Medichemie, Switz. Medichemie AG, Brühlstrasse, 4107 Ettingen, Switzerland.

Medici Domus, Ital. Medici Domus s.r.l., Via Parini 3, 20028 S. Vittore Olona, Italy.

Medici, Ital. Lab. Farm. Dr Medici s.r.l., Via F.lli Ruspoli 14, 00198 Rome, Italy.

Médicia, Fr. Laboratoires Médicia, 36 rue Jules-Verne, 69003 Lyon, France.

Medicina, Switz. Medicina S.A., 19 rue de la Croix d'Or, 1204 Geneva, Switzerland.

Medico-Biological Laboratories, UK. Medico-Biological Laboratories Ltd, Kingsend House, 44 Kingsend, Ruislip, Middx HA4 7DA, England.

Medicoteknik, Denm. Palle Medicoteknik A/S, Bjerringbrovej 124, 2610 Rødovre, Denmark.

Medics, USA. Medics Pharmaceutical Corporation, 203 Rio Circle, Decatur GA 30030, USA.

Medidenta, Switz. Medidenta AG, Nüschelerstrasse 31, 8021 Zurich, Switzerland.

Medidroga, Spain. Medidroga, Spain.

Medimpex, Hung. Medimpex, Hungarian Trading Co. for Pharmaceutical Products, 4 Vorosmarty Ter, P.O. Box 126, Budapest 5, Hungary.

Medinova, Switz. Medinova AG, Eggbühlstrasse 14, 8050 Zurich, Switzerland.

Medinsa, Spain. Medinsa, Carr Vicalvaro 37, Madrid 22, Spain.

Medital, Ital. Medital Specialità Medicinali s.r.l., Via Tito Speri 10, 00040 Pomezia (Roma), Italy.

Medix, Spain. Medix, Spain.

Medo Chemicals, UK. Medo Chemicals Ltd, The Limes, 130 High St, Chesham, Bucks HP5 1EF, England.

Medosan, Ital. Medosan, Industrie Biochimiche Riunite s.p.a., Via Cino da Pistoia 28, 00152 Rome, Italy.

Meiji, Jap. Meiji Seika Kaisha Ltd, 4-16 Kyobashi 2-chome, Chuo-ku, Tokyo 104, Japan.

Mekos, Norw. Medisinkompaniet A/S Mekos, Drammensvn. 342, Postboks 188, 1324 Lysaker, Norway.

Mekos, Swed. AB Mekos, Box 944, 251 09 Helsingborg, Sweden.

Melusin, Ger. Melusin Schwarz GmbH, Mittelstrasse 11-13, Postfach: 27, 4019 Monheim/Rhld., W. Germany.

Menarini, Belg. Lab. Menarini, ave E. Demolder 128, 1030 Brussels, Belgium.

Menarini, Ital. A. Menarini s.a.s., Via Sette Santi 3, 50131 Firenze, Italy.

Menarini, Spain. Laboratorios Menarini SA, Alfonso XII 587, Badalona (Barcelona), Spain.

Mendell, USA. EMCO International Corporation, Route 52, Carmel NY 10512, USA.

Menley & James, UK. Menley & James Laboratories Ltd, Mundells, Welwyn Garden City, Herts AL7 1EY, England.

Mentholatum, UK. The Mentholatum Co. Ltd, Longfield Rd, Twyford, Berks, England.

Mepha, Switz. Mepha AG, Postfach 28, 4143 Dornach, Switzerland.

Mepros, Neth. Handelsonderneming Mepros, Industrieweg 1, 5531 AD Bladel, Netherlands.

Méram, Fr. Laboratoires Méram, 4 blvd Malesherbes, 75008 Paris, France.

Merchant, USA. W.F. Merchant Pharmaceutical Co. Inc., P.O. Box 2600, Laurel MD 20811, USA.

Merck, Arg. Merck Química Argentina S.A.I.C., Rosetti 1084, 1427 Buenos Aires, Argentina.

Merck, Aust. Austro-Merck GmbH, Zimbagasse 5, 1147 Vienna, Austria.

Merck, Belg. Merck S.A., ave Brugmann 24, 1060 Brussels, Belgium.

Merck-Clévenot, Fr. Laboratoires Merck-Clévenot, 5 rue Anquetil, 94130 Nogent-sur-Marne, France.

Merck-Clévenot, Switz. See *Diethelm, Switz.*

Merck, S.Afr. Merck Pharmaceuticals (SA) (Pty) Ltd, P.O. Box 3497, Johannesburg 2000, S. Africa.

Merck Sharp & Dohme, Arg. Merck Sharp & Dohme (Argentina) S.A.I.yC., Belgrano 1364, 1093 Buenos Aires, Argentina.

Merck Sharp & Dohme, Austral. Merck Sharp & Dohme (Australia) Pty Ltd, 54-68 Ferndell St, South Granville NSW 2142, Australia.

Merck Sharp & Dohme, Canad. Merck Sharp & Dohme Canada Ltd, P.O. Box 1005, Pointe Claire, Dorval, Quebec H9R 4P8, Canada.

Merck Sharp & Dohme-Chibret, Fr. Laboratoires Merck Sharp & Dohme-Chibret, 200 blvd Etienne-Clémentel, 63100 Clermont-Ferrand, France.

Merck Sharp & Dohme, Denm. Merck Sharp & Dohme, Marielundvej 46 C, 2730 Herlev, Denmark.

Merck Sharp & Dohme, Ger. MSD Sharp & Dohme GmbH, Leuchtenbergring 20, Postfach: 80 1649, 8000 Munich 80, W. Germany.

Merck Sharp & Dohme, Neth. See *Chibret, Neth.* and *MSD, Neth.*

Merck Sharp & Dohme, Norw. MSD (Norge) A/S, Solbakken 1, 3000 Drammen, Norway.

Merck Sharp & Dohme, S.Afr. Merck Sharp & Dohme (Pty) Ltd, Private Bag 3, Halfway House 1685, S. Africa.

Merck Sharp & Dohme, Spain. Merck Sharp & Dohme SA, Pedro Teixeira 8, Madrid, Spain.

Merck Sharp & Dohme, Switz. Merck Sharp & Dohme, Utoquai 55, 8008 Zurich, Switzerland.

Merck Sharp & Dohme, UK. Merck Sharp & Dohme Ltd, Hertford Rd, Hoddesdon, Herts EN11 9BU, England.

Merck Sharp & Dohme, USA. Merck Sharp & Dohme, Division of Merck & Co. Inc., West Point PA 19486, USA.

Merckle, Ger. L. Merckle GmbH & Co., Dr-Georg-Spohn-Strasse 7, Postfach: 1161, 7902 Blaubeuren, W. Germany.

Mérieux, Fr. Institut Mérieux, 17 rue Bourgelat, 69002 Lyon, France.

Merrell, Austral. William S. Merrell Co., 9 Help St, Chatswood NSW 2067, Australia.

Merrell, Canad. The Wm S. Merrell Co., Division of Richardson-Merrell (Canada) Ltd, 2 Norelco Drive, Weston, Ontario M9L 1R9, Canada.

Merrell, Ger. Merrell Pharma, Zweigniederlassung der Richardson-Merrell GmbH, H.-S.-Richardson-Strasse 1, Postfach: 1661, 6080 Gross-Gerau, W. Germany.

Merrell, Ital. Merrell s.p.a., Via Bargoni 78, 00153 Rome, Italy.

Merrell-National, USA. Merrell-National Laboratories, Division of Richardson-Merrell Inc., 2110 E. Galbraith Rd, Cincinnati OH 45215, USA.

Merrell, Switz. See *Doetsch, Grether, Switz.* and *Richardson-Merrell, Switz.*

Merrell Toraude, Belg. Division de Richardson-Merrell S.A., chaussée de Waterloo 868/870, 1180 Brussels, Belgium.

Merrell Toraude, Fr. Merrell Toraude, 168 rue de Rivoli, 75044 Paris Cedex 01, France.

Merrell, UK. Merrell Pharmaceuticals Ltd, Rusham Park, Whitehall Lane, Egham, Surrey TW20 9NW, England.

Mertens, Arg. Esp. Med. Mertens S.A., Gorostiaga 1650, 1426 Buenos Aires, Argentina.

Merz, Ger. Merz & Co., GmbH & Co., Eckenheimer Landstrasse 100, 6000 Frankfurt (Main) 1, W. Germany.

Merz, Neth. See *Roussel, Neth.*

Merz, Switz. See *Adroka, Switz.* and *Medidenta, Switz.*

Métadier, Fr. Laboratoires Paul Métadier, 37000 Tours, France.

Meuse, Belg. Laboratoires de la Meuse S.A., rue Hanesse 36/40, 5220 Andenne, Belgium.

Meyer, USA. Meyer Laboratories Inc., 1900 West Commercial Blvd, Fort Lauderdale FL 33309, USA.

Michels, Fr. Laboratoires Michels, 4 bis rue du Colonel-Moll, 75017 Paris, France.

Midelfart, Norw. Midelfart & Co. A/S, Amtmannsvingen 2, 3000 Drammen, Norway.

Midy, Fr. Laboratoires Clin Midy, Dépt. Midy, 20 rue des Fossés-St-Jacques, 75240 Paris Cedex 05, France.

Midy, Ital. Midy s.p.a., Via Piranesi 38, 21037 Milan, Italy.

Midy, Switz. See *Clin-Midy, Switz.* and *Galenica, Switz.*

Midyfarm, Fr. Midyfarm, 20 rue des Fossés-St-Jacques, 75240 Paris Cedex 05, France.

Migra, Arg. Esp. Med. Migra, Argerich 265, 1406 Buenos Aires, Argentina.

Miles, Canad. Miles Pharmaceuticals, Division of Miles Laboratories Ltd, 77 Belfield Rd, Rexdale, Ontario M9W 1G6, Canada.

Miles, Norw. See *Remed, Norw.*

Miles, UK. Miles Laboratories Ltd, Stoke Court, Stoke Poges, Slough, Berks SL2 4LY, England.

Miles, USA. Miles Laboratories Inc., 1127 Myrtle St, Elkhart IN 46514, USA.

Miller of Golden Square, UK. Miller of Golden Square Ltd, 13 Golden Square, London W1R 3AG, England.

Miller Pharmacal, USA. Miller Pharmacal, 1425 Melody Dr., Metairie LA 70002, USA.

Miller, USA. Miller Laboratories Inc., 2303 Schuetz Rd, St Louis MO 63141, USA.

Millet, Arg. Lab. Millet S.A.C.eI., Montevideo 160, 1019 Buenos Aires, Argentina.

Millipore, UK. Millipore (UK) Ltd, 11 Peterborough Rd, Harrow, Middx HA1 2YH, England.

Millot-Solac, Fr. Laboratoires Millot-Solac, 16 ave George-V, 75008 Paris, France.

Milupa, UK. Milupa Ltd, Western House, Hercies Rd, Hillingdon, Middx UB10 9NA, England.

Miluy, Spain. Miluy, Spain.

Minden, Ger. Chemische Werke Minden GmbH, Karlstrasse 42, Postfach: 1180, 4950 Minden, W. Germany.

Minnesota, UK. Minnesota 3M Laboratories Ltd, Morley St, Loughborough, Leics LE11 1EP, England.

Misemer, USA. Misemer Pharmaceuticals Inc., 4553 South Campbell St, Springfield MO 65804, USA.

Mission Pharmacal, USA. Mission Pharmacal Co., 1325 East Durango St, P.O. Box 1676, San Antonio TX 78296, USA.

Mitchum, UK. Mitchum Thayer Ltd, 86 Brook St, London W1Y 2BA, England.

Mitim, Ital. Mitim Farmaceutici di Dott. Aurora Giangrasso e C. s.n.c., Via S.M. Battaglia 40, 10042 Nichelino, Italy.

Modern Health Products, UK. Modern Health Products Ltd, Davis Rd, Chessington, Surrey, England.

Molteni, Ital. Molteni L. & C. dei F.Ui Alitti Società Esercizio s.p.a., Via Pisana 458, 50018 Scandicci, Italy.

Monal, Fr. Laboratoires Monal, 5 rue Salvador-Allende, 91120 Palaiseau, France.

Monico, Ital. Monico Jacopo, Casa Fondata nel 1883, Via Orlanda, Ponte P. 10, 30173 Mestre, Italy.

Monsanto, UK. Monsanto Ltd, Monsanto House, 10 Victoria St, London SW1, England.

Monsanto, USA. Monsanto Chemical Co., 800 North Lindbergh Blvd, St Louis MO 63166, USA.

Monserrat, Arg. Lab. Monserrat Eclair, V. Cevallos 1625, 1135 Buenos Aires, Argentina.

Montavit, Switz. See *Lucchini, Switz.*

Montedison, Arg. Montedison Farmaceutica S.A.C.I.F.I.A., Arcos 2626, 1428 Buenos Aires, Argentina.

Montedison, Belg. Montedison Farmaceutica Benelux, Blvd Reyers 155, 1040 Brussels, Belgium.

Montedison, Denm. Montedison Skandinavien A/S, Vester Søgade 10, 1601 Copenhagen V, Denmark.

Montedison, Norw. Montedison Legemidler, Informasjonskontor Norge, Billingstadsletta 72, 1360 Nesbru, Norway.

Montedison, Spain. Montedison Farmacéutica SA, Barcelona, Spain.

Montefarmaco, Ital. Montefarmaco s.p.a., Via G. Galilei 7, 20016 Pero, Italy.

Montpellier, Arg. Química Montpellier S.A., Virrey Liniers 667, 1220 Buenos Aires, Argentina.

Morgens, Spain. Morgens, Vizconde de Matamala 7, Madrid, Spain.

Morishita, Jap. Morishita Pharmaceutical Co. Ltd, 29 Doshomachi 4-chome, Higashi-ku, Osaka 541, Japan.

Morrith, Spain. Laboratorios Morrith SA, Miguel Yuste, Madrid 17, Spain.

Morson, UK. Thomas Morson Pharmaceuticals, Division of Merck Sharp & Dohme Ltd, Hertford Rd, Hoddesdon, Herts EN11 9BU, England.

MPS Lab., S.Afr. See *Dumex, S.Afr.*

MSD, Neth. Merck Sharp & Dohme B.V., Waarderweg 39, 2031 BN Haarlem, Netherlands.

Mucos, Ger. Mucos Emulsionsgesellschaft mbH, Alpenstrasse 29, Postfach: 1380, 8192 Geretsried 1, W. Germany.

Muir & Neil, Austral. Muir & Neil Pty Ltd, 479 Kent St, Sydney NSW 2000, Australia.

Müller/Göppingen, Ger. Chemische-Pharmazeutische Fabrik Göppingen Carl Müller, Apotheker, GmbH u. Co. KG, Bahnhofstrasse 33-35 u. 40, Postfach: 869, 7320 Göppingen, W. Germany.

Mulli, Ger. Dr Kurt Mulli Nachf. GmbH & Co. KG, Schulterblatt 58, 2000 Hamburg 6, W. Germany.

Multi-Pharma, Neth. Multi-Pharma B.V., Eemmeerlaan 3, 1382 KA Weesp, Netherlands.

Multilan, Denm. See *Organon, Denm.*

Multipharmax, Switz. Multipharmax Ets., Case postale 38, 1211 Geneva 9, Switzerland.

Mundipharma, Denm. See *Ringsted & Semler, Denm.*

Mundipharma, Switz. Mundipharma AG, St Alban-Vorstadt 94, 4052 Basel, Switzerland.

Møller, Denm. A. Møller & Co. ApS, Virumgade 41, 2830 Virum, Denmark.

Nadrol, Ger. Nadrol-Chemie-Pharma Keizer KG, Mönkedieckstrasse 3, Postfach: 3207, 4500 Osnabrück, W. Germany.

NAF, Norw. NAF-Laboratoriene A/S, Sven Oftedals vei 8, Oslo 9, Norway.

Nagel, Ital. Nagel Medizin Werke s.r.l., Strada Rivoltana 14, 20060 Milano-Liscate, Italy.

Nakataki, Jap. Nakataki, Japan.

Napa, UK. Napa Products Ltd, Queens House, Paragon St, Hull HU1 3NQ, England.

Napp, Denm. See *Helge Kjelstrup, Denm.*

Napp, UK. Napp Laboratories Ltd, Cambridge Science Park, Milton Rd, Cambridge CB4 4BH, England.

National Institutes of Health, USA. National Institutes of Health, Bethesda MD 20205, USA.

Nativelle, Belg. Nativelle, ave Franklin Roosevelt 138, 1050 Brussels, Belgium.

Nativelle, Fr. Laboratoires Nativelle S.A., 27 rue de la Procession, 75737 Paris Cedex 15, France.

Nativelle, Ital. Istituto Farmochimico Nativelle s.p.a., Via P. Filargo 34, 20143 Milan, Italy.

Nativelle, Switz. See *Biphar, Switz.* and *Cevep, Switz.*

Natrapharm, Ger. Natrapharm Arzneimittel GmbH, Nattermannallee 1, Postfach: 350120, 5000 Cologne 30, W. Germany.

Natterman, Neth. See *Therapeuticon, Neth.*

Nattermann, Ger. A. Nattermann & Cie. GmbH, Nattermannallee 1, Postfach: 350120, 5000 Cologne 30, W. Germany.

ND & K, Denm. See *Nordisk Droge, Denm.*

Nella, UK. Nella Pharmaceutical Products Ltd, 63 Jenkin Rd, Sheffield 9, England.

Nelson, Austral. Nelson Laboratories Pty Ltd, Australia.

Nemi, Arg. Nemi S.A.C.I.F.I., Lavalle 710 1°D, 1047 Buenos Aires, Argentina.

Neo, Canad. Neo Drug Co., 5476 Upper Lachine Rd, Montreal, Quebec H4A 2A4, Canada.

Neo Laboratories, UK. Neo Laboratories Ltd, 1a Frognal, London NW3 6AN, England.

Neomed, Switz. Neomed AG, Bahnhofstrasse, 3185 Schmitten, Switzerland.

Neopharmed, Ital. Neopharmed s.p.a., Via Pordoi 18, 20021 Baranzate di Bollate, Italy.

Nessa, Spain. Nessa, Spain.

Nestlé, Norw. A/S Nestlé-Findus, Postboks 595, 1301 Sandvika, Norway.

Nestlé, UK. The Nestlé Co. Ltd, St George's House, Croydon, Surrey CR9 1NR, England.

New Era Laboratories, UK. New Era Laboratories Ltd, 39 Wales Farm Rd, London W3 6XH, England.

Newark, Arg. Esp. Med. Newark S.R.L., Av. Federico Lacroze 3065, 1426 Buenos Aires, Argentina.

Newton, UK. Newton Chemical Ltd, 2 Mansfield Rd, South Croydon, Surrey CR2 6HN, England.

Nezel, Spain. Nezel SA, Independencia 317, Barcelona, Spain.

Nicholas, Austral. Nicholas Pty Ltd, 699 Warrigal Rd, Chadstone Vic. 3148, Australia.

Nicholas, Fr. Laboratoires Nicholas S.A., 74240 Gaillard, France.

Nicholas, Ger. Nicholas GmbH, Hauptstrasse 108, Postfach: 1240, 6231 Sulzbach/Ts., W. Germany.

Nicholas, Neth. Nicholas B.V., A. Dudok van Heelstraat 7, 1096 BE Amsterdam, Netherlands.

Nicholas, Norw. See *Henry Christenson, Norw.*

Nicholas, Switz. See *Doetsch, Grether, Switz.* and *Sauter, Switz.*

Nicholas, UK. Nicholas Laboratories Ltd, 225 Bath Rd, Slough SL1 4AU, England.

Nigy, Fr. Laboratoires Nigy, 82 rue Marius-Sidobre, 94110 Arcueil, France.

Nikken, Jap. Nikken Chemicals Co. Ltd, 4-14 Tsukiji 5-chome, Chuo-ku, Tokyo 104, Japan.

Nipa, UK. Nipa Laboratories Ltd, Nipa Industrial Estate, Llantwit Fardre, near Pontypridd, Mid Glam CF38 2SN, Wales.

Nippon Kayaku, Jap. Nippon Kayaku Co. Ltd, 2-1 Marunouchi 1-chome, Chiyoda-ku, Tokyo 100, Japan.

Nippon Roussel, Jap. Nippon Roussel Co. Ltd, Kinsan Bldg, 5 Nihonbashi Muromachi 4-chome, Chuo-ku, Tokyo 103, Japan.

Nippon Shinyaku, Jap. Nippon Shinyaku Co. Ltd, 14 Kisshoin Nishinosho Monguchicho, Minami-ku, Kyoto 601, Japan.

Norcliff Thayer, UK. Norcliff Thayer, Division of Berk Pharmaceuticals Ltd, St Leonard's House, St Leonard's Rd, Eastbourne, East Sussex BN21 3YG, England.

Nordex, Norw. See *Ingeborg Vidnes, Norw.*

Nordic, Canad. Nordic Pharmaceuticals Ltd, 2775 Bovet St, Laval, Quebec H7S 2A4, Canada.

Nordic, UK. Nordic Pharmaceuticals Ltd, 11 Mount Rd, Feltham, Middx TW13 6JG, England.

Nordisk Droge, Denm. Nordisk Droge Afdl. for farmaceutiske specialiteter, Ragnagade 9, 2100 Copenhagen Ø, Denmark.

Nordisk Insulin, Denm. Nordisk Insulinlaboratorium, Niels Steensensvej 1, 2820 Gentofte, Denmark.

Nordisk-UK, UK. Nordisk-UK, Highview House, Tattenham Crescent, Epsom, Surrey KT18 5QJ, England.

Nordmark, Belg. See *Labaz, Belg.*

Nordmark, Switz. See *Knoll, Switz.*

Nordmark-Werke, Ger. Nordmark-Werke GmbH Hamburg, Pinnau-Allee, Postfach: 1244, 2082 Uetersen/Holstein 1, W. Germany.

Norgan, Fr. Laboratoires Norgan, 21 rue de Madrid, 75008 Paris, France.

Norgesplaster, Norw. Norgesplaster A/S, Skøyen, Oslo 2, Norway.

Norgine, UK. Norgine Ltd, 59 High Holborn, London WC1V 6EB, England.

Noristan, S.Afr. Noristan Laboratories (Pty) Ltd, Private Bag X516, Silverton, Pretoria, S. Africa.

Norka, Spain. Norka, Spain.

Norma, UK. Norma Chemicals Ltd, 1a Frognal, London NW3 6AN, England.

Normon, Spain. Laboratorios Normon SA, Nieremberg, Madrid 2, Spain.

Northia, Arg. Esp. Med. Northia, Madero 135, 1408 Buenos Aires, Argentina.

Norton, UK. H.N. Norton & Co. Ltd, Patman House, George Lane, South Woodford, London E18, England.

Norwich Eaton, Arg. Norwich Eaton Arg. S.A.I.yC., Recuerdos de Provincia 4572, 1407 Buenos Aires, Argentina.

Norwich Eaton, Neth. Norwich Eaton N.V., Europalaan 101, 3526 KR Utrecht, Netherlands.

Norwich-Eaton, UK. Norwich-Eaton Pharmaceuticals Ltd, Regent House, The Broadway, Woking, Surrey GU21 5AP, England.

Norwich-Eaton, USA. Norwich-Eaton Pharmaceuticals, Division of Morton-Norwich, 13 Eaton Ave, Norwich NY 13815, USA.

Nourypharma, Neth. Nourypharma B.V./Nourypharma Nederland B.V., Wethouder van Eschstraat 1, 5340 AB Oss, Netherlands.

Nova-Drug, Canad. Nova-Drug Ltd, 5865 blvd St Michel, Montreal, Quebec H1Y 2E3, Canada.

Novo, Belg. See *Alcon-Couvreur, Belg.*

Novo, Denm. Novo Industri A/S, Hillerødgade 31, 2200 Copenhagen N, Denmark.

Novo, Ger. Novo Industrie GmbH Pharmaceutika, Kantstrasse 2, Postfach: 2840, 6500 Mainz, W. Germany.

Novo, Neth. Novo Industri B.V., Linnaeusparkweg 220, 1098 ER Amsterdam, Netherlands.

Novo, Norw. Novo Industri A/S, Gamle Drammensv. 48, 1320 Stabekk, Norway.

Novo, Swed. Novo Industri AB, Box 69, 201 20 Malmo 1, Sweden.

Novo, Switz. See *Aldepha, Switz.*

Novo, UK. Novo Laboratories Ltd, Ringway House, Bell Rd, Daneshill East, Basingstoke, Hants RG24 0QN, England.

Novocol Chemical, USA. Novocol Chemical Mfg Co. Inc., 2911 Atlantic Ave, Brooklyn NY 11207, USA.

Novopharma, Switz. Novopharma S.A., ch. Grand-Puits 28, Meyrin, Switzerland.

Noxell, UK. Noxell Corporation (UK) Ltd, North House, 9 St Edward Way, Romford, Essex RM1 1UJ, England.

N.T. Pharm, Denm. N.T. Pharm ApS (Søren Juhl & Co.), Schleppegrellsgade 3, 2200 Copenhagen N, Denmark.

Nuovo, Ital. Nuovo Consorzio Sanitario Nazionale di Malizia Dr Paolo, Via Svetonio 6, 00136 Rome, Italy.

Nutona, UK. Nutona Ltd, Unit 2, Castlefield Estate, Crossflatts, Bingley, West Yorkshire, England.

Nutricia, Neth. Nutricia N.V., Zoetermeer, Netherlands.

Nutrition Control Products, USA. Nutrition Control Products, Division of Pharmex Inc., 2113 Lincoln St, P.O. Box 151, Hollywood FL 33022, USA.

Nutrition House Products, UK. Nutrition House Products (UK) Ltd, 64 Sedlescombe Road North, St Leonards-on-Sea, East Sussex TN37 7TD, England.

Nyco, Denm. NycoMed A/S, Mose Alle 10 A, 2610 Rødovre, Denmark.

Nyco, Norw. Nyegaard & Co. A/S, Nycovn. 2, Postboks 4220 Torshov, Oslo 4, Norway.

Nyegaard, UK. Nyegaard (UK) Ltd, Mylen House, 11 Wagon Lane, Sheldon, Birmingham B26 3DU, England.

O'Neal, Canad. See *Seaway Midwest, Canad.*

O'Neal, USA. O'Neal, Jones & Feldman Inc., 2510 Metro Blvd, Maryland Heights MO 63043, USA.

Oberlin, Fr. Laboratoires Oberlin, 128 rue Danton, 92500 Rueil-Malmaison, France.

Oberval, Fr. Laboratoires Oberval, 115 ave Lacassagne, 69003 Lyon, France.

OFF, Ital. Officina Farmaceutica Fiorentina Istituto Biochimico, Quart. Varignano 12, 55049 Viareggio (Lucca), Italy.

Oftalmiso, Spain. Oftalmiso, Spain.

Ohio Medical, USA. Ohio Medical, Division of Air Reduction Co. Inc., 3030 Airco Drive, Madison WI 53701, USA.

Ohta, Jap. Ohta Pharmaceutical Co. Ltd, 28-2 Kamijujo 2-chome, Kita-ku, Tokyo 114, Japan.

Olin, USA. Olin Corporation, 120 Long Ridge Rd, Stamford CT 06904, USA.

Om, Switz. Laboratoire Om S.A., rue du Bois-du-Lan 22, 1217 Meyrin, Switzerland.

Omega, Arg. Esp. Med. Omega, Castillo 760, 1414 Buenos Aires, Argentina.

Omegin, Ger. Omegin Dr Schmidgall GmbH & Co. KG, Nürtinger Strasse 48, Postfach: 8, 7316 Köngen a.N., W. Germany.

Ono, Jap. Ono Pharmaceutical Co. Ltd, 14 Doshomachi 2-chome, Higashi-ku, Osaka 541, Japan.

Opfermann, Ger. Opfermann Arzneimittel GmbH, Hauptstrasse 1-9, Postfach: 20 07 20, 5060 Bergisch Gladbach 2, W. Germany.

Opochimiothérapie, Fr. Laboratoires d'Opochimiothérapie, 62 blvd des Récollets, 31030 Toulouse Cedex, France.

Opodex, Fr. Opodex S.A., 18 rue Raymond-Ridel, 92250 La Garenne-Colombes, France.

Opopharma, Switz. Opopharma AG, Kirchgasse 42, 8001 Zurich, Switzerland.

Optrex, UK. Optrex Ltd, City Wall House, Basing View, Basingstoke, Hants RG21 2JP, England.

Orapharm, Austral. Orapharm, Australia.

Orfi, Spain. Orfi Farma SA, Baronesa de la Malda 73, Esplugas de Llobregat (Barcelona), Spain.

Organon, Arg. Organón Arg. S.A., Charcas 3666, 1425 Buenos Aires, Argentina.

Organon, Austral. Organon (Australia) Pty Ltd, 34 Hotham Parade, Artarmon NSW 2064, Australia.

Organon, Belg. See *Organon Belge, Belg.* and *Organon Teknica, Belg.*

Organon Belge, Belg. Organon Belge S.A., ave Marnix 13, 1050 Brussels, Belgium.

Organon, Canad. Organon Canada Ltd, 565 Coronation Drive, West Hill, Ontario M1E 4S2, Canada.

Organon, Denm. Organon ApS, Literbuen 9-11, 2740 Skovlunde, Denmark.

Organon, Fr. Organon, B.P. 144, 93204 Saint-Denis Cedex 01, France.

Organon, Ger. Organon GmbH/Organon Teknika Medizinische Produkte GmbH, Mittenheimer Strasse 62, 8042 Oberschleissheim, W. Germany.

Organon, Neth. Organon Nederland B.V./Organon Teknika Nederland B.V., Wethouder van Eschstraat 1, 5340 AB Oss, Netherlands.

Organon, Norw. Organon A/S, Postboks 325, 1371 Asker, Norway.

Organon, Spain. Organon Española SA, Poligono Las Salinas, San Baudilio de Llobregat (Barcelona), Spain.

Organon, Swed. Organon AB, Box 5076, 421 05 Västra Frölunda, Sweden.

Organon, Switz. See *Opopharma, Switz.*

Organon Teknica, Belg. Organon Teknica S.A., Toekomstlaan 10, 2060 Merksem, Belgium.

Organon Teknika, UK. Organon Teknika Ltd, Teknika House, Cromwell Rd, St Neots, Huntingdon, Cambs PE19 2HS, England.

Organon, UK. Organon Laboratories Ltd, Crown House, London Rd, Morden, Surrey SM4 5DZ, England.

Organon, USA. Organon Pharmaceuticals, 375 Mount Pleasant Ave, West Orange NJ 07052, USA.

Orion, Denm. See *Erco, Denm.*

Orravan, Spain. Orravan, Spain.

Ortho-Cilag, UK. Ortho-Cilag Pharmaceutical Ltd, P.O. Box 79, Saunderton, High Wycombe, Bucks HP14 4HJ, England.

Ortho, Denm. See *Mecobenzon, Denm.*

Ortho Diagnostics, UK. Ortho Diagnostic Systems Ltd, Denmark House, Denmark St, High Wycombe, Bucks HP11 2ER, England.

Ortho, Norw. See *Cilag-Chemie, Norw.*

Ortho, USA. Ortho Pharmaceutical Corporation, Raritan NJ 08869, USA.

Oscar Brandenberger, Switz. Oscar Brandenberger AG, Fröbelstrasse 22, 8032 Zurich, Switzerland.

Osiris, Arg. Lab. Osiris S.A.I.C.F.I., Canalejas 1647, 1406 Buenos Aires, Argentina.

Österreichische Stickstoffwerke, Switz. See *Agpharm, Switz.* and *Globopharm, Switz.*

Otsuka, Jap. Otsuka Pharmaceutical Co. Ltd, 9 Kanda Tsukasacho 2-chome, Chiyoda-ku, Tokyo 101, Japan.

Otto Broe, Denm. Otto Broe A/S, Formervangen 9, 2600 Glostrup, Denmark.

Otto Jann, Switz. See *Doetsch, Grether, Switz.*

Ottosen, Denm. G.R. Ottosen, Romancevej 31, 2730 Herlev, Denmark.

Owen, Canad. Owen Laboratories, Division of Alcon Laboratories Ltd, 6500 Kitimat Rd, Mississauga, Ontario L5N 2B8, Canada.

Oxoid, UK. Oxoid Ltd, Wade Rd, Basingstoke, Hants RG24 0PW, England.

Padil, Ital. Farmaco Italiano Padil s.p.a., Via Prealpi 8, 20032 Cormano, Italy.

Padro, Spain. Padro, Spain.

Pages Maruny, Spain. Pages Maruny, Spain.

Paines & Byrne, UK. Paines & Byrne Ltd, Pabryn Laboratories, 177 Bilton Rd, Perivale, Greenford, Middx UB6 7HG, England.

Pan-American Pharmaceuticals, UK. Pan-American Pharmaceuticals Ltd, Jedburgh House, Jedburgh Rd, London E13 9LQ, England.

Pan Química Farmac., Spain. Pan Química Farmacéutica SA, Rufino Gonzalez 50, Madrid 17, Spain.

Panpharma, Switz. Panpharma AG, Untermattweg 8, 3027 Bern, Switzerland.

Panray, USA. Panray Pharmaceuticals, Division of Ormont Drug & Chemical Co. Inc., 16600 NW 54th Ave, Miami FL 33014, USA.

Panther-Osfa, Ital. Panther Osfa Chemie, Industria Farmaco Biologica e di Ricerche, Via Doberdò 16, 20126 Milan, Italy.

Panthox & Burck, Ital. Panthox & Burck s.p.a., Istituto Biochimico Italo Svizzero, Via Beldiletto 1, 20142 Milan, Italy.

Para-Pharma, Switz. Para-Pharma AG, Löwenstrasse 59, 8001 Zurich, Switzerland.

Paramed, Switz. Paramed AG, Brunnmattstrasse 12, 5400 Baden, Switzerland.

Parcor, Belg. See *Codali, Belg.*

Parkdale, USA. Parkdale, San Antonio, USA.

Parke, Davis, Arg. Parke, Davis & Cía. de Arg. S.A.I.yC., Sanabria 2353, 1417 Buenos Aires, Argentina.

Parke, Davis, Austral. Parke, Davis & Co., 32 Cawarra Rd North, Caringbah NSW 2229, Australia.

Parke, Davis, Belg. Parke, Davis et Cie S.A., ave Wielemans Ceuppens 45, 1190 Brussels, Belgium.

Parke, Davis, Canad. Parke, Davis & Co. Ltd, Box 633, Station A, Scarborough, Ontario M1K 5C5, Canada.

Parke, Davis, Denm. Parke-Davis, Rosenkaeret 22 B, 2860 Søborg, Denmark.

Parke, Davis, Fr. Parke-Davis (Division des Laboratoires Substantia), 11 ave Dubonnet, 92407 Courbevoie Cedex, France.

Parke, Davis, Ger. Parke, Davis & Co., Mooswaldallee 1-9, Postfach: 5620, 7800 Freiburg, W. Germany.

Parke, Davis, Ital. Parke Davis s.p.a., Via C. Colombo 1, 20020 Lainate (Milano), Italy.

Parke, Davis, Neth. Parke-Davis, Oderweg 1, 1043 AG Amsterdam, Netherlands.

Parke, Davis, Norw. Parke, Davis & Co. Informasjonsavd. Norge, Gamle Grav vei 32, 1340 Bekkestua, Norway.

Parke, Davis, S.Afr. Parke-Davis Laboratories, Division of Chamberlains (Pty) Ltd, 702 Foretrust Building, Martin Hammerschlag Way, Cape Town 8001, S. Africa.

Parke, Davis, Spain. Laboratorios Parke-Davis SA, Emilio Vargas 6, Madrid, Spain.

Parke, Davis, Swed. See *Warner-Lambert, Swed.*

Parke, Davis, Switz. See *Cosmopharm, Switz.*

Parke, Davis, UK. Parke, Davis & Co. Ltd, Usk Rd, Pontypool, Gwent NP4 0YH, Wales.

Parke, Davis, USA. Parke-Davis, Division Warner-Lambert Inc., 201 Tabor Rd, Morris Plains NJ 07950, USA.

Parkinsons, UK. Parkinsons Ltd, P.O. Box 8, Curzon St, Burnley, Lancs BB11 1BD, England.

Pasadena Research Labs, USA. Pasadena Research Labs Inc., 2107 E. Villa St, Pasadena CA 91107, USA.

Pascoe, Ger. Pascoe Pharmazeutische Präparate GmbH, Schiffenberger Weg 55, Postfach:6140, 6300 Giessen, W. Germany.

Patentex, Denm. See *Helge Kjelstrup, Denm.*

Paton, UK. F.C. Paton (Southport) Ltd, 43a Old Park Lane, Southport, Merseyside PR9 7BC, England.

Paul Dupin, Arg. Establecimiento Paul Dupin S.A. Quimica e Indust., Av. Gral. Paz 13284, 1429 Buenos Aires, Argentina.

Paylos, Arg. Lab. Paylos S.R.L., Dardo Rocha 202, 1870 Avellaneda, Argentina.

Pearson, Ger. Pearson & Co. (GmbH & Co.), Basshorn 15, 2082 Uetersen, W. Germany.

Pearson, UK. William Pearson Ltd, Clough Rd, Hull, North Humberside HU6 7QA, England.

Pechiney, UK. Pechiney Ugine Kuhlmann Ltd, Chemicals Division, Smith's Rd, Bolton, England.

Pedersen, Norw. O. Chr. Pedersen A/S Farm. Kjemisk Laboratorium, Trondheimsvn. 139, Oslo 5, Norway.

Pennwalt, USA. Pennwalt Pharmaceutical Division, Pennwalt Corporation, 755 Jefferson Rd, Rochester NY 14623, USA.

Pensa, Spain. Pensa Laboratorios, Literato Azorin 20, Valencia 6, Spain.

Pentagone, Canad. Pentagone Laboratories Ltd, 1000 blvd Roche, Vaudreuil, Quebec J7V 6B3, Canada.

Pental, Spain. Pental, Spain.

Perez Jimenez, Spain. Perez Jimenez, Spain.

Perga, Spain. Perga, Spain.

Permicutan, Ger. Permicutan-KG Dr Euler, Schulze-Delitzsch-Strasse 2, Postfach: 2270, 4790 Paderborn, W. Germany.

Perrier, Switz. See *Lucchini, Switz.*

Person & Covey, USA. Person & Covey Inc., 616 Allen Ave, Glendale CA 91201, USA.

Petersen, S.Afr. Petersen Ltd, P.O. Box 5787, Johannesburg, S. Africa.

Petri, Denm. Chr. F. Petri's Eftf. I/S Kemisk Fabrik, Apollovej 33, 2720 Vanløse, Denmark.

Pfanstiehl, USA. Pfanstiehl Laboratories Inc., 1219 Glen Rock Ave, Waukegan IL 60085, USA.

Pfister Chemical, USA. Pfister Chemical Inc., Linden Ave, Ridgefield NJ 07657, USA.

Pfizer, Arg. Pfizer S.A.C.I., Miñones 2177, 1428 Buenos Aires, Argentina.

Pfizer, Aust. Pfizer Corporation Austria GmbH, Mondscheingasse 16, 1071 Vienna VII, Austria.

Pfizer, Austral. Pfizer Pty Ltd, Wharf Rd, North Ryde NSW 2114, Australia.

Pfizer, Belg. Pfizer S.A., rue Léon Théodor 102, 1090 Brussels, Belgium.

Pfizer, Braz. Pfizer Quimica Ltda, Rodovia Presidente Dutra Km 391, Guarulhos, Brazil.

Pfizer, Canad. Pfizer Canada Inc., P.O. Box 800, Pointe Claire, Dorval, Quebec H9R 4V2, Canada.

Pfizer, Denm. Pfizer A/S, Vestre Gade 18, 2650 Hvidovre, Denmark.

Pfizer, Fr. Laboratoires Pfizer, 86 rue de Paris, B.P. 60, 91400 Orsay, France.

Pfizer, Ger. Pfizer GmbH, Pfizerstrasse 1, Postfach: 4949, 7500 Karlsruhe 1, W. Germany.

Pfizer, Hong Kong. Pfizer Corp., 4th Floor, Block A, Taikoo Trading Estate, Hong Kong.

Pfizer, Ital. Pfizer Italiana s.p.a., Via del Fornetto 85, 00149 Rome, Italy.

Pfizer, Neth. Pfizer B.V., Koningslaan 200, 3067 TG Rotterdam, Netherlands.

Pfizer, Norw. Pfizer A/S, Sofiesgt. 60, Oslo 1, Norway.

Pfizer, S.Afr. Pfizer Laboratories (Pty) Ltd, P.O. Box 3720, Sandton 2146, S. Africa.

Pfizer, Spain. Pfizer SA, Francisco Silvela 110, Madrid 6, Spain.

Pfizer, Swed. Pfizer AB, Box 3053, 183 03 Täby, Sweden.

Pfizer, Switz. Pfizer AG, Militärstrasse 84, 8004 Zurich, Switzerland.

Pfizer Taito, Jap. Pfizer Taito Co. Ltd, Shinjuku-Mitsui Bldg, 1-1 Nishi-shinjuku 2-chome, Shinjuku-ku, Tokyo 160, Japan.

Pfizer, UK. Pfizer Ltd, Sandwich, Kent CT13 9NJ, England.

Pfizer, USA. Pfizer Inc., 235 East 42nd St, New York NY 10017, USA.

Pfleger, Ger. Dr R. Pfleger Chemische Fabrik GmbH, Dr-Robert-Pfleger-Strasse 12, Postfach: 2240, 8600 Bamberg 1, W. Germany.

Pfrimmer, Denm. See *Otto Broe, Denm.*

Pfrimmer, Ger. Pfrimmer & Co., Pharmazeutische Werke Erlangen GmbH, Hofmannstrasse 26, Postfach: 2840, 8520 Erglangen, W. Germany.

Pfrimmer, Norw. See *Meda, Norw.*

Pharbil, Belg. Pharbil SID S.A., rue des Palais 112, 1030 Brussels, Belgium.

Pharbil, Neth. Pharbil B.V., Wijnhaven 44, 3011 WS Rotterdam, Netherlands.

Pharma-Medica, Denm. pHarma-Medica a-s, Farmaceutisk-teknisk laboratorium, Vesterlundvej 19, 2730 Herlev, Denmark.

Pharma-Medica, Norw. See *AFI, Norw.*

pHarma-medica, UK. pHarma-medica Ltd, Moreton-in-Marsh, Gloucestershire, England.

Pharma-Produits, Belg. Pharma-Produits, ave Louis Lepoutre 87, 1060 Brussels, Belgium.

Pharma-Schwarz, Ger. Pharma-Schwarz GmbH, Mittelstrasse 11, Postfach: 27, 4019 Monheim/Rhld, W. Germany.

Pharma-Schwarz, Switz. See *Adrosanol, Switz.*

Pharmac-Service, Switz. Pharmac-Service S.A., rue Micheli-du-Crest 4, 1205 Geneva, Switzerland.

Pharmacal, Switz. Pharmacal S.A., rue de la Scie 4-6, 1207 Geneva, Switzerland.

Pharmacare, USA. Pharmacare Generic Drugs Inc., 3227 Morganford Rd, St Louis MO 63116, USA.

Pharmaceutical Mfg, UK. Pharmaceutical Manufacturing Co., Westhoughton, Bolton BL5 3SL, England.

Pharmachemie, Neth. Pharmachemie B.V., Nijverheidsweg 48-50, 2031 CP Haarlem, Netherlands.

Pharmacia, Denm. Pharmacia AS, Herredsvejen 2, 3400 Hillerød, Denmark.

Pharmacia, Ger. Deutsche Pharmacia GmbH, Munzinger Strasse 9, Postfach: 5480, 7800 Freiburg, W. Germany.

Pharmacia, Neth. See *Nourypharma, Neth.*

Pharmacia, Norw. Norsk Pharmacia A/S, Postboks 2005 Grünerløkka, Oslo 5, Norway.

Pharmacia, Swed. Pharmacia AB, Box 181, 751 04 Uppsala, Sweden.

Pharmacia, Switz. See *Opopharma, Switz.*

Pharmacia, UK. Pharmacia (Great Britain) Ltd, Prince Regent Rd, Hounslow, Middx TW3 1NE, England.

Pharmacodex, Ger. Pharmacodex Gesellschaft zum Vertrieb pharmaz. Erzeugnisse mbH, Georg-Kalb-Strasse 7, Postfach: 710 769 München 71, 8023 Grosshesselohe bei München, W. Germany.

Pharmacolor, Switz. Pharmacolor AG, Hardstrasse 28, 4052 Basel, Switzerland.

Pharmafrica, S.Afr. Pharmafrica, S. Africa.

Pharmagen, UK. Pharmagen Ltd, West Lane, Runcorn, Cheshire WA7 2PE, England.

Pharmainvesti, Spain. Pharmainvesti SA, Modesto Lafuente 32, Madrid, Spain.

Pharmakon, Switz. Pharmakon AG, Bürglistrasse 39, 8304 Wallisellen, Switzerland.

Pharmaton, Switz. Pharmaton S.A., Lab. chimico-farmaceutici, 6934 Bioggio, Switzerland.

Pharmax, Denm. See *Nordisk Droge, Denm.*

Pharmax, Norw. See *Ingeborg Vidnes, Norw.*

Pharmax, UK. Pharmax Ltd, Bourne Rd, Bexley, Kent DA5 1NX, England.

Pharmethic, Belg. Pharmethic S.A., rue du Vivier 89-93, 1040 Brussels, Belgium.

Pharmexport, Neth. Pharmexport B.V., Oudeweg 147, 2031 CC Haarlem, Netherlands.

Pharmos, Switz. Pharmos S.A., rue St-Jean 92, 1201 Geneva, Switzerland.

Pharmuka, Belg. Pharmuka Benelux, chaussée d'Alsemberg 1001, 1180 Brussels, Belgium.

Pharnova, Switz. Pharnova S.A., Petit-Chêne 36, 1003 Lausanne, Switzerland.

Phial, Austral. Phial Pty Ltd, Australia.

Philip Harris, UK. Philip Harris Medical Ltd, Hazelwell Lane, Birmingham B30 2PS, England.

Philips-Duphar, Belg. See *Duphar, Belg.*

Philips Roxane, USA. Philips Roxane Laboratories Inc., 330 Oak St, Columbus OH 43216, USA.

Phillips Yeast, UK. Phillips Yeast Products Ltd, Park Royal Rd, London NW10 7JX, England.

Phoenix, Arg. Laboratorio Phoenix, Córdoba 3162, 1187 Buenos Aires, Argentina.

Phyteia, Switz. Phyteia AG, St Gallerstrasse 63, 9102 Herisau, Switzerland.

Piam, Ital. Vecchi & Piam s.a.s., Istituto Maragliano, Via Padre G. Semeria 5, 16131 Genoa, Italy.

Pickles, UK. J. Pickles & Sons, Pickles House, Knaresborough, North Yorkshire, England.

Pidefé, Spain. Pidefé, Spain.

Pierre Bardin, Arg. Lab. Pierre Bardin S.A.I.yC., Junin 508, 1026 Buenos Aires, Argentina.

Pierrel, Ital. Pierrel s.p.a., Via Comelico 39/41, 20134 Milan, Italy.

Pilsworth, UK. Pilsworth Manufacturing Co. Ltd, 252A Newchurch Rd, Stacksteads, Bacup, Lancs, England.

Pinewood, Eire. Pinewood Laboratories Ltd, Ballymacarbry, Clonmel, Co. Tipperary, Eire.

Piror, Spain. Piror, Spain.

Playtex-Wallco, Norw. Playtex-Wallco A/S, Postboks 1, 1473 Skårer, Norway.

Plough, UK. Plough (UK) Ltd, Penarth St, London SE15 1TT, England.

Poen, Arg. Lab. Poen S.A.C.I.F.I., Av. Gaona 5120/24, 1407 Buenos Aires, Argentina.

Pohl, Denm. See *Tjellesen, Denm.*

Pohl, Ger. G. Pohl-Boskamp GmbH & Co. KG, Breite Strasse 41, Postfach: 80, 2214 Hohenlockstedt, W. Germany.

Polcrome, UK. Polcrome Ltd, 11 Mount Rd, Feltham, Middx TW13 6JG, England.

Polfa, Pol. Ciech-Polfa Pharmaceutical Products Division, Wapolna 4, 00-505 Warsaw, Poland.

Poli, Ital. Poli Industria Chimica s.p.a., Piazza Agrippa 1, 20141 Milan, Italy.

Poli, Neth. See *Multi-Pharma, Neth.*

Poli, Switz. See *Galenica, Switz.* and *Iromedica, Switz.*

Polifarma, Ital. Polifarma s.p.a., Via Tor Sapienza 138, 00155 Rome, Italy.

Pons, Spain. Pons, Spain.

Porcher-Lavril, Fr. Laboratoires Clin Midy, Dépt. Porcher-Lavril, 20 rue des Fossés-St-Jacques, 75240 Paris Cedex 05, France.

Potter & Clarke, UK. Potter & Clarke Ltd, 415 Limpsfield Rd, The Green, Warlingham, Surrey CR3 9YS, England.

Potter's Herbal Supplies, UK. Potter's (Herbal Supplies) Ltd, Leyland Mill Lane, Wigan, Lancs WN1 2SB, England.

Poythress, USA. Wm. P. Poythress & Co. Inc., 16 North 22nd St, P.O. Box 26946, Richmond VA 23261, USA.

Pradel, Spain. Laboratorio Pradel SA, Madrid, Spain.

Prats, Spain. Prats, Spain.

Prem, Spain. Laboratorios Prem SA, Barcelona, Spain.

Princes Foods, UK. Princes Foods Ltd, Wilson Rd, Huyton, Liverpool, England.

Priory Laboratories, UK. Priory Laboratories Ltd, Hill Farm Ave, Watford WD2 7RA, England.

Procea, Eire. Procea Ltd, Alexandra Rd, Dublin 1, Eire.

Procter & Gamble, USA. Procter & Gamble, P.O. Box 171, Cincinnati OH 45201, USA.

Proctor & Gamble, UK. Proctor & Gamble Ltd, Gosforth, Newcastle-on-Tyne NE99 1EE, England.

Prodes, Spain. Laboratorio Prodes SA, Trabajo s/n, San Justo Desvern (Barcelona), Spain.

Prodotti Erma, Ital. Prodotti E.R.M.A. s.r.l., Via Colombo 1, 21010 Muceno P. Valtravaglia, Italy.

Prof. Pharm. Corp., Canad. Professional Pharmaceutical Corporation, 2795 Bates Rd, Montreal, Quebec H3S 1B6, Canada.

Promeco, Arg. Laboratorio Promeco S.A., Av. del Libertador 7208, 1429 Buenos Aires, Argentina.

Promedica, Fr. Laboratoires Promedica, 41 rue Camille-Pelletan, 92305 Levallois-Perret, France.

Promedica, Switz. See *Pharmac-Service, Switz.*

Promesa, Spain. Promesa SA, Arturo Soria 228, Madrid 33, Spain.

Promonta, Belg. See *Byk, Belg.*

Promonta, Ger. Chemische Fabrik Promonta GmbH, Hammer Landstrasse 162, Postfach: 260661, 2000 Hamburg 26, W. Germany.

Propan, S.Afr. Propan Ethicals (Pty) Ltd, P.O. Box 10534, Johannesburg 2000, S. Africa.

Prophin, Ital. Prophin s.p.a., Via A. Binda 21, 20143 Milan, Italy.

Propper, UK. Chance Propper Ltd, Spon Lane, Smethwick, Warley, West Midlands, England.

Prosana, Austral. Prosana Laboratories Pty Ltd, 22 Daisy St, Revesby NSW 2212, Australia.

Prospa, Belg. Prospa, rue de Brabant 107, 1030 Brussels, Belgium.

Protea, Austral. Protea Pharmaceuticals Pty Ltd, 13 Glebe St, Glebe NSW 2037, Australia.

Proter, Ital. Proter s.p.a., Via Lambro 38, 20090 Opera (Milano), Italy.

Protina, Ger. Protina, Chemische GmbH, Werner-Friedmann-Bogen 7, Postfach: 500470, 8000 Munich 50, W. Germany.

Provita, Switz. Provita S.A., La Route-Neuve, 1920 Martigny, Switzerland.

Pulitzer, Ital. Pulitzer Italiana s.p.a., Via Tiburtina 1004, 00156 Rome, Italy.

Purdue Frederick, Canad. The Purdue Frederick Co. (Canada) Ltd, 123 Sunrise Ave, Toronto, Ontario M4A 1A9, Canada.

Purdue Frederick, USA. The Purdue Frederick Co., 50 Washington St, Norwalk CT 06856, USA.

Pure Plant Products, UK. Pure Plant Products, Sandy Lane, Irby, Wirral, Merseyside, England.

Purissimus, Arg. Inst. de Terap. Purissimus S.A., Juan F. Seguí 4635, 1425 Buenos Aires, Argentina.

PVO International, USA. PVO International Inc., 416 Division St, Boonton NJ 07005, USA.

Quaker, USA. Quaker City Pharmacal Co., 129 North 4th St, Philadelphia PA 19106, USA.

Quimia, Spain. Quimia, Spain.

Químicos, Spain. Laboratorio Químicos Unidos SA, Azcona 48, Madrid 28, Spain.

Quimpe, Spain. Quimpe, Spain.

Quinoderm, UK. Quinoderm Ltd, Manchester Rd, Hollinwood, Oldham, Lancs OL8 4PB, England.

R. Rius, Spain. R. Rius, Spain.

Radiol, UK. Radiol Chemicals Ltd, Stepfield, Witham, Essex CM8 3AG, England.

Radiumfarma, Ital. Radiumfarma s.r.l., Laboratori Farmaco Biologici (ex Radiumfarm), Via Cavour 57, 20063 Cernusco S/N (Milano), Italy.

Raffo, Arg. Lab. Prof. Raffo S.A.I.C.yF., Viamonte 1770, 1055 Buenos Aires, Argentina.

Ragionieri, Ital. Dr R.R. Ragionieri s.p.a, Via Gramsci 356, 50019 Sesto Fiorentino, Italy.

Ralay, Spain. Ralay, Spain.

Ranbaxy, Ind. Ranbaxy Laboratories Ltd, 78 Nehru Place, New Delhi - 110 019, India.

Rapide, Spain. Rapide, Spain.

Ratiopharm, Ger. Ratiopharm GmbH Arzneimittel, Im Gehrn, Postfach: 1156, 7902 Blaubeuren, W. Germany.

Ravasini, Ital. Ravasini Dr R. & C.ia s.p.a., Via Ostilia 15, 00184 Rome, Italy.

Ravensberg, Belg. See *Pharmethic, Belg.*

Ravensberg, Ger. Ravensberg GmbH Chemische Fabrik, Steinstrasse 27, Postfach: 1228, 7750 Constance, W. Germany.

Ravizza, Belg. See *Therapeutica, Belg.*

Ravizza, Ital. Ravizza s.p.a., Via Europa 35, 20053 Muggiò, Italy.

Raymos, Arg. Raymos S.A.I.C., Cuba 2760, 1055 Buenos Aires, Argentina.

RBS Pharma, Ital. RBS Pharma (Roger Bellon Schoum) s.p.a., Via A. Kuliscioff 6, 20152 Milan, Italy.

Recip, Swed. AB Recip, Lindhagensgatan 133, 112 87 Stockholm, Sweden.

Reckitt & Colman, Austral. Reckitt & Colman Pharmaceutical Division, 44 Wharf Rd, West Ryde NSW 2114, Australia.

Reckitt & Colman, Neth. Reckitt & Colman Farma, divisie van R. & C. Nederland B.V., Hermesweg 5, 3741 GP Baarn, Netherlands.

Reckitt & Colman, Norw. See *Collett, Norw.*

Reckitt & Colman Pharmaceuticals, UK. Reckitt & Colman Pharmaceutical Division, Dansom Lane, Kingston-upon-Hull HU8 7DS, England.

Reckitt & Colman, S.Afr. Reckitt & Colman Pharmaceuticals, P.O. Box 1097, Cape Town 8000, S. Africa.

Reckitt Products, UK. Reckitt Products, Reckitt House, Stoneferry Rd, Hull HU8 8DD, England.

Reckitts, Austral. Reckitts Pty Ltd, 44 Wharf Rd, West Ryde NSW 2114, Australia.

Recordati, Belg. See *de Bournonville, Belg.*

Recordati, Ital. Recordati Industria Chimica e Farmaceutica s.p.a., Via Civitali 1, 20148 Milan, Italy.

Recordati, Switz. See *Galenica, Switz.*

Reddish Detergents, UK. Reddish Detergents Ltd, Stanley Rd, Cheadle Hulme, Cheadle, Cheshire, England.

Redel, Ger. Julius Redel Cesra-Arzneimittelfabrik GmbH & Co., Bahnhofstrasse 64, Postfach: 740, 7570 Baden-Baden 19, W. Germany.

Reder, Spain. Reder, Spain.

Reed & Carnrick, USA. Reed & Carnrick, 30 Boright Ave, Kenilworth NJ 07033, USA.

Regent Laboratories, UK. Regent Laboratories Ltd, Cunard Rd, London NW10 6PN, England.

Reid-Provident, USA. Reid-Provident Laboratories Inc., 640 Tenth St, Atlanta GA 30318, USA.

Reig Jofré, Spain. Reig Jofré, Spain.

Reiss, Ger. Dr Rudolf Reiss Chemische Werke GmbH & Co. KG (Schwarzhaupt-Gruppe), Erasmusstrasse 20/24, 1000 Berlin 21, W. Germany.

Remed, Norw. A/S Remed, Postboks 7658 Skil., Oslo 2, Norway.

Remedia, S.Afr. Remedia (Pty) Ltd, 7 Baldwin Rd, Village Deep, Johannesburg, S. Africa.

Remifarm, Norw. Remifarm A/S, Postboks 7658 Skil., Oslo 2, Norway.

Renapharm, Switz. Renapharm S.A., rue du Bourg de l'Auge, 1636 Broc, Switzerland.

Rendell, UK. W.J. Rendell Ltd, Ickleford Manor, Hitchin, Herts SG5 3XE, England.

Rentokil, UK. Rentokil Ltd, Products Division, Felcourt, East Grinstead, West Sussex RH19 2JY, England.

Research Industries Corp., USA. Research Industries Corporation, Pharmaceutical Division, 1847 West 2300 South, Salt Lake City UT 84119, USA.

Resfar, Ital. Resfar s.r.l., Italy.

Restan, S.Afr. Restan Laboratories (Pty) Ltd, Craighall Mews, Jan Smuts Ave, Craighall Park, Johannesburg, S. Africa.

Rether, Spain. Rether SA, Juan XXIII 15-19, Esplugas (Barcelona), Spain.

Revit, Switz. Revit AG, Seefeldstrasse 11, 6008 Luzern, Switzerland.

Revlon, UK. Revlon International Corporation, 86 Brook St, London W1Y 2BA, England.

Rewo, UK. Rewo Chemicals Ltd, Crown House, London Rd, Morden, Surrey SM4 5DU, England.

Rhein-Pharma, Ger. Rhein-Pharma Arzneimittelwerk GmbH, Brauereistrasse, 6831 Plankstadt, W. Germany.

RHM Foods, UK. RHM Foods Ltd, Birling Rd, Ashford, Kent, England.

Rhodia, Arg. Rhodia S.A., 1° Junta 525, 1879 Quilmes, Argentina.

Rhodia-Pharm, Switz. Rhodia-Pharm S.A., rue du Lièvre 2-4, 1211 Geneva, Switzerland.

Rhodia, Spain. Rhodia Iberica SA, San Salvador 29, Barcelona, Spain.

Rhône-Poulenc, Canad. Rhône-Poulenc Pharma Inc., 8580 Esplanade Ave, Montreal, Quebec H2P 2R9, Canada.

Rhone-Poulenc, Denm. Rhone-Poulenc Pharma Norden A/S, Topstykket 12, 3460 Birkerød, Denmark.

Rhône-Poulenc, Fr. Rhône-Poulenc, France.

Rhône-Poulenc, Ger. Rhône-Poulenc Pharma GmbH, Mühlenweg 131, Postfach: 1909, 2000 Norderstedt, W. Germany.

Rhône-Poulenc, Neth. Rhône-Poulenc Nederland B.V., Draaistroom 1, 1181 VT Amstelveen, Netherlands.

Rhône-Poulenc, Norw. Rhône-Poulenc, Medisinsk Informasjonskontor, Skårervn. 150, Postboks 20, 1473 Skårer, Norway.

Ricar, Arg. Lab. Ricar S.A., Guayaquil 623, 1424 Buenos Aires, Argentina.

Richards & Appleby, UK. Richards & Appleby Ltd, Gerrard Place, East Gillibrands, Skelmersdale, Lancs WN8 9SU, England.

Richardson-Merrell, Switz. Richardson-Merrell AG, Wallstrasse 14, 4002 Basel, Switzerland.

Richardson-Vicks, UK. Richardson-Vicks Ltd, Rusham Park, Whitehall Lane, Egham, Surrey TW20 9NW, England.

Richet, Arg. Lab. Richet S.A., Gaona 2028, Buenos Aires, Argentina.

Richter, Denm. See *Baungaard, Denm.*

Richter, Ital. Ormonoterapia Richter (Gruppo Lepetit s.p.a.), Via R. Lepetit 8, 20124 Milan, Italy.

Riddell, UK. Riddell Products Ltd, 70 Colliers Water Lane, Thornton Heath, Surrey CR4 7LB, England.

Riedel, Arg. Riedel y Levalle S.R.L., Dr Juen F. Aranguren 2955, 1406 Buenos Aires, Argentina.

Riker, Arg. Laboratorio Riker S.A., Av. del Trabajo 5820, 1439 Buenos Aires, Argentina.

Riker, Austral. Riker Laboratories Australia Pty Ltd, 9 Chilvers Rd, Thornleigh NSW 2120, Australia.

Riker, Canad. Riker Canada Inc., 3057 Mainway, Burlington, Ontario L7M 1A1, Canada.

Riker, Denm. Riker Pharmaceuticals A/S 3M, Fabriksparken 15, 2600 Glostrup, Denmark.

Riker, Fr. Laboratoires Riker, ave du 11-Novembre, Zone Industrielle, 45300 Pithiviers, France.

Riker, Norw. Riker Laboratories, Informasjonskontoret for Norge, Hvamvn. 6, Postboks 100, 2013 Skjetten, Norway.

Riker, UK. Riker Laboratories, 1 Morley St, Loughborough, Leics LE11 1EP, England.

Riker, USA. Riker Laboratories Inc., Subsidiary of 3M Co., 19901 Nordhoff St, Northridge CA 91324, USA.

Rimmer, UK. Rimmer Brothers, 18 Aylesbury St, London EC1R 0DD, England.

Ringsted & Semler, Denm. Ringsted & Semler A/S, N. Farimagsgade 13, 1364 Copenhagen K, Denmark.

Rinver, Spain. Rinver, Spain.

Rio, S.Afr. Rio Ethicals, A division of Adcock-Ingram Laboratories Ltd, 50 Commando Rd, Industria West, Johannesburg, S. Africa.

Riom, Fr. Riom Laboratoires, 63203 Riom Cedex, France.

Rioplatense, Arg. Lab. Rioplatense S.A.C.I.yI., Aguero 1843, 1425 Buenos Aires, Argentina.

Ripari-Gero, Ital. Istituto Farmaco Biologico Ripari Gero s.r.l., Via Chiantigiana 84, 53035 Monteriggioni, Italy.

RIT, Belg. R.I.T., rue du Tilleul 13, 1320 Genval, Belgium.

Rivero, Arg. P.L. Rivero & Cía. S.A.I.yC., Av. Boyacá 419, 1406 Buenos Aires, Argentina.

Robapharm, Switz. Robapharm AG, St Alban-Rheinweg 174, 4052 Basel, Switzerland.

Robeco Chemicals, USA. Robeco Chemicals Inc., 99 Park Ave, New York NY 10016, USA.

Robert & Carriere, Belg. Laboratoires Robert & Carriere, rue Roosendael 125, 1190 Brussels, Belgium.

Robert et Carrière, Fr. Laboratoires Robert et Carrière, 1 bis ave de Villars, 75341 Paris Cedex 07, France.

Robert et Carrière, Switz. See *Actipharm, Switz.*

Robert, Spain. Laboratorios Robert SA, Avda. San Antonio Maria Claret 158-164, Barcelona, Spain.

Roberts & Sheppey, UK. Roberts & Sheppey Ltd, Manor Farm House, Ickford, Bucks, England.

Robilliart, Fr. Laboratoires Michel Robilliart, 121 rue de Paris, 91570 Bièvres, France.

Robin, Ital. Boehringer Biochemia Robin s.p.a., Via S. Uguzzone 5, 20126 Milan, Italy.

Robins, Austral. A.H. Robins Pty Ltd, 4 Charles St, Canterbury NSW 2193, Australia.

Robins, Canad. A.H. Robins Canada Inc., 5950 Côte de Liesse Rd, Montreal, Quebec H4T 1E2, Canada.

Robins Consumer Products, UK. A.H. Robins Consumer Products, Redkiln Way, Horsham, West Sussex RH13 5QP, England.

Robins, Denm. See *Meda, Denm.*

Robins, Norw. See *Andersen, Norw.*

Robins, UK. A.H. Robins Co. Ltd, Redkiln Way, Horsham, West Sussex RH13 5QP, England.

Robins, USA. A.H. Robins Co., 1407 Cummings Dr., Richmond VA 23220, USA.

Robugen, Ger. Robugen GmbH Pharmazeutische Fabrik, Alleenstrasse 22, Postfach: 266, 7300 Esslingen-Zell 1, W. Germany.

Robugen, Switz. See *Renapharm, Switz.*

Rocador, Spain. Rocador SA, Calle J.A. Clave 98, Esplugas de Llobregat, Barcelona, Spain.

Roche, Arg. Productos Roche S.A. Química e Industrial, C. Correo 1893, 1000 Buenos Aires, Argentina.

Roche, Austral. Roche Products Pty Ltd, Inman Rd, Dee Why NSW 2099, Australia.

Roche, Belg. Produits Roche S.A., ave du Roi 157, 1060 Brussels, Belgium.

Roche, Braz. Produtos Roche Quimicos e Farmaceuticos S.A., Rua General Canabarro 666, Rio de Janeiro, Brazil.

Roche, Canad. Hoffmann-La Roche Ltd, 1000 blvd Roche, Vaudreuil, Quebec J7V 6B3, Canada.

Roche, Denm. Roche A/S, Industriholmen 59, 2650 Hvidovre, Denmark.

Roche, Fr. Produits Roche S.A., 52 blvd du Parc, 92521 Neuilly-sur-Seine Cedex, France.

Roche, Ger. Hoffmann-La Roche Aktiengesellschaft, Emil-Barell-Strasse 1, Postfach: 1380, 7889 Grenzach-Wyhlen 1, W. Germany.

Roche, Ital. Prodotti Roche s.p.a., Piazza Durante 11, 20131 Milan, Italy.

Roche, Neth. Hoffmann-La Roche B.V., Nijverheidsweg 38, 3641 RR Mijdrecht, Netherlands.

Roche, Norw. F. Hoffmann-La Roche & Co. AG, Informasjonskontor, Mustads vei 1, Postboks 66 Lilleaker, Oslo 2, Norway.

Roche, S.Afr. Roche Products (Pty) Ltd, P.O. Box 4589, Johannesburg 2000, S. Africa.

Roche, Spain. Productos Roche SA, Ruíz de Alarcon 23, Madrid 14, Spain.

Roche, Swed. Roche-Produkter AB, Box 250, 127 25 Skärholmen 1, Sweden.

Roche, Switz. F. Hoffmann-La Roche & Co. AG, Grenzacherstrasse 124, 4058 Basel, Switzerland.

Roche, UK. Roche Products Ltd, P.O. Box 8, Welwyn Garden City, Herts AL7 3AY, England.

Roche, USA. Roche Laboratories, Division of Hoffmann-La Roche Inc., Roche Park, Nutley NJ 07110, USA.

Rodeca, Canad. Rodeca Inc., 8480 St Lawrence Blvd, Montreal, Quebec H2P 2M6, Canada.

Roemmers, Arg. Roemmers S.A.I.C.F., México 1661-P.B., 1100 Buenos Aires, Argentina.

Roerig, Belg. See *Pfizer, Belg.*

Roerig, Neth. Roerig B.V., Koningslaan 117-119, 3067 TG Rotterdam, Netherlands.

Roerig, Switz. See *Pfizer, Switz.*

Roerig, USA. J.B. Roerig & Co., Division of Pfizer Pharmaceuticals, 235 East 42nd St, New York NY 10017, USA.

Roger, Spain. Laboratorios Roger SA, Corcega 541, Barcelona, Spain.

Roger, USA. Roger Pharmacal Inc., P.O. Box 011022, Miami FL 33010, USA.

Rohm & Haas, UK. Rohm & Haas (UK) Ltd, Lennig House, 2 Mason's Ave, Croydon CR9 3NB, England.

Röhm, Ger. Röhm Pharma GmbH, Dr-Otto-Röhm-Strasse 2-4, Postfach: 4347, 6100 Darmstadt 1, W. Germany.

Roland, Ger. Roland Arzneimittel GmbH, Bargkoppelweg 66, Postfach: 730 820, 2000 Hamburg 73, W. Germany.

Roland-Marie, Fr. Laboratoires Roland-Marie S.A., 15 rue Michelet, 93100 Montreuil, France.

Roland-Marie, Switz. See *Servier, Switz.*

Rona, Denm. See *Meda, Denm.*

Rona, Norw. See *Meda, Norw.*

Rona, S.Afr. See *Propan, S.Afr.*

Rona, UK. Rona Laboratories Ltd, Cadwell Lane, Hitchin, Herts SG4 0SF, England.

Ronchèse, Fr. Institut Ronchèse, 23 ave Morane-Saulnier, 92360 Meudon-la-Forêt, France.

Roner, Austral. Roner, Australia.

Ronsheim & Moore, UK. Ronsheim & Moore Ltd, Castleford, West Yorkshire WF10 2JT, England.

Roques, Fr. Laboratoires Roques, 31 rue Jules-Guesde, 92130 Issy-les-Moulineaux, France.

Rorer, Denm. See *Nordisk Droge, Denm.*

Rorer, Ital. Rorer Italiana s.p.a., Industria Chimica Farmaceutica Biologica, Via Valosa di Sopra 3, 20050 S. Fruttuoso Monza, Italy.

Rorer, UK. Rorer Pharmaceuticals, Stepfield, Witham, Essex CM8 3AG, England.

Rorer, USA. William H. Rorer Inc., 500 Virginia Dr., Fort Washington PA 19034, USA.

Rosa-Phytopharma, Fr. Laboratoires Rosa-Phytopharma S.A., 55 rue Jules-Auffret, 93502 Pantin, France.

Rosco, Denm. A/S Rosco, Farmaceutisk Industri, Tåstrupgårdsvej 30, 2630 Tåstrup, Denmark.

Rosco, Norw. See *Andersen, Norw.*

Ross, USA. Ross Laboratories, Division of Abbott Laboratories, 625 Cleveland Ave, Columbus OH 43216, USA.

Roter, Belg. See *Roterpharma, Belg.*

Roter, Neth. Pharm. Fabr. Roter C.V., Arendstraat 3, 1223 RE Hilversum, Netherlands.

Roterpharma, Belg. Roterpharma, Bosmanlei 35, 2000 Antwerpen, Belgium.

Roterpharma, UK. Roterpharma Ltd, Unit C, Dolphin Trading Estate, Windmill Rd, Sunbury-on-Thames, Middx, England.

Rotta, Ital. Rotta Farmaceutici s.p.a., Via Valosa di Sopra 3, 20050 San Fruttuoso Monza, Italy.

Rougier, Canad. Rougier Inc., 8480 St Lawrence Blvd, Montreal, Quebec H2P 2M6, Canada.

Roussel-Amor Gil, Spain. Roussel-Amor Gil SA, San Rafael s/n, Alcobendas (Madrid), Spain.

Roussel, Arg. Roussel-Lutetia S.A.C.eI., Avellaneda 2202, 1636 Olivos, Argentina.

Roussel, Austral. Roussel Pharmaceuticals Pty Ltd, Gladstone Rd, Castle Hill NSW 2154, Australia.

Roussel, Belg. Roussel S.A., ave Adolphe Lacomblé 59-61, 1040 Brussels, Belgium.

Roussel, Canad. Roussel (Canada) Inc., 4045 Côte Vertu, Montreal, Quebec H4R 2E8, Canada.

Roussel, Denm. See *Hoechst, Denm.*

Roussel, Fr. Laboratoires Roussel, 35 blvd des Invalides, 75323 Paris Cedex 07, France.

Roussel Maestretti, Ital. Roussel Maestretti s.p.a., Viale Gran Sasso 18, 20131 Milan, Italy.

Roussel, Neth. Roussel Laboratoria B.V., Bijenvlucht 30, 3871 JJ Hoevelaken, Netherlands.

Roussel, Norw. See *Hoechst, Norw.*

Roussel, S.Afr. Roussel Laboratories (Pty) Ltd, 5th St, Marlboro Ext. 1, Sandton 2199, Transvaal, S. Africa.

Roussel, Switz. See *Hoechst, Switz.*

Roussel-UCLAF, USA. Roussel-UCLAF, USA.

Roussel, UK. Roussel Laboratories Ltd, Roussel House, Wembley Park, Middx HA9 0NF, England.

Roux-Ocefa, Arg. Lab. Roux Ocefa S.A., Montevideo 79/81, 1019 Buenos Aires, Argentina.

Rovafarm, Arg. Rovafarm Argentina S.A., Paraná 720 3er. piso, 1017 Buenos Aires, Argentina.

Rovi, Spain. Laboratorios Farmacéuticos Rovi SA, Julian Camarillo 35, Madrid 17, Spain.

Rowa, Eire. See *Pinewood, Eire.*

Rowa, S.Afr. See *Holpro, S.Afr.*

Rowa-Wagner, Ger. Rowa-Wagner KG, Arzneimittelfabrik, Frankenforster Strasse 77, Postfach: 169, 5060 Bergisch Gladbach 1 (Bensberg), W. Germany.

Rowell, USA. Rowell Laboratories Inc., 210 Main St West, Baudette MN 56623, USA.

Roy, Canad. C.A. Roy Ltd, 102 Industrial Drive, Whitby, Ontario L1N 5Z8, Canada.

R.P. Drugs, UK. R.P. Drugs Ltd, R.P.D. House, Yorkdale Industrial Park, Braithwaite St, Leeds LS11 9XE, England.

Rubio, Spain. Rubio SA, Berlines 39, Barcelona, Spain.

Rutara, Switz. Rutara GmbH, Bürglistrasse 39, 8304 Wallisellen, Switzerland.

Rutin Products, UK. Rutin Products Ltd, 8 Union St, Pocklington, York YO4 2JL, England.

Rybar, UK. Rybar Laboratories Ltd, 25 Sycamore Rd, Amersham, Bucks HP6 5PQ, England.

Rycovet, UK. Rycovet Ltd, 127 Houldsworth St, Glasgow G3 8JT, Scotland.

Rystan, USA. Rystan Co. Inc., 470 Mamaroneck Ave, White Plains NY 10605, USA.

S. Chobet, Arg. Soubeiran Chobet S.R.L., Sarmiento 2748, 1045 Buenos Aires, Argentina.

Saarstickstoff-Fatol, Ger. Saarstickstoff-Fatol GmbH, Robert-Koch-Strasse, Postfach: 12 60, 6685 Schiffweiler, W. Germany.

Saba, Ital. Saba, Via Salbertrand 21, 10146 Torino, Italy.

Sabex, Canad. Sabex International (1980) Ltd, 977 Pierre-Duprey, Longueuil, Quebec J4K 1A1, Canada.

Saet, Spain. Saet, Spain.

Sagitta, Ger. Sagitta-Werk Arzneimittelfabrik GmbH, Frühlingstrasse 7, Postfach: 1260, 8152 Feldkirchen-Westerham 1, W. Germany.

Sainsbury, UK. J. Sainsbury Ltd, Stamford House, Stamford St, London SE1 9LL, England.

SAIS, Ital. S.A.I.S., Laboratorio Farmaco Biologico, Via Grazioli 2, 30174 Venezia Mestre, Italy.

Saita, Ital. Saita s.r.l., Biofarmaceutici, Via dei Giovi 131, 20037 Paderno Dugnano, Italy.

Salfa, Ital. Salfa, Biochimici dr. Ferranti s.a.s., Piazza Rosselli 2, 60100 Ancona, Italy.

Salsbury, UK. Salsbury Laboratories, 1 Cremyll Rd, Reading, Berks, England.

Salt, UK. Salt & Son Ltd, 220 Corporation St, Birmingham B4 6QR, England.

Salvat, Spain. Laboratorio Salvat SL, Valencia 230, Barcelona, Spain.

SAM, Ital. SAM, Officine Farmaceutiche Mariani s.r.l., Via Mandelli 4, 27058 Voghera (Pavia), Italy.

Samil, Ital. Samil s.r.l., Via Gerano 5, 00156 Rome, Italy.

San Carlo, Ital. S. Carlo Farmaceutici s.p.a., Tor Maggiore, 00040 S. Palomba Pomezia (Roma), Italy.

Sanders-Probel, Belg. Laboratoires Sanders-Probel, rue H. Wafelaerts 47/51, 1060 Brussels, Belgium.

Sandersons, UK. Sandersons (Chemists) Ltd, Highbank House, Marshdale Rd, Bolton BL1 4AQ, England.

Sandoz, Arg. Sandoz Argentina S.A.I.C., Hipolito Yrigoyen 1628, 1344 Buenos Aires, Argentina.

Sandoz, Aust. Sandoz GmbH, Brunnerstrasse 59, Objekt 4, 1235 Wien-Liesing, Austria.

Sandoz, Austral. Sandoz Australia Pty Ltd, 54 Waterloo Rd, North Ryde NSW 2113, Australia.

Sandoz, Canad. Sandoz Pharmaceuticals, Division of Sandoz (Canada) Ltd, 385 Bouchard Blvd, Dorval, Quebec H9R 4P5, Canada.

Sandoz, Denm. Sandoz A/S, Titangade 9 A, 2200 Copenhagen N, Denmark.

Sandoz, Eire. Sandoz Products (Ireland) Ltd, Airton Rd, Off Greenhills Rd, Tallaght, Co. Dublin, Eire.

Sandoz, Fr. Laboratoires Sandoz S.A.R.L., 14 blvd Richelieu, 92500 Rueil-Malmaison, France.

Sandoz, Ger. Sandoz AG, Deutschherrnstrasse 15, 8500 Nürnberg 1, W. Germany.

Sandoz, Greece. Sandoz (Hellas) S.A.C.I., 57 rue Deligiorgi, Place Karaiskaki, Athens 107, Greece.

Sandoz, Ital. Sandoz s.p.a., Via C. Arconati 1, 20135 Milan, Italy.

Sandoz, Neth. Sandoz B.V., Loopkantstraat 25, 5405 AC Uden, Netherlands.

Sandoz, Norw. Sandoz-informasjon, Økernveien 121, Boks 237 Økern, Oslo 5, Norway.

Sandoz, S.Afr. Sandoz Products (Pty) Ltd, P.O. Box 371, Randburg 2125, S. Africa.

Sandoz, Spain. Sandoz SA, Avda. José Antonio 764, Barcelona, Spain.

Sandoz, Swed. Sandoz AB, Box 122, 183 22 Täby, Sweden.

Sandoz, Switz. Sandoz Produkte (Schweiz) AG, Missionsstrasse 60, 4012 Basel, Switzerland.

Sandoz, UK. Sandoz Products Ltd, Sandoz House, 98 The Centre, Feltham, Middx TW13 4EP, England.

Sandoz, USA. Sandoz Pharmaceuticals, Division of Sandoz Inc., Route 10, East Hanover NJ 07936, USA.

Sandoz-Wander, Belg. Sandoz-Wander S.A., chaussée de Haecht 226, 1030 Brussels, Belgium.

Sangers Agencies, UK. Sangers Agencies Ltd, Ramsbury House, High St, Hungerford, Berks, England.

Sanico, Belg. Sanico, Stationstraat 60, 2300 Turnhout, Belgium.

Sanitas, Arg. Inst. Sanitas Argentina, Teodoro Vilardebó 2855/65, 1417 Buenos Aires, Argentina.

Sanitas, UK. Sanitas Group Sales Ltd, Sanitas House, 15 Stockwell Green, London SW9 9JJ, England.

Sanken, Jap. Sanwa Kagaku Kenkyusho Co. Ltd, 3 Higashi-sotoboricho 2-chome, Higashi-ku, Nagoya 461, Japan.

Sankyo, Jap. Sankyo Co. Ltd, 7-12 Ginza 2-chome, Chuo-ku, Tokyo 104, Japan.

Sanol, Ger. Sanol Schwarz GmbH, Mittelstrasse 11, Postfach: 27, 4019 Monheim/Rhld, W. Germany.

Sanol Schwarz, UK. Sanol Schwarz Pharmaceuticals Ltd, The Limes, 130 High St, Chesham, Bucks HP5 1EF, England.

Sanorania, Ger. Sanorania, Dr Gerhard Strohscheer, Düsterhauptstrasse 30, 1000 Berlin 28, W. Germany.

Santen, Jap. Santen Pharmaceutical Co. Ltd, 163 Shimoshinjocho 2-chome, Higashi Yodogawa-ku, Osaka 533, Japan.

Santos, Spain. Santos, Madrid, Spain.

SAPDC, S.Afr. SAPDC, S. Africa.

Saphar, S.Afr. Saphar Laboratories Ltd, Stephen Rd, Ophirton, Johannesburg, S. Africa.

Sapos, Neth. See *Roussel, Neth.*

Sapos, Switz. Sapos S.A., rue G. Moynier 5, 1202 Geneva, Switzerland.

Sarbach, Belg. See *Triosol, Belg.*

Sarbach, Fr. Laboratoires de Thérapeutique Moderne, Sarbach, 42 rue Rouget de Lisle, 92151 Suresnes Cedex, France.

Sarbach, Switz. See *Uhlmann-Eyraud, Switz.*

Sarein, Fr. Laboratoires Sarein, 65 rue Falguière, 75015 Paris, France.

Sarein, Neth. See *ICN, Neth.*

Sarep-Pharmeurop, Fr. S.A.R.E.P.-Pharmeurop, 3 impasse de la Montjoie, 93210 La Plaine-St-Denis, France.

Sarget, Fr. Laboratoires Sarget, ave J.-F. Kennedy, 33701 Mérignac, France.

Sarm, Ital. Sarm s.r.l., Soc. An. Ritrovati Medicinali, Via Tiburtina 1496, 00131 Rome, Italy.

Saron, USA. Saron Pharmacal Corporation, 1640 Central Ave, St Petersburg FL 33712, USA.

Sarva, Belg. Sarva, chaussée de Charleroi 18, 1060 Brussels, Belgium.

Sarva, Neth. Sarva-Nederland, Leeghwaterplein 24B, 2521 CV 's-Gravenhage, Netherlands.

Sas, UK. Sas Pharmaceuticals Ltd, Victoria House, Vernon Place, London WC1B 4DF, England.

Sasse, Ger. Dr Friedrich Sasse, Zweigniederlassung der Gödecke AG Berlin, Mooswaldallee 1-9, Postfach: 14 23, 7800 Freiburg, W. Germany.

Sastre, Spain. Sastre, Spain.

Sauba, Fr. Laboratoires Sauba, 260 rue de Rosny, 93104 Montreuil, France.

Sauflon, UK. Sauflon Pharmaceuticals Ltd, 16 Childs Place, London SW5, England.

Saunier-Daguin, Fr. Laboratoires Saunier-Daguin, 89 rue Lauriston, 75116 Paris, France.

Sauter, Switz. Lab. Sauter S.A., av. de l'Etang 46, 1211 Geneva 28, Switzerland.

Savage, USA. Savage Laboratories, Division of Byk-Gulden Inc., 1000 Main St, P.O. Box 1000, Missouri City TX 77459, USA.

Savio, Ital. Istituto Biochimico Nazionale Savio s.p.a., Via del Commercio 46, 16167 Genova Nervi, Italy.

Savory & Moore, UK. Savory & Moore Ltd, 177 Preston Rd, Brighton, England.

Savoy Laboratories, UK. Savoy Laboratories (International) Ltd, Prospect House, 146 Kilburn High Rd, London NW6, England.

Sawai, Jap. Sawai Pharmaceutical Co. Ltd, 4-25 Akagawacho 1-chome, Asahi-ku, Osaka 535, Japan.

Scalari, Ital. Istituto Farmaceutico Scalari s.r.l., Via L. da Vinci 168, 20090 Trezzano S.N., Italy.

Schaper & Brümmer, Ger. Schaper & Brümmer GmbH & Co. KG, Bahnhofstrasse 35, Postfach: 61 1160, 3320 Salzgitter 61 (Ringelheim), W. Germany.

Scharper, Ital. Scharper s.p.a. per l'industria Farmaceutica, Via Montenapoleone 27, 20121 Milan, Italy.

Scherag, S.Afr. Scherag (Pty) Ltd, P.O. Box 46, Isando 1600, Transvaal, S. Africa.

Scherer, USA. Scherer Laboratories Inc., 14335 Gills Rd, P.O. Drawer 400009, Dallas TX 75240, USA.

Schering AG, Norw. Schering AG, Gamle Drammensv. 48, Postboks 180, 1321 Stabekk, Norway.

Schering AG, NZ. Schering (NZ) Ltd, P.O. Box 66-011, Beachhaven, Auckland 10, New Zealand.

Schering, Arg. Schering Argentina S.A.I.C., Monroe 1378, 1405 Buenos Aires, Argentina.

Schering, Austral. See *Schering Corp., Austral.* and *Schering Pty, Austral.*

Schering, Belg. See *Coles, Belg.* and *Essex, Belg.*

Schering, Canad. Schering Canada Inc., 3535 Trans-Canada, Pointe Claire, Quebec H9R 1B4, Canada.

Schering Corp., Austral. Schering Corporation, 11 Gibbon Rd, Baulkham Hills NSW 2153, Australia.

Schering Corp., Spain. Schering Corp., Delg Av. Generalisimo 61, Madrid 16, Spain.

Schering, Denm. See *Essex, Denm.* and *Schering Kemi, Denm.*

Schering España, Spain. Schering España SA, Mendez Alvaro 55, Madrid 7, Spain.

Schering, Fr. Laboratoires Schering, rue de Toufflers, 59390 Lys-lez-Lannoy, France.

Schering, Ger. Schering AG, Müllerstrasse 170, Postfach: 650311, 1000 Berlin 65, W. Germany.

Schering, Ital. Schering s.p.a., Via Cassanese, 20090 Segrate, Italy.

Schering Kemi, Denm. Schering Kemi AS, Energivej 2, 2750 Ballerup, Denmark.

Schering, Neth. Schering Nederland B.V., Flevolaan 28, 1382 JZ Weesp, Netherlands.

Schering Nordiska, Swed. Schering Nordiska AB, Box 152, 131 06 Nacka, Sweden.

Schering, Norw. See *Schering AG, Norw.* and *Sentipharm, Norw.*

Schering, NZ. See *Essex, NZ* and *Schering AG, NZ.*

Schering-Prebbles, UK. Schering-Prebbles Ltd, St John's Rd, Bootle, Merseyside L20 8NJ, England.

Schering Pty, Austral. Schering Pty Ltd, Wood St, Tempe NSW 2044, Australia.

Schering, S.Afr. See *Berlimed, S.Afr.* and *Scherag, S.Afr.*

Schering, Spain. See *Schering Corp., Spain* and *Schering España, Spain.*

Schering, Swed. See *Essex, Swed.* and *Schering Nordiska, Swed.*

Schering, Switz. Schering Zürich AG, Hermetschloostr. 75, 8048 Zurich, Switzerland.

Schering, UK. Schering Pharmaceuticals Ltd, The Brow, Burgess Hill, West Sussex RH15 9NE, England.

Schering, USA. Schering Corporation, Galloping Hill Rd, Kenilworth NJ 07033, USA.

Scheurich, Ger. E. Scheurich, Pharmwerk GmbH, Strassburger Strasse 77, Postfach: 1140, 7604 Appenweier/Baden, W. Germany.

Schiapparelli, Ital. Schiapparelli Farmaceutici s.p.a., Corso Belgio 86, 10153 Torino, Italy.

Schmidgall, Switz. See *Iromedica, Switz.*

Schmidt, Neth. C.N. Schmidt B.V., Jan Rebelstraat 8, 1069 CB Amsterdam, Netherlands.

Schmitz, Arg. Lab. Schmitz C.I.S.A., Arengreen 611, 1405 Buenos Aires, Argentina.

Scholl, UK. Scholl (UK) Ltd, 182 St John St, London EC1P 1DH, England.

Schürholz, Ger. Schürholz Arzneimittel GmbH, Fritz-Berne-Strasse 47, Postfach: 280, 8000 Munich 60, W. Germany.

Schütz, Switz. P. Schütz, Labor. By-Tanol, 4900 Langenthal, Switzerland.

Schwab, Ger. Dr Schwab GmbH, Leopoldstrasse 16, Postfach: 400128, 8000 Munich 40, W. Germany.

Schwabe, Ger. Dr Willmar Schwabe, Willmar-Schwabe-Strasse 4, Postfach: 410925, 7500 Karlsruhe 41, W. Germany.

Schwabe, Neth. See *Willmar-Schwabe, Neth.*

Schwarz, Belg. See *Byk, Belg.*

Schwarzhaupt, Ger. Schwarzhaupt KG, Sachsenring 37, 5000 Cologne 1, W. Germany.

Schweiz. Serum & Impfinstitut, Switz. Schweiz. Serum & Impfinstitut, Postfach 2707, 3001 Bern, Switzerland.

Scientific Hospital Supplies, UK. Scientific Hopsital Supplies Ltd, 38 Queensland St, Liverpool L7 3JG, England.

Sclavo, USA. Sclavo Inc., 5 Mansard Court, Wayne NJ 07470, USA.

Scotia, UK. Scotia Pharmaceutical Products, 558 Cathcart Rd, Glasgow G42, Scotland.

SCS, S.Afr. SCS Pharmalab (Pty) Ltd, Private Bag X516, Silverton 0127, S. Africa.

Seaford, UK. Seaford Laboratories Ltd, Cradle Hill Industrial Estate, Seaford, Sussex BN25 3JE, England.

Searle, Arg. G.D. Searle International C.A., Lavalle 2107, 1026 Buenos Aires, Argentina.

Searle, Austral. Searle Laboratories, 8 West St, North Sydney NSW 2060, Australia.

Searle, Belg. Laboratoires Searle, ave A. Madoux 99, 1150 Brussels, Belgium.

Searle, Canad. G.D. Searle and Co. of Canada Ltd, 400 Iroquois Shore Rd, Oakville, Ontario L6H 1M5, Canada.

Searle, Denm. G.D. Searle A/S, H.C. Ørstedsvej 4, 5 sal, 1879 Copenhagen V, Denmark.

Searle, Fr. Laboratoires Searle, 7 blvd Romain-Rolland, 92128 Montrouge, France.

Searle, Neth. Searle Farmaca, Noordhollandstraat 71, 1081 AS Amsterdam, Netherlands.

Searle, Norw. Searle Norge A/S, Trondheimsvn. 137, Postboks 6594 Rodeløkka, Oslo 5, Norway.

Searle, S.Afr. G.D. Searle (SA) (Pty) Ltd, P.O. Box 391157, Bramley 2018, S. Africa.

Searle, Switz. See *Diethelm, Switz.*

Searle, UK. Searle Pharmaceuticals, Division of G.D. Searle & Co. Ltd, P.O. Box 53, Lane End Rd, High Wycombe, Bucks HP12 4HL, England.

Searle, USA. Searle Pharmaceuticals Inc., P.O. Box 5110, Chicago IL 60680, USA.

Seatrace, USA. The Seatrace Co., P.O. Box 363, Gadsden AL 35902, USA.

Seaway Midwest, Canad. Seaway Midwest Ltd, 1255 Fewster Dr., Mississauga, Ontario L4W 1A3, Canada.

Sebamat Chemie, Ger. Sebamat Chemie GmbH, Postfach: 80, 5404 Bad Salzig/Rhein, W. Germany.

Seber, Belg. Seber-Benelux, rue de Bomel 29a, 5000 Namur, Belgium.

Seber, Spain. Seber Española SA, Paseje Gomis 4-6, Barcelona, Spain.

Seclo, Fr. Laboratoires Seclo, 3 Impasse Dumur, 92110 Clichy, France.

Sedaph, Fr. Sedaph (Societé d'Applications Pharmaceutiques), 35 quai du Moulin de Cage, B.P. 59, 92234 Gennevilliers, France.

Seid, Spain. Seid SA, Carr Sabadell a Granollers Km 15, Llissa de Vall (Barcelona), Spain.

Sella, Ital. Sella A. Lab. Chim. Farm. s.r.l., Via Vicenza 2, 36015 Schio (Vicenza), Italy.

Selvi, Ital. Selvi & C. s.p.a., Via Gallarate 184, 20151 Milan, Italy.

Semar, Spain. Laboratorios Semar SA, Barcelona, Spain.

Senju, Jap. Senju Pharmaceutical Co. Ltd, 28 Hiranomachi 3-chome, Higashi-ku, Osaka 541, Japan.

Sentipharm, Norw. Sentipharm AG, Informasjonsavdelingen Norge, Aslakvn. 14B, Oslo 7, Norway.

Septa, Spain. Septa SA, Arroyo de la Elipa 9, Madrid 17, Spain.

Seres, USA. Seres Laboratories Inc., 2325 Third St, San Francisco CA 94107, USA.

Serono, Ital. Istituto Farmacologico Serono s.p.a., Via Casilina 125, 00176 Rome, Italy.

Serono, UK. Serono Laboratories (UK) Ltd, 2 Tewin Court, Welwyn Garden City, Herts AL7 1AU, England.

Serpero, Ital. Serpero, Industria Galenica Milanese s.p.a., Viale L. Majno 40, 20129 Milan, Italy.

Serumwerk, Belg. See *Kela, Belg.*

Servier, Canad. Servier Canada Inc., 243 Place Frontenac, Pointe-Claire, Quebec H9R 4Z7, Canada.

Servier, Denm. See *Armedic, Denm.*

Servier, Fr. Laboratoires Servier, 22 rue Garnier, 92200 Neuilly, France.

Servier, Ital. Servier Italia s.p.a., Via degli Aldobrandeschi 13, 00163 Rome, Italy.

Servier, Neth. Servier Nederland B.V., Storkstraat 5, 2722 NN Zoetermeer, Netherlands.

Servier, Spain. Laboratorios Servier SA España, Calle Xaudaro s/n Fuencarral, Madrid 34, Spain.

Servier, Switz. Servier S.A., rue Hugo de Senger 10, 1205 Geneva, Switzerland.

Servier, UK. Servier Laboratories Ltd, Fulmer Hall, Windmill Rd, Fulmer, Nr Slough, Bucks SL3 6HH, England.

Sestri, UK. Sestri (Sales) Ltd, Kingsend House, 44 Kingsend, Ruislip, Middx HA4 7DA, England.

Seton, UK. Seton Products Ltd, Tubiton House, Medlock St, Oldham OL1 3HS, England.

Sévenet, Fr. Laboratoires Sévenet, 56 rue du Chanoine-Porée, 27300 Bernay, France.

Shell Chemicals. Shell Chemicals UK Ltd, Villiers House, 41 Strand, London WC2N 5JE, England.

Shionogi, Jap. Shionogi & Co. Ltd, 12 Doshomachi 3-chome, Higashi-ku, Osaka 541, Japan.

Sideta, Spain. Sociedad Ibérica de Estudios Terapéuticos Aplicados, Madrid, Spain.

Sidus, Arg. Instituto Sidus S.A., Larrea 926, 1117 Buenos Aires, Argentina.

Sidus, Ital. Sidus Istituto Biochimico Nazionale s.p.a., Via Tiburtina n. 1496, 00131 Rome, Italy.

Siegfried, Belg. See *Triosol, Belg.*

Siegfried, Ger. Siegfried GmbH, Fabrik für chemisch-pharmazeutische Produkte, Mumpfer Fährstrasse 68, Postfach: 1141, 7880 Bad Säckingen, W. Germany.

Siegfried, Switz. Siegfried AG, 4800 Zofingen, Switzerland.

Sierochimica, Ital. Sierochimica-Labatori Biochimica s.r.l., Via C. Porta 14, 20090 Trezzano S/Naviglio, Italy.

SIFI, Ital. Società Industria Farmaceutica Italiana s.p.a., Via N. Coviello 15/B, 95128 Catania, Italy.

SIFSA, Spain. SIFSA, Spain.

Sigma, Austral. Sigma Co. Ltd, 1408 Centre Rd, Clayton Vic. 3168, Australia.

Sigma, UK. Sigma London Chemical Co. Ltd, Fancy Rd, Poole, Dorset BH17 7NH, England.

Sigmatau, Ital. Sigma Tau s.p.a., Via Pontina Km. 30.400, 00040 Pomezia, Italy.

Sigurtà, Ital. Sigurtà s.p.a., Viale Certosa 210, 20156 Milan, Italy.

Simes, Austral. Simes Australia Pty Ltd, Australia.

Simes, Ital. Simes s.p.a., Via Bellerio 41, 20161 Milan, Italy.

Simonsen & Weels, Denm. Simonsen & Weels eftf. A/S, Roskildevej 14, 2620 Albertslund, Denmark.

Simpkin, UK. A.L. Simpkin & Co. Ltd, Hunter Rd, Sheffield S6 4LD, England.

Simpla, UK. Simpla Plastics Ltd, Phoenix Estate, Caerphilly Rd, Cardiff, Wales.

Sinclair, UK. Sinclair Pharmaceuticals Ltd, Borough Rd, Godalming, Surrey GU7 2AB, England.

Sintesa, Belg. Sintesa S.A., rue Antoine Court 15, 1080 Brussels, Belgium.

Sintesina, Arg. Sintesina S.A., Tte. Gral. Uriburu 4194, 1663 San Miguel, Argentina.

Sintetica, Switz. La Sintetica S.A., Via F. Soave 9, 6830 Chiasso, Switzerland.

Sintex, Spain. Sintex SA, Av. Rep Argentina 54-56, Barcelona, Spain.

Sintyal, Arg. Laboratorio Sintyal, Carlos Berg 3669, 1437 Buenos Aires, Argentina.

SIRT-BBP, Ital. S.I.R.T.-B.B.P., Laboratori Farmaceutici, Via A. Marinuzzi 124, 90129 Palermo, Italy.

SIT, Ital. Specialità Igienico Terapeutiche s.p.a., Via Cavour 78, 27035 Mede (Pavia), Italy.

Skånska Bomullskrut, Swed. Skånska Bomullskrutfabriks AB, 240 23 Dösjebro, Sweden.

Smaller, Spain. Smaller, Azcona 25, Madrid 28, Spain.

SMB, Belg. S.M.B., rue de la Pastorale 26-28, 1080 Brussels, Belgium.

Smith & Hill, UK. Smith & Hill Ltd, 53 Cresswell Rd, Sheffield S9 4JZ, England.

Smith & Nephew, Denm. Smith & Nephew Scandinavia A/S, Naerum Hovedgade 2, 2850 Naerum, Denmark.

Smith & Nephew, Norw. See *Weiders, Norw.*

Smith & Nephew Pharmaceuticals, UK. Smith & Nephew Pharmaceuticals Ltd, Bampton Rd, Harold Hill, Romford, Essex RM3 8SL, England.

Smith & Nephew Toiletries, UK. Smith & Nephew Toiletries Ltd, Welwyn Garden City, Herts, England.

Smith & Nephew, UK. Smith & Nephew Ltd, Bessemer Rd, Welwyn Garden City, Herts, England.

Smith & Walker, UK. Smith & Walker Ltd, Linby St, Bulwell, Nottingham, England.

Smith Kendon, UK. Smith Kendon Ltd, Waterton, Bridgend, Wales.

Smith Kline & French, Arg. Smith Kline & French Inter., Bolívar 391 2°piso, 1006 Buenos Aires, Argentina.

Smith Kline & French, Austral. Smith Kline & French Laboratories (Australia) Ltd, Cnr Warringah and Allambie Rds, French's Forest NSW 2086, Australia.

Smith Kline & French, Canad. Smith Kline & French Canada Ltd, 1940 Argentia Rd, Mississauga, Ontario L5N 2V7, Canada.

Smith Kline & French, Denm. Smith Kline & French, Halmtorvet 29, 1700 Copenhagen V, Denmark.

Smith Kline & French, Fr. Laboratoires Smith Kline & French, 15 rue Jean-Jaurès, 92807 Puteaux Cedex, France.

Smith Kline & French, Ital. Smith Kline & French s.p.a., Viale Ortles 12, 20139 Milan, Italy.

Smith Kline & French, Neth. Smith Kline & French B.V., Koningin Julianaplein 30-5A, 2595 AA 's-Gravenhage, Netherlands.

Smith Kline & French, Norw. Smith Kline & French Informasjon Norge, Astrids vei 3, 1473 Skårer, Norway.

Smith Kline & French, S.Afr. Smith Kline & French Laboratories, P.O. Box 38, Isando 1600, S. Africa.

Smith Kline & French, Spain. Smith Kline & French SAE, Juan Bravo 3C, Madrid, Spain.

Smith Kline & French, UK. Smith Kline & French Laboratories Ltd, Welwyn Garden City, Herts AL7 1EY, England.

Smith Kline & French, USA. Smith Kline & French Laboratories, Division of SmithKline Corporation, 1500 Spring Garden St, P.O. Box 7929, Philadelphia PA 19101, USA.

Sobio, Fr. Laboratoires Sobio, 25 blvd de l'Amiral Bruix, 75782 Paris Cedex 16, France.

Sobio, Switz. See *Sodip, Switz.*

Society for Cancer Research, Switz. Society for Cancer Research, Arlesheim, Switzerland.

Sodip, Switz. Sodip S.A., rue Chandieu 44, 1202 Geneva, Switzerland.

Solac, Switz. See *Lucchini, Switz.*

Solco, Ger. Solco GmbH, Pharm. Spezialitäten, Salzwerkstrasse 7, Postfach: 110, 7889 Grenzach-Wyhlen 2, W. Germany.

Sopar, Belg. Sopar S.A., rue Jules Besme 124, 1080 Brussels, Belgium.

Southon-Horton, UK. Southon-Horton Laboratories Ltd, LRC House, Thames Rd, Crayford, Kent DA1 4SJ, England.

SPA, Ital. Società Prodotti Antibiotici s.p.a., Via Biella 8, 20143 Milan, Italy.

SPA, Switz. See *Diethelm, Switz.*

Spearhead, UK. Spearhead Chemicals Ltd, 3 Mount Rd, Hampton Rd West, Hanworth, Middx TW13 6AR, England.

Specia, Belg. Specia S.A. (Societé Parisienne d'Expansion Chimique), ave Carton de Wiart, 128/Bte 1, 1090 Brussels, Belgium.

Specia, Fr. Specia S.A., 16 rue Clisson, 75646 Paris Cedex 13, France.

Specia, Neth. See *Rhône-Poulenc, Neth.*

Specia, Switz. See *Rhodia-Pharm, Switz.*

Spedrog-Caillon, Arg. Spedrog Caillon S.A.I.yC., Venezuela 1600, 1095 Buenos Aires, Argentina.

Spemsa, Ital. Spemsa, Specialità Medicinali s.p.a., Via D. da Castiglione 7, 50125 Firenze, Italy.

Spencer, UK. Brian G. Spencer Ltd, Station Rd, Shenstone, Lichfield, Staffs WS14 0NP, England.

Speywood, UK. Speywood Laboratories Ltd, Chancel House, East St, Bingham, Nottingham NG13 8DR, England.

Spitzner, Ger. W. Spitzner, Arzneimittelfabrik GmbH, Bunsenstrasse 6-10, Postfach: 1654, 7505 Ettlingen, W. Germany.

Spodefell, UK. Spodefell Ltd, 5 Inverness Mews, London W2 3JQ, England.

Spofa, Cz. Spofa, Staré Město, Dlouhá tř. 11, Prague, Czeckoslovakia.

Spret-Mauchant, Fr. Spret-Mauchant, B.P. 110, 92232 Gennevilliers, France.

Spret, Switz. See *Biomed, Switz.*

Spyfarma, Spain. Spyfarma SA, Carr Sevilla-Malaga Km 9.500, Alcala de Guadaira (Sevilla), Spain.

Squibb, Arg. Squibb S.A.I.C., Av. Sir Alexander Fleming 1653, 1640 Martinez, Argentina.

Squibb, Austral. E.R. Squibb & Sons Pty Ltd, 556 Princes Highway, Noble Park Vic. 3174, Australia.

Squibb, Belg. Squibb, ave Louise 130a, 1050 Brussels, Belgium.

Squibb, Canad. Squibb Canada Inc., 2365 Côte de Liesse Rd, Montreal, Quebec H4N 2M7, Canada.

Squibb, Denm. Squibb ApS, Hanebred 2, 2720 Vanløse, Denmark.

Squibb, Fr. Laboratoires Squibb, 28 blvd du Parc, 92521 Neuilly-sur-Seine, France.

Squibb, Ital. Squibb s.p.a., Via Paolo di Dono 73, 00143 Rome, Italy.

Squibb, Neth. Squibb B.V., J.C. van Markenlaan 3, 2285 VL Rijswijk, Netherlands.

Squibb, Norw. Squibb Informasjon Norge, Sorgenfrigt. 11, Postboks 5084 Majorstua, Oslo 3, Norway.

Squibb, NZ. E.R. Squibb & Sons (NZ) Ltd, P.O. Box 6273, Auckland, New Zealand.

Squibb, S.Afr. Squibb Laboratories (Pty) Ltd, P.O. Box 48, Isando, Transvaal, S. Africa.

Squibb Surgicare, UK. Squibb Surgicare Ltd, Reeds Lane, Moreton, Wirral, Merseyside L46 1QW, England.

Squibb, Switz. See *Biochimica, Switz.*

Squibb, UK. E.R. Squibb & Sons Ltd, Squibb House, 141 Staines Rd, Hounslow, Middx TW3 3JA, England.

Squibb, USA. E.R. Squibb & Sons Inc., P.O. Box 4000, Princeton NJ 08540, USA.

S.S. White, UK. S.S. White Ltd, 51 St Ann's Rd, Harrow, Middx, England.

Stada-Chemie, Ger. Stada-Chemie GmbH, Stada-Strasse 2-18, Postfach: 1260, 6368 Bad Vilbel 4, W. Germany.

Stada, Ger. Stada-Arzneimittel AG, Stada-Strasse 2-18, Postfach: 1260, 6368 Bad Vilbel 4, W. Germany.

Stafford-Miller, UK. Stafford-Miller Ltd, Stafford-Miller House, The Common, Hatfield, Herts AL10 0NZ, England.

Stago, Fr. Laboratoires Stago, 6 ter rue Denis-Papin, 92600 Asnières, France.

Standard Laboratories, UK. Standard Laboratories Ltd, Windmill Rd, Sunbury-on-Thames, Middx, England.

STD Pharmaceutical Products, UK. STD Pharmaceutical Products Ltd, Field's Yard, Plough Lane, Hereford HR4 0EL, England.

Stecker, USA. Stecker, USA.

Steetley Mfg, UK. Steetley Chemicals Ltd, Chemicals Manufacturing Division, Canning Rd, London E15 3NX, England.

Steetley Minerals, UK. Steetley Minerals Ltd, P.O. Box 2, Carlton Rd, Worksop, Notts S81 7QG, England.

Steetley Trading, UK. Steetley Chemicals Ltd, Chemicals Trading Division, Berk House, P.O. Box 56, Basing View, Basingstoke, Hants RG21 2EG, England.

Steiner, UK. Steiner Marketing Ltd, Steiner House, 66 Grosvenor St, London W1X 0AX, England.

Sterling Health. Sterling Health, Sterling-Winthrop House, Surbiton, Surrey KT6 4PH, England.

Sterling Industrial, UK. Sterling Industrial, Chapeltown, Sheffield S30 4YP, England.

Sterling Research, UK. Sterling Research Laboratories, Sterling-Winthrop House, Surbiton, Surrey KT6 4PH, England.

Sterwin, Spain. Sterwin Española SA, Avda. General Peron 27-4, Madrid 20, Spain.

Stholl, Ital. Stholl s.r.l., Via Giardini 1271, 41100 Modena, Italy.

Stickley, Canad. E.L. Stickley & Co. Ltd, P.O. Box 1748, Brantford, Ontario N3T 5V7, Canada.

Stiefel, UK. Stiefel Laboratories (UK) Ltd, Wellcroft Rd, Slough SL1 4AQ, England.

STIP, Ital. STIP, Lab. Chim. Biol. di Micheletti R., Lungarno Gambacorti 55, 56100 Pisa, Italy.

Stotzer, Switz. Stotzer AG, Breitenrainplatz 40, 3014 Bern, Switzerland.

Strenol, UK. Strenol Products Ltd, Pearl House, 746 Finchley Rd, London NW11 7TH, England.

Streuli, Switz. G. Streuli & Co. AG, 8730 Uznach, Switzerland.

Stroschein, Ger. Pharma Stroschein GmbH, Frohmestrasse 110, Postfach: 61 04 25, 2000 Hamburg 61, W. Germany.

Stuart Pharmaceuticals, USA. Stuart Pharmaceuticals, Division of ICI Americas Inc., Wilmington DE 19897, USA.

Stuart, UK. Stuart Pharmaceuticals Ltd, Carr House, Carrs Rd, Cheadle, Cheshire SK8 2EG, England.

Substancia, Spain. Laboratorio Substancia SA, Poligono Industrial Manso Mateu, Prat de Llobregat (Barcelona), Spain.

Substantia, Belg. Laboratoires Substantia S.A., avenue Wielemans Ceuppens 45, 1190 Brussels, Belgium.

Substantia, Fr. Laboratoires Substantia, 11 ave Dubonnet, 92407 Courbevoie Cedex, France.

Substantia, Neth. B.V. Substantia, Oderweg 1, 1043 AG Amsterdam, Netherlands.

Sudamfos, Arg. Sudamfos S.A.V.A.C., Departamento Farmacéutico, Av. del Trabjo 5251, 1439 Buenos Aires, Argentina.

Südmedica, Denm. See *Tjellesen, Denm.*

Südmedica, Ger. Südmedica GmbH, Chemisch-pharmazeutische Fabrik, Ehrwalder Strasse 21, Postfach: 701669, 8000 Munich 70, W. Germany.

Sumitomo, Jap. Sumitomo Chemical Co. Ltd, Pharmaceutical Division, 40 Doshomachi 2-chome, Higashi-ku, Osaka 541, Japan.

Superol, Neth. Superol B.V., Handelsdwarsstraat 10, 6905 DJ Zevenaar, Netherlands.

Superol, S.Afr. See *SAPDC, S.Afr.*

Surf Ski International, UK. Surf Ski International, St Ouens' Bay, Jersey, Channel Islands.

Surgikos, UK. Surgikos, Kirkton Campus, Livingston, Scotland.

Swiss-Pharma, Ger. Swiss-Pharma GmbH, Basler Strasse 112, Postfach: 22 71, 7850 Lörrach, W. Germany.

Swiss Serum and Vaccine Institute, UK. Swiss Serum and Vaccine Institute, c/o Mr K.W. Blakey, 1 Camden Terrace, Camden Rd, Bath BA1 5HZ, England.

Syncro, Arg. Syncro (Arg.) S.A.Q.I.C.I.F., Muñiz 230, 1212 Buenos Aires, Argentina.

Synlab, Fr. Laboratoires Synlab, 21800 Quétigny, France.

Synmedic, Switz. Synmedic AG, Seebahnstrasse 85, 8003 Zurich, Switzerland.

Syntetic, Denm. A/S Syntetic, Edwin Rahrs Vej, 8220 Brabrand, Denmark.

Syntetic, Norw. See *AFI, Norw.*

Syntex, Austral. Syntex Australia Ltd, 275 North Alfred St, North Sydney NSW 2060, Australia.

Syntex, Belg. See *Sarva, Belg.*

Syntex, Denm. Astra-Syntex Terapeutika ApS, C.F. Richsvej 103, 2000 Copenhagen F, Denmark.

Syntex, Fr. Laboratoires Syntex, 25 rue du Dr-Finlay, 75015 Paris, France.

Syntex, Switz. Syntex Pharm AG, Binningerstrasse 95, 4123 Allschwil, Switzerland.

Syntex, UK. Syntex Pharmaceuticals, St Ives House, St Ives Rd, Maidenhead, Berks SL6 1RD, England.

Syntex, USA. Syntex Laboratories Inc., 3401 Hillview Ave, Stanford Industrial Park, Palo Alto CA 94304, USA.

Synthelabo, Fr. Synthelabo, 1 bis ave de Villars, 75341 Paris Cedex 07, France.

Szabó, Arg. Szabó Hnos. Kessler Cía. S.R.L., Humahuaca 4065, 1192 Buenos Aires, Argentina.

Szama, Arg. Lab. Dr Herbert Szama S.A.C.eI., J.M. Moreno 354, 1424 Buenos Aires, Argentina.

TAD, Ger. TAD Pharmazeutisches Werk GmbH, Heinz-Lohmann-Strasse 5, Postfach: 720, 2190 Cuxhaven, W. Germany.

Taiho, Jap. Taiho Pharmaceutical Co. Ltd, 9 Kanda Tsukasacho 2-chome, Chiyoda-ku, Tokyo 101, Japan.

Taisho, Jap. Taisho Pharmaceutical Co. Ltd, 24-1 Takata 3-chome, Toshima-ku, Tokyo 171, Japan.

Takeda, Jap. Takeda Chemical Industries Ltd, 27 Doshomachi 2-chome, Higashi-ku, Osaka 541, Japan.

Takeda, Neth. See *Pharbil, Neth.*

Tanabe, Jap. Tanabe Seiyaku Co. Ltd, 21 Doshomachi 3-chome, Higashi-ku, Osaka 541, Japan.

Tanabe, S.Afr. See *Noristan, S.Afr.*

Tanabe-Seiyaku, Neth. See *ICN, Neth.*

Tanabe, Switz. See *Biochimica, Switz.*

Taranto, Arg. Taranto & Cía. S.R.L., Callao 702, 1023 Buenos Aires, Argentina.

Tasman, UK. Tasman Vaccine Laboratory (UK) Ltd, Eastern Way, Bury St Edmunds, Suffolk IP32 7AL, England.

Tecfar, Spain. Tecfar, Spain.

Techni-Pharma, Mon. Techni-Pharma (Groupe Laphal), 7 rue de l'Industrie, B.P. 324, Monaco.

Teikoku, Jap. Teikoku Hormone Mfg Co. Ltd, 5-1 Akasaka 2-chome, Minato-ku, Tokyo 107, Japan.

Tell, UK. Tell Products Ltd, 93 Cobbold Rd, London NW10 9SU, England.

Temana, UK. Temana Bees Ltd, Sealand, Chester CH1 6BA, England.

Temis, Arg. Temis S.A.C.I.A., Humberto 1° 1860, 1229 Buenos Aires, Argentina.

Temmler, Denm. See *Nordisk Droge, Denm.*

Temmler, Ger. Temmler-Werke Vereinigte Chemische Fabriken Hermann Temmler GmbH & Co. KG, Temmlerstrasse 2, Postfach: 2269, 3550 Marburg/Lahn 1, W. Germany.

Temmler, Switz. See *Doetsch, Grether, Switz.*

Tempelhof, Ger. Chemische Fabrik Tempelhof Preuss & Temmler GmbH & Co., Oberlandstrasse 65, 1000 Berlin 42, W. Germany.

Tendo-Haco, Neth. Tendo-Haco Farmacie B.V., Kloosterweg 43, 8191 JA Wapenveld, Netherlands.

Tenneco, UK. Tenneco Organics Ltd, Rockingham Works, Avonmouth, Bristol BS11 0YT, England.

Terapeutico M.R., Ital. Labor. Terapeutico M.R. s.r.l., Via Buffalmacco 9, 50133 Firenze, Italy.

Terapia, Roum. The Terapia Medicinal Drugs Enterprise, Cluj-Napoca, Roumania.

Tetra, Arg. Prodte S.A.C.I.yF., Helguera 254/8, 1406 Buenos Aires, Argentina.

Tettamanti, Switz. Tettamanti AG, Stampfenbachstrasse 75, 8006 Zurich, Switzerland.

Teva, Israel. Teva Pharmaceutical Industries Ltd, P.O. Box 1142, Jerusalem, Israel.

Texcan, Canad. Texcan Pharmaceuticals Ltd, 705 Progress Ave, Unit No. 5, Scarborough, Ontario M1H 2X1, Canada.

Thackray, UK. Raymed Division of Chas. F. Thackray Ltd, Viaduct Rd, Leeds LS4 2BR, England.

Thames, UK. Thames Laboratories Ltd, Thames Building, 206 Upper Richmond Rd West, London SW14 8AH, England.

Théramex, Fr. Laboratoires Théramex, 11 blvd Lannes, 75116 Paris, France.

Théranol, Fr. Laboratoires Théranol, 180 rue de Vaugirard, 75015 Paris, France.

Therapeutica, Belg. Therapeutica S.A., chaussée de Charleroi 115, Jodoigne, Belgium.

Therapeuticon, Neth. Therapeuticon, Industrieweg 1, 5531 AD Bladel, Netherlands.

Therapex-Unik, Canad. Therapex-Unik Inc., 7961 Alfred, Ville d'Anjou, Quebec H1J 1J3, Canada.

Therapia, Spain. Therapia, Spain.

Theraplix, Belg. Theraplix S.A., ave Carton de Wiart 128/Bte 2, 1090 Brussels, Belgium.

Théraplix, Fr. Théraplix S.A., 46 rue Albert, 75640 Paris Cedex 13, France.

Théraplix, Neth. See *Rhône-Poulenc, Neth.*

Théraplix, Switz. See *Rhodia-Pharm, Switz.*

Thiemann, Ger. Dr Thiemann GmbH, Chem. pharm. Fabrik, Stadttorstrasse 3, Postfach: 2080, 4670 Lünen, W. Germany.

Thiemann, Switz. See *Medinova, Switz.* and *Pharmakon, Switz.*

Thilo, Ger. Dr Thilo & Co. GmbH, Rudolf-Diesel-Ring 21, Postfach: 1180, 8029 Sauerlach b. München, W. Germany.

Thomae, Ger. Dr Karl Thomae GmbH, Chemisch-pharmazeutische Fabrik, Birkendorfer Strasse 65, Postfach: 720, 7950 Biberach an der Riss 1, W. Germany.

Thomas, UK. Hubert A.C. Thomas & Co., Copperworks Rd, New Dock, Llanelli, Dyfed, Wales.

Thompson Medical, UK. Thompson Medical Co. Ltd, P.O. Box 365, London SW1P 1AA, England.

Thomson & Joseph, UK. Thomson & Joseph Ltd, Castle House, 21 Davey Place, Norwich NR2 1PJ, England.

Thornton & Ross, UK. Thornton & Ross Ltd, Linthwaite, Huddersfield, England.

Thyssen, Denm. O. Vilsoet Thyssen, Kemisk fabrik og laboratorium, Dr Olgas Vej 28, 2000 Copenhagen F, Denmark.

Tiber, Ital. Tiber s.r.l., Prodotti Chimico Biologici, Via Prenestina 707, 00155 Roma-Tor Sapienza, Italy.

Ticen, Eire. Ticen Ltd, 2 Church Lane, Dublin 2, Eire.

Tidebrook, UK. Tidebrook Chemical Products Ltd, 36 Parkside Rd, Leeds LS6 4QG, England.

Tika, Denm. See *Astra, Denm.*

Tika, Norw. See *Astra, Norw.*

Tika, Swed. AB Tika, Box 1100, 221 04 Lund 1, Sweden.

Tillotts, UK. Tillotts Laboratories, Henlow Trading Estate, Henlow, Beds SG16 6DS, England.

Tió, Spain. Tió, Spain.

Tjellesen, Denm. E. Tjellesen ApS, Blokken 81, 3460 Birkerød, Denmark.

Toa Eiyo, Jap. Toa Eiyo Kagaku Kogyo Co. Ltd, 1-2 Kyobashi 3-chome, Chuo-ku, Tokyo 104, Japan.
Toho, Jap. Toho Pharmaceutical Ind. Co. Ltd, 14 Awajimachi 1-chome, Higashi-ku, Osaka 541, Japan.
Torbet Laboratories, UK. Torbet Laboratories Ltd, 24 Great King St, Edinburgh EH3 6QH, Scotland.
Torch Laboratories, USA. Torch Laboratories Inc., 1619 F. St, P.O. Box 869, So. Belmar NJ 07719, USA.
Torlan, Spain. Laboratorios Torlan SA, Ballester 46, Barcelona, Spain.
Torrens Torrents, Spain. Torrens Torrents, Spain.
Tosara, UK. Tosara Products (UK) Ltd, 59 Crosby Rd North, Liverpool L22 4QD, England.
Tosi, Ital. Istituto Franco Tosi s.p.a., Via Bertola da Novate 14, 20157 Milan, Italy.
Tosi-Novara, Ital. Tosi Dr A. Farmaceutici s.a.s., Via Monte Nero 35, 28100 Novara, Italy.
Tosse, Ger. E. Tosse & Co. mbH, Friedrich-Ebert-Damm 101, Postfach: 70 16 48, 2000 Hamburg 70, W. Germany.
Toyama, Jap. Toyama Chemical Co. Ltd, 2-5 Nishi-shinjuku 3-chome, Shinjuku-ku, Tokyo 160, Japan.
Toyo Pharmar, Jap. Toyo Pharmar Co. Ltd, 65 Bakuro-machi 1-chome, Higashi-ku, Osaka 541, Japan.
Tramedico, Neth. Tramedico B.V., Flevolaan 19C, 1382 JX Weesp, Netherlands.
Trans-Canada Dermapeutics, Canad. Trans-Canada Dermapeutics Ltd, 3300 Sartelon, St Laurent, Quebec H4R 1E3, Canada.
Travenol, Denm. See *Simonsen & Weels, Denm.*
Travenol, Norw. Travenol Laboratorier A/S, Postboks 130, 1751 Halden, Norway.
Travenol, UK. Travenol Laboratories Ltd, Caxton Way, Thetford, Norfolk IP24 3SE, England.
Travenol, USA. Travenol Laboratories Inc., One Baxter Parkway, Deerfield IL 60015, USA.
Trenka, Aust. F. Trenka, Chem.-pharm. Fabrik, Staudgasse 35, 1181 Vienna XVIII, Austria.
Trenker, Belg. Laboratoires Trenker, ave Dolez 480-482, 1180 Brussels, Belgium.
Trentham, UK. Trentham Laboratories Ltd, Lavender House, Seymour Rd, London E10, England.
Treupha, Switz. Treupha AG, Postfach 59, 5401 Baden, Switzerland.
Trianon, Canad. Trianon Laboratories Inc., 715 Halperm, Dorval, Quebec H9P 1G5, Canada.
Trimen, USA. Trimen Laboratories Inc., 80-26th St, Pittsburgh PA 15222, USA.
Triosol, Belg. Triosol, rue Grande 243, 7458 Maisières, Belgium.
Trommsdorff, Ger. H. Trommsdorff Arzneimittelfabrik, Trommsdorffstrasse 2, 5110 Alsdorf/Rhl. 1, W. Germany.
Tropon, Ger. Troponwerke GmbH & Co. KG, Berliner Strasse 156, Postfach: 80 10 60, 5000 Cologne 80, W. Germany.
Tubi Lux, Ital. Tubi Lux Farma, Istituto Farmaco Oftalmico, Via del Mare 97, 00040 Pomezia (Roma), Italy.
Tudor, UK. Tudor Trading Co., 1 Laburnum Gardens, London N21 3HU, England.
Turon, Spain. Turon, Spain.
Turro, Spain. Turro, Spain.
Tutag, USA. Tutag Pharmaceuticals, Division of Reid-Provident, 640 Tenth St, Atlanta GA 30318, USA.
Typharm, UK. Typharm Ltd, 45 East St, Blandford, Dorset, England.
UAD, USA. UAD Laboratories Inc., 1400 Commerce St, Minden LA 71055, USA.
UCB, Arg. Unión Científica Belga Arg. S.A., Av. V. Salfield 5855, 1605 Munro, Argentina.
UCB, Belg. UCB, rue Berkendael 68, 1060 Brussels, Belgium.
UCB, Denm. See *Nordisk Droge, Denm.*
UCB, Fr. UCB, 21 rue de Neuilly, 92003 Nanterre, France.
UCB, Ger. UCB Chemie GmbH, Hüttenstrasse, Postfach: 1340, 5014 Kerpen, W. Germany.
UCB, Ital. Laboratori UCB s.p.a., Via S. Clemente 8, 10143 Torino, Italy.
UCB, Neth. UCB-Nederland, Leeghwaterplein 24B, 2521 CV 's-Gravenhage, Netherlands.
UCB, Norw. See *Mekos, Norw.*
UCB-Pevya, Spain. UCB-Pevya SA, Ramón y Cajal 6, Molins de Rey (Barcelona), Spain.
UCB, S.Afr. UCB (Pty) Ltd, P.O. Box 30136, Braamfontein 2017, S. Africa.
UCB, Swed. UCB Nordiska AB, Box 474, 124 04 Bandhagen 4, Sweden.
UCB, Switz. See *Diethelm, Switz.* and *Girod, Switz.*
UCM-Difme, Ital. Unione Chimica Medicamenti Difme s.p.a., Via Sabaudia 44, 10095 Grugliasco, Italy.
Uhlmann-Eyraud, Switz. F. Uhlmann-Eyraud S.A., ch. du Grand-Puits 28, 1217 Geneva, Switzerland.
Ulmer, USA. The Ulmer Pharmacal Co., 2440 Fernbrook Lane, Minneapolis MN 55441, USA.
Unichem, UK. Unichem Ltd, Crown House, Morden, Surrey, England.
Unichema, UK. Unichema Chemicals Ltd, Bebington, Wirral, Merseyside L62 4UF, England.
Unicliffe, UK. Unicliffe Ltd, 5 Trident Way, International Trading Estate, Brent Rd, Southall, Middx UB2 5LF, England.
Unifa, Arg. Unifa S.A.Q.eI., Av. San Martin 1750, 1602 Florida, Argentina.
Unigreg, UK. Unigreg Ltd, 15 Worple Rd, London SW19 4JS, England.
Unilabo, Fr. Laboratoires Unilabo, 92 rue Baudin, 92307 Levallois, France.
Unimed, UK. Unimed Pharmaceuticals Ltd, 24 Steynton Ave, Bexley, Kent DA5 3HP, England.
Unimed, USA. Unimed Inc., 35 Columbia Rd, Somerville NJ 08876, USA.
Union Carbide, USA. Union Carbide Corporation, 270 Park Ave, New York NY 10017, USA.
Unipharma, Switz. Unipharma S.A., 6911 Barbengo, Switzerland.
United Laboratories, Austral. United Laboratories Pty Ltd, Australia.
Universal Emulsifiers, UK. Universal Emulsifiers Ltd, Invicta Works, 157 Mill St, East Malling, Maidstone, Kent, England.
UPB, Belg. Union Pharmaceutique Belge S.A., rue aux Fleurs 30-38, 1000 Brussels, Belgium.
Upjohn, Arg. Laboratorio Upjohn S.A.I.C., Cuba 1833 5°Piso, 1428 Buenos Aires, Argentina.
Upjohn, Austral. Upjohn Pty Ltd, 55 Kirby St, Rydalmere NSW 2116, Australia.
Upjohn, Canad. The Upjohn Co. of Canada, 865 York Mills Rd, Don Mills, Ontario M3B 1Y6, Canada.
Upjohn, Denm. Upjohn S.A. Denmark Branch, Vangede Bygade 65, 2820 Gentofte, Denmark.
Upjohn, Fr. Laboratoires Upjohn, Tour Franklin, Cedex 11, 92081 Paris La Défense, France.
Upjohn, Ger. Upjohn GmbH, Humboldstrasse 10, Postfach: 449, 6148 Heppenheim, W. Germany.
Upjohn, Ital. Upjohn s.p.a., Via G.E. Upjohn 2, 20040 Caponago, Italy.
Upjohn, Neth. Upjohn-Nederland, Morsestraat 15, 6716 AH Ede, Netherlands.
Upjohn, Norw. Upjohn Informasjon, Postboks 10, 1310 Blommenholm, Norway.
Upjohn, S.Afr. Upjohn (Pty) Ltd, P.O. Box 246, Isando, Transvaal, S. Africa.
Upjohn, Swed. Upjohn AB, Box 289, 433 25 Partille, Sweden.
Upjohn, UK. Upjohn Ltd, Fleming Way, Crawley, West Sussex RH10 2NJ, England.
Upjohn, USA. The Upjohn Co., Portage Rd, Kalamazoo MI 49001, USA.
UPSA, Fr. UPSA, 128 rue Danton, 92500 Rueil-Malmaison, France.
UPSA, Switz. See *Sapos, Switz.*
Upsher-Smith, USA. Upsher-Smith Laboratories Inc., 14905 23rd Ave North, Minneapolis MN 55441, USA.
Uquifa, Spain. Uquifa, Union Químico Farmacéutica SAE, Av. Marques de Argentera 21, Barcelona, Spain.
Uriach, Spain. J. Uriach & Cia SA, Calle Bruch 49, Barcelona, Spain.
Ursula-Ruth, UK. Ursula-Ruth, 73 Church Rd, London NW4 4DP, England.
US Ethicals, Canad. See *Nova-Drug, Canad.*
US Ethicals, Denm. See *Helge Kjelstrup, Denm.*
US Ethicals, Norw. See *Midelfart, Norw.*
US Ethicals, USA. US Ethicals Inc., 37-02 48th Ave, Long Island City NY 11101, USA.
US Vitamin, Arg. Laboratorio de la U.S. Vitamin & Pharmaceutical Corp. de Arg. S.R.L., Hipolito Yrigoyen 3171, 1208 Buenos Aires, Argentina.
Usafarma, Ital. Usafarma s.r.l., Via Schiaparelli 1, 20125 Milan, Italy.
USV, Canad. USV Canada Inc., 2501 Stanfield Rd, Mississauga, Ontario L4Y 1R9, Canada.
USV Pharmaceutical Corp., USA. USV Pharmaceutical Corporation, 1 Scarsdale Rd, Tuckahoe NY 10707, USA.
Vaillant-Defresne, Fr. Laboratoires Vaillant-Defresne, 65 rue Falguière, 75739 Paris Cedex 15, France.
Vaillant-Defresne, Switz. See *Uhlmann-Eyraud, Switz.*
Vaillant, Ital. Laboratori Italiani Vaillant s.r.l., Via Melzi d'Eril 32, 20154 Milan, Italy.
Valderrama, Spain. Valderrama SA, San Cristobal 33, Derio-Bilbao, Spain.
Valeas, Ital. Valeas s.p.a., Via Vallisneri 10, 20133 Milan, Italy.
Valette, Arg. Casa Valette & Cía, Pueyrredon 211, 1650 San Martín Pcia Bs.As., Argentina.
Valpan, Fr. Laboratoires Valpan, B.P. 8, 77350 Le Mée-sur-Seine, France.
Van Dyk, USA. Van Dyk & Co. Inc., Main and William Sts, Belleville NJ 07109, USA.
Vanderbilt, USA. R.T. Vanderbilt Co. Inc., 30 Winfield St, Norwalk CT 06855, USA.
Vandos, Austral. Vandos, Australia.
Veride, Belg. Veride, Mommaertslaan 14, 1920 Machelen (Diegem), Belgium.
Verla, Ger. Verla-Pharm, Arzneimittelfabrik, Apotheker H.J. v. Ehrlich GmbH & Co. KG, Hauptstrasse 98, Postfach: 135, 8132 Tutzing, W. Germany.
Vernin, Fr. Laboratoires Vernin, 311 ave du Colonel-Fabien, 77190 Dammarie-les-Lys, France.
Vessen, UK. Vessen Ltd, 320 London Rd, Hazel Grove, Stockport, Cheshire SK7 4RF, England.
Vestric, UK. Vestric Ltd, West Lane, Runcorn, Cheshire WA7 2PE, England.
Vifor, Switz. Lab. Vifor S.A., rte d'Annecy 48, 1227 Carouge, Switzerland.
Villette, Fr. Laboratoires H. Villette, 5 rue Paul-Barruel, 75015 Paris, France.
Vinas, Spain. Laboratorios Vinas SA, Barcelona, Spain.
Vincent, UK. L.E. Vincent & Partners, 16 Eaton Square, London SW1, England.
Vine Chemicals, UK. Vine Chemicals Ltd, Lugsdale Rd, Widnes, Cheshire WA8 6ND, England.
Vine Products, UK. Vine Products Ltd, The Winery, Villiers Rd, Kingston-upon-Thames, Surrey KT1 3AS, England.
Vines Biocrin, UK. Vines Biocrin Ltd, 111 Clarence Rd, London E5 8EE, England.
Vir, Spain. Vir SA, Cardenal Mendoza 42, Madrid, Spain.
Virax, Austral. Virax Ethicals Ltd, 77 Market St, South Melbourne Vic. 3205, Australia.
Virgiliano, Ital. Istituto Farmaco Virgiliano s.p.a. (IFV), Via Chiesanuova 1, 46100 Mantova, Italy.
Vis, Ital. Vis Farmaceutici s.p.a., Istituto Scientifico delle Venezie, Viale dell'industria 54, 35100 Padova, Italy.
Vister, Ital. Vister s.p.a., Via Don Rossi, 22064 Casatenovo Brianza (Como), Italy.
Vister, S.Afr. See *Warner, S.Afr.*
Vita, Ital. Vita Farmaceutici s.p.a., Via Boucheron 14, 10122 Torino, Italy.
Vita, Spain. Laboratorios Vita SA, Barcelona, Spain.
Vitabiotics, UK. Vitabiotics Ltd, 122 Mount Pleasant, Alperton, Middx HA0 1UG, England.
Vitrum, Denm. See *KabiVitrum, Denm.*
Vitrum, Norw. See *KabiVitrum, Norw.*
Vitrum, Swed. Vitrum AB, Box 12170, 102 24 Stockholm 12, Sweden.
Vögelin, Switz. Dr H. Vögelin, 3123 Belp, Switzerland.
Voigt, Ger. Dr med. Hans Voigt, Pharmazeutische Fabrik GmbH, Mundipharmstrasse 4, Postfach: 350, 6250 Limburg/Lahn, W. Germany.
Volpino, Arg. Lab. Volpino S.A.C.I., Posadas 1564, 1112 Buenos Aires, Argentina.
Von Boch, Ital. Von Boch Arzneimittel s.r.l. Istituto Farmacobiologico, Via Rovigo 1, 00161 Rome, Italy.
Voxsan, UK. Voxsan Ltd, Church Street North, Church St, London E15 4DY, England.
Wacker Chemicals, UK. Wacker Chemicals UK Ltd, The Clock Tower, Mount Felix, Bridge St, Walton on Thames, Surrey KT12 1AS, England.
Wacker-Chemie, Ger. Wacker-Chemie GmbH, Prinzregentenstrasse 22, 8000 Munich 22, W. Germany.
Waco, Arg. Lab. Waco S.A.C.eI., Guemes 2045, 1602 Florida, Argentina.
Wade, UK. Wade Pharmaceuticals Ltd, Stepfield, Witham, Essex CM8 3AG, England.

Wahl, USA. William Wahl Corporation, 12908 Panama St, Los Angeles CA 90066, USA.

Wallace, Cameron, UK. Wallace, Cameron & Co. Ltd, Ultra House, Drakemire Drive, Castlemilk Industrial Estate, Glasgow G45 9SU, Scotland.

Wallace Mfg Chem., UK. Wallace Manufacturing Chemists Ltd, 1a Frognal, London NW3 6AN, England.

Wallace, USA. Wallace Laboratories, Division of Carter-Wallace Inc., Half Acre Rd, Cranbury NJ 08512, USA.

Wallis, UK. The Wallis Laboratory (Dayol Products Ltd), 11 Camford Way, Sundon Park, Luton, Beds LU3 3AN, England.

Wander, Belg. See *Sandoz-Wander, Belg.*

Wander, Ger. Wander Pharma GmbH, Deutschherrnstrasse 15, 8500 Nürnberg 1 1, W. Germany.

Wander, Neth. Wander-Pharma, afdeling van Sandoz B.V., Loopkantstraat 25, 5405 AC Uden, Netherlands.

Wander, Norw. See *Cortec, Norw.*

Wander, S.Afr. Wander Ltd (Division Sandoz Products), P.O. Box 371, Randburg 2125, S. Africa.

Wander, Switz. Wander AG, Eigerplatz 2, 3007 Bern, Switzerland.

Wander, UK. Wander Pharmaceuticals, 98 The Centre, Feltham, Middx TW13 4EP, England.

Warne, UK. E.E. Warne & Co., White Lion Rd, Amersham, Bucks, England.

Warner, Arg. William R. Warner & Cía. S.A., Sarmiento 3401, 1196 Buenos Aires, Argentina.

Warner, Austral. William R. Warner & Co. Pty Ltd, 32 Cawarra Rd, North Caringbah NSW 2229, Australia.

Warner, Ger. W.R. Warner & Co. GmbH, Mooswaldallee 1-9, Postfach: 1727, 7800 Freiburg im Breisgau, W. Germany.

Warner-Lambert, Swed. Warner-Lambert Sweden AB, Box 4130, 171 04 Solna, Sweden.

Warner-Lambert, UK. Warner-Lambert Health Care Division, Southampton Rd, Eastleigh, Hants SO5 5RY, England.

Warner-Lambert, USA. Warner-Lambert Co., 201 Tabor Rd, Morris Plains NJ 07950, USA.

Warner, Norw. See *Parke, Davis, Norw.*

Warner, NZ. Warner-Lambert (NZ) Ltd, (incorporating Wm R. Warner & Co. Ltd), P.O. Box 430, Auckland, New Zealand.

Warner, S.Afr. Warner Pharmaceuticals, Division of Chamberlains (Pty) Ltd, P.O. Box 1718, Cape Town 8000, S. Africa.

Warner, UK. William R. Warner & Co. Ltd, Medical Division, Usk Rd, Pontypool, Gwent NP4 0YH, Wales.

Warrick, Neth. Warrick (Nederland) B.V., Bankrashof 3, 1183 NP Amstelveen, Netherlands.

Washington, Ital. Washington, Via Passione 8, 20122 Milan, Italy.

Wassen, UK. Wassen Developments Ltd, Yale House, Thames St, Walton-on-Thames, Surrey, England.

Wassermann, Spain. Wassermann, Avda. San Antonio M. Claret 173, Barcelona, Spain.

Waterhouse, UK. J. Waterhouse & Co. Ltd, Church St, Ashton-under-Lyne, Lancs OL6 6XG, England.

Watson, USA. T.E. Watson Co., P.O. Box 3829, Sarasota FL 33578, USA.

Watson Victor, Austral. Watson Victor Ltd, Australia.

WB Pharmaceuticals, UK. WB Pharmaceuticals Ltd, P.O. Box 23, Bracknell, Berks RG12 4YS, England.

Webcon, USA. Webcon Pharmaceuticals, Division of Alcon Laboratories Inc., P.O. Box 1629, Fort Worth TX 76101, USA.

Weddel, UK. Weddel Pharmaceuticals Ltd, 14 West Smithfield, London EC1A 9HY, England.

Weiders, Norw. Weiders Farmasøytiske A/S, Hausmannsgt. 6, Postboks 9113 Vaterland, Oslo 1, Norway.

Weimer, Ger. Waldermar Weimer, Chemisch-pharmazeutische Fabrik, Schlackenwerther Strasse 8, Postfach: 2220, 7550 Rastatt (Baden), W. Germany.

Welbeck, UK. Welbeck Medical Distributors Ltd, Sanofi UK Ltd, Regent House, Heaton Lane, Stockport, Cheshire SK4 1AG, England.

Welcker-Lyster, Canad. Welcker-Lyster Ltd, 8480 St Lawrence Blvd, Montreal, Quebec H2P 2M6, Canada.

Weleda, UK. Weleda (UK) Ltd, Heanor Rd, Ilkeston, Derbyshire DE7 8DR, England.

Welfare Foods, UK. Welfare Foods (Stockport) Ltd, 63 London Road South, Poynton, Stockport, Cheshire SK12 1LA, England.

Wellcome, Arg. Burroughs Wellcome & Cía, Av. Leandro N Alén 619 2ºPiso, 1001 Buenos Aires, Argentina.

Wellcome, Austral. Burroughs Wellcome & Co. (Australia) Ltd, Phillips St, Concord NSW 2137, Australia.

Wellcome, Belg. Wellcome S.A., Industriezone III, 9440 Erembodegem, Belgium.

Wellcome, Canad. Burroughs Wellcome Inc., Wellcome Medical Division, 60 Riverview Ave, LaSalle, Quebec H8R 3S1, Canada.

Wellcome Consumer Division, UK. Wellcome Consumer Sales Division, Crewe Hall, Crewe, Cheshire CW1 1UB, England.

Wellcome, Denm. The Wellcome Foundation Ltd, Nyvej 16, 1851 Copenhagen V, Denmark.

Wellcome, Fr. Laboratoires Wellcome S.A., 159 rue Nationale, 75640 Paris Cedex 13, France.

Wellcome, Ital. Wellcome Italia s.p.a., Via del Mare 36, 00040 Pomezia (Roma), Italy.

Wellcome, Norw. The Wellcome Foundation Ltd, Informasjonsavdeling i Norge, Drammensvn. 230, Oslo 2, Norway.

Wellcome Reagents, UK. Wellcome Reagents Ltd, 299 Hither Green Lane, London SE13, England.

Wellcome, S.Afr. Wellcome (Pty) Ltd, P.O. Box 653, Kempton Park 1620, S. Africa.

Wellcome, Switz. Wellcome AG, Holeestrasse 87, 4015 Basel, Switzerland.

Wellcome, UK. Wellcome Medical Division, The Wellcome Foundation Ltd, Crewe Hall, Crewe, Cheshire CW1 1UB, England.

Wellcome, USA. Burroughs Wellcome Co., 3030 Cornwallis Rd, Research Triangle Park NC 27709, USA.

Wells, Ital. Wells Farmaceutici s.r.l. (Gruppo Panunion), XIV Strada, 20020 Cesate, Italy.

Westbrook, UK. Westbrook Lanolin Co., Argonaut Works, Laisterdyke, Bradford BD4 8AU, England.

Westminster, Reckitt & Colman Pharmaceuticals, UK. Westminster Laboratories, Reckitt & Colman Pharmaceutical Division, Dansom Lane, Kingston-upon-Hull HU8 7DS, England.

Westone, UK. Westone Products Ltd, 104 Marylebone Lane, London W1M 5FU, England.

Westwood, Canad. Westwood Pharmaceuticals, 200 Adam St, Belleville, Ontario K8N 5E9, Canada.

Westwood, USA. Westwood Pharmaceuticals Inc., 468 Dewitt St, Buffalo NY 14213, USA.

Whaley, UK. Whaley Pharmaceuticals, 7 Sheep St, Rugby, Warwickshire, England.

Whatman, Belg. See *Christiaens, Belg.*

Whatman, Switz. See *Arco, Switz.*

Whatman, UK. Whatman Ltd, Springfield Mill, Maidstone, Kent ME14 2LE, England.

White, J.F., UK. See *J.F. White, UK.*

White, S.S., UK. See *S.S. White, UK.*

Whitelaw, UK. Robert Whitelaw (Newcastle) Ltd, Klintex House, Industry Rd, Heaton, Newcastle upon Tyne NE6 5XE, England.

Wiedenmann, Switz. Wiedenmann AG, 4127 Birsfelden, Switzerland.

Wigglesworth, UK. Wigglesworth Ltd, Westhoughton, Bolton BL5 3SL, England.

Wilcox, UK. Wilcox Laboratories Ltd, Calgary House, Tobermory, Isle of Mull, Scotland.

Wild, Switz. Dr Wild & Co., Lange Gasse 4, 4052 Basel, Switzerland.

Will-Pharma, Belg. Will Pharma Benelux, ave Monplaisir 33, 1030 Brussels, Belgium.

Will-Pharma, Neth. Will-Pharma B.V., 2e Weteringplantsoen 3, 1017 ZD Amsterdam, Netherlands.

Willen, USA. Willen Drug Co., 18 North High St, Baltimore MD 21202, USA.

William Davies, UK. William Davies (Health Care High Fibre Foods), 135 Eign St, Hereford, England.

Williams, USA. The J.B. Williams Co. Inc., 750 Walnut Ave, Cranford NJ 07016, USA.

Willmar-Schwabe, Neth. Dr Willmar-Schwabe B.V., Westzijde 116, 1506 EJ Zaandam, Netherlands.

Wingfield, UK. Wingfield Industrial Co. Ltd, Havenville, Poynders Rd, London SW4 8PS, England.

WinPharm, UK. WinPharm, Winthrop Pharmaceuticals, Sterling-Winthrop House, Surbiton, Surrey KT6 4PH, England.

Winston, USA. Winston Pharmaceuticals Inc., 4706 Kirk Rd, Winston-Salem NC 27103, USA.

Winthrop, Arg. Farmasa Farmacéutica Argentina, Av. Libertador 6796, 1429 Buenos Aires, Argentina.

Winthrop, Austral. Winthrop Laboratories, Division of Sterling Pharmaceuticals Pty Ltd, 75 Atkins Rd, Ermington NSW 2115, Australia.

Winthrop, Belg. Winthrop, rue Franz Merjay 103, 1060 Brussels, Belgium.

Winthrop, Canad. Winthrop Laboratories, Division of Sterling Drug Ltd, Aurora, Ontario L4G 3H6, Canada.

Winthrop, Denm. Sterling-Winthrop A/S, Østerbrogade 165 B, 2100 Copenhagen Ø, Denmark.

Winthrop, Fr. Laboratoires Winthrop, 92 blvd Victor-Hugo, 92115 Clichy, France.

Winthrop, Norw. Sterling-Winthrop A/S, Postboks 7603 Skil., Oslo 2, Norway.

Winthrop, S.Afr. Winthrop, Division of Sterling Drug (SA) (Pty) Ltd, 1446 South Coast Rd, Mobeni, 4060 Durban, Natal, S. Africa.

Winthrop, Switz. Winthrop AG, Byfangweg 1a, 4051 Basel, Switzerland.

Winthrop, UK. Winthrop Laboratories, Sterling-Winthrop House, Surbiton, Surrey KT6 4PH, England.

Winthrop, USA. Winthrop Laboratories, 90 Park Ave, New York NY 10016, USA.

Winzer, Ger. Dr Winzer, Chem.-pharm. Fabrik, Mainaustrasse 146, Postfach: 5126, 7750 Constance, W. Germany.

Wisconsin Pharmacal, USA. Wisconsin Pharmacal Co., 2535 South 170th St, New Berlin WI 53151, USA.

Witco, UK. Witco Chemical Ltd, Union Lane, Droitwich, Worcs WR9 9BB, England.

Woelm, Denm. See *Dansk Dental Depot, Denm.*

Woelm, Ger. Woelm Pharma GmbH & Co., Max-Woelm-Strasse, Postfach: 840, 3440 Eschwege, W. Germany.

Woelm, Norw. See *Remed, Norw.*

Woelm, Switz. See *Heineking, Switz.*

Wolfs, Belg. Laboratoires Wolfs S.P.R.L., Haantjeslei 70, 2000 Antwerp, Belgium.

Wolins, USA. Wolins Pharmacal Corporation, 75 Marcus Dr., Melville NY 11746, USA.

Wolner, Spain. Wolner SL, Actor Tallavi, Melilla, Spain.

Woods, Austral. H.W. Woods Pty Ltd, 10 Clifford St, Huntingdale Vic. 3166, Australia.

Woodward, UK. G.O. Woodward & Co. Ltd, Larkhall Laboratories, Putney Bridge Rd, London SW15 2PY, England.

Wright Layman & Umney, UK. Wright Layman & Umney Ltd, Sanitas House, 15 Stockwell Green, London SW9 9JJ, England.

Wulfing, Belg. Wulfing, rue de l'Intendant 65, 1020 Brussels, Belgium.

Wülfing, Switz. See *Beecham, Switz.*

Wyeth, Arg. John Wyeth Laborat. S.A., Reconquista 1011 1ºpiso, 1003 Buenos Aires, Argentina.

Wyeth, Austral. Wyeth Pharmaceuticals Pty Ltd, Gregory Place, Parramatta NSW 2150, Australia.

Wyeth, Belg. Wyeth S.A., bd de la Cambre 33-39, 1050 Brussels, Belgium.

Wyeth, Canad. Wyeth Ltd, 4455 Chesswood Dr., Downsview, Ontario M3J 2C2, Canada.

Wyeth, Denm. See *Ferrosan, Denm.*

Wyeth, Neth. Wyeth Laboratoria B.V., Rengerskerkestraat 5-7, 1069 HT Amsterdam, Netherlands.

Wyeth, Switz. See *Doetsch, Grether, Switz.*

Wyeth, UK. Wyeth Laboratories, Huntercombe Lane South, Taplow, Maidenhead, Berks SL6 0PH, England.

Wyeth, USA. Wyeth Laboratories, P.O. Box 8299, Philadelphia PA 19101, USA.

Wyngood, UK. Wyngood (Birmingham) Ltd, Wyngood House, 1206 Stratford Rd, Hall Green, Birmingham B28 8HN, England.

Yamanouchi, Belg. See *Sarva, Belg.*

Yamanouchi, Jap. Yamanouchi Pharmaceutical Co. Ltd, 5 Nihonbashi Honcho 2-chome, Chuo-ku, Tokyo 103, Japan.

Yer, Spain. Yer, Spain.

York, Arg. Laboratorios York S.A., México 1477, 1097 Buenos Aires, Argentina.

Yoshitomi, Jap. Yoshitomi Pharmaceutical Industries Ltd, 35 Hiranomachi 3-chome, Higashi-ku, Osaka 541, Japan.

Ysatfabrik, Ger. Johannes Bürger Ysatfabrik GmbH, Herzog-Julius-Strasse 83, Postfach: 167, 3388 Bad Harzburg 1, W. Germany.

Zambeletti, Ital. Zambeletti dr L., Via Zambeletti, 20021 Baranzate, Italy.

Zambeletti, Spain. Zambeletti España SA, Poligono Industrial, Coslada (Madrid), Spain.

Zambon, Ital. Zambon Farmaceutici s.p.a., Via Lillo del Duca 12, 20091 Bresso, Italy.

Zambon, Spain. Zambon SA, Carr Nacional 11 Km 607.3, S. Vicenc dels Horts (Barcelona), Spain.

Zanardi, Ital. Zanardi Farmaceutici s.r.l., Via della Villa 17-19, 40127 Bologna, Italy.

Zarri, Ital. Laboratorio Zarri di Vauzini dr comm. Pietro, Via S. Carlo 12-14, 40121 Bologna, Italy.

Zilliken, Ital. Zilliken & Co. s.a.s., Via F. Nullo 23, 16147 Genova Quarto, Italy.

Zirkulin, Ger. Zirkulin Werke GmbH Chem.-pharm. Fabrik, Wetterstrasse 33-37, Postfach: 465, 5804 Herdecke/Ruhr, W. Germany.

Zoecon, USA. Zoecon Corporation, Palo Alto, USA.

Zoja, Ital. Zoja Giorgio s.p.a., Viale Lombardia 20, 20131 Milan, Italy.

Zyma-Blaes, Denm. See *Zyma, Denm.*

Zyma, Denm. A/S Zyma Pharma, Lyngbyvej 172, 2100 Copenhagen Ø, Denmark.

Zyma-Galen, Belg. Zyma-Galen, rue de Wand 209-213, 1020 Brussels, Belgium.

Zyma, Ger. Zyma GmbH, Zielstattstrasse 40, Postfach: 701980, 8000 Munich 70, W. Germany.

Zyma, Ital. Zyma s.p.a., Corso Italia 13, 21047 Saronno, Italy.

Zyma, Neth. B.V. Zyma-Nederland, Energieweg 4, 3641 RT Mijdrecht, Netherlands.

Zyma, Norw. See *Ciba, Norw.*

Zyma, S.Afr. Zyma, S. Africa.

Zyma, Spain. Zyma Ibérica SA, Marco Aurelio 3, Barcelona, Spain.

Zyma, Switz. Zyma S.A., 1260 Nyon, Switzerland.

Zyma, UK. Zyma (UK) Ltd, Hurdsfield Industrial Estate, Macclesfield, Cheshire SK10 2LY, England.

Index to Clinical Uses
Mentioned in Parts 1 and 2

This index is only a guide to the uses described in the text; it is not a comprehensive therapeutic index. The drugs or groups of drugs under each heading are arranged by order of page number and not by order of preference.
Synonyms for diseases are given where these may be helpful. However, in some cases related conditions are also given because they may be treated similarly.

Index to Martindale Identity Numbers

Each monograph and chapter introduction has an identity number. This index lists the identity number followed by the relevant monograph or chapter title and the page on which it appears.

General Index

Entries are arranged alphabetically in word-by-word order. Where an entry is followed by more than one page reference, the principal reference is printed in **bold** type.

B

C

G

H

I

M

N

O

Q

T

W

X